CPS at a Glance

AF894985

CPS is color-coded to help you find the information you need quickly and easily. For more information, see How to Use *CPS* on the next page.

Brand and Generic Name Index

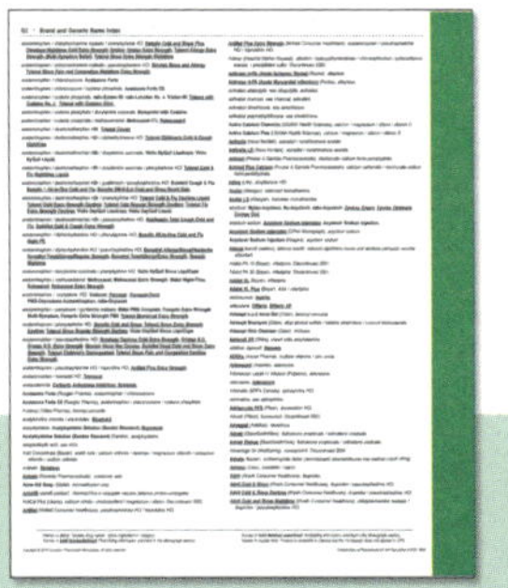

This section is an alphabetical, cross-referenced index of brand and generic names of products available in Canada including CPhA monographs. Also integrated in this section are discontinued products from 2000 to 2010.

Therapeutic Guide

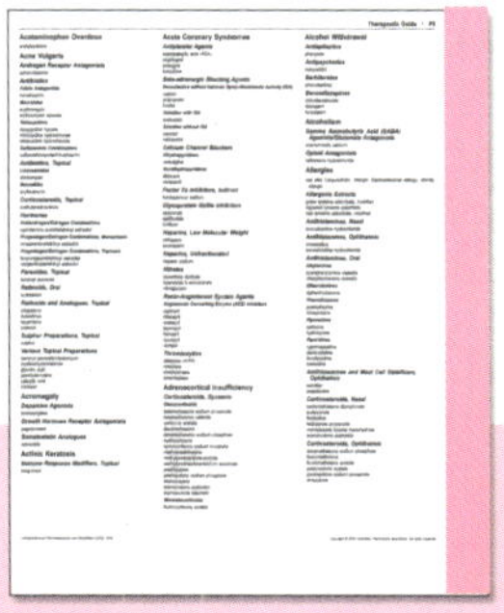

A listing of diseases or conditions and the generic names of drugs used to treat them. For listings of brand names, consult the Brand and Generic Name Index.

Clin-Info

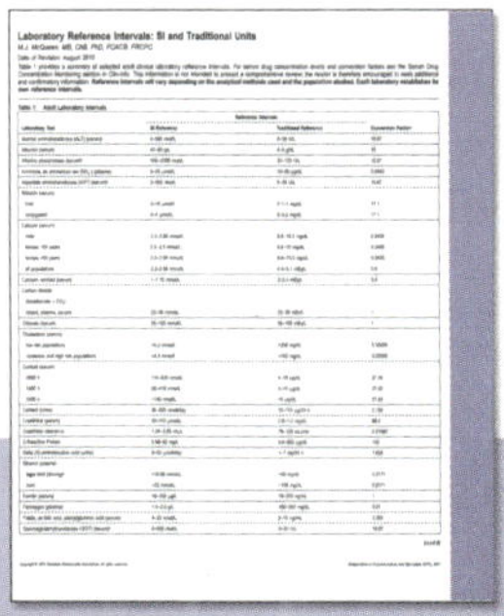

Valuable clinical information and practice tools to assist health care professionals use drugs safely and effectively.

Directory

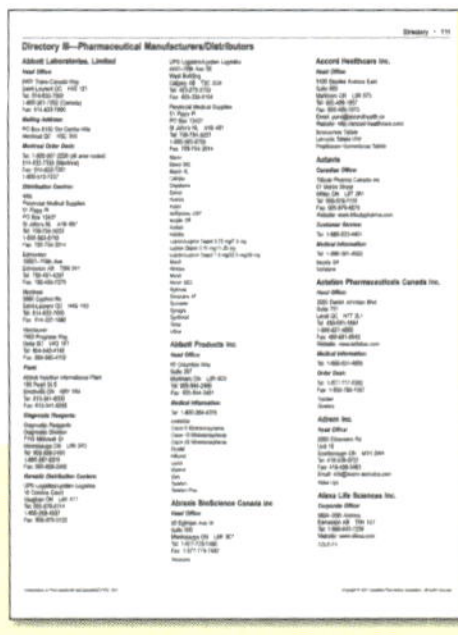

Contact information for:

- Poison Control Centres
- Health Organizations
- Pharmaceutical Manufacturers (includes product listings)

Product Monographs

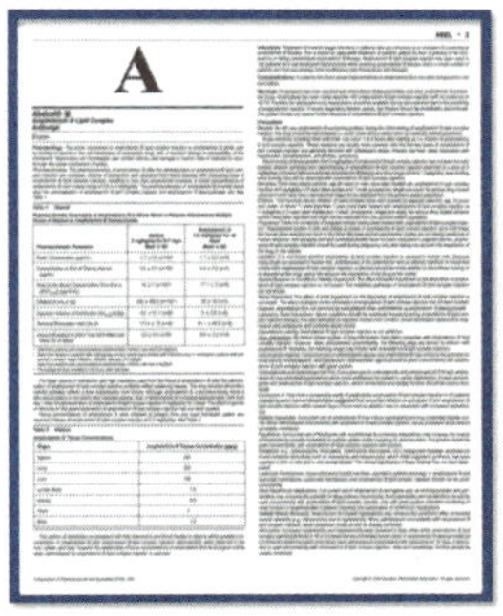

More than 2000 pharmaceutical product monographs appear in alphabetical order by brand name. The monographs are prepared by the manufacturers and approved by the Therapeutic Products Directorate, Health Canada. This edition has 145 new product monographs.

CPhA Monographs

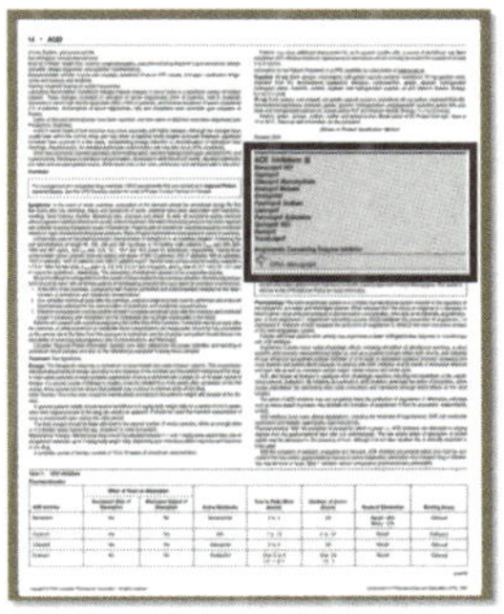

The CPhA Monograph titles are shaded in grey to distinguish them from the manufacturers' product monographs. These individual drug or drug class monographs are written by our editorial staff and reviewed by expert physicians and pharmacists. The 143 CPhA monograph titles appear in alphabetical order by generic or class name. New monographs include bisoprolol, dantrolene and propafenone. For a complete list see the CPhA Monographs Index.

Product Identification

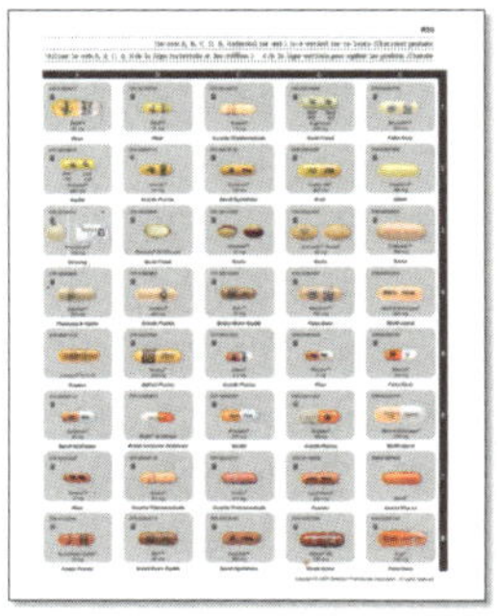

Full-color reproductions of products selected by manufacturers whose monographs appear in the Product Monograph section. This is a vital tool for accurate identification of pharmaceutical products.

Appendices

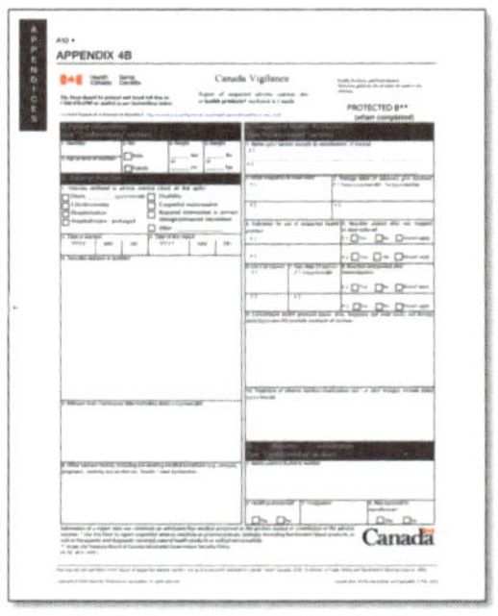

Health Canada drug regulatory and monitoring programs' reporting and request forms can be found in the Appendices.

Glossaries

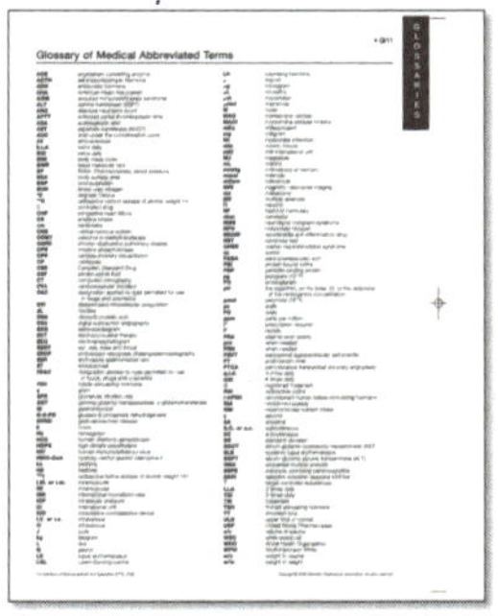

Glossaries of medical, Latin and microorganism abbreviations are located after the Appendices.

www.pharmacists.ca/products to order additional copies
www.pharmacists.ca/e-cps to subscribe to e-CPS
1-800-917-9489 ext. 300 to contact us

New **How to Use Guides** at the start of most sections.

How to Use *CPS*

CPS is composed of six main sections plus appendices and glossaries. See also the new How to Use Guides at the start of most sections. The following questions will guide you in locating specific types of information using this structure.

How do I find information about a drug when I know only the generic name, e.g., diltiazem?

Turn to the Brand and Generic Name Index (green section). Locate *diltiazem* (printed in light face italics). Although several brand names are listed (bold print) following diltiazem, only some are underlined. In the Monograph section (white section), which is organized alphabetically, you will find a complete product monograph for the underlined brand name. Brand names that are not underlined are accompanied by availability (supplied) information only.

Note: You will also see that information about diltiazem can be found in the CPhA monograph, **Calcium Channel Blockers** (bold and underlined). A complete list of all 143 CPhA monographs, written by CPhA editors, can be found in the front pages of *CPS*.

How do I find information about a brand name drug such as Xarelto?

Turn to the Brand and Generic Name Index (green section). **Xarelto** is printed in bold and underlined, indicating that complete prescribing information can be located alphabetically in the Monograph section (white section). A brand name that is printed in light face is available in Canada but a monograph does not appear in *CPS* or the product has been discontinued (the year the product was discontinued is indicated at the end of each listing).

How do I find what a drug looks like?

There are two ways to do this: 1) The product monograph contains a description in the Supplied section at the end of the monograph (e.g., Xarelto is available as light red tablets). If there is a photo of the dosage form in the Product Identification Section (glossy white pages), "Shown in Product Identification Section" will appear at the end of the monograph. 2) Check the index at the beginning of the Product Identification section to determine the specific location of the photo of Xarelto.

How do I find which drugs may be used to treat a certain disease or condition before recommending or prescribing for my patient, e.g., anticonvulsants?

Turn to the Therapeutic Guide (pink section) which is organized by medical indication. The index will guide you to "Epilepsy," where you will find a generic list of drugs organized by class (e.g., barbiturates, benzodiazepines, hydantoin derivatives).

How do I find clinical information, such as how to monitor serum drug concentration of phenytoin, its use in pregnancy or when to administer in relation to food?

The Clin-Info section (lilac section) contains quick reference information and dosing tools related to the drug or condition in question. Consult the Table of Contents (first page) or the Index (last page) of that section to find relevant information.

How do I find information on Poison Control Centres, Health Organizations or Pharmaceutical Manufacturers/ Distributors?

Turn to the first page of the Directory (yellow section).

How do I find information about Health Canada programs and the forms for reporting adverse drug reactions (ADRs)?

The Appendices at the end of the book contain information about narcotics and other targeted substances, the Special Access Programme and forms for reporting adverse events associated with drugs and vaccines.

What's New in *CPS*?

A table listing new products, new indications and other useful information is available at www.pharmacists.ca. On the CPhA Website, select "products" and choose *CPS* English from the navigation on the left. On the *CPS* page, click *CPS* Drug Updates to obtain the latest *CPS* drug update information.

How do I find discontinued products?

A listing of products discontinued from 2000-2010 is included in the Brand and Generic Name Index (green section). You only have to look in one place — the green section of *CPS*.

CPS 2011

Compendium of Pharmaceuticals and Specialties

The Canadian Drug Reference for Health Professionals

Published annually by: Canadian Pharmacists Association, Ottawa, Ontario, Canada

CPS Print Edition:
The *Compendium of Pharmaceuticals and Specialties (CPS)* is available in print in English and French.

CPS Online (www.e-cps.ca):
e-CPS is also available in English and French by subscription. For more information visit www.pharmacists.ca/e-CPS. For enterprise licences or more information contact the Canadian Pharmacists Association at service@pharmacists.ca.

Published by:
Canadian Pharmacists Association
1785 Alta Vista Drive
Ottawa ON K1G 3Y6
Canada
Tel: (613) 523-7877, 1-800-917-9489
Fax: (613) 523-0445, 1-800-601-1904
Website: www.pharmacists.ca

Comments/Inquiries:
Canadian Pharmacists Association
service@pharmacists.ca

Advertising Sales by:
Marg Churchill
Executive Vice President
Keith Communications Inc.
1599 Hurontario Street
Mississauga ON L5G 4S1
Canada
Tel: (905) 278-6700 ext. 13, 1-800-661-5004
Fax: (905) 278-4850
mchurchill@keithhealthcare.com

PAAB ccab

Printed in Canada by:
Webcom Inc.
3480 Pharmacy Avenue
Toronto ON M1W 2S7
Canada
Website: www.webcomlink.com

Library and Archives Canada Cataloguing in Publication

Compendium of pharmaceuticals and specialties.
9th ed. (1974)-
Issued also in French with title: Compendium des produits et spécialités pharmaceutiques.
Published in: Ottawa, 1980– .
ISSN 0069-7966
ISBN 978-1-894402-54-5 (2011 edition)

1. Pharmacopoeias—Canada—Periodicals. I. Canadian Pharmacists Association II. Title: CPS.

RS141.23.C612   615/.11/71

FSC www.fsc.org MIX Paper from responsible sources FSC® C004071

Table of Contents

CPhA Monographs Index

The CPhA monographs are compiled by the editorial staff of the Canadian Pharmacists Association and reviewed by expert physicians and pharmacists. They are presented alphabetically within the Monograph section by generic name or class name. The titles are lightly shaded in gray to distinguish them from manufacturers' product monographs. Readers should be aware that the text may contain information different from that found in Health Canada-approved product monographs. The term "non-approved indication" refers to indications not approved by Health Canada. The *CPS* Editorial Policy may be consulted for more information.

The following is a list of all CPhA monographs.

(cont'd)

Editorial Advisory Commitee

Participating Pharmaceutical Manufacturers/Distributors

The Canadian Pharmacists Association gratefully acknowledges the participation in *CPS* of the following manufacturers and distributors. The product monographs, submitted by the pharmaceutical manufacturers and distributors for inclusion in this book, have been approved by the Therapeutic Products Directorate, Health Canada and compiled and produced by the editorial staff of the Canadian Pharmacists Association.

Abbott Laboratories, Limited
Abbott Products Inc.
Abraxis BioScience Canada inc
Accord Healthcare Inc.
Actavis
Actelion Pharmaceuticals Canada Inc.
Adrem Inc.
Afexa Life Sciences Inc.
Alcon Canada Inc.
Alexion Pharma Canada
Allergan Inc.
Alveda Pharmaceuticals Inc.
Amgen Canada Inc.
Amphastar Pharmaceuticals, Inc.
Apotex Inc.
Astellas Pharma Canada, Inc.
AstraZeneca Canada Inc.
Aton Pharma
Awareness Corporation/dba AwarenessLife
Axcan Pharma Inc.
Bausch & Lomb Canada
Baxter Corporation
Bayer Inc.
Bayer Inc., Consumer Care
Biogen Idec Canada Inc.
Biovail Pharmaceuticals Canada
BLES Biochemicals Inc.
Boehringer Ingelheim (Canada) Ltd.
Bristol Laboratories of Canada
Bristol-Myers Squibb Canada
Canderm Pharma Inc.
Cangene Corporation
Chattem Canada
Church & Dwight Canada Corp.
Cobalt Pharmaceuticals Inc.
CSL Behring Canada
Cytex Pharmaceuticals Inc.
Dormer Laboratories Inc.
Duchesnay Inc.
Eli Lilly Canada Inc.
EMD Canada Inc.
Ethypharm, Inc.
Ferring Inc.
Fournier Pharma Inc.
Fresenius Kabi Canada
Fresenius Medical Care North America
Functional Nutrients International
Galderma Canada Inc.
Generic Medical Partners
GenMed
Genzyme Canada Inc.
Germiphene Corporation
Gilead Sciences Canada, Inc.
GlaxoSmithKline Consumer Healthcare Inc.
GlaxoSmithKline Inc.
GlaxoSmithKline Shire Canada
Glenwood Laboratories Canada Ltd.
Graceway Pharmaceuticals
GW Pharma
Helix Biopharma Corp.
Hill Dermaceuticals, Inc.
Hoffmann-La Roche Limited
Hospira Healthcare Corporation
ID Biomedical
Immunotec Inc
Insight Pharmaceuticals
Iroko Cardio (UK) Ltd.
Iroko International LP
Jacobus Pharmaceutical Company, Inc.
Janssen-Ortho Inc.
Johnson & Johnson Inc.
Johnson & Johnson • Merck Consumer Pharmaceuticals
King Pharmaceuticals Canada Inc.
Labopharm Inc.
Laboratoire HRA Pharma
Laboratoire Riva Inc.
Laboratoires Trianon Inc.
LEO Pharma Inc.
Lundbeck Canada Inc.
McNeil Consumer Healthcare
Mead Johnson Nutrition
Meda Valeant Pharma Canada Inc.
Medexus Inc.
Medical Futures Inc.
Merck Frosst Canada Ltd.
Merck Frosst-Schering Pharma, G.P.
Merz Pharma Canada Ltd.
MM Therapeutics Inc.
Mylan Pharmaceuticals ULC
Novartis Consumer Health Canada inc
Novartis Pharmaceuticals Canada Inc.
Novo Nordisk Canada Inc.
Nu-Pharm Inc.
Nycomed Canada Inc.
Octapharma Pharmazeutika Produktionsges m.b.H.
Odan Laboratories Ltd.
Paladin Labs Inc.
Pediapharm Inc.
PendoPharm
Pfizer Canada Inc.
Pfizer Consumer Healthcare
Pharmascience Inc.
Pierre Fabre Pharma Canada Inc.
Procter & Gamble Inc.
Purdue Pharma
Ranbaxy Pharmaceuticals Canada Inc.
ratiopharm
Rougier Pharma
Sandoz Canada Inc.
sanofi-aventis Canada Inc.
sanofi pasteur
Schering-Plough Canada Inc.
Sepracor Pharmaceuticals, Inc.
Servier Canada Inc.
Shire Canada Inc.
Sigma-Tau Pharmaceuticals, Inc.
Stellar Pharmaceuticals Inc.
SteriMax Inc.
Stiefel, a GSK company
Takeda Canada, Inc.
Takeda Pharmaceuticals America, Inc.
Talecris Biotherapeutics Ltd.
Tanta Pharmaceuticals Inc.
TaroPharma
Taro Pharmaceuticals Inc.
Teva Canada
Teva Canada Innovation
Theramed Corporation
Triton Pharma Inc.
tyco Healthcare
UCB Canada Inc.
USANA Health Sciences, Inc.
Valeant Canada Ltd
Valeo Pharma Inc.
ViiV Healthcare ULC
Warner Chilcott Canada Co.
WellSpring Pharmaceutical Canada Corp.

Reviewers

The Canadian Pharmacists Association gratefully acknowledges the participation of the following individuals in all CPhA publications.

David R. Anderson, *MD, FRCPC*
Professor of Medicine, Pathology and Community Health & Epidemiology
Dalhousie University
Head, Division of Hematology and Deputy Head Department of Medicine
Capital Health
Halifax, NS

Helen Anyoti, *MD*
Vaccine Safety Officer
Canadian AEFI Surveillance (CAEFIS/SSESAV) Vaccine Safety Section
Centre of Immunization and Respiratory Infections Division (CIRID)
Public Health Agency of Canada
Ottawa, ON

David G. Bailey, *BScPhm, MSc, PhD*
Scientist, Lawson Health Research Institute
London Health Sciences Centre
Professor, Physiology & Pharmacology and Medicine
University of Western Ontario
London, ON

Jennifer Blake, *BSc, MD, FRCSC*
Obstetrics and Gynecology
Women's College Hospital
University of Toronto
Toronto, ON

P. Joan Bobyn, *BSP, PhD*
Greystone Co-op Pharmacy Saskatoon
Adjunct Professor
College of Pharmacy and Nutrition
University of Saskatchewan
Saskatoon, SK

Marie-Sophie Brochet, *BPharm, MSc*
Pharmacy Department
Ste-Justine Hospital/University of Montreal
Montreal, QC

Gary Butterworth, *BScPharm, OD*
Optometrist
Winnipeg, MB

Roxane Carr, *BSc(Pharm), PharmD, BCPS, FCSHP*
Children's and Women's Health Centre of British Columbia
Assistant Professor, University of British Columbia
Vancouver, BC

John C. Chen, *MD, CM, MBA*
Associate Professor
Department of Ophthalmology
McGill University
Medical Director
Montreal Retina Institute
Montreal, QC

Alice Yuk-Yan Cheng, *MD, FRCPC*
Department of Medicine
Credit Valley Hospital
Mississauga, ON

Alex H.Y. Cho, *BSc(Pharm)*
Skin Care Centre Pharmacy
Vancouver General Hospital
Vancouver, BC

Paul J. Daeninck, *MD, MSc, FRCPC*
Symptom Management Group
CancerCare Manitoba
Director, Palliative Medicine Fellowship Program
Assistant Professor, Internal Medicine and Family Medicine
University of Manitoba
Winnipeg, MB

Orna Diav-Citrin, *MD*
The Israeli Teratology Information Service
Jerusalem, Israel

John M. Esdaile, *MD, MPH, FRCPC, FCAHS*
Scientific Director
Arthritis Research Centre of Canada
Vancouver, BC
Arthur J.E. Child Chair in Rheumatology Research
Professor of Medicine
University of Calgary
Calgary, AB

Barb Evans, *BSP, ACPR, MSc, FCSHP*
Clinical Manager, Pharmacy Services
Saskatoon Health Region
Clinical Assistant Professor
College of Pharmacy and Nutrition
University of Saskatchewan
Saskatoon, SK

David Gardner, *BScPharm, ACPR, PharmD, MSc*
Professor
Department of Psychiatry and College of Pharmacy
Dalhousie University
Halifax, NS

Alfred S. Gin, *BScPharm, PharmD, FCSHP*
Clinical Pharmacist, Infectious Diseases
Health Sciences Centre
Assistant Professor, Faculty of Medicine
University of Manitoba
Winnipeg, MB

Helen Grad, *MScPhm*
Assistant Professor
Faculty of Dentistry and Faculty of Medicine
University of Toronto
Toronto, ON

Daniel A. Haas, *DDS, PhD, FRCDC*
Associate Dean and Professor, Faculty of Dentistry
Professor, Faculty of Medicine
University of Toronto
Toronto, ON

Antony J. Ham Pong, *MBBS, FRCPC*
Consultant, Allergy & Immunology
Clinical Lecturer in Pediatrics, Children's Hospital of Eastern Ontario
Expert Content Advisor, Foundations Unit, University of Ottawa School of Medicine
Ottawa, ON

Brian G. Hardy, *BSc, BScPharm, ACPR, PharmD, FCSHP, FCCP*
Coordinator, Education and Clinical Programs
Department of Pharmacy
Sunnybrook Health Sciences Centre
Associate Professor, Faculty of Pharmacy
University of Toronto
Toronto, ON

Shinya Ito, *MD, ABCP, FRCPC*
Professor and Head
Division of Clinical Pharmacology & Toxicology
Department of Pediatrics
Hospital for Sick Children
University of Toronto
Toronto, ON

(cont'd)

Derek Jorgenson, *BSP, PharmD*
Assistant Professor
College of Pharmacy and Nutrition
University of Saskatchewan
Saskatoon, SK

David N. Juurlink, *BPhm, MD, PhD, FRCPC*
Attending Physician, Division of General Internal Medicine, Sunnybrook Health Sciences Centre
Director, Division of Clinical Pharmacology and Toxicology, University of Toronto
Medical Toxicologist, Ontario Poison Centre
Associate Professor of Medicine, Pediatrics, and Health Policy
Toronto, ON

Heather Kertland, *PharmD*
Clinical Pharmacy Specialist/Leader
St. Michael's Hospital
Assistant Professor
Leslie Dan Faculty of Pharmacy, University of Toronto
Toronto, ON

Sandra Knowles, *RPh, ACPR, BScPhm*
Drug Safety Pharmacist
Sunnybrook Health Sciences Centre
Toronto, ON

Gideon Koren, *MD, FRCPC, FACMT*
Professor & Director, Motherisk Program
The Hospital for Sick Children and University of Toronto
The Ivey Chair in Molecular Toxicology
The University of Western Ontario
Toronto, ON

Alka I. Kurichh, *BSc, Bed, MSc Dipl*
Senior Scientific Regulatory Officer, Population Health
Special Access Programme
Therapeutic Products Directorate
Health Canada
Ottawa, ON

Michael Libman, *MD, FRCPC*
Director, Division of Infectious Disease
Department of Microbiology
McGill University Health Centre
Montreal, QC

Mark J. Makowsky, *BSP, PharmD, ACPR*
Assistant Professor, Faculty of Pharmacy and Pharmaceutical Sciences
University of Alberta
Edmonton, AB

Anne Massicotte, *BPharm, MSc*
Drug Information Pharmacist
The Ottawa Hospital, Civic Campus
Ottawa, ON

Doreen Matsui, *MD, FRCPC*
Department of Pediatrics
Children's Hospital, London Health Sciences Centre
University of Western Ontario
London, ON

P.J. McLeod, *MD, FRCP, FACP*
Professor, Medicine and Pharmacology
McGill University
Montreal, QC

Matthew J. McQueen, *MB, ChB, PhD, FCACB, FRCPC*
Director, Lipid Research Clinic
Director, Clinical Trials Clinical Research Laboratory
Hamilton General Hospital
McMaster University
Hamilton, ON

Loran McVittie, *BScPharm*
Clinical Information Specialist
Poison and Drug Information Service
Calgary, AB

Michelle Mezei, *BSc(Pharm), MDCM, FRCPC*
Division of Neurology
University of British Columbia
Vancouver, BC

Scott J. Murray, *MD, FRCPC*
Division of Dermatology
Dalhousie University
Halifax, NS

Tania Mysak, *BSP, PharmD*
Clinical Practice Manager, Pharmacy Services
Clinical Adjunct Professor, Faculty of Pharmacy and Pharmaceutical Sciences
University of Alberta
Edmonton, AB

Leslie Phillips, *BSc(Pharm), PharmD*
Associate Director & Associate Professor
Memorial University of Newfoundland
St. John's, NL

C. Jane Richardson, *BSP, PhD, FCSHP*
Coordinator, Clinical Pharmacy Services
Saskatoon Health Region
Clinical Assistant Professor
College of Pharmacy and Nutrition
University of Saskatchewan
Saskatoon, SK

Neil Skjodt, *MD, MSc, FRCPC, FCCP, DABSM, FAASM*
Specialist in Internal, Respiratory & Critical Care Medicine
Adjunct Professor of Physiology
University of Alberta
Edmonton, AB

Kathy Slayter, *BScPharm, PharmD, FCSHP*
Clinical Pharmacy Specialist, Division of Infectious Diseases
Clinical Coordinator, General Medicine and Infectious Diseases
Department of Pharmacy
Capital Health
Halifax, NS

Laura Targownik, *MD, FRCPC, MS(Health Services)*
Associate Professor
Section of Gastroenterology
University of Manitoba
Winnipeg, MB

Peter Thomson, *BSc(Pharm), PharmD*
Clinical Resource Pharmacist
Winnipeg Regional Health Authority
Winnipeg, MB

Nese Yuksel, *BScPharm, PharmD, ACPR, FCSHP, NCMP*
Associate Professor
Faculty of Pharmacy and Pharmaceutical Sciences
University of Alberta
Edmonton, AB

Editor's Message

The Canadian Pharmacists Association has been serving Canadian health care professionals with a centralized source of Health Canada–approved product monographs since 1960. This 46th edition of the *Compendium of Pharmaceuticals and Specialties (CPS)* and its electronic counterpart e-CPS are simply the most comprehensive Canadian drug information databases available.

The **Brand and Generic Index** informs of the brand and generic names of drug products in Canada, whether marketed or discontinued and the manufacturer of the product. This index (green section) is the key to the white section (product monographs and CPhA monographs), but it also lists brand names that are not submitted to *CPS*. **Discontinued Products** from 2000 to 2010 have been integrated into this index. You only have to look in one place now—the green section of *CPS*.

The **Monograph** section when used with Brand and Generic Index points to full prescribing information, either a product monograph or a CPhA monograph. The **pharmaceutical manufacturers** (see Directories) submit Health Canada-approved **product monographs** for publication so that the most complete information is available to health care professionals who seek and apply that information in patient care.

CPhA monographs are evidence-based drug monographs that fill gaps in drug information when manufacturers do not submit/maintain a monograph for an older drug that may have been genericized. CPhA monographs are written by drug information pharmacists and reviewed by expert Canadian physicians and pharmacists. There are 143 such monographs in this edition. To find them, check the Brand and Generic Name Index (green section) by generic name or the listing following the Table of Contents. It is a rare occasion that you will not find information on a drug available in Canada. If you cannot, please let us know.

Clin-Info offers quick reference calculations and clinical tools to help the busy practitioner use drugs safely and effectively: the use of drugs in special patients (pregnancy, breastfeeding) and situations (dentistry, immunization), drug and food considerations, interactions with grapefruit, serum drug concentration monitoring and how to find reliable information about nonmedicinal ingredients and latex. We recommend that you familiarize yourself with this section so you can reference it quickly when you need it.

The very popular **Therapeutic Guide** lists diseases or conditions and the drugs and drug classes that are used to treat the condition. This section incorporates the conditions addressed in *Therapeutic Choices*, e-Therapeutics and *Patient Self-Care* and is enhanced every year. There's a reason why our users can't do without these pages. Therapeutic Guide is availabe only in the print version of *CPS*.

The **Product Identification** section is the go-to reference for Canadian product images. The consistency and quality of more than 1200 images are well recognized by health care professionals in Canada.

The 2011 edition also boasts:

- 145 new products
- 3 new CPhA drug monographs (bisoprolol, dantrolene, propafenone)
- 87 new images in the Product Identification Section
- New updates in all the Clin-Info articles.

The print version of *CPS* has been accompanied by e-CPS since 2004. **Information for the Patient** and **What's New in *CPS*** appear in the online version only. Health Canada Advisories and Warnings are linked to the relevant product monographs in e-CPS. The manufacturers' dates of preparation and revision (if applicable) are included at the top of new and recently revised monographs.

CPhA practices a rigorous editorial process. The 10 members of the **Editorial Advisory Committee**, chaired by Dr. Peter McLeod (see the front pages) advise us on the many issues pertinent to such a complex drug information reference. The expert **Reviewers** are well regarded pharmacists and physicians and dedicated clinicians (see front pages) who ensure that content is accurate and relevant for patient care.

The publication of *CPS* is possible because of the skill and dedication of CPhA's team of editors, information technologists, designers, managers and administrators.

We are always grateful to our subscribers for your support and constructive criticism. We are proud of *CPS* 2011 and always welcome your feedback.

Carol Repchinsky
Editor-in-Chief

Editorial Policy

General

CPS contains information on proprietary and nonproprietary products intended for human use. Product monographs are organized alphabetically by brand names that are the registered trademarks of the company whose name, in full or abbreviated form, immediately follows the trademark. CPhA monographs are shown in the monograph section under the generic name or class. Titles of CPhA monographs are shaded in gray.

The *CPS* Monograph section is not comprehensive of drug products available in Canada. The editorial staff of the Canadian Pharmacists Association compile and format monographs that have been submitted by the manufacturer for inclusion in the book. The inclusion of a manufacturer's product monograph in the *CPS* does not imply that the editors or the CPhA Editorial Advisory Committee accept, endorse or recommend these preparations as being clinically superior to similar products of any other manufacturer.

Great care has been taken to ensure the accuracy and completeness of the information contained in the *CPS*. However, the editors and publisher are not responsible for errors or any consequences arising from the use of the information published herein.

CPS users are advised that the information provided in the *CPS* is not exhaustive. Other sources may contain additional necessary information for safe use of the product.

Changes received by the publisher after established deadlines are not included in this edition.

Monograph Section

Product Monographs:

CPS provides the Product Monograph prepared by the pharmaceutical manufacturers and approved by the Therapeutic Products Directorate (TPD), Health Canada. Included are those products and medical devices with a drug component available for use in Canada. Product information as published in *CPS* is a direct equivalent of the prescribing information contained and described in Sections 2.2 to 2.12 of the Drugs Directorate, Health Protection Branch Guidelines for Product Monographs (1989) and in the document *Guidance for Industry: Product Monograph.* A revised product monograph template was implemented by Health Canada in October, 2003. Product monographs for new drugs and supplemental new drug submissions as well as drugs with notifiable changes since that date appear in the new format. Older products remain in the previous format. Editorial changes are limited to those required for consistency of style, clarity and presentation.

Product monographs approved by the TPD and containing the same therapeutic ingredient(s) may differ in their indications, contraindications, warnings, precautions, adverse effects, dosing regimens and constituents. *CPS* users are encouraged to consult the specific product monograph to ensure accurate information.

The product monographs contain listings of nonmedicinal ingredients. This information has been submitted voluntarily by the manufacturers and compiled by the editors. A statement may appear in the "Supplied/ Dosage Forms, Composition and Packaging" sections indicating the presence or absence of a specific nonmedicinal ingredient in the product. The lack of a statement indicates no information was available to the editorial staff regarding a specific nonmedicinal ingredient. *CPS* users are urged to consult the product monograph of the product dispensed (see Clin-Info Section for further discussion on this topic).

Some monographs contain boxed text indicating that the product has been approved under the Notice of Compliance with Conditions (NOC/c) policy of Health Canada. An NOC/c is a form of market approval granted to a product on the basis of promising evidence of clinical effectiveness following review of the submission by Health Canada. Products approved under this policy are intended for the treatment, prevention or diagnosis of a serious, life-threatening or severely debilitating illness. They have demonstrated promising benefit, are of high quality and possess an acceptable safety profile based on a benefit/risk assessment. In addition, they either respond to a serious unmet medical need in Canada or have demonstrated a significant improvement in the benefit/risk profile over existing therapies. Health Canada has provided access to this product on the condition that sponsors carry out additional clinical trials to verify the anticipated benefit within an agreed-upon time frame.

We request that manufacturers submit the most recent version of the product monograph for publication in print *CPS*. With the availability of e-CPS, we are able to publish the most recent version of the monograph as soon as it is available. The Date of Preparation and the Date of Revision (if applicable) are included for new or recently revised monographs. These dates will appear both in print *CPS* and e-CPS, the latter being the most current publication.

Risk Factors for Drug Use During Pregnancy:

See Glossary at the end of the book for definitions on risk factors (A, B, C, D, X) for drug use during pregnancy.

CPhA Monographs:

The CPhA monographs, titles shaded in gray and bearing the CPhA logo, are developed by the editorial staff of the Canadian Pharmacists Association. They are based on the best available information from independent literature sources including currently accepted clinical practice guidelines, primary literature and the originator's Product Monograph. CPhA monographs are reviewed by expert physicians and pharmacists for accuracy and appropriateness with respect to current medical practice. Readers should be aware that the text may contain information different from that found in Health Canada-approved Product Monographs. The term "Uses not approved in Canada" refers to indications not approved by Health Canada.

Clin-Info Section

The Clin-Info section contains quick reference clinical information and practice tools for health care professionals. Although the information is not intended to be all inclusive, the editors, authors and publisher have tried to ensure its accuracy at the time of publication. Readers should be aware that the text may contain information different from that approved by the Therapeutic Products Directorate and that the pharmaceutical manufacturers' approval has not been requested.

Erratum Policy

In spite of our careful review process, should a major error occur, it will be corrected immediately on www.e-cps.ca and posted on CPhA's website: http://www.pharmacists.ca/errata. All errors will be corrected in the next print edition of *CPS*.

Brand and Generic Name Index

About Brand and Generic Name Index

The Brand and Generic Name index is an alphabetical, cross-referenced listing of brand and generic names enabling you to find a product by either of its names. This index includes all drugs in the Monograph section (both product and CPhA monographs) as well as brand names for monographs not provided by the manufacturer and for products discontinued since 2000.

CPhA Monograph names are listed alphabetically within this index. CPhA monographs are written by the editorial staff of the Canadian Pharmacists Association, are based on the best available evidence and are reviewed by expert physicians and pharmacists. For a complete list of CPhA monographs, see front pages of *CPS*.

Online Updates

New and revised product listings and notice of discontinued products received by the publisher after the print deadlines are published in e-CPS, CPhA's online *CPS*. e-CPS is updated bi-weekly. For more information or to subscribe to e-CPS, visit www.pharmacists.ca/e-CPS.

How to Use the Brand and Generic Name Index

You can locate the listing by either the brand name or generic name. The listings are presented in the following format:

- Names in "**bold face/underlined**" identify the brand name for full prescribing information provided in the Monograph section. Each time this listing appears, it is followed by the manufacturer's name (or CPhA Monograph when CPhA is the author of the monograph) and the *generic name*.
- Names in "**bold face/not underlined**" identify the brand name for availability information provided in the Monograph section (e.g. dosage forms, composition and packaging information). Each time this listing appears, it is followed by the manufacturer's name and the *generic name*.
- "Names in regular face" identify the brand name for which the monograph is not provided by the manufacturer or identify a product discontinued. Each time this listing appears, it is followed by the manufacturer's name and *generic name*.
- Names in *italics* identify the *generic name*. Each time the generic name appears, it is followed by an alphabetical listing of brand names (and CPhA Monograph names when applicable). When the *generic name* is not available, a category of use is listed. Categories include dermatological preparations, disposable needles, electrolytes, fibrin sealant, insulin, multiple vitamins and minerals, nonmedicated soap, sea water.

If you cannot find the listing you are looking for, the product may have been recently introduced or discontinued. We suggest you consult e-CPS or consult the CPS Drug Updates table available at www.pharmacists.ca (on the Website, select "products" and select CPS English from the navigation menu then click on CPS Drug Updates to obtain the latest information).

#

1,25-dihydroxycholecalciferol. see *calcitriol.*

1,25-dihydroxyvitamin D_3. see *calcitriol.*

1α-hydroxycholecalciferol. see *alfacalcidol.*

1α-hydroxyvitamin D_3. see *alfacalcidol.*

5-ASA. **Asacol 800**; Asacol; **Mesasal**; **Mezavant**; **Pentasa**; **Salofalk, Rectal Suspension**; **Salofalk, Suppositories**; **Salofalk, Tablets**; **Teva-5 ASA**.

5-fluorouracil. **Fluorouracil Injection**; **Fluorouracil Injection USP**.

5-fluorouracil. see *fluorouracil.*

5-FU. see *fluorouracil.*

6-thioguanine. see *thioguanine.*

10 Benzagel Acne Gel (Dermik). *benzoyl peroxide.* Discontinued 2005.

222 Tablets (Johnson & Johnson • Merck). *ASA / caffeine citrate / codeine phosphate.*

282 (PendoPharm). *ASA / caffeine citrate / codeine phosphate.*

282 MEP (PendoPharm). *ASA / caffeine citrate / codeine phosphate / meprobamate.*

292 (PendoPharm). *ASA / caffeine citrate / codeine phosphate.*

3TC (ViiV Healthcare ULC). *lamivudine.*

A

α-tocopherol. see *vitamin E.*

A.C. and C (Pharmascience). *ASA / caffeine / codeine phosphate.*

A.P.L. (Wyeth-Ayerst). *chorionic gonadotropin.* Discontinued 2001.

abacavir sulfate. **Ziagen**.

abacavir sulfate / lamivudine. **Kivexa**.

abacavir sulfate / lamivudine / zidovudine. **Trizivir**.

abatacept. **Orencia**.

Abbokinase (Abbott). *urokinase.* Discontinued 2010.

abciximab. **ReoPro**.

Abelcet (Sigma-Tau). *amphotericin B lipid complex.*

Abilify (Bristol-Myers Squibb). *aripiprazole.*

Abraxane (Abraxis BioScience). *paclitaxel.*

Abreva (GlaxoSmithKline Consumer Healthcare). *docosanol.*

acamprosate calcium. **Campral**.

acarbose. **Glucobay**.

Accolate (AstraZeneca). *zafirlukast.*

Accupril (Pfizer). *quinapril HCl.*

Accuretic (Pfizer). *hydrochlorothiazide / quinapril HCl.*

Accutane Roche (Roche). *isotretinoin.*

acebutolol HCl. **Apo-Acebutolol**; **Nu-Acebutolol**; **Rhotral**; **Sectral**.

ACE Inhibitors (CPhA Monograph).

Acel-P (Wyeth-Ayerst). *acellular pertussis vaccine adsorbed.* Discontinued 2001.

acenocoumarin. see *acenocoumarol.*

acenocoumarin. see *nicoumalone.*

acenocoumarol. **Sintrom**.

acenocoumarol. see *nicoumalone.*

acenocoumarol / nicoumalone . **Nicoumalone**.

ACET 120 (PendoPharm). *acetaminophen.*

ACET 160 (PendoPharm). *acetaminophen.*

ACET 325 (PendoPharm). *acetaminophen.*

ACET 650 (PendoPharm). *acetaminophen.*

Acetaminophen (CPhA Monograph). *acetaminophen.*

Acetaminophen (Riva). *acetaminophen.*

acetaminophen. **ACET 120**; **ACET 160**; **ACET 325**; **ACET 650**; **Acetaminophen**; Acetaminophen; **Atasol Preparations**; Pediatrix; **Tempra**; **Tylenol Regular Strength Tablets, Caplets**; **Tylenol Extra Strength Tablets, Caplets, Gelcaps**; **Tylenol Arthritis Pain Extended Release Tablets**; **Tylenol Muscle Aches & Body Pain Extended Release Tablets**; **Tylenol Junior Strength Tablets "Meltaways"**; **Tylenol Children's Tablets "Meltaways" and Suspension**; **Tylenol Infants' Suspension Drops**; **Vicks Custom Care Body Aches**.

acetaminophen / caffeine. **Tylenol Ultra Relief Migraine Pain**.

acetaminophen / caffeine / codeine phosphate. **ratio-Lenoltec No. 1, 2 & 3**; **Tylenol No. 1**; **Tylenol with Codeine No. 2**; **Tylenol with Codeine No. 3**.

acetaminophen / caffeine / pyrilamine maleate. **Midol Menstrual Complete**; **Midol Teen Complete**.

acetaminophen / caffeine citrate / codeine phosphate. **Atasol-8, -15, -30**; **Triatec-8**; **Triatec-8 Strong**.

acetaminophen / chlorpheniramine maleate / codeine phosphate / pseudoephedrine HCl. **Sinutab with Codeine**.

acetaminophen / chlorpheniramine maleate / dextromethorphan HBr. **Tylenol Children's Cough & Runny Nose**.

acetaminophen / chlorpheniramine maleate / dextromethorphan HBr / guaifenesin / pseudoephedrine HCl. **Benylin 1 All-in-One Cold and Flu Nightime**.

acetaminophen / chlorpheniramine maleate / dextromethorphan HBr / phenylephrine HCl. **Tylenol Cold Extra Strength Nighttime**; **Tylenol Cold Regular Strength Nighttime**; **Tylenol Flu Extra Strength Nighttime**.

acetaminophen / chlorpheniramine maleate / dextromethorphan HBr / pseudoephedrine HCl. **Robitussin Total Extra Strength Nighttime, Cough Cold and Flu**; **Tylenol Children's and Junior Strength Cold DM**.

acetaminophen / chlorpheniramine maleate / phenylephrine HCl. **Benylin Cold and Sinus Plus**; **Dristan**; **Dristan Extra Strength**; **Tylenol Allergy Extra Strength (Multi-Symptom Relief)**; **Tylenol Sinus Extra Strength Nighttime**.

acetaminophen / chlorpheniramine maleate / pseudoephedrine HCl. **Sinutab Sinus and Allergy**; **Tylenol Sinus Pain and Congestion Nighttime Extra Strength**.

acetaminophen / chlorzoxazone. **Acetazone Forte**.

acetaminophen / chlorzoxazone / codeine phosphate. **Acetazone Forte C8**.

acetaminophen / codeine phosphate. **ratio-Emtec-30**; **ratio-Lenoltec No. 4**; **Triatec-30**; **Tylenol with Codeine No. 4**; **Tylenol with Codeine Elixir**.

acetaminophen / codeine phosphate / doxylamine succinate. **Mersyndol with Codeine**.

acetaminophen / codeine phosphate / methocarbamol. **Methoxacet-C⅛**; **Robaxacet-8**.

acetaminophen / dextromethorphan HBr. **Tylenol Cough**.

acetaminophen / dextromethorphan HBr / diphenhydramine HCl. **Tylenol Children's Cold & Cough Nighttime**.

acetaminophen / dextromethorphan HBr / doxylamine succinate. **Vicks NyQuil Liquicaps**; **Vicks NyQuil Liquid**.

acetaminophen / dextromethorphan HBr / doxylamine succinate / phenylephrine HCl. **Tylenol Cold & Flu Nighttime Liquid**.

acetaminophen / dextromethorphan HBr / guaifenesin / pseudoephedrine HCl. **Balminil Cough & Flu**; **Benylin 1 All-in-One Cold and Flu**; **Benylin DM-D-E-A Cold and Sinus Rapid Gels**.

acetaminophen / dextromethorphan HBr / phenylephrine HCl. **Tylenol Cold & Flu Daytime Liquid**; **Tylenol Cold Extra Strength Daytime**; **Tylenol Cold Regular Strength Daytime**; **Tylenol Flu Extra Strength Daytime**; **Vicks DayQuil Liquicaps**; **Vicks DayQuil Liquid**.

acetaminophen / dextromethorphan HBr / pseudoephedrine HCl. **Robitussin Total Cough Cold and Flu**; **Sudafed Cold & Cough Extra Strength**.

acetaminophen / diphenhydramine HCl / phenylephrine HCl. **Benylin All-in-One Cold and Flu Night PE**.

acetaminophen / diphenhydramine HCl / pseudoephedrine HCl. **Benadryl Allergy/Sinus/Headache**; **Benadryl Total/Allergy/Regular Strength**; **Benadryl Total/Allergy/Extra Strength**; **Sinutab Nightime**.

acetaminophen / doxylamine succinate / phenylephrine HCl. **Vicks NyQuil Sinus LiquiCaps**.

acetaminophen / methocarbamol. **Methoxacet**; **Methoxacet Extra Strength**; **Midol Night-Time**; **Robaxacet**; **Robaxacet Extra Strength**.

acetaminophen / oxycodone HCl. **Endocet**; **Percocet**; **Percocet-Demi**; **ratio-Oxycocet**.

acetaminophen / pamabrom / pyrilamine maleate. **Midol PMS Complete**; **Pamprin Extra Strength Multi-Symptom**; **Pamprin Extra Strength PMS**; **Tylenol Menstrual Extra Strength**.

acetaminophen / phenylephrine HCl. **Benylin Cold and Sinus**; **Tylenol Sinus Extra Strength Daytime**; **Tylenol Sinus Regular Strength Daytime**; **Vicks DayQuil Sinus LiquiCaps**.

Names in *italics*: Generic drug names, active ingredient or category.
Names in **bold face/underlined**: Prescribing information provided in the Monograph section.
Names in **bold face/not underlined**: Availability information provided in the Monograph section.
Names in regular face: Product is available in Canada but the monograph does not appear in *CPS*.

Names in *italics*: Generic drug names, active ingredient or category.
Names in **bold face/underlined**: Prescribing information provided in the Monograph section.
Names in **bold face/not underlined**: Availability information provided in the Monograph section.
Names in regular face: Product is available in Canada but the monograph does not appear in *CPS*.

Names in *italics*: Generic drug names, active ingredient or category.
Names in **bold face/underlined**: Prescribing information provided in the Monograph section.
Names in **bold face/not underlined**: Availability information provided in the Monograph section.
Names in regular face: Product is available in Canada but the monograph does not appear in *CPS*.

Names in *italics*: Generic drug names, active ingredient or category.
Names in **bold face/underlined**: Prescribing information provided in the Monograph section.
Names in **bold face/not underlined**: Availability information provided in the Monograph section.
Names in regular face: Product is available in Canada but the monograph does not appear in *CPS*.

Names in *italics*: Generic drug names, active ingredient or category.
Names in **bold face/underlined**: Prescribing information provided in the Monograph section.
Names in **bold face/not underlined**: Availability information provided in the Monograph section.
Names in regular face: Product is available in Canada but the monograph does not appear in *CPS*.

Names in *italics*: Generic drug names, active ingredient or category.
Names in **bold face/underlined**: Prescribing information provided in the Monograph section.
Names in **bold face/not underlined**: Availability information provided in the Monograph section.
Names in regular face: Product is available in Canada but the monograph does not appear in *CPS*.

Aviane 21 (Apotex). *ethinyl estradiol / levonorgestrel.*

Aviane 28 (Apotex). *ethinyl estradiol / levonorgestrel.*

Avirax (Fabrigen). *acyclovir.* Discontinued 2002.

Avlosulfon (Wyeth-Ayerst). *dapsone.* Discontinued 2001.

avobenzone / hydroquinone / octocrylene / oxybenzone. **Glyquin XM**.

Avodart (GlaxoSmithKline). *dutasteride.*

Avonex (Biogen Idec). *interferon beta-1a.*

Avonex PS (Biogen Idec). *interferon beta-1a.*

Axert (McNeil Consumer Healthcare). *almotriptan malate.*

Azarga (Alcon). *brinzolamide / timolol maleate.*

azathioprine. **Imuran Tablets**.

azathioprine sodium. **Imuran Injection**.

azelaic acid. **Finacea**.

azidothymidine. see zidovudine.

Azilect (Teva Canada Innovation). *rasagiline mesylate.*

azithromycin dihydrate. **Z-PAK (Zithromax)**; **Zithromax**.

azithromycin monohydrate. **CO Azithromycin**; **Sandoz Azithromycin Powder for Oral Suspension**.

azithromycin monohydrate hemiethanolate. **PMS-Azithromycin**; **ratio-Azithromycin**; **Sandoz Azithromycin Tablets**.

Azmacort (Aventis Pharma). *triamcinolone acetonide.* Discontinued 2001.

Azopt (Alcon). *brinzolamide.*

AZT. see zidovudine.

aztreonam. **Cayston**.

B

B_6, B_{12} & Folic Acid Multi-Vitamin (Jamieson). *cyanocobalamin / folic acid / pyridoxine HCl.*

Bacid (ERFA Canada). *Lactobacillus rhamnosus.*

Baciguent (Johnson & Johnson • Merck). *bacitracin.* Discontinued 2008.

BaciJect (SteriMax). *bacitracin.*

Bacillus Calmette-Guérin. **BCG Vaccine (Freeze-Dried)**.

Bacillus Calmette-Guérin (BCG), strain TICE. **OncoTICE**.

Bacillus Calmette-Guérin (BCG), substrain Connaught. **ImmuCyst**.

Bacitracin (Pfizer). *bacitracin.*

bacitracin. **BaciJect**; **Bacitracin**.

bacitracin / lidocaine HCl / polymyxin B sulfate. **Ozonol Antibiotic Plus**.

bacitracin / polymyxin B sulfate. **Polytopic Ointment**.

bacitracin zinc / gramicidin / lidocaine / polymyxin B sulfate. **Polysporin Complete Antibiotic Ointment**.

bacitracin zinc / gramicidin / polymyxin B sulfate. **Polysporin Triple Antibiotic Ointment**; **Triple Antibiotic Ointment**.

bacitracin zinc / hydrocortisone / neomycin sulfate / polymyxin B sulfate. **Cortisporin Ointment**; **Sandoz Cortimyxin Ophthalmic Ointment**.

bacitracin zinc / neomycin sulfate / polymyxin B sulfate. **Neosporin Ointment**.

bacitracin zinc / polymyxin B sulfate. **Optimyxin Ophthalmic Ointment**; **Polyderm**; **Polysporin Antibiotic Ointment**; **Polysporin Ophthalmic Ointment**.

Backaid (Rougier Pharma). *acetaminophen / chlorzoxazone.*

baclofen. **Lioresal Intrathecal**; **Lioresal Oral**; **ratio-Baclofen**.

Bacteriostatic Sodium Chloride Diluent for Inhalation (Bioniche). *sodium chloride.* Discontinued 2003.

Bacteriostatic Water for Injection (Hospira). *irrigation solution / solvents and diluting agents.*

Bactigras (Smith & Nephew). *chlorhexidine acetate.*

Bactine (Bayer Consumer Care). *benzalkonium chloride / lidocaine HCl.*

Bactrim Roche (Roche). *sulfamethoxazole / trimethoprim.* Discontinued 2000.

Bactroban Cream (GlaxoSmithKline Consumer Healthcare). *mupirocin calcium.*

Bactroban Ointment (GlaxoSmithKline). *mupirocin.*

Balanced Salt Solution (Hospira). *calcium chloride / magnesium chloride / potassium chloride / sodium acetate / sodium chloride / sodium citrate.*

Balminil Cough & Flu (Rougier Pharma). *acetaminophen / dextromethorphan HBr / guaifenesin / pseudoephedrine HCl.*

Balminil DM (Rougier Pharma). *dextromethorphan HBr.*

Balminil DM+Decongestant (Rougier Pharma). *dextromethorphan HBr / pseudoephedrine HCl.*

Balminil DM+Decongestant+Expectorant (Rougier Pharma). *dextromethorphan HBr / guaifenesin / pseudoephedrine HCl.*

Balminil DM+Expectorant (Rougier Pharma). *dextromethorphan HBr / guaifenesin.*

Balminil DM Children (Rougier Pharma). *dextromethorphan HBr.*

Balminil Expectorant (Rougier Pharma). *guaifenesin.*

Balminil Nasal Decongestant (Rougier Pharma). *xylometazoline HCl.*

Balminil Nasal Ointment (Rougier). *camphor / chlorobutanol / ephedrine HCl / eucalyptol / menthol.* Discontinued 2000.

Balminil Night-Time (Rougier Pharma). *ammonium chloride / dextromethorphan HBr / diphenhydramine HCl.*

Balminil Suppositories (Rougier). *eucalyptus oil / menthol / oil of niaouli / sodium dibunate.* Discontinued 2006.

Balnetar (Westwood-Squibb). *coal tar.* Discontinued 2009.

Baraclude (Bristol-Myers Squibb). *entecavir.*

Barbiturates (CPhA Monograph).

Barriere (WellSpring). *dimethylpolysiloxane.*

Barriere-HC (PendoPharm). *hydrocortisone / silicone.* Discontinued 2010.

basiliximab. **Simulect**.

Baxedin (Omega Laboratories). *chlorhexidine gluconate.*

Baycol (Bayer). *cerivastatin sodium.* Discontinued 2001.

BCAA (Baxter). *isoleucine / leucine / valine.*

BCG Vaccine (Freeze-Dried) (sanofi pasteur). *Bacillus Calmette-Guérin.*

Beano (GlaxoSmithKline Consumer Healthcare). *alpha-D-galactosidase.*

becaplermin. **Regranex**.

Beclodisk (Glaxo Wellcome). *beclomethasone dipropionate.* Discontinued 2000.

Beclodisk Diskhaler (Glaxo Wellcome). *beclomethasone dipropionate.* Discontinued 2000.

Becloforte (Glaxo Wellcome). *beclomethasone dipropionate.* Discontinued 2000.

beclomethasone dipropionate. **Corticosteroids: Eye Ear Nose**; **Corticosteroids: Inhaled**; **Mylan-Beclo AQ.**; **Propaderm**; **Qvar**; **Rivanase AQ.**

Beclovent Inhaler (Glaxo Wellcome). *beclomethasone dipropionate.* Discontinued 2000.

Beclovent Rotacaps (Glaxo Wellcome). *beclomethasone dipropionate.* Discontinued 2000.

Beclovent Rotahaler (Glaxo Wellcome). *beclomethasone dipropionate.* Discontinued 2000.

Beconase Aq (Glaxo Wellcome). *beclomethasone dipropionate.* Discontinued 2000.

Bedoz (Nadeau). *cyanocobalamin.* Discontinued 2002.

belladonna / ergotamine tartrate / phenobarbital. **Bellergal Spacetabs**.

Bellergal Spacetabs (Triton Pharma). *belladonna / ergotamine tartrate / phenobarbital.*

Benadryl Allergy/Sinus/Headache (McNeil Consumer Healthcare). *acetaminophen / diphenhydramine HCl / pseudoephedrine HCl.*

Benadryl Preparations (McNeil Consumer Healthcare). *diphenhydramine HCl.*

Benadryl Spray (McNeil Consumer Healthcare). *diphenhydramine HCl / zinc acetate.*

Benadryl Stick (McNeil Consumer Healthcare). *diphenhydramine HCl / zinc acetate.*

Benadryl Total/Allergy/Extra Strength (McNeil Consumer Healthcare). *acetaminophen / diphenhydramine HCl / pseudoephedrine HCl.*

Benadryl Total/Allergy/Regular Strength (McNeil Consumer Healthcare). *acetaminophen / diphenhydramine HCl / pseudoephedrine HCl.*

benazepril HCl. **ACE Inhibitors**; **Lotensin**.

BeneFIX (Pfizer). *coagulation factor IX (recombinant) (nonacog alfa).*

Benemid (Merck Frosst). *probenecid.* Discontinued 2000.

Bengay Arthritis Extra Strength (Johnson & Johnson). *menthol / methyl salicylate.*

Bengay Muscle Pain No Odour (Johnson & Johnson). *triethanolamine salicylate.*

Bengay Muscle Pain Regular Strength (Original) (Johnson & Johnson). *menthol / methyl salicylate.*

Bengay Muscle Pain Ultra Strength (Johnson & Johnson). *camphor / menthol / methyl salicylate.*

Benoxyl 5% (Stiefel, a GSK company). *benzoyl peroxide.*

Benoxyl 10% and 20% (Stiefel, a GSK company). *benzoyl peroxide.*

benserazide HCl / levodopa. **Prolopa**.

Bentylol (Axcan Pharma). *dicyclomine HCl.*

Names in *italics*: Generic drug names, active ingredient or category.
Names in **bold face/underlined**: Prescribing information provided in the Monograph section.
Names in **bold face/not underlined**: Availability information provided in the Monograph section.
Names in regular face: Product is available in Canada but the monograph does not appear in *CPS*.

Benuryl (Valeant). *probenecid.*

Benylin 1 All-in-One Cold and Flu (McNeil Consumer Healthcare). *acetaminophen / dextromethorphan HBr / guaifenesin / pseudoephedrine HCl.*

Benylin 1 All-in-One Cold and Flu Nightime (McNeil Consumer Healthcare). *acetaminophen / chlorpheniramine maleate / dextromethorphan HBr / guaifenesin / pseudoephedrine HCl.*

Benylin 2 All-in-One Cold and Flu with Codeine (Non-prescription) (McNeil Consumer Healthcare). *codeine phosphate / guaifenesin / pseudoephedrine HCl.*

Benylin All-in-One Cold and Flu Night PE (McNeil Consumer Healthcare). *acetaminophen / diphenhydramine HCl / phenylephrine HCl.*

Benylin Cold and Sinus (McNeil Consumer Healthcare). *acetaminophen / phenylephrine HCl.*

Benylin Cold and Sinus Plus (McNeil Consumer Healthcare). *acetaminophen / chlorpheniramine maleate / phenylephrine HCl.*

Benylin DM (McNeil Consumer Healthcare). *dextromethorphan HBr.*

Benylin DM 12 Hour (Nightime) (McNeil Consumer Healthcare). *dextromethorphan polistirex.*

Benylin DM-D (Adult) (McNeil Consumer Healthcare). *dextromethorphan HBr / pseudoephedrine HCl.*

Benylin DM-D-E-A Cold and Sinus Rapid Gels (McNeil Consumer Healthcare). *acetaminophen / dextromethorphan HBr / guaifenesin / pseudoephedrine HCl.*

Benylin DM-D-E Extra Strength with Menthactin (McNeil Consumer Healthcare). *dextromethorphan HBr / guaifenesin / menthol / pseudoephedrine HCl.*

Benylin DM-D for Children (McNeil Consumer Healthcare). *dextromethorphan HBr / pseudoephedrine HCl.*

Benylin DM-E (McNeil Consumer Healthcare). *dextromethorphan HBr / guaifenesin.*

Benylin DM-E Extra Strength with Menthactin (McNeil Consumer Healthcare). *dextromethorphan HBr / guaifenesin / menthol.*

Benylin DM for Children (McNeil Consumer Healthcare). *dextromethorphan HBr.*

Benylin DM for Children 12 Hour (Bedtime) (McNeil Consumer Healthcare). *dextromethorphan polistirex.*

Benylin E Extra Strength with Menthactin (McNeil Consumer Healthcare). *guaifenesin / menthol.*

Benylin Energy Boosting (Pfizer Consumer Healthcare). *siberian ginseng (eleutherococcus senticosus).* Discontinued 2004.

Benylin First Defense (Pfizer Consumer Healthcare). *echinacea / menthol.* Discontinued 2004.

Benylin Night Cough (McNeil Consumer Healthcare). *diphenhydramine HCl.*

Benzac AC 5 (Galderma). *benzoyl peroxide.*

Benzac AC 10 (Galderma). *benzoyl peroxide.*

BenzaClin (sanofi-aventis). *benzoyl peroxide / clindamycin phosphate.*

Benzac W5 (Galderma). *benzoyl peroxide.*

Benzac W Wash 5 (Galderma). *benzoyl peroxide.*

Benzac W Wash 10 (Galderma). *benzoyl peroxide.*

benzalkonium chloride / lidocaine HCl. **Bactine.**

Benzamycin (sanofi-aventis). *benzoyl peroxide / erythromycin.*

benzethonium chloride / aluminum acetate. **Buro-Sol Otic Solution**; **Buro-Sol Powder.**

benzocaine. **Anbesol Gel**; **Anbesol Gel Extra Strength**; **Anbesol Liquid Extra Strength**; **Anbesol Baby Grape Gel.**

benzocaine / antipyrine. **Auralgan.**

benzocaine / cetylkonium chloride. **Bionet.**

benzocaine / hydrocortisone acetate / zinc sulfate monohydrate. **Rectogel HC.**

benzocaine / magnesium sulfate. **Osmopak Plus.**

benzocaine / zinc sulfate monohydrate. **Rectogel.**

Benzodiazepines (CPhA Monograph).

benzoyl peroxide. **Adasept b.p.5 Acne Gel**; **Benoxyl 5%**; **Benoxyl 10% and 20%**; **Benzac AC 5**; **Benzac AC 10**; **Benzac W Wash 5**; **Benzac W Wash 10**; **Benzac W5**; **Panoxyl 5% Wash**; **Panoxyl 5%**; **Panoxyl 10% and 20%**; **Panoxyl Antibacterial Acne Creamy Wash**; **Panoxyl Aquagel 2.5% and 5%**; **Solugel 4**; **Solugel 8.**

benzoyl peroxide / clindamycin phosphate. **BenzaClin**; **Clindoxyl.**

benzoyl peroxide / erythromycin. **Benzamycin.**

Benztropine Mesylate (CPhA Monograph). *benztropine mesylate.*

benztropine mesylate. **Benztropine Mesylate.**

Benztropine Omega (Omega Laboratories). *benztropine mesylate.*

Benzydamine (CPhA Monograph). *benzydamine HCl.*

benzydamine HCl. **Apo-Benzydamine**; **Benzydamine.**

benzylpenicillin potassium. see penicilin G potassium.

beractant. **Survanta.**

Berinert (CSL Behring). *human C1 esterase inhibitor.*

Berotec Inhalation Aerosol (Boehringer Ingelheim). *fenoterol HBr.* Discontinued 2007.

Berotec Inhalation Solution (Boehringer Ingelheim). *fenoterol HBr.* Discontinued 2008.

besifloxacin. **Besivance**; **Fluoroquinolones.**

Besivance (Bausch & Lomb). *besifloxacin.*

Betacaine (Canderm Pharma). *lidocaine.*

beta-carotene. see vitamin A.

Betaderm (Taro). *betamethasone valerate.*

Betadine Topical Preparations (Purdue Pharma). *povidone-iodine.*

Betadine Vaginal Preparations (Purdue Pharma). *povidone-iodine.* Discontinued 2002.

Betagan (Allergan). *levobunolol HCl.*

betahistine dihydrochloride. **Serc**; **Teva-Betahistine.**

betaine amphoteric / alkyl alcohol sulfate / coconut alkanolamide. **Adasept Shampoo.**

Betaject (Sandoz). *betamethasone acetate / betamethasone sodium phosphate.*

Betaloc (AstraZeneca). *metoprolol tartrate.*

betamethasone acetate / betamethasone sodium phosphate. **Betaject**; **Celestone Soluspan.**

betamethasone dipropionate. **Corticosteroids: Topical**; **Diprolene Glycol**; **Diprosone**; **ratio-Topilene**; **ratio-Topisone**; **Taro-Sone.**

betamethasone dipropionate / calcipotriol. **Dovobet**; **Xamiol.**

betamethasone dipropionate / clotrimazole. **Lotriderm.**

betamethasone dipropionate / salicylic acid. **Diprosalic**; **ratio-Topisalic.**

betamethasone sodium phosphate. **Betnesol**; **Corticosteroids: Eye Ear Nose**; **Corticosteroids: Systemic**; **Corticosteroids: Topical.**

betamethasone sodium phosphate / betamethasone acetate. **Betaject**; **Celestone Soluspan.**

betamethasone sodium phosphate / gentamicin sulfate. **Garasone Ophthalmic/Otic Solution**; **Garasone Ophthalmic Ointment.**

betamethasone valerate. **Betaderm**; **Corticosteroids: Topical**; **Prevex B**; **ratio-Ectosone**; **Valisone Scalp Lotion.**

betamethasone valerate / gentamicin sulfate. **Valisone-G.**

Betaseron (Bayer). *interferon beta-1b.*

Betaxin (Hospira). *thiamine HCl.* Discontinued 2005.

betaxolol HCl. **Betoptic S.**

bethanechol chloride. **Duvoid.**

Betnesol (Paladin). *betamethasone sodium phosphate.*

Betoptic S (Alcon). *betaxolol HCl.*

bevacizumab. **Avastin.**

Bextra (Pfizer). *valdecoxib.* Discontinued 2005.

Bexxar Therapy (GlaxoSmithKline). *iodine I 131 tositumomab / tositumomab.*

bezafibrate. **Bezalip SR.**

Bezalip SR (Actavis). *bezafibrate.*

Biaxin (Abbott). *clarithromycin.*

Biaxin BID (Abbott). *clarithromycin.*

Biaxin XL (Abbott). *clarithromycin.*

bicalutamide. **Bicalutamide Tablets**; **Casodex**; **CO Bicalutamide**; **ratio-Bicalutamide**; **Sandoz Bicalutamide.**

Bicalutamide Tablets (Accord Healthcare). *bicalutamide.*

Bichloracetic Acid (Glenwood). *dichloroacetic acid.* Discontinued 2000.

Bicillin L-A (King Pharmaceuticals). *penicillin G benzathine.*

BiCNU (Bristol-Myers Squibb). *carmustine.*

bilberry / lutein / zeaxanthin. **Visionex.**

Biltricide (Bayer). *praziquantel.*

bimatoprost. **Lumigan RC**; **Lumigan.**

Biobase (Odan). *ethyl alcohol.*

Biobase-G (Odan). *ethyl alcohol / glycolic acid.*

Names in *italics*: Generic drug names, active ingredient or category.
Names in **bold face/underlined**: Prescribing information provided in the Monograph section.
Names in **bold face/not underlined**: Availability information provided in the Monograph section.
Names in regular face: Product is available in Canada but the monograph does not appear in *CPS*.

Names in *italics*: Generic drug names, active ingredient or category.
Names in **bold face/underlined**: Prescribing information provided in the Monograph section.
Names in **bold face/not underlined**: Availability information provided in the Monograph section.
Names in regular face: Product is available in Canada but the monograph does not appear in *CPS*.

Names in *italics*: Generic drug names, active ingredient or category.
Names in **bold face/underlined**: Prescribing information provided in the Monograph section.
Names in **bold face/not underlined**: Availability information provided in the Monograph section.
Names in regular face: Product is available in Canada but the monograph does not appear in *CPS*.

Names in *italics*: Generic drug names, active ingredient or category.
Names in **bold face/underlined**: Prescribing information provided in the Monograph section.
Names in **bold face/not underlined**: Availability information provided in the Monograph section.
Names in regular face: Product is available in Canada but the monograph does not appear in *CPS*.

Names in *italics*: Generic drug names, active ingredient or category.
Names in **bold face/underlined**: Prescribing information provided in the Monograph section.
Names in **bold face/not underlined**: Availability information provided in the Monograph section.
Names in regular face: Product is available in Canada but the monograph does not appear in *CPS*.

Names in *italics*: Generic drug names, active ingredient or category.
Names in **bold face/underlined**: Prescribing information provided in the Monograph section.
Names in **bold face/not underlined**: Availability information provided in the Monograph section.
Names in regular face: Product is available in Canada but the monograph does not appear in *CPS*.

codeine phosphate / acetaminophen / doxylamine succinate. **Mersyndol with Codeine**.

codeine phosphate / acetaminophen / methocarbamol. **Methoxacet-C⅛**; **Robaxacet-8**.

codeine phosphate / ammonium chloride / diphenhydramine HCl. **Calmylin Original with Codeine**.

codeine phosphate / ASA / butalbital / caffeine. **Fiorinal-C ¼, ½**; **ratio-Tecnal C¼, C½**; **Trianal C¼, C½**.

codeine phosphate / ASA / caffeine citrate. **222 Tablets**; **282**; **292**.

codeine phosphate / ASA / caffeine citrate / meprobamate. **282 MEP**.

codeine phosphate / ASA / methocarbamol. **Methoxisal-C⅛**; **Methoxisal-C¼**; **Methoxisal-C½**; **Robaxisal-C**.

codeine phosphate / brompheniramine maleate / guaifenesin / phenylephrine HCl. **Dimetane Expectorant-C**.

codeine phosphate / brompheniramine maleate / phenylephrine HCl. **Dimetapp-C Syrup**.

codeine phosphate / guaifenesin / pheniramine maleate. **Robitussin AC**.

codeine phosphate / guaifenesin / pseudoephedrine HCl. **Benylin 2 All-in-One Cold and Flu with Codeine (Non-prescription)**; **Calmylin PSE with Codeine**.

codeine phosphate / guaifenesin / pseudoephedrine HCl / triprolidine HCl. **CoActifed Expectorant**; **ratio-Cotridin Expectorant**.

codeine phosphate / pseudoephedrine HCl / triprolidine HCl. **CoActifed Syrup**; **CoActifed Tablets**; **ratio-Cotridin**.

codeine sulfate trihydrate / codeine monohydrate. **Codeine Contin**.

Cod Liver Oil (Novopharm). *vitamin A / vitamin D.* Discontinued 2009.

CO Enalapril (Cobalt). *enalapril maleate.*

CO Etidrocal (Cobalt). *calcium carbonate / etidronate disodium.*

CO Etidronate (Cobalt). *etidronate disodium.*

CO Famciclovir (Cobalt). *famciclovir.*

CO Fluconazole (Cobalt). *fluconazole.*

CO Fluoxetine (Cobalt). *fluoxetine HCl.*

CO Fluvoxamine (Cobalt). *fluvoxamine maleate.*

CO Gabapentin (Cobalt). *gabapentin.*

Cogentin (Merck Frosst). *benztropine mesylate.* Discontinued 2004.

Colace (WellSpring). *docusate sodium.*

colchicine. **Colchicine-Odan**; **Colchicine: Oral**.

Colchicine: Oral (CPhA Monograph). *colchicine.*

Colchicine-Odan (Odan). *colchicine.*

COLD-FX (Afexa Life Sciences). *North American ginseng (Panax quinquefolius).*

Cold Sore Lotion (Rougier Pharma). *benzoin / camphor / menthol.*

colecalciferol. see *cholecalciferol.*

Colestid (Pfizer). *colestipol HCl.*

colestipol HCl. **Colestid**.

CO Levetiracetam (Cobalt). *levetiracetam.*

CO Levofloxacin (Cobalt). *levofloxacin.*

CO Lisinopril (Cobalt). *lisinopril.*

Colistimethate for Injection U.S.P. (SteriMax). *sodium colistimethate.*

Colorless Antiseptic (Rougier Pharma). *chloroxylenol.*

CO Lovastatin (Cobalt). *lovastatin.*

Colprone (Wyeth-Ayerst). *medrogestone.* Discontinued 2001.

Coly-Mycin M Parenteral (ERFA Canada). *sodium colistimethate.*

Colyte (PendoPharm). *electrolytes / polyethylene glycol.*

Combantrin (McNeil Consumer Healthcare). *pyrantel pamoate.*

Combigan (Allergan). *brimonidine tartrate / timolol maleate.*

combined diphtheria and tetanus toxoids, acellular pertussis, hepatitis B (recombinant), inactivated poliomyelitis and adsorbed conjugated H. influenzae type b vaccine. **Infanrix hexa**.

combined diphtheria, tetanus, acellular pertussis (adsorbed) vaccine. **Boostrix**.

combined hepatitis A and hepatitis B vaccine. **Twinrix**.

combined purified Vi polysaccharide typhoid and inactivated hepatitis A vaccine. **ViVAXIM**.

Combivent Inhalation Aerosol (Boehringer Ingelheim). *ipratropium bromide / salbutamol sulfate.* Discontinued 2007.

Combivent UDV (Boehringer Ingelheim). *ipratropium bromide / salbutamol sulfate.*

Combivir (ViiV Healthcare ULC). *lamivudine / zidovudine.*

CO Meloxicam (Cobalt). *meloxicam.*

CO Memantine (Cobalt). *memantine HCl.*

CO Metformin Coated (Cobalt). *metformin HCl.*

Complete Multi-Adult (Jamieson). *multiple vitamins and minerals.* Discontinued 2010.

Comtan (Novartis Pharmaceuticals). *entacapone.*

Concentrated Milk of Magnesia—Cascara Suspension (Genpharm). *cascara / magnesium hydroxide.* Discontinued 2000.

Concerta (Janssen-Ortho). *methylphenidate HCl.*

Condyline (Canderm Pharma). *podofilox.*

Congest (Trianon). *conjugated estrogens.* Discontinued 2003.

conjugated estrogens. **C.E.S.**; **Premarin Intravenous**; **Premarin Tablets**; **Premarin Vaginal Cream**.

conjugated estrogens + medroxyprogesterone acetate. **Premplus**.

CO Norfloxacin (Cobalt). *norfloxacin.*

Conray 30 (tyco Healthcare). *iothalamate meglumine.*

Conray 43 (tyco Healthcare). *iothalamate meglumine.*

Conray 60 (tyco Healthcare). *iothalamate meglumine.*

Contac Chest Congestion, Non Drowsy, Regular Strength (GlaxoSmithKline Consumer Healthcare). *acetaminophen / guaifenesin / phenylephrine HCl.* Discontinued 2010.

Contac Cold & Sore Throat, Nighttime, Extra Strength (GlaxoSmithKline Consumer Healthcare). *acetaminophen / chlorpheniramine maleate / phenylephrine HCl.*

Contac Cold & Sore Throat, Non Drowsy, Extra Strength (GlaxoSmithKline Consumer Healthcare). *acetaminophen / phenylephrine HCl.*

Contac Cold 12 Hour Relief Extra Strength (SmithKline Beecham Consumer Healthcare). *chlorpheniramine maleate / phenylpropanolamine HCl.* Discontinued 2001.

Contac Complete – Cough, Cold & Flu, Nighttime, Extra Strength (GlaxoSmithKline Consumer Healthcare). *acetaminophen / chlorpheniramine maleate / dextromethorphan HBr / phenylephrine HCl.*

Contac Complete – Cough, Cold & Flu, Non Drowsy, Extra Strength (GlaxoSmithKline Consumer Healthcare). *acetaminophen / dextromethorphan HBr / phenylephrine HCl.*

CO Olanzapine (Cobalt). *olanzapine.*

CO Olanzapine ODT (Cobalt). *olanzapine.*

CO Ondansetron (Cobalt). *ondansetron HCl dihydrate.*

CO Pantoprazole (Cobalt). *pantoprazole sodium.*

CO Paroxetine (Cobalt). *paroxetine.*

Copaxone (Teva Canada Innovation). *glatiramer acetate.*

Cophylac (Valeo Pharma). *normethadone HCl / p-hydroxyephedrine HCl.*

CO Pioglitazone (Cobalt). *pioglitazone HCl.*

copper / ascorbic acid / lycopene / selenium / vitamin B complex / vitamin E / zinc. **Stresstabs for Men**.

copper / ascorbic acid / vitamin B complex / vitamin E / zinc. **Stresstabs Z-BEC**.

copper / calcium carbonate / magnesium / manganese / vitamin D / zinc. **Caltrate Plus**.

Coppertone Continuous Spray SPF 30 (Schering-Plough). *avobenzone / homosalate / octisalate / oxybenzone.*

Coppertone Kids Colorblock Spray SPF 30 (Schering-Plough). *homosalate / octinoxate / octisalate / oxybenzone.* Discontinued 2010.

Coppertone Kids Spray Lotion SPF 30 (Schering-Plough). *homosalate / octinoxate / octisalate / oxybenzone.* Discontinued 2010.

Coppertone Mist SPF 4 (Schering-Plough). *homosalate / oxybenzone.* Discontinued 2010.

Coppertone Oil Free Faces SPF 30 (Schering-Plough). *avobenzone / homosalate / octisalate / octocrylene / oxybenzone.*

Coppertone Sport Continuous Spray SPF 15 & 30 (Schering-Plough). *homosalate / octinoxate / octisalate / oxybenzone.*

Coppertone Sunscreen Lotion SPF 8 (Schering-Plough). *octinoxate / oxybenzone.*

Coppertone Sunscreen Lotion SPF 15 (Schering-Plough). *avobenzone / homosalate / octisalate / octocrylene.*

Coppertone Sunscreen Lotion SPF 30 & 60 (Schering-Plough). *avobenzone / homosalate / octisalate / octocrylene / oxybenzone.*

Coppertone Suntan Lotion SPF 4 (Schering-Plough). *octinoxate / oxybenzone.* Discontinued 2010.

Coppertone Waterbabies Sunblock Lotion SPF 60 (Schering-Plough). *avobenzone / homosalate / octisalate / octocrylene / oxybenzone.*

Names in *italics*: Generic drug names, active ingredient or category.
Names in **bold face/underlined**: Prescribing information provided in the Monograph section.
Names in **bold face/not underlined**: Availability information provided in the Monograph section.
Names in regular face: Product is available in Canada but the monograph does not appear in *CPS*.

CO Pramipexole (Cobalt). *pramipexole dihydrochloride*.

CO Pravastatin (Cobalt). *pravastatin sodium*.

CO Quetiapine (Cobalt). *quetiapine fumarate*.

Coquinone Coenzyme Q-10 (USANA Health Sciences). *ubidecarenone*.

CO Ramipril (Cobalt). *ramipril*.

CO Ranitidine (Cobalt). *ranitidine HCl*.

Cordarone (Pfizer). *amiodarone HCl*.

Coreg (GlaxoSmithKline). *carvedilol*. Discontinued 2006.

Coricidin II Cold and Flu (Schering-Plough). *acetaminophen / chlorpheniramine maleate*.

Coricidin II Cold and Flu Extra Strength (Schering-Plough). *acetaminophen / chlorpheniramine maleate / dextromethorphan HBr*.

Coricidin II Cough and Cold (Schering-Plough). *chlorpheniramine maleate / dextromethorphan HBr*.

Coricidin Non-Drowsy (Schering). *ASA / phenylpropanolamine*. Discontinued 2000.

CO Risperidone (Cobalt). *risperidone*.

Coristine-DH (Technilab). *hydrocodone bitartrate / phenylephrine HCl*. Discontinued 2002.

CO Ropinirole (Cobalt). *ropinirole HCl*.

Correctol (Schering-Plough). *bisacodyl*. Discontinued 2010.

Cortamed (Sandoz). *hydrocortisone acetate*.

Cortate (Schering-Plough). *hydrocortisone*.

Cortef Cream (Johnson & Johnson). *hydrocortisone acetate*.

Cortef Tablets (Pfizer). *hydrocortisone*.

Cortenema (Axcan Pharma). *hydrocortisone*.

Corticosteroids: Eye Ear Nose (CPhA Monograph).

Corticosteroids: Inhaled (CPhA Monograph).

Corticosteroids: Systemic (CPhA Monograph).

Corticosteroids: Topical (CPhA Monograph).

Corticreme (Rougier). *hydrocortisone acetate*. Discontinued 2000.

Cortifoam (Paladin). *hydrocortisone acetate*.

Cortisone Acetate (Valeant). *cortisone acetate*.

cortisone acetate. **Corticosteroids: Systemic**; **Cortisone Acetate**.

Cortisporin Eye/Ear Suspension Sterile (GlaxoSmithKline). *hydrocortisone / neomycin sulfate / polymyxin B sulfate*. Discontinued 2006.

Cortisporin Ointment (GlaxoSmithKline). *bacitracin zinc / hydrocortisone / neomycin sulfate / polymyxin B sulfate*.

Cortisporin Otic Solution Sterile (GlaxoSmithKline). *hydrocortisone / neomycin sulfate / polymyxin B sulfate*.

Cortoderm (Taro). *hydrocortisone*.

Cortone (Merck Frosst). *cortisone acetate*. Discontinued 2002.

Cortrosyn (Amphastar). *cosyntropin*.

Corvert (Pfizer). *ibutilide fumarate*.

CO Sertraline (Cobalt). *sertraline HCl*.

CO Simvastatin (Cobalt). *simvastatin*.

Cosmegen (Ovation). *dactinomycin*.

Cosopt (Merck Frosst). *dorzolamide HCl / timolol maleate*.

CO Sotalol (Cobalt). *sotalol HCl*.

CO Sumatriptan (Cobalt). *sumatriptan succinate*.

cosyntropin. **Cortrosyn**.

cosyntropin / zinc hydroxide. **Synacthen Depot**.

Cotazym (Schering-Plough). *pancrelipase*.

CO Temazepam (Cobalt). *temazepam*.

CO Terbinafine (Cobalt). *terbinafine HCl*.

CO Topiramate (Cobalt). *topiramate*.

cotrimoxazole. see *sulfamethoxazole-Trimethoprim*.

Coumadin (Bristol-Myers Squibb). *warfarin sodium*.

CO Valacyclovir (Cobalt). *valacyclovir HCl*.

CO Venlafaxine XR (Cobalt). *venlafaxine HCl*.

Covera-HS (Pfizer). *verapamil HCl*. Discontinued 2010.

Coversyl (Servier). *perindopril erbumine*.

Coversyl Plus (Servier). *indapamide / perindopril erbumine*.

Coversyl Plus HD (Servier). *indapamide / perindopril erbumine*.

Coversyl Plus LD (Servier). *indapamide / perindopril erbumine*.

Cozaar (Merck Frosst). *losartan potassium*.

CO Zopiclone (Cobalt). *zopiclone*.

Creon 5 Minimicrospheres (Abbott Products). *pancreatic enzymes*.

Creon 10 Minimicrospheres (Abbott Products). *pancreatic enzymes*.

Creon 25 Minimicrospheres (Abbott Products). *pancreatic enzymes*.

Creo-Rectal (Sandoz). *camphor / diphenylpyraline HCl / guaiacol carbonate*.

Crestor (AstraZeneca). *rosuvastatin calcium*.

Crinone (EMD Canada). *progesterone*.

Crixivan (Merck Frosst). *indinavir sulfate*.

Cromolyn (PendoPharm). *sodium cromoglycate*.

cromolyn sodium. see *sodium cromoglycate*.

Crystapen (Alveda). *penicillin G sodium*.

CTP 30 (Sepracor). *citalopram HBr*.

Cubicin (Sepracor). *daptomycin*.

Cucurbita pepo / Curcuma longa / Helianthus annus / Linum usitatissimum / Olea europaea / Rosmarinus officinalis. **Optomega**.

Cuplex (TCD). *lactic acid / salicylic acid*. Discontinued 2000.

Cuprimine (Aton Pharma). *penicillamine*.

Curcuma longa / Cucurbita pepo / Helianthus annus / Linum usitatissimum / Olea europaea / Rosmarinus officinalis. **Optomega**.

Cutivate (GlaxoSmithKline Consumer Healthcare). *fluticasone propionate*. Discontinued 2007.

cyanocobalamin. **Vitamin B12**; **Vitamin B_{12} Injection**.

Cyclen (Janssen-Ortho). *ethinyl estradiol / norgestimate*.

Cyclobenzaprine (CPhA Monograph). *cyclobenzaprine HCl*.

cyclobenzaprine HCl. **Cyclobenzaprine**; **ratio-Cyclobenzaprine**.

Cyclocort (Stiefel, a GSK company). *amcinonide*.

Cyclogyl (Alcon). *cyclopentolate HCl*.

Cyclomen (sanofi-aventis). *danazol*.

cyclopentasiloxane / polysilicone-11 / dimethicone / phenyl trimethicone / polymethylsilsesquioxane / tetrahexyldecyl ascorbate. **Dermatix Ultra**.

Cyclopentolate (CPhA Monograph). *cyclopentolate HCl*.

cyclopentolate HCl. **Cyclogyl**; **Cyclopentolate**.

cyclophosphamide. **Procytox**.

cyclosporine. **Neoral**; **Sandimmune I.V.**; **Restasis**; **Sandoz Cyclosporine**.

CyEstra-35 (Pharmascience). *cyproterone acetate / ethinyl estradiol*.

Cyklokapron (Pfizer). *tranexamic acid*.

Cymbalta (Lilly). *duloxetine HCl*.

cyproterone acetate. **Androcur**; **Androcur Depot**.

cyproterone acetate / ethinyl estradiol. **CyEstra-35**; **Diane-35**.

Cystistat (Alveda). *sodium hyaluronate*.

Cysto-Conray (Mallinckrodt). *iothalamate meglumine*. Discontinued 2002.

Cysto-Conray II (tyco Healthcare). *iothalamate meglumine*.

cytarabine. **Cytarabine Injection**; **Cytosar**.

Cytarabine Injection (Hospira). *cytarabine*.

CytoGam (CSL Behring). *cytomegalovirus immune globulin intravenous (human)*.

cytomegalovirus immune globulin intravenous (human). **CytoGam**.

Cytomel (King Pharmaceuticals). *liothyronine sodium*.

Cytosar (Pfizer). *cytarabine*.

cytosine arabinoside. see *cytarabine*.

Cytotec (Pharmacia). *misoprostol*. Discontinued 2003.

Cytovene (Roche). *ganciclovir sodium*.

Cytoxan (Bristol-Myers Squibb). *cyclophosphamide*. Discontinued 2008.

Names in *italics*: Generic drug names, active ingredient or category.
Names in **bold face/underlined**: Prescribing information provided in the Monograph section.
Names in **bold face/not underlined**: Availability information provided in the Monograph section.
Names in regular face: Product is available in Canada but the monograph does not appear in *CPS*.

D

Names in *italics*: Generic drug names, active ingredient or category.
Names in **bold face/underlined**: Prescribing information provided in the Monograph section.
Names in **bold face/not underlined**: Availability information provided in the Monograph section.
Names in regular face: Product is available in Canada but the monograph does not appear in *CPS*.

Names in *italics*: Generic drug names, active ingredient or category.
Names in **bold face/underlined**: Prescribing information provided in the Monograph section.
Names in **bold face/not underlined**: Availability information provided in the Monograph section.
Names in regular face: Product is available in Canada but the monograph does not appear in *CPS*.

Digibind (GlaxoSmithKline). *digoxin immune Fab (ovine).*

digoxin. **Digoxin Injection C.S.D.**; **Digoxin Pediatric Injection C.S.D.**; **Lanoxin**; **Toloxin**.

digoxin immune Fab (ovine). **Digibind**.

Digoxin Injection C.S.D. (Sandoz). *digoxin.*

Digoxin Pediatric Injection C.S.D. (Sandoz). *digoxin.*

digoxin-specific antibody fragments. see *digoxin immune Fab (ovine).*

dihydrocodeinone bitartrate. see *hydrocodone bitartrate.*

Dihydroergotamine (DHE) (SteriMax). *dihydroergotamine mesylate.*

dihydroergotamine mesylate. **Dihydroergotamine (DHE)**; **Dihydroergotamine Mesylate Injection USP**; **Migranal**.

Dihydroergotamine Mesylate Injection USP (Sandoz). *dihydroergotamine mesylate.*

dihydrohydroxycodeinone. see *oxycodone HCl.*

dihydromorphinone HCl. see *hydromorphone HCl.*

diiodohydroxyquin. see *iodoquinol.*

diiodohydroxyquinolone. see *iodoquinol.*

Dilantin-30 Suspension (Pfizer). *phenytoin.*

Dilantin-125 Suspension (Pfizer). *phenytoin.*

Dilantin Capsules (Pfizer). *phenytoin sodium.*

Dilantin Infatabs (Pfizer). *phenytoin.*

Dilaudid (Purdue Pharma). *hydromorphone HCl.*

Dilaudid-HP (Purdue Pharma). *hydromorphone HCl.*

Dilaudid-HP-Plus (Purdue Pharma). *hydromorphone HCl.*

Dilaudid Sterile Powder (Purdue Pharma). *hydromorphone HCl.*

Dilaudid-XP (Purdue Pharma). *hydromorphone HCl.*

diltiazem HCl. **Calcium Channel Blockers**; **Cardizem CD**; **Diltiazem Hydrochloride Injection**; **Nu-Diltiaz-CD**; **Nu-Diltiaz**; **ratio-Diltiazem CD**; **Sandoz Diltiazem CD**; **Sandoz Diltiazem T**; **Teva-Diltiazem**; **Teva-Diltiazem CD**; **Tiazac XC**; **Tiazac**.

Diltiazem Hydrochloride Injection (Sandoz). *diltiazem HCl.*

Dimenhydrinate (Sandoz). *dimenhydrinate.*

dimenhydrinate. **Dimenhydrinate**; **Gravol Preparations**.

Dimenhydrinate Injection USP (Alveda). *dimenhydrinate.*

Dimetane (Whitehall-Robins). *brompheniramine maleate.* Discontinued 2000.

Dimetane Expectorant (Whitehall-Robins). *brompheniramine maleate / guaifenesin / phenylephrine HCl / phenylpropanolamine HCl.* Discontinued 2001.

Dimetane Expectorant-C (Pfizer Consumer Healthcare). *brompheniramine maleate / codeine phosphate / guaifenesin / phenylephrine HCl.*

Dimetane Expectorant-DC (Pfizer Consumer Healthcare). *brompheniramine maleate / guaifenesin / hydrocodone bitartrate / phenylephrine HCl.*

Dimetapp-A Sinus (Whitehall-Robins). *acetaminophen / phenylephrine HCl / phenylpropanolamine HCl.* Discontinued 2001.

Dimetapp Chewables (Whitehall-Robins). *brompheniramine maleate / phenylpropanolamine HCl.* Discontinued 2001.

Dimetapp Chewables for Kids (Pfizer Consumer Healthcare). *brompheniramine maleate / phenylephrine HCl.*

Dimetapp Clear (Whitehall-Robins). *brompheniramine maleate / phenylpropanolamine HCl.* Discontinued 2001.

Dimetapp Cough & Cold Liqui-Gels (Whitehall-Robins). *brompheniramine maleate / dextromethorphan HBr / phenylpropanolamine HCl.* Discontinued 2001.

Dimetapp-C Syrup (Pfizer Consumer Healthcare). *brompheniramine maleate / codeine phosphate / phenylephrine HCl.*

Dimetapp Daytime Cold Extra Strength (Wyeth Consumer Healthcare). *acetaminophen / pseudoephedrine HCl.* Discontinued 2010.

Dimetapp DM Cough & Cold Liquid (Pfizer Consumer Healthcare). *brompheniramine maleate / dextromethorphan HBr / phenylephrine HCl.*

Dimetapp Extra Strength DM Cough & Cold Liquid (Pfizer Consumer Healthcare). *brompheniramine maleate / dextromethorphan HBr / phenylephrine HCl.*

Dimetapp Extra Strength Liquid (Pfizer Consumer Healthcare). *brompheniramine maleate / phenylephrine HCl.*

Dimetapp Liquid (Pfizer Consumer Healthcare). *brompheniramine maleate / phenylephrine HCl.*

Dimetapp Liqui-Gels (Whitehall-Robins). *brompheniramine maleate / phenylpropanolamine HCl.* Discontinued 2001.

Dimetapp Nighttime Cold Extra Strength (Wyeth Consumer Healthcare). *acetaminophen / chlorpheniramine maleate / phenylephrine HCl.* Discontinued 2010.

dimethicone / polysilicone-11 / cyclopentasiloxane / phenyl trimethicone / polymethylsilsesquioxane / tetrahexyldecyl ascorbate. **Dermatix Ultra**.

dimethylpolysiloxane. **Barriere**.

dimethyl sulfoxide. **Dimethyl Sulfoxide Irrigation USP**; **Rimso-50**.

Dimethyl Sulfoxide Irrigation USP (Sandoz). *dimethyl sulfoxide.*

dinoprostone. **Cervidil**; **Prepidil**; **Prostin E2 Tablets**; **Prostin E2 Vaginal Gel**.

dioctyl calcium sulfosuccinate. see *docusate calcium.*

dioctyl sodium sulfosuccinate. see *docusate sodium.*

Diodoquin (Glenwood). *iodoquinol.*

Diofluor Strips (Dioptic). *fluorescein sodium.* Discontinued 2004.

Diophenyl-T (Sandoz). *phenylephrine HCl / tropicamide.*

Diopred (Sandoz). *prednisolone acetate.*

Diovan (Novartis Pharmaceuticals). *valsartan.*

Diovan-HCT (Novartis Pharmaceuticals). *hydrochlorothiazide / valsartan.*

Diovol (Church & Dwight). *aluminum hydroxide / magnesium hydroxide.*

Diovol Ex (Church & Dwight). *aluminum hydroxide / magnesium hydroxide.* Discontinued 2007.

Diovol Plus (Church & Dwight). *aluminum hydroxide / magnesium hydroxide / simethicone.*

Diovol Plus AF (Church & Dwight). *calcium carbonate / magnesium hydroxide / simethicone.*

Dipentum (UCB). *olsalazine sodium.*

diphenhydramine HCl. **Allernix**; **Benadryl Preparations**; **Benylin Night Cough**; **Diphenhydramine Hydrochloride Injection USP**; **Nytol Extra Strength**; **Unisom**.

diphenhydramine HCl / acetaminophen / dextromethorphan HBr. **Tylenol Children's Cold & Cough Nighttime**.

diphenhydramine HCl / acetaminophen / phenylephrine HCl. **Benylin All-in-One Cold and Flu Night PE**.

diphenhydramine HCl / acetaminophen / pseudoephedrine HCl. **Benadryl Allergy/Sinus/Headache**; **Benadryl Total/Allergy/Regular Strength**; **Benadryl Total/Allergy/Extra Strength**; **Sinutab Nightime**.

diphenhydramine HCl / ammonium chloride / codeine phosphate. **Calmylin Original with Codeine**.

diphenhydramine HCl / ammonium chloride / dextromethorphan HBr. **Balminil Night-Time**.

diphenhydramine HCl / zinc acetate. **Benadryl Spray**; **Benadryl Stick**.

Diphenhydramine Hydrochloride Injection USP (Sandoz). *diphenhydramine HCl.*

Diphenist (Omega Laboratories). *diphenhydramine HCl.* Discontinued 2010.

diphenoxylate HCl / atropine sulfate. **Lomotil**.

diphenylhydantoin. see *phenytoin.*

diphtheria and tetanus toxoids and acellular pertussis vaccine adsorbed combined with inactivated poliomyelitis vaccine. **Quadracel**.

diphtheria and tetanus toxoids and acellular pertussis vaccine adsorbed combined with inactivated poliomyelitis vaccine and Haemophilus b conjugate vaccine (tetanus protein-conjugate). **Pediacel**.

Diphtheria Antitoxin Equine (Aventis Pasteur). *diphtheria antitoxin equine.* Discontinued 2003.

Diprivan (AstraZeneca). *propofol.*

Diprogen (Schering). *betamethasone dipropionate / gentamicin sulfate.* Discontinued 2001.

Diprolene Glycol (Schering-Plough). *betamethasone dipropionate.*

Diprosalic (Schering-Plough). *betamethasone dipropionate / salicylic acid.*

Diprosone (Schering-Plough). *betamethasone dipropionate.*

dipyridamole. **Persantine**.

dipyridamole / ASA. **Aggrenox**.

Disalcid (3M Pharmaceuticals). *salsalate.* Discontinued 2001.

Disipal (3M Pharmaceuticals). *orphenadrine HCl.* Discontinued 2001.

disopyramide. **Rythmodan**.

disposable needles. **NovoFine 32G Tip**; **NovoFine 30G**.

Ditropan (Janssen-Ortho). *oxybutynin chloride.* Discontinued 2009.

Ditropan XL (Janssen-Ortho). *oxybutynin chloride.*

divalproex sodium. **Epival**; **Nu-Divalproex**.

Names in *italics*: Generic drug names, active ingredient or category.
Names in **bold face/underlined**: Prescribing information provided in the Monograph section.
Names in **bold face/not underlined**: Availability information provided in the Monograph section.
Names in regular face: Product is available in Canada but the monograph does not appear in *CPS*.

Dixarit (Boehringer Ingelheim). *clonidine HCl.*

DMSO. see *dimethyl sulfoxide.*

Doak Oil (Stiefel, a GSK company). *isopropyl palmitate / mineral oil / tar distillate.*

Doak Oil Forte (Stiefel, a GSK company). *isopropyl palmitate / mineral oil / tar distillate.*

dobutamine HCl. **Dobutamine Injection**; **Dobutamine Injection USP**.

Dobutamine Injection (Hospira). *dobutamine HCl.*

Dobutamine Injection USP (Sandoz). *dobutamine HCl.*

docetaxel. **Taxotere**.

docosanol. **Abreva**.

docusate calcium. **ratio-Docusate Calcium**; **Soflax C**.

Docusate Sodium (Taro). *docusate sodium.*

docusate sodium. **Colace**; **Docusate Sodium**; **ratio-Docusate Sodium**; **Selax**; **Soflax**; **Soflax**.

docusate sodium / senna (standardized sennosides from senna concentrate CG). **Senokot•S**.

docusate sodium / sennosides. **Senna-S Tablets Peristaltic Stimulant-Surfactant**.

dolasetron mesylate. **Anzemet**.

Dolobid (Merck Frosst). *diflunisal.* Discontinued 2000.

Domperidone (CPhA Monograph). *domperidone maleate.*

domperidone maleate. **Domperidone**; **RAN-Domperidone**; **ratio-Domperidone**.

donepezil HCl. **Aricept**; **Aricept RDT**.

Donnagel-PG Capsules (Wyeth-Ayerst). *attapulgite / opium / pectin.* Discontinued 2001.

Donnagel-PG Suspension (Wyeth-Ayerst). *kaolin / opium / pectin.* Discontinued 2001.

Donnatal (Wyeth-Ayerst). *belladonna alkaloids / phenobarbital.* Discontinued 2001.

dopamine HCl / dextrose. **Dopamine HCl and 5% Dextrose Injection**; **Dopamine HCl and Dextrose Injection**.

Dopamine HCl and 5% Dextrose Injection (Baxter). *dextrose / dopamine HCl.*

Dopamine HCl and Dextrose Injection (Hospira). *dextrose / dopamine HCl.*

Dopram (Wyeth-Ayerst). *doxapram HCl.* Discontinued 2001.

Doribax (Janssen-Ortho). *doripenem.*

doripenem. **Doribax**.

Dormer 211 Cream SPF 15 (Dormer). *avobenzone / octinoxate / oxybenzone.*

Dormer 211 Cream SPF 30 (Dormer). *avobenzone / octinoxate / octisalate / oxybenzone / titanium dioxide.*

dornase alfa recombinant. **Pulmozyme**.

dorzolamide HCl. **Trusopt**.

dorzolamide HCl / timolol maleate. **Cosopt**.

Dostinex (Paladin). *cabergoline.*

Dovobet (LEO Pharma). *betamethasone dipropionate / calcipotriol.*

Dovonex (LEO Pharma). *calcipotriol.*

doxazosin mesylate. **Cardura-1**; **Cardura-2**; **Cardura-4**.

doxepin HCl. **Apo-Doxepin**.

doxercalciferol. **Vitamin D**.

doxorubicin HCl. **Adriamycin PFS**; **Doxorubicin HCl for Injection USP**.

Doxorubicin HCl for Injection USP (Hospira). *doxorubicin HCl.*

doxorubicin HCl, pegylated liposomal. **Caelyx**.

Doxycin (Riva). *doxycycline hyclate.*

doxycycline hyclate. **Doxycin**; **Nu-Doxycycline**; **Periostat**; **Tetracyclines**; **Vibramycin**; **Vibra-Tabs**.

doxylamine succinate. **Unisom-2**.

doxylamine succinate / acetaminophen / codeine phosphate. **Mersyndol with Codeine**.

doxylamine succinate / acetaminophen / dextromethorphan HBr. **Vicks NyQuil Liquicaps**; **Vicks NyQuil Liquid**.

doxylamine succinate / acetaminophen / dextromethorphan HBr / phenylephrine HCl. **Tylenol Cold & Flu Nighttime Liquid**.

doxylamine succinate / acetaminophen / phenylephrine HCl. **Vicks NyQuil Sinus LiquiCaps**.

doxylamine succinate / dextromethorphan hydrobromide. **Vicks NyQuil Cough Liquid**.

doxylamine succinate / etafedrine HCl / hydrocodone bitartrate. **ratio-Calmydone**.

doxylamine succinate / etafedrine HCl / hydrocodone bitartrate / sodium citrate. **Dalmacol**.

doxylamine succinate / pyridoxine HCl. **Diclectin**.

DPE (Alcon). *dipivefrin HCl.* Discontinued 2000.

Dr. Scholl's 2–Drop Corn & Callus Remedy (Schering-Plough). *salicylic acid.*

Dr. Scholl's Athlete's Foot Powder (Schering-Plough). *tolnaftate.*

Dr. Scholl's Athlete's Foot Spray Powder (Schering-Plough). *tolnaftate.*

Dr. Scholl's Clear Away Liquid Wart Remover (Schering-Plough). *salicylic acid.*

Dr. Scholl's Clear Away One Step Wart Remover System (Schering-Plough). *salicylic acid.*

Dr. Scholl's Clear Away Plantar Wart Remover System (Schering-Plough). *salicylic acid.*

Dr. Scholl's Clear Away Wart Remover System (Schering-Plough). *salicylic acid.*

Dr. Scholl's Medicated Powder (Schering-Plough). *zinc oxide.* Discontinued 2010.

Drisdol (sanofi-aventis). *ergocalciferol.*

Dristan (Pfizer Consumer Healthcare). *acetaminophen / chlorpheniramine maleate / phenylephrine HCl.*

Dristan Extra Strength (Pfizer Consumer Healthcare). *acetaminophen / chlorpheniramine maleate / phenylephrine HCl.*

Dristan Long Lasting Mentholated Nasal Spray (Wyeth Consumer Healthcare). *oxymetazoline HCl.* Discontinued 2006.

Dristan Long Lasting Nasal Mist/Spray (Pfizer Consumer Healthcare). *oxymetazoline HCl.*

Dristan Nasal Mist (Pfizer Consumer Healthcare). *pheniramine maleate / phenylephrine HCl.*

Dristan Sinus (Whitehall-Robins). *acetaminophen / ibuprofen / pseudoephedrine HCl.* Discontinued 2004.

Drixoral Cold & Sinus (Schering-Plough). *dexbrompheniramine maleate / pseudoephedrine sulfate*. Discontinued 2010.

Drixoral Decongestant Nasal Spray 0.05% (Schering-Plough). *oxymetazoline HCl.*

Drixoral ND Long Acting (Schering-Plough). *pseudoephedrine sulfate.* Discontinued 2010.

Drixoral No Drip Extra Moisturizing (Schering-Plough). *oxymetazoline HCl.*

Drixoral No Drip Original (Schering-Plough). *oxymetazoline HCl.*

Drixoral No Drip with Cooling Menthol (Schering-Plough). *oxymetazoline HCl.*

Drixoral SRT (Schering). *dexbrompheniramine maleate / pseudoephedrine sulfate.* Discontinued 2009.

dronedarone HCl. **Multaq**.

droperidol. **Droperidol Injection USP**.

Droperidol Injection USP (Sandoz). *droperidol.*

drospirenone / estradiol-17β. **Angeliq**.

drospirenone / ethinyl estradiol. **Yasmin 21**; **Yasmin 28**; **Yaz**.

drotrecogin alfa (activated). **Xigris**.

D-Tabs (Riva). *vitamin D.*

DTIC (Bayer). *dacarbazine.* Discontinued 2005.

DT Polio Adsorbed (Aventis Pasteur). *diphtheria and tetanus toxoids adsorbed and poliomyelitis vaccine.* Discontinued 2005.

Dukoral (sanofi pasteur). *oral, inactivated travellers' diarrhea and cholera vaccine.*

Dulcolax (Boehringer Ingelheim). *bisacodyl.*

duloxetine HCl. **Cymbalta**.

Duo-C.V.P (Rhône-Poulenc Rorer). *ascorbic acid.* Discontinued 2000.

Duofilm Gel for Kids (Stiefel). *salicylic acid.* Discontinued 2007.

Duofilm Liquid (Stiefel, a GSK company). *lactic acid / salicylic acid.*

Duofilm Patch (Stiefel, a GSK company). *salicylic acid.*

Duofilm Plantar Patch (Stiefel, a GSK company). *salicylic acid.*

Duoforte 27 (Stiefel, a GSK company). *salicylic acid.*

Duonalc (Valeant). *isopropyl alcohol.* Discontinued 2009.

Duonalc-E Mild (Valeant). *ethyl alcohol.* Discontinued 2009.

Duonalc-E Solution (Valeant). *ethyl alcohol / isopropyl alcohol.* Discontinued 2009.

Duoplant (Stiefel, a GSK company). *formalin / lactic acid / salicylic acid.*

DuoTrav (Alcon). *timolol maleate / travoprost.*

Duovent UDV (Boehringer Ingelheim). *fenoterol HBr / ipratropium bromide.*

Duragesic 12 (Janssen-Ortho). *fentanyl.* Discontinued 2010.

Duragesic 25 (Janssen-Ortho). *fentanyl.* Discontinued 2010.

Duragesic 50 (Janssen-Ortho). *fentanyl.* Discontinued 2010.

Duragesic 75 (Janssen-Ortho). *fentanyl.* Discontinued 2010.

Duragesic 100 (Janssen-Ortho). *fentanyl.* Discontinued 2010.

Names in *italics*: Generic drug names, active ingredient or category.
Names in **bold face/underlined**: Prescribing information provided in the Monograph section.
Names in **bold face/not underlined**: Availability information provided in the Monograph section.
Names in regular face: Product is available in Canada but the monograph does not appear in *CPS*.

Names in *italics*: Generic drug names, active ingredient or category.
Names in **bold face/underlined**: Prescribing information provided in the Monograph section.
Names in **bold face/not underlined**: Availability information provided in the Monograph section.
Names in regular face: Product is available in Canada but the monograph does not appear in *CPS*.

eplerenone. **Inspra**.

epoetin alfa. **Eprex**.

epoprostenol sodium. **Flolan for Injection**.

Eprex (Janssen-Ortho). *epoetin alfa.*

E-Prime (USANA Health Sciences). *vitamin E.*

eprosartan mesylate. **Teveten**.

eprosartan mesylate / hydrochlorothiazide. **Teveten Plus**.

Epsom Salts (Rougier Pharma). *magnesium sulfate.*

eptacog alfa (activated). **NiaStase RT**.

eptifibatide. **Integrilin**.

Equanil (Wyeth-Ayerst). *meprobamate.* Discontinued 2000.

Eraxis (Pfizer). *anidulafungin.*

Erbitux (Bristol-Myers Squibb/ImClone LLC). *cetuximab.*

Erdol (Odan). *ergocalciferol.*

Ergamisol (Janssen-Ortho). *levamisole HCl.* Discontinued 2003.

ergocalciferol. **Drisdol**; **Erdol**; **Vitamin D**.

Ergodryl (ERFA Canada). *caffeine citrate / diphenhydramine HCl / ergotamine tartrate.*

ergoloid mesylates. **Hydergine**.

Ergomar (Aventis Pharma). *ergotamine tartrate.* Discontinued 2001.

ergometrine maleate. see *ergonovine maleate.*

Ergonovine Maleate (CPhA Monograph). *ergonovine maleate.*

ergonovine maleate. **Ergonovine Maleate**.

Ergonovine Maleate Injection USP (Alveda). *ergonovine maleate.*

ergosterol. see *ergocalciferol.*

ergotamine tartrate / belladonna / phenobarbital. **Bellergal Spacetabs**.

ergotamine tartrate / caffeine. **Cafergot**.

erlotinib HCl. **Tarceva**.

ertapenem sodium. **Invanz**.

Eryc (Pfizer). *erythromycin.*

Erysol (Stiefel, a GSK company). *butyl methoxydibenzoylmethane / erythromycin / ethyl alcohol / octyl methoxycinnamate.*

Erythrocin I.V. (Methapharm). *erythromycin lactobionate.*

Erythromid (Abbott). *erythromycin.* Discontinued 2001.

erythromycin. **Eryc**; **Erythromycin**.

Erythromycin (CPhA Monograph).

erythromycin / benzoyl peroxide. **Benzamycin**.

erythromycin / butyl methoxydibenzoylmethane / ethyl alcohol / octyl methoxycinnamate. **Erysol**.

erythromycin / tretinoin. **Stievamycin Preparations**.

erythromycin estolate. **Erythromycin**; **Teva-Erythromycin Estolate**.

erythromycin ethylsuccinate. **Erythromycin**; **Teva-Erythromycin Ethylsuccinate**.

erythromycin lactobionate. **Erythromycin**.

erythromycin stearate. **Erythromycin**.

escitalopram oxalate. **Cipralex**; **Selective Serotonin Reuptake Inhibitors**.

esculin / cinchocaine HCl / framycetin sulfate / hydrocortisone. **Proctol**; **Proctosedyl**; **Sandoz Proctomyxin HC**.

esculin / cinchocaine HCl / framycetin sulfate / hydrocortisone acetate. **ratio-Proctosone**.

esmolol HCl. **Brevibloc**; **Brevibloc Premixed**.

esomeprazole magnesium trihydrate. **Nexium**.

esomeprazole magnesium trihydrate / amoxicillin / clarithromycin. **Nexium 1-2-3 A**.

Esoterica Facial Cream (Medicis). *hydroquinone / oxybenzone / padimate O.*

Esoterica Regular Cream (Medicis). *hydroquinone.*

Esoterica Sunscreen Fade Cream (Medicis). *hydroquinone / oxybenzone / padimate O.*

Esoterica Unscented (Medicis). *hydroquinone.* Discontinued 2010.

Estalis (Novartis Pharmaceuticals). *estradiol-17β / norethindrone acetate.*

Estar (Westwood-Squibb). *coal tar.* Discontinued 2005.

Estrace (Shire). *estradiol-17β (micronized).*

Estracomb (Novartis Pharmaceuticals). *estradiol-17β / norethindrone acetate+estradiol-17β.* Discontinued 2009.

Estraderm (Novartis Pharmaceuticals). *estradiol-17β.*

estradiol / norethindrone acetate. **Activelle LD**; **Activelle**.

estradiol-17β. **Climara**; **Estraderm**; **Estradot**; **Estring**; **Sandoz Estradiol Derm**; **Vagifem**.

estradiol-17β / drospirenone. **Angeliq**.

estradiol-17β / levonorgestrel. **Climara Pro**.

estradiol-17β / norethindrone acetate. **Estalis**.

estradiol-17β hemihydrate. **Estrogel**.

estradiol-17β (micronized). **Estrace**.

estradiol hemihydrate. **Oesclim**.

Estradot (Novartis Pharmaceuticals). *estradiol-17β.*

estramustine sodium phosphate. **Emcyt**.

Estring (Paladin). *estradiol-17β.*

Estrogel (Schering-Plough). *estradiol-17β hemihydrate.*

estrogens, conjugated. see *conjugated estrogens.*

estropipate. **Ogen**.

etafedrine HCl / doxylamine succinate / hydrocodone bitartrate. **ratio-Calmydone**.

etafedrine HCl / doxylamine succinate / hydrocodone bitartrate / sodium citrate. **Dalmacol**.

etanercept. **Enbrel**.

ethacrynate sodium. **Sodium Edecrin**.

ethacrynic acid. **Edecrin**.

Ethambutol (CPhA Monograph). *ethambutol HCl.*

ethambutol HCl. **Ethambutol**; **Etibi**.

ethinyl estradiol / cyproterone acetate. **CyEstra-35**; **Diane-35**.

ethinyl estradiol / desogestrel. **Apri 21**; **Apri 28**; **Linessa 21**; **Linessa 28**; **Marvelon**; **Ortho-Cept**.

ethinyl estradiol / drospirenone. **Yasmin 21**; **Yasmin 28**; **Yaz**.

ethinyl estradiol / ethynodiol diacetate. **Demulen 30**.

ethinyl estradiol / etonogestrel. **NuvaRing**.

ethinyl estradiol / levonorgestrel. **Alesse 21**; **Alesse 28**; **Aviane 21**; **Aviane 28**; **Min-Ovral 21**; **Min-Ovral 28**; **Portia 21**; **Portia 28**; **Seasonale**; **Triquilar 21**; **Triquilar 28**.

ethinyl estradiol / norelgestromin. **Evra**.

ethinyl estradiol / norethindrone. **Brevicon 0.5/35**; **Brevicon 1/35**; **Ortho 1/35**; **Ortho 0.5/35**; **Ortho 7/7/7**; **Select 1/35**; **Synphasic**.

ethinyl estradiol / norethindrone acetate. **femHRT**.

ethinyl estradiol / norgestimate. **Cyclen**; **Tri-Cyclen LO**; **Tri-Cyclen**.

ethinyl estradiol / norgestrel. **Ovral 21**.

Ethrane (Baxter). *enflurane.* Discontinued 2001.

ethyl alcohol. **Biobase**.

ethyl alcohol / butyl methoxydibenzoylmethane / erythromycin / octyl methoxycinnamate. **Erysol**.

ethyl alcohol / glycolic acid. **Biobase-G**.

ethyl aminobenzoate. see *benzocaine.*

ethynodiol diacetate / ethinyl estradiol. **Demulen 30**.

Etibi (Valeant). *ethambutol HCl.*

etidronate disodium. **Bisphosphonates: Oral**; **CO Etidronate**.

etidronate disodium / calcium carbonate. **CO Etidrocal**.

etodolac. **Apo-Etodolac**.

etonogestrel / ethinyl estradiol. **NuvaRing**.

etoposide. **Vepesid**.

Etoposide Injection USP (Mayne Pharma). *etoposide.* Discontinued 2007.

etravirine. **Intelence**.

eucalyptus / camphor / menthol. **Vicks VapoRub**.

eucalyptus oil / camphor / menthol / methyl salicylate. **Rub A-535 Antiphlogistine**.

Euflex (Schering-Plough). *flutamide.*

Eurax Cream (Columbia Laboratories). *crotamiton.*

everolimus. **Afinitor**.

Evista (Lilly). *raloxifene HCl.*

Names in *italics*: Generic drug names, active ingredient or category.
Names in **bold face/underlined**: Prescribing information provided in the Monograph section.
Names in **bold face/not underlined**: Availability information provided in the Monograph section.
Names in regular face: Product is available in Canada but the monograph does not appear in *CPS*.

F

Names in *italics*: Generic drug names, active ingredient or category.
Names in **bold face/underlined**: Prescribing information provided in the Monograph section.
Names in **bold face/not underlined**: Availability information provided in the Monograph section.
Names in regular face: Product is available in Canada but the monograph does not appear in *CPS*.

fluocinonide. **Corticosteroids: Topical**; **Lyderm**; **Tiamol**.

Fluoderm (Taro). *fluocinolone acetonide*. Discontinued 2004.

Fluoracaine (Innovo Medical Ophthalmics). *fluorescein sodium / proparacaine HCl*. Discontinued 2010.

Fluor-A-Day (PendoPharm). *sodium fluoride*.

fluorescein sodium. **Fluorescite**.

Fluorescite (Alcon). *fluorescein sodium*.

Fluorets (Novartis Ophthalmics). *fluorescein sodium*.

fluorometholone. **Corticosteroids: Eye Ear Nose**; **FML Forte**; **FML**.

fluorometholone acetate. **Corticosteroids: Eye Ear Nose**; **Flarex**.

Fluoroquinolones (CPhA Monograph).

fluorouracil. **Efudex**.

fluorouracil. see *5-fluorouracil*.

Fluorouracil Injection (Sandoz). *5-fluorouracil*.

Fluorouracil Injection USP (Hospira). *5-fluorouracil*.

Fluotic (sanofi-aventis). *sodium fluoride*. Discontinued 2007.

fluoxetine HCl. **CO Fluoxetine**; **FXT**; **Nu-Fluoxetine**; **PMS-Fluoxetine**; **Prozac**; **ratio-Fluoxetine**; **Selective Serotonin Reuptake Inhibitors**; **Teva-Fluoxetine**.

flupenthixol decanoate. **Fluanxol Depot**.

flupenthixol dihydrochloride. **Fluanxol**.

Fluphenazine (CPhA Monograph).

fluphenazine decanoate. **Fluphenazine**; **Modecate Concentrate**.

fluphenazine HCl. **Fluphenazine**.

flurazepam HCl. **Benzodiazepines**.

flurbiprofen. **Ansaid**.

flutamide. **Euflex**.

fluticasone furoate. **Avamys**.

fluticasone propionate. **Corticosteroids: Eye Ear Nose**; **Corticosteroids: Inhaled**; **Flonase**; **Flovent HFA**; **Flovent Diskus**; **ratio-Fluticasone**.

fluticasone propionate / salmeterol xinafoate. **Advair**; **Advair Diskus**.

fluvastatin sodium. **HMG-CoA Reductase Inhibitors**; **Lescol**; **Lescol XL**.

Fluviral (2010-2011) (ID Biomedical). *split-virion influenza virus vaccine trivalent, inactivated*.

fluvoxamine maleate. **CO Fluvoxamine**; **Luvox**; **ratio-Fluvoxamine**; **Selective Serotonin Reuptake Inhibitors**.

Fluzone (Aventis Pasteur). *influenza virus vaccine trivalent types A and B (zonal purified, subvirion), inactivated*. Discontinued 2003.

FML (Allergan). *fluorometholone*.

FML Forte (Allergan). *fluorometholone*.

folacin. see *folic acid*.

folate. see *folic acid*.

Folic Acid (CPhA Monograph). *folic acid*.

folic acid. **Folic Acid**.

folic acid / ascorbic acid / ferrous fumarate. **Palafer CF**.

folinic acid. see *calcium folinate*.

follitropin alpha. **Gonal-f Pen**.

follitropin alpha (rDNA origin). **Gonal-f**.

follitropin beta. **Puregon**.

Follow-Up (Nestlé). *infant formula (iron-fortified, cow's milk-based)*.

fomepizole. **Antizol**.

fondaparinux sodium. **Arixtra**.

Foradil (Novartis Pharmaceuticals). *formoterol fumarate*.

Forane (Baxter). *isoflurane*.

formalin / lactic acid / salicylic acid. **Duoplant**.

formoterol fumarate. **Foradil**.

formoterol fumarate dihydrate. **Oxeze Turbuhaler**.

formoterol fumarate dihydrate / budesonide. **Symbicort Turbuhaler**.

Fortamines 10 (Rougier). *minerals / multivitamins*. Discontinued 2000.

Fortaz (GlaxoSmithKline). *ceftazidime pentahydrate*.

Forteo (Lilly). *teriparatide (rDNA origin)*.

Fortovase Roche (Roche). *saquinavir*. Discontinued 2006.

Fosamax (Merck Frosst). *alendronate sodium*.

fosamprenavir calcium. **Telzir**.

fosaprepitant dimeglumine. **Emend IV**.

Fosavance (Merck Frosst). *alendronate sodium / cholecalciferol*.

fosinopril sodium. **ACE Inhibitors**; **Monopril**.

Fosrenol (Shire). *lanthanum carbonate*.

Fragmin (Pfizer). *dalteparin sodium*.

framycetin sulfate / cinchocaine HCl / esculin / hydrocortisone. **Proctol**; **Proctosedyl**; **Sandoz Proctomyxin HC**.

framycetin sulfate / cinchocaine HCl / esculin / hydrocortisone acetate. **ratio-Proctosone**.

framycetin sulfate / dexamethasone / gramicidin. **Sofracort**.

Fraxiparine (GlaxoSmithKline). *nadroparin calcium*.

Fraxiparine Forte (GlaxoSmithKline). *nadroparin calcium*.

free fatty acids / ceramides / cholesterol. **EpiCeram**.

Friar's Balsam (Rougier Pharma). *aloe / benzoin / myroxylon balsamum / storax*.

Froben (Abbott). *flurbiprofen*. Discontinued 2008.

Froben SR (Abbott). *flurbiprofen*. Discontinued 2008.

Frova (Teva Canada Innovation). *frovatriptan succinate*.

frovatriptan succinate. **Frova**.

frusemide. see *furosemide*.

FSME-IMMUN (Baxter). *tick-borne encephalitis virus vaccine, inactivated, with adjuvant*.

Fucidin Cream (LEO Pharma). *fusidic acid*.

Fucidin H (LEO Pharma). *fusidic acid / hydrocortisone acetate*.

Fucidin Ointment (LEO Pharma). *sodium fusidate*.

Fucidin Tablets (LEO). *sodium fusidate*. Discontinued 2009.

Fucithalmic (LEO Pharma). *fusidic acid*.

fulvestrant. **Faslodex**.

Fulvicin U/F (Schering). *griseofulvin*. Discontinued 2004.

Fungizone (Bristol-Myers Squibb). *amphotericin B*.

furosemide. **Furosemide Injection USP**; **Furosemide Special**; **Lasix Special**; **Lasix**.

Furosemide Injection USP (Sandoz). *furosemide*.

Furosemide Special (Sandoz). *furosemide*.

fusidate sodium. see *sodium fusidate*.

fusidic acid. **Fucidin Cream**; **Fucithalmic**.

fusidic acid / hydrocortisone acetate. **Fucidin H**.

Fuzeon (Roche). *enfuvirtide*.

FXT (Sepracor). *fluoxetine HCl*.

G

gabapentin. **CO Gabapentin**; **Neurontin**; **PMS-Gabapentin**; **ratio-Gabapentin**; **Teva-Gabapentin**.

gadobutrol. **Gadovist1.0**.

gadopentetate dimeglumine. **Magnevist**.

gadoversetamide. **OptiMARK**.

Gadovist1.0 (Bayer). *gadobutrol*.

gadoxetate disodium. **Primovist**.

galantamine HBr. **Reminyl ER**.

GamaSTAN S/D (Talecris). *immune globulin intramuscular (human)*.

Gamimune N (Bayer). *immune globulin intravenous (human)*. Discontinued 2005.

gamma benzene hexachloride. see *lindane*.

Gammagard Liquid (Baxter). *immune globulin intravenous (human)*.

Gammagard S/D (Baxter). *immune globulin intravenous (human)*.

Gamunex (Talecris). *immune globulin intravenous (human)*.

ganciclovir sodium. **Cytovene**.

ganirelix acetate. **Orgalutran**.

Names in *italics*: Generic drug names, active ingredient or category.
Names in **bold face/underlined**: Prescribing information provided in the Monograph section.
Names in **bold face/not underlined**: Availability information provided in the Monograph section.
Names in regular face: Product is available in Canada but the monograph does not appear in *CPS*.

Names in *italics*: Generic drug names, active ingredient or category.
Names in **bold face/underlined**: Prescribing information provided in the Monograph section.
Names in **bold face/not underlined**: Availability information provided in the Monograph section.
Names in regular face: Product is available in Canada but the monograph does not appear in *CPS*.

H

Names in *italics*: Generic drug names, active ingredient or category.
Names in **bold face/underlined**: Prescribing information provided in the Monograph section.
Names in **bold face/not underlined**: Availability information provided in the Monograph section.
Names in regular face: Product is available in Canada but the monograph does not appear in *CPS*.

Names in *italics*: Generic drug names, active ingredient or category.
Names in **bold face/underlined**: Prescribing information provided in the Monograph section.
Names in **bold face/not underlined**: Availability information provided in the Monograph section.
Names in regular face: Product is available in Canada but the monograph does not appear in *CPS*.

I

Names in *italics*: Generic drug names, active ingredient or category.
Names in **bold face/underlined**: Prescribing information provided in the Monograph section.
Names in **bold face/not underlined**: Availability information provided in the Monograph section.
Names in regular face: Product is available in Canada but the monograph does not appear in *CPS*.

J

K

Names in *italics*: Generic drug names, active ingredient or category.
Names in **bold face/underlined**: Prescribing information provided in the Monograph section.
Names in **bold face/not underlined**: Availability information provided in the Monograph section.
Names in regular face: Product is available in Canada but the monograph does not appear in *CPS*.

ketoprofen. **Apo-Keto**; **Apo-Keto-E**; **Apo-Keto SR**.

Ketorolac (CPhA Monograph). *ketorolac tromethamine.*

ketorolac tromethamine. **Acular**; **Acular LS**; **Ketorolac**; **Ketorolac Tromethamine Injection USP**; **ratio-Ketorolac**.

Ketorolac Tromethamine Injection USP (Sandoz). *ketorolac tromethamine.*

ketotifen fumarate. **Teva-Ketotifen**; **Zaditor**.

Kidrolase (EUSA Pharma SAS). *l-asparaginase.*

Kineret (Amgen). *anakinra.*

Kivexa (ViiV Healthcare ULC). *abacavir sulfate / lamivudine.*

Klean-Prep (Helix Biopharma). *electrolytes / polyethylene glycol.*

K-Lyte (WellSpring). *potassium citrate.*

Koffex DM (Rougier Pharma). *dextromethorphan HBr.*

Kogenate FS Supplied with BIO-SET Needle-less Reconstitution Set (Bayer). *antihemophilic factor (recombinant).*

Kwellada-P Creme Rinse (GlaxoSmithKline Consumer Healthcare). *permethrin.*

Kwellada-P Lotion (GlaxoSmithKline Consumer Healthcare). *permethrin.*

Kytril (Roche). *granisetron HCl.*

L

labetalol HCl. **Labetalol Hydrochloride Injection USP**; **Trandate**.

Labetalol Hydrochloride Injection USP (Sandoz). *labetalol HCl.*

Lacidofil (Institut Rosell). *Lactobacillus acidophilus / Lactobacillus rhamnosus.*

lacosamide. **Vimpat**.

Lacrisert (Aton Pharma). *hydroxypropyl cellulose.*

Lactaid (McNeil Consumer Healthcare). *lactase.*

lactase. **Dairy Free**; **Lactaid**.

Lactated Ringer's Injection (Hospira). *calcium chloride / potassium chloride / sodium chloride / sodium lactate.* Discontinued 2010.

lactic acid. **Dermalac**.

lactic acid / formalin / salicylic acid. **Duoplant**.

lactic acid / salicylic acid. **Duofilm Liquid**.

lactobacillus plantarum 299v. **TuZen**.

lactobacillus reuteri protectis. **BioGaia Chewable Tablets**; **BioGaia Drops**.

lactoflavin. see *riboflavin.*

Lactulose (CPhA Monograph). *lactulose.*

lactulose. **Apo-Lactulose**; **Lactulose**; **ratio-Lactulose**.

Lamictal (GlaxoSmithKline). *lamotrigine.*

Lamisil (Novartis Pharmaceuticals). *terbinafine HCl.*

lamivudine. **3TC**; **Heptovir**.

lamivudine / abacavir sulfate. **Kivexa**.

lamivudine / abacavir sulfate / zidovudine. **Trizivir**.

lamivudine / zidovudine. **Combivir**.

lamotrigine. **Lamictal**; **ratio-Lamotrigine**.

Lanohex (Rougier). *phenoxetol.* Discontinued 2000.

lanolin alcohols / mineral oil / white petrolatum. **Refresh Lacri-Lube S.O.P.**

Lanoxin (Pharmascience). *digoxin.*

lansoprazole. **Prevacid**; **Prevacid FasTab**; **Teva-Lansoprazole**.

lansoprazole / amoxicillin trihydrate / clarithromycin. **Hp-PAC**.

Lansoÿl (Aurium). *mineral oil.*

Lansoÿl Sugar-Free (Aurium). *mineral oil.*

lanthanum carbonate. **Fosrenol**.

Lantus (sanofi-aventis). *insulin glargine (rDNA origin).*

Lanvis (GlaxoSmithKline). *thioguanine.*

lapatinib ditosylate. **Tykerb**.

Largactil (sanofi-aventis). *chlorpromazine HCl.* Discontinued 2006.

Lariam (Roche). *mefloquine HCl.*

laronidase. **Aldurazyme**.

Lasix (sanofi-aventis). *furosemide.*

Lasix Special (sanofi-aventis). *furosemide.*

latanoprost. **Xalatan**.

latanoprost / timolol maleate. **Xalacom**.

Latisse (Allergan). *bimatoprost.*

Lax-A-Day (PendoPharm). *polyethylene glycol.*

Laxative Pills (Tanta). *sennosides.*

l-deprenyl hydrochloride. see *selegiline HCl.*

Lectopam (Roche). *bromazepam.*

Lederle Leucovorin (Pfizer). *calcium folinate.*

leflunomide. **Arava**; **Sandoz Leflunomide**.

l-epinephrine. see *epinephrine.*

lepirudin (rDNA). **Refludan**.

Leritine (Merck Frosst). *anileridine HCl.* Discontinued 2001.

Lescol (Novartis Pharmaceuticals). *fluvastatin sodium.*

Lescol XL (Novartis Pharmaceuticals). *fluvastatin sodium.*

Letrozole (Cobalt). *letrozole.*

letrozole. **Femara**; **Letrozole Tablets USP**; **Letrozole**; **MED-Letrozole**; **PMS-Letrozole**; **Sandoz Letrozole**.

Letrozole Tablets USP (Accord Healthcare). *letrozole.*

leucovorin calcium. see *calcium folinate.*

Leucovorin Calcium Injection USP (Hospira). *calcium folinate.*

Leukeran (GlaxoSmithKline). *chlorambucil.*

leuprolide acetate. **Eligard**; **Lupron Depot 3.75 mg/11.25 mg**; **Lupron**; **Lupron Depot 3.75 mg/7.5 mg**; **Lupron**; **Lupron Depot 7.5 mg/22.5 mg/30 mg**.

Leustatin (Janssen-Ortho). *cladribine.*

Levaquin (Janssen-Ortho). *levofloxacin.*

levarterenol bitartrate. see *norepinephrine bitartrate.*

Levemir (Novo Nordisk). *insulin detemir.*

levetiracetam. **CO Levetiracetam**; **Keppra**.

Levitra (Bayer). *vardenafil HCl.*

levobunolol HCl. **Betagan**; **ratio-Levobunolol**.

levocabastine HCl. **Livostin Eye Drops**; **Livostin Nasal Spray**.

levocarnitine. **Carnitor**.

levodopa / benserazide HCl. **Prolopa**.

levodopa / carbidopa. **Sinemet CR**; **Sinemet**.

levodopa / carbidopa / entacapone. **Stalevo**.

levofloxacin. **CO Levofloxacin**; **Fluoroquinolones**; **Levaquin**; **PMS-Levofloxacin**; **Sandoz Levofloxacin**.

levomepromazine maleate. see *methotrimeprazine maleate.*

levonorgestrel. **Mirena**; **NorLevo**; **Plan B**.

levonorgestrel / estradiol-17β. **Climara Pro**.

levonorgestrel / ethinyl estradiol. **Alesse 21**; **Alesse 28**; **Aviane 21**; **Aviane 28**; **Min-Ovral 21**; **Min-Ovral 28**; **Portia 21**; **Portia 28**; **Seasonale** ; **Triquilar 21**; **Triquilar 28**.

Levophed (Hospira). *norepinephrine bitartrate.*

Levotec (Technilab). *levothyroxine sodium.* Discontinued 2000.

levothyroxine sodium. **Eltroxin**; **Synthroid**.

Levovist (Berlex Canada). *galactose / palmitic acid.* Discontinued 2003.

Librax (Valeant). *chlordiazepoxide HCl / clidinium bromide.*

Lidemol (Medicis). *fluocinonide.* Discontinued 2010.

Lidex (Medicis). *fluocinonide.* Discontinued 2010.

lidocaine. **Lidodan Ointment**; **Xylocaine Endotracheal**; **Xylocaine Ointment 5%**.

lidocaine / bacitracin zinc / gramicidin / polymyxin B sulfate. **Polysporin Complete Antibiotic Ointment**.

lidocaine / prilocaine. **EMLA Cream**; **EMLA Patch**.

lidocaine HCl. **Lidocaine Parenteral (Antiarrhythmic Agent)**; **Lidodan Endotracheal**; **Lidodan Viscous**; **Xylocaine Jelly 2%**; **Xylocaine Parenteral Without Epinephrine**; **Xylocaine Topical 4%**; **Xylocaine Viscous 2%**; **Xylocard**.

Names in *italics*: Generic drug names, active ingredient or category.
Names in **bold face/underlined**: Prescribing information provided in the Monograph section.
Names in **bold face/not underlined**: Availability information provided in the Monograph section.
Names in regular face: Product is available in Canada but the monograph does not appear in *CPS*.

Names in *italics*: Generic drug names, active ingredient or category.
Names in **<u>bold face/underlined</u>**: Prescribing information provided in the Monograph section.
Names in **bold face/not underlined**: Availability information provided in the Monograph section.
Names in regular face: Product is available in Canada but the monograph does not appear in *CPS*.

Names in *italics*: Generic drug names, active ingredient or category.
Names in **bold face/underlined**: Prescribing information provided in the Monograph section.
Names in **bold face/not underlined**: Availability information provided in the Monograph section.
Names in regular face: Product is available in Canada but the monograph does not appear in *CPS*.

Names in *italics*: Generic drug names, active ingredient or category.
Names in **bold face/underlined**: Prescribing information provided in the Monograph section.
Names in **bold face/not underlined**: Availability information provided in the Monograph section.
Names in regular face: Product is available in Canada but the monograph does not appear in *CPS*.

Names in *italics*: Generic drug names, active ingredient or category.
Names in **bold face/underlined**: Prescribing information provided in the Monograph section.
Names in **bold face/not underlined**: Availability information provided in the Monograph section.
Names in regular face: Product is available in Canada but the monograph does not appear in *CPS*.

Names in *italics*: Generic drug names, active ingredient or category.
Names in **bold face/underlined**: Prescribing information provided in the Monograph section.
Names in **bold face/not underlined**: Availability information provided in the Monograph section.
Names in regular face: Product is available in Canada but the monograph does not appear in *CPS*.

N

Names in *italics*: Generic drug names, active ingredient or category.
Names in **bold face/underlined**: Prescribing information provided in the Monograph section.
Names in **bold face/not underlined**: Availability information provided in the Monograph section.
Names in regular face: Product is available in Canada but the monograph does not appear in *CPS*.

Names in *italics*: Generic drug names, active ingredient or category.
Names in **bold face/underlined**: Prescribing information provided in the Monograph section.
Names in **bold face/not underlined**: Availability information provided in the Monograph section.
Names in regular face: Product is available in Canada but the monograph does not appear in *CPS*.

Names in *italics*: Generic drug names, active ingredient or category.
Names in **bold face/underlined**: Prescribing information provided in the Monograph section.
Names in **bold face/not underlined**: Availability information provided in the Monograph section.
Names in regular face: Product is available in Canada but the monograph does not appear in *CPS*.

O

Names in *italics*: Generic drug names, active ingredient or category.
Names in **bold face/underlined**: Prescribing information provided in the Monograph section.
Names in **bold face/not underlined**: Availability information provided in the Monograph section.
Names in regular face: Product is available in Canada but the monograph does not appear in *CPS*.

P

Names in *italics*: Generic drug names, active ingredient or category.
Names in **bold face/underlined**: Prescribing information provided in the Monograph section.
Names in **bold face/not underlined**: Availability information provided in the Monograph section.
Names in regular face: Product is available in Canada but the monograph does not appear in *CPS*.

Pamprin Ultra Strength Ibuprofen Formula (Chattem). *ibuprofen.*

Panadol (GlaxoSmithKline). *acetaminophen.*

Pancrease (Janssen-Ortho). *pancrelipase.* Discontinued 2008.

Pancrease MT (Janssen-Ortho). *pancrelipase.*

pancreatic enzymes. **Creon 5 Minimicrospheres**; **Creon 10 Minimicrospheres**; **Creon 25 Minimicrospheres**.

pancrelipase. **Cotazym**; **Pancrease MT**; **Ultrase**; **Ultrase MT**; **Viokase**.

pancuronium bromide. **Pancuronium Bromide Injection**.

Pancuronium Bromide Injection (Sandoz). *pancuronium bromide.*

Pancuronium Bromide Injection (Hospira). *pancuronium bromide.* Discontinued 2005.

Panectyl (ERFA Canada). *trimeprazine tartrate.*

panitumumab. **Vectibix**.

Panoxyl 5% (Stiefel, a GSK company). *benzoyl peroxide.*

Panoxyl 5% Wash (Stiefel, a GSK company). *benzoyl peroxide.*

Panoxyl 10% and 20% (Stiefel, a GSK company). *benzoyl peroxide.*

Panoxyl Antibacterial Acne Creamy Wash (Stiefel, a GSK company). *benzoyl peroxide.*

Panoxyl Aquagel 2.5% and 5% (Stiefel, a GSK company). *benzoyl peroxide.*

Panoxyl Clear Acne Cleansing Gel (Stiefel, a GSK company). *salicylic acid / triclosan.*

PANTO IV (Nycomed). *pantoprazole sodium.*

Pantoloc (Nycomed). *pantoprazole sodium.*

pantoprazole magnesium. **Tecta**.

pantoprazole sodium. **CO Pantoprazole**; **PANTO IV**; **Pantoloc**; **Pantoprazole Sodium for Injection**; **PMS-Pantoprazole IV**; **PMS-Pantoprazole Tablets**; **RAN-Pantoprazole**; **ratio-Pantoprazole**; **Sandoz Pantoprazole**; **Teva-Pantoprazole**.

Pantoprazole Sodium for Injection (Sandoz). *pantoprazole sodium.*

Pantothenic Acid (CPhA Monograph). *pantothenic acid.*

pantothenic acid. **Pantothenic Acid**.

papaverine HCl. **Papaverine HCl Injection USP**.

Papaverine HCl Injection USP (Sandoz). *papaverine HCl.*

paracetamol. see *acetaminophen.*

paradichlorobenzene / chlorbutol / oil of turpentine. **Cerumol**.

Parafon Forte (Johnson & Johnson • Merck). *acetaminophen / chlorzoxazone.* Discontinued 2007.

Parafon Forte C8 (Johnson & Johnson • Merck). *acetaminophen / chlorzoxazone / codeine phosphate.* Discontinued 2000.

Paraldehyde Injection BP (Mayne Pharma). *paraldehyde.* Discontinued 2007.

Paraplatin-AQ (Bristol-Myers Squibb). *carboplatin.* Discontinued 2007.

paricalcitol. **Vitamin D**.

Pariet (Janssen-Ortho). *rabeprazole sodium.*

Parlodel (Novartis Pharmaceuticals). *bromocriptine mesylate.* Discontinued 2007.

Parnate (GlaxoSmithKline). *tranylcypromine sulfate.*

paroxetine. **CO Paroxetine**.

paroxetine HCl. **Paxil CR**; **Paxil**; **PMS-Paroxetine**; **ratio-Paroxetine**; **Selective Serotonin Reuptake Inhibitors**; **Teva-Paroxetine**.

Parsitan (ERFA Canada). *ethopropazine HCl.*

parsol MCX / butyl methoxydibenzoylmethane / tretinoin. **Retisol-A**.

Patanol (Alcon). *olopatadine HCl.*

Paxil (GlaxoSmithKline). *paroxetine HCl.*

Paxil CR (GlaxoSmithKline). *paroxetine HCl.*

pazopanib HCl. **Votrient**.

PCE (Abbott). *erythromycin.* Discontinued 2007.

Pediacel (sanofi pasteur). *diphtheria and tetanus toxoids and acellular pertussis vaccine adsorbed combined with inactivated poliomyelitis vaccine and Haemophilus b conjugate vaccine (tetanus protein-conjugate).*

Pedialyte (Abbott). *dextrose / electrolytes.*

Pediapred (sanofi-aventis). *prednisolone sodium phosphate.*

Pediasure (Abbott). *enteral nutrition.*

Pediatric Electrolyte (PendoPharm). *electrolytes.*

Pediatrix (Rougier Pharma). *acetaminophen.*

Pediazole (Abbott). *erythromycin ethylsuccinate / sulfisoxazole acetyl.* Discontinued 2008.

PEG 3350 / bisacodyl / electrolytes. **Bi-PegLyte**.

Pegalax (Medical Futures). *polyethylene glycol.*

pegaptanib sodium. **Macugen**.

Pegasys (Roche). *peginterferon alfa-2a.*

Pegasys RBV (Pegasys and Copegus) (Roche). *peginterferon alfa-2a / ribavirin.*

Pegetron (Schering-Plough). *peginterferon alfa-2b / ribavirin.*

pegfilgrastim. **Neulasta**.

peginterferon alfa-2a. **Pegasys**; **Unitron PEG**.

peginterferon alfa-2a / ribavirin. **Pegasys RBV (Pegasys and Copegus)**; **Pegetron**.

PegLyte (PendoPharm). *electrolytes / polyethylene glycol.*

pegvisomant. **Somavert**.

pemetrexed disodium. **Alimta**.

Penglobe (AstraZeneca). *bacampicillin HCl.* Discontinued 2003.

penicillamine. **Cuprimine**.

Penicillin G (CPhA Monograph).

penicillin G benzathine. **Bicillin L-A**; **Penicillin G**.

penicillin G sodium. **Penicillin G**.

Penicillin V (CPhA Monograph).

penicillin V potassium. **Penicillin V**.

Penlac (sanofi-aventis). *ciclopirox.*

Pennsaid (Paladin). *diclofenac sodium.*

Penta/3b (Sandoz). *vitamin B complex.*

Penta/3b+C (Sandoz). *ascorbic acid / vitamin B complex.*

Penta/3b Plus (Sandoz). *multiple vitamins.*

Pentacarinat (Aventis Pharma). *pentamidine isethionate.* Discontinued 2003.

Pentacel (sanofi pasteur). *Haemophilus b conjugate vaccine (tetanus protein-conjugate) reconstituted with component pertussis vaccine and diphtheria and tetanus toxoids adsorbed combined with inactivated poliomyelitis vaccine.* Discontinued 2009.

Pentamidine Isetionate for Injection BP (Hospira). *pentamidine isetionate.* Discontinued 2009.

Pentamycetin (Sandoz). *chloramphenicol.*

Pentamycetin/HC (Sandoz). *chloramphenicol / hydrocortisone acetate.*

Pentasa (Ferring). *5-ASA.*

Pentaspan (Bristol-Myers Squibb). *pentastarch.*

pentastarch. **Pentaspan**.

pentazocine HCl. **Opioids**; **Talwin Tablets**.

pentazocine lactate. **Opioids**; **Talwin Injection**.

pentobarbital sodium. **Barbiturates**.

pentosan polysulfate sodium. **Elmiron**.

Pentothal (Hospira). *thiopental sodium.*

pentoxifylline. **ratio-Pentoxifylline**; **Trental**.

Pepcid AC (Johnson & Johnson • Merck). *famotidine.*

Pepcid AC, Maximum Strength (Johnson & Johnson • Merck). *famotidine.*

Pepcid Complete (Johnson & Johnson • Merck). *calcium carbonate / famotidine / magnesium hydroxide.*

Pepcid Tablets (Merck Frosst). *famotidine.*

pepsin. **Fermentol**.

Pepto-Bismol Caplets (Procter & Gamble). *bismuth subsalicylate.*

Pepto-Bismol Chewable Tablets (Procter & Gamble). *bismuth subsalicylate / calcium carbonate.*

Pepto-Bismol Liquid (Procter & Gamble). *bismuth subsalicylate.*

Pepto-Bismol with InstaCool (Procter & Gamble). *bismuth subsalicylate.*

Percocet (Bristol-Myers Squibb). *acetaminophen / oxycodone HCl.*

Percocet-Demi (Bristol-Myers Squibb). *acetaminophen / oxycodone HCl.*

Percodan (Bristol-Myers Squibb). *ASA / oxycodone HCl.* Discontinued 2009.

Pergonal (Serono). *menotropins.* Discontinued 2004.

Periactin (Johnson & Johnson • Merck). *cyproheptadine HCl.* Discontinued 2003.

Names in *italics*: Generic drug names, active ingredient or category.
Names in **bold face/underlined**: Prescribing information provided in the Monograph section.
Names in **bold face/not underlined**: Availability information provided in the Monograph section.
Names in regular face: Product is available in Canada but the monograph does not appear in *CPS*.

Peri-Colace (WellSpring). *casanthranol / docusate sodium.* Discontinued 2004.

Peridex (Zila Pharmaceuticals). *chlorhexidine gluconate.*

perindopril erbumine. **ACE Inhibitors**; **Coversyl**.

perindopril erbumine / indapamide. **Coversyl Plus LD**; **Coversyl Plus**; **Coversyl Plus HD**.

Periostat (Pharmascience). *doxycycline hyclate.*

Permax (Lilly). *pergolide mesylate.* Discontinued 2007.

permethrin. **Kwellada-P Creme Rinse**; **Kwellada-P Lotion**; **Nix Creme Rinse**; **Nix Dermal Cream**.

Pernox (Westwood-Squibb). *salicylic acid / sulfur.* Discontinued 2007.

Persantine (Boehringer Ingelheim). *dipyridamole.*

pethidine HCl. **Demerol Tablets**; **Opioids**.

petrolatum. **Prevex Cream**.

PGE_2. see *dinoprostone.*

Pharma-Cal D 400 IU (Pharmascience). *calcium carbonate / vitamin D3.*

Pharmorubicin PFS (Pfizer). *epirubicin HCl.*

Phazyme (GlaxoSmithKline Consumer Healthcare). *simethicone.*

Phenaphen with Codeine (Wyeth-Ayerst). *ASA / codeine phosphate / phenobarbital.* Discontinued 2001.

Phenazo (Valeant). *phenazopyridine HCl.* Discontinued 2009.

Phenergan Injectable (Aventis Pharma). *promethazine HCl.* Discontinued 2003.

pheniramine maleate / codeine phosphate / guaifenesin. **Robitussin AC**.

pheniramine maleate / naphazoline HCl. **Visine Advance Allergy**.

pheniramine maleate / phenylephrine HCl. **Dristan Nasal Mist**.

phenobarbital. **PMS-Phenobarbital**.

phenobarbital / belladonna / ergotamine tartrate. **Bellergal Spacetabs**.

phenobarbital sodium. **Barbiturates**; **Phenobarbital Sodium Injection USP**.

Phenobarbital Sodium Injection USP (Sandoz). *phenobarbital sodium.*

phenobarbitone. see *phenobarbital.*

phenol / zinc oxide. **Ozonol Ointment**.

phenoxymethyl penicillin. see *penicillin V.*

phenoxymethyl penicillin potassium. see *penicillin V potassium.*

phentolamine mesylate. **Rogitine**.

phenylephrine HCl. **Mydfrin**; **Neo-Synephrine Hydrochloride USP**; **Sudafed PE Decongestant**.

phenylephrine HCl / acetaminophen. **Benylin Cold and Sinus**; **Tylenol Sinus Extra Strength Daytime**; **Tylenol Sinus Regular Strength Daytime**; **Vicks DayQuil Sinus LiquiCaps**.

phenylephrine HCl / acetaminophen / chlorpheniramine maleate. **Benylin Cold and Sinus Plus**; **Dristan**; **Dristan Extra Strength**; **Tylenol Allergy Extra Strength (Multi-Symptom Relief)**; **Tylenol Sinus Extra Strength Nighttime**.

phenylephrine HCl / acetaminophen / chlorpheniramine maleate / dextromethorphan HBr. **Tylenol Cold Extra Strength Nighttime**; **Tylenol Cold Regular Strength Nighttime**; **Tylenol Flu Extra Strength Nighttime**.

phenylephrine HCl / acetaminophen / dextromethorphan HBr. **Tylenol Cold & Flu Daytime Liquid**; **Tylenol Cold Extra Strength Daytime**; **Tylenol Cold Regular Strength Daytime**; **Tylenol Flu Extra Strength Daytime**; **Vicks DayQuil Liquicaps**; **Vicks DayQuil Liquid**.

phenylephrine HCl / acetaminophen / dextromethorphan HBr / doxylamine succinate. **Tylenol Cold & Flu Nighttime Liquid**.

phenylephrine HCl / acetaminophen / diphenhydramine HCl. **Benylin All-in-One Cold and Flu Night PE**.

phenylephrine HCl / acetaminophen / doxylamine succinate. **Vicks NyQuil Sinus LiquiCaps**.

phenylephrine HCl / ammonium chloride / hydrocodone bitartrate / pyrilamine maleate. **Hycomine**; **Hycomine-S**.

phenylephrine HCl / brompheniramine maleate. **Dimetapp Chewables for Kids**; **Dimetapp Extra Strength Liquid**; **Dimetapp Liquid**.

phenylephrine HCl / brompheniramine maleate / codeine phosphate. **Dimetapp-C Syrup**.

phenylephrine HCl / brompheniramine maleate / codeine phosphate / guaifenesin. **Dimetane Expectorant-C**.

phenylephrine HCl / brompheniramine maleate / dextromethorphan HBr. **Dimetapp DM Cough & Cold Liquid**; **Dimetapp Extra Strength DM Cough & Cold Liquid**.

phenylephrine HCl / brompheniramine maleate / guaifenesin / hydrocodone bitartrate. **Dimetane Expectorant-DC**.

phenylephrine HCl / dextromethorphan HBr. **Vicks Custom Care Nasal Congestion/Cough**.

phenylephrine HCl / hamamelis water. **Preparation H Cooling Gel**.

phenylephrine HCl / hydrocodone bitartrate. **Novahistex DH**; **Novahistine DH**; **ratio-Coristex-DH**.

phenylephrine HCl / pheniramine maleate. **Dristan Nasal Mist**.

phenylephrine HCl / tropicamide. **Diophenyl-T**.

phenyltoloxamine / hydrocodone bitartrate. **Tussionex**.

phenyl trimethicone / polysilicone-11 / cyclopentasiloxane / dimethicone / polymethylsilsesquioxane / tetrahexyldecyl ascorbate. **Dermatix Ultra**.

phenytoin. **Dilantin Infatabs**; **Dilantin-30 Suspension**; **Dilantin-125 Suspension**; **Phenytoin**; **Taro-Phenytoin**.

Phenytoin (CPhA Monograph).

phenytoin sodium. **Dilantin Capsules**; **Phenytoin**.

Phenytoin Sodium Injection, USP (Abbott). *phenytoin sodium.* Discontinued 2004.

Phillips' Preparations (Bayer Consumer Care). *magnesium hydroxide.*

pHisoHex (sanofi-aventis). *hexachlorophene.*

Phoslax (Odan). *sodium phosphates.*

PhosLo (Fresenius Medical Care). *calcium acetate.*

Phosphate-Novartis (Novartis Pharmaceuticals). *sodium acid phosphate.*

Phosphates Solution (PendoPharm). *sodium phosphates.*

Phospholine Iodide (Wyeth-Ayerst). *echothiophate iodide.* Discontinued 2001.

Photofrin (Axcan Pharma). *porfimer sodium.*

p-hydroxyephedrine HCl / normethadone HCl. **Cophylac**.

Phyllocontin (Purdue Pharma). *aminophylline.* Discontinued 2010.

Phyllocontin-350 (Purdue Pharma). *aminophylline.* Discontinued 2010.

Physioneal (Baxter). *glucose.*

phytomenadione. see *phytonadione.*

phytonadione. **Vitamin K_1**.

Phyto Soya (Arkopharma). *germinated soybean (Glycine max L.).* Discontinued 2010.

Pico-Salax (Ferring). *citric acid / magnesium oxide / picosulfate sodium.*

picosulfate sodium / citric acid / magnesium oxide. **Pico-Salax**; **Purg-Odan**.

pilocarpine HCl. **Isopto Carpine**; **Pilopine HS**; **Salagen**.

Pilopine HS (Alcon). *pilocarpine HCl.*

pimecrolimus. **Elidel**.

pimozide. **Apo-Pimozide**.

pinaverium bromide. **Dicetel**.

pindolol. **Nu-Pindol**; **Visken**.

pindolol / hydrochlorothiazide. **Viskazide**.

pioglitazone HCl. **Actos**; **CO Pioglitazone**; **Pioglitazone Hydrochloride Tablets**; **ratio-Pioglitazone**; **Sandoz Pioglitazone**.

Pioglitazone Hydrochloride Tablets (Accord Healthcare). *pioglitazone HCl.*

Piperacillin/Tazobactam for Injection (Pharmaceutical Partners). *piperacillin sodium / tazobactam sodium.* Discontinued 2009.

Piperacillin for Injection (Hospira). *piperacillin sodium.*

piperacillin sodium. **Piperacillin for Injection**.

piperacillin sodium / tazobactam sodium. **Piperacillin Sodium/Tazobactam Sodium Powder for Injection**; **Tazocin**.

Piperacillin Sodium/Tazobactam Sodium Powder for Injection (Sandoz). *piperacillin sodium / tazobactam sodium.*

piperazine estrone sulfate. see *estropipate.*

piperonyl butoxide / pyrethrins. **R & C Shampoo/Conditioner**.

Piportil L4 (sanofi-aventis). *pipotiazine palmitate.*

pipotiazine palmitate. **Piportil L4**.

Pipracil (Wyeth). *piperacillin sodium.* Discontinued 2003.

pipradrol HCl / vitamin B compound. **Alertonic**.

Pizotifen (CPhA Monograph). *pizotifen malate.*

pizotifen malate. **Pizotifen**; **Sandomigran**; **Sandomigran DS**.

pizotyline malate. see *pizotifen malate.*

Plan B (Paladin). *levonorgestrel.*

Plaquenil (sanofi-aventis). *hydroxychloroquine sulfate.*

Names in *italics*: Generic drug names, active ingredient or category.
Names in **bold face/underlined**: Prescribing information provided in the Monograph section.
Names in **bold face/not underlined**: Availability information provided in the Monograph section.
Names in regular face: Product is available in Canada but the monograph does not appear in *CPS*.

Names in *italics*: Generic drug names, active ingredient or category.
Names in **bold face/underlined**: Prescribing information provided in the Monograph section.
Names in **bold face/not underlined**: Availability information provided in the Monograph section.
Names in regular face: Product is available in Canada but the monograph does not appear in *CPS*.

Names in *italics*: Generic drug names, active ingredient or category.
Names in **bold face/underlined**: Prescribing information provided in the Monograph section.
Names in **bold face/not underlined**: Availability information provided in the Monograph section.
Names in regular face: Product is available in Canada but the monograph does not appear in *CPS*.

Names in *italics*: Generic drug names, active ingredient or category.
Names in **bold face/underlined**: Prescribing information provided in the Monograph section.
Names in **bold face/not underlined**: Availability information provided in the Monograph section.
Names in regular face: Product is available in Canada but the monograph does not appear in *CPS*.

Proflavanol C (USANA Health Sciences). *ascorbic acid.*

progesterone. **Crinone**; **Endometrin**; **Progesterone Injection USP**; **Prometrium**.

Progesterone Injection USP (Cytex). *progesterone.*

Proglycem (Schering-Plough). *diazoxide.*

Prograf (Astellas). *tacrolimus.*

proguanil HCl / atovaquone. **Malarone**; **Malarone Pediatric**.

Prolastin-C (Talecris). *alpha1-proteinase inhibitor (human), highly purified.*

Proleukin (Novartis Pharmaceuticals). *aldesleukin.*

Prolia (Amgen). *denosumab.*

Prolopa (Roche). *benserazide HCl / levodopa.*

Proloprim (GlaxoSmithKline). *trimethoprim.* Discontinued 2004.

Promatussin DM (Pangeo). *dextromethorphan HBr / promethazine HCl / pseudoephedrine.* Discontinued 2003.

Promazine Hydrochloride (Abbott). *promazine HCl.* Discontinued 2004.

Promethazine (CPhA Monograph). *promethazine HCl.*

promethazine HCl. **Promethazine**.

Prometrium (Schering-Plough). *progesterone.*

Pronestyl (Squibb). *procainamide HCl.* Discontinued 2002.

Pronestyl-SR (Squibb). *procainamide HCl.* Discontinued 2005.

Propaderm (Paladin). *beclomethasone dipropionate.*

Propafenone (CPhA Monograph). *propafenone HCl.*

propafenone HCl. **Propafenone**; **Rythmol**.

Propanthel (Valeant). *propantheline bromide.* Discontinued 2004.

proparacaine HCl. **Alcaine**.

Propecia (Merck Frosst). *finasteride.*

Propine (Allergan). *dipivefrin HCl.* Discontinued 2005.

propofol. **Diprivan**; **Propofol Injection**.

Propofol Injection (Hospira). *propofol.*

Propofol Injection (Teva Canada). *propofol.*

propoxyphene HCl. **Opioids**.

propoxyphene napsylate. **Opioids**.

Propranolol (CPhA Monograph). *propranolol HCl.*

propranolol HCl. **Inderal-LA**; **Propranolol**.

propylene glycol / polyethylene glycol. **Rhinaris Lubricating Nasal Gel/Nasal Mist**; **Secaris**.

propylene glycol / polyethylene glycol / sodium chloride. **Salinex Nasal Lubricant/Nasal Lubricant Gel**.

Propylthiouracil (CPhA Monograph). *propylthiouracil.*

propylthiouracil. **Propyl-Thyracil**; **Propylthiouracil**.

Propyl-Thyracil (Paladin). *propylthiouracil.*

Proscar (Merck Frosst). *finasteride.*

Pro-Sope (Rougier). *hydrophilic lanolin / sodium lauryl ether sulfate.* Discontinued 2000.

prostaglandin E_1. see *alprostadil.*

prostaglandin E_2. see *dinoprostone.*

Prostigmin (Valeant). *neostigmine bromide.*

Prostin E2 Tablets (Paladin). *dinoprostone.*

Prostin E2 Vaginal Gel (Paladin). *dinoprostone.*

Prostin VR (Pfizer). *alprostadil.*

protamine sulfate. **Protamine Sulfate Injection USP**.

Protamine Sulfate Injection USP (Sandoz). *protamine sulfate.*

protein isolate. **Immunocal**.

Protopam Chloride (Wyeth Canada). *pralidoxime chloride.* Discontinued 2006.

Protopic (Astellas). *tacrolimus.*

Protropin (Roche). *somatrem.* Discontinued 2004.

Provera (Pfizer). *medroxyprogesterone acetate.*

Proviodine (Rougier Pharma). *povidone-iodine.*

Provocholine (Methapharm). *methacholine chloride.*

proxymetacaine HCl. see *proparacaine HCl.*

Prozac (Lilly). *fluoxetine HCl.*

pseudoephedrine HCl. **Eltor 120**; **Pseudofrin**; **Sudafed Decongestant 12 Hour**.

pseudoephedrine HCl / acetaminophen. **Sinutab Sinus Non Drowsy**; **Sudafed Head Cold and Sinus Extra Strength**; **Tylenol Children's Decongestant**; **Tylenol Sinus Pain and Congestion Daytime Extra Strength**.

pseudoephedrine HCl / acetaminophen / chlorpheniramine maleate. **Sinutab Sinus and Allergy**; **Tylenol Sinus Pain and Congestion Nighttime Extra Strength**.

pseudoephedrine HCl / acetaminophen / chlorpheniramine maleate / codeine phosphate. **Sinutab with Codeine**.

pseudoephedrine HCl / acetaminophen / chlorpheniramine maleate / dextromethorphan HBr. **Robitussin Total Extra Strength Nighttime, Cough Cold and Flu**; **Tylenol Children's and Junior Strength Cold DM**.

pseudoephedrine HCl / acetaminophen / chlorpheniramine maleate / dextromethorphan HBr / guaifenesin. **Benylin 1 All-in-One Cold and Flu Nightime**.

pseudoephedrine HCl / acetaminophen / dextromethorphan HBr. **Robitussin Total Cough Cold and Flu**; **Sudafed Cold & Cough Extra Strength**.

pseudoephedrine HCl / acetaminophen / dextromethorphan HBr / guaifenesin. **Balminil Cough & Flu**; **Benylin 1 All-in-One Cold and Flu**; **Benylin DM-D-E-A Cold and Sinus Rapid Gels**.

pseudoephedrine HCl / acetaminophen / diphenhydramine HCl. **Benadryl Allergy/Sinus/Headache**; **Benadryl Total/Allergy/Regular Strength**; **Benadryl Total/Allergy/Extra Strength**; **Sinutab Nightime**.

pseudoephedrine HCl / acetaminophen / triprolidine HCl. **Actifed Plus Extra Strength**.

pseudoephedrine HCl / cetirizine HCl. **Reactine Allergy & Sinus**.

pseudoephedrine HCl / chlorpheniramine maleate / ibuprofen. **Advil Cold and Sinus Plus**; **Advil Cold and Sinus Nighttime**.

pseudoephedrine HCl / codeine phosphate / guaifenesin. **Benylin 2 All-in-One Cold and Flu with Codeine (Non-prescription)**; **Calmylin PSE with Codeine**.

pseudoephedrine HCl / codeine phosphate / guaifenesin / triprolidine HCl. **CoActifed Expectorant**; **ratio-Cotridin Expectorant**.

pseudoephedrine HCl / codeine phosphate / triprolidine HCl. **CoActifed Syrup**; **CoActifed Tablets**; **ratio-Cotridin**.

pseudoephedrine HCl / dextromethorphan HBr. **Balminil DM+Decongestant**; **Benylin DM-D (Adult)**; **Benylin DM-D for Children**; **Robitussin Children's Cough & Cold**.

pseudoephedrine HCl / dextromethorphan HBr / guaifenesin. **Balminil DM+Decongestant+Expectorant**; **Robitussin Cough & Cold**; **Robitussin Extra Strength Cough & Cold**.

pseudoephedrine HCl / dextromethorphan HBr / guaifenesin / menthol. **Benylin DM-D-E Extra Strength with Menthactin**.

pseudoephedrine HCl / fexofenadine HCl. **Allegra-D**.

pseudoephedrine HCl / guaifenesin. **Entex LA**.

pseudoephedrine HCl / ibuprofen. **Advil Cold & Sinus**; **Advil Cold & Sinus Daytime**; **Children's Advil Cold**; **Sudafed Sinus Advance**.

pseudoephedrine HCl / triprolidine HCl. **Actifed**.

pseudoephedrine sulfate / desloratadine. **Aerius Dual Action 12 Hour**.

pseudoephedrine sulfate / loratadine. **Claritin Allergy+Sinus Extra Strength**; **Claritin Allergy+Sinus**.

Pseudofrin (Trianon). *pseudoephedrine HCl.*

psyllium husk. **Metamucil Fibre Therapy Capsules**; **Metamucil Fibre Therapy Smooth Texture Pink Lemonade Flavour, Sugar-free**.

psyllium husk / calcium carbonate. **Metamucil Capsules plus Calcium**.

psyllium hydrophilic mucilloid. **Metamucil Preparations**.

pteroylglutamic acid. see *folic acid.*

Pulmicort Nebuamp (AstraZeneca). *budesonide.*

Pulmicort Turbuhaler (AstraZeneca). *budesonide.*

Pulmozyme (Roche). *dornase alfa recombinant.*

Pure Gardens (Awareness Corporation/dba AwarenessLife). *herbal compound.*

Puregon (Schering-Plough). *follitropin beta.*

PureTrim Mediterranean Wellness Shake (Awareness Corporation/dba AwarenessLife). *multiple vitamins and minerals.*

Purg-Odan (Odan). *citric acid / magnesium oxide / picosulfate sodium.*

Purinethol (Teva Canada). *mercaptopurine.*

PVF K (Pangeo). *penicillin V potassium.* Discontinued 2003.

Pylorid (Glaxo Wellcome). *ranitidine bismuth citrate.* Discontinued 2001.

Names in *italics*: Generic drug names, active ingredient or category.
Names in **bold face/underlined**: Prescribing information provided in the Monograph section.
Names in **bold face/not underlined**: Availability information provided in the Monograph section.
Names in regular face: Product is available in Canada but the monograph does not appear in *CPS*.

pyrantel pamoate. **Combantrin**.

pyrazinamide. **Tebrazid**.

pyrazinamide / isoniazid / rifampin. **Rifater**.

pyrethrins / piperonyl butoxide. **R & C Shampoo/Conditioner**.

Pyridium (Pfizer). *phenazopyridine HCl.* Discontinued 2003.

pyridostigmine bromide. **Mestinon**; **Mestinon-SR**.

pyridoxine HCl. **B-natal Lozenge**; **B-natal Therapop**; **Vitamin B_6**.

pyridoxine HCl / doxylamine succinate. **Diclectin**.

Pyridoxine Hydrochloride Injection, USP (Alveda). *pyridoxine HCl.*

pyrilamine maleate / acetaminophen / caffeine. **Midol Menstrual Complete**; **Midol Teen Complete**.

pyrilamine maleate / acetaminophen / pamabrom. **Midol PMS Complete**; **Pamprin Extra Strength Multi-Symptom**; **Pamprin Extra Strength PMS**; **Tylenol Menstrual Extra Strength**.

pyrilamine maleate / ammonium chloride / hydrocodone bitartrate / phenylephrine HCl. **Hycomine**; **Hycomine-S**.

pyrimethamine. **Daraprim**.

pyrithione disulfide / coal tar / menthol / salicylic acid. **Polytar AF**.

Q

Quadracel (sanofi pasteur). *diphtheria and tetanus toxoids and acellular pertussis vaccine adsorbed combined with inactivated poliomyelitis vaccine.*

quadrivalent human papillomavirus (types 6, 11, 16, 18) recombinant vaccine. **Gardasil**.

Quelicin Injection (Hospira). *succinylcholine chloride.*

Questran (Bristol). *cholestyramine resin.* Discontinued 2005.

Questran Light (Bristol). *cholestyramine resin.* Discontinued 2005.

quetiapine fumarate. **CO Quetiapine**; **PMS-Quetiapine**; **ratio-Quetiapine**; **Sandoz Quetiapine**; **Seroquel XR**; **Seroquel**; **Teva-Quetiapine**.

Quibron-T SR (Bristol). *theophylline.* Discontinued 2004.

quinagolide HCl. **Norprolac**.

quinalbarbitone. see *secobarbital sodium.*

quinapril HCl. **Accupril**; **ACE Inhibitors**.

quinapril HCl / hydrochlorothiazide. **Accuretic**.

Quinidex Extentabs (Wyeth-Ayerst). *quinidine sulfate.* Discontinued 2001.

Quinidine (CPhA Monograph).

quinidine gluconate. **Quinidine**.

quinidine sulfate. **Quinidine**.

Quinine-Odan (Odan). *quinine sulfate.*

Quinine Sulfate (CPhA Monograph). *quinine sulfate.*

quinine sulfate. **Quinine Sulfate**; **Quinine-Odan**.

Qvar (Graceway). *beclomethasone dipropionate.*

R

R & C Shampoo/Conditioner (GlaxoSmithKline Consumer Healthcare). *piperonyl butoxide / pyrethrins.*

RabAvert (Novartis Pharmaceuticals). *rabies vaccine.*

rabeprazole sodium. **Pariet**; **PMS-Rabeprazole EC**; **RAN-Rabeprazole**; **Sandoz Rabeprazole**; **Teva-Rabeprazole EC**.

rabies immune globulin (human). **HYPERRAB S/D**.

rabies immune globulin, pasteurized (human). **IMOGAM Rabies Pasteurized**.

rabies vaccine. **RabAvert**.

Rabies Vaccine Inactivated (Connaught). *rabies vaccine, inactivated, diploid cell origin.* Discontinued 2000.

rabies vaccine inactivated (DCO). **IMOVAX Rabies**.

Rafton Liquid (Ferring). *aluminum hydroxide / sodium alginate.* Discontinued 2002.

Rafton Tablets (Ferring). *alginic acid / aluminum hydroxide.* Discontinued 2002.

Ralivia (Biovail Pharmaceuticals). *tramadol HCl.*

raloxifene HCl. **Evista**.

raltegravir potassium. **Isentress**.

raltitrexed disodium. **Tomudex**.

ramipril. **ACE Inhibitors**; **Altace**; **CO Ramipril**; **RAN-Ramipril**; **ratio-Ramipril**; **Teva-Ramipril**.

ramipril / hydrochlorothiazide. **Altace HCT**.

RAN-Amlodipine (Ranbaxy). *amlodipine besylate.*

RAN-Atenolol (Ranbaxy). *atenolol.*

RAN-Atorvastatin (Ranbaxy). *atorvastatin calcium.*

RAN-Carvedilol (Ranbaxy). *carvedilol.*

RAN-Cefprozil (Ranbaxy). *cefprozil.*

RAN-Ciproflox (Ranbaxy). *ciprofloxacin HCl.*

RAN-Ciprofloxacin (Ranbaxy). *ciprofloxacin HCl.*

RAN-Citalo (Ranbaxy). *citalopram HBr.*

RAN-Citalopram (Ranbaxy). *citalopram HBr.* Discontinued 2009.

RAN-Domperidone (Ranbaxy). *domperidone maleate.*

RAN-Fentanyl Matrix Patch (Ranbaxy). *fentanyl.*

RAN-Fentanyl Transdermal System (Ranbaxy). *fentanyl.*

ranibizumab. **Lucentis**.

ranitidine HCl. **CO Ranitidine**; **Nu-Ranit**; **PMS-Ranitidine**; **Ranitidine Injection USP**; **ratio-Ranitidine**; **Zantac**; **Zantac**; **Zantac Maximum Strength Non-Prescription**.

Ranitidine Injection USP (Sandoz). *ranitidine HCl.*

RAN-Lisinopril (Ranbaxy). *lisinopril.*

RAN-Lovastatin (Ranbaxy). *lovastatin.*

RAN-Metformin (Ranbaxy). *metformin HCl.*

RAN-Ondansetron (Ranbaxy). *ondansetron HCl.*

RAN-Pantoprazole (Ranbaxy). *pantoprazole sodium.*

RAN-Pravastatin (Ranbaxy). *pravastatin sodium.*

RAN-Rabeprazole (Ranbaxy). *rabeprazole sodium.*

RAN-Ramipril (Ranbaxy). *ramipril.*

RAN-Risperidone (Ranbaxy). *risperidone.*

RAN-Ropinirole (Ranbaxy). *ropinirole HCl.*

RAN-Simvastatin (Ranbaxy). *simvastatin.*

RAN-Tamsulosin (Ranbaxy). *tamsulosin HCl.*

RAN-Zopiclone (Ranbaxy). *zopiclone.*

Rapamune (Pfizer). *sirolimus.*

Raptiva (EMD Serono). *efalizumab.* Discontinued 2009.

rasagiline mesylate. **Azilect**.

rasburicase. **Fasturtec**.

Rasilez (Novartis Pharmaceuticals). *aliskiren fumarate.*

Rasilez HCT (Novartis Pharmaceuticals). *aliskiren fumarate / hydrochlorothiazide.*

ratio-Aclavulanate (ratiopharm). *amoxicillin trihydrate / clavulanate potassium.*

ratio-Acyclovir (ratiopharm). *acyclovir.*

ratio-Alendronate (ratiopharm). *alendronate sodium.*

ratio-Amcinonide (ratiopharm). *amcinonide.*

ratio-Amiodarone (ratiopharm). *amiodarone HCl.*

ratio-Amlodipine (ratiopharm). *amlodipine besylate.*

ratio-Atenolol (ratiopharm). *atenolol.*

ratio-Atorvastatin (ratiopharm). *atorvastatin calcium.*

ratio-Azithromycin (ratiopharm). *azithromycin monohydrate hemiethanolate.*

ratio-Baclofen (ratiopharm). *baclofen.*

ratio-Beclomethasone AQ (ratiopharm). *beclomethasone dipropionate.* Discontinued 2009.

ratio-Benzydamine (ratiopharm). *benzydamine HCl.* Discontinued 2008.

ratio-Bicalutamide (ratiopharm). *bicalutamide.*

ratio-Bisacodyl (ratiopharm). *bisacodyl.*

ratio-Brimonidine (ratiopharm). *brimonidine tartrate.*

ratio-Bupropion SR (ratiopharm). *bupropion HCl.*

ratio-Buspirone (ratiopharm). *buspirone HCl.* Discontinued 2010.

ratio-Calmydone (ratiopharm). *doxylamine succinate / etafedrine HCl / hydrocodone bitartrate.*

ratio-Carvedilol (ratiopharm). *carvedilol.*

Names in *italics*: Generic drug names, active ingredient or category.
Names in **bold face/underlined**: Prescribing information provided in the Monograph section.
Names in **bold face/not underlined**: Availability information provided in the Monograph section.
Names in regular face: Product is available in Canada but the monograph does not appear in *CPS*.

ratio-Cefuroxime (ratiopharm). *cefuroxime axetil.*
ratio-Ciprofloxacin (ratiopharm). *ciprofloxacin HCl.*
ratio-Citalopram (ratiopharm). *citalopram HBr.*
ratio-Clarithromycin (ratiopharm). *clarithromycin.*
ratio-Clindamycin (ratiopharm). *clindamycin HCl.* Discontinued 2009.
ratio-Clobazam (ratiopharm). *clobazam.* Discontinued 2010.
ratio-Clobetasol (ratiopharm). *clobetasol 17-propionate.*
ratio-Clonazepam (ratiopharm). *clonazepam.*
ratio-Codeine (ratiopharm). *codeine phosphate.*
ratio-Coristex-DH (ratiopharm). *hydrocodone bitartrate / phenylephrine HCl.*
ratio-Cotridin (ratiopharm). *codeine phosphate / pseudoephedrine HCl / triprolidine HCl.*
ratio-Cotridin Expectorant (ratiopharm). *codeine phosphate / guaifenesin / pseudoephedrine HCl / triprolidine HCl.*
ratio-Cyclobenzaprine (ratiopharm). *cyclobenzaprine HCl.*
ratio-Dexamethasone (ratiopharm). *dexamethasone.*
ratio-Diltiazem CD (ratiopharm). *diltiazem HCl.*
ratio-Dipivefrin (ratiopharm). *dipivefrin HCl.* Discontinued 2005.
ratio-Docusate Calcium (ratiopharm). *docusate calcium.*
ratio-Docusate Sodium (ratiopharm). *docusate sodium.*
ratio-Domperidone (ratiopharm). *domperidone maleate.*
ratio-Ectosone (ratiopharm). *betamethasone valerate.*
ratio-Emtec-30 (ratiopharm). *acetaminophen / codeine phosphate.*
ratio-Enalapril (ratiopharm). *enalapril maleate.*
ratio-Fenofibrate MC (ratiopharm). *fenofibrate nanocrystals.*
ratio-Fentanyl (ratiopharm). *fentanyl.*
ratio-Finasteride (ratiopharm). *finasteride.*
ratio-Flunisolide (ratiopharm). *flunisolide.* Discontinued 2008.
ratio-Fluoxetine (ratiopharm). *fluoxetine HCl.*
ratio-Fluticasone (ratiopharm). *fluticasone propionate.*
ratio-Fluvoxamine (ratiopharm). *fluvoxamine maleate.*
ratio-Gabapentin (ratiopharm). *gabapentin.*
ratio-Gentamicin (ratiopharm). *gentamicin sulfate.*
ratio-Glimepiride (ratiopharm). *glimepiride.*
ratio-Glyburide (ratiopharm). *glyburide.*
ratio-Hemcort-HC (ratiopharm). *hydrocortisone acetate / zinc sulfate monohydrate.*
ratio-Heracline (ratiopharm). *adrenal cortical extract / cyanocobalamin / orchitic extract.* Discontinued 2006.
ratio-Indomethacin (ratiopharm). *indomethacin.*
ratio-Ipra Sal UDV (ratiopharm). *ipratropium bromide / salbutamol sulfate.*
ratio-Ipratropium (ratiopharm). *ipratropium bromide.*
ratio-Ipratropium UDV (ratiopharm). *ipratropium bromide.*
ratio-Ketorolac (ratiopharm). *ketorolac tromethamine.*
ratio-Lactulose (ratiopharm). *lactulose.*
ratio-Lamotrigine (ratiopharm). *lamotrigine.*
ratio-Lenoltec No. 1, 2 & 3 (ratiopharm). *acetaminophen / caffeine / codeine phosphate.*
ratio-Lenoltec No. 4 (ratiopharm). *acetaminophen / codeine phosphate.*
ratio-Levobunolol (ratiopharm). *levobunolol HCl.*
ratio-Lisinopril P (ratiopharm). *lisinopril.*
ratio-Lisinopril Z (ratiopharm). *lisinopril.*
ratio-Lovastatin (ratiopharm). *lovastatin.*
ratio-Meloxicam (ratiopharm). *meloxicam.*
ratio-Memantine (ratiopharm). *memantine HCl.*
ratio-Metformin (ratiopharm). *metformin HCl.*
ratio-Methotrexate Sodium (ratiopharm). *methotrexate sodium.*
ratio-Minocycline (ratiopharm). *minocycline HCl.*
ratio-Mirtazapine (ratiopharm). *mirtazapine.*
ratio-Mometasone (ratiopharm). *mometasone furoate.*
ratio-Morphine (ratiopharm). *morphine HCl.*
ratio-Morphine SR (ratiopharm). *morphine sulfate.*
ratio-Nystatin (ratiopharm). *nystatin.*
ratio-Omeprazole (ratiopharm). *omeprazole magnesium.*
ratio-Ondansetron (ratiopharm). *ondansetron HCl dihydrate.*
ratio-Oxycocet (ratiopharm). *acetaminophen / oxycodone HCl.*
ratio-Oxycodan (ratiopharm). *ASA / oxycodone HCl.*
ratio-Pantoprazole (ratiopharm). *pantoprazole sodium.*
ratio-Paroxetine (ratiopharm). *paroxetine HCl.*
ratio-Pentoxifylline (ratiopharm). *pentoxifylline.*
ratio-Pioglitazone (ratiopharm). *pioglitazone HCl.*
ratio-Pravastatin (ratiopharm). *pravastatin sodium.*
ratio-Prednisolone (ratiopharm). *prednisolone acetate.*
ratio-Proctosone (ratiopharm). *cinchocaine HCl / esculin / framycetin sulfate / hydrocortisone acetate.*
ratio-Quetiapine (ratiopharm). *quetiapine fumarate.*
ratio-Ramipril (ratiopharm). *ramipril.*
ratio-Ranitidine (ratiopharm). *ranitidine HCl.*
ratio-Risedronate (ratiopharm). *risedronate sodium hemi-pentahydrate.*
ratio-Risperidone (ratiopharm). *risperidone.* Discontinued 2008.
ratio-Rivastigmine (ratiopharm). *rivastigmine hydrogen tartrate.*
ratio-Salbutamol (ratiopharm). *salbutamol sulfate.*
ratio-Sertraline (ratiopharm). *sertraline HCl.*
ratio-Sildenafil R (ratiopharm). *sildenafil citrate.*
ratio-Simvastatin (ratiopharm). *simvastatin.*
ratio-Sotalol (ratiopharm). *sotalol HCl.*
ratio-Sumatriptan (ratiopharm). *sumatriptan succinate.* Discontinued 2010.
ratio-Tamsulosin (ratiopharm). *tamsulosin HCl.*
ratio-Tecnal (ratiopharm). *ASA / butalbital / caffeine.*
ratio-Tecnal C¼, C½ (ratiopharm). *ASA / butalbital / caffeine / codeine phosphate.*
ratio-Temazepam (ratiopharm). *temazepam.*
ratio-Terazosin (ratiopharm). *terazosin HCl.*
ratio-Theo-Bronc (ratiopharm). *guaifenesin / mepyramine maleate / potassium iodide / theophylline.*
ratio-Topilene (ratiopharm). *betamethasone dipropionate.*
ratio-Topiramate (ratiopharm). *topiramate.*
ratio-Topisalic (ratiopharm). *betamethasone dipropionate / salicylic acid.*
ratio-Topisone (ratiopharm). *betamethasone dipropionate.*
ratio-Trazodone (ratiopharm). *trazodone HCl.*
ratio-Triacomb (ratiopharm). *gramicidin / neomycin sulfate / nystatin / triamcinolone acetonide.*
ratio-Tryptophan (ratiopharm). *L-tryptophan.*
ratio-Valproic (ratiopharm). *valproic acid.*
ratio-Venlafaxine XR (ratiopharm). *venlafaxine HCl.*
ratio-Zopiclone (ratiopharm). *zopiclone.*
Raxar (Glaxo Wellcome). *grepafloxacin HCl.* Discontinued 2000.
Reactine (McNeil Consumer Healthcare). *cetirizine HCl.*
Reactine Allergy & Sinus (McNeil Consumer Healthcare). *cetirizine HCl / pseudoephedrine HCl.*
Readi-Cat (E-Z-EM Canada). *barium sulfate.* Discontinued 2010.
Rebetron (Schering). *interferon alfa-2b / ribavirin.* Discontinued 2004.
Rebif (EMD Canada). *interferon beta-1a.*
Recombinate (Baxter). *antihemophilic factor (recombinant).* Discontinued 2010.
Recombivax HB (Merck Frosst). *hepatitis B vaccine (recombinant).*
Recothrom (Bayer). *thrombin alfa (recombinant).*
Rectogel (Riva). *benzocaine / zinc sulfate monohydrate.*
Rectogel HC (Riva). *benzocaine / hydrocortisone acetate / zinc sulfate monohydrate.*
Red Away (Rivex Ophthalmics). *naphazoline HCl.* Discontinued 2000.
Redoxon (Bayer Consumer Care). *multiple vitamins and minerals.*
Refludan (Bayer). *lepirudin (rDNA).*

Names in *italics*: Generic drug names, active ingredient or category.
Names in **bold face/underlined**: Prescribing information provided in the Monograph section.
Names in **bold face/not underlined**: Availability information provided in the Monograph section.
Names in regular face: Product is available in Canada but the monograph does not appear in *CPS*.

Refresh (Allergan). *polyvinyl alcohol.*
Refresh Celluvisc (Allergan). *carboxymethylcellulose sodium.*
Refresh Contacts (Allergan). *carboxymethylcellulose sodium.*
Refresh Eye Allergy Relief (Allergan). *antazoline phosphate / naphazoline HCl.*
Refresh Lacri-Lube S.O.P. (Allergan). *lanolin alcohols / mineral oil / white petrolatum.*
Refresh Liquigel (Allergan). *carboxymethylcellulose sodium.*
Refresh Plus (Allergan). *carboxymethylcellulose sodium.*
Refresh Redness Relief (Allergan). *naphazoline HCl.*
Refresh Tears (Allergan). *carboxymethylcellulose sodium.*
Refresh Ultra (Allergan). *boric acid / castor oil / glycerin.*
Reglan (Wyeth-Ayerst). *metoclopramide HCl.* Discontinued 2001.
Regranex (Janssen-Ortho). *becaplermin.*
Rejuva-A (Stiefel, a GSK company). *tretinoin.*
Relafen (GlaxoSmithKline). *nabumetone.* Discontinued 2006.
Relaxophen (Tanta). *acetaminophen / methocarbamol.* Discontinued 2010.
Relefact TRH (Odan). *protirelin.* Discontinued 2009.
Relenza (GlaxoSmithKline). *zanamivir.*
Relistor (Pfizer). *methylnaltrexone bromide.*
Relpax (Pfizer). *eletriptan HBr.*
Remeron (Schering-Plough). *mirtazapine.*
Remeron RD (Schering-Plough). *mirtazapine.*
Remicade (Schering-Plough). *infliximab.*
remifentanil HCl. **Ultiva**.
Reminyl ER (Janssen-Ortho). *galantamine HBr.*
Renagel (Genzyme). *sevelamer HCl.*
Renamin (Baxter). *amino acids.*
Renedil (sanofi-aventis). *felodipine.*
Renova (Johnson & Johnson). *tretinoin.* Discontinued 2007.
ReoPro (Lilly). *abciximab.*
repaglinide. **GlucoNorm**.
Replagal (Paladin). *agalsidase alfa.*
Replens (WellSpring). *lubricant / vaginal moisturizer.*
Repronex (Ferring). *menotropins.*
ReQuip (GlaxoSmithKline). *ropinirole HCl.*
Rescriptor (ViiV Healthcare ULC). *delavirdine mesylate.*
Resonium Calcium (sanofi-aventis). *calcium polystyrene sulfonate.*
Restasis (Allergan). *cyclosporine.*
Restoril (Sepracor). *temazepam.*
Resultz (Nycomed). *isopropyl myristate.*
Retavase (Biovail Pharmaceuticals). *reteplase.* Discontinued 2009.
Retin-A (Johnson & Johnson). *tretinoin.*
Retin-A Micro (Johnson & Johnson). *tretinoin.*
retinol. see vitamin A.
Retisol-A (Stiefel, a GSK company). *butyl methoxydibenzoylmethane / parsol MCX / tretinoin.*
Retrovir (AZT) (ViiV Healthcare ULC). *zidovudine.*
Revatio (Pfizer). *sildenafil citrate.*
Reversa UV Anti-Wrinkle Cream SPF 15 (Dermtek). *avobenzone / glycolic acid / octinoxate / oxybenzone.*
Reversa UV Anti-Wrinkle Eye Contour Cream SPF 15 (Dermtek). *avobenzone / glycolic acid / octinoxate / octisalate.*
Reversa UV Anti-Wrinkle Fluid SPF 15 (Dermtek). *avobenzone / glycolic acid / octinoxate / oxybenzone.*
ReVia (Apotex). *naltrexone HCl.*
Revitalose-C-1000 (Rivex Pharma). *ascorbic acid.* Discontinued 2005.
Revlimid (Celgene). *lenalidomide.*
Reyataz (Bristol-Myers Squibb). *atazanavir sulfate.*
Rh$_0$(D) immune globulin. see immune globulin, Rh$_0$(D).
Rheumatrex (Wyeth-Ayerst). *methotrexate sodium.* Discontinued 2000.
Rhinaris CS Anti-allergic (PendoPharm). *sodium cromoglycate.*
Rhinaris Lubricating Nasal Gel/Nasal Mist (PendoPharm). *polyethylene glycol / propylene glycol.*
Rhinaris Nozoil (PendoPharm). *sesame oil.*
Rhinaris Saline Pediatric Drops/Saline Spray—Daily Hygiene (PendoPharm). *sodium chloride.*
Rhinaris Sinomarin (PendoPharm). *sea water.*
Rhinaris Sinus (PendoPharm). *sodium chloride.*
Rhinocort Aqua (AstraZeneca). *budesonide.*
Rhinocort Turbuhaler (AstraZeneca). *budesonide.*
Rhodacine (Sandoz). *indomethacin.* Discontinued 2006.
Rhodiaprox (Rhodiapharm). *naproxen.* Discontinued 2000.
Rhodis (Rhodiapharm). *ketoprofen.* Discontinued 2006.
Rhodis EC (Rhodiapharm). *ketoprofen.* Discontinued 2006.
Rho-Nitro Pumpspray (sanofi-aventis). *nitroglycerin.*
Rhotral (sanofi-aventis). *acebutolol HCl.*
Rhotrimine (Rhodiapharm). *trimipramine maleate.* Discontinued 2006.
Rhovail (Rhodiapharm). *ketoprofen.* Discontinued 2005.
Rhovane (sanofi-aventis). *zopiclone.*
ribavirin. **Virazole (Lyophilized)**.
ribavirin / peginterferon alfa-2a. **Pegasys RBV (Pegasys and Copegus)**; **Pegetron**.
riboflavin. **Vitamin B$_2$**.
riboflavin. see vitamin B$_2$.
Ridaura (Xediton). *auranofin.*
rifabutin. **Mycobutin**.
Rifadin (sanofi-aventis). *rifampin.*
rifampicin. see rifampin.
Rifampin (CPhA Monograph). *rifampin.*
rifampin. **Rifadin**; **Rifampin**; **Rofact**.
rifampin / isoniazid / pyrazinamide. **Rifater**.
Rifater (sanofi-aventis). *isoniazid / pyrazinamide / rifampin.*
Rilutek (sanofi-aventis). *riluzole.*
riluzole. **Rilutek**.
rimexolone. **Corticosteroids: Eye Ear Nose**; **Vexol**.
Rimso-50 (Alveda). *dimethyl sulfoxide.*
Ringers Injection (Paladin). *calcium chloride / potassium chloride / sodium chloride.* Discontinued 2010.
Riopan (Whitehall-Robins). *magaldrate.* Discontinued 2001.
Riopan Plus (Whitehall-Robins). *magaldrate / simethicone.* Discontinued 2001.
risedronate sodium hemi-pentahydrate. **Actonel**; **Bisphosphonates: Oral**; **PMS-Risedronate**; **ratio-Risedronate**.
Risperdal Consta (Janssen-Ortho). *risperidone.*
Risperdal M-Tab (Janssen-Ortho). *risperidone.*
Risperdal Oral Solution (Janssen-Ortho). *risperidone tartrate.*
Risperdal Tablets (Janssen-Ortho). *risperidone.*
risperidone. **CO Risperidone**; **PMS-Risperidone**; **RAN-Risperidone**; **Risperdal Consta**; **Risperdal Tablets**; **Risperdal M-Tab**.
risperidone tartrate. **Risperdal Oral Solution**.
Ritalin (Novartis Pharmaceuticals). *methylphenidate HCl.*
Ritalin SR (Novartis Pharmaceuticals). *methylphenidate HCl.*
ritonavir. **Norvir**; **Norvir SEC**.
ritonavir / lopinavir. **Kaletra**.
Rituxan (Roche). *rituximab.*
rituximab. **Rituxan**.
Riva-Dicyclomine (Riva). *dicyclomine HCl.*
Riva-Loperamide (Riva). *loperamide HCl.*
Rivanase AQ. (Riva). *beclomethasone dipropionate.*
rivaroxaban. **Xarelto**.

Names in *italics*: Generic drug names, active ingredient or category.
Names in **bold face/underlined**: Prescribing information provided in the Monograph section.
Names in **bold face/not underlined**: Availability information provided in the Monograph section.
Names in regular face: Product is available in Canada but the monograph does not appear in *CPS*.

Rivasol (Riva). *zinc sulfate monohydrate.*

Rivasol HC (Riva). *hydrocortisone acetate / zinc sulfate monohydrate.*

rivastigmine. **Exelon Patch 5**; **Exelon Patch 10**.

rivastigmine hydrogen tartrate. **Exelon**; **PMS-Rivastigmine**; **ratio-Rivastigmine**; **Sandoz Rivastigmine**.

Rivotril (Roche). *clonazepam.*

rizatriptan benzoate. **Maxalt**; **Maxalt RPD**.

Robaxacet (Pfizer Consumer Healthcare). *acetaminophen / methocarbamol.*

Robaxacet-8 (Pfizer Consumer Healthcare). *acetaminophen / codeine phosphate / methocarbamol.*

Robaxacet Extra Strength (Pfizer Consumer Healthcare). *acetaminophen / methocarbamol.*

Robaxin (Pfizer Consumer Healthcare). *methocarbamol.*

Robaxin-750 (Pfizer Consumer Healthcare). *methocarbamol.*

Robaxisal-C (Pfizer Consumer Healthcare). *ASA / codeine phosphate / methocarbamol.*

Robaxisal Extra Strength (Pfizer Consumer Healthcare). *ASA / methocarbamol.*

Robaxisal Tablets (Wyeth Consumer). *ASA / methocarbamol.* Discontinued 2006.

Robax Platinum (Pfizer Consumer Healthcare). *ibuprofen / methocarbamol.*

Robidone (Wyeth-Ayerst). *hydrocodone bitartrate.* Discontinued 2001.

Robinul-Robinul Forte (Wyeth-Ayerst). *glycopyrrolate.* Discontinued 2000.

Robitussin (Pfizer Consumer Healthcare). *guaifenesin.*

Robitussin AC (Pfizer Consumer Healthcare). *codeine phosphate / guaifenesin / pheniramine maleate.*

Robitussin Children's Cough & Cold (Pfizer Consumer Healthcare). *dextromethorphan HBr / pseudoephedrine HCl.*

Robitussin Cough & Cold (Pfizer Consumer Healthcare). *dextromethorphan HBr / guaifenesin / pseudoephedrine HCl.*

Robitussin DM (Pfizer Consumer Healthcare). *dextromethorphan HBr / guaifenesin.*

Robitussin DM Cough Control (Pfizer Consumer Healthcare). *dextromethorphan HBr / guaifenesin.*

Robitussin DM CoughGels (Pfizer Consumer Healthcare). *dextromethorphan HBr.*

Robitussin Extra Strength (Pfizer Consumer Healthcare). *guaifenesin.*

Robitussin Extra Strength Cough & Cold (Pfizer Consumer Healthcare). *dextromethorphan HBr / guaifenesin / pseudoephedrine HCl.*

Robitussin Extra Strength DM Cough Control (Pfizer Consumer Healthcare). *dextromethorphan HBr / guaifenesin.*

Robitussin Honey Cough & Cold (Whitehall-Robins). *dextromethorphan HBr / pseudoephedrine HCl.* Discontinued 2003.

Robitussin Honey Cough DM (Whitehall-Robins). *dextromethorphan HBr.* Discontinued 2003.

Robitussin Honey Flu (Whitehall-Robins). *acetaminophen / dextromethorphan HBr / pseudoephedrine HCl.* Discontinued 2003.

Robitussin Total Cough Cold and Flu (Pfizer Consumer Healthcare). *acetaminophen / dextromethorphan HBr / pseudoephedrine HCl.*

Robitussin Total Extra Strength Nighttime, Cough Cold and Flu (Pfizer Consumer Healthcare). *acetaminophen / chlorpheniramine maleate / dextromethorphan HBr / pseudoephedrine HCl.*

Robitussin with Codeine (Whitehall-Robins). *codeine phosphate / guaifenesin / pheniramine maleate.* Discontinued 2004.

Rocaltrol (Roche). *calcitriol.*

Rocephin (Roche). *ceftriaxone sodium.*

rocuronium bromide. **Rocuronium Bromide Injection**; **Rocuronium Bromide Injection**; **Zemuron**.

Rocuronium Bromide Injection (Sandoz). *rocuronium bromide.*

Rocuronium Bromide Injection (Hospira). *rocuronium bromide.*

Rofact (Valeant). *rifampin.*

Roferon-A (Roche). *interferon alfa-2a.* Discontinued 2004.

Rogaine (Johnson & Johnson). *minoxidil.*

Rogitine (Paladin). *phentolamine mesylate.*

romiplostim. **Nplate**.

ropinirole HCl. **CO Ropinirole**; **PMS-Ropinirole**; **RAN-Ropinirole**; **ReQuip**.

ropivacaine HCl. **Naropin**.

Rosasol (Stiefel, a GSK company). *metronidazole.*

rosiglitazone maleate. **Avandia**.

rosiglitazone maleate / glimepiride. **Avandaryl**.

rosiglitazone maleate / metformin HCl. **Avandamet**.

Rosmarinus officinalis / Cucurbita pepo / Curcuma longa / Helianthus annus / Linum usitatissimum / Olea europaea. **Optomega**.

rosuvastatin calcium. **Crestor**; **HMG-CoA Reductase Inhibitors**.

Rotarix (GlaxoSmithKline). *rotavirus vaccine, human, live, attenuated, oral.*

RotaTeq (Merck Frosst). *rotavirus vaccine, live, oral, pentavalent.*

rotavirus vaccine, human, live, attenuated, oral. **Rotarix**.

rotavirus vaccine, live, oral, pentavalent. **RotaTeq**.

Rougier Calcium (Rougier Pharma). *calcium glucoheptonate / calcium gluconate.* Discontinued 2009.

Rougier Clean Derm (Rougier Pharma). *chlorhexidine gluconate.*

Rougier Magnesium (Rougier Pharma). *magnesium glucoheptonate.*

Rougier Vap (Rougier Pharma). *chlorhexidine gluconate.*

Rouhex-G (Rougier). *chlorhexidine gluconate.* Discontinued 2000.

Rouphylline (Rougier). *oxtriphylline.* Discontinued 2000.

Rovamycine (Odan). *spiramycin.*

Royvac (Waymar). *bisacodyl / magnesium citrate.*

Rub A-535 Antiphlogistine (Church & Dwight). *camphor / eucalyptus oil / menthol / methyl salicylate.*

RUB A-535 Antiphlogistine Capsaicin (Church & Dwight). *capsaicin.*

Rub A-535 Antiphlogistine Ice (Church & Dwight). *menthol.*

Rub A-535 Antiphlogistine No Odour (Church & Dwight). *triethanolamine salicylate.*

Rub A-535 Extra Strength Arthritis Roll-On Lotion (Church & Dwight). *capsaicin / menthol / triethanolamine salicylate.*

Rubbing Alcohol Compound (Rougier Pharma). *ethanol.*

Rubramin (Squibb). *vitamin* B_{12}. Discontinued 2000.

Rylosol (ICN). *sotalol HCl.* Discontinued 2001.

Rythmodan (sanofi-aventis). *disopyramide.*

Rythmol (Abbott). *propafenone HCl.*

S

S.A.S. (ICN). *sulfasalazine.* Discontinued 2002.

Sabril (Lundbeck). *vigabatrin.*

Saccharomyces boulardii lyo. **Florastor**.

Saizen (EMD Canada). *somatropin.*

Saizen click.easy (EMD Canada). *somatropin.*

Salac (Medicis). *salicylic acid.* Discontinued 2000.

Salagen (Pfizer). *pilocarpine HCl.*

Salazopyrin (Pfizer). *sulfasalazine.*

Salazopyrin EN-tabs (Pfizer). *sulfasalazine.*

salbutamol sulfate. **Airomir**; **ratio-Salbutamol**; **Ventolin Diskus**; **Ventolin HFA**; **Ventolin I.V. Infusion Solution**; **Ventolin Respirator Solution**; **Ventolin Nebules P.F.**

salbutamol sulfate / ipratropium bromide. **Combivent UDV**; **ratio-Ipra Sal UDV**.

salicylazosulfapyridine. see *sulfasalazine.*

salicylic acid. **Duofilm Patch**; **Duofilm Plantar Patch**; **Duoforte 27**.

salicylic acid / betamethasone dipropionate. **Diprosalic**; **ratio-Topisalic**.

salicylic acid / cantharidin / podophyllin. **Canthacur-PS**; **Cantharone Plus**.

salicylic acid / coal tar. **Targel S.A.**

salicylic acid / coal tar / menthol / pyrithione disulfide. **Polytar AF**.

salicylic acid / coal tar / triclosan. **Tardan**.

salicylic acid / diflucortolone valerate. **Nerisalic**.

salicylic acid / formalin / lactic acid. **Duoplant**.

salicylic acid / lactic acid. **Duofilm Liquid**.

salicylic acid / triclosan. **Panoxyl Clear Acne Cleansing Gel**.

Saliject (Omega Laboratories). *sodium salicylate.*

Saline from Otrivin Nasal Drops (Novartis Consumer Health). *sodium chloride.*

Salinex Nasal Lubricant/Nasal Lubricant Gel (Sandoz). *polyethylene glycol / propylene glycol / sodium chloride.*

Salinex Nasal Spray/Nasal Drops/Nasal Mist (Sandoz). *sodium chloride.*

salmeterol xinafoate. **Serevent Diskhaler Disk**; **Serevent Diskus**.

Names in *italics*: Generic drug names, active ingredient or category.
Names in **bold face/underlined**: Prescribing information provided in the Monograph section.
Names in **bold face/not underlined**: Availability information provided in the Monograph section.
Names in regular face: Product is available in Canada but the monograph does not appear in *CPS*.

Names in *italics*: Generic drug names, active ingredient or category.
Names in **bold face/underlined**: Prescribing information provided in the Monograph section.
Names in **bold face/not underlined**: Availability information provided in the Monograph section.
Names in regular face: Product is available in Canada but the monograph does not appear in *CPS*.

Names in *italics*: Generic drug names, active ingredient or category.
Names in **bold face/underlined**: Prescribing information provided in the Monograph section.
Names in **bold face/not underlined**: Availability information provided in the Monograph section.
Names in regular face: Product is available in Canada but the monograph does not appear in *CPS*.

Names in *italics*: Generic drug names, active ingredient or category.
Names in **bold face/underlined**: Prescribing information provided in the Monograph section.
Names in **bold face/not underlined**: Availability information provided in the Monograph section.
Names in regular face: Product is available in Canada but the monograph does not appear in *CPS*.

Stelabid Preparations (GlaxoSmithKline). *isopropamide iodide / trifluoperazine HCl*. Discontinued 2002.

Stelara (Janssen-Ortho). *ustekinumab*.

Stelazine (SmithKline Beecham). *trifluoperazine HCl*. Discontinued 2001.

Stemetil (sanofi-aventis). *prochlorperazine mesylate*. Discontinued 2007.

Stemgen (Amgen). *ancestim*.

sterculia. **Normacol**.

Steri/Sol (Johnson & Johnson). *hexetidine*.

Stericide (Rougier). *glutaraldehyde*. Discontinued 2000.

Sterile Water for Injection (Alveda). *water*.

Stieprox (Stiefel, a GSK company). *ciclopirox olamine*.

Stieva-A (Stiefel, a GSK company). *tretinoin*.

Stievamycin Preparations (Stiefel, a GSK company). *erythromycin / tretinoin*.

Stilamin (EMD Canada). *somatostatin*.

stilboestrol. see *diethylstilbestrol sodium diphosphate*.

Stop Itch First Aid Lotion 3.5% (Schering-Plough). *homosalate / octinoxate / octisalate / oxybenzone*. Discontinued 2010.

Strattera (Lilly). *atomoxetine HCl*.

Strawberry Extract (Rougier Pharma). *extract of strawberry leaves / tannic acid*.

Strepsil (Schering-Plough). *amylmetracresol / dichlorobenzyl aclohol*.

Streptase (CSL Behring). *streptokinase*.

Streptokinase (CPhA Monograph). *streptokinase*.

streptokinase. **Streptase**; **Streptokinase**.

Streptomycin (CPhA Monograph). *streptomycin*.

streptomycin. **Streptomycin**; **Streptomycin Injection USP**.

Streptomycin Injection USP (SteriMax). *streptomycin*.

Streptomycin Sulfate (Pfizer). *streptomycin sulfate*. Discontinued 2001.

streptozocin. **Zanosar**.

Stress Formula (Jamp Pharma). *multiple vitamins and minerals*.

Stresstabs Allbee C-550 (Wyeth Consumer Healthcare). *ascorbic acid / vitamin B complex*. Discontinued 2006.

Stresstabs Beminal 500 (Wyeth Consumer Healthcare). *ascorbic acid / vitamin B complex*. Discontinued 2006.

Stresstabs for Men (Pfizer Consumer Healthcare). *ascorbic acid / copper / lycopene / selenium / vitamin B complex / vitamin E / zinc*.

Stresstabs for Women (Pfizer Consumer Healthcare). *ascorbic acid / iron / vitamin B complex / vitamin E*.

Stresstabs Plus (Pfizer Consumer Healthcare). *ascorbic acid / lycopene / selenium / vitamin B complex / vitamin E*.

Stresstabs Regular (Pfizer Consumer Healthcare). *ascorbic acid / vitamin B complex / vitamin E*.

Stresstabs Z-BEC (Pfizer Consumer Healthcare). *ascorbic acid / copper / vitamin B complex / vitamin E / zinc*.

strontium chloride. **Sensodyne Original**.

Suboxone (Schering-Plough). *buprenorphine HCl / naloxone HCl dihydrate*.

succinylcholine chloride. **Quelicin Injection**.

sucralfate. **Nu-Sucralfate**; **Sulcrate**; **Sulcrate Suspension Plus**.

Sudafed Cold & Cough Extra Strength (McNeil Consumer Healthcare). *acetaminophen / dextromethorphan HBr / pseudoephedrine HCl*.

Sudafed Decongestant 12 Hour (McNeil Consumer Healthcare). *pseudoephedrine HCl*.

Sudafed Head Cold and Sinus Extra Strength (McNeil Consumer Healthcare). *acetaminophen / pseudoephedrine HCl*.

Sudafed PE Decongestant (McNeil Consumer Healthcare). *phenylephrine HCl*.

Sudafed Sinus Advance (McNeil Consumer Healthcare). *ibuprofen / pseudoephedrine HCl*.

Sufenta (Janssen-Ortho). *sufentanil citrate*. Discontinued 2009.

sufentanil citrate. **Opioids**; **Sufentanil Citrate Injection USP**.

Sufentanil Citrate Injection USP (Sandoz). *sufentanil citrate*.

Sulcrate (Axcan Pharma). *sucralfate*.

Sulcrate Suspension Plus (Axcan Pharma). *sucralfate*.

sulfacetamide sodium. **Sodium Sulamyd**.

sulfacetamide sodium / prednisolone acetate. **Blephamide**.

sulfacetamide sodium / sulfur. **Sulfacet-R**.

Sulfacet-R (sanofi-aventis). *sulfacetamide sodium / sulfur*.

sulfamethoxazole / trimethoprim. **Nu-Cotrimox**; **Septra Injection**; **Sulfamethoxazole–Trimethoprim**; **Teva-Sulfamethoxazole Trimethoprim**; **Teva-Sulfamethoxazole Trimethoprim DS**.

Sulfamethoxazole–Trimethoprim (CPhA Monograph). *sulfamethoxazole / trimethoprim*.

Sulfapyridine (CPhA Monograph). *sulfapyridine*.

sulfapyridine. **Sulfapyridine**.

sulfasalazine. **PMS-Sulfasalazine**; **PMS-Sulfasalazine EC**; **Salazopyrin**; **Salazopyrin EN-tabs**.

Sulfinpyrazone (AA Pharma). *sulfinpyrazone*.

Sulfonylureas (CPhA Monograph).

Sulfoxyl (Stiefel). *benzoyl peroxide / sulfur*. Discontinued 2000.

sulfur / aluminum chlorhydroxide / methylprednisolone acetate. **Medrol Acne Lotion**.

sulfur / aluminum chlorhydroxide / methylprednisolone acetate / neomycin sulfate. **Neo-Medrol Acne Lotion**.

sulfur / sulfacetamide sodium. **Sulfacet-R**.

sulphasalazine. see *sulfasalazine*.

sulphinpyrazone. see *sulfinpyrazone*.

Sultrin (Janssen-Ortho). *triple sulfa*. Discontinued 2000.

sumatriptan hemisulfate. **Imitrex Nasal Spray**.

sumatriptan succinate. **CO Sumatriptan**; **Imitrex DF Tablets**; **Imitrex Injection/Autoinjector**; **Sandoz Sumatriptan**; **Teva-Sumatriptan**; **Teva-Sumatriptan DF**.

sunitinib malata. **Sutent**.

Supeudol (Sandoz). *oxycodone HCl*.

Suplasyn (Alveda). *sodium hyaluronate*.

Suplasyn m.d. (Alveda). *sodium hyaluronate*.

Suprane (Baxter). *desflurane*.

Suprax (sanofi-aventis). *cefixime*.

Suprefact (sanofi-aventis). *buserelin acetate*.

Suprefact Depot (sanofi-aventis). *buserelin acetate*.

Supres (Merck Frosst). *chlorothiazide / methyldopa*. Discontinued 2000.

Surgam (sanofi-aventis). *tiaprofenic acid*. Discontinued 2007.

Surgam SR (sanofi-aventis). *tiaprofenic acid*. Discontinued 2007.

Surmontil (Aventis Pharma). *trimipramine maleate*. Discontinued 2005.

Survanta (Abbott). *beractant*.

Sustiva (Bristol-Myers Squibb). *efavirenz*.

Sutent (Pfizer). *sunitinib malata*.

suxamethonium. see *succinylcholine chloride*.

Symbicort Turbuhaler (AstraZeneca). *budesonide / formoterol fumarate dihydrate*.

Symmetrel (Antiparkinson) (Bristol-Myers Squibb). *amantadine HCl*. Discontinued 2009.

Symmetrel (Antiviral) (Bristol-Myers Squibb). *amantadine HCl*. Discontinued 2009.

Synacthen Depot (Novartis Pharmaceuticals). *cosyntropin / zinc hydroxide*.

Synagis (Abbott). *palivizumab*.

Synalar (Valeo Pharma). *fluocinolone acetonide*. Discontinued 2010.

Synarel (Pfizer). *nafarelin acetate*.

Synergy Defense (Awareness Corporation/dba AwarenessLife). *enzyme blend*.

Synflex (AltiMed). *naproxen sodium*. Discontinued 2002.

Synflex DS (AltiMed). *naproxen sodium*. Discontinued 2002.

Synflorix (GlaxoSmithKline). *pneumococcal conjugate vaccine (non-typeable H. influenzae (NTHi) protein D, diphtheria or tetanus toxoid conjugates) adsorbed*.

Synovisol (Baxter). *glycerin*.

Synphasic (Pfizer). *ethinyl estradiol / norethindrone*.

Synthroid (Abbott). *levothyroxine sodium*.

Synvisc (Genzyme). *hylan G-F 20*.

Synvisc One (Genzyme). *hylan G-F 20*.

Systane (Alcon). *polyethylene glycol / propylene glycol*.

Names in *italics*: Generic drug names, active ingredient or category.
Names in **bold face/underlined**: Prescribing information provided in the Monograph section.
Names in **bold face/not underlined**: Availability information provided in the Monograph section.
Names in regular face: Product is available in Canada but the monograph does not appear in *CPS*.

T

Names in *italics*: Generic drug names, active ingredient or category.
Names in **bold face/underlined**: Prescribing information provided in the Monograph section.
Names in **bold face/not underlined**: Availability information provided in the Monograph section.
Names in regular face: Product is available in Canada but the monograph does not appear in *CPS*.

Names in *italics*: Generic drug names, active ingredient or category.
Names in **bold face/underlined**: Prescribing information provided in the Monograph section.
Names in **bold face/not underlined**: Availability information provided in the Monograph section.
Names in regular face: Product is available in Canada but the monograph does not appear in *CPS*.

Names in *italics*: Generic drug names, active ingredient or category.
Names in **bold face/underlined**: Prescribing information provided in the Monograph section.
Names in **bold face/not underlined**: Availability information provided in the Monograph section.
Names in regular face: Product is available in Canada but the monograph does not appear in *CPS*.

tramadol HCl. **Opioids**; **Ralivia**; **Tridural**; **Ultram**; **Zytram XL**.

tramadol HCl / acetaminophen. **Tramacet**.

Trandate (Paladin). *labetalol HCl*.

trandolapril. **ACE Inhibitors**; **Mavik**.

trandolapril / verapamil HCl. **Tarka**.

tranexamic acid. **Cyklokapron**.

Tranexamic Acid Injection BP (Sandoz). *tranexamic acid*.

Transderm-Nitro (Novartis Pharmaceuticals). *nitroglycerin*.

Transderm-V (Novartis Pharmaceuticals). *scopolamine*.

trans-retinoic acid. see *tretinoin*.

Tranxene (Abbott). *clorazepate dipotassium*. Discontinued 2002.

tranylcypromine sulfate. **Parnate**.

Trasicor (Novartis Pharmaceuticals). *oxprenolol HCl*. Discontinued 2007.

trastuzumab. **Herceptin**.

Trasylol (Bayer). *aprotinin*.

Travasol With Electrolytes (Baxter). *amino acids / dextrose / electrolytes*.

Travasol Without Electrolytes (Baxter). *amino acids / dextrose*.

Travatan Z (Alcon). *travoprost*.

travoprost. **Travatan Z**.

travoprost / timolol maleate. **DuoTrav**.

trazodone HCl. **Desyrel**; **Desyrel Dividose**; **PMS-Trazodone**; **ratio-Trazodone**.

Trazorel (ICN). *trazodone HCl*. Discontinued 2002.

Trelstar 3.75 mg (1 month slow-release) (Paladin). *triptorelin pamoate*.

Trelstar 11.25 mg (3 month slow-release) (Paladin). *triptorelin pamoate*.

Trelstar (Endometriosis) (Paladin). *triptorelin pamoate*.

Trental (sanofi-aventis). *pentoxifylline*.

tretinoin. **Rejuva-A**; **Retin-A Micro**; **Retin-A**; **Stieva-A**; **Vesanoid**; **Vitamin A Acid**.

tretinoin / butyl methoxydibenzoylmethane / parsol MCX. **Retisol-A**.

tretinoin / erythromycin. **Stievamycin Preparations**.

Triaderm (Taro). *triamcinolone acetonide*.

triamcinolone. **Corticosteroids: Systemic**.

triamcinolone acetonide. **Aristocort, Creams and Ointments**; **Corticosteroids: Eye Ear Nose**; **Corticosteroids: Systemic**; **Corticosteroids: Topical**; **Kenalog-10 Injection**; **Kenalog-40 Injection**; **Nasacort AQ**; **Oracort**; **Triaderm**; **Triamcinolone Acetonide Injectable Suspension USP**.

triamcinolone acetonide / gramicidin / neomycin sulfate / nystatin. **ratio-Triacomb**; **Viaderm-K.C.**

Triamcinolone Acetonide Injectable Suspension USP (Sandoz). *triamcinolone acetonide*.

triamcinolone diacetate. **Corticosteroids: Systemic**.

Triaminic Allergy Congestion (Novartis Consumer Health). *pseudoephedrine HCl*. Discontinued 2002.

Triaminic Cold & Night Time Cough (Novartis Consumer Health). *chlorpheniramine maleate / dextromethorphan HBr / pseudoephedrine HCl*.

Triaminic Cold, Cough & Fever (Novartis Consumer Health). *acetaminophen / chlorpheniramine maleate / dextromethorphan HBr / pseudoephedrine HCl*.

Triaminic Cough (Novartis Consumer Health). *dextromethorphan HBr / pseudoephedrine HCl*. Discontinued 2002.

Triaminic Softchews Cold & Allergy (Novartis Consumer Health). *chlorpheniramine maleate / pseudoephedrine HCl*.

Triaminic Softchews Cold & Cough (Novartis Consumer Health). *chlorpheniramine maleate / dextromethorphan HBr / pseudoephedrine HCl*.

Triaminic Softchews Cough (Novartis Consumer Health). *dextromethorphan HBr*. Discontinued 2002.

Triaminic Softchews Cough & Sore Throat (Novartis Consumer Health). *acetaminophen / dextromethorphan HBr*.

triamterene / hydrochlorothiazide. **Nu-Triazide**.

Trianal (Trianon). *ASA / butalbital / caffeine*.

Trianal C¼, C½ (Trianon). *ASA / butalbital / caffeine / codeine phosphate*.

Triatec-8 (Trianon). *acetaminophen / caffeine citrate / codeine phosphate*.

Triatec-8 Strong (Trianon). *acetaminophen / caffeine citrate / codeine phosphate*.

Triatec-30 (Trianon). *acetaminophen / codeine phosphate*.

Triavil (Merck Frosst). *amitriptyline HCl / perphenazine*. Discontinued 2004.

triazolam. **Benzodiazepines**.

triclosan. **Adasept Skin Cleanser**; **Tersaseptic**.

triclosan / coal tar / salicylic acid. **Tardan**.

triclosan / salicylic acid. **Panoxyl Clear Acne Cleansing Gel**.

Tri-Cyclen (Janssen-Ortho). *ethinyl estradiol / norgestimate*.

Tri-Cyclen LO (Janssen-Ortho). *ethinyl estradiol / norgestimate*.

Tridural (Labopharm). *tramadol HCl*.

triethanolamine salicylate. **Myoflex**; **Rub A-535 Antiphlogistine No Odour**.

triethanolamine salicylate / capsaicin / menthol. **Rub A-535 Extra Strength Arthritis Roll-On Lotion**.

Trifluoperazine (CPhA Monograph). *trifluoperazine*.

trifluoperazine. **Trifluoperazine**.

trifluridine. **Viroptic**.

Trihexyphenidyl (CPhA Monograph). *trihexyphenidyl HCl*.

trihexyphenidyl HCl. **Trihexyphenidyl**.

Trilafon (Schering). *perphenazine*. Discontinued 2006.

Trileptal (Novartis Pharmaceuticals). *oxcarbazepine*.

Trilisate (Purdue Pharma). *choline magnesium trisalicylate*. Discontinued 2002.

trimebutine maleate. **Modulon**.

Trimethoprim (CPhA Monograph). *trimethoprim*.

trimethoprim. **Trimethoprim**.

trimethoprim / sulfamethoxazole. **Nu-Cotrimox**; **Septra Injection**; **Sulfamethoxazole–Trimethoprim**; **Teva-Sulfamethoxazole Trimethoprim**; **Teva-Sulfamethoxazole Trimethoprim DS**.

trimethoprim sulfate / polymyxin B sulfate. **Polytrim**.

Trinalin (Schering-Plough). *azatadine maleate / pseudoephedrine sulfate*. Discontinued 2007.

Trinipatch (Paladin). *nitroglycerin*.

Triphasil 21 (Wyeth Canada). *ethinyl estradiol / levonorgestrel*. Discontinued 2008.

Triphasil 28 (Wyeth Canada). *ethinyl estradiol / levonorgestrel*. Discontinued 2008.

Triple Antibiotic Ointment (Taro). *bacitracin zinc / gramicidin / polymyxin B sulfate*.

triprolidine HCl / acetaminophen / pseudoephedrine HCl. **Actifed Plus Extra Strength**.

triprolidine HCl / codeine phosphate / guaifenesin / pseudoephedrine HCl. **CoActifed Expectorant**; **ratio-Cotridin Expectorant**.

triprolidine HCl / codeine phosphate / pseudoephedrine HCl. **CoActifed Syrup**; **CoActifed Tablets**; **ratio-Cotridin**.

triprolidine HCl / pseudoephedrine HCl. **Actifed**.

Triptil (Merck Frosst). *protriptyline HCl*. Discontinued 2001.

triptorelin pamoate. **Trelstar (Endometriosis)**; **Trelstar 3.75 mg (1 month slow-release)**; **Trelstar 11.25 mg (3 month slow-release)**.

Triquilar 21 (Bayer). *ethinyl estradiol / levonorgestrel*.

Triquilar 28 (Bayer). *ethinyl estradiol / levonorgestrel*.

Trisoralen (ICN). *trioxsalen*. Discontinued 2000.

Trisulfaminic (Shepherd). *pheniramine maleate / phenylpropanolamine HCl compound / triple sulfas*. Discontinued 2001.

Tri-Vi-Flor (Mead Johnson Nutritionals). *multiple vitamins*. Discontinued 2002.

Trizivir (ViiV Healthcare ULC). *abacavir sulfate / lamivudine / zidovudine*.

Tropicamide (Rivex Ophthalmics). *tropicamide*. Discontinued 2002.

tropicamide. **Mydriacyl**.

tropicamide / phenylephrine HCl. **Diophenyl-T**.

Trosec (Sepracor). *trospium chloride*.

trospium chloride. **Trosec**.

Trosyd AF (Pfizer Consumer Healthcare). *tioconazole*. Discontinued 2002.

Trosyd J (Pfizer Consumer Healthcare). *tioconazole*. Discontinued 2002.

Trovan I.V. (Pfizer). *alatrofloxacin mesylate*. Discontinued 2002.

Trovan Tablets (Pfizer). *trovafloxacin mesylate*. Discontinued 2002.

Trusopt (Merck Frosst). *dorzolamide HCl*.

Truvada (Gilead Sciences). *emtricitabine / tenofovir disoproxil fumarate*.

Tryptan (Valeant). *L-tryptophan*.

Names in *italics*: Generic drug names, active ingredient or category.
Names in **bold face/underlined**: Prescribing information provided in the Monograph section.
Names in **bold face/not underlined**: Availability information provided in the Monograph section.
Names in regular face: Product is available in Canada but the monograph does not appear in *CPS*.

U

V

Names in *italics*: Generic drug names, active ingredient or category.
Names in **bold face/underlined**: Prescribing information provided in the Monograph section.
Names in **bold face/not underlined**: Availability information provided in the Monograph section.
Names in regular face: Product is available in Canada but the monograph does not appear in *CPS*.

valacyclovir HCl. **CO Valacyclovir**; **PMS-Valacyclovir**; **Valtrex**.

Valcyte (Roche). *valganciclovir HCl.*

valganciclovir HCl. **Valcyte**.

Valisone-G (Valeo Pharma). *betamethasone valerate / gentamicin sulfate.*

Valisone Scalp Lotion (Valeo Pharma). *betamethasone valerate.*

Valium Roche Injection (Roche). *diazepam.* Discontinued 2000.

Valium Roche Oral (Roche). *diazepam.*

valproic acid. **Depakene**; **ratio-Valproic**.

valsartan. **Diovan**.

valsartan / hydrochlorothiazide. **Diovan-HCT**.

Valtrex (GlaxoSmithKline). *valacyclovir HCl.*

Val-Vanco (Valeo Pharma). *vancomycin HCl.*

Vamin N (Baxter). *amino acids / electrolytes.* Discontinued 2004.

Vancenase (Schering). *beclomethasone dipropionate.* Discontinued 2001.

Vancocin (Iroko). *vancomycin HCl.*

vancomycin HCl. **Val-Vanco**; **Vancocin**; **Vancomycin Hydrochloride, USP**.

Vancomycin Hydrochloride, USP (Hospira). *vancomycin HCl.*

Vancomycin Hydrochloride, USP, Sterile (Pharmaceutical Partners). *vancomycin HCl.*

Vaniqa (Triton Pharma). *eflornithine HCl.*

Vanquin (Pfizer Consumer Healthcare). *pyrvinium pamoate.* Discontinued 2004.

Vantas (Paladin). *histrelin acetate.* Discontinued 2007.

Vaponefrin (sanofi-aventis). *epinephrine HCl.* Discontinued 2007.

Vaqta (Merck Frosst). *hepatitis A vaccine, purified inactivated.*

vardenafil HCl. **Levitra**.

varenicline tartrate. **Champix**.

varicella virus vaccine, live, attenuated (Oka/Merck). **Varivax III**.

varicella virus vaccine, live, attenuated (Oka-strain). **Varilrix**.

varicella zoster immune globulin (human). **VariZIG**.

Varilrix (GlaxoSmithKline). *varicella virus vaccine, live, attenuated (Oka-strain).*

Varivax III (Merck Frosst). *varicella virus vaccine, live, attenuated (Oka/Merck).*

VariZIG (Cangene). *varicella zoster immune globulin (human).*

Vaseretic (Merck Frosst). *enalapril / hydrochlorothiazide.*

Vasocidin (Novartis Ophthalmics). *prednisolone sodium phosphate / sulfacetamide sodium.* Discontinued 2004.

Vasocon (Novartis Ophthalmics). *naphazoline HCl.* Discontinued 2006.

Vasocon-A (Novartis Ophthalmics). *antazoline phosphate / naphazoline HCl.* Discontinued 2005.

vasopressin. **Pressyn AR**; **Pressyn**.

Vasopressin Injection USP (Sandoz). *vasopressin.*

Vasotec (Merck Frosst). *enalapril.*

Vasotec IV (Sandoz). *enalaprilat.*

Vasovist (Bayer). *gadofosveset trisodium.*

Vasoxyl (Glaxo Wellcome). *methoxamine HCl.* Discontinued 2001.

Vaxigrip (sanofi pasteur). *inactivated influenza vaccine trivalent types A and B (split virion).*

Vectibix (Amgen). *panitumumab.*

Vecuronium (Schein Pharmaceutical). *vecuronium bromide.* Discontinued 2001.

Vecuronium Bromide for Injection (Abbott). *vecuronium bromide.* Discontinued 2004.

Velbe (Lilly). *vinblastine sulfate.* Discontinued 2000.

Velcade (Janssen-Ortho). *bortezomib mannitol boronic ester.*

venlafaxine HCl. **CO Venlafaxine XR**; **Effexor XR**; **PMS-Venlafaxine XR**; **ratio-Venlafaxine XR**; **Sandoz Venlafaxine XR**; **Teva-Venlafaxine XR**.

Venofer (Mylan). *iron sucrose.*

Ventolin Diskus (GlaxoSmithKline). *salbutamol sulfate.*

Ventolin HFA (GlaxoSmithKline). *salbutamol sulfate.*

Ventolin I.V. Infusion Solution (GlaxoSmithKline). *salbutamol sulfate.*

Ventolin Nebules P.F. (GlaxoSmithKline). *salbutamol sulfate.*

Ventolin Oral Liquid (GlaxoSmithKline). *salbutamol sulfate.* Discontinued 2009.

Ventolin Respirator Solution (GlaxoSmithKline). *salbutamol sulfate.*

Vepesid (Bristol-Myers Squibb). *etoposide.*

verapamil HCl. **Calcium Channel Blockers**; **Isoptin SR**; **Nu-Verap**; **Verapamil Hydrochloride Injection USP**.

verapamil HCl / trandolapril. **Tarka**.

Verapamil Hydrochloride Injection USP (Hospira). *verapamil HCl.*

Verelan (Wyeth-Ayerst). *verapamil HCl.* Discontinued 2001.

Vermox (Janssen-Ortho). *mebendazole.*

Versed (Roche). *midazolam.* Discontinued 2002.

Versel (Valeo Pharma). *selenium sulfide.*

verteporfin. **Visudyne**.

Vesanoid (Roche). *tretinoin.*

Vesicare (Astellas). *solifenacin succinate.*

Vexol (Alcon). *rimexolone.*

Vfend (Pfizer). *voriconazole.*

Viaderm-K.C. (Taro). *gramicidin / neomycin sulfate / nystatin / triamcinolone acetonide.*

Viagra (Pfizer). *sildenafil citrate.*

Vibramycin (Pfizer). *doxycycline hyclate.*

Vibra-Tabs (Pfizer). *doxycycline hyclate.*

Vicks Children's NyQuil (Procter & Gamble). *chlorpheniramine maleate / dextromethorphan HBr.*

Vicks Custom Care Body Aches (Procter & Gamble). *acetaminophen.*

Vicks Custom Care Chest Congestion/Cough (Procter & Gamble). *dextromethorphan HBr / guaifenesin.*

Vicks Custom Care Cough & Cold PM (Procter & Gamble). *acetaminophen / chlorpheniramine maleate / dextromethorphan HBr.* Discontinued 2010.

Vicks Custom Care Dry Cough (Procter & Gamble). *dextromethorphan HBr.*

Vicks Custom Care Nasal Congestion/Cough (Procter & Gamble). *dextromethorphan HBr / phenylephrine HCl.*

Vicks DayQuil Cough (Proctor & Gamble). *dextromethorphan hydrobromide.*

Vicks DayQuil Liquicaps (Procter & Gamble). *acetaminophen / dextromethorphan HBr / phenylephrine HCl.*

Vicks DayQuil Liquid (Procter & Gamble). *acetaminophen / dextromethorphan HBr / phenylephrine HCl.*

Vicks DayQuil Mucus Control (Procter & Gamble). *guaifenesin.*

Vicks DayQuil Mucus Control DM (Procter & Gamble). *dextromethorphan HBr / guaifenesin.*

Vicks DayQuil Sinus LiquiCaps (Procter & Gamble). *acetaminophen / phenylephrine HCl.*

Vicks NyQuil Cough Liquid (Proctor & Gamble). *dextromethorphan hydrobromide / doxylamine succinate.*

Vicks NyQuil Liquicaps (Procter & Gamble). *acetaminophen / dextromethorphan HBr / doxylamine succinate.*

Vicks NyQuil Liquid (Procter & Gamble). *acetaminophen / dextromethorphan HBr / doxylamine succinate.*

Vicks NyQuil Sinus LiquiCaps (Procter & Gamble). *acetaminophen / doxylamine succinate / phenylephrine HCl.*

Vicks Sinex (Procter & Gamble). *oxymetazoline HCl.* Discontinued 2009.

Vicks VapoDrops (Procter & Gamble). *menthol.*

Vicks VapoRub (Procter & Gamble). *camphor / eucalyptus / menthol.*

Vicks Vapour Inhaler (Procter & Gamble). *camphor / menthol.*

Vicks Vitamin C Orange Drops (Procter & Gamble). *ascorbic acid.*

Victoza (Novo Nordisk). *liraglutide.*

Videx (Bristol-Myers Squibb). *didanosine.* Discontinued 2008.

Videx EC (Bristol-Myers Squibb). *didanosine.*

Vigamox (Alcon). *moxifloxacin HCl.*

Vimpat (UCB). *lacosamide.*

Vinblastine (CPhA Monograph). *vinblastine sulfate.*

vinblastine sulfate. **Vinblastine**; **Vinblastine Sulfate Injection**.

Vinblastine Sulfate Injection (Hospira). *vinblastine sulfate.*

Vincristine (CPhA Monograph). *vincristine sulfate.*

vincristine sulfate. **Vincristine**; **Vincristine Sulfate Injection USP**.

Vincristine Sulfate Injection USP (Hospira). *vincristine sulfate.*

Names in *italics*: Generic drug names, active ingredient or category.
Names in **bold face/underlined**: Prescribing information provided in the Monograph section.
Names in **bold face/not underlined**: Availability information provided in the Monograph section.
Names in regular face: Product is available in Canada but the monograph does not appear in *CPS*.

W

Names in *italics*: Generic drug names, active ingredient or category.
Names in **bold face/underlined**: Prescribing information provided in the Monograph section.
Names in **bold face/not underlined**: Availability information provided in the Monograph section.
Names in regular face: Product is available in Canada but the monograph does not appear in *CPS*.

Warfilone (Merck Frosst). *warfarin sodium.* Discontinued 2000.

Wartec (Stiefel). *podofilox.*

Wellbutrin SR (Biovail Pharmaceuticals). *bupropion HCl.*

Wellbutrin XL (Biovail Pharmaceuticals). *bupropion HCl.*

Wellferon (Glaxo Wellcome). *interferon alpha-n1 [lns].* Discontinued 2000.

white petrolatum / lanolin alcohols / mineral oil. **Refresh Lacri-Lube S.O.P.**

white petrolatum / mineral oil. **Hypotears Eye Ointment.**

wilate (Octapharma). *human coagulation factor VIII (FVIII) / human von Willebrand factor (VWF).*

Winpred (Valeant). *prednisone.*

WinRho SDF (Cangene). *immune globulin, Rho (D) human.*

Witch Hazel (Rougier Pharma). *hamamelis virginiana.*

Wydase (Wyeth-Ayerst). *hyaluronidase.* Discontinued 2001.

X

Xalacom (Pfizer). *latanoprost / timolol maleate.*

Xalatan (Pfizer). *latanoprost.*

Xamiol (LEO Pharma). *betamethasone dipropionate / calcipotriol.*

Xanax (Pfizer). *alprazolam.*

Xanax TS (Pfizer). *alprazolam.*

Xarelto (Bayer). *rivaroxaban.*

Xatral (sanofi-aventis). *alfuzosin HCl.*

Xeloda (Roche). *capecitabine.*

Xenical (Roche). *orlistat.*

Xeomin (Merz Pharma). *Clostridium botulinum neurotoxin type A (150 kD), free from complexing proteins.*

Xigris (Lilly). *drotrecogin alfa (activated).*

Xolair (Novartis Pharmaceuticals). *omalizumab.*

X-Prep (Purdue Pharma). *senna (standardized sennosides from senna concentrate CG).* Discontinued 2007.

X-Tar (Dormer). *coal tar / menthol / salicylic acid.* Discontinued 2009.

Xylocaine 4% Sterile Solution (AstraZeneca). *lidocaine HCl.* Discontinued 2007.

Xylocaine CO2 (AstraZeneca). *lidocaine hydrocarbonate.* Discontinued 2005.

Xylocaine Endotracheal (AstraZeneca). *lidocaine.*

Xylocaine Jelly 2% (AstraZeneca). *lidocaine HCl.*

Xylocaine Ointment 5% (AstraZeneca). *lidocaine.*

Xylocaine Parenteral with Epinephrine (AstraZeneca). *epinephrine / lidocaine HCl.*

Xylocaine Parenteral Without Epinephrine (AstraZeneca). *lidocaine HCl.*

Xylocaine Spinal (AstraZeneca). *glucose / lidocaine HCl.* Discontinued 2004.

Xylocaine Topical 4% (AstraZeneca). *lidocaine HCl.*

Xylocaine Viscous 2% (AstraZeneca). *lidocaine HCl.*

Xylocard (AstraZeneca). *lidocaine HCl.*

Xylometazoline (CPhA Monograph). *xylometazoline HCl.*

xylometazoline HCl. **Balminil Nasal Decongestant**; **Xylometazoline.**

Xyntha (Pfizer). *antihemophilic factor (recombinant) [BDDrFVIII], plasma/albumin free (moroctocog alfa).*

Xyrem (Valeant). *sodium oxybate.*

Y

Yasmin 21 (Bayer). *drospirenone / ethinyl estradiol.*

Yasmin 28 (Bayer). *drospirenone / ethinyl estradiol.*

Yaz (Bayer). *drospirenone / ethinyl estradiol.*

YF-VAX (sanofi pasteur). *yellow fever vaccine.*

Yocon (Glenwood). *yohimbine HCl.* Discontinued 2008.

yohimbine HCl. **Yohimbine-Odan.**

Yohimbine-Odan (Odan). *yohimbine HCl.*

Yondelis (Janssen-Ortho). *trabectedin.*

Yutopar (Bristol). *ritodrine HCl.* Discontinued 2000.

Z

Zaditen (Paladin). *ketotifen fumarate.*

Zaditor (Novartis Pharmaceuticals). *ketotifen fumarate.*

zafirlukast. **Accolate.**

Zanaflex (Paladin). *tizanidine HCl.*

zanamivir. **Relenza.**

Zanosar (Pfizer). *streptozocin.*

Zantac (GlaxoSmithKline). *ranitidine HCl.*

Zantac (McNeil Consumer Healthcare). *ranitidine HCl.*

Zantac Maximum Strength Non-Prescription (McNeil Consumer Healthcare). *ranitidine HCl.*

Zap (PendoPharm). *star anise oil (Illicium verum).*

Zarontin (ERFA Canada). *ethosuximide.*

Zaroxolyn (sanofi-aventis). *metolazone.*

Zavesca (Actelion). *miglustat.*

ZeaSORB (Stiefel, a GSK company). *aluminum dihydroxyallantoinate / cellulose / chloroxylenol.*

ZeaSORB AF (Stiefel, a GSK company). *tolnaftate.*

zeaxanthin / bilberry / lutein. **Visionex.**

Zeftera (Janssen-Ortho). *ceftobiprole medocaril.* Discontinued 2010.

Zeldox (Pfizer). *ziprasidone HCl.*

Zelnorm (Novartis Pharmaceuticals). *tegaserod hydrogen maleate.* Discontinued 2007.

Zemplar (Abbott). *paricalcitol.* Discontinued 2010.

Zemuron (Schering-Plough). *rocuronium bromide.*

Zenapax (Roche). *daclizumab.* Discontinued 2009.

Zerit (Bristol-Myers Squibb). *stavudine.*

Zestoretic (AstraZeneca). *hydrochlorothiazide / lisinopril.*

Zestril (AstraZeneca). *lisinopril.*

Zetar (Dermik). *coal tar.* Discontinued 2003.

Zevalin (Bayer). *ibritumomab tiuxetan.*

Ziagen (ViiV Healthcare ULC). *abacavir sulfate.*

zidovudine. **Retrovir (AZT).**

zidovudine / abacavir sulfate / lamivudine. **Trizivir.**

zidovudine / lamivudine. **Combivir.**

Zinacef (GlaxoSmithKline). *cefuroxime sodium.* Discontinued 2007.

Zinaderm (Rougier Pharma). *zinc oxide.*

zinc / ascorbic acid / copper / lycopene / selenium / vitamin B complex / vitamin E. **Stresstabs for Men.**

zinc / ascorbic acid / copper / vitamin B complex / vitamin E. **Stresstabs Z-BEC.**

zinc / calcium carbonate / copper / magnesium / manganese / vitamin D. **Caltrate Plus.**

zinc acetate / diphenhydramine HCl. **Benadryl Spray**; **Benadryl Stick.**

zinc bacitracin. see *bacitracin zinc.*

Zincfrin (Alcon). *phenylephrine HCl / zinc sulfate.* Discontinued 2005.

Zincfrin-A (Alcon). *antazoline phosphate / naphazoline HCl / zinc sulfate.* Discontinued 2005.

zinc hydroxide / cosyntropin. **Synacthen Depot.**

Zincofax (PendoPharm). *zinc oxide.*

Zinc Ointment (Rougier Pharma). *zinc oxide.*

zinc oxide / multiple vitamins. **ADEKs.**

zinc oxide / phenol. **Ozonol Ointment.**

zinc pyrithione / menthol. **Z-Plus.**

zinc sulfate / tetrahydrozoline HCl. **Visine Allergy Eye Drops.**

zinc sulfate monohydrate. **Anusol**; **Rivasol**; **Sandoz Anuzinc.**

zinc sulfate monohydrate / benzocaine. **Rectogel.**

zinc sulfate monohydrate / benzocaine / hydrocortisone acetate. **Rectogel HC.**

zinc sulfate monohydrate / hydrocortisone acetate. **Anodan-HC**; **Anusol-HC**; **ratio-Hemcort-HC**; **Rivasol HC**; **Sandoz Anuzinc HC.**

zinc sulfate monohydrate / hydrocortisone acetate / pramoxine HCl. **Anugesic-HC**; **Proctodan-HC**; **Sandoz Anuzinc HC Plus.**

Names in *italics*: Generic drug names, active ingredient or category.
Names in **bold face/underlined**: Prescribing information provided in the Monograph section.
Names in **bold face/not underlined**: Availability information provided in the Monograph section.
Names in regular face: Product is available in Canada but the monograph does not appear in *CPS*.

Names in *italics*: Generic drug names, active ingredient or category.
Names in **bold face/underlined**: Prescribing information provided in the Monograph section.
Names in **bold face/not underlined**: Availability information provided in the Monograph section.
Names in regular face: Product is available in Canada but the monograph does not appear in *CPS*.

Therapeutic Guide

About Therapeutic Guide

Therapeutic Guide was adapted from the Canadian version of the World Health Organization's Anatomical Therapeutic Chemical (ATC) Classification Index to provide a practical clinical guide for the use of single entity drugs available in Canada. It has been expanded to include indications, conditions and recommended therapies addressed in CPhA's publications *Therapeutic Choices* and *Patient Self-Care*. Some nonprescription and combination products are included.

Drugs are listed under alphabetically arranged therapeutic indications (e.g., Acne, Diarrhea). Drugs may be further classified under pharmacologic or chemical subheadings within a therapeutic indication and may be listed under more than one section if used for more than one indication.

Users are cautioned that this guide is not exhaustive and a drug entity may not be listed under all of its indications. Users must exercise professional judgment when consulting the Therapeutic Guide.

How to Use Therapeutic Guide

- Consult the alphabetical index for the appropriate indication or condition.
- Also consult the "see" cross-references within in the index to help find the included indications.
- Cross-references ("see also's") listed under an indication refer users to other drugs that may be used for that therapeutic indication.
- To find the brand name of a drug or further information on drugs listed in the guide, please consult the Brand and Generic Name Index (Green pages).

Index

Acetaminophen Overdose
acetylcysteine

Acne Vulgaris
Androgen Receptor Antagonists
spironolactone
Antibiotics
Folate Antagonists
trimethoprim
Macrolides
erythromycin
erythromycin estolate
Tetracyclines
doxycycline hyclate
minocycline hydrochloride
tetracycline hydrochloride
Sulfonamide Combinations
sulfamethoxazole/trimethoprim
Antibiotics, Topical
Lincosamides
clindamycin
Macrolides
erythromycin
Corticosteroids, Topical
methylprednisolone
Hormones
Antiandrogen/Estrogen Combinations
cyproterone acetate/ethinyl estradiol
Progestogen/Estrogen Combinations, Monophasic
drospirenone/ethinyl estradiol
Progestogen/Estrogen Combinations, Triphasic
levonorgestrel/ethinyl estradiol
norgestimate/ethinyl estradiol
Peroxides, Topical
benzoyl peroxide
Retinoids, Oral
isotretinoin
Retinoids and Analogues, Topical
adapalene
isotretinoin
tazarotene
tretinoin
Sulphur Preparations, Topical
sulphur
Various Topical Preparations
benzoyl peroxide/clindamycin
erythromycin/tretinoin
glycolic acid
povidone-iodine
salicylic acid
triclosan

Acromegaly
Dopamine Agonists
bromocriptine
Growth Hormone Receptor Antagonists
pegvisomant
Somatostatin Analogues
octreotide

Actinic Keratosis
Immune Response Modifiers, Topical
imiquimod

Acute Coronary Syndromes
Antiplatelet Agents
acetylsalicylic acid (ASA)
clopidogrel
prasugrel
ticlopidine
Beta-adrenergic Blocking Agents
Nonselective without Intrinsic Sympathomimetic Activity (ISA)
nadolol
propranolol
timolol
Selective with ISA
acebutolol
Selective without ISA
atenolol
metoprolol
Calcium Channel Blockers
Dihydropyridines
amlodipine
Nondihydropyridines
diltiazem
verapamil
Factor Xa Inhibitors, Indirect
fondaparinux sodium
Glycoprotein IIb/IIIa Inhibitors
abciximab
eptifibatide
tirofiban
Heparins, Low Molecular Weight
dalteparin
enoxaparin
Heparins, Unfractionated
heparin sodium
Nitrates
isosorbide dinitrate
isosorbide-5-mononitrate
nitroglycerin
Renin-Angiotensin System Agents
Angiotensin Converting Enzyme (ACE) Inhibitors
captopril
cilazapril
enalapril
fosinopril
lisinopril
quinapril
ramipril
Thrombolytics
alteplase (rt-PA)
reteplase
streptokinase
tenecteplase

Adrenocortical Insufficiency
Corticosteroids, Systemic
Glucocorticoids
betamethasone sodium phosphate
betamethasone valerate
cortisone acetate
dexamethasone
dexamethasone sodium phosphate
hydrocortisone
hydrocortisone sodium succinate
methylprednisolone
methylprednisolone acetate
methylprednisolone sodium succinate
prednisolone
prednisolone sodium phosphate
triamcinolone
triamcinolone acetonide
triamcinolone diacetate
Mineralocorticoids
fludrocortisone acetate

Alcohol Withdrawal
Antiepileptics
phenytoin
Antipsychotics
haloperidol
Barbiturates
phenobarbital
Benzodiazepines
chlordiazepoxide
diazepam
lorazepam

Alcoholism
Gamma Aminobutyric Acid (GABA) Agonists/Glutamate Antagonists
acamprosate calcium
Opioid Antagonists
naltrexone hydrochloride

Allergies
see also Conjunctivitis, Allergic; Gastrointestinal Allergy; Rhinitis, Allergic
Allergenic Extracts
grass tyrosine adsorbate, modified
ragweed tyrosine adsorbate
tree tyrosine adsorbate, modified
Antihistamines, Nasal
levocabastine hydrochloride
Antihistamines, Ophthalmic
emedastine
levocabastine hydrochloride
Antihistamines, Oral
Alkylamines
brompheniramine maleate
chlorpheniramine maleate
Ethanolamines
diphenhydramine
Phenothiazines
promethazine
trimeprazine
Piperazines
cetirizine
hydroxyzine
Piperidines
cyproheptadine
desloratadine
fexofenadine
loratadine
Antihistamines and Mast Cell Stabilizers, Ophthalmic
ketotifen
olopatadine
Corticosteroids, Nasal
beclomethasone dipropionate
budesonide
flunisolide
fluticasone propionate
mometasone furoate monohydrate
triamcinolone acetonide
Corticosteroids, Ophthalmic
dexamethasone sodium phosphate
fluorometholone
fluorometholone acetate
prednisolone acetate
prednisolone sodium phosphate
rimexolone

Mast Cell Stabilizers, Inhaled
sodium cromoglycate
Mast Cell Stabilizers, Nasal
sodium cromoglycate
Mast Cell Stabilizers, Ophthalmic
lodoxamide tromethamine
nedocromil sodium
sodium cromoglycate
Moisturizers/Lubricants, Nasal
polyethylene glycol/propylene glycol
sea water
sodium chloride

Alzheimer's Disease
Cholinesterase Inhibitors
donepezil hydrochloride
galantamine hydrobromide
rivastigmine tartrate
N-methyl-D-aspartate Receptor Antagonists
memantine hydrochloride

Amebiasis, Intestinal
8-Hydroxyquinoline Derivatives
iodoquinol
Aminoglycosides
paromomycin sulfate
Nitroimidazole Derivatives
metronidazole

Anaphylaxis
Adrenergic Agents
epinephrine

Androgen Deficiency
Androgens, Oral
testosterone undecanoate
Androgens, Parenteral
testosterone cypionate
testosterone enanthate
Androgens, Topical
testosterone
Androgens, Transdermal
testosterone

Anemia
Erythropoietics
darbepoetin alfa
epoetin alfa
Iron Preparations
ferrous fumarate
ferrous gluconate
ferrous sulfate
heme iron polypeptide
iron dextran, parenteral
iron sucrose, parenteral
sodium ferric gluconate, parenteral
Vitamins
folic acid
Vitamin B_{12} Preparations
cyanocobalamin
hydroxocobalamin

Anesthesia, General
Barbiturates
thiopental sodium
Halogenated Hydrocarbons
desflurane
enflurane
isoflurane
sevoflurane
Opioid Anesthetics
alfentanil hydrochloride
fentanyl citrate
remifentanil hydrochloride
sufentanil citrate
Various General Anesthetics
ketamine hydrochloride
midazolam hydrochloride
propofol

Anesthesia, Local
see also Ophthalmic Local Anesthesia
Amides
articaine hydrochloride
bupivacaine hydrochloride
lidocaine
lidocaine hydrocarbonate
lidocaine hydrochloride
lidocaine/prilocaine
mepivacaine hydrochloride
prilocaine hydrochloride
ropivacaine hydrochloride
Esters of Aminobenzoic Acid
benzocaine
chloroprocaine hydrochloride
cocaine hydrochloride
procaine hydrochloride
tetracaine
tetracaine hydrochloride

Angina, Stable
see also Cardiovascular Disease Prevention, Secondary
Beta-adrenergic Blocking Agents
Nonselective with Intrinsic Sympathomimetic Activity (ISA)
pindolol
Nonselective without ISA
nadolol
propranolol
timolol
Selective with ISA
acebutolol
Selective without ISA
atenolol
metoprolol
Calcium Channel Blockers
amlodipine
diltiazem
nifedipine
verapamil
Nitrates
isosorbide dinitrate
isosorbide-5-mononitrate
nitroglycerin

Ankylosing Spondylitis
Corticosteroids
cortisone acetate
hydrocortisone
methylprednisolone
Disease Modifying Antirheumatic Drugs (DMARDs), Biologic
Tumor Necrosis Factor Alpha (TNF-α) Inhibitors
adalimumab
etanercept
golimumab
infliximab
Nonsteroidal Anti-inflammatory Drugs (NSAIDs)
celecoxib
flurbiprofen
indomethacin
naproxen

Anogenital Warts
Antimitotic Agents
dichloroacetic acid
podofilox
podophyllum resin
trichloroacetic acid
Biologic Response Modifiers
imiquimod
interferon alfa-2b

Anorexia and Cachexia
megestrol acetate

Anticoagulation
see also Venous Thromboembolism, Prophylaxis and Treatment
Heparinoids
danaparoid
Heparins
Heparins, Low Molecular Weight (LMWH)
dalteparin sodium
enoxaparin sodium
nadroparin calcium
tinzaparin sodium
Heparins, Unfractionated
heparin sodium
Thrombin Inhibitors, Direct
argatroban
bivalirudin
dabigatran
lepirudin
Vitamin K Antagonists
nicoumalone
warfarin
Various Anticoagulants
antithrombin III (human)

Antiseptics
Alcohols
ethyl alcohol
isopropyl alcohol
Bisbiguanides
chlorhexidine gluconate
Iodine Products
cadexomer iodine
povidone-iodine
Oxidizing Agents
hydrogen peroxide
Phenol Derivatives
phenol
triclosan
Quaternary Ammonium Compounds
benzalkonium compounds
cetrimide

Anxiety
Antihistamines
hydroxyzine
promethazine hydrochloride
Azaspirodecanedione Derivatives
buspirone hydrochloride
Benzodiazepines
alprazolam
bromazepam
chlordiazepoxide hydrochloride
clorazepate dipotassium
diazepam
lorazepam
oxazepam
Beta-adrenergic Blocking Agents
propranolol

Phenothiazines
trifluoperazine
Selective Serotonin Reuptake Inhibitors (SSRIs)
escitalopram
paroxetine
Selective (Type A) MAOIs
moclobemide
Serotonin-Norepinephrine Reuptake Inhibitors (SNRIs)
duloxetine hydrochloride
venlafaxine hydrochloride
Tricyclic Antidepressants
clomipramine

Aphthous Ulcers (Canker Sores)
see also Mouth Pain
Corticosteroids, Topical
triamcinolone acetonide

Appetite Enhancement
megestrol acetate
zinc gluconate

Arrhythmias
Antiarrhythmics
Cardiac Glycosides
digoxin
Class I, Type 1A Antiarrhythmics
disopyramide
disopyramide phosphate
procainamide hydrochloride
Class I, Type 1B Antiarrhythmics
lidocaine hydrochloride
mexiletine hydrochloride
Class I, Type 1C Antiarrhythmics
flecainide hydrochloride
propafenone hydrochloride
Class II Antiarrhythmics, Beta-adrenergic Blocking Agents
esmolol hydrochloride
propranolol hydrochloride
sotalol hydrochloride
Class III Antiarrhythmics
amiodarone hydrochloride
bretylium tosylate
dronedarone hydrochloride
ibutilide fumarate
Class IV Antiarrhythmics, Calcium Channel Blockers
diltiazem hydrochloride
verapamil hydrochloride
Various Antiarrhythmics
adenosine

Arthritis, Psoriatic
Corticosteroids
cortisone acetate
hydrocortisone
methylprednisolone acetate
Disease Modifying Antirheumatic Drugs (DMARDs), Biologic
Tumor Necrosis Factor Alpha (TNF-α) Inhibitors
adalimumab
etanercept
golimumab
infliximab
Disease Modifying Antirheumatic Drugs (DMARDs), Nonbiologic
Cytotoxics
methotrexate sodium
Gold Preparations
sodium aurothiomalate

Arthritis, Rheumatoid
Corticosteroids
betamethasone
cortisone acetate
dexamethasone
dexamethasone sodium phosphate
methylprednisolone acetate
prednisolone
prednisone
triamcinolone
triamcinolone diacetate
Disease Modifying Antirheumatic Drugs (DMARDs), Biologic
β-Cell Depleting Agents
rituximab
Interleukin-1 (IL-1) Receptor Antagonists
anakinra
Interleukin-6 (IL-6) Receptor Antagonists
tocilizumab
T-Cell Activation Inhibitors
abatacept
Tumor Necrosis Factor Alpha (TNF-α) Inhibitors
adalimumab
certolizumab pegol
etanercept
golimumab
infliximab
Disease Modifying Antirheumatic Drugs (DMARDs), Nonbiologic
Cytotoxics
azathioprine
methotrexate sodium
Gold Preparations
auranofin
sodium aurothiomalate
Immunomodulators
leflunomide
Immunosuppressants
cyclosporine
Various DMARDs
hydroxychloroquine sulfate
minocycline hydrochloride
penicillamine
sulfasalazine
Joint and Muscular Pain Therapy, Topical
capsaicin
menthol
methyl salicylate
triethanolamine salicylate

Ascites
Diuretics
amiloride
furosemide
metolazone
spironolactone

Asthma
Adrenergics, Inhaled
Beta-2-adrenergic Agonists, Selective
formoterol fumarate
formoterol fumarate dihydrate
salbutamol
salmeterol xinafoate
terbutaline sulfate
Adrenergics, Systemic
Alpha- and Beta-adrenergic Agonists
epinephrine hydrochloride
Beta-2-adrenergic Agonists, Selective
salbutamol
Beta-adrenergic Agonists, Nonselective
isoproterenol hydrochloride
orciprenaline sulfate
Anticholinergics, Inhaled
ipratropium bromide
tiotropium bromide monohydrate
Anti-inflammatory Agents, Inhaled
Corticosteroids
beclomethasone dipropionate
budesonide
ciclesonide
fluticasone propionate
Mast Cell Stabilizers
sodium cromoglycate
Combination Inhalation Products
fenoterol hydrobromide/ipratropium bromide
formoterol fumarate dihydrate/budenoside
ipratropium bromide/salbutamol sulfate
salmeterol xinafoate/fluticasone propionate
Anti-inflammatory Agents, Systemic
Corticosteroids
cortisone acetate
hydrocortisone
hydrocortisone sodium succinate
methylprednisolone sodium succinate
prednisolone sodium phosphate
prednisone
triamcinolone
Leukotriene Receptor Antagonists
montelukast sodium
zafirlukast
Xanthines
aminophylline
oxtriphylline
theophylline
Monoclonal Antibodies
omalizumab

Attention Deficit Hyperactivity Disorder
CNS Stimulants
dextroamphetamine
lisdexamfetamine
methylphenidate
mixed salts amphetamine
Norepinephrine Reuptake Inhibitors (NRIs)
atomoxetine

Bacterial Vaginosis
Antibiotics, Oral
clindamycin
metronidazole
Antibiotics, Topical
clindamycin phosphate
metronidazole

Bell's Palsy

Antivirals

acyclovir
famciclovir
valacyclovir

Corticosteroids

prednisone

Benign Prostatic Hyperplasia

5 Alpha-reductase Inhibitors

dutasteride
finasteride

Alpha-adrenergic Blocking Agents

alfuzosin
doxazosin
tamsulosin
terazosin

Benzodiazepine Overdose

flumazenil

Bipolar Disorder

Antipsychotics

aripiprazole
olanzapine
quetiapine fumarate
risperidone
ziprasidone

Mood Stabilizers

Antiepileptics

carbamazepine
divalproex sodium
lamotrigine
valproic acid

Lithium Salts

lithium carbonate
lithium citrate

Serotonin Precursors

L-tryptophan

Black Widow Spider Venom Poisoning

Immune Sera

black widow spider antivenin (equine)

Bladder Cancer

Anthracyclines

doxorubicin
valrubicin

Immunologics

bacillus Calmette-Guérin (BCG), strain TICE, intravesical
bacillus Calmette-Guérin (BCG), substrain Connaught, intravesical
bacillus Calmette-Guérin (BCG), substrain Montréal, intravesical

Bleeding Esophageal Varices

Somatostatin Analogues

octreotide

Vasopressin Receptor Agonists

vasopressin

Blepharospasm

botulinum toxin type A

Bone Metastases

Bisphosphonates

pamidronate
zoledronic acid

Botulism Poisoning

Immune Sera

botulism antitoxin trivalent types A, B and E (equine)

Bowel Evacuation

Osmotic Laxatives

magnesium citrate
polyethylene glycol/electrolytes

Stimulant/Osmotic Laxative Combinations

bisacodyl/magnesium citrate
picosulfate sodium/magnesium citrate

Bronchospasm

Adrenergic Agonists

epinephrine hydrochloride

Bulimia Nervosa

Selective Serotonin Reuptake Inhibitors (SSRIs)

fluoxetine hydrochloride

Serotonin-Norepinephrine Reuptake Inhibitors (SNRIs)

venlafaxine hydrochloride

Burns

Antibiotics, Topical

bacitracin
framycetin
fusidic acid
mupirocin
silver sulfadiazine

Antiseptics

povidone/iodine

Cancer Chemotherapy Induced Nausea and Vomiting

see also Nausea and Vomiting

Cannabinoids

nabilone

Dopamine Antagonists

metoclopramide

Neurokinin 1 (NK1) Receptor Antagonists

aprepitant
fosaprepitant

Serotonin Antagonists

dolasetron mesylate
granisetron hydrochloride
ondansetron

Cancer Chemotherapy Toxicity Prevention

Cardioprotective Agents

dexrazoxane

Cytoprotective Agents

amifostine

Folic Acid Metabolites

calcium folinate

Growth Factors

palifermin

Uricolytic Agents

rasburicase

Uroprotectants

mesna

Cancer, General

see also Bladder Cancer; Bone Metastases; Cancer Chemotherapy Toxicity Prevention; Kaposi's Sarcoma; Prostate Cancer

Alkylating Agents

Alkyl Sulphonates

busulfan

Ethyleneimines

thiotepa

Methylhydrazines

procarbazine hydrochloride

Nitrogen Mustard Analogues

chlorambucil
cyclophosphamide
estramustine sodium phosphate
ifosfamide
mechlorethamine hydrochloride
melphalan

Nitrosoureas

carmustine
lomustine
streptozocin

Platinum-containing Compounds

carboplatin
cisplatin
oxaliplatin

Triazenes

dacarbazine
temozolomide

Antimetabolites

Cytidine Analogues

gemcitabine hydrochloride

Folic Acid Analogues

methotrexate sodium
pemetrexed disodium
raltitrexed disodium

Purine Analogues

cladribine
fludarabine phosphate
mercaptopurine
nelarabine
pentostatin
thioguanine

Pyrimidine Analogues

capecitabine
cytarabine
cytarabine liposomal
fluorouracil

Urea Derivatives

hydroxyurea

Biologic Response Modifiers

aldesleukin
imiquimod
interferon alfa-2b

Cytotoxic Antibiotics

Actinomycins

dactinomycin

Anthracyclines

daunorubicin
doxorubicin hydrochloride
doxorubicin hydrochloride pegylated liposomal
epirubicin hydrochloride
idarubicin hydrochloride
valrubicin

Various Cytotoxic Antibiotics

bleomycin sulfate
mitomycin
mitotane
mitoxantrone hydrochloride

Histone Deacetylase Inhibitors

vorinostat

Hormone Antagonists

Antiandrogens

bicalutamide
cyproterone acetate
flutamide
nilutamide

Antiestrogens

fulvestrant
tamoxifen citrate

Nonsteroidal Aromatase Inhibitors

anastrozole
exemestane
letrozole

Hormones
Estrogens
diethylstilbestrol sodium diphosphate
Gonadotropin Releasing Hormone Analogues
buserelin acetate
goserelin acetate
leuprolide acetate
Luteinizing Hormone-releasing Hormone (LHRH) Analogues
triptorelin pamoate
Progestogens
medroxyprogesterone acetate
megestrol acetate
Immunomodulatory Thalidomide Derivatives
lenalidomide
mTOR Inhibitors
everolimus
temsirolimus
Monoclonal Antibodies
alemtuzumab
bevacizumab
cetuximab
ibritumomab tiuxetan
panitumumab
rituximab
tositumomab
trastuzumab
Multikinase Inhibitors
erlotinib
gefitinib
sorafenib tosylate
Photosensitizers, Protoporphyrin
methyl aminolevulinate
Plant Alkaloids and Various Natural Products
Camptothecin Derivatives
irinotecan hydrochloride
topotecan hydrochloride
Epipodophyllotoxins
etoposide
teniposide
Taxanes
docetaxel
paclitaxel
Vinca Alkaloids and Analogues
vinblastine sulfate
vincristine sulfate
vinorelbine tartrate
Proteasome Inhibitors
bortezomib
Protein Tyrosine Kinase Inhibitors
dasatinib
imatinib mesylate
lapatinib ditosylate monohydrate
nilotinib hydrochloride monohydrate
sunitinib malate
Various Antineoplastics
amsacrine
clofarabine
L-asparaginase
porfimer sodium
tretinoin (all-trans retinoic acid), systemic

Cardiac Decompensation
Cardiac Sympathomimetics
dobutamine hydrochloride
dopamine hydrochloride
epinephrine hydrochloride
isoproterenol
methoxamine hydrochloride
norepinephrine hydrochloride
phenylephrine hydrochloride

Cardiovascular Disease Prevention, Primary
HMG CoA Reductase Inhibitors
atorvastatin calcium
pravastatin sodium
rosuvastatin calcium
simvastatin

Cardiovascular Disease Prevention, Secondary
see also Post-myocardial Infarction
Platelet Antiaggregants
Adenosine Diphosphate Inhibitors
clopidogrel
prasugrel
sulfinpyrazone
ticlopidine hydrochloride
Antiplatelet Agents
acetylsalicylic acid (ASA)
Combination Antiplatelet Agents
dipyridamole/acetylsalicylic acid
Glycoprotein IIb/IIIa (GP IIb/IIIa) Receptor Inhibitors
abciximab
eptifibatide
tirofiban hydrochloride
Renin-Angiotensin System Agents
Angiotensin Converting Enzyme (ACE) Inhibitors
perindopril erbumine
ramipril
Angiotensin II Receptor Antagonists (ARBs)
telmisartan
valsartan

Carnitine Deficiency
Amino Acid Derivatives
levocarnitine

Cataract Surgery Post-operative Care
see also Infections, Bacterial (Eye); Glaucoma
Corticosteroids, Ophthalmic
dexamethasone
fluorometholone
loteprednol etabonate
prednisolone
rimexolone
Cycloplegics, Ophthalmic
cyclopentolate
Dilators, Ophthalmic
phenylephrine
Nonsteroidal Anti-inflammatory Drugs (NSAIDs), Ophthalmic
Acetic Acid Derivatives
diclofenac
ketorolac
nepafenac
Prostaglandin-$F_{2\alpha}$ Analogues, Ophthalmic
travoprost

Chlamydia Infection
Fluoroquinolones
levofloxacin
ofloxacin
Macrolides
azithromycin dihydrate
erythromycin
Penicillins
Aminopenicillins
amoxicillin trihydrate
Tetracyclines
doxycycline

Cholera Prevention
Vaccines
cholera vaccine (live, oral, attenuated)
traveller's diarrhea and cholera vaccine (oral, inactivated)

Cholestatic Liver Disease
Gallstone Solubilizing Agents
ursodiol

Chronic Obstructive Pulmonary Disease
Adrenergics, Inhaled
Beta-2-adrenergic Agonists, Selective
formoterol fumarate
formoterol fumarate dihydrate
salbutamol
salmeterol xinafoate
terbutaline sulfate
Adrenergics, Systemic
Beta-adrenergic Agonists, Nonselective
isoproterenol hydrochloride
orciprenaline sulfate
Anticholinergics, Inhaled
ipratropium bromide
tiotropium bromide monohydrate
Anti-inflammatory Agents, Systemic
Corticosteroids
cortisone acetate
hydrocortisone sodium succinate
methylprednisolone sodium succinate
prednisone
triamcinolone
Xanthines
aminophylline
oxtriphylline
theophylline
Combination Inhalation Products
fenoterol hydrobromide/ipratropium bromide
formoterol fumarate dihydrate/budesonide
salbutamol sulfate/ipratropium bromide
salmeterol xinafoate/fluticasone propionate

Congestion, Respiratory
Decongestants
Sympathomimetics, Nasal
oxymetazoline
phenylephrine hydrochloride
xylometazoline
Sympathomimetics, Systemic
phenylephrine hydrochloride
pseudoephedrine hydrochloride
pseudoephedrine sulfate

Conjunctivitis
see also Conjunctivitis, Allergic; Infections, Bacterial (Eye); Ophthalmic Lubrication
Corticosteroids, Ophthalmic
dexamethasone sodium phosphate
fluorometholone
fluorometholone acetate
loteprednol etabonate
prednisolone acetate
prednisolone sodium phosphate
rimexolone
Decongestants, Ophthalmic
naphazoline
oxymetazoline
phenylephrine hydrochloride
tetrahydrozoline hydrochloride
Nonsteroidal Anti-inflammatory Drugs (NSAIDs), Ophthalmic
diclofenac sodium
ketorolac tromethamine

Conjunctivitis, Allergic

Antihistamines, Ophthalmic

emedastine
levocabastine hydrochloride

Antihistamines and Mast Cell Stabilizers, Ophthalmic

ketotifen
olopatadine

Mast Cell Stabilizers, Ophthalmic

lodoxamide tromethamine
nedocromil sodium
sodium cromoglycate

Constipation

see also Bowel Evacuation

Bulk Forming Agents

psyllium hydrophillic mucilloid
sterculia gum

Hyperosmotic Laxatives

glycerin
sorbitol

Lubricant Laxatives

mineral oil

Osmotic Laxatives

lactulose
magnesium citrate
magnesium hydroxide
magnesium sulfate
polyethylene glycol
polyethylene glycol/electrolytes
sodium phosphates

Stimulant Laxatives

bisacodyl
cascara
castor oil
sennosides

Stool Softeners

docusate calcium
docusate sodium

μ-opioid Receptor Antagonists

methylnaltrexone bromide

Contraception

Hormonal Contraceptives, Injectable

Progestogens

medroxyprogesterone acetate

Hormonal Contraceptives, Intrauterine

Progestogens

levonorgestrel

Hormonal Contraceptives, Intravaginal

Estrogens and Progestogens

ethinyl estradiol/etonorgestrel

Hormonal Contraceptives, Oral

Estrogens and Progestogens, Biphasic

ethinyl estradiol/norethindrone

Estrogens and Progestogens, Monophasic

ethinyl estradiol/desogestrel
ethinyl estradiol/drospirenone
ethinyl estradiol/ethynodiol diacetate
ethinyl estradiol/levonorgestrel
ethinyl estradiol/norethindrone
ethinyl estradiol/norethindrone acetate
ethinyl estradiol/norgestimate

Estrogens and Progestogens, Triphasic

ethinyl estradiol/desogestrel
ethinyl estradiol/levonorgestrel
ethinyl estradiol/norethindrone
ethinyl estradiol/norgestimate

Progestogens

norethindrone

Hormonal Contraceptives, Transdermal

Estrogens and Progestogens

ethinyl estradiol/norelgestromin

Nonhormonal Contraceptives, Intrauterine

copper IUD

Spermicides, Vaginal

nonoxynol-9

Contraception, Emergency or Postcoital

Hormonal Contraceptives

Estrogens and Progestogens

ethinyl estradiol/levonorgestrel

Progestogens

levonorgestrel

Corns and Calluses

Keratolytic Agents

salicylic acid

Cough

Antitussives

Nonopioids

chlophedianol hydrochloride
dextromethorphan hydrobromide

Opioids

codeine phosphate
hydrocodone bitartrate

Expectorants

guaifenesin

Crohn's Disease

see also Inflammatory Bowel Disease

Biologic Response Modifiers

Tumor Necrosis Factor Alpha (TNF-α) Inhibitors

adalimumab
infliximab

Croup

Corticosteroids

budesonide
dexamethasone

Cryopyrin-Associated Periodic Syndromes

Interleukin-1 beta (IL-1ß) Antibodies

canakinumab

Cyanide Poisoning

sodium thiosulfate

Cystic Fibrosis

Mucolytics

acetylcysteine
dornase alfa, recombinant

Cystitis

Anti-inflammatory Agents, Intravesicular

dimethyl sulfoxide

Glycosaminoglycan Layer Replacements

pentosan polysulfate sodium
sodium hyaluronate

Cytomegalovirus Prophylaxis

Nucleoside Analogues

ganciclovir
valganciclovir

Cytomegalovirus Treatment

Nucleoside Analogues

ganciclovir
valganciclovir

Dandruff and Seborrhea

Shampoos

coal tar
ketoconazole
salicylic acid
selenium sulfide
sulfur
zinc pyrithione

Dehydration

oral electrolytes
sodium chloride

Delirium

Benzisoxazole Derivatives

risperidone

Butyrophenone Derivatives

haloperidol

Dibenzothiazepine Derivatives

quetiapine fumarate

Dibenzoxazepine Derivatives

loxapine

Thienobenzodiazepine Derivatives

olanzapine

Dental Caries Prophylaxis

sodium fluoride

Dental Hypersensitivity

Desensitizing Agents

potassium nitrate
stannous fluoride
strontium chloride

Depression

see also Seasonal Affective Disorder

Cyclic Antidepressants

Tetracyclic Antidepressants

maprotiline

Tricyclic Antidepressants

amitriptyline
clomipramine
desipramine
doxepin
imipramine
nortriptyline
trimipramine

Dibenzothiazepine Derivatives

quetiapine fumarate

Monoamine Oxidase Inhibitors (MAOIs)

Irreversible MAOIs

phenelzine
tranylcypromine sulfate

Reversible Inhibitors of MAO-A

moclobemide

Selective Serotonin Reuptake Inhibitors (SSRIs)

citalopram hydrobromide
escitalopram oxalate
fluoxetine hydrochloride
fluvoxamine maleate
paroxetine hydrochloride
sertraline hydrochloride

Serotonin-Norepinephrine Reuptake Inhibitors (SNRIs)

desvenlafaxine succinate
duloxetine hydrochloride
venlafaxine hydrochloride

Serotonin Precursors

L-tryptophan

Various Antidepressants

bupropion hydrochloride
mirtazapine
trazodone hydrochloride

Dermatitis, Atopic

Barrier Emulsions

ceramides/cholesterol/free fatty acids

Corticosteroids, Oral

methylprednisolone

Corticosteroids, Topical

amcinonide
betamethasone dipropionate
betamethasone valerate
clobetasol-17-propionate
clobetasone butyrate
desonide
desoximetasone
diflucortolone valerate
fluocinolone acetonide
fluocinonide
hydrocortisone
hydrocortisone acetate
hydrocortisone-17-valerate
mometasone furoate
prednicarbate
triamcinolone acetonide

Immunomodulators, Topical

pimecrolimus
tacrolimus

Dermatitis Herpetiformis

see also Pediculosis; Scabies; Warts

dapsone
sulfapyridine

Diabetes Insipidus

Antidiuretic Hormones and Analogues

desmopressin
vasopressin

Diabetes Mellitus

Antihyperglycemics, Oral

Alpha-glucosidase Inhibitors

acarbose

Biguanides

metformin hydrochloride

DPP-4 Inhibitors

saxagliptin hydrochloride
sitagliptin phosphate monohydrate

Gastrointestinal Lipase Inhibitors

orlistat

Meglitinides

nateglinide
repaglinide

Sulfonylureas

chlorpropamide
gliclazide
glimepiride
glyburide
tolbutamide

Thiazolidinediones

pioglitazone
rosiglitazone

Combination Agents

Biguanide and DPP-4 Inhibitor Combinations

metformin hydrochloride/sitagliptin phosphate monohydrate

Biguanide and Thiazolidinedione Combinations

metformin/rosiglitazone

Sulfonylurea and Thiazolidinedione Combinations

glimepiride/rosiglitazone

Antihyperglycemics, Parenteral

Human Glucagon Like Peptide-1 (GLP-1)

liraglutide

Insulins

Intermediate Acting Human Insulins

insulin lente, biosynthetic
insulin NPH, biosynthetic

Intermediate Acting Pork Insulins

insulin lente, biosynthetic
insulin NPH
insulin porcine, isophane

Long Acting Insulin Analogues

insulin detemir
insulin glargine

Mixed (Regular/NPH) Human Insulins

insulin (30/70), biosynthetic
insulin (40/60), biosynthetic
insulin (50/50), biosynthetic

Mixed Insulin Analogues

insulin lispro/lispro protamine (25/75)
insulin lispro/lispro protamine (50/50)

Rapid Acting Human Insulins

insulin regular, biosynthetic

Rapid Acting Pork Insulins

insulin, regular

Very Rapid Acting Insulin Analogues

insulin aspart
insulin glulisine
insulin lispro

Diagnostic Imaging

Paramagnetic Contrast Media

gadopentetate dimeglumine
gadoversetamide
gadoxetate disodium

Ultrasound Contrast Agents

galactose/palmitic acid
perflutren

Water Soluble, Nephrotropic, High Osmolar X-Ray Contrast Media, Ionated

diatrizoate meglumine
diatrizoate sodium
iothalamate meglumine

Water Soluble, Nephrotropic, Low Osmolar X-Ray Contrast Media, Ionated

iopromide
iotrolan
ioversol
ioxaglate meglumine
ioxaglate sodium

Diagnostic Testing

Adrenal Function

cosyntropin
dexamethasone sodium phosphate

Asthma (Bronchial) Diagnosis

methacholine chloride

Diabetes

dextrose
glucagon

Fertility Disturbances

gonadorelin acetate

Gastric Secretions

histamine sulfate
methylene blue

Glycosaminoglycan Bladder Permeability Defects

potassium chloride/sodium chondroitin sulfate

Lymphatic Vessels, Delineation

isosulfan blue

Methemoglobinemia

methylene blue

Ophthalmic Diagnosis

fluorescein sodium

Oral Cancer

toluidine blue

Pheochromocytoma

phentolamine

Renal Permeability

methylene blue

Thyroid Function

protirelin
thyrotropin alfa

Tuberculosis

tuberculin
tuberculin purified protein derivative (Mantoux)

Diaper Rash

Antifungal Agents

clotrimazole
miconazole
nystatin

Barrier Agents

dimethylpolysiloxane
petrolatum
zinc oxide

Corticosteroids

hydrocortisone

Combination Agents

cod liver oil/zinc oxide
lanolin/petrolatum

Diarrhea

Antiperistaltics

diphenoxylate hydrochloride/atropine sulfate
loperamide hydrochloride

Centrally Acting Antiadrenergic Agents

clonidine hydrochloride

Hydrophilic Bulking Agents

cholestyramine resin
psyllium hydrophilic mucilloid

Intestinal Adsorbants

attapulgite, activated
bismuth subsalicylate

Probiotics

bifidobacterium
lactobacillus
lactobacillus acidophilus
lactobacillus reuteri protectis
saccharomyces boulardii lyo

Opioids

codeine phosphate

Somatostatin Analogues

lanreotide acetate
octreotide
octreotide acetate

Digoxin Overdose

digoxin immune Fab (ovine)

Diphtheria and Tetanus Prevention

Toxoids

diphtheria and tetanus toxoids, adsorbed

Diphtheria Immunization

Immune Sera

diphtheria antitoxin (equine)

Diphtheria Prevention

Toxoids

diphtheria toxoid

Diphtheria, Tetanus and Pertussis Prevention

Combination Bacterial and Viral Vaccines

diphtheria and tetanus with pertussis vaccine

Diphtheria, Tetanus and Poliomyelitis Prevention

Combination Bacterial and Viral Vaccines

diphtheria, tetanus toxoids, poliomyelitis vaccine (DT Polio)

Diphtheria, Tetanus, Pertussis and Poliomyelitis Prevention

Combination Bacterial and Viral Vaccines

diphtheria, tetanus toxoids, pertussis vaccine and poliomyelitis vaccine (DPT Polio)

Diphtheria, Tetanus, Pertussis, Poliomyelitis and Haemophilus Type b Prevention

Combination Bacterial and Viral Vaccines

diphtheria, tetanus toxoids, pertussis vaccine, poliomyelitis vaccine and haemophilus b conjugate vaccine

Diphtheria, Tetanus, Pertussis, Poliomyelitis, Haemophilus Type b and Hepatitis B Prevention

Combination Bacterial and Viral Vaccines

diphtheria, tetanus toxoids, pertussis vaccine, poliomyelitis vaccine, haemophilus b conjugate vaccine, hepatitis B (recombinant) vaccine

Dry Mouth

Human Keratinocyte Growth Factor

palifermin

Saliva Substitutes

antibacterial enzymes solution
electrolyte solution

Sialogogues

anethole trithione
pilocarpine hydrochloride

Dry Mouth Prevention

Cytoprotective Agents

amifostine

Dry Skin

Barrier Emulsions

ceramides/cholesterol/free fatty acids

Silicone Products

dimethicone
silicone

Urea Products

urea

Various Emollients and Protectants

ammonium lactate
glycolic acid
lactic acid
mineral oil
petrolatum

Zinc Products

zinc oxide
zinc sulfate monohydrate

Dyslipidemias

Cholesterol Absorption Inhibitors

ezetimibe

Fibrates

bezafibrate
fenofibrate
gemfibrozil

HMG CoA Reductase Inhibitors

atorvastatin
fluvastatin
lovastatin
pravastastin
rosuvastatin
simvastatin

Niacin Derivatives

niacin

Resins

cholestyramine resin
colestipol hydrochloride

Dysmenorrhea

Nonsteroidal Anti-inflammatory Drugs (NSAIDs)

diclofenac potassium
diclofenac sodium
ibuprofen
indomethacin
ketoprofen
mefenamic acid
naproxen
naproxen sodium
piroxicam

Earwax, Impacted

Softening Agents, Oil-based

almond oil
glycerin
light mineral oil
olive oil
propylene glycol

Softening Agents, Water-based

chlorbutol
docusate sodium
hydrogen peroxide
sodium bicarbonate

Various Softening Agents

carbamide peroxide

Eczema, Hand

Retinoids, Oral

alitretinoin

Eczema Herpeticum

Nucleoside Analogues

acyclovir

Edema

Loop Diuretics

bumetanide
ethacrynate sodium
ethacrynic acid
furosemide

Osmotic Diuretics

mannitol

Potassium Sparing Diuretics

amiloride hydrochloride
spironolactone

Thiazides and Related Diuretics

chlorthalidone
hydrochlorothiazide
indapamide
indapamide hemihydrate
metolazone

Diuretic Combinations

amiloride/hydrochlorothiazide
spironolactone/hydrochlorothiazide
triamterene/hydrochlorothiazide

Endocarditis, Infective (Prevention)

Cephalosporins

Cephalosporins, 1st Generation

cefadroxil
cefazolin sodium
cephalexin

Cephalosporins, 2nd Generation

cefaclor
cefprozil
cefuroxime axetil

Cephalosporins, 3rd Generation

ceftriaxone

Lincosamides

clindamycin

Macrolides

azithromycin
clarithromycin

Penicillins

Aminopenicillins

amoxicillin
ampicillin

Endometriosis

see also Contraception; Infertility

Gonadotropin Inhibitors

danazol

Gonadotropin-releasing Hormone (GnRH) Analogues

buserelin acetate
goserelin acetate
leuprolide acetate
nafarelin acetate
triptorelin pamoate

Hormones

Progestogens

medroxyprogesterone acetate

Epilepsy

Barbiturates and Derivatives

phenobarbital
primidone

Benzodiazepines

clobazam
clonazepam
diazepam
lorazepam
nitrazepam

Carboxylic Acid Derivatives

divalproex sodium
valproic acid

Fructose Derivatives

topiramate

Functionalized Amino Acids

lacosamide

Gamma Aminobutyric Acid (GABA) Derivatives

gabapentin
vigabatrin

Hydantoin Derivatives
fosphenytoin sodium
phenytoin
phenytoin sodium

Iminostilbene Derivatives
carbamazepine
oxacarbazepine

Phenyltriazine Derivatives
lamotrigine

Pyrrolidine Derivatives
levetiracetam

Succinimide Derivatives
ethosuximide
methsuximide

Various Antiepileptics
magnesium sulfate

Erectile Dysfunction

Phosphodiesterase Type 5 (PDE5) Inhibitors
sildenafil
tadalafil
vardenafil

Prostaglandin E_1 (PGE_1) Analogues
alprostadil

Esophagitis, Reflux
see also Gastroesophageal Reflux

Histamine H_2–receptor Antagonists
cimetidine
famotidine
nizatidine
ranitidine

Proton Pump Inhibitors
dexlansoprazole
esomeprazole
lansoprazole
omeprazole
pantoprazole magnesium
pantoprazole sodium
rabeprazole

Ethylene Glycol Poisoning

Alcohol Dehydrogenase Inhibitors
fomepizole

Expectoration
guaifenesin

Fabry Disease

Enzymes
agalsidase alfa
agalsidase beta

Fever

Antipyretics
acetaminophen
acetylsalicylic acid (ASA)
ibuprofen
naproxen sodium

Fibromyalgia

Gamma Aminobutyric Acid (GABA) Derivatives
pregabalin

Selective Serotonin Reuptake Inhibitors (SSRIs)
fluoxetine hydrochloride

Serotonin-Norepinephrine Reuptake Inhibitors (SNRIs)
duloxetine hydrochloride

Tricyclic Antidepressants
amitriptyline

Tricyclic Derivatives
cyclobenzaprine

Friedreich's Ataxia

ATP Production Modulator
idebenone

Gastroesophageal Reflux
see also Esophagitis, Reflux; Gastrointestinal Motility and Spasticity Disorders

Antacids

Aluminum Containing Preparations
aluminum hydroxide

Aluminum/Magnesium Containing Preparations
aluminum hydroxide/magnesium hydroxide

Calcium Containing Preparations
calcium carbonate

Magnesium Containing Preparations
magnesium hydroxide
magnesium carbonate

Foaming Agents
alginic acid
sodium alginate

Histamine H_2–receptor Antagonists
cimetidine
famotidine
nizatidine
ranitidine

Proton Pump Inhibitors
dexlansoprazole
esomeprazole
lansoprazole
omeprazole
pantoprazole magnesium
pantoprazole sodium
rabeprazole

Gastrointestinal Allergy

Mast Cell Stabilizers
sodium cromoglycate

Gastrointestinal Gas
see also Infant Colic

Coalescing Agents
simethicone

Enzymes
alpha-d-galactosidase

Gastrointestinal Motility and Spasticity Disorders

Anticholinergic Agents

Natural Alkaloids, Tertiary Amines
atropine sulfate
hyoscine butylbromide

Synthetic Amines, Quaternary Ammonium Compounds
pinaverium bromide

Synthetic Amines, Tertiary Amine
dicyclomine

Lower Gastrointestinal Tract Motility Agents
trimebutine

Macrolides
erythromycin lactobionate

Upper Gastrointestinal Tract Motility Agents
domperidone maleate
metoclopramide hydrochloride

Gaucher's Disease

Enzyme Inhibitors
miglustat

Enzyme Replacements
imiglucerase

Gingivitis and Periodontitis

Antiseptics
cetylpyridinium chloride
chlorhexidine gluconate
essential oils
hexetidine
povidone-iodine
sodium perborate
triclosan

Glaucoma

Adrenergic Agents, Ophthalmic
apraclonidine hydrochloride
brimonidine tartrate

Beta-blocking Agents, Ophthalmic
betaxolol
levobunolol
timolol maleate

Carbonic Anhydrase Inhibitors, Ophthalmic
brinzolamide
dorzolamide

Carbonic Anhydrase Inhibitors, Systemic
acetazolamide
methazolamide

Carbonic Anhydrase Inhibitor/Beta-blocking Agent Combinations, Ophthalmic
brinzolamide/timolol maleate
dorzolamide/timolol maleate

Miotics, Parasympathomimetics, Ophthalmic
acetylcholine chloride
carbachol
pilocarpine hydrochloride

Prostaglandin-$F_{2\alpha}$ Analogues, Ophthalmic
bimatoprost
latanoprost
travoprost

Prostaglandin-$F_{2\alpha}$ Analogue/Beta-blocking Agent Combinations, Ophthalmic
latanoprost/timolol
travoprost/timolol

Gonorrhea

Cephalosporins
cefixime
ceftriaxone sodium

Fluoroquinolones
ciprofloxacin
ciprofloxacin hydrochloride
ofloxacin

Macrolides
azithromycin

Gout
see also Hyperuricemia; Pain

Antimitotics
colchicine

Corticosteroids
hydrocortisone sodium succinate
methylprednisolone acetate
prednisone
triamcinolone

Nonsteroidal Anti-Inflammatory Drugs (NSAIDs)
indomethacin
naproxen
sulindac

Xanthine Oxidase Inhibitors
allopurinol
febuxostat

Growth Hormone Deficiency

Growth Hormone Replacements
somatropin

Haemophilus Influenza Infection Prevention

Vaccines
haemophilus b polysaccharide conjugate vaccine (meningococcal protein conjugate)
haemophilus b polysaccharide conjugate vaccine (tetanus protein conjugate)

Hair Regrowth

5-alpha-reductase Inhibitors, Systemic
finasteride

Piperidinopyrimidines, Topical
minoxidil

Halitosis
see also Dry Mouth; Gingivitis and Periodontitis

Antiseptic Agents
cetylpyridinium chloride
chlorhexidine gluconate
hexetidine
hydrogen peroxide
povidone-iodine
triclosan

Antiseptic Combinations
eucalyptol/mentol/thymol
eucalyptol/mentol/thymol/zinc chloride

Headache
see also Migraine Treatment

Nonsteroidal Anti-inflammatory Drugs (NSAIDs)
Acetic Acid Derivatives
ketorolac
Propionic Acid Derivatives
ibuprofen
naproxen
naproxen sodium
Salicylic Acid Derivatives
acetylsalicylic acid (ASA)

Para-aminophenol Derivatives
Anilides
acetaminophen

Heart Failure

Aldosterone Antagonists
eplerenone
spironolactone

Beta-adrenergic Blocking Agents
Nonselective with Alpha-blocking activity
carvedilol
Selective without Intrinsic Sympathomimetic Activity (ISA)
bisoprolol

Diuretics
amiloride hydrochloride
bumetanide
chlorthalidone
ethacrynate sodium
ethacrynic acid
furosemide
hydrochlorothiazide
metolazone
triamterene

Inotropes
Cardiac Glycosides
digoxin
Various Inotropes
dobutamine hydrochloride
dopamine hydrochloride
milrinone lactate

Recombinant Human B-type Natriuretic Peptide (rhBNP)
nesiritide

Renin-Angiotensin System Agents
Angiotensin Converting Enzyme (ACE) Inhibitors
captopril
cilazapril
enalapril maleate
fosinopril sodium
lisinopril
perindopril erbumine
quinapril hydrochloride
ramipril
Angiotensin II Receptor Antagonists (ARBs)
candesartan cilexetil
valsartan

Helicobacter pylori Eradication

Proton Pump Inhibitor/Antibiotic Combinations
lansoprazole/clarithromycin/amoxicillin
omeprazole/clarithromycin/amoxicillin
omeprazole/clarithromycin/metronidazole

Hemophilia A

Antidiuretic Hormone Analogues
desmopressin acetate

Blood Coagulation Factors
antihemophilic factor
antihemophilic factor (recombinant)
antihemophilic factor (recombinant) (BDDRFVIII), plasma/albumin-free (moroctocog alfa)
antihemophilic factor/von Willebrand factor complex
eptacog alfa

Hemophilia B

Blood Coagulation Factors
coagulation factor IX
eptacog alfa

Hemorrhage, Postpartum
carboprost tromethamine

Hemorrhoids
see also Constipation

Anti-Inflammatory Agents
hydrocortisone acetate

Astringents
zinc sulfate

Protectants
2-QR polysaccharide complex
white petrolatum

Topical Anesthetics
dibucaine

Combination Agents
glycerin/hamamelis
hamamelis/phenylephrine hydrochloride
hydrocortisone acetate/pramoxine hydrochloride
hydrocortisone acetate/framycetin sulfate/dibucaine/esculin
shark liver oil/yeast
zinc sulfate/hydrocortisone acetate
zinc sulfate/hydrocortisone acetate/benzocaine
zinc sulfate/hydrocortisone acetate/pramoxine hydrochloride
zinc sulfate/pramoxine hydrochloride

Hemostasis
see also Hemorrhage, Postpartum

Antidiuretic Hormone Analogues
desmopressin acetate

Antifibrinolytics
Amino Acids
aminocaproic acid
tranexamic acid
Proteinase Inhibitors
aprotinin

Blood Coagulation Factors
antihemophilic factor (recombinant)
eptacog alfa (activated)
factor IX concentrate (human)
factor IX (recombinant)
moroctocog alfa

Local Hemostatics
gelatin, absorbable
thrombin (bovine)
thrombin alfa (recombinant)

Vitamin K Analogues
phytonadione

Heparin Overdose
protamine sulfate

Hepatic Encephalopathy
lactulose
metronidazole

Hepatitis, Alcoholic
pentoxifylline
prednisone

Hepatitis, Autoimmune
azathioprine
mycophenolate mofetil
prednisone

Hepatitis A and B Immunization

Viral Vaccines
hepatitis A (inactivated) and hepatitis B (recombinant) combined vaccines

Hepatitis A Immunization

Viral Vaccines
hepatitis A vaccine (inactivated)
hepatitis A vaccine (inactivated, purified)
hepatitis A vaccine (inactivated, virosome-formulated)

Hepatitis A Prevention
Immune Globulins
hepatitis A immune globulin (human)

Hepatitis B Prevention
Immune Globulins
hepatitis B immune globulin (human)
Viral Vaccines
hepatitis B vaccine, recombinant

Hepatitis B Treatment
Antivirals
adefovir dipivoxil
entecavir
lamivudine
telbivudine
tenofovir disoproxil fumarate
Interferons
interferon alfa-2b
peginterferon alfa-2a

Hepatitis C Treatment
Interferons
interferon alfa-2b
peginterferon alfa-2a
peginterferon alfa-2b
Interferon/Antiviral Combinations
peginterferon alfa-2a/ribavirin
peginterferon alfa-2b/ribavirin

Herpes Simplex Virus, Anal and Genital
Nucleoside Analogues
acyclovir
acyclovir sodium
famciclovir
valacyclovir

Herpes Simplex Virus, Encephalitis
Nucleoside Analogues
acyclovir sodium

Herpes Simplex Virus, Keratoconjunctivitis
Nucleoside Analogues
acyclovir
idoxuridine
trifluridine

Herpes Simplex Virus, Mouth and Orolabial
Nucleoside Analogues, Oral
acyclovir
acyclovir sodium
famciclovir
valacyclovir
Various Antivirals, Topical
docosanol

Herpes Zoster Prevention
Vaccines
varicella-zoster vaccine, live, attenuated (Oka/Merck)

Herpes Zoster Prevention, Post-exposure
Immune Globulins
varicella-zoster immune globulin

Herpes Zoster Treatment
Nucleoside Analogues
acyclovir
famciclovir
valacyclovir

Heterozygous Familial Hypercholesterolemia, Adult
see also Dyslipidemias
Cholesterol Absorption Inhibitors
ezetimibe
HMG CoA Reductase Inhibitors
atorvastatin
fluvastatin
rosuvastatin
simvastatin
Niacin Derivatives
niacin
Combination Agents
HMG CoA Reductase Inhibitors/Niacin Derivatives
lovastatin/niacin

Heterozygous Familial Hypercholesterolemia, Pediatric
see also Dyslipidemias
HMG CoA Reductase Inhibitors
atorvastatin
fluvastatin
rosuvastatin
simvastatin

Hiccoughs, Persistent
Dopamine Antagonists
chlorpromazine hydrochloride
haloperidol
metoclopramide hydrochloride
Muscle Relaxants
baclofen

Hirsutism
Ornithine Decarboxylase Inhibitors
eflornithine hydrochloride

HIV
see also Anemia; Kaposi's Sarcoma; Pneumocystis jirovecii Pneumonia
Entry Inhibitors
maraviroc
HIV-1 Fusion Inhibitors
enfuvirtide
Integrase Inhibitors
raltegravir potassium
Non-nucleoside Reverse Transcriptase Inhibitors (NNRTIs)
delaviridine mesylate
efavirenz
etavirine
nevirapine
Nucleoside Analogue Reverse Transcriptase Inhibitors (NRTIs)
abacavir sulfate
didanosine (ddl)
lamivudine (3TC)
stavudine (d4T)
zidovudine (AZT)
Nucleotide Analogue Reverse Transcriptase Inhibitors
tenofovir
Protease Inhibitors
atazanavir
darunavir ethanolate
fosamprenavir
indinavir sulfate
nelfinavir
ritonavir
ritonavir/lopinavir
saquinavir mesylate
tipranavir
Combination HIV Antivirals
abacavir/lamivudine
abacavir sulfate/lamivudine/zidovudine
efavirenz/emtricitabine/tenofovir disoproxil fumarate
emtricitabine/tenofovir disoproxil fumarate
lamivudine/zidovudine

Homocystinuria
betaine

Human Papillomavirus Infection Prevention
Viral Vaccines
human papillomavirus vaccine types 16 and 18 (recombinant, AS04 adjuvanted)
quadrivalent human papillomavirus (types 6, 11, 16, 18) recombinant vaccine

Hypercalcemia
Antiparathyroid Hormones
calcitonin salmon
Bisphosphonates
clodronate
etidronate
pamidronate
zoledronic acid
Calcimimetics
cinacalcet hydrochloride
Phosphate Preparations
sodium acid phosphate

Hyperhidrosis
Anticholinergics
oxybutynin
Antiperspirants
aluminum chloride
aluminum chlorohydrate
Neuromuscular Paralytic Agents
botulinum toxin type A

Hyperkalemia
Ion Exchange Resins
sodium polystyrene sulfonate
calcium polystyrene sulfonate

Hyperkeratosis
lactic acid
salicylic acid

Hypermelanosis
Depigmenting Agents
hydroquinone

Hyperparathyroidism
Calcimimetics
cinacalcet hydrochloride
Vitamin D Analogues
paricalcitol

Hyperphosphatemia
Phosphate Binders
aluminum hydroxide gel
calcium acetate
lanthanum carbonate hydrate
sevelamer hydrochloride

Hyperprolactinemia
Dopamine Receptor Agonists
bromocriptine
cabergoline
quinagolide hydrochloride

Hypertension

Adrenergic Blocking Agents

Alpha-1 and Beta-adrenergic Blocking Agents
labetalol hydrochloride

Alpha-1-adrenergic Blocking Agents
doxazosin mesylate
prazosin hydrochloride
terazosin hydrochloride dihydrate

Alpha-1 and Alpha-2-adrenergic Blocking Agents
phentolamine mesylate

Beta-adrenergic Blocking Agents, Nonselective with Intrinsic Sympathomimetic Activity (ISA)
pindolol

Beta-adrenergic Blocking Agents, Nonselective without ISA
nadolol
propranolol hydrochloride
timolol maleate

Beta-adrenergic Blocking Agents, Selective with ISA
acebutolol hydrochloride

Beta-adrenergic Blocking Agents, Selective without ISA
atenolol
bisoprolol fumarate
esmolol hydrochloride
metoprolol tartrate

Centrally Acting Antiadrenergic Agents
clonidine hydrochloride
methyldopa

Calcium Channel Blockers

Dihydropyridines
amlodipine besylate
felodipine
nifedipine

Nondihydropyridines
diltiazem hydrochloride
verapamil hydrochloride

Combination Agents

ACE Inhibitor/Calcium Channel Blocker Combinations
trandolapril/verapamil

ACE Inhibitor/Diuretic Combinations
cilazapril/hydrochlorothiazide
enalapril/hydrochlorothiazide
lisinopril/hydrochlorothiazide
perindopril/hydrochlorothiazide
quinapril/hydrochlorothiazide
ramipril/hydrochlorothiazide

ARB/Diuretic Combinations
candesartan/hydrochlorothiazide
eprosartan/hydrochlorothiazide
irbesartan/hydrochlorothiazide
losartan/hydrochlorothiazide
olmesartan/hydrochlorothiazide
telmisartan/hydrochlorothiazide
valsartan/hydrochlorothiazide

Beta-adrenergic Antagonist/Diuretic Combinations
atenolol/chlorthalidone
pindolol/hydrochlorothiazide

Calcium Channel Blocker/HMG CoA Reductase Inhibitor Combinations
amlodipine/atorvastatin

Centrally Acting Antiadrenergic/Diuretic Combinations
methyldopa/hydrochlorothiazide

Renin inhibitor/Diuretic Combinations
aliskiren fumarate/hydrochlorothiazide

Diuretics

Loop Diuretics
ethacrynate sodium
ethacrynic acid
furosemide

Osmotic Diuretics
mannitol

Thiazides and Related Agents
chlorthalidone
hydrochlorothiazide
indapamide
indapamide hemihydrate
metolazone

Diuretic Combinations
amiloride/hydrochlorothiazide
spironolactone/hydrochlorothiazide
triamterene/hydrochlorothiazide

Renin Inhibitors
aliskiren fumarate

Renin-Angiotensin System Agents

Angiotensin Converting Enzyme (ACE) Inhibitors
benazepril hydrochloride
captopril
cilazapril
enalapril maleate
enalaprilat
fosinopril sodium
lisinopril
perindopril erbumine
quinapril hydrochloride
ramipril
trandolapril

Angiotensin II Receptor Antagonists (ARBs)
candesartan cilexetil
eprosartan mesylate
irbesartan
losartan potassium
olmesartan medoxomil
telmisartan
valsartan

Vasodilators
diazoxide
epoprostenol sodium
hydralazine hydrochloride
minoxidil
nitroglycerin
sodium nitroprusside

Hyperthyroidism

Antithyroid Agents
methimazole
propylthiouracil

Beta-adrenergic Blocking Agents
atenolol
metoprolol
propranolol

Hyperuricemia
see also Cancer Chemotherapy Toxicity Prevention; Gout

Uricosurics
probenecid
sulfinpyrazone

Xanthine Oxidase Inhibitors
allopurinol
febuxostat

Hypoglycemia
dextrose (glucose)
glucagon

Hypokalemia

Potassium Sparing Diuretics
amiloride hydrochloride
spironolactone

Potassium Supplements
potassium chloride
potassium citrate
potassium gluconate
potassium phosphate

Hypophosphatemia

Phosphate Preparations
sodium acid phosphate

Hypopituitarism
cosyntropin/zinc hydroxide

Hypothyroidism

Thyroid Hormones
levothyroxine
liothyronine
thyroid, dessicated

Hypovolemia

Blood Derivatives
albumin (human)

Plasma Substitutes

Plasma Expanders
dextran
hetastarch
hydroxyethyl starch
pentastarch

Idiopathic Thrombocytopenic Purpura

Anti-Rho(D) Antibodies
immune globulin, Rho(D) human

IgG Antibodies
immune globulin

Thrombopoietic Peptide Mimetics
romiplostim

Immunization, Passive (General)

Immune Globulins Standard
immune globulin (human), IM

Immunodeficiency, Primary

Immune Globulins Standard
immune globulin (human), IV

Immunosuppression

Corticosteroids, Systemic
betamethasone sodium phosphate
cortisone acetate
dexamethasone
hydrocortisone
hydrocortisone sodium succinate
methylprednisolone
methylprednisolone sodium succinate
prednisolone
prednisone
triamcinolone diacetate

Cyclic Peptides
cyclosporine

Cytotoxic Agents
azathioprine

Immune Globulins
anti-thymocyte globulin (equine)

Monoclonal Antibodies
basiliximab

Various Immunosuppresive Agents
mycophenolate mofetil
sirolimus
tacrolimus

Infant Colic
see also Gastrointestinal Gas

Coalescing Agents
simethicone

Probiotics
bifidobacterium
lactobacillus reuteri protectis

Infections, Bacterial (Eye)

Antibiotics, Ophthalmic

besifloxacin
chloramphenicol
ciprofloxacin hydrochloride
erythromycin
framycetin
fusidic acid
gatifloxacin
gentamicin sulfate
gramicidin
moxifloxacin hydrochloride
neomycin sulfate
ofloxacin
polymyxin B sulfate
sulfacetamide sodium
tobramycin

Infections, Bacterial (Systemic)

Aminoglycosides

amikacin sulfate
gentamicin sulfate
paromomycin sulfate
streptomycin sulfate
tobramycin sulfate

Carbapenems

doripenem
ertapenem sodium
imipenem/cilastatin sodium
meropenem

Cephalosporins

Cephalosporins, 1st Generation

cefadroxil
cefazolin sodium
cephalexin

Cephalosporins, 2nd Generation

cefaclor
cefoxitin sodium
cefprozil
cefuroxime axetil
cefuroxime sodium

Cephalosporins, 3rd Generation

cefixime
cefotaxime sodium
ceftazidime
ceftazidime pentahydrate
ceftriaxone sodium

Cephalosporins, 4th Generation

cefepime hydrochloride

Cyclic Lipopeptides

daptomycin

Fluoroquinolones

ciprofloxacin
ciprofloxacin hydrochloride
levofloxacin
moxifloxacin hydrochloride
norfloxacin
ofloxacin

Folate Antagonists

trimethoprim

Glycopeptides

vancomycin hydrochloride

Glycylcyclines

tigecycline

Lincosamides

clindamycin hydrochloride
clindamycin palmitate hydrochloride
clindamycin phosphate
lincomycin hydrochloride monohydrate

Macrolides

azithromycin dihydrate
clarithromycin
erythromycin
erythromycin estolate
erythromycin ethylsuccinate
erythromycin lactobionate
erythromycin stearate
spiramycin

Monobactams

aztreonam

Nitroimidazoles

metronidazole

Oxazolidinones

linezolid

Penicillins

Aminopenicillins

amoxicillin trihydrate
ampicillin
ampicillin sodium
ampicillin trihydrate

Penicillins, Antipseudomonal

piperacillin sodium
ticarcillin disodium

Penicillins, Penicillinase-Resistant

cloxacillin sodium

Penicillins, Penicillinase-Susceptible

penicillin G benzathine
penicillin G sodium
penicillin V potassium

Penicillins, β-lactamase Inhibitor Combinations

amoxicillin trihydrate/clavulanate potassium
piperacillin sodium/tazobactam sodium
ticarcillin disodium/clavulanate potassium

Sulfonamide Combinations

sulfamethoxazole/trimethoprim

Tetracyclines

doxycycline hyclate
minocycline hydrochloride
tetracycline hydrochloride

Infections, Bacterial (Topical)

Antibiotics, Topical

bacitracin
bacitracin/neomycin/polymyxin B
bacitracin/polymyxin B
bacitracin zinc
chloramphenicol
chlorhexidine acetate
chlorhexidine gluconate
framycetin sulfate
fusidic acid
gentamicin sulfate
gramicidin/polymyxin B
mupirocin
mupirocin calcium
neomycin sulfate
polymyxin B sulfate
silver sulfadiazine
sodium fusidate

Infections, Fungal (Eye)

Photosensitizing Agents

verteporfin

Infections, Fungal (Systemic)

Antifungal Antibiotics

amphotericin B
amphotericin B lipid complex
amphotericin B liposomal

Glucan Synthesis Inhibitors

anidulafungin
caspofungin acetate
micafungin

Imidazoles

ketoconazole

Triazoles

fluconazole
itraconazole
posaconazole
voriconazole

Infections, Fungal (Topical)

Allylamines

naftifine hydrochloride
terbinafine hydrochloride

Imidazoles

clotrimazole
ketoconazole
miconazole nitrate

Polyenes

nystatin

Various Antifungals

ciclopirox olamine
clioquinol
selenium sulfide
tolnaftate
undecylenic acid

Infections, Fungal (Vaginal)

Imidazoles, Vaginal

butoconazole nitrate
clotrimazole
miconazole nitrate

Polyenes

nystatin

Triazoles, Oral

fluconazole

Triazoles, Vaginal

terconazole

Infections, Viral (Eye)

trifluridine

Infertility

Gonadotropin-releasing Hormone Antagonists

ganirelix acetate
cetrorelix acetate

Gonadotropins

follitropin alpha
follitropin alpha (rDNA origin)
follitropin beta
gonadorelin acetate
gonadotropin (human) chorionic
lutropin alpha
menotropins
urofollitropin

Ovulation Stimulants, Synthetic

clomiphene citrate

Progestogens, Vaginal

progesterone

Inflammatory Bowel Disease

5-Aminosalicylic Acid Derivatives
5-aminosalicylic acid (mesalamine)
olsalazine sodium
sulfasalazine

Biologic Response Modifiers
Tumor Necrosis Factor Alpha (TNF-α) Inhibitors
adalimumab
infliximab

Corticosteroids, Oral
budesonide
hydrocortisone sodium succinate
methylprednisolone sodium succinate
prednisone

Corticosteroids, Rectal
betamethasone sodium phosphate
budesonide
hydrocortisone
hydrocortisone acetate

Immunosuppressants
azathioprine
cyclosporine
mercaptopurine
methotrexate sodium

Influenza A Prophylaxis and Treatment

Cyclic Amines
amantadine

Neuraminidase Inhibitors
oseltamivir phosphate
zanamivir

Influenza A and B Prevention

Viral Vaccines
influenza vaccine, live attenuated
influenza vaccine, trivalent (inactivated)

Influenza B Prophylaxis and Treatment

Neuraminidase Inhibitors
oseltamivir phosphate
zanamivir

Insect Bites Prevention

Insect Repellents, Topical
citronella oil
deet
lavender oil
lemon eucalyptus oil (P-methane 3,8-diol)
soybean oil

Insect Bites Treatment

Adrenergic Agents, Injectable
epinephrine

Antihistamines, Oral
cetirizine
chlorpheniramine
diphehydramine
loratadine

Corticosteroids, Topical
clobetasone 17-butyrate
hydrocortisone

Insomnia and Sedation

Aldehydes and Derivatives
chloral hydrate

Antihistamines
diphenhydramine
doxylamine succinate
promethazine hydrochloride

Barbiturates
pentobarbital sodium
phenobarbital

Benzodiazepines
alprazolam
bromazepam
clorazepate dipotassium
diazepam
flurazepam hydrochloride
lorazepam
midazolam hydrochloride
nitrazepam
oxazepam
temazepam
triazolam

Cyclopyrrolones
zopiclone

Various Hypnotics and Sedatives
propofol

Iron Overload

Chelating Agents
deferasirox
deferoxamine mesylate

Irritable Bowel Syndrome

Antiperistaltics
loperamide hydrochloride

Antispasmodics
dicyclomine
pinaverium bromide
trimebutine

Bulk Forming Agents
calcium polycarbophil
psyllium hydrophillic mucilloid

Probiotics
lactobacillus plantarum 299v

Tricyclic Antidepressants
amitriptyline
desipramine

Various Natural Products
peppermint oil

Ischemic Stroke, Acute

Antiplatelet Agents
acetylsalicylic acid (ASA)

Plasminogen Activators
Proteins, Recombinant DNA Origin
alteplase

Ischemic Stroke Prevention, Secondary

Anticoagulants
nicoumalone
warfarin

Antiplatelet Agents
acetylsalicylic acid (ASA)
clopidogrel
ticlopidine

Thrombin Inhibitors, Direct
dabigatran

Combination Antiplatelet Agents
dipyridamole/acetylsalicylic acid

Japanese Encephalitis Prevention

Viral Vaccines
Japanese encephalitis virus vaccine (inactivated)

Kaposi's Sarcoma
daunorubicin, liposomal
doxorubicin hydrochloride (pegylated liposomes)
interferon alfa-2b
paclitaxel

Labour Induction

Ergot Alkaloids
ergometrine (ergonovine) maleate

Oxytocin Analogues
carbetocin
oxytocin

Prostaglandins
dinoprostone

Lactose Intolerance

Enzyme Replacements
lactase

Leprosy
dapsone
rifampin

Lymphogranuloma Venereum

Macrolides
azithromycin dihydrate
erythromycin

Tetracyclines
doxycycline hyclate

Macular Degeneration, Age-related

Benzoporphyrin Photosensitizers
verteporfin

Vascular Endothelial Growth Factor Antagonists
pegaptanib
ranibizumab

Vitamin and Mineral Combinations
beta-carotene/copper/vitamin C/vitamin E/zinc
copper/vitamin C/vitamin E/zinc

Malaria Prevention

Combination Antimalarials
atovaquone/proguanil

Quinoline Derivatives
chloroquine phosphate
hydroxychloroquine sulfate
mefloquine hydrochloride
primaquine phosphate

Tetracyclines
doxycycline

Malignant Hyperthermia

Skeletal Muscle Relaxants
dantrolene sodium

Measles and Rubella Prevention

Combination Viral Vaccines
measles, rubella virus vaccine (live, attenuated)

Measles, Mumps and Rubella Prevention

Combination Viral Vaccines
measles, mumps and rubella virus vaccine (live, attenuated)

Measles, Mumps, Rubella and Varicella Prevention

Combination Viral Vaccines
measles, mumps, rubella and varicella vaccine (live, attenuated)

Meningitis, Bacterial

Cephalosporins, 3rd Generation

cefotaxime sodium
ceftazidime
ceftazidime pentahydrate
ceftriaxone sodium

Glycopeptides

vancomycin hydrochloride

Penicillins

Aminopenicillins

ampicillin trihydrate

Penicillins, Penicillinase-Susceptible

penicillin G sodium

Meningococcal Disease Prevention

Bacterial Vaccines

meningococcal group C-CRM197 conjugate vaccine
meningococcal group C-TT conjugate vaccine
meningococcal oligosaccharide CRM197, groups A, C, Y, W-135
meningococcal polysaccharide vaccine, groups A, C, Y, W-135 combined
meningococcal polysaccharide vaccine, groups A, C, Y, W-135 diphtheria toxoid conjugate

Menopausal Flushing

Centrally Acting Antiadrenergic Agents

clonidine hydrochloride

Ergot Combinations

belladonna/ergotamine tartrate/phenobarbital

Menopause

see also Vaginal Dryness

Estrogen/Progestogen Replacements, Oral

conjugated estrogens/medroxyprogesterone
estradiol-17β/drospirenone
ethinyl estradiol/norethindrone acetate

Estrogen/Progestogen Replacements, Transdermal

estradiol-17β/norethindrone

Estrogens, Oral

conjugated estrogens
estradiol-17β
estropipate

Estrogens, Transdermal

estradiol-17β

Estrogens, Vaginal Preparations

conjugated estrogens
estradiol
estradiol-17β hemihydrate
estrone

Progestogens, Oral

medroxyprogesterone acetate
megestrol acetate
norethindrone
progesterone

Menorrhagia

Antifibrinolytics

tranexamic acid

Progestogens, Intrauterine

levonorgestrel

Metabolic Acidosis

Bicarbonate Supplements

sodium bicarbonate

Migraine Prophylaxis

Antiepileptics

topiramate

Calcium Channel Blocking Agents, Selective

flunarizine

Serotonin Antagonists

pizotifen malate (pizotyline)

Migraine Treatment

see also Headache

Barbiturate/Analgesic Compounds

butalbital/ASA/caffeine
butalbital/ASA/caffeine/codeine phosphate

Ergot Alkaloids

dihydroergotamine mesylate

Ergot Alkaloids Compounds

ergotamine/caffeine
ergotamine/caffeine/belladonna/pentobarbital
ergotamine/caffeine/diphenhydramine
ergotamine/belladonna/phenobarbital

Serotonin (5-HT$_1$) Receptor Agonists

almotriptan malate
eletriptan
frovatriptan
naratriptan hydrochloride
rizatriptan benzoate
sumatriptan hemisulfate
sumatriptan succinate
zolmitriptan

Mineral Supplementation

see also Anemia

Calcium

calcium carbonate
calcium chloride
calcium citrate
calcium glucoheptonate
calcium gluconate

Magnesium

magnesium glucoheptonate
magnesium hydroxide
magnesium oxide

Zinc

zinc gluconate
zinc sulfate

Mouth Pain

see also Toothache

Local Anesthetics

benzocaine
benzydamine
lidocaine

Mucopolysaccharidosis

Enzymes

idursulfase
laronidase

Mucositis

Human Keratinocyte Growth Factor

palifermin

Multiple Sclerosis

see also Muscle Spasticity

Biologic Response Modifiers

glatiramer acetate
interferon beta-1a
interferon beta-1b

Cannabinoids

delta-9-tetrahydrocannabinol

Corticosteroids

hydrocortisone
methylprednisolone
prednisone

Monoclonal Antibodies

natalizumab

Mumps Prevention

see also Measles, Mumps, Rubella and Varicella Prevention

Viral Vaccines

mumps virus vaccine (live, attenuated)

Muscle Spasticity

Centrally Acting Agents

Alpha-2-adrenergic Agonists

tizanidine

Antihistamine Derivatives

orphenadrine citrate

Benzodiazepines

clonazepam
diazepam

Carbamic Acid Esters

methocarbamol

Gamma Aminobutyric Acid (GABA) Derivatives

baclofen

Tricyclic Derivatives

cyclobenzaprine hydrochloride

Direct Acting Agents

dantrolene sodium

Peripherally Acting Agents

botulinum toxin type A

Myasthenia Gravis

Cholinesterase Inhibitors

neostigmine bromide
pyridostigmine bromide

Mycobacterium avium Complex, Prophylaxis

Macrolides

azithromycin
clarithromycin

Rifamycins

rifabutin
rifampin

Mycobacterium avium Complex, Treatment

Aminoglycosides

amikacin

Antimycobacterial Agents

ethambutol

Fluoroquinolones

ciprofloxacin
levofloxacin

Macrolides

azithromycin
clarithromycin

Rifamycins

rifabutin
rifampin

Mydriasis and Cycloplegia

Anticholinergics, Ophthalmic

atropine sulfate
cyclopentolate hydrochloride
homatropine
tropicamide

Sympathomimetics, Ophthalmic

phenylephrine hydrochloride

Myopia
Photosensitizing Agents
verteporfin

Narcolepsy
CNS Stimulants
dexamphetamine
methylphenidate
modafinil
Gamma Aminobutyric Acid (GABA) Derivatives
sodium oxybate

Nausea and Vomiting
Anticholinergics
scopolamine
Antihistamines
dimenhydrinate
diphenhydramine
hydroxyzine hydrochloride
meclizine
promethazine hydrochloride
Antihistamine and Vitamin Combinations
doxylamine succinate/pyridoxine hydrochloride
Butyrophenone Derivatives
droperidol
haloperidol
Cannabinoids
dronabinol
nabilone
Dopamine Antagonists
chlorpromazine hydrochloride
domperidone
metoclopramide hydrochloride
perphenazine
prochlorperazine
prochlorperazine mesylate
trifluoperazine hydrochloride
Neurokinin 1 Receptor Antagonists
aprepitant
fosaprepitant
Serotonin (5-HT_3) Antagonists
dolasetron mesylate
granisetron hydrochloride
ondansetron
ondansetron hydrochloride dihydrate

Neuromuscular Relaxation
Neuromuscular Blocking Agents
Depolarizing Agents, Choline Derivative
succinylcholine chloride
Nondepolarizing Agents, Quaternary Ammonium Compounds
atracurium besylate
cisatracurium besylate
doxacurium chloride
mivacurium chloride
pancuronium bromide
rocuronium bromide
vecuronium bromide
Neuromuscular Paralytic Agents
botulinum toxin type A

Neuropathic Pain
see also Pain
Antiepileptics
Carboxylic Acid Derivatives
divalproex sodium
valproic acid
Gamma Aminobutyric Acid (GABA) Derivatives
baclofen
gabapentin
pregabalin
Hydantoin Derivatives
phenytoin
Iminostilbene Derivatives
carbamazepine
oxcarbazepine
Benzodiazepines
clonazepam
Serotonin-Norepinephrine Reuptake Inhibitors (SNRIs)
duloxetine hydrochloride
venlafaxine hydrochloride
Tricyclic Antidepressants
amitriptyline
desipramine
nortriptyline

Neutropenia
Hematopoietics
ancestim
filgrastim
pegfilgrastim

Niemann-Pick Type C Disease
Glucosylceramide Synthase Inhibitors
miglustat

Nocturnal Leg Cramps
Cinchona Alkaloids
quinine sulfate

Obesity
Gastrointestinal Lipase Inhibitors
orlistat
Noradrenergic Agents
bupropion hydrochloride

Obsessive-Compulsive Disorder
Selective Serotonin Reuptake Inhibitors (SSRIs)
fluoxetine hydrochloride
fluvoxamine maleate
paroxetine hydrochloride
sertraline hydrochloride
Tricyclic Antidepressants
clomipramine hydrochloride

Ophthalmic Cleansing
Antiseptic Agents
witch hazel
Combination Agents
boric acid/domiphen bromide/miranol 2 MCT modified/ sodium borate
cocamidopropylamine oxide/disodium laureth sulfosuccinate
methylparaben/sodium borate
magnesium chloride/sodium chloride

Ophthalmic Local Anesthesia
proparacaine hydrochloride
tetracaine hydrochloride

Ophthalmic Lubrication
Artificial Tears
carbopol 940
hydroxypropyl cellulose (hyprolose)
hypromellose
petrolatum
polyethylene glycol 400
polysorbate 80
polyvinyl alcohol
sodium carboxymethylcellulose
sodium hyaluronate
Immunomodulators
cyclosporine
Combination Agents
dextran 70/hypromellose
glycerin/hypromellose
mineral oil/petrolatum

Ophthalmic Lubrication for Artificial Eyes
tyloxapol

Ophthalmic Surgery
see also Cataract Surgery, Post-operative Care
Enzymatic Preparations
chymotrypsin
Ophthalmic Surgical Implants
gelatin, absorbable film
Viscoelastic Preparations
sodium hyaluronate

Opioid Dependence
buprenorphine hydrochloride
buprenorphine hydrochloride/naloxone hydrochloride
methadone hydrochloride

Opioid Overdose
naloxone hydrochloride

Opioid-induced Respiratory Depression
Opioid Antagonists
naloxone hydrochloride

Orthostatic Intolerance
Alpha-agonists
midodrine
Alpha-blocking Agents
yohimbine
Electrolytes
sodium chloride
Mineralocorticoids
fludrocortisone

Osteoarthritis
see also Pain
Capsicum Derivatives, Topical
capsaicin
Corticosteroids, Intra-articular
betamethasone acetate/betamethasone sodium succinate
methylprednisolone acetate
triamcinolone acetonide
triamcinolone hexacetonide
Nonsteroidal Anti-inflammatory Drugs (NSAIDs), Topical
diclofenac sodium
methyl salicylate
triethanolamine salicylate
Synovial Fluid Replacements
hyaluronic acid sodium
hylan G-F 20
sodium hyaluronate

Osteomyelitis
Aminoglycosides
amikacin sulfate
gentamicin sulfate
Carbapenems
imipenem/cilastatin sodium
meropenem
Cephalosporins
Cephalosporins, 1st Generation
cefazolin sodium
cephalexin
Cephalosporins, 2nd Generation
cefuroxime sodium
Cephalosporins, 3rd Generation
cefotaxime sodium
ceftazidime
ceftazidime pentahydrate
ceftriaxone sodium

Fluoroquinolones
ciprofloxacin
ciprofloxacin hydrochloride
moxifloxacin hydrochloride

Glycopeptides
vancomycin hydrochloride

Lincosamides
clindamycin hydrochloride
clindamycin palmitate hydrochloride
clindamycin phosphate
lincomycin hydrochloride monohydrate

Penicillins
Aminopenicillins
amoxicillin trihydrate

Penicillins, Penicillinase-Resistant
cloxacillin sodium

Penicillins, Penicillinase-Susceptible
penicillin G sodium
penicillin V

Penicillins, β-lactam Inhibitor Combinations
amoxicillin trihydrate/clavulanate potassium
piperacillin sodium/tazobactam sodium

Sulfonamide Combinations
sulfamethoxazole/trimethoprim

Osteoporosis Prevention
Antiparathyroid Hormones
calcitonin salmon

Bisphosphonates
alendronate
etidronate
risedronate
zoledronic acid

Bisphosphonate/Supplement Combinations
alendronate/vitamin D
etidronate/calcium
risedronate/calcium

Selective Estrogen Receptor Modulators (SERMs)
Benzothiophenes
raloxifene hydrochloride

Osteoporosis Prevention (Glucocorticoid-Induced)
Bisphosphonates
alendronate
etidronate
risedronate
zoledronic acid

Bisphosphonate/Supplement Combinations
alendronate/vitamin D
etidronate/calcium
risedronate/calcium

Osteoporosis Treatment
Antiparathyroid Hormones
calcitonin salmon

Bisphosphonates
alendronate
etidronate
risedronate
zoledronic acid

Bisphosphonate/Supplement Combinations
alendronate/vitamin D
etidronate/calcium
risedronate/calcium

Calcium Supplements
calcium carbonate
calcium chloride
calcium citrate
calcium glucoheptonate
calcium gluconate

Parathyroid Hormones
teriparatide

RANK Ligand Inhibitors
denosumab

Selective Estrogen Receptor Modulators (SERMs)
Benzothiophenes
raloxifene hydrochloride

Otitis Externa
Antibiotics, Otic
gentamicin
polymyxin B sulfate/gramicidin
polymyxin B sulfate/gramicidin/neomycin

Combination Antibiotic/Corticosteroid Preparations, Otic
chloramphenicol/hydrocortisone
ciprofloxacin hydrochloride/dexamethasone
clioquinol/flumethasone pivalate
framycetin sulfate/gramicidin/dexamethasone
gentamicin/betamethasone
polymyxin B sulfate/neomycin/hydrocortisone

Corticosteroids, Otic
dexamethasone sodium
flumethasone pivalate

Otitis Media, Acute (Pediatric)
Combination Antibiotic/Corticosteroid Preparations, Otic
ciprofloxacin hydrochloride/dexamethasone

Cephalosporins
cefprozil
ceftriaxone
cefuroxime axetil

Macrolides
azithromycin dihydrate
clarithromycin

Penicillins
Aminopenicillins
amoxicillin trihydrate

Penicillins, β-lactamase Inhibitor Combinations
amoxicillin trihydrate/clavulanate potassium

Otosclerosis
sodium fluoride

Overdoses, Miscellaneous
see also Acetaminophen, Benzodiazepine, Digoxin, Heparin and Opioid Overdose

Adsorbents
activated charcoal

Paget's Disease of the Bone
Antiparathyroid Hormones
calcitonin salmon

Bisphosphonates
alendronate
clodronate
etidronate
pamidronate
risedronate
zoledronic acid

Phosphate Preparations
sodium acid phosphate

Pain
Gamma Aminobutyric Acid (GABA) Derivative
pregabalin

Nonsteroidal Anti-inflammatory Drugs (NSAIDs)
Acetic Acid Derivatives (including Indole Derivatives)
diclofenac potassium
diclofenac sodium
etodolac
indomethacin
ketorolac tromethamine
sulindac

Cyclooxygenase-2 (COX-2) Inhibitors
celecoxib

Fenamates
floctafenine
mefenamic acid

Napthylalkanones
nabumetone

Oxicams
meloxicam
piroxicam
tenoxicam

Propionic Acid Derivatives
fenoprofen calcium
flurbiprofen
ibuprofen
ketoprofen
naproxen
naproxen sodium
oxaprozin
tiaprofenic acid

Salicylic Acid Derivatives
acetylsalicylic acid (ASA)
diflunisal

Opioids
Aminomethylcyclohexanol Derivatives
tramadol hydrochloride

Benzomorphan Derivatives
pentazocine hydrochloride
pentazocine lactate

Morphinan Derivatives
butorphanol tartrate
nalbuphine hydrochloride

Natural Opium Alkaloids
buprenorphine
codeine phosphate
hydromorphone hydrochloride
morphine hydrochloride
morphine sulfate
oxycodone hydrochloride

Phenylheptylamine Derivatives
methadone

Phenylpiperidine Derivatives
alfentanil hydrochloride
fentanyl citrate
meperidine hydrochloride (pethidine)
sufentanil citrate

Opioid Antagonist/Natural Opium Alkaloids Combinations
naloxone hydrochloride/oxycodone hydrochloride

Para-aminophenol Derivatives
Anilides
acetaminophen

Pain Therapy, Topical
Capsicum Derivatives
capsaicin

Monoterpenes
camphor/menthol
menthol

Nonsteroidal Anti-inflammatory Drugs (NSAIDs)
diclofenac diethylamine
diclofenac sodium
methyl salicylate
triethanolamine salicylate

Panic Disorder

Benzodiazepines
alprazolam
clonazepam

Monoamine Oxidase Inhibitors (MAOIs)
phenelzine
tranylcypromine sulfate

Selective Serotonin Reuptake Inhibitors (SSRIs)
citalopram hydrobromide
escitalopram oxalate
fluoxetine hydrochloride
fluvoxamine maleate
paroxetine hydrochloride
sertraline

Tricyclic Antidepressants
clomipramine
desipramine
imipramine

Parkinson's Disease

Anticholinergic Agents
benztropine mesylate
ethopropazine hydrochloride
procyclidine hydrochloride
trihexyphenidyl hydrochloride

COMT Inhibitors
entacapone

Dopaminergic Agents

Dopamine Agonists
bromocriptine mesylate
pramipexole dihydrochloride
ropinirole hydrochloride

Dopamine Precursors
levodopa

Dopamine Precursors and Decarboxylase Inhibitors
levodopa/benserazide hydrochloride
levodopa/carbidopa

Monoamine Oxidase (MAO) Inhibitors, Selective (Type B)
rasagiline mesylate
selegiline hydrochloride

Various Dopaminergic Agents
amantadine hydrochloride

Paroxysmal Nocturnal Hemoglobinuria

Monoclonal Antibodies
eculizumab

Patent Ductus Arteriosus Closure

Nonsteroidal Anti-inflammatory Drugs (NSAIDs)
indomethacin

Patent Ductus Arteriosus, Patency Maintenance

Prostaglandins
alprostadil

Pediculosis
isopropyl myristate
lindane (gamma benzene hexachloride)
permethrin
piperonyl butoxide/pyrethrins
star anise oil (Illicium verum)

Peptic Ulcer
see also Helicobacter pylori eradication

Antacids
aluminum hydroxide
aluminum hydroxide/magnesium hydroxide
calcium carbonate

Cytoprotective Agents
sucralfate

Histamine H_2-receptor Antagonists
cimetidine
famotidine
nizatidine
ranitidine hydrochloride

Mucosal Protective Agents
misoprostol

Proton Pump Inhibitors
esomeprazole
lansoprazole
omeprazole
pantoprazole magnesium
pantoprazole sodium
rabeprazole

Peripheral Vascular Disease

Antiplatelet Agents
acetylsalicylic acid (ASA)
clopidogrel

Peripheral Vasodilators
nylidrin hydrochloride

Rheologic Modifiers
pentoxifylline

Peritonitis, Spontaneous Bacterial

Cephalosporins, 3rd Generation
cefotaxime sodium
ceftriaxone sodium

Fluoroquinolones
norfloxacin

Sulfonamide Combinations
sulfamethoxazole/trimethoprim

Perspiration
see also Hyperhidrosis

Antiperspirants
aluminum chloride
aluminum chlorohydrate
aluminum lactate
aluminum sesquichlorohydrate
aluminum zirconium pentachlorohydrex-glycine
aluminum zirconium tetrachlorohydrex-glycine
aluminum zirconium trichlorohydrex-glycine
aluminum zirconyl hydroxychloride complex
ammonium alum
potassium alum
zinc oxide

Pertussis Prevention

Bacterial Vaccines
pertussis vaccine (acellular, adsorbed)

Photodamaged Skin

Retinoids, Topical
tazarotene
tretinoin

Pneumocystis jirovecii Pneumonia Prophylaxis
atovaquone
dapsone
pentamidine isethionate
pyrimethamine
sulfamethoxazole/trimethoprim

Pneumocystis jirovecii Pneumonia Treatment
atovaquone
dapsone
pentamidine isethionate
primaquine phosphate
sulfamethoxazole/trimethoprim

Pneumonia, Community-Acquired

Carbapenems
doripenem
ertapenem sodium
imipenem/cilastatin sodium
meropenem

Cephalosporins

Cephalosporins, 1st Generation
cefazolin sodium

Cephalosporins, 2nd Generation
cefaclor
cefprozil
cefuroxime axetil
cefuroxime sodium

Cephalosporins, 3rd Generation
cefotaxime sodium
ceftriaxone sodium
ceftazidime
ceftazidime pentahydrate

Cephalosporins, 4th Generation
cefepime hydrochloride

Fluoroquinolones
ciprofloxacin
ciprofloxacin hydrochloride
levofloxacin
moxifloxacin hydrochloride

Glycopeptides
vancomycin hydrochloride

Glycylcyclines
tigecycline

Lincosamides
clindamycin hydrochloride

Macrolides

Azalides
azithromycin dihydrate

Ketolides
telithromycin

Various Macrolides
clarithromycin
erythromycin
erythromycin estolate
erythromycin ethylsuccinate
erythromycin lactobionate
erythromycin stearate

Nitroimidazoles
metronidazole

Oxazolidinones
linezolid

Penicillins

Aminopenicillins
amoxicillin trihydrate
ampicillin

Penicillins, Penicillinase-Resistant
cloxacillin sodium

Penicillins, Penicillinase-Susceptible
penicillin G
penicillin V

Penicillins, β-lactamase Inhibitor Combinations
amoxicillin trihydrate/clavulanate potassium
piperacillin sodium/tazobactam sodium
ticarcillin disodium/clavulanate potassium

Sulfonamide Combinations
sulfamethoxazole/trimethoprim

Tetracyclines
doxycycline hyclate

Poliomyelitis Prevention

see also Diphtheria, Tetanus and Poliomyelitis Prevention; Diphtheria, Tetanus, Pertussis and Poliomyelitis Prevention; Diphtheria, Tetanus, Pertussis, Poliomyelitis and Haemophilus Type b Prevention; Diphtheria, Tetanus, Pertussis, Poliomyelitis, Haemophilus Type b and Hepatitis B Prevention

Viral Vaccines

poliomyelitis vaccine (inactivated, diploid cell origin)
poliomyelitis vaccine (inactivated vero cell origin)

Polymyalgia Rheumatica and Giant-Cell Arteritis

Corticosteroids

prednisone

Polyneuropathy, Chronic Inflammatory Demyelinating

Immune globulins

immunoglobulin (human)

Post-myocardial Infarction

see also Acute Coronary Syndromes; Cardiovascular Disease Prevention, Secondary; Heart Failure

Aldosterone Antagonists

eplerenone

Antiplatelet Agents

acetylsalicylic acid (ASA)
clopidogrel
prasugrel
ticlopidine

Beta-adrenergic Blocking Agents

Beta-adrenergic Blocking Agents with Alpha Blocking Activity

carvedilol

Nonselective without Intrinsic Sympathomimetic Activity (ISA)

nadolol
propranolol
timolol

Selective with ISA

acebutolol

Selective without ISA

atenolol
bisoprolol
metoprolol

HMG CoA Reductase Inhibitors

atorvastatin
fluvastatin
lovastatin
pravastastin
rosuvastatin
simvastatin

Renin-Angiotensin System Agents

Angiotensin II Receptor Antagonists (ARBs)

candesartan cilexetil
valsartan

Angiotensin Converting Enzyme (ACE) Inhibitors

captopril
cilazapril
enalapril
fosinopril
lisinopril
perindopril
quinapril
ramipril
trandolapril

Combination Agents

acetylsalicylic acid/pravastatin sodium

Post-traumatic Stress Disorder

Selective Serotonin Reuptake Inhibitors (SSRIs)

fluoxetine
paroxetine
sertraline

Serotonin-Norepinephrine Reuptake Inhibitors (SNRIs)

venlafaxine

Precocious Puberty, Central

Gonadotropin-releasing Hormone Analogues

leuprolide acetate

Premenstrual Dysphoric Disorder

Selective Serotonin Reuptake Inhibitors (SSRIs)

paroxetine

Prostate Cancer

see also Cancer, General

Gonadotropin Releasing Hormone Antagonists

degarelix acetate

Pruritus

Anesthetics, Topical

benzocaine
chloroprocaine hydrochloride
dibucaine hydrochloride
lidocaine hydrochloride
tetracaine
tetracaine hydrochloride

Antihistamines, Systemic

Alkylamines

brompheniramine maleate
chlorpheniramine maleate
dexchlorpheniramine maleate

Ethanolamines

diphenhydramine hydrochloride

Phenothiazine Derivatives

promethazine hydrochloride
trimeprazine tartrate

Piperazine Derivatives

cetirizine hydrochloride
hydroxyzine hydrochloride

Piperidine Derivatives

cyproheptadine hydrochloride
desloratadine
fexofenadine
loratadine

Various Antihistamines

doxepin
ketotifen

Antihistamines, Topical

diphenhydramine
doxepin hydrochloride
promethazine

Astringents, Topical

aluminum acetate

Pruritus, Cholestatic

cholestyramine resin
naltrexone hydrochloride

Psoriasis

Anthracene Derivatives, Topical

anthralin

Biologic Response Modifiers

Fusion Proteins

alefacept

Interleukin Receptor Antagonists

ustekinumab

Tumor Necrosis Factor Alpha (TNF-α) Inhibitors

adalimumab
etanercept
infliximab

Corticosteroids, Topical

amcinonide
betamethasone dipropionate
betamethasone valerate
hydrocortisone
mometasone propionate

Cytotoxics, Systemic

methotrexate sodium

Immunosuppressants, Systemic

cyclosporine

Psoralens, Systemic

methoxsalen

Psoralens, Topical

methoxsalen

Retinoids, Systemic

acitretin

Retinoids, Topical

tazarotene

Tars, Topical

coal tar
fractar

Vitamin D Derivatives, Topical

calcitriol
calcipotriol

Various Psoriasis Therapy Agents, Topical

phenol
salicylic acid

Various Combination Psoriasis Therapy Agents, Topical

calcipotriol/betamethasone
diflucortolone valerate/salicylic acid

Psychoses

Benzisothiazoylylpiperazine Derivatives

ziprasidone

Benzisoxazole Derivatives

paliperidone
risperidone

Butyrophenone Derivatives

haloperidol
haloperidol decanoate

Dibenzodiazepine Derivatives

clozapine

Dibenzothiazepine Derivatives

quetiapine fumarate

Dibenzoxazepine Derivatives

loxapine

Diphenylbutylpiperidine Derivatives

pimozide

Phenothiazines

Phenothiazines, Aliphatic

chlorpromazine hydrochloride
methotrimeprazine maleate

Phenothiazines, Piperazine

fluphenazine decanoate
fluphenazine enanthate
fluphenazine hydrochloride
perphenazine
prochlorperazine
thioproperazine mesylate
trifluoperazine hydrochloride

Phenothiazines, Piperidine

pipotiazine palmitate

Quinolinone Derivatives

aripiprazole

Thienobenzodiazepine Derivatives

olanzapine

Thioxanthene Derivatives

flupenthixol decanoate
flupenthixol dihydrochloride
thiothixene
zuclopenthixol acetate
zuclopenthixol decanoate
zuclopenthixol dihydrochloride

Pulmonary Arterial Hypertension

Endothelin Receptor Antagonists

ambrisentan
bosentan
sitaxsentan sodium

Phosphodiesterase Type 5 (PDE5) Inhibitors

sildenafil
tadalafil

Prostaglandins

epoprostenol sodium

Rabies Immunization

Immune Globulins

rabies immune globulin (human)
rabies immune globulin (pasteurized, human)

Viral Vaccines

rabies vaccine inactivated (diploid cell origin)

Raynaud's Phenomenon

Adrenergic Blocking Agents

Alpha-1-adrenergic Blocking Agents

prazosin hydrochloride

Calcium Channel Blockers

Dihydropyridines

amlodipine besylate
felodipine
nifedipine

Nondihydropyridines

diltiazem hydrochloride

Respiratory Syncytial Virus (RSV) Infection

Nucleoside Analogues

ribavirin

Respiratory Syncytial Virus (RSV) Immunization

Humanized Monoclonal Antibodies

palivizumab

Restless Legs Syndrome

Dopamine Agonists

pramipexole dihydrochloride

Reversal of Nondepolarizing Skeletal Muscle Relaxants

Anticholinesterase Agents

edrophonium

Rh Immunization Prevention for Pregnant Rho (D) Negative Women

Immune Globulins

Rho(D) immune globulin (human)

Rhinitis, Allergic

see also Allergies; Rhinorrhea

Antihistamines, Nasal

levocabastine hydrochloride

Corticosteroids, Nasal

beclomethasone dipropionate
budesonide
ciclesonide
flunisolide
fluticasone furoate
fluticasone propionate
mometasone furoate monohydrate
triamcinolone acetonide

Leukotriene Receptor Antagonists, Oral

montelukast

Mast Cell Stabilizers, Nasal

sodium cromoglycate

Antihistamine/Decongestant Combinations, Oral

cetirizine/pseudoephedrine
fexofenadine/pseudoephedrine
loratadine/pseudoephedrine
triprolidine/pseudoephedrine

Rhinitis, Viral

see also Rhinorrhea

Decongestants, Oral

phenylephrine hydrochloride
pseudoephedrine hydrochloride

Decongestants, Topical

oxymetazoline
phenylephrine hydrochloride
xylometazoline

Rhinorrhea

see also Congestion, Respiratory

Anticholinergic Agent, Oral

ipratropium bromide

Rosacea

Antibiotics, Ophthalmic

fusidic acid

Antibiotics, Oral

Macrolides

erythromycin

Tetracyclines

doxycycline hyclate
minocycline
tetracycline

Antibiotics, Topical

azelaic acid
metronidazole

Retinoids, Oral

isotretinoin

Rotavirus Gastroenteritis Prevention

Vaccines

rotavirus vaccine, human, live oral attenuated
rotavirus vaccine, live oral pentavalent

Salmonella typhi Infection Prevention

Bacterial Vaccines

salmonella typhi Vi capsular polysaccharide vaccine

Scabies

crotamiton
lindane (gamma benzene hexachloride)
permethrin
sulfur

Scars

collagen
polysiloxane dioxide

Seasonal Affective Disorder

Antidepressants

bupropion hydrochloride

Sepsis

Activated Protein C

drotrecogin alfa (activated)

Aminoglycosides

amikacin sulfate
gentamicin sulfate
tobramycin sulfate

Carbapenems

imipenem/cilastatin sodium
meropenem

Cephalosporins

Cephalosporins, 3rd Generation

cefotaxime sodium
ceftazidime
ceftriaxone sodium

Cephalosporins, 4th Generation

cefepime hydrochloride

Cyclic Lipopeptides

daptomycin

Fluoroquinolones

ciprofloxacin
levofloxacin
moxifloxacin hydrochloride

Glycopeptides

vancomycin hydrochloride

Glycylcyclines

tigecycline

Lincosamides

clindamycin hydrochloride

Macrolides

azithromycin dihydrate

Nitroimidazoles

metronidazole

Oxazolidinones

linezolid

Penicillins

Penicillins, β-lactamase Inhibitor Combinations

piperacillin sodium/tazobactam sodium
ticarcillin disodium/clavulanate potassium

Sinusitis

Cephalosporins

Cephalosporins, 2nd Generation

cefprozil
cefuroxime axetil
cefuroxime sodium

Cephalosporins, 3rd Generation

cefixime

Corticosteroids, Nasal

mometasone furoate monohydrate

Decongestants, Nasal

oxymetazoline
phenylephrine
xylometazoline

Decongestants, Systemic

pseudoephedrine hydrochloride

Fluoroquinolones

ciprofloxacin
ciprofloxacin hydrochloride
levofloxacin
moxifloxacin hydrochloride

Lincosamides

clindamycin hydrochloride
clindamycin palmitate hydrochloride

Macrolides

azithromycin
clarithromycin

Penicillins

Aminopenicillins

amoxicillin trihydrate

Penicillins, β-lactamase Inhibitors

amoxicillin trihydrate/clavulanate potassium

Sulfonamide Combinations

sulfamethoxazole/trimethoprim

Tetracyclines

doxycycline hyclate
minocycline hydrochloride

Sleep Disorders

see also Insomnia and Sedation; Narcolepsy

CNS Stimulants

modafinil

Smoking Cessation

Antidepressants

bupropion hydrochloride

Nicotine Receptor Partial Agonists

varenicline tartrate

Nicotine Replacement Therapy

Nicotine Gum

nicotine polacrilex

Nicotine Inhaler

nicotine

Nicotine Lozenge

nicotine polacrilex

Nicotine Transdermal

nicotine

Snake Venom Poisoning

Immune Sera

crotalid antivenin, polyvalent (equine)

Social Anxiety Disorder

Monoamine Oxidase Inhibitors (MAOIs)

moclobemide

Selective Serotonin Reuptake Inhibitors (SSRIs)

citalopram hydrobromide
fluvoxamine maleate
fluoxetine hydrochloride
paroxetine
sertraline hydrochloride

Serotonin-Norepinephrine Reuptake Inhibitors (SNRIs)

venlafaxine hydrochloride

Status Epilepticus

diazepam
lorazepam
midazolam
phenobarbital
phenytoin
propofol

Strabismus

botulinum toxin type A

Streptococcal Pharyngitis

Cephalosporins

Cephalosporins, 1st Generation

cefadroxil
cephalexin

Cephalosporins, 2nd Generation

cefprozil
cefuroxime axetil

Cephalosporins, 3rd Generation

cefixime

Lincosamides

clindamycin hydrochloride

Macrolides

azithromycin dihydrate
clarithromycin
erythromycin estolate
erythromycin ethylsuccinate

Penicillins

Aminopenicillins

amoxicillin trihydrate

Penicillins, Penicillinase-Susceptible

penicillin V

Penicillins, β-lactamase Inhibitor Combinations

amoxicillin trihydrate/clavulanate potassium

Streptococcus pneumoniae Infection Prevention

Bacterial Vaccines

pneumococcal 7-valent conjugate vaccine (diphtheria CRM197 protein)
pneumococcal 10-valent conjugate vaccine
pneumococcal 13-valent conjugate vaccine (diphtheria CRM197 protein)
pneumococcal polysaccharide vaccine, polyvalent

Subacute Sclerosing Panencephalitis

inosine pranobex

Subarachnoid Hemorrhage

Calcium Channel Blocking Agents

nimodipine

Sunburn Prevention

Physical Agents

titanium dioxide
zinc oxide

UVA Absorbers (broad spectrum)

butyl methoxydibenzoylmethane (Parsol 1789)
dioxybenzone (benzophenone-8)
menthyl anthranilate
oxybenzone (benzophenone-3)
terephthalylidene dicamphor sulfonic acid (Mexoryl SX)

UVB Absorbers (narrow spectrum)

ethoxyethyl p-methoxycinnamate (Cinoxate)
homosalate (homomenthyl salicylate)
methylbenzylidene camphor (Parsol 5000)
octocrylene
octyl dimethyl PABA (Padimate O)
octyl methoxycinnamate (Parsol MCX) (octinoxate)
octyl salicylate (octisalate)
phenylbenzimidazole sulfonic acid (Parsol HS)
triethanolamine salicylate

Supraventricular Tachyarrhythmias

see also Arrhythmias

Beta-adrenergic Blocking Agents

Nonselective without Intrinsic Sympathomimetic Activity (ISA)

nadolol
propranolol

Selective without ISA

atenolol
metoprolol

Calcium Channel Blockers

Nondihydropyridines

diltiazem
verapamil

Inotropes

Cardiac Glycosides

digoxin

Syphilis

doxycycline hyclate
penicillin G
penicillin G benzathine

Teething

Analgesics, Oral

acetaminophen
ibuprofen

Anesthetics, Topical

benzocaine

Tetanus Immunization

see also Diphtheria, Tetanus and Pertussis Prevention; Diphtheria, Tetanus and Poliomyelitis Prevention; Diphtheria, Tetanus, Pertussis and Poliomyelitis Prevention; Diphtheria, Tetanus, Pertussis, Poliomyelitis and Haemophilus Type b Prevention; Diphtheria, Tetanus, Pertussis, Poliomyelitis, Haemophilus Type b and Hepatitis B Prevention

Immune Globulins, Specific

tetanus immune globulin (human)

Toxoids

tetanus toxoid, adsorbed

Thrombocythemia

Antiplatelet Agents

anagrelide hydrochloride

Thrombolysis

Plasminogen Activators

Natural Enzymes

urokinase

Proteins, Derived from Bacteria

reteplase
streptokinase

Proteins, Recombinant DNA Origin

alteplase
anistreplase
tenecteplase

Thyroid Storm

Antithyroid Agents

methimazole
propylthiouracil

Beta-adrenergic Blocking Agents

propranolol

Corticosteroids

dexamethasone

Iodine Preparations

iodine

Tick-borne Encephalitis

tick-borne encephalitis virus vaccine, inactivated

Toothache

see also Pain

Anesthetics, Topical

benzocaine

Toxoplasma gondii Prophylaxis

dapsone
sulfamethoxazole/trimethoprim

Toxoplasma gondii Treatment

pyrimethamine
sulfadiazine
sulfamethoxazole/trimethoprim

Traveller's Diarrhea and Cholera Prevention

traveller's diarrhea and cholera vaccine (oral, inactivated)

Traveller's Diarrhea Treatment

Antibiotics

Fluoroquinolones

ciprofloxacin hydrochloride
norfloxacin
ofloxacin

Glycopeptides

vancomycin hydrochloride

Macrolides

azithromycin

Nitroimidazoles

metronidazole

Sulfonamide Combinations

sulfamethoxazole/trimethoprim

Tetracyclines

doxycycline hyclate

Antiperistaltics

loperamide hydrochloride

Intestinal Adsorbants

bismuth subsalicylate

Trichomonas Infection

Nitroimidazoles

metronidazole

Tuberculosis Prevention

Vaccines

bacillus Calmette-Guérin (BCG) vaccine (live, attenuated)

Tuberculosis Prophylaxis

isoniazid
rifampin

Tuberculosis Treatment

Aminoglycosides

streptomycin

Antimycobacterial Agents

ethambutol hydrochloride
pyrazinamide

Combination Agents

isoniazid/pyrazinamide/rifampin

Fluoroquinolones

levofloxacin
moxifloxacin hydrochloride
ofloxacin

Hydrazides

isoniazid

Rifamycins

rifabutin
rifampin

Typhoid Infection Prevention

Bacterial Vaccines

typhoid vaccine Ty21a (live, oral, attenuated)

Upper Gastrointestinal Bleeding

see also Bleeding Esophageal Varices

Proton Pump Inhibitors

pantoprazole magnesium
pantoprazole sodium

Urinary Incontinence, Children

Anticholinergics

oxybutynin chloride
tolterodine L-tartrate extended release

Antidiuretic Hormone Analogues, Oral

desmopressin acetate

Urinary Incontinence, Urge

Anticholinergics

darifenacin hydrobromide
hyoscine butylbromide
oxybutynin chloride
solifenacin succinate
tolterodine L-tartrate
trospium chloride

Smooth Muscle Relaxants

flavoxate hydrochloride

Urinary Retention

Parasympathomimetic Agents

bethanechol

Urinary Tract Infection

Aminoglycosides

amikacin sulfate
gentamicin sulfate
tobramycin sulfate

Carbapenems

doripenem

Cephalosporins

Cephalosporins, 1st Generation

cefazolin sodium
cephalexin

Cephalosporins, 2nd Generation

cefaclor
cefuroxime axetil
cefuroxime sodium

Cephalosporins, 3rd Generation

cefixime
cefotaxime sodium
ceftazidime
ceftazidime pentahydrate
ceftriaxone sodium

Folate Antagonists

trimethoprim

Methenamine Salts

methenamine (hexamine)
methenamine mandelate

Nitrofuran Derivatives

nitrofurantoin

Penicillins

Aminopenicillins

amoxicillin trihydrate
ampicillin

Penicillins, Antipseudomonal

piperacillin sodium

Penicillins, β-lactamase Inhibitor Combinations

amoxicillin trihydrate/clavulanate potassium
ticarcillin disodium/clavulanate potassium

Quinolones and Fluoroquinolones

ciprofloxacin
ciprofloxacin hydrochloride
levofloxacin
norfloxacin
ofloxacin

Sulfonamide Combinations

sulfamethoxazole/trimethoprim

Vaginal Dryness

polycarbophil gel/water
polyglyceryl methacrylate/propylene glycol

Vaginitis, Non-Specific

see also Bacterial Vaginosis; Infections, Fungal (Vaginal)

Probiotics

lactobacillus bulgaricus/lactobacillus rhamnosus/streptococcus thermophilus

Varicella Virus Infection Prevention

see also Measles, Mumps, Rubella and Varicella Prevention

Viral Vaccines

varicella virus vaccine

Varicella Virus Infection Prevention, Post-exposure

Immune Globulins

varicella zoster immune globulin

Varicose Veins

Sclerosing Agents for Local Injection

sodium tetradecyl sulfate

Venous Thromboembolism Prophylaxis

Factor Xa Inhibitors, Direct

rivaroxaban

Factor Xa Inhibitors, Indirect

fondaparinux sodium

Heparinoids

danaparoid

Heparins

Heparins, Low Molecular Weight (LMWH)

dalteparin sodium
enoxaparin sodium
nadroparin calcium
tinzaparin sodium

Heparins, Unfractionated

heparin sodium

Thrombin Inhibitor, Direct

dabigatran

Vitamin K Antagonists

nicoumalone
warfarin

Venous Thromboembolism Treatment

see also Thrombolysis

Factor Xa Inhibitors, Indirect

fondaparinux sodium

Heparins

Heparins, Low Molecular Weight (LMWH)

dalteparin sodium
enoxaparin sodium
nadroparin calcium
tinzaparin sodium

Heparins, Unfractionated

heparin sodium

Vitamin K Antagonists

nicoumalone
warfarin

Vertigo

see also Nausea and Vomiting

Anticholinergics

scopolamine

Antihistamines

dimenhydrinate
promethazine

Histamine H_1 Agonists

betahistine

Piperazines

flunarizine
meclizine

Vitamin Supplementation

Vitamin A

vitamin A (beta-carotene)
vitamin A (retinol)

Vitamin B

vitamin B_1 (thiamine)
vitamin B_2 (riboflavin)
vitamin B_3 (niacin, niacinamide)
vitamin B_5 (pantothenic acid, calcium pantothenate)
vitamin B_6 (pyridoxine)
vitamin B_9 (folic acid)
vitamin B_{12} (cyanocobalamin, hydroxocobalamin)

Vitamin C

vitamin C (ascorbic acid)

Vitamin D Analogues

Vitamin D Analogues, Various

dihydrotachysterol
doxercalciferol

Vitamin D_2 Analogues

ergocalciferol (calciferol)

Vitamin D_3 Analogues

alfacalcidol
calcitriol
cholecalciferol
paricalcitol

Vitamin E

Tocopherol

alpha tocopherol

Vitamin K Analogues

phytonadione

Vitiligo

methoxsalen

Von Willebrand's Disease Type 1

Antidiuretic Hormone Analogues

desmopressin acetate

Blood Coagulation Factors

antihemophilic factor von Willebrand factor complex

Warts

see also Anogenital Warts
cantharidin
imiquimod
podofilox
podophyllum resin
salicylic acid

Wernicke's Encephalopathy

thiamine

Wilson's Disease

penicillamine

Worm Infestations

Anthelmintics

mebendazole
praziquantel
pyrantel pamoate

Wounds and Skin Ulcers

Debriding Agents

Proteolytic Enzymes

collagenase

Hyperosmotics

magnesium sulfate

Medicated Dressings

framycetin sulfate
povidone/iodine
sodium fusidate

Other Wound Agents

collagen

Wound Healing Agents

Growth Factor

becaplermin

Starch Polymer

cadexomer iodine

Yellow Fever Prevention

Viral Vaccines

yellow fever vaccine (live 17D virus)

Product Identification

About Product Identification

This section contains full-color reproductions of products selected for inclusion by manufacturers. For further information on products listed in this section, readers are encouraged to consult the *CPS* Monograph section (white pages).

The Drug Identification Number (DIN) and the Natural Product Number (NPN) are shown when provided by the manufacturer. The identification number is an eight-digit number assigned to each drug product marketed under the Food and Drug Regulations, Health Canada.

When comparing actual drug dosage forms on hand with the reproductions in this section, the following points should be borne in mind:

i. Color: Colors vary considerably according to the light in which the product is viewed. Colors may also vary from batch to batch of the manufactured product. The color and texture of certain products are sensitive to light and moisture; even those which are relatively stable may undergo color changes during storage.

ii. Markings: Very small or faint markings may not be clearly visible on the reproduction owing to the limitations of the printing process. Certain types of markings, particularly those on sugar-coated tablets, come off very easily when handled–this should be taken into account when examining tablets which have been in the possession of a patient.

iii. Size: Unless otherwise noted, all solid dosage forms reproduced in this section are actual size, but allowance must be made for the angle of perspective in certain cases. Refer to the Monograph section (white pages) where drug identification, in many cases, is facilitated by the "word picture" of the various dosage forms as supplied by the manufacturer.

iv. Not all dosage forms of products have necessarily been chosen for reproduction in this section by the participating manufacturers. The product monographs of the Monograph section (white pages) should be consulted for information relative to the range of product dosage forms available.

This section is made possible through the participation in *CPS* of the manufacturers whose products appear in it.

Online Updates

New and revised full-color reproductions of product images received by the publisher after the print deadlines are published in e-CPS, CPhA's online *CPS*. e-CPS is updated bi-weekly. For more information or to subscribe to e-CPS, visit www.pharmacists.ca/e-CPS.

How to Use the Product Identification Section

Product images in this section are arranged in order by color, size and shape. The page number as well as the vertical and horizontal bar code of each product's entry appear in the index of this section. Use letters A, B, C, D, E on the horizontal bar and numbers 1 to 8 on the vertical bar to locate illustrated products.

	Page	Code
Angeliq® Tablet	I19	D6
Ansaid® 50 mg Tablet	I13	A2
Ansaid® 100 mg Tablet	I26	C4
Anzemet® 50 mg Tablet	I21	E3
Anzemet® 100 mg Tablet	I23	D1
Aptivus® 250 mg Capsule	I29	E6
Arava® 10 mg Tablet	I9	D3
Arava® 20 mg Tablet	I16	C6
Arava® 100 mg Tablet	I10	D5
Aredia® 30 mg Vial	I33	B1
Aredia® 90 mg Vial	I32	E7
Aricept™ 5 mg Tablet	I9	E3
Aricept™ 10 mg Tablet	I16	B3
Aricept RDT™ 5 mg Tablet	I11	D3
Aricept RDT™ 10 mg Tablet	I16	D4
Arimidex® 1 mg Tablet	I8	B8
Aromasin™ 25 mg Tablet	I8	E2
Arthrotec® 50 mg Tablet	I11	A4
Arthrotec® 75 mg Tablet	I11	E6
Asacol® 400 mg Tablet	I24	D4
Asacol® 800 mg Tablet	I24	E4
Aspirin® 81 mg Tablet	I25	A7
Aspirin® 325 mg Caplet	I14	B8
Aspirin® 325 mg Tablet	I11	B1
Aspirin® Arthritis Pain Relief 325 mg Caplet	I16	D7
Aspirin® Arthritis Pain Relief Extra Strength 500 mg Caplet	I16	E8
Aspirin® Extra Strength 500 mg Tablet	I11	B5
Aspirin® Stomach Guard™ with Calcium Carbonate 325 mg Tablet	I11	A5
Aspirin® Stomach Guard™ with Calcium Carbonate 500 mg Caplet	I15	E4
Atacand® 4 mg Tablet	I9	C1
Atacand® 8 mg Tablet	I19	E8
Atacand® 16 mg Tablet	I20	A1
Atacand® 32 mg Tablet	I20	C2
Atacand® Plus 16 mg/12.5 mg Tablet	I20	B4
Atacand® Plus 32 mg/12.5 mg Tablet	I18	E3
Atacand® Plus 32 mg/25 mg Tablet	I20	C4
Atasol® 325 mg Tablet	I10	B8
Atasol® 500 mg Caplet	I14	D1
Atasol® 500 mg Tablet	I12	A3
Atasol®-8 Tablet	I20	A3
Atasol®-15 Tablet	I16	C4
Atasol®-30 Tablet	I25	A3
Ativan® 0.5 mg Sublingual Tablet	I24	D8
Ativan® 0.5 mg Tablet	I8	A2
Ativan® 1 mg Sublingual Tablet	I8	A1
Ativan® 1 mg Tablet	I14	A2
Ativan® 2 mg Sublingual Tablet	I25	A5
Ativan® 2 mg Tablet	I12	A6
Atrovent® HFA 20 µg Inhalation Aerosol	I36	B7
Avalide® 150/12.5 mg Tablet	I20	D6
Avalide® 300/12.5 mg Tablet	I21	D1
Avalide® 300/25 mg Tablet	I23	B4
Avamys® 27.5 µg Nasal Spray	I34	A7
Avandamet® 1 mg/500 mg Tablet	I18	D4
Avandamet® 2 mg/500 mg Tablet	I23	B1
Avandamet® 2 mg/1000 mg Tablet	I18	E6
Avandamet® 4 mg/500 mg Tablet	I20	C6
Avandamet® 4 mg/1000 mg Tablet	I23	A5
Avandaryl™ 4 mg/1 mg Tablet	I17	E8
Avandaryl™ 4 mg/2 mg Tablet	I19	A3
Avandaryl™ 4 mg/4 mg Tablet	I22	A4
Avandia® 2 mg Tablet	I22	E3
Avandia® 4 mg Tablet	I20	E3
Avandia® 8 mg Tablet	I24	A2
Avapro™ 75 mg Tablet	I12	D7
Avapro™ 150 mg Tablet	I13	B3
Avapro™ 300 mg Tablet	I13	E8
Avelox® 400 mg Tablet	I23	C3
Avodart® 0.5 mg Capsule	I28	D6
Axert™ 6.25 mg Tablet	I8	A4
Axert™ 12.5 mg Tablet	I8	B4
Azilect® 0.5 mg Tablet	I8	D5
Azilect® 1 mg Tablet	I9	C8
B		
Baraclude™ 0.5 mg Tablet	I12	D1
Bellergal® Spacetabs Tablet	I16	B4
Bentylol® 10 mg Tablet	I9	B3
Bentylol® 20 mg Tablet	I9	C3
Besivance™ 0.6 % Ophthalmic Preparation	I35	D1
Betaloc® 50 mg Tablet	I9	C7
Betaloc® 100 mg Tablet	I10	E7
Betaloc® Durules® 200 mg Tablet	I13	C3
Betaseron® Vial	I32	E8
Bezalip® SR 400 mg Tablet	I11	C4
Biaxin BID® 250 mg Tablet	I16	B8
Biaxin BID® 500 mg Tablet	I16	C8
Biaxin® XL 500 mg Tablet	I16	D8
Biltricide® 600 mg Tablet	I15	B7
BiOmega Capsule	I28	A6
Bionet® Lozenge	I11	D8
Biphentin® 10 mg Capsule	I30	A7
Biphentin® 15 mg Capsule	I28	D8
Biphentin® 20 mg Capsule	I28	A3
Biphentin® 30 mg Capsule	I31	D5
Biphentin® 40 mg Capsule	I29	E4
Biphentin® 50 mg Capsule	I30	E4
Biphentin® 60 mg Capsule	I28	C1
Biphentin® 80 mg Capsule	I29	B8
BLES™ Vial	I32	A7
Brevicon® 0.5/35 21 day Tablet	I36	A1
Brevicon® 0.5/35 28 day Tablet	I36	A2
Brevicon® 1/35 21 day Tablet	I36	B1
Brevicon® 1/35 28 day Tablet	I36	B2
Bricanyl® Turbuhaler® 0.5 mg Inhaler Device	I37	D2
Burinex® 1 mg Tablet	I9	E4
Burinex® 5 mg Tablet	I11	D1
Buscopan® 10 mg Tablet	I8	A6
BuTrans® 5 mg Transdermal Patch	I38	A8
BuTrans® 10 mg Transdermal Patch	I38	B8
BuTrans® 20 mg Transdermal Patch	I38	C8
C		
Caduet® 5 mg/10 mg Tablet	I12	C7
Caduet® 5 mg/20 mg Tablet	I13	C1
Caduet® 5 mg/40 mg Tablet	I13	E3
Caduet® 5 mg/80 mg Tablet	I13	B7
Caduet® 10 mg/10 mg Tablet	I26	E1
Caduet® 10 mg/20 mg Tablet	I26	C3
Caduet® 10 mg/40 mg Tablet	I26	D3
Caduet® 10 mg/80 mg Tablet	I26	E3
Cafergot® Tablet	I17	D6
Campral® 333 mg Tablet	I11	A1
Capoten™ 25 mg Tablet	I12	D3
Capoten™ 50 mg Tablet	I12	B8
Cardizem® CD 120 mg Capsule	I31	D3
Cardizem® CD 180 mg Capsule	I31	E3
Cardizem® CD 240 mg Capsule	I31	C4
Cardizem® CD 300 mg Capsule	I32	D3
Cardura-1™ 1 mg Tablet	I9	D1
Cardura-2™ 2 mg Tablet	I14	B4
Casodex® 50 mg Tablet	I8	C8
CeeNU® 10 mg Capsule	I27	D3
CeeNU® 40 mg Capsule	I30	D4
CeeNU® 100 mg Capsule	I30	E5
Ceftin® 125 mg/5 mL Powder for Reconstitution	I37	D5
Ceftin® 250 mg Tablet	I15	A1
Ceftin® 500 mg Tablet	I15	C4
Cefzil™ 250 mg Tablet	I20	D5
Cefzil™ 500 mg Tablet	I14	B1
Celebrex® 100 mg Capsule	I27	B5
Celebrex® 200 mg Capsule	I27	C5
Celexa® 20 mg Tablet	I12	A7
Celexa® 40 mg Tablet	I13	D1
CellCept® 250 mg Capsule	I32	A4
CellCept® 500 mg Tablet	I26	B8
Celsentri® 150 mg Tablet	I26	B5
Celsentri® 300 mg Tablet	I26	C5
Champix® 0.5 mg Tablet	I14	E2
Champix® 1 mg Tablet	I26	A2
Cialis® 10 mg Tablet	I17	C8
Cialis® 20 mg Tablet	I17	D8
Cipralex® 10 mg Tablet	I12	C6
Cipralex® 20 mg Tablet	I13	B2
Cipro® 250 mg Tablet	I16	E4
Cipro® 500 mg Tablet	I15	A5
Cipro® 750 mg Tablet	I15	B5
Cipro® XL™ 500 mg Tablet	I15	A6
Cipro® XL™ 1000 mg Tablet	I15	B6
Claritin® 10 mg Tablet	I12	E5
Claritin® Allergy+Sinus Tablet	I11	A3
Claritin® Allergy+Sinus Extra Strength Caplet	I13	E7
Claritin® Rapid Dissolve 10 mg Tablet	I11	B3
Clarus 10 mg Capsule	I30	B3
Clarus 40 mg Capsule	I30	E3
Clavulin®-200, 200 mg Powder for Reconstitution	I37	B5
Clavulin®-400, 400 mg Powder for Reconstitution	I37	C5
Clavulin®-875, 875 mg Tablet	I15	B4
Climara® 50 Transdermal Patch	I38	C5
Climara® 100 Transdermal Patch	I38	D5
Climara Pro® 45/15 µg Transdermal Patch	I38	E5
Clomid® 50 mg Tablet	I10	D6
Clopixol® 10 mg Tablet	I23	B7
Clopixol® 25 mg Tablet	I23	C7
Clozaril® 25 mg Tablet	I16	C1
Clozaril® 100 mg Tablet	I16	A4
CoActifed® Tablet	I10	A8
Codeine Contin® 50 mg Tablet	I25	E6
Codeine Contin® 100 mg Tablet	I17	D7
Codeine Contin® 150 mg Tablet	I23	C6
Codeine Contin® 200 mg Tablet	I19	A6
COLD-FX® 200 mg Capsule	I31	C6
COLD-FX® 300 mg Capsule	I31	A2
Colestid® 1 g Tablet	I17	B1
Combivir® 150 mg/300 mg Tablet	I15	D2
Comtan® 200 mg Tablet	I19	A5
Concerta® 18 mg Tablet	I18	B1
Concerta® 27 mg Tablet	I15	A8
Concerta® 36 mg Tablet	I14	A3
Concerta® 54 mg Tablet	I24	D3
Copaxone® Prefilled Syringe	I33	E8
Cordarone® 200 mg Tablet	I22	D1
Cortef® 10 mg Tablet	I10	B2
Cortef® 20 mg Tablet	I10	E2
Cotazym® Capsule	I27	A8
Cotazym®-65 B Capsule	I27	E7
Cotazym® ECS 4 Capsule	I29	B6
Cotazym® ECS 8 Capsule	I27	E3
Cotazym® ECS 20 Capsule	I28	E6
Coumadin® 1 mg Tablet	I21	C7
Coumadin® 2 mg Tablet	I26	A7
Coumadin® 2.5 mg Tablet	I25	D2
Coumadin® 3 mg Tablet	I24	C5
Coumadin® 4 mg Tablet	I25	D7
Coumadin® 5 mg Tablet	I20	A2
Coumadin® 6 mg Tablet	I25	C2
Coumadin® 10 mg Tablet	I10	D3
Coversyl® 2 mg Tablet	I8	E1
Coversyl® 4 mg Tablet	I25	A4
Coversyl® 8 mg Tablet	I25	E1
Coversyl® Plus 4 mg/1.25 mg Tablet	I14	C3
Coversyl® Plus HD 8 mg/2.5 mg Tablet	I9	D5
Coversyl® Plus LD 2 mg/0.625 mg Tablet	I14	D2
Cozaar® 25 mg Tablet	I12	B5
Cozaar® 50 mg Tablet	I12	A8
Cozaar® 100 mg Tablet	I13	A4

I

	Page	Code
Imdur® 60 mg Tablet	I18	C4
Imitrex DF™ 50 mg Tablet	I12	B2
Imitrex DF™ 100 mg Tablet	I22	D4
Imitrex® Vial	I32	C6
Imitrex® Kit	I34	A5
Imitrex® Auto-Injector	I34	D4
Imitrex® Prefilled Syringe	I34	E4
Imitrex® 20 mg Nasal Spray	I34	E5
Imovane® 5 mg Tablet	I8	C6
Imovane® 7.5 mg Tablet	I26	B2
Imuran® 50 mg Tablet	I16	E5
Imuran® 50 mg Vial	I32	B7
Inderal®-LA 60 mg Capsule	I30	C8
Inderal®-LA 80 mg Capsule	I31	A3
Inderal®-LA 120 mg Capsule	I31	B3
Inderal®-LA 160 mg Capsule	I31	C3
Influvac® 15 µg/0.5 mL Prefilled Syringe	I34	E3
Intelence™ 100 mg Tablet	I13	D4
Invega™ 3 mg Tablet	I14	D4
Invega™ 6 mg Tablet	I18	B3
Invega™ 9 mg Tablet	I20	D4
Invega® Sustenna™ 50 mg/0.5 mL Prefilled Syringe	I33	A8
Invega® Sustenna™ 75 mg/0.75 mL Prefilled Syringe	I33	B8
Invega® Sustenna™ 100 mg/1 mL Prefilled Syringe	I33	C8
Invega® Sustenna™ 150 mg/1.5 mL Prefilled Syringe	I33	D8
Invirase® 200 mg Capsule	I32	C2
Invirase® 500 mg Tablet	I19	B5
Iressa® 250 mg Tablet	I24	D1
Isentress® 400 mg Tablet	I20	D7
Isoptin® SR 120 mg Tablet	I10	A7
Isoptin® SR 180 mg Tablet	I23	A2
Isoptin® SR 240 mg Tablet	I25	D4

J

	Page	Code
Janumet™ 50 mg/500 mg Tablet	I20	E8
Janumet™ 50 mg/850 mg Tablet	I21	C1
Janumet™ 50 mg/1000 mg Tablet	I24	B8
Januvia® 100 mg Tablet	I17	C7

K

	Page	Code
K-Dur® 20 mmol Tablet	I15	C2
Keppra® 250 mg Tablet	I26	A4
Keppra® 500 mg Tablet	I18	B6
Keppra® 750 mg Tablet	I21	A1
Ketek® 400 mg Tablet	I18	E7
Kivexa® 600 mg/300 mg Tablet	I19	C6

L

	Page	Code
Lamictal® 25 mg Tablet	I12	A1
Lamictal® 100 mg Tablet	I22	D5
Lamictal® 150 mg Tablet	I16	A1
Lamictal® Chewable/Dispersible 2 mg Tablet	I8	D1
Lamictal® Chewable/Dispersible 5 mg Tablet	I14	B3
Lamisil® 250 mg Tablet	I11	D4
Lamisil® Cream	I34	A8
Lamisil® Spray	I34	B5
Lanvis® 40 mg Tablet	I16	A3
Lasix® 20 mg Tablet	I8	E5
Lasix® 40 mg Tablet	I16	C2
Lasix® Special 500 mg Tablet	I16	C5
Lescol® 20 mg Capsule	I32	A1
Lescol® 40 mg Capsule	I32	B1
Lescol® XL 80 mg Tablet	I17	E7
Leukeran® 2 mg Tablet	I24	A5
Levaquin® 250 mg Tablet	I23	E1
Levaquin® 500 mg Tablet	I23	D4
Levaquin® 750 mg Tablet	I15	E5
Levemir® 100 IU Cartridge	I33	A6
Levitra® 5 mg Tablet	I17	E2
Levitra® 10 mg Tablet	I17	B4
Levitra® 20 mg Tablet	I17	B5
Linessa® 21 Tablet	I35	A3
Linessa® 28 Tablet	I35	B3
Lioresal® 10 mg Tablet	I13	A1
Lioresal® D.S. 20 mg Tablet	I15	C3
Lioresal® Intrathecal 0.05 mg/mL Ampul	I33	A4
Lioresal® Intrathecal 0.5 mg/mL Ampul	I33	B4
Lioresal® Intrathecal 2 mg/mL Ampul	I33	C4
Lipidil™ EZ 48 mg Tablet	I18	B4
Lipidil™ EZ 145 mg Tablet	I13	A7
Lipidil Supra® 160 mg Tablet	I14	A1
Lipitor® 10 mg Tablet	I12	E6
Lipitor® 20 mg Tablet	I12	E8
Lipitor® 40 mg Tablet	I13	E4
Lipitor® 80 mg Tablet	I13	D8
Livostin® Nasal Spray	I34	D5
Lomotil® 2.5 mg Tablet	I8	C2
Loniten® 2.5 mg Tablet	I9	D2
Loniten® 10 mg Tablet	I8	C7
Lopid™ 300 mg Capsule	I29	D7
Lopid™ 600 mg Tablet	I14	C1
Lopresor® 50 mg Tablet	I23	C1
Lopresor® SR 100 mg Tablet	I17	E6
Lopresor® SR 200 mg Tablet	I16	C3
Losec® 10 mg Capsule	I29	C5
Losec® 10 mg Tablet	I19	C7
Losec® 20 mg Capsule	I31	C7
Losec® 20 mg Tablet	I23	D7
Lotemax™ 0.5 % Ophthalmic Preparation	I35	E1
Lotensin® 5 mg Tablet	I18	D3
Lotensin® 10 mg Tablet	I19	E3
Lotensin® 20 mg Tablet	I19	A8
Lozide® 1.25 mg Tablet	I19	E1
Lozide® 2.5 mg Tablet	I21	B3
Luvox® 50 mg Tablet	I10	D2
Luvox® 100 mg Tablet	I13	B5
Lyrica™ 25 mg Capsule	I27	A3
Lyrica™ 50 mg Capsule	I27	B3
Lyrica™ 75 mg Capsule	I29	C7
Lyrica™ 150 mg Capsule	I27	C3
Lyrica™ 300 mg Capsule	I29	C8

M

	Page	Code
Malarone® 250 mg/100 mg Tablet	I22	A3
Malarone® Pediatric 62.5 mg/25 mg Tablet	I19	E7
Marinol® 2.5 mg Capsule	I26	D8
Marinol® 5 mg Capsule	I31	D6
Marvelon® 21 day Tablet	I35	C3
Marvelon® 28 day Tablet	I35	D3
Maxalt® 5 mg Tablet	I22	D6
Maxalt® 10 mg Tablet	I22	C8
Maxalt RPD® 5 mg Wafer	I11	C1
Maxalt RPD® 10 mg Wafer	I11	A8
Medrol® 4 mg Tablet	I12	D5
Medrol® 16 mg Tablet	I13	B1
Mepron® Oral Suspension	I37	D7
Mersyndol® with Codeine Tablet	I11	E1
Mesasal® 500 mg Tablet	I19	E5
M-Eslon® 10 mg Capsule	I27	D7
M-Eslon® 15 mg Capsule	I28	B3
M-Eslon® 30 mg Capsule	I29	C4
M-Eslon® 60 mg Capsule	I28	E7
M-Eslon® 100 mg Capsule	I28	B1
M-Eslon® 200 mg Capsule	I29	E7
Mevacor® 20 mg Tablet	I25	C7
Mevacor® 40 mg Tablet	I25	A2
Mezavant® 1.2 g Tablet	I24	A8
Miacalcin® NS Nasal Spray	I34	C5
Micardis® 40 mg Tablet	I14	C7
Micardis® 80 mg Tablet	I15	D1
Micardis® Plus 80 mg/12.5 mg Tablet	I23	C5
Micardis® Plus 80 mg/25 mg Tablet	I18	A7
Micro-K Extencaps® 600 mg Capsule	I28	B7
Micronor® 28 day Tablet	I35	E8
Min-Ovral® 21 Tablet	I36	C3
Min-Ovral® 28 Tablet	I36	D3
Mirapex® 0.125 mg Tablet	I8	B3
Mirapex® 0.25 mg Tablet	I12	E7
Mirapex® 0.5 mg Tablet	I13	D2
Mirapex® 1 mg Tablet	I11	A2
Mirapex® 1.5 mg Tablet	I11	B2
Mirena® Intrauterine System	I36	A5
Mobicox™ 7.5 mg Tablet	I16	B2
Mobicox™ 15 mg Tablet	I16	D2
Modulon® 200 mg Tablet	I11	C6
Monopril™ 10 mg Tablet	I12	B3
Monopril™ 20 mg Tablet	I14	C6
MS Contin® 15 mg Tablet	I25	B1
MS Contin® 30 mg Tablet	I26	C6
MS Contin® 60 mg Tablet	I21	E2
MS Contin® 100 mg Tablet	I15	D7
MS Contin® 200 mg Tablet	I23	A7
MS•IR® 5 mg Tablet	I9	A2
MS•IR® 10 mg Tablet	I10	E1
MS•IR® 20 mg Tablet	I14	D3
MS•IR® 30 mg Tablet	I14	A4
Multaq™ 400 mg Tablet	I15	D3
Mycobutin® 150 mg Capsule	I30	E1
Myfortic® 180 mg Tablet	I25	E2
Myfortic® 360 mg Tablet	I20	D8
Myleran® 2 mg Tablet	I8	D8

N

	Page	Code
Nalcrom® 100 mg Capsule	I27	A4
Natrecor™ 1.5 mg Vial	I32	D6
Neoral® 10 mg Capsule	I26	C8
Neoral® 25 mg Capsule	I28	D1
Neoral® 50 mg Capsule	I27	C7
Neoral® 100 mg Capsule	I28	E1
Neoral® 100 mg Oral Solution	I37	D4
Neurontin® 100 mg Capsule	I27	A2
Neurontin® 300 mg Capsule	I28	A5
Neurontin® 400 mg Capsule	I28	A7
Neurontin® 600 mg Tablet	I13	A8
Neurontin® 800 mg Tablet	I13	B8
Nexavar® 200 mg Tablet	I24	A1
Nexium® 10 mg Powder for Reconstitution	I37	E5
Nexium® 20 mg Tablet	I23	B2
Nexium® 40 mg Tablet	I23	A6
Nimotop® 30 mg Tablet	I17	A8
Nitoman® 25 mg Tablet	I17	D2
Nitro-Dur® 0.2 mg/h Transdermal Patch	I38	A6
Nitro-Dur® 0.4 mg/h Transdermal Patch	I38	B6
Nitro-Dur® 0.6 mg/h Transdermal Patch	I38	C6
Nitro-Dur® 0.8 mg/h Transdermal Patch	I38	D6
Nitrostat™ 0.3 mg Tablet	I8	B1
Nitrostat™ 0.6 mg Tablet	I8	C1
Norvasc™ 5 mg Tablet	I12	E3
Norvasc™ 10 mg Tablet	I12	C4
NovoRapid® 100 IU Cartridge	I33	B6
NuvaRing Vaginal Ring	I36	A4

O

	Page	Code
Ogen® 0.75 mg Tablet	I16	B7
Ogen® 1.5 mg Tablet	I20	A6
Ogen® 3 mg Tablet	I26	B3
Olmetec® 20 mg Tablet	I9	B7
Olmetec® 40 mg Tablet	I14	D7
Olmetec Plus® 20 mg/12.5 mg Tablet	I17	E5
Olmetec Plus® 40 mg/12.5 mg Tablet	I18	E4
Olmetec Plus® 40 mg/25 mg Tablet	I20	A7
Omnaris™ 50 µg Nasal Spray	I34	B6
Onglyza™ 5 mg Tablet	I21	A6
Optomega Liquid	I37	B4
Ortho® 0.5/35 21 day Tablet	I35	C7
Ortho® 0.5/35 28 day Tablet	I35	C8
Ortho® 1/35 21 day Tablet	I35	D7
Ortho® 1/35 28 day Tablet	I35	D8

Use code A, B, C, D, E, horizontal bar and 1 to 8 vertical bar to locate illustrated products

Utiliser le code A, B, C, D, E de la ligne horizontale et les chiffres 1 à 8 de la ligne verticale pour repérer les produits illustrés

	A	B	C	D	E
1	DIN 02041464 TC 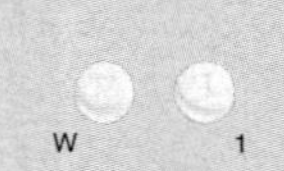 W 1 Ativan® Sublingual 1 mg **Pfizer**	DIN 00037613 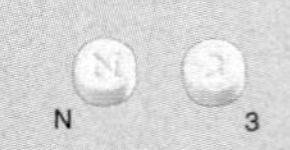 N 3 Nitrostat™ 0.3 mg **Pfizer**	DIN 00037621 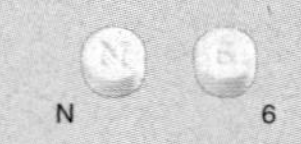 N 6 Nitrostat™ 0.6 mg **Pfizer**	DIN 02243803 Pr 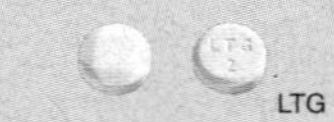 LTG 2 Lamictal® Chewable/Dispersible 2 mg **GlaxoSmithKline**	DIN 02123274 Pr  Coversyl® 2 mg **Servier**
2	DIN 02041413 TC 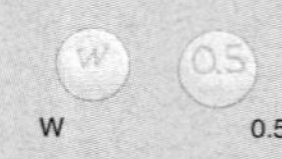 W 0.5 Ativan® 0.5 mg **Pfizer**	DIN 00015741 Pr 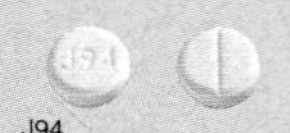 J94 Tapazole® 5 mg **Paladin**	DIN 00036323 Ⓝ 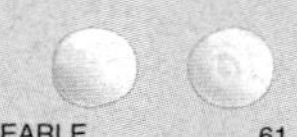 SEARLE 61 Lomotil® 2.5 mg **Pfizer**	DIN 02225190 Pr 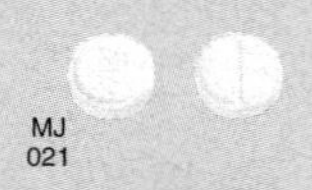 MJ 021 Estrace® 0.5 mg **Shire**	DIN 02242705 Pr 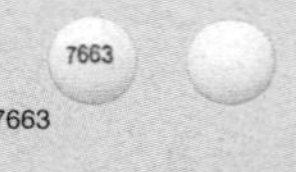 7663 Aromasin™ 25 mg **Pfizer**
3	DIN 02293129 Pr 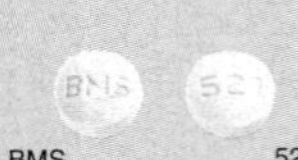 BMS 527 Sprycel™ 20 mg **Bristol-Myers Squibb**	DIN 02297256 Pr 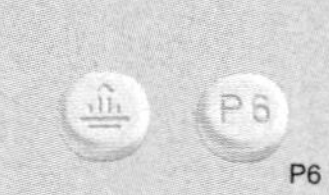 P6 Mirapex® 0.125 mg **Boehringer Ingelheim**	DIN 02224550 Pr 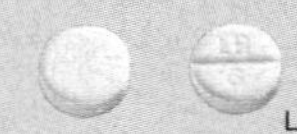 LB G Diabeta® 2.5 mg **sanofi-aventis**	DIN 01916599 Ⓝ 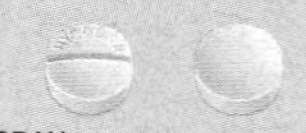 HYCODAN Hycodan® 5 mg **Bristol-Myers Squibb**	DIN 02230893 Pr 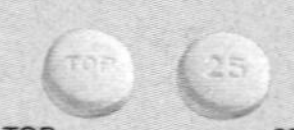 TOP 25 Topamax® 25 mg **Janssen-Ortho**
4	DIN 02248128 Pr 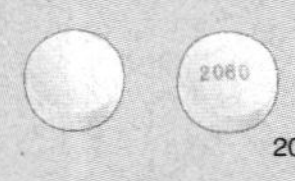 2080 Axert™ 6.25 mg **McNeil Consumer Healthcare**	DIN 02248129 Pr 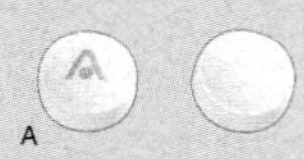 A Axert™ 12.5 mg **McNeil Consumer Healthcare**	DIN 02299194 Pr 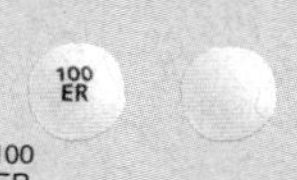 100 ER Ralivia™ 100 mg **Biovail Pharmaceuticals**	DIN 02239064 Pr 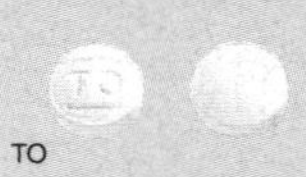 TO Detrol® 1 mg **Pfizer**	DIN 02239065 Pr  DT Detrol® 2 mg **Pfizer**
5	DIN 02269007 Pr 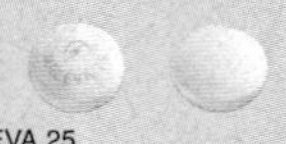 TARCEVA 25 Tarceva® 25 mg **Roche**	DIN 02213192 Pr 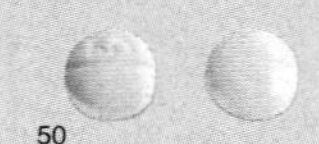 50 Eltroxin® 50 µg **Triton Pharma**	DIN 02086026 Pr 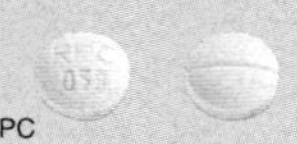 RPC 059 Florinef® 0.1 mg **Paladin**	DIN 02284642 Pr 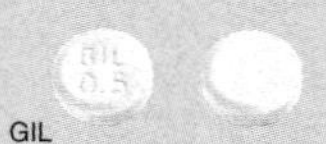 GIL 0.5 Azilect® 0.5 mg **Teva Canada Innovation**	DIN 02224690 Pr 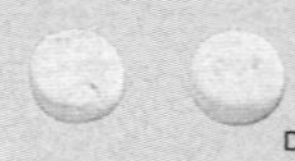 DLF Lasix® 20 mg **sanofi-aventis**
6	DIN 00363812 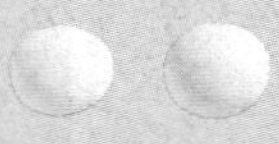 Buscopan® 10 mg **Boehringer Ingelheim**	DIN 02138018 Ⓝ 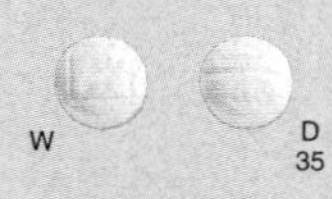 W D 35 Demerol® 50 mg **sanofi-aventis**	DIN 02216167 Pr 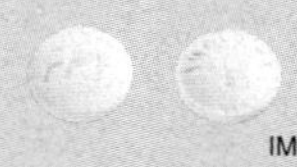 IMOVANE 5 Imovane® 5 mg **sanofi-aventis**	DIN 00010391 Pr 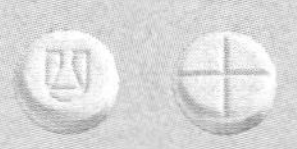 Sintrom® 4 mg **Paladin**	DIN 02229250 Pr 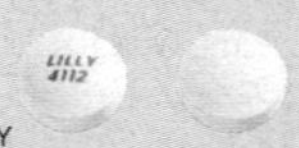 LILLY 4112 Zyprexa® 2.5 mg **Lilly**
7	DIN 00729973 Pr 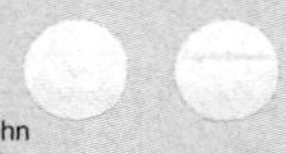 Upjohn 50 Provera® 10 mg **Pfizer**	DIN 02172070 Pr 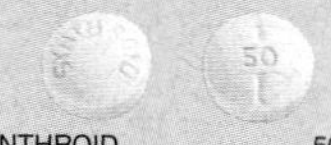 SYNTHROID 50 Synthroid® 50 µg **Abbott**	DIN 00514500 Pr 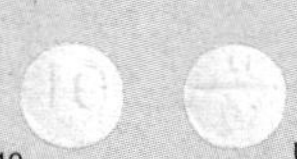 10 U 137 Loniten® 10 mg **Pfizer**	DIN 02296039 Pr 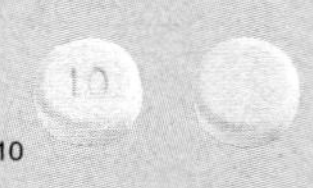 10 Tapazole® 10 mg **Paladin**	DIN 00417270 Pr 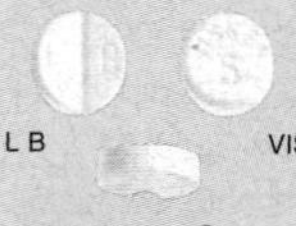 L B VISKEN 5 Visken® 5 mg **Novartis Pharmaceuticals**
8	DIN 02256460 Pr 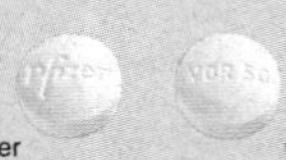 Pfizer VOR 50 Vfend™ 50 mg **Pfizer**	DIN 02224135 Pr 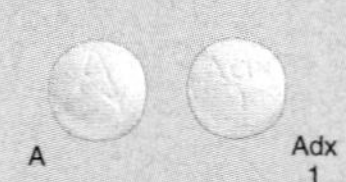 A Adx 1 Arimidex® 1 mg **AstraZeneca**	DIN 02184478 Pr 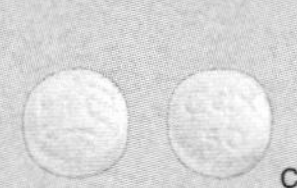 Cdx 50 Casodex® 50 mg **AstraZeneca**	DIN 00004618 Pr 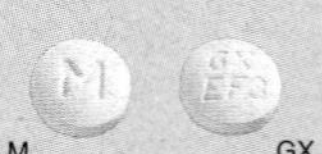 M GX EF3 Myleran® 2 mg **GlaxoSmithKline**	DIN 00004715 Pr 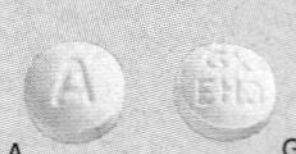 A GX EH3 Alkeran® 2 mg **GlaxoSmithKline**

* ILLUSTRATION LESS THAN ACTUAL SIZE / ILLUSTRATION RÉDUITE

Use code A, B, C, D, E, horizontal bar and 1 to 8 vertical bar to locate illustrated products

Utiliser le code A, B, C, D, E de la ligne horizontale et les chiffres 1 à 8 de la ligne verticale pour repérer les produits illustrés

1

A1 — DIN 02243045 — Pr
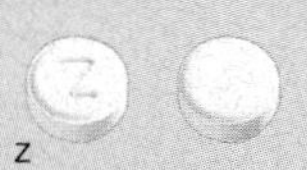
Z
Zomig Rapimelt® 2.5 mg
AstraZeneca

B1 — DIN 02216345 — Pr
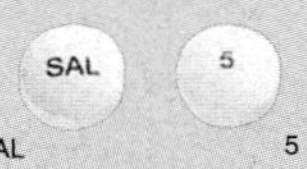
SAL / 5
Salagen® 5 mg
Pfizer

C1 — DIN 02239090 — Pr
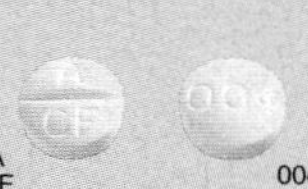
A CF / 004
Atacand® 4 mg
AstraZeneca

D1 — DIN 01958100 — Pr
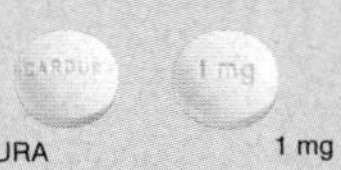
CARDURA / 1 mg
Cardura-1™ 1 mg
Pfizer

E1 — DIN 02279401 — Pr
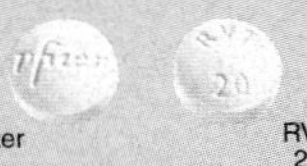
Pfizer / RVT 20
Revatio™ 20 mg
Pfizer

2

A2 — DIN 02014203 — N
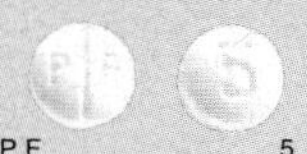
P F / 5
MS•IR® 5 mg
Purdue Pharma

B2 — DIN 02242572 — Pr
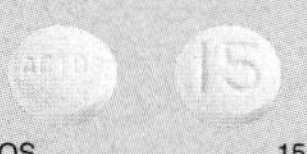
ACTOS / 15
Actos® 15 mg
Takeda Canada

C2 — DIN 02242573 — Pr
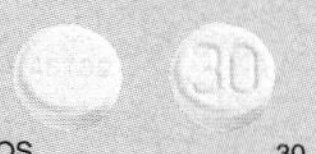
ACTOS / 30
Actos® 30 mg
Takeda Canada

D2 — DIN 00514497 — Pr
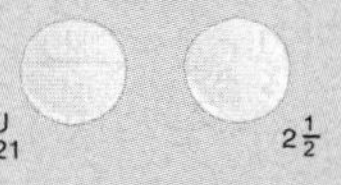
U 121 / 2½
Loniten® 2.5 mg
Pfizer

E2 — DIN 01926624 — Pr
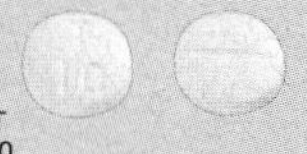
T 10
Tamofen® 10 mg
sanofi-aventis

3

A3 — DIN 02221861 — Pr
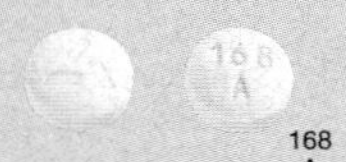
168 A
Anandron® 50 mg
sanofi-aventis

B3 — DIN 02103087
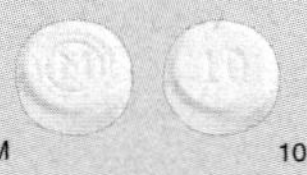
M / 10
Bentylol® 10 mg
Axcan Pharma

C3 — DIN 02103095
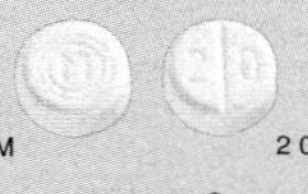
M / 2 0
Bentylol® 20 mg
Axcan Pharma

D3 — DIN 02241888 — Pr
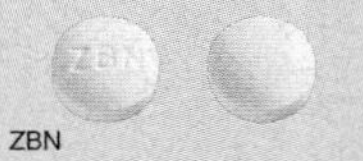
ZBN
Arava® 10 mg
sanofi-aventis

E3 — DIN 02232043 — Pr
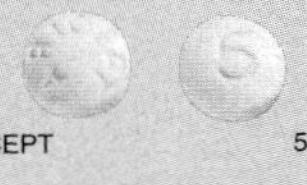
ARICEPT / 5
Aricept™ 5 mg
Pfizer

4

A4 — DIN 00632775 — C
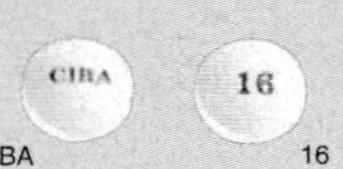
CIBA / 16
Ritalin® SR 20 mg
Novartis Pharmaceuticals

B4 — DIN 02202441 — N
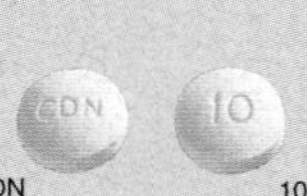
CDN / 10
OxyContin® 10 mg
Purdue Pharma

C4 — DIN 02229110 — Pr
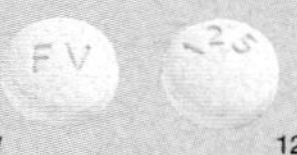
FV / 125
Famvir® 125 mg
Novartis Pharmaceuticals

D4 — DIN 00443948 — N
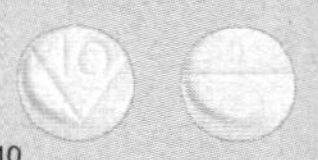
10 V
Supeudol® 10 mg
Sandoz

E4 — DIN 00728284 — Pr
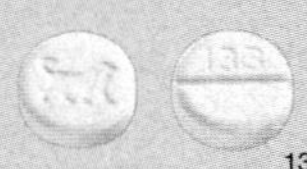
133
Burinex® 1 mg
LEO Pharma

5

A5 — DIN 02257084 — Pr
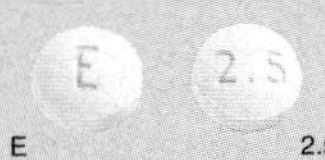
E / 2.5
Frova® 2.5 mg
Teva Canada Innovation

B5 — DIN 02231934 — N
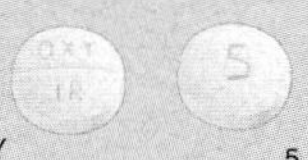
OXY IR / 5
Oxy•IR® 5 mg
Purdue Pharma

C5 — DIN 02275090 — Pr
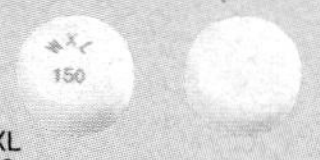
WXL 150
Wellbutrin® XL 150 mg
Biovail Pharmaceuticals

D5 — DIN 02321653 — Pr

Coversyl® Plus HD 8 mg/2.5 mg
Servier

E5 — DIN 02190885 — Pr
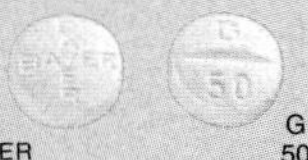
B A BAYER E R / G 50
Glucobay™ 50 mg
Bayer

6

A6 — DIN 02322412 — Pr
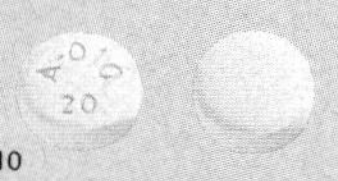
A-010 20
Abilify™ 20 mg
Bristol-Myers Squibb

B6 — DIN 00004774 — Pr
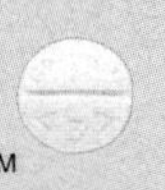
DARAPRIM A3A
Daraprim® 25 mg
GlaxoSmithKline

C6 — DIN 02299208 — Pr
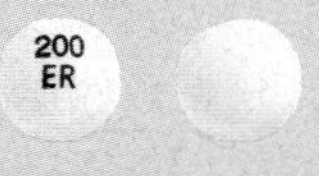
200 ER
Ralivia™ 200 mg
Biovail Pharmaceuticals

D6 — DIN 02049961 — Pr
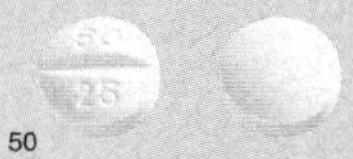
50 25
Tenoretic® 50 mg/25 mg
AstraZeneca

E6 — DIN 00443174 — Pr
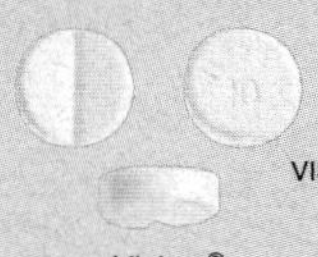
VISKEN 10
Visken® 10 mg
Novartis Pharmaceuticals

7

A7 — DIN 01926632 — Pr

T 20
Tamofen® 20 mg
sanofi-aventis

B7 — DIN 02318660 — Pr
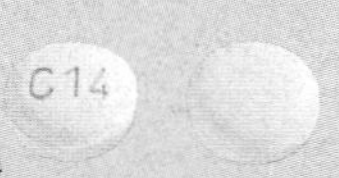
C14
Olmetec® 20 mg
Schering-Plough

C7 — DIN 00402605 — Pr
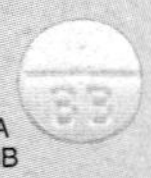
A BB
Betaloc® 50 mg
AstraZeneca

D7 — DIN 02039532 — Pr
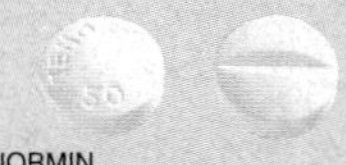
TENORMIN 50
Tenormin® 50 mg
AstraZeneca

E7 — DIN 02236606 — Pr
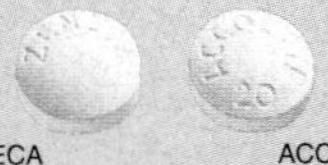
ZENECA / ACCOLATE 20
Accolate® 20 mg
AstraZeneca

8

A8 — DIN 00893722 — Pr
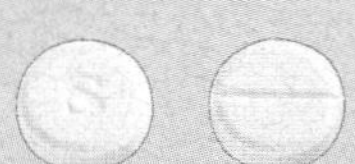
S
Serophene® 50 mg
EMD Canada

B8 — DIN 02045737 — Pr
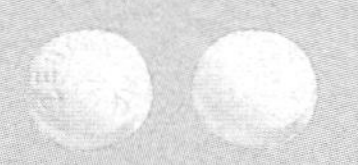
ZESTORETIC
Zestoretic® 20/12.5 mg
AstraZeneca

C8 — DIN 02284650 — Pr
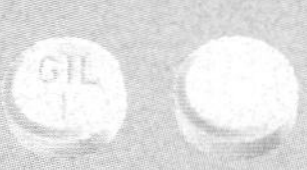
GIL 1
Azilect® 1 mg
Teva Canada Innovation

D8 — DIN 00765996 — Pr
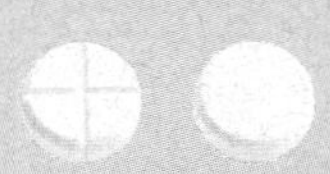
Diamicron® 80 mg
Servier

E8 — DIN 00030945 — Pr

U 467
Provera® 100 mg
Pfizer

* ILLUSTRATION LESS THAN ACTUAL SIZE / ILLUSTRATION RÉDUITE

Use code A, B, C, D, E, horizontal bar and 1 to 8 vertical bar to locate illustrated products

Utiliser le code A, B, C, D, E de la ligne horizontale et les chiffres 1 à 8 de la ligne verticale pour repérer les produits illustrés

	A	B	C	D	E
1	DIN 02229269 Pr 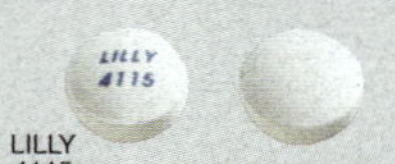 LILLY 4115 Zyprexa® 5 mg **Lilly**	DIN 00704431 Pr 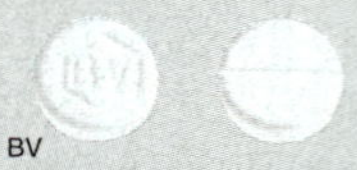 BV Androcur® 50 mg **Bayer**	DIN 02273217 Pr 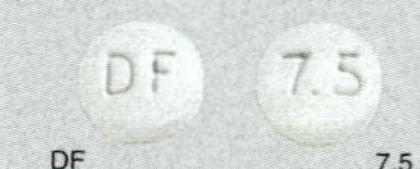 DF 7.5 Enablex® 7.5 mg **Novartis Pharmaceuticals**	DIN 02137984 (N) 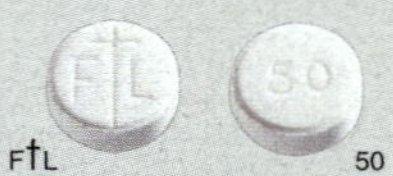 F†L 50 Talwin® 50 mg **sanofi-aventis**	DIN 02014211 (N) 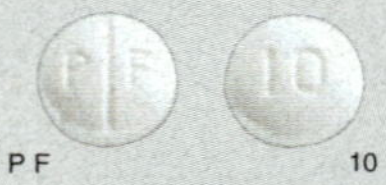 P F 10 MS•IR® 10 mg **Purdue Pharma**
2	DIN 02242574 Pr 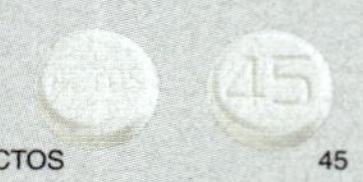 ACTOS 45 Actos® 45 mg **Takeda Canada**	DIN 00030910 Pr 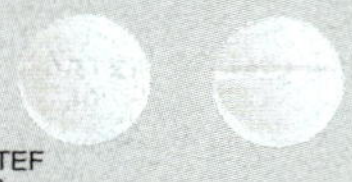 CORTEF 10 Cortef® 10 mg **Pfizer**	DIN 02239372 Pr 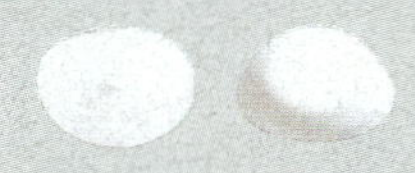 Zofran® ODT 4 mg **GlaxoSmithKline**	DIN 01919342 Pr 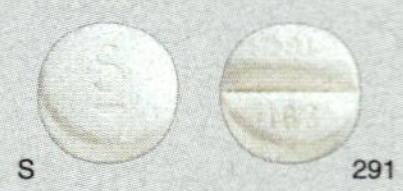 S 291 Luvox® 50 mg **Abbott Products**	DIN 00030929 Pr 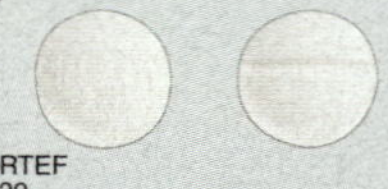 CORTEF 20 Cortef® 20 mg **Pfizer**
3	DIN 02229277 Pr 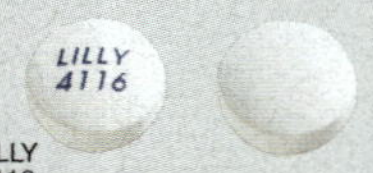 LILLY 4116 Zyprexa® 7.5 mg **Lilly**	DIN 02296381 Pr 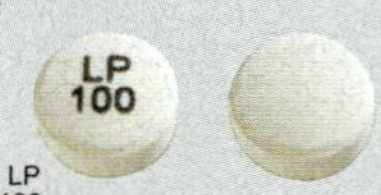 LP 100 Tridural® 100 mg **Labopharm**	DIN 02299216 Pr 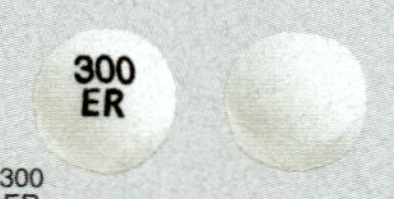 300 ER Ralivia™ 300 mg **Biovail Pharmaceuticals**	DIN 01918362 Pr 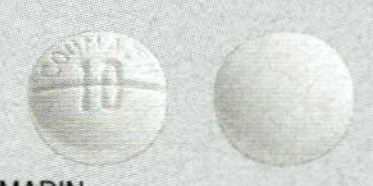 COUMADIN 10 Coumadin® 10 mg **Bristol-Myers Squibb**	DIN 00417289 Pr 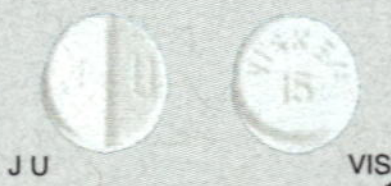 J U VISKEN 15 Visken® 15 mg **Novartis Pharmaceuticals**
4	DIN 02269015 Pr 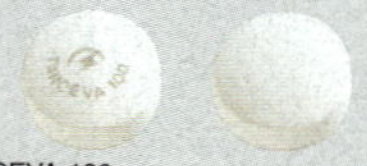 TARCEVA 100 Tarceva® 100 mg **Roche**	DIN 02293145 Pr 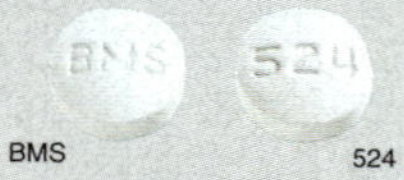 BMS 524 Sprycel™ 70 mg **Bristol-Myers Squibb**	DIN 02243878 Pr 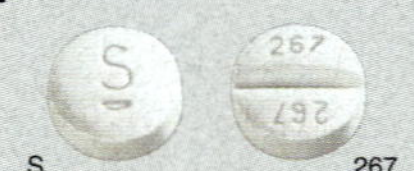 S 267 Serc® 16 mg **Abbott Products**	DIN 00010405 Pr 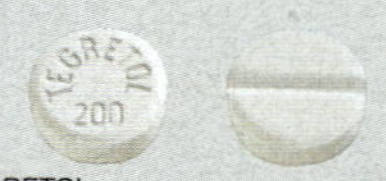 TEGRETOL 200 Tegretol® 200 mg **Novartis Pharmaceuticals**	DIN 02239170 Pr 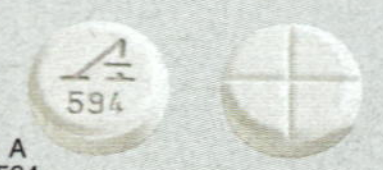 A 594 Zanaflex® 4 mg **Paladin**
5	DIN 00603708 Pr 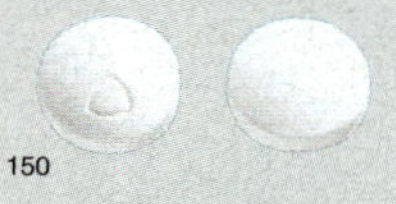 150 Rythmol® 150 mg **Abbott**	DIN 02049988 Pr 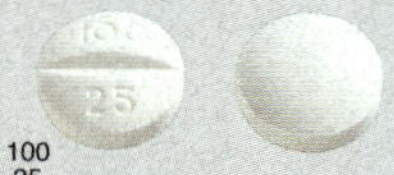 100 25 Tenoretic® 100 mg/25 mg **AstraZeneca**	DIN 02275104 Pr 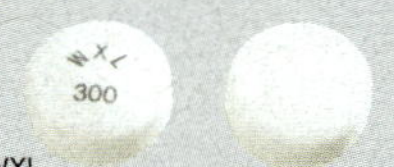 WXL 300 Wellbutrin® XL 300 mg **Biovail Pharmaceuticals**	DIN 02241890 Pr 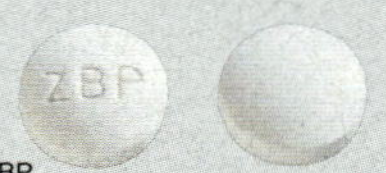 ZBP Arava® 100 mg **sanofi-aventis**	DIN 02190893 Pr 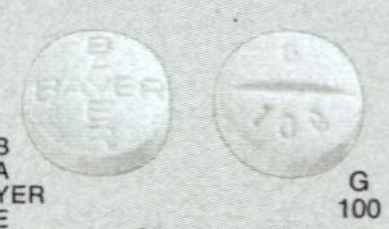 B A BAYER E R G 100 Glucobay™ 100 mg **Bayer**
6	DIN 02239665 Pr 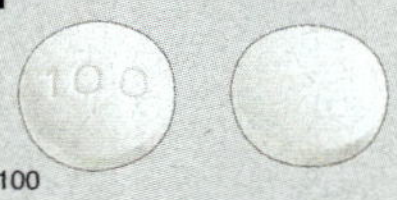 100 Alertec® 100 mg **Shire**	DIN 00369810 Pr 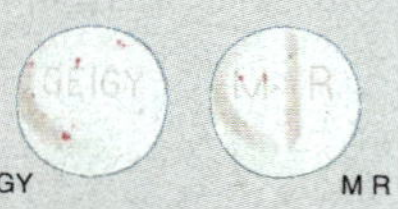 GEIGY M R Tegretol® 100 mg **Novartis Pharmaceuticals**	DIN 01947931 Pr 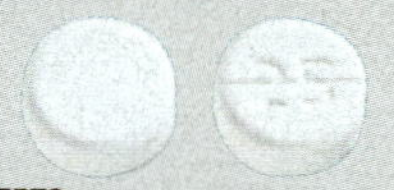 ROBERTS 102 25 Duvoid® 25 mg **Paladin**	DIN 02091879 Pr 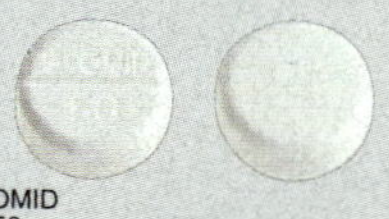 CLOMID 50 Clomid® 50 mg **sanofi-aventis**	DIN 02229285 Pr 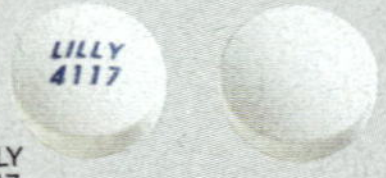 LILLY 4117 Zyprexa® 10 mg **Lilly**
7	DIN 01907123 Pr 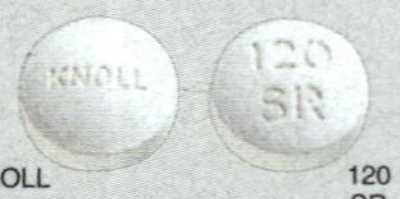 KNOLL 120 SR Isoptin® SR 120 mg **Abbott**	DIN 02296403 Pr 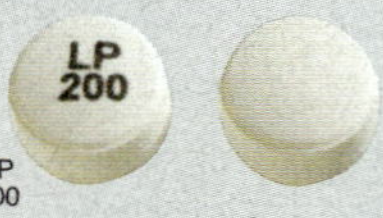 LP 200 Tridural® 200 mg **Labopharm**	DIN 02248542 Pr 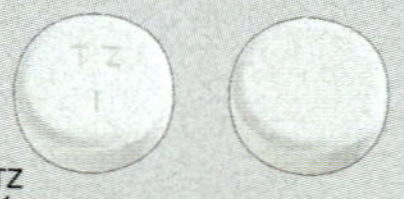 TZ 1 Remeron RD® 15 mg **Schering-Plough**	DIN 02212331 Pr 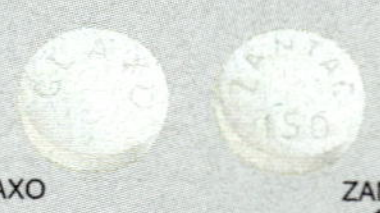 GLAXO ZANTAC 150 Zantac® 150 mg **GlaxoSmithKline**	DIN 00402540 Pr 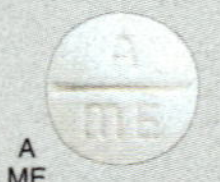 A ME Betaloc® 100 mg **AstraZeneca**
8	DIN 00068608 (N) 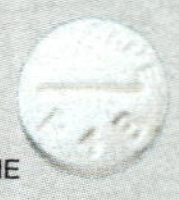 WELLCOME P4B CoActifed® **GlaxoSmithKline**	DIN 00293482 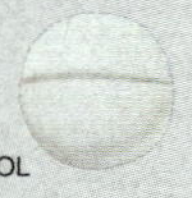 ATASOL Atasol® 325 mg **Church & Dwight**	DIN 02039540 Pr 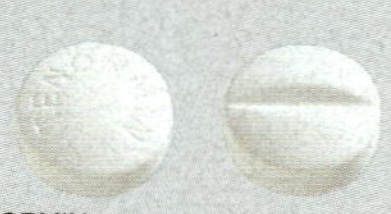 TENORMIN Tenormin® 100 mg **AstraZeneca**	DIN 02229129 Pr 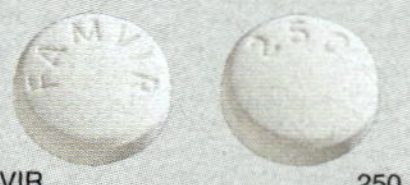 FAMVIR 250 Famvir® 250 mg **Novartis Pharmaceuticals**	DIN 02247998 Pr 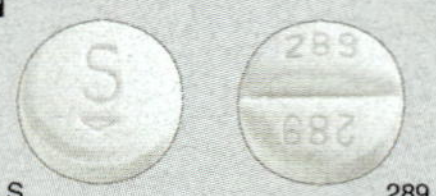 S 289 Serc® 24 mg **Abbott Products**

* ILLUSTRATION LESS THAN ACTUAL SIZE / ILLUSTRATION RÉDUITE

Use code A, B, C, D, E, horizontal bar and 1 to 8 vertical bar to locate illustrated products

Utiliser le code A, B, C, D, E de la ligne horizontale et les chiffres 1 à 8 de la ligne verticale pour repérer les produits illustrés

A B C D E

1

A1 — DIN 02293269

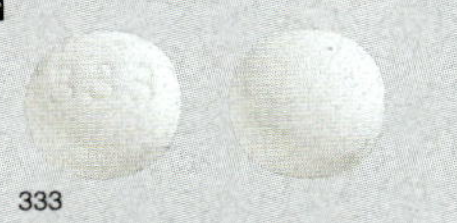

333

Campral® 333 mg

Mylan

B1 — DIN 02150328

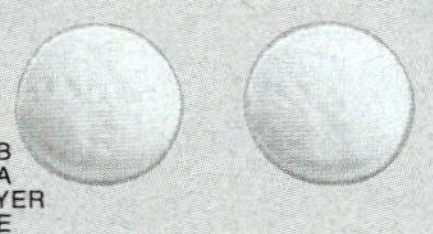

BAYER

Aspirin® 325 mg

Bayer Consumer Care

C1 — DIN 02240518

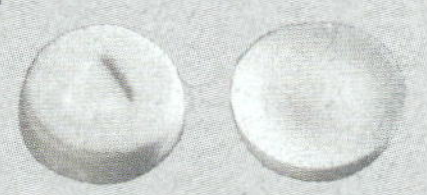

Maxalt RPD® 5 mg

Merck Frosst

D1 — DIN 00728276

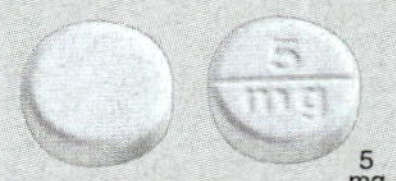

5 mg

Burinex® 5 mg

LEO Pharma

E1 — DIN 02047667 (N)

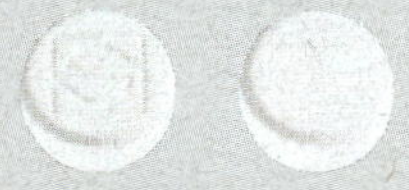

Mersyndol® with Codeine

sanofi-aventis

2

A2 — DIN 02237146

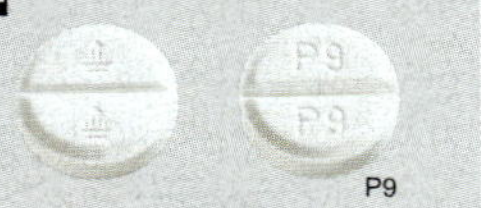

P9

Mirapex® 1 mg

Boehringer Ingelheim

B2 — DIN 02237147

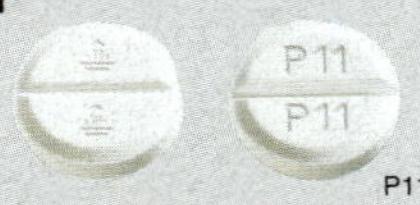

P11

Mirapex® 1.5 mg

Boehringer Ingelheim

C2 — DIN 02163934 (N)

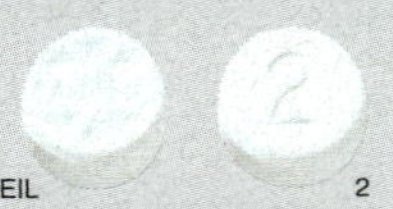

McNEIL 2

Tylenol® with Codeine No. 2 15 mg

Janssen-Ortho/ McNeil Consumer Healthcare

D2 — DIN 02163926 (N)

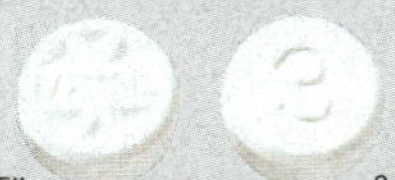

McNEIL 3

Tylenol® with Codeine No. 3 30 mg

Janssen-Ortho/ McNeil Consumer Healthcare

E2 — DIN 02163918 (N)

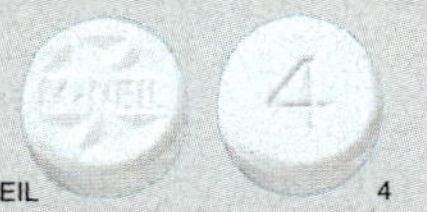

McNEIL 4

Tylenol® with Codeine No. 4 60 mg

Janssen-Ortho/ McNeil Consumer Healthcare

3

A3 — DIN01945157

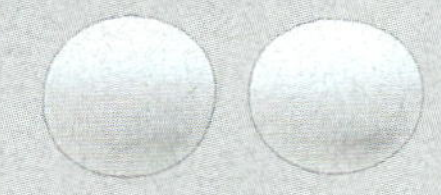

Claritin® Allergy+Sinus

Schering-Plough

B3 — DIN 02237734

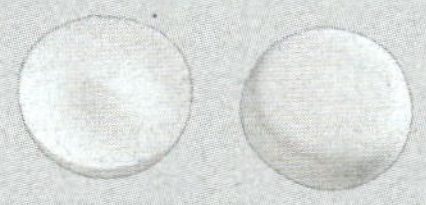

Claritin® Rapid Dissolve 10 mg

Schering-Plough

C3 — DIN 02269023

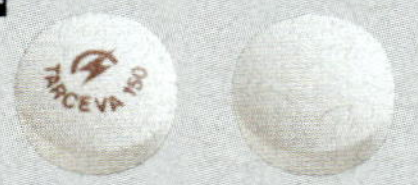

TARCEVA 150

Tarceva® 150 mg

Roche

D3 — DIN 02269457

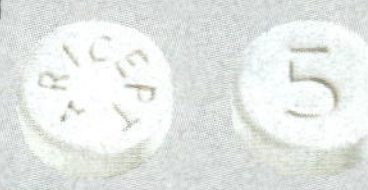

ARICEPT 5

Aricept RDT™ 5 mg

Pfizer

E3 — DIN 02014165

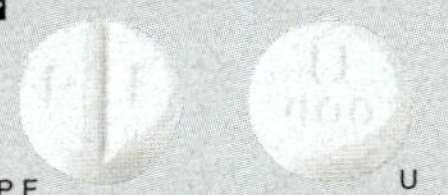

P F U 400

Uniphyl® 400 mg

Purdue Pharma

4

A4 — DIN 01917056

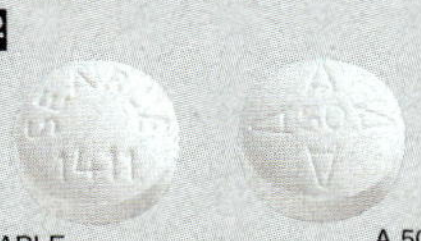

SEARLE 1411 A 50

Arthrotec® 50 mg

Pfizer

B4 — DIN 02239373

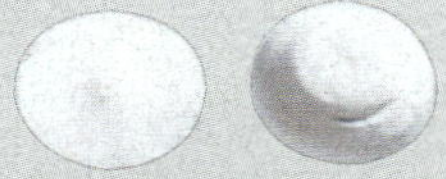

Zofran® ODT 8 mg

GlaxoSmithKline

C4 — DIN 02083523

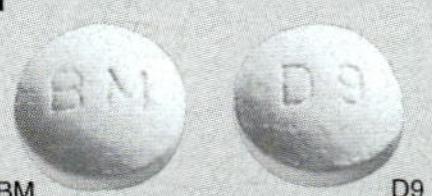

BM D9

Bezalip® SR 400 mg

Actavis

D4 — DIN 02031116

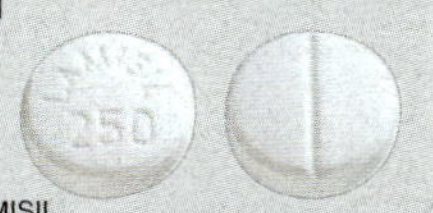

LAMISIL 250

Lamisil® 250 mg

Novartis Pharmaceuticals

E4 — DIN 00579378

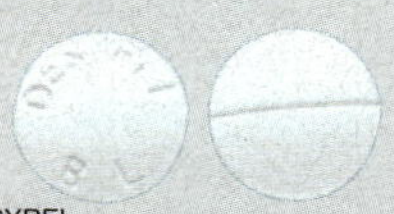

DESYREL B L

Desyrel® 100 mg

Bristol-Myers Squibb

5

A5 — DIN 02316889

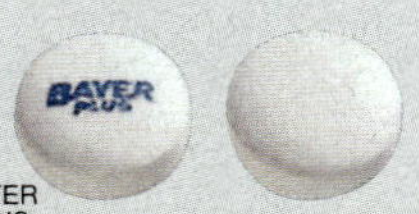

BAYER PLUS

Aspirin® Stomach Guard™ with Calcium Carbonate 325 mg

Bayer Consumer Care

B5 — DIN 02150336

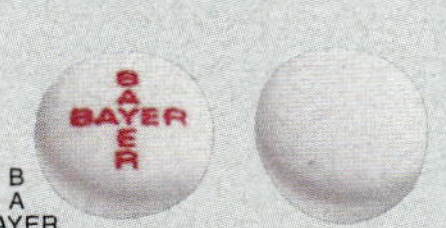

BAYER

Aspirin® Extra Strength 500 mg

Bayer Consumer Care

C5 — DIN 02236953

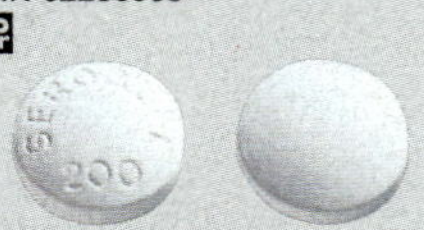

SEROQUEL 200

Seroquel® 200 mg

AstraZeneca

D5 — DIN 01916475 (N)

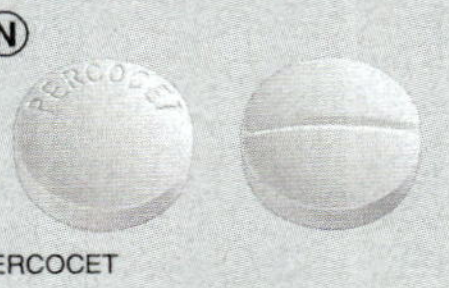

PERCOCET

Percocet®

Bristol-Myers Squibb

E5 — DIN 00603716

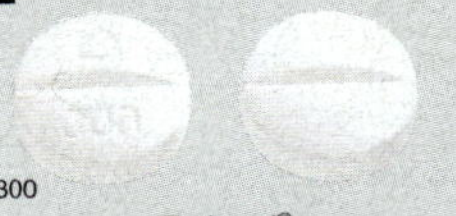

300

Rythmol® 300 mg

Abbott

6

A6 — DIN 00225819 *

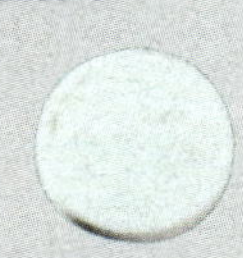

Phosphate-Novartis

Novartis Pharmaceuticals

B6 — DIN 02296411

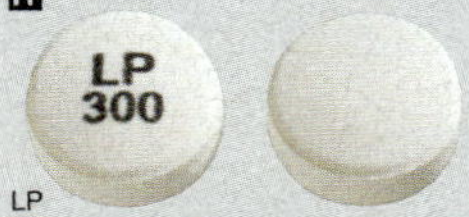

LP 300

Tridural® 300 mg

Labopharm

C6 — DIN 00803499

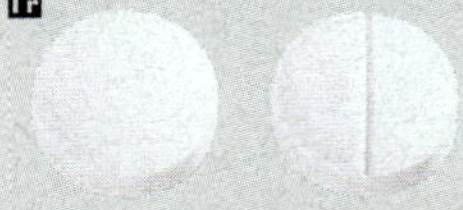

Modulon® 200 mg

Axcan Pharma

D6 — DIN 02248543

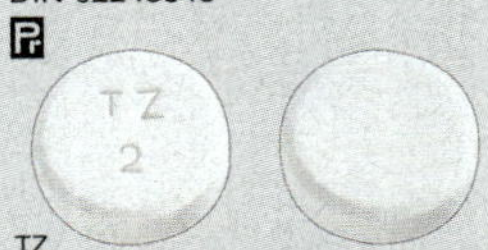

TZ 2

Remeron RD® 30 mg

Schering-Plough

E6 — DIN 02229837

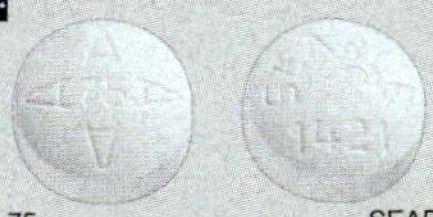

A 75 SEARLE 1421

Arthrotec® 75 mg

Pfizer

7

A7 — DIN 02099233

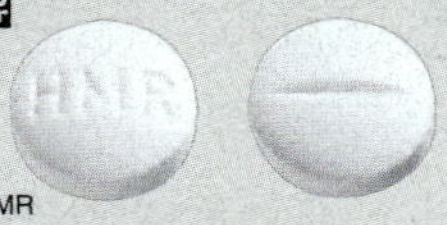

HMR

Glucophage® 500 mg

sanofi-aventis

B7 — DIN 02287420

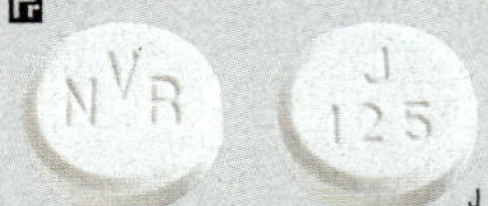

NVR J 125

Exjade® 125 mg

Novartis Pharmaceuticals

C7 — DIN 02287439 *

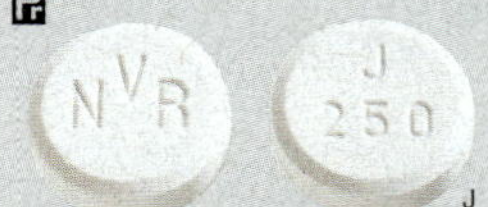

NVR J 250

Exjade® 250 mg

Novartis Pharmaceuticals

D7 — DIN 02287153

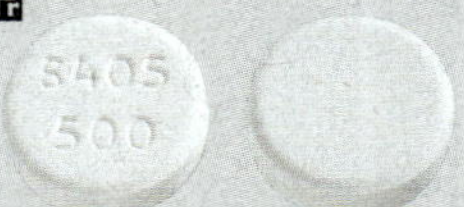

S405 500

Fosrenol® 500 mg

Shire

E7 — DIN 02229437

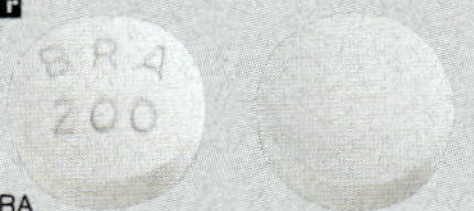

BRA 200

PhosLo® 667 mg

Fresenius Medical Care

8

A8 — DIN 02240519

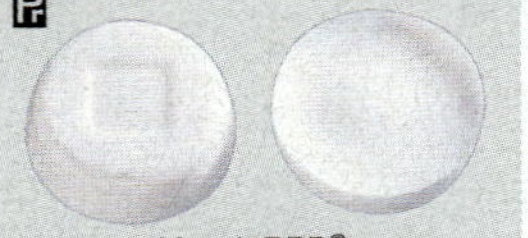

Maxalt RPD® 10 mg

Merck Frosst

B8 — DIN 02287447 *

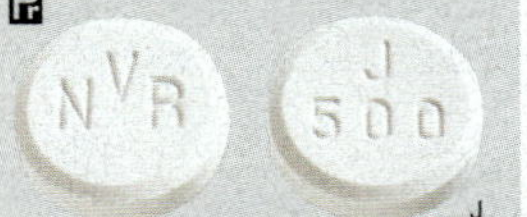

NVR J 500

Exjade® 500 mg

Novartis Pharmaceuticals

C8 — DIN 02248544

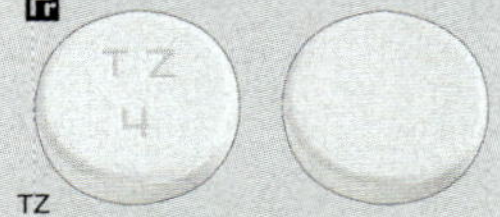

TZ 4

Remeron RD® 45 mg

Schering-Plough

D8 — DIN 00116785

Bionet®

Church & Dwight

E8 — DIN 02242531 *

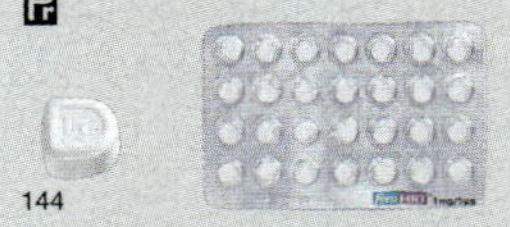

144

femHRT®

Warner Chilcott

* ILLUSTRATION LESS THAN ACTUAL SIZE / ILLUSTRATION RÉDUITE

Use code A, B, C, D, E, horizontal bar and 1 to 8 vertical bar to locate illustrated products

Utiliser le code A, B, C, D, E de la ligne horizontale et les chiffres 1 à 8 de la ligne verticale pour repérer les produits illustrés

1

A1 — DIN 02142082 Pr
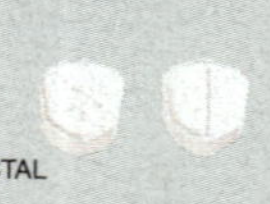
LAMICTAL 25
Lamictal® 25 mg
GlaxoSmithKline

B1 — DIN 02232565 Pr
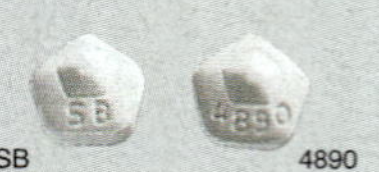
SB / 4890
ReQuip® 0.25 mg
GlaxoSmithKline

C1 — DIN 02201038 Pr
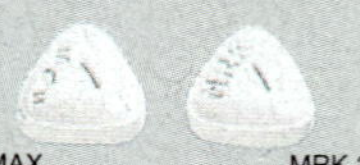
FOSAMAX / MRK 212
Fosamax® 40 mg
Merck Frosst

D1 — DIN 02282224 Pr
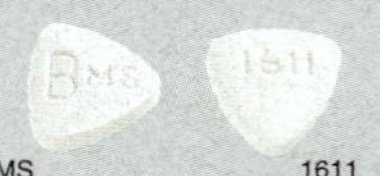
BMS / 1611
Baraclude™ 0.5 mg
Bristol-Myers Squibb

E1 — DIN 02247111 Pr
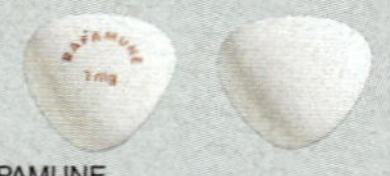
RAPAMUNE 1 mg
Rapamune® 1 mg
Pfizer

2

A2 — DIN 00708879 Pr
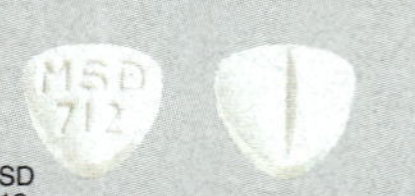
MSD 712
Vasotec® 5 mg
Merck Frosst

B2 — DIN 02212153 Pr
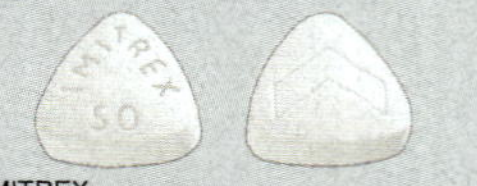
IMITREX 50
Imitrex DF™ 50 mg
GlaxoSmithKline

C2 — DIN 01926543 Pr
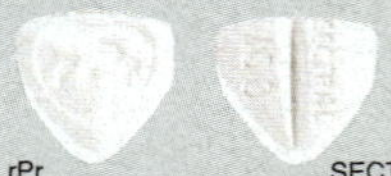
rPr / SECTRAL 100
Sectral® 100 mg
sanofi-aventis

D2 — DIN 01926578 Pr
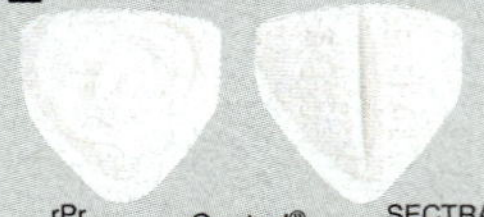
rPr / SECTRAL 400
Sectral® 400 mg
sanofi-aventis

E2 — DIN 00023698 Pr
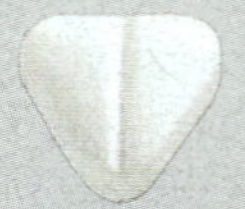
Dilantin® Infatab 50 mg
Pfizer

3

A3 — DIN 00013668

ATASOL FORTE
Atasol® 500 mg
Church & Dwight

B3 — DIN 01907107 Pr
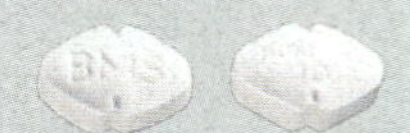
BMS / MONOPRIL 10
Monopril™ 10 mg
Bristol-Myers Squibb

C3 — DIN 02192683 Pr
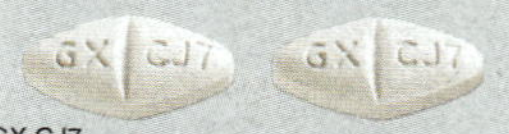
GX CJ7
3TC® 150 mg
ViiV Healthcare ULC

D3 — DIN 00546283 Pr
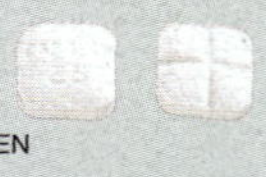
CAPOTEN 25
Capoten™ 25 mg
Bristol-Myers Squibb

E3 — DIN 00878928 Pr
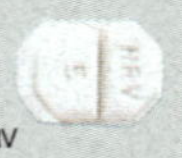
NRV 5
Norvasc™ 5 mg
Pfizer

4

A4 — DIN 02280132 Pr
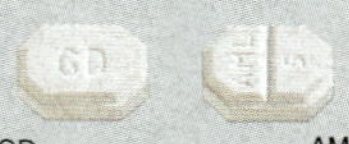
GD / AML 5
GD-amlodipine™ 5 mg
GenMed, a division of Pfizer

B4 — DIN 02280140 Pr
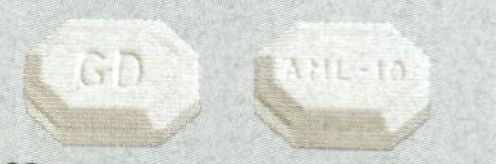
GD / AML-10
GD-amlodipine™ 10 mg
GenMed, a division of Pfizer

C4 — DIN 00878936 Pr
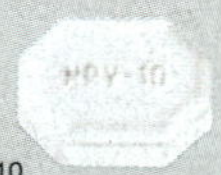
NRV-10
Norvasc™ 10 mg
Pfizer

D4 — DIN 02295695 N
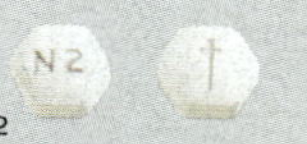
N2
Suboxone™ 2 mg/0.5 mg
Schering-Plough

E4 — DIN 02295709 N
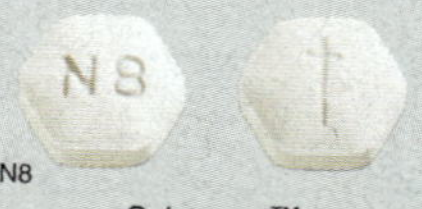
N8
Suboxone™ 8 mg/2 mg
Schering-Plough

5

A5 — DIN 02237820 Pr
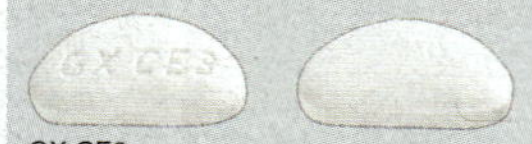
GX CE3
Amerge® 1 mg
GlaxoSmithKline

B5 — DIN 02182815 Pr
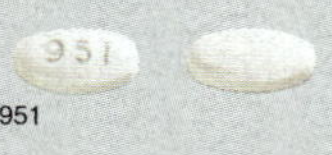
951
Cozaar® 25 mg
Merck Frosst

C5 — DIN 00839388 Pr
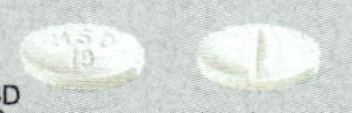
MSD 19
Prinivil® 5 mg
Merck Frosst

D5 — DIN 00030988 Pr
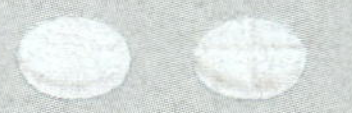
Medrol® 4 mg
Pfizer

E5 — DIN 00782696
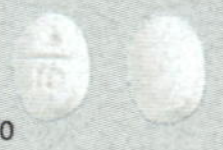
10
Claritin® 10 mg
Schering-Plough

6

A6 — DIN 02041448 TC

Ativan / 2
Ativan® 2 mg
Pfizer

B6 — DIN 00548359 TC
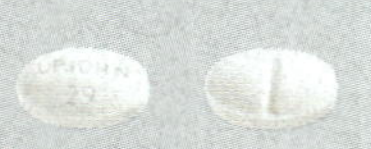
UPJOHN 29
Xanax® 0.25 mg
Pfizer

C6 — DIN 02263238 Pr
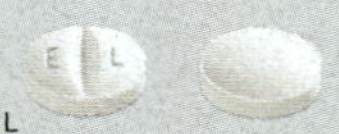
E L
Cipralex® 10 mg
Lundbeck

D6 — DIN 00851795 Pr
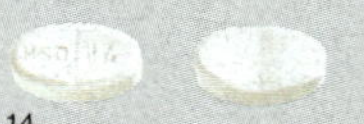
MSD 14
Vasotec® 2.5 mg
Merck Frosst

E6 — DIN 02230711 Pr
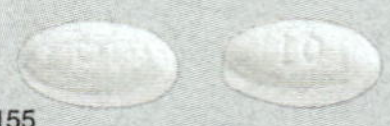
PD 155
Lipitor® 10 mg
Pfizer

7

A7 — DIN 02239607 Pr
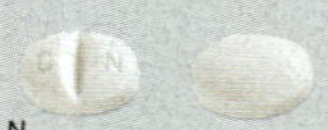
C N
Celexa® 20 mg
Lundbeck

B7 — DIN 02283174 Pr
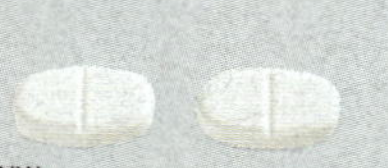
HNW
Altace® HCT 5/25 mg
sanofi-aventis

C7 — DIN 02273233 Pr
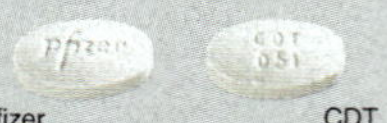
Pfizer / CDT 051
Caduet® 5 mg/10 mg
Pfizer

D7 — DIN 02237923 Pr
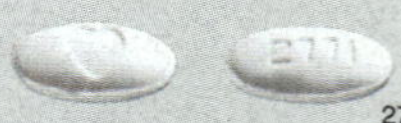
2771
Avapro™ 75 mg
Bristol-Myers Squibb/ sanofi-aventis

E7 — DIN 02237145 Pr
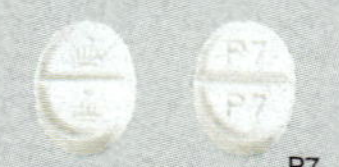
P7
Mirapex® 0.25 mg
Boehringer Ingelheim

8

A8 — DIN 02182874 Pr
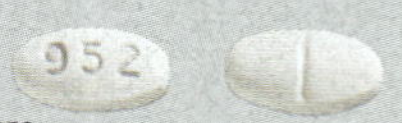
952
Cozaar® 50 mg
Merck Frosst

B8 — DIN 00546291 Pr
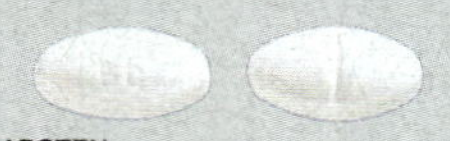
CAPOTEN 50
Capoten™ 50 mg
Bristol-Myers Squibb

C8 — DIN 02239028 Pr
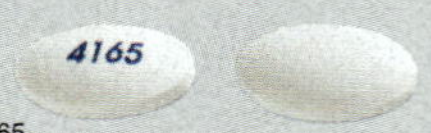
4165
Evista® 60 mg
Lilly

D8 — DIN 02293137 Pr
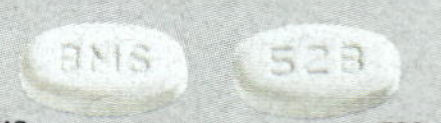
BMS / 528
Sprycel™ 50 mg
Bristol-Myers Squibb

E8 — DIN 02230713 Pr
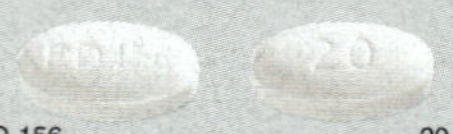
PD 156 / 20
Lipitor® 20 mg
Pfizer

* ILLUSTRATION LESS THAN ACTUAL SIZE / ILLUSTRATION RÉDUITE

Use code A, B, C, D, E, horizontal bar and 1 to 8 vertical bar to locate illustrated products

Utiliser le code A, B, C, D, E de la ligne horizontale et les chiffres 1 à 8 de la ligne verticale pour repérer les produits illustrés

	A	B	C	D	E
1	DIN 00455881 Pr 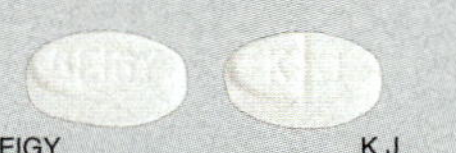 GEIGY K J Lioresal® 10 mg **Novartis Pharmaceuticals**	DIN 00036129 Pr 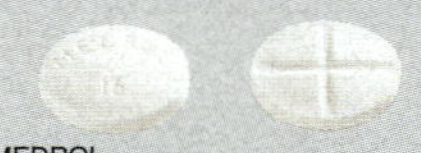 MEDROL 16 Medrol® 16 mg **Pfizer**	DIN 02273241 Pr 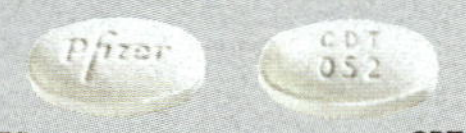 Pfizer CDT 052 Caduet® 5 mg/20 mg **Pfizer**	DIN 02239608 Pr 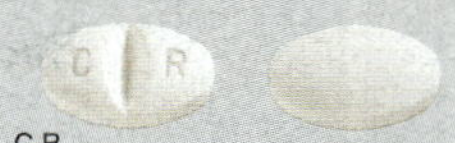 C R Celexa® 40 mg **Lundbeck**	DIN 02286424 Pr 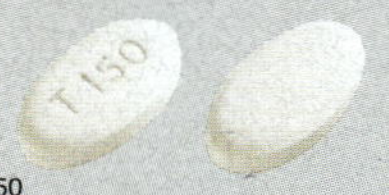 T150 Zytram XL® 150 mg **Purdue Pharma**
2	DIN 00647942 Pr 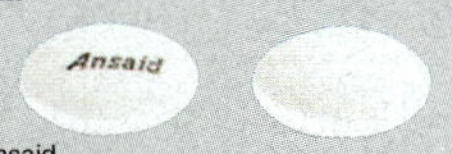 Ansaid Ansaid® 50 mg **Pfizer**	DIN 02263254 Pr 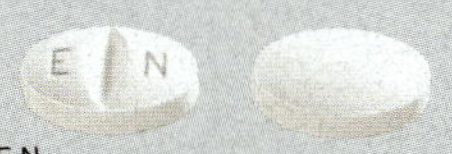 E N Cipralex® 20 mg **Lundbeck**	DIN 02262983 (N) 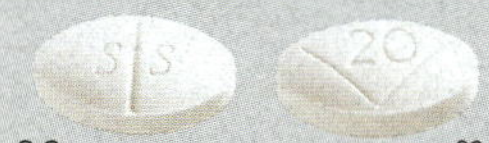 S S 20 Supeudol® 20 mg **Sandoz**	DIN 02241594 Pr 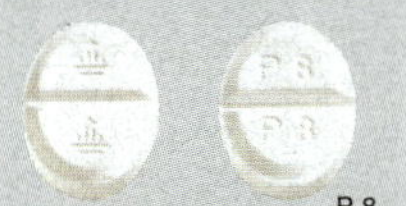 P 8 Mirapex® 0.5 mg **Boehringer Ingelheim**	DIN 02245329 Pr 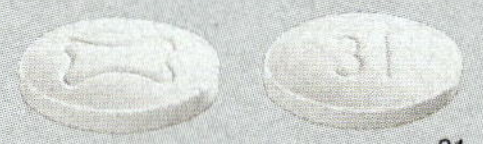 31 Fosamax® 70 mg **Merck Frosst**
3	DIN 02320193 Pr 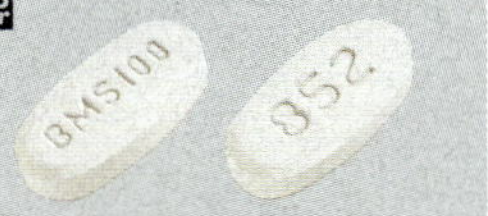 BMS100 852 Sprycel™ 100 mg **Bristol-Myers Squibb**	DIN 02237924 Pr 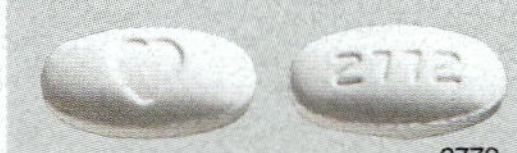 2772 Avapro™ 150 mg **Bristol-Myers Squibb/ sanofi-aventis**	DIN 00497827 Pr 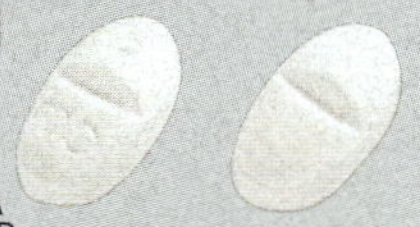 A MD Betaloc® Durules® 200 mg **AstraZeneca**	DIN 02297841 Pr 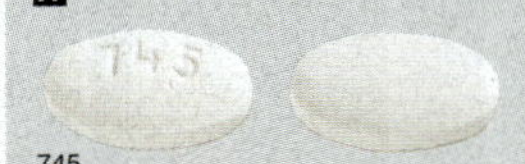 745 Hyzaar® 100/12.5 mg **Merck Frosst**	DIN 02273268 Pr 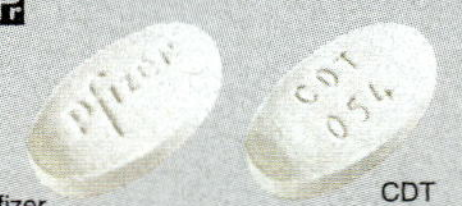 Pfizer CDT 054 Caduet® 5 mg/40 mg **Pfizer**
4	DIN 02182882 Pr 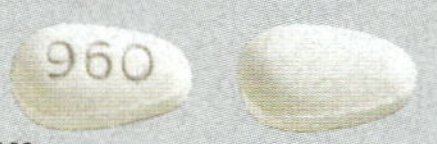 960 Cozaar® 100 mg **Merck Frosst**	DIN 02256479 Pr 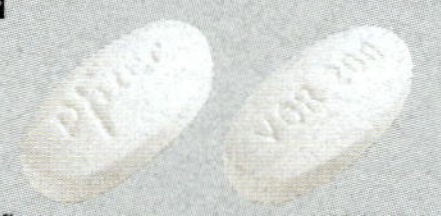 Pfizer VOR 200 Vfend™ 200 mg **Pfizer**	DIN 02231143 * Pr 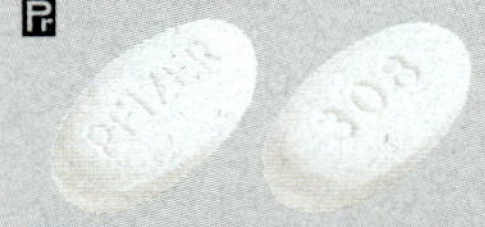 PFIZER 308 Zithromax™ 600 mg **Pfizer**	DIN 02306778 Pr 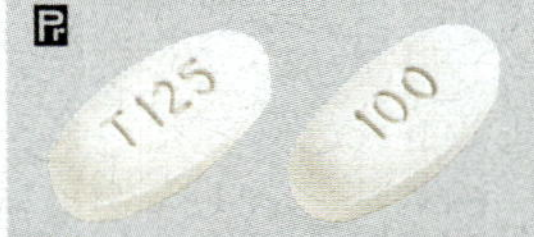 T125 100 Intelence™ 100 mg **Janssen-Ortho**	DIN 02230714 Pr 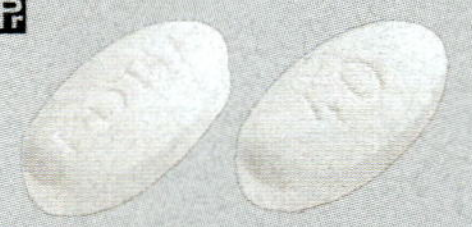 PD 157 40 Lipitor® 40 mg **Pfizer**
5	DIN 02238984 Pr 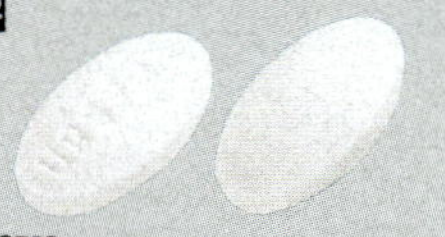 URS785 URSO® 250 mg **Axcan Pharma**	DIN 01919369 Pr 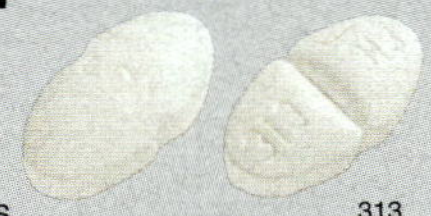 S 313 Luvox® 100 mg **Abbott Products**	DIN 02240132 (N) 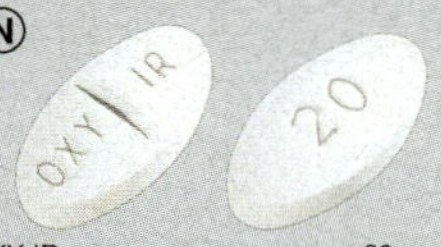 OXY IR 20 Oxy•IR® 20 mg **Purdue Pharma**	DIN 02248761 * Pr 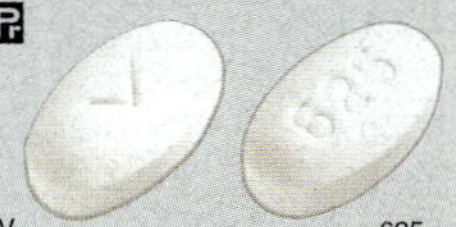 V 625 Viracept® 625 mg **Pfizer**	DIN 02245894 * Pr 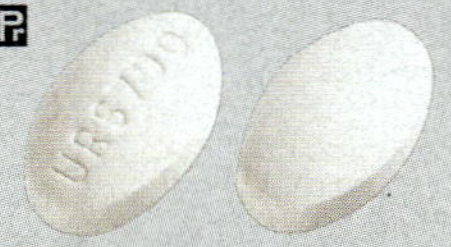 URS790 URSO DS® 500 mg **Axcan Pharma**
6	DIN 02286432 Pr 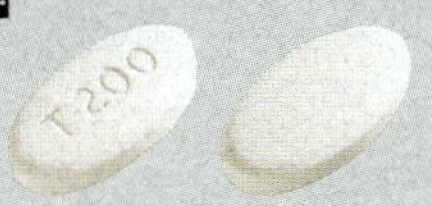 T200 Zytram XL® 200 mg **Purdue Pharma**	DIN 02286440 Pr 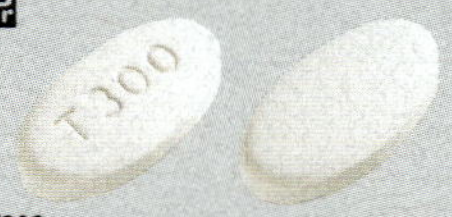 T300 Zytram XL® 300 mg **Purdue Pharma**	DIN 02286459 Pr 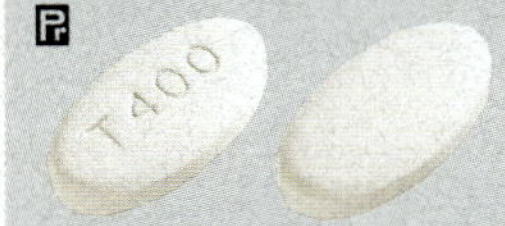 T400 Zytram XL® 400 mg **Purdue Pharma**	DIN 02268493 Pr 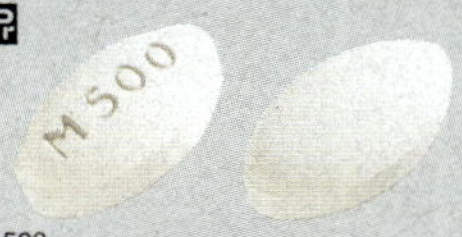 M 500 Glumetza® 500 mg **Biovail Pharmaceuticals**	DIN 00665088 * Pr 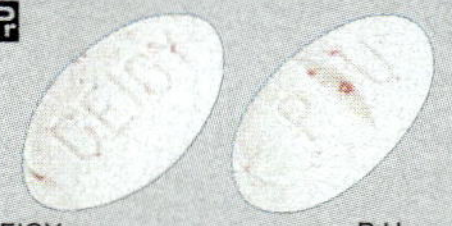 GEIGY P U Tegretol® 200 mg **Novartis Pharmaceuticals**
7	DIN 02269082 Pr 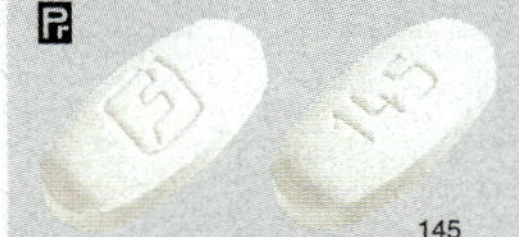 145 Lipidil™ EZ 145 mg **Fournier Pharma**	DIN 02273276 * Pr 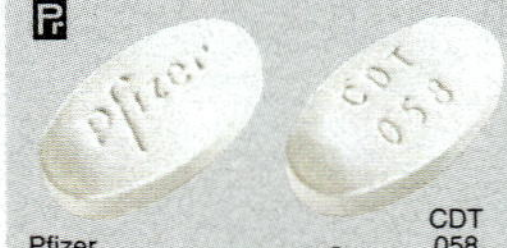 Pfizer CDT 058 Caduet® 5 mg/80 mg **Pfizer**	DIN 02300451 Pr 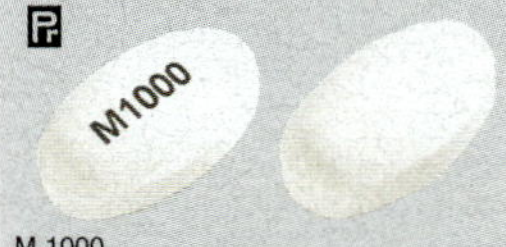 M 1000 Glumetza® 1000 mg **Biovail Pharmaceuticals**	DIN 02177102 Pr 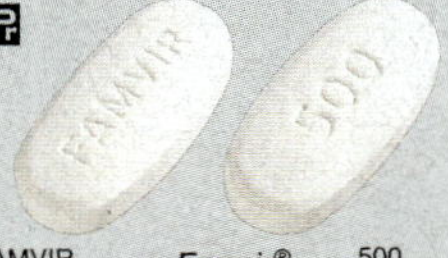 FAMVIR 500 Famvir® 500 mg **Novartis Pharmaceuticals**	DIN 02260557 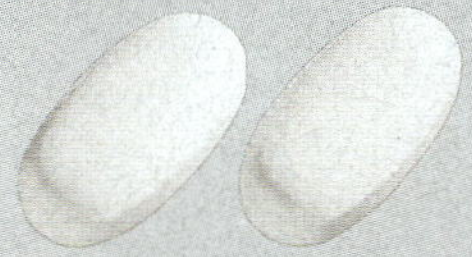 Claritin® Allergy+Sinus Extra Strength **Schering-Plough**
8	DIN 02239717 Pr 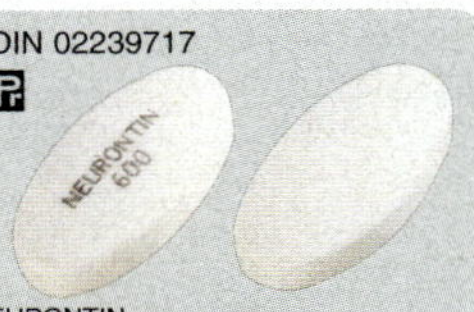 NEURONTIN 600 Neurontin® 600 mg **Pfizer**	DIN 02239718 * Pr 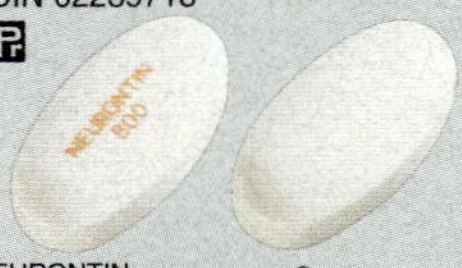 NEURONTIN 800 Neurontin® 800 mg **Pfizer**	DIN 02243684 * Pr 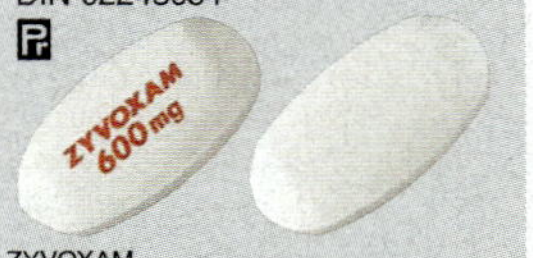 ZYVOXAM 600 mg Zyvoxam® 600 mg **Pfizer**	DIN 02243097 * Pr 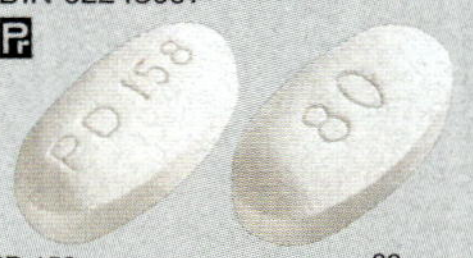 PD 158 80 Lipitor® 80 mg **Pfizer**	DIN 02237925 Pr 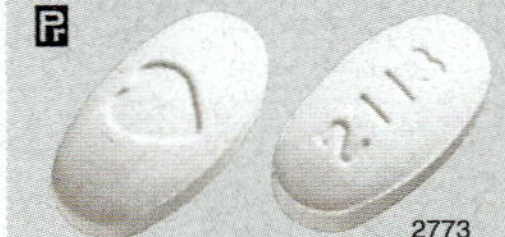 2773 Avapro™ 300 mg **Bristol-Myers Squibb/ sanofi-aventis**

* ILLUSTRATION LESS THAN ACTUAL SIZE / ILLUSTRATION RÉDUITE

Use code A, B, C, D, E, horizontal bar and 1 to 8 vertical bar to locate illustrated products

Utiliser le code A, B, C, D, E de la ligne horizontale et les chiffres 1 à 8 de la ligne verticale pour repérer les produits illustrés

1

A — DIN 02241602
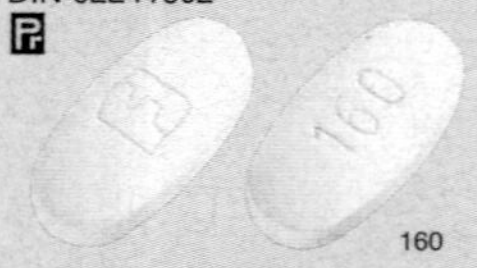
160
Lipidil Supra® 160 mg
Fournier Pharma

B — DIN 02163667
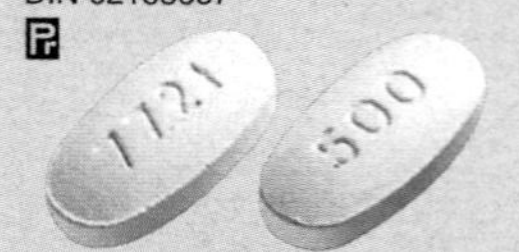
7721 / 500
Cefzil™ 500 mg
Bristol-Myers Squibb

C — DIN 00659606
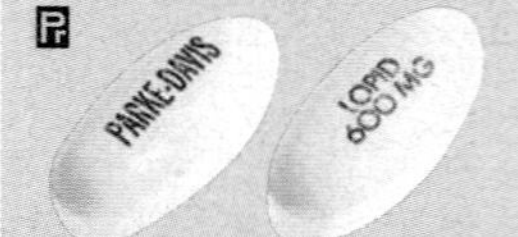
PARKE-DAVIS / LOPID 600 MG
Lopid™ 600 mg
Pfizer

D — DIN 00013668
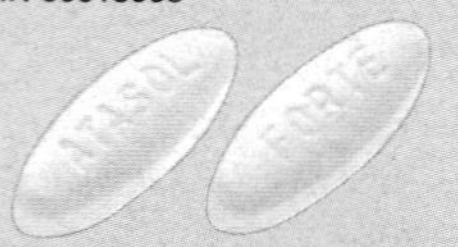
ATASOL / FORTE
Atasol® 500 mg
Church & Dwight

E — DIN 02238348
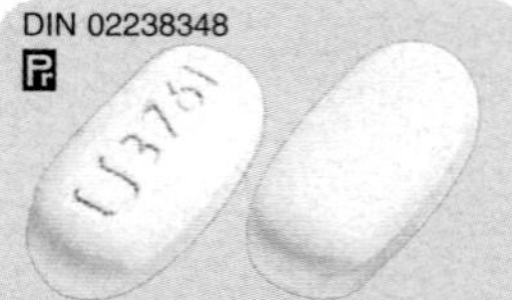
U 3761
Rescriptor® 100 mg
ViiV Healthcare ULC

2

A — DIN 02041421
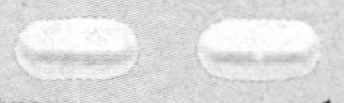
Ativan / 1
Ativan® 1 mg
Pfizer

B — DIN 02283131
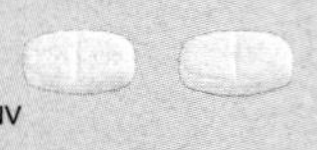
HNV
Altace® HCT 2.5/12.5 mg
sanofi-aventis

C — DIN 02242471
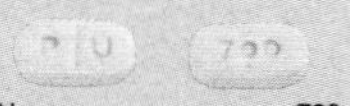
P U / 700
Dostinex™ 0.5 mg
Paladin

D — DIN 02246568
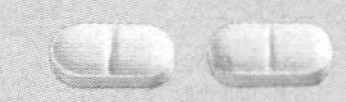
Coversyl® Plus LD 2 mg/0.625 mg
Servier

E — DIN 02291177
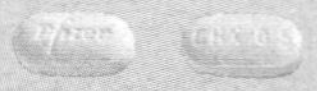
Pfizer / CHX 0.5
Champix® 0.5 mg
Pfizer

3

A — DIN 02247733
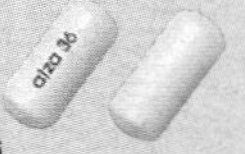
alza 36
Concerta® 36 mg
Janssen-Ortho

B — DIN 02240115
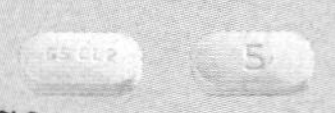
GS CL2 / 5
Lamictal® Chewable/Dispersible 5 mg
GlaxoSmithKline

C — DIN 02246569
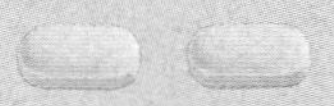
Coversyl® Plus 4 mg/1.25 mg
Servier

D — DIN 02014238
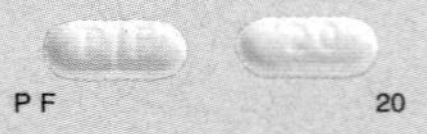
P F / 20
MS•IR® 20 mg
Purdue Pharma

E — DIN 02247521
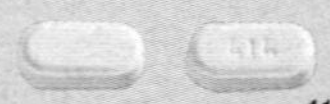
414
Ezetrol® 10 mg
Merck Frosst-Schering Pharma

4

A — DIN 02014254
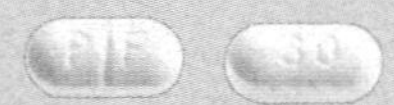
P F / 30
MS•IR® 30 mg
Purdue Pharma

B — DIN 01958097
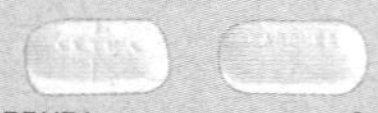
CARDURA / 2 mg
Cardura-2™ 2 mg
Pfizer

C — DIN 02242987
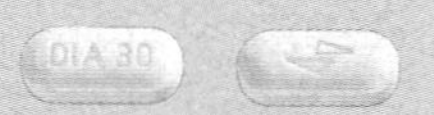
DIA 30
Diamicron® MR 30 mg
Servier

D — DIN 02300273
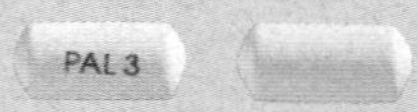
PAL 3
Invega™ 3 mg
Janssen-Ortho

E — DIN 02338432
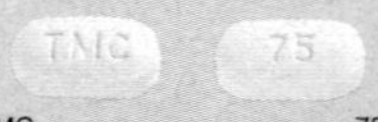
TMC / 75
Prezista® 75 mg
Janssen-Ortho

5

A — DIN 02025280
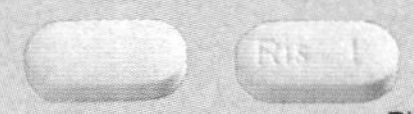
Ris 1
Risperdal® 1 mg
Janssen-Ortho

B — DIN 02242763
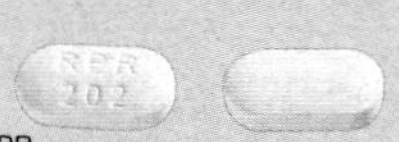
RPR 202
Rilutek® 50 mg
sanofi-aventis

C — DIN 02349469
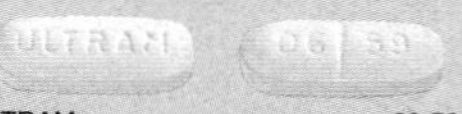
ULTRAM / 06 59
Ultram® 50 mg
Janssen-Ortho

D — DIN 00813958
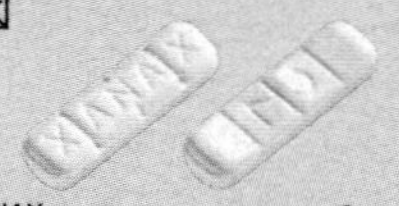
XANAX / 2
Xanax TS® 2 mg
Pfizer

E — DIN 02106280
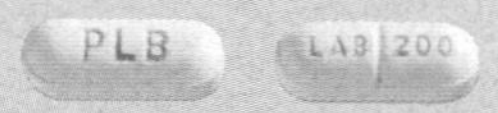
PLB / LAB 200
Trandate® 200 mg
Paladin

6

A — DIN 02224569
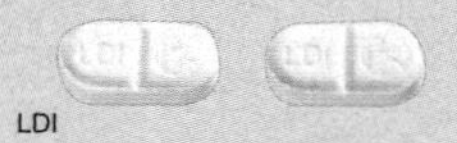
LDI
Diabeta® 5 mg
sanofi-aventis

B — DIN 02201011
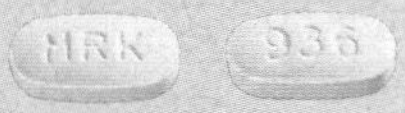
MRK / 936
Fosamax® 10 mg
Merck Frosst

C — DIN 01907115

BMS / MONOPRIL 20
Monopril™ 20 mg
Bristol-Myers Squibb

D — DIN 02239146
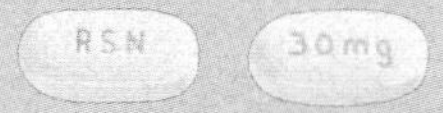
RSN / 30 mg
Actonel® 30 mg
Warner Chilcott

E — DIN 02017709
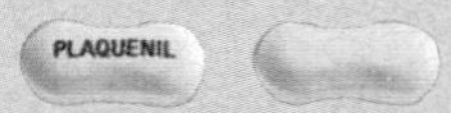
PLAQUENIL
Plaquenil® 200 mg
sanofi-aventis

7

A — DIN 02260638
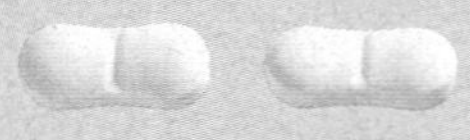
Ebixa® 10 mg
Lundbeck

B — DIN 02240131
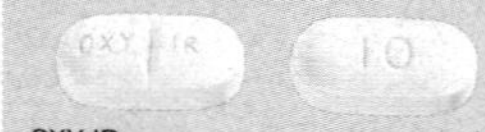
OXY IR / 10
Oxy•IR® 10 mg
Purdue Pharma

C — DIN 02240769
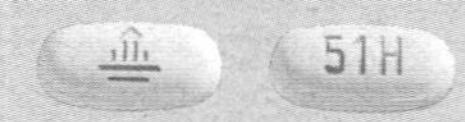
51H
Micardis® 40 mg
Boehringer Ingelheim

D — DIN 02318679
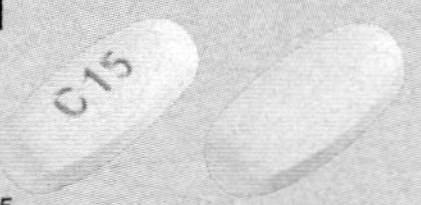
C15
Olmetec® 40 mg
Schering-Plough

E — DIN 02103109
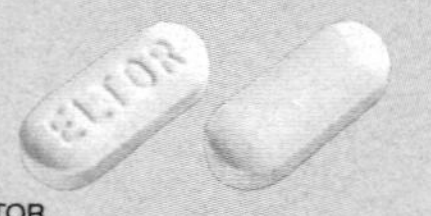
ELTOR
Eltor® 120
sanofi-aventis

8

A — DIN 02332728
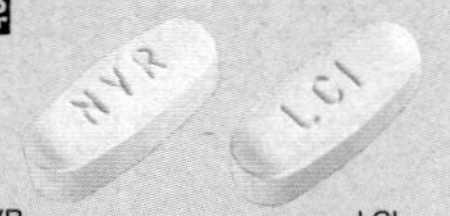
NVR / LCI
Rasilez HCT® 150 mg/12.5 mg
Novartis Pharmaceuticals

B — DIN 02150328
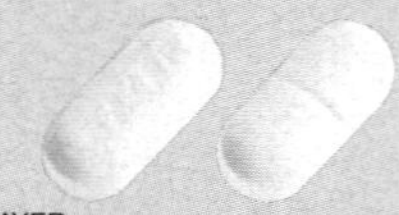
BAYER
Aspirin® 325 mg
Bayer Consumer Care

C — DIN 02256738
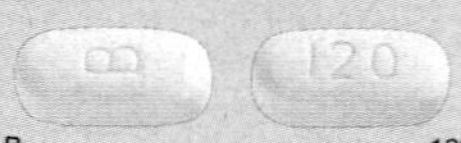
B / 120
Tiazac® XC 120 mg
Biovail Pharmaceuticals

D — DIN 02276429
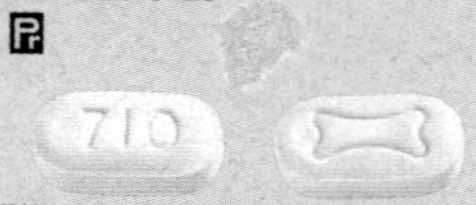
710
Fosavance® 70/2800
Merck Frosst

E — DIN 02314940
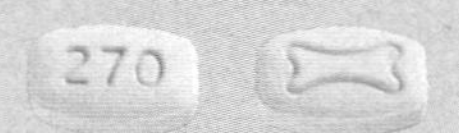
270
Fosavance® 70/5600
Merck Frosst

* ILLUSTRATION LESS THAN ACTUAL SIZE / ILLUSTRATION RÉDUITE

Use code A, B, C, D, E, horizontal bar and 1 to 8 vertical bar to locate illustrated products

Utiliser le code A, B, C, D, E de la ligne horizontale et les chiffres 1 à 8 de la ligne verticale pour repérer les produits illustrés

	A	B	C	D	E
1	DIN 02212277 Pr 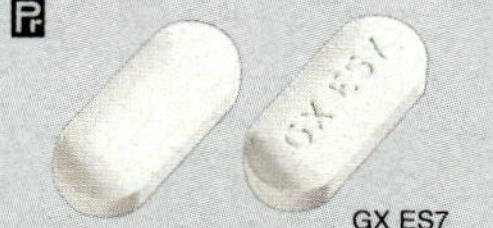 GX ES7 Ceftin® 250 mg **GlaxoSmithKline**	DIN 02256746 Pr 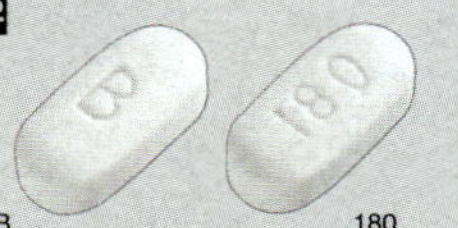 B 180 Tiazac® XC 180 mg **Biovail Pharmaceuticals**	DIN 02212358 Pr 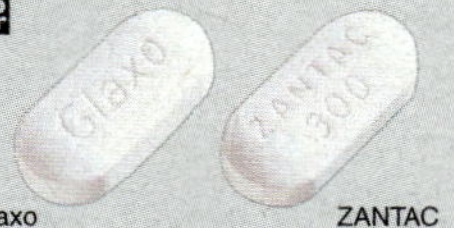 Glaxo ZANTAC 300 Zantac® 300 mg **GlaxoSmithKline**	DIN 02240770 Pr 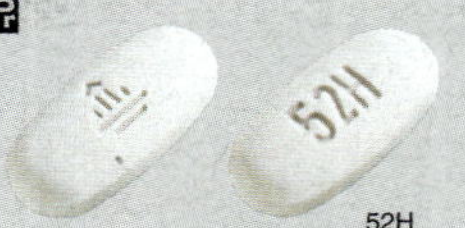 52H Micardis® 80 mg **Boehringer Ingelheim**	DIN 02246559 * Pr 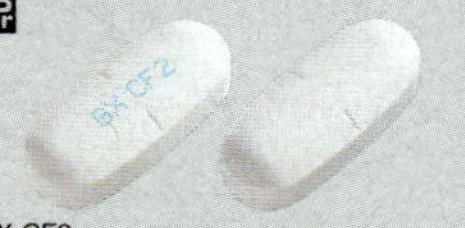 GX CF2 Valtrex® 1000 mg **GlaxoSmithKline**
2	DIN 02288389 Pr 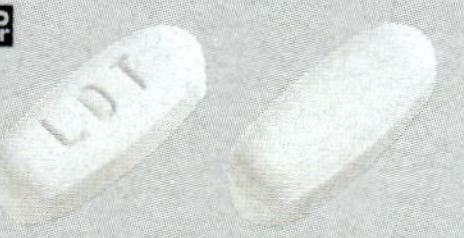 LDT Sebivo® 600 mg **Novartis Pharmaceuticals**	DIN 02321513 Pr 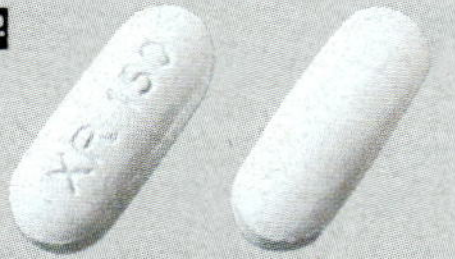 XR 150 Seroquel XR® 150 mg **AstraZeneca**	DIN 00713376 * 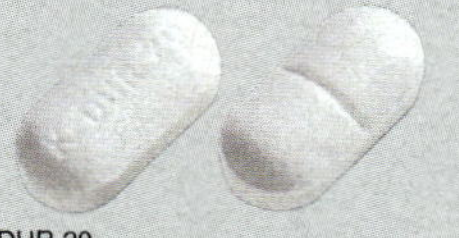 K-DUR 20 K-Dur® 20 mmol **Schering-Plough**	DIN 02239213 Pr 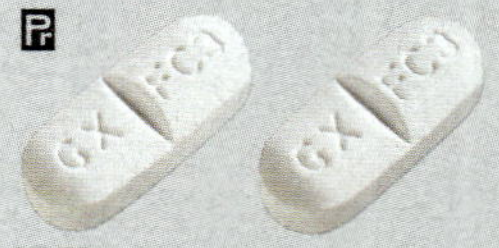 GX FC3 Combivir® 150 mg/300 mg **ViiV Healthcare ULC**	DIN 02238748 Pr 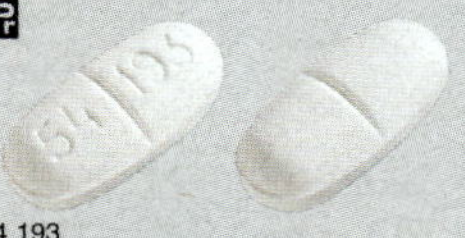 54 193 Viramune® 200 mg **Boehringer Ingelheim**
3	DIN 02256754 Pr 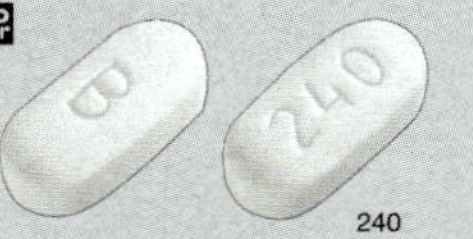 B 240 Tiazac® XC 240 mg **Biovail Pharmaceuticals**	DIN 02100622 * Pr 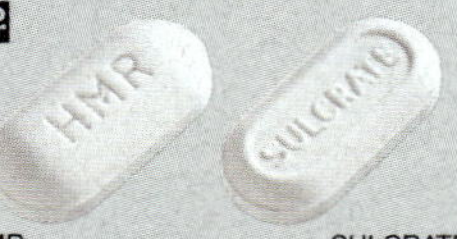 HMR SULCRATE Sulcrate® 1 g **Axcan Pharma**	DIN 00636576 Pr 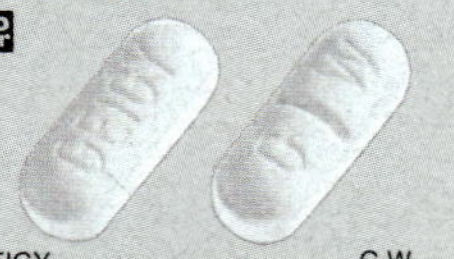 GEIGY G W Lioresal® D.S. 20 mg **Novartis Pharmaceuticals**	DIN 02330989 Pr 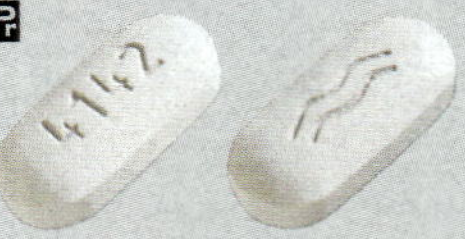 4142 Multaq™ 400 mg **sanofi-aventis**	DIN 02300214 Pr 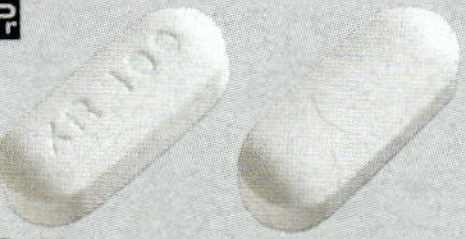 XR 400 Seroquel XR® 400 mg **AstraZeneca**
4	DIN 02064405 Pr 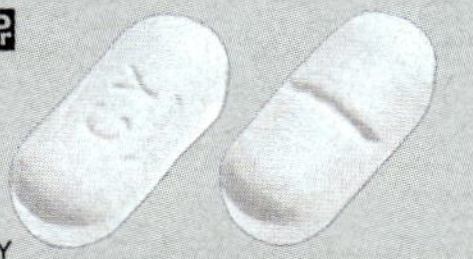 CY Cyklokapron® 500 mg **Pfizer**	DIN 02238829 Pr 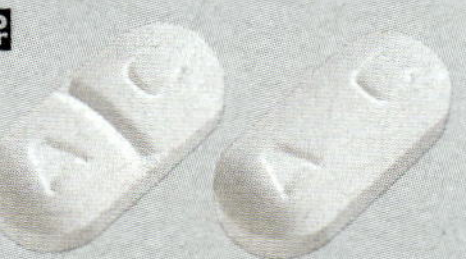 A C Clavulin®-875 **GlaxoSmithKline**	DIN 02212285 * Pr 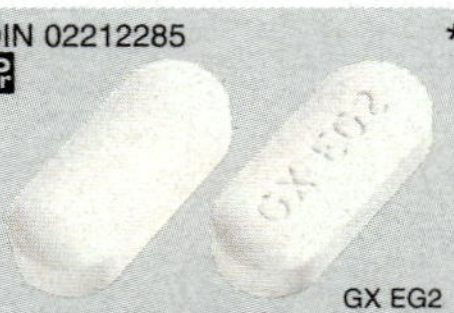 GX EG2 Ceftin® 500 mg **GlaxoSmithKline**	DIN 02244107 Pr 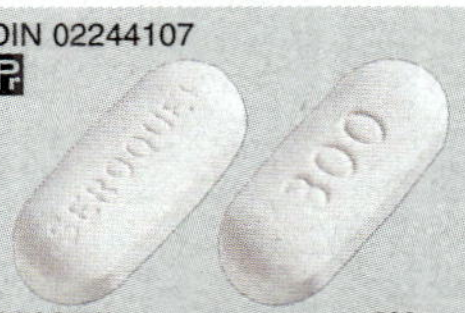 SEROQUEL 300 Seroquel® 300 mg **AstraZeneca**	DIN 02316897 BAYER PLUS 500 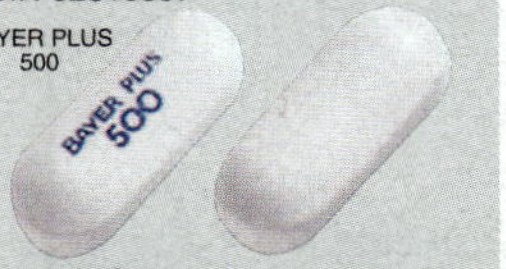 Aspirin® Stomach Guard™ with Calcium Carbonate 500 mg **Bayer Consumer Care**
5	DIN 02155966 Pr 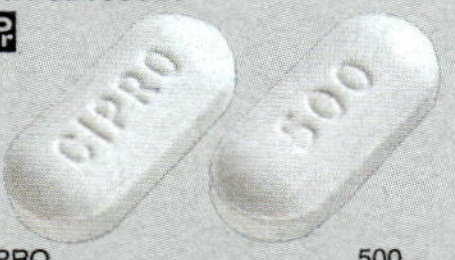 CIPRO 500 Cipro® 500 mg **Bayer**	DIN 02155974 Pr 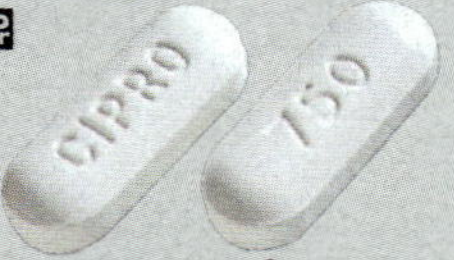 CIPRO 750 Cipro® 750 mg **Bayer**	DIN 02027860 * Pr 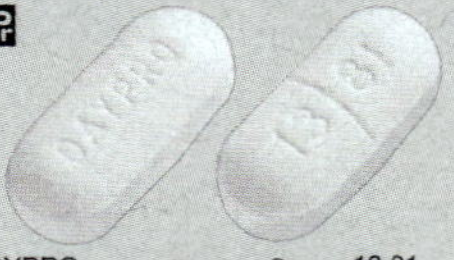 DAYPRO 13 81 Daypro® 600 mg **Pfizer**	DIN 02162849 * Pr 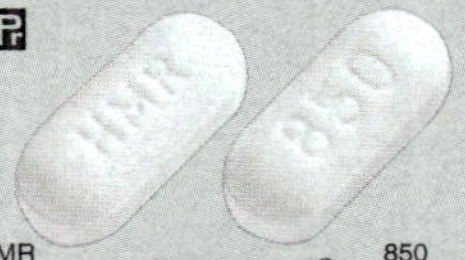 HMR 850 Glucophage® 850 mg **sanofi-aventis**	DIN 02246804 Pr 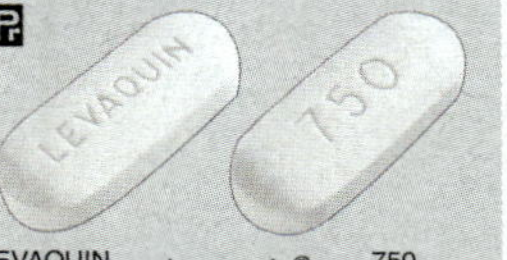 LEVAQUIN 750 Levaquin® 750 mg **Janssen-Ortho**
6	DIN 02247916 Pr 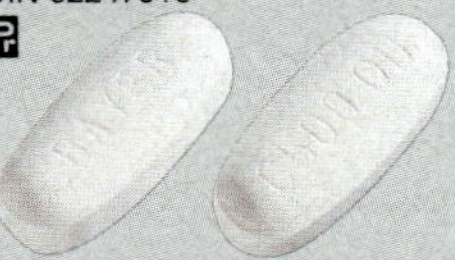 BAYER C500 QD Cipro® XL™ 500 mg **Bayer**	DIN 02251787 Pr 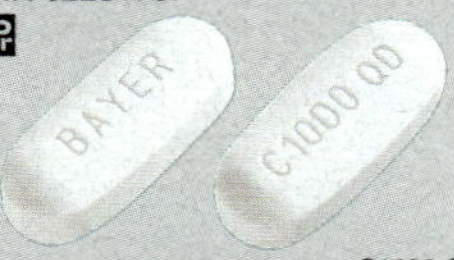 BAYER C1000 QD Cipro® XL™ 1000 mg **Bayer**	DIN 02256762 Pr 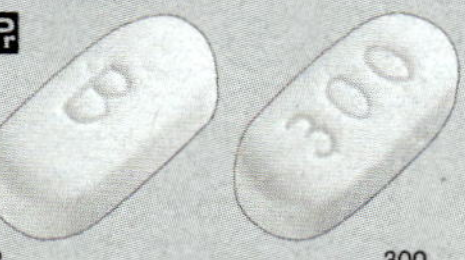 B 300 Tiazac® XC 300 mg **Biovail Pharmaceuticals**	DIN 02256770 Pr 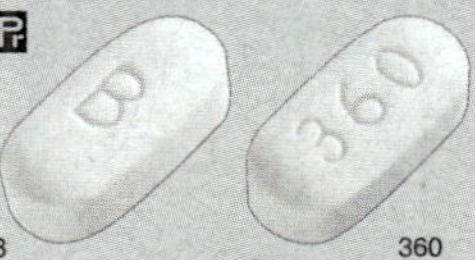 B 360 Tiazac® XC 360 mg **Biovail Pharmaceuticals**	DIN 02243942 Pr 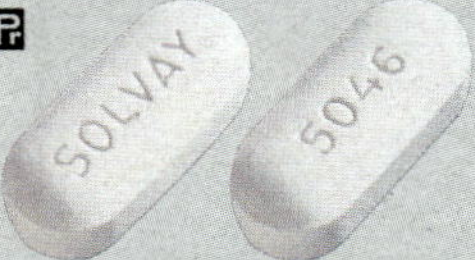 SOLVAY 5046 Teveten® 600 mg **Abbott Products**
7	DIN 00868981 Pr 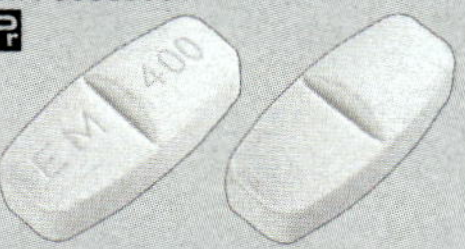 EM 400 Suprax® 400 mg **sanofi-aventis**	DIN 02230897 * Pr 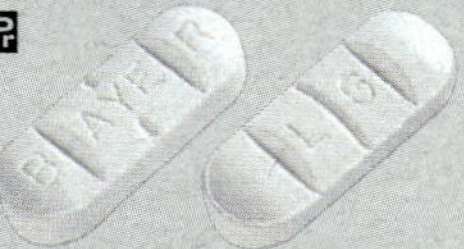 BAYER LG Biltricide® 600 mg **Bayer**	DIN 02014181 Pr 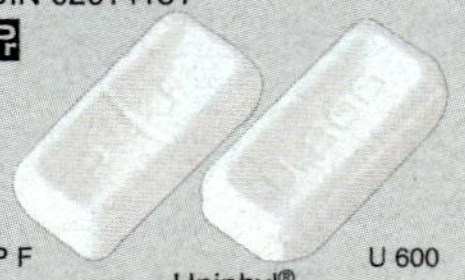 P F U 600 Uniphyl® 600 mg **Purdue Pharma**	DIN 02014319 Ⓝ 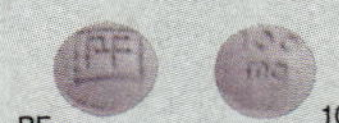 PF 100 mg MS Contin® 100 mg **Purdue Pharma**	DIN 02323192 Ⓝ 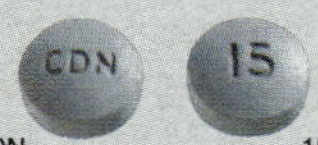 CDN 15 OxyContin® 15 mg **Purdue Pharma**
8	DIN 02250241 (C) 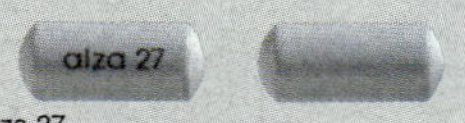 alza 27 Concerta® 27 mg **Janssen-Ortho**	DIN 02352303 Pr 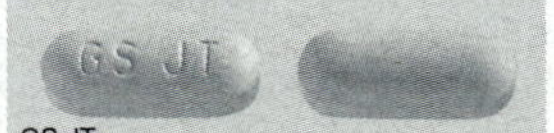 GS JT Votrient™ 200 mg **GlaxoSmithKline**	DIN 02172119 Pr 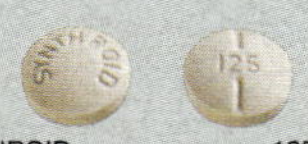 SYNTHROID 125 Synthroid® 125 µg **Abbott**	DIN 02277263 Pr 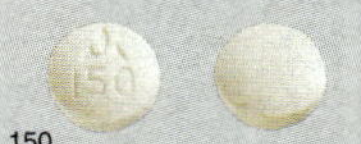 150 Vesicare® 5 mg **Astellas**	NPN 80003201 * 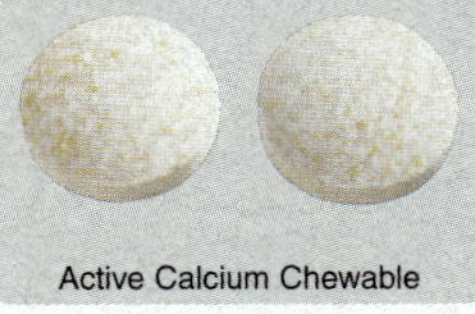 Active Calcium Chewable **USANA Health Sciences**

* ILLUSTRATION LESS THAN ACTUAL SIZE / ILLUSTRATION RÉDUITE

Use code A, B, C, D, E, horizontal bar and 1 to 8 vertical bar to locate illustrated products

Utiliser le code A, B, C, D, E de la ligne horizontale et les chiffres 1 à 8 de la ligne verticale pour repérer les produits illustrés

	A	B	C	D	E
1	DIN 02142112 Pr 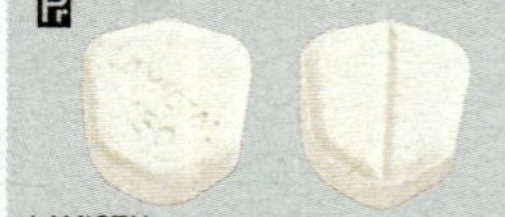 LAMICTAL 150 Lamictal® 150 mg **GlaxoSmithKline**	DIN 02213206 Pr 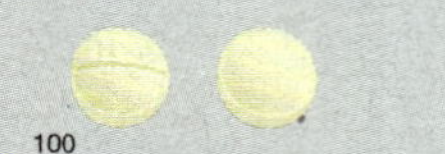 100 Eltroxin® 100 µg **Triton Pharma**	DIN 00894737 Pr 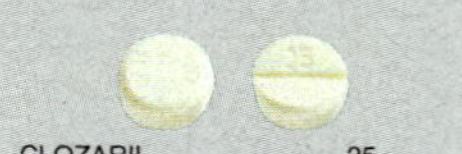 CLOZARIL 25 Clozaril® 25 mg **Novartis Pharmaceuticals**	DIN 02172100 Pr 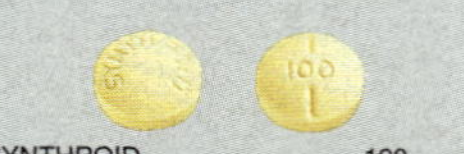 SYNTHROID 100 Synthroid® 100 µg **Abbott**	DIN 02238660 Pr 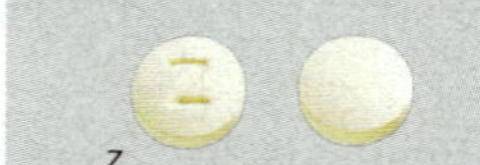 Z Zomig® 2.5 mg **AstraZeneca**
2	DIN 00005614 C 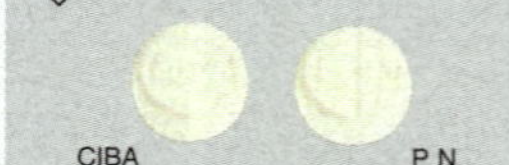 CIBA P N Ritalin® 20 mg **Novartis Pharmaceuticals**	DIN 02242785 Pr 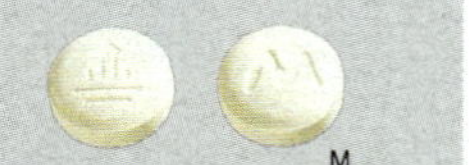 M Mobicox™ 7.5 mg **Boehringer Ingelheim**	DIN 02224704 Pr 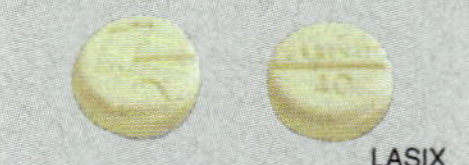 LASIX 40 Lasix® 40 mg **sanofi-aventis**	DIN 02242786 Pr 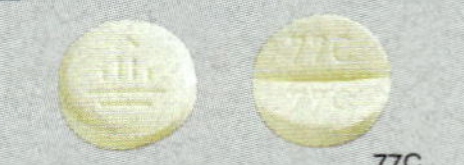 77C Mobicox™ 15 mg **Boehringer Ingelheim**	DIN 02245718 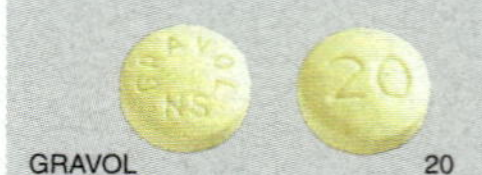 GRAVOL NS 20 Gravol® - Ginger - Natural Source **Church & Dwight**
3	DIN 00282081 Pr 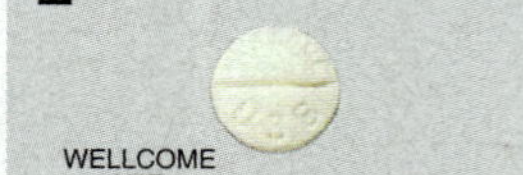 WELLCOME U3B Lanvis® 40 mg **GlaxoSmithKline**	DIN 02232044 Pr 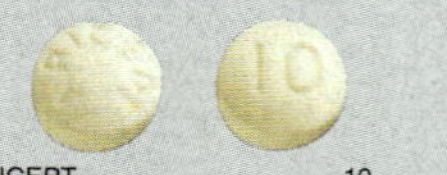 ARICEPT 10 Aricept™ 10 mg **Pfizer**	DIN 00534560 Pr 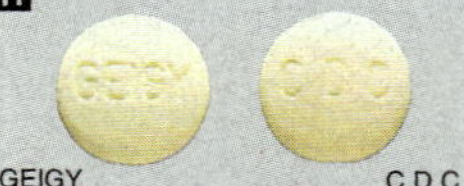 GEIGY C D C Lopresor® SR 200 mg **Novartis Pharmaceuticals**	DIN 02243086 Pr 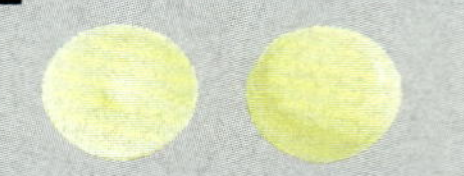 Zyprexa® Zydis® 5 mg **Lilly**	DIN 02243087 Pr 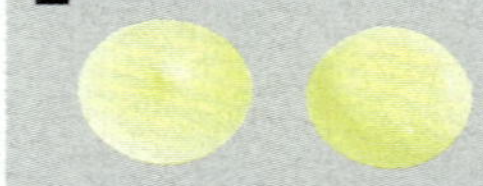 Zyprexa® Zydis® 10 mg **Lilly**
4	DIN 00894745 Pr 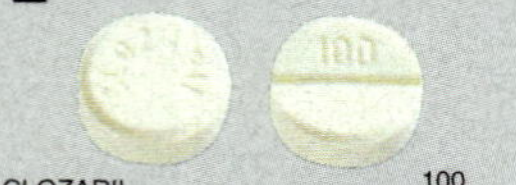 CLOZARIL 100 mg Clozaril® 100 mg **Novartis Pharmaceuticals**	DIN 00176141 C 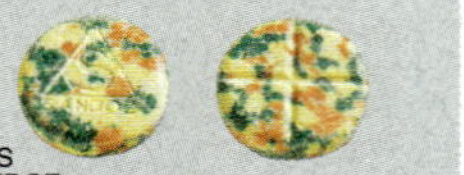 S SANDOZ Bellergal® Spacetabs **Triton Pharma**	DIN 00293504 N 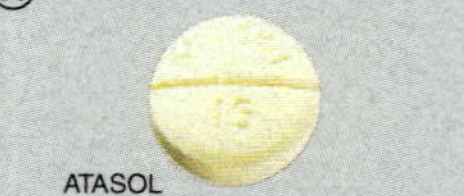 ATASOL 15 Atasol®-15 **Church & Dwight**	DIN 02269465 Pr 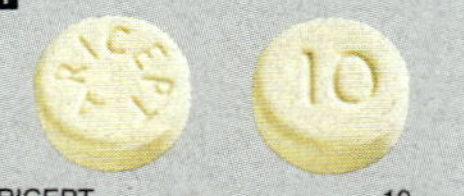 ARICEPT 10 Aricept RDT™ 10 mg **Pfizer**	DIN 02155958 Pr 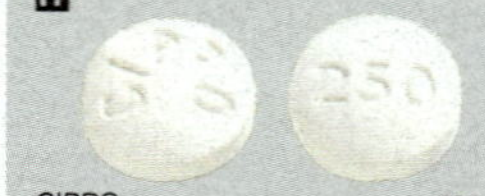 CIPRO 250 Cipro® 250 mg **Bayer**
5	DIN 02243088 Pr 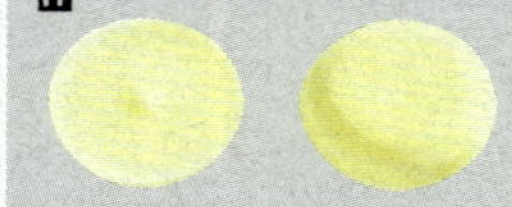 Zyprexa® Zydis® 15 mg **Lilly**	DIN 02243089 Pr 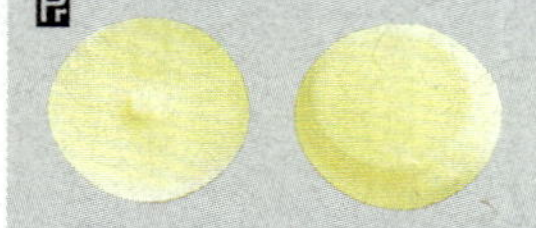 Zyprexa® Zydis® 20 mg **Lilly**	DIN 02224755 Pr 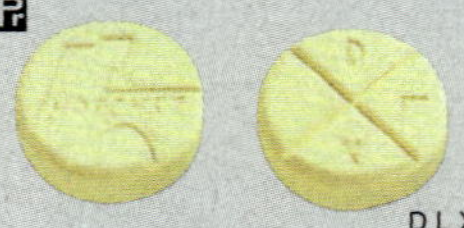 D L X Lasix® Special 500 mg **sanofi-aventis**	DIN 00637726 Pr 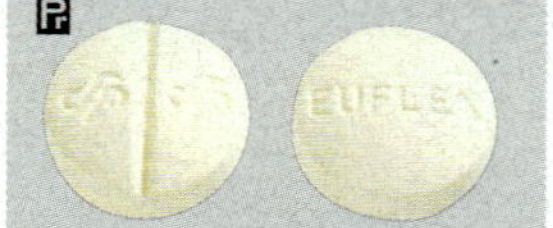 EUFLEX Euflex® 250 mg **Schering-Plough**	DIN 00004596 Pr 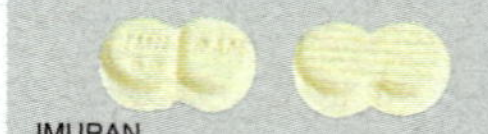 IMURAN 50 Imuran® 50 mg **Triton Pharma**
6	DIN 00893757 Pr 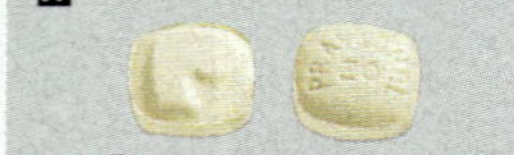 P PRAVACHOL 20 Pravachol® 20 mg **Bristol-Myers Squibb**	DIN 00884413 Pr 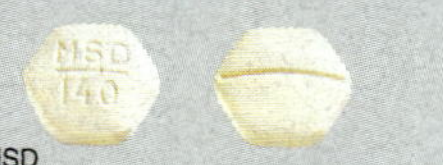 MSD 140 Prinzide® 20 mg/12.5 mg **Merck Frosst**	DIN 02241889 Pr 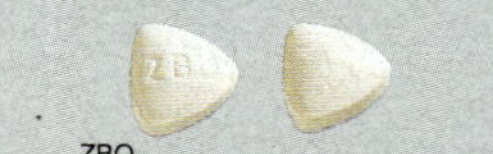 ZBO Arava® 20 mg **sanofi-aventis**	NPN 80013950 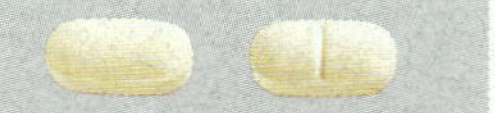 Vitamin D 25 µg **USANA Health Sciences**	DIN 00884324 Pr 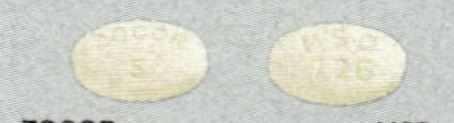 ZOCOR 5 MSD 726 Zocor® 5 mg **Merck Frosst**
7	DIN 02230047 Pr 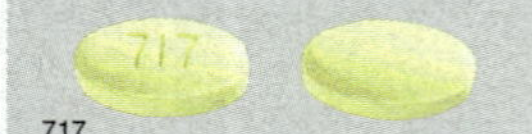 717 Hyzaar® 50/12.5 mg **Merck Frosst**	DIN 02089793 Pr 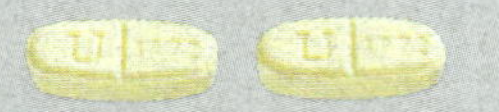 U 3772 Ogen® 0.75 mg **Pfizer**	DIN 02025302 Pr 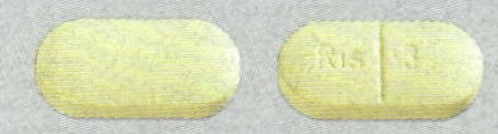 Ris 3 Risperdal® 3 mg **Janssen-Ortho**	DIN 02150417 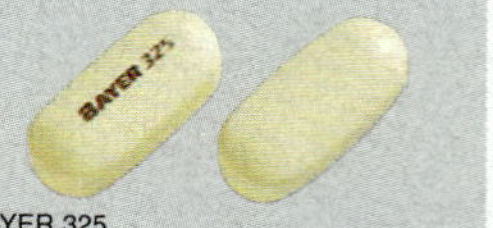 BAYER 325 Aspirin® Arthritis Pain Relief 325 mg **Bayer Consumer Care**	DIN 00513997 Pr 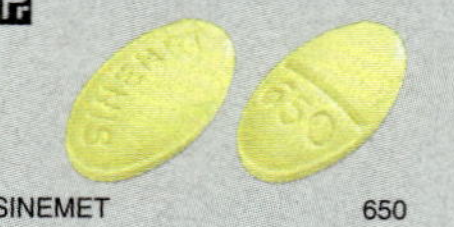 SINEMET 650 Sinemet® 100 mg/25 mg **Merck Frosst**
8	DIN 02241007 Pr 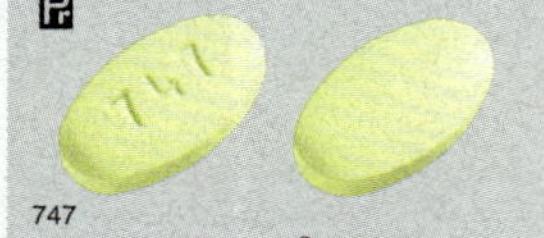 747 Hyzaar® DS 100/25 mg **Merck Frosst**	DIN 01984853 Pr 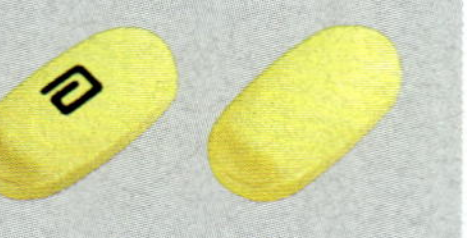 Biaxin BID® 250 mg **Abbott**	DIN 02126710 Pr 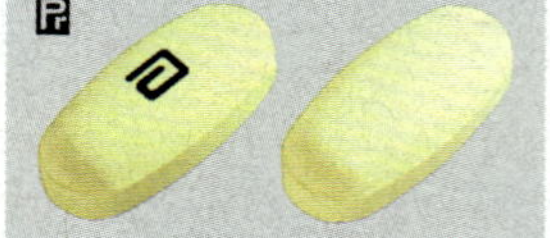 Biaxin BID® 500 mg **Abbott**	DIN 02244756 Pr 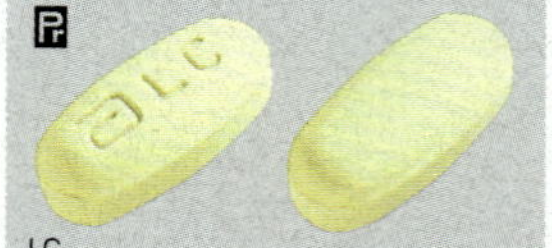 LC Biaxin® XL 500 mg **Abbott**	DIN 02150425 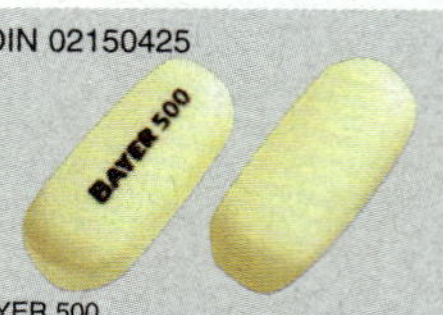 BAYER 500 Aspirin® Arthritis Pain Relief Extra Strength 500 mg **Bayer Consumer Care**

* ILLUSTRATION LESS THAN ACTUAL SIZE / ILLUSTRATION RÉDUITE

Use code A, B, C, D, E, horizontal bar and 1 to 8 vertical bar to locate illustrated products

Utiliser le code A, B, C, D, E de la ligne horizontale et les chiffres 1 à 8 de la ligne verticale pour repérer les produits illustrés

A | B | C | D | E

1

DIN 02246971
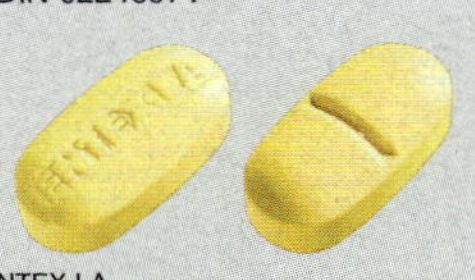
ENTEX LA
Entex® LA
Purdue Pharma

DIN 02132680 *
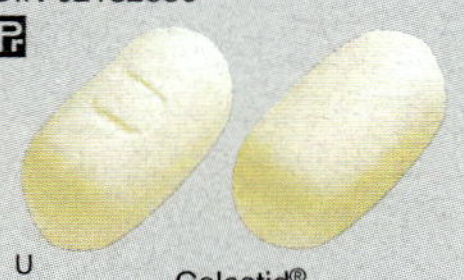
U
Colestid®
1 g
Pfizer

DIN 02244310 *
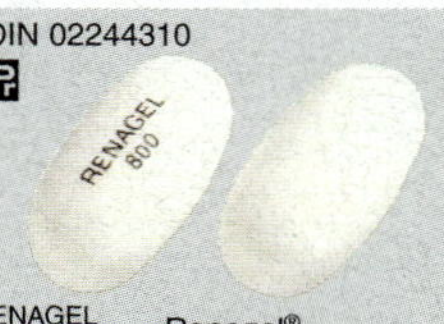
RENAGEL 800
Renagel®
800 mg
Genzyme

DIN 02233542
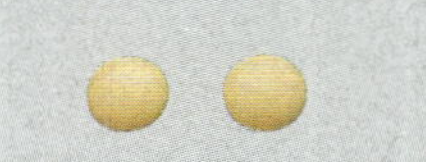
Diane®-35
Bayer

DIN 00254142
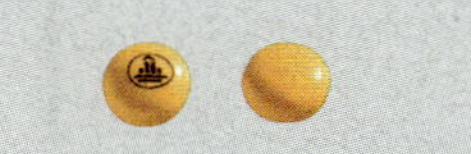
Dulcolax®
5 mg
Boehringer Ingelheim

2

DIN 02322404
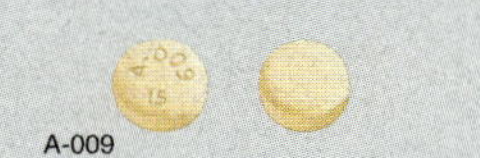
A-009 15
Abilify™
15 mg
Bristol-Myers Squibb

DIN 02231384
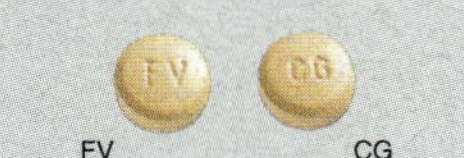
FV CG
Femara®
2.5 mg
Novartis Pharmaceuticals

DIN 02156008
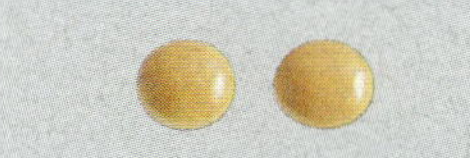
Fluanxol®
0.5 mg
Lundbeck

DIN 02199270
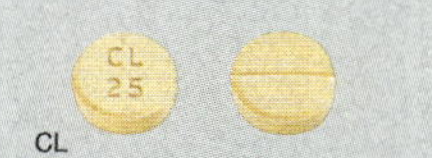
CL 25
Nitoman®
25 mg
Biovail Pharmaceuticals

DIN 02250462
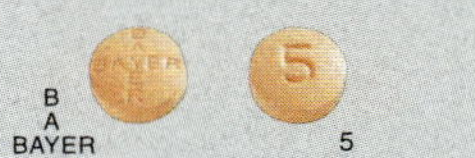
B A BAYER E R 5
Levitra®
5 mg
Bayer

3

DIN 02248503
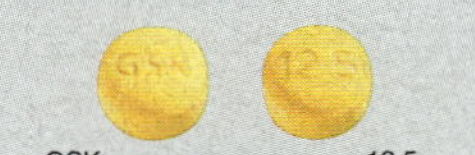
GSK 12.5
Paxil CR®
12.5 mg
GlaxoSmithKline

DIN 02265540
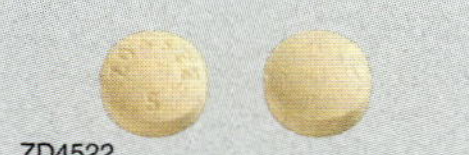
ZD4522 5
Crestor®
5 mg
AstraZeneca

DIN 02243797
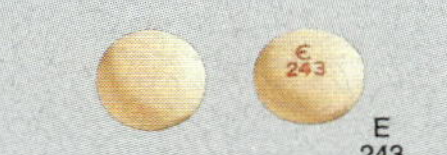
E 243
Pariet™
20 mg
Janssen-Ortho

DIN 02267233
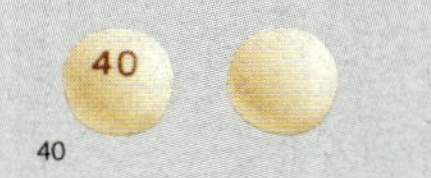
40
Tecta™
40 mg
Nycomed

DIN 02202476
Ⓝ
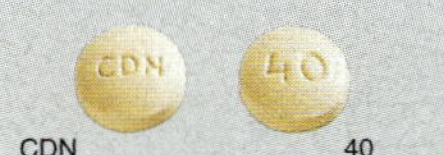
CDN 40
OxyContin®
40 mg
Purdue Pharma

4

DIN 02273578
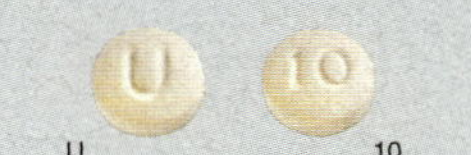
U 10
Uromax®
10 mg
Purdue Pharma

DIN 02250470
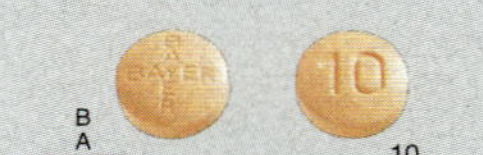
B A BAYER E R 10
Levitra®
10 mg
Bayer

DIN 00514012
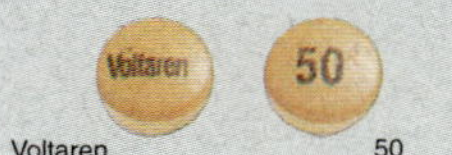
Voltaren 50
Voltaren®
50 mg
Novartis Pharmaceuticals

DIN 02243960
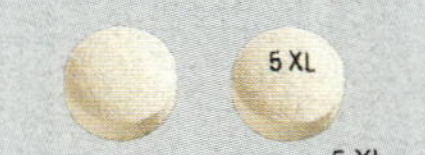
5 XL
Ditropan XL®
5 mg
Janssen-Ortho

DIN 02156016
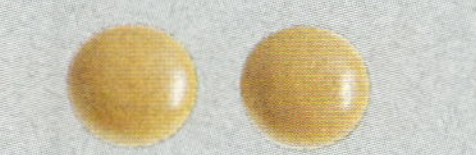
Fluanxol®
3 mg
Lundbeck

5

DIN 00028606
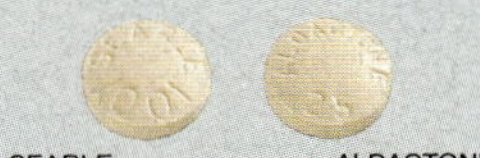
SEARLE 1001 ALDACTONE 25
Aldactone®
25 mg
Pfizer

DIN 02250489
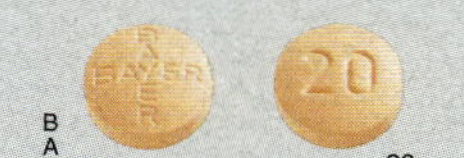
B A BAYER E R 20
Levitra®
20 mg
Bayer

DIN 00578452
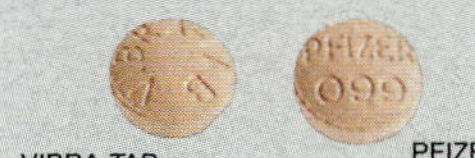
VIBRA-TAB PFIZER 099
Vibra-Tabs™
100 mg
Pfizer

DIN 02221985
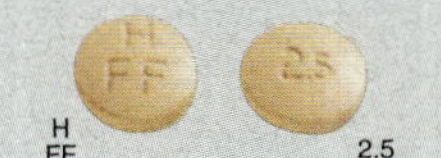
H FF 2.5
Renedil®
2.5 mg
sanofi-aventis

DIN 02319616
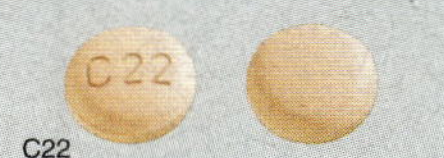
C22
Olmetec Plus®
20 mg/12.5 mg
Schering-Plough

6

DIN 02245565
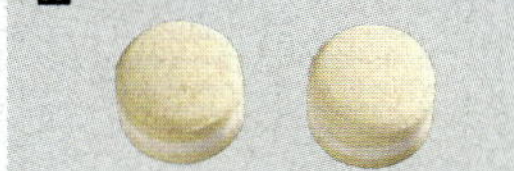
Xatral®
10 mg
sanofi-aventis

DIN 02057778
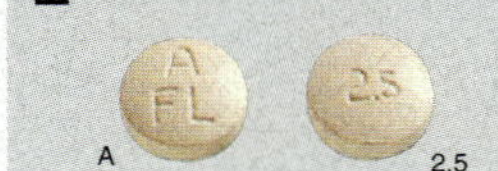
A FL 2.5
Plendil®
2.5 mg
AstraZeneca

DIN 02236952
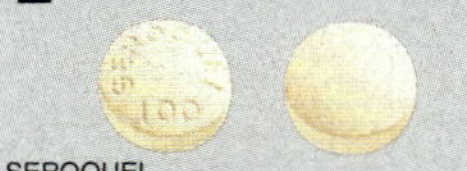
SEROQUEL 100
Seroquel®
100 mg
AstraZeneca

DIN 00176095
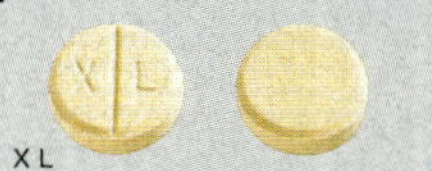
X L
Cafergot®
Novartis Pharmaceuticals

DIN 00658855
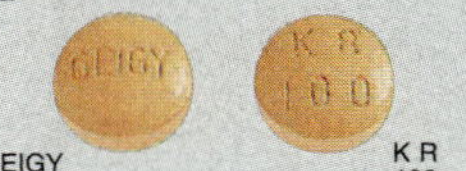
GEIGY K R 100
Lopresor® SR
100 mg
Novartis Pharmaceuticals

7

DIN 02270102
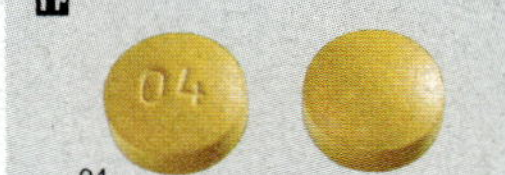
04
Flomax® CR
0.4 mg
Boehringer Ingelheim

DIN 02230894
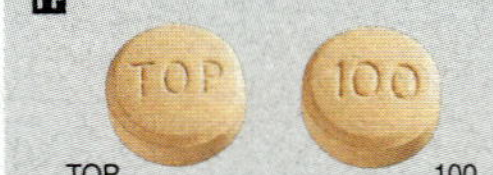
TOP 100
Topamax®
100 mg
Janssen-Ortho

DIN 02303922
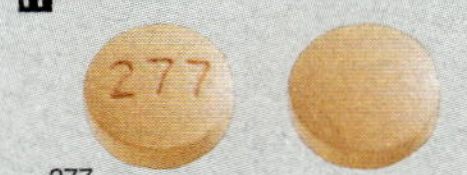
277
Januvia®
100 mg
Merck Frosst

DIN 02163748
Ⓝ
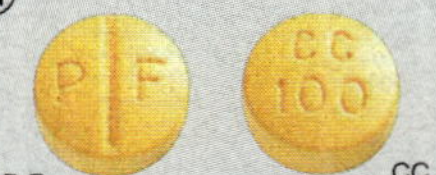
P F CC 100
Codeine Contin®
100 mg
Purdue Pharma

DIN 02250527
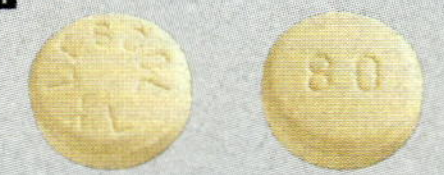
LESCOL XL 80
Lescol® XL
80 mg
Novartis Pharmaceuticals

8

DIN 02325926
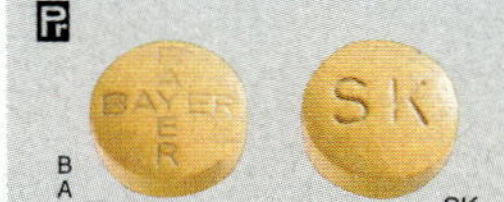
B A BAYER E R SK
Nimotop® Tablets
30 mg
Bayer

DIN 02064480
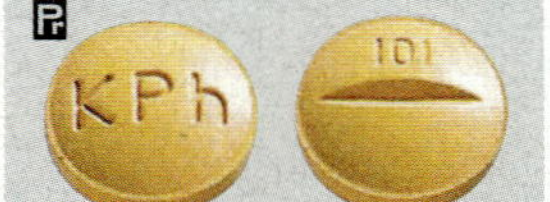
KPh 101
Salazopyrin®
500 mg
Pfizer

DIN 02248088
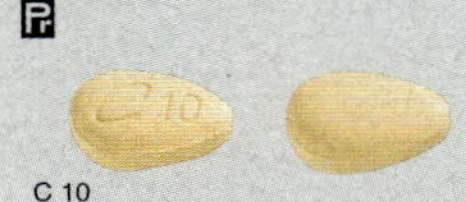
C 10
Cialis®
10 mg
Lilly

DIN 02248089
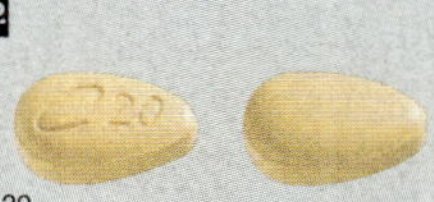
C 20
Cialis®
20 mg
Lilly

DIN 02258781
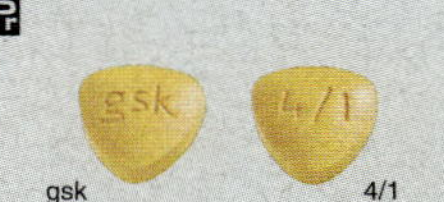
gsk 4/1
Avandaryl™
4 mg/1 mg
GlaxoSmithKline

* ILLUSTRATION LESS THAN ACTUAL SIZE / ILLUSTRATION RÉDUITE

Use code A, B, C, D, E, horizontal bar and 1 to 8 vertical bar to locate illustrated products

Utiliser le code A, B, C, D, E de la ligne horizontale et les chiffres 1 à 8 de la ligne verticale pour repérer les produits illustrés

1

A1 DIN 02283166 Pr
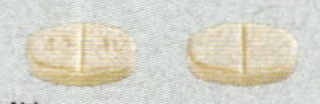
42 AV
Altace® HCT 10/12.5 mg
sanofi-aventis

B1 DIN 02247732 C
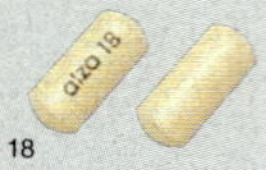
alza 18
Concerta® 18 mg
Janssen-Ortho

C1 DIN 02240551 Pr
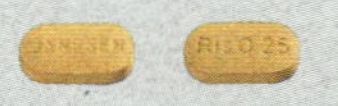
JANSSEN / Ris 0.25
Risperdal® 0.25 mg
Janssen-Ortho

D1 DIN 02270528 Pr
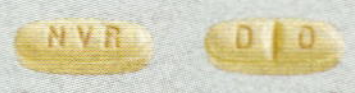
NVR / D O
Diovan® 40 mg
Novartis Pharmaceuticals

E1 DIN 02027887 Pr
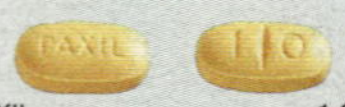
PAXIL / 1 0
Paxil® 10 mg
GlaxoSmithKline

2

A2 DIN 02106272 Pr
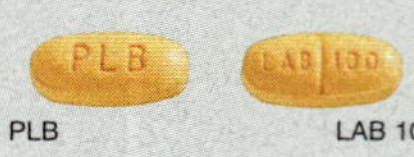
PLB / LAB 100
Trandate® 100 mg
Paladin

B2 DIN 02213567 Pr
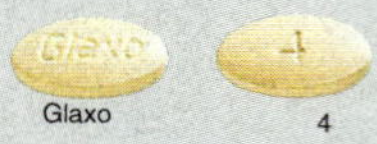
Glaxo / 4
Zofran® 4 mg
GlaxoSmithKline

C2 DIN 02241804 Pr
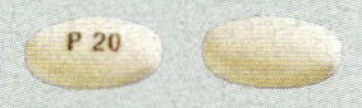
P 20
Pantoloc® 20 mg
Nycomed

D2 DIN 02229453 Pr
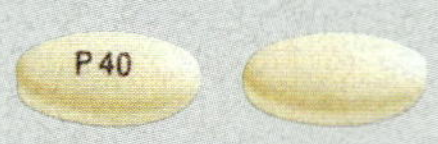
P 40
Pantoloc® 40 mg
Nycomed

E2 DIN 00839396 Pr
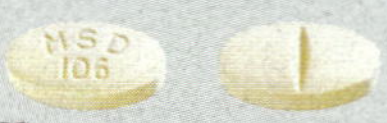
MSD 106
Prinivil® 10 mg
Merck Frosst

3

A3 DIN 02242067 Pr
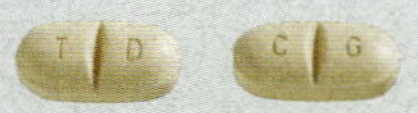
T D / C G
Trileptal® 150 mg
Novartis Pharmaceuticals

B3 DIN 02300281 Pr
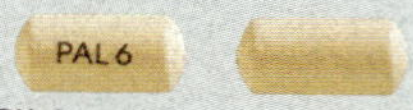
PAL 6
Invega™ 6 mg
Janssen-Ortho

C3 DIN 02242518 Pr
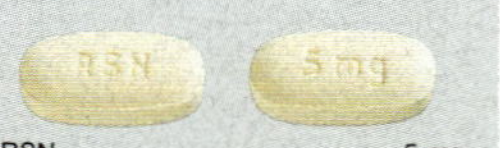
RSN / 5 mg
Actonel® 5 mg
Warner Chilcott

D3 DIN 00885835 Pr
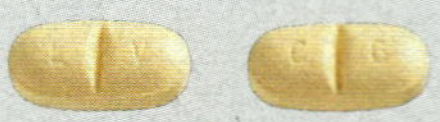
L V / C G
Lotensin® 5 mg
Novartis Pharmaceuticals

E3 DIN 02332922 Pr
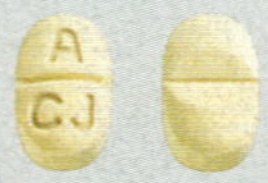
A CJ
Atacand® Plus 32 mg/12.5 mg
AstraZeneca

4

A4 DIN 02357623 Pr
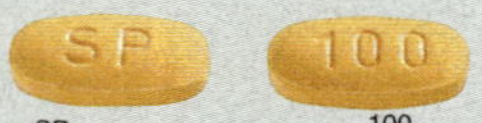
SP / 100
Vimpat™ 100 mg
UCB

B4 DIN 02269074 Pr
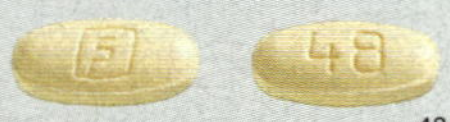
48
Lipidil™ EZ 48 mg
Fournier Pharma

C4 DIN 02126559
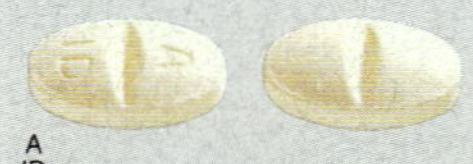
A ID
Imdur® 60 mg
AstraZeneca

D4 DIN 02247085 Pr
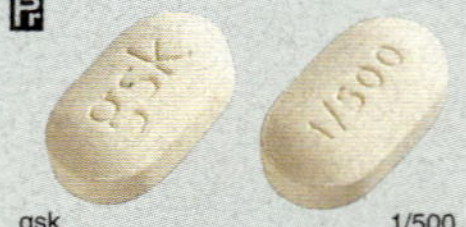
gsk / 1/500
Avandamet® 1 mg/500 mg
GlaxoSmithKline

E4 DIN 02319624 Pr
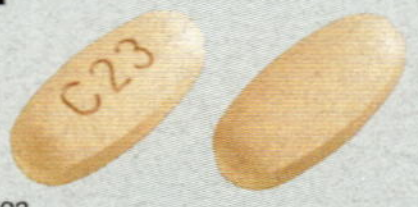
C23
Olmetec Plus® 40 mg/12.5 mg
Schering-Plough

5

A5 DIN 00870935 Pr
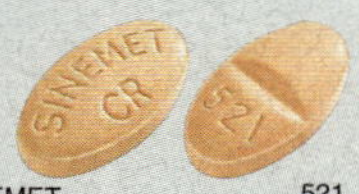
SINEMET CR / 521
Sinemet® CR 200 mg/50 mg
Merck Frosst

B5 DIN 02242068 Pr
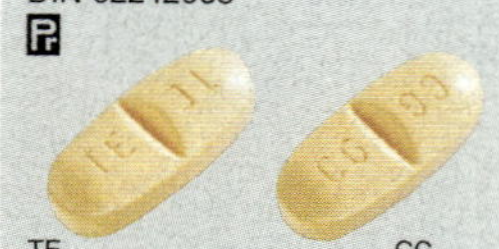
TE / CG
Trileptal® 300 mg
Novartis Pharmaceuticals

C5 DIN 02264846 Pr
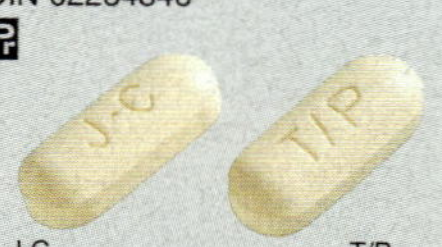
J-C / T/P
Tramacet® 37.5 mg/325 mg
Janssen-Ortho

D5 DIN 02300192 Pr
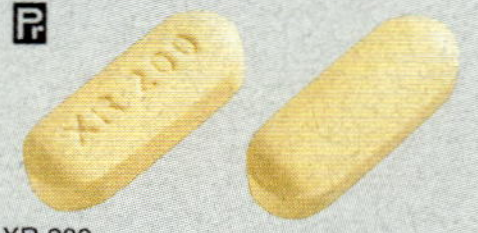
XR 200
Seroquel XR® 200 mg
AstraZeneca

E5 DIN 02300206 Pr
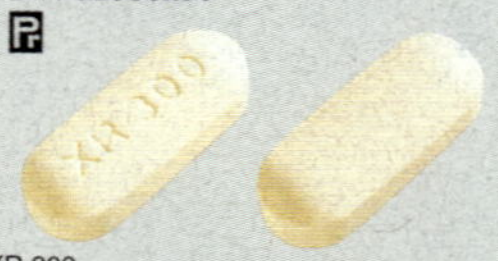
XR 300
Seroquel XR® 300 mg
AstraZeneca

6

A6 DIN 02332736 Pr
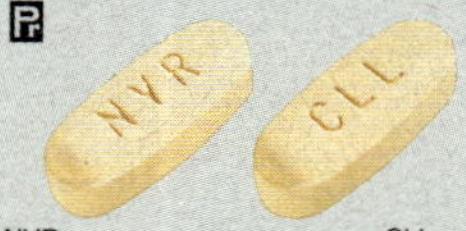
NVR / CLL
Rasilez HCT® 150 mg/25 mg
Novartis Pharmaceuticals

B6 DIN 02247028 Pr
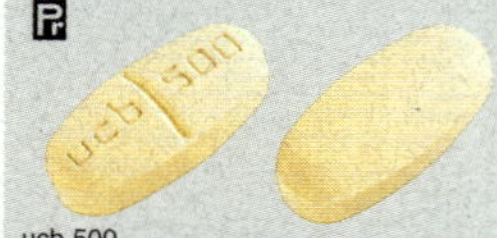
ucb 500
Keppra® 500 mg
UCB

C6 DIN 02253631 Pr
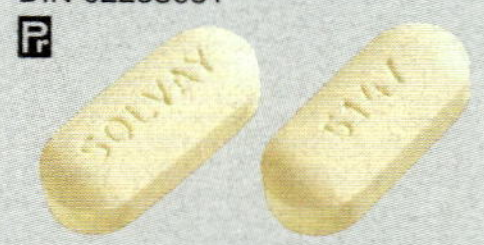
SOLVAY / 5147
Teveten® Plus 600/12.5 mg
Abbott Products

D6 DIN 02295636 Pr
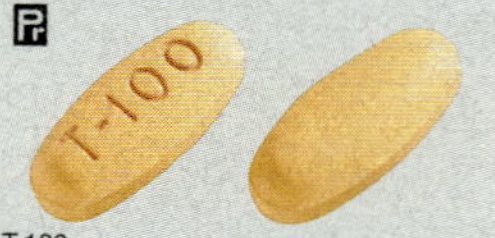
T-100
Thelin® 100 mg
Pfizer

E6 DIN 02248440 Pr
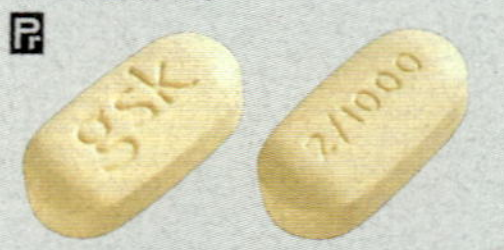
gsk / 2/1000
Avandamet® 2 mg/1000 mg
GlaxoSmithKline

7

A7 DIN 02318709 Pr
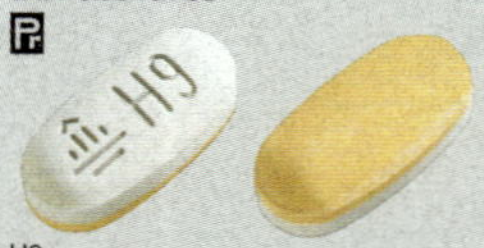
H9
Micardis® Plus 80 mg/25 mg
Boehringer Ingelheim

B7 DIN 02308916 Pr
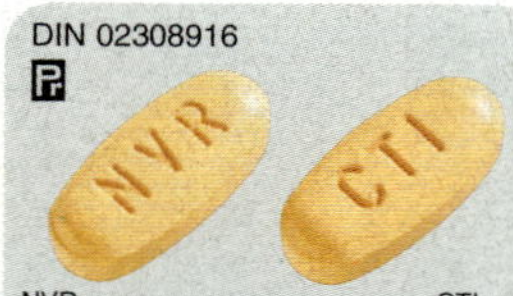
NVR / CTI
Diovan-HCT® 320/25 mg
Novartis Pharmaceuticals

C7 DIN 02245439 Pr
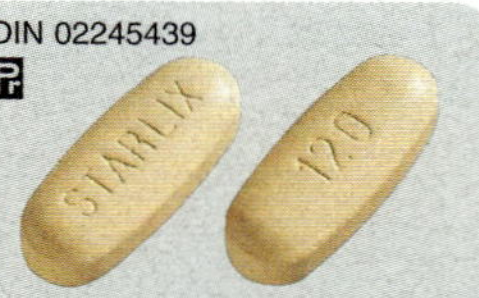
STARLIX / 120
Starlix® 120 mg
Novartis Pharmaceuticals

D7 DIN 02326442 Pr
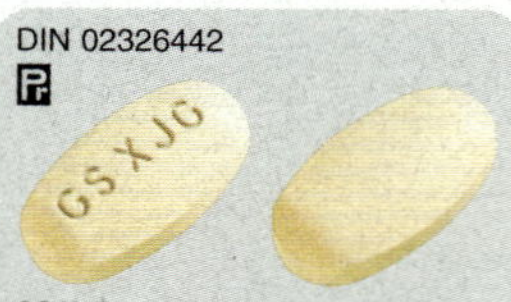
GS XJG
Tykerb™ 250 mg
GlaxoSmithKline

E7 DIN 02247520 Pr
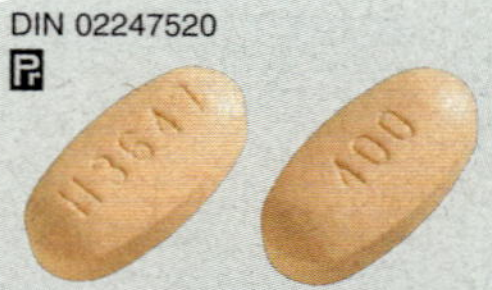
H3647 / 400
Ketek® 400 mg
sanofi-aventis

8

A8 DIN 02064472 Pr
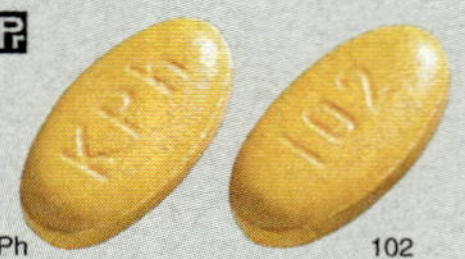
KPh / 102
Salazopyrin En-Tabs® 500 mg
Pfizer

B8 DIN 02112787 Pr
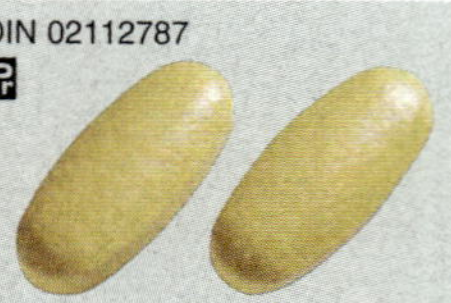
Salofalk® 500 mg
Axcan Pharma

C8 DIN 02240357 Pr
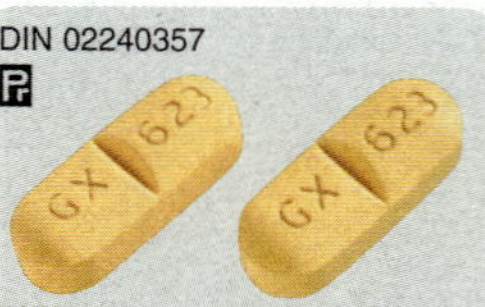
GX 623 / GX 623
Ziagen® 300 mg
ViiV Healthcare ULC

D8 DIN 02253283 Pr
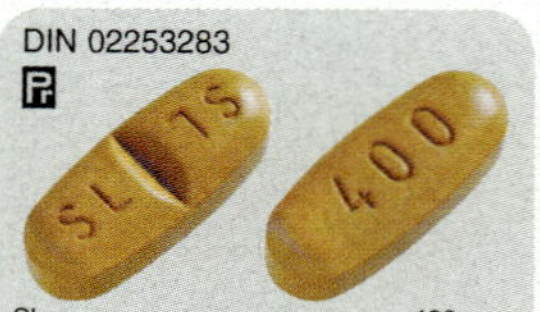
SL / 400
Gleevec® 400 mg
Novartis Pharmaceuticals

E8 DIN 02332752 Pr
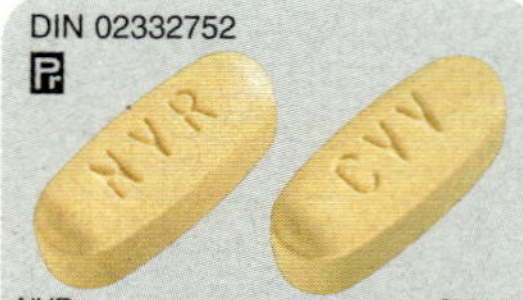
NVR / CVV
Rasilez HCT® 300 mg/25 mg
Novartis Pharmaceuticals

* ILLUSTRATION LESS THAN ACTUAL SIZE / ILLUSTRATION RÉDUITE

Use code A, B, C, D, E, horizontal bar and 1 to 8 vertical bar to locate illustrated products

Utiliser le code A, B, C, D, E de la ligne horizontale et les chiffres 1 à 8 de la ligne verticale pour repérer les produits illustrés

	A	B	C	D	E
1	DIN 02239853 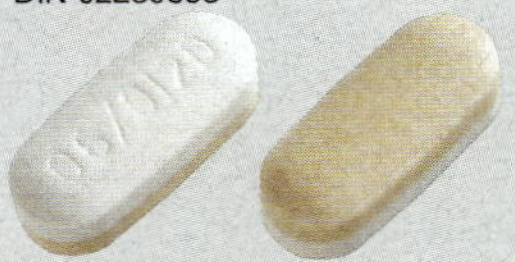 06/012D Allegra®-D 60 mg/120 mg **sanofi-aventis**	DIN 02246045 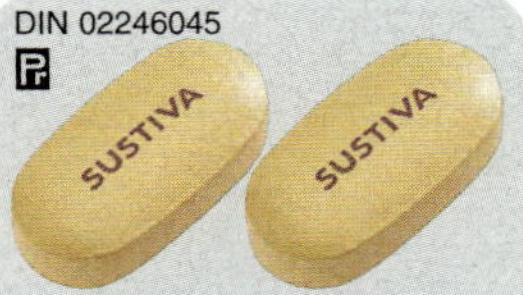 SUSTIVA Sustiva® 600 mg **Bristol-Myers Squibb**	DIN 02256290 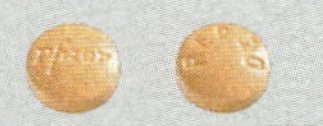 Pfizer REP 20 Relpax™ 20 mg **Pfizer**	DIN 01950592 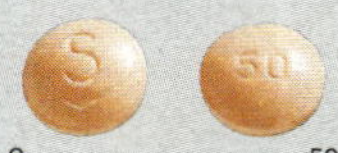 S 50 Dicetel® 50 mg **Abbott Products**	DIN 02179709 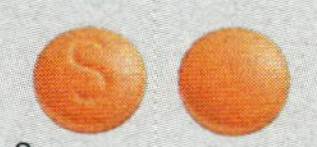 S Lozide® 1.25 mg **Servier**
2	DIN 02256304 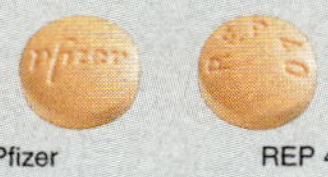 Pfizer REP 40 Relpax™ 40 mg **Pfizer**	DIN 00026123 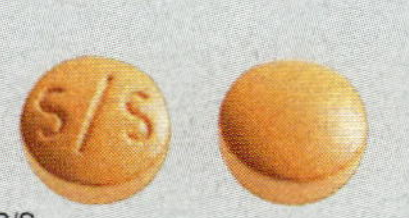 S/S Senokot®•S 8.6 mg/50 mg **Purdue Pharma**	DIN 00074225 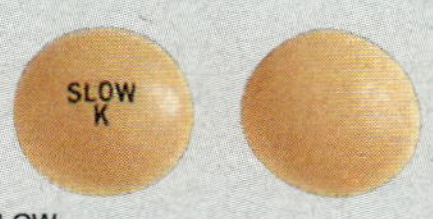 SLOW K Slow-K® 600 mg **Novartis Pharmaceuticals**	DIN 02230684 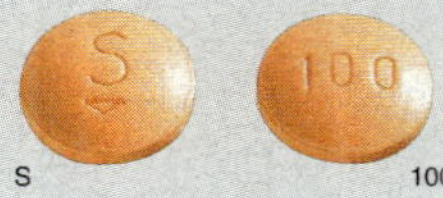 S 100 Dicetel® 100 mg **Abbott Products**	DIN 02338327 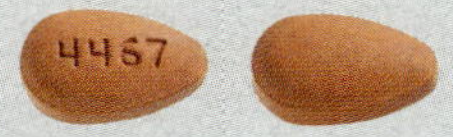 4467 Adcirca™ 20 mg **Lilly**
3	DIN 02258803 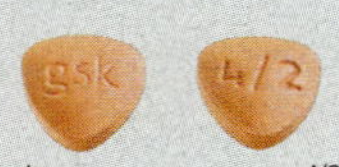 gsk 4/2 Avandaryl™ 4 mg/2 mg **GlaxoSmithKline**	DIN 01924516 © 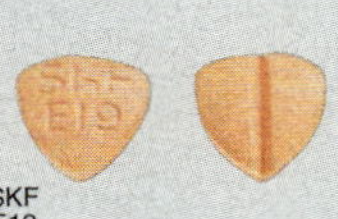 SKF E19 Dexedrine® 5 mg **Paladin**	DIN 00670928 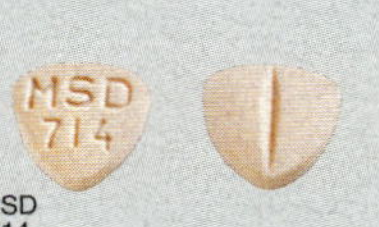 MSD 714 Vasotec® 20 mg **Merck Frosst**	DIN 02349124 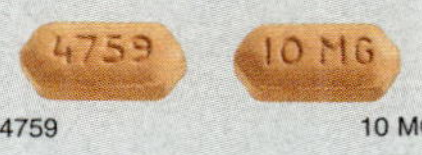 4759 10 MG Effient™ 10 mg **Lilly**	DIN 00885843 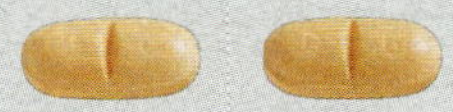 H O C G Lotensin® 10 mg **Novartis Pharmaceuticals**
4	DIN 02246896 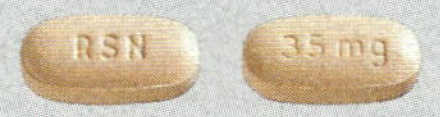 RSN 35 mg Actonel® 35 mg **Warner Chilcott**	DIN 02244782 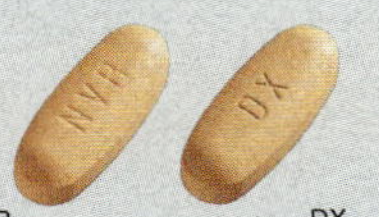 NVR DX Diovan® 160 mg **Novartis Pharmaceuticals**	DIN 02213575 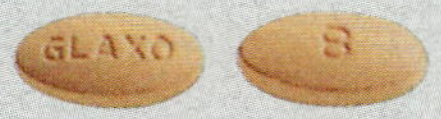 GLAXO 8 Zofran® 8 mg **GlaxoSmithKline**	DIN 00773611 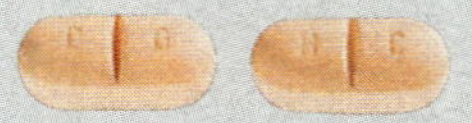 C G H C Tegretol® CR 200 mg **Novartis Pharmaceuticals**	DIN 02357631 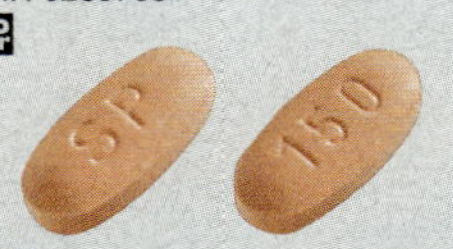 SP 150 Vimpat™ 150 mg **UCB**
5	DIN 02243763 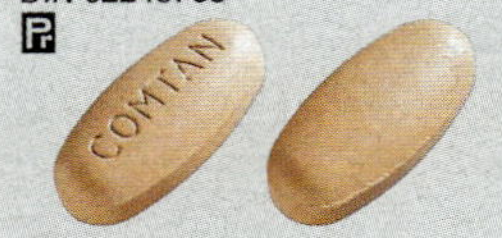 COMTAN Comtan® 200 mg **Novartis Pharmaceuticals**	DIN 02279320 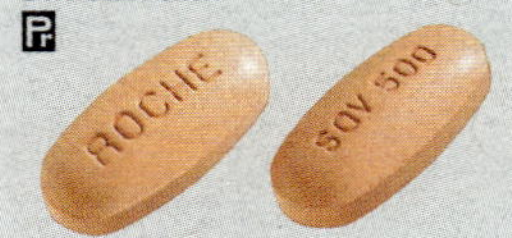 ROCHE SQV 500 Invirase® 500 mg **Roche**	DIN 02324016 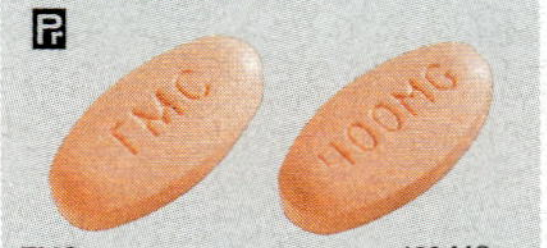 TMC 400 MG Prezista® 400 mg **Janssen-Ortho**	DIN 02324024 * 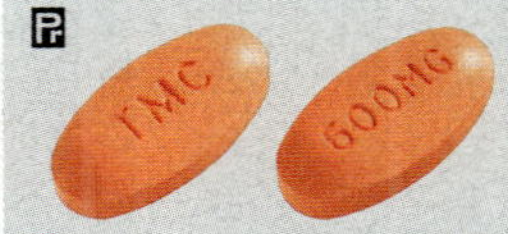 TMC 600 MG Prezista® 600 mg **Janssen-Ortho**	DIN 01914030 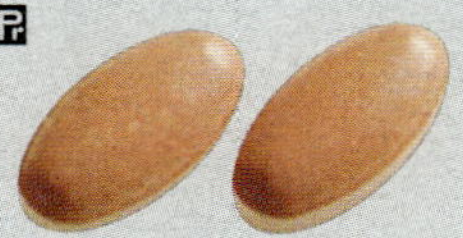 Mesasal® 500 mg **GlaxoSmithKline**
6	DIN 02163799 Ⓝ 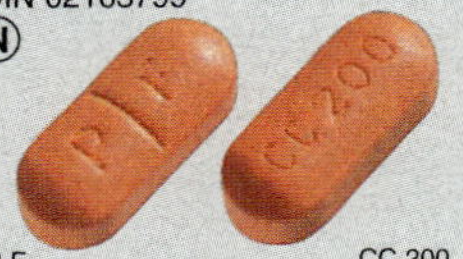 P F CC 200 Codeine Contin® 200 mg **Purdue Pharma**	DIN 02284057 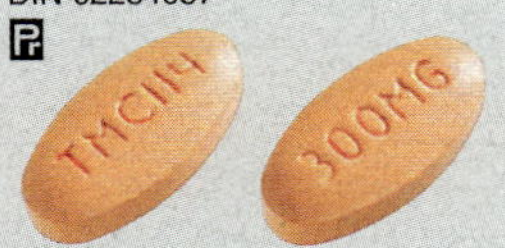 TMC114 300 MG Prezista® 300 mg **Janssen-Ortho**	DIN 02269341 * 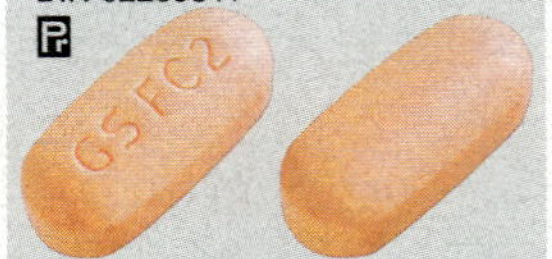 GS FC2 Kivexa® 600 mg/300 mg **ViiV Healthcare ULC**	DIN 02268825 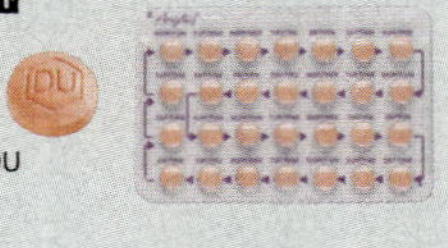 DU Angeliq® **Bayer**	DIN 02236951 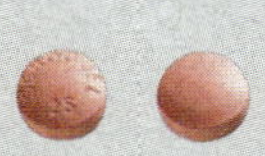 SEROQUEL 25 Seroquel® 25 mg **AstraZeneca**
7	DIN 02243796 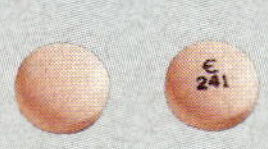 E 241 Pariet™ 10 mg **Janssen-Ortho**	DIN 00708917 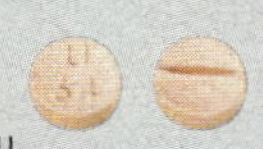 U 64 Provera® 2.5 mg **Pfizer**	DIN 02230737 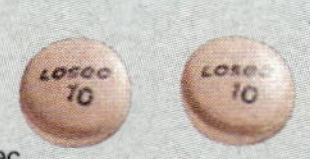 Losec 10 Losec® 10 mg **AstraZeneca**	DIN 02172062 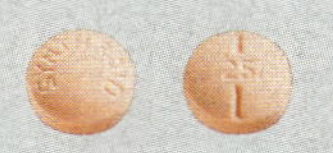 SYNTHROID 25 Synthroid® 25 µg **Abbott**	DIN 02264935 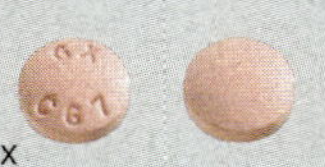 GX CG7 Malarone® Pediatric 62.5 mg/25 mg **GlaxoSmithKline**
8	DIN 00885851 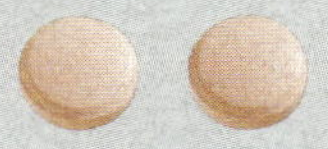 Lotensin® 20 mg **Novartis Pharmaceuticals**	DIN 02049376 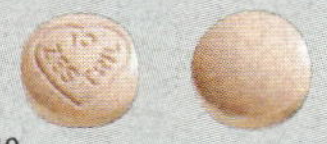 10 ZESTRIL Zestril® 10 mg **AstraZeneca**	DIN 02049384 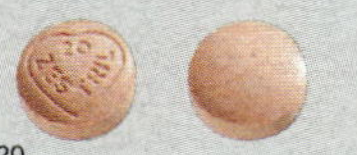 20 ZESTRIL Zestril® 20 mg **AstraZeneca**	DIN 00013803 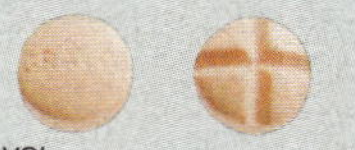 GRAVOL Gravol® 50 mg **Church & Dwight**	DIN 02239091 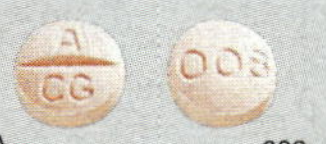 A CG 008 Atacand® 8 mg **AstraZeneca**

* ILLUSTRATION LESS THAN ACTUAL SIZE / ILLUSTRATION RÉDUITE

Use code A, B, C, D, E, horizontal bar and 1 to 8 vertical bar to locate illustrated products

Utiliser le code A, B, C, D, E de la ligne horizontale et les chiffres 1 à 8 de la ligne verticale pour repérer les produits illustrés

1

A — DIN 02239092

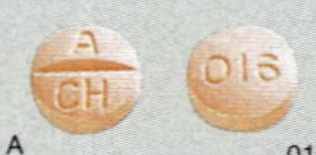

A CH · 016

Atacand® 16 mg

AstraZeneca

B — DIN 00568635

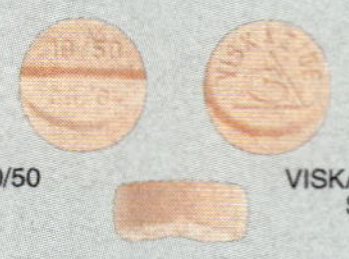

10/50 · VISKAZIDE S

Viskazide® 10/50

Novartis Pharmaceuticals

C — DIN 00180408

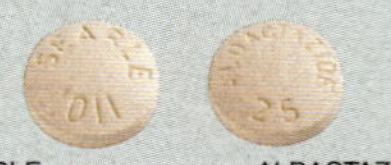

SEARLE 1011 · ALDACTAZIDE 25

Aldactazide 25®

Pfizer

D — DIN 02237369

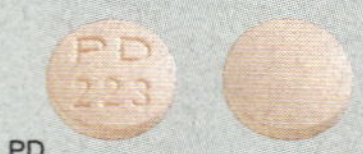

PD 223

Accuretic™ 20/25 mg

Pfizer

E — DIN 00579351

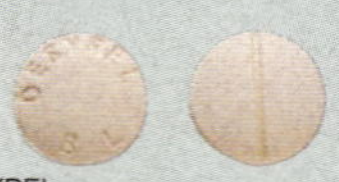

DESYREL B L

Desyrel® 50 mg

Bristol-Myers Squibb

2

A — DIN 01918354

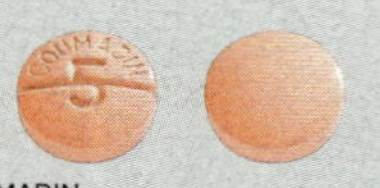

COUMADIN 5

Coumadin® 5 mg

Bristol-Myers Squibb

B — DIN 02222000

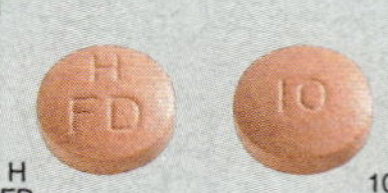

H FD · 10

Renedil® 10 mg

sanofi-aventis

C — DIN 02311658

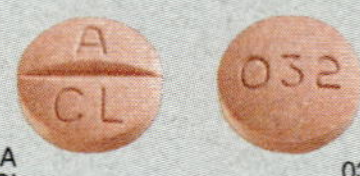

A CL · 032

Atacand® 32 mg

AstraZeneca

D — DIN 02247704

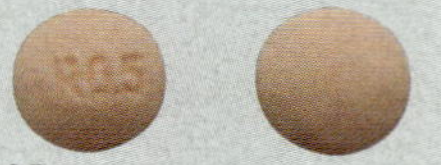

R 0.5

Risperdal® M-Tab® 0.5 mg

Janssen-Ortho

E — DIN 00285455

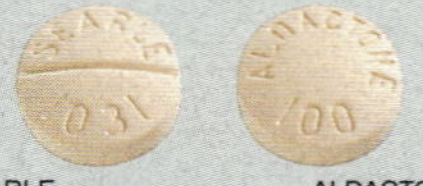

SEARLE 1031 · ALDACTONE 100

Aldactone® 100 mg

Pfizer

3

A — DIN 00293490

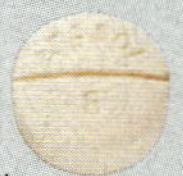

ATASOL 8

Atasol®-8

Church & Dwight

B — DIN 00013803

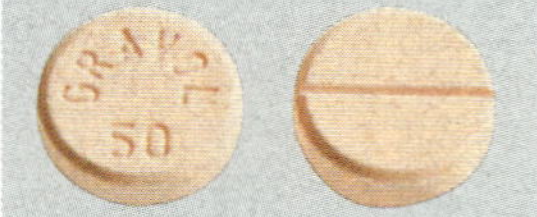

GRAVOL 50

Gravol® 50 mg

Church & Dwight

C — DIN 02247705

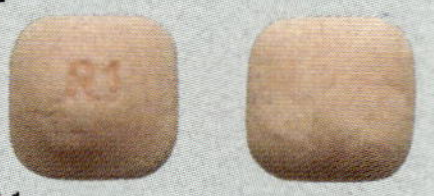

R 1

Risperdal® M-Tab® 1 mg

Janssen-Ortho

D — DIN 02232568

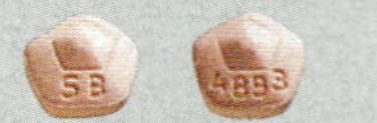

SB · 4893

ReQuip® 2 mg

GlaxoSmithKline

E — DIN 02241113

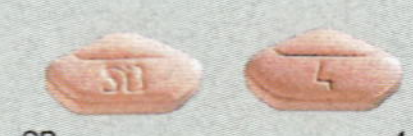

SB · 4

Avandia® 4 mg

GlaxoSmithKline

4

A — DIN 00548367

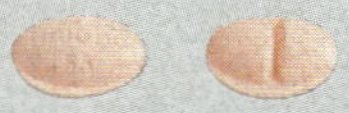

UPJOHN 55

Xanax® 0.5 mg

Pfizer

B — DIN 02244021

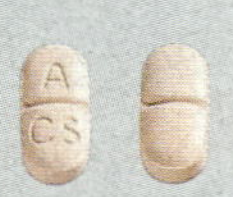

A CS

Atacand® Plus 16 mg/12.5 mg

AstraZeneca

C — DIN 02332957

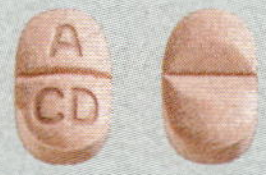

A CD

Atacand® Plus 32 mg/25 mg

AstraZeneca

D — DIN 02300303

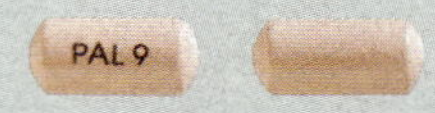

PAL 9

Invega™ 9 mg

Janssen-Ortho

E — DIN 00839418

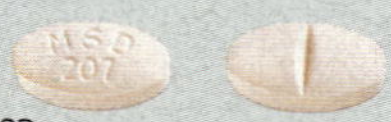

MSD 207

Prinivil® 20 mg

Merck Frosst

5

A — DIN 02231462

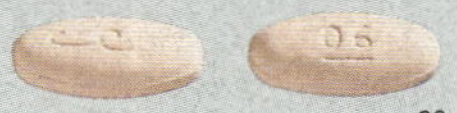

e · 06

Allegra® 12 Hour

sanofi-aventis

B — DIN 00884340

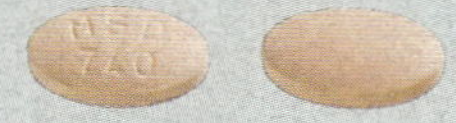

MSD 740

Zocor® 20 mg

Merck Frosst

C — DIN 02239193

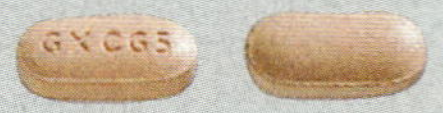

GX CG5

Heptovir® 100 mg

GlaxoSmithKline Shire Canada

D — DIN 02163659

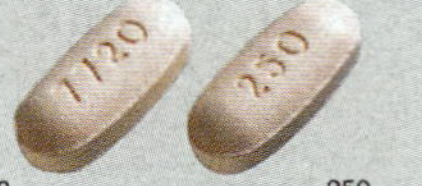

7720 · 250

Cefzil™ 250 mg

Bristol-Myers Squibb

E — DIN 02025299

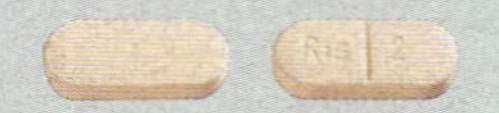

Ris 2

Risperdal® 2 mg

Janssen-Ortho

6

A — DIN 02089769

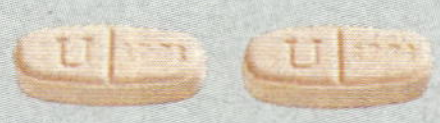

U 3773

Ogen® 1.5 mg

Pfizer

B — DIN 00594377

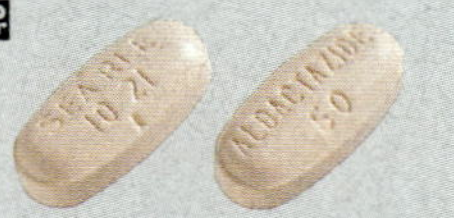

SEARLE 1021 · ALDACTAZIDE 50

Aldactazide 50®

Pfizer

C — DIN 02247087

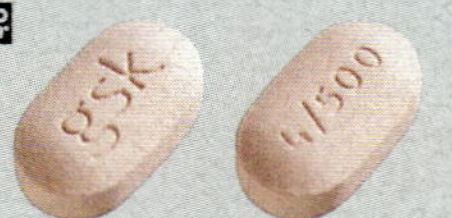

gsk · 4/500

Avandamet® 4 mg/500 mg

GlaxoSmithKline

D — DIN 02241818

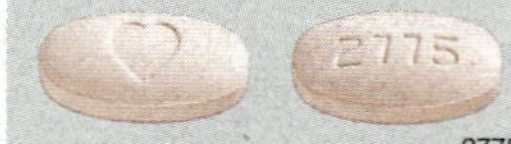

2775

Avalide® 150/12.5 mg

Bristol-Myers Squibb / sanofi-aventis

E — DIN 02242819

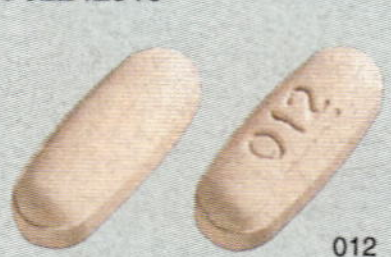

012

Allegra® 24 Hour

sanofi-aventis

7

A — DIN 02319632

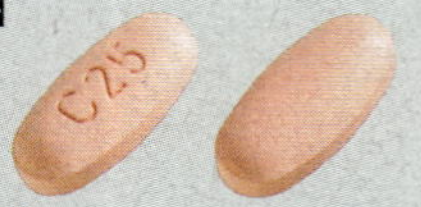

C25

Olmetec Plus® 40 mg/25 mg

Schering-Plough

B — DIN 02300184

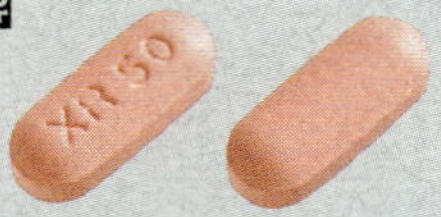

XR 50

Seroquel XR® 50 mg

AstraZeneca

C — DIN 00596426

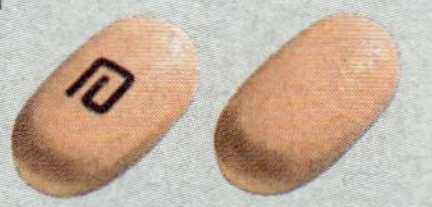

Epival® 250 mg

Abbott

D — DIN 02301881

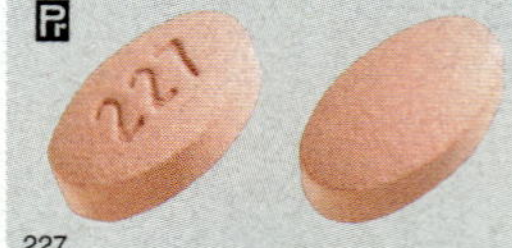

227

Isentress® 400 mg

Merck Frosst

E — DIN 02238454

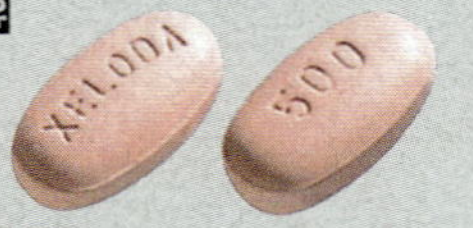

XELODA · 500

Xeloda® 500 mg

Roche

8

A — DIN 00702277

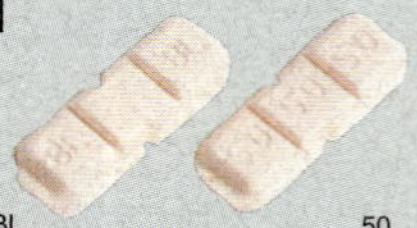

BL · 50

Desyrel® Dividose 150 mg

Bristol-Myers Squibb

B — DIN 00755583

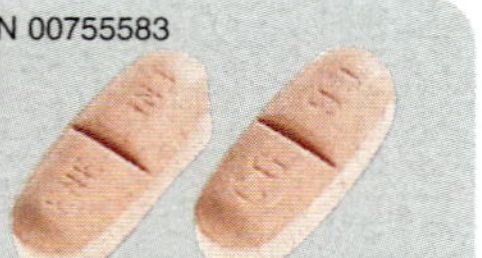

ENE · CG

Tegretol® CR 400 mg

Novartis Pharmaceuticals

C — DIN 02302071

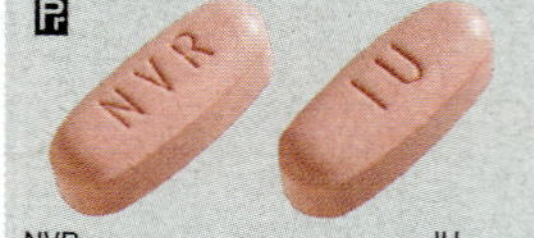

NVR · IU

Rasilez® 300 mg

Novartis Pharmaceuticals

D — DIN 02264579

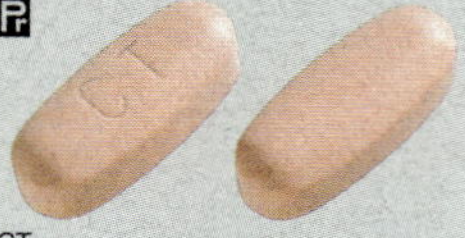

CT

Myfortic® 360 mg

Novartis Pharmaceuticals

E — DIN 02333856

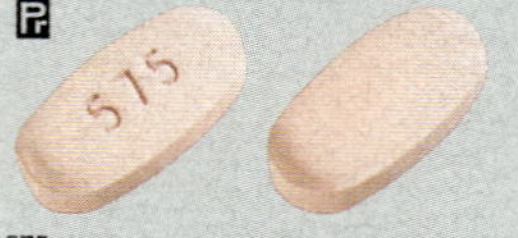

575

Janumet™ 50 mg/500 mg

Merck Frosst

* ILLUSTRATION LESS THAN ACTUAL SIZE / ILLUSTRATION RÉDUITE

Use code A, B, C, D, E, horizontal bar and 1 to 8 vertical bar to locate illustrated products

Utiliser le code A, B, C, D, E de la ligne horizontale et les chiffres 1 à 8 de la ligne verticale pour repérer les produits illustrés

A | B | C | D | E

1

DIN 02247029
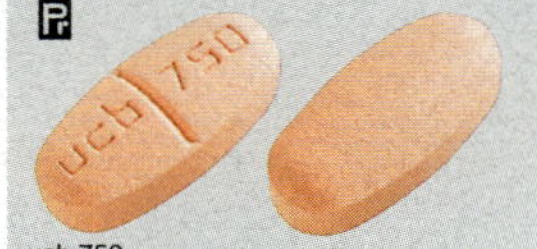
ucb 750
Keppra® 750 mg
UCB

DIN 02330555
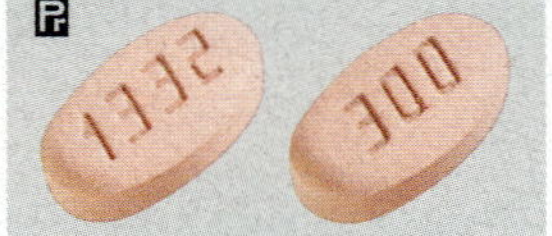
1332 300
Plavix® 300 mg
sanofi-aventis

DIN 02333864 *
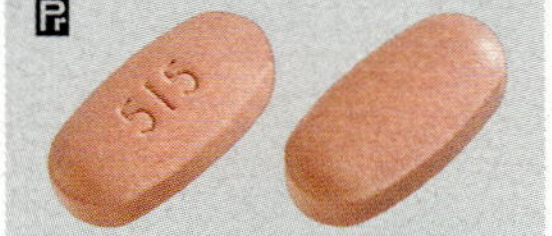
515
Janumet™ 50 mg/850 mg
Merck Frosst

DIN 02241819
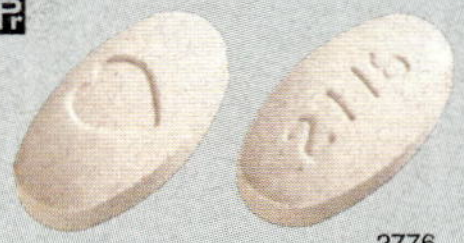
2776
Avalide® 300/12.5 mg
Bristol-Myers Squibb/ sanofi-aventis

DIN 00010383
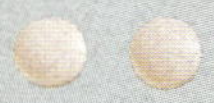
Sintrom® 1 mg
Paladin

2

DIN 02103729
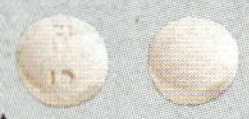
Zt 10
Zestoretic® 10/12.5 mg
AstraZeneca

DIN 02049333
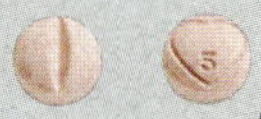
5
Zestril® 5 mg
AstraZeneca

DIN 02316986
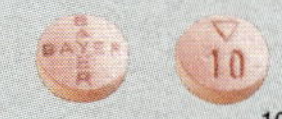
B A BAYER E R 10
Xarelto® 10 mg
Bayer

DIN 02244981
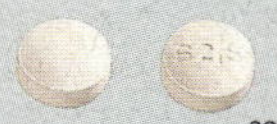
62.5
Tracleer® 62.5 mg
Actelion

DIN 02014300 Ⓝ
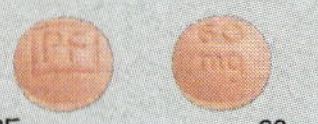
PF 60 mg
MS Contin® 60 mg
Purdue Pharma

3

DIN 02213222
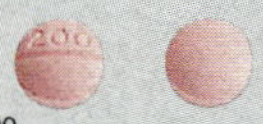
200
Eltroxin® 200 µg
Triton Pharma

DIN 00564966
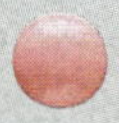
Lozide® 2.5 mg
Servier

DIN 02277271
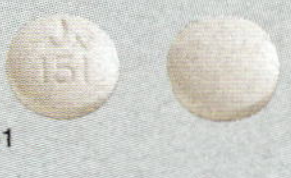
151
Vesicare® 10 mg
Astellas

DIN 00888400
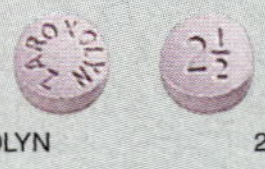
ZAROXOLYN 2 1/2
Zaroxolyn® 2.5 mg
sanofi-aventis

DIN 02231378
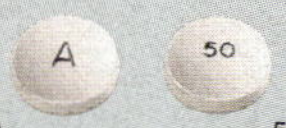
A 50
Anzemet® 50 mg
sanofi-aventis

4

DIN 02202468 Ⓝ
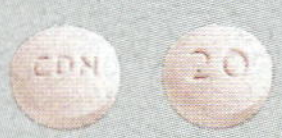
CDN 20
OxyContin® 20 mg
Purdue Pharma

DIN 02248504
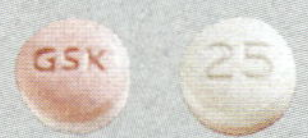
GSK 25
Paxil CR® 25 mg
GlaxoSmithKline

DIN 02247162
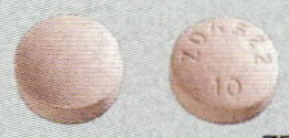
ZD4522 10
Crestor® 10 mg
AstraZeneca

DIN 02171228
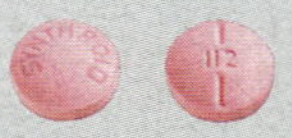
SYNTHROID 112
Synthroid® 112 µg
Abbott

DIN 02172143
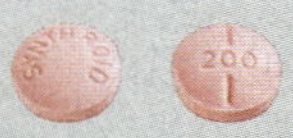
SYNTHROID 200
Synthroid® 200 µg
Abbott

5

DIN 02017776
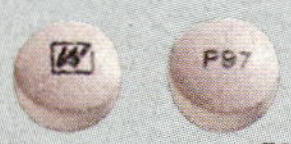
W P97
Primaquine 15 mg
sanofi-aventis

DIN 02243961
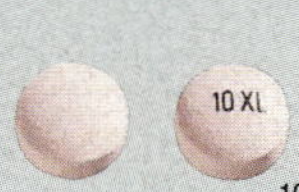
10 XL
Ditropan XL® 10 mg
Janssen-Ortho

DIN 02045729
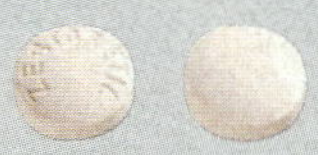
ZESTORETIC
Zestoretic® 20/25 mg
AstraZeneca

DIN 00568627
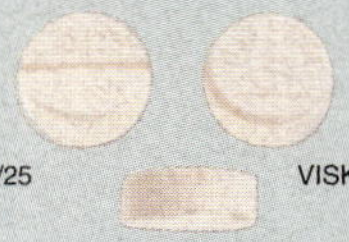
10/25 VISKAZIDE S
Viskazide® 10/25
Novartis Pharmaceuticals

DIN 02244781
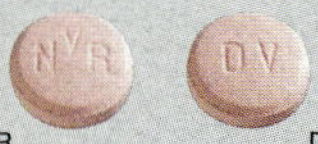
NVR DV
Diovan® 80 mg
Novartis Pharmaceuticals

6

DIN 02333554
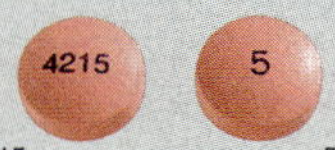
4215 5
Onglyza™ 5 mg
Bristol-Myers Squibb / AstraZeneca

DIN 02238682
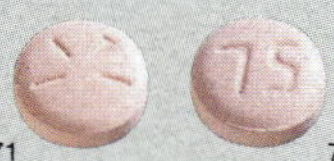
1171 75
Plavix® 75 mg
sanofi-aventis

DIN 02273225
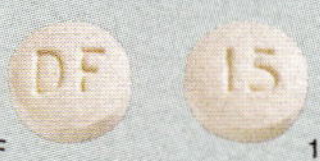
DF 15
Enablex® 15 mg
Novartis Pharmaceuticals

DIN 02313766 *
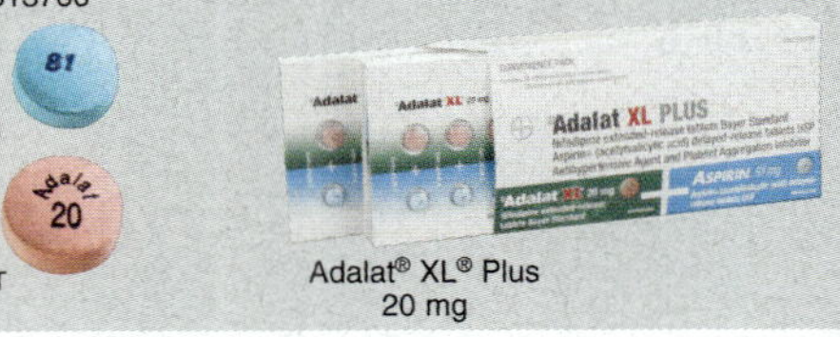

81
ADALAT 20
Adalat® XL® Plus 20 mg
Bayer

7

DIN 02221993
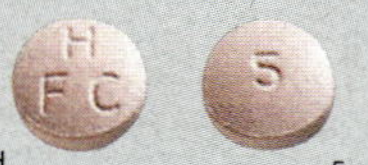
H F C 5
Renedil® 5 mg
sanofi-aventis

DIN 02247163
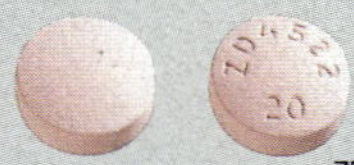
ZD4522 20
Crestor® 20 mg
AstraZeneca

DIN 01918311
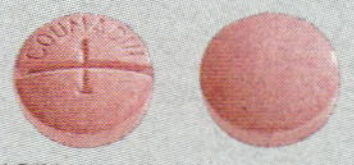
COUMADIN 1
Coumadin® 1 mg
Bristol-Myers Squibb

DIN 02313774 *
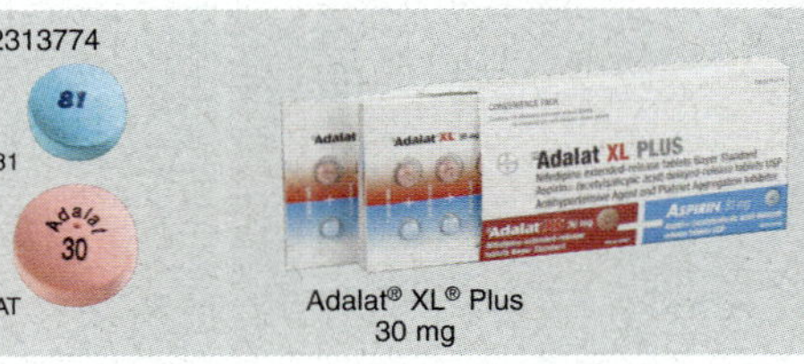

81
ADALAT 30
Adalat® XL® Plus 30 mg
Bayer

8

DIN 02237618
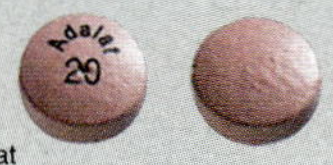
Adalat 20
Adalat® XL® 20 mg
Bayer

DIN 02155907
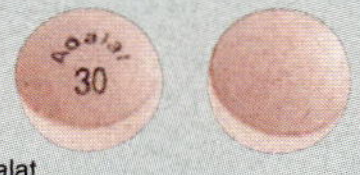
Adalat 30
Adalat® XL® 30 mg
Bayer

DIN 02155990
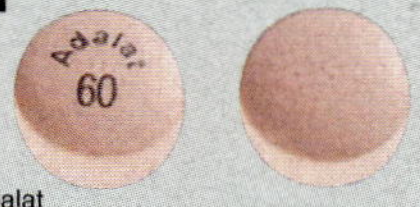
Adalat 60
Adalat® XL® 60 mg
Bayer

DIN 02313782 *
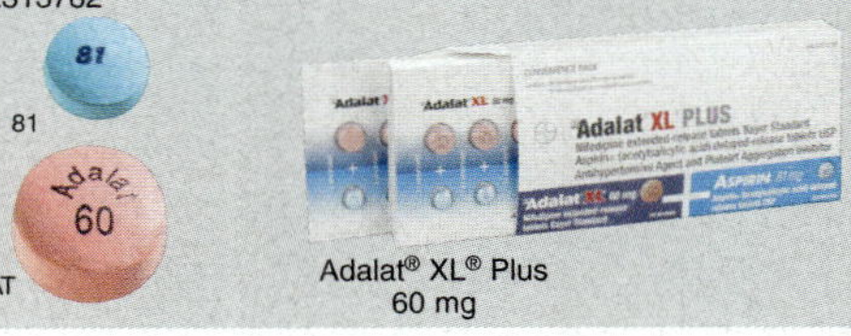

81
ADALAT 60
Adalat® XL® Plus 60 mg
Bayer

* ILLUSTRATION LESS THAN ACTUAL SIZE / ILLUSTRATION RÉDUITE

Use code A, B, C, D, E, horizontal bar and 1 to 8 vertical bar to locate illustrated products

Utiliser le code A, B, C, D, E de la ligne horizontale et les chiffres 1 à 8 de la ligne verticale pour repérer les produits illustrés

	A	B	C	D	E
1	DIN 02322455 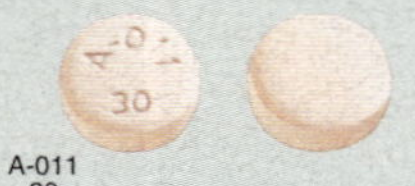 A-011 30 Abilify™ 30 mg **Bristol-Myers Squibb**	DIN 01947958 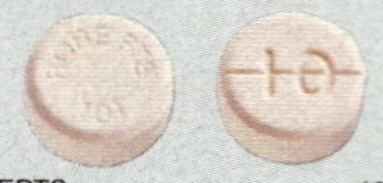 ROBERTS 101 · 10 Duvoid® 10 mg **Paladin**	DIN 01947923 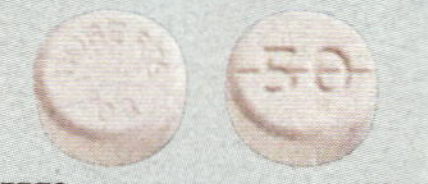 ROBERTS 103 · 50 Duvoid® 50 mg **Paladin**	DIN 02036282 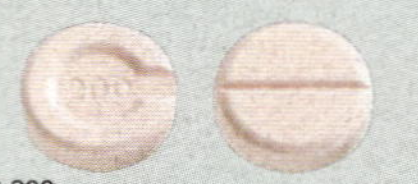 C 200 Cordarone® 200 mg **Pfizer**	DIN 00851779 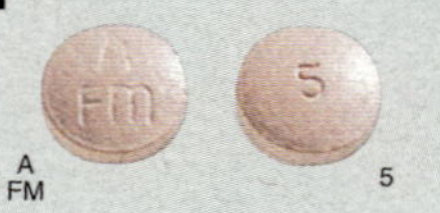 A FM · 5 Plendil® 5 mg **AstraZeneca**
2	DIN 02238216 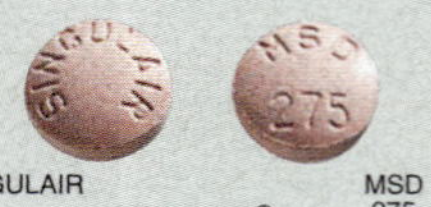 SINGULAIR · MSD 275 Singulair® 5 mg **Merck Frosst**	DIN 02245438 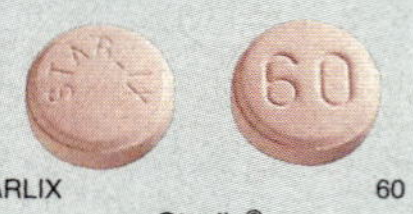 STARLIX · 60 Starlix® 60 mg **Novartis Pharmaceuticals**	DIN 00511196 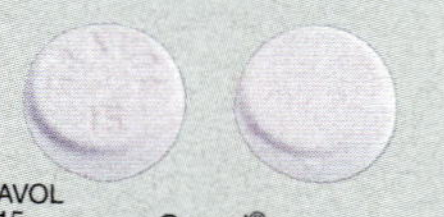 GRAVOL 15 Gravol® 15 mg **Church & Dwight**	DIN 02302063 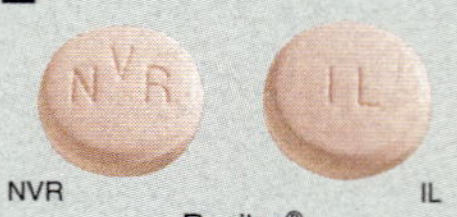 NVR · IL Rasilez® 150 mg **Novartis Pharmaceuticals**	DIN 02148625 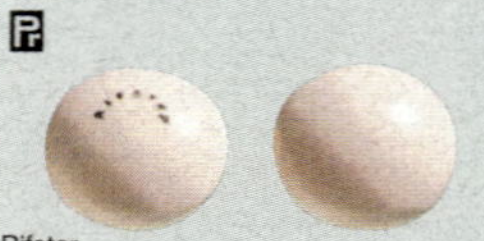 Rifater Rifater® **sanofi-aventis**
3	DIN 02238151 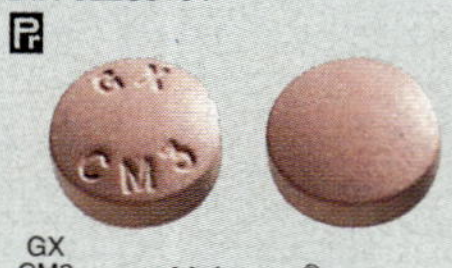 GX CM3 Malarone® 250 mg/100 mg **GlaxoSmithKline**	DIN 02268086 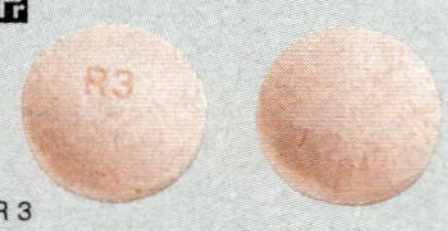 R 3 Risperdal® M-Tab® 3 mg **Janssen-Ortho**	DIN 02268094 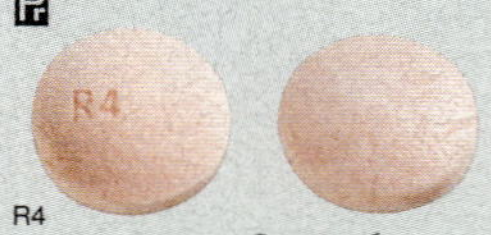 R4 Risperdal® M-Tab® 4 mg **Janssen-Ortho**	DIN 02247706 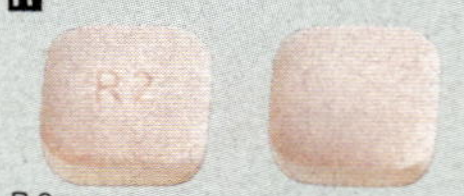 R 2 Risperdal® M-Tab® 2 mg **Janssen-Ortho**	DIN 02241112 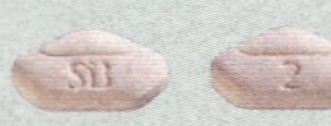 SB · 2 Avandia® 2 mg **GlaxoSmithKline**
4	DIN 02258811 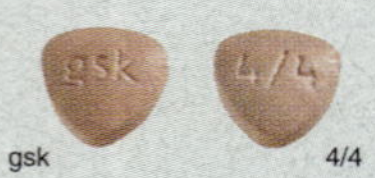 gsk · 4/4 Avandaryl™ 4 mg/4 mg **GlaxoSmithKline**	DIN 00782459 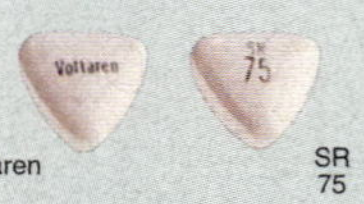 Voltaren · SR 75 Voltaren® SR 75 mg **Novartis Pharmaceuticals**	DIN 02237368 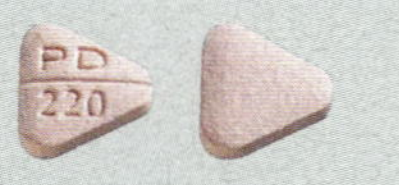 PD 220 Accuretic™ 20/12.5 mg **Pfizer**	DIN 02212161 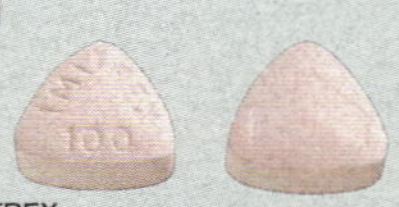 IMITREX 100 Imitrex DF™ 100 mg **GlaxoSmithKline**	DIN 00893749 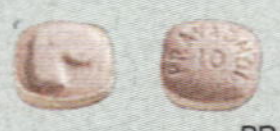 P · PRAVACHOL 10 Pravachol® 10 mg **Bristol-Myers Squibb**
5	DIN 02307065 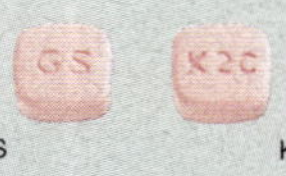 GS · K2C Volibris® 5 mg **GlaxoSmithKline**	DIN 00891800 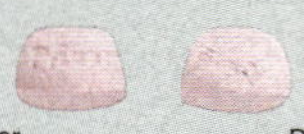 Pfizer · Diflucan 50 Diflucan™ 50 mg **Pfizer**	DIN 00891819 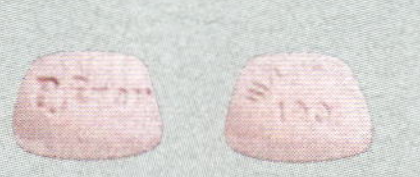 Pfizer · DIFLUCAN 100 Diflucan™ 100 mg **Pfizer**	DIN 02142104 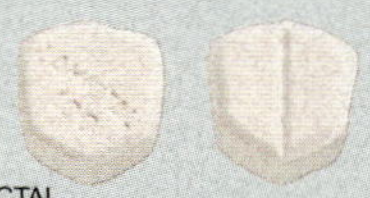 LAMICTAL 100 Lamictal® 100 mg **GlaxoSmithKline**	DIN 01911627 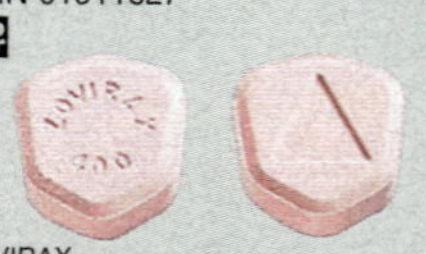 ZOVIRAX 400 Zovirax® 400 mg **GlaxoSmithKline**
6	DIN 02283158 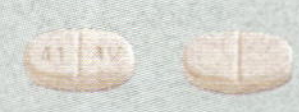 41 AV Altace® HCT 5/12.5 mg **sanofi-aventis**	DIN 02322390 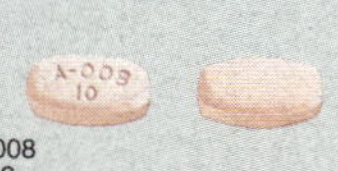 A-008 10 Abilify™ 10 mg **Bristol-Myers Squibb**	DIN 00884332 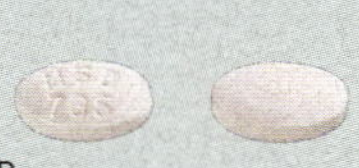 MSD 735 Zocor® 10 mg **Merck Frosst**	DIN 02240520 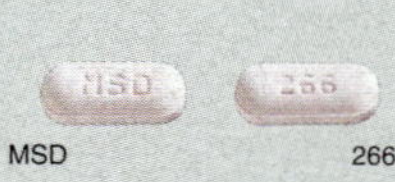 MSD · 266 Maxalt® 5 mg **Merck Frosst**	DIN 02357615 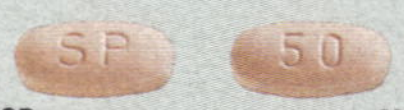 SP · 50 Vimpat™ 50 mg **UCB**
7	DIN 02237367 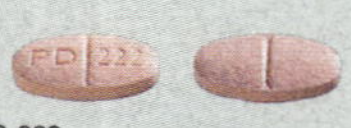 PD 222 Accuretic™ 10/12.5 mg **Pfizer**	DIN 02283182 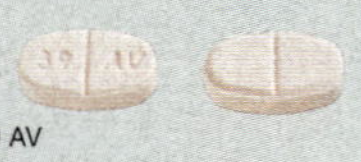 39 AV Altace® HCT 10/25 mg **sanofi-aventis**	DIN 02245272 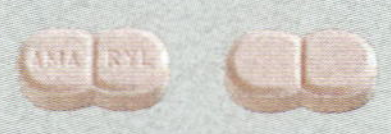 AMARYL Amaryl® 1 mg **sanofi-aventis**	DIN 02241900 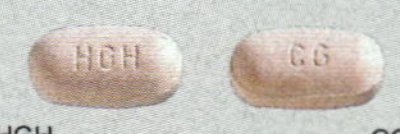 HGH · CG Diovan-HCT® 80 mg/12.5 mg **Novartis Pharmaceuticals**	DIN 02273586 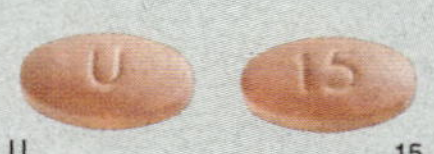 U · 15 Uromax® 15 mg **Purdue Pharma**
8	DIN 02244982 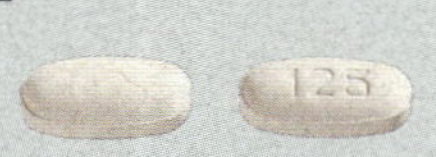 125 Tracleer® 125 mg **Actelion**	DIN 02238453 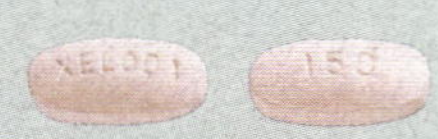 XELODA · 150 Xeloda® 150 mg **Roche**	DIN 02240521 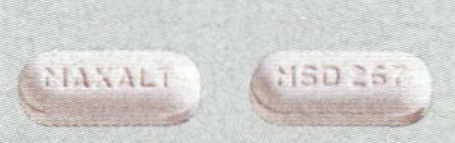 MAXALT · MSD 267 Maxalt® 10 mg **Merck Frosst**	DIN 02247164 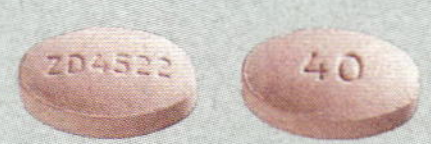 ZD4522 · 40 Crestor® 40 mg **AstraZeneca**	DIN 01940481 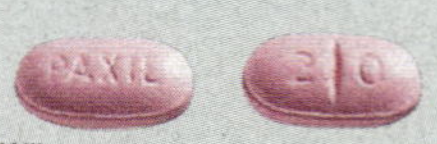 PAXIL · 2 0 Paxil® 20 mg **GlaxoSmithKline**

* ILLUSTRATION LESS THAN ACTUAL SIZE / ILLUSTRATION RÉDUITE

Use code A, B, C, D, E, horizontal bar and 1 to 8 vertical bar to locate illustrated products

Utiliser le code A, B, C, D, E de la ligne horizontale et les chiffres 1 à 8 de la ligne verticale pour repérer les produits illustrés

1

A1 DIN 02243602 Pr
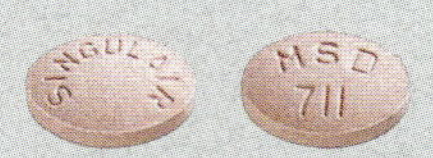
SINGULAIR / MSD 711
Singulair® 4 mg
Merck Frosst

B1 DIN 02247086 Pr
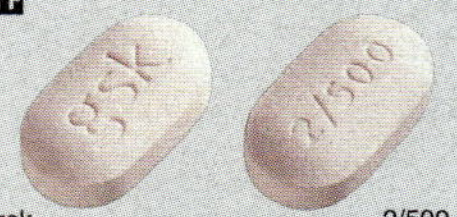
gsk / 2/500
Avandamet® 2 mg/500 mg
GlaxoSmithKline

C1 DIN 00397423 Pr
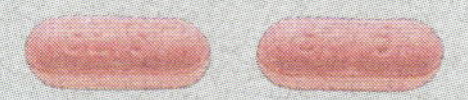
GEIGY / 51 51
Lopresor® 50 mg
Novartis Pharmaceuticals

D1 DIN 02231379 Pr
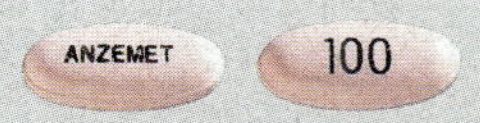
ANZEMET / 100
Anzemet® 100 mg
sanofi-aventis

E1 DIN 02236841 Pr
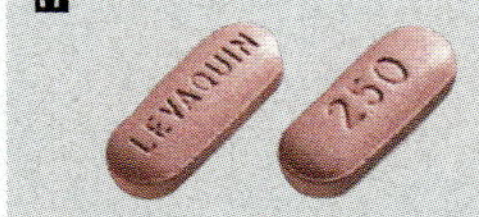
LEVAQUIN / 250
Levaquin® 250 mg
Janssen-Ortho

2

A2 DIN 01934317 Pr
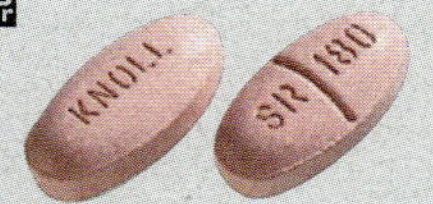
KNOLL / SR 180
Isoptin® SR 180 mg
Abbott

B2 DIN 02244521 Pr
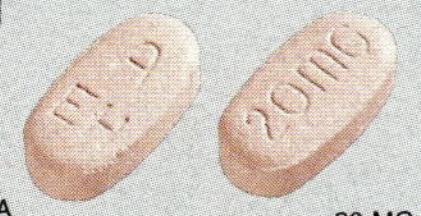
A EH / 20 MG
Nexium® 20 mg
AstraZeneca

C2 DIN 02254409
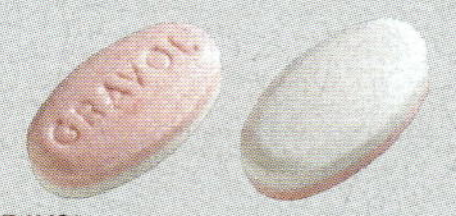
GRAVOL
Gravol® L/A 100 mg
Church & Dwight

D2 DIN 00884359 Pr
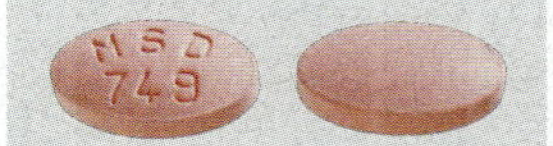
MSD 749
Zocor® 40 mg
Merck Frosst

E2 DIN 02028786 Pr
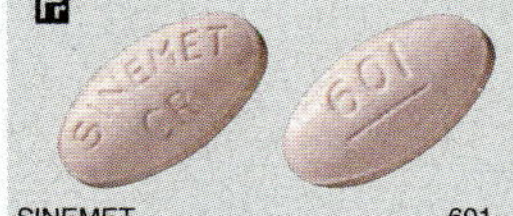
SINEMET CR / 601
Sinemet® CR 100 mg/25 mg
Merck Frosst

3

A3 DIN 02221977 Pr
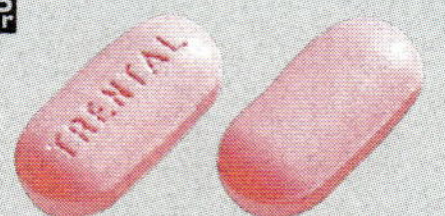
TRENTAL
Trental® 400 mg
sanofi-aventis

B3 DIN 02240332 Pr
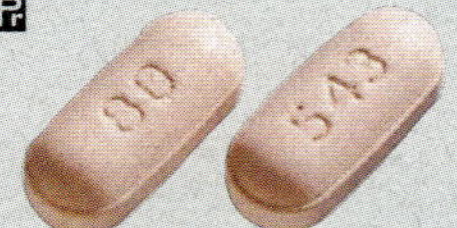
80 / 543
Zocor® 80 mg
Merck Frosst

C3 DIN 02242965 Pr
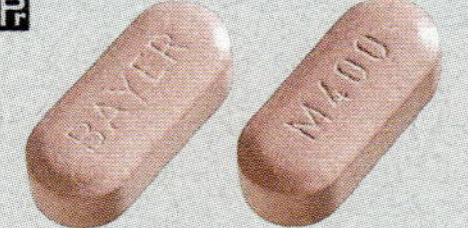
BAYER / M400
Avelox® 400 mg
Bayer

D3 DIN 02212021 Pr *
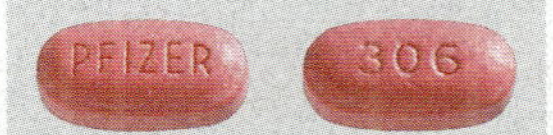
PFIZER / 306
Zithromax™ 250 mg
Pfizer

E3 DIN 02332744 Pr
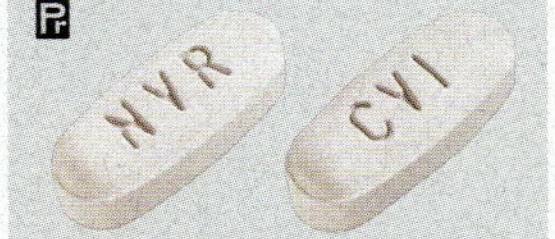
NVR / CVI
Rasilez HCT® 300 mg/12.5 mg
Novartis Pharmaceuticals

4

A4 DIN 02242069 Pr *
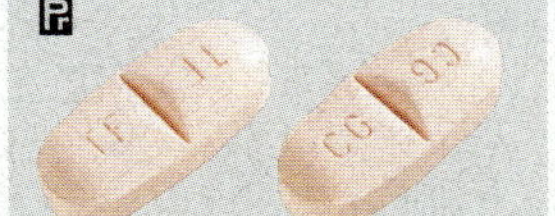
TF / CG
Trileptal® 600 mg
Novartis Pharmaceuticals

B4 DIN 02280213 Pr
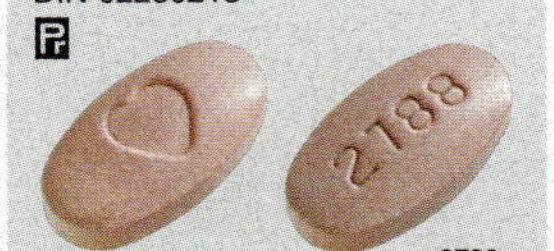
2788
Avalide® 300/25 mg
Bristol-Myers Squibb/ sanofi-aventis

C4 DIN 02245777 Pr
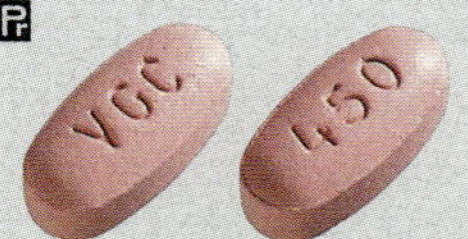
VGC / 450
Valcyte® 450 mg
Roche

D4 DIN 02236842 Pr
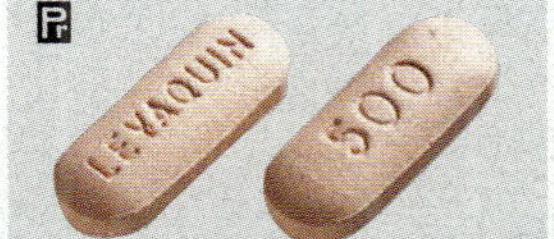
LEVAQUIN / 500
Levaquin® 500 mg
Janssen-Ortho

E4 DIN 02261545 Pr *
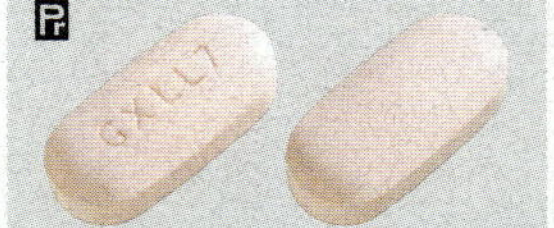
GX LL7
Telzir® 700 mg
ViiV Healthcare ULC

5

A5 DIN 02248441 Pr
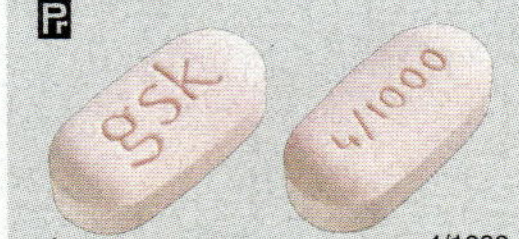
gsk / 4/1000
Avandamet® 4 mg/1000 mg
GlaxoSmithKline

B5 DIN 02308908 Pr
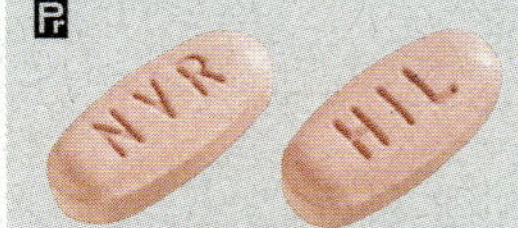
NVR / HIL
Diovan-HCT® 320/12.5 mg
Novartis Pharmaceuticals

C5 DIN 02244344 Pr
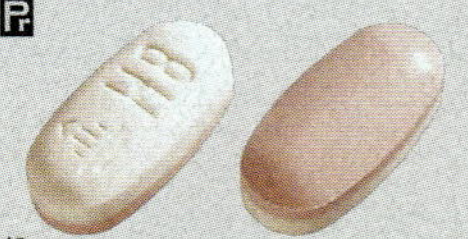
H8
Micardis® Plus 80 mg/12.5 mg
Boehringer Ingelheim

D5 DIN 02240432 Pr *
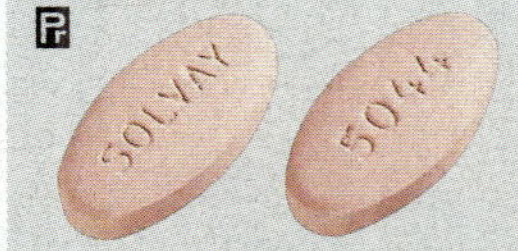
SOLVAY / 5044
Teveten® 400 mg
Abbott Products

E5 DIN 00596434 Pr
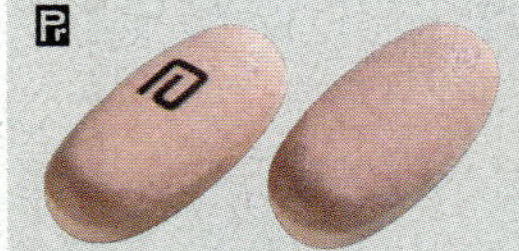
Epival® 500 mg
Abbott

6

A6 DIN 02244522 Pr
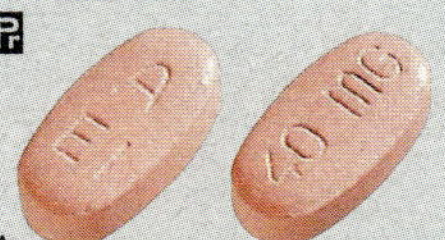
A EI / 40 MG
Nexium® 40 mg
AstraZeneca

B6 DIN 01919598 Pr
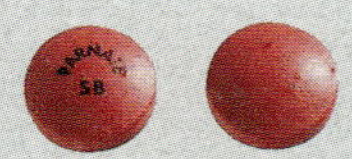
PARNATE SB
Parnate® 10 mg
GlaxoSmithKline

C6 DIN 02163780 N
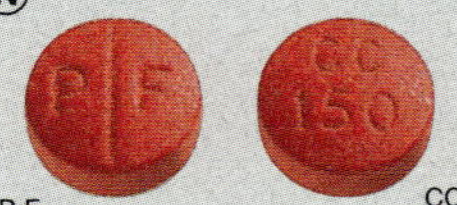
P F / CC 150
Codeine Contin® 150 mg
Purdue Pharma

D6 DIN 02307073 Pr
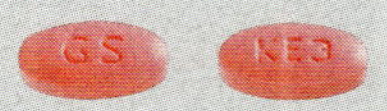
GS / KE3
Volibris® 10 mg
GlaxoSmithKline

E6 DIN 00596418 Pr
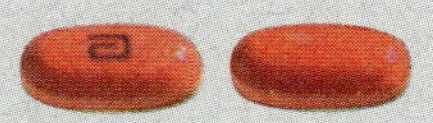
Epival® 125 mg
Abbott

7

A7 DIN 02014327 N
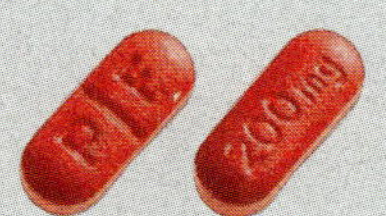
P F / 200 mg
MS Contin® 200 mg
Purdue Pharma

B7 DIN 02230402 Pr
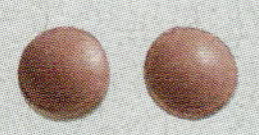
Clopixol® 10 mg
Lundbeck

C7 DIN 02230403 Pr
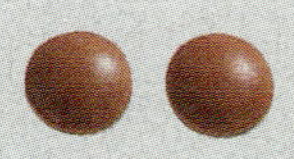
Clopixol® 25 mg
Lundbeck

D7 DIN 02190915 Pr
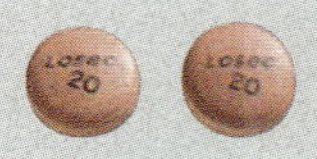
Losec 20
Losec® 20 mg
AstraZeneca

E7 DIN 02238213 Pr
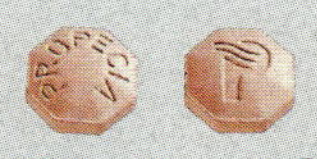
PROPECIA / P
Propecia® 1 mg
Merck Frosst

8

A8 DIN 00010480 Pr
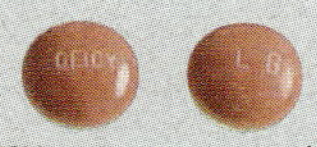
GEIGY / L B
Tofranil® 50 mg
Novartis Pharmaceuticals

B8 DIN 02323214 N
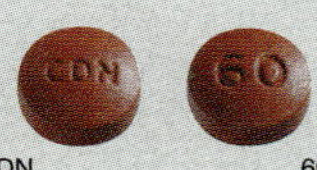
CDN / 60
OxyContin® 60 mg
Purdue Pharma

C8 DIN 00881635 Pr
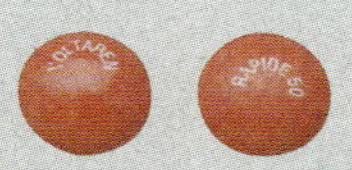
VOLTAREN / RAPIDE 50
Voltaren Rapide® 50 mg
Novartis Pharmaceuticals

D8 DIN 01947680 Pr
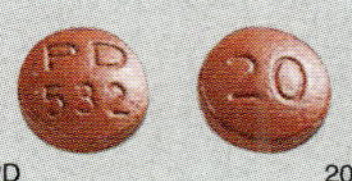
PD 532 / 20
Accupril™ 20 mg
Pfizer

E8 DIN 00851787 Pr
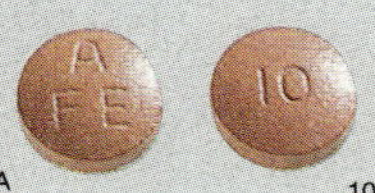
A FE / 10
Plendil® 10 mg
AstraZeneca

* ILLUSTRATION LESS THAN ACTUAL SIZE / ILLUSTRATION RÉDUITE

Use code A, B, C, D, E, horizontal bar and 1 to 8 vertical bar to locate illustrated products

Utiliser le code A, B, C, D, E de la ligne horizontale et les chiffres 1 à 8 de la ligne verticale pour repérer les produits illustrés

1

A1 DIN 02284227
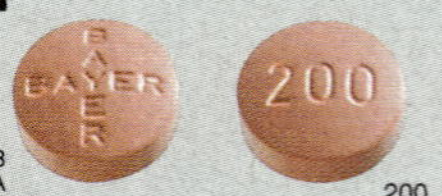
BAYER 200
Nexavar® 200 mg
Bayer

B1 DIN 02230896
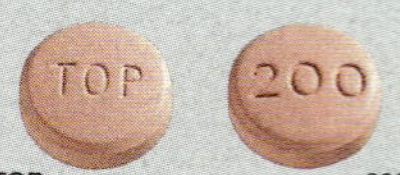
TOP 200
Topamax® 200 mg
Janssen-Ortho

C1 DIN 02305933
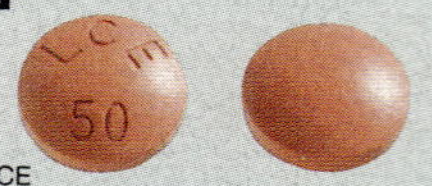
LCE 50
Stalevo™ 50 mg/12.5 mg/200 mg
Novartis Pharmaceuticals

D1 DIN 02248676
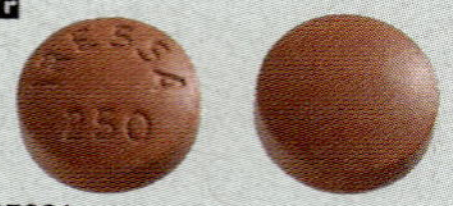
IRESSA 250
Iressa® 250 mg
AstraZeneca

E1 DIN 00710113
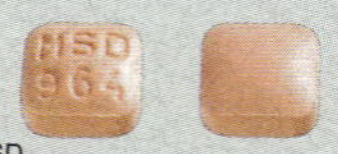
MSD 964
Pepcid® 40 mg
Merck Frosst

2

A2 DIN 02241114
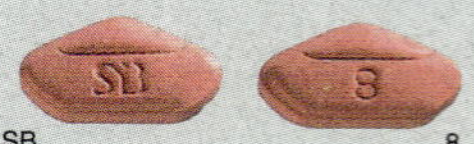
SB 8
Avandia® 8 mg
GlaxoSmithKline

B2 DIN 00670901
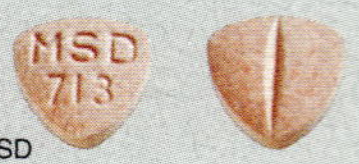
MSD 713
Vasotec® 10 mg
Merck Frosst

C2 DIN 01947672
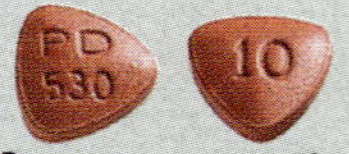
PD 530 10
Accupril™ 10 mg
Pfizer

D2 DIN 01947664
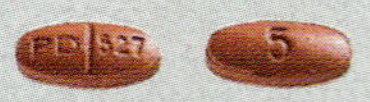
PD 527 5
Accupril™ 5 mg
Pfizer

E2 DIN 00657298
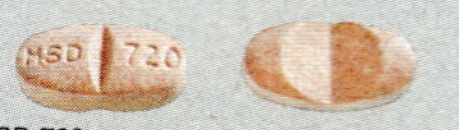
MSD 720
Vaseretic® 10/25 mg
Merck Frosst

3

A3 DIN 02240552
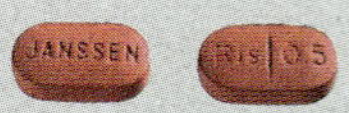
JANSSEN Ris 0.5
Risperdal® 0.5 mg
Janssen-Ortho

B3 DIN 02242878 *
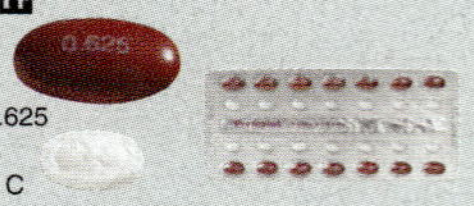
0.625 C
Premplus® 0.625 mg/2.5 mg
Pfizer

C3 DIN 02242879 *
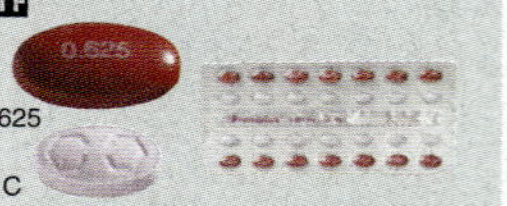
0.625 C
Premplus® 0.625 mg/5 mg
Pfizer

D3 DIN 02247734
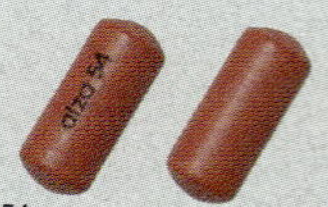
alza 54
Concerta® 54 mg
Janssen-Ortho

E3 DIN 02241901
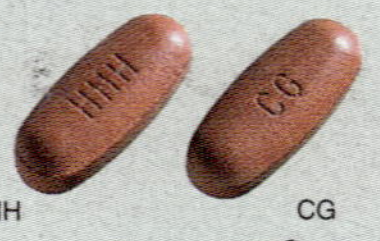
HHH CG
Diovan-HCT® 160 mg/12.5 mg
Novartis Pharmaceuticals

4

A4 DIN 01947699
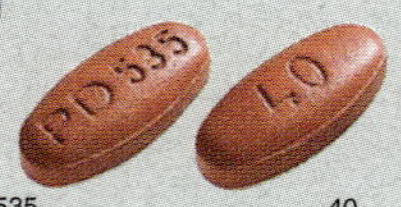
PD 535 40
Accupril™ 40 mg
Pfizer

B4 DIN 02337827
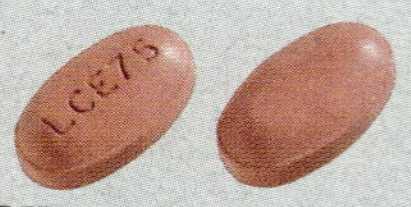
LCE 75
Stalevo™ 75 mg/18.75 mg/200 mg
Novartis Pharmaceuticals

C4 DIN 02337835
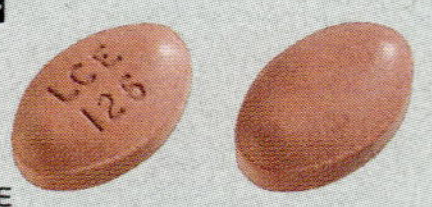
LCE 125
Stalevo™ 125 mg/31.25 mg/200 mg
Novartis Pharmaceuticals

D4 DIN 01997580
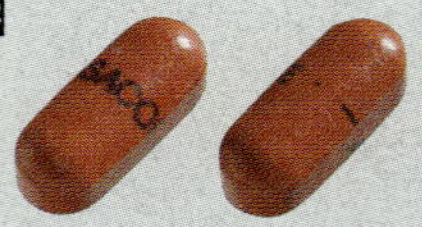
ASACOL NE - —
Asacol® 400 mg
Warner Chilcott

E4 DIN 02267217
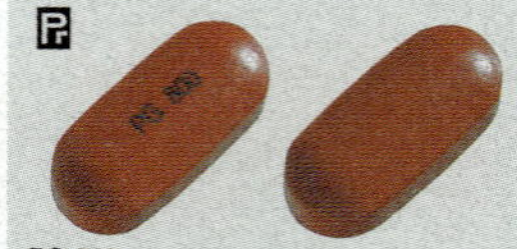
PG 800
Asacol® 800 mg
Warner Chilcott

5

A5 DIN 00004626
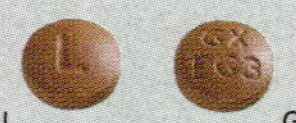
L GX EG3
Leukeran® 2 mg
GlaxoSmithKline

B5 DIN 02323206
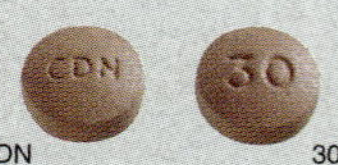
CDN 30
OxyContin® 30 mg
Purdue Pharma

C5 DIN 02240205
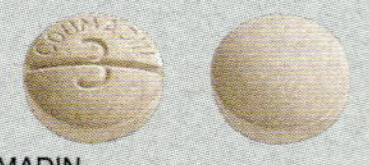
COUMADIN 3
Coumadin® 3 mg
Bristol-Myers Squibb

D5 DIN 02253275
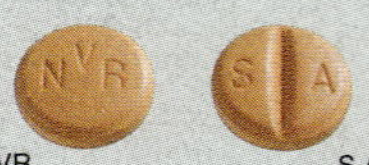
NVR S A
Gleevec® 100 mg
Novartis Pharmaceuticals

E5 DIN 00026158
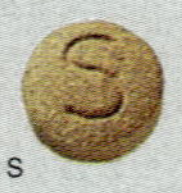
S
Senokot® 8.6 mg
Purdue Pharma

6

A6 DIN 02230019
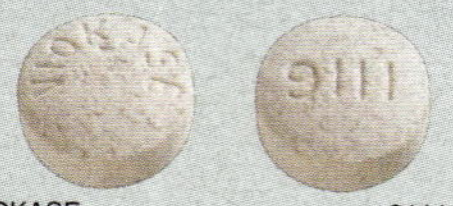
VIOKASE 9111
Viokase® 8
Axcan Pharma

B6 DIN 01916963
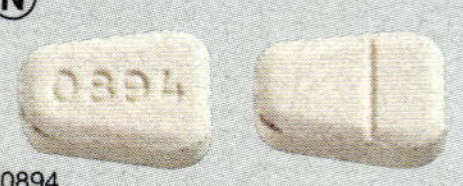
0894
Tussionex®
sanofi-aventis

C6 DIN 00710121
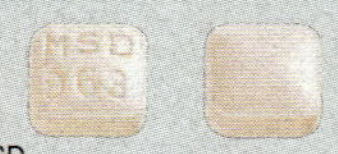
MSD 963
Pepcid® 20 mg
Merck Frosst

D6 DIN 02238217
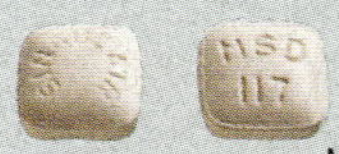
SINGULAIR MSD 117
Singulair® 10 mg
Merck Frosst

E6 DIN 02246955
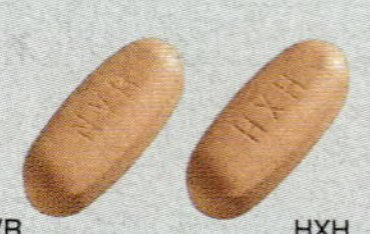
NVR HXH
Diovan-HCT® 160 mg/25 mg
Novartis Pharmaceuticals

7

A7 DIN 02243910
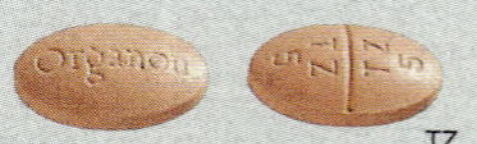
Organon TZ 5
Remeron® 30 mg
Schering-Plough

B7 DIN 02305941
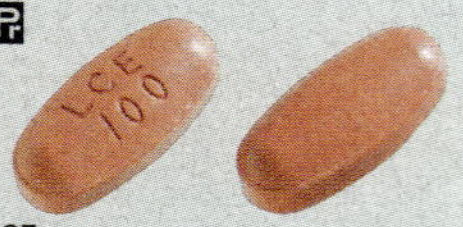
LCE 100
Stalevo™ 100 mg/25 mg/200 mg
Novartis Pharmaceuticals

C7 DIN 02305968
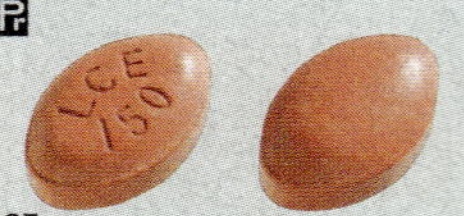
LCE 150
Stalevo™ 150 mg/37.5 mg/200 mg
Novartis Pharmaceuticals

D7 NPN 80002053
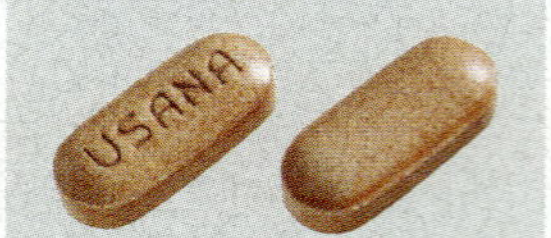
USANA
Proflavanol 90
USANA Health Sciences

E7 DIN 02031388
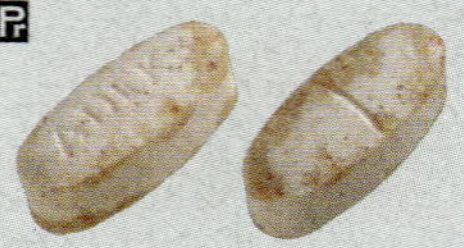
ADEKs
ADEKs®
Axcan Pharma

8

A8 DIN 02297558
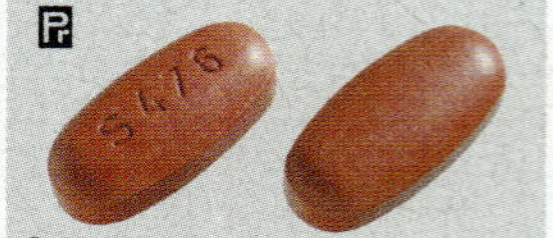
S476
Mezavant® 1.2 g
Shire

B8 DIN 02333872 *
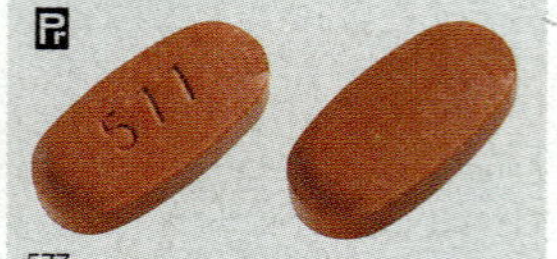
577
Janumet™ 50 mg/1000 mg
Merck Frosst

C8 DIN 02241933
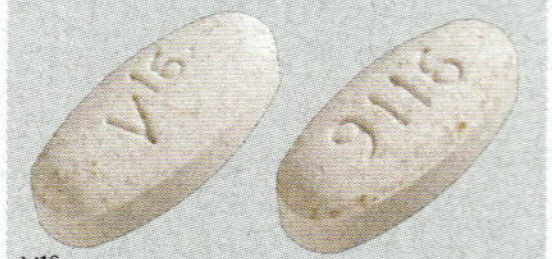
V16 9116
Viokase® 16
Axcan Pharma

D8 DIN 02041456
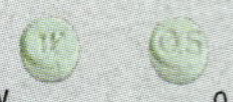
W 0.5
Ativan® 0.5 mg
Pfizer

E8 DIN 02148595
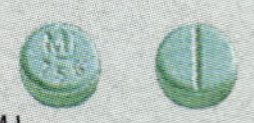
MJ 756
Estrace® 2 mg
Shire

* ILLUSTRATION LESS THAN ACTUAL SIZE / ILLUSTRATION RÉDUITE

Use code A, B, C, D, E, horizontal bar and 1 to 8 vertical bar to locate illustrated products

Utiliser le code A, B, C, D, E de la ligne horizontale et les chiffres 1 à 8 de la ligne verticale pour repérer les produits illustrés

	A	B	C	D	E
1	DIN 02213230 Pr 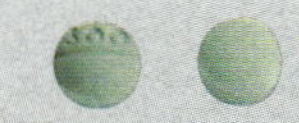 300 Eltroxin® 300 µg **Triton Pharma**	DIN 02015439 Ⓝ 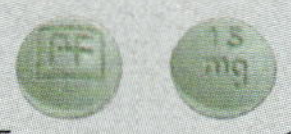 PF 15 mg MS Contin® 15 mg **Purdue Pharma**	DIN 02172097 Pr 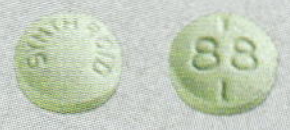 SYNTHROID 88 Synthroid® 88 µg **Abbott**	DIN 02172151 Pr 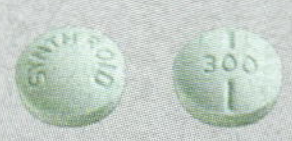 SYNTHROID 300 Synthroid® 300 µg **Abbott**	DIN 02246624 Pr 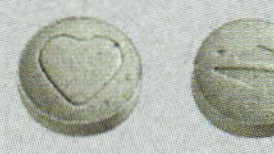 Coversyl® 8 mg **Servier**
2	DIN 00795852 Pr 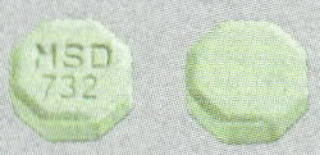 MSD 732 Mevacor® 40 mg **Merck Frosst**	DIN 02202484 Ⓝ 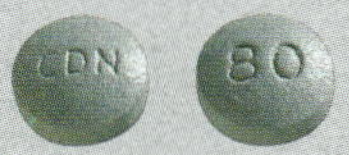 CDN 80 OxyContin® 80 mg **Purdue Pharma**	DIN 02240206 Pr 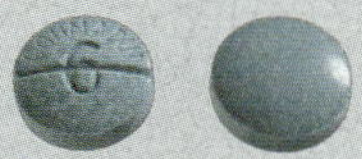 COUMADIN 6 Coumadin® 6 mg **Bristol-Myers Squibb**	DIN 01918346 Pr 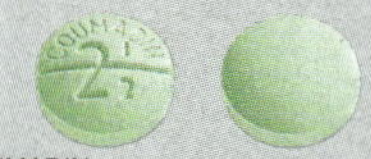 COUMADIN 2½ Coumadin® 2.5 mg **Bristol-Myers Squibb**	DIN 02264560 Pr 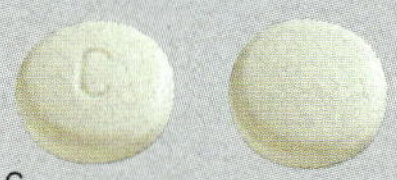 C Myfortic® 180 mg **Novartis Pharmaceuticals**
3	DIN 00293512 Ⓝ 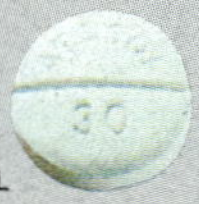 ATASOL 30 Atasol®-30 **Church & Dwight**	DIN 02222051 Pr 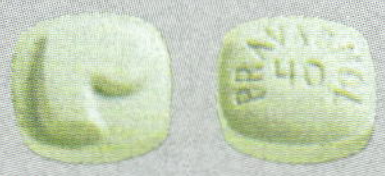 P PRAVACHOL 40 Pravachol® 40 mg **Bristol-Myers Squibb**	DIN 02232567 Pr 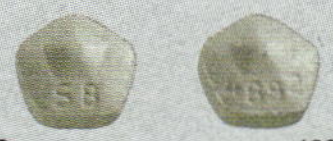 SB 4892 ReQuip® 1 mg **GlaxoSmithKline**	DIN 02237821 Pr 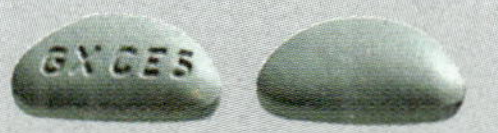 GX CE5 Amerge® 2.5 mg **GlaxoSmithKline**	DIN 02322374 Pr 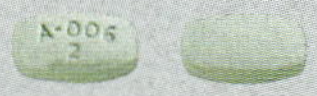 A-006 2 Abilify™ 2 mg **Bristol-Myers Squibb**
4	DIN 02123282 Pr 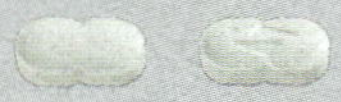 Coversyl® 4 mg **Servier**	DIN 02245273 Pr 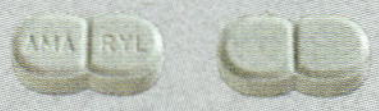 AMARYL Amaryl® 2 mg **sanofi-aventis**	DIN 02025310 Pr 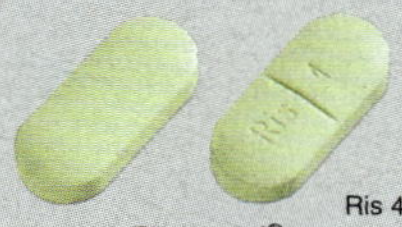 Ris 4 Risperdal® 4 mg **Janssen-Ortho**	DIN 00742554 * Pr 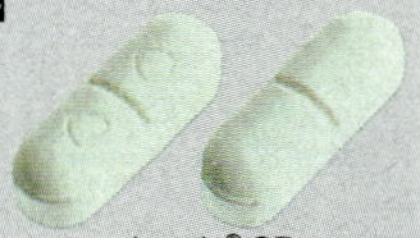 Isoptin® SR 240 mg **Abbott**	DIN 02244757 * Pr 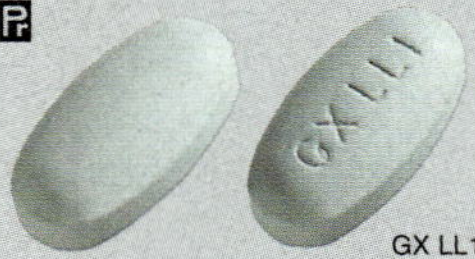 GX LL1 Trizivir® **ViiV Healthcare ULC**
5	DIN 02041472 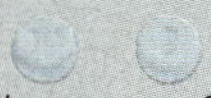 W 2 Ativan® Sublingual 2 mg **Pfizer**	DIN 02108194 Pr 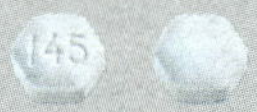 145 Prinzide® 10 mg/12.5 mg **Merck Frosst**	DIN 02213214 Pr 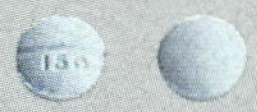 150 Eltroxin® 150 µg **Triton Pharma**	DIN 02243919 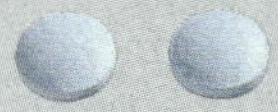 Aerius® 5 mg **Schering-Plough**	DIN 00030937 Pr 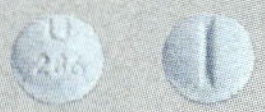 U 286 Provera® 5 mg **Pfizer**
6	DIN 02258129 Ⓝ 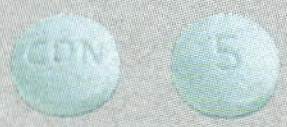 CDN 5 OxyContin® 5 mg **Purdue Pharma**	DIN 02233852 Pr 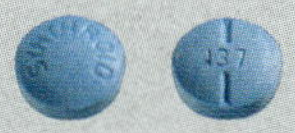 SYNTHROID 137 Synthroid® 137 µg **Abbott**	DIN 02172127 Pr 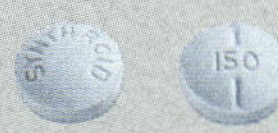 SYNTHROID 150 Synthroid® 150 µg **Abbott**	DIN 00005606 Ⓒ 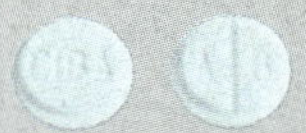 CIBA A B Ritalin® 10 mg **Novartis Pharmaceuticals**	DIN 02230302 Ⓝ 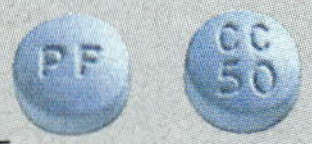 PF CC 50 Codeine Contin® 50 mg **Purdue Pharma**
7	DIN 02237726 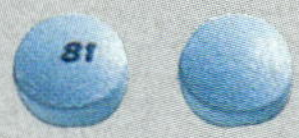 81 Aspirin® 81 mg **Bayer Consumer Care**	DIN 00789739 Ⓝ 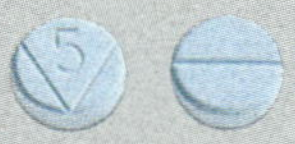 5 V Supeudol® 5 mg **Sandoz**	DIN 00795860 Pr 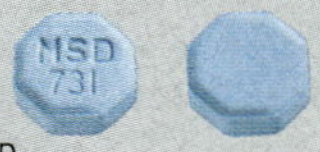 MSD 731 Mevacor® 20 mg **Merck Frosst**	DIN 02007959 Pr 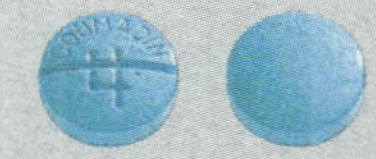 COUMADIN 4 Coumadin® 4 mg **Bristol-Myers Squibb**	DIN 01916491 Ⓝ 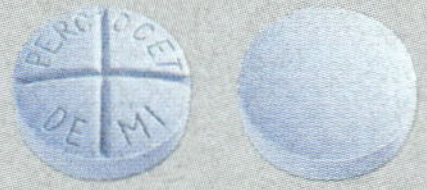 Percocet®-Demi **Bristol-Myers Squibb**
8	DIN 02010909 Pr 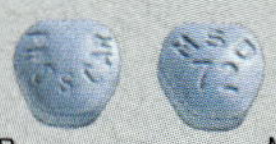 PROSCAR MSD 72 Proscar® 5 mg **Merck Frosst**	DIN 02232569 Pr 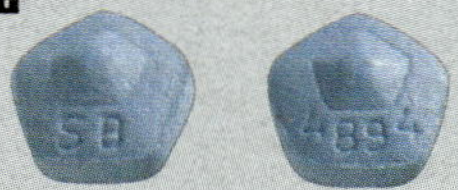 SB 4894 ReQuip® 5 mg **GlaxoSmithKline**	DIN 02239766 Pr 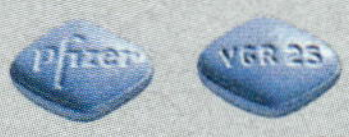 Pfizer VGR 25 Viagra™ 25 mg **Pfizer**	DIN 02239767 Pr 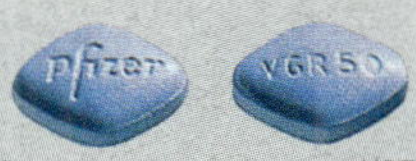 Pfizer VGR 50 Viagra™ 50 mg **Pfizer**	DIN 02239768 Pr 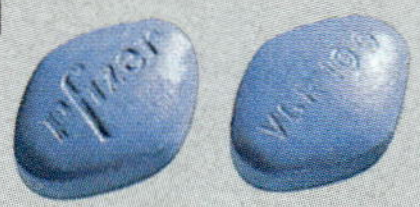 Pfizer VGR 100 Viagra™ 100 mg **Pfizer**

* ILLUSTRATION LESS THAN ACTUAL SIZE / ILLUSTRATION RÉDUITE

Use code A, B, C, D, E, horizontal bar and 1 to 8 vertical bar to locate illustrated products

Utiliser le code A, B, C, D, E de la ligne horizontale et les chiffres 1 à 8 de la ligne verticale pour repérer les produits illustrés

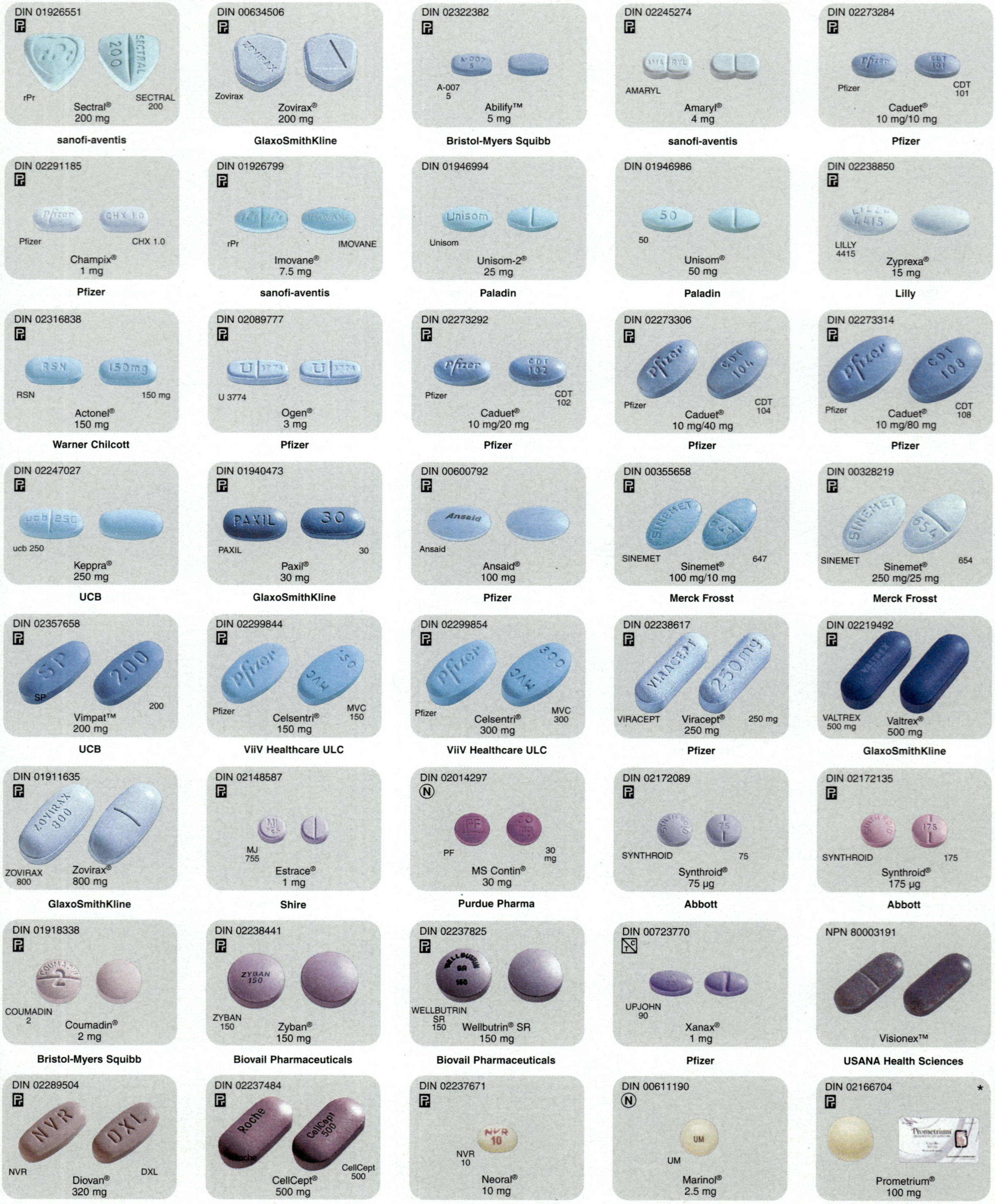

	A	B	C	D	E
1	DIN 01926551 Pr; rPr / SECTRAL 200; Sectral® 200 mg; **sanofi-aventis**	DIN 00634506 Pr; Zovirax; Zovirax® 200 mg; **GlaxoSmithKline**	DIN 02322382 Pr; A-007 5; Abilify™ 5 mg; **Bristol-Myers Squibb**	DIN 02245274 Pr; AMARYL; Amaryl® 4 mg; **sanofi-aventis**	DIN 02273284 Pr; Pfizer / CDT 101; Caduet® 10 mg/10 mg; **Pfizer**
2	DIN 02291185 Pr; Pfizer / CHX 1.0; Champix® 1 mg; **Pfizer**	DIN 01926799 Pr; rPr / IMOVANE; Imovane® 7.5 mg; **sanofi-aventis**	DIN 01946994 Pr; Unisom; Unisom-2® 25 mg; **Paladin**	DIN 01946986 Pr; 50; Unisom® 50 mg; **Paladin**	DIN 02238850 Pr; LILLY 4415; Zyprexa® 15 mg; **Lilly**
3	DIN 02316838 Pr; RSN / 150 mg; Actonel® 150 mg; **Warner Chilcott**	DIN 02089777 Pr; U 3774; Ogen® 3 mg; **Pfizer**	DIN 02273292 Pr; Pfizer / CDT 102; Caduet® 10 mg/20 mg; **Pfizer**	DIN 02273306 Pr; Pfizer / CDT 104; Caduet® 10 mg/40 mg; **Pfizer**	DIN 02273314 Pr; Pfizer / CDT 108; Caduet® 10 mg/80 mg; **Pfizer**
4	DIN 02247027 Pr; ucb 250; Keppra® 250 mg; **UCB**	DIN 01940473 Pr; PAXIL / 30; Paxil® 30 mg; **GlaxoSmithKline**	DIN 00600792 Pr; Ansaid; Ansaid® 100 mg; **Pfizer**	DIN 00355658 Pr; SINEMET / 647; Sinemet® 100 mg/10 mg; **Merck Frosst**	DIN 00328219 Pr; SINEMET / 654; Sinemet® 250 mg/25 mg; **Merck Frosst**
5	DIN 02357658 Pr; SP / 200; Vimpat™ 200 mg; **UCB**	DIN 02299844 Pr; Pfizer / MVC 150; Celsentri® 150 mg; **ViiV Healthcare ULC**	DIN 02299854 Pr; Pfizer / MVC 300; Celsentri® 300 mg; **ViiV Healthcare ULC**	DIN 02238617 Pr; VIRACEPT / 250 mg; Viracept® 250 mg; **Pfizer**	DIN 02219492 Pr; VALTREX 500 mg; Valtrex® 500 mg; **GlaxoSmithKline**
6	DIN 01911635 Pr; ZOVIRAX 800; Zovirax® 800 mg; **GlaxoSmithKline**	DIN 02148587 Pr; MJ 755; Estrace® 1 mg; **Shire**	DIN 02014297 N; PF / 30 mg; MS Contin® 30 mg; **Purdue Pharma**	DIN 02172089 Pr; SYNTHROID / 75; Synthroid® 75 µg; **Abbott**	DIN 02172135 Pr; SYNTHROID / 175; Synthroid® 175 µg; **Abbott**
7	DIN 01918338 Pr; COUMADIN 2; Coumadin® 2 mg; **Bristol-Myers Squibb**	DIN 02238441 Pr; ZYBAN 150; Zyban® 150 mg; **Biovail Pharmaceuticals**	DIN 02237825 Pr; WELLBUTRIN SR 150; Wellbutrin® SR 150 mg; **Biovail Pharmaceuticals**	DIN 00723770 TC; UPJOHN 90; Xanax® 1 mg; **Pfizer**	NPN 80003191; Visionex™; **USANA Health Sciences**
8	DIN 02289504 Pr; NVR / DXL; Diovan® 320 mg; **Novartis Pharmaceuticals**	DIN 02237484 Pr; CellCept 500; CellCept® 500 mg; **Roche**	DIN 02237671 Pr; NVR 10; Neoral® 10 mg; **Novartis Pharmaceuticals**	DIN 00611190 N; UM; Marinol® 2.5 mg; **Abbott Products**	DIN 02166704 Pr *; Prometrium® 100 mg; **Schering-Plough**

* ILLUSTRATION LESS THAN ACTUAL SIZE / ILLUSTRATION RÉDUITE

Use code A, B, C, D, E, horizontal bar and 1 to 8 vertical bar to locate illustrated products

Utiliser le code A, B, C, D, E de la ligne horizontale et les chiffres 1 à 8 de la ligne verticale pour repérer les produits illustrés

	A	B	C	D	E
1	DIN 02175991 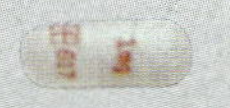 617 / 1 mg Prograf® 1 mg **Astellas**	DIN 02236859 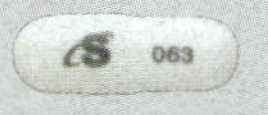 S / 063 Agrylin® 0.5 mg **Shire**	DIN 02250519 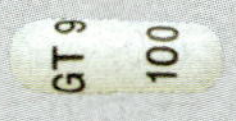 OGT 918 / 100 Zavesca® 100 mg **Actelion**	DIN 02262800 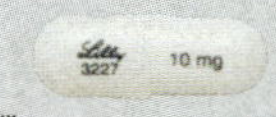 Lilly 3227 / 10 mg Strattera® 10 mg **Lilly**	DIN 02327619 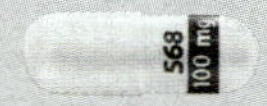 568 100 mg Zolinza® 100 mg **Merck Frosst**
2	DIN 02084260 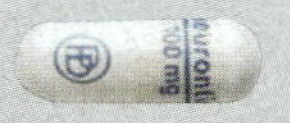 PD / Neurontin 100 mg Neurontin® 100 mg **Pfizer**	DIN 02266717 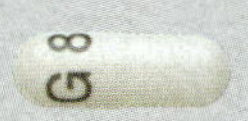 G 8 Reminyl® ER 8 mg **Janssen-Ortho**	DIN 02298619 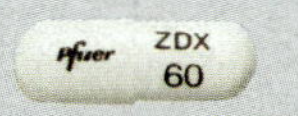 Pfizer / ZDX 60 Zeldox™ 60 mg **Pfizer**	DIN 02298791 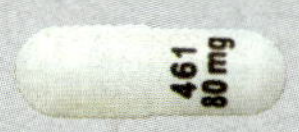 461 80 mg Emend® 80 mg **Merck Frosst**	DIN 02224828 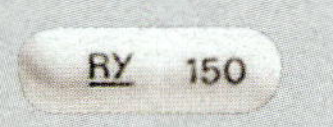 RY / 150 Rythmodan® 150 mg **sanofi-aventis**
3	DIN 02268418 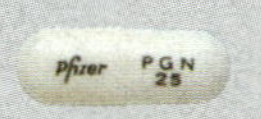 Pfizer / P G N 25 Lyrica™ 25 mg **Pfizer**	DIN 02268426 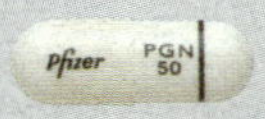 Pfizer / PGN 50 Lyrica™ 50 mg **Pfizer**	DIN 02268450 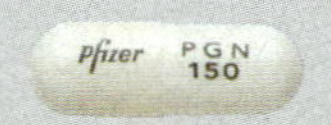 Pfizer / P G N 150 Lyrica™ 150 mg **Pfizer**	DIN 00360430 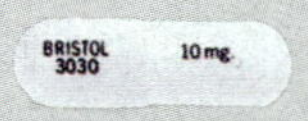 BRISTOL 3030 / 10 mg CeeNU® 10 mg **Bristol-Myers Squibb**	DIN 00502790 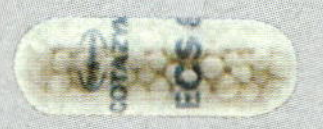 Organon COTAZYM / ECS 8 Cotazym® ECS 8 **Schering-Plough**
4	DIN 00500895 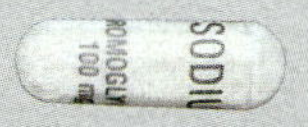 CROMOGLYCATE 100 mg / SODIUM Nalcrom® 100 mg **sanofi-aventis**	DIN 02244596 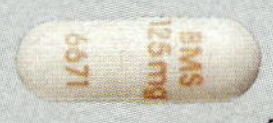 6671 / BMS 125 mg Videx™ EC 125 mg **Bristol-Myers Squibb**	DIN 02244597 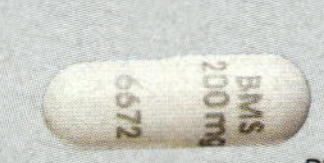 6672 / BMS 200 mg Videx™ EC 200 mg **Bristol-Myers Squibb**	DIN 02244598 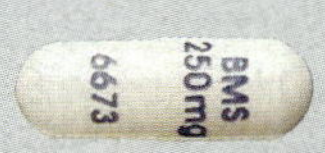 6673 / BMS 250 mg Videx™ EC 250 mg **Bristol-Myers Squibb**	DIN 02029448 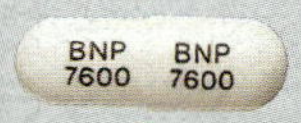 BNP 7600 Elmiron® 100 mg **Janssen-Ortho**
5	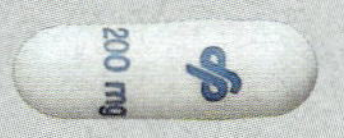 200 mg Pegetron® 200 mg **Schering-Plough**	DIN 02239941 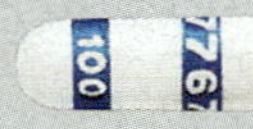 100 / 7767 Celebrex® 100 mg **Pfizer**	DIN 02239942 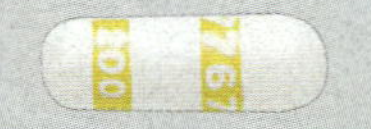 200 / 7767 Celebrex® 200 mg **Pfizer**	DIN 02239907 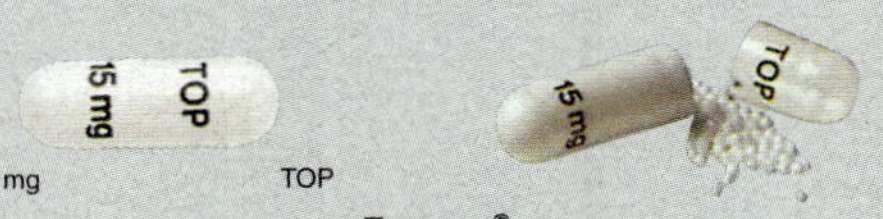 15 mg / TOP Topamax® 15 mg **Janssen-Ortho**	
6	DIN 01902660 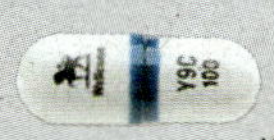 Wellcome / Y9C 100 Retrovir® (AZT™) 100 mg **ViiV Healthcare ULC**	DIN 02141442 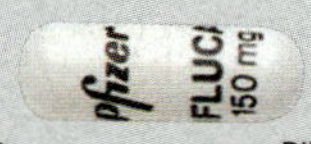 Pfizer / DIFLUCAN 150 mg Diflucan 150™ 150 mg **Pfizer**	DIN 02018160 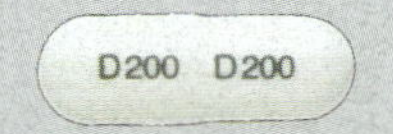 D 200 Cyclomen® 200 mg **sanofi-aventis**	DIN 02239908 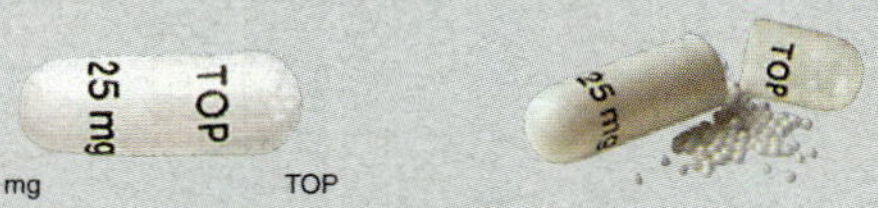 25 mg / TOP Topamax® 25 mg **Janssen-Ortho**	
7	DIN 02229161 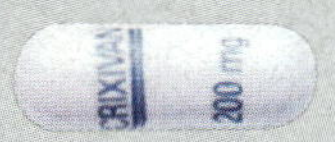 CRIXIVAN / 200 mg Crixivan® 200 mg **Merck Frosst**	DIN 02063794 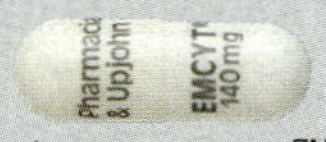 Pharmacia & Upjohn / EMCYT 140 mg Emcyt® 140 mg **Pfizer**	DIN 02150662 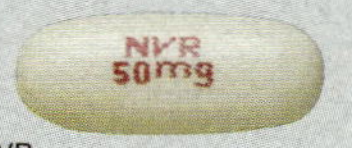 NVR 50 mg Neoral® 50 mg **Novartis Pharmaceuticals**	DIN 02019930 Ⓝ 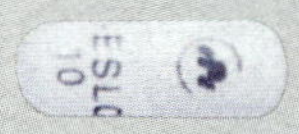 M-ESLON 10 / rPr M-Eslon® 10 mg **Ethypharm**	DIN 00456233 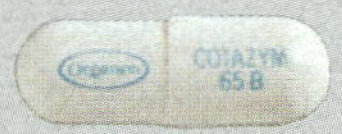 Organon / COTAZYM 65B Cotazym®-65 B **Schering-Plough**
8	DIN 00263818 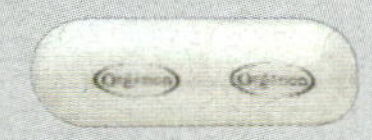 Organon Cotazym® **Schering-Plough**	DIN 02244599 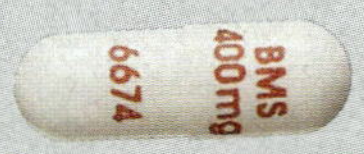 6674 / BMS 400 mg Videx™ EC 400 mg **Bristol-Myers Squibb**	DIN 02203324 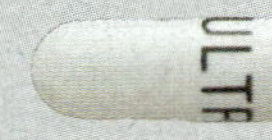 ULTRASE Ultrase® **Axcan Pharma**	DIN 02241096 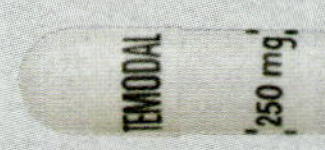 TEMODAL / 250 mg Temodal® 250 mg **Schering-Plough**	DIN 02229196 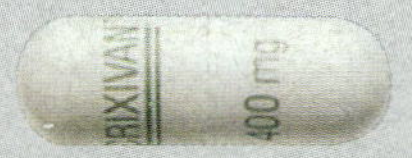 CRIXIVAN / 400 mg Crixivan® 400 mg **Merck Frosst**

* ILLUSTRATION LESS THAN ACTUAL SIZE / ILLUSTRATION RÉDUITE

Use code A, B, C, D, E, horizontal bar and 1 to 8 vertical bar to locate illustrated products

Utiliser le code A, B, C, D, E de la ligne horizontale et les chiffres 1 à 8 de la ligne verticale pour repérer les produits illustrés

	A	B	C	D	E
1	DIN 02018152 Pr 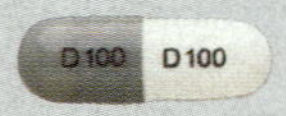 D 100 Cyclomen® 100 mg **sanofi-aventis**	DIN 02019965 (N) 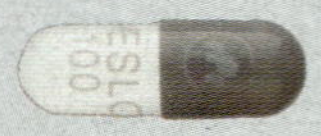 M-ESLON 100 rPr M-Eslon® 100 mg **Ethypharm**	DIN 02277204 (C) 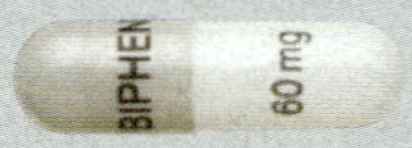 BIPHENTIN 60 mg Biphentin® 60 mg **Purdue Pharma**	DIN 02150689 Pr 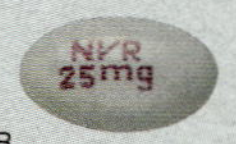 NVR 25 mg Neoral® 25 mg **Novartis Pharmaceuticals**	DIN 02150670 Pr 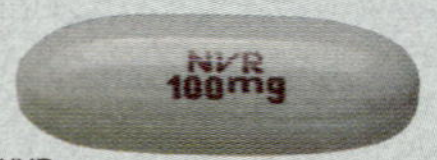 NVR 100 mg Neoral® 100 mg **Novartis Pharmaceuticals**
2	DIN 02125382 (N) 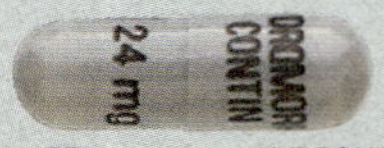 24 mg PF HYDROMORPH CONTIN Hydromorph Contin® 24 mg **Purdue Pharma**	DIN 02221829 Pr 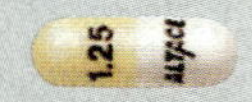 1.25 ALTACE Altace® 1.25 mg **sanofi-aventis**	DIN 00789445 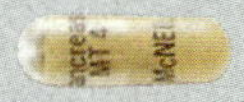 Pancrease MT 4 McNEIL Pancrease®MT 4 **Janssen-Ortho**	DIN 02239886 Pr 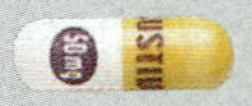 50 mg SUSTIVA Sustiva® 50 mg **Bristol-Myers Squibb**	DIN 02262819 Pr 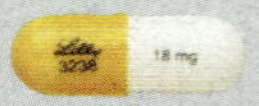 Lilly 3238 18 mg Strattera® 18 mg **Lilly**
3	DIN 02277158 (C) 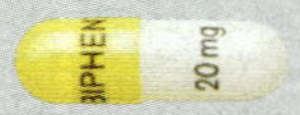 BIPHENTIN 20 mg Biphentin® 20 mg **Purdue Pharma**	DIN 02177749 (N) 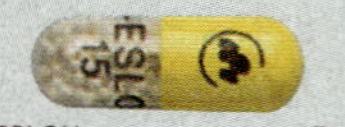 M-ESLON 15 rPr M-Eslon® 15 mg **Ethypharm**	DIN 02241094 Pr 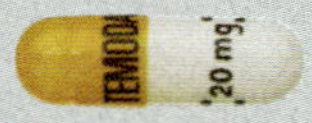 TEMODAL 20 mg Temodal® 20 mg **Schering-Plough**	DIN 02045834 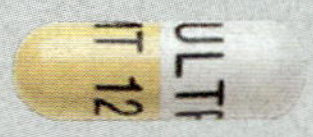 MT 12 ULTRASE Ultrase® MT12 **Axcan Pharma**	DIN 01962817 Pr 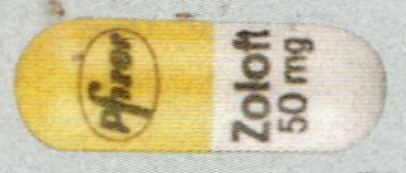 Pfizer Zoloft 50 mg Zoloft® 50 mg **Pfizer**
4	DIN 02243144 Pr  607 0.5 mg Prograf® 0.5 mg **Astellas**	DIN 02296462 Pr 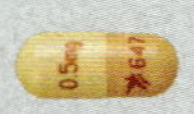 0.5 mg 647 Advagraf™ 0.5 mg **Astellas**	DIN 02132702 Pr 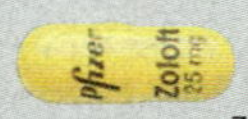 Pfizer Zoloft 25 mg Zoloft® 25 mg **Pfizer**	DIN 02242115 Pr 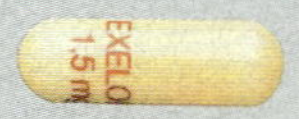 EXELON 1.5 mg Exelon® 1.5 mg **Novartis Pharmaceuticals**	DIN 02347156 (C) 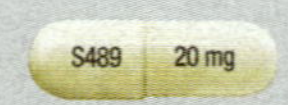 S489 20 mg Vyvanse® 20 mg **Shire**
5	DIN 02084279 Pr 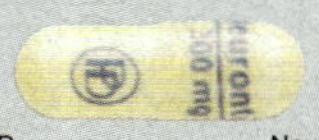 PD Neurontin 300 mg Neurontin® 300 mg **Pfizer**	DIN 02243562 (N) 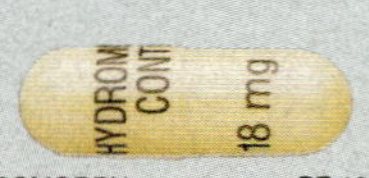 HYDROMORPH CONTIN PF 18 mg Hydromorph Contin® 18 mg **Purdue Pharma**	DIN 02043424 Pr 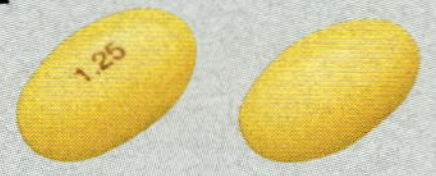 1.25 Premarin® 1.25 mg **Pfizer**	DIN 00582352 Pr 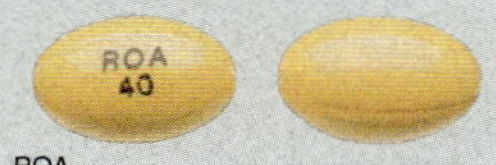 ROA 40 Accutane™ Roche® 40 mg **Roche**	DIN 00782327 (C) 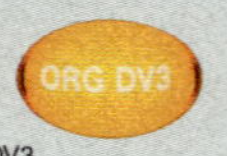 ORG DV3 Andriol® **Schering-Ploug**
6	NPN 80011054 * 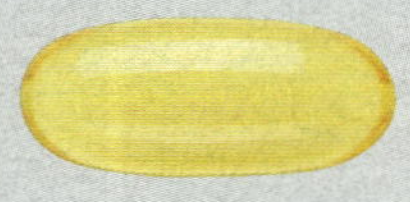 BiOmega **USANA Health Sciences**	DIN 02296470 Pr 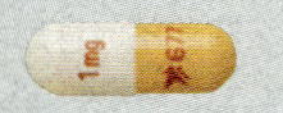 1 mg 677 Advagraf™ 1 mg **Astellas**	DIN 02242116 Pr 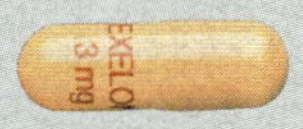 EXELON 3 mg Exelon® 3 mg **Novartis Pharmaceuticals**	DIN 02247813 Pr 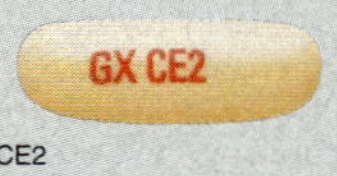 GX CE2 Avodart® 0.5 mg **GlaxoSmithKline**	DIN 00821373 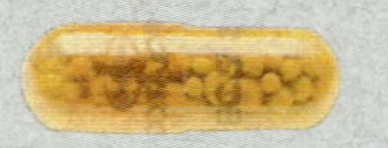 Organon COTAZYM ECS 20 Cotazym® ECS 20 **Schering-Plough**
7	DIN 02084287 Pr 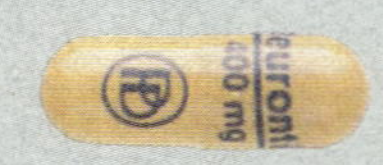 PD Neurontin 400 mg Neurontin® 400 mg **Pfizer**	NPN 02042304 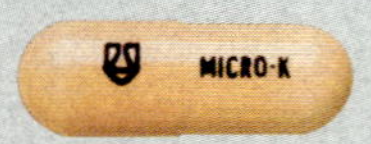 MICRO-K Micro-K Extencaps® 600 mg **Paladin**	DIN 02239888 Pr 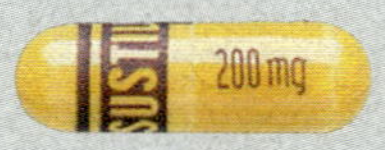 SUSTIVA 200 mg Sustiva® 200 mg **Bristol-Myers Squibb**	DIN 02315874 Pr 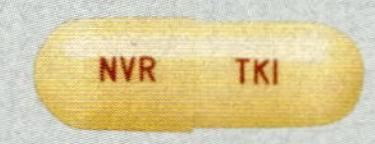 NVR TKI Tasigna® 200 mg **Novartis Pharmaceuticals**	DIN 02019957 (N) 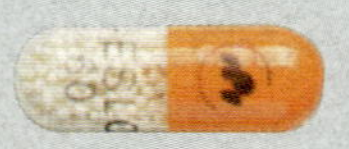 M-ESLON 60 rPr M-Eslon® 60 mg **Ethypharm**
8	DIN 00607142 Pr 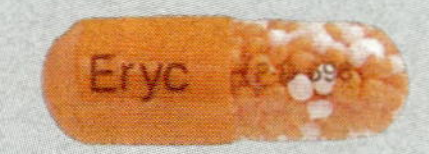 Eryc P-D 696 Eryc™ 250 mg **Pfizer**	DIN 02221837 Pr 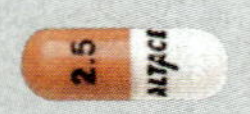 2.5 ALTACE Altace® 2.5 mg **sanofi-aventis**	DIN 02322951 (C) 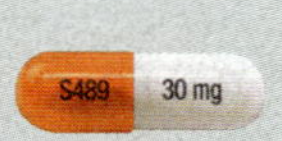 S489 30 mg Vyvanse® 30 mg **Shire**	DIN 02277131 (C) 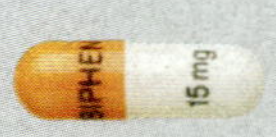 BIPHENTIN 15 mg Biphentin® 15 mg **Purdue Pharma**	DIN 00022780 Pr 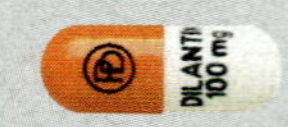 PD DILANTIN 100 mg Dilantin® 100 mg **Pfizer**

* ILLUSTRATION LESS THAN ACTUAL SIZE / ILLUSTRATION RÉDUITE

Use code A, B, C, D, E, horizontal bar and 1 to 8 vertical bar to locate illustrated products

Utiliser le code A, B, C, D, E de la ligne horizontale et les chiffres 1 à 8 de la ligne verticale pour repérer les produits illustrés

A | B | C | D | E

1

DIN 02248812 Ⓒ
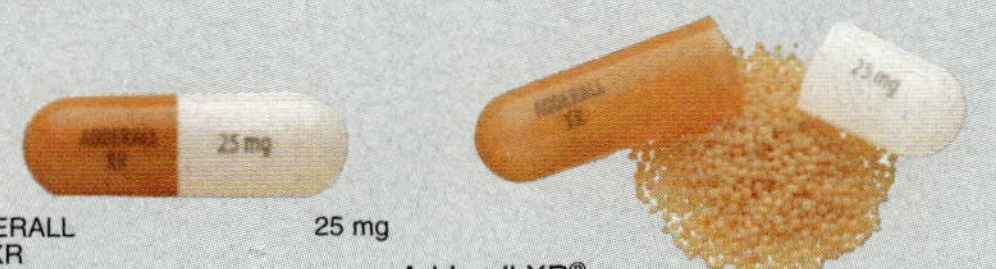
ADDERALL XR — 25 mg
Adderall XR® 25 mg
Shire

DIN 02175983 Pr
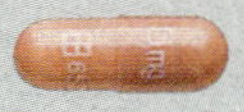
657 — 5mg
Prograf® 5 mg
Astellas

DIN 00503347 Pr
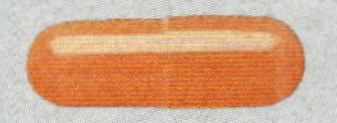
Proglycem® 100 mg
Schering-Plough

DIN 02125366 Ⓝ

12 mg PF — HYDROMORPH CONTIN
Hydromorph Contin® 12 mg
Purdue Pharma

2

DIN 02248813 Ⓒ
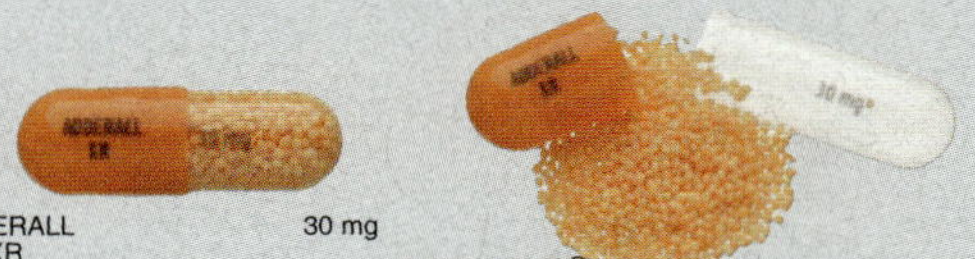
ADDERALL XR — 30 mg
Adderall XR® 30 mg
Shire

DIN 02216094 Pr
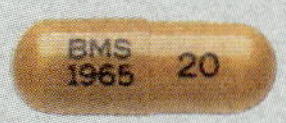
BMS 1965 — 20
Zerit™ 20 mg
Bristol-Myers Squibb

DIN 02216116 Pr
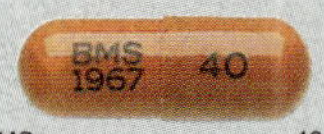
BMS 1967 — 40
Zerit™ 40 mg
Bristol-Myers Squibb

DIN 02242117 Pr
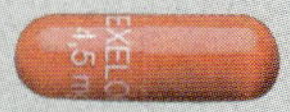
EXELON 4.5 mg
Exelon® 4.5 mg
Novartis Pharmaceuticals

3

DIN 02248811 Ⓒ
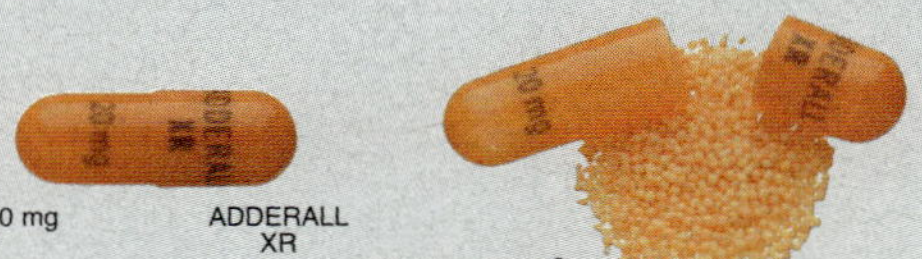
20 mg — ADDERALL XR
Adderall XR® 20 mg
Shire

DIN 02280817 Pr
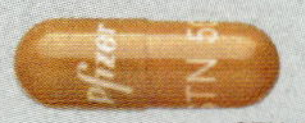
Pfizer — STN 50 mg
Sutent™ 50 mg
Pfizer

DIN 00443840 Pr
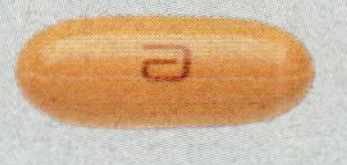
Depakene® 250 mg
Abbott

DIN 01962779 Pr
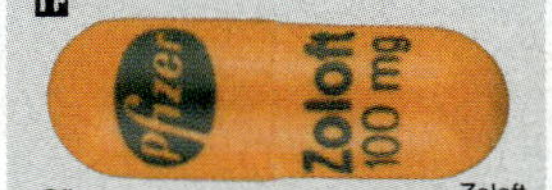
Pfizer — Zoloft 100 mg
Zoloft® 100 mg
Pfizer

4

DIN 00022772 Pr
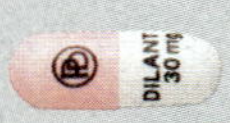
PD — Dilantin 30 mg
Dilantin® 30 mg
Pfizer

DIN 02298805 Pr
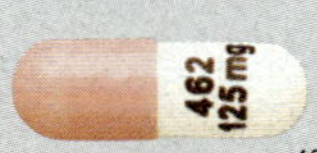
462 125 mg
Emend® 125 mg
Merck Frosst

DIN 02019949 Ⓝ
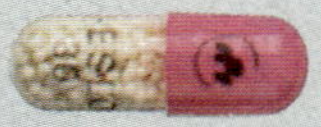
M-ESLON 30 — rPr
M-Eslon® 30 mg
Ethypharm

DIN 02241095 Pr
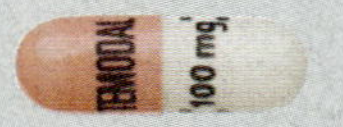
TEMODAL — 100 mg
Temodal® 100 mg
Schering-Plough

DIN 02277182 Ⓒ
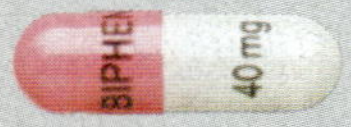
BIPHENTIN — 40 mg
Biphentin® 40 mg
Purdue Pharma

5

DIN 02125331 Ⓝ
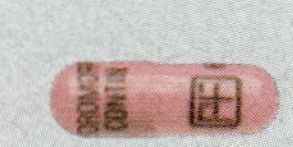
HYDROMORPH CONTIN — 6 mg PF
Hydromorph Contin® 6 mg
Purdue Pharma

DIN 02018144 Pr
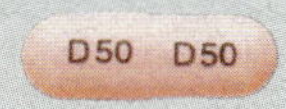
D 50
Cyclomen® 50 mg
sanofi-aventis

DIN 02119579 Pr
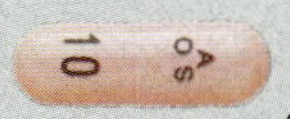
10 — A OS
Losec® 10 mg
AstraZeneca

DIN 02245867
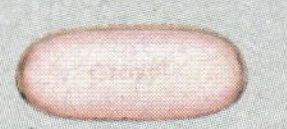
Gravol
Gravol® 50 mg
Church & Dwight

DIN 02266725 Pr
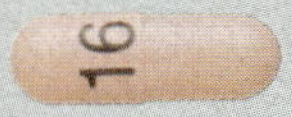
G 16
Reminyl® ER 16 mg
Janssen-Ortho

6

DIN 02237280 Pr
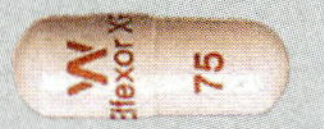
W Effexor XR — 75
Effexor® XR 75 mg
Pfizer

DIN 02181215
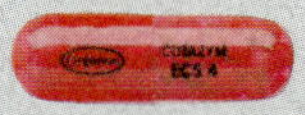
Organon — COTAZYM ECS 4
Cotazym® ECS 4
Schering-Plough

DIN 00789437
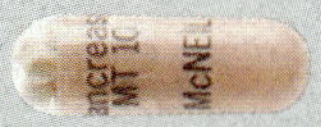
Pancrease MT 10 — McNEIL
Pancrease® MT 10
Janssen-Ortho

DIN 00789429

Pancrease MT 16 — McNEIL
Pancrease® MT 16
Janssen-Ortho

DIN 02273322 Pr *
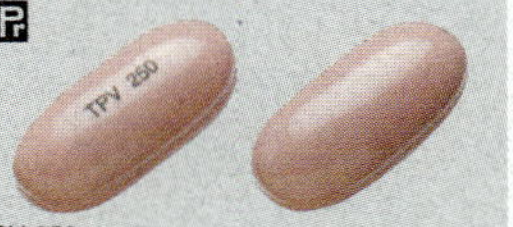
TPV 250
Aptivus® 250 mg
Boehringer Ingelheim

7

DIN 00616192 Pr
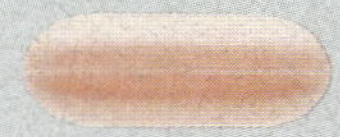
Vepesid® 50 mg
Bristol-Myers Squibb

DIN 02221845 Pr
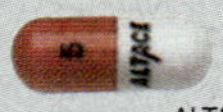
5 — ALTACE
Altace® 5 mg
sanofi-aventis

DIN 02268434 Pr
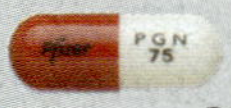
Pfizer — P G N 75
Lyrica™ 75 mg
Pfizer

DIN 00599026 Pr
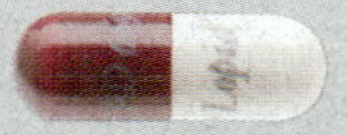
PD 669 — Lopid
Lopid™ 300 mg
Pfizer

DIN 02177757 Ⓝ
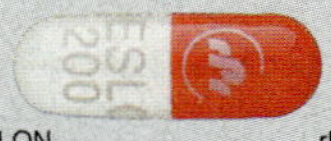
M-ESLON 200 — rPr
M-Eslon® 200 mg
Ethypharm

8

DIN 02239008
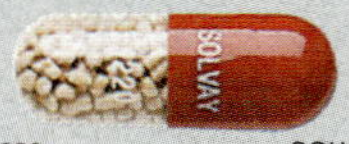
1220 — SOLVAY
Creon 20 Minimicrospheres®
Abbott Products

DIN 02277212 Ⓒ
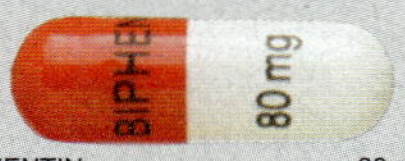
BIPHENTIN — 80 mg
Biphentin® 80 mg
Purdue Pharma

DIN 02268485 Pr
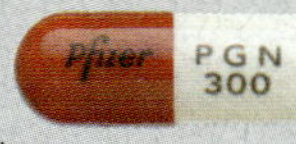
Pfizer — P G N 300
Lyrica™ 300 mg
Pfizer

DIN 01985205
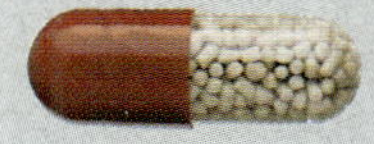
Creon 25 Minimicrospheres®
Abbott Products

DIN 02280795 Pr
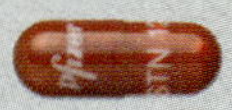
Pfizer — STN 12.5 mg
Sutent™ 12.5 mg
Pfizer

* ILLUSTRATION LESS THAN ACTUAL SIZE / ILLUSTRATION RÉDUITE

Use code A, B, C, D, E, horizontal bar and 1 to 8 vertical bar to locate illustrated products

Utiliser le code A, B, C, D, E de la ligne horizontale et les chiffres 1 à 8 de la ligne verticale pour repérer les produits illustrés

	A	B	C	D	E
1	DIN 02091887 Pr 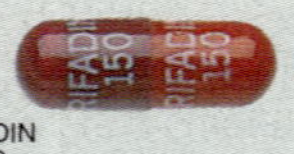 RIFADIN 150 Rifadin® 150 mg **sanofi-aventis**	DIN 02092808 Pr  RIFADIN 300 Rifadin® 300 mg **sanofi-aventis**	DIN 02237282 Pr 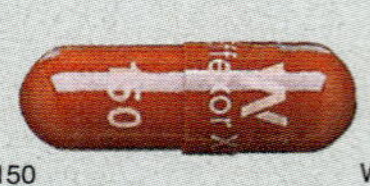 150 W Effexor XR Effexor®XR 150 mg **Pfizer**	DIN 02125390 Ⓝ 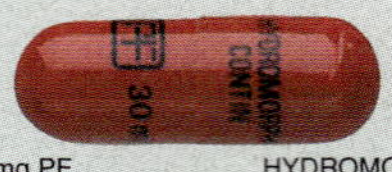 30 mg PF HYDROMORPH CONTIN Hydromorph Contin® 30 mg **Purdue Pharma**	DIN 02063786 Pr 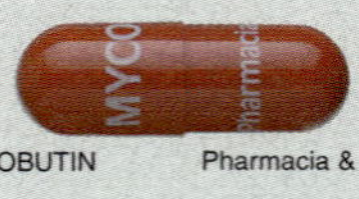 MYCOBUTIN Pharmacia & Upjohn Mycobutin® 150 mg **Pfizer**
2	DIN 02229293 Pr 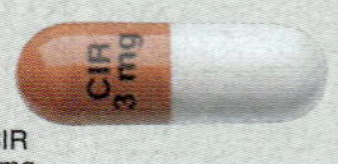 CIR 3 mg Entocort® 3 mg **AstraZeneca**	DIN 02279347 Pr 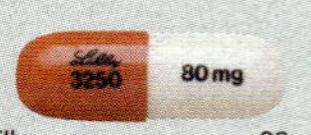 Lilly 3250 80 mg Strattera® 80 mg **Lilly**	DIN 02266733 Pr 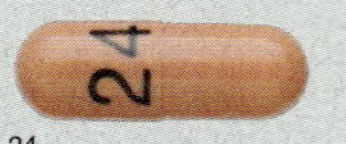 G 24 Reminyl® ER 24 mg **Janssen-Ortho**	DIN 02279355 Pr 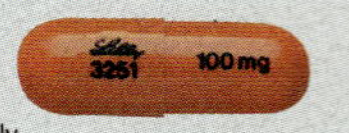 Lilly 3251 100 mg Strattera® 100 mg **Lilly**	DIN 00481823 Pr 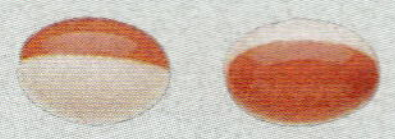 Rocaltrol® 0.25 µg **Roche**
3	DIN 02043408 Pr 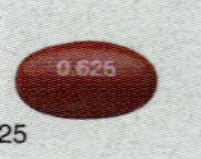 0.625 Premarin® 0.625 mg **Pfizer**	DIN 02257955 Pr 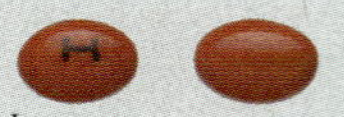 I Clarus 10 mg **Mylan**	DIN 00582344 Pr 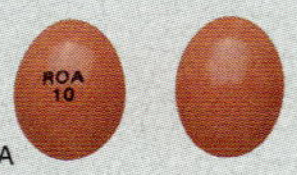 ROA 10 Accutane™ Roche® 10 mg **Roche**	DIN 00481815 Pr 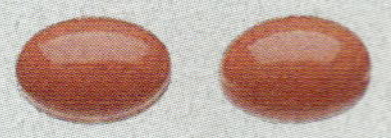 Rocaltrol® 0.50 µg **Roche**	DIN 02257963 Pr 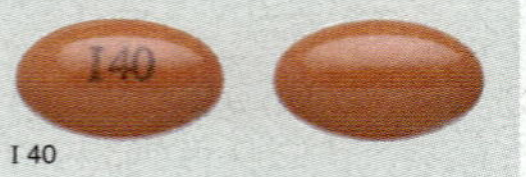 I 40 Clarus 40 mg **Mylan**
4	DIN 02070847 Pr 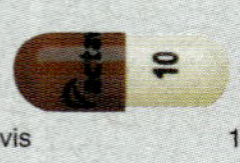 actavis 10 Soriatane® 10 mg **Actavis**	DIN 02200104 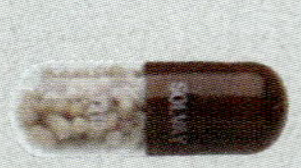 1210 SOLVAY Creon 10 Minimicrospheres® **Abbott Products**	DIN 02241093 Pr 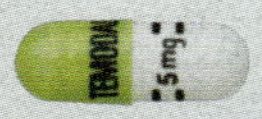 TEMODAL 5 mg Temodal® 5 mg **Schering-Plough**	DIN 00360422 Pr 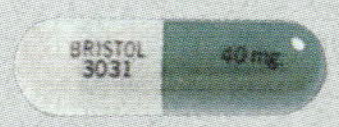 BRISTOL 3031 40 mg CeeNU® 40 mg **Bristol-Myers Squibb**	DIN 02277190 Ⓒ 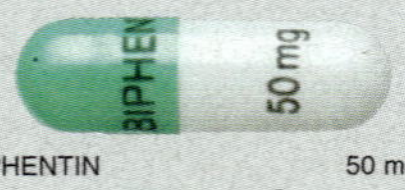 BIPHENTIN 50 mg Biphentin® 50 mg **Purdue Pharma**
5	DIN 02231151 Pr 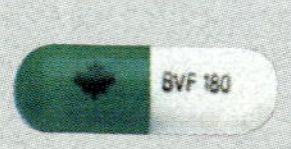 BVF 180 Tiazac® 180 mg **Biovail Pharmaceuticals**	DIN 02043394 Pr 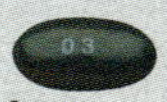 0.3 Premarin® 0.3 mg **Pfizer**	DIN 02244612 Pr 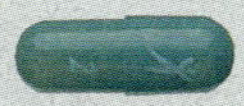 2 Detrol™ LA 2 mg **Pfizer**	DIN 02125323 Ⓝ 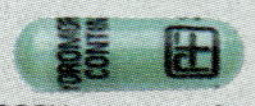 HYDROMORPH CONTIN 3 mg PF Hydromorph Contin® 3 mg **Purdue Pharma**	DIN 00360414 Pr 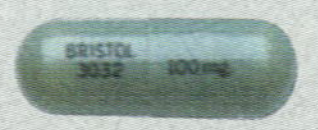 BRISTOL 3032 100 mg CeeNU® 100 mg **Bristol-Myers Squibb**
6	DIN 02231155 Pr 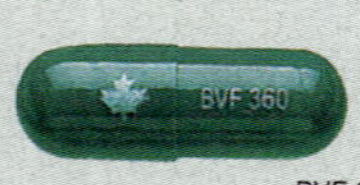 BVF 360 Tiazac® 360 mg **Biovail Pharmaceuticals**	DIN 02061597 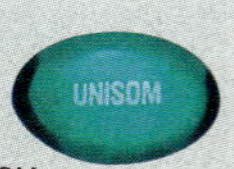 UNISOM Unisom® 50 mg **Paladin**	DIN 02221853 Pr 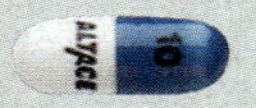 ALTACE 10 Altace® 10 mg **sanofi-aventis**	DIN 02248808 Ⓒ 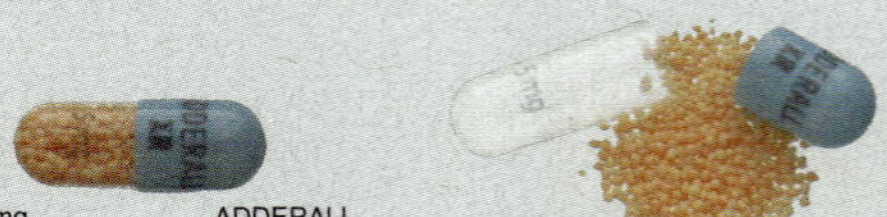 5 mg ADDERALL XR Adderall XR® 5 mg **Shire**	
7	DIN 02277166 Ⓒ 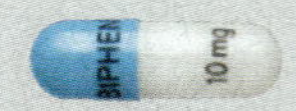 BIPHENTIN 10 mg Biphentin® 10 mg **Purdue Pharma**	DIN 02301482 Pr 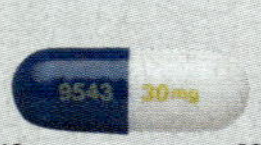 9543 30 mg Cymbalta™ 30 mg **Lilly**	DIN 02262827 Pr 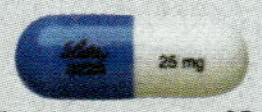 Lilly 3228 25 mg Strattera® 25 mg **Lilly**	DIN 02248810 Ⓒ 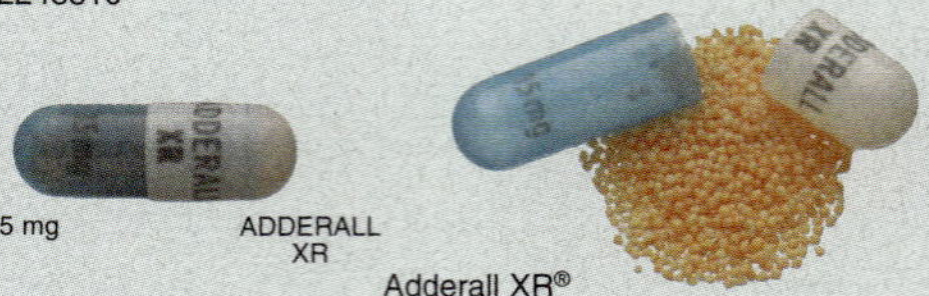 15 mg ADDERALL XR Adderall XR® 15 mg **Shire**	
8	DIN 02347164 Ⓒ 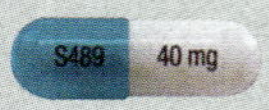 S489 40 mg Vyvanse® 40 mg **Shire**	DIN 02322978 Ⓒ 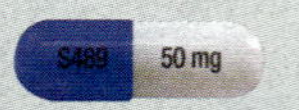 S489 50 mg Vyvanse® 50 mg **Shire**	DIN 02042231 Pr 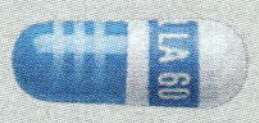 INDERAL-LA 60 Inderal®-LA 60 mg **Pfizer**	DIN 02248809 Ⓒ 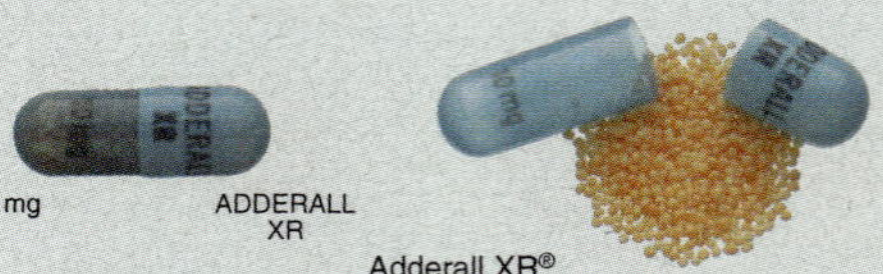 10 mg ADDERALL XR Adderall XR® 10 mg **Shire**	

* ILLUSTRATION LESS THAN ACTUAL SIZE / ILLUSTRATION RÉDUITE

Use code A, B, C, D, E, horizontal bar and 1 to 8 vertical bar to locate illustrated products

Utiliser le code A, B, C, D, E de la ligne horizontale et les chiffres 1 à 8 de la ligne verticale pour repérer les produits illustrés

1

A1 — DIN 02298597 Pr
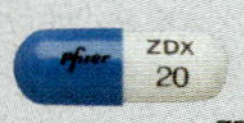
Pfizer / ZDX 20
Zeldox™ 20 mg
Pfizer

B1 — DIN 02298627 Pr
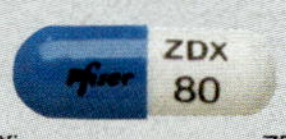
Pfizer / ZDX 80
Zeldox™ 80 mg
Pfizer

C1 — DIN 02312433 Pr
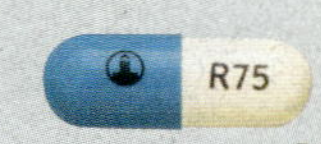
R75
Pradax™ 75 mg
Boehringer Ingelheim

D1 — DIN 02312441 Pr
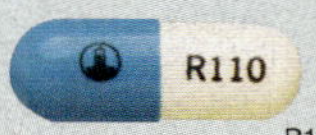
R110
Pradax™ 110 mg
Boehringer Ingelheim

E1 — DIN 00176192 Ⓝ
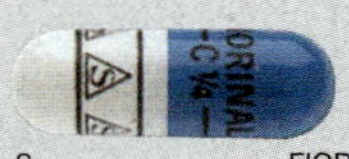
S / FIORINAL C ¼
Fiorinal®-C ¼ 50 mg
Novartis Pharmaceuticals

2

A2 — NPN 80015586 *
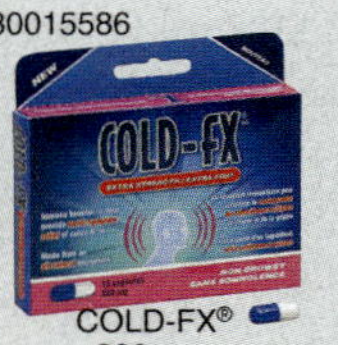
COLD-FX® 300 mg
Afexa Life Sciences

B2 — DIN 02298600 Pr
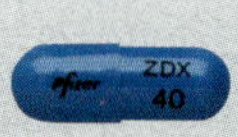
Pfizer / ZDX 40
Zeldox™ 40 mg
Pfizer

C2 — DIN 02262835 Pr
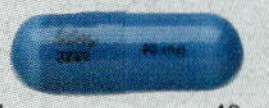
Lilly 3229 / 40 mg
Strattera® 40 mg
Lilly

D2 — DIN 02244613 Pr
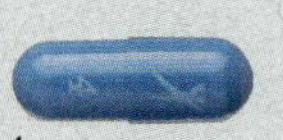
4
Detrol™ LA 4 mg
Pfizer

E2 — DIN 02347172 Ⓒ
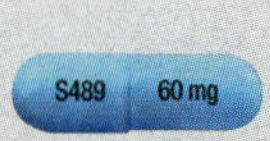
S489 / 60 mg
Vyvanse® 60 mg
Shire

3

A3 — DIN 02042258 Pr
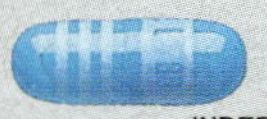
INDERAL-LA 80
Inderal®-LA 80 mg
Pfizer

B3 — DIN 02042266 Pr
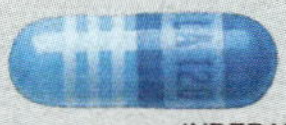
INDERAL-LA 120
Inderal®-LA 120 mg
Pfizer

C3 — DIN 02042274 Pr
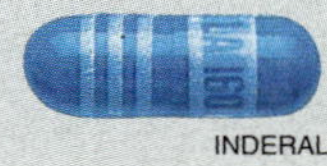
INDERAL-LA 160
Inderal®-LA 160 mg
Pfizer

D3 — DIN 02097249 Pr
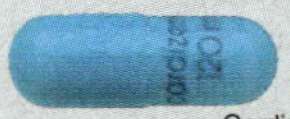
Cardizem CD 120 mg
Cardizem® CD 120 mg
Biovail Pharmaceuticals

E3 — DIN 02097257 Pr
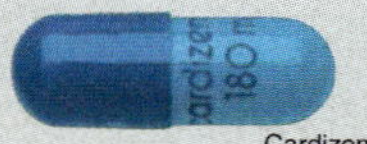
Cardizem CD 180 mg
Cardizem® CD 180 mg
Biovail Pharmaceuticals

4

A4 — DIN 02240325 Pr
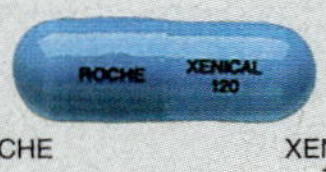
ROCHE / XENICAL 120
Xenical® 120 mg
Roche

B4 — DIN 00024368 Pr
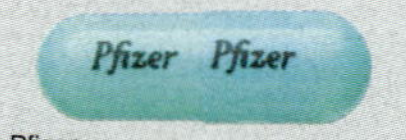
Pfizer
Vibramycin™ 100 mg
Pfizer

C4 — DIN 02097265 Pr
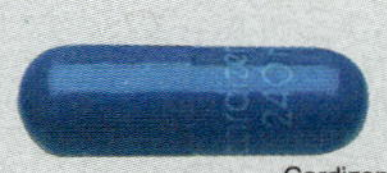
Cardizem CD 240 mg
Cardizem® CD 240 mg
Biovail Pharmaceuticals

D4 — DIN 02248610 Pr
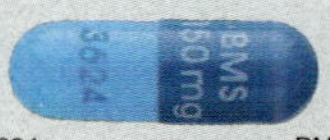
3624 / BMS 150 mg
Reyataz™ 150 mg
Bristol-Myers Squibb

E4 — DIN 02248611 Pr
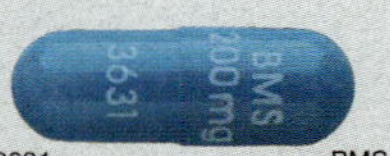
3631 / BMS 200 mg
Reyataz™ 200 mg
Bristol-Myers Squibb

5

A5 — DIN 00176206 Ⓝ
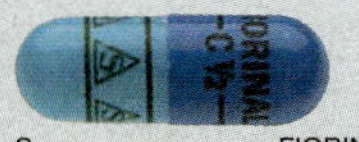
S / FIORINAL C ½
Fiorinal®-C ½ 50 mg
Novartis Pharmaceuticals

B5 — DIN 02182866 Pr *
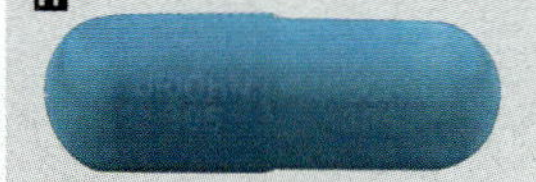
UPJOHN 395
Dalacin® C 300 mg
Pfizer

C5 — DIN 02231150 Pr
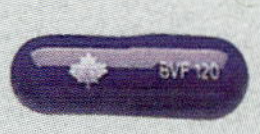
BVF 120
Tiazac® 120 mg
Biovail Pharmaceuticals

D5 — DIN 02277174 Ⓒ
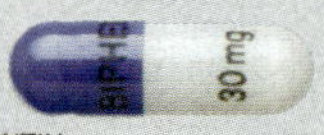
BIPHENTIN / 30 mg
Biphentin® 30 mg
Purdue Pharma

E5 — DIN 02231154 Pr
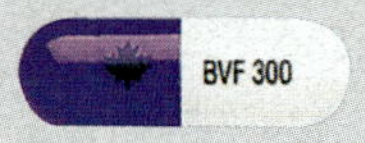
BVF 300
Tiazac® 300 mg
Biovail Pharmaceuticals

6

A6 — DIN 02141647 *
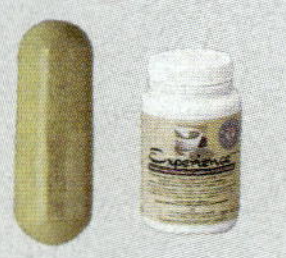
Experience™
Awareness Corporation/ Dba AwarenessLife

B6 — DIN 02243246 *
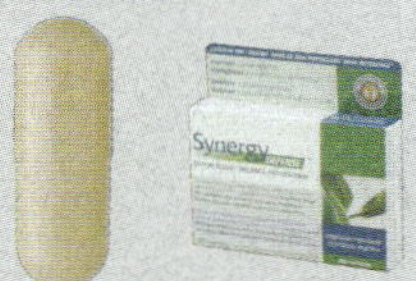
Synergy Defense™
Awareness Corporation

C6 — NPN 80002849 *
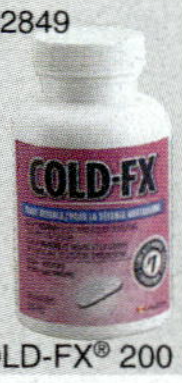
COLD-FX® 200 mg
Afexa Life Sciences

D6 — DIN 00611204 Ⓝ
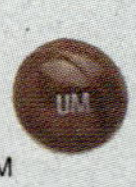
UM
Marinol® 5 mg
Abbott Products

E6 — DIN 02241472 Pr
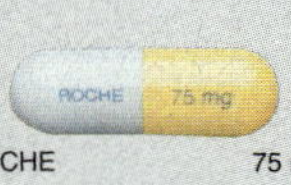
ROCHE / 75 mg
Tamiflu® 75 mg
Roche

7

A7 — DIN 02045869
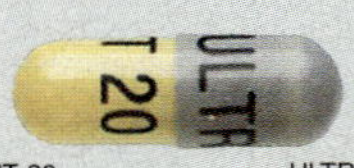
MT 20 / ULTRASE
Ultrase® MT20
Axcan Pharma

B7 — DIN 02237279 Pr
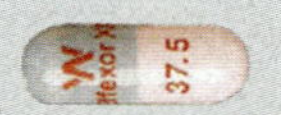
W Effexor XR / 37.5
Effexor® XR 37.5 mg
Pfizer

C7 — DIN 00846503 Pr
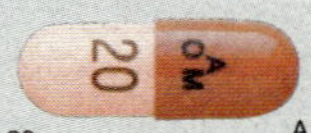
20 / A OM
Losec® 20 mg
AstraZeneca

D7 — DIN 02296489 Pr
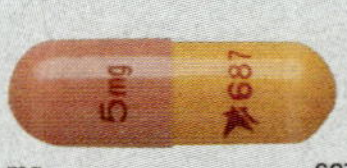
5 mg / 687
Advagraf™ 5 mg
Astellas

E7 — DIN 02216086 Pr
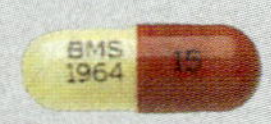
BMS 1964 / 15
Zerit™ 15 mg
Bristol-Myers Squibb

8

A8 — DIN 02242119 Pr
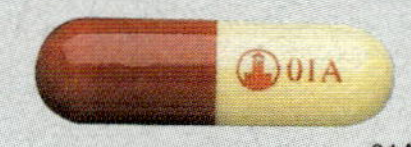
01A
Aggrenox® 200 mg/25 mg
Boehringer Ingelheim

B8 — DIN 00873454 Pr
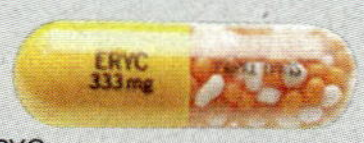
ERYC 333 mg / PARKE-DAVIS
Eryc™ 333 mg
Pfizer

C8 — DIN 02216108 Pr
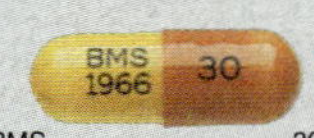
BMS 1966 / 30
Zerit™ 30 mg
Bristol-Myers Squibb

D8 — DIN 02280809 Pr
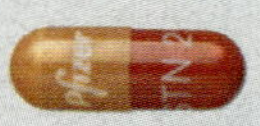
Pfizer / STN 25 mg
Sutent™ 25 mg
Pfizer

E8 — DIN 02242118 Pr
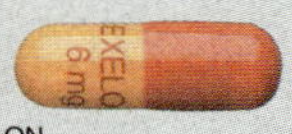
EXELON 6 mg
Exelon® 6 mg
Novartis Pharmaceuticals

* ILLUSTRATION LESS THAN ACTUAL SIZE / ILLUSTRATION RÉDUITE

Use code A, B, C, D, E, horizontal bar and 1 to 8 vertical bar to locate illustrated products

Utiliser le code A, B, C, D, E de la ligne horizontale et les chiffres 1 à 8 de la ligne verticale pour repérer les produits illustrés

	A	B	C	D	E
1	DIN 02061562 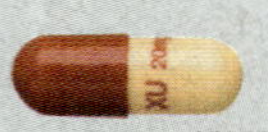 XU 20mg Lescol® 20 mg **Novartis Pharmaceuticals**	DIN 02061570 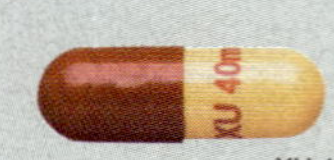 XU 40mg Lescol® 40 mg **Novartis Pharmaceuticals**	DIN 02145839 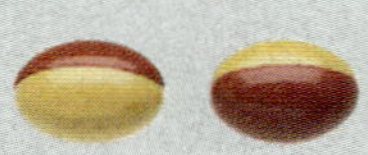 Vesanoid® 10 mg **Roche**	DIN 01924559 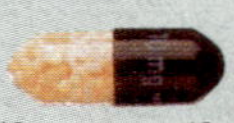 3513 10 mg SB Dexedrine® Spansule® 10 mg **Paladin**	DIN 01924567 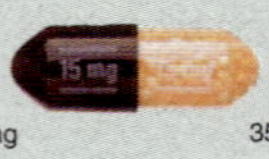 15 mg SB 3514 Dexedrine® Spansule® 15 mg **Paladin**
2	DIN 02070863 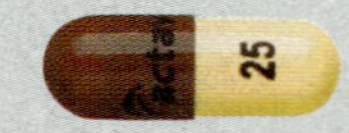 actavis 25 Soriatane® 25 mg **actavis**	DIN 02224801 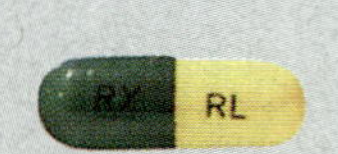 RY RL Rythmodan® 100 mg **sanofi-aventis**	DIN 02216965 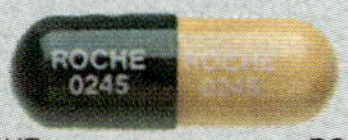 ROCHE 0245 ROCHE 0245 Invirase® 200 mg **Roche**	DIN 01926853 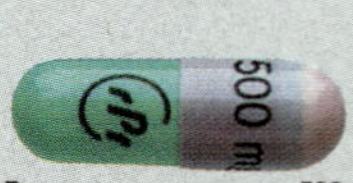 rPr 500 mg Flagyl® 500 mg **sanofi-aventis**	DIN 00465283 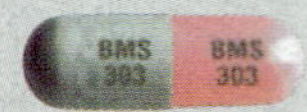 BMS 303 Hydrea® 500 mg **Bristol-Myers Squibb**
3	DIN 02231152 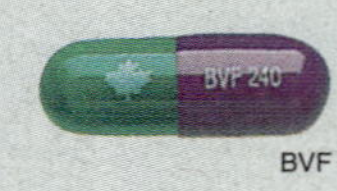 BVF 240 Tiazac® 240 mg **Biovail Pharmaceuticals**	DIN 00522597 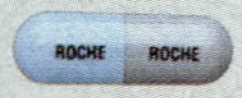 ROCHE Prolopa® 50 mg/12.5 mg **Roche**	DIN 02281112 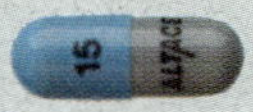 15 ALTACE Altace® 15 mg **sanofi-aventis**	DIN 02097273 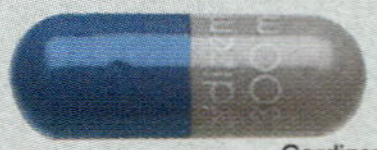 Cardizem CD 300 mg Cardizem® CD 300 mg **Biovail Pharmaceuticals**	DIN 02262843 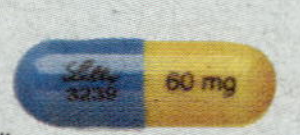 Lilly 3239 60 mg Strattera® 60 mg **Lilly**
4	DIN 02192748 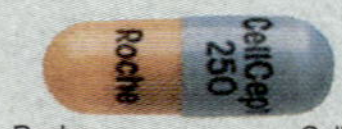 Roche CellCept 250 CellCept® 250 mg **Roche**	DIN 02047454 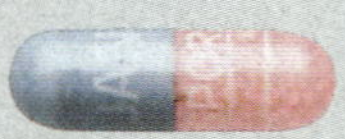 JANSSEN SPORANOX 100 Sporanox® 100 mg **Janssen-Ortho**	DIN 00386464 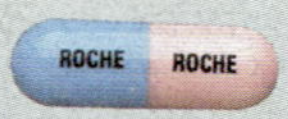 ROCHE Prolopa® 100 mg/25 mg **Roche**	DIN 00800430 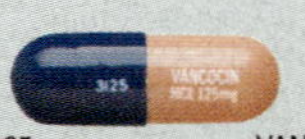 3125 VANCOCIN HCL 125 mg Vancocin® 125 mg **Iroko**	DIN 00788716 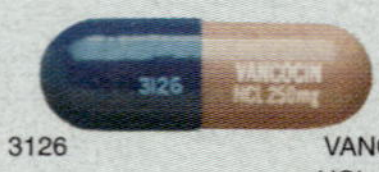 3126 VANCOCIN HCL 250 mg Vancocin® 250 mg **Iroko**
5	DIN 00030570 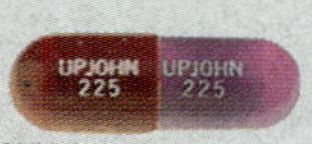 UPJOHN 225 Dalacin® C 150 mg **Pfizer**	DIN 02239007 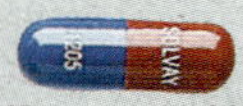 1205 SOLVAY Creon 5 Minimicrospheres® **Abbott Products**	DIN 00386472 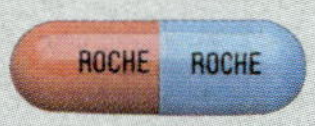 ROCHE Prolopa® 200 mg/50 mg **Roche**	DIN 02294176 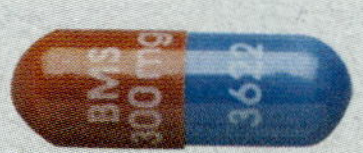 BMS 300 mg 3622 Reyataz™ 300 mg **Bristol-Myers Squibb**	DIN 02301490 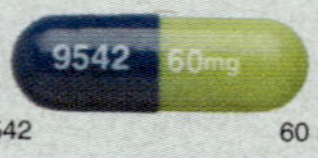 9542 60 mg Cymbalta™ 60 mg **Lilly**
6	DIN 02278057 * 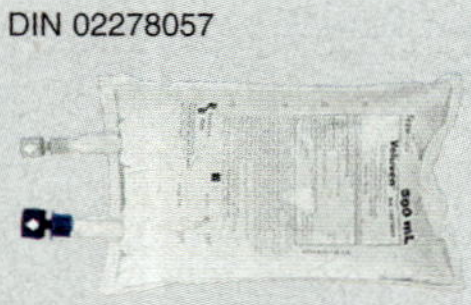 Voluven® **Fresenius Kabi**	DIN 00891835 * 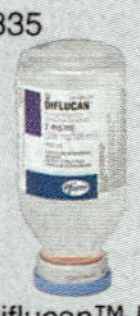 Diflucan™ I.V. 2 mg/mL **Pfizer**	DIN 02212188 * 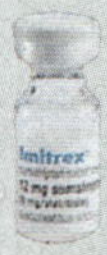 Imitrex® **GlaxoSmithKline**	DIN 02301393 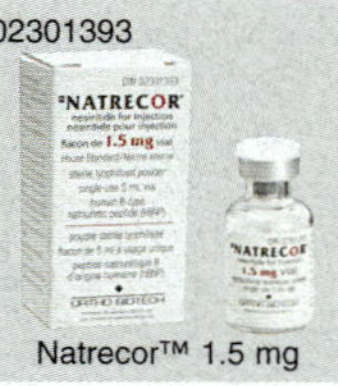 Natrecor™ 1.5 mg **Janssen-Ortho**	DIN 02213745 * 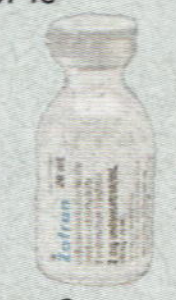 Zofran® 2 mg/mL **GlaxoSmithKline**
7	DIN 02245464 * 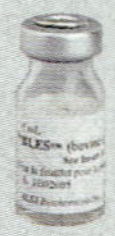 BLES™ **BLES**	DIN 02244895 * 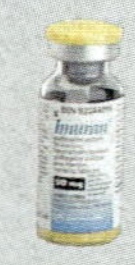 Imuran® 50 mg **Triton Pharma**	DIN 02248296 * 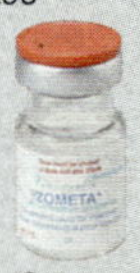 Zometa® Concentrate 4 mg/5 mL **Novartis Pharmaceuticals**	DIN 02049392 * 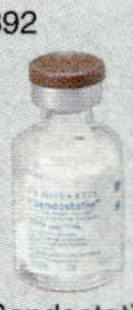 Sandostatin® 200 µg/mL **Novartis Pharmaceuticals**	DIN 02059789 * 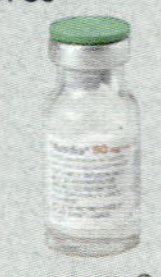 Aredia® 90 mg **Novartis Pharmaceuticals**
8	DIN 02206072 * 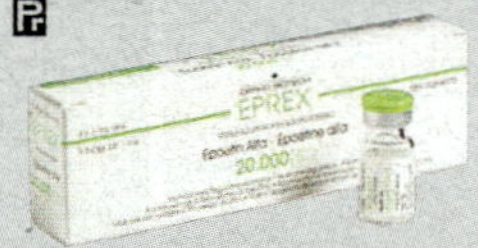 Eprex® 20 000 IU **Janssen-Ortho**	DIN 02320673 * 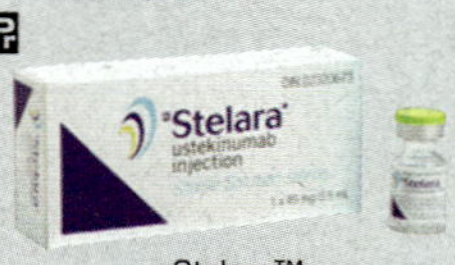 Stelara™ 45 mg/0.5 mL **Janssen-Ortho**	DIN 02239616 * 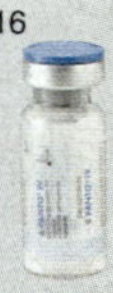 PANTO® IV 40 mg **Nycomed**	DIN 02242815 * 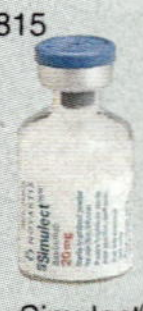 Simulect® 20 mg **Novartis Pharmaceuticals**	DIN 02169649 * 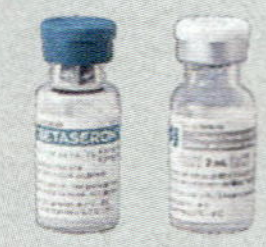 Betaseron® **Bayer**

* ILLUSTRATION LESS THAN ACTUAL SIZE / ILLUSTRATION RÉDUITE

Use code A, B, C, D, E, horizontal bar and 1 to 8 vertical bar to locate illustrated products

Utiliser le code A, B, C, D, E de la ligne horizontale et les chiffres 1 à 8 de la ligne verticale pour repérer les produits illustrés

	A	B	C	D	E
1	DIN 02260565 * 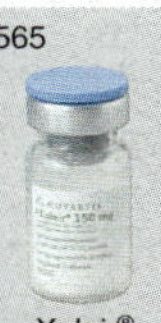 Xolair® 150 mg/5 mL **Novartis Pharmaceuticals**	DIN 02059762 * 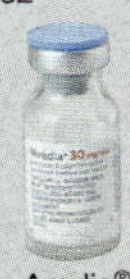 Aredia® 30 mg **Novartis Pharmaceuticals**	DIN 02262452 * 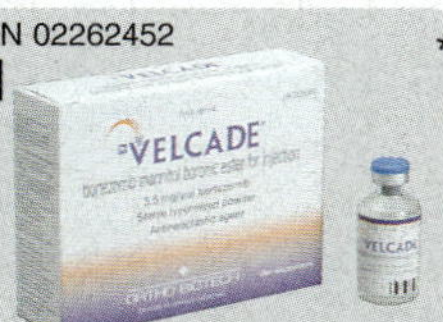 Velcade™ 3.5 mg **Janssen-Ortho**	DIN 02247099 * 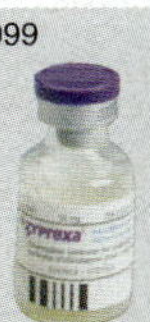 Zyprexa® IntraMuscular 10 mg **Lilly**	DIN 00464988 * 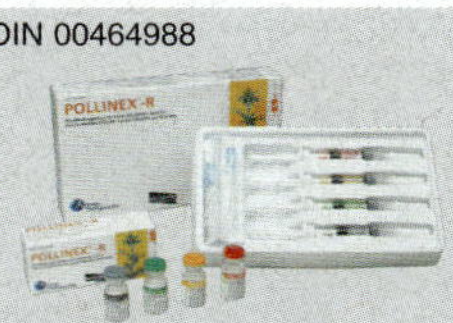 Pollinex®-R **Nycomed**
2	DIN 02298465 * 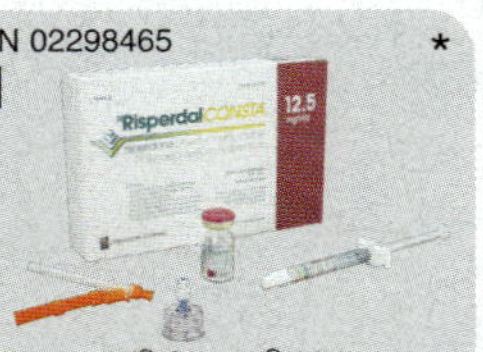 Risperdal® Consta® 12.5 mg **Janssen-Ortho**	DIN 02255707 * 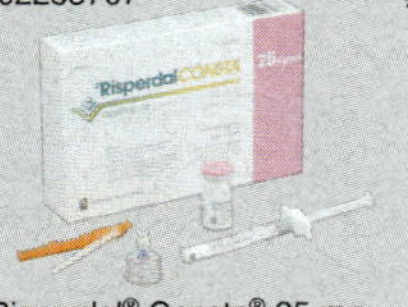 Risperdal® Consta® 25 mg **Janssen-Ortho**	DIN 02255723 * 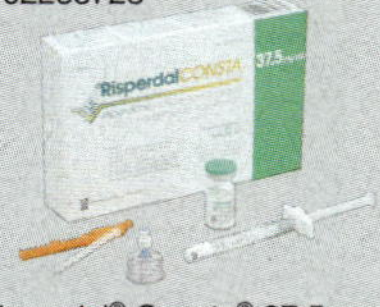 Risperdal® Consta® 37.5 mg **Janssen-Ortho**	DIN 02255758 * 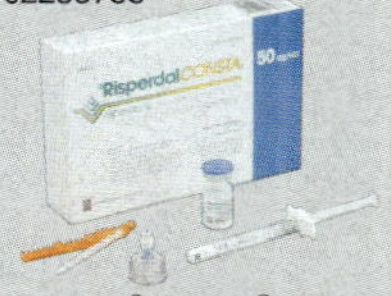 Risperdal® Consta® 50 mg **Janssen-Ortho**	DIN 02320673 * 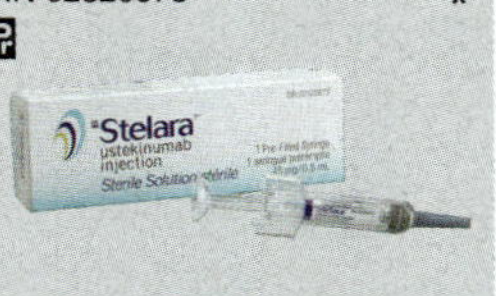 Stelara™ 45 mg/0.5 mL **Janssen-Ortho**
3	DIN 00839205 * 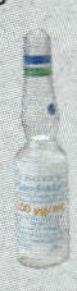 Sandostatin® 100 µg/mL **Novartis Pharmaceuticals**	DIN 00839213 * 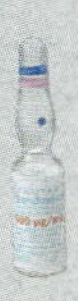 Sandostatin® 500 µg/mL **Novartis Pharmaceuticals**	DIN 02239323 * 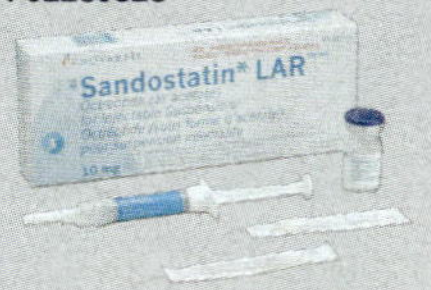 Sandostatin® LAR® 10 mg **Novartis Pharmaceuticals**	DIN 02239324 * 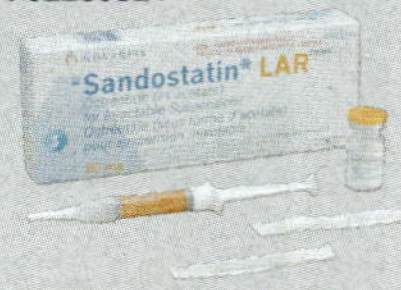 Sandostatin® LAR® 20 mg **Novartis Pharmaceuticals**	DIN 02239325 * 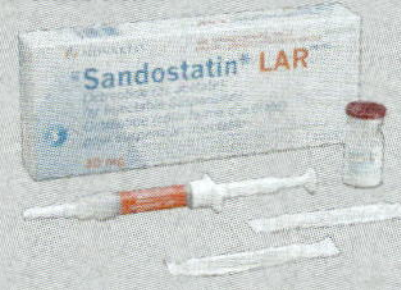 Sandostatin® LAR® 30 mg **Novartis Pharmaceuticals**
4	DIN 02131048 *  Lioresal® Intrathecal 0.05 mg/mL **Novartis Pharmaceuticals**	DIN 02131056 * 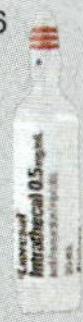 Lioresal® Intrathecal 0.5 mg/mL **Novartis Pharmaceuticals**	DIN 02131064 * 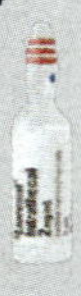 Lioresal® Intrathecal 2 mg/mL **Novartis Pharmaceuticals**	DIN 00593257 * 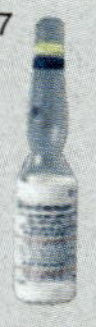 Sandimmune® I.V. 50 mg/1 mL **Novartis Pharmaceuticals**	DIN 00593257 * 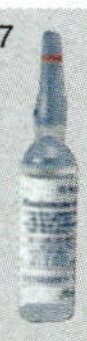 Sandimmune® I.V. 250 mg/5 mL **Novartis Pharmaceuticals**
5	DIN 02176009 * 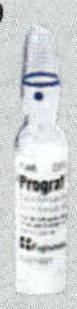 Prograf® 5 mg/1 mL **Astellas**	DIN 00839191 * 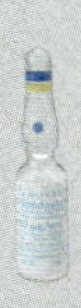 Sandostatin® 50 µg/mL **Novartis Pharmaceuticals**	DIN 00587737 * 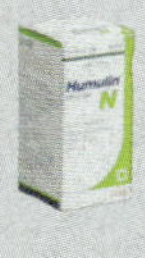 Humulin®-N 100 IU/mL **Lilly**	DIN 02241310 * 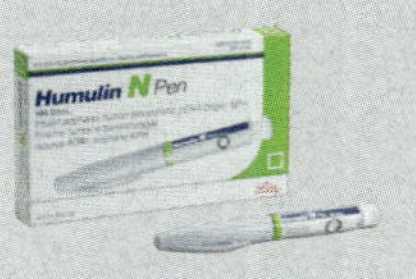 Humulin®-N 100 IU/mL **Lilly**	DIN 01959239 * 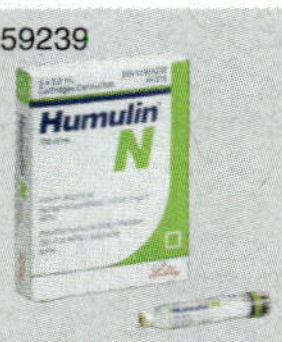 Humulin®-N 100 IU/mL **Lilly**
6	DIN 02271842 * 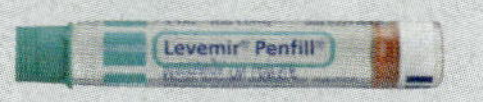 Levemir® 100 IU **Novo Nordisk**	DIN 02244353 * 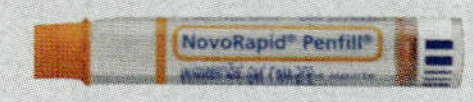 NovoRapid® 100 IU **Novo Nordisk**	DIN 02229704 * 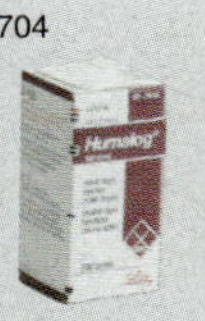 Humalog® 100 IU/mL **Lilly**	DIN 02229705 * 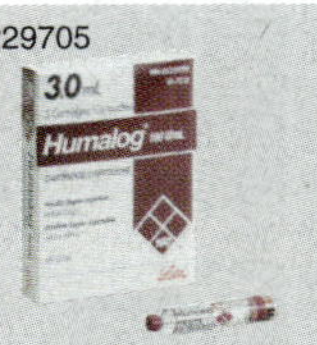 Humalog® 100 IU/mL **Lilly**	DIN 02241283 * 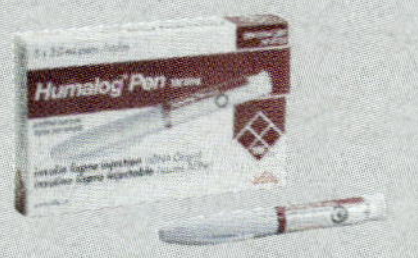 Humalog® 100 IU/mL **Lilly**
7	DIN 00509558 * 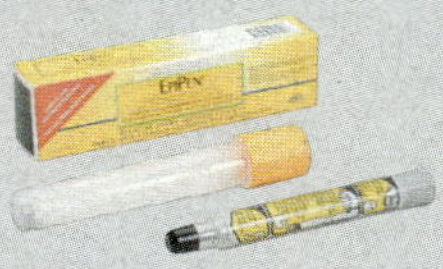 EpiPen® **King Pharmaceuticals**	DIN 00578657 * 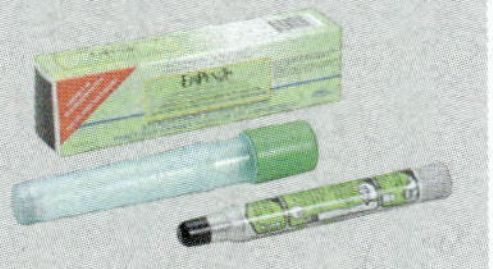 EpiPen® Jr. **King Pharmaceuticals**	DIN 02254689 * 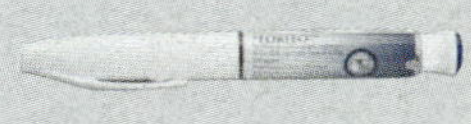 Forteo™ 250 µg/mL **Lilly**	DIN 02240294 * 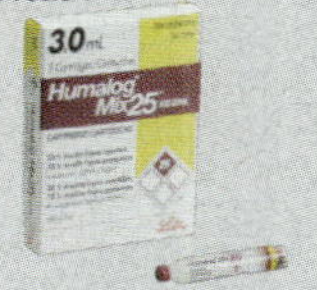 Humalog® Mix25® 100 IU/mL **Lilly**	DIN 02240295 * 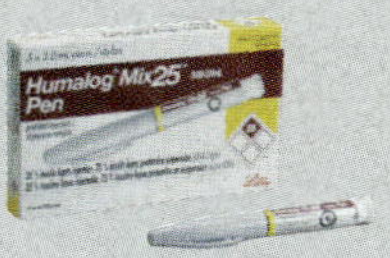 Humalog® Mix25® 100 IU/mL **Lilly**
8	DIN 02354217 * 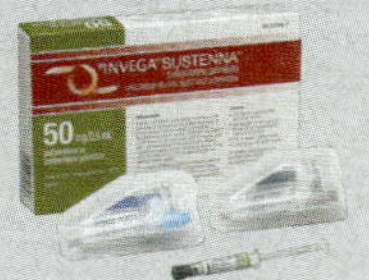 Invega® Sustenna™ 50 mg/0.5 mL **Janssen-Ortho**	DIN 02354225 * 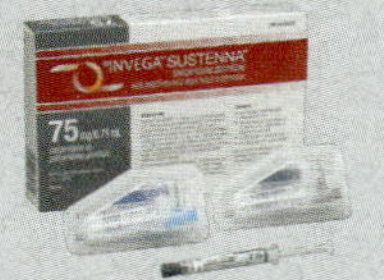 Invega® Sustenna™ 75 mg/0.75 mL **Janssen-Ortho**	DIN 02354233 * 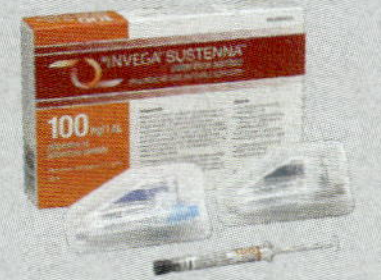 Invega® Sustenna™ 100 mg/1 mL **Janssen-Ortho**	DIN 02354241 * 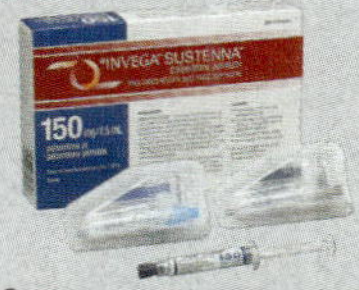 Invega® Sustenna™ 150 mg/1.5 mL **Janssen-Ortho**	DIN 02245619 * 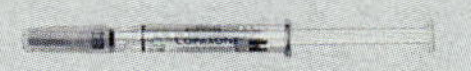 Copaxone® **Teva Canada Innovation**

* ILLUSTRATION LESS THAN ACTUAL SIZE / ILLUSTRATION RÉDUITE

Use code A, B, C, D, E, horizontal bar and 1 to 8 vertical bar to locate illustrated products

Utiliser le code A, B, C, D, E de la ligne horizontale et les chiffres 1 à 8 de la ligne verticale pour repérer les produits illustrés

1

A1 — DIN 02231583 *
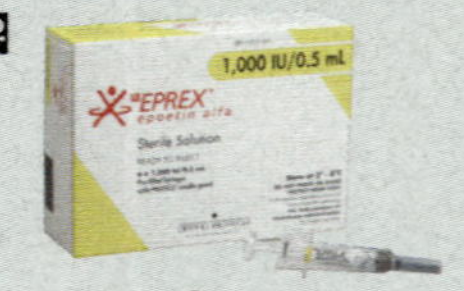
Eprex® 1000 IU
Janssen-Ortho

B1 — DIN 02231584 *
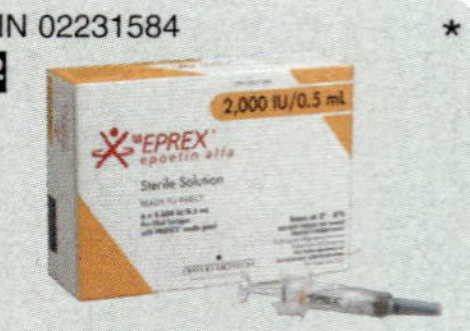
Eprex® 2000 IU
Janssen-Ortho

C1 — DIN 02231585 *
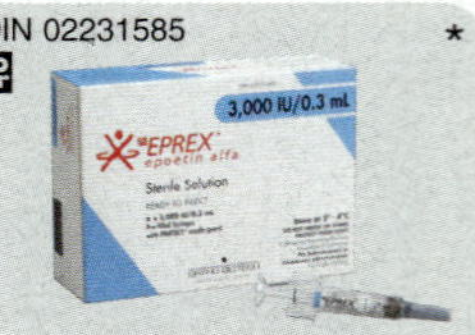
Eprex® 3000 IU
Janssen-Ortho

D1 — DIN 02231586 *
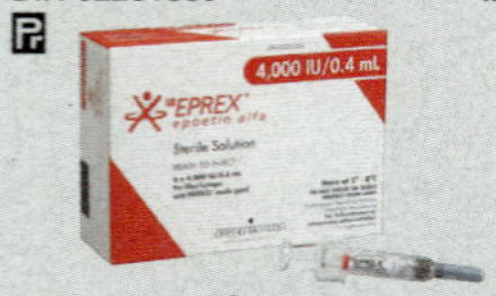
Eprex® 4000 IU
Janssen-Ortho

E1 — DIN 02243400 *
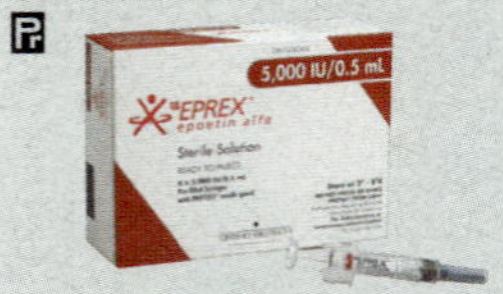
Eprex® 5000 IU
Janssen-Ortho

2

A2 — DIN 02243401 *
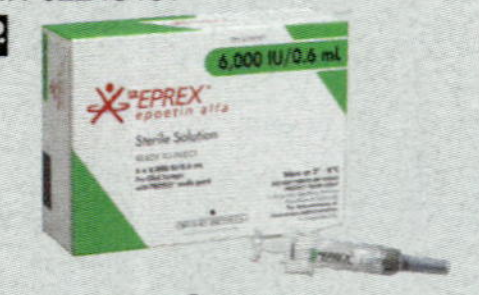
Eprex® 6000 IU
Janssen-Ortho

B2 — DIN 02243403 *
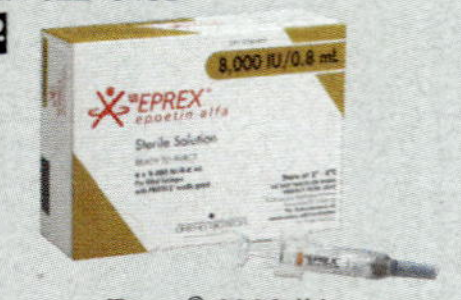
Eprex® 8000 IU
Janssen-Ortho

C2 — DIN 02231587 *
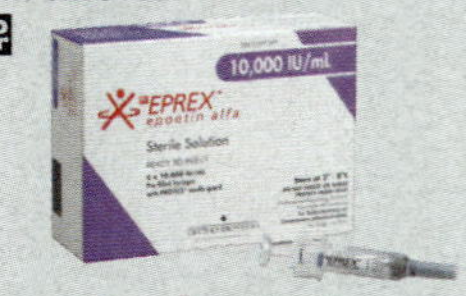
Eprex® 10 000 IU
Janssen-Ortho

D2 — DIN 02243239 *
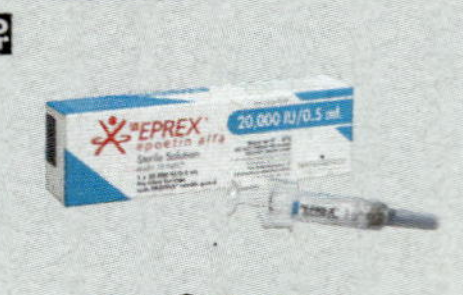
Eprex® 20 000 IU
Janssen-Ortho

E2 — DIN 02288680 *
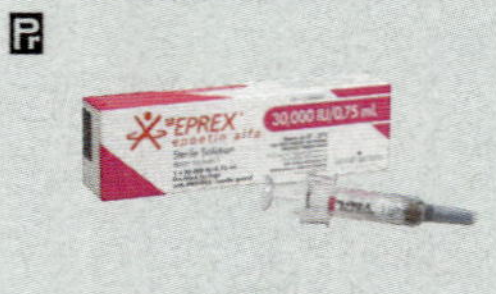
Eprex® 30 000 IU
Janssen-Ortho

3

A3 — DIN 02240722 *
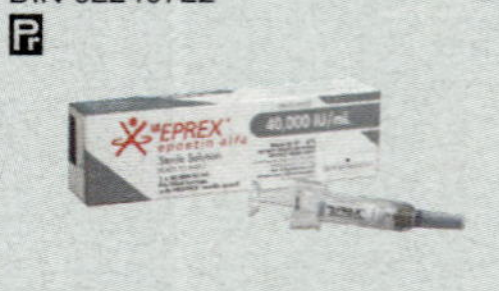
Eprex® 40 000 IU
Janssen-Ortho

B3 — DIN 02049325 *
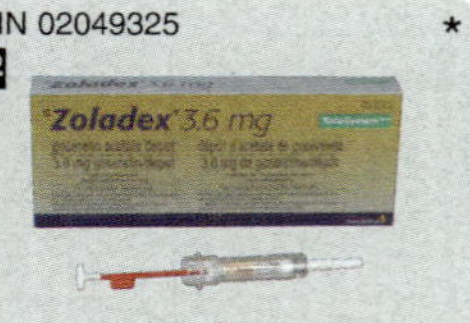
Zoladex® 3.6 mg
AstraZeneca

C3 — DIN 02225905 *
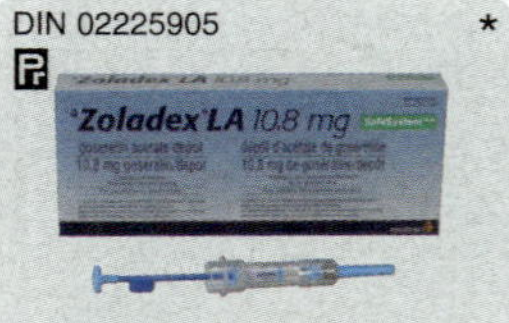
Zoladex® LA 10.8 mg
AstraZeneca

D3 — DIN 02248624 *
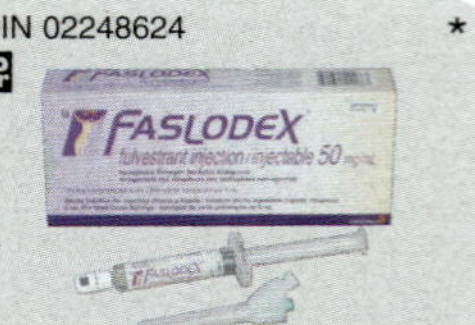
Faslodex® 250 mg/5 mL
AstraZeneca

E3 — DIN 02269562 *
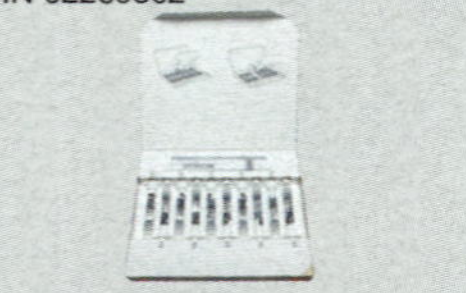
Influvac® 15 µg/0.5 mL
Abbott Products

4

A4 — *
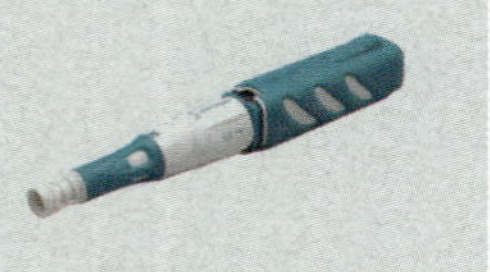
Rebif® Auto-Injector
EMD Canada

B4 — DIN 02237319 *
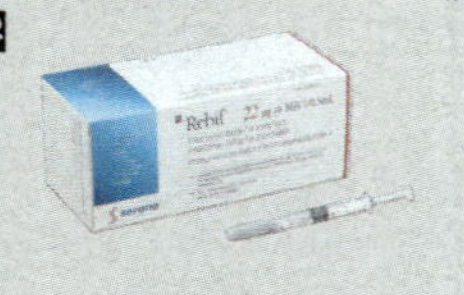
Rebif® 22 µg
EMD Canada

C4 — DIN 02237320 *
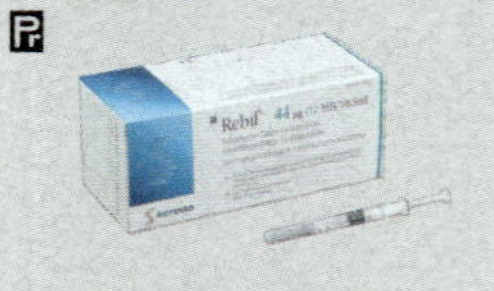
Rebif® 44 µg
EMD Canada

D4 — *
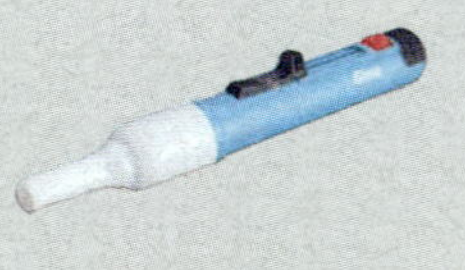
Imitrex® Auto-Injector
GlaxoSmithKline

E4 — DIN 02212188 *
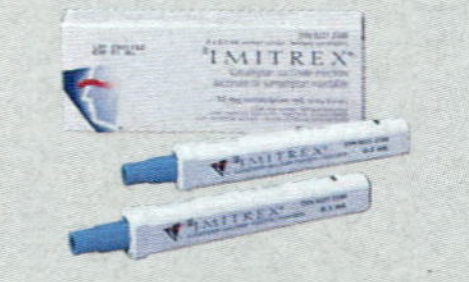
Imitrex® Prefilled Syringes
GlaxoSmithKline

5

A5 — DIN 02212188 *
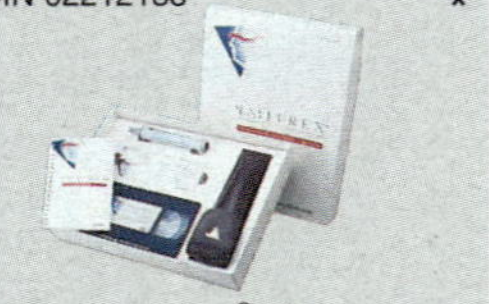
Imitrex® Kit
GlaxoSmithKline

B5 — DIN 02238703 *
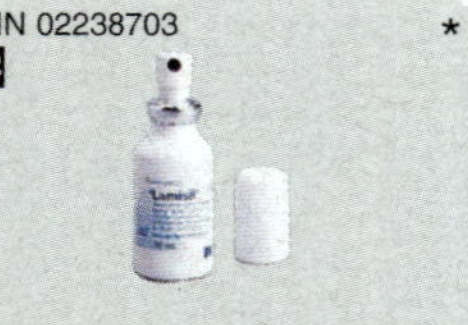
Lamisil®
Novartis Pharmaceuticals

C5 — DIN 02240775 *
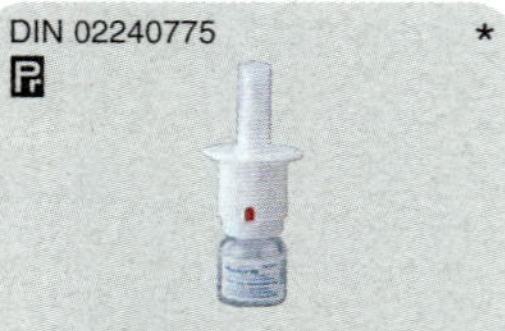
Miacalcin® NS
Novartis Pharmaceuticals

D5 — DIN 02020017 *
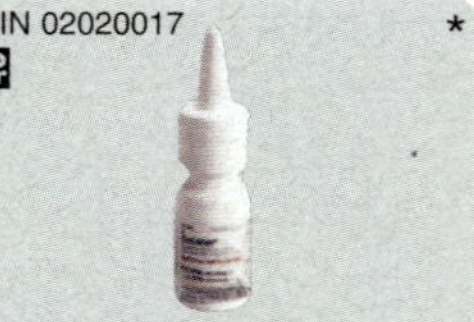
Livostin®
Janssen-Ortho

E5 — DIN 02230420 *
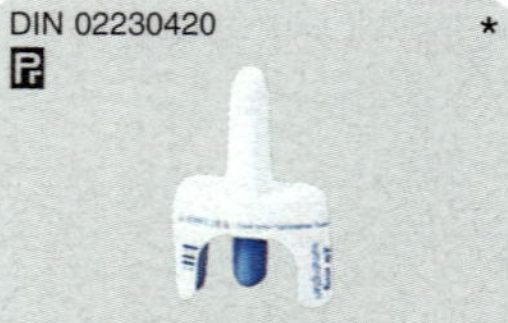
Imitrex® 20 mg
GlaxoSmithKline

6

A6 — DIN 02188783 *
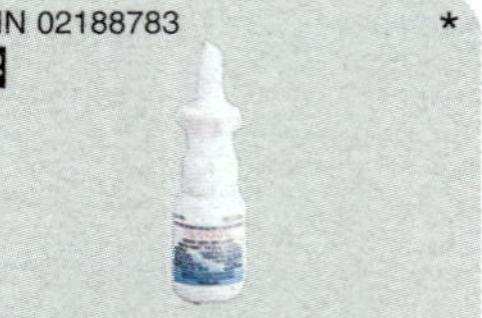
Synarel® 8 mL
Pfizer

B6 — DIN 02303671 *
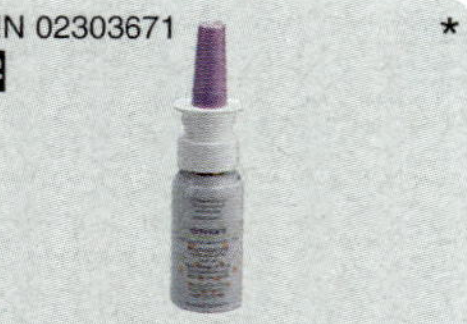
Omnaris™ 50 µg
Nycomed

C6 — DIN 02231923 *
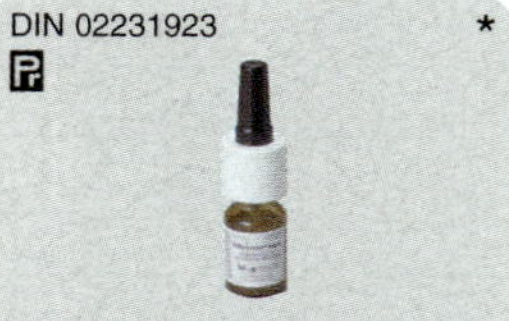
Rhinocort® Aqua 64 µg
AstraZeneca

D6 — DIN 02248993 *
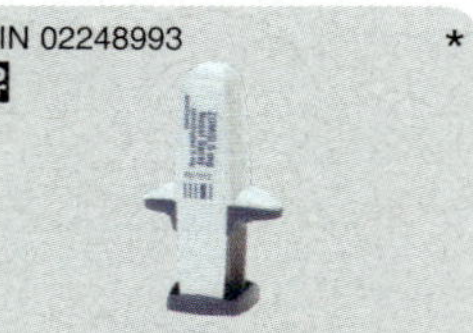
Zomig® 5 mg
AstraZeneca

E6 — DIN 02213672 *
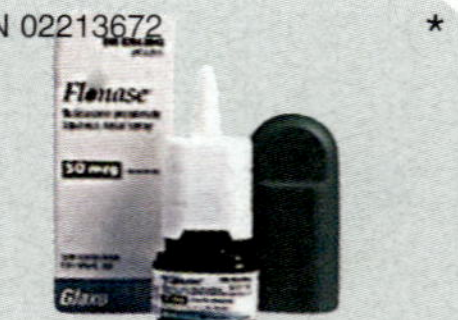
Flonase® 50 µg
GlaxoSmithKline

7

A7 — DIN 02298589 *
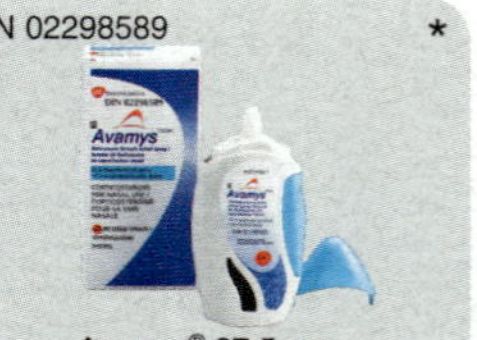
Avamys® 27.5 µg
GlaxoSmithKline

B7 — DIN 02112795 *
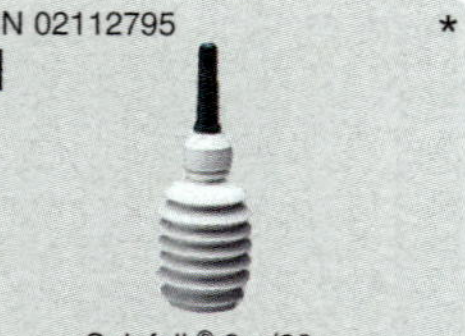
Salofalk® 2 g/60 g
Axcan Pharma

C7 — DIN 02052431 *
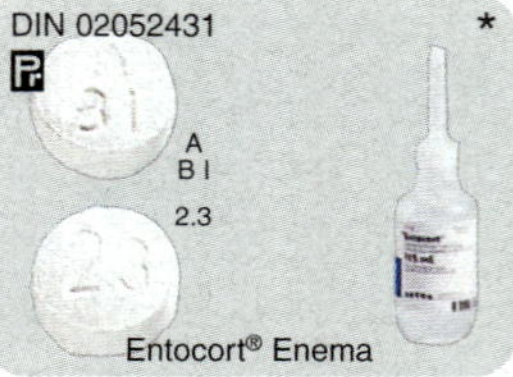
Entocort® Enema
AstraZeneca

D7 — DIN 02245345 *
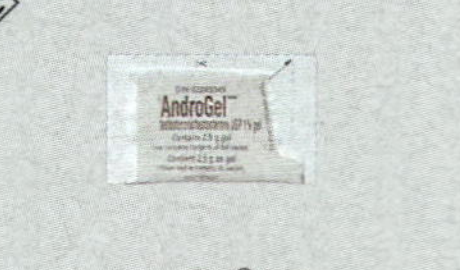
AndroGel® 2.5 g
Abbott Products

E7 — DIN 02245346 *
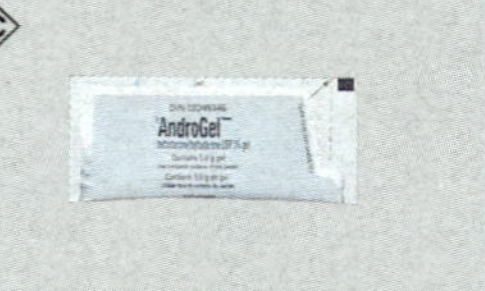
AndroGel® 5 g
Abbott Products

8

A8 — DIN 02031094 *
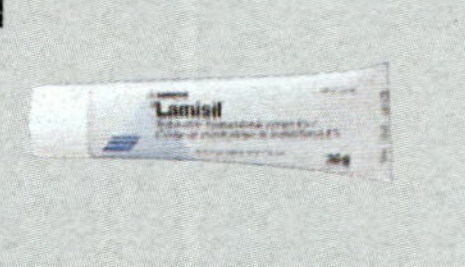
Lamisil®
Novartis Pharmaceuticals

B8 — DIN 02239405 *
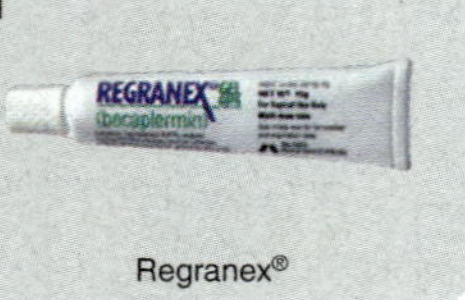
Regranex®
Janssen-Ortho

C8 — DIN 02247238 *
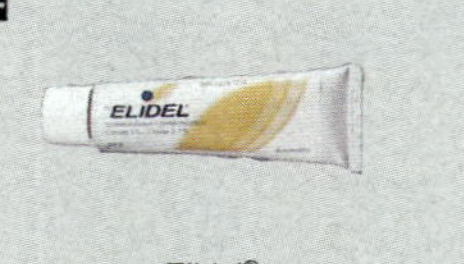
Elidel®
Novartis Pharmaceuticals

D8 — DIN 00886858 *
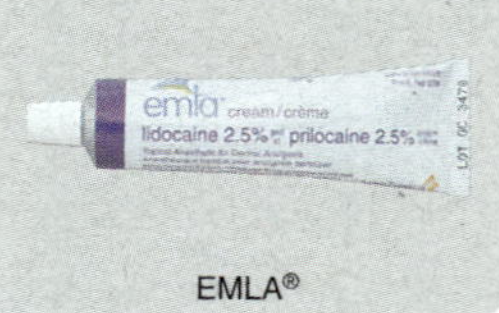
EMLA®
AstraZeneca

E8 — DIN 02249499 *
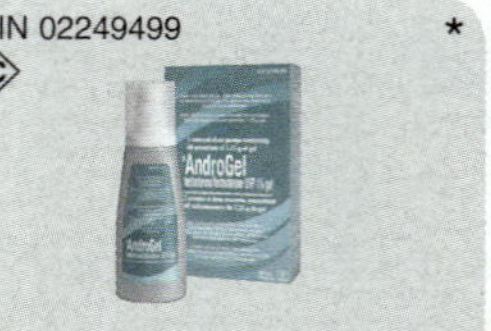
AndroGel®
Abbott Products

* ILLUSTRATION LESS THAN ACTUAL SIZE / ILLUSTRATION RÉDUITE

Use code A, B, C, D, E, horizontal bar and 1 to 8 vertical bar to locate illustrated products

Utiliser le code A, B, C, D, E de la ligne horizontale et les chiffres 1 à 8 de la ligne verticale pour repérer les produits illustrés

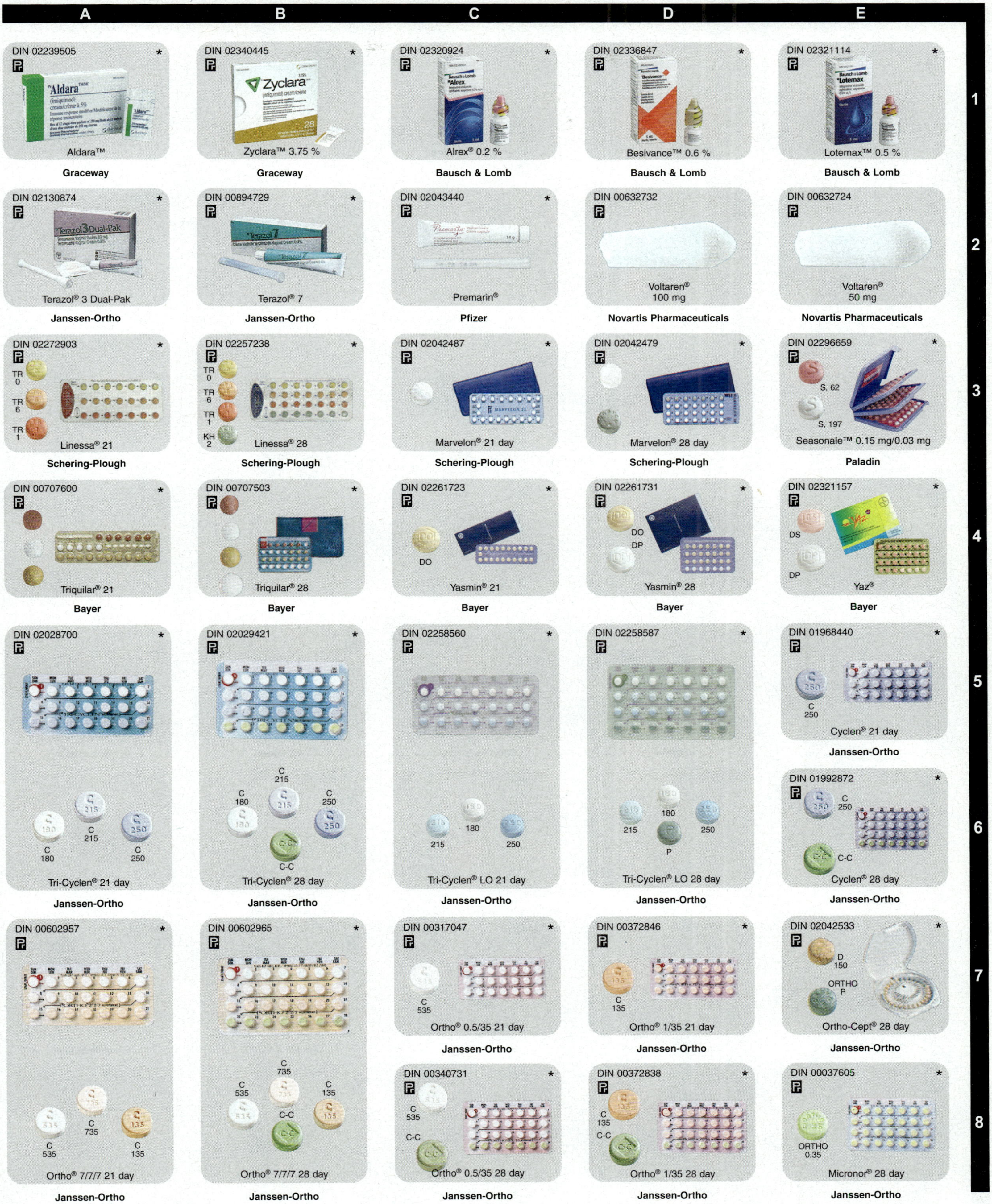

* ILLUSTRATION LESS THAN ACTUAL SIZE / ILLUSTRATION RÉDUITE

Use code A, B, C, D, E, horizontal bar and 1 to 8 vertical bar to locate illustrated products

Utiliser le code A, B, C, D, E de la ligne horizontale et les chiffres 1 à 8 de la ligne verticale pour repérer les produits illustrés

1

A — DIN 02187086 *
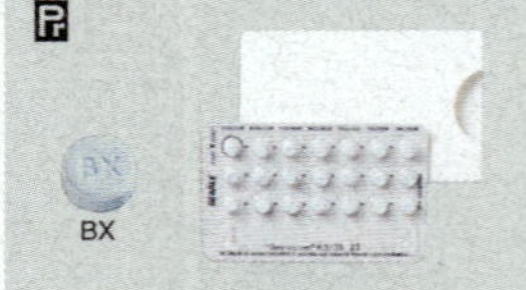

Brevicon® 0.5/35 21 day
Pfizer

B — DIN 02189054 *
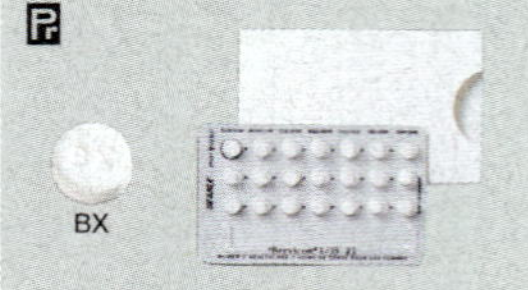

Brevicon® 1/35 21 day
Pfizer

C — DIN 00469327 *
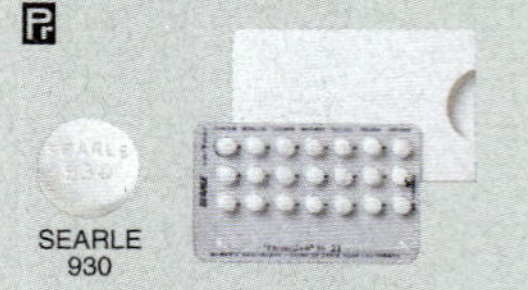

Demulen® 30 (21 day)
Pfizer

D — DIN 02187108 *
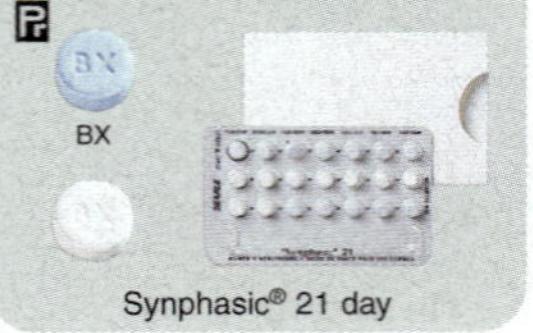

Synphasic® 21 day
Pfizer

E — DIN 02197502 *
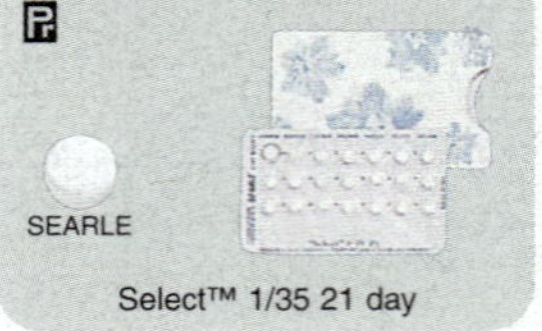

Select™ 1/35 21 day
Pfizer

2

A — DIN 02187094 *
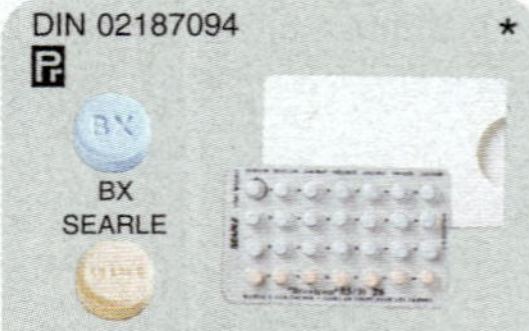

Brevicon® 0.5/35 28 day
Pfizer

B — DIN 02189062 *
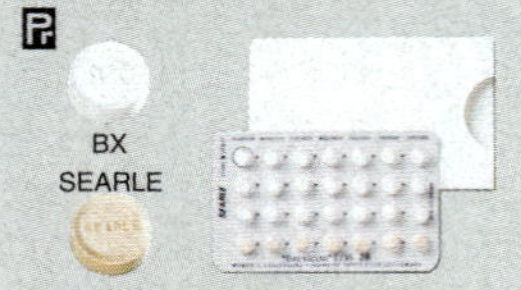

Brevicon® 1/35 28 day
Pfizer

C — DIN 00471526 *
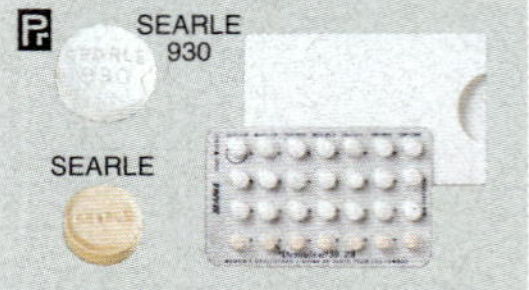

Demulen® 30 (28 day)
Pfizer

D — DIN 02187116 *
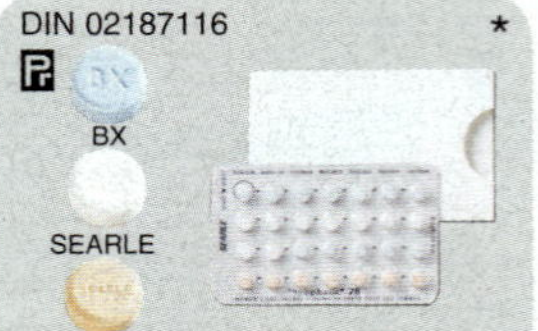

Synphasic® 28 day
Pfizer

E — DIN 02199297 *
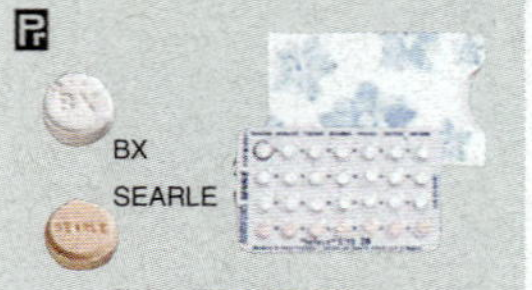

Select™ 1/35 28 day
Pfizer

3

A — DIN 02236974 *
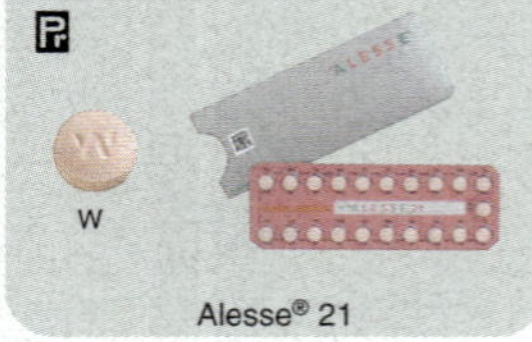

Alesse® 21
Pfizer

B — DIN 02236975 *
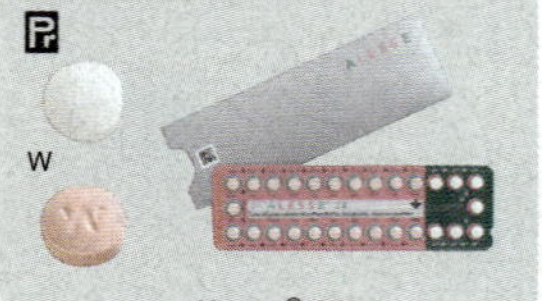

Alesse® 28
Pfizer

C — DIN 02042320 *
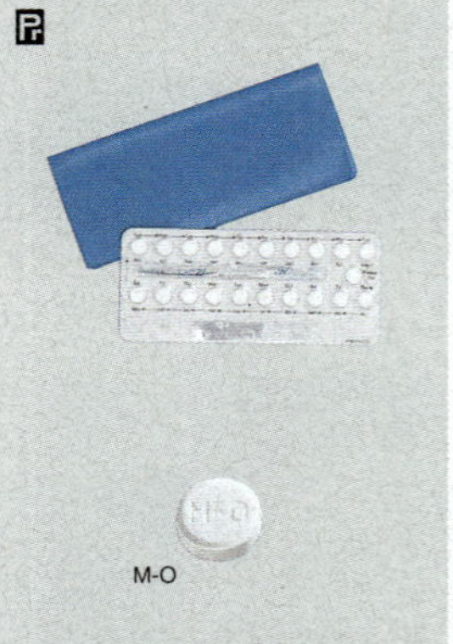

Min-Ovral® 21
Pfizer

D — DIN 02042339 *
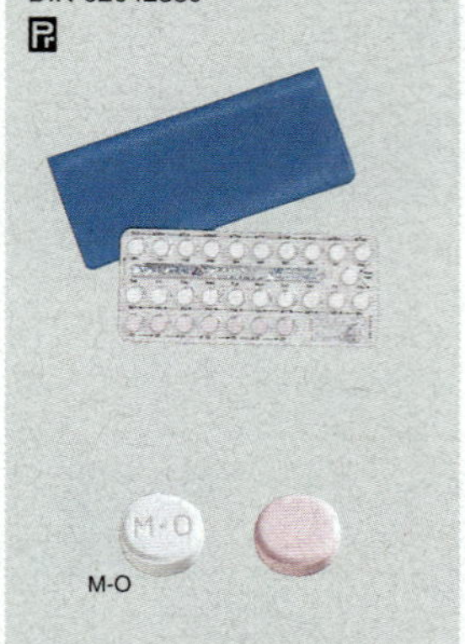

Min-Ovral® 28
Pfizer

E — DIN 02043033 *
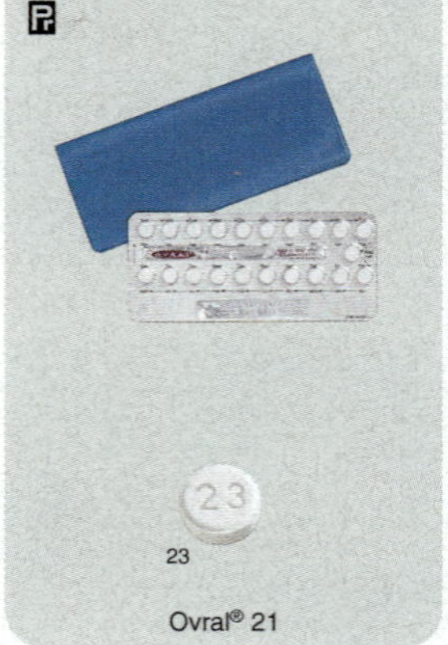

Ovral® 21
Pfizer

4

A — DIN 02253186 *

NuvaRing
Schering-Plough

B — DIN 02168898 *
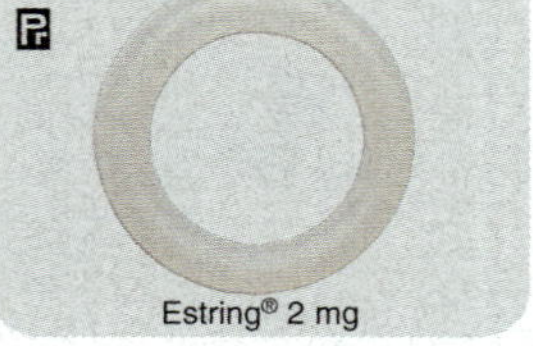
Estring® 2 mg
Paladin

5

A — DIN 02243005 *
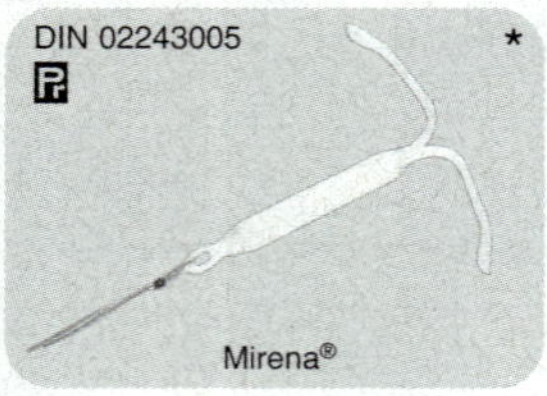
Mirena®
Bayer

B — DIN 02241674 *
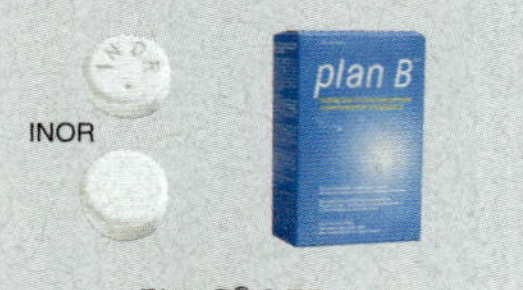

Plan B® 0.75 mg
Paladin

C — DIN 02244291 *
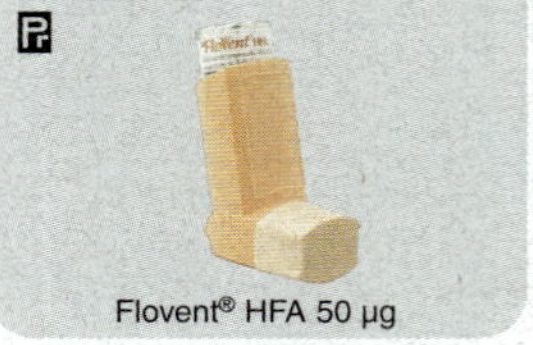
Flovent® HFA 50 µg
GlaxoSmithKline

D — DIN 02285606 *
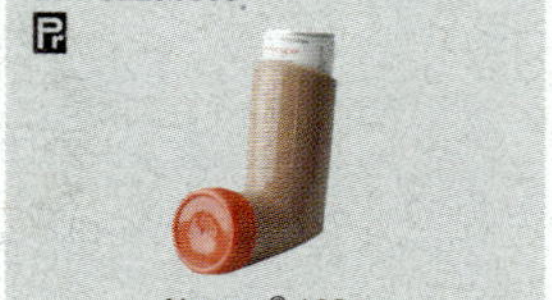
Alvesco® 100 µg
Nycomed

E — DIN 02285614 *
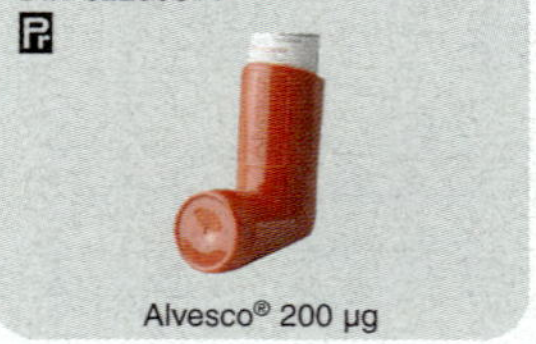
Alvesco® 200 µg
Nycomed

6

A — DIN 02245126 *
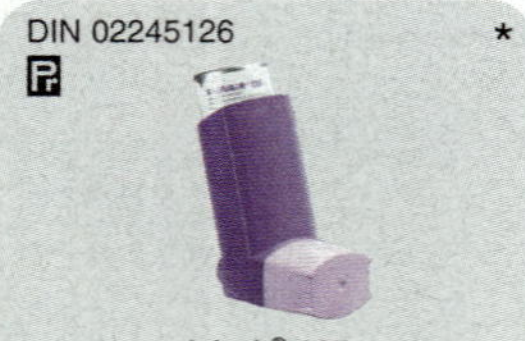
Advair® 125
GlaxoSmithKline

B — DIN 02244292 *
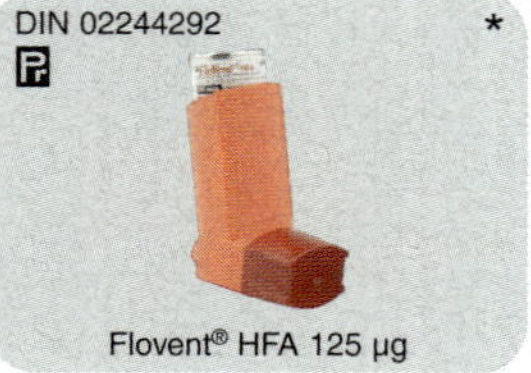
Flovent® HFA 125 µg
GlaxoSmithKline

C — DIN 02244293 *
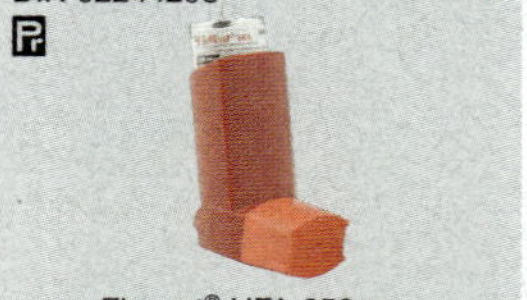
Flovent® HFA 250 µg
GlaxoSmithKline

D — DIN 02242029 *
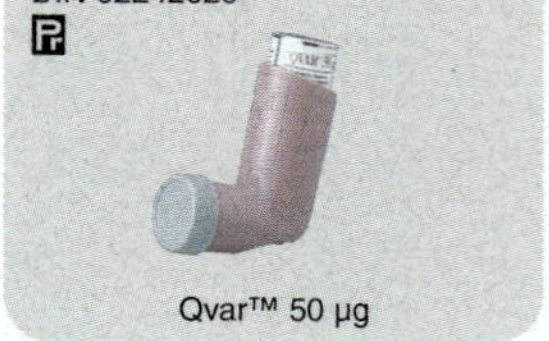
Qvar™ 50 µg
Graceway

E — DIN 02242030 *
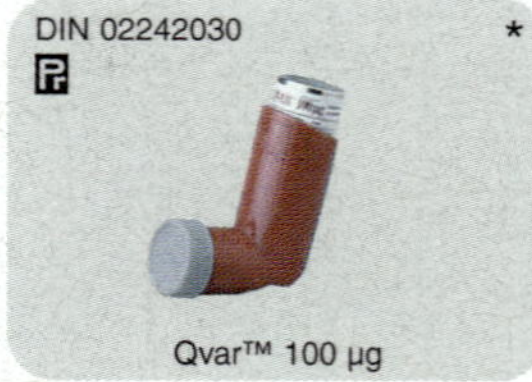
Qvar™ 100 µg
Graceway

7

A — DIN 02245127 *
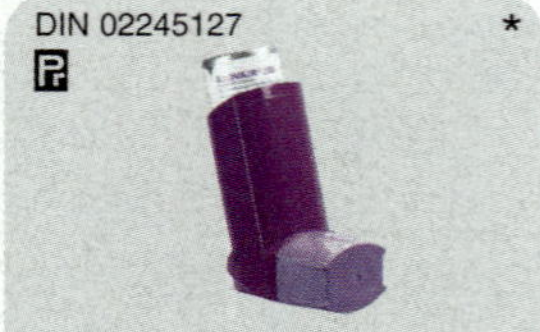
Advair® 250
GlaxoSmithKline

B — DIN 02247686 *
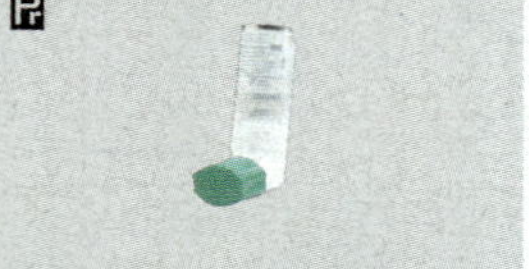
Atrovent® HFA 20 µg
Boehringer Ingelheim

C — DIN 02241497 *
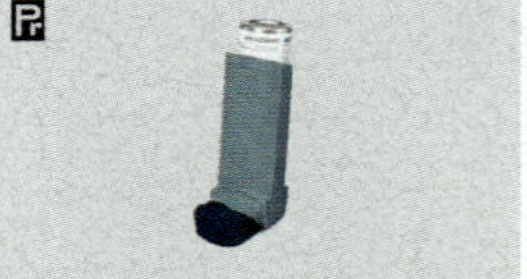
Ventolin® HFA 100 µg
GlaxoSmithKline

D — DIN 02214261 *
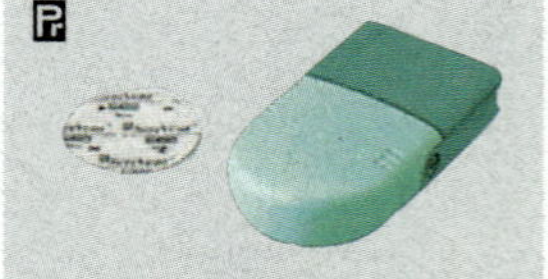
Serevent® Diskhaler®
GlaxoSmithKline

E — DIN 02240863 *
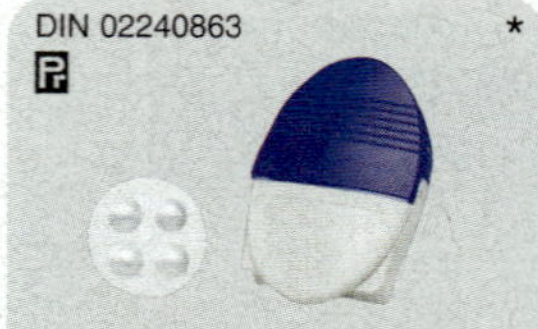
Relenza® Rotadisk 5 mg
GlaxoSmithKline

8

A — DIN 02237246 *
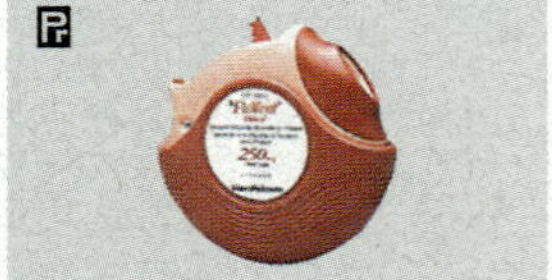
Flovent® Diskus® 250 µg
GlaxoSmithKline

B — DIN 02231129 *
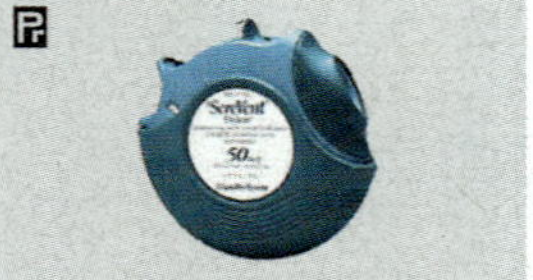
Serevent® Diskus® 50 µg
GlaxoSmithKline

C — DIN 02240835 *
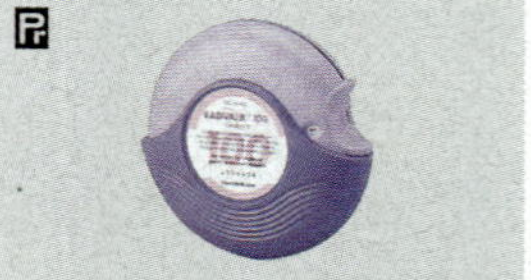
Advair® Diskus® 100 µg
GlaxoSmithKline

D — DIN 02240836 *
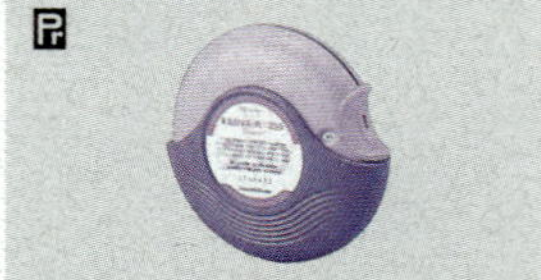
Advair® Diskus® 250 µg
GlaxoSmithKline

E — DIN 02240837 *
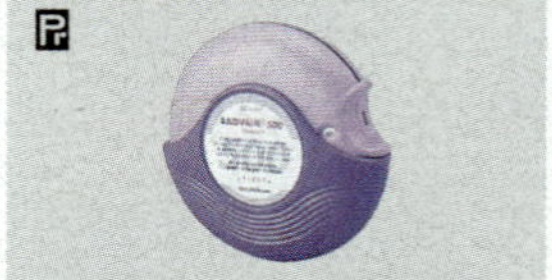
Advair® Diskus® 500 µg
GlaxoSmithKline

* ILLUSTRATION LESS THAN ACTUAL SIZE / ILLUSTRATION RÉDUITE

Use code A, B, C, D, E, horizontal bar and 1 to 8 vertical bar to locate illustrated products

Utiliser le code A, B, C, D, E de la ligne horizontale et les chiffres 1 à 8 de la ligne verticale pour repérer les produits illustrés

1

A1 — DIN 02237225 *
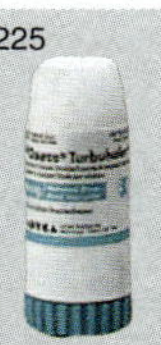
Oxeze® Turbuhaler® 6 µg
AstraZeneca

B1 — DIN 02237224 *
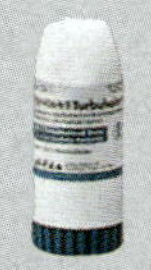
Oxeze® Turbuhaler® 12 µg
AstraZeneca

C1 — DIN 02035324 *
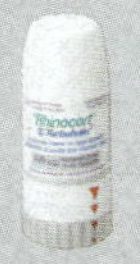
Rhinocort® Turbuhaler® 100 µg
AstraZeneca

D1 — DIN 02245385 *
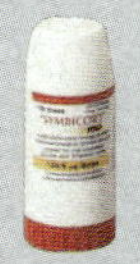
Symbicort® Turbuhaler® 100 µg
AstraZeneca

E1 — DIN 02245386 *
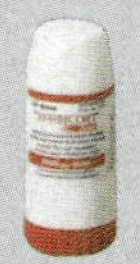
Symbicort® Turbuhaler® 200 µg
AstraZeneca

2

A2 — DIN 00852074 *
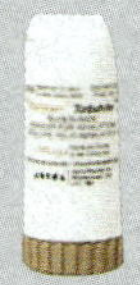
Pulmicort® Turbuhaler® 100 µg
AstraZeneca

B2 — DIN 00851752 *
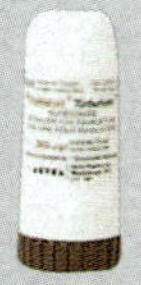
Pulmicort® Turbuhaler® 200 µg
AstraZeneca

C2 — DIN 00851760 *
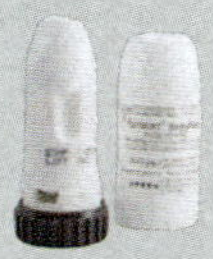
Pulmicort® Turbuhaler® 400 µg
AstraZeneca

D2 — DIN 00786616 *
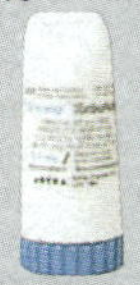
Bricanyl® Turbuhaler® 0.5 mg
AstraZeneca

E2 — DIN 02230898 *
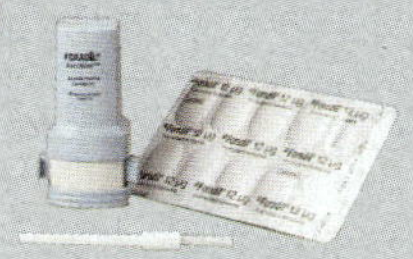
Foradil® 12 µg
Novartis Pharmaceuticals

3

A3 — DIN 02229099 *
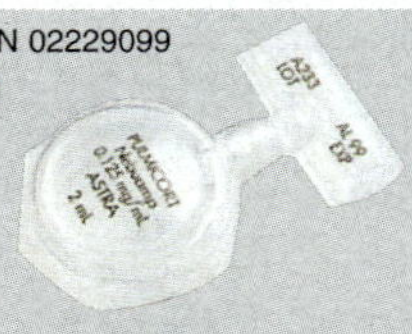
Pulmicort® Nebuamp® 0.125 mg/mL
AstraZeneca

B3 — DIN 01978918 *
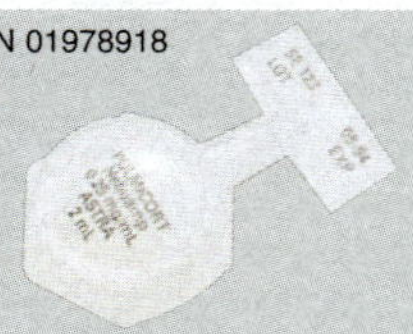
Pulmicort® Nebuamp® 0.25 mg/mL
AstraZeneca

C3 — DIN 01978926 *
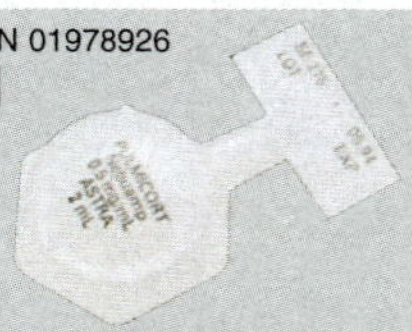
Pulmicort® Nebuamp® 0.5 mg/mL
AstraZeneca

D3 — DIN 02246793 *
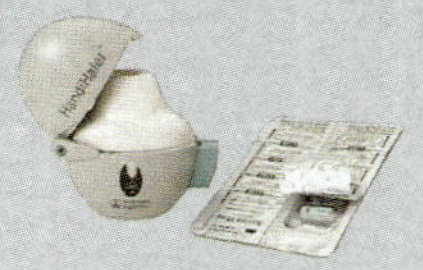
Spiriva® 18 µg
Boehringer Ingelheim

E3 — DIN 02239630 *
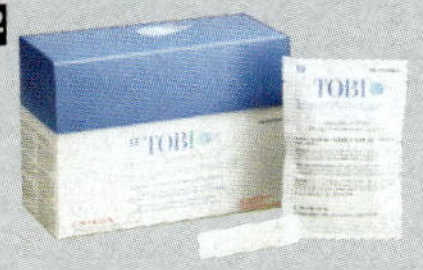
TOBI® Inhalation Solution
Novartis Pharmaceuticals

4

A4 — DIN 02237544 *
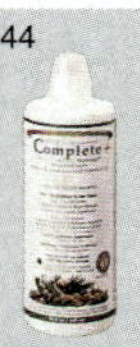
Daily Complete™
Awareness Corporation

B4 — NPN 80004785 *
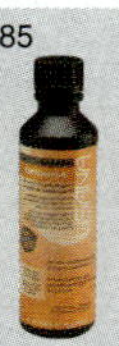
Optomega
USANA Health Sciences

C4 — DIN 02245240 *
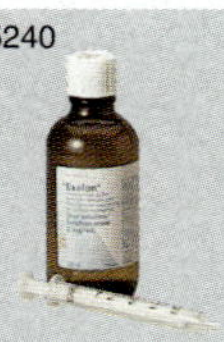
Exelon® 2 mg/mL
Novartis Pharmaceuticals

D4 — DIN 02150697 *
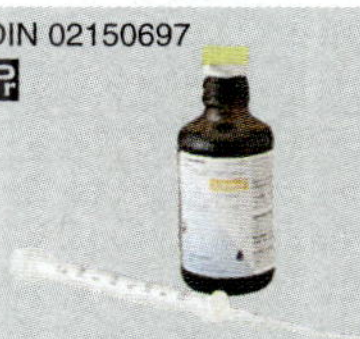
Neoral® 100 mg
Novartis Pharmaceuticals

E4 — DIN 02247997
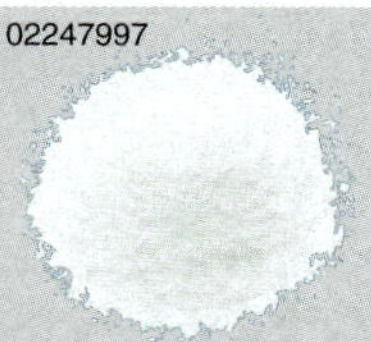
Singulair® 4 mg
Merck Frosst

5

A5–6 — DIN 02236950 *
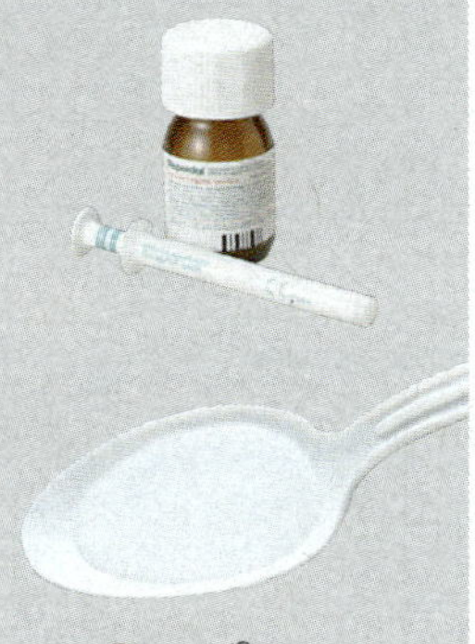
Risperdal® 1 mg
Janssen-Ortho

B5 — DIN 02238831
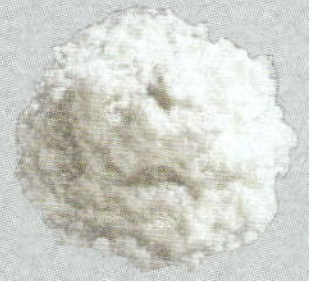
Clavulin®-200
GlaxoSmithKline

C5 — DIN 02238830
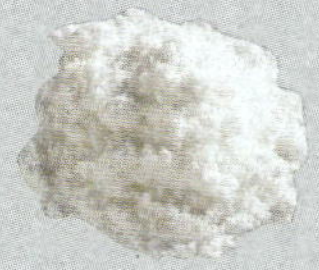
Clavulin®-400
GlaxoSmithKline

D5 — DIN 02212307
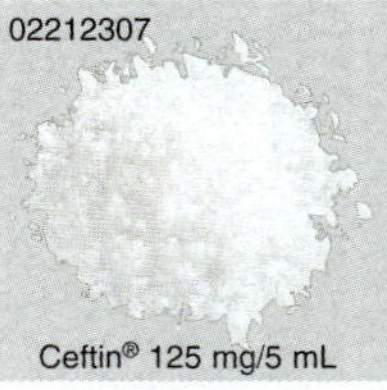
Ceftin® 125 mg/5 mL
GlaxoSmithKline

E5 — DIN 02300524
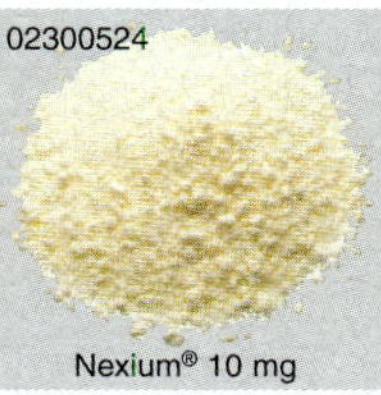
Nexium® 10 mg
AstraZeneca

6

B6 — DIN 02192691

3TC® 10 mg/mL
ViiV Healthcare ULC

C6 — DIN 02229639

Zofran® 4 mg/5 mL
GlaxoSmithKline

D6 — DIN 02240358
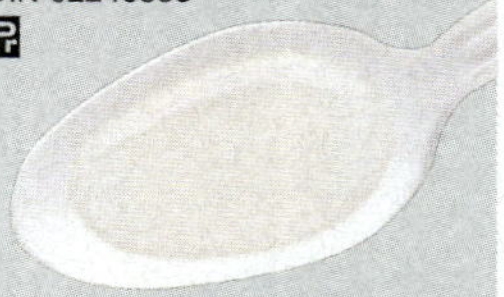
Ziagen® 20 mg
ViiV Healthcare ULC

E6 — DIN 02244673
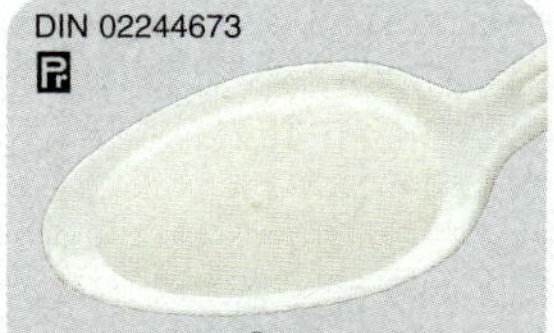
Trileptal® 60 mg/mL
Novartis Pharmaceuticals

7

A7–8 — DIN 02231347 *
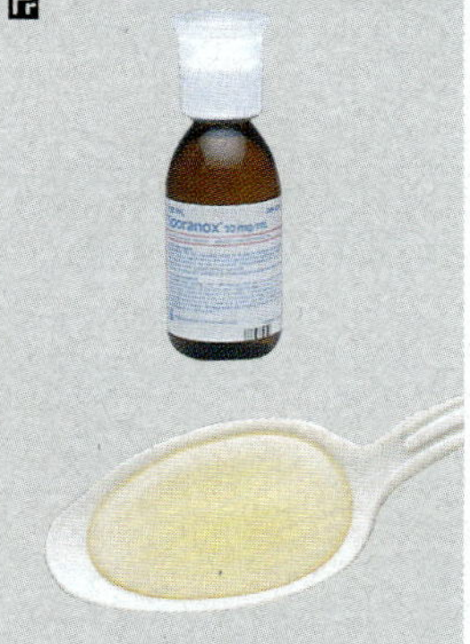
Sporanox® 10 mg
Janssen-Ortho

B7–8 — DIN 02163942 Ⓝ *
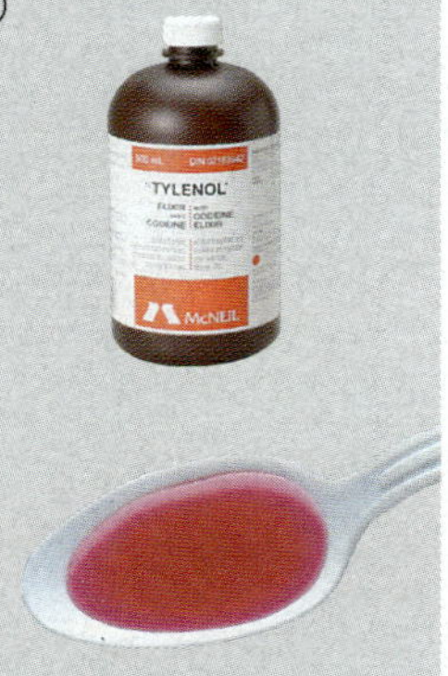
Tylenol® with Codeine
Janssen-Ortho/McNeil Consumer Healthcare

C7 — DIN 02212374

Zantac® 15 mg/mL
GlaxoSmithKline

D7 — DIN 02217422
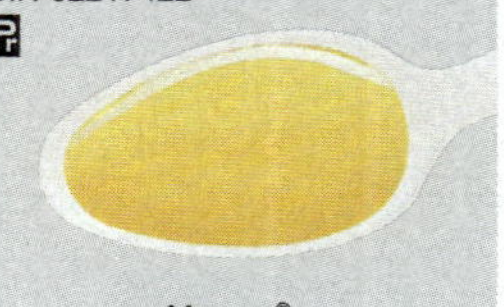
Mepron®
GlaxoSmithKline

E7 — DIN 02194333
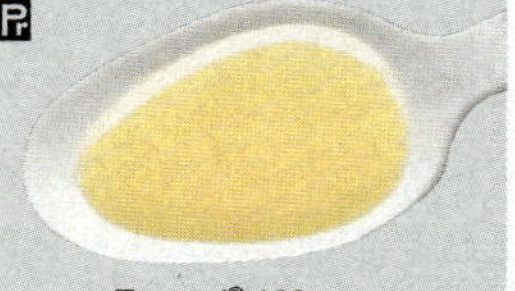
Tegretol® 100 mg
Novartis Pharmaceuticals

8

C8 — DIN 01916564 Ⓝ
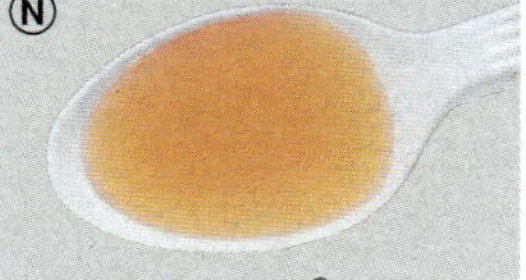
Hycomine®
Bristol-Myers Squibb

D8 — DIN 01916580 Ⓝ
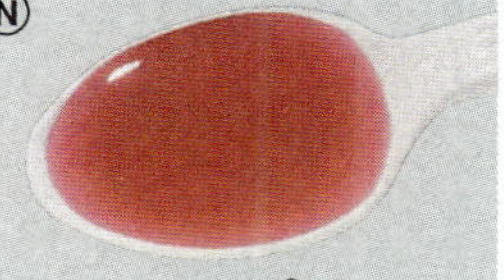
Hycodan®
Bristol-Myers Squibb

E8 — DIN 01916521 Ⓝ
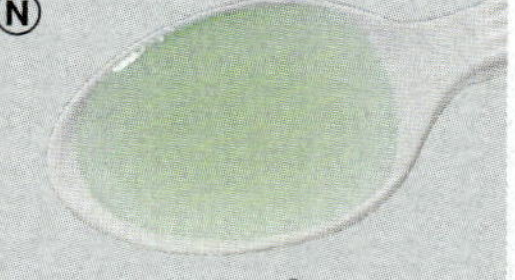
Hycomine®-S
Bristol-Myers Squibb

* ILLUSTRATION LESS THAN ACTUAL SIZE / ILLUSTRATION RÉDUITE

Use code A, B, C, D, E, horizontal bar and 1 to 8 vertical bar to locate illustrated products

Utiliser le code A, B, C, D, E de la ligne horizontale et les chiffres 1 à 8 de la ligne verticale pour repérer les produits illustrés

	A	B	C	D	E
1	DIN 02223716 * 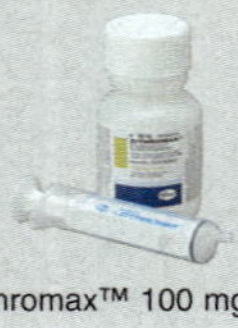 Zithromax™ 100 mg/5 mL **Pfizer**	DIN 02223724 * 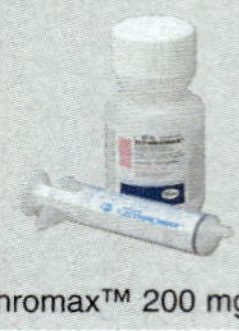 Zithromax™ 200 mg/5 mL **Pfizer**	DIN 02024152 * 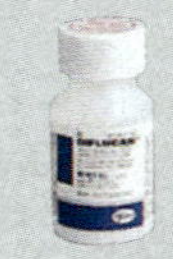 Diflucan™ **Pfizer**	* 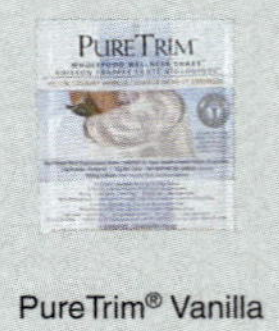 PureTrim® Vanilla **Awareness Corporation**	* 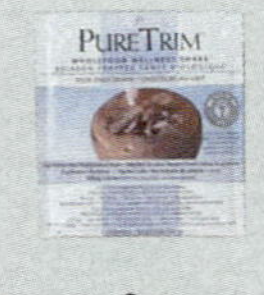 PureTrim® Chocolate **Awareness Corporation**
2	DIN 00756849 * 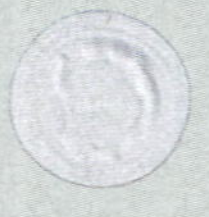 Estraderm® 25 µg **Novartis Pharmaceuticals**	DIN 00756792 * 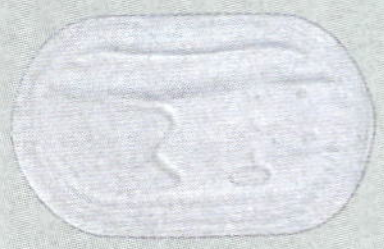 Estraderm® 100 µg **Novartis Pharmaceuticals**	DIN 02230732 * 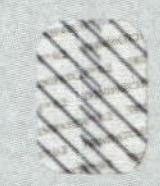 Trinipatch™ 0.2 mg/hour **Paladin**	DIN 02230733 * 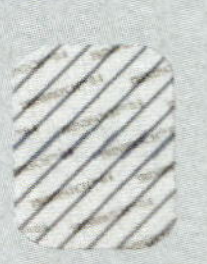 Trinipatch™ 0.4 mg/hour **Paladin**	DIN 02230734 * 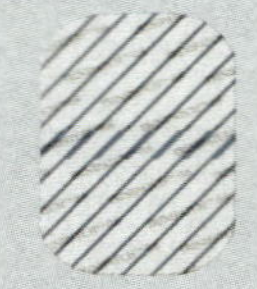 Trinipatch™ 0.6 mg/hour **Paladin**
3	DIN 02245676 *  Estradot® 25 µg **Novartis Pharmaceuticals**	DIN 02243999 * 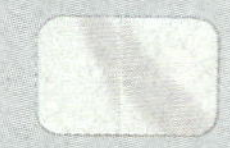 Estradot® 37.5 µg **Novartis Pharmaceuticals**	DIN 02244000 * 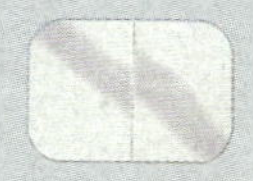 Estradot® 50 µg **Novartis Pharmaceuticals**	DIN 02244001 * 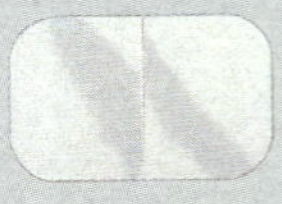 Estradot® 75 µg **Novartis Pharmaceuticals**	DIN 02244002 *  Estradot® 100 µg **Novartis Pharmaceuticals**
4	DIN 02302845 * 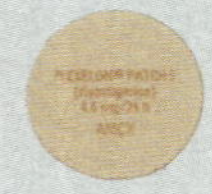 Exelon® Patch 5 **Novartis Pharmaceuticals**	DIN 02302853 * 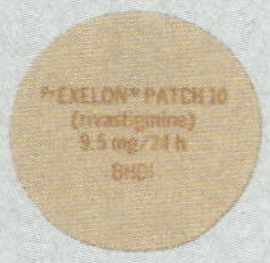 Exelon® Patch 10 **Novartis Pharmaceuticals**	DIN 00584223 * 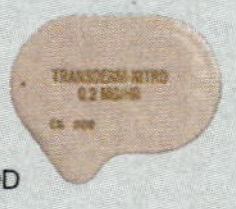 CG DOD Transderm-Nitro® 0.2 mg/hour **Novartis Pharmaceuticals**	DIN 00852384 * 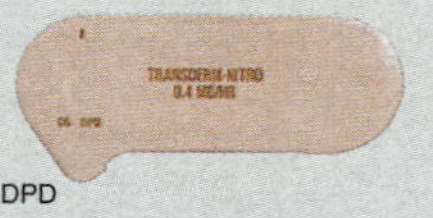 CG DPD Transderm-Nitro® 0.4 mg/hour **Novartis Pharmaceuticals**	DIN 02046156 * 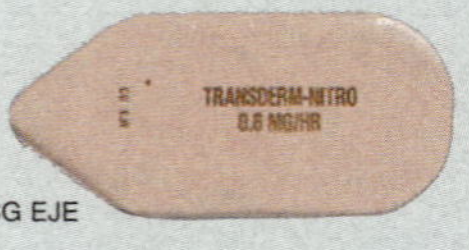 CG EJE Transderm-Nitro® 0.6 mg/hour **Novartis Pharmaceuticals**
5	DIN 02241835 * 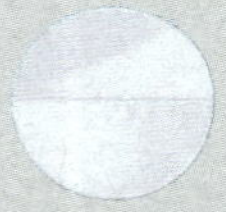 Estalis® 140/50 µg **Novartis Pharmaceuticals**	DIN 02241837 * 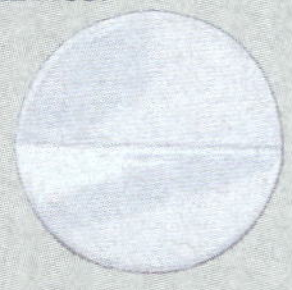 Estalis® 250/50 µg **Novartis Pharmaceuticals**	DIN 02231509 * 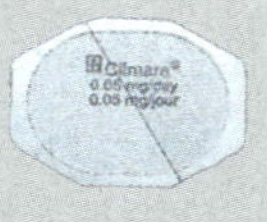 Climara® 50 **Bayer**	DIN 02231510 * 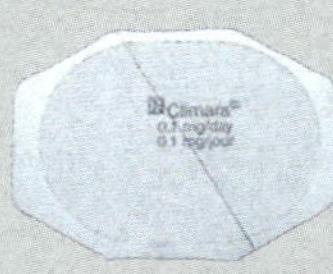 Climara® 100 **Bayer**	DIN 02250616 * 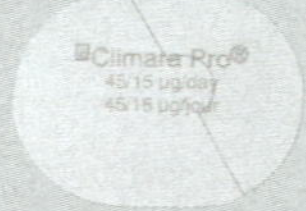 Climara Pro® 45/15 µg **Bayer**
6	DIN 01911910 * 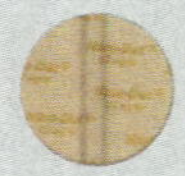 Nitro-Dur® 0.2 mg/h **Schering-Plough**	DIN 01911902 * 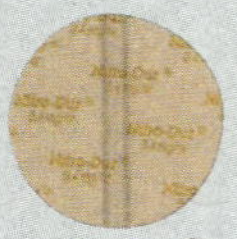 Nitro-Dur® 0.4 mg/h **Schering-Plough**	DIN 01911929 * 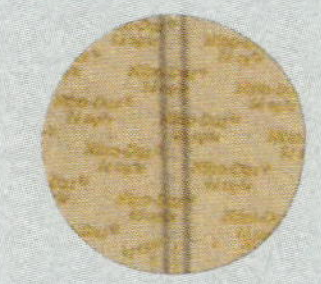 Nitro-Dur® 0.6 mg/h **Schering-Plough**	DIN 02011271 * 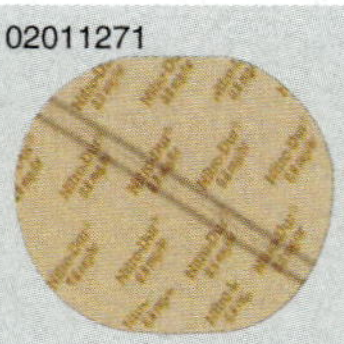 Nitro-Dur® 0.8 mg/h **Schering-Plough**	DIN 02057794 * 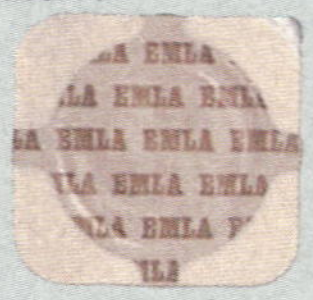 EMLA® **AstraZeneca**
7	DIN 02248297 * 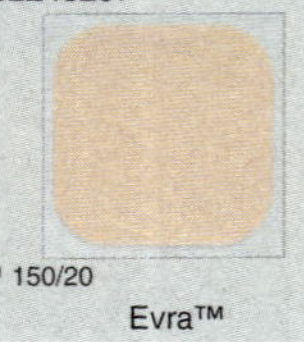 EVRA™ 150/20 Evra™ **Janssen-Ortho**	DIN 02275813 * 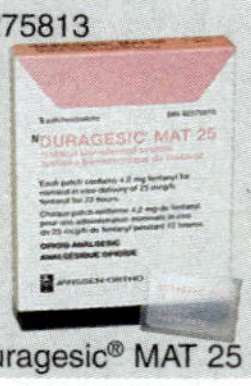 Duragesic® MAT 25 µg **Janssen-Ortho**	DIN 02275821 * 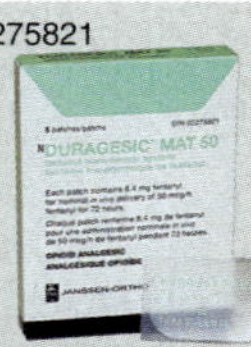 Duragesic® MAT 50 µg **Janssen-Ortho**	DIN 02275848 * 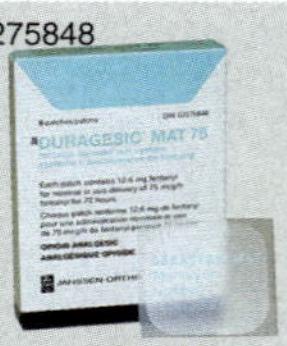 Duragesic® MAT 75 µg **Janssen-Ortho**	DIN 02275856 * 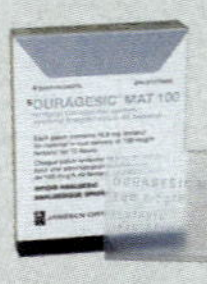 Duragesic® MAT 100 µg **Janssen-Ortho**
8	DIN 02341174 * 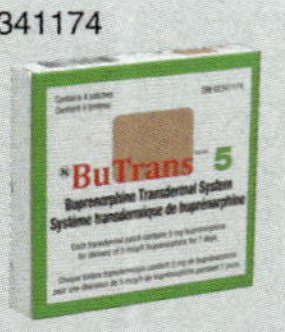 BuTrans® 5 mg **Purdue Pharma**	DIN 02341212 * 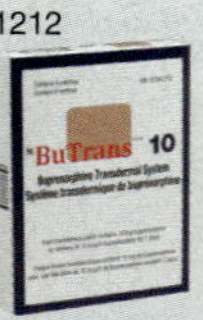 BuTrans® 10 mg **Purdue Pharma**	DIN 02341220 * 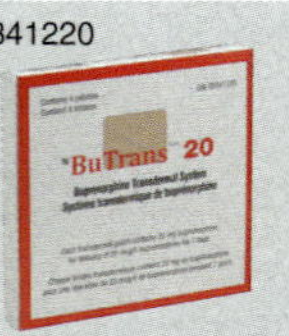 BuTrans® 20 mg **Purdue Pharma**		

* ILLUSTRATION LESS THAN ACTUAL SIZE / ILLUSTRATION RÉDUITE

Clin-Info

About Clin-Info

The Clin-Info section provides quick-reference clinical information and practice tools to assist health care professionals in the safe and effective use of drugs. It is reviewed annually. Although the information is not intended to be all inclusive, the editors, contributors and publisher have tried to ensure its accuracy at the time of publication. Readers should be aware that the text may contain information different from that approved by the Health Products and Food Branch, Health Canada, and that the pharmaceutical manufacturers' approval has not been sought for such information.

Drug therapy is constantly changing; consequently, it is the responsibility of the health care professional to seek additional and confirmatory information, to evaluate its appropriateness as it relates to the actual clinical situation, and to consider new developments.

Online Updates

Updates to Clin-Info content after the print deadline are published in e-cps, CPhA's online *CPS*. The e-CPS provides health care professionals with online access to the most current Canadian drug information available. It also includes links to Health Canada advisories, printable information for patients, searchable product images, an intuitive interface and time-saving features. e-CPS is updated bi-weekly. For more information or to subscribe to e-CPS, visit www.pharmacists.ca/e-CPS.

Table of Contents

Calculations and Dosing Tools

Body Surface Area (BSA):[1]

$$\text{BSA (m}^2) = \left[\frac{\text{height (cm)} \times \text{weight (kg)}}{3600}\right]^{0.5}$$

Body Surface Area in Infants, Children or Adults:[2]

$$\text{BSA (m}^2) = \text{weight (kg)}^{0.5378} \times \text{height (cm)}^{0.3964} \times 0.024265$$

Ideal Body Weight (IBW):

IBW (kg, males) = 50 kg + 2.3 × (height in inches – 60)
IBW (kg, females) = 45.5 kg + 2.3 × (height in inches – 60)

Adjusted Body Weight (ABW):

ABW (kg) = IBW (kg) + 0.4 × (total body weight in kg – IBW)

ABW has been recommended for dosing aminoglycosides in obese individuals (i.e., if total body weight is >25% above the IBW)[3,4]

Creatinine Clearance (ClCr):

Estimate using the Cockcroft-Gault equation:

$$\text{ClCr (mL/min)} = \frac{1.2\ (140 - \text{age})\ (\text{weight in kg})}{\text{Serum creatinine } (\mu\text{mol/L})}$$

For females, multiply result by 0.85.

References
1. Mosteller RD. Simplified calculation of body surface area. *N Engl J Med* 1987;317(17):1098.
2. Haycock GB, Schwartz GJ, Wisotsky DH. Geometric method for measuring body surface area: a height-weight formula validated in infants, children, and adults. *J Pediatr* 1978;93(1):62-6.
3. Green B, Duffull SB. What is the best size descriptor to use for pharmacokinetic studies in the obese? *Br J Clin Pharmacol* 2004;58(2):119-33.
4. Traynor AM, Nafziger AN, Bertino JS. Aminoglycoside dosing weight correction factors for patients of various body sizes. *Antimicrob Agents Chemother* 1995;39(2):545-8.

Laboratory Reference Intervals: SI and Traditional Units

M.J. McQueen, MB, ChB, PhD, FCACB, FRCPC

Date of Revision: August 2010

Table 1 provides a summary of selected adult clinical laboratory reference intervals. For serum drug concentration levels and conversion factors see the Serum Drug Concentration Monitoring section in Clin-Info. This information is not intended to present a comprehensive review; the reader is therefore encouraged to seek additional and confirmatory information. **Reference intervals will vary depending on the analytical methods used and the population studied. Each laboratory establishes its own reference intervals.**

Table 1: Adult Laboratory Intervals

	Reference Intervals		
Laboratory Test	SI Reference	Traditional Reference	Conversion Factor[a]
Alanine aminotransferase (ALT) (serum)[b]	0–585 nkat/L	0–35 U/L	16.67
Albumin (serum)	40–60 g/L	4–6 g/dL	10
Alkaline phosphatase (serum)[c]	500–2000 nkat/L	30–120 U/L	16.67
Ammonia, as ammonium ion (NH_4^+) (plasma)	5–50 µmol/L	10–85 µg/dL	0.5543
Aspartate aminotransferase (AST) (serum)[b]	0–585 nkat/L	0–35 U/L	16.67
Bilirubin (serum)			
total	2–18 µmol/L	0.1–1 mg/dL	17.1
conjugated	0–4 µmol/L	0–0.2 mg/dL	17.1
Calcium (serum)			
male	2.2–2.58 mmol/L	8.8–10.3 mg/dL	0.2495
female <50 years	2.2–2.5 mmol/L	8.8–10 mg/dL	0.2495
female >50 years	2.2–2.56 mmol/L	8.8–10.2 mg/dL	0.2495
all populations	2.2–2.56 mmol/L	4.4–5.1 mEq/L	0.5
Calcium, ionized (serum)	1–1.15 mmol/L	2–2.3 mEq/L	0.5
Carbon dioxide			
(bicarbonate + CO_2)			
(blood, plasma, serum)	22–28 mmol/L	22–28 mEq/L	1
Chloride (serum)	95–105 mmol/L	95–105 mEq/L	1
Cholesterol (serum)			
low risk populations	<5.2 mmol/L	<200 mg/dL	0.02586
moderate and high risk populations	<4.2 mmol/L	<162 mg/dL	0.02586
Cortisol (serum)			
0800 h	110–520 nmol/L	4–19 µg/dL	27.59
1600 h	50–410 nmol/L	2–15 µg/dL	27.59
2400 h	<140 nmol/L	<5 µg/dL	27.59
Cortisol (urine)	30–300 nmol/day	10–110 µg/24 h	2.759
Creatinine (serum)	50–110 µmol/L	0.6–1.2 mg/dL	88.4
Creatinine clearance	1.24–2.08 mL/s	75–125 mL/min	0.01667
C-Reactive Protein	0.68–82 mg/L	6.8–820 µg/dL	100
Delta (5)-aminolevulinic acid (urine)	8–53 µmol/day	1–7 mg/24 h	7.626
Ethanol (plasma)			
legal limit (driving)[d]	<10.86 mmol/L	<50 mg/dL	0.2171
toxic	>22 mmol/L	>100 mg/dL	0.2171
Ferritin (serum)	18–300 µg/L	18–300 ng/mL	1
Fibrinogen (plasma)	1.5–3.5 g/L	150–350 mg/dL	0.01
Folate, as folic acid, pteroylglutamic acid (serum)	4–22 nmol/L	2–10 ng/mL	2.266
Gammaglutamyltransferase (GGT) (serum)[b]	0–500 nkat/L	0–30 U/L	16.67

(cont'd)

Table 1: Adult Laboratory Intervals *(cont'd)*

Laboratory Test	Reference Intervals		Conversion Factor[a]
	SI Reference	Traditional Reference	
Gases (arterial blood)			
pO_2	10–13.3 kPa	75–100 mmHg	0.1333
pCO_2	4.7–6 kPa	35–45 mmHg	0.1333
Glucose, fasting (plasma)	3.9–6.1 mmol/L	70–110 mg/dL	0.05551
Glucose (CSF)	2.8–4.4 mmol/L	50–80 mg/dL	0.05551
Hematocrit			
male	0.39–0.49	39–49%	
female	0.33–0.43	33–43%	
Hemoglobin (blood)			
male	140–180 g/L	14–18 g/dL	10
female	115–155 g/L	11.5–15.5 g/dL	10
Hemoglobin A_{1c}	0.038–0.064	3.8–6.4%	0.01
Insulin, fasting (plasma, serum)	35–145 pmol/L	5–20 µU/mL	7.175
Iron (serum)			
male	14–32 µmol/L	80–180 µg/dL	0.1791
female	11–29 µmol/L	60–160 µg/dL	0.1791
Iron binding capacity (serum)	45–82 µmol/L	250–460 µg/dL	0.1791
Lipoproteins, high density (HDL) cholesterol (serum)	>1.3 mmol/L	>50 mg/dL	0.02586
Lipoproteins, low density (LDL) cholesterol (serum)			
low risk populations	<3.2 mmol/L	<125 mg/dL	0.02586
moderate and high risk populations	<2.0 mmol/L	<77 mg/dL	0.02586
Magnesium (serum)	0.8–1.2 mmol/L	1.8–3 mg/dL	0.4114
	0.8–1.2 mmol/L	1.6–2.4 mEq/L	0.5
Mean corpuscular volume (MCV) (blood)	76–100 fL	76–100 µm³	1
Mean corpuscular hemoglobin concentration (MCHC) (blood)	330–370 g/L	33–37 g/dL	10
Mean corpuscular hemoglobin (MCH) (blood)	27–33 pg	27–33 pg	1
Methanol (plasma)	0 mmol/L	0 mg/dL	0.3121
Osmolality (plasma)	280–300 mmol/kg	280–300 mOsm/kg	1
Osmolality (urine)	50–1200 mmol/kg	50–1200 mOsm/kg	1
Phosphate, as inorganic phosphorus (serum)	0.8–1.6 mmol/L	2.5–5 mg/dL	0.3229
Platelet count (blood)	130–400 × 10^9/L	130 000–400 000/mm³	0.001
Porphobilinogen (urine)	0–8.8 µmol/day	0–2 mg/24 h	4.42
Potassium (serum)	3.5–5 mmol/L	3.5–5 mEq/L	1
Red cell count, erythrocytes (Ercs)			
male	4.3–5.9 × 10^{12}/L	4.3–5.9 × 10^6/mm³	1 × 10^6
female	3.5–5 × 10^{12}/L	3.5–5 × 10^6/mm³	1 × 10^6
Reticulocyte count (blood)	10–75 × 10^9/L	10 000–75 000/mm³	0.001
Sodium (serum)	135–147 mmol/L	135–147 mEq/L	1
Thyroid tests (serum)			
Free thyroxine (free T_4)	10–36 pmol/L	0.8–2.8 ng/dL	12.87
Total serum thyroxine (T_4)	51–142 nmol/L	4–11 µg/dL	12.87
Total serum triiodothyroxine (T_3)	1.2–3.0 nmol/L	78–195 ng/dL	0.015
TSH	0.3–5.0 mU/L	0.3–5.0 µU/mL	1
Triglycerides	<1.70 mmol/L	<150 mg/dL	0.01129
Troponin T	0–0.1 µg/L	0–0.1 ng/mL	1

(cont'd)

Table 1: Adult Laboratory Intervals *(cont'd)*

Laboratory Test	Reference Intervals		Conversion Factor[a]
	SI Reference	Traditional Reference	
Urate, as uric acid (serum)[b]	120–420 µmol/L	2–7 mg/dL	59.48
Urea (serum)	3–6.5 mmol/L	8–18 mg/dL	0.357
Vitamin B_{12} (plasma, serum)	150–750 pmol/L	200–1000 pg/mL	0.7378
White cell count, WBC (blood)	3.2–9.8 × 10^9/L	3200–9800/mm^3	0.001
Zinc (serum)	11.5–18.5 µmol/L	75–120 µg/dL	0.153

[a] To convert from traditional to SI units, multiply the traditional value by the conversion factor. To convert from SI to traditional units, divide the SI value by the conversion factor.
[b] Male and female reference intervals should be established for the method in use by the laboratory.
[c] There is a wide range of alkaline phosphatase activities which are dependent on gender, age and laboratory method.
[d] Varies in different jurisdictions and may also be lower according to the age and experience of the driver.

References

1. Health and Welfare Canada. *SI manual in health care.* 3rd rev. ed. Ottawa (ON): Health Canada; 1986.
2. Kratz A, Lewandrowski KB. Case records of the Massachusetts General Hospital. Weekly clinicopathological exercises. Normal reference laboratory values. *N Engl J Med* 1998;339(15):1063-72.
3. Traub SL, editor. *Basic skills in interpreting laboratory data.* 2nd ed. Bethesda (MD): American Society of Health-System Pharmacists; 1996.

Serum Drug Concentration Monitoring

B. Hardy, PharmD, FCSHP, FCCP

Date of Revision: August 2010

The following is an overview of serum drug concentration monitoring. This information is not intended to present a comprehensive review; the reader is therefore encouraged to seek additional and confirmatory information. Individual patient management requires clinical judgment in the interpretation of the serum drug concentration. Therapeutic ranges vary widely according to drug assay methods and specific laboratory references.

Serum drug concentration monitoring (SDCM), also known as therapeutic drug monitoring, pharmacokinetic monitoring or clinical pharmacokinetics, is applying information from serum drug concentration data in light of the patient's clinical status, to optimize drug therapy.[1]

Collaboration of the hospital laboratory, physicians, nurses, iv technicians and pharmacists is essential for a successful SDCM service.

Uses of SDCM

- Determine or adjust a dosage regimen
- Evaluate a drug response
- Aid in the assessment of toxicity
- Check compliance
- Decrease the risk associated with medical-legal problems

If the serum drug concentration is to be fully utilized, results must be interpreted in light of the complete clinical situation. The clinician must be aware of patient-specific factors that affect the drug's disposition. Patient's age, diet, smoking habits, concurrent drugs, metabolic/excretory ability and changing disease states are some of the variables to consider in association with the serum drug concentration.[1]

The Modified Cockcroft and Gault equation[2] is a commonly used formula to estimate **creatinine clearance** (ClCr) using a stable serum creatinine level and patient demographics (e.g., age, gender).

$$\text{ClCr (mL/min)} = \frac{1.2\,(140-\text{age})\,(\text{weight in kg})}{\text{Serum creatinine } (\mu\text{mol/L})}$$

For females, multiply the result by 0.85.

Modification of creatinine clearance estimates may be required in some patients. The accuracy of using the serum creatinine value to predict creatinine clearance is influenced by diseases (e.g., cirrhosis), clinical conditions (e.g., malnutrition, obesity, spinal cord injuries) and dietary intake (e.g., high consumption of meat).

Which drugs are most appropriate for SDCM? (Table 1)

There are a number of characteristics common to drugs that are routinely monitored using serum concentrations:[1]

- Narrow therapeutic index
- Significant consequences associated with therapeutic failure or toxicity
- Wide interpatient pharmacokinetic variability
- Unpredictable dose-response relationship
- Serum drug concentrations available to the prescriber within a reasonable time frame

Table 1 presents information on SDCM for selected drugs. Information is gathered from results in average adult individuals for the most part. A drug's half-life may be prolonged in patients with renal or hepatic disease or may vary due to demographic differences (e.g., age, gender). Steady-state concentrations assume that the dosage has remained the same for four to five half-lives and that doses have not been missed.

Table 2 provides factors for conversion of serum drug concentrations between SI and traditional units.

When should drug concentrations be obtained?

Awareness of the sampling time relative to the last dose is critical for the proper interpretation of a drug level. In most cases, the serum sample should be obtained after the absorption and distribution phases are complete (e.g., trough level) and the drug has reached steady state (e.g., after administration of the same fixed dose for four to five half-lives). Levels obtained before a steady state concentration exists may be erroneously low or high; adjusting the dosage based on such a result could produce toxic or subtherapeutic concentrations, respectively.[1] In cases where toxicity is a concern or is suspected, sampling can be undertaken even if steady state has not been reached.

Table 1: Recommendations for Serum Drug Concentration Monitoring for Selected Drugs

Drug	Route	Sampling Time	Drug Concentration	Monitoring Considerations
Acetaminophen	Oral	Overdose: at least 4 h after ingestion.[3] For extended-release preparations, draw 2 levels, the first at 4 h post-ingestion (or as soon as possible thereafter) and the second 4–6 h later.[4]	For interpretation, refer to the Matthew-Rumack nomogram for acute acetaminophen poisoning in the Acetaminophen monograph written by CPhA in the product monograph section of CPS.	Half-life about 2–4 h. Delayed absorption occurs with long-acting formulations. In suspected overdose with these formulations, a second sample is necessary to take into account the delayed release of acetaminophen.
Amikacin	IV	Peak: 30 min after 30-min infusion. Trough: within 15 min prior to next dose.	Peak: 20–30 mg/L. Trough: less than 10 mg/L. For once daily amikacin, peaks of ≥40 mg/L have been suggested.[5]	Dosage should be stable for at least 3–4 half-lives prior to sampling. Usually obtain peak and trough levels. Half-life about 2–3 h in patients with normal renal function.[6]
	IM	Peak: 1 h after administration. Trough: within 15 min of the next dose.		
Amitriptyline	Oral	Trough: 12 h after the dose. For suspected toxicity, sample anytime.	430–900 nmol/L (parent drug + demethylated metabolite, nortriptyline).	Half-life 9–46 h. Routine monitoring as a therapeutic guideline is not warranted, but may be useful to assess noncompliance, nonresponders, suspected toxicity, drug interactions, elderly patients and children.[7]
Carbamazepine	Oral	Trough: for periodic monitoring, sample just before the next dose. For suspected toxicity, sample anytime.	17–50 µmol/L	Induces its own metabolism for up to 2–4 wk. Half-life with chronic dosing 15–25 h.[8]
Cyclosporine	Oral and iv	Trough: for periodic monitoring, sample just before the next dose. For suspected toxicity, sample anytime. Oral peak: within 2–4 h after the dose.	12 h trough values of 150–400 µg/L in whole blood (monoclonal specific RIA) or 50–125 µg/L in plasma (monoclonal specific RIA).	Half-life 10–27 h. Some institutions recommend a different therapeutic range for a specific transplant population. The ranges listed are intended for the early post-transplant period.[9]
Desipramine	Oral	Trough: 12 h after the dose. For suspected toxicity, sample anytime.	430–675 nmol/L	Half-life 12–28 h. Routine monitoring as a therapeutic guideline is not warranted but may be useful to assess noncompliance, nonresponders, suspected toxicity, drug interactions, elderly patients and children.[7]

(cont'd)

Table 1: Recommendations for Serum Drug Concentration Monitoring for Selected Drugs *(cont'd)*

Drug	Route	Sampling Time	Drug Concentration	Monitoring Considerations
Digoxin	Oral and iv	Post-load: at least 6 h after last dose of loading regimen (iv or po). For periodic monitoring, sample just before next dose. For suspected toxicity, sample anytime.	1–2.5 nmol/L	Dosage should be stable for 5–7 days in patients with normal renal function. Half-life 35–40 h. Time to steady state prolonged in patients with decreased renal function. Levels taken within 6 h of dose may be artificially elevated.[10]
Ethosuximide	Oral	Trough: for periodic monitoring, sample just before the next dose. For suspected toxicity, sample anytime.	280–710 µmol/L	Dosage should be stable for 8 days in adults and 5 days in children. Half-life 40–60 h in adults and 26–36 h in children.[11]
Fosphenytoin	Maintenance dose: im and iv	Trough: for periodic monitoring or suspected inadequate dose, sample just before the next dose. For suspected toxicity, sample anytime once conversion of fosphenytoin to phenytoin is complete (see Monitoring Considerations).	40–80 µmol/L phenytoin or 4–8 µmol/L free (unbound) phenytoin.	Dosage strength of fosphenytoin is expressed in terms of phenytoin equivalents. After absorption, phenytoin is cleaved enzymatically from the prodrug fosphenytoin. Phenytoin concentrations should not be measured until conversion of fosphenytoin to phenytoin is complete (i.e., 2 h after end of iv infusion and 4 h after im injection).[12]
	IM or iv loading dose (iv route preferred)	2 h after end of iv infusion; 4 h after im injection (see Monitoring Considerations).		
Gentamicin	IV	Peak: 15 min after 1-h infusion; 30 min after 30-min infusion. Trough: within 5 min of the next dose.	Peak: 5–10 mg/L. For serious gram-negative infections, 10–12 mg/L. Trough: less than 2 mg/L. For once daily gentamicin, peaks ≥20 mg/L have been suggested.[13]	Dosage should be stable for at least 3–4 half-lives prior to sampling. Usually obtain peak and trough levels. Half-life about 2 h in adults with normal renal function.[6]
	IM	Peak: 1 h after administration. Trough: within 5 min of the next dose.		
Imipramine	Oral	Trough: 12 h after the dose. For suspected toxicity, sample anytime.	550–1015 nmol/L (parent drug + demethylated metabolite, desipramine).	Half-life 6–28 h. Routine monitoring as a therapeutic guideline is not warranted but may be useful to assess noncompliance, nonresponders, suspected toxicity, drug interactions, elderly patients and children.[7]
Lithium	Oral	12 h after the last dose. For suspected toxicity, sample anytime.	0.8–1.2 mmol/L for acute therapy. 0.6–0.8 mmol/L for maintenance. 0.4–0.6 mmol/L for maintenance in the elderly.	Dosage should be stable for at least 3 days before a 12 h standard level is obtained. Half-life 18–27 h, varies with renal function.[14]
Nortriptyline	Oral	Trough: 12 h after the dose. For suspected toxicity, sample anytime.	170–495 nmol/L	Half-life 18–56 h. Routine monitoring as a therapeutic guideline is not warranted but may be useful to assess noncompliance, nonresponders, suspected toxicity, drug interactions, elderly patients and children.[7]
Phenobarbital	Oral, iv, im	For periodic monitoring, sample just before the dose. For suspected toxicity, sample anytime.	65–170 µmol/L	Time to steady state about 10–25 days in adults, 8–15 days in children. Half-life 75–126 h in adults, 37–73 h in children.[15]
Phenytoin	Maintenance dose: oral and iv	Trough: for periodic monitoring or suspected inadequate dose, sample just before the next dose. For suspected toxicity, sample anytime.	40–80 µmol/L phenytoin or 4–8 µmol/L free (unbound) phenytoin (adults, children, infants >3 mo). 25–55 µmol/L phenytoin (pre-term and term neonates 2 wk–3 mo).	Time to steady state is highly variable, 1–8 wk. Phenytoin kinetics are nonlinear and saturable, resulting in highly variable concentrations with even minor dosage changes. Free fraction (active) may increase in patients with renal or hepatic failure and/or hypoalbuminemia; lower dosages are usually necessary.[16]
	IV loading dose	60 min after end of infusion.		
Primidone	Oral	Trough: for periodic monitoring, sample just before the next dose. For suspected toxicity, sample anytime.	23–55 µmol/L	Time to steady state about 2 days. Half-life 6–18 h. Primidone is metabolized, in part, to phenobarbital.[17]
Procainamide	Oral: regular release	Peak: 2.5 h after the dose. For periodic monitoring or suspected inadequate dose, sample just before the next dose. For suspected toxicity, sample anytime.	17–43 µmol/L. Limited data suggests that plasma concentrations as high as 43–85 µmol/L may be required.	Dosage should be stable for 1–2 days. Half-life 2.4–3.6 h in patients with normal renal function and increases to 6–13 h in patients with reduced renal function.
	Oral: sustained release	Peak: 4 h after the dose. For periodic monitoring or suspected inadequate dose, sample just before the next dose. For suspected toxicity, sample anytime.		
	IV continuous infusion	2 h after the beginning of the maintenance infusion. For suspected toxicity, sample anytime.		
NAPA (n-acetyl-procainamide), active procainamide metabolite		For suspected toxicity, sample anytime.	<115 µmol/L (procainamide + NAPA).	Half-life about 6–10 h in patients with normal renal function and increases to 10–40 h in patients with reduced renal function. Routine monitoring for therapeutic efficacy is not warranted; measure in patients with moderate to severe renal impairment to identify those at increased risk for toxicity.[18]
Quinidine	Oral, iv, im	Trough: for periodic monitoring, sample just before the next dose. For suspected toxicity, sample anytime.	6–15 µmol/L	Dosage should be stable for 2 days. Half-life 6–9 h. Levels may be useful to assess compliance or toxicity.[19]
Salicylate	Oral	Peak: 1–2 h after the dose. Trough: sample just before the next dose. Overdose: at least 6 h post-ingestion.	1.1–2.2 mmol/L therapeutic for anti-inflammatory effect. The Done nomogram may be used to assess toxicity in acute overdose.[20]	Half-life is dose-dependent: low doses (e.g., 325 mg ASA), 2–3 h; higher doses (10–20 g), 15–30 h. Time to steady state 5–7 days.[21]

(cont'd)

Table 1: Recommendations for Serum Drug Concentration Monitoring for Selected Drugs *(cont'd)*

Drug	Route	Sampling Time	Drug Concentration	Monitoring Considerations
Tacrolimus	Oral	Trough: sample just before the next dose.	5–20 µg/L (or ng/mL) in whole blood	Range may vary slightly depending on the type of transplantation.[22]
	IV continuous infusion	No recommendations available.		
Theophylline	Oral: sustained release	Peak: twice-daily products—about 4 h after the dose; once-daily products—about 10 h after the dose. Consult individual product monographs. Trough: sample just before the next dose. For suspected toxicity, sample anytime.	55–110 µmol/L. For neonatal apnea, 28–55 µmol/L (higher levels may be tolerated).	Dosage should be stable for 48 h before sampling. Half-life varies greatly. Monitor peak levels to assess suspected toxicity. Trough levels may be monitored to assess efficacy at the end of the dosing interval.[23]
	Liquid and plain uncoated tablets	Peak: 2 h after the tablet dose. 1–2 h after the liquid dose. Trough: sample just before the next dose. For suspected toxicity, sample anytime.		
	IV loading dose	Sample 30 min after an iv loading dose.		
	Followed by iv continuous infusion	Sample 24–48 h after the start of the maintenance infusion. For suspected toxicity, sample anytime.		
Tobramycin	IV	Peak: 15 min after 1-h infusion; 30 min after 30-min infusion. Trough: within 5 min of the next dose.	Peak: 5–10 mg/L. For serious gram-negative infections, 10–12 mg/L. Trough: less than 2 mg/L. For once daily tobramycin, peaks of ≥20 mg/L have been suggested.[13]	Dosage should be stable for at least 3 doses prior to sampling. Usually obtain peak and trough levels. Half-life about 2–2.5 h in patients with normal renal function.[6]
	IM	Peak: 1 h after administration. Trough: within 5 min of the next dose.		
Valproic Acid	Oral and iv	Trough: for periodic monitoring, sample just before the next dose. Peak: 2–3 h after the dose. For suspected toxicity, sample anytime.	350–700 µmol/L	Dosage should be stable for at least 2 days. Half-life 8–19 h. Free fraction (active) may increase in the elderly and in patients with renal or hepatic failure and/or hypoalbuminemia; lower doses are usually necessary.[15]
Vancomycin	IV	Peak: 30 min–2 h after 1-h infusion. Trough: within 5 min of the next dose.	Peak: 25–40 mg/L. Trough: 15–20 mg/L.[24]	Dosage should be stable for 20–30 h. Half-life about 6 h in patients with normal renal function. Usually obtain trough levels. The association of peak and trough concentrations with efficacy and toxicity remains controversial.[25,26]

Table 2: Conversion Factors for Serum Drug Concentrations[27]

Drug	SI Units	Traditional Units	Conversion Factor[a]	Drug	SI Units	Traditional Units	Conversion Factor[a]
Amitriptyline	nmol/L	ng/mL	3.605	Phenytoin	µmol/L	mg/L	3.964
Carbamazepine	µmol/L	mg/L	4.233	Primidone	µmol/L	mg/L	4.582
Desipramine	nmol/L	ng/mL	3.754	Procainamide	µmol/L	mg/L	4.249
Digoxin	nmol/L	ng/mL	1.281	NAPA (n-acetylprocainamide)	µmol/L	mg/L	3.606
Ethosuximide	µmol/L	mg/mL	7.084	Quinidine	µmol/L	mg/L	3.082
Imipramine	nmol/L	ng/mL	3.566	Salicylate	mmol/L	mg/100 mL	0.0724
Lithium	mmol/L	mg/100 mL	1.441	Theophylline	µmol/L	mg/L	5.55
Nortriptyline	nmol/L	ng/mL	3.797	Valproic Acid	µmol/L	mg/L	6.934
Phenobarbital	µmol/L	mg/L	4.306				

[a] To convert from traditional to SI units, multiply the traditional value by the conversion factor. To convert from SI to traditional units, divide the SI value by the conversion factor.

References

1. Hardy B. Therapeutic drug monitoring. In: Cornish P, Knowles S, eds. *Focus on the literature.* Metro Toronto Hospitals Drug Information Service (MetroDIS) 1989;88(3):1-6.
2. Cockcroft DW, Gault MH. Prediction of creatinine clearance from serum creatinine. *Nephron* 1976;16(1):31-41.
3. Rumack BH, Matthew H. Acetaminophen poisoning and toxicity. *Pediatrics* 1975;55(6):871-6.
4. Cetaruk EW, Dart DC, Hurlbut KM et al. Tylenol Extended Relief overdose. *Ann Emerg Med* 1997;30(1):104-8.
5. Beaucaire G, Leroy O, Beuscart C et al. Clinical and bacteriological efficacy, and practical aspects of amikacin given once daily for severe infections. *J Antimicrob Chemother* 1991;27(Suppl C):91-103.
6. Schentag JJ, Meagher AK, Jelliffe RW. Aminoglycosides. In: Burton ME, Shaw LM, Schentag JJ et al., eds. *Applied pharmacokinetics and pharmacodynamics: principles of therapeutic drug monitoring.* 4th ed. Philadelphia (PA): Lippincott Williams & Wilkins; 2006. p. 285-327.
7. DeVane CL. Cyclic antidepressants. In: Burton ME, Shaw LM, Schentag JJ et al., eds. *Applied pharmacokinetics and pharmacodynamics: principles of therapeutic drug monitoring.* 4th ed. Philadelphia (PA): Lippincott Williams & Wilkins; 2006. p. 781-97.
8. Loiseau P, Duche B. Carbamazepine. Clinical use. In: Levy RH, Mattson RH, Meldrum BS, eds. *Antiepileptic drugs.* 4th ed. New York (NY): Raven Press; 1995. p. 555-66.
9. Johnston A, Holt DW. Cyclosporine. In: Burton ME, Shaw LM, Schentag JJ et al., eds. *Applied pharmacokinetics and pharmacodynamics: principles of therapeutic drug monitoring.* 4th ed. Philadelphia (PA): Lippincott Williams & Wilkins; 2006. p. 512-28.
10. Schentag JJ, Bang AJ, Kozinski-Tober JL. Digoxin. In: Burton ME, Shaw LM, Schentag JJ et al., eds. *Applied pharmacokinetics and pharmacodynamics: principles of therapeutic drug monitoring.* 4th ed. Philadelphia (PA): Lippincott Williams & Wilkins; 2006. p. 410-39.
11. Sherwin AL. Ethosuximide. Clinical use. In: Levy RH, Mattson RH, Meldrum BS, eds. *Antiepileptic drugs.* 4th ed. New York (NY): Raven Press; 1995. p. 667-73.
12. Meek PD, Davis SN, Collins DM et al. Guidelines for nonemergency use of parenteral phenytoin products: proceedings of an expert panel consensus process. *Arch Intern Med* 1999;159(22):2639-44.
13. Nicolau DP, Freeman CD, Belliveau PP et al. Experience with a once-daily aminoglycoside program administered to 2,184 adult patients. *Antimicrob Agents Chemother* 1995;39(3):650-5.
14. Bettinger TL, Crismon ML. Lithium. In: Burton ME, Shaw LM, Schentag JJ et al., eds. *Applied pharmacokinetics and pharmacodynamics: principles of therapeutic drug monitoring.* 4th ed. Philadelphia (PA): Lippincott Williams & Wilkins; 2006. p. 789-812.
15. Garnett WR, Anderson GD, Collins RJ. Antiepileptic drugs. In: Burton ME, Shaw LM, Schentag JJ et al., eds. *Applied pharmacokinetics and pharmacodynamics: principles of therapeutic drug monitoring.* 4th ed. Philadelphia (PA): Lippincott Williams & Wilkins; 2006. p. 491-511.
16. Winter ME, Tozer TN. Phenytoin. In: Burton ME, Shaw LM, Schentag JJ et al., eds. *Applied pharmacokinetics and pharmacodynamics: principles of therapeutic drug monitoring.* 4th ed. Philadelphia. (PA):Lippincott Williams & Wilkins; 2006. p. 463-90.
17. Smith DB, DeToledo J. Primidone. Clinical use. In: Levy RH, Mattson RH, Meldrum BS, eds. *Antiepileptic drugs.* 4th ed. New York (NY): Raven Press; 1995. p. 477-85.
18. Coyle JD, Lima JJ. Procainamide. In: Evans WE, Schentag JJ, Jusko WJ, eds. *Applied pharmacokinetics: principles of therapeutic drug monitoring.* 3rd ed. Vancouver (WA): Applied Therapeutics; 1992. p. 22-1, 22-33.
19. Bauman JL, Takahashi H, Fischer JH. Clinical pharmacokinetics of oral antiarrhythmic drugs. In: Burton ME, Shaw LM, Schentag JJ et al., eds. *Applied pharmacokinetics and pharmacodynamics: principles of therapeutic drug monitoring.* 4th ed. Philadelphia (PA): Lippincott Williams & Wilkins; 2006. p. 440-62.
20. Done AK. Salicylate intoxication. Significance of measurements of salicylate in blood in cases of acute ingestion. *Pediatrics* 1960;26:800-7.
21. Dromgoole SH, Furst DE. Salicylates. In: Evans WE, Schentag JJ, Jusko WJ, eds. *Applied pharmacokinetics: principles of therapeutic drug monitoring.* 3rd ed. Vancouver (WA): Applied Therapeutics; 1992. p. 32-1, 32-34.
22. Bauer LA. Tacrolimus (FK 506). In: Bauer LA, ed. *Applied clinical pharmacokinetics.* 1st ed. New York (NY): McGraw-Hill, Medical Publishing Division; 2001. p. 626-50.
23. Edwards DJ, Zarowitz BJ, Slaughter RL. Theophylline. In: Evans WE, Schentag JJ, Jusko WJ, eds. *Applied pharmacokinetics: principles of therapeutic drug monitoring.* 3rd ed. Vancouver (WA): Applied Therapeutics; 1992. p. 13-1, 13-38.

24. Rybak MJ, Lomaestro BM, Rotscahfer JC et al. Vancomycin therapeutic guidelines: a summary of consensus recommendations from the infectious diseases Society of America, the American Society of Health-System Pharmacists, and the Society of Infectious Diseases Pharmacists. *Clin Infect Dis* 2009;49(3):325-7.
25. Moise-Broder PA. Vancomycin. In: Burton ME, Shaw LM, Schentag JJ et al., eds. *Applied pharmacokinetics and pharmacodynamics: principles of therapeutic drug monitoring.* 4th ed. Philadelphia (PA): Lippincott Williams & Wilkins; 2006. p. 328-40.
26. Rybak MJ. The pharmacokinetic and pharmacodynamic properties of vancomycin. *Clin Infect Dis* 2006;42(Suppl 1):S35-9.
27. Health and Welfare Canada. *SI manual in health care.* 3rd rev. ed. Ottawa (ON): Health Canada; 1986.

Drug Use During Pregnancy

Orna Diav-Citrin, MD and Gideon Koren, MD, FRCPC

Date of Revision: November 2010

The following is an overview of drug use during pregnancy. This information is not intended to be a comprehensive review; the reader is therefore encouraged to seek additional and confirmatory information.

Principles of Prescribing in Pregnancy

Many pregnant women are exposed to a variety of medications that may exert therapeutic, toxic or teratogenic effects on the fetus. Since the thalidomide disaster, many physicians and pregnant women tend to withhold any medication during pregnancy, although the risk of teratogenic effect from most drugs in therapeutic doses is nonexistent. Major congenital defects occur in 1% to 3% of the general population at birth. Of the major defects, about 25% are of genetic origin (genetically inherited diseases, new mutations and chromosomal abnormalities) and 65% are of unknown etiology (multifactorial, polygenic, spontaneous errors of development and synergistic interactions of teratogens). Only 2% to 3% of malformations are thought to be associated with drug treatment. The remaining defects are related to other environmental exposures including infectious agents, maternal disease states, mechanical problems and irradiation.[1]

Proper prescribing in pregnancy is a challenge and should provide maximal safety to the fetus as well as therapeutic benefit to the mother. To date, very few drugs are proven teratogens in humans. However, drug-induced malformations are important because they are potentially preventable.

Maternal physiologic changes during pregnancy may alter the pharmacokinetics of drugs. Clearance rates of many drugs increase during late pregnancy due to increases in both renal and hepatic elimination (e.g., digoxin, phenytoin), while in others the clearance rate decreases (e.g., theophylline). Generally, little is known about the relationship between maternal serum drug concentration and risk of teratogenicity.

The importance of **timing of drug exposure** is better understood; the effect produced by a teratogenic agent depends upon the developmental stage in which the conceptus is exposed. Several important phases in human development are recognized:

- The **"all or none" period**, the time from conception until somite formation, which corresponds to the first 17 days after conception. Insults to the embryo in this phase are likely to result in death and miscarriage or intact survival. The embryo is undifferentiated, and repair and recovery are possible through multiplication of the still totipotential cells. Exposure to teratogens during the presomitic stage usually does not cause congenital malformations unless the agent persists in the body beyond this period.
- The **embryonic period**, from 18 to 60 days after conception when the basic steps in organogenesis occur. This is the period of maximum sensitivity to teratogenicity since tissues are differentiating rapidly and damage becomes irreparable. Exposure to teratogenic agents during this period has the greatest likelihood of causing a structural anomaly. The pattern of anomalies produced depends on which systems are differentiating at the time of teratogenic exposure.
- The **fetal phase**, from the end of the embryonic stage to term, when growth and functional maturation of formed organs and systems occurs. Teratogen exposure in this period will affect fetal growth (e.g., intrauterine growth restriction) and the size or function of an organ, rather than cause gross structural anomalies. The term **fetal toxicity** is commonly used to describe such an effect.

The potential effect of psychoactive agents (e.g., antidepressants, antiepileptics, alcohol and other drugs of abuse) on the developing central nervous system has led to the new field of behavioural teratology.

Many organ systems continue structural and functional maturation long after birth. Most of the adenocarcinomas associated with first trimester exposure to diethylstilbestrol occurred many years later.

Teratogens must reach the developing conceptus in sufficient amounts to cause their effects. Large molecules with a molecular weight greater than 1000 (e.g., heparin) do not easily cross the placenta into the embryonic-fetal bloodstream. Other factors influencing the rate and extent of placental transfer of drugs include polarity, lipid solubility and the existence of a specific carrier protein (e.g., P-glycoprotein).

In an attempt to provide the practitioner with a better assessment of fetal risk, the US Food and Drug Administration (FDA) developed a classification of fetal risk in 1979.[2] These categories initially appeared logical but are not helpful in counselling individual patients. Drug manufacturers may have legal rather than scientific reasons for assigning particular designations. The classification frequently results in ambiguity and even false alarm. For example, oral contraceptives are denoted as X (contraindicated in pregnancy), despite failure of two meta-analyses to show increased teratogenic risk. In 1994 the Teratology Society stated that the FDA ratings are inappropriate and should be replaced by narrative statements that summarize and interpret available data regarding hazards of developmental toxicity and provide estimates of teratogenic risk. During the last few years the FDA has begun a process to change the present system.

Teratology Counselling[3]

- Ascertain the clinical facts regarding the nature of the exposure: the length, dosage and timing during pregnancy, as well as other exposures of concern (e.g., alcohol, cigarette smoking, herbal remedies).
- Collect all available current data regarding the agent and the risk of exposure.
- Counselling should include background human baseline risk for major malformations, whether the fetus is at increased risk, which anomaly has been associated with the agent in question, a risk assessment, methods of prenatal detection when available, limitations in our knowledge and limitations of prenatal diagnostic capabilities.
- Additional considerations include the potential risk of the medical condition for which a drug is prescribed, known interactions between the disease state and the pregnancy, and preventive measures when applicable (e.g., folic acid supplementation in carbamazepine exposure).
- Because more than 50% of pregnancies are unplanned, teratogenic risk assessment should be started prior to pregnancy.

Table 1 lists Drugs with sufficient evidence to prove their teratogenic effect in humans are listed in . Use an alternative in pregnancy when possible.Table 2 lists possible teratogenic drugs with insufficient evidence as yet for teratogenicity in humans.

Drugs of Choice During Pregnancy

Table 3 presents drugs of choice during gestation for common maternal conditions.

Note: Antenatal drug/chemical risk counselling or information on safety of drug use during breastfeeding is available from the Motherisk Program, Hospital for Sick Children, Toronto, Ontario. Tel.: (416) 813-6780; email: momrisk@sickkids.on.ca; web site: www.motherisk.org.

Table 1: Proven Teratogenic Drugs in Humans[3]

Drug	Adverse Effects
Angiotensin Converting Enzyme Inhibitors (ACEI) and Angiotensin II Antagonists	Adverse effects relate to hemodynamic effects of ACEI and angiotensin II antagonists on the fetus. In late pregnancy, ACEI fetopathy: intrauterine renal insufficiency, neonatal hypotension, oliguria with renal failure, hyperkalemia, complications of oligohydramnios (fetal limb contractures, lung hypoplasia and craniofacial anomalies), prematurity, intrauterine growth restriction and fetal death. 1st trimester exposure: questionable teratogenic risk of cardiovascular and CNS malformations. Several cohort studies suggest the observed risk may be associated with the underlying maternal conditions.[4]
Antineoplastic Agents	A significant increase in the incidence of various fetal malformations and early miscarriages following 1st trimester exposure.
Carbamazepine	1st trimester exposure: 1% risk of neural tube defects (10 × baseline risk) and an increased risk of cardiovascular malformations. A pattern of malformations similar to the fetal hydantoin syndrome has also been associated.
Cocaine	Abruptio placenta, prematurity, fetal loss, decreased birth weight, microcephaly, limb defects, urinary tract malformations and poorer neurodevelopmental performance. Methodological problems make the findings difficult to interpret. Cocaine abuse is often associated with poly-drug abuse, alcohol consumption, smoking, malnutrition and poor prenatal care. Human epidemiology indicates the risk of major malformation from cocaine is probably low, but the anomalies may be severe.
Corticosteroids (systemic)	1st trimester exposure: <1% increased risk of oral clefts.

(cont'd)

Table 1: Proven Teratogenic Drugs in Humans[3] *(cont'd)*

Drug	Adverse Effects
Coumarin Anticoagulants	1st trimester exposure (6–9 wk gestation): fetal warfarin syndrome (nasal hypoplasia and calcific stippling of the epiphyses). Intrauterine growth restriction and developmental delay (CNS damage), eye defects and hearing loss. Warfarin embryopathy is found in up to 1/3 of the cases where a coumarin derivative was given throughout pregnancy. Associated with high rate of miscarriage. Risk of CNS damage due to hemorrhage after the 1st trimester.
Diethylstilbestrol	Vaginal clear cell adenocarcinoma in offspring exposed in utero before 18th wk (>90% of the cancers occurred after 14 y of age). High incidence of benign vaginal adenosis. Increased miscarriage rate and preterm delivery. In males exposed in utero: no signs of malignancy but genital lesions in 27% and pathologic changes in spermatozoa in 29%. The drug is not currently available in Canada.
Ethanol	Fetal alcohol syndrome: growth impairment, developmental delay and dysmorphic facies. Cleft palate and cardiac anomalies may occur. Full expression of the syndrome occurs with chronic daily ingestion of 2 g alcohol per kg (8 drinks/day) in about 1/3 of offspring and partial effects in ¾ of offspring.
Folic Acid Antagonists: aminopterin and methotrexate	Fetal aminopterin-methotrexate syndrome: CNS defects, craniofacial anomalies, abnormal cranial ossification, abnormalities in first branchial arch derivatives, intrauterine growth restriction and mental retardation after 1st trimester exposure. Maternal dose of methotrexate needed to induce defects is probably above 10 mg/wk with a critical period of 6–8 wk postconception.
Hydantoins (phenytoin)	Fetal hydantoin syndrome: craniofacial dysmorphology, anomalies and hypoplasia of distal phalanges and nails, growth restriction, mental deficiency and cardiac defects.
Lithium	Small increase in risk for cardiac teratogenesis in early gestation (1%). The risk of Ebstein's anomaly (a congenital heart defect, characterized by anterior displacement of the tricuspid valve, enlarged right chambers, often with atrial septal defect and arrhythmias) exceeds spontaneous rate of occurrence. Fetal echocardiography if exposed in 1st trimester.
Misoprostol	1st trimester exposure: limb defects and Moebius sequence (a congenital facial palsy with impairment of ocular abduction, as a result of dysfunction of cranial nerves VI and VII). Absolute teratogenic risk: probably low. Uterine contraction inducing activity.
Retinoids (acitretin, isotretinoin) and megadoses of Vitamin A	Systemic exposure: potent human general and behavioural teratogens. Retinoic acid embryopathy: craniofacial anomalies, cardiac defects, abnormalities in thymic development and alterations in CNS development. Risk for associated miscarriage: 40%.
Tetracyclines	Discolouration of the teeth after 17 wk gestation when deciduous teeth begin to calcify. Close to term: crowns of permanent teeth may be stained. Oxytetracycline and doxycycline associated with a lower incidence of enamel staining.
Thalidomide	Malformations limited to tissues of mesodermal origin, primarily limbs (reduction defects), ears, cardiovascular system and gut musculature. Critical period: 34–50th day after the beginning of the last menstrual period. A single dose of <1 mg/kg has produced the syndrome. Embryopathy found in about 20% of pregnancies exposed in the critical period.
Valproic acid	1st trimester exposure: neural tube defects with 1–2% risk of meningomyelocele, primarily lumbar or lumbosacral, cardiovascular malformations and hypospadias. Fetal valproate syndrome: craniofacial dysmorphology, cardiovascular defects, long fingers and toes, hyperconvex fingernails and cleft lip, has been delineated by some investigations. Neurobehavioural teratogen.

Table 2: Possible Teratogenic Drugs in Humans[a,5]

Drug	Adverse Effects
Diazepam	A questionable small increase in the incidence of cleft lip and palate (small studies). Larger studies did not confirm the association.
Fluconazole	High-dose treatment: multiple synostosis, congenital heart defects, skeletal anomalies and recognizable dysmorphic facial features (case reports).
HMG-CoA Reductase Inhibitors (statins)	A questionable increase in the risk of CNS and limb anomalies (retrospective data), not confirmed by several prospective cohort studies.
Lamotrigine	A questionable increase in the risk of isolated oral clefts (<1%), not confirmed by several registries.
Methimazole	Scalp defects such as aplasia cutis congenita suggested through case reports and an epidemiological study in which methimazole had been added to animal feeds as a weight enhancer; methimazole embryopathy (choanal and esophageal atresia, scalp defects, minor facial anomalies and psychomotor delay).
Mycophenolate mofetil	Case series of ear, eye and craniofacial malformations, oral clefts, cardiac, finger, urogenital, gastrointestinal, CNS and skeletal malformations.
Paroxetine	A questionable increase in the risk of cardiac malformations, not confirmed by meta-analysis.
Penicillamine	High-dose treatment: connective tissue disorders (cutis laxa) (case reports).
Sulfamethoxazole/trimethoprim	Possible increased risk of neural tube and cardiovascular defects and oral clefts with 1st trimester exposure. Folic acid supplementation may reduce these risks.

[a] This list is not exhaustive.

Table 3: Drugs of Choice for Select Conditions During Pregnancy[3]

Condition	Drugs of Choice	Alternative	Comments
Allergy	Antihistamines: chlorpheniramine, desloratadine, diphenhydramine, dimenhydrinate, loratadine	Intranasal preparations of sodium cromoglycate, beclomethasone, budesonide, fluticasone; cetirizine, fexofenadine	
Anticoagulation	Heparin and low molecular weight heparins		
Anxiety	Benzodiazepines		Short or intermediate-acting agents (e.g., lorazepam, oxazepam) may be preferred if needed for regular use near term. Watch neonate for possible withdrawal or "floppy" infant when high doses used close to term. For diazepam, there is a questionable small increase in the incidence of cleft lip and palate (small studies). Larger studies did not confirm the association.
Asthma	Inhaled bronchodilators (salbutamol, terbutaline or ipratropium bromide) and inhaled corticosteroids (beclomethasone, budesonide, fluticasone)	Systemic corticosteroids and theophylline	
Bacterial Infections	Penicillins, cephalosporins, clindamycin, erythromycin	Aminoglycosides (amikacin, gentamicin, tobramycin), azithromycin, clarithromycin, quinolones	

(cont'd)

Table 3: Drugs of Choice for Select Conditions During Pregnancy[3] *(cont'd)*

Condition	Drugs of Choice	Alternative	Comments
Bipolar Disorder	Lithium	Carbamazepine, lamotrigine	With lithium, monitor using fetal echocardiography. Avoid valproic acid when possible, especially in the first trimester (if not possible to avoid, limit dose to <600–1000 mg/day). With carbamazepine and valproic acid, prescribe periconceptional folate supplementation: 5 mg po daily beginning before pregnancy and continuing at least in the first trimester. Monitor using level II ultrasound for prevention of neural tube defects.
Constipation	Bulk-forming agents (e.g., methylcellulose, psyllium hydrophilic mucilloid)	Docusate sodium, glycerin suppository, lactulose, mineral oil	Long term use of mineral oil can decrease absorption of lipid soluble vitamins A, D, E and K.
Cough	Antihistamines (in the case of cough due to rhinitis or allergy), codeine (when indicated)	Dextromethorphan	Avoid high doses of codeine close to term (risk of neonatal opioid withdrawal).
Depression	Tricyclic antidepressants, citalopram, fluoxetine, sertraline	Other selective serotonin reuptake inhibitors, bupropion, venlafaxine	Neonatal withdrawal may occur when used in 3rd trimester. There is a questionable association between paroxetine exposure in pregnancy and cardiac malformations.
Diabetes Mellitus	Human insulin	Metformin in gestational diabetes in 3rd trimester, glyburide	Important to achieve strict glycemic control before conception and during the 1st trimester.
Diarrhea	Bulk-forming agents (e.g., methylcellulose, psyllium hydrophilic mucilloid), kaolin pectin	Loperamide	
Dyspepsia	Alginic acid compound, antacids—numerous aluminum hydroxide combinations	H_2-antagonists (famotidine, ranitidine), omeprazole	
Epilepsy[6,7]	Carbamazepine, lamotrigine	Benzodiazepines (e.g., clonazepam) (see "Anxiety"), phenobarbital, phenytoin, valproic acid	The drug of choice for epilepsy in pregnancy should be the drug that best controls the seizures; monotherapy should be favoured. Use the lowest effective dose. Valproic acid dose should be <600–1000 mg/day whenever possible. With carbamazepine and valproic acid, prescribe periconceptional folate supplementation: 5 mg po daily beginning before pregnancy and continuing at least in the first trimester. Monitor using level II ultrasound for prevention of neural tube defects. Vitamin K (phytonadione) 10 to 20 mg/day to be given to women on antiepileptics (e.g., carbamazepine, phenytoin, phenobarbital) from 36 weeks of pregnancy on, to prevent hemorrhagic disease of the newborn.
Fever and Pain	Acetaminophen	ASA, NSAIDs	Avoid full anti-inflammatory dose of NSAIDs in 3rd trimester due to the risk of oligohydramnios and premature closure of ductus arteriosus.
Herpetic Infections	Acyclovir, valacyclovir		
Hypertension[8]	Hydralazine, methyldopa	Beta-blockers, calcium channel blockers	With beta-blockers, reduced birth weight and persistent beta-blockade possible in newborn. Monitor growth using serial ultrasounds in the 3rd trimester. Monitor newborn for hypoglycemia, bradycardia, hypotension and respiratory problems during the first 24–48 h.
Hyperthyroidism	Propylthiouracil		Perform fetal ultrasound near term for goitre detection.
Migraine (abortive therapy)	Acetaminophen	ASA, NSAIDs, sumatriptan	Avoid full anti-inflammatory dose of NSAIDs in 3rd trimester due to the risk of oligohydramnios and premature closure of ductus arteriosus.
Nausea/Vomiting	Doxylamine/pyridoxine (Diclectin)	Dimenhydrinate, metoclopramide	
Schizophrenia	Phenothiazines	Haloperidol, risperidone	Watch neonate for possible adverse effects if taken close to term. Continue present antipsychotic if the woman is stable and unplanned pregnancy occurs. Monitor the woman for metabolic complications (weight gain, hyperglycemia, hyperlipidemia), especially with atypical antipsychotics.
Vaginal Candidiasis	Vaginal: clotrimazole, miconazole, nystatin Topical azoles are preferred.[9,10]	Fluconazole: single systemic dose of 150 mg	

References

1. Koren G, Pastuszak A, Ito S. Drugs in pregnancy. *N Engl J Med* 1998;338(16):1128-37.
2. Briggs GG, Freeman RK, Yaffe SJ. *Drugs in pregnancy and lactation: a reference guide to fetal and neonatal risk.* 8th ed. Philadelphia (PA): Wolters Kluwer; Lippincott Williams & Wilkins; 2008.
3. Koren G. *Medication safety in pregnancy and breastfeeding.* New York (NY): McGraw-Hill; 2007.
4. Cooper WO, Hernandez-Diaz S, Arbogast PG et al. Major congenital malformations after first-trimester exposure to ACE inhibitors. *N Engl J Med* 2006;354(23):2443-51.
5. Motherisk. Toronto (ON): Hospital for Sick Children. Available from: www.motherisk.org/women/index.jsp. Accessed September 2010.
6. Battino D, Tomson T. Management of epilepsy during pregnancy. *Drugs* 2007;67(18):2727-46.
7. Harden CL, Meador KJ, Pennell PB et al. Management issues for women with epilepsy—Focus on pregnancy (an evidence-based review): II. Teratogenesis and perinatal outcomes: Report of the Quality Standards Subcommittee and Therapeutics and Technology Subcommittee of the American Academy of Neurology and the American Epilepsy Society. *Epilepsia* 2009;50(5):1237-46.
8. Society of Obstetricians and Gynaecologists of Canada. Diagnosis, evaluation and management of the hypertensive disorders of pregnancy. *J Obstet Gynaecol Can* 2008;30(3 Suppl 1):1-49. Available from: www.sogc.org/guidelines/documents/gui206CPG0803_001.pdf. Accessed November 16, 2010.
9. Expert Working Group on the Canadian Guidelines on Sexually Transmitted Infections. *Updates to the Canadian guidelines on sexually transmitted infections.* Ottawa (ON): Public Health Agency of Canada; 2008. Available from: www.phac-aspc.gc.ca/std-mts/sti_2006/pdf/Guidelines_Eng_complete_06-26-08.pdf. Accessed September 2010.
10. Young GL, Jewell D. Topical treatment for vaginal candidiasis (thrush) in pregnancy. *Cochrane Database Syst Rev* 2001;(4):CD000225.

Drug Use During Breastfeeding

S. Ito, MD, FRCPC and M.S. Brochet, BPharm, MSc

Date of Preparation: November 2010

The following is an overview of drug use during breastfeeding. This information is not intended to be a comprehensive review; the reader is therefore encouraged to seek additional and confirmatory information.

Principles of Drug Use During Breastfeeding

Clinicians can use the following general principles to manage cases where drug exposure in a breast-fed infant is questioned:

- Almost all drugs are excreted to some degree in breast milk.
- Breast milk/feeding has tangible medical and other benefits compared to formula.[1,2,3]
- Even when the breast milk:maternal plasma concentration ratio approaches or exceeds 1.0, the amount of drug ingested by the infant rarely attains therapeutic levels.
- A short exposure to a drug, as might be expected in the case of analgesics given to relieve postpartum pain, is usually of less concern than a drug given for long periods of time. The amount of drug ingested by the infant can, on occasion, be minimized by feeding the infant just before or at the time of maternal dosing.
- In the case of chronic drug therapy, the infant is usually exposed to lower concentrations of the drug while breastfeeding than while the fetus is in utero. Nevertheless, in most cases the long-term consequences of chronic exposure to subtherapeutic levels of medications are not known.
- Recommendations about breastfeeding where maternal medications are indicated depends on knowing if small amounts of the drug (subtherapeutic amounts) taken for even short periods of time may be associated with the following:
  - causing idiosyncratic reactions, e.g., chloramphenicol
  - interfering with genetically abnormal metabolic pathways, e.g., nitrofurantoin in patients with G-6-PD deficiencies
  - acting synergistically with drugs the infant receives therapeutically, e.g., caffeine in coffee and tea may enhance effects of therapeutic caffeine or aminophylline in the neonate

The clinician requires a reasonable knowledge of pharmacology and therapeutics in the newborn as well as a knowledge of the amount of drug excreted in the breast milk.

There are a number of reviews about drug excretion in breast milk and recommendations for breastfeeding during maternal therapy. One of the most reliable and authoritative web-based resources is the Drugs and Lactation database, LactMed [toxnet.nlm.nih.gov/cgi-bin/sis/htmlgen?LACT], which is free of charge and run by the United States National Library of Medicine.[4] LactMed is housed within the TOXNET [toxnet.nlm.nih.gov/] web site.

There are several important questions the clinician should consider when a breastfeeding mother starts drug therapy:

- Is the drug absorbed from the GI tract?
- Is the drug ever given directly to infants for therapeutic reasons?
- Does the estimated dose delivered by milk approach a therapeutic quantity?
- Are the effects of the drug easily recognized in the infant?
- Are there idiosyncratic or allergic reactions to the drug that are not dose-related?
- Are there less toxic alternatives for maternal therapy?
- Is there a potential for drug accumulation during prolonged therapy?
- Could subtherapeutic doses of the drug mask early signs of medical conditions in the infant?
- Is the risk posed by the drug substantial enough to outweigh the significant proven benefits of breastfeeding?

Drugs Compatible with Breastfeeding

The drugs considered compatible with breastfeeding far outnumber the drugs considered contraindicated during breastfeeding. Table 1 discusses some examples of drugs considered to be compatible with breastfeeding.

Table 1: Drugs Compatible with Breastfeeding[a]

Therapeutic Class	Drugs/Drug Classes Compatible with Breastfeeding	Comments
Analgesics	Acetaminophen, morphine	• For most **narcotic analgesics**, the amount of drug excreted in breast milk is small, and short-term use should be of no major concern. If the use is longer than 3 days the infant should be more closely monitored. **Meperidine** is an exception; in neonates, the long half-lives of meperidine (13 hours) and normeperidine (63 hours) may result in accumulation in plasma, possibly leading to neurobehavioural depression.[5,6] • In addition, use **codeine** with caution at the lowest effective dose for the shortest period of time. Mothers with ultra-rapid metabolizer CYP2D6 genotype may experience intensified effects from a regular dosing regimen of codeine due to increased conversion of codeine to morphine, causing morphine toxicity. Resultant high levels of morphine in maternal serum could cause relatively high morphine levels in milk. Monitor baby for signs and symptoms of drowsiness, sedation, difficulty breathing, difficulty breastfeeding, decreased tone.[7] Mothers showing morphine toxicity, whether it is due to this genotype or a morphine overdose, should not breastfeed. Postpartum codeine use should be limited to less than 3–4 days. • Data for **tramadol** is lacking. Low excretion in breast milk, therefore unlikely to affect healthy babies. Short-term use may be a concern due to its long half-life (7 hours for tramadol and 8.5 hours for the active metabolite in newborns) especially in premature infants: monitor for increased sleepiness. An exclusively breast-fed infant would receive about 14% of the therapeutic dose for a child.[8]
Antibiotics	Aminoglycosides, cephalosporins, clindamycin, macrolides, metronidazole, nitrofurantoin, penicillins, sulfonamides	• For many of the drugs, the amounts ingested by a breast-fed infant will be below therapeutic levels (e.g., **penicillins**, **cephalosporins**), but might be sufficient to result in idiosyncratic reactions (e.g., **chloramphenicol**) or cause anemia in an infant with G-6-PD deficiency (e.g., **nitrofurantoin, sulfonamides**). Other potential problems are modifications to the normal GI flora leading to thrush and diarrhea. However, clinical significance of these risks is usually not high enough to justify discontinuation of breastfeeding. • The **aminoglycosides** are excreted in breast milk when administered im and iv to the mother; because the drugs are poorly absorbed from the GI tract, it is unlikely that renal toxicity or ototoxicity would occur in the infant. • Only small amounts of oral **clindamycin** are excreted in breast milk (2% to 6% of the recommended pediatric dosage). It is unlikely that these quantities would be clinically relevant but at least one case of bloody stools has been reported in the breast-fed infant of a mother receiving clindamycin. Topical clindamycin (not used in the nipple area) is generally associated with lower maternal systemic drug levels and lower milk excretion compared to systemic use.[9] • **Erythromycin** is excreted in milk in low amounts and is compatible with breastfeeding. Limited data regarding **clarithromycin** and **azithromycin** demonstrate that these drugs are excreted in breast milk in small amounts but the amount of drug ingested by a breast-fed infant is likely below therapeutic pediatric levels.[10,11] No data are available regarding the excretion of **telithromycin** in breast milk. • **Metronidazole** use during breastfeeding has raised some concerns based on reports that it is mutagenic in bacteria and carcinogenic in rodents during life-long ingestion. Specific untoward effects in a nursing infant as a result of metronidazole ingestion have not been reported. Without more direct evidence of the harmful effects of short-term use in humans, it seems overly conservative to withhold the drug or discontinue breastfeeding in patients with symptomatic infections. For the treatment of trichomoniasis with a single oral dose of metronidazole 2 g, some clinicians now recommend an interruption of breastfeeding for 12 to 24 hours, especially with young babies.[5] Topical metronidazole (as long as it not used in the nipple area) is considered compatible with breastfeeding since blood levels and excretion into breast milk are lower than with maternal systemic metronidazole use. • Fluoroquinolones have traditionally not been used in infants because of concerns regarding adverse effects on joint development. Studies indicate little risk. Short-term use of **ciprofloxacin, levofloxacin, norfloxacin** or **ofloxacin** is acceptable in nursing mothers. These quinolones are excreted in breast milk in small amounts which do not result in significant serum concentrations in breast-fed infants.[12] The calcium in breast milk may also decrease quinolone absorption in the infant.[9] There are no data available for **moxifloxacin**. Maternal use of **gatifloxacin** eye drops presents negligible risk for the nursing infant.[9]

(cont'd)

Table 1: Drugs Compatible with Breastfeeding[a] *(cont'd)*

Therapeutic Class	Drugs/Drug Classes Compatible with Breastfeeding	Comments
		• The **sulfonamides** are excreted in breast milk in small amounts. **Nitrofurantoin** excretion is also small. In each case, there are concerns about these drugs causing anemia in an infant with G-6-PD deficiency which is more common in those of African, Greek, middle-eastern and south-east Asian origin. Use with caution in mothers breastfeeding premature infants or neonates with hyperbilirubinemia.[5] Use alternatives unless the infection is not responding to other therapy. • Some reviews classify **tetracyclines** as contraindicated in breastfeeding based on concerns of staining of dental enamel or bone deposition. Available data indicate that harm is unlikely with short-term use of tetracyclines. Milk levels are low and calcium in breast milk limits absorption of tetracyclines. However, as a theoretical precaution prolonged or repeated courses should be avoided during breastfeeding.[9]
Anticoagulants	Warfarin, heparin (unfractionated and low molecular weight)	• **Heparin**, administered parenterally for acute short-term therapy of thrombophlebitis, has not been shown to be excreted in breast milk. Heparin is a large polysaccharide molecule that is inactivated in the GI tract when taken orally. Its transfer into breast milk and risk to a breast-fed infant are considered negligible.[5] • Few data are available regarding the effects of **low molecular weight heparins** during breastfeeding. There is a case report of 12 full-term neonates being breast-fed by mothers treated with 20 or 40 mg of **enoxaparin** injected subcutaneously daily.[13] No anticoagulant effects, as measured by anti-Xa activity levels, were detected in the babies. It is thought that with the relatively high molecular weight of enoxaparin and its inactivation in the GI tract if orally ingested, its transfer into breast milk and risk to a breast-fed infant should be considered negligible.[5] No drug was found in breast milk of two patients who received 5000 to 10 000 IU of **dalteparin**.[14] In a study of 15 lactating mothers after once daily routine dalteparin 2500 IU sc no quantitative correlation was noted between anti-Xa activities in plasma and milk.[15] There are no data available on excretion into milk of **nadroparin** or **tinzaparin**; however based on their molecular weight and inactivation by the GI tract, excretion into breast milk is expected to be negligible. • Among breast-fed infants whose mothers were taking **warfarin**, the drug was undetectable in plasma and the bleeding time was not affected.[16]
Antidepressants	Tricyclic antidepressants, selective serotonin reuptake inhibitors, venlafaxine	• Except for **doxepin** there are no reports of untoward effects of any of the **tricyclic antidepressants** in breast-fed infants.[17] • **Sertraline** is transferred into breast milk resulting in an estimated infant dose of between 0.5% and 5% of the weight-adjusted maternal dose[b]. There are no case reports of adverse events in the infants.[18,19,20,21] • **Paroxetine** is transferred into breast milk resulting in an estimated infant dose of between 0.1% and 4.3% of the weight-adjusted maternal dose[b]. In these studies, paroxetine was not detected in the serum of the majority of infants (in whom it was measured) and no adverse effects were reported.[22,23,24,25,26] • The amount of **fluoxetine** excreted in breast milk is 2% to 18% of the weight-adjusted maternal dose[b,18,19,20,21,22,23,24,25,26,27] Nearly therapeutic serum concentrations were reported in some symptomatic infants.[28,29,30,31,32,33,34,35,36] Also, infants breast-fed by mothers on fluoxetine had poorer weight gain, although the significance is unclear.[32] A few cases of colic have been associated with fluoxetine.[29,33] • Excretion of **fluvoxamine** seems to be low and no adverse effects were reported in the few available cases.[22,37] • The amount of **citalopram** excreted in breast milk is approximately 0.7% to 9% of the weight-adjusted maternal dose[b]. In one study, a single infant presented an "uneasy" sleep pattern which improved when maternal dose was decreased.[38,39,40,41] The amount of **escitalopram** excreted in breast milk is less than 8% of the weight-adjusted maternal dose[b] and no adverse effects were reported in the available cases.[9] • **Venlafaxine** and its metabolites are excreted in breast milk in approximately 5% to 9% of the weight-adjusted maternal dose[b]. In one study of seven infants the active metabolite O-desmethylvenlafaxine was detected in the plasma of four infants. No adverse effects were reported in the infants.[42,43,44] • No published information is available on the use of **duloxetine** during breastfeeding; however, the amount excreted into breast milk seems to be low. The excretion of duloxetine metabolites, which are inactive, into breast milk was not studied.[45] • Although **bupropion, moclobemide** and **mirtazapine** have not been studied extensively, for each of these drugs the amount excreted in breast milk is less than 2% of the weight-adjusted maternal dose.[b] No adverse effects were reported[9,46,47,48,49,50,51] except for bupropion (two case reports of possible seizure) although the significance is unclear.[52,53] Limited data indicate that excretion of **trazodone** into breast milk is low but data on its active metabolites are lacking.[54,55,56,57] • Overall, no significant short-term effect has been reported for the commonly used antidepressants such as tricyclics and SSRIs. Clinical significance of reported adverse events remains unclear. Base the choice of antidepressants on the maternal condition and response. No matter what drug is used, use caution until more experience is gained.
Antiepileptics	Carbamazepine, clonazepam, phenytoin, valproic acid	• The excretion into milk is low: approximately 5% and 2% of the weight-adjusted maternal dose[b] for **carbamazepine** and its epoxide metabolite, less than 4% for **valproic acid**, and less than 8% for **phenytoin**. Limited data for **clonazepam** indicate that the weight adjusted maternal dose is <3% therefore risk for toxicity is expected to be low.[9] However the long half-life and lipophilicity of clonazepam could be a concern. Despite sporadic case reports of adverse effects, these antiepileptics are believed to be compatible with breastfeeding.[5,58] • **Phenobarbital**, **ethosuximide** and **primidone** may warrant more caution because the infant's exposure may reach therapeutic levels. The infant exposure levels for phenobarbital, ethosuximide and primidone are estimated at 100%, 50% and >10%, respectively, of the levels expected when the drug is given directly to an infant in a therapeutic dose.[58] Whether this high-level exposure precludes breastfeeding or not depends on various factors in each individual case. In selected cases, regular monitoring of clinical signs (e.g., lethargy, poor feeding, sedation) and of drug concentrations in breast milk and/or in infant's plasma may guide breastfeeding. • **Lamotrigine** plasma levels as high as 50% of maternal serum levels were found in breast-fed infants whose mothers were taking lamotrigine. Many infants have been breast-fed without adverse reactions but this drug may be of concern.[9] • Newer antiepileptic drugs such as **clobazam**, **gabapentin**, **levetiracetam**, **oxcarbazepine** and **topiramate** have not been extensively studied and their use during breastfeeding should be evaluated on a case-by-case basis.
Antifungals	Amphotericin B, caspofungin, fluconazole, ketoconazole, topical antifungals	• Data on **amphotericin B** are lacking. However, it is virtually unabsorbed orally and is commonly used in pediatrics.[59,60] • Although data are lacking on topical fungicidal agents like **clotrimazole**, **miconazole**, **terconazole** and **nystatin** in breastfeeding, systemic absorption in the mother is very poor. Milk levels are probably too low to be clinically relevant. Most of these topical antifungals are used in pediatrics. • Data on **caspofungin** in breastfeeding are lacking but it has poor oral bioavailability. • **Fluconazole** excretion into milk is low after an oral administration of 150 mg, amounting to 16% of the weight-adjusted maternal dose[b] and less than 6% of a daily pediatric dose. There are no case reports of adverse effects in the infants. Data on larger doses are lacking. However, breastfeeding must be continued for yeast mastitis treated with fluconazole including doses of 100 to 200 mg for two to three weeks. This amount of drug in milk is insufficient as an infant therapeutic dose.[9] • Data regarding **itraconazole** and **voriconazole** are lacking; fluconazole is preferred.[5] • Less than 1% of the weight-adjusted maternal dose[b] is excreted in breast milk after an oral dose of **ketoconazole** 200 mg. This amount is also less than the daily pediatric dose. Maternal systemic absorption after shampoo application is considered negligible.[9,59,61]

(cont'd)

Table 1: Drugs Compatible with Breastfeeding[a] *(cont'd)*

Therapeutic Class	Drugs/Drug Classes Compatible with Breastfeeding	Comments
Antihistamines	Loratadine, desloratadine, fexofenadine	• **Loratadine** and **fexofenadine** (based on terfenadine data) result in infant exposure levels of <1% of the therapeutic dose standardized by weight.[62,63] • **Desloratadine** is the active metabolite of loratadine. The calculated maximum expected dose of desloratadine in milk is 0.46% of the maternal weight-adjusted dose[b] of loratadine.[62] • Other antihistamines may be given, but data on the concentrations of these drugs in breast milk are lacking. Infants should be monitored for irritability or drowsiness.[64] • Antihistamines are not usually contraindicated during breastfeeding. Alternatives to oral antihistamines that may be considered during breastfeeding include nasally administered steroids or cromolyn.
Antihypertensives	Labetalol, metoprolol, propranolol, ACE inhibitors, calcium channel blockers, diuretics	• Beta-blockers that are safe to use even in the neonatal period are **labetalol**, **metoprolol** and **propranolol**.[58,65,66] • **Acebutolol**, **atenolol**, and **sotalol** (although the latter is not indicated as an antihypertensive agent) may cause relatively high exposure levels, 10%, 25% and 20%, respectively, of those expected when the drug is given directly to an infant in a therapeutic dose. This may not be a problem in post-neonatal infants. However, exercise caution in the early neonatal period because newborns may have low clearance of atenolol and sotalol as a result of immature renal function (low GFR). Signs of beta-blockade have been reported in a breast-fed infant of a woman taking atenolol (bradycardia, cyanosis, hypotension, hypothermia) and acebutolol (hypotension, bradycardia, tachypnea, drowsiness).[67,68,69] • **Diuretics, methyldopa**, some **calcium channel blockers** (**diltiazem, nifedipine** and **verapamil**) and some **angiotensin-converting enzyme inhibitors** (**benazepril, captopril, enalapril** and **ramipril**) are not excreted into breast milk in clinically significant amounts and are considered compatible with breastfeeding.[12,70,71] Data concerning the use of **angiotensin II receptor antagonists** during lactation are lacking. Use with caution in breastfeeding mothers.[5]
Antimalarial Agents (Prophylactic)	Chloroquine, mefloquine, proguanil	• The very small amount of **chloroquine**, **mefloquine** and **proguanil** excreted in breast milk is not thought to be harmful to a nursing infant.[5] • There is no information on the amount of **primaquine** that enters into human breast milk but the drug may cause severe hemolysis in G-6-PD-deficient individuals. Because data are not yet available on the safety and efficacy of **atovaquone/proguanil** in infants weighing <11 kg, the medication should not be given to a woman who is breastfeeding an infant less than this weight unless the potential benefit to the woman outweighs the potential risk to the infant. Consider mefloquine. • Quantity of antimalarial medication transferred in breast milk is insufficient to provide adequate protection against malaria. Infants who require chemoprophylaxis should receive the recommended dosages of appropriate antimalarial drugs.[72,73]
Antimanic Agents		• **Lithium** should be used with caution in breastfeeding mothers. Lithium is excreted in breast milk, occasionally in quantities sufficient to produce infant serum levels ranging from 10–50% of maternal serum levels. In an infant exposed to lithium in utero and through breastfeeding, cyanosis, T-wave abnormalities and decreased muscle tone were reported. Other studies have reported no adverse effects.[5,74] • Monitoring of drug concentrations in milk and/or infant's serum may be justified.[75] Consider periodic thyroid evaluation of the infant as lithium can reduce thyroxine production. Monitor changes in infant hydration carefully as hydration status can greatly alter lithium serum levels.[5]
Antivirals	Acyclovir, valacyclovir	• **Acyclovir** and **valacyclovir** (which is almost entirely transformed to acyclovir) excretion into milk are low (less than 1% of the maximal daily pediatric dosage). No adverse effects were reported in breast-fed infants.[76] • No studies have been reported on the excretion of **amantadine** in human milk. However, amantadine is a dopamine agonist. Clinical studies using amantadine concurrently with neuroleptic medications have demonstrated a decrease of prolactin and galactorrhea induced by neuroleptic drugs. The maternal prolactin level in a mother with established lactation may not affect her ability to breastfeed.[77,78] • Data on **famciclovir** in breastfeeding and pediatrics are lacking. Acyclovir and valacyclovir are preferred.[9]
	Oseltamivir	• Even though the amount of **oseltamivir** excreted in breast milk seems to be low (less than 1% of the usual pediatric dosage and 0.5% of the weight-adjusted maternal dose[b] after 75 mg twice daily for 5 days in a 9 months postpartum nursing mother), it would not be expected to cause any adverse effects in breast-fed infants, especially if the infant is older than 2 months.[79,80] • No data are available regarding the excretion of **zanamivir** in breast milk, but due to the poor inhaled absorption and very low plasma levels, it would not be expected to cause any adverse effects in breast-fed infants.[80]
Anxiolytics and Sedatives	Lorazepam, oxazepam	• If used occasionally as a sedative, **benzodiazepines** are not contraindicated during breastfeeding. Benzodiazepines with shorter half-lives, lower lipophilicity and no active metabolites are preferred in breastfeeding mothers (e.g., oxazepam, lorazepam). • Benzodiazepines taken over a longer period of time to treat chronic maternal conditions may be of concern. The benzodiazepines and their metabolites are excreted in breast milk, are poorly metabolized by the neonate, and have been associated with drowsiness in nursing infants. Consequently, discourage the chronic use of a benzodiazepine in breastfeeding mothers unless the infant's condition is closely monitored.
Decongestants, oral	Pseudoephedrine	• 5.5% of the weight-adjusted maternal dosage[b] is excreted in breast milk after a single oral dose of 60 mg of **pseudoephedrine**. Decreased milk production was reported at same dosage. Irritability was reported in infants exposed to pseudoephedrine in one study of breastfeeding mothers.[64,81] Use should be limited to a few days and discontinued if a decrease in milk production is observed. No data are available on the use of **phenylephrine** during breastfeeding, therefore an alternate drug may be preferred, especially while nursing a newborn or preterm infant.
Diabetes Therapy	Insulin, metformin	• Human **insulin** is normally found in breast milk. Amount of synthetic insulin secreted into breast milk is unknown but, if secreted, this peptide would be destroyed in the infant's GI tract with no significant absorption.[5] • **Metformin** levels in milk are low and infants would receive less than 0.5% of their mother's weight-adjusted dosage. It is sometimes detectable in low levels in the serum of breast-fed infants but no adverse effects in breast-fed infants were reported in one study. Metformin should be used with caution while nursing newborn and premature infants and those with renal impairment.[9] • The amount of **glyburide** excreted in breast milk seems to be low (less than 1% of the weight-adjusted maternal dose[b]): no adverse effects on breast-fed infant's blood glucose have been reported but data are limited.[82] • No data are available regarding the excretion of **acarbose** into breast milk. However less than 2% of a dose of acarbose is absorbed from the mother's gastrointestinal tract making it unlikely that any drug reaches the infant through breast milk.[83] • No data are available regarding the excretion of **gliclazide, glimepiride, nateglinide, pioglitazone, repaglinide, rosiglitazone** in breast milk. An alternate drug may be preferred, especially while nursing a newborn or preterm infant. Some experts recommend monitoring the breast-fed infant's blood glucose during maternal therapy with hypoglycemic agents.[83]
Gastrointestinal Drugs	Antacids, sucralfate	• **Aluminum**, **calcium** and **magnesium antacids** and **sucralfate** are partially or poorly absorbed orally and are considered safe to use.[5]
	H_2 Antagonists	• Though considered safe for use by breastfeeding mothers, **cimetidine** and **ranitidine** may concentrate in milk whereas **famotidine** and **nizatidine** have the lowest concentrations, making them preferable choices.[5,16] Ranitidine has been widely used in pediatrics primarily for gastroesophageal reflux. Adverse effects have not been reported in nursing infants but the potential for inhibition of gastric acid secretion and enzyme metabolizing capability exist and may be of concern.

(cont'd)

Table 1: Drugs Compatible with Breastfeeding[a] *(cont'd)*

Therapeutic Class	Drugs/Drug Classes Compatible with Breastfeeding	Comments
	Proton Pump Inhibitors	• **Proton pump inhibitors** are unstable in an acid milieu and, when ingested via milk, would probably be destroyed in the infant's stomach prior to absorption.[5] **Pantoprazole** and **omeprazole** are excreted in milk in small quantities.[84,85] **Esomeprazole** is the s-enantiomer of omeprazole and therefore would also not be expected to cause any adverse effects in breast-fed infants.[85]
	Laxatives	• **Psyllium** is acceptable to use during breastfeeding because it is not absorbed from the gastrointestinal tract. There have been no cases of loose stools reported in breast-fed infants.[9] • **Docusate, bisacodyl** and **magnesium hydroxide** are not appreciably absorbed from the gastrointestinal tract and therefore these drugs are unlikely to be found in the maternal serum or breast milk. One postpartum patient receiving a laxative containing docusate in a dose of 120 mg daily in addition to danthron 100 mg daily stated that diarrhea occurred in her breast-fed infant.[5,9] • Usual doses of **senna** are acceptable to use during breastfeeding. However, a laxative effect was observed in a few case reports. **Cascara** was qualitatively detected in milk after a 5 mL dose, and some breast-fed infants appeared to have loose stools after administration of 1.2 mL of **cascara sagrada** fluid extract to their postpartum mothers.[5,9] • No data are available regarding the excretion of **lactulose** into breast milk; however less than 3% of a dose of lactulose is absorbed from the mother's GI tract, making it unlikely that any drug reaches the infant through breast milk.[86]
	Antidiarrheals	• Use of **loperamide** during breastfeeding is unlikely to affect the infant as it is minimally absorbed orally. Based on its chemical and pharmacological similarity to narcotics, occasional small doses of **diphenoxylate** may be acceptable while breastfeeding an older infant, but alternatives are preferred, especially while nursing a newborn.[5,9]
	GI Motility Agents	• The excretion into milk of **domperidone** and **metoclopramide** are less than 0.05% and 6% respectively of a daily pediatric dose. No adverse events are reported for domperidone but intestinal discomfort was reported in 2 breast-fed infants of mothers taking metoclopramide.[5,9] Domperidone is used to increase milk production in some women who do not respond to a nonpharmacologic approach.
Glucocorticoids	Prednisolone and prednisone	• The amount of **prednisolone** that the infant would ingest in breast milk is less than 0.1% of the therapeutic dose for an infant, standardized by weight.[16,87] This corresponds to less than 10% of the infant's endogenous cortisol production.
Insecticides, Pediculicides	Permethrin	• **Permethrin** cream is the treatment of choice. Although its excretion in breast milk is unknown after topical use, absorption through the skin is low. Permethrin is rapidly metabolized to inactive metabolites and excreted in urine. Overt toxicity is very unlikely. Avoid application on nipples.[5,88] • **Lindane** is not recommended because it is absorbed through the mother's skin and excreted into milk fat. Direct contact of lindane with neonatal skin results in significant absorption. Direct exposure is potentially toxic in infants with reports of elevated liver enzymes, seizure disorders and hypersensitivity. It may also have estrogenic effects that could affect lactation.[9,88]
Migraine Therapy	Sumatriptan, eletriptan	• Occasional use of **sumatriptan** and **eletriptan** seems to be acceptable because the amount of these drugs excreted into milk is low (3.5% and 0.02% of the weight-adjusted maternal dosage,[b] respectively). Data on **almotriptan, naratriptan, rizatriptan** and **zolmitriptan** are lacking.[5] • Because there is limited published experience with **ergotamine, dihydroergotamine** and **methysergide** during breastfeeding, and adverse effects in the infant cannot be ruled out, most authorities consider these drugs to be undesirable to use while nursing.[5,12]
Muscle Relaxants	Cyclobenzaprine, methocarbamol	• The excretion of **cyclobenzaprine**, **methocarbamol** and **orphenadrine** into milk has not been reported. However, occasional cyclobenzaprine and methocarbamol exposures are acceptable because of cyclobenzaprine's structural similarities to amitriptyline (see "Antidepressants") and the very short half-life of methocarbamol. No adverse events have been published, but infants (especially those that are newborn or premature) should be monitored for sedation while nursing.[5]
Nonsteroidal Anti-inflammatory Drugs (NSAIDs)	Diclofenac, ibuprofen, indomethacin, flurbiprofen, naproxen	• Most NSAIDs have been shown to be present in breast milk in small amounts and are considered safe to use. The use of short-acting drugs, such as **ibuprofen** and **flurbiprofen**, may be preferred over those with a longer half-life such as **naproxen**.[5] • The amount of **indomethacin** excreted in breast milk is less than 4% of a typical neonatal dose and it is considered safe to use while breastfeeding. However, other agents with more published information on use during breastfeeding may be preferable especially while nursing a newborn or preterm infant.[5] • Data on **celecoxib** are limited to a few infants but milk levels were low and adverse effects were not noted when taken short term.[5] More data are needed to determine risk since the drug has a long half-life and high oral absorption.
Oral Contraceptives	Progestin-only formulations	• **Progestin-only contraceptives** are preferred to estrogen-containing ones because the latter, even in low-dose formulations, can decrease milk yield. Oral contraceptives should not be started until breastfeeding is fully established (approximately 6 wk).[89]
Smoking Cessation		• Data on **nicotine patches** are limited but the amount of nicotine and cotinine excreted in breast milk seem to be less than 8% of the weight-adjusted maternal dose[b]. With a 21 mg transdermal patch, nicotine passes into breast milk in amounts equivalent to smoking 17 cigarettes daily. Lower patch strengths of 7 and 14 mg provide proportionately lower amounts of nicotine to the breast-fed infant. No studies on nicotine spray or nicotine gum use in nursing mothers have been reported. Nicotine gum may produce large variations in peak levels when gum is chewed rapidly: fluctuations similar to smoking itself. Some clinicians recommend to wait 2–3 hours after using the gum before breastfeeding.[90] • Data on **varenicline** are lacking but transfer is possible and effect on CNS is a concern.[5]
Thyroid Agents	Thyroid Hormones	• **Levothyroxine** is compatible with breastfeeding. Thyroid hormones cross into breast milk in low amounts. Their presence is not likely to affect the infant's thyroid.[16]
	Antithyroid Agents	• The estimated level of exposure to **propylthiouracil** in breastfeeding infants is less than 1% of the therapeutic dose standardized by weight, and the thyroid function of the infant is not affected.[91] **Methimazole** in doses up to 20 mg/day has been documented not to affect the infant's thyroid function.[92,93,94] For either drug, no adverse effects in breast-fed infants have been reported so far and monitoring of infants' thyroid function is not necessary if development is progressing normally.[94]
Vaccines		• Breastfeeding does not adversely affect immunization of the infant with either live or killed vaccines and may, in fact, improve the immune response to some vaccines. Lactating mothers may safely be given vaccines against rubella, measles, mumps, tetanus, diphtheria, influenza, *Streptococcus pneumoniae*, hepatitis A, hepatitis B, polio and varicella. Inactivated polio vaccine may be safely given to breastfeeding mothers who have not previously been immunized or who are travelling to a highly endemic area.[95]

[a] This list is not exhaustive or definitive. Drugs not listed in the table are not necessarily contraindicated. Individualized risk assessment is required when prescribing any medication to a breastfeeding woman.

[b] Weight-adjusted maternal dose is a mother's dose based on body weight (e.g., mg/kg). Experts recommend that an amount of drug received by the infant via breast milk which is >10% of the weight-adjusted maternal dose should be a theoretical level of concern when considering the acceptability of drug exposure. The estimated amount of drug received by the infant via breast milk is calculated by multiplying the standard milk intake (150 mL/kg/day) by the drug concentration in breast milk.

Abbreviation: GFR = glomerular filtration rate.

Drugs for Nonmedical Use (e.g., Alcohol, Tobacco) (Table 2)

Tobacco smoking and alcohol ingestion are the most common and socially acceptable sources of nonmedicinal drug exposure to breast-fed infants in Canada. Because they so often occur in the same individual, it is difficult to study their independent effects. Increasingly, these drugs are used together with other less fashionable and even illicit drugs such as marijuana and cocaine.

Table 2: Breastfeeding and Nonmedical Use of Drugs

Drug	Comments on Breastfeeding
Alcohol	• Not compatible with breastfeeding. The alcohol metabolizing capacity (alcohol and aldehyde dehydrogenase) is premature throughout the neonatal and infantile period. Overall, motor development is slightly slower in infants breast-fed by mothers who regularly drink alcohol. Chronic or heavy consumers of alcohol should not breastfeed.[5] • Short-term alcohol consumption by nursing mothers reportedly has an immediate effect on the odour characteristics of the milk and the feeding behaviour of their infants, resulting in less consumption of milk.[96] To avoid exposure of the infant to alcohol, breastfeeding mothers should not consume alcohol or should consume no more than one drink 2–3 h before breastfeeding.[5]
Caffeine	• Hypothetically, a nursing infant ingests 0.11% of the maternal dose after the mother drinks 1–2 cups of coffee. This is an insignificant amount of the drug, but it must be remembered that the half-life of caffeine is 80 h in the term newborn and 97.5 h in a premature infant (20–30 times that of an adult). Therefore, repeated ingestion might lead to accumulation of caffeine in the infant during the first 2 wk of postnatal life. This has yet to be studied.
Recreational or Street Drugs	• No systematic studies of recreational or street drug (or drug metabolite) excretion exist.
Tobacco	• Discourage during breastfeeding because there are well-documented health risks to the mother and infant from second-hand smoke. Infant exposure to nicotine is largely through inhalation of second-hand smoke. In mothers unwilling to stop smoking during breastfeeding, it should be noted that breast-fed babies of mothers who continue to smoke have better immunity and less respiratory infections than bottle-fed babies of mothers who continue to smoke.[97] • Nicotine is concentrated in human breast milk.[98,99] One study suggests that cigarette smoking significantly reduces breast milk production.[100] • Encourage nursing mothers to speak to their health care providers regarding options for smoking cessation.

References

1. Kramer MS, Aboud F, Mironova E et al. Breastfeeding and child cognitive development: new evidence from a large randomized trial. *Arch Gen Psychiatry* 2008;65(5):578-84.
2. Verhasselt V, Milcent V, Cazareth J et al. Breast milk-mediated transfer of an antigen induces tolerance and protection from allergic asthma. *Nat Med* 2008;14(2):170-5.
3. Breastfeeding and the use of human milk. American Academy of Pediatrics. Work Group on Breastfeeding. *Pediatrics* 1997;100(6):1035-9.
4. Akus M, Bartick M. Lactation safety recommendations and reliability compared in 10 medication resources. *Ann Pharmacother* 2007;41(9):1352-60.
5. Hale TW. *Medications and mothers' milk.* 13th ed. Amarillo (TX): Pharmasoft Medical Publishing; 2008.
6. Wittels B, Scott DT, Sinatra RS. Exogenous opioids in human breast milk and acute neonatal neurobehavior: a preliminary study. *Anesthesiology* 1990;73(5):864-9.
7. Health Canada; Janssen-Ortho. Important safety information about use of Tylenol with Codeine No. 2, 3, 4 and elixir in nursing mothers and ultra-rapid metabolizers of codeine; October 6, 2008. Available from: www.hc-sc.gc.ca/dhp-mps/alt_formats/hpfb-dgpsa/pdf/medeff/tylenol_codeine_hpc-cps-eng.pdf. Accessed November 15, 2010.
8. Ilett KF, Paech MJ, Page-Sharp M et al. Use of a sparse sampling study design to assess transfer of tramadol and its O-desmethyl metabolite into transitional breast milk. *Br J Clin Pharmacol* 2008;65(5):661-6.
9. Drugs and Lactation Database (LactMed). Bethesda (MD): U.S. National Library of Medicine. Available from: toxnet.nlm.nih.gov/cgi-bin/sis/htmlgen?LACT. Accessed November 1, 2010.
10. Sedlmayr T, Peters F, Raasch W et al. [Clarithromycin, a new macrolide antibiotic. Effectiveness in puerperal infections and pharmacokinetics in breast milk]. *Geburtshilfe Frauenheilkd* 1993;53(7):488-91. German.
11. Kelsey JJ, Moser LR, Jennings JC et al. Presence of azithromycin breast milk concentrations: a case report. *Am J Obstet Gynecol* 1994;170(5 Pt 1):1375-6.
12. American Academy of Pediatrics Committee on Drugs. Transfer of drugs and other chemicals into human milk. *Pediatrics* 2001;108(3):776-89. This policy is a revision of the policy posted on January 1, 1994. A statement of retirement for this policy was published on August 1, 2010.
13. Guillonneau M, de Crepy A, Aufrant C et al. [Breast-feeding is possible in case of maternal treatment with enoxaparin]. *Arch Pediatr* 1996;3(5):513-4. French.
14. Harenberg J, Leber G, Zimmermann R et al. [Prevention of thromboembolism with low-molecular weight heparin in pregnancy]. *Geburtshilfe Frauenheilkd* 1987;47(1):15-8. German.
15. Richter C, Sitzmann J, Lang P et al. Excretion of low molecular weight heparin in human milk. *Br J Clin Pharmacol* 2001;52(6):708-10.
16. Briggs GG, Freeman RK, Yaffe SJ. *Drugs in pregnancy and lactation: a reference guide to fetal and neonatal risk.* 8th ed. Baltimore (MD): Lippincott Williams & Wilkins; 2008.
17. Frey OR, Scheidt P, von Brenndorff AI. Adverse effects in a newborn infant breast-fed by a mother treated with doxepine. *Ann Pharmacother* 1999;33(6):690-3.
18. Birnbaum CS, Cohen LS, Bailey JW et al. Serum concentrations of antidepressants and benzodiazepines in nursing infants: a case series. *Pediatrics* 1999;104(1):e11.
19. Stowe ZN, Hostetter AL, Owens MJ et al. The pharmacokinetics of sertraline excretion into human breast milk: determinants of infant serum concentrations. *J Clin Psychiatry* 2003;64(1):73-80.
20. Dodd S, Stocky A, Buist A et al. Sertraline in paired blood plasma and breast-milk samples from nursing mothers. *Hum Psychopharmacol* 2000;15(4):161-264.
21. Epperson N, Czarkowski KA, Ward-O'Brien D et al. Maternal sertraline treatment and serotonin transport in breast-feeding mother-infant pairs. *Am J Psychiatry* 2001;158(10):1631-7.
22. Hendrick V, Fukuchi A, Altshuler L et al. Use of sertraline, paroxetine and fluvoxamine by nursing women. *Br J Psychiatry* 2001;179:163-6.
23. Begg EJ, Duffull SB, Saunders DA et al. Paroxetine in human milk. *Br J Clin Pharmacol* 1999;48(2):142-7.
24. Ohman R, Hagg S, Carleborg L et al. Excretion of paroxetine into breast milk. *J Clin Psychiatry* 1999;60(8):519-23.
25. Stowe ZN, Cohen LS, Hostetter A et al. Paroxetine in human breast milk and nursing infants. *Am J Psychiatry* 2000;157(2):185-9.
26. Misri S, Kim J, Riggs KW et al. Paroxetine levels in postpartum depressed women, breast milk, and infant serum. *J Clin Psychiatry* 2000;61(11):828-32.
27. Epperson CN, Jatlow P, Czarkowski K et al. Maternal fluoxetine treatment in the postpartum period: effects on platelet serotonin and plasma drug levels in breastfeeding mother-infant pairs. *Pediatrics* 2003;112(5):e425-9.
28. Moretti ME, Sharma A, Bar-Oz B et al. Fluoxetine and its effects on the nursing infant: a prospective cohort study. *Clin Pharmacol Ther* 1999;65(2):141.
29. Kristensen JH, Ilett KF, Hackett LP et al. Distribution and excretion of fluoxetine and norfluoxetine in human milk. *Br J Clin Pharmacol* 1999;48(4):521-7.
30. Taddio A, Ito S, Koren G. Excretion of fluoxetine and its metabolite, norfluoxetine, in human breast milk. *J Clin Pharmacol* 1996;36(1):42-7.
31. Yoshida K, Smith B, Craggs M et al. Fluoxetine in breast-milk and developmental outcome of breast-fed infants. *Br J Psychiatry* 1998;172:175-8.
32. Chambers CD, Anderson PO, Thomas RG et al. Weight gain in infants breast-fed by mothers who take fluoxetine. *Pediatrics* 1999;104(5):e61.
33. Lester BM, Cucca J, Andreozzi L et al. Possible association between fluoxetine hydrochloride and colic in an infant. *J Am Acad Child Adolesc Psychiatry* 1993;32(6):1253-5.
34. Hale TW, Shum S, Grossberg M. Fluoxetine toxicity in a breast-fed infant. *Clin Pediatr (Phila)* 2001;40(12):681-4.
35. Suri R, Stowe ZN, Hendrick V et al. Estimates of nursing infant daily dose of fluoxetine through breast milk. *Biol Psychiatry* 2002;52(5):446-51.
36. Piontek CM, Wisner KL, Perel JM. Serum fluvoxamine levels in breastfed infants. *J Clin Psychiatry* 2001;62(2):111-3.
37. Kristensen JH, Hackett LP, Kohan R et al. The amount of fluvoxamine in milk is unlikely to be a cause of adverse effects in breastfed infants. *J Hum Lact* 2002;18(2):139-43.
38. Rampono J, Kristensen JH, Hackett LP et al. Citalopram and demethylcitalopram in human milk; distribution, excretion and effects in breast fed infants. *Br J Clin Pharmacol* 2000;50(3):263-8.
39. Schmidt K, Olesen OV, Jensen PN. Citalopram and breast-feeding: serum concentration and side effects in the infant. *Biol Psychiatry* 2000;47(2):164-5.
40. Spigset O, Carieborg L, Ohman R et al. Excretion of citalopram in breast milk. *Br J Clin Pharmacol* 1997;44(3):295-8.
41. Heikkinen T, Ekblad U, Kero P et al. Citalopram in pregnancy and lactation. *Clin Pharmacol Ther* 2002;72(2):184-91.
42. Hendrick V, Altshuler L, Wertheimer A et al. Venlafaxine and breast-feeding. *Am J Psychiatry* 2001;158(12):2089-90.
43. Ilett KF, Hackett LP, Dusci LJ et al. Distribution and excretion of venlafaxine and O-desmethylvenlafaxine in human milk. *Br J Clin Pharmacol* 1998;45(5):459-62.
44. Ilett KF, Kristensen JH, Hackett LP et al. Distribution of venlafaxine and its O-desmethyl metabolite in human milk and their effects in breastfed infants. *Br J Clin Pharmacol* 2002;53(1):17-22.
45. Lobo ED, Loghin C, Knadler MP et al. Pharmacokinetics of duloxetine in breast milk and plasma of healthy postpartum women. *Clin Pharmacokinet* 2008;47(2):103-9.
46. Briggs GG, Samson JH, Ambrose PJ et al. Excretion of bupropion in breast milk. *Ann Pharmacother* 1993;27(4):431-3.
47. Baab SW, Peindl KS, Piontek CM et al. Serum bupropion levels in 2 breastfeeding mother-infant pairs. *J Clin Psychiatry* 2002;63(10):910-1.
48. Haas JS, Kaplan CP, Barenboim D et al. Bupropion in breast milk: an exposure assessment for potential treatment to prevent post-partum tobacco use. *Tob Control* 2004;13(1):52-6.
49. Aichhorn W, Whitworth AB, Weiss U et al. Mirtazapine and breast-feeding. *Am J Psychiatry* 2004;161(12):2325.
50. Kristensen JH, Ilett KF, Rampono J et al. Transfer of antidepressant mirtazapine into breast milk. *Br J Clin Pharmacol* 2007;63(3):322-7.
51. Buist A, Dennerstein L, Maguire KP et al. Plasma and human milk concentrations of moclobemide in nursing mothers. *Human Psychopharmacol Clin Exp* 1998;13(8):579-82.
52. Chaudron LH, Schoenecker CJ, Bupropion and breastfeeding: a case of a possible infant seizure. *J Clin Psychiatry* 2004;65(6):881-2.
53. Corriveau D. *Utilisation de Wellbutrin SR chez la femme enceinte et chez la femme allaitant.* In: GlaxoSmithKline, Personal Communication; 2001.
54. Verbeek RK, Ross SG, McKenna EA. Excretion of trazodone in breastmilk. *Br J Clin Pharmacol* 1986;22(3);367-70.
55. Misri S, Corral M, Wardrop AA et al. Quetiapine augmentation in lactation: a series of case reports. *J Clin Psychopharmacol* 2006;26(5):508-11.
56. Misri S, Sivertz K. Tricyclic drugs in pregnancy and lactation: a preliminary report. *Int J Psychiatry Med* 1991;21(2):157-71.
57. Newport DJ, Ritchie JC, Knight BT et al. Venlafaxine in human breast milk and nursing infant plasma: determination of exposure. *J Clin Psychiatry* 2009;70(9):1304-10.
58. Ito S. Drug therapy for breast-feeding women. *N Engl J Med* 2000;343(2):118-26.
59. Mactal-Haaf C, Hoffman M, Kuchta A. Use of anti-infective agents during lactation, Part 3: Antivirals, antifungals, and urinary antiseptics. *J Hum Lact* 2001;17(2):160-6.
60. Ilett KF, Kristensen JH. Drug use and breastfeeding. *Expert Opin Drug Saf* 2005;4(4):745-68.
61. Reed BR. Dermatologic drug use during pregnancy and lactation. *Dermatol Clin* 1997;15(1):197-206.
62. Hilbert J, Radwanski E, Affrime MB et al. Excretion of loratadine in human breast milk. *J Clin Pharmacol* 1988;28(3):234-9.
63. Lucas BD, Purdy CY, Scarim SK et al. Terfenadine pharmacokinetics in breast milk in lactating women. *Clin Pharmacol Ther* 1995;57(4):398-402.
64. Ito S, Blajchman A, Stephenson M et al. Prospective follow-up of adverse reactions in breast-fed infants exposed to maternal medication. *Am J Obstet Gynecol* 1993;168(5):1393-9.
65. Sandstrom B, Regardh CG. Metoprolol excretion into breast milk. *Br J Clin Pharmacol* 1980;9(5):518-9.
66. Ho TK, Moretti ME, Schaeffer IJ et al. Maternal beta-blocker usage and breast feeding in the neonate. *Pediatr Res* 1999;45(4):67A.
67. Schimmel MS, Eidelman AI, Wilschanski MA et al. Toxic effects of atenolol consumed during breast feeding. *J Pediatr* 1989;114(3):476-8.
68. Dumez Y, Tchobroutsky C, Hornych H et al. Neonatal effects of maternal administration of acebutolol. *Br Med J (Clin Res Ed)* 1981;283(6299):1077-9.
69. Boutroy MJ, Bianchetti G, Dubruc C et al. To nurse when receiving acebutolol: is it dangerous for the neonate? *Eur J Clin Pharmacol* 1986;30(6):737-9.
70. Jones HM, Cummings AJ. A study of the transfer of alpha-methyldopa to the human foetus and newborn infant. *Br J Clin Pharmacol* 1978;6(5):432-4.
71. White WB, Andreoli JW, Cohn RD. Alpha-methyldopa disposition in mothers with hypertension and in their breast-fed infants. *Clin Pharmacol Ther* 1985;37(4):387-90.
72. Committee to Advise on Tropical Medicine and Travel (CATMAT). Canadian recommendations for the prevention and treatment of malaria among international travellers. *Can Commun Dis Rep* 2004;30(Suppl 1):1-62. Available from: www.phac-aspc.gc.ca/publicat/ccdr-rmtc/04vol30/30s1/page4-eng.php. Accessed November 15, 2010.
73. Recommendations for the prevention of malaria among travelers. *MMWR Recomm Rep* 1990;39(RR-3):1-10. Available from: www.cdc.gov/mmwr/preview/mmwrhtml/00001584.htm. Accessed November 15, 2010.
74. Viguera AC, Newport DJ, Ritchie J et al. Lithium in breast milk and nursing infants: clinical implications. *Am J Psychiatry* 2007;164(2):342-5.
75. Tunnessen WW, Hertz CG. Toxic effects of lithium in newborn infants: a commentary. *J Pediatr* 1972;81(4):804-7.

76. Sheffield JS, Fish DN, Hollier LM et al. Acyclovir concentrations in human breast milk after valaciclovir administration. *Am J Obstet Gynecol* 2002;186(1):100-2.
77. Siever LJ. The effect of amantadine on prolactin levels and galactorrhea on neuroleptic-treated patients. *J Clin Psychopharmacol* 1981;1(1):2-7.
78. Correa N, Opler LA, Kay SR et al. Amantadine in the treatment of neuroendocrine side effects of neuroleptics. *J Clin Psychoharmacol* 1987;7(2):91-5.
79. Wentges-van Holthe N, van Eijkeren M, van der Laan JW. Oseltamivir and breastfeeding. *Int J Infect Dis* 2008;12(4):451.
80. Tanaka T, Nakajima K, Murashima A et al. Safety of neuraminidase inhibitors against novel influenza A (H1N1) in pregnant and breastfeeding women. *CMAJ* 2009;181(1-2):55-8.
81. Aljazaf K, Hale TW, Ilett KF et al. Pseudoephedrine: effects on milk production in women and estimation of infant exposure via breastmilk. *Br J Clin Pharmacol* 2003;56(1):18-24.
82. Feig DS, Briggs GG, Kraemer JM et al. Transfer of glyburide and glipizide into breast milk. *Diabetes Care* 2005;28(8):1851-5.
83. Everett JA. Use of oral antidiabetic agents during breastfeeding. *J Hum Lact* 1997;13(4):319-21.
84. Plante L, Ferron GM, Unruh M et al. Excretion of pantoprazole in human breast. *J Reprod Med* 2004;49(10):825-7.
85. Marshall JK, Thompson AB, Armstrong D. Omeprazole for refractory gastroesophageal reflux disease during pregnancy and lactation. *Can J Gastroenterol* 1998;12(3):225-7.
86. Ferreira E. *Grossesse et allaitement: guide thérapeutique*. Montréal (QC): CHU Sainte Justine; 2007.
87. Ost L, Wettrell G, Bjorkhem I et al. Prednisolone excretion in human milk. *J Pediatr* 1985;106(6):1008-11.
88. Porto I. Antiparasitic drugs and lactation: focus on anthelmintics, scabicides, and pediculicides. *J Hum Lact* 2003;19(4):421-5.
89. Black A, Francoeur D, Rowe T et al. Canadian contraception consensus. *J Obstet Gynaecol Can* 2004;26(4):347-87, 389-436.
90. Ilett KF, Hale TW, Page-Sharp M et al. Use of nicotine patches in breast-feeding mothers: transfer of nicotine and cotinine into human milk. *Clin Pharmacol Ther* 2003;74(6):516-24.
91. Kampmann JP, Johansen K, Hansen JM et al. Propylthiouracil in human milk. Revision of a dogma. *Lancet* 1980;1(8171):736-7.
92. Azizi F. Effect of methimazole treatment of maternal thyrotoxicosis on thyroid function in breast-feeding infants. *J Pediatr* 1996;128(6):855-8.
93. Azizi F, Khoshniat M, Bahrainian M et al. Thyroid function and intellectual development of infants nursed by mothers taking methimazole. *J Clin Endocrinol Metab* 2000;85(9):3233-8.
94. Mandel SJ, Cooper DS. The use of antithyroid drugs in pregnancy and lactation. *J Clin Endocrinol Metab* 2001;86(6):2354-9.
95. National Advisory Committee on Immunization (NACI). *Canadian immunization guide*. 7th ed. Ottawa (ON): Public Health Agency of Canada, Infectious Disease and Emergency Preparedness Branch, Centre for Infectious Disease and Control; 2006. Available from: www.phac-aspc.gc.ca/publicat/cig-gci/pdf/cig-gci-2006_e.pdf. Accessed November 15, 2010.
96. Mennella JA, Beauchamp GK. The transfer of alcohol to human milk. Effects on flavor and the infant's behavior. *N Engl J Med* 1991;325(14):981-5.
97. Dorea JG. Maternal smoking and infant feeding: breastfeeding is better and safer. *Matern Child Health J* 2007;11(3):287-91.
98. Luck W, Nau H. Nicotine and cotinine concentrations in serum and milk of nursing smokers. *Br J Clin Pharmacol* 1984;18(1):9-15.
99. Hardee GE, Stewart T, Capomacchia AC. Tobacco smoke xenobiotic compound appearance in mothers' milk after involuntary smoke exposures. I. Nicotine and cotinine. *Toxicol Lett* 1983;15(2-3):109-12.
100. Hopkinson JM, Schanler RJ, Fraley JK et al. Milk production by mothers of premature infants: influence of cigarette smoking. *Pediatrics* 1992;90(6):934-8.

Drugs in Dentistry

D.A. Haas, DDS, PhD, FRCDC

Date of Preparation: September 2007

Date of Revision: October 2010

The following is a summary of the use of analgesics, anti-infectives, anesthetics and medical emergency drugs in dentistry. This information is not intended to present a comprehensive review; the reader is therefore encouraged to seek additional and confirmatory information.

Analgesics[1,2,3] (Figure 1)

Consider the following points in the use of analgesics:

- Eliminate the source of pain, if possible.
- Individualize regimens.
- Optimize dose and frequency before switching.
- Maximize the nonopioid before adding the opioid.
- Consider a loading dose and/or a preoperative dose for nonsteroidal anti-inflammatory drugs (NSAIDs).
- Avoid chronic use of any analgesic.
- Reduce the dose in older individuals.

Be aware of the contraindications and cautions for NSAIDs, including ASA (see also individual product monographs and CPhA monographs as well as comprehensive drug interaction references):

- Allergic reaction to any NSAID, including ASA
- ASA-induced asthma and nasal polyps
- Gastrointestinal inflammatory or ulcerative disease
- History of bleeding disorder or concurrent use of anticoagulants
- Concurrent use of ACE inhibitors, loop diuretics or beta-blockers, particularly in patients with heart failure (avoid NSAIDs or limit use to ≤4 days)
- Concurrent use of antineoplastic doses of methotrexate
- Concurrent use of lithium
- Concurrent use of digoxin in older individuals or those with renal disease
- For ASA: concurrent use of sulfonylurea oral hypoglycemics.

Be aware of the contraindications and cautions for opioids:

- Severe respiratory disease
- Severe inflammatory bowel disease
- Concurrent use of alcohol or other CNS depressants.

Table 1 and Table 2 list common analgesics and corresponding pediatric and adult doses recommended to treat orofacial pain.

Figure 1: Management of Acute Postoperative Dental Pain in Adults

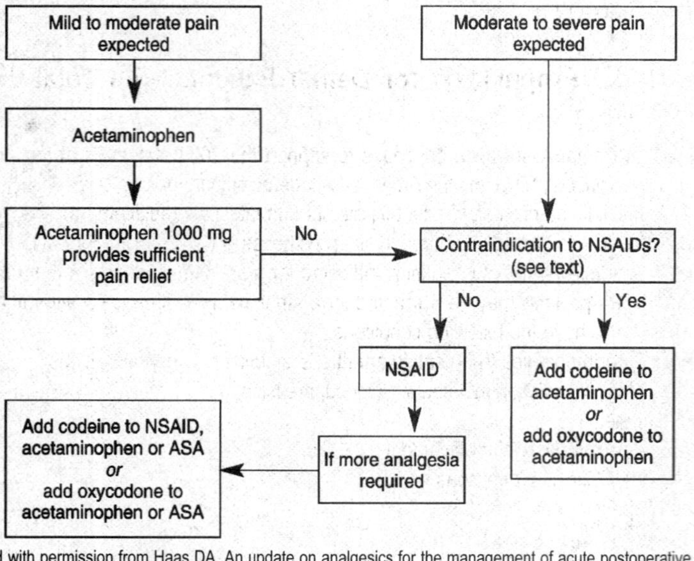

Adapted with permission from Haas DA. An update on analgesics for the management of acute postoperative dental pain. *J Can Dent Assoc* 2002;68(8):476-82.

Table 1: Analgesics for Orofacial Pain: Pediatric Doses

Drug	Pediatric Dose	Daily Maximum[a]
Acetaminophen	10–15 mg/kg Q4–6H po	65 mg/kg or 2600 mg
Codeine	0.5–1 mg/kg Q4–6H po	3 mg/kg[b]
Ibuprofen	10 mg/kg Q6–8H po	40 mg/kg or 2400 mg

[a] Maximum doses are for acute pain only.
[b] Do not exceed 60 mg/dose.

Table 2: Analgesics for Orofacial Pain: Adult Doses

Drug	Adult Dose	Daily Maximum[a]
Nonopioids		
Simple Analgesics		
Acetaminophen	325–1000 mg Q4–6H po	4000 mg
NSAIDs[b]		
ASA	325–1000 mg Q4–6H po	4000 mg
Celecoxib	200 mg daily to BID po	400 mg
Diflunisal	1000 mg × 1 dose po, then 500 mg Q12H	1500 mg
Etodolac	200–400 mg Q6–8H po	1200 mg
Floctafenine	200–400 mg Q6–8H po	1200 mg
Flurbiprofen	50–100 mg Q4–6H po	300 mg
Ibuprofen	400 mg Q4–6H po	2400 mg
Ketoprofen	25–50 mg Q6–8H po	300 mg
Ketorolac	10 mg Q4–6H po	40 mg
Naproxen	500 mg × 1 dose po, then 250 mg Q6–8H	1250 mg
Naproxen sodium	550 mg × 1 dose po, then 275 mg Q6–8H	1375 mg
Opioids[c]		
Codeine	30–60 mg Q4–6H po	[d]
Oxycodone	5–10 mg Q4–6H po	[d]

[a] Maximum doses are for acute pain only.
[b] Use for shortest possible time.
[c] In combination with a nonopioid.
[d] Maximum doses for opioids are not established. Base dosing on individual response and side effects.

Anti-infectives[4]

Consider the following points when using antibiotics:

- Use only when there is an indication.
- Use only when the risk-benefit ratio is favourable.
- They are not a substitute for establishing adequate drainage.
- Choose an effective agent with the narrowest spectrum of activity.
- Prescribe a therapeutic dose.
- Consider a loading dose.
- Prescribe at an appropriate frequency.
- Prescribe for an appropriate duration.
- Choose the drug with the fewest side effects.
- Consider laboratory culture and sensitivity tests to target specific bacteria with antibiotics identified as effective.
- Recognize that antibiotics encourage development of resistance if used for too long and/or at suboptimal doses.
- In superficial infections, consider alternatives to antibiotics such as topical debridement and application of topical antiseptics when appropriate.
- Consider individual patient factors such as age, allergies and drug interactions (especially with erythromycin, clarithromycin, metronidazole, tetracyclines and azole antifungals, e.g., ketoconazole, fluconazole, itraconazole); consult individual product monographs and drug interaction references.
- Consider cost.

Table 3 lists common antibiotics and corresponding adult doses recommended for orofacial infections.

Table 4 lists antifungals and corresponding adult doses recommended for the treatment of oral candidiasis.

Table 3: Antibacterial Dosages for Orofacial Infections[2]

Drug	Recommended Adult Dose
Amoxicillin	250–500 mg TID po
Amoxicillin/clavulanate	250–500 mg (amoxicillin) TID po
Cephalexin	250–500 mg QID po
Clarithromycin	250–500 mg BID po
Clindamycin	150–300 mg QID po
Doxycycline	100 mg once daily or BID po
Erythromycin	250–500 mg QID po
Metronidazole	250–500 mg TID po
Penicillin V	300–600 mg QID po

Table 4: Antifungals for the Treatment of Oral Candidiasis[5]

Drug	Adult Dose
Immunocompetent Patients	
Nystatin oral suspension	Swish and swallow 400 000–600 000 units QID × 14 days
Immunocompromised Patients	
Nystatin oral suspension	Swish and swallow 500 000–1 000 000 units QID × 14 days
Fluconazole	100 mg once daily po × 1–2 wk
Itraconazole	200 mg once daily po × 1–2 wk
Ketoconazole	200–400 mg once daily po × 1–2 wk

Endocarditis Prophylaxis[6]

Table 5 lists cardiac conditions associated with the highest risk of adverse outcome from infective endocarditis, in which antibacterial coverage is considered reasonable for patients undergoing certain dental procedures.[6]

Table 5: Cardiac Conditions Associated with the Highest Risk of Adverse Outcome from Endocarditis for which Prophylaxis with Dental Procedures is Reasonable

Prosthetic cardiac valve, or prosthetic material used for cardiac valve repair

Previous infective endocarditis

Congenital heart disease (CHD)[a]

- Unrepaired cyanotic CHD, including palliative shunts and conduits
- Completely repaired congenital heart defect with prosthetic material or device, whether placed by surgery or by catheter intervention, during the first 6 months after the procedure
- Repaired CHD with residual defects at the site or adjacent to the site of a prosthetic patch or prosthetic device[b]

Cardiac transplantation recipients who develop cardiac valvulopathy

[a] Except for conditions listed above, antibacterial prophylaxis is no longer recommended for any other form of CHD.
[b] Prophylaxis is reasonable because endothelialization of prosthetic material occurs within 6 months following the procedure.

Antibacterial prophylaxis is reasonable for patients with cardiac conditions listed in Table 5 who are undergoing certain dental procedures (see Table 6).[6]

Table 6: Dental Procedures for which Endocarditis Prophylaxis is Reasonable for Patients with Cardiac Conditions in Table 5

Endocarditis prophylaxis is **reasonable** for all dental procedures that involve manipulation of gingival tissue or the periapical region of teeth or perforation of the oral mucosa

Endocarditis prophylaxis is **not required** for the following dental procedures:

- routine local anesthetic injections (nonintraligamentary) through noninfected tissue
- placement of removable prosthodontic or orthodontic appliances
- fluoride treatments
- taking of oral radiographs
- orthodontic appliance adjustment
- placement of orthodontic brackets
- shedding of primary teeth
- bleeding from trauma to the lips or oral mucosa

The recommended antibacterial regimens for endocarditis prophylaxis in dental procedures[6] are listed in Table 7.

Table 7: Antibacterial Regimens for Endocarditis Prophylaxis in Dental Procedures[a]

Drug	Adult Dose (30–60 minutes before procedure)	Pediatric Dose[b] (30–60 minutes before procedure)
Standard Regimen		
Amoxicillin	2 g po	50 mg/kg po
Unable to Take Oral Medications		
Ampicillin	2 g im[c] or iv	50 mg/kg im[c] or iv
or		
Cefazolin	1 g im[c] or iv	50 mg/kg im[c] or iv
or		
Ceftriaxone	1 g im[c] or iv	50 mg/kg im[c] or iv
Allergic to Penicillins		
Clindamycin	600 mg po	20 mg/kg po
or		
Cephalexin[d,e]	2 g po	50 mg/kg po
or		
Clarithromycin	500 mg po	15 mg/kg po
or		
Azithromycin	500 mg po	15 mg/kg po
Allergic to Penicillins and Unable to Take Oral Medications		
Clindamycin	600 mg im[c] or iv	20 mg/kg iv
or		
Cefazolin[e]	1 g im[c] or iv	50 mg/kg im[c] or iv
or		
Ceftriaxone[e]	1 g im[c] or iv	50 mg/kg im[c] or iv

[a] See Table 5 and Table 6.
[b] Pediatric dose should not exceed adult dose.
[c] Avoid im injections in anticoagulated patients.
[d] Or other first- or second-generation oral cephalosporin in equivalent adult or pediatric dosage.
[e] Cephalosporins should not be used in individuals with immediate-type hypersensitivity reaction (urticaria, angioedema or anaphylaxis) to penicillins.

Antibacterial Prophylaxis for Dental Patients with Total Joint Replacements

The Canadian Dental Association continues to support the 2003 statement of the American Dental Association (ADA) and the American Academy of Orthopaedic Surgeons (AAOS) concerning antibiotic prophylaxis for dental patients with total joint replacements.[7,8] Antibacterial administration to prevent infection of joint prostheses is not indicated for patients with pins, plates and screws, nor is it routinely indicated for most dental patients with total joint replacements. Prophylaxis may be warranted for a small number of patients with total joint replacements who have the following conditions:

- Inflammatory arthropathies (rheumatoid arthritis, systemic lupus erythematosus)
- Disease-, drug- or radiation-induced immunosuppression
- Type 1 diabetes
- First two years following joint placement
- Previous prosthetic joint infections
- Malnourishment
- Hemophilia
- HIV infection
- Malignancy

Refer to Table 6 for dental procedures requiring antibacterial prophylaxis and to Table 8 for antibacterial regimens that may be used in these cases. Practitioners must use clinical judgment in selecting antibacterial prophylaxis for dental patients with total joint replacements.

Table 8: Antibacterial Prophylaxis for Dental Patients with a Total Joint Prosthesis

Drug	Adult Dose
Standard Regimen	
Amoxicillin or cephalexin[a]	2 g po to be taken 1 h before procedure
Penicillin Allergy	
Clindamycin	600 mg po to be taken 1 h before procedure
Unable to Take Oral Medications	
Standard Regimen	
Ampicillin	2 g im or iv to be given 1 h before procedure
or	
Cefazolin[a]	1 g im or iv to be given 1 h before procedure
Penicillin Allergy	
Clindamycin	600 mg iv to be given 1 h before procedure

[a] Cephalosporins should not be used in individuals with a history of immediate-type hypersensitivity reactions (urticaria, angioedema or anaphylaxis) to penicillins.

Local Anesthetics

Potential Interactions with Epinephrine or Levonordefrin:[9,10,11] Adding epinephrine or levonordefrin to the local anesthetic formulation improves the depth and duration of the local anesthetic block. However, exercise caution if a patient has a history of significant cardiovascular disease or is concomitantly taking any of the following drugs:

- **Nonselective beta-blockers** such as nadolol, pindolol, propranolol, sotalol or timolol (may result in increased blood pressure)
- **Tricyclic antidepressants** (may result in increased blood pressure and cardiac dysrhythmias).

In these cases, use the lowest effective dose of epinephrine and consider a maximum of <40 µg.[12] The administration of levonordefrin is contraindicated in individuals taking tricyclic antidepressants. For those with cardiovascular disease or taking nonselective beta-blockers, use the lowest effective dose of levonordefrin and consider a maximum of <200 µg.

Avoid epinephrine altogether in patients who have ingested **cocaine** within the previous 24 hours, as there is increased risk of cardiac dysrhythmias and increased blood pressure.

The vasoconstrictor dose per 1.8 mL dental cartridge is as follows:

1 cartridge of 1:200 000 epinephrine = 9 µg

1 cartridge of 1:100 000 epinephrine = 18 µg

1 cartridge of 1:50 000 epinephrine = 36 µg

1 cartridge of 1:20 000 levonordefrin = 90 µg.

The maximum recommended doses of local anesthetics and their expected duration of action are listed in Table 9 and Table 10, respectively.

Table 9: Maximum Recommended Doses of Local Anesthetics[13,14,15,16]

Drug	Maximum Dose (mg/kg)	Maximum Number of Cartridges[a]
Articaine 4% with epinephrine 1:100 000 or 1:200 000	7	7
Bupivacaine[b] 0.5% with epinephrine 1:200 000	2	10
Lidocaine 2% with epinephrine 1:50 000 or 1:100 000	7	13
Mepivacaine 2% with levonordefrin 1:20 000	6.6	11
Mepivacaine 3% plain	6.6	7
Prilocaine 4% plain	8	8
Prilocaine 4% with epinephrine 1:200 000	8	8

[a] 1.8 mL volume
[b] Not recommended for children.

Table 10: Expected Duration of Action (minutes) of Local Anesthetics[13,14,15,16]

	Maxillary Infiltration		Inferior Alveolar Block	
Drug	Tooth Pulp	Soft Tissue	Tooth Pulp	Soft Tissue
Articaine 4% with epinephrine 1:100 000 or 1:200 000	60	170	90	220
Bupivacaine 0.5% with epinephrine 1:200 000	40	340	240	440
Lidocaine 2% with epinephrine 1:50 000 or 1:100 000	60	170	85	190
Mepivacaine 2% with levonordefrin 1:20 000	50	130	75	185
Mepivacaine 3% plain	25	90	40	165
Prilocaine 4% plain	20	105	55	190
Prilocaine 4% with epinephrine 1:200 000	40	140	60	220

Medical Emergencies[17,18,19,20]

Treatment of a medical emergency in a dental office begins with assessment and, if necessary, treatment of airway, breathing and circulation (cardiopulmonary resuscitation). Most often, only after these basics are addressed should the drugs listed in Table 11 be considered. They should, however, be readily available for such emergencies. A sugar source such as orange juice or nondiet soft drink should be readily available for use in the management of hypoglycemic reactions. Additional agents may be appropriate depending on the nature of the dental practice.

Table 11: Drugs for Medical Emergencies

Drug	Indication	Initial Adult Dose	Initial Pediatric Dose[a]
Oxygen	Most medical emergencies	100% inhalation	100% inhalation
Epinephrine[b]	Anaphylaxis	0.3–0.5 mg im or 0.1 mg iv	0.01 mg/kg im or iv
	Asthmatic bronchospasm unresponsive to salbutamol	0.3–0.5 mg im or 0.1 mg iv	0.01 mg/kg im or iv
	Cardiac arrest	1 mg iv	0.01 mg/kg iv
ASA	Suspected MI or unstable angina	160[c]–325 mg orally; chewing is preferable to just swallowing (single dose). Enteric-coated ASA is not recommended unless it is chewed.	N/A
Diphenhydramine	Allergic reactions	25–50 mg iv or im	1 mg/kg iv or im
Nitroglycerin	Angina pectoris	0.3–0.6 mg sublingually	N/A
Salbutamol	Asthmatic bronchospasm	200 µg (2 puffs) by metered dose inhaler	100 µg (1 puff) by metered dose inhaler

[a] The total pediatric dose should not exceed the recommended adult dose.
[b] The dose suggested for the im route is also appropriate for intralingual or sublingual injection.
[c] For 160 mg dose, 2 × 80 mg children's chewable tablets may be used.
Abbreviations: MI = myocardial infarction; N/A = not applicable.

Suggested Readings

1. Malamed SF. *Handbook of local anesthesia*. 5th ed. St. Louis (MO): Mosby; 2004.
2. Malamed SF, Robbins KS. *Medical emergencies in the dental office*. 6th ed. St. Louis (MO): Mosby; 2007.
3. Pallasch TJ. Antibiotics for acute orofacial infections. *J Calif Dent Assoc* 1993;21(2):34-44.
4. Peterson LJ. Principles of antibiotic therapy. In: Topazian RG, Goldberg MH. *Oral and maxillofacial infections*. 3rd ed. Philadelphia (PA): Saunders; 1994.
5. Yagiela JA, Dowd FJ, Johnson BS, editors. *Pharmacology and therapeutics for dentistry*. 6th ed. St. Louis (MO): Mosby/Elsevier; 2011.

References

1. Haas DA. Adverse drug interactions in dental practice: interactions associated with analgesics, Part III in a series. *J Am Dent Assoc* 1999;130(3):397-407.
2. United States Pharmacopeial Convention. *USP DI Volume 1: Drug information for the health care professional.* 24th ed. Englewood (CO): Micromedex; 2004.
3. Haas DA. An update on analgesics for the management of acute postoperative dental pain. *J Can Dent Assoc* 2002;68(8):476-82.
4. Haas DA, Epstein JB, Eggert FM. Antimicrobial resistance: dentistry's role. *J Can Dent Assoc* 1998;64(7):496-502.
5. Levine M, Lexchin J, Pellizzari R, editors. *Drugs of choice: a formulary for general practice.* 3rd ed. Ottawa (ON): Canadian Medical Association; 1998. p. 78.
6. Wilson W, Taubert KA, Gewitz M et al. Prevention of infective endocarditis: guidelines from the American Heart Association: a guideline from the American Heart Association Rheumatic Fever, Endocarditis, and Kawasaki Disease Committee, Council on Cardiovascular Disease in the Young, and the Council on Clinical Cardiology, Council on Cardiovascular Surgery and Anesthesia, and the Quality of Care and Outcomes Research Interdisciplinary Working Group. *Circulation* 2007;116(15):1736-54.
7. American Dental Association; American Academy of Orthopedic Surgeons. Antibiotic prophylaxis for dental patients with total joint replacements. *J Am Dent Assoc* 2003;134(7):895-9.
8. Canadian Dental Association. *CDA's response to updated AAOS statement on antibiotic prophylaxis.* Ottawa (ON): CDA. Available from: www.cda-adc.ca/en/cda/news_events/media/dentistry_news/2009/06_09_09_aaos_statement.asp. Accessed October 4, 2010.
9. Becker DE. Drug interactions in dental practice: a summary of facts and controversies. *Compendium* 1994;15(10):1228-44.
10. Perusse R, Goulet JP, Turcotte JY. Contraindications to vasoconstrictors in dentistry: Part I. Cardiovascular diseases. *Oral Surg Oral Med Oral Pathol* 1992;74(5):679-86.
11. Yagiela JA. Adverse drug interactions in dental practice: interactions associated with vasoconstrictors. Part V of a series. *J Am Dent Assoc* 1999;130(5):701-9.
12. Malamed SF. *Handbook of local anesthesia.* 5th ed. St. Louis (MO): Mosby; 2004.
13. Jastak JT, Yagiela JA, Donaldson D, editors. *Local anesthesia of the oral cavity.* Philadelphia (PA): Saunders; 1995.
14. Yagiela JA, Dowd FJ, Johnson BS, editors. *Pharmacology and therapeutics for dentistry.* 6th ed. St. Louis (MO): Mosby/Elsevier; 2011.
15. Haas DA. An update on local anesthetics in dentistry. *J Can Dent Assoc* 2002;68(9):546-51.
16. Yagiela J. Local anesthetics. In: Dionne RA, Phero JC, Becker DE, editors. *Management of pain & anxiety in the dental office.* Philadelphia (PA): Saunders; 2002. p. 78-96.
17. 2005 American Heart Association guidelines for cardiopulmonary resuscitation and emergency cardiovascular care. Part 7.2: Management of cardiac arrest. *Circulation* 2005;112(24 Suppl):IV58-66. Available from: circ.ahajournals.org/cgi/reprint/112/24_suppl/IV-58. Accessed October 4, 2010.
18. Ewan PW. Anaphylaxis. *BMJ* 1998;316(7142):1442-5.
19. Malamed SF, Robbins KS. *Medical emergencies in the dental office.* 6th ed. St. Louis (MO): Mosby; 2007.
20. Haas DA. Emergency drugs. *Dent Clin North Am* 2002;46(4):815-30.

Routine Immunization Schedules

K. Slayter, PharmD

Date of Revision: November 2010

The following is an overview of routine immunization schedules for infants and children (Table 1) and adults (Table 2, Table 3). This information is not intended to present a comprehensive review; the reader is therefore encouraged to seek additional and confirmatory information. Each province/territory establishes its own routine immunization program and the reader should contact local public health authorities for details.

The ease and value of routine immunization make it an effective preventive measure against infectious diseases. Immunization carried out as recommended in the following schedules provide basic protection for most people against the diseases listed.

Following a standard schedule ensures complete and adequate protection. However, modifications to the recommended schedule may be necessary because of missed appointments or intercurrent illness. Interruption of a recommended series does not require starting the series over again, regardless of the interval elapsed.

Similar vaccines are available from different manufacturers but may not be identical. It is therefore essential to read the manufacturer's package insert. For further information consult the *Canadian Immunization Guide*, 7th ed. [www.phac-aspc.gc.ca/publicat/cig-gci/pdf/cig-gci-2006_e.pdf] and supplementary statements published by the National Advisory Committee on Immunization.[1]

Table 1: Routine Immunization Schedules for Infants and Children[1]

		Vaccine or Toxoid											
	Age/Timing	DTaP[a]	IPV[a]	Hib[a,b]	MMR	Td[c] or Tdap[c]	HBV[d] (3 doses)	Varicella[e,f]	PCV[g]	MCV[h]	Flu[i]	HPV[j]	Rotavirus[k]
Infants and Children	2 months	X	X	X			Infancy		X[l]	X[m]			Infancy
	4 months	X	X	X					X	X			
	6 months	X	X[n]	X			or		X[o]	X[p]	X[q]		
	12 months				X			X	X	X[r]			
	18 months	X	X	X	X[t] or			X[e] or					
	4–6 years	X[s]	X[s]		X[t]			X[e]					
	14–16 years					X	9–13 years[d]			X[u]		9–26 years[j]	
Children <7 Years of Age Not Immunized in Early Infancy	1st visit	X	X	X	X[v]			X	X[l]	X[m]			
	2 months after 1st visit	X	X	X[w]	X[t]			X	X[l]	X[m]			
	2 months after 2nd visit	X	X[n]						X[l]				
	6–12 months after 3rd visit	X	X	X[w]									
	4–6 years of age[w]	X[s]	X[s]										
	14–16 years of age					X	9–13 years[d]						
Children ≥7 Years of Age Not Immunized in Early Infancy	1st visit		X	X[x]	X	X		X		X			
	2 months after 1st visit		X		X[t]	X		X[e]					
	6–12 months after 2nd visit		X			X							
	10 years after 3rd visit					X	9–13 years[d]						

[a] It is preferable to use products in which diphtheria toxoid is combined with acellular pertussis vaccine and tetanus toxoid (DTaP), with or without inactivated poliomyelitis vaccine and *Haemophilus influenzae* b conjugate vaccine.

[b] Hib schedule shown is for PRP-T (Act-HIB) vaccine. If PRP-OMP is used (PedVax HIB), give at 2, 4 and 12 months of age.

[c] Td and Tdap combined, adsorbed, "adult type" preparations for use in persons ≥7 years of age contain less diphtheria toxoid and pertussis antigens than preparations given to younger children and are less likely to cause reactions in older persons.

[d] Hepatitis B vaccine can be routinely given to infants, children and preadolescents (9–13 years); three doses at 0-, 1- and 6-month intervals are preferred. Administer the second dose at least 1 month after the first dose. The third dose should be administered at least 2 months after the second dose. Alternatively, adolescents 11–15 years of age may be given a two-dose regimen of adult formulation Recombivax HB (10 µg/dose). The second dose is administered 4–6 months after the first dose.

[e] Varicella-susceptible healthy children aged 12 months to 12 years should receive two doses of varicella vaccine. The doses should be given at least 6 weeks to 3 months apart depending on vaccines used. Providers may find it optimal to administer the first dose at 12–15 months and the second dose at 18 months or at school entry (4–6 years) depending on the provincial/territorial policy. This can be given as MMRV combined vaccine. Varicella-susceptible individuals ≥13 years of age should receive two doses at least 6 weeks apart. MMRV is only licensed for use in children ≤12 years of age.[2,3]

[f] Live vaccines such as the MMR and varicella can be given concurrently but at separate sites. If not given concurrently, then they should be given at least 4 weeks apart.

[g] A pneumococcal conjugate vaccine (PCV7, PCV10, PCV13)[4] should be used for children <2 years of age because the pneumococcal polysaccharide vaccine is ineffective in this age group. Either type of vaccine may be used for children >2 years old; however, the conjugate vaccines are preferred for children up to the age of 5.

[h] The meningococcal C conjugate vaccine (MCV1) should be used for children <2 years of age because the meningococcal polysaccharide vaccine (MPSV4) is relatively ineffective in this age group. The polysaccharide vaccine is effective in children >2 years old; however, the conjugate vaccine provides better protection and is recommended for routine childhood immunization. Meningococcal polysaccharide diphtheria toxoid conjugate vaccine (MCV4) is recommended in children ≥2 years in high-risk groups such as those with asplenia and complement deficiencies.[5] In addition to the routine use of MCV1 in children <2 years, high-risk children (e.g., those with primary antibody deficiency) should receive MCV4 after their second birthdays.[5,6] For children 2–10 years in high-risk groups, MCV4 is recommended followed by the administration of MCV1 given 1 month later.[5]

[i] Priority should be given to the following children who are at high risk: healthy children aged 6 months to 4 years of age,[7] children with chronic cardiac, pulmonary (e.g., cystic fibrosis and asthma) or other chronic disorders (e.g., diabetes), children and adolescents (6 mo–18 years) with conditions treated for long periods with ASA. (See Table 2 for information on Adults).

[j] For females aged 9–13 years or older (<26 years), give 3 doses at 0-, 2- and 6-month intervals (Gardasil — quadrivalent HPV vaccine).[8] Gardasil is also indicated in males aged 9–13 years or older (<26 years) but this is not yet addressed by the National Advisory Committee on Immunization. A bivalent vaccine (Cervarix) is also available and indicated for females 10–25 years of age and administered as 3 doses at 0-, 1- and 6-month intervals.

(cont'd)

Table 1: Routine Immunization Schedules for Infants and Children[1] *(cont'd)*

[k] The live, oral, rotavirus vaccines can be routinely given to infants. Administer 2 or 3 doses, depending on the preparation used, with the first dose given between 6 and 15 weeks of age. Each subsequent dose should be administered at least 4 weeks apart. All doses should be administered by 32 weeks of age.[9,10] Avoid in immunocompromised infants.
[l] One to four doses depending on the age at first dose. For recommended schedule and number of doses refer to the current *Update on the Use of Conjugate Pneumococcal Vaccines in Childhood*[11] or the individual product monographs in the monograph section of *CPS*.
[m] One to three doses depending on the age at first dose. Infants <4 months old should receive three doses given at least 4 weeks apart. Children aged 4–11 months who have not previously received the vaccine should be immunized with two doses given at least 4 weeks apart. Children ≥12 months should receive one dose. Although these recommendations differ from the product monograph, they have been shown to be effective.
[n] This dose of polio vaccine is not needed routinely, but can be included for convenience.
[o] For PCV-7, a 3-dose schedule may be considered with doses given at 2, 4 and 11–12 months of age.
[p] Omit this dose if NeisVac-C is used. The schedule approved for infants from 2 to 12 months of age is two doses given two or more months apart.
[q] Children 6 months to <9 years of age require 2 doses 1 month apart if previously unvaccinated. If the child has received one or more doses during a previous vaccination season, the second dose is not needed. Live attenuated influenza vaccine (FluMist) should only be administered to children ≥2 years of age.
[r] If meningococcal C conjugate vaccine is given to infants <12 months, a booster should be given in the second year of life (age 12–23 months).
[s] Omit this dose if the fourth dose of DTaP and polio was given after the fourth birthday.
[t] A second dose of MMR is recommended, at least 1 month after the first dose given for better measles protection. It is usually given at 18 months of age or with school entry vaccinations at 4–6 years of age (depending on the provincial/territorial policy). Can be given as the combined MMRV vaccine.
[u] A dose should be given in early adolescence, ideally around 12 years of age, to ensure protection in the peak period for infection beyond infancy.[6] For routine immunization of adolescents 11–24 years of age, MCV1 or MCV4 can be used.[5]
[v] MMR should be given shortly after the first birthday.
[w] Recommended schedule and number of doses depend on the product used and the age of the child when vaccination is begun (see the current *Canadian Immunization Guide* or the product monograph for specific recommendations). Not required past age 5.
[x] Recommended in immunocompromised children >5 years of age who are at increased risk of invasive Hib infection, e.g., asplenia (see the current *Canadian Immunization Guide* for specific recommendations).

Abbreviations: DTaP = diphtheria, tetanus and acellular pertussis; HBV = hepatitis B virus; Hib = Haemophilus influenzae type b; HPV = human papillomavirus; IPV = inactivated poliovirus; MCV = meningococcal conjugate vaccine; MCV1 = meningococcal serogroup C conjugate vaccine; MCV4 = meningococcal serogroups A/C/Y/W-135 conjugate vaccine; MPSV4 = meningococcal serogroups A/C/Y/W-135 polysaccharide vaccine; MMR = measles, mumps and rubella; MMRV = measles, mumps, rubella and varicella; PCV = pneumococcal 7, 10 or 13 valent conjugate vaccine; PRP-OMP = polyribosylribitol phosphate capsular polysaccharide of Hib-outer membrane protein [meningococcal protein conjugate]; PRP-T = PRP-tetanus protein conjugate; Td = tetanus and diphtheria, adult formulation; Tdap = tetanus, diphtheria and acellular pertussis, adult formulation

Canadian Immunization Guide, Public Health Agency of Canada, 2006©. Adapted and reproduced with the permission of the Minister of Public Works and Government Services Canada, 2010.

Table 2: Routine Immunization for Adults[1]

Vaccine or Toxoid	Indication and Schedule	Comments
Diphtheria (adult preparation)	All adults.	• The need for regular boosters during adult life has not been established.
	Give every 10 years[a]. Preferably given with tetanus toxoid as Td.	• Acceptable options for adult booster doses are 10-year intervals or, as a minimum, review immunization status at least once during adult life and offer a single dose of Td to those who have not had one within the previous 10 years. • In addition, persons who are travelling to areas where they are likely to be exposed to diphtheria may be offered a booster dose of Td if more than 10 years have elapsed since their most recent booster. Close contacts of an active case of diphtheria who are not known to be immunized or have not received a booster within the last 10 years may also be offered a booster dose.
	For adults that have not previously received a dose of acellular pertussis vaccine, it is recommended that a single Td booster dose be replaced by combined Tdap.	• Usually given with tetanus toxoid as Td. See comments in Tetanus section for recommendation in pregnant women.
Haemophilus	For adults at risk of invasive *Haemophilus influenzae* type b infection.	• Individuals at risk include: - persons with functional and anatomic asplenia, congenital immunodeficiency (e.g., defects in antibody production, complement deficiencies, cell-mediated defects); persons with chronic renal disease or on dialysis; persons undergoing solid organ transplantation, bone marrow transplantation; persons with HIV/AIDS. See the current *Canadian Immunization Guide* for specific recommendations.
Hepatitis A	For individuals at risk of infection or at increased risk of severe Hepatitis A. Give two doses 6 months apart.	• Individuals at risk include: - travellers to endemic areas such as Canadian armed forces and emergency relief workers; residents in communities with high endemic rates; injection drug users; MSM; patients with chronic liver disease; patients who receive hepatotoxic drugs; patients with hemophilia who receive clotting factors from plasma; workers such as veterinarians and zoo-keepers who handle non-human primates; researchers such as vaccine developers who are exposed to hepatitis A; patients with disease conditions that necessitate future use of hepatotoxic drugs.
Hepatitis B	For individuals at risk of infection or at increased risk of severe Hepatitis B. Give 3 doses in total at 0, 1 and 6 months.	• Individuals at risk include: - **high risk individuals** such as: those who may or will be exposed to virus-containing blood, blood products and body fluids such as health care workers, police and firefighters; MSM, injection drug users; those who have unprotected sex with new partners or who have multiple sex partners; patients with hemophilia who receive clotting factors from plasma; patients on hemodialysis; household contacts of patients with acute HBV or who are HBV carriers; residents in communities with high endemic rates; travellers to endemic areas; immigrants from areas of high prevalence of HBV; residents and staffs of institutions, e.g., correctional facilities. - **others:** patients with chronic liver disease; patients who receive hepatotoxic drugs; patients with disease conditions that necessitate future use of hepatotoxic drugs; patients undergoing hematopoietic stem cell transplantation. • Anyone not in the above groups who wishes to protect themselves from HBV should be encouraged to receive the vaccine.
Herpes Zoster[12]	For adults ≥60 years	• Zostavax should be administered to patients for whom the vaccine is indicated irrespective of a prior history of chickenpox or documented prior varicella infection. • Avoid in pregnancy or immunocompromised patients. • Individuals who inadvertently receive systemic antiviral therapy active against VZV within 2 days before and 14 days after Zostavax injection may benefit from a second dose of vaccine 42 days or later and after discontinuing antiviral therapy. • Trivalent influenza vaccine may be administered concomitantly with Zostavax at a different injection site. Pneumococcal polysaccharide vaccine and Zostavax should be administered at least 4 weeks apart.
Human Papillomavirus[8]	For females <26 years who have not been previously immunized.	• Give three doses in total at 0, 1–2 and 6 months. • Not recommended for pregnant women. • Safe in breast-feeding women. • Gardasil (HPV-4) indicated for males <26 years but not yet addressed by the National Advisory Committee on Immunization.

(cont'd)

Table 2: Routine Immunization for Adults[1] *(cont'd)*

Vaccine or Toxoid	Indication and Schedule	Comments
Influenza[7]	All adults ≥65 years; adults <65 years of age at high risk of influenza-related complications, including pregnant women. Give every year using current vaccine formulation. Live attenuated influenza vaccine (FluMist) should not be administered to adults >59 years of age.	• Priority should be given to the following adults (see Table 1 for information on Infants and Children). - **high risk individuals** such as: those with chronic cardiac or pulmonary disorders (e.g., cystic fibrosis and asthma) or other chronic conditions (e.g., diabetes mellitus, cancer, immunodeficiency, immunosuppression, renal disease, anemia and hemoglobinopathy; conditions that compromise the management of respiratory secretions and are associated with an increased risk of aspiration); residents of nursing homes and other chronic care facilities; all persons ≥65 years old; persons with HIV; persons with morbid obesity; aboriginal persons; those at high risk of influenza complications travelling to foreign destinations where the virus is likely to be circulating. - **individuals capable of transmitting influenza to those at high risk**, e.g., health care workers, household contacts of high risk individuals (see list above) including household contacts of infants <6 months of age and those expecting a newborn during the influenza season, providers of regular care to children <24 months of age, persons providing services to high risk individuals within closed and relatively closed settings (e.g., crew on airplanes). - **others:** persons who provide essential community services, persons in direct contact with avian influenza-infected poultry during culling operations. • Anyone not in the above groups who wishes to protect themselves from influenza should be encouraged to receive the vaccine. • Safe in pregnant and breast-feeding women; **all pregnant women** regardless of trimester should receive the influenza vaccine.[7] • Ideal time for influenza vaccination is from October to mid-November, but can still be given later.
Measles	All adults born in 1970 or later who are susceptible to measles. May be given as MMR.	• Give one dose of measles vaccine to all adults born since 1970 who have not already received two doses or had natural measles infection. • Offer one additional dose to the following high risk adults: travellers to a measles endemic area, health care workers, students at post-secondary institutions and military recruits. • Avoid in pregnant women and immunocompromised patients.
Meningococcal quadrivalent conjugate (MCV4), conjugate-C (MCV1) and polysaccharide (MPSV4)[5,6,13]	Adults at increased risk of meningococcal disease	• Give MCV4 to the following high risk adults: those with functional or anatomic asplenia, those with complement, properdin or factor D deficiencies, those who are routinely exposed to *N. meningitidis* such as clinical laboratory personnel, military recruits, those travelling to endemic regions and close contacts of persons with invasive meningococcal disease (A, Y, W135). Consider for individuals with HIV. • Repeat dose once after 5 years for persons at increased risk of meningococcal disease. • An alternate approach is to administer MCV1 and MPSV4; both are required if MCV4 is not available and additional protection is required for A, Y and W-135. Give MCV1 then MPSV4 after 2 weeks. If MPSV4 is given first, then wait 6 months to give MCV1.
Mumps[14]	Mumps-susceptible adults. May be given as MMR.	• Give 2 doses of mumps-containing vaccine to the following groups unless there is laboratory evidence of immunity or laboratory confirmed evidence of mumps or if they were born before 1970: students at educational institutions, health care workers (if born before 1970, consider a single dose of MMR) and military personnel (if born before 1970, consider a single dose of MMR). • Avoid in pregnant women and immunocompromised patients.
Pertussis[15] (adolescent/adult preparation)	All adults. Preferably given as Tdap.	• For adults who have not previously received a dose of acellular pertussis vaccine, it is recommended that a single Td booster dose be replaced by the combined Tdap vaccine.
Pneumococcal polysaccharide	Adults ≥65 years; adults <65 years of age with conditions that increase the risk of pneumococcal disease.	• Give pneumococcal vaccine to the following high risk adults: all persons ≥65 years old; those with asplenia, splenic dysfunction or sickle-cell disease; homeless persons;[16] those with chronic cardiorespiratory disease (except asthma), cirrhosis, alcoholism, chronic renal disease, nephrotic syndrome, diabetes mellitus, chronic cerebrospinal fluid leak, HIV infection and other conditions associated with immunosuppression. • At present, routine revaccination is not recommended but should be considered in the following: functional or anatomic asplenia or sickle-cell disease; hepatic cirrhosis; chronic renal failure or nephrotic syndrome; HIV infection; and immunosuppression related to disease or therapy. A single revaccination is recommended after five years. Need for subsequent doses remains to be determined. • Consider giving pneumococcal vaccine to persons who use illicit drugs, i.e., injection drugs and crack cocaine.[16] • Not contraindicated in pregnant and breast-feeding women.
Rubella	Rubella-susceptible women of child-bearing age and health care workers. May be given as MMR.	• Rubella vaccine should be given to all women of child-bearing age unless they have proof of immunity (documented evidence of having received the vaccine, or laboratory evidence of immunity). Particular emphasis should be placed on the following: foreign-born women from countries that do not routinely immunize against rubella, staff and students in educational institutions, women found to be susceptible during pregnancy (give postpartum) and female health care workers. In addition, the vaccine should be given to susceptible persons of either gender who may, through frequent face-to-face contact, expose pregnant women to rubella. • If a vaccination is required one dose using measles-rubella containing vaccine should be given, as a high proportion of rubella-susceptible women may also be susceptible to measles. • Avoid in pregnant women.
Tetanus	All adults. Give every 10 years[a]. Preferably given as Td. For adults that have not previously received a dose of acellular pertussis vaccine, it is recommended that a single Td booster dose be replaced by combined Tdap.	• All Canadians should be immunized against tetanus, even patients who have recovered from this disease, because infection does not confer protective immunity. • Booster doses, administered as Td, are recommended at 10-year intervals. • Immunization status should be reviewed at least once during adult life, and a dose of Td given to everyone who has not had one within the previous 10 years. • Booster immunization should also be considered in the event of tetanus-prone wounds (refer to the *Canadian Immunization Guide* for Post-exposure prevention of Tetanus in the context of Wound Management). • In pregnant women, it is recommended to wait until the second trimester to administer a routinely required dose, unless the woman has experienced a tetanus-prone wound or has never received a primary series of immunization.
Varicella	Susceptible adults should receive 2 doses 28 days apart.	• Screen and immunize: health care workers, women of child-bearing age, household contacts of immunocompromised patients, susceptible adults with occupational exposure. • Avoid in pregnant women and immunocompromised patients. May be considered in susceptible HIV-infected adults and adolescents with CD4 cell count ≥200 x 10^6/L and percentage ≥15%.[17] Give 2 doses 3 months apart in this population.

[a] These recommendations assume that complete primary immunization has been performed.

Abbreviations: HBV = hepatitis B virus; HIV = human immunodeficiency virus; HPV-4 = quadrivalent human papilloma virus vaccine; MSM = men who have sex with men; Td = tetanus and diphtheria; Tdap = tetanus, diphtheria and acellular pertussis, adult formulation; VZV = varicella zoster virus

Canadian Immunization Guide, Public Health Agency of Canada, 2006©. Adapted and reproduced with the permission of the Minister of Public Works and Government Services Canada, 2010.

Table 3: Routine Immunization Schedule for Adults

Vaccine or Toxoid	Age				
	19–26 years	27–49 years	50–59 years	60–64 years	≥65 years
Tetanus, diphtheria, pertussis (Td/Tdap)	Boost with Td every 10 years; substitute with Tdap once in adulthood for pertussis protection[a]				
Human papillomavirus	3 doses[a]	No recommendation			
Varicella	2 doses[a]				
Herpes zoster	No recommendation			1 dose[a]	
Measles, mumps, rubella	1 or 2 doses[a]				
Influenza	1 dose annually[b]				1 dose annually[a]
Pneumococcal polysaccharide vaccine	1 or 2 doses[b]				1 dose[a]
Hepatitis A	2 doses[b]				
Hepatitis B	3 doses[b]				
Meningococcal	1 or more doses[b]				
Haemophilus	1 dose[b]				

[a] For all patients in this age category.
[b] Recommended if risk factor(s) present (e.g., based on medical, occupation, lifestyle or other indications).

References

1. National Advisory Committee on Immunization (NACI). *Canadian immunization guide*. 7th ed. Ottawa (ON): Public Health Agency of Canada, Infectious Disease and Emergency Preparedness Branch, Centre for Infectious Disease and Control; 2006. Available from: www.phac-aspc.gc.ca/publicat/cig-gci/pdf/cig-gci-2006_e.pdf. Accessed November 17, 2010.
2. National Advisory Committee on Immunization (NACI). An Advisory Committee Statement (ACS). Varicella vaccination two-dose recommendations. *Can Commun Dis Rep* 2010;36(ACS-8):1-26. Available from: www.phac-aspc.gc.ca/publicat/ccdr-rmtc/10vol36/acs-8/index-eng.php. Accessed October 19, 2010.
3. National Advisory Committee on Immunization (NACI). An Advisory Committee Statement (ACS). Statement on measles-mumps-rubella-varicella vaccine. *Can Commun Dis Rep* 2010;36(ACS-9):1-37. Available from: www.phac-aspc.gc.ca/publicat/ccdr-rmtc/10vol36/acs-9/index-eng.php. Accessed October 19, 2010.
4. National Advisory Committee on Immunization (NACI). An Advisory Committee Statement (ACS). Update on pediatric invasive pneumococcal disease and recommended use of conjugate pneumococcal vaccine. *Can Commun Dis Rep* 2010;36(ACS-3):1-30. Available from: www.phac-aspc.gc.ca/publicat/ccdr-rmtc/10vol36/acs-3/index-eng.php. Accessed July 12, 2010.
5. National Advisory Committee on Immunization (NACI). An Advisory Committee Statement (ACS). Statement on conjugate meningococcal vaccine for serogroups A, C, Y and W135. *Can Commun Dis Rep* 2007;33(ACS-3):1-23. Available from: www.phac-aspc.gc.ca/publicat/ccdr-rmtc/07pdf/acs33-03.pdf. Accessed November 17, 2010.
6. National Advisory Committee on Immunization (NACI). An Advisory Committee Statement (ACS). Update on the invasive meningococcal disease and meningococcal vaccine conjugate recommendations. *Can Commun Dis Rep* 2009;36(ACS-3):1-40. Available from: www.phac-aspc.gc.ca/publicat/ccdr-rmtc/09pdf/acs-dcc-3.pdf. Accessed November 17, 2010.
7. National Advisory Committee on Immunization (NACI). An Advisory Committee Statement (ACS). Statement on Seasonal Trivalent Inactivated Influenza Vaccine (TIV) for 2010-2011. *Can Commun Dis Rep* 2010;36(ACS-6):1-49. Available from: www.phac-aspc.gc.ca/publicat/ccdr-rmtc/10vol36/acs-6/index-eng.php. Accessed September 12, 2010.
8. National Advisory Committee on Immunization (NACI). An Advisory Committee Statement (ACS). Statement on human papillomavirus vaccine. *Can Commun Dis Rep* 2007;33(ACS-2):1-32. Available from: www.phac-aspc.gc.ca/publicat/ccdr-rmtc/07pdf/acs33-02.pdf. Accessed November 17, 2010.
9. National Advisory Committee on Immunization (NACI). An Advisory Committee Statement (ACS). Statement on the recommended use of pentavalent human-bovine reassortant rotavirus vaccine. *Can Commun Dis Rep* 2008; 34(ACS-1):1-33. Available from: www.phac-aspc.gc.ca/publicat/ccdr-rmtc/08pdf/acs-1.pdf. Accessed November 17, 2010.
10. National Advisory Committee on Immunization (NACI). An Advisory Committee Statement (ACS). Updated statement on the use of rotavirus vaccines. *Can Commun Dis Rep* 2010;36(ACS-4):1-37. Available from: www.phac-aspc.gc.ca/publicat/ccdr-rmtc/10vol36/acs-4/index-eng.php. Accessed August 23, 2010.
11. National Advisory Committee on Immunization (NACI). An Advisory Committee Statement (ACS). Update on the use of conjugate pneumococcal vaccines in childhood. *Can Commun Dis Rep* 2010;36(ACS-12):1-21. Available from: www.phac-aspc.gc.ca/publicat/ccdr-rmtc/10vol36/acs-12/index-eng.php. Accessed November 15, 2010.
12. National Advisory Committee on Immunization (NACI). An Advisory Committee Statement (ACS). Statement on the recommended use of herpes zoster vaccine. *Can Commun Dis Rep* 2010;36(ACS-1):1-13. Available from: www.phac-aspc.gc.ca/publicat/ccdr-rmtc/10vol36/acs-1/index-eng.php. Accessed July 12, 2010.
13. National Advisory Committee on Immunization (NACI). An Advisory Committee Statement (ACS). Statement on recommended use of meningococcal vaccines. *Can Commun Dis Rep* 2001;27(ACS-6):1-36. Available from: www.phac-aspc.gc.ca/publicat/ccdr-rmtc/01vol27/27sup/acs6.html. Accessed November 17, 2010.
14. National Advisory Committee on Immunization (NACI). An Advisory Committee Statement (ACS). Statement on mumps vaccine. *Can Commun Dis Rep* 2007;33(ACS-8):1-10. Available from: www.phac-aspc.gc.ca/publicat/ccdr-rmtc/07pdf/acs33-08.pdf. Accessed November 17, 2010.
15. National Advisory Committee on Immunization (NACI). An Advisory Committee Statement (ACS). Prevention of pertussis in adolescents and adults. *Can Commun Dis Rep* 2003;29(ACS-5,6):1-12. Available from: www.phac-aspc.gc.ca/publicat/ccdr-rmtc/03pdf/acs-dcc-29-5-6.pdf. Accessed November 17, 2010.
16. National Advisory Committee on Immunization (NACI). An Advisory Committee Statement (ACS). Statement on the recommended use of pneumococcal 23-valent polysaccharide vaccine in homeless persons and injection drug users. *Can Commun Dis Rep* 2008;34(ACS-5):1-12. Available from: www.phac-aspc.gc.ca/publicat/ccdr-rmtc/08vol34/acs-5/index-eng.php. Accessed November 17, 2010.
17. National Advisory Committee on Immunization (NACI). An Advisory Committee Statement (ACS). Updated recommendations for the use of varicella and MMR vaccines in HIV-infected individuals. *Can Commun Dis Rep* 2010;36(ACS-7):1-19. Available from: www.phac-aspc.gc.ca/publicat/ccdr-rmtc/10vol36/acs-7/index-eng.php. Accessed October 19, 2010.

Drug Administration and Food

Date of Revision: November 2010

Table 1 provides an overview of current recommendations for administration of oral drugs with respect to food. This information is not intended to present a comprehensive review; the reader is therefore encouraged to seek additional and confirmatory information.

Adherence to medication regimens can be encouraged by scheduling drug administration to coincide with routine activities such as meal times. Foods and beverages may interact with medications affecting bioavailability, metabolism or excretion. While such interactions can influence the effectiveness of a drug by altering the anticipated therapeutic effect, the clinical significance of most food–drug interactions is not clear. (See also Drug Administration and Grapefruit in the Clin-Info section.)

The following recommendations for drug administration in relation to food are compiled from drug information references,[1,2] as well as the product monograph provided by manufacturers. When tablets may be chewed or crushed and which capsules may be opened and sprinkled onto food has also been noted. The table is not meant to be exhaustive.

The recommendations made in this table are not absolute; clinical judgment must be used in their interpretation. More important is the consistency of drug administration to facilitate adherence and prevent fluctuations in the therapeutic effect of the drug.

The headings used in the table are described as follows:

- **Empty Stomach**—one hour before or two hours after meals with a full glass of liquid, usually water.
- **Before Meals**—usually 15 to 30 minutes before meals.
- **Empty Stomach Preferably**—as for Empty Stomach (above); however, may be taken with food if gastric upset occurs.
- **With or After Meals**
- **With or Without Food**—may be given without regard to meals. The notation "be consistent" in the comments column indicates that the drug should be taken consistently with or without food, as presence or absence of food may alter bioavailability.
- **Do Not Crush or Chew**—crushing enteric-coated, extended-release, sublingual and buccal formulations can render the drug ineffective and/or increase the risk of adverse events and toxicity. Other considerations regarding crushing may be the likelihood of the crushed drug to irritate mucosal tissue or be potentially carcinogenic.

Table 1: Drug Administration and Food

Drug Name	Empty Stomach	Before Meals	Empty Stomach Preferably	With or After Meals	With or Without Food	Do Not Crush or Chew	Comments
5-Aminosalicylic Acid		•				•	With a glass of water. Enteric-coated/delayed release
Abacavir					•		
Acamprosate					•	•	Be consistent. Swallow whole. Do not split tablets; enteric-coated
Acarbose				•			With first bite of a main meal
Acebutolol					•		
Acetaminophen — tablets					•		
Acetaminophen — ER	•					•	
Acetazolamide					•		Food decreases GI side effects
Acitretin				•			Food optimizes absorption
Acyclovir					•		
Adefovir					•	•	
Alendronate		•				•	In the morning at least 30 min before any food, beverage or other medication with a full glass of plain water only to prevent oropharyngeal ulceration; swallow whole
Alfacalcidol				•			With a glass of water or milk
Alfuzosin				•		•	Prolonged release
Alginic Acid					•		Chew tablets; follow with drink of water or milk
Aliskiren					•		Be consistent. See also Drug Administration and Grapefruit section in Clin-Info
Allopurinol				•			Food decreases GI side effects
Almotriptan					•		
Alpha-D-Galactosidase				•			Swallow, chew or crumble onto food; add only to food cool enough to eat
Alprazolam					•		
Altretamine				•		•	
Aluminum Hydroxide					•		
Amantadine					•		
Ambrisentan					•		
Amiloride				•			Food decreases GI side effects; avoid large quantities of potassium-rich foods
Aminobenzoate — capsules				•			After meals and at bedtime with a snack; with a glass of water
Aminobenzoate — powder				•			Add to a glass of chilled water or juice; stir to dissolve and drink after eating meal or snack

(cont'd)

Table 1: Drug Administration and Food *(cont'd)*

Drug Name	Empty Stomach	Before Meals	Empty Stomach Preferably	With or After Meals	With or Without Food	Do Not Crush or Chew	Comments
Aminobenzoate — tablets				•			Crush tablets and add to a glass of chilled water or juice; stir thoroughly and drink after eating meal or snack
Amiodarone					•		Be consistent; food decreases GI side effects. See also Drug Administration and Grapefruit section in Clin-Info
Amitriptyline					•		
Amlodipine					•		
Amoxicillin					•		
Amoxicillin/Clavulanic Acid					•	•	Food decreases GI side effects
Amphetamines, Mixed Salts (Adderall XR)					•	•	Can sprinkle contents of capsule on applesauce; do not chew or crush contents
Ampicillin	•						
Amprenavir — capsules					•		Decreased absorption with a high-fat meal
Amprenavir — liquid					•		Decreased absorption with a high-fat meal
Anagrelide					•		See also Drug Administration and Grapefruit section in Clin-Info
Anastrozole					•	•	With a glass of water
Aprepitant					•		See also Drug Administration and Grapefruit section in Clin-Info
Aripiprazole					•		
ASA — EC					•	•	With a glass of water
ASA — plain				•			Food decreases GI side effects
Atazanavir				•			Swallow whole; do not open capsules. Food enhances absorption
Atenolol					•		See also Drug Administration and Grapefruit section in Clin-Info
Atomoxetine					•	•	
Atorvastatin					•		See also Drug Administration and Grapefruit section in Clin-Info
Atovaquone				•			Food increases bioavailability
Atovaquone/Proguanil				•			Daily dose should be taken with food or a milky drink; absorption reduced when fasting
Attapulgite, Activated — suspension					•		
Attapulgite, Activated — tablets, regular strength					•	•	With a glass of water
Auranofin				•			
Azathioprine					•	•	Food decreases GI side effects
Azithromycin — suspension					•		
Azithromycin — tablets					•		
Baclofen					•		
Benazepril					•		
Benztropine					•		Food decreases GI side effects
Betahistine				•			Food decreases GI side effects
Betaine					•		Dissolve dose in 120–180 mL of water, juice, milk, formula or mix with food for immediate ingestion
Bethanechol	•						Avoid taking with meals, nausea and vomiting may occur soon after eating
Bezafibrate				•		•	With a glass of water. Sustained release
Bicalutamide					•	•	With a glass of water
Bisacodyl	•					•	With a glass of water; do not take with milk. Enteric-coated
Bisoprolol					•		
Bosentan					•		
Bromazepam					•		

(cont'd)

Table 1: Drug Administration and Food *(cont'd)*

Drug Name	Empty Stomach	Before Meals	Empty Stomach Preferably	With or After Meals	With or Without Food	Do Not Crush or Chew	Comments
Bromocriptine				•			Food decreases GI side effects
Budesonide		•				•	With a glass of water; swallow whole (controlled ileal release). See also Drug Administration and Grapefruit section in Clin-Info
Bumetanide					•		
Buprenorphine/Naloxone						•	Sublingual. Place under tongue until dissolved; takes 5 to 10 minutes for the tablet to dissolve; do not swallow
Bupropion					•	•	Food decreases GI side effects; with a glass of water. Do not divide; sustained release
Buspirone					•		See also Drug Administration and Grapefruit section in Clin-Info
Busulfan					•	•	If nausea occurs take on an empty stomach; take care when halving tablets to not contaminate hands or inhale the drug (antineoplastic)
Cabergoline					•		
Calcitriol					•		
Calcium Salts				•			Food increases absorption
Candesartan					•		With a glass of water
Candesartan/ Hydrochlorothiazide					•	•	
Capecitabine				•		•	With meal or within 30 min after end of a meal; with a glass of water
Captopril		•					1 h before meals preferred; may take with food but be consistent
Carbamazepine — CR				•		•	See also Drug Administration and Grapefruit section in Clin-Info
Carbamazepine — regular				•			Food decreases GI side effects. See also Drug Administration and Grapefruit section in Clin-Info
Carvedilol				•		•	Food slows rate of absorption and incidence of orthostatic effects especially during dose titration; take with a glass of water. See also Drug Administration and Grapefruit section in Clin-Info
Cefaclor					•		Food decreases GI side effects
Cefadroxil					•		Food decreases GI side effects
Cefixime					•		Food decreases GI side effects
Cefprozil					•		Food decreases GI side effects
Cefuroxime Axetil — suspension					•		Food increases absorption; may add to cold milk, lemonade, apple, orange or grape juice before administration, drink immediately
Cefuroxime Axetil — tablets					•	•	Food increases absorption; with a glass of water. Bitter taste if chewed or crushed
Celecoxib					•		
Cephalexin					•		Maximum peak levels when taken on an empty stomach
Cetirizine					•		
Chlophedianol					•		
Chloral Hydrate					•		Dilute with 120 mL of water or other liquid, e.g., fruit juice, to reduce gastric irritation
Chlorambucil					•	•	Do not divide tablets (antineoplastic)
Chloramphenicol			•				
Chlordiazepoxide					•		
Chlordiazepoxide/Clidinium		•					30 to 60 min before meals to maximize absorption
Chloroquine				•			Food decreases GI side effects
Chlorpheniramine					•		
Chlorpromazine					•	•	
Chlorpropamide					•		Long half-life
Chlorthalidone					•		Food decreases GI side effects
Cholecalciferol					•		May mix liquid with formula, fruit juice or other foods

(cont'd)

Table 1: Drug Administration and Food *(cont'd)*

Drug Name	Empty Stomach	Before Meals	Empty Stomach Preferably	With or After Meals	With or Without Food	Do Not Crush or Chew	Comments
Cholera Vaccine and Traveller's Diarrhea — Inactivated	•						Avoid food and drink 1 h before and after vaccine administration; vaccine is acid labile. Dissolve supplied effervescent granules of sodium hydrogen carbonate buffer in a glass of water (~150 mL). Mix vaccine with sodium hydrogen carbonate solution and drink the mixture within 2 h. Can also store mixture at room temperature (<27°C) for up to 2 h
Cholestyramine		•					Mix with water, milk, fruit juice or other noncarbonated beverage; may also be mixed with highly fluid soups or pulpy fruits with high moisture content, e.g., applesauce, crushed pineapple
Cilazapril					•		Be consistent
Cimetidine					•		Multiple doses—with meals and at bedtime
Cinacalcet				•		•	
Ciprofloxacin — liquid					•	•	Do not chew the microcapsules. Food decreases GI side effects; faster absorption on empty stomach; with a glass of water; avoid excessive caffeine intake; stagger dosing or reduce intake of dairy products. See also Drug Administration and Grapefruit section in Clin-Info
Ciprofloxacin — tablets, regular					•		Food decreases GI side effects; faster absorption on empty stomach; with a glass of water; avoid excessive caffeine intake; stagger dosing or reduce intake of dairy products. See also Drug Administration and Grapefruit section in Clin-Info
Ciprofloxacin — tablets, XL					•	•	See also Drug Administration and Grapefruit section in Clin-Info
Citalopram					•		With a glass of water
Clarithromycin — suspension					•		
Clarithromycin — tablets, regular					•		
Clarithromycin — tablets, XL				•		•	Food increases bioavailability
Clindamycin					•		With a glass of water to avoid esophageal irritation
Clobazam					•		
Clodronate	•						Check specific product monograph. At least 1 to 2 h before or after food; food decreases absorption. Avoid concomitant use of milk, antacids or drugs containing calcium, magnesium, iron or aluminum. With a glass of water; swallow whole
Clomiphene					•		
Clomipramine					•		Food decreases GI side effects. See also Drug Administration and Grapefruit section in Clin-Info
Clonazepam					•		
Clonidine					•		
Clopidogrel					•		See also Drug Administration and Grapefruit section in Clin-Info
Clorazepate					•		
Cloxacillin	•						
Clozapine					•		
Codeine					•		
Codeine — tablets, controlled release					•	•	All Codeine Contin strengths may be halved except 50 mg
Colchicine					•		
Colestipol — granules				•			Add to water, milk, flavoured drink, juice, carbonated beverage or any other liquid; may also add to hot or cold cereals, soups (avoid chunky soups), yogurt, pudding, cottage cheese or pulpy fruits, e.g., crushed pineapple, pears
Colestipol — tablets				•		•	With a glass of water or any liquid; do not cut
Cortisone Acetate				•			Food decreases GI side effects
Cyclobenzaprine					•		
Cyclophosphamide					•	•	Food decreases GI side effects
Cyclosporine — capsules					•	•	Be consistent; swallow whole. See also Drug Administration and Grapefruit section in Clin-Info

(cont'd)

Table 1: Drug Administration and Food *(cont'd)*

Drug Name	Empty Stomach	Before Meals	Empty Stomach Preferably	With or After Meals	With or Without Food	Do Not Crush or Chew	Comments
Cyclosporine — liquid					•		Be consistent; mix with any room temperature beverage excluding grapefruit juice; be consistent with beverage used. See also Drug Administration and Grapefruit section in Clin-Info
Cyproheptadine					•		
Cyproterone				•			
Dabigatran					•		
Danazol					•		
Dantrolene					•		
Darifenacin					•	•	Sustained release. See also Drug Administration and Grapefruit section in Clin-Info
Darunavir				•		•	
Dasatinib					•	•	Swallow whole; do not cut. See also Drug Administration and Grapefruit section in Clin-Info
Deferasirox	•					•	At least 30 min prior to first meal of the day. Do not swallow whole. Completely disperse tablets by stirring in noncarbonated water, orange juice or apple juice only until a fine suspension is obtained. Disperse doses of <1 g in 100 mL and doses of >1 g in 200 mL
Delavirdine					•		If achlorhydria or on acid secretion suppressor, take with acidic beverage, e.g., orange or cranberry juice; may be dissolved in water for easier swallowing
Delta-9-Tetrahydrocannabinol					•		
Desipramine					•		
Desloratadine					•		
Desloratadine/Pseudoephedrine					•	•	
Desmopressin Acetate					•		
Desvenlafaxine					•	•	Swallow whole
Dexamethasone				•			Food decreases GI side effects
Dexlansoprazole					•		
Dextroamphetamine — spansules					•	•	Swallow whole
Dextroamphetamine — tablets					•		
Dextromethorphan					•		
Diazepam					•		See also Drug Administration and Grapefruit section in Clin-Info
Diazoxide					•		Be consistent
Diclofenac				•		•	Food decreases GI side effects; with a glass of water or milk. EC or SR dosage forms; local irritation if regular dosage form is crushed or chewed
Dicyclomine					•		
Didanosine — EC	•					•	At least 30 min before a meal or 2 h after eating; swallow whole
Diflunisal				•		•	Food decreases GI side effects; with a glass of water or milk
Digoxin					•		Meals high in bran fibre may reduce amount of drug absorbed
Diltiazem — regular		•					
Diltiazem — SR or CD					•	•	Swallow whole
Diltiazem — XC					•	•	Once daily at bedtime
Dimenhydrinate					•		
Diphenhydramine					•		
Dipyridamole		•					1 h before meals preferred; may take with milk to reduce GI side effects
Dipyridamole/ASA					•	•	With a glass of water; swallow whole; extended-release dipyridamole pellets
Disopyramide — regular					•		

(cont'd)

Table 1: Drug Administration and Food *(cont'd)*

Drug Name	Empty Stomach	Before Meals	Empty Stomach Preferably	With or After Meals	With or Without Food	Do Not Crush or Chew	Comments
Divalproex Sodium — regular, EC					•	•	Food decreases GI side effects
Docusate Calcium					•		With a glass of water; swallow whole
Docusate Sodium — capsules					•	•	With a glass of water; swallow whole
Docusate Sodium — drops/syrup					•		Dilute with milk, fruit juice or infant formula to mask bitter taste
Dolasetron					•		
Domperidone		•					See also Drug Administration and Grapefruit section in Clin-Info
Donepezil					•		
Doxazosin					•		
Doxepin					•		
Doxercalciferol					•		
Doxycycline				•		•	Food decreases GI side effects; with a glass of water to avoid esophageal ulceration. Avoid concomitant use of milk, antacids or drugs containing aluminum, calcium, magnesium or iron
Doxylamine/Pyridoxine					•		
Dronedarone				•			With morning and evening meal. See also Drug Administration and Grapefruit section in Clin-Info
Duloxetine					•	•	Swallow whole. Do not sprinkle contents on food or mix with liquids; enteric coated/delayed release
Dutasteride					•	•	Swallow whole
Efavirenz	•					•	With a glass of water preferably at bedtime; swallow whole
Efavirenz/Emtricitabine/Tenofovir	•					•	With a glass of water preferably at bedtime; swallow whole
Eletriptan					•	•	With a glass of water; swallow whole
Emtricitabine/Tenofovir					•		
Enalapril					•		
Entacapone					•	•	
Entacavir	•						At least 2 h after meals and 2 h before the next meal
Eplerenone					•		
Eprosartan					•		Be consistent
Ergocalciferol					•		
Ergoloid Mesylates				•			
Erlotinib	•						With a glass of water. See also Drug Administration and Grapefruit section in Clin-Info
Erythromycin — base			•			•	If enteric-coated, do not crush or chew. See also Drug Administration and Grapefruit section in Clin-Info
Erythromycin — estolate					•		Food decreases GI side effects. See also Drug Administration and Grapefruit section in Clin-Info
Erythromycin — ethylsuccinate					•		Preferably immediately after meals for maximum absorption. See also Drug Administration and Grapefruit section in Clin-Info
Erythromycin — stearate			•				See also Drug Administration and Grapefruit section in Clin-Info
Escitalopram					•		
Esomeprazole — granules					•		
Esomeprazole — tablets					•	•	With a glass of water; may disperse in 120 mL of non-carbonated water—no other liquids should be used as the enteric coating may be dissolved, stir until tablet disintegrates, drink the liquid with the pellets within 30 min, rinse the glass with 120 mL of water and drink; the pellets must not be crushed or chewed
Estramustine	•					•	With a glass of water; swallow whole; do not take with milk or calcium-containing drugs

(cont'd)

Table 1: Drug Administration and Food *(cont'd)*

Drug Name	Empty Stomach	Before Meals	Empty Stomach Preferably	With or After Meals	With or Without Food	Do Not Crush or Chew	Comments
Estrogens					•		Food decreases GI side effects. See also Drug Administration and Grapefruit section in Clin-Info
Ethacrynic Acid				•			
Ethambutol					•		Food decreases GI side effects
Ethopropazine					•		
Ethosuximide					•		Food decreases GI side effects
Etidronate	•						At least 2 h before or after a meal; with a glass of water; swallow whole. Avoid concomitant use of milk, antacids or drugs containing aluminum, calcium, magnesium or iron within 2 h of dosing
Etodolac				•			Food decreases GI side effects; with a glass of water or milk
Etoposide	•					•	See also Drug Administration and Grapefruit section in Clin-Info
Etravirine				•		•	Swallow whole; should be taken following meals. If patient cannot swallow tablets, disperse in 100 mL of cold water until a homogenous, white, cloudy suspension is obtained; drink immediately. Rinse glass with water several times; swallow each rinse to ensure entire dose is ingested. See also Drug Administration and Grapefruit section in Clin-Info
Everolimus			•			•	May be taken with a light fat-free meal. Decreased absorption with a high-fat meal. See also Drug Administration and Grapefruit section in Clin-Info
Exemestane				•			
Ezetimibe					•		
Famciclovir					•	•	With a glass of water
Famotidine					•		15 min before meals for prevention of acid-related symptoms associated with food/beverage consumption
Febuxostat					•		
Felodipine					•	•	With a glass of water; avoid meals rich in carbohydrate or fat—significant increase in C_{max}. See also Drug Administration and Grapefruit section in Clin-Info
Fenofibrate				•			Food increases absorption
Fenofibrate — microcoated				•			With largest meal of the day; food optimizes absorption
Fenofibrate — micronized				•			With largest meal of the day; food optimizes absorption
Fenofibrate — nanocrystals					•		
Fentanyl citrate						•	Buccal film. Do not cut or tear. May drink liquids 5 minutes after application. Do not eat food until film is completely dissolved, generally within 15–30 minutes after application
Feverfew				•			With a glass of water
Fexofenadine					•		See also Drug Administration and Grapefruit section in Clin-Info
Fexofenadine/Pseudophedrine					•	•	Swallow whole
Finasteride					•		Crushed or broken tablets should not be handled by women who are or may become pregnant
Flavoxate				•			Food decreases GI side effects
Flecainide					•		
Floctafenine				•			Food decreases GI side effects; with a glass of water or milk
Fluconazole					•		
Fludarabine					•	•	
Fludrocortisone				•			
Flunarizine					•		
Fluoxetine					•		
Flupenthixol					•		
Fluphenazine					•		
Flurazepam					•		

(cont'd)

Table 1: Drug Administration and Food *(cont'd)*

Drug Name	Empty Stomach	Before Meals	Empty Stomach Preferably	With or After Meals	With or Without Food	Do Not Crush or Chew	Comments
Flurbiprofen — regular				•			Food decreases GI side effects; with a glass of water or milk
Flurbiprofen — SR				•		•	With a glass of water or milk; swallow whole
Flutamide					•		
Fluvastatin — regular					•	•	Be consistent. Can be taken at bedtime if once daily
Fluvastatin — XL					•	•	Be consistent. With a glass of water; swallow whole
Fluvoxamine					•	•	With a glass of water. See also Drug Administration and Grapefruit section in Clin-Info
Folic Acid					•		
Fosamprenavir — suspension	•						
Fosamprenavir — tablets					•		
Fosinopril					•		
Frovatriptan					•	•	Swallow whole with fluids
Furosemide					•		Be consistent
Gabapentin					•		
Galantamine — ER				•		•	Preferably with morning meal
Ganciclovir				•		•	Food maximizes bioavailability
Gefitinib					•		See also Drug Administration and Grapefruit section in Clin-Info
Gemfibrozil		•					30 min before morning and evening meal
Gliclazide — regular				•			
Gliclazide — MR				•		•	With a glass of cool water
Glimepiride				•			With breakfast or first main meal
Glyburide				•			With breakfast or first main meal
Granisetron					•		
Guaifenesin					•		
Haloperidol					•		
Hydralazine					•		
Hydrochlorothiazide					•		
Hydrocodone				•			
Hydrocortisone				•			Food decreases GI side effects
Hydromorphone — regular					•		
Hydromorphone — SR					•	•	Swallow whole; may sprinkle contents of capsule onto soft food but do not chew the beads
Hydroxychloroquine				•			Food decreases GI side effects
Hydroxyurea					•	•	With a glass of water; may empty contents of capsule into a glass of water and take immediately. Do not allow powder onto hands and do not inhale powder
Hydroxyzine					•		
Ibuprofen				•			Food decreases GI side effects; with a glass of water or milk
Imatinib				•			Food decreases GI side effects; with a glass of water. If patient cannot swallow tablets, disperse tablet in a glass of water or apple juice as per directions in product monograph. See also Drug Administration and Grapefruit section in Clin-Info
Imipramine					•		
Indapamide					•		
Indinavir			•				With a glass of water, skim milk, juice, coffee or tea; may take with a light meal; a meal high in calories, fat or protein reduces absorption
Indomethacin				•		•	Food decreases gastric irritation; with a glass of water or milk
Iodoquinol				•			

(cont'd)

Table 1: Drug Administration and Food *(cont'd)*

Drug Name	Empty Stomach	Before Meals	Empty Stomach Preferably	With or After Meals	With or Without Food	Do Not Crush or Chew	Comments
Irbesartan					•		Be consistent
Iron Salts — capsules/tablets			•			•	Food, especially dairy products, coffee and tea, decreases absorption and GI side effects
Iron Salts — liquid			•				Dilute dose with water or juice (not milk)
Isoniazid			•				Food decreases absorption
Isosorbide Dinitrate — regular	•						With a glass of water
Isosorbide Dinitrate — SL					•	•	Do not eat or drink while tablet dissolving
Isosorbide Dinitrate — SR					•	•	
Isosorbide Mononitrate					•	•	With a glass of water; may break tablet in half along the scored line
Isotretinoin				•		•	Food increases bioavailability
Itraconazole — capsules				•		•	Swallow whole; with cola beverage if achlorhydria or on acid secretion suppressor. See also Drug Administration and Grapefruit section in Clin-Info
Itraconazole — liquid	•						Swish and swallow; do not rinse after swallowing. Not with grapefruit juice; see also Drug Administration and Grapefruit section in Clin-Info
Ketoconazole				•			With cola beverage if achlorhydria or on acid secretion suppressor
Ketoprofen — EC or SR			•			•	With a glass of water
Ketoprofen — regular				•			Food decreases GI side effects; with a glass of water
Ketorolac				•			Food decreases GI side effects; with a glass of water or milk; high-fat meal decreases rate but not extent of absorption
Ketotifen — tablets					•		
Ketotifen — syrup					•		
Labetalol				•			Food increases bioavailability
Lacosamide					•		
Lactase — caplets				•		•	Immediately before meals that contains lactose
Lactase — drops					•		Add to milk
Lactase — tablets				•			Immediately before meals that contain lactose; can be chewed
Lactobacillus rhamnosus				•			Preferably with milk or lactose; may add contents of capsule to semi-solid food if unable to swallow
Lactulose					•		With a glass of water
Lamivudine — liquid					•		
Lamivudine — tablets					•	•	With a glass of water
Lamivudine/Zidovudine					•	•	
Lamotrigine — chewable/dispersible tablets					•		With a glass of water; may be chewed, dissolved in liquid or swallowed whole; dosing is based on whole tablets; do not divide tablets
Lamotrigine — tablets					•		
Lansoprazole — capsules, delayed release		•				•	Before breakfast and/or meals; with a glass of water; swallow whole; delayed-release capsules can be opened and the intact granules can be sprinkled on a tablespoon of applesauce and swallowed immediately; do not chew or crush granules; granules can also be mixed in juice for nasogastric administration (stable for up to 30 min)
Lansoprazole — tablets, delayed release		•				•	Do not swallow intact tablets; place tablet on tongue and swallow when all disintegrated; do not chew granules
Lanthanum carbonate				•			Do not swallow intact tablets; chew completely before swallowing
Lapatinib	•						Take at least 1 h before or 1 h after a low fat meal. See also Drug Administration and Grapefruit section in Clin-Info
Leflunomide					•	•	Be consistent; with a glass of water
Letrozole					•		With a glass of water
Levetiracetam					•		
Levocarnitine — liquid				•			May mix into drinks or other liquid foods; consume slowly to maximize tolerance

(cont'd)

Table 1: Drug Administration and Food *(cont'd)*

Drug Name	Empty Stomach	Before Meals	Empty Stomach Preferably	With or After Meals	With or Without Food	Do Not Crush or Chew	Comments
Levocarnitine — tablets					•		
Levodopa/Benserazide					•	•	Be consistent; swallow whole—do not open or dissolve; food decreases GI side effects; protein-rich foods may decrease levodopa absorption
Levodopa/Carbidopa — CR					•	•	200/50 strength tablets may be halved; food decreases GI side effects; protein-rich foods may decrease levodopa absorption
Levodopa/Carbidopa — regular					•		Be consistent; food decreases GI side effects; protein-rich foods may decrease levodopa absorption
Levodopa/Carbidopa/ Entacapone					•	•	Be consistent; food decreases GI side effects; protein-rich foods may decrease levodopa absorption
Levofloxacin					•		With a glass of water
Levonorgestrel					•		
Levothyroxine					•		Be consistent; can be crushed and suspended in water or mixed with soft food, e.g., applesauce; however, do not use foods with a large amount of soybean, fibre or iron for administration
Linezolid					•		Avoid foods or beverages with high tyramine content
Liothyronine					•		
Lisdexamfetamine					•		May dissolve contents of capsule in a glass of water and consume immediately
Lisinopril					•		With a glass of water
Lithium Salts — regular					•		Food decreases GI side effects
Lithium Salts — SR					•	•	Tablet may be broken in half
Lomustine					•		As a single dose—nausea may be minimized if given at bedtime on an empty stomach
Loperamide					•		
Lopinavir/Ritonavir — capsules, solution				•			Food enhances bioavailability
Lopinavir/Ritonavir — tablets					•	•	
Loratadine — syrup, regular tablet					•		
Loratadine — rapid dissolve tablet	•						May be taken without water
Loratadine/Pseudoephedrine					•	•	Swallow whole
Lorazepam					•		
Losartan					•		Be consistent
Lovastatin				•			With evening meal. See also Drug Administration and Grapefruit section in Clin-Info
Loxapine					•		
L-tryptophan				•			Food decreases GI side effects; best taken with protein-low, carbohydrate-rich snack or meal
Magnesium Salts				•			With a glass of water
Maprotiline					•		
Maraviroc					•	•	See also Drug Administration and Grapefruit section in Clin-Info
Mebendazole					•		Must chew tablets
Medroxyprogesterone					•		
Mefenamic Acid				•			Food decreases GI side effects; with a glass of water or milk
Mefloquine				•			Food increases absorption; with a glass of water; do not chew; may crush and suspend in a small amount of water, milk or other beverage
Megestrol					•		
Meloxicam					•		
Melphalan					•	•	
Memantine					•		

(cont'd)

Table 1: Drug Administration and Food *(cont'd)*

Drug Name	Empty Stomach	Before Meals	Empty Stomach Preferably	With or After Meals	With or Without Food	Do Not Crush or Chew	Comments
Meprobamate					•		
Mercaptopurine					•	•	
Metformin — regular				•			Food decreases GI side effects
Metformin — ER				•		•	Must be taken with food—optimizes absorption and ensures complete release of metformin
Methadone					•		
Methazolamide					•		Food decreases GI side effects
Methenamine				•			Food decreases GI side effects; avoid excessive intake of alkalinizing foods, e.g., milk products; with a glass of water
Methimazole					•		
Methocarbamol					•		
Methotrexate					•	•	
Methotrimeprazine					•		
Methoxsalen				•			Avoid the following foods for 24 h before and after administration and exposure to UVA radiation due to increased risk of burns: carrots, celery, figs, limes, mustard, parsley, parsnips
Methsuximide					•		Food decreases GI side effects
Methyldopa					•		
Methylphenidate — regular				•			Food increases rate of absorption and reduces GI side effects
Methylphenidate — SR or ER tablet				•		•	
Methylphenidate — CR capsule				•		•	May be sprinkled on soft food; do not crush or chew pellets
Methylprednisolone				•			See also Drug Administration and Grapefruit section in Clin-Info
Metoclopramide		•					
Metolazone					•		
Metoprolol — regular					•		Be consistent; food may increase bioavailability
Metoprolol — SR					•	•	
Metronidazole — ER	•					•	Food increases rate of absorption
Metronidazole — regular					•		Food decreases GI side effects
Mexiletine				•			With a glass of water
Midodrine					•		
Miglustat					•	•	Food decreases rate of absorption but no effect on extent of absorption; swallow whole
Mineral Oil	•						Not within 2 h of meal as it may interfere with digestion and absorption of nutrients and vitamins
Minocycline					•		Avoid concomitant use of milk, antacids or drugs containing aluminum, calcium, magnesium or iron
Minoxidil					•		With a glass of water
Mirtazapine — tablets					•	•	With a glass of water
Mirtazapine — RD tablets					•		Rapidly disintegrates on tongue; swallow with saliva; do not split tablets
Misoprostol				•		•	Swallow whole
Moclobemide				•			No MAOI dietary restrictions as long as taken after meals
Modafinil					•		
Montelukast Sodium — tablets					•		
Montelukast Sodium — chewables					•		
Montelukast Sodium — granules					•	•	Can be taken directly in the mouth. May mix granules with a spoonful of cold or room temperature food, e.g., applesauce; do not chew granules
Morphine — regular					•		

(cont'd)

Table 1: Drug Administration and Food *(cont'd)*

Drug Name	Empty Stomach	Before Meals	Empty Stomach Preferably	With or After Meals	With or Without Food	Do Not Crush or Chew	Comments
Morphine — SR					•	•	With a glass of water; only 200 mg SR tablet (MS Contin) may be halved along scored line; may open SR capsule and sprinkle contents onto soft food, e.g., applesauce; do not chew the pellets
Moxifloxacin					•	•	With a glass of water
Multivitamins					•		
Mycophenolate — capsules/tablets	•					•	Swallow whole
Mycophenolate — liquid	•						Dispense directly into mouth; do not mix with any other liquid before taking
Nabilone					•		
Nabumetone					•	•	Food decreases GI side effects; with a glass of water or milk
Nadolol					•		
Naltrexone					•		
Naproxen — regular				•			Food decreases GI side effects; with a glass of water or milk
Naproxen — SR				•		•	With a glass of water or milk
Naratriptan					•	•	With a glass of water
Nateglinide		•					1 min before main meal
Nelfinavir				•			Food increases absorption
Nevirapine					•		
Niacin — regular					•		With meals as antihyperlipidemic; food decreases GI side effects
Niacin — ER				•		•	After a low-fat snack at bedtime; swallow whole
Niacin/Lovastatin				•		•	After a low-fat snack at bedtime; swallow whole
Nicoumalone (acenocoumarol)					•		Be consistent; avoid abrupt changes in diet to maintain constant vitamin K intake
Nifedipine — regular					•		See also Drug Administration and Grapefruit section in Clin-Info
Nifedipine — XL					•	•	Do not divide. See also Drug Administration and Grapefruit section in Clin-Info
Nilotinib	•					•	Swallow whole with a glass of water; must not be taken with food. See also Drug Administration and Grapefruit section in Clin-Info
Nilutamide		•					Before breakfast
Nimodipine					•	•	See also Drug Administration and Grapefruit section in Clin-Info
Nitrazepam					•		
Nitrofurantoin				•		•	Food increases bioavailability and decreases GI side effects
Nitroglycerin					•	•	Do not crush, chew or swallow
Nizatidine					•		
Norfloxacin	•						With a glass of water; do not take with milk; avoid excessive caffeine intake
Normethadone				•			
Nortriptyline					•		
Nylidrin					•		
Nystatin					•		Sparingly absorbed
Ofloxacin					•	•	With a glass of water
Olanzapine — tablets					•	•	With a glass of water
Olanzapine — tablets, orally disintegrating					•		May stir into 125 mL of water, milk, coffee, orange juice or apple juice, consume immediately
Olmesartan					•		
Olsalazine				•		•	Food decreases GI side effects
Omeprazole — capsules					•	•	Swallow whole
Omeprazole — MUPS tablets					•	•	Swallow whole

(cont'd)

Table 1: Drug Administration and Food *(cont'd)*

Drug Name	Empty Stomach	Before Meals	Empty Stomach Preferably	With or After Meals	With or Without Food	Do Not Crush or Chew	Comments
Omeprazole — tablets					•	•	With a glass of water
Ondansetron					•		
Orciprenaline					•		
Orlistat				•		•	Up to 1 h after a meal; with a glass of water
Orphenadrine					•		
Oseltamivir					•		Food decreases GI side effects
Oxaprozin				•			Food decreases GI side effects; with a glass of water or milk
Oxazepam					•		
Oxcarbazepine					•		
Oxtriphylline — liquid/regular			•				With a glass of water
Oxybutynin — regular					•		
Oxybutynin — XL					•	•	With a glass of water
Oxycodone — regular					•		
Oxycodone — SR					•	•	
Paliperidone					•	•	Swallow whole. Do not divide; extended release
Pancreatic Enzymes — capsules with EC granules				•		•	With each meal or snack; with a glass of water; swallow whole; may open capsule and sprinkle onto soft food, e.g., applesauce, do not chew granules, take immediately after sprinkling
Pancreatic Enzymes — regular tab/cap or powder				•			With each meal or snack
Pantoprazole					•	•	With a glass of water
Paromomycin				•			Poorly absorbed
Paroxetine — regular					•	•	With a glass of water
Paroxetine — CR					•	•	
Pazopanib	•					•	See also Drug Administration and Grapefruit section in Clin-Info
Penicillamine	•						With a glass of water; do not take with milk
Penicillin V					•		
Pentazocine				•			
Pentosan Polysulfate	•						With a glass of water
Pentoxifylline				•		•	Swallow whole
Pepsin				•			
Perindopril	•						
Perphenazine					•		
Pethidine					•		
Phenelzine					•		Follow MAOI diet
Phenobarbital					•		Absorption faster on an empty stomach
Phenytoin				•		•	Food decreases GI side effects; not with an enteral feeding preparation
Phosphates Solution	•						May take up to 30 min before a meal; dilute dose in 120 mL water and follow dose with a glass of water
Pilocarpine					•	•	
Pimozide					•		See also Drug Administration and Grapefruit section in Clin-Info
Pinaverium				•			With a glass of water to avoid esophageal irritation
Pindolol				•			
Pioglitazone					•		
Piroxicam				•			Food decreases GI side effects; with a glass of water or milk
Pizotifen					•		

(cont'd)

Table 1: Drug Administration and Food *(cont'd)*

Drug Name	Empty Stomach	Before Meals	Empty Stomach Preferably	With or After Meals	With or Without Food	Do Not Crush or Chew	Comments
Posaconazole				•			Oral suspension; administer with food or nutritional supplement (if cannot tolerate food) to enhance oral absorption
Potassium Salts — liquid				•			Potassium chloride—dilute dose with water, citrus fruit juice or citrated soft drink
Potassium Salts — regular				•			Food decreases GI side effects
Potassium Salts — SR capsules				•		•	With a glass of water; swallow whole; may sprinkle contents of capsule onto soft food, e.g., applesauce, and swallow without chewing
Potassium Salts — SR tablets				•		•	With a glass of water; may break tablet in half for K-Dur; may also disintegrate tablet in half glass of water, stir and swallow immediately, rinse any residue on glass with more water and swallow
Pramipexole					•		Food decreases GI side effects
Prasugrel					•		
Pravastatin					•		
Praziquantel				•		•	With a glass of water; tablet may be halved. See also Drug Administration and Grapefruit section in Clin-Info
Prazosin					•		
Prednisone				•			Food decreases GI side effects
Pregabalin					•		
Primaquine					•		Food decreases GI side effects. See also Drug Administration and Grapefruit section in Clin-Info
Primidone					•		Food decreases GI side effects
Probenecid					•		Food decreases GI side effects
Procainamide — regular					•		
Procainamide — SR					•	•	
Procarbazine					•	•	Follow MAOI diet; capsules should not be opened
Prochlorperazine					•		
Procyclidine				•			
Propafenone					•		Manufacturer recommends administration with food but bioavailability was not significantly affected by food in multi-dose studies
Propoxyphene					•		
Propranolol — LA					•	•	Swallow whole
Propranolol — regular					•		Be consistent; food may increase bioavailability
Propylthiouracil					•		
Pseudoephedrine					•		
Psyllium — granules					•	•	With a glass of water
Psyllium — powder					•		With meals for cholesterol-lowering effect; mix dose into water, juice or other suitable liquid; follow dose with additional glass of liquid
Pyrantel					•		
Pyridostigmine — regular					•	•	Tablets may be cut in half. Do not crush or chew as may increase side effects
Pyridostigmine — SR					•	•	Do not divide
Pyridoxine					•		
Pyrimethamine				•			Food decreases GI side effects
Quetiapine					•		
Quetiapine — XR					•	•	Swallow whole. Do not divide; extended release
Quinagolide				•			Given at bedtime with a snack
Quinapril					•		
Quinidine Salts — regular				•			Food decreases GI side effects
Quinidine Salts — CR				•		•	Food decreases GI side effects; with a glass of water; may be cut in half

(cont'd)

Table 1: Drug Administration and Food *(cont'd)*

Drug Name	Empty Stomach	Before Meals	Empty Stomach Preferably	With or After Meals	With or Without Food	Do Not Crush or Chew	Comments
Quinine				•		•	Food decreases GI side effects
Rabeprazole					•	•	Enteric coated; swallow whole
Raloxifene					•		
Raltegravir					•	•	If crushed, may cause rapid release of the drug. Bitter taste
Ramipril					•		
Ranitidine					•		
Rasagiline Mesylate					•		
Repaglinide		•					See also Drug Administration and Grapefruit section in Clin-Info
Ribavirin				•			Be consistent
Riboflavin					•		
Rifabutin					•		Food decreases GI side effects
Rifampin			•				
Riluzole	•						Food decreases bioavailability
Risedronate	•					•	In the morning at least 30 min before first food, beverage, or other medication with a glass of plain water only to prevent oropharyngeal ulceration; swallow whole
Risperidone — liquid					•		Compatible with water, coffee, orange juice and low-fat milk; not compatible with cola or tea
Risperidone — tablets, regular					•		
Risperidone — tablets, oral disintegrating						•	Do not split in halves
Ritonavir — capsules				•			
Ritonavir — liquid				•			May mix with chocolate milk or Ensure within 1 h of dosing
Rivaroxaban					•	•	See also Drug Administration and Grapefruit section in Clin-Info
Rivastigmine				•			Food decreases GI side effects
Rizatriptan — tablets					•		With a glass of water
Rizatriptan — wafers					•		Place wafer on tongue to dissolve and swallow with saliva
Ropinirole					•	•	Food decreases GI side effects; with a glass of water; give morning dose without food in severely fluctuating patients to avoid delay in time to take effect
Rosiglitazone					•		
Rosuvastatin					•		
Rotavirus Vaccine, human					•		
Salbutamol					•		
Sapropterin				•			Food increases absorption. May be dissolved in 120–224 mL of water or apple juice and taken within 15 min
Saquinavir Mesylate				•		•	Within 2 h of a meal or substantial snack; with a glass of water; swallow whole. See also Drug Administration and Grapefruit section in Clin-Info
Saxagliptin					•		See also Drug Administration and Grapefruit section in Clin-Info
Selegiline				•			MAOI diet restrictions not required at the recommended dosage level of 10 mg/day
Sennosides					•		With a glass of water
Sertraline				•			Food increases bioavailability. See also Drug Administration and Grapefruit section in Clin-Info
Sevelamer				•		•	Immediately prior to or with meals; swallow whole; do not break into pieces
Sildenafil					•	•	With a glass of water; avoid high-fat meal (decreases absorption). See also Drug Administration and Grapefruit section in Clin-Info
Simethicone				•			

(cont'd)

Table 1: Drug Administration and Food *(cont'd)*

Drug Name	Empty Stomach	Before Meals	Empty Stomach Preferably	With or After Meals	With or Without Food	Do Not Crush or Chew	Comments
Simvastatin					•		With evening meal or at bedtime. See also Drug Administration and Grapefruit section in Clin-Info
Sirolimus					•		Be consistent; dilute dose with at least 60 mL of water or orange juice; stir vigorously for 1 min and drink; refill the container with at least 120 mL of water or orange juice; stir vigorously again and drink the rinse solution; do not use apple juice, grapefruit juice or other liquids for dilution. See also Drug Administration and Grapefruit section in Clin-Info
Sitagliptin					•		
Sitaxsentan					•		May be taken without regard to time of day
Sodium Bicarbonate					•		
Sodium Cromoglycate		•					Dissolve contents of capsule in warm water
Sodium Fluoride				•		•	
Sodium Oxybate	•						Food decreases bioavailability. First dose taken at bedtime, at least 2 h after last meal. Second dose is given 2.5 to 4 h later
Solifenacin					•		See also Drug Administration and Grapefruit section in Clin-Info
Sorafenib	•						Food decreases bioavailability; 1 h before or 2 h after meals
Sotalol	•						Preferably 1–2 h before meal
Spiramycin					•		
Spironolactone					•		Food increases absorption; avoid large quantities of potassium-rich foods
Stavudine					•		
Sterculia Gum					•	•	With a glass of water
Sucralfate	•						1 h before meals
Sulfadiazine/Trimethoprim				•			Food decreases GI side effects; with a glass of water
Sulfamethoxazole/Trimethoprim					•		Food decreases GI side effects; with a glass of water
Sulfasalazine — EC					•	•	With a glass of water
Sulfasalazine — regular				•		•	Food decreases GI side effects; with a glass of water
Sulfinpyrazone				•			Food decreases GI side effects
Sulindac				•			Food decreases GI side effects; with a glass of water or milk
Sumatriptan					•	•	With a glass of water
Sunitinib					•		See also Drug Administration and Grapefruit section in Clin-Info
Tacrolimus					•	•	Be consistent. See also Drug Administration and Grapefruit section in Clin-Info
Tadalafil					•		See also Drug Administration and Grapefruit section in Clin-Info
Tamoxifen					•		
Tamsulosin					•	•	Controlled release. See also Drug Administration and Grapefruit section in Clin-Info
Telbivudine					•		
Telithromycin					•	•	Bitter taste if crushed or chewed
Telmisartan					•		Be consistent
Temazepam					•		
Temozolomide	•					•	May take with food, but administration on empty stomach may decrease incidence of nausea and vomiting; be consistent; with a glass of water; swallow whole—do not open capsules (antineoplastic)
Tenofovir					•		
Tenoxicam				•			Food decreases GI side effects; with a glass of water or milk
Terazosin					•		
Terbinafine					•		Food slightly increases bioavailability
Terbutaline					•		Food decreases GI side effects

(cont'd)

Table 1: Drug Administration and Food *(cont'd)*

Drug Name	Empty Stomach	Before Meals	Empty Stomach Preferably	With or After Meals	With or Without Food	Do Not Crush or Chew	Comments
Testosterone Undecanoate				•		•	
Tetrabenazine					•		With a glass of water
Tetracycline	•						With a glass of water; do not take with milk
Theophylline — liquid			•				With a glass of water
Theophylline — SR tablets (except Uniphyl)					•	•	Be consistent; with a glass of water
Theophylline — Uniphyl				•		•	With or shortly after evening meal; with a glass of water; tablet may be halved
Thiamine					•		
Thioproperazine					•		
Thiothixene					•		
Thyroid, dessicated					•		Be consistent
Tiaprofenic Acid — regular				•			With a glass of water or milk
Ticlopidine				•			Food decreases GI side effects
Timolol					•		
Tipranavir				•			Avoid aluminum and magnesium based antacids—absorption of tipranavir decreased
Tizanidine					•		
Tolbutamide		•					Short half-life
Tolterodine — ER					•	•	Swallow whole
Tolterodine — regular					•		
Topiramate — capsules					•	•	Swallow whole; may sprinkle contents of capsule onto soft food, e.g., applesauce, swallow without chewing
Topiramate — tablets					•	•	With a glass of water
Tramadol					•		
Tramadol — XL					•	•	Swallow whole
Trandolapril					•		
Trandolapril/Verapamil				•		•	Do not split
Tranexamic Acid					•		
Tranylcypromine					•		Follow MAOI diet
Trazodone				•			Food decreases incidence of adverse effects (GI and dizziness)
Triamterene				•			Food decreases GI side effects; avoid large quantities of potassium-rich foods
Triamterene/ Hydrochlorothiazide				•			Food decreases GI side effects
Triazolam					•		See also Drug Administration and Grapefruit section in Clin-Info
Trifluoperazine					•		
Trihexyphenidyl					•		Food decreases GI side effects
Trimebutine		•					
Trimeprazine				•			Food promotes more gradual absorption and decreases incidence of drowsiness
Trimethoprim					•		Food decreases GI side effects
Trimipramine					•		
Trospium	•						At least 1 h prior to meals; food decreases absorption
Tryptophan — see L-tryptophan							
Typhoid Vaccine — capsules		•				•	1 h before a meal with a cold or lukewarm drink; swallow whole
Ursodiol				•			
Valacyclovir					•		

(cont'd)

Table 1: Drug Administration and Food *(cont'd)*

Drug Name	Empty Stomach	Before Meals	Empty Stomach Preferably	With or After Meals	With or Without Food	Do Not Crush or Chew	Comments
Valerian Root					•		
Valganciclovir				•		•	Food increases bioavailability
Valproic Acid					•	•	Food decreases GI side effects. Swallow whole with a glass of water; minimize local irritation of mouth and throat
Valsartan					•		Be consistent
Vancomycin					•		Not absorbed
Vardenafil					•		High fat meal decreases rate of absorption by 1 h. See also Drug Administration and Grapefruit section in Clin-Info
Varenicline				•			
Venlafaxine — XR				•		•	With a glass of water; swallow whole
Verapamil — regular				•			See also Drug Administration and Grapefruit section in Clin-Info
Verapamil — SR				•		•	240 mg scored tablet may be halved. See also Drug Administration and Grapefruit section in Clin-Info
Vigabatrin — powder					•		Dissolve in water, juice, milk or formula
Vigabatrin — tablets					•		
Vitamin A					•		
Vitamin B_{12}					•		
Vitamin C				•			With a glass of water
Vitamin D_3 – see Cholecalciferol							
Vitamin E					•	•	Swallow whole
Voriconazole	•						At least 1 h before or 2 h following meals
Vorinostat				•			Drink at least 2 L/day of fluid to prevent dehydration
Warfarin					•		Avoid abrupt changes in diet to maintain constant vitamin K intake
Yohimbine					•		
Zafirlukast	•						
Zidovudine					•		
Zinc			•				
Ziprasidone				•		•	Administration with food increases absorption. See also Drug Administration and Grapefruit section in Clin-Info
Zolmitriptan					•		
Zopiclone					•		
Zuclopenthixol					•		

Empty Stomach = 1 h before or 2 h after meals with a full glass of liquid, usually water; **Before Meals** = usually 15 to 30 min before meals; **Empty Stomach Preferably** = may be taken with food if gastric upset occurs; **With or Without Food** = may be given without regard to meals

Abbreviations: CD = controlled delivery; CR = controlled release; EC = enteric coating; ER = extended release; LA = long acting; MR = modified release; RD = rapid dissolve; SL = sublingual; SR = sustained release; XC = extended release delivery system; XL, XR = extended release

References

1. *Drug facts and comparisons*. St. Louis (MO): Facts and Comparisons; 2010.
2. McEvoy GK, editor. *AHFS drug information*. Bethesda (MD): American Society of Health-System Pharmacists; 2010.

Drug Administration and Grapefruit

D.G. Bailey, BScPhm, MSc, PhD

Date of Revision: November 2010

The following is an overview of drug administration and grapefruit consumption. This information is not intended to present a comprehensive review; the reader is therefore encouraged to seek additional and confirmatory information.

The following table outlines known pharmacokinetic and pharmacodynamic effects of concurrent grapefruit and drug administration as well as management options. The information is based on product monographs in *CPS* and the references listed at the conclusion of this document. Do not assume that drugs not appearing in the table do not interact.

Grapefruit acts as an irreversible inhibitor of the intestinal drug metabolizing enzyme, CYP3A4, to increase the systemic concentration of drugs normally undergoing first-pass metabolism. The clinical effect of grapefruit on P-glycoprotein is currently not clear. Grapefruit mainly affects drugs administered orally. As little as a single quantity of 200 mL of grapefruit juice can institute a significant clinical interaction. Repeated consumption of a normal amount of grapefruit during the day can enhance the magnitude of the interaction. Since there is prolonged inhibitory effect on intestinal CYP3A4-mediated drug metabolism, separating administration of drug from ingestion of grapefruit will not prevent an interaction. Moreover, the magnitude of the interaction is normally markedly variable among individuals and cannot be predicted prior to exposure. For these two reasons, avoidance of grapefruit entirely for all persons receiving therapy with affected medications is recommended. Although most studies have used grapefruit juice prepared from frozen concentrate, all forms of grapefruit (fresh juice and whole fruit) have the potential to inactivate intestinal CYP3A4 activity.[1,2,3,4,5]

The constituents in grapefruit responsible for the interaction appear to be the combined action of several furanocoumarins. They are not found in sweet orange juice, which does not produce the interaction. However, they are present in bitter (Seville) orange, lime and pomelo, which do cause the effect.

The clinical significance of the interaction is determined by the grapefruit-induced change in drug bioavailability relative to the therapeutic range for the individual drug (i.e., drugs with a wide therapeutic index may be less affected than drugs with a narrow therapeutic index) and the individual's susceptibility (e.g., patients with hepatic insufficiency or pre-existing medical conditions). Most of the reported studies of interactions with grapefruit juice are single-dose studies in healthy volunteers. Published case reports of grapefruit-associated adverse drug reactions of overdose/toxicity generally occurred in patients taking a stabilized drug regimen in whom grapefruit was added to their diet. These happened after repeated daily grapefruit ingestion for several days and were associated with usual or high amount of grapefruit consumption.

Individuals over 50 years of age commonly consume grapefruit, and are commonly prescribed the affected drugs. If they have a marked pharmacokinetic interaction they are less able to compensate for excessive systemic drug concentrations and thus are a particularly vulnerable population.

Little or no effect is observed when usual amounts of grapefruit are ingested concomitantly with parenterally administered drugs (e.g., iv midazolam and cyclosporine). Also, no interaction would be expected with the use of transdermal dosage forms (e.g., estradiol-17β patch) since usual amounts of grapefruit have little effect on hepatic CYP3A4. Large amounts of grapefruit juice administered under experimental conditions (e.g., 200 mL double-strength juice three times daily) have been shown to inhibit hepatic CYP3A4.

Grapefruit, orange and/or apple juices can also act by a different mechanism than that described above to decrease absorption of some drugs. Flavonoid-mediated inhibition of the intestinal drug uptake transporter, organic anion transporting polypeptide 1A2 (OATP1A2), appears to be involved. This interaction has the potential to occur in patients who take their medication with a fruit juice but may be avoided with an interval of 4 hours between consumption of juice and administration of drug.[6,7,8,9,10] Recent research supports that grapefruit may inhibit OATP2B1.[11] Further studies are needed to establish significance of these interactions.

If a drug is not listed in the table, there may be no information or inconclusive information about the interaction. Also, drugs that have been studied and found not to interact have not been included. The recommendations in the table are not absolute. Interpretation of the information requires clinical judgment and evaluation of the interaction using other sources.

Table 1: Drug Administration and Grapefruit

Drug	Grapefruit Effect	Management
Aliskiren	• May decrease systemic bioavailability of aliskiren, due to OATP2B1 inhibition. • Evaluated in an open randomized crossover study of 11 healthy subjects; markedly reduced C_{max} and AUC.[11]	• Avoid consumption of grapefruit and/or orange juice within 4 hours of intake of aliskiren. • Administer aliskiren with a glass of water on an empty stomach.
Amiodarone	• Repeated doses of grapefruit juice markedly increase amiodarone levels. • Evaluated in controlled studies in healthy volunteers; increased AUC and C_{max}.	• Avoid grapefruit. Seville orange, lime and pomelo may also cause the interaction. • If grapefruit consumed during drug therapy, monitor for adverse effects associated with increased serum levels of amiodarone (e.g., bradycardia, prolonged QTc interval, torsades de pointes, elevation of liver enzymes).
Anagrelide	• May increase anagrelide serum levels.	• Avoid grapefruit. Seville orange, lime and pomelo may also cause the interaction. • If grapefruit consumed during drug therapy, close clinical supervision of the patient is required, especially monitoring of platelet count for thrombocytopenia.
Aprepitant	• May increase aprepitant serum levels.	• Avoid grapefruit. Seville orange, lime and pomelo may also cause the interaction. • If grapefruit consumed during drug therapy, monitor for adverse effects associated with aprepitant (e.g., drowsiness, headache).
Atenolol	• Decreased atenolol serum levels inferred from studies with orange juice. • May be due to OATP1A2 inhibition. • Evaluated in a study of 10 healthy subjects; orange juice reduced C_{max} and AUC.[12]	• Avoid consumption of grapefruit or orange juice within 4 hours of intake of atenolol.
Atorvastatin	• Grapefruit juice may increase plasma levels of HMG-CoA reductase inhibitors metabolized by CYP3A4. • Atorvastatin appears to be affected to a lesser extent than lovastatin and simvastatin.	• Avoid grapefruit. Seville orange, lime and pomelo may also cause the interaction. • Consider choosing an HMG-CoA reductase inhibitor not metabolized by CYP3A4 (e.g., pravastatin and fluvastatin). • If grapefruit consumed during drug therapy, monitor for adverse effects associated with increased serum levels of atorvastatin (e.g., myopathy, rhabdomyolysis, acute renal failure).
Benzodiazepines, see Diazepam, Triazolam		
Budesonide	• Substantial intake of grapefruit juice may increase systemic exposure to orally administered budesonide. • Single oral dose of budesonide controlled release capsule following grapefruit juice 200 mL three times daily for 4 days produced double the bioavailability of that with water in 8 healthy men.[13]	• Avoid grapefruit. Seville orange, lime and pomelo may also cause the interaction. • If grapefruit consumed during drug therapy, monitor for adverse effects associated with the use of glucocorticoids (e.g., hyperglycemia, Cushingoid features).

(cont'd)

Table 1: Drug Administration and Grapefruit *(cont'd)*

Drug	Grapefruit Effect	Management
Buspirone	• Repeated doses of grapefruit juice markedly increase buspirone plasma levels. • Evaluated in a randomized, 2-phase crossover study in 10 healthy volunteers; increased mean peak plasma concentration, increased AUC and delayed time to C_{max}.[14]	• Avoid grapefruit. Seville orange, lime and pomelo may also cause the interaction. • If grapefruit consumed during drug therapy, monitor for adverse effects associated with increased plasma levels of buspirone (e.g., sedation and psychomotor impairment).
Calcium Channel Blockers, see Felodipine, Nifedipine, Nimodipine		
Carbamazepine	• May increase carbamazepine serum levels. • Evaluated in small controlled study of epileptic patients; increased AUC, peak and trough concentrations.[15]	• Avoid grapefruit. Seville orange, lime and pomelo may also cause the interaction. • If grapefruit consumed during drug therapy, monitor for signs of carbamazepine toxicity (e.g., drowsiness, dizziness, headache, unsteadiness on the feet, diplopia, nausea, vomiting).
Carvedilol	• Can result in higher plasma levels of carvedilol due to reduced drug metabolism. • Evaluated in controlled studies; increased AUC.	• Evidence of this interaction is limited. • If grapefruit consumed during drug therapy, monitor for adverse effects associated with increased serum levels of carvedilol (e.g., low blood pressure and bradycardia).
Ciprofloxacin	• Decreased ciprofloxacin serum levels inferred from studies with orange juice. • May be due to OATP1A2 inhibition. • Evaluated in a study of 15 healthy subjects; orange juice reduced AUC and C_{max}.[16]	• Avoid consumption of grapefruit or orange juice within 4 hours of intake of ciprofloxacin.
Clomipramine	• May increase clomipramine serum levels. • The interaction between grapefruit juice and other tricyclic antidepressants has not been established.	• Avoid grapefruit. Seville orange, lime and pomelo may also cause the interaction. • If grapefruit consumed during drug therapy, monitor for adverse effects associated with increased serum levels of clomipramine (e.g., drowsiness, hypotension, respiratory depression, cardiovascular disturbances, anticholinergic effects, agitation).
Clopidogrel	• May decrease plasma levels of active metabolite, thus weakening its ability to inhibit platelet aggregation.	• Avoid grapefruit. Seville orange, lime and pomelo may also cause the interaction.
Colchicine	• May increase systemic oral bioavailability of colchicine, due to inhibition of P-gp. • Case report of near fatal colchicine toxicity in a child following high chronic consumption of grapefruit juice.[17]	• Avoid grapefruit. Seville orange, lime and pomelo may also cause the interaction. • If high amount of grapefruit is consumed during drug therapy, monitor for serious adverse reactions (vomiting, alopecia, heart failure, pancytopenia, atonic falls).
Cyclophosphamide	• The manufacturer of Procytox does not recommend the concomitant administration of grapefruit juice with Procytox. • May impair activation of cyclophosphamide to its active metabolites resulting in reduced effectiveness.	• Avoid grapefruit. Seville orange, lime and pomelo may also cause the interaction.
Cyclosporine	• May increase plasma levels of cyclosporine. • Evaluated in controlled studies; increased AUC and increased plasma concentration.	• Avoid grapefruit. Seville orange, lime and pomelo may also cause the interaction. • If grapefruit consumed during drug therapy, monitor for symptoms of toxicity (e.g., nephrotoxicity, hepatotoxicity, increased immunosuppression). • Monitor cyclosporine effect particularly when grapefruit juice is initiated, discontinued or the interval between drug and grapefruit juice ingestion changes. • Lower doses of cyclosporine may be required.
Darifenacin	• May increase darifenacin serum levels.	• Avoid grapefruit. Seville orange, lime and pomelo may also cause the interaction. • If grapefruit consumed during drug therapy, monitor for excessive antimuscarinic effects (dry mouth, constipation) and serious effect of acute urinary retention.
Dasatinib	• May increase dasatinib serum levels.	• Avoid grapefruit. Seville orange, lime and pomelo may also cause the interaction. • If grapefruit consumed during drug therapy, close clinical monitoring is required, especially for myelosuppression, bleeding, prolongation of QTc interval and torsades de pointes.
Diazepam	• May increase diazepam levels. • Evaluated in controlled studies in healthy volunteers; increased AUC and C_{max}.	• Clinical importance is unknown. • It is likely that some patients would be adversely affected, especially those in whom diazepam levels are likely to be elevated (e.g., older individuals, those with liver impairment or concurrent use of other cytochrome P450 inhibitors). • Avoid grapefruit. Seville orange, lime and pomelo may also cause the interaction. • If grapefruit consumed during drug therapy, monitor for increased sedation.
Domperidone	• Interaction between grapefruit juice and domperidone has not been studied. • Potential for increased bioavailability of domperidone resulting in QTc prolongation and risk of serious cardiac arrhythmia (torsades de pointes).	• Avoid grapefruit. Seville orange, lime and pomelo may also cause the interaction.
Dronedarone	• Repeated doses of 300 mL of grapefruit juice three times daily resulted in a 3-fold increase in dronedarone serum levels.[18]	• Avoid grapefruit. Seville orange, lime and pomelo may also cause the interaction. • If grapefruit consumed during drug therapy, caution and close clinical monitoring for serious adverse effects associated with increased serum levels of dronedarone (prolonged QTc interval, torsades de pointes) are warranted.
Eplerenone	• Grapefruit juice produced a modest increase (mean 25% higher, range not reported) in eplerenone serum levels.[19]	• Avoid grapefruit. Seville orange, lime and pomelo may also cause the interaction. • If grapefruit consumed during drug therapy, caution and close clinical monitoring for serious adverse effects (hyperkalemia, serious arrhythmias, hypotension, abnormal renal function, dizziness) are warranted.
Ergotamine	• May increase ergotamine levels and risk of serious toxicity.	• Avoid grapefruit. Seville orange, lime and pomelo may also cause the interaction.

(cont'd)

Table 1: Drug Administration and Grapefruit *(cont'd)*

Drug	Grapefruit Effect	Management
Erlotinib	• May increase erlotinib serum levels.	• Avoid grapefruit. Seville orange, lime and pomelo may also cause the interaction. • If grapefruit consumed during drug therapy, close monitoring is required, especially for myelosuppression and bleeding.
Erythromycin	• Grapefruit juice may increase serum concentrations of erythromycin. • Evaluated in an open crossover study in 6 healthy subjects; increased C_{max} and AUC.[20]	• Avoid grapefruit. Seville orange, lime and pomelo may also cause the interaction. • If grapefruit consumed during drug therapy, monitor for adverse effects that may be associated with erythromycin.
Ethinyl estradiol	• Appears to increase serum concentrations of ethinyl estradiol. • Theoretically, grapefruit juice may affect the metabolism of other estrogens. • Case report of massive deep vein thrombosis following grapefruit consumption for 3 days.[21]	• Avoid grapefruit. Seville orange, lime and pomelo may also cause the interaction. • If grapefruit consumed during drug therapy, suggest maintaining a consistent interval between drug and grapefruit juice ingestion when possible.
Etoposide	• May decrease systemic bioavailability of etoposide. • May be due to OATP1A2 inhibition. • Evaluated in a small randomized crossover study in 6 patients with relapsed small cell lung cancer or with poor prognosis; markedly reduced oral bioavailability.[22]	• Avoid consumption of grapefruit within 4 hours of intake of etoposide. • Apple and orange juices may have effects similar to those of grapefruit juice.
Etravirine	• May increase etravirine serum levels.	• Avoid grapefruit. Seville orange, lime and pomelo may also cause the interaction. • If grapefruit consumed during drug therapy, monitor for adverse effects associated with etravirine (e.g., skin rash).
Everolimus	• The manufacturer of Afinitor advises that grapefruit and grapefruit juice should be avoided during everolimus therapy. • May increase everolimus concentration and risk of toxicity.	• Avoid grapefruit. Seville orange, lime and pomelo may also cause the interaction. • If grapefruit consumed during drug therapy, monitor for symptoms of serious toxicity (renal, hematopoietic, gastrointestinal and cardiac toxicities).
Felodipine	• Can significantly increase felodipine plasma levels. • Can increase plasma levels and intensify the clinical effects of some 1,4-dihydropyridine calcium channel blockers. • May be affected to a greater extent than other dihydropyridine calcium channel blockers.	• Avoid grapefruit. Seville orange, lime and pomelo may also cause the interaction. • If grapefruit consumed during drug therapy, monitor for adverse effects associated with increased serum concentrations of felodipine (e.g., decreased diastolic blood pressure, increased heart rate, flushing, headache, peripheral edema and lightheadedness).
Fexofenadine	• Can decrease fexofenadine serum levels, due to OATP1A2 inhibition. • Evaluated in several crossover studies in healthy volunteers; markedly lower AUC and C_{max}.	• Avoid consumption of grapefruit within 4 hours of intake of fexofenadine. • Apple and orange juices had effects similar to those of grapefruit juice. • If grapefruit consumed during drug therapy, monitor for decreased effectiveness of fexofenadine.
Fluvoxamine	• May increase plasma concentrations of fluvoxamine. • Evaluated in randomized crossover design in 10 healthy male subjects; increased AUC and C_{max}.[23]	• Avoid grapefruit. Seville orange, lime and pomelo may also cause the interaction.
HMG-CoA Reductase Inhibitors, see Atorvastatin, Lovastatin, Simvastatin		
Imatinib	• The manufacturer of Gleevec recommends caution when administering Gleevec with grapefruit juice. • May increase imatinib concentrations.	• Avoid grapefruit. Seville orange, lime and pomelo may also cause the interaction. • If grapefruit is consumed during drug therapy, caution and close monitoring for serious adverse reactions (heart failure, hemorrhage, fluid retention) are warranted.
Itraconazole	• May decrease itraconazole serum levels. • May be due to OATP1A2 inhibition. • Evaluated in controlled study in healthy volunteers; decreased AUC and C_{max}.[24] This effect has not been consistently shown in all studies.	• Avoid consumption of grapefruit within 4 hours of intake of itraconazole. • Apple and orange juices may have effects similar to those of grapefruit juice. • If grapefruit consumed during drug therapy, monitor patient for loss of efficacy.
Lapatinib	• May markedly increase lapatinib serum levels.	• Avoid grapefruit. Seville orange, lime and pomelo may also cause the interaction. • If grapefruit consumed during drug therapy, caution and close monitoring for serious adverse reactions (hepatotoxicity, decreased left ventricular ejection fraction, QTc prolongation, torsades de pointes, diarrhea) are warranted.
Losartan	• May decrease formation of major active metabolite. • Evaluated in an open study in 9 healthy subjects; decreased AUC of metabolite.[25]	• Clinical significance is not established. • Avoid grapefruit. Seville orange, lime and pomelo may also cause the interaction. • If grapefruit consumed during drug therapy, monitor for signs of decreased effect (e.g., increased blood pressure).
Lovastatin	• Repeated doses may result in markedly increased lovastatin serum concentrations. • Simvastatin appears to be similarly affected by grapefruit juice; however, atorvastatin is not as greatly affected.	• Avoid grapefruit. Seville orange, lime and pomelo may also cause the interaction. • Consider choosing an HMG-CoA reductase inhibitor not metabolized by CYP3A4 (i.e., fluvastatin and pravastatin). • If grapefruit consumed during drug therapy, monitor for signs of adverse effects associated with increased serum concentrations of lovastatin (e.g., myopathy, rhabdomyolysis, acute renal failure).
Maraviroc	• May increase maraviroc serum levels.	• Avoid grapefruit. Seville orange, lime and pomelo may also cause the interaction. • If grapefruit consumed during drug therapy, close monitoring is required, especially for postural hypotension and syncope.

(cont'd)

Table 1: Drug Administration and Grapefruit *(cont'd)*

Drug	Grapefruit Effect	Management
Methadone	• May increase bioavailability of methadone. • One small study (n=8) in patients undergoing methadone maintenance treatment demonstrated an increase in mean AUC of 17% (range: 3% to 29%) when grapefruit juice was administered 30 minutes prior to and during methadone administration.[26]	• Avoid grapefruit. Seville orange, lime and pomelo may also cause the interaction. • May cause a marked and clinically relevant interaction in susceptible individuals. • If grapefruit consumed during drug therapy, monitor for signs of adverse effects associated with increased serum concentration of methadone (e.g., shallow or decreased breathing, slow heart rate, small pupils).
Methylprednisolone	• Grapefruit juice may increase serum concentrations and half-life of methylprednisolone. • Evaluated in a crossover study in 10 healthy subjects; repeated administration of double-strength grapefruit juice increased AUC, C_{max} and half-life of methylprednisolone. Clinical significance unknown. The effect on half-life shown in this study is likely a function of the large doses of grapefruit juice administered.[27]	• Avoid grapefruit. Seville orange, lime and pomelo may also cause the interaction. • If grapefruit consumed during drug therapy, monitor for adverse effects that may be associated with the use of corticosteroids (e.g., hyperglycemia, Cushingoid features).
Nifedipine	• May lead to increased serum levels of nifedipine. • Evaluated in single dose controlled studies in healthy volunteers.	• Avoid grapefruit. Seville orange, lime and pomelo may also cause the interaction. • If grapefruit consumed during drug therapy, monitor for signs of adverse effects associated with increased serum concentrations of nifedipine (e.g., decreased diastolic blood pressure, increased heart rate, flushing, headache, peripheral edema and lightheadedness).
Nilotinib	• May markedly increase nilotinib serum levels. • Single oral dose of nilotinib with grapefruit juice produced mean C_{max} and AUC that were 60% and 29% higher respectively, than those with water, in 21 healthy male volunteers.[28]	• Avoid grapefruit. Seville orange, lime and pomelo may also cause the interaction.. • If grapefruit consumed during drug therapy, caution and close clinical monitoring for serious adverse effects associated with increased serum levels of nilotinib (prolonged QTc interval, torsades de pointes, neutropenia, thrombocytopenia) are warranted.
Nimodipine	• May increase plasma concentrations of nimodipine. • Pharmacokinetics after a single dose of grapefruit juice are altered. • Pharmacodynamic effects may be augmented.	• Avoid grapefruit. Seville orange, lime and pomelo may also cause the interaction. • If grapefruit consumed during drug therapy, monitor for increased hypotensive effect and side effects such as headache.
Pazopanib	• May increase pazopanib serum levels. • The manufacturer of Votrient advises avoidance of grapefruit and other foods known to affect CYP3A4 and P-gp activity during therapy.	• Avoid grapefruit. Seville orange, lime and pomelo may also cause the interaction. • If grapefruit is consumed during drug therapy, caution and close monitoring for serious adverse reactions (hepatotoxicity, hypertension, QTc prolongation and torsades de pointes, arterial thrombotic events, hemorrhage, gastrointestinal perforation and fistula) are warranted.
Phosphodiesterase Inhibitors, see Sildenafil, Tadalafil, Vardenafil		
Pimozide	• Can result in elevated levels due to decreased drug metabolism. • Elevated levels may enhance the risk of QTc prolongation.	• Avoid grapefruit. Seville orange, lime and pomelo may also cause the interaction. • If grapefruit consumed during drug therapy, monitor for signs of adverse effects associated with increased serum levels of pimozide (e.g., torsades de pointes, extrapyramidal symptoms, hypotension).
Praziquantel	• May increase praziquantel levels. • Evaluated in controlled studies in healthy volunteers; increased C_{max} and AUC.	• Clinical significance unknown.
Primaquine	• Evaluated in random, open-label, crossover study in healthy volunteers; increased geometric mean AUC and C_{max}.[29] • Marked interindividual differences in the increase in primaquine AUC and C_{max} were demonstrated with concomitant consumption of a single amount (300 mL) of half-strength grapefruit juice. • Magnitude of increase in certain individuals was sufficient to be potentially clinically important. • Pharmacokinetics of this interaction is not predictable.	• Avoid grapefruit. Seville orange, lime and pomelo may also cause the interaction. • If grapefruit consumed during drug therapy, monitor for adverse effects associated with increased plasma concentrations of primaquine (e.g., hematologic disturbances such as agranulocytosis, leukopenia, leukocytosis).
Propafenone	• May increase plasma levels of propafenone. • Effect likely to occur in 5–7% of population who are poor CYP2D6 metabolizers.	• Avoid grapefruit. Seville orange, lime and pomelo may also cause the interaction. • If grapefruit consumed during drug therapy, monitor closely for bradycardia, conduction disorders (sinoatrial, atrioventricular or intraventricular block), and proarrhythmic effects (tachycardia, ventricular fibrillation).
Protease Inhibitors, see Saquinavir mesylate		
Quinidine	• Grapefruit juice may increase quinidine levels. • Evaluated in controlled studies in healthy volunteers.	• Avoid grapefruit. Seville orange, lime and pomelo may also cause the interaction.
Repaglinide	• Elevated levels may enhance blood glucose-lowering effect and increase risk of hypoglycemia. • Modestly elevated repaglinide levels occurred in a crossover study of 36 healthy male subjects; no major change in blood glucose was noted.[30]	• Avoid grapefruit. Seville orange, lime and pomelo may also cause the interaction. • If grapefruit consumed during drug therapy, monitor for adverse effects associated with increased repaglinide serum levels (e.g., hypoglycemia).
Rivaroxaban	• May increase rivaroxaban serum levels.	• Avoid grapefruit. Seville orange, lime and pomelo may also cause the interaction. • If grapefruit consumed during drug therapy, close clinical monitoring is required, especially for bleeding.
Saquinavir mesylate	• Can increase absorption of saquinavir. • Coadministration with normal strength grapefruit juice increased AUC of saquinavir by 30% in a single dose study. AUC was doubled with coadministration of double strength grapefruit juice and saquinavir.[31] • No change in AUC has been reported with indinavir; effect on ritonavir has not been studied.	• Since saquinavir is generally well tolerated, clinical significance of interaction is unknown.

(cont'd)

Table 1: Drug Administration and Grapefruit *(cont'd)*

Drug	Grapefruit Effect	Management
Saxagliptin	• May give rise to modest increases in plasma levels of saxagliptin.	• If grapefruit consumed during drug therapy, monitor for possible excessive drug effect (hypoglycemia).
Sertraline	• Grapefruit juice may increase serum concentrations of sertraline. • Evaluated in an open controlled study in 5 patients being treated for depression with 50–75 mg/day of sertraline; increased the mean trough concentration of sertraline. No subject was withdrawn from the study due to adverse effects or mood changes.[32]	• Clinical significance unknown. • Avoid grapefruit. Seville orange, lime and pomelo may also cause the interaction. • If grapefruit consumed during drug therapy, monitor for adverse effects associated with increased serum levels of sertraline (e.g., insomnia or somnolence, tremor, dizziness).
Sildenafil	• Grapefruit juice may increase plasma concentrations and delay absorption of sildenafil. • Evaluated in crossover study in 24 healthy men; no major changes in heart rate or blood pressure were observed.[33]	• Avoid grapefruit. Seville orange, lime and pomelo may also cause the interaction. • If grapefruit consumed during drug therapy, monitor for both delayed effect and adverse effects associated with increased serum concentrations of sildenafil (e.g., hypotension, tachycardia).
Simvastatin	• May markedly increase simvastatin serum concentrations. • Lovastatin bioavailability is similarly increased by grapefruit juice; however, atorvastatin is not as greatly affected.	• Avoid grapefruit. Seville orange, lime and pomelo may also cause the interaction. • Consider choosing an HMG-CoA reductase inhibitor not metabolized by CYP3A4 (i.e., fluvastatin and pravastatin). • If grapefruit consumed during drug therapy, monitor for signs of adverse effects associated with increased serum concentrations of simvastatin (e.g., myopathy, rhabdomyolysis, acute renal failure).
Sirolimus	• Grapefruit juice may have the potential to increase sirolimus blood concentrations.	• Avoid grapefruit. Seville orange, lime and pomelo may also cause the interaction. The manufacturer of Rapamune specifically recommends taking Rapamune with either water or orange juice. • If grapefruit consumed during drug therapy, monitor for increased blood concentrations and for adverse effects associated with increased serum concentrations of sirolimus (e.g., thrombocytopenia, hyperlipidemia).
Solifenacin	• May increase solifenacin serum levels.	• Avoid grapefruit. Seville orange, lime and pomelo may also cause the interaction. • If grapefruit consumed during drug therapy, monitor for prolongation of QTc interval, dry mouth and constipation.
Sunitinib	• May increase sunitinib and active metabolite serum levels. • Steady state sunitinib followed by grapefruit juice 200 mL three times daily for 3 days produced an oral bioavailability that was 11% greater than that with water in 8 cancer patients on monotherapy.[34]	• Avoid grapefruit. Seville orange, lime and pomelo may also cause the interaction. • If grapefruit consumed during drug therapy, monitor for prolongation of QTc interval.
Tacrolimus	• May have the potential to increase tacrolimus blood concentrations.	• Avoid grapefruit. Seville orange, lime and pomelo may also cause the interaction. • If grapefruit consumed during drug therapy, monitor for increased blood levels and symptoms of toxicity (e.g., nephrotoxicity, hepatotoxicity, increased immunosuppression).
Tadalafil	• Grapefruit juice may increase plasma concentrations of tadalafil.	• Avoid grapefruit as per sildenafil. Seville orange, lime and pomelo may also cause the interaction.
Tamsulosin	• May increase tamsulosin levels.	• Avoid grapefruit. Seville orange, lime and pomelo may also cause the interaction. • If grapefruit consumed during drug therapy, monitor for symptoms of orthostatic hypotension (e.g., dizziness, weakness, syncope).
Triazolam	• May increase triazolam serum levels. • Evaluated in controlled studies in healthy volunteers; increased AUC and C_{max} and small increase in psychomotor impairment.	• It is likely that some patients would be adversely affected, especially those in whom triazolam levels are likely to be elevated (e.g., older individuals, those with liver impairment or concurrent use of other cytochrome P450 inhibitors). • Avoid grapefruit. Seville orange, lime and pomelo may also cause the interaction. • If grapefruit consumed during drug therapy, monitor for increased sedation. Significant increase in drowsiness has been reported.
Vardenafil	• Grapefruit juice may increase plasma concentrations of vardenafil.	• Avoid grapefruit. Seville orange, lime and pomelo may also cause the interaction. • If grapefruit consumed during drug therapy, monitor for both delayed effect and adverse effects associated with increased serum concentrations of vardenafil (e.g., hypotension, tachycardia).
Verapamil	• Several small studies in healthy volunteers have shown increases in verapamil serum concentrations and AUC under conditions of repeated grapefruit juice administration.[35,36] • One small study in hypertensive patients (n=10) taking verapamil chronically showed no significant effect of a single dose of grapefruit juice.[37] • Case report of toxic serum levels of verapamil/norverapamil (complete heart block, marked bradycardia and hypotension) with substantial grapefruit consumption in prior week.[38]	• Avoid grapefruit. Seville orange, lime and pomelo may also cause the interaction. • If grapefruit consumed during drug therapy, monitor for adverse effects of verapamil (e.g., bradycardia, hypotension).
Ziprasidone	• May increase ziprasidone serum levels.	• Avoid grapefruit. Seville orange, lime and pomelo may also cause the interaction. • If grapefruit consumed during drug therapy, close clinical monitoring is required, especially for prolongation of QTc interval, torsades de pointes and orthostatic hypotension.

Abbreviations: AUC = area under curve; C_{max} = maximum concentration; OATP1A2 = organic anion transporting polypeptide 1A2; P-gp = P-glycoprotein

References

1. Bailey DG, Malcolm J, Arnold O et al. Grapefruit juice-drug interactions. *Br J Clin Pharmacol* 1998;46(2):101-10.
2. Hansten PD, Horn JR. *Drug interactions analysis and management*. St. Louis (MO): Wolters Kluwer Health; Facts and Comparisons; 2010.
3. Bailey DG. Grapefruit and other fruit juices interactions with medicines. In: Boullata JI, Armenti VT, editors. *Handbook of drug-nutrient interactions*. 2nd ed. Totowa (NJ): Humana Press; 2009. p. 267-302.
4. Bailey DG, Dresser GK. Interactions between grapefruit juice and cardiovascular drugs. *Am J Cardiovasc Drugs* 2004;4(5):281-97.
5. Wilkinson GR. Drug metabolism and variability among patients in drug response. *N Engl J Med* 2005;352(21):2211-21.
6. Dresser GK, Bailey DG, Leake BF et al. Fruit juices inhibit organic anion transporting polypeptide-mediated drug uptake to decrease the oral availability of fexofenadine. *Clin Pharmacol Ther* 2002;71(1):11-20.

7. Dresser GK, Kim RB, Bailey DG. Effect of grapefruit juice volume on the reduction of fexofenadine bioavailability: possible role of organic anion transporting polypeptides. *Clin Pharmacol Ther* 2005;77(3):170-7.
8. Glaeser H, Bailey DG, Dresser GK et al. Intestinal drug transporter expression and the impact of grapefruit juice in humans. *Clin Pharmacol Ther* 2007;81(3):362-70.
9. Bailey DG, Dresser GK, Leake BF et al. Naringin is a major and selective clinical inhibitor of organic anion-transporting polypeptide 1A2 (OATP1A2) in grapefruit juice. *Clin Pharmacol Ther* 2007;81(4):495-502.
10. Bailey DG. Fruit juice inhibition of uptake transport: a new type of food-drug interaction. *Br J Clin Pharmacol* 2010;70(5):645-55.
11. Tapaninen T, Neuvonen PJ, Niemi M. Grapefruit juice greatly reduces the plasma concentrations of the OATP2B1 and CYP3A4 substrate aliskiren. *Clin Pharmacol Ther* 2010;88(3):339-42.
12. Lilja JJ, Raaska K, Neuvonen PJ. Effects of orange juice on the pharmacokinetics of atenolol. *Eur J Clin Pharmacol* 2005;61(5-6):337-40.
13. Seidegard J, Randvall G, Nyberg L et al. Grapefruit juice interaction with oral budesonide: equal effect on immediate-release and delayed-release formulations. *Pharmazie* 2009;64(7):461-5.
14. Lilja JJ, Kivisto KT, Backman JT et al. Grapefruit juice substantially increases plasma concentrations of buspirone. *Clin Pharmacol Ther* 1998;64(6):655-60.
15. Garg SJ, Kumar N, Bhargava VK et al. Effect of grapefruit juice on carbamazepine bioavailability in patients with epilepsy. *Clin Pharmacol Ther* 1998;64(3):286-8.
16. Neuhofel AL, Wilton JH, Victory JM et al. Lack of bioequivalence of ciprofloxacin when administered with calcium-fortified orange juice: a new twist on an old interaction. *J Clin Pharmacol* 2002;42(4):461-6.
17. Goldbart A, Press J, Sofer S et al. Near fatal acute colchicine intoxication in a child. A case report. *Eur J Pediatr* 2000;159(12):895-7.
18. Drug-food interactions: grapefruit juice. In: *Multaq (dronedarone HCl)* [product monograph]. Bridgewater (NJ): sanofi-aventis; July 31, 2009.
19. *Inspra (eplerenone)* [product monograph]. New York (NY): Pfizer; February 2009.
20. Kanazawa S, Ohkubo T, Sugawara K. The effects of grapefruit juice on the pharmacokinetics of erythromycin. *Eur J Clin Pharmacol* 2001;56(11):799-803.
21. Grande LA, Mendez RD, Krug RT et al. Attention—grapefruit! *Lancet* 2009;373(9670):1222.
22. Reif S, Nicolson MC, Bisset D et al. Effect of grapefruit juice intake on etoposide bioavailability. *Eur J Clin Pharmacol* 2002;58(7):491-4.
23. Hori H, Yoshimura R, Ueda N et al. Grapefruit juice-fluvoxamine interaction--is it risky or not. *J Clin Pyschopharmacol* 2003;23(4):422-4.
24. Kawakami M, Suzuki K, Ishizuka T et al. Effect of grapefruit juice on pharmacokinetics of itraconazole in health subjects. *Int J Clin Pharmacol Ther* 1998;36(6):306-8.
25. Zaidenstein R, Soback S, Gips M et al. Effect of grapefruit juice on the pharmacokinetics of losartan and its active metabolite E3174 in healthy volunteers. *Ther Drug Monit* 2001;23(4):369-73.
26. Benmebarek M, Devaud C, Gex-Fabry M et al. Effects of grapefruit juice on the pharmacokinetics of the enantiomers of methadone. *Clin Pharmacol Ther* 2004;76(1):55-63.
27. Varis T, Kivisto KT, Neuvonen PJ. Grapefruit juice can increase the plasma concentrations of oral methylprednisolone. *Eur J Clin Pharmacol* 2000;56(6-7):489-93.
28. Yin OQ, Gallagher N, Li A et al. Effect of grapefruit juice on the pharmacokinetics of nilotinib in healthy participants. *J Clin Pharmacol* 2010;50(2):188-94.
29. Cuong BT, Binh VQ, Dai B et al. Does gender, food or grapefruit juice alter the pharmacokinetics of primaquine in healthy subjects? *Br J Clin Pharmacol* 2006;61(6):682-9.
30. Bidstrup TB, Damkier P, Olsen AK et al. The impact of CYP2C8 polymorphism and grapefruit juice on the pharmacokinetics of repaglinide. *Br J Clin Pharmacol* 2006;61(1):49-57.
31. Kupferschmidt HH, Fattinger KE, Ha HR et al. Grapefruit juice enhances the bioavailability of the HIV protease inhibitor saquinavir in man. *Br J Clin Pharmacol* 1998;45(4):355-9.
32. Lee AJ, Chan WK, Harralson AF et al. The effects of grapefruit juice on sertraline metabolism: an in vitro and in vivo study. *Clin Ther* 1999;21(11):1890-9.
33. Jetter A, Kinzig-Schippers M, Walchner-Bonjean M et al. Effects of grapefruit juice on the pharmacokinetics of sildenafil. *Clin Pharmacol Ther* 2002;71(1):21-9.
34. van Erp NP, Baker SD, Zandvliet AS et al. Marginal increase of sunitinib exposure by grapefruit juice. *Cancer Chemother Pharmacol* 2010 May 29. [Epub ahead of print].
35. Ho PC, Ghose K, Saville D et al. Effect of grapefruit juice on pharmacokinetics and pharmacodynamics of verapamil enantiomers in healthy volunteers. *Eur J Clin Pharmacol* 2000;56(9-10):693-8.
36. Fuhr U, Muller-Peltzer H, Kern R et al. Effects of grapefruit juice and smoking on verapamil concentrations in steady state. *Eur J Clin Pharmacol* 2002;58(1):45-53.
37. Zaidenstein R, Dishi V, Gips M et al. The effect of grapefruit juice on the pharmacokinetics of orally administered verapamil. *Eur J Clin Pharmacol* 1998;54(4):337-40.
38. Pillai U, Muzaffar J, Sen S et al. Grapefruit juice and verapamil: a toxic cocktail. *South Med J* 2009;102(3):308-9.

Latex

Reviewed by Antony J Ham Pong, MBBS, FRCPC

Date of Revision: September 2010

Natural rubber latex (NRL), or latex allergy, has become an important health concern, especially for health care workers and patients who undergo multiple surgeries. Reactions to NRL products range from mild to life-threatening. The severity is dependent on individual susceptibility and the route of NRL-allergen exposure. Mucosal, visceral and parenteral exposures are associated with the greatest risk for severe systemic reactions.[1] These reactions can be divided into three groups:[2,3]

Nonallergic irritant contact dermatitis: a nonimmunologic reaction caused by mechanical irritation and characterized by redness, scaling, cracking, dryness, itching and vesicle formation on exposed areas.

Allergic contact dermatitis: a delayed, type IV allergic reaction to rubber chemicals used in the manufacturing of NRL products. Typical presentation occurs 24 to 48 hours after contact and is characterized by redness, itching and vesicle formation. Repeated contact may cause the skin to become dry, cracked and thickened.

Allergic Immunoglobulin E (IgE)-mediated reaction: an immediate, type I allergic reaction due to residual NRL proteins in NRL products. Urticaria, flushing, edema, rhinitis, conjunctivitis, asthma and anaphylaxis can occur within minutes of exposure.

The risk of NRL allergy seems to increase with early and repeated exposure to NRL products. High-risk individuals include patients with spina bifida or other congenital abnormalities that require multiple surgical interventions (especially children). Other groups at risk include health care workers, rubber industry workers and atopic individuals.[2,4,5] The following characteristics may be used to screen for adults and children who may be sensitive to NRL:[2]

- Contact urticaria, rhinoconjunctivitis, swelling, asthma or anaphylaxis after contact with NRL products, e.g., gloves, condoms, balloons
- History of eczema or atopic diseases
- Allergic reaction during medical, dental or surgical procedures
- Allergies to foods, especially tropical fruits (banana, avocado, papaya, kiwi) and chestnut

Patients who have high risk factors for NRL allergy should be referred to a specialist for consultation and confirmatory tests.[6]

Management and prevention of NRL allergy involves completely avoiding NRL products.[7,8] Precautions must be taken during preparation and administration of parenteral products. Review all materials (e.g., vials, syringes, tip caps, evacuated containers, tubing, minibags, infusion sets, gloves) for NRL content and select NRL-free products when available.

The risk of exposure to trace amounts of NRL from medication vial stoppers is unclear.[8] NRL vial stoppers are dry NRL products which have less residual NRL protein and have been reported to elicit allergic reactions less frequently than dipped NRL products (medical gloves, condoms, catheters).[1] However, due to isolated reports of rubber vial stoppers causing allergic reactions,[9,10] many health care institutions have adopted guidelines to prepare NRL-safe parenteral products. Two examples are:

- Remove the vial stopper. The benefit must be weighed against the potential for dosing errors, dilution problems, contamination and waste.[4]
- One-stick policy. Limit vial access to one puncture for any vial closure. Once the drug is withdrawn, change the needle before administration.[1,11,12]

These procedures do not eliminate the possibility that NRL proteins may leach from NRL vial stoppers into the drug solution during storage.[1] It is best to use latex-free products if possible.

How to Find Information About Latex in Product Monographs

Information about latex content in specific products can be located in the following sections of individual *CPS* product monographs:

- Summary Product Information
- Contraindications
- Dosage Forms, Composition and Packaging or Supplied

Users of e-CPS can also search for latex within a product monograph or across multiple product monographs, using the Advanced Search link.

Do not assume latex is not present if it is not listed in the manufacturer's monograph. CPhA strongly recommends that you contact the manufacturer directly for confirmatory information (see Manufacturers Directory).

References

1. Primeau MN, Adkinson NF, Hamilton RG. Natural rubber pharmaceutical vial closures release latex allergens that produce skin reactions. *J Allergy Clin Immunol* 2001;107(6):958-62.
2. Brehler R, Kutting B. Natural rubber latex allergy: a problem of interdisciplinary concern in medicine. *Arch Intern Med* 2001;161(8):1057-64.
3. Society of Gastroenterology Nurses and Associates, Inc. Guidelines for preventing sensitivity and allergic reactions to natural rubber latex in the workplace. *Gastroenterol Nurs* 2004;27(4):191-7.
4. Thomsen DJ, Burke TG. Lack of latex allergen contamination of solutions withdrawn from vials with natural rubber stoppers. *Am J Health Syst Pharm* 2000;57(1):44-7.
5. Bousquet J, Flahault A, Vandenplas O et al. Natural rubber latex allergy among health care workers: a systematic review of the evidence. *J Allergy Clin Immunol* 2006;118(2):447-54.
6. Sussman GL, Beezhold DH. Allergy to latex rubber. *Ann Intern Med* 1995;122(1):43-6.
7. LaMontagne AD, Radi S, Elder DS et al. Primary prevention of latex related sensitisation and occupational asthma: a systematic review. *Occup Environ Med* 2006;63(5):359-64.
8. Elliott BA. Latex allergy: the perspective from the surgical suite. *J Allergy Clin Immunol* 2002;110(2 Suppl):S117-20.
9. Towse A, O'Brien M, Twarog FJ et al. Local reaction secondary to insulin injection. A potential role for latex antigens in insulin vials and syringes. *Diabetes Care* 1995;18(8):1195-7.
10. Vassallo SA, Thurston TA, Kim SH et al. Allergic reaction to latex from stopper of a medication vial. *Anesth Analg* 1995;80(5):1057-8.
11. Children's Hospital of Eastern Ontario. *Latex precautions.* Ottawa (ON): CHEO; 1999.
12. Ottawa Hospital. *Pharmacy procedures for latex allergic patients.* Ottawa (ON): Civic Campus; 2002.

Nonmedicinal Ingredients

Reviewed by Antony J Ham Pong, MBBS, FRCPC

Date of Revision: September 2010

In addition to the active drug, products may also contain nonmedicinal ingredients (NMIs) used as diluents, binders, lubricants, buffers, antioxidants, fillers, preservatives, flavours, colouring agents and sweeteners. Examples of NMIs are alcohol, gluten, lactose, peanut oil, soybean oil, soya lecithin, sulfites and tartrazine. Some raw materials used in the manufacturing process are obtained from sources other than the pharmaceutical industry; therefore, the drug manufacturer may be unaware of unlabelled NMIs. For example, agents used to whiten powders may contain traces of sulfites, and dyes used to imprint names on capsules may contain traces of tartrazine or sulfites.

A small percentage of individuals with the propensity to allergic reactions or particular sensitivities may experience adverse effects to some NMIs. Adverse effects may range from general discomfort to those which are life-threatening.

How to Find Information About Nonmedicinal Ingredients (NMIs) in Product Monographs

Information about nonmedicinal ingredients in specific products can be located in the following sections of individual *CPS* product monographs:

- Summary Product Information
- Contraindications
- Dosage Forms, Composition and Packaging or Supplied

Consult the appropriate clinical information provided here for each nonmedicinal ingredient for synonyms (e.g., FD&C Yellow No. 5 for tartrazine). Do not assume the ingredient is not present if it is not listed in the manufacturer's monograph. CPhA strongly recommends that you contact the manufacturer directly for confirmatory information (See Manufacturers Directory).

Users of e-CPS can also search for a specific NMI within a product monograph or across multiple product monographs, using the Advanced Search link.

Ethanol

Awareness of the ethanol (also called absolute alcohol, anhydrous alcohol, dehydrated alcohol, ethyl alcohol, ethyl hydrate, ethyl hydroxide) content of pharmaceuticals assists the health professional in providing advice on product selection for both prescription and over-the-counter medications. Ethanol is often used as a preservative and solvent in pharmaceutical preparations.

Certain medications and conditions influence the need for awareness of the ethanol content of pharmaceuticals. "Disulfiram-like" reactions characterized by flushing, headache, nausea, sweating and/or tachycardia may occur when ethanol is taken with chlorpropamide, metronidazole or procarbazine.

Ethanol is a CNS depressant. When taken with drugs such as hypnotics, antihistamines, opioid analgesics, antiepileptics, antidepressants, antipsychotics or sedatives, the CNS effects of ethanol may be enhanced.

Ethanol content of oral products should be assessed in individuals with diabetes. Avoidance of ethanol, or use of low-ethanol-content products, is preferred for children.

Gluten

Gluten, a mixture of two proteins namely gliadin and glutenin, is present in wheat, barley and rye. Gluten is not present in rice, corn or oats; however, oats are avoided because of gluten cross-contamination during processing.

Celiac disease is a hypersensitivity reaction to the gliadin fraction of ingested gluten, resulting in immunologically mediated inflammatory damage to the lining of the small intestine in genetically predisposed individuals. The inflammation may lead to malabsorption by reducing the amount of surface area available for absorption of nutrients, fluids and electrolytes. Depending on the extent and severity of the mucosal inflammation, patients may be asymptomatic or exhibit a wide range of gastrointestinal (e.g., diarrhea, vomiting, abdominal pain, discomfort) symptoms and nongastrointestinal effects (e.g., iron-deficiency anemia, osteoporosis, dermatitis herpetiformis). The treatment for celiac disease is a strict, lifetime avoidance of gluten ingestion. Even a small amount of gluten, as in a gluten-containing medication administered orally or rectally, can be problematic for the individual with celiac disease.

In the Supplied section of the *CPS* product monographs, the statement "contains gluten" refers to the gluten derived from wheat, barley and rye for only the nonmedicinal ingredients. This does not refer to gluten if it is inherent in the active ingredient.

Lactose

Lactose is used as a diluent, bulking agent, filler and excipient for tablets and capsules. Medications that use lactose as a filler may cause symptoms of lactose intolerance in those who take multiple lactose-containing medications. Lactose intolerance occurs in individuals with a deficiency of the intestinal enzyme lactase and leads to symptoms including abdominal cramps, diarrhea, distension and flatulence. Drug-induced diarrhea due to lactose intolerance has been reported as a result of the lactose in pharmaceutical formulations.

Temporary or permanent lactose intolerance may also occur in individuals who have had an intestinal infection, gastric surgery or following the use of medications, particularly antibiotics or some anti-inflammatory agents. Administration of the enzyme lactase can increase lactose tolerance of lactose-intolerant individuals. Lactase is available as drops, tablets or caplets. For more information, consult individual lactase product monographs within *CPS*. Lactose is also contraindicated in individuals with the fructose-galactose malabsorption syndrome called galactosemia.

Peanut Oil, Soybean Oil or Soya Lecithin

Peanuts are the most common food trigger for anaphylaxis. The incidence and prevalence of peanut allergy is increasing. Peanut allergy tends to present earlier in life and is not usually outgrown. There are many allergens in peanuts that provoke the immunoglobulin E (IgE)-mediated type 1 hypersensitivity reactions and can cause allergic reactions. The most important are the seed storage proteins identified as Ara h1, Ara h2 and Ara h3. In highly sensitized individuals, trace quantities of these allergens can induce an allergic reaction; though most IgE mediated reactions occur within 60 minutes, some occur up to 4 hours after ingestion.

Risk factors for peanut allergy include atopy and family history of peanut allergy. Maternal consumption of peanuts, infant consumption of peanuts or peanut oil, use of maternal breast creams containing peanut oil and consumption of soya milk or soya formula by infants have also been implicated; however, there is increasing evidence that these factors do not play an important role.

Soya and peanuts both belong to the legume family and there may be potential for cross-reactivity. Peanut-allergic individuals may develop a soya allergy in 5 to 15% of cases. **Soya lecithin** and **soybean oil**, ingredients found in some pharmaceuticals, may contain small amounts of soya protein. Medications that contain soya lecithin and soybean oil should be avoided in individuals with a severe soya allergy unless otherwise advised by their doctor. However, peanut allergy is not a contraindication to use of soya products unless there is a co-existing soya allergy.

Avoidance of heat-refined **arachis oil** or **peanut oil** by peanut-allergic sufferers remains controversial since there is conflicting evidence on whether residual proteins in these oils can provoke allergic reactions. Heat-refined, protein-free arachis oil or peanut oil should not cause allergic reactions in peanut-allergy sufferers; however, medications that contain peanut oil should be avoided whenever possible because if not properly refined, traces of peanut protein may still be present.

Management of anaphylactic peanut allergies involves completely avoiding medications that contain **peanut products** and **arachis oil**. It is crucial to recognize early signs of allergic reactions and when and how to use a self-administered epinephrine auto-injector such as EpiPen or Twinject. Early treatment with epinephrine can prevent fatal allergic reactions. Antihistamines (e.g., diphenhydramine) may be given in addition, but they do not prevent or treat anaphylaxis. A trip to the emergency department is vital. A written action plan regarding management of a peanut allergy is good practice.

Sulfites

The term sulfites (sulphites) includes sodium or potassium bisulfite, sodium or potassium metabisulfite, sodium sulfite and sulfur dioxide. Sulfiting agents are used as antioxidants in the preservation of foods and drugs.

Hypersensitivity reactions such as urticaria, nausea, diarrhea, wheezing and dyspnea have been reported most frequently after ingestion of restaurant foods treated with sulfites, but they also occur after exposure to drug products containing sulfites. The concentration of sulfites in pharmaceuticals is usually low but adverse reactions to sulfites are not always dose related. Adverse reactions to sulfites, particularly in asthmatics, may be life-threatening. In asthmatics, sensitivity is more common to inhaled rather than ingested sulfites.

Many patients may have sulfite sensitivity rather than "food" or "drug allergy." Patients known to be sensitive to sulfites should carefully read the label of purchased food to determine if there are any sulfites in the product. Health professionals must be alert to the possible presence of sulfites in drug formulations.

Tartrazine

Tartrazine (FD&C Yellow No. 5) is a dye used to produce a yellow colour or in combination with other dyes produce red or green colour in food, beverages and drugs. It is a member of the azo dye compounds which are most commonly implicated in dye-induced toxicity. The most common reactions to tartrazine are asthma or urticaria. Although the overall sensitivity to tartrazine is low, it may occur more frequently in ASA-sensitive and NSAID-sensitive individuals.

Suggested Readings

1. European Medicines Agency. Evaluation of Medicines for Human Use. *Working party on herbal medicinal products. Final position paper on the allergenic potency of herbal medicinal products containing soya or peanut protein.* London (GB): EMEA; June 11, 2004. Available from: www.ema.europa.eu/docs/en_GB/document_library/Position_statement/2009/12/WC500018029.pdf. Accessed August 24, 2010.
2. Golightly LK, Smolinske SS, Bennett ML et al. Pharmaceutical excipients. Adverse effects associated with inactive ingredients in drug products (Part I). *Med Toxicol Adverse Drug Exp* 1988;3(2):128-65.
3. Green PH, Cellier C. Celiac disease. *N Engl J Med* 2007;357(17):1731-43.
4. Heyman MB; Committee on Nutrition. Lactose intolerance in infants, children, and adolescents. *Pediatrics* 2006;118(3):1279-86.
5. Hill ID, Dirks MH, Liptak GS et al. Guideline for the diagnosis and treatment of celiac disease in children: recommendations of the North American Society for Pediatric Gastroenterology, Hepatology and Nutrition. *J Pediatr Gastroenterol Nutr* 2005;40(1):1-19.
6. Klemola T, Kalimo K, Poussa T et al. Feeding a soy formula to children with cow's milk allergy: the development of immunoglobulin E-mediated allergy to soy and peanuts. *Pediatr Allergy Immunol* 2005;16(8):641-6.
7. Lack G, Fox D, Northstone K et al. Factors associated with the development of peanut allergy in childhood. *N Engl J Med* 2003;348(11):977-85.
8. Miyata M, Schuster B, Schellenberg R. Sulfite-containing Canadian pharmaceutical products available in 1991. *CMAJ* 1992;147(9):1333-8.
9. Napke E. Excipients, adverse drug reactions and patients' rights. *CMAJ* 1994;151(5):529-33.
10. Napke E. Additional hidden hazards in drug products. *Can Pharm J* 1995;128(2):23-5.
11. "Inactive" ingredients in pharmaceutical products: update (subject review). American Academy of Pediatrics Committee on Drugs. *Pediatrics* 1997;99(2):268-78.
12. Olszewski A, Pons L, Moutete F et al. Isolation and characterization of proteic allergens in refined peanut oil. *Clin Exp Allergy* 1998;28(7):850-9.
13. Parker WA, MacLachlan RA. Hypersensitivity to sodium bisulfite in Normosol-M with Dextrose. *Can J Hosp Pharm* 1987;40(4):139-40, 152.
14. Sampson HA. Clinical practice. Peanut allergy. *N Engl J Med* 2002;346(17):1294-9.
15. Scurlock AM, Burks AW. Peanut allergenicity. *Ann Allergy Asthma Immunol* 2004;93(5 Suppl 3):S12-8.
16. Smith JM, Dodd TRP. Adverse reactions to pharmaceutical excipients. *Adv Drug Reac Ac Pois Rev* 1982;1:98-142.
17. Vadas P, Wai Y, Burks W et al. Detection of peanut allergens in breast milk of lactating women. *JAMA* 2001;285(13):1746-8.
18. van Heel DA, West J. Recent advances in coeliac disease. *Gut* 2006;55(7):1037-46.
19. Yamamoto A, Wright D, Campbell J. We have a little list. *Rev Pharm Can* 1988;121(10):642-7.

Clin-Info

Index

Directory

I About Poison Control Centres

This directory provides contact information for Poison Control Centres across Canada and is arranged alphabetically by province/territory. Note that poison treatment is available in the emergency departments of most active treatment hospitals. In case of an emergency, contact the Poison Control Centre by telephone (and not by fax).

II About Health Organizations

This directory provides contact information for various health organizations that provide information for health professionals, health consumers or both. A brief overview of the organization is found in the mission statement. The organizations are listed alphabetically by disease state or subject. The list is not exhaustive; therefore, the reader is encouraged to seek additional references.

III About Pharmaceutical Manufacturers/Distributors

This directory provides contact information for manufacturers and Canadian distributors of pharmaceutical preparations listed in *CPS*. For further information on products listed in this directory, readers are encouraged to consult the Monographs Section.

Online Updates

Updates to the Poison Control Centres, Health Organizations and Pharmaceutical Manufacturers/Distributors received by the publisher after the print deadline are published in e-CPS, CPhA's online *CPS*. e-CPS is updated bi-weekly. For more information or to subscribe to e-CPS, visit www.pharmacists.ca/e-CPS.

Directory I—Poison Control Centres

Alberta
Poison and Drug Information Service
Foothills Hospital
1403–29th St NW
Calgary AB T2N 2T9
Tel: 1-800-332-1414
403-944-1414
Fax: 403-944-1472

British Columbia
B.C. Drug and Poison Information Centre
1081 Burrard St
Vancouver BC V6Z 1Y6
Tel: 1-800-567-8911 (remainder of Province)
604-682-5050 (Lower Mainland)
Fax: 604-806-8262

Manitoba
Manitoba Poison Control Centre
Children's Hospital
840 Sherbrook St
Winnipeg MB R3A 1S1
Tel: 204-787-2591
Fax: 204-787-5008

New Brunswick
Clinidata division of Sykes Assistance Services Corporation
Poison Information Centre
774 Main St 6th floor
Moncton NB E1C 9Y3
Tel: 911 (within New Brunswick)
Fax: 506-867-3259

Newfoundland
Poison Information Centre
The Janeway Child Health Centre
300 Prince Philip Dr
St. John's NL A1B 3V6
Tel: 709-722-1110
Fax: 709-726-0830

Northwest Territories
Telecare Health Line
Tel: 1-888-255-1010

Nova Scotia
Poison Information Centre
The IWK Health Centre
PO Box 3070
Halifax NS B3J 3G9
Tel: 1-800-565-8161 (Nova Scotia and Prince Edward Island)
902-470-8161 (remainder of Provinces)
Fax: 902-470-7213

Nunavut
Baffin (Qikiqtani) Regional Hospital
Box 1000
Iqaluit NU X0A 0H0
Tel: 867-975-8600
Fax: 867-975-8634

Cambridge Bay (Ikaluktutiak) Health Centre
Box 53
Cambridge Bay NU X0B 0C0
Tel: 867-983-4500
Fax: 867-983-4509

Rankin Inlet (Kangiqliniq) Health Centre
Bag 008
Rankin Inlet NU X0C 0G0
Tel: 867-645-8300
Fax: 867-645-8389

Ontario
Ontario Poison Centre
The Hospital for Sick Children
555 University Ave
Toronto ON M5G 1X8
Tel: 1-800-268-9017
416-813-5900
Fax: 416-813-7489

Prince Edward Island
Poison Information Centre
The IWK Health Centre
PO Box 3070
Halifax NS B3J 3G9
Tel: 1-800-565-8161

Quebec
Centre antipoison du Québec
Pavillon Jeffery Hale
1270, chemin Sainte-Foy, 4e étage
Quebec QC G1S 2M4
Tel: 1-800-463-5060
Fax: 418-654-2747

Saskatchewan
Poison and Drug Information Service
Foothills Hospital
1403–29th St NW
Calgary AB T2N 2T9
Tel: 1-866-454-1212

Yukon Territory
Emergency Department
Whitehorse General Hospital
5 Hospital Rd
Whitehorse YT Y1A 3H7
Tel: 867-393-8700
Fax: 867-393-8762

Directory II—Health Organizations

Acupuncture Foundation of Canada Institute
The AFCI enhances the health and healing impact of acupuncture for Canadians through: provision of competency-based continuing education in acupuncture for multidisciplinary, regulated health professionals; collaboration with government, regulators, consumers and insurers for access to, and funding for, acupuncture services; promotion of best practices and research in acupuncture; public outreach and education regarding the holistic benefits of acupuncture; and provision of ongoing support, website and administrative services to members.
204–2131 Lawrence Ave E
Scarborough ON M1R 5G4
Tel: 416-752-3988
Fax: 416-752-4398
Email: afciweb@afcinstitute.com
Website: www.afcinstitute.com

Adolescent Health, Canadian Association for
The CAAH is a non-profit organization which concentrates its efforts: to promote health and the well-being of adolescents, particularly those between 10 and 19 years old; to set standards in healthcare and services for adolescents; to promote cooperation between healthcare professionals and organizations working in the field.
CAAH
Section médecine de l'adolescence
Ste-Justine Hospital
3175 ch de la Côte Ste-Catherine
7th floor, 2nd block
Montreal QC H3T 1C5
Tel: 514-345-9959
Fax: 514-345-4778
Email: acsacaah@globetrotter.net
Website: www.acsa-caah.ca

AIDS Society, Canadian
The CAS is a national coalition of over 120 community-based AIDS organizations across Canada. We are dedicated to strengthening the response to HIV/AIDS across all sectors of society and to enriching the lives of people and communities living with HIV/AIDS.
800–190 O'Connor St
Ottawa ON K2P 2R3
Tel: 613-230-3580
1-800-499-1986
Fax: 613-563-4998
Email: casinfo@cdnaids.ca
Website: www.cdnaids.ca
See also AIDS Treatment Information Exchange, Canadian

AIDS Treatment Information Exchange, Canadian
The CATIE champions and supports innovation and excellence in knowledge exchange for the prevention of HIV transmission, and the care, treatment and support of people with HIV.
505–555 Richmond St W
PO Box 1104
Toronto ON M5V 3B1
Tel: 1-800-263-1638
Fax: 416-203-8284
Email: info@catie.ca
Website: www.catie.ca
See also AIDS Society, Canadian

Allergy/Asthma Information Association
The AAIA's mission is to create safer environments and improve quality of life for Canadians affected by allergy, asthma and anaphylaxis by empowering individuals and providing education, leadership, and a national voice.
118–295 The West Mall
Toronto ON M9C 4Z4
Tel: 416-621-4571
1-800-611-7011
Fax: 416-621-5034
Email: admin@aaia.ca
Website: www.aaia.ca
See also Asthma Society of Canada; Lung Association, Canadian

Alpha-1 Canada
Alpha-1 Canada's mission is to provide information, education and support to Canadians affected by alpha-1 antitrypsin deficiency; inform and educate the medical community about alpha-1 antitrypsin deficiency; and generate broad awareness about this genetic liver, lung and skin disease.
1638 Northway Ave
Windsor ON N9B 3L9
Tel: 519-258-1444
1-888-669-4583
Fax: 519-258-1614
Email: info@alpha1canada.ca
Website: www.alpha1canada.ca/

Alzheimer Society of Canada
The Society identifies, develops and facilitates national priorities that enable its members to effectively alleviate the personal and social consequences of Alzheimer's and related diseases, promotes research and leads the search for a cure.
1600–20 Eglinton Ave W
Toronto ON M4R 1K8
Tel: 416-488-8772
1-800-616-8816
Fax: 416-322-6656
Email: info@alzheimer.ca
Website: www.alzheimer.ca

Amyotrophic Lateral Sclerosis Society of Canada
(Lou Gehrig's Disease)
The ALS Society is committed to: support research towards a cure for ALS; support provincial ALS societies in their provision of quality care for persons living with ALS; build public awareness of ALS and its impact.
200–3000 Steeles Ave E
Markham ON L3R 4T9
Tel: 905-248-2052
1-800-267-4257
Fax: 905-248-2019
Website: www.als.ca

Anxiety Disorders Association of Canada
The ADAC is a registered Canadian non-profit organization whose aim is to promote the prevention, treatment and management of anxiety disorders and to improve the lives of people who suffer from them.
PO Box 117
Station Côte St-Luc
Montreal QC H4V 2Y3
Tel: 514-484-0504
1-888-223-2252
Fax: 514-484-7892
Email: contactus@anxietycanada.ca
Website: www.anxietycanada.ca
See also Mental Health Association, Canadian

Aplastic Anemia and Myelodysplasia Association of Canada
The Association's mandate is to inform the public about aplastic anemia, myelodysplasia (MDS) and paroxysmal nocturnal hemoglobinuria (PNH); to provide a nation-wide support network for patients and their families; to educate and advocate; to raise funds for medical research; to promote Canadian Blood Services and Héma-Québec blood programs and the unrelated bone marrow donor registry, OneMatch.
321–11181 Yonge St
Richmond Hill ON L4S 1L2
Tel: 905-780-0698
1-888-840-0039 (English)
Fax: 905-780-1648
Email: info@aamac.ca
Website: www.aamac.ca

Arthritis Society
The Arthritis Society is Canada's only not-for-profit organization devoted solely to funding and promoting arthritis research, programs and patient care.
National Office
1700–393 University Ave
Toronto ON M5G 1E6
Tel: 416-979-7228
Fax: 416-979-8366
Email: info@arthritis.ca
Website: www.arthritis.ca

Asthma Society of Canada
The Society's mission is supporting Canadians to achieve symptom-free asthma through the delivery of accredited and relevant asthma self-management education and certified asthma counselling.
2306–4950 Yonge St
Toronto ON M2N 6K1
Tel: 416-787-4050
1-866-787-4050
Fax: 416-787-5807
Email: info@asthma.ca
Website: www.asthma.ca
See also Allergy/Asthma Information Association; Lung Association, Canadian

Attention Deficit Disorder Canada Inc., Children and Adults with
CH.A.D.D. Canada is a charitable organization that aims to help support, educate, and ultimately better the lives of individuals with ADHD, and those who are for them.
CHADD Canada Inc.
PO Box 23043
Citadel RPO
St. Albert AB T8N 6Z9
Email: chaddcanada@hotmail.com
Website: www.chaddcanada.org

Blind, Canadian National Institute for the
CNIB is a nation-wide, community-based, registered charity committed to research, public education and vision health for all Canadians. CNIB provides the services and support necessary for people to enjoy a good quality of life while living with vision loss.
1929 Bayview Ave
Toronto ON M4G 3E8
Tel: 416-486-2500
1-800-563-2642
416-480-8645 (TTY)
Fax: 416-480-7700
Email: info@cnib.ca
Website: www.cnib.ca

Brain Tumour Foundation of Canada
The Brain Tumour Foundation of Canada is a national, not-for-profit organization dedicated to reaching every person in Canada affected by a brain tumour through support, education, information, and research.
301–620 Colborne St
London ON N6B 3R9
Tel: 519-642-7755
1-800-265-5106
Fax: 519-642-7192
Email: braintumour@braintumour.ca
Website: www.braintumour.ca

Breast Cancer Foundation, Canadian
The Foundation works collaboratively to fund, support and advocate for: relevant and innovative research; meaningful education and awareness programs; early diagnosis and effective treatment; and a positive quality of life for those living with breast cancer.
375 University Ave
6th floor
Toronto ON M5G 2J5
Tel: 416-596-6773
1-800-387-9816
Fax: 416-596-7857
Email: connect@cbcf.org
Website: www.cbcf.org
See also Cancer Society, Canadian; Women's Health Network, Canadian

Breastfeeding, Drug exposure during
See Motherisk

Cancer Society, Canadian
The Canadian Cancer Society is a national, community-based organization of volunteers, whose mission is the eradication of cancer and the enhancement of the quality of life of people living with cancer.
National Office
200–10 Alcorn Ave
Toronto ON M4V 3B1
Tel: 416-961-7223
Fax: 416-961-4189
Email: ccs@cancer.ca
Website: www.cancer.ca

Celiac Association, Canadian
The Canadian Celiac Association is a national organization dedicated to providing services and support to persons with celiac disease and dermatitis herpetiformis through programs of awareness, advocacy, education and research.
204–5170 Dixie Rd
Mississauga ON L4W 1E3
Tel: 905-507-6208
1-800-363-7296
Fax: 905-507-4673
Email: info@celiac.ca
Website: www.celiac.ca
See also Digestive Health Foundation, Canadian

Child Health, Canadian Institute of
Dedicated to promoting and protecting the health, well-being and rights of children and youth through monitoring education and advocacy.
300–384 Bank St
Ottawa ON K2P 1Y4
Tel: 613-230-8838
Fax: 613-230-6654
Email: cich@cich.ca
Website: www.cich.ca

Childhood Cancer Foundation Candlelighters Canada
The Childhood Cancer Foundation Candlelighters Canada is a national, volunteer governed, charitable organization dedicated to improving the quality of life for children with cancer and their families. We will achieve our mission through undertaking and supporting national initiatives resulting in the increased survival and wellbeing of our children, and ultimately a cure for all childhood cancers.
801–21 St. Clair Ave E
Toronto ON M4T 1L9
Tel: 416-489-6440
1-800-363-1062
Fax: 416-489-9812
Email: info@childhoodcancer.ca
Website: www.childhoodcancer.ca

Chronic fatigue syndrome
See ME/FM Action Network, National

Chronic Pain Association of Canada
The goals of the Association are to provide a meeting place for the consideration and discussion of questions concerning pain that affects the interests of the community. To provide information to the general public concerning the treatment of chronic pain. To work towards establishing multidisciplinary Pain Centres that use all the methods of treating and managing pain. To improve the way the medical profession is educated about the treatment and management of pain.
Mailing address:
Box 66017
Heritage Postal Station
Edmonton AB T6J 6T4
Tel: 780-482-6727
Fax: 780-433-3128
Email: cpac@chronicpaincanada.com
Website: www.chronicpaincanada.com

Continence Foundation, Canadian
The Foundation's mission is to enhance the quality of life for people experiencing incontinence by helping, them and/or their caregivers, to confidently seek and access cures and treatment options. To this end, the Foundation will implement and encourage important public and professional education, support, advocacy and research to advance incontinence treatment and/or management.
PO Box 417
Peterborough ON K9J 6Z3
Tel: 705-750-4600
Fax: 705-750-1770
Email: help@canadiancontinence.ca
Website: www.canadiancontinence.ca

Crohn's and Colitis Foundation of Canada
The CCFC believes that a cure will be found for Crohn's disease and ulcerative colitis. To realize this, the CCFC is committed, first and foremost, to raise increasing funds for medical research. The CCFC also believes it is important to make all individuals with inflammatory bowel disease (IBD) aware of the Foundation, and educate these individuals, their families, health professionals and the general public about these diseases.
National Office
600–60 St Clair Ave E
Toronto ON M4T 1N5
Tel: 416-920-5035
1-800-387-1479
Fax: 416-929-0364
Email: ccfc@ccfc.ca
Website: www.ccfc.ca
See also Digestive Health Foundation, Canadian

Cystic Fibrosis Foundation, Canadian
The Foundation funds research towards the goal of a cure or control for CF, and supports high quality CF care; promotes public awareness of CF; and raises and allocates funds for these purposes.
601–2221 Yonge St
Toronto ON M4S 2B4
Tel: 416-485-9149
1-800-378-2233
Fax: 416-485-0960
416-485-5707
Email: info@cysticfibrosis.ca
Website: www.cysticfibrosis.ca

Deaf, Canadian Association of the
The CAD provides consultation and information on deaf needs and interests to the public, business, media, educators, governments and others. We conduct research and collect data regarding deaf issues; issue reports on these studies; and provide expertise on them; develop and implement pilot programs.
203–251 Bank St
Ottawa ON K2P 1X3
Tel: 613-565-2882
613-565-8882 (TTY)
Fax: 613-565-1207
Email: info@cad.ca
Website: www.cad.ca
See also Hearing Society, Canadian; Hard of Hearing Association, Canadian

Diabetes Association, Canadian
The Canadian Diabetes Association supports people affected by diabetes by providing information, support and referrals if required. We also work with municipal, provincial, territorial and federal governments and policy-makers to ensure they recognize diabetes as one of the most significant public health issues in Canada today, and take action to address it.
1400–522 University Ave
Toronto ON M5G 2R5
Tel: 416-363-0177
1-800-226-8464
Fax: 416-408-7117
Email: info@diabetes.ca
Website: www.diabetes.ca
See also Juvenile Diabetes Research Foundation Canada

Digestive Health Foundation, Canadian
The CDHF is focused on activities that will: reduce the incidence of digestive disease; improve the quality of life for people living with digestive disease; support those suffering from digestive diseases and the professionals who care for them; and, enhance Canadian digestive health research and education.
1500 Upper Middle Rd, Unit 3
PO Box 76059
Oakville ON L6M 3H5
Tel: 905-829-3949
Email: director@cdhf.ca
Website: www.cdhf.ca
See also Celiac Association, Canadian

Down Syndrome Society, Canadian
The CDSS is a resource linking parents and professionals through advocacy, education and information. The CDSS strives to create a proud Canada where all are welcome, we embrace diversity and we value everyone's genes equally and to ensure equitable opportunities for all Canadians with Down syndrome.
283–5005 Dalhousie Dr NW
Calgary AB T3A 5R8
Tel: 403-270-8500
1-800-883-5608
Fax: 403-270-8291
Email: info@cdss.ca
Website: www.cdss.ca

Drug abuse
See Substance Abuse, Canadian Centre on

Dystonia Medical Research Foundation Canada
The mission of the DMRF is to advance research for more treatments and ultimately a cure, to promote awareness and education and to support the needs and well being of affected individuals and families.
909–100 Adelaide St W
Toronto ON M5H 1S3
Tel: 416-488-6974
1-800-361-8061
Fax: 416-488-5878
Website: www.dystoniacanada.org/

Eating Disorder Information Centre, National
The NEDIC is a Canadian, non-profit organization, established in 1985 to provide information and resources on eating disorders and weight preoccupation. NEDIC's vision is a culture that promotes and supports individuals engaged in healthy lifestyles regardless of ascribed or inherent characteristics, physical appearance and social status.
Toronto General Hospital
ES 7-421, 200 Elizabeth St
Toronto ON M5G 2C4
Tel: 416-340-4156
1-866-633-4220
Fax: 416-340-4736
Email: nedic@uhn.on.ca
Website: www.nedic.ca
See also Nutrition, Canadian Council of Food and

Endometriosis Association (International)
An independent self-help organization of women with endometriosis, doctors, and others interested in the disease, it is a recognized authority in its field whose goal is to work toward finding a cure for the disease as well as providing education, support and research.
8585 N 76th Place
Milwaukee WI 53223
Tel: 414-355-2200
Fax: 414-355-6065
Website: www.endometriosisassn.org
See also Women's Health Network, Canadian

Epilepsy Canada
Epilepsy Canada is the only national non-profit organization whose mission is to enhance the quality of life for persons affected by epilepsy through promotion and support of research and facilitation of education and awareness initiatives that build understanding and acceptance of epilepsy.
336–2255B Queen St E
Toronto ON M4E 1G3
Tel: 1-877-734-0873
Fax: 905-764-1231
Email: epilepsy@epilepsy.ca
Website: www.epilepsy.ca

Gerontology, Canadian Association on
The CAG is a national, multidisciplinary scientific and educational association established to provide leadership in matters related to the aging population.
CAG National Office
106–222 College St
Toronto ON M5T 3J1
Tel: 416-978-7977
Fax: 416-978-4771
Email: contact@cagacg.ca
Website: www.cagacg.ca

Hard of Hearing Association, Canadian
The CHHA is the national voice of all hard of hearing Canadians. Its mission is to raise public awareness concerning issues that are important for persons who are hard of hearing, to promote their integration in Canadian society, to remove any barriers to their participation and to generally make every community in Canada a better place for persons who are hard of hearing.
205–2415 Holly Lane
Ottawa ON K1V 7P2
Tel: 613-526-1584
613-526-2692 (TTY)
1-800-263-8068
Fax: 613-526-4718
Email: chhanational@chha.ca
Website: www.chha.ca
See also Hearing Society, Canadian; Deaf, Canadian Association of the

Headaches, Help for
Help For Headaches is a non-profit organization, and a registered Canadian charity that is committed to educational services for those suffering from and treating headaches.
515 Richmond St
PO Box 1568 Stn B
London ON N6A 5M3
Tel: 519-434-0008
Email: brent@helpforheadaches.org
Website: www.headache-help.org

Hearing Society, Canadian
The Canadian Hearing Society is the leading provider of services, products, and information that: remove barriers to communication; advance hearing health; promote equity for people who are culturally deaf, oral deaf, deafened, and hard of hearing.
Head Office
271 Spadina Rd
Toronto ON M5R 2V3
Tel: 416-928-2500
416-964-0023 (TTY)
1-877-347-3427
1-877-347-3429 (TTY)
Fax: 416-928-2506
Email: info@chs.ca
Website: www.chs.ca
See also Hard of Hearing Association, Canadian; Deaf, Canadian Association of the

Heart and Stroke Foundation
The Foundation, a volunteer-based health charity, leads in eliminating heart disease and stroke and reducing their impact through the advancement of research and its application, the promotion of healthy living and advocacy.
1402–222 Queen St
Ottawa ON K1P 5V9
Tel: 613-569-4361
Fax: 613-569-3278
Website: www.heartandstroke.com

Hemochromatosis Society, Canadian
The Society was established to create awareness about this little-known, but common disorder so that early diagnosis would become the rule rather than the exception and needless suffering and premature death from undiagnosed hemochromatosis would become a thing of the past. In the meantime, we are here to provide information and support to those adversely affected by iron overload.
272–7000 Minoru Blvd
Richmond BC V6Y 3Z5
Tel: 604-279-7135
1-877-223-4766
Fax: 604-279-7138
Email: office@toomuchiron.ca
Website: www.cdnhemochromatosis.ca

Hemophilia Society, Canadian
The Canadian Hemophilia Society strives to improve the health and quality of life for all people with inherited bleeding disorders and to find a cure.
400–1255 University St
Montreal QC H3B 3B6
Tel: 514-848-0503
1-800-668-2686
Fax: 514-848-9661
Email: chs@hemophilia.ca
Website: www.hemophilia.ca

Huntington Society of Canada
The Huntington Society of Canada aspires to a world free from Huntington disease. The Society maximizes the quality of life of people living with HD by: delivering services; enabling others to understand the disease and; furthering research to slow and to prevent Huntington disease.
400–151 Frederick St
Kitchener ON N2H 2M2
Tel: 519-749-7063
1-800-998-7398
Fax: 519-749-8965
Email: info@huntingtonsociety.ca
Website: www.huntingtonsociety.ca

Infertility Awareness Association of Canada
The IAAC provides assistance to Canadians who are experiencing difficulty conceiving or carrying a pregnancy. For these people, the inability to conceive a child may be the most profound medical and emotional challenge they ever face.
342–2100 Marlowe Ave
Montreal QC H4A 3L5
Tel: 514-484-2891
1-800-263-2929
Fax: 514-484-0454
Email: info@iaac.ca
Website: www.iaac.ca

International Association for Medical Assistance to Travellers
The IAMAT is a non-profit organization established in 1960. Our aim is to advise travellers about health risks, the geographical distribution of diseases worldwide, immunization requirements for all countries, and to make competent medical care available to travellers by western-trained doctors who speak English besides their mother tongue.
2162 Gordon St
Guelph ON N1L 1G6
Tel: 519-836-0102
Fax: 519-836-3412
Email: info@iamat.org
Website: www.iamat.org

Juvenile Diabetes Research Foundation Canada
The mission of JDRF is to find a cure for diabetes and its complications through the support of research.
Head Office
800–2550 Victoria Park Ave
Toronto ON M2J 5A9
Tel: 647-789-2000
1-877-CURE-533
Fax: 416-491-2111
Email: general@jdrf.ca
Website: www.jdrf.ca
See also Diabetes Association, Canadian

Kidney Foundation of Canada
The Foundation is the national volunteer organization committed to reducing the burden of kidney disease through: funding and stimulating innovative research; providing education and support; promoting access to high quality healthcare; and increasing public awareness and commitment to advancing kidney health and organ donation.
National Office
300–5165 Sherbrooke St W
Montreal QC H4A 1T6
Tel: 514-369-4806
1-800-361-7494
Fax: 514-369-2472
Email: info@kidney.ca
Website: www.kidney.ca

La Leche League Canada
Encourages, promotes, and provides mother-to-mother breast-feeding support, and educational opportunities as an important contribution to the health of children, families and society.
National Administration
PO Box 700
Winchester ON K0C 2K0
Tel: 613-774-4900
1-800-665-4324
Fax: 613-774-2798
Email: ofm@LLLC.ca
Website: www.lllc.ca/

Lactation, Drug exposure during
See Motherisk

Liver Foundation, Canadian
Provides support for research and education into the causes, diagnosis, prevention, and treatment of liver disease.
1500–2235 Sheppard Ave E
Toronto ON M2J 5B5
Tel: 416-491-3353
1-800-563-5483
Fax: 416-491-4952
Email: clf@liver.ca
Website: www.liver.ca

Lung Association, Canadian
The mission of the Canadian Lung Association is to lead nationwide and international lung health initiatives, prevent lung disease, help people manage lung disease and promote lung health.
300–1750 Courtwood Cr
Ottawa ON K2C 2B5
Tel: 613-569-6411
1-888-566-5864
Fax: 613-569-8860
Email: info@lung.ca
Website: www.lung.ca
See also Allergy/Asthma Information Association; Asthma Society of Canada

Lupus Canada
Lupus Canada is a national voluntary organization dedicated to improving the lives of people living with lupus through advocacy, education, public awareness, support and research.
3555–14th Ave
Unit #3
Markham ON L3R 0H5
Tel: 905-513-0004
1-800-661-1468
Fax: 905-513-9516
Email: info@lupuscanada.org
Website: www.lupuscanada.org

Marfan Association, Canadian
The Canadian Marfan Association is dedicated to saving lives and enabling promising futures for those living with Marfan syndrome through access to education; improved systems of health care and support; research.
Centre Plaza Postal Outlet
128 Queen St S
PO Box 42257
Mississauga ON L5M 4Z0
Tel: 905-826-3223
1-866-722-1722
Fax: 905-826-2125
Email: info@marfan.ca
Website: www.marfan.ca

MedicAlert Foundation, Canadian
MedicAlert is the leading provider of medical information services linked to customized medical bracelets, necklets and watches.
800–2005 Sheppard Ave E
Toronto ON M2J 5B4
Tel: 416-696-0267
1-800-668-1507 (English)
1-800-668-6381 (French)
Fax: 1-800-392-8422
Email: medinfo@medicalert.ca
Website: www.medicalert.ca

ME/FM Action Network, National
(Myalgic Encephalomyelitis/Chronic Fatigue Syndrome and Fibromyalgia)
The Network is a Canadian, registered, non-profit organization dedicated to advancing the recognition and understanding of Myalgic Encephalomyelitis/Chronic Fatigue Syndrome (ME/CFS) and Fibromyalgia Syndrome (FMS) through education, advocacy, support, and research.
512–33 Banner Rd
Nepean ON K2H 8V7
Tel: 613-829-6667
Fax: 613-829-8518
Email: mefmaction@ncf.ca
Website: www.mefmaction.net

Mental Health Association, Canadian
The Canadian Mental Health Association is a nation-wide, charitable organization that promotes the mental health of all and supports the resilience and recovery of people experiencing mental illness.
Phenix Professional Building
303–595 Montreal Rd
Ottawa ON K1K 4L2
Tel: 613-745-7750
Fax: 613-745-5522
Email: info@cmha.ca
Website: www.cmha.ca
See also Anxiety Disorders of Canada; Schizophrenia Society of Canada

Motherisk
Motherisk is a clinical, research and teaching program dedicated to antenatal drug, chemical, and disease risk counselling. It provides evidence-based information and guidance about the safety or risk to the developing fetus or infant, of maternal exposure to drugs, chemicals, diseases, radiation and environmental agents.
Hospital for Sick Children
555 University Ave
Toronto ON M5G 1X8
Tel: 1-877-327-4636—Alcohol and Substance
1-800-436-8477—Morning Sickness
1-888-246-5840—HIV and HIV Treatment
416-813-6780—Motherisk's Home Line
Website: www.motherisk.org

Mucopolysaccharide and Related Diseases Inc., Canadian Society for
Provides support for families whose children are affected with lysosomal storage diseases; brings about more public awareness of lysosomal storage diseases, and raises funds to further research in the hopes of finding a cure for these diseases.
PO Box 30034
RPO Parkgate
North Vancouver BC V7H 2Y8
Tel: 604-924-5130
1-800-667-1846
Fax: 604-924-5131
Email: info@mpssociety.ca
Website: www.mpssociety.ca

Multiple Sclerosis Society of Canada
Acts as a leader in finding a cure for multiple sclerosis and enabling people affected by MS to enhance their quality of life.
700–175 Bloor St E, North Tower
Toronto ON M4W 3R8
Tel: 416-922-6065
1-800-268-7582
Fax: 416-922-7538
Email: info@mssociety.ca
Website: www.mssociety.ca

Muscular Dystrophy Canada
Muscular Dystrophy Canada raises funds and works hard to support the independence and full participation of Canadians with neuromuscular disorders, funds research to find a cure and improve the quality of life of people with neuromuscular disorders, assists our clients to participate in the decisions that affect them, and collaborates with others for social change.
900–2345 Yonge St
Toronto ON M4P 2E5
Tel: 1-866-MUSCLE-8
Fax: 416-488-7523
Email: info@muscle.ca
Website: www.muscle.ca

Nutrition, Canadian Council of Food and
The CCFN is a national, non-profit organization which acts as a catalyst in advancing the nutritional health and well being of all Canadians by: championing evidence-based solutions to key nutritional issues affecting the nutritional health of Canadians; advocating for evidence-based nutrition policy in Canada; promoting public understanding of food and nutrition issues.
2810 Matheson Blvd E
1st floor
Mississauga ON L4W 4X7
Tel: 905-625-5746
Email: info@ccfn.ca
Website: www.ccfn.ca
See also Eating Disorder Information Centre, National

Occupational Health and Safety, Canadian Centre for
The CCOHS promotes health and safety in the workplace in Canada to facilitate consultation and cooperation among federal, provincial and territorial jurisdictions and participation by labour and management; to assist in the development and maintenance of policies and programs; to serve as a national centre for information relating to occupational health and safety.
135 Hunter St E
Hamilton ON L8N 1M5
Tel: 905-572-2981
1-800-668-4284
Fax: 905-572-2206
Email: clientservices@ccohs.ca
Website: www.ccohs.ca

Osteoporosis Canada
Educates, empowers, and supports individuals and communities the risk-reduction and treatment of osteoporosis.
301–1090 Don Mills Rd
Toronto ON M3C 3R6
Tel: 416-696-2663
1-800-463-6842 (English)
1-800-977-1778 (French)
Fax: 416-696-2673
Email: info@osteoporosis.ca
Website: www.osteoporosis.ca
See also Women's Health Network, Canadian

Palliative Care Association, Canadian Hospice
The CHPCA is the national voice for hospice palliative care in Canada. Advancing and advocating for quality end-of-life/hospice palliative care in Canada, its work includes public policy, public education and awareness.
Annex B, Saint-Vincent Hospital
60 Cambridge St N
Ottawa ON K1R 7A5
Tel: 613-241-3663
1-800-668-2785
Fax: 613-241-3986
Email: info@chpca.net
Website: www.chpca.net

Paraplegic Association, Canadian
Assists persons with spinal cord injuries and other physical disabilities to achieve independence, self-reliance and full community participation.
CPA National Office
230–1101 Prince of Wales Dr
Ottawa ON K2C 3W7
Tel: 613-723-1913
Fax: 613-723-1060
Email: info@canparaplegic.org
Website: www.canparaplegic.org

Parkinson Society Canada
The Society's purpose it to ease the burden and find a cure through: support services and education, research and advocacy.
316–4211 Yonge St
Toronto ON M2P 2A9
Tel: 416-227-9700
1-800-565-3000
Fax: 416-227-9600
Email: general.info@parkinson.ca
Website: www.parkinson.ca

Porphyria, Canadian Association for
The Canadian Association for Porphyria envisions a time when porphyric individuals, their families, health professionals, and the general public are educated and aware of the disease porphyria and the Association.
487 Walker Ave
PO Box 1206
Neepawa MB R0J 1H0
Tel: 204-476-2800
Fax: 204-476-2800
Website: www.cpf-inc.ca

Pregnancy, Drug exposure during
See Motherisk

Psoriasis Society of Canada
Assists those who have psoriasis by providing up-to-date information on treatment, programs and services; forms support groups across Canada; increases awareness of psoriasis among health care professionals and the public; consults with Government to assist with programs and services; encourages research programs to find the cause and cure for psoriasis.
PO Box 25015
Halifax NS B3M 4H4
Tel: 1-800-656-4494
Fax: 902-443-2073
Website: www.psoriasissociety.org

Rare Disorders, Canadian Organization for
CORD is Canada's national network for organizations representing all those with rare disorders. CORD provides a strong common voice to advocate for health policy and a healthcare system that works for those with rare disorders. CORD works with governments, researchers, clinicians and industry to promote research, diagnosis, treatment and services for all rare disorders in Canada.
National Office
600–151 Bloor St W
Toronto ON M5S 1S4
Tel: 416-969-7464
1-877-302-7273
Fax: 416-969-7420
Email: info@raredisorders.ca
Website: www.raredisorders.ca

Schizophrenia Society of Canada
The Schizophrenia Society of Canada exists to improve the quality of life for those affected by schizophrenia and psychosis through education, support programs, public policy and research.
100–4 Fort St
Winnipeg MB R3C 1C4
Tel: 204-786-1616
1-800-263-5545
Fax: 204-783-4898
Email: info@schizophrenia.ca
Website: www.schizophrenia.ca/
See also Mental Health Association, Canadian

Seniors
See Gerontology, Canadian Association on

Spina Bifida and Hydrocephalus Association of Canada
Works to improve the quality of life of all individuals with spina bifida and/or hydrocephalus, and their families, through awareness, education and research and advocacy.
647–167 Lombard Ave
Winnipeg MB R3B 0V3
Tel: 204-925-3650
1-800-565-9488
Fax: 204-925-3654
Email: info@sbhac.ca
Website: www.sbhac.ca

Sport, Canadian Centre for Ethics in
The mission of the CCES is to foster ethical sport for all Canadians. The CCES achieves this mission through research, promotion and education relevant to ethics in sport, including fair play and drug-free sport. As well, the CCES administers Canada's domestic anti-doping program, while at the same time exercising international leadership in advancing a doping-free, fair and ethical environment for sport worldwide.
350–955 Green Valley Cr
Ottawa ON K2C 3V4
Tel: 613-521-3340
1-800-672-7775
Fax: 613-521-3134
Email: info@cces.ca
Website: www.cces.ca

Substance Abuse, Canadian Centre on
The CCSA has a legislated mandate to provide national leadership and evidence-informed analysis and advice to mobilize collaborative efforts to reduce alcohol- and other drug-related harms.
500–75 Albert St
Ottawa ON K1P 5E7
Tel: 613-235-4048
Fax: 613-235-8101
Email: info@ccsa.ca
Website: www.ccsa.ca

Thyroid Foundation of Canada
The Foundation is a non-profit registered volunteer organization whose mission is to support thyroid patients across Canada through awareness, education and research.
263 MCG Building, Labrosse Ave
Pointe-Claire QC H9R 1A3
Tel: 1-800-267-8822
Fax: 519-630-9815
Website: www.thyroid.ca

Tourette Syndrome Foundation of Canada
The only national voluntary non-profit organization assisting individuals affected by Tourette Syndrome (TS) and its associated disorders. They are dedicated to improving the quality of life for those with, or affected by Tourette Syndrome through programs of education, advocacy, self-help and the promotion of research.
195–5945 Airport Rd
Mississauga ON L4V 1R9
Tel: 905-673-2255
1-800-361-3120
Fax: 905-673-2638
Email: tsfc@tourette.ca
Website: www.tourette.ca/

Travel
See International Association for Medical Assistance to Travellers

Turner Syndrome Society of Canada
Provides support services for individuals with TS and their families and disseminates up-to-date medical information to families, physicians and the general public.
30 Cleary Ave
Room 9
Ottawa ON K2A 4A1
Tel: 613-321-2267
1-800-465-6744
Fax: 613-321-2268
Email: info@turnersyndrome.ca
Website: www.turnersyndrome.ca

Women's Health Network, Canadian
Voluntary national organization to improve the health and lives of girls and women in Canada and the world by collecting, producing, distributing and sharing knowledge, ideas, education, information, resources, strategies and inspirations.
203–419 Graham Ave
Winnipeg MB R3C 0M3
Tel: 204-942-5500
1-888-818-9172
Fax: 204-989-2355
Email: cwhn@cwhn.ca
Website: www.cwhn.ca
See also Breast Cancer Foundation, Canadian; Endometriosis Association (International); Osteoporosis Canada

Directory III—Pharmaceutical Manufacturers/Distributors

Abbott Laboratories, Limited

Head Office:

8401 Trans-Canada Hwy
Saint-Laurent QC H4S 1Z1
Tel: 514-832-7000
1-800-361-7852 (Canada)
Fax: 514-832-7800

Mailing Address:

PO Box 6150 Stn Centre-Ville
Montreal QC H3C 3K6

Montreal Order Desk:

Tel: 1-800-567-2226 (all area codes)
514-832-7333 (Montreal)
Fax: 514-832-7251
1-800-513-7337

Distribution Centres:

Nfld:
Provincial Medical Supplies
51 Pippy Pl
PO Box 13427
St John's NL A1B 4B7
Tel: 709-754-3033
1-800-563-8755
Fax: 709-754-3014

Edmonton:
16607–116th Ave
Edmonton AB T5M 3V1
Tel: 780-451-4297
Fax: 780-455-7275

Montreal:
5685 Cypihot Rd
Saint-Laurent QC H4S 1R3
Tel: 514-832-7000
Fax: 514-337-1986

Vancouver:
7403 Progress Way
Delta BC V4G 1E7
Tel: 604-940-4148
Fax: 604-940-4102

Plant:

Abbott Nutrition International Plant
198 Pearl St E
Brockville ON K6V 1R4
Tel: 613-341-6000
Fax: 613-341-6056

Diagnostic Reagents:

Diagnostic Reagents
Diagnostic Division
7115 Millcreek Dr
Mississauga ON L5N 3R3
Tel: 905-858-2450
1-800-387-8378
Fax: 905-858-2462

Narcotic Distribution Centers:

UPS Logistics/Lynden Logistics
10 Corinne Court
Vaughan ON L4K 4T7
Tel: 905-879-0114
1-800-268-4937
Fax: 905-879-0123

UPS Logistics/Lynden Logistics
4441–76th Ave SE
West Building
Calgary AB T2C 2G8
Tel: 403-279-2700
Fax: 403-236-9104

Provincial Medical Supplies
51 Pippy Pl
PO Box 13427
St John's NL A1B 4B7
Tel: 709-754-3033
1-800-563-8755
Fax: 709-754-3014

Biaxin
Biaxin BID
Biaxin XL
Calcijex
Depakene
Epival
Humira
Hytrin
Isoflurane, USP
Isoptin SR
Kadian
Kaletra
Lupron/Lupron Depot 3.75 mg/7.5 mg
Lupron Depot 3.75 mg/11.25 mg
Lupron/Lupron Depot 7.5 mg/22.5 mg/30 mg
Mavik
Nimbex
Norvir
Norvir SEC
Rythmol
Sevorane AF
Survanta
Synagis
Synthroid
Tarka
Ultiva

Abbott Products Inc.

Head Office:

60 Columbia Way
Suite 207
Markham ON L3R 0C9
Tel: 905-944-2480
Fax: 905-944-2481

Medical Information:

Tel: 1-800-268-4276

AndroGel
Creon 5 Minimicrospheres
Creon 10 Minimicrospheres
Creon 25 Minimicrospheres
Dicetel
Influvac
Luvox
Marinol
Serc
Teveten
Teveten Plus

Abraxis BioScience Canada inc

Head Office:

30 Eglinton Ave W
Suite 500
Mississauga ON L5R 3E7
Tel: 1-877-779-7480
Fax: 1-877-779-7482

Abraxane

Accord Healthcare Inc.

Head Office:

3100 Steeles Avenue East
Suite 605
Markham ON L3R 8T3
Tel: 905-489-1957
Fax: 905-489-1973
Email: purvi@accordhealth.ca
Website: http://accord-healthcare.com/

Bicalutamide Tablets
Letrozole Tablets USP
Pioglitazone Hydrochloride Tablets

Actavis

Canadian Office:

Tribute Pharma Canada Inc.
57 Martin Street
Milton ON L9T 2R1
Tel: 905-876-1118
Fax: 905-876-4675
Website: www.tributepharma.com

Customer Service:

Tel: 1-888-333-4401

Medical Information:

Tel: 1-866-391-4503

Bezalip SR
Soriatane

Actelion Pharmaceuticals Canada Inc.

Head Office:

2550 Daniel Johnson Blvd
Suite 701
Laval QC H7T 2L1
Tel: 450-681-1664
1-866-531-4885
Fax: 450-681-9545
Website: www.actelion.com

Medical Information:

Tel: 1-866-531-4885

Order Desk:

Tel: 1-877-717-8382
Fax: 1-800-786-1967

Tracleer
Zavesca

Adrem Inc.

Head Office:

2000 Ellesmere Rd
Unit 16
Scarborough ON M1H 2W4
Tel: 416-438-6727
Fax: 416-438-3463
Email: info@nucro-technics.com

Wake Ups

Afexa Life Sciences Inc.

Corporate Office:

9604–20th Avenue
Edmonton AB T6N 1G1
Tel: 1-888-843-7239
Website: www.afexa.com

COLD-FX

Alcon Canada Inc.

Head Office:

2665 Meadowpine Blvd
Mississauga ON L5N 8C7
Tel: 905-826-6700
1-800-268-4574
1-800-387-8184 (french)
Fax: 905-826-1448
Website: www.alcon.ca

Medical Information:

Tel: 1-800-613-2245

Alcaine
Alomide
Azarga
Azopt
Betoptic S
Ciloxan
Ciprodex
Cyclogyl
DuoTrav
Emadine
Enuclene
Flarex
Fluorescite
Iopidine 0.5%
Iopidine 1%
Isopto Atropine
Isopto Carbachol
Isopto Carpine
Isopto Homatropine
Maxidex
Maxitrol
Miostat
Mydfrin
Mydriacyl
Naphcon Forte
Nevanac
Patanol
Pilopine HS
Tobradex
Tobrex
Travatan Z
Vexol
Vigamox

Alexion Pharma Canada

Head Office:

400 Applewood Crescent
Vaughan ON L4K 0C3

Soliris

Allergan Inc.

Head Office:

85 Enterprise Blvd
Suite 500
Markham ON L6G 0B5
Tel: 905-940-1660
Fax: 905-940-1902

Medical Information:

Tel: 1-877-ALLERGN (255-3746)

Order Desk:

Tel: 1-800-668-6427 (Ontario and Quebec)
1-800-668-6477 (other areas)

Acular
Acular LS
Alocril
Alphagan
Alphagan P
Betagan
Blephamide
Botox
Botox Cosmetic
Combigan
FML
FML Forte
Lumigan
Lumigan RC
Ocuflox
Opticrom
Polytrim
Pred Forte
Pred Mild
Refresh
Refresh Celluvisc
Refresh Contacts
Refresh Eye Allergy Relief
Refresh Lacri-Lube S.O.P.
Refresh Liquigel
Refresh Plus
Refresh Redness Relief
Refresh Tears
Refresh Ultra
Restasis
Tazorac Cream
Tazorac Gel
Tears Plus
Zymar

Alveda Pharmaceuticals Inc.

Head Office:

40 Holly St
Suite 801
Toronto ON M4S 3C3
Tel: 416-485-6995

Rimso-50

Amgen Canada Inc.

Head Office:

6775 Financial Dr
Suite 100
Mississauga ON L5N 0A4
Tel: 1-800-665-4273
Fax: 1-866-912-6436

Medical Information:

Tel: 1-866-50AMGEN (502-6436)
Fax: 1-866-472-6436
Email: MedinfoCanada@amgen.com

Customer Care:

Tel: 1-800-563-9798
Fax: 1-800-495-3187

Aranesp
Enbrel
Neulasta
Neupogen
Nplate
Prolia
Sensipar
Vectibix

Amphastar Pharmaceuticals, Inc.

Head Offices:

2000 Ellesmere Rd
Suite 16
Scarborough ON M1H 2W4
Tel: 416-438-6727
Fax: 416-438-3463

11570 Sixth St
Rancho Cucamonga CA 91730
USA
Tel: 1-800-423-4136 (Jacob Liawatidewi)

Cortrosyn

Apotex Inc.

Head Office:

150 Signet Dr
Weston ON M9L 1T9
Tel: 1-800-268-4623
Fax: 1-800-609-9444
Website: www.apotex.com/ca/en/products

DISpedia (Drug Information Service):

Tel: 1-800-667-4708
Fax: 416-401-3915
Email: dispedia@apotex.com

National Customer Contact Information:

Tel: 1-877-427-6839
Fax: 1-800-665-2854
Email: orderdesk@apotex.com

Apo-Acebutolol
Apo-Amiloride
Apo-Benzydamine
Apo-Bromazepam
Apo-Bromocriptine
Apo-Butorphanol
Apo-Carvedilol
Apo-Doxepin
Apo-Etodolac
Apo-Fenofibrate
Apo-Feno-Micro
Apo-Flavoxate
Apo-Floctafenine
Apo-Granisetron
Apo-Hydralazine
Apo-Hydro
Apo-Hydro (12.5 mg)
Apo-Keto
Apo-Keto-E
Apo-Keto SR
Apo-Lactulose
Apo-Methazolamide
Apo-Misoprostol
Apo-Moclobemide
Apo-Orciprenaline
Apo-Pimozide
Apo-Prazo
Apo-Prochlorazine
Apo-Sotalol
Apo-Tenoxicam
Apo-Timol
Apri 21
Apri 28
Aviane 21
Aviane 28
Cefazolin for Injection
Ceftriaxone for Injection USP
Portia 21
Portia 28
ReVia

Astellas Pharma Canada, Inc.

Head Office:

675 Cochrane Dr
Suite 500 – West Tower
Markham ON L3R 0B8
Tel: 905-470-7990
Fax: 905-470-7799

Customer Service:

Tel: 1-800-668-8641

Medical Information:

Tel: 1-888-338-1824

Adenocard
Advagraf
AmBisome
Amevive
Mycamine

Prograf
Protopic
Vesicare

AstraZeneca Canada Inc.

Head Office:

1004 Middlegate Rd
Mississauga ON L4Y 1M4
Tel: 905-277-7111
1-800-565-5877
Fax: 905-270-3248
Website: www.astrazeneca.ca

Medical Information:

Tel: 1-800-668-6000 (english)
1-800-461-3787 (french)
Fax: 905-277-3556
1-866-250-1909
Email: medinfo.Canada@astrazeneca.com

After Hours Service:

Tel: 1-800-818-4380

Compassionate Use Program:

Tel: 905-566-4015 (local)
1-800-668-6000 (english)
1-800-461-3787 (french)
Fax: 905-896-4745
1-800-268-0774

Customer Relations:

Tel: 905-566-4015 (local)
1-800-668-6000 (english)
1-800-461-3787 (french)
Fax: 905-896-4745
1-800-268-0774
Email: customer.relations1@astrazeneca.ca

Trading Partner Relations:

Tel: 905-804-4900 (local, bilingual)
1-888-669-2987 (bilingual)
Fax: 905-615-8119 (local)
1-888-697-9886

Accolate
Arimidex
Atacand
Atacand Plus
Betaloc
Bricanyl Turbuhaler
Casodex
Crestor
Diprivan
EMLA Cream
EMLA Patch
Entocort Capsules
Entocort Enema
Faslodex
FluMist
Imdur
Iressa
Losec 1-2-3 A
Losec 1-2-3 M
Losec Capsules
Losec Tablets
Merrem
Naropin
Nesacaine-CE
Nexium
Nexium 1-2-3 A
Nolvadex-D
Oxeze Turbuhaler
Plendil
Pulmicort Nebuamp
Pulmicort Turbuhaler
Rhinocort Aqua
Rhinocort Turbuhaler
Sensorcaine
Sensorcaine with Epinephrine
Seroquel
Seroquel XR
Symbicort Turbuhaler
Tenoretic
Tenormin
Xylocaine Endotracheal
Xylocaine Jelly 2%
Xylocaine Ointment 5%
Xylocaine Parenteral with Epinephrine
Xylocaine Parenteral Without Epinephrine
Xylocaine Topical 4%
Xylocaine Viscous 2%
Xylocard
Zestoretic
Zestril
Zoladex 3.6 mg
Zoladex LA
Zomig
Zomig Nasal Spray
Zomig Rapimelt

Aton Pharma

Canadian Office:

Valeo Pharma Inc.
16 667 Hymus Blvd
Kirkland QC H9H 4R9
Tel: 514-694-0150
1-866-694-0150
Fax: 514-694-0865
Email: info@valeopharma.com

Cuprimine
Edecrin
Lacrisert
Sodium Edecrin

Awareness Corporation/dba AwarenessLife

Head Office:

25 S Arizona Place
Suite 320
Chandler AZ 85225
USA

Canada Office:

210–9087B–198th St
Langley BC V1M 3B1
Tel: 1-800-69AWARE (692-9273)

Daily Complete
Experience
PureTrim Mediterranean Wellness Shake
Synergy Defense

Axcan Pharma Inc.

Head Office:

597 Laurier Blvd
Mont-Saint-Hilaire QC J3H 6C4
Tel: 450-467-5138
1-800-565-3255
Fax: 450-464-9979
Email: axcan@axcan.com
Website: www.axcan.com

Customer Service:

Tel: 1-800-809-4950
Fax: 450-467-0153

ADEKs
Bentylol
Cortenema
Modulon
Photofrin
Proctosedyl
Salofalk, Rectal Suspension
Salofalk, Suppositories
Salofalk, Tablets
Sulcrate
Sulcrate Suspension Plus
URSO
URSO DS
Ultrase
Ultrase MT
Viokase

Bausch & Lomb Canada

Head Office:

520 Applewood Cres.
Vaughan ON L4K 4B4
Tel: 905-695-7700
Fax: 905-695-7656
1-800-668-7510
Website: www.bausch.ca

Alrex
Besivance
Lotemax

Baxter Corporation

Head Office:

4 Robert Speck Parkway
Suite 700
Mississauga ON L4Z 3Y4
Tel: 905-270-1125
1-800-387-8399
Fax: 905-281-6560
Website: www.baxter.com

Customer Service:

Tel: 1-888-719-9955

Medical Information:

For Brevibloc, Enlon, Forane and Suprane:
Tel: 1-800-262-3784

For Procytox, Ifex and Uromitexan:
Tel: 1-888-922-2296

For FSME-Immun:
McKesson Canada
Tel: 1-877-211-3582

For All Other Drug/Biologic Products:
Tel: 1-888-719-9955

Adverse Event (ADR) Reporting (For All Drug/Biologic Products):

Tel: 1-800-387-8399 ext 6622/6626

Advate
Brevibloc
Brevibloc Premixed
Buminate
Dopamine HCl and 5% Dextrose Injection
Fluconazole Injection
Gammagard Liquid
Gammagard S/D
Gentamicin Sulfate Injection in 0.9% Sodium Chloride
Heparin Sodium and 0.9% Sodium Chloride Injection
Heparin Sodium in 5% Dextrose Injection
Ifex
Lidocaine HCl 0.2%, 0.4% and 0.8% in 5% Dextrose for I.V. Infusion
Metronidazole 500 mg/100 mL Injection
Nitroglycerin in 5% Dextrose Injection
Osmitrol
Procytox
Suprane
Tisseel Kit VH
Uromitexan

Bayer Inc.

Head Office:

77 Belfield Rd
Toronto ON M9W 1G6
Tel: 1-800-622-2937
Fax: 1-866-232-0565

Medical Information:

Tel: 1-800-265-7382
Fax: 1-866-232-0565
Email: canada.medinfo@bayer.com

Adverse Event Reporting:

Tel: 1-800-265-7382
Fax: 1-866-232-0565
Email: canada.medinfo@bayer.com

Special Access Program:

Tel: 1-800-265-7382
Fax: 1-866-232-0565

Adalat XL
Adalat XL Plus
Androcur
Androcur Depot
Angeliq
Avelox
Avelox I.V.
Betaseron
Biltricide
Bonefos
Cipro I.V.
Cipro Oral Suspension
Cipro Tablets
Cipro XL
Climara
Climara Pro
Diane-35
Finacea
Gadovist 1.0
Glucobay
Kogenate FS Supplied with BIO-SET Needle-less Reconstitution Set
Levitra
Magnevist
Mirena
Nexavar
Nimotop Tablets
Primovist
Recothrom
Refludan
Trasylol
Triquilar 21
Triquilar 28
Ultravist 240
Ultravist 300
Ultravist 370
Xarelto
Yasmin 21
Yasmin 28
Yaz
Zevalin

Bayer Inc., Consumer Care

Head Office:

77 Belfield Rd
Toronto ON M9W 1G6
Tel: 1-800-622-2937

Medical Information:

Tel: 1-800-265-7382
Fax: 416-248-3066
Email: Med.info.b@bayer.com

Adverse Event Reporting:

Tel: 1-800-265-7382
Fax: 416-248-3066
Email: Med.info.b@bayer.com

Customer Service:

Tel: 1-800-268-1432
Fax: 1-800-567-1710

Aleve
Alka-Seltzer
Alka-Seltzer Flavoured
Aspirin
Bactine
Bugs Bunny and friends
CanesOral
CanesOral Combi-Pak
Canesten Topical
Canesten Vaginal
Coated Aspirin
Flintstones
Midol Menstrual Complete
Midol Night-Time
Midol PMS Complete
Midol Teen Complete
Myoflex
One A Day
Ozonol Antibiotic Plus
Ozonol Ointment
Phillips' Preparations
Redoxon

Biogen Idec Canada Inc.

Head Office:

90 Burnhamthorpe Road West
Suite 1100
Mississauga ON L5B 3C3
Tel: 905-804-1444
1-866-359-2502
Fax: 905-897-3222

Drug Safety and Medical Information:

Tel: 1-866-477-3462

Order Desk:

Tel: 1-800-268-4937

Avonex
Avonex PS
Tysabri

Biovail Pharmaceuticals Canada

Head Office:

7150 Mississauga Rd
Mississauga ON L5N 8M5
Tel: 905-286-3100
Fax: 905-286-3150
Website: www.biovail.com

Medical Information:

Tel: 1-866-825-8120
Fax: 1-866-270-6437
Email: medinfo@biovail.com

Compassionate Care:

Fax: 1-866-205-8131

Ordering Centre:

Tel: 1-888-214-6000 (from 8:30 am-5:00 pm Est)
Fax: 905-286-3127 (24 hrs a day)

Cardizem CD
Glumetza
Nitoman
Ralivia
Tiazac
Tiazac XC
Wellbutrin SR
Wellbutrin XL
Zyban

BLES Biochemicals Inc.

Head Office:

8–60 Pacific Court
London ON N5V 3K4
Tel: 519-457-2537
Fax: 519-457-7470
Email: bles@wwdc.com

BLES

Boehringer Ingelheim (Canada) Ltd.

Head Office:

5180 South Service Rd
Burlington ON L7L 5H4
Tel: 905-639-0333
1-800-263-9107
Fax: 905-639-3769
Website: www.boehringer-ingelheim.ca

Medical Information:

Tel: 905-631-4633 (4-MED)
1-800-263-5103 ext 4633 (4-MED)

Customer Service:

Tel: 1-800-263-BICL (2425)
Fax: 905-634-4421
1-800-665-3405
Email: rxinquiry@bur.boehringer-ingelheim.com

Adverse Event Reporting:

Tel: 905-631-4603
1-800-263-5103 ext: 4603

Aggrenox
Aptivus
Atrovent HFA Inhalation Aerosol
Atrovent Inhalation Solution
Atrovent Nasal Spray
Buscopan
Catapres
Combivent UDV
Dixarit
Dulcolax
Duovent UDV
Flomax CR
Micardis
Micardis Plus
Mirapex
Mobicox
Persantine
Pradax
Spiriva
Viramune

Bristol Laboratories of Canada

Head Office:

Bristol-Myers Squibb Canada
2344 Alfred-Nobel
Suite 300
St-Laurent QC H4S 0A4
Tel: 514-333-3200
1-800-267-1088
Fax: 514-335-4102

Medical Information:

Tel: 1-866-463-6267
Fax: 1-888-267-6211

After Hours Emergency:

Tel: 514-333-3200

Customer Service:

Tel: 1-800-BMS-0005 (267-0005)
Fax: 1-800-463-6334

Order Desk:

Tel: 1-800-BMS-0005 (267-0005)
Fax: 1-800-463-6334

Blenoxane

Bristol-Myers Squibb Canada

Head Office:

2344 Alfred-Nobel
Suite 300
St-Laurent QC H4S 0A4
Tel: 514-333-3200
1-800-267-1088
Fax: 514-335-4102

Medical Information:

Tel: 1-866-463-6267
Fax: 1-888-267-6211

After Hours Emergency:

Tel: 514-333-3200

Customer Service:

Tel: 1-800-BMS-0005 (267-0005)
Fax: 1-800-463-6334

Order Desk:

Tel: 1-800-BMS-0005 (267-0005)
Fax: 1-800-463-6334

Abilify
Avalide
Avapro
Baraclude
BiCNU
Capoten
CeeNU
Cefzil
Coumadin
Desyrel
Desyrel Dividose
Endocet
Erbitux
Fungizone
Hycodan
Hycomine
Hycomine-S
Hydrea
Kenalog-10 Injection
Kenalog-40 Injection
Lysodren
Maxipime
Megace OS
Modecate Concentrate
Monopril
Onglyza
Orencia
Pentaspan
Percocet
Percocet-Demi
Pravachol
Reyataz
Sprycel
Sustiva
Taxol
Tempra
Vepesid
Videx EC
Vumon Parenteral
Zerit

Canderm Pharma Inc.

Head Office:

5353 Thimens Blvd
Saint-Laurent QC H4R 2H4
Tel: 514-334-3835
Fax: 514-334-7078
Email: mail@canderm.com

Medical Information:

Tel: 514-334-1364
1-800-465-3376

Condyline

Cangene Corporation

Head Office:

155 Innovation Dr
Winnipeg MB R3T 5Y3
Tel: 204-275-4200
1-877-CANGENE (226-4363)
Fax: 204-269-7003
Website: www.cangene.com

HepaGam B
VariZIG
WinRho SDF

Chattem Canada

Head Office:

2220 Argentia Rd
Mississauga ON L5N 2K7
Tel: 905-821-4975
Fax: 905-821-0544

Pamprin Extra Strength Multi-Symptom
Pamprin Extra Strength PMS
Pamprin Ultra Strength Ibuprofen Formula

Church & Dwight Canada Corp.

Head Office:

635 Secretariat Court
Mississauga ON L5S 0A5
Tel: 905-696-6570
1-800-387-2130
Fax: 905-564-0356
Website: www.churchdwight.ca

Medical Information:

Tel: 514-731-3931 ext 2314
1-800-361-5541 ext 2314
Fax: 514-738-5509

Customer Service:

Tel: 905-696-6599
1-800-472-8658
Fax: 905-564-1202
1-800-786-8516
Website: www.churchdwight.ca

Commercial Office:

Tel: 905-696-6570
1-800-387-2130
1-800-268-3186
Fax: 905-564-0356
1-800-786-8516

Sales Office:

Tel: 905-696-6570
1-800-472-8658
Fax: 905-564-1202
1-800-786-8516

Plant:

5485 Ferrier St
Montreal QC H4P 1M6
Tel: 514-731-3931
1-800-361-5541
Fax: 514-738-5509

Atasol-8, -15, -30
Atasol Preparations
Bionet
Carters Little Pills
Diovol
Diovol Plus
Diovol Plus AF
Fermentol
Gravol - Ginger - Natural Source
Gravol Preparations
Infantol
Maltlevol-12
Ovol Preparations
Rub A-535 Antiphlogistine
RUB A-535 Antiphlogistine Capsaicin
Rub A-535 Antiphlogistine Ice
Rub A-535 Antiphlogistine No Odour
Rub A-535 Extra Strength Arthritis Roll-On Lotion

Cobalt Pharmaceuticals Inc.

Head Office:

6500 Kitimat Rd
Mississauga ON L5N 2B8
Tel: 905-814-1820
1-866-254-6111
Fax: 905-814-8722
1-866-510-8722
Email: info@cobaltpharma.com

CO Alendronate
CO Amlodipine
CO Atenolol
CO Atorvastatin
CO Azithromycin
CO Bicalutamide
CO Cabergoline
CO Cilazapril
CO Ciprofloxacin
CO Citalopram
CO Clomipramine
CO Clonazepam
CO Enalapril
CO Etidrocal
CO Etidronate
CO Famciclovir
CO Fluconazole
CO Fluoxetine
CO Fluvoxamine
CO Gabapentin
CO Levetiracetam
CO Levofloxacin
CO Lisinopril
CO Lovastatin
CO Meloxicam
CO Memantine
CO Metformin Coated
CO Norfloxacin
CO Olanzapine
CO Olanzapine ODT
CO Ondansetron
CO Pantoprazole
CO Paroxetine
CO Pioglitazone
CO Pramipexole
CO Pravastatin
CO Quetiapine
CO Ramipril
CO Ranitidine
CO Risperidone
CO Ropinirole

CO Sertraline
CO Simvastatin
CO Sotalol
CO Sumatriptan
CO Temazepam
CO Terbinafine
CO Topiramate
CO Valacyclovir
CO Venlafaxine XR
CO Zopiclone
Letrozole

CSL Behring Canada

Head Office:

55 Metcalfe St
Suite 1460
Ottawa ON K1P 6L5
Tel: 613-232-3111
Fax: 613-232-5031
Website: www.cslbehring.com

Alburex 25
Alburex 5
Berinert
CytoGam
Helixate FS
Humate-P
Privigen
Streptase
Vivaglobin

CV Technologies Inc.

see Afexa Life Sciences Inc.

Cytex Pharmaceuticals Inc.

Head Office:

5545 Macara St
Halifax NS B3K 1W1
Tel: 902-453-1230
1-888-453-1230
Fax: 902-453-5753
Email: cytex@eastlink.ca

Progesterone Injection USP

Dormer Laboratories Inc.

Head Office:

91 Kelfield St
Unit 5
Toronto ON M9W 5A3
Tel: 416-242-6167
1-800-363-5040
Fax: 416-242-9487
Email: info@dormer.com
Website: www.dormer.com

Cantharone
Cantharone Plus
Z-Plus

Duchesnay Inc.

Head Office:

950 Michèle-Bohec Blvd
Blainville QC J7C 5E2
Tel: 450-433-PREG (7734)
1-877-833-PREG (7734)
Fax: 450-433-2211
1-888-588-8508
Email: info@duchesnay
Website: www.duchesnay.com

Medical Information:

Tel: 1-888-666-0611
Email: medicalinfo@duchesnay.com

Diclectin
PregVit
PregVit folic 5
Proctofoam-HC

Eli Lilly Canada Inc.

Head Office:

3650 Danforth Ave
Toronto ON M1N 2E8
Tel: 416-694-3221
1-800-268-4446
Fax: 416-699-7274
Website: www.lilly.ca

Customer Response Centre:

Tel: 416-693-3510
1-888-545-5972
Fax: 1-888-898-2961

Adcirca
Alimta
Cialis
Cymbalta
Effient
Evista
Forteo
Gemzar
Glucagon Injection
Humalog
Humalog Mix25
Humalog Mix50
Humatrope
Humulin (30/70)
Humulin-N
Humulin-R
Prozac
ReoPro
Strattera
Xigris
Zyprexa
Zyprexa IntraMuscular
Zyprexa Zydis

EMD Canada Inc.

Head Office:

2695 North Sheridan Way
Suite 200
Mississauga ON L5K 2N6
Tel: 905-919-0200
1-888-737-6668
Fax: 905-919-0299

Cetrotide
Crinone
Gonal-f
Gonal-f Pen
Luveris
Ovidrel
Rebif
Saizen
Saizen click.easy
Serophene
Serostim
Stilamin

Ethypharm, Inc.

Canada Office:

1000 de la Gauchetière Ouest
Suite 2400
Montréal QC H3B 4W5
Tel: 450-973-7500
Fax: 450-973-7503
Email: tiganos.evangelos@ethypharmamerica.com
Website: www.ethypharm.com

Customer Service/Medical Information/Pharmacovigilance:

Tel: 1-800-265-7927

M-Eslon

Ferring Inc.

Head Office:

200 Yorkland Blvd
Suite 800
Toronto ON M2J 5C1
Tel: 416-490-0121
1-800-263-4057
Fax: 416-493-1692

Quebec Office:

7333 Place des Roseraies
Suite 100
Anjou QC H1M 2X6
Tel: 514-354-3677
1-866-354-3677
Fax: 514-352-6090

Order Desk:

Ontario including Metro Toronto:
Tel: 1-800-268-4937
Fax: 905-879-0123

Metropolitan Montreal:
Tel: 514-956-0768
Fax: 514-956-0325

Quebec:
Tel: 1-800-361-3362
Fax: 514-956-0325

Atlantic Provinces:
Tel: 1-800-268-4937
Fax: 905-879-0123

Western Canada:
Tel: 1-800-661-1237
Fax: 403-236-9104

Calgary:
Tel: 403-236-1787
Fax: 403-236-9104

Mail Orders:

Ferring Inc.
PO Box 4500
Concord ON L4K 1B6

BioGaia Chewable Tablets
BioGaia Drops
B-natal Lozenge
B-natal Therapop
Bravelle
Caltine
Cervidil
DDAVP Injection
DDAVP Melt
DDAVP Rhinyle Nasal Solution
DDAVP Spray
DDAVP Tablets
Duratocin
Endometrin
Firmagon
Florazole ER
Gynazole•1
Lutrepulse
Menopur
Minirin
Norprolac
Octostim
Pentasa
Pico-Salax
Pressyn
Pressyn AR
Repronex
TuZen

Fournier Pharma Inc.

Head Office:

Abbott Products Inc.
60 Columbia Way
Suite 207
Markham ON L3R 0C9
Tel: 905-944-2480
Fax: 905-944-2481

Medical Information:

Tel: 1-800-268-4276

Lipidil EZ
Lipidil Supra

Fresenius Kabi Canada

A Division of Calea Ltd.

Head Office:

2785 Skymark Avenue
Unit 2
Mississauga ON L4W 4Y3
Tel: 1-877-953-9002
Fax: 905-624-9330
Website: www.fresenius-kabi.ca

Voluven

Fresenius Medical Care North America

Head Office:

920 Winter St
Waltham MA 02451-1457
USA
Tel: 781-699-9000
1-800-662-1237
Website: www.fmcna.com

PhosLo

Functional Nutrients International

Head Office:

104-5863 Leslie Street
Toronto ON M2H 1J8
Tel: 416-760-3777
1-877-444-4080
Fax: 416-760–3722
Email: info@functionalnutrients.com
Website: www.functionalnutrients.com

MAP Master Amino Acid Pattern (MAP)

Galderma Canada Inc.

Head Office:

105 Commerce Valley Dr W
Suite 300
Thornhill ON L3T 7W3
Tel: 905-762-2500
1-800-467-2081
Fax: 905-762-2505
Email: GaldermaCanada@galderma.com
Website: www.galderma.ca

Customer Service:

6090 White Hart Lane
Mississauga ON L5R 3Y4
Tel: 905-712-7232
1-800-847-7696
Fax: 1-800-786-1967

Benzac AC 10
Benzac AC 5
Benzac W5
Benzac W Wash 10
Benzac W Wash 5
Capex
Clobex Lotion
Clobex Shampoo
Clobex Spray
Desocort
Differin
Differin XP
MetroCream
MetroGel
MetroLotion
Metvix
Silkis

Generic Medical Partners

Head Office:

451 DuPont Street
Toronto ON M5R 1W5
Tel: 416-444-4GMP or 4467
Fax: 800-786-1967
Website: www.GMPRx.com

MED-Letrozole

GenMed

A division of Pfizer Canada Inc.

Head Office:

Pfizer Canada Inc.
17 300 Trans-Canada Hwy
Kirkland QC H9J 2M5
Website: http://www.pfizer.ca/en/

Mailing Address:

PO Box 800
Pointe-Claire-Dorval QC H9R 4V2
Tel: 514-695-0500
Fax: 514-426-7529

Medical Information:

Tel: 1-800-463-6001

Customer Service:

Tel: 1-800-387-4974
Fax: 1-800-420-2019

Distribution Centre:

2400 Skymark Ave
Unit 3
Mississauga ON L4W 5L7
Tel: 1-877-633-2001 (press 0)
Fax: 905-219-2731

Plant:

Pfizer Canada Inc.
PO Box 3003
Arnprior ON K7S 3K2
Tel: 613-623-4221
Fax: 613-623-1259

GD-amlodipine

Genpharm ULC

see Mylan Pharmaceuticals ULC

Genzyme Canada Inc.

Head Office:

800–2700 Matheson Blvd E
West Tower
Mississauga ON L4W 4V9
Tel: 905-625-0011
1-877-220-8918
Fax: 905-625-7811
Website: www.genzyme.ca

Medical Information:

500 Kendall St
Cambridge MA 02142
USA
Tel: 1-800-745-4447
Fax: 617-591-7178

Customer Service:

10 Corrine Court
Vaughan ON L4K 4T7
Tel: 905-879-0114
1-888-333-0506
Fax: 905-879-0123

Aldurazyme
Cerezyme
Clolar
Fabrazyme
MabCampath
Myozyme
Renagel
Synvisc
Synvisc One
Thymoglobulin
Thyrogen

Germiphene Corporation

Head Office:

1379 Colborne St E
Brantford ON N3T 5M1
Tel: 519-759-7100
Fax: 519-759-1625
Website: www.germiphene.com

ORO-Clense

Gilead Sciences Canada, Inc.

Head Office:

6711 Mississauga Rd
Suite 202
Mississauga ON L5N 2W3
Tel: 905-363-8008
1-866-565-5409
Fax: 905-363-8049
1-866-809-0406
Email: Canada_info@gilead.com
Website: www.gilead.ca

Medical Information & Adverse Event Reporting:

Tel: 905-363-8009
1-866-207-4267
Fax: 905-363-8049
1-866-809-0406
Email: medicalinformation@gilead.com

Customer Enquiries:

Tel: 905-363-8008
1-866-565-5409

Atripla
Cayston
Hepsera
Truvada
Viread

GlaxoSmithKline Inc.

Head Office:

7333 Mississauga Rd
Mississauga ON L5N 6L4
Tel: 905-819-3000
Fax: 905-819-3099
Website: www.gsk.ca

Quebec Office:

8455 route Transcanadienne
Saint-Laurent QC H4S 1Z1
Tel: 1-800-463-6314

Medical Information:

Tel: 1-800-387-7374
Fax: 1-800-565-2935
Email: cacsu@gsk.com

Customer Service:

Tel: 1-800-387-7374

Credit and Accounts Receivable Management:

Tel: 1-888-224-1050
Fax: 1-800-367-9609

Advair
Advair Diskus
Alkeran
Amerge
Arixtra
Atriance
Avamys
Avandamet
Avandaryl
Avandia
Avodart
Bactroban Ointment
Bexxar Therapy
Boostrix
Ceftin
Cervarix
Clavulin
CoActifed Expectorant
CoActifed Syrup
CoActifed Tablets
Cortisporin Ointment
Cortisporin Otic Solution Sterile
Daraprim
Digibind
Engerix-B
Flolan for Injection
Flonase
Flovent Diskus
Flovent HFA
Fortaz
Fraxiparine
Fraxiparine Forte
Havrix
Hycamtin
Imitrex DF Tablets
Imitrex Injection/Autoinjector
Imitrex Nasal Spray
Infanrix hexa
K-10
Lamictal
Lanvis
Leukeran
Malarone
Malarone Pediatric
Mepron
Mesasal
Myleran
NeisVac-C
Neosporin Cream
Neosporin Eye and Ear Solution
Neosporin Irrigating Solution
Neosporin Ointment
Parnate
Paxil
Paxil CR
Priorix
Priorix-Tetra
Relenza
ReQuip
Rotarix
Septra Injection
Serevent Diskhaler Disk
Serevent Diskus
Synflorix
Timentin
Twinrix
Tykerb
Typherix
Valtrex
Varilrix
Ventolin Diskus
Ventolin HFA
Ventolin I.V. Infusion Solution
Ventolin Nebules P.F.
Ventolin Respirator Solution
Volibris
Votrient
Zantac
Zofran
Zofran ODT
Zovirax Cream
Zovirax Ointment
Zovirax Oral

GlaxoSmithKline Consumer Healthcare Inc.

Head Office:

7333 Mississauga Road
4th Floor
Mississauga ON L5N 6L4
Tel: 905-819-3000
1-800-461-7096
Fax: 905-819-3096

Medical Information:

Tel: 1-800-250-8866

Adverse Event Reporting:

Tel: 1-800-250-8866
Fax: 905-819-3096

Customer Service:

Tel: 905-814-3686
905-814-2014
1-800-461-7096

Abreva
Beano
Gaviscon Heartburn & Acid Reflux Relief Formula Liquid
Gaviscon Heartburn & Acid Reflux Relief Formula Tablets
Gaviscon MAXRELIEF Heartburn & Acid Reflux Formula Tablets
Kwellada-P Creme Rinse
Kwellada-P Lotion
Nix Dermal Cream
Nytol Extra Strength
Palafer
Palafer CF
R & C Shampoo/Conditioner
Sensodyne
Sensodyne-F Iso-Active
Sensodyne Original
Sensodyne ProNamel
Sensodyne ProNamel for Children
Spectro EczemaCare Medicated Cream
Spectro Jel
Tums Tablets

GlaxoSmithKline Shire Canada

Head Office:

7333 Mississauga Rd
Mississauga ON L5N 6L4
Tel: 905-819-3000
Fax: 905-819-3099
Website: www.gsk.ca

Quebec Office:

8455 route Transcanadienne
Saint-Laurent QC H4S 1Z1
Tel: 1-800-463-6314

Medical Information:

Tel: 1-800-387-7374
Fax: 1-800-565-2935
Email: cacsu@gsk.com

Customer Service:

Tel: 1-800-387-7374

Credit and Accounts Receivable Management:

Tel: 1-888-224-1050
Fax: 1-800-367-9609

Heptovir

Glenwood Laboratories Canada Ltd.

Head Office:

2392 Speers Rd
Oakville ON L6L 5M2
Tel: 905-825-8244
Fax: 905-825-9543

Diodoquin
Potaba

Graceway Pharmaceuticals

Head Office:

252 Pall Mall Street
Suite 302
London ON N6A 5P6
Tel: 519-432-7373
1-866-272-1661
Fax: 519-432-8097
Website: www.gracewaypharma.ca

Distribution Centre:

McKesson Logistics
6090 White Hart Lane
Mississauga ON L5R 3Y4

Airomir
Aldara
Minitran
NidaGel
Norflex
Qvar
Tambocor
Theolair
Ulone
Zyclara

GW Pharma

Head Office:

Bayer Inc.
77 Belfield Rd
Toronto ON M9W 1G6
Tel: 1-800-622-2937
Fax: 1-866-232-0565

Medical Information:

Tel: 1-800-265-7382
Fax: 1-866-232-0565
Email: canada.medinfo@bayer.com

Adverse Event Reporting:

Tel: 1-800-265-7382
Fax: 1-866-232-0565
Email: canada.medinfo@bayer.com

Special Access Program:

Tel: 1-800-265-7382
Fax: 1-866-232-0565

Sativex

Helix Biopharma Corp.

Head Office:

3–305 Industrial Pky S
Aurora ON L4G 6X7

Medical Information:

Tel: 905-841-2300 ext 243
1-800-784-0975 ext 243
Fax: 905-841-2244

Customer Service:

Tel: 905-825-4677
1-866-220-4043
Fax: 905-825-9292

Imunovir
Klean-Prep
Monovisc
Normacol
OrthoVisc

Hill Dermaceuticals, Inc.

Distributor:

Hill Dermaceuticals, Inc.
Mississauga ON L4X 2X6

Manufacturer:

Hill Dermaceuticals, Inc.
Sanford FL 32773
USA
Tel: 407-323-1887
1-800-344-5707
Website: www.hillderm.com

Derma-Smoothe/FS
DermOtic Oil Ear Drops

Hoffmann-La Roche Limited

Head Office:

2455 Meadowpine Blvd
Mississauga ON L5N 6L7
Tel: 905-542-5555
1-800-561-1759
Fax: 905-542-7130
Website: www.rochecanada.com

Customer Service:

Tel: 905-542-5500
1-800-268-0440
Fax: 1-800-436-3481

Medical Information:

Tel: 905-542-5537
1-888-762-4388
Fax: 905-542-5610
Email: mississauga.canada_medinfo@roche.com

Accutane Roche
Actemra
Activase rt-PA (Acute Ischemic Stroke)
Activase rt-PA (Acute Myocardial Infarction)
Anexate
Avastin
Cathflo
CellCept
CellCept i.v.
Cytovene
Fuzeon
Herceptin
Inhibace
Inhibace Plus
Invirase
Kytril
Lariam
Lectopam
Naprosyn
Nutropin
Nutropin AQ
Nutropin AQ Pen Cartridge
Pegasys
Pegasys RBV (Pegasys and Copegus)
Prolopa
Pulmozyme
Rituxan
Rivotril
Rocaltrol
Rocephin
Tamiflu
Tarceva
TNKase
Valcyte
Valium Roche Oral
Vesanoid
Xeloda
Xenical

Hospira Healthcare Corporation

Head Office:

1111 Dr.-Frederik-Philips Blvd
Suite 600
Saint Laurent QC H4M 2X6
Tel: 514-905-2600
Fax: 514-331-4685

Acyclovir Sodium Injection
Aminophylline
Atropine Sulfate Injection, USP
Bleomycin Sulphate for Injection USP
Calcium Chloride
Carbocaine
Carboplatin Injection
Cefotaxime Sodium for Injection, BP
Ceftriaxone Sodium for Injection, BP
Ciprofloxacin Injection USP
Cisplatin Injection
Cytarabine Injection
Dacarbazine For Injection BP
Desferrioxamine Mesilate for Injection BP
Dobutamine Injection
Dopamine HCl and Dextrose Injection
Doxorubicin HCl for Injection USP
Ephedrine Sulfate Injection USP
Epinephrine
Epirubicin Hydrochloride for Injection
Epirubicin Hydrochloride Injection
Fentanyl Citrate Injection USP
Fluorouracil Injection USP
Gemcitabine for Injection, USP
Gentamicin Sulfate in 0.9% Sodium Chloride Injection
Heparin Lock Flush
Heparin Sodium in 5% Dextrose Injection
Irinotecan Hydrochloride Trihydrate for Injection
Leucovorin Calcium Injection USP
Levophed
Lidocaine Parenteral (Antiarrhythmic Agent)
Mannitol
Marcaine
Marcaine E
Marcaine Spinal
Methotrexate Injection USP
Methotrexate Tablets USP
Metronidazole Injection USP
Mitoxantrone Injection USP
Morphine Sulfate
Neo-Synephrine Hydrochloride USP
Nipride
Oxytocin Injection, USP
Paclitaxel for Injection
Pamidronate Disodium for Injection
Pentothal
Piperacillin for Injection
Pontocaine
Potassium Chloride
Precedex
Propofol Injection
Quelicin Injection
Rocuronium Bromide Injection
Scopolamine Hydrobromide
Sodium Bicarbonate Injection
Sodium Chloride Injection, USP
Sodium Thiosulfate Injection USP
Talwin Injection
Tomudex
Vancomycin Hydrochloride, USP
Verapamil Hydrochloride Injection USP
Vinblastine Sulfate Injection
Vincristine Sulfate Injection USP
Vinorelbine Tartrate for Injection

HRA Pharma

see Laboratoire HRA Pharma

ID Biomedical

dba GlaxoSmithKline Biologicals North America

Head Office:

525 West Cartier Blvd
Laval QC H7V 3S8
Tel: 450-978-9136
Fax: 450-978-7866

Customer Service:

UPS SCS
8455 route Transcanadienne
Saint-Laurent QC H4S 1Z1
Tel: 1-800-387-7374
Fax: 1-800-565-2935
Email: cacsu@gsk.com
Website: www.gsk.com

Fluviral (2010-2011)

Immunotec Inc

Head Office:

300 Joseph Carrier
Vaudreuil-Dorion QC J7V 5V5
Tel: 450-424-9992
Fax: 450-424-9993
Email: info@immunotec.com
Website: www.immunotec.com

Immunocal

Insight Pharmaceuticals

Head Office:

Associated National Brokerage Inc.
199 Matthew Boyd Cres
Newmarket ON L3X 3C7
Tel: 905-953-9777
Fax: 905-953-9223
Email: customerservice@anbcanada.com
Website: www.anbcanada.com

Nix Creme Rinse

Iroko International LP

Head Office:

Navy Yard Corporate Center
One Crescent Dr
Suite 400
Philadelphia PA 19112
USA
Tel: 267-546-3003
Fax: 267-546-3004

Distributor:

Accuristix
6090 White Hart Lane
Mississauga ON L5R 3Y4

Medical Information:

Tel: 1-866-396-5676

Customer Service:

Tel: 1-866-554-7656

Vancocin

Iroko Cardio (UK) Ltd.

Head Office:

201 Bishopsgate
London EC2M 3AF
United Kingdom
Tel: + 44 (0) 207-873-2494
Fax: + 44 (0) 207-788-9666

Distributor:

Innomar Strategies Inc.
3450 Harvester Road
Burlington ON L7N 3M7

Medical Information:

Tel: 1-866-396-5676

Customer Service:

Tel: 1-866-949-9916

Aggrastat

Jacobus Pharmaceutical Company, Inc.

Head Office:

2000 Ellesmere Rd
Unit 16
Scarborough ON M1H 2W4
Tel: 416-438-6727
Fax: 416-438-3463

Dapsone

Janssen-Ortho Inc.

Head Office:

19 Green Belt Dr
Toronto ON M3C 1L9
Tel: 416-449-9444
1-800-387-8781
Fax: 416-449-2658
Website: www.jansseninc.ca

Medical Information:

Tel: 1-800-567-3331
Website: www.joimedicalinformation.com

Drug Safety and Surveillance:

Tel: 1-800-567-3331
Fax: 416-382-5982
1-866-767-5865

Concerta
Cyclen
Ditropan XL
Doribax
Duragesic MAT
Elmiron
Eprex
Evra
Intelence
Invega
Invega Sustenna
Jurnista
Leustatin
Levaquin
Livostin Nasal Spray
Micronor
Natrecor
Ortho 0.5/35
Ortho 1/35
Ortho 7/7/7
Ortho-Cept
Pancrease MT
Pariet
Prezista
Regranex
Reminyl ER
Risperdal Consta
Risperdal M-Tab
Risperdal Oral Solution
Risperdal Tablets
Sporanox Capsules
Sporanox Oral Solution
Stelara
Terazol
Topamax
Tramacet
Tri-Cyclen
Tri-Cyclen LO
Tylenol No. 1
Tylenol with Codeine Elixir
Tylenol with Codeine No. 2
Tylenol with Codeine No. 3
Tylenol with Codeine No. 4
Ultram
Velcade
Vermox
Yondelis

Johnson & Johnson Inc.

Head Office:

88 McNabb St
Markham ON L3R 5L2
Tel: 905-968-2000
Fax: 905-968-2174

Consumer Information Line:

Tel: 1-800-361-8068

Customer Service Centre:

Tel: 1-800-361-8990
Fax: 1-800-563-2013

Monistat 1 Combination Pack
Monistat 1 Vaginal Ovule
Monistat 3 Dual-Pak Package (Combination Packs)
Monistat 3 Vaginal Cream
Monistat 3 Vaginal Ovules
Monistat 7 Dual-Pak Package (Combination Packs)
Monistat 7 Vaginal Cream
Monistat Derm Cream
Nizoral Shampoo
Polysporin Antibiotic Cream
Polysporin Antibiotic Ointment
Polysporin Antibiotic Plus Pain Relief Cream
Polysporin Complete Antibiotic Ointment
Polysporin Eye/Ear Drops
Polysporin For Kids Cream
Polysporin Ophthalmic Ointment
Polysporin Plus Pain Relief Ear Drops
Polysporin Triple Antibiotic Ointment
Retin-A
Retin-A Micro
Rogaine
Visine Advance Allergy
Visine Advance Triple Action
Visine Advance True Tears
Visine Allergy Eye Drops
Visine Contact Lens Eye Drops
Visine Cool Eye Drops
Visine Original Eye Drops
Visine Workplace Eye Drops

Johnson & Johnson • Merck Consumer Pharmaceuticals

Head Office:

88 McNabb St
Markham ON L3R 5L2
Tel: 905-968-2000
Fax: 905-968-2174

Consumer Information Line:

Tel: 1-800-730-4636

Customer Service Centre:

Tel: 1-800-361-8990
Fax: 1-800-563-2013

222 Tablets
Fleet Enema
Fleet Enema Mineral Oil
Pepcid AC
Pepcid AC, Maximum Strength
Pepcid Complete

King Pharmaceuticals Canada Inc.

Head Office:

2915 Argentia Road
Unit 7
Mississauga ON L5N 8G6
Tel: 905-812-9911
Fax: 905-812-9916

Bicillin L-A
Cytomel
EpiPen
EpiPen Jr

Labopharm Inc.

Head Office:

480 Armand-Frappier Blvd
Laval QC H7V 4B4
Tel: 1-800-686-1017
Email: medinfo@labopharm.com
Website: www.labopharm.com

Tridural

Laboratoire HRA Pharma

Head Office:

15, rue Béranger
75003 Paris
France
Tel: 011 +33 (0) 1 40 33 11 30
Fax: 011 +33 (0) 1 40 33 12 31
Website: www.hra-pharma.com

NorLevo

Laboratoire Riva Inc.

Head Office:

660 Industriel Blvd
Blainville QC J7C 3V4
Tel: 450-434-7482
1-800-363-7988
Fax: 450-434-2500

Acetaminophen
Calcite 500 + D 400
Calcite 500 + D 800
Calcite D 500
Dalmacol
Doxycin
Rectogel
Rectogel HC
Riva-Dicyclomine
Riva-Loperamide
Rivanase AQ.
Rivasol
Rivasol HC
Vita 3B
Vita 3B+C

Laboratoires Trianon Inc.

Head Office:

660 Industriel Blvd
Blainville QC J7C 3V4
Tel: 450-434-7482
1-800-363-7988
Fax: 450-434-2500

Calcium 500
Calcium D 500
Codéine
Pseudofrin

Trianal
Trianal C¼, C½
Triatec-30
Triatec-8
Triatec-8 Strong

LEO Pharma Inc.

Head Office:

123 Commerce Valley Dr E
Suite 400
Thornhill ON L3T 7W8
Tel: 905-886-9822
1-800-668-7234
Fax: 905-886-6622
Website: www.leo-pharma.com/canada

Medical Information:

Tel: 1-800-263-4218

Order Depots:

Acurristix
Advancing Health Care Logistics
2844 Bristol Circle
Oakville ON L6H 6G4
Tel: 905-712-7254
1-800-590-6259

Burinex
Dovobet
Dovonex
Fucidin Cream
Fucidin H
Fucidin Ointment
Fucithalmic
Heparin LEO
Innohep
One-Alpha
Xamiol

Lilly

see Eli Lilly Canada Inc.

Lundbeck Canada Inc.

Subsidiary of H. Lundbeck A/S

Head Office:

1000 de la Gauchetière
Suite 500
Montréal QC H3B 4W5
Tel: 514-844-8515
1-800-586-2325
Fax: 514-844-5495

Medical Information:

Tel: 514-844-8088
1-866-880-4636
Fax: 514-844-8125
Email: canadamedicalinformation@lundbeck.com

Customer Service:

Tel: 514-844-8338
1-866-610-8338
Fax: 514-844-0711
1-866-722-0711
Email: canadacustomerservice@lundbeck.com

Celexa
Cipralex
Clopixol
Clopixol-Acuphase
Clopixol Depot
Ebixa
Fluanxol
Fluanxol Depot

McNeil Consumer Healthcare

Head Office:

88 McNabb St
Markham ON L3R 5L2
Tel: 905-968-2000
Fax: 905-968-2174
Email: cpr@mccca.jnj.com
Website: www.mcneilcanada.com

Medical Information:

Tel: 1-800-611-5889
Fax: 519-826-6205
Email: cpr@mccca.jnj.com

Consumer Information Line:

Tel: 1-800-265-7323

Nicorette Call it Quits Line:

Tel: 1-866-311-5655

Nicoderm Call it Quits Line:

Tel: 1-866-311-5659

Customer Service Centre:

Tel: 1-800-361-8990
Fax: 1-800-563-2013

Actifed
Actifed Plus Extra Strength
Anugesic-HC
Anusol
Anusol-HC
Anusol Plus
Axert
Benadryl Allergy/Sinus/Headache
Benadryl Preparations
Benadryl Spray
Benadryl Stick
Benadryl Total/Allergy/Extra Strength
Benadryl Total/Allergy/Regular Strength
Benylin 1 All-in-One Cold and Flu
Benylin 1 All-in-One Cold and Flu Nightime
Benylin 2 All-in-One Cold and Flu with Codeine (Non-prescription)
Benylin All-in-One Cold and Flu Night PE
Benylin Cold and Sinus
Benylin Cold and Sinus Plus
Benylin DM
Benylin DM 12 Hour (Nightime)
Benylin DM-D (Adult)
Benylin DM-D-E-A Cold and Sinus Rapid Gels
Benylin DM-D-E Extra Strength with Menthactin
Benylin DM-D for Children
Benylin DM-E
Benylin DM-E Extra Strength with Menthactin
Benylin DM for Children
Benylin DM for Children 12 Hour (Bedtime)
Benylin E Extra Strength with Menthactin
Benylin Night Cough
Combantrin
Imodium Advanced
Imodium Caplets
Imodium Oral Solution
Imodium Quick-Dissolve
Lactaid
Microlax
Motrin (Children's)
Motrin IB
Motrin IB Extra Strength
Motrin IB Liquid Gels
Motrin IB Super Strength
Nicoderm
Nicorette Gum
Nicorette Inhaler
Nicorette Lozenge
Nicorette Patch
Reactine
Reactine Allergy & Sinus
Sinutab Nightime
Sinutab Sinus and Allergy
Sinutab Sinus Non Drowsy
Sinutab with Codeine
Sudafed Cold & Cough Extra Strength
Sudafed Decongestant 12 Hour
Sudafed Head Cold and Sinus Extra Strength
Sudafed PE Decongestant
Sudafed Sinus Advance
Tylenol Allergy Extra Strength (Multi-Symptom Relief)
Tylenol Arthritis Pain Extended Release Tablets
Tylenol Children's and Junior Strength Cold DM
Tylenol Children's Cold & Cough Nighttime
Tylenol Children's Cough & Runny Nose
Tylenol Children's Decongestant
Tylenol Children's Tablets "Meltaways" and Suspension
Tylenol Cold & Flu Daytime Liquid
Tylenol Cold & Flu Nighttime Liquid
Tylenol Cold Extra Strength Daytime
Tylenol Cold Extra Strength Nighttime
Tylenol Cold Regular Strength Daytime
Tylenol Cold Regular Strength Nighttime
Tylenol Cough
Tylenol Extra Strength Tablets, Caplets, Gelcaps
Tylenol Flu Extra Strength Daytime
Tylenol Flu Extra Strength Nighttime
Tylenol Infants' Suspension Drops
Tylenol Junior Strength Tablets "Meltaways"
Tylenol Menstrual Extra Strength
Tylenol Muscle Aches & Body Pain Extended Release Tablets
Tylenol Regular Strength Tablets, Caplets
Tylenol Sinus Extra Strength Daytime
Tylenol Sinus Extra Strength Nighttime
Tylenol Sinus Pain and Congestion Daytime Extra Strength
Tylenol Sinus Pain and Congestion Nighttime Extra Strength
Tylenol Sinus Regular Strength Daytime
Tylenol Ultra Relief Migraine Pain
Zantac
Zantac Maximum Strength Non-Prescription

Mead Johnson Nutrition

Head Office:

535 Legget Drive
Suite 900
Kanata ON K2K 3B8
Tel: 613-567-3536
1-800-263-7464

Hospital Resource Center:

Tel: 1-800-263-1143
Fax: 1-800-263-1142
Website: www.enfamil.ca/medical

Customer Resource Center:

Tel: 1-800-361-6323
Fax: 1-800-263-1142
Website: www.enfamil.ca

D-Vi-Sol
Fer-In-Sol

Meda Valeant Pharma Canada Inc.

Head Offices:

Meda Valeant Pharma Canada Inc.
4787 Levy Street
Montreal QC H4R 2P9
Canada
Tel: 514-744-6792
1-800-361-1448

Medical Information (General):

Tel: 514-744-6792
1-800-361-1448
Fax: 514-744-6272
1-800-361-4266
Email: custserv.canada@valeant.com

Medical Information (ONSOLIS):

Tel: 1-888-966-7654
Email: onsolismedinfo@solutionsinhealth.com

Drug Safety (General):

Tel: 514-744-6792
1-800-361-1448
Fax: 514-744-6272
1-800-361-4266
Email: custserv.canada@valeant.com

Drug Safety (ONSOLIS):

Tel: 1-888-966-7654
Email: onsolismedinfo@solutionsinhealth.com

Customer Service:

Tel: 514-744-6792
1-800-361-4261
Fax: 514-744-1842
1-800-361-4266
Email: custserv.canada@valeant.com

Order Desk:

Tel: 514-744-6792
1-800-361-4261
Fax: 514-744-1842
1-800-361-4266
Email: custserv.canada@valeant.com

Credit and Account Receivable:

Tel: 514-744-6792
1-800-361-1448
Fax: 514-744-1842
1-800-361-4266

Manerix

Medexus Inc.

Head Office:

4–7895 Tranmere Dr
Mississauga ON L5S 1V9
Tel: 1-877-MEDEXUS (633-3987)
Website: www.medexus.ca

Metoject

Medical Futures Inc.

Head Office:

16 Sims Cres
Suite 29
Richmond Hill ON L4B 2P1
Tel: 905-731-0294 ext. 212
Fax: 905-731-2873
Website: www.medfutures.com

Florastor
Pegalax
Proferrin

Merck Frosst Canada Ltd.

Head Office:

16 711 Trans-Canada Hwy
Kirkland QC H9H 3L1
Website: www.merckfrosst.com

Mailing Address:

PO Box 1005
Pointe-Claire-Dorval QC H9R 4P8
Tel: 514-428-7920

Customer Information Centre:

Tel: 1-800-567-2594 (Canada)
Fax: 1-877-428-8675
Email: servicesmt_customer@merck.com

Orders:

Tel: 1-800-463-7251 (Canada)
Fax: 1-800-563-7251

Cancidas
Cosopt
Cozaar
Crixivan
Emend
Emend IV
Fosamax
Fosavance
Gardasil
Hyzaar
Hyzaar DS
Invanz
Isentress
Janumet
Januvia
Maxalt
Maxalt RPD
Mevacor
M-M-R II
Pepcid Tablets
Pneumovax 23
Primaxin
Prinivil
Prinzide
Propecia
Proscar
Recombivax HB
RotaTeq
Sinemet
Sinemet CR
Singulair
Timoptic
Timoptic-XE
Trusopt
Vaqta
Varivax III
Vaseretic
Vasotec
Zocor
Zolinza
Zostavax

Merck Frosst-Schering Pharma, G.P.

Head Office:

16 711 Trans-Canada Hwy
Kirkland QC H9H 3L1
Website: www.merckfrosst.com

Mailing Address:

PO Box 1005
Pointe-Claire-Dorval QC H9R 4P8
Tel: 514-428-7920

Customer Information Centre:

Tel: 1-800-567-2594 (Canada)
Fax: 1-877-428-8675
Email: servicesmt_customer@merck.com

Orders:

Tel: 1-800-463-7251 (Canada)
Fax: 1-800-563-7251

Ezetrol

Merz Pharma Canada Ltd.

Head Office:

4145 North Service Road
Suite 200
Burlington ON L7L 6A3
Tel: 905-315-1193
Fax: 905-315-1194

Order Desk:

Tel: 1-877-336-4008

Medical Information:

Tel: 1-866-815-8715

Xeomin

MM Therapeutics Inc.

Head Office:

6111 Royalmount Ave
Suite 100
Montreal QC H4P 2T4
Tel: 1-888-668-1004
Fax: 1-888-668-1006

Medical Information:

Tel: 1-877-454-4149
Email: med.info@scientificaffairs.ca

Toloxin

Mylan Pharmaceuticals ULC

Head Office:

85 Advance Rd
Etobicoke ON M8Z 2S6
Tel: 416-236-4170
1-800-575-1379
Fax: 416-236-8766
1-888–745-7373
Email: customerservice@mylan.ca
Website: www.mylan.ca

Campral
Clarus
Gen-Clozapine
Mylan-Beclo AQ.
Mylan-Budesonide AQ.
Mylan-Nifedipine Extended Release
Mylan-Nitro

Novartis Consumer Health Canada inc

Head Office:

2233 Argentia Rd
West Tower, Unit 205
Mississauga ON L5N 2X7
Tel: 905-812-4100
Fax: 905-821-4936
Website: www.novartis.ca

Habitrol
Voltaren Emulgel
Voltaren Emulgel Joint Pain

Novartis Pharmaceuticals Canada Inc.

Head Office:

385 Bouchard Blvd
Dorval QC H9S 1A9
Tel: 514-631-6775
1-877-631-6775
Fax: 514-631-1867
Website: www.novartis.ca

Customer Relations:

385 Bouchard Blvd
Dorval QC H9S 1A9
Tel: 1-800-465-2244
Fax: 1-800-435-4423

Medical Information:

Tel: 514-631-6775
1-800-363-8883
Fax: 514-633-7054
1-866-633-7054

Clozaril Support and Assistance Network (CSAN):

Tel: 514-631-6775
1-800-267-2726
Fax: 1-800-465-1312

Special Access Program (Dorval, Quebec):

Tel: 514-631-6775
1-800-263-6775
Fax: 1-888-400-5151

Novartis Ophthalmics:

385 Bouchard Blvd
Dorval QC H9S 1A9
Tel: 514-631-6775
1-877-631-6775
Fax: 514-631-1867
Website: www.norvatis.ca

Order Desk:

Tel: 1-866-393-6337

Aclasta
Afinitor
Agriflu
Aredia
Cafergot
Clozaril
Comtan
Desferal
Diovan
Diovan-HCT
Elidel
Enablex
Estalis
Estraderm
Estradot
Exelon
Exelon Patch 5
Exelon Patch 10
Exjade
Extavia
Famvir
Femara
Fiorinal
Fiorinal-C ¼, ½
Foradil
Genteal
Genteal Gel Drops
Gleevec
Hypotears Eye Ointment
Hypotears Ophthalmic Solution
Ilaris
Ixiaro
Lamisil
Lescol
Lescol XL
Lioresal Intrathecal
Lioresal Oral
Livostin Eye Drops
Lopresor
Lotensin
Lucentis
Menjugate
Menveo
Miacalcin NS
Miochol-E
Myfortic
Neoral
Phosphate-Novartis
Proleukin
RabAvert
Rasilez
Rasilez HCT
Ritalin
Ritalin SR
Sandimmune I.V.
Sandostatin
Sandostatin LAR
Sebivo
Simulect
Slow-K
Stalevo
Starlix
Synacthen Depot
Tasigna
Tegretol
TOBI Tobramycin Inhalation Solution, USP
Tofranil
Transderm-Nitro
Transderm-V
Trileptal
Viskazide
Visken
Visudyne
Voltaren Ophtha
Vitalux AREDS
Vitalux-S
Vitalux Time Release
Voltaren
Voltaren Rapide
Voltaren SR
Xolair
Zaditor
Zometa Concentrate

Novo Nordisk Canada Inc.

Head Office:

300–2680 Skymark Ave
Mississauga ON L4W 5L6
Tel: 905-629-4222
1-800-465-4334
Fax: 905-629-8662
Website: www.novonordisk.ca

Activelle
Activelle LD
GlucaGen
GlucaGen HypoKit
GlucoNorm
Levemir
NiaStase RT
NovoFine 30G
NovoFine 32G Tip
Novolinge (30/70, 40/60, 50/50)
Novolinge NPH
Novolinge Toronto
Novolin-Pen 4
NovoMix 30
NovoRapid
Vagifem
Victoza

Novopharm Limited

see Teva Canada

Nu-Pharm Inc.

Head Office:

50 Mural St
Units 1 & 2
Richmond Hill ON L4B 1E4
Tel: 905-886-2344
1-800-267-1438 (Canada)
Fax: 905-886-0564

Nu-Acebutolol
Nu-Acyclovir
Nu-Amilzide
Nu-Amoxi
Nu-Cephalex
Nu-Cimet
Nu-Cotrimox
Nu-Diclo
Nu-Diclo-SR
Nu-Diltiaz
Nu-Diltiaz-CD
Nu-Divalproex
Nu-Doxycycline
Nu-Famotidine
Nu-Fluoxetine
Nu-Glyburide
Nu-Indo
Nu-Lovastatin
Nu-Metformin
Nu-Metoclopramide
Nu-Metop
Nu-Moclobemide
Nu-Naprox
Nu-Oxybutyn
Nu-Pindol
Nu-Pravastatin
Nu-Ranit
Nu-Sertraline
Nu-Sucralfate
Nu-Tetra
Nu-Ticlopidine
Nu-Triazide
Nu-Verap

Nycomed Canada Inc.

Head Office:

435 North Service Rd W
1st Floor
Oakville ON L6M 4X8
Tel: 905-469-9333
1-888-367-3331
Fax: 905-469-4883
Website: www.nycomed.ca

Medical Information:

Tel: 1-866-295-4636

Alvesco
Omnaris
PANTO IV
Pantoloc
Pollinex-R
Resultz
Tecta

Octapharma Pharmazeutika Produktionsges m.b.H.

Head Office:

Oberlaaer Strasse 235
A-1100 Vienna
Austria

Octapharma S.A.S.
70-72 Rue Du Maréchal Foch, BP-33
F-67381 Lingolsheim
France
Website: www.octapharma.com

Distributor:

Octapharma Canada Inc.
326 – 171 East Liberty St.
Toronto ON M6K 3P6
Tel: 416-531-5533
Fax: 416-531-8891
Email: info@octapharma.ca

octaplex
wilate

Odan Laboratories Ltd.

Head Office:

325 Stillview Ave
Pointe-Claire QC H9R 2Y6
Tel: 514-428-1628
Fax: 514-428-9783
Email: odan@odanlab.com
Website: www.odanlab.com

Customer Service:

Tel: 1-800-387-9342
Fax: 1-800-FAX-ODAN

Consumer Information:

Tel: 1-888-666-ODAN

Adasept b.p.5 Acne Gel
Adasept Shampoo
Adasept Skin Cleanser
Alertonic
Anodan-HC
Asatab
Biobase
Biobase-G
Chloral Hydrate-Odan
Citalopram-Odan
Citrodan
Colchicine-Odan
Erdol
Ferodan Infant Drops
Ferodan Syrup
Ferodan Tablets
Hexit Lotion
Hexit Shampoo
Lidodan Endotracheal
Lidodan Ointment
Lidodan Viscous
Liquor Carbonis Detergens
Magnesium-Odan
Ni-odan Extended Release Formula
Nu-Cal
Nu-Cal D
Nu-Cal D 400
Odan K-20
Ondansetron-Odan
Phoslax
Proctodan-HC
Proctol
Purg-Odan
Quinine-Odan
Rovamycine
Selax
Tardan
Targel
Targel S.A.
Urisec
Urisec-10
Urisec-40
Yohimbine-Odan

Organon Canada Ltd.

see Schering-Plough Canada Inc.

Oryx Pharmaceuticals Inc.

see Sepracor Pharmaceuticals, Inc.

Paladin Labs Inc.

Head Office:

100 Blvd. Alexis Nihon
Suite 600
Saint-Laurent QC H4M 2P2
Tel: 514-340-1112
1-888-376-7830
Fax: 514-344-4675
Email: info@paladin-labs.com
Website: www.paladinlabs.com

Medical Information:

For All Paladin Products:
Tel: 514-344-0764
1-888-550-6060
Fax: 514-340-0164
Email: medinfo@paladin-labs.com

Customer Service:

For All Paladin Products:
Tel: 1-866-340-1112
Fax: 514-340-7221
1-800-340-7221
Email: CustomerService@paladin-labs.com

Anbesol Baby Grape Gel
Anbesol Gel
Anbesol Gel Extra Strength
Anbesol Liquid Extra Strength
Androderm
Antizol
Auralgan
Betnesol
Canthacur
Canthacur-PS
Cerumol
Cortifoam
Dalacin Vaginal Cream
Darvon-N
Dexedrine
Dostinex
Duvoid
Elaprase
Estring
Florinef
Kaopectate
Locacorten Vioform Cream
Locacorten Vioform Eardrops
Metadol
Micro-K Extencaps
MUSE
Nitrol
Oxytrol
Pennsaid
Plan B
Podofilm
Prepidil
Propaderm
Propyl-Thyracil
Prostin E2 Tablets
Prostin E2 Vaginal Gel
Replagal
Rogitine
Sandomigran
Sandomigran DS
Seasonale
Sintrom
Statex
Tapazole
Testim 1%
Trandate
Trelstar (Endometriosis)
Trelstar 11.25 mg (3 month slow-release)
Trelstar 3.75 mg (1 month slow-release)
Trinipatch
Twinject 0.15 mg Auto-Injector
Twinject 0.3 mg Auto-Injector
Unisom
Unisom-2
Vioform Hydrocortisone
Zanaflex

Pediapharm Inc.

Head Office:

1 Du Commerce Pl,
Suite 225
Verdun QC H3E 1A2
Tel: 514-762-2626
Fax: 514-762-2336
Website: www.pedia-pharm.com
www.epiceram.ca

EpiCeram

PendoPharm

Division of Pharmascience Inc.

Head Office:

5950 chemin de la Côte-de-Liesse
Mont-Royal QC H4T 1E2
Tel: 514-340-1114
Fax: 514-733-9684

Medical Information:

Tel: 1-888-550-6060

Customer Service:

Tel: 1-866-926-7653
Fax: 1-866-926-7654
Website: www.pendopharm.com

282
282 MEP
292
ACET 120
ACET 160
ACET 325
ACET 650
Bi-PegLyte
Colyte
Cromolyn
Entrophen
Fluor-A-Day
Lax-A-Day
Pediatric Electrolyte
PegLyte
Phosphates Solution
PMS-Lindane
Rhinaris CS Anti-allergic
Rhinaris Lubricating Nasal Gel/Nasal Mist
Rhinaris Nozoil
Rhinaris Saline Pediatric Drops/Saline Spray—Daily Hygiene
Rhinaris Sinomarin
Rhinaris Sinus
Secaris
Soflax
Soflax C
Zap

Pfizer Canada Inc.

Head Office:

17 300 Trans-Canada Hwy
Kirkland QC H9J 2M5
Website: http://www.pfizer.ca/en/

Mailing Address:

PO Box 800
Pointe-Claire-Dorval QC H9R 4V2
Tel: 514-695-0500
Fax: 514-426-7529

Medical Information:

Tel: 1-800-463-6001

Customer Service:

Tel: 1-800-387-4974
Fax: 1-800-420-2019

Distribution Centre:

2400 Skymark Ave
Unit 3
Mississauga ON L4W 5L7
Tel: 1-877-633-2001 (press 0)
Fax: 905-219-2731

Plant:

Pfizer Canada Inc.
PO Box 3003
Arnprior ON K7S 3K2
Tel: 613-623-4221
Fax: 613-623-1259

Accupril
Accuretic
Adriamycin PFS
Aldactazide 25
Aldactazide 50
Aldactone
Alesse 21
Alesse 28
Ansaid

Aricept
Aricept RDT
Aromasin
Arthrotec
Atgam
Ativan
Bacitracin
BeneFIX
Brevicon 0.5/35
Brevicon 1/35
Caduet
Camptosar
Cardura-1
Cardura-2
Cardura-4
Caverject
Celebrex
Champix
Colestid
Cordarone
Cortef Tablets
Corvert
Cyklokapron
Cytosar
Dalacin C
Dalacin C Flavored Granules
Dalacin C Phosphate Sterile Solution
Dalacin T Topical Solution
Daypro
Demulen 30
Depo-Medrol
Depo-Medrol with Lidocaine
Depo-Provera
Depo-Testosterone
Detrol
Detrol LA
Diazemuls
Diflucan
Diflucan 150
Dilantin-125 Suspension
Dilantin-30 Suspension
Dilantin Capsules
Dilantin Infatabs
Effexor XR
Emcyt
Eraxis
Eryc
Fragmin
Gelfoam Powder
Gelfoam Sponge
Hemabate
Idamycin
Idamycin PFS
Inderal-LA
Inspra
Lederle Leucovorin
Lincocin
Lipitor
Lomotil
Loniten
Lopid
Lyrica
Macugen
Medrol
Medrol Acne Lotion
Meningitec
Methotrexate
Min-Ovral 21
Min-Ovral 28
Mycobutin
Neo-Medrol Acne Lotion
Neurontin
Nitrostat
Norvasc
Ogen
Ovral 21
Pharmorubicin PFS
Premarin Intravenous
Premarin Tablets
Premarin Vaginal Cream
Premplus
Prevnar
Prevnar 13
Pristiq
Prostin VR
Provera
Rapamune
Relistor
Relpax
Revatio
Salagen
Salazopyrin
Salazopyrin EN-tabs
Select 1/35
Solu-Cortef
Solu-Medrol
Somavert
Sutent
Synarel
Synphasic
Tazocin
Thelin
Torisel
Tygacil
Vfend
Viagra
Vibramycin
Vibra-Tabs
Viracept
Xalacom
Xalatan
Xanax
Xanax TS
Xyntha
Zanosar
Zeldox
Zinecard
Zithromax
Zoloft
Z-PAK (Zithromax)
Zyvoxam
Zyvoxam I.V.

Pfizer Consumer Healthcare

A division of Pfizer Canada Inc.

Head Office:

5975 Whittle Rd
Mississauga ON L4Z 3M6
Tel: 905-507-7000
1-800-387-8647
Fax: 905-507-7111
Email: Pfizerinfo@healthconnect.ca

Orders Desk:

Tel: 905-507-7000
1-800-387-8647

Medical Information:

Tel: 1-888-275-9938

Drug Safety:

Tel: 1-888-275-9938

Advil
Advil Cold & Sinus
Advil Cold & Sinus Daytime
Advil Cold and Sinus Nighttime
Advil Cold and Sinus Plus
Caltrate
Caltrate Plus
Caltrate Select
Caltrate with Vitamin D
Centrum
Centrum Advantage
Centrum Cardio
Centrum Forte
Centrum Junior Complete
Centrum Materna
Centrum Performance
Centrum Protegra
Centrum Select
Centrum Select Chewables
Children's Advil Cold
Dimetane Expectorant-C
Dimetane Expectorant-DC
Dimetapp Chewables for Kids
Dimetapp-C Syrup
Dimetapp DM Cough & Cold Liquid
Dimetapp Extra Strength DM Cough & Cold Liquid
Dimetapp Extra Strength Liquid
Dimetapp Liquid
Dristan
Dristan Extra Strength
Dristan Long Lasting Nasal Mist/Spray
Dristan Nasal Mist
Preparation H Cooling Gel
Preparation H Cream
Preparation H Ointment
Preparation H Suppositories
Robaxacet
Robaxacet-8
Robaxacet Extra Strength
Robaxin
Robaxin-750
Robaxisal-C
Robaxisal Extra Strength
Robax Platinum
Robitussin
Robitussin AC
Robitussin Children's Cough & Cold
Robitussin Cough & Cold
Robitussin DM
Robitussin DM Cough Control
Robitussin DM CoughGels
Robitussin Extra Strength
Robitussin Extra Strength Cough & Cold
Robitussin Extra Strength DM Cough Control
Robitussin Total Cough Cold and Flu
Robitussin Total Extra Strength Nighttime, Cough Cold and Flu
Stresstabs for Men
Stresstabs for Women
Stresstabs Plus
Stresstabs Regular
Stresstabs Z-BEC

Pharmascience Inc.

Head Office:

6111 Royalmount Ave
Suite 100
Montreal QC H4P 2T4
Tel: 514-340-1114
1-800-363-8805
Fax: 514-342-7764
Website: www. pharmascience.com

Medical Information:

Tel: 514-344-0764
1-888-550-6060
Email: medinfo@pharmascience.com

Asaphen
Asaphen E.C.
CyEstra-35
Lanoxin
Periostat
PMS-Alendronate FC
PMS-Amiodarone
PMS-Amlodipine
PMS-Atenolol
PMS-Atorvastatin
PMS-Azithromycin

PMS-Carvedilol
PMS-Cetirizine
PMS-Cholestyramine
PMS-Citalopram
PMS-Clonazepam
PMS-Desmopressin
PMS-Desonide
PMS-Dexamethasone Elixir/Tablets
PMS-Dexamethasone Injection
PMS-Finasteride
PMS-Fluoxetine
PMS-Gabapentin
PMS-Hydrocodone
PMS-Hydromorphone
PMS-Letrozole
PMS-Levofloxacin
PMS-Loxapine
PMS-Memantine
PMS-Metformin
PMS-Methylphenidate
PMS-Metoprolol-L
PMS-Mirtazapine
PMS-Naproxen
PMS-Naproxen EC
PMS-Nizatidine
PMS-Olanzapine
PMS-Olanzapine ODT
PMS-Omeprazole
PMS-Omeprazole DR
PMS-Ondansetron
PMS-Oxybutynin
PMS-Oxycodone
PMS-Pantoprazole IV
PMS-Pantoprazole Tablets
PMS-Paroxetine
PMS-Phenobarbital
PMS-Pravastatin
PMS-Quetiapine
PMS-Rabeprazole EC
PMS-Ranitidine
PMS-Risedronate
PMS-Risperidone
PMS-Rivastigmine
PMS-Ropinirole
PMS-Sertraline
PMS-Simvastatin
PMS-Sulfasalazine
PMS-Sulfasalazine EC
PMS-Testosterone
PMS-Topiramate
PMS-Trazodone
PMS-Ursodiol C
PMS-Valacyclovir
PMS-Venlafaxine XR
PMS-Zopiclone
Soflax

Pierre Fabre Pharma Canada Inc.

Head Office:

1400 Marie-Victorin
Suite 207
St-Bruno-de-Montarville QC J3V 6B9

Medical Information:

Tel: 450-441-2011
1-877-441-2011
Fax: 450-441-6811
1-877-441-6811

Navelbine

Prempharm Inc.

see Mylan Pharmaceuticals ULC

Prestwick Pharmaceuticals Canada Inc.

see Biovail Pharmaceuticals Canada

Procter & Gamble Inc.

Head Office:

PO Box 355 Stn A
Toronto ON M5W 1C5
Tel: 416-730-4711
1-800-983-4237
Fax: 416-730-4415

Metamucil Capsules plus Calcium
Metamucil Fibre Therapy Capsules
Metamucil Fibre Therapy Smooth Texture Pink Lemonade Flavour, Sugar-free
Metamucil Preparations
Pepto-Bismol Caplets
Pepto-Bismol Chewable Tablets
Pepto-Bismol Liquid
Pepto-Bismol with InstaCool
Vicks Children's NyQuil
Vicks Custom Care Body Aches
Vicks Custom Care Chest Congestion/Cough
Vicks Custom Care Dry Cough
Vicks Custom Care Nasal Congestion/Cough
Vicks DayQuil Cough
Vicks DayQuil Liquicaps
Vicks DayQuil Liquid
Vicks DayQuil Mucus Control
Vicks DayQuil Mucus Control DM
Vicks DayQuil Sinus LiquiCaps
Vicks NyQuil Cough Liquid
Vicks NyQuil Liquicaps
Vicks NyQuil Liquid
Vicks NyQuil Sinus LiquiCaps
Vicks VapoDrops
Vicks VapoRub
Vicks Vapour Inhaler
Vicks Vitamin C Orange Drops

Procter & Gamble Pharmaceuticals Canada, Inc.

see Warner Chilcott Canada Co.

Purdue Pharma

Head Office:

575 Granite Court
Pickering ON L1W 3W8
Tel: 905-420-6400
1-800-387-5349
Fax: 905-420-0385
Website: www.purdue.ca

Medical Information:

Tel: 1-800-387-5349
Fax: 905-420-2503
Email: MedInfo@purdue.ca

Customer Service:

Tel: 905-420-4955
1-800-387-4501
Fax: 905-420-0385
Email: customerservice@purdue.ca

Betadine Topical Preparations
Biphentin
BuTrans 10
BuTrans 20
BuTrans 5
Codeine Contin
Dilaudid
Dilaudid-HP
Dilaudid-HP-Plus
Dilaudid Sterile Powder
Dilaudid-XP
Entex LA
Hydromorph Contin
MS Contin
MS•IR
Oxy·IR
OxyContin
Senokot Preparations
Senokot•S
Uniphyl
Uromax
Zytram XL

Ranbaxy Pharmaceuticals Canada Inc.

Head Office:

2680 Matheson Blvd E
Suite 200
Mississauga ON L4W 0A5
Tel: 905-219-8820
1-866-840-1340
Fax: 905-602-4216
Website: www.ranbaxy.ca

RAN-Amlodipine
RAN-Atenolol
RAN-Atorvastatin
RAN-Carvedilol
RAN-Cefprozil
RAN-Ciproflox
RAN-Citalo
RAN-Domperidone
RAN-Fentanyl Matrix Patch
RAN-Fentanyl Transdermal System
RAN-Lisinopril
RAN-Lovastatin
RAN-Metformin
RAN-Ondansetron
RAN-Pantoprazole
RAN-Pravastatin
RAN-Rabeprazole
RAN-Ramipril
RAN-Risperidone
RAN-Ropinirole
RAN-Simvastatin
RAN-Tamsulosin
RAN-Zopiclone

ratiopharm

Corporate Head Office:

30 Novopharm Court
Toronto ON M1B 2K9
Canada
Tel: 1-800-268-4127 (toll-free)
Website: www.tevacanada.com

Drug Information Inquiries:

Tel: 1-800-268-4127 ext. 5005 (english inquiries)
1-877-777-9117 (french inquiries)
Fax: 1-416-335-4472 (english and french inquiries)
Email: druginfo@tevacanada.com

Reporting Side Effects and Lack-of-Efficacy Complaints:

Tel: 1-800-268-4127 ext. 5005 (all inquiries)
Fax: 1-416-335-4472
Email: phv@tevacanada.com

Customer Care:

Tel: 1-800-268-4129 (toll-free)
Fax: 1-800-387-4733 (toll-free)
Email: customer.service@tevacanada.com

ratio-Aclavulanate
ratio-Acyclovir
ratio-Alendronate
ratio-Amcinonide
ratio-Amiodarone
ratio-Amlodipine
ratio-Atenolol
ratio-Atorvastatin
ratio-Azithromycin
ratio-Baclofen
ratio-Bicalutamide

ratio-Bisacodyl
ratio-Brimonidine
ratio-Bupropion SR
ratio-Calmydone
ratio-Carvedilol
ratio-Cefuroxime
ratio-Ciprofloxacin
ratio-Citalopram
ratio-Clarithromycin
ratio-Clobetasol
ratio-Clonazepam
ratio-Codeine
ratio-Coristex-DH
ratio-Cotridin
ratio-Cotridin Expectorant
ratio-Cyclobenzaprine
ratio-Dexamethasone
ratio-Diltiazem CD
ratio-Docusate Calcium
ratio-Docusate Sodium
ratio-Domperidone
ratio-Ectosone
ratio-Emtec-30
ratio-Enalapril
ratio-Fenofibrate MC
ratio-Fentanyl
ratio-Finasteride
ratio-Fluoxetine
ratio-Fluticasone
ratio-Fluvoxamine
ratio-Gabapentin
ratio-Gentamicin
ratio-Glimepiride
ratio-Glyburide
ratio-Hemcort-HC
ratio-Indomethacin
ratio-Ipra Sal UDV
ratio-Ipratropium
ratio-Ipratropium UDV
ratio-Ketorolac
ratio-Lactulose
ratio-Lamotrigine
ratio-Lenoltec No. 1, 2 & 3
ratio-Lenoltec No. 4
ratio-Levobunolol
ratio-Lisinopril P
ratio-Lisinopril Z
ratio-Lovastatin
ratio-Meloxicam
ratio-Memantine
ratio-Metformin
ratio-Methotrexate Sodium
ratio-Minocycline
ratio-Mirtazapine
ratio-Mometasone
ratio-Morphine
ratio-Morphine SR
ratio-Nystatin
ratio-Omeprazole
ratio-Ondansetron
ratio-Oxycocet
ratio-Oxycodan
ratio-Pantoprazole
ratio-Paroxetine
ratio-Pentoxifylline
ratio-Pioglitazone
ratio-Pravastatin
ratio-Prednisolone
ratio-Proctosone
ratio-Quetiapine
ratio-Ramipril
ratio-Ranitidine
ratio-Risedronate
ratio-Rivastigmine
ratio-Salbutamol
ratio-Sertraline
ratio-Sildenafil R
ratio-Simvastatin
ratio-Sotalol
ratio-Tamsulosin
ratio-Tecnal
ratio-Tecnal C¼, C½
ratio-Temazepam
ratio-Terazosin
ratio-Theo-Bronc
ratio-Topilene
ratio-Topiramate
ratio-Topisalic
ratio-Topisone
ratio-Trazodone
ratio-Triacomb
ratio-Tryptophan
ratio-Valproic
ratio-Venlafaxine XR
ratio-Zopiclone

Riva

see Laboratoire Riva Inc.

Roche

see Hoffmann-La Roche Limited

Rougier Pharma

Division of Teva Canada

Corporate Head Office:

30 Novopharm Court
Toronto ON M1B 2K9
Canada
Tel: 1-800-268-4127 (toll-free)
Website: www.tevacanada.com

Drug Information Inquiries:

Tel: 1-800-268-4127 ext. 5005 (english inquiries)
1-877-777-9117 (french inquiries)
Fax: 1-416-335-4472 (english and french inquiries)
Email: druginfo@tevacanada.com

Reporting Side Effects and Lack-of-Efficacy Complaints:

Tel: 1-800-268-4127 ext. 5005 (all inquiries)
Fax: 1-416-335-4472
Email: phv@tevacanada.com

Customer Care:

Tel: 1-800-268-4129 (toll-free)
Fax: 1-800-387-4733 (toll-free)
Email: customer.service@tevacanada.com

Acetazone Forte
Acetazone Forte C8
Allernix
Balminil Cough & Flu
Balminil DM
Balminil DM+Decongestant
Balminil DM+Decongestant+Expectorant
Balminil DM+Expectorant
Balminil DM Children
Balminil Expectorant
Balminil Nasal Decongestant
Balminil Night-Time
Bismutal
Calmylin Original with Codeine
Calmylin PSE with Codeine
CaVit D
Citro-Mag
Glucodex
Glycerin Suppositories
Hydrosone
Koffex DM
Limonade Asepta
Methoxacet
Methoxacet-C⅛
Methoxacet Extra Strength
Methoxisal
Methoxisal-C¼
Methoxisal-C½
Methoxisal-C⅛
Methoxisal Extra Strength
Milk of Magnesia USP
Neo-Laryngobis
Osmopak Plus
Pediatrix
Proviodine
Rougier Clean Derm
Rougier Magnesium
Rougier Vap

Sandoz Canada Inc.

Head Office:

145 Jules-Léger St
Boucherville QC J4B 7K8
Tel: 514-596-0000
1-800-361-3062
Fax: 514-596-0003
Website: www.sandoz.com

Medical Information:

Tel: 450-641-4903 ext 4636
1-800-343-8839 ext 4636
Email: medinfo@sandoz.com

Acetylcysteine Solution (Sandoz Standard)
Alfentanil Injection USP
Amikacin Sulfate Injection USP
Amiodarone Hydrochloride for Injection Sandoz Standard
Atracurium Besylate Injection
Atropine Sulfate Injection USP
Betaject
Bretylium Tosylate Injection USP
Cefazolin for Injection USP
Ceftriaxone for Injection BP
Ciprofloxacin Intravenous Infusion BP
Clindamycin Injection USP
Cocaine Hydrochloride Topical Solution
Dehydrated Alcohol Injection USP
Dexamethasone Sodium Phosphate Injection USP
Diazepam Injection USP
Digoxin Injection C.S.D.
Digoxin Pediatric Injection C.S.D.
Dihydroergotamine Mesylate Injection USP
Diltiazem Hydrochloride Injection
Dimenhydrinate
Dimethyl Sulfoxide Irrigation USP
Diophenyl-T
Diopred
Diphenhydramine Hydrochloride Injection USP
Dobutamine Injection USP
Droperidol Injection USP
Ephedrine Sulfate Injection USP
Fentanyl Citrate Injection USP
Fluconazole Injection
Flumazenil Injection
Fluorouracil Injection
Furosemide Injection USP
Furosemide Special
Gemcitabine Hydrochloride for Injection
Gentamicin Injection USP
Glycopyrrolate Injection USP
Granisetron Hydrochloride Injection
Haloperidol Injection USP
Haloperidol LA
Heparin Sodium Injection USP
Hydromorphone HP 10
Hydromorphone HP 20
Hydromorphone HP 50
Hydromorphone HP Forte
Hydromorphone Hydrochloride Injection USP
Hyoscine Butylbromide Injection
Infufer
Irinotecan Hydrochloride Trihydrate Injection
Isoproterenol HCl Injection USP

Ketamine Hydrochloride Injection USP
Ketorolac Tromethamine Injection USP
Labetalol Hydrochloride Injection USP
Lorazepam Injection USP
Loxapac IM
Medroxyprogesterone Acetate Injectable Suspension USP
Meperidine Hydrochloride Injection USP
Methylprednisolone Acetate Injectable Suspension USP
Metoclopramide Hydrochloride Injection
Metoprolol Tartrate Injection USP
Midazolam Injection (Sandoz Standard)
Milrinone Lactate Injection
Morphine HP Injection
Morphine LP Epidural
Morphine Sulfate Injection USP
Naloxone Hydrochloride Injection USP
Neostigmine Methylsulfate Injection USP
Norepinephrine Bitartrate Injection USP
Nubain
Omnitrope
Ondansetron Injection USP
Optimyxin Eye/Ear Solution
Optimyxin Ophthalmic Ointment
Optimyxin Plus Eye/Ear Solution
Pamidronate Disodium for Injection
Pancuronium Bromide Injection
Pantoprazole Sodium for Injection
Papaverine HCl Injection USP
Penta/3b
Penta/3b+C
Penta/3b Plus
Pentamycetin
Pentamycetin/HC
Phenobarbital Sodium Injection USP
Piperacillin Sodium/Tazobactam Sodium Powder for Injection
Polytopic Cream
Polytopic Ointment
Prochlorperazine Mesylate Injection
Protamine Sulfate Injection USP
Ranitidine Injection USP
Rocuronium Bromide Injection
Salinex Nasal Lubricant/Nasal Lubricant Gel
Salinex Nasal Spray/Nasal Drops/Nasal Mist
Sandoz Alfuzosin
Sandoz Amiodarone
Sandoz Amlodipine
Sandoz Anagrelide
Sandoz Anuzinc
Sandoz Anuzinc HC
Sandoz Anuzinc HC Plus
Sandoz Atorvastatin
Sandoz Azithromycin Powder for Oral Suspension
Sandoz Azithromycin Tablets
Sandoz Bicalutamide
Sandoz Bisoprolol
Sandoz Bupropion SR
Sandoz Calcitonin NS
Sandoz Carbamazepine
Sandoz Cefprozil
Sandoz Clarithromycin
Sandoz Clonazepam
Sandoz Cortimyxin Ophthalmic Ointment
Sandoz Cortimyxin Otic Solution
Sandoz Cyclosporine
Sandoz Diclofenac
Sandoz Diclofenac Rapide
Sandoz Diclofenac SR
Sandoz Diltiazem CD
Sandoz Diltiazem T
Sandoz Estradiol Derm
Sandoz Famciclovir
Sandoz Felodipine
Sandoz Fenofibrate S
Sandoz Fentanyl Patch
Sandoz Finasteride
Sandoz Glimepiride
Sandoz Glyburide
Sandoz Leflunomide
Sandoz Letrozole
Sandoz Levofloxacin
Sandoz Lisinopril
Sandoz Lisinopril HCT
Sandoz Metformin FC
Sandoz Methylphenidate SR
Sandoz Metoprolol (Type L)
Sandoz Metoprolol SR
Sandoz Minocycline
Sandoz Mirtazapine
Sandoz Naratriptan
Sandoz Nitrazepam
Sandoz Olanzapine ODT
Sandoz Omeprazole
Sandoz Orphenadrine
Sandoz Pantoprazole
Sandoz Pioglitazone
Sandoz Pramipexole
Sandoz Pravastatin
Sandoz Prednisolone
Sandoz Prochlorperazine Suppository
Sandoz Proctomyxin HC
Sandoz Quetiapine
Sandoz Rabeprazole
Sandoz Rivastigmine
Sandoz Sotalol
Sandoz Sumatriptan
Sandoz Tamsulosin
Sandoz Terbinafine
Sandoz Topiramate
Sandoz Venlafaxine XR
Sandoz Zopiclone
Sodium Sulamyd
Sufentanil Citrate Injection USP
Supeudol
Testosterone Cypionate Injection USP
Tobramycin Injection USP
Topotecan for Injection
Triamcinolone Acetonide Injectable Suspension USP
Vitamin B12 Injection

sanofi-aventis Canada Inc.

Head Office:

2150 Saint-Elzear Blvd W
Laval QC H7L 4A8
Tel: 514-331-9220
1-800-363-6364
Fax: 514-334-8016

Customer Service/Medical Information/Pharmacovigilance:

Tel: 1-800-265-7927
Fax: 1-800-268-3846

Allegra 12 Hour
Allegra 24 Hour
Allegra-D
Altace
Altace HCT
Amaryl
Anandron
Anzemet
Apidra
Arava
BenzaClin
Benzamycin
Calcimar
Claforan
Clomid
Cyclomen
Demerol Tablets
Dermatop
Diabeta
Drisdol
Eligard
Eloxatin
Eltor 120
Fasturtec
Flagyl
Flagystatin
Gastrolyte
Glucophage
Imovane
Kayexalate
Ketek
Lantus
Lasix
Lasix Special
Loprox
Lovenox
Lovenox HP
Mersyndol with Codeine
Multaq
Myochrysine
Nalcrom
Nasacort AQ
Nitrolingual Pumpspray
Noritate
Novahistex DH
Novahistine DH
Nozinan
Pediapred
Penlac
pHisoHex
Piportil L4
Plaquenil
Plavix
Primaquine
Renedil
Resonium Calcium
Rho-Nitro Pumpspray
Rhotral
Rhovane
Rifadin
Rifater
Rilutek
Rythmodan
Sectral
Sofracort
Sulfacet-R
Suprax
Suprefact
Suprefact Depot
Talwin Tablets
Tamofen
Taxotere
Topicort Preparations
Trental
Tussionex
Vitamin A Acid
Xatral
Zaroxolyn

sanofi pasteur

Head Office:

Connaught Campus
1755 Steeles Ave W
Toronto ON M2R 3T4
Website: www.sanofipasteur.ca

Product Orders:

Tel: 416-667-2611
1-800-268-4171
Fax: 416-667-2998
1-877-311-9741

Vaccine Information Service:

Tel: 416-667-2779
1-888-621-1146
Fax: 416-667-2629

Act-HIB
Adacel

Avaxim
Avaxim-Pediatric
BCG Vaccine (Freeze-Dried)
Dukoral
ImmuCyst
IMOGAM Rabies Pasteurized
IMOVAX Polio
IMOVAX Rabies
Intanza
Menactra
Menomune-A/C/Y/W-135
Pediacel
Pneumo 23
Quadracel
Td Adsorbed
Td Polio Adsorbed
Tubersol
Typhim Vi
Vaxigrip
ViVAXIM

Schering-Plough Canada Inc.

Now part of Merck

Head Office:

16750 route Transcanadienne
Kirkland QC H9H 4M7
Tel: 514-426-7300
Fax: 514-695-7641

Medical Information and Adverse Event Reporting:

Tel: 1-800-463-5442
Fax: 1-800-369-3090
Email: Medical.services@spcorp.com

Customer Service:

17700 route Transcanadienne
Kirkland QC H9J 3A3

Montreal:
Tel: 514-426-7344 (english)
514-426-7340 (french)
Fax: 514-428-7400

Province of Quebec:
Tel: 1-800-361-2431
Fax: 1-888-428-7400

Western Canada, Ontario and Maritimes:
Tel: 1-800-361-6550
Fax: 1-888-428-7400

Aerius
Aerius Dual Action 12 Hour
Aerius Kids
Andriol
Caelyx
Celestone Soluspan
Claritin
Claritin Allergic Congestion Relief
Claritin Allergy+Sinus
Claritin Allergy+Sinus Extra Strength
Claritin Kids
Claritin Skin Itch Relief
Cotazym
Diprolene Glycol
Diprosalic
Diprosone
Elocom
Estrogel
Euflex
Garamycin Ophthalmic Drops
Garamycin Ophthalmic Ointment
Garamycin Otic Drops
Garasone Ophthalmic/Otic Solution
Garasone Ophthalmic Ointment
Hepalean
hydraSense
Integrilin
Intron A
K-Dur
Linessa 21
Linessa 28
Lotriderm
Marvelon
Nasonex
Nitro-Dur
NuvaRing
Olmetec
Olmetec Plus
OncoTICE
Orgalutran
Orgaran (HIT)
Orgaran-DVT
Pegetron
Posanol
Proglycem
Prometrium
Puregon
Remeron
Remeron RD
Remicade
Simponi
Suboxone
Temodal
Unitron PEG
Zemuron

Sepracor Pharmaceuticals, Inc.

Head Office:

6790 Century Ave.
Suite 100
Mississauga ON L5N 2V8
Tel: 905-814-9145
1-866-260-6291
Fax: 905-363-0162
Website: www.sepracorpharma.ca

Medical Information:

Tel: 905-814-9145 (press 2)
1-866-260-6291 (press 2)
Fax: 905-363-0162
Email: medinfo-ca@sepracor.com

Advicor
Anafranil
Angiomax
Clasteon
CTP 30
Cubicin
FXT
Naprelan
Niaspan
Niaspan FCT
Restoril
Trosec

Servier Canada Inc.

Head Office:

235 Armand-Frappier Blvd
Laval QC H7V 4A7
Tel: 450-978-9700
1-800-663-0839

Medical Information:

Tel: 450-978-9700
1-800-663-0839
Fax: 450-781-1430

Orders Desk:

Tel: 450-978-9700
1-800-363-6093
Fax: 450-978-9772

Coversyl
Coversyl Plus
Coversyl Plus HD
Coversyl Plus LD
Diamicron
Diamicron MR
Lozide

Shire Canada Inc.

Head Office:

2250 Alfred-Nobel Blvd
Suite 500
Saint-Laurent QC H4S 2C9
Tel: 514-787-2300
1-866-397-4473
Fax: 514-787-2427
Website: www.shire.com

Medical Information:

Tel: 1-800-268-2772
Fax: 514-787-5149
Email: medinfoglobal@shire.com

Orders and Customer Information:

Atlantic Provinces, Quebec and Ottawa Valley:
Lynden International Logistics Co.
Tel: 514-956-0768
1-800-361-3362
Fax: 514-956-0325

Ontario:
Lynden International Logistics Co.
10 Corinne Court
Vaughan ON L4K 4T7
Tel: 1-800-268-4937
Fax: 905-879-0123

Western Canada:
Lynden International Logistics Co.
Tel: 403-236-1787
1-800-661-1237
Fax: 403-236-9104

Adderall XR
Agrylin
Alertec
Estrace
Fosrenol
Mezavant
Vyvanse

Sigma-Tau Pharmaceuticals, Inc.

Head Office:

2000 Ellesmere Rd
Unit 16
Scarborough ON M1H 2W4
Tel: 416-438-6727
Fax: 416-438-3463
Website: www.sigma-tau.com

Abelcet
Carnitor
Matulane

Solvay Pharma Inc.

see Abbott Products Inc.

Stellar Pharmaceuticals Inc.

Head Office:

544 Egerton St
London ON N5W 3Z8
Tel: 519-434-1540
1-800-639-0643
Fax: 519-434-4382
Website: www.stellarpharma.com

NeoVisc
Uracyst

SteriMax Inc.

Head Office:

2735 Matheson Blvd. E.
Suite 1
Mississauga ON L4W 4M8
Tel: 905-890-0661
1-800-881-3550
Fax: 905-890-0298
Email: info@sterimaxinc.com
Website: www.sterimaxinc.com

Apresoline
BaciJect
Colistimethate for Injection U.S.P.
Dairy Free
Dihydroergotamine (DHE)
Hydergine
Migranal
Orfenace
Streptomycin Injection USP
Tobramycin for Injection USP

Stiefel, a GSK company

8455 Route Transcanadienne Hwy.
Saint-Laurent QC H4S 1Z1
Tel: 1-800-363-2862
Website: www.stiefel.ca

GSK Head Office:

7333 Mississauga Rd
Mississauga ON L5N 6L4
Tel: 905-819-3000
Fax: 905-819-3099

Medical Information:

Tel: 1-800-387-7374
Fax: 1-800-565-2935
Email: cacsu@gsk.com

Acne-Aid Soap
Benoxyl 10% and 20%
Benoxyl 5%
Buro-Sol Powder
Buro-Sol Otic Solution
Clindasol
Clindets
Clindoxyl
Cyclocort
Doak Oil
Doak Oil Forte
Duofilm Liquid
Duofilm Patch
Duofilm Plantar Patch
Duoforte 27
Duoplant
Emo-Cort
Erysol
Minocin
Nerisalic
Nerisone
Oilatum Dermatological Shower and Bath Oil
Panoxyl 10% and 20%
Panoxyl 5%
Panoxyl 5% Wash
Panoxyl Antibacterial Acne Creamy Wash
Panoxyl Aquagel 2.5% and 5%
Panoxyl Clear Acne Cleansing Gel
Polytar
Polytar AF
Prevex B
Prevex Cream
Prevex HC
Rejuva-A
Retisol-A
Rosasol
Sarna HC
Sarna-P
Solugel 4
Solugel 8
Stieprox
Stieva-A
Stievamycin Preparations
Tersaseptic
Tersa-Tar
Uremol 10
Uremol 20
Uremol HC
ZeaSORB
ZeaSORB AF

Takeda Pharmaceuticals America, Inc.

Head Office:

Abbott Laboratories, Limited
8401 Trans-Canada Hwy
Saint-Laurent QC H4S 1Z1
Tel: 514-832-7000
1-800-361-7852 (Canada)
Fax: 514-832-7800

Mailing Address:

PO Box 6150 Stn Centre-Ville
Montreal QC H3C 3K6

Montreal Order Desk:

Tel: 1-800-567-2226 (all area codes)
514-832-7333 (Montreal)
Fax: 514-832-7251
1-800-513-7337

Hp-PAC
Prevacid
Prevacid FasTab

Takeda Canada, Inc.

Head Office:

6750 Century Ave
Suite 400
Mississauga ON L5N 2V8
Website: www.takedacanada.com

Medical Information:

Tel: 1-888-825-3321
Fax: 905-814-2484
Email: medicalinformation@takedacanada.com

Adverse Event Reporting:

Tel: 1-888-825-3321
Fax: 905-814-2484
Email: medicalinformation@takedacanada.com

Actos
Dexilant
Uloric

Talecris Biotherapeutics Ltd.

Head Office:

5800 Explorer Dr
Unit 300
Mississauga ON L4W 5K9
Tel: 1-866-482-5226
Fax: 905-614-5590
Website: www.talecris.ca

Medical Information/Adverse Event Reporting:

Tel: 1-866-482-5226
Fax: 1-877-252-8510

Order Desk:

Tel: 1-866-482-5226

Ottawa Office:

1785 Alta Vista Dr
Suite 103
Ottawa ON K1G 3Y6
Tel: 613-730-3900
Fax: 613-730-3910

GamaSTAN S/D
Gamunex
HyperHEP B S/D
HYPERRAB S/D
HYPERTET S/D
Plasbumin-25
Plasbumin-5
Prolastin-C

Tanta Pharmaceuticals Inc.

Head Office:

1009 Burns St E
Whitby ON L1N 6A6
Tel: 905-430-8440
1-800-668-2682
Fax: 905-430-8449
Email: info@tanta.ca

Senna Laxative Pills Extra Strength Peristaltic Stimulant
Senna Laxative Pills Regular Strength Peristaltic Stimulant
Senna-S Tablets Peristaltic Stimulant-Surfactant
Senna Tablets Peristaltic Stimulant

Tap Pharmaceuticals

see Takeda Pharmaceuticals America, Inc.

TaroPharma

Head Office:

130 East Dr
Brampton ON L6T 1C1
Tel: 905-791-8276
1-800-268-1975
Fax: 905-458-8792
Website: www.taropharma.ca

Dermalac
Dermovate
HydroVal
Ketoderm
Lyderm
Tiamol

Taro Pharmaceuticals Inc.

Head Office:

130 East Dr
Brampton ON L6T 1C1
Tel: 905-791-8276
1-800-268-1975
Fax: 905-458-8792
Website: www.taro.ca

Betaderm
Clotrimaderm
Cortoderm
Docusate Sodium
Hyderm
Micozole
Nyaderm
Oracort
Polyderm
Taro-Amcinonide
Taro-Carbamazepine
Taro-Clindamycin
Taro-Clobetasol
Taro-Mometasone
Taro-Mupirocin
Taro-Phenytoin
Taro-Sone
Taro-Terconazole
Taro-Warfarin

Triaderm
Triple Antibiotic Ointment
Viaderm-K.C.

Teva Canada

Corporate Head Office:

30 Novopharm Court
Toronto ON M1B 2K9
Canada
Tel: 1-800-268-4127 (toll-free)
Website: www.tevacanada.com

Drug Information Inquiries:

Tel: 1-800-268-4127 ext. 5005 (english inquiries)
1-877-777-9117 (french inquiries)
Fax: 1-416-335-4472 (english and french inquiries)
Email: druginfo@tevacanada.com

Reporting Side Effects and Lack-of-Efficacy Complaints:

Tel: 1-800-268-4127 ext. 5005 (all inquiries)
Fax: 1-416-335-4472
Email: phv@tevacanada.com

Customer Care:

Tel: 1-800-268-4129 (toll-free)
Fax: 1-800-387-4733 (toll-free)
Email: customer.service@tevacanada.com

Purinethol
Teva-5 ASA
Teva-Alendronate
Teva-Amlodipine
Teva-Amoxicillin
Teva-Ampicillin
Teva-Atenolol
Teva-Betahistine
Teva-Cephalexin
Teva-Chloroquine
Teva-Chlorpromazine
Teva-Citalopram
Teva-Diltiazem
Teva-Diltiazem CD
Teva-Enalapril
Teva-Enalapril/HCTZ
Teva-Erythromycin Estolate
Teva-Erythromycin Ethylsuccinate
Teva-Fentanyl
Teva-Fluoxetine
Teva-Gabapentin
Teva-Ketotifen
Teva-Lansoprazole
Teva-Maprotiline
Teva-Metoprolol
Teva-Mexiletine
Teva-Naproxen
Teva-Naproxen-EC
Teva-Naproxen Sodium
Teva-Naproxen Sodium DS
Teva-Olanzapine
Teva-Pantoprazole
Teva-Paroxetine
Teva-Pravastatin
Teva-Quetiapine
Teva-Rabeprazole EC
Teva-Ramipril
Teva-Sertraline
Teva-Simvastatin
Teva-Spironolactone
Teva-Spironolactone HCTZ
Teva-Sulfamethoxazole Trimethoprim
Teva-Sulfamethoxazole Trimethoprim DS
Teva-Sumatriptan
Teva-Sumatriptan DF
Teva-Topiramate
Teva-Venlafaxine XR

Teva Canada Innovation

Head Office:

999 de Maisonneuve W
Suite 550
Montreal QC H3A 3L4
Tel: 1-866-329-0095
Fax: 514-878-0798

Medical Information:

For Azilect and Frova:
Tel: 1-866-530-6065

For Copaxone:
Tel: 1-800-283-0034

Customer Service:

For Azilect, Copaxone and Frova:
Tel: 1-800-268-4129
Fax: 1-800-387-4733

Azilect
Copaxone
Frova

Teva Neuroscience G.P.-S.E.N.C.

see Teva Canada Innovation

Theramed Corporation

Head Office:

6891 Edwards Blvd
Mississauga ON L5T 2T9
Tel: 905-564-5009
1-800-305-4441
Fax: 905-564-4776
1-888-633-3644
Email: theramed@theramed.com
Website: www.theramed.com

After Hours Emergency:

Tel: 416-410-0590
1-888-556-7276

Delatestryl
Viroptic

Trans CanaDerm Inc.

see Stiefel, a GSK company

Trianon

see Laboratoires Trianon Inc.

Triton Pharma Inc.

Head Office:

665 Millway Ave
Suite 31B
Concord ON L4K 3T8
Tel: 416-543-5430
1-866-429-9707
Email: info@tritonpharma.ca
Website: www.tritonpharma.ca

Bellergal Spacetabs
Eltroxin
Imuran Injection
Imuran Tablets
Oesclim
Vaniqa

tyco Healthcare

Head Office:

7500 Trans-Canada Hwy
Pointe-Claire QC H9R 5H8
Tel: 514-695-1220
1-877-664-8926
Fax: 514-695-1889
Email: dawn.boyce@tycohealthcare.com
Website: www.tyco.com

After Hours Emergency:

Tel: 514-695-1220 ext 638

Conray 30
Conray 43
Conray 60
Cysto-Conray II
OptiMARK
Optiray
Technetium Tc 99m Sestamibi Injection, Kit for the Preparation of
Telebrix 38 Oral

UCB Canada Inc.

Head Office:

2060 Winston Park Drive
Suite 401
Oakville ON L6H 5R7

Medical Information:

Tel: 1-866-709-8444

Cimzia
Dipentum
Keppra
Vimpat

USANA Health Sciences, Inc.

Head Office:

3838 West Parkway Blvd
Salt Lake City UT 84120-6336
USA
Tel: 801-954-7100
Fax: 801-954-7300
Website: www.usana.com

Active Calcium Chewable
Biomega
Optomega
Proflavanol 90
Visionex
Vitamin D

Valeant Canada Ltd

Head Offices:

Valeant Pharmaceuticals International, Inc.
7150 Mississauga Rd.
Mississauga ON L5N 8M5
Canada
Tel: 905-286-3100
Fax: 905-286-3150
Website: www.valeant.com

Valeant Canada Ltd
4787 Lévy St
Montreal QC H4R 2P9
Tel: 514-744-6792
1-800-361-1448
Fax: 514-744-6272
1-800-361-4266

Medical Information:

Tel: 514-744-6792
1-800-361-1448
Fax: 514-744-6272
1-800-361-4266
Email: custserv.canada@valeant.com

Drug Safety:

Tel: 514-744-6792
1-800-361-1448
Fax: 514-744-6272
1-800-361-4266
Email: custserv.canada@valeant.com

Customer Service:

Tel: 514-744-6792
1-800-361-4261
Fax: 514-744-1842
1-800-361-4266
Email: custserv.canada@valeant.com

Order Desk:

Tel: 514-744-6792
1-800-361-4261
Fax: 514-744-1842
1-800-361-4266
Email: custserv.canada@valeant.com

Credit and Account Receivable:

Tel: 514-744-6792
1-800-361-1448
Fax: 514-744-1842
1-800-361-4266

Benuryl
C.E.S.
Carbolith
Cesamet
Cortisone Acetate
Dermatix Ultra
Dexasone
Diastat
Efudex
Etibi
Glyquin XM
Hycort
Isotamine
Librax
M.O.S.
M.O.S.-SR
M.O.S.-Sulfate
Mestinon
Mestinon-SR
Mogadon
Nitrazadon
Prostigmin
Rofact
Tebrazid
Tryptan
Ultravate
Virazole (Lyophilized)
Winpred
Xyrem

Valeo Pharma Inc.

Head Office:

16 667 Hymus Blvd
Kirkland QC H9H 4R9
Tel: 514-694-0150
1-866-694-0150
Fax: 514-694-0865
Email: info@valeopharma.com

Aristocort, Creams and Ointments
Cophylac
Valisone-G
Valisone Scalp Lotion
Val-Vanco

ViiV Healthcare ULC

Head Office Canada:

8455, route Transcanadienne
Saint-Laurent Quebec H4S 1Z1
Tel: 1-877-393-8448
Fax: 514-956-3183
Website: www.viivhealthcare.com

3TC
Celsentri
Combivir
Kivexa
Rescriptor
Retrovir (AZT)
Telzir
Trizivir
Ziagen

Warner Chilcott Canada Co.

Head Office:

PO Box 4367 Station A
Toronto ON M5W 3N7
Tel: 416-572-3805

Medical Information:

Tel: 1-800-565-0814
Fax: 1-866-566-0019

Order Desk:

Tel: 1-800-265-8676

Actonel
Asacol
Asacol 800
femHRT
MacroBID

WellSpring Pharmaceutical Canada Corp.

Head Office:

400 Iroquois Shore Rd
Oakville ON L6H 1M5
Tel: 905-337-4500
1-866-337-4500
Fax: 905-337-3539
Website: www.wellspringpharm.com

Medical Information:

Tel: 1-866-337-4500

Customer Service:

Tel: 1-866-337-4500

Barriere
Colace
Dequadin Preparations
Glaxal Base
K-Lyte
Micatin
Mucomyst

Westwood-Squibb

see Bristol-Myers Squibb Canada

Wyeth Canada

see Pfizer Canada Inc.

Wyeth Consumer Healthcare Inc. (a Pfizer Company)

see Pfizer Consumer Healthcare

A

#
A

On the Abilify road...

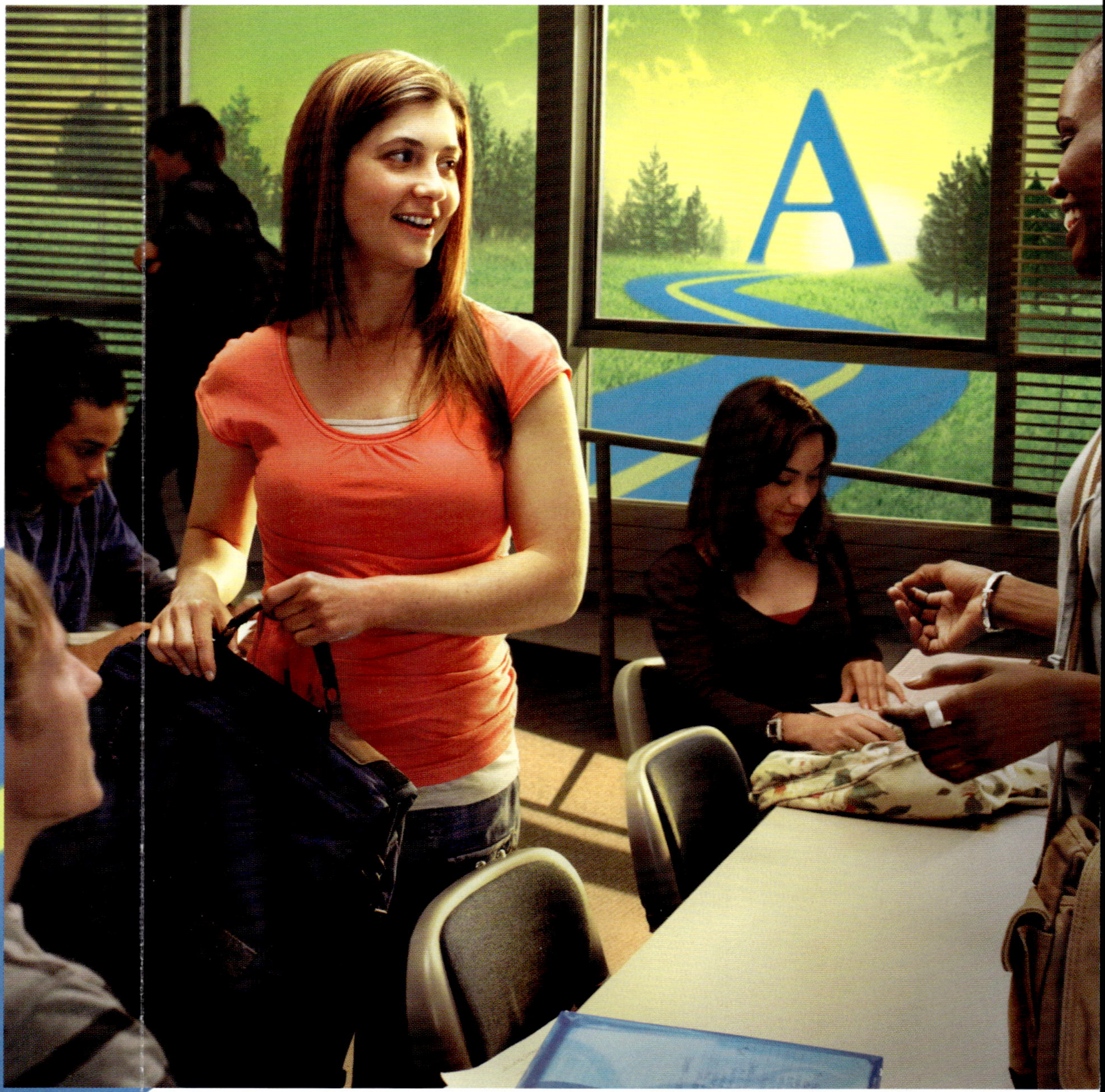

Monographs

About Product Monographs

The Monograph section contains more than 2000 product monographs for pharmaceutical products listed alphabetically by brand name. The product monographs are voluntarily submitted for publication by the pharmaceutical manufacturers. All product monographs have been approved by the Therapeutic Products Directorate, Health Canada. The editorial staff of the Canadian Pharmacists Association (CPhA) compile and produce the monographs. No changes are made to content. While the *CPS* is not an exhaustive listing of all pharmaceutical products available in Canada, by consulting the brand and generic name index, information on most Canadian products can be found. Consult the *CPS* Editorial Policy for more information.

The decision to include either Full Prescribing Information or an Availability Listing (shortened "Supplied" version) is the decision of the manufacturer. Products discontinued from *CPS* since 2000 appear in the Brand and Generic Name Index (green section).

About CPhA Monographs (titles are shaded in gray)

The monograph section contains 143 CPhA monographs that are written by the editorial staff of the Canadian Pharmacists Association, are based on the best available evidence and are reviewed by expert physicians and pharmacists. Readers should be aware that the text might contain information different from that found in Health Canada-approved product monographs. The term "non-approved indication" refers to indications not approved by Health Canada. The *CPS* Editorial Policy may be consulted for more information.

The CPhA monographs fill gaps in drug information when manufacturers do not submit a monograph for an older drug that may have been genericized. The CPhA monograph titles are lightly shaded in gray to distinguish them from manufacturers' product monographs and are presented alphabetically by generic name or drug class name within the monograph section. The CPhA Monographs Index is located in the Front Pages of *CPS*, following the Table of Contents.

Online Updates

New products, revised product monographs and notice of discontinued products received by the publisher after the print deadline are published in e-CPS, CPhA's online *CPS*. The e-CPS provides health care professionals with online access to the most current Canadian drug information available. It also includes links to Health Canada advisories, printable information for patients, searchable product images, an intuitive interface and time-saving features. e-CPS is updated bi-weekly. For more information or to subscribe to e-CPS, visit www.pharmacists.ca/e-CPS.

How to Use the Monograph Section

- The product monographs appear alphabetically by brand name.
- The CPhA monographs appear alphabetically by generic name or drug class name. The CPhA Monographs Index is located in the Front Pages of *CPS*, following the Table of Contents.
- If the product you are looking for does not appear in the Monograph section, you will find your information by checking the Brand and Generic Name Index:

  i) Names in regular face: The monograph is not provided by the manufacturer. You may find information by locating the generic name of the product.

  ii) Names in regular face, discontinued: Product is discontinued. You may find information by locating the generic name of the product.

  iii) Names in italics: Generic drug name or active ingredient. Searching on the generic name(s) will tell you what entries include that drug.

  If you cannot find the listing your are looking for, please let us know.

See illustrative entry on the back of this page
(Full Prescribing Information and Availability Listing)

Full Prescribing Information
—Product Monograph—

A revised product monograph template was implemented by Health Canada in October 2003. Product monographs for new drugs and supplemental new drug submissions as well as drugs with notifiable changes since that date appear in the new format. Older products remain in the previous format. Information within each drug monograph is divided into the following sections (subsections are not listed):

Brand Name scheduling symbol (e.g. Ⓟ, ©, Ⓝ, ☒)
generic name(s) or active ingredient
Therapeutic class(es)

Manufacturer Name

Date of Preparation and/or Date of Revision

Revised Format:

-SUMMARY PRODUCT INFORMATION
-DESCRIPTION
-INDICATIONS AND CLINICAL USE
-WARNINGS AND PRECAUTIONS
-ADVERSE REACTIONS
-DRUG INTERACTIONS
-DOSAGE AND ADMINISTRATION
-OVERDOSAGE
-ACTION AND CLINICAL PHARMACOLOGY
-STORAGE AND STABILITY
-SPECIAL HANDLING INSTRUCTIONS
-INFORMATION FOR THE PATIENT (available on e-CPS when applicable)
-DOSAGE FORMS, COMPOSITION AND PACKAGING

Previous Format:

-PHARMACOLOGY
-INDICATIONS
-CONTRAINDICATIONS
-WARNINGS
-PRECAUTIONS
-*Drug Interactions*
-ADVERSE EFFECTS
-OVERDOSE: Symptoms, Treatment
-DOSAGE
-INFORMATION FOR THE PATIENT (available on e-CPS when applicable)
-SUPPLIED

Full Prescribing Information
—CPhA Monograph—

The CPhA Monograph name may appear by generic name, e.g. Acetaminophen or drug class name, e.g. Calcium Channel Blockers. Information within each CPhA monograph is divided into the following sections and may appear in either the revised format or the previous format (subsections are not listed):

CPhA Monograph Name scheduling symbol (e.g. Ⓟ, ©, Ⓝ, ☒)
generic name(s) or active ingredient
Therapeutic class(es)

CPhA Monograph

Date of Preparation and/or Date of Revision

This monograph has been compiled by CPhA and reviewed by experts. It may contain information different from that found in Health Canada-approved Product Monographs. The reader is referred to the *CPS* Editorial Policy for more information.

Availability Listing
—Supplied section of the Product Monograph—

An availability listing includes the dosage form, dosage strength, nonmedicinal ingredients and packaging. The color, shape, product markings and storage information is included when provided by the manufacturer. (No additional data supplied by the manufacturer.)

Brand Name scheduling symbol (e.g. Ⓟ, ©, Ⓝ, ☒)
generic name(s) or active ingredient
Therapeutic class(es)

Manufacturer Name

SUPPLIED: Each pink, round, biconvex tablet, embossed with "R-200" on one side and scored on the other side, contains: amiodarone HCl 200 mg. Nonmedicinal ingredients: anhydrous colloidal silica, colloidal silicon dioxide, corn starch, erythrosine, lactose, magnesium stearate and polyvidone. HDPE bottles of 100. Store at room temperature (15 to 30°C). Protect from light.

#

222® Tablets Ⓝ

ASA—caffeine citrate—codeine phosphate
Analgesic—Antipyretic

Johnson & Johnson • Merck

INDICATIONS: For the symptomatic relief of mild to moderate pain, fever and inflammation such as headaches, pain due to cold symptoms, toothache, pain or menstrual cramps, arthritic pain and the pain caused by muscle strains and sprain.

CONTRAINDICATIONS: Patients with a history of blood coagulation defects, or receiving anticoagulant drugs or with severe anemia.

Gastrointestinal ulceration and sensitivity to any of the components or to other nonsteroidal anti-inflammatory drugs (NSAIDs).

Patients who had a bronchospastic reaction, generalized urticaria, angioedema, severe rhinitis, laryngeal edema or shock precipitated by ASA or nonsteroidal anti-inflammatory drugs.

Pregnancy: Because of the potential for increased maternal blood loss and possible adverse effects on the neonate, ASA should be avoided during the last 3 months of pregnancy or when nursing. Pregnant women should be advised not to take ASA during the last trimester of pregnancy unless prescribed and monitored by a physician.

Lactation: See Pregnancy.

Persons with hypersensitivity to caffeine (risk of allergic reaction).

Persons with hypersensitivity to codeine, pre-existing respiratory depression.

WARNINGS: This product has the potential for being abused and for being habit forming.

Excessive and prolonged therapy has been associated with nephropathy.

ASA is one of the most frequent causes of accidental poisoning in toddlers and infants. ASA containing preparations should therefore be kept well out of the reach of all children.

PRECAUTIONS: ASA: General: Salicylates should be administered with caution to patients with asthma and other allergic conditions, with bleeding tendencies, or with hypoprothrombinemia or in patients prone to dyspepsia or known to have a lesion of the gastric mucosa. It should not be administered to patients with hemophilia or other hemorrhagic disorders or to those with an intolerance to ASA (especially ASA-sensitive asthmatics). Caution is necessary when renal or hepatic function is impaired.

Salicylates can produce changes in the thyroid function tests.

ASA may precipitate or worsen attacks of gout.

Discontinue use of 222 tablets 5 to 7 days prior to surgery.

Geriatrics: The elderly may be more susceptible to the toxic effects of salicylates, possibly because of decreased renal function. Inhibiting production of renal prostaglandins by ASA and other nonsteroidal anti-inflammatory agents can result in an acute reduction in renal blood flow with subsequent deterioration of renal function.

Certain prostaglandins may act as renal vasodilators if renal blood flow is reduced. Individuals at risk are those with pre-existing renal dysfunction, heart failure, and liver cirrhosis and ascites. The first two conditions occur more commonly in the elderly and may also depend on renal prostaglandins to act as vasodilators.

Opioids may increase the risk of adverse effects especially respiratory depression.

Children: Salicylates: Use of ASA may be associated with the development of Reye's Syndrome in children and teenagers with acute febrile illnesses, especially influenza and varicella. Although a direct causal relationship has not been established, salicylates should not be administered to, or used by, children or teenagers who have chickenpox or manifest flu symptoms before a physician or pharmacist is consulted about Reye's Syndrome, a rare but serious illness.

Caffeine: Pediatric patients are especially susceptible to overdose of caffeine and its adverse CNS effects.

Pregnancy: ASA does not appear to have any teratogenic effects. High doses (3 g daily) of ASA during pregnancy may lengthen the gestation and parturition time. This effect has also been described with nonsteroidal anti-inflammatory agents which inhibit prostaglandin synthesis.

Labor and Delivery: Chronic, high-dose salicylate therapy late in pregnancy may result in prolonged labor, complicated deliveries, and increased risk of maternal or fetal hemorrhage.

Lactation: Salicylate is excreted in breast milk, in moderate amounts, with chronic high-dose use, intake by the infant may be high enough to cause adverse effects.

Drug Interactions: Salicylates increase the effects of oral anticoagulants. Caution is necessary when salicylates and anticoagulants are prescribed concurrently. Also, salicylates may depress the concentration of prothrombin in the plasma.

Salicylates may potentiate sulfonylurea hypoglycemic agents. Large doses of salicylates may have a hypoglycemic action, and thus, affect the insulin requirements of diabetics.

Although salicylates in large doses are uricosuric agents, smaller amounts may depress uric acid clearance, and thus, decrease the uricosuric effects of probenecid, sulfinpyrazone and phenylbutazone.

Sodium excretion produced by spironolactone may be decreased in the presence of salicylates.

Salicylates also retard the renal elimination of methotrexate.

Concomitant use of salicylates and alcohol or other nonsteroidal anti-inflammatory drugs (NSAIDs), may predispose to gastric bleeding, including ulceration.

Concurrent use of other NSAIDs with ASA may also increase the risk of bleeding at sites other than the gastrointestinal tract because of additive inhibition of platelet aggregation.

Caution is necessary when cefamandole, cefoperazone, cefotetan, moxalactam, plicamycin or, valproic acid are prescribed concurrently with ASA as these medications may cause hypoprothrombinemia.

Salicylates may potentiate ototoxic agents (vancomycin, others). Concurrent or sequential administration of these medications with a salicylate should be avoided because hearing loss may occur and may progress to deafness even after discontinuation of the medication; although these effects may be reversible, but usually are permanent.

Salicylates decrease the clearance of zidovudine, leading to potentiation of zidovudine toxicity; concurrent use of ASA and zidovudine should be avoided.

Codeine: Care should be observed in the use of codeine although tolerance and addiction to its use are rare.

Codeine should be given with caution to patients with severe respiratory depression. The depressant effect of codeine may be enhanced by the concurrent administration of sedatives and tranquilizers.

ADVERSE EFFECTS: Gastrointestinal: dyspepsia, heartburn, nausea, vomiting, constipation, diarrhea, abdominal pain, gastrointestinal ulceration and bleeding.

Otic: tinnitus, hearing loss, dizziness.

Hematologic: anemia, leukopenia, thrombocytopenia, hypoprothrombinemia, purpura.

Dermatologic and Hypersensitivity: urticaria, angioedema, pruritus, various skin eruptions, asthma and anaphylaxis.

Hepatic: reversible hepatotoxicity particularly in patients with juvenile rheumatoid arthritis and systemic lupus erythematosus.

Miscellaneous: mental confusion, headache, drowsiness, sweating and thirst, palpitation, excessive diuresis.

CNS Depression: coma, cardiovascular collapse, respiratory failure, vertigo, muscle tremor, sensory disturbances, nervousness, insomnia.

The potential for habituation may occur.

OVERDOSE:

Symptoms: In mild overdosage, these may include rapid and deep breathing, severe drowsiness, nausea, vomiting (leading to alkalosis), stomach pain, diarrhea, headache, hyperpnea, vertigo, tinnitus, flushing, sweating, thirst and tachycardia. (High blood levels of ASA lead to acidosis.) Severe cases may show fever, hemorrhage, bloody urine, excitement, confusion, hallucinations, severe nervousness, convulsions or coma, and respiratory failure.

Codeine and related narcotic analgesics depress respiration by an action on the brain stem respiratory centres.

Other symptoms of overdose may include euphoria, dysphoria, and visual disturbances.

Treatment: Treatment is essentially symptomatic and supportive. Administer water, activated charcoal and ipecac syrup unless the patient is comatose, and remove by gastric lavage or emesis. Patients with mild intoxication should be encouraged to drink plenty of fluids. In patients with more severe intoxication, forced alkaline diuresis may be required. Plasma electrolytes, especially potassium, and the acid-base balance should be monitored regularly. In the presence of cardiac or renal impairment or in very severe intoxication, hemodialysis or hemoperfusion may need to be considered.

Respiratory depression may require intubation measures aimed at supporting respiration and the administration of a narcotic antagonist, e.g., naloxone.

> For management of a suspected drug overdose, CPhA recommends that you contact your **regional Poison Control Centre**. See the *CPS* Directory section for a list of Poison Control Centres.

DOSAGE: Adults: 1 or 2 tablet(s), 1 to 3 times daily (every 4 to 8 hours), as required. **Not recommended for use in children.** Do not exceed 4 g ASA (10 tablets) a day.

Children: **Warning: Do not administer** to children or teenagers who have chickenpox or flu symptoms before a physician or pharmacist is consulted about Reye's Syndrome, a rare and serious illness. When recommended by a physician or dentist: 10 to 14 years: 1 tablet, 1 to 3 times daily (every 4 to 8 hours).

INFORMATION FOR THE PATIENT: Published in e-CPS, available by subscription at www.e-cps.ca.

SUPPLIED: Each white tablet, engraved 222 contains: ASA 375 mg, caffeine 15 mg (equivalent to 30 mg caffeine citrate) and codeine phosphate 8 mg. Nonmedicinal ingredients: cornstarch, disodium edetate, ethylcellulose, hydrogenated vegetable oil, microcrystalline cellulose, sodium carboxymethylcellulose and sodium lauryl sulfate. Plastic bottles (with safety seal under cap) of 40 (child-resistant package), 100 and 250.

282® Ⓝ

ASA—codeine phosphate—caffeine citrate
Analgesic—Antipyretic

PendoPharm

SUPPLIED: Each orangy-yellow, round, biconvex tablet, debossed with "ø" on one side and scored on the other side, contains: ASA 375 mg, caffeine citrate 30 mg (equivalent to 15 mg caffeine) and codeine phosphate 15 mg. Bottles of 500. Store at room temperature between 15 and 30°C. Protect from light and moisture.

282 MEP® Ⓝ

ASA—caffeine citrate—codeine phosphate—meprobamate
Analgesic—Muscle Relaxant—Anxiolytic

PendoPharm

SUPPLIED: Each white, round, biconvex tablet, debossed with "ø" on one side and "282 MEP" on the other side, contains: ASA 350 mg, caffeine citrate 30 mg (equivalent to 15 mg caffeine), codeine phosphate 15 mg and meprobamate 200 mg. Bottles of 50 and 500.

292® Ⓝ

ASA—codeine phosphate—caffeine citrate
Analgesic—Antipyretic

PendoPharm

SUPPLIED: Each orange, round, biconvex tablet, debossed with "ø" on one side and "292" on the other side, contains: ASA 375 mg, caffeine citrate 30 mg (equivalent to 15 mg caffeine) and codeine phosphate 30 mg. Bottles of 50 and 500. Store at room temperature between 15 and 30°C. Protect from light and moisture.

3TC® Pr

lamivudine
Antiretroviral Agent

ViiV Healthcare ULC

Date of Revision: April 23, 2010

SUMMARY PRODUCT INFORMATION:

Route of Administration	Dosage Form/ Strength	Clinically Relevant Nonmedicinal Ingredients
Oral	Tablets/150 mg	Hydroxypropyl methylcellulose, magnesium stearate, microcrystalline cellulose, polyethylene glycol, polysorbate 80, sodium starch glycolate and titanium dioxide
	Tablets/300 mg	Black iron oxide, hydroxypropyl methylcellulose, magnesium stearate, microcrystalline cellulose, polyethylene glycol, polysorbate 80, sodium starch glycolate and titanium dioxide
	Oral Solution/10 mg/mL	Artificial strawberry and banana flavours, citric acid (anhydrous), hydrochloric acid, methylparaben, propylparaben, propylene glycol, sodium citrate (dihydrate), sodium hydroxide, sucrose and water

INDICATIONS AND CLINICAL USE: 3TC (lamivudine) in combination with other antiretroviral agents is indicated for:

- the treatment of HIV infection.

CONTRAINDICATIONS:

- 3TC (lamivudine) is contraindicated in patients with previously demonstrated clinically significant hypersensitivity to any of the components of the products (see Dosage Forms, Composition and Packaging).

WARNINGS AND PRECAUTIONS:

Serious Warnings and Precautions

- **Lactic Acidosis and Severe Hepatomegaly with Steatosis:** Lactic acidosis and severe hepatomegaly with steatosis, including fatal cases, have been reported with the use of nucleoside analogues alone or in combination, including 3TC and other antiretrovirals. A majority of these cases have been in women. Obesity and prolonged nucleoside exposure may be risk factors. However, cases have also been reported in patients with no known risk factors. Treatment with 3TC should be suspended in any patient who develops clinical or laboratory findings suggestive of lactic acidosis or pronounced hepatotoxicity (which may include hepatomegaly and steatosis even in the absence of marked transaminase elevations).
- **Post-Treatment Exacerbation of Hepatitis:** It is recommended that all patients with HIV be tested for the presence of chronic hepatitis B virus (HBV) before initiating antiretroviral therapy. 3TC is not indicated for the treatment of chronic HBV infection and the safety and efficacy of 3TC have not been established in patients coinfected with HBV and HIV. Exacerbations of hepatitis B have been reported in patients after the discontinuation of antiretroviral therapy. Patients coinfected with HIV and HBV should be closely monitored with both clinical and laboratory follow-up for at least several months after stopping treatment with 3TC.
- **Pancreatitis in Pediatric Patients:** In pediatric patients with a history of prior antiretroviral nucleoside exposure, a history of pancreatitis, or other significant risk factors for the development of pancreatitis, 3TC should be used with caution. Treatment with 3TC should be stopped immediately if clinical signs, symptoms, or laboratory abnormalities suggestive of pancreatitis occur (see Adverse Reactions).

General: The safety profile of combination therapy with 3TC (lamivudine) and other antiretroviral agents reflects the individual safety profile of each component. The individual product monographs for each drug in the combination regimen should be consulted before combination therapy is initiated.

Evidence for once-daily dosing using the 300 mg tablets is mainly in antiretroviral naive patients.

Trough levels of lamivudine in plasma and of intracellular triphosphate were lower with once-daily dosing than with twice-daily dosing. Furthermore, the C_{max} levels of lamivudine in plasma were higher with once-daily dosing than with twice-daily dosing (see Action and Clinical Pharmacology). The clinical significance of these observations is not known.

The clinical status of the patient and the adverse event profile of 3TC should be borne in mind when considering the patient's ability to drive or operate machinery.

Endocrine and Metabolism: Fat Redistribution: Redistribution/accumulation of body fat including central obesity, dorsocervical fat enlargement ("buffalo hump"), peripheral wasting, facial wasting, breast enlargement, and "cushingoid appearance" have been observed in patients receiving antiretroviral therapy. The mechanism and long-term consequences of these events are currently unknown. A causal relationship has not been established.

Clinical examination should include evaluation for physical signs of fat redistribution. Consideration should be given to the measurement of serum lipids and blood glucose. Lipid disorders should be managed as clinically appropriate.

Hematologic: Very rare occurrences of pure red cell aplasia have been reported with lamivudine use. Discontinuation of lamivudine has resulted in normalization of hematologic parameters in patients with suspected lamivudine-induced pure red cell aplasia.

Hepatic/Biliary/Pancreatic: Pancreatitis has been observed in some patients receiving lamivudine. However it is unclear whether this was due to treatment with the medicinal product or to the underlying HIV disease. Pancreatitis must be considered whenever a patient develops abdominal pain, nausea, vomiting or elevated biochemical markers. Discontinue use of lamivudine until diagnosis of pancreatitis is excluded.

Use With Interferon- and Ribavirin-Based Regimens: In vitro studies have shown ribavirin can reduce the phosphorylation of pyrimidine nucleoside analogues such as lamivudine. Although no evidence of a pharmacokinetic or pharmacodynamic interaction (e.g., loss of HIV/HCV virologic suppression) was seen when ribavirin was coadministered with lamivudine in HIV/HCV co-infected patients, hepatic decompensation (some fatal) has occurred in HIV/HCV co-infected patients receiving combination antiretroviral therapy for HIV and interferon alfa with or without ribavirin. Patients receiving interferon alfa with or without ribavirin and 3TC should be closely monitored for treatment-associated toxicities, especially hepatic decompensation. Discontinuation of 3TC should be considered as medically appropriate.

Lactic Acidosis/Severe Hepatomegaly with Steatosis: Lactic acidosis and severe hepatomegaly with steatosis, including fatal cases, have been reported with the use of antiretroviral nucleoside analogues either alone or in combination, including lamivudine. A majority of these cases have been in women. Clinical features which may be indicative of the development of lactic acidosis include generalized weakness, anorexia and sudden unexplained weight loss, gastrointestinal symptoms and respiratory symptoms (dyspnea and tachypnea).

Caution should be exercised when administering 3TC to any patient, and particularly to those with known risk factors for liver disease. Treatment with 3TC should be suspended in any patient who develops clinical or laboratory findings suggestive of lactic acidosis or hepatotoxicity (which may include hepatomegaly and steatosis even in the absence of marked transaminase elevations).

Patients Co-infected with Hepatitis B Virus: Clinical trials and marketed use of 3TC have shown that some patients with chronic hepatitis B virus (HBV) disease may experience clinical or laboratory evidence of recurrent hepatitis upon discontinuation of 3TC, which may have more severe consequences in patients with decompensated liver disease. If 3TC is discontinued in a patient with HIV and HBV coinfection, periodic monitoring of both liver function tests and markers of HBV replication should be considered.

Immune: Patients receiving 3TC or any other antiretroviral therapy may continue to develop opportunistic infections and other complications of HIV infection. Therefore, patients should remain under close observation by physicians experienced in the treatment of patients with HIV-associated diseases.

Immune Reconstitution: During the initial phase of treatment, patients responding to antiretroviral therapy may develop an inflammatory response to indolent or residual opportunistic infections (such as MAC, CMV, PCP, and TB) which may necessitate further evaluation and treatment.

Renal: Patients with Impaired Renal Function: Patients with impaired renal function may be at a greater risk of toxicity from 3TC due to decreased renal clearance of the drug. Consideration should be given to appropriate reduction in the dose of lamivudine (see Dosage and Administration).

Special Populations: Pregnant Women: There are no adequate and well-controlled studies in pregnant women.

Consistent with passive transmission of the drug across the placenta, lamivudine concentrations in infant serum at birth were similar to those in maternal and cord serum. There have been reports of mild, transient elevations in serum lactate levels, which may be due to mitochondrial dysfunction, in neonates and infants exposed in utero or peri partum to nucleoside reverse transcriptase inhibitors (NRTIs). The clinical relevance of transient elevations in serum lactate is unknown. There have also been very rare reports of developmental delay, seizures and other neurological disease. However, a causal relationship between these events and NRTI exposure in utero or peri partum has not been established. These findings do not affect current recommendations to use antiretroviral therapy in pregnant women to prevent vertical transmission of HIV. Reproductive studies in animals have not shown evidence of teratogenicity, and have shown no effect on male or female fertility. Lamivudine induced early embryolethality when administered to pregnant rabbits at exposure levels comparable to those achieved in man. Because animal reproductive toxicity studies are not always predictive of the human response, lamivudine should be used during pregnancy only if the potential benefits outweigh the potential risks.

Antiretroviral Pregnancy Registry: To monitor maternal-fetal outcomes of pregnant women exposed to 3TC, an Antiretroviral Pregnancy Registry has been established. Physicians are encouraged to register patients by calling ViiV Healthcare ULC's Drug Safety Department (1-877-393-8448).

Nursing Women: Following oral administration lamivudine was excreted in breast milk at similar concentrations to those found in serum (1 to 8 μg/mL). It is recommended that mothers taking lamivudine do not breastfeed to avoid risking postnatal transmission of HIV infection and potential adverse effects from lamivudine in nursing infants.

Pediatrics: The safety and pharmacokinetic properties of 3TC in combination with other antiretroviral agents have not been established in pediatric patients who are less than 3 months of age.

ADVERSE REACTIONS: Clinical Trial Adverse Drug Reactions: Because clinical trials are conducted under very specific conditions the adverse reaction rates observed in the clinical trials may not reflect the rates observed in practice and should not be compared to the rates in the clinical trials of another drug. Adverse drug reaction information from clinical trials is useful for identifying drug-related adverse events and for approximating rates.

Adults: Selected clinical adverse events in therapy naive patients receiving either 3TC (lamivudine) 300 mg once daily or 3TC 150 mg twice daily in combination with RETROVIR 300 mg twice daily and efavirenz 600 mg once daily are listed in Table 1 and Table 2. The most frequent clinical adverse events (≥5% frequency) reported during therapy with 3TC 150 mg b.i.d. plus RETROVIR (AZT) 600 mg per day compared with RETROVIR (AZT) are listed in Table 3.

Table 1: 3TC

Most Common Adverse Events (>10%)[a] Occurring in Subjects in EPV20001 Safety Population During 48 Weeks

Adverse Event	3TC 300 mg q.d. plus RETROVIR plus Efavirenz (n=272) %	3TC 150 mg b.i.d. plus RETROVIR plus Efavirenz (n=273) %
At Least One Adverse Event	94	97
Nausea	39	44
Dizziness	30	36
Fatigue	31	31
Dreams	26	24
Headaches	25	22
Rashes	24	20
Viral Respiratory Infections	22	21
Diarrhea	20	21
Ear, Nose, & Throat Infections	15	21
Sleep Disorders	17	19
Vomiting	14	16
Abdominal Pain	10	19
Anorexia	13	9
Mood Disorders	12	10
Musculoskeletal Pain	7	14
Sinus Disorders	9	10
Fever	7	12

a >10% of subjects in either treatment group.

Table 2: 3TC

Severe Adverse Events (Grade 3/4) Occurring in More Than One Subject[a] in EPV20001 Safety Population During 48 Weeks

Adverse Event	3TC 300 mg q.d. plus RETROVIR plus Efavirenz (n=272) %	3TC 150 mg b.i.d. plus RETROVIR plus Efavirenz (n=273) %
At Least One Severe Adverse Event	24	26
Increased Creatine Phosphokinase Levels	3	4
Nausea	3	3
Increased Liver Function Tests	2	3
Decreased White Cells	2	2
Fatigue	1	2
Hypertriglyceridemia	2	1
Dizziness	1	1
Vomiting	1	<1
Sleep Disorders	1	1
Abdominal Pain	1	<1
Dreams	<1	1
Increased Amylase Levels	1	<1
Anxiety	1	<1
Rashes	0	2
Anemia	<1	1
Depressive Disorders	<1	1
Mood Disorders	1	<1
Skin Infections	<1	<1
Ear, Nose, & Throat Infections	<1	<1
Diarrhea	<1	<1
Headaches	<1	<1
Suicide & Attempted Suicide	<1	<1

(cont'd)

Table 2: 3TC *(cont'd)*

Severe Adverse Events (Grade 3/4) Occurring in More Than One Subject[a] in EPV20001 Safety Population During 48 Weeks

Adverse Event	3TC 300 mg q.d. plus RETROVIR plus Efavirenz (n=272) %	3TC 150 mg b.i.d. plus RETROVIR plus Efavirenz (n=273) %
Viral Respiratory Infections	<1	<1
Confusion	<1	<1
Migraines	<1	<1
General Signs & Symptoms	<1	<1
Malaise	0	<1
Viral Infection	<1	0
Lower Respiratory Infections	<1	<1
Hypotension	0	<1

[a] More than one subject in any treatment group.

Table 3: 3TC

Most Frequent Clinical Adverse Events (≥5% Frequency) Reported in Four Controlled Clinical Trials (NUCA3001, NUCA3002, NUCB3001 and NUCB3002)

Adverse Event	3TC 150 mg b.i.d. plus RETROVIR (AZT) (n=251) %	RETROVIR (AZT) (n=230) %
Body as a Whole		
Headache	35	27
Malaise and Fatigue	27	23
Fever or Chills	10	12
Digestive		
Nausea	33	29
Diarrhea	18	22
Nausea and Vomiting	13	12
Anorexia and/or Decreased Appetite	10	7
Abdominal Pain	9	11
Abdominal Cramps	6	3
Dyspepsia	5	5
Nervous		
Neuropathy	12	10
Dizziness	10	7
Insomnia and Other Sleep Disorders	11	4
Depressive Disorders	9	4
Respiratory		

(cont'd)

Table 3: 3TC *(cont'd)*

Most Frequent Clinical Adverse Events (≥5% Frequency) Reported in Four Controlled Clinical Trials (NUCA3001, NUCA3002, NUCB3001 and NUCB3002)

Adverse Event	3TC 150 mg b.i.d. plus RETROVIR (AZT) (n=251) %	RETROVIR (AZT) (n=230) %
Nasal Signs and Symptoms	20	11
Cough	18	13
Skin and Appendages		
Skin Rashes	9	6
Musculoskeletal		
Musculoskeletal Pain	12	10
Myalgia	8	6
Arthralgia	5	5

Other clinical adverse events reported in controlled clinical trials in association with 3TC 150 mg b.i.d. plus RETROVIR (AZT) 600 mg per day in at least 1% of patients were:

Gastrointestinal: abdominal discomfort and pain (3%), abdominal distension (3%), dyspepsia (2%), gastrointestinal discomfort and pain (3%), gastrointestinal gas (4%), hyposalivation (2%), oral ulceration (1%).
Musculoskeletal: muscle atrophy/weakness/tiredness (1%), muscle pain (2%).
Neurological: mood disorders (1%), sleep disorders (4%), taste disturbances (1%).
Other: breathing disorders (2%), general signs and symptoms (1%), pain (2%), sexual function disturbances (1%), temperature regulation disturbance (1%).
Skin: pruritus (1%), skin rashes (1%), sweating (1%).

Pancreatitis was observed in 9 of 2613 adult patients (0.3%) in controlled clinical trials EPV20001, NUCA3001, NUCB3001, NUCA3002, NUCB3002, and B3007.

Six percent (6%) of patients treated with 3TC 150 mg b.i.d. plus RETROVIR (AZT) 200 mg t.i.d. in controlled clinical trials permanently discontinued treatment due to an investigator-attributed drug-related adverse event, compared with 7% of patients receiving monotherapy with RETROVIR (AZT) and 13% of patients receiving RETROVIR (AZT) plus zalcitabine. The most frequent adverse events necessitating such permanent discontinuation of therapy with 3TC 150 mg b.i.d. plus RETROVIR (AZT) 200 mg t.i.d. were nausea (2%), malaise and fatigue (1%), and anemia (1%).

The frequencies of selected laboratory abnormalities (Grades 3 and 4) during therapy are listed in Table 4.

Pediatric Patients: Selected clinical adverse events and physical findings with a ≥5% frequency during therapy with 3TC 4 mg/kg twice daily plus RETROVIR (AZT) 160 mg/m^2 three times daily compared with didanosine in patients without, or with, minimal (≤56 days) prior antiretroviral therapy are listed in Table 5.

Selected laboratory abnormalities experienced by patients without or minimal (≤56 days) prior antiretroviral therapy are listed in Table 6.

Pancreatitis, which has been fatal in some cases, has been observed in antiretroviral nucleoside-experienced pediatric patients receiving 3TC alone or in combination with other antiretroviral agents. In an open-label dose-escalation study (NUCA2002), 14 patients (14%) developed pancreatitis while receiving monotherapy with 3TC. Three of these patients died of complications of pancreatitis. In a second open-label study (NUCA2005), 12 patients (18%) developed pancreatitis. In Study ACTG300, pancreatitis was not observed in 236 patients randomized to 3TC plus RETROVIR (AZT). Pancreatitis was observed in one patient in this study who received open-label 3TC in combination with RETROVIR (AZT) and ritonavir following discontinuation of didanosine monotherapy.

Paresthesias and peripheral neuropathies were reported in 15 patients (15%) in Study NUCA2002, six patients (9%) in Study NUCA2005, and two patients (<1%) in Study ACTG300.

Post-Market Adverse Drug Reactions: The following additional adverse experiences have been reported in post-marketing experience without regard to causality. Because they are reported voluntarily from a population of unknown size, estimates of frequency cannot be made. These events have been chosen for inclusion due to either their seriousness, frequency of reporting, potential causal connection to lamivudine, or a combination of these factors.
Body as a Whole: anaphylaxis, fatigue, fever, malaise, redistribution/accumulation of body fat (see Warnings and Precautions, Fat Redistribution), weakness.
Digestive: stomatitis.
Endocrine/Metabolic: hyperglycemia, hyperlactatemia, lactic acidosis and hepatic steatosis (see Warnings and Precautions).
Gastrointestinal: diarrhea, nausea, pancreatitis, rises in serum amylase, upper abdominal pain, vomiting.
Hematological: pure red cell aplasia.
Hepatic: transient rises in liver enzymes.
Hemic and Lymphatic: anemia, lymphadenopathy, neutropenia, splenomegaly, thrombocytopenia.
Musculoskeletal: arthralgia, muscle disorders including very rarely rhabdomyolysis.
Nervous: headache, paresthesia, peripheral neuropathy.
Other: alopecia.
Skin: pruritus, rash, urticaria.

Table 4: 3TC

Selected Laboratory Abnormalities in Studies of 3TC in Adults

	24-Week Surrogate Endpoint Studies (NUCA3001, NUCA3002, NUCB3001, NUCB3002)		Clinical Endpoint Study[a] (B3007)		Study EPV20001[a]	
Test (Abnormal Level)	**3TC Plus RETROVIR %**	**RETROVIR %**	**3TC Plus Current Therapy[b] %**	**Placebo Plus Current Therapy[b] %**	**3TC 300 mg q.d.[c] %**	**3TC 150 mg b.i.d.[c] %**
Neutropenia (ANC <750/mm^3)	7	5	15	13	6	6
Anemia (Hgb <8.0 g/dL)	3	2	2	3	<1	<1
Thrombocytopenia (platelets <50 000/mm^3)	<1	1	3	4	0	<1
ALT (>5.0×ULN)	4	4	4	2	3	5
AST (>5.0×ULN)	2	2	4	2	2	4
Bilirubin (>2.5×ULN)	<1	<1	ND	ND	0	<1
Amylase (>2.0×ULN)	4	2	2	1	3	2

[a] The median duration on study was 12 months.
[b] Current therapy was either zidovudine, zidovudine plus didanosine, or zidovudine plus zalcitabine.
[c] Therapy was 3TC plus Retrovir plus efavirenz.
Legend: ULN=upper limit of normal; ANC=absolute neutrophil count; ND=not done.

Table 5: 3TC

Selected Clinical Adverse Events and Physical Findings (≥5% Frequency) in Pediatric Patients in Study ACTG300

Adverse Event	3TC plus RETROVIR (AZT) (n=236) %	Didanosine (n=235) %
Body as a Whole		
Fever	25	32
Digestive		
Hepatomegaly	11	11
Nausea and Vomiting	8	7
Diarrhea	8	6
Stomatitis	6	12
Splenomegaly	5	8
Respiratory		
Cough	15	18
Abnormal Breath Sounds/Wheezing	7	9
Ear, Nose and Throat		
Signs or Symptoms of Ears[a]	7	6
Nasal Discharge or Congestion	8	11
Other		
Skin Rashes	12	14
Lymphadenopathy	9	11

[a] Includes pain, discharge, erythema, or swelling of an ear.

Table 6: 3TC

Frequencies of Selected Laboratory Abnormalities in Pediatric Patients in Study ACTG300

Test (Abnormal Level)	3TC plus RETROVIR (AZT) %	Didanosine %
Neutropenia (ANC <400/mm³)	8	3
Anemia (Hgb <7.0 g/dL)	4	2
Thrombocytopenia (platelets <50 000/mm³)	1	3
ALT (>10×ULN)	1	3
AST (>10×ULN)	2	4
Lipase (>2.5×ULN)	3	3
Total Amylase (>2.5×ULN)	3	3

Legend: ULN=upper limit of normal; ANC=absolute neutrophil count.

DRUG INTERACTIONS: Overview: Lamivudine is predominantly eliminated by active organic cationic secretion. The possibility of interactions with other drugs administered concurrently should be considered, particularly when the main route of elimination is renal.

Drug-Drug Interactions: See Table 7.

Table 7: 3TC

Established or Potential Drug-Drug Interactions

Proper Name	Effect	Clinical Comment
Trimethoprim	Administration of trimethoprim, a constituent of co-trimoxazole, causes a 40% increase in lamivudine plasma levels.	However, unless the patient has renal impairment, no dosage adjustment of lamivudine is necessary. Lamivudine has no effect on the pharmacokinetics of co-trimoxazole. Administration of co-trimoxazole with the 3TC/RETROVIR (AZT) combination in patients with renal impairment should be carefully assessed. The effect of co-administration of 3TC with higher doses of co-trimoxazole for the treatment of *P. carinii* pneumonia and toxoplasmosis has not been studied.
Zalcitabine	Lamivudine may inhibit the intracellular phosphorylation of zalcitabine when the two medicinal products are used concurrently.	3TC is not recommended to be used in combination with zalcitabine.
Zidovudine	Zidovudine has no effect on the pharmacokinetics of lamivudine (see Action and Clinical Pharmacology).	A modest increase in C_{max} (28%) was observed for zidovudine when administered with lamivudine, however overall exposure (AUC) was not significantly altered. Zidovudine plasma levels are not significantly altered when coadministered with 3TC.

DOSAGE AND ADMINISTRATION: 3TC therapy should be initiated by a physician experienced in the management of HIV infection.

Recommended Dose and Dosage Adjustment: 3TC can be taken with or without food.

Adults and Adolescents: The recommended oral dose of 3TC (lamivudine) for adults and adolescents who are at least 12 years old is 300 mg daily, administered as either 150 mg twice daily or 300 mg once daily, in combination with other antiretroviral agents (see Action and Clinical Pharmacology and Warnings and Precautions).

Pediatric Patients Aged ≥3 Months to 12 Years: The recommended oral dose of 3TC for pediatric patients is 4 mg/kg twice daily (up to a maximum of 150 mg twice a day), administered in combination with other antiretroviral agents.

Pediatric Patients Less Than 3 Months of Age: The limited data available are insufficient to propose specific dosage recommendations (see Action and Clinical Pharmacology, Pharmacokinetics).

Dose Adjustment: Patients with impaired renal function have increases in C_{max} and half-life of lamivudine with diminishing creatinine clearance. In addition, apparent total oral clearance of lamivudine decreases as creatinine clearance decreases. Doses of 3TC may be adjusted, as shown in Table 8 and Table 9, in accordance with creatinine clearance.

No dose adjustment is necessary in patients with moderate or severe hepatic impairment unless accompanied by renal impairment.

For adults with low body weight (less than 50 kg), the recommended oral dose of 3TC is 2 mg/kg twice daily administered in combination with other antiretrovirals.

Table 8: 3TC

Adjustment of Dosage of 3TC in Accordance with Creatinine Clearance in Adults and Adolescents >12 Years of Age

Creatinine Clearance (mL/min)	Recommended Dosage of 3TC
≥50	150 mg twice daily or 300 mg once daily
30–50	150 mg once daily
15–29	150 mg first dose, then 100 mg once daily
5–14	150 mg first dose, then 50 mg once daily
<5	50 mg first dose, then 25 mg once daily

Table 9: 3TC

Adjustment of Dosage of 3TC in Accordance with Creatinine Clearance in Children Aged 3 Months to 12 Years

Creatinine Clearance (mL/min)	Recommended Dosage of 3TC
30–50	4 mg/kg once daily
15–29	4 mg/kg first dose then 2.6 mg/kg once daily
5–14	4 mg/kg first dose then 1.3 mg/kg once daily
<5	1.3 mg/kg first dose then 0.7 mg/kg once daily

Missed Dose: If you forget to take your medicine, take it as soon as you remember. Then continue as before.

OVERDOSAGE:

There is no known antidote for 3TC (lamivudine).

If overdosage occurs the patient should be monitored, and standard supportive treatment applied as required. Although no data is available, administration of activated charcoal may be used to aid in the removal of unabsorbed drug. Because a negligible amount of lamivudine was removed via (4-hour) hemodialysis, continuous ambulatory peritoneal dialysis, and automated peritoneal dialysis, it is not known if continuous hemodialysis would provide clinical benefit in a lamivudine overdose event.

Limited data are available on the consequences of ingestion of acute overdoses in humans. No fatalities occurred, and the patients recovered. No specific signs or symptoms have been identified following such overdose.

One case of acute overdose in an adult ingesting 6 g of 3TC was reported; there were no clinical signs or symptoms noted and hematologic tests remained normal. One other adult patient in error ingested lamivudine 1200 mg per day plus zidovudine 1200 mg per day for approximately 2 weeks; he had a Grade 3 decrease in absolute neutrophil count that resolved upon reduction of doses of lamivudine and zidovudine. Two cases of pediatric overdose were reported in ACTG300. One case was a single dose of 7 mg/kg of 3TC; the second case involved the use of 5 mg/kg of 3TC twice daily for 30 days. There were no clinical signs or symptoms noted in either case.

In Phase I studies, lamivudine was administered at doses up to 20 mg/kg per day (i.e., approximately five times the usual recommended dose in adults) without serious consequences.

> For management of a suspected drug overdose, CPhA recommends that you contact your **regional Poison Control Centre**. See the *CPS* Directory section for a list of Poison Control Centres.

ACTION AND CLINICAL PHARMACOLOGY: Mechanism of Action: Lamivudine is a potent, selective inhibitor of HIV-1 and HIV-2 replication in vitro. Lamivudine is the (-) enantiomer of a dideoxy analogue of cytidine. The sugar ring of lamivudine is novel in that it contains a sulphur at the 3′ position as a second heteroatom. Intracellularly, lamivudine is phosphorylated to its active 5′-triphosphate metabolite (lamivudine triphosphate or L-TP), which has an intracellular half-life of approximately 10.5 to 15.5 hours. The principal mode of action of lamivudine is inhibition of HIV reverse transcription via viral DNA chain termination. In addition, L-TP inhibits both the RNA- and DNA-dependent DNA polymerase activities of reverse transcriptase (RT), and is a weak inhibitor of mammalian α, β, and γ DNA polymerases.

Pharmacokinetics: The pharmacokinetic properties of lamivudine have been studied in asymptomatic, HIV-infected adult patients after administration of single oral, multiple oral and intravenous (IV) doses ranging from 0.25 to 10 mg/kg. After oral administration of 2 mg/kg, the peak plasma lamivudine concentration (C_{max}) was 1.5±0.5 µg/mL (mean±S.D.) and half-life was 2.6±0.5 hours. There were no significant differences in half-life across the range of single doses (0.25 to 8 mg/kg). The area under the plasma concentration versus time curve (AUC) and C_{max} increased in proportion to dose over the range from 0.25 to 10 mg/kg.

The steady-state pharmacokinetic properties of the 3TC 300 mg tablet once daily for 7 days compared to the 3TC 150 mg tablet twice daily for 7 days were assessed in a crossover study in 60 healthy volunteers. 3TC 300 mg once daily resulted in lamivudine exposures that were similar to 3TC 150 mg twice-daily with respect to plasma $AUC_{24,ss}$; however, $C_{max,ss}$ was 66% higher and the trough value was 53% lower compared to the 150 mg twice-daily regimen. Intracellular lamivudine triphosphate exposures in peripheral blood mononuclear cells were also similar with respect to $AUC_{24,ss}$ and $C_{max24,ss}$; however, trough values were lower compared to the 150 mg twice-daily regimen.

The clinical significance of observed differences for both plasma lamivudine concentrations and intracellular lamivudine triphosphate concentrations is not known.

Lamivudine is well absorbed from the gut, and the bioavailability of oral lamivudine in adults is normally between 80 and 85%. Following oral administration, the mean time (t_{max}) to maximal serum concentrations (C_{max}) is about an hour.

No dose adjustment is needed when coadministered with food as lamivudine bioavailability is not altered, although a delay in t_{max} and reduction in C_{max} have been observed. Lamivudine exhibits linear pharmacokinetics over the therapeutic dose range and displays limited binding to the major plasma protein albumin.

Coadministration of zidovudine results in a 13% increase in AUC_{∞} for zidovudine and a 28% increase in peak plasma levels. This is not considered to be of significance to patient safety and therefore no dosage adjustments are necessary.

STORAGE AND STABILITY: 3TC tablets should be stored between 2 and 30°C.

3TC oral solution should be stored between 2 and 25°C.

SPECIAL HANDLING INSTRUCTIONS: Not applicable.

INFORMATION FOR THE PATIENT: Published in e-CPS, available by subscription at www.e-cps.ca.

DOSAGE FORMS, COMPOSITION AND PACKAGING: Oral Solution: Each mL of colorless to pale yellow, strawberry-banana flavoured, clear liquid contains: lamivudine 10 mg. Nonmedicinal ingredients: artificial strawberry and banana flavours, citric acid (anhydrous), hydrochloric acid, methylparaben, propylene glycol, propylparaben, sodium citrate (dihydrate), sodium hydroxide, sucrose and water. Each 150 mg (15 mL) contains 3 g of sucrose. Plastic bottles of 240 mL.

Tablets: 150 mg: Each, white, modified diamond-shaped, scored, film-coated tablet, imprinted with "GX CJ7" on both faces, contains: lamivudine 150 mg. Nonmedicinal ingredients: hydroxypropyl methylcellulose, magnesium stearate, microcrystalline cellulose, polyethylene glycol, polysorbate 80, sodium starch glycolate and titanium dioxide. Plastic bottles of 60.

300 mg: Each grey, modified diamond-shaped, film-coated tablet, imprinted with "GX EJ7" on one face contains: lamivudine 300 mg. Nonmedicinal ingredients: black iron oxide, hydroxypropyl methylcellulose, magnesium stearate, microcrystalline cellulose, polyethylene glycol, polysorbate 80, sodium starch glycolate and titanium dioxide. Plastic bottles of 30.

(Shown in Product Identification Section)

A

Abelcet® Ⓟ

amphotericin B lipid complex

Antifungal

Sigma-Tau

Date of Revision: March 29, 2010

PHARMACOLOGY: The active component in Amphotericin B Lipid Complex Injection is amphotericin B which acts by binding to sterols in the cell membrane of susceptible fungi, with a resultant change in permeability of the membrane. Mammalian cell membranes also contain sterols, and damage to human cells is believed to occur through the same mechanism of action.

Pharmacokinetics: The pharmacokinetics of amphotericin B after the administration of ABELCET are nonlinear. Volume of distribution and clearance from blood increase with increasing dose of ABELCET, resulting in less than proportional increases in blood concentrations of amphotericin B over a dose range of 0.6-5 mg/kg/day. The pharmacokinetics of amphotericin B in whole blood after the administration of ABELCET and amphotericin B desoxycholate are shown in Table 1.

Table 1: ABELCET

Pharmacokinetic Parameters of Amphotericin B in Whole Blood in Patients Administered Multiple Doses of ABELCET or Amphotericin B Desoxycholate

Pharmacokinetic Parameter	ABELCET 5 mg/kg/day for 5-7 days Mean ± SD	Amphotericin B 0.6 mg/kg/day for 42 days[a] Mean ± SD
Peak Concentration (μg/mL)	1.7±0.8 (n=10)[b]	1.1± 0.2 (n=5)
Concentration at End of Dosing Interval (μg/mL)	0.6±0.3 (n=10)[b]	0.4±0.2 (n=5)
Area Under Blood Concentration-Time Curve (AUC_{0-24h}) (μg·h/mL)	14±7(n=14)[b,c]	17.1±5 (n=5)
Clearance (mL/h·kg)	436±188.5 (n=14)[b,c]	38±15 (n=5)
Apparent Volume of Distribution (Vd_{area}) (L/kg)	131±57.7 (n=8)[c]	5±2.8 (n=5)
Terminal Elimination Half-Life (h)	173.4±78 (n=8)[c]	91.1±40.9 (n=5)
Amount Excreted in Urine Over 24 h After Last Dose (% of dose)[d]	0.9±0.4 (n=8)[c]	9.6±2.5 (n=8)

[a] Data from patients with mucocutaneous leishmaniasis. Infusion rate was 0.25 mg/kg/h.

[b] Data from studies in patients with cytologically proven cancer being treated with chemotherapy or neutropenic patients with presumed or proven fungal infection. Infusion rate was 2.5 mg/kg/h.

[c] Data from patients with mucocutaneous leishmaniasis. Infusion rate was 4 mg/kg/h.

[d] Percentage of dose excreted in 24 hours after last dose.

The large volume of distribution and high clearance value from the blood of amphotericin B after the administration of ABELCET probably reflect uptake by tissues. The long terminal elimination half-life probably reflects a slow redistribution from tissues. Although amphotericin B is excreted slowly, there is little accumulation in the blood after repeated dosing. AUC of amphotericin B increased approximately 34% from day 1 after the administration of Amphotericin B Lipid Complex Injection 5 mg/kg/day for 7 days. The effect of gender or ethnicity on the pharmacokinetics of Amphotericin B Lipid Complex Injection has not been studied.

Tissue concentrations of amphotericin B were obtained at autopsy from one heart transplant patient who received three doses of Amphotericin B Lipid Complex Injection at 5.3 mg/kg/day. The results are shown in Table 2.

Table 2: ABELCET

Amphotericin B Tissue Concentrations

Organ	Amphotericin B Tissue Concentration (μg/g)
Spleen	290
Lung	222
Liver	196
Lymph Node	7.6
Kidney	6.9
Heart	5
Brain	1.6

This pattern of distribution is consistent with that observed in preclinical studies in dogs in which greatest concentrations of amphotericin B after ABELCET administration were observed in the liver, spleen, and lung; however, the relationship of tissue concentrations of amphotericin B to its biological activity when administered as Amphotericin B Lipid Complex Injection is unknown.

INDICATIONS AND CLINICAL USE: ABELCET (Amphotericin B Lipid Complex Injection) is indicated for the treatment of invasive fungal infections in patients who are refractory to or intolerant of conventional amphotericin B therapy. This is based on open-label treatment of patients judged by their physicians to be intolerant to or failing conventional amphotericin B therapy. ABELCET has been used in 162 patients who had developed nephrotoxicity while receiving amphotericin B therapy and in a small number of patients who had pre-existing renal insufficiency (see Precautions and Dosage and Administration).

CONTRAINDICATIONS: ABELCET (Amphotericin B Lipid Complex Injection) is contraindicated in patients who have shown hypersensitivity to amphotericin B or any other component in the formulation.

WARNINGS: Anaphylaxis has been reported with amphotericin B desoxycholate and other amphotericin B-containing drugs. Anaphylaxis has been rarely reported with ABELCET (Amphotericin B Lipid Complex Injection) with an incidence of <0.1%. Facilities for cardiopulmonary resuscitation should be available during administration due to the possibility of anaphylactoid reaction. If severe respiratory distress occurs, the infusion should be immediately discontinued. The patient should not receive further infusions of ABELCET.

PRECAUTIONS: General: As with any amphotericin B-containing product, during the initial dosing of ABELCET, the drug should be administered intravenously under close clinical observation by medically trained personnel.

Acute reactions including fever and chills may occur 1 to 2 hours after starting an intravenous infusion of ABELCET. These reactions are usually more common with the first few doses of ABELCET and generally diminish with subsequent doses. Infusion has been rarely associated with hypotension, bronchospasm, arrhythmias, and shock.

Renal toxicity of doses greater than 5 mg/kg/day of ABELCET has not been formally studied. Despite generally less nephrotoxicity of ABELCET observed at a dose of 5 mg/kg/day compared with conventional amphotericin B therapy at a dose range of 0.6-1 mg/kg/day, dose limiting renal toxicity may still be observed with ABELCET.

Geriatrics: Forty-nine elderly patients, age 65 years or over, have been treated with ABELCET at 5 mg/kg/day in two open-label studies and one small, prospective, single-arm study. No serious drug related adverse events have been reported that might not be expected from the general patient population.

Children: One hundred eleven children (2 were enrolled twice and counted as separate patients) age 16 years and under, of whom 11 were less than 1 year, have been treated with ABELCET at 5 mg/kg/day in two open-label studies and one small, prospective, single-arm study. No serious drug related adverse events have been reported that might not be expected from the general patient population.

Pregnancy: There are no reports of pregnant women having been treated with ABELCET. Reproductive studies in rats and rabbits at doses of ABELCET up to 0.64 times the human dose revealed no harm to the fetus. Because animal reproductive studies are not always predictive of human response, and adequate and well-controlled studies have not been conducted in pregnant women, ABELCET should be used during pregnancy only after taking into account the importance of the drug to the mother.

Lactation: It is not known whether ABELCET is excreted in human milk. Because many drugs are excreted in human milk, and because of the potential for serious adverse reactions in breast-fed infants from ABELCET, a decision should be made whether to discontinue nursing or to discontinue the drug, taking into account the importance of the drug to the mother.

Patients with Special Diseases or Conditions: Hepatic Impairment: The effect of hepatic impairment on the disposition of ABELCET is not known. The metabolic pathways of ABELCET are not known.

Renal Impairment: The effect of renal impairment on the disposition of ABELCET is not known. The effect of dialysis on the elimination of ABELCET has not been studied; however, amphotericin B is not removed by hemodialysis when administered as amphotericin B desoxycholate.

Laboratory Tests: Serum creatinine should be monitored frequently during ABELCET therapy. It is also advisable to regularly monitor liver function, serum electrolytes (particularly magnesium and potassium), and complete blood counts.

Dependence Liability: ABELCET is not addictive.

Drug Interactions: No formal clinical studies of drug interactions have been conducted with ABELCET. However, when administered concomitantly, the following drugs are known to interact with amphotericin B; therefore, the following drugs may interact with ABELCET:

Antineoplastic Agents: Concurrent use of antineoplastic agents and amphotericin B may enhance the potential for renal toxicity, bronchospasm, and hypotension. Antineoplastic agents should be given concomitantly with ABELCET with great caution.

Corticosteroids and Corticotropin (ACTH): Concurrent use of corticosteroids and corticotropin (ACTH) with amphotericin B may potentiate hypokalemia which could predispose the patient to cardiac dysfunction. If used concomitantly with ABELCET, serum electrolytes and cardiac function should be closely monitored.

Cyclosporin A: Data from a prospective study of prophylactic ABELCET in 22 patients undergoing bone marrow transplantation suggested that concurrent initiation of cyclosporin A and ABELCET within several days of bone marrow ablation may be associated with increased nephrotoxicity.

Digitalis Glycosides: Concurrent use of amphotericin B may induce hypokalemia and may potentiate digitalis toxicity. When administered concomitantly with ABELCET, serum potassium levels should be closely monitored.

Flucytosine: Concurrent use of flucytosine with amphotericin B-containing preparations may increase the toxicity of flucytosine by possibly increasing its cellular uptake and/or impairing its renal excretion. Flucytosine should be given concomitantly with ABELCET with caution.

Imidazoles (e.g., ketoconazole, miconazole, clotrimazole, fluconazole, etc.): Antagonism between amphotericin B and imidazole derivatives such as miconazole and ketoconazole, which inhibit ergosterol synthesis, has been reported in both in vitro and in vivo animal studies. The clinical significance of these findings has not been determined.

Leukocyte Transfusions: Acute pulmonary toxicity has been reported in patients receiving intravenous amphotericin B and leukocyte transfusions. Leukocyte transfusions and ABELCET should not be given concurrently.

Other Nephrotoxic Medications: Concurrent use of amphotericin B and agents such as aminoglycosides and pentamidine may enhance the potential for drug-induced renal toxicity. Aminoglycosides and pentamidine should be used concomitantly with ABELCET only with great caution. Intensive monitoring of renal function is recommended in patients requiring any combination of nephrotoxic medications.

Skeletal Muscle Relaxants: Amphotericin B-induced hypokalemia may enhance the curariform effect of skeletal muscle relaxants (e.g., tubocurarine) due to hypokalemia. When administered concomitantly with ABELCET, serum potassium levels should be closely monitored.

Zidovudine: Increased myelotoxicity and nephrotoxicity were observed in dogs when either ABELCET (at doses 0.16 or 0.5 times the recommended human dose) or amphotericin B desoxycholate (at 0.5 times the recommended human dose) were administered concomitantly with zidovudine for 30 days. If zidovudine is used concomitantly with ABELCET, renal and hematologic function should be closely monitored.

ADVERSE EFFECTS: The total safety data base is composed of 921 patients treated with ABELCET (Amphotericin B Lipid Complex Injection), (5 patients were enrolled twice and counted as separate patients), of whom 775 were treated with 5 mg/kg/day. Of these 775 patients, 194 patients were treated in four comparative studies, 25 were treated in open-label, non-comparative studies, and 556 patients were treated in an open-label, emergency-use program. These 556 patients were treated for their invasive fungal infections, and were refractory to or intolerant of conventional amphotericin B therapy. Most had underlying hematologic neoplasms, and many were receiving multiple concomitant medications. Of the 556 patients treated with ABELCET, 9% of ABELCET patients discontinued treatment due to adverse events, regardless of presumed relationship to drug.

In general, the adverse events most commonly reported with ABELCET were transient chills and fever during infusion of the drug. Table 3 lists the most frequently reported adverse events.

Table 3: ABELCET

Adverse Events[a] with Incidence Rates ≥3% (N=556)

Adverse Event	Percentage (%) of Patients
Chills	18
Fever	14
Increased Serum Creatinine	11
Multiple Organ Failure	11
Nausea	9
Hypotension	8
Respiratory Failure	8
Vomiting	8
Dyspnea	7

(cont'd)

Table 3: ABELCET *(cont'd)*

Adverse Events[a] with Incidence Rates ≥3% (N=556)

Adverse Event	Percentage (%) of Patients
Sepsis	7
Diarrhea	6
Headache	6
Heart Arrest	6
Hypertension	5
Hypokalemia	5
Infection	5
Kidney Failure	5
Pain	5
Thrombocytopenia	5
Abdominal Pain	4
Anemia	4
Bilirubinemia	4
Gastrointestinal Hemorrhage	4
Leukopenia	4
Rash	4
Respiratory Disorder	4
Chest Pain	3
Nausea and Vomiting	3

[a] The causal association between adverse events and ABELCET is uncertain.

The following adverse events have also been reported in patients using ABELCET in open-label, uncontrolled clinical studies. The causal association between these adverse events and ABELCET is uncertain:
Body as a whole: anorexia, malaise, weight loss, deafness, injection site reaction including inflammation.
Allergic: bronchospasm, wheezing, asthma, anaphylactoid and other allergic reactions.
Cardiopulmonary: cardiac failure, pulmonary edema, shock, myocardial infarction, hemoptysis, tachypnea, thrombophlebitis, pulmonary embolus, cardiomyopathy, pleural effusion, arrhythmias including ventricular fibrillation.
Dermatological: maculopapular rash, pruritus, exfoliative dermatitis, erythema multiforme.
Gastrointestinal: acute liver failure, hepatitis, jaundice, melena, anorexia, dyspepsia, cramping, epigastric pain, veno-occlusive liver disease, diarrhea, hepatomegaly, cholangitis, cholecystitis.
Hematologic: coagulation defects, leukocytosis, blood dyscrasias including eosinophilia.
Musculoskeletal: myasthenia, including bone, muscle, and joint pains.
Neurologic: convulsions, tinnitus, visual impairment, hearing loss, peripheral neuropathy, tremors, transient vertigo, diplopia, encephalopathy, cerebral vascular accident, extrapyramidal syndrome and other neurologic symptoms.
Urogenital: oliguria, decreased renal function, anuria, renal tubular acidosis, impotence, dysuria.
Altered Laboratory Findings: Serum electrolyte abnormalities: hypomagnesemia, hyperkalemia, hypocalcemia, hypercalcemia.
Liver function test abnormalities: increased AST, ALT, alkaline phosphatase, LDH.
Renal function test abnormalities: increased BUN.
Other test abnormalities: acidosis, hyperamylasemia, hypoglycemia, hyperglycemia, hyperuricemia, hypophosphatemia.

OVERDOSE:

Symptoms and Treatment: Amphotericin B desoxycholate overdose has been reported to result in cardio-respiratory arrest. Twelve patients have been reported to have received two or more doses of ABELCET between 7-13 mg/kg. None of these patients had a serious acute reaction to ABELCET. If an overdose is suspected, discontinue therapy, monitor the patient's clinical status, and administer supportive therapy as required. ABELCET **is not hemodialyzable.**

> For management of a suspected drug overdose, CPhA recommends that you contact your **regional Poison Control Centre**. See the *CPS* Directory section for a list of Poison Control Centres.

DOSAGE AND ADMINISTRATION: The recommended daily dosage for adults and children (see Precautions) is 5 mg/kg given as a single infusion. ABELCET (Amphotericin B Lipid Complex Injection) should be administered by intravenous infusion at a rate of 2.5 mg/kg/h. If the infusion time exceeds 2 hours, resuspend the contents by shaking the infusion bag every 2 hours. Facilities for cardiopulmonary resuscitation should be available during administration due to the possibility of anaphylactoid reaction.

The median and mean duration of ABELCET treatment was 22 days and 33 days, respectively. ABELCET has been administered for as long as 17 months, and cumulative doses have been as high as 56.6 g.

Renal Impairment: Renal toxicity of ABELCET, as measured by serum creatinine levels, has been shown to be dose dependent. There are no firm guidelines for dose adjustment based on laboratory test results and decisions about dose adjustments should be made only after taking into account the overall clinical condition of the patient (see Precautions and Overdose:Symptoms and Treatment). Some patients with elevated serum creatinine levels have improved renal function while on Abelcet treatment.

Hepatic Impairment: No dose adjustment is required for patients with hepatic impairment.

Stability and Storage Conditions: Prior to admixture, ABELCET should be stored at 2 to 8°C and protected from exposure to light. Do not freeze. ABELCET should be retained in the carton until time of use.

The admixed ABELCET and 5% Dextrose Injection may be stored for up to 48 hours at 2 to 8ºC and an additional 6 hours at room temperature. Do not freeze. Any unused material should be discarded.

Preparation of Admixture for Infusion: Shake the vial gently until there is no evidence of any yellow sediment at the bottom. Withdraw the appropriate dose of ABELCET from the required number of vials into one or more sterile syringes using an 18-gauge needle. Remove the needle from each syringe filled with ABELCET and replace with the 5-micron filter needle supplied with each vial. Each filter needle may be used to filter the contents of up to four 100 mg vials. Insert the filter needle of the syringe into an IV bag containing 5% Dextrose Injection USP, and empty the contents of the syringe into the bag. The final infusion concentration should be 1 to 2 mg/mL. Do not use the admixture after dilution with 5% Dextrose Injection if there is any evidence of foreign matter. Vials are for single use. Unused material should be discarded. Aseptic technique must be strictly observed throughout handling of ABELCET since no bacteriostatic agent or preservative is present.

Do not dilute with saline solutions or mix with other drugs or electrolytes as the compatibility of ABELCET with these materials has not been established. An existing intravenous line should be flushed with 5% Dextrose Injection before infusion of ABELCET, or a separate infusion line should be used. **Do not use an in-line filter.**

The diluted ready-for-use admixture is stable for up to 48 hours at 2 to 8°C and an additional 6 hours at room temperature.

SUPPLIED: Liposomal encapsulation or incorporation in a lipid complex can substantially affect a drug's functional properties relative to those of the unencapsulated or nonlipid-associated drug. In addition, different liposomal or lipid-complexed products with a common active ingredient may vary from one another in the chemical composition and physical form of the lipid component. Such differences may affect functional properties of these drug products.

ABELCET (Amphotericin B Lipid Complex Injection) is a sterile, pyrogen-free suspension for intravenous infusion. While ABELCET consists of amphotericin B combined with two phospholipids in roughly a 1:1 drug-to-lipid weight ratio, the stoichiometry of the molecular complex that forms between amphotericin B and lipid is near a 1:1 drug-to-lipid molar ratio. ABELCET is yellow and opaque in appearance, with a pH of 5-7.

Each mL of sterile, opaque suspension contains: amphotericin B USP 5 mg. Nonmedicinal ingredients: L-α-dimyristoylphosphatidylcholine (DMPC), L-α-dimyristoylphosphatidylglycerol (DMPG), sodium chloride USP and water for Injection USP. Glass single-use vials of 20 mL along with 5-micron filter needles are individually packaged.

Abilify™ Pr

aripiprazole

Antipsychotic

Bristol-Myers Squibb

Date of Preparation: July 3, 2009
Date of Revision: August 18, 2010

SUMMARY PRODUCT INFORMATION:

Route of Administration	Dosage Form/Strength	Nonmedicinal Ingredients
Oral	Tablet, 2 mg, 5 mg, 10 mg, 15 mg, 20 mg and 30 mg	Cornstarch, hydroxypropyl cellulose, lactose monohydrate, magnesium stearate, and microcrystalline cellulose and coloring agents (2 mg: FD&C Blue No. 2 Aluminum Lake and iron oxide Yellow; 5 mg: FD&C Blue No. 2 Aluminum Lake; 10 mg and 30 mg: iron oxide red; 15 mg: iron oxide yellow)

INDICATIONS AND CLINICAL USE: Schizophrenia: ABILIFY (aripiprazole) is indicated for the treatment of schizophrenia and related psychotic disorders. In controlled clinical trials, ABILIFY was found to improve both positive and negative symptoms.

ABILIFY has been shown to be more effective than placebo in maintaining clinical improvement for up to 26 weeks.

Bipolar Disorder: ABILIFY (aripiprazole) is indicated for the acute treatment of manic or mixed episodes in Bipolar I Disorder. ABILIFY may be used as acute monotherapy or cotherapy with lithium or divalproex sodium when there is an insufficient acute response to these agents alone.

The physician who elects to use ABILIFY for extended periods should periodically re evaluate the long term usefulness of the drug for the individual patient.

Geriatrics (≥65 years of age): ABILIFY is not indicated in elderly patients with dementia. (See Warnings and Precautions, Serious Warnings and Precautions and Special Populations.) The safety and efficacy of ABILIFY in patients 65 years of age or older has not been established. Caution should be used when treating geriatric patients. (See Warnings and Precautions, Special Populations and Action and Clinical Pharmacology.)

Pediatrics (<18 years of age): Safety and efficacy of ABILIFY in pediatric and adolescent patients have not been established. ABILIFY is not indicated for the treatment of pediatric and adolescent patients.

CONTRAINDICATIONS: ABILIFY (aripiprazole) is contraindicated in those patients with a known hypersensitivity to this drug or the excipients of the product. For a complete listing, see Dosage Forms, Composition and Packaging.

WARNINGS AND PRECAUTIONS:

> **Serious Warnings and Precautions**
> **Increased Mortality in Elderly Patients with Dementia: Elderly patients with dementia treated with atypical antipsychotic drugs are at an increased risk of death compared to placebo. Analyses of thirteen placebo-controlled trials with various atypical antipsychotics (modal duration of 10 weeks) in these patients showed a mean 1.6-fold increase in the death rate in the drug-treated patients. Although the causes of death were varied, most of the deaths appeared to be either cardiovascular (e.g., heart failure, sudden death) or infectious (e.g., pneumonia) in nature (see Warnings and Precautions, Special Populations, Use in Elderly Patients with Dementia).**

General: Body Temperature Regulation: Disruption of the body's ability to reduce core body temperature has been attributed to antipsychotic agents. Appropriate care is advised when prescribing ABILIFY for patients who will be experiencing conditions which may contribute to an elevation in core body temperature, (eg, exercising strenuously, exposure to extreme heat, receiving concomitant medication with anticholinergic activity, or being subject to dehydration) (see Adverse Reactions).

Cardiovascular: Orthostatic Hypotension: Aripiprazole may be associated with orthostatic hypotension, perhaps due to its α1-adrenergic receptor antagonism. ABILIFY may induce orthostatic hypotension, tachycardia, dizziness, and sometimes syncope, especially at the initiation of treatment. The incidence of orthostatic hypotension-associated events from short-term, placebo-controlled trials of patients on oral ABILIFY (n=2096) included (aripiprazole incidence, placebo incidence): orthostatic hypotension (1.1%, 0.4%), postural dizziness (0.5%, 0.3%), and syncope (0.4%, 0.5%). The risk of orthostatic hypotension may be reduced by more gradual titration to the target dose.

The incidence of a significant orthostatic change in blood pressure (defined as a decrease in systolic blood pressure ≥20 mmHg accompanied by an increase in heart rate ≥25 bpm when comparing standing to supine values) for oral aripiprazole was not statistically different from placebo (aripiprazole incidence, placebo incidence): 4.6%, 3.0%.

Aripiprazole should be used with caution in patients with known cardiovascular disease (e.g., history of myocardial infarction or ischemic heart disease, heart failure or conduction abnormalities), cerebrovascular disease, or conditions which would predispose patients to hypotension (e.g., dehydration, hypovolemia, and treatment with antihypertensive medications). Patients with a history of clinically significant cardiovascular disorders were excluded from clinical trials.

QT Interval: In clinical trials with aripiprazole, the incidence of QT prolongation was comparable to placebo. In post-marketing experience, QT prolongation has been reported very rarely with ABILIFY treatment. As with other antipsychotics, caution should be exercised when ABILIFY is prescribed in patients with a history of cardiac arrhythmias, in patients with congenital or family history of long QT syndrome, and in concomitant use with drugs known to prolong the QT interval (see Adverse Reactions, Post-Market Adverse Drug Reactions).

Dependence/Tolerance: Aripiprazole has not been systematically studied in humans for its potential for abuse, tolerance, or physical dependence. In physical dependence studies in monkeys, withdrawal symptoms were observed upon abrupt cessation of dosing. While the clinical trials did not reveal any tendency for any drug-seeking behavior, these observations were not systematic and it is not possible to predict on the basis of this limited experience the extent to which a CNS-active drug will be misused, diverted, or abused once marketed. Consequently, patients should be evaluated carefully for a history of drug abuse, and such patients should be observed closely for signs of ABILIFY misuse or abuse (eg, development of tolerance, increases in dose, drug-seeking behavior).

Endocrine and Metabolism: Hyperglycemia and Diabetes Mellitus: As with some other antipsychotics, exacerbation of pre-existing diabetes and hyperglycemia have been reported rarely and diabetic ketoacidosis and diabetic coma including some fatal cases, have been reported very rarely during the use of ABILIFY (see Adverse Reactions).

Assessment of the relationship between atypical antipsychotic use and glucose abnormalities is complicated by the possibility of an increased background risk of diabetes mellitus in patients with schizophrenia and the increasing incidence of diabetes mellitus in the general population. Given these confounders, the relationship between atypical antipsychotic use and hyperglycemia-related adverse events is not completely understood. However, epidemiological studies which did not include ABILIFY suggest an increased risk of treatment-emergent hyperglycemia-related adverse events in patients treated with the atypical antipsychotics. Because ABILIFY was not marketed at the time these studies were performed, it is not known if ABILIFY is associated with this increased risk. Precise risk estimates for hyperglycemia-related adverse events in patients treated with atypical antipsychotics are not available.

Any patient treated with atypical antipsychotics should be monitored for symptoms of hyperglycemia including polydipsia, polyuria, polyphagia, and weakness. Patients who develop symptoms of hyperglycemia during treatment with atypical antipsychotics should undergo fasting blood glucose testing. In some cases, hyperglycemia has resolved when the atypical antipsychotic was discontinued; however, some patients required continuation of anti-diabetic treatment despite discontinuation of the suspect drug. Patients with risk factors for diabetes mellitus (eg, obesity, family history of diabetes) who are starting treatment with atypical antipsychotics should undergo fasting blood glucose testing at the beginning of treatment and periodically during treatment. Patients with an established diagnosis of diabetes mellitus who are started on atypical antipsychotics should be monitored regularly for worsening of glucose control.

Genitourinary: Priapism: Rare cases of priapism have been reported with ABILIFY. This adverse reaction, as with other psychotropic drugs, did not appear to be dose-dependent and did not correlate with the duration of treatment. The most likely mechanism of action of priapism is a relative decrease in sympathetic tone.

Hematologic: Infrequent cases of leukopenia have been reported with ABILIFY. In case of symptoms of infection, WBC count and differential count should be considered.

Neurologic: Neuroleptic Malignant Syndrome (NMS): Neuroleptic malignant syndrome is a potentially fatal symptom complex that has been reported in association with antipsychotic drugs, including aripiprazole.

Clinical manifestations of NMS are hyperpyrexia, muscle rigidity, altered mental status, and evidence of autonomic instability (irregular pulse or blood pressure, tachycardia, diaphoresis, and cardiac dysrhythmia). Additional signs may include elevated creatine phosphokinase, myoglobinuria (rhabdomyolysis), and acute renal failure.

In arriving at a diagnosis, it is important to identify cases where the clinical presentation includes both serious medical illness (e.g., pneumonia, systemic infection, etc.), and untreated or inadequately treated extrapyramidal signs and symptoms (EPS). Other important considerations in the differential diagnosis include central anticholinergic toxicity, heat stroke, drug fever, and primary central nervous system pathology.

The management of NMS should include 1) immediate discontinuation of all antipsychotic drugs including ABILIFY and other drugs not essential to therapy; 2) intensive symptomatic treatment and medical monitoring; and 3) treatment of any concomitant serious medical problems for which specific treatments are available. There is no general agreement about specific pharmacological treatment for uncomplicated NMS.

If a patient requires antipsychotic drug treatment after recovery from NMS, the potential re-introduction of therapy should be very carefully considered. The patient should be carefully monitored, since recurrence of NMS has been reported.

Tardive Dyskinesia: A syndrome of potentially irreversible, involuntary, dyskinetic movements may develop in patients treated with antipsychotic drugs. Although the prevalence of the syndrome is highest among the elderly, especially elderly women, it is impossible to rely upon prevalence estimates to predict, at the inception of antipsychotic treatment, which patients are likely to develop the syndrome. Whether antipsychotic drug products differ in their potential to cause tardive dyskinesia is unknown.

The risk of developing tardive dyskinesia and the likelihood that it will become irreversible increase as the duration of treatment and the total cumulative dose of antipsychotic drugs administered to the patient increase. However, the syndrome can develop, although much less commonly, after relatively brief treatment periods at low doses.

There is no known treatment for established cases of tardive dyskinesia, although the syndrome may remit, partially or completely, if antipsychotic treatment is withdrawn. Antipsychotic treatment, itself, however, may suppress (or partially suppress) the signs and symptoms of the syndrome and, thereby, may possibly mask the underlying process. The effect that symptomatic suppression has upon the long-term course of the syndrome is unknown.

Given these considerations, ABILIFY should be prescribed in a manner that is most likely to minimize the occurrence of tardive dyskinesia. Chronic antipsychotic treatment should generally be reserved for patients who suffer from a chronic illness that (1) is known to respond to antipsychotic drugs and (2) for whom alternative, equally effective, but potentially less harmful treatments are not available or appropriate. In patients who do require chronic treatment, the smallest dose and the shortest duration of treatment producing a satisfactory clinical response should be sought. The need for continued treatment should be reassessed periodically.

If signs and symptoms of tardive dyskinesia appear in a patient on ABILIFY, drug discontinuation should be considered. However, some patients may require treatment with ABILIFY despite the presence of the syndrome.

Seizure/Convulsion: In short-term, placebo-controlled trials of patients treated with oral aripiprazole, seizures/convulsions occurred in 0.1% (3/2096) of patients. There were confounding factors that may have contributed to the occurrence of seizures in some of these patients.

As with other antipsychotic drugs, aripiprazole should be used cautiously in patients with a history of seizures or with conditions that lower the seizure threshold. Conditions that lower the seizure threshold may be more prevalent in a population of 65 years or older.

Potential for Cognitive and Motor Impairment: Like other antipsychotics drugs, ABILIFY has the potential to impair judgment, thinking, or motor skills. Somnolence was a commonly reported adverse event in patients treated with ABILIFY in clinical trials.

Because ABILIFY may cause somnolence, and impair motor skills, patients should be cautioned about performing activities requiring mental alertness, such as operating hazardous machinery, including motor vehicles, until they are reasonably certain that ABILIFY therapy does not affect them adversely.

Psychiatric: Suicide: The possibility of a suicide attempt is inherent in psychotic illnesses and bipolar disorder, and close supervision and appropriate clinical management of high-risk patients should accompany drug therapy.

Special Populations: Pregnant Women: There are no adequate and well-controlled studies in pregnant women. It is not known whether aripiprazole can cause fetal harm when administered to a pregnant woman or can affect reproductive capacity. In animal studies, aripiprazole demonstrated developmental toxicity, including possible teratogenic effects in rats and rabbits. Aripiprazole should be used during pregnancy only if the potential benefit outweighs the potential risk to the fetus.

Labor and Delivery: The effect of aripiprazole on labor and delivery in humans is unknown.

Nursing Women: Aripiprazole was excreted in milk of rats during lactation. It is not known whether aripiprazole or its metabolites are excreted in human milk. It is recommended that women receiving aripiprazole should not breast-feed.

Pediatrics (<18 years of age): Safety and efficacy in children under the age of 18 years of age have not been established. ABILIFY is not indicated for the treatment of pediatric and adolescent patients.

Geriatrics (≥65 years of age): In formal single-dose pharmacokinetic studies (with aripiprazole given in a single dose of 15 mg), aripiprazole clearance was 20% lower in elderly (≥65 years) subjects compared to younger adult subjects (18 to 64 years). There was no detectable age effect, however, in the population pharmacokinetic analysis in schizophrenia patients. Also, the pharmacokinetics of aripiprazole after multiple doses in elderly patients appeared similar to that observed in young, healthy subjects (see Warnings and Precautions, Serious Warnings and Precautions and Dosage and Administration, Geriatric (≥65 years of age)).

Placebo-controlled studies of oral aripiprazole in schizophrenia or bipolar mania did not include sufficient numbers of subjects aged 65 and over to determine whether they respond differently from younger subjects.

Nevertheless, geriatric patients generally have decreased cardiac, hepatic and renal function, and more frequent use of concomitant medication. The presence of multiple factors that might increase the pharmacodynamic response to aripiprazole, or cause poorer tolerance or orthostasis, should lead to consideration of a lower starting dose, slower titration, and careful monitoring during the initial dosing period for elderly patients.

Use in Elderly Patients with Dementia: Studies of elderly patients with Alzheimer's disease have suggested that there may be a different tolerability profile in this population compared to younger patients with schizophrenia (see Warnings and Precautions, Serious Warnings and Precautions). The safety and efficacy of ABILIFY in the treatment of patients with Alzheimer's disease has not been established. If the prescriber elects to treat such patients with ABILIFY, vigilance should be exercised.

Overall Mortality: Elderly patients with dementia treated with atypical antipsychotic drugs showed increased mortality compared to placebo in a meta-analysis of 13 placebo-controlled trials of various atypical antipsychotic drugs. In three placebo-controlled studies of aripiprazole in elderly patients with Alzheimer's disease (n=938; mean age: 82.4 years; range: 56-99 years), the rate of death in aripiprazole-treated patients was 3.5%, compared to a rate of 1.7% in the placebo group during or within 30 days after termination from the double-blind phase of the studies. Although the causes of death were varied, most of the deaths appeared to be either cardiovascular (eg, heart failure, sudden death) or infectious (eg, pneumonia) in nature. ABILIFY is not indicated for the treatment of patients with dementia (see Serious Warnings and Precautions).

Dysphagia: Esophageal dysmotility and aspiration have been associated with antipsychotic drug use, including ABILIFY. Aspiration pneumonia is a common cause of morbidity and mortality in elderly patients, in particular those with advanced Alzheimer's dementia. Aripiprazole and other antipsychotic drugs should be used cautiously in patients at risk for aspiration pneumonia (see Adverse Reactions).

Cerebrovascular Adverse Events, Including Stroke in Elderly Patients with Dementia: In placebo-controlled clinical studies (two flexible dose and one fixed dose study) of elderly patients with dementia, there was an increased incidence of cerebrovascular adverse events (e.g., stroke, transient ischemic attack), including fatalities, in aripiprazole-treated patients. In the fixed-dose study, there was a statistically significant dose response relationship for cerebrovascular adverse events in patients treated with aripiprazole. Aripiprazole is not indicated for the treatment of patients with dementia (see Warnings and Precautions, Serious Warnings and Precautions).

Safety Experience in Elderly Patients with Alzheimer's Disease: In three, 10-week, placebo-controlled studies of aripiprazole in elderly patients with Alzheimer's disease (n=938; mean age: 82.4 years; range: 56-99 years), the treatment-emergent adverse events that were reported at an incidence of ≥3% and aripiprazole incidence at least twice that for placebo were lethargy [placebo 2%, aripiprazole 5%], somnolence (including sedation) [placebo 3%, aripiprazole 8%], and incontinence (primarily, urinary incontinence) [placebo 1%, aripiprazole 5%], excessive salivation (placebo 0%, aripiprazole 4%), and lightheadedness (placebo 1%, aripiprazole 4%).

The safety and efficacy of ABILIFY in the treatment of patients with dementia have not been established. If the prescriber elects to treat such patients with ABILIFY, vigilance should be exercised, particularly for the emergence of difficulty swallowing or excessive somnolence, which could predispose to accidental injury or aspiration (see Warnings and Precautions, Serious Warnings and Precautions).

Use in Patients with Renal Impairment: No dosage adjustment is required in subjects with renal impairment (see Action and Clinical Pharmacology, Special Populations and Conditions, Renal Insufficiency).

Use in Patients with Hepatic Impairment: No dosage adjustment is required in subjects with hepatic impairment (see Action and Clinical Pharmacology, Special Populations and Conditions, Hepatic Insufficiency).

Use in Patients with Concomitant Illness: Clinical experience with ABILIFY in patients with certain concomitant systemic illnesses is limited. ABILIFY has not been evaluated or used to any appreciable extent in patients with a recent history of myocardial infarction or unstable heart disease. Patients with these diagnoses were excluded from pre-marketing clinical studies (see Warnings and Precautions, Cardiovascular, Orthostatic Hypotension).

Gender: Cmax and AUC of aripiprazole and its active metabolite, dehydro-aripiprazole, are 30 to 40% higher in women than in men, and correspondingly, the apparent oral clearance of aripiprazole is lower in women. These differences, however, are largely explained by differences in body weight (25%) between men and women. No dosage adjustment is recommended based on gender.

Race: Although no specific pharmacokinetic study was conducted to investigate the effects of race on the disposition of aripiprazole, population pharmacokinetic evaluation did not demonstrate important race-related differences in the pharmacokinetics of aripiprazole. No dosage adjustment is recommended based on race.

Lactose: ABILIFY tablets contain lactose (70 mg, 67 mg, 62 mg, 57 mg, 124 mg and 187 mg for the 2 mg, 5 mg, 10 mg, 15 mg, 20 mg and 30 mg tablets respectively). Patients with rare hereditary problems of galactose intolerance or glucose-galactose malabsorption should not take ABILIFY.

ADVERSE REACTIONS: Adverse Drug Reaction Overview: Aripiprazole was evaluated for safety in 13 543 patients who participated in multiple-dose, clinical trials in schizophrenia, bipolar disorder, major depression, dementia of the Alzheimer's type, Parkinson's disease, and alcoholism, and who had approximately 7619 patient-years of exposure to oral aripiprazole and 749 patients with exposure to aripiprazole injection. A total of 3390 patients were treated with oral aripiprazole for at least 180 days and 1933 patients treated with oral aripiprazole had at least 1 year of exposure.

The conditions and duration of treatment with aripiprazole (monotherapy or adjunctive therapy with antidepressants or mood stabilizers) included (in overlapping categories) double-blind, comparative and noncomparative open-label studies, inpatient and outpatient studies, fixed- and flexible-dose studies, and short- and longer-term exposure.

Adverse events during exposure were obtained by collecting volunteered adverse events, as well as results of physical examinations, vital signs, weights, laboratory analyses, and ECG. Adverse events were recorded by clinical investigators using terminology of their own choosing. In the tables and tabulations that follow, MedDRA dictionary terminology has been used to classify reported adverse events into a smaller number of standardized event categories, in order to provide a meaningful estimate of the proportion of individuals reporting adverse events.

The stated frequencies of adverse events represent the proportion of individuals who reported at least once, a treatment-emergent adverse event of the type listed. An event was considered treatment emergent if it occurred for the first time or worsened while receiving therapy following baseline evaluation. There was no attempt to use investigator causality assessments; i.e. all events meeting the defined criteria, regardless of investigator causality are included.

Clinical Trial Adverse Drug Reactions: Because clinical trials are conducted under very specific conditions the adverse reaction rates observed in the clinical trials may not reflect the rates observed in practice and should not be compared to the rates in the clinical trials of another drug. Adverse drug reaction information from clinical trials is useful for identifying drug-related adverse events and for approximating rates.

Short-Term, Placebo-Controlled Trials of Patients with Schizophrenia: The following findings are based on a pool of five placebo-controlled trials (four 4-week and one 6-week) in which aripiprazole was administered orally in doses ranging from 2 to 30 mg/day.

Adverse Events Associated with Discontinuation of Treatment: Overall, there was little difference in the incidence of discontinuation due to adverse events between aripiprazole-treated (7%) and placebo-treated (9%) patients. The types of adverse events that led to discontinuation were similar between the aripiprazole and placebo-treated patients.

Commonly Reported Adverse Events: The only commonly observed adverse event associated with the use of aripiprazole in patients with schizophrenia (incidence of 5% or greater and aripiprazole incidence at least twice that for placebo) was akathisia (placebo 4%; aripiprazole 8%).

Short-Term, Placebo-Controlled Trials of Aripiprazole in Patients with Bipolar Mania: The following findings are based on a pool of 3-week, placebo-controlled, bipolar mania trials in which aripiprazole was administered orally at doses of 15 or 30 mg/day.

Adverse Events Associated with Discontinuation of Treatment: Overall, in patients with bipolar mania, there was little difference in the incidence of discontinuation due to adverse events between aripiprazole-treated (11%) and placebo-treated (10%) patients. The types of adverse events that led to discontinuation were similar between the aripiprazole and placebo-treated patients. Akathisia, the most common adverse event leading to discontinuation in the aripiprazole group, led to withdrawal of 2% of aripiprazole-treated patients and 0.3% of patients on placebo.

Commonly Reported Adverse Events: Commonly reported adverse events associated with the use of aripiprazole in patients with bipolar mania (incidence of 5% or greater and aripiprazole incidence at least twice that for placebo) are shown in Table 1.

Table 1: ABILIFY

Commonly Reported Adverse Events in Short-Term, Placebo-Controlled Trials of Patients with Bipolar Mania Treated with ABILIFY

	Percentage of Patients Reporting Event	
Preferred Term	**Aripiprazole (n=917)**	**Placebo (n=753)**
Akathisia	13	4
Sedation	8	3
Restlessness	6	2
Extrapyramidal Disorder	5	2

Adverse Events Reported at an Incidence of 2% or More Among Aripiprazole-Treated Patients and Greater than Placebo in Short-Term, Schizophrenia and Bipolar Mania Placebo-Controlled Trials : Table 2 enumerates the pooled incidence, rounded to the nearest percent, of treatment-emergent adverse events that were reported during acute therapy (up to 6 weeks in schizophrenia and up to 3 weeks in bipolar mania), including only those events that were reported in 2% or more of patients treated with aripiprazole (doses ≥2 mg/day) and for which the incidence in patients treated with aripiprazole was greater than the incidence in patients treated with placebo in the combined dataset.

An examination of population subgroups did not demonstrate a difference in the incidence of adverse events based on age, gender, or race.

Table 2: ABILIFY

Treatment-Emergent Adverse Events in Short-Term, Placebo-Controlled Trials in Patients with Schizophrenia[a] and Bipolar Mania[b] Treated with Oral ABILIFY

System Organ Class Preferred Term	Percentage of Patients Reporting Event[c] Aripiprazole (n=1843)	 Placebo (n=1166)
Eye Disorders		
Blurred Vision	3	1
Gastrointestinal Disorders		
Nausea	15	11
Constipation	11	7
Vomiting	11	6
Dyspepsia	9	7
Dry Mouth	5	4
Toothache	4	3
Abdominal Discomfort	3	2
Stomach Discomfort	3	2
General Disorders and Administration Site Conditions		
Fatigue	6	4
Pain	3	2
Musculoskeletal and Connective Tissue Disorders		
Musculoskeletal Stiffness	4	3
Pain in Extremity	4	2
Myalgia	2	1
Muscle Spasms	2	1
Nervous System Disorders		
Headache	27	23
Dizziness	10	7
Akathisia	10	4
Sedation	7	4
Extrapyramidal Disorder	5	3
Tremor	5	3
Somnolence	5	3
Psychiatric Disorders		
Agitation	19	17
Insomnia	18	13
Anxiety	17	13
Restlessness	5	3
Respiratory, Thoracic, and Mediastinal Disorders		
Pharyngolaryngeal Pain	3	2
Cough	3	2

[a] 926 aripiprazole-treated patients and 413 placebo treated patients.
[b] 917 aripiprazole-treated patients and 753 placebo-treated patients.
[c] Events reported by at least 2% of patients treated with oral aripiprazole, except events which had an incidence equal to or less than placebo.

Short-Term, Placebo-Controlled Trial of Adjunctive Therapy in Patients with Bipolar Mania: In a placebo-controlled trial of patients with bipolar mania who were already tolerating either lithium or valproate as monotherapy, aripiprazole was administered orally for 6 weeks at doses of 15 or 30 mg as adjunctive therapy with lithium or valproate. The adverse events reported in that study were generally similar to the adverse events listed in Table 1 from clinical trials in which aripiprazole was used as monotherapy. Akathisia and tremor were reported more frequently when aripiprazole was used as adjunctive therapy. Akathisia was reported in 19% of patients treated with aripiprazole as adjunctive therapy compared to 5% of patients who received placebo as adjunctive therapy. In the lithium subgroup, the incidence of akathisia was 28% in patients treated with aripiprazole as adjunct and 4% in patients treated with placebo. In the valproate subgroup akathisia was reported in 12% of patients treated with aripiprazole as adjunctive therapy compared to 6% treated with placebo as adjunctive therapy. The incidence of tremor was 9% for patients treated with aripiprazole as adjunctive therapy and 6% for patients who received placebo as adjunctive therapy. Other commonly reported adverse events in this trial were insomnia 8% vs 4% and extrapyramidal disorder 5% vs 1%, in aripiprazole-treated patients and placebo-treated patients, respectively.

Discontinuation rates due to adverse events were 12% for patients treated with adjunctive aripiprazole compared to 6% for patients treated with adjunctive placebo. Akathisia, the most common adverse event leading to discontinuation in the aripiprazole group, led to withdrawal of 5% of aripiprazole-treated patients and 1% of patients on placebo.

Dose-Related Adverse Events: Dose response relationships for the incidence of treatment-emergent adverse events were evaluated from four trials in patients with schizophrenia comparing various fixed oral doses (2, 5, 10, 15, 20, or 30 mg/day) of aripiprazole to placebo. This analysis, stratified by study, indicated that the only adverse event to have a possible dose response relationship, and then most prominent only with 30 mg, was somnolence [including sedation]; (incidences were placebo, 7.4%; 10 mg, 8.5%; 15 mg, 8.7%; 20 mg, 7.5%; 30 mg, 12.6%). In two clinical trials in patients with bipolar mania comparing fixed doses of 15 or 30 mg of oral aripiprazole to placebo, no dose response relationship for treatment-emergent adverse events was found.

Extrapyramidal Symptoms: Table 3 provides the percentage of patients reporting treatment-emergent extrapyramidal symptoms in short-term placebo-controlled trials.

Table 3: ABILIFY

Percentage of Patients Reporting Treatment-Emergent Extrapyramidal Symptoms in Short-Term Placebo-Controlled Trials

	Percentage of Patients Reporting Event					
	Schizophrenia		Bipolar Mania Monotherapy		Bipolar Mania Cotherapy	
	Aripiprazole	Placebo	Aripiprazole	Placebo	Aripiprazole	Placebo
EPS-Related AEs (excluding akathisia)	14	14	16	8	15	8
Akathisia-Related Events	8	4	13	4	19	5

Table 4 provides the mean change from baseline to endpoint score on the Simpson Angus Rating Scale (for EPS) (SAS), Barnes Akathisia Scale (for akathisia), and the Assessments of Involuntary Movement Scales (for dyskinesia) (AIMS) from short-term, placebo-controlled trials.

Table 4: ABILIFY

Mean Change From Baseline to Endpoint Score on the SAS, Barnes Akathisia Scale, and AIMS From Short-Term Placebo-Controlled Trials

	Mean Change from Baseline to Endpoint Score					
	Schizophrenia		Bipolar Mania Monotherapy		Bipolar Mania Cotherapy	
	Aripiprazole	Placebo	Aripiprazole	Placebo	Aripiprazole	Placebo
SAS	−0.06	−0.08	0.50[c]	−0.01	0.73[a]	0.07
Barnes	0.08	−0.05	0.21[c]	−0.05	0.30[b]	0.11
AIMS	−0.44[a]	−0.02	−0.02	−0.06	0.08	−0.10

[a] $p \le 0.01$.
[b] $p \le 0.05$.
[c] $p \le 0.001$.
A negative score indicates improvement.

In a long-term (26-week), placebo-controlled trial of schizophrenia, data on the Simpson Angus Rating Scale (for EPS), the Barnes Akathisia Scale (for akathisia), and the Assessments of Involuntary Movement Scales (for dyskinesias) did not show a difference between aripiprazole and placebo.

Weight Gain: In 4- to 6-week trials in schizophrenia, there was a slight difference in mean weight gain between aripiprazole and placebo patients (+0.7 kg vs −0.05 kg, respectively) and also a statistically significant difference in the proportion of patients meeting a weight gain criterion of ≥7% of body weight [aripiprazole (8%) compared to placebo (3%)].

In 3-week trials in bipolar mania, the mean weight gain for aripiprazole and placebo patients was 0.1 kg vs. 0.0 kg, respectively. The proportion of patients meeting a weight gain criterion of ≥7% of body weight was aripiprazole 2% compared to placebo 3%. In the 6-week trial in mania in which aripiprazole or placebo was used as adjunctive therapy with either lithium or valproate, the mean weight gain for aripiprazole and placebo patients was 0.6 kg vs 0.2 kg, respectively. The proportion of patients meeting a weight gain criterion of ≥7% of body weight with adjunctive aripiprazole was 3% compared to adjunctive placebo 4%.

In a long-term (26-week) placebo-controlled study of aripiprazole, a categorization of patients with schizophrenia at baseline on the basis of body mass index [BMI<23 ("low"); 23-27 ("normal"); >27 ("high")] revealed mean weight losses in patients treated with aripiprazole and patients on placebo ("low" BMI, −0.5 kg weight loss in both treatment groups; "normal" BMI, mean weight loss of −1.3 kg in aripiprazole-treated patients and −0.6 kg in placebo-treated patients; "high" BMI, mean weight loss of −2.1 kg in aripiprazole-treated patients and −1.5 kg in placebo-treated patients).

In a long-term (52-week) study of aripiprazole and haloperidol, a categorization of patients with schizophrenia at baseline on the basis of BMI revealed the greatest mean weight gain in patients with low BMI compared to normal or overweight patients in both groups (patients with "low" BMI, mean weight gain 2.6 kg in aripiprazole-treated patients and 1.5 kg in haloperidol-treated patients; "normal" BMI, a mean weight gain of 1.4 kg in aripiprazole-treated patients and 0.2 kg in haloperidol-treated patients; "high" BMI, weight loss of −1.2 kg in aripiprazole-treated patients and −0.8 kg in haloperidol-treated patients).

In both studies, the highest incidence of clinically significant weight gain (>7% of body weight) was in patients with a low BMI (<23) compared to normal (23-27) or overweight patients (>27).

ECG Changes: Between group comparisons for a pooled analysis of placebo-controlled trials in patients with schizophrenia or bipolar mania, revealed no significant differences between oral aripiprazole and placebo in the proportion of patients experiencing potentially important changes in ECG parameters. Aripiprazole was associated with a median increase in heart rate of 2 beats per minute compared to no increase among placebo patients.

Additional Findings Observed in Clinical Trials: Adverse Events in Long-Term, Double-Blind, Placebo-Controlled Trials: The adverse events reported in a 26-week, double-blind trial comparing oral ABILIFY and placebo in patients with schizophrenia were generally consistent with those reported in the short-term, placebo-controlled trials, except for a higher incidence of tremor [8% (12/153) for ABILIFY vs 2% (3/153) for placebo]. In this study, the majority of the cases of tremor were of mild intensity (8/12 mild and 4/12 moderate), occurred early in therapy (9/12 ≤49 days), and were of limited duration (7/12 ≤10 days). Tremor infrequently led to discontinuation (<1%) of ABILIFY. In addition, in a long-term (52-week), active-controlled study, the incidence of tremor for ABILIFY was 5% (40/859).

A similar adverse event profile was observed in a long-term, 26-week placebo-controlled study in bipolar mania.

Other Adverse Events Observed During the Pre-Marketing Evaluation of Oral Aripiprazole: Following is a list of MedDRA terms that reflect treatment-emergent adverse events as defined in the introduction to the Adverse Reactions section reported by patients treated with oral aripiprazole at multiple doses ≥2 mg/day during any phase of a trial within the database of 13 543 patients. All events assessed as possible adverse drug reactions have been included. In addition, medically/clinically meaningful events particularly those that are likely to be useful to the prescriber or that have pharmacologic plausibility, have been included. Events already listed in Table 2, Table 3, or Table 4, or other parts of the Adverse Reactions section have been excluded. Although the events reported occurred during treatment with aripiprazole, they were not necessarily caused by it.

Events are further categorized by MedDRA system organ class and listed in order of decreasing frequency according to the following definitions: frequent adverse events are defined as those occurring on 1 or more occasions in at least 1/100 patients (only those not already listed in the tabulated results from placebo-controlled trials appear in this listing); infrequent adverse events are those occurring in less than 1/100 but at least 1/1000 patients; rare events are those occurring in less than 1/1000.

Blood and Lymphatic System Disorders: Infrequent: leukopenia, neutropenia, thrombocytopenia.

Cardiac Disorders: Infrequent: bradycardia, palpitations, cardiopulmonary failure, myocardial infarction, cardio-respiratory arrest, atrioventricular block, extrasystoles, sinus tachycardia, atrial fibrillation, angina pectoris, myocardial ischemia; Rare: atrial flutter, supraventricular tachycardia, ventricular tachycardia.

Endocrine Disorders: Infrequent: diabetes mellitus (including blood insulin increased, carbohydrate tolerance decreased, diabetes mellitus non-insulin-dependent, glucose tolerance impaired, glycosuria, glucose urine, glucose urine present), hyperglycemia, hypoglycemia, polydipsia; Rare: diabetic ketoacidosis, diabetic hyperosmolar coma.

Eye Disorders: Infrequent: photophobia, diplopia, eyelid edema, photopsia.

Gastrointestinal Disorders: Infrequent: gastroesophageal reflux disease, dysphagia, swollen tongue, esophagitis; Rare: pancreatitis.
General Disorders and Administration Site Conditions: Frequent: asthenia, peripheral edema, pyrexia, irritability, chest pain; Infrequent: feeling jittery, face edema, thirst, angioedema; Rare: hypothermia.
Hepatobiliary Disorders: Rare: hepatitis, jaundice.
Immune System Disorders: Infrequent: hypersensitivity.
Injury, Poisoning, and Procedural Complications: Frequent: fall; Infrequent: self mutilation; Rare: heat stroke.
Investigations: Frequent: weight decreased, creatine phosphokinase increased; Infrequent hepatic enzyme increased (increased ALT, increased AST), blood glucose increased, blood prolactin increased, blood urea increased, electrocardiogram QT prolonged, blood creatinine increased, blood bilirubin increased; Rare: blood lactate dehydrogenase increased, glycosylated hemoglobin increased, gamma-glutamyl transferase (GGT) increased.
Metabolism and Nutrition Disorders: Frequent: decreased appetite; Infrequent: hyperlipidemia, anorexia, hypokalemia, hyponatremia.
Musculoskeletal and Connective Tissue Disorders: Frequent: arthralgia; Infrequent muscle rigidity, muscular weakness, muscle tightness, mobility decreased; Rare: rhabdomyolysis.
Nervous System Disorders: Frequent: coordination abnormal; Infrequent: speech disorder, dyskinesia, parkinsonism, dystonia, memory impairment, cogwheel rigidity, cerebrovascular accident, convulsion, hypokinesia, tardive dyskinesia, hypotonia, myoclonus, hypertonia, akinesia, bradykinesia; Rare: Grand Mal convulsion, choreoathetosis, neuroleptic malignant syndrome.
Psychiatric Disorders: Frequent: suicidal ideation; Infrequent: aggression, loss of libido, suicide attempt, hostility, libido increased, anger, anorgasmia, delirium, intentional self injury, completed suicide, tic, homicidal ideation; Rare: catatonia, sleep walking.
Renal and Urinary Disorders: Infrequent: urinary incontinence, urinary retention, polyuria, nocturia.
Reproductive System and Breast Disorders: Infrequent: menstruation irregular, erectile dysfunction, amenorrhea, breast pain; Rare: gynaecomastia, priapism.
Respiratory, Thoracic, and Mediastinal Disorders: Frequent: nasal congestion, dyspnea, pneumonia aspiration.
Skin and Subcutaneous Tissue Disorders: Frequent: rash (including erythematous, exfoliative, generalized, macular, maculopapular, papular rash; acneiform, allergic, contact, exfoliative, seborrheic dermatitis, neurodermatitis, and drug eruption), hyperhydrosis; Infrequent: pruritus, photosensitivity reaction, alopecia, urticaria.
Vascular Disorders: Frequent: hypertension; Infrequent: hypotension, syncope.
Abnormal Hematologic and Clinical Chemistry Findings: A between-group comparison for 3- to 6-week, placebo-controlled trials in patients with bipolar mania and schizophrenia revealed no differences between the aripiprazole and placebo groups in the proportions of patients experiencing clinically important changes in most routine serum chemistry, hematology, or urinalysis parameters (including changes in prolactin, fasting glucose, triglyceride, HDL, LDL and total cholesterol measurements).

Similarly, there were no differences in the incidence of discontinuations for changes in serum chemistry, hematology, or urinalysis.

In a long-term (26-week), placebo-controlled trial there were no clinically important differences between the aripiprazole and placebo patients in the mean change from baseline in prolactin, fasting glucose, triglyceride, HDL, LDL, and total cholesterol measurements.

Higher percentages of elevated creatine phosphokinase were observed in aripiprazole-treated patients compared to placebo-treated patients in short-term and long-term clinical trials. The most common AEs that were temporally associated with elevated CPK levels were musculoskeletal stiffness, myalgia, chest pain, fall, and muscle rigidity.
Post-Market Adverse Drug Reactions: The adverse reactions presented in Table 5 were reported during the post-marketing use of aripiprazole. Because these reactions are reported voluntarily from a population of uncertain size, it is not always possible to reliably estimate their frequency or establish a causal relationship to drug exposure.

Table 5: ABILIFY

Post-Introduction Treatment-Emergent Adverse Drug Reactions

Investigations	Very rare: weight increased, blood glucose fluctuation
Skin and Subcutaneous Tissue Disorders	Very rare: allergic reaction (eg, anaphylactic reaction, angioedema, laryngospasm, oropharyngeal spasm)
Gastrointestinal Disorders	Very rare: diarrhea

As with other antipsychotics, sudden death, torsades de pointes, ventricular tachycardia, arrhythmia, cardiopulmonary arrest and QT prolongation have been reported during treatment with ABILIFY. These events during ABILIFY treatment have been very rare or isolated. Many of the patients had pre-existing cardiovascular disease, were on concomitant medications known to prolong the QT interval, had risk factors for QT prolongation, took an overdose of ABILIFY, and/or were morbidly obese. Very rarely, QT prolongation has been reported in the absence of confounding factors.

DRUG INTERACTIONS: Drug-Drug Interactions: Potential for Other Drugs to Affect ABILIFY: Aripiprazole is not a substrate of CYP1A1, CYP1A2, CYP2A6, CYP2B6, CYP2C8, CYP2C9, CYP2C19, or CYP2E1 enzymes. Aripiprazole also does not undergo direct glucuronidation. This suggests that an interaction of aripiprazole with inhibitors or inducers of these enzymes, or other factors, like smoking, is unlikely.

Both CYP3A4 and CYP2D6 are responsible for aripiprazole metabolism (see Action and Clinical Pharmacology).

Agents that induce CYP3A4 (eg, carbamazepine) could cause an increase in aripiprazole clearance and lower blood levels. Inhibitors of CYP3A4 (e.g. ketoconazole) or CYP2D6 (e.g. quinidine, fluoxetine, or paroxetine) can inhibit aripiprazole elimination and cause increased blood levels.

Approximately 8% of Caucasians lack the capacity to metabolize CYP2D6 substrates and are classified as poor metabolizers (PM), whereas the rest are extensive metabolizers (EM). CYP2D6 metabolizing capacity should be considered when aripiprazole is co-administered with drugs that inhibit CYP2D6.
Ketoconazole and Other CYP3A4 Inhibitors: Coadministration of ketoconazole (200 mg/day for 14 days) with a 15-mg single dose of aripiprazole increased the AUC of aripiprazole and its active metabolite by 63% and 77%, respectively. The effect of a higher ketoconazole dose (400 mg/day) has not been studied. When ketoconazole is administered concomitantly with aripiprazole, aripiprazole dose should be reduced to one-half of its normal dose. Other strong inhibitors of CYP3A4 (itraconazole) would be expected to have similar effects and require similar dose reductions; weaker inhibitors (erythromycin, grapefruit juice) have not been studied. When the CYP3A4 inhibitor is withdrawn from the combination therapy, the aripiprazole dose should be increased.
Quinidine and Other CYP2D6 Inhibitors: Coadministration of quinidine (166 mg/day for 13 days), a potent inhibitor of CYP2D6, with a 10-mg single dose of aripiprazole increased the AUC of aripiprazole by 107% but decreased the AUC of its active metabolite, dehydro-aripiprazole, by 32%. The dose of aripiprazole should be reduced to one-half of its normal dose when quinidine is administered concomitantly with aripiprazole.

Concomitant administration of other significant inhibitors of CYP2D6, such as fluoxetine or paroxetine, would be expected to have similar effects and, therefore, should be accompanied by similar dose reductions. When the CYP2D6 inhibitor is withdrawn from the combination therapy, the aripiprazole dose should be increased.
Carbamazepine: Coadministration of carbamazepine (200 mg BID), a potent CYP3A4 inducer, with aripiprazole (30 mg QD) resulted in an approximate 70% decrease in Cmax and AUC values of both aripiprazole and its active metabolite, dehydro-aripiprazole. When carbamazepine is added to aripiprazole therapy, the dose of aripiprazole should be doubled. Additional dose increases should be based on clinical evaluation. When carbamazepine is withdrawn from the combination therapy, the aripiprazole dose should be reduced.
Potential for ABILIFY to Affect Other Drugs: Aripiprazole is unlikely to cause clinically important pharmacokinetic interactions with drugs metabolized by cytochrome P450 enzymes. In in vivo studies, 10-mg/day to 30-mg/day doses of aripiprazole had no significant effect on metabolism by CYP2D6 (dextromethorphan), CYP2C9 (warfarin), CYP2C19 (omeprazole, warfarin), and CYP3A4 (dextromethorphan) substrates. Additionally, aripiprazole and dehydro-aripiprazole did not show potential for altering CYP1A2-mediated metabolism in vitro.

Due to its alpha-1 adrenergic receptor antagonist activity, aripiprazole has the potential to enhance the effect of certain antihypertensive agents.

Drugs having no clinically important interactions with ABILIFY: Famotidine: Co-administration of aripiprazole (given in a single dose of 15 mg) with a 40-mg single dose of the H2 antagonist famotidine, a potent gastric acid blocker, decreased the solubility of aripiprazole and, hence, its rate of absorption. The Cmax of aripiprazole and dehydro-aripiprazole, was reduced by 37% and 21%, respectively. The extent of absorption (AUC) of aripiprazole and dehydro-aripiprazole, was reduced by 13% and 15%, respectively. No dosage adjustment of aripiprazole is required when administered concomitantly with famotidine.
Valproate: When valproate (500-1500 mg/day) and aripiprazole (30 mg/day) were co-administered, at steady state the Cmax and AUC of aripiprazole were decreased by 25%. No dosage adjustment of aripiprazole is required when administered concomitantly with valproate.

When aripiprazole (30 mg/day) and valproate (1000 mg/day) were co-administered, at steady state there were no clinically important changes in the Cmax or AUC of valproate. No dosage adjustment of valproate is required when administered concomitantly with aripiprazole.
Lithium: A pharmacokinetic interaction of aripiprazole with lithium is unlikely because lithium is not bound to plasma proteins, is not metabolized, and is almost entirely excreted unchanged in urine. Co-administration of therapeutic doses of lithium (1200-1800 mg/day) for 21 days with aripiprazole (30 mg/day) did not result in clinically important changes in the pharmacokinetics of aripiprazole or its active metabolite, dehydro-aripiprazole (Cmax and AUC increased by less than 20%). No dosage adjustment of aripiprazole is required when administered concomitantly with lithium.

Co-administration of aripiprazole (30 mg/day) with lithium (900 mg/day) did not result in clinically important changes in the pharmacokinetics of lithium. No dosage adjustment of lithium is required when administered concomitantly with aripiprazole.
Lamotrigine: Co-administration of 10 to 30 mg daily oral doses of aripiprazole for 14 days to subjects with bipolar I disorder had no effect on the steady-state pharmacokinetics 100 to 400 mg once daily lamotrigine, a UDP-glucuronosyltransferase 1A4 substrate. No dosage adjustment of lamotrigine is required if aripiprazole and lamotrigine are administered concomitantly. Dosing recommendations for lamotrigine should be followed closely if valproate is also to be administered.
Venlafaxine: Co-administration of 10 to 20 mg daily oral doses of aripiprazole for 14 days to healthy subjects had no effect on the steady-state pharmacokinetics of venlafaxine and O-desmethylvenlafaxine following 75 mg once daily venlafaxine XR, a CYP2D6 substrate. No dosage adjustment of venlafaxine is required if aripiprazole is administered concomitantly with venlafaxine.
Escitalopram: Co-administration of 10 mg daily oral doses of aripiprazole for 14 days to healthy subjects had no effect on the steady-state pharmacokinetics of 10 mg once daily escitalopram, a substrate of CYP2C19 and CYP3A4. No dosage adjustment of escitalopram is required if aripiprazole and escitalopram are administered concomitantly.
Dextromethorphan: Aripiprazole at doses of 10 to 30 mg per day for 14 days had no effect on dextromethorphan's O-dealkylation to its major metabolite, dextrorphan, a pathway dependent on CYP2D6 activity. Aripiprazole also had no effect on dextromethorphan's N-demethylation to its metabolite 3-methyoxymorphan, a pathway dependent on CYP3A4 activity. No dosage adjustment of dextromethorphan is required when administered concomitantly with aripiprazole.
Warfarin: Aripiprazole 10 mg per day for 14 days had no effect on the pharmacokinetics of R- and S-warfarin or on the pharmacodynamic end point of International Normalized Ratio, indicating the lack of a clinically relevant effect of aripiprazole on CYP2C9 and CYP2C19 metabolism or the binding of highly protein-bound warfarin. No dosage adjustment of warfarin is required when administered concomitantly with aripiprazole.
Omeprazole: Co-administration of aripiprazole (10 mg per day for 15 days) and a single 20-mg dose of omeprazole, a CYP2C19 substrate, had no effect on the pharmacokinetics of omeprazole in healthy subjects. No dosage adjustment of omeprazole is required when administered concomitantly with aripiprazole.
Lorazepam: Co-administration of oral lorazepam (2 mg) and oral aripiprazole (15 mg) to healthy subjects (n=24 males; ages 18-43 years old) did not result in clinically important changes in the pharmacokinetics of either drug. No dosage adjustment of either drug is required when they are administered concomitantly. However, the intensity of sedation was greater with the combination as compared to that observed with aripiprazole alone and the incidence of orthostatic hypotension observed was greater with the combination as compared to that observed with lorazepam alone (see Warnings and Precautions).
Drug-Food Interactions: ABILIFY can be administered with or without food (see Action and Clinical Pharmacology).
Drug-Herb Interactions: Interactions with herbal products have not been studied.
Drug-Laboratory Test Interactions: Interactions with laboratory tests have not been identified.
Drug-Lifestyle Interactions: Alcohol/CNS Drugs: Given the primary CNS effects of aripiprazole, as with most psychoactive medications, combination use of aripiprazole with alcohol or other CNS drugs with overlapping undesirable effects such as sedation, should be avoided.
Smoking: Aripiprazole is metabolised by multiple pathways involving the CYP2D6 and CYP3A4 enzymes but not CYP1A enzymes. Thus, no dosage adjustment is required for smokers.

DOSAGE AND ADMINISTRATION: Dosing Considerations: The efficacy and safety of ABILIFY, at doses greater than 30 mg/day, have not been established.
Schizophrenia: Usual Dose in Adults: The recommended starting and target dose for ABILIFY is 10 or 15 mg/day administered on a once-a-day schedule without regard to meals. Doses in the range of 10 to 30 mg/day have been established as effective in clinical trials. However, greater efficacy has not been demonstrated at doses higher than 10 mg/day. Dosage increases, if needed, should only be made after 2 weeks, the time needed to achieve steady state. The maximum daily dose should not exceed 30 mg/day.

Patients should be maintained on the lowest effective dose that provides optimal clinical response and tolerability and should be periodically reassessed to determine the need for maintenance treatment.
Switching from Other Antipsychotics: There are no systematically collected data to specifically address switching patients with schizophrenia from other antipsychotics to ABILIFY or concerning concomitant administration with other antipsychotics. While immediate discontinuation of the previous antipsychotic treatment may be acceptable for some patients with schizophrenia, more gradual discontinuation may be most appropriate for others. In all cases, the period of overlapping antipsychotic administration should be minimized.
Bipolar Disorder: Usual Dose in Adults: The recommended starting dose for ABILIFY as acute monotherapy or as cotherapy with lithium or valproate is 15 mg given once a day, without regard to meals. The dose can be increased to 30 mg/day based on clinical response.

Patients should be treated with the lowest effective dose that provides optimal clinical response and tolerability. The maximum daily dose should not exceed 30 mg/day.
Dosing Considerations in Special Populations: Pediatric (<18 years of age): Safety and efficacy of ABILIFY in pediatric and adolescent patients have not been established. ABILIFY is not indicated for the treatment of pediatric and adolescent patients.
Geriatric (≥65 years of age): Safety and efficacy of ABILIFY in the treatment of schizophrenia and Bipolar I Disorder in patients 65 years of age or older have not been established. Given the greater sensitivity of this population, a lower starting dose may be considered when clinical factors warrant (see Warnings and Precautions, Special Populations, Geriatrics (≥65 years of age)).
Patients with Hepatic Impairment: No dosage adjustment is required for patients with hepatic impairment.
Patients with Renal Impairment: No dosage adjustment is required in patients with renal impairment.
Gender: No dosage adjustment is required for female patients as compared to male patients.
Smoking Status: No dosage adjustment is required for smokers (see Drug Interactions, Drug-Lifestyle Interactions).

Refer to Drug Interactions section for dosage adjustment in patients taking aripiprazole concomitantly with strong CYP3A4 inhibitors (such as ketoconazole or clarithromycin), with potential CYP2D6 inhibitors (such as quinidine, fluoxetine, or paroxetine) or with potential CYP3A4 inducers (such as carbamazepine).
Missed Dose: If a patient misses a dose by a few hours, the patient should be advised to take their dose as soon as he/she remembers. If most of the day has passed, he/she should be advised to wait until the next scheduled dose. Patients should be advised to not take 2 doses of ABILIFY at once.

OVERDOSAGE:
Human Experience: In clinical studies, no deaths were associated with accidental or intentional acute overdosage of aripiprazole alone. In clinical trials, in the patient taking the largest confirmed amount of aripiprazole, 1080 mg, ingested with alcohol, the only symptom reported was vomiting.

In post-marketing experience, there is a single case of death that was possibly associated with accidental or intentional acute overdosage of aripiprazole alone. The patient ingested 900 mg of aripiprazole, was hospitalized in the intensive care unit for 10 to 14 days and died. The patient's medical history included excessive alcohol use, although it is unclear whether alcohol was present at the time of overdosage. In the patient taking the largest confirmed amount of aripiprazole, 1680 mg, the only symptoms reported were vomiting, fatigue, and dizziness. In addition, a report of non-fatal accidental overdose with aripiprazole alone (up to 195 mg) in a 2.5 year old child has been received. Vomiting, somnolence, lethargy, transient loss of consciousness and CNS depression were reported for this patient. Other potentially medically important signs and symptoms that have been observed during overdose included blood pressure increased and tachycardia. In the patients who were evaluated in hospital settings, there were no reported observations indicating clinically important adverse change in vital signs, laboratory assessments, or electrocardiogram.

Management of Overdosage: No specific information is available on the treatment of overdose with aripiprazole. Management of overdose should concentrate on supportive therapy, maintaining an adequate airway, oxygenation and ventilation, and management of symptoms. The possibility of multiple drug involvement should be considered. Therefore, cardiovascular monitoring should commence immediately and should include continuous electrocardiographic monitoring to detect possible arrhythmias. Following any confirmed or suspected overdose with aripiprazole, close medical supervision and monitoring should continue until the patient recovers.

Charcoal: In the event of an overdose of ABILIFY, an early charcoal administration may be useful in partially preventing the absorption of aripiprazole. Administration of 50 g of activated charcoal, one hour after a single 15-mg oral dose of aripiprazole, decreased the mean AUC and Cmax of aripiprazole by 50%.

Hemodialysis: Although there is no information on the effect of hemodialysis in treating an overdose with aripiprazole, hemodialysis is unlikely to be useful in overdose management since aripiprazole is highly bound to plasma proteins.

For management of a suspected drug overdose, contact your regional Poison Control Centre. See the *CPS* Directory section for a list of Poison Control Centres.

ACTION AND CLINICAL PHARMACOLOGY: Mechanism of Action: The mechanism of action of aripiprazole, as with other drugs having efficacy in schizophrenia and bipolar disorder is unknown. However, it has been proposed that the efficacy of aripiprazole may be mediated through a combination of partial agonist activity at D2 and 5-HT1A receptors and antagonist activity at 5-HT2A receptors; however, the clinical relevance of these interactions has not been established. Actions at receptors other than D2, 5-HT1A, and 5-HT2A may explain some of the other clinical effects of aripiprazole (eg, the orthostatic hypotension observed with aripiprazole may be explained by its antagonist activity at adrenergic alpha1 receptors). The clinical relevance of these receptor interactions with aripiprazole is unknown.

Pharmacodynamics: Aripiprazole exhibits high affinity for dopamine D2 and D3, serotonin 5-HT1A and 5-HT2A receptors (Ki values of 0.34, 0.8, 1.7, and 3.4 nM, respectively), moderate affinity for dopamine D4, serotonin 5-HT2C and 5-HT7, alpha1-adrenergic and histamine H1 receptors (Ki values of 44, 15, 39, 57, and 61 nM, respectively), and moderate affinity for the serotonin reuptake site (Ki=98 nM). Aripiprazole has no appreciable affinity for cholinergic muscarinic receptors (IC50>1000 nM). Aripiprazole functions as a partial agonist at the dopamine D2 and the serotonin 5-HT1A receptors, and as an antagonist at serotonin 5-HT2A receptor. The clinical relevance of these receptor interactions with aripiprazole is unknown.

Pharmacokinetics: ABILIFY activity is presumably primarily due to the parent drug, aripiprazole, and to a lesser extent, to its major metabolite, dehydro-aripiprazole, which has affinities for D2 receptors similar to the parent drug and represents 40% of the parent drug exposure in plasma. The mean elimination half-lives are about 75 hours and 94 hours for aripiprazole and dehydro-aripiprazole, respectively. Steady-state concentrations are attained within 14 days of dosing for both active moieties. Aripiprazole accumulation is predictable from single-dose pharmacokinetics. At steady state, the pharmacokinetics of aripiprazole are dose-proportional. Elimination of aripiprazole is mainly through hepatic metabolism involving two P450 isozymes, CYP2D6 and CYP3A4.

Absorption: Aripiprazole is well absorbed after oral administration of the tablet, with peak plasma concentrations occurring within 3 to 5 hours; the absolute oral bioavailability of the tablet formulation is 87%. ABILIFY can be administered with or without food. Administration of a 15-mg ABILIFY Tablet with a standard high-fat meal did not significantly affect the Cmax or AUC of aripiprazole or its active metabolite, dehydro-aripiprazole, but delayed Tmax by 3 hours for aripiprazole and 12 hours for dehydro-aripiprazole.

Distribution: The steady-state volume of distribution of aripiprazole following intravenous administration is high (404 L or 4.9 L/kg), indicating extensive extravascular distribution. At therapeutic concentrations, aripiprazole and its major metabolite are greater than 99% bound to serum proteins, primarily to albumin. In healthy human volunteers administered 0.5 to 30 mg/day aripiprazole for 14 days, there was dose-dependent D2 receptor occupancy. The clinical relevance of this receptor occupancy by aripiprazole is unknown.

Metabolism and Excretion: Aripiprazole is metabolized primarily by three biotransformation pathways: dehydrogenation, hydroxylation, and N-dealkylation. Based on in vitro studies, CYP3A4 and CYP2D6 enzymes are responsible for dehydrogenation and hydroxylation of aripiprazole, and N-dealkylation is catalyzed by CYP3A4. Aripiprazole is the predominant drug moiety in the systemic circulation. At steady state, dehydro-aripiprazole, the active metabolite, represents about 40% of aripiprazole AUC in plasma.

Approximately 8% of Caucasians lack the capacity to metabolize CYP2D6 substrates and are classified as poor metabolizers (PM), whereas the rest are extensive metabolizers (EM). PMs have about an 80% increase in aripiprazole exposure and about a 30% decrease in exposure to the active metabolite compared to EMs, resulting in about a 60% higher exposure to the total active moieties from a given dose of aripiprazole compared to EMs. Co-administration of ABILIFY with known inhibitors of CYP2D6, like quinidine in EMs, results in a 112% increase in aripiprazole plasma exposure, and dose adjustment is needed (see Drug Interactions). The mean elimination half-life for aripiprazole is about 75 hours in EMs and 146 hours in PMs. Aripiprazole does not inhibit or induce the CYP2D6 pathway.

Following a single oral dose of [14C]-labeled aripiprazole, approximately 25% and 55% of the administered radioactivity was recovered in the urine and feces, respectively. Less than 1% of unchanged aripiprazole was excreted in the urine and approximately 18% of the oral dose was recovered unchanged in the feces.

Special Populations and Conditions: Geriatrics: In formal single-dose pharmacokinetic studies (with aripiprazole given in a single dose of 15 mg), clearance of aripiprazole was 20% lower in elderly (≥65 years) subjects compared to younger adult subjects (18 to 64 years). However, there was no effect of age in the population pharmacokinetic analysis in schizophrenia patients. Also, the pharmacokinetics of aripiprazole after multiple doses in elderly patients appeared similar to that observed in young, healthy subjects (see Warnings and Precautions, Special Populations, Geriatrics (≥65 years of age) and Dosage and Administration).

Gender: Cmax and AUC of aripiprazole and its active metabolite, dehydro-aripiprazole, are 30 to 40% higher in women than in men, and correspondingly, the apparent oral clearance of aripiprazole is lower in women. However, these differences are largely explained by differences in body weight (25%) between men and women. No dosage adjustment is recommended based on gender.

Race: Although no specific pharmacokinetic study was conducted to investigate the effects of race on the disposition of aripiprazole, population pharmacokinetic evaluation did not demonstrate clinically important race-related differences in the pharmacokinetics of aripiprazole. No dosage adjustment is recommended based on race.

Hepatic Insufficiency: In a single-dose study (15 mg of aripiprazole) in subjects with varying degrees of liver cirrhosis (Child-Pugh Classes A, B, and C), the AUC of aripiprazole, compared to healthy subjects, increased 31% in mild HI, increased 8% in moderate HI, and decreased 20% in severe HI. None of these differences would require dose adjustment.

Renal Insufficiency: In patients with severe renal impairment (creatinine clearance <30 mL/min), Cmax of aripiprazole (given in a single dose of 15 mg) and dehydro-aripiprazole increased by 36% and 53%, respectively, but AUC was 15% lower for aripiprazole and 7% higher for dehydro-aripiprazole. Renal excretion of both unchanged aripiprazole and dehydro-aripiprazole is less than 1% of the dose. No dosage adjustment is required in subjects with renal impairment.

Smoking: Based on studies utilizing human liver enzymes in vitro, aripiprazole is not a substrate for CYP1A2 and also does not undergo direct glucuronidation. Smoking should, therefore, not have an effect on the pharmacokinetics of aripiprazole. Consistent with these in vitro results, population pharmacokinetic evaluation did not demonstrate any significant pharmacokinetic differences between smokers and nonsmokers. No dosage adjustment is recommended based on smoking status.

STORAGE AND STABILITY: Store tablets at 15 to 30°C.

INFORMATION FOR THE PATIENT: Published in e-CPS, available by subscription at www.e-cps.ca.

DOSAGE FORMS, COMPOSITION AND PACKAGING: 2 mg: Each green, modified rectangle tablet, imprinted with "A-006" and "2" contains: aripiprazole 2 mg. Nonmedicinal ingredients: cornstarch, hydroxypropyl cellulose, lactose monohydrate, magnesium stearate and microcrystalline cellulose; coloring agents: FD&C Blue No. 2 Aluminum Lake and Iron Oxide Yellow. Bottles of 30.

5 mg: Each blue, modified rectangle tablet, imprinted with "A-007" and "5" contains: aripiprazole 5 mg. Nonmedicinal ingredients: cornstarch, hydroxypropyl cellulose, lactose monohydrate, magnesium stearate and microcrystalline cellulose; coloring agents: FD&C Blue No. 2 Aluminum Lake. Bottles of 30.

10 mg: Each pink, modified rectangle tablet, imprinted with "A-008" and "10" contains: aripiprazole 10 mg. Nonmedicinal ingredients: cornstarch, hydroxypropyl cellulose, lactose monohydrate, magnesium stearate and microcrystalline cellulose; coloring agents: iron oxide red. Bottles of 30.

15 mg: Each yellow, round tablet, imprinted with "A-009" and "15" contains: aripiprazole 15 mg. Nonmedicinal ingredients: cornstarch, hydroxypropyl cellulose, lactose monohydrate, magnesium stearate and microcrystalline cellulose; coloring agents: iron oxide yellow. Bottles of 30.

20 mg: Each white, round tablet, imprinted with "A-010" and "20" contains: aripiprazole 20 mg. Nonmedicinal ingredients: cornstarch, hydroxypropyl cellulose, lactose monohydrate, magnesium stearate and microcrystalline cellulose. Bottles of 30.

30 mg: Each pink, round tablet, imprinted with "A-011" and "30" contains: aripiprazole 30 mg. Nonmedicinal ingredients: cornstarch, hydroxypropyl cellulose, lactose monohydrate, magnesium stearate and microcrystalline cellulose; coloring agents: iron oxide red. Bottles of 30.

(Shown in Product Identification Section)

Abraxane® Ⓟ

paclitaxel

Antineoplastic

Abraxis BioScience

Date of Revision: February 23, 2010

SUMMARY PRODUCT INFORMATION:

Route of Administration	Dosage Form/ Strength	Clinically Relevant Nonmedicinal Ingredients
Intravenous infusion	Lyophilized powder, 100 mg paclitaxel per single use vial	Human albumin

INDICATIONS AND CLINICAL USE: ABRAXANE for Injectable Suspension (paclitaxel powder for injectable suspension) (nanoparticle, albumin-bound [nab] paclitaxel) is indicated for:

- the treatment of metastatic breast cancer.

ABRAXANE should be administered under the supervision of a physician experienced in the use of cancer chemotherapeutic agents and in the management of breast cancer. Appropriate management of therapy and complications is only possible when adequate diagnostic and treatment facilities are readily available.

No premedication to prevent hypersensitivity reactions is required prior to administration of ABRAXANE.

Note: An albumin form of paclitaxel may substantially affect a drug's functional properties relative to those of drug in solution. **Do not substitute with or for other paclitaxel formulations.**

Geriatrics (>65 years of age): Evidence from clinical studies suggests that use in the geriatric population is not associated with notably more frequent toxicities among elderly patients who received ABRAXANE. A brief discussion can be found in Warnings and Precautions.

Pediatrics (≤16 years of age): The safety and effectiveness of ABRAXANE in pediatric patients have not been evaluated.

CONTRAINDICATIONS:

- Patients who are hypersensitive to this drug or to any ingredient in the formulation or component of the container. For a complete listing of ingredients, see Dosage Forms, Composition and Packaging.
- ABRAXANE for Injectable Suspension (paclitaxel powder for injectable suspension) (nanoparticle, albumin-bound [nab] paclitaxel) should not be used in patients who have baseline neutrophil counts of <1500 cells/mm³.

WARNINGS AND PRECAUTIONS:

Serious Warnings and Precautions

- ABRAXANE for Injectable Suspension (paclitaxel powder for injectable suspension) (nanoparticle, albumin-bound [nab] paclitaxel) should be administered under the supervision of a physician experienced in the use of cancer chemotherapeutic agents. Appropriate management of complications is possible only when adequate diagnostic and treatment facilities are readily available.
- ABRAXANE therapy should not be administered to patients with metastatic breast cancer who have baseline neutrophil counts of less than 1500 cells/mm³. In order to monitor the occurrence of bone marrow suppression, primarily neutropenia, which may be severe and result in infection, it is recommended that frequent peripheral blood cell counts be performed on all patients receiving ABRAXANE (see Hematologic).
- **Note:** An albumin form of paclitaxel may substantially affect a drug's functional properties relative to those of drug in solution. **Do not substitute with or for other paclitaxel formulations.** In the treatment of metastatic breast cancer ABRAXANE has been evaluated as a single agent only.

General: Albumin (Human): ABRAXANE for Injectable Suspension (paclitaxel powder for injectable suspension) (nanoparticle, albumin-bound [nab] paclitaxel) contains albumin (human), a derivative of human blood and is a nanoparticle albumin-bound (nab) form of paclitaxel. Based on effective donor screening and product manufacturing processes, it carries an extremely remote risk for transmission of viral diseases. A theoretical risk for transmission of Creutzfeldt-Jakob Disease (CJD) is also considered extremely remote. No cases of transmission of viral diseases or CJD have ever been identified for albumin.

Carcinogenesis and Mutagenesis: The carcinogenic potential of ABRAXANE has not been studied.

Paclitaxel has been shown to be clastogenic in vitro (chromosome aberrations in human lymphocytes) and in vivo (micronucleus test in mice). Paclitaxel injection was not mutagenic in the Ames test or the CHO/HGPRT gene mutation assay.

Hematologic: Bone marrow suppression (primarily neutropenia) is dose-dependent and a dose limiting toxicity. ABRAXANE therapy should not be administered to patients with baseline neutrophil counts of less than 1500 cells/mm³. In order to monitor the occurrence of myelotoxicity, it is recommended that frequent peripheral blood cell counts be performed on all patients receiving ABRAXANE. Patients should not be retreated with subsequent cycles of ABRAXANE until neutrophils recover to a level >1500 cells/mm³ and platelets recover to a level >100 000 cells/mm³. In the case of severe neutropenia (<500 cells/mm³ for seven days or more) during a course of ABRAXANE therapy, a dose reduction for subsequent courses of therapy is recommended (see Dosage and Administration).

Hepatic/Biliary/Pancreatic: The use of ABRAXANE has not been studied in patients with hepatic dysfunction. In the randomized controlled trial, patients were excluded for baseline serum bilirubin >15 mg/L.

Neurologic: Sensory neuropathy occurs frequently with ABRAXANE. The occurrence of grade 1 or 2 sensory neuropathy does not generally require dose modification. If grade 3 sensory neuropathy develops, treatment should be withheld until resolution to grade 1 or 2 followed by a dose reduction for all subsequent courses of ABRAXANE (see Dosage and Administration).

Renal: The use of ABRAXANE has not been studied in patients with renal dysfunction. In the randomized controlled trial, patients were excluded for baseline serum creatinine >20 mg/L.

Sexual Function/Reproduction: Men should be advised to not father a child while receiving treatment with ABRAXANE. Administration of paclitaxel powder for injectable suspension to male rats at 42 mg/m² on a weekly basis (approximately 16% of the daily maximum recommended human exposure on a mg/m² basis) for 11 weeks prior to mating with untreated female rats resulted in significantly reduced fertility accompanied by decreased pregnancy rates and increased loss of embryos in mated females. A low incidence of skeletal and soft tissue fetal anomalies was also observed at doses of 3 and 12 mg/m²/week in this study (approximately 1 to 5% of the daily maximum recommended human exposure on a mg/m² basis). Testicular atrophy/degeneration has also been observed in single-dose toxicology studies in rodents administered paclitaxel powder for injectable suspension at 54 mg/m² and dogs administered 175 mg/m².

Injection Site Reactions: Injection site reactions can occur with ABRAXANE. Given the possibility of extravasation, it is advisable to closely monitor the infusion site for possible infiltration during drug administration.

Special Populations: Pregnant Women/Teratogenic Effects: ABRAXANE can cause fetal harm when administered to a pregnant woman. Administration of paclitaxel powder for injectable suspension to rats on gestation days 7-17 at doses of 6 mg/m² (approximately 2% of the daily maximum recommended human dose on a mg/m² basis) caused embryo- and fetotoxicity, as indicated by intrauterine mortality, increased resorptions (up to 5-fold), reduced numbers of litters and live fetuses, reduction in fetal body weight and increase in fetal anomalies. Fetal anomalies included soft tissue and skeletal malformations, such as eye bulge, folded retina, microphthalmia, and dilation of brain ventricles. A lower incidence of soft tissue and skeletal malformations was also exhibited at 3 mg/m² (approximately 1% of the daily maximum recommended human dose on a mg/m² basis).

There are no adequate and well-controlled studies in pregnant women using ABRAXANE. If this drug is used during pregnancy, or if the patient becomes pregnant while receiving this drug, the patient should be apprised of the potential hazard to the fetus. Women of childbearing potential should be advised to avoid becoming pregnant while receiving treatment with ABRAXANE.

There was no exposure in pregnancy in the clinical trials.

Nursing Women: It is not known whether paclitaxel is excreted in human milk. In rats, following intravenous administration of carbon-14 labeled paclitaxel on days 9 to 10 postpartum, concentrations of radioactivity in milk were higher than in plasma and declined in parallel with the plasma concentrations. Because many drugs are excreted in human milk and because of the potential for serious adverse reactions in nursing infants, it is recommended that nursing be discontinued when receiving ABRAXANE therapy.

Pediatrics (≤16 years of age): The safety and effectiveness of ABRAXANE in pediatric patients have not been evaluated.

Geriatrics (>65 years of age): Of the 229 patients in the randomized study who received ABRAXANE, 13% were at least 65 years of age and <2% were 75 years or older. No toxicities occurred notably more frequently among elderly patients who received ABRAXANE.

Ability to Drive and Use Machines: Adverse events such as fatigue, weakness and malaise may affect the ability to drive and use machines.

Monitoring and Laboratory Tests: In order to monitor the occurrence of bone marrow suppression, primarily neutropenia, which may be severe and result in infection, it is recommended that frequent peripheral blood cell counts be performed on all patients receiving ABRAXANE. Patients should not be retreated with subsequent cycles of ABRAXANE until neutrophils recover to a level >1500 cells/mm^3 and platelets recover to a level >100 000 cells/mm^3. In the case of severe neutropenia (<500 cells/mm^3 for seven days or more) during a course of ABRAXANE therapy, a dose reduction for subsequent courses of therapy is recommended (see Dosage and Administration).

ADVERSE REACTIONS: Adverse Drug Reaction Overview: In the Phase III study, the adverse events which were very common were those expected for paclitaxel and included alopecia (90%), neutropenia (80%), leukopenia (72%), sensory neuropathy (71%), asthenia (47%), arthralgia/myalgia (44%), AST elevations (39%), alkaline phosphatase elevations (36%), abnormal ECG [all patients (60%) and patients with normal baseline (35%)], anemia in patients with normal baseline (20%), nausea (30%), vomiting (18%), infections (24%), diarrhea (27%), dyspnea (12%), and fluid retention/edema (10%).

In the Phase III study, twenty-seven percent of patients receiving ABRAXANE on a 3 weekly regimen experienced serious adverse events (SAEs). The events occurring in greater than 10 patients were Grade 4 neutropenia (9%), infection (3%), and increased GGT (3%).

Clinical Trial Adverse Drug Reactions: Because clinical trials are conducted under very specific conditions, the adverse reaction rates observed in the clinical trials may not reflect the rates observed in practice and should not be compared to the rates in the clinical trials of another drug. Adverse drug reaction information from clinical trials is useful for identifying drug-related adverse events and for approximating rates.

Table 1 shows the frequency of common important adverse events for the patients who received single-agent ABRAXANE for Injectable Suspension (paclitaxel powder for injectable suspension) (nanoparticle, albumin-bound [nab] paclitaxel) or Paclitaxel Injection for the treatment of metastatic breast cancer in the randomized comparative phase III trial.

Table 1: ABRAXANE

Frequency[a] of Common Important Treatment Emergent Adverse Events in the Randomized Study

	ABRAXANE for Injectable Suspension[b] 260 mg/m²/30 minutes n=229 (%)	Paclitaxel Injection[b] 175 mg/m²/3 hours n=225 (%)
Bone Marrow		
Neutropenia		
<2.0×10⁹/L	80	82
<0.5×10⁹/L	9	22
Leukopenia		
<4.0×10⁹/L	72	79
<1.0×10⁹/L	0	1
Thrombocytopenia		
<100×10⁹/L	2	3
<50×10⁹/L	<1	1
Anemia (normal at baseline) (Hb)		
<110 g/L	33	25
<80 g/L	1	<1
Infections	24	20
Febrile Neutropenia	2	1
Bleeding	2	2
Hypersensitivity Reaction[c]		
All	4	12
Severe[d]	0	2
Cardiovascular		
Vital Sign Changes[e]		
Bradycardia	<1	<1
Hypotension	5	5
Severe Cardiovascular Events[d]	3	4
Abnormal ECG		
All patients	60	52
Patients with Normal Baseline	35	30
Respiratory		
Cough	7	6

(cont'd)

Table 1: ABRAXANE *(cont'd)*

Frequency[a] of Common Important Treatment Emergent Adverse Events in the Randomized Study

	ABRAXANE for Injectable Suspension[b] 260 mg/m²/30 minutes n=229 (%)	Paclitaxel Injection[b] 175 mg/m²/3 hours n=225 (%)
Dyspnea	12	9
Sensory Neuropathy		
Any Symptoms	71	56
Severe Symptoms[d]	1	<1
Myalgia/Arthralgia		
Any Symptoms	44	49
Severe Symptoms[d]	8	4
Fluid Retention/Edema		
Any Symptoms	10	8
Severe Symptoms[d]	0	1
Gastrointestinal		
Nausea—Any Symptoms	30	22
Vomiting—Any Symptoms	18	10
Diarrhea—Any Symptoms	27	15
Mucositis—Any Symptoms	7	6
Alopecia	90	94
Asthenia		
Any Symptoms	47	39
Severe Symptoms[d]	8	3
Hepatic (Patients with Normal Baseline)		
Bilirubin Elevations	7	7
Alkaline Phosphatase Elevations	36	31
AST Elevations	39	32
Injection Site Reaction	<1	1
Skin/Dermatology		
Nail changes	1	0

[a] Based on worst grade.
[b] Paclitaxel injection patients received premedication.
[c] Includes treatment-related events related to hypersensitivity (e.g., flushing, dyspnea, chest pain, hypotension) that began on a day of dosing.
[d] Severe events are defined as at least grade 3 toxicity.
[e] During study drug dosing. Bradycardia defined as pulse <50 bpm and hypotension defined as diastolic blood pressure <40 mmHg or decrease in systolic blood pressure of ≥30 mmHg.

Adverse Event Experiences by Body System: Unless otherwise noted, the following discussion refers to the primary safety database of 229 patients with metastatic breast cancer treated with single-agent ABRAXANE in the randomized controlled trial. The frequency and severity of important clinically relevant adverse events for the study are presented above in tabular form. In some instances, rare severe events observed with paclitaxel injection may be expected to occur with ABRAXANE. Refer to Less Common Clinical Trial Adverse Drug Reactions (<1%) for the adverse events that occurred at a rate of less than 1%.

Hematologic: Neutropenia, the most important hematologic toxicity, was dose-dependent and generally rapidly reversible. Among patients with metastatic breast cancer in the randomized trial, neutrophil counts declined below 500 cells/mm^3 (Grade 4) in 9% of the patients treated with ABRAXANE at a dose of 260 mg/m^2 compared to 22% in patients receiving Cremophor-based paclitaxel injection at a dose of 175 mg/m^2.

In the randomized metastatic breast cancer study, infectious episodes were reported in 24% of the patients treated with a dose of 260 mg/m^2 given as a 30 minute infusion. Oral candidiasis, respiratory tract infections and pneumonia were the most frequently reported infectious complications. Febrile neutropenia was reported in 2% of patients in the ABRAXANE arm and 1% of patients in the paclitaxel injection arm. Fever occurring at any time during the treatment course was reported in 14% of patients in the ABRAXANE arm.

Thrombocytopenia was almost never severe (<50×10^9/L). Two percent of patients treated with ABRAXANE in the randomized trial experienced a decrease in their platelet count below 100×10^9/L at least once while on treatment. In the randomized metastatic breast cancer study, bleeding episodes were reported in 2% of the patients in each treatment arm.

Anemia (Hb <110 g/L) in patients with normal baseline was observed in 20% of patients treated with ABRAXANE in the randomized trial and was severe (Hb <80 g/L) in 1% of the patients with normal baseline hemoglobin. Red cell transfusions were required in 2% of patients in the Phase III study, and in 1% of those with normal baseline hemoglobin levels.

Hypersensitivity Reactions (HSRs): Hypersensitivity reactions to ABRAXANE were observed in 4% of all patients. None of these reactions were severe. In the Phase III study, the minor hypersensitivity reactions (i.e., those related to hypersensitivity and occurring on the day of dosing) consisted of dyspnea (1%) and flushing, hypotension, chest pain, and arrhythmia (all <1%). The use of ABRAXANE in patients previously exhibiting hypersensitivity to paclitaxel injection or human albumin has not been studied.

Cardiovascular: Hypotension, during the 30-minute infusion, occurred in 5% of patients treated with ABRAXANE in the randomized metastatic breast cancer trial. This vital sign change most often caused no symptoms and required neither specific therapy nor treatment discontinuation.

Severe cardiovascular events possibly related to single-agent ABRAXANE occurred in approximately 3% of patients in the randomized trial. These events included chest pain, cardiac arrest, supraventricular tachycardia, edema, thrombosis, pulmonary thromboembolism, pulmonary emboli, and hypertension.

Electrocardiogram (ECG) abnormalities were common among patients at baseline. ECG abnormalities on study did not usually result in symptoms, were not dose-limiting, and required no intervention. ECG abnormalities were noted in 60% of patients treated with ABRAXANE in the metastatic breast cancer randomized trial. Among patients with a normal ECG prior to study entry, 35% of patients treated with ABRAXANE developed an abnormal tracing while on study. The most frequently reported ECG modifications were non-specific repolarization abnormalities, sinus bradycardia, and sinus tachycardia.

Respiratory: Dyspnea (12%) and cough (7%) were reported after treatment with ABRAXANE in the randomized trial.

Neurologic: The frequency and severity of neurologic manifestations were influenced by prior and/or concomitant therapy with neurotoxic agents.

In general, the frequency and severity of neurologic manifestations were dose-dependent in patients receiving single-agent ABRAXANE. In the randomized trial, sensory neuropathy was observed in 71% of patients (10% severe) in the ABRAXANE arm and in 56% of patients (2% severe) in the paclitaxel injection arm. The frequency of sensory neuropathy increased with cumulative dose. Sensory neuropathy was the cause of discontinuation in 7/229 (3%) patients receiving ABRAXANE in the randomized trial. Severe sensory symptoms have typically improved in a median of 22 days after interrupting ABRAXANE therapy. No incidences of grade 4 sensory neuropathies were reported in the clinical trials. Reports of autonomic neuropathy resulting in paralytic ileus have been received as part of the continuing surveillance of paclitaxel injection safety.

Ocular/Visual Disturbances: Thirteen percent (13%) of all patients (n=366) treated with ABRAXANE in single arm and randomized trials reported ocular/visual disturbances and 1% were severe. The severe cases (keratitis and blurred vision) were reported in patients in a single arm study who received higher doses than those recommended (300 or 375 mg/m²). These effects generally have been reversible. However, rare reports in the literature of abnormal visual evoked potentials in patients treated with paclitaxel injection have suggested persistent optic nerve damage.

Arthralgia/Myalgia: Forty-four percent (44%) of patients treated with ABRAXANE in the randomized trial experienced arthralgia/myalgia; 8% experienced severe symptoms. The symptoms were usually transient, occurred two or three days after ABRAXANE administration, and resolved within a few days. There was no consistent relationship between dose of ABRAXANE and the frequency of arthralgia/myalgia.

Hepatic: Among patients with normal baseline liver function treated with ABRAXANE in the randomized trial, 7%, 36%, 39%, 36% and 50% had elevations in bilirubin, alkaline phosphatase, AST, ALT and GGT respectively. Grade 3 or 4 elevations in GGT were reported for 14% of patients treated with ABRAXANE and 10% of patients treated with paclitaxel injection in the randomized trial. Prolonged exposure to ABRAXANE was not associated with cumulative hepatic toxicity.

Renal: Eleven percent (11%) of patients treated with ABRAXANE in the randomized trial experienced creatinine elevation, <1% severe. No discontinuations, dose reductions, or dose delays were caused by renal toxicities.

Gastrointestinal (GI): Nausea, vomiting, diarrhea, and mucositis were reported by 30%, 18%, 27%, and 7% of patients treated with ABRAXANE in the randomized trial. These manifestations were usually mild to moderate. The frequency and severity of GI adverse events were not obviously dose-related. Infrequent reports of esophagitis were reported in the clinical trials. Dehydration was reported commonly in clinical trials. Constipation and anorexia were considered very common.

Injection Site Reactions: Injection site reactions were reported in 1% of patients treated with ABRAXANE and included reactions secondary to extravasation, which were usually mild and included erythema.

Asthenia: Asthenia was reported in 47% of patients (8% severe) treated with ABRAXANE in the randomized trial. Asthenia included reports of asthenia, fatigue, weakness, lethargy and malaise.

Alopecia: Alopecia was observed in almost all of the patients.

Skin: Nail changes (changes in pigmentation or discolouration of nail bed) occurred in 1% of patients treated with ABRAXANE in the randomized trial. Transient skin changes (rash 9%; flushing 2%; pruritus 6%) were observed in the randomized trial. No other skin adverse events were significantly associated with ABRAXANE administration.

Less Common Clinical Trial Adverse Drug Reactions (<1%): Cardiovascular: Bradycardia, during the 30-minute infusion, occurred in <1% of patients in the phase III study. Cases of cardiac ischemia/infarction and thrombosis/embolism possibly related to ABRAXANE treatment were uncommon. Cases of cerebrovascular attacks (strokes) and transient ischemic attacks were uncommon.

Gastrointestinal: Rare reports of intestinal obstruction, intestinal perforation, pancreatitis, and ischemic colitis have been received as part of the continuing surveillance of paclitaxel injection safety and may occur following ABRAXANE treatment. Rare reports of neutropenic enterocolitis (typhlitis), despite the coadministration of G-CSF, were observed in patients treated with paclitaxel injection alone and in combination with other chemotherapeutic agents.

Hepatic: Rare reports of hepatic necrosis and hepatic encephalopathy leading to death have been received as part of the continuing surveillance of paclitaxel injection safety and may occur following ABRAXANE treatment.

Hypersensitivity Reactions: Flushing, hypotension, chest pain, and arrhythmia occurring on the day of dosing were all reported at <1%.

Injection Site Reactions: Rare reports of more severe events such as phlebitis, cellulitis, induration, skin exfoliation, necrosis, and fibrosis have been received as part of the continuing surveillance of paclitaxel injection safety. In some cases the onset of the injection site reaction in paclitaxel injection patients either occurred during a prolonged infusion or was delayed by a week to ten days. Recurrence of skin reactions at a site of previous extravasation following administration of paclitaxel injection at a different site, i.e., "recall", has been reported rarely.

Given the possibility of extravasation, it is advisable to closely monitor the infusion site for possible infiltration during drug administration.

Neurologic: Uncommon serious neurologic events following ABRAXANE administration have included ischemic stroke, metabolic encephalopathy, confusion, dizziness/light-headedness, and mood alteration/depression.

Respiratory: Reports (<1%) of pneumothorax were uncommon after treatment with ABRAXANE in the randomized trial. Rare reports of interstitial pneumonia, lung fibrosis, and pulmonary embolism have been received as part of the continuing surveillance of paclitaxel injection safety and may occur following ABRAXANE treatment. Rare reports of radiation pneumonitis have been received in paclitaxel injection patients receiving concurrent radiotherapy. There is no experience with the use of ABRAXANE with concurrent radiotherapy.

Post-Market Adverse Drug Reactions: The following rare adverse events have been reported as part of the continuing surveillance of paclitaxel injection safety and **may** occur following ABRAXANE treatment: skin abnormalities related to radiation recall as well as reports of Stevens-Johnson syndrome, toxic epidermal necrolysis, conjunctivitis, and increased lacrimation. Scleroderma-like changes preceded by chronic edema have been reported with solvent-based paclitaxel injection. Because these events have been reported during clinical practice, true estimates of frequency cannot be made and a causal relationship to the events has not been established.

As part of the continuing surveillance of ABRAXANE, skin reactions including generalized or maculo-papular rash, erythema, and pruritus have been observed. Additionally, there have been case reports of photosensitivity reactions, radiation recall phenomenon, and in some patients previously exposed to capecitabine, reports of palmar-plantar erythrodyaesthesiae. Because these events have been reported during clinical practice, true estimates of frequency cannot be made and a causal relationship to the events has not been established.

During post-marketing surveillance, rare occurrences of severe hypersensitivity reactions have been reported with ABRAXANE. Patients who experience a severe hypersensitivity reaction to ABRAXANE should not be rechallenged with the drug.

Cranial nerve palsies, pleural effusion and vocal cord paresis have been reported during post-marketing surveillance of ABRAXANE. Because these events have been reported during clinical practice, true estimates of frequency cannot be made and a causal relationship to the events has not been established. Only one incident of motor neuropathy (grade 2) was observed in either arm of the controlled trial.

DRUG INTERACTIONS: Overview: No drug interaction studies have been conducted with ABRAXANE for Injectable Suspension (paclitaxel powder for injectable suspension) (nanoparticle, albumin-bound [nab] paclitaxel).

The metabolism of paclitaxel is catalyzed by CYP2C8 and CYP3A4. In the absence of formal clinical drug interaction studies, caution should be exercised when administering ABRAXANE concomitantly with medicines known to inhibit (e.g. ketoconazole and other imidazole antifungals, erythromycin, fluoxetine, gemfibrozil, cimetidine, ritonavir, saquinavir, indinavir, and nelfinavir) or induce (e.g. rifampicin, carbamazepine, phenytoin, efavirenz, nevirapine) either CYP2C8 or CYP3A4 (see Action and Clinical Pharmacology).

Drug-Drug Interactions: Interactions with other drugs have not been established.

Drug-Food Interactions: Interactions with food have not been established.

Drug-Herb Interactions: Interactions with herbal products have not been established.

Drug-Laboratory Test Interactions: Interactions with laboratory tests have not been established.

DOSAGE AND ADMINISTRATION: Dosing Considerations: No premedication to prevent hypersensitivity reactions is required prior to administration of ABRAXANE for Injectable Suspension (paclitaxel powder for injectable suspension) (nanoparticle, albumin-bound [nab] paclitaxel).

Do not substitute for or with other paclitaxel formulations.

Recommended Dose and Dosage Adjustment: For the treatment of metastatic breast cancer, the recommended regimen for ABRAXANE is 260 mg/m² administered intravenously over 30 minutes every 3 weeks. Dose levels of mg/m² refer to mg of paclitaxel in ABRAXANE.

Dose Reduction: Patients who experience severe neutropenia (neutrophil <500 cells/mm³ for a week or longer) or severe sensory neuropathy during ABRAXANE therapy should have dosage reduced to 220 mg/m² for subsequent courses of ABRAXANE. For recurrence of severe neutropenia or severe sensory neuropathy, an additional dose reduction should be made to 180 mg/m². For grade 3 sensory neuropathy, hold treatment until resolution to grade 1 or 2, followed by a dose reduction for all subsequent courses of ABRAXANE.

Hepatic Impairment: The appropriate dose of ABRAXANE for patients with bilirubin greater than 15 mg/L is not known.

Missed Dose: ABRAXANE is administered every three weeks. In the event that the next scheduled dose is missed, dosing should occur as soon as possible, consistent with good medical practice, after the missed dose.

Administration: Given the possibility of extravasation, it is advisable to closely monitor the infusion site for possible infiltration during drug administration. Limiting the infusion of ABRAXANE to 30 minutes, as directed, reduces the likelihood of infusion-related reactions (see Warnings and Precautions, Injection Site Reactions).

Each mL of the reconstituted formulation will contain 5 mg/mL paclitaxel. Calculate the exact total dosing volume of 5 mg/mL suspension required for the patient: Dosing volume (mL)=Total dose (mg)/5 (mg/mL).

Inject the appropriate amount of reconstituted ABRAXANE into an empty, sterile, intravenous infusion bag (plasticized polyvinyl chloride (PVC) containers, PVC or non-PVC type i.v. bag). No further dilution is required. The use of specialized DEHP-free solution containers or administration sets is not necessary to prepare or administer ABRAXANE infusions. The use of an in-line filter is not recommended.

Do not mix any other drugs with the ABRAXANE infusion.

Reconstitution: ABRAXANE is supplied as a sterile lyophilized powder for reconstitution before use. **Avoid errors, read entire preparation instructions prior to reconstitution.**

Vial Size	Volume of Diluent to be Added to Vial	Approximate Available Volume	Nominal Concentration per mL
50 mL	20 mL 0.9% Sodium Chloride Injection USP	20 mL	5 mg/mL

1. Aseptically, reconstitute each vial by injecting 20 mL of 0.9% Sodium Chloride Injection, USP.
2. Slowly inject the 20 mL of 0.9% Sodium Chloride Injection, USP, over a minimum of 1 minute, using the sterile syringe to direct the solution flow onto the **inside wall of the vial**.
3. **Do not inject** the 0.9% Sodium Chloride Injection, USP, directly onto the lyophilized cake as this will result in foaming.
4. Once the injection is complete, allow the vial to sit for a minimum of 5 minutes to ensure proper wetting of the lyophilized cake/powder.
5. Gently swirl and/or invert the vial slowly for at least 2 minutes until complete dissolution of any cake/powder occurs. Avoid generation of foam.
6. If foaming or clumping occurs, stand solution for at least 15 minutes until foam subsides.

The reconstituted suspension should be milky and homogenous without visible particulates. If particulates or settling are visible, the vial should be **gently** inverted again to ensure complete resuspension prior to use. Discard the reconstituted suspension if precipitates are observed. Discard any unused portion.

Neither freezing nor refrigeration adversely affects the stability of the product.

Stability of Reconstituted Suspension in the Vial: ABRAXANE reconstituted in the vial should be used immediately, but may be refrigerated at 2 to 8°C for a maximum of 8 hours if necessary. If not used immediately, each vial of reconstituted suspension should be replaced in the original carton to protect it from bright light. Discard any unused portion. Some settling of the reconstituted suspension may occur. Ensure complete resuspension by mild agitation before use. Discard the reconstituted suspension if precipitates are observed.

Inject the appropriate amount of reconstituted ABRAXANE into an empty, sterile, polyvinyl chloride (PVC) intravenous infusion bag. No further dilution is required. The use of specialized DEHP-free solution containers or administration sets may also be used but are not required to prepare or administer ABRAXANE infusions. The use of an in line filter is not recommended.

Stability of Reconstituted Suspension in the Infusion Bag: The suspension for infusion prepared as recommended is stable in an infusion bag at ambient temperature (approximately 20 to 25°C) and lighting conditions for up to 8 hours.

Parenteral drug products should be inspected visually for particulate matter and discolouration prior to administration whenever solution and container permit.

ABRAXANE is a cytotoxic anticancer drug and, as with other potentially toxic paclitaxel compounds, caution should be exercised in handling ABRAXANE. The use of gloves is recommended. If ABRAXANE (lyophilized cake or reconstituted suspension) contacts the skin, wash the skin immediately and thoroughly with soap and water. Following topical exposure to paclitaxel, events may include tingling, burning and redness. If ABRAXANE contacts mucous membranes, the membranes should be flushed thoroughly with water.

OVERDOSAGE:

There is no known antidote for ABRAXANE for Injectable Suspension (paclitaxel powder for injectable suspension) (nanoparticle, albumin-bound [nab] paclitaxel) overdosage. The primary anticipated complications of overdosage would consist of bone marrow suppression, sensory neurotoxicity, and mucositis.

For management of a suspected drug overdose, CPhA recommends that you contact your **regional Poison Control Centre**. See the *CPS* Directory section for a list of Poison Control Centres.

ACTION AND CLINICAL PHARMACOLOGY: Mechanism of Action: Paclitaxel, the active pharmaceutical ingredient in ABRAXANE for Injectable Suspension (paclitaxel powder for injectable suspension) (nanoparticle, albumin-bound [nab] paclitaxel), is an antimicrotubule agent that promotes the assembly of microtubules from tubulin dimers and stabilizes microtubules by preventing depolymerization. This stability results in the inhibition of the normal dynamic reorganization of the microtubule network that is essential for vital interphase and mitotic cellular functions. Paclitaxel induces abnormal arrays or "bundles" of microtubules throughout the cell cycle and multiple asters of microtubules during mitosis.

Pharmacodynamics: In preclinical models, ABRAXANE resulted in higher intra-tumour concentrations of paclitaxel compared to paclitaxel injection. Albumin is known to mediate endothelial transcytosis of plasma constituents and, based on in vitro data, it is hypothesized that albumin-bound paclitaxel facilitates the transport of paclitaxel across the endothelial cell via an albumin-receptor (gp60) mediated pathway.

Pharmacokinetics: See Table 2.

Table 2: ABRAXANE

Summary of Pharmacokinetic Parameters in Patients with Metastatic Breast Cancer

	C_{max} (ng/mL)	$t_{1/2}$ (h)	$AUC_{0-\infty}$ (h·ng/mL)	Clearance (L/h/m²)	Volume of Distribution (L/m²)
Single dose mean	18 741	27.4	17 940	15.2	632

Absorption and Distribution: The pharmacokinetics of total paclitaxel following 30- and 180-minute infusions of paclitaxel powder for injectable suspension at dose levels of 80-375 mg/m² were determined in clinical studies. Following intravenous administration of paclitaxel powder for injectable suspension, paclitaxel plasma concentrations declined in a biphasic manner, the initial rapid decline representing distribution to the peripheral compartment and the slower second phase representing drug elimination. The terminal half-life was about 27 hours.

The drug exposure (AUCs) was dose proportional over 80 to 300 mg/m² and the pharmacokinetics of paclitaxel for paclitaxel powder for injectable suspension were independent of the duration of administration. At the recommended clinical dose, 260 mg/m², the mean maximum concentration of paclitaxel, which occurred at the end of the infusion, was 18 741 ng/mL. The mean total clearance was 15 L/h/m². The mean volume of distribution was 632 L/m²; the large volume of distribution indicates extensive extravascular distribution and/or tissue binding of paclitaxel.

The pharmacokinetic data of 260 mg/m² paclitaxel powder for injectable suspension administered over 30 minutes was compared to the pharmacokinetics of 175 mg/m² paclitaxel injection over 3 hours. The volume of distribution and clearance of paclitaxel powder for injectable suspension were greater (by 53% and 43% respectively) than for paclitaxel injection. Differences in C_{max} and C_{max} corrected for dose, reflected differences in total dose and rate of infusion. There were no differences in terminal half-lives (approximately 21 hours for each).

In vitro studies of binding to human serum proteins, using paclitaxel concentrations ranging from 0.1 to 50 µg/mL, indicate that between 89-98% of drug is bound; the presence of cimetidine, ranitidine, dexamethasone, or diphenhydramine did not affect protein binding of paclitaxel.

Metabolism: In vitro studies with human liver microsomes and tissue slices showed that paclitaxel was metabolized primarily to 6α-hydroxypaclitaxel by CYP2C8; and to two minor metabolites, 3'-p-hydroxypaclitaxel and 6α, 3'-p-dihydroxypaclitaxel, by CYP3A4. In vitro, the metabolism of paclitaxel to 6α-hydroxypaclitaxel was inhibited by a number of agents (ketoconazole, verapamil, diazepam, quinidine, dexamethasone, cyclosporin, teniposide, etoposide, and vincristine), but the concentrations used exceeded those found in vivo following normal therapeutic doses. Testosterone, 17α-ethinyl estradiol, retinoic acid, and quercetin, a specific inhibitor of CYP2C8, also inhibited the formation of 6α-hydroxypaclitaxel in vitro. The pharmacokinetics of paclitaxel may also be altered in vivo as a result of interactions with compounds that are substrates, inducers, or inhibitors of CYP2C8 and/or CYP3A4 (see Drug Interactions). The effect of renal or hepatic dysfunction on the disposition of paclitaxel powder for injectable suspension has not been investigated.

Excretion: After a 30-minute infusion of 260 mg/m² doses of paclitaxel powder for injectable suspension, the mean values for cumulative urinary recovery of unchanged drug (4%) indicated extensive non-renal clearance. Less than 1% of the total administered dose was excreted in urine as the metabolites 6α-hydroxypaclitaxel and 3'-p-hydroxypaclitaxel. Fecal excretion was approximately 20% of the total dose administered.

Possible interactions of paclitaxel with concomitantly administered medications have not been formally investigated.

STORAGE AND STABILITY: Store the vials of ABRAXANE for Injectable Suspension (paclitaxel powder for injectable suspension) (nanoparticle, albumin-bound [nab] paclitaxel) in original cartons at 20 to 25°C. Retain in the original package to protect from bright light.

Neither freezing nor refrigeration adversely affects the stability of the product.

ABRAXANE reconstituted in the original vial should be used immediately, but may be refrigerated at 2 to 8°C for a maximum of 8 hours if necessary. If not used immediately, each vial of reconstituted suspension should be replaced in the original carton to protect it from bright light. Discard any unused portion. Some settling of the reconstituted suspension may occur. Ensure complete resuspension by mild agitation before use. Discard the reconstituted suspension if precipitates are observed.

The suspension for infusion prepared as recommended is stable in an infusion bag at ambient temperature (approximately 20 to 25°C) and ambient lighting conditions for up to 8 hours.

SPECIAL HANDLING INSTRUCTIONS: ABRAXANE for Injectable Suspension (paclitaxel powder for injectable suspension) (nanoparticle, albumin-bound [nab] paclitaxel) is a cytotoxic anticancer drug and, as with other potentially toxic paclitaxel compounds, caution should be exercised in handling ABRAXANE. The use of gloves is recommended.

Handling and Disposal: Procedures for proper handling and disposal of anticancer drugs should be considered. Several guidelines on this subject have been published. There is no general agreement that all of the procedures recommended in the guidelines are necessary or appropriate.

Accidental Exposure: No reports of accidental exposure to ABRAXANE have been received. However, upon inhalation of paclitaxel, dyspnea, chest pain, burning eyes, sore throat, and nausea have been reported. Following topical exposure, events have included tingling, burning, and redness. If ABRAXANE (lyophilized cake or reconstituted suspension) contacts the skin, wash the skin immediately and thoroughly with soap and water. Following topical exposure to paclitaxel, events may include tingling, burning and redness. If ABRAXANE contacts mucous membranes, the membranes should be flushed thoroughly with water.

INFORMATION FOR THE PATIENT: Published in e-CPS, available by subscription at www.e-cps.ca.

DOSAGE FORMS, COMPOSITION AND PACKAGING: ABRAXANE for Injectable Suspension (paclitaxel powder for injectable suspension) (nanoparticle, albumin-bound [nab] paclitaxel) is supplied as a white to yellow, sterile, lyophilized cake for reconstitution with 20 mL of 0.9% Sodium Chloride Injection, USP prior to intravenous infusion. Paclitaxel exists in the particle in a non-crystalline, amorphous state. Each single use vial contains: 100 mg of paclitaxel and approximately 900 mg of human albumin. Each mL of reconstituted suspension contains: 5 mg paclitaxel. ABRAXANE is free of solvents. Single use glass vials with a latex free stopper, individually packaged in a carton.

Abreva®

docosanol

Viral Entry Blocking Agent

GlaxoSmithKline Consumer Healthcare

PHARMACOLOGY: Mechanism of Action: The predominant mechanism for the anti-HSV activity of docosanol appears to be inhibition of fusion between the plasma membrane and the HSV envelope and, as a result, the blocking of entry and subsequent viral replication. This is in contrast to the mode of action of currently available antiviral agents. This mechanism of action explains the effectiveness of docosanol against all tested lipid-enveloped viruses that employ fusion as the sole or major means of entry into the cell and contrasts its mode of action to other antiviral agents that target a single viral protein.

Pharmacokinetics: Under conditions reflecting normal clinical use of ABREVA (docosanol cream 10%), the active ingredient could not be quantified (LOQ=10 ng/mL) in the plasma of treated patients. Ten women with active oral-facial herpes simplex lesions were treated with ABREVA, applied as a single dose (Day 1), and as multiple topical doses (five times daily, Days 2 and 3). Blood samples were withdrawn up to 24 hours after treatment and analyzed for docosanol. Of the 209 plasma samples analyzed, the docosanol level was below the limit of quantitation in 208 and exactly 10 ng/mL in the other.

n-Docosanoic acid, the major metabolite of docosanol, is an endogenous component of cell membranes in man, particularly in erythrocytes, brain, nerve myelin sheath, lung and kidney.

INDICATIONS: ABREVA (docosanol cream 10%) is indicated for the treatment of acute episodes of recurrent oral-facial herpes simplex (fever blisters or cold sores) in adults.

CONTRAINDICATIONS: ABREVA (docosanol cream 10%) is contraindicated in patients with known hypersensitivity to the product or any of its components.

WARNINGS: See Precautions.

Table 1: ABREVA

Local Adverse Reactions Reported in North American Phase 2/3 Clinical Trials

Description	ABREVA (N=1008) %	Placebo (N=989) %
Application site reaction	2.9	2.3
Rash	0.5	0.8
Pruritus	0.4	0.2
Dry skin	0.4	0.2
Acne	0.3	0.0

PRECAUTIONS: ABREVA should only be used to treat cold sores on the lips and face. Care should be taken to avoid application in or near the eyes since it may cause irritation; if contact occurs, rinse thoroughly with water. If excessive skin irritation develops or increases, discontinue use and consult a doctor. It should not be taken orally.

Children: The safety and effectiveness has not been established. ABREVA is not recommended for children under 12 years of age.

Pregnancy: No evidence of impaired fertility or harm to the fetus due to docosanol administered in oral doses of 10, 500, 1000, or 2000 mg/kg/day was observed in reproduction studies performed in rat and rabbits. Based on the lack of absorption of topically applied docosanol, these tested doses are a thousand-fold higher than the human dose. There are no adequate and well-controlled studies in pregnant women. ABREVA should be used during pregnancy only if clearly needed once the benefits and risk have been considered.

Lactation: It is not known whether docosanol is excreted in human milk. Because many drugs are excreted in human milk, caution should be exercised when ABREVA is administered to a nursing woman.

ADVERSE EFFECTS: In controlled clinical trials with ABREVA the most frequently reported adverse event was headache, which occurred in 10.4% of the patients treated with ABREVA and 10.7% of the patients treated with placebo. One or more local adverse reactions (application site reaction, rash, pruritus, dry skin, acne) were reported by 4.4% of patients treated with ABREVA and 3.2% of placebo treated patients. No evidence of contact sensitization or photoallergy was observed. See Table 1.

OVERDOSE:

Adverse reactions related to overdosage by topical application of ABREVA (docosanol cream 10%) are unlikely because of limited transcutaneous absorption. Similarly, poor oral absorption makes the occurrence of adverse reactions unlikely following ingestion of docosanol.

For management of a suspected drug overdose, CPhA recommends that you contact your **regional Poison Control Centre**. See the *CPS* Directory section for a list of Poison Control Centres.

DOSAGE: ABREVA (docosanol cream 10%) should be applied topically 5 times/day as soon as possible, preferably at the prodrome or erythema stages, until the lesion is healed, up to a maximum of 10 days. Treatment is most effective if applied at the first symptoms (pain, itching, burning or tingling) or sign, (redness), prior to the formation of a papule (bump) or a blister. Apply with clean finger, rub in gently, wash hands following application. Avoid contaminating tip of tube.

SUPPLIED: Each g of cream contains: docosanol 100 mg (10%) in a cream base. Nonmedicinal ingredients: benzyl alcohol, light mineral oil, propylene glycol, purified water and sucrose stearate (and) sucrose distearate. Tubes of 2 g. Store between 15 and 25°C. Do not freeze.

Accolate® Ⓟ

zafirlukast

Leukotriene Receptor Antagonist

AstraZeneca

Date of Preparation: January 19, 2000
Date of Revision: January 15, 2010

PHARMACOLOGY: Zafirlukast is a selective and competitive receptor antagonist of leukotriene D_4 and E_4 (LTD_4 and LTE_4), components of slow-reacting substance of anaphylaxis (SRSA). Cysteinyl leukotriene production and receptor occupation have been correlated with the pathophysiology of asthma, including airway edema, smooth muscle constriction, and altered cellular activity associated with the inflammatory process, which contribute to the signs and symptoms of asthma. Patients with asthma were found in one study to be 25 to 100 times more sensitive to the bronchoconstricting activity of inhaled LTD_4 than nonasthmatic subjects.

In vitro studies demonstrated that zafirlukast antagonized the contractile activity of 3 leukotrienes (LTC_4, LTD_4 and LTE_4) in conducting airway smooth muscle from laboratory animals and humans. Zafirlukast prevented intradermal LTD_4-induced increases in cutaneous vascular permeability and inhibited inhaled LTD_4-induced influx of eosinophils into animal lungs. Inhalational challenge studies in sensitized sheep showed that zafirlukast suppressed the airway responses to antigen; this included both the early- and late-phase response and the nonspecific hyperresponsiveness.

In humans, zafirlukast inhibited bronchoconstriction caused by several kinds of inhalational challenges. Pretreatment with single oral doses of zafirlukast inhibited the bronchoconstriction caused by sulfur dioxide and cold air in patients with asthma. Pretreatment with single doses of zafirlukast attenuated the early- and late-phase reaction caused by inhalation of various antigens such as grass, cat dander, ragweed, and mixed antigens in patients with asthma. Zafirlukast also attenuated the increase in bronchial hyperresponsiveness to inhaled histamine that followed inhaled allergen challenge.

Clinical Studies: Three double-blind, randomized, placebo-controlled, 13-week clinical trials in 1380 patients with mild to moderate asthma demonstrated that zafirlukast improved daytime asthma symptoms, nighttime awakenings, mornings with asthma symptoms, rescue β_2-agonist use, FEV_1, and morning peak expiratory flow rate (PEFR). In these studies, the patients had a mean baseline FEV_1 of approximately 75% of predicted normal and a mean baseline β-agonist requirement of approximately 4 to 5 puffs of salbutamol/day. The results of the largest of the trials are shown in Table 1.

Table 1: Accolate

Mean Change from Baseline at Study Endpoint

Parameter		Accolate 20 mg twice daily N=514	Placebo N=248
Daytime Asthma Symptom Score	(0–3 scale)	−0.44[a]	−0.25
Nighttime Awakenings	(number/week)	−1.27[a]	−0.43
Mornings with Asthma Symptoms	(days/week)	−1.32[a]	−0.75
Rescue β_2-agonist use	(puffs/day)	−1.15[a]	−0.24
FEV_1	(L)	+0.15[a]	+0.05
Morning PEFR	(L/min)	+22.06[a]	+7.63
Evening PEFR	(L/min)	+13.12	+10.14

[a] $p<0.05$, compared to placebo.

In a second and smaller study, the effect of zafirlukast on most efficacy parameters was comparable to the active control (inhaled sodium cromoglycate 1600 µg 4 times/day) and superior to placebo at endpoint for decreasing rescue β-agonist use. See Figure 1.

In these trials, improvement in asthma symptoms occurred within 1 week of initiating treatment with zafirlukast. The role of zafirlukast in the management of patients with more severe asthma, patients receiving antiasthma therapy other than as-needed, inhaled β_2-agonists, or as an oral or inhaled corticosteroid-sparing agent remains to be fully characterized.

Pharmacokinetics: Absorption: Zafirlukast is rapidly absorbed following oral administration. The absolute bioavailability of zafirlukast is unknown. Peak plasma concentrations are achieved 3 hours after dosing. In 2 separate studies, one using a high fat and the other a high protein meal, administration of zafirlukast with food reduced the mean bioavailability by approximately 40%.

Figure 1: Accolate

Effect of Accolate on Rescue Medication Use

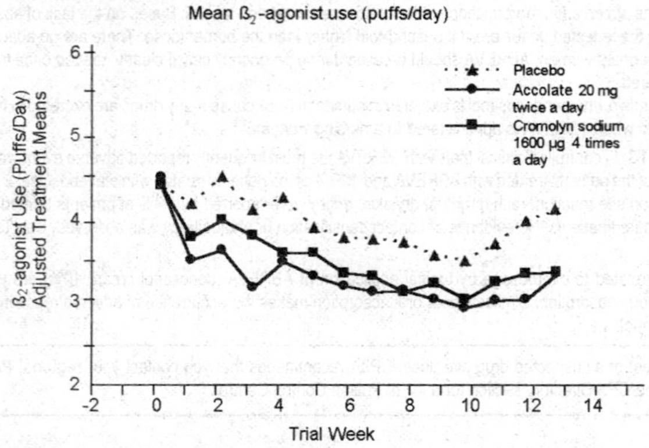

Plasma Kinetics and Disposition: The mean terminal elimination half-life of zafirlukast is approximately 10 hours in both normal subjects and patients with asthma. Steady-state plasma concentrations of zafirlukast are proportional to the dose and predictable from single dose pharmacokinetic data. In the concentration range of 0.25 to 10 µg/mL, zafirlukast is >99% bound to plasma proteins, predominantly albumin.

Biotransformation: Zafirlukast is extensively metabolized. Following oral administration of a radiolabeled dose, urinary excretion accounts for approximately 10% of the dose and the remainder is excreted in feces. Unmetabolized zafirlukast is not detected in urine. In vitro studies using human liver microsomes showed that the hydroxylated metabolites of zafirlukast are formed through the cytochrome P450 2C9 (CYP2C9) enzyme pathway. Additional in vitro studies utilizing human liver microsomes show that zafirlukast inhibits the cytochrome P450 CYP3A4 and CYP2C9 isoenzymes at concentrations close to the clinically achieved plasma concentrations. The metabolites of zafirlukast found in plasma are at least 90 times less potent as LTD_4 receptor antagonists than zafirlukast in a standard in vitro test of activity.

Special Populations: Elderly: Cross-study comparisons in patients ranging from 7 years to greater than 65 years of age show that mean dose (mg/kg) normalized AUC and C_{max} increase and plasma clearance (CL) decreases with increasing age. In patients above 65 years of age, there is an approximately 2-3 fold greater C_{max} and AUC compared to young adult patients.

Hepatic Impairment: In a study of patients with hepatic impairment (biopsy-proven cirrhosis), there was a 50 to 60% greater C_{max} and AUC compared to normal subjects.

Renal Impairment: Based on a cross-study comparison, there are no apparent differences in the pharmacokinetics of zafirlukast between renally impaired patients and normal subjects.

INDICATIONS: For the prophylaxis and chronic treatment of asthma in adults and children 12 years of age and older.

Zafirlukast should be considered to be an add-on therapy following initial management with an "as needed" short-acting beta-agonist, an inhaled corticosteroid, or inhaled corticosteroid together with a long-acting beta agonist in patients who continue to experience asthma symptoms.

The clinical decision to use zafirlukast must be based on assessing its risks and benefits for each individual patient.

CONTRAINDICATIONS: Zafirlukast is contraindicated in patients who have previously experienced hypersensitivity to the product or any of its ingredients.

Zafirlukast is also contraindicated in patients with hepatic impairment including hepatic cirrhosis and patients in whom zafirlukast is discontinued due to hepatotoxicity where no other attributable cause is identified.

WARNINGS: Zafirlukast is not indicated for use in the reversal of bronchospasm in acute asthma attacks, including status asthmaticus.

Warfarin Interaction: Warfarin coadministration with zafirlukast produces clinically significant increases in prothrombin time (PT). Patients on oral warfarin anticoagulant therapy and zafirlukast should have their prothrombin times monitored closely and anticoagulant dose adjusted accordingly (see Precautions, Drug Interactions).

Hepatic Effects: Clinical Trials: Rarely, elevations of one or more liver enzymes have occurred in patients receiving zafirlukast in controlled clinical trials. In clinical trials, most of these cases have been observed in asymptomatic patients at doses four times higher than the recommended dose.

Post-Marketing Experience: The reporting rates of adverse events from the post-marketing experience are generally considered to significantly underestimate the incidence of the events.

Elevations in serum transaminases can occur during treatment with zafirlukast. These were usually asymptomatic and transient but could represent early evidence of hepatotoxicity and have very rarely (less than 1 case/10 000 patient years) been associated with more severe hepatocellular injury, fulminant hepatitis and liver failure resulting in some cases of liver transplantation and death. **In some post-marketing cases of more severe hepatic injury, no clinical symptoms or signs suggestive of liver dysfunction were reported to precede these observations.** The following hepatic events (which have occurred predominantly in females) have been reported from post-marketing adverse event surveillance of patients who have received the recommended dose of zafirlukast (40 mg/day): very rare (less than 1 case/10 000 patient years) cases of symptomatic hepatitis (with or without hyperbilirubinemia) without other attributable cause; and very rarely, hyperbilirubinemia without other elevated liver function tests. In most, but not all, post-marketing reports, the patient's symptoms abated and the liver enzymes returned to normal or near normal after stopping zafirlukast.

In very rare (less than 1 case/100 000 patient years) cases, patients have progressed to fulminant hepatitis and/or hepatic failure despite early detection of liver enzyme elevations or signs and symptoms and/or discontinuation of zafirlukast.

Table 2 lists the number and the main outcomes of post-marketing reports of specific hepatic events in patients receiving zafirlukast through 23 December 2003 only and is not an illustration of any causality assessments of these outcomes. The reports are listed irrespective of pre-existing conditions and/or of concomitant therapies that may have contributed to the outcomes.

Table 2: Accolate

Number and Main Outcomes of Post-Marketing Reports of Specific Hepatic Events in Patients Receiving Accolate through 23 December 2003

Type of Hepatic Event	Number of Reports	Recovered	Resolving/Not fully recovered at the time of the report	Death	Transplant	Unknown
Liver Failure[a]	14	2	4	5	2 (1 died)	1
Hepatitis[b]	46	16	22	1	0	7
Other significant liver dysfunction	59	20	20	1	0	18

[a] Includes 3 reports of fulminant hepatitis that progressed to liver failure; Two of these patients have died and one was not fully recovered at the time of the report.

[b] Hepatitis includes: hepatitis, hepatitis acute, hepatitis cholestatic, possible autoimmune hepatitis, hepatitis chronic active and chronic hepatitis.

For all patients who are to be treated with zafirlukast, serum transaminase testing should be done at baseline and periodically during the treatment. However, note that periodic serum transaminase testing has not proven to prevent idiosyncratic liver injury. Particular caution should be used when patients are using a combination of zafirlukast and concomitant medications known to be hepatotoxic. Such patients should be closely monitored for possible hepatotoxicity.

It is important that physicians be informed and subsequently inform their patients to be alert to the signs and symptoms of hepatic injury [e.g., right upper quadrant abdominal pain (enlarged liver), nausea, vomiting, fatigue, lethargy, pruritus, jaundice, "flu-like" symptoms, anorexia, dark urine, discoloured and/or pale stools], and to seek immediate medical attention if these signs or symptoms develop. The appearance of signs and symptoms of hepatotoxicity or development of abnormal aminotransferase and/or bilirubin levels while on treatment is an indication for immediate termination of zafirlukast treatment and close monitoring of patient. The serum transaminases, in particular serum ALT, should be measured immediately and the patient managed accordingly. **In very rare (less than 1 case/100 000 patient years) cases, patients have progressed to fulminant hepatitis and/or hepatic failure despite early detection of liver enzyme elevations or signs and symptoms and/or discontinuation of zafirlukast.** If liver function tests are consistent with hepatic dysfunction, zafirlukast therapy should not be resumed. Patients in whom zafirlukast is discontinued due to hepatotoxicity where no other attributable cause is identified, should not be re-exposed to zafirlukast. Zafirlukast is contraindicated for patients with hepatic impairment including hepatic cirrhosis (see Contraindications).

PRECAUTIONS: General: Zafirlukast should be taken regularly as prescribed, even during symptom-free periods. Zafirlukast therapy can be continued during acute exacerbations of asthma.

Zafirlukast is not a bronchodilator and should not be used to treat acute episodes of asthma.

Patients receiving zafirlukast should be instructed not to decrease the dose or stop taking any other antiasthma medications unless instructed by a physician.

Eosinophilic Conditions: In rare cases, patients with asthma on anti-leukotriene medications, including zafirlukast may present with systemic eosinophilia, eosinophilic pneumonia or clinical features of systemic vasculitis consistent with Churg-Strauss syndrome, a condition which is often treated with systemic corticosteroid therapy. These events usually, but not always, have been associated with the reduction and/or withdrawal of steroid therapy.

Presentations may involve various body systems including vasculitic rash, worsening pulmonary symptoms, cardiac complications, and/or neuropathy presenting in their patients. The possibility that leukotriene receptor antagonists, including zafirlukast, may be associated with the emergence of Churg-Strauss syndrome can neither be excluded nor established (see Adverse Effects).

Hepatic Effects: See Warnings.

Pediatric Use: The efficacy and safety of zafirlukast in children under 12 years have not been established.

Carcinogenesis and Mutagenicity: In 2-year oral carcinogenicity studies, zafirlukast was administered at daily doses of 10 to 300 mg/kg to mice and 40 to 2000 mg/kg to rats. At 300 mg/kg/day male mice had an increased incidence of hepatocellular adenomas and female mice showed an increased incidence of whole body histocytic sarcomas as compared to concurrent controls. The plasma concentrations at these tumorigenic doses were approximately 220 times maximum recommended human daily oral dose. Male and female rats given 2000 mg/kg/day had an increased incidence of urinary bladder transitional cell papillomas as compared to concurrent controls. The plasma concentrations at these tumorigenic doses were approximately 200 times the plasma concentrations in humans at the maximum recommended human daily oral dose. The data for both the mouse and rat demonstrate: large safety margins, a clear threshold over the no-effect level, and findings that are applicable or restricted to only one species. Further, zafirlukast has no evident genotoxic potential. The bladder tumor induction seen in rats and liver tumor induction seen in mice are therefore unlikely to be relevant to humans.

No mutagenic potential was evident in point mutation assays or chromosomal aberrations clastogenic assays.

Reproduction and Fertility: Reproduction and fertility studies in rats showed no effect on fertility due to zafirlukast at doses up to 2000 mg/kg (approximately 400 times the maximum recommended human daily oral dose on mg/m^2 basis). In the 1-year toxicity studies in dogs, zafirlukast produced an increase in absolute and relative uterine and ovarian weights at an oral dose of 150 mg/kg, resulting in approximately 85 times the systemic exposure (AUC_{0-12h}) in humans at the maximum recommended human oral daily dose.

Pregnancy: The safety of zafirlukast in human pregnancy has not been established. The potential risks should be weighed against the benefits of continuing therapy during pregnancy; zafirlukast should be used only if clearly needed.

No teratogenicity was observed in the following species for the given oral doses (the approximate equivalence to the maximum recommended human daily oral dose on a mg/m^2 basis is given in brackets): mice 1600 mg/kg/day (160 times); rats 2000 mg/kg/day (400 times); cynomolgus monkeys 2000 mg/kg/day (800 times).

At these doses, maternal toxicity was manifested in rats (as deaths and increased incidence of early fetal resorption), and cynomolgus monkeys (as spontaneous abortions). There are no adequate and well-controlled trials in pregnant women. Because animal reproduction studies are not always predictive of human response, zafirlukast should be used during pregnancy only if clearly needed.

Lactation: Zafirlukast is excreted in human breast milk. Following repeated 40 mg twice-a-day dosing in healthy women, average steady-state concentrations of zafirlukast in breast milk were 50 ng/mL compared to 255 ng/mL in plasma. Because of the potential for tumorigenicity shown for zafirlukast in mouse and rat studies and the enhanced sensitivity of neonatal rats and dogs to the adverse effects of zafirlukast, Accolate should not be administered to mothers who are breast-feeding.

Geriatrics: A total of 8094 patients were exposed to zafirlukast in North American and European short-term placebo-controlled clinical trials. Of these, 243 patients were elderly (age 65 years and older). No overall difference in adverse events was seen in the elderly patients, except for an increase in the frequency of infection among zafirlukast treated elderly patients compared to placebo treated elderly patients (7.0% vs 2.9%). The infections were not severe, occurred mostly in the lower respiratory tract, and did not necessitate withdrawal of therapy.

An open-label, uncontrolled, 4-week trial of 3759 asthma patients compared the safety and efficacy of zafirlukast 20 mg given twice daily in 3 patient age groups, adolescents (12 to 17 years), adults (18 to 65 years), and elderly (greater than 65 years). A higher percentage of elderly patients (n=384) reported adverse events when compared to adults and adolescents. These elderly patients showed less improvement in efficacy measures. In the elderly patients, adverse events occurring in greater than 1% of the population included headache (4.7%), diarrhea and nausea (1.8%) and pharyngitis (1.3%). The elderly reported the lowest percentage of infections of all three age groups in this study.

Drug Interactions: Zafirlukast may be administered with other therapies routinely used in the management of asthma and allergy. Examples of agents which have been coadministered with zafirlukast without adverse interaction include inhaled steroids, inhaled and oral bronchodilator therapy, antihistamines and antibiotics.

Coadministration with:

- erythromycin will result in decreased plasma levels of zafirlukast. In a drug interaction study in 11 asthmatic patients, coadministration of a single dose of zafirlukast (40 mg) with erythromycin (500 mg 3 times daily for 5 days) to steady-state resulted in decreased mean plasma levels of zafirlukast by approximately 40% due to a decrease in zafirlukast bioavailability.
- ASA (e.g., Aspirin) may result in increased plasma levels of zafirlukast. Coadministration of zafirlukast (40 mg/day) with ASA (650 mg 4 times daily) resulted in mean increased plasma levels of zafirlukast by approximately 45%.
- theophylline may result in decreased plasma levels of zafirlukast, without effect on plasma theophylline levels. Coadministration of zafirlukast (80 mg/day) at steady-state with a single dose of a liquid theophylline preparation (6 mg/kg) in 13 asthmatic patients resulted in decreased mean plasma levels of zafirlukast by approximately 30%, but no effect on plasma theophylline levels was observed. Paradoxically, postmarketing surveillance revealed rare cases of patients experiencing increased theophylline levels (with or without theophylline toxicity symptoms) when zafirlukast was coadministered. The mechanism of action for this interaction is unknown.
- terfenadine decreases zafirlukast AUC, but has no effect on plasma terfenadine levels. In a drug interaction study in 16 healthy male volunteers, coadministration of zafirlukast (320 mg/day), with terfenadine (60 mg twice daily) to steady-state resulted in a decrease in the mean C_{max} (-66%) and AUC (-54%) of zafirlukast. No effect of zafirlukast on terfenadine plasma concentrations or ECG parameters (i.e., QTc interval) was seen. No formal drug-drug interaction studies between zafirlukast and other drugs known to be metabolized by the P450 3A4 (CYP 3A4) isoenzymes have been conducted (see Cytochrome P450 Enzyme Inhibition).
- warfarin increases in prothrombin time by approximately 35%. In a drug interaction study in 16 healthy male volunteers, coadministration of multiple doses of zafirlukast (160 mg/day) to steady-state with a single 25 mg dose of warfarin resulted in a significant increase in the mean AUC (+63%) and half-life (+36%) of S-warfarin. The mean prothrombin time (PT) increased by approximately 35%. This interaction is probably due to an inhibition by zafirlukast of the cytochrome P450 2C9 isoenzyme system. Patients on oral warfarin anticoagulant therapy and zafirlukast should have their prothrombin times monitored closely and anticoagulant dose adjusted accordingly (see Warnings).

Oral contraceptives may be administered with zafirlukast without adverse interaction. In a single-blind, parallel-group, 3-week study in 39 healthy female subjects taking oral contraceptives, 40 mg twice daily of zafirlukast had no significant effect on ethinyl estradiol plasma concentrations or contraceptive efficacy.

Cytochrome P450 Enzyme Inhibition: Aside from warfarin and terfenadine, no formal zafirlukast drug-drug interaction studies have been conducted with other drugs known to be metabolized by cytochrome P450 isoenzymes. However, care should be exercised when zafirlukast is coadministered with metabolised drugs such as: tolbutamide, phenytoin, carbamazepine (isozyme 2C9); dihydropyridine calcium channel blockers, cyclosporine, cisapride, astemizole (isozyme CYP 3A4).

Food Interaction: Zafirlukast bioavailability may be altered when taken with a meal (see Pharmacology, Pharmacokinetics).

ADVERSE EFFECTS: The adverse drug reactions that have been associated with Accolate (zafirlukast) treatment in adults and children (12 years of age and older) are in Table 3. Frequencies are based on pooled data from 45 randomized, double-blind, placebo-controlled studies and post-marketing data. The clinical trials involved more than 12 000 patients treated with either Accolate or placebo.

Table 3: ACCOLATE

Adverse Drug Reactions

Frequency	System Organ Class	Reaction
Very common ≥10% (>1/10)	Infections and Infestations	Infection
Common 1% to 10% (>1/100, <1/10)	Gastrointestinal Disorders	Nausea Vomiting Diarrhoea Abdominal Pain
	Hepatobiliary Disorders	Elevations in transaminase levels
	Musculoskeletal and Connective Tissue Disorders	Myalgia
	Nervous System Disorders	Headache
	Skin and Subcutaneous Tissue Disorders	Rash[a]
Uncommon 0.1% to 1% (>1/1000, <1/100)	General Disorders and Administration Site Conditions	Oedema[a] Malaise[a]
	Immune System Disorders	Hypersensitivity[a]
	Hepatobiliary Disorders	Hyperbilirubinemia
	Musculoskeletal and Connective Tissue Disorders	Arthralgia
	Psychiatric Disorders	Insomnia[a]
	Skin and Subcutaneous Tissue Disorders	Pruritus[a] Urticaria[a]
Rare ≥0.01% to <0.1% (>1/10 000, <1/1000)	Hepatobiliary Disorders	Hepatitis
	Immune System Disorders	Angioedema[a]
	Injury, Poisoning and Procedural Complications	Bruising[a]
	Skin and Subcutaneous Tissue Disorders	Blister[a]
	Vascular Disorders	Bleeding disorders[a] (including thrombocytopenia, haemoptysis, haematemesis, haemorrhage and rectal bleeding)
Very rare <0.01% (<1/10 000)	Blood and Lymphatic System Disorders	Agranulocytosis[a,b]
	Hepatobiliary Disorders	Fulminant hepatitis[b] Hepatic failure[b]

[a] These reactions have usually resolved following cessation of therapy.
[b] Frequency is based on post-marketing data.

Hepatic Effects: Elevations of one or more liver enzymes have occurred in patients receiving ACCOLATE in controlled clinical trials. In clinical trials, most of these cases have been observed in asymptomatic patients at doses four times higher than the recommended dose. Hepatic events (which have occurred predominantly in females) have been reported from post-marketing adverse event surveillance of patients (total exposure of more than 2.6 million patient years) who have received the recommended dose of Accolate (40 mg/day). Rarely reports of symptomatic hepatitis (with or without hyperbilirubinemia) have been associated with the use of Accolate. In most, but not all, post-marketing reports, the patient's symptoms abated and the liver enzymes returned to normal or near normal after stopping Accolate. In very rare cases, patients have progressed to fulminant hepatitis and/or hepatic failure in some cases resulting in liver transplantation and/or death (see Warnings).

Infections and Age: In placebo-controlled clinical trials, an increased incidence of infection has been observed in elderly patients given Accolate. These infections were mostly mild in intensity and predominantly affected the respiratory tract and did not necessitate withdrawal from Accolate therapy.

Eosinophilic Conditions: In rare cases, patients with asthma on anti-leukotriene medications, including Accolate, may present with systemic eosinophilia, eosinophilic pneumonia or clinical features of systematic vasculitis consistent with Churg-Strauss syndrome, a condition which is often treated with systemic corticosteroid therapy. These events usually, but not always, have been associated with the reduction and/or withdrawal of steroid therapy. Physicians should be alert to eosinophilia, vasculitic rash, worsening pulmonary symptoms, cardiac complications, and/or neuropathy presenting in their patients. The possibility that leukotriene receptor antagonists, including Accolate, may be associated with the emergence of Churg-Strauss syndrome can neither be excluded nor established (see Precautions).

OVERDOSE:

Symptoms: No deaths occurred at oral zafirlukast doses of 2000 mg/kg in mice (approximately 200 times the maximum recommended human daily oral dose on a mg/m² basis), 2000 mg/kg in rats (approximately 400 times the maximum recommended human daily oral dose on a mg/m² basis), and 500 mg/kg in dogs (approximately 330 times the maximum recommended human daily oral dose on a mg/m² basis).

Treatment: Reports of overdose with zafirlukast have been received. In reports with excessive zafirlukast doses, no significant symptoms have been observed. It is reasonable to employ the usual supportive measures in the event of an overdose; e.g., remove unabsorbed material from the gastrointestinal tract, employ clinical monitoring, and institute supportive therapy, if required.

For management of a suspected drug overdose, CPhA recommends that you contact your **regional Poison Control Centre**. See the *CPS* Directory section for a list of Poison Control Centres.

DOSAGE: Zafirlukast is indicated for the chronic treatment of asthma and should be taken regularly as prescribed, even during symptom-free periods.

Zafirlukast is not a bronchodilator, and should not be used to treat acute episodes of asthma.

Patients receiving zafirlukast should be instructed not to decrease the dose or stop taking any other antiasthma medications unless instructed by a physician.

Adults and Children Aged 12 Years and Over: The recommended dose is 20 mg, twice daily for a total daily dose of 40 mg.

Since food reduces the bioavailability of zafirlukast, the drug should be taken at least 1 hour before or 2 hours after meals.

Elderly: The clearance of zafirlukast is reduced in patients 65 years of age and older such that C_{max} and AUC are approximately 2- to 3-fold greater than those of younger patients. However, accumulation of zafirlukast is not evident in elderly patients.

No overall difference in adverse events was seen in the elderly patients, except for an increase in the frequency of infection among zafirlukast-treated elderly patients compared to placebo-treated elderly patients (7.0% vs 2.9%). The infections were not severe, occurred mostly in the lower respiratory tract and did not necessitate withdrawal of therapy (see also Precautions and Pharmacology).

Children: The safety and efficacy in children under 12 years have not been established.

Renal Impairment: Dosage adjustment is not required in patients with renal impairment.

Hepatic Impairment: Zafirlukast is contraindicated in patients with hepatic impairment, including hepatic cirrhosis.

The clearance of zafirlukast is reduced in patients with stable alcoholic cirrhosis such that C_{max} and AUC are approximately 50 to 60% greater than those of normal adults.

INFORMATION FOR THE PATIENT: Published in e-CPS, available by subscription at www.e-cps.ca.

SUPPLIED: Each white to off-white, round, biconvex, film-coated, intagliated tablet contains: zafirlukast 20 mg. Nonmedicinal ingredients: croscarmellose sodium, hypromellose, lactose monohydrate, magnesium stearate, microcrystalline cellulose, povidone and titanium dioxide. Packs of 60. Store between 15 and 30°C.

(Shown in Product Identification Section)

The reader is invited to consult CPhA's monograph **ACE Inhibitors**.

Accupril™

quinapril HCl

Angiotensin Converting Enzyme Inhibitor

Pfizer

Date of Preparation: January 5, 2001
Date of Revision: September 3, 2009

PHARMACOLOGY: ACCUPRIL (quinapril hydrochloride) is a nonpeptide, nonsulphydryl inhibitor of angiotensin converting enzyme (ACE), which is used in the treatment of hypertension.

Angiotensin converting enzyme (ACE) is a peptidyl dipeptidase that catalyzes the conversion of angiotensin I to the vasoconstrictor angiotensin II. After absorption, quinapril is rapidly de-esterified to quinaprilat (quinapril diacid), its principal active metabolite. Its primary mode of action is to inhibit circulating and tissue ACE, thereby decreasing vasopressor activity and aldosterone secretion. Although the decrease in aldosterone is small, it results in a small increase in serum K^+ (see Precautions). Removal of angiotensin II negative feedback on renin secretion leads to increased plasma renin activity. Although ACCUPRIL had antihypertensive activity in all races studied, black hypertensive patients (usually a low-renin hypertensive population) had a smaller average response to ACE inhibitor monotherapy than non-black patients.

ACE is identical to kininase II. Thus, quinapril may interfere with the degradation of bradykinin, a potent peptide vasodilator. However, it is not known whether this system contributes to the therapeutic effects of ACCUPRIL.

The antihypertensive effect of quinapril outlasts its inhibitory effect on circulating ACE in animal studies. Tissue ACE inhibition more closely correlates with the duration of antihypertensive effects and this may be related to enzyme binding characteristics as shown for quinapril on purified tissue ACE from human kidney and heart.

Pharmacokinetics: Following oral administration of ACCUPRIL, peak plasma concentrations of quinapril occur within one hour. Based on the recovery of quinapril and its metabolites in urine, the extent of absorption is at least 60%. Following absorption, quinapril is de-esterified to its major active metabolite, quinaprilat (quinapril diacid) a potent ACE inhibitor, and to minor inactive metabolites. Quinapril has an apparent half-life in plasma of approximately one hour. Peak plasma quinaprilat concentrations occur approximately 2 hours after an oral dose of ACCUPRIL. Quinaprilat is eliminated primarily by renal excretion and has an effective accumulation half-life of approximately 3 hours. Quinaprilat has an elimination half-life in plasma of approximately 2 hours with a prolonged terminal phase of 25 hours. Approximately 97% of either quinapril or quinaprilat circulating in plasma is bound to proteins.

Pharmacokinetic studies in patients with end-stage renal disease on chronic hemodialysis or continuous ambulatory peritoneal dialysis indicate that dialysis has little effect on the elimination of quinapril and quinaprilat.

The disposition of quinapril and quinaprilat in patients with renal insufficiency is similar to that in patients with normal renal function until creatinine clearance is 60 mL/min or less. With creatinine clearance less than 60 mL/min, peak and trough quinaprilat concentrations increase, apparent half-life increases, and time to steady state may be delayed. The elimination of quinaprilat may be reduced in elderly patients (>65 years) and in those with heart failure; this reduction is attributable to decrease in renal function (see Dosage). Quinaprilat concentrations are reduced in patients with alcoholic cirrhosis due to impaired de-esterification of quinapril.

The rate and extent of quinapril absorption are diminished moderately (approximately 25-30%) when ACCUPRIL tablets are administered during a high-fat meal. However, no effect on quinapril absorption occurs when taken during a regular meal.

Studies in rats indicate that quinapril and its metabolites do not cross the blood-brain barrier.

Pharmacodynamics: Administration of 10 to 40 mg of ACCUPRIL to patients with essential hypertension results in a reduction of both sitting and standing blood pressure with minimal effect on heart rate. Antihypertensive activity commences within one hour with peak effects usually achieved by 2 to 4 hours after dosing. Achievement of maximum blood pressure lowering effects may require 2 weeks of therapy in some patients. At the recommended doses, antihypertensive effects are maintained throughout the 24-hour dosing interval in most patients. While the dose response relationship is relatively flat, a dose of 40 mg was somewhat more effective at trough than 10-20 mg, and twice daily dosing tended to give a somewhat lower blood pressure than once daily dosing with the same total daily dose. The antihypertensive effect of ACCUPRIL was maintained during long-term therapy with no evidence of loss of effectiveness.

Hemodynamic assessments in patients with essential hypertension indicate that blood pressure reduction produced by quinapril is accompanied by a reduction in total peripheral resistance and renal vascular resistance with little or no change in heart rate and cardiac index. There was an increase in renal blood flow which was not significant. Little or no change in glomerular filtration rate or filtration fraction was observed.

Quinapril has been shown to reduce microalbuminuria in patients with essential hypertension independently of changes in systemic blood pressure.

When ACCUPRIL is given together with thiazide-type diuretics, the antihypertensive effects are approximately additive.

Administration of ACCUPRIL to patients with congestive heart failure (CHF) reduces peripheral vascular resistance, systolic and diastolic blood pressure, pulmonary capillary wedge pressure, and increases cardiac output. The onset of effects was observed within one hour and maximal effects occurred at 1.25 to 4 hours after administration of ACCUPRIL. Peak hemodynamic effects correlated well with peak plasma levels of quinaprilat (1 to 4 hours after administration).

Exercise tolerance was improved with ACCUPRIL therapy.

The effect of ACCUPRIL on survival in patients with heart failure has not been evaluated.

Therapeutic effects appear to be the same for elderly (>65 years of age) and younger adult patients given the same daily dosages, with no increase in adverse events in elderly patients.

The antihypertensive effect of angiotensin converting enzyme inhibitors is generally lower in black patients than in non-blacks.

INDICATIONS: Hypertension: ACCUPRIL (quinapril hydrochloride) is indicated in the treatment of essential hypertension. It is usually administered in association with other drugs, particularly thiazide diuretics.

In using ACCUPRIL, consideration should be given to the risk of angioedema (see Warnings).

ACCUPRIL should normally be used in those patients in whom treatment with a diuretic or a beta-blocker was found ineffective or has been associated with unacceptable adverse effects. ACCUPRIL can also be tried as an initial agent in those patients in whom use of diuretics and/or beta-blockers is contraindicated or in patients with medical conditions in which these drugs frequently cause serious adverse effects.

The safety and efficacy of ACCUPRIL in renovascular hypertension has not been established; therefore, use in this condition is not recommended.

Congestive Heart Failure: ACCUPRIL is indicated in the treatment of congestive heart failure as adjunctive therapy when added to diuretics and/or digitalis glycosides.

Treatment with ACCUPRIL should be initiated under close medical supervision.

CONTRAINDICATIONS: ACCUPRIL (quinapril hydrochloride) is contraindicated in patients who are hypersensitive to this product, and in patients with a history of angioedema related to previous treatment with an ACE inhibitor.

Published data suggest that quinapril is contraindicated in women who are pregnant, intend to become pregnant, or of child-bearing potential who are not using adequate contraceptive measures. Quinapril should be administered to women of childbearing age only when such patients are highly unlikely to conceive and have been informed of the potential hazards to the fetus (see Warnings and Adverse Effects).

WARNINGS:

Serious Warnings and Precautions
When used in pregnancy, angiotensin converting enzyme (ACE) inhibitors can cause injury or even death of the developing fetus. When pregnancy is detected, ACCUPRIL should be discontinued as soon as possible.

Head and Neck Angioedema: Head and neck angioedema has been reported in patients treated with ACCUPRIL (quinapril hydrochloride). Angioedema associated with laryngeal involvement may be fatal. If laryngeal stridor or angioedema of the face, tongue, or glottis occurs, ACCUPRIL should be discontinued immediately, the patient treated appropriately in accordance with accepted medical care, and carefully observed until the swelling disappears. In instances where swelling is confined to the face and lips, the condition generally resolves without treatment, although antihistamines may be useful in relieving symptoms. Where there is involvement of the tongue, glottis or larynx, likely to cause airway obstruction, appropriate therapy (including but not limited to 0.3 to 0.5 mL of subcutaneous epinephrine solution 1:1000) should be administered promptly (see Adverse Effects).

The incidence of angioedema during ACE inhibitor therapy has been reported to be higher in black than in non-black patients.

Patients with a history of angioedema unrelated to ACE inhibitor therapy may be at increased risk of angioedema while receiving an ACE inhibitor (see Contraindications).

Intestinal Angioedema: Intestinal angioedema has been reported in patients treated with ACE inhibitors. These patients presented with abdominal pain (with or without nausea or vomiting); in some cases there was no prior history of facial angioedema and C-1 esterase levels were normal. The angioedema was diagnosed by procedures including abdominal CT scan or ultrasound, or at surgery, and symptoms resolved after stopping the ACE inhibitor. Intestinal angioedema should be included in the differential diagnosis of patients on ACE inhibitors presenting with abdominal pain.

Hypotension: Symptomatic hypotension has occurred after administration of ACCUPRIL, usually after the first or second dose or when the dose was increased. It is more likely to occur in patients who are volume depleted by diuretic therapy, dietary salt restriction, dialysis, diarrhea, or vomiting. In patients with ischemic heart or cerebrovascular disease, an excessive fall in blood pressure could result in a myocardial infarction or cerebrovascular accident (see Adverse Effects). Because of the potential fall in blood pressure in these patients, therapy with ACCUPRIL should be started under close medical supervision (see Dosage). Such patients should be followed closely for the first weeks of treatment and whenever the dose of ACCUPRIL is increased. In patients with severe congestive heart failure, with or without associated renal insufficiency, excessive hypotension has been observed and may be associated with oliguria and/or progressive azotemia, and rarely with acute renal failure and/or death.

If hypotension occurs, the patient should be placed in supine position and, if necessary, receive an intravenous infusion of 0.9% sodium chloride. A transient hypotensive response is not a contraindication to further doses which usually can be given without difficulty once the blood pressure has increased after volume expansion. However, lower doses of ACCUPRIL and/or reduced concomitant diuretic therapy should be considered.

Neutropenia/Agranulocytosis: Agranulocytosis and bone marrow depression have been caused by ACE inhibitors. Agranulocytosis did occur during ACCUPRIL treatment in one patient with a history of neutropenia during previous captopril therapy. Periodic monitoring of white blood cell counts should be considered, especially in patients with collagen vascular disease and/or renal disease.

Pregnancy: Quinapril is contraindicated in pregnancy (see Contraindications and Adverse Effects). ACE inhibitors can cause fetal and neonatal morbidity and mortality when administered to pregnant women. Several dozen cases have been reported in the world literature. When pregnancy is detected, ACCUPRIL should be discontinued as soon as possible.

The use of ACE inhibitors during the second and third trimesters of pregnancy has been associated with fetal and neonatal injury including hypotension, neonatal skull hypoplasia, anuria, reversible or irreversible renal failure, and death. Oligohydramnios has also been reported, presumably resulting from decreased fetal renal function; oligohydramnios in this setting has been associated with fetal limb contractures, craniofacial deformation, and hypoplastic lung development.

Prematurity, and patent ductus arteriosus and other structural cardiac malformations, as well as neurologic malformations have also been reported, following exposure in the first trimester of pregnancy.

Infants with a history of in utero exposure to ACE inhibitors should be closely observed for hypotension, oliguria, and hyperkalemia. If oliguria occurs, attention should be directed toward support of blood pressure and renal perfusion. Exchange transfusion or dialysis may be required as a means of reversing hypotension and/or substituting for impaired renal function, however; limited experience with those procedures has not been associated with significant clinical benefit.

Hemodialysis and peritoneal dialysis have little effect on the elimination of quinapril and quinaprilat.

If oligohydramnios is observed, a non-stress test (NST), and/or a biophysical profiling (BPP) may be appropriate, depending upon the week of pregnancy. If concerns regarding fetal well-being still persist, a contraction stress testing (CST) should be considered. Patients and physicians should be aware, however, that oligohydramnios may not appear until after the fetus has sustained irreversible injury.

Animal Data: No fetotoxic or teratogenic effects were observed in rats at doses as high as 300 mg/kg/day (180 times the maximum daily human dose), despite maternal toxicity at 150 mg/kg/day. Offspring body weights were reduced in rats treated late in gestation and during lactation with doses of 25 mg/kg/day or more. Quinapril hydrochloride was not teratogenic in rabbits; however, maternal and embryo toxicity were seen in some rabbits at 1 mg/kg/day.

No adverse effects on fertility or reproduction were observed in rats at dose levels up to 100 mg/kg/day (60 times the maximum daily human dose).

PRECAUTIONS: Renal Impairment: As a consequence of inhibiting the renin-angiotensin-aldosterone system, changes in renal function have been seen in susceptible individuals. In patients whose renal function may depend on the activity of the renin-angiotensin-aldosterone system, such as patients with bilateral renal artery stenosis, unilateral renal artery stenosis to a solitary kidney, or severe congestive heart failure, treatment with agents that inhibit this system has been associated with oliguria, progressive azotemia, and rarely, acute renal failure and/or death. In susceptible patients, concomitant diuretic use may further increase risk (see Adverse Effects and Dosage).

Use of ACCUPRIL (quinapril hydrochloride) should include appropriate assessment of renal function (see Adverse Effects and Dosage).

Anaphylactoid Reactions during Membrane Exposure: Anaphylactoid reactions have been reported in patients dialysed with high-flux membranes (e.g.: polyacrylonitrile [PAN]) and treated concomitantly with an ACE inhibitor. Dialysis should be stopped immediately if symptoms such as nausea, abdominal cramps, burning, angioedema, shortness of breath and severe hypotension occur. Symptoms are not relieved by antihistamines. In these patients consideration should be given to using a different type of dialysis membrane or a different class of antihypertensive agents.

Anaphylactoid Reactions during LDL Apheresis: Rarely, patients receiving ACE inhibitors during low density lipoprotein apheresis with dextran sulfate have experienced life-threatening anaphylactoid reactions. These reactions were avoided by temporarily withholding the ACE inhibitor therapy prior to each apheresis.

Anaphylactoid Reactions during Desensitization: There have been isolated reports of patients experiencing sustained life threatening anaphylactoid reactions while receiving ACE inhibitors during desensitizing treatment with hymenoptera (bees, wasps) venom. In the same patients, these reactions have been avoided when ACE inhibitors were temporarily withheld for at least 24 hours, but they have reappeared upon inadvertent rechallenge to an ACE inhibitor.

Hyperkalemia and Potassium-Sparing Diuretics: Elevated serum potassium (greater than 5.7 mEq/L) was observed in approximately 2% of patients receiving ACCUPRIL. In most cases these were isolated values which resolved despite continued therapy. Hyperkalemia was a cause of discontinuation of therapy in less than 0.1% of hypertensive patients. Risk factors for the development of hyperkalemia may include renal insufficiency, diabetes mellitus, and the concomitant use of agents to treat hypokalemia (see Precautions, Drug Interactions and Adverse Effects).

Hypoglycemia and Diabetes: ACE inhibitors may reduce insulin resistance and may lead to hypoglycemia in diabetic patients on insulin or oral hypoglycemic agents; closer monitoring of diabetic patients may be required.

Valvular Stenosis: There is concern on theoretical grounds that patients with aortic stenosis might be at particular risk of decreased coronary perfusion when treated with vasodilators because they do not develop as much afterload reduction.

Surgery/Anaesthesia: In patients undergoing major surgery or during anaesthesia with agents that produce hypotension, ACCUPRIL will block angiotensin II formation secondary to compensatory renin release. If hypotension occurs and is considered to be due to this mechanism, it can be corrected by volume expansion.

Patients with Impaired Liver Function: Hepatitis (hepatocellular and/or cholestatic), elevations of liver enzymes and/or serum bilirubin have occurred during therapy with other ACE inhibitors in patients with or without pre-existing liver abnormalities. In most cases the changes were reversed on discontinuation of the drug.

Elevations of liver enzymes and/or serum bilirubin have been reported for ACCUPRIL (see Adverse Effects). Should the patient receiving ACCUPRIL experience any unexplained symptoms particularly during the first weeks or months of treatment, it is recommended that a full set of liver function tests and any other necessary investigation be carried out. Discontinuation of ACCUPRIL should be considered when appropriate.

There are no adequate studies in patients with cirrhosis and/or liver dysfunction. ACCUPRIL should be used with particular caution in patients with pre-existing liver abnormalities. In such patients baseline liver function tests should be obtained before administration of the drug and close monitoring of response and metabolic effects should apply.

Quinapril, when combined with a diuretic should be used with caution in patients with impaired hepatic function or progressive liver disease, since minor alterations of fluid and electrolyte balance may precipitate hepatic coma. The metabolism of quinapril to quinaprilat is normally dependant upon hepatic esterase. Quinaprilat concentrations are reduced in patients with alcoholic cirrhosis due to impaired deesterification of quinapril.

Cough: Cough has been reported with the use of ACE inhibitors, including quinapril. Characteristically, the cough is dry and persistent and usually disappears only after withdrawal or lowering of the dose of ACCUPRIL. ACE inhibitor-induced cough should be considered as part of the differential diagnosis of the cough.

Lactation: The presence of concentrations of ACE inhibitor have been reported in human milk. Use of ACE inhibitors is not recommended during breast-feeding.

Children: The safety and effectiveness of ACCUPRIL in children have not been established, therefore use in this age group is not recommended.

Geriatrics: Of the total number of subjects in clinical studies of ACCUPRIL, 21% were 65 and over. (There was no distinction between patients over 65 or over 75 years.) No overall differences in safety or effectiveness were observed between these subjects and younger subjects, and other reported clinical experience has not identified differences in responses between the elderly and younger patients, but greater sensitivity of some older individuals cannot be ruled out.

This drug is known to be substantially excreted by the kidney, and the risk of toxic reactions to this drug may be greater in patients with impaired renal function. Because elderly patients are more likely to have decreased renal function, care should be taken in dose selection, and it may be useful to monitor renal function (see Adverse Effects and Dosage).

Elderly patients exhibited increased area under the plasma concentration time curve and peak levels for quinaprilat compared to values observed in younger patients; this appeared to relate to decreased renal function rather than to age itself.

Occupational Hazards: Driving and Operating Machinery: The ability to engage in activities such as operating machinery or operating a motor vehicle may be impaired, especially when initiating quinapril therapy.

Drug Interactions: Concomitant Diuretic Therapy: Patients concomitantly taking ACE inhibitors and diuretics, and especially those in whom diuretic therapy was recently instituted, may occasionally experience an excessive reduction of blood pressure after initiation of therapy. The possibility of hypotensive effects after the first dose of ACCUPRIL can be minimized by either discontinuing the diuretic or increasing the salt intake (except in patients with heart failure), prior to initiation of treatment with ACCUPRIL. If it is not possible to discontinue the diuretic, the starting dose of ACCUPRIL should be reduced and the patient should be closely observed for several hours following initial dose and until blood pressure has stabilized (see Warnings and Dosage).

Agents Increasing Serum Potassium: Since ACCUPRIL decreases aldosterone production, elevation of serum potassium may occur. Potassium sparing diuretics such as spironolactone, triamterene or amiloride, or potassium supplements should be given only for documented hypokalemia and with caution and frequent monitoring of serum potassium, since they may lead to a significant increase in serum potassium. Salt substitutes which contain potassium should also be used with caution.

Agents Causing Renin Release: The antihypertensive effect of ACCUPRIL is augmented by antihypertensive agents that cause renin release (e.g. diuretics).

Agents Affecting Sympathetic Activity: Agents affecting sympathetic activity (e.g. ganglionic blocking agents or adrenergic neuron blocking agents) may be used with caution. Beta-adrenergic blocking drugs add some further antihypertensive effect to ACCUPRIL.

Tetracycline: Concomitant administration of tetracycline with ACCUPRIL reduced the absorption of tetracycline in healthy volunteers (by 28-37%) due to the presence of magnesium carbonate as an excipient in the formulation. This interaction should be considered with concomitant use of ACCUPRIL and tetracycline or other drugs which interact with magnesium.

Lithium: As with other drugs which eliminate sodium, the lithium elimination may be reduced. Therefore, the serum lithium levels should be monitored carefully if lithium salts are to be administered.

Other Agents: In single dose pharmacokinetic studies, no important changes in pharmacokinetic parameters were observed when ACCUPRIL was used concomitantly with propranolol, hydrochlorothiazide, digoxin, or cimetidine. No change in prothrombin time occurred when ACCUPRIL and warfarin were given together.

Information to Be Provided to the Patient:

Serious Warnings and Precautions
ACCUPRIL should not be used during pregnancy. Patients should be advised to stop medication and contact their physician as soon as possible if they discover that they are pregnant while taking ACCUPRIL.

Note: As with many other drugs, certain advice to patients being treated with ACCUPRIL is warranted. This information is intended to aid in the safe and effective use of this medication. It is not a disclosure of all possible adverse or intended effects.

Angioedema: Angioedema, including laryngeal edema, may occur especially following the first dose of ACCUPRIL. Patients should be so advised and told to report immediately any signs or symptoms suggesting angioedema, such as swelling of face, extremities, eyes, lips, tongue, difficulty in swallowing or breathing. They should immediately stop taking ACCUPRIL and consult with their physician.

Hypotension: Patients should be cautioned to report light-headedness, especially during the first few days of ACCUPRIL therapy. If actual syncope occurs, the patients should be told to discontinue the drug and consult with their physician.

All patients should be cautioned that excessive perspiration and dehydration may lead to an excessive fall in blood pressure because of reduction in fluid volume. Other causes of volume depletion such as vomiting or diarrhea may also lead to a fall in blood pressure; patients should be advised to consult with their physician.

Agranulocytosis/Neutropenia: Patients should be told to report promptly to their physician any indication of infection (e.g. sore throat, fever), as this may be a sign of neutropenia.

Impaired Liver Function: Patients should be advised to return to the physician if he/she experiences any symptoms possibly related to liver dysfunction. This would include "viral-like symptoms" in the first weeks to months of therapy (such as fever, malaise, muscle pain, rash or adenopathy which are possible indicators of hypersensitivity reactions), or if abdominal pain, nausea or vomiting, loss of appetite, jaundice, itching or any other unexplained symptoms occur during therapy.

Hyperkalemia: Patients should be told not to use salt substitutes containing potassium without consulting their physician.

Surgery: Patients planning to undergo surgery and/or anesthesia should be told to inform their physician that they are taking an ACE inhibitor.

Pregnancy and Breast-Feeding: Taking ACCUPRIL during pregnancy can cause injury and even death to the developing fetus. This medicine should not be used by women who are pregnant, intend to become pregnant, or could become pregnant and who are not using adequate contraceptive measures (see Contraindications, Warnings and Adverse Effects). Patients should be advised to stop medication and report to their physician as soon as possible if they become pregnant while taking ACCUPRIL. It is possible that ACCUPRIL passes into breast milk. Patients should be advised not to breast-feed while taking ACCUPRIL.

ADVERSE EFFECTS: Hypertension: ACCUPRIL (quinapril hydrochloride) monotherapy has been evaluated for safety in 2005 hypertensive patients enrolled in placebo-controlled clinical trials. These trials included 313 elderly patients. There was no increase in the incidence of adverse events in elderly patients given the same daily dosages. ACCUPRIL has been evaluated for long-term safety in over 1100 patients treated for one year or more. Adverse events were usually mild and transient in nature.

The most serious adverse event was angioedema (0.1%). Renal insufficiency (1 case), agranulocytosis (1 case) and mild azotemia (2 cases in CHF patients) have been reported. Myocardial infarction and cerebrovascular accident occurred, possibly secondary to excessive hypotension in high risk patients (see Warnings and Precautions).

The most frequent adverse events in controlled clinical trials were headache (8.1%), dizziness (4.1%), cough (3.2%), fatigue (3.2%), rhinitis (3.2%), nausea and/or vomiting (2.3%), and abdominal pain (2.0%).

Discontinuation of therapy because of adverse events was required in 4.7% of patients treated with ACCUPRIL in placebo controlled trials.

Congestive Heart Failure (CHF): At least one adverse event was experienced by 605 (55%) of the 1108 patients with congestive heart failure. Five hundred twenty five of these patients were evaluated for safety in controlled clinical trials. The frequencies of adverse events were similar for both sexes as well as for younger (< 65 years) and older (≥ 65 years) patients.

The most serious non-fatal adverse events/reactions were angioedema (0.1%), chest pain of unknown origin (0.8%), angina pectoris (0.4%), hypotension (0.1%), and impaired renal function (see Precautions). Myocardial infarct, and cerebrovascular accident occurred (see Warnings). Rare cases of eosinophilic pneumonitis have been reported. Hepatitis or hepatic failure have rarely been observed with other ACE inhibitors.

The most frequent adverse events in controlled clinical trials were dizziness (11.2%), cough (7.6%), chest pain (6.5%), dyspnea (5.5%), fatigue (5.1%), and nausea/vomiting (5.0%).

Discontinuation due to adverse events in controlled clinical trials was required for 41 (8.0%) patients. Hypotension (0.8%) and cough (0.8%) were the most common reasons for withdrawal.

Adverse events occurring in ≥ 0.5% of 2005 hypertensive patients treated with ACCUPRIL monotherapy and in 525 patients with congestive heart failure treated with ACCUPRIL as adjunctive therapy, in controlled clinical trials, are presented in Table 1.

Table 1: ACCUPRIL

Adverse Events in Patients (≥ 0.5%) with Hypertension and Congestive Heart Failure in Controlled Clinical Trials (Irrespective of Causal Relationship)

	Hypertension[a] % Patients (N=2005)	Congestive Heart Failure[b] % Patients (N=525)
Body as a Whole		
Chest Pain	1.2	6.5
Fatigue	3.2	5.1
Headache	8.1	3.2
Back Pain	1.3	1.7
Asthenia	1.0	1.7
Peripheral Edema	0.9	1.5
Generalized Edema	0.7	0.2
Cardiovascular System		
Hypotension	1.0	3.4
Angina Pectoris	0.2	2.3
Palpitation	0.4	1.3
Tachycardia	0.2	1.1
Myocardial Infarct	—	0.6
Arrhythmia	0.1	0.6
Digestive System		
Nausea and/or vomiting	2.3	5.0
Abdominal pain	2.0	2.5
Diarrhea	1.9	3.4
Dyspepsia	1.9	1.5
Dry mouth or throat	0.4	0.8
Musculoskeletal System		
Myalgia	1.7	2.9
Nervous System		
Dizziness	4.1	11.2
Insomnia	1.3	1.1
Paresthesia	1.0	1.3
Nervousness	1.0	0.2
Somnolence	0.9	0.6
Syncope	0.3	0.6
Vertigo	0.4	0.8
Depression	0.6	1.0
Respiratory		
Cough	3.2	7.6
Dyspnea	0.9	5.5
Hemoptysis	—	0.6
Rhinitis	3.2	2.5
Skin and Appendages		
Rash	0.6	1.9

(cont'd)

Table 1: ACCUPRIL *(cont'd)*

Adverse Events in Patients (≥ 0.5%) with Hypertension and Congestive Heart Failure in Controlled Clinical Trials (Irrespective of Causal Relationship)

	Hypertension[a] % Patients (N=2005)	Congestive Heart Failure[b] % Patients (N=525)
Sweating increased	0.8	1.1
Pruritus	0.6	0.4
Urogenital System		
Impotence	0.5	0.2
Special Senses		
Amblyopia	0.3	1.3
Unusual Taste	0.1	0.8
Abnormal Vision	0.1	0.6
Taste Loss	0.2	0.6

[a] ACCUPRIL monotherapy.
[b] ACCUPRIL as adjunctive therapy to diuretic and/or digitalis.

Adverse events occurring in <0.5% of patients with hypertension or congestive heart failure include:
Body as a whole: allergy, face edema, chill, weight increase, dehydration.
Cardiovascular: vasodilatation, cerebrovascular accident, heart failure, ventricular tachycardia, atrial flutter.
Digestive System: constipation, tongue edema, GI hemorrhage, anorexia, bloody stools.
Hemic and Lymphatic System: anemia, including hemolytic anemia, agranulocytosis.
Nervous System: confusion, amnesia, anxiety, arthralgia.
Musculoskeletal System: arthritis.
Respiratory System: asthma, hoarseness.
Skin and Appendages: dermatitis, urticaria, eczema, Stevens-Johnson syndrome.
Urogenital system: dysuria, polyuria, impaired renal function.
Special Senses: tinnitus.
Laboratory Deviations: hematuria, WBC decreased, elevated BUN, hyperglycemia, azotemia.
Clinical adverse experiences probably, possibly, or definitely related, or of uncertain relationship to therapy occurring in 0.5% to ≤ 1.0% of the patients treated with quinapril (with or without concomitant diuretic) in controlled or uncontrolled clinical trials and less frequent events seen in clinical trials or post-marketing experience (indicated by a *) included:
Body as a Whole: anaphylactoid reaction*; photosensitivity reaction*.
Cardiovascular: postural hypotension*, syncope*, vasodilation.
Gastrointestinal: flatulence, pancreatitis*.
Hemic and Lymphatic: thrombocytopenia*.
Integumentary: alopecia*, exfoliative dermatitis*, pemphigus*.
Urogenital: urinary tract infection.
Congenital and Familial/Genetic Disorders: See Contraindications, Warnings, Pregnancy.
Other: athralgia, edema (peripheral and generalized), hemolytic anemia*.
Clinical Laboratory Test Findings: Hematology: See Warnings.
Hyperkalemia: See Precautions.
Creatinine and Blood Urea Nitrogen: Increases (>1.25 times the upper limit of normal) in serum creatinine and blood urea nitrogen were observed in 2% and 2%, respectively, of patients treated with ACCUPRIL alone. Increases are more likely to occur in patients receiving concomitant diuretic therapy than in those on ACCUPRIL alone (see Precautions). These increases often reversed on continued therapy. In controlled studies of heart failure, increases in blood urea nitrogen and serum creatinine were observed in 11% and 8%, respectively, of patients treated with ACCUPRIL. Most often these patients were receiving diuretics with or without digitalis.
Hepatic: Elevations of liver enzymes and/or serum bilirubin have occurred (see Precautions).

OVERDOSE:

Symptoms: No data are available regarding overdosage of ACCUPRIL (quinapril hydrochloride) in humans. The most likely clinical manifestation would be symptoms attributable to severe hypotension, which should be normally treated by intravenous volume expansion with 0.9% sodium chloride. Hemodialysis and peritoneal dialysis have little effect on the elimination of quinapril and quinaprilat.

Treatment: See Symptoms.

For management of a suspected drug overdose, CPhA recommends that you contact your **regional Poison Control Centre**. See the *CPS* Directory section for a list of Poison Control Centres.

DOSAGE: Dosage of ACCUPRIL (quinapril hydrochloride) must be individualized.
Hypertension: Initiation of therapy requires consideration of recent antihypertensive drug treatment, the extent of blood pressure elevation and salt restriction. The dosage of other antihypertensive agents being used with ACCUPRIL may need to be adjusted.
Monotherapy: The recommended initial dose of ACCUPRIL in patients not on diuretics is 10 mg once daily. An initial dose of 20 mg once daily can be considered for patients without advanced age, renal impairment, or concomitant heart failure and who are not volume depleted (see Warnings, Hypotension). Dosage should be adjusted according to blood pressure response, generally at intervals of two to four weeks. A dose of 40 mg daily should not be exceeded.

In some patients treated once daily, the antihypertensive effect may diminish towards the end of the dosing interval. This can be evaluated by measuring blood pressure just prior to dosing to determine whether satisfactory control is being maintained for 24 hours. If it is not, either twice daily administration with the same total daily dose, or an increase in dose should be considered. If blood pressure is not controlled with ACCUPRIL alone, a diuretic may be added. After the addition of a diuretic, it may be possible to reduce the dose of ACCUPRIL.

Concomitant Diuretic Therapy: Symptomatic hypotension occasionally may occur following the initial dose of ACCUPRIL and is more likely in patients who are currently being treated with a diuretic. The diuretic should, if possible, be discontinued for two to three days before beginning therapy with ACCUPRIL to reduce the likelihood of hypotension (see Warnings). If the diuretic cannot be discontinued, an initial dose of 5 mg ACCUPRIL should be used with careful medical supervision for several hours and until blood pressure has stabilized. The dosage of ACCUPRIL should subsequently be titrated (as described above) to the optimal response.

Dosing Adjustment in Renal Impairment: See Precautions and Adverse Effects section for use in hemodialysis patients.

Starting doses should be reduced according to the following guidelines in Table 2.

Patients should subsequently have dosage titrated (as described above) to the optimal response.

Dosage in the Elderly (over 65 years): The recommended initial dosage of ACCUPRIL is 10 mg once daily (depending on renal function), followed by titration (as described above) to the optimal response.

Congestive Heart Failure: ACCUPRIL is indicated as adjunctive therapy to diuretics, and/or cardiac glycosides. Therapy should be initiated under close medical supervision. Blood pressure and renal function should be monitored, both before and during treatment with ACCUPRIL, because severe hypotension and, more rarely, consequent renal failure have been reported (see Warnings and Precautions).

Table 2: ACCUPRIL
Dosing Guideline in Renal Impairment

Creatinine Clearance (mL/min)	Maximum Recommended Initial Dose (mg)
>60	10
30–60	5
10–30	2.5
<10	Insufficient data for dosage recommendation

Initiation of therapy requires consideration of recent diuretic therapy and the possibility of severe salt/volume depletion. If possible, the dose of diuretic should be reduced before beginning treatment, to reduce the likelihood of hypotension. Serum potassium should also be monitored (see Precautions, Drug Interactions).

The recommended starting dose is 5 mg once daily, to be administered under close medical supervision to determine the initial effect on blood pressure. After the initial dose, the patient should be observed for at least two hours, or until the pressure has stabilized for at least an additional hour (see Warnings, Hypotension). This dose may improve symptoms of heart failure, but increases in exercise duration have generally required higher doses. Therefore, if the initial dosage of ACCUPRIL is well tolerated or after effective management of symptomatic hypotension following initiation of therapy, the dose should then be increased gradually to 10 mg once daily, then 20 mg once daily, and to 40 mg per day given in 2 equally divided doses, depending on the patient's response. The maximum daily dose is 40 mg.

The dose titration may be done at weekly intervals, as indicated by the presence of residual signs or symptoms of heart failure. Renal Impairment or Hyponatremia: Kinetic data indicate that ACCUPRIL elimination is dependent on the level of renal function. The recommended initial dose of ACCUPRIL is 5 mg in patients with a creatinine clearance of 30 to 60 mL/min and 2.5 mg in patients with a creatinine clearance of 10 to 30 mL/min. There is insufficient data for dosage recommendation in patients with a creatinine clearance less than 10 mL/min. If the initial dose is well tolerated, ACCUPRIL may be administered the following day as a twice daily regimen. In the absence of excessive hypotension or significant deterioration of renal function, the dose may be increased at weekly intervals based on clinical and hemodynamic response (see Precautions and Adverse Effects).

INFORMATION FOR THE PATIENT: Published in e-CPS, available by subscription at www.e-cps.ca.

SUPPLIED: 5 mg: Each scored, brown, film-coated, elliptical tablet, debossed "PD/527" on one side and "5" on the other, contains: quinapril hydrochloride 5 mg. Nonmedicinal ingredients: candelilla wax, crospovidone, gelatin, hydroxypropylcellulose, hydroxypropylmethylcellulose, lactose, magnesium carbonate, magnesium stearate, polyethylene glycol, synthetic red iron oxide and titanium dioxide. Bottles of 90. Store at controlled room temperature, 15-30°C. Protect from moisture. Dispense in well-closed containers.

10 mg: Each brown, film-coated, triangular tablet, debossed "PD/530" on one side and "10" on the other, contains: quinapril hydrochloride 10 mg. Nonmedicinal ingredients: candelilla wax, crospovidone, gelatin, hydroxypropylcellulose, hydroxypropylmethylcellulose, lactose, magnesium carbonate, magnesium stearate, polyethylene glycol, synthetic red iron oxide and titanium dioxide. Bottles of 90. Store at controlled room temperature, 15-30°C. Protect from moisture. Dispense in well-closed containers.

20 mg: Each brown, film-coated, round tablet, debossed "PD/532" on one side and "20" on the other, contains: quinapril hydrochloride 20 mg. Nonmedicinal ingredients: candelilla wax, crospovidone, gelatin, hydroxypropylcellulose, hydroxypropylmethylcellulose, lactose, magnesium carbonate, magnesium stearate, polyethylene glycol, synthetic red iron oxide and titanium dioxide. Bottles of 90. Store at controlled room temperature, 15-30°C. Protect from moisture. Dispense in well-closed containers.

40 mg: Each brown, film-coated, elliptical tablet, debossed "PD/535" on one side and "40" on the other, contains: quinapril hydrochloride 40 mg. Nonmedicinal ingredients: candelilla wax, crospovidone, gelatin, hydroxypropylcellulose, hydroxypropylmethylcellulose, lactose, magnesium carbonate, magnesium stearate, polyethylene glycol, synthetic red iron oxide and titanium dioxide. Bottles of 90. Store at controlled room temperature, 15-30°C. Protect from moisture. Dispense in well-closed containers.

(Shown in Product Identification Section)

The reader is invited to consult CPhA's monograph **ACE Inhibitors**.

Accuretic™

quinapril HCl—hydrochlorothiazide
Angiotensin Converting Enzyme Inhibitor—Diuretic

Pfizer

Date of Preparation: January 5, 2001
Date of Revision: September 3, 2009

PHARMACOLOGY: Accuretic is a fixed-combination tablet which combines the antihypertensive actions of an angiotensin converting enzyme (ACE) inhibitor, quinapril HCl, and a diuretic, hydrochlorothiazide. In clinical studies, administration of this combination produced greater reductions in blood pressure than the single agents given alone.

Pharmacokinetics: Quinapril: Following oral administration of quinapril, peak plasma concentrations of quinapril occur within 1 hour. Based on the recovery of quinapril and its metabolites in urine, the extent of absorption is at least 60%. Following absorption, quinapril is de-esterified to its major active metabolite, quinaprilat (quinapril diacid), a potent ACE inhibitor, and to minor inactive metabolites. Quinapril has an apparent half-life in plasma of approximately 1 hour. Peak plasma quinaprilat concentrations occur approximately 2 hours after an oral dose of quinapril. Quinaprilat is eliminated primarily by renal excretion and has an effective accumulation half-life of approximately 3 hours. Quinaprilat has an elimination half-life in plasma of approximately 2 hours with a prolonged terminal phase of 25 hours. Approximately 97% of either quinapril or quinaprilat circulating in plasma is bound to proteins.

Pharmacokinetic studies in patients with end-stage renal disease or chronic hemodialysis or continuous ambulatory peritoneal dialysis indicate that dialysis has little effect on the elimination of quinapril and quinaprilat.

The disposition of quinapril and quinaprilat in patients with renal insufficiency is similar to that in patients with normal renal function until creatinine clearance is 60 mL/min or less. With creatinine clearance less than 60 mL/min, peak and trough quinaprilat concentrations increase, apparent half-life increases, and time to steady-state may be delayed. The elimination of quinaprilat may be reduced in elderly patients (>65 years of age) and in those with heart failure; this reduction is attributable to decrease in renal function (see Dosage). Quinaprilat concentrations are reduced in patients with alcoholic cirrhosis due to impaired de-esterification of quinapril.

The rate and extent of quinapril absorption are diminished moderately (approximately 25 to 30%) when administered during a high-fat meal. However, no effect on quinapril absorption occurs when taken during a regular meal.

Studies in rats indicate that quinapril and its metabolites do not cross the blood-brain barrier.

Hydrochlorothiazide: After oral administration of hydrochlorothiazide, diuresis begins within 2 hours, peaks in about 4 hours, and lasts about 6 to 12 hours; the extent of absorption is approximately 50 to 80%. Hydrochlorothiazide is excreted unchanged by the kidney. When plasma levels have been followed for at least 24 hours, the plasma half-life has been observed to vary between 4 to 15 hours. At least 61% of the oral dose is eliminated unchanged within 24 hours. Hydrochlorothiazide crosses the placental but not the blood-brain barrier.

Quinapril/Hydrochlorothiazide: Concomitant administration of quinapril and hydrochlorothiazide has little or no effect on the bioavailability or the pharmacokinetics of either drug.

Pharmacodynamics: Quinapril: Quinapril is a nonpeptide, nonsulphydryl ACE inhibitor. ACE is a peptidyl dipeptidase that catalyzes the conversion of angiotensin I to the vasoconstrictor angiotensin II. After absorption, quinapril is rapidly de-esterified to quinaprilat (quinapril diacid), its principal active metabolite. Its primary mode of action is to inhibit circulating and tissue ACE, thereby decreasing vasopressor activity and aldosterone secretion. Although the decrease in aldosterone is small, it results in a small increase in serum K^+ (see Precautions). Removal of edtensin II negative feedback on renin secretion leads to increased plasma renin activity.

ACE is identical to kininase II. Thus, quinapril may interfere with the degradation of bradykinin, a potent peptide vasodilator. However, it is not known whether this system contributes to the therapeutic effects of quinapril.

The antihypertensive effect of quinapril outlasts its inhibitory effect on circulating ACE in animal studies. Tissue ACE inhibition more closely correlates with the duration of antihypertensive effects and this may be related to enzyme-binding characteristics as shown for quinapril on purified tissue ACE from human kidney and heart.

Administration of 10 to 40 mg of quinapril to patients with essential hypertension results in a reduction of both sitting and standing blood pressure with minimal effect on heart rate. Antihypertensive activity commences within 1 hour with peak effects usually achieved by 2 to 4 hours after dosing. Achievement of maximum blood pressure lowering effects may require 2 to 4 weeks of therapy in some patients. At the recommended doses, antihypertensive effects are maintained throughout the 24-hour dosing interval in most patients. While the dose response relationship is relatively flat, a dose of 40 mg was somewhat more effective at trough than 10 to 20 mg, and twice-daily dosing tended to give a somewhat lower blood pressure than once-daily dosing with the same total daily dose. The antihypertensive effect of quinapril was maintained during long-term therapy with no evidence of loss of effectiveness.

Hemodynamic assessments in patients with essential hypertension indicate that blood pressure reduction produced by quinapril is accompanied by a reduction in total peripheral resistance and renal vascular resistance with little or no change in heart rate and cardiac index. There was an increase in renal blood flow that was not significant. Little or no change in glomerular filtration rate or filtration fraction was observed.

Therapeutic effects appear to be the same for elderly (>65 years of age) and younger adult patients given the same daily dosages, with no increase in adverse events in elderly patients.

The antihypertensive effect of angiotensin converting enzyme inhibitors is generally lower in black patients than in non-blacks. Hydrochlorothiazide: Hydrochlorothiazide acts directly on the kidney to increase excretion of sodium and chloride and an accompanying volume of water. Hydrochlorothiazide also increases the excretion of potassium and bicarbonate and decreases calcium excretion.

As a result of its diuretic effect, hydrochlorothiazide increases plasma renin activity, increases aldosterone secretion, decreases serum potassium and increases urinary potassium loss. Administration of quinapril inhibits the renin-angiotensin-aldosterone axis and tends to attenuate the potassium decrease associated with hydrochlorothiazide.

The mechanism underlying the antihypertensive activity of diuretics is unknown. During chronic administration, peripheral vascular resistance is reduced; however, this may be secondary to changes in sodium balance.

Quinapril/Hydrochlorothiazide: When quinapril and hydrochlorothiazide are given together, the antihypertensive effects are approximately additive.

INDICATIONS: For the treatment of essential hypertension in patients for whom combination therapy is appropriate.

In using Accuretic, consideration should be given to the risk of angioedema (see Warnings, Angioedema).

Quinapril should normally be used in those patients in whom treatment with a diuretic or a beta-blocker was found ineffective or has been associated with unacceptable adverse effects. Quinapril can also be tried as an initial agent in those patients in whom use of diuretics and/or beta-blockers is contraindicated or in patients with medical conditions in which these drugs frequently cause serious adverse effects.

Accuretic is not indicated for initial therapy. Patients in whom quinapril and hydrochlorothiazide are initiated simultaneously can develop symptomatic hypotension (see Warnings, Hypotension and Precautions, Drug Interactions).

Patients should be titrated on the individual drugs. If the fixed combination represents the dosage determined by this titration, the use of Accuretic may be more convenient in the management of patients. If during maintenance therapy dosage adjustment is necessary, it is advisable to use individual drugs.

CONTRAINDICATIONS: Patients who are hypersensitive to any component of this product (see Supplied) and patients with a history of angioedema related to previous treatment with an ACE inhibitor.

Because of the hydrochlorothiazide component, this product is contraindicated in patients with anuria or hypersensitivity to other sulfonamide-derived drugs.

Published data suggest that Quinapril is contraindicated in women who are pregnant, intend to become pregnant, or of childbearing potential who are not using adequate contraceptive measures. Quinapril should be administered to women of childbearing age only when such patients are highly unlikely to conceive and have been informed of the potential hazards to the fetus (see Warnings and Adverse Effects).

WARNINGS:

Serious Warnings and Precautions
When used in pregnancy, angiotensin converting enzyme (ACE) inhibitors can cause injury or even death of the developing fetus. When pregnancy is detected, Accuretic should be discontinued as soon as possible.

Angioedema: Angioedema has been reported in patients treated with ACE inhibitors, including quinapril. Angioedema associated with laryngeal involvement may be fatal. If laryngeal stridor or angioedema of the face, tongue, or glottis occurs, treatment with Accuretic should be discontinued immediately, the patient treated appropriately in accordance with accepted medical care and carefully observed until the swelling disappears. In instances where swelling is confined to the face and lips, the condition generally resolves without treatment, although antihistamines may be useful in relieving symptoms. Where there is involvement of the tongue, glottis or larynx likely to cause airway obstruction, appropriate therapy (including but not limited to 0.3 to 0.5 mL of s.c. epinephrine solution 1:1000) should be administered promptly (see Adverse Effects).

The incidence of angioedema during ACE inhibitor therapy has been reported to be higher in black than in non-black patients.

Patients with a history of angioedema unrelated to ACE inhibitor therapy may be at increased risk of angioedema while receiving an ACE inhibitor (see Contraindications).

Hypotension: Symptomatic hypotension has occurred after administration of quinapril, usually after the first or second dose or when the dose was increased. It is more likely to occur in patients who are volume-depleted by diuretic therapy, dietary salt restriction, dialysis, diarrhea, or vomiting. In patients with ischemic heart or cerebrovascular disease, an excessive fall in blood pressure could result in a myocardial infarction or cerebrovascular accident (see Adverse Effects). Because of the potential fall in blood pressure in these patients, therapy with Accuretic should be started under close medical supervision. Such patients should be followed closely for the first weeks of treatment and whenever the dose of Accuretic is increased. In patients with severe congestive heart failure, with or without associated renal insufficiency, excessive hypotension has been observed and may be associated with oliguria and/or progressive azotemia and rarely with acute renal failure and/or death.

If hypotension occurs, the patient should be placed in supine position and, if necessary, receive an i.v. infusion of 0.9% sodium chloride. A transient hypotensive response is not a contraindication to further doses which usually can be given without difficulty once the blood pressure has increased after volume expansion. If symptoms persist, the dosage should be reduced or the drug discontinued.

Neutropenia/Agranulocytosis: Agranulocytosis and bone marrow depression have been caused by ACE inhibitors. Agranulocytosis did occur during quinapril treatment in one patient with a history of neutropenia during previous captopril therapy. Periodic monitoring of white blood cell counts should be considered, especially in patients with collagen vascular disease and/or renal disease.

Azotemia: Azotemia may be precipitated or increased by hydrochlorothiazide. Cumulative effects of the drug may develop in patients with impaired renal function. If increasing azotemia and oliguria occur, Accuretic should be discontinued.

Impairment of Liver Function: Hepatitis (hepatocellular and/or cholestatic), elevations of liver enzymes and/or serum bilirubin have occurred during therapy with other ACE inhibitors in patients with or without pre-existing liver abnormalities. In most cases the changes were reversed on discontinuation of the drug.

Elevations of liver enzymes and/or serum bilirubin have been reported for Accuretic (see Adverse Effects). Should the patient receiving Accuretic experience any unexplained symptoms particularly during the first weeks or months of treatment, it is recommended that a full set of liver function tests and any other necessary investigation be carried out. Discontinuation of Accuretic should be considered when appropriate.

There are no adequate studies in patients with cirrhosis and/or liver dysfunction. Accuretic should be used with particular caution in patients with pre-existing liver abnormalities. In such patients baseline liver function tests should be obtained before administration of the drug and close monitoring of response and metabolic effects should apply.

Hypersensitivity to Hydrochlorothiazide: Sensitivity reactions to hydrochlorothiazide may occur in patients with or without a history of allergy or bronchial asthma. Exacerbation or activation of systemic lupus erythematosus has been reported in patients treated with hydrochlorothiazide.

Pregnancy: Quinapril is contraindicated in pregnancy (see Contraindications and Adverse Effects). ACE inhibitors can cause fetal and neonatal morbidity and mortality when administered to pregnant women. Several dozen cases have been reported in the world literature. When pregnancy is detected, Accuretic should be discontinued as soon as possible.

The use of ACE inhibitors during the second and third trimesters of pregnancy has been associated with fetal and neonatal injury including hypotension, neonatal skull hypoplasia, anuria, reversible or irreversible renal failure, and death. Oligohydramnios has also been reported, presumably resulting from decreased fetal renal function; oligohydramnios in this setting has been associated with fetal limb contractures, craniofacial deformation, and hypoplastic lung development.

Prematurity, and patent ductus arteriosus and other structural cardiac malformations, as well as neurological malformations, have also been reported following exposure in the first trimester of pregnancy.

Infants with a history of in utero exposure to ACE inhibitors should be closely observed for hypotension, oliguria and hyperkalemia. If oliguria occurs, attention should be directed toward support of blood pressure and renal perfusion. Exchange transfusion or dialysis may be required as a means of reversing hypotension and/or substituting for impaired renal function; however, limited experience with those procedures has not been associated with significant clinical benefit.

Hemodialysis and peritoneal dialysis have little effect on the elimination of quinapril and quinaprilat. If oligohydramnios is observed, a non-stress test (NST), and/or a biophysical profiling (BPP) may be appropriate, depending upon the week of pregnancy. If concerns regarding fetal well-being still persist, a contraction stress test (CST) should be considered. Patients and physicians should be aware, however, that oligohydramnios may not appear until after the fetus has sustained irreversible injury.

Thiazides cross the placental barrier and appear in cord blood. Although studies in humans have not been done, effects to the fetus may include fetal or neonatal jaundice, thrombocytopenia and possibly other adverse reactions which have occurred in the adult.

Animal Data: No fetotoxic or teratogenic effects were observed in rats at quinapril doses as high as 300 mg/kg/day (180 times the maximum daily human dose) despite maternal toxicity at 150 mg/kg/day. Offspring body weights were reduced in rats treated late in gestation and during lactation with doses of 25 mg/kg/day or more. Quinapril was not teratogenic in rabbits; however, maternal and embryo toxicity were seen in some rabbits at doses as low as 0.5 mg/kg/day and 1 mg/kg/day, respectively.

No adverse effects on fertility or reproduction were observed in rats at quinapril dose levels up to 100 mg/kg/day (60 times the maximum daily human dose).

PRECAUTIONS: Renal Impairment: As a consequence of inhibiting the renin-angiotensin-aldosterone system, changes in renal function have been seen in susceptible individuals. In patients whose renal function may depend on the activity of the renin-angiotensin- aldosterone system, such as patients with bilateral renal artery stenosis, unilateral renal artery stenosis to a solitary kidney, or severe congestive heart failure, treatment with agents that inhibit this system has been associated with oliguria, progressive azotemia and, rarely, acute renal failure and/or death. In susceptible patients, concomitant diuretic use may further increase risk (see Adverse Effects and Dosage).

Use of Accuretic should include appropriate assessment of renal function (see Adverse Effects and Dosage).

Thiazides may not be appropriate diuretics for use in patients with renal impairment and are ineffective at creatinine clearance values of 30 mL/min or below (i.e., moderate or severe renal insufficiency) (see Adverse Effects and Dosage).

Hyperkalemia: Elevated serum potassium (greater than 5.7 mEq/L) was observed in approximately 2% of patients receiving quinapril. In most cases these were isolated values which resolved despite continued therapy. Hyperkalemia was a cause of discontinuation of therapy in less than 0.1% of hypertensive patients. Risk factors for the development of hyperkalemia may include renal insufficiency, diabetes mellitus, and the concomitant use of agents to treat hypokalemia (see Precautions, Drug Interactions: Agents Increasing Serum Potassium, and Adverse Effects). The addition of a potassium-sparing diuretic to Accuretic, which contains a diuretic, is not recommended.

Patients with Impaired Liver Function: Accuretic should be used with caution in patients with impaired hepatic function or progressive liver disease, since minor alterations of fluid and electrolyte balance may precipitate hepatic coma. Also, since the metabolism of quinapril to quinaprilat is normally dependent upon hepatic esterase, patients with impaired liver function could develop markedly elevated plasma levels of quinapril.

Valvular Stenosis: There is concern on theoretical grounds that patients with aortic stenosis might be at particular risk of decreased coronary perfusion when treated with vasodilators because they do not develop as much afterload reduction.

Metabolism: Hyperuricemia may occur, or acute gout may be precipitated, in certain patients receiving thiazide therapy.

Thiazides may decrease serum PBI levels without signs of thyroid disturbance.

Increase in cholesterol, triglyceride and glucose levels may be associated with thiazide diuretic therapy. Overt diabetes may be precipitated in susceptible individuals.

Initial and periodic determination of serum electrolytes should be performed at appropriate intervals to detect possible electrolyte imbalance.

As with other ACE inhibitors, patients on quinapril alone may have increased serum potassium levels (see Precautions, Hyperkalemia). Conversely, treatment with thiazide diuretics has been associated with hypokalemia. The opposite effects of hydrochlorothiazide and quinapril on serum potassium may approximately balance each other in many patients so that no net effect will be seen. In other patients, one or the other effect may be dominant.

In addition to hypokalemia, treatment with thiazide diuretics has also been associated with hyponatremia and hypochloremic alkalosis. These disturbances have sometimes been manifest as one or more of the following: dryness of mouth, thirst, weakness, lethargy, drowsiness, restlessness, muscle pain or cramps, muscular fatigue, hypotension, oliguria, tachycardia, nausea, confusion, seizures and vomiting. Hypokalemia can also sensitize or exaggerate the response of the heart to the toxic effects of digitalis. The risk of hypokalemia is greatest in patients with cirrhosis of the liver, in patients experiencing a brisk diuresis, in patients who are receiving inadequate oral intake of electrolytes, and in patients receiving concomitant therapy with corticosteroids or ACTH. Chloride deficits secondary to thiazide therapy are generally mild and require specific treatment only under extraordinary circumstances (e.g., in liver disease or renal disease). Dilutional hyponatremia may occur in edematous patients, especially in hot weather; appropriate therapy is water restriction rather than administration of salt, except when the hyponatremia is life-threatening. In actual salt depletion, replacement of salt is the therapy of choice.

Thiazides may decrease calcium excretion. Thiazides may cause intermittent and slight elevation of serum calcium in the absence of known disorders of calcium metabolism. Marked hypercalcemia may be evidence of hidden hypoparathyroidism. In a few patients on prolonged thiazide therapy, pathological changes in the parathyroid gland have been observed with hypercalcemia and hypophosphatemia. More serious complications of hyperparathyroidism (renal lithiasis, bone resorption and peptic ulceration) have not been seen. Thiazides should be discontinued before performing tests for parathyroid function.

Thiazides increase the urinary excretion of magnesium and hypomagnesemia may result.

Surgery/Anesthesia: In patients undergoing major surgery or during anesthesia with agents that produce hypotension, ACE inhibitors will block angiotensin II formation secondary to compensatory renin release. If hypotension occurs and is considered to be due to this mechanism, it can be corrected by volume expansion.

Systemic Lupus Erythematosus: Thiazide diuretics have been reported to cause exacerbation or activation of systemic lupus erythematosus.

Cough: A dry, persistent cough, which usually disappears only after withdrawal or lowering of the dose of quinapril, has been reported. Such possibility should be considered as part of the differential diagnosis of the cough.

Lactation: The presence of concentrations of ACE inhibitor have been reported in human milk. Thiazides appear in human milk. Use of ACE inhibitors is not recommended during breast-feeding.

Children: The safety and effectiveness of Accuretic in children have not been established; therefore, use in this age group is not recommended.

Anaphylactoid Reactions during Membrane Exposure: Anaphylactoid reactions have been reported in patients dialysed with high-flux membranes (e.g., polyacrylonitrile [PAN]) and treated concomitantly with an ACE inhibitor. Dialysis should be stopped immediately if symptoms such as nausea, abdominal cramps, burning, angioedema, shortness of breath and severe hypotension occur. Symptoms are not relieved by antihistamines. In these patients, consideration should be given to using a different type of dialysis membrane or a different class of antihypertensive agent.

Anaphylactoid Reactions during LDL Apheresis: Rarely, patients receiving ACE inhibitors during low density lipoprotein apheresis with dextran sulfate have experienced life-threatening anaphylactoid reactions. These reactions were avoided by temporarily withholding the ACE inhibitor therapy prior to each apheresis.

Anaphylactoid Reactions during Desensitization: There have been isolated reports of patients experiencing sustained life-threatening anaphylactoid reactions while receiving ACE inhibitors during desensitizing treatment with hymenoptera (bees, wasps) venom. In the same patients, these reactions have been avoided when ACE inhibitors were temporarily withheld for at least 24 hours, but they have reappeared upon inadvertent rechallenge to an ACE inhibitor.

Drug Interactions: Concomitant Diuretic Therapy: Patients concomitantly taking ACE inhibitors and diuretics, and especially those in whom diuretic therapy was recently instituted, may occasionally experience an excessive reduction of blood pressure after initiation of therapy. The possibility of hypotensive effects after the first dose of quinapril can be minimized by either discontinuing the diuretic or increasing the salt intake (except in patients with heart failure) prior to initiation of treatment with quinapril. If it is not possible to discontinue the diuretic, the starting dose of quinapril should be reduced and the patient should be closely observed for several hours following initial dose and until blood pressure has stabilized (see Warnings and Dosage).

Agents Increasing Serum Potassium: Since quinapril decreases aldosterone production, elevation of serum potassium may occur. Potassium-sparing diuretics, such as spironolactone, triamterene or amiloride, or potassium supplements, should be given only for documented hypokalemia and with caution and frequent monitoring of serum potassium since they may lead to a significant increase in serum potassium. Salt substitutes which contain potassium should also be used with caution.

Agents Affecting Sympathetic Activity: Agents affecting sympathetic activity (e.g., ganglionic blocking agents or adrenergic neuron blocking agents) may be used with caution. Beta-adrenergic blocking drugs add some further antihypertensive effect to quinapril.

Tetracycline: Concomitant administration of tetracycline with quinapril reduced the absorption of tetracycline in healthy volunteers (by 28 to 37%) due to the presence of magnesium carbonate as an excipient in the formulation. This interaction should be considered with concomitant use of Accuretic and tetracycline or other drugs which interact with magnesium.

Lithium: In general, lithium should not be given with diuretics or ACE inhibitors. Diuretic agents and ACE inhibitors reduce the renal clearance of lithium and add a high risk of lithium toxicity.

Cardiac Glycosides: Thiazide diuretics may enhance digitalis toxicity associated with hypokalemia or hypomagnesemia.

Alcohol, Barbiturates, or Narcotics: Potentiation of orthostatic hypotension may occur in the presence of hydrochlorothiazide.

Antidiabetic Drugs: Dosage adjustment of oral hypoglycemic agents and insulin may be required.

Other Antihypertensive Agents: Additive effects may occur.

Corticosteroids, ACTH: Intensified electrolyte depletion, particularly hypokalemia, may occur when administered with hydrochlorothiazide.

Pressor Amines (e.g., norepinephrine): Possible decreased response to pressor amines may occur in the presence of a thiazide diuretic, but is not sufficient to preclude their use.

Nondepolarizing Neuromuscular Blocking Agents (e.g., d-tubocurarine): Hydrochlorothiazide may increase responsiveness to these drugs.

Nonsteroidal Anti-inflammatory Drugs: In some patients, the administration of a nonsteroidal anti-inflammatory agent can reduce the diuretic, natriuretic and antihypertensive effects of loop, potassium-sparing and thiazide diuretics. Therefore, when Accuretic and nonsteroidal anti-inflammatory agents are used concomitantly, the patient should be observed closely to determine if the desired effect of Accuretic is obtained.

Anion Exchange Resins: Absorption of hydrochlorothiazide is impaired in the presence of anion exchange resins, such as cholestyramine and colestipol. Single doses of the resins bind the hydrochlorothiazide and reduce its absorption from the gastrointestinal tract by up to 85% and 43%, respectively.

Information to Be Provided to the Patient:

> Serious Warning and Precautions
> Accuretic should not be used during pregnancy. Patients should be advised to stop the medication and contact their physician as soon as possible if they discover that they are pregnant while taking Accuretic.

Note: As with many other drugs, certain advice to patients being treated with Accuretic is warranted. This information is intended to aid in the safe and effective use of this medication. It is not a disclosure of all possible adverse or intended effects.

Angioedema: Angioedema, including laryngeal edema, may occur with ACE inhibitors, especially following the first dose. Patients should be so advised and told to report immediately any signs or symptoms suggesting angioedema, such as swelling of face, extremities, eyes, lips, tongue, difficulty in swallowing or breathing. They should immediately stop taking Accuretic and consult with their physician.

Pregnancy and Breast-feeding: Taking Accuretic during pregnancy can cause injury and even death to the developing fetus. This medicine should not be used by women who are pregnant, intend to become pregnant, or could become pregnant and who are not using adequate contraceptive measures (see Contraindications, Warnings and Adverse Effects). Patients should be advised to stop the medication and report to their doctor as soon as possible if they become pregnant while taking Accuretic. It is possible that Accuretic passes into breast milk. Patients should be advised not to breast-feed while taking Accuretic.

Hypotension: Patients should be cautioned to report light-headedness, especially during the first few days of Accuretic therapy. If actual syncope occurs, patients should be told to discontinue the drug and consult with their physician.

All patients should be cautioned that excessive perspiration and dehydration may lead to an excessive fall in blood pressure because of reduction in fluid volume. Other causes of volume depletion such as vomiting or diarrhea may also lead to a fall in blood pressure; patients should be advised to consult with their physician.

Agranulocytosis/Neutropenia: Patients should be told to report promptly to their physician any indication of infection (e.g., sore throat, fever) as this may be a sign of neutropenia.

Impaired Liver Function: Patients should be advised to return to their physician if they experience any symptoms possibly related to liver dysfunction. This would include "viral-like symptoms" in the first weeks to months of therapy (such as fever, malaise, muscle pain, rash or adenopathy which are possible indicators of hypersensitivity reactions) or if abdominal pain, nausea or vomiting, loss of appetite, jaundice, itching or any other unexplained symptoms occur during therapy.

Hyperkalemia: Patients should be told not to use salt substitutes containing potassium without consulting their physician.

Surgery: Patients planning to undergo surgery and/or anesthesia should be told to inform their physician that they are taking an ACE inhibitor.

ADVERSE EFFECTS: Accuretic has been evaluated for safety in 1571 patients with essential hypertension, including 943 patients in controlled studies (see Table 1), 345 patients in placebo-controlled trials and 517 patients who were treated with Accuretic for at least 1 year. Adverse reactions have been limited to those reported previously with quinapril or hydrochlorothiazide when used separately for the treatment of hypertension.

Serious or clinically significant adverse reactions observed in less than 0.2% of patients treated with quinapril and hydrochlorothiazide were: hematemesis, gout, syncope and angioedema. Therapy was discontinued in 2.1% of patients due to an adverse event. Headache (0.5%) and dizziness (0.3%) were the most frequent reasons for withdrawal.

The most frequent adverse experiences in controlled trials were headache (6.7%), dizziness (4.8%), cough (3.2%) and fatigue (2.9%). The cough is characteristically nonproductive, persistent and resolves after discontinuation of therapy (see Warnings, Angioedema and Hypotension).

Table 1: Accuretic

Adverse Events in ≥1% of Quinapril/Hydrochlorothiazide Patients in Controlled Clinical Studies

Adverse Events	Quinapril/HCTZ N=943 (% Patients)	Quinapril N=799 (% Patients)
Body as a Whole		
Asthenia	1.1	1.2
Fatigue	2.9	2.0
Headache	6.7	4.8
Back pain	1.5	0.7
Chest pain	1.0	1.2
Viral infection	1.9	2.0
Cardiovascular		
Vasodilation	1.0	0.4
Digestive		
Dyspepsia	1.2	1.9

(cont'd)

Table 1: Accuretic *(cont'd)*

Adverse Events in ≥1% of Quinapril/Hydrochlorothiazide Patients in Controlled Clinical Studies

Adverse Events	Quinapril/HCTZ N=943 (% Patients)	Quinapril N=799 (% Patients)
Nausea and/or vomiting	1.8	2.0
Diarrhea	1.4	1.7
Abdominal pain	1.7	1.6
Musculoskeletal		
Myalgia	2.4	0.9
Nervous System		
Dizziness	4.8	2.7
Insomnia	1.2	1.5
Somnolence	1.2	0.9
Vertigo	1.0	0.3
Respiratory		
Pharyngitis	1.1	1.4
Rhinitis	2.0	3.0
Bronchitis	1.2	1.3
Coughing	3.2	2.7
Upper respiratory infection	1.3	1.1

Clinical adverse events, regardless of relationship to therapy, occurring in ≥0.5% to <1% of patients treated with quinapril plus hydrochlorothiazide in controlled and uncontrolled trials and less frequent clinically significant events seen in clinical trials or in postmarketing experience included:
Cardiovascular: tachycardia, hypotension, palpitations.
Gastrointestinal: flatulence, dry mouth or throat, pancreatitis.
Respiratory: dyspnea, sinusitis.
Integumentary: erythema multiforme, exfoliative dermatitis, alopecia, pemphigus, pruritus, rash.
Nervous/Psychiatric: paresthesia, nervousness.
Urogenital: impotence, urinary tract infection.
Other: arthralgia, peripheral edema, hemolytic anemia.

Rare adverse events, not listed above, which have been reported with either hydrochlorothiazide, quinapril, or the combination, include:
Cardiovascular: cerebrovascular accident, heart failure, atrial flutter, vasodilation, necrotizing angiitis, myocardial ischemia, heart arrest, transient ischemic attack. Orthostatic hypotension may occur, especially in elderly patients with reduced plasma volume, and may be potentiated by alcohol, barbiturates, or narcotics.
Gastrointestinal: anorexia, gastric irritation, cramping, constipation, jaundice (intrahepatic cholestatic), pancreatitis, sialadenitis, gastrointestinal hemorrhage, bloody stools.
Respiratory: respiratory distress including pneumonitis, asthma, hoarseness.
Integumentary: photosensitivity, rash, urticaria, Stevens-Johnson syndrome, eczema.
Nervous System: paresthesias, xanthopsia, confusion, amnesia, anxiety, facial paralysis, polyneuritis.
Hematological: leukopenia, thrombocytopenia, agranulocytosis, aplastic anemia, hemolytic anemia, purpura.
Urogenital: dysuria, polyuria, impaired renal function, hematuria, glycosuria.
Special Senses: tinnitus, transient blurred vision, taste disturbance.
Congenital and Familial/Genetic Disorders: See Contraindications and Warnings, Pregnancy.
Other: muscle spasm, weakness, restlessness, chill, weight increase, dehydration, arthritis, allergy, face edema, fever, anaphylactic reactions, fracture.
Laboratory Deviations: WBC decreased, hyperglycemia, azotemia, transient hyperlipidemia, hyperuricemia.
Clinical Laboratory Test Findings: Creatinine, Blood Nitrogen: Increases (>1.25 times the upper limit of normal) in serum creatinine and blood urea nitrogen were observed in 3% and 4% respectively of patients treated with Accuretic (see Precautions and Dosage).
Hepatic: Elevations of liver enzymes and/or serum bilirubin have occurred (see Precautions).
Glucose: Elevations in glucose values have occurred (see Precautions).
Triglyceride: Elevations in triglyceride values have occurred (see Precautions).
Serum Uric Acid: Elevations in serum uric acid values have occurred (see Precautions).
Hematology: Possibly clinically important increases and decreases in hematology parameters have occurred (see Warnings).

Other laboratory test values with clinically important deviations during controlled and uncontrolled trials included: magnesium, cholesterol, PBI, parathyroid function tests and calcium (see Precautions); hematology (see Warnings).

OVERDOSE:

Symptoms: No data are available regarding overdosage of Accuretic or quinapril in humans. The most likely clinical manifestation would be symptoms attributable to severe hypotension, which should be normally treated by i.v. volume expansion with 0.9% sodium chloride. Hemodialysis and peritoneal dialysis have little effect on the elimination of quinapril and quinaprilat.

The most common signs and symptoms observed for hydrochlorothiazide monotherapy overdosage are those caused by electrolyte depletion (hypokalemia, hypochloremia, hyponatremia) and dehydration resulting from excessive diuresis. If digitalis has also been administered, hypokalemia may accentuate cardiac arrhythmias.

Treatment: See Symptoms.

> For management of a suspected drug overdose, CPhA recommends that you contact your **regional Poison Control Centre**. See the *CPS* Directory section for a list of Poison Control Centres.

DOSAGE: Dosage must be individualized. The fixed combination is not for initial therapy. The dose of Accuretic should be determined by titration of the individual components.

Once the patient has been successfully titrated with the individual components as described below, Accuretic may be substituted if the titrated doses and dosing schedule can be achieved by the fixed combination (see Indications and Warnings). In some patients, a twice daily administration may be required.

Patients do not generally require hydrochlorothiazide in excess of 50 mg daily, particularly when combined with other antihypertensive agents.

Monotherapy: The recommended initial dose of quinapril in patients not on diuretics is 10 mg once daily. An initial dose of 20 mg once daily can be considered for patients without advanced age, renal impairment, or concomitant heart failure and who are not volume-depleted (see Precautions, Hypotension). Dosage should be adjusted according to blood pressure response, generally at intervals of 2 to 4 weeks. A dose of 40 mg daily should not be exceeded.

In some patients treated once daily, the antihypertensive effect may diminish towards the end of the dosing interval. This can be evaluated by measuring blood pressure just prior to dosing to determine whether satisfactory control is being maintained for 24 hours. If it is not, either twice daily administration with the same total daily dose, or an increase in dose should be considered. If blood pressure is not controlled with quinapril alone, a diuretic may be added. After the addition of a diuretic, it may be possible to reduce the dose of quinapril.

Concomitant Diuretic Therapy: Symptomatic hypotension occasionally may occur following the initial dose of quinapril and is more likely in patients who are currently being treated with a diuretic. The diuretic should, if possible, be discontinued for 2 to 3 days before beginning therapy with quinapril to reduce the likelihood of hypotension (see Warnings). If the diuretic cannot be discontinued, an initial dose of 5 mg of quinapril should be used with careful medical supervision for several hours and until blood pressure has stabilized. The dosage of quinapril should subsequently be titrated (as described above) to the optimal response.

Dosage Adjustment in Renal Impairment: For use in hemodialysis patients (see Precautions and Adverse Effects, Anaphylactoid Reactions during Membrane Exposure). Quinapril should be administered on days when dialysis is not performed.

Starting doses should be reduced according to the guidelines in Table 2.

Table 2: Accuretic

Dosage Adjustment in Renal Impairment

Creatinine Clearance (mL/min)	Maximum Recommended Initial Dose (mg)
>60	10
30–60	5
10–30	2.5
<10	Insufficient data for dosage recommendation

Patients should subsequently have dosage titrated (as described above) to the optimal response as described under Monotherapy.

When concomitant diuretic therapy is required in patients with severe renal impairment, a loop diuretic rather than a thiazide is preferred for use with quinapril. Therefore, for patients with severe renal dysfunction, Accuretic is not recommended.

Geriatrics: The recommended initial dosage of quinapril is 10 mg once daily (depending on renal function) followed by titration to the optimal response as described above under Monotherapy.

SUPPLIED: 10/12.5: Each pink, oval, biconvex, film-coated tablet, with bisecting score on both sides and PD222 on one side contains: quinapril 10 mg and hydrochlorothiazide 12.5 mg. Nonmedicinal ingredients: candelilla wax, crospovidone, lactose, magnesium carbonate, magnesium stearate, povidone, synthetic red iron oxide, synthetic yellow iron oxide and titanium dioxide. Blisters of 28. Store at controlled room temperature 15 to 25°C. Dispense in well-closed containers.

20/12.5: Each pink, triangular, biconvex, film-coated tablet, with bisecting score and PD220 on one side contains: quinapril 20 mg and hydrochlorothiazide 12.5 mg. Nonmedicinal ingredients: candelilla wax, crospovidone, lactose, magnesium carbonate, magnesium stearate, povidone, synthetic red iron oxide, synthetic yellow iron oxide and titanium dioxide. Blisters of 28. Store at controlled room temperature 15 to 25°C. Dispense in well-closed containers.

20/25: Each pink, round, biconvex, film-coated tablet with PD223 on one side contains: quinapril 20 mg and hydrochlorothiazide 25 mg. Nonmedicinal ingredients: candelilla wax, crospovidone, lactose, magnesium carbonate, magnesium stearate, povidone, synthetic red iron oxide, synthetic yellow iron oxide and titanium dioxide. Blisters of 28. Store at controlled room temperature 15 to 25°C. Dispense in well-closed containers.

(Shown in Product Identification Section)

Accutane™ Roche® Ⓟ

isotretinoin

Nodular/Inflammatory and Conglobate Acne Therapy

Roche

Date of Preparation: November 25, 1982
Date of Revision: April 21, 2010

SUMMARY PRODUCT INFORMATION:

Route of Administration	Dosage Form/ Strength	Clinically Relevant Nonmedicinal Ingredients
Oral	Capsule/10 mg	Glycerol, mannitol, peanut oil (see Contraindications), sorbitol, soybean oil (see Contraindications)
	Capsule/40 mg	Glycerol, methylparaben (see Contraindications), propylparaben (see Contraindications), soybean oil (see Contraindications), Sunset Yellow FCF
For a complete listing of nonmedicinal ingredients see Dosage Forms, Composition and Packaging section.		

INDICATIONS AND CLINICAL USE: ACCUTANE ROCHE (isotretinoin) is indicated for the treatment of:

- Severe Nodular and/or Inflammatory Acne
- Acne Conglobata
- Recalcitrant Acne

Because of significant side effects associated with its use, ACCUTANE should be reserved for patients where the conditions listed above are unresponsive to conventional first line therapies.

ACCUTANE should only be prescribed by physicians knowledgeable in the use of retinoids systemically, who understand the risk of teratogenicity in females of child bearing age and who are experienced in counselling young adults for whom ACCUTANE is generally indicated (see Contraindications and Warnings and Precautions, Serious Warnings and Precautions and Special Populations, Pregnant Women).

A careful assessment of the patient's mental state should be made, including whether or not they have a history of previous psychiatric illness (see Warnings and Precautions, Serious Warnings and Precautions, Psychiatric).

It is strongly recommended that each ACCUTANE prescription be limited to a one-month supply in order to encourage patients to return for follow-up to monitor side-effects.

Pediatrics: The use of ACCUTANE in pediatric patients less than 12 years of age is not recommended. The use of ACCUTANE for the treatment of severe recalcitrant nodular acne in pediatric patients ages 12 to 17 years should be given careful consideration, especially for those patients where a known metabolic or structural bone disease exists (see Warnings and Precautions, Special Populations, Pediatrics).

Geriatrics: Clinical studies of ACCUTANE did not include sufficient numbers of subjects aged 65 years and over to determine whether they respond differently from younger subjects. Although reported clinical experience has not identified differences in responses between elderly and younger patients, effects of aging might be expected to increase some risks associated with isotretinoin therapy.

CONTRAINDICATIONS:

- **ACCUTANE (isotretinoin) is contraindicated in pregnancy.**
  - Females must not become pregnant while taking ACCUTANE or for at least one month after its discontinuation. ACCUTANE causes severe birth defects in a very high percentage of infants born to women who became pregnant during treatment with ACCUTANE in any amount, even for a short period of time. Potentially any exposed fetus can be affected. There are no accurate means of determining whether an exposed fetus has been affected (see Warnings and Precautions, Special populations, Pregnant Women).
  - If pregnancy does occur during treatment with ACCUTANE or for one month after its discontinuation, ACCUTANE treatment must be immediately stopped and the physician and patient should discuss the desirability of continuing the pregnancy.
- ACCUTANE should only be prescribed by physicians knowledgeable in the use of retinoids systemically (see Indications and Clinical Use).

ACCUTANE is also contraindicated in the following conditions:

- breastfeeding women,
- hepatic and renal insufficiency,
- hypervitaminosis A,
- patients with excessively elevated blood lipid values,
- patients taking tetracyclines (see Warnings and Precautions, Serious Warnings and Precautions, Neurologic and Drug Interactions, Drug-Drug Interactions).
- patients who are sensitive to isotretinoin, or to any of the excipients. ACCUTANE capsules contain hydrogenated soybean oil, parabens, partially hydrogenated soybean oil, peanut oil (component of canthaxanthin), and soybean oil (see Dosage Forms, Composition and Packaging).

WARNINGS AND PRECAUTIONS:

Serious Warnings and Precautions

- **Pregnancy Prevention:** ACCUTANE (isotretinoin) is a known teratogen contraindicated in pregnancy (see boxed Contraindications). Physicians should **only** prescribe ACCUTANE to females of childbearing potential if **all** the conditions described below under Conditions of Use are met.

  In addition, when prescribing this drug to female patients of childbearing potential, physicians **must** use Hoffmann-La Roche Limited's Pregnancy Prevention Program, which includes comprehensive information about the potential risks of this drug, a checklist for criteria which **must** be met prior to prescribing this drug to female patients of childbearing potential, detailed information on birth control options, a patient informed consent for review and signature, and monthly pregnancy reminders for physicians to use at each patient visit during the treatment period.
- **Psychiatric:** Some patients treated with ACCUTANE have become depressed and some attempted or committed suicide. Although a causal relationship has not been established, all patients should be screened and monitored for signs of depression during therapy (see Warnings and Precautions, Monitoring and Laboratory Tests). Before starting therapy with ACCUTANE physicians should determine whether the patient may be depressed or has a history of depression including a family history of major depression before starting therapy with ACCUTANE. If symptoms of depression develop or worsen during treatment with ACCUTANE, the drug should be discontinued promptly and the patient referred for appropriate psychiatric treatment as necessary. However, discontinuation of ACCUTANE may not alleviate symptoms and therefore further psychiatric or psychological evaluation may be necessary.
- **Neurologic:** ACCUTANE use has been associated with a number of cases of pseudotumor cerebri (benign intracranial hypertension), some of which involved concomitant use of tetracyclines (see Contraindications and Drug Interactions, Drug-Drug Interactions). Early symptoms of pseudotumor cerebri include headache, nausea and vomiting, and visual disturbances. Patients with these symptoms should be screened for papilledema and, if present, the drug should be discontinued immediately and the patient referred to a neurologist for diagnosis and care. Concomitant treatment with tetracyclines should be avoided (see Contraindications and Drug Interactions, Drug-Drug Interactions).

Serious Skin Reactions: There have been very rare post-marketing reports of severe skin reactions (e.g., erythema multiforme (EM), Stevens-Johnson syndrome (SJS), and toxic epidermal necrolysis (TEN)) associated with ACCUTANE use. These events may be serious and result in hospitalization, life threatening events, disfiguration, disability and/or death. ACCUTANE treatment should be discontinued if the patient develops any of the following reactions: rash, especially if associated with fever and/or malaise, conjunctivitis (red or inflamed eyes); blisters on legs, arms or face and/or sores in mouth, throat, nose or eyes; peeling skin or other serious skin reactions.

Conditions of Use: ACCUTANE is contraindicated in females of childbearing potential unless **all** of the following conditions apply:

1. The patient has severe disfiguring nodular and/or inflammatory acne, acne conglobata or recalcitrant acne that has not responded to standard therapy, including systemic antibiotics.
2. The patient is reliable in understanding and carrying out instructions.
3. The patient is able and willing to comply with the mandatory effective contraceptive measures.
4. The patient has received, and acknowledged understanding of, a careful oral and printed explanation of the hazards of fetal exposure to ACCUTANE and the risk of possible contraception failure. This explanation may include showing a line drawing to the patient of an infant with the characteristic external deformities resulting from ACCUTANE exposure during pregnancy.
5. The patient has been informed and understands the need to rapidly consult her physician if there is a risk of pregnancy.
6. The patient understands the need for rigorous follow-up on a monthly basis.
7. The patient uses effective contraception without any interruption for one month before beginning ACCUTANE therapy, during ACCUTANE therapy and for one month following discontinuation of ACCUTANE therapy. It is recommended that two reliable forms of contraception be used simultaneously (see Warnings and Precautions, Special Populations, Pregnant Women).
8. The patient has had two negative pregnancy tests before starting ACCUTANE therapy with the first pregnancy test conducted at initial assessment when the patient is qualified for ACCUTANE therapy by the physician. The patient has had a second serum or urine pregnancy test with a sensitivity of at least 25 mIU/mL with a negative result, performed in a licensed laboratory, within 11 days prior to initiating therapy. The patient has had two or three days of the next normal menstrual period before ACCUTANE therapy is initiated.
9. In the event of relapse treatment, the patient must also use the same uninterrupted and effective contraceptive measures one month prior to, during and for one month after ACCUTANE.

(Re items 2 to 9 see Warnings and Precautions, Special Populations, Pregnant Women).

Even female patients who normally do not employ contraception due to a history of infertility, or claim absence of sexual activity should be advised to employ contraception while taking ACCUTANE, following the above guidelines. Even female patients who have amenorrhea must follow all the advice on effective contraception.

Information concerning the Pregnancy Prevention Program (see boxed Serious Warnings and Precautions) has also been provided directly to patients via the ACCUTANE compliance packaging (see Information for the Patient). This "Patient Information" asks female patients of childbearing potential, who have not been counseled using Hoffmann-La Roche Limited's Pregnancy Prevention Program, to contact their physician for further information.

Patients should also be informed that confidential contraception counseling (provided by a health care professional) is available from Hoffmann-La Roche Limited.

Special Populations: Pregnant Women: There is an extremely high risk (25% or greater) that major human fetal abnormalities will occur if pregnancy occurs during treatment with ACCUTANE or up to one month following its discontinuation. Potentially any exposed fetus can be affected. These abnormalities, associated with ACCUTANE administration during pregnancy, have been reported and include: CNS (hydrocephalus, hydranecephaly, microcephaly, posterior fossa abnormalities, cranial nerve dysfunction, cerebellar malformation); craniofacial (anotia, microtia, low set ears, small or absent external auditory canals, microphthalmia, facial dysmorphia, cleft palate); cardiac (septal defects, aortic arch abnormalities, tetralogy of Fallot); thymus gland abnormalities; and parathyroid hormone deficiency. Cases of IQ scores less than 85 with or without other abnormalities have been reported.

Pregnancy Tests: Female patients of childbearing potential must not be given ACCUTANE until pregnancy is excluded. The patient must have two negative pregnancy tests before starting ACCUTANE therapy with the first pregnancy test conducted at initial assessment when the patient is qualified for ACCUTANE therapy by the physician. A second pregnancy test must be performed within 11 days prior to starting ACCUTANE treatment. ACCUTANE treatment should start on the second or third day of the next normal menstrual period following this negative pregnancy test.

It is mandatory that all female patients of childbearing potential treated with ACCUTANE have regular monthly pregnancy tests during treatment and one month after the discontinuation of treatment. The dates and results of pregnancy tests should be documented. These pregnancy tests will:

a. Serve primarily to reinforce to the patient the necessity of avoiding pregnancy.
b. In the event of accidental pregnancy, provide the physician and patient an immediate opportunity to discuss the serious risk to the fetus from this exposure to ACCUTANE and the desirability of continuing the pregnancy in view of the potential teratogenic effect of ACCUTANE (see Contraindications).

Contraception: Effective contraception must be used for at least one month before starting ACCUTANE treatment, during treatment and for at least one month following the discontinuation of ACCUTANE treatment. It is recommended that two reliable forms of contraception be used simultaneously. At least 1 of these forms of contraception must be a primary form, unless the patient has undergone a hysterectomy. Effective forms of contraception include: tubal ligation, partner's vasectomy, intrauterine devices, birth control pills, and topical/injectable/insertable hormonal birth control products. Barrier forms of contraception include diaphragms, latex condoms, and cervical caps; each must be used with a spermicide. Any birth control method can fail. Therefore, it is critically important that women of childbearing potential use 2 effective forms of contraception simultaneously (see Drug Interactions, Drug-Drug Interactions).

Pregnancy occurring during treatment with ACCUTANE and for one month after its discontinuation, carries the risk of fetal malformation and the increased risk of spontaneous abortion (see Contraindications). ACCUTANE, treatment must be stopped and the patient should be fully counselled on the serious risk to the fetus should they become pregnant while undergoing treatment. If pregnancy does occur during this time the physician and patient should discuss the desirability of continuing the pregnancy.

Nursing Women: It is not known whether isotretinoin is excreted in human milk. As isotretinoin is highly lipophilic, the passage of the drug in human milk is very likely. Because of the potential for adverse effects, women should not breast feed if they are receiving ACCUTANE (see Contraindications).

Pediatrics: The long term safety of ACCUTANE, in prepubertal children (**< 12 years of age**), has not been established.

In studies with ACCUTANE, adverse reactions reported in pediatric patients ages 12 to 17 years were similar to those described in adults except for the increased incidence of back pain and arthralgia (both of which were sometimes severe) and myalgia in pediatric patients (see Adverse Reactions).

Pediatric patients and their caregivers should be informed that approximately 29% (104/358) of pediatric patients treated with ACCUTANE developed back pain. Back pain was severe in 13.5% (14/104) of the cases and occurred at a higher frequency in female patients than male patients. Arthralgias were experienced in 22% (79/358) of pediatric patients. Arthralgias were severe in 7.6% (6/79) of patients. Appropriate evaluation of the musculoskeletal system should be done in patients who present with these symptoms during or after a course of ACCUTANE. Consideration should be given to discontinuation of ACCUTANE if any significant abnormality is found.

Geriatrics (>65 years of age): Clinical studies of isotretinoin did not include sufficient numbers of subjects aged 65 years and over to determine whether they respond differently from younger subjects.

Special Patient Groups: In high risk patients (with diabetes, obesity, alcoholism or lipid metabolism disorder) undergoing treatment with ACCUTANE, more frequent checks of serum values for lipids (see Warnings and Precautions, Endocrine and Metabolism and Hepatic/Biliary/Pancreatic) and/or blood glucose may be necessary.

Male Patients: The available data suggest that the level of maternal exposure from the semen of the patients receiving ACCUTANE is not of a sufficient magnitude to be associated with the teratogenic effects of ACCUTANE. The threshold dose of isotretinoin exposure causing birth defects is not known. Postmarketing reports through 20 years include 4 with isolated defects compatible with features of retinoid exposed fetus; however 2 of these reports were incomplete, and 2 had other possible explanations for the defects observed.

Male patients should be reminded that they must not share their medication with anyone, particularly not females.

Isotretinoin, in therapeutic dosages, does not affect the number, motility and morphology of sperm.

Both male and female patients should be given a copy of the Consumer Information (Part III), see Information for the Patient.

Blood Donation: It is recommended that blood donation for transfusion purposes be deferred during therapy with ACCUTANE and for one month after discontinuation of treatment. Theoretically, blood from such donors could present a small risk to the fetus if transfused to a pregnant mother during the first trimester of pregnancy.

Cardiovascular: Approximately 25% of patients receiving ACCUTANE experienced an elevation in plasma triglycerides. Approximately 15% developed a decrease in high density lipoproteins and about 7% showed an increase in cholesterol levels. These effects on triglycerides, HDL and cholesterol were reversible upon reduction of the dose or cessation of ACCUTANE therapy (see Adverse Reactions, Laboratory Abnormalities).

Patients with increased tendency to develop hypertriglyceridemia include those with diabetes mellitus, obesity, increased alcohol intake and familial history.

The cardiovascular consequences of hypertriglyceridemia are not well understood, but may increase the patient's risk status. Therefore, every attempt should be made to control significant triglyceride elevation (see Warnings and Precautions, Monitoring and Laboratory Tests). Some patients have been able to reverse triglyceride elevation by reduction in weight, restriction of dietary fat and alcohol, and reduction in dose while continuing ACCUTANE. An obese male patient with Darier's disease developed elevated triglycerides and subsequent eruptive xanthomas.

Ear/Nose/Throat: Impaired hearing at certain frequencies has been reported in some patients treated with ACCUTANE. Patients who experience tinnitus or hearing impairment should discontinue ACCUTANE treatment and be referred for specialized care for further evaluation.

Endocrine and Metabolism: Patients with diabetes or a family history of diabetes may experience problems with the control of their blood sugar during ACCUTANE therapy. Therefore, known or suspected diabetics should have periodic blood sugar determinations. Although no causal relationship has been established, elevated fasting blood sugars have been reported, and new cases of diabetes have been diagnosed during ACCUTANE therapy (see Adverse Reactions, Clinical Trial and Post-Market Adverse Reactions, Laboratory Abnormalities).

Gastrointestinal: ACCUTANE has been temporally associated with inflammatory bowel disease (including regional ileitis, colitis and hemorrhage) in patients without a prior history of intestinal disorders. Patients experiencing abdominal pain, rectal bleeding or severe diarrhea should discontinue ACCUTANE immediately.

Hepatic/Biliary/Pancreatic: Liver function tests should be monitored before treatment and at regular intervals during treatment (one month after the start of treatment and at least three month intervals thereafter) unless more frequent monitoring is clinically indicated. Several cases of clinical hepatitis have been noted which are considered to be possibly or probably related to ACCUTANE therapy. Additionally, mild to moderate elevations of liver enzymes have been observed in approximately 15% of individuals treated during clinical trials, some of which normalized with dosage reduction or continued administration of the drug. If normalization does not readily occur, or if hepatitis is suspected during treatment with ACCUTANE, the drug should be discontinued and the etiology further investigated (see Warnings and Precautions, Monitoring and Laboratory Tests).

There have been some reports of acute pancreatitis, which is known to be potentially fatal. This is sometimes associated with elevation of serum triglycerides in excess of 800 mg/dL or 9 mmol/L (see Adverse Reactions, Clinical Trial and Post-Market Adverse Drug Reactions, Laboratory Abnormalities). Therefore, every attempt should be made to control significant triglyceride elevation (see Warnings and Precautions, Cardiovascular). ACCUTANE should be discontinued if uncontrolled hypertriglyceridemia or symptoms of pancreatitis occur.

Immune: Anaphylactic reactions have been reported. These reactions were more serious after prior exposure to topical retinoids. Allergic cutaneous reactions and serious cases of allergic vasculitis, often with purpura (bruises and red patches) of the extremities and extracutaneous involvement have been reported. Severe allergic reactions necessitate interruption of therapy and careful monitoring.

Musculoskeletal: Effects of multiple courses of ACCUTANE on the developing musculoskeletal system are unknown. There is some evidence that long-term, high-dose, or multiple courses of therapy with isotretinoin have more of an effect than a single course of therapy on the musculoskeletal system (see also Warnings and Precautions, Special Populations, Pediatrics).

In an open-label clinical trial (N=217) of a single course of therapy with ACCUTANE for severe recalcitrant nodular acne in pediatric patients 12 to 17 years, bone density measurements at several skeletal sites were not significantly decreased (lumbar spine change >−4% and total hip change>−5%) or were increased in the majority of patients. One patient had a decrease in lumbar spine bone mineral density >4% based on unadjusted data. Sixteen (7.9%) patients had decreases in lumbar spine bone mineral density >4%, and all the other patients (92%) did not have significant decreases or had increases (adjusted for body mass index). Nine patients (4.5%) had a decrease in total hip bone mineral density >5% based on unadjusted data. Twenty-one (10.6%) patients had decreases in total hip bone mineral density >5%, and all the other patients (89%) did not have significant decreases or had increases (adjusted for body mass index). Follow-up studies performed in 8 of the patients with decreased bone mineral density for up to 11 months thereafter demonstrated increasing bone density in 5 patients at the lumber spine, while the other 3 patients had lumbar spine bone density measurements below baseline values. Total hip bone mineral densities remained below baseline (range −1.6% to −7.6%) in 5 of 8 patients (62.5%).

In this clinical trial transient elevations in CPK were observed in 12% of patients, including those undergoing strenuous physical activity in association with reported musculoskeletal adverse events such as back pain, arthralgia, limb injury, or muscle sprain. In these patients, approximately half of the CPK elevations returned to normal within 2 weeks and half returned to normal within 4 weeks. No cases of rhabdomyolysis were reported in this trial.

In a separate open-label extension study of 10 patients, ages 13-18 years, who started a second course of ACCUTANE 4 months after the first course, two patients showed a decrease in mean lumbar spine bone mineral density up to 3.25%.

Spontaneous reports of osteoporosis, osteopenia, bone fractures, and delayed healing of bone fractures have been seen in the ACCUTANE population. While causality to ACCUTANE has not been established, an effect cannot be ruled out. Longer term effects have not been studied. It is important that ACCUTANE be given at the recommended doses for no longer than the recommended duration.

Although an effect of ACCUTANE on bone loss is not established, physicians should use caution when prescribing ACCUTANE to patients with a genetic predisposition for age-related osteoporosis, a history of childhood osteoporosis conditions, osteomalacia, or other disorders of bone metabolism. This would include patients diagnosed with anorexia nervosa and those who are on chronic drug therapy that causes drug-induced osteoporosis/osteomalacia and/or affects vitamin D metabolism, such as systemic corticosteroids and any anticonvulsant. Patients may be at increased risk when participating in sports with repetitive impact where the risks of spondylolisthesis with and without pars fractures and hip growth plate injuries in early and late adolescence are known. There are spontaneous reports of fractures and/or delayed healing in patients while on treatment with ACCUTANE or following cessation of treatment with ACCUTANE while involved in these activities. While causality to ACCUTANE has not been established, an effect cannot be ruled out.

Hyperostosis: Due to possible occurrence of bone changes, a careful evaluation of the risk/benefit ratio should be carried out in every patient and ACCUTANE administration should be restricted to severe cases of acne. Bone changes including, premature epiphyseal closure, hyperostosis and calcification of tendons and ligaments have occurred after several years of administration at high doses for treating disorders of keratinization. The dose levels, duration of treatment and total cumulative dose in these patients generally far exceeded those recommended for the treatment of acne.

In clinical trials of disorders of keratinization, with a mean dose of 2.24 mg/kg/day, a high prevalence of skeletal hyperostosis was noted. Two children showed x ray findings suggestive of premature closure of the epiphysis. Additionally, skeletal hyperostosis was noted in six of eight patients in a prospective study of disorders of keratinization.

Minimal skeletal hyperostosis and calcification of tendons have also been observed by x-rays in prospective studies of cystic acne patients treated with a single course of therapy at recommended doses. There are spontaneous reports of premature epiphyseal closure in acne patients receiving recommended doses of ACCUTANE. The effect of multiple courses of ACCUTANE on epiphyseal closure is unknown.

In a clinical study of 217 pediatric patients (12 to 17 years) with severe recalcitrant nodular acne, hyperostosis was not observed after 16 to 20 weeks of treatment with approximately 1 mg/kg/day of ACCUTANE given in two divided doses. Hyperostosis may require a longer time frame to appear. The clinical course and significance remain unknown.

Myalgia and arthralgia (mild to moderate) may occur and may be associated with reduced tolerance to vigorous exercise (see Adverse Reactions, Clinical Trial and Post-Market Adverse Drug Reactions, Musculoskeletal). Instances of raised serum creatine phosphokinase (CPK) values have been reported in patients receiving ACCUTANE, particularly those undertaking vigorous physical activity. Discontinuation of ACCUTANE may be required.

Ophthalmologic: Corneal opacities have occurred in patients receiving ACCUTANE for acne and more frequently when higher drug dosages were used in patients with disorders of keratinization. Dry eyes, corneal opacities, decreased night vision, keratitis, blepharitis and conjunctivitis usually resolve after discontinuation of therapy. Due to the possible occurrence of keratitis, patients with dry eyes should be monitored. All ACCUTANE patients experiencing visual difficulties should discontinue the drug and have an ophthalmological examination (see Adverse Reactions, Clinical Trial and Post-Market Adverse Drug Reactions, Ophthalmologic). Dry eyes, can be helped by the application of a lubricating eye ointment or by the application of tear replacement therapy. Intolerance to contact lenses may occur which may necessitate the patient to wear glasses during treatment.

A number of cases of decreased night vision have occurred during ACCUTANE therapy and in rare instances have persisted after therapy (see Adverse Reactions, Clinical Trial and Post-Market Adverse Drug Reactions, Ophthalmologic). Because the onset in some patients was sudden, patients should be advised of this potential problem and warned to be cautious when driving or operating any vehicle at night. ACCUTANE patients experiencing visual impairment should discontinue treatment and have an ophthalmological examination. Visual problems should be carefully monitored.

Skin: Acute exacerbation of acne is occasionally seen during the initial period but this subsides with continued treatment, usually 7-10 days, and usually does not require dose adjustment.

Exposure to intense sunlight or to UV rays should be avoided. When necessary a sun-protection product with a high protection factor of a least SPF 15 should be used.

It is recommended that aggressive chemical dermabrasion and cutaneous laser treatment be avoided in patients on ACCUTANE and for a period of 5-6 months after the end of treatment because of the risk of hypertrophic scarring in atypical areas, and more rarely hyper- or hypo-pigmentation in treated areas.

It is recommended that wax epilation be avoided in patients on ACCUTANE therapy and for a period of 5-6 months after treatment because of the risk of epidermal stripping, scarring or dermatitis.

Concurrent administration of ACCUTANE with keratolytic or exfoliative anti-acne agents should be avoided as local irritation may increase.

Patients should be advised to use a skin-moisturizing ointment or cream and a lip balm from the start of treatment as ACCUTANE is likely to cause dryness of the skin and lips.

There have been post-marketing reports of severe skin reactions (see Warnings and Precautions, Serious Skin Reactions).

Monitoring and Laboratory Tests: Pregnancy Tests: The patient should have two negative pregnancy tests (β-hCG in urine or serum) before starting ACCUTANE therapy with the first pregnancy test conducted at initial assessment when the patient is qualified for ACCUTANE therapy by the physician. The patient then should have a second pregnancy test with a sensitivity of at least 25 mIU/mL with a negative result, performed in a licensed laboratory, within 11 days prior to initiating therapy. The patient has had two or three days of the next normal menstrual period before ACCUTANE therapy is initiated. **Pregnancy test must be repeated monthly for pregnancy detection** during ACCUTANE treatment and at one month after discontinuation of treatment. The dates and results of the pregnancy tests should be documented.

Signs of Depression: Sad mood, hopelessness, feeling of guilt, worthlessness or helplessness, loss of pleasure or interest in activities, fatigue, difficulty concentrating, changes in sleep pattern, change in weight or appetite, suicidal thoughts or attempts, restlessness, irritability, acting on dangerous impulses, and persistent physical symptoms unresponsive to treatment If symptoms of depression develop or worsen during treatment with ACCUTANE, the drug should be discontinued promptly and the patient referred for appropriate psychiatric treatment.

The following tests are required before starting ACCUTANE, at first month, then as clinically indicated:

- Serum blood lipid determinations (under fasting conditions) should be performed before ACCUTANE is given and then at intervals (one month after the start of therapy) until the lipid response to ACCUTANE is established (which usually occurs within four weeks), and also at the end of treatment.
- Complete blood count and differential: for early detection of leukopenia, neutropenia, thrombocytopenia and anemia.
- Liver function tests: Increases in about 15% of ALT, AST, ALP baseline levels have been reported. Liver function tests should be monitored before treatment and at regular intervals during treatment (one month after the start of treatment and at least three month intervals thereafter) unless more frequent monitoring is clinically indicated.
- Blood glucose levels: all patients and in particular patients with known or suspected diabetes should have periodic blood sugar determinations.

ADVERSE REACTIONS: Adverse Drug Reaction Overview: The adverse reactions listed below reflect the experience from clinical studies of ACCUTANE (isotretinoin), and the post-marketing experience. The relationship of some of these events to ACCUTANE therapy is unknown.

Many of the side effects and adverse reactions seen or expected in patients receiving ACCUTANE are similar to those described in patients taking high doses of vitamin A.

Clinical Trial and Post-Market Adverse Drug Reactions: Dose Relationship and Duration: Cheilitis and hypertriglyceridemia are usually dose related.

Adverse reactions were generally reversible when therapy was discontinued; however, some have persisted after cessation of therapy.

The most common side effects are mucocutaneous or dermatologic. The common side effects include: cheilitis (96%), facial erythema/dermatitis (55%), dry nose (51%), desquamation (50%), pruritus (30%), dry skin (22%), conjunctivitis (19%), alopecia (13%), irritation of the eyes (11%), rash (<10%). Dryness of the nasal mucosa and pharynx may be associated with mild epistaxis and hoarseness, respectively. Mild to moderate conjunctivitis may be alleviated by use of an ophthalmic ointment. In rare cases, hair loss persisted after treatment was completed.

Approximately 13% of patients experience joint pain during treatment.

Peeling of palms and soles, skin infections, increased susceptibility to sunburn, nonspecific urogenital symptoms, nonspecific gastrointestinal symptoms, headache, fatigue occured in approximately 5% of patients.

Body as a Whole: weight loss, anemia, lymphadenopathy, vasculitis including Wegener's granulomatosis, allergic vasculitis, allergic responses, and systemic hypersensitivity.

Cardiovascular: edema, transient pain in the chest, palpitations, tachycardia, vascular thrombotic disease, stroke.

Endocrine and Metabolism: new cases of diabetes (see Warnings and Precautions, Endocrine and Metabolism)

Gastrointestinal: nausea, severe diarrhea, mild gastrointestinal bleeding, rectal bleeding, abdominal pain, inflammatory bowel disease (including regional ileitis, colitis and hemorrhage) (see Warnings and Precautions, Gastrointestinal).

Hearing Disorders: tinnitus, impaired hearing at certain frequencies.

Hepatic/Biliary/Pancreatic: Patients treated with ACCUTANE especially those with high triglyceride levels are at risk of developing pancreatitis. Rare cases of fatal pancreatitis and several cases of clinical hepatitis have been reported (see Warnings and Precautions, Hepatic/Biliary/Pancreatic).

Mucocutaneous and Dermatologic: flushing, changes in skin pigment, urticaria, bruising, disseminated herpes simplex, hair problems (other than thinning), hirsutism, erythema nodosum, paronychia, nail dystrophy, pyogenic granuloma, bleeding and inflammation of the gums, acne fulminans, exanthema, sweating, increased formation of granulation tissue, photoallergic/photosensitizing reactions, skin fragility. Acne flare occurs at the start of treatment and persists for several weeks.

During the post-marketing period, erythema multiforme (EM), Stevens-Johnson syndrome (SJS), and toxic epidermal necrolysis (TEN) have been reported to be associated with ACCUTANE (see Warning and Precautions, Serious Skin Reactions).

Musculoskeletal: arthritis, muscle pain (myalgia; elevations of serum CPK values), arthralgia, calcification of ligaments, tendon and tendinitis, reduced bone density, back pain, epiphyses, premature fusion, hyperostosis (see Warnings and Precautions, Musculoskeletal and Hyperostosis).

There have been rare postmarketing reports of rhabdomyolysis, some associated with strenuous physical activity. However, there is insufficient information to suggest an association between treatment with ACCUTANE and the development of rhabdomyolysis.

Neurologic: seizures, dizziness, nervousness, drowsiness, malaise, weakness, insomnia, lethargy, paresthesia, benign intracranial hypertension (see Warnings and Precautions, Serious Warnings and Precautions, Neurologic).

Ophthalmologic: optic neuritis, photophobia, eye lid inflammation, lenticular cataracts, keratitis, blurred vision, blepharitis, conjunctivitis, papilledema as sign of benign intracranial hypertension and colour vision disturbances. Dry eyes and/or decreased tolerance to contact lenses have also been reported during therapy. In some instances these conditions have persisted after cessation of therapy.

Of 72 patients who had normal pre-treatment ophthalmological examinations, five developed corneal opacities while taking ACCUTANE (all five patients had a disorder of keratinization). Corneal opacities have also been reported in nodular and/or inflammatory acne patients treated with ACCUTANE (see Warnings and Precautions, Ophthalmologic). Decrease in night vision has been reported and in rare instances has persisted (see Warnings and Precautions, Ophthalmologic). Cataracts and visual disturbances have also been reported.

Psychiatric Disorders: depression, psychotic symptoms and, rarely, suicide attempts, suicide, and aggressive and/or violent behaviours (see Warnings and Precautions, Serious Warnings and Precautions, Psychiatric). Depression has been reported during and after therapy. In some of these patients, depression has subsided with discontinuation of therapy and recurred when ACCUTANE therapy was reintroduced. Emotional instability has been reported with ACCUTANE.

Respiratory: respiratory infections. Bronchospasm has been rarely reported; sometimes in patients with pre-history of asthma.

Reproductive System: abnormal menses.

Urinary System: glomerulonephritis.

Laboratory Abnormalities: ACCUTANE therapy induces changes in serum lipids in a significant number of treated subjects. These changes consisted of: elevation of serum triglycerides (25% of patients), mild to moderate decrease in serum high density lipoprotein (HDL) (16% of patients), and minimal elevations of serum cholesterol (7% of patients). Abnormalities of serum triglycerides, HDL and cholesterol were reversible upon cessation of ACCUTANE therapy.

A rise in serum levels of liver enzymes may occur, especially with higher dosages. Although the changes have usually been within the normal range, and may return to baseline levels despite continued treatment, significant increases have occurred in a few cases, necessitating dosage reduction or discontinuation of ACCUTANE (see Warnings and Precautions, Hepatic/Biliary/Pancreatic). An elevated erythrocyte sedimentation rate may also occur (40% of patients).

Other less commonly reported laboratory abnormalities were: Elevated fasting blood sugar, elevated CPK, and hyperuricemia. Decreases in red blood cell parameters, decreases in white blood cell counts, elevated sedimentation rates, elevated platelet counts, thrombocytopenia and anemia. White blood cells in the urine, proteinuria, and red blood cells in the urine.

DRUG INTERACTIONS: Drug-Drug Interactions: Tetracyclines: Rare cases of benign intracranial hypertension "pseudotumor cerebri" have been reported after use of ACCUTANE (isotretinoin) and/or tetracyclines. Therefore, concomitant treatment with tetracyclines must be avoided (see Warnings and Precautions, Serious Warnings and Precautions, Neurologic).

Vitamin A: Because of the relationship of ACCUTANE to vitamin A, patients should be advised against taking vitamin supplements containing vitamin A, to avoid additive toxic effects.

Phenytoin: ACCUTANE has not been shown to alter the pharmacokinetics of phenytoin in a study in seven healthy volunteers. These results are consistent with the in vitro finding that neither isotretinoin nor its metabolites induce or inhibit the activity of the CYP 2C9 human hepatic P450 enzyme. Phenytoin is known to cause osteomalacia. No formal clinical studies have been conducted to assess if there is an interactive effect on bone loss between phenytoin and ACCUTANE. Therefore, caution should be exercised when using these drugs together.

Norethindrone/Ethinyl Estradiol: In a study of 31 premenopausal women with severe recalcitrant nodular acne receiving OrthoNovum 7/7/7 Tablets as an oral contraceptive agent, ACCUTANE at the recommended dose of 1 mg/kg/day, did not induce clinically relevant changes in the pharmacokinetics of ethinyl estradiol and norethindrone and in the serum levels of progesterone, follicle-stimulating hormone (FSH) and luteinizing hormone (LH). A drug interaction that decreases effectiveness of hormonal contraceptives has not been entirely ruled out for ACCUTANE.

Microdosed progesterone preparations (minipills) are not a suitable method of contraception during ACCUTANE therapy.

Systemic Corticosteroids: Systemic corticosteroids are known to cause osteoporosis. No formal clinical studies have been conducted to assess if there is an interactive effect on bone loss between systemic corticosteroids and ACCUTANE. Therefore, caution should be exercised when using these drugs together.

Drug-Food Interactions: Due to its lipophilic properties, absorption of ACCUTANE is increased when taken with food. Therefore, the recommended dose is to be taken with food (see Dosage and Administration, Recommended Dose and Dosage Adjustment).

Drug-Herb Interactions: St. John's Wort: ACCUTANE use is associated with depression in some patients (see Warnings and Precautions, Serious Warnings and Precautions, Psychiatric and Adverse Reactions, Psychiatric Disorders). Patients should be prospectively cautioned not to self-medicate with the herbal supplement St. John's Wort because a possible interaction has been suggested with hormonal contraceptives based on reports of breakthrough bleeding on oral contraceptives shortly after starting St. John's Wort. Pregnancies have been reported by users of combined hormonal contraceptives who also used some form of St. John's Wort.

DOSAGE AND ADMINISTRATION: Dosing Considerations: The therapeutic response to ACCUTANE (isotretinoin) is dose related and varies between patients. This necessitates individual adjustment of dosage according to the response of the condition and the patient's tolerance of the drug. In most cases, complete or near complete suppression of acne is achieved with a single 12 to 16 week course of therapy. If a second course of therapy is needed, it can be initiated eight or more weeks after completion of the first course, since experience has shown that patients may continue to improve while off the drug.

Recommended Dose and Dosage Adjustment: Initial Therapy: The initial dose of ACCUTANE should be individualized according to the patient's weight and severity of the disease.

In general, patients initially should receive ACCUTANE 0.5 mg/kg body weight daily for a period of two to four weeks, when their responsiveness to the drug will usually be apparent. It should be noted that transient exacerbation of acne is occasionally seen during this initial period.

The daily dosage should be taken with food in the nearest number of whole capsules, either as a single dose or in two divided doses during the day, whichever is more convenient.

Maintenance Therapy: Maintenance dose should be adjusted between 0.1 and 1 mg/kg body weight daily and, in exceptional instances, up to 2 mg/kg body weight daily, depending upon individual patient response and tolerance to the drug.

A complete course of therapy consists of 12-16 weeks of ACCUTANE administration.

Patients may show additional improvement for up to several months after a course of ACCUTANE has been completed. With effective treatment, appearance of new lesions will not normally be evident for a period of at least three to six months.

OVERDOSAGE:
In the event of acute ACCUTANE (isotretinoin) overdose evacuation of the stomach should be considered during the first few hours after this overdose. Signs and symptoms of acute overdose have been associated with headache, vomiting, facial flushing, cheilitis, abdominal pain, dizziness and ataxia. To date, all symptoms have quickly resolved without apparent residual effects and usually without treatment. Elevated intracranial pressure has been reported with patients receiving therapeutic doses of ACCUTANE. Patients with an ACCUTANE overdose should be monitored closely for signs of increased intracranial pressure. Signs of hypervitaminosis A could appear in cases of overdose.

Limited data exists on the pharmacokinetic characteristics of isotretinoin in an overdose situation. Following the oral administration of single 80, 160, 240 and 340 mg doses to 12 healthy male subjects C_{max} was 366, 820, 1056 and 981 ng/mL, and $t_{1/2}$ was 13.6, 14.1, 14.4 and 16.5 hours for isotretinoin, respectively. Twenty three compromised cancer patients received weekly oral doses of 200 (3 patients); 400 (7 patients); 660 (2 patients); 1000 (3 patients); 1400 (6 patients) and 1800 (1 patient) mg/m². Normal body surface area for healthy subjects is 1.73 m². After the first dose, C_{max} was 1.5, 3.8, 3.5, 2.5, 2.7 and 4.6 μg/mL, and $t_{1/2}$ was 45, 9.1, 14.5, 57, 13.1 and 6.1 hours for isotretinoin, respectively. The absorption of isotretinoin appears to be a saturable process.

Since it is difficult to extrapolate from the results of these studies to the overdose situation, the following precautions should be taken with all female patients of childbearing potential who have taken an overdose of ACCUTANE.

1. At the time of the overdose, a pregnancy test must be performed and a blood sample collected for the determination of isotretinoin and metabolite concentrations.
2. One complete menstrual cycle after the overdose, a second pregnancy test must be performed and a second blood sample collected for the determination of isotretinoin and metabolite concentrations.
3. Effective contraception must be used for at least one complete menstrual cycle after the overdose and continued longer, if necessary until isotretinoin and its metabolites are no longer measurable in the blood.

Patients who present with a positive pregnancy test at the time of the overdose, one complete menstrual cycle after the overdose, or while isotretinoin or metabolite blood concentrations are measurable, should be fully counselled on the serious risk to the fetus from this exposure to ACCUTANE and the physician and patient should discuss the desirability of continuing the pregnancy. (See Contraindications and Warnings and Precautions, Special Populations, Pregnant Women.)

Canadian Regional Poison Information Centres have been advised on the proper collection and handling of ACCUTANE blood samples and also on the laboratory(s) equipped to assay these samples.

For management of a suspected drug overdose, contact your regional Poison Control Centre. See the *CPS* Directory section for a list of Poison Control Centres.

ACTION AND CLINICAL PHARMACOLOGY: Mechanism of Action: The mechanism of action of isotretinoin is unknown. Vitamin A is important for functional integrity of the skin and is known to affect the keratinization process. In acne patients, improvement occurs in association with a reduction in sebum secretion. The decrease in sebum secretion is temporary and is related to either the dose or duration of ACCUTANE administration and reflects a reduction in sebaceous gland size and an inhibition of sebaceous gland differentiation.

Pharmacokinetics: Absorption: Following oral administration of 80 mg, peak plasma concentrations ranged from 167 to 459 ng/mL (mean 256 ng/mL) with a mean time to peak of 3.2 hours in volunteers, while in acne patients peak plasma concentrations ranged from 98 to 535 ng/mL (mean 262 ng/mL) with a mean time to peak of 2.9 hours.

When isotretinoin is taken with food, the bioavailability is doubled relative to fasting conditions (see Dosage and Administration).

Distribution: Isotretinoin is 99.9% protein bound in human plasma, almost exclusively to albumin.

Metabolism: The major metabolite identified in blood and urine was 4-oxo-isotretinoin. Tretinoin and 4-oxo-tretinoin were also observed. The apparent half life for elimination of the 4 oxo isotretinoin ranged from 11 to 50 hours, with a mean of 28 hours. Following 80 mg of isotretinoin administered orally, maximum plasma concentrations of the 4-oxo-isotretinoin was 87 to 399 ng/mL and maxima were observed between 6 and 20 hours. The blood concentration of the major metabolite generally exceeded that of isotretinoin after 6 hours. The data suggest that both isotretinoin and the major metabolite are excreted in the bile and reabsorbed.

The mean minimum steady state blood concentrations of isotretinoin were 160 ng/mL in 10 patients receiving 40 mg twice daily doses. After single and multiple doses, the mean ratio of areas under the curves of 4-oxo-isotretinoin to isotretinoin was between 3 and 3.5.

Excretion: The mean terminal elimination half life of isotretinoin in patients with acne has a mean value of 19 hours. Following oral administration of ^{14}C-isotretinoin, ^{14}C activity in blood declined with a mean half life of 90 hours. Approximately equal amounts of radioactivity were recovered in the urine and feces, with 65-83% of the dose recovered.

Special Populations and Conditions: Pediatrics: The pharmacokinetics of isotretinoin were evaluated after single and multiple doses in 38 pediatric patients (12 to 15 years) and 19 adult patients (≥18 years) who received ACCUTANE for the treatment of severe recalcitrant nodular acne. In both age groups, 4-oxo-isotretinoin was the major metabolite; tretinoin and 4-oxo-tretinoin were also observed. The dose-normalized pharmacokinetic parameters for isotretinoin following single and multiple doses are summarized in Table 1 for pediatric patients. There were no statistically significant differences in the pharmacokinetics of isotretinoin between pediatric and adult patients.

Table 1: ACCUTANE ROCHE

Pharmacokinetic Parameters of Isotretinoin Following Single and Multiple Dose Administration in Pediatric Patients, 12 to 15 Years of Age Mean (±SD), N=38[a]

Parameter	Isotretinoin (Single Dose)	Isotretinoin (Steady-State)
C_{max} (ng/mL)	573.25 (278.79)	731.98 (361.86)
$AUC_{(0-12)}$ (ng·h/mL)	3033.37 (1394.17)	5082.00 (2184.23)
$AUC_{(0-24)}$ (ng·h/mL)	6003.81 (2885.67)	—
T_{max} (h)[b]	6.00 (1.00–24.60)	4.00 (0–12.00)
Css_{min} (ng/mL)	—	352.32 (184.44)
$T_{1/2}$ (h)	—	15.69 (5.12)
CL/F (L/h)	—	17.96 (6.27)

a The single and multiple dose data in this table were obtained following a non standardized meal (non high-fat meal).
b Median (range).

In pediatric patients (12 to 15 years), the mean±SD elimination half-lives (t1/2) of isotretinoin and 4-oxo-isotretinoin were 15.7±5.1 hours and 23.1±5.7 hours, respectively. The accumulation ratios of isotretinoin ranged from 0.46 to 3.65 for pediatric patients.

STORAGE AND STABILITY: ACCUTANE (isotretinoin) 10 mg and 40 mg capsules: Store at 15-30°C. Store in the original package. Protect from exposure to moisture, heat and light.

Keep in a safe place out of the reach of children.

SPECIAL HANDLING INSTRUCTIONS: The release of pharmaceuticals in the environment should be minimized. Medicines should not be disposed of via wastewater and disposal through household waste should be avoided. Use established "collection systems" if available in your location.

Return any unused ACCUTANE (isotretinoin) capsules to the pharmacist.

INFORMATION FOR THE PATIENT: Published in e-CPS, available by subscription at www.e-cps.ca.

DOSAGE FORMS, COMPOSITION AND PACKAGING: 10 mg: Each brown-red, opaque, oval-shaped, soft gelatin capsule, imprinted ROA 10 contains: isotretinoin 10 mg. Nonmedicinal ingredients: beeswax, black iron oxide, gelatin, glycerol, hydrogenated hydrolysed starch, hydrogenated soybean oil, mannitol, partially hydrogenated soybean oil, propylene glycol, red iron oxide, shellac, sorbitol, soybean oil and titanium dioxide. Blister packs of 30.

40 mg: Each yellow, opaque, oval-shaped, soft gelatin capsule, imprinted ROA 40 contains: isotretinoin 40 mg. Nonmedicinal ingredients: beeswax, black iron oxide, gelatin, glycerol, hydrogenated soybean oil, methylparaben, partially hydrogenated soybean oil, propylene glycol, propylparaben, quinoline yellow WS, shellac, soybean oil, sunset yellow FCF and titanium dioxide. Blister packs of 30.

(Shown in Product Identification Section)

ACE Inhibitors ℞

benazepril HCl
captopril
cilazapril monohydrate
enalapril maleate
enalaprilat
fosinopril sodium
lisinopril
perindopril erbumine
quinapril HCl
ramipril
trandolapril

Angiotensin Converting Enzyme Inhibitor

CPhA Monograph

Date of Revision: October 2006

This monograph has been compiled by CPhA and reviewed by experts. It may contain information different from that found in Health Canada-approved Product Monographs. The reader is referred to the *CPS* Editorial Policy for more information.

PHARMACOLOGY: The renin-angiotensin system is a complex neuroendocrine system involved in the regulation of hemodynamics and water and electrolyte balance. When renin is released from the kidney in response to a decrease in blood volume, renal perfusion pressure or plasma sodium concentration, it acts on its substrate, angiotensinogen, to form angiotensin I. Angiotensin converting enzyme (ACE) catalyzes the conversion of angiotensin I to angiotensin II. Inhibitors of ACE suppress the production of angiotensin II, which is the most vasoactive product of the renin-angiotensin system.

Patients with low plasma renin activity may experience a lesser antihypertensive response to monotherapy with ACE inhibitors.

Angiotensin II exerts many physiologic effects, including stimulation of aldosterone secretion, direct systemic and coronary vasoconstriction and a positive inotropic effect, both directly, and indirectly through enhanced sympathetic outflow. Inhibition of ACE decreases systemic arteriolar resistance and mean diastolic and systolic blood pressure. In patients with HF, inhibition of ACE decreases afterload and heart rate and increases cardiac output, stroke volume and stroke work.

ACE, also known as kininase II, catalyzes the breakdown of the vasodilating autocoid, bradykinin. By inhibiting its inactivation, ACE inhibitors potentiate the action of bradykinin, which causes vasodilation (by stimulating nitric oxide production) and natriuresis (through direct effects on the renal tubules).

The action of ACE inhibitors may not completely block the production of angiotensin II. Tissue-based chymases may facilitate the formation of angiotensin II from its precursors, independently of ACE.

ACE inhibitors have many clinical applications, including the treatment of hypertension, HF, left ventricular dysfunction and diabetic nephropathy (see Indications).

Pharmacokinetics: With the exception of enalaprilat, which is given i.v., ACE inhibitors are absorbed to varying degrees from the gastrointestinal tract after oral administration. The rate and/or extent of absorption of certain agents may be decreased in the presence of food, although it is not clear whether this is clinically important in every case.

With the exception of captopril, enalaprilat and lisinopril, ACE inhibitors are prodrug esters that must be converted in the liver and/or gastrointestinal mucosa to active metabolites. Elimination of unchanged drug or metabolites may be renal or fecal. The pharmacokinetic properties of ACE inhibitors are summarized in Table 1.

Other pharmacokinetic properties that may differentiate ACE inhibitors include: lipophilicity and tissue binding; drug-receptor affinity and rate of dissociation of the drug-receptor complex; peak—trough ratio (ideally, at least 50% of the peak effect should remain at the end of the dosing interval). Further study is needed to establish the potential clinical significance of these pharmacokinetic differences.

INDICATIONS: ACE inhibitors are used as first-line agents in the management of hypertension.

ACE inhibitors slow the progression of nephropathy in diabetic patients with or without proteinuria and in nondiabetic nephropathy. This renoprotective effect is thought to involve mechanisms independent of blood pressure reduction, and occurs in both hypertensive and normotensive diabetic patients.

ACE inhibitors are considered standard therapy in post- MI patients, to reduce afterload and preload and to prevent complications such as left ventricular remodeling and HF. They have been shown to reduce cardiovascular morbidity (e.g. hospitalization for cardiac causes) and mortality post-MI. ACE inhibitors are also considered to be first-line agents in the treatment of systolic heart failure.

Whether there is a class effect with respect to the clinical efficacy of ACE inhibitors for indications other than uncomplicated hypertension is controversial. Differences among the agents are discussed in relevant sections of the monograph. An evidence-based approach to drug selection is considered prudent. It should be noted that the approved indications may not reflect the most current evidence or standard practice with respect to these agents. The approved indications for each of the agents available in Canada are presented in Table 2.

The i.v. formulation of enalaprilat is indicated for the treatment of hypertension when the oral route is not practical.

CONTRAINDICATIONS: In patients with known hypersensitivity to a particular ACE inhibitor, the specific agent in question is contraindicated. All ACE inhibitors are contraindicated in patients with a history of angioedema related to previous use of any member of this class. Products containing a fixed combination of an ACE inhibitor and a thiazide diuretic are contraindicated in anuric patients and those with hypersensitivity to thiazides or other sulfonamide-derived drugs.

WARNINGS: *Pregnancy* (see Precautions, Pregnancy): **Exposure to ACE inhibitors during the first trimester of pregnancy has been associated with an increased risk of major congenital malformations. When used during the second and third trimesters of pregnancy, ACE inhibitors may cause significant fetal morbidity or mortality. ACE inhibitors should be discontinued as soon as possible if pregnancy is detected.**

Angioedema: Angioedema has been reported with the use of ACE inhibitors. Involvement of the larynx may be fatal. If swelling is limited to the face and lips, discontinuation of the ACE inhibitor is usually the only corrective measure required. However, if there is involvement of the tongue, glottis or larynx, appropriate therapy (e.g., epinephrine) should be instituted as life-threatening airway obstruction may occur. Patients should be advised that swelling in the mouth or facial area or difficulty breathing or swallowing may be signs of angioedema and that they should discontinue the ACE inhibitor and contact their physician immediately if any of these symptoms occur.

Hypotension: Severe hypotension may occur with the use of ACE inhibitors, particularly in patients who are volume depleted, hyponatremic, receiving concomitant diuretics or on dialysis. ACE inhibitors should be used with caution in patients with cerebrovascular disease or ischemic heart disease, as severe hypotension could have serious consequences in these patients. In patients with severe heart failure with or without pre-existing renal insufficiency, ACE inhibitors may cause excessive hypotension with oliguria, azotemia and potentially fatal renal failure. In these patient groups, ACE inhibitors should be initiated under close medical supervision and monitored closely for the first few weeks of therapy and whenever the dose is increased.

Table 1: ACE Inhibitors

Pharmacokinetics

ACE Inhibitor	Effect of Food on Absorption: Decreased Rate of Absorption	Effect of Food on Absorption: Decreased Extent of Absorption	Active Metabolite	Time to Peak Effect (hours)	Duration of Action (hours)	Route of Elimination	Binding Group
Benazepril	Yes	No	Benazeprilat	2 to 4	24[a]	Renal[b]: 88% Biliary: 12%	Carboxyl
Captopril	Yes	Yes	NA[c]	1 to 1.5	6 to 12[d]	Renal[b]	Sulfhydryl
Cilazapril	Yes	Yes	Cilazaprilat	2 to 4	24[a]	Renal[b]	Carboxyl
Enalapril	No	No	Enalaprilat	Oral: 4 to 6 I.V.: 1 to 4	Oral: 24[a] I.V.: 6	Renal[b]	Carboxyl
Fosinopril	Yes	No	Fosinoprilat	2 to 6	24[a]	Renal: 50% Fecal: 50%	Phosphinyl
Lisinopril	No	No	NA[c]	6	24[a]	Renal[b]	Carboxyl
Perindopril	No	No[e]	Perindoprilat	6	24[a]	Renal[b]	Carboxyl
Quinapril	Yes[f]	No	Quinaprilat	2 to 24	24[d]	Renal[b]: 60% Fecal: 40%	Carboxyl
Ramipril	Yes	No	Ramiprilat	4 to 6.5	24[a]	Renal[b]: 60% Fecal: 40%	Carboxyl
Trandolapril	Yes	No	Trandolaprilat	2 to 4	24[a]	Renal: 33% Fecal: 67%	Carboxyl

[a] Some patients may not have adequate blood pressure control at the end of a 24-hour dosing interval and may require dosage adjustment (see Dosage).
[b] Dosage adjustment is recommended in patients with renal failure.
[c] Not applicable.
[d] Dose-related.
[e] The extent of biotransformation to perindoprilat may be decreased in the presence of food, resulting in slightly decreased pharmacodynamic effect.
[f] Especially high fat meals.

Patients taking ACE inhibitors should be advised that vomiting, diarrhea, excessive perspiration or dehydration due to low fluid intake may cause an exaggerated decrease in blood pressure and that they should inform their physician if any of these conditions occur.

Neutropenia/Agranulocytosis: Neutropenia and bone marrow depression have occurred during therapy with ACE inhibitors. Periodic monitoring of white blood cell count is suggested, especially in patients with risk factors such as collagen vascular disease, renal failure or drug therapy that may cause immunosuppression. ACE inhibitors should be used with caution in these patients. Patients should be advised to report any symptoms of infection, such as sore throat or fever, to their physician

Table 2: ACE Inhibitors

Labeled Indications[a]

ACE Inhibitor	Hypertension	Heart Failure	Left Ventricular Dysfunction	Diabetic Nephropathy	Prevention of Cardiovascular Events
Benazepril	Yes	—	—	—	—
Captopril	Yes	Yes	Yes[b]	Yes	—
Cilazapril	Yes	Yes	—	—	—
Enalapril	Yes	Yes	Yes	—	—
Enalaprilat	Yes	—	—	—	—
Fosinopril	Yes	Yes	—	—	—
Lisinopril[c]	Yes	Yes	[c]	—	—
Perindopril	Yes	Yes	—	—	Yes[d]
Quinapril	Yes	Yes	—	—	—
Ramipril[e]	Yes	—	Yes[b]	—	Yes[e]
Trandolapril	Yes	—	Yes[b]	—	—

[a] See Indications, above.
[b] Following acute MI.
[c] Lisinopril is approved for use in hemodynamically stable patients within 24 hours of acute MI, to improve survival. To be reassessed after 6 weeks if no LVD.
[d] Perindopril is approved to reduce the risk of cardiovascular death, nonfatal MI and cardiac arrest in mild or moderately hypertensive patients with stable coronary artery disease (CAD), or in patients with previous (> 3 months ago) MI and stable CAD when administered as an add-on to conventional treatment.
[e] Ramipril is approved to reduce the risk of MI, stroke or cardiovascular death in patients over 55 years of age who have a history of CAD, stroke, peripheral artery disease or diabetes that is accompanied by at least one other cardiovascular risk factor.

PRECAUTIONS: Impaired Renal Function: Renal function should be evaluated prior to the initiation of ACE inhibitor therapy. Patients with impaired renal function, particularly those with bilateral or unilateral renal artery stenosis, may experience further deterioration of renal function, including acute renal failure, while taking ACE inhibitors. Patients with HF or those receiving concomitant diuretic therapy may be at increased risk. Reducing the dose of the ACE inhibitor or discontinuing the diuretic may be sufficient to restore adequate renal perfusion.

Although ACE inhibitors have been found to slow the progression of diabetic nephropathy in type I diabetic patients with documented proteinuria, some patients with pre-existing renal disease may be at increased risk of developing proteinuria while on ACE inhibitor therapy.

Hypersensitivity: Sudden, life-threatening anaphylactoid reactions have occurred during therapy with ACE inhibitors in patients undergoing hemodialysis with polyacrylonitrile (PAN) high-flux membranes and in patients being desensitized to hymenoptera venom (i.e., bees, wasps). Dialysis should be stopped immediately if symptoms such as nausea, abdominal cramps, burning, angioedema or shortness of breath occur, and appropriate treatment initiated. Antihistamines generally do not provide symptomatic relief in these situations.

Hyperkalemia: Increases in serum potassium can occur during therapy with ACE inhibitors. Clinically significant hyperkalemia usually occurs in patients with impaired renal function, HF or diabetes, and those who are taking drugs that increase serum potassium such as potassium-sparing diuretics (amiloride, spironolactone, triamterene), and/or potassium supplements.

Impaired Liver Function: Increases in serum transaminase and/or bilirubin levels, cholestatic jaundice and cases of hepatocellular injury with or without cholestasis have occurred during ACE inhibitor therapy, even in patients with no pre-existing liver disease. In most cases, these changes were reversible upon discontinuation of the drug. Patients reporting symptoms such as abdominal pain, muscle aches, vomiting, loss of appetite, etc., should be investigated for possible hepatic adverse effects. ACE inhibitors should be used with caution in these patients and baseline liver function tests should be performed prior to initiation of treatment.

Cough: A persistent, dry cough occurs in some patients after initiating treatment with an ACE inhibitor. Inhibition of kininase II and accumulation of kinins in tissues of the respiratory tract is thought to cause the cough. The overall incidence has been reported to range from 5 to 35%, is more common in women, patients with HF, nonsmokers and those of Chinese heritage. The onset of cough has been reported to occur within hours of the first dose of medication to weeks or months after initiating treatment.

Cough is associated with all ACE inhibitors, is not dose related and rarely improves upon switching to a different agent in the class. To determine whether ACE inhibitor is the cause of a chronic cough, therapy should be discontinued regardless of the temporal relationship between the initiation of the ACE inhibitor and the onset of the cough. ACE-inhibitor induced cough usually resolves within 1 to 4 weeks of cessation of the drug, although in some patients this may not occur for up to 3 months. For patients with a compelling indication for an ACE inhibitor, and in whom the cough resolves after withdrawal of the drug, a repeat trial with a different agent may be attempted.

The only uniformly effective treatment for ACE inhibitor-induced cough is discontinuation of therapy. When the cough is persistent or intolerable, therapy should be changed, when indicated, to an angiotensin II receptor antagonist or another agent. Many drugs have been tried to attenuate ACE inhibitor induced cough (e.g., inhaled sodium cromolyn), although the size of the trials has generally been small and the quality of evidence is poor.

Pregnancy: Pregnancy (see Warnings): ACE inhibitors should not be taken during pregnancy. The results of a large cohort study showed that exposure to ACE inhibitors during the first trimester of pregnancy was associated with an increased risk of major congenital malformations of the cardiovascular and central nervous systems compared with both exposure to other antihypertensive agents and no exposure to antihypertensive agents. Exposure to ACE inhibitors during the second and third trimesters of pregnancy has resulted in serious neonatal complications including hypotension, reversible or irreversible renal failure, anuria, skull hypoplasia and/or death. Oligohydramnios, which may be associated with contractures of the limbs, craniofacial deformities, lung hypoplasia and intrauterine growth retardation, has also occurred. ACE inhibitors should be discontinued in women planning to become pregnant and as soon as possible if pregnancy is detected.

Lactation: Detectable levels of various ACE inhibitors have been found in breast milk. Although the respective manufacturers generally advise not to breast feed while taking ACE inhibitors, there is no evidence to date of harmful effects in nursing infants.

Children: Although there is limited experience with the use of captopril in infants and children, safety and efficacy of ACE inhibitors in the pediatric population have not been established. There appear to be specific risks associated with their use in neonates and infants, such as oliguria and neurologic abnormalities, possibly caused by decreased renal and cerebral perfusion due to prolonged, excessive hypotension. Most manufacturers advise against the use of their product in children. The manufacturer of captopril recommends its use only when other measures for controlling blood pressure have not been successful.

Geriatrics: ACE inhibitors are presumed to be more effective in the treatment of hypertensive patients with high or normal plasma renin activity. Although renin activity may decrease with advancing age, an age-related decline in renal function may result in a higher area under the concentration-time curve for ACE inhibitors. The net effect is that no significant differences in blood pressure response or adverse effects have been reported in elderly patients taking ACE inhibitors, compared with the general population. However, the possibility of increased sensitivity to the hypotensive effects of these drugs in some elderly patients should be borne in mind.

__Drug Interactions:__ Some of the drug interactions involving ACE inhibitors are class effects, while others are specific to one or more individual agents.

Agents Causing Renin Release: The antihypertensive effect of ACE inhibitors is augmented by antihypertensive agents which cause renin release, such as thiazide diuretics.

Agents Increasing Serum Potassium: ACE inhibitors decrease aldosterone production which may increase potassium retention by the kidney. When ACE inhibitors are combined with potassium-sparing diuretics, potassium supplements or potassium-containing salt substitutes, severe hyperkalemia may occur. Frequent monitoring of serum potassium is recommended when these agents are used concomitantly with an ACE inhibitor. Patients with diabetes, impaired renal function or HF are at increased risk of hypokalemia.

Allopurinol: Although a causal relationship has not been proven, a small number of patients taking captopril or enalapril experienced severe hypersensitivity reactions including anaphylaxis and fatal Stevens-Johnson syndrome, when allopurinol was added to their therapeutic regimen. Other factors may have contributed to the reactions. It is not known whether all ACE inhibitors increase the risk of allopurinol hypersensitivity reactions. A cautious approach is recommended until more information is available.

Alpha-blocking Agents: Patients taking ACE inhibitors may experience an exaggerated hypotensive response to the first dose of an alpha-blocker (e.g., doxazosin, prazosin, terazosin). These drugs should be introduced at a low initial dosage, and used with caution.

Diuretics: Patients on severe dietary salt restriction or those on diuretic therapy, especially if the diuretic was recently instituted, may experience excessive hypotension when ACE inhibitor therapy is initiated. This effect may be minimized by increasing salt intake or discontinuing the diuretic 2 to 7 days prior to introduction of the ACE inhibitor. If this is not feasible, the initial dose of the ACE inhibitor should be reduced and the patient's blood pressure carefully monitored after the first dose. If hypotension occurs, the patient should be placed in a supine position, and i.v. normal saline may be given if necessary. Hypotension should subside once volume expansion occurs and is a not a contraindication to further ACE inhibitor therapy.
Iron: ACE inhibitor therapy may augment the systemic adverse effects of i.v. iron, such as fever, arthralgia and hypotension, possibly by decreasing the metabolism of kinins. This does not seem to be the case with oral iron salts. Concomitant ACE inhibitor and i.v. iron therapy should be avoided whenever possible.
Lithium: Lithium toxicity, including CNS symptoms, ECG changes and renal failure, has occurred in patients taking ACE inhibitors. Proposed mechanisms include decreased renal elimination of lithium due to decreased aldosterone secretion or decreased renal function. Frequent monitoring of lithium levels is recommended in patients taking these agents concurrently.
NSAIDs (including COX-2 inhibitors): There is some evidence that the antihypertensive effect of ACE inhibitors may be antagonized by NSAIDs. Patients taking these agents concurrently should be monitored for signs of worsening heart failure or renal function or loss of blood pressure control.
Tetracyclines: The absorption of tetracyclines may be reduced when taken concurrently with quinapril, due to the presence of magnesium carbonate as an excipient in its pharmaceutical formulation.

ADVERSE EFFECTS: Cardiovascular: Hypotension may occur in patients taking ACE inhibitors, particularly during initial therapy and in patients with other risk factors (see Warnings). Rarely, other cardiovascular effects such as chest pain, tachycardia, palpitations, angina and MI have occurred.
Dermatologic: A maculopapular rash has occurred in patients taking ACE inhibitors and is more frequent in patients with renal impairment. It usually appears within the first month of therapy and may disappear on its own, with a dosage reduction or discontinuation of the ACE inhibitor, or with oral antihistamine therapy. It has been postulated that this rash is mediated by kinins.

Photosensitivity and pemphigoid lesions have occurred in patients taking ACE inhibitors.
Hematologic: Neutropenia, agranulocytosis and other blood dyscrasias have occurred during therapy with ACE inhibitors, especially in patients with additional risk factors (see Warnings). Patients should be advised to report symptoms such as sore throat or fever to their physician.
Hypersensitivity: Angioedema (see Warnings), serum sickness and bronchospasm have been reported. Anaphylactoid reactions have occurred in patients undergoing hemodialysis with PAN membranes or desensitization to hymenoptera venom (see Precautions).
Renal: Deterioration of renal function has occurred during therapy with ACE inhibitors, particularly in patients with predisposing conditions (see Precautions). Proteinuria, potentially progressing to nephrotic syndrome, has also been reported.
Respiratory: A persistent, dry cough has been associated with the use of ACE inhibitors (see Precautions).
Taste Disturbances: Although more common with captopril, all ACE inhibitors may decrease taste acuity or alter taste perception (e.g., metallic or salty taste). Taste disturbance usually occurs during the first 3 months of therapy and is usually reversible over 2 to 3 months, even if the ACE inhibitor is continued. Weight loss may accompany loss of taste.

OVERDOSE:

For management of a suspected drug overdose, CPhA recommends that you contact your **regional Poison Control Centre**. See the *CPS* Directory section for a list of Poison Control Centres.

DOSAGE: **Oral:** The initial dosage of an ACE inhibitor must be individualized, because of the risk of hypotension, taking into consideration factors such as renal and/or hepatic dysfunction, HF, diuretic therapy, volume depletion or hyponatremia. Patients at increased risk of hypotension should receive lower initial doses, with the first dose given under close medical supervision. Observation of the patient should continue for at least 2 hours following administration, or until blood pressure has been stable for 1 hour.

Once therapy has been initiated, the dosage should be gradually titrated to achieve the desired effect, depending on the indication for use. Table 3 lists dosage recommendations for ACE inhibitors in the treatment of hypertension, including initial, maintenance and maximum dosages. Table 4 lists dosage recommendations for ACE inhibitors in the treatment of HF. More detailed information may be found in individual product monographs, including specific dosage recommendations for different indications, titration guidelines and dosage adjustment in patients with renal or hepatic dysfunction.

Table 3: ACE Inhibitors

Oral Dosage for Hypertension

Drug	Usual Initial Dosage[a]	Usual Maintenance Dosage[a]	Recommended Maximum Daily Dose
Benazepril[b]	10 mg once daily	20 mg once daily[c]	40 mg
Captopril[b]	25 mg 2 to 3 times daily[d]	50 mg 2 to 3 times daily	450 mg
Cilazapril[b]	2.5 mg once daily	2.5 to 5 mg once daily[c]	10 mg
Enalapril[b]	5 mg once daily	10 to 40 mg daily in one single or two divided doses	40 mg
Fosinopril[e]	10 mg once daily	20 mg once daily[c]	40 mg
Lisinopril[b]	10 mg once daily	10 to 40 mg once daily[c]	80 mg
Perindopril[b]	4 mg once daily	4 to 8 mg once daily[c]	8 mg
Quinapril[b]	10 mg once daily	10 to 20 mg once daily[c]	40 mg
Ramipril[b]	2.5 mg once daily	2.5 to 10 mg once daily[c]	20 mg
Trandolapril[f]	1 mg once daily	1 to 2 mg once daily[c]	4 mg

[a] As monotherapy in the treatment of hypertension, in patients with no additional risk factors such as renal failure, HF or concomitant diuretic therapy (see Warnings and Precautions).
[b] Dosage and/or interval require adjustment in renal dysfunction (see individual product monographs).
[c] Some patients may experience a diminished antihypertensive effect toward the end of a 24-hour dosing interval. Splitting the daily dose into two equal 12-hourly doses or increasing the once daily dose may be considered (see individual product monographs).
[d] The manufacturer of captopril recommends that doses be taken 1 hour before meals.
[e] No dosage adjustment necessary in patients with renal failure and normal hepatic function, and vice versa.
[f] Dosage adjustment required in renal or hepatic failure.

Table 4: ACE Inhibitors

Oral Dosage for HF

Drug	Initial Dosage	Target Dosage
Captopril[a,b]	6.25–12.5 mg three times daily	50 mg three times daily
Cilazapril[a]	0.5 mg once daily	2.5 mg once daily
Enalapril[a]	1.25–2.5 mg twice daily	10 mg twice daily
Lisinopril[a]	2.5–5 mg once daily	20–35 mg once daily
Perindopril[a]	2 mg once daily	4 mg once daily
Quinapril[a]	5–10 mg once daily	40 mg once daily or 20 mg twice daily
Ramipril[a]	1.25–2.5 mg twice daily	5 mg twice daily or 10 mg once daily

(cont'd)

Table 4: ACE Inhibitors *(cont'd)*

[a] Dosage and/or interval require adjustment in renal dysfunction (see individual product monographs).
[b] The manufacturer of captopril recommends doses be taken one hour before meals.

I.V.: When the oral route is not feasible, the usual initial dosage of enalaprilat in the treatment of hypertension is 1.25 mg every 6 hours, administered i.v., either undiluted or mixed with up to 50 mL compatible diluent, over a period of at least 5 minutes (see product monograph). When converting from i.v. enalaprilat to oral enalapril, the initial dose should be 5 mg once daily, with subsequent adjustments as necessary.

Patients on diuretic therapy should receive a lower initial i.v. enalaprilat dosage of 0.625 mg over 5 minutes, with a second dose after 1 hour if an inadequate response is seen. Additional doses may be repeated at 6-hour intervals.

ACET 120
acetaminophen
Analgesic—Antipyretic

PendoPharm

ACET 160
acetaminophen
Analgesic—Antipyretic

PendoPharm

ACET 325
acetaminophen
Analgesic—Antipyretic

PendoPharm

ACET 650
acetaminophen
Analgesic—Antipyretic

PendoPharm

SUPPLIED: 120 mg: Each cone shaped suppository contains: acetaminophen USP 120 mg. Nonmedicinal ingredients: triglycerides. Individually sealed and available in boxes of 4 and 12. Store below 22°C.
160 mg: Each cone shaped suppository contains: acetaminophen USP 160 mg. Nonmedicinal ingredients: triglycerides. Individually sealed and available in boxes of 4 and 12. Store below 22°C.
325 mg: Each cone shaped suppository contains: acetaminophen USP 325 mg. Nonmedicinal ingredients: triglycerides. Individually sealed and available in boxes of 4 and 12. Store below 22°C.
650 mg: Each cone shaped suppository contains: acetaminophen USP 650 mg. Nonmedicinal ingredients: triglycerides. Individually sealed and available in boxes of 4 and 12. Store below 22°C.

Acetaminophen
Analgesic—Antipyretic

CPhA Monograph

Date of Revision: October 2009

This monograph has been compiled by CPhA and reviewed by experts. It may contain information different from that found in Health Canada-approved Product Monographs. The reader is referred to the *CPS* Editorial Policy for more information.

SUMMARY PRODUCT INFORMATION:

Route of Administration	Dosage Form	Strength
Oral	Immediate-release tablet	325 mg, 500 mg
	Immediate-release caplet	325 mg, 500 mg
	Extended-release caplet	650 mg
	Gelcap	500 mg
	Chewable tablet	80 mg, 160 mg
	Rapidly-dissolving tablet	80 mg, 160 mg
	Liquid	80 mg/mL, 32 mg/mL (160 mg/5 mL)
Rectal	Suppository	160 mg, 325 mg, 650 mg

PHARMACOLOGY: Acetaminophen, also known as paracetamol, is a synthetic derivative of p-aminophenol. It is also an active metabolite of two other p-aminophenol derivatives, phenacetin and acetanilid, which were withdrawn from the market because of unacceptable nephrotoxicity.

Acetaminophen is an analgesic and antipyretic agent, similar in potency and efficacy to salicylates. Acetaminophen does not share the anti-inflammatory or uricosuric effects of ASA and does not cause gastrointestinal ulceration or inhibit platelet aggregation.

The mechanism of acetaminophen's antipyretic action may involve a direct effect on the heat-regulating centres in the hypothalamus, leading to increased heat dissipation through vasodilation and sweating.

The proposed mechanism of acetaminophen's analgesic action is through inhibition of prostaglandin synthetase in the CNS. Acetaminophen has minimal effect on peripheral prostaglandin synthesis, which may explain its relative lack of anti-inflammatory effect compared to ASA.

Pharmacokinetics: Acetaminophen is rapidly and completely absorbed from the gastrointestinal tract. A mean peak plasma concentration of 100 µmol/L is reached approximately 0.8 hours following a 1000 mg oral dose of immediate-release acetaminophen tablets. Rectal absorption is slower and less complete, with peak plasma concentrations occurring in roughly 2-5 hours in children. The plasma half-life ranges from 1 to 4 hours but may be prolonged in acute overdose.

Extended-release bilayer tablets contain a total of 650 mg acetaminophen, with 325 mg in an immediate-release layer and 325 mg in a slow-release matrix. Following a 1300 mg oral dose, a mean peak concentration of 60 µmol/L is reached in approximately 1.5 hours. The half-life is similar to that of immediate-release formulations.

Up to 95% of a dose of acetaminophen is conjugated in the liver, mainly with glucuronic acid and to a lesser extent sulfuric acid, then excreted renally. A small percentage is either excreted in the urine unchanged or oxidized by hepatic CYP2E1 yielding N-acetyl-p-benzoquinoneimine (NAPQI), a toxic metabolite that is subsequently conjugated with glutathione and excreted by the kidney. However, when glutathione is depleted following a high dose of acetaminophen, NAPQI accumulates and is believed to be the cause of acetaminophen-induced liver necrosis (see Overdose).

INDICATIONS: Acetaminophen is indicated for treatment of mild to moderate pain and the reduction of fever; it is considered the drug of first choice for the management of osteoarthritis and for fever in children.

CONTRAINDICATIONS: Hypersensitivity to acetaminophen or any component of the formulation; acetaminophen-induced liver disease.

WARNINGS: Acetaminophen is one of the most frequent causes of accidental poisoning in infants and toddlers. Acetaminophen-containing products should be kept well out of reach of children. Because acetaminophen is an ingredient in many combination products, health practitioners and caregivers must be vigilant to prevent unintended overdosage through administration of multiple acetaminophen-containing products to the same patient. See also Precautions.

PRECAUTIONS: Potentially fatal hepatotoxicity can result from acetaminophen overdose (see Overdose). However, hepatotoxicity has occurred in patients receiving high or excessive doses with therapeutic intent. Certain patients may be more susceptible to acetaminophen hepatotoxicity, e.g., chronic alcoholics, patients with liver disease or those who are malnourished or taking other drugs that induce hepatic enzymes (see also Children and Drug Interactions).

Because of the risk of hepatotoxicity, patients should be cautioned against the inadvertent administration of excessive doses of acetaminophen that can occur through concomitant use of multiple acetaminophen-containing products, such as cough and cold remedies, analgesic or arthritis formulations, antipyretics or products for relief of menstrual symptoms or muscle spasm. Administration of acetaminophen to children may be especially prone to error due to the many concentrations and strengths of products available. To avoid dosing errors, all product labels should be checked carefully to ensure accurate calculation of the amount of acetaminophen to be given.

Drug Interactions: Anticoagulants, Oral: Administration of acetaminophen may potentiate the anticoagulant effect of warfarin. This interaction may be more likely with higher doses of acetaminophen but may occur with short-term use of lower doses. Patients stabilized on oral anticoagulants should be made aware of this potential interaction and additional monitoring of INR may be indicated.

ASA: Concurrent long-term use of analgesic-antipyretic agents with ASA may be associated with analgesic nephropathy (papillary necrosis and tubulointerstitial inflammation).

Cholestyramine: Cholestyramine reduces the absorption of acetaminophen. Oral doses of cholestyramine and acetaminophen should be given at least 1 hour apart.

Enzyme Inducers: Barbiturates and other enzyme inducers such as carbamazepine, isoniazid, phenytoin or rifampin may enhance the metabolism of acetaminophen. This can result in increased clearance and diminished therapeutic effect of acetaminophen, or increased hepatotoxicity. Appropriate monitoring (for therapeutic effect and hepatotoxicity) is indicated if these agents are used concurrently. Patients taking enzyme-inducing drugs should limit self-medication with acetaminophen.

Ethanol: Ethanol is both a substrate and inducer of CYP2E1, the enzyme responsible for the formation of acetaminophen's toxic metabolite NAPQI. The relationship between acute or chronic ethanol use or recent abstinence and susceptibility to acetaminophen toxicity from either therapeutic use or overdose is complex and controversial. There is insufficient evidence on which to base firm conclusions about the differential risk of hepatotoxicity conferred by ethanol use or recent abstinence.

Drug-Food Interactions: Food delays the absorption of acetaminophen. For rapid onset of action, avoid taking acetaminophen with food, particularly carbohydrates.

Lactation: Acetaminophen passes into breast milk but is not likely to have an adverse effect on the infant at therapeutic doses. Peak concentrations in the milk occur 1 to 2 hours after a dose.

Pregnancy: Acetaminophen crosses the placenta and is considered safe for short-term use when therapeutic doses are used.

Children: Dosages of acetaminophen for children should be calculated on a mg/kg basis. Liquid dosage forms should be measured with a calibrated measuring device, as household spoons vary significantly with respect to volume.

No more than 75 mg/kg of acetaminophen should be given to a child in a 24-hour period. Children under two years old who have received 120 mg/kg/day or more of acetaminophen for more than one day and who are acutely malnourished and dehydrated may be at higher risk for hepatotoxicity.

ADVERSE EFFECTS: Chronic use of high doses of acetaminophen may produce significant toxicity (see Precautions).

Dermatologic: Although uncommon, cutaneous reactions have been reported with acetaminophen.

Hematologic: Neutropenia and thrombocytopenia purpura have been reported and rarely agranulocytosis.

Hepatic: See Precautions.

Hypersensitivity: Reactions including laryngeal edema, angioedema, bronchospasm and/or anaphylaxis have occurred rarely. Dose-dependent cross-sensitivity to acetaminophen is reported to occur in up to 34% of ASA-sensitive asthmatic patients. Low initial doses of acetaminophen (less than 1000 mg) are recommended in these patients, with monitoring for about 3 hours following initial doses.

Renal: Nephropathy, including papillary renal failure has been reported following consumption of large amounts of acetaminophen. Renal tubular necrosis has been associated occasionally with hepatic injury produced by acetaminophen overdose.

OVERDOSE:

In adults, hepatotoxicity may occur after ingestion of a single dose of more than 7.5 g (adults) or 150 mg/kg (children) of acetaminophen; a dose of 10 g or more is potentially fatal. However, reports have indicated hepatic necrosis with a single dose of 6 g and death occurring with a single dose of 13 g. Nonfatal overdoses of 12.5 to 31.5 g have also been reported (see also Precautions).

Symptoms: Early symptoms (nausea, vomiting, weakness, diaphoresis) usually occur after acute ingestion of an acetaminophen overdose large enough to cause hepatic toxicity. However, since some patients may exhibit few or none of these early signs, in cases of suspected acetaminophen overdose, antidotal therapy should begin as soon as possible. A latent period of 24 to 36 hours exists between ingestion and the onset of symptoms of hepatic injury. Laboratory evidence usually appears within 24 to 48 hours if severe hepatotoxicity is to occur. Therefore, liver function tests (AST or ALT) should be monitored for up to 48 hours after an acute ingestion. Following the latent period, vomiting, pain in the upper right quadrant and manifestations of hepatic failure including the onset of coma, may ensue. Maximum hepatic necrosis appears 2 to 5 days following overdose. Signs include gross elevation of ALT, AST, increased bilirubin, hypoglycemia and increased prothrombin time. Renal dysfunction following acetaminophen overdose is rare overall but quite common in cases where liver injury or failure occurs.

In addition to hepatic and renal damage, there are rare reports of pancreatitis, clotting defects, and myocardial damage with ST segment abnormalities, T wave flattening and pericarditis.

Treatment: In cases of acute overdose, consultation with a Poison Control Centre is recommended. In cases of hepatotoxicity associated with subacute acetaminophen overdose, consultation with a toxicologist is recommended.

Treatment of acute acetaminophen overdose includes supportive measures, gut decontamination with activated charcoal, and prompt administration of acetylcysteine as an antidote. Laboratory determinations include plasma acetaminophen levels, AST, ALT, prothrombin time, bilirubin, creatinine, urea, blood glucose and electrolyte concentrations.

A single dose of activated charcoal is recommended, ideally within 1 hour of ingestion of overdose, and may be of benefit if given up to 4 hours postingestion.

Properly timed plasma acetaminophen levels are key prognosticators in determining a patient's risk of hepatotoxicity. The first level should be drawn at least 4 hours postingestion as peak concentrations may not be reached before this time. The Matthew-Rumack Nomogram for Acetaminophen Poisoning [*Pediatrics* 1975;55(6):871–6] should be used when acetaminophen levels are drawn between 4 and 24 hours following acute single ingestion, to determine the probability of hepatotoxicity and need for acetylcysteine therapy. For immediate-release acetaminophen formulations, when serum levels are above the lower treatment line (above 990 µmol/L at 4 hours, above 460 µmol/L at 8 hours or above 260 µmol/L at 12 hours postingestion), acetylcysteine therapy should be instituted to minimize hepatic toxicity.

Even in the absence of acetaminophen serum level determinations, therapy with acetylcysteine should be promptly instituted if a massive acetaminophen overdose is suspected (i.e., >7.5 g in adults or >150 mg/kg in children) and 24 hours or less have elapsed since ingestion. In the case of overdose with immediate-release formulations, maintenance doses of acetylcysteine may be discontinued if the initial acetaminophen serum level is nontoxic and the time of ingestion is known with some certainty. Subsequent levels are not predictive of toxicity and should not be used as criteria for acetylcysteine discontinuation.

Antidotal therapy with acetylcysteine is most effective if initiated within 8 hours following acetaminophen overdose. However, acetylcysteine therapy may improve outcomes even in patients presenting more than 24 hours postingestion with hepatic injury, including those in fulminant hepatic failure with encephalopathy.

Acetylcysteine Dosing in Acetaminophen Overdose: Oral: Loading Dose: 140 mg/kg. Maintenance Dose: 70 mg/kg every 4 hours for a total of 17 doses. Each oral dose should be diluted to a final concentration of 5% acetylcysteine (i.e., 3 mL of soft drinks, fruit juice or water added for each mL of 20% acetylcysteine solution) and consumed within 1 hour of preparation. If vomiting occurs within 1 hour following any oral dose, the entire dose should be repeated.

IV: Acetylcysteine may be given by the iv route if necessary. Loading Dose: 150 mg/kg in 5% dextrose over 15 minutes. Extending the infusion time to 30-60 minutes may reduce risk of infusion reactions. Maintenance Infusion: 12.5 mg/kg/hour for 4 hours, followed by 6.25 mg/kg/hour for 16 hours (consult acetylcysteine product monograph or other specialized references for details pertaining to dilution and infusion).

Hemodialysis may be helpful in certain cases, e.g., massive overdoses or acute renal failure.

For management of a suspected drug overdose, CPhA recommends that you contact your **regional Poison Control Centre**. See the *CPS* Directory section for a list of Poison Control Centres.

DOSAGE: Acetaminophen should not be used in adults or children for self-medication of marked fever (greater than 39.5°C), fever persisting longer than 3 days, or recurrent fever, unless directed by a physician, since such fevers may indicate serious illness requiring prompt medical attention.

Acetaminophen should not be used for self-medication of pain for longer than 10 days in adults or 5 days in children, unless directed by a physician, since pain of such intensity and duration may indicate a pathological condition requiring medical evaluation.

Immediate-release Dosage Forms (oral or rectal): Adults: 325 to 650 mg every 4 to 6 hours, not to exceed 4000 mg/24 hours. Children (see Warnings and Precautions, Children): 10 to 15 mg/kg po/pr every 4 to 6 hours, not to exceed 65 mg/kg/24 hours. Alternatively, see Table 1.

Because of the risk of toxicity, dosing for children must not exceed 5 doses in 24 hours unless under the advice of a physician.

Table 1: Acetaminophen

Pediatric Dosing: PO/PR

Age	Single Dose (mg)	Maximum Daily Dose (mg)
6[a] to under 12 months	80	400
12 to under 24 months	120	600
2 to under 4 years	160	800
4 to under 6 years	240	1200
6 to under 9 years	320	1600
9 to under 11 years	400	2000
11 to under 12 years	480	2400

[a] The Canadian Paediatric Society recommends consultation with a physician for infants under 6 months.

Note: Acetaminophen in oral drop formulations may be more concentrated than other liquid formulations. Careful attention must be paid to acetaminophen concentration when dosage volumes are calculated for liquid preparations.

Extended-release Caplets: Adults and Children Over 12 Years: 1300 mg every 8 hours, to a maximum of 4000 mg daily. Caplets should be swallowed whole and taken with water on an empty stomach.

Acetaminophen

acetaminophen

Analgesic—Antipyretic

Riva

SUPPLIED: Tablets: 160 mg (Cephanol): Each white, round, scored tablet contains: acetaminophen USP 160 mg. Nonmedicinal ingredients: hydroxypropyl methylcellulose, polyethylene glycol, polyvinylpyrrolidone, starch and stearic acid. Alcohol-, gluten-, lactose-, sulfite- and tartrazine-free. Bottles of 20.

325 mg: Each white tablet (round, caplet) contains: acetaminophen USP 325 mg. Nonmedicinal ingredients: polyvinylpyrrolidone, starch and stearic acid. Gluten-, lactose- and tartrazine-free. Bottles of 1 000.

500 mg: Each white tablet (round, caplet or "blazon" shape) contains: acetaminophen USP 500 mg. Nonmedicinal ingredients: polyvinylpyrrolidone, starch and stearic acid. Gluten-, lactose- and tartrazine-free. Bottles of 1 000.

Chewable Tablets: 80 mg: Each purple children's tablet contains: acetaminophen USP 80 mg. Nonmedicinal ingredients: aspartame, cellulose, compressible sugar, FD&C Blue, FD&C Red, flavoring, magnesium stearate and mannitol. Gluten- and tartrazine-free. Bottles of 24.

160 mg: Each purple children's tablet contains: acetaminophen USP 160 mg. Nonmedicinal ingredients: aspartame, cellulose, compressible sugar, FD&C Blue, FD&C Red, flavoring, magnesium stearate and mannitol. Gluten- and tartrazine-free. Bottles of 20.

Acetazolamide Ⓟ

CPhA Monograph

see *Carbonic Anhydrase Inhibitors: Systemic*

Acetazone Forte

chlorzoxazone—acetaminophen

Muscle Relaxant—Analgesic

Rougier Pharma

Acetazone Forte C8 Ⓝ

chlorzoxazone—acetaminophen—codeine phosphate

Muscle Relaxant—Analgesic

Rougier Pharma

SUPPLIED: Acetazone Forte: Each round, uncoated, green biplane tablet with beveled edges, imprinted with a horizontal line on one side and "rph" on the reverse, contains: chlorzoxazone USP 250 mg and acetaminophen USP 300 mg. Nonmedicinal ingredients: cornstarch, crospovidone, D&C yellow #10 aluminum lake, FD&C blue #1 aluminum lake, magnesium stearate, microcrystalline cellulose, povidone, pregelatinized cornstarch, sodium benzoate and sodium docusate, sodium croscarmellose and stearic acid. Bottles of 100. Blister packs of 20. Keep the bottle tightly closed. Store between 15-30°C. Protect from light.
Acetazone Forte C8: Each round, uncoated, pink and white biconvex, speckled tablet, imprinted with a horizontal line on one side and "TEC" on the reverse, contains: chlorzoxazone USP 250 mg, acetaminophen USP 300 mg and codeine phosphate USP 8 mg. Nonmedicinal ingredients: artificial coloring, cornstarch, crospovidone, magnesium stearate, microcrystalline cellulose, povidone, pregelatinized cornstarch, sodium benzoate and sodium docusate, sodium croscarmellose and stearic acid. Blister packs of 20. Keep the bottle tightly closed. Store between 15-30°C. Protect from light.

Acetylcysteine Solution (Sandoz Standard)

acetylcysteine

Mucolytic—Antidote for Acetaminophen Poisoning

Sandoz

SUPPLIED: Each mL contains: acetylcysteine 200 mg, disodium edetate 0.5 mg, sodium hydroxide to adjust pH and water for injection. Preservative-free. Lacquered rubber stoppered glass vials of 10 and 30 mL, boxes of 1. Store between 15 and 30°C. Protect from light. For i.v. use: Discard unused portion. For oral and inhalation use: Store opened vials in refrigerator between 2 and 8°C; use within 96 hours.

Acetylsalicylic Acid

CPhA Monograph

see *ASA*

Aclasta® Pr

zoledronic acid

Bone Metabolism Regulator

Novartis Pharmaceuticals

Date of Preparation: June 30, 2005
Date of Revision: September 21, 2009

SUMMARY PRODUCT INFORMATION:

Route of Administration	Dosage Form/ Strength	Clinically Relevant Nonmedicinal Ingredients
Intravenous infusion	5 mg/100 mL[a]	Mannitol, sodium citrate, water for injection

[a] One bottle with 100 mL solution contains 5.330 mg of zoledronic acid monohydrate, equivalent to 5 mg zoledronic acid on an anhydrous basis.

INDICATIONS AND CLINICAL USE: ACLASTA (zoledronic acid 5 mg/100 mL) is indicated for:

- The treatment of osteoporosis in postmenopausal women, as a once-yearly intravenous infusion, to reduce the incidence of hip, vertebral and non-vertebral fractures.
- The treatment to increase bone mineral density in men with osteoporosis, as a once-yearly intravenous infusion.
- The treatment and prevention of glucocorticoid-induced osteoporosis, to increase bone mineral density, as a once-yearly intravenous infusion.
- The prevention of postmenopausal osteoporosis in women with osteopenia as a single intravenous infusion.
- The treatment of Paget's disease of the bone in men and women, as a single-dose intravenous infusion. Treatment is indicated in patients with Paget's disease of bone with elevations in serum alkaline phosphatase (SAP) of at least two times the upper limit of the age-specific normal reference range, or those who are symptomatic, or those at risk for complications from their disease to induce remission (normalization of serum alkaline phosphatase). The effectiveness of ACLASTA is based on serum alkaline phosphatase (SAP) levels.

Geriatrics (>65 years of age): No overall differences in safety and efficacy were observed according to age (see Warnings and Precautions, Special Populations).
Pediatrics (<18 years of age): Safety and efficacy in children and growing adolescents have not been established. ACLASTA should not be given to this patient population.

CONTRAINDICATIONS:

- Patients who are hypersensitive to this drug or to any ingredient in the formulation, or to any bisphosphonates or component of the container. For a complete listing, see Dosage Forms, Composition and Packaging.
- Pregnancy and nursing mothers.
- Non-corrected hypocalcemia at the time of infusion.

WARNINGS AND PRECAUTIONS: General: ACLASTA contains the same active ingredient that is found in ZOMETA (zoledronic acid). Patients being treated with ZOMETA should not be treated with ACLASTA.
Patients being treated with ACLASTA should not be treated with other bisphosphonates concomitantly.
Infusion Duration: The 5 mg single dose of ACLASTA (zoledronic acid 5 mg/100 mL) should be infused in **no less than 15 minutes**.
Cardiovascular: Overall incidence of atrial fibrillation in the 3-year postmenopausal osteoporosis trial (HORIZON-PFT) using ACLASTA (zoledronic acid) 5 mg dose yearly, was 2.5% (96 out of 3862) and 1.9% (75 out of 3852) in patients receiving zoledronic acid and placebo, respectively. The rate of atrial fibrillation serious adverse events was 1.3% (51 out of 3862) and 0.6% (22 out of 3852) in patients receiving zoledronic acid and placebo, respectively. The overall incidence of atrial fibrillation in the 2-year male osteoporosis trial was 3.3 % (5 out of 153) for zoledronic acid-treated patients compared to 2% (3 out of 148) for alendronate-treated patients. The rate of atrial fibrillation serious adverse events was 0% for zoledronic acid-treated patients compared to 0.7% (1/148) for alendronate-treated patients. The overall incidence of atrial fibrillation in the 1-year glucocorticoid induced-osteoporosis trial was 0.7 % (3 out of 416) for zoledronic acid-treated patients compared to 0.0% (0 out of 417) for risedronate-treated patients. The rate of atrial fibrillation serious adverse events was 0% for zoledronic acid-treated patients and 0% for risedronate-treated patients. This increased incidence of atrial fibrillation was not observed in clinical trials conducted in Paget's disease, in the HORIZON-RFT trial in post-hip fracture patients, or in the trial for the prevention of postmenopausal osteoporosis. The mechanism behind the increased incidence of atrial fibrillation is unknown.
Endocrine and Metabolism: Hypocalcemia: It is recommended that all patients should have their serum calcium levels and vitamin D levels assessed before treatment with ACLASTA (e.g., as part of their annual examination). Pre-existing hypocalcemia must be treated by adequate administration of calcium and vitamin D before initiating ACLASTA (see Contraindications). Other disturbances of mineral metabolism (e.g., diminished parathyroid reserve; thyroid surgery, parathyroid surgery, intestinal calcium malabsorption) must also be effectively treated.

It is strongly advised that patients receive adequate calcium and vitamin D supplementation. All patients should be counseled regarding the importance of calcium and vitamin D supplementation in maintaining serum calcium levels and on the symptoms of hypocalcemia. The recommended daily vitamin D supplement should be determined by the treating physician based on the patient's individual needs. In the postmenopausal osteoporosis trial (HORIZON-PFT), patients received 1000 to 1500 mg of elemental calcium plus 400 to 1200 IU of vitamin D supplements per day.
Renal: Patients must be appropriately hydrated prior to administration of ACLASTA, and this is especially important for patients receiving diuretic therapy (see Dosage and Administration). On the day of infusion, it is recommended that patients eat and drink normally, which includes drinking at least 2 glasses of fluids (500 mL or 2 cups), such as water, before and after the administration of ACLASTA (see Information to Be Provided to the Patient).
It is recommended that all patients have their renal function assessed before treatment with ACLASTA (e.g., as part of their annual examination).
Renal Dysfunction: Zoledronic acid, has been associated with renal dysfunction manifested as deterioration in renal function (i.e., increased serum creatinine), and in rare cases, acute renal failure. Renal deterioration, progression to renal failure (some with fatal outcome) and dialysis have been reported very rarely in oncology patients (e.g., those with hypercalcemia of malignancy and/or pre-existing renal disease), after the initial dose or a single dose of zoledronic acid (4 mg dose, every 3-4 weeks) (see Adverse Reactions).
Renal Insufficiency: ACLASTA is not recommended for use in patients with severe renal impairment (creatinine clearance <30 mL/min) due to lack of adequate clinical experience in this population (see Dosage and Administration). It is recommended that all patients have their serum creatinine measured before treatment with ACLASTA (e.g., as part of their annual examination).
Osteonecrosis of the Jaw: Osteonecrosis of the jaw (ONJ) has been reported rarely in the treatment of postmenopausal osteoporosis with zoledronic acid as well as with other oral and intravenous bisphosphonates. The condition currently termed Osteonecrosis of the jaw has unknown etiology and pathogenesis, and may or may not originate in the bone. ONJ has been reported in patients with cancer receiving treatment regimens that include bisphosphonates such as zoledronic acid. Many of these patients were also receiving chemotherapy and corticosteroids. The majority of reported cases have been associated with invasive dental procedures, such as root canal or dental extraction. Many had signs of local infection including osteomyelitis. A causal relationship between bisphosphonate use and ONJ has not been established.
A routine dental examination with appropriate preventive dentistry should be performed prior to treatment with bisphosphonates, such as ACLASTA, in patients with possible risk factors (e.g., cancer, chemotherapy, head and neck radiotherapy, corticosteroids, poor oral hygiene). While receiving treatment, these patients should avoid invasive dental procedures, if possible, but should continue with regular dental cleaning and oral hygiene. For patients requiring oral surgery, there are no data available to suggest whether discontinuation of bisphosphonate treatment reduces the risk of ONJ. In patients who develop ONJ while on bisphosphonate therapy, surgery at the affected area may exacerbate the condition. Clinical judgment of the treating physician should guide the management plan of each patient based on individual benefit/risk assessment.
Musculoskeletal Pain: In post-marketing experience with multiple dose regimen bisphosphonates, including ACLASTA, severe and occasionally incapacitating bone, joint, and/or muscle pain has been reported in patients. The time to onset of symptoms varied from one day to several months after starting the drug. A subset of patients had recurrence of symptoms when rechallenged with the same drug or another bisphosphonate.
Respiratory: While not observed in clinical trials with ACLASTA, there have been reports of bronchoconstriction in ASA (acetylsalicylic acid) sensitive patients receiving bisphosphonates. ACLASTA must be used with caution in ASA-sensitive patients.
Special Populations: Pregnant Women: ACLASTA should not be used during pregnancy as zoledronic acid may cause fetal harm when administered to a pregnant woman. In reproductive studies in the pregnant rat, subcutaneous doses equivalent to 2.0 or 4.5 times the human systemic exposure (an i.v. dose of 5 mg based on an AUC comparison) resulted in pre- and post-implantation losses, decreases in viable fetuses and fetal skeletal, visceral and external malformations.
There are no studies in pregnant women using zoledronic acid. If the patient becomes pregnant while taking this drug, the patient should be apprised of the potential harm to the fetus. Women of childbearing potential should be advised to avoid becoming pregnant.
Nursing Women: It is not known whether ACLASTA is excreted in human milk. Because many drugs are excreted in human milk, it should not be administered to a nursing woman.
Pediatrics (<18 years of age): The safety and effectiveness of ACLASTA in pediatric patients have not been established.
Geriatrics (>65 years of age): The combined osteoporosis trials (HORIZON-PFT and HORIZON-RFT) included 4,761 ACLASTA-treated patients who were at least 65 years of age, while 2083 patients were at least 75 years old. No overall differences in safety and efficacy were observed according to age.
The osteoporosis study in men included 59 (38.3%) ACLASTA-treated patients who were at least 65 years of age, while 24 (15.6%) patients were at least 75 years old. No overall differences in safety and efficacy were observed according to age.
The glucocorticoid-induced osteoporosis trial included 116 (27.9%) ACLASTA-treated patients who were at least 65 years of age, while 29 (7.0%) patients were at least 75 years old. No overall differences in safety and efficacy were observed according to age.
Phase 3 studies of ACLASTA in the treatment of Paget's disease of bone included 132 (75.5%) ACLASTA-treated patients who were at least 65 years of age, while 68 (37.4%) ACLASTA-treated patients were at least 75 years old. No overall differences in efficacy or safety were observed between these patients and younger patients.
Information to Be Provided to the Patient: Physicians should instruct their patients to read the Patient Information before starting therapy with ACLASTA (zoledronic acid 5 mg/100 mL).

- ACLASTA is given as one single infusion into a vein by a nurse or a doctor, and the infusion time must **not be less than 15 minutes**.
- Before being given ACLASTA patients should tell their doctor if they have kidney problems and what medications they are taking (see Adverse Reactions, Renal Dysfunction).
- ACLASTA should not be given if the patient is taking ZOMETA, which contains the same active ingredient as in ACLASTA.
- ACLASTA should not be given if the patient is pregnant or plans to become pregnant, or if they are breast-feeding (see Contraindications and Warnings and Precautions).
- If the patient had surgery to remove some or all of the parathyroid glands or thyroid gland in their neck, or had sections of their intestine removed, or are unable to take calcium supplements, they should tell the doctor.
- It is strongly advised that patients receive adequate calcium **and** vitamin D supplementation in order to maintain normal blood calcium levels. Supplementation of both calcium and vitamin D is especially important in the days before and following ACLASTA administration. The recommended daily vitamin D supplement should be determined by the treating physician based on the patient's individual needs.
- On the day of infusion, it is recommended that patients eat and drink normally, which includes drinking at least 2 glasses of fluids (500 mL or 2 cups) such as water, before and after the administration of ACLASTA.
- Patients should also be aware of the most common side effects. Patients may experience one or more side effects that could include: fever and chills; muscle, bone or joint pain; nausea; fatigue; and headache. Most of these side effects are mild to moderate and occur within 3 days after taking ACLASTA. They usually go away within 3 days after they start, but may last for up to 7-14 days. The incidence of post-dose symptoms occurring within the first 3 days after administration of ACLASTA, can be reduced with the administration of acetaminophen or ibuprofen shortly following ACLASTA administration.
- Some patients experienced hypocalcemia. Hypocalcemia is usually asymptomatic, but symptoms may include numbness or tingling sensations, especially in the area around the mouth, muscle cramps or muscle spasms. Patients should consult their physician immediately if they develop these symptoms of hypocalcemia after ACLASTA treatment (see Adverse Reactions).
- Redness, swelling and or pain at the infusion site may occur. Redness, itching, or pain to the eyes may occur.
- There have been some reports of persistent pain and/or a non-healing sore of the mouth or jaw, if you experience these symptoms tell your doctor or dentist.

Monitoring and Laboratory Tests: Hypocalcemia: Serum calcium levels and vitamin D levels should be assessed for all patients before treatment with ACLASTA (e.g., as part of their annual examination). The recommended daily vitamin D supplement should be determined by the treating physician based on the patient's individual needs.
Renal: Renal function should be assessed and serum creatinine should be measured before every treatment with ACLASTA (e.g., as part of their annual examination).

ADVERSE REACTIONS: Adverse Drug Reaction Overview: Postmenopausal Osteoporosis: In the postmenopausal osteoporosis trial (HORIZON-PFT), Phase III randomized, double-blind, placebo-controlled, multinational study of 7736 women aged 65-89 years, there were no significant differences in the overall incidence of serious adverse events compared to placebo and most adverse events were mild to moderate. The duration of the trial was three years with 3862 patients exposed to ACLASTA and 3852 patients exposed to placebo administered once annually as a single 5 mg dose in 100 mL solution infused over at least 15 minutes, for a total of three doses. All women received 1000 to 1500 mg of elemental calcium plus 400 to 1200 IU of vitamin D supplementation per day.

The incidence of all-cause mortality was: 3.4% in the ACLASTA group and 2.9% in the placebo group. The incidence of serious adverse events was similar between treatment groups 29.2% in the ACLASTA group and 30.1% in the placebo group. The percentage of patients who withdrew from the study due to adverse events was 2.1% and 1.8% for the ACLASTA and placebo groups, respectively. The rate of atrial fibrillation serious adverse events was 1.3% (51 out of 3862) and 0.6% (22 out of 3852) in patients receiving ACLASTA (zoledronic acid) and placebo, respectively.

ACLASTA has been most commonly associated with the following post-dose symptoms: fever (18.1%), myalgia (9.4%), flu-like symptoms (7.8%), arthralgia (6.8%) and headache (6.5%), the majority of which occur within the first 3 days following ACLASTA administration. The majority of these symptoms were mild to moderate in nature and resolved within 3 days of the event onset. The incidence of these symptoms decreased markedly with subsequent doses of ACLASTA.

The incidence of post-dose symptoms occurring within the first 3 days after administration of ACLASTA, can be reduced with the administration of acetaminophen or ibuprofen shortly following ACLASTA administration.

In the HORIZON-RFT trial, a randomized, double-blind, placebo-controlled, multinational endpoint study of 2127 osteoporotic patients aged 50-95 years with a recent (within 90 days) low-trauma hip fracture, 1054 patients were exposed to ACLASTA (zoledronic acid) and 1057 patients were exposed to placebo. ACLASTA was administered once annually as a single 5 mg dose in 100 mL solution infused over at least 15 minutes. All participants received 1000 to 1500 mg of elemental calcium plus 800 to 1200 IU of vitamin D supplementation per day.

The incidence of all-cause mortality was 9.6% in the ACLASTA-treated group compared to 13.3% in the placebo group. The incidence of serious adverse events was 38% in the ACLASTA group and 41% in the placebo group. The percentage of patients who withdrew from the study due to adverse events was 2.0% and 1.7% for the ACLASTA and placebo groups, respectively.

Osteoporosis in Men: In general, ACLASTA was well tolerated in the male osteoporosis trial as assessed in a two-year randomized, multicentre, double-blind, active-controlled group study of 302 men aged 25-86 years. 153 patients were exposed to ACLASTA administered once annually as a single 5 mg dose in 100 mL solution infused over 15 minutes for a total of two doses and 148 patients were exposed to oral alendronate 70 mg weekly for two years. All participants received 1000 mg elemental calcium plus 800 to 1000 IU vitamin D supplementation per day.

The incidence of serious adverse events was similar between the ACLASTA and alendronate treatment groups (17.6% vs. 20.9%, respectively). The percentage of patients who withdrew from the study due to serious adverse events was 4.6% and 3.4% for the ACLASTA and alendronate groups, respectively. The percentage of patients experiencing at least one adverse event was comparable between the ACLASTA and alendronate treatment groups (93.5% compared to 93.2%), with the exception of a higher incidence of post-dose symptoms in the ACLASTA group that occurred within 3 days after infusion. The incidence of these post-dose symptoms were reported as follow for ACLASTA and alendronate, respectively: myalgia (17.1% vs. 2.7%), fever (15.7% vs. 1.4%), fatigue (12.4% vs. 1.4%), arthralgia (11.1% vs. .7%), pain (10.5% vs. 2.7%), chills (9.8% vs. 0.7%), headache (9.8% vs. 2.0%), influenza-like illness (8.5% vs. 2.0%), malaise (5.2% vs. 0.7%), and back pain (3.3% vs. 0.7%).

Glucocorticoid-Induced Osteoporosis: In general, ACLASTA was well tolerated in the glucocorticoid-induced osteoporosis trial.

The duration of the trial was one year, with 416 patients exposed to ACLASTA administered once as a single infusion 5 mg dose in 100 mL solution infused over 15 minutes and 417 patients exposed to oral risedronate 5 mg daily for one year. All participants received 1000 mg elemental calcium plus 400 to 1000 IU vitamin D supplementation per day.

The overall percentage of adverse events was higher for the zoledronic acid group compared to the risedronate group (77.4% vs. 66.9%, respectively) driven by a higher incidence of post-dose symptoms in the ACLASTA group that occurred within 3 days after infusion. The most common post-dose symptoms were reported as follows for ACLASTA and risedronate, respectively: pyrexia (12.7% vs. 3.6%), arthralgia (9.9% vs. 7.4%), nausea (9.6% vs. 8.4%), myalgia (9.1% vs. 3.4%), and influenza-like illness (6% vs. 1%).

The incidence of serious adverse events was similar between the ACLASTA and risedronate treatment groups (14.7% vs. 14.4%, respectively). The percentage of patients who withdrew from the study due to adverse events was 7.9% for the ACLASTA group and 5.3% for the risedronate group.

Prevention of Postmenopausal Osteoporosis: The safety of ACLASTA in postmenopausal women with osteopenia (low bone mass) was assessed in a 2-year randomized, double-blind, placebo-controlled trial of postmenopausal women aged 45 years or older. 181 women were exposed to ACLASTA as a single 5 mg dose administered at randomisation and 202 patients were exposed to placebo for two years. All women received 500 to 1200 mg elemental calcium plus 400 to 800 IU vitamin D supplementation per day.

The incidence of serious adverse events was 9.4% and 11.4% for the zoledronic acid and the placebo groups, respectively. The percentage of patients who withdrew from the study due to adverse events was 1.7% and 0.5% for the zoledronic acid and the placebo groups, respectively.

The incidence of the most frequent treatment-emergent adverse events for the zoledronic acid group was reported as follows: myalgia (22.7%), pyrexia (21%), headache (20.4%), chills (18.2%), pain in extremity (16%), pain (14.9%), nausea (11.6%), fatigue (9.9%), influenza (8.3%), non-cardiac chest pain (7.7%), dizziness (6.1%), hypercholesterolemia (5.5%), sciatica (5%), bone pain (3.3%), asthenia (2.8), and hypoesthesia (2.2%).

Paget's Disease of Bone: In general, ACLASTA (zoledronic acid 5 mg/100 mL) was well-tolerated in Paget's disease trials. Consistent with intravenous administration of bisphosphonates, ACLASTA has been most commonly associated with the following signs and symptoms, the majority of which occur within 3 days following the administration: influenza-like illness (transient post-dose symptoms), pyrexia, myalgia, arthralgia, and bone pain. In Paget's disease trials, one or more of these events which were suspected to be related to drug were reported in 25% of patients in the ACLASTA-treated group compared to 8% in the risedronate-treated group within the first 3 days following the ACLASTA administration. After the first 3 days, rates for these symptoms were reduced to 3% for ACLASTA-treated patients and 3% for risedronate-treated patients. The majority of these symptoms resolved within 3 days of their onset.

Clinical Trial Adverse Drug Reactions: Because clinical trials are conducted under very specific conditions the adverse reaction rates observed in the clinical trials may not reflect the rates observed in practice and should not be compared to the rates in the clinical trials of another drug. Adverse drug reaction information from clinical trials is useful for identifying drug-related adverse events and for approximating rates.

Postmenopausal Osteoporosis: Adverse reactions reported in at least 2.0% of the postmenopausal osteoporosis patients, and more frequently in the ACLASTA-treated patients than placebo-treated patients are shown in Table 1.

Table 1: ACLASTA

Adverse Reactions Occurring in ≥2.0% of Postmenopausal Osteoporosis Patients Receiving ACLASTA (5 mg i.v. infusion once yearly) and More Frequently than in Placebo-Treated Patients Over 3 Years

System Organ Class	5 mg IV ACLASTA Once Per Year % (N=3862)	Placebo Once Per Year % (N=3852)
Blood and the Lymphatic System Disorders		
Anemia	4.4	3.6
Metabolism and Nutrition Disorders		
Anorexia	2.0	1.1
Nervous System Disorders		
Headache	12.4	8.1
Dizziness	7.6	6.7
Vascular Disorders		
Hypertension	12.7	12.4
Ear and Labyrinth Disorders		
Vertigo	4.3	4.0
Cardiac Disorders		
Atrial fibrillation	2.4	1.9
Gastrointestinal Disorders		
Nausea	8.5	5.2
Diarrhea	6.0	5.6
Vomiting	4.6	3.2
Abdominal pain upper	4.6	3.1
Dyspepsia	4.3	4.0
Musculoskeletal, Connective Tissue and Bone Disorders		
Arthralgia	23.8	20.4
Myalgia	11.7	3.7
Pain in extremity	11.3	9.9
Shoulder pain	6.9	5.6
Bone pain	5.8	2.3
Neck pain	4.4	3.8
Muscle spasms	3.7	3.4
General Disorders and Administrative Site Conditions		
Pyrexia	17.9	4.6
Influenza-like illness	8.8	2.7
Fatigue	5.4	3.5
Chills	5.4	1.0
Asthenia	5.3	2.9
Peripheral edema	4.6	4.2
Pain	3.3	1.3
Malaise	2.0	1.0

The incidence of post-dose symptoms decreased after each annual infusion. Table 2 presents the overall incidence of adverse events by time of onset from infusion by first, second and third infusion.

Table 2: ACLASTA

Overall Incidence of Adverse Events in the Postmenopausal Osteoporosis Trial by Infusion and Time of Onset (safety population)

Infusion	1st Infusion		2nd Infusion		3rd Infusion	
	ACLASTA n (%)	Placebo n (%)	ACLASTA n (%)	Placebo n (%)	ACLASTA n (%)	Placebo n (%)
Total no. of patients with infusion	3862	3852	3409	3517	3106	3190
Time of onset ≤3 days	1726 (44.69)	571 (14.82)	570 (16.72)	462 (10.29)	316 (10.17)	270 (8.46)

Table 3: ACLASTA

Adverse Reactions Occurring in At Least 2% of Men and Women with a Low Trauma Hip Fracture Receiving ACLASTA (5 mg i.v. infusion once yearly) and Greater Than Placebo

System Organ Class	5 mg IV ACLASTA Once Per Year % (N=1054)	Placebo Once Per Year % (N=1057)
Nervous System Disorders		
Headache	3.8	2.5
Vascular Disorders		

(cont'd)

Table 3: ACLASTA *(cont'd)*

Adverse Reactions Occurring in at Least 2% of Men and Women with a Low Trauma Hip Fracture Receiving ACLASTA (5 mg i.v. infusion once yearly) and Greater Than Placebo

System Organ Class	5 mg IV ACLASTA Once Per Year % (N=1054)	Placebo Once Per Year % (N=1057)
Hypertension	6.8	5.4
Musculoskeletal, Connective Tissue and Bone Disorders		
Pain in extremity	5.9	4.8
Myalgia	4.9	2.6
Bone pain	3.2	1.0
Musculoskeletal pain	3.1	1.2
General Disorders and Administrative Site Conditions		
Pyrexia	8.7	3.1
Edema peripheral	5.5	5.3
Hyperthermia	2.2	0.3
Fatigue	2.1	1.2
Injury, Poisoning, and Procedural Complications		
Post procedure complication	3.8	3.3
Osteoarthritis	5.7	4.5
Cataracts	3.0	2.3
Urinary tract infection	10.6	9.6

Osteoporosis in Men: The overall safety and tolerability profile of ACLASTA in male osteoporosis was similar to that reported in the ACLASTA postmenopausal osteoporosis trial (HORIZON-PFT). Adverse events reported in at least 2% of men with osteoporosis that were either not reported in the postmenopausal osteoporosis trial (HORIZON-PFT) or reported more frequently in the osteoporosis trial in men are presented in Table 4.

Glucocorticoid-Induced Osteoporosis: The overall safety and tolerability profile of ACLASTA in the glucocorticoid-induced osteoporosis trial was similar to that reported in the ACLASTA postmenopausal osteoporosis clinical trial (HORIZON-PFT). Adverse events reported in at least 2% of patients that were either not reported in the postmenopausal osteoporosis trial (HORIZON-PFT) or reported more frequently in the glucocorticoid-induced osteoporosis trial included the following: abdominal pain* (ACLASTA 7.5%; risedronate 5.0%), and musculoskeletal pain† (ACLASTA 3.1%; risedronate 1.7%). In addition, the following adverse events occurred more frequently than in the postmenopausal osteoporosis trial: nausea (ACLASTA 9.6%; risedronate 8.4%), rheumatoid arthritis (ACLASTA 6.3%; risedronate 5%), dyspepsia (ACLASTA 5.5%; risedronate 4.3%), urinary tract infection (ACLASTA 5%; risedronate 4.1%) and back pain (ACLASTA 4.3%; risedronate 6.2%).

In the one-year glucocorticoid-induced osteoporosis trial, arrhythmia and tachycardia were reported in 1% (4 out of 416) of zoledronic acid-treated patients compared to 0.0% arrhythmia and 0.5% (2 out of 417) tachycardia in the risedronate-treated patients.

Prevention of Postmenopausal Osteoporosis: See Table 5.

Paget's Disease of Bone: Adverse reactions suspected (investigator assessment) to be drug related and occurring in at least 2% of the Paget's patients receiving ACLASTA (single, 5 mg, intravenous infusion) or risedronate (30 mg, oral, daily dose for 2 months) over a 6-month study period are listed by system organ class in Table 6.

Local Reactions: In the postmenopausal osteoporosis trial, local reactions at the infusion site such as itching, redness and/or pain have been reported in 0.7% of patients following the administration of ACLASTA and 0.5% of patients following the administration of placebo. In the male osteoporosis trial, the event rate was 2.6% in the zoledronic acid treatment group and 1.4% in the alendronate treatment group. In the prevention of postmenopausal osteoporosis trial, the event rate was 1.1% in ACLASTA-treated patients compared to 2.0% in placebo treated patients.

Iritis/Uveitis/Episcleritis/Conjunctivitis: Cases of iritis/uveitis/episcleritis/conjunctivitis have been reported in patients treated with bisphosphonates, including zoledronic acid. In the postmenopausal osteoporosis trial, 9 (0.2%) patients treated with ACLASTA and 1 (<0.1%) patient treated with placebo developed iritis/uveitis/episcleritis. Of the ocular conditions known to be related to bisphosphonate use, one case of iritis in a zoledronic acid-treated patient was reported in the HORIZON-RFT trial. In the male osteoporosis trial, two cases of conjunctivitis and one case of eye pain were reported in zoledronic acid-treated patients. In addition, one case of iritis was reported in the alendronate group. One case of conjunctivitis in a zoledronic acid-treated patient was reported in the glucocorticoid-induced osteoporosis trial. In the prevention of postmenopausal osteoporosis trial, conjunctivitis was reported in two patients (1.1%) in the zoledronic acid group. Uveitis/iritis was reported in 3 patients (1.7%) in the zoledronic acid group and in no patients (0%) in the placebo group.

Renal Dysfunction: In the postmenopausal osteoporosis HORIZON-PFT trial, zoledronic acid has been associated with renal dysfunction manifested as deterioration in renal function (i.e. increased serum creatinine) and in rare cases acute renal failure (see Table 8). In the clinical trial for postmenopausal osteoporosis, patients with baseline creatinine clearance <30 mL/min, urine dipstick ≥2+ protein or increase in serum creatinine of >0.5 mg/dL (44.2 μmol/L) during the screening visits were excluded. Overall, there was a transient increase in serum creatinine observed within 10 days of dosing in 42 (1.8%) ACLASTA-treated patients versus 19 (0.8%) placebo-treated patients which resolved without specific therapy. Severe renal dysfunction was rarely reported, and in most of these patients recovery was not achieved by the end of the trial. Adjudicated changes in renal function and renal adverse events over the 3 year trial are described in Table 8 and Table 9.

In the HORIZON-RFT trial, the change in creatinine clearance (measured annually prior to dosing), and the incidence of renal failure and impairment was comparable for both the ACLASTA and placebo treatment groups over 3 years.

In the male osteoporosis trial, the incidence of confirmed renal adverse events was higher in the zoledronic acid group (4.6%) relative to the alendronate group (1.4%). There was a transient increase in serum creatinine from baseline (>0.5 mg/dL) observed 9-11 days post-infusion in 7 (4.6%) zoledronic acid-treated patients versus 1 (0.7%) alendronate-treated patient which subsequently decreased to baseline or near baseline levels. Adjudicated changes in renal function and renal adverse events over the 2 year trial are described in Table 10 and Table 11.

In the glucocorticoid-induced osteoporosis trial, the incidence of confirmed renal adverse events was 2.2% for zoledronic acid-treated patients versus 1.4% for risedronate-treated patients. There was a greater incidence of confirmed increases in serum creatinine from baseline (>0.5% mg/dL) observed in 9 (2.2%) zoledronic acid-treated patients compared to 3 (0.7%) risedronate-treated patients. Adjudicated laboratory changes in renal function and renal adverse events over the one year trial are described in Table 12. In addition, the incidence of renal failure was 0.7% in the zoledronic acid patients and 0.0% in the risedronate patients and the incidence of acute renal failure was 0.2% in the zoledronic acid patients and 0.5% in the risedronate patients.

* Combined abdominal pain, abdominal pain upper, and abdominal pain lower as one ADR.
† Combined musculoskeletal pain and musculoskeletal chest pain as one ADR.

In the prevention of postmenopausal osteoporosis trial, one zoledronic acid-treated patient (0.6%) reported a creatinine clearance value of <30 mL/min. One zoledronic acid-treated patient (0.6%) reported a creatinine clearance value of <30 mL/min and a ≥30% decline in CrCl during the study from a baseline value of ≤60 mL/min. One zoledronic acid-treated patient (0.6%) had renal failure confirmed by adjudication. No patients in the placebo group had renal failure, acute renal failure, or decreased CrCl.

Bronchoconstriction in ASA (acetylsalicylic acid) Sensitive Asthma Patients: While not observed in clinical trials with ACLASTA there have been previous reports of bronchoconstriction in ASA-sensitive patients receiving bisphosphonates.

Osteonecrosis of the Jaw (ONJ): In the postmenopausal osteoporosis trial (HORIZON-PFT) in 7736 patients, symptoms consistent with ONJ occurred in one patient treated with ACLASTA and one patient treated with placebo. Both cases resolved after appropriate treatment. ONJ has not been observed in the HORIZON-RFT, the male osteoporosis, the glucocorticoid-induced osteoporosis, the prevention of postmenopausal osteoporosis, or the Paget's disease trials with ACLASTA.

Avascular Necrosis and Delayed Fracture Union/Non-Union: In the postmenopausal osteoporosis trial, 3 cases (2 zoledronic acid, 1 placebo patients) were confirmed to be cases of delayed union of fracture, one of which occurred in a patient with fracture that pre-existed at baseline. 7 cases of avascular necrosis (zoledronic acid=4, placebo=3) were reported (6 cases occurred in the hip region and 1 case was in the knee region). In the HORIZON-RFT trial, 3 (0.3%) patients had confirmed events of delayed union/non-union in the zoledronic acid group (2 incident hip and 1 humerus) and 3 (0.3%) patients had confirmed events in the placebo group (1 incident hip, 1 contralateral hip, and 1 shoulder). Six (0.6%) patients in the zoledronic acid group and 3 (0.3%) patients in the placebo group had confirmed events of avascular necrosis, all of which involved the hip. In the glucocorticoid-induced osteoporosis trial, 5 cases of avascular necrosis (zoledronic acid=2 and risedronate=3) were reported.

Table 4: ACLASTA

Adverse Reactions Occurring in ≥2%[a] of Patients with Male Osteoporosis Receiving ACLASTA (5-mg i.v. infusion once yearly) or 70 mg Once Weekly of Alendronate Over 24 Months

System Organ Class	5 mg IV ACLASTA Once Per Year % (N=153)	Alendronate 70 mg/ Once Weekly % (N=148)
Nervous System Disorders		
Headache	15.0	6.1
Lethargy	3.3	1.4
Eye Disorders		
Eye pain	2.0	0.0
Cardiac Disorders		
Atrial fibrillation	3.3	2.0
Palpitations	2.6	0.0
Gastrointestinal Disorders		
Abdominal pain[b]	7.9	4.1
Respiratory, Thoracic and Mediastinal Disorders		
Dyspnea	6.5	4.7
Skin and Subcutaneous Tissue Disorders		
Hyperhidrosis	2.6	2.0
Rash	2.0	2.7
Musculoskeletal, Connective Tissue and Bone Disorders		
Myalgia	19.6	6.8
Musculoskeletal pain[c]	12.4	10.8
Musculoskeletal stiffness	4.6	0.0
Back pain	12.4	17.6
Renal and Urinary Disorders		
Blood creatinine increased	2.0	0.7
General Disorders and Administrative Site Conditions		
Fatigue	17.6	6.1
Pain	11.8	4.1
Chills	9.8	2.7
Influenza-like illness	9.2	2.0
Malaise	7.2	0.7
Acute phase reaction	3.9	0.0
Investigations		
C-reactive protein increased	4.6	1.4

[a] Includes adverse reactions that occurred in ≥2% of patients which were either not reported in the postmenopausal osteoporosis trial or reported more frequently in the trial of men with osteoporosis.
[b] Combined abdominal pain, abdominal pain upper, and abdominal pain lower as one ADR.
[c] Combined musculoskeletal pain and musculoskeletal chest pain as one ADR.

Table 5: ACLASTA

Adverse Reactions Occurring in at Least 2% of Women with Osteopenia Receiving ACLASTA 5 mg IV Infusion (administered as a single dose at randomisation) and Greater Than Placebo in the Prevention of Postmenopausal Osteoporosis Trial Over 2 Years

System Organ Class	ACLASTA 5 mg IV % (N=181)	Placebo % (N=202)
Endocrine Disorders		
Hypothyroidism	2.8	1.5
Gastrointestinal Disorders		
Nausea	11.6	7.9
Constipation	7.2	6.9
Dyspepsia	6.6	5.0
Vomiting	5.0	4.5
Vascular Disorders		
Hypertension	8.3	6.9
Musculoskeletal, Connective Tissue and Bone Disorders		
Myalgia	22.7	6.9
Back pain	16.6	11.9
Pain in extremity	16.0	9.9
Neck pain	6.6	5.0
Musculoskeletal pain	5.5	5.4
Pain in jaw	3.9	2.5
Bone pain	3.3	1.0
Arthritis	2.2	1.5
General Disorders and Administrative Site Conditions		
Pyrexia	21.0	4.5
Chills	18.2	3.0
Pain	14.9	3.5
Fatigue	9.9	4.0
Non-cardiac chest pain	7.7	3.0
Edema peripheral	3.9	3.5
Influenza-like illness	3.3	2.0
Asthenia	2.8	1.0
Malaise	2.2	0.5
Immune System Disorders		
Seasonal allergy	2.8	1.5
Infections and Infestations		
Influenza	8.3	5.9
Tooth infection	2.8	1.0
Injury, Poisoning, and Procedural Complications		
Joint sprain	2.8	1.5
Post-traumatic pain	2.8	2.5
Metabolism and Nutrition Disorders		
Hypercholesterolemia	5.5	2.0
Nervous System Disorders		
Headache	20.4	11.4
Dizziness	6.1	3.5
Sciatica	5.0	2.0
Hypoesthesia	2.2	2.0
Reproductive System and Breast Disorders		
Vulvovaginal dryness	2.2	2.0

(cont'd)

Table 5: ACLASTA *(cont'd)*

Adverse Reactions Occurring in at Least 2% of Women with Osteopenia Receiving ACLASTA 5 mg IV Infusion (administered as a single dose at randomisation) and Greater Than Placebo in the Prevention of Postmenopausal Osteoporosis Trial Over 2 Years

System Organ Class	ACLASTA 5 mg IV % (N=181)	Placebo % (N=202)
Respiratory, Thoracic and Mediastinal Disorders		
Cough	6.1	5.0
Pharyngolaryngeal pain	3.9	2.5
Nasal congestion	2.2	2.0

Table 6: ACLASTA

Adverse Reactions Suspected[a] to be Drug Related Occurring in at Least 2% of Paget's Patients Receiving ACLASTA (single 5 mg i.v. infusion) or Risedronate (oral 30 mg daily for 2 months) Over a 6-Month Follow-up Period

System Organ Class	Single 5 mg i.v. ACLASTA Administration % (N=177)	30 mg/day × 2 Months Risedronate % (N=172)
Metabolism and Nutrition Disorders		
Hypocalcemia	3	1
Nervous System Disorders		
Headache	7	4
Lethargy	4	1
Gastrointestinal Disorders		
Diarrhea	2	0
Nausea	6	2
Dyspepsia	2	2
Infections and Infestations		
Influenza	3	0
Musculoskeletal, Connective Tissue and Bone Disorders		
Myalgia	6	4
Bone pain	5	1
Arthralgia	4	2
General Disorders and Administrative Site Conditions		
Influenza-like illness	9	5
Pyrexia	7	1
Rigors	7	1
Fatigue	5	2
Pain	3	2
Asthenia	2	1
Respiratory, Thoracic and Mediastinal Disorders		
Dyspnea	2	0

[a] Investigator assessment.

Table 7: ACLASTA

Most Frequent Adverse Reactions Occurring in at Least 5% of Paget's Patients in any Group Receiving ACLASTA (single 5 mg i.v. infusion) or Risedronate (oral 30 mg daily for 2 months) by Time of Occurrence

System Organ Class	AE Occurrence ≤3 Days After Treatment Initiation		AE Occurrence >3 Days After Treatment Initiation	
	Single 5 mg i.v. ACLASTA Administration % (N=177)	30 mg/day × 2 Months Risedronate % (N=172)	Single 5 mg i.v. ACLASTA Administration % (N=177)	30 mg/day × 2 Months Risedronate % (N=172)
Nervous System Disorders				
Headache	7	4	4	6
Dizziness	3	1	5	3
Gastrointestinal Disorders				
Diarrhea	2	1	4	5

(cont'd)

Table 7: ACLASTA *(cont'd)*

Most Frequent Adverse Reactions Occurring in at Least 5% of Paget's Patients in any Group Receiving ACLASTA (single 5 mg i.v. infusion) or Risedronate (oral 30 mg daily for 2 months) by Time of Occurrence

	AE Occurrence ≤3 Days After Treatment Initiation		AE Occurrence >3 Days After Treatment Initiation	
System Organ Class	**Single 5 mg i.v. ACLASTA Administration % (N=177)**	**30 mg/day × 2 Months Risedronate % (N=172)**	**Single 5 mg i.v. ACLASTA Administration % (N=177)**	**30 mg/day × 2 Months Risedronate % (N=172)**
Nausea	6	2	3	5
Infections and Infestations				
Nasopharyngitis	1	0	5	8
Musculoskeletal, Connective Tissue and Bone Disorders				
Myalgia	7	4	1	1
Bone pain	5	1	4	4
Arthralgia	5	0	5	11
Back pain	2	1	2	7
Pain in extremity	0	1	7	7
General Disorders and Administrative Site Conditions				
Influenza-like illness	10	4	1	2
Pyrexia	7	1	1	1
Rigors	7	1	1	1
Fatigue	7	2	2	2

Table 8: ACLASTA

Adverse Renal Events Associated with Change in Renal Function Confirmed by Adjudication, Regardless of Study Drug Relationship, by Preferred Term (safety population of the HORIZON-PFT trial)

Preferred Term	ACLASTA (N=3862) n (%)	Placebo (N=3852) n (%)
Total	90 (2.33)	74 (1.92)
Creatinine decreased renal clearance	29 (0.75)	33 (0.86)
Blood creatinine increased	22 (0.57)	6 (0.16)
Renal failure	16 (0.41)	14 (0.36)
Renal impairment	11 (0.28)	20 (0.52)
Proteinuria	9 (0.23)	6 (0.16)
Renal failure acute	9 (0.23)	2 (0.05)
Renal failure chronic	1 (0.03)	2 (0.05)
Azotemia	4 (0.10)	0 (0.00)

Table 9: ACLASTA

Change in Renal Function Confirmed by Adjudication, Safety Population of the HORIZON-PFT Trial

	Zoledronic Acid (N=3862) n (%)	Placebo (N=3852) n (%)
Overall	178 (4.6)	157 (4.1)
Renal adverse event	175 (4.5)	154 (4.0)
Increase in serum creatinine >0.5 mg/dL	55 (1.4)	41 (1.1)
Calculated creatinine clearance <30 mL/min	62 (1.6)	57 (1.5)
Baseline calculated creatinine clearance ≤60 mL/min and declined by ≥30%	114 (3.0)	115 (3.0)

Legend: N=the number of patients in the analysis population; n=the number of patients with the event; (%)=n/N *100.

Table 10: ACLASTA

Change in Renal Function Confirmed by Adjudication, Safety Population of Male Osteoporosis Trial

	Zoledronic Acid N=153 n (%)	Alendronate N=148 n (%)
Overall	7 (4.6)	2 (1.4)
Renal adverse event	7 (4.6)	2 (1.4)
Increase in serum creatinine >0.5 mg/dL	7 (4.6)	1 (0.7)
Creatinine clearance <30 mL/min	2 (1.3)	1 (0.7)
Baseline calculated creatinine clearance ≤60 and declined ≥30%	5 (3.3)	1 (0.7)
Significant proteinuria	1 (0.7)	0 (0.0)

Legend: N=the number of patients in the analysis population; n=the number of patients with the event; (%)=n/N *100.

Table 11: ACLASTA

Adverse Renal Events Associated with Change in Renal Function, Regardless of Study Drug Relationship, by Preferred Term (safety population of male osteoporosis trial)

Preferred Term	ACLASTA (N=153) n (%)	Alendronate (N=148) n (%)
Total	7 (4.6)	6 (4.1)
Blood creatinine increased	3 (2.0)	1 (0.7)
Renal impairment	2 (1.3)	1 (0.7)
Azotemia	1 (0.7)	0
Proteinuria	1 (0.7)	0
Renal failure	1 (0.7)	1 (0.7)
Creatinine renal clearance decreased	0	2 (1.4)
Renal failure acute	0	1 (0.7)

Table 12: ACLASTA

Renal Laboratory Criteria Confirmed as a Significant Renal Adverse Event by Adjudication (GIO safety population)

	Zoledronic Acid N=416 n (%)	Risedronate N=417 n (%)
Overall	9 (2.2)	6 (1.4)
Renal adverse event[a]	9 (2.2)	6 (1.4)
Increase in serum creatinine >0.5 mg/dL (1)	9 (2.2)	3 (0.7)
Creatinine clearance <30 mL/min	1 (0.2)	0 (0.0)
Baseline CrCl ≤60 and declined ≥30%	0 (0.0)	1 (0.2)
Significant proteinuria	3 (0.7)	2 (0.5)

[a] The adjudication committee determined that a clinically significant renal adverse event had occurred independent of an event being reported by the investigator.

Legend: N=the number of patients in the analysis population; n=the number of patients with the event; (%)=100*n/N.

Abnormal Hematologic and Clinical Chemistry Findings: Serum Creatinine and Creatinine Clearance: Postmenopausal Osteoporosis: A transient increase in serum creatinine (>0.5 mg/dL (44.2 µmol/L)) was observed within 10 days following administration in 42 (1.8%) ACLASTA-treated patients versus 19 (0.8%) placebo-treated patients (see Adverse Reactions, Renal Dysfunction).

Severe renal dysfunction was rarely reported, and in most of these patients recovery was not achieved by the end of the trial. Adjudicated changes in renal function and renal adverse events over the 3 year trial are described in Table 8 and Table 9 (see Adverse Reactions).

Osteoporosis in Men: There was a transient increase in serum creatinine from baseline (>0.5 mg/dL) observed 9-11 days post-infusion in 7 (4.6%) zoledronic acid-treated patients versus 1 (0.7%) alendronate-treated patient which subsequently decreased to baseline or near baseline levels. Adjudicated changes in renal function and renal adverse events over the two year trial are described in Table 10 and Table 11 (see Adverse Reactions).

Glucocorticoid-Induced Osteoporosis: Confirmed increases in serum creatinine from baseline (>0.5% mg/dL) were observed in 9 (2.2%) zoledronic acid-treated patients compared to 3 (0.7%) risedronate-treated patients. Adjudicated laboratory changes in renal function and renal adverse events over the one year trial are described in Table 12.

Paget's Disease of Bone: No clinically significant changes in serum creatinine have occurred in the Paget's disease trials.

Hypocalcemia: Postmenopausal Osteoporosis: In the postmenopausal osteoporosis trial (HORIZON-PFT), mild, transient, asymptomatic decrease in calcium levels, have been observed with ACLASTA primarily after the first dose. Approximately 0.2% of patients had notable declines of serum calcium levels (less than 1.87 mmol/L) following ACLASTA administration. No symptomatic cases of hypocalcaemia were observed. In this trial, patients received supplemental daily doses of elemental calcium (1000 to 1500 mg) and vitamin D (400 to 1200 IU).

In the prevention of postmenopausal osteoporosis trial, one patient (0.5%) treated with ACLASTA (administered at randomization and at Month 12) had a confirmed event of hypocalcemia with a notable decline of calcium level of 1.70 mmol/L from a screening value of 2.17 mmol/L one month following the first infusion of ACLASTA.

Paget's Disease of Bone: In the Paget's disease trials, early, transient decreases in serum calcium and phosphate levels, that were usually asymptomatic, have been observed. Approximately 21% of subjects had serum calcium levels <2.1 mmol/L (<8.4 mg/dL) 9-11 days following ACLASTA infusion. In the Paget's disease trials, symptomatic hypocalcemia was observed in approximately 1% of patients, all of which resolved.

In the HORIZON-RFT, the male osteoporosis, or the glucocorticoid induced-osteoporosis trials, there were no patients who had treatment emergent serum calcium levels below 1.87 mmol/L.

Post-Market Adverse Drug Reactions: Because these events are reported voluntarily from a population of uncertain size, it is not always possible to reliably estimate their frequency or clearly establish a causal relationship to ACLASTA exposure.

The following adverse reactions have been identified during the post approval use of this drug: hypocalcaemia, arthralgia, myalgia, flu-like symptoms, fever and headache. Hypersensitivity reactions including rare cases of bronchoconstriction, urticaria and angioedema, and very rare cases of anaphylactic reactions/shock have also been reported.

DRUG INTERACTIONS: Overview: ACLASTA is not metabolized in humans. Zoledronic acid is eliminated by renal excretion.

Drug-Drug Interactions: No in vivo drug interaction studies have been performed for ACLASTA. In vitro and ex vivo studies showed low affinity of zoledronic acid for the cellular components of human blood. In vitro mean zoledronic acid protein binding in human plasma ranged from 28% at 200 ng/mL to 53% at 50 ng/mL. In vivo studies showed that zoledronic acid is not metabolized, and is excreted into the urine as the intact drug. See Table 13.

(cont'd)

Table 13: ACLASTA

Established or Potential Drug-Drug Interactions

Zoledronic Acid	Ref	Effect	Clinical Comment
Aminoglycosides	T	↓ serum calcium level	Caution is advised when bisphosphonates, including zoledronic acid, are administered with aminoglycosides, since these agents may have an additive effect to lower serum calcium level for prolonged periods. This effect has not been reported in zoledronic acid clinical trials.
Loop Diuretics	T	↑ risk of hypocalcemia	Caution should also be exercised when ACLASTA is used in combination with loop diuretics due to an increased risk of hypocalcemia.
Nephrotoxic Drugs	T		Caution is indicated when ACLASTA is used with other potentially nephrotoxic drugs such as nonsteroidal anti-inflammatory drugs.

Legend: CT=clinical trial; T=theoretical.

Drug-Food Interactions: The interaction of zoledronic acid has not been studied with regards to food.
Drug-Herb Interactions: The interaction of zoledronic acid with herbal medications or supplements has not been studied.
Drug-Laboratory Test Interactions: No data suggest that zoledronic acid interferes with laboratory tests.
Drug-Lifestyle Interactions: Specific drug-lifestyle interaction studies have not been conducted with zoledronic acid.

DOSAGE AND ADMINISTRATION: Recommended Dose and Dosage Adjustment:

- **Treatment of postmenopausal osteoporosis**
  The recommended dose is a once yearly single intravenous infusion of ACLASTA.
- **Treatment to increase bone mineral density in men with osteoporosis**
  The recommended dose is a once yearly single intravenous infusion of ACLASTA.
- **Treatment and prevention of glucocorticoid-induced osteoporosis, to increase bone mineral density**
  The recommended dose is a once yearly single intravenous infusion of ACLASTA.
- **Prevention of postmenopausal osteoporosis**
  The recommended dose is a single intravenous infusion of ACLASTA.
  Re-treatment for prevention of postmenopausal osteoporosis
  Specific re-treatment data after 24 months are not available. After one treatment with ACLASTA 5 mg intravenous infusion in the prevention of postmenopausal osteoporosis trial, the effect on lumbar spine BMD was observed for up to 24 months. There are no clinical efficacy data available beyond the 24 months' duration of the trial.
- **Treatment of Paget's disease of bone**
  The recommended dose is a single intravenous infusion of ACLASTA.
  ACLASTA (5 mg in 100 mL ready to infuse solution) is administered intravenously via a vented infusion line.
  Patients should be advised to be appropriately hydrated before the administration of ACLASTA.

The infusion time **must not be less than 15 minutes** (see Warnings and Precautions) and the infusion rate should be constant. ACLASTA should only be given by intravenous infusion. The total volume of the ACLASTA solution should be infused. ACLASTA must never be given as a bolus injection.

Renal: Zoledronic acid is not recommended for use in patients with severe renal impairment (creatinine clearance <30 mL/min). No dosage adjustment is necessary in patients with a creatinine clearance ≥30 mL/min. Patients must be appropriately hydrated prior to administration of ACLASTA, and this is especially important for patients receiving diuretic therapy (see Warnings and Precautions).

Calcium and Vitamin D Intake: It is strongly advised that patients receive adequate calcium and vitamin D supplementation especially in the days before and following ACLASTA administration (see Warnings and Precautions). All patients should be counseled regarding the importance of calcium and vitamin D supplementation in maintaining serum calcium levels, and on the symptoms of hypocalcemia. The recommended daily vitamin D supplement should be determined by the treating physician based on the patient's individual needs. In the postmenopausal osteoporosis trial (HORIZON-PFT), patients received 1000 to 1500 mg of elemental calcium plus 400 to 1200 IU of vitamin D supplements per day.

Post-Infusion Management: About 25% of patients experienced transient post-dose symptoms within the first 3 days of their ACLASTA infusion (see Adverse Reactions). Symptomatic management can be considered on an individual basis. No anaphylactic reactions have been observed in the clinical trials but good medical practice dictates caution (see Contraindications).

Re-treatment of Paget's Disease: Specific re-treatment data are not available. After one treatment with ACLASTA in Paget's disease an extended remission period of up to 19 months was observed in 98% (143/146) of patients.

OVERDOSAGE:
Clinical experience with acute overdose with ACLASTA is limited. Patients who have received doses higher than those recommended should be carefully monitored. In the event of clinically significant hypocalcemia, reversal may be achieved with supplemental oral calcium and vitamin D and/or an infusion of calcium gluconate.

> For management of a suspected drug overdose, CPhA recommends that you contact your **regional Poison Control Centre**. See the *CPS* Directory section for a list of Poison Control Centres.

ACTION AND CLINICAL PHARMACOLOGY: Mechanism of Action: ACLASTA belongs to the class of nitrogen containing bisphosphonates and acts primarily on bone in order to protect the bone against excessive and abnormal osteoclastic and osteoblastic activity. It is an inhibitor of osteoclast-mediated bone resorption.

The selective action of bisphosphonates on bone is based on their high affinity for mineralized bone. Intravenously administered zoledronic acid rapidly partitions to bone and, as with other bisphosphonates, localizes preferentially at sites of high bone turnover. The main molecular target of zoledronic acid in the osteoclast is the enzyme farnesyl pyrophosphate synthase (FPP) which is critical for the regulation of a variety of cell processes important for osteoclast function, but this does not exclude other inhibitory mechanisms. In vitro assays have demonstrated that zoledronic acid has the highest potency to inhibit FPP synthase amongst available nitrogen containing bisphosphonates. This higher inhibition of FPP synthase correlated with a greater anti-resorptive potency as observed in vivo in rats. The relatively long duration of action of zoledronic acid is attributable to its high binding affinity for the active site of farnesyl pyrophosphate (FPP) synthase and its strong binding affinity to bone mineral.

Pharmacodynamic Effects: In long-term animal studies, zoledronic acid inhibits bone resorption without adversely affecting bone formation, mineralization or mechanical properties of bone. Histomorphometric data from long-term rat and monkey studies showed the typical response of bone to an anti-resorptive agent with a dose-dependent reduction in osteoclastic activity and in activation frequency of new remodeling sites in both trabecular and haversian bone. Continuing bone remodeling was observed in bone samples from all animals treated with clinically relevant doses of zoledronic acid. There was no evidence of a mineralizing defect, no aberrant accumulation of osteoid, and no woven bone in treated animals.

Bone Histology and Bone Markers: Postmenopausal Osteoporosis: Dynamic bone histomorphometry was evaluated in 93 postmenopausal patients with osteoporosis after being treated with 3 annual doses of ACLASTA. These results showed bone of normal quality with no evidence of impaired bone remodeling and no evidence of mineralization defects. Microcomputed tomography analysis demonstrated preservation of trabecular bone architecture in patients treated with ACLASTA compared to placebo. In summary, the bone biopsies and biomarkers indicate ongoing bone remodeling with qualitatively normal bone.

In the osteoporosis treatment trial, the effect of ACLASTA treatment on markers of bone resorption (serum beta-C-telopeptides (b-CTx)) and bone formation (bone specific alkaline phosphatase (BSAP), serum N-terminal propeptide of type I collagen (P1NP)) was evaluated in patients (subsets ranging from 517 to 1246 patients) at periodic intervals. Treatment with a 5 mg annual dose of ACLASTA reduces bone turnover markers to the pre-menopausal range with an approximate 55% reduction in b-CTx, a 29% reduction in BSAP and a 52 % reduction in P1NP over 36 months. There was no progressive reduction of bone turnover markers with repeated annual dosing.

ACLASTA treatment rapidly reduced the rate of bone turnover from elevated postmenopausal levels with the nadir for resorption markers observed at 7 days, and for formation markers at 12 months. Thereafter bone markers stabilized within the pre-menopausal range. There was no progressive reduction of bone turnover markers with repeated annual dosing.

Glucocorticoid-Induced Osteoporosis: Bone biopsy specimens were obtained at month 12 from 23 patients treated with either an annual dose of ACLASTA or daily oral risedronate (12 in the ACLASTA treatment group and 11 in the risedronate treatment group). All biopsies were adequate for qualitative histomorphometry assessment. Qualitative and quantitative assessments showed bone of normal architecture and quality without mineralization defects.

Paget's Disease: Bone histology was evaluated in 7 patients with Paget's disease 6 months after being treated with ACLASTA. Bone biopsy results showed bone of normal quality with no evidence of impaired bone remodeling and no evidence of mineralization defect. These results were consistent with biochemical marker evidence of normalization of bone turnover.

Pharmacokinetics: Pharmacokinetic data in patients with postmenopausal osteoporosis, osteoporosis and Paget's disease of bone are not available.

Distribution: Single or multiple (q 28 days) 5-minute or 15-minute infusions of 2, 4, 8 or 16 mg zoledronic acid were given to 64 cancer patients. The post-infusion decline of zoledronic acid concentrations in plasma was consistent with a triphasic process showing a rapid decrease from peak concentrations at end-of-infusion to <1% of C_{max} 24 hours post infusion with population half-lives of $t_{1/2\alpha}$ 0.24 hours and $t_{1/2\beta}$ 1.87 hours for the early disposition phases of the drug. The terminal elimination phase of zoledronic acid was prolonged, with very low concentrations in plasma between days 2 and 28 post infusion, and an estimated terminal elimination half-life $t_{1/2\gamma}$ of 146 hours. The area under the plasma concentration versus time curve (AUC_{0-24h}) of zoledronic acid was dose proportional from 2 to 16 mg. The accumulation of zoledronic acid measured over three cycles was low, with mean AUC_{0-24h} ratios for cycles 2 and 3 versus 1 of 1.13±0.30 and 1.16±0.36, respectively.

In vitro and ex vivo studies showed low affinity of zoledronic acid for the cellular components of human blood. Binding to human plasma proteins was approximately 43-55% at 50 ng/mL, a concentration of zoledronic acid within the range observed after 15 minute infusion of the 5 mg dose. It was only slightly less (about 43%) at 500 ng/mL a concentration of zoledronic acid greater than the expected C_{max}. Therefore, interactions resulting from displacement of highly protein-bound drugs are unlikely.

Metabolism: Zoledronic acid is not metabolized in humans. It was found to have little or no capacity as a direct acting and/or irreversible metabolism-dependent inhibitor of P450 enzymes. Therefore, zoledronic acid is unlikely to reduce the metabolic clearance of substances which are metabolized via the cytochrome P450 enzyme systems. In animal studies, <3% of the administered intravenous dose was found in the feces, with the balance either recovered in the urine or taken up by bone, indicating that the drug is eliminated intact via the kidney.

Excretion: In 64 patients, on average 39±16% (±SD) of the administered zoledronic acid dose was recovered in the urine within 24 hours with only trace amounts of drug found in urine after 48 hours. The cumulative percentage of drug excreted in the urine over 0-24 hours was independent of dose. The balance of drug not recovered in urine over 0-24 hours, representing drug presumably bound to bone, is slowly released back into the systemic circulation, giving rise to the observed prolonged low plasma concentrations. The 0-24 hour renal clearance of zoledronic acid was 3.7±2.0 L/h (±SD).

Zoledronic acid clearance was independent of dose but dependent upon the patient's creatinine clearance. In a study with patients, increasing the infusion time of a 4 mg dose of zoledronic acid from 5 minutes (n=5) to 15 minutes (n=7) resulted in a 34% decrease in the zoledronic acid plasma concentration at the end of the infusion ([mean±SD] 403±118 ng/mL vs. 264±86 ng/mL) and a 10% increase in the total AUC (378±116 ng×h/mL vs. 420±218 ng×h/mL). The difference between the AUC means was not statistically significant.

Special Populations and Conditions: Pediatrics: Pharmacokinetic data of zoledronic acid in pediatric patients are not available.

Geriatrics: The pharmacokinetics of zoledronic acid were not affected by age in patients who ranged in age from 38 years to 84 years.

Gender: The pharmacokinetics of zoledronic acid were not affected by gender.

Race: The pharmacokinetics of zoledronic acid were not affected by race.

Hepatic Insufficiency: No clinical studies were conducted to evaluate the effect of hepatic impairment on the pharmacokinetics of zoledronic acid. Zoledronic acid does not inhibit human P450 enzymes in vitro, shows no biotransformation, suggesting no relevant role of liver function in the pharmacokinetics of zoledronic acid and no required dosage adjustment. Following an intravenous dose of 20 nCi 14C-zoledronic acid in a patient with cancer and bone metastases, only a single radioactive species with chromatographic properties identical to those of parent drug was recovered in urine, which suggests that zoledronic acid is not metabolized.

Renal Insufficiency: The pharmacokinetic studies conducted in 64 patients represented typical clinical populations with normal to moderately impaired renal function. Compared to patients with normal renal function (creatinine clearance >80 mL/min, N=37), patients with mild renal impairment (creatinine clearance=50 to 80 mL/min, N=15) showed an average increase in plasma AUC of 15%, whereas patients with moderate renal impairment (creatinine clearance=30 to 50 mL/min, N=11) showed an average increase in plasma AUC of 43%. No dosage adjustment is required in patients with a creatinine clearance of ≥30 mL/min. Based on population PK/PD modeling, the risk of renal deterioration appears to increase with AUC, the risk is doubled at a creatinine clearance of 10 mL/min. Zoledronic acid is not recommended for patients with severe renal impairment (creatinine clearance <30 mL/min) due to lack of adequate clinical experience in this population (see Warnings and Precautions).

STORAGE AND STABILITY: Store ACLASTA at room temperature between 15-30°C. The ACLASTA bottle is for single use only. ACLASTA should be used immediately and the entire volume in the bottle should be administered. Any unused solution should be discarded.

SPECIAL HANDLING INSTRUCTIONS: Note: Parenteral drug products should be inspected visually for particulate matter and discoloration prior to administration, whenever solution and container permit.

- Solution does not need to be diluted before administration.
- Strict adherence to the intravenous route is recommended for the parenteral administration of ACLASTA.
- The entire volume in the bottle should be administered.

Compatibility:

- ACLASTA must not be allowed to come in contact with any calcium- or other divalent cations-containing solutions, and it should be administered as a single dose through a separate vented infusion line.
- ACLASTA is considered to be compatible with the typical vented infusion line materials polyvinylchloride (PVC), polyurethane (PUR) and polyethylene (PE).

INFORMATION FOR THE PATIENT: Published in e-CPS, available by subscription at www.e-cps.ca.

DOSAGE FORMS, COMPOSITION AND PACKAGING: Each bottle of ready-to-use sterile solution for intravenous infusion, contains: zoledronic acid monohydrate 5.330 mg (equivalent to 5 mg zoledronic acid on an anhydrous basis). pH between 6.0 to 7.0. Nonmedicinal ingredients: mannitol, sodium citrate and water for injection. Plastic bottles of 100 mL. The colorless plastic bottle is sealed with a rubber stopper which is held in place with an aluminum cap with flip component. The stopper is made of bromobutyl rubber coated with fluorocarbon polymer and contains no latex. The ACLASTA plastic bottle comes with a convenient plastic hanger to facilitate the infusion set-up.

Acne-Aid® Soap

nonmedicated soap

Acne Therapy

Stiefel, a GSK company

SUPPLIED: Each bar consists of a hypoallergenic blend of neutral soap and surfactant, containing sulfonated oil 6.3%. Nonmedicinal ingredients: mineral oil light, oilytex, purified water, quaternium-15, soap chips and tetrasodium HEDTA. Bars of 100 g.

Actemra™ Pr

tocilizumab

Interleukin Receptor Inhibitor

Roche

Date of Preparation: April 30, 2010

ACTEMRA (tocilizumab) should be prescribed by and administered under the supervision of health care professionals who are experienced in the use of biologics in the management of patients with moderate to severe rheumatoid arthritis and who have fully familiarized themselves with the efficacy and safety profile of ACTEMRA.

SUMMARY PRODUCT INFORMATION:

Route of Administration	Dosage Form/ Strength	Clinically Relevant Nonmedicinal Ingredients
Intravenous	20 mg/mL concentrate solution for infusion	For a complete listing see Dosage Forms, Composition and Packaging.

DESCRIPTION: ACTEMRA (tocilizumab) is a recombinant humanized anti-human interleukin 6 (IL-6) receptor monoclonal antibody of the immunoglobulin (Ig) IgG1 subclass with a H2L2 polypeptide structure.

INDICATIONS AND CLINICAL USE: ACTEMRA (tocilizumab) is indicated for:

- reducing signs and symptoms in adult patients with moderately to severely active rheumatoid arthritis who have inadequate response to one or more disease modifying anti-rheumatic drugs (DMARDs) and/or tumour necrosis factor (TNF) antagonists.

General use of ACTEMRA in DMARD-inadequate responder (IR) patients is not recommended at this time. Physicians may consider the use of ACTEMRA in the DMARD-IR population on a case by case basis dependent on disease and patient characteristics, experience with the drug, and the benefits and risks of ACTEMRA as compared to other therapeutic options available.

CONTRAINDICATIONS: ACTEMRA (tocilizumab) should not be administered to patients with known hypersensitivity to tocilizumab or any of its components. For a complete listing, see Dosage Forms, Composition and Packaging.

WARNINGS AND PRECAUTIONS:

Serious Warnings and Precautions

RISK OF SERIOUS INFECTIONS: Serious infections including sepsis, tuberculosis (TB), invasive fungal, and other opportunistic infections have been observed with the use of biologics agents, including ACTEMRA. Hospitalization or fatal outcomes associated with infections have been reported.

Most patients who developed these infections were taking concomitant immunosuppressants such as methotrexate or corticosteroids, that, in addition to their rheumatoid arthritis could predispose them to infections.

Before starting treatment with ACTEMRA, all patients should be evaluated for both active and latent tuberculosis.

Treatment with ACTEMRA should not be initiated in patients with active infections including chronic or localized infections.

If a serious infection develops, interrupt ACTEMRA until the infection is controlled. Patients should be closely monitored for the development of signs and symptoms of infection during and after treatment with ACTEMRA, including the possible development of tuberculosis in patients who tested negative for latent tuberculosis infection prior to initiating therapy.

Concurrent therapy with ACTEMRA and another biologic agent is not recommended. When transitioning from another biologic therapy to ACTEMRA, patients should be monitored for signs of infection. In the clinical trials, a higher incidence of infections was observed in patients previously exposed to a TNF inhibitor.

Serious Infections: Serious infections including sepsis, tuberculosis (TB), invasive fungal, and other opportunistic infections have been observed. Patients should be closely monitored for the development of signs and symptoms of infection during and after treatment with ACTEMRA. Most patients who developed these infections were taking concomitant immunosuppressants such as methotrexate or corticosteroids, that, in addition to their rheumatoid arthritis could predispose them to infections.

Treatment with ACTEMRA should not be initiated in patients with active infections including chronic or localized infections. Administration of ACTEMRA should be interrupted if a patient develops a serious infection until the infection is controlled (see Dosage and Administration, Dosing Considerations). Physicians should exercise caution when considering the use of ACTEMRA in patients with a history of recurring infection or with underlying conditions (e.g. diverticulitis, diabetes) which may predispose patients to infections or who have resided in regions where tuberculosis and histoplasmosis are endemic.

Vigilance for the timely detection of serious infection is recommended for patients receiving biologic treatments for rheumatoid arthritis, as signs and symptoms of acute inflammation may be lessened, associated with suppression of the acute phase reactants. Patients should be instructed to contact a physician immediately when any symptoms suggesting infection appear, in order to assure rapid evaluation and appropriate treatment.

Tuberculosis: As recommended for other biologic therapies in rheumatoid arthritis, patients should be screened for latent tuberculosis infection prior to starting ACTEMRA therapy. Patients with latent tuberculosis should be treated with standard antimycobacterial therapy before initiating ACTEMRA.

Viral Reactivation: Treatment with TNF inhibitors has been associated with reactivation of hepatitis B and C. Therefore screening for viral hepatitis should be performed in accordance with published guidelines before starting therapy with ACTEMRA. In clinical studies with ACTEMRA, patients who screened positive for hepatitis were excluded from the study.

Gastrointestinal Perforations: Events of diverticular perforations as complications of diverticulitis have been reported. ACTEMRA should be used with caution in patients with previous history of intestinal ulceration or diverticulitis. Patients presenting with symptoms potentially indicative of complicated diverticulitis, such as abdominal pain, should be evaluated promptly for early identification of gastrointestinal perforation. In clinical studies with ACTEMRA, patients with a history of diverticulitis, chronic ulcerative lower GI disease such as Crohn's disease, ulcerative colitis or other symptomatic lower GI conditions were excluded.

Laboratory Abnormalities: Neutrophils: Treatment with ACTEMRA was associated with a higher incidence of neutropenia (see Adverse Reactions, Abnormal Hematologic and Clinical Chemistry Findings, Hematology Abnormalities).

Caution should be exercised when considering initiation of treatment with ACTEMRA in patients with a low neutrophil count i.e. absolute neutrophil count (ANC) $<2\times10^9$/L. In patients with an absolute neutrophil count $<0.5\times10^9$/L treatment is not recommended.

Neutrophils should be monitored 4 to 8 weeks after start of therapy and thereafter according to good clinical practice (see Action and Clinical Pharmacology, Pharmacodynamics). For recommended modifications based on ANC results, see Dosage and Administration.

Platelets: Treatment with ACTEMRA was associated with a reduction in platelet counts.

Caution should be exercised when considering initiation of ACTEMRA treatment in patients with a platelet counts below 100×10^3/μL. In patients with a platelet count $<50\times10^3$/μL treatment is not recommended.

Platelets should be monitored 4 to 8 weeks after start of therapy and thereafter according to good clinical practice. For recommended modifications based on platelet counts, see Dosage and Administration.

Liver Function Tests: Treatment with ACTEMRA particularly when administered concomitantly with methotrexate, may be associated with elevations in hepatic transaminases (see Adverse Reactions, Abnormal Hematologic and Clinical Chemistry Findings, Liver Enzyme Elevations), therefore caution should be exercised when considering treatment of patients with active hepatic disease or hepatic impairment.

In clinical trials, mild and moderate elevations of hepatic transaminases have been observed with tocilizumab treatment, without progression to hepatic injury (see Adverse Reactions, Abnormal Hematologic and Clinical Chemistry Findings). Increased frequency of these elevations was observed when potential hepatotoxic drugs (e.g. methotrexate (MTX)) were used in combination with tocilizumab.

Caution should be exercised when considering initiation of ACTEMRA treatment in patients with elevated transaminases: ALT or AST >1.5×ULN. In patients with elevated ALT or AST >5×ULN treatment is not recommended.

ALT and AST should be monitored 4 to 8 weeks after start of therapy and thereafter according to good clinical practice. For recommended modifications based on transaminases, see Dosage and Administration.

Lipids: Lipid levels in untreated RA patients tend to be lower compared to the general population as it relates to the increase in systemic inflammation in patients with RA. Elevations of lipid parameters such as total cholesterol, triglycerides, low density lipoprotein (LDL) cholesterol, and/or cholesterol have been observed (see Adverse Reactions, Abnormal Hematologic and Clinical Chemistry Findings, Elevations in Lipid Parameters).

Assessment of lipid parameters should be performed 4 to 8 weeks following initiation of ACTEMRA therapy. Patients should be managed according to local clinical guidelines for management of hyperlipidaemia.

Cardiovascular Risk: RA patients have an increased risk for cardiovascular disorders and should have risk factors (e.g. hypertension, hyperlipidaemia) managed as part of usual standard of care. Adverse events of hypertension have been observed with ACTEMRA treated patients in clinical trials (see Adverse Reactions). Most events were transitory.

Malignancies: The impact of treatment with ACTEMRA on the development of malignancies is not known but malignancies were observed in clinical studies (see Adverse Reactions, Adverse Drug Reaction Overview, Malignancies). ACTEMRA is an immunosuppressant, and treatment with immunosuppressants may result in an increased risk of malignancies.

Carcinogenesis and Mutagenesis: No long-term animal studies have been performed to establish the carcinogenicity potential of ACTEMRA. Standard genotoxicity studies with tocilizumab in both prokaryotic and eukaryotic cells were all negative.

Hypersensitivity Reactions: Serious hypersensitivity reactions have been reported in association with infusion of ACTEMRA (see Adverse Reactions, Adverse Drug Reaction Overview, Infusion Reactions). Appropriate treatment should be available for immediate use in the event of an anaphylactic reaction during administration of ACTEMRA.

Demyelinating Disorders: The impact of treatment with ACTEMRA on demyelinating disorders is not known, but multiple sclerosis and chronic inflammatory demyelinating polyneuropathy were reported rarely in clinical studies. Patients should be closely monitored for signs and symptoms potentially indicative of demyelinating disorders. Prescribers should exercise caution in considering the use of ACTEMRA in patients with preexisting or recent onset demyelinating disorders.

Active Hepatic Disease and Hepatic Impairment: Treatment with ACTEMRA is not recommended in patients with active hepatic disease or hepatic impairment.

Immunization: Live and live attenuated vaccines should not be given concurrently with ACTEMRA as clinical safety has not been established. No data are available on the secondary transmission of infection from persons receiving live vaccines to patients receiving ACTEMRA.

Dependence/Tolerance: No studies on the effects on the potential for ACTEMRA to cause dependence have been performed. However, there is no evidence from the available data that ACTEMRA treatment results in dependence.

Effects on Ability to Drive and Use Machines: No studies on the effects on the ability to drive and use machinery have been performed. However, there is no evidence from the available data that treatment with ACTEMRA affects the ability to drive and use machines.

Special Populations: Pregnant Women: There are no adequate data from the use of ACTEMRA in pregnant women. A study in monkeys did not indicate any dysmorphogenic potential but has yielded a higher number of spontaneous abortions/embryo-foetal deaths at a high dose. The relevance of these data for humans is unknown.

ACTEMRA should be used during pregnancy only if the potential benefit justifies the potential risk to the fetus.

Pregnancy Registry: To monitor the outcomes of pregnant women exposed to ACTEMRA, a pregnancy registry has been established. Physicians are encouraged to register patients and pregnant women are encouraged to register themselves by calling 1-877-311-8972.

Nursing Women: Excretion of a murine analogue of tocilizumab into the milk of lactating mice has been observed, however, it is unknown whether tocilizumab is excreted in human breast milk. A decision on whether to continue/discontinue breast-feeding or to continue/discontinue therapy with tocilizumab should be made taking into account the benefit of breast-feeding to the child and the benefit of tocilizumab therapy to the woman.

Pediatrics (<18 years of age): Safety and effectiveness of ACTEMRA in pediatric patients have not been established.

Geriatrics (>65 years of age): Of the 2644 patients who received ACTEMRA in studies, a total of 435 rheumatoid arthritis patients were 65 years of age and older, including 50 patients 75 years and older. The frequency of serious infection among ACTEMRA treated subjects 65 years of age and older was higher than those under the age of 65. There is a higher incidence in infections in the elderly population in general, therefore, caution should be used when treating the elderly with ACTEMRA.

Hepatic Impairment: The safety and efficacy of ACTEMRA has not been studied in patients with hepatic impairment.

Renal Impairment: No dose adjustment is required in patients with mild renal impairment. ACTEMRA has not been studied in patients with moderate to severe renal impairment.

ADVERSE REACTIONS: Adverse Drug Reaction Overview: The ACTEMRA data described below includes 5 double-blind, controlled, multicenter studies. In these studies, patients received doses of ACTEMRA 8 mg/kg monotherapy (288 patients), ACTEMRA 8 mg/kg in combination with DMARDs (including methotrexate) (1582 patients), or ACTEMRA 4 mg/kg in combination with methotrexate (774 patients).

The all exposure population includes all patients in registration studies who received at least one dose of ACTEMRA. Of the 4009 patients in this population, 3577 received treatment for at least 6 months, 3296 for at least one year; 2806 received treatment for at least 2 years and 1222 for 3 years.

All patients in these studies had moderately to severely active rheumatoid arthritis. The study population had a mean age of 52 years, 82% were female and 74% were Caucasian.

The most commonly reported adverse events in 6-month controlled studies (occurring in ≥5% of patients treated with monotherapy or in combination with traditional DMARDs) were upper respiratory tract infections, nasopharyngitis, headache, hypertension and increased alanine amino transferase (ALT).

Infections: In the 6-month controlled studies, the rate of all infections reported in the 4 mg/kg and 8 mg/kg ACTEMRA plus traditional DMARD treatment was 133 and 127 events per 100 patient years, respectively, compared to 112 events per 100 patient years in the placebo plus traditional DMARD group. The overall rate of infections with ACTEMRA in the all exposure population was 108 events per 100 patient years exposure.

Serious Infections: In the 6-month controlled clinical studies, the rate of serious infections in the 4 mg/kg and 8 mg/kg ACTEMRA plus traditional DMARDs was 4.4 and 5.3 events per 100 patient years, respectively, compared to 3.9 events per 100 patient years exposure in the placebo plus traditional DMARD group. In the monotherapy study the rate of serious infections was 3.6 events per 100 patient years of exposure in the ACTEMRA group and 1.5 events per 100 patient years of exposure in the MTX group.

In the all exposure population, the overall rate of serious infections observed with ACTEMRA plus traditional DMARD treatment was 4.7 events per 100 patient years exposure. Reported serious infections, some with fatal outcome, included pneumonia, urinary tract infection, herpes zoster, gastroenteritis, diverticulitis, sepsis and bacterial arthritis. Cases of opportunistic infections have been reported.

Gastrointestinal Perforation: During the 6-month controlled clinical trials, the incidence of gastrointestinal perforation was 0.26 events per 100 patient-years with tocilizumab therapy. In the long-term exposure population the overall rate of gastrointestinal perforation was 0.28 events per 100 patient years. Reports of gastrointestinal perforation on tocilizumab were primarily reported as complications of diverticulitis including generalized purulent peritonitis, lower GI perforation, fistula and abscess. Most patients who developed gastrointestinal perforations were taking concomitant nonsteroidal anti-inflammatory medications (NSAIDs), corticosteroids, or methotrexate (see Warnings and Precautions, Gastrointestinal Perforations). The relative contribution of these concomitant medications versus ACTEMRA to the development of GI perforations is not known.

Infusion Reactions: In the 6-month controlled clinical studies, adverse events associated with infusion (occurring during or within 24 hours of infusion) were reported in 8% and 7% of patients in the 4 mg/kg and 8 mg/kg ACTEMRA plus DMARD group, respectively, compared to 5% of patients in the placebo plus DMARD group. The most frequently reported event on the 4 mg/kg and 8 mg/kg dose during the infusion was hypertension (1% for both doses), while the most frequently reported event occurring within 24 hours of finishing an infusion were headache (1% for both doses) and skin reactions (1% for both doses), including rash, pruritus and urticaria. These events were not treatment limiting. No premedication were administered in the clinical trials.

Clinically significant hypersensitivity reactions (e.g., anaphylactoid and anaphylactic reactions) associated with ACTEMRA and requiring treatment discontinuation were reported 0.1% (3/2644) in the 6-month, controlled trials and in 0.2% (9/4009) in the all-exposure population. These reactions were generally observed during the second to fourth infusion of ACTEMRA (see Warnings and Precautions, Hypersensitivity Reactions).

Immunogenicity: In 6-month controlled clinical studies, a total of 2876 patients have been tested for anti-tocilizumab antibodies. Forty six patients (1.6%) developed positive anti-tocilizumab antibodies of whom 5 had an associated medically significant hypersensitivity reaction leading to withdrawal. Thirty patients (1.1%) developed neutralizing antibodies.

Malignancies: During the 6-month controlled period of the studies, 15 malignancies were diagnosed in patients receiving ACTEMRA, compared to 8 malignancies in patients in the control groups. Exposure-adjusted incidence was similar in the ACTEMRA groups (1.32 events per 100 patient years) and in the placebo plus DMARD group (1.37 events per 100 patient years). In the all-exposure population, the rate of malignancies remained consistent (1.10 events per 100 patient years) with the rate observed in the 6-month, controlled period.

Clinical Trial Adverse Drug Reactions: Because clinical trials are conducted under very specific conditions the adverse reaction rates observed in the clinical trials may not reflect the rates observed in practice and should not be compared to the rates in the clinical trials of another drug. Adverse drug reaction information from clinical trials is useful for identifying drug-related adverse events and for approximating rates.

Table 1 below lists the adverse events (regardless of causality) occurring in ≥1% of patients treated with ACTEMRA during placebo-controlled double-blind rheumatoid arthritis studies.

Table 1: ACTEMRA

Adverse Events Reported by ≥1% of Patients Treated with ACTEMRA Dosed Every 4 Weeks During Phase III Rheumatoid Arthritis Placebo-Controlled Studies

Body System/ Adverse Event	ACTEMRA 8 mg/kg Monotherapy N=288 (%)	MTX N=284 (%)	ACTEMRA 4 mg/kg + MTX N=774 (%)	ACTEMRA 8 mg/kg + DMARDS N=1582 (%)	Placebo + DMARDs N=1170 (%)
Infections and Infestations					
Upper respiratory tract infection	7.3	5.3	6.2	7.8	6.1
Nasopharyngitis	6.9	6.0	4.3	5.6	4.4
Urinary tract infection	4.2	4.6	2.2	3.4	3.3
Sinusitis	3.1	3.9	2.1	2.9	2.1
Bronchitis	3.1	2.1	4.3	3.2	3.2
Pharyngitis	2.4	2.1	1.7	1.6	1.7
Influenza	1.7	2.8	2.8	2.5	2.6
Gastroenteritis	1.4	3.2	2.3	1.5	1.5
Oral herpes	0.7	0.7	1.2	1.4	0.6
Pneumonia	1.0	0.4	1.0	1.0	0.9
Gastroenteritis viral	1.7	1.4	0.9	0.8	0.6
Herpes zoster	0.3	—	0.8	1.1	0.7
Rhinitis	0.7	2.1	1.4	0.6	0.5
Cellulitis	0.3	0.4	0.3	1.1	0.7
Cystitis	0.7	0.7	1.2	0.6	0.3
Gastrointestinal Disorders					
Nausea	6.3	12.0	4.3	4.0	3.8
Diarrhea	5.2	5.3	4.0	3.9	3.2
Dyspepsia	3.5	4.2	2.2	2.6	2.0
Mouth ulceration	2.1	2.1	1.3	2.0	0.5
Abdominal pain, upper	1.7	2.1	2.7	2.5	1.5
Vomiting	2.1	3.2	2.1	1.7	1.6
Abdominal pain	3.8	2.1	1.7	1.3	1.3
Gastritis	1.0	1.8	1.2	1.8	0.8
Constipation	1.4	1.4	1.0	1.2	0.9
Stomatitis	1.4	1.8	0.5	0.8	0.3
Abdominal discomfort	1.0	—	0.3	0.2	0.2
Skin and Subcutaneous Tissue Disorders					
Rash	2.4	1.4	3.9	3.3	1.3
Pruritus	2.8	1.1	1.4	1.6	0.9
Alopecia	2.1	2.8	0.8	1.0	0.5
Musculoskeletal and Connective Tissue Disorders					
Back pain	2.4	1.1	2.1	3.3	2.4
Rheumatoid arthritis	0.7	2.1	3.0	2.1	4.1
Arthralgia	2.4	1.4	1.4	1.1	2.0
Musculoskeletal pain	1.0	0.4	0.8	0.4	0.4
Osteoarthritis	1.4	—	0.3	0.3	0.3
Nervous System Disorders					
Headache	7.3	2.5	5.8	5.3	3.4
Dizziness	3.1	1.4	1.9	3.1	1.7
Paraesthesia	1.0	—	0.4	0.6	0.5
Hypoaesthesia	1.0	0.4	0.5	0.3	0.3
Investigations					

(cont'd)

Table 1: ACTEMRA *(cont'd)*

Adverse Events Reported by ≥1% of Patients Treated with ACTEMRA Dosed Every 4 Weeks During Phase III Rheumatoid Arthritis Placebo-Controlled Studies

Body System/ Adverse Event	ACTEMRA 8 mg/kg Monotherapy N=288 (%)	MTX N=284 (%)	ACTEMRA 4 mg/kg + MTX N=774 (%)	ACTEMRA 8 mg/kg + DMARDS N=1582 (%)	Placebo + DMARDs N=1170 (%)
Alanine aminotransferase increased	5.6	3.9	2.8	3.2	0.9
Transaminases increased	1.0	4.6	1.7	2.3	0.5
Hepatic enzyme increased	2.1	2.8	1.2	1.5	0.6
Weight increased	1.7	0.4	0.6	0.8	0.2
Aspartate aminotransferase Increased	1.7	0.4	0.4	0.3	<0.1
Neutrophil count decreased	1.0	—	0.3	0.3	—
Blood triglycerides increased	1.0	—	—	0.3	
Vascular Disorders					
Hypertension	5.6	2.1	4.1	4.4	2.7
Flushing	1.0	0.4	0.6	0.3	0.3
General Disorders and Administration Site Conditions					
Fatigue	1.7	3.2	1.4	2.4	2.1
Oedema peripheral	1.7	—	1.3	2.1	1.5
Pyrexia	0.3	1.1	1.3	0.6	1.6
Asthenia	0.7	0.7	1.0	0.5	0.6
Chest pain	1.4	1.1	0.8	0.5	0.5
Respiratory, Thoracic and Mediastinal Disorders					
Cough	2.8	0.4	2.1	2.3	1.9
Pharyngolaryngeal pain	2.4	1.1	1.9	1.7	1.1
Dyspnoea	0.3	0.4	1.0	0.8	0.3
Injury, Poisoning and Procedural Complications					
Fall	0.3	—	1.0	0.7	0.9
Reproductive System and Breast Disorders					
Menorrhagia	1.0	0.4	0.3	0.3	0.3
Renal and Urinary Disorders					
Dysuria	1.7	0.4	0.4	0.4	0.7
Ear and Labyrinth Disorders					
Vertigo	0.7	0.4	1.2	0.7	1.0
Blood and Lymphatic System Disorders					
Leukopenia	1.4	—	0.5	1.2	<0.1
Anaemia	0.3	2.5	0.8	1.0	1.9
Neutropenia	1.4	—	0.4	1.1	—
Metabolism and Nutrition Disorders					
Hypercholesterolaemia	0.3	0.4	0.3	1.1	—
Hyperlipidaemia	1.4	—	0.4	0.2	0.3
Psychiatric Disorders					
Insomnia	2.1	1.1	2.1	1.0	1.3
Depression	2.1	0.7	1.0	1.3	1.2
Anxiety	2.4	0.7	0.6	0.8	0.8
Eye Disorders					
Conjunctivitis	1.4	0.4	0.6	0.9	0.5

Less Common Clinical Trial Adverse Drug Reactions (<1%): Other infrequent adverse drug reactions occurring at an incidence of less than 1% in rheumatoid arthritis patients treated with ACTEMRA in placebo-controlled trials were:

Blood and Lymphatic System Disorders: neutropenia, anaemia, thrombocytopenia, lymphopenia, lymphadenopathy, eosinophilia, leukaemoid reaction, hypocomplementaemia, haemolysis.

Cardiac Disorders: palpitations, tachycardia, acute coronary syndrome, supraventricular tachycardia, sinus tachycardia, left ventricular hypertrophy, extrasystoles, bundle branch block left.

Congenital, Familial and Genetic Disorders: pyloric stenosis.
Ear and Labyrinth Disorders: vertigo, motion sickness, ear pain, tinnitus, hypoacusis, cerumen impaction.
Endocrine Disorders: hypothyroidism, goitre.
Eye Disorders: conjunctivitis, vision blurred, eyelid oedema, eye oedema, dry eye, blepharitis, eye pain, glaucoma, lacrimation increased, ocular hyperaemia, conjunctivitis allergic, xerophthalmia, vitreous floaters, visual disturbance, Sicca syndrome, scleritis, punctate keratitis, keratitis interstitial, foreign body sensation in eyes, eyelids pruritus, eye pruritus, eye irritation, extraocular muscle paresis, dacryoadenitis acquired, conjunctival haemorrhage, cataract.
Gastrointestinal Disorders: abdominal pain, gastritis, aphthous stomatitis, stomatitis, constipation, gastrooesophageal reflux disease, abdominal discomfort, abdominal distension, flatulence, gingival bleeding, glossodynia, toothache, gastric ulcer, gingival pain, gingivitis, haematochezia, oesophagitis, dry mouth, frequent bowel movements, gastritis erosive, hiatus hernia, abdominal pain lower, epigastric discomfort, gastrointestinal disorder, oral pain, pancreatitis, rectal haemorrhage, tongue ulceration, dysphagia, enteritis, hypoaesthesia oral, irritable bowel syndrome, lip ulceration, odynophagia, reflux oesophagitis, abdominal tenderness, anal inflammation, anorectal disorder, stomach discomfort, oral mucosal blistering, oral soft tissue disorder, erosive oesophagitis, tongue exfoliation, tongue disorder, tongue blistering, sigmoiditis, periodontitis, pancreatitis chronic, oral soft tissue disorder, oral discomfort, melaena, malabsorption, lip oedema, large intestine perforation, haemorrhoids, gingival ulceration, gastrointestinal motility disorder, gastrointestinal pain, gastrointestinal perforation, erosive esophagitis, dental caries, colitis, cheilitis, change of bowel habit, gastric disorder.
General Disorders and Administration Site Conditions: oedema peripheral, pyrexia, asthenia, chills, chest pain, infusion related reaction, chest discomfort, pain, impaired healing, malaise, influenza like illness, injection site reaction, face oedema, oedema, infusion site reaction, injection site haematoma, feeling hot and cold, inflammation, pitting oedema, thirst, temperature intolerance, swelling, sensation of foreign body, secretion discharge, mucosal ulceration, mucosal inflammation, local swelling, injection site pain, injection site pruritus, injection site swelling, infusion site pain, hypothermia, gravitational oedema, generalised oedema, feeling hot, feeling cold, drug withdrawal syndrome, drug intolerance.
Hepatobiliary Disorders: hepatotoxicity, hyperbilirubinaemia, hepatic steatosis, liver disorder, hepatomegaly, hepatic function abnormal, cytolytic hepatitis, cholelithiasis, cholecystitis acute, biliary colic.
Immune System Disorders: hypersensitivity, anaphylactic reaction, antiphospholipid syndrome, autoimmune disorder, immunodeficiency, drug hypersensitivity.
Infections and Infestations: oral herpes, herpes zoster, influenza, pneumonia, gastroenteritis, cellulitis, cystitis, rhinitis, folliculitis, respiratory tract infection, tonsillitis, tinea pedis, viral upper respiratory tract infection, herpes simplex, ear infection, localised infection, vulvovaginal mycotic infection, abscess limb, furuncle, laryngitis, lower respiratory tract infection, paronychia, viral infection, eye infection, acute sinusitis, nail infection, onychomycosis, otitis media, rash pustular, tooth abscess, fungal skin infection, body tinea, candidiasis, cervicitis, gastroenteritis viral, genital herpes, labyrinthitis, pharyngitis streptococcal, Pseudomonas infection, subcutaneous abscess, tracheitis, chronic sinusitis, conjunctivitis bacterial, erysipelas, gastrointestinal infection, giardiasis, infection, infection parasitic, osteomyelitis, otitis media acute, postoperative wound infection, sepsis, sialoadenitis, tooth infection, herpes virus infection, oral candidiasis, purulent discharge, pyelonephritis chronic, tinea versicolour, vulvovaginitis, acarodermatitis, alveolar osteitis, anal candidiasis, arthritis bacterial, vaginal candidiasis, parasitic infection intestinal, perianal abscess, viral pharyngitis, vaginitis Gardnerella, wound infection, tracheobronchitis, tinea capitis, staphylococcal skin infection, staphylococcal infection, skin Candida, septic arthritis staphylococcal, respiratory tract infection viral, pyoderma, pyelonephritis acute, pyelonephritis, peridiverticular abscess, perianal abscess, parotitis, oral bacterial infection, nipple infection, pneumonia necrotizing, *P. jiroveci* pneumonia, nasal vestibulitis, nasal abscess, nail bed infection, myringitis, *M. avium* Complex infection, mediastinitis, keratitis herpetic, keratitis bacterial, infected skin ulcer, infected insect bite, hordeolum, herpes simplex ophthalmic, hand-foot-and-mouth disease, gastrointestinal candidiasis, fungal infection, erythrasma, enterobiasis, endocarditis enterococcal, diarrhoea infectious, dermatitis infected, conjunctivitis viral, cellulitis staphylococcal, bursitis infective.
Injury, Poisoning and Procedural Complications: contusion, procedural hypertension, traumatic haematoma, sunburn, stress fracture, spinal fracture, skin laceration, skin injury, postoperative wound complication, hip fracture, foot fracture, fall, drug toxicity.
Investigations: liver function test abnormal, weight increased, aspartate aminotransferase increased, blood bilirubin increased, blood pressure increased, neutrophil count decreased, platelet count decreased, white blood cell count decreased, blood triglycerides increased, haemoglobin decreased, low density lipoprotein increased, blood pressure decreased, blood cholesterol increased, weight decreased, alanine aminotransferase abnormal, blood creatinine increased, alanine aminotransferase, blood alkaline phosphatase increased, blood bilirubin unconjugated increased, weight abnormal, white blood cells urine positive, serum ferritin decreased, neutrophil count abnormal, heart rate increased, electrocardiogram repolarisation abnormality, electrocardiogram QT prolonged, cardiac murmur, body temperature increased, blood urine present, blood urea increased, blood pressure diastolic increased, blood pressure abnormal, blood glucose increased, blood count abnormal.
Metabolism and Nutrition Disorders, Hypernatremia: hypercholesterolaemia, hyperlipidaemia, hypertriglyceridaemia, dyslipidaemia, hyperuricaemia, hypokalaemia, diabetes mellitus, hypoglycaemia, fluid retention, anorexia, lipid metabolism disorder, increased appetite, dehydration, decreased appetite, hypernatremia.
Musculoskeletal and Connective Tissue Disorders: back pain, rheumatoid arthritis, arthralgia, muscle spasms, myalgia, pain in extremity, joint swelling, arthritis, musculoskeletal chest pain, musculoskeletal pain, rheumatoid nodule, bursitis, muscular weakness, neck pain, osteoarthritis, tendonitis, costochondritis, nodule on extremity, rotator cuff syndrome, synovitis, osteopenia, muscle atrophy, limb discomfort, exostosis.
Neoplasms Benign, Malignant and Unspecified (incl cysts and polyps): lung neoplasm, angiolipoma, benign salivary gland neoplasm, uterine leiomyoma, thyroid adenoma, skin papilloma, meningioma, hepatic neoplasm, cervix carcinoma stage 0.
Nervous System Disorders: paraesthesia, hypoaesthesia, dysgeusia, migraine, somnolence, burning sensation, tremor, carpal tunnel syndrome, haemorrhagic stroke, lethargy, restless legs syndrome, amnesia, tension headache, syncope, sinus headache, neuropathy peripheral, neuralgia, lumbar radiculopathy, ischaemic cerebral infarction, grand mal convulsion, facial palsy, dyslexia, dysaesthesia, dementia, cerebrovascular accident.
Psychiatric Disorders: insomnia, anxiety, depression, libido decreased, neurosis, nervousness, major depression.
Renal and Urinary Disorders: dysuria, haematuria, nephrolithiasis, pollakiuria, renal failure, renal cyst, polyuria, micturition urgency, leukocyturia, hypertensive nephropathy.
Reproductive System and Breast Disorders: menorrhagia, amenorrhoea, breast pain, uterine haemorrhage, vulval ulceration, vaginal ulceration, vaginal discharge, vaginal burning sensation, ovarian cyst, metrorrhagia, menstruation irregular, menstrual disorder, hypomenorrhoea, genital haemorrhage, breast swelling.
Respiratory, Thoracic and Mediastinal Disorders: dyspnoea, epistaxis, rhinitis allergic, nasal congestion, sinus congestion, asthma, rhinorrhoea, chronic obstructive pulmonary disease, interstitial lung disease, nasal ulcer, nasal discomfort, nasal dryness, respiratory tract congestion, vasomotor rhinitis, sinusitis noninfective, rhinitis atrophic, respiratory tract irritation, respiratory disorder, pleuritic pain, pleurisy, pleural effusion, pharyngeal inflammation, nasal septum perforation, idiopathic pulmonary fibrosis, dysphonia.
Skin and Subcutaneous Tissue Disorders: alopecia, hyperhidrosis, rash papular, urticaria, rash erythematous, skin ulcer, dermatitis, increased tendency to bruise, dermatitis allergic, eczema, rash pruritic, erythema, night sweats, petechiae, rash macular, blister, dry skin, ecchymosis, drug eruption, acne, pruritus generalised, rosacea, skin lesion, swelling face, cold sweat, erythema nodosum, ingrowing nail, rash maculo-papular, skin fragility, skin nodule, stasis dermatitis, vasculitic rash, angioedema, cutaneous vasculitis, dyspnoea exertional, hyperkeratosis, photosensitivity reaction, pityriasis, psoriasis, purpura, skin hyperpigmentation, acrodermatitis, acute febrile neutrophilic dermatosis, urticaria generalised, urticaria generalised, skin exfoliation, skin discolouration, skin atrophy, scab, rash vesicular, rash generalized, pruritus allergic, pityriasis rosea, perivascular dermatitis, panniculitis, palpable purpura, livedo reticularis, leukocytoclastic vasculitis, hypoaesthesia facial, erythema multiforme, erythema annulare, dyshidrosis, dermatitis contact, dermatitis bullous, decubitus ulcer, blood blister.
Vascular Disorders: flushing, hypotension, hot flush, vasculitis, haematoma, varicose vein, Raynaud's phenomenon, phlebitis, orthostatic hypotension, essential hypertension, thrombophlebitis superficial.
Abnormal Hematologic and Clinical Chemistry Findings: Hematology Abnormalities: In 6-month controlled clinical studies, decreases in neutrophil counts below 1×10⁹/L occurred in 1.8% and 3.4% of patients in the 4 mg/kg and 8 mg/kg ACTEMRA plus DMARD group, respectively, compared to 0.1% of patients in the placebo plus DMARD group (see Table 2). Approximately half of the instances of ANC <1×10⁹/L occurred within 8 weeks of starting therapy. Decreases below 0.5×10⁹/L were reported in 0.4% and 0.3% of patients in the 4 mg/kg and 8 mg/kg ACTEMRA plus DMARD, respectively, compared to 0.1% of patients in the placebo plus DMARD group (see Warnings and Precautions, Laboratory Abnormalities). In the all exposure population, the pattern and incidence of decreases in neutrophil counts remained consistent with what was seen in the 6-month controlled clinical studies.

In 6-month controlled clinical studies, decreases in platelet counts below 100×10³/μL occurred in 1.3% and 1.7% of patients on 4 mg/kg and 8 mg/kg ACTEMRA plus DMARD, respectively, compared to 0.5% of patients on placebo plus DMARD (see Table 3). In the all exposure population, the pattern and incidence of decreases in platelet counts remained consistent with what was seen in the 6-month controlled clinical studies.

Table 2: ACTEMRA

Clinically Significant Changes in Hematological Laboratory Values in the 6 Month Controlled Period

Laboratory Parameter	ACTEMRA 8 mg/kg Monotherapy N=288 (%)	Methotrexate N=284 (%)	ACTEMRA 4 mg/kg + DMARDs N=774 (%)	ACTEMRA 8 mg/kg + DMARDs N=1582 (%)	Placebo + DMARDs N=1170 (%)
Neutropenia					
Grade 3/4 (<1×10⁹/L)	9 (3.1%)	1 (0.4%)	14 (1.8%)	54 (3.4%)	1 (0.1%)
Thrombocytopenia					
<100×10³/μL	4 (1.4%)	1 (0.4%)	10 (1.3%)	27 (1.7%)	6 (0.5%)

Liver Enzyme Elevations: In 6-month controlled trials, transient elevations in ALT/AST >3×ULN were observed in 4.9% of patients on MTX compared to 2.1% of patients on ACTEMRA 8 mg/kg and in 5.9% and 6.5% of patients who received 4 mg/kg and 8 mg/kg ACTEMRA plus traditional DMARDs, respectively, compared to 1.5% of patients on placebo plus traditional DMARDs. The addition of potentially hepatotoxic drugs (e.g. MTX), to ACTEMRA monotherapy resulted in increased frequency of these elevations. Elevations of ALT/AST >5×ULN were observed in 0.7% of ACTEMRA monotherapy patients and 1.4% of ACTEMRA plus traditional DMARD patients, the majority of whom were discontinued from ACTEMRA treatment. These elevations were not associated with any clinically relevant increase in direct bilirubin, nor were they associated with clinical evidence of hepatitis or hepatic insufficiency. Increases in indirect bilirubin greater than the upper limit of normal, collected as a routine laboratory parameter, were observed in 0% of patients on MTX compared to 4.5% of patients on ACTEMRA 8 mg/kg, and in 3.5% and 6.1% of patients who received 4 mg/kg and 8 mg/kg ACTEMRA plus traditional DMARDs, respectively, compared to 0.8% of patients on placebo plus traditional DMARDs. In the all exposure population, the pattern and incidence of elevations in ALT/AST remained consistent with what was seen in the 6 month controlled clinical trials.

Table 3: ACTEMRA

Incidence of ALT/AST in the 6-Month Controlled Period

	ACTEMRA 8 mg/kg Monotherapy N=288 n (%)	Methotrexate N=284 n (%)	ACTEMRA 4 mg/kg + DMARDs N=774 n (%)	ACTEMRA 8 mg/kg + DMARDs N=1582 n (%)	Placebo + DMARDs N=1170 n (%)
ALT (U/L)					
>ULN to 3×ULN	105 (36)	95 (33)	349 (45)	763 (48)	269 (23)
>3×ULN to 5×ULN	4 (1.4)	11 (3.9)	36 (4.7)	80 (5.1)	15 (1.3)
>5×ULN	2 (0.7)	3 (1.1)	10 (1.3)	23 (1.5)	3 (0.3)
AST (U/L)					
>ULN to 3×ULN	64 (22)	74 (26)	264 (34)	646 (41)	194 (17)
>3×ULN to 5×ULN	1 (0.3)	5 (1.8)	8 (1.0)	29 (1.8)	3 (0.3)
>5×ULN	2 (0.7)	1 (0.4)	1 (0.1)	3 (0.2)	1 (<0.1)

Legend: ULN=upper limit of normal.

Elevations in Lipid Parameters: During the 6-month controlled trials, elevations in lipid parameters (total cholesterol, LDL, HDL, triglycerides) were observed 6 weeks following initiation of ACTEMRA and remained stable thereafter. Increases in triglycerides to levels above 5.64 mmol/L were rarely observed. Approximately 24% of patients receiving ACTEMRA in clinical trials experienced sustained elevations in total cholesterol >6.2 mmol/L, with 15% experiencing a sustained increase in LDL to ≥4.1 mmol/L. Changes in lipid parameters from baseline to week 24 were evaluated and are summarized below:

- Mean LDL increased by 0.34 mmol/L in the TCZ 4 mg/kg + DMARD arm, 0.52 mmol/L in the TCZ 8 mg/kg + DMARD, and 0.65 mmol/L in TCZ 8 mg/kg monotherapy.
- Mean HDL increased by 0.08 mmol/L in the TCZ 4 mg/kg + DMARD arm, 0.13 mmol/L in the TCZ 8 mg/kg + DMARD, and 0.10 mmol/L in TCZ 8 mg/kg monotherapy.
- Mean LDL/HDL ratio increased by an average of 0.004 mmol/L in the TCZ 4 mg/kg + DMARD arm, 0.004 mmol/L in the TCZ 8 mg/kg + DMARD, and 0.007 mmol/L in TCZ 8 mg/kg monotherapy.

In the majority of patients there was no increase in atherogenic indices, and elevations in total cholesterol responded to treatment with lipid-lowering agents.

In the all exposure population, the pattern and incidence of elevations in lipid parameters remained consistent with what was seen in the 6 month controlled clinical trials.

DRUG INTERACTIONS: Drug-Drug Interactions: Population pharmacokinetic analyses did not detect any effect of methotrexate, non-steroidal anti-inflammatory drugs or corticosteroids on tocilizumab clearance. Concomitant administration of a single dose of 10 mg/kg ACTEMRA with 10-25 mg methotrexate once weekly had no clinically significant effect on methotrexate exposure.

ACTEMRA has not been studied in combination with other biological DMARDs.

Treatment with ACTEMRA in combination with azathioprine, cyclophosphamide, or chlorambucil is limited or has not been studied, therefore the benefits and risks of such combinations are unknown.

Interactions with CYP450 Substrates: The expression of hepatic CYP450 enzymes is suppressed by the pro-inflammatory cytokines such as IL-6. Thus, it is expected that for any drug with a potent anti-cytokine inhibition,such as ACTEMRA, CYP450 suppression may be reversed when introduced in patients with rheumatoid arthritis.

In vitro data suggested that IL-6 reduced mRNA expression for several CYP450 isoenzymes including CYP1A2, CYP2B6, CYP2C9, CYP2C19, CYP2D6 and CYP3A4, and this reduced expression was reversed by co-incubation with tocilizumab at clinically relevant concentrations. Accordingly, inhibition of IL-6 signaling in RA patients treated with tocilizumab may restore CYP450 activities to higher levels than those in the absence of tocilizumab leading to increased metabolism of drugs that are CYP450 substrates. Its effect on CYP2C8 or transporters (e.g., P-gp) is unknown. This is clinically relevant for CYP450 substrates with a narrow therapeutic index, where the dose is individually adjusted. Upon initiation of ACTEMRA, in patients being treated with these types of medicinal products, therapeutic monitoring of the effect (e.g., warfarin) or drug concentration (e.g., cyclosporine or theophylline) should be performed and the individual dose of the medicinal product adjusted as needed. Caution should be exercised when ACTEMRA is coadministered with drugs where decrease in effectiveness is undesirable, e.g., oral contraceptives (CYP3A4 substrates).

When starting or stopping therapy with tocilizumab, patients taking medicinal products which are individually adjusted and are metabolised via CYP450 3A4, 1A2, 2C9 or 2C19 (e.g. atorvastatin, calcium channel blockers, theophylline, warfarin, phenytoin, ciclosporin, or benzodiazepines) should be monitored as doses may need to be increased to maintain therapeutic effect. Given the elimination half-life ($t_{½}$=13 days), the effect of tocilizumab on CYP450 enzyme activity may persist for several weeks after stopping therapy.

Simvastatin: Simvastatin is a CYP3A4 and OATP1B1 substrate. In 12 RA patients, not treated with ACTEMRA, receiving 40 mg simvastatin, exposures of simvastatin and its metabolite, simvastatin acid, was 4- to 10-fold and 2-fold higher, respectively, than the exposures observed in healthy subjects. One week following administration of a single infusion of ACTEMRA (10 mg/kg), exposure of simvastatin and simvastatin acid decreased by 57% and 39%, respectively, to exposures that were similar or slightly higher than those observed in healthy subjects. Exposures of simvastatin and simvastatin acid increased upon withdrawal of ACTEMRA in RA patients. Selection of a particular dose of simvastatin in RA patients should take into account the potentially lower exposures that may result after initiation of ACTEMRA (due to normalization of CYP3A4) or higher exposures after discontinuation of ACTEMRA.

Omeprazole: Omeprazole is a CYP2C19 and CYP3A4 substrate. In RA patients receiving 10 mg omeprazole, exposure to omeprazole was approximately 2 fold higher than that observed in healthy subjects. In RA patients receiving 10 mg omeprazole, before and one week after ACTEMRA infusion (8 mg/kg), the omeprazole AUCinf decreased by 12% for poor (N=5) and intermediate metabolizers (N=5) and by 28% for extensive metabolizers (N=8) and were slightly higher than those observed in healthy subjects.

Dextromethorphan: Dextromethorphan is a CYP2D6 and CYP3A4 substrate. In 13 RA patients receiving 30 mg dextromethorphan, exposure to dextromethorphan was comparable to that in healthy subjects. However, exposure to its metabolite, dextrorphan (a CYP3A4 substrate), was a fraction of that observed in healthy subjects. One week following administration of a single infusion of ACTEMRA (8 mg/kg), dextromethorphan exposure was decreased by approximately 5%. However, a larger decrease (29%) in dextrorphan levels was noted after ACTEMRA infusion.

DOSAGE AND ADMINISTRATION: Dosing Considerations:

- It would be prudent not to use ACTEMRA in patients who are using azathioprine or cyclophosphamide.
- ACTEMRA has not been studied in combination with biological DMARDs such as TNF antagonists.
- Treatment with biological DMARDs such as TNF inhibitors has been associated with reactivation of Hepatitis B and C. Therefore screening for viral hepatitis should be performed in accordance with published guidelines before starting therapy with ACTEMRA. In clinical studies with ACTEMRA, patients who screened positive for hepatitis were excluded from the study.
- ACTEMRA treatment should be interrupted if a patient develops a serious infection until the infection is controlled.

Recommended Dose and Dosage Adjustment: Recommended Dose: ACTEMRA should be given in combination with methotrexate (MTX) or other DMARDs. ACTEMRA may also be given as monotherapy in cases of intolerance to MTX or where treatment with MTX is not appropriate. The recommended dose of ACTEMRA for adult patients with rheumatoid arthritis given once every 4 weeks as an intravenous infusion over 1 hour is:

Recommended Adult Dosage Every 4 Weeks	
Patients who have had an inadequate response to one or more DMARDs and/or TNF antagonists.	**When used in combination with DMARDs or as monotherapy the recommended starting dose is 4 mg/kg followed by an increase to 8 mg/kg based on clinical response.**

In clinical trials with ACTEMRA, patients with the following laboratory parameter were not initiated: Platelet count <100 000/mm³, hemoglobin (Hb) <8.5 g/dL, WBC <3000/mm³, ANC <2.0×10⁹/L, absolute lymphocyte count <500/mm³, ALT or AST > 1.5× upper limit of normal (ULN), total bilirubin >ULN, Triglycerides (TG) >10 mmol/L (>900 mg/dL), Serum creatinine >1.4 mg/dL in female patients and >1.6 mg/dL in male patients.

For individuals whose body weight is more than 100 kg, doses exceeding 800 mg per infusion are not recommended.

Dose Adjustments: The following dose adjustments are recommended for management of certain dose-related laboratory changes including elevated liver enzymes, neutropenia, and thrombocytopenia. See Table 4, Table 5 and Table 6.

Table 4: ACTEMRA

Liver Enzyme Abnormalities

Lab Value	Action
>1 to 3×ULN	Dose modify concomitant DMARDs if appropriate. For persistent increases in this range, reduce tocilizumab dose to 4 mg/kg or interrupt tocilizumab until ALT/AST have normalized.
>3 to 5×ULN (confirmed by repeat testing)	Interrupt tocilizumab dosing until <3×ULN and follow recommendations above for >1 to 3×ULN. For persistent increases >3×ULN, discontinue tocilizumab.
>5×ULN	Discontinue tocilizumab.

Table 5: ACTEMRA

Low Absolute Neutrophil Count (ANC)

Lab Value (cells×10⁹/L)	Action
ANC >1	Maintain dose.
ANC 0.5 to 1	Interrupt tocilizumab dosing. When ANC >1×10⁹/L resume tocilizumab at 4 mg/kg and increase to 8 mg/kg as clinically appropriate
ANC <0.5	Discontinue tocilizumab.

Table 6: ACTEMRA

Low Platelet Count

Lab Value (cells×10³/μL)	Action
50 to 100	Interrupt tocilizumab dosing. When platelet count is >100×10³/μL resume tocilizumab at 4 mg/kg and increase to 8 mg/kg as clinically appropriate.
<50	Discontinue tocilizumab.

Special Dosage Instructions: Pediatric: The safety and efficacy of ACTEMRA in children have not been established.

Geriatric: As with all biologics, there is a higher incidence of infections in the elderly population in general, therefore, caution should be used when treating the elderly.

Renal impairment: No dose adjustment is required in patients with mild renal impairment (see Action and Clinical Pharmacology, Special Populations and Conditions, Renal Insufficiency). ACTEMRA has not been studied in patients with moderate to severe renal impairment.

Hepatic impairment: The safety and efficacy of ACTEMRA has not been studied in patients with hepatic impairment (see Warnings and Precautions, Active Hepatic Disease and Hepatic Impairment). Therefore, no dose recommendations can be made.

Administration: ACTEMRA concentrate for intravenous infusion should be diluted to 100 mL by a healthcare professional using aseptic technique as follows:

- Withdraw the required amount of ACTEMRA for a dose of 4 mg/kg or 8 mg/kg (equivalent to 0.2 mL/kg or 0.4 mL/kg, respectively).
- Withdraw the same amount of sterile, non-pyrogenic 0.9% w/v sodium chloride solution from the infusion bag and discard.
- Slowly add the withdrawn ACTEMRA concentrate into the infusion bag. **The final volume in the infusion bag should total 100 mL.**
- To mix the solution, gently invert the bag to avoid foaming.
- Allow the fully diluted ACTEMRA solution to reach room temperature prior to infusion.
- The infusion should be administered over 60 minutes, and must be administered with an infusion set. **Do not administer as an intravenous push or bolus.**

For Prepared Infusion Solution: ACTEMRA does not contain preservatives, therefore reconstitution and dilution of the product should be performed under aseptic conditions. The prepared infusion solution of tocilizumab is physically and chemically stable in 0.9% w/v sodium chloride solution at 2-8°C or 30°C for 24 hours. From a microbiological point of view, the prepared infusion should be used immediately (see Storage and Stability).

Parenteral drug products should be inspected visually for particulate matter and discoloration prior to administration, whenever solution and container permit. ACTEMRA is a colorless to pale yellow liquid. If particulates and discolorations are noted, the product should not be used. Fully diluted ACTEMRA solutions are compatible with polypropylene, polyethylene and polyvinyl chloride infusion bags and polypropylene, polyethylene and glass infusion bottles.

ACTEMRA should not be infused concomitantly in the same intravenous line with other drugs. No physical or biochemical compatibility studies have been conducted to evaluate the co-administration of ACTEMRA with other drugs.

OVERDOSAGE:
There are limited data available on overdosage with ACTEMRA (tocilizumab). One case of accidental overdose was reported in which a patient with multiple myeloma received a single dose of 40 mg/kg. No adverse drug reactions were observed. No serious adverse drug reactions were observed in healthy volunteers who received a single dose up to 28 mg/kg, although dose-limiting neutropenia was observed.

In case of an overdose, it is recommended that the patient be monitored for signs and symptoms of adverse reactions. Patients who develop adverse reactions should receive appropriate symptomatic treatment.

> For management of a suspected drug overdose, contact your regional Poison Control Centre. See the *CPS* Directory section for a list of Poison Control Centres.

ACTION AND CLINICAL PHARMACOLOGY: Mechanism of Action: Tocilizumab binds specifically to both soluble and membrane-bound IL-6 receptors (sIL-6R and mIL-6R), and has been shown to inhibit sIL-6R and mIL-6R-mediated signaling through these receptors. IL-6 is a pleiotropic pro-inflammatory cytokine produced by a variety of cell types including T- and B-cells, lymphocytes, monocytes and fibroblasts. IL-6 has been shown to be involved in diverse physiological processes such as T-cell activation, induction of immunoglobulin secretion, initiation of hepatic acute phase protein synthesis, and stimulation of hematopoietic precursor cell proliferation and differentiation. IL-6 is the most abundantly produced cytokine by synovial and endothelial cells leading to local production of IL-6 in joints affected by inflammatory processes such as rheumatoid arthritis.

Pharmacodynamics: In clinical studies of ACTEMRA (tocilizumab), decreases in levels of C-reactive protein (CRP) to within normal ranges were seen as early as week 2 and were maintained while on treatment. Decreases in rheumatoid factor (RF), erythrocyte sedimentation rate (ESR) and serum amyloid A (SAA) were also observed in the clinical studies. Improvement in hemoglobin were observed, through tocilizumab decreasing the IL-6 driven effects on hepcidin production to increase iron availability.

In healthy subjects administered tocilizumab in doses from 2 to 28 mg/kg, absolute neutrophil counts decreased to the nadir 3 to 5 days following administration. Thereafter, neutrophils recovered towards baseline in a dose dependent manner. Rheumatoid arthritis patients demonstrated a similar pattern of absolute neutrophil counts following tocilizumab administration (see Warnings and Precautions, Laboratory Abnormalities, Neutrophils).

Pharmacokinetics: The pharmacokinetics characterized in healthy subjects and RA patients suggested that PK is similar between the two populations. The clearance (CL) of tocilizumab decreased with increased doses. At the 10 mg/kg single dose in RA patients, mean CL was 0.29±0.10 mL/hr/kg and mean apparent terminal $t_{½}$ was 151±59 hours (6.3 days).

The pharmacokinetics of tocilizumab were determined using a population pharmacokinetic analysis on a database composed of 1793 rheumatoid arthritis patients treated with tocilizumab 4 and 8 mg/kg every 4 weeks for 24 weeks. The pharmacokinetic parameters of tocilizumab did not change with time. A more than dose-proportional increase in area under the curve (AUC) and trough concentration (C_{min}) was observed for doses of 4 and 8 mg/kg every 4 weeks. Maximum concentration (C_{max}) increased dose-proportionally. At steady-state, predicted AUC and C_{min} were 2.7 and 6.5 fold higher at 8 mg/kg as compared to 4 mg/kg, respectively.

The following parameters are valid for a dose of 4 mg/kg tocilizumab given every 4 weeks. Predicted mean (±SD) steady-state AUC, C_{min} and C_{max} of tocilizumab were 13 000±5800 μg·h/mL, 1.49±2.13 μg/mL, and 88.3±41.4 μg/mL, respectively. The accumulation ratios for AUC and C_{max} were small; 1.11 and 1.02, respectively. The accumulation ratio was higher for C_{min} (1.96). Steady-state was reached following the first administration for C_{max} and AUC, respectively, and after 16 weeks for C_{min}.

The following parameters are valid for a dose of 8 mg/kg tocilizumab given every 4 weeks. Predicted mean (±SD) steady-state AUC, C_{min} and C_{max} of tocilizumab were 35 000±15 500 h·μg/mL, 9.74±10.5 μg/mL, and 183±85.6 μg/mL, respectively. The accumulation ratios for AUC and C_{max} were small; 1.22 and 1.06, respectively. The accumulation ratio was higher for C_{min} (2.35), which was expected based on the nonlinear clearance contribution at lower concentrations. Steady-state was reached following the first administration and after 8 and 20 weeks for C_{max}, AUC, and C_{min}, respectively. Tocilizumab AUC, C_{min} and C_{max} increased with increase of body weight. At body weight >100 kg, the predicted mean (±SD) steady state AUC, C_{min} and C_{max} of tocilizumab were 55 500±14 100 μg·h/mL, 19.0±12.0 μg/mL, and 269±57 μg/mL, respectively, which are higher than mean exposure values for the patient population. Therefore, tocilizumab doses exceeding 800 mg per infusion are not recommended in patients ≥100 kg.

Distribution: Following IV dosing, tocilizumab undergoes biphasic elimination from the circulation. In rheumatoid arthritis patients the central volume of distribution was 3.5 L, the peripheral volume of distribution was 2.9 L resulting in a volume of distribution at steady state of 6.4 L.

Excretion: The total clearance of tocilizumab was concentration-dependent and is the sum of the linear clearance and the nonlinear clearance. The linear clearance was estimated as a parameter in the population pharmacokinetic analysis and was 12.5 mL/h. The concentration-dependent nonlinear clearance plays a major role at low tocilizumab concentrations. Once the nonlinear clearance pathway is saturated, at higher tocilizumab concentrations, clearance is mainly determined by the linear clearance.

The $t_{½}$ of tocilizumab is concentration-dependent. The concentration-dependent apparent $t_{½}$ is 11 days for 4 mg/kg and up to 13 days for 8 mg/kg every 4 weeks at steady state.

Special Populations and Conditions: Pediatrics: ACTEMRA is not recommended for use in children below 18 years of age due to a lack of data on safety and efficacy.

Hepatic Insufficiency: No formal study of the effect of hepatic impairment on the pharmacokinetics of ACTEMRA was conducted.

Renal Insufficiency: No formal study of the effect of renal impairment on the pharmacokinetics of ACTEMRA was conducted.

Most of the patients in the population pharmacokinetic analysis had normal renal function or mild renal impairment. Mild renal impairment (creatinine clearance based on Cockcroft-Gault <80 mL/min and ≥50 mL/min) did not impact the pharmacokinetics of ACTEMRA.

Other Special Populations: Population analyses evaluated the potential effects of demographic characteristics on the pharmacokinetics of ACTEMRA in adult rheumatoid arthritis patients. Results of these analyses showed that no adjustment of the dose is necessary for age, gender, or race.

Population pharmacokinetic analyses in adult rheumatoid arthritis patients showed that age, gender and race did not affect the pharmacokinetics of tocilizumab. Linear clearance was found to increase with body size. The body weight-based dose (8 mg/kg) resulted in approximately 86% higher exposure in patients who are greater than 100 kg in comparison to patients who are less than 60 kg.

STORAGE AND STABILITY: ACTEMRA (tocilizumab) vials should be stored in a refrigerator at 2 to 8°C. Do not freeze. Keep the vial in the outer carton to protect it from light. Do not use beyond expiration date stated on the vial and carton.

For prepared infusion solution: ACTEMRA does not contain preservatives, therefore reconstitution and dilution of the product should be performed under aseptic conditions. The prepared infusion solution of tocilizumab is physically and chemically stable in 0.9% w/v sodium chloride solution at 2-8°C or 30°C for 24 hours. From a microbiological point of view, the prepared infusion should be used immediately.

ACTEMRA solutions do not contain preservatives; therefore, unused product remaining in the vials should not be used.

INFORMATION FOR THE PATIENT: Published in e-CPS, available by subscription at www.e-cps.ca.

DOSAGE FORMS, COMPOSITION AND PACKAGING: Each mL of sterile concentrate solution for intravenous infusion contains: tocilizumab 20 mg. Preservative-free. Nonmedicinal ingredients: disodium phosphate dodecahydrate, polysorbate 80, sodium dihydrogen phosphate dihydrate, sucrose and water for injections. Type I glass single use vials of 4 mL with a stopper (butyl rubber). Packs of 1 and 4. Type I glass single use vials of 10 mL with a stopper (butyl rubber). Packs of 1 and 4. Type I glass single use vials of 20 mL with a stopper (butyl rubber). Packs of 1 and 4.

Act-HIB®

Haemophilus b conjugate vaccine (tetanus protein-conjugate)

Active Immunizing Agent

sanofi pasteur

Date of Revision: July 2006

SUMMARY PRODUCT INFORMATION:

Route of Administration	Dosage Form/ Strength	Clinically Relevant Nonmedicinal Ingredients
Intramuscular injection	Reconstituted Product for Injection Each 0.5 mL dose of vaccine contains: 10 µg purified capsular polysaccharide of *H. influenzae* type b covalently bound to 20 µg of tetanus protein	Sucrose, trometamol, sodium chloride solution For a complete listing see Dosage Forms, Composition and Packaging.

DESCRIPTION: Act-HIB [Haemophilus b Conjugate Vaccine (Tetanus Protein–Conjugate)] is a freeze-dried powder and diluent for intramuscular administration.

Act-HIB is prepared from *H. influenzae* type b (Hib) strain cultures and *C. tetani* cultures. Hib strains are precipitated with cetrimide and capsular polysaccharide (PRP) is extracted. PRP is then purified and activated. At the same time, the preparation of *C. tetani* strains is precipitated with ammonium sulphate and detoxified to obtain tetanus protein, which is concentrated. Activated PRP and concentrated tetanus protein are conjugated by carbodiimide group reaction to produce the drug substance (PRP-T), which is then formulated with excipients (final bulk product) that is then freeze-dried.

The diluent for reconstitution is a 0.4% saline solution. After reconstitution the vaccine appears clear and colourless and does not contain a preservative.

INDICATIONS AND CLINICAL USE: Act-HIB [Haemophilus b Conjugate Vaccine (Tetanus Protein–Conjugate)] is indicated for the active immunization of persons 2 months of age and older for the prevention of invasive disease caused by *H. influenzae* type b.

This vaccine is indicated for routine immunization against invasive disease caused by *H. influenzae* type b in infants and children starting at 2 months of age.

Older children and adults with asplenia or hyposplenism (including sickle cell anemia, thalassemia major, essential thrombocytopenia, celiac disease and inflammatory bowel disease); those with defects in antibody production (e.g., agammaglobulinemia, isotype and IgG subclass deficiencies and hyper-IgM syndromes), complement deficiencies; and those with lymphoreticular or hematopoietic malignancies, bone marrow transplantation, HIV infection and alcoholism are at increased risk of infections due to encapsulated bacteria, including *H. influenzae* and should receive Act-HIB.

Candidates for and recipients of cochlear implants should receive Act-HIB.

Children in whom invasive Hib disease develops before 24 months of age should still receive vaccine as recommended, since natural disease may not induce protection.

Premature infants whose clinical condition is satisfactory should be immunized with full doses of vaccine at the same chronological age and according to the same schedule as full-term infants, regardless of birth weight.

Before the introduction of Haemophilus b conjugate vaccines in Canada, *H. influenzae* type b (Hib) was the most common cause of bacterial meningitis and a leading cause of other serious infections in young children. About 55% to 65% of affected children had meningitis, the remainder suffering from epiglottitis, bacteremia, cellulitis, pneumonia or septic arthritis. The case-fatality rate of meningitis is about 5%. Severe neurologic sequelae occur in 10% to 15% of survivors and deafness in 15% to 20% (severe in 3% to 7%). The risk of Hib meningitis is at least twice as high for children attending full-time day care as for children cared for at home. The risk is also greater among children with splenic dysfunction (e.g., sickle cell disease, asplenia) or antibody deficiency, and among Inuit children.

Before 1988, there were an estimated 2000 cases of Hib disease annually in Canada. Since then the overall incidence has fallen by more than 99%. After 1996, when routine infant immunization with Act-HIB began, only 8-10 cases a year were reported. In 1998-99 over 600 000 Canadian infants completed primary immunization with Act-HIB (contained in PENTACEL) and over 200 000 completed a four-dose series including a booster in the second year of life. Only one single case of Hib infection in a child fully vaccinated with PENTACEL was reported to Canada's nation-wide vaccine surveillance system in 1999. In 2000, case reports of Haemophilus b meningitis reached an historical low with only 4 cases reported, a reduction of 99% from pre-vaccine levels.

H. influenzae is also commonly associated with otitis media, sinusitis, bronchitis and other respiratory tract disorders. However, since type b organisms seldom cause these disorders, Hib vaccines have not affected their incidence.

CONTRAINDICATIONS: Allergy to any component of Act-HIB [Haemophilus b Conjugate Vaccine (Tetanus Protein–Conjugate)] (see components listed in Description), including tetanus protein, or an allergic or anaphylactic reaction to a previous dose of Act-HIB are contraindications to vaccination. When Act-HIB is reconstituted with Sanofi Pasteur Limited's TRIPACEL or QUADRACEL the contraindications for TRIPACEL or QUADRACEL must also be considered.

Immunization with Act-HIB should be deferred in the presence of any acute illness, including febrile illness, to avoid superimposing adverse effects from the vaccine on the underlying illness or mistakenly attributing to the vaccine a manifestation of the underlying illness. A minor afebrile illness such as mild upper respiratory infection is not usually reason to defer immunization.

WARNINGS AND PRECAUTIONS: As with any vaccine, immunization with Act-HIB [Haemophilus b Conjugate Vaccine (Tetanus Protein–Conjugate)] may not protect 100% of susceptible individuals.

Do not inject into a blood vessel.

Aseptic technique must be used. Use a separate sterile needle and syringe, or a sterile disposable unit, for each individual dose to prevent disease transmission. Needles should not be recapped and should be disposed of in accordance with biohazardous waste recommendations.

Before administration, take all appropriate precautions to prevent adverse reactions. This includes a review of the patient's history concerning possible hypersensitivity to the vaccine or similar vaccine, previous immunization history, the presence of any contraindications to immunization and current health status.

Before administration of Act-HIB, health-care providers should inform the patient, parent or guardian of the benefits and risks of immunization, inquire about the recent health status of the patient and comply with any local requirements regarding information to be provided to the patient before immunization and the importance of completing the immunization series.

Because the vaccine will not protect against non-typeable strains of *H. influenzae*, which cause recurrent upper respiratory disease, otitis media and sinusitis, the vaccine is not recommended for these conditions.

Carcinogenesis and Mutagenesis: No evaluation of Act-HIB has been made with respect to its potential for carcinogenesis or mutagenesis.

Hematologic: Because of the risk of bleeding and hematoma formation following any intramuscular injection, Act-HIB should be given with caution in persons with any bleeding disorder, such as hemophilia or thrombocytopenia, or persons on anticoagulant therapy.

Immune: As with other products, Epinephrine Hydrochloride Solution (1:1000) and other appropriate agents should be available for immediate use in case an anaphylactic or acute hypersensitivity reaction occurs. Health-care providers should be familiar with current recommendations for the initial management of anaphylaxis in non-hospital settings, including proper airway management. For instructions on recognition and treatment of anaphylactic reactions, see the current edition of the Canadian Immunization Guide or visit the Health Canada website.

When Act-HIB is reconstituted with Sanofi Pasteur Limited's TRIPACEL or QUADRACEL, the possibility of allergic reactions to the components of these vaccines must also be evaluated.

Immunocompromised persons (whether from disease or treatment) may not obtain the expected immune response. If possible, consideration should be given to delaying routine vaccination until after the completion of any immunosuppressive treatment. However, the vaccination of subjects with chronic immunosupression, such as HIV infection, asplenia or sickle cell disease, is recommended even though there is a risk of suboptimal immune response.

In patients <10 years of age with functional or anatomic asplenia it may be prudent to verify the presence of antibodies directed against *H. influenzae* and re-immunize as needed.

Individuals who have received multiple doses of products containing tetanus toxoid show no differences in reaction rates when immunized with this vaccine.

Recipients of Haemophilus b vaccine are not protected against Hib disease in the week after vaccination, before the onset of the protective effects of the vaccine.

Peri-Operative Considerations: Act-HIB along with other recommended vaccines should be administered if possible at least 2 weeks before removal of the spleen.

Special Populations: Pregnant Women: Vaccination of adults against Hib is uncommon. Data on the use of this vaccine in pregnant women are limited, therefore, the administration of the vaccine during pregnancy is not recommended. Act-HIB should be given to pregnant women only if clearly needed and following an assessment of the risks and benefits.

Animal reproduction studies have not been conducted with Act-HIB. It is also not known whether Act-HIB or the diluent can cause fetal harm when administered to a pregnant woman or can affect reproduction capacity.

Nursing Women: Vaccination of adults against Hib is uncommon. It is not known whether this vaccine is excreted in human milk; therefore, the risk and benefits should be carefully considered before administering Act-HIB to a nursing mother.

NACI states that lactating mothers who have not received the recommended immunizations may safely be given vaccines.

ADVERSE REACTIONS: Adverse Drug Reaction Overview: Pain, redness, swelling or induration at the injection site, are seen in 5-30% of vaccinees. It is generally early, transient, and of moderate intensity. Systemic reactions including fever, irritability, drowsiness, prolonged or abnormal crying, anorexia and vomiting have occurred after immunization with Act-HIB [Haemophilus b Conjugate Vaccine (Tetanus Protein–Conjugate)] in conjunction with whole-cell or acellular DPT-containing vaccines. The rates of reactions observed were generally comparable to those usually reported following the concomitant vaccine given alone.

Adverse events presented in this section are listed using MedDRA terminology (system organ classes and terms). Within each system organ class, the adverse events are ranked under headings of frequency (most frequent reactions first), using the following convention: very common: ≥10%, common: ≥1% and <10% , uncommon: ≥0.1% and <1%, rare: ≥0.01% and <0.1%, very rare: <0.01%, including isolated reports.

Clinical Trial Adverse Drug Reactions: Act-HIB has been administered during clinical trials to over 110 000 infants and children in Canada, the United States, Finland, France, Chile, Israel, and the United Kingdom using local immunization schedules, almost always in conjunction with whole-cell or acellular DPT vaccines and has been used widely in immunization programs. In controlled studies, when Act-HIB was administered in conjunction with DPT vaccines, the rate and type of subsequent systemic reactions were not different from those seen with DPT administered alone.

Adverse events, possibly related, observed during clinical studies in more than 1% of patients after immunization (i.e., "common" to "very common") are presented in this section, categorized by frequency. They usually occur soon after the administration of the vaccine (within 6-24 hours), are transient, and have a mild to moderate intensity.

No increase in the incidence or severity of these events was seen with subsequent doses of the primary vaccination series.

The most common reactions occurring after Act-HIB administration were local reactions at the injection site, fever and irritability.

Gastrointestinal Disorders: Vomiting: common.

General Disorders and Application Site Conditions: General Disorders: pyrexia (fever): common (above 39°C: uncommon). Application Site Conditions: injection site reactions such as pain, erythema, swelling and/or inflammation, induration: common to very common.

Psychiatric Disorders: Irritability: very common. Crying (uncontrollable or abnormal): uncommon to common.

Post-Market Adverse Drug Reactions: Safety data from post-marketing surveillance: Act-HIB post-marketing surveillance is based on extensive experience. Since the product launch, several million doses have been administered worldwide.

Adverse events reported in clinical studies are also observed in post-marketing surveillance.

The following additional adverse events were reported during the commercial use of Act-HIB with frequencies of less than 0.01% (very rare). This calculation is based on the number of adverse event reports per estimated number of vaccinated patients.

General Disorders and Application Site Conditions: Edema of lower limbs: These are edematous reactions with cyanosis or transient purpura within the first few hours following the vaccination and resolving quickly and spontaneously without sequelae. These reactions are not associated with cardio-respiratory signs. They were mainly reported when the vaccine was administered in conjunction with another vaccine (such as DPT-containing vaccines).

Immune System Disorders: hypersensitivity reactions.

Nervous System Disorders: convulsions (with or without fever).

Skin and Subcutaneous Tissue Disorders: urticaria, rash, pruritus. Face edema, laryngeal edema (suggestive of a possible hypersensitivity reaction): exceptional.

Potential Adverse Events: Other adverse events reported with administration of other Haemophilus b conjugate vaccines include renal failure and Guillain-Barré syndrome (GBS). A cause and effect relationship among any of these events and the vaccination has not been established.

When Act-HIB is reconstituted with another vaccine, the product monograph of that other vaccine must be carefully reviewed.

Physicians should be familiar with the adverse reactions associated with whatever vaccine is used to reconstitute Act-HIB and read carefully the direction leaflet which accompanies each such vaccine.

Physicians, nurses and pharmacists should report any adverse occurrences temporally associated with the administration of the product in accordance with local requirements and to the Global Pharmacovigilance Department, Sanofi Pasteur Limited, 1755 Steeles Avenue West, Toronto, ON, M2R 3T4, Canada. 1-888-621-1146 (phone) or 416-667-2435 (fax).

DRUG INTERACTIONS: Act-HIB [Haemophilus b Conjugate Vaccine (Tetanus Protein–Conjugate)] may be reconstituted with the diluent provided or with QUADRACEL or TRIPACEL.

Once reconstituted, this vaccine must not be mixed with other vaccine or medicinal products.

Act-HIB may be administered simultaneously with whole-cell DPT, DT, whole-cell DPT Polio, IPV, QUADRACEL or TRIPACEL at separate sites with separate syringes and with OPV.

Act-HIB may also be given simultaneously with measles, mumps, rubella, hepatitis B, pneumococcal and meningococcal vaccines at separate sites with separate syringes.

Because simultaneous administration of common childhood vaccines is not known to affect the efficacy or safety of any of the routine recommended childhood vaccines, if the return of a vaccine recipient for further immunization is doubtful, simultaneous administration of all vaccines appropriate for age and previous vaccination status at separate sites with separate syringes is indicated.

Immunosuppressive therapies, including irradiation, antimetabolites, alkylating agents, cytotoxic drugs and corticosteroids (used in greater than physiologic doses), may reduce the immune response to vaccines. (See Warnings and Precautions, Immune.)

Drug-Laboratory Test Interactions: Capsular polysaccharide antigen can be detected in the urine of vaccinees for up to 2 weeks following immunization with conjugate vaccines. This phenomenon should not be confused with invasive Hib infections.

DOSAGE AND ADMINISTRATION: Recommended Dose and Dosage Adjustment: Each dose is a single injection of 0.5 mL given intramuscularly.

1. **Routine:** Act-HIB [Haemophilus b Conjugate Vaccine (Tetanus Protein–Conjugate)] is indicated for the routine immunization of all children between **2 and 59 months** of age. In infants, three injections are to be given intramuscularly at **2, 4 and 6 months** of age, followed by a booster at **18* months** of age.
2. a) Infants starting their primary immunization series between the age of **3 and 6 months** should receive three doses at two month intervals with a booster dose at **18* months** of age. (While an interval of 2 months between doses is recommended, an interval as short as 1 month is acceptable.)
   b) For infants between the age of **7 and 11 months**, two doses should be given at an interval of two months, followed by a booster at **18* months** of age.
   c) Children between **12 and 14 months** of age who have not previously received any Haemophilus b vaccine should receive one dose of the vaccine followed by a booster at or after **18 months*** of age.
   d) Unvaccinated children between **15 and 59 months** of age should receive a single dose of vaccine.
3. Older children or adults with chronic conditions associated with increased risk of invasive Hib disease (see Indications and Clinical Use) should be immunized with a single dose of the vaccine.

It is preferable, when possible, to use the same product for all doses in the primary series. However, available data suggest that a primary immunization series consisting of three doses of different Hib conjugate vaccine product results in adequate antibody responses. When use of a different product is unavoidable, the specific vaccine given for each of the primary series injections should be carefully documented.

Missed Dose: If a dose is missed, it can be given any time.

Administration: Sanofi Pasteur Limited's QUADRACEL may be used for the reconstitution of lyophilized Act-HIB in place of the saline diluent. This provides an efficient means of administering routine immunization against diphtheria, tetanus, pertussis, poliomyelitis and *H, influenzae* type b in a single injection at a single visit.

* The booster dose may be given as early as 15 months of age provided that at least 2 months have elapsed since the previous dose.

Sanofi Pasteur Limited's TRIPACEL may be used for the reconstitution of lyophilized Act-HIB in place of the saline diluent. This provides an efficient means of administering routine immunization against diphtheria, tetanus, pertussis and *H. influenzae* type b in a single injection at a single visit.

Reconstitution: Reconstitution of Freeze-Dried Product and Withdrawal from Stoppered Vial: Reconstitute the vaccine using only the diluent supplied, Sanofi Pasteur Limited's TRIPACEL or QUADRACEL. The use of any other vaccine or diluent to reconstitute Act-HIB is **not** recommended.

Do not remove the stopper from the vial.

Apply a **sterile** piece of cotton moistened with a suitable antiseptic to the surface of the stopper of the vial of vaccine. Withdraw the diluent into a syringe. Holding the plunger of the syringe containing the diluent steady, pierce the center of the stopper in the vial and **slowly** inject the 0.5 mL of diluent into the freeze-dried vaccine. Do not try to force all of the diluent into the vial at once as this will create pressure. It is necessary to allow air to escape gradually into the syringe by intermittently aspirating air from the vial while injecting the diluent into the vial. Do not remove the needle from the stopper until the required volume of diluent has been injected. Shake the vial gently until a clear, colourless solution results. **Avoid foaming** since this will prevent withdrawal of the proper dose. Withdraw the entire contents of the reconstituted vaccine into the syringe and inject the total volume (about 0.5 mL). Aseptic technique must be used for withdrawal of each dose. (See Warnings and Precautions.)

When Sanofi Pasteur Limited's TRIPACEL or QUADRACEL is used for the reconstitution of Act-HIB, **shake the single dose vial well** to distribute uniformly the suspension before withdrawing entire contents (about 0.5 mL). Do not remove either the stopper or the metal seal holding it in place. Inject all the TRIPACEL or QUADRACEL into the vial of Act-HIB vaccine. Swirl the vial until a cloudy, uniform suspension results. Avoid foaming since this will prevent withdrawal of the proper dose. Use a sterile needle and syringe to withdraw the entire contents for one dose.

Upon reconstitution the vaccine should be used immediately.

Administer the vaccine **intramuscularly**. The preferred site is into the anterolateral aspect of the mid-thigh (vastus lateralis muscle) or into the deltoid muscle. In children >1 year of age, the deltoid is the preferred site since use of the anterolateral thigh results in frequent complaints of limping due to muscle pain.

Do not inject intravenously.

Each person who is immunized should be given a permanent personal immunization record. In addition, it is essential that the physician or nurse record the immunization history in the permanent medical record of each patient. This permanent office record should contain the name of the vaccine, date given, dose, manufacturer and lot number. If Act-HIB is reconstituted with QUADRACEL or TRIPACEL, the lot numbers of both vaccines should be recorded.

ACTION AND CLINICAL PHARMACOLOGY: Pharmacodynamics: Hib conjugate vaccines are the second generation of vaccines against Hib disease, having replaced earlier polysaccharide vaccines. Polysaccharide-protein conjugate antigens have the advantage of producing greater immune response in infants and young children than purified polysaccharide vaccine. The latter stimulates only B-cells, whereas the former activates macrophages, T-helper cells and B-cells, resulting in greatly enhanced antibody responses and establishment of immunologic memory.

Immunogenicity studies in infants ≥2 months of age given a primary series demonstrated that almost all developed anti-PRP antibody titre ≥0.15 µg/mL, and approximately 90% had a titre ≥1 µg/mL after the 3rd dose. A booster dose administered 8 to 12 months later induced a very significant increase in the mean titre of the PRP antibodies. A serum level of 0.15 µg/mL is considered to indicate a positive response to conjugated vaccine. A level of >1.0 µg/mL indicates long-term protection.

Pharmacokinetics: No pharmacokinetic studies have been performed.

Duration of Effect: In children who received four doses of Act-HIB (at 2, 4, 6 and 18 months), anti-PRP antibodies remained above 0.15 µg/mL at 4-5 years of age in 99%, and all responded vigorously to restimulation, consistent with persistent immune memory.

STORAGE AND STABILITY: Store at 2 to 8°C. **Do not freeze.** Product which has been exposed to freezing should not be used. The vaccine should be used immediately after reconstitution.

Do not use after the expiration date.

INFORMATION FOR THE PATIENT: Published in e-CPS, available by subscription at www.e-cps.ca.

DOSAGE FORMS, COMPOSITION AND PACKAGING: Each 0.5 mL dose contains: *H. influenzae* type b polysaccharide conjugated to tetanus protein 10 µg, tetanus protein 20 µg, trometamol 0.6 mg, sucrose 42.5 mg. Diluent: saline solution 0.4%.

Packages containing five single dose vials of Act-HIB and five × 0.5 mL (single dose vials) of Sanofi Pasteur Limited's diluent, 0.4% Saline for reconstitution of Act-HIB. Also supplied in packages containing five single dose vials of Act-HIB and five × 0.5 mL (single dose) vial of Sanofi Pasteur Limited's QUADRACEL to be used for reconstitution in place of the Act-HIB diluent and sold under the tradename PENTACEL. Also supplied in one or five dose packages containing either one or five single dose vials of Act-HIB and one or five × 0.5 mL (single dose) vials of Sanofi Pasteur Limited's TRIPACEL to be used for reconstitution in place of the Act-HIB diluent and sold under the tradename ACTACEL. The vial stoppers supplied with this product do not contain dry natural latex rubber.

Actifed®

triprolidine HCl—pseudoephedrine HCl

Antihistamine—Decongestant

McNeil Consumer Healthcare

Date of Revision: May 2008

INDICATIONS: The prophylaxis and treatment of symptoms associated with the common cold, acute and subacute sinusitis, acute eustachian salpingitis, serous otitis media with eustachian tube congestion, aerotitis media and croup; in allergic conditions which respond to antihistamines, including hay fever, pollenosis, allergic and vasomotor rhinitis.

CONTRAINDICATIONS: Hypersensitivity to triprolidine or pseudoephedrine. Should not be administered to patients receiving MAO inhibitors or who have taken them within the preceding 2 weeks. Patients with severe hypertension or severe coronary artery disease.

WARNINGS: No data supplied by the manufacturer.

PRECAUTIONS: Occupational Hazards: Patients should be cautioned not to operate vehicles or hazardous machinery until their response to the drug has been determined.

Since the depressant effects of antihistamines are additive to those of other drugs affecting the CNS, patients should avoid drinking alcoholic beverages or taking hypnotics, sedatives, psychotherapeutic agents or other drugs with CNS depressant effects during antihistamine therapy.

Hypertension and unconsciousness following the ingestion of 60 mg pseudoephedrine by a normotensive individual has been reported and should be regarded as an extremely rare example of pseudoephedrine intolerance.

As with other sympathomimetic agents and decongestants, this product should be used with caution in patients with prostatic enlargement, in hypertensive and diabetic patients, patients with latent or clinically recognized angle closure glaucoma, coronary artery disease, congestive heart failure, hyperthyroidism, and urinary retention. In severe hepatic or renal dysfunction, this product should be given at less than the usual recommended dose and the patient's response used as a guide to the dosage requirement for further administration.

Pregnancy: Use with caution.

Lactation: Use with caution. Pseudoephedrine and triprolidine have been reported to be excreted into breast milk of lactating women.

Drug Interactions: Concomitant use of this product with sympathomimetic agents such as decongestants, appetite suppressants, and amphetamine-like psychostimulants or with monoamine oxidase inhibitors may occasionally cause a rise in blood pressure.

The antibacterial agent, furazolidone, is known to cause a dose-related inhibition of MAO. Although there are no reports of a hypertensive crisis caused by the concurrent administration of pseudoephedrine and furazolidone, they should not be taken together.

Because of its pseudoephedrine component, this product may partially reverse the hypotensive action of drugs which interfere with sympathetic activity including bretylium, bethanidine, guanethidine, debrisoquine, methyldopa, beta and/or alpha adrenergic blocking agents.

ADVERSE EFFECTS: Some patients may exhibit mild sedation or mild stimulation. Sleep disturbance and rarely hallucinations have been reported.

Urinary retention may occasionally occur in male subjects where prostatic enlargement is present. Fixed drug eruption due to pseudoephedrine and lichenoid skin eruption due to triprolidine have been reported but both these reactions should be regarded as rare events.

OVERDOSE:

Symptoms: Insomnia, tremors, tachycardia, difficulty in micturition, irritability, drowsiness, lethargy, dizziness, ataxia, weakness, hypotonicity, respiratory depression, dryness of the skin and mucous membranes, hypertension, hyperpyrexia, hyperactivity, convulsions.

Treatment: There is no specific antidote for triprolidine or pseudoephedrine. General measures to eliminate the drug and reduce its absorption should be undertaken. Gastric lavage should be performed up to 3 hours after ingestion if indicated. If desired the elimination of pseudoephedrine can be accelerated by urine acidification. If respiratory depression is severe, intubation and artificial respiration should be used. Convulsions should be treated with diazepam. Maintain blood pressure through fluid replacement and supportive measures. Catheterization of the bladder may be necessary. Hypertension may be controlled with alpha-adrenoceptor blocking drugs and tachycardia with beta-adrenoceptor blocking drugs.

> For management of a suspected drug overdose, CPhA recommends that you contact your **regional Poison Control Centre**. See the *CPS* Directory section for a list of Poison Control Centres.

DOSAGE: To be given every 4 to 6 hours. Do not exceed 4 doses in 24 hours. Adults and children 12 years of age and over: 1 tablet. Children 6 to 11 years of age: ½ tablet.

Persons over 65 or under 6 years, use as directed by a physician.

INFORMATION FOR THE PATIENT: Published in e-CPS, available by subscription at www.e-cps.ca.

SUPPLIED: Each white, biconvex tablet, with code number ACTIFED M2A on same side as score mark, contains: triprolidine HCl 2.5 mg and pseudoephedrine HCl 60 mg. Nonmedicinal ingredients: cornstarch, gelatin, lactose and magnesium stearate. Blister packages of 24 and 48. Store at 15 to 30°C. Protect from light. Keep dry.

Actifed™ Plus Extra Strength

acetaminophen—pseudoephedrine HCl—triprolidine HCl

Analgesic—Antipyretic—Antihistamine—Decongestant

McNeil Consumer Healthcare

Date of Revision: May 2008

INDICATIONS: The prophylaxis and treatment of symptoms associated with the common cold, acute and subacute sinusitis; in allergic conditions which respond to antihistamines, including hay fever, pollenosis, allergic and vasomotor rhinitis. Relieves nasal congestion, runny nose, sneezing, sinus pain, headache and fever.

CONTRAINDICATIONS: Hypersensitivity to triprolidine, pseudoephedrine or acetaminophen. Should not be administered to patients receiving MAO inhibitors or who have taken them within the preceding 2 weeks. Patients with severe hypertension or severe coronary artery disease.

WARNINGS: Massive acetaminophen overdose can be toxic and potentially fatal. In adults, hepatotoxicity from acetaminophen is unlikely to occur with overdoses of less than 10 g ingested at one time and fatalities are unlikely to occur with overdoses of less than 15 g ingested at one time.

PRECAUTIONS: Occupational Hazards: Patients should be cautious not to operate vehicles or hazardous machinery until their response to the drug has been determined.

Since the depressant effects of antihistamines are additive to those of other drugs affecting the CNS, patients should avoid drinking alcoholic beverages or taking hypnotics, sedatives, psychotherapeutic agents or other drugs with CNS depressant effects during antihistamine therapy.

Hypertension and unconsciousness following the ingestion of 60 mg pseudoephedrine by a normotensive individual has been reported and should be regarded as an extremely rare example of pseudoephedrine intolerance.

As with other sympathomimetic agents and decongestants, this product should be used with caution in patients with prostatic enlargement, in hypertensive and diabetic patients, patients with latent or clinically recognized angle closure glaucoma, coronary artery disease, congestive heart failure, hyperthyroidism, and urinary retention. In severe hepatic or renal dysfunction, this product should be given at less than the usual recommended dose and the patient's response used as a guide to the dosage requirement for further administration.

Pregnancy: Use with caution.

Lactation: Use with caution. Pseudoephedrine and triprolidine have been reported to be excreted into breast milk of lactating women.

Drug Interactions: Concomitant use of this product with sympathomimetic agents such as other decongestants, appetite suppressants, and amphetamine-like psychostimulants or with MAO inhibitors may occasionally cause a rise in blood pressure.

The antibacterial agent, furazolidone, is known to cause a dose-related inhibition of MAO. Although there are no reports of a hypertensive crisis caused by the concurrent administration of pseudoephedrine and furazolidone, they should not be taken together.

Because of its pseudoephedrine component, this product may partially reverse the hypotensive action of drugs which interfere with sympathetic activity including bretylium, bethanidine, guanethidine, debrisoquine, methyldopa, beta and/or alpha adrenergic blocking agents.

ADVERSE EFFECTS: Some patients may exhibit mild sedation or mild stimulation. Sleep disturbances and rarely hallucinations have been reported.

Urinary retention may occasionally occur in male subjects where prostatic enlargement is present. Fixed drug eruption due to pseudoephedrine and lichenoid skin eruption due to triprolidine have been reported but both these reactions should be regarded as rare events.

OVERDOSE:

Symptoms: Insomnia, tremors, tachycardia, difficulty in micturition, irritability, drowsiness, lethargy, dizziness, ataxia, weakness, hypotonicity, respiratory depression, dryness of the skin and mucous membranes, hypertension, hyperpyrexia, hyperactivity and convulsions.

Treatment: There is no specific antidote for triprolidine or pseudoephedrine. General measures to eliminate the drug and reduce its absorption should be undertaken. Gastric lavage should be performed up to 3 hours after ingestion if indicated. If desired the elimination of pseudoephedrine can be accelerated by urine acidification. If respiratory depression is severe, intubation and artificial respiration should be used. Convulsions should be treated with diazepam. Maintain blood pressure through fluid replacement and supportive measures. Catheterization of the bladder may be necessary. Hypertension may be controlled with alpha-adrenoceptor blocking drugs and tachycardia with beta-adrenoceptor blocking drugs.

> For management of a suspected drug overdose, CPhA recommends that you contact your **regional Poison Control Centre**. See the *CPS* Directory section for a list of Poison Control Centres.

DOSAGE: Adults and children 12 years and over: 1 caplet every 4 to 6 hours. Do not exceed 4 doses in 24 hours. Children 12 years and under: use only as directed by a physician.

Geriatrics: Persons over 65: use only as directed by a physician.

INFORMATION FOR THE PATIENT: Published in e-CPS, available by subscription at www.e-cps.ca.

SUPPLIED: Each white caplet, engraved "A" on one side and "WL02" on the other, contains: triprolidine HCl 2.5 mg, pseudoephedrine HCl 60 mg and acetaminophen 500 mg. Nonmedicinal ingredients: celluloses, magnesium stearate and povidone. Blister packages of 24. Store between 15 and 30°C. Protect from light and keep dry.

Activase® rt-PA (Acute Ischemic Stroke)

alteplase

Fibrinolytic Agent

Roche

Date of Revision: April 10, 2001

Acute Ischemic Stroke Indication: Health Canada has issued a conditional marketing authorization under the Notice of Compliance with Conditions policy to reflect the promising nature of the clinical evidence for the use of alteplase in the treatment of stroke. It is expected that clinical experience will validate which patients will benefit most from treatment with alteplase. Alteplase can cause bleeding, including intracranial hemorrhage. Acute stroke patients should be advised of the potential risks as well as the benefits of this therapy.

PHARMACOLOGY: Acute Ischemic Stroke: Alteplase is a serine protease which has the property of fibrin-enhanced conversion of plasminogen to plasmin. Alteplase produces minimal conversion of plasminogen in the absence of fibrin; and when introduced into the systemic circulation, alteplase binds to fibrin in a thrombus and converts the entrapped plasminogen to plasmin. This initiates local fibrinolysis with minimal systemic effects. Following administration of alteplase, there is a decrease (20 to 30%) in circulating fibrinogen. Decreases in plasminogen and α_2-antiplasmin are also evident.

Alteplase is cleared rapidly from circulating plasma with an initial half-life of less than 5 minutes. The plasma clearance of alteplase is approximately 500 mL/min. The clearance is mediated primarily by the liver.

INDICATIONS: Management of Acute Ischemic Stroke: (For information on use in acute myocardial infarction, please consult the product monograph for the acute myocardial infarction indication.)

Alteplase is indicated for the management of acute ischemic stroke in adults for improving neurological recovery and reducing the incidence of disability.

Treatment should only be initiated within 3 hours after the onset of stroke symptoms, and after exclusion of intracranial hemorrhage by a cranial computerized tomography (CT) scan or other diagnostic imaging method sensitive for the presence of hemorrhage.

Patients should be advised of the potential risk as well as the benefits of the use of alteplase for this indication.

NINDS Study Summary: The National Institute of Neurological Disorders and Stroke (NINDS) acute ischemic stroke study randomized 624 patients to a double-blind, placebo controlled trial using i.v. t-PA in a dose of 0.9 mg/kg t-PA to a maximum of 90 mg, with 10% of the total dose given as a bolus over 1 to 2 minutes and the remainder of the dose infused over 60 minutes. Patients were treated within 3 hours of a well defined symptom onset after exclusion of the presence of intracranial hemorrhage (ICH) by cranial computerized tomography (CT) scan. Additional exclusion criteria were included in the protocol (see Contraindications).

Efficacy outcomes at 3 months as measured by the outcome scales follow (see Table 1).

Table 1: Activase rt-PA (Acute Ischemic Stroke)

The NINDS t-PA Stroke Trial, Part 2 3-month Efficacy Outcomes

	Frequency of Favorable Outcome[a]		
Analysis	**Placebo (n=165)**	**Activase (n=168)**	**Absolute Difference (95% CI)**
Barthel Index	37.6%	50.0%	12.4% (3.0, 21.9)
Modified Rankin Scale	26.1%	38.7%	12.6% (3.7, 21.6)
Glasgow Outcome Scale	31.5%	44.0%	12.5% (3.3, 21.8)
NIHSS	20.0%	31.0%	11.0% (2.6, 19.3)

[a] Favorable outcome is defined as recovery with minimal or no disability.

The NINDS protocol required close patient monitoring and blood pressure management to maintain systolic blood pressure below 185 mmHg and diastolic pressure less than 110 mmHg for 24 hours. Blood pressure was monitored during the hospital stay. I.V. labetalol using 10 mg boluses over 1 to 2 minutes repeated every 10 to 20 minutes has been recommended as part of the NINDS protocol for blood pressures above these limits to reduce the risk of intracranial hemorrhage.

The risks of alteplase therapy must be weighed against potential benefits in patients in the following circumstances: Patients with severe neurological deficits at presentation (e.g., NIH Stroke Scale >20). There is an increased risk of intracerebral hemorrhage in these patients (odds ratio 1.8; 95% CI, 1.2 to 1.9). Patients with substantial brain edema (acute hypodensity) or mass effect on CT before treatment. Major CT changes of an early infarct are associated with increased risk of intracerebral bleeding.

CONTRAINDICATIONS: Acute Ischemic Stroke: In the following situations because of an increased risk of bleeding, which could result in significant disability or death: symptom onset greater than 3 hours; evidence of intracranial hemorrhage on pretreatment evaluation; suspicion of subarachnoid hemorrhage on pretreatment evaluation; recent (within 3 months) intracranial surgery or intraspinal surgery, serious head trauma or recent previous stroke; history of intracranial hemorrhage; uncontrolled hypertension at time of treatment (e.g., >185 mmHg systolic or >110 mmHg diastolic); seizure at the onset of stroke; active internal bleeding; intracranial neoplasm, arteriovenous malformation, or aneurysm; known bleeding diathesis including but not limited to: current use of oral anticoagulants (e.g., warfarin sodium) or an International Normalized Ratio (INR) >1.7 or a prothrombin time (PT) >15 seconds, administration of heparin within 48 hours preceding the onset of stroke and an elevated activated partial thromboplastin time (aPTT) at presentation, platelet count <100 000/mm^3.

WARNINGS: Acute Ischemic Stroke: **Alteplase is a drug known to cause severe bleeding and an increased incidence of intracranial hemorrhage. Use of alteplase for the treatment of stroke is limited to physicians experienced in acute stroke management, who are treating patients in a hospital setting equipped with appropriate laboratory facilities to follow the neurological (CT scan) and hematological status of the patient.**

Two European studies have been conducted by the European Collaborative Acute Stroke Study Group, referred to as ECASS I and ECASS II, using another alteplase product, Actilyse.

The ECASS I study suggested that doses greater than 0.9 mg/kg may be associated with increased risk of ICH. **The dose of 0.9 mg/kg (maximum 90 mg) should not be exceeded in the management of acute ischemic stroke.**

The results of the ECASS II study indicated a trend towards efficacy when the treatment was initiated within 6 hours or less after the onset of the event, although the results do not confirm a statistical benefit for alteplase. It was concluded that despite the increased risk for ICH, thrombolysis with alteplase may lead to a clinically relevant improvement in outcome in selected patients and in experienced centres.

Based on burden of evidence, treatment of patients with acute ischemic stroke more than 3 hours after symptom onset is not recommended (see Contraindications). The risks of alteplase therapy to treat acute ischemic stroke may be increased in the following conditions and should be weighed against the anticipated benefits: Patients with severe neurological deficit (e.g., NIHSS >22) at presentation. There is an increased risk of intracranial hemorrhage in these patients. Patients with major early infarct signs on a computerized cranial tomography (CT) scan (e.g., substantial edema, mass effect, or midline shift).

In patients without recent use of oral anticoagulants or heparin, alteplase treatment can be initiated prior to the availability of coagulation study results. However, infusion should be discontinued if either a pretreatment International Normalized Ratio (INR) >1.7 or a prothrombin time (PT) >15 seconds or an elevated activated partial thromboplastin time (aPTT) is identified.

Treatment must be limited to facilities that can provide appropriate evaluation and management of ICH.

Due to the increased risk for misdiagnosis of acute ischemic stroke, special diligence is required in making this diagnosis in patients whose blood glucose values are <50 mg/dL or >400 mg/dL. The safety and efficacy of treatment with alteplase in patients with minor neurological deficit or with rapidly improving symptoms prior to the start of alteplase administration has not been evaluated. Therefore, treatment of patients with minor neurological deficit or with rapidly improving symptoms is not recommended.

Antithrombotics: The concomitant use of heparin or ASA during the first 24 hours following symptom onset were prohibited in The NINDS t-PA Stroke Trial. The safety of such concomitant use with alteplase for the management of acute ischemic stroke is unknown.

General: Bleeding: The most common complication encountered during therapy with alteplase is bleeding. The type of bleeding associated with thrombolytic therapy can be divided into 2 broad categories: internal bleeding involving the gastrointestinal tract, genitourinary tract, respiratory tract, retroperitoneal or intracranial sites; and superficial or surface bleeding, observed mainly at invaded or disturbed sites (e.g., venous cutdowns, arterial punctures, sites of recent surgical intervention).

Fibrin will be lysed during the infusion of alteplase and bleeding from recent puncture sites may occur. Therefore, therapy with alteplase, as with other thrombolytic agents, requires careful attention to all potential bleeding sites (including catheter insertion sites, arterial and venous puncture sites, cutdown sites and needle puncture sites).

I.M. injections and nonessential handling of the patient should be avoided during and immediately following treatment with alteplase. Venipunctures should be performed carefully and only as required.

Should an arterial puncture be necessary during an infusion of alteplase, it is preferable to use an upper extremity vessel that is accessible to manual compression. Pressure should be applied for at least 30 minutes, a pressure dressing applied and the puncture site checked frequently for evidence of bleeding.

Should serious bleeding in a critical location (not controllable by local pressure) occur, the infusion of alteplase and any other concomitant anticoagulant should be discontinued immediately and treatment initiated (see Overdose, Symptoms and Treatment).

In the following conditions, the risks of alteplase therapy may be increased and should be weighed against the anticipated benefits: recent (within 10 days) major surgery, e.g., coronary artery bypass graft, obstetrical delivery, organ biopsy, previous puncture of noncompressible vessels; clinical evidence or history of transient ischemic attacks; recent gastrointestinal or genitourinary bleeding (within 10 days); recent trauma (within 10 days); hypertension: systolic BP ≥ 175 mmHg and/or diastolic BP ≥ 110 mmHg; a history or clinical evidence of hypertensive disease in a patient over 70 years old; advanced age, e.g., over 75 years old; high likelihood or known presence of left heart thrombus, e.g., mitral stenosis with atrial fibrillation; apical MI, with thrombus; acute pericarditis; subacute bacterial endocarditis; hemostatic defects including those secondary to severe hepatic or renal disease; significant liver dysfunction, e.g., prolonged prothrombin time; pregnancy; diabetic hemorrhagic retinopathy, or other hemorrhagic ophthalmic conditions; septic thrombophlebitis or occluded AV cannula at seriously infected site; patients currently receiving oral anticoagulants, e.g., warfarin sodium; any other condition in which bleeding constitutes a significant hazard or would be particularly difficult to manage because of its location.

Cholesterol Embolization: Cholesterol embolization has been reported rarely in patients treated with all types of thrombolytic agents; the true incidence is unknown. This serious condition, which can be lethal, is also associated with invasive vascular procedures (e.g., cardiac catheterization, angiography, vascular surgery) and/or anticoagulant therapy. Clinical features of cholesterol embolism include livedo reticularis, "purple toe" syndrome, acute renal failure, gangrenous digits, hypertension, pancreatitis, myocardial infarction, cerebral infarction, spinal cord infarction, retinal artery occlusion, bowel infarction, and rhabdomyolysis.

PRECAUTIONS: Acute Ischemic Stroke: Alteplase must be administered in a hospital setting where the appropriate diagnostic and monitoring techniques are readily available.

Noncompressible arterial puncture must be avoided. Arterial and venous punctures should be minimized. In the event of serious bleeding, alteplase and heparin should be discontinued immediately. Heparin effects can be reversed by protamine.

Drug Interactions: The interaction of alteplase with other drugs has not been studied. In addition to bleeding associated with heparin and warfarin, drugs that alter platelet function (such as ASA) may increase the risk of bleeding if administered prior to, during or after alteplase infusion.

Orolingual angioedema has been observed after alteplase administration in patients receiving concomitant ACE inhibitor therapy. However, the significance of this observation has not been determined (see Adverse Effects, Allergic Reactions section).

Laboratory Tests: During alteplase infusion, coagulation tests and/or measures of fibrinolytic activity may be performed if desired. However, routine measurements of fibrinogen as well as fibrinogen degradation products are unreliable, and should not be undertaken unless specific precautions are taken to prevent in vitro artifacts. Alteplase is a serine protease that when present in blood in pharmacologic concentrations remains active under in vitro conditions. This can lead to degradation of fibrinogen in a blood sample removed for analysis. Collection of blood samples on aprotinin (150 to 200 units/mL) can to some extent mitigate this phenomenon.

Geriatrics: The risks of therapy may be increased in the elderly (see Warnings).

In alteplase-treated patients (NINDS study) of advanced age (e.g., >77 years of age), the trend toward increased risk for symptomatic ICH within the first 36 hours was more prominent. Similar trends were also seen for total ICH and for all-cause 90-day mortality. Analyses for efficacy suggested a reduced but still favorable clinical outcome for these patients.

Children: Safety and effectiveness of alteplase in children has not been established. Therefore treatment of such patients is not recommended.

Pregnancy: Alteplase has been shown to have an embryocidal effect in rabbits when i.v. administered in doses of approximately 2 times (3 mg/kg) the human dose for AMI. No maternal or fetal toxicity was evident at 0.65 times (1 mg/kg) the human dose in pregnant rats and rabbits dosed during the period of organogenesis. There are no adequate and well controlled studies in pregnant women. Alteplase should be used during pregnancy only if the potential benefit justifies the potential risk to the fetus.

Lactation: It is not known whether alteplase is excreted in human milk. Because many drugs are excreted in human milk, caution should be exercised when alteplase is administered to a nursing woman.

Readministration: There has been little documentation of readministration of alteplase. Readministration should be undertaken with caution. Less than 0.5% of patients receiving single courses of alteplase therapy have experienced transient antibody formation. Nevertheless, if an anaphylactoid reaction occurs, the infusion should be discontinued immediately and appropriate therapy initiated.

ADVERSE EFFECTS: Acute Ischemic Stroke: The incidence of ICH, especially symptomatic ICH, in patients with acute ischemic stroke was higher in alteplase-treated patients than placebo patients.

The incidences of ICH, and new ischemic stroke following alteplase treatment compared to placebo are presented in Table 2 as a combined safety analysis (n=624) for Parts 1 and 2. These data indicated a significant increase in ICH following alteplase treatment, particularly symptomatic ICH within 36 hours. Symptomatic ICH within 36 hours was experienced by 2 of 312 (0.6%) of placebo-treated patients and 20 of 312 (6.4%) alteplase-treated patients (p<0.01). Potential predictors of symptomatic ICH within 36 hours of study drug administration were baseline values of NIHSS score, fibrinogen (<200 mg/dL), and platelet count (<150 000/μL). These predictors were the same in both treatment groups.

Table 2: Activase rt-PA (Acute Ischemic Stroke)

The NINDS t-PA Stroke Trial Safety Outcome

	Part 1 and Part 2 Combined		
	Placebo (n=312)	**Activase (n=312)**	**p-Value[b]**
Total ICH[a]	20 (6.4%)	48 (15.4%)	<0.01
Symptomatic	4 (1.3%)	25 (8.0%)	<0.01
Asymptomatic	16 (5.1%)	23 (7.4%)	0.32
Symptomatic ICH within 36 hours	2 (0.6%)	20 (6.4%)	<0.01
New Ischemic Stroke (3 months)	17 (5.4%)	18 (5.8%)	1.00

[a] Within trial follow-up period. Symptomatic ICH was defined as the occurrence of sudden clinical worsening followed by subsequent verification of ICH on CT scan. Asymptomatic ICH was defined as ICH detected on a routine repeat CT scan without preceding clinical worsening.

[b] Fisher's Exact Test.

Table 3 displays the incidences of all-cause 90-day mortality and mortality rates and odds ratios by baseline NIHSS subgroup. In alteplase-treated patients, there were no increases compared to placebo in the incidences of 90-day mortality or severe disability but all-cause 90-day mortality rates increased in both treatment groups with higher baseline NIHSS score category. As with any subgroup analysis, these results should be viewed with caution. However, there appeared to be a (nonsignificant) trend toward higher mortality for alteplase rt-PA patients with baseline NIHSS scores >20. Only 22% of the NINDS study patients were in this subgroup, and the observed proportions are therefore based on small denominators. Whilst the interpretation of any subgroup should be undertaken with caution, these figures are included to assist physicians in the assessment of the risk-benefit ratio for a particular patient.

Table 3: Activase rt-PA (Acute Ischemic Stroke)

All-cause 90-day Mortality for Baseline NIHSS Subgroups

Baseline NIHSS Score	Placebo (n=312)	Activase (n=312)	Odds Ratio and 95% CI
All-cause 90-day mortality	64 (20.5%)	54 (17.3%)	p-Value 0.36
0–10	9/99 (9.1%)	2/110 (1.8%)	5.40 (1.14, 25.63)[a]
1–20	26/136 (19.1%)	22/139 (15.8%)	1.26 (0.67, 2.35)
1 >20	29/77 (37.7%)	30/63 (47.6%)	0.67 (0.34, 1.31)

[a] Significant difference ($p<0.05$).
Odds ratios >1 indicate benefit for Activase patients. (Where 95% CIs include 1, difference is nonsignificant on this sample size.)

Bleeding: General: The most frequent adverse reaction associated with alteplase is bleeding. The type of bleeding associated with thrombolytic therapy can be divided into 2 broad categories: internal bleeding, involving the gastrointestinal tract, genitourinary tract, respiratory tract, retroperitoneal or intracranial sites; and superficial or surface bleeding due to lysis of fibrin in the hemostatic plug. Therefore, alteplase therapy requires careful attention to potential bleeding sites such as venous cutdowns, catheter insertion sites, arterial puncture sites, and any site of recent surgical intervention.

Bleeding events other than ICH were noted in the studies of acute ischemic stroke and were consistent with the general safety profile of alteplase. In the NINDS t-PA Stroke Trial (Parts 1 and 2), the frequency of bleeding requiring red blood cell transfusions was 6.4% for alteplase-treated patients compared to 3.8% for placebo (p=0.19, using Mantel-Haenszel Chi-Square).

Allergic Reactions: Allergic-type reactions, e.g., anaphylactoid reaction, laryngeal edema, orolingual angioedema, rash and urticaria have been reported. A cause and effect relationship to alteplase therapy has not been established.

Other Adverse Reactions: The following adverse reactions have been reported among patients receiving alteplase in clinical trials and in postmarketing experience. These reactions are frequent sequelae of the underlying disease and the effect of alteplase on the incidence of these events is unknown.

Use in Acute Ischemic Stroke: cerebral edema, cerebral herniation, seizure, new ischemic stroke. These events may be life threatening and may lead to death.

OVERDOSE:

Symptoms : Acute Ischemic Stroke: Overdosage could lead to serious bleeding.

Treatment: Should serious bleeding occur in a critical location, the infusion of alteplase and any other concomitant anticoagulant should be discontinued immediately. If necessary, blood loss and reversal of the bleeding tendency can be managed with whole blood or packed red cells. In the event of clinically significant fibrinogen depletion, fresh frozen plasma or cryoprecipitate can be infused.

For management of a suspected drug overdose, CPhA recommends that you contact your **regional Poison Control Centre**. See the *CPS* Directory section for a list of Poison Control Centres.

DOSAGE: Acute Ischemic Stroke: Alteplase is intended for i.v. use only. It should be given via a dedicated i.v. line with an infusion pump. Extravasation of alteplase infusion can cause ecchymosis and/or inflammation. Management consists of terminating the infusion at the i.v. site and application of local therapy.

The recommended dose is 0.9 mg/kg (maximum of 90 mg) infused over 60 minutes with 10% of the total dose administered as an initial i.v. bolus over 1 minute.

Blood pressure should be monitored frequently and controlled during and following administration of alteplase administration.

The safety and efficacy of this regimen with concomitant administration of heparin and ASA during the first 24 hours after symptom onset has not been investigated.

The dose for treatment of acute ischemic stroke should not exceed 90 mg.

A. The bolus dose may be prepared in one of the following ways: 1. By removing the appropriate volume from the vial of reconstituted (1 mg/mL) alteplase using a syringe and needle. If this method is used with the 50 mg vials, the syringe should not be primed with air and the needle should be inserted into the alteplase-vial stopper. If the 100 mg vial is used, the needle should be inserted away from the puncture mark made by the transfer device. 2. By removing the appropriate volume from a port (second injection site) on the infusion line after the infusion set is primed. 3. By programming an infusion pump to deliver the appropriate volume as a bolus at the initiation of the infusion. B. The remainder of the alteplase dose may be administered as follows: **50 mg Vials:** Administer using either a polyvinyl chloride bag or glass vial and infusion set. **100 mg Vials:** Remove from the vial any quantity of drug in excess of that specified for patient treatment. Insert the spike end of an infusion set through the same puncture site created by the transfer device in the stopper of the vial of reconstituted alteplase. Hang the alteplase vial from the plastic molded capping attached to the bottom of the vial.

Reconstitution and Dilution: Alteplase should be reconstituted by aseptically adding to the vial, the appropriate volume of Sterile Water for Injection, USP [SWFI] (50 mL for 50 mg vials, 100 mL for 100 mg vials). It is important that alteplase be reconstituted only with Sterile Water for Injection, USP, without preservatives. Do not use Bacteriostatic Water for Injection. The reconstituted preparation results in a colorless to pale yellow transparent solution containing alteplase 1.0 mg/mL at a pH of 7.3. The osmolality of this solution is approximately 215 mOsm/kg.

Before further dilution or administration, parenteral drug products should be visually inspected for particulate matter and discoloration prior to administration whenever solution and container permit. Because alteplase contains no preservatives, it should be reconstituted immediately before use (see Stability and Storage).

The reconstituted solution may be diluted further immediately before administration to yield concentrations as low as 0.5 mg/mL in 0.9% Sodium Chloride Injection, USP or 5% Dextrose Injection, USP. Excessive agitation during dilution should be avoided; mixing should be accomplished with gentle swirling and/or slow inversion. Do not use other infusion solutions e.g., Sterile Water for Injection, USP, or preservative containing solutions for further dilution.

No other medication should be added to alteplase solution. Solutions should be administered as described above. Unused infusion solution should be immediately discarded.

50 mg Vials: Using a large bore needle (e.g., 18 gauge), **and the accompanying 50 mL Sterile Water for Injection, USP,** direct the stream of Sterile Water for Injection, USP into the lyophilized cake. **Do not use if vacuum is not present.** Slight foaming upon reconstitution is not unusual; standing undisturbed for several minutes is usually sufficient to allow dissipation of any large bubbles. Excessive or vigorous shaking should be avoided.

100 mg Vials: Using the transfer device provided, the contents of the accompanying 100 mL vial of Sterile Water for Injection, USP should be added to the contents of the 100 mg vial of alteplase powder. Slight foaming upon reconstitution is not unusual; standing undisturbed for several minutes is usually sufficient to allow dissipation of any large bubbles. **No vacuum is present in 100 mg vials.** Please refer to the accompanying instructions for Reconstitution and Administration of the 100 mg vials:

1. Use aseptic technique throughout.
2. Remove the protective flip-caps from 1 vial of alteplase and 1 vial of Sterile Water for Injection, USP [SWFI].
3. Open the package containing the transfer device by peeling the paper label off the package.
4. Remove the protective cap from one end of the transfer device and keeping the vial of SWFI upright, insert the piercing pin vertically into the centre of the stopper of the vial of SWFI.
5. Remove the protective cap from the other end of the transfer device. **Do not invert the vial of SWFI.**
6. Holding the vial of alteplase upside-down, position it so that the centre of the stopper is directly over the exposed piercing pin of the transfer device.
7. Push the vial of alteplase down so that the piercing pin is inserted through the centre of the alteplase stopper.
8. Invert the 2 vials so that the vial of alteplase is on the bottom (upright) and the vial of SWFI is upside-down, allowing the SWFI to flow down through the transfer device. Allow the entire contents of the vial of SWFI to flow into the alteplase vial (approximately 0.5 mL of SWFI will remain in the diluent vial). Approximately 2 minutes are required for this procedure.
9. Remove the transfer device and the empty SWFI vial from the alteplase vial. Safely discard both the transfer device and the empty diluent vial according to institutional procedures.
10. Swirl gently to dissolve the alteplase powder. **Do not shake.**

Stability and Storage: Lyophilized alteplase is stable up to the expiration date stamped on the vial when stored at controlled temperatures between 2 and 30°C. Protect the lyophilized material during extended storage from excessive exposure to light.

Unused reconstituted alteplase (in the vial) may be stored at 2 to 30°C for up to 8 hours. After that time, any unused portion of the reconstituted material should be discarded. During the period of reconstitution and infusion, protection from light is not necessary.

SUPPLIED: 50 mg: Each vial of sterile, white to off-white, lyophilized powder contains: alteplase 50 mg. Nonmedicinal ingredients: L-arginine, phosphoric acid, polysorbate 80. Phosphoric acid and/or sodium hydroxide may be used prior to lyophilization for pH adjustment. Vials of 50 mg **with vacuum** present. Boxes of 1 vial of Activase rt-PA 50 mg (29×10^6 IU), and 1 vial of Sterile Water for Injection, USP 50 mL, for preparing a sterile solution of Activase rt-PA.

100 mg: Each vial of sterile, white to off-white, lyophilized powder contains: alteplase 100 mg. Nonmedicinal ingredients: L-arginine, phosphoric acid, polysorbate 80. Phosphoric acid and/or sodium hydroxide may be used prior to lyophilization for pH adjustment. Vials of 100 mg with **no vacuum** present. Boxes of 1 vial of Activase rt-PA 100 mg (58×10^6 IU), and 1 vial of Sterile Water for Injection, USP 100 mL, and 1 transfer device for preparing a sterile solution of Activase rt-PA.

Biological potency is determined by an in vitro clot lysis assay and is expressed in International Units (58×10^4 IU/mg alteplase).

Lyophilized alteplase is stable up to the expiration date stamped on the vial when stored at controlled temperatures between 2 and 30°C. Protect the lyophilized material during extended storage from excessive exposure to light.

Activase® rt-PA (Acute Myocardial Infarction)

alteplase

Fibrinolytic Agent

Roche

Date of Revision: April 10, 2001

PHARMACOLOGY: Acute Myocardial Infarction: Alteplase is a serine protease which has the property of fibrin-enhanced conversion of plasminogen to plasmin. It produces minimal conversion of plasminogen in the absence of fibrin; and when introduced into the systemic circulation, alteplase binds to fibrin in a thrombus and converts the entrapped plasminogen to plasmin. This initiates local fibrinolysis with minimal systemic effects. Following administration of alteplase there is a decrease (20 to 30%) in circulating fibrinogen. Decreases in plasminogen and α_2-antiplasmin are also evident.

Alteplase is cleared rapidly from circulating plasma with an initial half-life of less than 5 minutes. There is no difference in the dominant initial plasma half-life between the 3-hour and accelerated regimens for acute myocardial infarction (AMI). The plasma clearance of alteplase is approximately 500 mL/min. The clearance is mediated primarily by the liver.

An occlusive thrombus is present in the infarct-related coronary artery in approximately 80% of patients experiencing a transmural myocardial infarction evaluated within 4 hours of onset of symptoms.

Acute Myocardial Infarction Patients Studies: Two alteplase dose regimens have been studied in patients experiencing AMI: accelerated infusion, and 3-hour infusion. The comparative efficacy of these two regimens has not been evaluated.

There is no difference in the dominant initial plasma half-life between the 3-hour and accelerated regimens for acute myocardial infarction (AMI).

90-Minute Accelerated Infusion in Patients with Acute Myocardial Infarction: Accelerated infusion of alteplase was studied in an international, multicentre trial (GUSTO) where 41 021 patients with acute myocardial infarction were randomized to 4 thrombolytic regimens: accelerated infusion of alteplase (<100 mg over 90 minutes) plus i.v. heparin; streptokinase (1.5×10^6 units over 60 minutes) plus i.v. heparin; streptokinase (1.5×10^6 units over 60 minutes) plus s.c. heparin; or combined alteplase (1.0 mg/kg over 60 minutes) plus streptokinase (1.0×10^6 units over 60 minutes). ASA was administered daily. The results are shown in Table 1. The 30-day mortality for the accelerated infusion of alteplase was 1% lower (14% relative risk reduction) than for streptokinase (i.v. or s.c. heparin). In addition, the combined incidence of 30-day mortality or nonfatal stroke for accelerated alteplase was 1% lower (12% relative risk reduction) than for streptokinase (i.v. heparin) and 0.8% lower (10% relative risk reduction) than for streptokinase (s.c. heparin). One year follow-up data suggest a sustained mortality benefit.

Table 1: Activase rt-PA (Acute Myocardial Infarction)

Accelerated Infusion in Patients with Myocardial Infarction

Event	Accelerated Activase rt-PA (i.v. heparin)	Streptokinase (i.v. heparin)	p-value[a]	Streptokinase (s.c. heparin)	p-value[a]
30-Day Mortality	6.3%	7.3%	0.003	7.3%	0.007
30-Day Mortality or Nonfatal Stroke	7.2%	8.2%	0.006	8.0%	0.036
24-Hour Mortality	2.4%	2.9%	0.009	2.8%	0.029

[a] Two-tailed p-value is for comparison of accelerated infusion of alteplase to the respective streptokinase control arm.

Subgroup analysis of patients by age, infarct location, and time from symptom onset to thrombolytic treatment showed consistently lower 30-day mortality for the group receiving the accelerated infusion of alteplase. For patients who were over 75 years of age, a predefined subgroup consisting of 12% of patients enrolled, the incidence of stroke was 4.0% for the group receiving the accelerated infusion of alteplase, 2.8% for streptokinase (i.v. heparin), and 3.2% for streptokinase (s.c. heparin); the incidence of combined 30-day mortality or nonfatal stroke was 20.6% for accelerated infusion of alteplase, 21.5% for streptokinase (i.v. heparin), and 22.0% for streptokinase (s.c. heparin).

In-hospital events in the overall patient population, as well as events in patients who survived beyond 30 days are shown in Table 2.

Table 2: Activase rt-PA (Acute Myocardial Infarction)

In-Hospital Clinical Events/Procedures[a]

	Overall			30-Day Survivors[b]		
	SK (pooled) %		Activase %	SK (pooled) %		Activase %
Reinfarction	3.9		4.1	3.4		3.6
Cardiogenic Shock	6.5	***	5.0	3.2	***	2.3
CABG	8.3		9.0	8.6		9.2
PTCA (IRA)[c]	14.3		14.6	14.8		15.2
CHF or Pulmonary Edema	16.7	***	15.0	14.3	**	13.1
Recurrent Ischemia	20.3		19.7	20.1		19.6
Sustained Hypotension	12.8	***	10.0	9.4	***	7.0
2° or 3° Atrioventricular Block	8.9	***	7.3	7.6	***	6.2
Ventricular Tachycardia	6.5	*	5.7	4.8		4.4

(cont'd)

Table 2: Activase rt-PA (Acute Myocardial Infarction) *(cont'd)*

In-Hospital Clinical Events/Procedures[a]

	Overall			30-Day Survivors[b]		
	SK (pooled) %		Activase %	SK (pooled) %		Activase %
Ventricular Fibrillation	6.9	*	6.2	5.0		4.6
Asystole	6.0	**	5.1	1.9		1.7
Atrial Fibrillation/Flutter	9.9	**	8.7	9.1	**	8.0
Acute Mitral Regurgitation	1.5		1.3	1.3		1.1
Swan-Ganz Catheter	12.6	**	11.5	11.5		10.7
Cardioversion	9.8	**	8.6	7.4	*	6.7
Angiography	55.0	*	56.5	57.4	*	58.9

[a] Events other than death, stroke and bleeding.
[b] Patients alive at 30-day timepoint.
[c] IRA=Infarct-Related Artery.
Legend:
*p<0.05.
**p<0.01.
***p<0.001.

An angiographic substudy of the GUSTO trial provided data on infarct-related artery patency. Results are shown in Table 3. Reocclusion rates were similar for all 3 treatment regimens.

Table 3: Activase rt-PA (Acute Myocardial Infarction)

Data on Infarct-Related Artery Patency

	Accelerated Activase rt-PA			Streptokinase (i.v. heparin)			Streptokinase (s.c. heparin)		
Patency	TIMI 2 or 3	TIMI 3	(N)	TIMI 2 or 3	TIMI 3	(N)	TIMI 2 or 3	TIMI 3	(N)
90-Minute	81.3%[a]	54.8%[a]	(272)	59.0%	30.7%	(261)	53.5%	27.3%	(260)
180-Minute	76.3%	41.3%	(80)	72.4%	38.2%	(76)	71.6%	34.7%	(95)
24 Hours	88.9%	39.5%	(81)	87.5%	47.2%	(72)	82.1%	56.7%	(67)
5–7 Day	83.3%	63.9%	(72)	90.9%	67.5%	(77)	78.7%	58.7%	(75)

[a] p<0.001 compared to streptokinase with i.v. heparin and s.c. heparin. No other treatment groups were significantly different.

3-Hour Infusion in Patients with Acute Myocardial Infarction: In patients studied with coronary angiography prior to and following infusion of alteplase, the use of alteplase resulted in reperfusion of documented obstructed vessels within 90 minutes after the commencement of thrombolytic therapy in approximately 70% of patients. In 2 studies involving 145 patients, alteplase produced reperfusion in 73% of patients who received 70 to 100 mg (40.6 to 58×10^{6} IU) over 90 minutes. In 2 double blind randomized controlled trials in patients with AMI, the patients infused with 80 to 100 mg of alteplase experienced improved ventricular function and reduced incidence of clinical congestive heart failure compared to those treated with placebo.

In a double-blind study involving 5013 patients (ASSET Study) where patients were infused with either alteplase or placebo within 5 hours of onset of symptoms of AMI, improved 30-day survival was shown in patients receiving alteplase compared to placebo. At 1 month, the overall mortality rates were 7.2% for the alteplase-treated group and 9.8% for the placebo-treated group (p=0.001). This benefit was maintained at 6 months (10.4% and 13.1% for alteplase and placebo-treated patients respectively, p=0.008).

In the LATE study involving 5711 patients where patients were infused with either alteplase (100 mg over 3 hours) or placebo within 6 to 24 hours of onset of AMI symptoms, the 35-day mortality rates were 8.9% for Activase rt-PA treated patients and 10.3% for placebo-treated patients (p=not significant). Prespecified survival analysis according to treatment within 12 hours of symptom onset showed a significant reduction in mortality for the alteplase treated patients, 8.9% versus 12.0% for the placebo-treated patients (p=0.0229).

INDICATIONS: Acute Myocardial Infarction: (For information on use in acute ischemic stroke, please consult the product monograph for the acute ischemic stroke indication.) For i.v. use in adults for: the lysis of suspected occlusive coronary artery thrombi associated with evolving transmural myocardial infarction; and the reduction of mortality associated with AMI, the improvement of ventricular function following AMI and the reduction in the incidence of congestive heart failure.

Treatment should be initiated as soon as possible after the onset of acute myocardial symptoms. Greater benefit appears to be associated with earlier treatment of alteplase, following the onset of symptoms.

Alteplase is effective in patients in whom therapy is initiated within 6 hours of onset of symptoms for the accelerated infusion regimen or up to 12 hours after onset of symptoms for the 3-hour infusion regimen. The GUSTO study was designed to enrol patients within a 6-hour period following the onset of myocardial infarct symptoms. The data available from this trial are insufficient to support a recommendation for use of the accelerated infusion regimen in patients presenting more than 6 hours after the onset of symptoms.

CONTRAINDICATIONS: Acute Myocardial Infarction: In the following situations because of an increased risk of bleeding: active internal bleeding; history of stroke; patients receiving other i.v. thrombolytic agents; recent (within 2 months) intracranial, or intraspinal surgery or trauma (see Warnings); intracranial neoplasm, arteriovenous malformation, or aneurysm; known bleeding diathesis; severe uncontrolled hypertension, i.e., diastolic BP≥ 110 mmHg and/or systolic BP≥ 180 mmHg; recent traumatic cardiopulmonary resuscitation; recent severe trauma.

WARNINGS: Acute Myocardial Infarction: Bleeding: The most common complication encountered during therapy with alteplase is bleeding. The type of bleeding associated with thrombolytic therapy can be divided into 2 broad categories: internal bleeding involving the gastrointestinal tract, genitourinary tract, respiratory tract, retroperitoneal or intracranial sites; superficial or surface bleeding, observed mainly at invaded or disturbed sites (e.g., venous cutdowns, arterial punctures, sites of recent surgical intervention).

The concomitant use of heparin anticoagulation contributes to the risk of bleeding.

Fibrin will be lysed during the infusion of alteplase and bleeding from recent puncture sites may occur. Therefore, therapy with alteplase, as with other thrombolytic agents, requires careful attention to all potential bleeding sites (including catheter insertion sites, arterial and venous puncture sites, cutdown sites and needle punctures sites).

I.M. injections and nonessential handling of the patient should be avoided during and immediately following treatment with alteplase. Venipunctures should be performed carefully and only as required.

Should an arterial puncture be necessary during an infusion of alteplase, it is preferable to use an upper extremity vessel that is accessible to manual compression. Pressure should be applied for at least 30 minutes, a pressure dressing applied and the puncture site checked frequently for evidence of bleeding.

Should serious bleeding in a critical location (not controllable by local pressure) occur, the infusion of alteplase and any other concomitant anticoagulant should be discontinued immediately and treatment initiated (see Overdose: Symptoms and Treatment).

In the following conditions, the risks of alteplase therapy may be increased and should be weighed against the anticipated benefits: recent (within 10 days) major surgery, e.g., coronary artery bypass graft, obstetrical delivery, organ biopsy, previous puncture of noncompressible vessels; clinical evidence or history of transient ischemic attacks; recent gastrointestinal or genitourinary bleeding (within 10 days); recent trauma (within 10 days); hypertension: systolic BP≥ 175 mmHg and/or diastolic BP≥ 110 mmHg; a history or clinical evidence of hypertensive disease in a patient over 70 years old; advanced age, e.g., over 75 years old; high likelihood or known presence of left heart thrombus, e.g., mitral stenosis with atrial fibrillation; apical MI, with thrombus; acute pericarditis; subacute bacterial endocarditis; hemostatic defects including those secondary to severe hepatic or renal disease; significant liver dysfunction, e.g., prolonged prothrombin time; pregnancy; diabetic hemorrhagic retinopathy, or other hemorrhagic ophthalmic conditions; septic thrombophlebitis or occluded AV cannula at seriously infected site; patients currently receiving oral anticoagulants, e.g., warfarin sodium; any other condition in which bleeding constitutes a significant hazard or would be particularly difficult to manage because of its location.

In a small subgroup of AMI patients who are at low risk for death from cardiac causes (i.e., no previous myocardial infarction, Killip class I) and who have high blood pressure at the time of presentation, the risk for stroke may offset the survival benefit produced by thrombolytic therapy.

Cholesterol Embolization: Cholesterol embolization has been reported rarely in patients treated with all types of thrombolytic agents; the true incidence is unknown. This serious condition, which can be lethal, is also associated with invasive vascular procedures (e.g., cardiac catheterization, angiography, vascular surgery) and/or anticoagulant therapy. Clinical features of cholesterol embolism include livedo reticularis, "purple toe" syndrome, acute renal failure, gangrenous digits, hypertension, pancreatitis, myocardial infarction, cerebral infarction, spinal cord infarction, retinal artery occlusion, bowel infarction, and rhabdomyolysis.

Arrhythmias: Coronary thrombolysis may result in arrhythmias associated with reperfusion. These arrhythmias (such as sinus bradycardia, accelerated idioventricular rhythm, ventricular premature depolarizations, ventricular tachycardia) are not different from those often seen in the ordinary course of AMI and may be managed with standard antiarrhythmic measures. It is recommended that antiarrhythmic therapy for bradycardia and/or ventricular irritability be available when infusions of alteplase are administered.

Use of Antithrombotics: ASA and heparin may be administered concomitantly with and following infusions of alteplase. Because either heparin, ASA or alteplase alone may cause bleeding complications, careful monitoring for bleeding is advised, especially at arterial puncture sites.

PRECAUTIONS: Acute Myocardial Infarction: General: Alteplase should be administered in a hospital setting where the appropriate diagnostic and monitoring techniques are readily available.

Routine management of myocardial infarction should not be deferred after evidence of successful thrombolysis is seen. Evaluation and management of underlying atherosclerotic heart disease should be carried out as clinically indicated.

Noncompressible arterial puncture must be avoided. Arterial and venous punctures should be minimized. In the event of serious bleeding, alteplase and heparin should be discontinued immediately. Heparin effects can be reversed by protamine.

Drug Interactions: The interaction of alteplase with other drugs has not been studied. In addition to bleeding associated with heparin and warfarin, drugs that alter platelet function (such as ASA) may increase the risk of bleeding if administered prior to, during or after alteplase infusion.

Laboratory Tests: During alteplase infusion, coagulation tests and/or measures of fibrinolytic activity may be performed if desired. However, routine measurements of fibrinogen as well as fibrinogen degradation products are unreliable, and should not be undertaken unless specific precautions are taken to prevent in vitro artifacts. Alteplase is a serine protease that when present in blood in pharmacologic concentrations remains active under in vitro conditions. This can lead to degradation of fibrinogen in a blood sample removed for analysis. Collection of blood samples on aprotinin (150 to 200 units/mL) can to some extent mitigate this phenomenon.

Geriatrics: The risks of therapy may be increased in the elderly (see Pharmacology, Warnings and Adverse Effects).

Children: Safety and effectiveness of alteplase in children has not been established. Therefore treatment of such patients is not recommended.

Pregnancy: Alteplase has been shown to have an embryocidal effect in rabbits when i.v. administered in doses of approximately 2 times (3 mg/kg) the human dose for AMI. No maternal or fetal toxicity was evident at 0.65 times (1 mg/kg) the human dose in pregnant rats and rabbits dosed during the period of organogenesis. There are no adequate and well controlled studies in pregnant women. Alteplase should be used during pregnancy only if the potential benefit justifies the potential risk to the fetus.

Lactation: It is not known whether alteplase is excreted in human milk. Because many drugs are excreted in human milk, caution should be exercised when alteplase is administered to a nursing woman.

Readministration: There has been little documentation of readministration of alteplase. Readministration should be undertaken with caution. Less than 0.5% of patients receiving single courses of alteplase therapy have experienced transient antibody formation. Nevertheless, if an anaphylactoid reaction occurs, the infusion should be discontinued immediately and appropriate therapy initiated.

ADVERSE EFFECTS: Acute Myocardial Infarction: Bleeding: The most frequent adverse reaction associated with alteplase is bleeding. The type of bleeding associated with thrombolytic therapy can be divided into 2 broad categories: internal bleeding, involving the gastrointestinal tract, genitourinary tract, respiratory tract, retroperitoneal or intracranial sites; superficial or surface bleeding, observed mainly at invaded or disturbed sites (e.g., venous cutdowns, arterial punctures, sites of recent surgical intervention).

Reported Incidence of Bleeding During Alteplase Treatment: The incidence of all strokes for the accelerated alteplase (90 minute) infusion regimen in the GUSTO trial was 1.6%, while the incidence of nonfatal stroke was 0.9%. The incidence of hemorrhagic stroke was 0.7%, not all of which were fatal. Data from previous trials utilizing a 3-hour infusion indicate that the incidence of total stroke in 6 randomized double-blind placebo controlled trials was 1.2% (37/3 161) in alteplase-treated patients (≤100 mg) compared with 0.9% (27/3 092) in placebo-treated patients.

Although the incidence of all strokes, as well as that for hemorrhagic stroke, increased with increasing age, treatment with accelerated regimen of alteplase was still shown to reduce mortality in older patients. For patients who were over 75 years of age, a predefined subgroup consisting of 12% of patients enrolled, the incidence of stroke was 4.0% for the accelerated regimen of alteplase group, 2.8% for streptokinase (i.v. heparin), and 3.2% for streptokinase (s.c. heparin) (see Table 4). However, combined 30-day mortality or nonfatal stroke was 20.6% for accelerated regimen of alteplase, 21.5% for streptokinase (i.v. heparin) and 22.0% for streptokinase (s.c. heparin) in the GUSTO study.

The following incidence of significant internal bleeding (estimated as ≥250 mL blood loss) has been reported in studies involving over 1300 patients treated at all doses of alteplase, administered as a 3-hour infusion regimen: gastrointestinal 5%, genitourinary 4%.

The following incidence of moderate or severe bleeding was reported when ≤100 mg alteplase was administered by accelerated infusion to >10 000 patients [GUSTO study]: gastrointestinal 1.5%, genitourinary 0.5%.

Incidence of ≤1% of ecchymosis, retroperitoneal bleeding, epistaxis and gingival bleeding has been reported in clinical studies involving alteplase.

The incidence of intracranial bleeding in patients treated with up to 120 mg alteplase (3-hour infusion) has been 0.4%. At doses in excess of 120 mg (120 to 180 mg) the incidence of intracranial bleeding increased to 1.3%. The incidence of intracranial bleeding in patients treated ≤100 mg alteplase (accelerated infusion, weight adjusted) was 0.7%. The maximum total dose of alteplase used in the treatment of acute myocardial infarction should not exceed 100 mg.

Death and permanent disability have been reported in patients who have experienced stroke and other serious bleeding episodes.

Table 4: Activase rt-PA (Acute Myocardial Infarction)

Incidence of Stroke and Intracranial Hemorrhage

	rt-PA%	SK (i.v.)		SK (s.c.)	
	%	%	p-value	%	p-value
Stroke	1.6%	1.4%	0.32	1.2%	0.03
Intracranial hemorrhage	0.7%	0.6%	0.22	0.5%	0.02
Stroke in >75 yrs	4.0%	2.8%	0.09	3.2%	0.27
Intracranial hemorrhage >75 yrs	2.0%	1.1%	0.06	1.3%	0.17

p-value is for pairwise comparison to rt-PA.

Table 5: Activase rt-PA (Acute Myocardial Infarction)
Accelerated Regimen: Infusion Chart

Patient Weight		Bolus	Volume of rt-PA Added to Empty PVC Bag or Glass Vial	0.75 mg/kg over 30 Minutes			0.50 mg/kg over 60 Minutes			rt-PA Total Dose (mg) (bolus+ maintenance) (maximum dose =100 mg)
(lb)	(kg)	Volume 15 mg[a] (15 mL) over 2 Minutes	(mL)	Infusion Dose (mg) (max dose =50 mg)	Infusion Rate (mL/h)	Volume to be Infused (mL)	Infusion Dose (mg) (max dose =35 mg)	Infusion Rate (mL/h)	Volume to be Infused (mL)	
90–94	41–42	15	52	31	62	31	21	21	21	67
95–97	43–44	15	54	32	64	32	22	22	22	69
98–104	45–47	15	57	34	68	34	23	23	23	72
105–109	48–49	15	60	36	72	36	24	24	24	75
110–114	50–51	15	63	38	75	38	25	25	25	78
115–119	52–54	15	65	39	78	39	26	26	26	80
120–124	55–56	15	68	41	82	41	27	27	27	83
125–129	57–58	15	71	43	86	43	28	28	28	86
130–134	59–60	15	73	44	88	44	29	29	29	88
135–139	61–63	15	76	46	92	46	30	30	30	91
140–144	64–65	15	80	48	96	48	32	32	32	95
145–149	66–67	15	83	50	100	50	33	33	33	98
>149	>67	15	85	50	100	50	35	35	35	100

[a] 1 mg=1 mL.

Allergic Reactions: Allergic-type reactions, e.g., anaphylactoid reaction, laryngeal edema, orolingual angioedema, rash and urticaria have been reported very rarely (<0.02%). A cause and effect relationship to alteplase therapy has not been established.

Other Adverse Reactions: The following adverse reactions have been reported among patients receiving alteplase in clinical trials and in postmarketing experience. These reactions are frequent sequelae of the underlying disease and the effect of alteplase on the incidence of these events is unknown.

Patients with myocardial infarction can experience disease-related events such as cardiogenic shock, arrhythmias, AV block, pulmonary edema, heart failure, cardiac arrest, recurrent ischemia, myocardial reinfarction, myocardial rupture, mitral regurgitation, pericardial effusion, pericarditis, cardiac tamponade, venous thrombosis and embolism, and electromechanical dissociation. These events may lead to death. Other adverse reactions have been reported, principally nausea and/or vomiting, hypotension, and fever.

OVERDOSE:

Symptoms: Acute Myocardial Infarction: Overdosage could lead to serious bleeding.

Treatment: Should serious bleeding occur in a critical location, the infusion of alteplase and any other concomitant anticoagulant should be discontinued immediately. If necessary, blood loss and reversal of the bleeding tendency can be managed with whole blood or packed red cells. In the event of clinically significant fibrinogen depletion, fresh frozen plasma or cryoprecipitate can be infused.

For management of a suspected drug overdose, CPhA recommends that you contact your **regional Poison Control Centre**. See the *CPS* Directory section for a list of Poison Control Centres.

DOSAGE: Acute Myocardial Infarction: Alteplase is intended for i.v. use only. It should be given via a dedicated i.v. line with an infusion pump. Extravasation of alteplase infusion can cause ecchymosis and/or inflammation. Management consists of terminating the infusion at the i.v. site and application of local therapy.

Administer alteplase as soon as possible after the onset of symptoms.

There are 2 dose regimens for alteplase for use in the management of AMI. The comparative efficacy of these two regimens has not been evaluated.

90-Minute Accelerated Infusion: See Table 5. The recommended total dose is based upon patient weight, not to exceed 100 mg. For patients weighing >67 kg, the recommended dose is 100 mg, administered as a 15 mg i.v. bolus, followed by 50 mg infused over 30 minutes and then 35 mg infused over the next 60 minutes.

For patients weighing <67 kg, the recommended dose is 15 mg administered as an i.v. bolus, followed by 0.75 mg/kg to a maximum of 50 mg, infused over the next 30 minutes, and then 0.50 mg/kg to a maximum of 35 mg infused over the next 60 minutes.

This 90-minute infusion regimen is recommended for use up to 6 hours after onset of AMI symptoms.

Preparation and Administration: The alteplase dose administered by accelerated infusion may be prepared and administered as follows: A) The bolus dose may be prepared in one of the following ways:

1) By removing 15 mL from the vial of reconstituted (1 mg/mL) alteplase using a syringe and needle. For 50 mg vials, the syringe should not be primed with air and the needle should be inserted into the alteplase vial stopper. If the 100 mg vial is used, the needle should be inserted away from the puncture mark made by the transfer device. 2) By removing 15 mL from a port (second injection site) on the infusion line after the infusion set is primed. 3) By programming an infusion pump to deliver a 15 mL (1 mg/mL) bolus at the initiation of the infusion. B) The remainder of the alteplase dose may be administered as follows: **50 mg vials:** Administer using either a polyvinyl chloride bag or glass vial and infusion set. **100 mg vials:** Insert the spike end of an infusion set through the same puncture site created by the transfer device in the stopper of the vial of reconstituted alteplase. Hang the vial of alteplase from the plastic molded capping attached to the bottom of the vial.

3-Hour Infusion: The recommended dose is 100 mg administered as 60 mg in the first hour, of which 6 to 7 mg is administered as a bolus over the first 1 to 2 minutes and the remainder is administered by continuous infusion, 20 mg by continuous infusion during the second hour, and 20 mg by continuous infusion over the following 1 to 4 hours. For smaller patients (<65 kg), a dose of 1.25 mg/kg may be warranted. This 3-hour regimen is recommended for use up to 12 hours after onset of AMI symptoms.

Preparation and Administration: A) The bolus dose may be prepared in one of the following ways:

1) By removing 6 to 10 mL from the vial of reconstituted (1 mg/mL) alteplase using a syringe and needle. For 50 mg vials, the syringe should not be primed with air and the needle should be inserted into the alteplase vial stopper. If the 100 mg vial is used, the needle should be inserted away from the puncture mark made by the transfer device. 2) By removing 6 to 10 mL from a port (second injection site) on the infusion line after the infusion set is primed. 3) By programming an infusion pump to deliver a 6 to 10 mL (1 mg/mL) bolus at the initiation of the infusion. B) The remainder of the alteplase dose may be administered as follows: **50 mg vials:** Administer using either a polyvinyl chloride bag or glass vial and infusion set. **100 mg vials:** Insert the spike end of an infusion set through the same puncture site created by the transfer device in the stopper of the vial of reconstituted alteplase. Hang the vial of alteplase from the plastic molded capping attached to the bottom of the vial.

Anticoagulation During and After Treatment with Alteplase: To date, heparin has been administered concomitantly in more than 90% of patients given alteplase. Adjunctive i.v. heparin administration is recommended to obtain a therapeutic partial thromboplastin time (PTT). The infusion of heparin should be initiated prior to the termination of the infusion of alteplase.

Reconstitution and Dilution: Alteplase should be reconstituted by aseptically adding to the vial, the appropriate volume of Sterile Water for Injection, USP [SWFI] (50 mL for 50 mg vials, 100 mL for 100 mg vials). It is important that alteplase be reconstituted only with Sterile Water for Injection, USP, without preservatives. Do not use Bacteriostatic Water for Injection. The reconstituted preparation results in a colourless to pale yellow transparent solution containing alteplase 1 mg/mL at a pH of 7.3. The osmolality of this solution is approximately 215 mOsm/kg.

Before further dilution or administration, parenteral drug products should be visually inspected for particulate matter and discoloration prior to administration whenever solution and container permit. Because alteplase contains no preservatives, it should be reconstituted immediately before use (see Stability and Storage).

The reconstituted solution may be diluted further immediately before administration to yield concentrations as low as 0.5 mg/mL in 0.9% Sodium Chloride for Injection, USP or 5% Dextrose for Injection, USP. Excessive agitation during dilution should be avoided; mixing should be accomplished with gentle swirling and/or slow inversion. Do not use other infusion solutions e.g., Sterile Water for Injection, USP, or preservative containing solutions for further dilution.

No other medication should be added to alteplase solution. Solutions should be administered as described above. Unused infusion solution should be immediately discarded.

50 mg vials: Using a large bore needle (e.g., 18 gauge), **and the accompanying 50 mL Sterile Water for Injection, USP,** direct the stream of Sterile Water for Injection, USP into the lyophilized cake. **Do not use if vacuum is not present.** Slight foaming upon reconstitution is not unusual; standing undisturbed for several minutes is usually sufficient to allow dissipation of any large bubbles. Excessive or vigorous shaking should be avoided.

100 mg vials: Using the transfer device provided, the contents of the accompanying 100 mL vial of Sterile Water for Injection, USP should be added to the contents of the 100 mg vial of alteplase powder. Slight foaming upon reconstitution is not unusual; standing undisturbed for several minutes is usually sufficient to allow dissipation of any large bubbles. **No vacuum is present in 100 mg vials.** Please refer to the accompanying instructions for Reconstitution and Administration of the 100 mg vials:

1. Use aseptic technique throughout.
2. Remove the protection flip-caps from 1 vial of alteplase and 1 vial of Sterile Water for Injection, USP [SWFI].
3. Open the package containing the transfer device by peeling the paper label off the package.
4. Remove the protective cap from one end of the transfer device and keeping the vial of Sterile Water for Injection upright, insert the piercing pin vertically into the centre of the stopper of the vial of Sterile Water for Injection.
5. Remove the protective cap from the other end of the transfer device. **Do not invert the vial of Sterile Water for Injection.**
6. Holding the vial of alteplase upside-down, position it so that the centre of the stopper is directly over the exposed piercing pin of the transfer device.
7. Push the vial of alteplase down so that the piercing pin is inserted through the centre of the alteplase stopper.
8. Invert the 2 vials so that the vial of alteplase is on the bottom (upright) and the vial of Sterile Water for Injection is upside-down, allowing the Sterile Water for Injection to flow down through the transfer device. Allow the entire contents of the vial of Sterile Water for Injection to flow into the alteplase vial (approximately 0.5 mL of Sterile Water for Injection will remain in the diluent vial). Approximately 2 minutes are required for this procedure.
9. Remove the transfer device and the empty Sterile Water for Injection vial from the alteplase vial. Safely discard both the transfer device and the empty diluent vial according to institutional procedures.
10. Swirl gently to dissolve the alteplase powder. **Do not shake.**

Stability and Storage: Lyophilized alteplase is stable up to the expiration date stamped on the vial when stored at controlled temperatures between 2 and 30°C. Protect the lyophilized material during extended storage from excessive exposure to light.

Unused reconstituted alteplase (in the vial) may be stored at 2 to 30°C for up to 8 hours. After that time, any unused portion of the reconstituted material should be discarded. During the period of reconstitution and infusion, protection from light is not necessary.

SUPPLIED: 50 mg: Each vial of sterile, white to off-white, lyophilized powder contains: alteplase 50 mg. Nonmedicinal ingredients: L-arginine, phosphoric acid, polysorbate 80. Phosphoric acid and/or sodium hydroxide may be used prior to lyophilization for pH adjustment. Vials of 50 mg **with vacuum** present. Boxes of 1 vial of Activase rt-PA 50 mg (29×10⁶ IU), and 1 vial of Sterile Water for Injection, USP 50 mL, for preparing a sterile solution of Activase rt-PA.

100 mg: Each vial of sterile, white to off-white, lyophilized powder contains: alteplase 100 mg. Nonmedicinal ingredients: L-arginine, phosphoric acid, polysorbate 80. Phosphoric acid and/or sodium hydroxide may be used prior to lyophilization for pH adjustment. Vials of 100 mg with **no vacuum** present. Boxes of 1 vial of Activase rt-PA 100 mg (58 × 10⁶ IU) and 1 vial of Sterile Water for Injection, USP 100 mL, and 1 transfer device for preparing a sterile solution of Activase rt-PA.

Biological potency is determined by an in vitro clot lysis assay and is expressed in International Units (58×10⁴ IU/mg alteplase).

Lyophilized alteplase is stable up to the expiration date stamped on the vial when stored at controlled temperatures between 2 and 30°C. Protect the lyophilized material during extended storage from excessive exposure to light.

Activated Charcoal

CPhA Monograph

see *Charcoal, Activated*

Active Calcium Chewable

calcium—magnesium—vitamin D—silicon

Mineral Supplement

USANA Health Sciences

SUPPLIED: Each tablet contains: calcium (citrate, carbonate) 200 mg, magnesium (oxide, citrate) 100 mg, vitamin D_3 (cholecalciferol) 2.5 µg, and silicon (calcium silicate) 2.25 mg. Nonmedicinal ingredients: citric acid, fructose, guar gum, honey powder, malic acid, maltodextrin, natural flavour, rice protein hydrolysate, soy lecithin, vegetable stearic acid and xylitol. Bottles of 112. Safety seal under cap. Store below 25°C.

(Shown in Product Identification Section)

Activelle® Ⓟ

estradiol—norethindrone acetate

Estrogenic Hormones—Progestin

Novo Nordisk

Date of Preparation: March 6, 2008

SUMMARY PRODUCT INFORMATION:

Route of Administration	Dosage Form/ Strength	Clinically Relevant Nonmedicinal Ingredients
Oral	Film-coated tablet Estradiol 1 mg (as hemihydrate) and norethisterone acetate 0.5 mg	Lactose monohydrate For a complete listing see Dosage Forms, Composition and Packaging.

INDICATIONS AND CLINICAL USE: Activelle (1 mg Estradiol 0.5 mg Norethindrone acetate) is indicated for:
- Treatment of moderate to severe vasomotor symptoms occurring in naturally or surgically induced estrogen deficiency states.
- Treatment of vulvar or vaginal atrophy associated with menopause.

Activelle is recommended only in women with intact uteri since the regimen includes a progestogen to prevent endometrial hyperplasia.

CONTRAINDICATIONS:
- Patients with known hypersensitivity to this drug or any ingredient in the formulation or components of the container. For complete listing, see Dosage Forms, Composition and Packaging.
- Liver dysfunction or disease as long as liver function tests have failed to return to normal.
- Known or suspected estrogen-dependent or progestin-dependent malignant neoplasia (e.g. endometrial cancer).
- Endometrial hyperplasia.
- Known, suspected, or past history of breast cancer.
- Undiagnosed abnormal genital bleeding.
- Known or suspected pregnancy.
- Active or past history of arterial thromboembolic disease (e.g. stroke, myocardial infarction, coronary heart disease).
- Active or past history of confirmed venous thromboembolism (such as deep vein thrombosis or pulmonary embolism) or active thrombophlebitis.
- Partial or complete loss of vision from ophthalmic vascular disease.
- Porphyria.
- Classical migraine.
- Lactation.

WARNINGS AND PRECAUTIONS:

Serious Warnings and Precautions

The Women's Health Initiative (WHI) trial examined the health benefits and risks of oral combined estrogen plus progestin therapy (n=16 608) and oral estrogen-alone therapy (n=10 739) in postmenopausal women aged 50 to 79 years.

The estrogen plus progestin arm of the WHI trial (mean age 63.3 years) indicated an increased risk of myocardial infarction (MI), stroke, invasive breast cancer, pulmonary emboli and deep vein thrombosis in postmenopausal women receiving treatment with combined conjugated equine estrogens (CEE, 0.625 mg/day) and medroxyprogesterone acetate (MPA, 2.5 mg/day) for 5.2 years compared to those receiving placebo.

The estrogen-alone arm of the WHI trial (mean age 63.6 years) indicated an increased risk of stroke and deep vein thrombosis in hysterectomized women treated with CEE-alone (0.625 mg/day) for 6.8 years compared to those receiving placebo.

Therefore, the following should be given serious consideration at the time of prescribing:
- Estrogens with or without progestins **should not** be prescribed for primary or secondary prevention of cardiovascular diseases.
- Estrogens with or without progestins should be prescribed at the **lowest effective dose** for the approved indication.
- Estrogens with or without progestins should be prescribed for the **shortest period** possible for the approved indication.

General: For the treatment of postmenopausal symptoms, HRT should only be initiated for symptoms that adversely affect quality of life. In all cases, a careful appraisal of the risks and benefits should be undertaken at least annually and HRT should only be continued as long as the benefit outweighs the risk.

Carcinogenesis and Mutagenesis: Breast Cancer: Available epidemiological data indicate that the use of combined estrogen plus progestin by postmenopausal women is associated with an increased risk of invasive breast cancer. In the estrogen plus progestin arm of the WHI trial, among 10 000 women over a one-year period, there were:
- 8 more cases of invasive breast cancer (38 on combined HRT versus 30 on placebo).

The WHI study also reported that the invasive breast cancers diagnosed in the estrogen plus progestin group were similar in histology but were larger (mean [SD], 1.7 cm [1.1] vs 1.5 cm [0.9], respectively; P=0.04) and were at a more advanced stage compared with those diagnosed in the placebo group. The percentage of women with abnormal mammograms (recommendations for short-interval follow-up, a suspicious abnormality, or highly suggestive of malignancy) was significantly higher in the estrogen plus progestin group versus the placebo group. This difference appeared at year one and persisted in each year thereafter.

In the estrogen-alone arm of the WHI trial, there was no statistically significant difference in the rate of invasive breast cancer in hysterectomized women treated with conjugated equine estrogens versus women treated with placebo.

It is recommended that estrogens with or without progestins not be given to women with existing breast cancer or those with a previous history of the disease (see Contraindications).

There is a need for caution in prescribing estrogens with or without progestins for women with known risk factors associated with the development of breast cancer, such as strong family history of breast cancer (first degree relative) or who present a breast condition with an increased risk (abnormal mammograms and/or atypical hyperplasia at breast biopsy).

Other known risk factors for the development of breast cancer such as nulliparity, obesity, early menarche, late age at first full term pregnancy and at menopause should also be evaluated.

It is recommended that women undergo mammography prior to the start of HRT treatment and at regular intervals during treatment, as deemed appropriate by the treating physician and according to the perceived risks for each patient.

The overall benefits and possible risks of hormone replacement therapy should be fully considered and discussed with patients. It is important that the modest increased risk of being diagnosed with breast cancer after 4 years of treatment with combined estrogen plus progestin HRT (as reported in the results of the WHI trial) be discussed with the patient and weighed against its known benefits.

Instructions for regular self-examination of the breasts should be included in this counseling.

Endometrial Hyperplasia and Endometrial Carcinoma: The risk of endometrial hyperplasia and carcinoma is increased when estrogens are administered alone for prolonged periods to women with intact uteri.

The role of a progestin, when combined with estrogen, is to prevent endometrial hyperplasia/carcinoma in women with intact uteri. The addition of progestin for at least 12 days per cycle in non-hysterectomised women greatly reduces this risk.

In the WHI study, endometrial cancer rates were low and were not increased by 5 years of estrogen plus progestin exposure (hazard ratio 0.83 [adjusted 95% CI 0.29-2.32]). Because endometrial cancer has a relatively low incidence rate, the incidence of endometrial hyperplasia is used as a surrogate endpoint in clinical studies.

In a 12 month prospective, double-blind, randomized, multicentre clinical trial of 1176 postmenopausal women (age range 44 to 82), who were randomized to one of four arms: 1 mg estradiol unopposed (n=296), 1 mg E_2 + 0.1 mg NETA (n=294), 1 mg E_2 + 0.25 mg NETA (n=291), and Activelle 1.0 mg/0.5 mg (n=295). At the end of the study, endometrial biopsy results were available for 988 subjects and the incidence of endometrial hyperplasia with Activelle was 0.4% (one simple hyperplasia without atypia) compared with 14.6% with 1 mg unopposed estradiol.

All women taking estrogen/progestin combination should undergo clinical surveillance for endometrial abnormalities. Adequate diagnostic measures, including endometrial sampling, should be performed in all cases of undiagnosed persistent or recurring abnormal genital bleeding.

Ovarian Cancer: Recent epidemiologic studies have found the use of hormone replacement therapy (estrogen-alone and estrogen plus progestin therapies), in particular for five or more years, has been associated with an increased risk of ovarian cancer.

Cardiovascular: The results of the Heart and Estrogen/progestin Replacement Studies (HERS and HERS II) and the Women's Health Initiative (WHI) trial indicate that the use of estrogen plus progestin is associated with an increased risk of coronary heart disease (CHD) in postmenopausal women. The results of the WHI trial indicate that the use of estrogen-alone and estrogen plus progestin is associated with an increased risk of stroke in postmenopausal women.

WHI Trial Findings: In the combined estrogen plus progestin arm of the WHI trial, among 10 000 women over a one-year period, there were:
- 8 more cases of stroke (29 on combined HRT versus 21 on placebo)
- 7 more cases of CHD (37 on combined HRT versus 30 on placebo).

In the estrogen-alone arm of the WHI trial of women with prior hysterectomy, among 10 000 women over a one-year period, there were/was:
- 12 more cases of stroke (44 on estrogen-alone therapy versus 32 on placebo)
- no statistically significant difference in the rate of CHD.

HERS and HERS II Findings: In the Heart and Estrogen/progestin Replacement Study (HERS) of postmenopausal women with documented heart disease (n=2763, average age 66.7 years), a randomized placebo-controlled clinical trial of secondary prevention of coronary heart disease (CHD), treatment with 0.625 mg/day oral conjugated equine estrogen (CEE) plus 2.5 mg oral medroxyprogesterone acetate (MPA) demonstrated no cardiovascular benefit. Specifically, during an average follow-up of 4.1 years, treatment with CEE plus MPA did not reduce the overall rate of CHD events in postmenopausal women with established coronary heart disease. There were more CHD events in the hormone-treated group than in the placebo group in year 1, but not during the subsequent years.

From the original HERS trial, 2321 women consented to participate in an open label extension of HERS known as HERS II. Average follow-up in HERS II was an additional 2.7 years, for a total of 6.8 years overall. After 6.8 years, hormone therapy did not reduce the risk of cardiovascular events in women with CHD.

Blood Pressure: Women using hormone replacement therapy sometimes experience increased blood pressure. Blood pressure should be monitored with HRT use. Elevation of blood pressure in previously normotensive or hypertensive patients should be investigated and HRT may have to be discontinued.

Ear/Nose/Throat: Estrogens should be used with caution in patients with otosclerosis.

Endocrine and Metabolism: Glucose and Lipid Metabolism: A worsening of glucose tolerance and lipid metabolism have been observed in a significant percentage of peri- and post-menopausal patients. Therefore, diabetic patients or those with a predisposition to diabetes should be observed closely to detect any alterations in carbohydrate or lipid metabolism, especially in triglyceride blood levels.

In 38 randomized postmenopausal women (age range 53 to 70) with type 2 diabetes included in a 6-month randomised, parallel, double-blind, single-center trial randomized to one of two arms: 1 mg E_2 (n=19) and 1 mg E_2 + 0.5 mg NETA (n=19) showed no change over time in glycemic control as measured by fasting glucose, serum free insulin, HBA1c or fructosamine. In post menopausal women with type 2 diabetes after 6 months of treatment, diabetic women receiving Activelle had a significant decrease over time in total cholesterol, LDL-cholesterol and lipoprotein (a), without modifying triglycerides or HDL-cholesterol levels.

Women with familial hyperlipidemias need special surveillance. Lipid-lowering measures are recommended additionally, before treatment is started. Women with pre-existing hypertriglyceridemia should be followed closely during estrogen replacement or hormone replacement therapy, since rare cases of large increases of plasma triglycerides leading to pancreatitis have been reported with estrogen therapy in this condition.

Calcium and Phosphorus Metabolism: Because the prolonged use of estrogens with or without progestins influences the metabolism of calcium and phosphorus, estrogens with or without progestins should be used with caution in patients with metabolic and malignant bone diseases associated with hypercalcemia and in patients with renal insufficiency.

Hypothyroidism: Patients who require thyroid hormone replacement therapy and who are also taking estrogen should have their thyroid function monitored regularly to assure that thyroid hormone levels remain in an acceptable range (see Drug Interactions, Drug-Laboratory Test Interactions).

Other Conditions: Activelle contains lactose. In patient with rare hereditary galactose intolerance, lactase deficiency or glucose-galactose malabsorption, the severity of the condition should be taken into careful consideration before prescribing Activelle. The patients should be closely monitored.

Gastrointestinal: No specific information available.

Genitourinary: Vaginal Bleeding: Breakthrough bleeding and spotting may occur during the first months of treatment. Abnormal vaginal bleeding, such as breakthrough bleeding or spotting due to its prolongation, irregularity or heaviness, occurring during therapy should prompt appropriate diagnostic measures, which may include endometrial biopsy to rule out the possibility of uterine malignancy and the treatment should be re-evaluated. If breakthrough bleeding or spotting appears after some time on therapy, or continues after treatment has been discontinued, the reason should be investigated, which may include endometrial biopsy to exclude endometrial malignancy.

Uterine Leiomyomata: Pre-existing uterine leiomyomata may increase in size during estrogen use. Growth, pain or tenderness of uterine leiomyomata requires discontinuation of medication and appropriate investigation.

Endometriosis: Symptoms and physical findings associated with a previous diagnosis of endometriosis may reappear or become aggravated with estrogen use.

Hematologic: Venous Thromboembolism: Available epidemiological data indicate that use of estrogen with or without progestin by postmenopausal women is associated with an increased risk of developing venous thromboembolism (VTE).

In the estrogen plus progestin arm of the WHI trial, among 10 000 women on combined HRT over a one-year period, there were 18 more cases of venous thromboembolism, including 8 more cases of pulmonary embolism.

In the estrogen-alone arm of the WHI trial, among 10 000 women on estrogen therapy over a one-year period, there were 7 more cases of venous thromboembolism, although there was no statistically significant difference in the rate of pulmonary embolism.

Generally recognized risk factors for VTE include a personal history, a family history (the occurrence of VTE in a direct relative at a relatively early age may indicate genetic predisposition), severe obesity (body mass index >30 kg/m²) and systemic lupus erythematosus. The risk of VTE also increases with age and smoking.

The risk of VTE may be temporarily increased with prolonged immobilization, major surgery or trauma. In women on HRT, attention should be given to prophylactic measures to prevent VTE following surgery. Also, patients with varicose veins should be closely supervised. The physician should be alert to the earliest manifestations of thrombotic disorders (thrombophlebitis, retinal thrombosis, cerebral embolism and pulmonary embolism). If these occur or are suspected, hormone therapy should be discontinued immediately, given the risks of long-term disability or fatality.

If feasible, estrogens with or without progestins should be discontinued at least 4 weeks before major surgery which may be associated with an increased risk of thromboembolism, or during periods of prolonged immobilization.

Hepatic/Biliary/Pancreatic: Gallbladder Disease: A 2- to 4-fold increase in the risk of gallbladder disease requiring surgery in women receiving postmenopausal estrogens has been reported.

Jaundice: Caution is advised in patients with a history of liver and/or biliary disorders. If cholestatic jaundice develops during treatment, the treatment should be discontinued and appropriate investigations carried out.

Liver Function Tests: Liver function tests should be done periodically in subjects who are suspected of having hepatic disease. For information on endocrine and liver function tests, see Monitoring and Laboratory Tests.

Liver Disorders: Patients who have or have previously had liver disorder such as liver adenoma should be closely supervised as this condition may recur or be aggravated during treatment with Activelle.

Immune: Systemic Lupus Erythematosus: Particular caution is indicated in women with systemic lupus erythematosus, as HRT may cause an exacerbation of this condition.

Neurologic: Cerebrovascular Insufficiency: Patients who develop visual disturbances, classical migraine, transient aphasia, paralysis or loss of consciousness should discontinue medication.

Patients with a previous history of classical migraine and who develop a recurrence or worsening of migraine symptoms should be reevaluated.

Dementia: Available epidemiological data indicate that the use of combined estrogen plus progestin in women age 65 and over may increase the risk of developing probable dementia.

The Women's Health Initiative Memory Study (WHIMS), a clinical substudy of the WHI, was designed to assess whether postmenopausal hormone replacement therapy (oral estrogen plus progestin or oral estrogen-alone) reduces the risk of dementia in women aged 65 and over (age range 65-79 years) and free of dementia at baseline.

In the estrogen plus progestin arm of the WHIMS (n=4532), women with intact uteri were treated with daily 0.625 mg conjugated equine estrogens (CEE) plus 2.5 mg medroxyprogesterone acetate (MPA) or placebo for an average of 4.05 years. The results, when extrapolated to 10 000 women treated over a one-year period showed:

- 23 more cases of probable dementia (45 on combined HRT versus 22 on placebo).

In the estrogen-alone arm of the WHIMS (n=2947), women with prior hysterectomy were treated with daily 0.625 mg CEE or placebo for an average of 5.21 years. The results, when extrapolated to 10 000 women treated over a one-year period showed:

- 12 more cases of probable dementia (37 on estrogen-alone versus 25 on placebo), although this difference did not reach statistical significance.

When data from the estrogen plus progestin arm of the WHIMS and the estrogen-alone arm of the WHIMS were combined, as per the original WHIMS protocol, in 10 000 women over a one-year period, there were:

- 18 more cases of probable dementia (41 on estrogen plus progestin or estrogen-alone versus 23 on placebo).

It is unknown whether these findings apply to younger postmenopausal women.

Epilepsy: Particular caution is indicated in women with epilepsy, as HRT may cause an exacerbation of this condition.

Ophthalmologic: See Contraindications and Warnings and Precautions, Neurologic.

Psychiatric: No specific information is available.

Renal: Fluid Retention: Estrogens with or without progestins may cause fluid retention. Therefore, particular caution is indicated in cardiac or renal dysfunction or asthma. If, in any of the above-mentioned conditions, a worsening of the underlying disease is diagnosed or suspected during treatment, the benefits and risks of treatment should be reassessed based on the individual case.

Respiratory: No specific information available.

Sensitivity/Resistance: See Contraindications.

Sexual Function/Reproduction: See Warnings and Precautions, Special Populations.

Skin: No specific information available.

Special Populations: Pregnant Women: Activelle is contraindicated during pregnancy.

If pregnancy occurs during medication with Activelle, treatment should be withdrawn immediately.

Data on a limited number of exposed pregnancies indicate adverse effects of norethindrone on the fetus. At doses higher than normally used in Oral Contraceptives (OC) and HRT formulations masculinisation of female fetuses was observed.

The results of most epidemiological studies to date relevant to inadvertent fetal exposure to combinations of estrogens and progestins indicate no teratogenic or fetotoxic effect.

Nursing Women: Activelle is contraindicated during lactation.

Pediatrics: Activelle is not indicated for use in a pediatric population. Safety and effectiveness in pediatric patients have not been established.

Geriatrics (>65 years of age): Experience in treating women older than 65 years is limited.

Monitoring and Laboratory Tests: Before Activelle is administered, the patient should have a complete physical examination including a blood pressure determination. Breasts and pelvic organs should be appropriately examined and a Papanicolaou smear should be performed. Endometrial biopsy should be done only when indicated. Baseline tests should include mammography, measurements of blood glucose, calcium, triglycerides and cholesterol, and liver function tests.

The first follow-up examination should be done within 3-6 months after initiation of treatment to assess response to treatment. Thereafter, examinations should be made at intervals at least once a year. Appropriate investigations should be arranged at regular intervals as determined by the physician.

The importance of regular self-examination of the breasts should be discussed with the patient.

ADVERSE REACTIONS: Adverse Drug Reaction Overview: See Warnings and Precautions regarding potential induction of malignant neoplasms and adverse effects similar to those of oral contraceptives.

The following adverse reactions have been reported with other estrogen/progestin combinations in general:

Blood and Lymphatic System Disorders: altered coagulation tests (see Drug Interactions, Drug-Laboratory Test Interactions).

Cardiac Disorders: palpitations; increase in blood pressure (see Warnings and Precautions); coronary thrombosis.

Endocrine Disorders: increased blood sugar levels; decreased glucose tolerance.

Eye Disorders: neuro-ocular lesions (e.g. retinal thrombosis, optic neuritis); visual disturbances; steepening of the corneal curvature; intolerance to contact lenses.

Gastrointestinal Disorders: nausea; vomiting; abdominal discomfort (cramps, pressure, pain, bloating).

General Disorders and Administration Site Conditions: fatigue; changes in appetite; changes in body weight; change in libido.

Hepatobiliary Disorders: gallbladder disorder; asymptomatic impaired liver function; cholestatic jaundice.

Musculoskeletal and Connective Tissue Disorders: musculoskeletal pain including leg pain not related to thromboembolic disease (usually transient, lasting 3-6 weeks) may occur.

Nervous System Disorders: aggravation of migraine episodes; headaches; dizziness; neuritis.

Psychiatric Disorders: mental depression; nervousness; irritability.

Renal and Urinary Disorders: cystitis; dysuria; sodium retention; edema.

Reproductive System and Breast Disorders: breakthrough bleeding; spotting; change in menstrual flow; dysmenorrhea; vaginal itching/discharge; dyspareunia; endometrial hyperplasia; pre-menstrual-like syndrome; reactivation of endometriosis; changes in cervical erosion and amount of cervical secretion; breast swelling and tenderness.

Skin and Subcutaneous Tissue Disorders: chloasma or melasma, which may persist when drug is discontinued; erythema multiforme; erythema nodosum; hemorrhagic eruption; loss of scalp hair; hirsutism and acne.

Vascular Disorders: isolated cases of: thrombophlebitis; thromboembolic disorders.

Clinical Trial Adverse Drug Reactions: Because clinical trials are conducted under very specific conditions the adverse reaction rates observed in the clinical trials may not reflect the rates observed in practice and should not be compared to the rates in the clinical trials of another drug. Adverse drug reaction information from clinical trials is useful for identifying drug-related adverse events and for approximating rates.

Adverse events reported by investigators in the Activelle Phase 3 studies regardless of causality assessment are shown in Table 1.

Table 1: Activelle

All Treatment-emergent Adverse Events Regardless of Relationship Reported at a Frequency of ≥1% with Activelle

	Activelle (n=371) %	Placebo (n=82) %
Body as a Whole, General Disorders		
Back pain	5.7	3.7
Abdominal pain	4.0	—[a]
Pain NOS	3.8	4.9
Hot flushes	3.5	4.9
Fatigue	2.2	1.2
Influenza-like symptoms	1.6	1.2
Allergic reaction	1.3	—[a]
Chest pain	1.3	1.2
Oedema peripheral	1.3	—[a]
Leg pain	1.1	2.4
Cardiovascular Disorders, General		
Hypertension	1.9	4.9
Central and Peripheral Nervous Systems Disorders		
Headache	15.6	11.0
Dizziness	1.1	1.2
Paraesthesia	1.1	—[a]
Gastrointestinal System Disorders		
Nausea	4.9	—[a]
Flatulence	3.8	3.7
Diarrhoea	3.5	1.2
Constipation	2.7	3.7
Abdominal pain	2.4	2.4
Dyspepsia	2.4	3.7
Gastroenteritis	2.2	2.4
Vomiting	1.1	
Hearing and Vestibular Disorders		
Ear disorder NOS	1.1	
Metabolic and Nutritional Disorders		
Weight increase	1.1%	3.7
Musculoskeletal System Disorders		
Arthralgia	4.3	3.7
Fracture bone	2.2	2.4
Myalgia	1.6	—[a]
Neoplasms		
Uterine fibroid	4.9	4.9
Ovarian cyst	2.7	4.9
Cervical uterine polyp	2.4	2.4
Breast neoplasm benign female	1.3	0.0
Psychiatric Disorders		
Insomnia	4.9	6.1
Depression	3.8	—[a]
Emotional lability	1.3	—[a]
Nervousness	1.3	1.2
Reproductive Disorders, Female		
Breast pain female	22.9	4.9
Post-menopausal bleeding	6.2	1.2
Breast enlargement	3.2	—[a]
Breast disorder NOS	3.0	1.2
Abdominal pain	2.2	1.2
Cervical smear test positive	2.2	—[a]
Leukorrhoea	1.6	2.4
Vaginitis	1.1	2.4
Resistance Mechanism Disorders		

(cont'd)

Table 1: Activelle *(cont'd)*

All Treatment-emergent Adverse Events Regardless of Relationship Reported at a Frequency of ≥1% with Activelle

	Activelle (n=371) %	Placebo (n=82) %
Infection NOS	2.2	1.2
Infection viral	3.8	4.9
Moniliasis genital	3.8	—[a]
Respiratory System Disorders		
Upper respiratory tract infection	17.0	13.4
Sinusitis	8.1	6.1
Bronchitis	3.2	1.2
Rhinitis	2.7	1.2
Pharyngitis	1.9	2.4
Coughing	1.3	2.4
Secondary Terms		
Injury accidental	5.9	2.4
Other evens	5.1	2.4
Cyst NOS	2.2	1.2
Skin and Appendages Disorders		
Rash	2.2	2.4
Pruritus genital	1.6	—[a]
Acne	1.3	1.2
Pruritus	1.1	2.4
Urinary System Disorders		
Haematuria	1.1	1.2
Urinary tract infection	1.1	2.4

[a] No adverse events reported.

The most frequently reported adverse events in the clinical trials with Activelle were breast pain/tenderness and headache reported in approximately 10-20% of patients.

There were no significant changes in mean body weight from baseline to the end of the trial (3 months or 12 months) in any Activelle study.

Less Common Clinical Trial Adverse Drug Reactions (<1%): Gastrointestinal: abdominal distension.
Immune System: hypersensitivity, see also Skin and Subcutaneous Tissue Disorders.
Metabolism and Nutrition: fluid retention.
Musculoskeletal, Connective Tissue and Bone: leg cramps.
Nervous System Disorders: migraine.
Skin and Subcutaneous Tissue: alopecia.
Vascular Disorders: thrombophlebitis superficial/deep; pulmonary embolism.
Abnormal Hematologic and Clinical Chemistry Findings: None of the observed changes with regard to hematology and clinical chemistry in clinical studies of Activelle were clinically relevant.
Post-Market Adverse Drug Reactions: The following events have been spontaneously reported during five years experience (i.e. 1998-2002) with Activelle in clinical practice representing a total of 2 301 955 woman-years and a reporting rate of <1/10 000 patient years.
Neoplasm Benign and Malignant: endometrial cancer.
Psychiatric Disorders: insomnia, anxiety, libido decreased, libido increased.
Nervous System Disorders: dizziness.
Eye Disorders: visual disturbances.
Vascular Disorders: hypertension aggravated.
Gastrointestinal Disorders: dyspepsia, vomiting.
Hepatobiliary Disorders: gallbladder disease, cholelithiasis, cholelithiasis aggravated, cholelithiasis re-occurrence.
Skin and Subcutaneous Disorders: seborrhea, rash, angioneurotic edema.
Reproductive System and Breast Disorders: hyperplasia endometrial, vulvovaginal pruritus.
Investigations: weight decreased, blood pressure increased.

DRUG INTERACTIONS: Overview: Estrogens are partially metabolized by cytochrome P450 3A4 (CYP3A4) as shown in vitro and in vivo studies. Therefore, estrogen drug metabolism may be affected by inducers or inhibitors of CYP3A4.

Estrogens may diminish the effectiveness of anticoagulant, antidiabetic and antihypertensive agents.

Preparations inducing liver enzymes (eg, barbiturates, hydantoins, carbamazepine, meprobamate, phenylbutazone or rifampin) may interfere with the activity of orally administered estrogens.
Drug-Drug Interactions: See Table 2.

Table 2: Activelle

Established or Potential Drug-Drug Interactions

Drug Class	Ref	Effect	Clinical comment
Anticonvulsants (e.g. phenobarbital, phenytoin, carbamazepine), anti-infectives (e.g. rifampicin, rifabutin, nevirapine, efavirenz)	C	Reduce plasma concentrations of estrogens	Therapeutic monitoring is recommended
Protease inhibitors (e.g. ritonavir, nelfinavir)	C	Increase plasma concentrations of estrogens	Therapeutic monitoring is recommended
Imidazoles (e.g. ketoconazole)	C	Increase plasma concentration of estrogens	Therapeutic monitoring is recommended

Legend: C=Case Study; CT=Clinical Trial; T=Theoretical.

Drug-Food Interactions: A single dose-study in 24 healthy postmenopausal women was conducted to investigate any potential impact of administration of Activelle with and without food.

Administration of Activelle with food did not modify the bioavailability of E_2, although food increased AUC_{0-72} for NET by 19% and decreased C_{max} for NET by 36%.

Grapefruit juice may increase plasma concentrations of estrogen.
Drug-Herb Interactions: It was found that some herbal products (e.g. St. John's wort) which are available as over-the-counter (OTC) products might interfere with steroid metabolism, and therefore alter the efficacy and safety of estrogen/progestin products.

Physicians and other health care providers should be aware of other non-prescription products concomitantly used by the patient, including herbal and natural products, obtained from the widely spread health stores.
Drug-Laboratory Test Interactions: The results of certain endocrine and liver function tests may be affected by estrogen-containing products:

- increased sulfobromophthalein retention;
- increased prothrombin time and partial thromboplastin time; increased levels of fibrinogen and fibrinogen activity; increased coagulation factors VII, VIII, IX, X; increased norepinephrine-induced platelet aggregability; decreased antithrombin III;
- increased thyroxin-binding globulin (TBG), leading to increased circulating total thyroid hormone (T_4) as measured by column or radioimmunoassay; free T_3 resin uptake is decreased, reflecting the elevated TBG; free T_4 concentration is unaltered;
- other binding proteins may be elevated in serum (eg, corticosteroid binding globulin (CBG), sex-hormone binding globulin (SHBG), leading to increased circulating corticosteroids and sex steroids respectively; free or biologically active hormone concentrations are unchanged;
- impaired glucose tolerance;
- increased serum triglycerides and phospholipids concentration.

The results of the above laboratory tests should not be considered reliable unless therapy has been discontinued for two to four weeks.

The pathologist should be informed that the patient is receiving hormone replacement therapy when relevant specimens are submitted.
Drug-Lifestyle Interactions: None identified.

DOSAGE AND ADMINISTRATION: Dosing Considerations: Activelle is a continuous combined hormone replacement therapy intended for use in women with intact uteri. For initiation and continuation of treatment of postmenopausal symptoms, the lowest effective dose for the shortest duration should be used.

In women with amenorrhea and not taking HRT or women transferring from another continuous combined HRT product, treatment with Activelle may be started on any convenient day. In women transferring from sequential HRT regimens, treatment should start right after their withdrawal bleeding has ended.
Recommended Dose and Dosage Adjustment: For the treatment of moderate to severe vasomotor symptoms, one tablet of Activelle (1 mg Estradiol and 0.5 mg Norethindrone Acetate 0.5 mg) should be taken orally once a day without interruption, preferably at the same time every day. Patients should be re-evaluated within 3-6 months after initiation of treatment, to assess response to treatment.
Missed Dose: If the patient has forgotten to take a tablet, the tablet should be taken as soon as possible within the next twelve hours. After 12 hours the tablet should be discarded and next dose taken at the normal time. Forgetting a dose may increase the likelihood of breakthrough bleeding and spotting.

OVERDOSAGE:
Symptoms of Overdose: Numerous reports of ingestion of large doses of estrogen products and estrogen-containing oral contraceptives by young children have not revealed acute serious ill effects. Over dosage with estrogen may cause nausea, breast discomfort, fluid retention, bloating or vaginal bleeding in women. Progestin (e.g. norethindrone acetate) overdosage has been characterized by depressed mood, tiredness, acne and hirsutism.
Treatment of Overdose: Overdose may be manifested by nausea and vomiting. Symptomatic treatment should be given.

> For management of a suspected drug overdose, contact your **regional Poison Control Centre**. See the *CPS* Directory section for a list of Poison Control Centres.

ACTION AND CLINICAL PHARMACOLOGY: Mechanism of Action: Estradiol: The active ingredient, synthetic estradiol, is chemically and biologically identical to endogenous human estradiol.
Norethindrone Acetate: Because estrogens promote the growth of the endometrium, unopposed estrogens increase the risk of endometrial hyperplasia and cancer. The addition of a progestin may reduces the estrogen-induced risk of endometrial hyperplasia in non-hysterectomised women.
Pharmacodynamics: Estrogen Pharmacology: Estradiol, E_2, is chemically and biologically identical to the endogenous human hormone. It is the major estrogenic hormone secreted by the human ovary which is also produced in small quantities (<20 pg/mL) in the postmenopausal woman. Among numerous effects, E_2, is responsible for the development and maintenance of the female reproductive system and secondary sex characteristics. By a direct action, it causes growth and development of the uterus, fallopian tubes, and vagina. With other hormones, such as pituitary hormones and progesterone, it causes enlargement of the breasts through promotion of ductal growth, stromal development, and the accretion of fat.

E_2 is intricately involved with other hormones, especially progesterone, in the processes of the ovulatory menstrual cycle and pregnancy and affect the release of pituitary gonadotropins. It also contributes to the shaping of the skeleton, maintenance of tone and elasticity of urogenital structures, changes in the epiphyses of the long bone that allow for the pubertal growth spurt and its termination, and pigmentation of the nipples and genitals.

Estrogen replacement therapy acts through a negative feedback pathway to reduce elevated circulating levels of luteinizing hormone (LH) and follicle-stimulating hormone (FSH) observed in postmenopausal women.
Progestin Pharmacology: Norethindrone Acetate, NETA, is a progestogen that essentially mimics the biological effects of progesterone. NETA enhances cellular differentiation and generally opposes the actions of estrogen, by decreasing estrogen receptor levels, increasing local metabolism of estrogen to less active metabolites, or by inducing gene products that blunt cellular responses to estrogen.

NETA exerts its effect in target cells by binding to specific progesterone receptors which interact with progesterone response elements in target genes. Progesterone receptors have been identified in the female reproductive tract, breast, pituitary, hypothalamus and central nervous system. NETA produces similar endometrial changes to those of the naturally occurring hormone progesterone.

Unopposed estrogen therapy in women with intact uteri is associated with an increased risk of endometrial hyperplasia and endometrial carcinoma. The concomitant use of an appropriate dose of a progestogen for an adequate time period reduces the incidence of endometrial hyperplasia and carcinoma in women with intact uteri who are receiving estrogen replacement therapy.
Pharmacokinetics: See Table 3.

Table 3: Activelle

Pharmacokinetic Parameters of Activelle After Single Dose

Component/ Metabolite	1 mg E_2/0.5 mg NETA Arithmetic Mean SD n=25
17β-estradiol (E_2)[a]	
AUC (pg/mL·h)	706±252
C_{max} (pg/mL)	29.7±9.4
t_{max} (h)	6.8±2.9
$t_{½}$ (h)	13.2 ± 4.7

(cont'd)

Table 3: Activelle *(cont'd)*

Pharmacokinetic Parameters of Activelle After Single Dose

Component/ Metabolite	1 mg E_2/0.5 mg NETA Arithmetic Mean SD n=25
Estrone (E_1)[a]	
AUC (pg/mL·h)	3741±1446
C_{max} (pg/mL)	230±89
t_{max} (h)	5.7±1.4
$t_{½}$ (h)	12.2±4.6
Norethindrone (NET)	
AUC (pg/mL·h)	23681±9023 (n=24)
C_{max} (pg/mL)	5308±1510
t_{max} (h)	1.0±0.0
$t_{½}$ (h)	11.4±2.7

[a] Baseline adjusted.

Absorption and Distribution: E_2 is well absorbed through the gastrointestinal tract. When given orally, E_2 is extensively metabolized (first pass effect) to estrone sulfate. E_2 circulates bound to sex-hormone-binding globulin (SHBG) (37%) and to albumin (61%), while only approximately 1-2% is unbound. The half-life of E_2 is about 12-14 hours following single administration. See Table 3. After oral administration NETA (norethindrone acetate) is rapidly absorbed and transformed to norethindrone (NET). The terminal half-life of NET is about 8-11 hours. NET binds to SHBG (36%) and albumin (61%).

Metabolism and Excretion: Metabolism of E_2, occurs mainly in the liver and gut but also in target organs. Complex metabolic processes result in a dynamic equilibrium of circulating conjugated and unconjugated estrogenic forms which are continually interconverted, especially between E_1 and E_2 and between esterified and nonesterified forms. A significant proportion of the circulating estrogen exists as a circulating reservoir for the formation of more active estrogenic species. A certain proportion of the estrogen is excreted into the bile and then reabsorbed from the intestine. During this enterohepatic recirculation, estrogens are desulfated and resulfated and undergo thorough conversion to less active estrogens (estriol and other estrogens), oxidation to nonestrogenic substances (catecholestrogens, which interact with catecholamine metabolism, especially in the central nervous system), and conjugation with glucuronic acids (which are then rapidly excreted in the urine). Following oral administration of Activelle, a peak plasma concentration is reached within 5-8 hours. The most important metabolites of norethindrone are isomers of 5α-dihydro-NET and of tetrahydro-NET, which are excreted mainly in the urine as sulfate or glucuronide conjugates. NETA undergoes first-pass metabolism in the liver and other enteric organs, and reaches a peak plasma concentration within 0.5-1.5 hours.

The pharmacokinetics of estradiol are not influenced by NET.

Special Populations and Conditions: Pediatrics: Activelle is not indicated for use in pediatric populations. Safety and effectiveness in pediatric patients have not been established.

Geriatrics: Experience in treating women older than 65 years is limited. The pharmacokinetics in the elderly has not been studied.

Gender: Activelle is not indicated for use in male population.

Race: No specific information available.

Hepatic Insufficiency: No specific information available.

Renal Insufficiency: No specific information available.

Genetic Polymorphism: No specific information available.

STORAGE AND STABILITY: Keep out of reach of children. Store in a dry place, protected from light. Store between 15-25°C. Do not refrigerate.

INFORMATION FOR THE PATIENT: Published in e-CPS, available by subscription at www.e-cps.ca.

DOSAGE FORMS, COMPOSITION AND PACKAGING: Each white, round, biconvex, film-coated tablet, engraved with NOVO 288 on one side and APIS on the other side, contains: estradiol 1 mg (as the hemihydrate) and norethindrone acetate 0.5 mg. Nonmedicinal ingredients: tablet core: crospovidone, lactose monohydrate, magnesium stearate, maize starch and talc; film-coating: hypromellose, talc and triacetin. Calendar dial packs of 1×28 tablets and 3×28 tablets.

Activelle® LD ℞

estradiol—norethindrone acetate

Estrogenic Hormones—Progestin

Novo Nordisk

Date of Preparation: December 31, 2007

Date of Revision: April 17, 2008

SUMMARY PRODUCT INFORMATION:

Route of Administration	Dosage Form/ Strength	Clinically Relevant Nonmedicinal Ingredients
Oral	Film-coated tablet 0.5 mg Estradiol (as hemihydrate) and 0.1 mg norethindrone acetate	Lactose monohydrate For a complete listing see Dosage Forms, Composition and Packaging.

INDICATIONS AND CLINICAL USE: Activelle LD (estradiol/norethindrone acetate) is indicated for:

- The treatment of moderate to severe vasomotor symptoms occurring in naturally or surgically induced estrogen deficiency states associated with menopause.
- The efficacy of Activelle LD in the treatment of menopausal symptoms has been studied in controlled clinical trials. As menopausal and postmenopausal symptoms tend to decrease with time, even in the absence of hormone replacement therapy, patients should be re-evaluated on a regular basis by their physicians, considering the risks and benefits of the treatment as well as effective alternatives.

Activelle LD is recommended only in women with intact uteri since the regimen includes a progestin to prevent endometrial hyperplasia.

CONTRAINDICATIONS:

- Patients with known hypersensitivity to this drug or to any ingredient in the formulation or component of the container. For a complete listing, see Dosage Forms, Composition and Packaging.
- Liver dysfunction or disease as long as liver function tests have failed to return to normal.
- Known or suspected estrogen-dependent or progestin-dependent malignant neoplasia (e.g. endometrial cancer).
- Endometrial hyperplasia.
- Known, suspected, or past history of breast cancer.
- Undiagnosed abnormal genital bleeding.
- Known or suspected pregnancy.
- Active or past history of arterial thromboembolic disease (e.g. stroke, myocardial infarction, coronary heart disease).
- Active or past history of confirmed venous thromboembolism (such as deep vein thrombosis or pulmonary embolism) or active thrombophlebitis.
- Partial or complete loss of vision due to ophthalmic vascular disease.
- Porphyria.

WARNINGS AND PRECAUTIONS:

Serious Warnings and Precautions

The Women's Health Initiative (WHI) trial examined the health benefits and risks of oral combined estrogen plus progestin therapy (n=16 608) and oral estrogen-alone therapy (n=10 739) in postmenopausal women aged 50 to 79 years.

The estrogen plus progestin arm of the WHI trial (mean age 63.3 years) indicated an increased risk of myocardial infarction (MI), stroke, invasive breast cancer, pulmonary emboli and deep vein thrombosis in postmenopausal women receiving treatment with combined conjugated equine estrogens (CEE, 0.625 mg/day) and medroxyprogesterone acetate (MPA, 2.5 mg/day) for 5.2 years compared to those receiving placebo.

The estrogen-alone arm of the WHI trial (mean age 63.3 years) indicated an increased risk of stroke and deep vein thrombosis in hysterectomized women treated with CEE-alone (0.625 mg/day) for 6.8 years compared to those receiving placebo.

Therefore, the following should be given serious consideration at the time of prescribing:

- Estrogens with or without progestins **should not** be prescribed for primary or secondary prevention of cardiovascular diseases.
- Estrogens with or without progestins should be prescribed at **the lowest effective dose** for the approved indication.
- Estrogens with or without progestins should be prescribed for **the shortest period** possible for the approved indication.

General: For the treatment of postmenopausal symptoms, HRT should only be initiated for symptoms that adversely affect quality of life. In all cases, a careful appraisal of the risks and benefits should be undertaken at least annually and HRT should only be continued as long as the benefit outweighs the risk.

Carcinogenesis and Mutagenesis: Breast Cancer: Available epidemiological data indicate that the use of combined estrogen plus progestin by postmenopausal women is associated with an increased risk of invasive breast cancer.

In the estrogen plus progestin arm of the WHI trial, among 10 000 women over a one-year period, there were:

- 8 more cases of invasive breast cancer (38 on combined HRT versus 30 on placebo).

The WHI study also reported that the invasive breast cancers diagnosed in the estrogen plus progestin group were similar in histology but were larger (mean [SD], 1.7 cm [1.1] vs 1.5 cm [0.9], respectively; P=0.04) and were at a more advanced stage compared with those diagnosed in the placebo group. The percentage of women with abnormal mammograms (recommendations for short-interval follow-up, a suspicious abnormality, or highly suggestive of malignancy) was significantly higher in the estrogen plus progestin group versus the placebo group. This difference appeared at year one and persisted in each year thereafter.

In the estrogen-alone arm of the WHI trial, there was no statistically significant difference in the rate of invasive breast cancer in hysterectomized women treated with conjugated equine estrogens versus women treated with placebo.

It is recommended that estrogens with or without progestins not be given to women with existing breast cancer or those with a previous history of the disease (see Contraindications).

There is a need for caution in prescribing estrogens with or without progestins for women with known risk factors associated with the development of breast cancer, such as strong family history of breast cancer (first degree relative) or who present a breast condition with an increased risk (abnormal mammograms and/or atypical hyperplasia at breast biopsy).

Other known risk factors for the development of breast cancer such as nulliparity, obesity, early menarche, late age at first full term pregnancy and at menopause should also be evaluated.

It is recommended that women undergo mammography prior to the start of HRT treatment and at regular intervals during treatment, as deemed appropriate by the treating physician and according to the perceived risks for each patient.

The overall benefits and possible risks of hormone replacement therapy should be fully considered and discussed with patients. It is important that the modest increased risk of being diagnosed with breast cancer after 4 years of treatment with combined estrogen plus progestin HRT (as reported in the results of the WHI trial) be discussed with the patient and weighed against its known benefits.

Instructions for regular self-examination of the breasts should be included in this counselling.

Endometrial Hyperplasia and Endometrial Carcinoma: The risk of endometrial hyperplasia and carcinoma is increased when estrogens are administered alone for prolonged periods to women with intact uteri. The role of a progestin, when combined with estrogen, is to prevent endometrial hyperplasia/carcinoma in women with intact uteri. The addition of a progestin for at least 12 days per cycle in non-hysterectomised women greatly reduces this risk.

In the WHI study, endometrial cancer rates were low and were not increased by 5 years of estrogen plus progestin exposure (hazard ratio 0.83 [adjusted 95% CI 0.29-2.32]). Because endometrial cancer has a relatively low incidence rate, the incidence of endometrial hyperplasia is used as a surrogate endpoint in clinical studies.

In a double-blind, randomised, multi-center study, 1176 healthy postmenopausal women aged 44 years and older without evidence of endometrial abnormalities were given 12 months of treatment with continuous combined regimens of 1 mg E2 with three different doses of norethindrone acetate (NETA; 0.1 mg, 0.25 mg, 0.5 mg). All three doses, have shown similar incidences of endometrial hyperplasia at the end of 12 month study, and were significantly better at reducing the incidence of endometrial hyperplasia relative to E2 alone (p<0.001), based on 988 endometrial biopsies.

A second study assessed the endometrial thickness resulting from treatment with Activelle LD (0.5 mg E2/0.1 mg NETA; n=185) versus a formulation containing 0.5 mg E2/0.25 mg NETA (n=173) or placebo (n=177). At 24 weeks, there were no differences between the groups in mean change of endometrial thickness, as evaluated by transvaginal ultrasound.

Ovarian Cancer: Some recent epidemiologic studies have found that the use of hormone replacement therapy (estrogen-alone and estrogen plus progestin therapies), in particular for five or more years, has been associated with an increased risk of ovarian cancer.

Cardiovascular: The results of the Heart and Estrogen/progestin Replacement Studies (HERS and HERS II) and the Women's Health Initiative (WHI) trial indicate that the use of estrogen plus progestin is associated with an increased risk of coronary heart disease (CHD) in postmenopausal women. The results of the WHI trial indicate that the use of estrogen-alone and estrogen plus progestin is associated with an increased risk of stroke in postmenopausal women.

WHI Trial Findings: In the combined estrogen plus progestin arm of the WHI trial, among 10 000 women over a one-year period, there were:

- 8 more cases of stroke (29 on combined HRT versus 21 on placebo)
- 7 more cases of CHD (37 on combined HRT versus 30 on placebo).

In the estrogen-alone arm of the WHI trial of women with prior hysterectomy, among 10 000 women over a one-year period, there were/was:

- 12 more cases of stroke (44 on estrogen-alone therapy versus 32 on placebo)
- no statistically significant difference in the rate of CHD.

HERS and HERS II Findings: In the Heart and Estrogen/progestin Replacement Study (HERS) of postmenopausal women with documented heart disease (n=2763, average age 66.7 years), a randomized placebo-controlled clinical trial of secondary prevention of coronary heart disease (CHD), treatment with 0.625 mg/day oral conjugated equine estrogen (CEE) plus 2.5 mg oral medroxyprogesterone acetate (MPA) demonstrated no cardiovascular benefit. Specifically, during an average follow-up of 4.1 years, treatment with CEE plus MPA did not reduce the overall rate of CHD events in postmenopausal women with established coronary heart disease. There were more CHD events in the hormone-treated group than in the placebo group in year 1, but not during the subsequent years.

From the original HERS trial, 2321 women consented to participate in an open label extension of HERS known as HERS II. Average follow-up in HERS II was an additional 2.7 years, for a total of 6.8 years overall. After 6.8 years, hormone therapy did not reduce the risk of cardiovascular events in women with CHD.

Blood Pressure: Women using hormone replacement therapy sometimes experience increased blood pressure. Blood pressure should be monitored with HRT use. Elevation of blood pressure in previously normotensive or hypertensive patients should be investigated and HRT may have to be discontinued.

Ear/Nose/Throat: Estrogens should be used with caution in patients with otosclerosis.

Endocrine and Metabolism: Glucose and Lipid Metabolism: A worsening of glucose tolerance and lipid metabolism have been observed in a significant percentage of peri- and post-menopausal patients. Therefore, diabetic patients or those with a predisposition to diabetes should be observed closely to detect any alterations in carbohydrate or lipid metabolism, especially in triglyceride blood levels.

Women with familial hyperlipidemias need special surveillance. Lipid-lowering measures are recommended additionally, before treatment is started. Women with pre-existing hypertriglyceridemia should be followed closely during estrogen replacement or hormone replacement therapy, since rare cases of large increases of plasma triglycerides leading to pancreatitis have been reported with estrogen therapy in this condition.

Calcium and Phosphorus Metabolism: Because the prolonged use of estrogens with or without progestins influences the metabolism of calcium and phosphorus, estrogens with or without progestins should be used with caution in patients with metabolic and malignant bone diseases associated with hypercalcemia and in patients with renal insufficiency.

Hypothyroidism: Patients who require thyroid hormone replacement therapy and who are also taking estrogen should have their thyroid function monitored regularly to assure that thyroid hormone levels remain in an acceptable range (see Drug Interactions, Drug-Laboratory Test Interactions).

Other Conditions: Activelle LD contains lactose. In patient with rare hereditary galactose intolerance, lactase deficiency or glucose-galactose malabsorption, the severity of the condition should be taken into careful consideration before prescribing Activelle LD tablets. The patients should be closely monitored.

Gastrointestinal: No specific information available.

Genitourinary: Vaginal Bleeding: Breakthrough bleeding and spotting may occur during the first months of treatment. Abnormal vaginal bleeding, such as breakthrough bleeding or spotting due to its prolongation, irregularity or heaviness, occurring during therapy should prompt appropriate diagnostic measures, which may include endometrial biopsy to rule out the possibility of uterine malignancy and the treatment should be re-evaluated. If breakthrough bleeding or spotting appears after some time on therapy, or continues after treatment has been discontinued, the reason should be investigated, which may include endometrial biopsy to exclude endometrial malignancy.

Uterine Leiomyomata: Pre-existing uterine leiomyomata may increase in size during estrogen use. Growth, pain or tenderness of uterine leiomyomata requires discontinuation of medication and appropriate investigation.

Endometriosis: Symptoms and physical findings associated with a previous diagnosis of endometriosis may reappear or become aggravated with estrogen use.

Hematologic: Venous Thromboembolism: Available epidemiological data indicate that use of estrogen with or without progestin by postmenopausal women is associated with an increased risk of developing venous thromboembolism (VTE).

In the estrogen plus progestin arm of the WHI trial, among 10 000 women on combined HRT over a one-year period, there were 18 more cases of venous thromboembolism, including 8 more cases of pulmonary embolism.

In the estrogen-alone arm of the WHI trial, among 10 000 women on estrogen therapy over a one-year period, there were 7 more cases of venous thromboembolism, although there was no statistically significant difference in the rate of pulmonary embolism.

Generally recognized risk factors for VTE include a personal history, a family history (the occurrence of VTE in a direct relative at a relatively early age may indicate genetic predisposition), severe obesity (body mass index >30 kg/m^2) and systemic lupus erythematosus. The risk of VTE also increases with age and smoking.

The risk of VTE may be temporarily increased with prolonged immobilization, major surgery or trauma. In women on HRT, attention should be given to prophylactic measures to prevent VTE following surgery. Also, patients with varicose veins should be closely supervised. The physician should be alert to the earliest manifestations of thrombotic disorders (thrombophlebitis, retinal thrombosis, cerebral embolism and pulmonary embolism). If these occur or are suspected, hormone therapy should be discontinued immediately, given the risks of long-term disability or fatality.

If feasible, estrogens with or without progestins should be discontinued at least 4 to 6 weeks before major surgery which may be associated with an increased risk of thromboembolism such as abdominal or orthopaedic surgery to lower limbs, or during periods of prolonged immobilization. Treatment should not be restarted until the woman is completely mobilised.

Hepatic/Biliary/Pancreatic: Gallbladder Diseases: A 2- to 4-fold increase in the risk of gallbladder disease requiring surgery in women receiving postmenopausal estrogens has been reported.

Jaundice: Caution is advised in patients with a history of liver and/or biliary disorders. If cholestatic jaundice develops during treatment, the treatment should be discontinued and appropriate investigations carried out.

Liver Function Tests: Liver function tests should be done periodically in subjects who are suspected of having hepatic disease. For information on endocrine and liver function tests, see Monitoring and Laboratory Tests.

Liver Disorders: Patients who have or have previously had liver disorder such as liver adenoma should be closely supervised as this condition may recur or be aggravated during treatment with Activelle LD.

Immune: Systemic Lupus Erythematosus: Particular caution is indicated in women with systemic lupus erythematosus, as HRT may cause an exacerbation of this condition.

Neurologic: Cerebrovascular Insufficiency: Patients who develop visual disturbances, classical migraine, transient aphasia, paralysis or loss of consciousness should discontinue medication.

Patients with a previous history of classical migraine and who develop a recurrence or worsening of migraine symptoms should be reevaluated.

Dementia: Available epidemiological data indicate that the use of combined estrogen plus progestin in women age 65 and over may increase the risk of developing probable dementia.

The Women's Health Initiative Memory Study (WHIMS), a clinical substudy of the WHI, was designed to assess whether postmenopausal hormone replacement therapy (oral estrogen plus progestin or oral estrogen-alone) reduces the risk of dementia in women aged 65 and over (age range 65-79 years) and free of dementia at baseline.

In the estrogen plus progestin arm of the WHIMS (n=4532), women with intact uteri were treated with daily 0.625 mg conjugated equine estrogens (CEE) plus 2.5 mg medroxyprogesterone acetate (MPA) or placebo for an average of 4.05 years. The results, when extrapolated to 10 000 women treated over a one-year period showed:

- 23 more cases of probable dementia (45 on combined HRT versus 22 on placebo).

In the estrogen-alone arm of the WHIMS (n=2947), women with prior hysterectomy were treated with daily 0.625 mg CEE or placebo for an average of 5.21 years. The results, when extrapolated to 10 000 women treated over a one-year period showed:

- 12 more cases of probable dementia (37 on estrogen-alone versus 25 on placebo), although this difference did not reach statistical significance.

When data from the estrogen plus progestin arm of the WHIMS and the estrogen-alone arm of the WHIMS were combined, as per the original WHIMS protocol, in 10 000 women over a one-year period, there were:

- 18 more cases of probable dementia (41 on estrogen plus progestin or estrogen-alone versus 23 on placebo).

It is unknown whether these findings apply to younger postmenopausal women.

Epilepsy: Particular caution is indicated in women with epilepsy, as HRT may cause an exacerbation of this condition.

Ophthalmologic: See Contraindications and Warnings and Precautions, Neurologic.

Psychiatric: No specific information available.

Renal: Fluid Retention: Estrogens with or without progestins may cause fluid retention. Therefore, particular caution is indicated in cardiac or renal dysfunction or asthma. If, in any of the above-mentioned conditions, a worsening of the underlying disease is diagnosed or suspected during treatment, the benefits and risks of treatment should be reassessed based on the individual case.

Respiratory: No specific information available.

Sensitivity/Resistance: See Contraindications.

Sexual Function/Reproduction: See Warnings and Precautions, Special Populations.

Skin: No specific information available.

Special Populations: Pregnant Women: Activelle LD is contraindicated during pregnancy.

If pregnancy occurs during medication with Activelle LD tablets, treatment should be withdrawn immediately.

Data on a limited number of exposed pregnancies indicate adverse effects of norethindrone on the fetus. At doses higher than normally used in Oral Contraceptives (OC) and HRT formulations masculinisation of female fetuses was observed.

The results of most epidemiological studies to date relevant to inadvertent fetal exposure to combinations of estrogens and progestins indicate no teratogenic or fetotoxic effect.

Nursing Women: Activelle LD should not be used during lactation.

Pediatrics: Activelle LD tablets are not indicated for use in a pediatric population. Safety and effectiveness in pediatric patients have not been established.

Geriatrics (>65 years of age): Experience in treating women older than 65 years is limited.

Monitoring and Laboratory Tests: Before Activelle LD is administered, the patient should have a complete physical examination including a blood pressure determination. Breasts and pelvic organs should be appropriately examined and a Papanicolaou smear should be performed. Endometrial biopsy should be done only when indicated. Baseline tests should include mammography, measurements of blood glucose, calcium, triglycerides and cholesterol, and liver function tests.

The first follow-up examination should be done within 3-6 months after initiation of treatment to assess response to treatment. Thereafter, examinations should be made at intervals at least once a year. Appropriate investigations should be arranged at regular intervals as determined by the physician.

The importance of regular self-examination of the breasts should be discussed with the patient.

ADVERSE REACTIONS: Adverse Drug Reaction Overview: See Warnings and Precautions regarding potential induction of malignant neoplasms and adverse effects similar to those of oral contraceptives.

The following adverse reactions have been reported with estrogen/progestin combination in general:

Blood and Lymphatic System Disorders: Altered coagulation tests (see Warnings and Precautions and Drug Interactions, Drug-Laboratory Test Interactions).

Cardiac Disorders: palpitations; increase in blood pressure (see Warnings and Precautions); coronary thrombosis.

Endocrine Disorders: increased blood sugar levels; decreased glucose tolerance.

Eye Disorders: neuro-ocular lesions (e.g. retinal thrombosis, optic neuritis); visual disturbances; steepening of the corneal curvature; intolerance to contact lenses.

Gastrointestinal Disorders: nausea; vomiting; abdominal discomfort (cramps, pressure, pain, bloating).

General Disorders and Administration Site Conditions: fatigue; changes in appetite; changes in body weight; change in libido.

Hepatobiliary Disorders: gallbladder disorder; asymptomatic impaired liver function; cholestatic jaundice.

Musculoskeletal and Connective Tissue Disorders: Musculoskeletal pain including leg pain not related to thromboembolic disease (usually transient, lasting 3-6 weeks) may occur.

Nervous System Disorders: aggravation of migraine episodes; headaches; dizziness; neuritis.

Psychiatric Disorders: mental depression; nervousness; irritability.

Renal and Urinary Disorders: cystitis; dysuria; sodium retention; edema.

Reproductive System and Breast Disorders: breakthrough bleeding; spotting; change in menstrual flow; dysmenorrhea; vaginal itching/discharge; dyspareunia; endometrial hyperplasia; pre-menstrual-like syndrome; reactivation of endometriosis; changes in cervical erosion and amount of cervical secretion; breast swelling and tenderness.

Skin and Subcutaneous Tissue Disorders: chloasma or melasma, which may persist when drug is discontinued; erythema multiforme; erythema nodosum; hemorrhagic eruption; loss of scalp hair; hirsutism and acne.

Vascular Disorders: Isolated cases of: thrombophlebitis; thromboembolic disorders.

Clinical Trial Adverse Drug Reactions: Because clinical trials are conducted under very specific conditions the adverse drug reaction rates observed in the clinical trials may not reflect the rates observed in practice and should not be compared to the rates in the clinical trials of another drug. Adverse drug reaction information from clinical trials is useful for identifying drug-related adverse events and for approximating rates.

Adverse events reported by investigators in the Activelle LD pivotal trial at a frequency of ≥1% are shown in Table 1. The regimens evaluated Activelle LD over a 6-month treatment period.

Table 1: Activelle LD

Treatment-emergent Adverse Events with Possible or Probable Relationship Reported at a Frequency of ≥1% with Activelle LD

	Activelle LD (n=194) %	Placebo (n=200) %
Gastrointestinal Disorders		
Nausea	3	2
Dyspepsia	2	—[a]
Abdominal distension	1	—[a]
Abdominal pain	1	2
Diarrhea	1	—[a]
Musculoskeletal and Connective Tissue		
Back pain	1	—[a]
Nervous System		
Headache	11	8
Dizziness	1	—[a]
Vascular Disorders		
Vaginal hemorrhage	25	12
Hot flush	2	3
Urogenital/Reproductive System		
Endometrial thickening	9	4
Uterine leiomyoma	3	2
Ovarian cyst	2	—[a]
Vaginal discharge	1	—[a]
Breast pain	1	—[a]
Vulvovaginal mycotic infection	1	—[a]
Uterine polyp	1	—[a]

[a] No adverse events reported.

The most frequently reported adverse events in the clinical trials with Activelle LD tablets were vaginal hemorrhage (any release of blood from uterus), endometrial thickening (double layer measured at ≥5 mm) and headache. The majority of AEs occurred with similar frequency in the treatment groups and were classified as mild or moderate in severity. As expected, the incidence of vaginal bleeding was higher in the continuous combined treatment groups Activelle LD (25%) than in the placebo group (12%).

There were no reports of thromboembolic events in any treatment group. Clinically important symptoms related to the breast (breast discomfort, breast pain and tenderness) were reported by <2% of subjects treated with the Activelle LD regimens, which was comparable with the placebo group.

Less Common Clinical Trial Adverse Drug Reactions (<1%): Gastrointestinal: abdominal pain upper; constipation; epigastric discomfort; gastritis; stomach discomfort.

General and Administration Site Conditions: malaise; suprapubic pain.

Musculoskeletal, Connective Tissue and Bone: musculoskeletal stiffness; neck pain; pain in extremity.

Nervous System Disorders: migraine; disturbance in attention; mental impairment; restless legs syndrome; stress incontinence.

Reproductive System and Breast: breast tenderness; breast discomfort; vulvovaginal dryness; cervical cyst.

Skin and Subcutaneous Tissue: pruritus genital; acne; skin irritation.

Cardiac Disorders: chest discomfort; chest pain.

Vascular Disorders: hypertension; varicose vein.

Respiratory, Thoracic and Mediastinal Disorders: epistaxis.

Renal and Urinary Disorders: fluid retention; urinary retention.
Infections and Infestations: salpingitis; vaginal candidiasis.
Other: post procedural haemorrhage; liver function test abnormal.
Abnormal Hematologic and Clinical Chemistry Findings: None of the observed changes with regard to hematology and clinical chemistry in clinical studies of Activelle LD were clinically relevant.
Post-Market Adverse Drug Reactions: No data is available.

If adverse symptoms persist, the prescription of HRT should be re-considered.

DRUG INTERACTIONS: Overview: Estrogens are partially metabolized by cytochrome P450 3A4 (CYP3A4) as shown in vitro and in vivo studies. Therefore, estrogen drug metabolism may be affected by inducers or inhibitors of CYP3A4.

Estrogens may diminish the effectiveness of anticoagulant, antidiabetic and antihypertensive agents.

Preparations inducing liver enzymes (e.g. barbiturates, hydantoins, carbamazepine, meprobamates, phenylbutazone or rifampicin) may interfere with the activity of orally administered estrogens.
Drug-Drug Interactions: See Table 2.

Table 2: Activelle LD

Established or Potential Drug-Drug Interactions

Drug Class	Ref	Effect	Clinical Comment
Anticonvulsants (e.g. phenobarbital, phenytoin, carbamazepine), anti-infectives (e.g. rifampicin, rifabutin, nevirapine, efavirenz)	C	Reduce plasma concentrations of estrogens	Therapeutic monitoring is recommended
Protease inhibitors (e.g. ritonavir, nelfinavir)	C	Increase plasma concentrations of estrogens	Therapeutic monitoring is recommended
Imidazoles (e.g. ketoconazole)	C	Increase plasma concentration of estrogens	Therapeutic monitoring is recommended

Legend: C=case study; CT=clinical trial; T=theoretical.

Drug-Food Interactions: Grapefruit juice may increase plasma concentrations of estrogen.
Drug-Herb Interactions: It was found that some herbal products (e.g. St. John's wort) which are available as over-the-counter (OTC) products might interfere with steroid metabolism and therefore alter the efficacy and safety of estrogen/progestin products.

Physicians and other health care providers should be made aware of other non-prescription products concomitantly used by the patient, including herbal and natural products obtained from the widely spread health stores.
Drug-Laboratory Test Interactions: The results of certain endocrine and liver function tests may be affected by estrogen-containing products:

- increased prothrombin time and partial thromboplastin time; increased levels of fibrinogen and fibrinogen activity; increased coagulation factors VII, VIII, IX, X; increased norepinephrine-induced platelet aggregability; decreased antithrombin III;
- increased thyroxine-binding globulin (TBG), leading to increased circulating total thyroid hormone (T4) as measured by column or radioimmunoassay; T3 resin uptake is decreased, reflecting the elevated TBG; free T4 concentration is unaltered;
- other binding proteins may be elevated in serum i.e., corticosteroid binding globulin (CBG), sex-hormone binding globulin (SHBG), leading to increased circulating corticosteroids and sex steroids respectively; free or biologically active hormone concentrations are unchanged;
- impaired glucose tolerance;
- increased serum triglycerides and phospholipids concentration.

The results of the above laboratory tests should not be considered reliable unless therapy has been discontinued for two to four weeks.

The pathologist should be informed that the patient is receiving hormone replacement therapy (HRT) when relevant specimens are submitted.
Drug-Lifestyle Interactions: None identified.

DOSAGE AND ADMINISTRATION: Dosing Considerations: Activelle LD tablet is a low dose continuous combined hormone replacement therapy intended for use in women with intact uteri. For initiation and continuation of treatment of post-menopausal symptoms, the lowest effective dose for the shortest duration should be used.

In women with amenorrhea and not taking HRT or women transferring from another continuous combined HRT product, treatment with Activelle LD tablets may be started on any convenient day. In women transferring from sequential HRT regimens, treatment should start right after their withdrawal bleeding has ended.
Recommended Dose and Dosage Adjustment: For the treatment of moderate to severe vasomotor symptoms, one tablet of Activelle LD (estradiol 0.5 mg and norethindrone acetate 0.1 mg) should be taken orally once a day without interruption, preferably at the same time every day. Patients should be re-evaluated within 3-6 months after initiation of treatment, to assess response to treatment.
Missed Dose: If the patient has forgotten to take a tablet, the tablet should be taken as soon as possible within the next twelve hours. After 12 hours the tablet should be discarded and next dose taken at the normal time. Forgetting a dose may increase the likelihood of breakthrough bleeding and spotting.

OVERDOSAGE:
Symptoms of Overdose: Numerous reports of ingestion of large doses of estrogen products and estrogen-containing oral contraceptives by young children have not revealed acute serious ill effects. Over dosage with estrogen may cause nausea, breast discomfort, fluid retention, bloating or vaginal bleeding in women. Progestin (e.g. norethindrone acetate) overdosage has been characterized by depressed mood, tiredness, acne and hirsutism.
Treatment of Overdose: Overdose may be manifested by nausea and vomiting. Treatment should be symptomatic.

For management of a suspected drug overdose, contact your **regional Poison Control Centre**. See the *CPS* Directory section for a list of Poison Control Centres.

ACTION AND CLINICAL PHARMACOLOGY: Mechanism of Action: Estradiol: The active ingredient, synthetic estradiol, is chemically and biologically identical to endogenous human estradiol.
Norethindrone Acetate: Because estrogens promote the growth of the endometrium, unopposed estrogens increase the risk of endometrial hyperplasia and cancer. The addition of a progestin may reduce the estrogen-induced risk of endometrial hyperplasia in non-hysterectomised women.
Pharmacodynamics: Estrogen Pharmacology: Estradiol, E_2, is chemically and biologically identical to the endogenous human hormone. It is the major estrogenic hormone secreted by the human ovary which is also produced in small quantities (<20 pg/mL) in the postmenopausal woman. Among numerous effects, E_2, is responsible for the development and maintenance of the female reproductive system and secondary sex characteristics. By a direct action, it causes growth and development of the uterus, fallopian tubes, and vagina. With other hormones, such as pituitary hormones and progesterone, it causes enlargement of the breasts through promotion of ductal growth, stromal development, and the accretion of fat. E_2 is intricately involved with other hormones, especially progesterone, in the processes of the ovulatory menstrual cycle and pregnancy and affect the release of pituitary gonadotropins. It also contributes to the shaping of the skeleton, maintenance of tone and elasticity of urogenital structures, changes in the epiphyses of the long bone that allow for the pubertal growth spurt and its termination, and pigmentation of the nipples and genitals.

Estrogen replacement therapy acts through a negative feedback pathway to reduce elevated circulating levels of luteinizing hormone (LH) and follicle-stimulating hormone (FSH) observed in postmenopausal women.
Progestin Pharmacology: Norethindrone Acetate, NETA, is a progestogen that essentially mimics the biological effects of progesterone. NETA enhances cellular differentiation and generally opposes the actions of estrogen, by decreasing estrogen receptor levels, increasing local metabolism of estrogen to less active metabolites, or by inducing gene products that blunt cellular responses to estrogen.

NETA exerts its effect in target cells by binding to specific progesterone receptors which interact with progesterone response elements in target genes. Progesterone receptors have been identified in the female reproductive tract, breast, pituitary, hypothalamus and central nervous system. NETA produces similar endometrial changes to those of the naturally occurring hormone progesterone.

Unopposed estrogen therapy in women with intact uteri is associated with an increased risk of endometrial hyperplasia and endometrial carcinoma. The concomitant use of an appropriate dose of a progestogen for an adequate time period reduces the incidence of endometrial hyperplasia and carcinoma in women with intact uteri who are receiving estrogen replacement therapy.
Pharmacokinetics: See Table 3.

Table 3: Activelle LD

Pharmacokinetic Parameters After Administration of 2 Tablets of Activelle LD to Healthy Postmenopausal Women

	2 × Activelle LD (n=24) Mean[a] (% CV)[b]
Estradiol[c] (E_2)	
AUC_{0-t} (pg/mL·h)	697.3 (53)
C_{max} (pg/mL)	26.5 (37)
t_{max} (h): median (range)	6.5 (0.5–16.0)
$t_{1/2}$ (h)[d]	14.5[e] (27)
Estrone[c] (E_1)	
AUC_{0-t} (pg/mL·h)	4469.1 (48)
C_{max} (pg/mL)	195.5 (37)
t_{max} (h): median (range)	6.0 (1.0–9.0)
$t_{1/2}$ (h)[d]	10.7 (44)[f]
Norethindrone (NET)	
AUC_{0-t} (pg/mL·h)	8407.2 (43)
C_{max} (pg/mL)	2375.4 (41)
t_{max} (h): median (range)	0.8 (0.7–1.3)
$t_{1/2}$ (h)	11.4 (36)[g]

[a] Geometric mean.
[b] Geometric % coefficient of variation.
[c] Baseline unadjusted data.
[d] Baseline adjusted data.
[e] n=16.
[f] n=13.
[g] n=21.
Legend: AUC=area under the curve, 0=last quantifiable sample; C_{max}=maximum plasma concentration; t_{max}=time at maximum plasma concentration; $t_{1/2}$=half-life.

Absorption and Distribution: Following oral administration of Activelle LD tablets, estradiol in micronized form, rapid absorption from the gastrointestinal tract occurs. The half-life of estradiol is about 15 hours. It circulates bound to sex hormone binding globulin (SHBG) (37%) and to albumin (61%), while only approximately 1-2% is unbound.

After oral administration of an Activelle LD tablet, norethindrone acetate is rapidly absorbed and transformed to norethindrone (NET). The terminal half-life of NET is about 9-11 hours. NET binds to SHBG (36%) and to albumin (61%).
Metabolism and Excretion: After rapid absorption from the gastrointestinal tract, estradiol undergoes a first-pass metabolism in the liver and other enteric organs, and reaches a peak plasma concentration of approximately 24 pg/mL (CV 38 %) (after administration of two Activelle LD tablets) within 5-8 hours.

Metabolism of estradiol, occurs mainly in the liver and gut but also in target organs, and involves the formation of less active or inactive metabolites, including estrone, catecholestrogens and several estrogen sulphates and glucuronides. Estrogens are excreted with the bile, where they are hydrolysed and reabsorbed (enterohepatic circulation), and mainly in urine in biologically inactive form.

After absorption, norethindrone undergoes first-pass metabolism in the liver and other enteric organs, and reaches a peak plasma concentration of approximately 2.4 ng/mL (CV 41 %) (after administration of two Activelle LD tablets) within 0.5-1.5 hour. The most important metabolites of norethindrone are isomers of 5α-dihydro-NET and of tetrahydro-NET, which are excreted mainly in the urine as sulfate or glucuronide conjugates.

The pharmacokinetics of estradiol are not influenced by NET.
Special Populations and Conditions: Pediatrics: Activelle LD tablets are not indicated for use in a pediatric population. Safety and effectiveness in pediatric patients have not been established.
Geriatrics: Experience in treating women older than 65 years is limited. The pharmacokinetics in the elderly has not been studied.
Gender: Activelle LD tablets are not indicated for use in a male population.
Race: No specific information available.
Hepatic Insufficiency: No specific information available.
Renal Insufficiency: No specific information available.
Genetic Polymorphism: No specific information available.
STORAGE AND STABILITY: Keep out of reach of children. Store in a dry place, protected from light. Store between 15-25°C. Do not refrigerate.
INFORMATION FOR THE PATIENT: Published in e-CPS, available by subscription at www.e-cps.ca.
DOSAGE FORMS, COMPOSITION AND PACKAGING: Each white, round, biconvex, film-coated tablet, engraved with NOVO 291 on one side and APIS on the other side, contains: estradiol 0.5 mg (as the hemihydrate) and norethindrone acetate 0.1 mg. Nonmedicinal ingredients: tablet core: hydroxypropylcellulose, lactose monohydrate, magnesium stearate, maize starch and talc; film-coating: hypromellose, talc and triacetin. Calendar dial packs of 1×28 tablets and 3×28 tablets.

The reader is invited to consult CPhA's monograph **Bisphosphonates: Oral.**

Actonel® Pr

risedronate sodium hemi-pentahydrate

Bone Metabolism Regulator

Warner Chilcott

Date of Revision: February 16, 2010

SUMMARY PRODUCT INFORMATION:

Route of Administration	Dosage Form/ Strength	Clinically Relevant Nonmedicinal Ingredients
Oral	Tablet 5 mg, 30 mg, 35 mg, 75 mg and 150 mg	Lactose monohydrate (5 mg, 30 mg, and 35 mg only) For a complete listing see Dosage Forms, Composition and Packaging.

INDICATIONS AND CLINICAL USE: ACTONEL (risedronate sodium hemi-pentahydrate) is indicated for:
- the treatment and prevention of osteoporosis in post-menopausal women
- the treatment of osteoporosis in men, to improve bone mineral density
- the treatment and prevention of glucocorticoid-induced osteoporosis in men and women
- Paget's disease of bone

Postmenopausal Osteoporosis: In the treatment of osteoporosis in postmenopausal women, ACTONEL prevents vertebral and nonvertebral osteoporosis-related fractures and increases bone mineral density (BMD) at all measured skeletal sites of clinical importance for osteoporotic fractures, including spine, hip, and wrist.

Osteoporosis may be confirmed by the presence or history of osteoporotic fracture, or by the finding of low bone mass (e.g., at least 2 standard deviation [SD] below the premenopausal mean).

For the prevention of osteoporosis in postmenopausal women who are at risk of developing osteoporosis, ACTONEL preserves or increases BMD at sites of clinical importance.

ACTONEL may be considered in postmenopausal women who are at risk of developing osteoporosis and for whom the desired clinical outcome is to maintain bone mass and to reduce the risk of fracture.

Factors such as family history of osteoporosis (particularly maternal history), previous fracture, smoking, moderately low BMD, high bone turnover, thin body frame, Caucasian or Asian race, and early menopause are associated with an increased risk of developing osteoporosis and fractures.

Paget's Disease of Bone: ACTONEL is indicated for patients with Paget's disease of bone (osteitis deformans) having alkaline phosphatase levels at least two times the upper limit of normal, or who are symptomatic, or who are at risk for future complications from their disease, to induce remission (normalization of serum alkaline phosphatase).

Geriatrics: In the daily, weekly and monthly postmenopausal osteoporosis dosing studies, 35-43% of patients who received ACTONEL were between 65 and 75 years of age and 12-23% were over 75 years of age. The corresponding proportions were 26% and 11% in glucocorticoid-induced osteoporosis trials. In the male osteoporosis study, 27% of patients receiving ACTONEL were between 65 and 75 years of age and 10% were ≥75 years.

Based upon the above study populations, no overall differences in efficacy or safety were observed between these patients and younger patients (<65 years).

Pediatrics: Safety and efficacy in children and growing adolescents have not been established.

CONTRAINDICATIONS:
- Patients who are hypersensitive to this drug or to any ingredient in the formulation. For a complete listing, see Dosage Forms, Composition and Packaging.
- Hypocalcemia (see Warnings and Precautions, General).

WARNINGS AND PRECAUTIONS: General: Hypocalcemia and other disturbances of bone and mineral metabolism should be effectively treated before starting ACTONEL (risedronate sodium) therapy.

Adequate intake of calcium and vitamin D is important in all patients, especially in patients with Paget's disease in whom bone turnover is significantly elevated (see Drug Interactions).

Osteonecrosis of the Jaw: In post-marketing reporting, osteonecrosis of the jaw has been reported in patients treated with bisphosphonates. The majority of reports occurred following dental procedures such as tooth extractions and have involved cancer patients treated with intravenous bisphosphonates, but some occurred in patients receiving oral treatment for postmenopausal osteoporosis and other diagnoses. Many had signs of local infection, including osteomyelitis. Osteonecrosis has other well documented multiple risk factors. It is not possible to determine if these events are related to bisphosphonates, to concomitant drugs or other therapies, to the patient's underlying disease or to other co-morbid risk factors (e.g. anemia, infection, pre-existing oral disease). A dental examination with appropriate preventative dentistry should be considered prior to treatment with bisphosphonates in patients with concomitant risk factors (e.g., cancer, immune suppression, head and neck radiotherapy or poor oral hygiene). While on treatment, these patients should avoid invasive dental procedures if possible. For patients requiring dental procedures, there are no data available to suggest whether discontinuation of bisphosphonate treatment prior to the procedure reduces the risk of osteonecrosis of the jaw. Clinical judgment, based on individual risk assessment, should guide the management of patients undergoing dental procedures.

Musculoskeletal: In postmarketing experience, severe and occasionally incapacitating bone, joint and/or muscle pain has been reported in patients taking bisphosphonates (see Adverse Reactions). The time to onset of symptoms varied from one day to several months after starting the drug. Most patients had relief of symptoms after stopping the medication. A subset of patients had recurrence of symptoms when rechallenged with the same drug or another bisphosphonate. Consider discontinuing use if severe symptoms develop.

Gastrointestinal: Bisphosphonates may cause upper gastrointestinal (GI) disorders such as dysphagia, esophagitis, esophageal ulcer, and gastric ulcer (see Adverse Reactions). Since some bisphosphonates have been associated with esophagitis and esophageal ulcerations, to facilitate delivery to the stomach and minimize the risk of these events, patients should take ACTONEL while in an upright position (i.e., sitting or standing) and with sufficient plain water (≥120 mL). Patients should not lie down for at least 30 minutes after taking the drug. Health professionals should be particularly careful to emphasize the importance of the dosing instructions to patients with a history of esophageal disorders (e.g., inflammation, stricture, ulcer, or disorders of motility).

Renal: ACTONEL is not recommended for use in patients with severe renal impairment (creatinine clearance <30 mL/min).

Special Populations: Pregnant Women: ACTONEL is not intended for use during pregnancy. There are no studies of ACTONEL in pregnant women.

Nursing Women: ACTONEL is not intended for use with nursing mothers. It is not known whether risedronate is excreted in human milk. Risedronate was detected in feeding pups exposed to lactating rats for a 24-hour period post-dosing, indicating a small degree of lacteal transfer. Since many drugs are excreted in human milk and because of the potential for serious adverse reactions in nursing infants from bisphosphonates, a decision should be made whether to discontinue nursing or to discontinue the drug, taking into account the importance of the drug to the mother.

Pediatrics: The safety and efficacy of ACTONEL in children and growing adolescents have not been established.

ADVERSE REACTIONS: Adverse Drug Reaction Overview: Bisphosphonates may cause upper gastrointestinal disorders such as dysphagia, esophagitis, esophageal ulcer and gastric ulcer. It is therefore important to follow the recommended dosing instructions (see Dosage and Administration).

Musculoskeletal pain, rarely severe, has been reported as a common adverse event in patients who received ACTONEL (risedronate sodium) for all indications.

In postmenopausal and glucocorticoid-induced osteoporosis studies with ACTONEL, the most commonly reported adverse reactions were abdominal pain, dyspepsia and nausea. In addition, upper abdominal pain and diarrhea were the most commonly reported adverse reactions for the highest ACTONEL monthly dose.

In Paget's disease studies with ACTONEL the most commonly reported adverse reactions were diarrhea, nausea, abdominal pain and headache.

Clinical Trial Adverse Drug Reactions: Because clinical trials are conducted under very specific conditions the adverse reaction rates observed in the clinical trials may not reflect the rates observed in practice and should not be compared to the rates in the clinical trials of another drug. Adverse drug reaction information from clinical trials is useful for identifying drug-related adverse events and approximate rates of occurrence.

Treatment and Prevention of Postmenopausal Osteoporosis: ACTONEL 5 mg daily has been studied for up to 3 years in over 5000 women enrolled in Phase III clinical trials for treatment or prevention of postmenopausal osteoporosis. Most adverse events reported in these trials were either mild or moderate in severity, and did not lead to discontinuation from the study. The distribution of severe adverse events was similar across treatment groups. In addition, the overall incidence of adverse events (AEs) was found to be comparable amongst ACTONEL and placebo-treated patients.

Table 1 lists adverse events considered possibly or probably drug-related, reported in ≥1% of ACTONEL 5 mg daily-treated patients, in Phase III postmenopausal osteoporosis trials. Discontinuation of therapy due to serious clinical adverse events occurred in 5.5 % of ACTONEL 5 mg daily-treated patients and 6.0% of patients treated with placebo.

Table 1: ACTONEL

Drug-Related[a] Adverse Events Reported in ≥1% of ACTONEL 5 mg Daily-Treated Patients in Combined Phase III Postmenopausal Osteoporosis Trials

Adverse Event	ACTONEL 5 mg N=1742 (%)	Placebo Control N=1744 (%)
Body as a Whole		
Abdominal Pain	4.1	3.3
Headache	2.5	2.3
Asthenia	1.0	0.7
Digestive System		
Dyspepsia	5.2	4.8
Nausea	4.8	5.0
Constipation	3.7	3.6
Diarrhea	2.9	2.5
Flatulence	2.1	1.8
Gastritis	1.1	0.9
Skin and Appendages		
Rash	1.4	0.9
Pruritus	1.0	0.5

[a] Considered to be possibly or probably causally related by clinical study Investigators.

Once-a-Week Dosing: In the 1-year, double-blind, multicentre study comparing ACTONEL 35 mg Once-a-Week to ACTONEL 5 mg daily for the treatment of osteoporosis in postmenopausal women, the overall safety and tolerability profiles of the 2 oral dosing regimens were similar.

The proportion of patients who experienced an upper gastrointestinal adverse event and the pattern of those events were found to be similar between the ACTONEL 35 mg Once-a-Week and ACTONEL 5 mg daily-treated groups. In addition to the previously described adverse reactions reported in ACTONEL osteoporosis clinical trials, arthralgia (ACTONEL 35 mg, 2.1%; ACTONEL 5 mg, 1.3%) was reported in ≥1% of patients and in more ACTONEL 35 mg weekly treated patients than ACTONEL 5 mg daily.

In the 1-year, double-blind, multicentre study comparing ACTONEL 35 mg Once-a-Week to placebo for the prevention of osteoporosis in postmenopausal women, the overall safety and tolerability profiles of the two groups were comparable with the exception of "arthralgia". Specifically, 1.5% of patients taking ACTONEL 35 mg Once-a-Week experienced arthralgia compared to 0.7% of placebo patients. The overall safety profile observed in this study showed no substantive difference from that observed in the ACTONEL 5 mg daily versus ACTONEL 35 mg Once-a-Week treatment study.

Monthly Dosing: (Two Consecutive Days per Month): In a 1-year, double-blind, multicenter study for the treatment of osteoporosis in postmenopausal women comparing ACTONEL 75 mg on two consecutive days per month to ACTONEL 5 mg daily, the overall safety profiles of the dosing regimens were similar. The proportion of patients who experienced an upper gastrointestinal adverse event and the pattern of those events were found to be similar between the ACTONEL 75 mg two consecutive days per month and the ACTONEL 5 mg daily treated groups. In addition to the previously described adverse reactions reported in ACTONEL osteoporosis clinical trials, arthralgia (ACTONEL 75 mg, 1.5%; ACTONEL 5 mg, 1.0%), vomiting (ACTONEL 75 mg, 1.1%; ACTONEL 5 mg daily, 1.0%) and gastritis erosive (ACTONEL 75 mg, 1.0%; ACTONEL 5 mg, 0.3%) was reported in ≥1% of patients and in more ACTONEL 75 mg-treated patients than ACTONEL 5 mg daily.

Symptoms consistent with acute phase reactions have been reported. Based on reporting of any 33 acute phase reaction-like symptoms (without regard to causality) within the first 5 days of first dose, the overall incidence of acute phase reaction was 7.6% of patients on ACTONEL 75mg two consecutive days per month and 3.6% of patients on ACTONEL 5 mg daily. Fever or influenza-like illness (without regard to causality) occurring within the first 5 days of first dose were reported by 0.6% of patients in the ACTONEL 75 mg two consecutive days per month and 0.0% in the ACTONEL 5 mg daily groups.

(Once-a-Month): In a 1-year, double-blind, multicentre study for the treatment of osteoporosis in postmenopausal women comparing ACTONEL 150 mg Once-a-Month to ACTONEL 5 mg daily, the overall safety profiles of dosing regimens were similar. The proportion of patients who experienced an upper gastrointestinal adverse event and the pattern of those events were found to be similar between ACTONEL 150 mg Once-a-Month and the ACTONEL 5 mg daily treated groups. In addition to the previously described adverse reactions reported in ACTONEL osteoporosis clinical trials, diarrhea (ACTONEL 150 mg, 3.1%; ACTONEL 5 mg, 0.5), vomiting (ACTONEL 150 mg, 1.5%; ACTONEL 5 mg, 0.6%), arthralgia (ACTONEL 150 mg, 1.5%; ACTONEL 5 mg, 0.9%) and myalgia (ACTONEL 150 mg, 1.1%; ACTONEL 5 mg, 0.3%) were reported in ≥1% of patients and in more ACTONEL 150 mg treated patients than ACTONEL 5 mg daily.

Symptoms consistent with acute phase reactions have been reported. Based on reporting of any 33 acute phase reaction-like symptoms (without regard to causality) within the first 3 days of first dose and lasting less than 7 days, the overall incidence of acute phase reaction was 5.2% of patients in the ACTONEL 150 mg Once-a-Month group and 1.1% in the ACTONEL 5 mg daily group. Fever or influenza-like illness (without regard to causality) occurring within the first 3 days of first dose and lasting less than 7 days was reported by 1.4% of patients in the ACTONEL 150 mg Once-a-Month group and 0.2% of patients in the ACTONEL 5 mg daily group.

Treatment of Osteoporosis in Men, to Improve Bone Mineral Density: In a 2 year, double-blind, multicentre study using ACTONEL 35 mg Once-a-Week (n=191) and placebo (n=93) in men with osteoporosis, the overall safety and tolerability profiles of the two treatment groups were similar.

Patients with active or a history of upper gastrointestinal disorders at baseline and those taking acetylsalicylic acid (ASA), non-steroidal anti-inflammatory drugs (NSAIDs) or drugs traditionally used for the treatment of peptic ulcers were not specifically excluded from participating in the 2-year male osteoporosis study. The proportion of patients who experienced an upper gastrointestinal adverse event and the pattern of those events were higher in placebo (18%) than in ACTONEL 35 mg Once-a-Week treated patients (8%).

In addition to the previously described adverse events reported in ACTONEL osteoporosis clinical trials, the following adverse events were reported in ≥2% of patients and in more ACTONEL-treated patients than placebo-treated patients in the male osteoporosis study (events are included without attribution of causality): hypoaesthesia (ACTONEL 35 mg, 2%; placebo, 1%), nephrolithiasis (ACTONEL 35 mg, 3%; placebo, 0%), benign prostatic hyperplasia (ACTONEL 35 mg, 5%; placebo, 3%), and arrhythmia (ACTONEL 35 mg, 2%; placebo 0%).

Glucocorticoid-Induced Osteoporosis: ACTONEL 5 mg daily has been studied in two Phase III glucocorticoid-induced osteoporosis trials enrolling more than 500 patients. The adverse event profile of this population was similar to that seen in postmenopausal osteoporosis trials.

The overall incidence of adverse events was found to be comparable between the ACTONEL 5 mg daily and placebo treatment groups, with the exception of back and joint pain. Back pain was reported in 8.8% of placebo-treated patients and 17.8% of ACTONEL-treated patients; joint pain occurred in 14.7% of placebo patients and 24.7% of ACTONEL patients. Most adverse experiences reported were either mild or moderate in severity, and did not lead to discontinuation from the study. Discontinuation of therapy due to serious clinical adverse events occurred in 2.9% of ACTONEL 5 mg daily-treated patients and 5.3% of patients treated with placebo. The occurrence of adverse events does not appear to be related to patient age, gender or race.

Table 2 lists adverse events considered possibly or probably drug-related, reported in ≥1% of ACTONEL 5 mg daily-treated patients, in Phase III glucocorticoid-induced osteoporosis studies.

Table 2: ACTONEL

Drug-Related[a] Adverse Events Reported in ≥1% of ACTONEL 5 mg Daily-Treated Patients in the Phase III Glucocorticoid-induced Osteoporosis Trials

Adverse Event	ACTONEL 5 mg N=174 (%)	Placebo Control N=170 (%)
Body as a Whole		
Abdominal Pain	4.0	4.7
Headache	1.1	1.2
Digestive System		
Dyspepsia	5.7	2.9
Nausea	5.7	5.3
Constipation	2.9	3.5
Diarrhea	2.9	3.5
Dry Mouth	1.1	0.6
Duodenitis	1.1	0.0
Esophagitis	1.1	0.0
Flatulence	1.1	1.8
Gastrointestinal Disorder	1.1	0.0
Nervous System		
Dizziness	1.1	1.2
Skin and Appendages		
Rash	1.1	2.4
Skin Disorder	1.1	0.0

[a] Considered to be possibly or probably causally related by clinical study Investigators.

Endoscopic Findings: ACTONEL 5 mg daily clinical studies enrolled over 5700 patients for the treatment and prevention of postmenopausal and glucocorticoid-induced osteoporosis, many with pre-existing gastrointestinal disease and concomitant use of NSAIDs or ASA. Investigators were encouraged to perform endoscopies in any patients with moderate-to-severe gastrointestinal complaints while maintaining the blind. These endoscopies were ultimately performed on equal numbers of patients between the treated and placebo groups (75 ACTONEL; 75 placebo).

Across treatment groups, the percentage of patients with normal esophageal, gastric, and duodenal mucosa on endoscopy was similar (21% ACTONEL; 20% placebo). Positive findings on endoscopy were also generally comparable across treatment groups. There were a higher number of reports of mild duodenitis in the ACTONEL group; however, there were more duodenal ulcers in the placebo group. Clinically important findings (perforations, ulcers or bleeding) among this symptomatic population were similar between groups (39% ACTONEL; 51% placebo).

In the 1-year study comparing ACTONEL 35 mg Once-a-Week to ACTONEL 5 mg daily in the treatment of postmenopausal osteoporosis, endoscopies performed during the study revealed no dose dependent pattern in the number of patients with positive endoscopic findings or in the anatomical location of abnormalities detected.

In two, 1-year studies for the treatment of osteoporosis in postmenopausal women comparing ACTONEL 75 mg on two consecutive days per month and ACTONEL 150 mg Once-a-Month respectively to ACTONEL 5 mg daily, a similar percentage of patients for each of the intermittent regimens had at least one abnormal endoscopic finding when compared to the daily regimen (ACTONEL 75 mg, 3.2%; ACTONEL 5 mg, 3.1% and ACTONEL 150 mg, 3.4%; ACTONEL 5 mg, 4.2%).

Paget's Disease of Bone: ACTONEL has been studied in over 390 patients with Paget's disease of bone. The adverse experiences reported have usually been mild or moderate and generally have not required discontinuation of treatment. The occurrence of adverse experiences does not appear to be related to patient age, gender or race.

In a Phase III clinical study, ACTONEL and Didronel (etidronate disodium tablets) showed similar adverse event profiles: 6.6% (4/61) of the patients treated with ACTONEL 30 mg daily for 2 months discontinued treatment due to adverse experiences, compared with 8.2% (5/61) of the patients treated with Didronel 400 mg daily for 6 months.

Table 3 lists adverse events considered possibly or probably drug related, reported in ≥1% of ACTONEL 30 mg daily-treated patients, in Phase III Paget's trial.

Table 3: ACTONEL

Drug-Related[a] Adverse Events Reported in ≥1% of ACTONEL 30 mg Daily-Treated Patients in the Phase III Paget's Trial

Adverse Event	ACTONEL 30 mg/day×2 months N=61 (%)	Didronel 400 mg/day×6 months N=61 (%)
Body as a Whole		
Abdominal Pain	6.6	3.3
Headache	4.9	6.6
Infection	3.3	6.6
Flu Syndrome	1.6	0.0
Neck Rigidity	1.6	1.6
Neoplasm	1.6	0.0
Pain	1.6	8.2
Chest Pain	1.6	0.0
Digestive System		
Diarrhea	13.1	9.8
Nausea	8.2	4.9
Constipation	3.3	1.6
Flatulence	3.3	4.9
Colitis	1.6	0.0
Metabolic and Nutritional		
Peripheral Edema	1.6	0.0
Hypocalcemia	1.6	0.0
Weight Decreased	1.6	0.0
Musculoskeletal System		
Arthralgia	9.8	8.2
Leg Cramps	1.6	0.0
Myasthenia	1.6	0.0
Bone Pain	1.6	0.0
Nervous System		
Dizziness	1.6	0.0
Respiratory System		
Apnea	1.6	0.0
Bronchitis	1.6	0.0
Sinusitis	1.6	0.0
Skin		
Rash	1.6	0.0
Special Senses		
Amblyopia	1.6	0.0
Corneal Lesion	1.6	0.0
Dry Eyes	1.6	0.0
Ear Pain	1.6	1.6
Tinnitus	1.6	0.0
Urogenital System		
Nocturia	1.6	0.0

[a] Considered to be possibly or probably causally related by clinical study Investigators.

In the Phase III comparative study versus Didronel, patients with a history of upper GI disease or abnormalities were not excluded. Patients were also not excluded based on NSAID or ASA use. The proportion of ACTONEL 30 mg daily-treated patients with mild or moderate upper GI experiences was similar to that in the Didronel-treated group, with no severe upper GI experiences observed in either treatment group.

Less Common Clinical Trial Adverse Drug Reactions: The following adverse drug reactions were reported in ≤1% of patients who received ACTONEL for all indications. Uncommon (0.1-1.0%): duodenitis, iritis. Rare (<0.1%): abnormal liver function tests, glossitis.

Abnormal Hematologic and Clinical Chemistry Findings: Asymptomatic mild decreases in serum calcium and phosphorus levels have been observed in some patients (see Action and Clinical Pharmacology, Pharmacodynamics).

Rare cases of leukemia have been reported following therapy with bisphosphonates. Any causal relationship to either the treatment or to the patients' underlying disease has not been established.

Post-Market Adverse Drug Reactions: Hypersensitivity and Skin Reactions: Reported rarely, angioedema, generalized rash and bullous skin reactions, some severe.

Osteonecrosis of the Jaw: Osteonecrosis of the jaw has been reported rarely (see Warnings and Precautions).

Ophthalmologic: Reported rarely, iritis and uveitis.

DRUG INTERACTIONS: Overview: No specific drug-drug interaction studies were performed. Animal studies have demonstrated that risedronate is highly concentrated in bone and is retained only minimally in soft tissue. No metabolites have been detected systemically or in bone. The binding of risedronate to plasma proteins in humans is low (24%), resulting in minimal potential for interference with the binding of other drugs. In an additional animal study, there was also no evidence of hepatic microsomal enzyme induction. In summary, ACTONEL (risedronate sodium) is not systemically metabolized, does not induce cytochrome P450 enzymes and has low protein binding. ACTONEL is therefore not expected to interact with other drugs based on the effects of protein binding displacement, enzyme induction or metabolism of other drugs.

Drug-Drug Interactions: Patients in the clinical trials were exposed to a wide variety of commonly used concomitant medications (including NSAIDs, H_2-blockers, proton pump inhibitors, antacids, calcium channel blockers, beta-blockers, thiazides, glucocorticoids, anticoagulants, anticonvulsants, cardiac glycosides) without evidence of clinically relevant interactions.

The drugs listed in Table 4 are based on either drug interaction case reports or predicted interactions due to the expected magnitude and seriousness of the interaction (i.e., those identified as contraindicated).

Table 4: ACTONEL

Established or Predicted Drug-Drug Interactions with ACTONEL

Risedronate Sodium	Reference	Effect	Clinical Comment
Antacids/supplements which contain polyvalent cations (e.g., calcium, magnesium, aluminum and iron)	T	Interference with the absorption of ACTONEL	Such medications should be administered at a different time of the day (see Dosage and Administration).
Hormone replacement therapy	CT	No clinically significant effect	If considered appropriate, ACTONEL may be used concomitantly with hormone replacement therapy.
H_2-blockers and proton pump inhibitors (PPIs)	CT	Among H_2-blockers and PPIs users, the incidence of upper gastrointestinal adverse events was similar between the ACTONEL-treated patients and placebo-treated patients.	Of over 5700 patients enrolled in the ACTONEL 5 mg daily Phase III osteoporosis studies, 21% used H_2-blockers and/or PPIs.
		Among H_2-blockers and PPIs users, the incidence of upper gastrointestinal adverse experiences was found to be similar between the weekly- and daily-treated groups.	In the 1-year study comparing ACTONEL Once-a-Week and daily dosing regimens in postmenopausal women with osteoporosis, at least 9% of patients in the ACTONEL 35 mg Once-a-Week and 5 mg daily groups used H_2-blockers and/or PPIs.

Legend: CT=Clinical Trial; T=Theoretical.

Of over 5700 patients enrolled in the ACTONEL 5 mg daily Phase III osteoporosis studies, ASA use was reported by 31% of patients and NSAID use by 48%. Among these ASA or NSAID users, the incidence of upper gastrointestinal adverse events was similar between the ACTONEL-treated patients and placebo-treated patients.

In the 1-year study comparing ACTONEL 35 mg Once-a-Week to ACTONEL 5 mg daily, ASA use was reported by 56% and NSAID use by 41%. The incidence of upper gastrointestinal adverse events was similar between the ACTONEL weekly- and daily-treated groups.

In two, 1-year studies comparing ACTONEL 75 mg two consecutive days per month or ACTONEL 150 mg once-a-month to ACTONEL 5 mg daily in postmenopausal women, 55% (75 mg) and 46% (150 mg) of patients reported the use of ASA and/or NSAIDs. Among these ASA or NSAID users, the incidence of upper gastrointestinal adverse events was similar in the ACTONEL monthly-treated groups when compared to the daily-treated groups respectively.

Drug-Food Interactions: Clinical benefits may be compromised by failure to take ACTONEL on an empty stomach. For dosing information see Dosage and Administration.

Drug-Herb Interactions: Interactions with herbs have not been studied.

Drug-Laboratory Test Interactions: Bisphosphonates are known to interfere with the use of bone-imaging agents. Specific studies with ACTONEL have not been performed.

DOSAGE AND ADMINISTRATION: Dosing Considerations:

- Patients should receive supplemental calcium and vitamin D if dietary intake is inadequate (see Warnings and Precautions, General).
- Food and medications containing polyvalent cations (e.g., calcium, magnesium, aluminum, and iron) can interfere with the absorption of ACTONEL (risedronate sodium). Therefore, food and other medications should be administered at a different time of the day (see Recommended Dose and Dosage Adjustment).
- Each tablet should be swallowed whole while the patient is in an upright position and with sufficient plain water (≥120 mL) to facilitate delivery to the stomach. Patients should not lie down for at least 30 minutes after taking the medication (see Warnings and Precautions, General).

Recommended Dose and Dosage Adjustment: For all indications and doses: The patient should be informed to pay particular attention to the dosing instructions as clinical benefits may be compromised by failure to take the drug according to instructions. Specifically, ACTONEL should be taken on an empty stomach at least 30 minutes before consuming the first food, drink (other than plain water) and/or any other medication of the day. Each tablet should be swallowed whole—do not chew.

Treatment of Postmenopausal Osteoporosis: The recommended regimens are daily (5 mg), weekly (35 mg Once-a-Week), monthly duet (75 mg on two consecutive days per month, on the same calendar days each month), or monthly (1 tablet of 150 mg Once-a-Month on the same calendar day each month), taken orally.

Prevention of Postmenopausal Osteoporosis: The recommended regimens are daily (5 mg) or weekly (35 mg Once-a-Week), taken orally.

Treatment of Osteoporosis in Men, to Improve Bone Mineral Density: The recommended regimen is 35 mg once-a-week, taken orally.

Treatment and Prevention of Glucocorticoid-induced Osteoporosis: The recommended regimen is 5 mg daily, taken orally.

Treatment of Paget's Disease of Bone: The recommended regimen is 30 mg daily for 2 months, taken orally. Re-treatment may be considered (following post-treatment observation of at least 2 months) if relapse has occurred, or if treatment fails to normalize serum alkaline phosphatase. For re-treatment, the dose and duration of therapy are the same as for initial treatment. There are no data available on more than one course of re-treatment.

Renal Impairment: No dosage adjustment is necessary in patients with a creatinine clearance ≥30 mL/min or in the elderly. Not recommended for use in patients with severe renal impairment (creatinine clearance <30 mL/min).

Geriatrics: No dosage adjustment is necessary in elderly patients (see Indications and Clinical Use, Geriatrics).

Missed Dose: Daily: Patients should be instructed that if they miss a dose of ACTONEL 5 mg or 30 mg, they should take 1 tablet of ACTONEL as they normally would for their next dose. Patients should not double their next dose or take 2 tablets on the same day.

Weekly: Patients should be instructed that if they miss a dose of ACTONEL 35 mg Once-a-Week on their regularly scheduled day, they should take 1 tablet of Actonel on the day they first remember missing their dose. Patients should then return to taking 1 tablet once a week as originally scheduled on their chosen day. Patients should not take 2 tablets on the same day.

Monthly Duet: If one or both tablets of ACTONEL 75 mg monthly duet are missed, and the next month's scheduled doses are more than 7 days away, the patient should be instructed as follows:

- If both tablets are missed, take 1 ACTONEL 75 mg tablet in the morning after the day it is remembered and then the other tablet on the next consecutive morning.
- If only 1 ACTONEL 75 mg tablet is missed, take the missed tablet in the morning after the day it is remembered.

Patients should then return to taking their ACTONEL 75 mg monthly duet on two consecutive days each month as originally scheduled. Patients should not take more than two 75 mg tablets within 7 days. If one or both tablets of ACTONEL 75 mg are missed, and the next month's scheduled doses are within 7 days, patients should wait until their next month's scheduled doses and then continue taking ACTONEL 75 mg monthly duet on two consecutive days each month as originally scheduled.

Once-a-Month: Patients should be instructed that if they miss a 150 mg dose of ACTONEL (1 tablet of 150 mg), and the next month's scheduled dose is more than 7 days away, they should take the missed tablet in the morning after the day it is remembered. Patients should then return to taking their ACTONEL 150 mg as originally scheduled.

If a dose of ACTONEL 150 mg is missed, and the next month's scheduled dose is within 7 days, patients should be instructed to wait until their next month's scheduled dose and then continue taking ACTONEL 150 mg. Patients should not take more than 150 mg of ACTONEL within 7 days.

OVERDOSAGE:

Decreases in serum calcium following substantial overdose may be expected in some patients. Signs and symptoms of hypocalcemia may also occur in some of these patients.

Administration of milk or antacids containing calcium may be helpful to chelate ACTONEL (risedronate sodium) and reduce absorption of the drug. In cases of substantial overdose, gastric lavage may be considered to remove unabsorbed drug if performed within 30 minutes of ingestion. Standard procedures that are effective for treating hypocalcemia, including the administration of calcium intravenously, would be expected to restore physiologic amounts of ionized calcium and to relieve signs and symptoms of hypocalcemia.

> For management of a suspected drug overdose, contact your **regional Poison Control Centre**. See the *CPS* Directory section for a list of Poison Control Centres.

ACTION AND CLINICAL PHARMACOLOGY: Mechanism of Action: Risedronate sodium, a pyridinyl-bisphosphonate in the form of hemi-pentahydrate with small amounts of monohydrate, inhibits osteoclast bone resorption and modulates bone metabolism. Risedronate has a high affinity for hydroxyapatite crystals in bone and is a potent antiresorptive agent. At the cellular level, risedronate inhibits osteoclasts. The osteoclasts adhere normally to the bone surface, but show evidence of reduced active resorption (e.g., lack of ruffled border). Histomorphometry in rats, dogs, minipigs and humans showed that risedronate treatment reduces bone turnover (i.e., activation frequency, the rate at which bone remodelling sites are activated) and bone resorption at remodelling sites.

Pharmacodynamics: Treatment and Prevention of Osteoporosis in Postmenopausal Women: Osteoporosis is a degenerative and debilitating bone disease characterized by decreased bone mass and increased fracture risk at the spine, hip, and wrist. The diagnosis can be confirmed by the finding of low bone mass, evidence of fracture on x-ray, a history of osteoporotic fracture, or height loss or kyphosis indicative of vertebral fracture. Osteoporosis occurs in both men and women but is more common among women following menopause.

In healthy humans, bone formation and resorption are closely linked; old bone is resorbed and replaced by newly-formed bone. In postmenopausal osteoporosis, bone resorption exceeds bone formation, leading to bone loss and increased risk of bone fracture. After menopause, the risk of fractures of the spine and hip increases dramatically; approximately 40% of 50-year-old women will experience an osteoporosis-related fracture of the spine, hip, or wrist during their remaining lifetimes. After experiencing one osteoporosis-related fracture, the risk of future fracture increases 5-fold compared to the risk among a non-fractured population. One in five men older than 50 years will have an osteoporotic fracture, most commonly at the spine, hip and wrist.

ACTONEL (risedronate sodium) treatment decreases the elevated rate of bone turnover and corrects the imbalance of bone resorption relative to bone formation that is typically seen in postmenopausal osteoporosis. In clinical trials, administration of ACTONEL to postmenopausal women resulted in dose-dependent decreases in biochemical markers of bone turnover, including urinary markers of bone resorption and serum markers of bone formation, at doses as low as 2.5 mg daily. At the 5 mg daily dose, decreases in resorption markers were evident within 14 days of treatment. Changes in bone formation markers were observed later than changes in resorption markers, as expected, due to the coupled nature of bone formation and bone resorption; decreases in bone formation of about 20% were evident within 3 months of treatment. Bone turnover markers (BTMs) reached a nadir of about 40% below baseline values by the sixth month of treatment and remained stable with continued treatment for up to 3 years.

These data demonstrate that ACTONEL 5 mg administered daily to postmenopausal women produces a rapid reduction in bone resorption without over-suppression of bone formation. Bone turnover is decreased as early as 2 weeks and maximally within about 6 months of treatment, with achievement of a new steady-state which more nearly approximates the rate of bone turnover seen in premenopausal women.

In weekly and monthly ACTONEL postmenopausal osteoporosis dosing studies, consistent decreases in bone resorption (50-60%) and bone formation (30-40%) markers were observed at Month 12.

As a result of the inhibition of bone resorption, asymptomatic and usually transient decreases from baseline in serum calcium (about 2%) and serum phosphate levels (about 5%) and compensatory increases in serum parathyroid hormone (PTH) levels were observed within 6 months in ACTONEL 5 mg daily-treated patients in postmenopausal osteoporosis trials. No further decreases in serum calcium or phosphate, or increases in PTH were observed in postmenopausal women treated for up to 3 years. In two 1-year studies for the treatment of osteoporosis in postmenopausal women comparing ACTONEL 35 mg Once-a-Week and ACTONEL 150 mg Once-a-Month respectively to ACTONEL 5 mg daily, similar mean changes from baseline in serum calcium, phosphate and PTH were found for each of the intermittent regimens when compared to the daily dosage regimen. In the 1-year study comparing ACTONEL 75 mg on two consecutive days per month to ACTONEL 5 mg daily, the mean percent changes from baseline were for serum calcium (0.8% and 0.2%), phosphate (−1.1% and −1.9%) and PTH (−11.7% and −3.0%), respectively.

Consistent with the effects of ACTONEL on biochemical markers of bone turnover, daily oral doses as low as 2.5 mg produced dose dependent, significant increases in lumbar spine bone mineral density (BMD) (ACTONEL 2.5 mg, 3% to 3.7%; ACTONEL 5 mg, 4% to 4.5%) after 12 months of treatment in large-scale postmenopausal osteoporosis trials. A dose-dependent response to treatment was also observed in the BMD of the femoral neck over the same time (ACTONEL 2.5 mg, 0.7% to 0.9%; ACTONEL 5 mg, 1.5% to 2%). In three 1-year weekly and monthly dosing studies for the treatment of osteoporosis in postmenopausal women, comparing ACTONEL 35 mg Once-a-Week, ACTONEL 75 mg on two consecutive days per month and ACTONEL 150 mg Once-a-Month respectively to ACTONEL 5 mg daily, similar mean changes from baseline in BMD of the lumbar spine, total proximal femur, femoral neck and femoral trochanter were found for each of the intermittent regimens when compared to the daily regimen.

Treatment of Osteoporosis in Men, to Improve Bone Mineral Density: In a 2-year clinical trial in the treatment of osteoporosis in men, ACTONEL 35 mg once a week decreased urinary collagen cross-linked N-telopeptide (NTX) (a marker of bone resorption), and serum bone specific alkaline phosphatase (BAP) (a marker of bone formation) by approximately 40% and 30%, below baseline values, respectively, within 12 months. The BTMs all had statistically significant decreases in bone turnover from baseline compared to placebo at all time points. The decreases in bone turnover were observed within 3 months after initiation of therapy and maintained throughout the 2-year study.

Glucocorticoid-Induced Osteoporosis: Chronic exposure to glucocorticoids (≥7.5 mg/day prednisone or its equivalent) induces rapid bone loss by decreasing bone formation and increasing bone resorption. The bone loss occurs most rapidly during the first 6 months of therapy with persistent but slowing bone loss for as long as glucocorticoid therapy continues.

Glucocorticoid-induced osteoporosis is characterized by low bone mass that leads to an increased risk of fracture (especially vertebral, hip, and rib). It occurs in both men and women, and approximately 50% of patients on chronic glucocorticoid treatment will experience fractures. The relative risk of a hip fracture in patients on >7.5 mg/day prednisone is more than doubled (RR=2.27); the relative risk of vertebral fracture is increased five-fold (RR=5.18).

ACTONEL treatment decreases bone resorption without directly inhibiting bone formation. In 1-year clinical trials in the treatment and prevention of glucocorticoid-induced osteoporosis, ACTONEL 5 mg daily produced rapid and statistically significant reductions in biochemical markers of bone turnover, similar to those seen in postmenopausal osteoporosis. Urinary collagen cross-linked N-telopeptide (a marker of bone resorption) and serum bone specific alkaline phosphatase (a marker of bone formation) were decreased by 50% to 55% and 25% to 30%, respectively, within 3 to 6 months after initiation of therapy. The reduction was evident within 14 days and BTMs remained decreased throughout the duration of ACTONEL treatment.

Consistent with the changes in biochemical markers of bone turnover, ACTONEL 5 mg daily provides a beneficial effect on bone mineral density and reduces the risk of vertebral fractures by approximately 70% when compared to placebo.

Paget's Disease of Bone: Paget's disease of bone is a chronic focal skeletal disorder characterized by greatly increased and disordered bone remodelling. Excessive osteoclastic bone resorption is followed by osteoblastic new bone formation, leading to the replacement of the normal bone architecture by disorganized, enlarged and weakened bone structure.

Clinical manifestations of Paget's disease range from no symptoms to severe morbidity due to bone pain, bone deformity, pathological fractures, and neurological and other complications. Serum alkaline phosphatase, the most frequently used biochemical marker of disease activity, provides an objective measure of disease severity and response to therapy.

ACTONEL is a bisphosphonate that acts primarily to inhibit bone resorption. This effect is related to its inhibitory effect on osteoclasts. In the Phase III clinical trial, ACTONEL 30 mg daily for 2 months produced significant (p<0.001) reductions of 81% to 88% in serum alkaline phosphatase excess, as well as significant reductions in bone-specific serum alkaline phosphatase (Ostase, 67% to 70%) and urinary deoxypyridinoline/creatinine (47% to 51%). Reductions were evident as early as 1 month after the start of treatment, and progressively increased in magnitude (following completion of the 2 month treatment) when measured at monthly intervals over a 6 month period. Clinically meaningful reductions in serum alkaline phosphatase were observed starting at 1 month with levels maintained through 12 months.

Asymptomatic and mild decreases in serum calcium and phosphorus levels have been observed in some patients. These decreases in calcium are associated with increases in serum intact PTH and 1,25-dihydroxy vitamin D, resulting in an increase in tubular reabsorption of calcium.

Markers of bone resorption (such as urinary deoxypyridinoline/creatinine or hydroxyproline/creatinine) usually decrease before markers of bone formation (such as serum alkaline phosphatase). This difference is indicative of the primary antiresorptive effect of ACTONEL.

Bone turnover marker levels continue to decrease when ACTONEL treatment is stopped. Therefore, to assess the full effect of response, patients should be followed for at least 2 months following the 2 month treatment period.

Pharmacokinetics:

Table 5: ACTONEL

Summary of Pharmacokinetic Parameters of Risedronate

	C_{max} (ng/mL)	t_{max} (h)	$t_{1/2}$, z (h)	$AUC_{0-\infty}$ (ng·h/mL)	Clearance (L/h/kg)	V_z (L/kg)
5 mg tablet; single dose	0.85	0.93[a]	206.1	3.45	19.94	5542
30 mg tablet; single dose	4.2	0.87[a]	226.1	17.1	23.60	7542
35 mg tablet; multiple dose[b], steady state	10.6	0.49	nd	53.3	12.9	nd
75 mg tablet, multiple dose[c], steady state	19.3[d]	0.66[a]	299.7[d]	180.7[d]	14.8[a]	nd
150 mg tablet, single dose	74.8[d]	0.66[d]	349.6[d]	332.4[d]	6.94[d]	3118[d]

[a] Arithmetic mean.
[b] Administered weekly.
[c] Administered on two consecutive days per month (150 mg total monthly dose).
[d] Geometric mean.

Legend: $t_{1/2}$, z: is the half-life of the terminal exponential phase; V_Z: is the terminal volume of distribution uncorrected for bioavailability; nd=: not determined.

Absorption: Absorption after an oral dose is relatively rapid (t_{max} ~1 hour) and occurs throughout the upper gastrointestinal tract. Absorption is independent of dose over the range studied (single dose, from 2.5 to 30 mg; multiple dose, from 2.5 mg/day to 75 mg two consecutive days per month and 35 and 50 mg weekly); systemic exposure increases disproportionally at 150 mg (about 2 fold greater than expected based on dose). Steady-state conditions in the serum are observed within 57 days of daily dosing. Mean oral bioavailability of the tablet is 0.63% and is bioequivalent to a solution. Extent of absorption when administered 30 minutes before breakfast is reduced by 55% compared to dosing in the fasting state (i.e., no food or drink for 10 hours prior to or 4 hours after dosing). Dosing 1 hour prior to breakfast reduces extent of absorption by 30% compared to dosing in the fasting state. Dosing either 30 minutes prior to breakfast or 2 hours after a meal results in a similar extent of absorption.

Distribution: The mean steady-state volume of distribution is 6.3 L/kg in humans. Human plasma protein binding of drug is about 24%. Preclinical studies in rats and dogs dosed intravenously with single doses of [^{14}C] risedronate indicate that approximately 60% of the dose is distributed to bone. The remainder of the dose is excreted in the urine. After multiple oral dosing in rats, the uptake of risedronate in soft tissues was found to be minimal (in the range of 0.001% to 0.01%), with drug levels quickly decreasing after the final dose.

Metabolism: There is no evidence that risedronate is systemically metabolized.

Excretion: Approximately half of the absorbed dose is excreted in urine within 24 hours, and 85% of an intravenous dose is recovered in the urine over 28 days. Mean renal clearance is 105 mL/min (CV=34%) and mean total clearance is 122 mL/min (CV=19%), with the difference primarily reflecting non-renal clearance or clearance due to adsorption to bone. The renal clearance is not concentration dependent, and there is a linear relationship between renal clearance and creatinine clearance. Unabsorbed drug is eliminated unchanged in feces. Once risedronate is absorbed, the serum concentration-time profile is multi-phasic with an initial half-life of about 1.5 hours and a terminal exponential half-life of 480 hours. Although the elimination rate of bisphosphonates from human bone is unknown, the 480 hour half-life is hypothesized to represent the dissociation of risedronate from the surface of bone.

Special Populations and Conditions: Pediatrics: Risedronate pharmacokinetics have not been studied in patients <18 years of age.

Geriatrics: Bioavailability and disposition are similar in elderly (>65 years of age) and younger subjects. No dosage adjustment is necessary.

Gender: Bioavailability and disposition following oral administration are similar in men and women.

Race: Pharmacokinetic differences due to race have not been studied.

Hepatic Insufficiency: No studies have been performed to assess risedronate's safety or efficacy in patients with hepatic impairment. Risedronate is not metabolized in rat, dog, and human liver preparations. Insignificant amounts (<0.1% of intravenous dose) of drug are excreted in the bile in rats. Therefore, dosage adjustment is unlikely to be needed in patients with hepatic impairment.

Renal Insufficiency: Risedronate is excreted intact primarily via the kidney. Patients with mild-to-moderate renal impairment (creatinine clearance >30 mL/min) do not require a dosage adjustment. Exposure to risedronate was estimated to increase by 44% in patients with creatinine clearance of 20 mL/min. ACTONEL is not recommended for use in patients with severe renal impairment (creatinine clearance <30 mL/min) because of a lack of clinical experience.

Genetic Polymorphism: No data are available.

STORAGE AND STABILITY: Store at controlled room temperature (20-25°C).

INFORMATION FOR THE PATIENT: Published in e-CPS, available by subscription at www.e-cps.ca.

DOSAGE FORMS, COMPOSITION AND PACKAGING: 5 mg: Each film-coated, oval-shaped, yellow tablet for oral administration with "RSN" engraved on one face and "5 mg" engraved on the other, contains the equivalent of: anhydrous risedronate sodium 5 mg in the form of the hemi-pentahydrate with small amounts of monohydrate. Nonmedicinal ingredients: crospovidone, ferric oxide yellow, hydroxypropyl cellulose, hypromellose, lactose monohydrate, magnesium stearate, microcrystalline cellulose, polyethylene glycol, silicon dioxide and titanium dioxide. Cartons of 28 blister packaged tablets.

30 mg: Each film-coated, oval-shaped, white tablet for oral administration with "RSN" engraved on one face and "30 mg" engraved on the other, contains the equivalent of: anhydrous risedronate sodium 30 mg in the form of the hemi-pentahydrate with small amounts of monohydrate. Nonmedicinal ingredients: crospovidone, hydroxypropyl cellulose, hypromellose, lactose monohydrate, magnesium stearate, microcrystalline cellulose, polyethylene glycol, silicon dioxide and titanium dioxide. Bottles of 30 tablets.

35 mg: Each film-coated, oval-shaped, orange tablet for oral administration with "RSN" engraved on one face and "35 mg" engraved on the other, contains the equivalent of: anhydrous risedronate sodium 35 mg in the form of the hemi-pentahydrate with small amounts of monohydrate. Nonmedicinal ingredients: crospovidone, ferric oxide red, ferric oxide yellow, hydroxypropyl cellulose, hypromellose, lactose monohydrate, magnesium stearate, microcrystalline cellulose, polyethylene glycol, silicon dioxide and titanium dioxide. Cartons of 4 blister packaged tablets.

75 mg: Each film-coated, oval-shaped, pink tablet for oral administration with "RSN" engraved on one face and "75 mg" engraved on the other, contains the equivalent of: anhydrous risedronate sodium 75 mg in the form of the hemi-pentahydrate with small amounts of monohydrate. Nonmedicinal ingredients: crospovidone, ferric oxide red, hydroxypropyl cellulose, hypromellose, magnesium stearate, microcrystalline cellulose, polyethylene glycol, silicon dioxide and titanium dioxide. Cartons of 2 blister packaged tablets.

150 mg: Each film-coated, oval-shaped, blue tablet for oral administration with "RSN" engraved on one face and "150 mg" engraved on the other, contains the equivalent of: anhydrous risedronate sodium 150 mg in the form of the hemi-pentahydrate with small amounts of monohydrate. Nonmedicinal ingredients: crospovidone, hydroxypropyl cellulose, hypromellose, indigo carmine, magnesium stearate, microcrystalline cellulose, polyethylene glycol, silicon dioxide and titanium dioxide. Cartons of 1 blister packaged tablet.

(Shown in Product Identification Section)

Actos® ℞

pioglitazone HCl

Antidiabetic—Insulin Resistance Reducing Agent

Takeda Canada

Date of Preparation: August 15, 2000
Date of Revision: October 22, 2009

SUMMARY PRODUCT INFORMATION:

Route of Administration	Dosage Form/ Strength	Clinically Relevant Nonmedicinal Ingredients
Oral	Tablets/15 mg, 30 mg, 45 mg	Lactose monohydrate For a complete listing see Dosage Forms, Composition and Packaging.

INDICATIONS AND CLINICAL USE: Indications: ACTOS (pioglitazone hydrochloride) is indicated as monotherapy in patients not controlled by diet and exercise alone, to decrease insulin resistance and blood glucose levels in patients with type 2 diabetes mellitus (non-insulin dependent diabetes mellitus, NIDDM).

ACTOS is indicated for use in combination with a sulfonylurea or metformin when diet and exercise plus the single agent do not result in adequate glycemic control.

Clinical Use: It is recommended that patients be treated for an adequate period of time to evaluate change in HbA_{1c} unless glycemic control deteriorates.

Management of type 2 diabetes should also include nutritional counselling, weight reduction as needed, and exercise. These efforts are important not only in the primary treatment of type 2 diabetes, but also to maintain the efficacy of drug therapy.

Geriatrics (≥65 years of age): No significant differences in effectiveness and safety were observed between patients over 65 years of age and younger patients in ACTOS clinical trials.

Pediatrics (<18 years of age): Safety and effectiveness of ACTOS in pediatric patients have not been established. Use in patients under 18 years of age is not recommended.

CONTRAINDICATIONS: ACTOS (pioglitazone hydrochloride) is contraindicated in:

- New York Heart Association (NYHA) Class I to IV cardiac status.
- known hypersensitivity to this drug or any of its components;
- serious hepatic impairment (see Warnings and Precautions, Hepatic/Biliary/Pancreatic);
- pregnancy. Insulin is recommended during pregnancy to control blood glucose levels. Oral antidiabetic agents should not be given (see Warnings and Precautions, Special Populations, Pregnant Women).

WARNINGS AND PRECAUTIONS: General: The effect of ACTOS (pioglitazone hydrochloride) on morbidity and mortality has not been established.

ACTOS exerts its antihyperglycemic effect only in the presence of insulin. Therefore, ACTOS should not be used in patients with type 1 diabetes or for the treatment of diabetic ketoacidosis.

The use of ACTOS in combination with insulin is not indicated. The use of ACTOS in combination with metformin AND a sulfonylurea (triple therapy) is not indicated.

Weight Gain: ACTOS may be associated with weight gain. Mean weight gain in controlled monotherapy studies ranged from 0.5 to 2.8 kg. In controlled combination therapy studies, the mean weight gain ranged from 0.95 to 3.0 kg. Treatment should be re-evaluated in patients with excessive weight gain (see Action and Clinical Pharmacology, Pharmacodynamics).

Fractures: In a pooled analysis of randomized, controlled double-blind clinical studies, an increased incidence of bone fracture was observed in female patients taking ACTOS versus non-TZD comparator drugs or placebo (2.6% versus 1.7%). The majority of these fractures were in the distal upper limb or distal lower limb. The risk of fracture should be considered in the care of female patients treated with ACTOS, and attention given to assessing and maintaining bone health according to current standards of care.

Cardiovascular: Congestive Heart Failure: Thiazolidinediones, like ACTOS, alone or in combination with other antidiabetic agents, can cause fluid retention, which can lead to congestive heart failure. The fluid retention may very rarely present as rapid and excessive weight gain. All patients should be monitored for signs and symptoms of adverse reactions relating to fluid retention and heart failure. In particular, patients who are at risk for heart failure including those receiving concurrent therapy which increases insulin levels (i.e. sulfonylureas) should be closely monitored (see Adverse Reactions).

Treatment with thiazolidinediones, like ACTOS, has been associated with cases of congestive heart failure, some of which were difficult to treat unless medication was discontinued. ACTOS should be discontinued if any deterioration in cardiac status occurs.

Since patients experiencing acute coronary syndrome (ACS) are at an increased risk of developing heart failure, and in view of the potential for pioglitazone to cause or exacerbate heart failure, initiation of pioglitazone in patients experiencing an acute coronary event is not recommended. Furthermore, discontinuation of pioglitazone during the acute phase should be considered.

ACTOS is contraindicated in patients with NYHA Class I, II, III, and IV heart failure. Patients with severe heart failure (including NYHA Class III and IV cardiac status) were not studied during clinical trials.

Edema: ACTOS should be used with caution in patients with edema. In placebo-controlled clinical studies, the incidence of edema is increased with ACTOS relative to the control groups and may be dose-related (see Adverse Reactions). For information on macular edema, see Warnings and Precautions, Ophthalmologic.

Endocrine and Metabolism: Hypoglycemia: During the administration of ACTOS as monotherapy, documented hypoglycemia has not been observed, nor would it be expected based on the mechanism of action. Patients receiving ACTOS in combination with other hypoglycemic agents (e.g. insulin secreting agents) may be at risk for hypoglycemia, and a reduction in the dose of either agent may be necessary.

Hematologic: Across all clinical studies, mean hemoglobin values declined by 2% to 4% in ACTOS-treated patients but remained within normal limits at all times (including up to 18 months of continuous therapy). In all studies, patients were excluded if they had a hemoglobin of less than 120 g/L for males or 100 g/L for females. In the monotherapy studies, the mean hemoglobin declined from 151 to 147 g/L, with the range in the bottom 10% of hemoglobin values 111 to 125 g/L. In a long-term, open-label follow-up monotherapy study of an additional 84 weeks, the change in hemoglobin remained small, declining from 151 to 143 g/L. In the combination studies, the mean hemoglobin declined from 147 to 142 g/L, with the range in the bottom 10% of hemoglobin values 100 to 124 g/L. In a long-term, open-label follow up combination study, after an additional 72 weeks, the change in hemoglobin remained small, declining from 147 to 138 g/L. These changes may be related to increased plasma volume and have not been associated with any significant hematologic clinical effects (see Adverse Reactions, Abnormal Hematologic and Clinical Chemistry Findings).

Hepatic/Biliary/Pancreatic: Rare cases of severe hepatocellular injury have been reported associated with thiazolidinediones. **Therapy with ACTOS should not be initiated in patients with increased baseline liver enzyme levels (ALT >2.5 times the upper limit of normal).**

Although available data from clinical studies show no evidence of ACTOS-induced hepatotoxicity or ALT elevations, pioglitazone has a common thiazolidinedione structure to troglitazone, which has been associated with idiosyncratic hepatotoxicity and rare cases of liver failure, liver transplants, and death. In post-marketing experience with ACTOS, reports of hepatitis, hepatic enzyme elevations 3 or more times the upper limit of normal, and hepatic failure with and without fatal outcome have been received. It is recommended that patients treated with ACTOS undergo periodic monitoring of liver enzymes. Liver enzymes should be checked prior to the initiation of therapy with ACTOS in all patients. In patients with normal baseline liver enzymes, following initiation of therapy with ACTOS, it is recommended that liver enzymes be monitored periodically thereafter, per the clinical judgement of the healthcare professional. Patients with mildly elevated liver enzymes (ALT levels one to 2.5 times the upper limit of normal) at baseline or during therapy with ACTOS should be evaluated to determine the cause of the liver enzyme elevation. Initiation of, or continuation of therapy with ACTOS in patients with mild liver enzyme elevations should proceed with caution and include appropriate close clinical follow-up, including more frequent liver enzyme monitoring, to determine if the liver enzyme elevations resolve or worsen. If at any time ALT levels increase to >3 times the upper limit of normal in patients on therapy with ACTOS, liver enzymes should be rechecked as soon as possible. If ALT levels remain >3 times the upper limit of normal, or the patient is jaundiced, therapy with ACTOS should be discontinued (see Dosage and Administration). (For Use in Patients with Hepatic Insufficiency, see under Special Populations and Conditions.)

Ophthalmologic: New onset and/or worsening macular edema with decreased visual acuity has been reported rarely in post-marketing experience with ACTOS. In some cases, the visual events resolved or symptoms improved following discontinuation of ACTOS. Physicians should consider the possibility of macular edema if a patient reports disturbances in visual acuity (see Adverse Reactions, Post-Market Adverse Drug Reactions).

Sexual Function/Reproduction: In premenopausal anovulatory patients with insulin resistance, treatment with thiazolidinediones, including ACTOS, may result in resumption of ovulation. These patients may be at risk for pregnancy if adequate contraception is not used.

Special Populations: Pregnant Women: There are no adequate and well-controlled studies in pregnant women. ACTOS is contraindicated during pregnancy. Current information strongly suggests that abnormally high blood glucose levels during pregnancy are associated with a higher incidence of congenital anomalies as well as increased neonatal morbidity and mortality. Most experts recommend that insulin be used during pregnancy to maintain blood glucose levels as close to normal as possible.

Nursing Women: Pioglitazone is secreted in the milk of lactating rats. It is not known whether ACTOS is secreted in human milk. Because many drugs are excreted in human milk, ACTOS should not be administered to a breast-feeding woman.

Pediatrics (<18 years of age): Safety and effectiveness of ACTOS in pediatric patients have not been established. Use in patients under 18 years of age is not recommended.

Geriatrics (≥65 years of age): Approximately 500 patients in placebo-controlled clinical trials of ACTOS were 65 and over. No significant differences in effectiveness and safety were observed between these patients and younger patients.

Monitoring and Laboratory Tests: FPG and HbA_{1c} measurements should be performed periodically to monitor glycemic control and the therapeutic response to ACTOS. Liver enzyme monitoring is recommended prior to initiation of therapy with ACTOS in all patients and periodically thereafter per the clinical judgment of the health care professional (see Warnings and Precautions, Hepatic/Biliary/Pancreatic and Adverse Reactions, Abnormal Hematologic and Clinical Chemistry Findings).

ADVERSE REACTIONS: Adverse Drug Reaction Overview: In worldwide clinical trials, over 3700 patients with type 2 diabetes have been treated with ACTOS (pioglitazone hydrochloride). For most clinical adverse events the incidence was similar for groups treated with ACTOS monotherapy and those treated in combination with sulfonylureas and metformin.

Controlled Clinical Trials: The overall incidence and types of adverse events reported in placebo-controlled clinical trials of ACTOS monotherapy at doses of 7.5 mg, 15 mg, 30 mg, or 45 mg once daily are shown in Table 1.

Table 1: ACTOS

Placebo-Controlled Clinical Studies of ACTOS Monotherapy: Adverse Events Reported at a Frequency ≥5% of ACTOS-treated Patients

	(% of Patients)	
	Placebo n=259	**ACTOS n=606**
Upper respiratory tract infection	8.5	13.2
Headache	6.9	9.1
Sinusitis	4.6	6.3
Myalgia	2.7	5.4
Tooth disorder	2.3	5.3
Diabetes mellitus aggravated	8.1	5.1
Pharyngitis	0.8	5.1

In addition, 4.8% of patients on ACTOS experienced edema, compared with 1.2% on placebo. In a long-term, open-label follow-up study of monotherapy, a cumulative incidence of edema of 6.0% has been reported with ACTOS. Chest pain was reported in 2.3% of patients taking ACTOS monotherapy compared with 1.5% on placebo. Heart rate and rhythm disorders were reported in 1.0% of patients taking ACTOS monotherapy compared with 1.2% on placebo. Hypoglycemia was experienced by 1.2% of patients on ACTOS monotherapy compared to none on placebo.

Adverse drug reactions reported commonly (frequency >1%, <10%) and at least 0.5% in excess of placebo in double-blind placebo-controlled studies for ACTOS monotherapy were: visual disturbance, upper respiratory tract infection, weight increased and hypoaesthesia.

The types of clinical adverse events reported when ACTOS was used in combination with sulfonylureas (N=373) or metformin (N=168) were generally similar to those reported during ACTOS monotherapy. The most commonly reported adverse events from the combination therapy studies with sulfonylureas or metformin are shown in Table 2.

Table 2: ACTOS

Placebo-Controlled Clinical Studies of ACTOS in Combination With a Sulfonylurea or Metformin: Adverse Events Reported at a Frequency ≥5% in any Group

	(% of Patients)			
Combination Therapy	**Sulfonylurea**		**Metformin**	
Treatment Group	**Placebo n=187**	**ACTOS n=373**	**Placebo n=160**	**ACTOS n=168**
Upper respiratory tract infection	15.5	16.6	15.6	15.4
Accidental injury	8.6	3.5	3.8	4.2
Peripheral edema	2.1	5.1	2.5	4.2
Diarrhea	3.7	1.6	6.3	4.8
Headache	3.7	4.8	1.9	6.0

Mild to moderate hypoglycemia was reported during combination therapy with sulfonylurea. In double-blind, combination therapy studies with a sulfonylurea the incidence of hypoglycemia was higher for patients initiated with ACTOS 30 mg than for those receiving placebo or ACTOS 15 mg (Table 3).

Edema also occurred more frequently in patients receiving ACTOS 30 mg (Table 3; see also Warnings and Precautions, Weight Gain, Edema).

During an open-label extension study, ACTOS was added to the patient's sulfonylurea or metformin, and the dose titrated based on the HbA_{1c} response. Selected adverse events that occurred during this long-term study are shown in Table 4. However, the study did not include a placebo group to control for the background rate of adverse events.

The incidence of withdrawals from clinical trials due to an adverse event other than hyperglycemia was similar for patients treated with placebo (2.8%) or ACTOS (3.3%).

Weight gain was observed in all clinical trials, including two patients withdrawn due to excessive weight gain (see Action and Clinical Pharmacology, Pharmacodynamics, and Warnings and Precautions).

Abnormal Hematologic and Clinical Chemistry Findings: Hematologic: Across all clinical studies, mean hemoglobin values declined by 2% to 4% in ACTOS-treated patients. These changes generally occurred within the first 4 to 12 weeks of therapy and remained relatively stable thereafter. These changes may be related to increased plasma volume associated with ACTOS therapy and have not been associated with any significant hematologic clinical effects. Values remained within normal limits at all times (including up to 18 months of continuous therapy).

Table 3: ACTOS

Selected Adverse Events During Controlled, Combination Therapy Studies

	Sulfonylurea			Metformin	
Combination Therapy	**Placebo**	**ACTOS 15 mg**	**ACTOS 30 mg**	**Placebo**	**ACTOS 30 mg**
N	187 (%)	184 (%)	189 (%)	160 (%)	168 (%)
Hypoglycemia	1 (0.5)	0	7 (3.7)	1 (0.6)	1 (0.6)
Edema[a]	4 (2.1)	3 (1.6)	25 (13.2)	4 (2.5)	10 (6.0)
Hypertension	2 (1.1)	2 (1.1)	4 (2.1)	2 (1.3)	3 (1.79)
Cardiac disorders[b]	4 (2.1)	7 (3.8)	6 (3.2)	3 (1.9)	1 (0.6)
Ischemia[c]	3 (1.6)	1 (0.5)	5 (2.5)	0	1 (0.6)

[a] Edema and peripheral edema.
[b] Chest pain and abnormal ECG.
[c] Angina pectoris, myocardial infarction, myocardial ischemia and transient ischemic attacks.

Table 4: ACTOS

Selected Adverse Events During Open Label, Combination Therapy Study (67.6 Weeks Median Duration)

	Sulfonylurea			Metformin		
Combination Therapy	**15 mg**	**30 mg**	**45 mg**	**15 mg**	**30 mg**	**45 mg**
N	46 (%)	81 (%)	109 (%)	5 (%)	75 (%)	74 (%)
Hypoglycemia	6 (13.0)	9 (11.1)	4 (3.7)	1 (20.0)	1 (1.3)	3 (4.1)
Edema[a]	8 (17.4)	17 (20.9)	24 (22.0)	0	13 (17.3)	11 (14.9)
Hypertension	2 (4.3)	5 (6.2)	9 (8.3)	0	5 (6.7)	3 (4.1)
Cardiac disorders[b]	4 (8.7)	8 (9.9)	12 (11.0)	0	5 (6.7)	7 (9.5)
Ischemia[c]	3 (6.5)	0	3 (2.8)	0	3 (4.0)	2 (2.7)

[a] Edema and peripheral edema.
[b] Chest pain and abnormal ECG.
[c] Angina pectoris, myocardial infarction, myocardial ischemia and transient ischemic attacks.

CPK Levels: During required laboratory testing in clinical trials, sporadic, transient elevations in creatine phosphokinase levels (CPK) were observed. An isolated elevation to greater than 10 times the upper limit of normal was noted in 9 patients (values of 2150 to 11400 IU/L. Six of these patients continued to receive ACTOS, two patients had completed receiving study medication at the time of the elevated value and one patient discontinued study medication due to the elevation. These elevations resolved without any apparent clinical sequelae. The relationship of these events to ACTOS therapy is unknown.

Serum Transaminase Levels: A total of 4 of 1526 (0.26%) ACTOS-treated patients and 2 of 793 (0.25%) placebo-treated patients had ALT values ≥3 times the upper limit of normal in double-blind, randomized clinical trials. During all clinical studies in the US, 11 of 2561 (0.43%) ACTOS-treated patients had ALT values ≥3 times the upper limit of normal. All patients with follow-up values had reversible elevations in ALT. In the population of patients treated with ACTOS, mean values for bilirubin, AST, ALT, alkaline phosphatase, and GGT were decreased at the final visit compared with baseline. Fewer than 0.12% of ACTOS-treated patients were withdrawn from clinical trials due to abnormal liver function tests.

In pre-approval clinical trials, there were no cases of idiosyncratic drug reactions leading to hepatic failure.

Post-Market Adverse Drug Reactions: Findings from post-market experience with ACTOS are reported below, including spontaneously reported adverse drug reactions. Because the latter are reported voluntarily from a population of uncertain size, it is not always possible to reliably estimate their frequency or clearly establish a causal relationship to ACTOS exposure.

In post-marketing experience with ACTOS, cases of congestive heart failure and pulmonary edema have been reported.

Cases of hepatitis and of hepatic enzyme elevations to 3 or more times the upper limit of normal have been received. Very rarely, these reports have involved hepatic failure with and without fatal outcome, although causality has not been established.

Postmarketing reports of new onset or worsening (diabetic) macular edema with decreased visual acuity have been reported rarely with the use of pioglitazone as monotherapy or in combination therapy. Affected patients also frequently reported concurrent peripheral edema. In some cases, symptoms improved following discontinuation of pioglitazone.

In a pooled analysis of randomized, controlled double-blind clinical studies, an increased incidence of bone fracture was observed in female patients taking ACTOS versus metformin, sulfonylureas or placebo (2.6% versus 1.7%). The majority of these fractures were in the distal upper limb or distal lower limb.

Postmarketing reports of bladder cancer have been reported very rarely with the use of pioglitazone.

DRUG INTERACTIONS: Overview: Pioglitazone neither induced nor inhibited P450 activity when tested following chronic administration to rats or when incubated with human P450 liver microsomes, indicating minimal effects of ACTOS on metabolic pathways of the liver. The cytochrome P450 isoform CYP3A4 is partially responsible for the metabolism of pioglitazone.

Patients on drugs metabolized by cytochrome P450 enzymes including calcium channel blockers and HMG-CoA reductase inhibitors were permitted in clinical trials.

Drug-Drug Interactions: The following drugs were studied in healthy volunteers with a coadministration of ACTOS. Listed below are the results:

Oral Contraceptives: Coadministration of ACTOS (45 mg once daily) and an oral contraceptive (1 mg norethindrone plus 0.035 mg ethinyl estradiol once daily) for 21 days, resulted in least square mean (90% CI) values for ethinyl estradiol of 0.87 (0.78-0.96) for C_{max} and 0.89 (0.83-0.96) for $AUC_{(0-24)}$. There were no significant changes in norethindrone $AUC_{(0-24)}$ and C_{max}. In view of the high variability of ethinyl estradiol pharmacokinetics, the clinical significance of this finding is unknown.

Glipizide: In healthy volunteers, coadministration of ACTOS (45 mg once daily) and glipizide (5.0 mg once daily) for 7 days did not alter the steady-state pharmacokinetics of glipizide.

Digoxin: In healthy volunteers, coadministration of ACTOS (45 mg once daily) with digoxin (0.25 mg once daily) for 7 days did not alter the steady-state pharmacokinetics of digoxin.

Warfarin: In healthy volunteers, coadministration of ACTOS (45 mg once daily) for 7 days with warfarin did not alter the steady-state pharmacokinetics of warfarin. In addition, ACTOS has no clinically significant effect on prothrombin time when administered to patients receiving chronic warfarin therapy.

Metformin: In healthy volunteers, coadministration of metformin (1000 mg) and ACTOS after 7 days of ACTOS (45 mg once daily) did not alter the pharmacokinetics of the single dose of metformin.

Fexofenadine HCl: Coadministration of ACTOS (45 mg once daily) for 7 days with 60 mg fexofenadine administered orally twice daily resulted in no significant effect on pioglitazone pharmacokinetics. ACTOS had no significant effect on the pharmacokinetics of fexofenadine administered in the AM. However, coadministration of ACTOS with fexofenadine administered in the PM resulted in least square mean (90% CI) values for fexofenadine of 1.37 (1.14-1.63) for C_{max} and 1.30 (1.15-1.46) for AUC_{0-t}. The clinical significance of this AM/PM variation is unknown.

Midazolam: Administration of ACTOS (45 mg once daily) for 15 days followed by a single 7.5 mg dose of midazolam syrup resulted in least square mean (90% CI) values for unchanged midazolam of 0.74 (0 66-0.84) for C_{max} and 0.74 (0.65-0.83) for $AUC_{(0-\infty)}$.

Ranitidine HCl: Coadministration of ACTOS (45 mg once daily) for 7 days with ranitidine administered orally twice daily for either 4 or 7 days resulted in no significant effect on pioglitazone pharmacokinetics. ACTOS showed no significant effect on ranitidine pharmacokinetics.

Nifedipine ER: Coadministration of ACTOS (45 mg once daily) for 7 days with 30 mg nifedipine ER administered orally once daily for 4 days to male and female volunteers did not affect the pharmacokinetics of nifedipine in females, but resulted in least square mean (90% CI) values for unchanged nifedipine of 0.75 (0.62-0.91) for C_{max} and 0.78 (0.69-0.88) for $AUC_{0-τ}$ in males. In view of the high variability of nifedipine pharmacokinetics, the clinical significance of this finding is unknown.

Ketoconazole: Coadministration of ACTOS (45 mg once daily) for 7 days with ketoconazole 200 mg administered twice daily resulted in least square mean (90% CI) values for total pioglitazone of 1.17 (1.10-1.24) for C_{max}, 1.21 (1.16-1.25) for $AUC_{(0-24)}$ and 1.29 (1.23-1.35) for C_{min}. These changes are not expected to have any significant effect on the clinical efficacy of ACTOS.

Atorvastatin Calcium: Coadministration of ACTOS (45 mg once daily) for 7 days with atorvastatin calcium (LIPITOR) 80 mg once daily resulted in least square mean (90% CI) values for total pioglitazone of 0.78 (0.70-0.88) for C_{max}, 0.80 (0.73-0.88) for $AUC_{(0-24)}$ and 0.89 (0.82-0.96) for C_{min}. For total atorvastatin the least square mean (90% CI) values were 0.76 (0.65-0.89) for C_{max}, 0.87 (0.80-0.95) for $AUC_{(0-24)}$ and 0.96 (0.88-1.04) for C_{min}.

Theophylline: Coadministration of ACTOS (45 mg once daily) for 7 days with theophylline 400 mg administered twice daily resulted in no change in the pharmacokinetics of either drug.

Gemfibrozil: Coadministration of ACTOS 30 mg with gemfibrozil 600 mg twice daily (an inhibitor of CYP2C8) was reported to result in a 3-fold increase in AUC of pioglitazone. Given the potential for dose-related adverse events, a decrease in dose may be needed when ACTOS is coadministered with gemfibrozil. Close monitoring of glycemic control should be considered.

Rifampicin: Coadministration of ACTOS 30 mg with rifampicin 600 mg once daily (an inducer of CYP2C8) was reported to result in a 54% decrease in AUC of pioglitazone. The dose of ACTOS may need to be increased when the drug is coadministered with rifampicin. Close monitoring of glycemic control should be considered.

Drug-Food Interactions: ACTOS may be taken without regard to meals. Food slightly delays the time to peak serum concentration but does not alter the extent of absorption.

Drug-Herb Interactions: There is no evidence of drug-herb interactions.

Drug-Laboratory Test Interactions: There is no evidence of drug-laboratory interactions.

DOSAGE AND ADMINISTRATION: Dosing Considerations: The management of antidiabetic therapy should be individualized. Ideally, the response to therapy should be evaluated using HbA_{1c}, which is a better indicator of long-term glycemic control than FBG alone. HbA_{1c} reflects glycemia over the past two to three months. In clinical use, it is recommended that patients be treated with ACTOS for a period of time adequate to evaluate change in HbA_{1c} unless glycemic control deteriorates.

Liver enzymes should be checked prior to the initiation of therapy with ACTOS in all patients. ACTOS is contraindicated in patients with severe hepatic impairment. Therapy with ACTOS should not be initiated if a patient exhibits clinical evidence of active liver disease or increased serum transaminase levels (ALT >2.5 times upper limit of normal). If ALT levels remain >3 times the upper limit of normal, therapy with ACTOS should be discontinued. See Warnings and Precautions, Hepatic/Biliary/Pancreatic. In cases where therapy is to be initiated, dose adjustment in patients with hepatic disease is not required (see Actions and Clinical Pharmacology, Special Populations and Conditions).

Dose adjustment in patients with renal insufficiency is not required (see Actions and Clinical Pharmacology, Special Populations and Conditions).

As adverse events such as edema and weight gain appear to be dose-related, the smallest effective dose should be used.

Recommended Dose and Dosage Adjustment: ACTOS should be taken once daily without regard to meals.

The dose of ACTOS (pioglitazone hydrochloride) should not exceed 45 mg once daily since doses higher than 45 mg once daily have not been studied in placebo-controlled clinical studies.

Monotherapy: ACTOS in patients not adequately controlled with diet and exercise may be initiated at 15 mg or 30 mg once daily. For patients who respond inadequately to the initial dose of ACTOS, the dose can be increased in increments up to 45 mg once daily.

Combination Therapy: In patients not adequately controlled with a sulfonylurea or metformin, ACTOS may be initiated at 15 or 30 mg once daily. For patients who do not respond adequately to the initial dose, ACTOS may be increased in increments up to 45 mg once daily.

In patients receiving a sulfonylurea, the dose of the sulfonylurea may need to be decreased if hypoglycemia occurs (see Adverse Reactions). It is unlikely that the metformin dose will require adjustment because of hypoglycemia.

OVERDOSAGE:

During controlled clinical trials, one case of overdose with ACTOS (pioglitazone hydrochloride) was reported. A male patient took 120 mg per day for four days, then 180 mg per day for seven days. The patient denied any clinical symptoms during this period.

In the event of overdosage, appropriate supportive treatment should be initiated according to the patient's clinical signs and symptoms.

For management of a suspected drug overdose, contact your regional Poison Control Centre. See the *CPS Directory* section for a list of Poison Control Centres.

ACTION AND CLINICAL PHARMACOLOGY: Mechanism of Action: ACTOS (pioglitazone hydrochloride) is a thiazolidinedione antidiabetic agent that depends on the presence of insulin for its mechanism of action. ACTOS decreases insulin resistance in the periphery and liver, resulting in increased insulin-dependent glucose disposal and decreased hepatic glucose output respectively.

ACTOS improves glycemic control while reducing circulating insulin levels. Unlike sulfonylureas, ACTOS is not an insulin secretagogue. ACTOS is a potent and highly selective agonist for peroxisome proliferator-activated receptor-gamma (PPARγ). PPARγ receptors are found in tissues important for insulin action such as adipose tissue, skeletal muscle, and liver. Activation of PPARγ nuclear receptors modulates the transcription of a number of insulin responsive genes involved in the control of glucose and lipid metabolism, and in the maturation of preadipocytes, predominantly of subcutaneous origin.

Insulin resistance is a primary feature characterizing the pathogenesis of type 2 diabetes. ACTOS results in increased responsiveness of insulin-dependent tissues. ACTOS significantly improves hepatic and peripheral (muscle) tissue sensitivity to insulin in patients with type 2 diabetes. ACTOS also results in significant reductions in markers of beta cell hyperstimulation, such as fasting insulin and fasting C-peptide. In short term clinical studies of 16 weeks duration, ACTOS has also been shown to significantly improve biochemical markers of pancreatic beta cell function.

In clinical studies in patients with type 2 diabetes, ACTOS reduces the hyperglycemia and hyperinsulinemia characteristic of insulin-resistant states, including type 2 diabetes. ACTOS significantly reduces hemoglobin A_{1c} (HbA_{1c}, a marker for long term glycemic control), and fasting blood glucose (FBG) in patients with type 2 diabetes.

Low HDL-C and elevated triglycerides are common in patients with type 2 diabetes. ACTOS significantly increases high density lipoprotein cholesterol (HDL-C) and reduces triglycerides in patients with type 2 diabetes. It also increases the particle size of low density lipoprotein.

ACTOS significantly reduces carotid arterial intimal medial thickness. It also results in modest, but significant, reductions in blood pressure. In addition, ACTOS significantly decreases microalbuminuria in patients with type 2 diabetes.

Since ACTOS enhances the effects of circulating insulin (by decreasing insulin resistance), it does not lower blood glucose in animal models that lack endogenous insulin.

Pharmacodynamics: Clinical studies demonstrate that ACTOS improves insulin sensitivity in insulin-resistant patients. ACTOS enhances cellular responsiveness to insulin, increases insulin-dependent glucose disposal, improves hepatic sensitivity to insulin, and improves dysfunctional glucose homeostasis. In patients with type 2 diabetes, the decreased insulin resistance produced by ACTOS results in significantly lower blood glucose concentrations, lower plasma insulin levels, and lower HbA_{1c} values. Based on results from open-label extension studies, the glucose lowering effects of ACTOS are sustained for more than 1 year, but some patients require titration to higher doses to maintain the response. The effect of ACTOS occurs in the absence of weight loss.

ACTOS exerts its antihyperglycemic effect in the presence of insulin. Because ACTOS does not stimulate insulin secretion, hypoglycemia would not be expected in patients treated with ACTOS alone.

In pharmacodynamic studies of both monotherapy and combination therapy, treatment with ACTOS was associated with decreases in free fatty acids.

In a 26-week, placebo-controlled, dose-ranging study, mean triglyceride levels decreased in the 15 mg, 30 mg, and 45 mg ACTOS dose groups compared to a mean increase in the placebo group. Mean HDL-C levels increased to a greater extent in the ACTOS-treated patients than in the placebo-treated patients. There were no consistent differences for low density lipoprotein cholesterol (LDL-C) and total cholesterol in ACTOS-treated patients compared to placebo (see Table 5).

Table 5: ACTOS

Lipids in a 26-Week, Multicentre, Placebo-Controlled Dose-Ranging Study

	Placebo	ACTOS 15 mg Once Daily	ACTOS 30 mg Once Daily	ACTOS 45 mg Once Daily
Triglycerides (mmol/L)	N=79	N=79	N=84	N=77
Baseline (mean)	2.97	3.2	2.95	2.93
Percent change from baseline (mean)	4.8%	−9.0%	−9.6%	−9.3%
HDL Cholesterol (mmol/L)	N=79	N=79	N=83	N=77
Baseline (mean)	1.08	1.04	1.06	1.05
Percent change from baseline (mean)	8.1%	14.1%	12.2%	19.1%
LDL Cholesterol (mmol/L)	N=65	N=63	N=74	N=62
Baseline (mean)	3.59	3.41	3.51	3.28
Percent change from baseline (mean)	4.8%	7.2%	5.2%	6.0%
Total Cholesterol (mmol/L)	N=79	N=79	N=84	N=77
Baseline (mean)	5.81	5.69	5.76	5.53
Percent change from baseline (mean)	4.4%	4.6%	3.3%	6.4%

In two other monotherapy studies (study duration 24 weeks and 16 weeks), the results were generally consistent with the data above. For ACTOS-treated patients, the placebo-corrected mean changes from baseline decreased by 21 to 23% for triglycerides, and increased by 5 to 13% for HDL-C.

Statistically significant increases in HDL-C and reductions in triglycerides were also observed with ACTOS in 2 controlled, combination therapy studies (each 16 weeks duration), in which patients with type 2 diabetes who were receiving therapy with a sulfonylurea or metformin were randomized to placebo or combination therapy with ACTOS.

Patients taking statins were not excluded from clinical trials. In these patients, the mean increases in HDL-C and reductions of triglycerides with ACTOS were observed in addition to the effects of the statin.

ACTOS is also associated with weight gain (see Warnings and Precautions, and Adverse Reactions). In addition, ACTOS significantly decreases visceral (abdominal) fat stores while increasing extra-abdominal fat. The reduction in visceral fat correlates with improved hepatic and peripheral tissue insulin sensitivity.

Figure 1 plots the change in body weight for patients who had completed 48 weeks of treatment with pioglitazone in an open-label trial.

Figure 1: ACTOS

Mean Change from Baseline for Body Weight by Visit, for Patients who Completed 48 Weeks of Open-Label Treatment

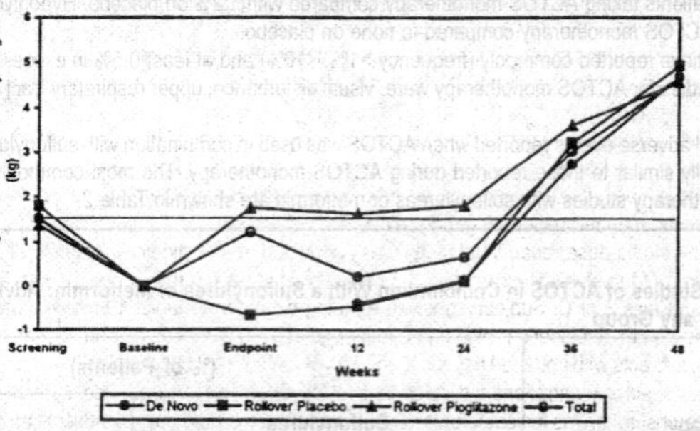

As indicated in Figure 1, at Week 48 the mean change from baseline in body weight was 5.55 kg for the de novo group (newly diagnosed patients), 6.34 kg for the roll-over placebo group (double-blind placebo treatment followed by open-label pioglitazone), and 5.36 kg for the roll-over pioglitazone group (double-blind pioglitazone treatment followed by open-label pioglitazone). For the total patient group, the mean change from baseline in body weight was 5.56 kg. The maximum and minimum weight changes observed up to Week 48 from time of entry into this open-label trial for the total patient group were 21.77 kg and −19.86 kg, respectively (median weight change: 4.54 kg).

Two patients were withdrawn from the study due to reported weight increases of 15.6 kg and 20.8 kg respectively. For the first patient, the investigator believed the weight gain was due to edema, and for the second, a dose of 60 mg of pioglitazone was used, and the patient had dietary factors that could have also contributed to the weight gain. Any abnormally large weight gain experienced by some patients may be due to fluid retention. (See Warnings and Precautions, Edema.)

During two placebo-controlled, 16 week, combination therapy studies the mean weight increased for all ACTOS treatment groups: for the sulfonylurea combination therapy study the mean increases with ACTOS 15 mg and 30 mg were 1.9 and 2.9 kg, respectively; for the metformin combination therapy study, the mean increase with ACTOS 30 mg was 0.95 kg.

However, the individual weight change was highly variable. The range of weight changes during the studies is shown in Table 6 (see Warnings and Precautions, Weight Gain).

Table 6: ACTOS

Change in Weight During Double-Blind, Combination Therapy Studies

	Sulfonylurea			Metformin	
Combination Therapy:	**Placebo**	**ACTOS 15 mg**	**ACTOS 30 mg**	**Placebo**	**ACTOS 30 mg**
N	160 (%)	157 (%)	168 (%)	112 (%)	137 (%)
>10 kg loss	1 (0.6)	—	—	—	1 (0.6)
5 to 10 kg loss	13 (8.1)	2 (1.3)	4 (2.4)	15 (13.4)	9 (6.6)

(cont'd)

Table 6: ACTOS *(cont'd)*

Change in Weight During Double-Blind, Combination Therapy Studies

Combination Therapy:	Sulfonylurea Placebo	Sulfonylurea ACTOS 15 mg	Sulfonylurea ACTOS 30 mg	Metformin Placebo	Metformin ACTOS 30 mg
0 to <5 kg loss	76 (47.5)	23 (14.6)	16 (9.5)	54 (48.2)	21 (15.3)
0 kg	19 (11.9)	5 (3.2)	4 (2.4)	9 (8.0)	10 (7.3)
0 to 5 kg gain	49 (30.6)	110 (70.0)	106 (63.1)	33 (29.5)	81 (59.1)
>5 to 10 kg gain	2 (1.3)	16 (10.2)	36 (21.4)	1 (0.9)	15 (10.9)
>10 kg gain	—	1 (0.6)	2 (1.2)	—	—

In patients receiving long-term combination therapy with sulfonylurea or metformin, median weight gain (5.40 kg after at least 60 weeks ACTOS therapy) was similar to that with ACTOS monotherapy (median weight gain 4.54 kg after 48 weeks).

Pharmacokinetics: Serum concentrations of total pioglitazone (pioglitazone plus active metabolites) remain elevated 24 hours after once-daily dosing. Steady-state serum concentrations of both pioglitazone and total pioglitazone are achieved within 7 days. At steady state, two of the pharmacologically active metabolites of pioglitazone, Metabolites III (M-III) and IV (M-IV), reach serum concentrations equal to or greater than pioglitazone. At steady state, in both healthy volunteers and in patients with type 2 diabetes, pioglitazone comprises approximately 30% to 50% of the peak total pioglitazone serum concentrations and 20% to 25% of the total area under the serum concentration-time curve (AUC).

Maximum serum concentration (C_{max}), AUC, and trough serum concentrations (C_{min}) for both pioglitazone and total pioglitazone increase proportionally at doses of 15 mg and 30 mg per day. There is a slightly less than proportional increase for pioglitazone and total pioglitazone at a dose of 60 mg per day.

Absorption: Following oral administration, in the fasting state, pioglitazone is first measurable in serum within 30 minutes, with peak concentrations observed within 2 hours. Food slightly delays the time to peak serum concentration to 3 to 4 hours, but does not alter the extent of absorption.

Distribution: The mean apparent volume of distribution (Vd/F) of pioglitazone following single-dose administration is 0.63±0.41 (mean±SD) L/kg of body weight. Pioglitazone is extensively protein bound (>99%) in human serum, principally to serum albumin. Pioglitazone also binds to other serum proteins, but with lower affinity. Metabolites M-III and M-IV also are extensively bound (>98%) to serum albumin.

Metabolism: Pioglitazone is extensively metabolized by hydroxylation and oxidation; the metabolites also partly convert to glucuronide or sulfate conjugates. Metabolites M-II and M-IV (hydroxy derivatives of pioglitazone) and M-III (keto derivative of pioglitazone) are pharmacologically active in animal models of type 2 diabetes. In addition to pioglitazone, M-III and M-IV are the principal drug-related species found in human serum following multiple dosing.

Pioglitazone incubated with expressed human P450 or human liver microsomes results in the formation of M-IV and to a much lesser degree, M-II. The major cytochrome P450 isoforms involved in the hepatic metabolism of pioglitazone are CYP2C8 and CYP3A4 (>50% of metabolism) with contributions from a variety of other isoforms including the mainly extrahepatic CYP1A1. Ketoconazole inhibited up to 85% of hepatic pioglitazone metabolism in vitro at an equimolar concentration to pioglitazone. At higher than therapeutic concentrations, pioglitazone had no effect on the reactions mediated by human liver microsomes expressing cytochrome P450 isoforms including CYP2C8 and CYP3A4. The potential induction or inhibition of CYP3A4 by pioglitazone has been observed in vivo (see Drug Interactions, Drug-Drug Interactions).

Excretion: Following oral administration, approximately 15 to 30% of the pioglitazone dose is recovered in the urine as metabolites. Renal elimination of unchanged pioglitazone is negligible, and the drug is excreted primarily as metabolites and their conjugates. It is presumed that most of the oral dose is excreted into the bile either unchanged or as metabolites and eliminated in the feces.

The mean serum half-life of pioglitazone and total pioglitazone ranges from 3 to 7 hours and 16 to 24 hours, respectively. Pioglitazone has an apparent clearance, CL/F, calculated to be 5 to 7 L/hr.

Special Populations and Conditions: Pediatrics: Pharmacokinetic data in the pediatric population are not available. ACTOS is not recommended for patients under 18 years of age.

Geriatrics: In healthy elderly subjects, peak serum concentrations of pioglitazone and total pioglitazone are not significantly different, but AUC values are slightly higher and the terminal half-life values slightly longer than for younger subjects. These changes were not of a magnitude that would be considered clinically relevant.

Gender: ACTOS improved glycemic control in both males and females. In controlled clinical trials the mean C_{max} and AUC values were increased 20 to 60% in females. HbA_{1c} decreases from baseline were generally greater for females than for males (average mean absolute difference in HbA_{1c} 0.005). Since therapy should be individualized for each patient to achieve glycemic control, no dose adjustment is recommended based on gender alone.

Hepatic Insufficiency: A single-dose, open-label study was conducted to investigate the effects of impaired hepatic function on pioglitazone. A group of 24 subjects was enrolled; 12 with normal hepatic function and 12 with abnormal hepatic function classified as Childs-Pugh Class B or C. Subjects received a 30 mg pioglitazone tablet 10 minutes after a diet-controlled meal, and changes in the serum pharmacokinetic profile and urinary excretion of pioglitazone and its metabolites were then studied. Compared with controls, subjects with impaired hepatic function have a 45% reduction in pioglitazone and total (pioglitazone plus active metabolites) mean peak concentrations but no change in the mean AUC values. The findings of this study showed that the extent of pioglitazone absorption, as indicated by $AUC_{(0-24)}$, was similar in both normal subjects and individuals with impaired hepatic function. No adverse events attributable to pioglitazone were reported in either group, and no clinically significant changes in baseline laboratory tests, including liver function tests, were observed.

Although no adverse events attributed to drug were noted in any group, ACTOS should be used with caution in patients with hepatic disease. Therapy with ACTOS should not be initiated if a patient exhibits clinical evidence of active liver disease or increased serum transaminase levels (ALT >2.5 times upper limit of normal) at baseline (see Warnings and Precautions, Hepatic/Biliary/Pancreatic).

Renal Insufficiency: The serum elimination half-life of pioglitazone, M-III, and M-IV remains unchanged in patients with moderate (creatinine clearance 0.5 to 1.0 mL/s [30 to 60 mL/min]) to severe (creatinine clearance <0.5 mL/s [30 mL/min]) renal impairment when compared to normal subjects. No dose adjustment in patients with renal dysfunction is recommended.

STORAGE AND STABILITY: ACTOS (pioglitazone hydrochloride) tablets may be stored at controlled room temperature (15-30°C). Keep container tightly closed and protect from moisture.

INFORMATION FOR THE PATIENT: Published in e-CPS, available by subscription at www.e-cps.ca.

DOSAGE FORMS, COMPOSITION AND PACKAGING: 15 mg: Each white to off-white, round, convex, non-scored tablet, with "ACTOS" printed on one side and "15" on the other, contains: pioglitazone HCl equivalent to pioglitazone 15 mg. Nonmedicinal ingredients: carboxymethylcellulose calcium, hydroxypropylcellulose, lactose monohydrate and magnesium stearate. Bottles of 90.

30 mg: Each white to off-white, round, flat, non-scored tablet, with "ACTOS" printed on one side and "30" on the other, contains: pioglitazone HCl equivalent to pioglitazone 30 mg. Nonmedicinal ingredients: carboxymethylcellulose calcium, hydroxypropylcellulose, lactose monohydrate and magnesium stearate. Bottles of 90.

45 mg: Each white to off-white, round, flat, non-scored tablet, with "ACTOS" printed on one side and "45" on the other, contains: pioglitazone HCl equivalent to pioglitazone 45 mg. Nonmedicinal ingredients: carboxymethylcellulose calcium, hydroxypropylcellulose, lactose monohydrate and magnesium stearate. Bottles of 90.

(Shown in Product Identification Section)

Acular® Pr

ketorolac tromethamine

Topical Nonsteroidal Anti-inflammatory Agent

Allergan

Acular® LS Pr

ketorolac tromethamine

Topical Nonsteroidal Anti-inflammatory Agent

Allergan

Date of Preparation: February 10, 1992
Date of Revision: January 6, 2004

PHARMACOLOGY: Mechanism of Action: Ketorolac tromethamine is a nonsteroidal, anti-inflammatory agent demonstrating analgesic and anti-inflammatory activity mediated by peripheral effects. Ketorolac inhibits the synthesis of prostaglandins through inhibition of the cyclo-oxygenase enzyme system. Prostaglandins play a critical role in many inflammatory processes of the eye and appear to play a role in the miotic response during ocular surgery. At concentrations of 0.02% - 0.5%, ketorolac tromethamine solution did not irritate the eyes of rats, dogs or monkeys. Up to 4.0% concentrations were nonirritating in albino rabbits.

Ketorolac tromethamine has demonstrated anti-inflammatory activity when applied topically in several animal models of ocular inflammation. The compound significantly inhibited the inflammatory responses to silver nitrate-induced cauterization of the corneas of rat eyes at concentrations of 0.25% and 0.5%. Concentrations of ketorolac ranging from 0.02% to 0.5% blocked vascular permeability changes caused by endotoxin-induced uveitis in the eyes of rabbits. Using the same model, ketorolac also blocked endotoxin-induced elevation of aqueous humor PGE2. It prevented the development of increased intraocular pressure induced in rabbits with topically applied arachidonic acid. Ketorolac did not inhibit rabbit lens aldose reductase in vitro.

Applications of a 0.5% ketorolac solution did not delay the healing of experimental corneal wounds in rabbits. This solution did not enhance the spread of experimental ocular infections induced in rabbits with *C. albicans*, Herpes simplex virus type one, or *P. aeruginosa*.

Pharmacokinetics: Absorption: In human studies, penetration of the drug is rapid after application to the eye. The relationship between the concentrations of solution administered and the amount of drug that penetrates the cornea is roughly linear.

Two drops (0.1 mL) of 0.5% ketorolac tromethamine ophthalmic solution, instilled into the eyes of patients 12 hours and 1 hour prior to cataract extraction, achieved measurable levels in 8 of 9 patients' eyes. The mean ketorolac concentration was 95 ng/mL in the aqueous humor and the range was 40 ng/mL to 170 ng/mL. The mean concentration of PGE2 was 80 pg/mL in the aqueous humor of eyes receiving vehicle and 28 pg/mL in the eyes receiving 0.5% ketorolac tromethamine ophthalmic solution.

One drop (0.05 mL) of 0.5% ketorolac tromethamine ophthalmic solution was instilled into one eye and one drop of the vehicle into the other eye t.i.d. for 21 days in 26 healthy subjects. Only 5 of 26 subjects had detectable amount of ketorolac in their plasma (range 10.7 ng/mL and 22.5 ng/mL) when tested 15 minutes after the morning dose on day 10.

When ketorolac is given systemically to relieve pain, the average plasma level following chronic systemic treatment was approximately 850 ng/mL.

Distribution: Animal studies have shown that ^{14}C-labelled ophthalmic solution 0.5% was found to be extensively distributed in ocular tissues with major portions retained in the cornea and sclera.

Metabolism: Although no studies have been conducted regarding the sites of metabolism for ophthalmic ketorolac, studies of systemic administration have shown that the drug is metabolized in the liver.

Excretion: Results of studies in rabbits and cynomolgus monkeys suggest that the major route of drug elimination from the eye is probably through intraocular blood flow after distribution from the aqueous humor to the iris-ciliary body.

Pharmacodynamics: Ketorolac tromethamine given systemically does not cause pupil constriction. Results from clinical studies indicate that ketorolac tromethamine ophthalmic solution has no significant effect upon intraocular pressure, although changes in intraocular pressure may occur following refractive surgery.

Clinical Studies: In two double-masked, multi-centered, parallel-group studies, 313 patients who had undergone photorefractive keratectomy received Acular LS (ketorolac tromethamine) ophthalmic solution 0.4% or its vehicle QID for up to 4 days. Significant differences favored Acular LS for the treatment of ocular pain and the ocular symptoms of foreign body sensation, burning/stinging, tearing, and photophobia.

INDICATIONS: Acular (ketorolac tromethamine) ophthalmic solution 0.5% is indicated for the prophylaxis and the relief of postoperative ocular inflammation in patients undergoing cataract extraction with or without implantation of an intraocular lens.

Acular LS (ketorolac tromethamine) ophthalmic solution 0.4% is indicated for the reduction of ocular pain and ocular symptoms of foreign body sensation, burning/stinging, tearing, and photophobia following refractive surgery.

CONTRAINDICATIONS: Ketorolac tromethamine ophthalmic solutions should not be used in patients who have previously exhibited hypersensitivity to any of the ingredients in the formulation.

WARNINGS: General: With some nonsteroidal anti-inflammatory drugs, there exists the potential for increased bleeding time due to interference with thrombocyte aggregation. There have been reports that ocularly applied nonsteroidal anti-inflammatory drugs may cause increased bleeding of ocular tissues (including hyphemas) in conjunction with ocular surgery.

Lactation: Ketorolac tromethamine ophthalmic solutions are not recommended for treatment of nursing mothers. Secretion of ketorolac tromethamine in human milk after systemic administration is limited. The milk-to-plasma ratio of ketorolac tromethamine concentrations ranged between 0.015 and 0.037 in a study of 10 women.

PRECAUTIONS: General: It is recommended that ketorolac tromethamine ophthalmic solutions be used with caution in surgical patients with known bleeding tendencies or who are receiving other medications which may prolong bleeding time.

All topical nonsteroidal anti-inflammatory drugs (NSAIDs) may slow or delay wound healing. Postmarketing experiences suggest that topical nonsteroidal anti-inflammatories (NSAIDs) used by patients with complicated ocular surgeries, corneal denervation, corneal epithelial defects, diabetes mellitus, ocular surface disease, rheumatoid arthritis, or repeat ocular surgeries within a short period of time may be at an increased risk of corneal adverse events. These may include keratitis, epithelial breakdown, corneal thinning, corneal errosion, corneal ulceration or corneal perforation.

The potential for cross sensitivity to acetylsalicylic acid, phenylacetic acid, and other nonsteroidal anti-inflammatory drugs exists. Ketorolac tromethamine ophthalmic solutions therefore should be used with caution in patients who have previously exhibited sensitivities to these drugs.

Pregnancy: Pregnancy, Labor, and Delivery: Use of ketorolac tromethamine ophthalmic solutions is not recommended during pregnancy, labor or delivery.

Because of the known effects of prostaglandin-inhibiting drugs on the fetal cardiovascular system of rats (closure of the ductus arteriosus), the use of ketorolac tromethamine ophthalmic solutions during late pregnancy should be avoided.

Drug Interactions: There have been no reports of interactions of ketorolac tromethamine ophthalmic solution 0.5% with topical or injectable drugs used in ophthalmology pre-, intra, or post-operatively, including antibiotics (e.g., gentamicin, tobramycin, neomycin, polymyxin), sedatives (e.g., diazepam, hydroxyzine, lorazepam, promethazine HCl), miotics, mydriatics, cycloplegics (e.g., acetylcholine, atropine, epinephrine, physostigmine, phenylephrine, timolol maleate), hyaluronidase, local anesthetics (e.g., bupivacaine HCl, cyclopentolate HCl, lidocaine HCl, tetracaine), or corticosteroids.

Carcinogenesis, Mutagenesis, and Impairment of Fertility: Long-term studies in mice and rats have shown no evidence of carcinogenicity, teratogenicity, or impairment of fertility, with ketorolac tromethamine. No mutagenic potential of ketorolac was found in the Ames bacterial or the micronucleus test for mutagenicity.

Children: Safety and effectiveness of ketorolac tromethamine ophthalmic solutions in pediatric patients below the age of 3 have not been established.

Geriatrics: No overall differences in safety or effectiveness have been observed between elderly and younger patients.

Ophthalmology: Blurred and/or diminished vision has been reported with the use of ketorolac tromethamine ophthalmic solution and other nonsteroidal anti-inflammatory drugs. These symptoms should diminish over time. However, if they persist, this drug should be discontinued and an ophthalmic examination should be performed.

ADVERSE EFFECTS: Since other nonsteroidal anti-inflammatory drugs have been known to irritate the eye upon topical application, ketorolac tromethamine was studied for its ocular irritation potential in animals and man.

In two multi-dose studies in healthy volunteers, one drop of 0.5% ketorolac tromethamine ophthalmic solution was applied three times daily for 21 days. Mild to moderate transient ocular burning/stinging was reported.

Most ocular complaints reported in clinical studies with Acular (ketorolac tromethamine) ophthalmic solution 0.5% could not be distinguished from adverse events caused by the trauma of cataract surgery and the insertion of an intraocular lens.

Up to two drops (0.1 mL or 0.5 mg) of 0.5% ketorolac ophthalmic solution per eye every 6 to 8 hours have been administered postsurgically.

The most frequent adverse reactions were conjunctivitis (redness, scratchiness, foreign body sensation, 10%) eye pain (pain, ache and burn, 6%), ptosis (5%) and keratitis (corneal edema, 3%). Iritis, corneal lesion, eye disorder, photophobia, pupillary disorder, blepharitis and elevated intraocular pressure were each reported with a prevalence of 2%.

In the controlled clinical trials with Acular LS (ketorolac tromethamine) ophthalmic solution 0.4%, the most frequently reported adverse reactions occurring in approximately 1 to 5 % of the overall study population were conjunctival hyperemia, corneal infiltrates, eye edema, eye pain, and headache (see Table 1).

Table 1: Acular

Number (%) of Patients with Treatment-Related Adverse Events Reported During Treatment Period in the Pooled Phase 3 Studies

Body System Preferred Term	Ketorolac N=156 (%)	Vehicle N=157 (%)
Body as a Whole		
Headache	1 (0.6%)	3 (1.9%)
Digestive System		
Nausea	0 (0.0%)	1 (0.6%)
Vomiting	0 (0.0%)	1 (0.6%)
Special Senses		
Pain eye	2 (1.3%)	4 (2.5%)
Corneal Infiltrates	1 (0.6%)	1 (0.6%)
Edema Eye	1 (0.6%)	0 (0.0%)
Conjunctival Hyperemia (NOS)	1 (0.6%)	0 (0.0%)
Irritation	0 (0.0%)	1 (0.6%)

None of the typical adverse reactions reported with the systemic nonsteroidal anti-inflammatory agents or ketorolac tromethamine have been observed at the doses used in topical ophthalmic therapy.

OVERDOSE:

Symptoms: The absence of experience with acute overdosage systemically or topically precludes characterization of sequelae and assessment of antidotal efficacy at this time. If ingested accidentally, drink fluids to dilute.

Treatment: See Symptoms.

> For management of a suspected drug overdose, CPhA recommends that you contact your regional Poison Control Centre. See the *CPS* Directory section for a list of Poison Control Centres.

DOSAGE: The recommended dose of Acular (ketorolac tromethamine) ophthalmic solution 0.5% is one to two drops (0.25 mg - 0.5 mg) every six to eight hours beginning 24 hours before surgery and continuing for three to four weeks for prophylaxis and relief of postoperative ocular inflammation.

The recommended dose of Acular LS (ketorolac tromethamine) ophthalmic solution 0.4% is one drop four times a day for up to four days in the affected eye.

Information to Be Provided to the Patient: Contact lenses should be removed prior to instillation of ketorolac tromethamine ophthalmic solutions and may be re-inserted 15 minutes following administration. Patients should be advised that Acular and Acular LS both contain benzalkonium chloride, which may discolor soft contact lenses.

Patients should be instructed to avoid allowing the tip of the dispensing container to contact the eye, surrounding structures, fingers, or any other surface in order to avoid contamination of the solution by common bacteria known to cause ocular infections. Based on the pharmacodynamic profile, ketorolac is not expected to influence a patient's ability to drive or operate machinery. As with any ocular medication, if transient blurred vision occurs at instillation, the patient should wait until the vision clears before driving or using machinery.

INFORMATION FOR THE PATIENT: Published in e-CPS, available by subscription at www.e-cps.ca.

SUPPLIED: Acular: Each bottle of sterile ophthalmic solution contains: ketorolac tromethamine 0.5%. Nonmedicinal ingredients: benzalkonium chloride NF, edetate disodium, USP, octoxynol 40, purified water, sodium chloride, USP and sodium hydroxide and/or hydrochloric acid to adjust the pH to 7.4. White opaque plastic bottles of 5 and 10 mL with a controlled dropper tip. Store in the original container at 25°C, with excursions to 15-30°C. Protect from light. **Discard** 28 days after opening.

Acular LS: Each bottle of sterile ophthalmic solution contains: ketorolac tromethamine 0.4%. Nonmedicinal ingredient: benzalkonium chloride 0.006%, edetate disodium, hydrochloric acid and/or sodium hydroxide to adjust the pH to 7.4, octoxynol 40, purified water and sodium chloride. White opaque plastic bottles of 5 mL with a controlled dropper tip. Store in the original container at 25°C, with excursions to 15-30°C. Protect from light. **Discard** 28 days after opening.

Acyclovir Sodium Injectable 🄿
Antiviral

CPhA Monograph

Date of Preparation: March 2008

> This monograph has been compiled by CPhA and reviewed by experts. It may contain information different from that found in Health Canada-approved Product Monographs. The reader is referred to the *CPS* Editorial Policy for more information.

SUMMARY PRODUCT INFORMATION:

Route of Administration	Dosage Form	Strength
IV	Powder for solution	500 mg
IV	Solution	25 mg/mL (20 mL)
IV	Solution	50 mg/mL (10, 20 mL)

INDICATIONS AND CLINICAL USE: Acyclovir sodium is indicated for:

- treatment of serious initial and recurrent infections with susceptible herpesviruses including herpes simplex virus (HSV-1 and HSV-2) and varicella-zoster virus (VZV) in immunocompromised adults and children;
- treatment of HSV encephalitis and neonatal HSV infections;
- treatment of severe or disseminated herpesvirus infections in pregnancy.

Immunocompromised patients are at increased risk of herpesvirus infections and tend to experience more frequent and more severe bouts of HSV and VZV infection. With the exception of severe infections, such as encephalitis or herpesvirus infections in neonates, oral formulations of acyclovir or famciclovir or valganciclovir are preferred for the treatment of initial and recurrent infections with HSV-1, HSV-2 and VZV in immunocompetent individuals.

Intravenous acyclovir decreases the duration of viral shedding, the duration of itching and pain and the time required for lesions to heal in immunocompromised patients with HSV infection.

Intravenous acyclovir is the treatment of choice for profoundly immunocompromised patients with VZV infection including:

- recipients of allogeneic hematopoietic stem cell transplants;
- recipients of hematopoietic stem cell transplants with moderate to severe graft-versus-host disease;
- recipients of any organ transplant who require aggressive anti-rejection therapy;
- recipients of transplants with suspected visceral dissemination of VZV (e.g., pneumonitis, encephalitis [*Clin Infect Dis* 2007;44(suppl 1):S1-26].

VZV is less susceptible to acyclovir than HSV; thus, higher dosages are recommended for treatment of VZV infections.

The antiviral spectrum of acyclovir is restricted to herpesviruses and includes HSV-1, HSV-2, and VZV. The drug has progressively less activity against Epstein-Barr virus, cytomegalovirus (CMV) and human herpesvirus 6. Acyclovir has been used clinically against CMV, although it has been superseded by ganciclovir (and valganciclovir) for this indication because of the superior activity of ganciclovir against this entity.

Acyclovir is ineffective against latent virus present in ganglia, which is by definition not actively replicating.

Geriatrics: Lower doses of acyclovir may be required in elderly patients because of the age-related decline in renal function.

Pediatrics: Intravenous acyclovir is used to treat severe herpesvirus infections in neonates and children. Oral therapy is not recommended in neonates with HSV infection.

CONTRAINDICATIONS:

- Patients who are hypersensitive to acyclovir or to any ingredient in the formulation.

WARNINGS AND PRECAUTIONS:

> **Serious Warnings and Precautions**
> - Use with caution in patients with renal dysfunction including elderly patients.
> - Use with caution in combination with other nephrotoxic drugs.

Neurologic: CNS toxicity: Patients with pre-existing renal insufficiency, those receiving high doses of acyclovir and those with high serum levels of the drug are at increased risk. Confusion and altered mental status due to acyclovir may be difficult to assess when the drug is being used to treat encephalitis.

Renal: Renal insufficiency: Patients with pre-existing renal insufficiency, those receiving high doses of acyclovir and those with high serum levels of the drug are at increased risk. Rapid infusion of the drug, dehydration and inadequate urine flow elevate the risk further. Keeping a patient well hydrated can potentially prevent this complication.

Reversible renal dysfunction occurs in approximately 5% of patients and is related to elevated levels of acyclovir in urine and crystalline nephropathy. Symptoms include nausea, emesis, flank pain and elevated BUN levels.

Sensitivity/Resistance: Repeated treatment of recurrent infections with acyclovir may select resistant viral strains, although this has been documented most often in severely immunocompromised patients.

Special Populations: Pregnant Women: Acyclovir crosses the placenta, is detectable in amniotic fluid and, after iv administration, the drug concentration is higher in cord blood compared with maternal serum. Intravenous acyclovir is the treatment of choice for women with severe or disseminated herpesvirus infections during pregnancy. The drug has been administered during all stages of pregnancy with no evidence of an increased rate of congenital malformations, although it must be noted that the formal studies have not been conducted in pregnancy.

Nursing Women: Acyclovir is distributed into human breast milk and is absorbed by nursing infants. The American Academy of Pediatrics considers acyclovir to be compatible with breast-feeding.

Pediatrics: Acyclovir is used to treat herpesvirus infections in neonates, infants and children of all ages.

Geriatrics: The elderly may experience more marked CNS adverse effects of acyclovir. Moreover, elderly patients may require dosage reductions because of the age-related decrease in renal function.

ADVERSE REACTIONS: Adverse Drug Reactions Overview: Dose-limiting adverse events of iv acyclovir include renal insufficiency and central nervous system adverse events. Patients predisposed to these events are those with pre-existing renal insufficiency and those receiving high doses and/or concomitant nephrotoxic drugs. See Table 1.

Table 1: Acyclovir Sodium Injectable

More Common Adverse Drug Reactions (≥1%)

Body System	Effect	Clinical Comment
Cutaneous	Injection site reactions (9%)	Avoid extravasation and im injections
Gastrointestinal	Nausea, vomiting (7%)	
Renal	Nephrotoxicity (5%) including increased urea and serum creatinine	Patients with renal dysfunction are predisposed. Rapid infusion rates, dehydration and inadequate urine flow elevate the risk. Usually resolves on cessation and volume expansion.
Neurologic	Headache (2%)	

Less Common Adverse Drug Reactions (<1%): Cardiovascular: hypotension.

Central Nervous System/Neurologic: agitation, confusion, coma, delirium, diaphoresis, dizziness, lethargy, hallucinations, lightheadedness, obtundation, psychosis, seizures, somnolence, tremors.

Allergic/Dermatologic: rash, pruritus, urticaria.

Gastrointestinal: anorexia, diarrhea.

Hematologic: anemia, disseminated intravascular coagulation, hemoglobinemia, hemolysis, leukocytosis, leucopenia, lymphadenopathy, neutropenia, neutrophilia, thrombocytopenia, thrombocytosis.

Hepatobiliary: elevated liver enzymes, hyperbilirubinemia, jaundice.

Immune: anaphylaxis, Stevens-Johnson syndrome, erythema multiforme, toxic epidermal necrolysis.

Abnormal Hematologic and Clinical Chemistry Findings: See Table 2.

Table 2: Acyclovir Sodium Injectable

Abnormal Hematologic and Clinical Chemistry Findings

Test	Effect	Clinical Comment
Serum creatinine	Increased	Usually resolves on cessation and volume expansion.
Neutrophil count	Decreased	May be more common in neonates.

DRUG INTERACTIONS: Overview: Acyclovir does not undergo hepatic metabolism and thus has a very low potential for drug-drug interactions involving cytochrome P450 isoenzymes or other metabolic pathways. Drugs that alter active tubular secretion of drugs may alter the pharmacokinetics of acyclovir; conversely, acyclovir may interfere with tubular secretion of other agents excreted in this manner. Other possible clinically significant interactions are those that potentiate acyclovir-induced renal toxicity.

Drug-Drug Interactions: See Table 3.

Table 3: Acyclovir Sodium Injectable

Drug-Drug Interactions

Interacting Drug	Effect	Clinical Comment
Amphotericin B	Increased risk of renal toxicity	Avoid if possible. Monitor renal function and adjust drug dosages.

(cont'd)

Table 3: Acyclovir Sodium Injectable *(cont'd)*

Drug-Drug Interactions

Interacting Drug	Effect	Clinical Comment
Probenecid	Probenecid decreases tubular secretion, increases the elimination $t_{1/2}$ and elevates serum levels of acyclovir. Increased potential for acyclovir toxicity	Avoid if possible. Monitor renal function. Adjust acyclovir dosage.
Tenofovir	Acyclovir decreases tubular secretion, increases the elimination $t_{1/2}$ and elevates serum levels of tenofovir.	Monitor patients for signs of tenofovir excess.

DOSAGE AND ADMINISTRATION: Dosing Considerations: IV acyclovir should be administered by slow infusion at a constant rate over at least 1 hour. The drug should not be administered by im injection. The iv formulation should not be applied topically to the eye. For obese patients, calculated dose should be based on ideal body weight.

Recommended Dose and Dosage Adjustment: Adults: See Table 4.

Table 4: Acyclovir Sodium Injectable

Dose in Adult Patients

Indication	Route	Usual Dose	Clinical Comment
Severe primary genital HSV infection [Canadian Guidelines on Sexually Transmitted Infections. 2006. Public Health Agency of Canada]	IV	5 mg/kg Q8H	Switch to an oral antiviral formulation and complete 7 to 10 days of therapy.
Moderate to severe mucocutaneous HSV lesions in HIV-infected adults and adolescents	IV	5 mg/kg Q8H	Switch to an oral antiviral formulation when lesions start to regress and continue until all lesions have healed.
HSV encephalitis in HIV-infected adults and adolescents	IV	10 mg/kg Q8H×14–21 days	
Severe or disseminated HSV infection in pregnancy [*Obstet Gynecol* 2007;109(6):1489-98]	IV	5–10 mg/kg Q8H×2–7 days	Switch to an oral antiviral formulation and complete 10 days of therapy.
VZV disease in severely immunocompromised patients [*Clin Infect Dis* 2007;44(suppl 1):S1-26]	IV	10 mg/kg (or 500 mg/m²) Q8H	Switch to oral medication when the infection is controlled. VZV disease in HIV-positive patients should be treated until all lesions have healed, which is often longer than the 7 to 10 day standard course of treatment.
VZV retinitis (acute retinal necrosis) in immunocompetent patients [*Clin Infect Dis* 2007;44(suppl 1):S1-26]	IV	10–15 mg/kg Q8H×10–14 days	Switch to oral therapy (e.g., valacyclovir 1 g TID) for 4 to 6 weeks.

Neonates: The rate of survival was significantly higher in neonates with CNS or disseminated HSV infection who received a 21-day course of acyclovir 60 mg/kg/day compared with historical controls treated with 30 mg/kg/day [*Pediatrics* 2001;108(2):230-8]. Transient neutropenia occurred in 6 of 29 (21%) neonates treated with high dose acyclovir in the trial; however, the absolute neutrophil count recovered without incident. Treatment with acyclovir does not interfere with the development of an adequate antibody response in neonates. See Table 5.

Table 5: Acyclovir Sodium Injectable

Dose in Neonates

Indication	Route	Age/Weight	Dose	Clinical Comment
CNS or disseminated HSV infection	IV	Post-conceptional age >32 weeks weight ≥1200 g	20 mg/kg Q8H×21 days	Maintain hydration and urine output. Oral therapy is not recommended in neonates. Monitor CBC and differential weekly in infants receiving dosages >30 mg/kg/day. Adjust dose in renal impairment.

Pediatrics: See Table 6.

Table 6: Acyclovir Sodium Injectable

Dose in Pediatric Patients

Indication	Route	Age/Weight	Dose	Clinical Comment
HSV encephalitis	IV	1 month to 12 years	20 mg/kg Q8H×14–21 days	Maintain hydration and urine output (≥1 mL/kg/h) Avoid use of nephrotoxic agents Adjust dose in renal impairment
		>12 years	10 mg/kg Q8H×14–21 days	
HSV infections (other than encephalitis)	IV		5–10 mg/kg Q8H (maximum 1000 mg/day)	

Renal Impairment: See Table 7.

Table 7: Acyclovir Sodium Injectable

Dose in Adult Patients with Renal Impairment

Route	Creatinine Clearance (mL/min)	Dosage	Clinical Comment
IV	>50	5–10 mg/kg Q8H	Patients with renal dysfunction are at increased risk of neurotoxicity and renal toxicity
IV	>25–50	5–10 mg/kg Q12H	
IV	10–25	5–10 mg/kg Q24H	
IV	<10	2.5–5 mg/kg Q24H	

Dialysis: Acyclovir is removed by hemodialysis; thus, a supplemental dose should be administered after dialysis. In patients receiving continuous renal replacement therapy, iv acyclovir should be administered at a dose of 5 to 10 mg/kg Q24H. An appropriate dosage for patients on peritoneal dialysis is equivalent to that recommended for patients with a ClCr of <10 mL/min.

Administration: Infuse the drug at a constant rate over at least 1 hour to minimize the risk of renal toxicity.

OVERDOSAGE:

For management of a suspected drug overdose, CPhA recommends that you contact your **regional Poison Control Centre**. See the *CPS* Directory section for a list of Poison Control Centres.

ACTION AND CLINICAL PHARMACOLOGY: Mechanism of Action: Acyclovir is an acyclic guanine nucleoside analogue that must undergo intracellular phosphorylation by viral thymidine kinases and host cell kinases to form the active triphosphate moiety. The requirement for a viral kinase to catalyse the first step in the activation of the drug means that little or no drug is activated in uninfected cells.

Acyclovir triphosphate is a competitive inhibitor of viral DNA polymerase. When incorporated into the primer strand during viral DNA replication, acyclovir triphosphate causes chain termination and forms an inactive complex with viral DNA polymerase. Acyclovir triphosphate is approximately 30 to 50 times as potent in inhibiting viral DNA polymerase as compared with human DNA polymerase alpha.

Resistance to acyclovir arises most often as the result of absent or deficient thymidine kinase activity, and, rarely, because of changes in the viral DNA polymerase. Resistant HSV variants occur naturally.

Pharmacokinetics: Adults: Distribution: Plasma concentrations of acyclovir increase linearly with the administered dose. When administered at an iv dose of 5 or 10 mg/kg Q8H peak acyclovir concentrations of 9.8 and 20.7 µg/mL have been obtained. The drug is distributed widely in body fluids and penetrates aqueous humour and cerebrospinal fluid.

Acyclovir crosses the placenta and penetrates breast milk. The ratio of the concentration of acyclovir in cord blood to maternal serum is reported to range from 1.25 to 1.4 after iv administration.

Acyclovir concentrations in breast milk have been reported to exceed those in maternal serum after administration of acyclovir iv 300 mg Q8H for 5 days. Acyclovir was detectable in breast milk for 88 hours after administration of the last dose [*J Am Acad Dermatol* 1995;32(6):1053-5].

Metabolism: The intracellular half-life of acyclovir triphosphate (measured in vitro) is 1-2 hours.

Excretion: Acyclovir is eliminated primarily by glomerular filtration and tubular secretion. The mean elimination half-life ($t_{1/2}$) of acyclovir has been estimated to be 2.5 (range 1.5 to 6 hours) in adults with normal renal function. In anuric patients the $t_{1/2}$ is 20 hours.

Special Populations: Pediatrics: The mean steady-state C_{max} of acyclovir was 18.82±5.22 µg/mL (range 9.82-28.25 µg/mL) and the mean C_{min} was 3.18±2.62 µg/mL (range 0.60-9.95 µg/mL) in neonates aged ≤28 days treated with a dose of 15 mg/kg Q8H. The mean $t_{1/2}$ was 3.03±1.06 hours and the mean CL was 4.42±1.57 mL/min/kg [*Pediatrics* 2001;108(2):230-8].

Acyclovir Sodium Injection ℞

acyclovir sodium

Antiviral Agent

Hospira

SUPPLIED: Each vial of sterile aqueous solution contains: acyclovir sodium equivalent to acyclovir 500 mg as a 25 mg/mL solution. Hydrochloric acid or sodium hydroxide may be used for pH adjustment. Preservative-free. Single use vials of 20 mL, cartons of 1. Store between 15 and 25°C. Protect from light. Discard unused portion.

Adacel®

tetanus toxoid, reduced diphtheria toxoid and acellular pertussis vaccine adsorbed

Active Immunizing Agent

sanofi pasteur

Date of Revision: August 2009

SUMMARY PRODUCT INFORMATION:

Route of Administration	Dosage Form/ Strength	Clinically Relevant Nonmedicinal Ingredients
Intramuscular Injection	Suspension for Injection Each 0.5 mL is formulated to contain: Active Ingredients: Tetanus toxoid, diphtheria toxoid, acellular pertussis [pertussis toxoid (PT), filamentous haemagglutinin (FHA), pertactin (PRN), fimbriae types 2 and 3 (FIM)]	Excipients: Aluminum phosphate (adjuvant), 2-phenoxyethanol. Manufacturing process residuals: Formaldehyde and glutaraldehyde are present in trace amounts. For a complete listing see Dosage Forms, Composition and Packaging.

DESCRIPTION: ADACEL (Tetanus Toxoid, Reduced Diphtheria Toxoid and Acellular Pertussis Vaccine Adsorbed) is a sterile, uniform, cloudy, white suspension of tetanus and diphtheria toxoids adsorbed separately on aluminum phosphate, combined with acellular pertussis vaccine and suspended in water for injection. The acellular pertussis vaccine is composed of 5 purified pertussis antigens (PT, FHA, PRN and FIM).

INDICATIONS AND CLINICAL USE: ADACEL is indicated for active booster immunization for the prevention of tetanus, diphtheria and pertussis (whooping cough) as a single dose in persons 4 to 64 years of age.

In children 4 to 6 years of age, ADACEL may be considered as an alternative for the fifth dose of tetanus, diphtheria and acellular pertussis vaccine (DTaP). These children should also receive a separate booster with Inactivated Poliomyelitis Vaccine (IPV) to complete the vaccination series for this age, when indicated.

Persons who have had tetanus, diphtheria or pertussis should still be immunized since these clinical infections do not always confer immunity. Human Immunodeficiency Virus (HIV)-infected persons, both asymptomatic and symptomatic, should be immunized against tetanus, diphtheria and pertussis according to standard schedules.

ADACEL is not to be used for the treatment of disease caused by *B. pertussis*, *C. diphtheriae* or *C. tetani* infections.

Pediatrics: ADACEL is not indicated for immunization of children below the age of 4 years.

Geriatrics: Clinical data are not available for use of the product in persons above the age of 64 years.

Tetanus Prophylaxis in Wound Management: The need for active immunization with a tetanus toxoid-containing preparation such as Td Adsorbed vaccine or ADACEL, with or without passive immunization with Tetanus Immune Globulin, depends on both the condition of the wound and the patient's vaccination history. (See Dosage and Administration.)

CONTRAINDICATIONS: Hypersensitivity: Known systemic hypersensitivity reaction to any component of ADACEL or a life-threatening reaction after previous administration of the vaccine or a vaccine containing one or more of the same components are contraindications to vaccination. (See Summary Product Information.) Because of uncertainty as to which component of the vaccine may be responsible, none of the components should be administered. Alternatively, such persons may be referred to an allergist for evaluation if further immunizations are considered.

Acute Neurological Disorders: Encephalopathy (e.g., coma, decreased level of consciousness, prolonged seizures) within 7 days of a previous dose of a pertussis-containing vaccine not attributable to another identifiable cause is a contraindication to vaccination with any pertussis-containing vaccine, including ADACEL.

WARNINGS AND PRECAUTIONS: General: Before administration of ADACEL, health-care providers should inform the recipient or the parent or guardian of the recipient of the benefits and risks of immunization, inquire about the recent health status of the recipient, review the recipient's history concerning possible hypersensitivity to the vaccine or similar vaccine, previous immunization history, the presence of any contraindications to immunization and comply with any local requirements regarding information to be provided to the recipient/guardian before immunization.

It is extremely important that the recipient, parent or guardian be questioned concerning any signs or symptoms of an adverse reaction after a previous dose of vaccine. (See Contraindications and Adverse Reactions.)

The rates and severity of adverse events in recipients of tetanus toxoid are influenced by the number of prior doses and level of pre-existing antitoxins.

As with any vaccine, ADACEL may not protect 100% of vaccinated persons.

Administration Route Related Precautions: Do not administer ADACEL by intravascular injection: ensure that the needle does not penetrate a blood vessel.

Intradermal or subcutaneous routes of administration are not to be utilized.

ADACEL should not be administered into the buttocks.

Febrile and Acute Disease: Vaccination should be postponed in cases of an acute or febrile disease. However, a disease with low-grade fever should not usually be a reason to postpone vaccination.

Hematologic: Because any intramuscular injection can cause an injection site hematoma in persons with any bleeding disorders, such as hemophilia or thrombocytopenia, or in persons on anticoagulant therapy, intramuscular injections with ADACEL should not be administered to such persons unless the potential benefits outweigh the risk of administration. If the decision is made to administer any product by intramuscular injection to such persons, it should be given with caution, with steps taken to avoid the risk of hematoma formation following injection.

Immune: The possibility of allergic reactions in persons sensitive to components of the vaccine should be evaluated. Hypersensitivity reactions may occur following the use of ADACEL even in persons with no prior history of hypersensitivity to the product components.

As with all other products, epinephrine hydrochloride solution (1:1000) and other appropriate agents should be available for immediate use in case an anaphylactic or acute hypersensitivity reaction occurs. Health-care providers should be familiar with current recommendations for the initial management of anaphylaxis in non-hospital settings, including proper airway management. For instructions on recognition and treatment of anaphylactic reactions, see the current edition of the Canadian Immunization Guide or visit the Health Canada website.

Immunocompromised persons (whether from disease or treatment) may not achieve the expected immune response. If possible, consideration should be given to delaying vaccination until after the completion of any immunosuppressive treatment. Nevertheless, vaccination of persons with chronic immunodeficiency such as HIV infection is recommended even if the immune response might be limited.

Neurologic: ADACEL should not be administered to individuals with progressive or unstable neurological disorders, uncontrolled epilepsy or progressive encephalopathy until a treatment regimen has been established, the condition has stabilized and the benefit clearly outweighs the risk.

A review by the US Institute of Medicine (IOM) found evidence for a causal relation between tetanus toxoid and both brachial neuritis and Guillain-Barré syndrome (GBS). If GBS occurred within 6 weeks of receipt of prior vaccine containing tetanus toxoid, the decision to give ADACEL or any vaccine containing tetanus toxoid should be based on careful consideration of the potential benefits and possible risks.

A few cases of demyelinating diseases of the central nervous system, peripheral mononeuropathies and cranial mononeuropathies have been reported following vaccines containing tetanus and/or diphtheria toxoids, although the IOM concluded that the evidence is inadequate to accept or reject a causal relation between these conditions and vaccination.

Special Populations: Pregnant Women: The effect of ADACEL on the development of the embryo and fetus has not been assessed. Vaccination in pregnancy is not recommended unless there is a definite risk of acquiring pertussis. As the vaccine is inactivated, risk to the embryo or the fetus is improbable. The benefits versus the risks of administering ADACEL during pregnancy should be carefully evaluated when there is a high probable risk of exposure to a household contact or during an outbreak in the community.

Nursing Women: The effect of administration of ADACEL during lactation has not been assessed. As ADACEL is inactivated, any risk to the mother or the infant is improbable. However, the effect on breast-fed infants of the administration of ADACEL to their mothers has not been studied. The risks and benefits of vaccination should be assessed before making the decision to immunize a nursing woman.

ADVERSE REACTIONS: Clinical Trial Adverse Drug Reactions: Because clinical trials are conducted under widely varying conditions, adverse reaction rates observed in the clinical trials of a vaccine cannot be directly compared to rates in the clinical trials of another vaccine and may not reflect rates observed in practice. The adverse reaction information from clinical trials does, however, provide a basis for identifying the adverse events that appear to be related to vaccine use and for approximating rates of those events.

The safety of ADACEL was evaluated in a total of 4648 participants who received a single dose of ADACEL in 5 clinical trials (298 children ≥4 years of age, 1508 adolescents and 2842 adults).

Pain at the injection site was the most common solicited injection site reaction. Most injection site reactions occurred within 3 days following vaccination and their mean duration was less than 3 days. The most frequent systemic reaction was tiredness in children and headache in adolescents and adults. Fever was reported in less than 10% of vaccinees. These reactions were usually transient and of mild to moderate intensity. In addition, in adolescents and adults the incidence of injection site and systemic reactions following ADACEL was comparable to those observed with a Td vaccine booster. In children the observed frequencies of injection site reactions and fever following ADACEL were significantly lower than those observed with QUADRACEL (DTaP-IPV) when administered as a booster at 4 to 6 years of age. Except for fever, the observed rates for the systemic reactions were comparable between the two vaccines. The frequency of the solicited injection site and systemic reactions reported in two clinical trials are shown in Table 1.

Table 1: ADACEL

Frequency (%) of Solicited Reactions Observed Within 0 to 14 Days in Clinical Trials in Children, Adolescents and Adults, Following a Single Dose with ADACEL

Solicited Reactions	Children (N=298)	Adolescents (N=1184)	Adults (N=1752)
Injection Site Reactions			
Pain	39.6	77.8	65.7
Swelling	24.2	20.9	21.0
Erythema	34.6	20.8	24.7
Systemic Reactions			
Fever (≥38.0°C)	8.7	5.0	1.4
Headache	16.4	43.7	33.9
Nausea	9.4	13.3	9.2
Diarrhea	14.4	10.3	10.3
Vomiting	8.1	4.6	3.0
Rash	8.4	2.7	2.0
Anorexia	21.5	N.S[a]	N.S[a]
Body Ache or Muscle Weakness	6.4	30.4	21.9
Sore or Swollen Joints	4.0	11.3	9.1
Tiredness	31.5	30.2	24.3

(cont'd)

Table 1: ADACEL *(cont'd)*

Frequency (%) of Solicited Reactions Observed Within 0 to 14 Days in Clinical Trials in Children, Adolescents and Adults, Following a Single Dose with ADACEL

Solicited Reactions	Children (N=298)	Adolescents (N=1184)	Adults (N=1752)
Chills	7.1	15.1	8.1
Axillary Lymph Node Swelling	5.4	6.6	6.5

[a] Not solicited.

Data from Post-Marketing Experience: The following additional adverse events have been spontaneously reported during the post-marketing use of ADACEL. Because these events are reported voluntarily from a population of uncertain size, it is not always possible to reliably estimate their frequency or establish a causal relationship to vaccine exposure. Decisions to include these events in labelling were based on one or more of the following factors: 1) severity of the event, 2) frequency of reporting, or 3) strength of causal connection to ADACEL.

Immune System Disorders: hypersensitivity (anaphylactic) reaction (angioedema, edema, rash, hypotension).

Nervous System Disorders: paraesthesia, hypoesthesia, Guillain-Barré syndrome, brachial neuritis, facial palsy, convulsion, syncope, myelitis.

Cardiac Disorders: myocarditis.

Skin and Subcutaneous Tissue Disorders: pruritus, urticaria.

Musculoskeletal and Connective Tissue Disorders: myositis, muscle spasm.

General Disorders and Administration Site Conditions: Large injection site reactions (>50 mm) and extensive limb swelling from the injection site beyond one or both joints have been reported after administration of ADACEL in adolescents and adults. These reactions usually start within 24-72 hours after vaccination, may be associated with erythema, warmth, tenderness or pain at the injection site and resolve spontaneously within 3-5 days. The risk appears to be dependent on the number of prior doses of acellular pertussis containing vaccine.

Injection site bruising, sterile abscess.

Physicians, nurses, and pharmacists should report any adverse occurrences temporally related to the administration of the product in accordance with local requirements and to the Global Pharmacovigilance Department, Sanofi Pasteur Limited, 1755 Steeles Avenue West, Toronto, ON, M2R 3T4 Canada. 1-888-621-1146 (phone) or 416-667-2435 (fax).

DRUG INTERACTIONS: Vaccine-Drug Interactions: Immunosuppressive treatments may interfere with the development of the expected immune response. (See Warnings and Precautions.)

Concomitant Vaccine Administration: ADACEL may be administered concurrently with a dose of trivalent inactivated influenza vaccine and with a dose of hepatitis B vaccine in 11 to 12 year-olds.

The concomitant use of ADACEL and trivalent inactivated influenza vaccine was evaluated in a clinical trial involving 696 adults 19 to 64 years of age. The safety and immunogenicity profiles in adults that received the vaccines concomitantly were comparable to those observed when the vaccines were given on separate occasions one month apart.

The concomitant use of ADACEL and hepatitis B vaccine was evaluated in a clinical trial involving 269 adolescents 11 to 12 years of age. The safety and immunogenicity profiles in adolescents that received the vaccines concomitantly were comparable to those observed when the vaccines were given on separate occasions one month apart. No interference was observed in the immune responses to any of the vaccine antigens when ADACEL and hepatitis B vaccines were given concurrently or separately.

Vaccines administered simultaneously should be given using separate syringes at separate sites and preferably in separate limbs. ADACEL should not be mixed in the same syringe with other parenterals.

DOSAGE AND ADMINISTRATION: Recommended Dose: ADACEL should be administered as a single injection of 1 dose (0.5 mL) by the intramuscular route. The preferred site is into the deltoid muscle.

Fractional doses (doses <0.5 mL) should not be given. The effect of fractional doses on the safety and efficacy has not been determined.

Health-care professionals should refer to the NACI guidelines for tetanus prophylaxis in routine wound management shown in Table 2.

Table 2: ADACEL

NACI Recommended Use of Immunizing Agents in Wound Management

History of Tetanus Immunization	Clean, Minor Wounds		All Other Wounds	
	Td[a]	TIG[b] (Human)	Td[a]	TIG[b] (Human)
Uncertain or <3 doses of an immunization series[c]	Yes	No	Yes	Yes
≥3 doses received in an immunization series[c]	No[d]	No	No[e]	No[f]

[a] Adult-type tetanus and diphtheria toxoid.
[b] Tetanus immune globulin, given at a separate site from Td.
[c] Primary immunization is at least 3 doses at age appropriate intervals.
[d] Yes, if >10 years since last booster.
[e] Yes, if >5 years since last booster.
[f] Yes, if persons are known to have a significant humoral immune deficiency state (eg, HIV, agammaglobulinemia) since immune response to tetanus toxoid may be suboptimal.

A thorough attempt must be made to determine whether a patient has completed primary immunization. Persons who have completed primary immunization against tetanus and who sustain wounds that are minor and uncontaminated, should receive a booster dose of a tetanus toxoid-containing preparation if they have not received tetanus toxoid within the preceding 10 years. For tetanus-prone wounds (eg, wounds contaminated with dirt, feces, soil and saliva, puncture wounds, avulsions and wounds resulting from missiles, crushing, burns or frostbite), a booster is appropriate if the patient has not received a tetanus toxoid-containing preparation within the preceding 5 years.

For adults who have not previously received a dose of acellular pertussis vaccine, a single diphtheria-tetanus (Td) booster dose be replaced by the combined tetanus-diphtheria-acellular pertussis (Tdap) vaccine.

Administration: Inspect for extraneous particulate matter and/or discolouration before use. (See Description.) If these conditions exist, the product should not be administered.

Shake the vial well until a uniform, cloudy, suspension results. Cleanse the vial stopper with a suitable germicide prior to withdrawing the dose. Do not remove either the stopper or the metal seal holding it in place. Aseptic technique must be used. Use a separate sterile needle and syringe, or a sterile disposable unit for each individual recipient, to prevent disease transmission. Needles should not be recapped but should be disposed of according to biohazard waste guidelines. (See Warnings and Precautions.)

Before injection, the skin over the site to be injected should be cleansed with a suitable germicide. Administer the total volume of 0.5 mL **intramuscularly** (IM). The preferred site of injection is the deltoid muscle.

Give the patient a permanent personal immunization record. In addition, it is essential that the physician or nurse record the immunization history in the permanent medical record of each patient. This permanent office record should contain the name of the vaccine, date given, dose, manufacturer and lot number.

ACTION AND CLINICAL PHARMACOLOGY: Tetanus and Diphtheria: Tetanus is an acute and often fatal disease caused by an extremely potent neurotoxin produced by *C. tetani*. The toxin causes neuromuscular dysfunction, with rigidity and spasms of skeletal muscles. Protection against disease attributable to *C. tetani* is due to the development of neutralizing antibodies to tetanus toxin. A serum tetanus antitoxin level of at least 0.01 IU/mL, measured by neutralization assay, is considered the minimum protective level. A tetanus antitoxin level of at least 0.1 IU/mL as measured by the ELISA used in clinical studies of ADACEL is considered as protective for tetanus. Levels of 1.0 IU/mL have been associated with long-term protection.

Strains of *C. diphtheriae* that produce diphtheria toxin can cause severe or fatal illness characterized by membranous inflammation of the upper respiratory tract and toxin-induced damage to the myocardium and nervous system. Protection against disease attributable to *C. diphtheriae* is due to the development of neutralizing antibodies to diphtheria toxin. A serum diphtheria antitoxin level of 0.01 IU/mL is the lowest level giving some degree of protection. Antitoxin levels of at least 0.1 IU/mL are generally regarded as protective. Levels of 1.0 IU/mL have been associated with long-term protection.

Pertussis: Pertussis (whooping cough) is a respiratory disease caused by *B. pertussis*. This Gram-negative coccobacillus produces a variety of biologically active components, though their role in either the pathogenesis of, or immunity to, pertussis has not been clearly defined. The mechanism of protection from *B. pertussis* disease is not well understood. However, in a clinical trial in Sweden (Sweden I Efficacy Trial), the same pertussis components as in ADACEL (i.e., PT, FHA, PRN and FIM) have been shown to prevent pertussis in infants with a protective efficacy of 85.2% using the World Health Organization (WHO) case definition (≥21 consecutive days of paroxysmal cough with culture or serologic confirmation or epidemiological link to a confirmed case). In the same study, the protective efficacy against mild disease was 77.9%.

Minimum serum antibody levels to specific pertussis vaccine components that confer protection against the development of clinical pertussis have not been identified. Nevertheless, a number of studies have demonstrated a correlation between the presence of serum antibody responses to pertussis vaccine components and protection against clinical disease. In ADACEL clinical trials, post-vaccination Geometric Mean Concentrations (GMCs) for all pertussis antibodies in both adolescents and adults were consistently above those of TRIPACEL in the Sweden I Efficacy Trial.

Duration of Effect: Long-term follow-up of serum antibody levels in adolescents and adults who received a single dose of ADACEL show that protective levels for tetanus antitoxin (≥0.01 EU/mL) and diphtheria antitoxin (≥0.01 IU/mL) persist in 100% and 93.3% of participants, respectively, after at least 5 years. While protective levels against pertussis have not yet been clearly defined, pertussis antibody levels remain 2 to 9 fold higher than pre-immunization levels after 5 years. Tetanus and diphtheria toxoid boosters are recommended every 10 years, however, the optimal interval for administering subsequent booster doses with ADACEL has not been determined.

STORAGE AND STABILITY: Store at 2 to 8°C. **Do not freeze.** Discard product if exposed to freezing.

Do not use after expiration date.

INFORMATION FOR THE PATIENT: Published in e-CPS, available by subscription at www.e-cps.ca.

DOSAGE FORMS, COMPOSITION AND PACKAGING: Each dose (0.5 mL) of a sterile, uniform, cloudy, white suspension contains: tetanus toxoid 5 Lf, diphtheria toxoid 2 Lf, pertussis toxoid (PT) 2.5 μg, filamentous haemagglutinin (FHA) 5 μg, pertactin (PRN) 3 μg, fimbriae types 2 and 3 (FIM) 5 μg, aluminum phosphate (adjuvant) 1.5 mg and 0.6% (v/v) 2-phenoxyethanol. Manufacturing process residuals: formaldehyde and glutaraldehyde are present in trace amounts. The container closure system is free of latex (natural rubber). Single dose Type 1 glass vials of 0.5 mL, packages of 1 and 5.

The reader is invited to consult CPhA's monograph **Calcium Channel Blockers**.

Adalat® XL®
nifedipine
Antianginal—Antihypertensive
Bayer

Date of Preparation: March 26, 1992
Date of Revision: December 8, 2009

DESCRIPTION: System Components and Performance: Adalat XL extended release tablets, while similar in appearance to a conventional tablet, nonetheless consist of a semipermeable membrane surrounding an osmotically active drug core. The core itself is divided into 2 layers: an "active" layer containing the drug, and a "push" layer containing pharmacologically inert, but osmotically active components. As water from the gastrointestinal tract enters the tablet, pressure increases in the osmotic layer and "pushes" against the drug layer, forcing drug through the orifice in the active layer.

Drug delivery is essentially constant as long as the osmotic gradient remains constant, and then gradually falls to zero as drug is exhausted from the tablet. Upon swallowing, the biologically inert components of the tablet remain intact during gastrointestinal transit and are eliminated in the feces as an insoluble shell.

PHARMACOLOGY: Nifedipine is a calcium ion influx inhibitor (calcium channel blocker or calcium ion antagonist).

The antianginal and antihypertensive actions of nifedipine are believed to be related to a specific cellular action of selectively inhibiting transmembrane influx of calcium ions into cardiac muscle and vascular smooth muscle. The contractile processes of these tissues are dependent upon the movement of extracellular calcium into the cells through specific ion channels. Nifedipine selectively inhibits the transmembrane influx of calcium through the slow channel without affecting, to any significant degree, the transmembrane influx of sodium through the fast channel. This results in a reduction of free calcium ions available within the muscle cells and an inhibition of the contractile processes. Nifedipine does not alter total serum calcium.

The specific mechanisms by which nifedipine relieves angina and reduces blood pressure have not been fully determined but are believed to be brought about largely by its vasodilatory action.

Nifedipine dilates the main coronary arteries and coronary arterioles both in normal and ischemic regions resulting in an increase in blood flow and hence in myocardial oxygen delivery.

Nifedipine by its vasodilatory action on peripheral arterioles, reduces the total peripheral vascular resistance. This reduces the workload of the heart and thus reduces myocardial energy consumption and oxygen requirements which probably accounts for the effectiveness of nifedipine in chronic stable angina.

The mechanism by which nifedipine reduces arterial blood pressure involves peripheral arterial vasodilation and subsequent reduction in peripheral vascular resistance. The increased peripheral vascular resistance that is an underlying cause of hypertension results from an increase in active tension in the vascular smooth muscle. Studies have demonstrated that the increase in active tension reflects an increase in cytosolic free calcium.

The negative inotropic effect of nifedipine is usually not of major clinical significance because at therapeutic doses, nifedipine's vasodilatory property evokes a baroreceptor mediated reflex tachycardia which tends to counterbalance this negative inotropic effect. Continued administration of nifedipine to hypertensive patients has shown no significant increase in heart rate.

Although nifedipine causes a slight depression of sinoatrial node function and AV conduction in isolated myocardial preparations, such effects have not been seen in studies in intact animals or in man. In formal electrophysiologic studies, predominantly in patients with normal conduction systems, nifedipine has had no tendency to prolong AV conduction or sinus node recovery time, or to slow sinus rate.

The International Nifedipine GITS Study Intervention as a Goal in Hypertension Treatment trial called INSIGHT was a prospective double-blind trial with dynamic randomisation which enrolled mainly white hypertensive men and women. The primary endpoint was a composite of death from any cardiovascular or cerebrovascular cause, together with non-fatal stroke, myocardial infarction, and heart failure. The secondary endpoint included total mortality, death from a vascular cause, and non-fatal vascular events including transient ischemic attacks, angina (new or worsening) and renal failure. INSIGHT was designed to establish the superiority of Adalat XL over the diuretic combination co-amilozide (hydrochlorothiazide and amiloride). When the results of the Swedish Trial in Old Patients with Hypertension-2 study (STOP-2) became known and because these results suggested that calcium-channel blockade and diuretic treatment had similar efficacy in preventing complications, but before the patient code in INSIGHT was broken, a secondary, non-inferiority analysis was added.

INSIGHT randomized 6575 mild to moderate essential hypertensive or isolated systolic hypertensive patients, 55-80 years of age, with at least one other cardiovascular risk factor to nifedipine and co-amilozide. Patients were excluded if they had heart failure with low ejection fraction (< 40%), unstable angina, PTCA (Percutaneous Transluminal Coronary Angioplasty) or CABG (Coronary Artery Bypass Grafting) within 6 months prior to study start, or myocardial infarction or stroke in the 12 months prior to study start. Doses of each drug were titrated to achieve a target blood pressure of 140/90 mmHg (or drop of 20/10 mmHg) and if that target was not reached additional drugs could be added (atenolol and subsequently enalapril). On average patients were treated for 3.5 years. After placebo washout, the baseline blood pressure was 173/99 mmHg and decreased to 138/82 mmHg by the end of the trial in both groups. Heart rate was not different between the groups. At the end of the study 69 and 72% of patients on Adalat XL and hydrochlorothiazide/amiloride, respectively, were on monotherapy. All endpoints were assessed and adjudicated by the Critical Events Committee. The overall results of the study in Table 1 show that Adalat XL was not inferior to the diuretic combination co-amilozide.

Table 1: Adalat XL
Results of the INSIGHT Study

	Adalat XL	Hydrochlorothiazide/ Amiloride	Odds Ratio (95% CI)	p-value
Primary Outcomes Composite	200 (6.3%)	182 (5.8%)	1.11 (0.90–1.36)	0.34
Secondary Outcomes Composite	383 (12.1%)	397 (12.5%)	0.96 (0.83–1.12)	0.62
Total Mortality	153 (4.8%)	152 (4.8)	1.01 (0.80–1.27)	0.95
All Adverse Events	1546 (49%)	1327 (42%)	N/A	<0.001
Serious Adverse Events	796 (25%)	880 (28%)	N/A	0.02

Pharmacokinetics: Nifedipine is completely absorbed after oral administration. Plasma drug concentrations rise at a gradual, controlled rate exhibiting zero-order absorption kinetics after nifedipine administration and reach a plateau at approximately 6 hours after the first dose. For subsequent doses, relatively constant plasma concentrations at this plateau are maintained with minimal fluctuations over the 24-hour dosing interval. About a 4-fold higher fluctuation index (ratio of peak to trough plasma concentration) was observed with the conventional immediate release Adalat capsule at t.i.d. dosing than with once daily Adalat XL tablets. At steady state the bioavailability of the Adalat XL tablet is 86% relative to Adalat capsules. Administration of the Adalat XL tablet in the presence of food slightly alters the early rate of drug absorption, but does not influence the extent of drug bioavailability. Markedly reduced gastrointestinal retention time over prolonged periods (i.e., short bowel syndrome), however, may influence the pharmacokinetic profile of the drug which could potentially result in lower plasma concentrations. Pharmacokinetics of Adalat XL tablets are linear over the dose range of 30 to 180 mg in that plasma drug concentrations are proportional to dose administered. There was no evidence of dose dumping either in the presence or absence of food. The bioavailability of the 20 mg tablet is directly proportional to the 30 mg tablet.

Nifedipine is extensively metabolized to highly water-soluble, inactive metabolites accounting for 60 to 80% of the dose excreted in the urine. The remainder is excreted in the feces in metabolized form, most likely as a result of biliary excretion. The main metabolite (95%) is the hydroxycarbolic acid derivative, the remaining 5% is the corresponding lactone. Only traces (less that 0.1% of the dose) of unchanged nifedipine can be detected in the urine. Thus, the pharmacokinetics of nifedipine are not significantly influenced by the degree of renal impairment. Patients in hemodialysis or CAPD (continuous ambulatory peritoneal dialysis) have not reported significantly altered pharmacokinetics of nifedipine.

Since hepatic biotransformation is the predominant route for the disposition of nifedipine, the pharmacokinetics may be altered in patients with chronic liver disease. Pharmacokinetic studies in patients with hepatic cirrhosis showed a clinically significant prolongation of elimination half-life and a decrease in total clearance of nifedipine. The degree of serum protein binding of nifedipine is high (92 to 98%). Protein binding may be greatly reduced in patients with renal or hepatic impairment (see Precautions).

Nifedipine is metabolized by the cytochrome P450 enzyme system, predominantly via CYP3A4, but also by CYP1A2 and CYP2A6 isoenzymes.

Compounds found in grapefruit juice inhibit the cytochrome P450 system, especially CYP3A4. In a grapefruit juice-nifedipine interaction study in healthy male volunteers, pharmacokinetics of nifedipine showed significant alteration. Following administration of a single dose of nifedipine 10 mg with 250 mL of grapefruit juice, the mean value of nifedipine AUC increased by 34% and the t_{max} increased from 0.8 to 1.2 hours, as compared to water (see Precautions, Interaction with Grapefruit Juice).

INDICATIONS: Chronic Stable Angina: In the management of chronic stable angina (effort-associated angina) without evidence of vasospasm in patients who remain symptomatic despite adequate doses of beta-blockers and/or nitrates, or who cannot tolerate these agents.

May be used in combination with beta-blocking drugs in patients with chronic stable angina. However, available information is not sufficient to predict with confidence the effects of concurrent treatment, especially in patients with compromised left ventricular function or cardiac conduction abnormalities. When introducing such concomitant therapy, care must be taken to monitor blood pressure closely, since severe hypotension can occur from the combined effects of the drugs (see Warnings).

Hypertension: In the management of mild to moderate essential hypertension. Should normally be used in those patients in whom treatment with diuretics or beta-blockers has been ineffective, or has been associated with unacceptable adverse effects.

It can be tried as an initial agent in those patients in whom the use of diuretics and/or beta-blockers is contraindicated, or in patients with medical conditions in which these drugs frequently cause serious adverse effects.

Combination of Adalat XL with a diuretic has been found compatible and has shown added antihypertensive effect. Concurrent administration of low doses of Adalat XL and enalapril has been shown to produce an enhanced antihypertensive effect with no additional safety concerns when compared to that observed with either of the monotherapies.

Safety of concurrent use of Adalat XL with other antihypertensive agents has not been established.

CONTRAINDICATIONS: *Pregnancy:* Nifedipine is contraindicated in pregnancy, during lactation, and in women of childbearing potential. Fetal malformations and adverse effects on pregnancy have been reported in animals.

An increase in the number of fetal mortalities and resorptions occurred after the administration of 30 and 100 mg/kg of nifedipine to pregnant mice, rats and rabbits. Fetal malformations occurred after the administration of 30 and 100 mg/kg nifedipine to pregnant mice and 100 mg/kg to pregnant rats.

Lactation: See Pregnancy.

In patients with hypersensitivity to nifedipine.

In patients with severe hypotension or cardiovascular shock.

Nifedipine must not be used in combination with rifampicin because insufficient plasma levels of nifedipine may result due to enzyme induction.

WARNINGS: Excessive Hypotension in Patients with Angina: Since nifedipine lowers peripheral vascular resistance and blood pressure, it should be used cautiously in patients with angina who are prone to develop hypotension and those with a history of cerebrovascular insufficiency. Occasional patients have had excessive and poorly tolerated hypotension. Syncope has been reported (see Adverse Effects). These responses have usually occurred during initial titration or at the time of subsequent upward dosage adjustment, and may be more likely in patients on concomitant beta-blockers. If excessive hypotension occurs, dosage should be lowered or the drug should be discontinued (see Contraindications).

Severe hypotension and/or increased fluid volume requirements have been reported in patients receiving nifedipine, with a beta-blocker, who underwent coronary artery bypass surgery using high dose fentanyl anesthesia. The interaction with high dose fentanyl appears to be due to the combination of nifedipine and a beta-blocker, but the possibility that it may occur with nifedipine alone, with low doses of fentanyl in other surgical procedures, or with other narcotic analgesics cannot be ruled out. In nifedipine-treated patients where surgery using high dose fentanyl anesthesia is contemplated, the physician should be aware of these potential problems and if the patient's condition permits, sufficient time (at least 36 hours), should be allowed for nifedipine to be washed out of the body prior to surgery.

The following information should be taken into account in those patients who are being treated for hypertension as well as angina.

Increased Angina and/or Myocardial Infarction: Rarely, patients, particularly those who have severe obstructive coronary artery disease have developed well-documented increased frequency, duration and/or severity of angina or acute myocardial infarction on starting nifedipine or at the time of dosage increase. The mechanism of the response is not established.

Since there has not been a study of Adalat XL in acute myocardial infarction reported, similar effects of Adalat XL to that of immediate-release nifedipine cannot be excluded. Immediate-release nifedipine is contraindicated in acute myocardial infarction.

Beta-blocker Withdrawal: Patients with angina recently withdrawn from beta-blockers may develop a withdrawal syndrome with increased angina, probably related to increased sensitivity to catecholamines. Initiation of treatment with nifedipine will not prevent this occurrence and might be expected to exacerbate it by provoking reflex catecholamine release. There have been occasional reports of increased angina in a setting of beta-blocker withdrawal and initiation of nifedipine. It is important to taper beta-blockers if possible, rather than stopping them abruptly before beginning nifedipine.

Patients with Heart Failure: There have been isolated reports of severe hypotension and lowering of cardiac output following administration of nifedipine to patients with severe heart failure. Thus, nifedipine should be used cautiously in patients with severe heart failure. Rarely, patients usually receiving a beta-blocker, have developed heart failure after beginning nifedipine therapy.

In patients with severe aortic stenosis, nifedipine will not produce its usual afterload reducing effects and there is a possibility that an unopposed negative inotropic action of the drug may produce heart failure if the end-diastolic pressure is raised. Caution should therefore be exercised when using nifedipine in patients with these conditions.

Patients with Pre-existing Gastrointestinal Narrowing: Since the Adalat XL delivery system contains a nondeformable material, caution should be used when administering it in patients with pre-existing severe gastrointestinal narrowing (pathologic or iatrogenic). There have been rare reports of obstructive symptoms in patients with known strictures in association with the ingestion of Adalat XL tablets. In single cases, obstructive symptoms have been described without known history of gastrointestinal disorders. Bezoars can occur in very rare cases and may require surgical intervention. Adalat XL must not be used in patients with a Kock pouch (ileostomy after proctocolectomy).

When doing barium contrast X-ray, Adalat XL may cause false positive effects (e.g., filling defects interpreted as polyp).

PRECAUTIONS: Hypotension/Heart Rate: Because nifedipine is an arterial and arteriolar vasodilator, hypotension and a compensatory increase in heart rate may occur. Thus, blood pressure and heart rate should be monitored carefully during nifedipine therapy. Close monitoring is especially recommended for patients who are prone to develop hypotension, those with a history of cerebrovascular insufficiency, and those who are taking medications that are known to lower blood pressure (see Warnings).

Peripheral Edema: Mild to moderate peripheral edema, typically associated with arterial vasodilation and not due to left ventricular dysfunction, has been reported to occur in patients treated with nifedipine (see Adverse Effects). This edema occurs primarily in the lower extremities and may respond to diuretic therapy. with patients whose angina or hypertension is complicated by congestive heart failure, care should be taken to differentiate this peripheral edema from the effects of increasing left ventricular dysfunction.

Male Fertility: In some cases of in vitro fertilization, nifedipine has been associated with reversible spermatozoal biochemical changes. In vitro studies have shown that nifedipine may inhibit expression of mannose-ligand receptors, thus preventing the spermatozoa from attaching to the zona pellucida and impairing sperm function. In those men who are repeatedly unsuccessful in fathering a child by in vitro fertilization, and where no other explanation could be found, nifedipine should be considered as a possible cause.

Geriatrics: Nifedipine should be administered cautiously to elderly patients, especially to those with a history of hypotension or cerebral vascular insufficiency.

Diabetic Patients: The use of nifedipine in diabetic patients may require adjustment for their control.

Patients with Impaired Liver Function: Nifedipine should be used with caution in patients with impaired liver function (see Pharmacology). A dose reduction, particularly in severe cases, may be required. Close monitoring of response and metabolic effect should apply.

Occupational Hazards: Ability to Drive and Use Machines: Reactions to the drug, which vary in intensity from individual to individual, can impair the ability to drive or to operate machinery, particularly at the start of the treatment, upon changing the medication, or in combination with alcohol.

Interaction with Grapefruit Juice: Published data indicate that through inhibition of cytochrome P450, flavonoids present in the grapefruit juice can increase plasma levels and augment pharmacodynamic effects of some dihydropyridine calcium channel blockers, including nifedipine (see Pharmacology). Therefore, the administration of nifedipine with grapefruit juice should be avoided.

Drug Interactions: As with all drugs, care should be exercised when treating patients with multiple medications. Dihydrophyridine calcium channel blockers undergo biotransformation by the cytochrome P450 system, mainly via the CYP3A4 isoenzyme. Coadministration of nifedipine with other drugs which follow the same route of biotransformation may result in altered bioavailability. Dosages of similarly metabolized drugs, particularly those of low therapeutic ratio, and especially in patients with renal and/or hepatic impairment, may require adjustment when starting or stopping concomitantly administered nifedipine to maintain optimum therapeutic blood levels. If necessary, a reduction in the dose of nifedipine may be considered.

Drugs known to be inhibitors of the cytochrome P450 system include: azole antifungals (ketoconazole, itraconazole, fluconazole), cimetidine, cyclosporine, erythromycin, fluoxetine, HIV protease inhibitors (amprenavir, indinavir, nelfinavir, ritonavir, saquanavir), nefazodone, quinidine, terfenadine and warfarin.

Drugs known to be inducers of the cytochrome P450 system include: phenobarbital, phenytoin and rifampicin.

Drugs known to be biotransformed via cytochrome P450 include: benzodiazepines, cisapride, flecainide, tacrolimus, theophylline, imipramine and propafenone.

Beta Adrenergic Blocking Agents: Concomitant administration of nifedipine and beta-blocking agents is usually well tolerated but there have been occasional literature reports suggesting that the combination may increase the likelihood of congestive heart failure, severe hypotension, or exacerbation of angina. Therefore, caution and careful monitoring of patients on concomitant therapy is recommended (see Indications and Warnings).

Diltiazem: Diltiazem decreases the clearance of nifedipine. The combination of both drugs should be administered with caution, and a reduction of the nifedipine dose may be considered.

Long-acting Nitrates: Nifedipine may be safely coadministered with nitrates, but there have been no controlled studies to evaluate the antianginal effectiveness of this combination.

Digoxin: Administration of nifedipine with digoxin may lead to reduced digoxin clearance, and therefore, an increase in the plasma digoxin level. It is recommended that digoxin levels be monitored when initiating, adjusting and discontinuing nifedipine to avoid possible "under-" or "over-" dosing with digitalis.

Coumarin Anticoagulants: There have been rare reports of increased prothrombin time in patients taking coumarin anticoagulants to whom nifedipine was administered. However, the relationship to nifedipine therapy is uncertain.

Carbamazepine: No formal studies have been performed to investigate the potential interaction between nifedipine and carbamazepine. As carbamazepine has been shown to reduce the plasma concentrations of the structurally similar calcium channel blocker nimodipine due to enzyme induction, a decrease in nifedipine plasma concentrations and hence a reduction in efficacy cannot be excluded.

Quinidine: The addition of nifedipine to a stable quinidine regimen may reduce the quinidine by 50%, an enhanced response to nifedipine may also occur. The addition of quinidine to a stable nifedipine regimen may result in elevated nifedipine concentrations and a reduced response to quinidine. Some patients have experienced elevated quinidine levels when nifedipine was discontinued. Therefore, patients receiving concomitant therapy of nifedipine and quinidine, or those who had their nifedipine discontinued while still receiving quinidine, should be closely monitored, including determination of plasma levels of quinidine. Consideration should be given to dosage adjustment.

Quinupristin/Dalfopristin: Simultaneous administration of quinupristin/dalfopristin and nifedipine may lead to increased plasma concentrations of nifedipine. Upon co-administration of both drugs, blood pressure should be monitored and, if necessary, a reduction of the nifedipine dose should be considered.

Cimetidine and Ranitidine: Pharmacokinetic studies have shown that concurrent administration of cimetidine or ranitidine with nifedipine results in significant increases in nifedipine plasma levels (ca. 80% with cimetidine, and 70% with ranitidine). Patients receiving either of these drugs concomitantly with nifedipine should be monitored carefully for the possible exacerbation of effects of nifedipine, such as hypotension. Adjustment of nifedipine dosage may be necessary.

Cisapride: Simultaneous administration of cisapride and nifedipine may lead to increased plasma concentrations of nifedipine. Upon co-administration of both drugs, the blood pressure should be monitored and, if necessary, a reduction of the nifedipine dose considered.

Valproic Acid: No formal studies have been performed to investigate the potential interaction between nifedipine and valproic acid. As valproic acid has been shown to increase the plasma concentrations of the structurally similar calcium channel blocker nimodipine due to enzyme inhibition, an increase in nifedipine plasma concentrations and hence an increase in efficacy cannot be excluded.

ADVERSE EFFECTS: Angina: In 257 chronic stable angina patients treated in controlled and long-term open studies, adverse effects were reported in 30% of patients and required discontinuation of therapy in 8.5% of patients.

The most common adverse effects were: edema (10.1%), headache (3.1%) and angina pectoris (3.1%).

The following adverse effects were also reported. Incidences greater than 1% are given in parenthesis:

Cardiovascular: palpitation (2.3%), tachycardia, myocardial infarction, ventricular arrhythmia, extrasystoles, dyspnea, chest pain.

In patients with angina, rarely, and possibly due to tachycardia, nifedipine has been reported to have precipitated an angina pectoris attack. In addition, more serious events were occasionally observed, not readily distinguishable from the natural history of the disease in these patients. It remains possible, however, that some or many of these events were drug related. These events include myocardial infarction, congestive heart failure or pulmonary edema, and ventricular arrhythmias or conduction disturbances.

Central Nervous System: dizziness (2.3%), hypoesthesia (1.2%), confusion, insomnia, somnolence, nervousness, asthenia, hyperkinesia.

Gastrointestinal : constipation (1.9%), dyspepsia (1.2%), abdominal pain (1.2%), diarrhea, nausea, melena.

Genitourinary: impotence, hematuria, polyuria, dysuria.

Musculoskeletal: leg cramps, paresthesia, myalgia, arthralgia.

Dermatologic: rash, pruritus.

Other: fatigue (1.2%), pain, periorbital edema.

Hypertension: In 661 hypertensive patients treated in controlled trials with nifedipine, adverse effects were reported in 54% of patients and required discontinuation of therapy in 11.9% of patients. The majority of adverse effects reported occurred within the first 3 months of therapy.

The most common adverse effects reported were edema, which was dose related and ranged in frequency from approximately 10 to 30% in the 30 to 120 mg dose range, headache (16.6%), fatigue (6.2%), dizziness (4.4%), constipation (3.5%) and nausea (3.5%).

The following adverse effects were also reported. Incidences greater than 1% are given in parenthesis:

Cardiovascular: flushing (2.4%), palpitation (2.3%), tachycardia (1.2%), chest pain (1.1%), ventricular arrhythmia, hypotension, syncope.

Central Nervous System: insomnia (1.8%), nervousness (1.8%), somnolence (1.5%), depression, tremor, decreased libido, migraine, vertigo, amnesia, anxiety, impaired concentration, twitching, ataxia, hypertonia, paresthesia, hypoesthesia.

Gastrointestinal: dyspepsia (1.5%), flatulence (1.5%), abdominal pain (1.4%), dry mouth (1.1%), diarrhea, vomiting, thirst, melena, eructation, weight increase.

Genitourinary: impotence (1.5%), polyuria (1.5%), dysuria, nocturia, oliguria, urinary incontinence, urinary frequency, menstrual disorder.

Musculoskeletal : arthralgia, back pain, myalgia.

Special Senses: abnormal vision, abnormal lacrimation, taste disturbance, conjunctivitis, tinnitus.

Dermatologic: rash (2.3%), pruritus (1.1%), erythematous rash, alopecia.

Respiratory: dyspnea (1.7%), bronchospasm, pharyngitis, upper respiratory tract infection, epistaxis.

Other: leg cramps (2.7%), pain (2.7%), asthenia (2.0%), face edema, gout, allergy, fever, breast pain.

An open, nonrandomized postmarketing surveillance study (EXACT), involving 1700 mild to moderate hypertensive patients, was conducted in the offices of general practitioners across Canada. Patients were enrolled in the study if they had been previously treated with either single or dual antihypertensive therapy and the physician considered Adalat XL an appropriate monotherapy. Patients were to be started on Adalat XL 30 mg. If after 3 or 6 weeks of therapy with Adalat XL 30 mg, blood pressure was uncontrolled (i.e., sitting diastolic blood pressure was >95 mmHg), then the patient was given 60 mg Adalat XL at the physician's discretion. Twelve patients were started immediately on Adalat XL 60 mg. Patients were followed for 20 weeks. Adverse events were reported in 605/1700 patients (35.6%). These adverse events were typical of those seen with the dihydropyridine class of calcium channel blockers (edema, headache, dizziness) and are related to the vasodilatory properties of this class of compounds.

The following is a summary of adverse effects which occurred with a frequency of ≥1% during this 20-week study. See Table 2.

Table 2: Adalat XL

Adverse Effects

Adverse Effect	All Patients (n=1700) %	(n)
Patients with ≥1 Adverse Effect	35.6	(605)
Headache	12.2	(207)
Peripheral Edema	8.1	(137)
Dizziness	2.9	(50)
Asthenia	2.8	(48)
Vasodilatation	2.5	(43)
Constipation	2.4	(40)
Palpitations	1.7	(29)
Nausea	1.5	(26)
Anxiety	1.2	(20)
Dyspepsia	1.1	(18)
Insomnia	1.1	(18)
Tachycardia	1.0	(17)

Table 3 illustrates the time period during which the adverse effects in the preceding table occurred. The majority of the adverse effects occurred during the first 3 weeks that the patients received Adalat XL. The incidence rate of adverse effects continued to diminish as the length of exposure to Adalat XL increased.

Table 3: Adalat XL

Adverse Effects Occurring During Each Time Period

	Unknown		0-3 Weeks		3-6 Weeks		6-12 Weeks		12-20 Weeks	
Adverse Events	n	(%)	n	(%)	n	(%)	n	(%)	n	(%)
Headache	7	(0.7)	148	(13.8)	41	(3.8)	22	(2.1)	6	(0.6)
Peripheral Edema	2	(0.2)	56	(5.2)	42	(3.9)	33	(3.1)	18	(1.7)
Dizziness	2	(0.2)	27	(2.5)	11	(1.0)	7	(0.7)	4	(0.4)
Asthenia	2	(0.2)	23	(2.1)	15	(1.4)	9	(0.8)	0	(0)
Vasodilatation	2	(0.2)	27	(2.5)	5	(0.5)	4	(0.4)	6	(0.6)
Constipation	0	(0)	25	(2.3)	8	(0.7)	5	(0.5)	3	(0.3)
Palpitations	1	(0.1)	17	(1.6)	6	(0.6)	2	(0.2)	4	(0.4)
Nausea	0	(0)	21	(2.0)	4	(0.4)	2	(0.2)	0	(0)
Anxiety	2	(0.2)	5	(0.5)	6	(0.6)	2	(0.2)	6	(0.6)

(cont'd)

Table 3: Adalat XL *(cont'd)*

Adverse Effects Occurring During Each Time Period

	Unknown		0-3 Weeks		3-6 Weeks		6-12 Weeks		12-20 Weeks	
Adverse Events	**n**	**(%)**	**n**	**(%)**	**n**	**(%)**	**n**	**(%)**	**n**	**(%)**
Dyspepsia	1	(0.1)	5	(0.5)	5	(0.5)	5	(0.5)	2	(0.2)
Insomnia	1	(0.1)	6	(0.6)	3	(0.3)	3	(0.3)	6	(0.6)
Tachycardia	1	(0.1)	5	(0.5)	3	(0.3)	6	(0.6)	3	(0.3)

The following adverse events have been reported with nifedipine rarely.

Rare instances of allergic hepatitis, cholestasis with, or without jaundice have been reported in patients treated with nifedipine.

Gingival hyperplasia similar to that caused by phenytoin has been reported in patients treated with nifedipine. The lesions usually regressed on discontinuation of the drug. However on occasion, gingivectomy was necessary.

Gynecomastia has been observed rarely in older men on long-term therapy, but has so far always regressed completely on discontinuation of the drug.

Isolated cases of angioedema have been reported. Angioedema may be accompanied by breathing difficulty. Anaphylaxis has been reported rarely.

In postmarketing experience, there have been rare reports of exfoliative dermatitis and Stevens-Johnson syndrome. Gastrointestinal irritation and gastrointestinal bleeding were also reported; however, the causal relationship is uncertain.

Laboratory Tests: Rare, usually transient, but occasionally significant elevations of enzymes such as CPK, AST and ALT have been noted. The relationship to drug therapy is uncertain in most cases, but probable in some. These laboratory abnormalities have rarely been associated with clinical symptoms, however, cholestasis with or without jaundice has been reported.

An increase (5.4%) in mean alkaline phosphatase was noted in patients treated with nifedipine. This was an isolated finding not associated with clinical symptoms and rarely resulted in values which exceeded the upper limit of the normal range.

Serum potassium was unchanged in patients receiving nifedipine in the absence of concomitant diuretic therapy, and slightly decreased in patients receiving concomitant diuretics.

Nifedipine decreases platelet aggregation in vitro. Limited clinical studies have demonstrated a moderate but statistically significant decrease in platelet aggregation and increase in bleeding time in some nifedipine treated patients. This is thought to be a function of inhibition of calcium transport across the platelet membrane. No clinical significance for these findings has been demonstrated.

Positive direct Coombs' tests, with or without associated hemolytic anemia, have been reported but a causal relationship between nifedipine administration and positivity of this laboratory test, including hemolysis, could not be determined.

Rare reversible elevations in BUN and serum creatinine have been reported in patients with pre-existing chronic renal insufficiency. The relationship to therapy with nifedipine is uncertain in most cases, but probable in some.

OVERDOSE:

Symptoms: There are several well documented cases of nifedipine overdosage. The following symptoms are observed in cases of severe nifedipine intoxication: disturbance of consciousness to the point of coma, a drop in blood pressure, tachycardia/bradycardia, hyperglycemia, metabolic acidosis, hypoxia, cardiogenic shock with pulmonary edema.

Treatment: As far as treatment is concerned, elimination of the active substance and the restoration of stable cardiovascular conditions have priority. After oral ingestion, thorough gastric lavage is indicated, if necessary in combination with irrigation of the small intestine. Particularly in cases of intoxication with slow-release products like Adalat XL, elimination must be as complete as possible including the small intestine to prevent the otherwise inevitable subsequent absorption of the active substance. Hemodialysis serves no purpose, as nifedipine is not dialyzable, but plasmapheresis is advisable (high plasma protein binding, relatively low volume of distribution).

Clinically significant hypotension calls for active cardiovascular support including monitoring of cardiac and respiratory function including elevation of extremities and attention to circulating fluid volume and urine output.

Hypotension as a result of arterial vasodilation can also be treated with calcium (10 mL of 10% calcium gluconate solution administered slowly via i.v. route and repeated if necessary). As a result, the serum calcium can reach the upper normal range to slightly elevated levels. If an insufficient increase in blood pressure is achieved with calcium, vasoconstricting sympathomimetics such as dopamine or norepinephrine are additionally administered as a last resort only in patients without cardiac arrhythmia or ischemic heart disease and when other safer measures have failed. The dosage of these drugs is determined solely by the effect obtained. Additional liquid or volume must be administered with caution because of the danger of overloading the heart.

Bradycardia and/or bradyarrhythmias have been observed in some cases of nifedipine overdosage. Appropriate clinical measures, according to the nature and severity of the symptoms, should be applied.

> For management of a suspected drug overdose, contact your **regional Poison Control Centre**. See the *CPS* Directory section for a list of Poison Control Centres.

DOSAGE: Dosage should be individualized depending on patient tolerance and response.

Adalat XL tablets must be swallowed whole and should not be bitten or divided.

In general, titration steps should proceed over a 7 to 14 day period so that the physician can assess the response to each dose level before proceeding to higher doses. Since steady-state plasma levels are achieved on the second day of dosing, if symptoms so warrant, titration may proceed more rapidly provided that the patient is closely monitored.

Angina: Therapy should normally be initiated with 30 mg once daily. Experience with doses greater than 90 mg daily in patients with angina is limited; therefore, doses greater than 90 mg daily are not recommended.

Angina patients controlled on Adalat capsules alone or in combination with beta-blockers may be safely switched to Adalat XL tablets at the nearest equivalent daily dose. Subsequent titration to higher or lower doses may be necessary and should be initiated as clinically warranted.

Hypertension: Therapy should normally be initiated with 20 or 30 mg once daily. The usual maintenance dose is 30 to 60 mg once daily. Doses greater than 90 mg are not recommended.

Patients switched from Adalat PA 10 or 20 to Adalat XL therapy should receive an initial dosage of Adalat XL no higher than 30 mg once daily, based on previously prescribed dosing regimen. If clinically warranted, the dosage of Adalat XL should be increased to 60 mg once daily. Blood pressure and patient symptoms should be monitored closely following the switch from Adalat PA to Adalat XL.

No "rebound effect" has been observed upon discontinuation of Adalat XL. However, if discontinuation of nifedipine is necessary, sound clinical practice suggests that the dosage should be decreased gradually under close physician supervision.

INFORMATION FOR THE PATIENT: Published in e-CPS, available by subscription at www.e-cps.ca.

SUPPLIED: 20 mg: Each dusty rose, extended-release tablet, imprinted with "ADALAT 20" on one side, contains: nifedipine 20 mg. Nonmedicinal ingredients: cellulose acetate, hydroxypropylcellulose, hydroxypropyl methylcellulose 2910, magnesium stearate, pharmaceutical shellac, polyethylene glycol 3350, polyethylene oxide, propylene glycol, red ferric oxide, sodium chloride, synthetic black iron oxide and titanium dioxide. Lactose-free. Blister packs of 28 and 98. Store between 15 and 30°C. Protect from light and humidity.

30 mg: Each dusty rose, extended-release tablet, imprinted with "ADALAT 30" on one side, contains: nifedipine 30 mg. Nonmedicinal ingredients: cellulose acetate, hydroxypropylcellulose, hydroxypropyl methylcellulose 2910, magnesium stearate, pharmaceutical shellac, polyethylene glycol 3350, polyethylene oxide, propylene glycol, red ferric oxide, sodium chloride, synthetic black iron oxide and titanium dioxide. Lactose-free. Blister packs of 28 and 98. Store between 15 and 30°C. Protect from light and humidity.

60 mg: Each dusty rose, extended-release tablet, imprinted with "ADALAT 60" on one side, contains: nifedipine 60 mg. Nonmedicinal ingredients: cellulose acetate, hydroxypropylcellulose, hydroxypropyl methylcellulose 2910, magnesium stearate, pharmaceutical shellac, polyethylene glycol 3350, polyethylene oxide, propylene glycol, red ferric oxide, sodium chloride, synthetic black iron oxide and titanium dioxide. Lactose-free. Blister packs of 28 and 98. Store between 15 and 30°C. Protect from light and humidity.

(Shown in Product Identification Section)

> The reader is invited to consult CPhA's monograph **Calcium Channel Blockers**.

Adalat® XL® Plus ℞

nifedipine—ASA

Antihypertensive—Platelet Aggregation Inhibitor

Bayer

Date of Revision: March 31, 2009

SUMMARY PRODUCT INFORMATION:

Route of Administration	Dosage Form/ Strength	Clinically Relevant Nonmedicinal Ingredients
ADALAT XL (nifedipine extended-release tablets Bayer Standard)		
Oral	Extended-release tablets 20, 30, and 60 mg	For a complete listing see Dosage Forms, Composition and Packaging.
ASPIRIN 81 mg (acetylsalicylic acid delayed-release tablets USP)		
Oral	Delayed-release, enteric coated tablets 81 mg	Lactose For a complete listing see Dosage Forms, Composition and Packaging.

INDICATIONS AND CLINICAL USE: ADALAT XL PLUS (nifedipine extended-release tablets and acetylsalicylic acid delayed-release tablets) is indicated in patients for whom treatment with both ADALAT XL and ASPIRIN 81 mg is appropriate. Please refer to ADALAT XL and ASPIRIN Product Monographs for additional information concerning approved indications.

ADALAT XL PLUS is not indicated for initial therapy. The dose of ADALAT XL should be determined by titration before the switch to ADALAT XL PLUS. If the fixed combination represents the dose and dosing frequency determined by this titration, the use of ADALAT XL PLUS may be more convenient in the management of patients.

If during maintenance therapy dosage adjustment is necessary, it is advisable to use the individual drugs.

CONTRAINDICATIONS:

- ADALAT XL PLUS (nifedipine extended-release tablets and acetylsalicylic acid delayed-release tablets) should not be given to patients who are hypersensitive to nifedipine, acetylsalicylic acid, or to any ingredient in the formulation or component of the container. For a complete listing, see Dosage Forms, Composition and Packaging.
- ADALAT XL PLUS is contraindicated in pregnancy, during lactation, and in women of childbearing potential. Fetal malformations and adverse effects on pregnancy have been reported in animals (see Warnings and Precautions, Special Populations).
- ADALAT XL PLUS is contraindicated in children.
- ADALAT XL PLUS is contraindicated in patients with severe hypotension or cardiovascular shock.
- ADALAT XL PLUS must not be used in combination with rifampicin because insufficient plasma levels of nifedipine may result due to enzyme induction.
- ADALAT XL PLUS should not be used in combination with methotrexate at doses of 15 mg/week or more.
- ADALAT XL PLUS is contraindicated in patients with a history of asthma induced by the administration of salicylates or substances with a similar action, notably a nonsteroidal anti-inflammatory drug.
- ADALAT XL PLUS should not be used in patients with hemorrhagic diathesis.
- ADALAT XL PLUS should not be used in patients with active peptic ulcer.

WARNINGS AND PRECAUTIONS:

> **Serious Warnings and Precautions**
> - Increased angina and/or myocardial infarction in patients with severe obstructive coronary artery disease (see Warnings and Precautions, Increased Angina and/or Myocardial Infarction).
> - Severe hypotension and lowering of cardiac output in patients with severe heart failure (see Warnings and Precautions, Patients with Heart Failure).

General: ASA (acetylsalicylic acid) is one of the most frequent causes of accidental poisonings in toddlers and infants. ADALAT XL PLUS (nifedipine extended-release tablets and acetylsalicylic acid delayed-release tablets) and its constituents should be kept well out of the reach of children.

ADALAT XL PLUS should be administered cautiously to patients with the following:

- hypersensitivity to anti-inflammatory or antirheumatic drugs or other allergens;
- impaired renal function or hepatic function;
- a history of chronic or recurrent gastrointestinal ulcerations and bleeds;
- a history of bleeding tendencies, significant anemia and/or hypothrombinemia.

Cardiovascular: Excessive Hypotension in Patients with Angina: Since ADALAT XL (nifedipine extended-release tablets) lowers peripheral vascular resistance and blood pressure, ADALAT XL PLUS should be used cautiously in patients with angina who are prone to develop hypotension and those with a history of cerebrovascular insufficiency.

Occasionally patients have had excessive and poorly tolerated hypotension. Syncope has been reported (see Adverse Reactions). These responses have usually occurred during initial titration or at the time of subsequent upward dosage adjustment and may be more likely in patients on concomitant beta blockers. If excessive hypotension occurs, dosage should be lowered or the drug should be discontinued (see Contraindications).

Severe hypotension and/or increased fluid volume requirements have been reported in patients receiving nifedipine with a beta blocker, who underwent coronary artery bypass surgery using high-dose fentanyl anesthesia. The interaction with high-dose fentanyl appears to be due to the combination of nifedipine and a beta blocker, but the possibility that it may occur with nifedipine alone, with low doses of fentanyl in other surgical procedures, or with other narcotic analgesics cannot be ruled out. In nifedipine-treated patients where surgery using high-dose fentanyl anesthesia is contemplated, the physician should be aware of these potential problems, and if the patient's condition permits, sufficient time (at least 36 hours) should be allowed for nifedipine to be washed out of the body prior to surgery.

Increased Angina and/or Myocardial Infarction: Rarely, patients, particularly those who have severe obstructive coronary artery disease have developed well-documented increased frequency, duration and/or severity of angina or acute myocardial infarction on starting nifedipine or at the time of dosage increase. The mechanism of the response is not established.

Since there has not been a study of ADALAT XL in acute myocardial infarction reported, similar effects of ADALAT XL to that of immediate-release nifedipine cannot be excluded. Immediate-release nifedipine is contraindicated in acute myocardial infarction.

Beta-Blocker Withdrawal: Patients with angina recently withdrawn from beta blockers may develop a withdrawal syndrome with increased angina, probably related to increased sensitivity to catecholamines. Initiation of treatment with ADALAT XL will not prevent this occurrence and might be expected to exacerbate it by provoking reflex catecholamine release. There have been occasional reports of increased angina in a setting of beta-blocker withdrawal and initiation of nifedipine. It is important to taper beta blockers if possible, rather than stopping them abruptly before beginning ADALAT XL.

Patients with Heart Failure: There have been isolated reports of severe hypotension and lowering of cardiac output following administration of nifedipine to patients with severe heart failure. Thus, ADALAT XL should be used cautiously in patients with severe heart failure. Rarely have patients usually receiving a beta blocker developed heart failure after beginning nifedipine therapy.

In patients with severe aortic stenosis, nifedipine will not produce its usual afterload reducing effects, and there is a possibility that an unopposed negative inotropic action of the drug may produce heart failure if the end-diastolic pressure is raised. Caution should therefore be exercised when using ADALAT XL in patients with these conditions.

Peripheral Edema: Mild to moderate peripheral edema, typically associated with arterial vasodilation and not due to left ventricular dysfunction, has been reported to occur in patients treated with ADALAT XL (see Adverse Reactions, ADALAT XL). This edema occurs primarily in the lower extremities and may respond to diuretic therapy. With patients whose angina or hypertension is complicated by congestive heart failure, care should be taken to differentiate this peripheral edema from the effects of increasing left ventricular dysfunction.

Gastrointestinal: Patients with Pre-Existing Gastrointestinal Narrowing: Since the ADALAT XL delivery system contains a nondeformable material, caution should be used when administering ADALAT XL in patients with pre-existing severe gastrointestinal narrowing (pathologic or iatrogenic). There have been rare reports of obstructive symptoms in patients with known strictures in association with the ingestion of ADALAT XL tablets. In single cases, obstructive symptoms have been described without known history of gastrointestinal disorders. Bezoars can occur in very rare cases and may require surgical intervention. ADALAT XL must not be used in patients with a Kock pouch (ileostomy after proctocolectomy).

When doing barium contrast X-ray, ADALAT XL may cause false positive effects (e.g., filling defects interpreted as polyp).

Hypersensitivity: Acetylsalicylic acid may precipitate bronchospasm and induce asthma attacks or other hypersensitivity reactions. Risk factors are present bronchial asthma, hay fever, nasal polyps, or chronic respiratory disease. This applies also for patients showing allergic reactions (e.g., cutaneous reactions, itching, urticaria) to other substances.

Hematologic: Due to effect on platelet aggregation, acetylsalicylic acid may be associated with an increased risk of bleeding. Caution is necessary when salicylates and anticoagulants are prescribed concurrently, as salicylates can depress the concentration of prothrombin in the plasma.

Peri-Operative Considerations: Due to its inhibitory effect on platelet aggregation, acetylsalicylic acid may lead to an increased bleeding tendency during and after surgical operations (including minor surgeries, e.g., dental extractions).

Sexual Function/Reproduction: Male Fertility: In some cases of in vitro fertilization, nifedipine has been associated with reversible spermatozoal biochemical changes. In vitro studies have shown that nifedipine may inhibit expression of mannose-ligand receptors, thus preventing the spermatozoa from attaching to the zona pellucida and impairing sperm function. In those men who are repeatedly unsuccessful in fathering a child by in vitro fertilization and where no other explanation could be found, nifedipine should be considered as a possible cause.

Special Populations: Pregnant Women: The use of ADALAT XL PLUS is contraindicated during pregnancy (see Contraindications).

There are no adequate and well-controlled studies of ADALAT XL in pregnant women. An increase in the number of fetal mortalities and resorptions occurred after the administration of 30 and 100 mg/kg nifedipine to pregnant mice, rats, and rabbits. Fetal malformations occurred after the administration of 30 and 100 mg/kg nifedipine to pregnant mice and 100 mg/kg to pregnant rats (see Contraindications).

Use of salicylates in the first 3 months of pregnancy has been associated in several epidemiological studies with an elevated risk of malformations (cleft palate, heart malformations). After normal therapeutic doses this risk seems to be low: a prospective study with exposure of about 32 000 mother-child pairs has not yielded any association with the risk of malformations.

In the last 3 months of pregnancy, administration of salicylates in high doses (>300 mg/day) can lead to prolongation of the gestation period, premature closure of the arterial duct, and inhibition of uterine contractions. An increased hemorrhagic tendency has been observed in both mother and child.

Administration of acetylsalicylic acid in high doses (>300 mg/d) shortly before birth can lead to intracranial hemorrhages, particularly in premature babies.

Nursing Women: The use of nifedipine is contraindicated during lactation (see Contraindications).

ASA and its metabolites pass into breast milk in small quantities. Since no adverse effects on the infant have been observed after occasional use, interruption of breast-feeding is usually unnecessary. However, on regular use or on intake of high doses, breast-feeding should be discontinued early.

Pediatrics: ADALAT XL PLUS should not be used in children (see Contraindications).

Geriatrics: ADALAT XL should be administered cautiously to elderly patients, especially to those with a history of hypotension or cerebral vascular insufficiency.

Diabetic Patients: The use of ADALAT XL in diabetic patients may require adjustment for their control.

Hepatic Insufficiency: ADALAT XL should be used with caution in patients with impaired liver function (see Action and Clinical Pharmacology, Special Populations and Conditions, Hepatic Insufficiency). A dose reduction, particularly in severe cases, may be required. Close monitoring of response and metabolic effect should apply.

Low Uric Acid Excretion: At low doses, ASA reduces excretion of uric acid. This can trigger gout in patients who already tend to have low uric acid excretion.

Monitoring and Laboratory Tests: Hypotension/Heart Rate: Because ADALAT XL is an arterial and arteriolar vasodilator, hypotension and a compensatory increase in heart rate may occur. Thus, blood pressure and heart rate should be monitored carefully during nifedipine therapy. Close monitoring is especially recommended for patients who are prone to develop hypotension, those with a history of cerebrovascular insufficiency, and those who are taking medications that are known to lower blood pressure (see Warnings and Precautions, Cardiovascular).

Thyroid Function Tests: Salicylates can produce changes in thyroid function tests.

Liver Function Tests: Isolated cases of liver function disturbances (transaminases increase) have been described following administration of ASA.

ADVERSE REACTIONS: Formal clinical trials to examine the safety of combination use of ADALAT XL (nifedipine extended-release tablets) and ASPIRIN 81 mg (acetylsalicylic acid delayed-release tablets) have not been conducted. The following sections summarize the safety information derived from clinical trials and postmarketing use of the individual drugs.

ADALAT XL: Hypertension: In 661 hypertensive patients treated in controlled trials with ADALAT XL, adverse effects were reported in 54.0% of patients and required discontinuation of therapy in 11.9% of patients. The majority of adverse effects reported occurred within the first three months of therapy.

The most common adverse effects reported with ADALAT XL were edema, which was dose related and ranged in frequency from approximately 10 to 30% in the 30 to 120 mg dose range, headache (16.6%), fatigue (6.2%), dizziness (4.4%), constipation (3.5%), and nausea (3.5%).

The following adverse effects were also reported. Incidences greater than 1% are given in parenthesis:

Cardiovascular: flushing (2.4%), palpitation (2.3%), tachycardia (1.2%), chest pain (1.1%), ventricular arrhythmia, hypotension, syncope.

Central Nervous System: insomnia (1.8%), nervousness (1.8%), somnolence (1.5%), depression, tremor, decreased libido, migraine, vertigo, amnesia, anxiety, impaired concentration, twitching, ataxia, hypertonia, paresthesia, hypoesthesia.

Gastrointestinal: dyspepsia (1.5%), flatulence (1.5%), abdominal pain (1.4%), dry mouth (1.1%), diarrhea, vomiting, thirst, melena, eructation, weight increase.

Genitourinary: impotence (1.5%), polyuria (1.5%), dysuria, nocturia, oliguria, urinary incontinence, urinary frequency, menstrual disorder.

Musculoskeletal: arthralgia, back pain, myalgia.

Special Senses: abnormal vision, abnormal lacrimation, taste disturbance, conjuctivitis, tinnitus.

Dermatologic: rash (2.3%), pruritus (1.1%), erythematous rash, alopecia.

Respiratory: dyspnea (1.7%), bronchospasm, pharyngitis, upper respiratory tract infection, epistaxis.

Other: leg cramps (2.7%), pain (2.7%), asthenia (2.0%), face edema, gout, allergy, fever, breast pain.

Angina: In 257 chronic stable angina patients treated in controlled and long-term open studies with ADALAT XL, adverse effects were reported in 30.0% of patients and required discontinuation of therapy in 8.5% of patients.

The most common adverse effects were: edema (10.1%), headache (3.1%), angina pectoris (3.1%).

The following adverse effects were also reported. Incidences greater than 1% are given in parenthesis:

Cardiovascular: palpitation (2.3%), tachycardia, myocardial infarction, ventricular arrhythmia, extrasystoles, dyspnea, chest pain.

In patients with angina, rarely, and possibly due to tachycardia, nifedipine has been reported to have precipitated an angina pectoris attack. In addition, more serious events were occasionally observed, not readily distinguishable from the natural history of the disease in these patients. It remains possible, however, that some or many of these events were drug related. These events include myocardial infarction, congestive heart failure or pulmonary edema, and ventricular arrhythmias or conduction disturbances.

Central Nervous System: dizziness (2.3%), hypoesthesia (1.2%), confusion, insomnia, somnolence, nervousness, asthenia, hyperkinesia.

Gastrointestinal: constipation (1.9%), dyspepsia (1.2%), abdominal pain (1.2%), diarrhea, nausea, melena.

Genitourinary: impotence, hematuria, polyuria, dysuria.

Musculoskeletal: leg cramps, paresthesia, myalgia, arthralgia.

Dermatologic: rash, pruritus.

Other: fatigue (1.2%), pain, periorbital edema.

Other Adverse Effects: The following adverse events have been reported with nifedipine rarely.

Rare instances of allergic hepatitis and cholestasis with or without jaundice have been reported in patients treated with nifedipine.

Gingival hyperplasia similar to that caused by diphenylhydantoin has been reported in patients treated with nifedipine. The lesions usually regressed on discontinuation of the drug. However, on occasion gingivectomy was necessary.

Gynecomastia has been observed rarely in older men on long-term therapy, but has so far always regressed completely on discontinuation of the drug.

Isolated cases of angioedema have been reported. Angioedema may be accompanied by breathing difficulty. Anaphylaxis has been reported rarely.

In postmarketing experience, there have been rare reports of exfoliative dermatitis and Stevens-Johnson Syndrome. Gastrointestinal irritation and gastrointestinal bleeding were also reported; however, the causal relationship is uncertain.

Abnormal Hematologic and Clinical Chemistry Findings: Rare, usually transient, but occasionally significant elevations of enzymes such as CPK, AST, and ALT have been noted. The relationship to drug therapy is uncertain in most cases, but probable in some. These laboratory abnormalities have rarely been associated with clinical symptoms; however, cholestasis with or without jaundice has been reported.

An increase (5.4%) in mean alkaline phosphatase was noted in patients treated with ADALAT XL. This was an isolated finding not associated with clinical symptoms and rarely resulted in values which exceeded the upper limit of the normal range.

Serum potassium was unchanged in patients receiving ADALAT XL in the absence of concomitant diuretic therapy and slightly decreased in patients receiving concomitant diuretics.

Nifedipine decreases platelet aggregation in vitro. Limited clinical studies have demonstrated a moderate but statistically significant decrease in platelet aggregation and increase in bleeding time in some nifedipine-treated patients. This is thought to be a function of inhibition of calcium transport across the platelet membrane. No clinical significance for these findings has been demonstrated.

Positive direct Coombs tests, with or without associated hemolytic anemia, have been reported but a causal relationship between nifedipine administration and positivity of this laboratory test, including hemolysis, could not be determined.

Rare reversible elevations in BUN and serum creatinine have been reported in patients with pre-existing chronic renal insufficiency. The relationship to therapy with ADALAT XL is uncertain in most cases, but probable in some.

ASPIRIN 81 mg: Many adverse reactions due to ASPIRIN ingestion are dose related. Table 1 lists adverse reactions that have been reported in the literature and from both clinical and postmarketing experience.

Table 1: ADALAT XL PLUS

ASPIRIN Adverse Drug Reactions Reported in Clinical and Postmarketing Experience

Gastrointestinal	Nausea, vomiting, diarrhea, gastrointestinal bleeding and/or ulceration, dyspepsia, heartburn, hematemesis, melena (the frequency and severity of these adverse effects are dose related)
Ear	Tinnitus, vertigo, hearing loss
Hematologic	Leukopenia, thrombocytopenia, purpura, anemia
Dermatologic and Hypersensitivity	Urticaria, angioedema, pruritus, skin eruptions, asthma, anaphylaxis, Quincke edema
Miscellaneous	Mental confusion, drowsiness, sweating, thirst

DRUG INTERACTIONS: Drug-Drug Interactions: General: Biotransformation by Cytochrome P450 System: As with all drugs, care should be exercised when treating patients with multiple medications. Dihydrophyridine calcium channel blockers, including ADALAT XL (nifedipine extended-release tablets), undergo biotransformation by the cytochrome P450 system, mainly via the CYP3A4 isoenzyme. Coadministration of nifedipine with other drugs which follow the same route of biotransformation may result in altered bioavailability. Dosages of similarly metabolized drugs, particularly those of low therapeutic ratio, and especially in patients with renal and/or hepatic impairment, may require adjustment when starting or stopping concomitantly administered nifedipine to maintain optimum therapeutic blood levels. If necessary, a reduction in the dose of nifedipine may be considered.

Drugs known to be inhibitors of the cytochrome P450 system include: azole antifungals (ketoconazole, itraconazole, fluconazole), cimetidine, cyclosporine, erythromycin, fluoxetine, HIV protease inhibitors (amprenavir, indinavir, nelfinavir, ritonavir, saquanavir), nefazodone, quinidine, terfenadine, and warfarin.

Drugs known to be inducers of the cytochrome P450 system include: phenobarbital, phenytoin, and rifampicin.

Drugs known to be biotransformed via cytochrome P450 include: benzodiazepines, cisapride, flecainide, tacrolimus, theophylline, imipramine, and propafenone.

ADALAT XL PLUS (nifedipine extended-release tablets and acetylsalicylic acid delayed-release tablets) should be used with caution with other products that have anticoagulation or antiplatelet effects, as these effects may be potentiated. Drugs that bind to protein binding sites should also be used cautiously since ASA may displace drugs from their protein binding site.

Angiotensin-Converting Enzyme (ACE) Inhibitors: The hyponatremic and hypotensive effects of ACE inhibitors **may** be diminished by the concomitant administration of ASA due to its indirect effect on the renin-angiotensin conversion pathway. The potential interaction may be related to the dose of ASA (3 g/day or more).

Anticoagulants: There have been rare reports of increased prothrombin time in patients taking coumarin anticoagulants to whom nifedipine was administered. However, the relationship to nifedipine therapy is uncertain.

Caution is necessary when salicylates and anticoagulants are prescribed concurrently, as salicylates can depress the concentration of prothrombin in the plasma.

ASA and Other NSAIDs: The use of other nonsteroidal anti-inflammatory drugs with salicylates at high doses (≥3 g/day) may increase the risk of ulcers and gastrointestinal bleeding due to a synergistic effect with ASPIRIN (acetylsalicylic acid tablets).

Beta Adrenergic Blocking Agents: Concomitant administration of nifedipine and beta blocking agents is usually well tolerated, but there have been occasional literature reports suggesting that the combination may increase the likelihood of congestive heart failure, severe hypotension, or exacerbation of angina. Therefore, caution and careful monitoring of patients on concomitant therapy is recommended (see Indications and Clinical Use and Warnings and Precautions, Cardiovascular).

Carbamazepine: No formal studies have been performed to investigate the potential interaction between nifedipine and carbamazepine. As carbamazepine has been shown to reduce the plasma concentrations of the structurally similar calcium channel blocker, nimodipine, due to enzyme induction, a decrease in nifedipine plasma concentrations and hence a decrease in efficacy cannot be excluded.

Cimetidine and Ranitidine: Pharmacokinetic studies have shown that concurrent administration of cimetidine or ranitidine with nifedipine results in significant increases in nifedipine plasma levels (ca. 80% with cimetidine and 70% with ranitidine). Patients receiving either of these drugs concomitantly with nifedipine should be monitored carefully for the possible exacerbation of effects of nifedipine, such as hypotension. Adjustment of nifedipine dosage may be necessary.

Cisapride: Simultaneous administration of cisapride and nifedipine may lead to increased plasma concentrations of nifedipine. Upon coadministration of both drugs, the blood pressure should be monitored and, if necessary, a reduction of the nifedipine dose considered.

Coadministration with ASPIRIN: The safety, pharmacodynamic effects, and pharmacokinetics of coadministration of ADALAT XL 60 mg and acetylsalicylic acid (100 mg enteric-coated tablet) were studied in a multiple-dose, randomized, double-blind, placebo-controlled, three-treatment crossover study in healthy male volunteers. The results of this clinical pharmacology study showed that concomitant administration of nifedipine and acetylsalicylic acid has no clinically relevant effect on the pharmacokinetics of the two drugs. Coadministration of nifedipine did not alter the effect of acetylsalicylic acid on platelet aggregation and bleeding time.

Digoxin: Administration of nifedipine with digoxin may lead to reduced digoxin clearance and therefore an increase in the plasma digoxin level. It is recommended that digoxin levels be monitored when initiating, adjusting, and discontinuing nifedipine to avoid possible "underdosing" or "overdosing" with digitalis.

Plasma concentrations of digoxin are increased due to a decrease in renal excretion with concomitant usage of ASPIRIN.

Diuretics: Sodium excretion produced by spironolactone may be decreased by salicylate administration.

Diltiazem: Diltiazem decreases the clearance of nifedipine. The combination of both drugs should be administered with caution, and a reduction of the nifedipine dose may be considered.

Glucocorticoids (Systemic), Except Hydrocortisone Used as Replacement Therapy in Addison's Disease: Decreased blood salicylate levels during corticosteroid treatment and risk of salicylate overdose after this treatment is stopped via increased elimination of salicylates by corticosteroids.

Ibuprofen: Ibuprofen may interfere with the cardioprotective effects and platelet aggregation inhibitory properties of ASPIRIN. Patients should talk to their doctor if they are on an ASPIRIN regimen and take ibuprofen for pain. Studies have shown that single doses and multiple doses of ibuprofen may interfere with the antiplatelet effects of low-dose ASPIRIN.
Long-Acting Nitrates: Nifedipine may be safely coadministered with nitrates, but there have been no controlled studies to evaluate the antianginal effectiveness of this combination.
Methotrexate, Used at 15 mg/week or Less: Salicylates may retard the elimination of methotrexate by decreasing renal clearance of methotrexate, displacing methotrexate from protein binding sites, and thereby increasing its hematological toxicity.
Oral Hypoglycemics: Large doses of salicylates have a hypoglycemic action and may enhance the effect of oral hypoglycemic agents. Diabetics receiving concurrent salicylate and hypoglycemic therapy should be monitored closely: reduction of the sulfonylurea hypoglycemic drug dosage may be necessary.
Quinidine: The addition of nifedipine to a stable quinidine regimen may reduce the quinidine by 50%; an enhanced response to nifedipine may also occur. The addition of quinidine to a stable nifedipine regimen may result in elevated nifedipine concentrations and a reduced response to quinidine. Some patients have experienced elevated quinidine levels when nifedipine was discontinued. Therefore, patients receiving concomitant therapy of nifedipine and quinidine, or those who had their nifedipine discontinued while still receiving quinidine, should be closely monitored, including determination of plasma levels of quinidine. Consideration should be given to dosage adjustment.
Quinupristin/Dalfopristin: Simultaneous administration of quinupristin/dalfopristin and nifedipine may lead to increased plasma concentrations of nifedipine. Upon coadministration of both drugs, blood pressure should be monitored and, if necessary, a reduction of the nifedipine dose should be considered.
Uricosuric Agents: Salicylates in large doses are uricosuric agents; smaller amounts may depress uric acid clearance and thus decrease the uricosuric effects of other drugs.
Valproic Acid: No formal studies have been performed to investigate the potential interaction between nifedipine and valproic acid (VPA). As VPA has been shown to increase the plasma concentrations of the structurally similar calcium channel blocker nimodipine due to enzyme inhibition, an increase in nifedipine plasma concentrations and hence an increase in efficacy cannot be excluded.

Salicylates may alter VPA metabolism and may displace VPA from protein binding sites, possibly intensifying the effects of VPA. Caution is recommended when VPA is administered concomitantly with salicylates.

Drug-Food Interactions: Published data indicate that through inhibition of cytochrome P450, flavonoids present in the grapefruit juice can increase plasma levels and augment pharmacodynamic effects of some dihydropyridine calcium channel blockers, including nifedipine (see Action and Clinical Pharmacology, Pharmacokinetics). Therefore, the administration of nifedipine with grapefruit juice should be avoided.

Interactions with food have not been established for ASPIRIN.

Drug-Herb Interactions: Interactions with herbal products have not been established.
Drug-Laboratory Test Interactions: Salicylates can produce changes in thyroid function tests.
Drug-Lifestyle Interactions: Reactions to the drug, which vary in intensity from individual to individual, can impair the ability to drive or to operate machinery, particularly at the start of the treatment, upon changing the medication, or in combination with alcohol.

Patients taking ASA daily are at an increased risk of developing gastrointestinal bleeding following the ingestion of alcohol.

DOSAGE AND ADMINISTRATION: **Dosing Considerations:** See Warnings and Precautions, Special Populations and Drug Interactions, Drug-Drug Interactions.
Administration: ADALAT XL PLUS (nifedipine extended-release tablets and acetylsalicylic acid delayed-release tablets) is not indicated for initial therapy. The dose of nifedipine should be determined by titration before the switch to ADALAT XL PLUS.

Dosage should be individualized depending on patient tolerance and response. Once the dose of nifedipine has been established, patients should take 1 tablet of ADALAT XL (nifedipine extended-release tablets) and 1 tablet of ASPIRIN 81 mg (acetylsalicylic acid delayed-release tablets) daily.

Therapy for hypertension should normally be initiated with 20 or 30 mg of nifedipine extended-release tablets once daily. The usual maintenance dose is 30 to 60 mg once daily. Doses greater than 90 mg daily are not recommended.

No "rebound effect" has been observed upon discontinuation of ADALAT XL. However, if discontinuation of nifedipine is necessary, sound clinical practice suggests that the dosage should be decreased gradually under close physician supervision.

ADALAT XL and ASPIRIN 81 mg tablets must be swallowed whole and should not be bitten or divided. Both tablets should preferably be taken after meals, with plenty of liquid.

OVERDOSAGE:
ADALAT XL: There are several well-documented cases of ADALAT XL (nifedipine extended-release tablets) overdosage. The following symptoms are observed in cases of severe nifedipine intoxication: disturbance of consciousness to the point of coma, a drop in blood pressure, tachycardia/bradycardia, hyperglycemia, metabolic acidosis, hypoxia, and cardiogenic shock with pulmonary edema.

As far as treatment is concerned, elimination of the active substance and the restoration of stable cardiovascular conditions have priority. After oral ingestion, thorough gastric lavage is indicated, if necessary in combination with irrigation of the small intestine. Particularly in cases of intoxication with slow-release products like ADALAT XL, elimination must be as complete as possible, including the small intestine, to prevent the otherwise inevitable subsequent absorption of the active substance. Hemodialysis serves no purpose, as nifedipine is not dialysable, but plasmapheresis is advisable (high plasma protein binding, relatively low volume of distribution).

Clinically significant hypotension calls for active cardiovascular support including monitoring of cardiac and respiratory function including elevation of extremities and attention to circulating fluid volume and urine output.

Hypotension as a result of arterial vasodilation can also be treated with calcium (10 mL of 10% calcium gluconate solution administered slowly via intravenous route and repeated if necessary). As a result, the serum calcium can reach the upper normal range to slightly elevated levels. If an insufficient increase in blood pressure is achieved with calcium, vasoconstricting sympathomimetics such as dopamine or noradrenaline are additionally administered as a last resort only in patients without cardiac arrhythmia or ischemic heart disease and when other safer measures have failed. The dosage of these drugs is determined solely by the effect obtained. Additional liquid or volume must be administered with caution because of the danger of overloading the heart.

Bradycardia and/or bradyarrhythmias have been observed in some cases of nifedipine overdosage. Appropriate clinical measures, according to the nature and severity of the symptoms, should be applied.
ASPIRIN 81 mg: See Table 2.

Table 2: ADALAT XL PLUS

Symptoms of ASPIRIN (Acetylsalicylic Acid Tablets) Overdose

Mild Overdose or Early Poisoning	Burning in the mouth, lethargy, nausea, vomiting, tinnitus, sweating, thirst, tachycardia or dizziness
Moderate Overdose	All of the symptoms from mild overdose plus tachypnea, hyperpyrexia, dehydration, loss of coordination, restlessness, mental confusion
Severe Overdose	All of the symptoms from moderate overdose plus hypotension, hallucinations, stupor, hypoglycemia, convulsions, cerebral edema, oliguria, renal failure, cardiovascular failure, coma, metabolic acidosis, respiratory alkalosis and/or failure

Emergency Management:
1. Immediate transfer to hospital and maintain cardiovascular and respiratory support.
2. Gastric lavage, administration of activated charcoal.
3. Check of acid-base balance and correct if necessary.
4. Alkaline diuresis so as to obtain urine pH between 7.5 and 8 should be considered when plasma salicylate concentration is greater than 500 mg/L (3.6 mmol/L) in adults or 300 mg/L (2.2 mmol/L) in children.
5. Hemodialysis should be considered in severe poisoning 800 mg/L (5.8 mmol/L) in adults and 700 mg/L (5.0 mmol/L) in children, as renal elimination of salicylates may be slow due to the presence of acidic urine and renal failure. Hemodialysis should also be considered if the patient is experiencing severe systemic metabolic acidosis (arterial pH <7.2), acute renal failure, pulmonary edema, or CNS symptoms such as: drowsiness, agitation, coma, or convulsions.
6. Fluid losses should be replaced with hypotonic solution (eg, half-saline) and supplemented with glucose 50 to 100 g/L.
7. Symptomatic treatment.

Fatal Dose: The fatal dose varies from 10 to 30 g of ASA. However, (in one case) 130 g of ASA was ingested without fatal outcome.

> For management of a suspected drug overdose, CPhA recommends that you contact your **regional Poison Control Centre**. See the *CPS* Directory section for a list of Poison Control Centres.

ACTION AND CLINICAL PHARMACOLOGY: ADALAT XL: Mechanism of Action: ADALAT XL (nifedipine extended-release tablets) is a calcium ion influx inhibitor (calcium channel blocker or calcium ion antagonist).

ADALAT XL, while similar in appearance to a conventional tablet, nonetheless consists of a semipermeable membrane surrounding an osmotically active drug core. The core itself is divided into two layers: an "active" layer containing the drug, and a "push" layer containing pharmacologically inert but osmotically active components. As water from the gastrointestinal tract enters the tablet, pressure increases in the osmotic layer and "pushes" against the drug layer, forcing drug through the orifice in the active layer.

Drug delivery is essentially constant as long as the osmotic gradient remains constant and then gradually falls to zero as drug is exhausted from the tablet. Upon swallowing, the biologically inert components of the tablet remain intact during gastrointestinal transit and are eliminated in the feces as an insoluble shell.

The antianginal and antihypertensive actions of nifedipine are believed to be related to a specific cellular action of selectively inhibiting transmembrane influx of calcium ions into cardiac muscle and vascular smooth muscle. The contractile processes of these tissues are dependent upon the movement of extracellular calcium into the cells through specific ion channels. Nifedipine selectively inhibits the transmembrane influx of calcium through the slow channel without affecting, to any significant degree, the transmembrane influx of sodium through the fast channel. This results in a reduction of free calcium ions available within the muscle cells and an inhibition of the contractile processes. Nifedipine does not alter total serum calcium.

The specific mechanisms by which nifedipine relieves angina and reduces blood pressure have not been fully determined but are believed to be brought about largely by its vasodilatory action.

Pharmacodynamics: Nifedipine dilates the main coronary arteries and coronary arterioles both in normal and ischemic regions resulting in an increase in blood flow and hence in myocardial oxygen delivery.

Nifedipine by its vasodilatory action on peripheral arterioles, reduces the total peripheral vascular resistance. This reduces the workload of the heart and thus reduces myocardial energy consumption and oxygen requirements which probably accounts for the effectiveness of nifedipine in chronic stable angina.

The mechanism by which nifedipine reduces arterial blood pressure involves peripheral arterial vasodilation and subsequent reduction in peripheral vascular resistance. The increased peripheral vascular resistance that is an underlying cause of hypertension results from an increase in active tension in the vascular smooth muscle. Studies have demonstrated that the increase in active tension reflects an increase in cytosolic free calcium.

The negative inotropic effect of nifedipine is usually not of major clinical significance because at therapeutic doses, nifedipine's vasodilatory property evokes a baroreceptor mediated reflex tachycardia which tends to counterbalance this negative inotropic effect. Continued administration of nifedipine to hypertensive patients has shown no significant increase in heart rate.

Although nifedipine causes a slight depression of sinoatrial node function and atrioventricular conduction in isolated myocardial preparations, such effects have not been seen in studies in intact animals or in man. In formal electrophysiologic studies, predominantly in patients with normal conduction systems, nifedipine has had no tendency to prolong atrioventricular conduction or sinus node recovery time, or to slow sinus rate.

Pharmacokinetics: Absorption: Nifedipine is completely absorbed after oral administration. Plasma drug concentrations rise at a gradual, controlled rate exhibiting zero-order absorption kinetics after ADALAT XL administration and reach a plateau at approximately six hours after the first dose. For subsequent doses, relatively constant plasma concentrations at this plateau are maintained with minimal fluctuations over the 24-hour dosing interval. About a four-fold higher fluctuation index (ratio of peak to trough plasma concentration) was observed with the conventional immediate-release nifedipine capsule at t.i.d. dosing than with once-daily ADALAT XL tablets. At steady state the bioavailability of the ADALAT XL tablet is 86% relative to nifedipine capsules. Administration of the ADALAT XL tablet in the presence of food slightly alters the early rate of drug absorption but does not influence the extent of drug bioavailability. Markedly reduced GI retention time over prolonged periods (i.e., short bowel syndrome), however, may influence the pharmacokinetic profile of the drug which could potentially result in lower plasma concentrations. Pharmacokinetics of ADALAT XL tablets are linear over the dose range of 30 to 180 mg in that plasma drug concentrations are proportional to dose administered. There was no evidence of dose dumping either in the presence or absence of food. The bioavailability of the 20 mg tablet is directly proportional to the 30 mg tablet.

Metabolism: Nifedipine is metabolized by the cytochrome P450 enzyme system, predominantly via CYP3A4, but also by CYP1A2 and CYP2A6 isoenzymes.

Compounds found in grapefruit juice inhibit the cytochrome P450 system, especially CYP3A4. In a grapefruit-juice-nifedipine interaction study in healthy male volunteers, pharmacokinetics of nifedipine showed significant alteration. Following administration of a single dose of nifedipine 10 mg with 250 mL grapefruit juice, the mean value of nifedipine AUC increased by 34% and the t_{max} increased from 0.8 hours to 1.2 hours as compared to water (see Drug Interactions, Drug-Food Interactions).

Excretion: Nifedipine is extensively metabolized to highly water-soluble, inactive metabolites accounting for 60 to 80% of the dose excreted in the urine. The remainder is excreted in the feces in metabolized form, most likely as a result of biliary excretion. The main metabolite (95%) is the hydroxycarbolic acid derivative; the remaining 5% is the corresponding lactone. Only traces (less than 0.1% of the dose) of unchanged nifedipine can be detected in the urine.

Special Populations and Conditions: Hepatic Insufficiency: Since hepatic biotransformation is the predominant route for the disposition of nifedipine, the pharmacokinetics may be altered in patients with chronic liver disease. Pharmacokinetic studies in patients with hepatic cirrhosis showed a clinically significant prolongation of elimination half-life and a decrease in total clearance of nifedipine. The degree of serum protein binding of nifedipine is high (92-98%). Protein binding may be greatly reduced in patients with hepatic impairment (see Warnings and Precautions, Special Populations, Hepatic Insufficiency).

Renal Insufficiency: Patients in hemodialysis or CAPD (continuous ambulatory peritoneal dialysis) have not reported significantly altered pharmacokinetics of nifedipine.

The pharmacokinetics of nifedipine are not significantly influenced by the degree of renal impairment.

ASPIRIN 81 mg: Mechanism of Action: ASPIRIN (acetylsalicylic acid tablets) interferes with the production of prostaglandins in various organs and tissues through acetylation of the enzyme cyclo-oxygenase. Prostaglandins are themselves powerful irritants and produce headaches and pain on injection in man. Prostaglandins also appear to sensitize pain receptors to other noxious substances such as histamine and bradykinin. By preventing the synthesis and release of prostaglandins in inflammation, ASPIRIN may avert the sensitization of pain receptors.

The antipyretic activity of ASPIRIN is due to its ability to interfere with the production of prostaglandin E_1 in the brain. Prostaglandin E_1 is one of the most powerful pyretic agents known.

The inhibition of platelet aggregation by ASPIRIN is due to its ability to interfere with the production of thromboxane A_2 within the platelet. Thromboxane A_2 is largely responsible for the aggregating properties of platelets.

In vitro studies have shown that ASPIRIN enhances the activity of the Nitric oxide (NO)-cGMP system and heme oxygenase-1 (HO-1) by acting on the endothelial NO synthase site.

Pharmacokinetics: Absorption: When ASPIRIN is taken orally, it is rapidly absorbed from the stomach and proximal small intestine. The gastric mucosa is permeable to the nonionized form of acetylsalicylic acid, which passes through the stomach wall by a passive diffusion process.

Optimum absorption of salicylate in the human stomach occurs in the pH range of 2.15 to 4.10. Absorption in the small intestine occurs at a significantly faster rate than in the stomach. After an oral dose of 0.65 g ASPIRIN, the plasma acetylsalicylate concentration in man usually reaches a level between 0.6 and 1.0 mg % in 20 minutes after ingestion and drops to 0.2 mg % within an hour. Within the same period of time, half or more of the ingested dose is hydrolyzed to salicylic acid by esterases in the gastrointestinal mucosa and the liver, the total plasma salicylate concentration reaching a peak between one or two hours after ingestion, averaging between 3 and 7 mg %. Many factors influence the speed of absorption of ASA in a particular individual at a given time; tablet disintegration, solubility, particle size, gastric emptying time, psychological state, physical condition, nature and quantity of gastric contents, etc—all affect absorption.

Distribution: Distribution of salicylate throughout most body fluids and tissues proceeds at a rapid rate after absorption. Aside from the plasma itself, fluids which have been found to contain substantial amounts of salicylate after oral ingestion include spinal, peritoneal and synovial fluids, saliva, and milk. Tissues containing high concentrations of the drug are the kidney, liver, heart, and lungs. Concentrations in the brain are usually low, and are minimal in feces, bile and sweat.

The drug readily crosses the placental barrier. At clinical concentrations, from 50% to 90% of the salicylate is bound to plasma proteins especially albumin, while acetylsalicylic acid itself is bound to only a very limited extent. However, ASA has the capacity of acetylating various proteins, hormones, DNA, platelets, and hemoglobin, which at least partly explains its wide-ranging pharmacological actions.

Metabolism: The liver appears to be the principal site for salicylate metabolism, although other tissues may also be involved. The three chief metabolic products of ASPIRIN or salicylic acid are salicyluric acid, the ether or phenolic glucuronide, and the ester or acyl glucuronide. A small fraction is also converted to gentisic acid and other hydroxybenzoic acids. The half-life of ASPIRIN in the circulation is from 13 to 19 minutes so that the blood level drops quickly after absorption is complete. However, the half-life of the salicylate ranges between 3.5 and 4.5 hours, which means that 50% of the ingested dose leaves the circulation within that time.

Excretion: Excretion of salicylates occurs principally via the kidney, through a combination of glomerular filtration and tubular excretion, in the form of free salicylic acid, salicyluric acid, as well as phenolic and acyl glucuronides. Salicylate can be detected in the urine shortly after its ingestion but the full dose requires up to 48 hours for complete elimination. The rate of excretion of free salicylate is extremely variable, reported recovery rates in human urine ranging from 10% to 85%, depending largely on urinary pH. In general, it can be stated that acid urine facilitates reabsorption of salicylate by renal tubules, while alkaline urine promotes excretion of the drug.

With the administration of 325 mg, elimination of ASPIRIN is linear following a first order kinetics. At higher doses, elimination half-life increases.

Special Populations and Conditions: Absorption and clearance of salicylates are not affected by gender or age.

STORAGE AND STABILITY: Store between 15 and 30°C. Protect from light and humidity.

INFORMATION FOR THE PATIENT: Published in e-CPS, available by subscription at www.e-cps.ca.

DOSAGE FORMS, COMPOSITION AND PACKAGING: ADALAT XL PLUS (nifedipine extended-release tablets and acetylsalicylic acid delayed-release tablets) is available in cartons containing 28 ASPIRIN 81 mg tablets (acetylsalicylic acid delayed-release tablets) packed with 28 (either 20 mg, 30 mg, or 60 mg) ADALAT XL tablets (nifedipine extended-release tablets). The tablets are packaged in clear blisters and are arranged side by side. Due to the clear nature of the blister package and the difference in color of the two products, they are readily distinguishable from each other. Each carton contains two blister packs of 14 ADALAT XL tablets and 14 ASPIRIN 81 mg tablets.

ADALAT XL: 20 mg: Each dusty rose, extended-release tablet, imprinted with "ADALAT 20" on one side contains: nifedipine 20 mg. Nonmedicinal ingredients: cellulose acetate, hydroxypropyl cellulose, hydroxypropyl methylcellulose 2910, magnesium stearate, pharmaceutical shellac, polyethylene glycol 3350, polyethylene oxide, propylene glycol, red ferric oxide, sodium chloride, synthetic black iron oxide and titanium dioxide.

30 mg: Each dusty rose, extended-release tablet, imprinted with "ADALAT 30" on one side contains: nifedipine 30 mg. Nonmedicinal ingredients: cellulose acetate, hydroxypropyl cellulose, hydroxypropyl methylcellulose 2910, magnesium stearate, pharmaceutical shellac, polyethylene glycol 3350, polyethylene oxide, propylene glycol, red ferric oxide, sodium chloride, synthetic black iron oxide and titanium dioxide.

60 mg: Each dusty rose, extended-release tablet, imprinted with "ADALAT 60" on one side contains: nifedipine 60 mg. Nonmedicinal ingredients: cellulose acetate, hydroxypropyl cellulose, hydroxypropyl methylcellulose 2910, magnesium stearate, pharmaceutical shellac, polyethylene glycol 3350, polyethylene oxide, propylene glycol, red ferric oxide, sodium chloride, synthetic black iron oxide and titanium dioxide.

ASPIRIN: Each pale blue, delayed-release, enteric-coated tablet, imprinted with "81" in dark blue ink on one side contains: ASA 81 mg. Nonmedicinal ingredients: carnauba wax, corn starch, croscarmellose sodium, FD&C Blue #1, FD&C Blue #2, hypromellose, lactose monohydrate, methacrylic acid copolymer, microcrystalline cellulose, polysorbate 80, powdered cellulose, pregelatinized starch, propylene glycol, shellac, sodium lauryl sulfate, titanium dioxide and triacetin.

(Shown in Product Identification Section)

Adasept® b.p.5 Acne Gel

benzoyl peroxide

Acne Therapy

Odan

Adasept® Shampoo

alkyl alcohol sulfate—betaine amphoteric—coconut alkanolamide

Acne Therapy

Odan

Adasept® Skin Cleanser

triclosan

Acne Therapy

Odan

SUPPLIED: b.p.5 Acne Gel: Each bottle contains: benzoyl peroxide 5%. Nonmedicinal ingredients: alcohol denat, butylparaben, carbomer, disodium PEG-12 dimethicone sulfosuccinate, ethylparaben, methylparaben, phenoxyethanol, propylparaben, sodium hydroxide and water. Color- and oil-free. Plastic applicator bottles of 50 mL.

Shampoo: Each bottle of dermatological shampoo for oily hair contains: alkyl alcohol sulfate, betaine amphoteric and coconut alkanolamide. Nonmedicinal ingredients: ammonium lauryl sulfate, ammonium laureth sulfate, diazolidinyl urea, FD&C Yellow No. 6, fragrance, lauramide diethanolamine, lauryl glucoside, methylparaben, propylene glycol, propylparaben, sodium chloride, sodium hydroxide and water. Acid pH. Plastic applicator bottles of 250 and 500 mL.

Skin Cleanser: Each bottle contains: triclosan 0.5% in a blend of amphoteric and anionic surfactants. Nonmedicinal ingredients: cocamide diethanolamine, diazolidinyl urea, disodium cocoamphodiacetate, FD&C Blue No. 1, FD&C Yellow No. 6, lactic acid, methylparaben, PEG-120 methyl glucose dioleate, fragrance, propylene glycol, propylparaben, sodium laureth sulfate and water. Acid pH. Plastic bottles of 250 and 500 mL with dispensing pump applicator.

Adcirca™ Ⓟ

tadalafil

cGMP-Specific Phosphodiesterase Type 5 Inhibitor—Treatment of Pulmonary Arterial Hypertension

Lilly

Date of Preparation: May 10, 2010

SUMMARY PRODUCT INFORMATION:

Route of Administration	Dosage Form/Strength	All Nonmedicinal Ingredients
Oral	Tablet/20 mg	Croscarmellose sodium, hydroxypropyl cellulose, hydroxypropyl methylcellulose, iron oxide, lactose monohydrate, magnesium stearate, microcrystalline cellulose, sodium lauryl sulfate, talc, titanium dioxide, and triacetin

INDICATIONS AND CLINICAL USE: ADCIRCA (tadalafil) is indicated for the treatment of idiopathic ("primary") pulmonary arterial hypertension (PAH) or PAH associated with connective tissue disease, congenital heart disease or anorexigen use in patients with WHO functional class II or III who have not responded to conventional therapy.

CONTRAINDICATIONS:

- Administration of ADCIRCA to patients who are using any form of organic nitrate (e.g., oral, sublingual, transdermal, by inhalation), either regularly and/or intermittently, is contraindicated, due to the risk of developing potentially severe hypotension.
- Patients who are hypersensitive to this drug or to any ingredient in the formulation or component of the container (see Dosage Forms, Composition and Packaging).

WARNINGS AND PRECAUTIONS: Cardiovascular: Physicians should discuss with patients the appropriate action in the event that they experience anginal chest pain requiring nitroglycerin following intake of ADCIRCA. In such a patient, who has taken ADCIRCA, where nitrate administration is deemed medically necessary for a life-threatening situation, at least 48 hours should have elapsed after the last dose of ADCIRCA before nitrate administration is considered. In such circumstances, nitrates should still only be administered under close medical supervision with appropriate hemodynamic monitoring. Therefore, patients who experience anginal chest pain after taking ADCIRCA should seek immediate medical attention.

As with other PDE5 inhibitors, tadalafil has mild systemic vasodilatory properties that may result in transient decreases in blood pressure. While this effect should not be of consequence in most patients, prior to prescribing ADCIRCA, physicians should carefully consider whether their patients with underlying cardiovascular disease could be affected adversely by such vasodilatory effects. Patients with severely impaired autonomic control of blood pressure may be particularly sensitive to the actions of vasodilators, including PDE5 inhibitors.

Patients with left ventricular outflow obstruction, (e.g., aortic stenosis and idiopathic hypertrophic subaortic stenosis) can be sensitive to the action of vasodilators, including PDE5 inhibitors.

Pulmonary Veno-Occlusive Disease: Administration to patients with pulmonary veno-occlusive disease is not recommended. Pulmonary vasodilators may significantly worsen the cardiovascular status of patients with pulmonary veno-occlusive disease (PVOD). Since there are no clinical data on administration of ADCIRCA to patients with veno-occlusive disease, administration of ADCIRCA to such patients is not recommended. Should signs of pulmonary edema occur when ADCIRCA is administered, the possibility of associated PVOD should be considered.

The following groups of patients with cardiovascular disease were excluded in the PAH clinical trials:

- Patients with clinically significant aortic and mitral valve disease
- Patients with pericardial constriction
- Patients with restrictive or congestive cardiomyopathy
- Patients with significant left ventricular dysfunction
- Patients with life-threatening arrhythmias
- Patients with symptomatic coronary artery disease
- Patients with hypotension (<90/50 mm Hg), or uncontrolled hypertension

Ophthalmologic: Physicians should advise patients to seek immediate medical attention in the event of a sudden loss of vision in one or both eyes. Such an event may be a sign of non-arteritic anterior ischemic optic neuropathy (NAION), a cause of decreased vision, including permanent loss of vision that has been reported rarely postmarketing in temporal association with the use of all PDE5 inhibitors. It is not possible to determine whether these events are related directly to the use of PDE5 inhibitors or other factors. Physicians should also discuss with patients the increased risk of NAION in individuals who have already experienced NAION in one eye, including whether such individuals could be adversely affected by use of vasodilators such as PDE5 inhibitors (see Adverse Reactions).

- There is evidence that patients at risk for NAION may have abnormal optic discs (e.g. crowded disc) prior to development of the condition. Causal association between the use of ADCIRCA (a PDE5 inhibitor) and NAION in patients with abnormal discs has not been established. If physicians are concerned about the overall risk of NAION, they should consider discussing these concerns with an ophthalmologist.
- Administration of ADCIRCA to patients with previously diagnosed NAION is not recommended. Physicians treating patients with previous NAION should consult an ophthalmologist prior to initiating ADCIRCA.

Patients with known hereditary degenerative retinal disorders, including retinitis pigmentosa, were not included in the clinical trials, and use in these patients is not recommended.

Otologic: Physicians should advise patients to seek immediate medical attention in the event of sudden decrease or loss of hearing. These events, which may be accompanied by tinnitus and dizziness, have been reported in temporal association to the intake of PDE5 inhibitors, including ADCIRCA. It is not possible to determine whether these events are related directly to the use of PDE5 inhibitors or to other factors (see Adverse Reactions, Post-Market Adverse Drug Reactions).

Reproduction/Urogenital: ADCIRCA should be used with caution in patients with anatomical deformation of the penis (such as angulation, cavernosal fibrosis, or Peyronie's disease), or in patients who have conditions which may predispose them to priapism (such as sickle cell anemia, multiple myeloma, or leukemia).

Long-term human studies with subjects 45 years or older have shown that tadalafil therapy may decrease sperm concentration in some patients, but the clinical relevance of this to human fertility is unknown.

Special Populations: Pregnant Women: There are no adequate and well controlled studies of ADCIRCA use in pregnant women. Animal reproduction studies in rats and mice revealed no evidence of fetal harm.

Non-Teratogenic Effects: Animal reproduction studies showed no evidence of teratogenicity, embryotoxicity, or fetotoxicity when tadalafil was given to pregnant rats or mice at unbound tadalafil exposures up to 9 times the maximum recommended human dose (MRHD) of 40 mg/day during organogenesis.

Nursing Women: It is not known whether tadalafil or its metabolites are excreted into human breast milk. Since many drugs are excreted in human milk, caution should be used when ADCIRCA is administered to nursing women.

Pediatrics: The pharmacokinetics, safety or effectiveness of ADCIRCA in pediatric patients has not been established.

Geriatrics (>65 years of age): Of the total number of subjects in the clinical study of tadalafil for pulmonary arterial hypertension, 28 percent were 65 and over, while 8 percent were 75 and over. No overall differences in safety were observed between subjects over 65 years of age compared to younger subjects or over 75 years of age. No dose adjustment is warranted based on age alone. However, a greater sensitivity to medications in some older individuals should be considered.

Use in Patients with Hepatic Impairment:

- **In patients with mild to moderate hepatic cirrhosis (Child-Pugh Class A and B):** See Dosage and Administration.
- **In patients with severe hepatic cirrhosis (Child-Pugh Class C):** Patients with severe hepatic cirrhosis have not been studied and therefore dosing of ADCIRCA is not recommended.

Use in Patients with Renal Impairment:

- **In patients with mild to moderate renal insufficiency:** See Dosage and Administration.
- **In patients with severe renal insufficiency:** The use of ADCIRCA is not recommended due to increased tadalafil exposure (AUC), limited clinical experience, and the lack of ability to influence clearance by dialysis (see Dosage and Administration).

Information to Be Provided to the Patient: Physicians should discuss with patients the contraindication of ADCIRCA with regular and/or intermittent use of organic nitrates.

Physicians should advise patients to seek immediate medical attention in the event of a sudden loss of vision in one or both eyes. Such an event may be a sign of non-arteritic anterior ischemic optic neuropathy (NAION), a cause of decreased vision including permanent loss of vision, that has been reported rarely post-marketing in temporal association with the use of all PDE5 inhibitors when used in the treatment of male erectile dysfunction. It is not possible to determine whether these events are related directly to the use of PDE5 inhibitors or to other factors. Should the vision loss be diagnosed as NAION, continued use of ADCIRCA is not recommended (see Warnings and Precautions, Ophthalmologic).

ADVERSE REACTIONS: Adverse Drug Reaction Overview: ADCIRCA was administered to 402 patients with PAH during clinical trials worldwide. In trials of ADCIRCA, a total of 266 patients were treated for at least 182 days, and 110 patients were treated for at least 360 days. Adverse events (AEs) were reported with greater incidence in subjects taking tadalafil 40 mg; however, the rate of discontinuation due to AEs other than events related to worsening of PAH was similar in the tadalafil treatment group (3.8%) and in placebo (4.9%).

Clinical Trial Adverse Drug Reactions: Because clinical trials are conducted under widely varying conditions, adverse reaction rates observed in the clinical trials of a drug cannot be directly compared to rates in the clinical trials of another drug and may not reflect the rates observed in practice.

Table 1: ADCIRCA

Treatment Emergent Adverse Events Reported by ≥3% of Patients in ADCIRCA 40 mg group and More Frequent than Placebo

Event	Placebo (%) (N=82)	Tadalafil 40 mg (%) (N=79)
Headache	15	42
Myalgia	4	14
Nasopharyngitis	7	13

(cont'd)

Table 1: ADCIRCA *(cont'd)*

Treatment Emergent Adverse Events Reported by ≥3% of Patients in ADCIRCA 40 mg group and More Frequent than Placebo

Event	Placebo (%) (N=82)	Tadalafil 40 mg (%) (N=79)
Flushing	2	13
Respiratory Tract Infection (upper and lower)	6	13
Pain in Extremity	2	11
Diarrhea	10	11
Nausea	6	11
Back Pain	6	10
Dyspepsia	2	10
Nasal Congestion (including sinus congestion)	1	9
Chest Pain	1	6
Dyspnea	4	6
Fatigue	4	6
Vomiting	1	6
Upper Respiratory Tract Infection	4	6
Bronchitis	0	5
Gastroesophageal Reflux Disease	4	5
Edema	1	5
Rash	3	5
Constipation	1	4
Hot Flush	2	4
Insomnia	2	4
Menorrhagia (including increased uterine bleeding)[a]	0	4
Musculoskeletal Stiffness	0	4
Non-Cardiac Chest Pain	0	4
Urinary Tract Infection	0	4
Abdominal Discomfort	0	3
Abdominal Pain	2	3
Abdominal Pain Lower	1	3
Abdominal Pain Upper	1	3
Sinusitis	0	3
Muscle Spasms	2	3
Vision Blurred	1	3

[a] Clinical non-MedDRA term to include reports of abnormal/excessive menstrual bleeding conditions such as menorrhagia, metrorrhagia or menometrorrhagia.

In the placebo controlled study, one subject (receiving tadalafil 10 mg) reported changes in colour vision. In the long-term extension study, no patients reported changes in colour vision.

Less Common Clinical Trial Adverse Drug Reactions: The following section identifies additional, less frequent events reported in the controlled clinical trial of ADCIRCA occurring in at least two subjects in the 40 mg treatment group, and greater than placebo. A causal relationship of these events to ADCIRCA is uncertain:

Blood and Lymphatic Disorders: Increased International Normalized Ratio.
Body as a Whole: chills, herpes zoster, onychomycosis, pain.
Digestive: abdominal discomfort, abdominal pain (lower and upper), gastritis, stomach discomfort.
Metabolic and Nutrition Disorders: hypercholesterolemia.
Musculoskeletal: arthralgia, joint sprain, limb discomfort/pain.
Nervous: hypesthesia, paresthesia.
Psychiatric Disorders: depression.
Ophthalmologic: lacrimation increased, eyelid edema/swelling.
Otologic: vertigo.
Respiratory: lower respiratory tract infection, pharyngolaryngeal pain, rhinitis.
Reproductive System: vaginal hemorrhage.

Post-Market Adverse Drug Reactions: In post-marketing surveillance, adverse events that have been reported very rarely in temporal association in patients taking tadalafil include:

Body as a Whole: hypersensitivity reactions including rash, urticaria, facial edema, Stevens-Johnson syndrome and exfoliative dermatitis.

Cardiovascular and Cerebrovascular: Serious cardiovascular events, including myocardial infarction, sudden cardiac death, unstable angina pectoris, ventricular arrhythmia, stroke, transient ischemic attacks, chest pain, palpitations and tachycardia.

Hypotension (more commonly reported when tadalafil is given to patients who are already taking antihypertensive agents), hypertension and syncope.

Skin and Subcutaneous Tissues: hyperhidrosis (sweating).
Gastrointestinal: abdominal pain and gastroesophageal reflux.
Nervous System: migraine, transient global amnesia.
Respiratory System: epistaxis (nose bleed).
Special Senses: blurred vision, nonarteritic anterior ischemic optic neuropathy, retinal vein occlusion, visual field defect.

Otologic: Cases of sudden decrease or loss of hearing have been reported postmarketing in temporal association with the use of PDE5 inhibitors, including tadalafil. In many cases, medical follow-up information was limited.
Urogenital: priapism, prolonged erection.

DRUG INTERACTIONS: Potential for Pharmacodynamic Interactions with ADCIRCA: Nitrates: Administration of ADCIRCA to patients who are using any form of organic nitrate, is contraindicated. In clinical pharmacology studies, ADCIRCA was shown to potentiate the hypotensive effect of nitrates. In a patient who has taken ADCIRCA, where nitrate administration is deemed medically necessary in a life-threatening situation, at least 48 hours should elapse after the last dose of ADCIRCA before nitrate administration is considered. In such circumstances, nitrates should still only be administered under close medical supervision with appropriate hemodynamic monitoring (see Contraindications and Action and Clinical Pharmacology).

Alpha-Blockers: Caution is advised when PDE5 inhibitors are coadministered with alpha-blockers. PDE5 inhibitors, including ADCIRCA, and alpha-adrenergic blocking agents are both vasodilators with blood-pressure-lowering effects. When vasodilators are used in combination, an additive effect on blood pressure may be anticipated. Clinical pharmacology studies have been conducted with coadministration of tadalafil with doxazosin, alfuzosin or tamsulosin (see Action and Clinical Pharmacology).

Combination with Other PDE5 Inhibitors: Tadalafil is also marketed as CIALIS for treatment of male erectile dysfunction. The safety and efficacy of combinations of ADCIRCA with CIALIS or other PDE5 inhibitors have not been studied. Therefore, the use of such combinations is not recommended.

Antihypertensives: PDE5 inhibitors, including ADCIRCA, are mild systemic vasodilators. Clinical pharmacology studies were conducted to assess the effect of tadalafil on the potentiation of the blood-pressure-lowering effects of selected antihypertensive medications (amlodipine, angiotensin II receptor blockers, bendrofluazide, enalapril, and metoprolol). Small reductions in blood pressure occurred following coadministration of tadalafil with these agents compared with placebo (see Action and Clinical Pharmacology).

Physicians should discuss with patients the potential for ADCIRCA to augment the blood pressure lowering effect of alpha-blockers and antihypertensive medications (see Action and Clinical Pharmacology).

In some patients, concomitant use of PDE5 inhibitors and alpha-blockers can lower blood pressure significantly, which may lead to symptomatic hypotension (e.g., fainting). Consideration should be given to the following:

- Patients should be stable on alpha-blocker therapy prior to initiating treatment with ADCIRCA. Patients who demonstrate hemodynamic instability on alpha-blocker therapy alone are at increased risk of symptomatic hypotension with concomitant use of PDE5 inhibitors.
- In those patients already taking an optimized dose of PDE5 inhibitor, alpha-blocker therapy should be initiated at the lowest dose. Stepwise increase in alpha-blocker dose may be associated with further lowering of blood pressure when taking a PDE5 inhibitor.
- Safety of combined use of PDE5 inhibitors and alpha-blockers may be affected by other variables, including intravascular volume depletion and other antihypertensive drugs.

Alcohol: PDE5 inhibitors, including tadalafil, are vasodilators and may augment the blood-pressure-lowering effect of alcohol.

Tadalafil did not affect alcohol concentrations, and alcohol did not affect tadalafil concentrations. At high doses of alcohol (0.7 g/kg, mean maximum blood concentration 0.08%), the addition of tadalafil 10 or 20 mg did not induce statistically significant mean blood pressure decreases. In some subjects, postural dizziness and orthostatic hypotension were observed. When ADCIRCA was administered with lower doses of alcohol (0.6 g/kg), hypotension was not observed and dizziness occurred with similar frequency to alcohol alone.

Potential for Other Drugs to Affect ADCIRCA: Cytochrome P450 Inducers: Studies have shown that drugs that induce CYP3A4 can decrease tadalafil exposure. For patients chronically taking potent inducers of CYP3A4, such as rifampicin, the use of tadalafil is not recommended (see Dosage and Administration).

Rifampin (600 mg daily), a CYP3A4 inducer, reduced tadalafil 10 mg single-dose exposure (AUC) by 88% and C_{max} by 46%, relative to the values for tadalafil 10 mg alone.

Bosentan (125 mg twice daily), a substrate of CYP2C9 and CYP3A4 and a moderate inducer of CYP3A4, CYP2C9 and possibly CYP2C19, reduced tadalafil (40 mg once per day) systemic exposure by 42% and C_{max} by 27% following multiple-dose co-administration.

Although specific interactions have not been studied, other CYP3A4 inducers, such as carbamazepine, phenytoin, and phenobarbital, would likely decrease tadalafil exposure.

Cytochrome P450 Inhibitors: Tadalafil is metabolized predominantly by CYP3A4. In patients taking potent inhibitors of CYP3A4 such as ketoconazole, itraconazole or ritonavir, the use of ADCIRCA is not recommended (see Dosage and Administration). Studies have shown that drugs that inhibit CYP3A4 can increase tadalafil exposure.

Ketoconazole (400 mg daily), a selective and potent inhibitor of CYP3A4, increased tadalafil 20 mg single-dose exposure (AUC) by 312% and C_{max} by 22%, relative to the values for tadalafil 20 mg alone. Ketoconazole (200 mg daily) increased tadalafil 10 mg single-dose exposure (AUC) by 107% and C_{max} by 15%, relative to the values for tadalafil 10 mg alone (see Dosage and Administration).

Although specific interactions have not been studied, other CYP3A4 inhibitors, such as erythromycin and itraconazole would likely increase tadalafil exposure.

HIV Protease inhibitor: Ritonavir (500 mg or 600 mg twice daily at steady state), an inhibitor of CYP3A4, CYP2C9, CYP2C19, and CYP2D6, increased tadalafil 20 mg single-dose exposure (AUC) by 32% with a 30% reduction in C^{max}, relative to the values for tadalafil 20 mg alone. Ritonavir (200 mg twice daily), increased tadalafil 20 mg single-dose exposure (AUC) by 124% with no change in C_{max}, relative to the values for tadalafil 20 mg alone. Although specific interactions have not been studied, other HIV protease inhibitors would likely increase tadalafil exposure (see Dosage and Administration).

Antacids: Simultaneous administration of an antacid (magnesium hydroxide/aluminum hydroxide) and tadalafil (10 mg) reduced the apparent rate of absorption of tadalafil without altering exposure (AUC) to tadalafil.

H2 Antagonists (e.g. Nizatidine): An increase in gastric pH resulting from administration of nizatidine had no significant effect on tadalafil (10 mg) pharmacokinetics.

Potential for ADCIRCA to Affect Other Drugs: Cytochrome P450 Substrates: Tadalafil is not expected to cause clinically significant inhibition or induction of the clearance of drugs metabolized by cytochrome P450 (CYP) isoforms.

CYP1A2 (e.g. Theophylline): Tadalafil (10 mg once per day) had no significant effect on the pharmacokinetics of theophylline. When tadalafil was administered to subjects taking theophylline, a small augmentation (3 beats per minute) of the increase in heart rate associated with theophylline was observed.

CYP2C9 (e.g. Warfarin): Tadalafil (10 mg and 20 mg once per day) had no significant effect on exposure (AUC) to S-warfarin or R-warfarin, nor did tadalafil affect changes in prothrombin time induced by warfarin.

CYP3A4 (e.g. Midazolam, Lovastatin or Bosentan): Tadalafil (10 mg and 20 mg once per day) had no significant effect on exposure (AUC) to midazolam or lovastatin. Tadalafil (40 mg once per day) had no clinically significant effect on exposure (AUC and C_{max}) of bosentan, a substrate of CYP2C9 and CYP3A4, or its metabolites.

Aspirin: Tadalafil (10 mg and 20 mg once per day) did not potentiate the increase in bleeding time caused by aspirin.

P-glycoprotein (e.g. Digoxin): Coadministration of tadalafil (40 mg once per day) for 10 days did not have a significant effect on the steady-state pharmacokinetics of digoxin (0.25 mg/day) in healthy subjects.

Combined Oral Contraceptives: At steady-state, tadalafil (40 mg once per day) increased ethinylestradiol exposure (AUC) by 26% and C_{max} by 70% relative to oral contraceptive administered with placebo. There was no statistically significant effect of tadalafil on levonorgestrel.

Drug-Food Interactions: Grapefruit juice being a weak inhibitor of CYP3A4 gut wall metabolism, may give rise to modest increases in plasma levels of tadalafil.

Drug-Herb Interactions: Interaction with herbal products has not been established.

Drug-Laboratory Test Interactions: Interaction with laboratory tests has not been established.

DOSAGE AND ADMINISTRATION: Dosing Considerations:

- ADCIRCA may be taken without regard to food.
- No dose adjustment is required in patients >65 years of age.

Recommended Dose and Dosage Adjustment: The recommended dose of ADCIRCA is 40 mg taken once daily. Dividing the dose (40 mg) over the course of the day is not recommended.

Patients with Renal Insufficiency:

- **Mild (creatinine clearance 51 to 80 mL/min) and moderate (creatinine clearance 30 to 50 mL/min):** A starting dose of 20 mg once per day is recommended, the dose may be increased to 40 mg once per day based on individual efficacy and tolerability.
- **Severe (creatinine clearance <30 mL/min):** The use of ADCIRCA is not recommended (see Warnings and Precautions).

Patients with Hepatic Impairment:

- **Mild or moderate (Child Pugh Class A or B):** Due to limited clinical experience in patients with mild to moderate hepatic cirrhosis, a starting dose of 20 mg once per day is recommended. If ADCIRCA is prescribed, a careful individual benefit/risk evaluation should be undertaken by the prescribing physician.

- **Severe (Child Pugh Class C):** Patients with severe hepatic cirrhosis have not been studied and therefore dosing of ADCIRCA is not recommended (see Warnings and Precautions).

OVERDOSAGE:
Single doses of up to 500 mg tadalafil have been given to healthy subjects, and multiple doses of 100 mg/day for 21 days have been given to patients with erectile dysfunction. Adverse events (e.g., headache, dyspepsia) were similar to those seen at lower doses. Doses greater than 40 mg have not been studied in patients with pulmonary arterial hypertension.

In cases of overdose, standard supportive measures should be adopted as required. Hemodialysis contributes negligibly to elimination, as tadalafil is highly bound to plasma proteins.

> For management of a suspected drug overdose, contact your regional Poison Control Centre. See the *CPS* Directory section for a list of Poison Control Centres.

ACTION AND CLINICAL PHARMACOLOGY: ADCIRCA (tadalafil), an oral treatment for pulmonary arterial hypertension, is a potent, selective, reversible inhibitor of cyclic guanosine monophosphate (cGMP)-specific phosphodiesterase type 5 (PDE5).
Mechanism of Action: Tadalafil is a potent and selective inhibitor of phosphodiesterase type 5 (PDE5), the enzyme responsible for the degradation of cyclic guanosine monophosphate (cGMP). Pulmonary arterial hypertension is associated with impaired release of nitric oxide by the vascular endothelium and consequent reduction of cGMP concentrations within in the pulmonary vascular smooth muscle. PDE5 is the predominant phosphodiesterase in the pulmonary vasculature. Inhibition of PDE5 by tadalafil increases the concentrations of cGMP resulting in relaxation of the pulmonary vascular smooth muscle cell and vasodilation of the pulmonary vascular bed.
Pharmacodynamics: Effects on Blood Pressure and Heart Rate: Tadalafil 20 mg administered to healthy male subjects produced no significant difference compared to placebo in supine systolic and diastolic blood pressure (difference in the mean maximal decrease of 1.6/0.8 mm Hg, respectively) and in standing systolic and diastolic blood pressure (difference in the mean maximal decrease of 0.2/4.6 mm Hg, respectively). In addition, there was no significant effect on heart rate.
Nitrates: In clinical pharmacology studies, tadalafil (5 to 20 mg) was shown to potentiate the hypotensive effect of nitrates. Therefore, the use of ADCIRCA in patients taking any form of nitrates is contraindicated (see Contraindications).
Antihypertensives: When tadalafil and certain oral antihypertensive medications (amlodipine, enalapril, metoprolol, bendrofluazide, angiotensin II receptor blockers) were assessed in drug interaction studies, tadalafil 10 or 20 mg doses did not result in clinically significant augmentation of the antihypertensive effects of those medications (see Drug Interactions). Analysis of Phase 3 clinical trial data also showed no difference in adverse events in patients taking tadalafil with or without antihypertensive medications.
Alpha-Blockers: The potential hemodynamic interactions of tadalafil with a non-selective alpha-blocker (doxazosin 4, 8 mg), a selective [1A] alpha-blocker (tamsulosin 0.4 mg) and a selective [1] alpha-blocker (alfuzosin 10 mg) were investigated in randomized, double-blind, crossover design studies. Blood pressure (BP) and heart rate were recorded before dosing and for 24 hours after dosing.

Tadalafil 20 mg augmented the hypotensive effect of 8 mg doxazosin by producing a mean maximal decrease in standing systolic BP (SBP) that was significantly greater than placebo (a mean difference of 9.8 mm Hg). Analysis of BP outliers showed that the number of subjects with a standing SBP of less than 85 mm Hg was greater after doxazosin plus tadalafil (28%) versus doxazosin plus placebo (6%). A further clinical pharmacology study was performed in order to investigate the lower dose of 4 mg doxazosin. The changes produced in that study were comparable to those observed in the earlier study. An additional study carried out with doxazosin (up to 4 mg daily) added to tadalafil (5 mg daily) also showed an augmentation of response, and symptoms associated with a decrease in blood pressure.

In subjects on tamsulosin, tadalafil 10 and 20 mg produced mean maximal decreases in standing SBP that were similar to placebo (mean difference of 1.7 and 2.3 mm Hg, respectively). No subject taking tamsulosin had a decrease in standing SBP less than 85 mm Hg. An additional study carried out with tamsulosin (0.4 mg) added to tadalafil (5 mg daily) also showed similar results with only two of the 37 subjects showing significantly low systolic and diastolic blood pressure following the administration of tadalafil and tamsulosin. In subjects receiving alfuzosin, tadalafil 20 mg also produced a maximal decrease in SBP that was not significantly different from that after placebo (mean difference of 4.35 mm Hg). One subject taking alfuzosin had an asymptomatic SBP of less than 85 mm Hg.

No vasodilatory adverse events were observed when tadalafil was administered with tamsulosin or alfuzosin. Dizziness, vertigo and syncope were reported following administration of tadalafil with doxazosin.
Effects on Other Cardiac/Hemodynamic Parameters: In patients with stable coronary artery disease (CAD) and demonstrable ischemia with exercise, tadalafil 10 mg was non-inferior to placebo with respect to effect on time to ischemia. In a separate double-blind, placebo-controlled study to evaluate the effects of ADCIRCA on myocardial perfusion in patients with CAD, tadalafil 20 mg had no significant effect on myocardial blood flow, both at rest and during pharmacological stress with dobutamine.

Tadalafil at doses up to 500 mg did not significantly change cardiac output and did not significantly impact patients' hemodynamic response to exercise.

No tadalafil-related changes in electrocardiographic measures, including QTc interval, were observed following administration of tadalafil single doses up to 500 mg and multiple doses of up to 100 mg once-daily for 21 days, to healthy subjects or patients with ED. ECGs were obtained pre- and post-dose, spanning the period from the expected T_{max} of tadalafil (2 hours) to the expected T_{max} of the primary metabolite (methylcatechol glucuronide, 24 hours).

The effect of a single 100 mg dose of tadalafil (2.5 times the recommended dose) on the QT interval was evaluated at the time of peak tadalafil concentration in a randomized, double-blinded, placebo, and active (intravenous ibutilide)-controlled crossover study in 90 healthy males aged 18 to 53 years. The mean change in QTc (Fridericia QT correction) for tadalafil, relative to placebo, was 3.5 milliseconds (two-sided 90% CI=1.9, 5.1). The mean change in QTc (individual QT correction) for tadalafil, relative to placebo, was 2.8 milliseconds (two-sided 90% CI=1.2, 4.4). In this study, the mean increase in heart rate associated with a 100 mg dose of tadalafil compared to placebo was 3.1 beats per minute.

In clinical pharmacology studies, tadalafil 10 and 20 mg had no clinically significant effect on acetylsalicylic acid-induced prolongation of bleeding time or warfarin-induced changes in prothrombin time (see Drug Interactions).
Effects on Vision: In a study to assess the effects of a single dose of tadalafil 40 mg on vision, no impairment of colour discrimination (blue/green) was detected using the Farnsworth-Munsell 100-hue test. This finding is consistent with the low affinity of tadalafil for PDE6 compared to PDE5 (see Action and Clinical Pharmacology, Mechanism of Action). In addition, no effects were observed on visual acuity, electroretinograms, intraocular pressure, or pupillometry. Across all clinical studies with tadalafil 10 or 20 mg, reports of changes in colour vision were rare (<0.1% of patients).
Effects on Sperm Characteristics: Three studies were conducted in men, ages 45-70 years, to assess the potential effect on spermatogenesis of tadalafil 10 mg (one 6-month study) and 20 mg (one 6-month and one 9-month study) administered once daily. In all 3 studies, there were no adverse effects on sperm morphology or sperm motility. There were also no significant changes in mean concentrations of the reproductive hormones, testosterone, luteinizing hormone or follicle-stimulating hormone with either 10 or 20 mg of tadalafil compared to placebo. No decrease in sperm concentration was observed in the study of tadalafil 20 mg taken for 6 months. In the study of tadalafil 10 mg for 6 months and the study of tadalafil 20 mg for 9 months, results showed a statistically significant decrease in mean sperm concentration relative to placebo. The clinical relevance of this to human fertility is unknown. In the 9 month study (n=125 [tadalafil 20 mg], n=128 [placebo]), decreases in sperm concentration were in a few patients (but not all) associated with higher ejaculatory frequency, which may have resulted from tadalafil-related improvement in sexual function.
Exposure-Response Relationship: An analysis of tadalafil exposure and 6-minute walk distance in subjects with PAH in the Phase 3 Study, generated a model-predicted increase in 6-minute walk distance from baseline of 35.6 meters (30.5, 39.6 meters) and 38.09 meters (33.52, 43.20 meters) at 16 weeks of 20 mg and 40 mg daily administration, assuming the median (10th and 90th percentiles) steady-state tadalafil exposures.
Pharmacokinetics: Over a dose range of 2.5 to 20 mg, tadalafil exposure (AUC) increases proportionally with dose in healthy subjects. Between 20 to 40 mg, an approximate 1.5-fold greater AUC is observed indicating a less than proportional increase in exposure over the entire dose range of 2.5 to 40 mg. During tadalafil 20 and 40 mg once-daily dosing, steady-state plasma concentrations are attained within 5 days, and exposure is approximately 1.3-fold than that after a single dose.
Absorption: Tadalafil is rapidly absorbed after oral administration and the maximum observed plasma concentration is achieved at a median time of 4 hours after dosing. The absolute bioavailability of tadalafil has not been determined.

The rate and extent of absorption of tadalafil are not influenced by food, thus ADCIRCA may be taken with or without food.
Distribution: The mean apparent volume of distribution is approximately 77 L at steady-state, indicating that tadalafil is distributed into tissues. At therapeutic concentrations, 94% of tadalafil in plasma is bound to proteins. Protein binding is not affected by impaired renal function.
Metabolism: Tadalafil is predominantly metabolized by the cytochrome P450 (CYP) 3A4 isoform. The major circulating metabolite is the methylcatechol glucuronide. This metabolite is at least 13 000-fold less potent than tadalafil for PDE5. Consequently, it is not expected to be clinically active at observed metabolite concentrations.
Excretion: The mean oral clearance for tadalafil is 3.4 L/hr and the mean terminal half-life is 15 hours in healthy subjects. Tadalafil is excreted predominantly as inactive metabolites, mainly in the feces (approximately 61% of the dose) and to a lesser extent in the urine (approximately 36% of the dose).
Population Pharmacokinetics: In patients with pulmonary hypertension not receiving concomitant bosentan, the average tadalafil exposure at steady-state following 40 mg was 26% higher when compared to those of healthy volunteers. There were no clinically relevant differences in C_{max} compared to healthy volunteers. The results suggest a lower clearance of tadalafil in patients with pulmonary hypertension compared to healthy volunteers.
Special Populations and Conditions: Geriatrics: The mean AUC value (4881 µg·h/L for 10 mg dose) in male subjects aged 65 to 78 years was approximately 25% higher than AUC (3896 µg·h/L) for subjects aged 19 to 45 years, while age had negligible effect on C_{max} values. This effect of age is not clinically significant and does not require a dose adjustment (see Warnings and Precautions, Special Populations, Geriatrics (>65 years of age)).
Pediatrics: Tadalafil has not been evaluated in individuals less than 18 years old.
Hepatic Insufficiency: In a clinical pharmacology study using tadalafil 10 mg, tadalafil exposure (AUC) in subjects with mild and moderate hepatic impairment (Child-Pugh Class A and B) was comparable to exposure in healthy subjects (see Warnings and Precautions, Special Populations, Use in Patients with Hepatic Impairment and Dosage and Administration).
Renal Insufficiency: In clinical pharmacology studies using single-dose ADCIRCA 5 to 20 mg, tadalafil exposure (AUC) approximately doubled in subjects with mild (creatinine clearance 51 to 80 mL/min) or moderate (creatinine clearance 31 to 50 mL/min) renal insufficiency, and in subjects with end-stage renal disease on dialysis. In dialysis patients, C^{max} was 41% higher than that observed in healthy subjects. Hemodialysis contributed negligibly to tadalafil elimination. (See Warnings and Precautions, Special Populations, Use in Patients with Renal Impairment and Dosage and Administration.)
Patients with Diabetes: Tadalafil exposure (AUC 3454 µg·h/L for a 10 mg dose) in patients with diabetes was 19% lower, and the mean maximum plasma concentration (C_{max} of 184 µg/L) was 5% lower than that observed in healthy subjects. This difference in exposure does not require a dose adjustment.
Race: Pharmacokinetic studies have included subjects and patients from different ethnic groups, and no differences in the typical exposure to tadalafil have been identified. No dose adjustment is warranted.
Gender: In healthy female and male subjects following single and multiple-doses of tadalafil, no clinically relevant differences in exposure (AUC and C_{max}) were observed. No dose adjustment is warranted.

STORAGE AND STABILITY: Store at controlled room temperature, 15-30°C.

INFORMATION FOR THE PATIENT: Published in e-CPS, available by subscription at www.e-cps.ca.

DOSAGE FORMS, COMPOSITION AND PACKAGING: Each orange, film-coated, almond-shaped tablet, debossed with "4467" contains: tadalafil 20 mg. Nonmedicinal ingredients: croscarmellose sodium, hydroxypropyl cellulose, hydroxypropyl methylcellulose, iron oxide, lactose monohydrate, magnesium stearate, microcrystalline cellulose, sodium lauryl sulfate, talc, titanium dioxide and triacetin. Blisters of 56.

(Shown in Product Identification Section)

Adderall XR® Ⓒ
mixed salts amphetamine
CNS Stimulant

Shire

Date of Revision: September 30, 2009

PHARMACOLOGY: Amphetamines are non-catecholamine sympathomimetic amines with CNS stimulant activity. The mode of therapeutic action in Attention Deficit Hyperactivity Disorder (ADHD) is not known. Amphetamines are thought to block the reuptake of norepinephrine and dopamine into the presynaptic neuron and increase the release of these monoamines into the extraneuronal space.
Pharmacokinetics: Pharmacokinetic studies of ADDERALL XR (mixed salts amphetamine extended-release capsules) have been conducted in healthy adult and pediatric (aged 6-12 years) subjects, and adolescent (aged 13-17 years) and pediatric patients with ADHD. ADDERALL XR capsules contain dextroamphetamine (d-amphetamine) and levoamphetamine (l-amphetamine) salts in the ratio of 3:1.

ADDERALL XR demonstrates linear pharmacokinetics over the dose range of 20 to 60 mg in adults and adolescents aged 13 to 17 years weighing greater than 75 kg, over the dose range of 10 to 40 mg in adolescents weighing less than or equal to 75 kg and 5 to 30 mg in children aged 6 to 12 years. There was no unexpected accumulation at steady state.

Comparison of the pharmacokinetics of d- and l-amphetamine after oral administration of ADDERALL XR in pediatric (aged 6-12 years) and adolescent (aged 13-17 years) ADHD patients and healthy adult volunteers indicates that body weight is the primary determinant of apparent differences in the pharmacokinetics of d- and l-amphetamine across the age range. Systemic exposure measured by area under the curve to infinity (AUC_{∞}) and maximum plasma concentration (C_{max}) decreased with increases in body weight, while oral volume of distribution (V_z/F), oral clearance (CL/F), and elimination half-life ($t_{1/2}$) increased with increases in body weight.
Pharmacokinetic Results in Healthy Adult and Pediatric Subjects: Following oral administration of a single dose of ADDERALL XR in healthy adult subjects, peak plasma concentrations (C_{max}) of 28.1 ng/mL and 8.7 ng/mL occurred in about 7 hours for d-amphetamine and 8 hours for l-amphetamine, respectively. The $AUC_{0\text{-}inf}$ for d-amphetamine and l-amphetamine were 567 ng·hr/mL and 203 ng·hr/mL, respectively.

The mean elimination half-life is 1 hour shorter for d-amphetamine and 2 hours shorter for l-amphetamine in children aged 6 to 12 years compared to that in adults ($t_{1/2}$ is 10 hours for d-amphetamine and 13 hours for l-amphetamine in adults, and 9 hours and 11 hours, respectively, for children). Children had higher systemic exposure to amphetamine (C_{max} and AUC) than adults for a given dose of ADDERALL XR, which was attributed to the higher dose administered to children on a mg/kg body weight basis compared to adults. Upon dose normalization on a mg/kg basis, children showed 30% less systemic exposure compared to adults.
Pharmacokinetic Results in Children and Adolescents with ADHD: In a 20 mg single dose study in 51 children (aged 6-12 years) with ADHD, the mean T_{max} for d-amphetamine was 6.8 hours and the mean C_{max} was 48.8 ng/mL. The corresponding mean T_{max} and C_{max} values for l-amphetamine were 6.9 hours and 14.8 ng/mL, respectively. The mean elimination half-life for d-amphetamine and l-amphetamine was 9.5 and 10.9 hours, respectively. Following dosing of children with ADHD to steady state with ADDERALL XR 10, 20 and 30 mg, the mean d-amphetamine C_{max} (ng/mL) in plasma for ADDERALL XR was 28.8 (10 mg), 54.6 (20 mg) and 89.0 (30 mg). For l-amphetamine, the mean C_{max} values for the three ADDERALL XR doses were 8.8, 17.2 and 28.1 ng/mL, respectively.

In adolescents aged 13-17 years and weighing less than or equal to 75 kg, the mean elimination half-life for d-amphetamine is 11 hours, and 13-14 hours for l-amphetamine.
Metabolism: Amphetamine is reported to be oxidized at the 4 position of the benzene ring to form 4-hydroxyamphetamine, or on the side chain α or β carbons to form alpha-hydroxy-amphetamine or norephedrine, respectively. Norephedrine and 4-hydroxy-amphetamine are both active and each is subsequently oxidized to form 4-hydroxy-norephedrine. Alpha-hydroxy-amphetamine undergoes deamination to form phenylacetone, which ultimately forms benzoic acid and its glucuronide and the glycine conjugate hippuric acid. Although the enzymes involved in amphetamine metabolism have not been clearly defined, CYP2D6 is known to be involved with formation of 4-hydroxy-amphetamine. Since CYP2D6 is genetically polymorphic, population variations in amphetamine metabolism are a possibility.

Amphetamine is known to inhibit monoamine oxidase, whereas the ability of amphetamine and its metabolites to inhibit various P450 isozymes and other enzymes has not been adequately elucidated. In vitro experiments with human microsomes indicate minor inhibition of CYP2D6 by amphetamine and minor inhibition of CYP1A2, 2D6, and 3A4 by one or more metabolites. However, due to the probability of auto-inhibition and the lack of information on the concentration of these metabolites relative to in vivo concentrations, no predications regarding the potential for amphetamine or its metabolites to inhibit the metabolism of other drugs by CYP isozymes in vivo can be made.
Excretion: With normal urine pHs approximately half of an administered dose of amphetamine is recoverable in urine as derivatives of alpha-hydroxy-amphetamine and approximately another 30-40% of the dose is recoverable in urine as amphetamine itself. Since amphetamine has a pKa of 9.9, urinary recovery of amphetamine is highly dependent on pH and urine flow rates. Alkaline urine pHs result in less ionization and reduced renal elimination, and acidic pHs and high flow rates result in increased renal elimination with clearances greater than glomerular filtration rates, indicating the involvement of active secretion. Urinary recovery of amphetamine has been reported to range from 1% to 75%, depending on urinary pH, with the remaining fraction of the dose hepatically metabolized. Consequently, both hepatic and renal dysfunction have the potential to inhibit the elimination

of amphetamine and result in prolonged exposures. In addition, drugs that effect urinary pH are known to alter the elimination of amphetamine, and any decrease in amphetamine's metabolism that might occur due to drug interactions or genetic polymorphisms is more likely to be clinically significant when renal elimination is decreased, (see Precautions, Drug Interactions).

Food Effect Study in Healthy Adult Subjects: A single dose study compared the relative bioavailability of d-amphetamine and l-amphetamine following administration of a single 30 mg dose of ADDERALL XR fasted, fed (high fat meal) and sprinkled on food (otherwise fasted) in 21 healthy adult subjects. Food does not affect the extent of absorption of ADDERALL XR capsules, but prolongs T_{max} by 2.5 hours (from 5.2 hrs at fasted state to 7.7 hrs after a high-fat meal). Opening the capsule and sprinkling the contents on applesauce results in comparable absorption to the intact capsule taken in the fasted states.

Clinical Trials: Children: A double-blind, randomized, placebo-controlled, parallel-group study of 584 children aged 6 to 12 years who met DSM-IV criteria for ADHD (either combined type or hyperactive-impulsive type) was conducted in a naturalistic setting. Patients were randomized to fixed dose treatment groups receiving final doses of 10, 20, or 30 mg/day of ADDERALL XR or placebo. ADDERALL XR or placebo was taken once daily in the morning for three weeks. Significant improvements in patient behavior, based upon teacher and parent ratings of attention and hyperactivity, were observed for all ADDERALL XR doses compared to patients who received placebo, for all three weeks, including the first week of treatment, when all ADDERALL XR subjects were receiving a titration dose of 10 mg/day. Patients who received ADDERALL XR showed behavioral improvements within the first week of treatment (p<0.001) and in both morning (p<0.001) and afternoon (p<0.001) compared to patients on placebo.

A double-blind, randomized, placebo- and active-controlled crossover study of 51 children aged 6 to 12 years with ADHD was conducted in a classroom laboratory setting. In comparison to placebo, ADDERALL XR 10, 20, and 30 mg/day showed rapid improvement and continued significant efficacy (p<0.05) up to 12 hours post-dose for all cognitive and behavioral measures.

In these two clinical trials conducted in different settings, ADDERALL XR taken once in the morning demonstrated efficacy in the treatment of ADHD (either combined type or hyperactive-impulsive type) for at least 12 hours.

Adolescents: A double-blind, randomized, multi-center, parallel-group, placebo-controlled study was conducted in adolescents aged 13-17 years (N=327) who met DSM-IV criteria for ADHD. The primary cohort of patients (n=287, weighing ≤75 kg) was randomized to fixed dose treatment groups and received four weeks of treatment. Patients were randomized to receive final doses of 10 mg, 20 mg, 30 mg, and 40 mg ADDERALL XR or placebo once daily in the morning; patients randomized to doses greater than 10 mg were titrated to their final doses by 10 mg each week. The secondary cohort consisted of 40 subjects weighing >75 kg who were randomized to fixed dose treatment groups receiving final doses of 50 mg and 60 mg ADDERALL XR or placebo once daily in the morning for 4 weeks. The primary efficacy variable was the ADHD-RS-IV total scores for the primary cohort. Improvements in the primary cohort were statistically significantly greater in all four primary cohort active treatment groups (ADDERALL XR 10 mg, 20 mg, 30 mg, and 40 mg) compared with the placebo group. ADDERALL XR at doses of 10-40 mg is effective in the treatment of ADHD in adolescents weighing ≤75 kg. There was not adequate evidence that doses greater than 20 mg/day conferred additional benefit.

Adults: A double-blind, randomized, placebo-controlled, parallel-group study of 255 adults who met DSM-IV criteria for ADHD was conducted. Patients were randomized to fixed dose treatment groups receiving final doses of 20, 40 or 60 mg/day of ADDERALL XR or placebo. ADDERALL XR or placebo was taken once daily in the morning for four weeks. Significant improvements in patient symptoms of inattention and impulsivity/hyperactivity, based upon the 18-item total ADHD symptom score, were observed at endpoint for all ADDERALL XR doses compared to patients who received placebo for all four weeks (p<0.001). There was not adequate evidence that doses greater than 20 mg/day conferred additional benefit.

A long-term, open-label extension of the above-mentioned clinical study was conducted in 223 adult patients. At 12 months, all patients showed continuing symptomatic improvement as measured by the 18-item total ADHD symptom score.

INDICATIONS: ADDERALL XR (mixed salts amphetamine extended-release capsules) is indicated for the treatment of Attention Deficit Hyperactivity Disorder (ADHD).

A diagnosis of ADHD (DSM-IV) implies the presence of hyperactive-impulsive or inattentive symptoms that caused impairment and that were present before age 7 years. The symptoms must be persistent, must be more severe than is typically observed in individuals at a comparable level of development, must cause clinically significant impairment e.g., in social, academic, or occupational functioning), and must be present in two or more settings (e.g., school or work, and at home). The symptoms must not be better accounted for by another mental disorder. For the Inattentive Type, at least six of the following symptoms must have persisted for at least six months: lack of attention to details/careless mistakes, lack of sustained attention, poor listener, failure to follow through on tasks, poor organization, avoids tasks requiring sustained mental effort, loses things, easily distracted, forgetful. For the Hyperactive-Impulsive Type, at least six of the following symptoms must have persisted for at least six months: fidgeting/squirming, leaving seat, inappropriate running/climbing, difficulty with quiet activities, "on the go", excessive talking, blurting answers, can't wait turn, intrusive. For a Combined Type diagnosis, both inattentive and hyperactive-impulsive criteria must be met.

Special Diagnostic Considerations: The specific etiology of ADHD is unknown, and there is no single diagnostic test. Adequate diagnosis requires the use not only of medical but of special psychological, educational, and social resources. Learning may or may not be impaired. The diagnosis must be based upon a complete history and evaluation of the patient and not solely on the presence of the required number of DSM-IV characteristics.

Need for Comprehensive Treatment Program: ADDERALL XR is indicated as an integral part of a total treatment program for ADHD that may include other measures (psychological, educational, social) for patients with this syndrome. Drug treatment may not be indicated for all patients with this syndrome. Drug treatment is not intended for use in the patient who exhibits symptoms secondary to environmental factors and/or other primary psychiatric disorders, including psychosis. Appropriate educational placement is essential in patients with this diagnosis and psychosocial intervention is often helpful. When remedial measures alone are insufficient, the decision to prescribe drug treatment will depend upon the physician's assessment of the chronicity and severity of the patient's symptoms.

Long-Term Use: The effectiveness of ADDERALL XR for long-term use, i.e., for more than 3 weeks in children aged 6 to 12 years and 4 weeks in adolescents aged 13 to 17 years, and adults, has not been systematically evaluated in controlled trials. Therefore, the physician who elects to use ADDERALL XR for extended periods should periodically re-evaluate the long-term usefulness of the drug for the individual patient (see Dosage).

CONTRAINDICATIONS: Advanced arteriosclerosis, symptomatic cardiovascular disease, moderate to severe hypertension, hyperthyroidism, known hypersensitivity or idiosyncrasy to the sympathomimetic amines, glaucoma, allergy to amphetamines or to components of ADDERALL XR (mixed salts amphetamine extended-release capsules) or its container.

Agitated states.

Patients with a history of drug abuse.

Administration of ADDERALL XR during or within 14 days following the administration of monoamine oxidase inhibitors may result in hypertensive crises (see Precautions, Drug Interactions).

WARNINGS: Misuse and Serious Cardiovascular Adverse Events: The misuse of amphetamines may cause serious cardiovascular adverse events and sudden deaths.

Pre-Existing Structural Cardiac Abnormalities or Other Serious Heart Problems and Sudden Death: Sudden death has been reported with sympathomimetic drugs used for ADHD treatment at therapeutic doses in children/adolescents with structural cardiac abnormalities or other serious heart problems. Although some serious heart problems alone carry an increased risk of sudden death, ADDERALL XR (mixed salts amphetamine extended-release capsules) generally should not be used in children/adolescents with known serious structural cardiac abnormalities or other serious heart problems (e.g., cardiomyopathy, serious heart rhythm abnormalities) that may place them at increased vulnerability to the sympathomimetic effects of ADHD drugs (see also Contraindications).

Adults: Sudden deaths, stroke, and myocardial infarction have been reported in adults taking stimulant drugs at usual doses for ADHD. Although the role of stimulants in these adult cases is also unknown, adults have a greater likelihood than children of having serious structural cardiac abnormalities, cardiomyopathy, serious heart rhythm abnormalities, coronary artery disease, or other serious cardiac problems. Adults with such abnormalities should also generally not be treated with stimulant drugs (see Contraindications).

Hypertension and Other Cardiovascular Conditions: Sympathomimetic medications can cause a modest increase in average blood pressure and average heart rate and individuals may have larger increases. While the mean changes alone would not be expected to have short-term consequences, all patients should be monitored for larger changes in heart rate and blood pressure. Caution is indicated in treating patients whose underlying medical conditions might be compromised by increases in blood pressure or heart rate, e.g., those with pre-existing hypertension, heart failure, recent myocardial infarction, or ventricular arrhythmia (see also Contraindications). Blood pressure and pulse should be monitored at appropriate intervals in patients taking ADDERALL XR, especially patients with hypertension.

General: Children: Theoretically there exists a pharmacological potential for all ADHD drugs to increase the risk of sudden/cardiac death. Although confirmation of an incremental risk for adverse cardiac events arising from treatment with ADHD medications is lacking, prescribers should consider this potential risk.

All drugs with sympathomimetic effects prescribed in the management of ADHD should be used with caution in patients who: a) are involved in strenuous exercise or activities b) use other sympathomimetic drugs or c) have a family history of sudden/cardiac death. Prior to the initiation of treatment with sympathomimetic medications, a personal and family history (including assessment for a family history of sudden death or ventricular arrhythmia) and physical exam should be obtained to assess for the presence of cardiac disease. In patients with relevant risk factors and based on the clinician's judgment, further cardiovascular evaluation may be considered (e.g., electrocardiogram and echocardiogram). Patients who develop symptoms such as exertional chest pain, unexplained syncope, or other symptoms suggestive of cardiac disease during ADHD treatment should undergo a prompt cardiac evaluation.

Long-Term Suppression of Growth: In a controlled trial of ADDERALL XR in adolescents aged 13 to 17 years, mean weight change from baseline within the initial 4 weeks of therapy was −1.1 lbs. and −2.8 lbs., respectively, for patients receiving 10 mg and 20 mg ADDERALL XR. Higher doses were associated with greater weight loss within the initial 4 weeks of treatment.

Published data for other stimulants report that in children aged 7-10 years, there is a temporary slowing in growth rate without evidence of growth rebound on treatment. Data are inadequate to determine whether the chronic use of amphetamines, in children may be causally associated with suppression of growth. Therefore, growth should be monitored during treatment, and patients who are not growing or gaining weight as expected may need to have their treatment interrupted.

Pre-Existing Psychosis: Clinical experience suggests that in psychotic patients, administration of stimulants may exacerbate symptoms of behavior disturbance and thought disorder.

Emergence of New Psychotic or Manic Symptoms: Treatment emergent psychotic or manic symptoms, e.g., hallucinations, delusional thinking, or mania in children without a prior history of psychotic illness or mania can be caused by stimulants at therapeutic doses. If such symptoms occur, consideration should be given to a possible causal role of the stimulant, and discontinuation of treatment may be appropriate (see also Contraindications).

Bipolar Illness: Particular care should be taken in using stimulants to treat ADHD in patients with comorbid bipolar disorder because of concern for possible induction of a mixed/manic episode in such patients. Prior to initiating treatment with a stimulant, patients with comorbid depressive symptoms should be adequately screened to determine if they are at risk for bipolar disorder; such screening should include a detailed psychiatric history, including a family history of suicide, bipolar disorder, and depression.

Aggression: Aggressive behavior or hostility is often observed in children with ADHD, and has been reported in clinical trials and the postmarketing experience of some medications indicated for the treatment of ADHD. Although there is no systematic evidence that stimulants cause aggressive behavior or hostility, patients beginning treatment for ADHD should be monitored for the appearance of or worsening of aggressive behavior or hostility.

Seizures: There is some clinical evidence that stimulants may lower the convulsive threshold in patients with prior history of seizures, in patients with prior EEG abnormalities in absence of seizures, and, very rarely, in patients without a history of seizures and no prior EEG evidence of seizures. In the presence of seizures, the drug should be discontinued.

Visual Disturbance: Difficulties with accommodation and blurring of vision have been reported with stimulant treatment (see Contraindications).

PRECAUTIONS: General: The least amount of amphetamine feasible should be prescribed or dispensed at one time in order to minimize the possibility of overdosage. ADDERALL XR should be used with caution in patients who use other sympathomimetic drugs.

Tics: Amphetamines have been reported to exacerbate motor and phonic tics in Tourette's syndrome. Therefore, careful clinical evaluation for tics in Tourette's syndrome in children and their families should precede use of stimulant medications.

Pregnancy: Teratogenic Effect: Amphetamine, in the enantiomer ratio present in ADDERALL XR (d- to l- ratio of 3:1), had no apparent effect on embryofetal morphological development or survival when orally administered to pregnant rats and rabbits throughout the period of organogenesis at doses up to 6 and 16 mg/kg/day, respectively. These doses are approximately 1.5 and 8 times the maximum recommended human dose of 30 mg/day on a mg/m² body surface area basis. Fetal malformations and death have been reported in mice following parenteral administration of d-amphetamine doses of 50 mg/kg/day (approximately 6 times the maximum recommended human dose of 30 mg/day on a mg/m² basis) or greater to pregnant animals. Administration of these doses was also associated with severe maternal toxicity.

A number of studies in rodents indicate that prenatal or early postnatal exposure to amphetamine (d- or d,l-), at doses similar to those used clinically in children, can result in long-term neurochemical and behavioral alterations. Reported behavioral effects include learning and memory deficits, altered locomotor activity, and changes in sexual function.

There are no adequate and well-controlled studies with ADDERALL XR in pregnant women. There has been one report of severe congenital bony deformity, tracheoesophageal fistula, and anal atresia (VATER association) in a baby born to a woman who took d-amphetamine sulfate with lovastatin during the first trimester of pregnancy.

Non-Teratogenic Effects: Infants born to mothers dependent on amphetamines have an increased risk of premature delivery and low birth weight. Also, these infants may experience symptoms of withdrawal as demonstrated by dysphoria, including agitation, and significant lassitude.

Amphetamines should be used during pregnancy only if the potential benefit justifies the potential risk to the fetus.

Lactation: Amphetamines are excreted in human milk. Mothers taking amphetamines should be advised to refrain from nursing.

Geriatrics: ADDERALL XR has not been studied in the geriatric population.

Children: ADDERALL XR is indicated for use in children 6 years of age and older. The long-term effects of amphetamines in children have not been well established. Amphetamines are not recommended for use in children with ADHD under 6 years of age.

Carcinogenesis/Mutagenesis and Impairment of Fertility: No evidence of carcinogenicity was found in studies in which d,l-amphetamine (enantiomer ratio of 1:1) was administered to mice and rats in the diet for 2 years at doses of up to 30 mg/kg/day in male mice, 19 mg/kg/day in female mice, and 5 mg/kg/day in male and female rats. These doses are approximately 2.4, 1.5, and 0.8 times, respectively, the maximum recommended human dose of 30 mg/day on a mg/m² body surface area basis.

Amphetamine, in the enantiomer ratio present in ADDERALL XR (d- to l- ratio of 3:1), was not clastogenic in the mouse bone marrow micronucleus test in vivo and was negative when tested in the *E. coli* component of the Ames test in vitro. d,l-Amphetamine (1:1 enantiomer ratio) has been reported to produce a positive response in the mouse bone marrow micronucleus test, an equivocal response in the Ames test, and negative responses in the in vitro sister chromatid exchange and chromosomal aberration assays.

Amphetamine, in the enantiomer ratio present in ADDERALL XR (d- to l- ratio of 3:1), did not adversely affect fertility or early embryonic development in the rat at doses of up to 20 mg/kg/day (approximately 5 times the maximum recommended human dose of 30 mg/day on a mg/m² body surface area basis).

Dependence Liability: ADDERALL XR is a Schedule III drug under the Controlled Drugs and Substances Act (CDSA).

Amphetamines have been extensively abused (see Warnings). Tolerance, extreme psychological dependence, and severe social disability have occurred. There are reports of patients who have increased the dosage to levels many times higher than recommended. Abrupt cessation following prolonged high dosage administration results in extreme fatigue and mental depression; changes are also noted on the sleep EEG. Careful supervision is therefore recommended during drug withdrawal. Manifestations of chronic intoxication with amphetamines may include severe dermatoses, marked insomnia, irritability, hyperactivity, and personality changes. The most severe manifestation of chronic intoxication is psychosis, often clinically indistinguishable from schizophrenia.

Drug Interactions: Acidifying Agents: Gastrointestinal acidifying agents (e.g. guanethidine, reserpine, glutamic acid HCl, ascorbic acid, etc.) may lower absorption of amphetamines.

Urinary Acidifying Agents: (ammonium chloride, sodium acid phosphate, etc.) increase the concentration of the ionized species of the amphetamine molecule, thereby increasing urinary excretion. Both groups of agents lower blood levels and efficacy of amphetamines.

Adrenergic Blockers: As expected by their pharmacologic action, adrenergic blockers are inhibited by amphetamines.

Alkalinizing Agents: Gastrointestinal alkalinizing agents (sodium bicarbonate, etc.), may increase absorption of amphetamines. Co-administration of ADDERALL XR and gastrointestinal alkalinizing agents, such as antacids, should be avoided. Urinary alkalinizing agents (acetazolamide, some thiazides) increase the concentration of the non-ionized species of the amphetamine molecule, thereby decreasing urinary excretion. Both groups of agents increase blood levels and therefore potentiate the actions of amphetamines.

Proton Pump Inhibitors: Proton pump inhibitors act on proton pumps by blocking acid production thereby reducing gastric acidity. In the presence of a proton pump inhibitor, the median T_{max} of ADDERALL XR was shortened from 5 hours to 2.75 hours. Therefore, co-administration of ADDERALL XR and proton pump inhibitors should be avoided.

Antidepressants, Tricyclic: Amphetamines may enhance the activity of tricyclic antidepressant or sympathomimetic agents; d-amphetamine with desipramine or protriptyline and possibly other tricyclics cause striking and sustained increases in the concentration of d-amphetamine in the brain; cardiovascular effects can be potentiated.

MAO Inhibitors: Monoamine oxidase inhibitor antidepressants, as well as a metabolite of furazolidone, slow amphetamine metabolism. This slowing potentiates amphetamines, increasing their effect on the release of norepinephrine and other monoamines from adrenergic nerve endings; this can cause headaches and other signs of hypertensive crisis. A variety of neurological toxic effects and malignant hyperpyrexia can occur, sometimes with fatal results.
Antihistamines: Amphetamines may counteract the sedative effect of some antihistamines.
Antihypertensives: Amphetamines may antagonize the hypotensive effects of antihypertensives.
Chlorpromazine: Chlorpromazine blocks dopamine and norepinephrine receptors, thus inhibiting the central stimulant effects of amphetamines, and can be used to treat amphetamine poisoning.
Ethosuximide: Amphetamines may delay intestinal absorption of ethosuximide.
Haloperidol: Haloperidol blocks dopamine receptors, thus inhibiting the central stimulant effects of amphetamines.
Lithium Carbonate: The anorectic and stimulatory effects of amphetamines may be inhibited by lithium carbonate.
Meperidine: Amphetamines potentiate the analgesic effect of meperidine.
Methenamine Therapy: Urinary excretion of amphetamines is increased, and efficacy is reduced, by acidifying agents used in methenamine therapy.
Norepinephrine: Amphetamines enhance the adrenergic effect of norepinephrine.
Phenobarbital: Amphetamines may delay intestinal absorption of phenobarbital; co-administration of phenobarbital may produce a synergistic anticonvulsant action.
Phenytoin: Amphetamines may delay intestinal absorption of phenytoin; co-administration of phenytoin may produce a synergistic anticonvulsant action.
Propoxyphene: In cases of propoxyphene overdosage, amphetamine CNS stimulation is potentiated and fatal convulsions can occur.
Veratrum Alkaloids: Amphetamines inhibit the hypotensive effect of veratrum alkaloids.
Laboratory Tests: Amphetamines can cause a significant elevation in plasma corticosteroid levels. This increase is greatest in the evening. Amphetamines may interfere with urinary steroid determinations.

ADVERSE EFFECTS: In a single-dose pharmacokinetic study in 23 adolescents aged 13 to 17 years, isolated increases in systolic blood pressure (above the upper 95% CI for age, gender and stature) were observed in 2/17 (12%) and 8/23 (35%), subjects administered 10 mg and 20 mg ADDERALL XR, respectively. Higher single doses were associated with a greater increase in systolic blood pressure. All increases were transient, appeared maximal at 2 to 4 hours post dose and not associated with symptoms.

The pre-marketing development program for ADDERALL XR (mixed salts amphetamine extended-release capsules) included exposures in a total of 1315 participants in clinical trials (635 pediatric patients aged 6 to 12 years, 350 adolescent patients aged 13-17 years, 248 adult patients, 82 healthy adult subjects). The 635 pediatric patients were evaluated in two controlled clinical studies, one open-label clinical study, and two single-dose clinical pharmacology studies (n=40). The 248 adult patients were evaluated in one controlled clinical study and one open-label clinical study. The 350 adolescent patients were evaluated in one controlled clinical study and one pharmacokinetic study. Safety data on all patients are included in the discussion that follows. Adverse reactions were assessed by collecting adverse events, results of physical examinations, vital signs, weights, laboratory analyses, and ECGs.

Adverse Events Associated with Discontinuation of Treatment: In two placebo-controlled studies of up to 5 weeks duration in children aged 6 to 12 years with ADHD, 2.4% (10/425) of ADDERALL XR treated patients discontinued due to adverse events (including 3 patients with loss of appetite, one of whom also reported insomnia) compared to 2.7% (7/259) receiving placebo. The most frequent adverse events associated with discontinuation of ADDERALL XR in controlled and uncontrolled, multiple-dose clinical trials (n=595) are presented in Table 1. Over half of these patients were exposed to ADDERALL XR for 12 months or more.

Table 1: ADDERALL XR

Most Frequent Adverse Events Resulting in Discontinuation (>0.5%)

Adverse Event	% of Pediatric Patients Discontinuing (n=595)
Anorexia (loss of appetite)	2.9
Insomnia	1.5
Weight loss	1.2
Emotional lability	1.0
Depression	0.7

In a separate placebo-controlled 4-week study in adolescents aged 13 to 17 years with ADHD, eight patients (3.4%) discontinued treatment due to adverse events among ADDERALL XR-treated patients (N=233). Three patients discontinued due to insomnia and one patient each for depression, motor tics, headaches, light-headedness, and anxiety.

In one placebo-controlled, 4-week study in adults with ADHD, the most frequent adverse events resulting in discontinuation (>0.5%) in ADDERALL XR treated patients (n=191) were for nervousness including anxiety and irritability (3.1%); for insomnia (2.6%); and for headache, palpitation, and somnolence (1% each). In an open-label extension of the trial (n=223), at 12 months, the only adverse event leading to discontinuation that was reported by at least 2% of patients was depression (4.9%).

Adverse events leading to discontinuations for ADDERALL XR trials in adults were consistent with those reported in ADDERALL XR trials in children and were also consistent with the known side effects for amphetamines.

Adverse Events Occurring in a Controlled Trial: Adverse events reported in a controlled fixed dose clinical study of pediatric patients treated with ADDERALL XR at doses up to 30 mg/day, or placebo, for up to 3 weeks are presented in Table 2.

Table 2: ADDERALL XR

Adverse Events Reported by More Than 1% of Children Aged 6 to 12 Years Receiving Fixed Doses of ADDERALL XR (up to final doses of 10, 20 or 30 mg/day) with an Incidence Greater Than Placebo in a Controlled Clinical Study

Body System	Adverse Event	ADDERALL XR (n=374)	Placebo (n=210)
General	Abdominal pain (stomach ache)	14%	10%
	Accidental injury	3%	2%
	Asthenia (fatigue)	2%	0%
	Fever	5%	2%
	Infection	4%	2%
	Viral infection	2%	0%
Digestive System	Loss of appetite	22%	2%
	Diarrhea	2%	1%
	Dyspepsia	2%	1%
	Nausea	5%	3%
	Vomiting	7%	4%
Nervous System	Dizziness	2%	0%
	Emotional lability	9%	2%
	Insomnia	17%	2%
	Nervousness	6%	2%
Metabolic/Nutritional	Weight loss	4%	0%

Adverse events reported in a 4-week clinical trial in adolescents aged 13 to 17 years treated with ADDERALL XR at doses up to 40 mg/day in adolescents weighing ≤75 kg, or placebo are presented in Table 3.

Table 3: ADDERALL XR

Adverse Events Reported by ≥1%[a] or More of Adolescents Weighing ≤75 kg Receiving ADDERALL XR with Higher Incidence than Placebo in a Forced Weekly-Dose Titration Study[a]

Body System	Adverse Event	ADDERALL XR (n=233)	Placebo (n=54)
General	Abdominal pain (stomach ache)	11%	2%
	Asthenia	3%	0%
Cardiovascular	Tachycardia	1%	0%
Digestive	Diarrhea	2%	0%
	Dry mouth	4%	0%
	Dyspepsia	3%	0%
	Loss of appetite[b]	36%	2%
	Nausea	3%	0%
	Vomiting	1%	0%
Nervous	Depression	1%	0%
	Emotional lability	3%	0%
	Insomnia[b]	12%	4%
	Nervousness	6%	6%[c]
	Somnolence	5%	4%
	Twitching	1%	0%
Metabolic/Nutritional	Weight loss[b]	9%	0%
Skin and Appendages	Herpes simplex	1%	0%
Urogenital	Albuminuria	2%	0%
	Dysmenorrhea	1%	0%

[a] Included doses up to 40 mg.
[b] Dose-related adverse events.
[c] Appears the same due to rounding.

Adverse events reported in a controlled fixed dose clinical study of adult patients treated with ADDERALL XR at doses up to 60 mg/day, or placebo, for up to 4 weeks are presented in Table 4.

Table 4: ADDERALL XR

Adverse Events Reported by ≥1% or More of Adults Receiving Fixed Doses of ADDERALL XR (up to final doses of 20, 40 or 60 mg/day) with an Incidence Greater than Placebo in a Controlled Clinical Trial

Body System	Adverse Event	ADDERALL XR (n=191)	Placebo (n=64)
General	Asthenia	6%	5%
	Chills	2%	0%
	Headache	26%	13%
	Infection	4%	2%
	Fungal infection	2%	0%
	Neck pain	2%	0%
	Pain	5%	5%[a]
	Photosensitivity reaction	3%	0%
Digestive System	Constipation	4%	0%
	Diarrhea	6%	0%

(cont'd)

Table 4: ADDERALL XR *(cont'd)*

Adverse Events Reported by ≥1% or More of Adults Receiving Fixed Doses of ADDERALL XR (up to final doses of 20, 40 or 60 mg/day) with an Incidence Greater than Placebo in a Controlled Clinical Trial

Body System	Adverse Event	ADDERALL XR (n=191)	Placebo (n=64)
	Dry mouth	35%	5%
	Loss of appetite	33%	3%
	Nausea	8%	3%
	Gastroenteritis	1%	0%
	Thirst	1%	0%
	Tooth disorder	3%	2%
	Vomiting	1%	0%
Nervous System	Agitation	8%	5%
	Amnesia	1%	0%
	Anxiety	8%	5%
	Dizziness	7%	0%
	Insomnia	27%	13%
	Depersonalization	1%	0%
	Emotional lability	3%	2%
	Hyperkinesia	4%	3%
	Libido decreased	4%	0%
	Libido increased	1%	0%
	Nervousness	13%	13%[a]
	Somnolence	3%	2%
	Speech disorder	2%	0%
Cardiovascular System	Hypertension	2%	0%
	Palpitation	4%	0%
	Tachycardia	6%	3%
	Vasodilation	1%	0%
Metabolic/Nutritional	Bilirubinemia	1%	0%
	AST increased	1%	0%
	ALT increased	1%	0%
	Weight loss	11%	0%
Musculoskeletal	Arthralgia	1%	0%
	Myalgia	2%	2%[a]
	Twitching	3%	0%
Respiratory	Cough increased	1%	0%
	Dyspnea	3%	0%
	Sinusitis	1%	0%
Skin and Appendages	Rash	2%	0%
	Sweating	3%	0%
Special Senses	Taste perversion	2%	0%
Urogenital System	Dysmenorrhea	2%	0%
	Impotence	2%	0%
	Oliguria	1%	0%
	Urinary tract disorder	1%	0%
	Urinary tract infection	5%	0%
	Urination impaired	1%	0%

[a] Appears the same due to rounding.

The following adverse reactions have also been associated with the use of amphetamine, or mixed salt amphetamines:
Cardiovascular: elevation of blood pressure, sudden death, myocardial infarction, stroke, palpitations, tachycardia; there have been isolated reports of cardiomyopathy associated with chronic amphetamine use.
Digestive: anorexia, constipation, diarrhea, dryness of the mouth, unpleasant taste, other gastrointestinal disturbances.
Metabolic and Nutritional: weight loss.
Nervous System: depression, dizziness, dyskinesia, dysphoria, euphoria, headache, insomnia, change in libido, overstimulation, psychotic and manic episodes at recommended doses (e.g., hallucinations, delusional thinking, and mania), restlessness, tremor, exacerbation of phonic and motor tics and Tourette's syndrome, seizures, aggressive behavior, hostility.
Skin and Appendages: urticaria, rash, hypersensitivity reactions including angioedema and anaphylaxis, serious skin rashes, including Stevens Johnson Syndrome and toxic epidermal necrolysis have been reported.
Urogenital: impotence.

OVERDOSE:
Individual patient response to amphetamines varies widely. Toxic symptoms may occur idiosyncratically at low doses.

Symptoms: Manifestations of acute overdosage with amphetamines include restlessness, tremor, hyperreflexia, rapid respiration, confusion, assaultiveness, hallucinations, panic states, hyperpyrexia and rhabdomyolysis. Fatigue and depression usually follow the central nervous system stimulation. Cardiovascular effects include arrhythmias, hypertension or hypotension and circulatory collapse. Gastrointestinal symptoms include nausea, vomiting, diarrhea, and abdominal cramps. Fatal poisoning is usually preceded by convulsions and coma.

Treatment: Treatment of overdosage consists of appropriate supportive measures. Consult with a Certified Poison Control Center for up to date guidance and advice. Management of acute amphetamine intoxication is largely symptomatic and includes gastric lavage, administration of activated charcoal, administration of a cathartic and sedation. Experience with hemodialysis or peritoneal dialysis is inadequate to permit its recommendation in this regard. Acidification of the urine increases amphetamine excretion, but is believed to increase risk of acute renal failure if myoglobinuria is present. If acute severe hypertension complicates amphetamine overdosage, administration of intravenous phentolamine has been suggested. However, a gradual drop in blood pressure will usually result when sufficient sedation has been achieved. Chlorpromazine antagonizes the central stimulant effects of amphetamines and can be used to treat amphetamine intoxication.

The prolonged release of mixed salts amphetamine from ADDERALL XR capsules should be considered when treating patients with overdose.

Animal Toxicology: Acute administration of high doses of amphetamine (d- or d,l-) has been shown to produce long-lasting neurotoxic effects, including irreversible nerve fiber damage, in rodents. The significance of these findings to humans is unknown.

For management of a suspected drug overdose, CPhA recommends that you contact your **regional Poison Control Centre**. See the *CPS* Directory section for a list of Poison Control Centres.

DOSAGE: Dosing Considerations: ADDERALL XR (mixed salts amphetamine extended-release capsules) is a once-a-day capsule administered orally in the morning. ADDERALL XR dosage should be individualized according to the needs and response of the patient.

ADDERALL XR should be administered starting at the lowest possible dose. Dosage should then be individually and slowly adjusted, to the lowest effective dosage, since individual patient response to ADDERALL XR varies widely.

ADDERALL XR should not be used in patients with symptomatic cardiovascular disease including coronary artery disease in adults and should generally not be used in patients with known serious structural cardiac abnormalities or other serious heart problems (e.g., cardiomyopathy, serious heart rhythm abnormalities) that may place them at increased vulnerability to the sympathomimetic effects of ADHD drugs (see Contraindications and Warnings).

Theoretically there exists a pharmacological potential for all ADHD drugs to increase the risk of sudden/cardiac death. Although confirmation of an incremental risk for adverse cardiac events arising from treatment with ADHD medications is lacking, prescribers should consider this potential risk.

All drugs with sympathomimetic effects prescribed in the management of ADHD should be used with caution in patients who: a) are involved in strenuous exercise or activities b) use other sympathomimetic drugs or c) have a family history of sudden/cardiac death. Prior to the initiation of treatment with sympathomimetic medications, a personal and family history (including assessment for a family history of sudden death or ventricular arrhythmia) and physical exam should be obtained to assess for the presence of cardiac disease. In patients with relevant risk factors and based on the clinician's judgment, further cardiovascular evaluation may be considered (e.g., electrocardiogram and echocardiogram). Patients who develop symptoms such as exertional chest pain, unexplained syncope, or other symptoms suggestive of cardiac disease during ADHD treatment should undergo a prompt cardiac evaluation.

Patients who are considered to need extended treatment with ADDERALL XR should undergo periodic evaluation of their cardiovascular status (see Warnings).

ADDERALL XR is a once-a-day capsule for the treatment of ADHD containing immediate-release and delayed-release pellets. Capsules may be taken whole in the morning, or the capsule may be opened and the entire contents sprinkled on applesauce. If using the sprinkle administration method, the sprinkled applesauce should be consumed immediately and not stored. Patients should eat the applesauce with sprinkled beads in its entirety and refrain from chewing. The dose of a single capsule should not be divided—the contents of the entire capsule should be taken. Afternoon doses should be avoided because of the long-acting nature of the drug, including the potential for insomnia.

Where possible, drug administration should be interrupted occasionally to determine if there is a recurrence of behavioral symptoms sufficient to require continued therapy.

Children (6 to 12 years of age): **Amphetamines are not recommended for children under 6 years of age.** When in the judgement of the clinician a lower dose is appropriate, patients may begin treatment with 5 mg once daily in the morning. The usual starting dose is 10 mg daily. The daily dosage may be adjusted in increments of 5 mg to 10 mg at weekly intervals, as determined by clinical response and tolerability up to the maximum recommended dose of 30 mg per day.

Adolescents (13 to 17 years of age) and Adults (over 18 years of age): In adolescents and adults with ADHD who are either starting treatment for the first time or switching from another stimulant medication, start with 10 mg once daily in the morning; daily dosage may be adjusted in increments of 5 to 10 mg at weekly intervals up to a usual maximum of 20 mg. In some cases, higher doses not to exceed 30 mg/day may be required, as determined by clinical response and tolerability.

INFORMATION FOR THE PATIENT: Published in e-CPS, available by subscription at www.e-cps.ca.

SUPPLIED: 5 mg: Each clear/blue extended-release capsule, imprinted "ADDERALL XR" on one end and "5 mg" on the other, contains: 5 mg of mixed salts amphetamine. Nonmedicinal ingredients: FD&C Blue #2, hydroxypropyl methylcellulose, methacrylic acid copolymer, opadry beige, starch, sugar spheres, talc and triethyl citrate; gelatin capsule: edible inks, kosher gelatin and titanium dioxide. Bottles of 100. Dispense in a tight, light-resistant container as defined in the USP. Store at 25°C. Excursions permitted to 15-30°C.

10 mg: Each blue/blue extended-release capsule, imprinted "ADDERALL XR" on one end and "10 mg" on the other, contains: 10 mg of mixed salts amphetamine. Nonmedicinal ingredients: FD&C Blue #2, hydroxypropyl methylcellulose, methacrylic acid copolymer, opadry beige, starch, sugar spheres, talc and triethyl citrate; gelatin capsule: edible inks, kosher gelatin and titanium dioxide. Bottles of 100. Dispense in a tight, light-resistant container as defined in the USP. Store at 25°C. Excursions permitted to 15-30°C.

15 mg: Each blue/white extended-release capsule, imprinted "ADDERALL XR" on one end and "15 mg" on the other, contains: 15 mg of mixed salts amphetamine. Nonmedicinal ingredients: FD&C Blue #2, hydroxypropyl methylcellulose, methacrylic acid copolymer, opadry beige, starch, sugar spheres, talc and triethyl citrate; gelatin capsule: edible inks, kosher gelatin and titanium dioxide. Bottles of 100. Dispense in a tight, light-resistant container as defined in the USP. Store at 25°C. Excursions permitted to 15-30°C.

20 mg: Each orange/orange extended-release capsule, imprinted "ADDERALL XR" on one end and "20 mg" on the other, contains: 20 mg of mixed salts amphetamine. Nonmedicinal ingredients: hydroxypropyl methylcellulose, methacrylic acid copolymer, opadry beige, red iron oxide, starch, sugar spheres, talc, triethyl citrate and yellow iron oxide; gelatin capsule: edible inks, kosher gelatin and titanium dioxide. Bottles of 100. Dispense in a tight, light-resistant container as defined in the USP. Store at 25°C. Excursions permitted to 15-30°C.

25 mg: Each orange/white extended-release capsule, imprinted "ADDERALL XR" on one end and "25 mg" on the other, contains: 25 mg of mixed salts amphetamine. Nonmedicinal ingredients: hydroxypropyl methylcellulose, methacrylic acid copolymer, opadry beige, red iron oxide, starch, sugar spheres, talc, triethyl citrate and yellow iron oxide; gelatin capsule: edible inks, kosher gelatin and titanium dioxide. Bottles of 100. Dispense in a tight, light-resistant container as defined in the USP. Store at 25°C. Excursions permitted to 15-30°C.

30 mg: Each clear/orange extended-release capsule, imprinted "ADDERALL XR" on one end and "30 mg" on the other, contains: 30 mg of mixed salts amphetamine. Nonmedicinal ingredients: hydroxypropyl methylcellulose, methacrylic acid copolymer, opadry beige, red iron oxide, starch, sugar spheres, talc, triethyl citrate and yellow iron oxide; gelatin capsule: edible inks, kosher gelatin and titanium dioxide. Bottles of 100. Dispense in a tight, light-resistant container as defined in the USP. Store at 25°C. Excursions permitted to 15-30°C.

(Shown in Product Identification Section)

ADEKs® Ⓟ
multiple vitamins—zinc oxide
Multivitamin Supplement—Zinc

Axcan Pharma

Date of Revision: March 6, 2008

PHARMACOLOGY: Deficiencies of one or more of the fat-soluble vitamins may occur in the presence of steatorrhea or other malabsorption, hepatic dysfunction, protein malnutrition, zinc deficiency, and very low fat diets. As with all vitamins, adequate levels are essential to good health and proper growth. Early nutritional intervention in disease such as cystic fibrosis appears crucial to growth and long-term outcome of these patients. Deficiencies lead to a wide variety of pathologies.

Vitamin A is essential for growth and bone development, vision, reproduction and maintenance of the integrity of mucosal and epithelial surfaces. Vitamin A deficiencies may lead to xerophthalmia, epithelial metaplasia of mucous membranes, decreased resistance to infection (characteristic change in epithelium of eye), night blindness and hyperkeratosis of the skin.

Vitamin D is essential for the absorption and utilization of calcium and phosphate and aids in the mobilization of bone calcium and maintenance of serum calcium concentrations.

Vitamin E is considered an essential element of human nutrition. Many of its actions are related to its antioxidant properties. Vitamin E deficiency rarely causes clinical symptoms in adults. In premature neonates, irritability, edema, thrombosis, and hemolytic anemia may be caused by vitamin E deficiency.

Vitamin K is necessary for synthesis in the liver of factor II (prothrombin), factor VII (proconvertin), factor IX (thromboplastin), and factor X. Deficiency of vitamin K or disturbances of liver function lead to deficiencies of these factors, with either latent or manifest hemorrhage. Vitamin K deficiency may occur in patients with biliary obstruction or other conditions limiting absorption of vitamin K such as celiac disease, ulcerative colitis, sprue, regional enteritis, cystic fibrosis, and intestinal resection and in patients receiving drugs that may affect liver function or intestinal flora.

INDICATIONS: ADEKs tablets are specially formulated to provide nutritional supplementation in individuals with malabsorptive conditions. ADEKs tablets use water-miscible forms of the fat-soluble vitamins to improve absorption in these individuals. It also provides vitamin C, B complex vitamins, and other vitamins plus zinc to supplement dietary intake. ADEKs tablets are indicated for nutritional supplementation in individuals with deficient diets or difficulty in absorbing fat-soluble vitamins such as may occur in cystic fibrosis. For use solely under medical supervision.

CONTRAINDICATIONS: None known.

PRECAUTIONS: General: Do not exceed recommended dose. Pernicious anemia should be excluded before using this product since folic acid in doses above 0.1 mg daily may mask symptoms.

Pregnancy: Excessive amounts of vitamin A may be hazardous to the embryo or fetus when taken during pregnancy. Women of childbearing potential should consult their physicians regarding total vitamin A intake.

Drug Interactions: Vitamin K interferes with actions of anticoagulant drugs. Patients taking anticoagulants should consult their physicians before taking ADEKs tablets.

ADVERSE EFFECTS: None known.

OVERDOSE:

Symptoms: None known.

Treatment: None known.

For management of a suspected drug overdose, CPhA recommends that you contact your **regional Poison Control Centre**. See the *CPS* Directory section for a list of Poison Control Centres.

DOSAGE: Tablets: 4 to 10 years: 1 tablet daily; over 10 years: 2 tablets daily, or as directed by physician.

Tablets must be chewed or crushed thoroughly. Tablets may also be crushed and given with soft foods for children unable to chew tablets.

SUPPLIED: Each tan tablet contains: see Table 1.

Table 1: ADEKs

Composition

Vitamin A	5667 IU
Beta Carotene	29%[a,b] (5000 IU)
Vitamin A Palmitate	71%[b] (4000 IU)
Vitamin D (cholecalciferol)	400 IU
Vitamin E (succinate)	150 IU
Vitamin K (phytonadione)	0.15 mg
Vitamin C (ascorbic acid)	60 mg
Folic Acid	0.2 mg
Thiamine (vitamin B_1)	1.2 mg
Riboflavin (vitamin B_2)	1.3 mg
Niacin	10 mg
Vitamin B_6 (pyridoxine)	1.5 mg
Vitamin B_{12} (cyanocobalamin)	12 µg
Biotin	50 µg
Pantothenic Acid	10 mg
Zinc (oxide)	7.5 mg

[a] Beta carotene 29% (5000 IU, equivalent to 1667 IU of vitamin A). Calculations: In each ADEKs tablet there is 3 mg beta carotene (equivalent to 5000 IU beta carotene). Each IU of vitamin A is equivalent to 3 IU beta carotene (Canadian Vitamin and Labelling Standard). 5000 IU÷3=1667 IU (IU beta carotene expressed as equivalent IU of vitamin A). 4000 IU (IU vitamin A as vitamin A palmitate) + 1667 IU=5667 IU.

[b] Percentage expressed as % of total IU in vitamin A or equivalent of vitamin A. Calculations: (1667÷5667)×100%=29%; (4000÷5667)×100%=71%.

Nonmedicinal ingredients: dextrose with corn syrup solids, flavor, fructose, glycirrhizic acid, magnesium stearate, silicon dioxide and stearic acid. Bottles of 60. Dispense in tight, light-resistant containers. Store at 15 to 30°C.

(Shown in Product Identification Section)

Adenocard® Ⓟ
adenosine
Antiarrhythmic

Astellas

Date of Preparation: August 24, 2005
Date of Revision: June 9, 2010

PHARMACOLOGY: Adenosine is an endogenous nucleoside occurring in all cells of the body. When injected i.v. adenosine slows atrioventricular (AV) nodal conduction, can interrupt the reentry pathways through the AV node and can restore normal sinus rhythm in patients with paroxysmal supraventricular tachycardia (PSVT), including PSVT associated with Wolff-Parkinson-White syndrome.

Adenosine is antagonized competitively by methylxanthines such as caffeine and theophylline and potentiated by blockers of nucleoside transport such as dipyridamole. Adenosine is not blocked by atropine.

In controlled clinical trials, cumulative 60% and 92% of patients converted to normal sinus rhythm within 1 minute after 6 mg and 12 mg bolus doses of adenosine, respectively. In other controlled clinical trials with bolus doses of 3, 6, 9 and 12 mg some patients with paroxysmal supraventricular tachycardia converted to normal sinus rhythm on 3 mg of adenosine. Reports in the medical literature indicate success in treating PSVT in pediatric patients (including newborns) with adenosine in doses equivalent by weight to those used in adults.

Adenosine is not effective in converting rhythms other than PSVT, such as atrial flutter, atrial fibrillation, or ventricular tachycardia to normal sinus rhythm.

Hemodynamics: Adenosine is a potent vasodilator in most vascular beds, except in renal afferent arterioles and hepatic veins where it produces vasoconstriction. The i.v. bolus dose of 6 or 12 mg adenosine usually has no systemic hemodynamic effects. When larger doses are given by infusion, adenosine decreases blood pressure by decreasing peripheral resistance.

Pharmacokinetics: I.V. administered adenosine is rapidly cleared from the circulation via cellular uptake, primarily by erythrocytes and vascular endothelial cells, with a half-life of less than 10 seconds. Intracellular adenosine is rapidly metabolized either via phosphorylation to adenosine monophosphate by adenosine kinase, or via deamination to inosine by adenosine deaminase in the cytosol. Adenosine monophosphate formed by phosphorylation of adenosine is incorporated into the high-energy phosphate pool. Inosine formed by deamination of adenosine can leave the cell intact or can be metabolized to hypoxanthine, xanthine and ultimately uric acid.

Since neither the kidney nor the liver are required for the metabolism or elimination of adenosine, the activity of adenosine should be unaffected by hepatic or renal insufficiency.

INDICATIONS AND CLINICAL USE: Adenocard (adenosine) is indicated for the conversion to sinus rhythm of paroxysmal supraventricular tachycardia (PSVT), including that associated with accessory bypass tracts (Wolff-Parkinson-White Syndrome). When clinically advisable, appropriate vagal maneuvers (e.g. Valsalva maneuver) should be attempted prior to Adenocard administration.

Adenosine is indicated to aid in the diagnosis of broad or narrow complex supraventricular tachycardia. Although adenosine is not effective in converting atrial flutter, atrial fibrillation or ventricular tachycardia to sinus rhythm, the transient atrioventricular nodal block produced helps diagnosis of atrial activity.

It is essential to ascertain that adenosine actually reaches the systemic circulation (see Dosage and Administration).

Adenosine **does not** convert atrial flutter, atrial fibrillation or ventricular tachycardia to normal sinus rhythm.

Adenosine should only be used with appropriate cardiac monitoring.

CONTRAINDICATIONS: Adenocard (adenosine) is contraindicated in:

- Second or third degree AV block (except in patients with a functioning artificial pacemaker).
- Sick sinus syndrome (except in patients with a functioning artificial pacemaker).
- Symptomatic bradycardia (except in patients with a functioning artificial pacemaker).
- Known hypersensitivity to adenosine.

WARNINGS: Heart Block: Adenocard (adenosine) exerts its effect by decreasing conduction through the A-V node and may produce a short lasting first-, second- or third-degree heart block. Appropriate therapy should be instituted as needed. Patients who develop high level block on one dose of Adenocard should not be given additional doses. Because of the very short half-life of adenosine (<10 seconds), these effects are generally self-limiting. Appropriate resuscitative measures should be available.

Rarely, ventricular fibrillation/flutter has been reported following adenosine administration, including both resuscitated and fatal events. In most instances, these cases were associated with the concomitant use of digoxin **and, less frequently, with digoxin and verapamil**. Adenosine should be used with caution in patients receiving digoxin **or digoxin and verapamil in combination.**

Patients with atrial fibrillation/flutter and an accessory by-pass tract may develop increased conduction down the anomalous pathway.

Arrhythmias at Time of Conversion: At the time of conversion to normal sinus rhythm, a variety of new rhythms may appear on the electrocardiogram. They generally last only a few seconds without intervention, and may take the form of premature ventricular contractions, polymorphic ventricular tachycardia, torsades de pointes, atrial premature contractions, atrial fibrillation, sinus bradycardia, sinus tachycardia, skipped beats, and varying degrees of A-V nodal block. These arrhythmias and conduction disturbances were observed in about 55% of patients.

Asystole: Transient or prolonged episodes of asystole have been reported with fatal outcomes in some cases.

Bronchoconstriction: Adenosine has been administered to a limited number of patients with asthma and serious exacerbation of their symptoms has been reported in some patients. Respiratory compromise has occurred during adenosine infusion in patients with chronic obstructive pulmonary disease (COPD). Therefore, the use of adenosine should be avoided in patients with COPD or asthma.

Adenosine therapy should be discontinued in any patient who develops severe respiratory difficulties.

PRECAUTIONS: Pregnancy: Adenosine is a substance naturally present in the body and therefore no fetal effects would be anticipated. However, since it is not known whether adenosine can cause fetal harm when administered to pregnant women, it should not be used during pregnancy unless potential benefits outweigh the potential risks to the fetus.

Children: No controlled studies have been conducted in pediatric patients to establish the safety and efficacy of adenosine for the conversion of paroxysmal supraventricular tachycardia (PSVT). However, open-label studies carried out by independent investigators indicated that i.v. adenosine can be used safely in neonates, infants, children and adolescents (see Dosage, Pediatric Patients).

Geriatrics: Clinical studies of Adenocard did not include sufficient numbers of subjects aged 65 and over to determine whether they respond differently from younger subjects. Other reported clinical experience has not identified differences in responses between elderly and younger patients. In general, Adenocard in geriatric patients should be used with caution since this population may have a diminished cardiac function, nodal dysfunction, concomitant diseases or drug therapy that may alter hemodynamic function and produce severe bradycardia or AV block.

Drug Interactions:

1. **Cardioactive Drugs:** Adenosine has been effectively administered in the presence of other cardioactive drugs, such as quinidine, beta-adrenergic blocking agents, calcium channel blocking agents and angiotensin converting enzyme inhibitors, without any change in the adverse reaction profile. **Digoxin and verapamil use may be rarely associated with ventricular fibrillation when combined with adenosine (see Warnings).** Because of the synergistic depressant effects on the SA and AV nodes, adenosine should be used with caution in the presence of these agents.
2. **Methylxanthines:** The effects of adenosine are antagonized by methylxanthines (such as caffeine and theophylline). In the presence of methylxanthines, larger doses of adenosine may be required or adenosine may not be effective.
3. **Dipyridamole:** Adenosine effects are potentiated by dipyridamole. Thus, smaller doses of adenosine may be effective in the presence of dipyridamole.
4. **Carbamazepine:** Carbamazepine has been reported to increase the degree of heart block produced by other agents. Since the primary effect of adenosine is to decrease conduction through the AV node, higher degrees of heart block may be produced in the presence of carbamazepine.

ADVERSE EFFECTS: In controlled clinical trials 268 patients received adenosine. One hundred and two patients (38%) experienced one or more adverse events. These adverse events appeared immediately after administration of adenosine and usually lasted less than 1 minute. The most common adverse reactions were: facial flushing (18%), dyspnea (12%), chest pressure (7%) and nausea (3%).

Cardiovascular: facial flushing (18%), headache (2%), sweating, palpitations, chest pain, hypotension (less than 1%). A variety of arrhythmias and conduction disturbances were observed in about 55% of patients at the time of conversion to normal sinus rhythm.

Respiratory: shortness of breath/dyspnea (12%), chest pressure (7%), hyperventilation, head pressure (less than 1%).
Central Nervous System: lightheadedness (2%), dizziness, tingling in arms, numbness (1%), apprehension, blurred vision, burning sensation, heaviness in arms, neck and back pain (less than 1%).
Gastrointestinal: nausea (3%), metallic taste, tightness in throat, pressure in groin (less than 1%).

The following adverse events have been reported from marketing experience with Adenocard. Because these events are reported voluntarily from a population of uncertain size, are associated with concomitant diseases and multiple drug therapies and surgical procedures, it is not always possible to reliably estimate their frequency or establish a causal relationship to drug exposure. Decisions to include these events in labeling are typically based on one or more of the following factors: (1) seriousness of the event, (2) frequency of the reporting, (3) strength of causal connection to the drug, or a combination of these factors.
Cardiovascular: prolonged asystole, ventricular tachycardia, ventricular fibrillation, transient increase in blood pressure, bradycardia, atrial fibrillation, and Torsade de Pointes (see Warnings and Precautions).
Respiratory: bronchospasm.
Central Nervous System: convulsions, grand mal and tonic clonic seizures.

OVERDOSE:
No cases of overdosage associated with the use of adenosine have been reported. It is unlikely that the true overdosage will occur because adenosine has a short half-life (<10 seconds) and is dosed by a rapid bolus injection. If prolonged adverse events associated with the use of adenosine occur, treatment should be individualized and directed toward the specific event. To date, no patient has required administration of adenosine antagonists such as aminophylline to counteract adverse events associated with the use of adenosine.

In clinical studies on the use of adenosine as a diagnostic agent in imaging, less than 0.1% of the patients exposed to adenosine were described as having severe, prolonged, adverse events. These prolonged adverse events were treated with aminophylline after discontinuation of the adenosine infusion. The usual concentration of aminophylline used was 1.25 mg/mL (125 mg in 100 mL) administered i.v. over 5 to 6 minutes. An additional 1.25 mg/mL (125 mg in 100 mL) can be administered, but clinical experience has demonstrated that this is rarely required.

> For management of a suspected drug overdose, contact your regional Poison Control Centre. See the *CPS* Directory section for a list of Poison Control Centres.

DOSAGE AND ADMINISTRATION: Adenosine should only be used with appropriate cardiac monitoring.

Adenosine should be given as a rapid bolus i.v. injection. To be certain the solution reaches the systemic circulation, it should be administered either directly into a peripheral vein or, if given into an i.v. line, it should be given as close to the patient as possible and followed by a rapid saline flush.
Adult Patients: The recommended i.v. doses for adults are as follows: Initial dose: 6 mg administered as a rapid i.v. bolus given over a 1- to 2-second time period.
Additional Doses: If the initial dose does not terminate supraventricular tachycardia within 1 to 2 minutes, 12 mg dose should be given as a rapid i.v. bolus. This 12 mg dose may be repeated a second time if required. Single bolus injections greater than 12 mg are not recommended.
Pediatric Patients: Pediatric patients with a body weight <50 kg: Initial Dose: Give 0.05 to 0.1 mg/kg as a rapid i.v. bolus given either centrally or peripherally.
Additional Doses: If conversion of PSVT does not occur within 1 to 2 minutes, additional bolus injections of adenosine can be administered at incrementally higher doses, increasing the amount given by 0.05 to 0.1 mg/kg. Follow each bolus with a saline flush. This process should be continued until sinus rhythm is established or up to a maximum dose of 0.3 mg/kg.

For pediatric patients who require single i.v. doses less than 0.6 mg (0.2 mL), adenosine may be further diluted with normal saline to a final concentration range from 0.3 to 1 mg/mL.
Patient with a Body Weight ≥50 Kg: Administer the adult dose.

Single bolus injections greater than 12 mg are not recommended for adult or pediatric patients.
Note: Adenosine injection should be inspected visually for particulate matter and discoloration prior to administration.

Store at controlled room temperature 15 to 30°C. **Do not refrigerate** as crystallization may occur. If crystallization has occurred, dissolve crystals by warming to room temperature. The solution must be clear at the time of use.

SUPPLIED: Each mL of sterile solution for rapid bolus i.v. injection contains: adenosine 3 mg and sodium chloride 9 mg in water for injection. The pH of the solution is between 4.5 and 7.5. Additive-, color- and preservative-free. Single-dose flip-top vials of 2 mL. Prefilled sterile Ansyr plastic disposable syringes of 2 and 4 mL (may require needle or blunt). Any portion of the vial or syringe not used at once should be discarded.
Instructions for Syringe Use: The new Ansyr syringe delivery system, easily adapts to most peripheral line connection valves without the use of a needle. A needle is not provided with the Adenocard Ansyr syringe delivery system. Should you require the use of a needle to inject Adenocard directly into a vein, the adaptable Luer Lock tip can accomodate an 18 or 20 gauge needle. To use the syringe, remove luer cover. Hold plunger and push barrel forward to relieve any resistance that may be present. Pull the barrel down until air is expelled from the syringe. Adenocard is now ready to be administered. (See Dosage and Administration.) Syringes and vials, are intended for single use only. To prevent needle-stick injuries needles should not be recapped, purposely bent or broken by hand. Ansyr is a latex free, plastic delivery system and is a registered trademark of Hospira Inc. Any portion of the vial or syringe not used at once should be discarded. For additional information pertaining to the use of the Adenocard Ansyr syringe, please refer to the drug carton diagrams.

Adriamycin® PFS® Ⓟ
doxorubicin HCl
Antineoplastic

Pfizer

Date of Revision: January 8, 2010

Caution: ADRIAMYCIN (doxorubicin hydrochloride) is a potent drug and should be used only by physicians experienced with cancer chemotherapy drugs (see Warnings and Precautions). Blood counts and hepatic function tests should be performed regularly. Because of the experience with cardiac toxicity, it is not recommended to exceed a total dose of ADRIAMYCIN 550 mg/m² with the 21-day regimen and 700 mg/m² with the weekly regimen. Cardiac monitoring is advised in those patients who have received mediastinal radiotherapy, other anthracycline or anthracene therapy, with pre-existing cardiac disease, or who have received prior ADRIAMYCIN cumulative doses exceeding 400 mg/m² with the 21-day regimen and 550 mg/m² utilizing the weekly regimen.

SUMMARY PRODUCT INFORMATION:

Route of Administration	Dosage Form/ Strength	Clinically Relevant Nonmedicinal Ingredients
Parenteral and intravesical	Ready to use solution for injection 2 mg/mL (5 mL, 25 mL, 100 mL vials)	For a complete listing see Dosage Forms, Composition and Packaging.

INDICATIONS AND CLINICAL USE: ADRIAMYCIN (doxorubicin hydrochloride) has been used successfully both as a single agent and also in combination with other approved cancer chemotherapeutic agents to produce regression in neoplastic conditions such as acute lymphoblastic leukemia, acute myeloblastic leukemia, Wilms' tumor, neuroblastomas, soft tissue sarcomas, bone sarcomas, breast carcinoma, gynecologic carcinomas, testicular carcinomas, bronchogenic carcinoma, Hodgkin's disease, non-Hodgkin's lymphoma, thyroid carcinoma, bladder carcinomas, squamous cell carcinoma of the head and neck, and gastric carcinoma.

ADRIAMYCIN has also been used by instillation into the bladder for the topical treatment of superficial bladder tumors.

A number of other solid tumors have also shown some responsiveness to ADRIAMYCIN alone or in combination with other drugs (see Dosage and Administration). Studies to date have shown malignant melanoma, kidney carcinoma, large bowel carcinomas, brain tumors and metastases to the central nervous system not to be significantly responsive to ADRIAMYCIN therapy.

CONTRAINDICATIONS:
- Patients who are hypersensitive to this drug or to any ingredient in the formulation or component of the container. For a complete listing, see Dosage Forms, Composition and Packaging.
- Hypersensitivity to doxorubicin or any other component of the product, other anthracyclines or anthracenediones such as PHARMORUBICIN (epirubicin hydrochloride), daunorubicin hydrochloride, mitoxantrone or mitomycin C.
- Marked persistent myelosuppression induced by prior treatment with other antitumor agents or by radiotherapy;
- Severe hepatic impairment;
- Severe myocardial insufficiency;
- Recent myocardial infarction;
- Severe arrhythmias;
- History of severe cardiac disease;
- Previous treatment with maximum cumulative doses of doxorubicin, daunorubicin, epirubicin, idarubicin and/or other anthracyclines and anthracenediones (see Warnings and Precautions).

Contraindication for intravesical use:
- Hematuria;
- Urinary tract infections;
- Inflammation of the bladder.

WARNINGS AND PRECAUTIONS: Carcinogenesis and Mutagenesis and Impairment of Fertility: Secondary leukemia, with or without a preleukemic phase, has been reported in patients treated with topoisomerase-II inhibitors including the anthracyclines such as doxorubicin. Secondary leukemia is more common when anthracyclines are given in combination with DNA-damaging antineoplastic agents (0.5%) and/or in combination with radiotherapy (2.5 %) with a risk estimated at 1.5% at 10 years. Secondary leukemia can have a 1-3 year latency period, and can occur as late as 10 years following treatment.

Pediatric patients are also at risk of developing secondary AML.

Doxorubicin was genotoxic in a battery of in vitro or in vivo tests. An increase in the incidence of mammary tumors was reported in rats, and a trend for delay or arrest of follicular maturation was seen in female dogs.

In women, doxorubicin may cause infertility during the time of drug administration. Doxorubicin may cause amenorrhea. Ovulation and menstruation appear to return after termination of therapy, although premature menopause can occur.

Doxorubicin was toxic to male reproductive organs in animal studies, producing testicular atrophy, diffuse degeneration of the seminiferous tubules, and hypospermia.

Doxorubicin is mutagenic and can induce chromosomal damage in human spermatozoa. Oligospermia or azoospermia may be permanent; however, sperm counts have been reported to return to normospermic levels in some instances. This may occur several years after the end of therapy. Men undergoing doxorubicin treatment should use effective contraceptive methods.
Cardiovascular: Acute life-threatening arrhythmias have been reported to occur during or within a few hours after ADRIAMYCIN (doxorubicin hydrochloride) administration (see Adverse Reactions).
Cardiac Function: Cardiotoxicity is a risk of anthracycline treatment that may be manifested by early (i.e., acute) or late (i.e., delayed) events.
Early (i.e., Acute) Events: Early cardiotoxicity of doxorubicin consists mainly of sinus tachycardia and/or ECG abnormalities such as non-specific ST-T wave changes.

Tachyarrhythmias, including premature ventricular contractions and ventricular tachycardia, bradycardia, and atrioventricular and bundle-branch block also have been reported. Those effects usually do not predict subsequent development of delayed cardiotoxicity, are rarely of clinical importance and generally do not necessitate discontinuation of doxorubicin treatment.
Late (i.e., Delayed) Events: Delayed cardiotoxicity usually develops late in the course of therapy with doxorubicin or within 2 to 3 months after treatment termination, but later events, several months to years after completion of treatment, have also been reported. Delayed cardiomyopathy is manifested by reduced left ventricular ejection fraction (LVEF) and/or signs and symptoms of congestive heart failure (CHF) such as dyspnea, pulmonary edema, dependent edema, cardiomegaly and hepatomegaly, oliguria, ascites, pleural effusion and gallop rhythm. Subacute effects such as pericarditis/myocarditis also have been reported. Life-threatening CHF is the most severe form of anthracycline-induced cardiomyopathy and is the cumulative dose-limiting toxicity of anthracycline drugs.

The probability of developing CHF, estimated around 1% to 2% at a cumulative dose of 300 mg/m², slowly increases up to the total cumulative dose of 450-550 mg/m². Thereafter, the risk of developing CHF increases steeply (3 to 5% at 400 mg/m²; 5 to 8% at 450 mg/m², and 6 to 20% at 500 mg/m²). **It is recommended not to exceed a maximum cumulative dose of 550 mg/m² of ADRIAMYCIN.**

The total dose of ADRIAMYCIN administered to a patient should take into account: prior therapy with related compounds such as epirubicin and daunorubicin or anthracene derivatives; and/or radiotherapy to the mediastinal area.

Risk factors for cardiac toxicity include active or dormant cardiovascular disease, prior or concomitant radiotherapy to the mediastinal/pericardial area, previous therapy with other anthracyclines or anthracenediones, and concomitant use of drugs with the ability to suppress cardiac contractility or cardiotoxic drugs. Anthracyclines including doxorubicin should not be administered in combination with other cardiotoxic agents unless the patient's cardiac function is closely monitored.

Patients receiving anthracyclines after stopping treatment with other cardiotoxic agents, especially those with long half-lives such as trastuzumab, may also be at an increased risk of developing cardiotoxicity. The half-life of trastuzumab is approximately 28.5 days and may persist in the circulation for up to 24 weeks. Therefore, physicians should avoid anthracycline-based therapy for up to 24 weeks after stopping trastuzumab when possible. If anthracyclines are used before this time, careful monitoring of cardiac function is recommended.

Cardiac function must be carefully monitored in patients receiving high cumulative doses and in those with risk factors. While cardiotoxicity with doxorubicin may occur at lower cumulative doses whether or not cardiac risk factors are present, it may be more likely to occur at lower cumulative doses in patients with these risk factors.

New studies show that children and adolescents are at an increased risk for developing delayed cardiotoxicity following doxorubicin administration (up to 15 years). Females may be at greater risk than males. Follow-up cardiac evaluations such as ECHO LVEF/MUGA are recommended periodically to monitor for this effect (see Monitoring and Laboratory Tests).
Vascular Effects: Phlebosclerosis may result from an injection into a small vessel or from repeated injections into the same vein. Following the recommended administration procedures may minimize the risk of phlebitis/thrombophlebitis at the injection site (see Dosage and Administration). As with other cytotoxic agents, thrombophlebitis and thromboembolic phenomena, including pulmonary embolism (in some cases fatal), have been coincidentally reported with the use of doxorubicin.
Extravasation: Extravasation of doxorubicin during intravenous injection may produce local pain, severe tissue lesions (vesication, severe cellulitis) and necrosis. If any signs or symptoms of extravasation have occurred, the injection or infusion should be immediately stopped.
Immunosuppressant Effects/Increased Susceptibility to Infections: Administration of live or live-attenuated vaccines in patients immunocompromised by chemotherapeutic agents including doxorubicin, may result in serious or fatal infections. Vaccination with a live vaccine should be avoided in patients receiving doxorubicin. Killed or inactivated vaccines may be administered; however, the response to such vaccines may be diminished.
Gastrointestinal: Doxorubicin is emetogenic. Mucositis/stomatitis generally appears early after drug administration and, if severe, may progress over a few days to mucosal ulcerations. Most patients recover from this adverse event by the third week of therapy.

Necrotizing colitis manifested by typhlitis (cecal inflammation), bloody stools and severe, sometimes fatal, infections have been associated with a combination of ADRIAMYCIN given by IV push daily for 3 days and cytarabine given by continuous infusion daily for 7 or more days.
Genitourinary: ADRIAMYCIN PFS may impart a red coloration to the urine for 1 to 2 days after administration and patients should be advised to expect this during active therapy.
Hematologic: As with other cytotoxic agents, doxorubicin may produce myelosuppression. Hematologic profiles should be assessed before and during each cycle of therapy with doxorubicin, including differential white blood cell (WBC) counts. A dose-dependent, reversible leukopenia and/or granulocytopenia (neutropenia) is the predominant manifestation of doxorubicin hematologic toxicity and is the most common acute dose-limiting toxicity of this drug. Leukopenia and neutropenia generally reach the nadir between days 10 and 14 after drug administration; the WBC/neutrophil counts return to normal values in most cases by day 21. Thrombocytopenia and anemia may also occur. Clinical consequences of severe myelosuppression include fever, infections, sepsis/septicemia, septic shock, hemorrhage, tissue hypoxia, or death. Hematologic toxicity may require dose reduction or suspension or delay of ADRIAMYCIN therapy. Persistent severe myelosuppression may result in superinfection or hemorrhage. Secondary leukemia, with or without a preleukemic phase, has been reported in patients treated with anthracyclines (including doxorubicin, see Warnings and Precautions). Acute myeloblastic leukemia (AML) also occurs in children.
Hepatic/Biliary/Pancreatic: Doxorubicin is extensively metabolized by the liver and its major route of elimination is the hepatobiliary system. Toxicity to recommended doses of ADRIAMYCIN is enhanced by hepatic impairment, therefore prior to the individual dosing and during treatment, evaluation of hepatic function is recommended using conventional clinical laboratory

tests such as AST, ALT, alkaline phosphatase and bilirubin. Patients with elevated bilirubin may experience slower clearance of doxorubicin with an increase in overall toxicity. Lower doses of doxorubicin are recommended in these patients (see Dosage and Administration). Patients with severe hepatic impairment should not receive doxorubicin (see Contraindications).

Toxicities with Co-administration of Antineoplastic Agents: ADRIAMYCIN may potentiate the toxicity of other anticancer therapies. Exacerbation of cyclophosphamide induced hemorrhagic cystitis and enhancement of the hepatotoxicity of 6-mercaptopurine have been reported. Radiation-induced toxicity to the myocardium, mucosae, skin and liver has been reported to be increased by the administration of ADRIAMYCIN.

Patients should recover from acute toxicities of prior cytotoxic treatment (such as stomatitis, neutropenia, thrombocytopenia, and generalized infections) before beginning treatment with doxorubicin.

Additional Warnings and Precautions for Other Routes of Administration: Intravesical Route of Administration: Administration of doxorubicin by the intravesical route may produce symptoms of chemical cystitis (such as dysuria, polyuria, nocturia, stranguria, hematuria, bladder discomfort, necrosis of the bladder wall) and bladder constriction. Special attention is required for catheterization problems (e.g., uretheral obstruction due to massive intravesical tumors).

Special Populations: Pregnant Women: The embryotoxic potential of doxorubicin was confirmed in vitro and in vivo. When given to female rats before and during mating, pregnancy, and lactation, doxorubicin was toxic to both dams and fetuses.

Doxorubicin has been implicated in causing fetal harm when administered to a pregnant woman. If a woman receives doxorubicin during pregnancy or becomes pregnant while taking the drug, she should be informed of the potential hazard to the fetus.

Nursing Women: Doxorubicin is secreted into breast milk. Mothers should not breast-feed while undergoing chemotherapy with ADRIAMYCIN.

Pediatrics: Pediatric population is at a higher risk of Secondary Leukemia (AML included). Early and delayed cardiotoxicities have been described in children. On long-term follow-up, subclinical cardiac dysfunction may occur in over 20% of pediatric patients and 5% may develop congestive heart failure. This long-term cardiotoxicity may be related to the dose of doxorubicin.

Monitoring and Laboratory Tests: Initial treatment with ADRIAMYCIN PFS requires close observation of the patient and extensive laboratory monitoring. Like other cytotoxic drugs, ADRIAMYCIN PFS may induce hyperuricemia secondary to rapid lysis of neoplastic cells, particularly in patients with leukemia. The clinician should monitor the patient's serum chemistry and blood uric acid level and be prepared to use such supportive and pharmacologic measures as might be necessary to control this problem. Hydration, urine alkalinization and allopurinol administration will help to prevent or minimize potential complications of tumor-lysis syndrome.

The systemic clearance of doxorubicin has been found to be reduced in obese patients (i.e., >130% ideal body weight; see Dosage and Administration, Other Special Populations).

Cardiac function should be assessed before patients undergo treatment with doxorubicin and must be monitored throughout therapy to minimize the risk of incurring severe cardiac impairment. The risk may be decreased through regular monitoring of LVEF during the course of treatment with prompt discontinuation of doxorubicin at the first sign of impaired function. The appropriate quantitative method for repeated assessment of cardiac function (evaluation of LVEF) includes multi-gated radionuclide angiography (MUGA) or echocardiography (ECHO). A baseline cardiac evaluation with an ECG and either a MUGA scan or an ECHO is recommended, especially in patients with risk factors for increased cardiotoxicity. Repeated MUGA or ECHO determinations of LVEF should be performed, particularly with higher cumulative anthracycline doses (e.g. ≥450 mg/m²). The technique used for assessment should be consistent throughout follow-up.

ADRIAMYCIN PFS is not an anti-microbial agent.

ADVERSE REACTIONS: Adverse Drug Reaction Overview: The following adverse events have been reported in association with ADRIAMYCIN (doxorubicin hydrochloride) therapy:

Cardiovascular: sinus tachycardia, ECG abnormalities, tachyarrhythmias, atrio-ventricular and bundle branch block, asymptomatic reductions in left ventricular ejection fraction (LVEF), congestive heart failure, acute life-threatening arrhythmias during or within few hours after ADRIAMYCIN administration (see Warnings and Precautions, Cardiovascular: Maximum Cumulative Dose [550 mg/m²]).

Hematologic: leukopenia, neutropenia, anemia, thrombocytopenia, hemorrhage.

Gastrointestinal: anorexia, nausea/vomiting, dehydration, mucositis/stomatitis, hyperpigmentation of the oral mucosa, esophagitis, abdominal pain, gastric erosions, gastrointestinal tract bleeding, diarrhea, colitis.

Liver: changes in transaminase levels, hyperuricemia.

Endocrine: amenorrhea, hot flashes, oligospermia, azoospermia, weight gain.

Ocular: conjunctivitis/keratitis, lacrimation.

Skin: alopecia, local toxicity, rash/itch, skin changes, severe local tissue necrosis with intravenous injection, extravasation may occur, skin and nail hyperpigmentation, photosensitivity, hypersensitivity to irradiated skin ("radiation recall reaction"), urticaria, acral erythema, palmar plantar erythrodysesthesia.

Vascular: phlebitis, thrombophlebitis, thromboembolism.

Urological: red coloration of urine for 1 to 2 days after administration.

Bladder, local: pain, hemorrhage, and occasionally decreased bladder capacity upon instillation.

Local: severe cellulitis, vesication, tissue necrosis upon extravasation, erythematous streaking along the vein proximal to the site of the injection (see Dosage and Administration).

Other: anaphylaxis, infection, sepsis/septicemia, acute lymphocytic leukemia, acute myelogenous leukemia, malaise/asthenia, fever, chills, shock, cross sensitivity to lincomycin.

DRUG INTERACTIONS: ADRIAMYCIN (doxorubicin hydrochloride) is mainly used in combination with other cytotoxic drugs. Additive toxicity may occur especially with regard to bone marrow/hematologic and gastrointestinal effects (see Warnings and Precautions). The use of doxorubicin in combination chemotherapy with other potentially cardiotoxic drugs, as well as the concomitant use of other cardioactive compounds (e.g., calcium channel blockers), requires monitoring of cardiac function throughout treatment. Changes in hepatic function induced by concomitant therapies may affect doxorubicin metabolism, pharmacokinetics, therapeutic efficacy and/or toxicity.

Literature reports have also described the following drug interactions:

- Paclitaxel can cause increased plasma-concentrations of doxorubicin and/or its metabolites when given prior to doxorubicin. The pharmacokinetic drug interaction is dependent on the administration schedule, dose, sequence, infusion duration and time interval between administration. Certain data indicate that this effect is minor when this anthracycline is administrated prior to paclitaxel;
- Phenobarbital increases elimination of doxorubicin;
- Phenytoin levels may be decreased by doxorubicin;
- Streptozocin may inhibit hepatic metabolism of doxorubicin;
- Exacerbation of cyclophosphamide induced hemorrhagic cystitis;
- Enhancement of the hepatotoxicity of 6-mercaptopurine;
- Concomitant actinomycin-D therapy produces "recall" acute pneumonitis at variable times after local radiation therapy, in pediatric populations.
- Increases in the AUC of doxorubicin as high as 47% were observed in concomitant treatments with sorafenib 400 mg twice daily. The clinical significance of these findings is unknown. Adriamycin and sorafenib are not indicated for use in combination.

DOSAGE AND ADMINISTRATION: Refer to Special Handling Instructions.

Dosing Considerations: A variety of dose schedules has been used. The following recommendations are for use as a single agent only.

Intravenous (IV) Administration: The total ADRIAMYCIN (doxorubicin hydrochloride) dose per cycle may differ according to its use within a specific treatment regimen (e.g., given as a single agent or in combination with other cytotoxic drugs) and according to the indication.

The most commonly used dosage schedule is 60-75 mg/m² as a single intravenous injection administered at 21-day intervals. An alternative dose schedule is weekly doses of 20 mg/m², which has been reported to produce a lower incidence of congestive heart failure. A dose of 30 mg/m² on each of 3 successive days repeated every 4 weeks has also been used.

Hepatic Dysfunction: ADRIAMYCIN dosage must be reduced if the bilirubin is elevated as follows: Serum Bilirubin 1.2-3.0 mg/dL—give ½ of recommended starting dose, >3 mg/dL—give ¼ of recommended starting dose. Doxorubicin should not be administered to patients with severe hepatic impairment (see Contraindications).

Other Special Populations: Lower starting doses or longer intervals between cycles may need to be considered for heavily pretreated patients, children, elderly patients, obese patients, or patients with neoplastic bone marrow infiltration (see Warnings and Precautions).

Intravesical Administration: Intravesical administration is not suitable for the treatment of invasive tumors that have penetrated the muscular layer of the bladder wall. When ADRIAMYCIN PFS is instilled intravesically for the treatment of superficial bladder carcinomas, the usual dose employed ranges from 50-80 mg in a total volume of 50-100 mL of 0.9% Sodium Chloride Solution USP with a contact time of 1-2 hours. Care should be taken to ensure that the tip of the catheter is in the bladder cavity before instilling the ADRIAMYCIN solution. Instillation is repeated weekly for 4 weeks, and subsequently at monthly intervals. Therapy may continue for 1 year or longer as no significant systemic toxicity has been reported. Care should be exercised in the handling and disposal of the voided urine (refer to Special Handling Instructions). PVC gloves should be worn and the urine should be inactivated by decolorizing it with 10 mL or more of sodium hypochlorite solution (household bleach).

Other methods of administration have been investigated, including intra-arterial administration and also continuous or long-term intravenous infusion utilizing appropriate infusion pumps.

Clinical studies support the efficacy of ADRIAMYCIN used concurrently with other chemotherapeutic agents. Listed below are tumor types and drugs used concurrently with ADRIAMYCIN:

Acute lymphocytic leukemia in adults: ADRIAMYCIN with vincristine and prednisone or with cytosine arabinoside, vincristine and prednisone.

Acute lymphocytic leukemia in children: ADRIAMYCIN with L-asparaginase, vincristine and prednisone.

Acute non-lymphocytic leukemia: ADRIAMYCIN with cytosine arabinosyl or with arabinosyl cytosine, vincristine and prednisone.

Carcinoma of the breast: ADRIAMYCIN in treating early or advanced breast cancer in combination with 5-fluorouracil and/or cyclophosphamide or with vincristine with or without cyclophosphamide, or with taxane therapy.

Bronchogenic carcinoma, non-small cell: ADRIAMYCIN with cyclophosphamide, methotrexate and procarbazine or with cyclophosphamide and cisplatinum.

Bronchogenic carcinoma, small cell: ADRIAMYCIN with vincristine or etoposide (VP-16) and cyclophosphamide.

Hodgkin's disease: ADRIAMYCIN with bleomycin, vincristine and dacarbazine.

Non-Hodgkin's lymphoma: ADRIAMYCIN with cyclophosphamide, vincristine and prednisone, or bleomycin, cyclophosphamide, vincristine and prednisone.

Carcinoma of the ovary: ADRIAMYCIN with cisplatinum.

Soft tissue sarcoma: ADRIAMYCIN with dacarbazine, or with dacarbazine, cyclophosphamide and vincristine.

Carcinoma of the bladder: ADRIAMYCIN with methotrexate, vinblastine and cisplatinum or cisplatinum and cyclophosphamide or with 5-fluorouracil.

Carcinoma of the stomach: ADRIAMYCIN with 5-fluorouracil and mitomycin-C.

Administration: Intravenous (IV) Administration: Care in the administration of ADRIAMYCIN PFS will reduce the chance of perivenous infiltration. It may also decrease the chance of local reactions such as urticaria and erythematous streaking. On intravenous administration of ADRIAMYCIN PFS, extravasation may occur with or without an accompanying stinging or burning sensation even if the blood returns well on aspiration of the infusion needle. If any signs or symptoms of extravasation have occurred, the injection or infusion should be immediately terminated and restarted in another vein.

If it is known or suspected that subcutaneous extravasation has occurred, the following steps are recommended:

1. Attempt aspiration of the infiltrated ADRIAMYCIN solution.
2. Local intermittent application of ice for up to 3 days.
3. Elevation of the affected limb.
4. Close observation of the lesion.
5. Consultation with a plastic surgeon familiar with drug extravasations if local pain persists or skin changes progress after 3 to 4 days. If ulceration begins, early wide excision of the involved area should be considered.

ADRIAMYCIN PFS should be slowly administered into the tubing of a freely running intravenous infusion of Sodium Chloride Solution USP (0.9%) or 5% Dextrose Solution USP. The tubing should be attached to a Butterfly needle, or other suitable device and inserted preferably into a large vein. If possible, avoid veins over joints or in extremities with compromised venous or lymphatic drainage. The rate of administration is dependent on the size of the vein and the dosage, however, the dosage should be administered for not less than 3 minutes and not more than 10 minutes to minimize the risk of thrombosis or perivenous extravasation. Local erythematous streaking along the vein as well as facial flushing may be indicative of too rapid administration. A direct push injection is not recommended due to the risk of extravasation, which may occur even in the presence of adequate blood return upon needle aspiration (see Warnings and Precautions).

Unless specific compatibility data are available, the mixing of ADRIAMYCIN solutions with other drugs is not recommended. Precipitation occurs with 5-fluorouracil and heparin.

Intravesical Administration: Doxorubicin should be instilled using a catheter and retained intravesically for 1 to 2 hours. Care should be taken to ensure that the tip of the catheter is in the bladder cavity before instilling the ADRIAMYCIN solution. During instillation, the patient should be rotated to ensure that the vesical mucosa of the pelvis receives the most extensive contact with the solution. To avoid dilution with urine, the patient should be instructed not to drink any fluid in the 12 hours prior to instillation. The patient should be instructed to void at the end of the instillation.

OVERDOSAGE:

Acute overdosage with ADRIAMYCIN PFS (doxorubicin hydrochloride) enhances the toxic effects of mucositis, leukopenia and thrombocytopenia. Treatment of acute overdosage consists of treatment of the severely myelosuppressed patient with hospitalization, antibiotics, platelet and granulocyte transfusions and symptomatic treatment of mucositis.

Chronic overdosage with cumulative doses exceeding 550 mg/m² increases the risk of cardiomyopathy and resultant congestive heart failure. Treatment consists of vigorous management of congestive heart failure with digitalis preparations and diuretics. The use of peripheral vasodilators has been recommended.

For management of a suspected drug overdose, CPhA recommends that you contact your **regional Poison Control Centre**. See the *CPS* Directory section for a list of Poison Control Centres.

ACTION AND CLINICAL PHARMACOLOGY: Mechanism of Action: Though not completely elucidated, the mechanism of action of doxorubicin is related to its ability to bind to DNA and inhibit nucleic acid synthesis.

Pharmacodynamics: Cell culture studies have demonstrated rapid cell penetration and perinucleolar chromatin binding, rapid inhibition of mitotic activity and nucleic acid synthesis, mutagenesis and chromosomal aberrations. Animal studies have shown activity in a wide spectrum of experimental tumors, immunosuppression, carcinogenic properties in rodents, induction of a variety of toxic effects, including delayed and progressive cardiac toxicity, myelosuppression in all species and atrophy of testes in rats and dogs.

Pharmacokinetics: Pharmacokinetic studies show that the intravenous administration of normal or radiolabelled ADRIAMYCIN (doxorubicin hydrochloride) for injection is followed by rapid plasma clearance and significant tissue binding. Urinary excretion, as determined by fluorimetric methods, accounts for approximately 4-5% of the administered dose in 5 days. Biliary excretion represents the major excretion route, 40-50% of the administered dose being recovered in the bile or the feces in 7 days. Impairment of liver function results in slower excretion, and consequently, increased retention and accumulation in plasma and tissues. Doxorubicin does not cross the blood brain barrier.

STORAGE AND STABILITY: Store under refrigeration (2-8°C), protect from light and retain in carton until time of use. Discard unused solution.

Storage of the solution for injection at refrigerated conditions can result in the formation of a gelled product. This gelled product will likely return to a slightly viscous to a mobile solution after 2 hours to a maximum of 4 hours equilibration at controlled room temperature (15-25°C).

Dispensing from the Pharmacy Bulk Vial should be completed within 8 hours of initial entry because of the potential for microbial contamination. The contents of the syringes filled from the Pharmacy Bulk Vial should be used within 24 hours at room temperature or 48 hours when refrigerated **from the time of the initial entry into the Pharmacy Bulk Vial**.

SPECIAL HANDLING INSTRUCTIONS: Preparation and Handling:

1. Personnel should be trained in good techniques for reconstitution and handling. Pregnant staff should be excluded from working with this drug.
2. Preparation of antineoplastic solutions should be done in a vertical laminar flow hood (Biological Safety Cabinet-Class II). The work surface should be protected by disposable, plastic-backed absorbent paper.
3. Personnel handling ADRIAMYCIN (doxorubicin hydrochloride) solutions should wear PVC gloves, safety glasses and protective clothing such as disposable gowns and masks. If ADRIAMYCIN contacts the skin or mucosa, the area should be washed with soap and water or sodium bicarbonate immediately. Do not abrade the skin by using a scrub brush and always wash hands after removing gloves.
4. In case of contact with the eye(s), hold back the eyelid of the affected eye(s) and flush with copious amounts of water for at least 15 minutes; proceed to a physician for medical evaluation.
5. Personnel regularly involved in the preparation and handling of antineoplastics should have blood examinations on a regular basis.
6. **Directions for Dispensing from Pharmacy Bulk Vial:** The use of Pharmacy Bulk Vials is restricted to hospitals with a recognized intravenous admixture program. The Pharmacy Bulk Vial is intended for single puncture, multiple dispensing and for intravenous use only.

Entry into the vial must be made with a suitable, sterile transfer or dispensing device. Multiple use of a syringe with needle is not recommended since it may cause leakage as well as increasing the potential for microbial and particulate contamination.

In a suitable work area such as a laminar flow hood, swab the vial stopper with an antiseptic solution. Insert the device into the vial. Withdraw contents of the vial into sterile syringes using strict aseptic techniques. Dispensing from the Pharmacy Bulk Vial should be completed within 8 hours of the **initial entry** because of the potential for microbial contamination. Discard any unused portion. The contents of the syringes filled from the Pharmacy Bulk Vial should be used within 24 hours at room temperature or 48 hours when refrigerated **from the time of the initial entry into the Pharmacy Bulk Vial**.

Disposal:

1. Avoid contact with skin and inhalation of airborne particles by use of PVC gloves and disposable gowns and masks.
2. All needles, syringes, vials and other materials which have come in contact with doxorubicin should be segregated in plastic bags, sealed, and marked as hazardous waste. Incinerate at 1000°C or higher. Sealed containers may explode if a tight seal exists.
3. If incineration is not available, ADRIAMYCIN may be detoxified by adding sodium hypochlorite solution (household bleach) to the vial, in sufficient quantity to decolorize the doxorubicin, care being taken to vent the vial to avoid a pressure build-up of the chlorine gas which is generated. Dispose of detoxified vials in a safe manner.

Needles, Syringes, Disposable and Non-disposable Equipment: Rinse equipment with an appropriate quantity of sodium hypochlorite solution. Discard the solution in the sewer system with running water and discard disposable equipment in a safe manner. Thoroughly wash non-disposable equipment in soap and water.

Spillage/Contamination: Wear gloves, mask, and protective clothing. Treat spilled powder or liquid with dilute sodium hypochlorite solution (1% available chlorine). Carefully absorb solution with gauze pads or towels, wash area with water and absorb with gauze or towels again and place in polyethylene bag; seal, double bag and mark as hazardous waste. Dispose of waste by incineration or by other methods approved for hazardous materials. Personnel involved in clean-up should wash with soap and water.

INFORMATION FOR THE PATIENT: Published in e-CPS, available by subscription at www.e-cps.ca.

DOSAGE FORMS, COMPOSITION AND PACKAGING: Vials: 10 mg: Each single-dose vial of sterile, isotonic, nonpreserved solution contains: doxorubicin HCl USP 10 mg, sodium chloride USP 45 mg, water for injection USP and hydrochloric acid USP for pH adjustment. Glass vials or polypropylene vials of 5 mL, cartons of a single vial.

50 mg: Each single-dose vial of sterile, isotonic, nonpreserved solution contains: doxorubicin HCl USP 50 mg, sodium chloride USP 225 mg, water for injection USP and hydrochloric acid USP for pH adjustment. Glass vials or polypropylene vials of 25 mL, cartons of a single vial.

Pharmacy Bulk Vials (200 mg): Each vial of sterile, isotonic, nonpreserved solution contains: doxorubicin HCl USP 200 mg, sodium chloride USP 900 mg, water for injection USP and hydrochloric acid USP for pH adjustment. Pharmacy bulk glass vials or polypropylene vials of 100 mL, cartons of a single vial.

Note: The use of pharmacy bulk vials is restricted to hospitals with a recognized intravenous admixture program. The pharmacy bulk vial is intended for single puncture, multiple dispensing and for intravenous use only.

Incompatibility: Unless specific compatibility data are available, ADRIAMYCIN PFS should not be mixed with other drugs. Contact with alkaline solutions should be avoided since this can lead to hydrolysis of doxorubicin. Doxorubicin should not be mixed with heparin due to chemical incompatibility that may lead to precipitation. Precipitation also occurs with 5-fluorouracil.

Advagraf® ℞

tacrolimus

Immunosuppressant

Astellas

Date of Preparation: June 13, 2007
Date of Revision: August 10, 2009

SUMMARY PRODUCT INFORMATION:

Route of Administration	Dosage Form/ Strength	Clinically Relevant Nonmedicinal Ingredients
Oral	0.5 mg, 1 mg and 5 mg capsules	Lactose For a complete listing see Dosage Forms, Composition and Packaging.

INDICATIONS AND CLINICAL USE: Advagraf (tacrolimus extended release capsules) is indicated for prophylaxis of organ rejection in adult patients receiving allogeneic kidney transplants.

Advagraf is to be used concomitantly with adrenal corticosteroids and mycophenolate mofetil (MMF) in de novo renal transplant recipients. Antibody induction therapy should also be used in kidney transplant recipients.

Stable renal transplant patients may be converted from Prograf (twice daily) to Advagraf (once daily), in combination with adrenal corticosteroids and MMF, based on equivalent tacrolimus blood concentrations. Any changes in immunosuppressive therapy must be initiated by physicians experienced in immunosuppressive therapy and the management of transplant patients.

Geriatrics (≥65 years of age): Experience with Advagraf in patients older than 65 years of age is limited.

Pediatrics (<18 years of age): Experience with Advagraf in pediatric kidney transplant patients is limited.

CONTRAINDICATIONS: Advagraf (tacrolimus extended release capsules) is contraindicated in patients with hypersensitivity to tacrolimus or to any ingredient in the formulation or component of the capsules. For a complete listing, see Dosage Forms, Composition and Packaging.

WARNINGS AND PRECAUTIONS:

Serious Warnings and Precautions

- **Increased susceptibility to infection and the possible development of lymphoma may result from immunosuppression (see Warnings and Precautions, Carcinogenesis and Mutagenesis, and Immune/Infection).**
- **Only physicians experienced in immunosuppressive therapy and management of organ transplant should prescribe Advagraf (tacrolimus extended release capsules). Patients receiving the drug should be managed in facilities equipped and staffed with adequate laboratory and supportive medical resources. The physician responsible for maintenance therapy should have complete information requisite for the follow-up of the patient.**

General: Medication errors, including inadvertent, unintentional or unsupervised substitution of Prograf (immediate-release)—or Advagraf (extended-release) tacrolimus formulations, have been observed. This has led to serious adverse events, including graft rejection, or other side effects which could be a consequence of either under- or over-exposure to tacrolimus. Patients should be maintained on a single formulation of tacrolimus with the corresponding daily dosing regimen; alterations in formulation or regimen should only take place under the close supervision of a transplant specialist.

In de novo kidney transplant patients AUC_{0-24} of tacrolimus for Advagraf (extended-release formulation) on day 1 is significantly lower in comparison with that for Prograf (immediate-release formulation) at equivalent doses. By day 3, tacrolimus exposure as measured by trough levels is similar for both formulations. All patients in the clinical studies received antibody induction therapy. Advagraf is only approved to be used in combination with adrenal corticosteroids and MMF.

In clinical studies for stable patients converted from Prograf (immediate-release formulation) to Advagraf (extended-release formulation) on 1:1 (mg:mg) total daily dose basis, approximately one-third of patients required dose adjustment after conversion during the early conversion period due to dosing errors, adverse events, or levels outside the target range. Tacrolimus blood trough levels should be measured and closely monitored prior to and after conversion. Conversion to Advagraf (extended-release formulation) has primarily been studied from Prograf (immediate-release formulation) in combination with adrenal corticosteroids and MMF based on equivalent tacrolimus blood concentrations.

Carcinogenesis and Mutagenesis: An increased incidence of malignancy is a recognized complication of immunosuppression in recipients of organ transplants. The most common forms of neoplasms are non-Hodgkin's lymphomas and carcinomas of the skin. As with other immunosuppressive therapies, the risk of developing lymphomas and other malignancies, particularly of the skin, may be higher in Advagraf recipients than in the normal, healthy population. This risk appears to be related to the intensity and duration of immunosuppression rather than to the use of any specific agent.

Lymphoproliferative disorders associated with Epstein-Barr Virus infection have been seen with tacrolimus. It has been reported that reduction or discontinuation of immunosuppression may cause the lesions to regress.

No evidence of genotoxicity was seen in bacterial (Salmonella and *E. coli*) or mammalian (Chinese hamster lung-derived cells) in vitro assays of mutagenicity, the in vitro CHO/HGPRT assay of mutagenicity, or in vivo clastogenicity assays performed in mice; tacrolimus did not cause unscheduled DNA synthesis in rodent hepatocytes.

Carcinogenicity studies were carried out in male and female rats and mice. In the 80-week mouse study and in the 104-week rat study no relationship of tumor incidence to tacrolimus dosage was found. The highest doses used in the mouse and rat studies were 0.8-2.5 times (mice) and 3.5-7.1 times (rats) the recommended clinical dose range when corrected for body surface area.

Cardiovascular: Heart failure, myocardial hypertrophy and arrhythmia have been reported in association with the administration of Prograf (immediate-release formulation).

Hypertension is a common adverse effect of tacrolimus therapy (see Adverse Reactions). Mild or moderate hypertension is more frequently reported than severe hypertension. Antihypertensive therapy may be required; the control of blood pressure can be accomplished with any of the common antihypertensive agents. Since tacrolimus may cause hyperkalemia, potassium-sparing diuretics should be avoided. Tacrolimus should be discontinued in patients in whom hypertension and hyperkalemia cannot be controlled.

While calcium-channel blocking agents can be effective in treating tacrolimus-associated hypertension, care should be taken since interference with tacrolimus metabolism may require a dosage reduction (see Drug Interactions).

Myocardial hypertrophy has been reported in association with the administration of tacrolimus as Prograf (immediate-release formulation), and is generally manifested by echocardiographically demonstrated concentric increases in left ventricular posterior wall and interventricular septum thickness. Hypertrophy has been observed in infants, children and adults. This condition appears reversible in most cases following dose reduction or discontinuance of therapy. In a group of 20 patients with pre- and post-treatment echocardiograms who showed evidence of myocardial hypertrophy, mean tacrolimus whole blood concentrations during the period prior to diagnosis of myocardial hypertrophy ranged from 11 to 53 ng/mL in infants (n=10, age 0.4 to 2 years), 4 to 46 ng/mL in children (n=7, age 2 to 15 years) and 11 to 24 ng/mL in adults (n=3, age 37 to 53 years).

In patients who develop renal failure or clinical manifestations of ventricular dysfunction while receiving tacrolimus therapy, echocardiographic evaluation should be considered. If myocardial hypertrophy is diagnosed, dosage reduction or discontinuation of tacrolimus should be considered.

Hepatic/Biliary/Pancreatic: Tacrolimus has been associated with hyperglycemia and posttransplant diabetes mellitus. New onset glucose intolerance, defined as fasting plasma glucose ≥126 mg/dL, insulin use ≥30 days or oral hypoglycemic use, was determined in a 1-year prospective, comparative, phase III trial of Advagraf in de novo kidney transplant recipients (see Table 1 and Table 2).

Table 1: Advagraf

New Onset Glucose Intolerance in De Novo Kidney Transplant Recipients at 1 Year Posttransplant

	Advagraf (extended-release)/MMF (n=163)	Prograf (immediate-release)/MMF (n=150)	Neoral/MMF (n=152)
Fasting Plasma Glucose ≥126 mg/dL	56.4%	64.0%	52.6%
Insulin Use ≥30 Days	5.5%	6.0%	2.6%
Oral Hypoglycemic Use	14.1%	10.0%	3.3%

All regimens included corticosteroids. At risk population.

Table 2: Advagraf

New Onset Glucose Intolerance in De Novo Kidney Black Transplant Recipients at 1 Year Posttransplant

	Advagraf (extended-release)/MMF (n=35)	Prograf (immediate-release)/MMF (n=33)	Neoral/MMF (n=25)
Fasting Plasma Glucose ≥126 mg/dL	54.3%	54.5%	36.0%
Insulin Use ≥30 Days	8.6%	6.1%	4.0%
Oral Hypoglycemic Use	20.0%	12.1%	0

All regimens included corticosteroids. At risk population.

Immune/Infection: A lymphoproliferative disorder (LPD) related to Epstein-Barr Virus (EBV) infection has been reported in immunosuppressed organ transplant recipients. The risk of LPD appears greatest in young children who are at risk for primary EBV infection while immunosuppressed or who are switched to Advagraf following long-term immunosuppression therapy. Because of the danger of oversuppression of the immune system which can increase susceptibility to infection, combination immunosuppressant therapy other than corticosteroids and MMF is not recommended.

Immunosuppressed patients are at increased risk for opportunistic infections, including latent viral infections. These include BK virus associated nephropathy and JC virus associated progressive multifocal leukoencephalopathy (PML) which have been observed in patients receiving tacrolimus. These infections are often related to a high immunosuppressive burden and may lead to serious or fatal conditions that physicians should consider in the differential diagnosis in immunosuppressed patients with deteriorating renal function or neurological symptoms.

Neurologic: Tacrolimus can cause neurotoxicity, particularly when used in high doses.

Nervous system disorders, including tremor, headache, and other changes in motor function, mental status, and sensory function were reported in 63.1% of de novo kidney transplant recipients. Tremor occurred in 35.0% of Advagraf-treated kidney transplant patients compared to 19.8% of Neoral-treated kidney transplant patients. The incidence of other neurological events in kidney transplant patients was similar in the two treatment groups (see Adverse Reactions). Tremor and headache have been associated with high whole blood concentrations of tacrolimus and may respond to dosage adjustment. Seizures have occurred in adult and pediatric patients receiving tacrolimus as Prograf (immediate-release formulation). Coma and delirium also have been associated with high plasma concentrations of tacrolimus received as Prograf (immediate-release formulation).

Patients treated with tacrolimus have been reported to develop posterior reversible encephalopathy syndrome (PRES). Symptoms indicating PRES include headache, altered mental status, seizures, visual disturbances. Diagnosis should be confirmed by radiological procedure (e.g., MRI). If PRES is suspected or diagnosed, blood pressure and seizure control and immediate discontinuation of immunosuppression is advised. Most patients completely recover after appropriate measures are taken.

Renal: Tacrolimus can cause nephrotoxicity, particularly when used in high doses. Renal and urinary disorders were reported in 36.9% of de novo kidney transplantation patients receiving Advagraf. In de novo kidney transplant recipients, increased creatinine was reported in 18.7% of Advagraf-treated patients and 22.6% of Neoral-treated patients (see Adverse Reactions). More overt toxicity is seen early after transplantation, characterized by increasing serum creatinine and a decrease in urine output. Patients with impaired renal function should be monitored closely as the dosage of tacrolimus may need to be reduced. In patients with persistent elevations of serum creatinine who are unresponsive to dosage adjustments, consideration should be given to changing to another immunosuppressive therapy. Care should be taken in using tacrolimus with other nephrotoxic drugs. **In particular, to avoid excess nephrotoxicity, tacrolimus should not be used simultaneously with cyclosporine.**

Mild to severe hyperkalemia was reported in 22.0% of kidney de novo transplant recipients treated with Advagraf and may require treatment (see Adverse Reactions). **Serum potassium levels should be monitored and potassium-sparing diuretics should not be used during Advagraf therapy (see Warnings and Precautions, Cardiovascular and Monitoring and Laboratory Tests).**

Sexual Function/Reproduction: No impairment of fertility was demonstrated in studies of male and female rats. In reproduction studies in rats and rabbits, adverse effects on the fetus were observed mainly at dose levels that were toxic to dams. However, in female rats dosed during organogenesis, embryo toxicity (expressed as reduced pup weights) was seen at a dose which was one-third of the maternally toxic dose. At this same dose, when administered prior to mating and during gestation, tacrolimus was associated with adverse effects on female reproductive parameters and embryolethality. This dose was equivalent to 0.5× the clinical dose. (See Warnings and Precautions, Special Populations.)

Special Populations: Pregnant Women: There are no adequate and well-controlled studies in pregnant women. Tacrolimus is transferred across the placenta. The use of tacrolimus during pregnancy has been associated with neonatal hyperkalemia and renal dysfunction. Advagraf should be used during pregnancy only if the potential benefit to the mother justifies potential risk to the fetus.

Nursing Women: Since tacrolimus is excreted in human milk, nursing should be avoided.

Pediatrics (<18 years of age): Heart failure, cardiomegaly and increased thickness of the myocardium have been reported in patients taking tacrolimus.

Geriatrics (≥65 years of age): No formal studies have been performed to evaluate the effect of tacrolimus specifically in the geriatric population.

Forty-three patients have been treated with Advagraf in phase II and III studies in solid organs transplantation; there were no patient deaths or graft failures in these patients. Two of these 43 elderly patients experienced acute rejection. No overall differences in safety or effectiveness were observed between elderly patients and younger patients, but greater sensitivity of some older individuals cannot be ruled out. In general, dose selection for an elderly patient should be cautious, reflecting the greater frequency of decreased hepatic, renal, or cardiac function and of concomitant disease or other drug therapy.

Monitoring and Laboratory Tests: Serum creatinine, potassium, and fasting glucose should be assessed regularly. Routine monitoring of metabolic and hematologic systems should be performed as clinically warranted.

Blood Concentration Monitoring: Monitoring of tacrolimus blood levels in conjunction with other laboratory and clinical parameters is considered an essential aid to transplant patient management. During the immediate post-operative period trough blood concentrations should be measured every 1-3 days. In patients with hepatic or renal dysfunction or in those receiving or discontinuing concomitant interacting medications, more intensive monitoring may be required, since tacrolimus clearance may be affected under each of these circumstances. More frequent monitoring may also be required in patients early after transplantation since it is at this time patients experience the highest risk of rejection. Blood concentration monitoring is not a replacement for renal and liver function monitoring and tissue biopsies. Following discharge from the hospital, the frequency of patient monitoring will decrease with time post-transplant.

Methods commonly used for the assay of tacrolimus include high performance liquid chromatography with tandem mass spectrometric detection (HPLC/MS/MS), enzyme immunoassay (EIA), microparticle enzyme immunoassay (MEIA), and enzyme linked immunosorbent assay (ELISA). Comparison of the concentrations in published literature to patient concentrations using the current assays must be made with detailed knowledge of the assay methods and biological matrices employed. Whole blood is the matrix of choice and specimens should be collected into tubes containing ethylene diamine tetraacetic acid (EDTA) anti-coagulant. Heparin anti-coagulation is not recommended because of the tendency to form clots on storage. Samples which are not analyzed immediately should be stored at room temperature or in a refrigerator and assayed within 7 days; if samples are to be kept longer, they should be deep frozen at −20°C for up to 12 months.

Data from kidney transplant recipients receiving tacrolimus administered as Prograf (immediate-release formulation) indicate that trough concentrations of tacrolimus in whole blood, as measured by IMx MEIA (kidney), were most variable during the first week of dosing, and the relative risk of toxicity is increased with higher trough concentrations. Therefore, monitoring of whole blood trough concentrations is recommended to assist in the clinical evaluation of toxicity. Long-term posttransplant patients often are maintained at the low end of the recommended target range. For stable transplant recipients converted from Prograf (immediate-release formulation) to Advagraf (extended-release formulation), the same type of therapeutic monitoring can be used.

Data from the phase III Advagraf study indicate that trough concentrations of tacrolimus in whole blood were most variable during the first week of dosing. By month 2, 76% of the patients had trough concentrations between 7-16 ng/mL, and greater than 78% maintained concentrations between 5-15 ng/mL, from month 4 through 1 year.

ADVERSE REACTIONS: Adverse Drug Reaction Overview: The most common adverse reactions reported were infection, tremor, hypertension, decreased renal function, constipation, diarrhea, headache, abdominal pain and insomnia. Many of these adverse reactions were mild and responded to a reduction in dosage. Insulin-dependent post-transplant diabetes mellitus (PTDM) was related to increased whole blood trough concentrations of tacrolimus and higher doses of corticosteroids. The median time to onset of PTDM was 68 days.

Clinical Trial Adverse Drug Reactions: Because clinical trials are conducted under very specific conditions the adverse reaction rates observed in the clinical trials may not reflect the rates observed in practice and should not be compared to the rates in the clinical trials of another drug. Adverse drug reaction information from clinical trials is useful for identifying drug-related adverse events and for approximating rates.

In a large (n=668), phase III, randomized, comparative trial, de novo kidney transplant recipients received either Advagraf (extended-release formulation) plus mycophenolate mofetil (MMF) or Prograf (immediate-release formulation) plus MMF or Neoral plus MMF. All three regimens included corticosteroids and basiliximab induction. The incidence of adverse events that occurred in ≥15% of Advagraf-treated de novo kidney transplant recipients is shown in Table 3.

Table 3: Advagraf

De Novo Kidney Transplantation: Adverse Events Occurring in ≥15% of Advagraf (tacrolimus extended-release capsules) + MMF Treated Patients

	Prograf (immediate-release)+MMF N=212	Advagraf (extended-release)+MMF N=214	Neoral+MMF N=212
Gastrointestinal Disorders			
Diarrhea	44.3%	45.3%	25.5%
Nausea	38.7%	42.1%	46.7%
Constipation	35.8%	41.6%	41.0%
Vomiting	25.5%	26.2%	24.5%
Dyspepsia	17.9%	15.0%	15.1%
Injury, Poisoning and Procedural Complications			
Post Procedural Pain	28.8%	29.4%	27.4%
Incision Site Complication	28.3%	20.6%	23.1%
Metabolism and Nutritional Disorders			
Hypomagnesemia	28.3%	25.7%	22.2%
Hypophosphatemia	27.8%	23.8%	21.2%
Hyperkalemia	25.5%	22.0%	19.3%
Hyperglycemia	21.2%	19.2%	15.1%
Hyperlipidemia	17.5%	16.4%	24.5%
Hypokalemia	16.0%	15.9%	17.5%
Infections and Infestations			
Urinary Tract Infection	25.5%	15.9%	22.2%
General Disorders and Administration Site Conditions			
Edema Peripheral	34.9%	35.5%	45.8%
Fatigue	10.8%	15.9%	12.3%
Nervous System Disorders			
Tremor	34.4%	35.0%	19.8%
Headache	24.1%	21.5%	24.5%
Investigations			
Blood Creatinine Increased	23.1%	18.7%	22.6%
Blood and Lymphatic System Disorders			
Anemia	30.2%	33.6%	27.8%
Leukopenia	15.6%	16.4%	11.8%
Vascular Disorders			
Hypertension	32.1%	29.9%	34.9%
Musculoskeletal and Connective Tissue Disorders			
Back Pain	12.7%	15.0%	14.2%
Psychiatric Disorders			
Insomnia	30.2%	25.7%	21.2%

The following adverse events were also reported in clinical studies of solid organ transplant recipients who were treated with Advagraf at a frequency of ≥3% to <15%.

Cardiac Disorders: tachycardia.

Gastrointestinal Disorders: abdominal pain upper, flatulence.

General Disorders and Administration Site Conditions: asthenia, chest pain, edema, pyrexia, pain.

Infections and Infestations: cytomegalovirus infection, gastroenteritis, influenza, nasopharyngitis, sinusitis, upper respiratory tract infection.

Investigations: hepatic enzyme increased.

Metabolism and Nutrition Disorders: dehydration, diabetes mellitus, hypocalcemia, metabolic acidosis.

Musculoskeletal and Connective Tissue Disorders: arthralgia, muscle cramp, pain in extremity.

Nervous System Disorders: (see Warnings and Precautions): dizziness.

Psychiatric Disorders: anxiety, depression.

Skin and Subcutaneous Tissue Disorders: acne, pruritus.

Renal and Urinary Disorders: (see Warnings and Precautions): hematuria, renal impairment, renal insufficiency.

Respiratory, Thoracic and Mediastinal Disorders: cough, dyspnea, pharyngolaryngeal pain.

Vascular Disorders: hypotension.

Less Common Clinical Trial Adverse Drug Reactions (≥1% to <3%): The following adverse events were reported in clinical trials of solid organ transplant recipients treated with Advagraf at a frequency rate of ≥1% and <3%:

Blood and Lymphatic System Disorders: leukocytosis, neutropenia, polycythemia, thrombocytopenia.

Cardiac Disorders: atrial fibrillation.

Eye Disorders: vision blurred.

Gastrointestinal Disorders: abdominal discomfort, abdominal distension, abdominal pain lower, ascites, gastritis, gastroesophageal reflux disease, hemorrhoids, loose stools, oesophagitis, post procedural nausea, toothache.

General Disorders and Administration Site Conditions: anasarca, rigors.

Hepatobiliary Disorders: bile duct stenosis, cholestasis.

Infections and Infestations: bronchitis, cellulitis, Escherichia urinary tract infection, fungal infection, herpes simplex, herpes zoster, human polyomavirus infection, oral candidiasis, pharyngitis, pneumonia, pyelonephritis, sepsis, wound infection.

Injury, Poisoning, and Procedural Complications: complications of transplant surgery, contusion, incisional hernia, necrotic preservation injury of graft, post procedural discharge, therapeutic agent toxicity, wound dehiscence.

Investigations: blood glucose increased, blood magnesium decreased, blood phosphorus decreased, blood potassium decreased, cardiac murmur, liver function test abnormal, urine output decreased, weight decreased, weight increased.

Metabolism and Nutrition Disorders: acidosis, anorexia, diabetes mellitus non-insulin-dependant, dyslipidemia, fluid overload, gout, hypercalcemia, hypercholesterolemia, hyperhomocysteinemia, hyperphosphatemia, hyperuricemia, hypoalbuminemia, hypoglycemia, hyponatremia.

Musculoskeletal and Connective Tissue Disorders: myalgia, osteopenia, osteoporosis.

Nervous System Disorders: hypoesthesia, paraesthesia.

Psychiatric Disorders: agitation, confusional state.

Renal and Urinary Disorders: dysuria, oliguria, proteinuria, renal failure acute, urethral pain.

Reproductive System and Breast Disorders: erectile dysfunction.

Respiratory, Thoracic and Mediastinal Disorders: dyspnea exertional, epistaxis, nasal congestion, productive cough.

Skin and Subcutaneous Tissue Disorders: alopecia, ecchymosis, night sweats, rash, skin lesion.

Vascular Disorders: hematoma, hot flush, orthostatic hypotension.

Post-Market Adverse Drug Reactions: The following adverse events have been reported from worldwide marketing experience with tacrolimus (Advagraf [extended-release formulation] and/or Prograf [immediate-release formulation]). Because these events are reported voluntarily from a population of uncertain size, are associated with concomitant diseases and multiple drug therapies and surgical procedures, it is not always possible to reliably estimate their frequency or establish a causal relationship to drug exposure. Decisions to include these events in labeling are typically based on one or more of the following factors: (1) seriousness of the event, (2) frequency of the reporting, or (3) strength of causal connection to the drug:

Cardiovascular: atrial fibrillation, atrial flutter, cardiac arrhythmia, cardiac arrest, electrocardiogram t wave abnormal, flushing, myocardial infarction, myocardial ischaemia, pericardial effusion, QT prolongation with or without torsades de pointes, venous thrombosis deep limb, ventricular extrasystoles, ventricular fibrillation.

Gastrointestinal: bile duct stenosis, colitis, enterocolitis, gastroenteritis, gastroesophageal reflux disease, hepatic cytolysis, hepatic necrosis, hepatotoxicity, impaired gastric emptying, liver fatty, mouth ulceration, pancreatitis haemorrhagic, pancreatitis necrotizing, stomach ulcer, venoocclusive liver disease.
Hemic/Lymphatic: disseminated intravascular coagulation, neutropenia, pancytopenia, thrombocytopenic purpura, thrombotic thrombocytopenic purpura.
Infections and Infestations: JC virus associated progressive multifocal leukoencephalopathy (PML) and BK virus associated nephropathy.
Metabolic/Nutritional: glycosuria, increased amylase including pancreatitis, weight decreased.
Miscellaneous: feeling hot and cold, feeling jittery, hot flushes, multi-organ failure, primary graft dysfunction.
Nervous System: posterior reversible encephalopathy syndrome (PRES), carpal tunnel syndrome, cerebral infarction, hemiparesis, leukoencephalopathy, mental disorder, mutism, quadriplegia, speech disorder, syncope.
Respiratory: acute respiratory distress syndrome, interstitial lung disease, lung infiltration, respiratory distress, respiratory failure.
Skin: Stevens-Johnson syndrome, toxic epidermal necrolysis.
Special Senses: blindness, blindness cortical, hearing loss including deafness, photophobia.
Urogenital: albuminuria, acute renal failure, cystitis haemorrhagic, hemolytic-uremic syndrome, micturition disorder.

There have been rare spontaneous reports of myocardial hypertrophy associated with clinically manifested ventricular dysfunction in patients receiving Prograf (immediate-release formulation) therapy (see Warnings and Precautions).

There has been a report of pure red cell aplasia in a renal transplant recipient who was receiving tacrolimus. This condition was reversed upon termination of the administration of tacrolimus.

DRUG INTERACTIONS: Overview: Due to the potential for additive or synergistic impairment of renal function, care should be taken when administering Advagraf with drugs that may be associated with renal dysfunction. These include, but are not limited to, aminoglycosides, amphotericin B, and cisplatin. Initial clinical experience with the co-administration of Prograf (immediate-release formulation) and cyclosporine resulted in additive/synergistic nephrotoxicity.

Since tacrolimus is metabolized mainly by the CYP3A (cytochrome P450 IIIA) enzyme systems, substances known to inhibit these enzymes may decrease the metabolism or increase bioavailability of tacrolimus as indicated by increased whole blood or plasma concentrations. Drugs known to induce these enzyme systems may result in an increased metabolism of tacrolimus or decreased bioavailability as indicated by decreased whole blood or plasma concentrations. Monitoring of blood concentrations and appropriate dosage adjustments are essential when such drugs are used concomitantly.

Drug-Drug Interactions: In a study of 6 normal volunteers, a significant increase in tacrolimus (administered as Prograf [immediate-release formulation]) oral bioavailability (14±5% vs 30±8%) was observed with concomitant ketoconazole administration (200 mg). The apparent clearance of oral tacrolimus (administered as Prograf [immediate-release formulation]) during ketoconazole administration was significantly decreased compared to tacrolimus alone (0.430+0.129 L/hr/kg vs. 0.148+0.043 L/hr/kg). Overall, clearance of IV tacrolimus was not significantly changed by ketoconazole co-administration, although it was highly variable between patients.

In a single-dose crossover study in healthy volunteers, co-administration of tacrolimus (administered as Prograf [immediate-release formulation]) and magnesium-aluminium-hydroxide resulted in a 21% increase in the mean tacrolimus AUC and a 10% decrease in the mean tacrolimus C_{max} relative to tacrolimus administration alone.

Table 4: Advagraf

[a]Drugs That May Increase Tacrolimus Blood Concentrations

Antifungal Agents	Calcium Channel Blockers
clotrimazole fluconazole ketoconazole itraconazole voriconazole	diltiazem nicardipine nifedipine verapamil
Gastrointestinal Prokinetic Agents	**Macrolide Antibiotics**
cisapride[b] metoclopramide	erythromycin clarithromycin troleandomycin
Others	
bromocriptine cimetidine chloramphenicol cyclosporine danazol ethinyl estradiol	lansoprazole magnesium aluminum hydroxide methylprednisolone nefazodone omeprazole protease inhibitors

[a] This table is not all inclusive.
[b] Cisapride is no longer marketed in Canada.

In a study of 6 normal volunteers, a significant decrease in tacrolimus (administered as Prograf [immediate-release formulation]) oral bioavailability (14±6% vs 7±3%) was observed with concomitant rifampin administration (600 mg). In addition, there was a significant increase in tacrolimus clearance (0.036±0.008 L/hr/kg vs. 0.053±0.010 L/hr/kg) with concomitant rifampin administration. In a study of 9 normal volunteers, concomitantly administered 10 mL doses of aluminum hydroxide or milk of magnesia antacids did not affect the rate and extent of absorption of orally administered tacrolimus, as indicated by C_{max}, T_{max} and AUC_{0-t}.

Lansoprazole (CYP2C19, CYP3A4 substrate) may potentially inhibit CYP3A4-mediated metabolism of tacrolimus and thereby substantially increase tacrolimus whole blood concentrations, especially in transplant patients who are intermediate or poor CYP2C19 metabolizers, as compared to those patients who are efficient CYP2C19 metabolizers.

Following 14 days co-administration of tacrolimus (administered as Prograf [immediate-release formulation]) and sirolimus (2 mg/day or 5 mg/day) in stable renal transplant patients, tacrolimus AUC and C_{min} decreased approximately 30% relative to tacrolimus alone.

Based on a clinical study of 5 liver transplant recipients, co-administration of tacrolimus with nelfinavir increased blood concentrations of tacrolimus significantly.

Table 5: Advagraf

[a]Drugs That May Decrease Tacrolimus Blood Concentrations

Anticonvulsants	Antimicrobials
carbamazepine phenobarbital phenytoin	caspofungin rifabutin rifampin
Herbal Preparations	**Others**
St. John's wort	sirolimus

[a] This table is not all inclusive.

Immunosuppressants may affect vaccination. Therefore, during treatment with Advagraf, vaccination may be less effective. The use of live vaccines should be avoided; live vaccines may include, but are not limited to, measles, mumps, rubella, oral polio, BCG, yellow fever and TY 21a typhoid.

Tacrolimus may affect the pharmacokinetics of other drugs (e.g., phenytoin) and increase their concentration.

At a given mycophenolate mofetil (MMF) dose, mycophenolic acid (MPA) exposure is higher with tacrolimus (administered as Prograf [immediate-release formulation]) co-administration than with cyclosporine co-administration due to the inhibitory action of cyclosporine on biliary excretion of MPA-glucuronide by MRP-2 and the resulting reduction in enterohepatic recirculation of MPA. As a result, exposure to MPA when mycophenolate mofetil is given in combination with cyclosporine is approximately 30-40% lower than that observed when given alone or with tacrolimus. No effect on enterohepatic MPA-glucuronide recirculation is exerted by tacrolimus thus clinicians should be aware that there is a potential for increased MPA exposure after crossover from cyclosporine to tacrolimus in patients concomitantly receiving MMF or mycophenolate sodium (MPS). Conversely, there is a potential for decreased MPA exposure after crossover from tacrolimus to cyclosporine in patients concomitantly receiving MMF or MPS.

Drug-Food Interactions: Co-administered grapefruit juice has been reported to increase tacrolimus blood trough concentrations.

Drug-Herb Interactions: St. John's wort (Hypericum perforatum) induces CYP3A4 and P-glycoprotein. Since tacrolimus is a substrate for CYP3A4, there is the potential that the use of St. John's wort in patients receiving Advagraf could result in reduced tacrolimus levels.

Drug-Laboratory Test Interactions: Tacrolimus is not known to interfere with laboratory tests.

Drug-Lifestyle Interactions: As with other immunosuppressive agents, owing to the potential risk of malignant skin changes, exposure to sunlight and ultraviolet (UV) light should be limited by wearing protective clothing and using sunscreen with a high protection factor.

DOSAGE AND ADMINISTRATION: **Dosing Considerations:** Advagraf is a once-a-day oral formulation of tacrolimus. Advagraf therapy requires careful monitoring by adequately qualified and equipped personnel. The medicinal product should only be prescribed, and changes in immunosuppressive therapy initiated, by physicians experienced in immunosuppressive therapy and the management of transplant patients.

Inadvertent, unintentional or unsupervised switching of Prograf (immediate-release)—or Advagraf (extended-release) of tacrolimus is unsafe (see Warnings and Precautions, General). This can lead to graft rejection or increased incidence of side effects, including under- or overimmunosuppression, due to clinically relevant differences in systemic exposure to tacrolimus. Patients should be maintained on a single formulation of tacrolimus with the corresponding daily dosing regimen; alterations in formulation or regimen should only take place under the close supervision of a transplant specialist (see Dosage and Administration). Following conversion to any alternative formulation, therapeutic drug monitoring must be performed and dose adjustments made to ensure that systemic exposure to tacrolimus is maintained.

Patients converting from Prograf (immediate-release formulation) to Advagraf (extended-release formulation) should be administered a single daily morning dose of Advagraf equivalent to the patients' previous stable total daily dose of Prograf (immediate-release formulation). Subsequent doses of Advagraf should be adjusted in order to maintain trough concentrations similar to those prior to conversion.

Due to intersubject variability following dosing with tacrolimus, individualization of the dosing regimen is necessary for optimal therapy.

Advagraf is to be used concomitantly with adrenal corticosteroids and mycophenolate mofetil (MMF) in de novo renal transplant recipients. Antibody induction therapy should be used in kidney transplant recipients.

Patients with Hepatic or Renal Dysfunction: Advagraf (extended-release formulation) has not been studied in patients with hepatic or renal dysfunction, the following are based on experiences obtained from use of Prograf (immediate-release formulation).

Due to the reduced clearance and prolonged half-life, patients with severe hepatic impairment (Pugh ≥10) may require lower doses of Advagraf. Close monitoring of blood concentrations is warranted. Due to the potential for nephrotoxicity in patients with renal or hepatic impairment, these patients should receive doses at the lowest value of the recommended oral dosing range. Further reductions in dose below these ranges may be required.

Race: The data from Advagraf administration in de novo kidney transplant patients indicate that black patients required a higher dose to attain comparable trough concentrations compared to white patients.

Recommended Dose and Dosage Adjustment: Initial dosage and typical tacrolimus whole blood trough concentrations are shown in Table 6; blood concentration details are described under Warnings and Precautions, Monitoring and Laboratory Tests.

Table 6: Advagraf

Advagraf (tacrolimus extended-release capsules)—Summary of Initial Oral Dosage Recommendations and Typical Whole Blood Trough Concentrations

Patient Population	Recommended Initial Once Daily (AM) Oral Dose	Typical Whole Blood Trough Concentrations
Adult Kidney Transplant Patients	0.15–0.2 mg/kg/day	Month 1–3: 7–16 ng/mL Month 4–12: 5–15 ng/mL

The recommended starting oral dose of Advagraf for kidney transplant patients is 0.15 to 0.2 mg/kg administered once daily in the morning. The initial dose of Advagraf should be administered within 24 hours of transplantation. Dosing should be titrated to maintain the whole blood trough concentration levels noted above; blood concentration details are described under Warnings and Precautions, Monitoring and Laboratory Tests.

Stable kidney transplant recipients can be converted from Prograf (immediate-release formulation) twice daily to once-daily Advagraf (extended-release formulation) dosing on a 1:1 (mg:mg) total daily dose basis to achieve appropriate tacrolimus blood concentrations. The same target trough range and blood concentration monitoring should be used as with Prograf (immediate-release formulation) in order to maintain blood trough concentrations of tacrolimus similar to those prior to conversion.

In patients unable to take oral Advagraf (extended-release) capsules, therapy may be initiated with Prograf injection and the patient subsequently converted to oral Advagraf. The recommended starting dose of Prograf injection is 0.03-0.05 mg/kg/day (kidney) as a continuous IV infusion. Adult patients should receive doses at the lower end of the dosing range.

Patients converting from Prograf (immediate-release formulation) to Advagraf (extended-release formulation) should be administered a single daily morning dose of Advagraf (extended-release formulation) equivalent to the patients' previous stable total daily dose of Prograf (immediate-release formulation). Subsequent doses of Advagraf (extended-release formulation) should be adjusted in order to maintain trough concentrations similar to those prior to conversion.

The data from Advagraf (extended-release formulation) administration in kidney transplant patients indicate that black patients required a higher dose to attain comparable trough concentrations compared to white patients (see Table 7).

Table 7: Advagraf

Advagraf (tacrolimus extended-release capsules) Trough Concentrations in Kidney Transplant Patients

	White n=160		Black n=41	
Time After Transplant	Dose (mg/kg)	Mean Trough Concentration (ng/mL)	Dose (mg/kg)	Mean Trough Concentration (ng/mL)
Day 7	0.14	10.79	0.14	7.85
Month 1	0.14	11.11	0.18	10.83
Month 6	0.10	7.96	0.13	8.50
Month 12	0.09	7.54	0.12	7.52

Administration: Advagraf can be administered with or without food; however, doses should be administered in a consistent manner (see Action and Clinical Pharmacology).

OVERDOSAGE:
Activated charcoal may be administered to aid in the removal of unabsorbed drug. General supportive measures are recommended.

Limited overdosage experience with tacrolimus is available.

An overdosage of 5 times the intended dose has been reported with Advagraf, followed by an adverse event of hypomagnesaemia that was successfully treated with medication.

Acute overdosages of up to 30 times the intended dose have been reported with Prograf (immediate-release formulation). Almost all cases have been asymptomatic and all patients recovered with no sequelae. Occasionally, acute overdosage has been followed by adverse reactions consistent with those listed in the adverse reactions section except in one case where transient urticaria and lethargy were observed. Based on the poor aqueous solubility and extensive erythrocyte and plasma protein binding, it is anticipated that tacrolimus is not dialyzable to any significant extent; there is no experience with charcoal hemoperfusion. General supportive measures and treatment of specific symptoms should be followed in all cases of overdosage.

> For management of a suspected drug overdose, contact your **regional Poison Control Centre**. See the *CPS* Directory section for a list of Poison Control Centres.

ACTION AND CLINICAL PHARMACOLOGY: Mechanism of Action/Pharmacodynamics: Tacrolimus, the active ingredient in Advagraf, is a macrolide immunosuppressant produced by *S. tsukubaensis*.

Tacrolimus prolongs the survival of the host and transplanted graft in animal transplant models of liver, kidney, heart, bone marrow, small bowel and pancreas, lung and trachea, skin, cornea, and limb.

In animals, tacrolimus has been demonstrated to suppress some humoral immunity and, to a greater extent, cell-mediated reactions such as allograft rejection, delayed-type hypersensitivity, collagen-induced arthritis, experimental allergic encephalomyelitis, and graft versus host disease.

Tacrolimus inhibits T-lymphocyte activation, although the exact mechanism of action is not known. Experimental evidence suggests that tacrolimus binds to an intracellular protein, FKBP-12. A complex of tacrolimus-FKBP-12, calcium, calmodulin, and calcineurin is then formed and the phosphatase activity of calcineurin inhibited. This effect may prevent the dephosphorylation and translocation of nuclear factor of activated T-cells (NF-AT), a nuclear component thought to initiate gene transcription for the formation of lymphokines (such as interleukin-2, gamma interferon). The net result is the inhibition of T-lymphocyte activation (i.e., immunosuppression).

Pharmacokinetics: Tacrolimus activity is primarily due to the parent drug. The pharmacokinetic parameters of tacrolimus have been determined following oral administration of Advagraf in healthy volunteers, and in kidney transplant recipients (see Table 8).

Table 8: Advagraf

Pharmacokinetic Parameters of Advagraf (tacrolimus extended-release capsules)

Population	N	Dose	Day[c]	Pharmacokinetic Parameters		
				C_{max}[b] (ng/mL)	T_{max}[a] (hr)	AUC_{0-24}[b] (ng·hr/mL)
Healthy Volunteers	24	4 mg	Day 1 Day 10	6.2 11.6	2.0 2.0	74.3 155.0
Adult Kidney De Novo	34	0.19 mg/kg 0.20 mg/kg	Day 1 Day 14	18.2 29.9	3.0 2.0	231.9 363.9
Adult Kidney Conversion	66	5.8 mg 6.1 mg	Day 1 Day 14	14.8 14.2	2.0 2.0	204.6 197.6

[a] Median values.
[b] Arithmetic means.
[c] Day of Advagraf treatment.
Dose is the group mean once daily dose (transplant patients) or the actual administered dose (healthy volunteers). Conversion refers to 1:1 (mg:mg) conversion from Prograf (immediate-release formulation) to Advagraf (extended-release formulation) on a total daily dose basis.

There was a marked reduction of intra-subject variability for exposure (AUC_{0-24}) in black kidney transplant recipients at steady state after converting from Prograf (immediate-release formulation) (% coefficient of variation; %CV: 25.4%) to Advagraf (extended-release formulation) (%CV: 12.2%). In white kidney transplant recipients, the intra-subject variability for exposure at steady state was similar after converting from Prograf (immediate-release formulation) (% CV: 12.2%) to Advagraf (extended-release formulation) (% CV: 14.1%).

Due to intersubject variability in tacrolimus pharmacokinetics, individualization of dosing regimen is necessary for optimal therapy (see Dosage and Administration). Pharmacokinetic data indicate that whole blood concentrations rather than plasma concentrations serve as the more appropriate sampling compartment to describe tacrolimus pharmacokinetics.

Absorption: Absorption of tacrolimus from the gastrointestinal tract after oral administration is incomplete and variable.

In 20 healthy subjects, oral administration of an aqueous suspension of Advagraf was associated with a 5% higher AUC_{0-inf} and a 30% higher C_{max} compared with oral administration of intact capsules; administration of the aqueous suspension via nasogastric tube was associated with a 17% lower AUC_{0-inf} and 28% higher C_{max} compared with intact capsules.

Stable kidney transplant recipients can be converted from twice-daily Prograf (immediate-release formulation) to once-daily Advagraf (extended-release formulation) on a 1:1 (mg:mg) total daily dose basis to achieve appropriate tacrolimus blood concentrations (see Table 9).

Table 9: Advagraf

Relative Biopharmaceutics (AUC_{0-24}) at Steady State in Stable Transplant Recipients Converted from Prograf (immediate-release formulation) to Advagraf (extended-release formulation)

	N	Advagraf/Prograf	90% CI
Adult Kidney Transplant Recipients	66	95.0%	90.7%, 99.4%

CI: confidence interval Least square mean parameters were generated from ANOVA. The ratio of least square mean AUC_{0-24} and 90% confidence intervals consist of natural log-transformed values (expressed as a percent) transformed back to linear scale. For all adult studies, data represent a comparison of two steady state profiles for each drug.

There was a strong correlation between trough (C_{min}) and exposure (AUC_{0-24}) after Advagraf administration in de novo kidney (r=0.83) transplant recipients as well as postconversion to Advagraf in kidney (r=0.86) transplant recipients.

Food Effects: The presence of food affects the absorption of tacrolimus; the rate and extent of absorption is greatest under fasted conditions. In 24 healthy volunteers, administration of Advagraf immediately following a high fat meal (150 protein calories, 250 carbohydrate calories, and 500 to 600 fat calories) reduced C_{max}, AUC_{0-t}, and AUC_{0-inf} by approximately 25% compared with fasting values. Food delayed the median T_{max} from 2 hours in the fasted state to 4 hours in the fed state; however the terminal half-life remained 36 hours regardless of dosing conditions.

In 24 healthy volunteers, the time of the meal affected tacrolimus bioavailability. When Advagraf was administered immediately after consumption of a high-fat breakfast, tacrolimus AUC_{0-inf} was decreased approximately 25% relative to the fasted state. When Advagraf was administered 1.5 hours after consumption of a high-fat breakfast, tacrolimus exposure was decreased approximately 35%. Administration of Advagraf 1 hour prior to a high-fat breakfast reduced tacrolimus exposure by 10%.

In 23 healthy volunteers, a diurnal effect on the absorption of tacrolimus was observed. Evening dosing of Advagraf reduced AUC_{0-inf} by 35% relative to morning dosing.

Distribution: The apparent volume of distribution (based on whole blood concentrations) of tacrolimus is approximately 1.91 and 1.41 L/kg in healthy volunteers and kidney transplant patients, respectively (refer to Table 10).

Table 10: Advagraf

Distribution in Healthy Volunteers and Kidney Transplant Patients

Parameter	Volunteers (n=8)	Kidney Transplant Patients (n=26)
Mean IV Dose	0.025 mg/kg/4 hr	0.02 mg/kg/4 hr
V (L/kg)	1.91±0.31	1.41±0.66
Cl (L/hr/kg)	0.040±0.009	0.083±0.050

The plasma protein binding of tacrolimus is approximately 99% and is independent of concentration over a range of 5-50 ng/mL. Tacrolimus is bound to proteins, mainly albumin and alpha-1-acid glycoprotein, and has a high level of association with erythrocytes. The distribution of tacrolimus between whole blood and plasma depends on several factors, such as hematocrit, temperature at the time of plasma separation, drug concentration, and plasma protein concentration. In a U.S. study in which tacrolimus was administered as Prograf (immediate-release formulation), the ratio of whole blood concentration to plasma concentration averaged 35 (range 12 to 67).

Metabolism: Tacrolimus is extensively metabolized by the mixed-function oxidase system, primarily the cytochrome P-450 enzyme system (CYP3A). A metabolic pathway leading to the formation of 8 possible metabolites has been proposed. Demethylation and hydroxylation were identified as the primary mechanisms of biotransformation in vitro. The major metabolite identified in incubations with human liver microsomes is 13-demethyl tacrolimus. In in vitro studies, a 31-demethyl metabolite has been reported to have the same activity as tacrolimus; the 13-demethyl, 15-demethyl and 15- and 31- double-demethylated metabolites were shown to retain an activity of less than 10%.

Excretion: The mean clearance following IV administration of tacrolimus is 0.040 and 0.083 L/hr/kg in healthy volunteers and adult kidney transplant patients respectively. In man, less than 1% of the dose administered is excreted unchanged in urine.

Special Populations and Conditions: Pediatrics: Experience with tacrolimus in pediatric kidney transplant patients is limited.

Geriatrics: The pharmacokinetics of tacrolimus has not been established in the geriatric population.

Gender: Data from kidney transplant recipients converted from Prograf (immediate-release formulation) to Advagraf (extended-release formulation) in a phase II, open-label study showed equivalence in exposure for both male and female patients; the ratio of least square means (Advagraf:Prograf) for AUC_{0-24} at steady state was 92.0% [90% CI: 86.1%, 98.3%] for females (n=24) and 96.7% [90% CI: 90.9%, 102.9%] for males (n=42).

Race: The data from Advagraf administration in de novo kidney transplant patients indicate that black patients required a higher dose to attain comparable trough concentrations compared to white patients.

Black kidney transplant recipients (n=12) were converted from Prograf (immediate-release formulation) to Advagraf (extended-release formulation) on a 1:1 (mg:mg) total daily dose basis. The ratio of least square means (Advagraf:Prograf) for AUC_{0-24} at steady state was 109.8% [90% CI: 99.0%, 121.7%] for black patients. Intra-subject variability in exposure for black patients was reduced with Advagraf compared with Prograf.

Hepatic Insufficiency: The pharmacokinetics of tacrolimus administered as Prograf (immediate-release formulation) were determined in six subjects with mild hepatic dysfunction (mean Pugh score: 6.2) following single IV and oral administrations. The pharmacokinetic parameters obtained were as follows: see Table 11.

Table 11: Advagraf

Tacrolimus (immediate-release formulation) Pharmacokinetics in Patients with Mild Hepatic Impairment

Parameter (N=6)	Dose and Route	
	7.7 mg P.O.	1.3 mg IV
Age Range (yrs)	52–63	
Absolute Bioavailability (%)	22.3±11.4	—
C_{max} (ng/mL)	48.2±17.9	—
T_{max} (hr)	1.5±0.6	—
AUC_{0-72} (ng·hr/mL)	488±320	367±107
V (L/kg)	3.7±4.7[a]	3.1±1.6
Cl (L/hr/kg)	0.034±0.019[a]	0.042±0.020
$t_{½}$ (hr)	66.1±44.8	60.6±43.8

[a] Corrected for bioavailability.

The disposition of tacrolimus in patients with mild hepatic dysfunction was not substantially different from that in normal volunteers (see previous tables). In general, tacrolimus elimination half-life was longer and volume of distribution larger in patients with mild hepatic dysfunction compared to normal volunteers. The clearance in both populations was similar and since tacrolimus is extensively metabolized at multiple sites, patients with mild hepatic dysfunction may not require lower maintenance doses of tacrolimus than patients with normal hepatic function.

Tacrolimus pharmacokinetics were also studied in 6 subjects with severe hepatic dysfunction (mean Pugh score >10) administered Prograf (immediate-release formulation). The mean clearance was substantially lower in patients with severe hepatic dysfunction, irrespective of the route of administration. See Table 12.

Table 12: Advagraf

Tacrolimus (immediate-release formulation) Pharmacokinetics in Patients with Severe Hepatic Impairment

Route, N	Dose	AUC ng·hr/mL (0-t)	$T_{½}$ (hr)	V (L/kg)	Cl (L/hr/kg)
IV, n=6	0.02 mg/kg/4hr IV (n=2)	762 (t=120 hr)	198±158 Range: 81-436	—	—
	0.01 mg/kg/8hr IV (n=4)	289±117 (t=144 hr)		3.9±1.0	0.017±0.013
PO, n=5[a]	8 mg PO (n=1)	658 (t=120 hr)	119±35 Range: 85-178	3.1±3.4	0.016±0.011
	5 mg PO (n=4)	533±156 (t=144 hr)			
	4 mg PO (n=1)	—			

[a] 1 patient did not receive the PO dose.

Renal Insufficiency: The pharmacokinetics of tacrolimus following a single IV administration of Prograf were determined in 12 subjects (7 not on dialysis and 5 on dialysis). The pharmacokinetic parameters obtained are presented in Table 13.

Table 13: Advagraf
Tacrolimus Pharmacokinetics in Patients with Renal Insufficiency

Serum Creatinine (mg/dL)	3.9±1.6 (not on dialysis) 12.0±2.4 (on dialysis)
Age Range (yrs)	25–65
Route	IV
Dose (mg)	1.17±0.28
AUC_{0-60} (ng·hr/mL)	393 ±123
AUC_{0-inf} (ng·hr/mL)	499 ±155
V (L/kg)	1.07±0.20
Cl (L/hr/kg)	0.038±0.014
$t_{½}$(hr)	26.3±9.2

The disposition of tacrolimus in patients with renal dysfunction was not different from that in normal volunteers (see previous tables). The clearance was similar whereas volume of distribution was smaller and the mean terminal elimination half-life shorter than that of normal volunteers.

Diabetes: Stable kidney transplant recipients who had diabetes or new onset diabetes after transplant (NODAT) and were converted to Advagraf had ratios of least square means (Advagraf:Prograf) for AUC_{0-24} of 92.0% [90% CI: 84.8%, 99.7%] in kidney transplant recipients (n=13).

STORAGE AND STABILITY: Store and dispense at controlled room temperature, 15-30°C.

SPECIAL HANDLING INSTRUCTIONS: None required.

INFORMATION FOR THE PATIENT: Published in e-CPS, available by subscription at www.e-cps.ca.

DOSAGE FORMS, COMPOSITION AND PACKAGING:

0.5 mg: Each hard gelatin, extended-release oblong capsule, with a light yellow cap and an orange body, imprinted with red "✱647" on the capsule body and "0.5 mg" on the capsule cap, contains: the equivalent of 0.5 mg of anhydrous tacrolimus. Nonmedicinal ingredients: ethylcellulose, hydroxypropyl methylcellulose, lactose and magnesium stearate; capsule shell: ferric oxide, gelatin, titanium dioxide. The ingredients are directly proportional across all capsule strengths. Bottles of 50. Blister packs of 50 (10 capsules per card).

1 mg: Each hard gelatin, extended-release oblong capsule, with a white cap and an orange body, imprinted with red "✱677" on the capsule body and "1 mg" on the capsule cap contains: the equivalent of 1 mg of anhydrous tacrolimus. Nonmedicinal ingredients: ethylcellulose, hydroxypropyl methylcellulose, lactose and magnesium stearate; capsule shell: ferric oxide, gelatin, titanium dioxide. The ingredients are directly proportional across all capsule strengths. Bottles of 50. Blister packs of 50 (10 capsules per card).

5 mg: Each hard gelatin, extended-release oblong capsule, with a grayish-red cap and orange body, imprinted with red "✱687" on the capsule body and "5 mg" on the capsule cap contains: the equivalent of 5 mg of anhydrous tacrolimus. Nonmedicinal ingredients: ethylcellulose, hydroxypropyl methylcellulose, lactose and magnesium stearate; capsule shell: ferric oxide, gelatin, titanium dioxide. The ingredients are directly proportional across all capsule strengths. Bottles of 30. Blister packs of 50 (10 capsules per card).

(Shown in Product Identification Section)

Advair® Ⓟ

salmeterol xinafoate—fluticasone propionate

Bronchodilator—Corticosteroid for Oral Inhalation

GlaxoSmithKline

Advair® Diskus® Ⓟ

salmeterol xinafoate—fluticasone propionate

Bronchodilator—Corticosteroid for Oral Inhalation

GlaxoSmithKline

Date of Revision: July 8, 2010

SUMMARY PRODUCT INFORMATION:

Route of Administration	Dosage Form/Strength	Nonmedicinal Ingredients
Oral Inhalation	Dry Powder for inhalation/50 μg salmeterol/100, 250, 500 μg fluticasone propionate/blister	Lactose and milk protein
	Inhalation aerosol/25 μg salmeterol/125, 250 μg fluticasone propionate/metered dose	1,1,1,2-tetrafluoroethane (HFA-134a)

INDICATIONS AND CLINICAL USE: Asthma: ADVAIR (salmeterol xinafoate/fluticasone propionate) is indicated for:

- the maintenance treatment of asthma in patients with reversible obstructive airways disease where the use of a combination product is considered to be appropriate.

When treating asthma patients, ADVAIR/ADVAIR DISKUS should be used only in patients whose conditions are not adequately controlled using low- to medium-dose inhaled corticosteroids or the severity of whose disease clearly warrants the initiation of treatment with two maintenance therapies. ADVAIR/ADVAIR DISKUS is **not** indicated for patients whose asthma can be managed by occasional use of a rapid onset, short duration, inhaled $beta_2$-agonist or for patients whose asthma can be successfully managed by inhaled corticosteroids along with occasional use of a rapid onset, short duration, inhaled $beta_2$-agonist.

ADVAIR contains a long-acting $beta_2$-agonist and should not be used as a rescue medication. To relieve acute asthmatic symptoms, a rapid onset, short duration inhaled bronchodilator (e.g. salbutamol) should be used.

Chronic Obstructive Pulmonary Disease (COPD): ADVAIR 250 DISKUS and ADVAIR 500 DISKUS are indicated for:

- the maintenance treatment of COPD, including emphysema and chronic bronchitis, in patients where the use of a combination product is considered appropriate.

ADVAIR DISKUS should not be used as a rescue medication.

Physicians should reassess patients several months after the initiation of ADVAIR DISKUS and if symptomatic improvement has not occurred, ADVAIR DISKUS should be discontinued.

Geriatrics: There is no need to adjust the dose in elderly patients.

Pediatrics (<4 years of age): At present, there is insufficient clinical data to recommend the use of ADVAIR DISKUS in children younger than 4 years of age and the use of ADVAIR inhalation aerosol in children younger than 12 years of age.

CONTRAINDICATIONS:

- Patients who are hypersensitive to this drug or to any ingredient in the formulation or component of the container. For a complete listing, see Dosage Forms, Composition and Packaging.
- Patients with IgE mediated allergic reactions to lactose (which contains milk protein) or milk (ADVAIR DISKUS users only).
- Patients with cardiac tachyarrhythmias.
- Patients with untreated fungal, bacterial or tuberculous infections of the respiratory tract.
- In the primary treatment of status asthmaticus or other acute episodes of asthma, or in patients with moderate to severe bronchiectasis.

WARNINGS AND PRECAUTIONS: General: Information Concerning a Study Regarding Salmeterol, a Component of ADVAIR/ADVAIR DISKUS:

Serious Warnings and Precautions

Long-acting $beta_2$-adrenergic agonists, such as salmeterol, one of the active ingredients in ADVAIR/ADVAIR DISKUS, may increase the risk of asthma-related death. When treating asthma patients, ADVAIR/ADVAIR DISKUS should be used only in patients whose conditions are not adequately controlled using low- to medium- dose inhaled corticosteroids or the severity of whose disease clearly warrants the initiation of treatment with two maintenance therapies. Data from a large placebo-controlled US study (Salmeterol Multi-center Asthma Research Trial, also known as "SMART") comparing the safety of salmeterol (SEREVENT Inhalation Aerosol) to that of a placebo added to the original asthma therapy showed an increase in asthma-related deaths in patients receiving salmeterol (13 deaths out of 13,176 patients treated for 28 weeks on salmeterol versus 3 deaths out of 13, 179 patients on placebo). Data from this study also suggested that African American patients may be at greater risk of serious respiratory-related events or deaths when using salmeterol compared to placebo. It is not known if this was due to pharmacogenetic or other factors.

ADVAIR (salmeterol xinafoate/fluticasone propionate) should not be used to treat acute symptoms of asthma. It is crucial to inform patients of this and prescribe rapid onset, short duration inhaled bronchodilator (e.g., salbutamol) to relieve the acute symptoms of asthma. Patients should be clearly instructed to use rapid onset, short duration, inhaled $beta_2$-agonists only for symptomatic relief if they develop asthma symptoms while taking ADVAIR. When beginning treatment with ADVAIR, patients who have been taking rapid onset, short duration, inhaled $beta_2$-agonists on a regular basis (e.g., q.i.d) should be instructed to discontinue the regular use of these drugs and use them only for symptomatic relief if they develop acute symptoms of asthma while taking ADVAIR.

Discontinuance: Treatment with inhaled corticosteroids should not be stopped abruptly in patients with asthma due to risk of exacerbation. In this case, therapy should be titrated down gradually, under physician supervision. For patients with COPD, cessation of therapy may be associated with symptomatic decompensation and should be supervised by a physician.

Cardiovascular and Other Effects: Although clinically not significant, a small increase in QTc interval has been reported with therapeutic doses of salmeterol. It is not known if this becomes clinically significant when concomitant medications causing similar effects are prescribed and/or in the presence of heart diseases, hypokalemia, or hypoxia. Large doses of inhaled or oral salmeterol (12 to 20 times the recommended dose) have been associated with clinically significant prolongation of the QTc interval, which has the potential for producing ventricular arrhythmias.

Fatalities have been reported following excessive use of aerosol preparations containing sympathomimetic amines, the exact cause of which is unknown. Cardiac arrest was reported in several instances.

No clinically significant effect on the cardiovascular system is usually seen after the administration of inhaled salmeterol in recommended doses. Cardiovascular effects such as increased blood pressure and heart rate may occasionally be seen with all sympathomimetic drugs, especially at higher than therapeutic doses. Central nervous system effects (increased excitement) can occur after the use of salmeterol. Occurrence of cardiovascular or central nervous system effects may require discontinuation of the drug.

For this reason, salmeterol xinafoate/fluticasone propionate, like all sympathomimetic amines, should be used with caution in patients with cardiovascular disorders, especially coronary insufficiency, cardiac arrhythmias, and hypertension; in patients with convulsive disorders or thyrotoxicosis; and in patients who are unusually responsive to sympathomimetic amines.

In individual patients any $beta_2$-adrenergic agonist may have a clinically significant cardiac effect. As has been described with other beta-adrenergic agonist bronchodilators, clinically significant changes in systolic and/or diastolic blood pressure, pulse rate, and electrocardiograms have been seen infrequently in individual patients in controlled clinical studies with salmeterol.

Ear/Nose/Throat: Symptoms of laryngeal spasm, irritation, or swelling, such as stridor and choking, have been reported rarely in patients receiving salmeterol.

Also see Immune, Candidiasis.

Endocrine and Metabolism: Systemic Steroid Replacement by Inhaled Steroid: Particular care is needed in patients who are transferred from systemically active corticosteroids to inhaled corticosteroids because deaths due to adrenal insufficiency have occurred in patients with asthma during and after transfer. For the transfer of patients being treated with oral corticosteroids, inhaled corticosteroids should first be added to the existing oral steroid therapy which is then gradually withdrawn.

Patients with adrenocortical suppression should be monitored regularly and the oral steroid reduced cautiously. Some patients transferred from other inhaled steroids or oral steroids remain at risk of impaired adrenal reserve for a considerable time after transferring to inhaled fluticasone propionate.

After withdrawal from systemic corticosteroids, a number of months are required for recovery of hypothalamic-pituitary-adrenal (HPA) function. During this period of HPA suppression, patients may exhibit signs and symptoms of adrenal insufficiency when exposed to trauma, surgery or infections, particularly gastroenteritis. Although inhaled fluticasone propionate may provide control of asthmatic symptoms during these episodes, it does not provide the systemic steroid which is necessary for coping with these emergencies. The physician may consider supplying oral steroids for use in times of stress (e.g. worsening asthma attacks, chest infections, and surgery).

During periods of stress or a severe asthmatic attack, patients who have been withdrawn from systemic corticosteroids should be instructed to resume systemic steroids immediately and to contact their physician for further instruction. These patients should also be instructed to carry a warning card indicating that they may need supplementary systemic steroids during periods of stress or a severe asthma attack. To assess the risk of adrenal insufficiency in emergency situations, routine tests of adrenal cortical function, including measurement of early morning and evening cortisol levels, should be performed periodically in all patients. An early morning resting cortisol level may be accepted as normal only if it falls at or near the normal mean level.

Systemic Effects: Systemic effects may occur with any inhaled corticosteroid, particularly at high doses prescribed for long periods; these effects are much less likely to occur than with oral corticosteroids. Possible systemic effects include Cushing's syndrome, Cushingoid features, and adrenal suppression, growth retardation in children and adolescents, decrease in bone mineral density (BMD), cataract and glaucoma. It is important therefore, that the dose of inhaled corticosteroid is titrated to the lowest dose at which effective control is maintained (see Monitoring and Laboratory Tests).

The long-term effects of fluticasone propionate in human subjects are still unknown. The local effect of the drug on developmental or immunologic processes in the mouth, pharynx, trachea, and lungs is unknown. There is also no information about the possible long-term systemic effects of the agent (see Monitoring and Laboratory Tests).

Long-term use of orally inhaled corticosteroids may affect normal bone metabolism resulting in a loss of bone mineral density. In patients with major risk factors for decreased bone mineral content, such as chronic alcohol use, tobacco use, age, sedentary lifestyle, strong family history of osteoporosis, or chronic use of drugs that can reduce bone mass (e.g., anticonvulsants and corticosteroids), ADVAIR may pose an additional risk.

Effects of treatment with ADVAIR DISKUS 50/500 μg, fluticasone propionate 500 μg, salmeterol 50 μg, or placebo on BMD was evaluated in a subset of 658 patients (females and males 40 to 80 years of age) with COPD in a 3 year study (SCO30003). BMD evaluations were conducted at baseline and at 48, 108 and 158 weeks. There were no significant differences between any of the treatment groups at 3 years. A slight reduction in BMD measured at the hip was observed in all treatment groups (ADVAIR DISKUS −3.2%, fluticasone propionate −2.9%, salmeterol −1.7%, placebo −3.1%). Fracture risk was estimated for the entire population of patients with COPD in study SCO30003 (N=6184). There were no significant differences between any of the treatment groups. The probability of a fracture over 3 years was 6.3% for ADVAIR DISKUS, 5.4% for fluticasone propionate, 5.1% for salmeterol, and 5.1% for placebo.

During post-marketing use, there have been reports of clinically significant drug interactions in patients receiving intranasal or inhaled fluticasone propionate and ritonavir, resulting in systemic corticosteroid effects including Cushing's syndrome and adrenal suppression. Therefore, concomitant use of fluticasone propionate and ritonavir should be avoided, unless the potential benefit to the patient outweighs the risk of systemic corticosteroid side-effects (see Drug Interactions).

The results of a drug interaction study conducted in healthy subjects indicated that concomitant use of systemic ketoconazole (a strong cytochrome P450 3A4 inhibitor) increased exposure to salmeterol in some subjects. This increase in plasma salmeterol exposure may lead to prolongation in the QTc interval. Due to the potential increased risk of cardiovascular adverse events, the concomitant use of salmeterol with ketoconazole is not recommended (see Drug Interactions, and Action and Clinical Pharmacology, Pharmacokinetics). Caution should also be exercised when other CYP3A4 inhibitors are co-administered with salmeterol (e.g. ritonavir, atazanavir, clarithromycin, indinavir, itraconazole, nefazodone, nelfinavir, saquinavir, telithromycin).

Metabolic Effects: Doses of the related $beta_2$-adrenoceptor agonist salbutamol, when administered intravenously, have been reported to aggravate pre-existing diabetes mellitus and ketoacidosis. Administration of $beta_2$-adrenoceptor agonists may cause a decrease in serum potassium, possibly through intracellular shunting, which has the potential to increase the likelihood of arrhythmias. The effect is usually seen at higher therapeutic doses and the decrease is usually transient, not requiring supplementation. Therefore, salmeterol/fluticasone propionate should be used with caution in patients predisposed to low levels of serum potassium.

The possibility of impaired adrenal response should always be borne in mind in emergency and elective situations likely to produce stress and appropriate corticosteroid treatment must be considered.

Certain individuals can show greater susceptibility to the effects of inhaled corticosteroid than do most patients.

In common with other beta-adrenergic agents, salmeterol can induce reversible metabolic changes (hyperglycemia, hypokalemia). There have been very rare reports of increases in blood glucose levels and this should be considered when prescribing to patients with a history of diabetes mellitus.

There is an enhanced effect of corticosteroids on patients with hypothyroidism.

Hematologic: Eosinophilic Conditions: In rare cases, patients on inhaled fluticasone propionate may present with systemic eosinophilic conditions, with some patients presenting with clinical features of vasculitis consistent with Churg-Strauss syndrome, a condition that is often treated with systemic corticosteroid therapy. These events usually, but not always, have been associated with the reduction and/or withdrawal of oral corticosteroid therapy following the introduction of fluticasone propionate. Cases of serious eosinophilic conditions have also been reported with other inhaled corticosteroids in this clinical setting. Physicians should be alerted to eosinophilia, vasculitic rash, worsening pulmonary symptoms, cardiac complications, and/or neuropathy presenting in their patients. A causal relationship between fluticasone propionate and these underlying conditions has not been established.

Hepatic/Biliary/Pancreatic: There is an enhanced effect of corticosteroids on patients with cirrhosis.

Hypersensitivity: Immediate hypersensitivity reactions may occur after administration of salmeterol, as demonstrated by rare cases of urticaria, angioedema, rash and bronchospasm, and very rare cases of anaphylactic reactions, anaphylactic shock.

Immune: Candidiasis: Therapeutic dosages of fluticasone propionate frequently cause the appearance of *C. albicans* (thrush) in the mouth and throat. The development of pharyngeal and laryngeal candidiasis is a cause for concern because the extent of its penetration into the respiratory tract is unknown. Patients may find it helpful to rinse the mouth and gargle with water after using ADVAIR. Symptomatic candidiasis can be treated with topical anti-fungal therapy while continuing to use ADVAIR.

Infection: Corticosteroids may mask some signs of infection and new infections may appear. A decreased resistance to localised infection has been observed during corticosteroid therapy. This may require treatment with appropriate therapy or stopping the administration of fluticasone propionate until the infection is eradicated. Patients who are on drugs that suppress the immune system are more susceptible to infections than healthy individuals. Chickenpox and measles, for example, can have a more serious or even fatal course in susceptible children or adults on corticosteroids. In such children or adults who have not had these diseases, particular care should be taken to avoid exposure. How the dose, route, and duration of corticosteroid administration affect the risk of developing a disseminated infection is not known. The contribution of the underlying disease and/or prior corticosteroid treatment to the risk is also not known. If exposed to chickenpox, prophylaxis with varicella zoster immune globulin (VZIG) may be indicated. If exposed to measles, prophylaxis with intramuscular pooled immunoglobulin (IG) may be indicated. If chickenpox develops, treatment with antiviral agents may be considered.

For patients with asthma or COPD, consideration should be given to additional corticosteroid therapy and to antibiotics if an exacerbation is associated with an infection.

For COPD patients, it is important that even mild chest infections be treated immediately since these patients may be more susceptible to damaging lung infections than healthy individuals. Patients should be instructed to contact their physician as soon as possible if they suspect an infection.

Physicians should recommend that COPD patients receive an annual influenza vaccination.

In a 3 year study of 6,184 patients with COPD (SCO30003) there was an increased reporting of any adverse event of pneumonia in patients receiving ADVAIR 50/500 µg compared with placebo (16% on ADVAIR DISKUS 50/500 µg, 14% on fluticasone propionate 500 µg, 11% on salmeterol 50 µg and 9% on placebo). Physicians should remain vigilant for the possible development of pneumonia in patients with COPD as the clinical features of pneumonia and exacerbations frequently overlap (see Adverse Reactions, Clinical Trial Adverse Drug Reactions, COPD).

Ophthalmologic: For patients at risk, monitoring of ocular effects (cataract and glaucoma) should also be considered in patients receiving maintenance therapy with ADVAIR.

Effects of treatment with ADVAIR DISKUS 50/500 µg, fluticasone propionate 500 µg, salmeterol 50 µg, or placebo on development of cataracts or glaucoma was evaluated in a subset of 658 patients with COPD in a 3 year (SCO30003) study. Ophthalmic examinations were conducted at baseline and at 48, 108 and 158 weeks. The presence of cataracts and glaucoma at baseline was similar across treatment groups (61% to 71% and 5% to 8%, respectively). New cataracts were diagnosed in all treatment groups (26% on ADVAIR DISKUS 50/500 µg, 17% on fluticasone propionate, 15% on salmeterol, and 21% on placebo). A few new cases of glaucoma were diagnosed (2% on ADVAIR DISKUS 50/500 µg, 5% on fluticasone propionate, none on salmeterol, and 2% on placebo). There were no significant differences in the development of glaucoma or cataracts between any of the treatment groups.

Respiratory: As with other inhalation therapy, paradoxical bronchospasm may occur characterized by an immediate increase in wheezing after dosing. This should be treated immediately with a rapid onset, short duration inhaled bronchodilator (e.g. salbutamol) to relieve acute asthmatic symptoms. ADVAIR should be discontinued immediately, the patient assessed, and if necessary, alternative therapy instituted.

Special Populations: Pregnant Women: There are no adequate and well-controlled studies with ADVAIR in pregnant women. ADVAIR should be used during pregnancy only if the potential benefit justifies the potential risk to the fetus.

In animal studies, some effects on the fetus, typical for a beta-agonist, occurred at exposure levels substantially higher than those that occur with therapeutic use. Extensive use of other beta-agonists has provided no evidence that effects in animals are relevant to human use.

Like other glucocorticoids, fluticasone propionate is teratogenic to rodent species. Adverse effects typical of potent corticosteroids are only seen at high systemic exposure levels; administration by inhalation ensures minimal systemic exposure. The relevance of these findings to humans has not yet been established since well-controlled trials relating to fetal risk in humans are not available. Infants born of mothers who have received substantial doses of glucocorticoids during pregnancy should be carefully observed for hypoadrenalism.

Use in Labour and Delivery: There are no well-controlled human studies that have investigated effects of salmeterol on preterm labour or labour at term. Because of the potential for beta-agonist interference with uterine contractility, use of ADVAIR during labour should be restricted to those patients in whom the benefits clearly outweigh the risks.

Nursing Women: Plasma levels of salmeterol after inhaled therapeutic doses are very low (85 to 200 pg/mL) in humans and therefore levels in milk should be correspondingly low. Studies in lactating animals indicate that salmeterol is likely to be secreted in only very small amounts in breast milk.

Glucocorticoids are excreted in human milk. The excretion of fluticasone propionate into human breast milk has not been investigated. When measurable plasma levels were obtained in lactating laboratory rats following subcutaneous administration, there was evidence of fluticasone propionate in the breast milk. However, plasma levels in patients following inhaled fluticasone propionate at recommended doses are likely to be low.

Since there is no experience with use of ADVAIR by nursing mothers, a decision should be made whether to discontinue nursing or to discontinue the drug, taking into account the importance of the drug to the mother.

Pediatrics (≥4 years of age): In adolescents and children, the severity of asthma may vary with age and periodic reassessment should be considered to determine if continued maintenance therapy with ADVAIR is still indicated.

Also see Monitoring and Laboratory Tests.

The safety and efficacy of ADVAIR DISKUS in children younger than 4 years of age have not been established.

The safety and efficacy of ADVAIR inhalation aerosol in children younger than 12 years of age have not been established.

Geriatrics: As with other beta$_2$-agonists, special caution should be observed when using salmeterol in elderly patients who have concomitant cardiovascular disease that could be adversely affected by this class of drug. Based on available data, no adjustment of salmeterol dosage in geriatric patients is warranted.

Monitoring and Laboratory Tests: Monitoring Control of Asthma or COPD: ADVAIR should not be introduced in acutely deteriorating asthma or COPD, which is a potentially life threatening condition. Increasing use of rapid onset, short duration inhaled bronchodilators to control symptoms indicates deterioration of asthma control. Sudden and progressive deterioration in asthma control is potentially life-threatening and the treatment plan should be re-evaluated. Also, where current dosage of ADVAIR has failed to give adequate control of reversible obstructive airways disease the patient should be reviewed by a physician. Before introducing ADVAIR, adequate education should be provided to the patient on how to use the drug and what to do if asthma flares up.

During long-term therapy, HPA axis function and haematological status should be assessed periodically. For patients at risk, monitoring of bone and ocular effects (cataract and glaucoma) should also be considered in patients receiving maintenance therapy with ADVAIR. It is recommended that the height of children receiving prolonged treatment with inhaled corticosteroids is regularly monitored.

ADVERSE REACTIONS: Adverse Drug Reaction Overview: As with other inhalation therapy paradoxical bronchospasm may occur with an immediate increase in wheezing after dosing. This should be treated immediately with a rapid onset, short duration inhaled bronchodilator. ADVAIR (salmeterol xinafoate/fluticasone propionate) should be discontinued immediately, the patient assessed and alternative therapy instituted if necessary.

The type and severity of adverse reactions associated with salmeterol xinafoate and fluticasone propionate may be expected with ADVAIR. There is no incidence of additional adverse events following combined administration of the two compounds.

Salmeterol Xinafoate: The pharmacological side effects of beta$_2$-agonist treatment, such as tremor, subjective palpitations and headache, have been reported, but tend to be transient and reduce with regular therapy.

Cardiac arrhythmias (including atrial fibrillation, supraventricular tachycardia and extrasystoles) may occur in some patients.

There have been reports of arthralgia and hypersensitivity reactions, including rash, urticaria, bronchospasm, edema, angioedema, anaphylactic reaction and anaphylactic shock.

There have been reports of oropharyngeal irritations as well as common reports of muscle cramps.

Symptoms of laryngeal spasm, irritation, or swelling, such as stridor and choking, have been reported rarely in patients receiving salmeterol.

Clinically significant changes in blood glucose and/or serum potassium were seen rarely during clinical studies with long-term administration of salmeterol at recommended doses.

Fluticasone Propionate: In general, inhaled corticosteroid therapy may be associated with dose dependent increases in the incidence of ocular complications, reduced bone density, suppression of HPA axis responsiveness to stress, and inhibition of growth velocity in children. Such events have been reported rarely in clinical trials with fluticasone propionate.

Possible systemic effects include Cushing's syndrome, Cushingoid features and adrenal suppression.

Glaucoma may be exacerbated by inhaled corticosteroid treatment. In patients with established glaucoma who require long-term inhaled corticosteroid treatment, it is prudent to measure intraocular pressure before commencing the inhaled corticosteroid and to monitor it subsequently. In patients without established glaucoma, but with a potential for developing intraocular hypertension (e.g. the elderly), intraocular pressure should be monitored at appropriate intervals.

In elderly patients treated with inhaled corticosteroids, the prevalence of posterior subcapsular and nuclear cataracts is probably low but increases in relation to the daily and cumulative lifetime dose. Cofactors such as smoking, ultraviolet B exposure, or diabetes may increase the risk. Children may be less susceptible.

A reduction of growth velocity in children or teenagers may occur as a result of inadequate control of chronic diseases such as asthma or from use of corticosteroids for treatment. Physicians should closely follow the growth of children and adolescents taking corticosteroids by any route and weigh the benefits of corticosteroid therapy and asthma control against the possibility of growth suppression if any child's or adolescent's growth appears slowed.

Osteoporosis and fracture are the major complications of long-term treatment with parenteral or oral steroids. Inhaled corticosteroid therapy is also associated with dose-dependent bone loss although the degree of risk is very much less than with oral steroid. This risk may be offset by estrogen replacement in post-menopausal women, and by titrating the daily dose of inhaled steroid to the minimum required to maintain optimal control of respiratory symptoms. It is not yet known whether the peak bone density achieved during youth is adversely affected if substantial amounts of inhaled corticosteroid are administered prior to 30 years of age.

Failure to achieve maximal bone density during youth could increase the risk of osteoporotic fracture when those individuals reach 60 years of age and older.

Hoarseness and candidiasis (thrush) of the mouth and throat can occur in some patients receiving inhaled fluticasone propionate. These may be relieved by rinsing the mouth and gargling with water after use of ADVAIR. Symptomatic candidiasis can be treated with topical anti-fungal therapy while still continuing with ADVAIR (see Drug Interactions).

There have been uncommon reports of cutaneous hypersensitivity reactions. There have also been rare reports of hypersensitivity reactions manifesting as angioedema (mainly facial and oropharyngeal edema), respiratory symptoms (dyspnea and/or bronchospasm) and very rarely, anaphylactic reactions.

There have been very rare reports of anxiety, sleep disorders and behavioural changes, including hyperactivity and irritability (predominantly in children and adolescents).

Eosinophilic Conditions: In rare cases, patients on inhaled fluticasone propionate may present with systemic eosinophilic conditions, with some patients presenting with clinical features of vasculitis consistent with Churg-Strauss syndrome, a condition that is often treated with systemic corticosteroid therapy. These events usually, but not always, have been associated with the reduction and/or withdrawal of oral corticosteroid therapy following the introduction of fluticasone propionate. Cases of serious eosinophilic conditions have also been reported with other inhaled corticosteroids in this clinical setting. Physicians should be alerted to eosinophilia, vasculitic rash, worsening pulmonary symptoms, cardiac complications, and/or neuropathy presenting in their patients. A causal relationship between fluticasone propionate and these underlying conditions has not been established.

Asthma: Data from a large placebo-controlled US study comparing the safety of salmeterol to that of a placebo added to the original asthma therapy showed an increase in asthma-related deaths in patients receiving salmeterol. Data from this study also suggested that African American patients may be at greater risk of serious respiratory-related events or deaths when using salmeterol compared to placebo. It is not known if this was due to pharmacogenetic or other factors.

Clinical Trial Adverse Drug Reactions: Because clinical trials are conducted under very specific conditions the adverse reaction rates observed in the clinical trials may not reflect the rates observed in practice and should not be compared to the rates in the clinical trials of another drug. Adverse drug reaction information from clinical trials is useful for identifying drug-related adverse events and for approximating rates.

Asthma: Use in Adolescents and Adults: There have been very rare reports of anxiety, sleep disorders and behavioural changes including hyperactivity and irritability (predominantly in children and adolescents).

There have been uncommon reports of contusions (skin bruising).

ADVAIR DISKUS: In clinical trials involving 1824 adult and adolescent patients, the most commonly reported adverse events with the combination salmeterol xinafoate/fluticasone propionate DISKUS were: hoarseness/dysphonia, throat irritation, headache, candidiasis of mouth and throat and palpitations as detailed in Table 1.

Table 1: ADVAIR DISKUS

Number (and percentage) of Patients with Drug-Related Adverse Events (incidence ≥1%[a]) (Safety Population)

Adverse Events	Salmeterol Xinafoate/ Fluticasone Propionate Combination Product	Salmeterol Xinafoate and Fluticasone Propionate Concurrent Therapy	Fluticasone Propionate Alone	Salmeterol Xinafoate Alone	Placebo
Number of Patients	644	486	339	180	175
Any Event	110 (17%)	81 (17%)	50 (15%)	9 (5%)	5 (3%)
Hoarseness/ Dysphonia	15 (2%)	11 (2%)	8 (2%)	1 (<1%)	0
Throat Irritation	14 (2%)	10 (2%)	8 (2%)	1 (<1%)	1 (<1%)
Candidiasis of Mouth and Throat	15 (2%)	9 (2%)	5 (1%)	0	0
Headaches	16 (2%)	11 (2%)	3 (<1%)	0	0
Asthma[b]	9 (1%)	11 (2%)	3 (<1%)	0	0
Palpitations	7 (1%)	4 (<1%)	2 (<1%)	1 (<1%)	0
Cough	6 (<1%)	2 (<1%)	5 (1%)	1 (<1%)	0
Breathing Disorders	6 (<1%)	2 (<1%)	4 (1%)	0	0

(cont'd)

Table 1: ADVAIR DISKUS *(cont'd)*

Number (and percentage) of Patients with Drug-Related Adverse Events (incidence ≥1%[a]) (Safety Population)

Adverse Events	Salmeterol Xinafoate/ Fluticasone Propionate Combination Product	Salmeterol Xinafoate and Fluticasone Propionate Concurrent Therapy	Fluticasone Propionate Alone	Salmeterol Xinafoate Alone	Placebo
Candidiasis–Unspecified Site	6 (<1%)	3 (<1%)	4 (1%)	0	2 (1%)
Upper Respiratory Tract Infection	5 (<1%)	5 (1%)	2 (<1%)	0	0

[a] In any integrated treatment group.
[b] Asthma was not recorded as an adverse event in those studies which included treatment with salmeterol xinafoate alone or placebo (unless it was a serious adverse event).

In the ADVAIR DISKUS group, there was no apparent relationship to fluticasone propionate dose for drug-related adverse events (15% with 50/100 µg, 19% with 50/250 µg and 17% with 50/500 µg).

ADVAIR Inhalation Aerosol: In clinical trials, the most commonly reported adverse events with the combination salmeterol xinafoate/fluticasone propionate inhalation aerosol were: hoarseness/dysphonia, throat irritation and headache. All other adverse events with a reasonable possibility of being related to study drug were reported in ≤1% of subjects. See Table 2.

The incidence of drug-related adverse events for the MDI combination product groups was similar to the individual components.

Use in Children: A total of 257 pediatric patients participated in the clinical development programme and received either the combination 50 µg salmeterol xinafoate/100 µg fluticasone propionate DISKUS or concurrent therapy (with salmeterol and fluticasone propionate administered via separate inhalers). Only one drug-related adverse event, candidiasis, was reported with an incidence of 2% or more in the ADVAIR group. The combination product was generally well tolerated and the safety profile was comparable to that observed in the concurrent therapy group.

There have been very rare reports of anxiety, sleep disorders and behavioural changes including hyperactivity and irritability (predominantly in children and adolescents).

COPD: Clinical trial adverse drug reaction data is provided for two 24-week studies, a 52-week study and a 3-year study.

24-Week Studies: In clinical trials involving 2054 adults, the most commonly reported adverse events with ADVAIR DISKUS after 24 weeks were: upper respiratory tract infection, throat irritation, headache and musculoskeletal pain as detailed in Table 3. These adverse reactions were mostly mild to moderate in severity.

Table 3 includes all events (whether considered drug-related or non drug-related by the investigator) that occurred at a rate of 3% or greater in either of the groups receiving ADVAIR DISKUS and were more common than in the placebo group.

Other COPD Clinical Trial Adverse Drug Reactions (1-3%): Cardiovascular: arrhythmias, hypertension, palpitations.

Drug Interaction, Overdose and Trauma: contusions, fractures, hematomas, lacerations and wounds.

Ear/Nose/Throat: ear/nose/throat infections, ear/nose/throat signs and symptoms, ear signs and symptoms, epistaxis, laryngitis, nasal sinus disorders, pharyngitis/throat infections, rhinorrhea/post nasal drip, sputum abnormalities.

Endocrine and Metabolism: diabetes mellitus, hypothyroidism.

Gastrointestinal: constipation, dental discomfort and pain, diverticulosis, dyspeptic symptoms, gastrointestinal infections, gum signs and symptoms, hyposalivation, oral discomfort and pain; oral lesions, regurgitation and reflux.

Hepatic/Biliary/Pancreatic: abnormal liver function tests.

Immune: bacterial infections, candidiasis unspecified site, viral infections.

Neurologic: anxiety, situational disorders, sleep disorders, syncope, tremors, vertigo.

Non-Site Specific: bone and skeletal pain, edema and swelling, non-site specific pain, non-specific condition, soft tissue injuries.

Ophthalmologic: dry eyes, eye infections, lacrimal disorders, ocular pressure disorders, visual disturbances.

Peri-Operative Considerations: postoperative complications.

Respiratory: breathing disorders, bronchitis, lower respiratory hemorrhage, lower respiratory signs and symptoms, pneumonia.

Skin: fungal skin infections and skin infections.

Table 2: ADVAIR Inhalation Aerosol

Number (and percentage) of Patients with Drug-Related Adverse Events (Incidence ≥1%[a]) (Safety Population)

Adverse Events	Salmeterol Xinafoate/ Fluticasone Propionate MDI Combination Product	Fluticasone Propionate Alone	Salmeterol Xinafoate Alone	Placebo
Number of Patients	622	614	274	176
Any Event	67 (11%)	71 (11%)	29 (11%)	9 (5%)
Hoarseness/Dysphonia	13 (2%)	7 (1%)	3 (2%)	0 (0%)
Throat Irritation	13 (2%)	14 (2%)	10 (4%)	3 (2%)
Candidiasis of Mouth and Throat	8 (1%)	8 (1%)	0 (0%)	1 (<1%)
Headaches	11 (2%)	11 (2%)	5 (2%)	3 (2%)
Cough	3 (<1%)	3 (<1%)	6 (2%)	1 (<1%)
Hyposalivation	6 (1%)	2 (<1%)	1 (<1%)	0 (0%)

[a] In any integrated treatment group.
Legend: MDI=metered dose inhaler.

Table 3: ADVAIR DISKUS

Overall Adverse Experiences with ≥3% Incidence in Controlled Clinical Trials with ADVAIR DISKUS in Patients with COPD

Adverse Event	ADVAIR DISKUS 50/500 µg (n=169) %	ADVAIR DISKUS 50/250 µg (n=178) %	Fluticasone propionate 500 µg (n=391) %	Fluticasone propionate 250 µg (n=399) %	Salmeterol 50 µg (n=341) %	Placebo (n=576) %
Any Event	78	70	80	74	68	69
Ear, Nose, and Throat						
Upper Respiratory Tract Infection	17	12	18	16	11	15
Nasal Congestion/Blockage	4	3	7	4	4	3
Throat Irritation	11	8	9	9	7	6
Upper Respiratory Inflammation	9	2	7	5	5	5
Sinusitis	3	3	3	6	4	2
Sinusitis/Sinus Infection	4	2	2	2	1	2
Hoarseness/Dysphonia	3	5	5	5	<1	1
Candidiasis Mouth/Throat	7	10	12	6	2	<1
Lower Respiratory						
Viral Respiratory Infections	8	6	9	5	5	4
Neurology						
Dizziness	3	4	2	2	4	2
Headaches	18	16	17	13	14	11
Gastrointestinal						
Nausea & Vomiting	4	2	4	4	3	3
Non-Site Specific						
Fever	4	4	3	3	1	3
Musculoskeletal						
Malaise & Fatigue	4	3	3	3	2	3
Muscle Cramps & Spasms	8	3	2	2	3	1
Muscle Pain	4	0	3	2	1	<1
Musculoskeletal Pain	12	9	9	10	12	10

52-Week Study: After 52 weeks of treatment with ADVAIR DISKUS (50/500 μg), fluticasone propionate 500 μg, salmeterol 50 μg and placebo in 1465 patients with COPD, the most commonly reported drug related adverse event was candidiasis of the mouth and throat (ADVAIR DISKUS 50/500 μg, 6%; fluticasone propionate 500 μg, 6%; salmeterol 50 μg, 1%; placebo, 1%).

3-Year Study: Study SCO30003 provided safety data on 6184 patients with moderate to severe COPD who were randomised and received at least one dose of study medication and treated for up to 3 years; defined as the Safety population. The safety profile of ADVAIR over the three-year treatment period was comparable to that seen in previous studies of shorter duration, confirming the long-term tolerability of ADVAIR. All three active treatments were well tolerated and the adverse events reported were generally those expected based on clinical experience with these treatments, with the exception of pneumonia. The estimated 3 year probability of having pneumonia reported as an adverse event was 12.3% for placebo, 13.3% for salmeterol, 18.3% for fluticasone propionate and 19.6% for ADVAIR (Hazard ratio for ADVAIR vs placebo: 1.64, 95% CI: 1.33 to 2.01, p <0.001). There was no increase in pneumonia related deaths for ADVAIR; deaths while on treatment that were adjudicated as primarily due to pneumonia were 7 for placebo, 9 for salmeterol, 13 for fluticasone propionate and 8 for ADVAIR. There was no significant difference in probability of bone fracture (5.1% placebo, 5.1% salmeterol, 5.4% fluticasone propionate and 6.3% ADVAIR; Hazard ratio for ADVAIR versus placebo: 1.22, 95% CI: 0.87 to 1.72, p=0.248). The incidence of adverse events of eye disorders, bone disorders, and HPA axis disorders was low and there was no difference observed between treatments. There was no evidence of an increase in cardiac events for ADVAIR, salmeterol, and fluticasone propionate.

Post-Market Adverse Drug Reactions: There have been uncommon reports of cutaneous hypersensitivity reactions. There have also been rare reports of hypersensitivity reactions manifesting as angioedema (mainly facial and oropharyngeal edema), respiratory symptoms (dyspnea and/or bronchospasm) and very rarely, anaphylactic reactions, anaphylactic shock.

There have been very rare reports of anxiety, sleep disorders and behavioural changes, including hyperactivity and irritability (predominantly in children and adolescents). Very rarely, hyperglycemia and hypertension have been reported.

DRUG INTERACTIONS: Overview: Use ADVAIR (salmeterol xinafoate/fluticasone propionate) with caution in patients receiving other medications causing hypokalemia and/or increased QTc interval (diuretics, high dose steroids, anti-arrhythmics, astemizole, terfenadine) since cardiac and vascular effects may be potentiated.

Salmeterol Xinafoate: Co-administration of repeat dose ketoconazole (a cytochrome P450 3A4 inhibitor) and salmeterol in healthy subjects resulted in a significant increase in plasma salmeterol exposure (1.4-fold increase in C_{max} and 15-fold increase in AUC). This increase in plasma salmeterol exposure may cause a prolongation of the QTc interval (see Warnings and Precautions and Action and Clinical Pharmacology, Pharmacokinetics).

Fluticasone Propionate: Under normal circumstances, low plasma concentrations of fluticasone propionate are achieved after inhaled dosing, due to extensive first pass metabolism and high systemic clearance mediated by cytochrome P450 3A4 in the gut and liver. Hence, clinically significant drug interactions involving fluticasone propionate are unlikely.

A drug interaction study of intranasal fluticasone propionate in healthy subjects has shown that ritonavir (a highly potent cytochrome P450 3A4 inhibitor) can greatly increase fluticasone propionate plasma concentrations, resulting in markedly reduced serum cortisol concentrations. During post-marketing use, there have been reports of clinically significant drug interactions in patients receiving intranasal or inhaled fluticasone propionate and ritonavir, resulting in systemic corticosteroid effects including Cushing's syndrome and adrenal suppression. Therefore, concomitant use of fluticasone propionate and ritonavir should be avoided, unless the potential benefit to the patient outweighs the risk of systemic corticosteroid side-effects.

This study has shown that other inhibitors of cytochrome P450 3A4 produce negligible (erythromycin) and minor (ketoconazole) increases in systemic exposure to fluticasone propionate without notable reductions in serum cortisol concentrations. However, there have been a few case reports during world-wide post-market use of adrenal cortisol suppression associated with concomitant use of azole anti-fungals and inhaled fluticasone propionate. Therefore, care is advised when co-administering potent cytochrome P450 3A4 inhibitors (e.g. ketoconazole) as there is potential for increased systemic exposure to fluticasone propionate.

Drug-Drug Interactions: See Table 4.

Table 4: ADVAIR DISKUS

Established or Potential Drug-Drug Interactions

Proper Name	Ref	Effect	Clinical Comment
Sympathomimetic Agents	CT	May lead to deleterious cardiovascular effects.	Aerosol bronchodilators of the rapid onset, short duration adrenergic stimulant type may be used for relief of breakthrough symptoms while using salmeterol for asthma. Increasing use of such preparations to control symptoms indicates deterioration of disease control and the patient's therapy plan should be reassessed. The regular, concomitant use of salmeterol and other sympathomimetic agents is not recommended.
Mono amine Oxidase Inhibitors or Tricyclic Antidepressants	CS	Action of salmeterol on vascular system may be potentiated.	Salmeterol should be administered with extreme caution to patients being treated with monoamine oxidase inhibitors or tricyclic antidepressants, or within 2 weeks of discontinuation of such agents.
Methylxanthines	CT	Unknown	The concurrent use of intravenously or orally administered methylxanthines (e.g., aminophylline, theophylline) by patients receiving salmeterol has not been completely evaluated.
Beta-Blockers	CS	May antagonise the bronchodilating action of salmeterol.	Non-selective beta-blocking drugs should never be prescribed in asthma or COPD. Cardioselective beta-blocking drugs should be used with caution in patients with asthma or COPD.
Acetylsalicylic Acid	T		Use with caution in conjunction with corticosteroids in hypoprothrombinemia.
Ritonavir	CT & post-marketing	Systemic effects including Cushings syndrome and adrenal suppression.	Concomitant use of fluticasone propionate and ritonavir should be avoided. (See Drug Interactions, Overview.)
Other Inhibitors of Cytochrome P450 3A4	CT	Increased systemic exposure to salmeterol xinafoate and fluticasone propionate.	Caution is advised when co-administering potent cytochrome P450 3A4 inhibitors (e.g. ketoconazole). (See Drug Interactions, Overview, Warnings and Precautions and Action and Clinical Pharmacology, Pharmacokinetics.)

Legend: C=case study; CT=clinical trial; T=theoretical; CS=class statements.

DOSAGE AND ADMINISTRATION:

Dosing Considerations: When treating asthma patients, ADVAIR/ADVAIR DISKUS should be used only in patients whose conditions are not adequately controlled using low- to medium-dose inhaled corticosteroids or the severity of whose disease clearly warrants the initiation of treatment with two maintenance therapies. ADVAIR/ADVAIR DISKUS is **not** indicated for patients whose asthma can be managed by occasional use of a rapid onset, short duration, inhaled beta$_2$-agonist or for patients whose asthma can be successfully managed by inhaled corticosteroids along with occasional use of a rapid onset, short duration, inhaled beta$_2$-agonist.

ADVAIR (salmeterol xinafoate/fluticasone propionate) should not be used to treat acute symptoms of asthma or COPD. It is crucial to inform patients of this.

For asthma, a rapid onset, short duration beta$_2$-agonist should be prescribed for this purpose. Medical attention should be sought if patients find that rapid onset, short duration relief bronchodilator treatment becomes less effective or if they need more inhalations than usual. Sudden worsening of symptoms may require increased corticosteroid dosage, which should be administered under medical supervision.

As twice-daily regular treatment, ADVAIR provides twenty-four hour bronchodilation and can replace regular use of a rapid onset, short duration (4 hour) inhaled or oral bronchodilator (e.g. salbutamol). Rapid onset, short duration beta$_2$-agonists should be used only to relieve acute symptoms of asthma (see Warnings and Precautions).

Patients should be regularly reassessed so that the strength of ADVAIR they are receiving remains optimal and is only changed on medical advice. The dose should be titrated to the lowest dose of fluticasone propionate at which effective control of symptoms is maintained.

There is no need to adjust the dose in the otherwise healthy elderly or in patients with impaired renal function. Because salmeterol is predominantly cleared by hepatic metabolism, patients with hepatic disease should be closely monitored.

Recommended Dose and Dosage Adjustment: See Table 5 and Table 6.

Table 5: ADVAIR DISKUS

Recommended Dose and Dosage Adjustment

	Asthma		COPD	
	Children 4–11 Years of Age	Adults and Adolescents ≥12 Years of Age	Adults ≥18 Years of Age	
ADVAIR 100 DISKUS	One inhalation twice daily	One inhalation twice daily	—	or
ADVAIR 250 DISKUS	—	One inhalation twice daily	One inhalation twice daily	or
ADVAIR 500 DISKUS	—	One inhalation twice daily	One inhalation twice daily	

Table 6: ADVAIR Inhalation Aerosol

Recommended Dose and Dosage Adjustment

	Asthma	
	Adults and Adolescents ≥12 Years of Age	
ADVAIR 125	Two inhalations twice daily	or
ADVAIR 250	Two inhalations twice daily	

It is intended that each prescribed dose of ADVAIR Inhalation Aerosol be given by a minimum of two inhalations twice daily. However, the prescribed dose of ADVAIR DISKUS may be given by a single inhalation twice daily.

Use with Spacer Devices: Spacer devices may be used in patients who have difficulty coordinating the actuation of a metered dose inhaler (MDI) with inhalation. The dosage of ADVAIR inhalation aerosol should be adjusted according to individual response. For patients whose asthma has been stabilized without the use of a spacer device, continuation of therapy with a spacer may require a dosage adjustment.

Two small single dose pharmacokinetic studies were conducted in subjects with asthma to investigate the performance of various spacer devices. The studies showed that following the administration of ADVAIR inhalation aerosol, the exposure to both fluticasone propionate (FP) and salmeterol xinafoate (SAL) was significantly higher (up to 4 fold) when used with the AeroChamber Max spacer, compared to the MDI alone. Exposure to FP and SAL was also increased with the use of the AeroChamber Plus and Ventahaler spacers, but to a lesser degree than that seen with the AeroChamber Max spacer. The long term safety and clinical effect of using a spacer device with ADVAIR inhalation aerosol was not evaluated in these studies.

Missed Dose: If a single dose is missed, instruct the patient to take the next dose when it is due.

Administration: ADVAIR is to be administered by oral inhalation only.

The patient should be made aware that for optimum benefit ADVAIR should be taken regularly, even when asymptomatic.

As a general rule, rinsing the mouth and gargling with water after each inhalation can help in preventing the occurrence of candidiasis. Cleansing dentures has the same effect.

OVERDOSAGE:

ADVAIR (salmeterol xinafoate/fluticasone propionate) should not be used more frequently than twice daily (morning and evening) at the recommended dose. Fatalities have been reported in association with excessive use of inhaled sympathomimetic drugs (see Warnings and Precautions). Large doses of inhaled or oral salmeterol (12 to 20 times the recommended dose) have been associated with clinically significant prolongation of the QTc interval, which has the potential for producing ventricular arrhythmias.

There are no data available from clinical trials on overdose with ADVAIR (salmeterol xinafoate/fluticasone propionate), however data on overdose with individual drugs is given below.

The expected signs and symptoms of salmeterol overdosage are those typical of excessive beta$_2$-adrenergic stimulation, including tremor, headache, tachycardia, increases in systolic blood pressure, cardiac arrhythmias, hypokalemia, hypertension and, in extreme cases, sudden death. Treatment should be symptomatic; cardiac and respiratory function should be monitored and support provided if necessary. The preferred antidote is the judicious use of a cardioselective beta-blocking agent. Cardioselective beta-blocking drugs should be used with caution, bearing in mind the danger of inducing an asthmatic attack. Serum potassium level should be monitored. If ADVAIR therapy has to be withdrawn due to overdose of the beta-agonist component of the drug; provision of appropriate replacement steroid therapy should be considered.

Acute inhalation of fluticasone propionate doses in excess of those approved may lead to temporary suppression of the hypothalamic-pituitary-adrenal axis. This does not usually require emergency action, as normal adrenal function typically recovers within a few days.

If higher than approved doses are continued over prolonged periods, significant adrenocortical suppression is possible. There have been very rare reports of acute adrenal crisis occurring in children exposed to higher than approved dosages (typically 1000 μg daily and above), over prolonged periods (several months or years); observed features included hypoglycemia and sequelae of decreased consciousness and/or convulsions. Situations which would potentially trigger acute adrenal crisis include exposure to trauma, surgery or infection or any rapid reduction in dosage. Patients receiving higher than approved dosages should be managed closely and the dose reduced gradually.

For management of a suspected drug overdose, contact your regional Poison Control Centre. See the *CPS* Directory section for a list of Poison Control Centres.

ACTION AND CLINICAL PHARMACOLOGY: Mechanism of Action: ADVAIR (salmeterol xinafoate/fluticasone propionate) contains salmeterol xinafoate and fluticasone propionate which have differing modes of action for the treatment of COPD and reversible obstructive airways disease, including asthma. Salmeterol is a long-acting bronchodilator that prevents breakthrough symptoms of wheezing and chest tightness; fluticasone propionate is an inhaled anti-inflammatory agent that reduces airways irritability. ADVAIR can offer a more convenient regime for patients requiring concurrent long-acting beta$_2$-agonists and inhaled corticosteroid therapy. ADVAIR is designed to produce a greater improvement in pulmonary function and symptom control than either fluticasone propionate or salmeterol used alone at their recommended dosages. The respective mechanisms of action of both drugs are discussed below:

Salmeterol is a selective, long-acting (12 hours), slow onset (10-20 minutes) beta$_2$-adrenoceptor agonist with a long side-chain which binds to the exo-site of the receptor. Salmeterol offers more effective protection against histamine-induced bronchoconstriction and produces a longer duration of bronchodilation, lasting for at least 12 hours, than recommended doses of conventional rapid onset, short duration beta$_2$-agonists.

In vitro tests on human lung have shown that salmeterol is a potent and long-lasting inhibitor of the release of mast cell mediators, such as histamine, leukotrienes and prostaglandin D_2.

In man, salmeterol inhibits the early and late phase response to inhaled allergen. The late phase response is inhibited for over 30 hours after a single dose, when the bronchodilator effect is no longer evident. The full clinical significance of these findings is not yet clear. The mechanism is different from the anti-inflammatory effect of corticosteroids.

Fluticasone propionate is a highly potent glucocorticoid anti-inflammatory steroid. When administered by inhalation at therapeutic dosages, it has a direct potent anti-inflammatory action within the lungs, resulting in reduced symptoms and exacerbations of asthma, and less adverse effects than systemically administered corticosteroids.

In comparisons with beclomethasone dipropionate, fluticasone propionate has demonstrated greater topical potency.

Pharmacodynamics: The pharmacodynamic effects and pharmacokinetics of the combination product in the DISKUS powder inhaler were investigated in healthy adult male and female volunteers after single and repeat-dose administration.

Those studies showed that the systemic pharmacodynamic effects of salmeterol xinafoate and fluticasone propionate are essentially unchanged when the two drugs are administered in combination, when compared with the component drugs given alone or concurrently.

There was no evidence that the systemic exposure to salmeterol was altered by concomitant exposure to fluticasone propionate. In one study, the salmeterol plasma C_{max} and T_{max} were not significantly different when compared between the groups receiving salmeterol xinafoate 100 µg and fluticasone propionate 500 µg twice daily in the combination product (C_{max} 0.23 ng/mL) or salmeterol xinafoate 100 µg twice daily as a single agent (C_{max} 0.22 ng/mL).

When fluticasone propionate alone or the salmeterol xinafoate/fluticasone propionate product are administered at the same dosage, there is similar systemic exposure to fluticasone propionate.

Pharmacokinetics: There is no evidence in animal or human subjects that the administration of salmeterol xinafoate and fluticasone propionate together by the inhaled route affects the pharmacokinetics of either component. For pharmacokinetic purposes therefore each component can be considered separately.

Salmeterol Xinafoate: Salmeterol acts locally in the lung; therefore, plasma levels are not an indication of therapeutic effect. Because of the low therapeutic dose, systemic levels of salmeterol are low or undetectable after inhalation of recommended doses (50 µg twice daily). Salmeterol is predominantly cleared by hepatic metabolism; liver function impairment may lead to accumulation of salmeterol in plasma. Therefore, patients with hepatic disease should be closely monitored.

An in vitro study showed that salmeterol is extensively metabolised to α-hydroxysalmeterol (aliphatic oxidation) by cytochrome P450 3A4 (CYP3A4). A repeat dose study with salmeterol and erythromycin in healthy volunteers showed no clinically significant changes in pharmacodynamic effects at 500 mg three times daily doses of erythromycin. However, a salmeterol-ketoconazole interaction study resulted in a significant increase in plasma salmeterol exposure (see Warnings and Precautions, and Drug Interactions).

In a placebo-controlled, crossover drug interaction study in 15 healthy subjects, co-administration of salmeterol (50 µg twice daily inhaled) and the cytochrome P450 3A4 (CYP3A4) inhibitor, ketoconazole (400 mg once daily orally), for 7 days, resulted in a significant increase in plasma salmeterol exposure (1.4-fold C_{max} and 15-fold AUC). There was no increase in salmeterol accumulation with repeat dosing. Three subjects were withdrawn from salmeterol and ketoconazole co-administration due to QTc prolongation or palpitations with sinus tachycardia. In the remaining 12 subjects, co-administration of salmeterol and ketoconazole did not result in a clinically significant effect on heart rate, blood potassium or QTc duration (see Warnings and Precautions, and Drug Interactions).

Fluticasone Propionate: Following intravenous administration, the pharmacokinetics of fluticasone propionate are proportional to the dose. Fluticasone propionate is extensively distributed within the body. The volume of distribution at steady state is approximately 300 L and has a very high clearance which is estimated to be 1.1 L/min indicating extensive hepatic extraction.

Peak plasma fluticasone propionate concentrations are reduced by approximately 98% within 3-4 hours and only low plasma concentrations are associated with the terminal half-life, which is approximately 8 hours.

Following oral administration of fluticasone propionate, 87-100% of the dose is excreted in the faeces. Following doses of either 1 or 16 mg, up to 20% and 75% respectively, is excreted in the faeces as the parent compound. There is a non-active major metabolite. Absolute oral bioavailability is negligible (<1%) due to a combination of incomplete absorption from the gastrointestinal tract and extensive first-pass metabolism.

Following inhaled dosing in healthy volunteers, absolute systemic bioavailability of fluticasone propionate varies between approximately 10-30% of the nominal dose depending on the inhalation device used. Systemic absorption of fluticasone propionate occurs mainly through the lungs, and is initially rapid, then prolonged.

The plasma protein binding of fluticasone propionate is 91%. Fluticasone propionate is extensively metabolised by CYP3A4 enzyme to an inactive carboxylic acid derivative.

STORAGE AND STABILITY: ADVAIR DISKUS: Do not store ADVAIR DISKUS above 25°C. Keep in a dry place.

ADVAIR Inhalation Aerosol: Replace the mouthpiece cover firmly and snap it into position. Store ADVAIR inhalation aerosol between 15 and 25°C. Protect from frost and direct sunlight.

SPECIAL HANDLING INSTRUCTIONS: ADVAIR Inhalation Aerosol: Contents under pressure. Container may explode if heated. Do not place in hot water or near radiators, stoves, or other sources of heat. Even when apparently empty, do not puncture or incinerate container or store at temperatures over 25°C.

As with most inhaled medications in pressurized canisters, the therapeutic effect of this medication may decrease when the canister is cold.

INFORMATION FOR THE PATIENT: Published in e-CPS, available by subscription at www.e-cps.ca.

DOSAGE FORMS, COMPOSITION AND PACKAGING: ADVAIR DISKUS: ADVAIR 100 DISKUS: A plastic inhaler device containing a foil strip with 28 or 60 blisters. Each blister contains 50 µg of salmeterol (as the xinafoate salt) and 100 µg of fluticasone propionate. Nonmedicinal ingredients: lactose (milk sugar), including milk protein, which acts as the "carrier".

ADVAIR 250 DISKUS: A plastic inhaler device containing a foil strip with 28 or 60 blisters. Each blister contains 50 µg of salmeterol (as the xinafoate salt) and 250 µg of fluticasone propionate. Nonmedicinal ingredients: lactose (milk sugar), including milk protein, which acts as the "carrier".

ADVAIR 500 DISKUS: A plastic inhaler device containing a foil strip with 28 or 60 blisters. Each blister contains 50 µg of salmeterol (as the xinafoate salt) and 500 µg of fluticasone propionate. Nonmedicinal ingredients: lactose (milk sugar), including milk protein, which acts as the "carrier".

ADVAIR Inhalation Aerosol: ADVAIR 125: A pressurized metered-dose inhaler (MDI) consisting of an aluminum canister with a metering valve. Each canister is fitted into the supplied purple actuator/adaptor. A dust cap is fitted over the actuator's mouthpiece when not in use. It delivers: 25 µg salmeterol (as the xinafoate salt) and 125 µg fluticasone propionate per actuation. Nonmedicinal ingredients: HFA-134a (1,1,1,2-tetrafluoroethane). It contains no excipients. Formats of 120 doses.

ADVAIR 250: A pressurized metered-dose inhaler (MDI) consisting of an aluminum canister with a metering valve. Each canister is fitted into the supplied purple actuator/adaptor. A dust cap is fitted over the actuator's mouthpiece when not in use. It delivers: 25 µg salmeterol (as the xinafoate salt) and 250 µg fluticasone propionate per actuation. Nonmedicinal ingredients: HFA-134a (1,1,1,2-tetrafluoroethane). It contains no excipients. Formats of 120 doses.

(Shown in Product Identification Section)

Advate

antihemophilic factor (recombinant) plasma/albumin free method (rAHF-PFM)

Coagulant

Baxter

Date of Preparation: July 27, 2006
Date of Revision: March 6, 2009

SUMMARY PRODUCT INFORMATION:

Route of Administration	Dosage Form/ Strength	Clinically Relevant Nonmedicinal Ingredients
Intravenous	Powder for Intravenous injection/250, 500, 1000, 1500, 2000 and 3000 International Units (IU) per vial reconstituted in 5 mL of water for injection.	None are clinically relevant. For a complete listing see Dosage Forms, Composition and Packaging.

DESCRIPTION: ADVATE [Antihemophilic Factor (Recombinant), Plasma/Albumin-Free Method] is synthesized by a genetically engineered Chinese hamster ovary (CHO) cell line. In culture, the CHO cell line expresses recombinant antihemophilic factor (rAHF) into the cell culture medium. The rAHF is purified from the culture medium using a series of chromatography columns. The cornerstone of the purification process is an immunoaffinity chromatography step in which a monoclonal antibody directed against Factor VIII is employed to selectively isolate the rAHF from the medium. The rAHF synthesized by the CHO cells has the same biological effects as Antihemophilic Factor (Human) [AHF (Human)]. Structurally the recombinant protein has a similar combination of heterogeneous heavy and light chains as found in AHF (Human).

INDICATIONS AND CLINICAL USE: ADVATE is indicated for:

- prevention and control of bleeding episodes, in hemophilia A (classical hemophilia).
- peri-operative management of patients with hemophilia A.

ADVATE can be of therapeutic value in patients with Factor VIII inhibitors not exceeding 10 Bethesda Units (BU) per mL. However, in patients with a known or suspected inhibitor to Factor VIII, the plasma Factor VIII level should be monitored frequently and the dose of ADVATE should be adjusted accordingly. (See Warnings and Precautions.)

ADVATE is not indicated for treatment of von Willebrand's disease.

Geriatrics (>65 years of age): Insufficient data are available.

Pediatrics (<16 years of age): The safety and efficacy of ADVATE in pediatric patients are similar to that of adult patients. (See Dosage and Administration.)

CONTRAINDICATIONS: ADVATE is contraindicated in patients who have hypersensitivity reactions, including anaphylaxis, to the product or its components, including mouse or hamster proteins. For a complete listing, see Dosage Forms, Composition and Packaging.

WARNINGS AND PRECAUTIONS: General: Identification of the clotting defect as Factor VIII deficiency is essential before the administration of ADVATE. No benefit may be expected from this product in treating other coagulation factor deficiencies.

As with all Factor VIII products, the clinical response to ADVATE may vary. If bleeding is not controlled with the recommended dose, the plasma level of Factor VIII should be determined and a sufficient dose of ADVATE should be administered to achieve a satisfactory clinical response. If the patient's plasma Factor VIII level fails to increase as expected or if bleeding is not controlled after adequate dosing, the presence of an inhibitor (neutralizing antibodies) should be suspected and appropriate testing performed.

Carcinogenesis and Mutagenesis: No studies were conducted with the active ingredient in ADVATE to assess its mutagenic or carcinogenic potential. The CHO cell line employed in the production of ADVATE is derived from that used in the biosynthesis of RECOMBINATE rAHF. ADVATE has been shown to be comparable to RECOMBINATE rAHF with respect to its biochemical and physicochemical properties, as well as its non-clinical in vivo pharmacology and toxicology. By inference, RECOMBINATE rAHF and ADVATE would be expected to have equivalent mutagenic and carcinogenic potential.

RECOMBINATE rAHF was tested for mutagenicity at doses considerably exceeding plasma concentrations in vitro, and at doses up to ten times the expected maximal clinical dose in vivo. At that concentration, it did not cause reverse mutations, chromosomal aberrations, or an increase in micronuclei formation in bone marrow polychromatic erythrocytes. Studies in animals have not been performed to evaluate carcinogenic potential.

Immune: Hypersensitivity Reactions: Allergic type hypersensitivity reactions have been observed with ADVATE. Patients should be informed of the early signs of hypersensitivity reactions including hives, generalized urticaria, and tightness of the chest, wheezing, hypotension, and anaphylaxis. Patients should be advised to discontinue use of the product and contact their physician if these symptoms occur.

Formation of Antibodies to Mouse or Hamster Protein: ADVATE contains trace amounts of mouse immunoglobulin G (MuIgG; maximum of 0.1 ng/IU ADVATE rAHF-PFM) and hamster (CHO) proteins (maximum of 1.5 ng/IU ADVATE rAHF-PFM). As such, there exists a remote possibility that patients treated with this product may develop hypersensitivity to these non-human mammalian proteins.

Peri-Operative Considerations: ADVATE is also indicated in the peri-operative management of patients with hemophilia A. Careful control of replacement therapy is important, especially in cases of major surgery or life-threatening hemorrhages.

Sensitivity/Resistance: Formation of Inhibitors to Factor VIII: The formation of neutralizing antibodies, which are inhibitors of Factor VIII, is a known complication in the management of individuals with hemophilia A. Among previously untreated patients receiving rAHF products inhibitors occur in 15-32% of the population. The incidence among patients who have previously experienced >50 exposure days to rAHF is approximately 2 per 1000 patient-years. These inhibitors are invariably of the immunoglobulin G (IgG) isotype, and the Factor VIII inhibitory activity is expressed as BU per mL of plasma or serum. Patients treated with AHF products should be carefully monitored for the development of Factor VIII inhibitors by appropriate clinical observations and laboratory tests.

Special Populations: Pregnant Women: Animal reproduction studies have not been conducted with ADVATE. It is not known whether ADVATE can cause fetal harm when administered to a pregnant woman, or whether it can affect reproductive capacity. ADVATE should be given to a pregnant woman only if clearly needed.

Nursing Women: It is unknown if the drug is excreted in human milk. Because many drugs are excreted in human milk precaution should be exercised.

Pediatrics (<16 years of age): More frequent or larger doses should be considered for pediatric patients to account for the observed difference in adjusted recovery and terminal half-life between adult and pediatric patients (Table 5). Separate dosing guidelines have also been established for pediatric patients <6 years old (see Dosage and Administration).

Geriatrics (>65 years of age): Insufficient data are available.

Monitoring and Laboratory Tests: Although the dose can be estimated using calculations (see Dosage and Administration), it is highly recommended that, whenever possible, appropriate laboratory tests be performed on the patient's plasma at suitable intervals to assure that adequate Factor VIII levels have been reached and are maintained.

If the patient's plasma Factor VIII level fails to increase as expected or if bleeding is not controlled after adequate dosing, the presence of an inhibitor should be suspected. By performing the appropriate laboratory procedures, the presence of an inhibitor can be demonstrated and quantified in terms of the number of BU per mL (i.e., the amount of Factor VIII activity neutralized by one mL of patient plasma). If the inhibitor is present at levels less than 10 BU per mL, the administration of additional AHF concentrate may neutralize the inhibitor. Thereafter, the administration of additional AHF concentrate should elicit the predicted response. The close monitoring of plasma Factor VIII levels by laboratory assays is necessary in this situation.

Inhibitor titers above 10 BU per mL may make control of hemostasis with AHF concentrates either impossible or impractical because of the very large dose required. In addition, the inhibitor titer may rise following AHF infusion as a result of an anamnestic response to Factor VIII. The treatment or prevention of bleeding in such patients requires the use of alternative therapeutic approaches and agents.

ADVERSE REACTIONS: Adverse Drug Reaction Overview: The majority of the Adverse Events in the clinical trials appear to have been related to trauma, intercurrent mild respiratory or gastrointestinal disease, or well-described complications of hemophilia (see Warnings and Precautions).

Clinical Trial Adverse Drug Reactions: Because clinical trials are conducted under very specific conditions the adverse reaction rates observed in the clinical trials may not reflect the rates observed in practice and should not be compared to the rates in the clinical trials of another drug. Adverse drug reaction information from clinical trials is useful for identifying drug-related adverse events and for approximating rates.

The following information is based on data collected from clinical trials conducted under very specific controlled conditions. In the ADVATE clinical program, 234 treated subjects received a total of 84 539 784 IU of ADVATE from 47 lots in 44 926 infusions. Overall exposure was a total of 113 488 subject days and a total of 43 776 exposure days. A total of 2507 adverse events (AEs) were reported in 215 subjects treated with at least 1 of the study drugs. Only 59 AEs in 49 subjects were serious and all but 5 AEs were judged by the investigator to be unrelated to study drug. The 5 serious AEs considered related to study product were related to the development of FVIII inhibitors in 5 previously untreated patients. There were no deaths in any of the studies of ADVATE. Among the 2448 non-serious AEs, the majority were mild (n=1741; 85.9%) or moderate (n=649; 59.4%).

Of all AEs, only 56 were judged by the investigator to be possibly or probably related to the administration of ADVATE. None led to the discontinuation of study medication*. Among the AEs deemed product-related, no particular type of AE predominated; nearly all (53/56) were isolated events in subjects who had numerous subsequent infusions without recurrence. The adverse drug reactions that occurred in the greatest number of patients were anti-Factor VIII antibody and headache (5 patients each). Common adverse events with a frequency greater than 0.5% are reported in Table 1.

* One of the 5 previously untreated patients (PUPs) who developed a FVIII inhibitor underwent immune tolerance induction therapy with study product according to the protocol and discontinued from the study. This subject successfully completed an immune tolerance induction regimen using commercial ADVATE.

Table 1: ADVATE
Summary of Adverse Drug Reactions from the ADVATE Clinical Program [Frequency Greater than 0.5 % (n=234)]

MedDRA System Organ Class	MedDRA Preferred Term	Number of Patients	AE Rate (% Patients)[a]
Gastrointestinal Disorders	Diarrhoea	2	0.85%
General Disorders and Administrative Site Conditions	Pyrexia	3	1.28%
Investigations	Anti FVIII antibody positive	5[b]	2.14%
Nervous System Disorders	Dizziness	3	1.28%
	Headache	5	2.14%
Skin and Subcutaneous Tissue Disorders	Pruritus	2	0.85%
	Rash	2	0.85%

[a] Baxter clinical program included 234 unique, treated subjects from: completed studies 069901 (Pivotal), 060102 (Pivotal Continuation), BLB-200-01 (Japanese Pivotal), 060101 (Pediatric), and 069902 (Surgery), and ongoing study 060103 (PUPs) (database snapshot 27 March 2006).
[b] As specified in the protocol of Baxter clinical study 060103, a FVIII inhibitor titer ≥0.6 BU was reported as an SAE.

During clinical trials with ADVATE in 198 patients, diagnosed with severe to moderately severe hemophilia A (FVIII ≤2%) and with previous exposure to Factor VIII concentrates >150 days, only one subject developed a low-titer inhibitor (2.4 BU in the modified Bethesda assay) after 26 exposure days. Follow-up inhibitor tests performed for this subject after withdrawal from the study were negative (See Formation of Inhibitors for Factor VIII). Also, in 53 pediatric patients under the age of 6, also diagnosed with severe to moderately severe hemophilia A (FVIII ≤2%) and with previous exposure to Factor VIII concentrates >50 days, no inhibitor incidence was detected. Based on the results obtained so far in the ADVATE clinical program and the number of subjects enrolled and followed, the 95% confidence intervals for the risk of previously treated patients of developing inhibitors to Factor VIII is 0.026 to 2.91% for low titer (≤5.0 BU), 0 to 1.90% for high titer (>5.0 BU), and 0.026 to 2.91% for factor VIII inhibitor of any titer. The incidence of Factor VIII inhibitors in previously untreated patients (PUPs) is being assessed in an ongoing clinical study. The eligible patients should have no previous treatment experience with other FVIII concentrates at study entry and no more than 3 exposure days with ADVATE within 28 days prior to screening. Of the 25 subjects treated in the study, 5 thus far have developed inhibitors to factor VIII. The maximal titer was high (>5 BU) in 4 subjects and low (≤5 BU) in one.

Immunogenicity was also evaluated by the development of antibodies to heterologous proteins (i.e., CHO cell protein, murine IgG, and human VWF). Of 182 subjects who were treated and assessed for anti-CHO cell protein antibodies, 3 showed a statistically significant (p<0.01) upward trend by regression analysis and 4 showed sustained peaks or transient spikes. Of 182 subjects who were treated and assessed for anti-murine IgG antibodies, 10 showed a statistically significant upward trend and 2 showed a sustained peak or transient spike. Four of these subjects reported isolated events of urticaria, pruritus, rash, and slightly elevated eosinophil counts amongst numerous repeat study product exposures. None of the other subjects exhibited signs or symptoms indicative of an allergic or hypersensitivity response. Of the 181 subjects who were treated and assessed for the presence of anti-human VWF antibodies, none displayed laboratory evidence indicative of a positive serologic response.

Less Common Clinical Trial Adverse Drug Reactions (<0.5%): Less common clinical study adverse events observed in a single subject include: see Table 2.

Table 2: ADVATE
Less Common Clinical Study Adverse Events

MedDRA System Organ Class	MedDRA Preferred Term	Number of Patients	AE Rate (% Patients)[a]
Blood and Lymphatic System Disorders	Lymphangitis	1	0.43%
Eye Disorders	Eye inflammation	1	0.43%
Gastrointestinal Disorders	Abdominal pain upper	1	0.43%
	Nausea	1	0.43%
	Vomiting	1	0.43%
General Disorders and Administrative Site Conditions	Chest pain	1	0.43%
	Chills	1	0.43%
	Feeling abnormal	1	0.43%
	Oedema peripheral	1	0.43%
Infections and Infestations	Influenza	1	0.43%
	Laryngitis	1	0.43%
Injury, Poisoning and Procedural Complications	Post procedural complication	1	0.43%
	Post procedural haemorrhage	1	0.43%
	Procedural site reaction	1	0.43%
Investigations	Coagulation FVIII decreased	1[b]	0.43%
	Haematocrit decreased	1	0.43%
	Laboratory test abnormal	1	0.43%
Nervous System Disorders	Dysgeusia[c]	1	0.43%
	Migraine	1	0.43%
	Memory impairment	1	0.43%
	Tremor	1	0.43%
Respiratory, Thoracic and Mediastinal Disorders	Dyspnoea	1	0.43%
Skin and Subcutaneous Tissue Disorders	Dermatitis diaper	1	0.43%
	Hyperhidrosis	1	0.43%
Vascular Disorders	Haematoma	1	0.43%
	Hot flush[c]	1	0.43%
	Pallor	1	0.43%

(cont'd)

[a] The Baxter rAHF-PFM clinical program included 234 unique, treated subjects from: completed studies 069901 (Pivotal), 060102 (Pivotal Continuation), BLB-200-01 (Japanese Pivotal), 060101 (Pediatric), and 069902 (Surgery), and ongoing study 060103 (PUPs) (database snapshot 27 March 2006).
[b] The unexpected decreased coagulation FVIII levels in association with an infected central catheter occurred in 1 patient during continuous infusion of rAHF-PFM following surgery (postoperative days 10-14). Hemostasis was maintained at all times during this period and both plasma FVIII levels and clearance rates returned to appropriate levels by postoperative day 15. FVIII inhibitor assays performed after completion of continuous infusion and at study termination were negative.
[c] Dysgeusia was reported four times by a single patient and hot flushes occurred twice in another patient.

Abnormal Hematologic and Clinical Chemistry Findings: The abnormal hematologic and clinical chemistry findings that were observed in a single case each are; decrease in FVIII level, decrease in hematocrit and an abnormal laboratory test (see Table 2). Examination of the changes in laboratory parameters indicated no evidence of toxicity with ADVATE.

Post-Market Adverse Drug Reactions: A total of 293 adverse drug reaction reactions (ADR's) associated with the use of ADVATE were reported between 18 August 2003 and 30 September 2006. Of the 293 reports, 155 were serious and 138 were non-serious. During the period of time covered by these reports, 1.727 billion units of ADVATE were sold.

Adverse reactions identified during post-approval use of ADVATE can be found in Table 3. Because these reactions are reported voluntarily from a population of uncertain size, it is not always possible to reliably estimate their frequency or establish a causal relationship to drug exposure.

Table 3: ADVATE
Summary of Adverse Drug Reactions from ADVATE Post-Marketing Experience

MedDRA Standard System Organ Class (SOC)	MedDRA Preferred Term (PT)
Blood and Lymphatic System Disorders	Factor VIII inhibition
Immune System Disorders	Hypersensitivity
	Anaphylactic reaction
Nervous System Disorders	Headache
	Dizziness
	Paraesthesia
	Cerebral haemorrhage
Vascular Disorders	Flushing
	Haemorrhage
Respiratory, Thoracic and Mediastinal Disorders	Dyspnoea
	Wheezing
	Pharyngolaryngeal pain
	Bronchospasm
	Throat tightness
Gastrointestinal Disorders	Abdominal pain
	Nausea
Skin and Subcutaneous Disorders	Urticaria (generalized)
	Erythema
	Pruritus
	Rash (macular)
	Increased tendency to bruise
	Prurigo
General Disorders and Administration Site Conditions	Drug effect decreased
	Drug ineffective
	Pyrexia
	Chest discomfort
	Chest pain
	Chills
	Infusion site pain
	Asthenia
Musculoskeletal and Connective Tissue Disorders	Haemathrosis

A small cluster of lack of effect events were noted from Germany. More than 90% of these reports of decreased efficacy were received from one Haemophilia Center in Bonn, Germany. The age of the patients ranged between 5 and 52 years (median: 36 yrs). The majority of patients received prophylactic treatment. Period of factor VIII treatment documented prior to ADVATE ranged between 125 to 477 days (median 372 days) and after change to ADVATE between 11 to 340 days (median 133 days).

One third of these patients did not suffer from any bleeding events during ADVATE treatment, however, felt better protected with the previous Factor VIII concentrate. One third suffered from only 1 bleed (primarily spontaneous bleeding) under ADVATE and the remaining patients experienced between 2 and 5 bleeds under ADVATE. However, comparing the pre-ADVATE period with the period of ADVATE therapy, in none of the patients could a clearly increased bleeding incidence be demonstrated.

In three-quarters of the cases, no relevant results on inhibitor testing were available. In one-quarter of the reports, sporadic inhibitor tests were performed during ADVATE treatment; however, results were negative in all instances. No formal pharmacokinetic investigations (recovery, half-life testing) to exclude low factor VIII inhibitors were performed.

However, none of the patients reported a lack of efficacy or increased bleeding frequency with their previous product, observations that are consistent with the absence of inhibitor formation.

DRUG INTERACTIONS: No interaction of ADVATE with other medicinal products is known or has been established.

DOSAGE AND ADMINISTRATION: Dosing Considerations: Each vial of ADVATE is labeled with the rAHF activity expressed in IU per vial. This potency assignment employs a Factor VIII concentrate standard that is referenced to a WHO International Standard for Factor VIII Concentrates, and is evaluated by appropriate methodology to ensure accuracy of the results.

The expected in vivo peak increase in Factor VIII level expressed as IU/dL of plasma or percent of normal can be estimated by multiplying the dose administered per kg body weight (IU/kg) by two. This calculation is based on the findings of several pharmacokinetic studies of rAHF concentrates, and is supported by the data generated by 223 pharmacokinetic determinations with ADVATE in 107 Phase 2/3 pivotal study subjects. These pharmacokinetic data demonstrated a peak post-infusion recovery of approximately 2 IU/dL per IU/kg above the pre-infusion baseline.

Examples (assuming patient's baseline Factor VIII level is <1% of normal):

1. A dose of 1750 IU ADVATE administered to a 70 kg patient, i.e. 25 IU/kg (1750/70), should be expected to cause a peak post-infusion Factor VIII increase of 25×2 or 50 IU/dL (50% of normal).
2. A peak level of 70% is required in a 40 kg child. In this situation, the dose would be 70/2×40=1400 IU.

Although dose can be estimated by the calculations above, it is highly recommended that, whenever possible, appropriate laboratory tests including serial Factor VIII activity assays be performed on the patient's plasma at suitable intervals to assure that adequate Factor VIII levels have been reached and are maintained. The amount and frequency of administration should be adapted to the clinical response in the patient. Individual patients may vary in their response to Factor VIII, demonstrating different levels of Factor VIII in vivo recovery, half-life as well as clinical response to treatment.

Recommended Dose and Dosage Adjustment: Physician supervision of the treatment regimen is required. A guide for dosing in the treatment of hemorrhages is provided in Table 4.

Table 4: ADVATE

Guide to ADVATE Dosing for Treatment & Control of Bleeding Episodes

Degree of Hemorrhage	Required Peak Post-Infusion Factor VIII Activity in the Blood (as % of Normal or IU/dL)	Frequency of Infusion[a]
Early hemarthrosis, muscle bleeding episode, or oral bleeding episode	20–40	Begin infusions every 12 to 24 hours (8 to 24 hours for patients under the age of 6 years)[a] for one to three days until the bleeding episode is resolved (as indicated by relief of pain) or healing is achieved.
More extensive hemarthrosis, muscle bleeding episode, or hematoma	30–60	Repeat infusions every 12 to 24 hours (8 to 24 hours for patients under the age of 6 years)[a] for (usually) three days or more until pain and disability are resolved.
Life-threatening bleeding episodes such as head injury, throat bleeding episode, or severe abdominal pain	60–100	Repeat infusions every 8 to 24 hours (6 to 12 hours for patients under the age of 6 years)[a] until resolution of the bleeding episode has occurred.

[a] The frequency of infusion was adjusted for pediatric patients to compensate for the fact that the observed adjusted recovery and half-life were generally higher in adolescents and adults compared to infants and children (Table 6).

For prevention of bleeding episodes, dosing between 25 to 40 IU of Factor VIII per kg body weight every other day (3 to 4 times weekly) may be utilized. In patients under the age of 6, doses of 25 to 50 IU of Factor VIII per kg body weight 3 to 4 times weekly are recommended. The exact dose should be defined by the patient's clinical status and demonstrated Factor VIII in vivo recovery and half-life. Other treatment regimens have been proposed, such as that of Schimpf et al, which describes continuous maintenance therapy.

A guide for dosing in peri-operative management is provided in Table 5. Careful monitoring and control of replacement therapy is especially important in cases of major surgery or life-threatening hemorrhages.

Table 5: ADVATE

Guide to ADVATE Dosing for Peri-Operative Management

Type of Procedure	Required Peak Post-Infusion Factor VIII Activity in the Blood (as % of Normal or IU/dL)	Frequency of Infusion[a]
Minor surgery, including tooth extraction	60–100	A single bolus infusion plus 5–7 days of oral antifibrinolytic therapy (for dental extractions), beginning within one hour of the operation, is sufficient in most cases.
Major surgery	80–120 (pre- and post-operative)	For bolus infusion replacement, repeat infusions every 8 to 24 hours (6 to 24 hours for patients under the age of 6 years[a]), depending on the desired level of Factor VIII and state of wound healing. For continuous infusion replacement, begin infusion at 4-5 IU/kg/h after a loading dose, monitor levels of Factor VIII at least once per day, and modify the infusion rate according to the desired level of Factor VIII and the state of wound healing (see Administration by Continuous Infusion).

[a] The frequency of infusion was adjusted for pediatric patients to compensate for the fact that the observed adjusted recovery and half-life were generally higher in adolescents and adults compared to infants and children (Table 6).

Missed Dose:

- Double doses are generally not required to compensate for forgotten individual doses.
- Patients should be advised to proceed immediately with a regular administration of ADVATE and to continue treatment at regular intervals as required.

Administration: Administration by Bolus Infusion: Parenteral drug products should be inspected for particulate matter and discoloration prior to administration, whenever solution and container permit. A colorless appearance is acceptable for ADVATE. ADVATE should be administered at room temperature not more than 3 hours after reconstitution. Plastic syringes must be used with this product, since proteins such as ADVATE tend to stick to the surface of glass syringes. A dose of ADVATE should be administered over a period of ≤5 minutes (maximum infusion rate, 10 mL/min). The pulse rate should be determined before and during administration of ADVATE. Should a significant increase in pulse rate occur, reducing the rate of administration or temporarily halting the injection usually allows the symptoms to disappear promptly.

Administration by Continuous Infusion: There are limited safety and efficacy data to support the administration of ADVATE by continuous infusion.

The 3000, 2000, 1500, 1000, and 500 IU/vial nominal potencies of ADVATE are suitable for use in a continuous infusion mode of administration. Continuous infusion of ADVATE must employ either a syringe pump running at a rate of ≥0.4 mL/h, or a CADD-1 type infusion pump running at a rate of ≥1.5 mL/h. In vitro studies employing a syringe pump or a CADD-1 pump have demonstrated >80% recovery of the Hour 0 potency of ADVATE for up to 48 hours of continuous infusion. For sterility assurance purposes, a fresh supply of reconstituted ADVATE for continuous infusion should be replaced at bedside at no less frequently than every 12 hours. Either polyvinylchloride or polyethylene infusion tubing (microbore) may be used, and 2-5 IU heparin/mL reconstituted product can be added as a means to prevent thrombophlebitis at the infusion site. ADVATE reconstituted with 5 mL Sterile Water for Injection USP should never be further diluted. However, one of three "piggy-backed" intravenous solutions (normal saline, 0.45% saline, or 0.45% saline in 5% dextrose) may be infused concurrently with ADVATE through a "Y" connector. The post-reconstitution photostability of ADVATE is acceptable under the conditions of visible and ultra-violet light exposure anticipated in a clinical setting.

After administration of a loading dose to correct the plasma Factor VIII level to 80-120 IU/dL, begin infusion of ADVATE at a rate of 4 IU/kg/h for patients >12 years of age and 5 IU/kg/h for children between 5 and 12 years of age. The use of ADVATE by continuous infusion has not been evaluated in children under 5 years of age. Based on experience with other Factor VIII products, administration of ADVATE by continuous infusion, in a small number of subjects, was preceded by a loading bolus dose. After administration of a loading dose to correct the plasma Factor VIII level to 80-120 IU/dL, begin infusion of Factor VIII at a rate of 4 IU/kg/h for patients >12 years of age and 5 IU/kg/h for children between 5 and 12 years of age. It is highly recommended that plasma Factor VIII levels be checked within 3 to 6 hours after the initiation of continuous infusion in order to document that the desired Factor VIII levels are being maintained. Rates of infusion should be modified based on the levels of plasma Factor VIII activity measured at least once per day thereafter, and based on the desired level of Factor VIII.

Reconstitution: Reconstitution Using the BAXJECT II Device: Use Aseptic Technique :

1. Bring the ADVATE (dry factor concentrate) and Sterile Water for Injection USP (diluent) to room temperature.
2. Remove caps from the factor concentrate and diluent vials.
3. Cleanse stoppers with germicidal solution and allow to dry prior to use. Place the vials on a flat surface.
4. Open the BAXJECT II device package by peeling away the lid, without touching the inside. **Do not remove the device from the package.**
5. Turn the package over. Press straight down to fully insert the clear plastic spike through the diluent vial stopper.
6. Grip the BAXJECT II package at its edge and pull the package off the device. **Do not remove the blue cap from the BAXJECT II device.** Do not touch the exposed white plastic spike.
7. Turn the system over, so that the diluent vial is on top. Quickly insert the white plastic spike fully into the ADVATE vial stopper by pushing straight down. The vacuum will draw the diluent into the ADVATE vial.
8. Swirl gently until ADVATE is completely dissolved.
9. Remove the blue cap from the BAXJECT II device. Connect the syringe to the BAXJECT II device. **Do not inject air.**
10. Turn the system upside down (factor concentrate vial now on top). Draw the factor concentrate into the syringe by pulling the plunger back slowly.
11. Disconnect the syringe; attach a suitable needle and inject intravenously as instructed under Administration.
12. If a patient is to receive more than one vial of ADVATE, the contents of multiple vials may be drawn into the same syringe. **Please note that the BAXJECT II reconstitution device is intended for use with a single vial of ADVATE and Sterile Water for Injection USP only, therefore reconstituting and withdrawing a second vial into the syringe requires a second BAXJECT II device.**

Note: Do not refrigerate after reconstitution. If ADVATE is being prepared for administration by continuous infusion (see Administration by Continuous Infusion), it should be reconstituted and pooled in a laminar airflow environment in order to optimize the maintenance of sterility during infusion. A fresh supply of reconstituted ADVATE for continuous infusion should be replaced at the bedside at intervals of ≤12 hours.

OVERDOSAGE:

Of all infusions administered during clinical studies, 0.9% of infusions were >100 IU/kg. No subject received a dose >208 IU/kg in these studies. No safety concerns were identified in association with these infusions.

For management of a suspected drug overdose, CPhA recommends that you contact your **regional Poison Control Centre**. See the *CPS* Directory section for a list of Poison Control Centres.

ACTION AND CLINICAL PHARMACOLOGY: Mechanism of Action: ADVATE contains recombinant coagulation Factor VIII, a glycoprotein that has an amino acid sequence comparable to human Factor VIII, and post-translational modifications that are similar to those of the plasma-derived molecule. Activated Factor VIII acts as a cofactor for activated Factor IX, accelerating the conversion of Factor X to activated Factor X. Activated Factor X converts prothrombin to thrombin. Thrombin then converts fibrinogen into fibrin and a fibrin clot is formed.

Pharmacodynamics: Hemophilia A is a sex-linked hereditary disorder of blood coagulation due to decreased levels of Factor VIII activity and results in profuse bleeding into joints, muscles or internal organs, either spontaneously or as a result of accidental or surgical trauma. The plasma levels of Factor VIII are increased by replacement therapy, thereby enabling a temporary correction of the factor deficiency and correction of the bleeding tendency. The level required to achieve adequate hemostasis varies depending on anatomic location and severity of traumatic insult if present.

Pharmacokinetics: A total of 167 subjects are included in the determination of the pharmacokinetic parameters of ADVATE (Table 6). Of these 8 were infants, 55 children, 28 adolescents, and 76 adults. No neonates were included. Area-under-the-curve (AUC), incremental recovery, half-life, and mean residence time (MRT) were generally higher and clearance (CL) was generally lower in adolescents and adults compared to infants and children. Only minimal differences were observed in the volume of distribution at steady state (V_{ss}) among the different age groups. No age-related differences were observed in pharmacokinetic parameters among subjects who were older than 12 years of age.

Table 6: ADVATE

Summary of Pharmacokinetic Parameters of ADVATE per Age Group[a]

Parameter (Mean±Standard Deviation)	Infants (n=8)	Children (n=55)	Adolescents (n=28)	Adults (n=76)
Adjusted Recovery (IU/dL:IU/kg)	2.11±0.51	1.96±0.48	2.29±0.57	2.54±0.60
Half-life (h)	8.6±1.3	10.0±1.9	12.3±3.6	12.2±3.0
Total AUC (IU·h/dL)	1217±312	1254±468	1410±527	1717±497
Clearance (mL/(kg·h))	4.31±0.94	4.52±1.46	4.01±1.44	3.19±0.98
Mean Residence Time (h)	10.2±2.4	12.5±3.1	15.1±5.4	15.8±4.5
Volume of Distribution at Steady State (dL/kg)	0.43±0.09	0.53±0.12	0.55±0.11	0.48±0.10

[a] The summary pharmacokinetic parameters were calculated using data from completed studies in the Baxter ADVATE clinical program. This data set included 167 subjects from completed studies 069901 (Pivotal), 060102 (Pivotal Continuation), BLB-200-01 (Japanese Pivotal), and 060101 (Pediatric).

Absorption: Refer to Table 6 for a summary of the adjusted recovery, AUC, and V_{ss} in the infant, child, adolescent and adult populations.

Distribution: When infused into a hemophilia patient, ADVATE binds to endogenous von Willebrand factor in the patient's circulation. The Factor VIII/von Willebrand factor complex is distributed primarily in the intravascular space.

Metabolism: Not applicable.

Excretion: It is currently believed that Factor VIII clearance is mediated by vascular receptors, including low-density lipoprotein receptor-related protein (LPR) and heparin sulphate proteoglycans (HSPGs), by mechanisms that have not been fully elucidated.
Special Populations and Conditions: Pediatrics: A total of 126 pediatric patients (≤16 years old) diagnosed with severe to moderately severe hemophilia A (Factor VIII ≤2%) participated in a number of clinical studies. The safety and hemostatic efficacy of ADVATE in this population are similar to that of adult patients. Adjusted recovery was approximately 20% lower in the pediatric population compared to adults, which is consistent with the known higher plasma volume per kg body weight in younger patients. The terminal half-life was also approximately 20% lower in the pediatric population than in adults (see Pharmacokinetic Data, Table 6).

STORAGE AND STABILITY: ADVATE should be refrigerated (2-8°C). Avoid freezing to prevent damage to the diluent vial. ADVATE may be stored at room temperature (up to 28°C) for a period of up to six months not to exceed the expiration date. Do not place back in the refrigerator once removed from refrigerated storage. Do not use beyond the expiration date printed on the vial or six months after date noted on the carton, whichever is the earliest.

SPECIAL HANDLING INSTRUCTIONS:
- ADVATE reconstituted with 5 mL Sterile Water for Injection USP should never be further diluted.
- Do not refrigerate after reconstitution.
- ADVATE should be administered at room temperature not more than 3 hours after reconstitution.
- Parenteral drug products should be inspected for particulate matter and discoloration prior to administration, whenever solution and container permit.
- Plastic syringes must be used with this product, since proteins such as ADVATE tend to stick to the surface of glass syringes.

INFORMATION FOR THE PATIENT: Published in e-CPS, available by subscription at www.e-cps.ca.

DOSAGE FORMS, COMPOSITION AND PACKAGING: Single-dose vials that contain nominally 250, 500, 1000, 1500, 2000 and 3000 IU per vial. ADVATE is packaged with 5 mL of Sterile Water for Injection USP, a BAXJECT II device for reconstitution, butterfly infusion set, 10 mL sterile syringe, alcohol swab, bandage, one full prescribing physician insert, and one patient insert.

When reconstituted with the appropriate volume of diluent, ADVATE contains the following stabilizers, nonmedicinal ingredients, or excipients in target amounts: 3.2 % (w/v) mannitol, 0.8 % (w/v) α,α-trehalose, 90 mM sodium chloride, 10 mM histidine, 10 mM Tris (hydroxymethyl) aminomethane, 1.6 mM calcium chloride, 0.01 % (w/v) polysorbate 80, and 0.08 mg/mL reduced glutathione. Recombinant von Willebrand Factor (rVWF) is co-expressed with recombinant Factor VIII, and helps to stabilize it in culture. The final product contains no more than 2 ng rVWF/IU rAHF, which will not have any clinically relevant effect in patients with von Willebrand's Disease. The product contains no preservative.

Each vial of ADVATE is labeled with the AHF activity expressed in IU per vial. Biological potency is determined by an in vitro assay, which employs a Factor VIII concentrate standard that is referenced to a World Health Organization (WHO) International Standard for Factor VIII: C concentrates. The specific activity of ADVATE is 4000 to 10 000 IU per milligram of protein.

The reader is invited to consult CPhA's monograph **HMG-CoA Reductase Inhibitors.**

Advicor®

niacin—lovastatin

Lipid Metabolism Regulator

Sepracor

Date of Revision: July 6, 2010

SUMMARY PRODUCT INFORMATION:

Route of Administration	Dosage Form/ Strength	Clinically Relevant Nonmedicinal Ingredients
Oral	500/20 mg, 750/20 mg, 1000/20 mg and 1000/40 mg film-coated tablets	Hydroxypropyl methylcellulose, povidone, stearic acid, polyethylene glycol, titanium dioxide and polysorbate 80 For a complete listing see Dosage Forms, Composition and Packaging.

INDICATIONS AND CLINICAL USE: Therapy with lipid-altering agents should be only one component of multiple risk-factor intervention in individuals at significantly increased risk for atherosclerotic vascular disease due to hypercholesterolemia. Medical therapy is indicated as an adjunct to diet when the response to a diet restricted in saturated fat and cholesterol and other nonpharmacologic measures alone has been inadequate.

ADVICOR (extended-release niacin and lovastatin) is indicated for the treatment of primary hypercholesterolemia (heterozygous familial and nonfamilial) and mixed dyslipidaemia (Fredrickson Types IIa and IIb) in:
- Patients treated with lovastatin who require further triglyceride (TG) lowering or high-density lipoprotein (HDL)-raising who may benefit from niacin added to their regimen;
- Patients treated with extended-release niacin who require further LDL-lowering who may benefit from having lovastatin added to their regimen.

ADVICOR is not intended for initial therapy (see Dosage and Administration). The dose of ADVICOR should be determined by the titration of individual components. The use of ADVICOR should be reserved for patients in whom treatment with lovastatin or NIASPAN (extended-release niacin) monotherapy has not been adequate to meet treatment goals.

Pediatrics: No studies in patients under 18 years of age have been conducted with ADVICOR.

CONTRAINDICATIONS:
- Pregnant women and lactating mothers (see Warnings and Precautions, boxed Serious Warnings and Precautions).
- Patients with active liver disease or unexplained persistent elevations in serum transaminases (see Warnings and Precautions).
- Patients with active peptic ulcer, or active bleeding.
- Patients who are hypersensitive to niacin, lovastatin or to any ingredient in the formulation or component of the container (see Dosage Forms, Composition and Packaging).

WARNINGS AND PRECAUTIONS:

Serious Warnings and Precautions
- ADVICOR preparations should not be substituted for equivalent doses of immediate-release (crystalline) niacin or nicotinic acid (see General below).
- Cases of severe hepatic toxicity, including fulminant hepatic necrosis, have occurred in patients who have substituted sustained-release (modified-release, timed-release) niacin products for immediate-release (crystalline) niacin at equivalent doses (see Hepatic/Biliary/Pancreatic below).
- ADVICOR should be used with caution in patients who consume substantial quantities of alcohol.
- Active liver disease or unexplained transaminase elevations are contraindications to the use of ADVICOR.
- Myopathy (see Skeletal Muscle below).
- Cholesterol and other products of cholesterol biosynthesis pathway are essential components of fetal development, including synthesis of steroids and cell membranes. Because of the ability of lovastatin to decrease the synthesis of cholesterol and possibly other products of the cholesterol biosynthesis pathway, ADVICOR may cause harm when administered to pregnant women.

ADVICOR should be administered to women of childbearing potential only when such patients practice a reliable form of contraception (see Contraindications).

If the patient becomes pregnant, ADVICOR should be discontinued immediately and the patient should be informed of the potential hazard to the fetus.

Clinically significant warnings and precautions are listed below in alphabetical order.

General: Prior to initiating therapy with ADVICOR, secondary causes for elevation in plasma lipid levels should be excluded (e.g. poorly controlled diabetes mellitus, hypothyroidism, nephritic syndrome, dysproteinemias, obstructive liver disease, and alcoholism) and a lipid profile performed to measure total cholesterol, LDL-C, HDL-C and TG. For patients with TG<4.52 mmol/L (<400 mg/dL), LDL-C can be estimated using the following equation:

LDL-C (mmol)=total-C – [(0.37×TG)+HDL-C]

LDL-C (mg/dL)=total-C – [(0.2×TG)+HDL-C]

For patients with TG levels >4.52 mmol/L (>400 mg/dL), this equation is less accurate and LDL-C concentrations should be measured directly, or by ultracentrifugation.

ADVICOR should not be substituted for equivalent doses of immediate-release (crystalline) niacin or nicotinic acid. For patients switching from immediate-release niacin to NIASPAN, therapy with NIASPAN should be initiated with low doses (i.e., 500 mg once daily at bedtime) and the NIASPAN dose should then be titrated to the desired therapeutic response. Cases of severe hepatic toxicity, including fulminant hepatic necrosis, have occurred in patients who have substituted sustained release (modified release, timed release) niacin products for immediate release (crystalline niacin) at equivalent doses (see Dosage and Administration).

Before instituting therapy with a lipid-altering medication, an attempt should be made to control dyslipidaemia with appropriate diet, exercise, and weight reduction in obese patients, and to treat other underlying medical problems (see Indications and Clinical Use).

While pretreatment with acetylsalicylic acid (ASA) or other non-steroidal anti-inflammatory drugs (NSAIDs) may reduce flushing of the skin, some patients should not take these medications (e.g., patients who have peptic ulcer or active inflammatory disease of the gastrointestinal system or ASA hypersensitivity; refer to the Product Monograph for the NSAID product).

Niacin: Elevated uric acid levels have occurred with niacin therapy; therefore, in patients predisposed to gout, niacin therapy should be used with caution. Niacin is rapidly metabolized by the liver, and excreted through the kidneys. ADVICOR is contraindicated in patients with significant or unexplained hepatic dysfunction (see Contraindications and Warnings and Precautions, Hepatic/Biliary/Pancreatic) and should be used with caution in patients with renal dysfunction.

Lovastatin: Lovastatin may elevate creatine phosphokinase and transaminase levels (see Warnings and Precautions, Hepatic/Biliary/Pancreatic and Skeletal Muscle, and Adverse Reactions). This should be considered in the differential diagnosis of chest pain in a patient on therapy with lovastatin.

Cardiovascular: Data on the safety and efficacy of ADVICOR in patients with unstable angina or in the acute phase of myocardial infarction are not available. Therefore, caution should be used when ADVICOR is administered, particularly when such patients are also receiving vasodilator agents.

Carcinogenesis and Mutagenesis and Fertility Impairment: No studies have been conducted with ADVICOR regarding carcinogenesis, mutagenesis, or impairment of fertility.

Endocrine and Metabolism: Niacin: Elevated uric acid levels have occurred with niacin therapy, therefore use with caution in patients predisposed to gout.

In placebo-controlled trials, extended-release niacin tablets have been associated with small but statistically significant, dose-related reductions in phosphorus levels (mean of −13% with 2000 mg). Although these reductions were transient, phosphorus levels should be monitored periodically in patients at risk for hypophosphatemia.

Periodic serum creatine phosphokinase (CK) and potassium determinations should be carried out.

Lovastatin: HMG-CoA reductase inhibitors interfere with cholesterol synthesis and as such might theoretically blunt adrenal and/or gonadal steroid production. However, clinical studies have shown that lovastatin does not reduce basal plasma cortisol concentration or impair adrenal reserve, and does not reduce basal testosterone concentration. The effects of HMG-CoA reductase inhibitors on male fertility have not been studied in adequate numbers of male patients. The effects, if any, on the pituitary-gonadal axis in premenopausal women are unknown.

Patients treated with lovastatin who develop clinical evidence of endocrine dysfunction should be evaluated appropriately. Caution should also be exercised if an HMG-CoA reductase inhibitor or other agent used to lower cholesterol levels is administered to patients also receiving other drugs (e.g., ketoconazole, spironolactone, cimetidine) that may decrease the levels or activity of endogenous steroid hormones.

Gastrointestinal: Patients with a past history of jaundice or peptic ulcer should be observed closely during niacin therapy.

Hematologic: Extended-release niacin tablets have been associated with small, but statistically significant dose-related reductions in platelet count (mean of −11% with 2000 mg). In addition, extended-release niacin tablets have been associated with small but statistically significant increases in prothrombin time (PT) (mean of approximately +4% with 2000 mg); accordingly, patients undergoing surgery should be carefully evaluated. Caution should be observed when ADVICOR is administered concomitantly with anticoagulants; prothrombin time and platelet counts should be monitored closely in such patients.

It is recommended that in patients taking anticoagulants, PT be determined before starting ADVICOR and frequently enough during early therapy to ensure that no significant alteration of PT occurs. Once a stable PT has been documented, PT can be monitored at the intervals usually recommended for patients on coumarin anticoagulants. If the dose of ADVICOR is changed, the same procedure should be repeated.

In one long-term study of 106 patients treated with ADVICOR, elevations in prothrombin time (PT) >3×ULN occurred in 2 patients (2%) during study drug treatment. In a long-term study of 814 patients treated with ADVICOR, 7 patients were noted to have platelet counts <100 000 during study drug treatment. Four of these patients were discontinued, and one patient with a platelet count <100 000 had prolonged bleeding after a tooth extraction. Prior studies have shown that NIASPAN can be associated with dose-related reductions in platelet counts (mean of −11% with 2000 mg) and increases of PT (mean of approximately +4% with 2000 mg). Accordingly, patients undergoing surgery should be carefully evaluated.

Hepatic/Biliary/Pancreatic: No clinical studies have been carried out in patients with impaired liver function.

Patients with a past history of jaundice, hepatobiliary disease, or peptic ulcer should be observed closely during ADVICOR therapy. Frequent monitoring of liver function tests and blood glucose should be performed (see Contraindications). ADVICOR should be used in patients with liver impairment only if the benefits outweigh the risks.

ADVICOR should be used with caution in patients who consume substantial quantities of alcohol and/or have a past history of liver disease.

Niacin preparations and lovastatin preparations have been associated with abnormal liver tests. In studies using NIASPAN alone, 0.8% of patients were discontinued for transaminase elevations. In studies using lovastatin alone, 0.2% of patients were discontinued for transaminase levels.

In two double-blind controlled 28-week studies, the 48-week open-label extension of both trials, and one open-label 100-week trial, one percent of patients (10/1145 patients) with normal liver function treated with ADVICOR experienced reversible elevations in AST/ALT to more than 3 times the upper limit of normal (ULN). Three of 10 elevations occurred at doses outside the recommended dosing limit of 2000/40 mg. No patient receiving 1000/20 mg had 3-fold elevations in AST/ALT.

In clinical studies with ADVICOR, elevations in transaminases did not appear to be related to treatment duration. However, elevations in AST and ALT levels did appear to be dose related. Transaminase elevations were reversible upon discontinuation of ADVICOR.

Diabetic patients may experience a dose-related rise in fasting blood sugar (FBS). In clinical studies, which included 1028 patients exposed to ADVICOR (6 to 22% with diabetes type II at baseline), increases in FBS above normal occurred in 46-65% of patients during the study, and 1.4% of patients discontinued treatment. In patients treated with lovastatin or NIASPAN monotherapy, 24 to 41% and 43 to 58% of patients, respectively, had increases in FBS above normal.

Diabetic or potentially diabetic patients should be monitored closely during treatment with ADVICOR, and adjustment of diet and/or hypoglycemic therapy may be necessary.

Renal: No information is available on the safety of ADVICOR in patients with renal insufficiency. ADVICOR should be used with caution in patients with renal dysfunction.

Skeletal Muscle: Lovastatin: Lovastatin and other inhibitors of HMG-CoA reductase occasionally cause myopathy, which is manifested as muscle pain or weakness associated with grossly elevated creatinine kinase (>10 times ULN). Rhabdomyolysis, with or without acute renal failure secondary to myoglobinuria, has been reported rarely and can occur at any time.

Lovastatin is metabolised by the cytochrome P450 isoform 3A4. Drugs which share this metabolic pathway can raise the plasma level of lovastatin and may increase the risk of myopathy. These include cyclosporin, itraconazole, ketoconazole and other antifungal azoles, the macrolide antibiotics erythromycin and clarithromycin, HIV protease inhibitors, or grapefruit juice.

ADVICOR: Myopathy and/or rhabdomyolysis have been reported when lovastatin is used in combination with lipid-altering doses (≥1 g/day) of niacin. **Physicians contemplating the use of ADVICOR, a combination of lovastatin and extended-release niacin, should weigh the potential benefits and risks, and should carefully monitor patients for any signs and symptoms of muscle pain, tenderness, or weakness, particularly during the initial month of treatment or during any period of upward dosage titration of either drug.** Periodic CK determinations may be considered in such situations, but there is no assurance that such monitoring will prevent myopathy.

In clinical studies, 1 case of suspected myopathy and no cases of rhabdomyolysis were reported in 1145 patients treated with ADVICOR at doses up to 2000/40 mg for periods up to 2 years, however, cases of myopathy and rhabdomyolysis have been identified in post-market use of ADVICOR.

Patients starting therapy with ADVICOR should be advised of the risk of myopathy, and told to report promptly unexplained muscle pain, tenderness, or weakness. A CK level above 10 times ULN in a patient with unexplained muscle symptoms indicates myopathy. ADVICOR therapy should be discontinued if myopathy is diagnosed or suspected.

In patients with complicated medical histories predisposing to rhabdomyolysis, such as preexisting renal insufficiency, dose escalation requires caution. Also, as there are no known adverse consequences of brief interruption of therapy, treatment with ADVICOR should be stopped for a few days before elective major surgery and when any major acute medical or surgical condition supervenes. If ADVICOR therapy is discontinued for an extended period, reinstitution of therapy should include a titration period.

The risk of adverse muscle events with statins is dose related and the risk may be increased by concomitant use of statins with other lipid lowering drugs that can cause myopathy when given alone, including niacin. Accordingly, the higher doses of ADVICOR should be reserved for patients who require more aggressive lipid management. It is important that such patients be advised to report as soon as possible symptoms such as muscle ache or weakness. A baseline CK determination is recommended for patients who may require higher doses of ADVICOR.

Use of ADVICOR with other Drugs: The incidence and severity of myopathy may be increased by concomitant administration of ADVICOR with drugs that can cause myopathy when given alone, such as gemfibrozil and other fibrates. The use of ADVICOR in combination with fibrates should be avoided unless the benefit of further alterations in lipid levels is likely to outweigh the increased risk of this drug combination. In patients taking concomitant cyclosporine or fibrates, the dose of ADVICOR should generally not exceed 1000/20 mg (see Dosage and Administration), as the risk of myopathy may increase at higher doses. Interruption of ADVICOR therapy during a course of treatment with a systemic antifungal azole or a macrolide antibiotic should be considered.

Special Populations: Pregnant Women: ADVICOR is contraindicated in pregnancy. It should be administered to women of childbearing potential only if they practice a reliable method of contraception and have been informed of the potential hazard. Treatment should be immediately discontinued as soon as pregnancy is recognised (see Contraindications).

Niacin: Animal reproduction studies have not been conducted with niacin or ADVICOR. It is also not known whether niacin at doses used for lipid disorders can cause fetal harm when administered to pregnant women or whether it can affect reproductive capacity. If a woman receiving niacin or ADVICOR becomes pregnant, the drug should be discontinued.

Lovastatin: Lovastatin is contraindicated in pregnancy. Lovastatin has been shown to produce fetal skeletal malformations in mice and rats.

Nursing Women: Use of ADVICOR in nursing mothers is contraindicated (see Contraindications and Warnings and Precautions, Serious Warnings and Precautions).

Pediatrics (<18 years of age): Safety and effectiveness of ADVICOR therapy in pediatric patients have not been established. No studies in patients under 18 years of age have been conducted with ADVICOR.

Geriatrics (>65 years of age): No formal studies have been carried out in elderly patients. In controlled and open label studies, the safety and efficacy data in patients over 65 years of age treated with ADVICOR were comparable to data observed in younger patients.

Sex: Data indicate that in patients with primary hypercholesterolemia and dyslipidaemia treated with ADVICOR the changes in lipid concentrations are greater for women than for men.

Monitoring and Laboratory Tests: Liver tests should be performed on all patients during therapy with ADVICOR. Serum transaminase levels, including AST and ALT, should be monitored before treatment begins, every 6 to 12 weeks for the first year, and periodically thereafter (e.g., at 6 month intervals). Special attention should be paid to patients who develop elevated serum transaminase levels. In these patients, measurements should be repeated promptly and then performed more frequently. If the transaminase levels show evidence of progression, particularly if they rise to 3 times ULN and are persistent, or if they are associated with symptoms of nausea, fever, and/or malaise, the drug should be discontinued.

ADVERSE REACTIONS: Adverse Drug Reaction Overview: The most frequently-reported events with ADVICOR (extended-release niacin/lovastatin) are flushing episodes (i.e, warmth, redness, itching and/or tingling), which generally become less common as treatment progresses.

The most frequent adverse events observed in double blind controlled clinical trials were: flushing, infection, headache, pain, diarrhea, nausea and pruritus.

The following potentially serious adverse reactions have been reported in controlled clinical trials: cholecystitis, cholelithiasis and kidney stones.

Clinical Trial Adverse Drug Reactions: Because clinical trials are conducted under very specific conditions the adverse reaction rates observed in the clinical trials may not reflect the rates observed in practice and should not be compared to the rates in the clinical trials of another drug. Adverse drug reaction information from clinical trials is useful for identifying drug-related adverse events and for approximating rates.

Clinical studies enrolled 1028 patients; 214 in two controlled trials of 24 weeks duration and 814 in a long term open label study at doses up to 2000/40 mg. Doses were titrated up every 4 weeks up to a maximum of 2000/40 mg.

Controlled Clinical Trials: In two controlled clinical trials, ADVICOR has been evaluated for safety in 214 patients treated for hypercholesterolemia, 65 at doses of 2000/40 mg. Discontinuation due to adverse events occurred in 19% (40/214) of the patients, 18/214 (8%) due to flushing.

The adverse events that occurred at an incidence of 2% or greater are given in Table 1.

Table 1: ADVICOR

Treatment-emergent Adverse Events in Double Blind Controlled Trials, Irrespective of Causality, Occurring in Frequency of 2% or Greater in Patients Treated with ADVICOR

Adverse Event	ADVICOR	NIASPAN	Lovastatin
Total Number of Patients	214	92	94
Flushing	**71%**	**65%**	**18%**
Body as a Whole	**49%**	**54%**	**45%**
Asthenia	5%	7%	5%
Flu Syndrome	6%	8%	4%
Headache	9%	13%	5%
Infection	20%	15%	20%
Injury, Accidental	3%	4%	4%
Pain	8%	9%	10%
Pain, Abdominal	4%	1%	6%
Pain, Back	5%	5%	5%
Pain, Chest	2%	1%	3%
Cardiovascular System	**18%**	**14%**	**10%**
Hypertension	2%	2%	2%
Digestive System	**24%**	**28%**	**17%**
Diarrhea	6%	9%	2%

(cont'd)

Table 1: ADVICOR *(cont'd)*

Treatment-emergent Adverse Events in Double Blind Controlled Trials, Irrespective of Causality, Occurring in Frequency of 2% or Greater in Patients Treated with ADVICOR

Adverse Event	ADVICOR	NIASPAN	Lovastatin
Dyspepsia	3%	7%	4%
Flatulence	2%	1%	1%
Gastritis	2%	1%	0
Nausea	7%	12%	2%
Vomiting	3%	5%	0
Hemic and Lymphatic System	**3%**	**1%**	**3%**
Ecchymosis	2%	0	1%
Metabolic and Nutrit. System	**17%**	**13%**	**14%**
CK Increased	2%	1%	2%
Edema, Peripheral	4%	2%	3%
Hyperglycemia	4%	7%	6%
(AST) Increased	3%	0	1%
(ALT) Increased	2%	0	1%
Musculoskeletal System	**9%**	**10%**	**18%**
Arthritis	3%	0	3%
Myalgia	3%	5%	9%
Nervous System	**14%**	**12%**	**14%**
Dizziness	3%	3%	4%
Insomnia	4%	3%	4%
Paresthesia	2%	2%	1%
Respiratory System	**12%**	**15%**	**11%**
Cough Increased	4%	3%	1%
Rhinitis	2%	4%	2%
Sinusitis	4%	1%	2%
Skin and Appendages	**18%**	**21%**	**12%**
Pruritus	7%	8%	3%
Rash	5%	12%	3%
Rash, Maculopapular	2%	0	0
Urticaria	3%	2%	1%
Urogenital System	**9%**	**8%**	**12%**
Infection, Urinary Tract	3%	2%	2%

Less Common Clinical Trial Adverse Drug Reactions: The following adverse events have also been reported with niacin, lovastatin, and/or other HMG-CoA reductase inhibitors, but not necessarily with ADVICOR, either during clinical studies or in routine patient management.

Body as a Whole: face edema; peripheral chest pain; abdominal pain; generalized edema; chills; malaise.

Cardiovascular: atrial fibrillation; tachycardia; palpitations, and other cardiac arrhythmias; orthostasis; hypotension; syncope.

Eye: toxic amblyopia; cystoid macular edema; ophthalmoplegia; eye irritation.

Gastrointestinal: activation of peptic ulcers and peptic ulceration; dyspepsia; vomiting; anorexia; constipation; eructation; flatulence; pancreatitis; hepatitis; fatty change in liver; jaundice; and rarely, cirrhosis, fulminant hepatic necrosis, and hepatoma.

Metabolic: gout.

Musculoskeletal: muscle cramps; myopathy; rhabdomyolysis; arthralgia; myasthenia.

Nervous: dizziness; insomnia; dry mouth; paresthesia; anxiety; tremor; vertigo; memory loss; peripheral neuropathy; psychic disturbances; dysfunction of certain cranial nerves, leg cramps; nervousness.

Skin: hyper-pigmentation; acanthosis nigricans; urticaria; alopecia; dry skin; sweating; and a variety of skin changes (e.g., nodules, discoloration, dryness of mucous membranes, changes to hair/nails).

Respiratory: dyspnea; rhinitis.

Urogenital: gynecomastia; loss of libido; erectile dysfunction.

Hypersensitivity: An apparent hypersensitivity syndrome has been reported rarely, which has included one or more of the following features: anaphylaxis, angioedema, lupus erythematous-like syndrome, polymyalgia rheumatica, vasculitis, purpura, thrombocytopenia, leukopenia, hemolytic anemia, positive ANA, ESR increase, eosinophilia, arthritis, arthralgia, urticaria, asthenia, photosensitivity, fever, chills, flushing, malaise, dyspnea, toxic epidermal necrolysis, erythema multiforme, including Stevens-Johnson syndrome.

Other: migraine.

Abnormal Hematologic and Clinical Chemistry Findings: ADVICOR: Elevations in serum transaminases, creatinine kinase and fasting blood glucose, and a reduction in serum phosphorus have been observed.

Niacin: Extended-release niacin tablets have been associated with elevations in lactate dehydrogenase, uric acid, total bilirubin and amylase.

Extended-release niacin tablets have also been associated with reduction in platelet counts and prolongation of prothrombin time.

Lovastatin: Lovastatin has been associated with elevations in alkaline phosphatase, glutamyl transpeptidase and bilirubin, and thyroid function abnormalities (see Warnings and Precautions).

Open-label, Long-term Clinical Trial: In a 52-week, long-term, open-label study of 814 patients, 550 patients completed one-year of treatment and 454 patients continued into the 48-week extension phase of the trial. Of the 814 patients in the study, 610 received the 2000/40 mg dose and 376 patients remained on study medication for up to 104 weeks (85-88 wks at the 2000/40 mg dose). The mean treatment duration for all 814 patients was 66.2 weeks.

Discontinuations due to adverse events occurred in 25% (203/814 patients) during the first year of treatment and in 7% (32/454) during the second year. The most common adverse event that led to discontinuation was flushing (10% during the first year of treatment and 2% during the extension phase).

The adverse events that occurred at an incidence of 2% or greater, irrespective of causality, are given in Table 2.

Table 2: ADVICOR

Treatment-Emergent Adverse Events in Open-label, Long-Term Trial, Irrespective of Causality, Occurring in Frequency of 2% or Greater in Patients Treated in a Long Term Clinical Trial with ADVICOR

Adverse Event	ADVICOR
Total Number of Patients	814
Flushing	**65%**
Body as a Whole	**65%**
Allergic Reaction	4%
Asthenia	7%
Fever	3%
Flu Syndrome	9%
Headache	13%
Hernia	2%
Infection	28%
Infection, Fungal	3%
Injury, Accidental	10%
Pain	21%
Pain, Abdominal	7%
Pain, Back	8%
Pain, Chest	5%
Pain, Neck	2%
Cardiovascular System	**73%**
Angina Pectoris	2%
Cardiovascular Disease	3%
Hemorrhage	2%
Hypertension	4%
Occlusion, Coronary	2%
Palpitation	2%
Vascular Disorder	2%
Digestive System	**39%**
Abscess, Periodontal	2%
Anorexia	2%
Colitis	2%
Constipation	5%
Diarrhea	12%
Dyspepsia	9%
Flatulence	5%
Gastrointestinal Disorder	3%
Nausea	12%
Vomiting	7%
Hemic & Lymphatic System	**8%**
Anemia	2%
Ecchymosis	3%
Metabolic & Nutritional System	**26%**
Creatine PK Increased	5%
Diabetes, Mellitus	3%
Edema, Peripheral	6%

(cont'd)

Table 2: ADVICOR *(cont'd)*

Treatment-Emergent Adverse Events in Open-label, Long-Term Trial, Irrespective of Causality, Occurring in Frequency of 2% or Greater in Patients Treated in a Long Term Clinical Trial with ADVICOR

Adverse Event	ADVICOR
Glucose Tolerance Decreased	3%
Hyperglycemia	7%
Hypokalemia	2%
Musculoskeletal System	**19%**
Arthralgia	2%
Arthritis	3%
Bone Disorder	2%
Cramps, Leg	4%
Myalgia	5%
Tendon Disorder	2%
Nervous System	**30%**
Anxiety	3%
Depression	3%
Dizziness	7%
Dry Mouth	3%
Hypertonia	2%
Insomnia	5%
Paresthesia	5%

Post-Market Adverse Drug Reactions: In an open-label Phase IV study in over 4000 patients at doses of 1000/40 mg for 8 weeks, flushing was the most common adverse event leading to discontinuation of 6% of patients. Incidence of AST/ALT elevations >3×ULN was 0.24%, increases in CK >5×ULN occurred in 0.24% of patients and no cases of drug-induced myopathy were observed.

Anaphylactoid reaction, angioedema and thrombocytopenia have been observed during post-marketing use of ADVICOR. Rhabdomyolysis and/or myopathy have also been reported, albeit very rarely, during post-marketing use of ADVICOR. There were no differences in rates when compared with extended-release niacin or lovastatin used as monotherapy.

DRUG INTERACTIONS: Overview: Extended-Release Niacin: Antihypertensive Therapy: Niacin may potentiate the effects of ganglionic blocking agents and vasoactive drugs resulting in postural hypotension.
Acetylsalicylic Acid (ASA): Concomitant administration of ASA may decrease the metabolic clearance of niacin (see Warnings and Precautions, General).
Bile-Acid Sequestrants: An interval of 4 to 6 hours, or as great an interval as possible, should elapse between the ingestion of bile acid-binding resins and the administration of ADVICOR. An in vitro study showed that about 98% of available niacin was bound to colestipol, and 10 to 30% was bound to cholestyramine.
Other: Vitamins or other nutritional supplements containing large doses of niacin or related compounds such as nicotinamide may potentiate the adverse effects of ADVICOR.
Lovastatin: Serious skeletal muscle disorders, e.g., rhabdomyolysis, have been reported during concomitant therapy of lovastatin or other HMG-CoA reductase inhibitors with cyclosporine, itraconazole, ketoconazole, gemfibrozil, niacin, erythromycin, clarithromycin, nefazodone or HIV protease inhibitors (see Warnings and Precautions, Skeletal Muscle).
Coumarin Anticoagulants: Bleeding and/or increased prothrombin time (PT) have been reported in a few patients taking coumarin anticoagulants concomitantly with lovastatin (see Warnings and Precautions, Hematologic).
Antipyrine: Lovastatin had no effect on the pharmacokinetics of antipyrine or its metabolites. However, since lovastatin is metabolized by the cytochrome P450 isoform 3A4 enzyme system, this does not preclude an interaction with other drugs metabolized by the same isoform.
Propranolol: In normal volunteers, there was no clinically significant pharmacokinetic or pharmacodynamic interaction with concomitant administration of single doses of lovastatin and propranolol.
Digoxin: In patients with hypercholesterolemia, concomitant administration of lovastatin and digoxin resulted in no effect on digoxin plasma concentrations.
Oral Hypoglycemic Agents: In pharmacokinetic studies of lovastatin in hypercholesterolemic, non-insulin-dependent diabetic patients, there was no drug interaction with glipizide or with chlorpropamide.
Drug-Food Interactions: Concomitant consumption of alcohol or hot drinks may increase the side effects of flushing and pruritus and should be avoided around the time of ADVICOR ingestion.
Drug-Herb Interactions: Interactions with herbal products have not been studied.
Drug-Laboratory Test Interactions: Niacin may produce false elevations in some fluorometric determinations of plasma or urinary catecholamines. Niacin may also give false-positive reactions with cupric sulphate solution (Benedict's reagent) in urine glucose tests.

DOSAGE AND ADMINISTRATION: The dosage of ADVICOR (extended-release niacin/lovastatin) must be individualized. The fixed combination is not indicated for initial therapy. The dose of ADVICOR should be determined by titration of individual components (see Recommended Dose and Dosage Adjustment).

Patients should be placed on a standard cholesterol-lowering diet at least equivalent to the NCEP Adult Treatment Panel III TLC diet before receiving ADVICOR and should continue on this diet during treatment with ADVICOR. If appropriate, a program of weight control and physical exercise should be implemented.

Dosing Considerations:

- Equivalent doses of ADVICOR may be substituted for equivalent doses of NIASPAN but should not be substituted for other modified-release (sustained release or time-release) niacin preparations or immediate-release (crystalline) niacin preparations (see Warnings and Precautions). Patients previously receiving niacin products other than NIASPAN should be started on NIASPAN with the recommended NIASPAN titration schedule, and the dose should subsequently be individualized based on patient response.
- **ADVICOR tablet strengths are not interchangeable.**
- Women may respond at lower ADVICOR doses than men.
- Flushing of the skin may be reduced in frequency or severity by pretreatment with acetylsalicylic acid (see Warnings and Precautions, General).
- Avoid administration on an empty stomach
- ADVICOR is contraindicated in patients with significant or unexplained hepatic dysfunction.
- No information is available on the safety of ADVICOR in patients with renal insufficiency.
- ADVICOR tablets should be taken whole and should not be broken, crushed, or chewed before swallowing.

Recommended Dose and Dosage Adjustment: ADVICOR should be taken during the evening hours, before or at bedtime, after a low-fat snack. Doses should be individualized according to patient response with the goal being to achieve recommended target lipid levels at the lowest possible dose.

ADVICOR can be substituted if the titrated doses of individual components corresponds to ADVICOR fixed dose combination as shown below in Table 3.

Table 3: ADVICOR

NIASPAN and Lovastatin Dosing Table

NIASPAN Dose (mg)	Lovastatin Dose (mg)	Corresponding ADVICOR Dose (niacin extended release mg/lovastatin mg)
500	20	500/20
750	20	750/20
1000	20	1000/20
1000	40	500/20 (2 tablets) or 1000/40
1500	40	750/20 (2 tablets)
2000	40	1000/20 (2 tablets)

Note: A period of at least 4 weeks is recommended before increasing the dose during titration.

NIASPAN Monotherapy:

The tablet strengths of NIASPAN are not interchangeable. Do not alternate between different strengths to provide the same daily dosage. The physician should specify the tablet strengths that the patient should use during titration and continue to use for maintenance therapy.

The recommended starting dose for NIASPAN is 500 mg to be taken at bedtime after a low-fat snack. To reduce the incidence and severity of adverse effects, the dose may be increased after 4 weeks by no more than 500 mg and by 500 mg every 4 weeks thereafter to a maximum of 2000 mg per day, depending on patient response. Patients already receiving a stable dose of NIASPAN may be switched directly to a niacin equivalent dose of ADVICOR (see Table 3).

Lovastatin Monotherapy: The recommended starting dose of lovastatin is 20 mg once daily given with the evening meal. If required, the dose of lovastatin may be increased to a maximum of 40 mg once daily after at least an interval of 4 weeks. Patients already receiving a stable dose of lovastatin, for whom adding NIASPAN is considered appropriate, may receive concomitant dosing with NIASPAN, and switch to ADVICOR once a stable dose of NIASPAN has been reached as recommended for NIASPAN monotherapy above (see Table 3).

Doses of ADVICOR greater than 2000/40 mg daily are not recommended.

Dosage in Patients with Renal Insufficiency: Use of ADVICOR in patients with renal insufficiency has not been studied. No information is available regarding the safety of ADVICOR use in patients with renal insufficiency.

Dosage in Patients with Hepatic Insufficiency: Use of ADVICOR in patients with hepatic insufficiency has not been studied. ADVICOR is contraindicated in patients with significant or unexplained hepatic dysfunction (see Contraindications).

Missed Dose: If a dose of this medication is missed, it is not necessary to make up the missed dose. Skip the missed dose and continue with the next scheduled dose. Do not double dose.

If ADVICOR therapy is discontinued for an extended period (>7 days), reinstitution of therapy should begin with the lowest dose of ADVICOR.

OVERDOSAGE:

Supportive measures should be undertaken in the event of an overdose of ADVICOR. Monitor liver function and initiate appropriate therapy if required.

For management of a suspected drug overdose, CPhA recommends that you contact your **regional Poison Control Centre**. See the *CPS* Directory section for a list of Poison Control Centres.

ACTION AND CLINICAL PHARMACOLOGY: Mechanism of Action: Niacin: The mechanism by which niacin alters lipid profiles has not been well defined. It may involve several actions including partial inhibition of release of free fatty acids from adipose tissue, and increased lipoprotein lipase activity, which may increase the rate of chylomicron triglyceride removal from plasma. Niacin decreases the rate of hepatic synthesis of VLDL and LDL, and does not appear to affect fecal excretion of fats, sterols, or bile acids.

Lovastatin: Lovastatin is a specific inhibitor of 3-hydroxy-3-methylglutaryl-coenzyme A (HMG-CoA) reductase, the enzyme that catalyzes the conversion of HMG-CoA to mevalonate. The conversion of HMG-CoA to mevalonate is an early step in the biosynthetic pathway for cholesterol. Lovastatin is a prodrug and has little, if any, activity until hydrolyzed to its active beta-hydroxyacid form, lovastatin acid. The mechanism of the LDL-lowering effect of lovastatin may involve both reduction of VLDL-C concentration and induction of the LDL receptor, leading to reduced production and/or increased catabolism of LDL-C.

Pharmacodynamics: Epidemiologic, clinical and experimental studies have established that high LDL cholesterol (LDL-C), low High Density Lipoprotein cholesterol (HDL-C) and high plasma triglycerides (TG) promote human atherosclerosis and are risk factors for developing cardiovascular disease. Increased levels of HDL-C are associated with decreased cardiovascular risk.

ADVICOR: ADVICOR reduces LDL-C, TC, TG, Lp(a), Apo B, TC:HDL and LDL:HDL, and increases HDL-C and Apo A-1 due to the individual actions of extended-release niacin and lovastatin. The magnitude of individual lipid and lipoprotein responses may be influenced by the severity and type of underlying lipid abnormality.

Niacin: Niacin functions in the body after conversion to nicotinamide adenine dinucleotide (NAD) in the NAD coenzyme system. Niacin (but **not** nicotinamide) in gram doses reduces TC, LDL-C, Apo B, Lp(a) and TG, and increases HDL-C. The magnitude of individual lipid and lipoprotein responses may be influenced by the severity and type of underlying lipid abnormality. The increase in HDL-C is associated with an increase in apolipoprotein A-I (Apo A-I) and a shift in the distribution of HDL subfractions. These shifts include an increase in the HDL_2:HDL_3 ratio, and an elevation in lipoprotein A-I (Lp A-I, an HDL particle containing only Apo A-I). Niacin treatment also decreases serum levels of Apo B, the major protein component of the VLDL and LDL fractions, and of lipoprotein a (Lp(a)), a variant form of LDL independently associated with coronary risk.

In addition, niacin preparations (including extended-release niacin) have been shown to cause favourable transformations in LDL particle size subclass distribution, converting the pattern B phenotype (characterised by a predominance of triglyceride-rich, small dense LDL) to pattern A (characterised by a predominance of large buoyant LDL) or the intermediate AB phenotype. Pattern B LDL phenotype is one manifestation of what has been termed the Atherogenic Lipoprotein Profile (ALP), a Mendelian dominant inherited condition which also includes low levels of HDL-C, raised triglyceride, and insulin resistance.

Lovastatin: Lovastatin has been shown to reduce both normal and elevated LDL-C concentrations. Apo B also falls substantially during treatment with lovastatin. Since each LDL-C particle contains one molecule of Apo B, and since little Apo B is found in other lipoproteins, this strongly suggests that lovastatin does not merely cause cholesterol to be lost from LDL-C, but also reduces the concentration of circulating LDL particles. In addition, lovastatin can slightly increase HDL-C, and modestly reduce VLDL-C and plasma TG.

Pharmacokinetics: Absorption: ADVICOR: In single-dose studies of ADVICOR, rate and extent of niacin and lovastatin absorption were bioequivalent under fed conditions to that from NIASPAN (extended-release niacin) and lovastatin given alone. After administration of two ADVICOR 1000/20 mg tablets, approximately 72% of the niacin dose was absorbed as measured by the recovery of niacin and its metabolites in the urine, with peak concentrations of nicotinuric acid in plasma averaging approximately 18 µg/mL and occurring about 5 hours after dosing.

The extent of niacin absorption from ADVICOR was increased by administration with food. The administration of two ADVICOR 1000/20 mg tablets under low-fat or high-fat conditions resulted in a 22 to 30% increase in niacin bioavailability relative to dosing under fasting conditions. Lovastatin bioavailability is affected by food. Lovastatin C_{max} was increased 48% and 21% after a high- and a low-fat meal, respectively, but the lovastatin AUC was decreased 26% and 24% after a high- and a low-fat meal, respectively, compared to those under fasting conditions.

Following the administration of a single dose of 1000 mg extended-release niacin and 40 mg lovastatin as the 1000/40 mg ADVICOR tablet formulation versus two 500/20 mg ADVICOR tablets the pharmacokinetic profiles of niacin and its metabolites are different. As a result, ADVICOR tablets of different strengths are not interchangeable.

Lovastatin: Lovastatin appears to be incompletely absorbed after oral administration. Because of extensive hepatic extraction, the amount of lovastatin reaching the systemic circulation as active inhibitors after oral administration is low (<5%) and shows considerable inter-individual variation. Peak concentrations of active and total inhibitors occur within 2 to 4 hours after lovastatin administration.

Lovastatin absorption appears to be increased by at least 30% by grapefruit juice; however, the effect is dependent on the amount of grapefruit juice consumed and the interval between grapefruit juice and lovastatin ingestion.

With a once-a-day dosing regimen, plasma concentrations of total inhibitors over a dosing interval achieved a steady-state between the second and third days of therapy and were about 1.5 times those following a single dose of lovastatin.

Distribution: Niacin: Niacin is less than 20% bound to serum proteins and distribute into milk. Studies using radiolabeled niacin in mice showed that niacin and its metabolites concentrate in the liver, kidney and adipose tissue.

Lovastatin: Both lovastatin and its beta-hydroxyacid metabolite are highly bound (>95%) to human plasma proteins. Distribution of lovastatin or its metabolites into human milk is unknown; however, lovastatin distributes into milk in rats. In animal studies, lovastatin concentrated in the liver, and crossed the blood-brain and placental barriers.

Metabolism: Niacin: Niacin undergoes rapid and extensive first-pass metabolism that is dose-rate specific and, at the doses used to treat dyslipidaemia, saturable. In humans, one pathway is through a simple conjugation step with glycine to form nicotinuric acid (NUA). NUA is then excreted, although there may be a small amount of reversible metabolism back to niacin. The other pathway results in the formation of NAD. It is unclear whether nicotinamide is formed as a precursor to, or following the synthesis of, NAD. Nicotinamide is further metabolized to at least N-methylnicotinamide (MNA) and nicotinamide-N-oxide (NNO). MNA is further metabolized to two other compounds, N-methyl-2-pyridone-5-carboxamide (2PY) and N-methyl-4-pyridone-5-carboxamide (4PY). The formation of 2PY appears to predominate over 4PY in humans.

Lovastatin: Lovastatin undergoes extensive first-pass extraction and metabolism by cytochrome P450 3A4 in the liver, its primary site of action. The major active metabolites present in human plasma are the beta-hydroxyacid of lovastatin (lovastatin acid), its 6'-hydroxy derivative, and two additional metabolites.

Excretion: ADVICOR: Niacin is primarily excreted in urine mainly as metabolites. After a single dose of ADVICOR, at least 60% of the niacin dose was recovered in urine as unchanged niacin and its metabolites. The plasma half-life for lovastatin was about 4.5 hours in single-dose studies.

Niacin: The plasma half-life for niacin is about 20 to 48 minutes after oral administration and dependent on dose administered. Following multiple oral doses of NIASPAN, up to 12% of the dose was recovered in urine as unchanged niacin depending on dose administered. The ratio of metabolites recovered in the urine was also dependent on the dose administered.

Lovastatin: Lovastatin is excreted in urine and bile, based on studies of lovastatin. Following an oral dose of radiolabeled lovastatin in man, 10% of the dose was excreted in urine and 83% in feces. The latter represents absorbed drug equivalents excreted in bile, as well as any unabsorbed drug.

Special Populations and Conditions: Pediatrics: No studies in patients under 18 years of age have been conducted with ADVICOR.

Geriatrics: In patients who received ADVICOR in double blind and open label studies, responses in LDL-C, HDL-C and TG were similar in younger patients and patients over 65 years of age and older. No overall differences were observed in selected chemistry values between the two groups, except for serum amylase which was higher in older patients.

Gender: Steady-state plasma concentrations of niacin and metabolites after administration of niacin are generally higher in women than in men. Recovery of niacin and metabolites in urine, however, is generally similar for men and women, indicating that absorption is similar for both sexes. Data from the clinical trials suggest that women have a greater hypolipidaemic response than men at equivalent doses of NIASPAN and ADVICOR.

Hepatic Insufficiency: No studies have been performed in patients with hepatic insufficiency (see Contraindications and Warnings and Precautions, Hepatic/Biliary/Pancreatic).

Renal Insufficiency: There are no data available on the use of ADVICOR in patients with impaired renal function (see Warnings and Precautions).

STORAGE AND STABILITY: Temperature: Store at room temperature (15 to 30°C).

Other: Keep in a safe place out of the reach of children.

INFORMATION FOR THE PATIENT: Published in e-CPS, available by subscription at www.e-cps.ca.

DOSAGE FORMS, COMPOSITION AND PACKAGING: 500/20 mg: Each light yellow, unscored, capsule-shaped tablet, debossed "502" on one side, contains: 500 mg niacin in an extended-release formulation and 20 mg lovastatin in an immediate-release formulation. Nonmedicinal ingredients: hydroxypropyl methylcellulose, iron oxide red, iron oxide yellow, macrogol, polyethylene glycol, polysorbate 80, povidone, stearic acid and titanium dioxide. Bottles of 90. Blister-packs of 3.

750/20 mg: Each light orange, unscored, capsule-shaped tablet, debossed "752" on one side, contains: 750 mg niacin in an extended-release formulation and 20 mg lovastatin in an immediate-release formulation. Nonmedicinal ingredients: FD&C yellow No 615, hydroxypropyl methylcellulose, macrogol, polyethylene glycol, polysorbate 80, povidone, stearic acid and titanium dioxide. Bottles of 90.

1000/20 mg: Each dark pink/light purple, unscored, capsule-shaped tablet, debossed "1002" on one side, contains: 1000 mg niacin in an extended-release formulation and 20 mg lovastatin in an immediate-release formulation. Nonmedicinal ingredients: hydroxypropyl methylcellulose, iron oxide black, iron oxide red, iron oxide yellow, macrogol, polyethylene glycol, polysorbate 80, povidone, stearic acid and titanium dioxide. Bottles of 90.

1000/40 mg: Each reddish-brown/ brown, unscored, capsule-shaped tablet, debossed "1004" on one side, contains: 1000 mg niacin in an extended-release formulation and 40 mg lovastatin in an immediate-release formulation. Nonmedicinal ingredients: hydroxypropyl methylcellulose, iron oxide red, macrogol, polyethylene glycol, povidone, stearic acid and titanium dioxide. Bottles of 90.

Advil®

ibuprofen

Analgesic—Antipyretic

Pfizer Consumer Healthcare

PHARMACOLOGY: Actions: Ibuprofen, like all nonsteroidal anti-inflammatory drugs (NSAIDs), is an analgesic, antipyretic, and anti-inflammatory medication. There is strong evidence to support the view that the main mechanism of action of ibuprofen (like other NSAIDs) is related to decreasing prostaglandin biosynthesis.

Prostaglandins are naturally-occurring fatty acid derivatives that are widely distributed in the tissues. They are believed to be a common factor in the production of pain, fever, and inflammation. Prostaglandins are believed to sensitise tissues to pain- and inflammation-producing mediators such as histamine, 5-hydroxytryptamine, and kinins. The enzyme catalysing the committed step in prostaglandin biosynthesis is prostaglandin endoperoxide synthase, also know as cyclooxygenase. There is significant evidence that the main mechanism of analgesic/antipyretic action of NSAIDs is prostaglandin biosynthesis inhibition. Other pharmacologic effects such as lysosome and plasma membrane stabilisation have been observed, but the potential relevance of these effects to ibuprofen-induced analgesia and antipyresis is unclear.

Pharmacokinetics: Absorption: Ibuprofen is rapidly and almost completely absorbed. Peak serum concentration occurs within 1-2 hours in adults. Advil Liqui-Gels contain solubilized ibuprofen which has peak serum concentrations within 36-42 minutes. In febrile children ages 3 months to <12 years, the time of peak serum concentration was 1.60 and 1.54 hours for ibuprofen 5 mg/kg and 10 mg/kg, respectively. One study found a time to peak concentration of 1.1 and 1.2 hours for these respective doses. A similar study in febrile children which used an ibuprofen suspension showed a time of peak serum concentration of 1.3 and 1.7 hours for ibuprofen 5 mg/kg and 10 mg/kg, respectively. This study also found that mean ibuprofen plasma concentration at one hour was 21.7±6.7 and 28.4±15.2 µg/mL for 5 mg/kg and 10 mg/kg, respectively. Food decreases the rate but not the extent of absorption.

Distribution: The volume of distribution in adults after oral administration is 0.1-0.2 L/kg. In febrile children the volume of distribution is 0.18 and 0.22 L/kg for ibuprofen 5 mg/kg and 10 mg/kg, respectively.

At therapeutic concentrations ibuprofen is highly bound to whole human plasma and to site II of purified albumin. There is no appreciable plasma accumulation of ibuprofen or its metabolites with repeated doses.

Metabolism: Ibuprofen is a racemic mixture of R-(-) ibuprofen and S-(+) ibuprofen. R-(-) ibuprofen undergoes extensive enantiomeric conversion to S-(+) ibuprofen in humans, averaging between 53% and 65%. S-(+) ibuprofen is believed to be the pharmacologically more active enantiomer. Two major metabolites, 2-[4-(2-carboxypropyl)phenyl] propionic acid and 2-[4-(2-hydroxy-2-methylpropyl]propionic acid, have been identified in plasma and urine. The metabolites 1-hydroxyibuprofen and 3-hydroxy-ibuprofen have also been found in urine in very small concentrations. Cytochrome P450 (CYP) 2C9 has been identified as the most important catalyst for formation of all oxidative metabolites of R-(-) and S-(+) ibuprofen. Approximately 80% of a dose is recovered in urine, primarily as carboxymetabolites and conjugated hydroxymetabolites. Ibuprofen does not appear to induce the formation of drug metabolising enzymes in the rat.

Elimination: Ibuprofen's plasma half-life in adults is 1.5-2.0 hours. In febrile children the plasma half-life is 1.65 and 1.48 hours for ibuprofen 5 mg/kg and 10 mg/kg, respectively. Parent drug and metabolites are primarily excreted in the urine; bile and faeces are relatively minor elimination routes. Total recovery in urine is between 70% and 90% of the administered dose within 24 hours.

There is no evidence of a differential metabolism or elimination of ibuprofen in the elderly. A pharmacokinetic evaluation of ibuprofen in geriatric subjects (65 to 78 years) compared with young adult subjects (22 to 35 years) found that there was no clinically significant difference in the kinetic profiles of ibuprofen for these age groups. Furthermore, there was no statistically significant difference between the two populations in the urinary excretion pattern of the drug and its major metabolites.

The pharmacokinetics of ibuprofen have also been evaluated in children, in whom the metabolism has been shown to be similar to that reported for adults. A study found that for ibuprofen 10 mg/kg given to children under 12 years of age, peak plasma concentration occurred at 1.5 hours and then declined with a plasma half-life of 1.8 hours. Thus, ibuprofen appears to exhibit a similar pharmacokinetic profile in all age groups examined.

Breast Milk and Placental Transport: Ibuprofen excretion in breast milk following ingestion of one 400 mg ibuprofen tablet every 6 hours for five doses was below the level (i.e., 1 µg/mL) of detection. However, a later study using a more sensitive assay showed ibuprofen to be rapidly excreted in breast milk 30 minutes following oral ingestion of 400 mg of ibuprofen at a concentration of 13 ng/mL. A milk: plasma ratio of 1:126 was determined and the exposure of a suckling infant was calculated to be approximately 0.0008% of the maternal dose. It is not known whether ibuprofen crosses the placenta.

Comparative Bioavailability Advil Liqui-Gels (fasted) and Children's Advil Suspension (fasted): See Table 1.

Table 1: Advil

Summary Table of the Comparative Bioavailability Data

Advil Liqui-Gel Capsules (2×200 mg) From Measured Data			
Geometric Mean Arithmetic Mean (CV%)			
Parameter	**Test**	**Reference**[a]	**Ratio of least squares means**[c]
AUC_T (µg·h/mL)	135.17 138.05 (22.0%)	132.82 135.71 (22.7%)	99.3%
$AUC_{RefTmax}$ (µg·h/mL)	13.1745 14.767 (49.3%)	16.5162 18.138 (47.9%)	82.6%
AUC_1 (µg·h/mL)	136.52 139.63 (22.9%)	134.25 137.40 (23.8%)	99.2%
C_{max} (µg/mL)	47.33 47.6761 (12.1%)	42.47 42.8216 (13.2%)	111.1%
T_{max}[b] (h)	0.70 (35.2%)	0.81 (62.1%)	N/A
$T_{1/2}$[b](h)	2.44 (16.2%)	2.53 (16.2%)	N/A

[a] Reference product: Wyeth Consumer Healthcare Inc. (20 mg/mL) Children's Advil (ibuprofen) suspension, DIN 02232297.
[b] The T_{max} and $T_{1/2}$ parameters are expressed as the arithmetic means (CV%).
[c] The ratio of least-squares means is reported in order to compensate for the unbalanced number subjects/sequence in this study.

INDICATIONS: Adults and Children over 12 years: 200 mg ibuprofen tablets, caplets, gel caplets or liqui-gels, or 400 mg ibuprofen extra strength caplets or extra strength liqui-gels: For headaches and the temporary relief of menstrual pain (dysmenorrhea), toothache (dental pain), minor aches and pains in muscles, bones and joints and for reduction of fever and for temporary relief of mild to moderate pain. Consult your physician if the pain or fever persists for more than 5 days.

Liqui-Gels: Also indicated for temporary relief of mild to moderate migraine headaches including associated symptoms of nausea, and sensitivity to light and sound.

There is considerable evidence in the world literature documenting the efficacy of 200 to 400 mg doses of ibuprofen in the treatment of mild to moderate pain in a broad range of pain models.

Sore Throat Pain: A double-blind, randomized study showed that ibuprofen 400 mg relieved sore throat pain significantly better than placebo and acetaminophen.

Headache: A double-blind, randomized study showed that ibuprofen 400 mg relieved headache pain significantly better than acetaminophen 1000 mg and placebo. Another double-blind, placebo-controlled, randomized study showed that ibuprofen 400 mg began to exert a significant analgesic effect on headache within 30 minutes after dosing. A recent study confirmed that ibuprofen 400 mg provided a significantly faster onset of relief as measured by first perceptible relief, meaningful relief, per cent attaining complete relief, and superior overall analgesic efficacy compared to acetaminophen 1000 mg for relief of episodic tension-type headache.

Dental Pain: A double-blind, randomized study showed that ibuprofen 400 mg relieved dental pain following removal of impacted third molars significantly better than acetaminophen and placebo. Several other comparative dental studies have described similar results.

Muscle Aches: A double-blind, randomized study showed that ibuprofen 400 mg every four hours for a total of three doses relieved muscle soreness following exercise significantly better than acetaminophen 1000 mg and placebo every four hours.

Dysmenorrhea: Several studies demonstrate the significant effect of ibuprofen compared to placebo or other active analgesics on uterine pain and cramping.

Fever: The antipyretic efficacy of ibuprofen has been demonstrated in adult fever.

Children under 12 years: children's suspension, pediatric drops and junior strength chewable tablets: For children's fever and pain due to colds, sore throat, immunization and earache.

Fever: Multiple studies in the archival literature using ibuprofen doses ranging from 5 to 10 mg/kg have shown the drug's ability to lower fever in children.

Pain: Several studies have been conducted to evaluate the efficacy of ibuprofen in mild to moderate pain arising from sore throat, otitis media, migraine, dental, immunization, post-surgery, and, soft tissue injury.

CONTRAINDICATIONS: The following are contraindications to the use of Advil:

1. Active peptic ulcer, a history of recurrent ulceration or active inflammatory disease of the gastrointestinal system.
2. Known or suspected hypersensitivity to the drug or other nonsteroidal anti-inflammatory drugs. The potential for cross reactivity between different NSAIDs must be kept in mind.

   Advil should not be used in patients with the complete or partial syndrome of nasal polyps, or in whom asthma, anaphylaxis, urticaria, rhinitis or other allergic manifestations are precipitated by ASA or other nonsteroidal anti-inflammatory agents. Fatal anaphylactoid reactions have occurred in such individuals. As well, individuals with the above medical problems are at risk of a severe reaction even if they have taken NSAIDs in the past without any adverse effects.
3. Significant hepatic impairment or active liver disease.
4. Severely impaired or deteriorating renal function (creatinine clearance <30 mL/min). Individuals with lesser degrees of renal impairment are at risk of deterioration of their renal function when prescribed NSAIDs and must be monitored.
5. Ibuprofen is not recommended for use with other NSAIDs because of the absence of any evidence demonstrating synergistic benefits and the potential for additive side effects.
6. Children with kidney disease and children who have suffered significant fluid loss should not be given ibuprofen.
7. Serious GI toxicity, such as peptic ulceration, perforation and gastrointestinal bleeding, **sometimes severe and occasionally fatal**, can occur at any time, with or without symptoms in patients treated with NSAIDs including ibuprofen.
8. Do not use in the third trimester of pregnancy, because of risk of premature closure of the ductus arteriosus and prolonged parturition.

WARNINGS: General: Patients with heart disease, high blood pressure, diabetes, thyroid disease, narrow angle glaucoma, or difficulty in urination due to enlargement of the prostate gland should not take this drug unless directed by a physician.

Side effects may be minimized by using the smallest dose for the shortest duration of time.

As with other anti-inflammatory drugs, ibuprofen may mask the usual signs of infection.

If nervousness, dizziness, or sleeplessness occurs, use of Advil should be discontinued and a physician should be consulted. If symptoms do not improve within 5 days or are accompanied by fever, a physician should be consulted.

Gastrointestinal System (GI): Serious GI toxicity, such as peptic ulceration, perforation and gastrointestinal bleeding, **sometimes severe and occasionally fatal**, can occur at any time, with or without symptoms in patients treated with NSAIDs including ibuprofen.

Minor upper GI problems, such as dyspepsia, are common, usually developing early in therapy. Physicians should remain alert for ulceration and bleeding in patients treated with nonsteroidal anti-inflammatory drugs, even in the absence of previous GI tract symptoms.

In patients observed in clinical trials of such agents, symptomatic upper GI ulcers, gross bleeding, or perforation appear to occur in approximately 1% of patients treated for 3-6 months and in about 2-4% of patients treated for one year. The risk continues beyond one year and possibly increases. The incidence of these complications increases with increasing dose.

Advil should be given under close medical supervision to patients prone to gastrointestinal tract irritation, particularly those with a history of peptic ulcer, diverticulosis or other inflammatory disease of the gastrointestinal tract such as ulcerative colitis and Crohn's disease. In these cases the physician must weigh the benefits of treatment against the possible hazards.

Physicians should inform patients about the signs and/or symptoms of serious GI toxicity and instruct them to contact a physician immediately if they experience persistent dyspepsia or other symptoms or signs suggestive of gastrointestinal ulceration or bleeding. Because serious GI tract ulceration and bleeding can occur without warning symptoms, physicians should follow chronically treated patients by checking their haemoglobin periodically and by being vigilant for the signs and symptoms of ulceration and bleeding and should inform the patients of the importance of this follow-up. If ulceration is suspected or confirmed, or if GI bleeding occurs, Advil should be discontinued immediately, appropriate treatment instituted and the patient monitored closely.

No studies, to date, have identified any group of patients not at risk of developing ulceration and bleeding. A prior history of serious GI events and other factors such as excess alcohol intake, smoking, age, female gender and concomitant oral steroid and anticoagulant use have been associated with increased risk. Studies to date show that all NSAIDs can cause GI tract adverse events. Although existing data does not clearly identify differences in risk between various NSAIDs, this may be shown in the future.

Geriatrics: Patients older than 65 years and frail or debilitated patients are most susceptible to a variety of adverse reactions from nonsteroidal anti-inflammatory drugs (NSAIDs): the incidence of these adverse reactions increases with dose and duration of treatment. In addition, these patients are less tolerant to ulceration and bleeding. Most reports of fatal GI events are in this population. Older patients are also at risk of lower oesophageal ulceration and bleeding.

For such patients, consideration should be given to a starting dose lower than the one usually recommended, with individual adjustment when necessary and under close supervision. See Precautions for further advice.

Cross-Sensitivity: Patients sensitive to any one of the nonsteroidal anti-inflammatory drugs may be sensitive to any of the other NSAIDs also.

Aseptic Meningitis: In occasional cases, with some NSAIDs, the symptoms of aseptic meningitis (stiff neck, severe headaches, nausea and vomiting, fever or clouding of consciousness) have been observed. Patients with autoimmune disorders (systemic lupus erythematosus, mixed connective tissue diseases, etc.) seem to be pre-disposed. Therefore, in such patients, the physician must be vigilant to the development of this complication.

Pregnancy: Reproductive studies conducted in rats and rabbits have not demonstrated evidence of developmental abnormalities. However, animal reproduction studies are not always predictive of human response. Because of the known effects of NSAIDs on the fetal cardiovascular system, use of ibuprofen during late pregnancy should be avoided. As with other drugs known to inhibit prostaglandin synthesis, an increased incidence of dystocia and delayed parturition occurred in rats. Administration of ibuprofen is not recommended during pregnancy.

Breast Milk and Placental Transport: The high protein binding and lower pH of breast milk versus plasma tend to inhibit the excretion of ibuprofen into breast milk. One study showed an ibuprofen concentration of 13 ng/mL 30 minutes after ingesting 400 mg. The milk:plasma ratio was 1:126. This translates to an infant exposure of 0.0008% of the maternal dose. It is not known to what extent, if any, ibuprofen crosses the human placenta.

Children: Studies conducted to date have **not** demonstrated pediatric-specific problems that would limit the usefulness of ibuprofen in children 6 months and older.

Special Warnings: Skin: In rare cases, serious skin reactions such as Stevens-Johnson syndrome, toxic epidermal necrolysis, exfoliative dermatitis and erythema multiforme have been associated with the use of some NSAIDs. Because the rate of these reactions is low, they have usually been noted during post-marketing surveillance in patients taking other medications also associated with the potential development of these serious skin reactions. Thus, causality is **not** clear. These reactions are potentially life threatening but may be reversible if the causative agent is discontinued and appropriate treatment instituted. Patients should be advised that if they experience a skin rash, reddening or blisters they should discontinue their NSAID and contact their physician for assessment and advice, including which additional therapies to discontinue.

Other: Stop use and check with your physician if you vomit blood, have bloody or black stools, or experience any weakness.

Use with caution in the elderly.

PRECAUTIONS: Gastrointestinal System: There is no definitive evidence that the concomitant administration of histamine H2-receptor antagonists and/or antacids will either prevent the occurrence of gastrointestinal side effects or allow the continuation of Advil therapy when and if these adverse reactions appear.

Renal Function: Long-term administration of nonsteroidal anti-inflammatory drugs to animals has resulted in renal papillary necrosis and other abnormal renal pathology. In humans, there have been reports of acute interstitial nephritis with hematuria, proteinuria, and occasionally nephrotic syndrome.

A second form of renal toxicity has been seen in patients with prerenal conditions leading to the reduction in renal blood flow or blood volume, where the renal prostaglandins have a supportive role in the maintenance of renal perfusion. In these patients, administration of a nonsteroidal anti-inflammatory drug may cause a dose dependent reduction in prostaglandin formation and may precipitate overt renal decompensation. Patients at greatest risk of this reaction are those with impaired renal function, heart failure, liver dysfunction, those taking diuretics, and the elderly. Discontinuation of nonsteroidal anti-inflammatory therapy is usually followed by recovery to the pre-treatment state.

Ibuprofen and its metabolites are eliminated primarily by the kidneys; therefore the drug should be used with great caution in patients with impaired renal function. In these cases, utilisation of lower doses of Advil should be considered and patients carefully monitored.

During long-term therapy kidney function should be monitored periodically.

Genitourinary Tract: Some NSAIDs are known to cause persistent urinary symptoms (bladder pain, dysuria, urinary frequency), hematuria or cystitis. The onset of these symptoms may occur at any time after the initiation of therapy with an NSAID. Some cases have become severe on continued treatment. Should urinary symptoms occur, treatment with Advil **must be stopped immediately** to obtain recovery. This should be done before any urological investigations or treatments are carried out.

Hepatic Function: As with other nonsteroidal anti-inflammatory drugs, borderline elevations of one or more liver function tests may occur in up to 15% of patients. These abnormalities may progress, may remain essentially unchanged, or may be transient with continued therapy. A patient with symptoms and/or signs suggesting liver dysfunction, or in whom an abnormal liver test has occurred, should be evaluated for evidence of the development of more severe hepatic reaction while on therapy with this drug. Severe hepatic reactions including jaundice and cases of fatal hepatitis have been reported with nonsteroidal anti-inflammatory drugs.

Although such reactions are rare, if abnormal liver tests persist or worsen, if clinical signs and symptoms consistent with liver disease develop, or if systemic manifestations occur (e.g. eosinophilia, rash, etc.), this drug should be discontinued.

During long-term therapy, liver function tests should be monitored periodically. If there is a need to prescribe this drug in the presence of impaired liver function, it must be done under strict observation.

The frequency of acute liver injury among 625 307 people who received NSAIDs in England and Wales between 1987 and 1991, was examined. There were 311 716 patients who were prescribed ibuprofen. The incidence of acute liver injury among ibuprofen users was 1.6/100 000; this was the lowest incidence among the 8 NSAIDs studied and was significantly lower than the incidence among users of ketoprofen, piroxicam, fenbrufen, or sulindac. For NSAID users as a group, the only factors that had an independent effect on the occurrence of acute liver injury were the simultaneous use of hepatotoxic medication or the presence of rheumatoid arthritis. Based on these data, the short-term use of ibuprofen as an analgesic/antipyretic should not be of concern regarding the development of liver disease.

Fluid and Electrolyte Balance: Fluid retention and oedema have been observed in patients treated with ibuprofen. Therefore, as with many other nonsteroidal anti-inflammatory drugs, the possibility of precipitating congestive heart failure in elderly patients or those with compromised cardiac function should be borne in mind. Advil should be used with caution in patients with heart failure, hypertension or other conditions predisposing to fluid retention. With nonsteroidal anti-inflammatory treatment there is a potential risk of hyperkalemia, particularly in patients with conditions such as diabetes mellitus or renal failure; elderly patients; or in patients receiving concomitant therapy with B-adrenergic blockers, angiotensin converting enzyme inhibitors or some diuretics. Serum electrolytes should be monitored periodically during long-term therapy, especially in those patients who are at risk.

Haematology: Drugs inhibiting prostaglandin biosynthesis do interfere with platelet function to varying degrees; therefore, patients who may be adversely affected by such an action should be carefully observed when ibuprofen is administered.

Blood dyscrasias (such as neutropenia, leukopenia, thrombocytopenia, aplastic anaemia and agranulocytosis) associated with the use of nonsteroidal anti-inflammatory drugs are rare, but could occur with severe consequences.

Infection: In common with other anti-inflammatory drugs, ibuprofen may mask the usual signs of infection.

Ophthalmology: Blurred and/or diminished vision has been reported with the use of ibuprofen and other nonsteroidal anti-inflammatory drugs. If such symptoms develop this drug should be discontinued and an ophthalmologic examination performed; ophthalmic examination should be carried out at periodic intervals in any patient receiving this drug for an extended period of time.

Central Nervous System: Some patients may experience drowsiness, dizziness, vertigo, insomnia or depression with the use of ibuprofen. If patients experience these side effects, they should exercise caution in carrying out activities that require alertness.

Cardiovascular Function: Congestive heart failure in patients with marginal cardiac function, elevated blood pressure and palpitations.

Drug Interactions: Acetylsalicylic acid (ASA) or other NSAIDs: The use of Advil in addition to any other NSAID, including ASA, is not recommended due to the possibility of additive side effects. Animal studies show that aspirin given with NSAIDs, including ibuprofen, yields a net decrease in anti-inflammatory activity with lowered blood levels of the non-aspirin drug. Single-dose bioavailability studies in normal volunteers have failed to show an effect of aspirin on ibuprofen blood levels. Correlative clinical studies have not been conducted.

Acetaminophen: Although interactions have not been reported, concurrent use with Advil is not advisable: it may increase the risk of adverse renal effect.

Digoxin: Ibuprofen has been shown to increase serum digoxin concentration. Increased monitoring and dosage adjustments of digitalis glycoside may be necessary during and following concurrent ibuprofen therapy.

Coumarin Type: Numerous studies have shown that the concomitant use of NSAIDs and anticoagulants increases the risk of GI adverse events such as ulceration and bleeding. Because prostaglandins play an important role in hemostasis, and NSAIDs affect platelet function, concurrent therapy of ibuprofen with warfarin requires close monitoring to be certain that no change in anticoagulant dosage is necessary. Several short-term controlled studies failed to show that ibuprofen significantly affected prothrombin time or a variety of other clotting factors when administered to individuals on coumarin-type anticoagulants. Nevertheless, the physician, should be cautious when administering Advil to patients on anticoagulants.

Hypoglycaemic Agents: Ibuprofen may increase hypoglycaemic effects of oral antidiabetic agents and insulin.

Antihypertensives: Prostaglandins are an important factor in cardiovascular homeostasis and inhibition of their synthesis by NSAIDs may interfere with circulatory control. NSAIDs may elevate blood pressure in patients receiving antihypertensive medication. Two meta analyses have observed this relationship for NSAIDs as a class and for certain NSAIDs in particular, but ibuprofen did not significantly affect blood pressure in either meta analysis. Consistent with this lack of effect, a study showed that ibuprofen 1600 mg/day for 14 days did not attenuate the antihypertensive effect of two β-adrenergic blockers. Another study showed no effect of three weeks' therapy with ibuprofen on the antihypertensive efficacy of verapamil, but it is not known whether this lack of interaction extends to other classes of calcium channel blockers.

When renal perfusion pressure is reduced both prostaglandins and angiotensin II are important mediators of renal autoregulation. As a class, the combination of an NSAID and angiotensin converting enzyme inhibitor theoretically may have the potential to decrease renal function. One study found a clinically significant decrease in renal function in 4 of 17 patients treated with hydrochlorothioazide and fosinopril who received ibuprofen 2400 mg/day for one month. In contrast, another study found no effect on the antihypertensive effect of enalapril or on plasma renin or aldosterone following two days' treatment with ibuprofen 1200 mg/day.

The relationship of ibuprofen and antihypertensives is clearly not well defined. The benefits of concomitant medication should be analysed and compared to the potential risks before being prescribed. If ibuprofen is being recommended for **long-term** use, then periodic monitoring of blood pressure may be useful. Blood pressure monitoring is not necessary if ibuprofen is being recommended for **short-term** use as an **analgesic**.

Diuretics: Clinical studies, as well as random observations, have shown that ibuprofen can reduce the natriuretic effect of furosemide and thiazides in some patients. This response has been attributed to inhibition of renal prostaglandin synthesis. During concomitant therapy with ibuprofen, the patient should be observed closely for signs of renal failure as well as to assure diuretic efficacy.

Antacids: A bioavailability study has shown that there was no interference with the absorption of ibuprofen when given in conjunction with an antacid containing aluminium hydroxide and magnesium hydroxide.

H_2-Antagonists: In studies with human volunteers, coadministration of cimetidine or ranitidine with ibuprofen had no substantive effect on ibuprofen serum concentrations.

Methotrexate: Ibuprofen as well as other NSAIDs has been reported to competitively inhibit methotrexate accumulation in rabbit kidney slices. This may indicate that ibuprofen could enhance the toxicity of methotrexate. Caution should be used when ibuprofen is administered concomitantly with methotrexate.

Lithium: Ibuprofen produced an elevation of plasma lithium levels and a reduction in renal lithium clearance in a study of eleven normal volunteers. The mean minimum lithium concentration increased 15% and the renal clearance of lithium was decreased by 19% during this period of concomitant drug administration. This effect has been attributed to inhibition of renal prostaglandin synthesis by ibuprofen. Thus, when ibuprofen and lithium are administered concurrently, subjects should be observed carefully for signs of lithium toxicity.

Other Drugs: Although ibuprofen binds extensively to plasma proteins, interactions with other protein-bound drugs occur rarely. Nevertheless, caution should be observed when other drugs, also having a high affinity for protein binding sites, are used concurrently. No interactions have been reported when ibuprofen has been used in conjunction with probenecid, thyroxine, steroids, antibiotics or benzodiazepines.

ADVERSE EFFECTS: Prescription Experience: The following adverse reactions have been noted in patients treated with prescription doses (≥1200 mg/day).

Note: Reactions listed below under Causal Relationship Unknown are those which occurred under circumstances where a causal relationship could not be established. However, in these rarely reported events, the possibility of a relationship to ibuprofen cannot be excluded.

Gastrointestinal: The adverse reactions most frequently seen with prescribed ibuprofen therapy involve the gastrointestinal system.

Incidence 3 to 9%: nausea, epigastric pain, heartburn.

Incidence 1 to 3%: diarrhea, abdominal distress, nausea and vomiting, indigestion, constipation, abdominal cramps or pain, fullness of the gastrointestinal tract (bloating or flatulence).

Incidence less than 1%: gastric or duodenal ulcer with bleeding and/or perforation, gastrointestinal haemorrhage, melena, hepatitis, jaundice, abnormal liver function (AST, serum bilirubin and alkaline phosphatase).

Immune: Incidence less than 1%: anaphylaxis (see Contraindications).

Causal relationship unknown: fever, serum sickness, lupus erythematosus.

Central Nervous System: Incidence 3 to 9%: dizziness.

Incidence 1 to 3%: headache, nervousness.

Incidence less than 1%: depression, insomnia.

Causal relationship unknown: paresthesias, hallucinations, dream abnormalities.

Aseptic meningitis and meningoencephalitis, in one case accompanied by eosinophilia in the cerebrospinal fluid, have been reported in patients who took ibuprofen intermittently and did not have any connective tissue disease.

Integumentary: Incidence 3 to 9%: rash (including maculopapular type).

Incidence 1 to 3%: pruritus.

Incidence less than 1%: vesiculobullous eruptions, urticaria, erythema multiforme.

Causal relationship unknown: alopecia, Stevens-Johnson syndrome.

Cardiovascular: Incidence less than 1%: congestive heart failure in patients with marginal cardiac function, elevated blood pressure.

Causal relationship unknown: arrhythmias (sinus tachycardia, sinus bradycardia, palpitations).

Special Senses: Incidence 1 to 3%: tinnitus.

Incidence less than 1%: amblyopia (blurred and/or diminished vision, scotomata and/or changes in colour vision). Any patient with eye complaints during ibuprofen therapy should have an ophthalmological examination.

Causal relationship unknown: conjunctivitis, diplopia, optic neuritis.

Hematologic: Incidence less than 1%: leukopenia, and decreases in haemoglobin and hematocrit.

Causal relationship unknown: haemolytic anaemia, thrombocytopenia, granulocytopenia, bleeding episodes (e.g., purpura, epistaxis, hematuria, menorrhagia).

Renal: Causal relationship unknown: decreased creatinine clearance, polyuria, azotemia.

Like other nonsteroidal anti-inflammatory drugs, ibuprofen inhibits renal prostaglandin synthesis, which may decrease renal function and cause sodium retention. Renal blood flow and glomerular filtration rate decreased in patients with mild impairment of renal function who took 1200 mg/day of ibuprofen for one week. Renal papillary necrosis has been reported. A number of factors appear to increase the risk of renal toxicity (see Precautions).

Hepatic: Incidence less than 1%. Hepatitis, jaundice, abnormal liver function (AST, serum bilirubin, and alkaline phosphatase).

Endocrine: Causal relationship unknown: gynecomastia, hypoglycaemic reaction.

Menstrual delays of up to two weeks and dysfunctional uterine bleeding occurred in nine patients taking ibuprofen, 400 mg t.i.d., for three days before menses.

Metabolic: Incidence 1 to 3%: decreased appetite, oedema, fluid retention.

Fluid retention generally responds promptly to drug discontinuation (See Precautions).

Non-Prescription Experience: Literature (at dosages ≤1200 mg/day): One researcher conducted an extensive analysis of published data concerning the relative safety of non-prescription doses of ibuprofen and acetaminophen. Of a total of 96 randomized and blinded trials, there were 10 trials of seven days' duration or less where the safety of both drugs was directly compared. In three of these trials, the incidence of adverse events was higher with acetaminophen; there were no reported adverse events in six trials; and one trial reported a higher incidence with ibuprofen. In this subset of 10 studies, it was reported that gastrointestinal adverse events were found to be the most common type of event reported and were predominantly dyspepsia, nausea, or vomiting. None of the GI events appeared to warrant follow-up from which the author inferred there were no serious gastrointestinal events.

It was concluded: "Although we recognise that the above mentioned data are very selective and are based on information derived from a variety of trial designs and populations, it is nonetheless instructive for indicating a relatively low incidence of severe adverse reactions with both drugs when taken at their respective non-prescription dosages."

A double-blind, placebo-controlled study (N=1246) was conducted to prospectively evaluate the gastrointestinal tolerability, as compared to placebo, of the maximum non-prescription dose and duration (1200 mg/day for 10 consecutive days) of ibuprofen use in healthy subjects representative of a non-prescription analgesic user population. Gastrointestinal adverse experiences were similar in the placebo and ibuprofen groups (67 out of 413, 16% with placebo vs. 161 out of 833, 19% with ibuprofen). There was no difference between the two groups in the proportion of discontinuing due to a gastrointestinal event. Gastrointestinal adverse experiences reported by ≥1% of subjects were: dyspepsia, abdominal pain, nausea, diarrhea, flatulence, and constipation. Seventeen (1.4%) subjects had positive occult blood tests: their frequency was comparable between treatments. When used as directed to treat episodic pain, non-prescription ibuprofen at the maximum dose of 1200 mg/day for 10 days, is well-tolerated.

In two multitrial analyses a meta analysis, and a literature review, single doses of ibuprofen had a low incidence of gastrointestinal drug reactions, comparable to that of acetaminophen and placebo. Reports from spontaneous reporting systems in the United Kingdom, France and the United States, where a prescription is not needed for ibuprofen at a daily dose up to 1200 mg, confirm the medication's gastrointestinal safety and acceptability. A recently-completed large-scale randomised trial comparing non-prescription doses of acetylsalicylic acid, acetaminophen, and ibuprofen in 8677 adults found that the rates of significant adverse reactions were: aspirin 18.7%, ibuprofen 13.7%, and acetaminophen 14.5%. Ibuprofen was not statistically different from acetaminophen. Total gastrointestinal events (including dyspepsia) and abdominal pain were less frequent with ibuprofen (4% and 2.8%, respectively) than with acetaminophen (5.3% and 3.9%) or aspirin (7.1% and 6.8%) [all p<0.035]. It was concluded that "The overall tolerability of ibuprofen in this large-scale study was equivalent to that of paracetamol and better than that of [ASA]."

Other Ibuprofen Adverse Events: Health professionals should keep in mind other potential adverse events associated with ibuprofen use including: Crohn's disease, colitis, gastritis, hematemesis, mouth ulceration, abdominal distension, dyspepsia, abdominal pain upper, hypersensitivity, cerebrovascular accident, angioneurotic edema, dermatitis bullous, face edema, pupura, cardiac failure, myocardial infarction, angina pectoris, vertigo, visual disturbance, agranulocytosis, anemia, aplastic anemia, hematuria, interstitial nephritis, renal failure, nephrotic syndrome, proteinuria, and renal papillary necrosis, liver disorder, asthma, bronchospasm, dyspnea, wheezing, meningitis aseptic, meningitis, edema, swelling, and peripheral edema.

Experience in Children: Safety studies of ibuprofen suspension in children are among the largest prospective clinical trials ever conducted. Both the Children's Analgesic Medicine Project (CAMP) and the Boston Fever Study enrolled a wide age range of children, which supports the generalisability of these studies' findings. These large-scale studies focused on examining the potential risk in children of several rare events that can be related to the pharmacologic action of NSAIDs: GI bleeding, acute renal failure, and anaphylaxis. The Children's Analgesic Medicine Project (CAMP) was a multicenter, all-comers, open-label, prospective study to compare the safety of ibuprofen suspension with acetaminophen suspension in children with fever and/or pain. Four hundred twenty four (424) pediatricians enrolled 41 810 children (aged 1 month to 18 years old) at 69 US clinics. Safety data included information concerning medication use and adverse events summarised by severity and analysed by age groups (younger and older than 2 years). Among 30 238 children who took at least one dose of ibuprofen or acetaminophen, 14 281 were younger (<2 years) and 15 863 were older (≥2-<12 years. Within both age groups, the incidence rates for specific AEs, including abdominal pain, insomnia, and hyperkinesia were rare and generally <1% for both treatments. For younger children, fever, vomiting, diarrhea, rhinitis, rash and otitis media were the only AEs with an incidence rate >1% (in either treatment group). For older children, the only AEs with an incidence rate >1% in either group were rhinitis, pharyngitis and otitis media. AEs were generally mild to moderate for both treatments within the two age groups. There were no serious AEs, including anaphylaxis, Reye's syndrome, renal failure, GI bleeding/perforation or necrotizing fasciitis. Overall, ibuprofen exhibited an AE profile similar to acetaminophen in both younger and older children.

The Boston Fever Study was a large, randomized, double-blind study that assessed the risk of rare but serious adverse events following the use of ibuprofen suspension in febrile children between the ages of 6 months and 12 years of age. The study evaluated a total of 83 915 children enrolled by 1735 pediatricians, family physicians, and general practitioners in the U.S. Children were randomized to receive ibuprofen suspension 5 mg/kg (N=27 948), ibuprofen suspension 10 mg/kg (N=27 837) or acetaminophen suspension 12 mg/kg (N=28 130). Medications were given every 4-6 hours, as needed, up to five doses per day. The study focused on hospitalisations for acute GI bleeding, acute renal failure, and anaphylaxis, as well as monitoring for the occurrence of Reye syndrome. In the entire pediatric population, the authors found no significant difference between ibuprofen- and acetaminophen-treated children in the observed risk of GI bleeding, acute renal failure, or anaphylaxis. No cases of Reye syndrome were seen in febrile children.

The safety findings of the Boston Fever Study are concordant with those of the Children's Analgesic Medicine Project: ibuprofen is well tolerated in children at doses of 20-30 mg/kg/day and higher. No symptom or syndrome emerged in these trials that was not predictable from the drug's pharmacology or could not be anticipated based on ibuprofen's extensive use as an analgesic/antipyretic in adults.

OVERDOSE:

Symptoms: The toxicity of ibuprofen overdose is dependent upon the amount of drug ingested and the time elapsed since ingestion; individual responses may vary, thus making it necessary to evaluate each case separately. Although uncommon, serious toxicity and death have been reported with ibuprofen overdosage. The most frequently reported symptoms of ibuprofen overdose include abdominal pain, nausea, vomiting, lethargy, vertigo, drowsiness (somnolence), dizziness and insomnia. Other CNS symptoms include headache, loss of consciousness, tinnitus, CNS depression, convulsions and seizures. Metabolic acidosis, abnormal hepatic function, hyperkalemia, renal failure, dyspnea, respiratory depression, coma, acute renal failure, and apnea (primarily in very young pediatric patients) may rarely occur. Cardiovascular toxicity, including hypotension, bradycardia, tachycardia and atrial fibrillation, also have been reported.

Treatment: In cases of acute overdose, the stomach should be emptied through induction of emesis (in alert patients only) or gastric lavage. Emesis is most effective if initiated within 30 minutes of ingestion. Orally administered activated charcoal may help in reducing the absorption of ibuprofen when given less than 2 hours following ingestion. There is some evidence that repeated administration of activated charcoal may bind the medication that has diffused from the circulation. Inducing diuresis may be helpful. The treatment of acute overdose is primarily supportive. Management of hypotension, acidosis and gastrointestinal bleeding may be necessary.

In pediatric patients, the estimated amount of ibuprofen ingested per body weight may be helpful to predict the potential for development of toxicity although each case must be evaluated. Ingestion of less than 100 mg/kg is unlikely to produce toxicity. Pediatric patients ingesting 100 to 200 mg/kg may be managed with induced emesis and a minimal observation time of at least four hours. Pediatric patients ingesting 200 to 400 mg/kg of ibuprofen should have immediate gastric emptying and at least four hours observation. Pediatric patients ingesting greater than 400 mg/kg require immediate medical referral, careful observation and appropriate supportive therapy. Induced emesis is not recommended in overdoses greater than 400 mg/kg because of the risk for convulsions and the potential for aspiration of gastric contents.

In adult patients, the dose reportedly ingested does not appear to be predictive of toxicity. The need for referral and follow-up must be judged by the circumstances at the time of the overdose ingestion. Symptomatic adults should be carefully evaluated, observed and supported.

For management of a suspected drug overdose, CPhA recommends that you contact your **regional Poison Control Centre**. See the *CPS*Directory section for a list of Poison Control Centres.

DOSAGE: Adults and Children over 12 years: Take 1 or 2 tablets, caplets, gel caplets or liqui-gels or 1 extra strength caplet or extra strength liqui-gel every 4 hours as needed. Do not exceed 6 tablets, caplets, gel caplets or liqui-gels or 3 extra strength caplets or extra strength liqui-gels in 24 hours, unless directed by a physician.
Children under 12 years: Children's Advil Suspension: See Table 2.
Advil Pediatric Drops: See Table 3.
Advil Junior Strength Chewable Tablets: See Table 4.

Table 2: Advil

Dosage—Children's Advil Suspension 20 mg/mL (or 100 mg/5 mL)

Directions: If possible, use weight to dose; otherwise use age. Shake well and ensure that all the contents of the dosage cup are taken.
Doses below may be repeated every 6-8 hours while symptoms persist, up to 3 doses a day, or as directed by a physician.

Weight (kg)	Age (years)	Dose (tsp)
	Under 2	Use Advil Pediatric Drops
10.9–15.9	2–3	6.0 mL=1¼ tsp
16.0–21.3	4–5	10 mL=2 tsp
21.4–26.7	6–8	12.5 mL=2½ tsp
26.8–32.5	9–10	15 mL=3 tsp
32.6–43.0	11–12	19.0 mL=3¾ tsp

Note: Children's Advil Suspension may be administered to adults who have difficulty in swallowing tablets. Children over 12 and adults may take 2-4 teaspoons (200-400 mg) every 4 hours as needed. Do not exceed 12 teaspoons (1200 mg) in 24 hours, unless directed by a physician.

Table 3: Advil

Dosage—Advil Pediatric Drops 40 mg/mL (or 200 mg/5 mL)

Directions: If possible, use weight to dose; otherwise use age. Shake well. Use only with enclosed SURE-DOSE oral syringe.
Doses below may be repeated every 6-8 hours while symptoms persist, up to 3 doses a day, or as directed by a physician.

Weight (kg)	Age (months)	Dosage (mL)
2.5–5.4	0–3	5 mg/kg (0.125 mL/kg) To be Calculated
5.5–7.9	4–11	1.0 mL
8.0–10.8	12–23	1.4 mL
10.9–15.9	2–3 years	3.0 mL

Table 4: Advil

Advil Junior Strength Chewable Tablets 100 mg/Tablet

If possible, use weight to dose; otherwise use age.
Doses below may be repeated every 6-8 hours while symptoms persist, up to 4 doses a day, or as directed by a physician.

Weight (kg)	Age (years)	Dosage (tablets)
	Under 2	Recommend Advil Pediatric Drops
10.9–15.9	2–3	1
16.0–21.3	4–5	1½
21.4–26.7	6–8	2
26.8–32.5	9–10	2½
32.6–43.0	11–12	3

INFORMATION FOR THE PATIENT: Published in e-CPS, available by subscription at www.e-cps.ca.

SUPPLIED: Tablets/Caplets (Sugar-coated): Each brown, sugar-coated tablet/caplet contains: ibuprofen 200 mg. Nonmedicinal ingredients: acetylated monoglyceride, beeswax, carnauba wax, corn starch, croscarmellose sodium, ethoxyethanol, iron oxides, lecithin, microcrystalline cellulose, parabens, pharmaceutical glaze, pharmaceutical shellac, povidone, pregelatinized starch, silicon dioxide, simethicone, sodium benzoate, sodium lauryl sulfate, stearic acid, sucrose and titanium dioxide. Blisters of 8 and 10. Bottles of 24, 50, 100, 150 and 250 tablets. Professional sample pouches of 2 tablets. Bottles of 24, 50 and 100 caplets. Store in tightly closed containers under room temperature (15-30°C) conditions.

Gel Caplets: Each beige brown, gelatin-coated gel-caplet contains: ibuprofen 200 mg. Nonmedicinal ingredients: corn starch, croscarmellose sodium, FD&C Red No.40, FD&C Yellow No. 6, gelatin, glycerin, hypromellose, iron oxides, medium chain triglycerides, pregelatinized starch, propyl gallate, propylene glycol, silicon dioxide, sodium lauryl sulfate, stearic acid, titanium dioxide and triacetin. Bottles of 16, 32 and 72. Store in tightly closed containers under room temperature (15-30°C) conditions.
Liqui-Gels: Each green, transparent, gelatin capsule contains: ibuprofen 200 mg. Nonmedicinal ingredients: FD&C Green No. 3, gelatin, polyethylene glycol, polyvinyl acetate phthalate, potassium hydroxide, propylene glycol, purified water, sorbitan, sorbitol and titanium dioxide. Bottles of 16, 32, 72, and 165. Professional pouches of 2. Store in tightly closed containers under room temperature (15-30°C) conditions.
Extra Strength Caplets: Each brown film-coated caplet contains: ibuprofen 400 mg. Nonmedicinal ingredients: cornstarch, croscarmellose sodium, hydroxypropyl methylcellulose, iron oxides, lecithin, pharmaceutical shellac, polyethylene glycol, pregelatinized starch, silicon dioxide, simethicone, sodium lauryl sulfate, stearic acid, talc and titanium dioxide. Bottles of 16, 32, 72, and 165. Professional sample pouches of 1. Store in tightly closed containers under room temperature (15-30°C) conditions.
Extra Strength Liqui-Gels: Each yellow, transparent, gelatin capsule contains: ibuprofen 400 mg. Nonmedicinal ingredients: gelatin, iron oxide, lecithin, medium chain triglycerides, polyethylene glycol, polyvinyl acetate phthalate, potassium hydroxide, propylene glycol, purified water, sorbitan and sorbitol. Bottles of 12, 24, and 50. Store in tightly closed containers under room temperature (15-30 °C) conditions.
Pediatric Drops: Dye-Free: Each 5 mL of white to off-white suspension contains: ibuprofen 200 mg. Nonmedicinal ingredients: artificial flavours, citric acid, disodium EDTA, glycerin, microcrystalline cellulose, polysorbate 80, sodium benzoate, sodium carboxymethylcellulose, sorbitol, sucrose, water, and xanthan gum. Bottles of 15 and 24 mL with SURE-DOSE oral syringe. Professional samples of 15 mL. Store in tightly closed containers under room temperature (15-30°C) conditions.
Fruit Flavor: Each 5 mL of translucent red suspension with sweet fruity odour contains: ibuprofen 200 mg. Nonmedicinal ingredients: artificial flavors, citric acid, disodium EDTA, FD&C Red No. 40, glycerin, microcrystalline cellulose, polysorbate 80, sodium benzoate, sodium carboxymethylcellulose, sorbitol, sucrose, water, and xanthan gum. Bottles of 15 and 24 mL with SURE-DOSE oral syringe. Professional samples of 15 mL. Store in tightly closed containers under room temperature (15-30°C) conditions.
Grape Flavor: Each 5 mL of translucent purple suspension with sweet fruity odour contains: ibuprofen 200 mg. Nonmedicinal ingredients: artificial flavors, citric acid, disodium EDTA, FD&C Blue No. 1, FD&C Red No. 40, glycerin, microcrystalline cellulose, polysorbate 80, sodium benzoate, sodium carboxymethylcellulose sorbitol, sucrose, water, and xanthan gum. Bottles of 15 and 24 mL with SURE-DOSE oral syringe. Professional samples of 15 mL. Store in tightly closed containers under room temperature (15-30°C) conditions.
Children's Suspension: Blue Raspberry Flavor: Each 5 mL of translucent blue suspension with sweet fruity odor contains: ibuprofen 100 mg. Nonmedicinal ingredients: citric acid, disodium EDTA, FD&C Blue No. 1, glycerin, microcrystalline cellulose, natural and artificial flavors, polysorbate 80, sodium benzoate, sodium carboxymethylcellulose, sodium citrate, sorbitol, sucrose, water and xanthan gum. Bottles of 100 mL. Professional samples of 25 mL. Store in tightly closed containers under room temperature (15-30°C) conditions.
Dye-free: Each 5 mL of white to off-white suspension contains: ibuprofen 100 mg. Nonmedicinal ingredients: artificial flavors, citric acid, disodium EDTA, glycerin, microcrystalline cellulose, polysorbate 80, sodium benzoate, sodium carboxymethylcellulose, sorbitol, sucrose, water and xanthan gum. Bottles of 100 mL. Professional samples of 25 mL. Store in tightly closed containers under room temperature (15-30°C) conditions.
Fruit Flavor: Each 5 mL of translucent red suspension with sweet fruity odor contains: ibuprofen 100 mg. Nonmedicinal ingredients: artificial flavors, citric acid, disodium EDTA, FD&C Red No. 40, glycerin, microcrystalline cellulose, polysorbate 80, sodium benzoate, sodium carboxymethylcellulose, sorbitol, sucrose, water and xanthan gum. Bottles of 100 mL. Professional samples of 25 mL. Store in tightly closed containers under room temperature (15-30°C) conditions.
Grape Flavor: Each 5 mL of translucent purple suspension with sweet fruity odor contains: ibuprofen 100 mg. Nonmedicinal ingredients: artificial flavors, citric acid, disodium EDTA, FD&C Blue No. 1, FD&C Red No. 40, glycerin, microcrystalline cellulose, polysorbate 80, sodium benzoate, sodium carboxymethylcellulose, sorbitol, sucrose, water and xanthan gum. Bottles of 100 mL. Professional samples of 25 mL. Store in tightly closed containers under room temperature (15-30°C) conditions.
Junior Strength Tablets: Fruit Flavor: Each ½" round, mottled red, flat-faced, beveled edged tablet with "Advil 100" debossed on one side and a bisect on the other, contains: ibuprofen 100 mg. Nonmedicinal ingredients: aspartame (contains phenylalanine), cellulose acetate phthalate, D&C Red No. 27 Lake, FD&C Red No. 40 Lake, gelatin, magnasweet, magnesium stearate, mannitol, microcrystalline cellulose, natural and artificial flavors, silicon dioxide and sodium starch glycolate. Bottles of 20 and 40. Store at room temperature (20-25°C). Protect from moisture and excessive heat.
Grape Flavor: Each ½" round, mottled purple, flat-faced, beveled edged tablet with "Advil 100" debossed on one side and a bisect on the other, contains: ibuprofen 100 mg. Nonmedicinal ingredients: aspartame (contains phenylalanine), cellulose acetate phthalate, D&C Red No. 30 Lake, FD&C Blue No. 2 Lake, gelatin, magnasweet, magnesium stearate, mannitol, microcrystalline cellulose, natural and artificial flavors, silicon dioxide and sodium starch glycolate. Bottles of 20 and 40. Professional sample pouches of 2. Store at room temperature (20-25°C). Protect from moisture and excessive heat.
Blue Raspberry Flavour: Each ½" round, mottled blue, flat-faced, beveled edged tablet with "Advil 100" debossed on one side and a bisect on the other contains: ibuprofen 100 mg. Nonmedicinal ingredients: aspartame (contains phenylalanine), cellulose acetate phthalate, FD&C Blue No. 1 Lake, FD&C Blue No. 2 Lake, gelatin, magnasweet, magnesium stearate, mannitol, microcrystalline cellulose, natural and artificial flavors, silicon dioxide and sodium starch glycolate. Bottles of 20 and 40. Protect from moisture and excessive heat.

Advil® Cold & Sinus
ibuprofen—pseudoephedrine HCl
Analgesic—Antipyretic—Decongestant

Pfizer Consumer Healthcare

Advil® Cold & Sinus Daytime
ibuprofen—pseudoephedrine HCl
Analgesic—Antipyretic—Decongestant

Pfizer Consumer Healthcare

Children's Advil® Cold
ibuprofen—pseudoephedrine HCl
Analgesic—Antipyretic—Decongestant

Pfizer Consumer Healthcare

PHARMACOLOGY: Ibuprofen has exhibited analgesic and antipyretic activity in animal studies designed to specifically demonstrate these effects. Ibuprofen has been shown to have no glucocorticoid-like activity.

Pseudoephedrine is an orally effective nasal decongestant when administered in doses of 60 mg/dose, up to 240 mg/day. In order to comply with the flexible dosing schedule approved for nonprescription ibuprofen, clinical studies were conducted to demonstrate the efficacy of 30 mg pseudoephedrine when administered in the combination product and evidence of dose response between the 30 and 60 mg doses.

A 3-way bioavailability study of ibuprofen, pseudoephedrine and a combination of ibuprofen/pseudoephedrine indicated that the absorption and the disposition of the 2 drugs were not different, i.e., there was no pharmacokinetic interaction when the 2 drugs were combined.

In another 3-way bioequivalence comparison of ibuprofen, pseudoephedrine and a combination of the 2 drugs, no statistically significant differences were noted among the 3 treatments for any pharmacokinetic variables for ibuprofen or pseudoephedrine.

INDICATIONS: Advil Cold & Sinus and Advil Cold & Sinus Daytime: For the temporary relief of symptoms associated with the common cold, sinusitis or flu including sinus pain, nasal congestion, headache, fever and body aches and pains.
Children's Advil Cold: For the temporary relief of symptoms associated with the common cold, sinusitis or flu including nasal and sinus congestion, fever, stuffy nose, headache, sore throat and body aches and pains.
Consult a physician if pain or fever worsens or persists for more than 5 days.

CONTRAINDICATIONS: Patients who have previously exhibited hypersensitivity to it, or to its components (ibuprofen, pseudoephedrine), or individuals with the angioedema syndrome, nasal polyps or bronchospastic reactivity to ASA or other nonsteroidal anti-inflammatory agents.

Patients with hypertension, coronary artery disease and patients on MAO inhibitor therapy.

Do not use if monoamine oxidase inhibitors (MAOIs) have been taken in the last days for depression, psychiatric or emotional conditions.

Serious GI toxicity, such as peptic ulceration, perforation and gastrointestinal bleeding, **sometimes severe and occasionally fatal**, can occur at any time, with or without symptoms in patients treated with NSAIDs including ibuprofen.

Pregnancy: Do not use in the third trimester of pregnancy, because of risk of premature closure of the ductus arteriosus and prolonged parturition.

Advil Cold & Sinus and Advil Cold & Sinus Daytime should not be used during pregnancy because its safety under this condition has not been established.

Lactation: Advil Cold & Sinus and Advil Cold & Sinus Daytime should not be used in nursing mothers because its safety under this condition has not been established.

Children: Advil Cold & Sinus and Advil Cold & Sinus Daytime should not be used in pediatric patients because its safety under this condition has not been established.

Aseptic meningitis, fever and rash have been reported in connection with ibuprofen therapy in patients with systemic lupus erythematosus. Advil Cold & Sinus, Advil Cold & Sinus Daytime and Children's Advil Cold should not be used by patients with systemic lupus erythematosus except under a physician's supervision.

Advil Cold & Sinus, Advil Cold & Sinus Daytime and Children's Advil Cold should not be taken by patients with active peptic ulcer disease or gastrointestinal bleeding unless directed by a physician.

WARNINGS: Anaphylactoid reactions have occurred in patients with known ASA hypersensitivity.

Peptic ulcerations and gastrointestinal bleeding, sometimes severe, have been reported in patients receiving prescription doses of ibuprofen. Peptic ulcerations, perforation or severe gastrointestinal bleeding can have a fatal outcome, and although few such reports have been received with ibuprofen, a cause and effect relationship has not been established. Patients with a history of upper gastrointestinal tract disease should take Advil Cold & Sinus, Advil Cold & Sinus Daytime and Children's Advil Cold under the supervision of a physician.

Like other nonsteroidal anti-inflammatory agents, ibuprofen can inhibit platelet aggregation. However, compared to ASA, the effect is quantitatively less, of shorter duration, and reversible upon discontinuation of ibuprofen. Bleeding time has also been prolonged by ibuprofen though within the normal range in normal subjects. Because this effect on bleeding time may be exaggerated in patients with underlying hemostatic defects, Advil Cold & Sinus, Advil Cold & Sinus Daytime and Children's Advil Cold should be avoided by persons with intrinsic coagulation defects and those on anticoagulant therapy.

Patients with high blood pressure, heart disease, diabetes, narrow-angle glaucoma, thyroid disease, kidney or liver disease, or difficulty in urination due to enlargement of the prostate gland should take Advil Cold & Sinus, Advil Cold & Sinus Daytime and Children's Advil Cold only under the advice and supervision of a physician.

General: Side effects may be minimized by using the smallest dose for the shortest duration of time.

As with other anti-inflammatory drugs, ibuprofen may mask the usual signs of infection.

If nervousness, dizziness, or sleeplessness occurs, use of Advil should be discontinued and a physician should be consulted. If symptoms do not improve within 5 days or are accompanied by fever, a physician should be consulted.

Special Warnings: Skin: In rare cases, serious skin reactions such as Stevens-Johnson syndrome, toxic epidermal necrolysis, exfoliative dermatitis and erythema multiforme have been associated with the use of some NSAIDs. Because the rate of these reactions is low, they have usually been noted during post-marketing surveillance in patients taking other medications also associated with the potential development of these serious skin reactions. Thus, causality is **not** clear. These reactions are potentially life threatening but may be reversible if the causative agent is discontinued and appropriate treatment instituted. Patients should be advised that if they experience a skin rash, reddening or blisters they should discontinue their NSAID and contact their physician for assessment and advice, including which additional therapies to discontinue.

Other: Stop use and check with your physician if you vomit blood, have bloody or black stools, or experience any weakness.

Use with caution in the elderly.

PRECAUTIONS: Conditions associated with dehydration appear to increase the risk of renal toxicity. Advil Cold & Sinus, Advil Cold & Sinus Daytime and Children's Advil Cold should therefore be used with caution in patients with chronic renal failure, congestive heart failure or hypertension being treated chronically with diuretics. Caution should be observed in elderly patients, due to increased susceptibility to effects of sympathomimetic amines and increased risk of toxicity with ibuprofen, and patients with diminished renal function.

Patients on Advil Cold & Sinus, Advil Cold & Sinus Daytime or Children's Advil Cold should be cautioned to report to their physician any signs or symptoms of gastrointestinal ulceration or bleeding, blurred vision or other eye symptoms, skin rash, weight gain, edema, tinnitus, dizziness or respiratory difficulties.

If Advil Cold & Sinus, Advil Cold & Sinus Daytime or Children's Advil Cold is taken in conjunction with prolonged corticosteroid therapy and it is decided to discontinue the latter therapy, as under other circumstances, the corticosteroid dosage should be tapered slowly to avoid exacerbation of disease or adrenal insufficiency.

There is a possibility of insomnia if this medicine is taken before bedtime.

If the symptoms do not improve or are accompanied by a high fever, the patient should be advised to report to the physician.

ADVERSE EFFECTS: Ibuprofen: The following adverse reactions have been noted in patients treated with prescription regimens of ibuprofen.

Gastrointestinal: The adverse reactions most frequently seen with prescribed ibuprofen therapy involve the gastrointestinal system: nausea, epigastric pain, heartburn, diarrhea, abdominal distress, vomiting, indigestion, constipation, abdominal cramps, fullness of the gastrointestinal tract (bloating or flatulence).

Central Nervous System: dizziness, headache, nervousness.

Integumentary: rash (including maculopapular type), pruritus.

Special Senses: tinnitus.

Metabolic: decreased appetite, edema, fluid retention. Fluid retention generally responds promptly to drug discontinuation.

Pseudoephedrine: Pseudoephedrine may cause mild CNS stimulation, especially in patients who are hypersensitive to the effects of sympathomimetic drugs. Nervousness, excitability, restlessness, dizziness, weakness and insomnia may occur. Headache and drowsiness have also been reported. Large doses may cause lightheadedness, nausea and/or vomiting. In addition, the possibility of other adverse effects associated with sympathomimetic drugs, including fear, anxiety, tenseness, tremor, hallucinations, seizures, pallor, respiratory difficulty, dysuria and cardiovascular collapse should be considered.

Although oral administration of usual doses of pseudoephedrine to normotensive patients usually produced negligible pressor effects, the drug should be used with caution in hypertensive patients. Pseudoephedrine may increase the irritability of the heart muscle and may alter the rhythmic function of the ventricles, especially in large doses or when administered to patients who are hypersensitive to the myocardial effects of sympathomimetic drugs. Tachycardia or palpitation may occur.

Other Ibuprofen Adverse Events: Health professionals should keep in mind other potential adverse events associated with ibuprofen use including: Crohn's disease, colitis, gastritis, hematemesis, mouth ulceration, abdominal distension, dyspepsia, abdominal pain upper, hypersensitivity, cerebrovascular accident, angioneurotic edema, dermatitis bullous, face edema, pupura, cardiac failure, myocardial infarction, angina pectoris, vertigo, visual disturbance, agranulocytosis, anemia, aplastic anemia, hematuria, interstitial nephritis, renal failure, nephrotic syndrome, proteinuria, and renal papillary necrosis, liver disorder, asthma, bronchospasm, dyspnea, wheezing, meningitis aseptic, meningitis, edema, swelling, and peripheral edema.

OVERDOSE:

Treatment: Due to the rapid absorption of pseudoephedrine and ibuprofen from the gut, emetics and gastric lavage must be instituted within 4 hours of overdosage to be effective. Charcoal is useful only if given within 1 hour. Cardiac status should be monitored and the serum electrolytes measured. If there are signs of cardiac toxicity, propranolol may be administered i.v. A slow infusion of a dilute solution of potassium chloride should be initiated in the event of a drop in the serum potassium levels. Despite hypokalemia, the patient is unlikely to be potassium-depleted; therefore, overload must be avoided. Monitoring of the serum potassium is advisable for several hours after administration of the salt. For delirium or convulsions, i.v. administration of diazepam is indicated.

The toxicity of ibuprofen overdose is dependent upon the amount of drug ingested and the time elapsed since ingestion; individual responses may vary, thus making it necessary to evaluate each case separately. Although uncommon, serious toxicity and death have been reported with ibuprofen overdosage. The most frequently reported symptoms of ibuprofen overdose include abdominal pain, nausea, vomiting, lethargy, vertigo, drowsiness (somnolence), dizziness and insomnia. Other CNS symptoms include headache, loss of consciousness, tinnitus, CNS depression, convulsions and seizures. Metabolic acidosis, abnormal hepatic function, hyperkalemia, renal failure, dyspnea, respiratory depression, coma, acute renal failure, and apnea (primarily in very young pediatric patients) may rarely occur. Cardiovascular toxicity, including hypotension, bradycardia, tachycardia and atrial fibrillation, also have been reported.

> For management of a suspected drug overdose, CPhA recommends that you contact your **regional Poison Control Centre**. See the *CPS* Directory section for a list of Poison Control Centres.

DOSAGE: **Advil Cold & Sinus:** Adults and children over 12 years: Take 1 or 2 caplets or liqui-gels every 4 hours as needed. Do not exceed 6 caplets or liqui-gels in 24 hours, unless directed by a physician.

Do not give to children under 12 years of age.

Advil Cold & Sinus Daytime: Take 1 or 2 caplets every 4 hours as needed. Do not exceed 6 caplets in 24 hours, unless directed by a physician. Do not give to children under 12 years of age.

Children's Advil Cold Suspension: Administer every 6 hours. Do not exceed 4 doses in 24 hours, unless directed by a physician. Children 6 to 12 years/21.4-43 kg: 10 mL/dose (2 tsp); Children under 6 years: **Do not use.**

Do not use longer than 5 days.

SUPPLIED: Advil Cold & Sinus: Caplets: Each caplet contains: ibuprofen 200 mg and pseudoephedrine HCl 30 mg. Nonmedicinal ingredients: acetylated monoglyceride, carnauba wax, cellulose, cornstarch, croscarmellose sodium, ethoxyethanol, iron oxides, lecithin, parabens, pharmaceutical glaze, pharmaceutical shellac, povidone, pregelatinized starch, silicon dioxide, simethicone, sodium benzoate, sodium lauryl sulfate, stearic acid, sucrose and titanium dioxide. Blister packages of 10 and 20. Bottles of 40 and 72. Store at room temperature (15 to 30°C).

Liqui-Gels: Each liqui-gel contains: ibuprofen 200 mg and pseudoephedrine HCl 30 mg. Nonmedicinal ingredients: D&C Yellow no. 10, FD&C Red no. 40, fractionated coconut oil, gelatin, iron oxide, polyethylene glycol, polyvinyl acetate phthalate, potassium hydroxide, propylene glycol, purified water, sorbitan and sorbitol. Blister packages of 10 and 20. Bottles of 40. Store at room temperature (15 to 30°C).

Advil Cold & Sinus Daytime: Each caplet contains: ibuprofen 200 mg and pseudoephedrine HCl 30 mg. Nonmedicinal ingredients: acetylated monoglycerides, carnauba wax, cellulose, cornstarch, croscarmellose sodium, ethoxyethanol, iron oxides, lecithin, parabens, pharmaceutical glaze, pharmaceutical shellac, povidone, pregelatinized starch, silicon dioxide, simethicone, sodium benzoate, sodium lauryl sulfate, stearic acid, sucrose and titanium dioxide. Combination blister packages of 12 with 6 Advil Cold & Sinus Nighttime caplets and 24 with 12 Advil Cold & Sinus Nighttime caplets. Store at room temperature (15 to 30°C).

Children's Advil Cold GRAPE: Each 5 mL of grape-flavored, purple-colored liquid contains: ibuprofen 100 mg and pseudoephedrine HCl 15 mg. Nonmedicinal ingredients: carboxymethylcellulose sodium, citric acid, edetate disodium, FD&C Blue no. 1, FD&C Red no. 40, flavor, glycerin, microcrystalline cellulose, polysorbate 80, purified water, sodium benzoate, sorbitol solution, sucrose and xanthan gum. Bottles of 120 mL. Store at room temperature (15 to 30°C).

Advil® Cold and Sinus Plus

ibuprofen—pseudoephedrine HCl—chlorpheniramine maleate

Analgesic—Nasal Decongestant —Antihistamine

Pfizer Consumer Healthcare

Advil® Cold and Sinus Nighttime

ibuprofen—pseudoephedrine HCl—chlorpheniramine maleate

Analgesic—Nasal Decongestant—Antihistamine

Pfizer Consumer Healthcare

PHARMACOLOGY:

Pharmacokinetics: In a 4-way bioavailability study of ibuprofen, pseudoephedrine and chlorpheniramine and a two-caplet combination product of the 3 drugs, the rate and extent of absorption of the three drugs were **not different** (i.e., there was no pharmacokinetic interaction when the 3 drugs were combined).

In another bioavailability study of the 3 drug combination under fed and fasted conditions, the absorption of ibuprofen, pseudoephedrine and chlorpheniramine was not significantly affected by the administration of food.

In a randomized study, one caplet of the ibuprofen, pseudoephedrine and chlorpheniramine combination significantly relieved allergy-associated pain and other symptoms of seasonal allergic rhinitis more than the pseudoephedrine and chlorpheniramine combination alone.

Ibuprofen: Ibuprofen is an effective analgesic and antipyretic drug at non-prescription levels of 200 mg to 400 mg.

Pseudoephedrine: Pseudoephedrine is an orally effective nasal decongestant when administered in doses of 60 mg/dose, up to 240 mg/day. In order to comply with the flexible dosing schedule approved for nonprescription ibuprofen, clinical studies were conducted to demonstrate the efficacy of 30 mg pseudoephedrine when administered in the combination product and evidence of dose response between the 30 mg and 60 mg doses.

Chlorpheniramine: Chlorpheniramine is an orally effective antihistamine (H_1-receptor antagonist) when administered in doses of 2 to 4 mg/dose, up to 24 mg/day. Chlorpheniramine has antihistaminic and anticholinergic properties.

INDICATIONS: For temporary relief of the combined symptoms associated with allergies and sinusitis including runny nose, fever, sneezing, headache, itchy, watery eyes, nasal congestion, minor aches and pains, itching of the throat, sinus pain and pressure.

Consult a physician if pain or fever worsens or persists for more than 5 days.

CONTRAINDICATIONS: Patients who have previously exhibited hypersensitivity to this product, or to its components (ibuprofen, pseudoephedrine, chlorpheniramine), or individuals with angioedema syndrome, nasal polyps or bronchospastic reactivity to ASA or other nonsteroidal anti-inflammatory agents (see Warnings).

Patients with hypertension, coronary artery disease, and patients on monoamine oxidase (MAO) inhibitor therapy (see Precautions, Drug Interactions).

Serious GI toxicity, such as peptic ulceration, perforation and gastrointestinal bleeding, **sometimes severe and occasionally fatal**, can occur at any time, with or without symptoms in patients treated with NSAIDs including ibuprofen.

Pregnancy: Do not use in the third trimester of pregnancy, because of risk of premature closure of the ductus arteriosus and prolonged parturition.

Advil Cold & Sinus Plus and Advil Cold & Sinus Nighttime should not be used during pregnancy, in nursing mothers or in pediatric patients because its safety under these conditions has not been established.

Lactation: See Pregnancy.

Children: See Pregnancy.

Aseptic meningitis, fever and rash have been reported in connection with ibuprofen therapy in patients with systemic lupus erythematosus. Advil Cold & Sinus Plus and Advil Cold & Sinus Nighttime should not be used by patients with systemic lupus erythematosus except under a physician's supervision.

Advil Cold & Sinus Plus and Advil Cold & Sinus Nighttime should not be taken by patients with active peptic ulcer disease or gastrointestinal bleeding unless directed by a physician.

WARNINGS: Anaphylactoid reactions have occurred in patients with known ASA hypersensitivity (see Contraindications).

Peptic ulcerations, perforations and gastrointestinal bleeding, sometimes severe, have been reported in patients receiving prescription doses of ibuprofen. Peptic ulcerations, perforation or severe gastrointestinal bleeding can have a fatal outcome, and although few such reports have been received with ibuprofen, a cause and effect relationship has not been established. Patients with a history of upper gastrointestinal tract disease should take Advil Cold & Sinus Plus and Advil Cold & Sinus Nighttime under the supervision of a physician.

Like other nonsteroidal anti-inflammatory agents, ibuprofen can inhibit platelet aggregation. However, compared to ASA, the effect is quantitatively less, of shorter duration, and reversible upon discontinuation of ibuprofen. Bleeding time has also been prolonged by ibuprofen though within the normal range in normal subjects. Because this effect on bleeding time may be exaggerated in patients with underlying hemostatic defects, Advil Cold & Sinus Plus and Advil Cold & Sinus Nighttime should be avoided by persons with intrinsic coagulation defects and those on anticoagulant therapy.

Patients with high blood pressure, heart disease, diabetes, narrow-angle glaucoma, thyroid disease, kidney or liver disease or difficulty in urination due to enlargement of the prostate gland should take Advil Cold & Sinus Plus and Advil Cold & Sinus Nighttime only under the advice and supervision of a physician. Advil Cold & Sinus Plus and Advil Cold & Sinus Nighttime may cause drowsiness. Alcohol may increase this effect. Alcoholic beverages, driving a motor vehicle or operating machinery should be avoided while taking this drug. This drug should not be taken along with other antihistamines, sedatives or tranquilizers without first consulting a physician (see Precautions, Drug Interactions).

General: Patients with heart disease, high blood pressure, diabetes, thyroid disease, narrow angle glaucoma, or difficulty in urination due to enlargement of the prostate gland should not take this drug unless directed by a physician.

Side effects may be minimized by using the smallest dose for the shortest duration of time.

As with other anti-inflammatory drugs, ibuprofen may mask the usual signs of infection.

If nervousness, dizziness, or sleeplessness occurs, use of Advil should be discontinued and a physician should be consulted. If symptoms do not improve within 5 days or are accompanied by fever, a physician should be consulted.

Special Warnings: Skin: In rare cases, serious skin reactions such as Stevens-Johnson syndrome, toxic epidermal necrolysis, exfoliative dermatitis and erythema multiforme have been associated with the use of some NSAIDs. Because the rate of these reactions is low, they have usually been noted during post-marketing surveillance in patients taking other medications also associated with the potential development of these serious skin reactions. Thus, causality is **not** clear. These reactions are potentially life threatening but may be reversible if the causative agent is discontinued and appropriate treatment instituted. Patients should be advised that if they experience a skin rash, reddening or blisters they should discontinue their NSAID and contact their physician for assessment and advice, including which additional therapies to discontinue.

Other: Stop use and check with your physician if you vomit blood, have bloody or black stools, or experience any weakness.

Use with caution in the elderly.

PRECAUTIONS: Conditions associated with dehydration appear to increase the risk of renal toxicity. Advil Cold & Sinus Plus and Advil Cold & Sinus Nighttime should therefore be used with caution in patients with chronic renal failure, congestive heart failure or hypertension being treated chronically with diuretics. Caution should be observed in elderly patients, due to increased susceptibility to effects of sympathomimetic amines and increased risk of toxicity with ibuprofen, and patients with diminished renal function.

Patients on Advil Cold & Sinus Plus or Advil Cold & Sinus Nighttime should be cautioned to report to their physician any signs or symptoms of gastrointestinal ulceration, perforation, or bleeding, blurred vision or other eye symptoms, skin rash, weight gain, edema, tinnitus, dizziness or respiratory difficulties. Intraocular pressure may increase slightly in patients who have open-angle glaucoma.

If Advil Cold & Sinus Plus or Advil Cold & Sinus Nighttime is taken in conjunction with prolonged corticosteroid therapy and it is decided to discontinue the latter therapy, as under other circumstances, the corticosteroid dosage should be tapered slowly to avoid exacerbation of disease or adrenal insufficiency.

If the symptoms do not improve within 5 days or are accompanied by a high fever, the patient should be advised to report to the physician.

Drug Interactions: Acetylsalicylic acid (ASA) or Other NSAIDs: Not recommended due to the possibility of additive side effects.

Acetaminophen: Although interactions have not been reported, concurrent use with ibuprofen is not advisable; it may increase the risk of adverse renal effect.

Digoxin: Ibuprofen has been shown to increase serum digoxin concentration. Increased monitoring and dosage adjustments of digitalis glycoside may be necessary during and following concurrent ibuprofen therapy.

Coumarin-type Anticoagulants: Because prostaglandins play an important role in hemostasis, and NSAIDs affect platelet function, concurrent therapy of ibuprofen with warfarin requires close monitoring to be certain that no change in dosage is necessary.

Hypoglycemic Agents: Ibuprofen may increase hypoglycemic effects of oral antidiabetic agents and insulin.

Antihypertensives: Prostaglandins are an important factor in cardiovascular homeostasis and inhibition of their synthesis by NSAIDs may interfere with circulatory control. NSAIDs may elevate blood pressure in patients receiving antihypertensive medication. Blood pressure monitoring is not necessary during short-term ibuprofen use but is recommended during long-term use.

Diuretics: Clinical studies, as well as random observations, have shown that ibuprofen can reduce the natriuretic effect of furosemide and thiazides in some patients. This response has been attributed to inhibition of renal prostaglandin synthesis. During concomitant therapy with ibuprofen, the patient should be observed closely for signs of renal failure as well as to assure diuretic efficacy.

Antacids: A bioavailability study has shown that there was no interference with the absorption of ibuprofen when given in conjunction with an antacid containing aluminium hydroxide and titanium hydroxide.

H_2 Antagonists: In studies with human volunteers, coadministration of cimetidine or ranitidine with ibuprofen had no substantive effect on ibuprofen serum concentrations.

Methotrexate: Ibuprofen as well as other NSAIDs has been reported to competitively inhibit methotrexate accumulation in rabbit kidney slices. This may indicate that ibuprofen could enhance the toxicity of methotrexate. Caution should be used when ibuprofen is administered concomitantly with methotrexate.

Lithium: Ibuprofen produced an elevation of plasma lithium levels and a reduction in renal lithium clearance in a study of eleven normal volunteers. The mean lithium concentration increased by 15% and the renal clearance of lithium increased by 19% during this period of concomitant drug administration. This effect has been attributed to inhibition of renal prostaglandin synthesis by ibuprofen. When ibuprofen and lithium are administered concurrently, subjects should be observed carefully for signs of lithium toxicity.

Monoamine Oxidase Inhibitors: Advil Cold & Sinus Plus and Advil Cold & Sinus Nighttime should not be used concomitantly with MAO inhibitors. Hypertensive crisis and other serious adverse reactions have been reported in patients using pseudoephedrine or other sympathomimetic drugs in combination with or shortly after discontinuing MAO inhibitors.

Alcohol and Other CNS Depressant Drugs: Because of the possibility of additive CNS depressant effects, patients should avoid alcoholic beverages when taking Advil Cold & Sinus Plus or Advil Cold & Sinus Nighttime. Caution is necessary if Advil Cold & Sinus Plus or Advil Cold & Sinus Nighttime is used by patients who are taking sedatives or tranquilizers.

Phenytoin: Concomitant use of chlorpheniramine may delay the hepatic metabolism of phenytoin, potentially resulting in phenytoin toxicity.

Other Drugs: Although ibuprofen binds extensively to plasma proteins, interactions with other protein-bound drugs occur rarely. Caution should be observed when other drugs, with a high affinity for protein binding sites, are used concurrently. No interactions have been reported when ibuprofen has been used in conjunction with probenecid, thyroxine, steroids, antibiotics or benzodiazepines.

ADVERSE EFFECTS: Ibuprofen: The following adverse reactions have been noted in patients treated with prescription regimens of ibuprofen.

Gastrointestinal: The adverse reactions most frequently seen with prescribed ibuprofen therapy (above 1200 mg daily) involve the gastrointestinal system: nausea, epigastric pain, heartburn, diarrhea, abdominal distress, vomiting, indigestion, constipation, abdominal cramps, fullness of the gastrointestinal tract (bloating or flatulence).

CNS: dizziness, headache, nervousness.

Dermatologic: rash (including maculopapular type), pruritus.

Special Senses: tinnitus.

Metabolic: decreased appetite, edema, fluid retention. Fluid retention generally responds promptly to drug discontinuation.

Pseudoephedrine: Pseudoephedrine may cause mild CNS stimulation, especially in patients who are hypersensitive to the affects of sympathomimetic drugs. Nervousness, excitability, restlessness, dizziness, weakness and insomnia may occur. Headache and drowsiness have been reported. Large doses may cause lightheadedness, nausea and/or vomiting. In addition, the possibility of other adverse effects associated with sympathomimetic drugs, including fear, anxiety, tremor, hallucinations, seizures, pallor, respiratory difficulty, dysuria and cardiovascular collapse should be considered.

Although oral administration of usual doses of pseudoephedrine to normotensive patients usually produced negligible pressor effects, the drug should be used with caution in hypertensive patients. Pseudoephedrine may increase the irritability of the heart muscle and may alter the rhythmic function of the ventricles, especially in large doses or when administered to patients who are hypersensitive to the myocardial effects of sympathomimetic drugs. Tachycardia or palpitation may occur.

Chlorpheniramine: The most frequent side effect of first-generation H_1-receptor antagonists such as chlorpheniramine is sedation. Other adverse CNS effects include dizziness, tinnitus, lassitude, lack of coordination, fatigue, blurred vision, diplopia, euphoria, nervousness, insomnia, and tremors. Concurrent use of alcohol or other CNS depressants produces an additive effect that impairs motor skills.

Antihistamines frequently cause side effects involving the digestive tract, including loss of appetite, nausea, vomiting, epigastric distress, and constipation or diarrhoea. The incidence of gastrointestinal side effects may be reduced by taking the drug with meals.

Chlorpheniramine may also produce anticholinergic effects including dryness of the mouth and respiratory passages, urinary retention or frequency, and dysuria.

Other Ibuprofen Adverse Events: Health professionals should keep in mind other potential adverse events associated with ibuprofen use including: Crohn's disease, colitis, gastritis, hematemesis, mouth ulceration, abdominal distension, dyspepsia, abdominal pain upper, hypersensitivity, cerebrovascular accident, angioneurotic edema, dermatitis bullous, face edema, pupura, cardiac failure, myocardial infarction, angina pectoris, vertigo, visual disturbance, agranulocytosis, anemia, aplastic anemia, hematuria, interstitial nephritis, renal failure, nephrotic syndrome, proteinuria, and renal papillary necrosis, liver disorder, asthma, bronchospasm, dyspnea, wheezing, meningitis aseptic, meningitis, edema, swelling, and peripheral edema.

OVERDOSE:

Treatment: In case of accidental overdose, call a poison control centre, hospital, or doctor at once even if there are no symptoms.

Symptoms: The toxicity of ibuprofen overdose is dependent upon the amount of drug ingested and the time elapsed since ingestion; individual responses may vary, thus making it necessary to evaluate each case separately. Although uncommon, serious toxicity and death have been reported with ibuprofen overdosage. The most frequently reported symptoms of ibuprofen overdose include abdominal pain, nausea, vomiting, lethargy, vertigo, drowsiness (somnolence), dizziness and insomnia. Other CNS symptoms include headache, loss of consciousness, tinnitus, CNS depression, convulsions and seizures. Metabolic acidosis, abnormal hepatic function, hyperkalemia, renal failure, dyspnea, respiratory depression, coma, acute renal failure, and apnea (primarily in very young pediatric patients) may rarely occur. Cardiovascular toxicity, including hypotension, bradycardia, tachycardia and atrial fibrillation, also have been reported.

> For management of a suspected drug overdose, CPhA recommends that you contact your **regional Poison Control Centre**. See the *CPS* Directory section for a list of Poison Control Centres.

DOSAGE: Advil Cold & Sinus Plus and Advil Cold & Sinus Nighttime: Adults and children over 12: Take 1 or 2 caplets every 4 hours as needed. Do not exceed 6 caplets in 24 hours, unless directed by a physician. Do not give to children under 12.

SUPPLIED: Advil Cold & Sinus Plus: Each bright orange caplet, printed "Advil A/S" in black ink on one side contains: ibuprofen 200 mg, pseudoephedrine HCl 30 mg and chlorpheniramine maleate 2 mg. Nonmedicinal ingredients: carnauba wax, cornstarch, croscarmellose sodium, FD&C Red no. 40 aluminum lake, FD&C Yellow no. 6 aluminum lake, glyceryl behenate, hypromellose, iron oxide, microcrystalline cellulose, polydextrose, polyethylene glycol, propylene glycol, silicon dioxide and titanium dioxide. Blister packages of 10, 20 and 40. Bottles of 72. Pouches of 2. Store at room temperature (15-30°C).

Advil Cold & Sinus Nighttime: Each bright orange caplet, printed "Advil A/S" in black ink on one side contains: ibuprofen 200 mg, pseudoephedrine HCl 30 mg and chlorpheniramine maleate 2 mg. Nonmedicinal ingredients: carnauba wax, cornstarch, croscarmellose sodium, FD&C Red no. 40 aluminum lake, FD&C Yellow no. 6 aluminum lake, glyceryl behenate, hypromellose, iron oxide, microcrystalline cellulose, polydextrose, polyethylene glycol, propylene glycol, silicon dioxide and titanium dioxide. Combination blister packages of 6 with 12 Advil Cold & Sinus Daytime caplets and 12 with 24 Advil Cold & Sinus Daytime caplets. Store at room temperature (15-30°C).

Aerius®
desloratadine
Histamine H1-Receptor Antagonist

Schering-Plough

Aerius Kids®
desloratadine
Histamine H1-Receptor Antagonist

Schering-Plough

Date of Preparation: May 29, 2001
Date of Revision: October 22, 2007

SUMMARY PRODUCT INFORMATION:

Route of Administration	Dosage Form/ Strength	Clinically Relevant Nonmedicinal Ingredients
Oral	Tablet/5 mg Syrup/0.5 mg/mL	For a complete listing see Dosage Forms, Composition and Packaging.

INDICATIONS AND CLINICAL USE: AERIUS (desloratadine) tablets are indicated for:

- the fast relief of nasal and non-nasal symptoms associated with allergic rhinitis, including sneezing, nasal discharge and itching, congestion/stuffiness, itching of the palate, and coughing associated with these symptoms, as well as itching, tearing and redness of the eyes.
- the rapid relief of symptoms associated with chronic idiopathic urticaria, such as pruritus and hives.

AERIUS KIDS (desloratadine) syrup is indicated for:

- the fast relief of nasal and non-nasal symptoms associated with seasonal allergic rhinitis, including sneezing, nasal discharge and itching, congestion/stuffiness, itching of the palate, and coughing associated with these symptoms, as well as itching, tearing and redness of the eyes.
- the rapid relief of symptoms associated with chronic idiopathic urticaria, such as pruritus and hives.

CONTRAINDICATIONS:

- **Patients who are hypersensitive to this drug or to any ingredient in the formulation or component of the container. For a complete listing, see Dosage Forms, Composition and Packaging.**

WARNINGS AND PRECAUTIONS:

> **Serious Warnings and Precautions**
> In the case of severe hepatic or renal insufficiency, use with caution.

Hepatic/Biliary/Pancreatic: In a single-dose (7.5 mg) pharmacokinetic study, subjects with mild to severe hepatic dysfunction (n=4/group) had mean AUC and Cmax values up to 2.4 times higher than healthy subjects (n=8); however, these findings are not considered to be clinically relevant.

Desloratadine 5 mg was administered for 10 days to subjects with normal hepatic function (n=9) or moderate dysfunction (n=11). Subjects with hepatic dysfunction could experience a 3-fold increase in exposure (AUC) to desloratadine, but these findings are not considered to be clinically relevant.

Therefore no dosage modification is recommended in individuals with hepatic dysfunction.

Renal: In a single-dose (7.5 mg) pharmacokinetic study, subjects (n=25) with varying degrees of renal insufficiency (mild, moderate, severe and hemodialysis) had 1.7 to 2.5 fold increases in desloratadine mean AUC with minimal change in 3-hydroxy desloratadine concentrations. However, these findings are not considered to be clinically relevant.

In the case of severe renal insufficiency, AERIUS should be used with caution.

Respiratory: Use in Asthmatics: AERIUS has been safely administered to patients with mild to moderate asthma.

AERIUS did not cause exacerbation of asthma symptoms.

Special Populations: Pregnant Women: Since no clinical data on exposed pregnancies are available with desloratadine, the safe use of AERIUS during pregnancy has not been established. The use of AERIUS during pregnancy is therefore not recommended.

No overall effect on rat fertility was observed with desloratadine at an exposure that was 34 times higher than the exposure in humans at the recommended clinical dose. No teratogenic or mutagenic effects were observed in animal trials with desloratadine.

Nursing Women: Desloratadine passes into breast milk; therefore, breast-feeding is not recommended in lactating women taking AERIUS.

Pediatrics: (Tablets <12 years of age) and (Syrup <2 years of age): The efficacy and safety of AERIUS Tablets in children under 12 years of age and of AERIUS Syrup in children under 2 years of age have not been established.

Geriatrics (>65 years of age): In a multiple dose study with AERIUS 5 mg, subjects >65 years of age (n=17) had AUC and Cmax values 20% greater and plasma elimination half-life approximately 30% longer than in younger subjects; however, these changes are not considered to be clinically relevant and no dosage adjustment is warranted in this age subgroup.

ADVERSE REACTIONS: Adverse Drug Reaction Overview: No clinically relevant drug-related adverse effects including cardiovascular effects were observed with AERIUS in clinical trials.

Very rare cases of hypersensitivity reactions including anaphylaxis and rash have been reported during the marketing of desloratadine. In addition, cases of tachycardia, palpitations, psychomotor hyperactivity, seizures, elevations of liver enzymes, hepatitis, and increased bilirubin have been reported very rarely.

Clinical Trial Adverse Drug Reactions: Because clinical trials are conducted under very specific conditions the adverse reaction rates observed in the clinical trials may not reflect the rates observed in practice and should not be compared to the rates in the clinical trials of another drug. Adverse drug reaction information from clinical trials is useful for identifying drug-related adverse events and for approximating rates.

The frequency of reasonably related undesirable effects is presented as the excess incidence in 1866 patients who received AERIUS (desloratadine) 5 mg tablets compared to that seen in 1857 patients who received placebo in multiple-dose clinical trials evaluating the treatment of seasonal and allergic rhinitis and chronic idiopathic urticaria. The type and frequency of undesirable effects reported throughout the AERIUS allergic rhinitis and CIU clinical trials were comparable to those reported with placebo.

At the recommended dose of 5 mg daily, undesirable effects with AERIUS were reported in only 3% of patients in excess of those treated with placebo. No excess incidence of somnolence was reported in patients treated with AERIUS. Headache was reported in only 0.6% of patients in excess of those treated with placebo. The incidence of treatment-related adverse events reported by ≥1% of subjects treated with AERIUS 5 mg in multiple-dose clinical trials is presented in Table 1.

Table 1: AERIUS

Incidence of Treatment-related Adverse Events Reported by ≥2% of Subjects Treated with AERIUS 5 mg in Multiple-dose Seasonal Allergic Rhinitis and Chronic Idiopathic Urticaria Studies

	Number[a] (%) of Subjects	
	Desloratadine 5 mg (n=1866)	**Placebo (n=1857)**
No. of Subjects (%) with Any Related Adverse Event[b]	281 (15.1)	232 (12.5)
Autonomic Nervous System Disorders	**51 (2.7)**	**36 (1.9)**
Dry Mouth	49 (2.6)	34 (1.8)
Fatigue	33 (1.8)	12(0.6)
Body as a Whole—General Disorders	**124 (6.6)**	**88 (4.7)**
Headache	84 (4.5)	72 (3.9)
Psychiatric Disorders	**53 (2.8)**	**48 (2.6)**
Somnolence	36 (1.9)	35(1.9)

a Number of subjects reporting related adverse events at least once during the study. Some subjects may have reported more than 1 adverse event.

b Considered by the investigator to be possibly or probably related to treatment.

In pediatric clinical trials, 115 patients received desloratadine syrup and 116 received placebo. Possibly related undesirable effects were reported in only 1.7% (n=2) of subjects treated with desloratadine syrup. Both of these events (1 each of rash and headache) occurred among the 2-5 year old subjects (desloratadine 1.25 mg treatment group). There were no reports of reasonably related undesirable effects among the 6-11 year old subjects in either treatment group. A total of 11 treatment emergent adverse events (fever, headache, viral infection, Varicella, rash, and urinary tract infection) were reported in 8 subjects (0.8%) treated with 1.25 or 2.5 mg of desloratadine. Overall, there were no reports of somnolence, fatigue, paradoxical excitability, parakinesia, insomnia, or hyperkinesia.

Post-Market Adverse Drug Reactions: Very rare cases of hypersensitivity reactions, including anaphylaxis and rash have been reported during the marketing of desloratadine. In addition, cases of tachycardia, palpitations, psychomotor hyperactivity, seizures, elevations of liver enzymes, hepatitis, and increased bilirubin have been reported very rarely.

DRUG INTERACTIONS: Overview: AERIUS taken concomitantly with alcohol did not potentiate the performance impairing effects of alcohol.

Drug-Drug Interactions: No clinically relevant interactions with AERIUS were observed in clinical trials investigating the potential for interaction with azithromycin, erythromycin, ketoconazole, fluoxetine, and cimetidine.

Drug-Food Interactions: There was no effect of food or grapefruit juice on the disposition of desloratadine.

Drug-Herb Interactions: Interactions with herbal products have not been established.

Drug-Laboratory Interactions: Interactions with laboratory test have not been established.

Drug-Lifestyle Interactions: Effects on Ability To Drive and Use Machines: None.

DOSAGE AND ADMINISTRATION: Dosing Considerations: In the case of severe hepatic or renal insufficiency, AERIUS should be used with caution.

Recommended Dose and Dosage Adjustment: Tablets: Adults and Adolescents (12 years of age and older): One AERIUS (desloratadine) 5 mg tablet daily regardless of mealtime. For oral use.

Syrup: Adults and Adolescents (12 years of age and older): 10 mL (5 mg) AERIUS KIDS syrup once a day, regardless of mealtime.

Children 6 Through 11 years of Age: 5 mL (2.5 mg) AERIUS KIDS syrup once a day, regardless of mealtime.

Children 2 Through 5 years of Age: 2.5 mL (1.25 mg) AERIUS KIDS syrup once a day, regardless of mealtime.

Do not administer AERIUS KIDS to children between 2 to 12 years of age for longer than 14 days unless recommended by a physician.

OVERDOSAGE:

In the event of overdose, consider standard measures to remove unabsorbed active substance. Symptomatic and supportive treatment is recommended. AERIUS administered at a dose of 45 mg daily (nine times the clinical dose) for ten days showed no statistically or clinically relevant prolongation of the QTc interval. The mean changes in QTc were 0.3 msec and 4.3 msec for placebo and desloratadine, respectively (p=0.09; Lower confidence interval (LCI)=−0.6; Upper confidence interval (UCI)=8.7).

Desloratadine is not eliminated by hemodialysis; it is not known if it is eliminated by peritoneal dialysis.

For management of a suspected drug overdose, CPhA recommends that you contact your **regional Poison Control Centre**. See the *CPS* Directory section for a list of Poison Control Centres.

ACTION AND CLINICAL PHARMACOLOGY: Mechanism of Action: Desloratadine is a non-sedating long-acting antihistamine with selective peripheral H_1-receptor antagonist activity, which has demonstrated antiallergic, antihistaminic, and anti-inflammatory activity.

Desloratadine does not exacerbate asthma.

Pharmacodynamics: After oral administration, desloratadine selectively blocks peripheral histamine H_1-receptors as the drug is effectively excluded from entry into the central nervous system.

Wheal and Flare: Desloratadine 5 mg was significantly better than placebo, as measured by a reduction in histamine-induced wheal and flare areas for all days tested (1, 7, 14, 21, 28). There was no evidence of tachyphylaxis over the 28-day dosing period.

Psychomotor Pharmacodynamics: Clinical trials have demonstrated that there was no difference in the incidence of somnolence in subjects treated with AERIUS (desloratadine) 5 mg as compared to subjects treated with placebo.

No significant differences were found in the psychomotor test results between AERIUS and placebo groups, whether administered alone or with alcohol. Coadministration of alcohol with AERIUS did not increase the alcohol-induced impairment in performance or increase in sleepiness. No effects on the ability to drive and use machines have been observed. A single dose of AERIUS did not affect standard measures of flight performance including exacerbation of subjective sleepiness or tasks related to flying.

Cardiovascular Pharmacodynamics: In a multiple dose clinical trial, in which up to 20 mg of AERIUS was administered daily for 14 days to 49 healthy volunteers, no statistically or clinically relevant cardiovascular effects were observed. In another trial, AERIUS was administered at a dose of 45 mg daily (nine times the clinical dose) for ten days; no prolongation of the QTc interval was seen (see Overdosage).

The potential for desloratadine to interact with ketoconazole (N=24), erythromycin (N=24), azithromycin (N=90), fluoxetine (N=54), and cimetidine (N=36) was investigated in separate interaction studies. Ketoconazole coadministered with desloratadine increased Cmax and AUC values for desloratadine by 29% and 21% respectively, and 3-hydroxy desloratadine Cmax and AUC values by 77% and 110%, respectively. Erythromycin coadministered with desloratadine increased the Cmax and AUC values for desloratadine by 24% and 14%, respectively. The increases were 43% and 40%, respectively, for 3-hydroxy desloratadine. Azithromycin coadministered with desloratadine increased the Cmax and AUC values for desloratadine by 15% and 5%, respectively. The increases were 15% and 4%, respectively, for 3-hydroxy desloratadine. Fluoxetine coadministered with desloratadine resulted in no change in the AUC of desloratadine and an increase of 15% in the Cmax of desloratadine. The Cmax and AUC values for 3-hydroxy desloratadine were increased by 17% and 13% respectively. Cimetidine coadministered with desloratadine increased Cmax and AUC values by 12% and 19% respectively while the Cmax and AUC of 3-hydroxy desloratadine were reduced by 11.2% and 2.8% respectively. However, as there was no evidence of change in the safety profile of desloratadine throughout these studies, the increases in plasma concentrations are not considered to be clinically relevant. In addition, no clinically relevant changes in electrocardiographic pharmacodynamics (QTc) were observed.

Pharmacokinetics: Absorption: Desloratadine plasma concentrations can be detected within 30 minutes of desloratadine administration. Desloratadine is well absorbed with maximum concentrations achieved after approximately 3 hours; the mean elimination half-life is approximately 27 hours.

The bioavailability of desloratadine is dose proportional over the range of 5 mg to 20 mg. Equivalent exposure (AUC) to desloratadine, 3-hydroxy desloratadine, and 3-hydroxy desloratadine glucuronide was achieved after desloratadine 5 mg and loratadine 10 mg.

In a single dose crossover study of desloratadine, the tablet and syrup formulations were found to be bioequivalent.

In separate single dose studies, at the recommended doses, pediatric patients had comparable AUC and Cmax values of desloratadine to those in adults who received a 5 mg dose of desloratadine syrup or tablets.

Distribution: No information available.

Metabolism: Desloratadine is extensively metabolized. The results of metabolic profiling indicated that hydroxylation of desloratadine to 3-hydroxy desloratadine (3-OH desloratadine) followed by its subsequent glucuronidation was the major pathway of metabolism of desloratadine. The enzyme responsible for the metabolism of desloratadine has not been identified yet, and therefore some interactions with other drugs cannot be fully excluded. In-vivo studies with specific inhibitors of CYP3A4 and CYP2D6 have shown that these enzymes are not important in the metabolism of desloratadine. Desloratadine does not inhibit CYP3A4 and CYP2D6 and is neither a substrate nor an inhibitor of p-glycoprotein.

Data from clinical pharmacology studies indicate that a subset of the general adult and pediatric patient population has a decreased ability to form 3-hydroxydesloratadine. Ninety pediatric and 440 adult subjects were phenotyped for the polymorphism in clinical pharmacology studies. The incidence of the trait was approximately 8.6% in adults and 15.6% in pediatric subjects. In both pediatric and adult studies the slow metabolizer trait is more frequent in subjects of African descent than Caucasians. The desloratadine exposure (AUC) associated with the slow metabolizer phenotype has been well characterized (~4 times that of normal metabolizers) in single dose studies and is similar in pediatric and adult subjects at various doses. Median (range) AUC in pediatric normal and slow metabolizers was 31.9 (14-74) ng·h/mL and 116 (72-210) ng·hr/mL, respectively. The corresponding values for adult normal and slow metabolizers were 33.5 (8.7-99) ng·h/mL and 139 (82-393) ng·h/mL, respectively. In adults characterized as slow metabolizers, desloratadine exposure (AUC) after multiple doses has been demonstrated to be about six fold higher than that of normal metabolizers. The desloratadine exposure after multiple doses has not been documented for children. The safety profile of adult and pediatric slow metabolizers of desloratadine was not different from that of the general population.

Desloratadine is moderately bound (83% to 87%) to plasma proteins.

Following administration of desloratadine 5 mg for 28 days, the approximate two-fold degree of accumulation of desloratadine and 3-OH desloratadine is consistent with the half-life of DL and its active metabolite and a once daily dosing frequency. This accumulation is not clinically meaningful. The pharmacokinetics of desloratadine and 3-OH desloratadine do not change after daily dosing for 7 consecutive days.

There is no evidence of clinically relevant drug accumulation following once daily dosing of AERIUS (5 mg to 20 mg) for 14 days.

Results from a single dose trial of 7.5 mg AERIUS demonstrate that there was no effect of food (high-fat, high caloric breakfast) on the disposition of desloratadine. In another study, grapefruit juice had no effect on the disposition of desloratadine.

Excretion: A human mass balance study documented a recovery of approximately 87% of the ^{14}C-desloratadine dose, which was equally distributed in urine and feces as metabolic products.

STORAGE AND STABILITY: Temperature and Moisture: Tablets: Store between 15 and 30°C. Protect from excessive moisture.

Syrup: Store between 15 and 30°C.

Others: Keep in a safe place out of the reach of children.

SPECIAL HANDLING INSTRUCTIONS: None.

INFORMATION FOR THE PATIENT: Published in e-CPS, available by subscription at www.e-cps.ca.

DOSAGE FORMS, COMPOSITION AND PACKAGING: Syrup: Each mL of clear, orange colored liquid with bubblegum flavoring, contains: desloratadine 0.5 mg. Nonmedicinal ingredients: bubblegum flavor, citric acid anhydrous, disodium edetate, FD&C yellow No. 6, propylene glycol, purified water, sodium benzoate, sodium citrate dihydrate, sorbitol solution and sucrose. Amber glass bottles of 100 mL.

Tablets: Each blue, round, film-coated tablet for immediate release contains: desloratadine 5 mg. Nonmedicinal ingredients: carnauba wax, cornstarch, dibasic calcium phosphate dihydrate, FD&C Blue No. 2 lake, hydroxypropyl methylcellulose, lactose monohydrate, microcrystalline cellulose, polyethylene glycol, talc, titanium dioxide and white beeswax. PVC/aluminum blisters in boxes of 2 (professional sample), 10, 20, 30 and 50. HDPE bottles of 100.

(Shown in Product Identification Section)

Aerius® Dual Action 12 Hour™

desloratadine—pseudoephedrine sulfate

Histamine H1-Receptor Antagonist—Sympathomimetic Amine

Schering-Plough

Date of Preparation: June 3, 2009

SUMMARY PRODUCT INFORMATION:

Route of Administration	Dosage Form/ Strength	Clinically Relevant Nonmedicinal Ingredients
Oral	Extended release tablet[a]/ 2.5 mg desloratadine & 120 mg pseudoephedrine sulfate	For a complete listing see Dosage Forms, Composition and Packaging .

a Desloratadine is for immediate release and pseudoephedrine sulfate is for extended release, allowing for twice-daily oral administration.

INDICATIONS AND CLINICAL USE: AERIUS DUAL ACTION 12 HOUR (desloratadine/pseudoephedrine sulfate) is indicated for:

- The symptomatic treatment of seasonal allergic rhinitis including rhinorrhea, nasal itching and sneezing, itching/burning eyes, tearing/watering eyes, redness of the eyes, and itching of the ears or palate when accompanied by nasal congestion.

AERIUS DUAL ACTION 12 HOUR is not recommended for use in pregnant or lactating women.

AERIUS DUAL ACTION 12 HOUR is not recommended for use in patients with severe hepatic or renal impairment.

AERIUS DUAL ACTION 12 HOUR should be administered when the antihistaminic properties of desloratadine and the nasal decongestant activity of pseudoephedrine are desired.

Geriatrics (≥65 years of age): AERIUS DUAL ACTION 12 HOUR should be used with caution in patients 65 years of age and above.

Pediatrics (<12 years of age): AERIUS DUAL ACTION 12 HOUR is not recommended for use in children below the age of 12 years due to lack of data on safety and efficacy.

CONTRAINDICATIONS:

- Patients who are hypersensitive to this drug or to any ingredient in the formulation or component of the container. For a complete listing, see Dosage Forms, Composition and Packaging.
- Patients who are hypersensitive to adrenergic agents or to loratadine.
- Due to its pseudoephedrine content, it is also contraindicated in patients:
  - who are receiving irreversible monoamine oxidase (MAO) inhibitor therapy or during the 2 weeks following the stopping of such treatment (see Drug Interactions)
  - with narrow-angle glaucoma
  - with urinary retention
  - with cardiovascular diseases such as severe coronary artery disease, tachyarrhythmia and severe hypertension
  - with hyperthyroidism
  - with a history of haemorrhagic stroke or with risk factors which could increase the risk of haemorrhagic stroke.

WARNINGS AND PRECAUTIONS:

> **Serious Warnings and Precautions**
> AERIUS DUAL ACTION 12 HOUR is not recommended for use in patients with severe hepatic or renal impairment.

General: Do not exceed the recommended dosage and the duration of treatment.

Do not use concurrently with other over-the-counter antihistamines and decongestants.

Cardiovascular: Use with caution in patients with cardiovascular disease and hypertension. Treatment should be discontinued in case of hypertension, tachycardia, palpitations or cardiac arrhythmias.

Dependence/Tolerance: As with other CNS stimulants, pseudoephedrine sulfate carries the risk of abuse. Increased doses may ultimately produce toxicity. Continuous use can lead to tolerance and an increased risk of overdosing. Depression may follow rapid withdrawal.

Endocrine and Metabolism: Use with caution in patients with diabetes mellitus.

Gastrointestinal: Use with caution in patients with stenosing peptic ulcer and pyloroduodenal obstruction.

Genitourinary: Use with caution in patients with hypertrophy of the prostate or bladder neck obstruction.

Hepatic/Biliary/Pancreatic: The safety and efficacy of AERIUS DUAL ACTION 12 HOUR has not been established in patients with impaired hepatic function, and there are insufficient data to give adequate dose recommendations. The combination product is not recommended for use in patients with impaired hepatic function.

In a desloratadine single-dose (7.5 mg) pharmacokinetic study, subjects with mild to severe hepatic dysfunction had mean AUC and C_{max} values up to 2.4 times higher than healthy subjects. Desloratadine 5 mg was administered for 10 days to subjects with normal hepatic function or moderate dysfunction. Subjects with hepatic dysfunction could experience a 3-fold increase in exposure (AUC) to desloratadine. These findings are not considered to be clinically relevant.

Neurologic: Treatment should be discontinued in case of nausea or any other neurologic sign (such as headache or increased headache).

Ophthalmologic: Use with caution in patients with glaucoma and increased intraocular pressure.

Peri-Operative Considerations: If surgery is scheduled, discontinue treatment 24 hours before anaesthesia.

Renal: The safety and efficacy of AERIUS DUAL ACTION 12 HOUR has not been established in patients with impaired renal function, and there are insufficient data to give adequate dose recommendations. The combination product is not recommended for use in patients with impaired renal function.

In a desloratadine single-dose (7.5 mg) pharmacokinetic study, subjects (n=25) with varying degrees of renal insufficiency (mild, moderate, severe and hemodialysis) had 1.2 to 2.5 fold increases in desloratadine median AUC with minimal change in 3-hydroxy desloratadine concentrations. However, these findings are not considered to be clinically relevant.

Special Populations: Pregnant Women: The safe use of AERIUS DUAL ACTION 12 HOUR during pregnancy has not been established. The use of pseudoephedrine decreases maternal blood flow. The use of AERIUS DUAL ACTION 12 HOUR is not recommended for pregnant women.

Nursing Women: Desloratadine and pseudoephedrine are both excreted in breast milk, therefore the use of AERIUS DUAL ACTION 12 HOUR is not recommended for women who are breast-feeding.

Pediatrics* (<12 years of age): AERIUS DUAL ACTION 12 HOUR is not recommended for use in children below the age of 12 years due to lack of data on safety and efficacy.

Geriatrics* (≥65 years of age): The number of patients 65 years of age and above treated with AERIUS DUAL ACTION 12 HOUR were too limited to make any clinically relevant judgement regarding efficacy or safety of this drug product in this age group. Patients of 65 years or older are more likely to experience adverse reactions from sympathomimetic medicinal products. Therefore the combination product should be used with caution in patients above 65 years of age.

Athletes: Athletes should be informed that treatment with pseudoephedrine could lead to positive doping tests.

ADVERSE REACTIONS: Adverse Drug Reaction Overview: Very rare cases of hypersensitivity reactions including anaphylaxis and rash have been reported during the marketing of desloratadine. In addition, cases of tachycardia, palpitations, psychomotor hyperactivity, seizures, elevations of liver enzymes, hepatitis and increased bilirubin have been reported very rarely.

As with other sympathomimetic amines, central nervous system stimulation, muscular weakness, tightness in the chest and syncope may also be encountered with the use of pseudoephedrine sulfate.

Clinical Trial Adverse Drug Reactions: Because clinical trials are conducted under very specific conditions the adverse reaction rates observed in the clinical trials may not reflect the rates observed in practice and should not be compared to the rates in the clinical trials of another drug. Adverse drug reaction information from clinical trials is useful for identifying drug-related adverse events and for approximating rates.

A total of 1248 subjects, 12 years of age and older were randomized in two Phase-3 studies and received at least one dose of study drug. All subjects were included in the safety evaluation presented in Table 1, demonstrating adverse events ≥1%.

Table 1: AERIUS DUAL ACTION 12 HOUR

Incidence of Adverse Events Reported by ≥1% of Patients Receiving AERIUS DUAL ACTION 12 HOUR Extended Release Tablets

	DL 2.5 mg/PSE 120 mg QD n=414 (%)	DL, 5 mg QD n=412 (%)	PSE, 120 mg BID n=422 (%)
Gastrointestinal			
Abdominal pain	1	2	1
Anorexia	2	0	2
Constipation	2	0	1
Diarrhea	0	2	1
Dyspepsia	1	2	1
Nausea	2	1	3
Vomiting	0	1	0
General Disorders			
Back pain	1	1	1
Chest pain	0	1	1
Fatigue	4	2	2
Fever	1	1	0
Headache	8	8	9
Heart Rate and Rhythm Disorders			
Palpitation	1	0	2
Tachycardia	1	0	1
Musculoskeletal System			
Arthralgia	1	1	1
Myalgia	1	2	1
Nervous System			
Dry mouth	8	2	8
Dizziness	3	2	2
Psychomotor hyperactivity	2	1	1
Psychiatric			
Agitation	1	0	1
Insomnia	10	3	13
Nervousness	1	0	3
Sleep disorder	1	0	2
Somnolence	3	4	2
Reproductive System			
Dysmenorrhea	0	1	0
Vaginitis	0	1	0
Resistance Mechanism			
Infection viral	2	2	2
Respiratory System			
Coughing	2	1	1
Epistaxis	1	1	1
Pharyngitis	3	3	3
Sinusitis	<1	1	3
Upper respiratory tract infection	0	2	2
Urinary System			
Urinary tract infection	0	2	1
Vision			
Dry eyes	1	1	0

* **CNS stimulations with convulsions or cardiovascular collapse with accompanying hypotension may be produced by sympathomimetic amines. These effects may be more likely to occur in children or elderly patients.**

(cont'd)

Table 1: AERIUS DUAL ACTION 12 HOUR *(cont'd)*

Legend: DL=desloratadine; PSE=pseudoephedrine sulfate.

In all clinical studies conducted, AERIUS DUAL ACTION 12 HOUR was safe and well tolerated. In Phase-3 studies, the overall incidence of adverse events was similar in AERIUS DUAL ACTION 12 HOUR and pseudoephedrine treatment groups, but was lower in the desloratadine group. The most common treatment-emergent adverse events of AERIUS DUAL ACTION 12 HOUR were insomnia, headache and dry mouth.

Less Common Clinical Trial Adverse Drug Reactions (<1%) with AERIUS DUAL ACTION 12 HOUR: Cardiovascular: palpitation, premature atrial contractions.

Dermatological: pruritus.

Gastrointestinal: abdominal pain, gastroenteritis, nausea, stool abnormal.

General: aggravated headache, rigors.

Hepatobiliary: increased hepatic enzymes.

Metabolism and Nutrition: glycosuria, hyperglycemia, thirst.

Nervous System: hyperkinesias, hot flashes, confusion.

Ophthalmic: blurred vision, dry eyes.

Psychiatric: agitation, anxiety, irritability.

Renal and Urinary: dysuria, micturition disorder, altered micturition frequency.

Respiratory, Thoracic and Mediastinal: epistaxis, nasal irritation, rhinitis, rhinorrhea, sinusitis, dry throat, hyposmia.
Abnormal Hematologic and Clinical Chemistry Findings: None to report.
Post-Market Adverse Drug Reactions: Very rare cases of hypersensitivity reactions (including anaphylaxis and rash), tachycardia, palpitations, psychomotor hyperactivity, seizures, elevation of liver enzymes, hepatitis and increased bilirubin have been reported during the marketing of desloratadine.

DRUG INTERACTIONS: Overview: Concomitant administration of sympathomimetics and reversible MAO inhibitors are not recommended. Caution should be exercised in patients being treated with other sympathomimetics, including decongestants, anorexogenics or amphetamine-type psychostimulants, antihypertensive agents, tricyclic antidepressants and other antihistamines. Caution should be exercised in patients receiving digitalis.

Antacids increase the rate of pseudoephedrine sulfate absorption, kaolin decreases it.

Drug-Drug Interactions: Interaction studies with AERIUS DUAL ACTION 12 HOUR and other medicinal products have not been conducted, however no clinically relevant interactions were observed in clinical trials with desloratadine in which azithromycin, erythromycin, ketoconazole, fluoxetine or cimetidine were co-administered.

Table 2: AERIUS DUAL ACTION 12 HOUR
Established or Potential Drug-Drug Interactions

Proper Name	Ref	Effect	Clinical Comment
Reversible and irreversible MAO inhibitor(s)	T	May cause risk of vasoconstriction and increased blood pressure.	n/ap
Sympathomimetic medicines	T	May result in critical hypertension reactions.	n/ap
Bromocriptine, cabergoline, lisuride, pergolide	T	Risk of vasoconstriction and increase in blood pressure.	n/ap
Dihydroergotamine, ergotamine, methylergometrine	T	Risk of vasoconstriction and increase in blood pressure.	n/ap
Vasoconstrictors used as nasal decongestant	T	Risk of vasoconstriction.	n/ap

Legend: C=Case Study; CT=Clinical Trial; T=Theoretical.

Drug-Food Interactions: Food had no significant effect on the bioavailability (C_{max} and AUC) of desloratadine and pseudoephedrine.
Drug-Herb Interactions: Interactions with herbal products have not been established.
Drug-Laboratory Test Interactions: The administration of AERIUS DUAL ACTION 12 HOUR should be discontinued at least 48 hours before skin tests since antihistamines may prevent or reduce otherwise positive reactions to dermal reactivity index.

Athletes should be informed that treatment with pseudoephedrine could lead to positive doping tests.

Drug-Lifestyle Interactions: The interaction with AERIUS DUAL ACTION 12 HOUR and alcohol has not been established, however in a clinical pharmacology trial, desloratadine taken concomitantly with alcohol did not potentiate the performance impairing effects of alcohol.

No studies on the effects on the ability to drive and use machines have been performed with AERIUS DUAL ACTION 12 HOUR. However, in clinical trials that assessed the driving ability, no impairment occurred in patients receiving desloratadine. However, patients should be informed that very rarely some people experience drowsiness, which may affect their ability to drive or use machines.

It is not expected that pseudoephedrine sulfate impairs psychomotor performance.

DOSAGE AND ADMINISTRATION: Dosing Considerations: The duration of the treatment should be kept as short as possible and should not be continued after the symptoms have disappeared. It is advisable to limit treatment to about 14 days, as during chronic administration the activity of pseudoephedrine diminishes with time.

Recommended Dose and Dosage Adjustment: Adults and adolescents 12 years of age and over: The recommended dose of AERIUS DUAL ACTION 12 HOUR is one tablet twice a day, administered approximately 12 hours apart.

After improvement of the congestive condition of the mucosae of the upper airway, treatment may be maintained with desloratadine alone, if necessary.

Administration: The tablet may be taken with a full glass of water but must be swallowed whole (without crushing, breaking or chewing it). The tablet may be taken with or without a meal.

OVERDOSAGE:
Symptoms of overdose are mostly of a sympathomimetic nature. Symptoms may vary from CNS depression (sedation, apnoea, diminished mental alertness, cyanosis, coma, cardiovascular collapse) to CNS stimulation (insomnia, hallucination, tremors, convulsions) with possible fatal outcome. Other symptoms may include: headache, anxiety, micturition difficulty, muscle weakness and tenseness, euphoria, excitement, respiratory failure, cardiac arrhythmias, tachycardia, palpitations, thirst, perspiration, nausea, vomiting, precordial pain, dizziness, tinnitus, ataxia, blurred vision and hypertension or hypotension. CNS stimulation is particularly likely in children, as are atropine-like symptoms (dry mouth, fixed and dilated pupils, flushing, hyperthermia, and gastrointestinal symptoms). Some patients may present a toxic psychosis with delusions and hallucinations.

Treatment: In the event of overdose, consider standard measures to remove any unabsorbed drug. Symptomatic and supportive treatment is recommended. Adsorption of active substance remaining in the stomach may be attempted by administration of active charcoal suspended in water. Perform gastric lavage with physiologic saline solution, particularly in children. In adults, tap water can be used. Remove as much as possible of the amount administered before the next instillation. Desloratadine is not removed by haemodialysis and it is not known if it is eliminated by peritoneal dialysis. After emergency treatment, continue to monitor the patient medically.

AERIUS (desloratadine) administered at a dose of 45 mg daily (nine times the clinical dose) for ten days showed no statistically or clinically relevant prolongation of the QTc interval. The mean changes in QTc were 0.3 msec and 4.3 msec for placebo and desloratadine, respectively (p=0.09; Lower confidence interval (LCI)=−0.6; Upper confidence interval (UCI)=8.7).

Treatment of the pseudoephedrine overdosage is symptomatic and supportive. Stimulants (analeptics) must not be used. Hypertension can be controlled with an alpha-blocking agent and tachycardia with a beta-blocking agent. Short acting barbiturates, diazepam or paraldehyde may be administered to control seizures. Hyperpyrexia, especially in children, may require treatment with tepid water sponge baths or hypothermia blanket. Apnoea is treated with respiratory assistance.

> For management of a suspected drug overdose, CPhA recommends that you contact your **regional Poison Control Centre**. See the *CPS* Directory section for a list of Poison Control Centres.

ACTION AND CLINICAL PHARMACOLOGY: Mechanism of Action: Desloratadine is a non-sedating long acting antihistamine with selective peripheral histamine H_1-receptor antagonist activity, which has demonstrated antiallergic, antihistaminic and anti-inflammatory activity.

Pseudoephedrine sulfate is the synthetic salt of one of the naturally occurring dextrorotatory diastereomer of ephedrine and classified as an indirect sympathomimetic amine. It provides a nasal decongestant effect after oral administration due to its vasoconstrictive action and produces a gradual but sustained decongestant effect, facilitating shrinkage of congested mucosa in upper respiratory areas.

Pharmacodynamics: After oral administration, desloratadine selectively blocks peripheral histamine H_1-receptors as the drug is effectively excluded from entry into the central nervous system. Receptor binding data indicate that at a concentration of 2-3 ng/mL, desloratadine shows significant interaction with the human histamine H_1 receptor. Desloratadine inhibited histamine release from human mast cells in vitro.

Pseudoephedrine sulfate is a sympathomimetic agent with mostly α-adrenergic activity. It has an indirect sympathomimetic effect due primarily to the release of adrenergic mediators from the post-ganglionic nerve endings. Oral administration of pseudoephedrine at the recommended dose can cause other sympathomimetic effects, such as increased blood pressure, tachycardia or manifestations of central nervous system excitation.

Pharmacokinetics: Absorption: In a single dose pharmacokinetic study with AERIUS DUAL ACTION 12 HOUR, the mean time to maximum plasma concentrations (T_{max}) for desloratadine occurred at approximately 4-5 hours post dose and mean peak plasma concentrations (C_{max}) and area under the concentration-time curve (AUC) of approximately 1.09 ng/mL and 31.6 ng·hr/mL, respectively, were observed. For pseudoephedrine, the mean T_{max} occurred at 6-7 hours post dose and mean peak plasma concentrations (C_{max} and AUC) of approximately 263 ng/mL and 4,588 ng·hr/mL, respectively, were observed. Food had no effect on the bioavailability (C_{max} and AUC) of desloratadine or pseudoephedrine.

Following oral administrations of AERIUS DUAL ACTION 12 HOUR Extended Release Tablets twice daily for 14 days in normal healthy volunteers, steady-state conditions were reached on day 10 for desloratadine, 3-hydroxydesloratadine and pseudoephedrine. For desloratadine, mean steady state peak plasma concentrations (C_{max}) and area under the concentration-time curve (AUC 0-12 h) of approximately 1.7 ng/mL and 16 ng·hr/mL were observed, respectively. For pseudoephedrine, mean steady state peak plasma concentrations (C_{max}) and AUC (0-12 h) of 459 ng/mL and 4658 ng·hr/mL were observed. Similar values of DSL and PSE for AUC and C_{max} between the 0-12 hour and 12-24 hour intervals indicates a lack of diurnal variation.

In another pharmacokinetic study, food and grapefruit juice had no effect on the bioavailability (C_{max} and AUC) of desloratadine.

Distribution: Desloratadine is moderately bound, 83% to 87%, to plasma proteins. Protein binding of desloratadine and 3-hydroxydesloratadine was unaltered in subjects with impaired renal function.

Metabolism: Desloratadine is extensively metabolized. The results of metabolic profiling indicated that hydroxylation of desloratadine to 3-hydroxy desloratadine (3-OH desloratadine) followed by its subsequent glucuronidation was the major pathway of metabolism of desloratadine. The enzyme responsible for the metabolism of desloratadine has not been identified yet, and therefore some interactions with other drugs cannot be fully excluded. In-vivo studies with specific inhibitors of CYP3A4 and CYP2D6 have shown that these enzymes are not important in the metabolism of desloratadine. Desloratadine does not inhibit CYP3A4 and CYP2D6 and is neither a substrate nor an inhibitor of p-glycoprotein.

Data from clinical pharmacology studies indicate that a subset of the general adult and pediatric patient population has a decreased ability to form 3-hydroxydesloratadine. In pharmacokinetic and clinical trials in subjects between 2 and 70 years of age, 6% of the subjects were poor metabolizers of desloratadine and reached a higher desloratadine concentration (poor metabolizer defined as a subject with an AUC ratio of 3-hydroxydesloratadine to desloratadine less than 0.1, or a subject with a desloratadine half-life exceeding 50 hours). In this data, no difference in prevalence of poor metabolizers was noted across age groups, but the frequency was higher in Blacks (18%) compared to Caucasians (2%) or Hispanics (2%). Ninety pediatric and 440 adult subjects were phenotyped for the polymorphism in clinical pharmacology studies. The incidence of the trait was approximately 8.6% in adults and 15.6% in pediatric subjects. The desloratadine exposure (AUC) associated with the poor metabolizer phenotype has been well characterized (~4 times that of normal metabolizers) in single dose studies and is similar in pediatric and adult subjects at various doses. Median (range) AUC in pediatric normal and poor metabolizers was 31.9 (14-74) ng·hr/mL and 116 (72-210) ng·hr/mL, respectively. The corresponding values for adult normal and poor metabolizers were 33.5 (8.7-99) ng·hr/mL and 139 (82-393) ng·hr/mL, respectively. In adults characterized as poor metabolizers, desloratadine exposure (AUC) after multiple doses has been demonstrated to be about six fold higher than that of normal metabolizers. The desloratadine exposure after multiple doses has not been documented for children. The safety profile of adult and pediatric poor metabolizers of desloratadine was not different from that of the general population.

Following administration of desloratadine 5 mg for 28 days, the approximate two-fold degree of accumulation of desloratadine and 3-OH desloratadine is consistent with the half-life of DL and its active metabolite and a once daily dosing frequency. This accumulation is not clinically meaningful. The pharmacokinetics of desloratadine and 3-OH desloratadine do not change after daily dosing for 7 consecutive days.

There is no evidence of clinically relevant drug accumulation following once daily dosing of AERIUS (5 mg to 20 mg) for 14 days.

Excretion: A human mass balance study documented a recovery of approximately 87% of the ^{14}C-desloratadine dose, which was equally distributed in urine and feces as metabolic products.

The mean elimination half-life of pseudoephedrine is dependent on urinary pH. The elimination half-life is approximately 3-6 or 9-16 hours when the urinary pH is 5 or 8, respectively. The active substance and its metabolite are excreted in urine; 55-75% of the administered dose is excreted unchanged.

Special Populations and Conditions: Pediatrics: AERIUS DUAL ACTION 12 HOUR Extended Release Tablets are not an appropriate dosage form for use in pediatric patients below 12 years of age.

Geriatrics: The number of patients (n=10) 65 years of age and above treated with AERIUS DUAL ACTION 12 HOUR Extended Release Tablets was too limited to make any clinically relevant judgment regarding the efficacy or safety of this drug product in this age group.

Following multiple-dose administration of AERIUS (desloratadine) Tablets, the mean C_{max} and AUC values for desloratadine were 20% greater than in younger subjects (<65 years old). The oral total body clearance (CL/F) when normalized for body weight was similar between the two age groups. The mean plasma elimination half-life of desloratadine was 33.7 hr in subjects <65 years old. The pharmacokinetics for 3-hydroxydesloratadine appeared unchanged in older versus younger subjects. These age-related differences are unlikely to be clinically relevant and no dosage adjustment is recommended in elderly subjects.

Gender: No clinically significant gender-related differences were observed in the pharmacokinetic parameters of desloratadine, 3-hydroxydesloratadine or pseudoephedrine following administration of AERIUS DUAL ACTION 12 HOUR Extended Release Tablets. Female subjects treated for 14 days with AERIUS Tablets had 10% and 3% higher desloratadine C_{max} and AUC values, respectively, compared with male subjects. The 3-hydroxydesloratadine C_{max} and AUC values were also increased by 45% and 48%, respectively, in females compared with males. However, these apparent differences are not considered clinically relevant and therefore no dosage adjustment is recommended.

Race: No studies have been conducted to evaluate the effect of race on the pharmacokinetics of AERIUS DUAL ACTION 12 HOUR Extended Release Tablets. Following 14 days of treatment with AERIUS Tablets, the C_{max} and AUC values for desloratadine were 18% and 32% higher, respectively in Blacks compared with Caucasians. For 3-hydroxydesloratadine there was a corresponding 10% reduction in C_{max} and AUC values in Blacks compared to Caucasians. These differences are not considered to be clinically relevant and therefore no dose adjustment is recommended.

Hepatic Insufficiency: No studies with AERIUS DUAL ACTION 12 HOUR Extended Release Tablets or pseudoephedrine were conducted in patients with hepatic impairment.

Following a single oral dose of desloratadine, pharmacokinetics were characterized in patients with mild (n=4), moderate (n=4) and severe (n=4) hepatic impairment as defined by the Child-Pugh classification of hepatic impairment and 8 subjects with normal hepatic function. Patients with hepatic impairment, regardless of severity, had approximately a 2.4-fold increase in AUC as compared with normal subjects. The apparent oral clearance of desloratadine in subjects with mild, moderate, and severe hepatic impairment was 37%, 36%, and 28% of that in normal subjects, respectively. An increase in the mean elimination half-life of desloratadine in patients with hepatic impairment was observed. For 3-hydroxydesloratadine, the mean C_{max} and AUC values for subjects with hepatic impairment combined were not statistically significantly different from subjects with normal hepatic function.

AERIUS DUAL ACTION 12 HOUR Extended Release Tablets is not recommended in patients with severe hepatic impairment.

Renal Insufficiency: No studies with AERIUS DUAL ACTION 12 HOUR Extended Release Tablets were conducted in patients with renal impairment.

Following a single dose of desloratadine 7.5 mg pharmacokinetics were characterized in patients with mild (n=7; creatinine clearance 51-69 mL/min/1.73 m²), moderate (n=6; creatinine clearance 34-43 mL/min/1.73 m²) and severe (n=6; creatinine clearance 5-29 mL/min/1.73 m²) renal impairment or hemodialysis dependent (n=6) patients. In subjects with mild and moderate impairment, median C_{max} and AUC values increased by approximately 1.2 and 1.9-fold, respectively, relative to subjects with normal renal function. In patients with severe renal impairment or who were hemodialysis dependent, C_{max} and AUC values increased by approximately 1.7- and 2.5-fold, respectively. Minimal changes in 3-hydroxydesloratadine concentrations were observed. Desloratadine and 3-hydroxydesloratadine were poorly removed by hemodialysis. Plasma protein binding of desloratadine and 3-hydroxydesloratadine was unaltered by renal impairment.

Pseudoephedrine is primarily excreted unchanged in the urine as unchanged drug with the remainder apparently being metabolized in the liver. Therefore, pseudoephedrine may accumulate in patients with renal impairment.

AERIUS DUAL ACTION 12 HOUR Extended Release Tablets is not recommended in patients with severe renal impairment.

STORAGE AND STABILITY: Temperature and Moisture:
- Store between 15 and 30°C.
- Protect from excessive moisture.
- Protect from light.

Others: Keep in a safe place out of the reach of children.

SPECIAL HANDLING INSTRUCTIONS: Keep blister package in the outer carton.

INFORMATION FOR THE PATIENT: Published in e-CPS, available by subscription at www.e-cps.ca.

DOSAGE FORMS, COMPOSITION AND PACKAGING: Each blue and white bilayer oval extended release tablet with "D12" branded to the blue layer, contains: desloratadine 2.5 mg in the blue immediate-release layer and pseudoephedrine sulfate, USP 120 mg in the white extended-release layer which is released slowly. Nonmedicinal ingredients: citric acid anhydrous, corn starch, edetate disodium, FD&C Blue No. 2 aluminum lake dye, hypromellose, povidone, magnesium stearate, microcrystalline cellulose, silicon dioxide and stearic acid. Unit dose blisters comprised of laminate blister film and foil lidding. The blister is packaged in a folding carton. Packs of 2 (physician sample), 10 and 30 tablets.

Afinitor® 🅱

everolimus

Antineoplastic

Novartis Pharmaceuticals

Date of Preparation: December 11, 2009

SUMMARY PRODUCT INFORMATION:

Route of Administration	Dosage Form/ Strength	Clinically Relevant Nonmedicinal Ingredients
Oral	Tablet 5 mg and 10 mg	Butylated hydroxytoluene (E321), magnesium stearate, lactose monohydrate, hypromellose, crospovidone, lactose anhydrous. For a complete listing see Dosage Forms, Composition and Packaging.

INDICATIONS AND CLINICAL USE: AFINITOR (everolimus) is indicated for the treatment of patients with metastatic renal cell carcinoma (RCC) of clear cell morphology, after failure of initial treatment with either of the VEGF-receptor TKIs* sunitinib or sorafenib.

Approval of AFINITOR is based on progression-free survival (PFS). Prolongation of overall survival was not demonstrated for AFINITOR in RCC nor were quality-of-life differences shown between patients receiving AFINITOR versus placebo in the pivotal phase III trial.

Geriatrics (≥65 years of age): No differences in safety or efficacy were observed between older and younger patients.

Pediatrics (<18 years of age): AFINITOR is not recommended for use in paediatric cancer patients.

CONTRAINDICATIONS: AFINITOR is contraindicated in patients who are hypersensitive to the drug, to other rapamycin derivatives or to any of the excipients. For a complete listing, see Dosage Forms, Composition and Packaging (see also Warnings and Precautions).

WARNINGS AND PRECAUTIONS:

Serious Warnings and Precautions

AFINITOR (everolimus tablets) should be prescribed by a qualified healthcare professional who is experienced in the use of antineoplastic therapy.

AFINITOR has not been studied in patients with severe hepatic impairment (Child-Pugh class C).

The following are clinically significant adverse events:

- Non-infectious pneumonitis (see Respiratory)
- Infections (see Immune)

General: Drug-Drug Interactions: Co-administration with strong inhibitors of CYP3A4 or P-glycoprotein (PgP) should be avoided (see Dosage and Administration and Drug Interactions).

Use caution when administered in combination with moderate CYP3A4 or PgP inhibitors. If AFINITOR must be co-administered with a moderate CYP3A4 or PgP inhibitor, the patient should be carefully monitored for undesirable effects and the dose reduced (see Dosage and Administration and Drug Interactions).

Co-administration with strong inducers of CYP3A4 or PgP should be avoided due to the risk of reduced effectiveness of the drug.

Carcinogenesis and Mutagenesis: Genotoxicity studies showed no evidence of clastogenic or mutagenic activity. Administration of everolimus for up to 2 years did not indicate any oncogenic potential in mice and rats up to the highest doses, corresponding respectively to 4.3 and 0.2 times the estimated clinical exposure.

Endocrine and Metabolism: Hyperlipidaemia: Hypercholesterolaemia and hypertriglyceridaemia have been reported in clinical trials (see Adverse Reactions, Clinical Trial Adverse Drug Reactions). Monitoring of fasting lipid profile is recommended prior to the start of AFINITOR therapy and periodically thereafter (see Monitoring and Laboratory Tests).

Hyperglycaemia: Hyperglycaemia has been reported in clinical trials (see Adverse Reactions, Clinical Trial Adverse Drug Reactions). Monitoring of fasting serum glucose is recommended prior to the start of AFINITOR therapy and periodically thereafter (see Monitoring and Laboratory Tests). Optimal glycaemic control should be achieved before starting a patient on AFINITOR. New onset type 2 diabetes has occurred with AFINITOR treatment (see Adverse Reactions, Clinical Trial Adverse Drug Reactions).

Gastrointestinal: Mucositis (including stomatitis, aphthous stomatitis) is a common adverse event in patients treated with AFINITOR. Approximately half of the patients receiving AFINITOR experienced mucositis in the pivotal phase III trial.

For mouth ulcers, stomatitis and oral mucositis topical treatments are recommended, but alcohol- or peroxide-containing mouthwashes should be avoided as they may exacerbate the condition. Antifungal agents should not be used unless fungal infection has been diagnosed (see Drug Interactions).

Hematologic: Decreased haemoglobin, lymphocytes, neutrophils and platelets have been reported in clinical trials (see Adverse Reactions). Monitoring of complete blood count is recommended prior to the start of AFINITOR therapy and periodically thereafter.

Immune: Infections: AFINITOR has immunosuppressive properties and may predispose patients to bacterial, fungal, viral or protozoal infections, including infections with opportunistic pathogens (see Adverse Reactions). Localised and systemic infections, including pneumonia, other bacterial infections and invasive fungal infections, such as aspergillosis or candidiasis and viral infections including reactivation of hepatitis B virus have been described in patients taking AFINITOR. Some of these infections have been severe (e.g. leading to respiratory or hepatic failure) and occasionally have had a fatal outcome.

Physicians and patients should be aware of the increased risk of infection with AFINITOR. Pre-existing infections should be treated and fully resolved prior to starting treatment with AFINITOR. Be vigilant for signs and symptoms of infection; if a diagnosis of infection is made, institute appropriate treatment promptly and consider interruption or discontinuation of AFINITOR.

If a diagnosis of invasive systemic fungal infection is made, discontinue AFINITOR* and treat with appropriate antifungal therapy.

Vaccinations: The use of live vaccines and close contact with those who have received live vaccines should be avoided during treatment with AFINITOR (see Drug Interactions).

Peri-Operative Considerations: Impaired wound healing is a class effect of rapamycin derivatives, including AFINITOR. Caution should therefore be exercised with the use of AFINITOR in the peri-surgical period.

Renal: Elevations of serum creatinine, usually mild, have been reported in clinical trials (see Adverse Reactions). Monitoring of renal function, including measurement of blood urea nitrogen (BUN) or serum creatinine, is recommended prior to the start of AFINITOR therapy and periodically thereafter.

Respiratory: Non-Infectious Pneumonitis: Non-infectious pneumonitis is a class effect of rapamycin derivatives, including AFINITOR. Cases of non-infectious pneumonitis (including interstitial lung disease) were reported in 14% of patients treated with AFINITOR (see Adverse Reactions). Some of these have been severe and on rare occasions, a fatal outcome was observed.

A diagnosis of non-infectious pneumonitis should be considered in patients presenting with non-specific respiratory signs and symptoms such as hypoxia, pleural effusion, cough or dyspnoea, and in whom infectious, neoplastic and other non-medicinal causes have been excluded by means of appropriate investigations. Patients should be advised to report promptly any new or worsening respiratory symptoms.

Patients who develop radiological changes suggestive of non-infectious pneumonitis and have few or no symptoms may continue AFINITOR therapy without dose alteration. If symptoms are moderate, consideration should be given to interruption of therapy until symptoms improve. The use of corticosteroids may be indicated. AFINITOR may be reintroduced at 5 mg daily.

For cases where symptoms of non-infectious pneumonitis are severe, AFINITOR therapy should be discontinued and the use of corticosteroids may be indicated until clinical symptoms resolve. Therapy with AFINITOR may be re-initiated at a reduced dose of 5 mg daily depending on the individual clinical circumstances.

Sensitivity/Resistance: Hypersensitivity Reactions: Hypersensitivity reactions manifested by symptoms including, but not limited to, anaphylaxis, dyspnoea, flushing, chest pain or angio-oedema (e.g. swelling of the airways or tongue, with or without respiratory impairment) have been observed with everolimus (see Contraindications).

Special Populations: Pregnant Women: Foetal harm may occur when administered to pregnant women. Apprise women of potential harm to the foetus. Animal studies have shown post-implantation loss in rats and rabbits as well as foetal toxicity at below clinical exposures.

Nursing Women: It is not known whether everolimus is excreted in breast milk. However, in animal studies everolimus and/or its metabolites readily passed into the milk of lactating rats. Women taking AFINITOR should therefore not breast-feed.

Women of Childbearing Potential: Women of childbearing potential should be advised to use an effective method of contraception while receiving AFINITOR, and for up to 8 weeks after ending treatment.

Fertility: Based on non-clinical findings, male fertility may be compromised by treatment with AFINITOR.

Hepatic Impairment: AFINITOR is not recommended in patients with severe hepatic impairment (Child-Pugh class C) (see Dosage and Administration and Action and Clinical Pharmacology, Special Populations and Conditions, Hepatic Insufficiency).

Monitoring and Laboratory Tests: Evaluation of CBC and serum chemistries (including blood glucose, lipids, liver function tests, creatinine, electrolytes, magnesium, calcium and phosphate) should be performed at the beginning of treatment with AFINITOR and periodically thereafter.

ADVERSE REACTIONS: Adverse Drug Reaction Overview: The data described below reflect exposure to AFINITOR (n=274) and placebo (n=137) in a randomised phase III study for the treatment of metastatic renal cell carcinoma. In total, 165 patients were exposed to AFINITOR 10 mg/day for ≥4 months. The median age of patients was 61 years (range 27 to 85). The median duration of blinded study treatment was 141 days (range 19 to 451) for patients receiving AFINITOR and 60 days (range 21 to 295) for those receiving placebo.

The most common treatment-emergent adverse events irrespective of causality (incidence ≥30%) were stomatitis, anaemia, infections, asthenia, fatigue, cough and diarrhoea. The most common grade 3-4 adverse events (incidence ≥3%) were anaemia, infections, dyspnoea, hyperglycaemia, stomatitis, fatigue, dehydration, pneumonitis, abdominal pain, asthenia and hypercholesterolaemia.

The rates of treatment-emergent adverse events resulting in permanent discontinuation were 14% and 3% for the AFINITOR and placebo treatment groups, respectively. Most treatment-emergent adverse events were grade 1 or 2 in severity.

Table 1 compares the incidence of treatment-emergent adverse events reported with an incidence of ≥10% for patients receiving AFINITOR 10 mg/day versus placebo.

Treatment-emergent adverse events in Table 1 are listed according to MedDRA system organ class. Within each system organ class, the adverse events are ranked by frequency, with the most frequent events first.

Clinical Trial Adverse Drug Reactions:

Table 1: AFINITOR

Adverse Events, Irrespective of Causality, Reported in at Least 10% of Patients and at a Higher Rate in the AFINITOR Arm Than in the Placebo Arm

	AFINITOR 10 mg/day N=274			Placebo N=137		
	All grades %	**Grade 3 %**	**Grade 4 %**	**All grades %**	**Grade 3 %**	**Grade 4 %**
Any Adverse Event	**97**	**52**	**13**	**93**	**23**	**5**
Gastrointestinal Disorders						
Stomatitis[a]	44	4	<1	8	0	0
Diarrhoea	30	1	0	7	0	0
Nausea	26	1	0	19	0	0
Vomiting	20	2	0	12	0	0
Blood and Lymphatic System Disorders						
Anaemia	38	9	<1	15	4	<1
Infections and Infestations[b]	37	7	3	18	1	0
General Disorders and Administration Site Conditions						
Asthenia	33	3	<1	23	4	0
Fatigue	31	5	0	27	3	<1
Oedema peripheral	25	<1	0	8	<1	0
Pyrexia	20	<1	0	9	0	0
Mucosal inflammation	19	1	0	1	0	0
Respiratory, Thoracic and Mediastinal Disorders						
Cough	30	<1	0	16	0	0
Dyspnoea	24	6	1	15	3	0
Epistaxis	18	0	0	0	0	0
Pneumonitis[c]	14	4	0	0	0	0
Skin and Subcutaneous Tissue Disorders						
Rash	29	1	0	7	0	0
Pruritus	14	<1	0	7	0	0
Dry skin	13	<1	0	5	0	0
Metabolism and Nutrition Disorders						
Anorexia	25	1	0	14	<1	0
Hypercholesterolaemia	20	3	0	2	0	0

(cont'd)

* VEGF receptor TKIs=vascular endothelial growth factor receptor tyrosine kinase inhibitors.

Table 1: AFINITOR *(cont'd)*

Adverse Events, Irrespective of Causality, Reported in at Least 10% of Patients and at a Higher Rate in the AFINITOR Arm Than in the Placebo Arm

	AFINITOR 10 mg/day N=274			Placebo N=137		
	All grades %	Grade 3 %	Grade 4 %	All grades %	Grade 3 %	Grade 4 %
Hypertriglyceridaemia	15	1	0	2	0	0
Hyperglycaemia	12	6	0	2	1	0
Nervous System Disorders						
Headache	19	<1	<1	9	<1	0
Dysgeusia	10	0	0	2	0	0
Musculoskeletal and Connective Tissue Disorders						
Pain in extremity	10	1	0	7	0	0
Median Duration of Treatment (d)		**141**			**60**	

[a] Stomatitis (including aphthous stomatitis), and mouth and tongue ulceration.
[b] Includes all preferred terms within the 'infections and infestations' system organ class, the most common being nasopharyngitis (6%), pneumonia (6%), urinary tract infection (5%), bronchitis (4%), and sinusitis (3%), and also including aspergillosis (<1%), candidiasis (<1%), and sepsis (<1%).
[c] Includes pneumonitis, interstitial lung disease, lung infiltration, pulmonary alveolar haemorrhage, pulmonary toxicity, and alveolitis.
CTCAE Version 3.0.

Other notable treatment-emergent adverse events occurring more frequently with AFINITOR than with placebo, but with an incidence of <10% include:

Gastrointestinal Disorders: abdominal pain (9%), dry mouth (8%), haemorrhoids (5%), dysphagia (4%).
General Disorders and Administration Site Conditions: weight decreased (9%), chest pain (5%), chills (4%), impaired wound healing (<1%).
Investigations: blood creatinine increased (9%).
Blood and Lymphatic System Disorders: lymphopenia (8%), thrombocytopenia (7%), leucopenia (3%).
Respiratory, Thoracic and Mediastinal Disorders: pleural effusion (7%), pharyngolaryngeal pain (4%), rhinorrhoea (3%).
Skin and Subcutaneous Tissue Disorders: hand-foot syndrome (reported as palmar-plantar erythrodysaesthesia syndrome) (5%), nail disorder (5%), erythema (4%), onychoclasis (4%), skin lesion (4%), acneiform dermatitis (3%).
Metabolism and Nutrition Disorders: hypophosphataemia (5%), alanine aminotransferase increased (3%), aspartate aminotransferase increased (3%), hypocalcaemia (3%), exacerbation of pre-existing diabetes mellitus (2%), new-onset diabetes mellitus (<1%).
Psychiatric Disorders: insomnia (9%).
Nervous System Disorders: Dizziness (7%), paraesthesia (5%).
Eye Disorders: eyelid oedema (4%), conjunctivitis (2%).
Vascular Disorders: hypertension (4%).
Renal and Urinary Disorders: renal failure (3%).
Cardiac Disorders: tachycardia (3%), congestive cardiac failure (1%).
Musculoskeletal and Connective Tissue Disorders: jaw pain (3%).
Haematologic Disorders: haemorrhage (3%).
Abnormal Hematologic and Clinical Chemistry Findings: Key treatment-emergent laboratory abnormalities are presented in Table 2.

Table 2: AFINITOR

Key Laboratory Abnormalities Reported at a Higher Rate in the AFINITOR Arm Than in the Placebo Arm

	AFINITOR 10 mg/day N=274			Placebo N=137		
Laboratory Parameter	All grades %	Grade 3 %	Grade 4 %	All grades %	Grade 3 %	Grade 4 %
Haematology[a]						
Haemoglobin decreased	92	12	1	79	5	<1
Lymphocytes decreased	51	16	2	28	5	0
Platelets decreased	23	1	0	2	0	<1
Neutrophils decreased	14	0	<1	4	0	0
Clinical Chemistry						
Cholesterol increased	77	4	0	35	0	0
Triglycerides increased	73	<1	0	34	0	0
Glucose increased	57	15	<1	25	1	0
Creatinine increased	50	1	0	34	0	0
Phosphate decreased	37	6	0	8	0	0
Aspartate transaminase (AST) increased	25	<1	<1	7	0	0
Alanine transaminase (ALT) increased	21	1	0	4	0	0
Bilirubin increased	3	<1	<1	2	0	0

[a] Includes reports of anaemia, leucopenia, lymphopenia, neutropenia, pancytopenia, thrombocytopenia.
CTCAE Version 3.0.

Information from Further Clinical Trials: In clinical trials, everolimus has been associated with serious cases of hepatitis B reactivation, including fatal outcome. Reactivation of infections is an expected event during periods of immunosuppression.

DRUG INTERACTIONS: Overview: Everolimus is a substrate of CYP3A4, and also a substrate and moderate inhibitor of the multidrug efflux pump P-glycoprotein (PgP). Therefore, absorption and subsequent elimination of everolimus may be influenced by products that affect CYP3A4 and/or PgP.

In vitro, everolimus is a competitive inhibitor of CYP3A4 and a mixed inhibitor of CYP2D6.

Drug-Drug Interactions: Agents That May Increase Everolimus Blood Concentrations: Everolimus blood concentrations may be increased by substances that inhibit CYP3A4 activity and thus decrease everolimus metabolism.

Everolimus blood concentrations may be increased by inhibitors of PgP that may decrease the efflux of everolimus from intestinal cells.

Concurrent treatment with strong inhibitors of CYP3A4 or PgP (including but not limited to ketoconazole, itraconazole, voriconazole, ritonavir, clarithromycin and telithromycin) should be avoided.

There was a significant increase in exposure to everolimus (C_{max} and AUC increased by 3.9- and 15.0-fold, respectively) in healthy subjects when everolimus was co-administered with ketoconazole (a strong CYP3A4 inhibitor and PgP inhibitor).

Concomitant treatment with moderate inhibitors of CYP3A4 including, but not limited to, erythromycin, verapamil, cyclosporine, fluconazole, diltiazem, amprenavir, fosamprenavir, or aprepitant, and PgP requires caution. Reduce the AFINITOR dose if co-administered with moderate CYP3A4/PgP inhibitors (see Dosage and Administration and Warnings and Precautions).

There was an increase in exposure to everolimus in healthy subjects when everolimus was co-administered with:

- erythromycin (a moderate CYP3A4 inhibitor and a PgP inhibitor; C_{max} and AUC increased by 2.0- and 4.4-fold, respectively).
- verapamil (a moderate CYP3A4 inhibitor and a PgP inhibitor; C_{max} and AUC increased by 2.3-and 3.5-fold, respectively).
- cyclosporine (a CYP3A4 substrate and a PgP inhibitor; C_{max} and AUC increased by 1.8- and 2.7-fold, respectively).

Other moderate inhibitors of CYP3A4 and PgP that may increase everolimus blood concentrations include certain antifungal agents (e.g. fluconazole) and calcium channel blockers (e.g. diltiazem).

Agents That May Decrease Everolimus Blood Concentrations: Substances that are inducers of CYP3A4 or PgP may decrease everolimus blood concentrations by increasing metabolism or the efflux of everolimus from intestinal cells.

Concurrent treatment with strong inducers of CYP3A4 or PgP should be avoided.

Pre-treatment of healthy subjects with multiple doses of rifampicin (a CYP3A4 and PgP inducer) 600 mg daily for 8 days followed by a single dose of everolimus, increased everolimus oral-dose clearance nearly 3-fold and decreased C_{max} by 58% and AUC by 63%.

Other strong inducers of CYP3A4 that may increase the metabolism of everolimus and decrease everolimus blood levels include St. John's wort (Hypericum perforatum), corticosteroids (e.g. dexamethasone, prednisone, prednisolone), anticonvulsants (e.g. carbamazepine, phenobarbital, phenytoin) and anti-HIV agents (e.g. efavirenz, nevirapine).

Potential Pharmacokinetic Interactions Between Everolimus and Agents Which are CYP3A4 Substrates: Studies in healthy subjects indicate that there are no clinically significant pharmacokinetic interactions between AFINITOR and the HMG-CoA reductase inhibitors atorvastatin (a CYP3A4 substrate) and pravastatin (a non-CYP3A4 substrate) and population pharmacokinetic analyses also detected no influence of simvastatin (a CYP3A4 substrate) on the clearance of AFINITOR. However, these studies were carried out with a 2 mg oral dose of everolimus. The effects of a 10 mg dose have not been studied and therefore pharmacological interactions cannot be ruled out in this setting.

In vitro, everolimus competitively inhibited the metabolism of the CYP3A4 substrate cyclosporine and was a mixed inhibitor of the CYP2D6 substrate dextromethorphan. The mean steady-state of everolimus C_{max} with an oral dose of 10 mg daily or 70 mg weekly is more than 12- to 36-fold below the Ki-values of the in vitro inhibition. An effect of everolimus on the metabolism of CYP3A4 and CYP2D6 substrates is therefore unlikely.

Vaccinations: Immunosuppressants may affect the response to vaccination and vaccination during treatment with AFINITOR may therefore be less effective. The use of live vaccines should be avoided during treatment with AFINITOR (see Warnings and Precautions). Examples of live vaccines are: intranasal influenza, measles, mumps, rubella, oral polio, BCG, yellow fever, varicella, and TY21, a typhoid vaccine.

Drug-Food Interactions: Grapefruit, grapefruit juice and other foods that are known to affect cytochrome P450 and PgP activity should be avoided during treatment.

Drug-Herb Interactions: St. John's wort (Hypericum perforatum) is an inducer of CYP3A4 that may increase the metabolism of everolimus and decrease everolimus blood levels.

Drug-Laboratory Test Interactions: Interactions between AFINITOR and laboratory tests have not been studied.

DOSAGE AND ADMINISTRATION: Recommended Dose and Dosage Adjustment: The recommended dose for treatment of metastatic renal cell carcinoma is 10 mg.

AFINITOR should be administered orally once daily at the same time every day (preferably in the morning), either in a fasting state or after no more than a light fat-free meal (see Action and Clinical Pharmacology).

AFINITOR tablets should be swallowed whole with a glass of water. The tablets should not be chewed or crushed.

Treatment should continue as long as clinical benefit is observed or until unacceptable toxicity occurs.

Dosing Considerations: Management of severe and/or intolerable suspected adverse reactions may require temporary dose reduction and/or interruption of AFINITOR therapy. If dose reduction is required, the suggested dose is 5 mg daily (see Warnings and Precautions).

Moderate CYP3A4 or PgP Inhibitors: Use caution when administered in combination with moderate CYP3A4 or PgP inhibitors. If patients require co-administration of a moderate CYP3A4 or PgP inhibitor, reduce the dose to 5 mg daily. Further dose reduction to 5 mg every other day may be required to manage adverse reactions (see Warnings and Precautions and Drug Interactions).

Strong CYP3A4 or PgP Inducers: Avoid the use of concomitant strong CYP3A4 or PgP inducers, due to the risk of reduced effectiveness of the drug.

Elderly Patients (≥65 years): No dosage adjustment is required (see Action and Clinical Pharmacology, Special Populations and Conditions, Geriatrics).

Patients with Renal Impairment: No studies with AFINITOR in patients with impaired renal function have been carried out. However, given that renal metabolism and clearance of AFINITOR is minimal (<5% of total), no dosage adjustment is recommended (see Action and Clinical Pharmacology, Special Populations and Conditions, Renal Insufficiency).

Patients with Hepatic Impairment: For patients with moderate hepatic impairment (Child-Pugh class B), the dose should be reduced to 5 mg daily. Everolimus has not been evaluated in patients with severe hepatic impairment (Child-Pugh class C) and is not recommended for use in this patient population (see Warnings and Precautions and Action and Clinical Pharmacology, Special Populations and Conditions, Hepatic Insufficiency).

Missed Dose: AFINITOR can still be taken up to 6 hours after the time it is normally taken. After more than 6 hours, the dose should be skipped for that day. The next day, AFINITOR should be taken at its usual time. Double doses should not be taken to make up for the one that was missed.

OVERDOSAGE:
In animal studies, everolimus showed a low acute toxic potential. No lethality or severe toxicity was observed in either mice or rats given single oral doses of 2000 mg/kg (limit test).

Reported experience with overdose in humans is very limited. Single doses of up to 70 mg have been given with acceptable acute tolerability.

There is no specific treatment for AFINITOR overdose and general supportive care, including frequent monitoring of vital signs and close observation of the patient, is indicated.

> For management of a suspected drug overdose, contact your regional Poison Control Centre. See the *CPS* Directory section for a list of Poison Control Centres.

ACTION AND CLINICAL PHARMACOLOGY: Mechanism of Action: Everolimus is a signal transduction inhibitor targeting mTOR (mammalian target of rapamycin), or more specifically, mTORC1 (mammalian 'target of rapamycin' complex 1). mTOR is a key serine-threonine kinase playing a central role in the regulation of cell growth, proliferation and survival. The regulation of mTORC1 signalling is complex, being modulated by mitogens, growth factors, energy and nutrient availability. mTORC1 is an essential regulator of global protein synthesis downstream of the PI3K/AKT pathway, which is dysregulated in the majority of human cancers. Consistent with the central regulatory role of mTORC1, its inhibition by everolimus has been shown to reduce cell proliferation, glycolysis and angiogenesis in solid tumours in vivo, both through direct anti-tumour cell activity and inhibition of the tumour stromal compartment.

Pharmacodynamics: Everolimus exerts its activity through high affinity interaction with the intracellular receptor protein FKBP12. The FKBP12/everolimus complex binds to mTORC1, inhibiting its signalling capacity. mTORC1 signalling is effected through modulation of the phosphorylation of downstream effectors, the best characterised of which are the translational regulators S6 ribosomal protein kinase (S6K1) and eukaryotic elongation factor 4E-binding protein (4E-BP1). Disruption of S6K1 and 4E-BP1 function, as a consequence of mTORC1 inhibition, interferes with the translation of mRNAs encoding pivotal proteins involved in cell cycle regulation, glycolysis and adaptation to low oxygen conditions (hypoxia). This inhibits cell cycle progression and expression of hypoxia-inducible factors (e.g. HIF-1 transcription factor); the latter resulting in reduced expression of factors involved in the potentiation of tumour angiogenic processes (e.g. the vascular endothelial growth factor [VEGF] and platelet derived growth factor [PDGF]).

There was a moderate correlation between the decrease in the phosphorylation of 4E-BP1 (p4E-BP1) in tumour tissue and the average everolimus C_{min} at steady state in blood after daily administration of 5 or 10 mg everolimus. Further data suggest that the inhibition of phosphorylation of the S6 kinase is very sensitive to the mTOR inhibition by everolimus. Inhibition of phosphorylation of eIF-4G was complete at all C_{min} values after the 10 mg daily dose.

QT/QTc Interval Prolongation: A thorough QT study conducted in humans indicated that single doses of everolimus up to 50 mg had minimal effects on QTc prolongation (maximal mean changes from baselines were 4.1 ms for 20 mg and 4.3 ms for 50 mg) that are acceptable according to the current guidelines. The effect of multiple dosing in humans on QTc prolongation was not studied.

Pharmacokinetics: Absorption: In patients with advanced solid tumours, peak everolimus concentrations are reached 1 to 2 hours after administration of an oral dose of 5 to 70 mg everolimus under fasting conditions or with a light fat-free snack. C_{max} is dose-proportional between 5 and 10 mg in the daily and weekly regimens. At doses of 20 mg/week and higher, the increase in C_{max} is less than dose-proportional; however, AUC shows dose-proportionality over the 5 to 70 mg dose range. Steady-state was achieved within two weeks with the daily dosing regimen. There was a significant correlation between $AUC_{0-τ}$ and pre-dose trough concentration at steady-state on the daily regimen.

Table 3: AFINITOR

Summary Statistics of Main Pharmacokinetic Parameters of Everolimus in the Pivotal Phase III Trial

	C_{max} (ng/mL)	t_{max} (h)	C_{min} (ng/mL)	$AUC_{0-τ}$ (ng·h/mL)	CL/F (L/h)	CL/F (L/h/m²)
Day 1 (n=13)	68.1±29.8	1 (1–2)	7.9±3.4	455.0±168.5	—	—
CV	(43.7%)		(43.3%)	(37.0%)		
Day 15 (n=12)	76.7±39.3	1 (1–5)	19.8±12.3	729.1±262.7	15.4±5.3	7.5±2.3
CV	(51.2%)		(61.8%)	(36.0%)	(34.3%)	(30.1%)

Food effect: Based on data in healthy subjects taking 1 mg everolimus tablets, a high-fat meal reduced C_{max} and AUC by 60% and 16%, respectively. No data are available with AFINITOR 5 and 10 mg tablets, which have a different formulation from the 1 mg everolimus tablets used in this study.

Distribution: The blood-to-plasma ratio of everolimus, which is concentration-dependent over the range of 5 to 5000 ng/mL, is 17% to 73%. The amount of everolimus confined to the plasma is approximately 20% at blood concentrations observed in cancer patients given AFINITOR 10 mg/day. Plasma protein binding is approximately 74%, both in healthy subjects and in patients with moderate hepatic impairment.

Following intravenous administration in a rat model, everolimus was shown to cross the blood-brain barrier in a non-linear dose-dependent manner, suggesting saturation of an efflux pump at the blood-brain barrier. Brain penetration of everolimus has also been demonstrated in rats receiving oral doses of everolimus.

Metabolism: Everolimus is a substrate of CYP3A4 and PgP. Following oral administration, it is the main circulating component in human blood. Six main metabolites of everolimus have been detected in human blood, including three monohydroxylated metabolites, two hydrolytic ring-opened products, and a phosphatidylcholine conjugate of everolimus. These metabolites were also identified in animal species used in toxicity studies, and showed approximately 100-times less activity than everolimus itself. Hence, the parent substance is considered to contribute the majority of the overall pharmacological activity of everolimus.

Excretion: No specific excretion studies have been undertaken in cancer patients; however, data are available from the transplantation setting. Following the administration of a single dose of radio-labelled everolimus in conjunction with cyclosporine, 80% of the radioactivity was recovered from the faeces, while 5% was excreted in the urine over 10 days. The parent substance was not detected in urine or faeces.

Special Populations and Conditions: Pediatrics: There is no indication for use of AFINITOR in the paediatric population (see Indications and Clinical Use).

Geriatrics: In a population pharmacokinetic evaluation in cancer patients, no significant influence of age (27 to 85 years) on oral clearance (CL/F: range 4.8 to 54.5 L/hour) of everolimus was detected.

Gender: Analyses of efficacy and safety data in male and female subgroups suggest that no dose adjustments are necessary based on patient gender.

Race: Oral clearance (CL/F) is similar in Japanese and Caucasian cancer patients with similar liver functions. Based on analysis of population pharmacokinetics, oral clearance (CL/F) is on average 20% higher in black transplant patients.

Hepatic Insufficiency: The average AUC of everolimus in 8 subjects with moderate hepatic impairment (Child-Pugh class B) was twice that found in 8 subjects with normal hepatic function. AUC was positively correlated with serum bilirubin concentration and with prolongation of prothrombin time and negatively correlated with serum albumin concentration. The impact of severe hepatic impairment (Child-Pugh class C) has not been assessed (see Dosage and Administration and Warnings and Precautions).

Renal Insufficiency: In a population pharmacokinetic analysis of 170 patients with advanced cancer, no significant influence of creatinine clearance (25 to 178 mL/min) was detected on CL/F of everolimus. Post-transplant renal impairment (creatinine clearance range 11 to 107 mL/min) did not affect the pharmacokinetics of everolimus in transplant patients.

STORAGE AND STABILITY: Store at room temperature (15-30°C). Store in the original package to protect from light and moisture.

Keep in a safe place out of the reach of children and pets.

SPECIAL HANDLING INSTRUCTIONS: No special requirements.

INFORMATION FOR THE PATIENT: Published in e-CPS, available by subscription at www.e-cps.ca.

DOSAGE FORMS, COMPOSITION AND PACKAGING: 5 mg: Each elongated, white to slightly yellow tablet with a bevelled edge and no score, engraved with "5" on one side and "NVR" on the other, contains: everolimus 5 mg. Nonmedicinal ingredients: butylated hydroxytoluene, crospovidone, hypromellose, lactose anhydrous, lactose monohydrate and magnesium stearate. Blister packs (3 strips of 10 blisters/card, 3 cards/carton).

10 mg: Each elongated, white to slightly yellow tablet with a bevelled edge and no score, engraved with "UHE" on one side and "NVR" on the other, contains: everolimus 10 mg. Nonmedicinal ingredients: butylated hydroxytoluene, crospovidone, hypromellose, lactose anhydrous, lactose monohydrate and magnesium stearate. Blister packs (3 strips of 10 blisters/card, 3 cards/carton).

Aggrastat® Ⓟ

tirofiban HCl

Platelet Aggregation Inhibitor

Iroko Cardio

Date of Revision: January 4, 2010

PHARMACOLOGY: Mechanism of Action: Tirofiban is a reversible non-peptide antagonist of fibrinogen binding to the GP IIb/IIIa receptor, the major platelet surface receptor involved in platelet aggregation. When administered i.v., tirofiban inhibits ex vivo platelet aggregation in a dose and concentration dependent manner.

Pharmacodynamics: Tirofiban causes potent inhibition of platelet function as demonstrated by its ability to inhibit ex vivo adenosine phosphate (ADP) induced platelet aggregation and prolong bleeding time (BT) in healthy subjects and patients with coronary artery disease.

The time course of inhibition parallels the plasma concentration profile of the drug. Following discontinuation of an infusion of tirofiban, 0.1 µg/kg/min, ex vivo-platelet aggregation returns to near baseline in approximately 90% of patients with coronary artery disease in 4 to 8 hours. The addition of heparin to this regimen does not significantly alter the percentage of subjects with >70% inhibition of platelet aggregation (IPA), but does increase the average bleeding time, as well as the number of patients with bleeding times prolonged to >30 minutes.

In patients with unstable angina, a 2-staged i.v. infusion regimen of tirofiban (loading infusion of 0.4 µg/kg/min for 30 minutes followed by 0.1 µg/kg/min for up to 48 hours in the presence of heparin and ASA), produces approximately 90% inhibition of ex vivo ADP-induced platelet aggregation with a 2.9 fold prolongation of bleeding time during the infusion. Inhibition was achieved rapidly with the 30 minute loading infusion and was maintained over the duration of the infusion.

Pharmacokinetics: In healthy subjects, tirofiban is cleared from the plasma largely by renal excretion, with about 66% of a ^{14}C labeled tirofiban dose appearing in the urine and about 23% in the feces, mainly as unchanged tirofiban. The metabolism of tirofiban appears to be limited.

Tirofiban is not highly bound to plasma proteins and protein binding is concentration independent over the range of 0.01 to 25 µg/mL. Unbound fraction in human plasma is 35%. The steady-state volume of distribution of tirofiban ranges from 22 to 42 L.

In healthy subjects, the plasma clearance of tirofiban ranges from 213 to 314 mL/min. Renal clearance accounts for 39 to 69% of plasma clearance. Half-life ranges from 1.4 to 1.8 hours.

In patients with coronary artery disease, the plasma clearance of tirofiban ranges from 152 to 267 mL/min. Renal clearance accounts for 39% of plasma clearance. Half-life ranges from 1.9 to 2.2 hours.

Special Populations: Gender: Plasma clearance of tirofiban in patients with coronary artery disease is similar in males and females.

Geriatrics: Plasma clearance of tirofiban is about 19 to 26% lower in elderly (>65 years) patients with coronary artery disease compared to younger (≤65 years) patients.

Race: No difference in plasma clearance was detected in patients of different races.

Renal Insufficiency: Plasma clearance of tirofiban is lower to a clinically significant extent (>50%) in patients with creatinine clearance <30 mL/min, including patients requiring hemodialysis (see Dosage, Patients with Severe Renal Insufficiency). Tirofiban is removed by hemodialysis.

Clinical Trials: Unstable Angina/Non-Q-Wave Myocardial Infarction: In the multicentre, randomized, parallel, double-blind PRISM-PLUS trial (Platelet Receptor Inhibition in Ischemic Syndrome Management in Patients Limited by Unstable Signs and Symptoms), the use of tirofiban in combination with heparin (n=773) versus heparin alone (n=797) was compared in patients with documented unstable angina/non-Q-wave myocardial infarction within 12 hours of the last episode of chest pain before randomization. All patients with unstable angina/non-Q-wave myocardial infarction had cardiac ischemia documented by ECG or had elevated cardiac enzymes. The mean age of the population was 63 years; 32% of patients were female and approximately half of the population presented with non-Q-wave myocardial infarction. Patients were randomized to either tirofiban (30 minute loading infusion of 0.4 µg/kg/min followed by a maintenance infusion of 0.10 µg/kg/min) and heparin (bolus of 5000 units (U) followed by an infusion of 1000 U/h titrated to maintain an activated partial thromboplastin time (aPTT) of approximately 2 times control), or heparin alone (bolus of 5000 U followed by an infusion of 1000 U/h titrated to maintain an aPTT of approximately 2 times control). All patients received concomitant ASA unless contraindicated.

Comprehensive Management: Patients underwent 48 hours of medical stabilization on study drug therapy, after which they could undergo angiography and angioplasty (if indicated), while continuing on tirofiban. Tirofiban was generally administered for a minimum of 48 hours and was continued up to 108 hours; patients received tirofiban for 71.3 hours (average for all patients).

The primary endpoint of the study was a composite of refractory ischemia, new myocardial infarction and death at 7 days following initiation of tirofiban. At the primary endpoint, there was a 31.6% risk reduction in the overall composite, a 46.6% risk reduction in myocardial infarction, and a 42.8% risk reduction in the composite of myocardial infarction and death. The results are shown in Table 1.

Table 1: Aggrastat

Cardiac Ischemic Events (7 Days)

Endpoint	Aggrastat + Heparin (n=773) %	Heparin (n=797) %	Risk Reduction %	p-value
Composite Endpoint	12.9	17.9	31.6	0.004
Components				
Myocardial Infarction and Death	4.9	8.3	42.8	0.006
Myocardial Infarction	3.9	7.0	46.6	0.006
Death	1.9	1.9	—	—
Refractory Ischemia	9.3	12.7	29.6	0.023

The early clinical benefit seen at 7 days was maintained over time. At 30 days, the risk of the composite endpoint was reduced by 21.8% (p=0.029) and there was a 29.8% (p=0.027) reduction in the composite of myocardial infarction and death. At 6 months, the risk of the composite endpoint was reduced by 18.9% (p=0.024). In addition, there was a 22.5% (p=0.063) risk reduction in the composite of myocardial infarction and death. The risk reduction in the composite endpoint at 7 days, 30 days and 6 months is shown in the Kaplan-Meier curve (see Figure 1).

Figure 1: Aggrastat

Composite Endpoint—180-Day Follow-Up

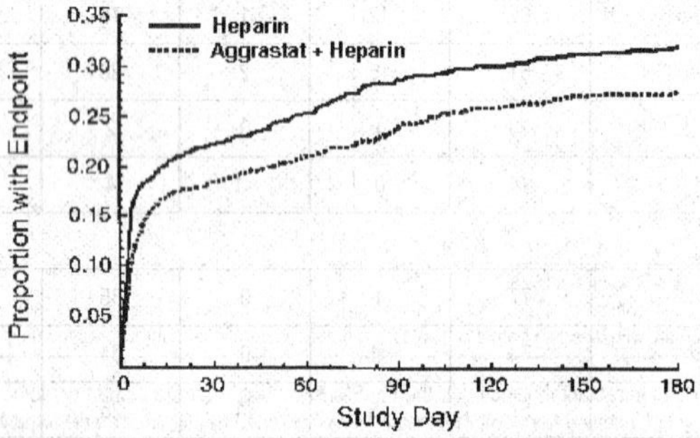

In the PRISM-PLUS study, 90% of patients underwent coronary angiography and 30% underwent angioplasty. The majority of these patients continued on study drug throughout these procedures. Tirofiban was continued for 12 to 24 hours (average 15 hours) after angioplasty.

Although the benefit of adding tirofiban to heparin was observed in all interventional subgroups used in the management of these patients [Percutaneous Transluminal Coronary Angioplasty (PTCA), Coronary Artery Bypass Graft (CABG) or medical management alone], a pre-specified analysis suggested that there was some amplification of the benefit in patients undergoing PTCA.

A sub-study in PRISM-PLUS of angiograms up to 96 hours found that there was a statistically significant decrease in the extent of angiographically apparent thrombus and increase in the blood flow in patients treated with tirofiban in combination with heparin compared to heparin alone.

In the PRISM-PLUS study, the benefit of tirofiban was consistent regardless of age or gender.

INDICATIONS: Tirofiban, in combination with heparin and ASA, is indicated in the management of patients with unstable angina or non-Q-wave myocardial infarction, including patients who may subsequently undergo PTCA, to decrease the rate of refractory ischemic conditions, new myocardial infarction and death.

CONTRAINDICATIONS: In patients with: known hypersensitivity to any component of the product; active internal bleeding or a history of bleeding diathesis; a history of intracranial hemorrhage or neoplasm, arteriovenous malformation, or aneurysm; who developed thrombocytopenia following prior exposure to tirofiban; known coagulopathy, platelet disorder or history of thrombocytopenia; stroke within 30 days prior to hospitalization or any history of hemorrhagic stroke; major surgical procedure or severe physical trauma within the previous month; history, symptoms or findings suggestive of aortic dissection; severe uncontrolled hypertension (systolic blood pressure >180 mmHg and/or diastolic blood pressure of >110 mmHg); concomitant use of another GP IIb/IIIa inhibitor; acute pericarditis; cirrhosis or clinically significant liver disease; and angina precipitated by obvious provoking factors (e.g., arrhythmia, severe anemia, hyperthyroidism or hypotension); recent epidural procedure.

WARNINGS: Tirofiban inhibits platelet aggregation and therefore caution should be employed when used with other drugs affecting hemostasis (see Precautions, Laboratory Monitoring; Adverse Effects and Postmarketing Experience).

Tirofiban should be used with caution in the following patients: recent (<1 year) bleeding, including a history of gastrointestinal bleeding, or genitourinary bleeding of clinical significance; platelet count <150 000 cells/mm³; history of cerebrovascular disease within 1 year; hemorrhagic retinopathy; chronic hemodialysis (see Dosage).

Pregnancy: Tirofiban has been shown to cross the placenta in pregnant rats and rabbits. However, there are no adequate and well-controlled studies in pregnant women. Tirofiban should be used during pregnancy only if clearly needed.

Lactation: It is not known whether tirofiban is excreted in human milk. However, significant levels of tirofiban are excreted in rat milk. Therefore, nursing should be discontinued during the period of drug administration and the milk discarded. Nursing may resume 24 hours after cessation of treatment with tirofiban.

Children: Safety and effectiveness in children have not been established.

PRECAUTIONS: Bleeding Precautions: Tirofiban inhibits platelet aggregation and therefore caution should be employed when it is used with other drugs that affect hemostasis (e.g., warfarin). The safety of tirofiban when used in combination with thrombolytic agents has not been established.

During therapy with tirofiban, patients should be monitored for potential bleeding. When bleeding cannot be controlled with pressure, infusion of tirofiban and heparin should be discontinued. Transfusions may be given if required.

Fatal bleedings have been reported (see Adverse Effects).

Femoral Artery Access Site: Tirofiban is associated with minor increases in bleeding rates particularly at the site of arterial access for femoral sheath placement. Care should be taken when attempting vascular access that only the anterior wall of the femoral artery is punctured [a Seldinger (through and through) technique for obtaining sheath access should be avoided]. Arterial sheaths should be removed when the patient's activated clotting time is <180 seconds or 2 to 6 hours following cessation of heparin.

Laboratory Monitoring: Baseline Evaluation: Should be performed on platelet count, hematocrit, hemoglobin and activated partial thromboplastin time (aPTT) prior to treatment.

Following the Loading Infusion: Monitor platelet count within 6 hours following the loading infusion and at least daily thereafter (or more frequently if there is evidence of significant decline). Acute decrease in platelet count to <20 000 cells/mm³ within 1 day after start of therapy with tirofiban has been reported postmarketing (see Adverse Effects, Postmarketing Experience, Thrombocytopenia).

In Patients Previously Exposed to GP IIb/IIIa Receptor Antagonists: Monitor platelet count earlier and more often. Platelet decreases have been observed in patients with no prior history of thrombocytopenia upon re-administration of GP IIb/IIIa receptor antagonists (see Adverse Effects, Postmarketing Experience).

If the Platelet Count Decreases to <90 000 Cells/mm³: Evaluate to exclude pseudothrombocytopenia. If thrombocytopenia is confirmed discontinue tirofiban and heparin and treat appropriately.

Monitor aPTT: Monitor aPTT frequently and adjust the dose of heparin accordingly. Potentially life-threatening bleeding may occur especially when heparin is administered with other products affecting hemostasis, such as GP IIb/IIIa receptor antagonists (see Dosage).

Renal Insufficiency: Patients with moderate (creatinine clearance <60 mL/min) and severe (creatinine clearance <30 mL/min) renal insufficiency should be monitored for bleeding complications. Since clinical studies showed a decreased plasma clearance of tirofiban in patients with severe renal insufficiency, the dosage should be reduced in these patients (see Dosage).

Geriatrics: In clinical studies the efficacy of tirofiban in the elderly (≥65 years) was comparable to that seen in younger patients (<65 years). Elderly patients receiving tirofiban with heparin or heparin alone had a higher incidence of bleeding complications than younger patients.

Drug Interactions: Tirofiban has been studied on a background of ASA and heparin.

The use of tirofiban, in combination with heparin and ASA, has been associated with an increase in bleeding compared to heparin and ASA alone (see Adverse Effects). Caution should be employed when tirofiban is used with other drugs that affect hemostasis (e.g., warfarin, ticlopidine) (see Precautions, Bleeding Precautions).

Tirofiban has been used concomitantly in clinical studies with β-blockers, calcium-channel blockers, NSAIDs and nitrate preparations without evidence of clinically significant adverse interactions.

Pharmacokinetics of tirofiban were not affected by a wide variety of drugs commonly administered to this patient population (e.g., antihypertensives, calcium-channel blockers, β-blockers, diuretics, antidiabetics, lipid-lowering agents, digitalis preparations, and agents for the control of gastric acidity).

ADVERSE EFFECTS: The most common drug-related adverse event reported during therapy with tirofiban when used concomitantly with heparin and ASA, was **bleeding** (usually reported by the investigators as oozing or mild). The incidences of major and minor bleeding using the TIMI Criteria in the PRISM-PLUS (Platelet Receptor Inhibition in Ischemic Syndrome Management in Patients Limited by Unstable Signs and Symptoms) study is shown in Table 2.

Table 2: Aggrastat

PRISM-PLUS[a] [Unstable Angina Pectoris (UAP)/Non-Q-Wave Myocardial Infarction (MI) Study]

Bleeding	Aggrastat + Heparin (n=773) %	Heparin (n=797) %
Major Bleeding (TIMI Criteria)[b]	1.4	0.8
Minor Bleeding (TIMI Criteria)[c]	10.5	8.0
Transfusions	4.0	2.8

a Patients received ASA unless contraindicated.
b Hemoglobin drop of >50 g/L with or without an identified site, intracranial hemorrhage, or cardiac tamponade.
c Hemoglobin drop of >30 g/L with bleeding from a known site, spontaneous gross hematuria, hematemesis or hemoptysis.

There were no reports of intracranial bleeding in the PRISM-PLUS study for tirofiban in combination with heparin or in the heparin control group (which received heparin). The incidences of retroperitoneal bleeding reported for tirofiban in combination with heparin, and for the heparin control group were 0% and 0.1%, respectively.

Female patients receiving tirofiban with heparin or heparin alone had a higher incidence of bleeding complications than male patients.

The overall incidence of **non-bleeding** adverse events was higher in female patients (compared to male patients) and older patients (compared to younger patients).

However, the incidences of non-bleeding adverse events in these patients were comparable between the tirofiban with heparin and the heparin alone groups (see Table 2 for bleeding adverse events).

The most frequent drug-related non-bleeding side effects reported with tirofiban, administered concomitantly with heparin, occurring at an incidence of >1% were nausea (1.7%), fever (1.5%), and headache (1.1%). The incidence of these side effects was similar in the heparin control group.

The incidences of adverse events were generally similar among different races, patients with or without hypertension, patients with or without diabetes mellitus, and patients with or without hypercholesterolemia.

Thrombocytopenia: Patients treated with tirofiban and heparin, experienced decreases in platelet counts (<90 000 cells/mm³) more often (1.5%) than the heparin control group (0.8%). The percentage of patients with a decrease of platelets to <50 000 cells/mm³ was 0.3%. There were 0.1% of patients who had platelet counts <20 000 cells/mm³. These decreases were reversible within 4 to 6 days after discontinuation of tirofiban.

Laboratory Test Findings: The most frequently observed laboratory adverse events in patients receiving tirofiban concomitantly with heparin were related to bleeding. Decreases in hemoglobin and hematocrit, and platelet count were observed. Increases in the presence of urine and fecal occult blood were also observed.

Postmarketing Experience: The following additional adverse reactions have been reported in postmarketing experience:

Bleeding: Intracranial bleeding, retroperitoneal bleeding and hemopericardium, pulmonary (alveolar) hemorrhage and spinal-epidural hematoma. Fatal bleedings have been reported.

Body as a Whole: Acute and/or severe decreases in platelet counts which may be associated with chills, low-grade fever, or bleeding complications (see above).

Hypersensitivity: Severe allergic reactions including anaphylactic reactions. The reported cases have occurred during the first day of tirofiban infusion, during initial treatment, and during readministration of tirofiban. Some cases have been associated with severe thrombocytopenia (platelet counts <10 000 cells/mm³).

Thrombocytopenia: Acute decreases in platelet counts to less than 20 000 cells/mm³ within 1 day after start of therapy with tirofiban have been reported (see Precautions, Laboratory Monitoring and Adverse Effects, Body as a Whole and Laboratory Test Findings).

OVERDOSE:

Symptoms: In clinical trials, inadvertent overdosage with tirofiban occurred in doses up to 5 times and 2 times the recommended dose for bolus administration and loading infusion, respectively. Inadvertent overdosage occurred in doses up to 9.8 times of the 0.15 µg/kg/min maintenance infusion rate.

The most frequently reported manifestation of overdosage was bleeding; primarily minor mucocutaneous bleeding events and minor bleeding at the sites of cardiac catheterization (see Precautions, Bleeding Precautions).

Treatment: Overdosage of tirofiban should be treated by assessment of the patient's clinical condition and cessation or adjustment of the drug infusion as appropriate.

Tirofiban is dialyzable.

For management of a suspected drug overdose, CPhA recommends that you contact your **regional Poison Control Centre**. See the *CPS* Directory section for a list of Poison Control Centres.

DOSAGE: Unstable Angina Pectoris or Non-Q-Wave Myocardial Infarction: Tirofiban should be administered i.v., in combination with heparin, at the initial infusion rate of 0.4 µg/kg/min for 30 minutes. Upon completion of the initial infusion, tirofiban should be continued at a maintenance infusion rate of 0.1 µg/kg/min.

Recommended Length of Infusion: For patients who do not exhibit any signs of refractory ischemic symptoms and do not proceed into angiography and angioplasty: at least 48 hours.

For patients proceeding into angiography and angioplasty the infusion should continue throughout both procedures and for at least 12 hours, and not more than 24 hours after angioplasty. Once a patient is clinically stable and no further coronary intervention is planned by the treating physician, the infusion should be discontinued. There are no safety data for total infusion time extended beyond 108 hours.

Directions for Use: See Table 3.

Table 3: Aggrastat

Directions for Use

	Most Patients			Severe Renal Impairment		
	30-minute Loading Infusion		Maintenance Infusion	30-minute Loading Infusion		Maintenance Infusion
Patient Weight (kg)	Rate[a] (mL/h)	Volume to Infuse Over 30 Minutes (mL)	Rate[a] (mL/h)	Rate[a] (mL/h)	Volume to Infuse Over 30 Minutes (mL)	Rate[a] (mL/h)
30–37	16	8	4	8	4	2
38–45	20	10	5	10	5	3
46–54	24	12	6	12	6	3
55–62	28	14	7	14	7	4
63–70	32	16	8	16	8	4
71–79	36	18	9	18	9	5
80–87	40	20	10	20	10	5
88–95	44	22	11	22	11	6
96–104	48	24	12	24	12	6
105–112	52	26	13	26	13	7
113–120	56	28	14	28	14	7
121–128	60	30	15	30	15	8
129–137	64	32	16	32	16	8
138–145	68	34	17	34	17	9
146–153	72	36	18	36	18	9

a Infusion rate based on a final concentration of 50 µg/mL.

Patients with Severe Renal Insufficiency: As specified in Table 3, the dosage of tirofiban should be decreased by 50% in patients with severe renal insufficiency (creatinine clearance <30 mL/min) (see Precautions, Renal Insufficiency and Pharmacology, Pharmacokinetics, Special Populations, Renal Insufficiency).

Other Patient Populations: No dosage adjustment is recommended for elderly patients or female patients.

Administration: Tirofiban is for i.v. use only using sterile equipment. Tirofiban may be coadministered with heparin through the same line.

Tirofiban is recommended for use with a calibrated infusion device. Care should be taken to avoid a prolonged loading infusion. In clinical studies, patients received ASA unless contraindicated.

Tirofiban may be administered in the same i.v. line as atropine sulfate, dobutamine, dopamine, epinephrine HCl, furosemide, lidocaine, midazolam HCl, morphine sulfate, nitroglycerin, Pepcid (famotidine), potassium chloride and propranolol HCl injection.

Tirofiban should not be administered in the same i.v. line as diazepam.

Solution for Infusion: Directions for Use—Solution for Infusion: Aggrastat—Solution for Infusion, supplied in IntraVia containers (PL 2408 plastic), is available as a 250 mL iso-osmotic solution premixed with 0.9% sodium chloride and is stable through the labeled expiration date when stored under the recommended conditions.

Directions for Use of IntraVia Containers: **Caution: Do not withdraw solution directly from the IntraVia container with a syringe.**

Do not use plastic containers in series connections. Such use could result in air embolism due to residual air being drawn from the primary container before administration of the fluid from the secondary container is completed.

To Open: Tear foil overpouch (250 mL Solution for Infusion) down side at slit and remove IntraVia container. Some opacity of the plastic due to moisture absorption during the sterilization process may be observed. This is normal and does not affect the solution quality or safety. The opacity will diminish gradually. Check for minute leaks by squeezing inner bag firmly. If leaks are found, discard solution as sterility may be impaired. Do not use unless solution is clear and seal is intact. Do not add supplementary medication or withdraw solution directly from the bag with a syringe.

Preparation for Administration: 1) Suspend container from eyelet support. 2) Remove plastic protector from outlet port at bottom of container. 3) Attach administration set. Refer to complete directions accompanying set. 4) Any unused solution should be discarded.

SUPPLIED: Each mL of solution for infusion (premixed, iso-osmotic solution) contains: tirofiban free base 0.05 mg (as tirofiban hydrochloride). Nonmedicinal ingredients: citric acid anhydrous, sodium chloride and sodium citrate dihydrate. The pH ranges from 5.5 to 6.5 and may have been adjusted with hydrochloric acid and/or sodium hydroxide. Nonpolyvinylchloride infusion bags of 250 mL. Store between 15-25°C. Do not freeze. Protect from light during storage.

Aggrenox® ℞

dipyridamole—ASA

Antiplatelet Agent

Boehringer Ingelheim

Date of Revision: September 25, 2008

SUMMARY PRODUCT INFORMATION:

Route of Administration	Dosage Form/ Strength	Clinically Relevant Nonmedicinal Ingredients
Oral	Capsules, 200 mg/25 mg	Nonmedicinal ingredients: acacia, aluminium stearate, colloidal silicon dioxide, corn starch, dimethicone, hydroxypropyl methylcellulose, hydroxypropyl methylcellulose phthalate, lactose monohydrate, methacrylic acid copolymer, microcrystalline cellulose, povidone, stearic acid, sucrose, talc, tartaric acid, titanium dioxide, and triacetin. The capsule shell contains gelatin, red iron oxide and yellow iron oxide, titanium dioxide and water.

INDICATIONS AND CLINICAL USE: AGGRENOX is indicated for:

- the prevention of stroke in patients who have had a previous stroke or a transient ischemic attack (TIA).

Pediatrics (<18 years of age): Safety and effectiveness of AGGRENOX in pediatric patients has not been studied. Therefore, AGGRENOX should not be used in pediatric patients.

ASA should not be used in children or teenagers for viral infections, with or without fever, because of the risk of Reye's syndrome with concomitant use of ASA in certain viral illnesses.

CONTRAINDICATIONS:

- Patients who are hypersensitive to this drug or to any ingredient in the formulation or component of the container. For a complete listing, see Dosage Forms, Composition and Packaging.
- Due to the ASA component, AGGRENOX is also contraindicated in patients with known allergy to nonsteroidal anti-inflammatory drug products and in patients with the syndrome of asthma, rhinitis and nasal polyps.
- Patients with rare hereditary problems of fructose intolerance and/or galactose intolerance (e.g. galactosaemia) should not take this medicine. AGGRENOX contains approximately 23 mg sucrose and 106 mg of lactose per maximum recommended daily dose.

WARNINGS AND PRECAUTIONS: General: Alcohol Warning: Patients who consume three or more alcoholic drinks every day should be counselled about the bleeding risks involved with chronic, heavy alcohol use while taking AGGRENOX, due to the ASA component.

If a patient is to undergo elective surgery, consideration should be given to discontinue AGGRENOX 10 days prior to surgery to allow for the reversal of the effect.

Headache or migraine-like headache which may occur especially at the beginning of AGGRENOX therapy should not be treated with analgesic doses of acetylsalicylic acid (see Dosage and Administration,Alternative Regimen in Case of Intolerable Headaches).

This product contains 106 mg of lactose and 22.5 mg sucrose per maximum recommended daily dose. Patients with rare hereditary problems of fructose intolerance and/or galactose intolerance e.g. galactosaemia should not take this medicine.

Major Hemorrhagic Events: As any antiplatelet agents, which cause bleeding, the use of AGGRENOX may increase the risk of bleeding such as skin haemorrhage, gastrointestinal bleeding and intracerebral haemorrhage. The addition of other antiplatelet agents (e.g. Clopidogrel, Ticlopidine) to AGGRENOX may further increase the risk of serious bleeding. Even though no study has been conducted, such combination is not recommended.

Due to the risk of bleeding, as with other antiplatelet agents, AGGRENOX should be used with caution in patients at increased bleeding risk and patients should be followed carefully for any signs of bleeding, including occult bleeding. In patients with recent transient ischaemic attack (TIA) or strokes who are at high risk of recurrent ischemic events, AGGRENOX has been shown to increase major hemorrhagic events and hemorrhagic strokes (see Adverse Reactions).

Due to the ASA component, the concomitant use of AGGRENOX with either selective serotonin reuptake inhibitors (SSRIs) or corticosteroids can increase the gastrointestinal bleeding.

Carcinogenesis and Mutagenesis: Carcinogenesis: In carcinogenicity studies in rats and mice with the combination of dipyridamole and ASA at the ratio of 1:6 over a period of 125 and 105 weeks respectively, no significant tumorigenic effect was observed at maximum doses of 450 mg/kg (corresponding to a share of 75 mg/kg of dipyridamole, 9 times the maximum recommended daily human dose for a 50 kg person on a mg/kg basis [or 1.5-2.1 times on a mg/m² basis]), and 375 mg/kg ASA, 375 times the maximum recommended daily human dose for a 50 kg person on a mg/kg basis (or 58-83 times on a mg/m² basis).

Cardiovascular: AGGRENOX should be used with caution in patients with severe coronary artery disease (e.g. unstable angina or recently sustained myocardial infarction), due to the vasodilatory effect of the dipyridamole component. Chest pain may be aggravated in patients with underlying coronary artery disease who are receiving dipyridamole. Patients being treated with AGGRENOX should not receive additional intravenous dipyridamole. If pharmacological stress testing with intravenous dipyridamole for coronary artery disease is considered necessary, then AGGRENOX should be discontinued twenty-four hours prior to testing, otherwise the sensitivity of the intravenous stress test could be limited.

For stroke or TIA patients for whom ASA is indicated to prevent recurrent myocardial infarction (MI) or angina pectoris, the dose of ASA in AGGRENOX has not been proven to provide adequate treatment for these cardiac indications.

Gastrointestinal: Peptic Ulcer Disease: Patients with a history of active peptic ulcer disease should avoid using AGGRENOX, which can cause gastric mucosal irritation, and bleeding, due to the ASA component.

GI side effects include stomach pain, heartburn, nausea, vomiting, diarrhoea, and gross GI bleeding. Although minor upper GI symptoms, such as dyspepsia, are common and can occur anytime during therapy, physicians should remain alert for signs of ulceration and bleeding, even in the absence of previous GI symptoms. Physicians should inform patients about the signs and symptoms of GI side effects and what steps to take if they occur.

Hematologic: AGGRENOX should be used with caution in patients with inherited (haemophilia) or acquired (liver disease or vitamin K deficiency) bleeding disorders, due to the fact that even low doses of ASA can inhibit platelet function leading to an increase in bleeding time.

Hepatic/Biliary/Pancreatic: Due to the ASA component, AGGRENOX should be avoided in patients with severe hepatic insufficiency.

Renal: Due to the ASA component, AGGRENOX should be avoided in patients with severe renal failure (glomerular filtration rate less than 10 mL/min).

Sexual Function/Reproduction: Fertility studies with dipyridamole revealed no evidence of impaired fertility in rats at oral dosages of up to 1250 mg/kg, 156 times the maximum recommended human dose on a mg/kg basis for a 50 kg person (or 35 times on a mg/m² basis). ASA inhibits ovulation in rats.

Special Populations: Pregnant Women: There are no adequate and well-controlled studies of AGGRENOX in pregnant women. Because animal reproduction studies are not always predictive of human response, AGGRENOX should be given during the first two trimesters of pregnancy only if the potential benefit to the mother justifies the potential risk to the fetus. Due to the ASA component, AGGRENOX should not be prescribed during the third trimester of pregnancy.

Nursing Women: Dipyridamole and ASA are excreted in human breast milk in low concentrations. Therefore, caution should be exercised when AGGRENOX is administered to a nursing woman.

Pediatrics (<18 years of age): Safety and effectiveness of AGGRENOX in pediatric patients has not been studied. Therefore, AGGRENOX should not be used in pediatric patients. ASA should not be used in children or teenagers for viral infections, with or without fever, because of the risk of Reye's syndrome with concomitant use of ASA in certain viral illnesses.

Monitoring and Laboratory Tests: ASA has been associated with elevated hepatic enzymes, blood urea nitrogen and serum creatinine, hyperkalemia, proteinuria and prolonged bleeding time. Over the course of the 24-month study (ESPS2), patients treated with AGGRENOX showed a decline (mean change from baseline) in hemoglobin of 0.25 g/dL, hematocrit of 0.75%, and erythrocyte count of 0.13×10⁶/mm³.

ADVERSE REACTIONS: Adverse Drug Reaction Overview: Two large scale trials (ESPS-2, PRoFESS) enrolling a total of 26 934 patients, thereof 11 831 patients treated with AGGRENOX (ESPS2: 1650, PRoFESS: 10, 055), were used to define the side effects profile of AGGRENOX. The duration of the trials was 24-months and 2.5 years for ESPS-2 and PRoFESS respectively. In addition, from spontaneous reporting also those events where facts and evidence qualified these as side effects have been included.

Serious adverse events from controlled clinical trials were bleeding disorders, clotting disorders, gastrointestinal disorders, syncope, headache, and hypotension. Bleeding events (major bleeding, hemorrhage intracranial and gastrointestinal hemorrhage) were reported in patients treated with AGGRENOX in both of these trials. In the PRoFESS trial, major hemorrhagic events were reported in 4.1% and 3.6% of patients in the AGGRENOX treatment group and the clopidogrel treatment group respectively. Any intracranial hemorrhage was reported in 1.4% (AGGRENOX) and 1.0% (clopidogrel) of patients (see Warnings and Precautions).

The most common adverse reactions were dizziness, dyspepsia, abdominal pain, anaemia, hypersensitivity, worsening of symptoms of CAD, epistaxis, gastrointestinal hemorrhage, headache, myalgia, vomiting, and nausea. Events that most commonly lead to discontinuation of AGGRENOX were headache, vomiting and nausea.

Clinical Trial Adverse Drug Reactions: Because clinical trials are conducted under very specific conditions the adverse reaction rates observed in the clinical trials may not reflect the rates observed in practice and should not be compared to the rates in the clinical trials of another drug. Adverse drug reaction information from clinical trials is useful for identifying drug-related adverse events and for approximating rates.

ESPS2: A 24-month, multicenter, double-blind, randomized study (ESPS2) was conducted to compare the efficacy and safety of AGGRENOX with placebo, extended release dipyridamole alone and ASA alone. The study was conducted in a total of 6602 male and female patients who had experienced a previous ischemic stroke or transient ischemia of the brain within three months prior to randomization. Discontinuation due to adverse events in ESPS2 was 27.8% for AGGRENOX, 28.2% for extended release dipyridamole, 23.2% for ASA, and 23.7% for placebo.

Table 1 presents the incidence of adverse events that occurred in 1% or more of patients treated with AGGRENOX where the incidence was also greater than those patients treated with placebo.

Table 1: AGGRENOX

Incidence of Adverse Events in ESPS2 Reported by >1% of Patients During AGGRENOX Treatment Where the Incidence was Greater Than Those Treated with Placebo

	Individual Treatment Group			
	AGGRENOX	**ER-DP Alone**	**ASA Alone**	**Placebo**
Total Number of Patients	**N=1650**	**N=1654**	**N=1649**	**N=1649**
Total Number (%) of Patients with at Least One On-Treatment Adverse Event	**1319 (79.9%)**	**1305 (78.9%)**	**1323 (80.2%)**	**1304 (79.1%)**
Body System/Preferred Term				
Any Bleeding[a] Severity of Bleeding:[b]				
Mild	84 (5.1%)	53 (3.2%)	82 (5.0%)	52 (3.2%)
Moderate	33 (2.0%)	18 (1.1%)	33 (2.0%)	15 (0.9%)
Severe	23 (1.4%)	4 (0.2%)	19 (1.2%)	5 (0.3%)
Fatal	4 (0.2%)	2 (0.1%)	1 (0.1%)	2 (0.1%)
Body as a Whole—General Disorders				
Pain	105 (6.4%)	88 (5.3%)	103 (6.2%)	99 (6.0%)
Fatigue	95 (5.8%)	93 (5.6%)	97 (5.9%)	90 (5.5%)
Back Pain	76 (4.6%)	77 (4.7%)	74 (4.5%)	65 (3.9%)
Accidental Injury	42 (2.5%)	24 (1.5%)	51 (3.1%)	37 (2.2%)
Malaise	27 (1.6%)	23 (1.4%)	26 (1.6%)	22 (1.3%)
Asthenia	29 (1.8%)	19 (1.1%)	17 (1.0%)	18 (1.1%)
Syncope	17 (1.0%)	13 (0.8%)	16 (1.0%)	8 (0.5%)
Cardiovascular Disorders, General				
Cardiac Failure	26 (1.6%)	17 (1.0%)	30 (1.8%)	25 (1.5%)
Central and Peripheral Nervous Systems Disorders				
Headache	647 (39.2%)	634 (38.3%)	558 (33.8%)	543 (32.9%)
Convulsions	28 (1.7%)	15 (0.9%)	28 (1.7%)	26 (1.6%)
Gastrointestinal System Disorders				
Dyspepsia	303 (18.4%)	288 (17.4%)	299 (18.1%)	275 (16.7%)
Abdominal Pain	289 (17.5%)	255 (15.4%)	262 (15.9%)	239 (14.5%)

(cont'd)

Table 1: AGGRENOX *(cont'd)*

Incidence of Adverse Events in ESPS2 Reported by >1% of Patients During AGGRENOX Treatment Where the Incidence was Greater Than Those Treated with Placebo

	Individual Treatment Group			
	AGGRENOX	**ER-DP Alone**	**ASA Alone**	**Placebo**
Nausea	264 (16.0%)	254 (15.4%)	210 (12.7%)	232 (14.1%)
Diarrhea	210 (12.7%)	257 (15.5%)	112 (6.8%)	161 (9.8%)
Vomiting	138 (8.4%)	129 (7.8%)	101 (6.1%)	118 (7.2%)
Hemorrhage Rectum	26 (1.6%)	22 (1.3%)	16 (1.0%)	13 (0.8%)
Melena	31 (1.9%)	10 (0.6%)	20 (1.2%)	13 (0.8%)
Hemorrhoids	16 (1.0%)	13 (0.8%)	10 (0.6%)	10 (0.6%)
GI Hemorrhage	20 (1.2%)	5 (0.3%)	15 (0.9%)	7 (0.4%)
Musculoskeletal System Disorders				
Arthralgia	91 (5.5%)	75 (4.5%)	91 (5.5%)	76 (4.6%)
Arthritis	34 (2.1%)	25 (1.5%)	17 (1.0%)	19 (1.2%)
Arthrosis	18 (1.1%)	22 (1.3%)	13 (0.8%)	14 (0.8%)
Myalgia	20 (1.2%)	16 (1.0%)	11 (0.7%)	11 (0.7%)
Neoplasm				
Neoplasm NOS	28 (1.7%)	16 (1.0%)	23 (1.4%)	20 (1.2%)
Platelet, Bleeding and Clotting Disorders				
Hemorrhage NOS	52 (3.2%)	24 (1.5%)	46 (2.8%)	24 (1.5%)
Epistaxis	39 (2.4%)	16 (1.0%)	45 (2.7%)	25 (1.5%)
Purpura	23 (1.4%)	8 (0.5%)	9 (0.5%)	7 (0.4%)
Psychiatric Disorders				
Amnesia	39 (2.4%)	40 (2.4%)	57 (3.5%)	34 (2.1%)
Confusion	18 (1.1%)	9 (0.5%)	22 (1.3%)	15 (0.9%)
Anorexia	19 (1.2%)	17 (1.0%)	10 (0.6%)	15 (0.9%)
Somnolence	20 (1.2%)	13 (0.8%)	18 (1.1%)	9 (0.5%)
Red Blood Cell Disorders				
Anemia	27 (1.6%)	16 (1.0%)	19 (1.2%)	9 (0.5%)
Respiratory System Disorders				
Coughing	25 (1.5%)	18 (1.1%)	32 (1.9%)	21 (1.3%)
Upper Respiratory Tract Infection	16 (1.0%)	9 (0.5%)	16 (1.0%)	14 (0.8%)

[a] Bleeding at any site, reported during follow-up and within 15 days after eventual stroke or treatment cessation.
[b] Severity of bleeding: mild=requiring no special treatment; moderate=requiring specific treatment but no blood transfusion; severe=requiring blood transfusion.
Note: ER-DP=Extended Release Dipyridamole 400 mg/day; ASA=Acetylsalicylic Acid 50 mg/day.
Note: The dosage regimen for all treatment groups is b.i.d.
Note: NOS=Not otherwise specified.

Less Common Clinical Trial Adverse Drug Reactions (<1%): Adverse reactions that occurred in less than 1% of patients treated with AGGRENOX in the ESPS2 study and that were medically judged to be possibly related to either dipyridamole or ASA are listed below.
Body as a Whole: allergic reaction, fever.
Cardiovascular: hypotension, flushing.
Central Nervous System: coma, dizziness, paraesthesia.
Gastrointestinal: gastritis, ulceration and perforation.
Hearing and Vestibular Disorders: tinnitus, and deafness. Patients with high frequency hearing loss may have difficulty perceiving tinnitus. In these patients, tinnitus cannot be used as a clinical indicator of salicylism.
Heart Rate and Rhythm Disorders: tachycardia, palpitation, arrhythmia, supraventricular tachycardia.
Liver and Biliary System Disorders: cholelithiasis, jaundice, abnormal hepatic function.
Metabolic and Nutritional Disorders: hyperglycemia, thirst.
Platelet, Bleeding and Clotting Disorders: haematoma, gingival bleeding, cerebral hemorrhage, intracranial hemorrhage, subarachnoid hemorrhage.
Note: There was one case of pancytopenia recorded in a patient within the AGGRENOX treatment group, from which the patient recovered without discontinuation of AGGRENOX.
Psychiatric Disorders: agitation.
Reproductive: uterine hemorrhage.
Respiratory: hypernea, asthma, bronchospasm, haemoptysis, pulmonary edema.
Special Senses: taste loss.
Skin and Appendages Disorders: pruritus, urticaria.
Urogenital: renal insufficiency and failure, hematuria.
Abnormal Hematologic and Clinical Chemistry Findings: Over the course of the 24-month study (ESPS2), patients treated with AGGRENOX showed a decline (mean change from baseline) in hemoglobin of 0.25 g/dL, hematocrit of 0.75%, and erythrocyte count of $0.13 \times 10^6/mm^3$.
Post-Market Adverse Drug Reactions: The following is a list of additional adverse reactions that have been reported either in the literature or are from post-marketing spontaneous reports for either dipyridamole or ASA.
Body as a Whole: hypothermia, migraine-like headache (especially at the beginning of treatment), pyrexia.
Cardiovascular: angina pectoris, worsening of symptoms of coronary heart disease, tachycardia, syncope, hypotension, hot flush, arrhythmia.
Central Nervous System: cerebral edema, dizziness, headache, also migraine-like headache (especially at the beginning of treatment), agitation, brain oedema, lethargy, convulsion.
Eye Disorders: eye haemorrhage.
Fluid and Electrolyte: hyperkalemia, metabolic acidosis, respiratory alkalosis.
Gastrointestinal: pancreatitis, vomiting, nausea, diarrhoea, dyspepsia, gastric ulcer, duodenal ulcer, gastritis erosive, gastrointestinal haemorrhage, abdominal pain, gastric ulcer perforation, duodenal ulcer perforation, melaena, haematemesis.
Hearing and Vestibular Disorders: hearing loss, tinnitus, deafness.
Hypersensitivity: acute anaphylaxis, laryngeal edema, hypersensitivity reactions including rash, urticaria, severe bronchospasm and angio-oedema, anaphylactic reactions (especially in patients with asthma).
Investigations: liver function test abnormal, blood uric acid increased (may lead to gout attacks), prothrombin time prolonged.
Liver and Biliary System Disorders: hepatitis, incorporated into gallstones, Reye's Syndrome.
Musculoskeletal: rhabdomyolysis, myalgia.
Metabolic and Nutritional Disorders: hypoglycaemia (children), dehydration, hyperglycaemia, thirst, hyperkaleamia, metabolic acidosis, respiratory alkalosis.
Psychiatric Disorders: confusional state.
Blood, Platelet, Bleeding and Clotting Disorders: prolongation of the prothrombin time, prolongation of bleeding time, operative haemorrhage (increased bleeding during surgery), post-procedural haemorrhage (increased bleeding after surgery), disseminated intravascular coagulation, coagulopathy, thrombocytopenia (reduction of platelet count), anaemia, iron deficiency anaemia due to occult gastrointestinal bleeding.
Reproductive: prolonged pregnancy and labour, stillbirths, lower birth weight infants, antepartum and postpartum bleeding, small for dates baby.
Respiratory: tachypnea, epistaxis, dyspnoea, gingival bleeding, laryngeal oedema, hyperventilation, pulmonary oedema, tachypnoea.
Skin and Appendages Disorders: rash, alopecia, angioedema, skin haemorrhages such as contusion, ecchymosis and haematoma, erythema exsudativum multiforme.
Urogenital: interstitial nephritis, renal failure, renal papillary necrosis, proteinuria.

DRUG INTERACTIONS: Drug-Drug Interactions: Overview: When AGGRENOX is used in combination with acetylsalicylic acid or with warfarin the statements regarding precautions, warnings and tolerance for these preparations must be observed. Because of the increased risk of bleeding, the concomitant administration of heparin, or warfarin with AGGRENOX should be undertaken with caution.

The drugs listed in Table 2 are based on either drug interaction case reports or studies, or potential interactions due to the expected magnitude and seriousness of the interaction (i.e., those identified as contraindicated).

Table 2: AGGRENOX

Established or Potential Drug-Drug Interactions

	Effect	Clinical comment
The following drug interactions are associated with the dipyridamole component of AGGRENOX:		
Adenosine	Dipyridamole has been reported to increase the plasma levels and cardiovascular effects of adenosine.	Adjustment of adenosine dosage may be necessary.
Cholinesterase Inhibitors	The dipyridamole component of AGGRENOX may counteract the anticholinesterase effect of cholinesterase inhibitors, thereby potentially aggravating myasthenia gravis.	Patients should be advised to consult a physician if any worsening of the disease occurs.
The following drug interactions are associated with the ASA component of AGGRENOX:		
Acetazolamide	Due to the ASA component, concurrent use of AGGRENOX and acetazolamide can lead to high serum concentrations of acetazolamide (and toxicity) due to competition at the renal tubule for secretion.	Adjustment of acetazolamide dosage may be necessary.
Alcohol Use (Chronic)	Gastrointestinal bleeding may increase when acetylsalicylic acid is administered concomitantly during chronic alcohol use.	Patients should be advised to consult a physician if any signs or symptoms of bleeding occur.
Angiotensin Converting Enzyme (ACE) Inhibitors	Due to the indirect effect of the ASA component on the renin-angiotensin conversion pathway, the hyponatremic and hypotensive effects of ACE inhibitors may be diminished by concomitant administration of AGGRENOX.	Patients should be advised to consult a physician if any signs or symptoms of decreased renal function such as oedema, or increase in blood pressure occur.
Anticoagulant Therapy (heparin and warfarin)	Patients on anticoagulation therapy are at increased risk for bleeding because of drug-drug interactions and effects on platelets. ASA can displace warfarin from protein binding sites, leading to prolongation of both the prothrombin time and the bleeding time. The ASA component of AGGRENOX can increase the anticoagulant activity of heparin, increasing bleeding risk. Acetylsalicylic acid has been shown to enhance the effect of anticoagulants (e.g. coumarin derivatives and heparin) which may result in an increased risk of bleeding.	Patients should be advised to consult a physician if any signs or symptoms of bleeding occur.
Antiplatelet Drugs (clopidogrel, ticlopidine)	Acetylsalicylic acid has been shown to enhance the effect of antiplatelet drugs (e.g. clopidogrel, ticlopidine) which may result in an increased risk of bleeding.	Patients should be advised to consult a physician if any signs or symptoms of bleeding occur.
Anticonvulsants	The ASA component of AGGRENOX can displace protein-bound phenytoin and valproic acid, leading to a decrease in the total concentration of phenytoin and an increase in serum valproic acid levels. Acetylsalicylic acid has been shown to enhance the effect of valproic acid which may result in an increased risk of rare, but often fatal hepatotoxicity.	Adjustment of phenytoin or valproic acid dosage may be necessary.
Beta blockers	The hypotensive effects of beta blockers may be diminished by the concomitant administration of AGGRENOX due to inhibition of renal prostaglandins by ASA, leading to decreased renal blood flow, and salt and fluid retention.	Patient should be advised to consult a physician if any signs or symptoms of decreased renal function such as oedema, or increase in blood pressure occur.
Corticosteroids	Gastrointestinal bleeding increase when acetylsalicylic acid is administered concomitantly with corticosteroids.	Patient should be advised to consult a physician if any signs or symptoms of bleeding occur.

(cont'd)

Table 2: AGGRENOX *(cont'd)*

Established or Potential Drug-Drug Interactions

	Effect	Clinical comment
Diuretics	The effectiveness of diuretics in patients with underlying renal or cardiovascular disease may be diminished by the concomitant administration of AGGRENOX due to inhibition of renal prostaglandins by ASA, leading to decreased renal blood flow and salt and fluid retention.	Patient should be advised to consult a physician if any signs or symptoms of decreased renal function such as oedema occur.
Ibuprofen	The concomitant administration of ibuprofen in healthy volunteers shortened the platelet aggregation inhibitory effect of ASA.	
Methotrexate	The ASA component of AGGRENOX can inhibit renal clearance of methotrexate, leading to bone marrow toxicity, especially in the elderly or renally impaired.	Adjustment of methotrexate dosage may be necessary.
Nonsteroidal Anti-inflammatory Drugs (NSAIDS)	Due to the ASA component, the concurrent use of AGGRENOX with other NSAIDs may increase bleeding or lead to decreased renal function. Gastrointestinal bleeding increases when acetylsalicylic acid is administered concomitantly with NSAIDs.	Patient should be advised to consult a physician if any signs or symptoms of bleeding occur.
Oral Hypoglycaemics	AGGRENOX may increase the effectiveness of oral hypoglycemic drugs, leading to hypoglycaemia.	Patient should be advised to consult a physician if any signs or symptoms of hypoglycaemia occur.
Selective Serotonin Reuptake Inhibitors (SSRIs)	Selective serotonin reuptake inhibitors (SSRIs) may increase the risk of bleeding.	Patient should be advised to consult a physician if any signs or symptoms of bleeding occur.
Uricosuric Agents (probenecid and sulfinpyrazone) and Natriuretic Agents	The ASA component of AGGRENOX antagonizes the uricosuric action of uricosuric agents. ASA decreased the natriuretic effect of spironolactone in healthy volunteers.	Patient should be advised to consult a physician if any signs or symptoms of decreased renal function such as oedema occur.

Drug-Herb Interactions: Pharmacokinetic studies to determine the effect of herb or food have not been conducted with AGGRENOX.
Drug-Laboratory Test Interactions: Pharmacokinetic studies to determine the effect of laboratory interactions have not been conducted with AGGRENOX.
Drug-Lifestyle Interactions: Pharmacokinetic studies to determine the effect of lifestyle have not been conducted with AGGRENOX.

DOSAGE AND ADMINISTRATION: Dosing Considerations: For oral administration.
Recommended Dose and Dosage Adjustment: The recommended dose of AGGRENOX is one capsule twice daily, one in the morning and one in the evening, with or without food.
Alternative Regimen in Case of Intolerable Headaches: In the event of intolerable headaches during treatment initiation, a regimen of one capsule of AGGRENOX at bedtime, along with low-dose (not 500-1000 mg) acetylsalicylic acid (ASA) alone in the morning may be used.

Since it is expected that headaches related to the vasodilatory properties of dipyridamole will subside over time, the standard twice-daily regimen of AGGRENOX may generally be resumed within a week or so.
Administration: The capsules should be swallowed whole without chewing.

OVERDOSAGE:
Because of the dose ratio of dipyridamole to ASA, overdosage of AGGRENOX is likely to be dominated by signs and symptoms of dipyridamole overdose. For real or suspected overdose, a Poison Control Center should be contacted immediately. Careful medical management is essential.
Dipyridamole: Symptoms: Based upon the known hemodynamic effects of dipyridamole, symptoms such as feeling warm, flushes, sweating, restlessness, feeling of weakness and dizziness may occur. A drop in blood pressure and tachycardia might also be observed.
Treatment: Symptomatic treatment is recommended, possibly including a vasopressor drug. Gastric lavage should be considered. Since dipyridamole is highly protein bound, dialysis is not likely to be of benefit.
ASA: Symptoms: In mild overdosage these may include rapid and deep breathing, nausea, vomiting, vertigo, tinnitus, flushing, sweating, thirst and tachycardia. In more severe cases acid base disturbances including respiratory alkalosis and metabolic acidosis can occur. Severe cases may show fever, hemorrhage, excitement, confusion, convulsion or coma, and respiratory failure.
Treatment: It consists of prevention and management of acid-base and fluid and electrolyte disturbances. Renal clearance is increased by increasing urine flow and by alkaline diuresis but care must be taken in this approach not to aggravate further the metabolic acidosis that develops and the hypokalemia. Acidemia should be prevented by administration of adequate sodium containing fluids and sodium bicarbonate. Hypoglycemia is an occasional accompaniment of salicylate overdosage and can be managed by administration of glucose solutions. If a hemorrhagic diathesis is evident, give vitamin K. Haemodialysis may be useful in complex acid base disturbances particularly in the presence of abnormal renal function.

> For management of a suspected drug overdose, CPhA recommends that you contact your **regional Poison Control Centre**. See the *CPS* Directory section for a list of Poison Control Centres.

ACTION AND CLINICAL PHARMACOLOGY: Mechanism of Action: Blood platelets participate actively in the pathogenesis of atherosclerotic lesions and thrombosis which is the principle cause of most strokes and transient ischemic attacks (TIAs). Platelets are believed to adhere to denuded, dysfunctional endothelium and to release mitogenic substances, such as platelet-derived growth factor (PDGF), that foster the lesion's progression to rupture and thrombosis. The antithrombotic action of AGGRENOX is the result of the additive antiplatelet effects of dipyridamole and acetylsalicylic acid (ASA).
Dipyridamole: Dipyridamole inhibits the uptake of adenosine into platelets, endothelial cells and erythrocytes in vitro and in vivo; the inhibition amounts to approximately 80% at C_{max} and occurs in a dose dependent manner at therapeutic plasma concentrations (0.5-1.9 µg/mL). This inhibition results in an increase in local concentrations of adenosine which acts on the platelet A2-receptor thereby stimulating platelet adenylate cyclase and increasing platelet cyclic-3', 5'-adenosine monophosphate (cAMP) levels. Via this mechanism, platelet aggregation is inhibited in response to various stimuli such as platelet activating factor (PAF), collagen and adenosine diphosphate (ADP). Reduced platelet aggregation reduces platelet consumption towards normal levels.

Dipyridamole also inhibits phosphodiesterase (PDE) in various tissues. While the inhibition of cAMP-PDE is weak, therapeutic levels of dipyridamole inhibit cyclic-3', 5'-guanosine monophosphate-PDE (cGMP-PDE), thereby augmenting the increase in cGMP produced by EDRF (endothelium-derived relaxing factor, now identified as nitric oxide).
ASA: ASA inhibits platelet aggregation by irreversible inhibition of platelet cyclo-oxygenase and thus inhibits the generation of thromboxane A2, a powerful inducer of platelet aggregation and vasoconstriction. In studies of platelet activity inhibition, 25 mg ASA was administered b.i.d. to 5 subjects for 2.5 days. Complete inhibition of collagen-induced aggregation was achieved by the 5th dose of ASA, and maximal effect persisted up to 2-3 days following stoppage of drug.
Pharmacokinetics: There are no significant interactions between ASA and dipyridamole. The kinetics of the components are unchanged by their co-administration as AGGRENOX. AGGRENOX is not interchangeable with the individual components of ASA and dipyridamole.

Dipyridamole: Absorption: The dissolution and absorption of dipyridamole from AGGRENOX capsules is independent of the pH of the gastrointestinal tract. Peak plasma levels are achieved in 1.5-2 hours after administration. The absolute bioavailability of dipyridamole from AGGRENOX is about 70%. With a daily maintenance dose of 400 mg of the extended release formulation, peak plasma levels at steady state are between 1.5-3 µg/mL and trough levels are between 0.4-0.8 µg/mL.

Pharmacokinetic studies to determine the effect of food have not been conducted with AGGRENOX.
Distribution: Due to its high lipophilicity, dipyridamole distributes to many organs; however it has been shown that the drug does not cross the blood brain barrier to any significant extent.
Metabolism: Dipyridamole is metabolized in the liver. In plasma, about 80% of the total amount is present as parent compound and 20% as monoglucuronide.
Excretion: Most of the glucuronide metabolite (about 95%) is excreted via bile into the feces, with some evidence of entero-hepatic circulation. Renal excretion of parent compound is negligible and urinary excretion of the glucuronide metabolite is low (about 5%). The dominant half-life for elimination after oral or intravenous administration is about 40 minutes.
Special Populations and Conditions: Geriatrics: Plasma concentrations (determined as area under the curve, AUC) of dipyridamole in healthy elderly subjects (>65 years) are about 30-50% higher than in subjects younger than 55 years, on treatment with AGGRENOX. The difference is caused mainly by reduced clearance.
Hepatic Insufficiency: Patients with mild to severe hepatic insufficiency show no change in plasma concentrations of dipyridamole compared to healthy volunteers, but show an increase in the pharmacologically inactive monoglucuronide metabolite. Dipyridamole can be dosed without restriction as long as there is no evidence of liver failure.
Renal Insufficiency: Renal excretion of dipyridamole is very low (about 5%). In patients with creatinine clearances ranging from about 15 mL/min to >100 mL/min, no changes were observed in the pharmacokinetics of dipyridamole or its glucuronide metabolite.
ASA: Absorption: The rate of absorption of ASA from the gastrointestinal tract is dependent on the dosage form, the presence or absence of food, gastric pH, and other physiologic factors. Since ASA produces its pharmacodynamic effect via the irreversible acetylating of platelets, the time course of its pharmacodynamic activity is not dependent on the pharmacokinetics of ASA but rather on the lifespan of the platelets (approximately 8-10 days). Therefore, small differences in the pharmacokinetics of ASA, such as variations in its absorption rate or in elimination, are largely irrelevant to its pharmacologic activity with chronic administration. ASA undergoes moderate hydrolysis to salicylic acid in the liver and the gastrointestinal wall, with 50%-75% of an administered dose reaching the systemic circulation as intact ASA. Peak plasma levels of ASA are achieved 0.5-1 hour after administration of a 50 mg ASA daily dose from AGGRENOX (given as 25 mg b.i.d.). Peak mean plasma concentration at steady state is 319 ng/mL (175-463 ng/mL).
Distribution: ASA is poorly bound to plasma proteins and its apparent volume of distribution is low (10 L). At low plasma concentrations (<100 µg/mL), approximately 90% of salicylic acid is bound to albumin. Salicylic acid is widely distributed to all tissues and fluids in the body including the central nervous system, breast milk, and fetal tissues. Early signs of salicylate overdose (salicylism), including tinnitus (ringing in the ears), occur at plasma concentrations approximating 200 µg/mL. (See Adverse Reactions and Overdosage.)
Metabolism: ASA is rapidly hydrolyzed in plasma to salicylic acid, with a half-life of 15-30 minutes. Plasma levels of ASA are essentially undetectable 1-2 hours after dosing and peak salicylic acid concentrations occur within 1-2 hours of administration of ASA. Salicylate metabolism is saturable and total body clearance decreases at higher serum concentrations due to the limited ability of the liver to form both salicyluric acid and phenolic glucuronide. Following toxic doses (10-20 g), the plasma half-life may be increased to over 20 hours.
Excretion: The elimination of salicylic acid follows first order kinetics at lower doses, with a resultant half-life of approximately 2-3 hours, which may rise to 30 hours at higher doses because of nonlinearity in metabolism and plasma protein binding. Renal excretion of unchanged drug depends upon urinary pH. As urinary pH rises above 6.5, the renal clearance of free salicylate increases from <5% to >80%. Alkalinization of the urine is a key concept in the management of salicylate overdose (see Overdosage). Following therapeutic doses, about 10% is excreted as salicylic acid and 75% as salicyluric acid, in urine.
Special Populations and Conditions: Hepatic Insufficiency: Due to the ASA component, AGGRENOX is to be avoided in patients with severe hepatic insufficiency.
Renal Insufficiency: Due to the ASA component, AGGRENOX is to be avoided in patients with severe renal failure (glomerular filtration rate less than 10 mL/min).

STORAGE AND STABILITY: Store at 15 to 30°C.

SPECIAL HANDLING INSTRUCTIONS: Protect from excessive moisture.

INFORMATION FOR THE PATIENT: Published in e-CPS, available by subscription at www.e-cps.ca.

DOSAGE FORMS, COMPOSITION AND PACKAGING: Each hard gelatin capsule, with a red cap and an ivory-colored body, imprinted in red with the Boehringer Ingelheim logo and with "01A", contains: dipyridamole 200 mg as extended-release pellets (a mixture of 2 release rate pellets) and ASA 25 mg as an immediate-release sugar-coated tablet. Nonmedicinal ingredients: acacia, aluminum stearate, colloidal silicon dioxide, corn starch, dimethicone, hydroxypropyl methylcellulose, hydroxypropyl methylcellulose phthalate, lactose monohydrate, methacrylic acid copolymer, microcrystalline cellulose, povidone, stearic acid, sucrose, talc, tartaric acid, titanium dioxide and triacetin; capsule shell: gelatin, red iron oxide, titanium dioxide, water and yellow iron oxide. Polypropylene tubes of 60.

(Shown in Product Identification Section)

Agriflu®

influenza vaccine, surface antigen, inactivated

Active Immunizing Agent for the Prevention of Influenza

Novartis Pharmaceuticals

Date of Preparation: June 10, 2010

SUMMARY PRODUCT INFORMATION:

Route of Administration	Dosage Form/ Strength	Clinically Relevant Nonmedicinal Ingredients
Intramuscular injection	Parenteral/Each 0.5 mL pre-filled syringe contains 15 µg of influenza virus haemagglutinin surface antigens from each of the three virus strains, types A and B (see Description)	Trace amounts of neomycin, kanamycin, egg proteins, formaldehyde, polysorbate 80, cetyltrimethylammonium bromide (CTAB) For a complete listing see Dosage Forms, Composition and Packaging.

DESCRIPTION: AGRIFLU is a trivalent, surface antigen, inactivated influenza virus vaccine prepared from virus propagated in the allantoic cavity of embryonated hens' eggs inoculated with a specific type of influenza virus suspension containing kanamycin and neomycin sulphate. Each of the influenza virus strains is harvested and clarified separately by centrifugation and filtration prior to inactivation with formaldehyde. The inactivated virus is concentrated and purified by zonal centrifugation. The surface antigens, hemagglutinin and neuraminidase, are obtained from the influenza virus particle by further centrifugation in the presence of cetyltrimethylammonium bromide (CTAB), a process which removes most of the internal proteins. The CTAB is removed from the surface antigen preparation.

AGRIFLU is a sterile clear aqueous suspension for an intramuscular use that has been formulated to contain a total of at least 45 µg hemagglutinin (HA) per 0.5 mL dose in the recommended ratio of 15 µg HA of each of the following three influenza strains recommended for the 2010/2011 influenza season: A/California/7/2009 (H1N1)-like virus (H1N1); A/Perth/16/2009 (H3N2)-like virus (H3N2); and B/Brisbane/60/2008-like virus, as recommended annually for immunization by the World Health Organisation (WHO) and the National Advisory Committee on Immunization (NACI).

INDICATIONS AND CLINICAL USE: AGRIFLU is an inactivated influenza virus vaccine indicated for active immunization of persons 6 months of age and older against influenza disease caused by influenza virus subtypes A and type B contained in the vaccine (see Dosage and Administration).

The National Advisory Committee on Immunization (NACI) encourages annual vaccine for all Canadians who have no contraindication.

Vaccine should be offered to both children and adults up to and even after influenza virus activity is documented in a community.

CONTRAINDICATIONS: AGRIFLU is contraindicated in persons with a known hypersensitivity to the active substances, to any of the excipients, and to eggs, chicken proteins, kanamycin and neomycin sulphate, formaldehyde, polysorbate 80 and cetyltrimethylammonium bromide (CTAB), or in anyone who has had a life-threatening reaction to previous influenza vaccination.

Patients who are hypersensitive to AGRIFLU or to any ingredient in the formulation or component of the container. For a complete listing, see Dosage Forms, Composition and Packaging.

WARNINGS AND PRECAUTIONS: General: AGRIFLU should under no circumstances be administered intravascularly.

Prior to administration of any dose of AGRIFLU, the vaccine recipient should be asked about personal history, family history, and recent health status, including immunization history, current health status, main allergies and any adverse event associated with previous immunizations.

Before the injection of any biological, the person responsible for administration should take all precautions known for the prevention of allergic or any other reactions. As with all injectable vaccines, appropriate medical treatment and supervision should always be readily available in case of a rare anaphylactic event following administration of the vaccine.

Immunization with AGRIFLU shall be postponed in patients with febrile illness or acute infections.

As with any vaccine, immunization with AGRIFLU may not protect 100% of individuals against influenza disease.

Hematologic: As with other intramuscular injections, administration of AGRIFLU requires careful consideration in patients with clinically significant bleeding disorders.

Immune: The immune response to AGRIFLU in immunocompromised persons, including individuals receiving immunosuppressive therapy, may be lower than in immunocompetent individuals. It is possible that antibody response in patients with endogenous or iatrogenic immunosuppression may be insufficient.

Neurologic: If Guillain-Barré syndrome has occurred within 6 weeks of receipt of prior influenza vaccine, the decision to give AGRIFLU should be based on careful consideration of the potential benefits and risks.

Immunization should be delayed in a patient with an active neurologic disorder, but should be considered when the disease process has been stabilized.

Special Populations: Pediatrics (≥6 months to 17 years of age): Results of clinical studies conducted in children aged 6 months to 17 years demonstrate that AGRIFLU was well tolerated and immunogenic. Immunogenicity and safety data are limited in 6 to 35 months old children. However, a post-marketing effectiveness study will be undertaken, in the near future, in 6 to 35 months-old children.

Geriatrics (≥65 years of age): Results of clinical studies conducted in healthy elderly adults demonstrate that AGRIFLU was well tolerated. Immune responses were generally lower in the geriatric population than in younger adult subjects, but they reached acceptable levels.

Pregnant Women: Based on reproductive toxicology data in rabbits, AGRIFLU is not predicted to increase the risk of developmental abnormalities. Limited data are available from vaccinations with AGRIFLU in pregnant women.

NACI considers influenza vaccination safe during pregnancy. NACI recommends influenza vaccination in pregnant women with high-risk conditions at any stage during pregnancy.

Nursing Women: No data are available from vaccinations with AGRIFLU in lactating women. Exposure to AGRIFLU is not predicted to affect the quantity and/or quality of human milk production. AGRIFLU is not expected to be present in human milk or to affect the breast-fed child.

Adults at Risk: NACI recommends influenza vaccination in adults with chronic health conditions.

A total of 180 adult subjects aged 18 to 60 years with underlying chronic respiratory, cardiovascular and/or metabolic diseases have received AGRIFLU in a randomized, controlled, observer-blind clinical trial performed during 2006-2007 Northern Hemisphere influenza season. The safety profile of AGRIFLU in this at risk population is consistent with that reported for healthy adults.

Monitoring and Laboratory Tests: Following influenza vaccination, false positive results in serology tests using the ELISA method to detect antibodies against HIV1, hepatitis C and, especially HTLV1 have been observed. The Western Blot technique disproves the results. The transient false positive reactions could be due to the IgM response by the vaccine.

ADVERSE REACTIONS: Adverse Drug Reaction Overview: Adverse event information is derived from both controlled and uncontrolled clinical trials and worldwide postmarketing experience.

Vaccination with AGRIFLU cannot cause influenza because the vaccine does not contain live virus.

Immediate, allergic-type responses, such as hives, allergic asthma, or systemic anaphylaxis occur extremely rarely. These reactions probably result from sensitivity to some vaccine component—most likely residual egg proteins (see Contraindications).

The most common AGRIFLU adverse drug reactions are pain at the injection site, and headache. Reactions are generally mild and of limited duration. Prophylactic acetaminophen may decrease the frequency of some side effects in adults.

Clinical Trial Adverse Drug Reactions: Because clinical trials are conducted under very specific conditions the adverse reaction rates observed in the clinical trials may not reflect the rates observed in practice and should not be compared to the rates in the clinical trials of another drug. Adverse drug reaction information from clinical trials is useful for identifying drug-related adverse events and for approximating rates.

The safety profile of AGRIFLU thimerosal-free formulation in adults, elderly, children and adolescents is based on data from 11 studies (five controlled and six uncontrolled studies mostly conducted for the annual strain composition update as required in European countries where AGRIFLU is currently marketed). In all studies solicited local (injection site) and systemic reactions were collected from subjects/subjects' parents who completed a symptom diary card for at least four days following vaccination.

Adults 18 to 64 Years of Age: Safety data for adults 18 to 64 years of age come from ten clinical trials: six open label and single arm, whereas four (Studies C, E, G and J) included an investigational vaccine as comparator. Reactogenicity data are presented individually by study in Table 1.

The most frequently reported solicited local adverse events within 4 days of vaccination were injection site pain, followed by induration, erythema, and swelling. Except for <1% of subjects reporting severe pain all solicited local adverse events were mild to moderate in intensity and generally transient.

The most frequently reported solicited systemic adverse events were headache, myalgia, malaise, and fatigue. Most reports of solicited systemic reactions were mild to moderate in intensity and generally transient, with 2% or less of subjects reporting a severe solicited systemic adverse event across all studies.

Adults 65 Years of Age and Older: Safety data for subjects 65 years of age and older come from eight clinical trials: six open label and single arm, whereas the remaining two (Studies C and E) included an investigational vaccine as comparator.

Reactogenicity data are provided individually by study (Table 2).

The most frequently reported solicited local adverse events within 4 days of vaccination were injection site pain, followed by erythema, induration and swelling. All solicited local adverse events were mild to moderate in intensity and generally transient, with no subjects reporting severe solicited local adverse events across all studies.

The most frequently reported solicited systemic adverse events were fatigue, headache, malaise, arthralgia and sweating. Most reports of solicited systemic reactions were mild to moderate in intensity and generally transient, with 2% or less of subjects reporting a severe solicited systemic adverse event across all studies.

Children and Adolescents (≥6 months to 17 years of age): Safety data for the pediatric population come from two controlled studies. Reactogenicity data are presented individually by study in Table 3.

Study K was an active controlled trial conducted in previously unvaccinated young children aged ≥6 to <36 months of age who received two half vaccine doses (i.e., 7.5 μg HA/strain) 4 weeks apart.

The most frequently observed solicited local and systemic adverse events in the young children were tenderness and irritability, respectively (Table 3). Solicited local and systemic reactions were of short duration and of generally mild or moderate intensity, with few solicited adverse events reported as severe (by 1% of subjects or less).

Study J in addition to enrolling adults also included 802 pediatric and adolescent subjects who received AGRIFLU (402 aged 3 to 18 years and 400 aged 9 to 17 years). AGRIFLU was generally well tolerated in these age groups and the safety profile was consistent with that reported for healthy adults with pain, headache and myalgia being the most frequently reported solicited local and systemic reactions, respectively. Severe solicited local or systemic reactions were reported by 1% of subjects or less and were generally transient.

Post-Market Adverse Drug Reactions: AGRIFLU was first licensed in Italy in 1986 for use in persons 6 months of age and older. The authorization was extended to other European Union countries in 1998 and currently AGRIFLU is registered for marketing authorization in many countries worldwide. The initial formulation contained the preservative thimerosal, and thimerosal was also used in the manufacturing process. Since 2003 AGRIFLU is thimerosal-free (see Dosage Forms, Composition and Packaging).

The postmarketing experience with AGRIFLU is extensive. Because postmarketing reporting is voluntary and from a population of uncertain size, it is not always possible to reliably estimate their frequency or establish a causal relationship to vaccine exposure.

The adverse events described below have been included because: a) they represent reactions that are known to occur following immunizations generally or influenza immunizations specifically; b) they are potentially serious; or c) of the frequency of reporting. The following adverse reactions have been the subject of spontaneous reports during post-approval use of AGRIFLU since 2003.

General Disorders and Administration Site Conditions: local injection site reactions including pain limiting limb movement, local lymphadenopathy, asthenia, and facial edema.

Immune System Disorders: hypersensitivity reactions (including throat and/or mouth edema, anaphylaxis, and anaphylactic shock).

Vascular Disorders: vasculitis (in rare cases associated with transient renal involvement), hot flush.

Table 1: AGRIFLU

Percentage of Subjects 18-64 Years of Age Reporting Solicited Adverse Events in Days 1-4 After Vaccination with AGRIFLU

	Percentage of Subjects with Adverse Events[a]									
	Study A 2003-04 N=79	Study B 2004-05 N=67	Study C 2004-05[a] N=841	Study D 2004-05 N=80	Study E 2005-06[a] N=662	Study F 2005-06 N=64	Study G 2005-06[a] N=171	Study H 2006-07 N=92	Study I 2007-08 N=68	Study J 2007-08[a] N=460
Local Reactions										
Injection Site Pain	18	31	15	13	16	20	8	22	21	25
Erythema	0	9	15	11	11	3	18	1	4	6
Induration	6	15	6	8	6	5	11	7	10	8
Swelling	3	9	4	4	3	5	8	3	0	6
Ecchymosis	1	3	3	5	4	2	6	0	3	5
Systemic Complaints										
Fatigue	6	13	11	10	7	6	11	11	4	10
Malaise	5	6	10	9	6	3	12	5	7	12
Chills	0	3	4	3	1	3	7	2	0	5
Fever (≥38°C)	0	0	<1	0	1	0	2	1	0	2
Musculoskeletal and Connective Tissue Disorders										
Myalgia	3	12	7	11	7	9	5	7	9	14
Arthralgia	4	9	4	8	3	6	1	2	4	7
Nervous System Disorders										
Headache	10	10	10	14	5	5	9	11	10	23
Skin and Subcutaneous Disorders										
Sweating	3	9	4	8	3	9	3	5	9	5

[a] Active-controlled trials.

Table 2: AGRIFLU

Percentage of Subjects ≥65 Years of Age Reporting Solicited Adverse Events in Days 1-4 After Administration of AGRIFLU[a]

	Percentage of Subjects with Adverse Events							
	Study A 2003-04 N=33	**Study B 2004-05 N=52**	**Study C 2004-05[a] N=483**	**Study D 2004-05 N=49**	**Study E 2005-06[a] N=469**	**Study F 2005-06 N=46**	**Study H 2006-07 N=32**	**Study I 2007-08 N=57**
Local Reactions								
Injection Site Pain	0	6	3	6	5	0	9	5
Erythema	0	2	10	4	5	2	0	0
Induration	0	6	4	6	2	4	0	2
Swelling	0	8	2	4	1	2	0	0
Ecchymosis	0	2	4	0	6	4	3	2
Systemic Complaints								
Fatigue	0	6	11	4	6	2	0	7
Malaise	0	2	8	6	6	7	3	4
Chills	0	2	2	4	1	2	0	5
Fever (≥38°C)	3	0	<1	0	<1	0	0	4
Musculoskeletal and Connective Tissue Disorders								
Myalgia	0	4	6	0	2	9	3	7
Arthralgia	0	2	5	6	3	9	0	12
Nervous System Disorders								
Headache	3	4	9	6	7	4	3	5
Skin and Subcutaneous Disorders								
Sweating	0	0	7	8	3	2	0	9

[a] Active-controlled trials.

Table 3: AGRIFLU

Summary of Solicited Local and Systemic Reactions (Days 1-4)—Children and Adolescents ≥6 Months to 17 Years of Age (Studies K and J)

	Percentages of Subjects with Adverse Events					
	Study K 2005-2006			**Study J 2007-2008**		
	Children 6–<36 Months			**Children 3–8 Years**		**Adolescents 9–17 Years**
Type of Reaction	**1st vacc. N=93**	**2nd vacc. N=89**	**Type of Reaction**	**1st vacc. N=402**	**2nd vacc. N=396**	**N=400**
Local Reactions						
Ecchymosis	2	0	Ecchymosis	4	3	2
Erythema	9	4	Erythema	2	1	2
Induration	0	1	Induration	2	3	7
Swelling	0	1	Swelling	5	3	7
Tenderness	19	17	Pain	17	14	29
Systemic Reactions[a]						
Change in Eating Habits	10	9	Headache	6	3	13
Sleepiness	10	9	Malaise	3	4	4
Irritability	25	15	Fatigue	3	2	6
Unusual Crying	4	3	Myalgia	4	5	8
Vomiting	1	0	Chills	2	1	4
Diarrhoea	2	6	Arthralgia	1	1	2
Fever ≥38°C	2	2	Sweating	1	1	1
			Fever ≥38°C	2	1	<1

[a] Categories present/not present.

Gastrointestinal Disorders: abdominal pain.
Blood and Lymphatic System Disorders: transient thrombocytopenia.
Eye Disorders: conjunctivitis, eyelid edema, eye redness.
Musculoskeletal and Connective Tissue Disorders: myasthenia.

Nervous System Disorders: syncope shortly after vaccination, dizziness, neuralgia, paraesthesia, convulsion, myelitis (including encephalomyelitis and transverse myelitis), neuropathy (including neuritis and brachial plexus neuropathy), paralysis (including Bell's Palsy and other cranial nerve paralyses), Guillain Barré Syndrome.
Respiratory, Thoracic and Mediastinal Disorders: dyspnea, chest pain, cough, sore throat.
Skin and Subcutaneous Tissue Disorders: angioedema, erythema multiforme, pruritus, urticaria, rash (including non-specific, maculopapular, and vesiculobulbous), leucocytoclastic vasculitis.

DRUG INTERACTIONS: Overview: No interaction between AGRIFLU and other vaccines or medication are known.
Drug-Drug Interactions: AGRIFLU may be given at the same time as other vaccines. AGRIFLU should not be mixed with any other vaccine in the same syringe. Immunisation should be carried out on separate limbs. It should be noted that the systemic adverse reactions may be intensified.

The immunological response may be diminished if the patient is undergoing immunosuppressant treatment.

Although a possible interaction has been suggested in the literature between influenza vaccination and the use of warfarin and theophylline, clinical studies have not shown any adverse effects attributable to these drugs in people receiving influenza vaccine.

DOSAGE AND ADMINISTRATION: Recommended Dose and Dosage Adjustment: Children From 6 to 35 Months: Children in this age group may receive one intramuscular dose of 0.25 mL. For children in this age group who have not previously been vaccinated, a second intramuscular dose should be given after an interval of at least 4 weeks.
Children From 3 to 8 Years: Children in this age group should receive a single intramuscular dose of 0.5 mL if they have been vaccinated previously with any influenza vaccine. For children who have not previously been vaccinated, a second intramuscular dose of 0.5 mL should be given with an interval of at least 4 weeks.
Children From 9 years and Adults: A single intramuscular dose of 0.5 mL should be administered.
Administration: Shake the contents of each syringe to aid inspection for the presence of particulate matter. If this condition exists, do not use the contents. Do not use the vaccine if it has been frozen.

The vaccine should be allowed to reach room temperature before use.

Before immunization, the skin over the site to be injected should be cleansed with a suitable germicide.

Do not inject intravascularly. AGRIFLU should be administered by intramuscular injection. The recommended site of vaccination is the deltoid muscle for adults and older children, and the anterolateral aspect of the thigh for infants and young children. The vaccine should not be injected in the gluteal region or areas where there may be a major nerve trunk.
Administration with Other Vaccines: AGRIFLU should not be mixed with other vaccines in the same syringe. Separate injection limbs should be used if more than one vaccine is being administered during the same visit.

OVERDOSAGE:

> For management of a suspected drug overdose, contact your regional Poison Control Centre. See the *CPS Directory* section for a list of Poison Control Centres.

ACTION AND CLINICAL PHARMACOLOGY: Mechanism of Action: Influenza illness and its complications follow infection with influenza viruses. Global surveillance of influenza identifies yearly antigenic variants. For example, since 1977, antigenic variants of influenza A (H1N1 and H3N2) viruses and influenza B viruses have been in global circulation. Specific levels of hemagglutination inhibition (HI) antibody titers induced by vaccination with inactivated influenza virus vaccine have not been correlated with protection from influenza illness. In some human studies, HI antibody titers of 1:40 or greater have been associated with protection from influenza illness in up to 50% of subjects.

Antibody against one influenza virus type or subtype confers limited or no protection against another. Furthermore, antibody to one antigenic variant of influenza virus might not protect against a new antigenic variant of the same type or subtype. Frequent development of antigenic variants through antigenic drift is the virologic basis for seasonal epidemics and the reason for the usual change of one or more new strains in each year's influenza vaccine. Therefore, inactivated influenza vaccines are standardized to contain the hemagglutinin of influenza virus strains (typically two type A and one type B), representing the influenza viruses likely to be circulating in Canada during the upcoming flu season, on the basis of the recommendations from the World Health Organization (WHO) and the National Advisory Committee on Immunization (NACI).

Annual revaccination with the current vaccine is recommended because immunity declines during the year after vaccination, and because circulating strains of influenza virus change from year to year.
Pharmacodynamics: Seroprotection is generally obtained within 2 to 3 weeks after vaccination.

Duration of Effect: The duration of post vaccination immunity to homologous strains or to strains closely related to the vaccine strains varies. Data from clinical studies with AGRIFLU indicated that the acceptable level of immune response was maintained up to 12 months after vaccination.

STORAGE AND STABILITY: Store AGRIFLU between +2 and +8°C. Do not freeze. Protect from light. Under the above storage conditions, the recommended shelf-life for AGRIFLU is 1 year. Do not use vaccine after expiration date.

INFORMATION FOR THE PATIENT: Published in e-CPS, available by subscription at www.e-cps.ca.

DOSAGE FORMS, COMPOSITION AND PACKAGING: Each 0.5 mL dose of sterile clear aqueous suspension for intramuscular injection contains: 15 µg per strain of haemagglutinin of influenza virus surface antigens, of each following strain: A/California/7/2009 (H1N1)-like virus; A/Perth/16/2009 (H3N2)-like virus; and B/Brisbane/60/2008-like virus. Nonmedicinal ingredients: calcium chloride, disodium phosphate dihydrate, magnesium chloride, potassium chloride, potassium dihydrogen phosphate, sodium chloride and water for injections. The vaccine may contain trace amounts of: barium (residual), citrates (residual), egg proteins (residual), formaldehyde (residual), kanamycin, neomycin, ovalbumin (residual) and polysorbate 80 or cetyltrimethylammonium bromide (CTAB) (residual). Single dose pre-filled glass syringes (Type I) of 0.5 mL, packages of 1 and 10. The syringe plunger does not contain latex. The syringe may be fitted alternatively with a Luer Lock system. AGRIFLU contains no thimerosal or other preservative. No thimerosal is used during the manufacture of AGRIFLU.

Agrylin® Ⓟ

anagrelide HCl

Platelet-reducing Agent

Shire

Date of Revision: July 9, 2010

SUMMARY PRODUCT INFORMATION:

Route of Administration	Dosage Form/Strength	Nonmedicinal Ingredients
Oral	Capsule 0.5 mg	Crospovidone, black iron oxide, gelatine, lactose anhydrous, lactose monohydrate, magnesium stearate, microcrystalline cellulose, povidone, silicone dioxide, sodium lauryl sulphate, titanium dioxide

INDICATIONS AND CLINICAL USE: AGRYLIN (anagrelide hydrochloride) capsules are indicated for:

- treatment of patients with thrombocythemia secondary to myeloproliferative disorders to reduce the elevated platelet count and the risk of thrombosis and to ameliorate associated symptoms, including thrombo-hemorrhagic events.

AGRYLIN is intended for chronic usage and has not been evaluated for treatment of the acute life threatening complications of thrombocytosis.

Geriatrics (>65 years of age): The safety and effectiveness of AGRYLIN have not been evaluated in studies specific to the elderly.

Pediatrics (<16 years of age): The safety and efficacy of AGRYLIN in patients under the age of 16 years have not been established.

CONTRAINDICATIONS:

- Patients who are hypersensitive to this drug or to any ingredient in the formulation or component of the container. For a complete listing, see Dosage Forms, Composition and Packaging.
- Anagrelide is contraindicated in patients with severe hepatic impairment. Use of anagrelide in patients with severe hepatic impairment has not been studied. Anagrelide must be used with caution in patients with moderate hepatic impairment as exposure to anagrelide is increased 8-fold in such patients (see Action and Clinical Pharmacology and Warnings and Precautions, Hepatic/Biliary/Pancreatic).

WARNINGS AND PRECAUTIONS: General: The decision to treat asymptomatic young adults with thrombocythemia secondary to myeloproliferative disorders should be individualized.

Sudden discontinuation or interruption of AGRYLIN (anagrelide hydrochloride) treatment is followed by an increase in platelet count. Following discontinuation, an increase in platelet count can be observed within four days.

Carcinogenesis and Mutagenesis: In a two-year rat carcinogenicity study, a higher incidence of uterine adenocarcinoma, relative to controls, was observed in females receiving the dose of 30 mg/kg/day (at least 174 times human AUC exposure after a 1 mg twice daily dose). Adrenal benign and malignant phaeochromocytomas were increased relative to controls in males at all dose levels (receiving 3 mg/kg/day and above), and in females receiving the doses of 10 and 30 mg/kg/day (at least 10 and 18 times respectively human AUC exposure after a 1 mg twice daily dose).

Anagrelide produced no detectable or reproducible increases in gene mutational activity in studies conducted in vitro with mutant strains of *S. typhimurium* in the Ames test, or in a mouse lymphoma mutagenesis assay, with or without a rat hepatic drug metabolising enzyme system.

In addition, no clastogenic activity was seen in vitro using cultured human peripheral lymphocytes or in vivo in a mouse bone marrow erythrocyte micronucleus assay. At the concentrations and doses employed in these studies, there was no indication that anagrelide was a potential mutagen either directly or after metabolic activation.

Cardiovascular: AGRYLIN should be used with caution in patients with known or suspected heart disease, and only if the potential benefits of therapy outweigh the potential risks. Because of the positive inotropic effects and side-effects of AGRYLIN, a pre-treatment cardiovascular examination is recommended along with careful monitoring during treatment. In humans, therapeutic doses of AGRYLIN may cause cardiovascular effects, including vasodilation, tachycardia, palpitations, and congestive heart failure.

Hepatic/Biliary/Pancreatic: Hepatic metabolism represents the major route of anagrelide clearance and liver function may therefore be expected to influence this process. AGRYLIN has not been studied in patients with severe hepatic impairment and is contraindicated (see Contraindications). Exposure to anagrelide is increased 8-fold in patients with moderate hepatic impairment (see Action and Clinical Pharmacology). It is recommended that patients with mild and moderate hepatic impairment receive AGRYLIN only if, in the physician's judgment, the potential benefits of therapy outweigh the potential risks. Patients with mild or moderate hepatic impairment should be carefully and regularly monitored for cardiovascular effects and hepatic toxicity while receiving AGRYLIN (see Warnings and Precautions,Cardiovascular and Adverse Reactions). In patients with moderate hepatic impairment, a dosage reduction is required (see Dosage and Administration, Recommended Dose and Dosage Adjustment).

Respiratory: Interstitial Lung Diseases: Interstitial lung diseases (including allergic alveolitis, eosinophilic pneumonia and interstitial pneumonitis) have been reported to be associated with the use of anagrelide in post-marketing reports. Most cases presented with progressive dyspnea associated with lung infiltrations. The time of onset ranges from 1 week to several years after initiating anagrelide. In most cases, the symptoms improved after discontinuation of anagrelide (see Adverse Reactions, Post-Market Adverse Drug Reactions).

Renal: It is recommended that patients with renal insufficiency (creatinine ≥2 mg/dL) receive AGRYLIN when, in the physician's judgment, the potential benefits of therapy outweigh the potential risks. These patients should be monitored closely for signs of renal toxicity while receiving AGRYLIN (see Adverse Reactions, Urogenital).

Special Populations: Pregnant Women: There are no adequate and well-controlled studies in pregnant women. AGRYLIN should be used during pregnancy only if the potential benefit justifies the potential risk to the foetus.

AGRYLIN is not recommended in women who are or may become pregnant. If this drug is used during pregnancy, or if the patient becomes pregnant while taking this drug, the patient should be apprised of the potential harm to the foetus. Women of child-bearing potential should be instructed that they must not be pregnant and that they should use contraception while taking AGRYLIN. AGRYLIN may cause foetal harm when administered to a pregnant woman.

Nursing Women: It is not known whether this drug is excreted in human milk. Because many drugs are excreted in human milk and because of the potential for serious adverse reaction in nursing infants from AGRYLIN, a decision should be made whether to discontinue nursing or to discontinue the drug, taking into account the importance of the drug to the mother.

Geriatrics (>65 years of age): Pharmacokinetic differences between elderly and younger patients with essential thrombocythemia (ET) have been observed (see Action and Clinical Pharmacology, Special Populations and Conditions, Geriatrics, and Dosage and Administration).

Pediatrics (<16 years of age): The safety and efficacy of AGRYLIN in patients under the age of 16 years have not been established. Myeloproliferative disorders are uncommon in pediatric patients and limited data are available in this population. An open-label study conducted in 17 pediatric patients 7-14 years of age and 18 adult patients (67% of which were elderly patients, i.e., 65 years of age and older) with essential thrombocythemia indicated that dose and body weight-normalized exposure, C_{max} and AUC of anagrelide were lower in children/adolescents compared to adults (C_{max} 48%, AUC_t 55%) (see Action and Clinical Pharmacology, Pharmacokinetics). AGRYLIN should be used in this patient group with caution.

Monitoring and Laboratory Tests: AGRYLIN therapy requires close clinical supervision of the patient. To monitor the effect of AGRYLIN and prevent the occurrence of thrombocytopenia, platelet counts should be performed every two days during the first week of treatment and at least weekly thereafter, until the maintenance dosage is reached. Typically, platelet count begins to respond within 7 to 14 days at the proper dosage. The time to complete response, defined as platelet count ≤600 000/µL, ranged from 4 to 12 weeks. Most patients will experience an adequate response at a dose of 1.5 to 3.0 mg/day. In case of overdose, close clinical supervision of the patient is required, including monitoring of the platelet count for thrombocytopenia. Dosage should be decreased or stopped as appropriate, until platelet count returns to within the normal range. However, in patients with hepatic insufficiency or renal insufficiency, liver function and kidney function tests should be performed at least once per month or when deemed necessary in the physician's judgement.

As cases of hepatitis have been reported from post-marketing surveillance, it is recommended that liver functions tests are performed before anagrelide treatment is initiated and at regular intervals thereafter.

ADVERSE REACTIONS: Adverse Drug Reaction Overview: Analysis of the adverse events in a population consisting of 942 patients diagnosed with myeloproliferative diseases of varying etiology [Essential Thrombocythemia (ET): 551; Polycythemia Vera (PV): 117; other myeloproliferative disorders (OMPD): 274] has shown that all disease groups have the same adverse event profile. While most reported adverse events during AGRYLIN (anagrelide hydrochloride) therapy have been mild in intensity and have decreased in frequency with continued therapy, serious adverse events reported were reported in these patients. These include the following: congestive heart failure, myocardial infarction, cardiomyopathy, cardiomegaly, complete heart block, atrial fibrillation, cerebrovascular accident, pericarditis, pericardial effusion, pleural effusion, pulmonary infiltrates, pulmonary fibrosis, pulmonary hypertension, pancreatitis, gastric/duodenal ulceration, and seizure.

The mean duration of AGRYLIN therapy for ET, PV, Chronic Myelogenous Leukemia (CML) and OMPD patients was 65, 67, 40 and 44 weeks, respectively. Of the 942 patients treated with AGRYLIN, 161 (17%) were discontinued from the study because of adverse events or abnormal laboratory test results. The most common adverse events for treatment discontinuation were headache, diarrhea, edema, palpitation, and abdominal pain. Overall, the occurrence rate of all adverse events was 17.9 per 1000 treatment days. The occurrence rate of adverse events increased at higher dosages of AGRYLIN.

Clinical Trial Adverse Drug Reactions: Because clinical trials are conducted under very specific conditions the adverse reaction rates observed in the clinical trials may not reflect the rates observed in practice and should not be compared to the rates in the clinical trials of another drug. Adverse drug reaction information from clinical trials is useful for identifying drug-related adverse events and for approximating rates.

The most frequently reported adverse reactions to AGRYLIN (in 5% or greater of 942 patients with myeloproliferative disease) in clinical trials are included in Table 1.

Table 1: AGRYLIN

Adverse Events with an Incidence of ≥5%

	AGRYLIN
Body as a Whole	Headache (43.5%)
	Asthenia (23.1%)
	Abdominal Pain (16.5%)
	Pain, other (15.0%)
	Fever (8.9%)
	Chest Pain (8.0%)
	Malaise (6.4%)
	Back Pain (5.9%)
Cardiovascular	Palpitations (26.1%)
	Tachycardia (7.5%)
Digestive	Diarrhea (25.7%)
	Nausea (17.1%)
	Flatulence (10.2%)
	Vomiting (9.7%)
	Anorexia (7.7%)
	Dyspepsia (5.2%)
Metabolic	Edema, other (20.6%)
	Peripheral Edema (8.5%)
Nervous	Dizziness (15.4%)
	Paresthesia (5.9%)
Respiratory	Dyspnea (11.9%)
	Pharyngitis (6.8%)
	Cough (6.3%)
Skin and Appendages	Pruritus (5.5%)
	Rash, including urticaria (8.3%)

Table 2: AGRYLIN

Adverse Events with an Incidence of 1% to <5%

	AGRYLIN
Body as a Whole	Chills, flu symptoms, infection, neck pain, accidental injury, photosensitivity, cellulites.
Cardiovascular	Arrhythmia, hemorrhage, cardiovascular disease, angina pectoris, heart failure, congestive heart failure, vasodilatation, postural hypotension, migraine, syncope, hypotension, thrombosis, hypertension.

(cont'd)

Table 2: AGRYLIN *(cont'd)*

Adverse Events with an Incidence of 1% to <5%

	AGRYLIN
Digestive	Constipation, GI hemorrhage, GI distress, melena, nausea and vomiting, gastritis, dysphagia, eructation, dry mouth.
Hemic and Lymphatic	Anemia, thrombocytopenia, ecchymosis, lymphadenoma. Platelet counts below 100 000/μL occurred in 84 patients (ET: 35; PV: 9; OMPD: 40) and reduction below 50 000/μL occurred in 44 patients (ET: 7; PV: 6; OMPD: 31) while on AGRYLIN therapy. Thrombocytopenia promptly recovered upon discontinuation of AGRYLIN.
Hepatic	Elevated liver enzymes were observed in 3 patients (ET: 2; OMPD: 1) during AGRYLIN therapy.
Musculoskeletal	Arthralgia, myalgia, leg cramps, arthritis, bone pain.
Nervous	Depression, somnolence, insomnia, confusion, nervousness, amnesia.
Nutritional Disorders	Weight loss, weight gain, oedema, dehydration.
Respiratory	Rhinitis, epistaxis, respiratory disease, sinusitis, pneumonia, bronchitis, asthma.
Skin and Appendages	Sweating, skin disease, alopecia, skin ulcer, skin discoloration.
Special Senses	Amblyopia, abnormal vision, ear disorder, conjunctivitis, visual field abnormality, tinnitus, eye disorder, diplopia.
Urogenital	Urinary tract disorder, urinary frequency, hematuria, urinary tract infection, dysuria, nocturia, urinary incontinence.

Renal abnormalities occurred in 15 patients (ET: 10; PV: 4; OMPD: 1). Six ET, 4 PV and 1 with OMPD experienced renal failure (approximately 1%) while on AGRYLIN treatment; in 4 cases, the renal failure was considered to be possibly related to AGRYLIN treatment. The remaining 11 were found to have pre-existing renal impairment and were successfully treated with AGRYLIN. Doses ranged from 1.5-6.0 mg/day, with exposure periods of 2 to 12 months. No dose adjustment was required because of renal insufficiency.

Post-Market Adverse Drug Reactions: In individual case reports, a causal relationship has been established between acute pulmonary reactions (severe hypersensitivity pneumonia "allergic alveolitis", pulmonary infiltrates/fibrosis, and dyspnea) and the use of anagrelide. AGRYLIN should be discontinued in patients showing acute pulmonary reactions. Congestive heart failure, cardiomyopathy and myocardial infarction have occurred in a small number of patients with the use of anagrelide. Hepatitis has also been reported in patients who have taken anagrelide treatment. The incidence of these events is not known.

DRUG INTERACTIONS: Overview: Anagrelide is an inhibitor of cyclic AMP PDE III. The effects of medicinal products with similar properties, such as the inotrope milrinone, may be exacerbated by anagrelide.

Drug-Drug Interactions: Limited pharmacokinetic and/or pharmacodynamic studies investigating possible interactions between anagrelide and other medicinal products have been conducted. In vivo interaction studies in humans have demonstrated that digoxin and warfarin do not affect the PK properties of anagrelide, nor does anagrelide affect the PK properties of digoxin or warfarin.

Apart from acetylsalicylic acid discussed further below, additional drug interaction studies have not been conducted, with the other most common medications used concomitantly with AGRYLIN (anagrelide hydrochloride) in clinical trials, which were acetaminophen, furosemide, iron, ranitidine, hydroxyurea, and allopurinol. The most frequently used concomitant cardiac medication has been digoxin. There is no clinical evidence to suggest that AGRYLIN interacts with any of these compounds.

Anagrelide is metabolized at least in part by CYP1A2. It is known that CYP1A2 is inhibited by several medicinal products, including fluvoxamine, and such medicinal products could theoretically adversely influence the clearance of anagrelide and its active metabolite BCH24426. Anagrelide demonstrates some limited inhibitory activity towards CYP1A2 which may present a theoretical potential for interaction with other co-administered medicinal products sharing that clearance mechanism e.g. theophylline. Drug-drug interactions with CYP1A2 substrates and inhibitors cannot be excluded.

There is a single case report which suggests that sucralfate may interfere with AGRYLIN absorption.

Two clinical interaction studies in healthy subjects, a single-dose study of co-administered anagrelide 1 mg and acetylsalicylic acid 900 mg and a repeat-dose dose study of co-administered anagrelide 1 mg once daily and acetylsalicylic acid 75 mg once daily, demonstrated greater anti-platelet aggregation effects than administration of acetylsalicylic acid alone. In the repeat-dose study, anagrelide alone had no effect on platelet aggregation, but did slightly enhance the inhibition of platelet aggregation by acetylsalicylic acid. There was a short-lived decrease in platelet aggregation beyond the effects of acetylsalicylic acid alone for the first 2 hours after administration. The clinical relevance of this interaction in essential thrombocythemia patients is unknown.

Co-administered anagrelide 1 mg and acetylsalicylic acid 900 mg single-dose was generally well tolerated. There was no effect on bleeding time, prothrombin time (PT) or activated partial thromboplastin time (aPTT). No clinically relevant pharmacokinetic interactions between anagrelide and acetylsalicylic acid were observed. In that same study, acetylsalicylic acid alone produced a marked inhibition in platelet aggregation ex vivo.

The potential risks and benefits of the concomitant use of anagrelide with acetylsalicylic acid should be assessed, particularly in patients with a high risk profile for haemorrhage and/or with a platelet count greater than 1000×10^9/L before treatment is commenced. The clinical relevance of the interaction between anagrelide and acetylsalicylic acid in essential thrombocythemia patients is unknown.

Drug-Food Interactions: Food decreased the C_{max} of anagrelide by 14%, but increased the $AUC_{0-\infty}$ by 20%. For both parameters, the exposure after food was not equivalent to that in the fasted state. Food decreased the C_{max} of the active metabolite BCH24426 by 29%, but had no effect on the $AUC_{0-\infty}$. The most marked effects of food were evident in a longer time lag before absorption (or appearance, in the case of BCH24426), a slower rate of absorption and a later time of peak for plasma concentration of both anagrelide and BCH24426.

Grapefruit juice has been shown to inhibit CYP1A2 and therefore could also reduce the clearance of anagrelide.

Drug-Herb Interactions: Interactions with herbal products have not been established.

Drug-Laboratory Test Interactions: Interactions with laboratory tests have not been established.

DOSAGE AND ADMINISTRATION: Recommended Dose and Dosage Adjustment: Treatment with AGRYLIN (anagrelide hydrochloride) Capsules should be initiated under close medical supervision. The recommended starting dosage of AGRYLIN is 0.5 mg qid or 1 mg bid, which should be maintained for at least one week. Dosage should then be adjusted to the lowest effective dosage required to reduce and maintain platelet count below 600 000/μL, and ideally to the normal range. The dosage should be increased by not more than 0.5 mg/day in any one week. Dosage should not exceed 10 mg/day or 2.5 mg in a single dose (see Warnings and Precautions, Monitoring and Laboratory Tests). The decision to treat asymptomatic young adults with thrombocythemia secondary to myeloproliferative disorders should be individualized.

It is recommended that patients with moderate hepatic impairment start anagrelide therapy at a dose of 0.5 mg/day and be maintained for a minimum of one week with careful and regular monitoring of cardiovascular effects and hepatic toxicity. The dosage increment must not exceed more than 0.5 mg/day in any one-week. The potential risks and benefits of anagrelide therapy in a patient with mild and moderate impairment of hepatic function should be assessed before treatment is commenced. Use of anagrelide in patients with severe hepatic impairment has not been studied. Use of anagrelide in patients with severe hepatic impairment is contraindicated (see Contraindications).

The observed pharmacokinetic differences between the elderly and younger patients with ET would not be expected to require alteration of the recommended dosing regimen of AGRYLIN (see Action and Clinical Pharmacology, Special Populations and Conditions, Geriatrics).

To monitor the effect of AGRYLIN and prevent the occurrence of thrombocytopenia, platelet counts should be performed every two days during the first week of treatment and at least weekly thereafter until the maintenance dosage is reached.

Typically, platelet count begins to respond within 7 to 14 days at the proper dosage. The time to complete response, defined as platelet count ≤600 000/μL, ranged from 4 to 12 weeks. Most patients will experience an adequate response at a dose of 1.5 to 3.0 mg/day. Patients with known or suspected heart disease, renal insufficiency, or hepatic dysfunction should be monitored closely.

OVERDOSAGE:

Acute Toxicity and Symptoms: There have been a small number of post-marketing case reports of intentional overdose with AGRYLIN (anagrelide hydrochloride). Reported symptoms include sinus tachycardia and vomiting. Symptoms resolved with conservative management. Platelet reduction from AGRYLIN therapy is dose related; therefore, thrombocytopenia, which can potentially cause bleeding, is expected from overdosage. Should overdosage occur, cardiac, and central nervous system toxicity can also be expected.

Management and Treatment: In case of overdosage, close clinical supervision of the patient is required; this especially includes monitoring of the platelet count for thrombocytopenia. Dosage should be decreased or stopped, as appropriate, until the platelet count returns to within the normal range.

> For management of a suspected drug overdose, contact your regional Poison Control Centre. See the *CPS* Directory section for a list of Poison Control Centres.

ACTION AND CLINICAL PHARMACOLOGY: Mechanism of Action: The mechanism by which AGRYLIN (anagrelide hydrochloride) reduces blood platelet count is still under investigation. Studies in patients support a hypothesis of dose-related reduction in platelet production resulting from a decrease in megakaryocyte hypermaturation. In blood withdrawn from normal volunteers treated with anagrelide, a disruption was found in the postmitotic phase of megakaryocyte development and a reduction in megakaryocyte size and ploidy. At therapeutic doses anagrelide does not produce significant changes in white cell counts or coagulation parameters, and may have a small, but clinically insignificant effect on red cell parameters.

Anagrelide was shown to inhibit phosphodiesterase III found in platelets and as a result raises cAMP levels, which in turn may explain the inhibitory effect on platelet aggregation. Platelet aggregation is inhibited in humans at doses higher than those required to reduce platelet count. Two major metabolites, one active and one inactive, have been identified. The active metabolite, BCH24426 or 3-hydroxy anagrelide, shows similar potency and efficacy than anagrelide in the platelet lowering effect. Exposure as measured by plasma AUC is approximately 2-fold higher for 3-hydroxy anagrelide (BCH24426) compared to anagrelide. The inactive metabolite, RL603 or 5,6-dichloro-3,4-dihydroquinazolin-2-ylamine, does not participate in the overall affect of AGRYLIN.

Pharmacodynamics: Oral administration of single and multiple doses of anagrelide in healthy volunteers caused dose-related reductions in platelet count during treatment. In addition, dose-related reductions occur in platelet aggregation. These effects were reversible following cessation of treatment. No clinically important changes in other study variables were noted, i.e., bleeding time, platelet survival time, bone marrow morphology, blood pressure, pulse rate, urinalysis, and EKG. Anagrelide is well tolerated at low doses. A 5 mg dose caused orthostatic hypotension and dizziness in healthy volunteers; doses of 1 to 2 mg/day were tolerable.

In most cases, the incidence of adverse effects is dose-related, intensity is mild, duration is transient, and treatment is unnecessary.

In 9 subjects receiving a single 5-mg dose of anagrelide, standing blood pressure decreased an average of 22/15 mm Hg, usually accompanied by dizziness. Only minimal changes in blood pressure were observed following a dose of 2 mg.

Pharmacological evaluation of anagrelide and its metabolites showed that 3-hydroxy anagrelide (BCH24426) had a comparable inhibitory effect to the parent drug on megakaryocytopoiesis—and therefore platelet formation—while RL603 was inactive. Anagrelide and 3-hydroxy anagrelide (BCH24426) were also found to be inhibitors of PDEIII although 3-hydroxy anagrelide (BCH24426) was almost forty times more potent than the parent drug while RL603 was again virtually inactive.

Pharmacokinetics: Absorption: Single oral-dose administration of either 1 or 2 mg of anagrelide resulted in C_{max} values ranging between 7 and 13 ng/mL, about 1 hour after administration.

Pharmacokinetic data obtained from healthy subjects comparing the pharmacokinetics of anagrelide in the fed and fasted states showed that administration of a 1 mg dose of anagrelide with food decreased the C_{max} by 14%, but increased the AUC by 20%. For both parameters, the exposure after food was not equivalent to that in the fasted state. Food decreased the C_{max} of the active metabolite BCH24426 by 29%, but had no effect on the $AUC_{0-\infty}$. The most marked effects of food were evident in a longer time lag before absorption (or appearance, in the case of BCH24426), a slower rate of absorption and a later time of peak for plasma concentration of both anagrelide and BCH24426.

Distribution: The available plasma concentration time data at the steady state in patients showed no evidence of anagrelide accumulation in plasma after repeated administration. Long-term oral administration (≥2 months to >5 years) of anagrelide at doses of 2 to 4 mg/day resulted in plasma levels within the range expected after a single dose.

Metabolism: The drug is extensively metabolized; less than 1% is recovered in the urine as anagrelide. At fasting and at a dose of 0.5 mg of anagrelide, the plasma half-life is 1.3 hours.

Excretion: Following oral administration of ^{14}C-anagrelide in humans, more than 70% of the radioactivity was recovered in urine. Urinary excretion was monophasic, while the plasma half-life of anagrelide was in the range of 1 to 2 hours. This pharmacokinetic half-life is consistent with the clinical dose frequency of 2 to 4 times per day. The plasma half-life of the pharmacologically active metabolite, 3-hydroxy anagrelide (BCH24426), was approximately 3 hours.

There was a statistically greater amount of anagrelide metabolite excreted in the urine during the 24-hour period after fasted administration of anagrelide, compared to after the fed state. These differences, however, were not considered to be clinically significant.

Long-term oral administration (≥2 months to >5 years) of anagrelide at doses of 2 to 4 mg/day resulted in mean excretion values for the major metabolite in the 24-hour urine sample similar to those values obtained following single oral-dose administration of 0.5 mg of anagrelide.

Special Populations and Conditions: Geriatrics: Pharmacokinetic data from fasting elderly patients with ET (age range 65-75 years) compared to fasting adult patients (age range 22-50 years) indicate that the C_{max} and AUC of anagrelide were 36% and 61% higher respectively in elderly patients, but that the C_{max} and AUC of the active metabolite, 3-hydroxy anagrelide, were 42% and 37% lower respectively in the elderly patients. These differences were likely caused by lower presystemic metabolism of anagrelide to 3-hydroxy anagrelide in the elderly patients.

Pediatrics: An open-label study conducted in 17 pediatric patients 7-14 years of age and 18 adult patients (67% of which were elderly patients, i.e., 65 years of age and older) with essential thrombocythemia indicated that dose and body weight-normalized exposure, C_{max} and AUC of anagrelide were lower in children/adolescents compared to adults (C_{max} 48%, AUC 55%).

Table 3: AGRYLIN

Summary of PK Parameters for Anagrelide and Metabolites in Adolescent/Adult and Pediatric/Adolescent Subjects on 0.5 mg bid Regimen

PK Parameter	Anagrelide AA (n=4) Mean (SD)	Anagrelide PA (n=4–6) Mean (SD)	BCH24426 AA (n=4) Mean (SD)	BCH24426 PA (n=4–6) Mean (SD)
T_{max} (h)	1.9 (1.5)	3.9 (3.1)	2.4 (1.1)	4.0 (3.1)
C_{max} (ng/mL)	3.1 (1.3)	1.9 (0.6)	4.5 (1.8)	5.5 (2.8)
C_{min} (ng/mL)	0	0.03 (0.04)	0.2 (0.1)	0.4 (0.2)
AUC (ng·h/mL)	8.6 (3.3)	8.2 (3.3)	19.9 (3.7)	24.4 (8.3)
$T_{½z}$ (h)	1.5 (0.5)	3.9 (3.7)	2.8 (0.7)	4.2 (1.6)
C_{avg} (ng/mL)	0.7 (0.3)	0.7 (0.3)	1.7 (0.3)	2.0 (1.7)
FI	4.3 (1.0)	3.2 (2.2)	2.5 (0.6)	1.1 (0.9)

(cont'd)

Table 3: AGRYLIN *(cont'd)*

Summary of PK Parameters for Anagrelide and Metabolites in Adolescent/Adult and Pediatric/Adolescent Subjects on 0.5 mg bid Regimen

PK Parameter	Anagrelide		BCH24426	
	AA (n=4) Mean (SD)	PA (n=4–6) Mean (SD)	AA (n=4) Mean (SD)	PA (n=4–6) Mean (SD)
Cl/F (mL/min)	1062 (315)	1169 (465)	429 (71)	1004 (455)

Legend: AA=adolescent/adult subject group; PA=pediatric/adolescent subject group.

Hepatic Insufficiency: Hepatic metabolism represents the major route of anagrelide clearance and liver function is expected to influence this process. Accordingly, an open label pharmacokinetic study has been performed on subjects with moderate hepatic impairment (and otherwise healthy) vs. healthy subjects. A single dose of 1 mg anagrelide was administered to each individual. Though a limited number of patients were enrolled for the study, the results show that $AUC_{0-\infty}$ was nearly 8 times higher in subjects with moderate hepatic impairment (n=10) than in healthy subjects (n=10). A strong correlation has been established between the AUC measurements and the Child-Pugh Score (indicator of hepatic impairment severity). Pharmacokinetic measurements performed on 3-hydroxy anagrelide (BCH24426, the active metabolite of anagrelide) and RL603 (the inactive metabolite of anagrelide) show approximately a doubling of AUC in patients with moderate hepatic impairment as compared to healthy subjects. No study has been performed either on patients with severe or on patients with mild hepatic impairment, therefore, no data are available.

STORAGE AND STABILITY: Store from 15 to 25°C in a light-resistant container.

INFORMATION FOR THE PATIENT: Published in e-CPS, available by subscription at www.e-cps.ca.

DOSAGE FORMS, COMPOSITION AND PACKAGING: Each white, opaque capsule, imprinted with Shire logo "S" and "063" in black ink, contains: anagrelide 0.5 mg as anagrelide hydrochloride. Nonmedicinal ingredients: black iron oxide, crospovidone, gelatine, lactose anhydrous, lactose monohydrate, magnesium stearate, microcrystalline cellulose, povidone, silicon dioxide, sodium lauryl sulfate and titanium oxide. Bottles of 100.

(Shown in Product Identification Section)

Airomir™

salbutamol sulfate

Bronchodilator—Beta2-adrenergic Stimulant

Graceway

PHARMACOLOGY: Salbutamol produces bronchodilation through stimulation of β_2-adrenergic receptors in bronchial smooth muscle, thereby causing relaxation of bronchial muscle fibers. This action results in improved pulmonary function as demonstrated by spirometric measurements. At therapeutic doses, salbutamol has little action on the β_1-adrenergic receptors in cardiac muscle.

Clinical experience has shown that inhaled salbutamol, like other β-adrenergic agonists, can produce significant cardiovascular effects in some patients, as measured by pulse rate, blood pressure and/or ECG changes. Other effects common to this class of drugs and probably mediated by β-adrenoreceptors are tremor and hypokalemia.

The time to onset of a 15% increase in FEV_1 is 5 to 15 minutes after inhalation of salbutamol and the time to peak effect occurs within 60 to 90 minutes. The mean duration of effect as measured by a 15% increase in FEV_1 is about 3 hours. In some patients, duration of effect is as long as 6 hours.

INDICATIONS: For the symptomatic relief and prevention of bronchospasm due to bronchial asthma, chronic bronchitis and other chronic bronchopulmonary disorders in patients in whom reversible bronchospasm is a complicating factor. In addition, salbutamol inhalation aerosol is indicated for the prevention of exercise-induced asthma.

CONTRAINDICATIONS: In patients hypersensitive to salbutamol or any of the components in the Airomir Inhalation Aerosol (see Supplied).

WARNINGS: Use of Anti-inflammatory Agents: In accordance with the present practice for asthma treatment, concomitant anti-inflammatory therapy (e.g., corticosteroids) should be part of the regimen if inhaled salbutamol needs to be used on a regular daily basis (see Dosage). It is essential that the physician instruct the patient in the need for further evaluation if the patient's asthma becomes worse.

Cardiovascular Effects: In individual patients, any β_2-adrenergic agonist, including salbutamol, may have a clinically significant cardiac effect. Care should be taken with patients suffering from cardiovascular disorders, especially coronary insufficiency, cardiac arrhythmias, and hypertension. Special care and supervision are required in patients with idiopathic hypertrophic subvalvular aortic stenosis, in whom an increase in the pressure gradient between the left ventricle and the aorta may occur, causing increased strain on the left ventricle.

Paradoxical Bronchospasm: With repeated excessive use of sympathomimetic inhalation preparations, some patients have been reported to have developed severe paradoxical bronchospasm, occasionally leading to death. The cause of either the refractory state or death is unknown. However, it is suspected in the fatal episodes that cardiac arrest occurred following the unexpected development of a severe acute asthmatic crisis and subsequent hypoxia.

Do Not Exceed the Recommended Dose: Fatalities have been reported in association with excessive use of inhaled sympathomimetic drugs. The exact cause of death is unknown, but cardiac arrest following the unexpected development of a severe acute asthmatic crisis and subsequent hypoxia is suspected.

Immediate Hypersensitivity Reactions: Immediate hypersensitivity reactions may occur after administration of salbutamol inhalation aerosol, as demonstrated by rare cases of urticaria, angioedema, rash, bronchospasm, anaphylaxis, and oropharyngeal edema.

Patients with Special Diseases and Conditions: Care should be taken in patients with convulsive disorders, hyperthyroidism, or in patients who are unusually responsive to sympathomimetic amines.

PRECAUTIONS: General: If salbutamol therapy does not produce a significant improvement or if the patient's condition worsens, medical advice must be sought to determine a new plan of treatment. In the case of acute or rapidly worsening dyspnea, a physician should be consulted immediately.

Failure to respond for at least 3 hours to a previously effective dose of salbutamol indicates a deterioration of the condition and the physician should be contacted promptly. Patients should be warned not to exceed the recommended dose. Increasing use of β_2-agonists to control symptoms is usually a sign of worsening asthma. In worsening asthma it is inadequate to increase β_2-agonist use only, especially over an extended period of time. Instead, a reassessment of the patient's therapy plan is required and concomitant anti-inflammatory therapy should be considered (see Dosage).

Geriatrics: As with other β_2-agonists, special caution should be observed when using salbutamol in elderly patients who have concomitant cardiovascular disease that could be adversely affected by this class of drug.

Children: Safety and effectiveness in children below the age of 6 years have not been established.

Pregnancy: Salbutamol has been in widespread use for many years in human beings without apparent ill consequence. However, there are no adequate or well-controlled studies in pregnant women, and there is little published evidence of its safety in the early stages of human pregnancy. Administration of any drug to pregnant women should only be considered if the anticipated benefits to the expectant woman are greater than any possible risks to the fetus.

A reproduction study in rats was performed with salbutamol inhalation aerosol and no teratogenic effects were observed. Studies of propellant HFA-134a in pregnant rats or rabbits have not shown any specific hazard.

Labor and Delivery: Although there have been no reports concerning the use of salbutamol inhalation aerosol during labor and delivery, it has been reported that high doses of salbutamol administered i.v. inhibit uterine contractions. Although this effect is extremely unlikely as a consequence of aerosol use, it should be kept in mind.

Lactation: Since salbutamol is likely excreted in breast milk, and because of the potential for tumorigenicity shown for salbutamol in animal studies, a decision should be made whether to discontinue nursing or to discontinue the drug, taking into account the importance of the drug to the mother. It is not known whether salbutamol in breast milk has a harmful effect on the neonate.

Patients with Special Diseases and Conditions: Large doses of i.v. salbutamol have been reported to aggravate pre-existing diabetes and ketoacidosis. Additionally, β-agonists, including salbutamol, given i.v. may cause a decrease in serum potassium possibly through intracellular shunting. The relevance of this observation to the use of salbutamol inhalation aerosol given at the recommended daily dosing is unknown, since the aerosol dose is much lower than doses given i.v.

Drug Interactions: MAO Inhibitors or Tricyclic Antidepressants: Salbutamol should be administered with extreme caution to patients being treated with MAO inhibitors or tricyclic antidepressants, or within 2 weeks of discontinuation of such agents, because the action of salbutamol on the cardiovascular system may be potentiated.

Other Inhaled Sympathomimetics/Epinephrine: Other inhaled sympathomimetic bronchodilators or epinephrine should not be used concomitantly with salbutamol. If additional adrenergic drugs are to be administered by any route to the patient using inhaled salbutamol, the adrenergic drugs should be used with caution to avoid deleterious cardiovascular effects. Such concomitant use must be individualized and not given on a routine basis. If regular coadministration is required, then alternative therapy must be considered.

β-Blockers: β-adrenergic receptor blocking agents, especially the noncardioselective ones, may effectively antagonize the action of salbutamol, and therefore salbutamol and nonselective β-blocking drugs, such as propranolol, should not usually be prescribed together.

Diuretics: The ECG changes and/or hypokalemia which may result from the administration of non-potassium sparing diuretics (such as loop or thiazide diuretics) can be acutely worsened by β-agonists, especially when the recommended dose of the β-agonist is exceeded. Although the clinical significance of these effects is not known, caution is advised in the coadministration of β-agonists with non-potassium sparing diuretics.

Digoxin: Mean decreases of 16 and 22% in serum digoxin levels were demonstrated after single dose i.v. and oral administration of salbutamol, respectively, to normal volunteers who had received digoxin for 10 days. The clinical significance of these findings for patients with obstructive airway disease who are receiving salbutamol and digoxin on a chronic basis is unclear; however, careful evaluation of serum digoxin levels is recommended in patients who are currently receiving digoxin and salbutamol.

Information to Be Provided to the Patient: Patients should be advised to always carry their salbutamol inhalation aerosol to use immediately if an episode of asthma is experienced.

See the illustrated Information for the Consumer insert that is dispensed with the product.

It is important that patients be instructed on how to use salbutamol inhalation aerosol correctly and how it should be used in relation to other medication they are taking. Patients should be given the following information: The action of salbutamol inhalation aerosol should last for 4 to 6 hours. Salbutamol inhalation aerosol should not be used more frequently than recommended. Do not increase the number of puffs or the frequency of doses of salbutamol inhalation aerosol without consulting your physician. If you find that treatment becomes less effective for symptomatic relief, your symptoms become worse, and/or you need to use the product more frequently than usual, seek medical attention immediately. While you are taking salbutamol inhalation aerosol, other inhaled drugs should be taken only as directed by your physician. If you are pregnant or nursing, contact your physician about the use of salbutamol inhalation aerosol. You may notice a different taste or spray force with Airomir compared to salbutamol aerosol inhalers that contain CFC propellants. Laboratory tests using instruments (not on people) show that Airomir Inhalation Aerosol delivers a softer spray force (less than 1/3 the maximum impact force) and warmer spray temperature (more than 30°C warmer) than salbutamol aerosol inhalers containing CFC propellants.

There is no tail-off phenomenon observed for Airomir since the propellant and drug exhaust simultaneously, providing consistent dosing from priming through to a few sprays beyond the planned maximum number of doses. Tail-off means that as most inhalers approach empty, the delivered dose becomes unpredictable and subject to wide variation (Tansey, BJCP 1995, (Suppl 79):14).

Common adverse effects of your treatment with inhaled salbutamol include palpitations, chest pain, rapid heart rate, tremor, or nervousness.

ADVERSE EFFECTS: A 12-week double-blind study compared Airomir Inhalation Aerosol, Ventolin inhaler (US source), and HFA-134a placebo in 565 asthmatic patients. Table 1 lists the incidence of all adverse events (whether considered drug-related or not related to drug by the investigator) from this study which occurred at a rate of at least 3% in the Airomir Inhalation Aerosol group. Only those adverse events which occurred more frequently in either the Airomir Inhalation Aerosol treatment group or the Ventolin treatment group than the placebo group are listed.

Table 1: Airomir

Adverse Experience Incidences (% of patients) in a Large 12-Week Clinical Trial[a]

Body System/Adverse Event (Preferred Term)	Airomir Inhalation Aerosol N=193	Ventolin (US)-I Inhaler N=186	HFA-134a Placebo Inhaler N=186
Application Site Disorders			
Inhalation Site Sensation	6	9	2
Inhalation Taste Sensation	4	3	3
Body as a Whole			
Allergic Symptoms	6	4	<1
Back Pain	4	2	3
Fever	6	2	5
Central and Peripheral Nervous System			
Dizziness	5	8	6
Tremor	7	8	2
Gastrointestinal System			
Nausea	10	9	5
Vomiting	7	2	3
Heart Rate and Rhythm Disorder			
Tachycardia	7	2	<1
Psychiatric Disorders			
Nervousness	7	9	3
Respiratory System Disorders			
Respiratory Disorder	6	4	5
Rhinitis	16	22	14
Upper Respiratory Tract Infection	21	20	18
Urinary System Disorder			
Urinary Tract Infection	3	4	2

[a] This table includes all adverse events (whether considered drug-related or not related to drug) which occurred at an incidence rate of at least 3% in the Airomir Inhalation Aerosol group and more frequently in the Airomir Inhalation Aerosol group than in the HFA-134a placebo inhaler group.

Adverse events reported by less than 3% of the patients receiving Airomir Inhalation Aerosol, and by a greater proportion of Airomir Inhalation Aerosol patients than placebo patients, which have the potential to be related to Airomir Inhalation Aerosol, include: dysphonia, contact dermatitis, increased sweating, dry mouth, chest pain, edema, rigors, ataxia, leg cramps, hyperkinesia, eructation, flatulence, tinnitus, diabetes mellitus, anxiety, depression, somnolence and rash.

In a small cumulative dose study, tremor, nervousness, and headache appeared to be dose-related. Palpitation has also been observed with Airomir.

Rare cases of urticaria, angioedema, rash, bronchospasm and oropharyngeal edema have been reported after the use of inhaled salbutamol. In addition, salbutamol, like other sympathomimetic agents, can cause adverse reactions such as hypertension, angina, vomiting, vertigo, CNS stimulation, insomnia, headache, unusual taste and drying or irritation of the oropharynx.

OVERDOSE:

Symptoms: Manifestations of overdosage may include anginal pain, hypertension, hypokalemia, tremor and tachycardia and exaggeration of other pharmacological effects as listed in Adverse Effects.

As with all sympathomimetic aerosol medications, cardiac arrest and even death may be associated with abuse.

The oral LD_{50} in male and female rats and mice was greater than 2000 mg/kg. The aerosol LD_{50} could not be determined.

Treatment: In the event of overdose, supportive therapy should be instituted. Dialysis is not appropriate treatment for overdosage of salbutamol inhalation aerosol. The judicious use of a cardioselective β-receptor blocker is suggested, bearing in mind the danger of inducing an asthmatic attack.

> For management of a suspected drug overdose, CPhA recommends that you contact your **regional Poison Control Centre**. See the *CPS* Directory section for a list of Poison Control Centres.

DOSAGE: Dosage should be individualized, and the patient's response should be monitored by the prescribing physician on an ongoing basis.

In accordance with the present practice for asthma treatment, if salbutamol is required for relief of symptoms more than twice a day on a regular daily basis or for an extended period of time, anti-inflammatory therapy (e.g., corticosteroids) should be part of the regimen.

Increasing demand for salbutamol preparations in bronchial asthma is usually a sign of worsening asthma and indicates that the treatment plan should be reviewed.

If a previously effective dose fails to provide the usual relief, or the effects of a dose last for less than 3 hours, patients should seek prompt medical advice since this is usually a sign of worsening asthma.

As there may be adverse effects associated with excessive dosing, the dosage or frequency of administration should only be increased on medical advice. However, if a more severe attack has not been relieved by the usual dose, additional doses may be required. In these cases, patients should immediately consult their doctors or the nearest hospital.

Acute Symptoms: Patients 12 years and older: 1 to 2 inhalations (100 to 200 μg). Children (6 to 11 years): 1 inhalation (100 μg).

If a more severe attack has not been relieved by the usual dose (1 to 2 inhalations), further inhalations may be required. In these cases, patients should immediately consult their doctors or the nearest hospital.

Intermittent and Long-term Treatment: If despite appropriate maintenance therapy, regular daily use of the inhalation aerosol remains necessary for the control of bronchospasm, the recommended dose is: Patients 12 years and older: 1 to 2 inhalations (100 to 200 μg) 3 to 4 times daily, not exceeding 8 inhalations (800 μg)/day. Children (6 to 11 years): 1 inhalation (100 μg), not exceeding 4 inhalations (400 μg)/day.

Prevention of Exercise-induced Asthma: Patients 12 years and older: 2 inhalations (200 μg) 30 minutes before exertion. Children (6 to 11 years of age): 1 inhalation (100 μg) 30 minutes before exertion.

Total Daily Dose Should Not Exceed: Patients 12 years and older: 8 inhalations (800 μg). Patients 6 to 11 years: 4 inhalations (400 μg).

INFORMATION FOR THE PATIENT: Published in e-CPS, available by subscription at www.e-cps.ca.

SUPPLIED: Each pressurized inhalation aerosol delivers salbutamol sulfate, USP equivalent to 120 ex-valve μg into the mouthpiece of the adapter. Nonmedicinal ingredients: ethanol, oleic acid and propellant HFA-134a. The inhalation aerosol contains a new propellant, HFA-134a, and does not contain chlorofluorocarbons (CFCs).

Ethanol has been previously used in inhaled medication as a cosolvent. The small amounts used in inhalers are not known to cause safety problems in asthmatics. A metered dose from Airomir Inhalation Aerosol delivers 0.0054 mL of ethanol per puff which is subject to evaporation as the aerosol expands and is diluted in body fluids as it expands.

Individual packages of 100- or 200-dose inhalers. The 200-dose product contains a minimum net content weight of 6.7 g and will provide a minimum of 200 inhalations. The 100-dose product (hospital pack) contains a minimum net content weight of 3.7 g and will provide a minimum of 100 inhalations.

Store between 15 and 30°C. Protect from direct sunlight and frost. **Prime the inhaler when new and after 2 or more weeks of non-use in any storage orientation by discharging a minimum of 4 sprays to the atmosphere.** Shake well before using. As the vial is pressurized no attempt should be made to puncture it or dispose of it by burning.

Alburex® 5

albumin (human)

Plasma Substitute/Blood Derivative

CSL Behring

Alburex® 25

albumin (human)

Plasma Substitute/Blood Derivative

CSL Behring

Date of Revision: February 10, 2010

SUMMARY PRODUCT INFORMATION:

Route of Administration	Dosage Form/ Strength	Clinically Relevant Nonmedicinal Ingredients
Intravenous	Solution for infusion: 5% (50 g/L) and 25% (250 g/L)	Sodium N-acetyltryptophanate, sodium caprylate, sodium chloride, water for injection See Dosage Forms, Composition and Packaging for a complete list of excipients.

DESCRIPTION: Alburex 5 and Alburex 25, Albumin (Human), are sterile aqueous solutions of albumin obtained from large pools of adult human venous plasma by low temperature controlled fractionation according to the Cohn process modified by Kistler Nitschmann. It is stabilized with sodium acetyltryptophanate and sodium caprylate and pasteurized at 60°C for at least 10 hours.

Alburex 5, Albumin (Human) solution for infusion is mildly hypooncotic to normal human plasma and contains, in each 100 mL, 5 grams of protein, of which at least 96% is human albumin.

Alburex 25, Albumin (Human) solution for infusion is hyperoncotic to normal human plasma and contains, in each 100 mL, 25 grams of protein, of which at least 96% is human albumin.

The pH of the solution is adjusted as needed with hydrochloric acid or sodium hydroxide. Approximate concentrations of significant electrolytes per liter are: sodium-130-150mEq; and potassium n.m.t. 2 mEq. The solution contains no preservative.

Alburex solutions should be administered intravenously.

This product has been prepared in accordance with the requirements established by the Food and Drug Administration and is in compliance with the standards of the United States Pharmacopoeia.

INDICATIONS AND CLINICAL USE: Alburex 5 and Alburex 25, Albumin (Human), are indicated for:

Restoring and maintaining circulating blood volume, based on albumin's oncotic and colloid-osmotic properties. The choice of albumin over artificial colloid and crystalloid solutions should be made according to current medical practice. Please refer to Dosage Forms, Composition and Packaging for concentration specific modes of administration.

Shock: Alburex is indicated in the emergency treatment of shock and in other similar conditions where the restoration of blood volume is urgent. In conditions associated mainly with a volume deficit, albumin is best administered as a 5% solution; but where there is an oncotic deficit, the 25% solution may be preferred. If there has been considerable loss of red blood cells, transfusion with packed red blood cells is indicated.

Burns: Alburex in combination with crystalloid solutions is used to maintain adequate plasma volume and protein content.

Hypoproteinemia With or Without Edema: Alburex is indicated in those clinical situations usually associated with a low concentration of plasma protein and a resulting decreased circulating blood volume. Measures of adequacy of circulating volume and not plasma albumin levels should be used to determine the dose required. Albumin (Human) is not indicated as nutrient in the treatment of chronic hypoproteinemia.

Pediatrics: No clinical studies using Alburex have been conducted in pediatric patients. Safety and effectiveness in pediatric patients have not been established. However, extensive experience in patients suggests that children respond to Alburex in the same manner as adults.

CONTRAINDICATIONS: Alburex 5 and Alburex 25, Albumin (Human), are contraindicated in patients who are hypersensitive to human albumin or to any ingredient in the formulation or component of the container. For a complete listing of ingredients, see Description.

Alburex is contraindicated in patients with severe anemia or cardiac failure.

WARNINGS AND PRECAUTIONS: General: Suspicion of allergic or anaphylactic type reactions requires immediate discontinuation of the infusion. In case of shock, standard medical treatment for shock should be implemented.

Alburex 5 and Alburex 25, Albumin (Human), should be used with caution in conditions where hypervolemia and its consequences or hemodilution could represent a special risk for the patient. Examples of such conditions are:

- decompensated cardiac insufficiency
- hypertension
- esophageal varices
- pulmonary edema
- hemorrhagic diathesis
- severe anemia
- renal and post-renal anuria

The colloid-osmotic effect of 250 g/L Albumin (Human) is approximately four times that of blood plasma. Therefore, when concentrated albumin is administered, care must be taken to assure adequate hydration of the patient. Patients should be monitored carefully to guard against circulatory overload and hyperhydration.

250 g/L Albumin (Human) solutions are relatively low in electrolytes compared to the 50 g/L Albumin (Human) solutions. When albumin is given, the electrolyte status of the patient should be monitored (see Dosage and Administration) and appropriate steps taken to restore or maintain the electrolyte balance.

Protein containing solutions such as Alburex must not be diluted with hypotonic solutions such as sterile water for injection, as this may result in severe hemolysis and acute renal failure. Please refer to the Dosage and Administration for information about the recommended diluents for Alburex, which are 5% glucose or 0.9% sodium chloride.

Alburex is made from human plasma. Standard measures to prevent infections resulting from use of medicinal products prepared from human blood or plasma include selection of donors, screening of individual donations and plasma pools for specific markers of infection and inclusion of effective manufacturing steps for inactivation/removal of viruses. Despite this, when medicinal products prepared from human blood or plasma are administered, the possibility of transmitting infective agents cannot be totally excluded (i.e. Parvovirus B19 which may affect pregnant women or immune compromised individuals). This also applies to unknown or emerging viruses and other pathogens.

The measures taken are considered effective for enveloped viruses such as HIV, HBV, HCV and for the non-enveloped viruses HAV and parvovirus B19.

A theoretical risk for transmission of variant Creutzfeldt Jacob disease (vCJD) is considered extremely remote.

There are no reports of proven virus transmissions with albumin manufactured to European or US pharmacopoeia specifications by established CSL processes.

Any infection thought by a physician to possibly have been transmitted by this product, should be reported by the physician or other healthcare provider to CSL Behring Canada, Inc. at 1-613-783-1892. The physician should discuss the risks and benefits of this product with the patient.

Effect on Ability to Drive and Use Machines: No effects on the ability to drive and use machines have been observed.

Hematologic: If comparatively large volumes are to be replaced, controls of coagulation and hematocrit are necessary care must be taken to ensure adequate substitution of other blood constituents (coagulation factors, electrolytes, platelets and erythrocytes).

Cardiovascular: The colloid-osmotic effect of 250 g/L Albumin (Human) is approximately four times that of blood plasma. Therefore, care must be taken to assure adequate hydration of the patient when administering Alburex. Patients should be monitored carefully to guard against circulatory overload and hyperhydration. Hypervolemia may occur if the dosage and infusion rate are not adjusted to the patient's circulatory situation.

Alburex should be administered with caution to patients with low cardiac reserve. At the first clinical signs of cardiovascular overload (headache, dyspnea, jugular vein congestion), or increased blood pressure, raised venous pressure and pulmonary edema, the infusion is to be stopped immediately and the patient's haemodynamic parameter carefully monitored.

Sexual Function/Reproduction: It is not known whether Alburex can affect reproduction capacity.

Special Populations: Pregnant Women: The safety of Alburex solutions for infusion, for use in human pregnancy has not been established in controlled clinical trials. However, clinical experience with albumin suggests that no harmful effects on the course of pregnancy, or on the foetus and neonate are to be expected. No animal reproduction studies have been conducted with Alburex solutions for infusion. However, human albumin is a normal constituent of human blood.

Alburex should only be used in pregnant woman when the benefits outweigh the risks associated with its use.

Nursing Women: Alburex should only be used in nursing woman when the benefits outweigh the risks associated with its use.

Pediatrics: No clinical studies using Alburex have been conducted in pediatric patients. Safety and effectiveness in pediatric patients have not been established. However, extensive experience in patients suggests that children respond to Alburex in the same manner as adults.

Monitoring and Laboratory Tests: Refer to Hematologic.

ADVERSE REACTIONS: Clinical Trial Adverse Drug Reactions: The Cochrane Collaboration examined 30 previously published albumin studies, involving a total of 1419 patients. The authors included randomized trials that enrolled critically-ill patients who were hypovolemic or hypoalbuminemic and treated with albumin, plasma protein fraction or crystalloids. The intent of the authors was to compare outcomes with the albumin and plasma protein fraction with that of crystalloids. The results, published in 1998 (BMJ 1998;317:235-40), suggested that the mortality rates were higher in the patient groups treated with albumin or plasma protein fraction than in the groups treated with crystalloids. However, this meta-analysis has been challenged due to the heterogeneity of the patient populations studied, the inclusion of poor-quality and old studies not reflecting current practice, and the use of studies with unpublished data and/or patient populations that were too small to be meaningful. In addition, this meta-analysis was not an appropriate tool to compare albumin vs. crystalloids, since this type of analysis are used to generate hypotheses, rather than to prove hypotheses.

A larger, rigorous meta-analysis by Wilkes and Navickis, published in 2001 (Ann Intern Med 2001;135:149-64), which included additional studies with larger patient populations did not reproduce the results of the Cochrane group and suggests on the contrary that albumin may reduce mortality.

The recent Saline versus Albumin Fluid Evaluation study (The SAFE Study Investigators, NEJM 2004;350:2247-56) was designed to provide a definitive answer to the questions raised by the Cochrane report. This was a double-blind study which effectively captured all critically-ill patients receiving volume resuscitation in Australia. The study randomized 6997 patients, of whom 3497 were treated with 4% albumin and 3500 with normal saline. The primary outcome measure was mortality at 28 days, but the authors also examined time spent in the ICU, time spent in hospital, requirements for mechanical ventilation and requirements for renal dialysis. The study found no significant differences in any study outcome in the first 28 days of stay in the intensive care unit. This study, by far the largest study ever done with albumin, showed that there was no additional mortality due to the use of albumin.

A greater number of patients with trauma involving brain injury died among those randomly assigned to albumin as opposed to saline (59 of 241 in the albumin group compared to 38 of 251 in the saline group with a relative risk of 1.62 and p=0.009). However, the overall number of these patients was relatively small. The study had insufficient power to detect differences in mortality among the predefined subgroups and the authors warn that the observed difference should be interpreted with caution.

Post-Market Adverse Drug Reactions: The incidence of untoward reactions to Alburex 5/Alburex 25, Albumin (Human) is low. Mild reactions such as flush, urticaria, fever and nausea occur rarely. These reactions normally disappear rapidly when the infusion rate is slowed down or the infusion is stopped. Reports have been received of anaphylaxis, which may be severe, and hypersensitivity reactions (including urticaria, skin rash, pruritus, edema, erythema, hypotension and bronchospasm). Very rarely, severe reactions such as shock may occur. In these cases, the infusion should be stopped immediately and an appropriate treatment should be initiated.

For safety with respect to transmissible agent, see Warnings and Precautions.

DRUG INTERACTIONS: No specific interactions of Alburex 5/Alburex 25, Albumin (Human) with other medicinal products are known. However, the effects of medicinal products with extensive binding to albumin may be impacted by changes in circulating albumin levels.

Incompatibilities: Alburex 5 and Alburex 25, Albumin (Human), solutions for infusion must not be mixed with other medicinal products (except those mentioned in Dosage and Administration) including whole blood and packed red cells.

DOSAGE AND ADMINISTRATION: Alburex, Albumin (Human) is a ready-to-use solution and should be administered by the intravenous route only. Alburex 25 can also be diluted in an isotonic solution of e.g. 5% glucose or 0.9% sodium chloride. Alburex 5/Alburex 25, Albumin (Human) solution for infusion must not be diluted with water for injection as this may cause hemolysis in recipients.

Recommended Dose, Dosage Adjustment and Administration: The concentration of the albumin preparation, dosage and the infusion-rate should be adjusted to the patient's individual requirements. The infusion rate should normally not exceed 5 mL/min for Alburex 5 or 1-2 mL/min for Alburex 25, Albumin (Human). Care must be taken to ensure adequate substitution of other blood components (coagulation factors, electrolytes, platelets and erythrocytes).

Alburex 5: Alburex 5, 50 g/L Albumin (Human) is a ready-to-use solution and should be administered by the intravenous route only. This concentration is approximately isotonic and iso-osmotic with citrated plasma. Albumin (Human) in this concentration provides additional fluid for plasma volume replacement. Therefore, when it is administered to patients with normal blood volume, the rate of infusion should be slow enough to prevent too rapid an increase of plasma volume.

The dose should be adjusted based on patient's body weight, severity of treated condition, and estimated fluid and protein loss as determined by monitoring hemodynamic parameters, circulating volume and plasma protein levels, to avoid complications related to potential hypervolemia.

Shock: Therapy should be guided by the patient's response.

Burns: In the treatment of burns an optimal regimen involving use of albumin, crystalloids, electrolytes and water has not been established. Suggested therapy during the first 24 hours includes administration of large volumes of crystalloid solution to maintain an adequate plasma volume. After the first 24 hours, the ratio of albumin to crystalloid may be increased to establish and maintain a plasma albumin level of about 2.5 g/100 mL or a total serum protein level of about 5.2 g/100 mL. Duration of treatment varies depending upon the extent of protein loss through renal excretion, denuded areas of skin and decreased albumin synthesis.

Hypoproteinemia: The infusion of Albumin (Human) as a nutrient in the treatment of chronic hypoproteinemia is not recommended. In acute hypoproteinemia, 50 g/L Albumin (Human) may be used in replacing the protein lost in hypoproteinemic conditions. However, if edema is present or if large amounts of albumin are lost, 250 g/L Albumin (Human) is preferred because of the greater amount of protein in the concentrated solution.

Alburex 25: Alburex 25, 250 g/L Albumin (Human) is a ready-to-use solution and should be administered by the intravenous route only. Alburex 25 can also be diluted in an isotonic solution of e.g. 5% glucose or 0.9% sodium chloride. 200 mL per liter gives a solution which is mildly hypooncotic and isoosmotic with citrated plasma. Alburex 25, Albumin (Human) solution for infusion, must not be diluted with water for injection as this may cause hemolysis in recipients.

When undiluted Alburex 25, Albumin (Human), solution for infusion is administered in patients with normal blood volume, the infusion rate should be slow enough (1-2 mL per minute) to prevent a too rapid expansion of plasma volume.

Shock: In the treatment of shock, the amount of albumin and duration of therapy must be based on the responsiveness of the patient as indicated by blood pressure, degree of pulmonary congestion, and hematocrit. The initial dose may be followed by additional albumin within 15-30 minutes if the response is deemed inadequate. If there is continued loss of protein, it may be desirable to give packed red blood cells.

The dose should be adjusted based on patient's body weight, severity of treated condition, and estimated fluid and protein loss as determined by monitoring hemodynamic parameters, circulating volume and plasma protein levels, to avoid complications related to potential hypervolemia.

Burns: In the treatment of burns an optimal regimen involving use of albumin, crystalloids, electrolytes and water has not been established. Suggested therapy during the first 24 hours includes administration of large volumes of crystalloid solution to maintain an adequate plasma volume. After the first 24 hours, the ratio of albumin to crystalloid may be increased to establish and maintain a plasma albumin level of about 2.5 g/100 mL or a total serum protein level of about 5.2 g/100 mL. Duration of treatment varies depending upon the extent of protein loss through renal excretion, denuded areas of skin and decreased albumin synthesis.

Hypoproteinemia: In the treatment of hypoproteinemia, 200 to 300 mL of 250 g/L Albumin (Human) may be required to reduce edema and to bring serum protein values to normal. Since such patients usually have approximately normal blood volume, doses of more than 100 mL of 250 g/L Albumin (Human) should not be given faster than 100 mL in 30 to 45 minutes to avoid circulatory embarrassment. If slower administration is desired, the product may be diluted as described in the first paragraph under Dosage and Administration.

Dosing Considerations: The dose required depends on the size of the patient, the severity of trauma or illness and on continuing fluid and protein losses. Measures of adequacy of circulating volume and not plasma albumin levels, as well as hemodynamic parameters should be used to determine the dose required.

If Albumin (Human) is to be administered, hemodynamic performance should be monitored regularly; this may include:

- arterial blood pressure and pulse rate
- central venous pressure
- pulmonary artery wedge pressure
- urine output
- electrolyte
- hematocrit/hemoglobin

Missed Dose: Not applicable.

Reconstitution: Not applicable. Alburex is a ready-to-use solution.

OVERDOSAGE:
Hypervolemia may occur if the dosage and infusion rate are too high. At the first clinical signs of cardiovascular overload (headache, dyspnea, jugular vein congestion) or increased blood pressure, raised central venous pressure and pulmonary edema, the infusion should be stopped immediately and the patient's hemodynamic parameters carefully monitored.

For management of a suspected drug overdose, CPhA recommends that you contact your **regional Poison Control Centre**. See the *CPS* Directory section for a list of Poison Control Centres.

ACTION AND CLINICAL PHARMACOLOGY: Mechanism of Action: The most important physiological functions of Albumin (Human) results from its contribution to oncotic pressure of the blood and transport function. Albumin stabilizes circulating blood volume and is a carrier of hormones, enzymes, medicinal products and toxins.

Pharmacodynamics: Albumin (Human) is active osmotically and is therefore important in regulating the volume of circulating blood. It is a valuable therapeutic aid for the treatment of conditions that will be benefited by its marked osmotic effect.

It is convenient to use since no cross matching is required and the absence of cellular elements removes the danger of sensitization with repeated infusions.

Pharmacokinetics: Under normal conditions, the total exchangeable albumin pool is 4-5 g/kg body weight of which 40-45% is present intravascularly and 55-60% in the extravascular space. Increased capillary permeability will alter albumin kinetics and abnormal distribution may occur in conditions such as severe burns or septic shock.

Under normal conditions, the average half-life of albumin is about 19 days. The balance between synthesis and breakdown is normally achieved by feedback regulation. Elimination is predominantly intracellular and due to liposome proteases.

In healthy subjects, less than 10% of infused albumin leaves the intravascular compartment during the first 2 hours following infusion. There is considerable individual variation in the effect on plasma volume. In some patients the plasma volume can remain increased for some hours. However, in critically ill patients, albumin can leak out of the vascular space in substantial amounts at an unpredictable rate.

When infused intravenously, 50 mL of 250 g/L Albumin (Human) draws approximately 175 mL of additional fluid into the circulation within 15 minutes, except in the presence of marked dehydration. This extra fluid reduces hemoconcentration and blood viscosity. The degree of volume expansion is dependent on the initial blood volume. When the circulating blood volume has been depleted, the hemodilution following albumin administration persists for many hours. In individuals with normal blood volume, it usually lasts only a few hours.

Duration of Effect: Refer to Pharmacokinetics.

STORAGE AND STABILITY: Alburex 5 and Alburex 25, Albumin (Human), solutions for infusion should be stored protected from light at controlled room temperature (15-30°C).

Keep the container in the outer carton in order to protect from light. Do not freeze.

Shelf-life: 3 years.

The product may not be used beyond the expiration date mentioned on the container label.

SPECIAL HANDLING INSTRUCTIONS: If large volumes are administered, the product should be warmed to room temperature before use.

Parenteral drug products should be inspected visually for particulate matter and discoloration prior to administration, whenever solution and container permit.

The solution should be clear or slightly opalescent. Do not use solutions which are cloudy or have deposits. This may indicate that the protein is unstable or that the solution has become contaminated.

Since this product contains no antimicrobial preservative, it should be used immediately once the stopper has been perforated. Any unused product should be disposed of in accordance with local requirements.

It is strongly recommended that every time Alburex 5/Alburex 25, Albumin (Human), is administered to a patient, the name and batch number of the product be recorded in order to maintain a link between the patient and the batch of the product.

INFORMATION FOR THE PATIENT: Published in e-CPS, available by subscription at www.e-cps.ca.

DOSAGE FORMS, COMPOSITION AND PACKAGING: Alburex 5: Each L of clear, slightly viscous liquid, almost colorless, yellow, amber, or green, sterile and non-pyrogenic solution for infusion contains: albumin of human origin 50 g (5%). At least 96% of the total protein is albumin. The product contains aggregates (≤10.0%) and trace amounts of immunoglobulins. The pH value of the ready-to-use solution is within the range of 6.4 to 7.4. Nonmedicinal ingredients: sodium N-acetyl-tryptophanate and sodium caprylate are included as stabilizers and sodium chloride is included as a tonicity agent. The solution may contain hydrochloric acid or sodium hydroxide as buffering agents. Preservative-free. The aluminum content of Alburex is below 200 µg/L, which respects current European Pharmacopoeia requirements. Infusion bottles, glass type II (Ph.Eur.) of 100 mL, 250 mL and 500 mL.

Alburex 25: Each L of clear, slightly viscous liquid, almost colorless, yellow, amber, or green, sterile and non-pyrogenic solution for infusion contains: albumin of human origin 250 g (25%). At least 96% of the total protein is albumin. The product contains aggregates (≤10.0%) and trace amounts of immunoglobulins. The pH value of the ready-to-use solution is within the range of 6.4 to 7.4. Nonmedicinal ingredients: sodium N-acetyl-tryptophanate and sodium caprylate are included as stabilizers and sodium chloride is included as a tonicity agent. The solution may contain hydrochloric acid or sodium hydroxide as buffering agents. Preservative-free. The aluminum content of Alburex is below 200 µg/L, which respects current European Pharmacopoeia requirements. Infusion bottles, glass type II (Ph.Eur.) of 50 mL and 100 mL.

Alcaine®
proparacaine HCl
Ophthalmic Anesthetic

Alcon

SUPPLIED: Each Drop-Tainer dispenser contains: proparacaine HCl 0.5%, preserved with benzalkonium chloride. Nonmedicinal ingredients: glycerin, hydrochloric acid, purified water and sodium hydroxide. Drop-Tainer dispensers of 15 mL. Refrigerate.

Aldactazide 25® Ⓟ
spironolactone—hydrochlorothiazide
Aldosterone Antagonist—Diuretic

Pfizer

Aldactazide 50® Ⓟ
spironolactone—hydrochlorothiazide
Aldosterone Antagonist—Diuretic

Pfizer

PHARMACOLOGY: A combination of two diuretic agents with different but complementary mechanisms and sites of action. The spironolactone component helps to minimize the potassium loss which may be induced by the thiazide component. Spironolactone is a specific pharmacologic antagonist of the adrenal mineralocorticoid, aldosterone, acting primarily through competitive binding with receptors at the aldosterone-dependent sodium/potassium exchange site in the distal convoluted renal tubule. Hydrochlorothiazide promotes excretion of sodium and water primarily by inhibiting their reabsorption by the cortical diluting segment of the renal tubule, in contrast to spironolactone which exerts its effect more distally. Both spironolactone and hydrochlorothiazide reduce exchangeable sodium and plasma volume.

The effects of hydrochlorothiazide will be observed on the day of administration, but the spironolactone component does not attain its maximal effect until the third day.

Spironolactone is rapidly and extensively metabolized. Sulfur-containing products are the predominant metabolites and are thought to be primarily responsible for the therapeutic effects of the drug. Approximately 25 to 30% of the dose administered is converted to canrenone, which attains peak serum levels 2 to 4 hours after single oral administration of spironolactone. In the dose range of 25 mg to 200 mg, an approximately linear relationship exists between a single dose of spironolactone and plasma levels of canrenone.

Plasma concentrations of canrenone decline in 2 distinct phases, the first phase lasting from 3 to 12 hours, being more rapid than the second phase lasting from 12 to 96 hours. Canrenone clearance data, following multiple doses of spironolactone, indicate that accumulation of canrenone in the body with 100 mg once a day would be lower than with 25 mg 4 times a day. Both spironolactone and canrenone are more than 90% bound to plasma proteins. The metabolites of spironolactone are excreted both in the urine (32 to 53%), and through biliary excretion in the feces (14 to 36%).

Hydrochlorothiazide is rapidly absorbed following oral administration, with onset of action occurring within 1 hour, and the duration of action is 6 to 12 hours. Plasma concentration attains a peak at 1 to 2 hours and declines with a half-life of 4 to 5 hours. Hydrochlorothiazide undergoes only slight metabolic alteration and is excreted in the urine. It is distributed throughout the extracellular space, with essentially no tissue accumulation except in the kidney. Hydrochlorothiazide is eliminated rapidly by the kidney.

INDICATIONS: Fixed-dose combination drugs are not indicated for initial therapy. Patients should be titrated on the individual drugs. If the fixed combination represents the dosage so determined, its use may be more convenient in patient management. If during maintenance therapy dosage adjustment is necessary, it is advisable to use the individual drugs.

Edematous Conditions for Patients with Congestive Heart Failure: For the management of edema and sodium retention when the patient is only partially responsive to, or is intolerant of, other therapeutic measures. The treatment of diuretic-induced hypokalemia in patients with congestive heart failure when other measures are considered inappropriate. The treatment of patients with congestive heart failure taking digitalis when other therapies are considered inadequate or inappropriate.

Cirrhosis of the Liver Accompanied by Edema and/or Ascites: Aldosterone levels may be exceptionally high in this condition. Aldactazide is indicated for maintenance therapy, together with bed rest and the restriction of fluid and sodium.

Nephrotic Syndrome: Aldactazide may be used in nephrotic patients who are not responsive to glucocorticoid therapy and who do not respond to other diuretics. However, Aldactazide has not been shown to affect the basic pathological process.

Essential Hypertension: In patients with essential hypertension in whom other measures are considered inadequate or inappropriate. In hypertensive patients for the treatment of a diuretic induced hypokalemia when other measures are considered inappropriate.

CONTRAINDICATIONS: Anuria, acute renal insufficiency, significant impairment of renal function, hyperkalemia, sensitivity to spironolactone and sensitivity to thiazides or other sulfonamide-derived drugs. Aldactazide may be contraindicated in patients with severe or progressive liver disease.

WARNINGS: Potassium (K^+) Supplementation: Do not give potassium supplementation (including dietary potassium) in conjunction with Aldactazide therapy.

Excessive potassium intake may cause hyperkalemia in patients receiving Aldactazide. Do not administer Aldactazide concurrently with other potassium-sparing diuretics.

Tumorigenicity: Spironolactone, in chronic toxicity studies, has been shown to be a tumorigen in rats.

Use Aldactazide only for conditions described under Indications.

PRECAUTIONS: Electrolyte Balance: Because of the diuretic action of Aldactazide, patients should be carefully evaluated for possible disturbance of fluid and electrolyte balance.

Hyperkalemia: Hyperkalemia may occur in patients treated with Aldactazide. This can cause cardiac irregularities, some of which may be fatal. Hyperkalemia may occur in the absence of excessive potassium intake, particulary in patients with impaired renal function, elderly patients, or patients with diabetes.

Consequently, no potassium supplementation should ordinarily be given with Aldactazide. Hyperkalemia can be treated promptly by rapid i.v. administration of glucose (20 to 50%) and regular insulin, using 0.25 to 0.5 units of insulin per gram of glucose. This is a temporary measure to be repeated if required. Aldactazide should be discontinued and potassium intake (including dietary potassium) restricted.

Hypokalemia: Hypokalemia may develop, especially with brisk diuresis, in severe cirrhosis or during concomitant use of loop diuretics, glucocorticoids, or ACTH. Digitalis therapy may exaggerate the metabolic effects of hypokalemia especially with reference to myocardial activity. If hypokalemia occurs, Aldactazide should be discontinued and consideration given to one of the following therapeutic regimens: use of hydrochlorothiazide alone with potassium supplementation as needed, or use of spironolactone (Aldactone) alone.

Hyponatremia: During the administration of Aldactazide, patients suffering from sodium depletion must be attentively monitored and signs of electrolyte imbalance must be carefully checked.

Aldactazide may, if administered concomitantly with other diuretics, cause or aggravate hyponatremia, as manifested by dryness of the mouth, thirst, lethargy and drowsiness.

A true low-salt syndrome may develop with Aldactazide therapy and may be manifested by increasing mental confusion similar to that observed with hepatic coma. This syndrome was differentiated from dilutional hyponatremia in that it does not occur with obvious fluid retention. Its treatment requires that diuretic therapy be discontinued and sodium administered.

Metabolic Effects: Hyperchloremic metabolic acidosis: Reversible hyperchloremic metabolic acidosis, usually in association with hyperkalemia, has been reported in decompensated hepatic cirrhosis, even in the presence of normal renal function.

Hypochloremic Alkalosis: Hypochloremic alkalosis occurs infrequently and is rarely severe. Unduly restricted dietary sodium may complicate therapy. A chloride deficit may be corrected by using ammonium chloride (except in renal or hepatic disease) and is largely prevented by a near-normal sodium/chloride intake.

Drug Interactions: Diuretics and Antihypertensives: Although Aldactazide may be administered concomitantly with diuretics and antihypertensives, the effect is additive. Thus, it is advisable to reduce the dose of these drugs. In particular, the dose of ganglionic blocking agents should be reduced by at least 50% when Aldactazide is included in the regimen.

Hyperkalemia has been associated with the use of angiotensin converting enzyme (ACE) inhibitors in combination with potassium-sparing diuretics.

Norepinephrine and Tubocurarine: Since hydrochlorothiazide and spironolactone each reduce vascular responsiveness to norepinephrine, caution should be exercised in the management of patients subjected to regional or general anesthesia. Thiazides may also increase responsiveness to tubocurarine. Consideration should be given to discontinuation of Aldactazide therapy prior to elective surgery.

Digoxin: Spironolactone has been shown to increase the half-life of digoxin. This may result in increased serum digoxin levels and subsequent digitalis toxicity. It may be necessary to reduce the maintenance dose of digoxin when Aldactazide is administered, and the patient should be carefully monitored to avoid over- or under-digitalization.

Carbenoxolone: Carbenoxolone may cause sodium retention and thus decrease the effectiveness of spironolactone. Concurrent use of the 2 agents should be avoided.

Nonsteroidal Anti-inflammatory Drugs: It has been reported that ASA, mefenamic acid, and indomethacin may interfere with the diuretic action of spironolactone. The mechanism may be due to the inhibition of intrarenal synthesis of prostaglandins. However, it has been shown that ASA does not alter the effect of spironolactone on blood pressure, serum electrolytes, urea nitrogen, or plasma renin activity in hypertensive patients.

Hyperkalemia has been associated with the use of indomethacin in combination with potassium-sparing diuretics.

Insulin: Insulin requirements in diabetics may be increased, decreased or unchanged. Hyperglycemia and glycosuria may be manifested in latent diabetics.

Gynecomastia: Gynecomastia may develop with the use of spironolactone and physicians should be advised of its possible occurrence. The development of gynecomastia appears to be related to both dosage and duration of therapy and is normally reversible when the drug is discontinued. If gynecomastia develops, discontinue the drug. In rare instances, some breast enlargement may persist.

Pregnancy: Spironolactone or its metabolites may, and thiazides do cross the placental barrier and appear in cord blood. When hydrochlorothiazide is used in women of childbearing age, the potential benefits of the drug should be weighed against the possible hazards to the fetus. These hazards include fetal or neonatal jaundice, thrombocytopenia, and possibly other adverse reactions which have occurred in the adult. In rats, feminization of the male fetus has been reported at high doses.

Lactation: Certain adverse reactions to thiazide therapy (e.g. hyperbilirubinemia, thrombocytopenia, altered carbohydrate metabolism) can occur in the newborn since thiazides have been demonstrated to appear in breast milk. Canrenone, a metabolite of spironolactone, also appears in breast milk. If use of these drugs is deemed essential, an alternative method of infant feeding should be instituted.

Laboratory Tests: General: Aldactazide therapy may result in a transient elevation of BUN, especially when azotemia exists at the beginning of treatment. This appears to represent a concentration phenomenon rather than renal toxicity, since the BUN returns to normal after Aldactazide is discontinued. Progressive elevation of BUN is suggestive of the presence of pre-existing renal impairment.

Several reports of possible interference with digoxin radioimmunoassays by spironolactone or its metabolites have appeared in the literature. Neither the extent nor the potential clinical significance of this interference (which may be assay-specific) has been fully established. Discontinue spironolactone for at least 4, and preferably 7, days prior to plasma cortisol determinations, **if they are to be done by the method of Mattingly**, that is, by fluorometric assay. No interference has been demonstrated with the competitive protein binding technique or radioimmunoassay technique.

Thiazides may decrease serum PBI levels without evidence of alteration of thyroid function.

Adrenal Vein Catheterization and Plasma Renin Activity: Discontinue spironolactone several days prior to adrenal vein catheterization for measurement of aldosterone concentrations and measurements of plasma renin activity.

Impaired Hepatic Function: Aldactazide should be used with caution in patients with impaired hepatic function, because minor alterations in electrolyte balance may precipitate hepatic coma. In the treatment of the edema/ascites of cirrhosis, when high doses are required, it is recommended that the drug dosage be decreased before diuresis is complete, in order to avoid dehydration. If mental confusion occurs, Aldactazide should be temporarily discontinued.

Miscellaneous: Orthostatic hypotension may occur and may be potentiated by alcohol, barbiturates or narcotics.

Pathological changes in the parathyroid gland, with resultant hypercalcemia and hypophosphatemia, have been observed in a few patients on prolonged thiazide therapy.

Exacerbation or activation of systemic lupus erythematosus has been reported for sulfonamide derivatives, including thiazides.

Caution is necessary in patients with hyperuricemia or a history of gout, because gout may be precipitated by thiazides.

ADVERSE EFFECTS: Spironolactone: The adverse reactions encountered most frequently with spironolactone are gynecomastia and gastrointestinal symptoms.

Gastrointestinal: nausea, cramping and diarrhea, vomiting, gastric bleeding, gastritis and ulceration.

Central Nervous System: drowsiness, dizziness, headache, mental confusion, ataxia, lethargy.

Dermatologic: maculopapular or erythematous cutaneous eruptions, urticaria.

Endocrinologic: gynecomastia, impotence, inability to achieve or maintain erection, abnormal semen (decreased motility and sperm count), irregular menses or amenorrhea and postmenopausal bleeding. Carcinoma of the breast has been reported in patients taking spironolactone, but a cause and effect relationship has not been established.

Miscellaneous: drug fever. A few cases of agranulocytosis have been reported in patients taking spironolactone.

Hydrochlorothiazide: Gastrointestinal: anorexia, gastric irritation, nausea, vomiting, cramps, diarrhea, constipation, jaundice (intrahepatic cholestatic), acute pancreatitis.

Central Nervous System: dizziness, vertigo, paresthesia, headache, xanthopsia.

Dermatologic: hypersensitivity, purpura, photosensitivity, rash, urticaria, necrotizing angiitis, pruritus and erythema multiforme.

Hematologic: leukopenia, thrombocytopenic purpura, agranulocytosis, aplastic anemia.

Cardiovascular: orthostatic hypotension may occur and may be potentiated by alcohol, barbiturates or narcotics.

Miscellaneous: muscle spasm, weakness, nitrogen retention, hypokalemia, hyperglycemia, glycosuria and hyperuricemia.

Adverse reactions due to Aldactazide are usually reversible upon discontinuation of Aldactazide. In rare instances, some gynecomastia may persist.

OVERDOSE:

Symptoms: There have been no reports of fatal overdose in man (except indirectly through hyperkalemia). Nausea and vomiting occurs, and (much more rarely) drowsiness, mental confusion, diarrhea, or a maculopapular or erythematous rash. These manifestations disappear promptly on discontinuation of medication. Hyperkalemia may be exacerbated. Thrombocytopenic purpura and granulocytopenia have occurred with thiazide therapy.

Treatment: No specific antidote. No persistent toxicity has occurred or is expected. Appearance of effects described above requires only discontinuation of drug. Induce vomiting and evacuate the stomach by lavage. For hyperkalemia, discontinue Aldactazide, reduce potassium intake, consider administration of potassium-excreting diuretics, i.v. glucose with regular insulin (see Precautions), ion-exchange resins, or dialysis. Treat fluid depletion and electrolyte imbalances appropriately if present.

For management of a suspected drug overdose, CPhA recommends that you contact your **regional Poison Control Centre**. See the *CPS* Directory section for a list of Poison Control Centres.

DOSAGE: Optimal dosage should be established by individual titration of the components.

Treatment should be continued for 2 weeks before optimal effectiveness can be assessed.

Adults: Edema (congestive heart failure, hepatic cirrhosis or nephrotic syndrome): Daily dosage of 2 to 4 tablets of Aldactazide 25 or 1 to 2 tablets of Aldactazide 50 in single or divided doses should be adequate for most patients, but may range from 2 to 8 tablets daily of Aldactazide 25 or 1 to 4 tablets of Aldactazide 50.

Children: Edema: The usual daily maintenance dose of Aldactazide should be that which provides 1.65 to 3.3 mg of spironolactone per kg of body weight.

Essential hypertension: In essential hypertension, a daily dosage of 2 to 4 Aldactazide 25 tablets or 1 to 2 Aldactazide 50 tablets in single or divided doses, will be adequate for most patients, but may range from 2 to 8 tablets of Aldactazide 25 or 1 to 4 tablets of Aldactazide 50.

Since Aldactazide increases the action of other antihypertensive drugs, especially the ganglionic blocking agents, the dosage of such drugs should be reduced by at least 50% when Aldactazide is added to the regimen.

INFORMATION FOR THE PATIENT: Published in e-CPS, available by subscription at www.e-cps.ca.

SUPPLIED: Aldactazide 25: Each light tan round biconvex film coated tablet, debossed "ALDACTAZIDE" and "25" on one side and "SEARLE" and "1011" on the other, peppermint odor, contains: spironolactone 25 mg and hydrochlorothiazide 25 mg. Nonmedicinal ingredients: calcium sulfate, cornstarch, magnesium stearate, peppermint flavoring, povidone, hypromellose, polyethylene glycol 400, carnauba wax, stearic acid and opaspray K-1-7076. Bottles of 100. Store at 15 to 25°C.

Aldactazide 50: Each light tan capsule-shaped film coated tablet debossed "ALDACTAZIDE" and "50" on one side and "SEARLE" and "1021" on the other, peppermint odor, contains: spironolactone 50 mg and hydrochlorothiazide 50 mg. Nonmedicinal ingredients: calcium sulfate, cornstarch, magnesium stearate, peppermint flavoring, povidone, hypromellose, polyethylene glycol 400, carnauba wax, stearic acid and opaspray K-1-7076. Bottles of 100. Store at 15 to 25°C.

(Shown in Product Identification Section)

Aldactone™ Ⓟ

spironolactone

Aldosterone Antagonist

Pfizer

Date of Revision: November 5, 2009

SUMMARY PRODUCT INFORMATION:

Route of Administration	Dosage Form/ Strength	Clinically Relevant Nonmedicinal Ingredients
Oral	Tablet 25 mg, 100 mg	Calcium sulfate, corn starch, magnesium stearate, peppermint flavouring, povidone, hypromellose, polyethylene glycol 400, carnauba wax, stearic acid, Opaspray M-1-2042 (25 mg), Opaspray M-1-2668 (100 mg)

INDICATIONS AND CLINICAL USE: ALDACTONE (spironolactone) is indicated for the following:

1. **Primary Hyperaldosteronism:** ALDACTONE (spironolactone) is a useful agent in the diagnosis of primary hyperaldosteronism. In the presence of hypokalemic alkalosis and hypertension, a diagnosis of primary hyperaldosteronism should be considered if both blood pressure (BP) and serum electrolytes return to normal following treatment with ALDACTONE.
   ALDACTONE is useful in the pre-operative treatment of patients with primary hyperaldosteronism and for the maintenance therapy of such patients who decline surgery, or who are unsuitable for surgery.
2. **Edematous Conditions:**
   a. **Congestive Heart Failure (CHF):** ALDACTONE is useful in the management of edema and sodium retention in CHF when the patient is only partially responsive to, or intolerant of, other therapeutic measures. ALDACTONE may be used alone or with thiazides. It is indicated in patients with CHF taking digitalis when other therapies are considered inappropriate.
   b. **Cirrhosis of the Liver Accompanied by Edema and/or Ascites:** Aldosterone levels may be exceptionally high in this condition. ALDACTONE is indicated for maintenance therapy, in combination with bed rest and the restriction of fluid and sodium.
   c. **The Nephrotic Syndrome:** ALDACTONE is useful for inducing a diuresis in patients not responsive to glucocorticoid therapy (for the nephrotic syndrome), and not responding to other diuretics. However, ALDACTONE has not been shown to affect the basic pathological process.
3. **Essential Hypertension:** ALDACTONE is indicated, usually in combination with other drugs, for patients who cannot be treated adequately with other agents or for whom other agents are considered inappropriate. ALDACTONE alone has mild to moderate antihypertensive activity.
4. **Hypokalemia:** ALDACTONE is indicated for treatment of hypokalemia, when other measures are considered inappropriate or inadequate. It is also indicated for the prophylaxis of hypokalemia in digitalis therapy when other measures are inadequate or inappropriate.

CONTRAINDICATIONS:

- Anuria
- Acute renal insufficiency
- Addison's disease
- Significant impairment of renal function
- Hyperkalemia
- Hypersensitivity to spironolactone or to any ingredient in the formulation. For a complete listing, see Dosage Forms, Composition and Packaging.

WARNINGS AND PRECAUTIONS: General: Use Only for "Indications": Use ALDACTONE (spironolactone) only for conditions described under Indications and Clinical Use.

Potassium (K^+) Supplementation: The concurrent administration of potassium supplements, a diet rich in potassium, or other K^+-sparing diuretics is not recommended as this may induce hyperkalemia.

Somnolence and Dizziness: Somnolence and dizziness have been reported to occur in some patients. Caution is advised when driving or operating machinery until the response to initial treatment has been determined.

Carcinogenesis and Mutagenesis: Tumorigenicity: Spironolactone, in chronic toxicity studies, has been shown to be a tumorigen in rats.

Endocrine and Metabolism: Gynecomastia: Gynecomastia may develop with the use of ALDACTONE and physicians should be advised of its possible occurrence. The development of gynecomastia appears to be related to both dosage and duration of therapy and is normally reversible when the drug is discontinued. If gynecomastia develops, discontinue the drug. In rare instances some breast enlargement may persist.

Hyperchloremic Metabolic Acidosis: Reversible hyperchloremic metabolic acidosis, usually in association with hyperkalemia, has been reported to occur in some patients with decompensated hepatic cirrhosis, even when renal function is normal.

Acidosis and Renal Function: Rare reports of acidosis have been reported with ALDACTONE.

Hematologic: Electrolyte Balance: Because of the diuretic action of ALDACTONE patients should be carefully evaluated for possible disturbance of fluid and electrolyte balance, due to the possibility of hyperkalemia, hypochloremic alkalosis, hyponatremia and possible BUN elevation, especially the elderly and/or patients with pre-existing impaired renal or hepatic function.

a. **Hyperkalemia:** Hyperkalemia may occur in patients treated with ALDACTONE if the potassium intake is excessive. This can cause cardiac irregularities, some of which may be fatal. Hyperkalemia may also occur even in the absence of potassium supplementation, particularly in patients with impaired renal function, elderly patients, or patients with diabetes. Consequently, no potassium supplementation should ordinarily be given with ALDACTONE. ALDACTONE should not be administered concurrently with other potassium-sparing diuretics. ALDACTONE, when used with angiotensin converting enzyme (ACE) inhibitors Angiotensin II antagonists, other aldosterone blockers or indomethacin, even in the presence of a diuretic, has been associated with severe hyperkalemia (see Drug Interactions).

   Hyperkalemia in Patients with Severe Heart Failure: As hyperkalemia may be fatal, it is critical to monitor and manage serum potassium in patients with severe heart failure receiving ALDACTONE. Avoid using other potassium-sparing diuretics. Avoid using oral potassium supplements in patients with serum potassium >3.5 mEq/L. No information is available regarding patients with serum creatinine >2.5 mg/dL or a recent increase in serum creatinine >25%. The recommended monitoring for potassium and creatinine is one week after initiation or increase in dose of ALDACTONE, monthly for the first 3 months, then quarterly for a year, and then every 6 months. Discontinue or interrupt treatment for serum potassium >5 mEq/L or for serum creatinine >4 mg/dL.

   Hyperkalemia can be treated promptly by rapid intravenous administration of glucose (20 to 50%) and regular insulin, using 0.25 to 0.5 units of insulin per gram of glucose. This is a temporary measure to be repeated if required. ALDACTONE should be discontinued and potassium intake (including dietary potassium) restricted.

b. **Hyponatremia:** During the administration of ALDACTONE patients suffering from sodium depletion must be attentively monitored and signs of electrolyte imbalance must be carefully checked.

   ALDACTONE may, if administered concomitantly with other diuretics, cause or aggravate hyponatremia, as manifested by dryness of the mouth, thirst, lethargy, and drowsiness.

Hepatic/Biliary/Pancreatic: Impaired Hepatic Function: ALDACTONE should be used with caution in patients with impaired hepatic function because minor alterations of fluid and electrolyte balance may precipitate hepatic coma.

Management of Cirrhosis: Although high doses of ALDACTONE are required to treat edema and ascites in patients with cirrhosis, the drug dosage may be decreased before diuresis is complete to avoid the possibility of dehydration.

Neurologic: Lithium generally should not be given with diuretics (see Drug Interactions).

Sexual Function/Reproduction: In a reproduction study in which female rats received dietary doses of 15 and 50 mg/kg/day spironolactone, there were no effects on mating or fertility, but there was a small increase in incidence of stillborn pups at the higher dose. When injected into female rats (100 mg/kg/day, 7 days i.p.) spironolactone was found to increase the length of the estrous cycle by prolonging diestrus during treatment and inducing constant diestrus during a two-week, post-treatment observation period. These effects were associated with retarded ovarian follicle development and a reduction in circulating estrogen levels, which would be expected to impair mating, fertility and fecundity. Spironolactone (100 mg/kg/day i.p.) administered to female mice decreased the number of mated mice that conceived, and decreased the number of implanted embryos in those that became pregnant; at 200 mg/kg/day it also increased the latency period to mating.

Special Populations: Pregnant Women: Spironolactone and its metabolites may cross the placental barrier. There are no studies in pregnant women. Therefore, the use of ALDACTONE requires that the potential benefits be weighed against the possible hazard to the mother and fetus.

Spironolactone was devoid of teratogenic effects in mice. Rabbits receiving spironolactone showed reduced conception rate, increased resorption rate, and lower number of live births. No embryotoxic effects were seen in rats administered high dosages, but limited, dose-related hypoprolactinemia and decreased ventral prostate and seminal vesicle weights in males, and increased leutinizing hormone secretion and ovarian and uterine weights in females were reported. Feminization of the external genitalia of male fetuses was reported in another rat study.

Nursing Women: Canrenone, a major (and active) metabolite of spironolactone, appears in human breast milk. Because of the unknown potential for adverse events on the breastfeeding infant, a decision should be made whether to discontinue breastfeeding or discontinue the drug, taking into account the importance of the drug to the mother.

Monitoring and Laboratory Tests: General: ALDACTONE therapy may cause transient elevation of BUN, especially in patients with pre existing renal impairment.

Several reports of possible interference with digoxin radioimmunoassays by spironolactone or its metabolites have appeared in the literature. Neither the extent nor the potential clinical significance of this interference (which may be assay specific) has been fully established.

Discontinue spironolactone for at least 4, and preferably 7, days prior to plasma cortisol determinations, **if they are to be done by the method of Mattingly**, that is, by fluorometric assay. No interference has been demonstrated with the competitive protein binding technique or radioimmunoassay technique.

Adrenal Vein Catheterization and Plasma Renin Activity: Discontinue spironolactone several days prior to adrenal vein catheterization for measurement of aldosterone concentrations and measurements of plasma renin activity.

ADVERSE REACTIONS: The following adverse reactions have been reported in association with ALDACTONE (spironolactone):

General Disorders and Administration Site Conditions: malaise.

Gastrointestinal Disorders: diarrhea and cramping, gastric bleeding, gastritis, nausea, ulceration, vomiting.

Blood and Lymphatic System Disorders: leukopenia (including agranulocytosis), thrombocytopenia, anemia.

Immune System Disorders: drug fever, urticaria, maculopapular or erythematous cutaneous eruptions, anaphylactic reactions, vasculitis, pruritus, rash.

Hepatobiliary Disorders: hepatic function disorder. A very few cases of mixed cholestatic/hepatocellular toxicity, with one reported fatality, have been reported with spironolactone administration.

Metabolism and Nutrition Disorders: electrolyte disturbances, hyperkalemia.

Musculoskeletal and Connective Tissue Disorders: leg cramps.

Nervous System/Psychiatric Disorders: mental confusion, ataxia, headache, drowsiness, lethargy, dizziness, change in libido.

Renal and Urinary Disorders: renal dysfunction (including acute renal failure).

Reproductive System and Breast Disorders: abnormal semen (decreased motility and sperm count), inability to achieve or maintain erection, irregular menses or amenorrhea, postmenopausal bleeding, benign breast neoplasm, breast pain, gynecomastia*.

Carcinoma of the breast has been reported in patients, including male patients, taking spironolactone, but a cause and effect relationship has not been established.

Respiratory, Thoracic and Mediastinal Disorders: dysphonia, dyspnea.

Skin and Subcutaneous Tissue Disorders: alopecia, hypertrichosis.

Adverse reactions are usually reversible upon discontinuation of the drug.

DRUG INTERACTIONS: Drug-Drug Interactions: See Table 1.

Drug-Food Interactions: Food increases the bioavailability of unmetabolized spironolactone (two 100 mg ALDACTONE tablets) by almost 100%. The clinical importance of this finding is not known.

Drug-Laboratory Test Interactions: Several reports of possible interference with digoxin radioimmunoassays by spironolactone, or its metabolites, have appeared in the literature. Neither the extent, nor the potential clinical significance of its interference (which may be assay specific) has been fully established.

* Gynecomastia may develop in association with the use of spironolactone. Development of gynecomastia is related to both dose and duration of therapy. Gynecomastia is usually reversible when spironolactone is discontinued, although in rare instances some breast enlargement may persist.

Spironolactone has been shown to increase the half life of digoxin. This may result in increased serum digoxin levels and subsequent digitalis toxicity (see Drug-Drug Interactions).

Table 1: ALDACTONE
Established or Potential Drug-Drug Interactions

ALDACTONE Drug Interaction	Effect	Clinical Comment
Alcohol, Barbiturates or Narcotics	Potentiation of orthostatic hypotension may occur.	
Antipyrine	Spironolactone enhances the metabolism of antipyrine.	
Cholestyramine/Ammonium Chloride	Hyperchloremic metabolic acidosis, frequently associated with hyperkalemia, has been reported in patients given spironolactone concurrently with ammonium chloride or cholestyramine.	
Corticosteroids, ACTH	Intensified electrolyte depletion, particularly hypokalemia, may occur.	
Diuretics and Antihypertensives	Although ALDACTONE may be administered concomitantly with diuretics and antihypertensives, the effect of ALDACTONE is additive. Hyperkalemia has been associated with the use of angiotensin converting enzyme (ACE) inhibitors, angiotensin II antagonists and aldosterone blockers in combination with spironolactone.	It is advisable to reduce the dose of these drugs. In particular, the dose of ganglionic blocking agents should be reduced by at least 50% when ALDACTONE is added to the regimen.
Lithium	Diuretic agents reduce the renal clearance of lithium and add a high risk of lithium toxicity.	Lithium generally should not be given with diuretics.
Norepinephrine	ALDACTONE reduces the vascular responsiveness to norepinephrine.	Caution should be exercised in the management of patients subjected to regional or general anaesthesia while being treated with spironolactone.
Digoxin	Spironolactone has been shown to increase the half-life of digoxin. This may result in increased serum digoxin levels and subsequent digitalis toxicity.	It may be necessary to reduce the maintenance dose of digoxin when spironolactone is administered, and the patient should be carefully monitored to avoid over- or underdigitalization.
Non-Steroidal Anti-Inflammatory Drugs	ASA, mefenamic acid, and indomethacin may attenuate the diuretic action of spironolactone due to inhibition of intrarenal synthesis of prostaglandins. Hyperkalemia has been associated with the use of indomethacin in combination with potassium-sparing diuretics.	However, it has been shown that ASA does not alter the effect of spironolactone on blood pressure, serum electrolytes, urea nitrogen, or plasma renin activity in hypertensive patients.

DOSAGE AND ADMINISTRATION:

1. **Diagnosis and Treatment of Primary Hyperaldosteronism:** As an initial diagnostic measure to provide presumptive evidence of primary hyperaldosteronism while patients are on normal diets:

   Long Test: Administer ALDACTONE at a daily dosage of 400 mg for 3-4 weeks. Correction of hypokalemia and hypertension provides presumptive evidence for the diagnosis of primary hyperaldosteronism.

   Short Test: Administer ALDACTONE at a daily dosage of 400 mg×4 days. If serum potassium increases or urinary potassium decreases during ALDACTONE administration, but reverts when ALDACTONE is discontinued, a presumptive diagnosis of primary hyperaldosteronism should be considered.

   After the diagnosis of primary hyperaldosteronism has been established by more definitive testing procedures, ALDACTONE may be administered in doses of 75 mg to 400 mg daily in preparation for surgery. For those unsuitable for surgery, spironolactone may be employed for long-term maintenance therapy at the lowest effective dosage determined for the individual.

2. **Edematous Disorders Associated with Congestive Heart Failure, Cirrhosis and the Nephrotic Syndrome:** When given as sole agent for diuresis, continue administration for at least 5 days. If an adequate response has been achieved within 5 days, continue dosage at the same level (or in selected patients, at a reduced dosage) in either single or divided daily doses. Some may respond adequately to a dosage of only 75 mg daily. If adequate diuresis is not obtained within 5 days, a second diuretic also should be given for additive effect. Occasionally for severe resistant edema, one may add a potent glucocorticoid to this combined therapy. Normally, an initial daily dosage of 100 mg (but may range from 25-200 mg daily) of ALDACTONE administered in either single or divided doses is recommended.

   Dosage in Children: The initial daily dosage should provide approximately 3 mg/kg of body weight administered in either single or divided doses. This dose should be reduced to 1-2 mg/kg for maintenance therapy or combination use with other diuretics.

3. **Essential Hypertension:** Usually in combination with other drugs, ALDACTONE is indicated for patients who cannot be treated adequately with other agents or for whom other agents are considered inappropriate. ALDACTONE has mild to moderate antihypertensive activity.

   For adults an initial daily dosage of 50-100 mg (in either single or divided doses) of ALDACTONE is recommended. ALDACTONE may also be given with diuretics that act more proximally in the renal tubule or with other antihypertensive agents. Since a stabilized response may not occur before 2 weeks, continue treatment in either single or divided daily doses for that duration of time. Subsequently, adjust dosage in response to patient's needs. Most patients will respond to doses not exceeding 200 mg/day.

4. **Hypokalemia:** ALDACTONE in dosage ranging from 25 mg to 100 mg daily is useful in treating a diuretic induced hypokalemia, when oral potassium supplements or other potassium-sparing regimens are inappropriate. See also Table 2 for a summary of dosage recommendations.

OVERDOSAGE:

Symptoms: There have been no reports of fatal overdose in man (except indirectly through hyperkalemia). Nausea and vomiting occurs, and (much more rarely) drowsiness, dizziness, mental confusion, diarrhea, or a maculopapular or erythematous rash. These manifestations disappear promptly on discontinuation of medication. Hyperkalemia may be exacerbated.

Treatment: No specific antidote. No persistent toxicity has occurred or is expected. Inducing vomiting and evacuating the stomach by lavage could be considered. Spironolactone use should be discontinued and potassium intake (including dietary sources) restricted.

For management of a suspected drug overdose, contact your **regional Poison Control Centre**. See the *CPS* Directory section for a list of Poison Control Centres.

Table 2: ALDACTONE

ALDACTONE Dosage[a]

Condition	Type of Test	In Single or Divided Daily Doses	
		Initial Dosage	Maximum Dosage
Primary Hyperaldosteronism			
	Long Test	400 mg/day×3–4 weeks	—
	Short Test	400 mg/day×4 days	—
In Preparation for Surgery:		100–400 mg/day	400 mg/day
Edematous Disorders			
Congestive Heart Failure	—	100 mg/day	200 mg/day
Cirrhosis	Urinary: Na^+/K^+ ratio >1	100 mg/day	100 mg/day
	Urinary: Na^+/K^+ ratio <1	200–400 mg/day	400 mg/day
Nephrotic Syndrome	—	100 mg/day	200 mg/day
Essential Hypertension	—	50–100 mg/day	200 mg/day
Hypokalemia	—	25–100 mg/day	100 mg/day

[a] Maintenance dosage should be individually determined and may be lower than the recommended initial dose.

ACTION AND CLINICAL PHARMACOLOGY: Mechanism of Action: ALDACTONE (spironolactone) is a specific pharmacologic antagonist of aldosterone, acting primarily through competitive binding of receptors at the aldosterone dependent, sodium potassium exchange site in the distal convoluted renal tubule. ALDACTONE causes increased amounts of sodium and water to be excreted, while potassium loss is minimized.

ALDACTONE acts both as a diuretic and as an antihypertensive drug by this mechanism. It may be given alone or with other diuretic agents which act more proximally in the renal tubule.

Pharmacodynamics: Increased levels of the mineralocorticoid, aldosterone, are present in primary and secondary hyperaldosteronism. Edematous states in which secondary aldosteronism is usually involved include congestive heart failure, hepatic cirrhosis, and nephrotic syndrome. By competing with aldosterone for receptor sites, ALDACTONE provides effective therapy for the edema and ascites in those conditions. ALDACTONE counteracts secondary aldosteronism induced by the volume depletion and associated sodium loss caused by diuretic therapy.

ALDACTONE is effective in lowering the systolic and diastolic blood pressure in patients with primary hyperaldosteronism. It is also effective in most cases of essential hypertension, despite the fact that aldosterone secretion may be within normal limits in benign essential hypertension.

Through its action in antagonizing the effect of aldosterone, ALDACTONE inhibits the exchange of sodium for potassium in the distal renal tubule and helps to prevent potassium loss.

ALDACTONE has not been demonstrated to elevate serum uric acid, to precipitate gout, or to alter carbohydrate metabolism.

Pharmacokinetics: Spironolactone is rapidly and extensively metabolized to a number of metabolites including canrenone and the sulfur-containing 7-thiomethylspirolactone, both of which are pharmacologically active. Approximately 25 to 30% of the dose administered is converted to canrenone, which attains peak serum levels 2-4 hours after single oral administration of spironolactone. In the dose range of 25 mg to 200 mg, an approximately linear relationship exists between a single dose of spironolactone and plasma levels of canrenone.

Plasma concentrations of canrenone decline in two distinct phases, the first phase lasting from 3 to 12 hours, being more rapid than the second phase lasting from 12 to 96 hours. Canrenone clearance data, following multiple doses of spironolactone, indicate that accumulation of canrenone in the body with 100 mg once a day would be lower than with 25 mg four times a day. Both spironolactone and canrenone are more than 90-percent bound to plasma proteins. The metabolites of spironolactone are excreted both in the urine (32-53%), and through biliary excretion in the feces (14-36%). See Table 3.

Table 3: ALDACTONE

Summary of ALDACTONE's Pharmacokinetic Parameters in Healthy Volunteers Administered 100 mg Daily for 15 Days

	Mean C_{max} (ng/mL)	Mean T_{max} (h)	Mean Post-Steady State $t_{½}$ (h)	Accumulation Factor: $AUC_{0\text{-}24\,h}$, Day 15/$AUC_{0\text{-}24\,h}$, Day 1
7-α-(thiomethyl) spirolactone (TMS)	391	3.2	13.8	1.25
6-β-hydroxy-7-α- (thiomethyl) spirolactone (HTMS)	125	5.1	15.0	1.5
Canrenone (C)	181	4.3	16.5	1.41
Spironolactone	80	2.6	~1.4 ($t_{½}$ β)	1.3

STORAGE AND STABILITY: Store at 15 to 25°C.

INFORMATION FOR THE PATIENT: Published in e-CPS, available by subscription at www.e-cps.ca.

DOSAGE FORMS, COMPOSITION AND PACKAGING: 25 mg: Each light yellow, round, biconvex, film-coated tablet, debossed "ALDACTONE" and "25" on one face and "SEARLE" and "1001" on the other face and with peppermint odour, contains: spironolactone 25 mg. Nonmedicinal ingredients: calcium sulfate, carnauba wax, cornstarch, hypromellose, magnesium stearate, opaspray M-1-2042, peppermint flavouring, polyethylene glycol 400, povidone and stearic acid. Bottles of 100.

100 mg: Each peach, round, biconvex, scored, film-coated tablet, debossed "ALDACTONE" and "100" on one face and "SEARLE" and "1031" on the other (scored) face and with peppermint odour, contains: spironolactone 100 mg. Nonmedicinal ingredients: calcium sulfate, carnauba wax, cornstarch, hypromellose, magnesium stearate, opaspray M-1-2668, peppermint flavouring, polyethylene glycol 400, povidone and stearic acid. Bottles of 100.

(Shown in Product Identification Section)

Aldara™

imiquimod

Immune Response Modifier

Graceway

Date of Preparation: March 29, 2007
Date of Revision: March 4, 2009

PHARMACOLOGY: In vitro studies have demonstrated that imiquimod induces the release of interferon alpha (IFN-α) and other cytokines from human monocytes/macrophages and keratinocytes. The panel of cytokines induced varied with the cell's tissue origin. Topical in vivo application of imiquimod cream on mouse skin resulted in increased concentrations of IFN and tumor necrosis factor (TNF) compared with skin of untreated mice. The cytokine inducing properties of imiquimod may be responsible for its activity against genital/perianal warts, as imiquimod does not have a direct antiviral activity in cell cultures. The clinical relevance of these findings is, however, unknown.

Pharmacodynamics: Superficial Basal Cell Carcinoma (sBCC): The mechanism of action of imiquimod in treating superficial basal cell carcinoma (sBCC) lesions is unknown. One clinical study in 6 subjects has suggested that imiquimod stimulates the infiltration of T-cell lymphocytes, dendritic cells, and macrophages into the basal cell carcinoma lesion.

Actinic Keratosis (AK): The mechanism of action of imiquimod in treating actinic keratosis (AK) lesions is unknown. While the following have been observed, the clinical significance of these observations in AK is not known. In a study of 58 patients with AK treated with imiquimod 3 times per week, the response of biomarkers sensitive to imiquimod after 16 weeks of dosing increased compared to the response after the first dose. For interleukin-1 antagonist, the median concentration observed following multiple dosing was <2-fold higher than that after single dose administration, for interferon-α was ≤3-fold, and for 2'5'-oligoadenylate synthetase was approximately 3-fold.

External Genital Warts (EGW): Imiquimod has no direct antiviral activity in cell culture. A study in 22 patients with genital/perianal warts comparing imiquimod and vehicle shows that imiquimod induces mRNA encoding cytokines including interferon-α at the treatment site. In addition HPVL1 mRNA and HPV DNA are significantly decreased following treatment. However, the clinical relevance of these findings is unknown.

Pharmacokinetics: Percutaneous absorption of imiquimod has been studied through intact healthy skin, the skin of genital warts, and lesions of sun damaged skin. Percutaneous absorption of [^{14}C] imiquimod was minimal in a study involving six healthy subjects treated with a single topical application (5 mg) of [^{14}C] imiquimod in cream formulation. No radioactivity was detected in the serum (lower limit of quantitation is 1 ng/mL) and <0.9% of the radiolabelled dose was excreted in the urine and feces following topical application.

Systemic absorption of imiquimod was observed across the affected skin of 12 patients with genital/perianal warts who were treated 3 times per week with sufficient 5% imiquimod cream to cover the affected wart area (average dose 4.6 mg imiquimod) for 16 weeks. Mean (median) peak drug concentrations of 0.3 (0.1) ng/mL were seen following week 16 dosing. Mean (median) urinary recoveries following the last dose of week 16, expressed as percent of the estimated applied dose, were 0.24 (0.09) and 2.52 (1.2) % of the dose for males and females, respectively, which may suggest a possible sex difference in absorption and/or excretion.

Similarly, systemic absorption of imiquimod across the affected skin of 58 patients with AK was observed with a dosing frequency of 3 applications per week for 16 weeks. Mean (median) peak serum drug concentrations at the end of week 16 were observed between 9 and 12 hours and were approximately 0.1 (0.1), 0.2 (0.2), and 3.5 (1.6) ng/mL for the applications to face (12.5 mg imiquimod, 1 single-use packet), scalp (25 mg, 2 packets) and hands/arms (75 mg, 6 packets), respectively. The application surface area was not controlled in the scalp and hands/arms groups. Dose proportionality was not observed, although the pharmacokinetic parameters (C_{max} and AUC) tended to increase with dose. It appears that systemic exposure may be more dependent on surface area of application than amount of applied dose. The apparent half-life following topical dosing was calculated as 26 hours, which is approximately 10 times greater than the 2 hour apparent half-life seen following subcutaneous dosing and suggests prolonged retention of drug in the skin. Mean (median) urinary recoveries at week 16 were 0.18 (0.14), 0.24 (0.24) and 0.12 (0.09) % of the applied dose following application to the face, scalp and hands/arms, respectively. The highest urinary recovery measured in any patient was less than 0.6% of the applied dose at week 16.

INDICATIONS: ALDARA (imiquimod) cream is indicated in immunocompetent adults for the following conditions:

- Treatment of biopsy-confirmed, primary **superficial** basal cell carcinoma (sBCC) with a maximum tumor diameter of 2.0 cm, located on the trunk (excluding anogenital skin), neck, or extremities (excluding hands and feet), otherwise amenable to simple surgical excision, in patients who, in consultation with their physician, choose not to have surgery and are willing to undergo regular follow-up. Note: Surgical excision is the usual treatment of choice for these sBCC tumors. While ALDARA has been shown to be effective in the short-term clearance of sBCC in ~75% of cases, there are no data directly comparing ALDARA to surgical excision.
- Treatment of clinically typical, nonhyperkeratotic, nonhypertrophic actinic keratosis on the face or balding scalp.
- Treatment of external genital and perianal warts/condyloma acuminata.

CONTRAINDICATIONS: ALDARA (imiquimod) cream is contraindicated in individuals with a history of sensitivity reactions to any of its components. It should be discontinued if hypersensitivity to any of its ingredients is noted.

WARNINGS: Patients with sBCC treated with ALDARA cream are required to have regular follow-up of the treatment site because the efficacy of imiquimod in the treatment of sBCC is generally less than that with surgery and, as well, because the long term efficacy and safety of imiquimod in the treatment of sBCC have not yet been established.

The histological diagnosis of **superficial** basal cell carcinoma should be established prior to treatment since ALDARA (imiquimod) cream has not been evaluated for the treatment of other types of basal cell carcinomas, including nodular, morpheaform (fibrosing or sclerosing) types and is not recommended for treatment of BCC subtypes other than the superficial variant.

ALDARA (imiquimod) cream has not been evaluated for the treatment of sBCC on the face, head, hands or feet, and anogenital area.

The efficacy of ALDARA in the prevention of squamous cell carcinoma (SCC) associated with AK has not been established. One subject who participated in a clinical trial of imiquimod and had complete clearance of AK lesions with imiquimod treatment developed a SCC in situ in the treatment area within 12 to 18 months of treatment.

ALDARA cream has not been evaluated for the treatment of urethral, intra-vaginal, cervical, rectal, or intra-anal human papilloma viral disease and is not recommended for these conditions.

Hypersensitivity reactions (urticaria) and erythema multiforme have been reported in patients receiving ALDARA cream. Causality has not been established and no other reports of similar cases have been reported in post-marketing surveillance. ALDARA cream should be discontinued immediately if these events occur.

Some reports of localised hypopigmentation and hyperpigmentation following use of ALDARA cream have been received. Post-marketing reporting suggests that these skin color changes may be permanent in some patients.

PRECAUTIONS: General: ALDARA cream administration is not recommended until skin or genital/perianal tissue is healed from any previous drug or surgical treatment. ALDARA cream has the potential to exacerbate inflammatory conditions of the skin.

Local skin reactions such as erythema, erosion, excoriation/flaking, and edema are common.

Should a severe local skin reaction occur, the cream should be removed by washing the treatment area with mild soap and water. Treatment with ALDARA can be resumed after the skin reaction has subsided.

The efficacy and safety of ALDARA cream have not been established for patients with Basal Cell Nevus Syndrome or Xeroderma Pigmentosum.

The safety of ALDARA cream applied to areas of skin greater than 25 cm² for the treatment of actinic keratosis has not been established.

The safety and efficacy of ALDARA cream in immunosuppressed patients have not been established.

Flu-like systemic signs and symptoms including malaise, fever, nausea, myalgias and rigors may occur. Dosing interruption may be required.

ALDARA cream should be used with caution in patients with pre-existing autoimmune conditions. Rare reports have been received of exacerbation of autoimmune conditions in patients treated with ALDARA.

Exposure to sunlight (including sunlamps) should be avoided or minimized during use of ALDARA cream because of concern for heightened sunburn susceptibility. Patients should be warned to use protective clothing (hat) when using ALDARA cream. Patients with sunburn should be advised not to use ALDARA cream until fully recovered. Patients who may have considerable sun exposure, e.g., due to their occupation, and those patients with inherent sensitivity to sunlight should exercise caution when using ALDARA cream. Phototoxicity has not been adequately assessed for ALDARA cream. The enhancement of ultraviolet carcinogenicity is not necessarily dependent on phototoxic mechanisms. Despite the absence of observed phototoxicity in humans, ALDARA cream shortened the time to skin tumor formation in an animal photoco-carcinogenicity study (see Carcinogenicity, Mutagenesis, and Impairment of Fertility). Therefore, it is prudent for patients to minimize or avoid natural or artificial sunlight exposure.

Carcinogenicity, Mutagenesis, and Impairment of Fertility: Two-year bioassays in Wistar rats (up to 3 mg/kg orally per day) and CD-1 mice (up to 4.5 mg/kg applied topically 3 times per week) showed no evidence of a carcinogenic effect in male and female rats and female mice. Liver tumors were increased in male mice exposed to the highest dose concentration, compared to the unexposed controls. However, the number of tumors was within the range seen historically for male CD-1 mice. It is generally accepted that an increase in liver tumors in male mice, in the absence of other neoplastic responses in mice or rats, is not indicative of a carcinogenic risk for humans.

In a photocarcinogenicity study in hairless mice, animals received ALDARA cream 3 times per week at imiquimod concentrations of 0.03%, 0.1% and 0.3% and were irradiated with solar ultraviolet light for 5 days each week for 40 weeks and observed an additional 12 weeks. Vehicle cream enhanced UVR-induced skin tumor development. ALDARA cream had no additional effect on tumor development beyond the vehicle effect (i.e., the addition of the active ingredient, imiquimod, to the vehicle cream did not result in an additional effect beyond the vehicle effect on tumor development).

Pregnancy: Imiquimod was not teratogenic in rat or rabbit teratology studies. In rats at a high maternally toxic dose (28 times human dose on a mg/m² basis), reduced pup weights and delayed ossification were observed. However, there are no adequate and well-controlled studies in pregnant women. Because animal reproduction studies are not always predictive of human response, this drug should be used during pregnancy only if clearly needed.

Lactation: It is not known whether topically applied imiquimod is excreted in breast milk.

Children: Safety and efficacy in patients below the age of 18 years have not been established.

Geriatrics: Although no overall differences in safety or effectiveness have been observed between elderly and younger patients, greater sensitivity of some older individuals cannot be ruled out. Of the 185 patients in the 5 times per week treatment groups of clinical studies evaluating the treatment of sBCC with ALDARA cream, 65 patients (35%) were 65 years and older, while 25 patients (14%) were 75 years and older. Of the 215 patients in the 2 times per week clinical studies evaluating the treatment of AK lesions with ALDARA cream, 127 patients (59%) were 65 years and older, while 60 patients (28%) were 75 years and older. No overall differences in safety or effectiveness were observed between these patients and younger patients. No other clinical experience has identified differences in responses between the elderly and younger patients.

ADVERSE EFFECTS: Superficial Basal Cell Carcinoma: The data described below reflect exposure to ALDARA cream or vehicle in 364 patients enrolled in two double-blind, vehicle-controlled studies in which subjects with sBCC applied ALDARA cream or vehicle to the target lesions 5×/week for 6 weeks. See Table 1.

Table 1: ALDARA

Summary of All Adverse Events Reported by >1% of Patients in the Combined 5×/Week Studies

Body System Preferred Term	Imiquimod 5×/Week (n=185)		Vehicle 5×/Week (n=179)	
Application Site Disorders				
Application Site Reaction	52	(28.1%)	5	(2.8%)
Body as a Whole—General Disorders				
Allergy Aggravated	2	(1.1%)	1	(0.6%)
Back Pain	7	(3.8%)	1	(0.6%)
Chest Pain	2	(1.1%)	0	(0.0%)
Fatigue	4	(2.2%)	2	(1.1%)
Fever	3	(1.6%)	0	(0.0%)
Pain	3	(1.6%)	2	(1.1%)
Cardiovascular Disorders, General				
Hypertension	5	(2.7%)	1	(0.6%)
Central & Peripheral Nervous Systems Disorders				
Dizziness	2	(1.1%)	1	(0.6%)
Headache	14	(7.6%)	4	(2.2%)
Gastrointestinal System Disorders				
Abdominal Pain	1	(0.5%)	2	(1.1%)
Diarrhea	1	(0.5%)	2	(1.1%)
Dyspepsia	3	(1.6%)	2	(1.1%)
Gastrointestinal Disorders NOS	1	(0.5%)	2	(1.1%)
Nausea	2	(1.1%)	0	(0.0%)
Tooth Disorder	0	(0.0%)	2	(1.1%)
Metabolic and Nutritional Disorders				
Gout	2	(1.1%)	0	(0.0%)
Musculoskeletal System Disorders				
Skeletal Pain	3	(1.6%)	2	(1.1%)
Psychiatric Disorders				
Anxiety	2	(1.1%)	1	(0.6%)
Resistance Mechanism Disorders				
Infection	1	(0.5%)	3	(1.7%)
Infection Fungal	2	(1.1%)	2	(1.1%)
Respiratory System Disorders				
Coughing	3	(1.6%)	1	(0.6%)
Pharyngitis	2	(1.1%)	1	(0.6%)
Rhinitis	5	(2.7%)	1	(0.6%)
Sinusitis	4	(2.2%)	1	(0.6%)
Upper Respiratory Tract Infection	6	(3.2%)	2	(1.1%)

(cont'd)

Table 1: ALDARA *(cont'd)*

Summary of All Adverse Events Reported by >1% of Patients in the Combined 5×/Week Studies

Body System Preferred Term	Imiquimod 5×/Week (n=185)		Vehicle 5×/Week (n=179)	
Secondary Terms				
Inflicted Injury	3	(1.6%)	3	(1.7%)
Procedural Site Reaction	2	(1.1%)	3	(1.7%)
Skin and Appendages Disorders				
Hyperkeratosis	3	(1.6%)	2	(1.1%)
Rash	3	(1.6%)	1	(0.6%)
Skin Disorder	1	(0.5%)	3	(1.7%)
White Cell and Resistance Disorders				
Lymphadenopathy	5	(2.7%)	1	(0.6%)

The most frequently reported adverse reactions were those of local skin and application site reactions including erythema, edema, induration, erosion, flaking/scaling, scabbing/crusting, itching and burning at the application site. The adverse reactions that most frequently resulted in clinical intervention (e.g., rest periods, withdrawal from study) were local skin and application site reactions; 10% (19/185) of patients received rest periods. The average number of doses not received per patient due to rest periods was 7 doses with a range of 2 to 22 doses; 79% of patients (15/19) resumed therapy after a rest period. Overall, in the clinical studies, 2% (4/185) of patients discontinued for local skin/application site reactions. The incidence of application site reactions reported by >1% of the subjects during the 6-week treatment period is summarized in Table 2.

Table 2: ALDARA

Summary of All Application Site Reactions Reported by >1% of Patients in the Combined 5×/Week Studies

Included Term	Imiquimod 5×/Week (n=185)		Vehicle 5×/Week (n=179)	
Itching at Target Site	30	(16.2%)	1	(0.6%)
Burning at Target Site	11	(5.9%)	2	(1.1%)
Pain at Target Site	6	(3.2%)	0	(0.0%)
Tenderness at Target Site	2	(1.1%)	0	(0.0%)
Erythema at Remote Site	3	(1.6%)	0	(0.0%)
Papule(s) at Target Site	3	(1.6%)	0	(0.0%)
Bleeding at Target Site	4	(2.2%)	0	(0.0%)
Tingling at Target Site	1	(0.5%)	2	(1.1%)
Infection at Target Site	2	(1.1%)	0	(0.0%)

Local skin reactions were collected independently of the adverse event "application site reaction" in an effort to provide a better picture of the specific types of local reactions that might be seen. The incidence and severity of local skin reactions that occurred during controlled studies are shown in Table 3.

Table 3: ALDARA

Most Intense Local Skin Reactions in the Treatment Area as Assessed by the Investigator (Percentage of Patients) 5×/Week Application

	Mild/Moderate		Severe	
Local Skin Reactions	**ALDARA Cream (n=184)**	**Vehicle (n=178)**	**ALDARA Cream (n=184)**	**Vehicle (n=178)**
Edema	71%	36%	7%	0%
Erosion	54%	14%	13%	0%
Erythema	69%	95%	31%	2%
Flaking/Scaling	87%	76%	4%	0%
Induration	78%	53%	6%	0%
Scabbing/Crusting	64%	34%	19%	0%
Ulceration	34%	3%	6%	0%
Vesicles	29%	2%	2%	0%

Adverse events judged to be probably or possibly related to ALDARA cream and reported by at least 1% of the patients included: Application Site Reactions: Target Site Reactions (itching, burning, pain, tenderness, bleeding, papules, infection, pimples); Remote Site Reactions (erythema); Body as a Whole: back pain; White Cell and Resistance Disorders: lymphadenopathy.

In the sBCC studies, 23 of 1266 (1.8%) imiquimod-treated patients developed treatment site infections that were treated with antibiotics; the majority of these patients required a rest period off ALDARA cream. In all vehicle controlled BCC studies, the adverse event lymphadenopathy was reported in 12 (1.8%) of the 672 imiquimod-treated patients. In all phase II/III BCC trials with 5×/week imiquimod dose groups, 9 (1.7%) of 518 patients with pre- and post-treatment laboratory tests developed a ≥2 toxicity grade level shift from baseline to end-of-treatment in absolute lymphocyte counts.

Actinic Keratosis: The data described below reflect exposure to ALDARA cream or vehicle in 436 patients enrolled in two double-blind, vehicle-controlled studies in which patients applied ALDARA cream or vehicle to a 25 cm² contiguous treatment area on the face or balding scalp 2 times per week for 16 weeks. See Table 4.

In controlled clinical studies, the most frequently reported adverse reactions were those of local skin and application site reactions including erythema, flaking/scaling/dryness, scabbing/crusting, itching and burning at the application site. The adverse reactions that most frequently resulted in clinical intervention (e.g., rest periods, withdrawal from study) were local skin and application site reactions: 16% (35/215) of patients received rest periods. The average number of doses not received per patient due to rest periods was 4 doses with a range of 1 to 11 doses: 91% of patients (32/35) resumed therapy after a rest period. Overall, in the clinical studies, 2% (5/215) of patients discontinued for local skin/application site reactions and one patient discontinued due to the development of urticaria. One patient developed a bacterial infection at the treatment site. See Table 5.

Table 4: ALDARA

Summary of All Adverse Events Reported by >1% of Patients in the Combined 2×/Week Studies

Body System Preferred Term	Imiquimod 2×/Week (n=215)		Vehicle 2×/Week (n=221)	
Application Site Disorders				
Application Site Reaction	71	(33.0%)	32	(14.5%)
Body as a Whole—General Disorders				
Back Pain	3	(1.4%)	2	(0.9%)
Fatigue	3	(1.4%)	2	(0.9%)
Fever	3	(1.4%)	0	(0.0%)
Headache	11	(5.1%)	7	(3.2%)
Hernia NOS	4	(1.9%)	1	(0.5%)
Influenza-like Symptoms	4	(1.9%)	4	(1.8%)
Pain	3	(1.4%)	3	(1.4%)
Rigors	3	(1.4%)	0	(0.0%)
Cardiovascular Disorders, General				
Chest Pain	1	(0.5%)	4	(1.8%)
Hypertension	3	(1.4%)	5	(2.3%)
Central & Peripheral Nervous Systems Disorders				
Dizziness	3	(1.4%)	1	(0.5%)
Gastrointestinal System Disorders				
Diarrhea	6	(2.8%)	2	(0.9%)
Dyspepsia	6	(2.8%)	4	(1.8%)
Gastroesophageal Reflux	3	(1.4%)	3	(1.4%)
Nausea	3	(1.4%)	3	(1.4%)
Vomiting	3	(1.4%)	1	(0.5%)
Heart Rate and Rhythm Disorders				
Fibrillation Atrial	3	(1.4%)	2	(0.9%)
Metabolic and Nutritional Disorders				
Hypercholesterolemia	4	(1.9%)	0	(0.0%)
Musculoskeletal System Disorders				
Arthralgia	2	(0.0%)	4	(1.8%)
Arthritis	2	(0.9%)	3	(1.4%)
Myalgia	3	(1.4%)	3	(1.4%)
Skeletal Pain	1	(0.5%)	3	(1.4%)
Neoplasm				
Basal Cell Carcinoma	5	(2.3%)	5	(2.3%)
Carcinoma Squamous	8	(3.7%)	5	(2.3%)
Resistance Mechanism Disorders	9	(4.2%)	11	(5.0%)
Herpes Simplex	4	(1.9%)	4	(1.8%)
Infection Viral	3	(1.4%)	2	(0.9%)
Respiratory System Disorders				
Bronchitis	2	(0.9%)	3	(1.4%)
Coughing	6	(2.8%)	10	(4.5%)
Pharyngitis	4	(1.9%)	4	(1.8%)
Pulmonary Congestion	1	(0.5%)	3	(1.4%)
Rhinitis	7	(3.3%)	8	(3.6%)
Sinusitis	16	(7.4%)	14	(6.3%)
Upper Respiratory Tract Infection	33	(15.3%)	27	(12.2%)

(cont'd)

Table 4: ALDARA *(cont'd)*

Summary of All Adverse Events Reported by >1% of Patients in the Combined 2×/Week Studies

Body System Preferred Term	Imiquimod 2×/Week (n=215)		Vehicle 2×/Week (n=221)	
Secondary Terms				
Abrasion NOS	7	(3.3%)	5	(2.3%)
Cyst NOS	0	(0.0%)	4	(1.8%)
Inflicted Injury	19	(8.8%)	21	(9.5%)
Post-operative Pain	3	(1.4%)	4	(1.8%)
Skin and Appendages Disorders	47	(21.9%)	42	(19.0%)
Alopecia	3	(1.4%)	0	(0.0%)
Dermatitis	3	(1.4%)	7	(3.2%)
Eczema	4	(1.9%)	3	(1.4%)
Hyperkeratosis	19	(8.8%)	12	(5.4%)
Photosensitivity Reaction	2	(0.9%)	4	(1.8%)
Pruritus	2	(0.9%)	3	(1.4%)
Rash	5	(2.3%)	5	(2.3%)
Skin Disorder	6	(2.8%)	7	(3.2%)
Verruca	1	(0.5%)	3	(1.4%)
Urinary System Disorders	8	(3.7%)	10	(4.5%)
Urinary Tract Infection	3	(1.4%)	1	(0.5%)
Vision Disorders				
Conjunctivitis	1	(0.5%)	3	(1.4%)
Eye Abnormality	4	(1.9%)	1	(0.5%)
Eye Infection	0	(0.0%)	3	(1.4%)

Table 5: ALDARA

Summary of All Application Site Reactions Reported by >1% of Patients in the Combined 2×/Week Studies

Included Term	Imiquimod 2×/Week (n=215)		Vehicle 2×/Week (n=221)	
Bleeding at Target Site	7	(3.3%)	1	(0.5%)
Burning at Remote Site	4	(1.9%)	0	(0.0%)
Burning at Target Site	12	(5.6%)	4	(1.8%)
Induration at Remote Site	3	(1.4%)	0	(0.0%)
Induration at Target Site	5	(2.3%)	3	(1.4%)
Irritation at Remote Site	3	(1.4%)	0	(0.0%)
Itching at Remote Site	7	(3.3%)	3	(1.4%)
Itching at Target Site	44	(20.5%)	15	(6.8%)
Pain at Target Site	5	(2.3%)	2	(0.9%)
Stinging at Target Site	6	(2.8%)	2	(0.9%)
Tenderness at Target Site	4	(1.9%)	3	(1.4%)

Table 6: ALDARA

Most Intense Local Skin Reactions in the Treatment Area as Assessed by the Investigator (Percentage of Patients) 2×/Week Application

	Mild/Moderate		Severe	
Event	ALDARA (n=215)	Vehicle (n=220)	ALDARA (n=215)	Vehicle (n=220)
Erythema	80%	91%	18%	2%
Edema	49%	10%	0%	0%
Weeping/Exudate	21%	1%	0%	0%
Vesicles	9%	1%	0%	0%
Erosion/Ulceration	46%	9%	2%	0%
Flaking/Scaling/Dryness	85%	87%	7%	3%
Scabbing/Crusting	70%	40%	8%	2%

Table 7: ALDARA
Wart Site Reactions as Assessed by Investigator (3×/Week Application)

	Mild/Moderate				Severe			
	Females		Males		Females		Males	
	ALDARA (n=114)	Vehicle (n=99)	ALDARA (n=156)	Vehicle (n=157)	ALDARA (n=114)	Vehicle (n=99)	ALDARA (n=156)	Vehicle (n=157)
Erythema	61%	21%	54%	22%	4%	0%	4%	0%
Erosion	30%	8%	29%	6%	1%	0%	1%	0%
Excoriation/Flaking	18%	8%	25%	8%	0%	0%	1%	0%
Edema	17%	5%	12%	1%	1%	0%	0%	0%
Induration	5%	2%	7%	2%	0%	0%	0%	0%
Ulceration	5%	1%	4%	1%	3%	0%	0%	0%
Scabbing	4%	0%	13%	3%	0%	0%	0%	0%
Vesicles	3%	0%	2%	0%	0%	0%	0%	0%

Local skin reactions were collected independently of the adverse event "application site reaction" in an effort to provide a better picture of the specific types of local reactions that might be seen. The most frequently reported local skin reactions were erythema, flaking/scaling/dryness, and scabbing/crusting. The prevalence and severity of local skin reactions that occurred during controlled studies are shown in Table 6.

External Genital Warts: In controlled clinical trials, the most frequently reported adverse reactions were those of local skin and application site reactions; some patients also reported systemic reactions. These reactions were usually mild to moderate in intensity; however, severe reactions were reported with 3 times per week application. **These reactions were more frequent and more intense with daily application than with 3 times per week application.** Overall, in the 3 times per week application clinical studies, 1.2% (4/327) of the patients discontinued due to local skin/application site reactions. The incidence and severity of local skin reactions during controlled clinical trials are shown in Table 7.

Remote site skin reactions were also reported in female and male patients treated 3 times a week with ALDARA cream. The severe remote site skin reactions reported for females were erythema (3%), ulceration (2%), and edema (1%); and for males, erosion (2%), and erythema, edema, induration, and excoriation/flaking (each 1%).

Adverse events judged to be probably or possibly related to ALDARA cream reported by more than 5% of patients are listed in Table 8; also included are soreness, influenza-like symptoms and myalgia.

Table 8: ALDARA
Adverse Events Probably or Possibly Related to ALDARA Cream (3×/Week Application)

	Females		Males	
	ALDARA (n=117)	Vehicle (n=103)	ALDARA (n=156)	Vehicle (n=158)
Application Site Disorders/Application Site Reactions				
Wart Site				
Itching	32%	20%	22%	10%
Burning	26%	12%	9%	5%
Pain	8%	2%	2%	1%
Soreness	3%	0%	0%	1%
Fungal Infection[a]	11%	3%	2%	1%
Systemic Reactions				
Headache	4%	3%	5%	2%
Influenza-like Symptoms	3%	2%	1%	0%
Myalgia	1%	0%	1%	1%

[a] Incidences reported without regard to causality with ALDARA cream.

Adverse events judged to be possibly or probably related to ALDARA cream and reported by more than 1% of patients include: Application Site Disorders: Wart Site Reactions (burning, hypopigmentation, irritation, itching, pain, rash, sensitivity, soreness, stinging, tenderness); Remote Site Reactions (bleeding, burning, itching, pain, tenderness, tinea cruris); Body as a Whole: fatigue, fever, influenza-like symptoms; Central and Peripheral Nervous System Disorders: headache; Gastrointestinal System Disorders: diarrhea; Musculoskeletal System Disorders: myalgia.

Post-Marketing Experience: Application Site Disorders (resulting from internal application): local skin reactions, pain and swelling, difficulty passing urine in female patients.

Rare reports have been received of either the onset or exacerbation of autoimmune conditions (including thyroiditis, multiple sclerosis, spondyloarthropathy, psoriasis, ulcerative colitis) in association with ALDARA therapy.

OVERDOSE:

Symptoms: Overdosage of ALDARA (imiquimod) cream in humans is unlikely due to minimal percutaneous absorption. Animal studies reveal a rabbit dermal lethal imiquimod dose of greater than 5000 mg/kg. Persistent **topical** overdosing of ALDARA cream could result in severe local skin reactions.

The most clinically serious adverse event reported following multiple oral imiquimod doses of ≥200 mg was hypotension which resolved following oral or intravenous fluid administration.

For management of a suspected drug overdose, CPhA recommends that you contact your **regional Poison Control Centre**. See the *CPS* Directory section for a list of Poison Control Centres.

DOSAGE: The application frequency for ALDARA (imiquimod) cream is different for each indication.

Superficial Basal Cell Carcinoma: ALDARA cream is to be applied to a biopsy-confirmed sBCC 5 times per week, prior to normal sleeping hours, and left on the skin for approximately 8 hours. The treatment area should include a 1 cm margin of skin around the tumor. The amount of cream to be applied depends upon the diameter of the target sBCC (see Table 9).

Table 9: ALDARA
Patient Dosing Guide

Target Tumor Diameter	Size of Cream Droplet to be Used (Diameter)	Approximate Amount of Cream to be Used
0.5 to <1.0 cm	4 mm	10 mg
≥1.0 to <1.5 cm	5 mm	25 mg
≥1.5 to 2.0 cm	7 mm	40 mg

Before applying the cream, the patient should wash the treatment area with mild soap and water and allow the area to dry thoroughly. The cream should be applied to cover the treatment area, including one centimetre of skin surrounding the tumor, and should be rubbed into the treatment area until the cream is no longer visible. Caution subjects to avoid contacting the cream in or near the eyes. Approximately 8 hours after applying ALDARA, cream should be removed by washing the area with mild soap and water. An example of a 5 times per week application schedule is to apply ALDARA cream once per day, Monday through Friday, prior to sleeping hours.

ALDARA cream treatment should continue for 6 weeks. Local skin reactions in the treatment area are common. Patients should contact their physician if they experience any sign or symptom in the treatment area that restricts or prohibits their daily activity or makes continued application of the cream difficult. A rest period of several days may be taken if required by the patient's discomfort or severity of the local skin reaction. However, the treatment period should not be extended beyond 6 weeks due to missed doses or rest periods.

The technique for proper dose administration should be demonstrated by the prescriber to maximize the benefit of ALDARA cream therapy. Hand washing before and after cream application is recommended. The application site is not to be occluded.

A follow-up visit at approximately 12 weeks post-treatment to assess the treatment site for clinical clearance is appropriate. Early clinical clearance cannot be adequately assessed until resolution of local skin reactions. If there is clinical evidence of persistent tumor at the 12-week post-treatment visit, a biopsy or other alternative intervention should be considered; the safety of and efficacy of a repeat course of ALDARA cream treatment have not been established. If any suspicious lesion arises in the treatment area at any time after 12 weeks, the patient should seek a medical evaluation.

ALDARA cream is packaged in single-use packets which contain 250 mg of the cream. No more than one sixth of a packet of ALDARA cream should be applied to the treatment area at each application. Partially-used packets should be discarded and not reused.

Actinic Keratosis: ALDARA cream is to be applied 2 times per week to a defined treatment area on the face or scalp no larger than 25 cm², prior to normal sleeping hours, and left on the skin for approximately 8 hours. Before applying the cream, the patient should wash the treatment area with mild soap and water and allow the area to dry thoroughly. The cream should be rubbed into the treatment area until the cream is no longer visible. Contact with the eyes, lips and nostrils should be avoided. Following the treatment period, cream should be removed by washing the area with mild soap and water. Examples of two times per week application schedules are Monday and Thursday, or Tuesday and Friday prior to sleeping hours.

ALDARA cream treatment should continue for 16 weeks. Local skin reactions in the treatment area are common. Patients should contact their physician if they experience any sign or symptom in the treatment area that restricts or prohibits their daily activity or makes continued application of the cream difficult. A rest period of several days may be taken if required by the patient's discomfort or severity of the local skin reaction. However, the treatment period should not be extended beyond 16 weeks due to missed doses or rest periods.

The technique for proper dose administration should be demonstrated by the prescriber to maximize the benefit of ALDARA cream therapy. Hand washing before and after cream application is recommended.

ALDARA cream is packaged in single-use packets. No more than one packet of ALDARA cream should be applied to the treatment area at each application. Partially-used packets should be discarded and not reused. The application site is not to be occluded.

External Genital Warts: ALDARA (imiquimod) cream is to be applied 3 times per week, prior to normal sleeping hours, and left on the skin for 6-10 hours. Following the treatment period cream should be removed by washing the treated area with mild soap and water. Examples of 3 times per week application schedules are: Monday, Wednesday, Friday; or Tuesday, Thursday, Saturday application prior to sleeping hours.

ALDARA cream treatment should continue until there is total clearance of the genital/perianal warts or for a maximum of 16 weeks. Local skin reactions (erythema) at the treatment site are common. A rest period of several days may be taken if required by the patient due to discomfort or severity of the local skin reaction. Treatment may resume once the reaction subsides. Non-occlusive dressings such as cotton gauze or cotton underwear may be used in the management of skin reactions.

The technique for proper dose administration should be demonstrated by the prescriber to maximize the benefit of ALDARA cream therapy. Hand washing before and after cream application is recommended.

ALDARA cream is packaged in single-use packets which contain sufficient cream to cover a wart area of up to 20 cm²; use of excessive amounts of cream should be avoided. Patients **self-administer** ALDARA cream by applying the cream to external genital and/or perianal warts. A **thin** layer is applied to the wart area and rubbed in until the cream is no longer visible. The application site is not to be occluded.

INFORMATION FOR THE PATIENT: Published in e-CPS, available by subscription at www.e-cps.ca.

SUPPLIED: Each g of cream contains: imiquimod 50 mg (5%) in an off-white oil-in-water vanishing cream base. Nonmedicinal ingredients: benzyl alcohol, cetyl alcohol, glycerin, isostearic acid, methylparaben, polysorbate 60, propylparaben, purified water, sorbitan monostearate, stearyl alcohol, white petrolatum and xanthan gum. Single-use packets of 250 mg, boxes of 12 or 24 packets. Store between 15-25°C. Avoid freezing.

(Shown in Product Identification Section)

Aldurazyme® Ⓟ

laronidase

Enzyme Replacement Therapy

Genzyme

Date of Preparation: May 31, 2004

SUMMARY PRODUCT INFORMATION:

Route of Administration	Dosage Form/Strength	Clinically Relevant Nonmedicinal Ingredients
Intravenous infusion	Sterile solution/0.58 mg/mL (100 Units/mL)[a]	There are no clinically relevant nonmedicinal ingredients. For a complete listing, see Dosage Forms, Composition and Packaging.

[a] Aldurazyme is supplied as a sterile solution in clear Type I glass 5 mL vials (2.9 mg laronidase per 5 mL). The closure consists of a siliconized butyl stopper and an aluminum seal with a plastic flip-off cap.

INDICATIONS AND CLINICAL USE: Aldurazyme (laronidase) is indicated for:

- long term enzyme replacement therapy in patients with Mucopolysaccharidosis I (MPS I; α-L-iduronidase deficiency) to treat the non-central nervous system manifestations of the disease.

CONTRAINDICATIONS: Patients who are severely hypersensitive to Aldurazyme (laronidase) or to any ingredient in the formulation or component of the container (see Warnings and Precautions: General). For a complete listing of the ingredients in the formulation and components of the container, refer to the table in the Summary Product Information section of the product monograph.

WARNINGS AND PRECAUTIONS: General: It is strongly recommended that patients receive antipyretics and/or antihistamines approximately 60 minutes prior to the start of the infusion. If an infusion-related reaction occurs, regardless of pre-treatment, decreasing the infusion rate, temporarily stopping the infusion, and/or administering additional antipyretics and/or antihistamines may ameliorate the symptoms.

If a severe hypersensitivity or anaphylactic reaction occurs, immediately discontinue the infusion of Aldurazyme (laronidase) and initiate appropriate treatment. Caution should be exercised if epinephrine is being considered for use in patients with MPS I due to the increased prevalence of coronary artery disease in these patients.

The risks and benefits of re-administering Aldurazyme following a severe hypersensitivity or anaphylactic reaction should be considered. Extreme care should be exercised, with appropriate resuscitation measures available, if the decision is made to re-administer the product.

Carcinogenesis and Mutagenesis: Studies to assess the carcinogenic and mutagenic potential of Aldurazyme have not been conducted.

Hepatic: The safety and efficacy of Aldurazyme in patients with hepatic insufficiency have not been evaluated and no dosage regimen can be recommended in these patients.

Immune: Patients treated with Aldurazyme may develop infusion-related hypersensitivity reactions (see General heading above and Adverse Reactions).

Renal: The safety and efficacy of Aldurazyme in patients with renal insufficiency have not been evaluated and no dosage regimen can be recommended in these patients.

Special Populations: All patients should be informed that a registry for MPS I patients has been established and should be encouraged to participate in order to better understand and continue to monitor and evaluate MPS I disease and treatments. This should apply to those special populations listed below treated with Aldurazyme (see Information for the Patient: MPS I registry). Information regarding the registry program may be found at www.MPSIregistry.com or by calling (800) 745-4447.

Pregnant Women: No experience. Reproduction studies have been performed in male and female rats at doses up to 6.2 times the human dose and have revealed no evidence of impaired fertility or harm to the fetus due to Aldurazyme. However, there are no adequate and well-controlled studies in pregnant women. Because animal reproduction studies are not always predictive of human response, Aldurazyme should be used during pregnancy only if clearly needed.

Nursing Women: It is not known whether the drug is excreted in human milk. Because many drugs are excreted in human milk, caution should be exercised when Aldurazyme is administered to a nursing woman.

Pediatrics (< 5 years of age): Patients younger than 5 were not included in the clinical studies because of inability to comply with efficacy outcome assessments. It is not known if children younger than 5 respond differently from older children.

Geriatrics (> 65 years of age): Clinical studies of Aldurazyme (laronidase) did not include patients aged 65 and over to determine whether they respond differently from younger patients.

Monitoring and Laboratory Test: Evaluation of bioactivity during the clinical studies included changes in urinary glycosaminoglycans (GAG) levels, which were shown to decrease in patients treated with Aldurazyme compared to those treated with placebo.

As seen in the clinical studies, it is expected that patients will develop antibodies to Aldurazyme. It is strongly recommended that patients be monitored periodically for IgG antibody formation.

ADVERSE REACTIONS: Adverse Drug Reaction Overview: The most serious adverse reaction reported with Aldurazyme (laronidase) was an anaphylactic reaction consisting of urticaria and airway obstruction, which occurred in one patient approximately three hours after the initiation of the infusion. This patient's pre-existing MPS I related upper airway obstruction may have contributed to the severity of this reaction (see Infusion-Related Reactions and Immunogenicity, and Warnings and Precautions: General).

The most common adverse reactions associated with Aldurazyme treatment in the clinical studies were upper respiratory tract infection, rash, and injection site reaction.

The most common adverse reactions requiring intervention were infusion-related reactions, particularly flushing. Most infusion-related reactions requiring intervention were ameliorated with slowing of the infusion rate, temporarily stopping the infusion, and/or administering additional antipyretics and/or antihistamines.

Clinical Trial Adverse Drug Reactions: Because clinical trials are conducted under very specific conditions the adverse reaction rates observed in the clinical trials may not reflect the rates observed in practice and should not be compared to the rates in the clinical trials of another drug. Adverse drug reaction information from clinical trials is useful for identifying drug-related adverse events and for approximating rates.

The data described below reflect exposure to 0.58 mg/kg of Aldurazyme for 26 weeks in a placebo-controlled double-blind study in 45 patients with MPS I (N=22 Aldurazyme, and N=23 placebo). All 45 patients continued into an open-label study of Aldurazyme treatment for an additional 36 weeks. An additional 10 patients participated in a Phase 1 open-label study with continued infusions for up to 3 years. The population in the placebo-controlled study was evenly distributed for gender (N=23 females and 22 males) and ranged in ages from 6 to 43 years. Of the 45 patients in the placebo-controlled study, 1 was clinically assessed as having Hurler form, 37 Hurler-Scheie, and 7 Scheie. All patients were treated with antipyretics and antihistamines prior to the infusions.

Table 1 enumerates adverse events and selected laboratory abnormalities that occurred during the placebo-controlled trial in at least 2 patients more in the Aldurazyme group than was observed in the placebo group. Reported adverse events have been classified using standard WHOART terms. Observed adverse events in the Phase 1 study and the open-label treatment period following the controlled study were not different in nature or severity.

Table 1: Aldurazyme

Number and (%) of Patients with Adverse Events and Selected Laboratory Abnormalities in the Placebo-Controlled Study

Adverse Event	Aldurazyme (N=22)	Placebo (N=23)
Respiratory System		
Upper respiratory tract infection	7 (32)	4 (17)
Body as a Whole		
Chest pain	2 (9)	0
Nervous System		
Hyperreflexia	3 (14)	0
Paresthesia	3 (14)	1 (4)
Skin and Appendages		
Rash	8 (36)	5 (22)
Resistance Mechanism		
Abscess	2 (9)	0
Liver and Biliary System		
Bilirubinemia	2 (9)	0
Vascular		
Vein disorder	3 (14)	1 (4)
Urinary System		
Facial edema	2 (9)	0
Cardiovascular, General		
Hypotension	2 (9)	0
Dependent edema	2 (9)	0
Vision		
Corneal opacity	2 (9)	0
Application Site		
Injection site pain	2 (9)	0
Injection site reaction	4 (18)	2 (9)
Platelet, Bleeding and Clotting		
Thrombocytopenia	2 (9)	0

Infusion-Related Reactions: Infusion-related reactions were reported in 7 of 22 patients treated with Aldurazyme. Infusion-related reactions were not significantly different between the Aldurazyme treatment group and the placebo (infusions of diluent and all nonmedicinal components of Aldurazyme) group. The most common infusion-related reactions included flushing, fever, headache and rash. Flushing occurred in 5 patients (23%) receiving Aldurazyme; the other reactions were less frequent. All reactions were mild to moderate in severity. The frequency of infusion-related reactions decreased with continued use during the open-label extended use period. There was one case of anaphylaxis during the open-label extension period (see Warnings and Precautions: General). Less common infusion-related reactions include cough, bronchospasm, dyspnea, urticaria, angioedema and pruritus.

Immunogenicity: Fifty of 55 patients (91%) treated with Aldurazyme were positive for antibodies to laronidase. The clinical significance of antibodies to Aldurazyme is not known, including the potential for product neutralization.

The data reflect the percentage of patients whose test results were considered positive for antibodies to Aldurazyme using an enzyme-linked immunosorbent assay (ELISA) for laronidase-specific IgG binding antibodies, and are highly dependent on the sensitivity and specificity of the assay. Additionally, the observed incidence of antibodies in an assay may be influenced by several factors including sample handling, timing of sample collection, concomitant medications, and underlying disease. For these reasons, comparison of the incidence of antibodies to Aldurazyme with the incidence of antibodies to other products may be misleading.

Four patients in the controlled study who experienced severe infusion-related reactions were tested for Aldurazyme specific IgE antibodies and complement activation. IgE testing was performed by ELISA and complement activation was measured by the Quidel Enzyme Immunoassay. One of the four patients had an anaphylactic reaction consisting of urticaria and airway obstruction and tested positive for both Aldurazyme specific IgE binding antibodies and complement activation (see Warnings and Precautions: General).

Other hypersensitivity reactions were also seen in patients receiving Aldurazyme (see Infusion-Related Reactions).

Post Market Adverse Drug Reactions: No further safety considerations have arisen during post market use of this drug.

DRUG INTERACTIONS: Drug-Drug Interactions: Interactions with other drugs have not been established. Physician monitoring is required for patients using medicinal products that contain chloroquine or procaine due to the potential risk of interference with the intracellular uptake of laronidase.

Drug-Food Interactions: Interactions with food have not been established.

Drug-Herb Interactions: Interactions with herbal products have not been established.

Drug-Laboratory Interactions: Interactions with laboratory tests have not been established.

DOSAGE AND ADMINISTRATION: Dosing Considerations:

- Aldurazyme treatment should be supervised by a physician experienced in the management of patients with MPS I or other inherited metabolic diseases.
- Administration of Aldurazyme must be carried out in a hospital setting where resuscitation equipment to manage medical emergencies is readily available.
- The safety and efficacy of Aldurazyme in children below the age of 5 years and in patients older than 65 years have not been established and no dosage regimen can be recommended in these patients.
- The safety and efficacy of Aldurazyme in patients with renal or hepatic insufficiency have not been evaluated and no dosage regimen can be recommended in these patients.

Recommended Dose and Dosage Adjustment: The recommended dosage regimen of Aldurazyme (laronidase) is 0.58 mg/kg body weight administered once weekly as an intravenous infusion.

Pretreatment with antipyretics and/or antihistamines is recommended 60 minutes prior to the start of the infusion (see Warnings and Precautions: General).

The initial infusion rate of 10 µg/kg/h may be incrementally increased every 15 minutes during the first hour, as tolerated, until a maximum infusion rate of 200 µg/kg/h is reached. The maximum rate is then maintained for the remainder of the infusion (2-3 hours).

The total volume of the infusion is determined by the patient's body weight and should be delivered over approximately 3 to 4 hours. Patients with a body weight of 20 kg or less should receive a total volume of 100 mL. Patients with a body weight of greater than 20 kg should receive a total volume of 250 mL.

The following tables provide infusion regimens and volumetric pump settings designed to administer the total volume over the recommended infusion time:

For Patients Weighing 20 kg or Less:

Total Volume of Aldurazyme Infusion=100 mL	
2 mL/h × 15 minutes	Obtain vital signs, if stable then increase the rate to…
4 mL/h × 15 minutes	Obtain vital signs, if stable then increase the rate to…
8 mL/h × 15 minutes	Obtain vital signs, if stable then increase the rate to…
16 mL/h × 15 minutes	Obtain vital signs, if stable then increase the rate to…
32 mL/h × ~3 hours	For the remainder of the infusion.

For Patients Weighing Greater than 20 kg:

Total Volume of Aldurazyme Infusion=250 mL	
5 mL/h × 15 minutes	Obtain vital signs, if stable then increase the rate to…
10 mL/h × 15 minutes	Obtain vital signs, if stable then increase the rate to…
20 mL/h × 15 minutes	Obtain vital signs, if stable then increase the rate to…
40 mL/h × 15 minutes	Obtain vital signs, if stable then increase the rate to…
80 mL/h × ~3 hours	For the remainder of the infusion.

Administration: Instructions for Use (With Aseptic Techniques and Sterile Preparation):

1. Determine the number of vials to be diluted based on the individual patient's weight and the recommended dose of 0.58 mg/kg:
   Patient's weight (kg) × 1 mL/kg of Aldurazyme = Total # mL of Aldurazyme
   Total # of mL of Aldurazyme ÷ 5 mL per Vial = Total # of Vials
   Round up to the nearest whole vial.
   Remove the required number of vials from the refrigerator to allow them to reach room temperature. Do not heat or microwave vials.
2. Before withdrawing the Aldurazyme from the vial, visually inspect each vial for particulate matter and discoloration. The Aldurazyme solution should be clear to slightly opalescent and colorless to pale yellow. A few translucent particles may be present. Do not use if the solution is discolored or if there is particulate matter in the solution.
3. Determine the total volume of the infusion to be used based on the patient's body weight. The total final volume should be either 100 mL (if weight is less than or equal to 20 kg) or 250 mL (if weight is greater than 20 kg).
4. Using the chart below, prepare an infusion bag of 0.1% Albumin (Human) in 0.9% Sodium Chloride Injection, USP. Remove and discard a volume of 0.9% Sodium Chloride Injection, USP equal to the volume of Albumin (Human) to be added to the infusion bag. Add the appropriate volume of Albumin (Human) to the infusion bag and gently rotate the infusion bag to ensure proper distribution of the Albumin.

Total Volume of Aldurazyme Infusion	Volume of Albumin (Human) 5% to be Added	Volume of Albumin (Human) 25% to be Added
100 mL	2 mL	0.4 mL
250 mL	5 mL	1 mL

5. Withdraw and discard a volume of the 0.1% Albumin (Human) in 0.9% Sodium Chloride Injection, USP from the infusion bag, equal to the volume of Aldurazyme concentrate to be added.
6. Slowly withdraw the calculated volume of Aldurazyme from the appropriate number of vials using caution to avoid excessive agitation. Do not use a filter needle, as this may cause agitation. Agitation may denature Aldurazyme, rendering it biologically inactive.
7. Slowly add the Aldurazyme solution to the 0.1% Albumin (Human) in 0.9% Sodium Chloride Injection, USP using care to avoid agitation of the solutions. Do not use a filter needle.
8. Gently rotate the infusion bag to ensure proper distribution of Aldurazyme. Do not shake the solution.

Aldurazyme does not contain any preservatives, therefore after dilution with saline in the infusion bags, any unused product or waste material should be discarded and disposed of in accordance with local requirements.

Aldurazyme must not be mixed with other medicinal products in the same infusion.

The compatibility of Aldurazyme in solution with other products has not been evaluated.

Storage and Stability: Store Aldurazyme (laronidase) under refrigeration at 2 to 8°C. **Do not freeze or shake. Do not use** Aldurazyme after the expiration date on the vial. This product contains no preservatives.

It is recommended that once Aldurazyme is diluted, the infusion should start immediately (within 3 hours) as there is no preservative in either Aldurazyme or in the infusion bag. Although not recommended, physicochemical stability studies have shown that the diluted solution may be stored at 2 to 8°C for up to 36 hours if aseptic technique is used throughout the procedure.

Special Handling Instructions: Do not use the vial more than one time. Aldurazyme should be prepared using PVC Containers and administered with a PVC infusion set equipped with an in-line, low protein binding 0.2 micrometer (µm) filter. There is no information on the compatibility of diluted Aldurazyme with glass containers.

OVERDOSAGE:

There is no experience with overdoses of Aldurazyme (laronidase).

> For management of a suspected drug overdose, CPhA recommends that you contact your **regional Poison Control Centre**. See the *CPS* Directory section for a list of Poison Control Centres.

ACTION AND CLINICAL PHARMACOLOGY: Mechanism of Action: Mucopolysaccharide storage disorders are caused by the deficiency of specific lysosomal enzymes required for the catabolism of glycosaminoglycans (GAGs). Mucopolysaccharidosis I (MPS I) is characterized by the deficiency of α-L-iduronidase, a lysosomal hydrolase which catalyses the hydrolysis of terminal α-L-iduronic acid residues of dermatan sulfate and heparan sulfate. Reduced or absent α-L-iduronidase activity results in the accumulation of the GAG substrates, dermatan sulfate and heparan sulfate, throughout the body and leads to widespread cellular, tissue, and organ dysfunction.

The rationale of Aldurazyme therapy in MPS I is to provide exogenous enzyme for uptake into lysosomes and increase the catabolism of GAG. Aldurazyme uptake by cells into lysosomes is most likely mediated by the mannose-6-phosphate-terminated oligosaccharide chains of laronidase binding to specific mannose-6-phosphate receptors.

Pharmacodynamics: Because many proteins in the blood are restricted from entry into the central nervous system by the blood brain barrier, effects of intravenously administered Aldurazyme on cells within the central nervous system (CNS) cannot be inferred from activity in sites outside the CNS. The ability of Aldurazyme to cross the blood brain barrier has not been evaluated in animal models or in clinical trials.

Pharmacokinetics: The pharmacokinetics of laronidase were evaluated in 12 patients with MPS I who received 0.58 mg/kg of Aldurazyme as a 4 hour infusion. After the 1st, 12th and 26th weekly infusions, the mean maximum plasma concentrations (C_{max}) ranged from 1.2 to 1.7 µg/mL for the 3 time points. The mean area under the plasma concentration-time curve (AUC_{∞}) ranged from 4.5 to 6.9 µg·hour/mL. The mean volume of distribution (V_z) ranged from 0.24 to 0.6 L/kg. Mean plasma clearance (CL) ranged from 1.7 to 2.7 mL/min/kg, and the mean elimination half-life ($t_{½}$) ranged from 1.5 to 3.6 hours.

Effects of Antibodies: Most patients who received once-weekly infusions of Aldurazyme developed antibodies to laronidase by week 12. Between weeks 1 and 12, increases in plasma clearance of laronidase were observed in some patients which appeared to be proportional to the antibody titer. At week 26, plasma clearance of laronidase was comparable to that at week 1, in spite of the continued and, in some cases, increased titers of antibodies.

INFORMATION FOR THE PATIENT: Published in e-CPS, available by subscription at www.e-cps.ca.

DOSAGE FORMS, COMPOSITION AND PACKAGING: Aldurazyme, for intravenous infusion, is supplied as a sterile, nonpyrogenic, colorless to pale yellow, clear to slightly opalescent solution, that must be diluted prior to administration in 0.9% Sodium Chloride Injection, USP, containing 0.1% Albumin (Human). The solution in each vial contains a nominal laronidase concentration of 0.58 mg/mL and a pH of approximately 5.5. The extractable volume of 5 mL from each vial provides 2.9 mg laronidase, 43.9 mg sodium chloride, 63.5 mg sodium phosphate monobasic monohydrate, 10.7 mg sodium phosphate dibasic heptahydrate, and 0.05 mg polysorbate 80. Nonmedicinal ingredients: polysorbate 80, sodium chloride, sodium phosphate dibasic heptahydrate, sodium phosphate monobasic monohydrate and water for injection. Does not contain preservatives; vials are for single use only. Viral Inactivation: The viral safety of Aldurazyme is confirmed by a combination of selection and qualification of vendors, raw material testing, cell bank characterization studies, validation of the viral removal and inactivation capacity of the rhIDU purification process, and routine in-process testing.

Alendronate ℞

CPhA Monograph

see *Bisphosphonates: Oral*

Alertec® ℞

modafinil

Central Nervous System Stimulant

Shire

Date of Preparation: February 26, 1999
Date of Revision: October 16, 2009

SUMMARY PRODUCT INFORMATION:

Route of Administration	Dosage Form/ Strength	Nonmedicinal Ingredients
Oral	Tablet 100 mg	Lactose, magnesium monosilicate, magnesium stearate, maize starch, polyvidone, sodium croscarmellose, talc

INDICATIONS AND CLINICAL USE: ALERTEC (modafinil) is indicated for the symptomatic treatment of excessive sleepiness in adult patients with narcolepsy, obstructive sleep apnea/hypopnea syndrome (OSAHS) and shift work sleep disorder (SWSD).

In OSAHS, ALERTEC is indicated as an adjunct to successful standard treatment(s) for the underlying obstruction, when excessive sleepiness persists. If continuous positive airway pressure (CPAP) is the treatment of choice for a patient with OSAHS, a maximal effort to treat with CPAP for an adequate period of time should be made prior to initiating ALERTEC. If ALERTEC is used adjunctively with CPAP, the encouragement of and periodic assessment of CPAP compliance is necessary.

ALERTEC (modafinil) is indicated for the symptomatic treatment of excessive sleepiness (as confirmed by multiple sleep latency test) in SWSD associated with loss of a normal sleep-wake pattern (as confirmed by polysomnography).

Daytime sleep (as measured by polysomnography) in SWSD is not affected by the use of ALERTEC.

The effect of ALERTEC on night-shift work performance, sleep deficit in SWSD, or performance following a night-shift have not been adequately evaluated in controlled studies.

The effectiveness of modafinil in long-term use (greater than 9 weeks in the narcolepsy clinical trials and 12 weeks in the OSAHS and SWSD clinical trials) has not been systematically evaluated in placebo-controlled trials. The physician who elects to prescribe ALERTEC for an extended time in patients with narcolepsy, OSAHS or SWSD should periodically reevaluate long-term usefulness for the individual patient.

In narcolepsy, ALERTEC has no significant effect on cataplexy.

ALERTEC should not be used for the treatment of normal fatigue states. The safety and efficacy of ALERTEC has not been studied in this patient population. See Warnings and Precautions.

There is no evidence that normal levels of alertness can be heightened by ALERTEC.

Geriatrics: Dyskinesias have been reported in the elderly with the use of ALERTEC. Elimination of modafinil and its metabolites may be reduced as a consequence of aging, and elderly patients have been found to be more sensitive to the effects of ALERTEC; these patients should be started at a lower dose. Caution should also be exercised when coadministration of modafinil and clomipramine is deemed necessary. See Drug Interactions, Dosage and Administration and Action and Clinical Pharmacology.

Pediatrics (<18 years of age): Safety and effectiveness in pediatric patients have not been established. Serious skin rashes, including erythema multiforme major (EMM) and Stevens-Johnson Syndrome (SJS) have been associated with modafinil use in pediatric patients (see Warnings and Precautions, Serious Rash, including Stevens-Johnson Syndrome).

ALERTEC is not approved for use in pediatric patients for any indication including Attention Deficit Hyperactivity Disorder.

CONTRAINDICATIONS: Patients who are hypersensitive to modafinil, armodafinil (the R enantiomer of modafinil; not marketed in Canada) or to any ingredient in the formulation or component of the container.

- ALERTEC is contraindicated in patients in agitated states and in patients with severe anxiety.

WARNINGS AND PRECAUTIONS: Serious Rash, including Stevens-Johnson Syndrome: Serious rash requiring hospitalization and discontinuation of treatment has been reported in adults and children in association with the use of modafinil.

Modafinil is not approved for use in pediatric patients for any indication.

In clinical trials of modafinil, the incidence of rash resulting in discontinuation was approximately 0.8% (13 per 1585) in pediatric patients (age <17 years); these rashes included 1 case of possible Stevens-Johnson Syndrome (SJS) and 1 case of apparent multi-organ hypersensitivity reaction. Several of the cases were associated with fever and other abnormalities (e.g., vomiting, leukopenia). The median time to rash that resulted in discontinuation was 13 days. No such cases were observed among 380 pediatric patients who received placebo. No serious skin rashes have been reported in adult clinical trials (0 per 4264) of modafinil.

Rare cases of serious or life-threatening rash, including SJS, Toxic Epidermal Necrolysis (TEN), and Drug Rash with Eosinophilia and Systemic Symptoms (DRESS) have been reported in adults and children in worldwide post-marketing experience. The reporting rate of TEN and SJS associated with modafinil use, which is generally accepted to be an underestimate due to underreporting, exceeds the background incidence rate. Estimates of the background incidence rate for these serious skin reactions in the general population range between 1 to 2 cases per million-person years.

There are no factors that are known to predict the risk of occurrence or the severity of rash associated with modafinil. Nearly all cases of serious rash associated with modafinil occurred within 1 to 5 weeks after treatment initiation. However, isolated cases have been reported after prolonged treatment (e.g., 3 months). Accordingly, duration of therapy cannot be relied upon as a means to predict the potential risk heralded by the first appearance of a rash.

Although benign rashes also occur with modafinil, it is not possible to reliably predict which rashes will prove to be serious. Accordingly, modafinil should ordinarily be discontinued at the first sign of rash, unless the rash is clearly not drug-related. Discontinuation of treatment may not prevent a rash from becoming life-threatening or permanently disabling or disfiguring.

Angioedema and Anaphylactoid Reactions: One serious case of angioedema and one case of hypersensitivity (with rash, dysphagia, and bronchospasm), were observed among 1595 patients treated in clinical trials with armodafinil (not marketed in Canada), the R enantiomer of modafinil (which is the racemic mixture). No such cases were observed in modafinil clinical trials.

Angioedema and anaphylactic reaction have been reported in postmarketing experience with modafinil.

Patients should be advised to discontinue therapy and immediately report to their physician any signs or symptoms suggesting angioedema or anaphylaxis (e.g., swelling of face, eyes, lips, tongue or larynx; difficulty in swallowing or breathing; hoarseness).

Multi-organ Hypersensitivity Reactions: Multi-organ hypersensitivity reactions, including at least one fatality in post-marketing experience, have occurred in close temporal association (median time to detection 13 days: range 4-33) to the initiation of modafinil.

Although there have been a limited number of reports, multi-organ hypersensitivity reactions may result in hospitalization or be life-threatening. There are no factors that are known to predict the risk of occurrence or the severity of multi-organ hypersensitivity reactions associated with modafinil. Signs and symptoms of this disorder were diverse; however, patients typically, although not exclusively, presented with fever and rash associated with other organ system involvement. Other associated manifestations included myocarditis, hepatitis, liver function test abnormalities, hematological abnormalities (e.g., eosinophilia, leukopenia, thrombocytopenia), pruritus, and asthenia. Because multi-organ hypersensitivity is variable in its expression, other organ system symptoms and signs, not noted here, may occur.

If a multi-organ hypersensitivity reaction is suspected, ALERTEC should be discontinued.

Although there are no case reports to indicate cross-sensitivity with other drugs that produce this syndrome, the experience with drugs associated with multi-organ hypersensitivity would indicate this to be a possibility.

Persistent Sleepiness: Patients with abnormal levels of sleepiness who take ALERTEC should be advised that their level of wakefulness may not return to normal. Patients with excessive sleepiness, including those taking ALERTEC, should be frequently reassessed for their degree of sleepiness and, if appropriate, advised to avoid driving or any other potentially dangerous activity.

Psychiatric Symptoms: Psychiatric adverse experiences have been reported in patients treated with ALERTEC. There have been reports of psychotic episodes associated with ALERTEC use. Postmarketing adverse events associated with the use of modafinil have included mania, delusions, hallucinations, and suicidal ideation and aggression, some resulting in hospitalization. Many, but not all, patients had a prior psychiatric history.

In the adult modafinil controlled trials database, psychiatric symptoms resulting in treatment discontinuation (at a frequency >0.3%) and reported more often in patients treated with modafinil compared to those treated with placebo were anxiety (1%), nervousness (1%), insomnia (<1%), confusion (<1%), agitation (<1%) and depression (<1%). Caution should be exercised when ALERTEC is given to patients with a history of psychosis, depression, or mania. Consideration should be given to the possible emergence or exacerbation of psychiatric symptoms in patients treated with ALERTEC. If psychiatric symptoms develop in association with ALERTEC administration, consider discontinuing ALERTEC.

In controlled clinical trials of pediatric patients with ADHD, adverse events categorized as signs and symptoms of psychosis or mania and/or suicidal ideation were reported in <1% of patients treated with modafinil and no patients treated with placebo. Aggression and violent behavior were reported in 1% of modafinil-treated patients and no placebo-treated patients in controlled clinical trials of pediatric patients with narcolepsy or OSAHS. There were no reports of psychosis or mania and/or suicidal ideation in clinical trials with this pediatric population.

Normal Fatigue States: ALERTEC should not be used for the treatment of normal fatigue states. One study in sleep-deprived subjects, employing a between-subject design (n=42) and a single dose (300 mg), suggests that ALERTEC causes an increased self-estimate of performance which is not commensurate with actual changes in performance (i.e., overconfidence). A subsequent study in sleep-deprived subjects, employing a within-subject design (n=6), using 100 mg administered three times over a period of 24 hours failed to demonstrate an adverse effect on the ability to judge one's own cognitive capabilities.

Occupational Hazards: Because of possible over-stimulation and overconfidence, ALERTEC may alter the ability of patients to perform hazardous activities. Patients should be cautioned about operating an automobile or other hazardous machinery until they are reasonably certain that ALERTEC therapy will not adversely affect their ability to engage in such activities.

CPAP Use in Patients with OSAHS: In OSAHS, ALERTEC is indicated as an adjunct to successful standard treatment(s) for the underlying obstruction. If continuous positive airway pressure (CPAP) is the treatment of choice for a patient, a maximal effort to treat with CPAP for an adequate period of time should be made prior to initiating ALERTEC. If ALERTEC is used adjunctively with CPAP, the encouragement of and periodic assessment of CPAP compliance is necessary.

Cardiovascular: The safety of ALERTEC has not been established in patients with coronary artery disease, a recent history of myocardial infarction, or unstable angina. Patients with these conditions were not included in the controlled clinical trials. Since transient increases in the blood pressure and heart rate may occur in the immediate period after dosing, the risks of using ALERTEC in patients with coronary artery disease, a recent history of myocardial infarction, or unstable angina should be carefully weighed against the potential therapeutic benefit.

In clinical studies of modafinil, signs and symptoms including chest pain, palpitations, dyspnea, and transient ischemic T-wave changes on ECG were observed in three subjects in association with mitral valve prolapse or left ventricular hypertrophy. It is recommended that ALERTEC not be used in patients with a history of left ventricular hypertrophy or in patients with ischemic ECG changes, chest pain, arrhythmia, or other clinically significant manifestations of mitral valve prolapse in association with CNS stimulant use. Such signs may include but are not limited to ischemic ECG changes, chest pain, or arrhythmia. If new onset of any of these symptoms occurs, consider cardiac evaluation.

Blood pressure monitoring in short-term (<3 months) controlled trials showed no clinically significant changes in mean systolic and diastolic blood pressure in patients receiving ALERTEC compared to placebo. However, a retrospective analysis of the use of antihypertensive medication in these studies showed that a greater proportion of patients on ALERTEC required new or increased use of antihypertensive medications (2.4%) compared to patients on placebo (0.7%). The differential was slightly larger when only studies on OSAHS were included, with 3.4% of patients on ALERTEC and 1.1% of patients on placebo requiring such alterations in the use of antihypertensive medication. Increased monitoring of blood pressure may be appropriate in patients on ALERTEC.

Cardiovascular adverse reactions increase significantly after single doses of 300 mg and after total daily doses of more than 400 mg.

Use in Combination with Other CNS Stimulants: Caution should be taken when ALERTEC is used in combination with amphetamines or other similar CNS stimulants, such as methylphenidate. Some CNS stimulants may cause increases in blood pressure and heart rate, and the concomitant use of these drugs may result in additive effects. Clinically important prolongation of the QTc interval may also occur within a few hours after simultaneous administration of modafinil and dextroamphetamine. ALERTEC and other CNS stimulants should not be taken at the same time. See Drug Interactions.

Patients Using Steroidal Contraceptives: The effectiveness of steroidal contraceptives may be reduced when used with ALERTEC and for one month after discontinuation of therapy (See Drug Interactions). Alternative or concomitant methods of contraception other than steroidal are recommended for patients treated with ALERTEC, and for one month after discontinuation of ALERTEC.

Patients Using Cyclosporine: The blood levels of cyclosporine may be reduced when used with ALERTEC (see Drug Interactions). Monitoring of circulating cyclosporine concentrations and appropriate dosage adjustment for cyclosporine should be considered when these drugs are used concomitantly.

Dependence/Tolerance: The potential for abuse should be considered when prescribing ALERTEC (see Action and Clinical Pharmacology, Mechanism of Action for pre-clinical results). Physicians should follow patients closely, especially those with a history of drug and/or stimulant (e.g., methylphenidate, amphetamine, or cocaine) abuse. Patients should be observed for signs of misuse (e.g., incrementation of doses or drug-seeking behavior).

In a study of 24 subjects with polysubstance abuse histories, ALERTEC doses of 200, 400, and 800 mg modafinil produced psychoactive and euphoric effects, alterations in mood, perception, thinking, and feelings typical of CNS stimulants versus placebo but showed lower abuse potential relative to methylphenidate (45 and 90 mg). ALERTEC did not produce a significant amphetamine score on the Addiction Research Center Inventory (ARCI) questionnaire.

ALERTEC was also clearly distinguishable from amphetamine on this scale in a study of 300 mg in 16 healthy volunteers. Subjective effects of ALERTEC differed markedly from those induced by 15 mg of d-amphetamine, and to a lesser extent, from those seen with placebo.

Withdrawal: The effects of modafinil withdrawal were monitored following 9 weeks of modafinil use in one Phase 3 controlled clinical trial. No specific symptoms of withdrawal were observed during 14 days of observation, although sleepiness returned in narcoleptic patients.

Endocrine and Metabolism: ALERTEC may cause induction of hepatic microsomal enzymes, especially at doses greater than 400 mg. The metabolism of oral anticoagulants, antidepressant, anticonvulsants, and oral contraceptives may be increased. Patients should be monitored closely for changes in their response to any of these therapies when treatment with ALERTEC is either initiated or discontinued.

Hepatic/Biliary/Pancreatic: Severe Hepatic Impairment: In patients with severe hepatic impairment, with cirrhosis (see Action and Clinical Pharmacology), the oral clearance of modafinil was decreased by about 60% and the steady state was doubled compared to normal patients. ALERTEC should be administered at a reduced dose in patients with severe hepatic impairment (see Dosage and Administration).

Liver Function Tests: In Phase 1, 2, and 3 studies, mean plasma levels of gamma glutamyltransferase (GGT) and alkaline phosphatase (AP) were found to be higher following administration of ALERTEC, but not placebo. Few subjects, however, had GGT or AP elevations outside of the normal range. Shifts to higher, but not clinically significantly abnormal, GGT and AP values appeared to increase with time in the population treated with ALERTEC in the Phase 3 clinical trials. No differences were apparent in alanine aminotransferase, aspartate aminotransferase, total protein, albumin, or total bilirubin.

Neurologic: Central nervous system adverse reactions increase significantly after single doses of 300 mg and after total daily doses of more than 400 mg.

Renal: Severe Renal Impairment : There is inadequate information to determine the safety and efficacy of dosing in patients with severe renal impairment.

In a single dose 200 mg modafinil study, compared to healthy individuals, modafinil plasma concentrations were unchanged in patients with severe chronic renal failure (creatinine clearance ≤20 mL/min). However, the renal clearance of the active metabolite, modafinil acid, was reduced, leading to a 9-fold increase in exposure. No adverse events were reported in this small number of patients. The clinical significance of increased modafinil acid plasma concentrations is unknown.

Special Populations: Pregnant Women: In studies conducted in rats and rabbits, development toxicity was observed at clinically relevant exposures. Embryotoxicity was observed in the absence of maternal toxicity when rats received oral modafinil (50, 100, or 200 mg/kg/day) throughout the period of organogenesis. At a dose 5 times the maximum recommended daily human dose of 400 mg on a mg/m^2 basis, there was an increase in resorption, hydronephrosis and skeletal variations. The higher no-effect dose for rat embryofetal developmental toxicity was associated with a plasma modafinil exposure approximately 0.25 to 0.5 times the AUC in humans at the recommended daily dose (RHD) of 200 to 400 mg. However, in a subsequent study of up to 480 mg/kg/day (plasma modafinil exposure approximately 1-2 times the AUC in humans at the RHD) no adverse effects on embryofetal development were observed.

Modafinil administered orally to pregnant rabbits throughout the period of organogenesis at doses of 45, 90, and 180 mg/kg/day increased the incidences of fetal structural alterations and embryofetal death at the highest dose. The highest no-effect dose for developmental toxicity was associated with a plasma modafinil AUC approximately equal to the AUC in humans at the RHD. Oral administration of armodafinil (the R-enantiomer of modafinil—not approved in Canada; 60, 200, or 600 mg/kg/day) to pregnant rats throughout the period of organogenesis resulted in increased incidences of fetal visceral and skeletal variations at the intermediate dose or greater and decreased fetal body weights at the highest dose. The no-effect dose for rat embryofetal developmental toxicity was associated with a plasma armodafinil exposure (AUC) approximately one-tenth times the AUC for armodafinil in humans treated with modafinil at the RHD.

Modafinil administration to rats throughout gestation and lactation at oral doses of up to 200 mg/kg/day resulted in decreased viability in the offspring at doses greater than 20 mg/kg/day (plasma modafinil AUC approximately 0.05 to 0.1 times the AUC in humans at the RHD). No effects on postnatal developmental and neurobehavioral parameters were observed in surviving offspring.

There are no adequate and well-controlled studies in pregnant women. Two cases of intrauterine growth retardation and one case of spontaneous abortion have been reported in association with armodafinil (the R enantiomer of modafinil; not marketed in Canada) and modafinil. Although the pharmacology of modafinil and armodafinil is not identical to that of the sympathomimetic amines, they do share some pharmacologic properties with this class. Certain of these drugs have been associated with intrauterine growth retardation and spontaneous abortions. Whether the cases reported are drug-related is unknown.

ALERTEC is not recommended during pregnancy.

The effect of modafinil on labor and delivery in humans has not been systematically investigated.

Nursing Women: It is not known whether modafinil is excreted in human milk. However, in rats, peak ^{14}C-modafinil concentrations appeared in the milk of lactating animals within one hour and at levels similar to the ones found in plasma. In the absence of human safety data ALERTEC is therefore not recommended during lactation.

Pediatrics (<18 years of age): Safety and effectiveness in pediatric patients have not been established. Serious skin rashes, including erythema multiforme major (EMM) and Stevens-Johnson Syndrome (SJS) have been associated with modafinil use in pediatric patients (see Serious Rash, including Stevens-Johnson Syndrome).

ALERTEC is not approved for use in pediatric patients for any indication including Attention Deficit Hyperactivity Disorder.

In a controlled 6-week study, 165 pediatric patients (aged 5-17 years) with narcolepsy were treated with modafinil (n=123), or placebo (n=42). There were no statistically significant differences favoring modafinil over placebo in prolonging sleep latency as measured by MSLT, or in perceptions of sleepiness as determined by the clinical global impression-clinician scale (CGI-C).

In the controlled and open-label clinical studies, treatment emergent adverse events of the psychiatric and nervous system included Tourette's syndrome, insomnia, hostility, increased cataplexy, increased hypnagogic hallucinations and suicidal ideation. Transient leucopenia, which resolved without medical intervention, was also observed.

In the controlled clinical study, 3 of 38 girls, ages 12 or older, treated with modafinil experienced dysmenorrheal compared to 0 of 10 girls who received placebo.

Geriatrics: Dyskinesias have been reported in the elderly with the use of ALERTEC. Elimination of modafinil and its metabolites may be reduced as a consequence of aging, and elderly patients have been found to be more sensitive to the effects of ALERTEC; these patients should be started at a lower dose. Caution should also be exercised when coadministration of modafinil and clomipramine is deemed necessary. See Drug Interactions.

ADVERSE REACTIONS: Adverse Drug Reaction Overview: The most commonly observed adverse events (≥5%) associated with the use of ALERTEC and observed more frequently than placebo-treated patients in the placebo-controlled clinical studies in primary disorders of sleep and wakefulness were headache, nausea, rhinitis, nervousness, diarrhea, back pain, anxiety, dizziness, dyspepsia, and insomnia. The adverse event profile was similar across these studies.

In the placebo-controlled clinical trials, 74 of the 934 patients (8%) who received ALERTEC discontinued due to an adverse experience compared to 3% of patients that received placebo. The most frequent reasons for discontinuation that occurred at a higher rate for ALERTEC than placebo patients were headache (2%), nausea, anxiety, dizziness, insomnia, chest pain and nervousness (each <1%).

Clinical Trial Adverse Drug Reactions: Because clinical trials are conducted under very specific conditions the adverse reaction rates observed in the clinical trials may not reflect the rates observed in practice and should not be compared to the rates in the clinical trials of another drug. Adverse drug reaction information from clinical trials is useful for identifying drug-related adverse events and for approximating rates.

Table 1 presents the adverse experiences that occurred at a rate of 1% or more and were more frequent in adult patients treated with ALERTEC than in placebo-treated patients in the principal, placebo-controlled clinical trials.

Less Common Clinical Trial Adverse Drug Reactions (<1%): In the narcolepsy pivotal clinical trials, adverse events occurring less frequently were:

Nervous System: CNS stimulation (1.0%), and twitch (0.7%).

Skin and Appendages: pruritus (1.0%).

Special Senses: conjunctivitis (1.0%).

Urogenital System: urinary frequency (0.7%).

Adverse events reported only once in the narcolepsy pivotal clinical trials include:

Body as a Whole: jaw pain (0.3%) and photosensitivity (0.3%).

Cardiovascular System: heart arrest (0.3%).

Digestive System: saliva increase (0.3%).

Hemic and Lymphatic System: leukocytosis (0.3%).

Musculoskeletal System: myasthenia (0.3%).

Nervous System: ataxia (0.3%), coordination abnormality (0.3%), dream abnormality (0.3%), libido increase (0.3%), personality disorder (0.3%).

Special Senses: decreased hearing (0.3%), hyperacusis (0.3%).

Urogenital System: cystitis (0.3%), and impotence (0.3%).

Dose Dependency of Adverse Events: In the adult placebo-controlled clinical trials which compared doses of 200, 300 and 400 mg/day of ALERTEC and placebo, the only adverse events that were clearly dose related were headache and anxiety.

Vital Sign Changes: While there was no consistent change in mean values of heart rate or systolic and diastolic blood pressure, the requirement for antihypertensive medication was slightly greater in patients on ALERTEC compared to placebo.

Weight Changes: There were no clinically significant differences in body weight change in patients treated with ALERTEC compared to placebo-treated patients in the placebo-controlled clinical trials.

Laboratory Changes: Clinical chemistry, hematology, and urinalysis parameters were monitored in Phase 1, 2, and 3 studies. In these studies, mean plasma levels of gamma glutamyltransferase (GGT) and alkaline phosphatase (AP) were found to be higher following administration of ALERTEC, but not placebo. Few subjects, however, had GGT or AP elevations outside of the normal range. Shifts to higher, but not clinically significantly abnormal, GGT and AP values appeared to increase with time in the population treated with ALERTEC in the Phase 3 clinical trials. No differences were apparent in alanine aminotransferase, aspartate aminotransferase, total protein, albumin, or total bilirubin.

ECG Changes: No treatment-emergent pattern of ECG abnormalities was found in placebo-controlled clinical trials following administration of ALERTEC. In a Canadian clinical trial, a 35 year-old obese narcoleptic male with a prior history of syncopal episodes experienced a 9-second episode of asystole after 27 days of modafinil treatment (300 mg/day in divided doses). (see Warnings and Precautions, Cardiovascular).

Post-Market Adverse Drug Reactions: In addition to the adverse events observed during clinical trials, the following adverse events have been identified during post-approval use of ALERTEC in clinical practice. Because these adverse effects are reported voluntarily from a population of uncertain size, reliable estimates of their frequency cannot be made.

Hematologic: agranulocytosis. The causality of the two cases reported could not be established due to concomitant use of Dyazide (hydrochlorothiazide/triamterene) in the first case and of omeprazole in the second case.

Central Nervous System: symptoms of psychosis, symptoms of mania.

Hypersensitivity: urticaria (hives), angioedema, anaphylactic reaction.

Dermatologic: rare reports of serious skin reactions [including cases of erythema multiforme, Stevens-Johnson syndrome, Drug Rash with Eosinophilia and Systemic Symptoms (DRESS) and toxic epidermal necrolysis].

Table 1: ALERTEC

Incidence of Treatment-emergent Adverse Experiences in Parallel-group, Placebo-controlled Clinical Trials[a] with ALERTEC in Adults with Narcolepsy and Obstructive Sleep Apnea/Hypopnea Syndrome and Shift Work Sleep Disorder with ALERTEC (200 mg, 300 mg and 400 mg)[b]

Body System	Preferred Term	Modafinil (n=934)	Placebo (n=567)
Body as a Whole	Headache	34%	23%
	Back Pain	6%	5%
	Flu Syndrome	4%	3%
	Chest Pain	3%	1%
	Chills	1%	0%
	Neck Rigidity	1%	0%
Cardiovascular	Hypertension	3%	1%
	Tachycardia	2%	1%
	Palpitations	2%	1%
	Vasodilatation	2%	0%
Digestive	Nausea	11%	3%
	Diarrhea	6%	5%
	Dyspepsia	5%	4%
	Dry Mouth	4%	2%
	Anorexia	4%	1%
	Constipation	2%	1%
	Abnormal Liver Function[c]	2%	1%
	Flatulence	1%	0%
	Mouth Ulceration	1%	0%
	Thirst	1%	0%
Hemic/Lymphatic	Eosinophilia	1%	0%
Metabolic/Nutritional	Edema	1%	0%
Nervous	Nervousness	7%	3%
	Insomnia	5%	1%
	Anxiety	5%	1%
	Dizziness	5%	4%
	Depression	2%	1%
	Paresthesia	2%	0%
	Somnolence	2%	1%
	Hypertonia	1%	0%
	Dyskinesia[d]	1%	0%
	Hyperkinesia	1%	0%
	Agitation	1%	0%
	Confusion	1%	0%
	Tremor	1%	0%
	Emotional Lability	1%	0%
	Vertigo	1%	0%
Respiratory	Rhinitis	7%	6%
	Pharyngitis	4%	2%
	Lung Disorder	2%	1%
	Epistaxis	1%	0%
	Asthma	1%	0%
Skin/Appendages	Sweating	1%	0%
	Herpes Simplex	1%	0%
Special Senses	Amblyopia	1%	0%
	Abnormal Vision	1%	0%
	Taste Perversion	1%	0%
	Eye Pain	1%	0%
Urogenital	Urine Abnormality	1%	0%
	Hematuria	1%	0%
	Pyuria	1%	0%

(cont'd)

Table 1: ALERTEC *(cont'd)*

Incidence of Treatment-emergent Adverse Experiences in Parallel-group, Placebo-controlled Clinical Trials[a] with ALERTEC in Adults with Narcolepsy and Obstructive Sleep Apnea/Hypopnea Syndrome and Shift Work Sleep Disorder with ALERTEC (200 mg, 300 mg and 400 mg)[b]

a Events reported by at least 1% of patients treated with ALERTEC that were more frequent than in the placebo group are included; incidence is rounded to the nearest 1%. The adverse experience terminology is coded using a standard modified COSTART Dictionary. Events for which the ALERTEC incidence was at least 1%, but equal to or less than placebo are not listed in the table. These events included the following: infection, pain, accidental injury, abdominal pain, hypothermia, allergic reaction, asthenia, fever, viral infection, neck pain, migraine, abnormal electrocardiogram, hypotension, tooth disorder, vomiting, periodontal abscess, increased appetite, ecchymosis, hyperglycemia, peripheral edema, weight loss, weight gain, myalgia, leg cramps, arthritis, cataplexy, thinking abnormality, sleep disorder, increased cough, sinusitis, dyspnea, bronchitis, rash, conjunctivitis, ear pain, dysmenorrhea*, urinary tract infection.

b Six double-blind, placebo controlled clinical studies in narcolepsy (200 and 400 mg), OSAHS (200 and 400 mg) and SWSD (200 mg and 300 mg).

c Elevated liver enzymes.

d Oro-facial dyskinesias.

DRUG INTERACTIONS: Drug-Drug Interactions: CNS Active Drugs: Methylphenidate: In a single-dose study in 21 healthy male volunteers, ages 21-37, coadministration of modafinil (200 mg) with methylphenidate (40 mg) did not cause any significant alterations in the pharmacokinetics of either drug. However, the absorption of modafinil may be delayed by approximately one hour when coadministered with methylphenidate. In a subsequent study, the effects of methylphenidate (20 mg per day) at steady state on the pharmacokinetics of modafinil (400 mg per day) at steady state were examined, with administration of the stimulant 8 hours after the daily dose of modafinil. No effects on the pharmacokinetic parameters of modafinil were observed.

Dextroamphetamine: In a single dose study in healthy volunteers, simultaneous administration of modafinil (200 mg) with dextroamphetamine (10 mg) did not cause any significant alterations in the pharmacokinetics of either drug. However, the absorption of ALERTEC may be delayed by approximately one hour when coadministered with dextroamphetamine. In a subsequent study, the effects of dextroamphetamine (20 mg per day) at steady state on the pharmacokinetics of modafinil (400 mg per day) at steady state were examined, with administration of the stimulant 7 hours after the daily dose of modafinil. No effects on the pharmacokinetic parameters of modafinil were observed. In the single-dose study, blood pressure and pulse rate were increased at a greater extent after administration of the two drugs combined than after administration of either drug alone. A mean increase in QTc interval of 15 ms, and individual prolonged QTc interval (including one result of clinical importance=507 ms) were also observed 2 hours after simultaneous administration of the two drugs at their minimum recommended dosage (see Warnings and Precautions). The same patient had an prolonged QTc interval of 480 ms when dexamphetamine was administered alone.

Patients who are receiving ALERTEC with drugs with CNS activity should be monitored closely. See Warnings and Precautions.

Clomipramine: In 18 healthy, male volunteers, ages 22-44, the coadministration of a single dose of clomipramine (50 mg) on the first of three days of treatment with modafinil (200 mg/day) did not appear to affect the pharmacokinetics of either drug. However, systolic blood pressure was significantly higher when the two drugs were administered together than following administration of either drug alone [mean increase above baseline 12.4 mmHg (combination) vs 5.7 mmHg (modafinil alone) vs 6.4 mmHg (clomipramine alone)]. Also, one incident of increased levels of clomipramine and its active metabolite desmethylclomipramine has been reported in a patient with narcolepsy during treatment with modafinil. The hypertensive effects of coadministration of higher than 50 mg doses of clomipramine and multiple doses of modafinil (200-400 mg daily) is unknown. Therefore, caution should be exercised when coadministration of modafinil and clomipramine is deemed necessary. See Warnings and Precautions.

Triazolam: In a pharmacodynamic study, single doses of modafinil (50, 100 or 200 mg) and triazolam (0.25 mg) were given to healthy, male volunteers, ages 19-26. No clinically important alterations in the safety profile of modafinil or triazolam were noted. However, the effects of concomitant administration of multiple doses of modafinil (200-400 mg daily) and 0.25 mg triazolam is unknown. In the drug interaction study between ALERTEC and ethinyl estradiol (EE_2), on the same days as those for the plasma sampling for EE_2 pharmacokinetics, a single dose of triazolam (0.125 mg) was also administered. Mean C_{max} and $AUC_{0-\infty}$ of triazolam were decreased by 42% and 59%, respectively, and its elimination half-life was decreased by approximately an hour after the modafinil treatment. Dosage adjustment for triazolam may be needed.

Monoamine Oxidase (MAO) Inhibitors: Interaction studies with monoamine oxidase inhibitors have not been performed. Therefore, caution should be used when concomitantly administering MAO inhibitors and modafinil.

Other Drugs: Warfarin: The following changes were observed in the pharmacokinetic profiles of S- warfarin: no changes in mean C_{max}, 20% increase in mean AUC for S-warfarin, in 13 healthy subjects given a single dose of racemic warfarin (5 mg) following chronic administration of modafinil (200 mg/day for 7 days followed by 400 mg/day for 27 days) relative to the profiles in 12 subjects given placebo. However, because multiple doses of warfarin in patients were not evaluated, the relevance of these findings in a clinical setting is unknown. For this reason, more frequent evaluations of prothrombin times/INR than the regular monitoring is advisable whenever ALERTEC is coadministered with warfarin.

Oral Contraceptives: Administration of modafinil to 16 female volunteers once daily at 200 mg/day for 7 days followed by 400 mg/day for 21 days resulted in a mean 11% decrease in C_{max} and 18% decrease in AUC_{0-24} of ethinyl estradiol (EE_2; 0.035 mg; administered orally with norgestimate). There was no apparent change in the elimination rate of ethinyl estradiol. However, higher individual decreases in the AUC_{0-24} of ethinyl estradiol and increased incidence of metrorrhagia were observed when modafinil and ethinyl estradiol were administered concomitantly. Also, one woman in the study had a decrease of 54% in the AUC_{0-24} of ethinyl estradiol during concomitant modafinil treatment. She had a negative pregnancy test at study completion, and a positive pregnancy test 25 days after she completed the study. She thereafter was lost to follow-up and further information on her pregnancy is not available. See Warnings and Precautions.

Cyclosporine: One case of an interaction between modafinil and cyclosporine, a substrate of CYP3A4, has been reported in a 41 years old woman who had undergone an organ transplant. After one month of administration of 200 mg/day of modafinil, cyclosporine blood levels were decreased by 50%. The interaction was postulated to be due to the increased metabolism of cyclosporine, since no other factor expected to affect the disposition of the drug had changed. Dosage adjustment for cyclosporine may be needed.

Concomitant use of ALERTEC and other agents that may elevate blood pressure has not been evaluated. Caution should be exercised when prescribing ALERTEC to patients already taking such agents.

* Incidence adjusted for gender.

Multi-dose treatment (twice daily, one at 8 a.m. and one at noon) with ALERTEC at 400 mg/day or higher for 7 days was shown to decrease the half-life of antipyrine. This finding suggests that chronic administration of ALERTEC at 400 mg or higher daily may induce the metabolism of other drugs.

Based on in vitro data, modafinil is metabolized partially by the 3A isoform subfamily of hepatic cytochrome P450 (CYP3A4). In addition, modafinil has the potential to inhibit CYP2C19, suppress CYP2C9, and induce CYP3A4, CYP2B6, and CYP1A2. Because modafinil and modafinil sulfone are reversible inhibitors of the drug-metabolizing enzyme CYP2C19, coadministration of modafinil with drugs such as diazepam, propranolol, phenytoin, or S-mephenytoin, which are largely eliminated via that pathway, may increase the circulating levels of those compounds and may require dosage reduction and monitoring for toxicity. In addition, in individuals deficient in the enzyme CYP2D6 (i.e., 7-10% of the Caucasian population; similar or lower in other populations), the levels of CYP2D6 substrates such as tricyclic antidepressants and selective serotonin reuptake inhibitors, which have ancillary routes of elimination through CYP2C19, may be increased by co administration of modafinil. Dose adjustments may be necessary for patients being treated with these and similar medications. An in vitro study demonstrated that armodafinil (one of the enantiomers of modafinil; not marketed in Canada) is a substrate of P-glycoprotein.

ALERTEC has a slight induction effect at the concentration of 10^{-5} M on CYP 3A, a hepatic enzyme associated with the metabolism of oral contraceptives. Chronic administration of modafinil 400 mg per day was found to decrease the systemic exposure to two CYP3A4 substrates, ethinyl estradiol and triazolam, after oral administration suggesting that CYP3A4 had been induced. Caution is therefore recommended with the combination of oral contraceptives and ALERTEC (see Warnings and Precautions). Chronic administration of modafinil can increase the elimination of substrates of CYP3A4. Dosage adjustment should be considered for concomitant medications that are substrates for CYP3A4, such as triazolam and cyclosporine.

In vitro studies using liver microsomes suggest that formation of the metabolite modafinil sulfone is primarily catalyzed by cytochrome CYP 3A. Potential inhibitors such as itraconazole or ketoconazole may therefore reduce the formation of modafinil sulfone. Because this pathway is of relatively minor importance in humans, such an interaction would not be expected to appreciably alter modafinil elimination.

The exposure of human hepatocytes to modafinil in vitro produced an apparent concentration-related suppression of expression of CYP2C9 activity suggesting that there is a potential for a metabolic interaction between modafinil and the substrates of this enzyme (e.g., S-warfarin and phenytoin). In a subsequent clinical study in healthy volunteers, chronic modafinil treatment resulted in a 20% increase in mean AUC on the single-dose pharmacokinetics of S-warfarin when compared to placebo. See Drug Interactions.

It should be noted that evaluation of drug interactions based on in vitro systems may not necessarily reflect those seen in vivo situations. This information should be used as a guide to assess the risks associated with the use of concomitant medications.

Drug-Food Interactions: Interactions with food have not been established.

Drug-Herb Interactions: Interactions with herbal products have not been established.

Drug-Laboratory Test Interactions: Interactions with laboratory tests have not been established.

DOSAGE AND ADMINISTRATION: **Dosing Considerations: The safety and efficacy of modafinil in children under the age of 18 has not been established. Therefore, modafinil is not indicated for use in pediatric patients** (see Indications and Clinical Use, Pediatrics (<18 years of age); Warnings and Precautions, Serious Rash, including Stevens-Johnson Syndrome).

Dosage adjustment should be considered for concomitant medications that are substrates for CYP3A4, such as triazolam and cyclosporine.

Because modafinil and modafinil sulfone are reversible inhibitors of the drug-metabolizing enzyme CYP2C19, coadministration of modafinil with drugs such as diazepam, propranolol, phenytoin, or S-mephenytoin, which are largely eliminated via that pathway, may increase the circulating levels of those compounds may have prolonged elimination upon coadministration with ALERTEC and may require dosage reduction and monitoring for toxicity.

Elderly: In elderly patients, elimination of ALERTEC and its metabolites may be reduced as a consequence of aging. Therefore, consideration should be given to the use of lower doses in this population. See Warnings and Precautions and Action and Clinical Pharmacology.

Severe Hepatic Impairment: In patients with severe hepatic impairment, the dose of ALERTEC should be reduced to one-half of the usual recommended dose See Warnings and Precautions.

Recommended Dose and Dosage Adjustment: Narcolepsy: The adult daily dosage of ALERTEC (modafinil) for patients with narcolepsy is between 200 to 400 mg, divided between morning and noon doses. The initial daily dose should be 200 mg in divided doses, increasing in increments of 100 mg as needed and tolerated.

The total daily dose can be divided according to the needs and response of the patient. The timing should be aimed to coincide with the periods of greatest excessive daytime sleepiness. The second dose should generally be taken no later than the early afternoon to minimize the risk of insomnia.

Although the occasional patient may need and tolerate daily doses of 500 mg, limited data from trials in healthy volunteers suggest that the number and type of side effects increase significantly after single doses of 300 mg and after total daily doses of more than 400 mg, compared to 100 and 200 mg doses b.i.d. Single doses of 300 mg or more, or total daily doses of more than 400 mg are therefore not recommended.

Obstructive Sleep Apnea/Hypopnea Syndrome: In OSAHS, ALERTEC is indicated as an adjunct to successful standard treatment(s) for the underlying obstruction (see Warnings and Precautions). For patients with OSAHS, the adult daily dosage of ALERTEC is 200 mg taken as a single dose in the morning.

Shift Work Sleep Disorder: For patients with SWSD, the adult daily dosage of ALERTEC is 200 mg taken approximately 1 hour prior to the start of their work shift.

Missed Dose: If a dose is missed, it can be taken when remembered, unless it is close to the time for the next dose. Taking the medication in the evening or the late afternoon may prevent from falling asleep at usual bedtime, and should, therefore, be avoided.

OVERDOSAGE:

Symptoms most often accompanying ALERTEC overdose, alone or in combination with other drugs have included: insomnia; central nervous system symptoms such as restlessness, disorientation, confusion, excitation and hallucination; digestive changes such as nausea and diarrhea; and cardiovascular changes such as tachycardia, bradycardia, hypertension, and chest pain.

For management of a suspected drug overdose, CPhA recommends that you contact your **regional Poison Control Centre**. See the *CPS* Directory section for a list of Poison Control Centres.

ACTION AND CLINICAL PHARMACOLOGY: Mechanism of Action: Modafinil is a central nervous system stimulant.

The precise mechanism(s) through which modafinil promotes wakefulness is unknown. Modafinil has wake-promoting actions similar to sympathomimetic agents like amphetamine and methylphenidate, although the pharmacologic profile is not identical to that of sympathomimetic amines.

Modafinil has weak to negligible interactions with receptors for norepinephrine, serotonin, dopamine, GABA, adenosine, histamine-3, melatonin, and benzodiazepines. Modafinil also does not inhibit the activities of MAO-B or phosphodiesterases II-V.

Modafinil-induced wakefulness can be attenuated by the α_1-adrenergic receptor antagonist prazosin; however, modafinil is inactive in other in vitro assay systems known to be responsive to α-adrenergic agonists, such as the rat vas deferens preparation.

Modafinil is not a direct- or indirect-acting dopamine receptor agonist. However, in vitro, modafinil binds to the dopamine transporter and inhibits dopamine reuptake. This activity has been associated in vivo with increased extracellular dopamine levels in some brain regions of animals. In genetically engineered mice lacking the dopamine transporter (DAT), modafinil lacked wake-promoting activity, suggesting that this activity was DAT-dependent. However, the wake-promoting effects of modafinil, unlike those of amphetamine, were not antagonized by the dopamine receptor antagonist haloperidol in cats. In addition, alpha-methyl-p-tyrosine, a dopamine synthesis inhibitor, blocks the action of dopamine, but does not block locomotor activity induced by modafinil.

EEG studies in man showed that modafinil increases high frequency α waves and decreases δ and θ waves, an effect consistent with increased alertness. When taken in the evening, modafinil 200 mg increases sleep latency and decreases total sleep time. Modafinil has weak peripheral sympathomimetic activity: single doses of 200 mg and total daily doses of 400 mg have minimal effect on hemodynamics. Higher doses cause blood pressure and heart rate to increase in a dose-dependent manner.

In the cat, equal wakefulness-promoting doses of methylphenidate and amphetamine increased neuronal activation throughout the brain. Modafinil at an equivalent wakefulness-promoting dose selectively and prominently increased neuronal activation in more discrete regions of the brain. The relationship of this finding in cats to the effects of modafinil in humans is unknown.

In addition to its wake-promoting effects and ability to increase locomotor activity in animals, modafinil produces psychoactive and euphoric effects, alterations in mood, perception, thinking, and feelings typical of other CNS stimulants in humans. Modafinil has reinforcing properties, as evidenced by its self-administration in monkeys previously trained to self-administer cocaine. Modafinil was also partially discriminated as stimulant-like.

The optical enantiomers of modafinil have similar pharmacological actions in animals. Two major metabolites of modafinil, modafinil acid and modafinil sulfone, do not appear to contribute to the CNS-activating properties of modafinil.

Pharmacokinetics: Modafinil is a racemic compound, whose enantiomers have different pharmacokinetics (e.g., the half-life of the l-isomer is approximately three times that of the d-isomer in adult humans). The enantiomers do not interconvert. At steady-state, total exposure to the l-isomer is approximately three times that for the d-isomer. The trough concentration (C_{minss}) of circulating modafinil after once daily dosing consists of 90% of the l-isomer and 10% of the d-isomer.

The effective elimination half-life of modafinil after multiple doses is about 15 hours. The enantiomers of modafinil exhibit linear kinetics upon multiple dosing of 200-600 mg/day once daily in healthy volunteers. Apparent steady states of total modafinil and l-(-)-modafinil are reached after 2-4 days of dosing.

Absorption: Absorption of ALERTEC tablets is rapid, with peak plasma concentrations occurring at 2-4 hours. The bioavailability of ALERTEC tablets is approximately equal to that of an aqueous suspension. The absolute oral bioavailability was not determined due to the aqueous insolubility (<1 mg/mL) of modafinil, which precluded intravenous administration. The C_{max} is slightly lower and the t_{max} slightly longer when ALERTEC is given after a meal but has no effect on overall ALERTEC bioavailability. Both the area under the plasma concentration curve (AUC), and the peak plasma concentration showed dose-proportionality in the 50 to 400 mg range.

Distribution: Modafinil is well distributed in body tissue with an apparent volume of distribution (~0.9 L/kg) larger than the volume of total body water (0.6 L/kg). In human plasma, in vitro, modafinil is moderately bound to plasma protein (~60%, mainly to albumin). At serum concentrations obtained at steady state after doses of 200 mg/day, modafinil exhibits no displacement of protein binding of warfarin, diazepam or propranolol. Even at much larger concentrations (1000 µM; >25 times the C_{max} of 40 µM at steady state at 400 mg/day), modafinil has no effect on warfarin binding. Modafinil acid at concentrations >500 µM decreases the extent of warfarin binding, but these concentrations are >35 times those achieved therapeutically.

Metabolism and Excretion: The major route of elimination is metabolism (~90%), primarily by the liver, with subsequent renal elimination of the metabolites. Urine alkalinization has no effect on the elimination of modafinil.

Metabolism occurs trough hydrolytic deamination, S-oxidation, aromatic ring hydroxylation, and glucuronic conjugation. Following oral administration of modafinil, less than 10% of the dose is found unchanged in the urine.

In a clinical study using radiolabeled modafinil, a total of 81% of the administered radioactivity was recovered in 11 days post-dose, predominantly in the urine (80% vs 1.0% in the feces). The largest fraction of the drug in urine was modafinil acid, but at least six other metabolites were present in lower concentrations. Only two metabolites reach appreciable concentrations in plasma, i.e., modafinil acid and modafinil sulfone. In preclinical models, modafinil acid, modafinil sulfone, 2-[(diphenylmethyl)sulfonyl]acetic acid and 4-hydroxy modafinil, were inactive or did not appear to mediate the arousal affects of modafinil.

In adults, decreases in though levels of modafinil have sometimes been observed after multiple weeks of dosing, suggesting auto-induction, but the magnitude of the decreases and the inconsistency of their occurrence suggest that their clinical significance is minimal. Significant accumulation of modafinil sulfone has been observed after multiple doses due to its long elimination half-life of 40 hours. Induction of metabolizing enzymes, most importantly cytochrome P-450 (CYP) 3A4, has also been observed in vitro after incubation of primary cultures of human hepatocytes with modafinil and in vivo after extended administration of modafinil at 400 mg/day. (For further discussion of the effects of modafinil on CYP enzyme activities, see Drug Interactions, Drug-Drug Interactions).

Special Populations and Conditions: Gender: The pharmacokinetics of modafinil are not effected by gender.

Age: A slight decrease (~20%) in the oral clearance (CL/F) of modafinil was observed in a single dose study at 200 mg in 12 subjects with a mean age of 63 years (range 53-72 years), but the change was considered not likely to be clinically significant. In a multiple dose study (300 mg/day) in 12 patients with a mean age of 82 years (range 67-87 years), the mean levels of modafinil in plasma were approximately two times those historically obtained in matched younger subjects. Due to potential effects from the multiple concomitant medications with which most of the patients were being treated, the apparent difference in modafinil pharmacokinetics may not be attributable solely to the effects of aging. However, the results suggest that the clearance of modafinil may be reduced in the elderly. See Dosage and Administration.

Race: The influence of race on the pharmacokinetics of modafinil has not been studied.

Renal Impairment: In a single dose 200 mg modafinil study, severe chronic renal failure (creatinine clearance ≤20 mL/min) did not significantly influence the pharmacokinetics of modafinil, but exposure to modafinil acid (an active metabolite) was increased 9-fold. See Warnings and Precautions.

Severe Hepatic Impairment: Pharmacokinetics and metabolism were examined in patients with cirrhosis of the liver (6 males and 3 females). Three patients had stage B or B+ cirrhosis (per the Child criteria) and 6 patients had stage C or C+ cirrhosis. Clinically 8 of 9 patients were icteric and all had ascites. In these patients, the oral clearance of modafinil was decreased by about 60% and the steady state concentration was doubled compared to normal patients. The dose of ALERTEC should be reduced in patients with hepatic impairment. See Warnings and Precautions.

STORAGE AND STABILITY: Store between 15 and 30°C.

INFORMATION FOR THE PATIENT: Published in e-CPS, available by subscription at www.e-cps.ca.

DOSAGE FORMS, COMPOSITION AND PACKAGING: Each white, round, convex tablet, engraved with "100" on one side, contains: modafinil 100 mg. Nonmedicinal ingredients: lactose, magnesium monosilicate, magnesium stearate, maize starch, polyvidone, sodium croscarmellose and talc. Blister strips of 10, packages of 3 strips.

(Shown in Product Identification Section)

Alertonic®

pipradrol HCl—vitamin B compound

Tonic

Odan

INDICATIONS: Short-term use in cases of vitamin B deficiencies accompanied by functional fatigue.

CONTRAINDICATIONS: In hyperactive, agitated, or anxious patients and depressive illness, obsessive-compulsive states or chorea.

WARNINGS: No data supplied by the manufacturer.

PRECAUTIONS: *Pregnancy:* Although animal reproductive studies have not indicated adverse effects, this drug should not be used during the first trimester of pregnancy unless in the opinion of the prescribing physician, the potential benefits outweigh the potential risks.

Dependence Potential: As with other CNS stimulant with dependence potential, pipradrol should not be administered for long periods or given to patients who are prone to drug dependence.

ADVERSE EFFECTS: CNS stimulation reported as agitation, insomnia, excitement, and irritability; allergic reactions usually related to the skin such as urticaria, rash, itching, and erythema; gastrointestinal disturbances manifested by gastritis, vomiting, nausea, abdominal distress, diarrhea, and constipation. Excessive overdosing has occurred in a few instances with severe reactions related to CNS stimulation and gastrointestinal disturbances.

OVERDOSE:

No data supplied by the manufacturer.

For management of a suspected drug overdose, CPhA recommends that you contact your **regional Poison Control Centre**. See the *CPS* Directory section for a list of Poison Control Centres.

DOSAGE: Adults, 15 mL (1 tablespoon) 3 times daily, 30 minutes before meals for limited periods only.

SUPPLIED: Each 45 mL of reddish-brown clear liquid with a characteristic date odor, contains: pipradrol HCl 2 mg, thiamine HCl 10 mg, riboflavin 5 mg, pyridoxine HCl 1.9 mg, niacinamide 50 mg, choline chloride 100 mg and inositol 100 mg. Nonmedicinal ingredients: alcohol, amaranth Red #2, butylparaben, caramel, cherry flavor, date flavor, FD&C Blue #1, hydrochloric acid, invert sugar, purified water, sodium hydroxide and sorbitol. Alcohol: 15%. Energy: 32 kJ (7.7 kcal)/15 mL. Sodium: <1 mmol (1.2 mg)/15 mL. Bottles of 500 mL. Store between 15 and 30°C. Dispense in a light resistant container.

Alesse® 21 ℞
levonorgestrel—ethinyl estradiol
Oral Contraceptive

Pfizer

Alesse® 28 ℞
levonorgestrel—ethinyl estradiol
Oral Contraceptive

Pfizer

Date of Revision: March 27, 2009

SUMMARY PRODUCT INFORMATION:

Route of Administration	Dosage Form/ Strength	Clinically Relevant Nonmedicinal Ingredients
Oral	Tablet, 100 µg levonorgestrel and 20 µg ethinyl estradiol	Lactose monohydrate For a complete listing see Dosage Forms, Composition and Packaging.

INDICATIONS AND CLINICAL USE: ALESSE Tablets are indicated for:
- Conception control
- Treatment of moderate acne vulgaris in women >14 years of age who, have no known contraindications to oral contraceptive therapy, desire contraception, and have achieved menarche.

Geriatrics (>65 years of age): ALESSE is not indicated for use in postmenopausal women.
Pediatrics (<16 years of age): Safety and efficacy of ALESSE tablets have been established in women of reproductive age. Use of this product before menarche is not indicated.

CONTRAINDICATIONS: Combination Oral Contraceptives (COCs) are contraindicated in the following:
- History of or actual thrombophlebitis or thromboembolic disorders.
- History of or actual cerebrovascular disorders.
- History of or actual myocardial infarction or coronary arterial disease.
- Deep vein thrombosis (current or history).
- Thrombogenic valvulopathies and Thrombogenic rhythm disorders.
- Hereditary or acquired thrombophilias.
- Migraine with focal neurological symptoms such as aura (current or history).
- Active liver disease, or history of or actual benign or malignant liver tumours.
- Known or suspected carcinoma of the breast.
- Known or suspected estrogen-dependent neoplasia.
- Undiagnosed abnormal vaginal bleeding.
- Any ocular lesion arising from ophthalmic vascular disease, such as partial or complete loss of vision or defect in visual fields.
- When pregnancy is suspected or diagnosed.
- Hypersensitivity to any of the components of ALESSE. For a complete listing, see Dosage Forms, Composition and Packaging.
- Diabetes with vascular involvement.
- Uncontrolled hypertension.

WARNINGS AND PRECAUTIONS:

Serious Warnings and Precautions
Cigarette smoking increases the risk of serious adverse effects on the heart and blood vessels. This risk increases with age and becomes significant in hormonal contraceptive users older than 35 years of age who smoke. Women should be counselled not to smoke (see Warnings and Precautions, Cardiovascular).

Patients should be counselled that birth control pills **do not protect** against sexually transmitted infections (STIs) including HIV/AIDS. For protection against STIs, it is advisable to use latex or polyurethane condoms **in combination with** birth control pills.

General: Physical Examination: Before COCs are used, a thorough history and physical examination should be performed, including a blood pressure determination. Breasts, liver, extremities and pelvic organs should be examined and a Papanicolaou smear should be taken if the patient has been sexually active.

The first follow-up visit should be three months after COCs are prescribed. Thereafter, examinations should be performed at least once a year or more frequently if indicated. At each annual visit, examination should include those procedures that were done at the initial visit as outlined above or per recommendations of the Canadian Workshop on Screening for Cancer of the Cervix. Their suggestion was that, for women who had two consecutive negative Pap smears, screening could be continued every three years to the age of 69.

Discontinue Medication at the Earliest Manifestation of the Following:

A. **Venous and Arterial Thrombosis and Thromboembolism:** Use of COCs is associated with an increased risk of venous and arterial thrombotic and thromboembolic events. For any particular estrogen/progestin combination, the dosage regimen prescribed should be one which contains the least amount of estrogen and progestin that is compatible with a low failure rate and the needs of the individual patient.

New users of COCs should be started on preparations containing less than 50 µg of estrogen.

Venous Thrombosis and Thromboembolism: Use of COCs increases the risk of venous thrombotic and thromboembolic events. Reported events include deep venous thrombosis, thrombophlebitis, pulmonary embolism and mesenteric thrombosis. For information on retinal vascular thrombosis see Warnings and Precautions, Ophthalmologic.

The use of any COCs carries an increased risk of venous thrombotic and thromboembolic events compared with no use. The excess risk is highest during the first year a woman ever uses a COC. This increased risk is less than the risk of venous thrombotic and thromboembolic events associated with pregnancy which is estimated as 60 cases per 100 000 woman-years. Venous thromboembolism is fatal in 1-2% of cases.

The risk of venous thrombotic and thromboembolic events is further increased in women with conditions predisposing for venous thrombosis and thromboembolism. Caution must be exercised when prescribing COCs for such women.

Arterial Thrombosis and Thromboembolism: The use of COCs increases the risk of arterial thrombotic and thromboembolic events. Reported events include myocardial infarction and cerebrovascular events (ischemic and hemorrhagic stroke, transient ischemic attack). For information on retinal vascular thrombosis see Warnings and Precautions, Ophthalmologic.

The risk of arterial thrombotic and thromboembolic event is further increased in women with underlying risk factors. Caution must be exercised when prescribing COCs for women with risk factors for arterial thrombotic and thromboembolic events.

B. **Conditions that Predispose to Venous Thrombosis and Thromboembolism:** (e.g. obesity, surgery or trauma with increased risk of thrombosis, immobilization after accidents or confinement to bed during long-term illness, recent delivery or second-trimester abortion [see Dosage and Administration, Administration]). Other nonhormonal methods of contraception should be used until regular activities are resumed. For use of oral contraceptives when surgery is contemplated, see Warnings and Precautions, Peri-Operative Considerations. Examples of risk factors for arterial thrombotic and thromboembolic events are smoking, hypertension, hyperlipidemias, obesity and increasing age.

C. **Visual Defects—Partial or Complete**

D. **Papilledema or Ophthalmic Vascular Lesions**

E. **Severe Headache of Unknown Etiology, Worsening of Pre-existing Migraine or Development of New Migraine** (particularly migraine with aura). Women with migraine who take COCs may be at increased risk of stroke

F. **Increase in Epileptic Seizures**

Carcinogenesis and Mutagenesis: Breast: A meta-analysis from 54 epidemiological studies reported that there is a slightly increased relative risk (RR=1.24) of having breast cancer diagnosed in women who are currently using COCs compared to never-users. The increased risk gradually disappears during the course of the 10 years after cessation of COC use. These studies do not provide evidence for causation. The observed pattern of increased risk of breast cancer diagnosis may be due to an earlier detection of breast cancer in COC users, the biological effects of COCs or a combination of both. Because breast cancer is rare in women under 40 years of age, the excess number of breast cancer diagnoses in current and recent COC users is small in relation to the lifetime risk of breast cancer. Breast cancers diagnosed in ever-users tend to be less advanced clinically than the cancers diagnosed in never-users.

Increasing age and a strong family history are the most significant risk factors for the development of breast cancer. Other established risk factors include obesity, nulliparity and late age for first full-term pregnancy. The identified groups of women that may be at increased risk of developing breast cancer before menopause are long-term users of COCs (more than eight years) and starters at early age. In a few women, the use of COCs may accelerate the growth of an existing but undiagnosed breast cancer. Since any potential increased risk related to COC use is small, there is no reason to change prescribing habits at present.

Women receiving COCs should be instructed in self-examination of their breasts. Their physicians should be notified whenever any masses are detected. A yearly clinical breast examination is also recommended because, if a breast cancer should develop, drugs that contain estrogen may cause a rapid progression.

Cervical Cancer: The most important risk factor for cervical cancer is persistent human papillomavirus infection. Some epidemiological studies have indicated that long-term use of COCs may further contribute to this increased risk but there continues to be controversy about the extent to which this finding is attributable to confounding effects, e.g., cervical screening and sexual behaviour including use of barrier contraceptives.

Hepatocellular Carcinoma: Hepatocellular carcinoma may be associated with COC use. The risk appears to increase with duration of COC use. However, the attributable risk (the excess incidence) of liver cancer in OC users is extremely small.

Cardiovascular: Predisposing Factors for Coronary Artery Disease: Cigarette smoking increases the risk of serious cardiovascular side effects and mortality from COC use. This risk increases with age and with the extent of smoking. Convincing data are available to support an upper age limit of 35 years for oral contraceptive use in women who smoke.

Other women who are independently at high risk for cardiovascular disease include those with diabetes, hypertension, abnormal lipid profile, obesity or a family history of these. Whether COCs accentuate this risk is unclear.

In low risk, non-smoking women of any age, the benefits of oral contraceptive use outweigh the possible cardiovascular risks associated with low dose formulations. Consequently, oral contraceptives may be prescribed for these women up to the age of menopause.

Hypertension: Patients with essential hypertension whose blood pressure is well-controlled may be given COCs but only under close supervision. If a significant elevation of blood pressure in previously normotensive or hypertensive subjects occurs at any time during the administration of the drug, cessation of medication is necessary.

Increases in blood pressure have been reported in women taking COCs. Elevated blood pressure associated with COC use will generally return to baseline after stopping COCs, and there appears to be no difference in the occurrence of hypertension among ever—and never—users.

Endocrine and Metabolism: Diabetes: Glucose intolerance has been reported in COC users. Current low-dose COCs exert minimal impact on glucose metabolism. Diabetic patients, or those with a family history of diabetes, should be observed closely to detect any worsening of carbohydrate metabolism. Women who are predisposed to diabetes, with impaired glucose tolerance or who have diabetes mellitus should be carefully monitored if using COCs. Young diabetic patients whose disease is of recent origin, well-controlled, and not associated with hypertension or other signs of vascular disease such as ocular fundal changes, should be monitored more frequently while using oral contraceptives.

Lipid and Other Metabolic Effects: A small proportion of women will have adverse lipid changes while taking oral contraceptives. Nonhormonal contraception should be considered in women with uncontrolled dyslipidemias. Persistent hypertriglyceridemia may occur in a small population of combination oral contraceptive users. Elevations of plasma triglycerides may lead to pancreatitis and other complications.

Women who are being treated for hyperlipidemias should be followed closely if they elect to use COCs.

Gastrointestinal: Absorption: Vomiting and/or diarrhea may reduce absorption of oral contraceptives resulting in decreased serum concentration and therefore may reduce contraceptive efficacy. Physicians should advise the patients of the need for a back-up contraceptive method in the case of such gastrointestinal symptoms.

Genitourinary: Vaginal Bleeding: Persistent irregular vaginal bleeding requires assessment to exclude underlying pathology.

Fibroids: Patients with fibroids (leiomyomata) should be carefully observed. Sudden enlargement, pain, or tenderness requires discontinuation of the use of COCs.

Hematologic: Venous Thrombosis and Thromboembolism: The use of any combined oral contraceptive carries an increased risk of VTE compared with no use. The excess risk of VTE is highest during the first year a woman ever uses a combined oral contraceptive. The increased risk is less than the risk of VTE associated with pregnancy, which is estimated as 60 cases per 100 000 woman years. VTE is fatal in 1-2% of cases.

Other Risk Factors for Venous Thromboembolism: Other generalized risk factors for venous thromboembolism include but are not limited to a personal history, a family history (the occurrence of VTE in a direct relative at a relatively early age may indicate genetic predisposition), severe obesity (body mass index >30 kg/m^2) and systemic lupus erythematosus. The risk of VTE also increases with age. The risk of VTE may be temporarily increased with prolonged immobilization, major surgery, or trauma. Also, patients with a leg cast should be closely supervised.

If a hereditary or acquired predisposition for venous thromboembolism is suspected, the woman should be referred to a specialist for advice before deciding on any COC use.

Hepatic/Biliary/Pancreatic: Hepatic Function: ALESSE is contraindicated in patients with active liver disease (see Contraindications and Drug Interactions, Drug-Laboratory Test Interactions).

Acute or chronic disturbances of liver function may necessitate the discontinuation of COC use until markers of liver function return to normal.

Jaundice: Patients who have had jaundice, should be given oral contraceptives only with great care and under close observation. Oral contraceptive-related cholestasis has been described in women with a history of pregnancy-related cholestasis. Women with a history of cholestasis may have the condition recur with subsequent hormonal contraceptive use, and in this instance, ALESSE should be discontinued.

The development of severe generalized pruritus or icterus requires that the medication be withdrawn until the problem is resolved.

If a patient develops jaundice that proves to be cholestatic in type, the use of oral contraceptives should not be resumed. In patients taking hormonal contraceptives, changes in the composition of the bile may occur and an increased incidence of gallstones has been reported.

Hepatic Nodules: Hepatic nodules (adenoma and focal nodular hyperplasia) have been reported, particularly in long-term users of oral contraceptives. Although these lesions are extremely rare, they have caused fatal intra-abdominal hemorrhage and should be considered in women presenting with an abdominal mass, acute abdominal pain, or evidence of intra-abdominal bleeding.

Hepatocellular injury has been reported with COC use. Early identification of drug-related hepatocellular injury can decrease the severity of hepatotoxicity when the drug is discontinued. If hepatocellular injury is diagnosed, patients should stop their COC, use a non-hormonal form of contraception and consult their doctor.

Pancreatic Function: Please see Warnings and Precautions, Endocrine and Metabolism, Lipid and Other Metabolic Effects.

Neurologic: Migraine and Headache: The onset or exacerbation of migraine or the development of headache of a new pattern that is recurrent, persistent or severe, requires discontinuation of COCs and evaluation of the cause (see Contraindications).

Women with migraine headaches who take oral contraceptives may be at increased risk of stroke (see Contraindications).

Ophthalmologic: Patients who are pregnant or are taking COCs, may experience corneal edema that may cause visual disturbances and changes in tolerance to contact lenses, especially of the rigid type. Soft contact lenses usually do not cause disturbances. If visual changes or alterations in tolerance to contact lenses occur, temporary or permanent cessation of wear may be advised.

With use of COCs, there have been reports of retinal vascular thrombosis which may lead to partial or complete loss of vision. If there are signs or symptoms such as visual changes, onset of proptosis or diplopia, papilledema, or retinal vascular lesions, the COC should be discontinued and the cause immediately evaluated.

Peri-Operative Considerations: Thromboembolic Complications—Post-Surgery: There is an increased risk of thromboembolic complications in COC users after major surgery. If feasible, COCs should be discontinued and an alternative method substituted at least one month prior to major elective surgery and during periods of prolonged immobilization. COC use should not be resumed for at least two weeks after major elective surgery, and only after the first menstrual period has occurred following hospital discharge.

Psychiatric: Patients with a history of emotional disturbances, especially the depressive type, may be more prone to have a recurrence of depression while taking COCs. Women with a history of depression who use COCs should be carefully observed and the drug discontinued if depression recurs to a serious degree. Patients becoming significantly depressed while taking COCs should stop the medication and use an alternate method of contraception in an attempt to determine whether the symptom is drug-related. Women with premenstrual syndrome (PMS) may have a varied response to oral contraceptives, ranging from symptomatic improvement to worsening of the condition.

Renal: Fluid Retention: Hormonal contraceptives may cause some degree of fluid retention.

Sexual Function/Reproduction: Return to Fertility: After discontinuing oral contraceptives therapy, the patient should delay pregnancy until at least one normal spontaneous menstrual cycle has occurred in order to date the pregnancy. An alternate contraceptive method should be used during this time.

Vaginal Bleeding: Breakthrough bleeding/spotting may occur in women taking COCs, especially during the first three months of use. If this bleeding persists or recurs, nonhormonal causes should be considered and adequate diagnostic measures may be indicated to rule out pregnancy, infection, malignancy, or other conditions. Persistent irregular vaginal bleeding requires assessment to exclude underlying pathology. If pathology has been excluded (see Warnings and Precautions, Cervical Cancer), continued use of the COC or a change to another formulation may solve the problem.

Amenorrhea: In some women, withdrawal bleeding may not occur during the tablet-free interval. If the COC has been taken according to directions, it is unlikely that the woman is pregnant. However, if the COC has not been taken according to directions prior to the first missed withdrawal bleed, or if two consecutive withdrawal bleeds are missed, tablet taking should be discontinued and a non-hormonal back-up method of contraception should be used until the possibility of pregnancy is excluded. Pregnancy must be ruled out before COC use is continued.

Women having a history of oligomenorrhea, secondary amenorrhea, or irregular cycles may remain anovulatory or become amenorrheic following discontinuation of estrogen-progestin combination therapy.

Amenorrhea, especially if associated with breast secretion, that continues for six months or more after withdrawal, warrants a careful assessment of hypothalamic-pituitary function.

Reduced Efficacy: The efficacy of COCs may be reduced in the event of missed tablets, gastro-intestinal disturbances or concomitant medication (see Drug Interactions).

Skin: Chloasma may occasionally occur with use of hormonal contraceptives, especially in women with a history of chloasma gravidarum. Women with a tendency to chloasma should protect the affected area from exposure to the sun or ultraviolet radiation while taking hormonal contraceptives.

Special Populations: Pregnant Women: Oral contraceptives should not be taken by pregnant women. If pregnancy occurs during treatment with ALESSE, further intake should be stopped. However, if conception accidentally occurs while taking the pill, there is no conclusive evidence that the estrogen and progestin contained in the oral contraceptive will damage the developing child.

Nursing Women: In breast-feeding women, the use of oral contraceptives results in the hormonal components being excreted in breast milk and may reduce its quantity and quality. Published studies have indicated that during lactation, 0.1% of the daily maternal dose of levonorgestrel and 0.02% of the daily maternal dose of ethinyl estradiol could be transferred to the newborn via milk.

Adverse effects on the child have been reported, including jaundice and breast enlargement. The nursing mother should be advised not to use oral contraceptives but to use other forms of contraception until she has completely weaned her child.

Pediatrics (<16 years of age): Safety and efficacy of ALESSE tablets have been established in women of reproductive age. Use of this product before menarche is not indicated.

Geriatrics (>65 years of age): ALESSE is not indicated for use in postmenopausal women.

Monitoring and Laboratory Tests: Physical Examination and Follow-up: Before oral contraceptives are used, a thorough history and physical examination should be performed, including a blood pressure determination and the family case history carefully noted. In addition, disturbances of the clotting system must be ruled out if any members of the family have suffered from thromboembolic diseases (e.g., deep vein thrombosis, stroke, myocardial infarction) at a young age. Breasts, liver, extremities and pelvic organs should be examined and a Papanicolaou (PAP) smear should be taken if the patient has been sexually active (see Warnings and Precautions, General).

Tissue Specimens: Pathologists should be advised of COC therapy when specimens obtained from surgical procedures and Pap smears are submitted for examination.

ADVERSE REACTIONS: Adverse Drug Reaction Overview: An increased risk of the following serious adverse reactions has been associated with the use of Combined Oral Contraceptives: arterial thromboembolism; being diagnosed with breast cancer; benign hepatic tumours (e.g. focal nodular hyperplasia, hepatic adenomas); cerebral hemorrhage; cerebral thrombosis; cervical cancer; cervical intraepithelial neoplasia; gallbladder disease, including gallstones*; hepatocellular carcinomas; hypertension; mesenteric thrombosis; myocardial infarction; neuro-ocular lesions (e.g. retinal thrombosis); pulmonary embolism; stroke; transient ischemic attach; thrombophlebitis; venous thrombosis.

The following adverse reactions also have been reported in patients receiving COCs: Nausea and vomiting, usually the most common adverse reaction, occurs in approximately 10 percent or fewer of patients during the first cycle. Other reactions, as a general rule, are seen less frequently or only occasionally.

The following adverse reactions have been reported in patients receiving COC and are believed to be drug related: amenorrhea; breakthrough bleeding; breast changes: pain, tenderness, enlargement, and secretion; change in cervical ectropion and secretion; change in corneal curvature (steepening); change in menstrual flow; change in weight (increase or decrease); chloasma (melasma) which may persist; cholestatic jaundice; diminution in lactation when given immediately postpartum; dysmenorrhea; fluid retention/edema; gastrointestinal symptoms (such as abdominal pain, cramps and bloating); headache, including migraines; hepatocellular injury (e.g., hepatitis, hepatic function abnormal); intolerance to contact lenses; mood changes, including depression; rash (allergic); reduced tolerance to carbohydrates; retinal vascular thrombosis; spotting; temporary infertility after discontinuance of treatment; vaginitis including candidiasis.

The following adverse reactions have been reported in users of COCs and the association has been neither confirmed nor refuted: acne; aggravation of varicose veins; anaphylactoid reactions, including very rare cases of urticaria, angioedema, and severe reactions with respiratory and circulatory symptoms); Budd-Chiari syndrome; cataracts; cerebrovascular disease with mitral valve prolapse; changes in appetite (increase or decrease); changes in libido; changes in serum lipid levels, including hypertriglyceridemia; colitis; congenital anomalies; cystitis-like syndrome; decrease in serum folate levels†; dizziness; erythema multiforme; erythema nodosum; exacerbation of chorea; exacerbation of porphyria; exacerbation of systemic lupus erythematosus; hemolytic uremic syndrome; hemorrhagic eruption; hepatic adenomas; hepatocellular carcinomas; hirsutism; impaired renal function; ischemic colitis; loss of scalp hair; lupus-like syndrome; nervousness; optic neuritis‡; pancreatitis; premenstrual syndrome; sickle-cell disease; vaginitis.

Clinical Trial Adverse Drug Reactions: Because clinical trials are conducted under very specific conditions the adverse reaction rates observed in the clinical trials may not reflect the rates observed in practice and should not be compared to the rates in the clinical trials of another drug. Adverse drug reaction information from clinical trials is useful for identifying drug-related adverse events and for approximating rates.

Oral Contraception: Treatment-emergent adverse events were analyzed for 1477 subjects exposed to the study drug for 7870 cycles. One or more treatment emergent adverse events were reported for 1106 (75%) subjects. Table 1 lists the frequency of treatment emergent adverse events that were reported by ≥2% of subjects.

A total of 133 (9%) subjects stopped taking the study medication because of adverse events. Some of the study events that led to subject discontinuation were considered by the medical monitor to be potentially serious: headache (21), hypertension (7), migraine (3), phlebitis (1), palpitations (1), varicose veins (1), vascular disorder (1), hypercholesterolemia/hyperlipidemia (6), depression/emotional lability (16), hypesthesia (1), abnormal vision (2), visual field defect (1), amenorrhea (8), dysmenorrhea (4), menorrhagia (6), irregular bleeding (1), menstrual bloating (1), irregular bleeding (1), fibroid growth (1).

No deaths occurred during the multicentre study.

Acne: In the two acne studies, the safety profile of ALESSE was compared with that of placebo. Treatment-emergent adverse events that were reported by ≥2% of patients in either treatment group are presented in Table 2.

As expected, menstrual-related events were more frequent in women treated with ALESSE than with placebo. However, other adverse events often associated with oral contraceptive use, including nausea, vomiting, breast pain, headache, migraine, and weight gain, occurred at similar rates in women treated with placebo or ALESSE.

* COCs may worsen existing gallbladder disease and may accelerate the development of this disease in previously asymptomatic women.

† Serum folate levels may be depressed by COC therapy.

‡ Optic neuritis may lead to partial or complete loss of vision.

Table 1: ALESSE

Frequency of Treatment-Emergent Adverse Events That Occurred in ≥2% of Subjects

Event	Number (%) of Subjects (n=1477)
Headache	400 (27)
Dysmenorrhea	210 (14)
Infection	200 (14)
Pharyngitis	146 (10)
Abdominal pain	134 (9)
Nausea	134 (9)
Metrorrhagia	123 (8)
Sinusitis	90 (6)
Flu syndrome	84 (6)
Vaginal moniliasis	71 (5)
Pain	71 (5)
Back pain	66 (4)
Breast pain	65 (4)
Accidental injury	64 (4)
Acne	62 (4)
Rhinitis	54 (4)
Emotional lability	50 (3)
Vaginitis	48 (3)
Urinary tract infection	41 (3)
Dizziness	40 (3)
Diarrhea	40 (3)
Bronchitis	37 (3)
Depression	36 (2)
Asthenia	35 (2)
Vomiting	34 (2)
Allergic reaction other than to study drug	33 (2)
Amenorrhea	30 (2)

Table 2: ALESSE

Percentage of Patients (≥2%) Reporting Treatment-Emergent Adverse Events in Either Treatment Group in Studies 0858A1-900, 901

Adverse Event	Number (%) of Subjects	
	ALESSE (n=349)	Placebo (n=355)
Headache	110 (31.5)	107 (30.1)
Metrorrhagia[a]	77 (21.8)	14 (3.9)
Nausea	49 (14.0)	40 (11.3)
Infection	48 (13.8)	49 (13.8)
Pharyngitis	46 (13.2)	58 (16.3)
Pain	31 (8.9)	36 (10.1)
Abdominal pain	27 (7.7)	24 (6.8)
Dysmenorrhea	27 (7.7)	39 (11.0)
Accidental injury	21 (6.0)	16 (4.5)
Menstrual disorder[a]	21 (6.0)	8 (2.3)
Flu syndrome	19 (5.4)	20 (5.6)
Allergic reaction[a]	16 (4.6)	6 (1.7)
Breast pain	16 (4.6)	11 (3.1)
Rhinitis	15 (4.0)	13 (3.7)
Sinusitis	14 (4.0)	2.0 (8)

(cont'd)

Table 2: ALESSE *(cont'd)*

Percentage of Patients (≥2%) Reporting Treatment-Emergent Adverse Events in Either Treatment Group in Studies 0858A1-900, 901

	Number (%) of Subjects	
Adverse Event	**ALESSE (n=349)**	**Placebo (n=355)**
Asthenia	13 (3.7)	5 (1.4)
Back pain	12 (3.4)	12 (3.4)
Dyspepsia	12 (3.4)	2.3 (8)
Weight gain	17 (3.4)	12 (2.3)
Emotional lability[a]	12 (3.4)	4 (1.1)
Acne	13 (3.4)	6 (1.4)
Migraine	11 (3.2)	8 (2.3)
Dizziness	11 (3.2)	10 (2.8)
Cough increased	10 (2.9)	8 (2.3)
Vomiting	10 (2.6)	6 (1.7)
Depression	9 (2.6)	11 (2.5)
Moniliasis	7 (2.0)	8 (2.3)
Myalgia	7 (2.0)	5 (1.4)
Bronchitis	7 (2.0)	7 (2.0)
Rash	7 (2.0)	7 (2.0)
Urticaria[a]	7 (2.0)	0
Allergic reaction other than drug	7 (2.0)	7 (2.0)
Diarrhea	6 (1.7)	10 (2.8)
Unintended pregnancy[a]	2 (0.6)	12 (3.1)

[a] Statistically significantly different between treatment groups (p<0.05).

DRUG INTERACTIONS: Overview: The concurrent administration of COCs with other substances may result in an altered response to either agent. Decreased ethinyl estradiol (EE) serum concentration may cause an increased incidence of breakthrough bleeding and menstrual irregularities and may possibly reduce efficacy of the COC. During concomitant use of EE containing products and substances that may lead to decreased EE serum concentration, it is recommended that a nonhormonal back-up method of birth control (such as condoms and spermicide) be used in addition to the regular intake of ALESSE. In the case of prolonged use of such substances COCs should not be considered the primary contraceptive.

After discontinuation of substances that may lead to decreased EE serum concentrations, use of a nonhormonal back-up method is recommended for at least 7 days. Longer use of a back-up method is advisable after discontinuation of substances that have led to induction of hepatic microsomal enzymes, resulting in decreased EE serum concentrations. It may sometimes take several weeks until enzyme induction has completely subsided, depending on dosage, duration of use and rate of elimination of the inducing substance.

Reduced effectiveness of the COC, should it occur, is more likely with the low-dose formulations. It is important to ascertain all drugs that a patient is taking, both prescription and non-prescription, before COCs are prescribed.

Examples of substances that may decrease serum EE concentrations:

- Any substance that reduces gastrointestinal transit time
- Hypericum perforatum, also known as St. John's wort and ritonovir (possibly by induction of hepatic microsomal enzymes)
- Substances that induce hepatic microsomal enzymes, such as rifampicin, rifabutin, barbiturates, primidone, phenylbutazone, phenytoin, dexamethasone, griseofulvin, topiramate, some protease inhibitors, modafinil
- Certain antibiotics (eg, ampicillin and other penicillins, tetracyclines), by a decrease of enterohepatic circulation of estrogens.

Examples of substances that may increase serum EE concentrations:

- Atorvastatin
- Competitive inhibitors for sulfation in the gastrointestinal wall, such as ascorbic acid (vitamin C) and acetaminophen (paracetamol).
- Substances that inhibit cytochrome P 450 3A4 isoenzymes such as indinavir, fluconazole and troleandomycin.
- Troleandomycin may increase the risk of intrahepatic cholestasis during coadministration with COCs.

EE may interfere with the metabolism of other drugs by inhibiting hepatic microsomal enzymes, or by inducing hepatic drug conjugation, particularly glucuronidation. Accordingly, plasma and tissue concentrations may either be increased (eg, cyclosporine, theophylline, corticosteroids) or decreased (eg, lamotrigine).

In patients treated with flunarizine, use of oral contraceptives has been reported to increase the risk of galactorrhea.

The prescribing information of concomitant medications should be consulted to identify potential interactions.

Drug-Drug Interactions: For possible drug interactions with COCs, see Table 3 and Table 4.

Table 3: ALESSE[a]

Drugs That May Decrease the Efficacy of Oral Contraceptives

Class of Compound	Drug	Proposed Mechanism	Suggested Management
Anticonvulsants	Carbamazepine Ethosuximide Phenobarbital Phenytoin Primidone	Induction of hepatic microsomal enzymes. Rapid metabolism of estrogen and increased binding of progestin and ethinyl estradiol to SHBG.	Use higher dose OCs (50 µg ethinyl estradiol), another drug or another method.
Antibiotics	Ampicillin Cotrimoxazole Penicillin	Enterohepatic circulation disturbance, intestinal hurry.	For short course, use additional method or use another drug.For long course, use another method.
	Rifampin	Increased metabolism of progestins. Suspected acceleration of estrogen metabolism.	Use another method.

(cont'd)

Table 3: ALESSE[a] *(cont'd)*

Drugs That May Decrease the Efficacy of Oral Contraceptives

Class of Compound	Drug	Proposed Mechanism	Suggested Management
	Chloramphenicol Metronidazole Neomycin Nitrofurantoin Sulfonamides Tetracyclines	Induction of hepatic microsomal enzymes. Also disturbance of enterohepatic circulation.	For short course, use additional method or use another drug. For long course, use another method.
	Troleandomycin	May retard metabolism of OCs, increasing the risk of cholestatic jaundice.	
Antifungals	Griseofulvin	Stimulation of hepatic metabolism of contraceptive steroids may occur.	Use another method.
Cholesterol Lowering Agents	Clofibrate	Reduces elevated serum triglycerides and cholesterol; this reduces OC efficacy.	Use another method.
Sedatives and Hypnotics	Benzodiazepines Barbiturates Chloral Hydrate Glutethimide Meprobamate	Induction of hepatic microsomal enzymes.	For short course, use additional method or another drug. For long course, use another method or higher dose of OCs.
Antacids		Decreased intestinal absorption of progestins.	Dose two hours apart.
Other Drugs	Phenylbutazone[b] Antihistamines[b] Analgesics[b] Antimigraine preparations[b] Vitamin E	Reduced OC efficacy has been reported. Remains to be confirmed.	

[a] Adapted from Dickey, RP, ed.: Managing Contraceptive Pill Patients, 5th edition, Creative Informatics Inc., Durant, OK, 1987.

[b] Refer to Oral Contraceptives 1994, A Report by the Special Advisory Committee on Reproductive Physiology to the Drugs Directorate, Health Protection Branch, Health Canada.

Table 4: ALESSE[a]

Modification of Other Drug Action by Oral Contraceptives

Class of Compound	Drug	Modification of Drug Action	Suggested Management
Alcohol		Possible increased levels of ethanol or acetaldehyde.	Use with caution.
Alpha-II Adrenoreceptor Agents	Clonidine	Sedation effect increased.	Use with caution.
Anticoagulants	All	OCs increase clotting factors, decrease efficacy. However, OCs may potentiate action in some patients.	Use another method.
Anticonvulsants	All	Fluid retention may increase risk of seizures.	Use another method.
Antidiabetic Drugs	Oral Hypoglycemics and Insulin	OCs may impair glucose tolerance and increase blood glucose.	Use low-dose estrogen and progestin OC or another method. Monitor blood glucose.
Antihypertensive Agents	Guanethidine and Methyldopa	Estrogen component causes sodium retention, progestin has no effect.	Use low-dose estrogen OC or use another method.
	Beta Blockers	Increased drug effect (decreased metabolism).	Adjust dose of drug if necessary. Monitor cardiovascular status.
Antipyretics	Acetaminophen	Increased metabolism and renal clearance.	Dose of drug may have to be increased.
	Antipyrine	Impaired metabolism.	Decrease dose of drug.
	ASA	Effects of ASA may be decreased by the short-term use of OCs.	Patients on chronic ASA therapy may require an increase in ASA dosage.
Aminocaproic Acid		Theoretically, a hypercoagulable state may occur because OCs augment clotting factors.	Avoid concomitant use.
Betamimetic Agents	Isoproterenol Agents	Estrogen causes decreased response to these drugs.	Adjust dose of drug as necessary. Discontinuing OCs can result in excessive drug activity.
Caffeine		The actions of caffeine may be enhanced as OCs may impair the hepatic metabolism of caffeine.	Use with caution.
Cholesterol Lowering Agents	Clofibrate	Their action may be antagonized by OCs. OCs may also increase metabolism of clofibrate.	May need to increase dose of clofibrate.
Corticosteroids	Prednisone	Markedly increased serum levels.	Possible need for decrease in dose.
Cyclosporine		May lead to an increase in cyclosporine levels and hepatotoxicity.	Monitor hepatic function. The cyclosporine dose may have to be decreased.

(cont'd)

Table 4: ALESSE[a] *(cont'd)*

Modification of Other Drug Action by Oral Contraceptives

Class of Compound	Drug	Modification of Drug Action	Suggested Management
Folic Acid		OCs have been reported to impair folate metabolism.	May need to increase dietary intake, or supplement.
Meperidine		Possible increased analgesia and CNS depression due to decreased metabolism of meperidine.	Use combination with caution.
Phenothiazine Tranquilizers	All Phenothiazines, Reserpine and similar drugs	Estrogen potentiates the hyperprolactinemia effect of these drugs.	Use other drugs or lower dose of OCs. If galactorrhea or hyperprolactinemia occurs, use other method.
Sedatives and Hypnotics	Chlordiazepoxide Lorazepam Oxazepam Diazepam	Increased effect (increased metabolism).	Use with caution.
Theophylline	All	Decreased oxidation, leading to possible toxicity.	Use with caution. Monitor theophylline levels.
Tricyclic Antidepressants	Clomipramine (possibly others)	Increased side effects: i.e., depression. Increased serum levels due to decreased clearance.	Use with caution.
Vitamin B_{12}		OCs have been reported to reduce serum levels of Vitamin B_{12}.	May need to increase dietary intake, or supplement.

[a] Adapted from Dickey, RP, ed.: Managing Contraceptive Pill Patients, 5th edition, Creative Informatics Inc., Durant, OK, 1987.

Drug-Food Interactions: No data is available.
Drug-Herb Interactions: Hypericum perforatum, also known as St. John's wort causes decrease in serum EE concentration possibly by induction of hepatic microsomal enzymes.
Drug-Laboratory Test Interactions: Results of laboratory tests should be interpreted in the light that the patient is on COCs. The following laboratory tests are modified:

Liver Function Tests	
Bromsulphthalein Retention Test (BSP)	Moderate increase
AST and GGT	Minor increase
Alkaline Phosphatase	Variable increase
Serum Bilirubin	Increased, particularly in conditions predisposing to or associated with hyperbilirubinemia
Coagulation Tests	
Factors II, VII, IX, X, XII and XIII	Increased
Factor VIII	Mild increase
Platelet aggregation and adhesiveness	Mild increase in response to common aggregating agents
Fibrinogen	Increased
Plasminogen	Mild increase
Antithrombin III	Mild decrease
Prothrombin Time	Increased
Thyroid Function Tests	
Protein-bound Iodine (PBI)	Increased
Total Serum Thyroxine (T3 and T4)	Increased
Thyroid Stimulating Hormone (TSH)	Unchanged
Free T3 Resin Uptake	Decreased
Adrenocortical Function Tests	
Plasma Cortisol	Increased
Cortisol Binding Globulin	Increased
Dehydroepiandrosterone sulfate (DHEAS)	Decreased
Renal Function	
Plasma Creatinine	Increased
Creatinine Clearance	Increased
Miscellaneous Tests	
Serum Folate	Occasionally decreased
Glucose Tolerance Test	Variable increase with return to normal after 6 to 12 months
Insulin Response	Mild to moderate increase
c-Peptide Response	Mild to moderate increase

Drug-Lifestyle Interactions: See Warnings and Precautions regarding cigarette smoking. The actions of caffeine may be enhanced as OCs may impair the hepatic metabolism of caffeine. Use with caution. There may be possible increased levels of ethanol or acetaldehyde when combined with alcohol. Use with caution.

Non-Contraceptive Benefits of Oral Contraceptives: Several health advantages other than contraception have been reported.
1. Combination oral contraceptives reduce the incidence of cancer of the endometrium and ovaries.
2. Oral contraceptives reduce the likelihood of developing benign breast disease and, as a result may decrease the incidence of breast biopsies.
3. Oral contraceptives reduce the likelihood of development of functional ovarian cysts.
4. Pill users have less menstrual blood loss and have more regular cycles, thereby reducing the chance of developing iron-deficiency anemia.
5. The use of oral contraceptives may decrease the severity of dysmenorrhea and premenstrual syndrome, and may improve acne vulgaris, hirsutism, and other androgen-mediated disorders.
6. Oral contraceptives decrease the incidence of acute pelvic inflammatory disease and reduce the incidence of ectopic pregnancy.
7. Oral contraceptives have potential effects on endometriosis.

DOSAGE AND ADMINISTRATION: Recommended Dose and Dosage Adjustment: Contraception: ALESSE 21 Tablets Regimen:

Each cycle consists of 21 days on medication and a 7-day interval without medication (three weeks on, one week off).

The dosage of ALESSE Tablets is one tablet daily for 21 consecutive days per menstrual cycle, according to prescribed schedule. For the first cycle of medication, the patient is instructed to take one ALESSE Tablet daily for 21 consecutive days beginning on Day 1 of her menstrual cycle, on Day 5, or on the first Sunday after her period begins. (For the first cycle only, the first day of menstrual flow is considered Day 1). The tablets are then discontinued for seven days (one week). Withdrawal bleeding should usually occur within three days following discontinuation of ALESSE.

The patient begins her next and all subsequent 21-day courses of ALESSE Tablets (following the same 21 days on, 7 days off) on the same day of the week that she began her first course. She begins taking her tablets seven days after discontinuation, regardless of whether or not withdrawal bleeding is still in progress.

ALESSE 28 Tablets Regimen: Each cycle consists of 21 days of pink ALESSE Tablets (active tablets) followed by 7 days of white inert tablets (three weeks on ALESSE, one week on inert tablets).

The dosage of ALESSE Tablets is one tablet daily for 21 consecutive days per menstrual cycle, according to prescribed schedule, followed by one inert tablet daily for 7 consecutive days according to prescribed schedule. For the first cycle of medication, the patient is instructed to take one pink tablet daily for 21 consecutive days beginning on Day 1 of her menstrual cycle, on Day 5, or on the first Sunday after her period begins. (For the first cycle only, the first day of menstrual flow is considered Day 1). One white tablet is taken daily for the following seven consecutive days. Withdrawal bleeding should usually occur within three days following the discontinuation pink ALESSE Tablets, i.e., during the week the patient is taking the white inert tablets.

The patient begins her next and all subsequent 28-day courses of tablets on the same day of the week that she began her first course. She continues her next course of 28 tablets immediately after the last course, regardless of whether or not a period of withdrawal bleeding is still in progress. There is no need for the patient to count days between cycles because there are no "off-tablet days".

Acne: The timing of initiation of ALESSE treatment for acne should follow the instructions for use of ALESSE for contraception (see Dosage and Administration information for oral contraception).

Missed Dose: The patient should be instructed to use the following chart if she misses one or more of her birth control pills (see Table 5). She should be told to match the number of pills with the appropriate starting time for her type of pill.

Table 5: ALESSE

What to Do if You Miss Pills

Sunday Start	Other Than Sunday Start
Miss One Pill	**Miss One Pill**
Take it as soon as you remember, and take the next pill at the usual time. This means that you might take two pills in one day.	Take it as soon as you remember, and take the next pill at the usual time. This means that you might take two pills in one day.
Miss Two Pills in a Row	**Miss Two Pills in a Row**
First two weeks: 1. Take two pills the day you remember and two pills the next day. 2. Then take one pill a day until you finish the pack. 3. Use a nonhormonal back-up method of birth control if you have sex in the seven days after you miss the pills. **Third week:** 1. Keep taking one pill a day until Sunday. 2. On Sunday, safely discard the rest of the pack and start a new pack that day. 3. Use a nonhormonal back-up method of birth control if you have sex in the seven days after you miss the pills. 4. You may not have a period this month. **If You Miss Two Periods in a Row, Call Your Doctor, Pharmacist or Clinic.**	**First two weeks:** 1. Take two pills the day you remember and two pills the next day. 2. Then take one pill a day until you finish the pack. 3. Use a nonhormonal back-up method of birth control if you have sex in the seven days after you miss the pills. **Third week:** 1. Safely dispose of the rest of the pill pack and start a new pack that same day. 2. Use a nonhormonal back-up method of birth control if you have sex in the seven days after you miss the pills. 3. You may not have a period this month. **If You Miss Two Periods in a Row, Call Your Doctor, Pharmacist or Clinic.**
Miss Three or More Pills in a Row	**Miss Three or More Pills in a Row**
Anytime in the cycle: 1. Keep taking one pill a day until Sunday. 2. On Sunday, safely discard the rest of the pack and start a new pack that day. 3. Use a nonhormonal back-up method of birth control if you have sex in the seven days after you miss the pills. 4. You may not have a period this month. **If You Miss Two periods in a Row, Call Your Doctor, Pharmacist or Clinic.**	**Anytime in the cycle:** 1. Safely dispose of the rest of the pill pack and start a new pack that same day. 2. Use a nonhormonal back-up method of birth control if you have sex in the seven days after you miss the pills. 3. You may not have a period this month. **If You Miss Two periods in a Row, Call Your Doctor, Pharmacist or Clinic.**

Contraceptive reliability may be reduced if active tablets are missed and particularly if the missed tablets extend the tablet-free interval. If active tablets were missed and intercourse took place in the week before the tablets were missed, the possibility of pregnancy should be considered.

Administration: Tablets for oral use.

Special Notes on Administration: Administration: It is recommended that ALESSE Tablets be taken at the same time each day, preferably after the evening meal or at bedtime.

ALESSE is effective from the first day of therapy if the tablets are begun on the first day of the menstrual cycle.

If ALESSE Tablets administration is initiated postpartum (no earlier than day 28 after delivery in the nonlactating mother) or after Day 1 of the first menstrual cycle, contraceptive reliance should not be placed on ALESSE until after the first seven consecutive days of administration. The possibility of ovulation and conception prior to initiation of medication should be considered. Therefore, nonhormonal methods of contraception (such as condoms and spermicide) should be used for the first 7 days of tablet taking.

If spotting or breakthrough bleeding occurs, the patient is instructed to continue on the same regimen. This type of bleeding usually is transient and without significance; however, if the bleeding is persistent or prolonged, the patient is advised to consult her physician.

Advice in Case of Vomiting: If vomiting occurs within 3-4 hours after tablet-taking, absorption may not be complete. In such event, advice concerning the Management of Missed Tablet is outlined in the above chart.

The woman must take the extra active tablet(s) needed from a backup pack.

No Hormonal Contraceptive Use in the Past Month: Tablet-taking should start on day 1 of the woman's natural cycle (ie, the first day of her menstrual bleeding). Starting on days 2-7 is allowed, but for the first 7 days of tablet-taking during the first cycle, a nonhormonal back-up method of birth control (such as condoms and spermicide) is recommended.

Changing from Another COC Pill: The woman should start ALESSE preferably on the day after the last active tablet of her previous COC, but at the latest, on the day following the usual tablet-free or inactive tablet interval of her previous COC.

Changing from a Progestin Only Method (progestin-only pill, injection, implant): The woman may switch any day from the progestin-only pill and should begin ALESSE the next day. She should start ALESSE on the day of an implant removal or, if using an injection, the day the next injection would be due. In all of these situations, the woman should be advised to use a nonhormonal back-up method for the first 7 days of tablet-taking.

Following First-Trimester Abortion: The woman may start ALESSE immediately. Additional contraceptive measures are not needed.

Following Delivery or Second-Trimester Abortion: Since the immediate post-partum period is associated with an increased risk of thromboembolism, oral contraceptives should be started no earlier than day 28 after delivery in the nonlactating mother or after second-trimester abortion. The woman should be advised to use a nonhormonal back-up method for the first 7 days of tablet-taking. However, if intercourse has already occurred, the possibility of pregnancy should be ruled out before the actual start of COC use or the woman must wait for her first menstrual period.

OVERDOSAGE:

Symptoms of COC overdosage in adults and children may include nausea, vomiting, breast tenderness, dizziness, abdominal pain, drowsiness/fatigue; withdrawal bleeding may occur in females. There is no specific antidote and further treatment of overdose, if necessary, is directed to the symptoms.

For management of a suspected drug overdose, contact your **regional Poison Control Centre**. See the *CPS* Directory section for a list of Poison Control Centres.

ACTION AND CLINICAL PHARMACOLOGY: Mechanism of Action: Oral Contraception: Although the primary mechanism of action is inhibition of ovulation, the effectiveness of ALESSE Tablets may also result from other mechanisms of action, such as hostility of the cervical mucus to sperm penetration and migration.

Acne: Acne is a disease of the pilosebaceous apparatus characterized by abnormal keratinization, increased sebum production, and bacterial colonization. While the etiology of acne is multifactorial, there is evidence that androgenic action, including stimulation of sebaceous glands, is necessary for the development of acne. The suppression of gonadotropins by ALESSE leads to decreased ovarian production of the androgens, including androstenedione. ALESSE also significantly reduces bioavailable serum testosterone by preserving the estrogen-induced increases in sex hormone binding globulin (SHBG). In addition, ALESSE decreases serum levels of 3β-androstanediol glucuronide (a marker of peripheral 5β-reductase activity). These biochemical changes produced by the coadministration of levonorgestrel and ethinyl estradiol are consistent with improvement of acne in otherwise healthy women.

Special Populations and Conditions: Pediatrics (<16 years of age): Safety and efficacy of ALESSE tablets have been established in women of reproductive age. Use of this product before menarche is not indicated.

Geriatrics (>65 years of age): ALESSE is not indicated for use in postmenopausal women.

STORAGE AND STABILITY: Store in original packaging between 15 and 30°C. Keep out of reach of children and pets.

ALESSE 21 and ALESSE 28 Tablets should be protected from light once opened using the protective covering provided.

Medications should not be disposed of via wastewater or household waste. Ask your pharmacist how to dispose of medications no longer required. These measures will help to protect the environment.

SPECIAL HANDLING INSTRUCTIONS: None.

INFORMATION FOR THE PATIENT: Published in e-CPS, available by subscription at www.e-cps.ca.

DOSAGE FORMS, COMPOSITION AND PACKAGING: ALESSE 21: Each pink tablet contains: levonorgestrel 100 µg and ethinyl estradiol 20 µg. Nonmedicinal ingredients: hydroxypropyl methylcellulose, lactose, magnesium stearate, microcrystalline cellulose, polacrilin potassium, polyethylene glycol, synthetic red iron oxide, titanium dioxide and wax E. Blister packs for the 21-day regimen.

ALESSE 28: Each pink tablet contains: levonorgestrel 100 µg and ethinyl estradiol 20 µg. The white tablets are inactive. Nonmedicinal ingredients: hydroxypropyl methylcellulose, lactose, magnesium stearate, microcrystalline cellulose, polacrilin potassium, polyethylene glycol, synthetic red iron oxide, titanium dioxide and wax E; white tablets: hydroxypropyl methylcellulose, lactose, magnesium stearate, microcrystalline cellulose, polacrilin potassium, polyethylene glycol, titanium dioxide and wax E. Blister packs for the 28-day regimen (21 active pink tablets and 7 inactive white tablets).

(Shown in Product Identification Section)

Aleve®

naproxen sodium

Nonsteroidal Anti-inflammatory Drug—Analgesic—Antipyretic

Bayer Consumer Care

Date of Revision: June 17, 2009

SUMMARY PRODUCT INFORMATION:

Route of Administration	Dosage Form/ Strength	Clinically Relevant Nonmedicinal Ingredients
Oral	Caplet, 220 mg	For a complete listing, see Dosage Forms, Composition and Packaging.

INDICATIONS AND CLINICAL USE: ALEVE (naproxen sodium) is indicated for the reduction of fever and the treatment of pain:

- ALEVE is clinically proven to relieve arthritis pain. ALEVE relieves the daily pain and stiffness of arthritis. ALEVE relieves morning stiffness and arthritis pain at rest, on passive motion, on weight bearing, pain experienced day or night due to arthritis.
- ALEVE helps relieve the night pain associated with arthritis.
- ALEVE relieves the pain of inflammation.
- ALEVE relieves the pain or stiffness of rheumatic or arthritic conditions.
- ALEVE relieves joint and body pain.
- ALEVE relieves muscular ache.
- ALEVE relieves the pain of muscle sprains and strains.
- ALEVE relieves backache.
- ALEVE relieves headache.
- ALEVE relieves migraine pain.
- ALEVE relieves the pain of menstrual cramps (dysmenorrhoea).
- ALEVE relieves the pain of minor surgery.
- ALEVE relieves toothache.
- ALEVE relieves the pain of dental extractions.
- ALEVE relieves minor aches and pain associated with the common cold.

CONTRAINDICATIONS: Naproxen sodium is contraindicated in patients:

- who have previously exhibited allergy to naproxen sodium.
- with known hypersensitivity to the active substance naproxen (including naproxen sodium) or any of the excipients in the caplets. For a complete listing, see Dosage Forms, Composition and Packaging.
- with a history of asthma, urticaria, or allergic-type reactions after taking acetylsalicylic acid (ASA) or other NSAIDs (i.e. complete or partial syndrome of ASA-intolerance—rhinosinusitis, urticaria/angioedema, nasal polyps, asthma). Fatal anaphylactoid reactions have occurred in such individuals. Individuals with the above medical problems are at risk of a severe reaction even if they have taken NSAIDs in the past without any adverse reaction.
- with active peptic ulcers, a history of recurrent ulceration, or active gastrointestinal bleeding.
- with inflammatory bowel disease.
- with severe liver impairment or active liver disease.
- with severe renal impairment (creatinine clearance <30 mL/min or 0.5 mL/sec) or deteriorating renal disease (individuals with lesser degrees of renal impairment are at risk of deterioration of their renal function when prescribed NSAIDs and must be monitored).
- in women in their third trimester of pregnancy because of risk of premature closure of the ductus arteriosus and prolonged parturition.

WARNINGS AND PRECAUTIONS: General: Patients who are taking any other analgesic or anti-inflammatory drugs (including naproxen or naproxen sodium), steroids, diuretics or drugs that influence hemostasis.

Cardiovascular: Patients with severe cardiac impairment and a history of hypertension.

Gastrointestinal: Patients with a medical history of gastrointestinal disease including peptic ulceration. Pain of gastrointestinal origin is not an indication for naproxen sodium.

Hematologic: Patients with coagulation disturbances. Numerous studies have shown that concomitant use of NSAIDs and anti-coagulants increases the risk of bleeding. Concurrent therapy of ALEVE with warfarin requires close monitoring of the international normalized ratio (INR). Even with therapeutic INR monitoring, increased bleeding may occur.

Neurologic: Some patients may experience drowsiness, dizziness, blurred vision vertigo, tinnitus, hearing loss, insomnia or depression with the use of NSAIDs such as ALEVE. If patients experience such adverse reactions, they should exercise caution in carrying out activities that require alertness, like driving or using machinery.

Respiratory: Patients with a medical history of asthma, rhinitis or nasal polyps.

Skin: Patients with a medical history of urticaria and angioedema.

Sexual Function/Reproduction: Naproxen, as with any drug known to inhibit cyclooxygenase/prostaglandin synthesis, may impair fertility and is not recommended in women attempting to conceive. In women who have difficulty conceiving or who are undergoing investigation of infertility, withdrawal of naproxen should be considered.

Special Populations: Geriatrics: Patients older than 65 years and frail or debilitated patients are more susceptible to a variety of adverse reactions from NSAIDs. The incidence of these adverse reactions increases with dose and duration of treatment. In addition, these patients are less tolerant to ulceration and bleeding. Most reports of fatal GI events are in this population. Older patients are also at risk of lower esophageal injury including ulceration and bleeding.

Pregnant Women: Caution should be exercised in prescribing ALEVE during the first and second trimesters of pregnancy. As with other drugs of this type, naproxen sodium produces delay in parturition in animals and also affects the human fetal cardiovascular system (closure of the ductus arteriosus). Therefore, naproxen sodium should not be used unless clearly needed and when directed to do so by a doctor. The use of naproxen sodium in the first and second trimesters of pregnancy requires cautious balancing of the possible benefits and risks to the mother and fetus, especially during the first trimester.

Inhibition of prostaglandin synthesis may adversely affect pregnancy and/or the embryo/fetal development. Data from epidemiological studies suggest an increased risk of miscarriage and of cardiac malformation after use of a prostaglandin synthesis inhibitor in early pregnancy. In animals, administration of a prostaglandin synthesis inhibitor has been shown to result in increased pre- and post-implantation loss and embryo-fetal lethality. In addition, increased incidences of various malformations, including cardiovascular, have been reported in animals given a prostaglandin synthesis inhibitor during the organogenetic period.

Nursing Women: Naproxen has been found in the milk of lactating mothers. The use of naproxen sodium should therefore be avoided in women who are breast feeding unless clearly needed and directed to do so by a doctor.

Pediatrics (<12 years of age): Children under 12 should not take this drug, unless directed by a doctor. The safety in pediatric use has not been established.

Persons on a Low Sodium Diet: One caplet contains 20 mg sodium, which is classified as low in sodium. A variety of Health Canada guidelines suggest that a diet low in sodium should be restricted to 2 g per day while the Sodium Collaborative Research group suggests that a low-sodium diet should be restricted to ≤1.2 g (50 mmol) per day.

Monitoring and Laboratory Tests: Naproxen sodium causes transient, dose-dependent modestly increased bleeding times. However, these values often do not exceed the upper limit of the reference range. Naproxen sodium may theoretically interfere with the urinary analyses of 17-ketogenic steroids and 5-hydroxy indoleacetic acid (5 HIAA).

ADVERSE REACTIONS: Clinical Trial Adverse Drug Reactions: Because clinical trials are conducted under very specific conditions the adverse reaction rates observed in the clinical trials may not reflect the rates observed in practice and should not be compared to the rates in the clinical trials of another drug. Adverse drug reaction information from clinical trials is useful for identifying drug-related adverse events and for approximating rates.

The safety profile of ALEVE was analysed through a meta-analysis of the clinical trials which were performed in the course of the ALEVE clinical development program. The meta-analysis included a total of 46 studies, which satisfied the criteria of being randomized, placebo controlled, double-blind and used ALEVE in single (SD, 220 mg or 440 mg pooled data), multiple (MD, 440 mg/day and 880 mg/day) or PRN (up to 880 mg/day) doses. In total 4623 subjects were treated with ALEVE while 2659 took placebo. Fifty-two percent of subjects participated in SD trials, 20 % in MD trials all lasting for 7 days and the remaining 28% in PRN trials. They were predominantly Caucasian, slightly more women with a mean age between the 20s and 30s with exception of 422 patients from the arthritis studies with a mean age in the low 60s. The occurrence of all adverse events did not differ between ALEVE and placebo, in the SD, MD or PRN trials. Moderate and severe events tended to occur less frequently in the subjects treated with ALEVE MD compared to placebo, presumably due to concomitant treatment of naturally occurring headache. The data in Table 1 show the frequencies of adverse events that are >1% from the meta-analysis. A thorough evaluation of gastrointestinal adverse events showed no difference between ALEVE and placebo. There was no serious gastrointestinal adverse event (bleeding or perforation) or any case of anaphylaxis.

Table 1: ALEVE

Adverse Events that Occurred with ALEVE (low dose short duration) with a Frequency >1% in Clinical Trials

	ALEVE n=4623 (%)	Placebo n=2659 (%)
Gastrointestinal		
Dyspepsia	1.9	1.8
Nausea	4.4	4.8
Vomiting	1.8	2.4
Nervous System		
Dizziness	2.0	2.1
Headache	4.9	6.8
Somnolence	2.4	1.5

Less Common Clinical Trial Adverse Drug Reactions (<1%): Gastrointestinal: constipation, diarrhea.

Other: allergic reactions, edema, rash/pruritus.

Post-Market Adverse Drug Reactions: See Table 2.

Severe allergic ADRs are very rare events, which are more likely to occur in subjects who have experienced allergic reactions previously. In short term use of naproxen sodium occurrence of GI ulcers/bleeding/perforation are rare events.

The adverse drug reactions seen during short term use of naproxen sodium are normally mild and disappear after discontinuing the drug. The most common ADRs for OTC naproxen sodium and/or solely for prescription doses (higher dose and or longer duration) are dizziness, headache, light-headedness, dyspepsia, nausea, heartburn, and abdominal pain. Uncommonly drowsiness, insomnia, and skin rashes are encountered. Peripheral edemas are rare events. Other ADRs are very rare and/or observed through isolated reports only. The adverse events are common to all NSAIDs as a class; there is no adverse event that is specific for naproxen alone.

Table 2: ALEVE

The Following Post-Marketing Adverse Drug Reactions Have Been Observed for OTC Naproxen Sodium and/or Solely for Prescription Dosages (higher dose and/or longer duration) of Naproxen/Naproxen Sodium

Immune System	Very rare <0.01% and isolated reports	anaphylaxis/anaphylactoid reactions
Blood	Very rare <0.01% and isolated reports	hematopoietic disturbances (leukopenia, thrombocytopenia, agranulocytosis, aplastic anemia, eosinophilia, hemolytic anemia)
Psychiatric	Very rare <0.01% and isolated reports	psychiatric disorders
Nervous	Common ≥1%–<10%	dizziness, headache, lightheadedness
	Uncommon ≥0.1 %–<1 %	drowsiness, insomnia, somnolence
	Very rare <0.01% and isolated reports	aseptic meningitis, cognitive dysfunction, convulsions
Eye	Very rare <0.01% and isolated reports	visual disturbance, corneal opacity, papillitis, retrobulbar optic neuritis, papilledema
Ear & Labyrinth	Uncommon ≥0.1 %–<1 %	vertigo
	Very rare <0.01% and isolated reports	hearing impairment, tinnitus
Cardiac	Very rare <0.01% and isolated reports	congestive heart failure, hypertension, pulmonary edema
Vascular	Very rare <0.01% and isolated reports	vasculitis
Respiratory	Very rare <0.01% and isolated reports	dyspnea, asthma, eosinophilic pneumonitis
Gastrointestinal	Common ≥1%–<10%	dyspepsia, nausea, heartburn, abdominal pain
	Uncommon ≥0.1 %–<1 %	diarrhea, constipation, vomiting
	Rare ≥0.01%–<0.1%	peptic ulcers without or with bleeding or perforation, gastrointestinal bleeding, hematemesis, melena
	Very rare <0.01% and isolated reports	pancreatitis, colitis, aphthous ulcers, stomatitis, esophagitis, intestinal ulcerations
Hepatobiliary	Very rare <0.01% and isolated reports	hepatitis, icterus
Skin & Subcutaneous Tissue	Uncommon ≥0.1–<1 %	exanthema (rash), pruritus, urticaria
	Rare ≥0.01%–0.1%	angioneurotic edema
	Very rare <0.01% and isolated reports	alopecia (usually reversible), photosensitivity, porphyria, exudative erythema multiforme, epidermal necrolysis, erythema nodosum, fixed drug eruption, lichen planus, pustular reaction, skin rashes, Systemic Lupus Erythematosus, Stevens-Johnson syndrome, photosensitivity reactions including porphyria cutanea tarda ("pseudoporphyria") or epidermolysis bullosa
Renal & Urinary	Rare ≥0.01%–<0.1%	renal impairment
	Very rare <0.01% and isolated reports	interstitial nephritis, renal papillary necrosis, nephrotic syndrome, renal failure, renal disease
Pregnancy	Very rare <0.01% and isolated reports	induction of labour
Congenital	Very rare <0.01% and isolated reports	closure of ductus arteriosus, orofacial clefts as an isolated report
Reproductive	Very rare <0.01% and isolated reports	female infertility
General Disorders	Rare ≥0.01%–<0.1%	peripheral edema, particular in patients with hypertension or kidney failure, pyrexia
Investigations	Very rare <0.01% and isolated reports	raised serum creatinine, abnormal liver function test

DRUG INTERACTIONS: Overview: During short term use of naproxen sodium, interactions with the following medications could be of clinical significance.

Drug-Drug Interactions: The drugs listed in Table 3 are based on either drug interaction case reports or studies.

In a recent (2005) American case-control study, labelled, short term use of OTC naproxen or OTC ibuprofen was not associated with GI risk nor was there any detectable interaction with ASA at this dose level; furthermore there was no difference between OTC naproxen or OTC ibuprofen. An increased risk could be attributed with concomitant use of ASA and high dose NSAIDs; however, the numbers of exposed cases were small.

Another recent (2006) American retrospective database study found an odds ratio of 2.07 (1.23-3.49) for GI complications with concomitant use of low dose ASA and OTC-dose naproxen; for comparison, this ratio was 3.36 (2.36-4.80) in subjects taking OTC-dose ibuprofen and low dose ASA; the corresponding ratio for naproxen as monotherapy was 1.54 (1.04-2.28) which is not significantly different from the combined therapy. The corresponding ratio for ibuprofen as monotherapy was 1.38 (1.07-1.78) which is significantly lower than the combined therapy of ibuprofen and low dose ASA therapy.

Due to the nature of the study, information regarding the duration of naproxen and ibuprofen intake could not be collected. The findings are consistent with previous study results indicating increased GI risk in patients taking OTC-NSAIDs for longer terms or prescription NSAIDs while on low dose ASA.

Labelled, short term use of OTC naproxen together with low dose ASA was not associated with a detectable GI-risk; longer term use (mainly >10 days) of NSAIDs in OTC doses and concomitant ASA can increase the relative risk a little, adding however only very little absolute risk.

During short term use of naproxen sodium interactions of clinical significance do not seem to be relevant for the following medications: antacids, antidiabetics, hydantoines, probenecid, zidovudine.

Drug-Food Interactions: The absorption may be slightly delayed with a meal.

Drug-Herb Interactions: Interactions with herbal products have not been established.

Drug-Laboratory Test Interactions: Naproxen sodium causes transient, dose-dependent modestly increased bleeding times. However, these values often do not exceed the upper limit of the reference range. Naproxen sodium may theoretically interfere with the urinary analyses of 17-ketogenic steroids and 5-hydroxy indoleacetic acid (5 HIAA).

Table 3: ALEVE

Established or Potential Drug-Drug Interactions

Proper Name	Effect	Clinical Comment
Cyclosporine	Cyclosporin concentrations may increase, which could induce nephrotoxicity	These patients should be monitored adequately.
Lithium	In some patients lithium concentrations may increase, which could induce nausea, polydipsia, polyuria, tremor, confusion	These patients should be monitored adequately.
Methotrexate	If weekly methotrexate intake exceeds 15 mg, methotrexate concentrations may increase which could induce blood dyscrasia, nephrotoxicity, mucosal ulcerations	These patients should be monitored adequately.
NSAIDs	Adds to the risk of gastrointestinal bleeding	Should be avoided; however, effects may be minimized by using the lowest effective dose for the shortest duration necessary.
Low dose ASA (81 mg to 325 mg daily, for cardiovascular protection e.g. ASPIRIN 81 mg)	Can add to the risk of gastrointestinal bleeding	These patients should be monitored adequately.
Anticoagulants	Adds to the risk of gastrointestinal bleeding	These patients should be monitored adequately.
Glucocorticoids	Adds to the risk of gastrointestinal bleeding	These patients should be monitored adequately.
Diuretics, antihypertensive drugs including ACE Inhibitors, β blockers	The diuretic and antihypertensive efficacy, particular in patients with pre-existing nephropathy, may be reduced	These patients should be monitored adequately. Concomitant use with diuretics may increase risk of congestive heart failure.

DOSAGE AND ADMINISTRATION: Dosing Considerations:

- In self-medication, ALEVE should only be used for a short term treatment period of up to five days for pain and 3 days for fever. Otherwise a doctor should be consulted.
- Each dose should be swallowed with a full glass of water and can be taken fasting or with meals and/or antacids. Absorption may be slightly delayed with meals.
- If symptoms change, a doctor should be consulted.
- The recommended dosage should be adhered to unless directed by a doctor.
- ALEVE is as safe on the stomach as Tylenol Extra Strength 500 mg and Advil 200 mg if the maximum daily dose and recommended length of use for each product is not exceeded.
- ALEVE provides non-prescription pain relief that lasts up to 12 hours with 1 pill.

Recommended Dose and Dosage Adjustment: Adults (12-65 years): 1 caplet every 8-12 hours. For individuals over 65 years, 1 caplet every 12 hours. Do not take more than 2 caplets in a 24 hour period. Drink a full glass of water with each dose.

Under 12 Years: Children under 12 should not take this drug. The safety in pediatric use has not been established.

OVERDOSAGE:

Significant overdose can be characterized by drowsiness, heartburn, indigestion, nausea and vomiting. A few patients have experienced convulsions but it is not clear if these were naproxen related. Some cases with acute, reversible renal failure have been described. It is not known what dose of the drug would be life-threatening.

Should a patient ingest a large quantity of naproxen sodium the stomach may be emptied and usual supportive measures like administration of activated charcoal employed. Hemodialysis does not decrease the plasma concentration of naproxen because of the high degree of its protein binding. There is no specific antidote.

For management of a suspected drug overdose, CPhA recommends that you contact your **regional Poison Control Centre**. See the *CPS* Directory section for a list of Poison Control Centres.

ACTION AND CLINICAL PHARMACOLOGY: Mechanism of Action: Naproxen like all other nonsteroidal anti-inflammatory drugs (NSAIDs) is an analgesic, antipyretic and anti-inflammatory medication. ALEVE works at both the site of pain and centrally. The principle mechanism of action relies on the inhibition of prostaglandin synthesis. Prostaglandins are naturally occurring fatty acids derivates that are widely distributed in the tissues, and are involved in the production of pain, fever and inflammation. NSAIDs inhibit prostaglandin synthesis through inhibition of the cyclo-oxygenase enzymes. The anti-inflammatory and analgesic activity of these drugs is based on the concept that prostaglandins sensitize the tissues to pain- and inflammation-producing mediators and the antipyretic activity is assumed to be due to inhibition of prostaglandin synthesis in the hypothalamus induced by infectious states such as the common cold.

Pharmacodynamics: In low dose, that is ≤660 mg naproxen sodium daily, the analgesic and antipyretic activities prevail, while higher doses mostly are necessary for a full anti-inflammatory activity response.

Pharmacokinetics:

Table 4: ALEVE

Summary of Naproxen Sodium's Pharmacokinetic Parameters in Healthy Subjects

Single Dose	C_{max} (µg/mL)	$t_{½}$ (hours)	$AUC_{0-\infty}$ (µg/mL·h)	Clearance (L/h)	Volume of Distribution (L)
220 mg	35	18	546	0.4	10
440 mg	66	18	1021	0.4	10.6

Absorption: Naproxen sodium promptly dissolves in the gastric juice to sodium and fine particles of naproxen. Naproxen is rapidly and completely absorbed from the gastrointestinal tract. Food can slightly delay the absorption but not the extent. More than 99% of the circulating Naproxen is albumin-bound, the kinetics being dose linear up to 550 mg naproxen sodium twice daily. Significant naproxen plasma levels and onset of pain relief can be obtained within 20 minutes of intake and peak levels (C_{max}) are attained in about 1 hour (T_{max}). The active component is free, non-bound circulating naproxen. Free naproxen plasma

concentrations from about 10 ng/mL exert analgesic action, corresponding to a total Naproxen plasma concentration of 15 µg/mL. Such plasma values can be detected within 15-30 minutes after intake of 440 and 220 mg respectively with corresponding C_{max} of 66 and 35 µg/mL reached 1-1½ hours after intake of naproxen sodium.
Distribution: The volume of distribution of naproxen is small, about 0.1 l/kg. Steady-state concentrations are obtained in two days, and no significant accumulation has been observed. The repeated dose kinetic study and pharmacokinetic simulation have shown that analgesic concentration levels can be achieved following one naproxen sodium 220 mg caplet or two caplets initially followed by a further caplet after twelve hours. ALEVE has the **strength to last up to 12 hours** because analgesia is maintained for up to 12 hours.
Metabolism: Naproxen is either metabolised (cytochrome P450) to 6-0-desmethyl naproxen (6-DMN) and conjugated to glucuronides or left un-metabolised. Naproxen does not induce metabolizing enzymes.
Excretion: Naproxen and its metabolites are primarily excreted via the kidneys (>95%). The elimination half-life of naproxen is about 14 hours. The rate of excretion has been found to coincide closely with the rate of drug disappearance from plasma.
Special Populations and Conditions: Geriatrics: There is no evidence of differential metabolism or excretion in the elderly.
Gender: There is no evidence of differential metabolism or excretion between genders.
Hepatic Insufficiency: In case of severe hepatic insufficiency circulating albumin is decreased giving rise to increased fractions of free and unbound naproxen.
Renal Insufficiency: In case of severe renal insufficiency protein binding is lower giving rise to increased fractions of free and unbound naproxen. In patients with severely reduced glomerular filtration, the rate of urinary excretion may be reduced. Naproxen, in contrast to its non-active metabolite 6-DMN, is not cleared from the body during haemodialysis.

STORAGE AND STABILITY: Store at room temperature (15-30°C).

SPECIAL HANDLING INSTRUCTIONS: No special requirements.

INFORMATION FOR THE PATIENT: Published in e-CPS, available by subscription at www.e-cps.ca.

DOSAGE FORMS, COMPOSITION AND PACKAGING: Each caplet contains: naproxen sodium 220 mg, of which 20 mg is sodium. Nonmedicinal ingredients: FD&C Blue No. 2, hypromellose, magnesium stearate, microcrystalline cellulose, polyethylene glycol, povidone, titanium dioxide and talc. Opaque HDPE bottles of 24 and 100.

Alfacalcidol Ⓟ

CPhA Monograph

see *Vitamin D*

Alfentanil Ⓝ

CPhA Monograph

see *Opioids*

Alfentanil Injection USP Ⓝ

alfentanil HCl

Opioid Analgesic—Adjunct to Anesthesia

Sandoz

SUPPLIED: Each mL of sterile, preservative-free solution contains: alfentanil (as hydrochloride) 500 µg. Nonmedicinal ingredients: hydrochloric acid and/or sodium hydroxide to adjust pH, sodium chloride for isotonicity and water for injection. Amber vials of 2 mL, boxes of 10. Store between 15 and 30°C. Protect from light. Discard unused portion.

Alimta® Ⓟ

pemetrexed disodium

Antineoplastic

Lilly

Date of Revision: May 10, 2010

SUMMARY PRODUCT INFORMATION:

Route of Administration	Dosage Form/ Strength	Clinically Relevant Nonmedicinal Ingredients
Intravenous	Lyophilized powder/100 mg or 500 mg pemetrexed per vial	Mannitol For a complete listing see Dosage Forms, Composition and Packaging.

INDICATIONS AND CLINICAL USE: Malignant Pleural Mesothelioma: ALIMTA (pemetrexed disodium) in combination with cisplatin is indicated for the first-line treatment of patients with malignant pleural mesothelioma whose disease is unresectable or who are otherwise not candidates for curative surgery.
First Line—Nonsquamous Non-Small Cell Lung Cancer—Combination with Cisplatin: ALIMTA (pemetrexed disodium) in combination with cisplatin therapy is indicated for the initial treatment of good performance status patients with locally advanced or metastatic nonsquamous non-small cell lung cancer.
Maintenance Therapy—Nonsquamous Non-Small Cell Lung Cancer—Monotherapy: ALIMTA (pemetrexed disodium) monotherapy is indicated for the maintenance treatment of locally advanced or metastatic nonsquamous non-small cell lung cancer, in good performance status patients without disease progression immediately following four cycles of first-line platinum doublet chemotherapy, excluding pemetrexed.
Second Line—Nonsquamous Non-Small Cell Lung Cancer—Monotherapy: ALIMTA (pemetrexed disodium) monotherapy is indicated as a treatment option for patients with locally advanced or metastatic nonsquamous non-small cell lung cancer after prior chemotherapy. Approval is based on similarity of the response rate, median survival rate and 1-year survival rate, for the overall study population, between ALIMTA and docetaxel.
Geriatrics (>65 years of age): The safety and effectiveness of ALIMTA in geriatric patients has been established (see Action and Clinical Pharmacology).
Pediatrics (<18 years of age): The safety and effectiveness of ALIMTA in pediatric patients have not been established.

CONTRAINDICATIONS:
- Hypersensitivity to pemetrexed or to any other ingredient used in the formulation. For a complete listing, see Dosage Forms, Composition and Packaging.
- Concomitant yellow fever vaccine (see Drug Interactions)

WARNINGS AND PRECAUTIONS:

Serious Warnings and Precautions
- ALIMTA (pemetrexed disodium) should only be administered by, or under the supervision of, a physician who is experienced in cancer chemotherapy and in the management of related toxicities.
- Hepatotoxicity: See Warnings and Precautions, Hepatic/Biliary/Pancreatic.

Carcinogenesis and Mutagenesis: No carcinogenicity studies have been conducted with pemetrexed. Pemetrexed was clastogenic in the in vivo micronucleus assay in mouse bone marrow but was not mutagenic in multiple in vitro tests (Ames assay, CHO cell assay). Pemetrexed administered at i.v. doses of 0.1 mg/kg/day or greater to male mice (about 1/1666 the recommended human dose on a mg/m² basis) resulted in reduced fertility, hypospermia, and testicular atrophy. Because pemetrexed may cause irreversible infertility, men are advised to seek counselling on sperm storage before starting treatment.
Cardiovascular: No thorough clinical QT/QTc study was performed to rule out the effect of ALIMTA on QT prolongation. Routine ECG assessments during clinical trials did not identify any concerns regarding QT prolongation. Serious cardiovascular and cerebrovascular events, including myocardial infarction, angina pectoris, cerebrovascular accident and transient ischemic attack have been uncommonly reported in clinical trials with ALIMTA, usually when given in combination with another cytotoxic agent. Most of the patients in whom these events have been observed had preexisting cardiovascular risk factors.
Gastrointestinal: Stomatitis, nausea, vomiting, and diarrhea are common in patients receiving ALIMTA with or without cisplatin. In rare cases gastrointestinal toxicity may lead to severe dehydration. Gastrointestinal toxicity should be vigorously managed (see Adverse Reactions, Clinical Trial Adverse Drug Reactions and Dosage and Administration, Nonhematologic Toxicities).
Hepatic/Biliary/Pancreatic: Serious hepatobiliary toxicity and rare cases of fatal hepatic failure, have been reported with ALIMTA alone or in association with other chemotherapeutic agents in clinical trials. Underlying risk factors for the development of hepatic toxicity including hepatic metastases and/or underlying hepatic disease have been present in some cases. A causal relationship between ALIMTA and these events has not been established.
Hematologic: ALIMTA can suppress bone marrow function, as manifested by neutropenia, thrombocytopenia, and anemia (or pancytopenia) (see Adverse Reactions); myelosuppression is usually the dose-limiting toxicity (see Laboratory Monitoring and Dose Reduction Recommendations under Dosage and Administration). Dose reductions for subsequent cycles are based on nadir Absolute Neutrophil Count (ANC), platelet count, and maximum nonhematologic toxicity seen in the previous cycle (see General Dose Reduction Recommendations under Dosage and Administration).

In the Phase 3 mesothelioma clinical trial, less overall toxicity and reductions in Grade 3/4 hematologic and nonhematologic toxicities such as neutropenia, febrile neutropenia and infection with Grade 3/4 neutropenia were reported when pre-treatment with folic acid and vitamin B_{12} was administered. Therefore, patients treated with ALIMTA must be instructed to take folic acid and vitamin B_{12} with ALIMTA as a prophylactic measure to reduce treatment-related toxicity (see Dosage and Administration).
Immune: Cases of hypersensitivity, including anaphylaxis, have been reported in patients treated with ALIMTA.
Renal: Serious renal events, including acute renal failure, have been reported with ALIMTA alone or in association with other chemotherapeutic agents. Most, but not all, of the patients in whom these serious renal events occurred had underlying risk factors for the development of renal events including dehydration or pre-existing hypertension or diabetes. A causal relationship between ALIMTA and these events has not been established.
Respiratory: Interstitial pneumonitis with respiratory insufficiency, sometimes fatal, has been reported in clinical trials. In patients with progressive dyspnea and cough, ALIMTA should be interrupted and prompt investigation initiated.

Cases of radiation pneumonitis have been reported in patients with radiation either prior to, during, or subsequent to their ALIMTA therapy.
Skin: Rare cases of bullous epidermolysis have been reported including Stevens-Johnson syndrome and Toxic epidermal necrolysis which in some cases were fatal.

Treatment-related adverse events of ALIMTA seen in clinical trials have been reversible. Skin rash has been reported in patients not pretreated with a corticosteroid in clinical trials. Pretreatment with dexamethasone (or equivalent) reduces the incidence and severity of cutaneous reaction (see Dosage and Administration).

Radiation recall dermatitis has been reported in patients on ALIMTA who have previously received radiotherapy. Severity of symptoms can vary from mild dermatitis to necrosis.
Third Space Fluid: The effect of third space fluid, such as pleural effusion and ascites, on ALIMTA is unknown. In patients with clinically significant third space fluid, consideration should be given to draining the effusion prior to ALIMTA administration.
Special Populations: Pregnant Women: ALIMTA may cause fetal harm when administered to a pregnant woman. ALIMTA clinical studies excluded pregnant women. Women of child bearing potential should have a negative serum pregnancy test prior to treatment with ALIMTA and should be advised to avoid becoming pregnant while on treatment with ALIMTA. Women should be advised to use effective contraceptive measures to prevent pregnancy during treatment with ALIMTA. If ALIMTA is used during pregnancy, or if the patient becomes pregnant while taking ALIMTA, the patient should be informed of the potential hazard to the fetus.
Nursing Women: It is not known whether pemetrexed or its metabolites are excreted in human milk. Because many drugs are excreted in human milk, and because of the potential for serious adverse reactions in nursing infants from pemetrexed, it is recommended that nursing be discontinued if the mother is treated with ALIMTA.
Men: Pemetrexed administered at i.v.doses of 0.1 mg/kg/day or greater to male mice (about 1/1666 the recommended human dose on a mg/m² basis) resulted in reduced fertility, hypospermia, and testicular atrophy. Because pemetrexed may cause irreversible infertility, men are advised to seek counselling on sperm storage before starting treatment.

Pemetrexed is clastogenic in the in vivo micronucleus assay in mouse bone marrow and can have genetically damaging effects. Men are advised to use effective contraceptive measures and thus not to father a child during treatment with ALIMTA and up to 6 months thereafter.
Pediatrics (<18 years of age): The safety and effectiveness of ALIMTA in pediatric patients have not been established.
Geriatrics (>65 years of age): Dose adjustments based on age other than those recommended for all patients have not been necessary. However, because renal function declines with age, and decreased renal function will result in reduced clearance of ALIMTA, older patients should be followed closely for toxicity.
Patients with Hepatic Impairment: Pemetrexed is not extensively metabolized by the liver. However, patients with hepatic impairment such as bilirubin >1.5 times the upper limit of normal (ULN) or transaminase >3 times the ULN (hepatic metastases absent) or >5 times the ULN (hepatic metastases present) have not been specifically studied.

For dose adjustments based on hepatic impairment, refer to Laboratory Monitoring and Dose Reduction Recommendations under Dosage and Administration.
Patients with Renal Impairment: ALIMTA is known to be primarily excreted by the kidney. There is limited clinical experience in patients with calculated creatinine clearance below 45 mL/min. Therefore, patients whose creatinine clearance is <45 mL/min should not receive ALIMTA. Decreased renal function will result in reduced clearance of ALIMTA compared with patients with normal renal function.

For dose adjustments based on renal impairment, refer to Laboratory Monitoring and Dose Reduction Recommendations under Dosage and Administration.
Use of Non-Steroidal Anti-Inflammatory Drugs in Mild to Moderate Renal Insufficiency: Caution should be used when administering ibuprofen concurrently with ALIMTA to patients with mild to moderate renal insufficiency (creatinine clearance from 45 to 79 mL/min). Other NSAIDS should also be used with caution (see Drug Interactions).
Monitoring and Laboratory Tests: All patients receiving ALIMTA should have frequent complete blood counts, including differential and platelets as well as periodic blood chemistry tests performed, including creatinine. Patients should not begin a new treatment cycle unless the absolute neutrophil count (ANC) is ≥1500 cells/mm³, the platelet count is ≥100 000 cells/mm³, and the creatinine clearance is ≥45 mL/min (see Dosage and Administration).

ADVERSE REACTIONS: Adverse Drug Reaction Overview: In clinical trials, the most common adverse reactions (incidence ≥10%) during therapy with ALIMTA as a single agent were fatigue, nausea, anorexia, anemia, vomiting, stomatitis/pharyngitis, rash/desquamation, diarrhea, leukopenia, and neutropenia. Additional common adverse reactions (incidence ≥10%) during therapy with ALIMTA when used in combination with cisplatin included thrombocytopenia, decreased creatinine clearance, constipation, alopecia, creatinine elevation, and sensory neuropathy.

In clinical trials, cases of gastrointestinal haemorrhage, ulceration, perforation and necrosis, sometimes fatal, have been reported uncommonly in patients treated with ALIMTA. Esophagitis/radiation esophagitis has also been uncommonly reported in clinical trials. Supplementation with folic acid and vitamin B_{12} during treatment with ALIMTA reduces the frequency and severity of hematologic and nonhematologic toxicities.
Clinical Trial Adverse Drug Reactions: Malignant Pleural Mesothelioma: Combination Use with Cisplatin: The following tables list adverse events, considered to be related to ALIMTA (pemetrexed disodium), reported in clinical trial patients with MPM treated with 500 mg/m² of ALIMTA and 75 mg/m² of cisplatin.

Overall, serious adverse events (SAEs) occurred significantly more frequently in patients on the pemetrexed plus cisplatin arm regardless of drug causality. This was expected because this regimen adds one drug (pemetrexed) to the control regimen (cisplatin). Among the fully supplemented (FS) subgroup, no single SAE, regardless of drug causality, occurred in >5% of patients in either arm. Most SAEs were hematologic or gastrointestinal and were expected effects of cytotoxic chemotherapy.

Table 1 displays the incidence (percentage of patients) of CTC Grade 3/4 toxicities in patients who received vitamin supplementation with daily folic acid and vitamin B_{12} from the time of enrolment in the study (fully supplemented) versus patients who never received vitamin supplementation (never supplemented) during the study in the ALIMTA plus cisplatin arm. Patients who received supplementation from the start of therapy experienced markedly less laboratory and nonlaboratory toxicity compared with patients who never received supplementation.

Table 1: ALIMTA

Selected Grade 3/4 Adverse Events Comparing Fully Supplemented versus Never Supplemented Patients in the ALIMTA plus Cisplatin Arm (% incidence)

Adverse Event Regardless of Causality[a] (%)	Fully Supplemented Patients (N=168)	Never Supplemented Patients (N=32)
Neutropenia	24	38
Thrombocytopenia	5	9
Nausea	12	31
Vomiting	11	34
Anorexia	2	9
Diarrhea without colostomy	4	9
Dehydration	4	9
Fever	0	6
Febrile neutropenia	1	9
Infection with Grade 3/4 neutropenia	1	6
Fatigue	17	25

[a] Refer to National Cancer Institute (NCI) Common Toxicity Criteria (CTC) criteria for laboratory values for each Grade of toxicity (Version 2.0).

Table 2 provides the frequency and severity of adverse events that have been reported in >5% of 168 patients with MPM who were randomly assigned to receive cisplatin and pemetrexed and 163 patients with mesothelioma randomly assigned to receive single agent cisplatin. In both treatment arms, these chemonaive patients were fully supplemented with folic acid and vitamin B_{12}.

Table 2: ALIMTA

Adverse Events[a] in Fully Supplemented Patients Receiving ALIMTA plus Cisplatin in MPM. CTC Grades (% incidence)

	All Reported Adverse Events Regardless of Causality					
	ALIMTA/Cisplatin (N=168)			Cisplatin (N=163)		
	All Grades	Grade 3	Grade 4	All Grades	Grade 3	Grade 4
Laboratory						
Hematologic						
Neutropenia	58	19	5	16	3	1
Leukopenia	55	14	2	20	1	0
Anemia	33	5	1	14	0	0
Thrombocytopenia	27	4	1	10	0	0
Renal						
Creatinine elevation	16	1	0	12	1	0
Renal failure	2	0	1	1	0	0
Clinical						
Constitutional Symptoms						
Fatigue	80	17	0	74	12	1
Fever	17	0	0	9	0	0
Other constitutional symptoms	11	2	1	8	1	1
Cardiovascular General						
Thrombosis/embolism	7	4	2	4	3	1
Gastrointestinal						
Nausea	84	11	1	79	6	0
Vomiting	58	10	1	52	4	1
Constipation	44	2	1	39	1	0
Anorexia	35	2	0	25	1	0
Stomatitis/pharyngitis	28	2	1	9	0	0
Diarrhea without colostomy	26	4	0	16	1	0
Dehydration	7	3	1	1	1	0
Dysphagia/esophagitis/odynophagia	6	1	0	6	0	0
Pulmonary						
Dyspnea	66	10	1	62	5	2
Pain						
Chest pain	40	8	1	30	5	1
Neurology						
Neuropathy/sensory	17	0	0	15	1	0
Mood alteration/depression	14	1	0	9	1	0
Infection/Febrile Neutropenia						
Infection without neutropenia	11	1	1	4	0	0
Infection with Grade 3 or Grade 4 neutropenia	6	1	0	4	0	0
Infection/febrile neutropenia—other	3	1	0	2	0	0
Febrile neutropenia	1	1	0	1	0	0
Immune						
Allergic reaction/hypersensitivity	2	0	0	1	0	0
Dermatology/Skin						
Rash/desquamation	22	1	0	9	0	0

[a] Refer to National Cancer Institute (NCI) Common Toxicity Criteria (CTC) (Version 2.0).

Drug related clinically relevant toxicity that was reported in ≥1% and ≤5% (common) of the patients that were randomly assigned to receive cisplatin and pemetrexed included: increased AST, ALT, and GGT, infection, febrile neutropenia, renal failure, chest pain, pyrexia and urticaria.

Drug related clinically relevant toxicity that was reported in <1% (uncommon) of the patients that were randomly assigned to receive cisplatin and pemetrexed included: arrhythmia and motor neuropathy.

Non-Small Cell Lung Cancer (NSCLC): Combination Use with Cisplatin: Table 3 provides the frequency and severity of adverse reactions that have been reported in >5% of 839 NSCLC patients who were randomized to study and received ALIMTA plus cisplatin and 830 NSCLC patients who were randomized to study and received gemcitabine plus cisplatin. All patients received study therapy as initial treatment for locally advanced or metastatic NSCLC and patients in both treatment groups were fully supplemented with folic acid and vitamin B_{12}.

Table 3: ALIMTA

Adverse Reactions in Fully Supplemented Patients Receiving ALIMTA plus Cisplatin in NSCLC[a]

	ALIMTA/cisplatin (N=839)		Gemcitabine/cisplatin (N=830)	
Reaction[b]	All Grades Toxicity (%)	Grades 3-4 Toxicity (%)	All Grades Toxicity (%)	Grades 3-4 Toxicity (%)
All Adverse Reactions	90	37	91	53
Laboratory				
Hematologic				
Anemia[c,d]	33	6	46	10
Neutropenia[c,d]	29	15	38	27
Leukopenia[c]	18	5	21	8
Thrombocytopenia[c,d]	10	4	27	13
Renal				
Creatinine elevation[d]	10	1	7	1
Clinical				
Constitutional Symptoms				
Fatigue	43	7	45	5
Gastrointestinal				
Nausea[c]	56	7	53	4
Vomiting	40	6	36	6
Anorexia[c]	27	2	24	1
Constipation	21	1	20	0
Stomatitis/pharyngitis	14	1	12	0
Diarrhea	12	1	13	2
Dyspepsia/heartburn	5	0	6	0

(cont'd)

Table 3: ALIMTA *(cont'd)*

Adverse Reactions in Fully Supplemented Patients Receiving ALIMTA plus Cisplatin in NSCLC[a]

Reaction[b]	ALIMTA/cisplatin (N=839)		Gemcitabine/cisplatin (N=830)	
	All Grades Toxicity (%)	Grades 3-4 Toxicity (%)	All Grades Toxicity (%)	Grades 3-4 Toxicity (%)
Neurology				
Neuropathy—sensory[c,d]	9	0	12	1
Taste disturbance	8	0[e]	9	0[e]
Dermatology/Skin				
Alopecia[d]	12	0[e]	21	1[e]
Rash/desquamation	7	0	8	1

a For the purpose of this table a cut off of 5% was used for inclusion of all events where the reporter considered a possible relationship to ALIMTA/cisplatin.
b Refer to NCI CTC Criteria version 2.0 for each Grade of toxicity.
c p<0.05 for Grades 3/4 toxicity.
d p<0.05 for any grade toxicity.
e According to NCI CTC Criteria version 2.0, this adverse event term should only be reported as Grade 1 or 2.

Drug related clinically relevant toxicity that was reported in ≥1% and ≤5% (common) of the patients that were randomly assigned to receive cisplatin and pemetrexed include: AST increase, ALT increase, infection, febrile neutropenia, renal failure, pyrexia, dehydration, conjunctivitis, and creatinine clearance decrease.

The incidence of febrile neutropenia was 1.7% on the ALIMTA/cisplatin arm compared to 4.1% on the gemcitabine/cisplatin arm. There were 4 patient deaths on the ALIMTA/cisplatin arm compared to 1 patient death on the gemcitabine/cisplatin arm due to sepsis.

Drug related clinically relevant toxicity that was reported in <1% (uncommon) of the patients that were randomly assigned to receive cisplatin and pemetrexed include: GGT increase, chest pain, arrhythmia, and motor neuropathy.

No clinically relevant differences in adverse reactions were seen in subpopulations based on gender, ethnicity, or histology. Patients aged ≥65 years generally experienced more toxicity (e.g., neutropenia, febrile neutropenia, thrombocytopenia, nausea, renal failure) than patients aged <65 years, regardless of treatment arm.

Maintenance: Table 4 provides the frequency and severity of adverse reactions that have been reported in >5% of 441 patients with NSCLC who were randomized to receive ALIMTA and 222 patients with NSCLC who were randomized to receive placebo. All patients without progressive disease received study therapy immediately following 4 cycles of platinum-based treatment for locally advanced or metastatic NSCLC. Patients in both study arms were fully supplemented with folic acid and vitamin B_{12}.

Table 4: ALIMTA

Adverse Reactions in Patients Randomized to ALIMTA versus Placebo in NSCLC[a]

Reaction[b]	ALIMTA (N=441)		Placebo (N=222)	
	All Grades Toxicity (%)	Grade 3-4 Toxicity (%)	All Grades Toxicity (%)	Grade 3-4 Toxicity (%)
All Adverse Reactions	66	16	37	4
Laboratory				
Hematologic				
Anemia	15	3	5	1
Neutropenia	6	3	0	0
Leukopenia	6	2	1	1
Hepatic				
Increased ALT	10	0	4	0
Increased AST	8	0	4	0
Clinical				
Constitutional Symptoms				
Fatigue	25	5	10	1
Gastrointestinal				
Nausea	19	1	5	1
Anorexia	19	2	5	0
Vomiting	9	0	1	0
Mucositis/stomatitis	7	1	2	0
Diarrhea	5	1	3	0
Infection	5	2	2	0
Neurology				
Neuropathy-sensory	9	1	4	0
Dermatology/Skin				
Rash/Desquamation	10	0	3	0

a For the purpose of this table a cut off of 5% was used for inclusion of all events where the reporter considered a possible relationship to ALIMTA.
b Refer to NCI CTCAE Criteria version 3.0 for each Grade of toxicity.

All-grade renal events were more frequent in patients ≥65 years of age than in patients <65 years of age (12.2% vs 6.8%). All-grade myelosuppression events were more frequent in patients ≥65 years of age than in patients <65 years of age (24.5% vs 16.7%).

No clinically relevant differences in Grade 3/4 adverse reactions were seen in patients based on age, gender, ethnic origin, or histology except a higher incidence of Grade 3/4 gastrointestinal events for patients ≥65 years of age compared to patients <65 years of age (7.5% vs 2.4%) and fatigue for Caucasian patients compared to non-Caucasian patients (6.5% versus 0.6%).

Safety was assessed by exposure for patients who were randomized and received at least one dose of ALIMTA (N=434). The incidence of adverse reactions was evaluated for patients who received ≤6 cycles of ALIMTA, and compared to patients who received >6 cycles of ALIMTA. Increases in adverse reactions (all grades) were observed with longer exposure; however no clinically relevant differences in Grade 3/4 adverse reactions were seen.

Consistent with the higher incidence of anemia (all grades) on the ALIMTA arm, use of transfusions (mainly RBC) and erythropoiesis stimulating agents (ESAs; erythropoietin and darbepoetin) were significantly higher in the ALIMTA arm compared to the placebo arm (transfusions 9.5% versus 3.2%, p=0.003; ESAs 5.9% versus 1.8%, p=0.017).

Drug related clinically relevant toxicity that was reported in ≥1% and ≤5% (common) of the patients that were randomly assigned to receive ALIMTA include: edema, fever (in the absence of neutropenia), constipation, thrombocytopenia, decreased creatinine clearance, increased creatinine, decreased glomerular filtration rate, alopecia, pruritus/itching, ocular surface disease (including conjunctivitis), and increased lacrimation.

Drug related clinically relevant toxicity that was reported in <1% (uncommon) of the patients that were randomly assigned to receive ALIMTA include: febrile neutropenia, allergic reaction/hypersensitivity, motor neuropathy, renal failure, supraventricular arrhythmia, and erythema multiforme.

After Prior Chemotherapy: ALIMTA has been evaluated for safety in 265 patients randomly assigned to receive single-agent ALIMTA with folic acid and vitamin B_{12} supplementation and 276 patients randomly assigned to receive single-agent docetaxel. All patients were diagnosed with locally advanced or metastatic NSCLC and had received prior chemotherapy. Drug-related adverse events that were reported in >1% of patients are listed in Table 5.

Table 5: ALIMTA

Selected Adverse Events (>1%) in Patients Receiving ALIMTA versus Docetaxel in NSCLC

Adverse Event	CTC Grades (% incidence)					
	ALIMTA (N=265)			Docetaxel (N=276)		
	All Grades (%)	Grade 3 (%)	Grade 4 (%)	All Grades (%)	Grade 3 (%)	Grade 4 (%)
Laboratory[a]						
Hematologic						
Hemoglobin	19.2	2.6	1.5	22.1	4.3	0
Leukocytes[c]	12.1	3.8	0.4	34.1	16.7	10.5
Neutrophils[c]	10.9	3.4	1.9	45.3	8.7	31.5
Platelets	8.3	1.9	0	1.1	0.4	0
Hepatic/Renal						
ALT elevation[d]	7.9	1.5	0.4	1.4	0	0
AST elevation	6.8	0.8	0.4	0.7	0	0
Decreased creatinine clearance	2	<1	0	<1	0	0
Creatinine elevation	2.3	0	0	0	0	0
Clinical[a]						
Constitutional Symptoms						
Fatigue	34.0	5.3	0	35.9	5.1	0.4
Fever	8.3	0	0	7.6	0	0
Alopecia[b]	6.4	0.4	0	37.7	1.4	0.7
Gastrointestinal						
Nausea	30.9	2.6	0	16.7	1.8	0
Anorexia	21.9	1.5	0.4	23.9	2.2	0.4
Vomiting	16.2	1.5	0	12.0	1.1	0
Stomatitis/pharyngitis	14.7	1.1	0	17.4	1.1	0
Diarrhea	12.8	0.4	0	24.3	2.5	0
Constipation	5.7	0	0	4.0	0	0
Pain						
Abdominal pain	2.6	0	0	3.3	1.1	0
Neurology						
Sensory—neuropathy	4.9	0	0	15.9	1.1	0
Neuropathy—motor	2.6	0.4	0	4.7	1.1	0
Infection/Febrile Neutropenia						
Infection without neutropenia	1.9	0.4	0	3.3	0	0.4
Febrile neutropenia[c]	1.9	1.1	0.8	13.8	10.1	2.5
Immune						

(cont'd)

Table 5: ALIMTA *(cont'd)*

Selected Adverse Events (>1%) in Patients Receiving ALIMTA versus Docetaxel in NSCLC

	CTC Grades (% incidence)					
	ALIMTA (N=265)			Docetaxel (N=276)		
Adverse Event	**All Grades (%)**	**Grade 3 (%)**	**Grade 4 (%)**	**All Grades (%)**	**Grade 3 (%)**	**Grade 4 (%)**
Allergic reaction/hypersensitivity	1.1	0	0	2.2	1.1	0
Dermatology/Skin						
Rash/desquamation	14.0	0	0	6.2	0	0
Pruritus	6.8	0.4	0	1.8	0	0
Erythema multiforme	1.1	0	0	2.5	0	0

[a] Refer to National Cancer Institute (NCI) Common Toxicity Criteria (CTC) for lab values for each Grade of toxicity (Version 2.0).
[b] According to NCI CTC Criteria (version 2.0), alopecia should only be reported as Grade 1 or 2.
[c] p<0.001 for Grades 3/4 toxicity.
[d] p=0.028 for Grades 3/4 toxicity.

There was a statistically significant difference between the ALIMTA treatment arm and docetaxel arm with respect to the incidence of any CTC Grade 3 or 4 laboratory toxicity (12.8% vs. 46.4%; p<0.001), largely due to the significantly higher rate of neutropenia in the docetaxel arm. The percentage of patients hospitalized for any adverse event was significantly lower in the ALIMTA arm than in the docetaxel arm (31.7% vs. 40.6%, p=0.032), particularly for drug-related febrile neutropenia (1.5% vs. 13.4%, p<0.001). However, the total number of days of hospitalization for any reason (i.e. drug administration, adverse events, protocol tests, social reasons) was higher in the ALIMTA arm than in the docetaxel arm (1722 vs. 1410 days).

Drug related clinically relevant CTC toxicity that was reported in <1% (uncommon) of the patients that were randomly assigned to pemetrexed include supraventricular arrhythmias.

The drug related clinically relevant Grade 3 and Grade 4 laboratory toxicities were similar between integrated Phase 2 results from three single agent pemetrexed studies (n=164, patients received vitamin supplementation) and the Phase 3 single agent pemetrexed study described above, with the exception of neutropenia (12.8% versus 5.3%, respectively) and alanine transaminase elevation (15.2% versus 1.9%, respectively). These differences were likely due to differences in the patient population, since the Phase 2 studies included chemonaive and heavily pretreated breast cancer patients with pre-existing liver metastases and/or abnormal baseline liver function tests.

There were no clinically relevant differences observed for the safety profile of ALIMTA within the histological subgroups.

Post-Market Adverse Drug Reactions: Gastrointestinal: Rare cases of colitis have been reported in patients treated with ALIMTA.

General Disorders and Administration Site Conditions: Rare cases of edema have been reported in patients treated with ALIMTA.

Peripheral ischaemia leading to extremity necrosis has been reported.

Hepatobiliary: Cases of hepatobiliary failure, sometimes fatal, have been reported very rarely.

Renal: Serious cases of acute renal failure have been reported rarely.

Respiratory: Rare cases of interstitial pneumonitis have been reported in patients treated with ALIMTA.

Injury, Poisoning and Procedural Complications: Rare cases of radiation recall have been reported in patients who have previously received radiotherapy.

Immune: Rare cases of haemolytic anemia have been reported in patients treated with ALIMTA.

DRUG INTERACTIONS: Drug-Drug Interactions: Pemetrexed is primarily eliminated unchanged renally as a result of glomerular filtration and tubular secretion. Concomitant administration of nephrotoxic drugs could result in delayed clearance of pemetrexed. Concomitant administration of substances that are also tubularly secreted (e.g., probenecid) could potentially result in delayed clearance of pemetrexed.

Ibuprofen: Although ibuprofen (400 mg qid) can be administered with ALIMTA in patients with normal renal function (creatinine clearance ≥80 mL/min), caution should be used when administering ibuprofen concurrently with ALIMTA to patients with mild to moderate renal insufficiency (creatinine clearance from 45 to 79 mL/min). Clinical trials have shown a decrease in pemetrexed clearance following co-administration of ibuprofen. It is recommended that patients with mild to moderate renal insufficiency should avoid taking NSAIDs with short elimination half-lives at least 2 days prior to, on the day of, and at least 2 days after administration of ALIMTA.

NSAIDs: In the absence of data regarding potential interaction between pemetrexed and NSAIDs with longer half-lives, all patients taking these NSAIDs should interrupt dosing for at least 5 days before, the day of, and at least 2 days following ALIMTA administration. If concomitant administration of an NSAID is necessary, patients should be monitored closely for toxicity, especially myelosuppression, renal and gastrointestinal toxicity.

Aspirin: Acetylsalicylic acid, administered in low to moderate doses (325 mg orally every 6 hours) does not affect the pharmacokinetics of pemetrexed.

Chemotherapeutic Agents: The pharmacokinetics of pemetrexed are not influenced by concurrently administered cisplatin or carboplatin. Similarly, the pharmacokinetics of total platinum are unaltered by pemetrexed.

Vitamins: Oral folic acid and intramuscular vitamin B_{12} supplementation do not affect the pharmacokinetics of pemetrexed.

Drugs Metabolized by Cytochrome P450 Enzymes: Pemetrexed undergoes limited hepatic metabolism. Results from in vitro studies with human liver microsomes predict that pemetrexed would not cause clinically significant inhibition of the metabolic clearance of drugs metabolized by CYP3A, CYP2D6, CYP2C9, and CYP1A2. No studies were conducted to determine the cytochrome P450 isozyme induction potential of pemetrexed, because ALIMTA used as recommended (once every 21 days) would not be expected to cause any significant enzyme induction.

Vaccines: Concomitant administration of yellow fever vaccine is contraindicated due to the risk of fatal generalised vaccinale disease (see Contraindications).

Concomitant administration of live attenuated vaccines (except yellow fever, for which concomitant use is contraindicated) is not recommended due to the risk of systemic, possibly fatal, disease. The risk is increased in subjects who are already immunosuppressed by their underlying disease. Use an inactivated vaccine where it exists (e.g., poliomyelitis).

Drug-Food Interactions: Interactions with food have not been established.

Drug-Herb Interactions: Interactions with herbal products have not been established.

Drug-Laboratory Test Interactions: Interactions with laboratory tests have not been established.

DOSAGE AND ADMINISTRATION:

Dosing Considerations: ALIMTA (pemetrexed disodium) is for intravenous infusion only. It should be administered under the supervision of a qualified physician experienced in the use of antineoplastic agents.

Recommended Dose and Dosage Adjustment: Malignant Pleural Mesothelioma (MPM): Combination Use with Cisplatin: The recommended dose of ALIMTA is 500 mg/m² administered as an intravenous infusion over 10 minutes on Day 1 of each 21-day cycle. The recommended dose of cisplatin is 75 mg/m² infused over 2 hours beginning approximately 30 minutes after the end of ALIMTA administration. Patients should receive appropriate hydration prior to and/or after receiving cisplatin. In clinical trials the median number of cycles was 6 (range=1 to 12 cycles).

Non-Small Cell Lung Cancer (NSCLC): Combination Use with Cisplatin: The recommended dose of ALIMTA is 500 mg/m² administered as an intravenous infusion over 10 minutes on Day 1 of each 21-day cycle. The recommended dose of cisplatin is 75 mg/m² infused over 2 hours beginning approximately 30 minutes after completion of the ALIMTA administration. Patients should receive appropriate hydration prior to and/or after receiving cisplatin. In the clinical trial, treatment was administered up to a total of 6 cycles of therapy, and the median number of cycles was 5 (range 1-7).

Single-Agent Use: The recommended dose of ALIMTA is 500 mg/m² administered as an intravenous infusion over 10 minutes on Day 1 of each 21-day cycle for both maintenance therapy and second line therapy. For both indications, patients were administered ALIMTA until progression. The median number of cycles was 5 (range 1-55) when used as maintenance therapy and 4 (range 1-20) when used as second line treatment.

Premedication Regimen for All Indications: Corticosteroid: Skin rash has been reported in patients not pretreated with a corticosteroid. Pretreatment with dexamethasone (or equivalent) reduces the incidence and severity of cutaneous reaction. In clinical trials, dexamethasone 4 mg was given by mouth twice daily the day before, the day of, and the day after ALIMTA administration.

Vitamin Supplementation: To reduce potential toxicity, patients treated with ALIMTA must be instructed to take a low-dose oral folic acid preparation or multivitamin with folic acid on a daily basis (see Table 6). At least 5 daily doses of folic acid (400 µg/day) must be taken during the 7-day period preceding the first dose of ALIMTA; and dosing should continue during the full course of therapy and for 21 days after the last dose of ALIMTA. Patients must also receive one (1) intramuscular injection of vitamin B_{12} (1000 µg) during the week preceding the first dose of ALIMTA and every 3 cycles thereafter. Subsequent vitamin B_{12} injections may be given the same day as ALIMTA. In clinical trials, the dose of folic acid studied ranged from 350 to 1000 µg, and the dose of vitamin B_{12} was 1000 µg. The most commonly used dose of oral folic acid in clinical trials was 400 µg (see Warnings and Precautions).

Table 6: ALIMTA

Vitamin Supplementation

Drug	Dose and Route	Timing
Folic acid	350 to 600 µg by mouth (may give 1000 µg but usual dose has been 400 µg).	Daily beginning 1 week prior to chemotherapy with ALIMTA (at least 5 of the 7 days prior to commencement of ALIMTA chemotherapy) and continuing daily until 3 weeks after the last dose of ALIMTA.
Vitamin B_{12}	1000 µg intramuscular injection	Beginning at least 1 week prior to the first dose of ALIMTA and continuing every 9 weeks from the previous dose until 3 weeks after the last dose of ALIMTA.

Laboratory Monitoring and Dose Reduction Recommendations: Monitoring: Complete blood cell counts, including platelets, and blood chemistries should be performed on all patients receiving ALIMTA. Patients should be monitored for nadir and recovery on days 8 and 15 of each cycle. Patients should not begin a new cycle of treatment unless the ANC is ≥1500 cell/mm³, platelet count ≥100 000 cells/mm³ and creatinine clearance ≥45 mL/min. Periodic chemistry tests should be collected to evaluate renal and hepatic function.

General Dose Reduction Recommendations: Dose adjustments at the start of a subsequent cycle should be based on nadir hematologic counts or maximum nonhematologic toxicity from the preceding cycle of therapy. Treatment may be delayed to allow sufficient time for recovery. Upon recovery, patients should be retreated using guidelines in Table 7, Table 8 and Table 9 which are suitable for using ALIMTA as a single agent or in combination with cisplatin. ALIMTA therapy should be discontinued if a patient experiences any Grade 3 or 4 toxicity after 2 dose reductions.

Hematologic Toxicities: In the event of hematologic toxicities, the recommended dose adjustments for ALIMTA and cisplatin are described in Table 7.

Table 7: ALIMTA

Dose Reduction for ALIMTA as Single-Agent or in Combination with Cisplatin—Hematologic Toxicities

Nadir ANC <500/mm³ and nadir platelets ≥50 000/mm³	75% of previous dose of ALIMTA and Cisplatin
Nadir platelets <50 000/mm³ regardless of nadir ANC	75% of previous dose of ALIMTA and Cisplatin
Nadir platelets <50 000/mm³ with bleeding[a], regardless of nadir ANC	50% of previous dose of ALIMTA and Cisplatin

[a] These criteria meet the CTC version 2.0 (NCI 1998) definition of ≥CTC Grade 2 bleeding.

Nonhematologic Toxicities: If patients develop nonhematologic toxicities (excluding neurotoxicity) ≥Grade 3, ALIMTA should be withheld until resolution to less than or equal to the patient's pre-therapy value. Treatment should be resumed according to guidelines in Table 8.

Table 8: ALIMTA

Dose Reduction for ALIMTA as Single-Agent or in Combination with Cisplatin—Nonhematologic Toxicities[a,b]

	Dose of ALIMTA (mg/m²)	Dose of Cisplatin (mg/m²)
Grade 3 or 4 mucositis	50% of previous dose	100% of previous dose
Any diarrhea requiring hospitalization (irrespective of Grade) or Grade 3 or 4 diarrhea	75% of previous dose	75% of previous dose
Any Grade 3 or 4 toxicities except mucositis	75% of previous dose	75% of previous dose

[a] NCI Common Toxicity Criteria (CTC).
[b] Guidelines for neurotoxicity are provided in Table 9.

Neurotoxicity: In the event of neurotoxicity, the recommended dose adjustments for ALIMTA and cisplatin are described in Table 9. Patients should immediately discontinue therapy if Grade 3 or 4 neurotoxicity is experienced.

Table 9: ALIMTA

Dose Reduction for ALIMTA as Single-Agent or in Combination with Cisplatin—Neurotoxicity

CTC Grade	Dose of ALIMTA (mg/m²)	Dose of Cisplatin (mg/m²)
0–1	100% of previous dose	100% of previous dose
2	100% of previous dose	50% of previous dose

Special Populations and Conditions: Geriatrics: In clinical trials, no dose reductions other than those recommended for all patients were specifically recommended for elderly patients. However, in the study comparing first-line ALIMTA/cisplatin with gemcitabine/cisplatin in NSCLC patients, those patients aged ≥65 years generally experienced more toxicity (e.g. neutropenia, febrile neutropenia, thrombocytopenia, nausea, renal failure) than patients aged <65 years, regardless of treatment arm. In the maintenance non-small cell lung cancer trial, patients ≥65 years of age experienced more myelosuppression and renal adverse events. Because renal function declines with age and decreased renal function results in reduced clearance of ALIMTA, older patients should be followed closely for toxicity.

Pediatrics: ALIMTA is not recommended for use in children as safety and efficacy have not yet been established in this group of patients.

Renally Impaired Patients: In clinical studies, patients with creatinine clearance ≥45 mL/min required no dose adjustments other than those recommended for all patients. Insufficient numbers of patients with creatinine clearance below 45 mL/min have been treated to make dosage recommendations for this group of patients. Therefore, ALIMTA should not be administered to patients whose creatinine clearance is <45 mL/min using the standard Cockcroft and Gault formula (below) or GFR measured by Tc99m-DPTA serum clearance method:

$$\text{Male:} \quad \frac{[140\text{-age in years}]\times\text{actual body weight (kg)}}{50\times\text{serum creatinine }(\mu\text{mol/L})} = \text{mL/sec}^{a}$$

Female: Estimated creatinine clearance for males×0.85

a To convert from SI (mL/sec) to (mL/min), multiply the mL/sec value by 60.

Caution should be exercised when administering ALIMTA concurrently with NSAIDs to patients whose creatinine clearance is <80 mL/min (see Drug Interactions).

Hepatically Impaired Patients: ALIMTA is not extensively metabolized by the liver. Dose adjustments based on hepatic impairment experienced during treatment with pemetrexed are provided in Table 8 (see Warnings and Precautions, Hepatic/Biliary/Pancreatic and Special Populations, Patients with Hepatic Impairment).

Missed Dose: If chemotherapy treatment is missed, physicians should advise patients to contact them in order to provide further instruction on the administration of folic acid and vitamin B_{12} (see Dosage and Administration).

Administration: ALIMTA (pemetrexed disodium) is for intravenous infusion only.

Preparation and Administration Precautions: As with other potentially toxic anticancer agents, care should be exercised in the handling and preparation of infusion solutions of ALIMTA. The use of gloves is recommended. If a solution of ALIMTA contacts the skin, wash the skin immediately and thoroughly with soap and water. If ALIMTA contacts the mucous membranes, flush thoroughly with water. Several published guidelines for handling and disposal of anticancer agents are available. There is no general agreement that all of the procedures recommended in the guideline are necessary or appropriate.

ALIMTA is not a vesicant. There is not a specific antidote for extravasation of ALIMTA. To date, there have been few reported cases of ALIMTA extravasation, which were not assessed as serious by the investigator. ALIMTA extravasation should be managed with local standard practice for extravasation as with other non-vesicants.

Reconstitution:

Vial Size	Volume of Diluent to be Added to Vial	Approximate Available Volume	Nominal Concentration per mL
10 mL (100 mg pemetrexed)	4.2 mL of 0.9% NaCl injection	Approximately 4.2 mL	25 mg/mL
50 mL (500 mg pemetrexed)	20 mL of 0.9% NaCl injection	Approximately 20 mL	25 mg/mL

The appropriate volume of reconstituted ALIMTA solution should be further diluted to a total volume of 100 mL with 0.9% Sodium Chloride Injection (preservative free) and administered as an intravenous infusion over 10 minutes.

Preparation for Intravenous Infusion Administration:

1. Use aseptic technique during the reconstitution and further dilution of ALIMTA for intravenous infusion administration.
2. Calculate the dose and the number of ALIMTA vials needed. Vials contain either 100 mg or 500 mg of pemetrexed. Each vial contains an excess of ALIMTA to facilitate delivery of label amount.
3. Reconstitute each 100 mg vial with 4.2 mL of 0.9% Sodium Chloride Injection (preservative free) to give a solution containing 25 mg/mL pemetrexed. Reconstitute each 500 mg vial with 20 mL of 0.9% Sodium Chloride Injection (preservative free) to give a solution containing 25 mg/mL of pemetrexed. Gently swirl each vial until the powder is completely dissolved. The resulting solution is clear and ranges in colour from colourless to yellow or green-yellow without adversely affecting product quality. The pH of the reconstituted ALIMTA solution is between 6.6 and 7.8. **Further dilution is required.**
4. As with all parenteral drug products, reconstituted vials and diluted admixtures should be inspected visually for clarity, particulate matter, precipitate, discolouration and leakage prior to administration. Solutions showing haziness, particulate matter, precipitate, discolouration or leakage should not be used. Discard unused portion.
5. The appropriate volume of reconstituted ALIMTA solution should be further diluted to a total volume of 100 mL with 0.9% Sodium Chloride Injection (preservative free) and administered as an intravenous infusion over 10 minutes.
6. Chemical and physical stability of reconstituted and infusion solutions of ALIMTA were demonstrated for up to 24 hours following initial reconstitution, when stored at refrigerated (2-8°C) or ambient room temperature (15-30°C) and lighting. When prepared as directed, reconstitution and infusion solutions of ALIMTA contain no antimicrobial preservatives. Discard any unused portion.

Reconstitution and further dilution prior to intravenous infusion is only recommended with 0.9% Sodium Chloride Injection (preservative free), USP. ALIMTA is physically incompatible with diluents containing calcium, including Lactated Ringer's Injection, USP and Ringer's Injection, USP, and therefore those should not be used. Coadministration of ALIMTA with other drugs and diluents has not been studied, and therefore is not recommended.

OVERDOSAGE:
There have been few cases of ALIMTA (pemetrexed disodium) overdose. Reported toxicities included neutropenia, anemia, thrombocytopenia, mucositis, and rash. Anticipated complications of overdose include bone marrow suppression as manifested by neutropenia, thrombocytopenia, and anemia. In addition, infection with or without fever, diarrhea, and mucositis may be seen. There is no known antidote for ALIMTA overdose. If an overdose occurs, general supportive measures should be instituted as deemed necessary by the treating physician.

The ability of pemetrexed to be dialyzed is unknown. In clinical trials, leucovorin was permitted for CTC Grade 4 leukopenia lasting ≥3 days, CTC Grade 4 neutropenia lasting ≥3 days, and immediately for CTC Grade 4 thrombocytopenia, bleeding associated with Grade 3 thrombocytopenia, or Grade 3 or 4 mucositis. The following intravenous doses and schedules of leucovorin were recommended for intravenous use: 100 mg/m², intravenously once, followed by leucovorin, 50 mg/m², intravenously every 6 hours for 8 days.

For management of a suspected drug overdose, contact your regional Poison Control Centre. See the *CPS* Directory section for a list of Poison Control Centres.

ACTION AND CLINICAL PHARMACOLOGY: Mechanism of Action: ALIMTA (pemetrexed disodium) is an antifolate antineoplastic agent that exerts its action by disrupting crucial folate-dependent metabolic processes essential for cell replication.

Pharmacodynamics: Pemetrexed is an antifolate containing the structurally novel pyrrolopyrimidine-based nucleus that exerts its antineoplastic activity by disrupting crucial folate-dependent metabolic processes that are essential for cell replication. In vitro studies have shown that pemetrexed behaves as a multi-targeted antifolate by inhibiting thymidylate synthase (TS), dihydrofolate reductase (DHFR), and glycinamide ribonucleotide formyltransferase (GARFT), which are key folate-dependent enzymes for the de novo bio-synthesis of thymidine and purine nucleotides. Pemetrexed is transported into cells by both the reduced folate carrier and membrane folate binding protein transport systems. Once in the cell, pemetrexed is rapidly and efficiently converted to polyglutamate forms by the enzyme folylpolyglutamate synthetase. The polyglutamate forms are retained in cells and are even more potent inhibitors of TS and GARFT. Polyglutamation is a time- and concentration-dependent process that occurs in tumor cells and, to a lesser extent, in normal tissues. Polyglutamated metabolites have an increased intracellular half-life resulting in prolonged drug action in malignant cells. Data indicate that overexpression of thymidylate synthase (TS) correlates with reduced sensitivity to pemetrexed in antifolate-resistant cell lines. Results in a recent study with specimens from chemonaive patients with NSCLC demonstrated lower levels of TS expression in adenocarcinoma as compared to squamous cell carcinoma tumors. Although these data suggest that pemetrexed may offer greater efficacy for patients with adenocarcinoma as compared to squamous carcinoma histology, this hypothesis requires further validation in studies that assess the predictive and prognostic value of TS expression in patients with NSCLC.

Pharmacokinetics: The pharmacokinetics of pemetrexed administered as a single-agent in doses ranging from 0.2 to 838 mg/m² infused over a 10-minute period have been evaluated in 426 cancer patients with a variety of solid tumors.

Absorption: Pemetrexed total systemic exposure (AUC) and maximum plasma concentration (C_{max}) increase proportionally with dose. The pharmacokinetics of pemetrexed are consistent over multiple treatment cycles.

Distribution: Pemetrexed has a steady-state volume of distribution of 16.1 L. In vitro studies indicate that pemetrexed is approximately 81% bound to plasma proteins. Binding is not affected by renal impairment.

Metabolism: Pemetrexed is not metabolized to an appreciable extent.

Excretion: Pemetrexed is primarily eliminated in the urine with 70% to 90% of the dose recovered unchanged within the first 24 hours following administration. Pemetrexed total systemic clearance is 91.8 mL/min and the elimination half-life from plasma is 3.5 hours in patients with normal renal function (creatinine clearance of 90 mL/min [calculated using the standard Cockcroft and Gault formula or measured glomerular filtration rate using the Tc99m-DPTA serum clearance method]). Between patient variability in clearance is moderate at 19.3%.

Absolute neutrophil counts (ANC) following single-agent administration of pemetrexed to patients not receiving folic acid and vitamin B_{12} supplementation were characterized using population pharmacodynamic analyses. Severity of hematologic toxicity, as measured by the depth of the ANC nadir, is inversely proportional to the systemic exposure of ALIMTA. It was also observed that lower ANC nadirs occurred in patients with elevated baseline cystathionine or homocysteine concentrations. The levels of these substances can be reduced by folic acid and vitamin B_{12} supplementation. There is no cumulative effect of pemetrexed exposure on ANC nadir over multiple treatment cycles.

Time to ANC nadir with pemetrexed systemic exposure (AUC), varied between 8 to 9.6 days over a range of exposures from 38.3 to 316.8 µg· hr/mL. Return to baseline ANC occurred 4.2 to 7.5 days after the nadir over the same range of exposures.

Special Populations and Conditions: The pharmacokinetics of pemetrexed in special populations were examined in about 400 patients in controlled and single arm studies.

Pediatrics: The safety and effectiveness of ALIMTA has not been established in pediatric patients.

Geriatrics: No effect of age on the pharmacokinetics of pemetrexed was observed over a range of 26 to 80 years.

Gender: The pharmacokinetics of pemetrexed were not different in male and female patients.

Race: The pharmacokinetics of pemetrexed were similar in Caucasians and patients of African descent. Insufficient data are available to compare pharmacokinetics for other ethnic groups.

Hepatic Insufficiency: There was no effect of elevated AST, ALT, or total bilirubin on the pharmacokinetics of pemetrexed. However, studies of hepatically impaired patients have not been conducted (see Warnings and Precautions).

Renal Insufficiency: Pharmacokinetic analyses of pemetrexed included 127 patients with reduced renal function. Plasma clearance of pemetrexed in the presence of cisplatin decreases as renal function decreases, with increase in systemic exposure. Patients with creatinine clearances of 45, 50, and 80 mL/min had 65%, 54%, and 13% increases, respectively in pemetrexed total systemic exposure (AUC) compared to patients with creatinine clearance of 100 mL/min (see Warnings and Precautions and Dosage and Administration).

STORAGE AND STABILITY: ALIMTA should be stored at controlled room temperature 25°C; excursions permitted to 15-30°C.

Chemical and physical stability of reconstituted and infusion solutions of ALIMTA were demonstrated for up to 24 hours following initial reconstitution, when stored refrigerated, 2-8°C, or at 25°C, excursions permitted to 15-30°C. When prepared as directed, reconstituted and infusion solutions of ALIMTA contain no antimicrobial preservatives and should be used immediately. Discard unused portion.

ALIMTA is not light sensitive.

SPECIAL HANDLING INSTRUCTIONS: Please see Dosage and Administration, Administration.

INFORMATION FOR THE PATIENT: Published in e-CPS, available by subscription at www.e-cps.ca.

DOSAGE FORMS, COMPOSITION AND PACKAGING: 100 mg: Each vial of white to either light yellowish or green-yellowish lyophilized powder for injection, contains: pemetrexed disodium equivalent to pemetrexed 100 mg and mannitol 106 mg. Hydrochloric acid and/or sodium hydroxide, may have been added to adjust pH. Sterile single use glass vials of 10 mL.

500 mg: Each vial of white to either light yellowish or green-yellowish lyophilized powder for injection, contains: pemetrexed disodium equivalent to pemetrexed 500 mg and mannitol 500 mg. Hydrochloric acid and/or sodium hydroxide, may have been added to adjust pH. Sterile single use glass vials of 50 mL.

Alka-Seltzer®
ASA—sodium bicarbonate—citric acid
Analgesic—Antacid

Bayer Consumer Care

Alka-Seltzer® Flavoured
ASA—sodium bicarbonate—citric acid
Analgesic—Antacid

Bayer Consumer Care

SUPPLIED: Alka-Seltzer: Each tablet contains: ASA 325 mg, sodium bicarbonate 1916 mg and citric acid 1000 mg. Packages of 12, 24 and 36.

Alka-Seltzer Flavoured: Each lemon-lime flavored tablet contains: ASA 325 mg, sodium bicarbonate 1700 mg and citric acid 1000 mg. Nonmedicinal ingredients: aspartame, docusate sodium, lemon and lime flavors, povidone and sodium benzoate. Packages of 24.

Alkeran® Ⓟ
melphalan
Antineoplastic

GlaxoSmithKline

Date of Revision: December 17, 2007

SUMMARY PRODUCT INFORMATION:

Route of Administration	Dosage Form/ Strength	Clinically Relevant Nonmedicinal Ingredients
Oral	Tablets/2 mg	Not applicable For a complete listing see Dosage Forms, Composition and Packaging.
Intravenous Perfusion	Injection/50 mg/vial	Ethanol For a complete listing see Dosage Forms, Composition and Packaging.

INDICATIONS AND CLINICAL USE: ALKERAN (melphalan) is indicated for:

- the palliative treatment of multiple myeloma.
- the palliation of nonresectable epithelial carcinoma of the ovary.
- ALKERAN for injection has been administered by hyperthermic isolated limb perfusion as an adjuvant to surgery in the treatment of malignant melanoma. However, there have been no prospective controlled or uncontrolled trials evaluating dose and its relationship to disease response and/or toxicity.

CONTRAINDICATIONS:

- Patients who are hypersensitive to this drug or to any ingredient in the formulation or component of the container. For a complete listing, see Dosage Forms, Composition and Packaging.
- ALKERAN (melphalan) should not be used in patients whose disease has demonstrated a prior resistance to this agent. Patients who have demonstrated hypersensitivity to melphalan should not be given the drug. There may be cross-sensitivity (skin rash) between melphalan and chlorambucil (LEUKERAN).
- Melphalan should not be given if other similar chemotherapeutic agents or radiotherapy have been administered to the patient recently, or if neutrophil and/or platelet counts are depressed.
- Melphalan should not be administered concurrently with radiotherapy.

WARNINGS AND PRECAUTIONS:

> **Serious Warnings and Precautions**
> ALKERAN (melphalan) should be administered in carefully adjusted dosages by or under the supervision of experienced physicians who are familiar with the drug's actions and the possible complications of its use.
> The major acute toxicities associated with melphalan are:
> - Hypersensitivity reactions including anaphylaxis (see Immune)
> - Bone marrow suppression (see Hematologic)
> - Pulmonary toxicity (see Respiratory and Overdosage)
> - Infertility (see Sexual Function/Reproduction)
> - Secondary malignancies (see Carcinogenesis and Mutagenesis)
> - Mutagenicity and teratogenicity (see Carcinogenesis and Mutagenesis)

General: ALKERAN should be administered in carefully adjusted dosages by or under the supervision of experienced physicians who are familiar with the drug's actions and the possible complications of its use. The drug should not be administered by hyperthermic isolated limb perfusion unless the clinician is experienced and well-trained in this technique.

In all instances where the use of ALKERAN for injection is considered for chemotherapy, the physician must evaluate the need and usefulness of the drug against the risk of adverse events. Melphalan should be used with extreme caution in patients whose bone marrow reserve may have been compromised by prior irradiation or chemotherapy, or whose marrow function is recovering from previous cytotoxic therapy. Dose reduction should be considered in patients with renal insufficiency receiving IV melphalan (see Hematologic and Renal).

Carcinogenesis and Mutagenesis: Secondary malignancies, including acute nonlymphocytic leukemia, myeloproliferative syndrome, and carcinoma, have been reported in patients with cancer treated with alkylating agents (including melphalan). Some patients also received other chemotherapeutic agents or radiation therapy. Precise quantitation of the risk of acute leukemia, myeloproliferative syndrome or carcinoma is not possible. Published reports of leukemia in patients who have received melphalan (and other alkylating agents) suggest that the risk of leukemogenesis increases with chronicity of treatment and with cumulative dose. In one study, the 10-year cumulative risk of developing acute leukemia or myeloproliferative syndrome after melphalan therapy was 19.5% for cumulative doses ranging from 730 mg to 9652 mg. In this same study, as well as in an additional study, the 10-year cumulative risk of developing acute leukemia or myeloproliferative syndrome after melphalan therapy was less than 2% for cumulative doses under 600 mg. This does not mean that there is a cumulative dose below which there is no risk of the induction of secondary malignancy. The potential benefits from melphalan therapy must be weighed on an individual basis against the possible risk of the induction of a second malignancy.

Melphalan has been shown to cause chromatid or chromosome damage in man.

Hematologic: As with other nitrogen mustard drugs, excessive dosage will produce marked bone marrow suppression. Bone marrow suppression is the most significant toxicity associated with ALKERAN for injection in most patients. Therefore, the following tests should be performed at the start of therapy and prior to each subsequent dose of ALKERAN: platelet count, hemoglobin, white blood cell count and differential. The occurrence of a platelet count below 50×10^9/L or an absolute neutrophil count below 0.5×10^9/L is an indication to withhold further therapy until the blood counts have sufficiently recovered. Frequent blood counts are essential to determine optimal dosage and to avoid toxicity.

If the leukocyte count falls below 3×10^9/L, or the platelet count below 100×10^9/L, the drug should be discontinued until the blood picture has had a chance to recover.

Blood counts may continue to fall for 6-8 weeks after initiation of treatment. So, at the first sign of abnormally large fall in leukocyte or platelet counts, treatment should be temporarily interrupted.

In one trial by Cornwell et al. (1982), melphalan administered intravenously without adjustment for renal failure increased incidence rates for severe leukopenia and thrombocytopenia by 35% in patients with renal insufficiency (BUN ≥30 mg/dL).

Immune: Acute hypersensitivity reactions, including anaphylaxis, have occurred infrequently (see Adverse Reactions). Treatment is symptomatic. The infusion should be terminated immediately, followed by the administration of volume expanders, pressor agents, corticosteroids, or antihistamines at the discretion of the physician.

Immunisation using a live organism vaccine has the potential to cause infection in immunocompromised hosts. Therefore, immunisations with live organism vaccines are not recommended.

Renal: Systemic exposure of melphalan was positively correlated to the degree of renal insufficiency following either route of administration. In one trial by Cornwell et al. (1982), increased incidence rate of bone marrow suppression has been associated with impaired renal function in patients with intravenous melphalan administration without dose adjustment for renal failure. Dose adjustments should be considered for patients with significant renal dysfunction (BUN ≥30 mg/dL) and these patients should be closely monitored for toxicity.

Respiratory: Rare reports of pulmonary fibrosis or interstitial pneumonitis (including fatal reports) have been seen in patients treated with ALKERAN.

Sexual Function/Reproduction: Melphalan causes suppression of ovarian function in premenopausal women, resulting in amenorrhea in a significant number of patients.

Reversible and irreversible testicular suppression have also been reported. There is evidence from some animal studies that melphalan can have an adverse effect on spermatogenesis.

Special Populations: Pregnant Women: Safe use of melphalan has not been established with respect to adverse effects on fetal development. Therefore, it should be used in women of childbearing potential and particularly during early pregnancy only when, in the judgment of the physician, the potential benefits outweigh the possible hazards.

Nursing Women: It is not known whether this drug is excreted in human milk. Because many drugs are excreted in human milk and because of the potential for serious adverse reactions in nursing infants from melphalan, a decision should be made whether to discontinue nursing or to discontinue the drug, taking into account the importance of the drug to the mother.

Pediatrics: The safety and effectiveness in children have not been established.

Geriatrics: Clinical experience with ALKERAN has not identified differences in responses between the elderly and younger patients. In general, dose selection for an elderly patient should be cautious, usually starting at the low end of the dosing range, reflecting the greater frequency of decreased hepatic, renal, or cardiac function, and of concomitant disease or other drug therapy.

Monitoring and Laboratory Tests: Periodic complete blood counts with differentials should be performed during the course of treatment with melphalan. At least one determination should be obtained prior to each dose. Patients should be observed closely for consequences of bone marrow suppression, which include severe infections, bleeding, and symptomatic anemia.

ADVERSE REACTIONS: Adverse Drug Reaction Overview: The following information on adverse reactions is based on data from both oral and intravenous administration of ALKERAN (melphalan) as a single agent, using several different dose schedules for treatment of a wide variety of malignancies.

For this product there is no modern clinical documentation which can be used as support for determining the frequency of undesirable effects. Undesirable effects may vary in their incidence depending on the indication and dose received and also when given in combination with other therapeutic agents.

Gastrointestinal: Gastrointestinal effects such as nausea and vomiting occur in up to 30% of patients receiving conventional oral doses of ALKERAN, and in up to 50% of patients receiving intravenous doses of ALKERAN. Diarrhea is noted to occur one week post high dose melphalan therapy. Oral ulceration and hepatic toxicity including veno-occlusive disease have been reported.

The incidence of diarrhea, vomiting and stomatitis becomes the dose-limiting toxicity in patients given high intravenous doses of melphalan in association with autologous bone marrow transplantation. Cyclophosphamide pretreatment appears to reduce the severity of gastrointestinal damage induced by high-dose melphalan and the literature should be consulted for details. Stomatitis at conventional doses is rare.

Hematologic: The most common side effect is bone marrow suppression leading to leukopenia, thrombocytopenia and anemia. Neutropenia and hemolytic anemia were also observed. Irreversible bone marrow failure has been reported. Bone marrow suppression is uncommon after limb perfusion.

Frequencies of severe myelosuppression and infections including fatal cases secondary to myelosuppression were much higher in patients with renal insufficiency (BUN ≥30 mg/dL) than those with normal renal function who were treated with intravenous melphalan (see Warnings and Precautions, Renal).

Hepatic: Hepatic disorders ranging from abnormal liver function tests to clinical manifestations such as hepatitis and jaundice have been reported. Veno-occlusive disease has been reported following high-dose intravenous treatment.

Elevation in liver function enzymes is usually mild.

Hyperthermic Isolated Limb Perfusion: Adverse reactions may be attributable to the surgical procedure as well as the heated perfusion with ALKERAN for Injection.

The local toxicity of hyperthermic perfusion appears to increase with increasing drug dose, duration of perfusion, and temperature. Muscle atrophy, muscle fibrosis, myalgia and increase in blood creatine phosphokinase were very commonly observed. Compartment syndrome has been commonly observed. Muscle necrosis and rhabdomyolysis have been seen at an unknown frequency. Severe nerve or muscle damage, severe skin or soft tissue reaction, or arterial thrombosis requiring amputation are rare, occurring in less than 1% of patients.

Systemic complications are uncommon, with reversible bone marrow suppression occurring in <5% of patients. Wound complications, such as delayed healing or infection, occur in 5 to 10% of patients.

Hypersensitivity: Acute hypersensitivity reactions, including anaphylaxis, were reported in 2.4% of 425 patients receiving ALKERAN for injection for myeloma (see Warnings and Precautions). These reactions were characterized by urticaria, pruritus, edema, skin rashes and in some patients, tachycardia, bronchospasm, dyspnea, and hypotension. Cardiac arrest had also been rarely reported in association with such events. These patients appeared to respond to antihistamine and corticosteroid therapy. Treatment with melphalan should be discontinued if a hypersensitivity reaction occurs.

Local Reactions: Mild pain and/or irritation at, or near, the site of injection occurred after approximately half of the infusions, resolving within few hours after the end of the injection, without a need for treatment. Skin ulceration at injection site and flushing were reported as well as subjective and transient sensation of warmth and/or tingling.

Miscellaneous: Other reported adverse reactions include: skin hypersensitivity, vasculitis, alopecia, allergic reaction, pulmonary fibrosis, stomatitis, maculopapular rashes and interstitial pneumonitis. Fatal reports of pulmonary fibrosis have been received. Flushing sensations were reported at high doses of melphalan.

Renal: Temporary significant elevation of the blood urea has been seen in the early stages of melphalan therapy in myeloma patients with renal damage. An increase in creatinine levels has been observed.

DRUG INTERACTIONS: Drug-Drug Interactions: See Table 1.

Table 1: ALKERAN

Established or Potential Drug-Drug Interactions

ALKERAN	Effect	Clinical comment
Nalidixic acid	Hemorrhagic enterocolitis	Nalidixic acid together with high-dose intravenous melphalan has caused deaths in children due to hemorrhagic enterocolitis.
Cyclosporine	Impaired renal function	In bone marrow transplant patients who were conditioned with high-dose intravenous melphalan and who subsequently received cyclosporine to prevent graft-versus-host disease.
Live Viral Vaccines	Potential to cause infection in immunocompromised hosts	Vaccinations with live organism vaccines are not recommended in immunocompromised individuals (See Warnings and Precautions).

Drug-Food Interactions: The oral administration of melphalan tablets immediately after food delayed the time to achieving peak plasma concentrations and reduced the area under the plasma concentration-time curves by between 39 and 45% (see Action and Clinical Pharmacology).

DOSAGE AND ADMINISTRATION: Recommended Dose and Dosage Adjustment: Oral: Multiple Myeloma: The usual oral dose is 6 mg (3 tablets) daily. The entire daily dose may be given at one time. It is adjusted, as required, on the basis of blood counts done at approximately weekly intervals. After 2-3 weeks of treatment, the drug should be discontinued for up to 4 weeks, during which time the blood count should be followed carefully. When the white blood cell and platelet counts are rising, a maintenance dose of 2 mg daily may be instituted. Because of the patient-to-patient variation in melphalan plasma levels following oral administration of the drug, several investigators have recommended that melphalan dosage be cautiously escalated until some myelosuppression is observed, in order to assure that potentially therapeutic levels of the drug have been reached.

Other dosage regimens have been used by various investigators. Osserman and Takatsuki have used an initial course of 10 mg/day for 7-10 days. They report that maximal suppression of the leukocyte and platelet counts occurs within 3-5 weeks and recovery within 4-8 weeks. Continuous maintenance therapy with 2 mg/day is instituted when the white blood cell count is greater than 4×10^9/L and the platelet count is greater than 100×10^9/L. Dosage is adjusted to between 1 and 3 mg/day depending upon the hematological response. It is desirable to try to maintain a significant degree of bone marrow depression so as to keep the leukocyte count in the range of 3 to 3.5×10^9/L. Hoogstraten et al. have started treatment with 0.15 mg/kg/day for 7 days. This is followed by a rest period of at least 14 days, but it may be as long as 5-6 weeks.

Maintenance therapy is started when the white blood cell and platelet counts are rising. The maintenance dose is 0.05 mg/kg/day or less and is adjusted according to the blood count.

Available evidence suggests that about one-third to one-half of the patients with multiple myeloma show a favorable response to oral administration of the drug.

It is to be emphasized that response may be very gradual over many months; it is important that repeated courses or continuous therapy be given since improvement may continue slowly over many months and the maximum benefit may be missed if treatment is abandoned too soon.

Epithelial Ovarian Cancer: One commonly employed regimen for the treatment of ovarian carcinoma has been to administer melphalan at a dose of 0.2 mg/kg P.O. daily for 5 days as a single course. Courses are repeated every 4-5 weeks depending upon hematologic tolerance.

Intravenous: Multiple Myeloma: The usual intravenous dose is 16 mg/m^2. Dosage reduction of up to 50% should be considered in patients with renal insufficiency (BUN =10.71 mmol/L [30 mg/dL]). The drug is administered in one dose and the length of infusion should be from 15 to 90 minutes. Melphalan is repeated at 2-week intervals initially for 4 doses, then at 4-week intervals after adequate recovery from toxicity. Available evidence suggests about one-third to one-half of the patients with multiple myeloma show a favorable response to the drug. Experience with oral melphalan suggests that repeated courses should be given since improvement may continue slowly over many months, and the maximum benefit may be missed if treatment is abandoned prematurely. Dose adjustment on the basis of blood cell counts at the nadir prior to each dose should be considered.

Perfusion Method: Malignant Melanoma: Only physicians experienced and well-trained in hyperthermic isolated limb perfusion should administer the drug in this fashion.

Administration: Preparation for Administration/Stability: Intravenous:

1. Reconstitute ALKERAN for injection, as directed, with 10 mL of the supplied diluent. This provides a 5 mg/mL solution of melphalan.
2. Immediately dilute the dose to be administered in 0.9% sodium chloride injection, USP, to a concentration not greater than 0.45 mg/mL.
3. Administer the diluted product over a minimum of 15 minutes.
4. Complete administration within 50 minutes of reconstitution.
5. Discard any reconstituted and diluted solutions remaining after 50 minutes of reconstitution.

The reconstituted product is stable for up to 2 hours at 30°C. A precipitate forms if the solution is stored at 5°C. **Do not refrigerate.**

Solutions diluted to a concentration of 0.1 mg/mL to 0.45 mg/mL in 0.9% sodium chloride injection are stable for up to 50 minutes at 30°C and 3 hours at 20°C.

Reconstitution: ALKERAN for injection must be reconstituted, at room temperature, by rapidly transferring 10 mL of the supplied solvent-diluent directly into the vial of lyophilized powder using a sterile needle (20 gauge or larger needle diameter) and syringe. Immediately shake vial vigorously until a clear solution is obtained. Rapid addition of the diluent followed by immediate vigorous shaking is important for proper dissolution. The pH of resulting solution is approximately 6.5. See Table 2.

ALKERAN injection solution has limited stability and should be prepared immediately before use. Any unused solution should be discarded. The reconstituted solution should be used immediately and should not be refrigerated as this will cause precipitation. It is stable for up to 2 hours at 30°C.

ALKERAN injection solution has reduced stability when further diluted in an infusion solution and the rate of degradation increases rapidly with rise in temperature. In that case, only sodium chloride infusion, 0.9% w/v should be used. Solutions diluted to a concentration of 0.1 mg/mL to 0.45 mg/mL in 0.9% sodium chloride infusion should be used immediately and are stable for up to 50 minutes at 30°C and 3 hours at 20°C.

Parenteral Products: Parenteral drug products should usually be inspected for particulate matter and discoloration prior to administration whenever solution and container permit. If either occurs, do not use this product.

Table 2: ALKERAN

Reconstitution

Vial Size	Volume of Diluent to be Added to Vial	Approximate Available Volume	Nominal Concentration per mL
50 mg	10 mL	10 mL	5 mg/mL

OVERDOSAGE:
Overdose as high as 290 mg/m² resulting in death has been reported. It has also been reported that a pediatric patient survived a 254 mg/m² overdose treated with standard supportive care. The immediate effects are severe nausea and vomiting. Decreased consciousness, convulsions, muscular paralysis and cholinomimetic effects are less frequently seen. Severe mucositis, stomatitis, colitis, diarrhea, and hemorrhage of the gastrointestinal tract occur at high doses (>100 mg/m²). Elevations in liver enzymes and veno-occlusive disease occur infrequently. Nephrotoxicity and adult respiratory distress syndrome have been reported rarely. The principal toxic effect is bone marrow suppression leading to leukopenia, thrombocytopenia and anemia. Hematologic parameters should be closely followed for 3 to 6 weeks. Administration of autologous bone marrow or hematopoietic growth factors (i.e., sargramostim, filgrastim) may shorten the period of pancytopenia. General supportive measures together with appropriate blood transfusions and antibiotics should be instituted as deemed necessary by the physician. This drug is not removed from plasma to any significant degree by hemodialysis or hemoperfusion.

> For management of a suspected drug overdose, CPhA recommends that you contact your **regional Poison Control Centre**. See the *CPS* Directory section for a list of Poison Control Centres.

ACTION AND CLINICAL PHARMACOLOGY: Mechanism of Action: ALKERAN (melphalan) is an alkylating agent of the bis-chloroethylamine type. As a result, its cytotoxicity appears to be related to the extent of its interstrand cross-linking with DNA, probably by binding at the N⁷ position of guanine. Like other bifunctional alkylating agents, it is active against both resting and rapidly dividing tumor cells.

Pharmacokinetics: Absorption: The absorption of oral melphalan is highly variable with respect to both the time to first appearance of the drug in plasma and peak plasma concentration. In studies of the absolute bioavailability of melphalan the mean absolute bioavailability ranged from 56 to 85%.

Mean (±SD) peak melphalan plasma concentrations in myeloma patients given melphalan intravenously at doses of 10 or 20 mg/m² were 1.2±0.4 and 2.8±1.9 µg/mL, respectively. Studies in children as young as 1 year showed results similar to adults.

The oral administration of melphalan tablets immediately after food delayed the time to achieving peak plasma concentrations and reduced the area under the plasma concentration-time curves by between 39 and 45% (see Drug Interactions).

Distribution: The steady-state volume of distribution of melphalan is 0.5 L/kg and approximates total body water. Penetration into cerebrospinal fluid (CSF) is low. The extent of melphalan binding to plasma proteins is ranging from 69% to 78%. There is evidence that the protein binding is linear in the range of plasma concentrations usually achieved at standard dose therapy, but that the binding may become concentration-dependent at the concentrations observed at high dose therapy. Serum albumin is the major binding protein, accounting for about 55% to 60% of the plasma protein binding, and 20% is bound to α_1-acid glycoprotein. In addition, melphalan binding studies have revealed the existence of an irreversible component attributable to the alkylation reaction with plasma proteins. Interactions with immunoglobulins have been found to be negligible.

Melphalan displays limited penetration of the blood-brain barrier. Melphalan was found at concentrations of approximately 10% of the corresponding plasma concentration in the cerebrospinal fluid samples following high-dose intravenous melphalan in two studies.

Metabolism: Melphalan is eliminated from plasma primarily by chemical hydrolysis to monohydroxy- and dihydroxy-melphalan. Aside from these hydrolysis products, no other melphalan metabolites have been observed in man.

Elimination: Following injection, drug plasma concentrations declined rapidly in a biexponential manner with distribution phase and terminal elimination phase half-lives of approximately 10 and 70 minutes, respectively. Estimates of average total body clearance varied among studies, but typical values of approximately 7 to 9 mL/min/kg (250 to 325 mL/min/m²) were observed.

Melphalan clearance may be decreased in renal impairment. An increase in AUC (i.e. melphalan systemic exposure) was observed in patients with renal impairment when melphalan was administered by either route. One study noted an increase in the occurrence of severe leukopenia in patients with elevated BUN after 10 weeks of therapy (see Warnings and Precautions, Hematologic).

The pharmacokinetics of melphalan administered by closed circuit limb perfusion have been studied by several investigators. Melphalan concentrations declined rapidly and biexponentially from circulating perfusate with average terminal half-lives reported from 26 min (n=4) to 53 min (n=48). Systemic exposure to melphalan during limb perfusion is generally very low. Peak melphalan concentrations in the closed circuit perfusate are typically 10 to 100 times greater than peak concentrations in plasma observed following standard dose systemic intravenous therapy for multiple myeloma.

STORAGE AND STABILITY: Tablets: Store in a refrigerator, 2-8°C.
Injection: Store at controlled room temperature (15-30°C). Protect from light.

SPECIAL HANDLING INSTRUCTIONS: As with other toxic compounds, caution should be exercised when handling and preparing the solution of ALKERAN. Skin reactions associated with accidental exposure may occur. The use of gloves is recommended. If the solution of ALKERAN contacts the skin or mucosa, immediately wash the skin or mucosa thoroughly with soap and water.

INFORMATION FOR THE PATIENT: Published in e-CPS, available by subscription at www.e-cps.ca.

DOSAGE FORMS, COMPOSITION AND PACKAGING: Injection: Each vial of sterile, white to cream-colored, freeze-dried powder contains: melphalan HCl equivalent to melphalan 50 mg and povidone 20 mg. Each vial of solvent-diluent provides 10 mL of buffer solution containing sodium citrate 0.20 g, ethanol 0.52 mL, propylene glycol 6 mL and water for injection, q.s. Component packs of 2 comprising a vial containing a freeze-dried powder and a vial of solvent-diluent.

Tablets: Each white to off-white, round, biconvex, film-coated tablet, imprinted with "A" on one side and on the other side "GX EH3", contains: melphalan 2 mg. Nonmedicinal ingredients: colloidal silicon dioxide, crospovidone, hydroxypropyl methylcellulose, magnesium stearate, microcrystalline cellulose, polyethylene glycol 400 and titanium dioxide. Bottles of 50.

(Shown in Product Identification Section)

Allegra® 12 Hour
fexofenadine HCl
Histamine H1-Receptor Antagonist

sanofi-aventis

Allegra® 24 Hour
fexofenadine HCl
Histamine H1-Receptor Antagonist

sanofi-aventis

Date of Revision: September 8, 2006

PHARMACOLOGY: Fexofenadine, the predominant human and animal active metabolite of terfenadine, is a selective histamine H_1-receptor antagonist. Both enantiomers of fexofenadine display approximately equipotent antihistaminic effects. In laboratory animals, there is no evidence of local anesthetic, analgesic, anticonvulsant, antidepressant, antidopaminergic, antiserotonergic, anticholinergic, sedative, H_2-receptor antagonist, α_1-adrenergic receptor or β-adrenergic receptor blocking activity. Fexofenadine inhibits antigen-induced bronchospasm in sensitized guinea pigs and histamine release from peritoneal mast cells of the rat. It does not cross the blood-brain barrier in the rat.

Fexofenadine inhibits histamine induced skin wheal and flare responses. Following single and twice daily oral dose administration, antihistaminic effects occur within 1 hour, achieve a maximum at 2 to 3 hours, and last a minimum of 12 hours. There is no evidence of tolerance to these effects after 28 days of dosing.

At steady-state with 60 mg b.i.d. dosing in adults, the average percent inhibition of skin wheal was 45.8% and 53.6% for fexofenadine and terfenadine, respectively. The average maximum inhibition and average area under effect curve was similar for both drugs at equivalent doses. Although higher doses, i.e., 180 mg b.i.d. produced somewhat greater inhibition, the average difference was only 10 to 12%. At 12 hours postdose, the average percent inhibition was approximately 30%.

Similar results were observed with the skin flare response, although the average percent inhibition was somewhat higher—69% and 75%, for 60 mg b.i.d. fexofenadine and terfenadine, respectively. Equivalent doses of both drugs produced comparable maximum inhibition and area under effect curve. The flare area was inhibited greater than 55% at 12 hours postdose.

There was no clear-cut relationship between plasma concentrations of fexofenadine and dose of either fexofenadine or terfenadine. Maximum inhibition was achieved at plasma fexofenadine concentrations of 200 ng/mL.

In randomized, double-blind, placebo-controlled trials, a daily dose of fexofenadine 60 mg b.i.d. and 120 mg once daily were shown to be effective in relieving the symptoms of seasonal allergic rhinitis (trees and grasses in the spring or ragweed pollen in the fall) and perennial allergic rhinitis (animal dander, dust mites and moulds). These symptoms consisted of sneezing, rhinorrhea, itchy nose/palate/throat and itchy, watery, red eyes. Fexofenadine also effectively relieved the signs and symptoms of chronic idiopathic urticaria, including pruritus and number of wheals (see Indications). There was no statistically significant difference in the treatment effect in subgroups defined by age, gender, race or weight.

There was no direct comparison with terfenadine. However, in studies with similar trial design, the effectiveness of fexofenadine appears to be comparable to that of the parent compound.

Preclinical and clinical evidence indicates that fexofenadine does not prolong the QT_c interval (the mechanism underlying the arrhythmias associated with elevated levels of terfenadine). The evidence is derived from in vitro electrophysiological studies, in vivo preclinical studies in dogs and rabbits and a number of clinical trials consisting of 2 definitive QT_c studies (n=24 and 40), 2 dose escalation studies (n=24 and 66), 2 drug interaction studies investigating the effects of erythromycin and ketoconazole (n=24 for each study), 2 randomized Phase III clinical trials in patients with fall allergic rhinitis (n=870 subjects treated with fexofenadine), 2 long-term safety studies (n=234 and 217 subjects treated with fexofenadine), and single dose (80 mg) studies in special populations (individuals over 65 years of age, patients with various degrees of renal and hepatic impairment).

Pharmacokinetics: Fexofenadine is rapidly absorbed following oral administration. The single and multiple dose pharmacokinetics of fexofenadine were linear for oral daily doses from 20 to 120 mg b.i.d. Following oral administration of a single dose of two 60 mg capsules to healthy, male volunteers, T_{max} occurred at approximately 2.6 hours. Following single dose oral administration of the 60 mg, 120 mg and 180 mg tablet to healthy, male volunteers, mean maximum plasma concentrations were 142, 289 and 494 ng/mL, respectively.

Following multiple dosing, fexofenadine has an apparent elimination half-life of 11 to 16 hours. Steady-state pharmacokinetic parameters following 60 mg b.i.d. dosing are: $AUC_{ss\,(0\text{-}12h)}$=1367 ng/mL·h, Cmax=299 ng/mL, Cmin=29 ng/mL, Tmax=1 h.

The pharmacokinetics of fexofenadine in seasonal allergic rhinitis patients and chronic idiopathic urticaria patients are similar to that of otherwise healthy subjects. Peak fexofenadine plasma concentrations were similar between adolescent (12 to 16 years of age) and adult patients.

Metabolism of fexofenadine is negligible. The methyl ester of fexofenadine (3.6% of the dose) and MDL 4829 (1.5% of the dose) were the only potential metabolites of fexofenadine detected.

Following a single 60 mg oral dose, 80% and 11% of the total [¹⁴C] fexofenadine dose is recovered in the feces and urine, respectively. The principal elimination pathways of fexofenadine are biliary and renal. Fecal excretion of fexofenadine is comprised of biliary excretion and gastrointestinal secretion processes as well as nonabsorbed drug. The contribution of each component is unknown.

The absolute bioavailability of fexofenadine has not been established but is estimated to be approximately 33%. The 60 mg capsule and tablet formulations are considered to be bioequivalent but the tablet formulation exhibits a greater food effect. The AUC and C_{max} of the 60 mg tablet formulation in the presence of food was reduced to 76% (83% for the capsule) and 75% (89% for the capsule) of the fasted values. The AUC and C_{max} of the 120 mg tablets in the presence of food was reduced to 85% (AUC) and 86% (C_{max}).

Current theory suggests that fexofenadine absorption is incomplete due to the "gate-keeping" function of the p-glycoprotein transport system in the intestinal epithelium which reduces both fexofenadine absorption, explaining the low bioavailability, as well as secretes absorbed drug back into the gastrointestinal tract. Since approximately 80% of an orally administered dose is recovered in the feces, primarily as unchanged drug, rather than 67% (100%−33%), this difference is believed to represent fexofenadine secretion from the systemic circulation into the gastrointestinal lumen.

Fexofenadine is 60 to 80% bound to plasma proteins, including serum albumin and α-acid glycoprotein. Protein binding is decreased to 56 to 68% and 56 to 75% in renally and hepatically impaired patients, respectively.

Special Populations: Pharmacokinetics in special populations were determined following a single 80 mg oral dose of fexofenadine. The pharmacokinetics were compared to those from normal subjects in a separate study of similar design. While subjects' weights were relatively uniform between the studies, the special population patients were older than the healthy, young volunteers. Thus, an age effect may be confounding the pharmacokinetic differences observed.

Renal Impairment: Following a single 80 mg oral dose, renal clearance is decreased to 68, 15 and 3% of the control value (3.63 L/h) in patients with mild to moderate impairment (creatinine clearance 41 to 80 mL/min; n=9), moderate to severe impairment (creatinine clearance 11 to 40 mL/min; n=10) and dialysis patients (creatinine clearance <10 mL/min; n=10). The corresponding $AUC_{0\text{-}\infty}$ and C_{max} were increased by 80, 154 and 88%, respectively (control value=1788.1 ng/mL·h), and by 58, 78 and 54%, respectively (control value= 248.7 ng/mL). The half-life increased from 13.7 h to 22.8, 24.8 and 18.9 h, respectively. Based on these increases in bioavailability and half-life, a dose of 60 mg once daily is recommended as the starting dose in patients with decreased renal function.

Hepatic Impairment: The pharmacokinetics of fexofenadine in 14 patients with hepatic disease (moderate, n=9; moderate to severe, n=5), did not differ substantially from that observed in healthy subjects. The lack of effect may be explained by the fact that none of the patients investigated suffered from complete biliary obstruction, as biliary excretion is one of the major elimination pathways for fexofenadine.

Effect of Age: The pharmacokinetics of fexofenadine in healthy elderly individuals (>65 years old, n=20) were different from those observed in healthy younger individuals following a single oral dose of 80 mg fexofenadine. Mean AUC was 63% higher (control value=1788 ng/mL·h), oral clearance 30% lower (control value=48 L/h), renal clearance 24% less (control value=3.6 L/h), C_{max} 68% higher (control value= 248.7 ng/mL) and half-life 10% longer (15.2 h).

Effect of Gender: The steady-state AUC and C_{max} values in female subjects (n=20) were 33% and 46% higher, respectively, than those observed in male subjects (n=20). Renal clearance was equivalent. There was no indication of any difference in safety or efficacy.

Drug Interactions: During multiple dose coadministration (fexofenadine 120 mg b.i.d. for 6.5 days plus erythromycin 500 mg t.i.d. for 6.33 days) erythromycin increased $AUC_{ss(0\text{-}12\,h)}$ of fexofenadine from 2422 to 5055 ng/mL·h (109%), reduced oral clearance by 51%, extended t_{max} from 2.2 to 3.7 hours and increased C_{max} from 410 to 744 ng/mL (80%) in 20 healthy volunteers. Renal clearance was increased from 3.6 to 4 L/h. Fexofenadine had no effect on the pharmacokinetics of erythromycin.

Ketoconazole coadministration (fexofenadine 120 mg b.i.d. plus ketoconazole 400 mg daily for 7 days) increased $AUC_{ss\,(0\text{-}12h)}$ of fexofenadine from 2100 to 5547 ng/mL·h (164%), reduced oral clearance by 61% and increased C_{max} from 388 to 914 ng/mL (136%) in 24 healthy volunteers. Fexofenadine had no effect on the pharmacokinetics of ketoconazole.

The increased systemic exposure to fexofenadine as a result of erythromycin or ketoconazole coadministration is below that observed with 240 or 400 mg b.i.d. doses (AUC_{ss} of 6935 and 13 578 ng/mL·h, respectively) of fexofenadine, neither of which was associated with any adverse effects.

INDICATIONS: Allergic Rhinitis: Allegra is indicated for the relief of symptoms associated with seasonal (Allegra 12 Hour, Allegra 24 Hour) and perennial (Allegra 12 Hour) allergic rhinitis, in adults and children 12 years of age and over.

Symptoms treated effectively include sneezing, rhinorrhea, lacrimation, itchy, red eyes and itchy nose/palate/throat. Allegra improves health-related quality of life and work/activity productivity.

Chronic Idiopathic Urticaria: Allegra 12 Hour is indicated for the relief of symptoms associated with chronic idiopathic urticaria in adults and children 12 years of age and older. Allegra 12 Hour significantly reduces the signs and symptoms of chronic idiopathic urticaria, the number of wheals and pruritus. Allegra 12 Hour improves health-related quality of life and work/activity productivity.

CONTRAINDICATIONS: In patients with known hypersensitivity to any of its ingredients.

PRECAUTIONS: *Drug Interactions:* Since fexofenadine does not undergo hepatic biotransformation, it is unlikely to interact with drugs that rely upon hepatic metabolism.

Allegra 12 Hour at twice the recommended dose (120 mg b.i.d.), has been safely coadministered with erythromycin (500 mg q8h) and ketoconazole (400 mg once daily) under steady-state conditions in healthy volunteers. No differences in adverse events were reported whether fexofenadine was administered alone or in combination. The coadministration of fexofenadine with erythromycin or ketoconazole resulted in no significant increases in daily mean or maximum QT_c interval when analyzed by machine or a cardiologist.

The mechanism of these interactions has been evaluated in in vitro, in situ, and in vivo animal models. These studies indicate that ketoconazole or erythromycin coadministration enhances fexofenadine gastrointestinal absorption. In vivo animal studies also suggest that in addition to enhancing absorption, ketoconazole decreases fexofenadine gastrointestinal secretion, while erythromycin may also decrease biliary excretion.

The administration of a single 20 mL dose of Maalox suspension followed 15 minutes later by a single oral dose of 120 mg fexofenadine resulted in a significant reduction in fexofenadine bioavailability (41% reduction in $AUC_{(0-30h)}$; 43% reduction in C_{max}). This interaction has been explained on the basis that up to 27.8% of fexofenadine is physically bound to Maalox in the stomach at pH of 4 or greater.

Pretreatment with omeprazole (20 mg 10 hours prior to and 40 mg 1 hour prior to a single dose of 120 mg fexofenadine) did not alter the bioavailability of fexofenadine.

Pregnancy: The reproduction toxicology data for fexofenadine rely solely upon those that have been obtained with terfenadine (Seldane) and linked by appropriate bridging pharmacokinetic studies.

There was no evidence of teratogenicity in rats or rabbits at fexofenadine plasma AUC values 4 and 37 times the human therapeutic value, respectively. Dose-related decreases in pup weight gain and survival were observed in rats exposed to fexofenadine plasma AUC values equal to or greater than 3 times the human therapeutic value (obtained at steady state with 60 mg b.i.d. dosing).

There are no adequate and well-controlled studies in pregnant women. Fexofenadine should be used during pregnancy only if the potential benefit justifies the potential risk to the fetus.

Lactation: There are no adequate and well controlled studies in women during lactation. However, when terfenadine was administered to nursing mothers, fexofenadine was found to cross into human breast milk. Therefore, fexofenadine is not recommended for breast-feeding women.

Children: The safety and effectiveness of fexofenadine in children under 12 years of age have not been established. In a randomized, controlled, clinical trial setting, a total of 205 subjects between the ages of 12 to 16 years were administered doses of fexofenadine ranging from 20 to 240 mg b.i.d. for 2 weeks. Adverse events were similar in this group compared to subjects above 16 years of age.

Geriatrics: In placebo-controlled trials 35 patients aged 65 to 74 years received fexofenadine doses of 20 to 240 mg b.i.d., and 4 patients 75 years and over received fexofenadine doses of 60 to 180 mg once daily. Adverse events were similar in this group compared to patients under 65 years of age. Nevertheless, the pharmacokinetics of fexofenadine are altered (increased bioavailability) in individuals over 65 years of age (see Pharmacology, Pharmacokinetics).

Special Populations: The pharmacokinetics of fexofenadine are altered in individuals with renal impairment (see Pharmacology, Pharmacokinetics). Based on increases in bioavailability and half-life, a dose of 60 mg once daily is recommended as the starting dose in patients with decreased renal function.

Moderate to severe hepatic disease does not affect the pharmacokinetics of fexofenadine substantially.

In surgically manipulated intestinal tissue (e.g., bowel resection) as well as in inflamed intestinal tissue, p-glycoprotein expression is actually increased. Thus, the oral bioavailability of fexofenadine could possibly be reduced in these disease states.

ADVERSE EFFECTS: In 4, 2-week, placebo-controlled seasonal allergic rhinitis trials with doses of 20 to 240 mg twice daily, adverse events were similar in fexofenadine and placebo-treated patients. There was no dose-related increase in adverse events, including drowsiness, when administered up to 4 times the recommended therapeutic dose. Adverse event rates were similar among subgroups defined by age, gender, and race. The rate of premature withdrawal because of adverse events was 2% (48/2346) with fexofenadine vs 3.2% (22/685) with placebo. See Table 1.

Table 1: Allegra

Percentage of Patients Reporting Adverse Events (≥1%) in Placebo-controlled Seasonal Allergic Rhinitis Clinical Trials (b.i.d. dosing)

Adverse Event	Placebo (n=671)	Allegra 60 mg b.i.d (n=679)	Total Allegra 20-240 mg b.i.d. (n=2319)
Headache	3.1	3.1	2.9
Nausea	1.0	1.3	0.8
Drowsiness	0.9	1.3	0.8
Fatigue	0.9	1.0	1.0

In addition to the above, the following infrequent (≥0.1 to <1%) adverse events were reported at rates similar to placebo in the controlled SAR studies with doses from 20 to 240 mg b.i.d. and have been reported rarely during postmarketing surveillance:

Body as a Whole: in rare cases, rash, urticaria, pruritus and hypersensitivity reactions with manifestations such as angioedema, chest tightness, dyspnea, flushing and systemic anaphylaxis.

Central and Peripheral Nervous Systems: insomnia, dizziness.

Gastrointestinal: diarrhea, dyspepsia, abdominal pain, flatulence, vomiting.

Respiratory: epistaxis, throat irritation.

Metabolic and Nutritional: thirst.

Psychiatric: appetite increase, nervousness, agitation, sleep disorders or paroniria.

Autonomic Nervous System: dry mouth, dryness of mucous membranes.

Skin and Appendages: pruritus, rash, urticaria

Urinary: urinary frequency.

Cardiovascular System: tachycardia, palpitation.

Infectious Disease: viral infection.

Vision: blurred vision.

Hearing and Vestibular: earache.

One 2-week, placebo-controlled trial evaluated once daily fexofenadine doses of 120 mg and 180 mg. Table 2 lists all adverse reactions reported by ≥1% of fexofenadine treated patients. The rate of premature withdrawal because of adverse events was 1.2% (7/570) with fexofenadine vs 1.4% (4/293) with placebo.

Table 2: Allegra

Percentage of Patients Reporting Adverse Reactions (≥1%) in Placebo-controlled Seasonal Allergic Rhinitis Clinical Trials (once daily dosing)

Adverse Event	Placebo (n=293)	Allegra 120 mg once daily (n=287)	Allegra 180 mg once daily (n=283)	Total Allegra 120–180 mg once daily (n=570)
Headache	1.4	1.7	3.9	2.8
Epistaxis	0.0	0.3	1.1	0.7
Abdominal Pain	0.3	0.7	1.1	0.9

In a 4-week trial conducted in perennial allergic rhinitis, the nature and incidence of adverse events observed were comparable for fexofenadine (60 mg b.i.d., 120 mg once daily) and placebo, and similar to those observed in the seasonal allergic rhinitis trials.

In 2, 4-week, placebo-controlled chronic idiopathic urticaria clinical trials evaluating doses of 20 to 240 mg twice daily, adverse reactions were similar in fexofenadine and placebo-treated patients, with no dose-related increase. Table 3 lists all adverse reactions reported by at least 1% of patients. The proportion of patients who withdrew prematurely because of adverse reactions was 3.6% (26/713) with fexofenadine vs 3.9% (7/178) with placebo.

Table 3: Allegra

Percentage of Patients Reporting Adverse Reactions (≥1%) in Placebo-controlled Chronic Idiopathic Urticaria Clinical Trials

Adverse Event	Placebo (n=178)	Allegra 60 mg b.i.d. (n=186)	Total Allegra 20–240 mg b.i.d. (n=713)
Headache	11.2	10.2	10.5
Diarrhea	0.6	1.6	0.8
Dyspepsia	2.2	1.6	2.0
Somnolence	0	1.6	1.5
Abdominal Pain	2.2	1.1	1.3
Dizziness	0.6	1.1	0.8
Dry Eyes	0.0	1.1	0.6
Insomnia	0.6	1.1	1.8
Nausea	3.9	1.1	3.1

In all studies, the frequency and magnitude of laboratory abnormalities were similar with fexofenadine and placebo.

Two double-blind, placebo-controlled, parallel group, long-term safety studies were conducted in healthy volunteers. In 1 study, 217 subjects received 60 mg fexofenadine b.i.d. for 6 months, and in the other, 234 subjects received 240 mg fexofenadine once daily for 12 months. The nature and incidence of adverse events observed were similar for fexofenadine and placebo, and the types of adverse events reported in these 2 long-term studies were not different from those observed in the Phase III clinical trials. There were no particular patterns observed in the occurrence of treatment related adverse events in demographic subgroups with respect to gender, age and race. There were no statistically significant changes in measured ECG parameters or vital signs from baseline to the last visit in subjects treated with fexofenadine vs placebo.

In U.S. postmarketing surveillance, 1 case of congestive heart failure has been reported. One case of atrial fibrillation has been reported in clinical studies. A definite cause and effect relationship has not been established.

OVERDOSE:

Symptoms: Most reports of fexofenadine overdose have been infrequent and contain limited information. However, dizziness, drowsiness, and dry mouth have been reported. Single doses of fexofenadine up to 800 mg and doses up to 690 mg b.i.d. for 1 month or 240 once daily for 1 year were investigated without the development of clinically significant adverse events as compared to placebo. The maximum tolerated dose of fexofenadine was not established. Overall, there was no evidence of QT_c prolongation at doses 11 times the recommended therapeutic dose.

Treatment: In the event of overdose, standard measures to remove any unabsorbed drug should be considered. Symptomatic and supportive treatment is recommended.

Hemodialysis did not effectively remove fexofenadine from blood (up to 1.7% removed) following terfenadine administration.

For management of a suspected drug overdose, CPhA recommends that you contact your **regional Poison Control Centre**. See the *CPS* Directory section for a list of Poison Control Centres.

DOSAGE: A dose of 60 mg once daily is recommended as the starting dose in patients with decreased renal function.

Safety and effectiveness of fexofenadine in children under the age of 12 have not been established.

Adults and Children, 12 years and older: Seasonal Allergic Rhinitis: Allegra 12 Hour: The recommended dose is 60 mg every 12 hours. Or Allegra 24 Hour: 120 mg tablet once daily.

Perennial Allergic Rhinitis: Allegra 12 Hour: The recommended dose is 60 mg every 12 hours.

Chronic Idiopathic Urticaria: Allegra 12 Hour: The recommended dose is 60 mg every 12 hours.

INFORMATION FOR THE PATIENT: Published in e-CPS, available by subscription at www.e-cps.ca.

SUPPLIED: Allegra 12 Hour: Each peach, oval, double convex tablet, engraved on one side with an "e" and with "06" on the other side, contains: fexofenadine HCl 60 mg. Nonmedicinal ingredients: croscarmellose sodium, hydroxypropyl methylcellulose, iron oxide, magnesium stearate, microcrystalline cellulose, polyethylene glycol, povidone, silicon dioxide, starch and titanium dioxide. Lactose-free. Blister packs of 12, 24 and 36.

Allegra 24 Hour: Each peach, oblong, double convex tablet, plain on one side and engraved on the other side with "012", contains: fexofenadine HCl 120 mg. Nonmedicinal ingredients: croscarmellose sodium, hydroxypropyl methylcellulose, iron oxide, magnesium stearate, microcrystalline cellulose, polyethylene glycol, povidone, silicon dioxide, starch and titanium dioxide. Lactose-free. Blister packs of 6, 12 and 18.

Store at 15 to 30°C in a dry place.

(Shown in Product Identification Section)

Allegra®-D

fexofenadine HCl—pseudoephedrine HCl

Histamine H1-Receptor Antagonist—Sympathomimetic Amine

sanofi-aventis

Date of Revision: March 5, 2010

PHARMACOLOGY: Allegra-D is a combination product containing a nonsedating antihistamine with selective peripheral H_1-receptor antagonist activity and an orally active sympathomimetic amine that exerts a decongestant action on the nasal mucosa.

Fexofenadine is the predominant human and animal active metabolite of terfenadine. Fexofenadine inhibits histamine induced skin wheal and flare responses. Following single and twice daily oral administration, antihistaminic effects occur within one hour, achieve a maximum at 2 to 3 hours, and last a minimum of 12 hours. There is no evidence of tolerance to these effects after 28 days of dosing.

Pseudoephedrine is an orally active sympathomimetic amine which exerts a decongestant action on the nasal mucosa. Pseudoephedrine is recognized as an effective agent for the relief of nasal congestion due to allergic rhinitis.

In randomized, double-blind, placebo-controlled trials, a daily dose of fexofenadine 60 mg b.i.d. was shown to be effective in relieving the symptoms of seasonal allergic rhinitis (trees and grasses in the spring or ragweed pollen in the fall). These symptoms consisted of sneezing, rhinorrhea, itchy nose/palate/throat and itchy, watery, red eyes.

In a randomized, double-blind, parallel-design safety and efficacy study, a daily dose of fexofenadine 60 mg/pseudoephedrine 120 mg b.i.d. was more effective than the decongestant alone (pseudoephedrine 120 mg b.i.d.) for histamine-mediated symptoms of seasonal allergic rhinitis, and more effective than the antihistamine component alone (fexofenadine 60 mg b.i.d.) for the nonhistamine-mediated symptoms of seasonal allergic rhinitis. Moreover, the combination therapy demonstrated higher improvement in the regular daily activities and work productivity than its components alone. There was no statistically significant difference in the treatment effect in subgroups defined by age, sex, race or weight.

Pharmacokinetics: Fexofenadine+Pseudoephedrine: Fexofenadine was rapidly absorbed following multiple dose administration of the 60 mg fexofenadine/120 mg pseudoephedrine caplet to healthy volunteers with a mean peak fexofenadine plasma concentration 233 ng/mL, which occurred 2.1 hours postdose. Pseudoephedrine, in the same study, produced a mean peak pseudoephedrine plasma concentration of 405 ng/mL which occurred 4.8 hours postdose.

Coadministration of Allegra-D with a high fat meal decreased fexofenadine bioavailability; however, the rate or extent of pseudoephedrine absorption was not affected. Allegra-D should be taken on an empty stomach.

Fexofenadine: Fexofenadine is rapidly absorbed following oral administration. The single and multiple dose pharmacokinetics of fexofenadine were linear from 20 mg to 120 mg doses. T_{max} occurs at approximately 2.6 hours and C_{max} is approximately 209 ng/mL following oral administration of a single 60 mg dose.

Following a single 60 mg oral dose, 80% of the total fexofenadine dose was recovered in the feces and 11% was recovered in the urine.

Following multiple dosing, fexofenadine has an apparent elimination half-life of 11 to 16 hours. Steady-state pharmacokinetic parameters following 60 mg b.i.d. dosing are: $AUC_{ss\,(0\text{-}12h)}$=1 367 ng/mL·h, Cmax=299 ng/mL, C_{min}=29 ng/mL, t_{max}=1 h.

The pharmacokinetics of fexofenadine in seasonal allergic rhinitis patients are similar to that of otherwise healthy subjects. Peak fexofenadine plasma concentrations were similar between adolescent (12 to 16 years of age) and adult patients.

Pseudoephedrine: Pseudoephedrine has been shown to have a mean elimination half-life of 4 to 8 hours which is dependent on urine pH. The elimination half-life is decreased at urine pH lower than 6 and may be increased at urine pH higher than 8. About 43 to 96% of an administered dose is excreted unchanged in the urine; the remainder is apparently metabolized in the liver.

Special Populations: There are no data available on special populations following the administration of Allegra-D. The following presentation is related to the pharmacokinetics in special populations following a single 80 mg oral dose of fexofenadine. The pharmacokinetics were compared to those from normal subjects in a separate study of similar design. While subjects' weights were relatively uniform between the studies, the special population patients were older than the healthy, young volunteers. Thus, an age effect may be confounding the pharmacokinetic differences observed.

Renal Impairment: Following a single 80 mg oral dose, renal clearance is decreased to 68, 15 and 3% of the control value (3.63 L/h) in patients with mild to moderate impairment (creatinine clearance 41 to 80 mL/min; n=9), moderate to severe impairment (creatinine clearance 11 to 40 mL/min; n=10) and dialysis patients (creatinine clearance <10 mL/min; n=10). The corresponding $AUC_{0\text{-}\infty}$ and C_{max} were increased by 80, 154 and 88%, respectively (control value=1 788.1 ng/mL·h), and by 58, 78 and 54%, respectively (control value=248.7 ng/mL). The half-life increased from 13.7 hours to 22.8, 24.8 and 18.9 hours, respectively.

Hepatic Impairment: The pharmacokinetics of fexofenadine in 14 patients with hepatic disease (moderate, n=9; moderate to severe, n=5), did not differ substantially from that observed in healthy subjects. The lack of effect may be explained by the fact that none of the patients investigated suffered from complete biliary obstruction, as biliary excretion is one of the major elimination pathways for fexofenadine.

Effect of Age: The pharmacokinetics of fexofenadine in healthy elderly individuals (>65 years old, n=20) were different from those observed in healthy younger individuals following a single oral dose of 80 mg fexofenadine. Mean AUC was 63% higher (control value=1 788 ng/mL.h), oral clearance 30% lower (control value= 48 L/h), renal clearance 24% less (control value=3.6 L/h), C_{max} 68% higher (control value=248.7 ng/mL) and half-life 10% longer (15.2 h).

Effect of Sex: The steady-state AUC and C_{max} values in female subjects (n=20) were 33% and 46% higher, respectively, than those observed in male subjects (n=20). Renal clearance was equivalent. There was no indication of any difference in safety or efficacy.

INDICATIONS: For the effective relief of sneezing, rhinorrhea, itchy nose/palate/throat, itchy/watery/red eyes, and temporary relief of nasal congestion associated with seasonal allergic rhinitis in adults and children 12 years of age and older.

Allegra-D is indicated for patients who may not receive complete relief from antihistamines alone and in whom both the antihistaminic properties of fexofenadine and the nasal decongestant properties of pseudoephedrine are desired.

CONTRAINDICATIONS: In patients with known hypersensitivity or idiosyncrasy to any of its ingredients, to adrenergic agents or to other drugs of similar chemical structures.

Allegra-D is also contraindicated in patients with severe hypertension, or severe coronary artery disease, narrow-angle glaucoma or urinary retention, and in patients receiving MAOI therapy or within 14 days of stopping such treatment. Patients who have shown sensitivity to adrenergic agents (manifestations include insomnia, dizziness, weakness, tremor, or arrhythmias).

WARNINGS: Pseudoephedrine, like other sympathomimetic amines, may produce CNS stimulation with convulsions or cardiovascular collapse.

PRECAUTIONS: General: Allegra-D should be used with caution in patients with hypertension, diabetes mellitus, ischemic heart disease, increased intraocular pressure, hyperthyroidism, renal impairment, prostatic hypertrophy, or hyperreactivity to ephedrine.

Sympathomimetics should be used with caution in patients receiving digitalis.

Sympathomimetics may cause CNS stimulation and convulsions or cardiovascular collapse with accompanying hypotension.

Pregnancy: There are no adequate and well controlled studies in pregnant women. Allegra-D should be used during pregnancy only if the potential benefit justifies the potential risk to the fetus.

Lactation: Allegra-D is not recommended for nursing women unless the potential benefit to the patient outweighs the potential risk to the infant. Following administration of terfenadine to nursing mothers, fexofenadine crosses into human breast milk and pseudoephedrine administered alone, distributes into breast milk.

Children: Safety and effectiveness of Allegra-D have not been established in children under 12 years of age.

Renal Impairment: Patients with decreased renal function should be given a lower initial dose, 1 caplet/day, due to the reduced elimination of fexofenadine and pseudoephedrine.

Geriatrics: The elderly are more likely to have adverse reactions to sympathomimetic amines.

Dependence Liability: There are no data available to indicate that abuse or dependency occurs with Allegra-D.

Drug Interactions: Fexofenadine has no effect on the pharmacokinetics of erythromycin and ketoconazole. The coadministration of fexofenadine with erythromycin or ketoconazole resulted in no significant increases in QT_c. No differences in adverse effects were reported whether this agent was administered alone or in combination with erythromycin or ketoconazole.

Since fexofenadine does not undergo hepatic biotransformation, it is unlikely to interact with drugs that rely upon hepatic metabolism.

The administration of a single 20 mL dose of Maalox suspension followed 15 minutes later by a single oral dose of 120 mg fexofenadine resulted in a significant reduction in fexofenadine bioavailability (41% reduction in $AUC_{(0\text{-}30h)}$; 43% reduction in C_{max}). This interaction has been explained on the basis that up to 27.8% of fexofenadine is physically bound to Maalox in the stomach at pH of 4 or greater (see Information for the Patient).

Concomitant use of pseudoephedrine with MAOIs and use within 14 days after stopping an MAOI are contraindicated.

Concomitant use of pseudoephedrine with antihypertensive drugs which interfere with sympathetic activity may reduce their antihypertensive effects.

Concomitant use of pseudoephedrine with sympathomimetic agents may have additive cardiovascular effects.

Drug/Laboratory Test Interactions: Allegra-D should be discontinued approximately 3 days prior to skin testing procedures since antihistamines may prevent or diminish otherwise positive reactions to dermal reactivity indications.

ADVERSE EFFECTS: Adverse events reported in the clinical trials were similar to adverse events reported in placebo-controlled clinical trials for fexofenadine and similar to effects attributable to pseudoephedrine.

Of the 651 patients that were enrolled in the safety and efficacy clinical trial and were evaluated for intent-to-treat, 218 received fexofenadine 60 mg, 218 received pseudoephedrine 120 mg, and 215 received fexofenadine 60 mg/pseudoephedrine 120 mg combination.

Of the 177 subjects enrolled in the pharmacokinetic studies, 21 were also exposed to fexofenadine 60 mg alone and 22 were exposed to pseudoephedrine 120 mg alone.

A total of 392 subjects have been exposed to Allegra-D and were evaluable for safety. Of these 392 subjects, 177 were healthy volunteers exposed to the treatment drug in 6 pharmacokinetic studies and 215 were patients suffering from seasonal allergic rhinitis (SAR) who were enrolled in a safety and efficacy clinical trial.

In clinical pharmacokinetic trials, subjects receiving Allegra-D reported adverse events similar to adverse events reported in placebo-controlled trials for fexofenadine and similar effects attributable to pseudoephedrine.

In the controlled clinical efficacy and safety study there were no statistically significant differences among the treatment groups with respect to sex, race, weight, height and years since first episode of seasonal (ragweed) allergic rhinitis (SAR) occurred. No statistically significant differences between treatment groups were found for baseline symptom assessments with the exception of sneezing.

Out of 651 patients evaluated for safety in the safety and efficacy trial, 280 patients (43%) experienced one or more adverse events. The most common adverse events were headache 14%, insomnia 10%, nausea 4%, dry mouth 3%, dizziness 2%.

Adverse events considered possibly or probably related to study medication in 17% of the patients receiving fexofenadine, 37% of the patients receiving pseudoephedrine and 35% of the patients who received the combination are presented in Table 1.

Table 1: Allegra-D
Adverse Events Possibly/Probably Related to Study Medication in the Clinical Trial

	Treatment Group			
System	**Fexofenadine n=218 n (%)**	**Pseudoephedrine n=218 n (%)**	**Allegra-D n=215 n (%)**	**Total n=651 n (%)**
Total Occurrence (patients with one or more adverse event)	36 (17)	80 (37)	75 (35)	191 (29)
Neurologic				
Headache	16 (7.3)	27 (12.4)	20 (9.3)	63 (9.7)
Dizziness	0 (0.0)	6 (2.8)	4 (1.9)	10 (1.5)
Psychomotor Hyperactivity	1 (0.5)	2 (0.9)	2 (0.9)	5 (0.8)
Drowsiness	0 (0.0)	3 (1.4)	1 (0.5)	4 (0.6)
Psychiatric				
Insomnia	4 (1.8)	28 (12.8)	24 (11.2)	56 (8.6)
Nervousness	1 (0.5)	4 (1.8)	3 (1.4)	8 (1.2)
Agitation	0 (0.0)	3 (1.4)	4 (1.9)	7 (1.1)
Anxiety	0 (0.0)	3 (1.4)	3 (1.4)	6 (0.9)
Restlessness	1 (0.5)	2 (0.9)	1 (0.5)	4 (0.6)
Gastrointestinal				
Nausea	1 (0.5)	10 (4.6)	12 (5.6)	23 (3.5)
Dry Mouth	1 (0.5)	12 (5.5)	6 (2.8)	19 (2.9)
Dyspepsia	1 (0.5)	1 (0.5)	4 (1.9)	6 (0.9)
Dry Throat	1 (0.5)	2 (0.9)	2 (0.9)	5 (0.8)
Respiratory				
Throat Irritation	2 (0.9)	0 (0.0)	3 (1.4)	5 (0.8)
Epistaxis	2 (0.9)	1 (0.5)	1 (0.5)	4 (0.6)
Sinus Headache	0 (0.0)	2 (0.9)	2 (0.9)	4 (0.6)
Body as a Whole				
Abdominal Pain	1 (0.5)	1 (0.5)	1 (0.5)	3 (0.5)
Fatigue	0 (0.0)	1 (0.5)	2 (0.9)	3 (0.5)
Cardiovascular				
Palpitation	0 (0.0)	2 (0.9)	4 (1.9)	6 (0.9)
Tachycardia	0 (0.0)	4 (1.8)	2 (0.9)	6 (0.9)
Dermatologic				
Rash	0 (0.0)	1 (0.5)	2 (0.9)	3 (0.5)
Acne	0 (0.0)	0 (0.0)	2 (0.9)	2 (0.3)

Clinical adverse events occurring in less than 1% of patients treated with Allegra-D in clinical trials which have been reported rarely during postmarketing surveillance, are listed below by body system:

Body as a Whole: In rare cases, rash, urticaria, pruritus, and hypersensitivity reactions with manifestations such as angioedema, chest tightness, dyspnea, flushing and systemic anaphylaxis, fatigue, chills, lassitude, neck pain, thoracic cage pain.

Hematologic: eosinophilia, leukocytosis, neutrophilia.

Respiratory: epistaxis, hemoptysis, nasal dryness, nasal irritation, pharyngitis, sinusitis, wheezing.

Cardiovascular: AV block, atrial arrhythmia, tachycardia, heart murmur, syncope.

Gastrointestinal: abdominal pain, constipation, dyspepsia, diarrhea, dry throat, dry lips, aphthous stomatitis.

Metabolic and Nutritional: hyperkalemia, hyperlipemia, hypoglycemia, hyperglycemia.

Hepatic and Biliary Systems: bilirubinemia, AST increased, ALT increased.

Ophthalmic: dry eyes.

Dermatologic: rash, urticaria, pruritus, acne, cold sweat, seborrhea.

Neurologic: drowsiness, psychomotor hyperactivity, somnolence, tremor.

Psychiatric: restlessness, irritability, anorexia, increased energy, depersonalization, sleep disorder or paroniria.

Musculoskeletal: myopathy, knee pain, tendon rupture.

Special Senses: taste perversion, taste metallic.

Pseudoephedrine has also been associated with other adverse effects such as anorexia, fear, anxiety, tenseness, weakness, pressor activity/hypertension, tremor, hallucinations, seizures, pallor, respiratory difficulty, difficulty in micturition, cardiac arrhythmia, cardiovascular collapse, and ischemic colitis. Pseudoephedrine may produce mild CNS stimulation.

Clinical Laboratory Test Findings: Statistically significant mean changes from baseline to endstudy were observed for ALT, albumin, hemoglobin, RBC, WBC, chloride and total cholesterol. However, these changes were not considered clinically significant.

OVERDOSE:

Symptoms: Fexofenadine: Most reports of fexofenadine overdose contain limited information. However, dizziness, drowsiness, and dry mouth have been reported. Single doses up to 800 mg and doses up to 690 mg b.i.d. for 1 month or 240 mg once daily for 1 year were studied in healthy subjects without the development of clinically significant adverse events as compared to placebo. The maximum tolerated dose of fexofenadine was not established.

Pseudoephedrine: Serious effects associated with pseudoephedrine overdosage include respiratory difficulty, convulsions, arrhythmias, hypertension and cardiovascular collapse.

Manifestations: These may vary from CNS depression (sedation, apnea, diminished mental alertness, cyanosis, coma, cardiovascular collapse) to stimulation (insomnia, hallucination, tremors or convulsions) to death. Other signs and symptoms may be euphoria, excitement, tachycardia, palpitations, thirst, perspiration, nausea, dizziness, tinnitus, ataxia, blurred vision and hypertension or hypotension. Stimulation is particularly likely in children, as are atropine-like signs and symptoms (dry mouth; fixed, dilated pupils; flushing; hyperthermia; and gastrointestinal symptoms).

In large doses, sympathomimetics may give rise to giddiness, headache, nausea, vomiting, sweating, thirst, tachycardia, precordial pain, palpitations, difficulty in micturition, muscular weakness and tenseness, anxiety, restlessness and insomnia. Many patients can present a toxic psychosis with delusions and hallucinations. Some may develop cardiac arrhythmias, circulatory collapse, convulsions, coma and respiratory failure.

Treatment: In the event of overdosage, treatment which should be started immediately, is symptomatic and supportive. Discontinuation of use, gastric lavage or induction of emesis (except in patients with impaired consciousness) and support of vital functions are advised.

The patient should be induced to vomit, even if emesis has occurred spontaneously. Pharmacologically-induced vomiting by the administration of ipecac syrup is a preferred method. However, vomiting should not be induced in patients with impaired consciousness. The action of ipecac is facilitated by physical activity and by the administration of 240 to 360 mL of water. If emesis does not occur within 15 minutes, the dose of ipecac should be repeated. Precautions against aspiration must be taken, especially in children. Following emesis, adsorption of any drugs remaining in the stomach may be attempted by the administration of activated charcoal as a slurry with water. If vomiting is unsuccessful, or contraindicated, gastric lavage should be performed. Physiologic saline solution is the lavage solution of choice, particularly in children. In adults, tap water can be used; however, as much as possible of the amount administered should be removed before the next instillation. Saline cathartics draw water into the bowel by osmosis and therefore may be valuable for their action in rapid dilution of bowel content.

Fexofenadine is not effectively cleared by hemodialysis from the blood. The effect of hemodialysis on pseudoephedrine is unknown.

Excretion of pseudoephedrine is increased by lowering the pH of the urine.

After emergency treatment, the patient should continue to be medically monitored.

Stimulants (analeptic agents) should not be used. Vasopressors may be used to treat hypotension. Short-acting barbiturates, diazepam or paraldehyde may be administered to control seizures. Hyperpyrexia, especially in children, may require treatment with tepid water sponge baths or hypothermic blanket. Apnea is treated with ventilatory support.

> For management of a suspected drug overdose, CPhA recommends that you contact your **regional Poison Control Centre**. See the *CPS* Directory section for a list of Poison Control Centres.

DOSAGE: Adults and Children 12 Years of Age and older: 1 caplet twice daily, swallowed whole on an empty stomach.
Children Under 12 Years of Age: Safety and effectiveness have not been established in this population.
Renal Impairment: A dose of 1 caplet once daily is recommended as a starting dose (see Precautions).

INFORMATION FOR THE PATIENT: Published in e-CPS, available by subscription at www.e-cps.ca.

SUPPLIED: Each caplet engraved with "06/012D" on the white layer contains: fexofenadine HCl 60 mg and pseudoephedrine HCl 120 mg. Available as a bi-layer clear film coated caplet (capsule-shaped tablet) with one half (lengthwise) white to off-white and the other half tan. The fexofenadine layer is an immediate-release formulation; the pseudoephedrine layer is a sustained-release formulation. Nonmedicinal ingredients: carnauba wax, cornstarch, croscarmellose sodium, hydroxypropyl methylcellulose, magnesium stearate, microcrystalline cellulose, polyethylene glycol, silicon dioxide and stearic acid. Blister packs of 10, 20 and 30. Store at 15 to 30°C. Protect from light and moisture.

(Shown in Product Identification Section)

Allernix
diphenhydramine HCl
Antihistamine

Rougier Pharma

SUPPLIED: Caplets: 25 mg: Each oblong, biconvex, white core caplet with a pink coating contains: diphenhydramine HCl USP 25 mg. Nonmedicinal ingredients: FD&C red #3 aluminum lake, hydroxypropyl methylcellulose, magnesium stearate, microcrystalline cellulose, polydextrose, polyethylene glycol, sodium croscarmellose, titanium dioxide and triacetin. Bottles of 100. Blister packs of 20. Keep bottle tightly closed and protect from light.
50 mg: Each oblong, biconvex, white core caplet with a white coating contains: diphenhydramine HCl USP 50 mg. Nonmedicinal ingredients: hydroxypropyl methylcellulose, magnesium stearate, microcrystalline cellulose, polydextrose, polyethylene glycol, sodium croscarmellose, titanium dioxide and triacetin. Bottles of 100. Blister packs of 20. Keep bottle tightly closed and protect from light.
Solution: Each 5 mL of pink, cinnamon-flavored solution contains: diphenhydramine HCl USP 12.5 mg. Nonmedicinal ingredients: alcohol, artificial coloring and flavoring, citric acid, glycerin, purified water, sodium benzoate and sucrose. Bottles of 100 and 450 mL. Keep bottle tightly closed and protect from light and freezing.
Store between 15 and 30°C.

Allopurinol Ⓟ
Xanthine Oxidase Inhibitor

CPhA Monograph

Date of Revision: October 2007

> This monograph has been compiled by CPhA and reviewed by experts. It may contain information different from that found in Health Canada-approved Product Monographs. The reader is referred to the *CPS* Editorial Policy for more information.

Summary Product Information:

Route of Administration[a]	Dosage Form[a]	Strength[a]
Oral	Tablet	100 mg, 200 mg, 300 mg

[a] For specific product information consult Health Canada's Drug Product Database http://www.hc-sc.gc.ca/dhp-mps/prodpharma/databasdon/index_e.html

PHARMACOLOGY: Allopurinol reduces uric acid concentrations in both serum and urine. Along with its active metabolite, oxypurinol, allopurinol inhibits xanthine oxidase, the enzyme responsible for the conversion of hypoxanthine to xanthine and of xanthine to uric acid. Inhibition of this enzyme accounts for the major pharmacologic effects of allopurinol. In addition, allopurinol increases reutilization of hypoxanthine and xanthine for nucleotide and nucleic acid synthesis, via an action involving the enzyme hypoxanthine-guanine phosphoribosyltransferase (HGPRTase). The resultant increase in nucleotide concentration leads to feedback inhibition of de novo purine synthesis.

Accompanying the decrease in uric acid produced by allopurinol is an increase in serum and urine concentrations of hypoxanthine and xanthine. Plasma concentrations of these oxypurines are only slightly increased, and renal clearance is rapid and greater than that of uric acid. In the absence of allopurinol, normal urinary output of oxypurines is almost solely in the form of uric acid. After administration of allopurinol, it is composed of hypoxanthine, xanthine and uric acid. Since each has its independent solubility, the concentration of uric acid in plasma is reduced without exposing the urinary tract to an excessive load of uric acid, thus decreasing the risk of crystalluria. By lowering the uric acid concentration in plasma to below its limit of solubility, allopurinol facilitates dissolution of tophi.

Pharmacokinetics: See Table 1.

Table 1: Allopurinol Pharmacokinetics

Absorption	80 to 90% of single 300 mg oral dose
Biotransformation	Hepatic[a]
Protein binding	None
Distribution	Distributed into total tissue water (except brain, where concentration is approximately 50% compared to other tissues).
Half-life	Allopurinol: 1 to 3 h Oxypurinol 12 to 30 h (average 15 h)[b]
Onset of action	2 to 3 days[c]
Time to peak serum concentrations	Allopurinol: 0.5 to 2 h Oxypurinol: 4.5 to 5 h
Time to peak effect	Decreases uric acid serum concentration to normal in 1 to 3 weeks.[d]
Duration of action	1 to 2 weeks after discontinuation of therapy.
Elimination	Renal: 5 to 7% as allopurinol, 70% as oxypurinol. Fecal: 20% within 48 to 72 h

[a] Approximately 70% of a dose is metabolized to the active metabolite, oxypurinol.
[b] May be prolonged in patients with renal impairment.
[c] Allopurinol's ability to lower serum uric acid appears dose-related.
[d] Because of continued mobilization of urate deposits, substantial decrease in uric acid may be delayed 6 to 12 months or may not occur in some patients, particularly those with tophaceous gout and those who are underexcretors of uric acid.

INDICATIONS: The treatment of gout, either primary, or secondary to hyperuricemia which occurs in polycythemia vera, myeloid metaplasia or other blood dyscrasias.

Allopurinol is also indicated in the treatment of primary or secondary uric acid nephropathy, with or without accompanying symptoms of gout.

Allopurinol may be given prophylactically to prevent tissue urate deposition or renal calculi as well as acute urate nephropathy and resultant renal failure in patients with leukemias, lymphomas or other malignancies who are receiving radiation therapy or antineoplastic drugs that will result in elevated serum uric acid concentrations.

To prevent the occurrence and recurrence of uric acid stones and renal calcium lithiasis in patients with hyperuricemia and/or hyperuricosuria.

CONTRAINDICATIONS: Allopurinol should not be given to patients who are hypersensitive to it or who have previously developed a severe reaction to this drug.

WARNINGS: Allopurinol should be discontinued at first appearance of skin rash or any sign of serious adverse reactions. Skin rash may sometimes be followed by more severe hypersensitivity reactions such as exfoliative, urticarial or purpuric lesions, as well as Stevens-Johnson syndrome (a sometimes fatal form of erythema multiforme) and, very rarely, generalized vasculitis which may lead to irreversible hepatotoxicity and death. Hypersensitivity reactions, frequently marked by fever and eosinophilia, usually begin 2 to 4 weeks after start of therapy and appear to be more common in patients with pre-existing renal dysfunction, elevated oxypurinol plasma levels and/or concurrent thiazide therapy.

In patients with cutaneous reactions to allopurinol for whom there is no therapeutic alternative, consideration should be given to desensitizing the patient to allopurinol.

Liver enzymes, renal function tests and complete blood counts should be performed before starting therapy then periodically during allopurinol therapy especially in patients with pre-existing liver disease, impaired renal function or diseases that may affect renal function. Alterations in liver enzymes, including transient elevations of serum alkaline phosphatase, AST and ALT, have occurred in some patients. Reversible hepatomegaly, hepatocellular damage (including necrosis), granulomatous changes, hepatitis and jaundice have also occurred.

Observe patients with impaired renal or hepatic function carefully during the early stages of allopurinol therapy and withdraw the drug if deterioration of hepatic or renal function occurs.

PRECAUTIONS: Allopurinol is not effective for the treatment of acute gouty attacks since it has no anti-inflammatory action and may intensify and prolong inflammation during the acute phase. However, allopurinol can be continued during acute attacks at the same dosage, in patients already established on allopurinol therapy.

When allopurinol therapy is initiated, acute gouty attacks may be precipitated, and these may continue even after serum uric acid concentrations begin to fall, usually for the first 6 to 12 months (see Dosage).

Although frequently selected before a uricosuric agent because of convenient once-daily dosing and effectiveness regardless of the cause of hyperuricemia, some rheumatologists recommend allopurinol be reserved for use in the following situations: when uricosurics cannot be used because of adverse effects, allergy, renal insufficiency or inadequate response; when there are visible tophi or radiographic evidence of uric acid deposits and stones; when urinary uric acid excretion is greater than 5.92 mmol/day (1000 mg/day); when serum urate concentrations are greater than 510 to 540 µmol/L (8.5 to 9 mg/100 mL) and there is a family history of tophi and low urate excretion.

In conditions where the body's miscible urate pool is greatly increased (e.g., malignant disease and its treatment, Lesch-Nyhan syndrome), the reduction of urate formation by allopurinol is accompanied by a relative rise in the xanthine and hypoxanthine fractions. In these circumstances, the absolute concentration of xanthine could rise to a level at which deposition in the urinary tract may occur. This risk may be minimized by adequate hydration to achieve maximum diuresis. Alkalinization of the urine can be of considerable benefit in the treatment of urate stones, but may be less effective in the presence of xanthine stones.

Drug Interactions: ACE Inhibitors: Isolated case reports indicate that concurrent administration of ACE inhibitors and allopurinol may increase the risk of hypersensitivity reactions, e.g., Stevens-Johnson syndrome, especially in patients with chronic renal failure. Patients already established on this combination should be monitored, and if a reaction occurs, the drugs should be discontinued.

Alcohol: Uricosuric effect of allopurinol may be decreased by alcohol.

Amoxicillin or Ampicillin: Concurrent ampicillin or amoxicillin and allopurinol therapy has resulted in an increased incidence of drug-induced skin rash. It is not clear whether this is due to allopurinol therapy.

Antacids: Concurrent administration of aluminum hydroxide-containing antacids with allopurinol may reduce gastrointestinal absorption of allopurinol. It is advisable that allopurinol be given at least 3 hours before the antacid.

Anticoagulants, Oral: Occasionally patients on oral anticoagulants and allopurinol develop an enhanced anticoagulant effect. INR should be monitored, and the oral anticoagulant dosage should be adjusted as needed.

Azathioprine and Mercaptopurine (Thiopurines): Allopurinol increases the pharmacologic and toxic effects of thiopurines by inhibiting their metabolism. Concomitant administration of azathioprine or mercaptopurine with allopurinol requires that initial thiopurine doses be reduced to 25% or 33% of the recommended initial dose. Subsequent doses should be adjusted according to clinical response.

Chlorpropamide: Allopurinol can compete with chlorpropamide for renal tubular secretion. When renal function is poor, the recognized risk of chlorpropamide's prolonged hypoglycemic activity may be increased if allopurinol is given concomitantly.

Co-trimoxazole: A few cases of thrombocytopenia have been reported in patients using this combination.

Cyclophosphamide: Concurrent cyclophosphamide and allopurinol therapy may increase the incidence of bone marrow depression as compared with cyclophosphamide alone, but the mechanism for this interaction is not known.

Diuretics: Thiazides and ethacrynic acid, when given with allopurinol, may increase serum oxypurinol concentrations and may thereby increase the risk of serious allopurinol toxicity, including hypersensitivity reactions, particularly in patients with decreased renal function.

Theophylline: Doses exceeding 600 mg/day of allopurinol may decrease theophylline clearance when both drugs are used for longer than 2 weeks. Since increases in serum theophylline concentrations of 25% have been reported, some patients may require monitoring for signs of possible theophylline toxicity and dosage adjustments during concurrent allopurinol therapy.

Uricosurics: Concomitant administration of a uricosuric agent, e.g., probenecid, and allopurinol may alter the disposition of both drugs. The combination usually results in an additive lowering of the serum uric acid level.
Occupational Hazards: Drowsiness may occur. Patients should be cautioned not to engage in activities where alertness is mandatory until their response to the drug is known.
Children: Allopurinol should not be given to children except those with hyperuricemia secondary to malignancy or with Lesch-Nyhan syndrome, because safety and effectiveness have not been established in other conditions.
Pregnancy: No adverse fetal outcomes attributable to allopurinol have been reported in humans. Assess risk versus benefit.
Lactation: Allopurinol and oxypurinol are distributed into breast milk. Limited data indicates that an exclusively breastfed infant would receive a near-therapeutic dose if allopurinol 300 mg daily were given to the lactating mother. Exclusively breastfed infants of mothers receiving allopurinol should be monitored for signs of allergic reaction such as rash. Also, perform periodic CBC and differential blood counts on infants whose mothers require treatment with allopurinol. Allopurinol is considered by the American Academy of Pediatrics to be compatible with breastfeeding.

ADVERSE EFFECTS: Dermatologic: Skin rash, usually maculopapular, is the most commonly reported adverse effect. Incidence of skin rash may be increased in the presence of renal disorders. In some instances, rashes have been followed by severe hypersensitivity reactions. Allopurinol should be discontinued immediately if such reactions occur (see Warnings). Exfoliative, urticarial or purpuric lesions, Stevens-Johnson syndrome (erythema multiforme), bullae and toxic epidermal necrolysis have also been reported. A few cases of alopecia with or without accompanying dermatitis have been reported. After recovery from *mild* reactions allopurinol may, if desired, be reintroduced at a low dose (e.g., 50 mg/day) and gradually increased. If the rash recurs, allopurinol should be discontinued permanently. The drug should not be reinstituted in patients who have had a severe reaction.
Gastrointestinal: Diarrhea, intermittent abdominal pain, nausea and vomiting have been reported. Gastrointestinal symptoms may be decreased by taking allopurinol with meals.
Generalized Hypersensitivity: Skin reactions associated with exfoliation, fever, chills, nausea and vomiting, lymphadenopathy, arthralgia and/or eosinophilia have occurred. These reactions may occur at any time during therapy and necessitate the immediate and permanent withdrawal of allopurinol. A generalized hypersensitivity vasculitis has rarely led to irreversible hepatotoxicity and death. Corticosteroids may be beneficial in managing such reactions.
When generalized hypersensitivity reactions have occurred, renal and/or hepatic dysfunction have usually been present.
Hematologic: There have been occasional reports of reduction in the number of circulating formed elements of the blood, including bone marrow suppression, granulocytopenia and thrombocytopenia, usually in association with renal and/or hepatic disorders or in whom concomitant drugs have been administered which have a potential for causing these reactions.
Miscellaneous: The following adverse effects have been reported occasionally: fever, general malaise, headache, vertigo, somnolence, taste perversion, hepatic necrosis, granulomatous hepatitis, abnormal liver function tests, rise in urea, hyperlipidemia, visual disorder, cataracts, macular changes, neuropathy, impotence, diabetes mellitus, furunculosis, hypertension, hematuria, edema, drowsiness, peripheral neuritis.

OVERDOSE:

For management of a suspected drug overdose, CPhA recommends that you contact your **regional Poison Control Centre**. See the *CPS* Directory section for a list of Poison Control Centres.

DOSAGE: Dosage of allopurinol varies with the severity of the disease and should be adjusted according to the response and tolerance of the patient. Allopurinol should not be started or stopped during an acute attack of gout but may be continued during acute attacks in patients already taking it (see Precautions).
Adults: Dosage range of 100 to 800 mg daily divided into 1 to 3 doses. Single dose should not exceed 300 mg. Allopurinol is better tolerated when taken with meals.
In all patients receiving allopurinol, a high fluid intake (e.g., 2.5 to 3 L daily) and the maintenance of a neutral or slightly alkaline urine are recommended.
Gout: Some investigators have reported an increase in acute attacks of gout during the early stages of allopurinol administration. Accordingly, allopurinol should be initiated at a dose of 100 to 200 mg daily and increased by 100 mg daily at weekly intervals, until a serum uric acid concentration of about 360 µmol/L (6 mg/dL) or less is attained, or until the maximum recommended dosage of 800 mg/day (in patients with normal renal function) is reached. In addition, concurrent administration of colchicine (0.6 mg twice daily) or an NSAID is recommended as prophylaxis during the first 3 to 6 months of allopurinol therapy. Serum urate concentrations are often reduced more slowly with allopurinol than with uricosuric agents, and minimum concentrations may not be reached for 1 to 3 weeks.
After serum urate concentrations are controlled, it may be possible to reduce dosage; the minimum effective dose is 100 to 200 mg/day. The average maintenance dosage is 200 to 300 mg/day for patients with mild gout, 400 to 600 mg/day for patients with moderately severe tophaceous gout, and 700 to 800 mg/day in severe conditions.
Dosage in Renal Impairment: Since allopurinol and its metabolites are excreted by the kidney, drug accumulation can occur if renal function is impaired; the initial dose of allopurinol should consequently be reduced. With a creatinine clearance of 0.33 to 0.17 mL/s, a daily dosage of 200 mg of allopurinol is suitable. When the creatinine clearance is less than 0.17 mL/s, the daily dosage should not exceed 100 mg. Some clinicians recommend the following maintenance dosages of allopurinol based on the patient's creatinine clearance (see Table 2). Refer to the Clin-Info Section for a formula for estimation of creatinine clearance.

Table 2: Allopurinol

Maintenance Dosage

Creatinine Clearance		
(mL/s)	(mL/min)	Dose
< 0.17	< 10	100 mg every 3 days
0.17	10	100 mg every 2 days
0.33	20	100 mg daily
0.67	40	150 mg daily
1.00	60	200 mg daily
1.33	80	250 mg daily
1.67	100	300 mg daily
2.00	120	350 mg daily
2.33	140	400 mg daily

Because allopurinol concentrations are difficult to determine and because serum concentrations may not adequately reflect the amount of drug bound to xanthine oxidase in the tissues, serum urate concentrations should be used to monitor therapy. The upper limit of normal is about 430 µmol/L for men and postmenopausal women and 345 µmol/L for premenopausal women. By selecting the appropriate dose of allopurinol and using uricosuric agents in certain patients, it is possible to reduce the serum uric acid concentration to normal and, if desired, to hold it as low as 120 to 180 µmol/L. Combined therapy of allopurinol and a uricosuric agent will often allow a dosage reduction of both agents.
In patients who are being treated with uricosuric agents, colchicine and/or NSAIDs, it is wise to continue this therapy while adjusting the allopurinol dosage until a normal serum uric acid concentration and freedom from acute attacks have been maintained for several months. If desired, the patient may then be maintained on allopurinol therapy exclusively. When a uricosuric agent is being withdrawn, dosage of the uricosuric agent should be tapered over several weeks.
Prevention of Uric Acid Nephropathy During Treatment of Neoplastic Disease: Allopurinol 600 to 800 mg daily for 2 or 3 days starting 1 or 2 days prior to chemotherapy or radiation therapy. When allopurinol is used with mercaptopurine or azathioprine, the dosage of the latter drugs must be reduced (see Precautions, Drug Interactions). Continue treatment at a dosage adjusted to the serum uric acid concentration until there is no longer a risk of hyperuricemia and hyperuricosuria.
Allopurinol treatment can be maintained during cancer treatment, for prophylaxis of hyperuricemia that may be secondary to cancer or cancer chemotherapy. In prolonged treatment, 300 to 400 mg of allopurinol daily is usually sufficient to control the serum uric acid concentration.
Prophylaxis of Renal Calcium Lithiasis: 200 to 300 mg daily. Therapy should be continued indefinitely. Some patients have received maintenance doses of 200 to 300 mg daily for more than 7 years. In some patients, the maintenance dose may be reduced to 100 to 200 mg daily.
Children: Children ≤ 10 years of age: 10 mg/kg/day in two to three divided doses. Maximum 800 mg/24 hours.
Alternatively in children < 6 years of age: 150 mg/day in three divided doses; 6 to 10 years of age: 300 mg/day in two to three divided doses.
For gout in children > 10 years of age and adults: 200 to 600 mg/day.
Response should be evaluated after approximately 48 hours by monitoring serum uric acid and/or urinary uric acid concentrations and adjusting the dose if necessary.

Alocril™ Ⓟ

nedocromil sodium

Antiallergic—Anti-inflammatory

Allergan

PHARMACOLOGY: Nedocromil displays specific antiallergic and anti-inflammatory properties.
The pharmacological actions of nedocromil in many respects resemble those of sodium cromoglycate, a compound which has been shown to have effects on both the symptoms of ocular allergic inflammation and the level of inflammatory mediators present in the tears. Nedocromil is not only an inhibitor of the immunological release of inflammatory mediators, but also extends this activity to mucosal mast cells, which are thought to play an important role in allergic inflammatory diseases. The conclusion that nedocromil sodium is an anti-inflammatory agent is supported by in vivo observations of its capacity to inhibit the late response to antigen challenge, microvascular leakage and platelet activating factor (PAF) induced bronchoconstriction and hyper-responsiveness. In the dog and guinea-pig, nedocromil sodium has been shown to modify sensory nerve responses, a possible mechanism for its observed inhibitory effects on reflex bronchoconstriction and cough.
When administered as 2% ophthalmic solution in human volunteers, up to 4% of a dose of nedocromil sodium is absorbed; absorption occurs primarily through the nasal mucosa since much of the dose of an ophthalmic solution will drain from the eye via the nasolacrimal duct. Approximately 4 to 8% of an intranasal dose and 2 to 3% of an oral dose of nedocromil sodium is absorbed.
Nedocromil is bound reversibly (up to 89%) to human proteins and to a lesser extent in animals. It is not metabolized in man or animals. In man it is excreted unchanged in the urine (approximately 70%) and in feces (approximately 30%). While the plasma concentration falls rapidly (i.e., 10% of peak levels in 8 hours) and urinary excretion is 90% within 12 hours, fecal eliminations may take up to 3 days to be completed.

INDICATIONS: For the treatment of seasonal allergic conjunctivitis.
It must be used regularly to ensure optimal control of symptoms.
Treatment should be initiated as closely as possible to the start of the symptoms.
Nedocromil may be used in conjunction with other antiallergic therapies, including topical ophthalmics, (xylometazoline, naphazoline, sodium cromoglycate) topical nasal solutions (xylometazoline, flunisolide, pseudoephedrine) and systemic therapies (e.g., oral antihistamine) as no interactions have been reported.

CONTRAINDICATIONS: Known hypersensitivity to nedocromil, disodium edetate or benzalkonium chloride.

WARNINGS: Patients who use soft contact lenses must not wear them during the treatment period with Alocril ophthalmic solution. Benzalkonium chloride, a constituent of the formulation, may accumulate in soft contact lenses. This preservative, when slowly released, could possibly irritate the cornea.
In patients who continue to wear hard or gas permeable contact lenses during nedocromil treatment, the lenses should be taken out of the eye prior to instillation of the drops. They should be inserted again not earlier than 5 minutes after administration, in order to allow an even conjunctival distribution of the solution.
To avoid contamination of the contents, patients should not touch the tip of the container or allow the tip of the bottle to come into contact with the eye.

PRECAUTIONS: Geriatrics: There is no evidence to suggest that a dose reduction in the elderly is required, as 2% nedocromil sodium ophthalmic solution appears to have a similar activity and safety profile in all groups of patient studied with allergic conjunctivitis. However there is limited clinical trial experience with nedocromil sodium ophthalmic solution, in the elderly.
Children: The safety and efficacy of nedocromil in children under 3 years of age has not yet been established.
Pregnancy: Safety in human pregnancy and the absence of adverse effects on the human reproductive process have not been established. Small amounts of nedocromil are known to cross the placenta but without effect in animals. In fact, in reproductive studies, nedocromil at dosage levels up to 100 mg/kg (more than 800 times the human maintenance dose) has shown no teratogenic or embryotoxic effects, nor has it been observed to interfere with reproductive performance, gestation, parturition, or lactation. Nedocromil has not affected male or female fertility nor has it altered the development of progeny.
Although there is no reason to suspect that nedocromil affects the fetus or mother, as with any drug caution must be exercised, especially during the first trimester. The benefits of treatment to the mother must be weighed against the potential risk to the fetus before proposing its use.
Lactation: Safety in breast-fed infants has not been established. Animal studies have indicated no toxicity of nedocromil in suckling newborns receiving drug from the parent or directly by injection. The concentrations of nedocromil in milk of animals were very low but have not been measured in human milk. The benefits of treating a nursing mother must be weighed against potential risk to the infant.
Drug Interactions: Nedocromil has been given to man in conjunction with other drugs with no apparent ill-effects. These included ophthalmic solutions such as xylometazoline, antazoline and naphazoline, pheniramine, sodium cromoglycate and dexamethasone; topical nasal therapies, such as xylometazoline, flunisolide, pseudoephedrine, chlorpheniramine and beclomethasone diproprionate, and oral antihistamines such as clemastine, astemizole, diphenhydramine, terfenadine, brompheniramine and promethazine.
Nedocromil by inhalation has also been used with inhaled and oral β_2-adrenergic agonists, inhaled and oral corticosteroids, theophylline and other methylxanthines and ipratropium bromide. No drug-drug interactions have been observed in humans or in animals.

ADVERSE EFFECTS: No major adverse events associated with nedocromil ophthalmic solution have been reported in any of the clinical trials. Only minor adverse effects were reported which were mostly mild and self-limiting.
Those adverse events reported with a frequency ≥ 1% in patients who received nedocromil in controlled therapeutic trials are displayed in Table 1.

Table 1: Alocril

Percentage of Patients Reporting Common Adverse Events in Controlled Therapeutic Trials (AEs reported with a frequency of ≥ 1% for the Total Nedocromil Sodium 2% Group)

Adverse Event	Total Nedocromil Sodium 2% (n=1 552)	Total Placebo (n=1 353)
Headache	10.9	9.3
Eye Burning	7.4[a]	4.2
Eye Stinging	6.0[a]	3.1
Taste Perversion	5.4[a]	0.6

(cont'd)

Table 1: Alocril *(cont'd)*

Percentage of Patients Reporting Common Adverse Events in Controlled Therapeutic Trials (AEs reported with a frequency of ≥ 1% for the Total Nedocromil Sodium 2% Group)

Adverse Event	Total Nedocromil Sodium 2% (n=1 552)	Total Placebo (n=1 353)
Eye Redness	2.3	1.8
Eye Itching	2.2	3.4
Rhinitis	1.9	2.3
Eye Watering	1.7	1.6
Eye Soreness	1.7	0.9
Pharyngitis	1.7	1.2
URI	1.7	1.1
Photophobia	1.2	1.1

[a] p <0.01.

OVERDOSE:

Treatment: There have been no reported cases of overdosage in humans. Animal studies have not shown evidence of toxic effects of nedocromil sodium even at high dosage. If overdosage is suspected, treatment should be supportive and directed to the control of the relevant symptoms.

For management of a suspected drug overdose, CPhA recommends that you contact your **regional Poison Control Centre**. See the *CPS* Directory section for a list of Poison Control Centres.

DOSAGE: The ophthalmic solution must be used regularly to ensure optimal control of symptoms.

Treatment should be initiated as closely as possible to the start of the symptoms.

Adults and Children (over 3 years of age): Seasonal Allergic Conjunctivitis: 1 drop into each eye twice daily.

Important: Soft contact lenses must not be worn during the treatment period. Benzalkonium chloride, a constituent of the formulation, may accumulate in soft contact lenses. This preservative, when slowly released, could possibly irritate the cornea.

In patients who continue to wear hard or gas permeable contact lenses during treatment, the lenses should be taken out of the eye prior to instillation of the drops. They should be inserted again not earlier than 5 minutes after administration, in order to allow an even conjunctival distribution of the solution.

To avoid contamination of the contents, do not touch any surface with the tip of the container.

INFORMATION FOR THE PATIENT: Published in e-CPS, available by subscription at www.e-cps.ca.

SUPPLIED: Each mL of sterile, aqueous, isotonic, preserved, stabilized, clear pale yellow ophthalmic solution, contains: nedocromil sodium 2% w/v. Nonmedicinal ingredients: benzalkonium chloride, disodium edetate (EDTA), purified water and sodium chloride. White opaque or translucent polyethylene dropper bottles of 5 mL. Store between 4 and 25°C. Protect from direct sunlight.

Alomide® Ⓟ

lodoxamide tromethamine

Antiallergic

Alcon

SUPPLIED: Each mL of sterile isotonic solution contains: lodoxamide 0.1% (lodoxamide tromethamine 0.178%) with benzalkonium chloride 0.007% (as preservative). Nonmedicinal ingredients: citric acid, edetate disodium, hydrochloric acid and/or sodium hydroxide (to adjust pH), hydroxypropyl methylcellulose, mannitol, purified water, sodium citrate and tyloxapol. Natural plastic ophthalmic Drop-Tainer dispensers of 10 mL. Store at room temperature (2-30°C).

Alphagan™ Ⓟ

brimonidine tartrate

Elevated Intraocular Pressure Therapy

Allergan

PHARMACOLOGY: Mechanism of Action: Brimonidine is a relatively selective alpha adrenergic receptor agonist that in radioligand binding assays and in functional assays, is approximately 1 000 times more selective for the alpha-2 adrenoceptor than the alpha-1 adrenoceptor. This selectivity results in the absence of vasoconstriction in microvessels associated with human retinal xenografts.

Topical administration of brimonidine decreases intraocular pressure (IOP) in humans. When used as directed, brimonidine ophthalmic solution reduces elevated IOP with minimal effect on cardiovascular parameters.

Brimonidine has a rapid onset of action, with the peak ocular hypotensive effect occurring at approximately 2 hours post-dosing. The duration of effect is 12 hours or greater.

Fluorophotometric studies in animals and humans suggest that brimonidine has a dual mechanism of action. Brimonidine lowers IOP by reducing aqueous humor production and increasing uveoscleral outflow.

Pharmacodynamics: Brimonidine has no effect on pulmonary function or exercise-induced tachycardia. The cardiovascular effects of brimonidine during exercise in normal volunteers were found to be limited to a slight suppression of systolic blood pressure, which was clinically insignificant, during the recovery period following a treadmill test.

Pharmacokinetics: After ocular administration of brimonidine 0.2% twice daily (both eyes) in humans for 10 days, plasma concentrations were low (mean C_{max}=0.06 ng/mL). Plasma brimonidine levels peaked within 1 to 4 hours and declined with a systemic half-life of approximately 3 hours.

In humans, brimonidine is eliminated rapidly via extensive systemic metabolism; there is no marked systemic accumulation after multiple dosing. It is metabolized primarily by the liver. Urinary excretion is the major route of elimination of the drug and its metabolites. Approximately 87% of an orally-administered radioactive dose was eliminated within 120 hours, with 74% found in the urine in the first 96 hours.

Clinical Studies: Brimonidine lowers intraocular pressure with minimal effect on cardiovascular parameters (heart rate, systolic and diastolic blood pressure) and no apparent effect on pulmonary parameters (spirometry, respiratory rate).

The long-term efficacy of brimonidine 0.2% dosed b.i.d. was demonstrated in two 1-year multicenter studies in subjects with open angle glaucoma or ocular hypertension. In these trials brimonidine 0.2% lowered IOP by mean values of 4.3 mm Hg at trough and 6.7 mm Hg at peak. IOP decreases were maintained for the duration of the studies in the majority of patients; no tachyphylaxis was observed. Nine percent of subjects were discontinued from the studies due to inadequately controlled intraocular pressure.

INDICATIONS: For the control of intraocular pressure in patients with chronic open-angle glaucoma or ocular hypertension.

CONTRAINDICATIONS: Patients with hypersensitivity to brimonidine or any component of this medication. It is also contraindicated in patients receiving monoamine oxidase (MAO) inhibitor therapy.

WARNINGS: For topical ophthalmic use only.

Children: **The use of brimonidine in pediatric patients is currently not recommended.** Several serious adverse reactions have been reported in association with the administration of brimonidine to infants in the age range of 28 days to 3 months (see Adverse Effects).

PRECAUTIONS: General: Brimonidine ophthalmic solution 0.2% should be used with caution in patients with known hypersensitivity to other alpha-adrenoceptor agonists.

Although brimonidine had minimal effect on blood pressure and heart rate of patients in clinical studies, caution should be exercised in treating patients with severe cardiovascular disease.

Brimonidine has not been studied in patients with hepatic or renal impairment; caution should be exercised in treating such patients.

Brimonidine should be used with caution in patients with depression, cerebral or coronary insufficiency, Raynaud's phenomenon, orthostatic hypotension or thromboangiitis obliterans.

Drug Interactions: Although specific drug interaction studies have not been conducted with brimonidine, the possibility of an additive or potentiating effect with CNS depressants (alcohol, barbiturates, opiates, sedatives, or anesthetics) should be considered.

Brimonidine did not have clinically significant effects on pulse and blood pressure in chronic clinical studies. However, since alpha-agonists, as a class, may reduce pulse and blood pressure, caution in the concomitant use of drugs such as beta-blockers (ophthalmic and/or systemic), antihypertensives and/or cardiac glycosides is advised.

Tricyclic antidepressants have been reported to blunt the hypotensive effect of systemic clonidine. It is not known whether the concurrent use of these agents with brimonidine can lead to an interference in IOP lowering effect. No data are available on the level of circulating catecholamines after brimonidine is instilled. Caution, however, is advised in patients taking tricyclic antidepressants which can affect the metabolism and uptake of circulating amines.

Carcinogenesis, Mutagenesis, Impairment of Fertility: No compound-related carcinogenic effects were observed in 21-month and 2-year studies in mice and rats given oral doses of 2.5 mg base/kg/day and 1.0 mg base/kg/day, respectively. These oral doses are approximately 830 and 330 times greater, respectively, than the maximum recommended human daily ophthalmic dosage for brimonidine (0.003 mg base/kg/day) based on a 60 kg human.

Brimonidine was not mutagenic or cytogenic in a series of in vitro and in vivo studies including the Ames test, host-mediated assay, chromosomal aberration assay in Chinese Hamster Ovary (CHO) cells, cytogenic studies in mice and dominant lethal assay.

Pregnancy: Teratogenicity studies showed no adverse effects in rats and rabbits when oral doses (1.65 mg base/kg/day and 3.33 mg base/kg/day) were administered at approximately 550 and 1110 times, respectively, the maximum recommended human daily ophthalmic dosage for brimonidine (based on a 60 kg human).

There are no studies of brimonidine in pregnant women; however, in animal studies, brimonidine crossed the placenta and entered into the fetal circulation to a limited extent (ratio of drug-related material in fetal:maternal blood = 0.1 to 0.3). Drug-derived material was eliminated from fetal tissues by 24 hours postdose. Brimonidine should be used during pregnancy only if the potential benefit to the mother justifies the potential risk to the fetus.

Lactation: It is not known whether brimonidine is excreted in human milk; although in animal studies, brimonidine has been shown to be excreted in breast milk. During treatment with brimonidine, a decision should be made whether to discontinue nursing or to discontinue the drug, taking into account the importance of the drug to the mother.

Children: **The use of brimonidine in pediatric patients is currently not recommended.** Several serious adverse reactions have been reported in association with the administration of brimonidine ophthalmic solution to infants in the age range of 28 days to 3 months (see Adverse Effects).

Information to Be Provided to the Patient: Occupational Hazards: Brimonidine, as with other similar medications, can potentially cause fatigue and/or drowsiness in some patients. Patients who engage in hazardous activities should be cautioned of the potential for a decrease in mental alertness.

The preservative in Alphagan, benzalkonium chloride, may be absorbed by soft contact lenses. Patients wearing soft contact lenses should be instructed to wait at least 15 minutes after instilling the product to insert soft contact lenses.

ADVERSE EFFECTS: In clinical studies including 717 patients on brimonidine, the most frequently reported adverse events were oral dryness [25.8%], ocular hyperemia [24.8%], burning and stinging [22.5%], blurring [17.3%], headache [16.3%], foreign body sensation [15.5%], fatigue/drowsiness [15.2%], corneal staining/erosion [10.0%], ocular allergic reactions [9.9%], and ocular pruritus [9.8%], and conjunctival follicles [9.6%].

Events occurring less frequently included photophobia [7.4%], ocular dryness [7.0%], eyelid erythema [6.1%], ocular ache/pain [6.0%], upper respiratory symptoms [6.0%], tearing [5.6%], conjunctival edema [5.3%], eyelid edema [4.9%], dizziness [4.2%], conjunctival blanching [3.8%], blepharitis [3.6%], ocular irritation [3.1%], gastrointestinal symptoms [3.1%], asthenia [2.8%], abnormal vision [2.6%], abnormal taste [1.4%], conjunctival discharge [1.4%] conjunctival papillae [1.0%], and nasal dryness [1.0%].

The following adverse reactions were reported infrequently (<1%): depression [0.8%], systemic allergic reactions [0.8%], and palpitations [0.4%].

Serious Reports of Adverse Reactions in Pediatric Patients: Several serious adverse reactions have been reported in association with the administration of brimonidine ophthalmic solution to infants in the age range of 28 days to 3 months. These reactions included: bradycardia, hypotension, hypothermia, hypotonia, apnea, dyspnea, hypoventilation, cyanosis and lethargy resulting in hospitalization. Upon discontinuation of brimonidine the infants recovered without sequelae.

OVERDOSE:

Treatment: No data are available on overdosage of brimonidine ophthalmic solution in humans. Treatment of an oral overdose includes supportive and symptomatic therapy; a patent airway should be maintained. Evacuation of the stomach should be considered during the first few hours after an overdosage.

For management of a suspected drug overdose, CPhA recommends that you contact your **regional Poison Control Centre**. See the *CPS* Directory section for a list of Poison Control Centres.

DOSAGE: The recommended dose is 1 drop of ophthalmic solution in the affected eye(s) twice daily (doses taken approximately 12 hours apart).

INFORMATION FOR THE PATIENT: Published in e-CPS, available by subscription at www.e-cps.ca.

SUPPLIED: Each mL of sterile ophthalmic solution contains: brimonidine tartrate 2 mg (0.2%). Nonmedicinal ingredients: benzalkonium chloride (as preservative), citric acid, hydrochloric acid and/or sodium hydroxide (to adjust pH), polyvinyl alcohol, purified water, sodium chloride and sodium citrate. White, opaque plastic dropper bottles of 5 and 10 mL b.i.d. (twice daily). Store at 15 to 25°C.

Alphagan® P Ⓟ

brimonidine tartrate

Elevated Intraocular Pressure Therapy

Allergan

Date of Preparation: November 12, 1997

Date of Revision: October 30, 2003

PHARMACOLOGY: Mechanism of Action: Brimonidine tartrate is a relatively selective alpha-2 adrenergic receptor agonist that, in radioligand binding assays and in functional assays, is approximately 1000 times more selective for the alpha-2 adrenoceptor than the alpha-1 adrenoceptor. This selectivity results in the absence of vasoconstriction in microvessels associated with human retinal xenografts.

Topical administration of brimonidine decreases intraocular pressure (IOP) in humans. When used as directed, brimonidine tartrate ophthalmic solutions reduce elevated IOP with minimal effect on cardiovascular parameters.

Brimonidine tartrate has a rapid onset of action, with the peak ocular hypotensive effect occurring at approximately two hours post-dosing. The duration of effect is 12 hours or greater.

Table 1: ALPHAGAN P

Intraocular Pressure Values (mm Hg) Phase 3 Studies (ITT LOCF Analysis)

		Study 190342-007		Study 190342-008	
		Alphagan P (0.15%) N=197	**Alphagan (0.2%) N=199**	**Alphagan P (0.15%) N=184**	**Alphagan (0.2%) N=184**
Baseline	**Hour-0** Mean	24.9	24.7	24.9	25.3
	Hour-2 Mean	23.1	23.0	23.6	24.1
	Hour-7 Mean	21.8	21.9	22.4	23.0
	Hour-9 Mean	21.7	21.6	22.4	23.1
Month-12	**Hour-0** Mean (mean change from baseline)	21.6 (−3.3)	21.3 (−3.4)	22.3 (−2.6)	22.7 (−2.6)
	CI[a]	(−0.61, 1.01)		(−1.44, 0.45)	
	Hour-2 Mean (mean change from baseline)	18.6 (−4.5)	18.1 (−4.9)	19.3 (−4.3)	19.3 (−4.8)
	CI[a]	(−0.35, 1.16)		(−0.62, 1.09)	
	Hour-7 Mean (mean change from baseline)	19.9 (−1.9)	19.6 (−2.3)	20.4 (−2.0)	21.0 (−2.0)
	CI[a]	(−0.59, 0.92)		(−1.09, 0.58)	
	Hour-9 Mean (mean change from baseline)	17.9 (−3.8)	17.4 (−4.2)	18.5 (−3.9)	18.5 (−4.6)
	CI[a]	(−0.27, 1.18)		(−0.41, 1.29)	

[a] = 95% confidence interval for difference between Alphagan P and Alphagan concentrations.
Legend: N = number of patients at baseline; CI = confidence interval.
Note: There was no statistical significance between Alphagan P and Alphagan for within group analysis of changes from baseline using a paired t-test (at all time points the p-value was <0.001).

Fluorophotometric studies in animals and humans suggest that brimonidine tartrate has a dual mechanism of action. ALPHAGAN P (brimonidine tartrate) ophthalmic solution 0.15% lowers IOP by reducing aqueous humor production and increasing uveoscleral outflow.

Pharmacodynamics: ALPHAGAN P has no effect on pulmonary function or exercise-induced tachycardia. The cardiovascular effects of ALPHAGAN P during exercise in normal volunteers were found to be limited to a slight suppression of systolic blood pressure, which was clinically insignificant, during the recovery period following a treadmill test.

Pharmacokinetics: After ocular administration of Brimonidine-Purite ophthalmic solution 0.1% or 0.2% (brimonidine tartrate 0.1% or 0.2% preserved with Purite), plasma concentrations peaked within 0.5 to 2.5 hours, and declined with a systemic half-life of approximately 2 hours.

In humans, brimonidine is eliminated rapidly via extensive systemic metabolism; there is no marked systemic accumulation after multiple dosing. It is metabolized primarily by the liver. Urinary excretion is the major route of elimination of the drug and its metabolites. Approximately 87% of an orally-administered radioactive dose was eliminated within 120 hours, with 74% found in the urine.

Clinical Studies: Brimonidine tartrate lowers intraocular pressure with minimal effect on cardiovascular parameters (heart rate, systolic and diastolic blood pressure) and no apparent effect on pulmonary parameters (spirometry, respiratory rate).

Two clinical studies (n=1,147) lasting for twelve months were conducted to evaluate the safety, efficacy, and acceptability of ALPHAGAN P and 0.2% Brimonidine-Purite™ compared with brimonidine tartrate ophthalmic solution 0.2% preserved with benzalkonium chloride (ALPHAGAN), administered three-times-daily in patients with glaucoma or ocular hypertension. The intraocular pressure values for the Baseline and Month-12 time points using ALPHAGAN P and ALPHAGAN, are summarized in Table 1.

Efficacy analyses from these two clinical trials indicated that ALPHAGAN P is non-inferior to ALPHAGAN and effectively lowered IOP in patients with glaucoma or ocular hypertension (mean values of at least 2.6 mm Hg at trough, and at least 4.3 mm Hg at peak) over the twelve months of the study. ALPHAGAN P was well tolerated, rated as comfortable by the majority of patients, and provided a superior safety profile when compared with ALPHAGAN. Among the most commonly reported adverse events (≥3.9% incidence) in the ALPHAGAN P group), the frequency of reports were generally fewer than with ALPHAGAN. There was a significantly smaller percentage of patients who experienced allergic conjunctivitis, oral dryness, asthenia, or somnolence in the ALPHAGAN P group. ALPHAGAN P was the lowest effective dose of brimonidine tartrate efficacy with the most favorable safety and tolerability profile.

INDICATIONS: ALPHAGAN P (brimonidine tartrate) ophthalmic solution 0.15% is indicated for the control of intraocular pressure in patients with chronic open-angle glaucoma or ocular hypertension.

CONTRAINDICATIONS: ALPHAGAN P (brimonidine tartrate) ophthalmic solution 0.15% is contraindicated in patients with hypersensitivity to brimonidine tartrate or any component of this medication. It is also contraindicated in patients receiving monoamine oxidase (MAO) inhibitor therapy.

WARNINGS: For topical ophthalmic use only.

The use of ALPHAGAN P (brimonidine tartrate) ophthalmic solution 0.15% in paediatric patients is currently not recommended. Several serious adverse reactions have been reported in association with the administration of brimonidine tartrate ophthalmic solution 0.2% to infants in the age range of 28 days to 3 months (see Adverse Effects).

PRECAUTIONS: General: ALPHAGAN P (brimonidine tartrate) ophthalmic solution 0.15% should be used with caution in patients with known hypersensitivity to other alpha-adrenoceptor agonists.

Use in Patients with Special Conditions: Although ALPHAGAN P had minimal effect on blood pressure and heart rate of patients in clinical studies, caution should be exercised in treating patients with severe cardiovascular disease.

ALPHAGAN P has not been studied in patients with hepatic or renal impairment; caution should be exercised in treating such patients.

ALPHAGAN P should be used with caution in patients with depression, cerebral or coronary insufficiency, Raynaud's phenomenon, orthostatic hypotension or thromboangiitis obliterans.

Drug Interactions: Although specific drug interaction studies have not been conducted with ALPHAGAN P, the possibility of an additive or potentiating effect with CNS depressants (alcohol, barbiturates, opiates, sedatives, or anesthetics) should be considered.

ALPHAGAN P did not have clinically significant effects on pulse and blood pressure in chronic clinical studies. However, since alpha-agonists, as a class, may reduce pulse and blood pressure, caution in the concomitant use of drugs such as beta-blockers (ophthalmic and/or systemic), antihypertensives and/or cardiac glycosides is advised.

Tricyclic antidepressants have been reported to blunt the hypotensive effect of systemic clonidine. It is not known whether the concurrent use of these agents with ALPHAGAN P can lead to an interference in IOP lowering effect. No data are available on the level of circulating catecholamines after ALPHAGAN P is instilled. Caution, however, is advised in patients taking tricyclic antidepressants which can affect the metabolism and uptake of circulating amines.

Carcinogenesis, Mutagenesis, Impairment of Fertility: No compound-related carcinogenic effects were observed in 21 month and 2 year studies in mice and rats given oral doses of 2.5 mg base/kg/day and 1.0 mg base/kg/day of brimonidine tartrate, respectively. These doses achieved 106 and 145 times, respectively, the plasma drug concentration estimated in humans treated with one drop of ALPHAGAN P into both eyes three times per day.

Brimonidine was not mutagenic or cytogenic in a series of in vitro and in vivo studies including the Ames test, host-mediated assay, chromosomal aberration assay in Chinese Hamster Ovary (CHO) cells, cytogenic studies in mice and dominant lethal assay.

Pregnancy: Teratogenicity studies showed no adverse effects in rats and rabbits when oral doses (1.65 mg base/kg/day and 3.33 mg base/kg/day of brimonidine tartrate) were administered during gestation days 6 through 15 in rats and days 6 through 18 in rabbits. These doses achieved AUC values 258- and 17-fold higher, respectively, than similar values estimated in humans treated with ALPHAGAN P given as one drop in both eyes three times per day.

There are no studies of ALPHAGAN P in pregnant women, however in animal studies, brimonidine crossed the placenta and entered into the fetal circulation to a limited extent (ratio of drug-related material in fetal:maternal blood = 0.1-0.3). Drug-derived material was eliminated from fetal tissues by 24 hours post-dose. ALPHAGAN P should be used during pregnancy only if the potential benefit to the mother justifies the potential risk to the fetus.

Lactation: It is not known whether brimonidine is excreted in human milk, although in animal studies, brimonidine has been shown to be excreted in breast milk. During treatment with ALPHAGAN P, a decision should be made whether to discontinue nursing or to discontinue the drug, taking into account the importance of the drug to the mother.

Children: **The use of ALPHAGAN P in paediatric patients is currently not recommended.** Several serious adverse reactions have been reported in association with the administration of brimonidine tartrate ophthalmic solution 0.2% to infants in the age range of 28 days to 3 months (see Adverse Effects).

Information to Be Provided to the Patient: ALPHAGAN P, as with other similar medications, can potentially cause fatigue and/or drowsiness in some patients. Patients who engage in hazardous activities should be cautioned of the potential for a decrease in mental alertness.

Patients should be advised to keep the dropper tip of the bottle from touching the eye or other surrounding structures, because of the potential for bacterial contamination.

Contact lenses should be removed prior to instillation of ALPHAGAN P and may be reinserted 15 minutes after its instillation.

ADVERSE EFFECTS: In clinical studies the most frequently reported adverse reactions (>1%) classified as treatment-related from the 12 month Phase III controlled clinical studies for patients (n=380) who received ALPHAGAN P (brimonidine tartrate) ophthalmic solution 0.15% were: conjunctival hyperemia (18.2%), allergic conjunctivitis (9.2%), eye pruritus (8.2%), visual disturbance (6.1%), conjunctival folliculosis (5.5%), oral dryness (5.3%), burning sensation in the eye (5.3%), eye dryness (2.9%), foreign body sensation (2.9%), epiphora (2.6%), headache (2.4%), eyelid edema (2.1%), eye pain (1.8%), asthenia (1.6%), blepharitis (1.6%), erythema eyelid (1.6%), irritation eye (1.6%), ocular stinging sensation (1.6%), photophobia (1.6%), conjunctival edema (1.3%), eye discharge (1.3%), follicular conjunctivitis (1.3%), superficial punctate keratitis (1.3%), rhinitis (1.1%), visual acuity worsened (1.1%).

Serious Reports of Adverse Reactions in Paediatric Patients: Several serious adverse reactions have been reported in association with the administration of brimonidine tartrate ophthalmic solution 0.2% to infants in the age range of 28 days to 3 months. These reactions included: bradycardia, hypotension, hypothermia, hypotonia, apnea, dyspnoea, hypoventilation, cyanosis and lethargy resulting in hospitalisation. Upon discontinuation of brimonidine tartrate ophthalmic solution 0.2% the infants recovered without sequelae.

OVERDOSE:

Treatment: No data are available on overdosage of ALPHAGAN P (brimonidine tartrate) ophthalmic solution 0.15% in humans. Treatment of an oral overdose includes supportive and symptomatic therapy; a patent airway should be maintained. Evacuation of the stomach should be considered during the first few hours after an overdosage.

For management of a suspected drug overdose, CPhA recommends that you contact your **regional Poison Control Centre**. See the *CPS* Directory section for a list of Poison Control Centres.

DOSAGE: The recommended dose is one drop of ALPHAGAN P (brimonidine tartrate) ophthalmic solution 0.15% in the affected eye(s) three times daily, approximately 8 hours apart.

INFORMATION FOR THE PATIENT: Published in e-CPS, available by subscription at www.e-cps.ca.

SUPPLIED: Each mL of ophthalmic solution contains: brimonidine tartrate 1.5 mg (0.15%). Nonmedicinal ingredients: boric acid, calcium chloride dihydrate, magnesium chloride hexahydrate, potassium chloride, purified water with hydrochloric acid or sodium hydroxide to adjust the pH, Purite 0.005% (Stabilized Oxychloro Complex (from chlorite, chlorate and chlorine dioxide)) as preservative, sodium borate decahydrate, sodium carboxymethylcellulose and sodium chloride. The pH range is 6.6 to 7.4. Teal, opaque plastic dropper bottles with a purple cap containing 3, 5 and 10 mL. Store at 15 to 25°C. Discard unused solution at the end of treatment.

Alprazolam

CPhA Monograph

see *Benzodiazepines*

Alrex®

loteprednol etabonate

Corticosteroid

Bausch & Lomb

Date of Preparation: December 22, 2008

SUMMARY PRODUCT INFORMATION:

Route of Administration	Dosage Form/ Strength	Clinically Relevant Nonmedicinal Ingredients
Ophthalmic	Suspension, 0.2% w/v	Benzalkonium Chloride For a complete listing see Dosage Forms, Composition and Packaging.

INDICATIONS AND CLINICAL USE: Alrex (loteprednol etabonate) Ophthalmic Suspension is indicated for:
- temporary short-term relief of the signs and symptoms of seasonal allergic conjunctivitis

Geriatrics (>65 years of age): Alrex should not be used in geriatric patients. The safety and efficacy of Alrex have not been established in patients >65 years of age.

Pediatrics (<18 years of age): Alrex should not be used in pediatric patients. The safety and efficacy of Alrex have not been studied in pediatric patients.

CONTRAINDICATIONS:
- Suspected or confirmed infection of the eye: viral diseases of the cornea and conjunctiva including epithelial herpes simplex keratitis (dendritic keratitis), vaccinia, and varicella; untreated ocular infection of the eye; mycobacterial infection of the eye and fungal diseases of ocular structures.
- Hypersensitivity to this drug or any ingredient in the formulation or container, or to other corticosteroids. For a complete listing, see Dosage Forms, Composition and Packaging.

WARNINGS AND PRECAUTIONS: General: For ophthalmic use only.

Alrex is indicated as a short-term treatment only (up to 14 days). The initial prescription and renewal of Alrex should be made by a physician only after appropriate ophthalmologic examination is performed. If signs and symptoms fail to improve after two days, the patient should be re-evaluated. If Alrex is used for 10 days or longer, intraocular pressure should be closely monitored. See Ophthalmologic.

Prolonged use of corticosteroids may result in cataract and/or glaucoma formation. Alrex should not be used in the presence of glaucoma or elevated intraocular pressure, unless absolutely necessary and close ophthalmologic monitoring is undertaken. Extreme caution should be exercised, and duration of treatment should be kept as short as possible. See Ophthalmologic.

Alrex should not be used in cases of existing (suspected or confirmed) ocular viral, fungal, or mycobacterial infections. Alrex may suppress the host response and thus increase the hazard of secondary ocular infections. The use of Alrex in patients with a history of herpes simplex requires great caution and close monitoring. See Ophthalmologic.

Alrex contains benzalkonium chloride. See Dosage and Administration.

Alrex has not been studied in pregnant or nursing women, but has been found to be teratogenic in animals. Alrex should not be used in pregnant or nursing women unless the benefits to the mother clearly outweigh the risk to the foetus or the nursing child. See Special Populations.

Carcinogenesis and Mutagenesis: Long-term animal studies have not been conducted to evaluate the carcinogenic potential of loteprednol etabonate. Loteprednol etabonate was not genotoxic in vitro in the Ames test, the mouse lymphoma tk assay, or in a chromosome aberration test in human lymphocytes, or in vivo in the single dose mouse micronucleus assay.

Endocrine and Metabolism: Glucocorticoids, mostly when systemic exposure occurs, decrease the hypoglycemic activity of insulin and oral hypoglycemics, so that a change in dose of the anti-diabetic drugs may be necessitated. In high doses, glucocorticoids also decrease the response to somatotropin. The usual doses of mineralocorticoids and large doses of some glucocorticoids cause hypokalemia and may exaggerate the hypokalemic effects of thiazides and high-ceiling diuretics. In combination with amphotericin-B, they also may cause hypokalemia. Glucocorticoids appear to enhance the ulcerogenic effects of non-steroidal anti-inflammatory drugs. They decrease the plasma levels of salicylates, and salicylism may occur on discontinuing steroids. Glucocorticoids may increase or decrease the effects of prothrombopenic anticoagulants. Estrogens, phenobarbital, phenytoin and rifampin increase the metabolic clearance of adrenal steroids and hence necessitate dose adjustments. However, given the very low systemic exposure to loteprednol etabonate when using Alrex as directed, these possible effects are not likely. See Action and Clinical Pharmacology.

Immune: Cortisol and the synthetic analogs of cortisol have the capacity to prevent or suppress the development of the local heat, redness, swelling, and tenderness by which inflammation is recognized. At the microscopic level, they inhibit not only the early phenomena of the inflammatory process (edema, fibrin deposition, capillary dilation, migration of leukocytes into the inflamed area, and phagocytic activity) but also the later manifestations, such as capillary proliferation, fibroblast proliferation, deposition of collagen, and, still later, cicatrisation.

Neurologic: Disturbances and suppression of the Hypothalamic-Pituitary-Adrenal (HPA) axis can occur with systemic exposure to corticosteroids. However, given the very low systemic exposure to loteprednol etabonate when using Alrex as directed, these possible effects are not likely. See Action and Clinical Pharmacology.

Ophthalmologic: Alrex should be used as a brief temporary treatment. If Alrex is used for 10 days or longer, intraocular pressure should be closely monitored. The initial prescription and renewal of Alrex should be made by a physician only after appropriate ophthalmologic examination is performed with the aid of magnification, such as slit lamp biomicroscopy and, where appropriate, fluorescein staining. If signs and symptoms fail to improve after two days, the patient should be re-evaluated.

Prolonged use of corticosteroids may result in glaucoma with damage to the optic nerve, defects in visual acuity and fields of vision, and in posterior subcapsular cataract formation. Alrex should not be used in the presence of glaucoma or elevated intraocular pressure, unless absolutely necessary and careful and close appropriate ophthalmologic monitoring (including intraocular pressure and lens clarity) is undertaken.

Fungal infections of the cornea are particularly prone to develop coincidentally with long-term local steroid application. Fungus invasion must be considered in any persistent corneal ulceration where a steroid has been used or is in use. Fungal cultures should be taken when appropriate.

Prolonged use of corticosteroids may suppress the host response and thus increase the hazard of secondary ocular infections. In those diseases causing thinning of the cornea or sclera, perforations have been known to occur with the use of topical steroids. In acute purulent conditions of the eye, steroids may mask infection or enhance existing infection.

Use of ocular steroids may prolong the course and may exacerbate the severity of many viral infections of the eye (including herpes simplex). Employment of a corticosteroid medication in the treatment of patients with a history of herpes simplex requires great caution.

Formulations with benzalkonium chloride should be used with caution in soft contact lens wearer. See Dosage and Administration, Administration.

Sexual Function/Reproduction: The effects of Alrex on sexual function and reproduction have not been studied in humans. Treatment of male and female rats with up to 50 mg/kg/day and 25 mg/kg/day of loteprednol etabonate, respectively (1000 and 500 times the Alrex clinical dose), prior to and during mating, was clearly harmful to the rats but did not impair their copulation performance and fertility (i.e., ability of females to become pregnant). However, these doses were highly toxic and had significant toxic effects on the pregnancies, and the survival and development of the offspring. Maternal toxicity, possible occurrence of abnormalities and growth retardation started at 10 times the Alrex clinical dose. See Special Populations, Pregnant Women.

Special Populations: Pregnant Women: Alrex should not be used in pregnant women, unless the benefit to the mother clearly outweighs the risks to the foetus. Studies in pregnant women have not been conducted. However, studies in animals have shown major reproductive and developmental toxicity when administered orally at ~100 times the Alrex clinical dose. At lower doses (10 times the Alrex clinical dose), maternal toxicity was demonstrated and, although there were no major teratogenic effects, growth retardation and a possible increase in the occurrence of some abnormalities were noted.

Nursing Women: Alrex should not be used in lactating women, unless the benefit to the mother clearly outweighs the risks to the nursing infant/child. Studies in lactating women have not been conducted. Systemic steroids appear in human milk and could suppress growth, interfere with endogenous corticosteroid production, or cause other untoward effects.

It is not known whether topical ophthalmic administration of corticosteroids could result in sufficient systemic absorption to produce detectable quantities in human milk.

Pediatrics: Alrex should not be used in pediatric patients. The safety and efficacy of Alrex have not been studied in pediatric patients.

Geriatrics (>65 years of age): Alrex should not be used in geriatric patients. The safety and efficacy of Alrex have not been established in patients >65 years of age.

Monitoring and Laboratory Tests: If Alrex is used for 10 days or longer, intraocular pressure should be monitored. See General.

ADVERSE REACTIONS: Adverse Drug Reaction Overview: Reactions associated with ophthalmic steroids include elevated intraocular pressure, which may be associated with optic nerve damage, visual acuity and field defects, posterior subcapsular cataract formation, secondary ocular infection from pathogens including herpes simplex, and perforation of the globe where there is thinning of the cornea or sclera.

In nineteen clinical trials ranging from 1 to 42 days in length, 1209 patients received various concentrations of loteprednol etabonate in topical ocular drops (0.005%, 0.05%, 0.1%, 0.2%, 0.5%). Adverse events related to loteprednol etabonate were generally, mild to moderate, non-serious and did not interrupt continuation in the studies. The most frequent ocular event reported as related to therapy was increased IOP: 6% (77/1209) in patients receiving loteprednol etabonate, as compared to 3% (25/806) in the placebo treated patients.

With the exception of elevations in IOP, the incidence of events in the LE group was similar to, or less than that of the placebo control groups. Itching was reported as related to therapy in 3% of the loteprednol treated eyes, injection, epiphora, burning/stinging other than at instillation, foreign body sensation, and burning/stinging at instillation were each reported for 2% of eyes. The most frequent non-ocular event reported as related to therapy was headache, reported for 1.2% of the loteprednol treated subjects and 0.6% of the placebo treated subjects.

Clinical Trial Adverse Drug Reactions: Because clinical trials are conducted under very specific conditions the adverse reaction rates observed in the clinical trials may not reflect the rates observed in practice and should not be compared to the rates in the clinical trials of another drug. Adverse drug reaction information from clinical trials is useful for identifying drug-related adverse events and for approximating rates.

Two phase III studies were designed to assess the safety and efficacy of Alrex in Seasonal Allergic Conjunctivitis (SAC). Both studies were randomized, double-masked, placebo controlled, multi-centre (3 and 4) parallel group studies. Patients with an IOP ≤21 mm Hg and no glaucoma were enrolled in study A (N=133) and study B (N=135). During these studies, 133 patients were exposed to Alrex.

Possibly or probably related adverse events are listed in Table 1.

Table 1: Alrex

Adverse Events

	Alrex 0.2%, N=133	Placebo, N=135
Special Senses (eye disorders)		
Intraocular Pressure		
elevation of 6 to 9 mm Hg[a]	2% to 12%[a]	0% to 6%[a]
elevation of ≥10 mm Hg	1 (1%)	1 (1%)
Chemosis	6 (5%)	7 (5%)
Vision, Abnormal or Blurred	4 (3%)	5 (4%)
Burning/Stinging On instillation	3 (2%)	6 (4%)
Itching, Eye	3 (2%)	3 (2%)
Dry Eyes	2 (2%)	4 (3%)
Burning/Stinging, not on instillation	2 (2%)	2 (1%)
Epiphora	1 (1%)	9 (7%)
Discharge	1 (1%)	3 (2%)
Foreign Body Sensation	1 (1%)	1 (1%)
Discomfort, Eye	1 (1%)	0 (0%)
Injection	1 (1%)	0 (0%)
Eye Pain	1 (1%)	0 (0%)
Sticky Eye	0 (0%)	7 (5%)
Erythema, Eyelids	0 (0%)	2 (1%)
Eye Disorder	0 (0%)	2 (1%)
Body as a Whole		
Face Edema (Head)	1 (1%)	0 (0%)
Allergic Reaction	1 (1%)	0 (0%)
Musculoskeletal System		
Twitching	0 (0%)	1 (1%)

[a] For IOP increase of 6 to 9 mm Hg, please see below.

One patient in the Alrex group and one patient in the placebo group experienced increases in IOP of ≥10 mm Hg. Among these, one in each group had an IOP increase of ≥15 mm Hg, reaching IOP values over 30 mm Hg.

In both studies, there were more patients with IOP increases of 6 to 9 mm Hg in the Alrex group than in the placebo group (see Table 2). In study A, among the patients with IOP increases of 6 to 9 mm Hg, four reached an IOP value of 22 to 23 mm Hg, and one patient reached 29 mm Hg and was discontinued (clinically significant increase in IOP). All these five patients were from the Alrex groups.

Table 2: Alrex

Incidence of IOP Increases of 6 to 9 mm Hg from Baseline (number of patients and percentages)

	Duration of treatment		
	Day 7	Day 14	Day 28
Alrex			
Study-A	6 (9%)	6 (9%)	8 (12%)
Study-B	3 (5%)	1 (2%)	4 (6%)
Placebo			
Study-A	0 (0%)	4 (6%)	1 (2%)
Study-B	0 (%)	0 (%)	0 (%)

Due to the sample size for each arm of the two phase III studies in SAC, all events captured are greater than 1% of n.

Adverse Reactions Reported in Other Controlled Randomized Trials: In nineteen clinical trials ranging from 1 to 42 days in length, 1209 patients received various concentrations of loteprednol etabonate in topical ocular drops (0.005%, 0.05%, 0.1%, 0.2%, 0.5%), the most frequent ocular event reported as related to therapy was increased intraocular pressure: 6% (77/1209) in patients receiving loteprednol etabonate, as compared to 3% (25/806) in the placebo population.

Ocular adverse reactions occurring in 5-15% of patients treated with loteprednol etabonate ophthalmic suspension (0.2%-0.5%) in clinical studies included abnormal vision/blurring, burning on instillation, chemosis, discharge, dry eyes, epiphora, foreign body sensation, itching, injection, and photophobia. Other ocular adverse reactions occurring in less than 5% of patients include conjunctivitis, corneal abnormalities, eyelid erythema, keratoconjunctivitis, ocular irritation/pain/discomfort, papillae, and uveitis. Some of these events were similar to the underlying ocular disease being studied.

Non-ocular adverse reactions occurred in less than 15% of patients. These include headache, rhinitis and pharyngitis.

In a summary of controlled, randomized studies of individuals treated for 28 days or longer with loteprednol etabonate, the incidence of significant elevation of intraocular pressure (≥10 mm Hg) was 2% (15/901) among patients receiving loteprednol etabonate and 0.5% (3/583) among patients receiving placebo.

Post-Market Adverse Drug Reactions: In over a decade of post-marketing experience, more than 8 million units of Alrex have been shipped globally. During that time four (4) adverse event reports that qualified as serious were received. Table 3 summarizes these events.

Table 3: Alrex

Alrex Serious Adverse Events Since 1998

Sex	Age	Event
M	12	Corneal perforation
M	58	Corneal disorder, Intraocular pressure increased
F	60	Visual field defect, Glaucoma
M	74	Corneal ulcer, Keratitis bacterial, Drug maladministration

One case of mild cataract has been reported during this time.

DRUG INTERACTIONS: Overview: No specific drug interaction studies have been conducted. There are no known drug interactions.

Alrex contains benzalkonium chloride which interacts with soft contact lens. See Dosage and Administration, Administration.

Drug-drug, drug-food, drug-herb, and drug-laboratory interactions have not been studied.

DOSAGE AND ADMINISTRATION: Recommended Dose and Dosage Adjustment: One drop instilled into the affected eye(s) four times daily for up to 14 days.

Missed Dose: If scheduled dose is missed, patient should be advised to wait until the next dose and then continue as before.

Administration: Shake vigorously before using. Instill one drop into the affected eye(s) four times daily.

Alrex should be stored upright between 15-25°C for up to 28 days after first opening.

The preservative in Alrex, benzalkonium chloride, may be absorbed by soft contact lenses, and can discolour soft contact lenses. Therefore, Alrex should not be used while the patient is wearing soft contact lenses. Patients who wear soft contact lenses and whose eyes are not red should wait ten to fifteen minutes after instilling Alrex before they insert their contact lenses.

Patients should be advised not to wear a contact lens if their eye is red. Alrex should not be used to treat contact lens related irritation.

OVERDOSAGE:

No cases of overdose have been reported.

For management of a suspected accidental oral ingestion or drug overdose, contact your **regional Poison Control Centre**. See the *CPS* Directory section for a list of Poison Control Centres.

ACTION AND CLINICAL PHARMACOLOGY: Mechanism of Action: There is no generally accepted explanation for the mechanism of action of ocular corticosteroids. However, corticosteroids are thought to act by the induction of phospholipase A_2 inhibitory proteins, collectively called lipocortins. It is postulated that these proteins control the biosynthesis of potent mediators of inflammation such as prostaglandins and leukotrienes by inhibiting the release of their common precursor arachidonic acid. Arachidonic acid is released from membrane phospholipids by phospholipase A_2. Corticosteroids are capable of producing a rise in intraocular pressure.

Pharmacodynamics: Corticosteroids inhibit the inflammatory response to a variety of inciting agents and probably delay or slow healing. They inhibit the edema, fibrin deposition, capillary dilation, leukocyte migration, capillary proliferation, fibroblast proliferation, deposition of collagen, and scar formation associated with inflammation.

Pharmacokinetics: Results from a bioavailability study in normal volunteers (8 females, 2 males; age range of 19-44 years) established that plasma levels of loteprednol etabonate and Δ^1 cortienic acid etabonate (PJ 91), its primary, inactive metabolite, were below the limit of quantitation (1 ng/mL) at all sampling times. The results were obtained following the ocular administration of one drop of 0.5% loteprednol etabonate ophthalmic suspension in each eye 8 times daily for 2 days or 4 times daily for 42 days.

STORAGE AND STABILITY: Store upright between 15-25°C. **Do not freeze. Keep out of reach of children.**

SPECIAL HANDLING INSTRUCTIONS: There is no special handling instruction for Alrex.

INFORMATION FOR THE PATIENT: Published in e-CPS, available by subscription at www.e-cps.ca.

DOSAGE FORMS, COMPOSITION AND PACKAGING: Loteprednol etabonate ophthalmic suspension 0.2% w/v is supplied in a white low density polyethylene plastic bottle with a white controlled drop tip and a pink polypropylene cap in the following size: 5 mL in a 7.5 mL bottle. Nonmedicinal ingredients: benzalkonium chloride, edetate disodium, glycerin, povidone, purified water and tyloxapol. Hydrochloric Acid and/or Sodium Hydroxide may be added to adjust the pH to 5.4-5.5.

(Shown in Product Identification Section)

The reader is invited to consult CPhA's monograph **ACE Inhibitors**.

Altace® Pr

ramipril

Angiotensin Converting Enzyme Inhibitor

sanofi-aventis

Date of Revision: December 3, 2009

SUMMARY PRODUCT INFORMATION:

Route of Administration	Dosage Form/ Strength	All Nonmedicinal Ingredients
Oral	Capsules: 1.25 mg, 2.5 mg, 5 mg, 10 mg, 15 mg	• 1.25 mg capsule: pre-gelatinized starch, gelatin, yellow iron oxide, titanium dioxide. • 2.5 mg capsule: pre-gelatinized starch, gelatin, yellow iron oxide, FD&C red no. 3, titanium dioxide • 5.0 mg capsule: pre-gelatinized starch, gelatin, FD&C blue no. 2, FD&C red no. 3, titanium dioxide. • 10.0 mg capsule: pre-gelatinized starch, gelatin, FD&C blue no. 2, FD&C red no. 3, black iron oxide, titanium dioxide. • 15.0 mg capsule: pre-gelatinized starch, gelatin, D&C red no. 28, FD&C blue no. 1, black iron oxide, titanium dioxide.

INDICATIONS AND CLINICAL USE: ALTACE (ramipril) is indicated for:

- **Essential Hypertension:** ALTACE is indicated in the treatment of essential hypertension. It may be used alone or in association with thiazide diuretics.

  ALTACE can also be tried as an initial agent in those patients in whom use of diuretics and/or beta blockers are contraindicated or in patients with medical conditions in which these drugs frequently cause serious adverse effects.

  The safety and efficacy of ALTACE in renovascular hypertension have not been established and therefore, its use in this condition is not recommended.

  The safety and efficacy of concurrent use of ALTACE with antihypertensive agents other than thiazide diuretics or calcium channel blocker felodipine have not been established.
- **Treatment Following Acute Myocardial Infarction:** ALTACE is indicated following acute myocardial infarction in clinically stable patients with signs of left ventricular dysfunction to improve survival and reduce hospitalizations for heart failure.

  Sufficient experience in the treatment of patients with severe (NYHA class IV) heart failure immediately after myocardial infarction is not yet available (see Warnings and Precautions, Cardiovascular, Hypotension).
- **Management of Patients at Increased Risk of Cardiovascular Events:** ALTACE may be used to reduce the risk of myocardial infarction, stroke or cardiovascular death in patients over 55 years of age who are at high risk of cardiovascular events because of a history of coronary artery disease, stroke, peripheral artery disease, or diabetes that is accompanied by at least one other cardiovascular risk factor such as hypertension, elevated total cholesterol levels, low high density lipoprotein levels, cigarette smoking, or documented microalbuminuria.

General: Geriatrics (>65 years of age): Although clinical experience has not identified differences in response between the elderly (>65 years) and younger patients, greater sensitivity of some older individuals cannot be ruled out (see Action and Clinical Pharmacology, Pharmacokinetics).

Pediatrics: The safety and effectiveness of ALTACE in children have not been established; therefore use in this age group is not recommended.

CONTRAINDICATIONS: ALTACE is contraindicated in:

- Patients who are hypersensitive to this drug, to any other ACE inhibitor, or to any ingredient in the formulation. For a complete listing of ingredients see Dosage Forms, Composition and Packaging.
- Patients who have a history of angioedema.
- During pregnancy
- In breast-feeding women
- In patients with haemodynamically relevant bilateral renal artery stenosis, or unilateral in the single kidney.
- Patients with hypotensive states

Concomitant use of ACE inhibitors and extracorporeal treatment leading to contact of blood with negatively charged surfaces must be avoided (see Warnings and Precautions, Immune).

WARNINGS AND PRECAUTIONS:

Serious Warnings and Precautions

When used in pregnancy, angiotensin converting enzyme (ACE) inhibitors can cause injury or even death of the developing fetus. When pregnancy is detected ALTACE should be discontinued as soon as possible.

General: Cough: A dry, persistent cough, which usually disappears only after withdrawal or lowering of the dose of ALTACE, has been reported. Such possibility should be considered as part of the differential diagnosis of cough (see Adverse Reactions).

Patient Alertness: ALTACE may lower the state of patient alertness and/or reactivity, particularly at the start of treatment (see Adverse Reactions).

Cardiovascular: Aortic Stenosis: There is concern, on theoretical grounds, that patients with aortic stenosis might be at particular risk of decreased coronary perfusion when treated with vasodilators because they do not develop as much afterload reduction.

Hypotension: Symptomatic hypotension has occurred after administration of ALTACE, usually after the first or second dose or when the dose was increased. It is more likely to occur in patients who are volume depleted by diuretic therapy, dietary salt restriction, dialysis, diarrhea, vomiting, or in other situations in which a significant activation of the renin-angiotensin system is to be anticipated such as in patients with severe, and particularly with malignant hypertension, in patients with haemodynamically relevant left-ventricular outflow impediment (e.g., stenosis of the aortic valve) or in patients with haemodynamically relevant renal artery stenosis.

In patients with ischemic heart disease or cerebrovascular disease, an excessive fall in blood pressure could result in a myocardial infarction or cerebrovascular accident (see Adverse Reactions, Clinical Trial Adverse Drug Reactions, Treatment Following Acute Myocardial Infarction, Management of Patients at Increased Risk of Cardiovascular Events and Less Common Clinical Trial Adverse Drug Reactions (<1%), Cardiovascular). Because of the potential fall in blood pressure in these patients, therapy with ALTACE should be started under close medical supervision. Such patients should be followed closely for the first weeks of treatment and whenever the dose of ALTACE is increased. In patients with severe congestive heart failure, with or without associated renal insufficiency, ACE inhibitor therapy may cause excessive hypotension and has been associated with oliguria, and/or progressive azotemia, and rarely, with acute renal failure and/or death.

Generally, it is recommended that dehydration, hypovolaemia or salt depletion be corrected before initiating treatment (in patients with heart failure, however, such corrective action must be carefully weighed against the risk of volume overload). When these conditions have become clinically relevant, treatment with ALTACE must only be started or continued if appropriate steps are taken concurrently to prevent an excessive fall in blood pressure and deterioration of renal function.

If hypotension occurs, the patient should be placed in a supine position and, if necessary, receive an intravenous infusion of 0.9% sodium chloride. A transient hypotensive response may not be a contraindication to further doses which usually can be given without difficulty once the blood pressure has increased after volume expansion in hypertensive patients. However, lower doses of ALTACE and/or reduced concomitant diuretic therapy should be considered. In patients receiving treatment following acute myocardial infarction, consideration should be given to discontinuation of ALTACE (see Adverse Reactions, Clinical Trial Adverse Drug Reactions, Treatment Following Acute Myocardial Infarction, Dosage and Administration, Recommended Dose and Dosage Adjustment, Treatment Following Acute Myocardial Infarction).

Hematologic: Hyperkalemia and Potassium-sparing Diuretics: Elevated serum potassium (greater than 5.7 mEq/L) was observed in approximately 1% of hypertensive patients in clinical trials treated with ALTACE. In most cases these were isolated values which resolved despite continued therapy. Hyperkalemia was not a cause of discontinuation of therapy in any hypertensive patient. Risk factors for the development of hyperkalemia may include renal insufficiency, diabetes mellitus, and the concomitant use of agents to treat hypokalemia or other drugs associated with increases in serum potassium (see Drug Interactions, Drug-Drug Interactions).

Neutropenia/Agranulocytosis: Agranulocytosis and bone marrow depression have been caused by ACE inhibitors. Several cases of agranulocytosis, neutropenia or leukopenia have been reported in which a causal relationship to ALTACE cannot be excluded. Current experience with the drug shows the incidence to be rare. Periodic monitoring of white blood cell counts should be considered especially in patients with collagen vascular disease and/or renal disease. (See Warnings and Precautions, Monitoring and Laboratory Tests, and Adverse Reactions, Less Common Adverse Drug Reactions, Hematologic.)

Hepatic/Biliary/Pancreatic: Hepatitis (hepatocellular and/or cholestatic), elevations of liver enzymes and/or serum bilirubin have occurred during therapy with ACE inhibitors in patients with or without pre-existing liver abnormalities. In most cases the changes were reversed on discontinuation of the drug.

Elevations of liver enzymes and/or serum bilirubin have been reported with ALTACE (see Adverse Reactions). Should the patient receiving ALTACE experience any unexplained symptoms particularly during the first weeks or months of treatment, it is recommended that a full set of liver function tests and any other necessary investigations be carried out. Discontinuation of ALTACE should be considered when appropriate.

There are no adequate studies in patients with cirrhosis and/or liver dysfunction. In patients with impaired liver function, response to the treatment with ALTACE may be either increased or reduced. In addition, in patients in whom severe liver cirrhosis with oedema and ascites is present, the renin-angiotensin system may be significantly activated. ALTACE should be used with particular caution in patients with pre-existing liver abnormalities. In such patients baseline liver function tests should be obtained before administration of the drug and close monitoring of response and metabolic effects should apply (see Action and Clinical Pharmacology, Special Populations and Conditions, Hepatic Insufficiency).

Rarely, ACE inhibitors, including ALTACE, have been associated with a syndrome that starts with cholestatic jaundice and progresses to fulminant hepatic necrosis and (sometimes) death. The mechanism of this syndrome is not understood. Patients receiving ACE inhibitors who develop jaundice or marked elevations of hepatic enzymes should discontinue the ACE inhibitor and receive appropriate medical follow-up.

Immune: Angioedema—Head and Neck: Angioedema has been reported in patients with ACE inhibitors including ALTACE. Angioedema associated with laryngeal involvement may be fatal. If laryngeal stridor or angioedema of the face, extremities, lips, tongue, or glottis occurs, ALTACE should be discontinued immediately, the patient treated appropriately in accordance with accepted medical care, and carefully observed until the swelling disappears. In instances where swelling is confined to the face and lips, the condition generally resolves without treatment, although antihistamines may be useful in relieving symptoms. Where there is involvement of tongue, glottis, or larynx, likely to cause airway obstruction, appropriate therapy (including, but not limited to 0.3 to 0.5 mL of subcutaneous epinephrine solution 1:1000) should be administered promptly (see Adverse Reactions, Clinical Trial Adverse Drug Reactions, Essential Hypertension; Less Common Clinical Trial Adverse Drug Reactions (<1%), Body as a Whole).

Angioedema—Intestinal: Intestinal angioedema has been reported in patients treated with ACE inhibitors. These patients presented with abdominal pain (with or without nausea or vomiting); in some cases facial angioedema also occurred. The intestinal angioedema symptoms resolved after stopping the ACE inhibitor.

The incidence of angioedema during ACE inhibitor therapy has been reported to be higher in black than in non-black patients.

Patients with a history of angioedema unrelated to ACE inhibitor therapy may be at increased risk of angioedema while receiving an ACE inhibitor (see Contraindications).

Angioedema, including laryngeal edema, may occur especially following the first dose of ALTACE.

Anaphylactoid Reactions During Membrane Exposure: Anaphylactoid reactions have been reported in patients dialyzed with high-flux membranes [e.g. polyacrylonitrile (PAN)] and treated concomitantly with an ACE inhibitor. Dialysis should be stopped immediately if symptoms such as nausea, abdominal cramps, burning, angioedema, shortness of breath and severe hypotension occur. Symptoms are not relieved by antihistamines. In these patients consideration should be given to using a different type of dialysis membrane or a different class of antihypertensive agents.

Anaphylactoid Reactions During LDL Apheresis: Rarely, patients receiving ACE inhibitors during low density lipoprotein apheresis with dextran sulfate have experienced life-threatening anaphylactoid reactions. These reactions were avoided by temporarily withholding the ACE inhibitor therapy prior to each apheresis.

Anaphylactoid Reactions During Desensitization: There have been isolated reports of patients experiencing sustained life threatening anaphylactoid reactions while receiving ACE inhibitors during desensitization treatment with hymenoptera (e.g. bees, wasps) venoma. In the same patients, these reactions have been avoided when ACE inhibitors were temporarily withheld for at least 24 hours, but they have reappeared upon inadvertent rechallenge.

Peri-operative Considerations: Surgery/Anesthesia: In patients undergoing surgery or anesthesia with agents producing hypotension, ALTACE may block angiotensin II formation secondary to compensatory renin release. If hypotension occurs and is considered to be due to this mechanism, it may be corrected by volume repletion.

Renal: As a consequence of inhibiting the renin-angiotensin-aldosterone system, changes in renal function have been seen in susceptible individuals. In patients whose renal function may depend on the activity of the renin-angiotensin-aldosterone system, such as patients with bilateral renal artery stenosis, unilateral renal artery stenosis to a solitary kidney, or severe congestive heart failure, treatment with agents that inhibit this system has been associated with oliguria, progressive azotemia, and rarely, acute renal failure and/or death. In susceptible patients, concomitant diuretic use may further increase risk; therefore, discontinuation of diuretic therapy may be required.

Use of ALTACE should include appropriate assessment of renal function.

ALTACE should be used with caution in patients with renal insufficiency as they may require reduced or less frequent doses (see Dosage and Administration). Close monitoring of renal function during therapy should be performed as deemed appropriate in patients with renal insufficiency.

Special Populations: Pregnant Women: ACE inhibitors can cause fetal and neonatal morbidity and mortality when administered to pregnant women. When pregnancy is detected, ALTACE should be discontinued as soon as possible.

The use of ACE inhibitors during the second and third trimesters of pregnancy has been associated with fetal and neonatal injury including hypotension, neonatal skull hypoplasia, anuria, reversible or irreversible renal failure, and death. Oligohydramnios has also been reported, presumably resulting from decreased fetal renal function, associated with fetal limb contractures, craniofacial deformation, and hypoplastic lung development.

Prematurity, and patent ductus arteriosus and other structural cardiac malformations, as well as neurologic malformations, have also been reported following exposure in the first trimester of pregnancy.

Infants with a history of in utero exposure to ACE inhibitors should be closely observed for hypotension, oliguria, and hyperkalemia. If oliguria occurs, attention should be directed toward support of blood pressure and renal perfusion. Exchange transfusion or dialysis may be required as a means of reversing hypotension and/or substituting for impaired renal function; however, limited experience with those procedures has not been associated with significant clinical benefit.

It is not known if ramipril or ramiprilat can be removed from the body by hemodialysis.

Animal Data: No teratogenic effects of ramipril were seen in studies of pregnant rats, rabbits, and cynomolgus monkeys. The doses used were: 10, 100, or 1000 mg/kg in rats (2500 times maximum human dose), 0.4, 1.0, or 2.5 mg/kg in rabbits (6.25 times maximum human dose), and 5, 50, or 500 mg/kg in cynomolgus monkeys (1250 times maximum human dose). In rats, the highest dose caused reduced food intake in the dams, with consequent reduced birth weights of the pups and weight development during the lactation period. In rabbits, maternal effects were mortalities (high and middle dose) and reduced body weight. In monkeys, maternal effects were mortalities (high and middle dose), vomiting, and reduced weight gain.

Nursing Women: The presence of concentrations of ACE inhibitor have been reported in human milk. The use of ALTACE is contraindicated during breast-feeding.

Pediatrics: The safety and effectiveness of ALTACE in children have not been established; therefore use in this age group is not recommended.

Geriatrics (>65 years of age): Although clinical experience has not identified differences in response between the elderly (>65 years) and younger patients, greater sensitivity of some older individuals cannot be ruled out (see Action and Clinical Pharmacology, Special Populations and Conditions, Geriatrics).

Monitoring and Laboratory Tests: Hematological Monitoring: Periodic monitoring of white blood cell counts should be considered to permit detection of a possible leukopenia. More frequent monitoring is advised in the initial phase of treatment and in patients with impaired renal function, those with concomitant collagen disease (e.g. lupus erythematosus or scleroderma) or those treated with other drugs that can cause changes in the blood picture (see Drug Interactions, Drug-Drug Interactions, Allopurinol, Immunosuppressants, Corticosteroids, Procainamide, Cytostatics and Other Substances That May Change the Blood Picture).

Renal Function Monitoring: Use of ALTACE should include appropriate assessment of renal function, particularly in the initial week's treatment with an ACE inhibitor. Close monitoring of renal function during therapy should be performed as deemed appropriate in patients with renal insufficiency.

Particularly careful monitoring is required in patients with: heart failure; renovascular disease, including patients with haemodynamically relevant unilateral renal artery stenosis. In the latter patient group, even a small increase in serum creatinine may be indicative of unilateral loss of renal function; impairment of renal function; kidney transplant.

Electrolyte Monitoring: It is recommended that serum potassium be monitored regularly. More frequent monitoring of serum potassium is necessary in patients with impaired renal function.

Driving a Vehicle or Performing Other Hazardous Tasks: Some adverse effects (e.g. some symptoms of a reduction in blood pressure such as lightheadedness, dizziness, syncope) may impair the patient's ability to concentrate and react and, therefore, constitute a risk in situations where these abilities are of particular importance (e.g. operating a vehicle or machinery).

Information to Be Provided to the Patient: Cardiovascular: Hypotension: Patients should be cautioned to report lightheadedness, especially during the first few days of ALTACE therapy. If actual syncope occurs, the patients should be told to discontinue the drug and consult with their physician.

All patients should be cautioned that excessive perspiration and dehydration may lead to an excessive fall in blood pressure because of reduction in fluid volume. Other causes of volume depletion such as vomiting or diarrhea may also lead to a fall in blood pressure, patients should be advised to consult with their physician.

Hematologic: Hyperkalemia and Potassium–sparing Diuretics: Patients should be told not to use salt substitutes containing potassium without consulting their physician.

Neutropenia/Agranulocytosis: Patients should be told to report promptly to their physician any indication of infection (e.g. sore throat, fever) as this may be a sign of neutropenia (see Adverse Reactions).

Hepatic/Biliary: Patients should be advised to return to their physician if they experience any symptoms possibly related to liver dysfunction. This would include "viral-like symptoms" in the first weeks to months of therapy (such as fever, malaise, muscle pain, rash or adenopathy which are possible indicators of hypersensitivity reactions), or if abdominal pain, nausea or vomiting, loss of appetite, jaundice, itching or any other unexplained symptoms occur during therapy.

Immune: Angioedema: Patients should be so advised and told to report immediately any signs or symptoms suggesting angioedema, such as swelling of face, extremities, eyes, lips, tongue, difficulty in swallowing or breathing. They should immediately stop taking ALTACE and consult with their physician.

Special Populations: Pregnancy: Since the use of ALTACE during pregnancy can cause injury and even death of the developing fetus, patients should be advised to report promptly to their physician if they become pregnant and the use of ALTACE should be stopped.

ADVERSE REACTIONS: Adverse Drug Reaction Overview: As ALTACE is an antihypertensive; the most common adverse reactions are effects secondary to its blood-pressure-lowering action.

The long-term safety of ramipril, as monotherapy was assessed in patients with hypertension. The most commonly reported serious adverse reactions were hypotension (0.1%); myocardial infarction (0.3%); cerebrovascular accident (0.1%); edema (0.2%); syncope (0.1%). Angioedema occurred in 0.1% patients treated with ramipril and a diuretic.

The most frequent adverse events occurring in these trials were: headache (15.1%); dizziness (3.7%); asthenia (3.7%); chest pain (2.0%); nausea (1.8%); peripheral edema (1.8%); somnolence (1.7%); impotence (1.5%); rash (1.4%); arthritis (1.1%); dyspnea (1.1%). Discontinuation of therapy due to clinical adverse events was required in 0.8% of patients treated with ALTACE. Approximately 1% of patients in North American controlled clinical trials have required discontinuation because of cough.

Post Acute Myocardial Infarction Adverse reactions (AIRE Study) considered possibly/probably related to study drug that occurred in more than 1% of patients and more frequently on ramipril were: Hypotension, Cough increased, Dizziness/Vertigo, Nausea/Vomiting, Angina pectoris, Postural hypotension, Syncope, Heart failure, Severe/resistant heart failure, Myocardial infarct, Vomiting, Headache, Abnormal kidney function, Abnormal chest pain and Diarrhea. Discontinuation of therapy due to adverse reactions was required in post-AMI patients taking ramipril (36.7%), compared to patients receiving placebo (40.8%).

The safety profile of ALTACE in patients at Increased Risk of Cardiovascular Events (HOPE Study) was consistent with the post-marketing surveillance experience. Reasons for discontinuation of therapy, were cough (ramipril 7.3%, placebo 1.8%), hypotension/dizziness (ramipril 1.9%, placebo 1.5%) and edema (ramipril 0.4%, placebo 0.2%).

Clinical Trial Adverse Drug Reactions: Because clinical trials are conducted under very specific conditions the adverse reaction rates observed in the clinical trials may not reflect the rates observed in practice and should not be compared to the rates in the clinical trials of another drug. Adverse drug reaction information from clinical trials is useful for identifying drug-related adverse events and for approximating rates.

Essential Hypertension: ALTACE has been evaluated for safety in over 4000 hypertensive patients. Almost 500 elderly patients have participated in controlled trials. Long-term safety has been assessed in almost 700 patients treated for 1 year or more. There was no increase in the incidence of adverse events in elderly patients given the same daily dose. The overall frequency of adverse events was not related to duration of therapy or total daily dose.

Serious adverse events occurring in North American placebo-controlled clinical trials with ramipril monotherapy in hypertension (n=972) were: hypotension (0.1%); myocardial infarction (0.3%); cerebrovascular accident (0.1%); edema (0.2%); syncope (0.1%). Among all North American ramipril patients (n=1244), angioedema occurred in 0.1% patients treated with ramipril and a diuretic.

The most frequent adverse events occurring in these trials with ALTACE monotherapy in hypertensive patients that were treated for at least one year (n=651) were: headache (15.1%); dizziness (3.7%); asthenia (3.7%); chest pain (2.0%); nausea (1.8%); peripheral edema (1.8%); somnolence (1.7%); impotence (1.5%); rash (1.4%); arthritis (1.1%); dyspnea (1.1%). Discontinuation of therapy due to clinical adverse events was required in 5 patients (0.8%).

In placebo-controlled trials, an excess of upper respiratory infection and flu syndrome was seen in the ramipril group. As these studies were carried out before the relationship of cough to ACE inhibitors was recognized, some of these events may represent ramipril-induced cough. In a later 1-year study, increased cough was seen in almost 12% of ALTACE patients, with about 4% of these patients requiring discontinuation of treatment. Approximately 1% of patients treated with ALTACE monotherapy in North American controlled clinical trials (n=972) have required discontinuation because of cough.

Treatment Following Acute Myocardial Infarction: 1004 post-AMI patients received ALTACE in a controlled clinical trial. In both the ramipril and placebo groups, myocardial infarction, heart failure, atrial fibrillation, peripheral vascular disease and urinary tract infection were more common in elderly than in younger patients. Gastrointestinal disturbances were more frequent in elderly patients on ramipril. Cough and hypotension were more frequent in women receiving ramipril.

Adverse events (except laboratory abnormalities) considered possibly/probably related to study drug that occurred in more than one percent of stabilized patients with clinical signs of heart failure treated with ALTACE following an acute myocardial infarction are shown below. The incidences represent the experiences from the AIRE (Acute Infarction Ramipril Efficacy) study. The follow-up time was between 6 and 48 months for this study (mean follow up=15 months). See Table 1 and Table 2.

Table 1: ALTACE

Percentage of Patients with Adverse Events Possibly/Probably Related to Study Drug Placebo-controlled (AIRE) Mortality Study

Adverse Event	ALTACE n=1004 %	Placebo n=982 %
Hypotension	10.7	4.7
Cough Increased	7.6	3.7
Dizziness/Vertigo	5.6	3.9
Nausea/Vomiting	3.8	1.9
Angina Pectoris	2.9	2.0
Postural Hypotension	2.2	1.4

(cont'd)

Table 1: ALTACE *(cont'd)*

Percentage of Patients with Adverse Events Possibly/Probably Related to Study Drug Placebo-controlled (AIRE) Mortality Study

Adverse Event	ALTACE n=1004 %	Placebo n=982 %
Syncope	2.1	1.4
Heart Failure	2.0	2.2
Severe/resistant Heart Failure	2.0	3.0
Myocardial Infarct	1.7	1.7
Vomiting	1.6	0.5
Headache	1.2	0.8
Abnormal Kidney Function	1.2	0.5
Abnormal Chest Pain	1.1	0.9
Diarrhea	1.1	0.4

Table 2: ALTACE

Percentage of Patients with Serious Adverse Events Possibly Related to Study Drug Placebo-controlled (AIRE) Mortality Study

Adverse Event	ALTACE n=1004 %	Placebo n=982 %
Hypotension	3.0	1.1
Angina Pectoris	2.0	1.2
Severe/resistant Heart Failure	1.9	2.9
Myocardial Infarct	1.7	1.7
Heart Failure	1.5	1.5
Syncope	1.3	0.8
Chest Pain	0.7	0.9
Nausea	0.6	0.5
Vomiting	0.5	0.1
Dizziness	0.5	0.5
Abnormal Kidney Function	0.5	0.2
Chest Infection	0.2	0.0
Postural Hypotension	0.2	0.2
Headache	0.1	0.0

Isolated cases of death have been reported with the use of ramipril that appear to be related to hypotension (including first dose effects), but many of these are difficult to differentiate from progression of underlying disease (see Warnings and Precautions, Cardiovascular, Hypotension).

Discontinuation of therapy due to adverse reactions was required in 368/1004 post-AMI patients taking ramipril (36.7%), compared to 401/982 patients receiving placebo (40.8%).

Management of Patients at Increased Risk of Cardiovascular Events: In the Heart Outcome Prevention Evaluation (HOPE) study, based on a total of 4645 patients treated with ramipril, the safety profile of ALTACE was consistent with the post-marketing surveillance experience. The reasons for stopping the treatment, where the incidence was greater in the ramipril than in the placebo group, were cough (ramipril 7.3%, placebo 1.8%), hypotension/dizziness (ramipril 1.9%, placebo 1.5%) and edema (ramipril 0.4%, placebo 0.2%).

Less Common Adverse Drug Reactions (<1%): Clinical adverse events occurring in less than 1% of patients treated with ALTACE in controlled clinical trials are listed below by body system:

Body as a Whole: angioedema.

Cardiovascular: symptomatic hypotension, flushing, syncope, angina pectoris, arrhythmia, chest pain, palpitations, tachycardia, myocardial infarction, disturbed orthostatic regulation, vascular stenosis, exacerbation of perfusion disturbances due to vascular stenoses.

CNS: anxiety, amnesia, confusion, convulsions, depression, impaired hearing, hearing loss, insomnia, sleep disturbances, nervousness, neuralgia, neuropathy, paresthesia, polyneuritis, somnolence, tinnitus, tremor, vertigo, vision disturbances (including blurred vision), disorders of balance, lightheadness, restlessness.

Dermatologic: apparent hypersensitivity reactions (with manifestations of urticaria, pruritus, or rash, with or without fever), photosensitivity, purpura.

In addition, the following cutaneous or mucosal reactions may occur: maculopapular rash, maculo-papular exanthema, psoriasiform exanthema, erythroderma/exfoliative dermatitis, and onycholysis.

Gastrointestinal: pancreatitis (cases of fatal outcome have been very exceptionally reported), abdominal pain (sometimes with enzyme changes suggesting pancreatitis), upper abdominal pain, gastritis, intestinal angioedema, glossitis, increased levels of pancreatic enzymes, anorexia, decreased appetite, constipation, diarrhea, digestive disturbances, dry mouth, dyspepsia, dysphagia, gastroenteritis, nausea, increased salivation, taste disturbance, vomiting, abdominal discomfort.

Rarely, ACE inhibitors, including ALTACE, have been associated with a syndrome that starts with cholestatic jaundice and progresses to fulminant hepatic necrosis and (sometimes) death.

Hematologic: agranulocytosis, leucopenia, eosinophilia, thrombocytopenia, (see Warnings and Precautions, Hematologic, Neutropenia/Agranulocytosis).

Renal: increases in blood urea nitrogen (BUN) and serum creatinine, impaired renal function, oliguria. Rarely, a deterioration of pre-existing proteinuria may develop (though ACE inhibitors usually reduce proteinuria) or an increase in urinary output (in connection with an improvement in cardiac performance).

Respiratory: increased cough, nasal congestion, sinusitis, bronchitis, and bronchospasm (including aggravated asthma).

Other: arthralgia, arthritis, dyspnea, edema, epistaxis, impotence, transient erectile impotence, increased sweating, malaise, myalgia, weight gain, conjunctivitis, muscle cramps, reduced libido, loss of taste, depressed mood.

A symptom complex has been reported which may include fever, vasculitis, myalgia, arthralgia/arthritis, elevated ESR, eosinophilia and leucocytosis. Rash, photosensitivity or other dermatologic manifestations may also occur.

Abnormal Hematologic and Clinical Chemistry Findings: Increased creatinine; increases in blood urea nitrogen (BUN); decreases in red blood cell count, hemoglobin or hematocrit; hyponatraemia; elevations of liver enzymes, serum bilirubin, uric acid, blood glucose; proteinuria and significant increases in serum potassium.

Post-Market Adverse Drug Reactions: Body as a Whole: anaphylactoid reactions, angioedema (cases of fatal outcome have been reported).

Cardiovascular: cerebrovascular disorders (including ischaemic stroke).

CNS: burning sensation (mainly to skin of face or extremities), smell disturbances, precipitation or intensification of Raynaud's phenomenon, impaired psychomotor skills (impaired reactions), attention disturbances.

Dermatologic: erythema multiforme, pemphigus, Stevens-Johnson syndrome, exacerbation of psoriasis, lichenoid exanthema, pemphigoid exanthema and enanthema, reversible alopecia, toxic epidermal necrolysis.

Gastrointestinal: hepatic failure, cholestatic jaundice, hepatitis (cases of fatal outcome have been very exceptionally reported), aphtous stomatitis; in isolated cases liver damage (including acute liver failure) may occur.

Haematologic: pancytopaenia, bone marrow depression and hemolytic anemia (see Warnings and Precautions, Hematologic, Neutropenia/Agranulocytosis).

Laboratory Test Findings: decrease in blood sodium.

Other: gynaecomastia, positive ANA.

DRUG INTERACTIONS: Drug-Drug Interactions: Concomitant Diuretic Therapy: Patients concomitantly taking ACE inhibitors and diuretics, and especially those in whom diuretic therapy was recently instituted, may occasionally experience an excessive reduction of blood pressure after initiation of therapy. The possibility of hypotensive effects after the first dose of ALTACE can be minimized by either discontinuing the diuretic or increasing the salt intake prior to initiation of treatment with ALTACE. If it is not possible to discontinue the diuretic, the starting dose of ALTACE should be reduced and the patient should be closely observed for several hours following the initial dose and until blood pressure has stabilized (see Warnings and Precautions and Dosage and Administration). Regular monitoring of serum sodium is recommended in patients undergoing concurrent diuretic therapy.

Other Substances with Antihypertensive Potential (e.g. nitrates): Potentiation of the antihypertensive effect is to be anticipated.

Vasopressor Sympathomimetics: These may reduce the antihypertensive effect of ALTACE. Particularly close blood pressure monitoring is recommended.

Agents Increasing Serum Potassium: Since ALTACE decreases aldosterone production, elevation of serum potassium may occur. Potassium sparing diuretics such as spironolactone, triamterene or amiloride, or potassium supplements should be given only for documented hypokalemia and with caution and frequent monitoring of serum potassium, since they may lead to a significant increase in serum potassium. Salt substitutes which contain potassium should also be used with caution. (See also Non-steroidal Anti-inflammatory Agents and Acetylsalicylic Acid.)

Agents Causing Renin Release: The antihypertensive effect of ALTACE is augmented by antihypertensive agents that cause renin release (e.g. diuretics).

Lithium: Increased serum lithium levels and symptoms of lithium toxicity have been reported in patients receiving ACE inhibitors during therapy with lithium. These drugs should be administered with caution, and frequent monitoring of serum lithium levels is recommended. If a diuretic is also used, the risk of lithium toxicity may be further increased.

Antacids: In one open-label, randomized, cross-over single dose study in 24 male subjects, it was determined that the bioavailability of ALTACE and the pharmacokinetic profile of ramiprilat were not affected by concomitant administration of the antacid, magnesium and aluminum hydroxides.

Digoxin: In one open-label study in 12 subjects, administered multiple doses of both ramipril and digoxin, no changes were found in serum levels of ramipril, ramiprilat, and digoxin.

Warfarin: The co-administration of ALTACE with warfarin did not alter the anticoagulant effects.

Acenocoumarol: In a multi-dose double-blind, placebo-controlled, pharmacodynamic interaction study with 14 patients with mild hypertension administered both ramipril and therapeutic doses of acenocoumarol, blood pressure, thrombotest time and coagulation factors were not significantly changed.

Non-steroidal Anti-inflammatory Agents and Acetylsalicylic Acid: The antihypertensive effects of ACE inhibitors may be reduced with concomitant administration of non-steroidal anti-inflammatory agents (e.g. indomethacin). Concomitant treatment of ACE inhibitors and Non-Steroidal Anti-Inflammatory drugs may lead to an increased risk of worsening of renal function and an increase in serum potassium. (See also Agents Increasing Serum Potassium.)

Heparin: Rise in serum potassium concentration possible.

Antidiabetic Agents (e.g. insulin and sulfonylurea derivates): ACE inhibitors may reduce insulin resistance. In isolated cases, such reduction may lead to hypoglycaemic reactions in patients concomitantly treated with antidiabetics. Particularly close blood glucose monitoring is, therefore, recommended in the initial phase of co-administration.

Allopurinol, Immunosuppressants, Corticosteroids, Procainamide, Cytostatics and Other Substances That May Change the Blood Picture: increased likelihood of haematological reactions.

Alcohol: increased vasodilatation. Alcohol may potentiate the effect of ALTACE.

Salt: increased dietary salt intake may attenuate the antihypertensive effect of ALTACE.

DOSAGE AND ADMINISTRATION: Recommended Dose and Dosage Adjustment: Essential Hypertension: Dosage of ALTACE must be individualized. Initiation of therapy requires consideration of recent antihypertensive drug treatment, the extent of blood pressure elevation and salt restriction. The dosage of other antihypertensive agents being used with ALTACE may need to be adjusted.

Monotherapy: The recommended initial dosage of ALTACE in patients not on diuretics is 2.5 mg once daily. Dosage should be adjusted according to blood pressure response, generally, at intervals of at least two weeks. The usual dose range is 2.5 to 10 mg once daily. A daily dose of 20 mg should not be exceeded.

In some patients treated once daily, the antihypertensive effect may diminish towards the end of the dosing interval. This can be evaluated by measuring blood pressure just prior to dosing to determine whether satisfactory control is being maintained for 24 hours. If it is not, either twice daily administration with the same total daily dose, or an increase in dose should be considered. If blood pressure is not controlled with ALTACE alone, a diuretic may be added. After the addition of a diuretic, it may be possible to reduce the dose of ALTACE.

Concomitant Diuretic Therapy: Symptomatic hypotension occasionally may occur following the initial dose of ALTACE and is more likely in patients who are currently being treated with a diuretic. The diuretic should, if possible, be discontinued for two to three days before beginning therapy with ALTACE to reduce the likelihood of hypotension (see Warnings and Precautions). If the diuretic cannot be discontinued, an initial dose of 1.25 mg ALTACE should be used with careful medical supervision for several hours and until blood pressure has stabilized. The dosage of ALTACE should subsequently be titrated (as described above) to the optimal response.

Use in Renal Impairment: For patients with a creatinine clearance below 40 mL/min/1.73 m^2 (serum creatinine above 2.5 mg/dL), the recommended initial dose is 1.25 mg ALTACE once daily. Dosage may be titrated upward until blood pressure is controlled or to a maximum total daily dose of 5 mg. In patients with severe renal impairment (creatinine clearance below 10 mL/min/1.73 m^2) the maximum total daily dose of 2.5 mg ALTACE should not be exceeded.

Treatment Following Acute Myocardial Infarction: Dosage of ALTACE must be individualized. Initiation of therapy requires consideration of concomitant medication and baseline blood pressure and should be instituted under close medical supervision, usually in a hospital, three to ten days following an acute myocardial infarction in haemodynamically stable patients with clinical signs of heart failure.

The recommended initial dosage of ALTACE is 2.5 mg given twice a day (b.i.d.), one in the morning and one in the evening. If tolerated, and depending on the patient's response, dosage may be increased by doubling at intervals of one to three days. The maximum daily dose of ALTACE should not exceed 5 mg twice daily (b.i.d.).

After the initial dose of ALTACE, the patient should be observed under medical supervision for at least two hours and until blood pressure has stabilized for at least an additional hour. If a patient becomes hypotensive at this dosage, it is recommended that the dosage be lowered to 1.25 mg b.i.d. following effective management of the hypotension (see Warnings and Precautions, Cardiovascular, Hypotension).

Patients who have been fluid or salt depleted, or treated with diuretics are at an increased risk of hypotension (see Warnings and Precautions, Cardiovascular, Hypotension). An excessive fall in blood pressure may occur particularly in the following: after the initial dose of ALTACE; after every first increase of dose of ALTACE; after the first dose of a concomitant diuretic and/or when increasing the dose of the concomitant diuretic. If appropriate, the dose of any concomitant diuretic should be reduced which may diminish the likelihood of hypotension (see Drug Interactions, Drug-Drug Interactions). Consideration should be given to reducing the initial dose to 1.25 mg of ALTACE in these patients.

Use in Renal Impairment: In patients with impaired renal function (creatinine clearance of 20-50 mL/min/1.73 m² body surface area), the initial recommended dosage is generally 1.25 mg of ALTACE once daily. This dosage may be increased with caution up to 1.25 mg of ALTACE twice daily, depending upon clinical response and tolerability.

Insufficient data is available concerning the use of ramipril following acute myocardial infarction in patients with heart failure and severe renal failure (see Action and Clinical Pharmacology, Pharmacokinetics and Warnings and Precautions, Renal).

Use in Hepatic Impairment: Insufficient data is available concerning the use of ramipril following acute myocardial infarction in patients with heart failure and hepatic dysfunction. Dose reduction and careful monitoring of these patients is required (see Actions and Clinical Pharmacology, Pharmacokinetics and Warnings and Precautions, Hepatic/Biliary/Pancreatic).

Management of Patients at Increased Risk of Cardiovascular Events: Recommended initial dose: 2.5 mg of ALTACE once daily. Depending on the tolerability, the dose is gradually increased. It is recommended to double the dose after one week of treatment and—after another three weeks—to increase it to 10 mg. Usual maintenance dose: 10 mg of ALTACE daily (see Action and Clinical Pharmacology and Warnings and Precautions).

Dosage recommendations for special risk groups such as patients with renal or hepatic impairment, or at an increased risk of hypotension (fluid or salt depletion, treated with diuretics) are to be followed as previously described (see Warnings and Precautions).

OVERDOSAGE:
Limited data are available regarding overdosage of ALTACE in humans. Two cases of overdosage have been reported.

In the case of an overdose with ramipril, the most likely clinical manifestation would be symptoms attributable to severe hypotension, which should normally be treated by intravenous volume expansion with normal saline.

Overdosage may cause excessive peripheral vasodilatation (with marked hypotension, shock), bradycardia, electrolyte disturbances, and renal failure.

Management: Primary detoxification by, for example, gastric lavage, administration of adsorbents, sodium sulfate; (if possible during the first 30 minutes). In the event of hypotension administration of α1-adrenergic agonists (e.g. norepinephrine, dopamine) or angiotensin II (angiotensinamide), which is usually available only in scattered research laboratories, must be considered in addition to volume and salt substitution.

No experience is available concerning the efficacy of forced diuresis, alteration in urine pH, haemofiltration, or dialysis in speeding up the elimination of ramipril or ramiprilat. If dialysis or haemofiltration is nevertheless considered, see also Warnings and Precautions, Immune, Anaphylactoid Reactions During Membrane Exposure.

> For management of a suspected drug overdose, contact your **regional Poison Control Centre**. See the *CPS* Directory section for a list of Poison Control Centres.

ACTION AND CLINICAL PHARMACOLOGY: Mechanism of Action: ALTACE is an angiotensin converting enzyme (ACE) inhibitor, which is used in the treatment of essential hypertension, following acute myocardial infarction in stabilized patients with clinically confirmed heart failure, and for the management of patients at increased risk of cardiovascular events.

Following oral administration, ALTACE is rapidly hydrolyzed to ramiprilat, its principal active metabolite.

Angiotensin-converting enzyme catalyzes the conversion of angiotensin I to the vasoconstrictor substance, angiotensin II. Angiotensin II also stimulates aldosterone secretion by the adrenal cortex. Inhibition of ACE activity leads to decreased levels of angiotensin II thereby resulting in decreased vasoconstriction and decreased aldosterone secretion. The latter decrease may result in a small increase in serum potassium (see Warnings and Precautions, Hematologic, Hyperkalemia and Potassium-sparing Diuretics). Decreased levels of angiotensin II and the accompanying lack of negative feedback on renal renin secretion result in increases in plasma renin activity.

ACE is identical to kininase II. Thus, ramipril may also block the degradation of the vasodepressor peptide bradykinin, which may contribute to its therapeutic effect.

Pharmacodynamics: Administration of ALTACE to patients with mild to moderate essential hypertension results in a reduction of both supine and standing blood pressure usually with little or no orthostatic change or change in heart rate. Symptomatic postural hypotension is infrequent, although this may occur in patients who are salt-and/or volume-depleted (see Warnings and Precautions).

In single dose studies, doses of 5-20 mg of ALTACE lowered blood pressure within 1-2 hours, with peak reductions achieved 3-6 hours after dosing. At recommended doses given once daily, antihypertensive effects have persisted over 24 hours.

The effectiveness of ALTACE appears to be similar in the elderly (over 65 years of age) and younger adult patients given the same daily doses.

In studies comparing the same daily dose of ALTACE given as a single morning dose or as a twice daily dose, blood pressure reductions at the time of morning trough blood levels were greater with the divided regimen.

While the mechanism through which ALTACE lowers blood pressure appears to result primarily from suppression of the renin-angiotensin-aldosterone system, ALTACE has an antihypertensive effect even in patients with low-renin hypertension.

The antihypertensive effect of ALTACE and thiazide diuretics used concurrently is greater than that seen with either agent used alone.

Abrupt withdrawal of ALTACE has not resulted in rapid increase in blood pressure.

Pharmacokinetics: See Table 3.

Table 3: ALTACE
Summary of Pharmacokinetic Parameters of Ramipril After Single Doses of 2.5 mg, 5 mg and 10 mg Capsules

Single Dose	Mean values±SD and (range) n=12 (11 subjects in 5 mg capsule data) C_{max} (ng/mL)	t_{max} (h)	$AUC_{(0-12)}$ (ng·h/mL)
2.5 mg capsule	10.40±6.93 (3.20–29.10)	0.69±0.22 (0.50–1.25)	13.23±9.34 (4.30–34.30)
5 mg capsule	21.54±8.10 (11.00–35.20)	0.70±0.31 (0.50–1.50)	31.71±20.57 (11.60–70.50)
10 mg capsule	50.96±22.24 (13.60–89.70)	0.79±0.42 (0.25–1.50)	70.78±33.65 (17.30–128.80)

Absorption: Following oral administration, ramipril is rapidly absorbed with peak plasma concentrations occurring within 1 hour. The extent of absorption of ramipril is 50-60% and is not significantly altered by the presence of food in the gastrointestinal tract, although the rate of absorption is reduced.

Following a single administration of up to 5 mg of ramipril, plasma concentrations of ramipril and ramiprilat increase in a manner that is greater than proportional to dose; after a single administration of 5 mg to 20 mg of ramipril the plasma concentrations for both are dose-proportional. The non-linear pharmacokinetics observed at the lower doses of ramipril can be explained by the saturable binding of ramiprilat to ACE. At steady-state, the 24-hour AUC for ramiprilat is dose-proportional over the recommended dose range. The absolute bioavailabilities of ramipril and ramiprilat were 28% and 44% respectively when 5 mg of oral ramipril was compared to 5 mg given intravenously.

Plasma concentrations of ramiprilat decline in a triphasic manner. The initial rapid decline, which represents distribution of the drug, has a half life of 2-4 hours. Because of its potent binding to ACE and slow dissociation from the enzyme, ramiprilat shows two elimination phases. The apparent elimination phase has a half-life of 9-18 hours, and the terminal elimination phase has a prolonged half-life of >50 hours. After multiple daily doses of ramipril 5-10 mg, the half-life of ramiprilat concentrations was 13-17 hours, but was considerably prolonged at 2.5 mg (27-36 hours).

After once daily dosing, steady state plasma concentrations of ramiprilat are reached by the fourth dose. Steady-state concentrations of ramiprilat are higher than those seen after the first dose of ALTACE especially at low doses (2.5 mg).

Distribution: Following absorption, ramipril is rapidly hydrolyzed in the liver to its active metabolite, ramiprilat. Peak plasma concentrations of ramiprilat are reached 2-4 hours after drug intake. The serum protein binding of ramipril is about 73% and that of ramiprilat is 56%.

Metabolism: Ramipril is almost completely metabolized to the active metabolite ramiprilat, and to the diketopiperazine ester, the diketopiperazine acid, and the glucuronides of ramipril and ramiprilat, all of which are inactive.

Excretion: After oral administration of ALTACE, about 60% of the parent drug and its metabolites is excreted in the urine, and about 40% is found in the feces. Drug recovered in the feces may represent both biliary excretion of metabolites and/or unabsorbed drug. Less than 2% of the administered dose is recovered in urine as unchanged ramipril.

Special Populations and Conditions: Geriatrics: A single dose pharmacokinetic study conducted in a limited number of elderly patients indicated that peak ramiprilat levels and the AUC for ramiprilat are higher in older patients (see Warnings and Precautions, Special Populations, Geriatrics (>65 years of age)).

Race: The antihypertensive effect of angiotension converting enzyme inhibitors is generally lower in black patients than in non-blacks.

Hepatic Insufficiency: In patients with impaired liver function, plasma ramipril levels increased about 3-fold, although peak concentrations of ramiprilat in these patients were not different from those seen in patients with normal hepatic function.

Renal Insufficiency: The urinary excretion of ramipril, ramiprilat, and their metabolites is reduced in patients with impaired renal function. In patients with creatinine clearance <40 mL/min/1.73 m², increases in C_{max} and AUC of ramipril and ramiprilat compared to normal subjects were observed following multiple dosing with 5 mg ramipril (see Dosage and Administration, Recommended Dose and Dosage Adjustment, Use in Renal Impairment).

STORAGE AND STABILITY: Store ALTACE in original container at room temperature, (15-30°C) and not beyond the date indicated on the container.

INFORMATION FOR THE PATIENT: Published in e-CPS, available by subscription at www.e-cps.ca.

DOSAGE FORMS, COMPOSITION AND PACKAGING: 1.25 mg: Each hard gelatin capsule size no. 4, with white opaque body, imprinted with "Altace" and yellow opaque cap, imprinted with "1.25", contains: ramipril 1.25 mg. Nonmedicinal ingredients: pregelatinized starch; capsule: gelatin, titanium dioxide and yellow iron oxide. Cartons of 30 (2×15 blister-packed capsules). White, high-density polyethylene (HDPE) bottles of 100.

2.5 mg: Each hard gelatin capsule size no. 4, with white opaque body, imprinted with "Altace" and orange opaque cap, imprinted with "2.5", contains: ramipril 2.5 mg. Nonmedicinal ingredients: pregelatinized starch; capsule: FD&C red No. 3, gelatin, titanium dioxide and yellow iron oxide. Cartons of 30 (2×15 blister-packed capsules). White, high-density polyethylene (HDPE) bottles of 100 and 500.

5 mg: Each hard gelatin capsule size no. 4, with white opaque body, imprinted with "Altace" and red opaque cap, imprinted with "5", contains: ramipril 5 mg. Nonmedicinal ingredients: pregelatinized starch; capsule: FD&C blue No. 2, FD&C red No. 3, gelatin and titanium dioxide. Cartons of 30 (2×15 blister-packed capsules). White, high-density polyethylene (HDPE) bottles of 100 and 500.

10 mg: Each hard gelatin capsule size no. 4, with white opaque body, imprinted with "Altace" and blue opaque cap, imprinted with "10", contains: ramipril 10 mg. Nonmedicinal ingredients: pregelatinized starch; capsule: black iron oxide, FD&C blue No. 2, FD&C red No. 3, gelatin and titanium dioxide. Cartons of 30 (2×15 blister-packed capsules). White, high-density polyethylene (HDPE) bottles of 100 and 500.

15 mg: Each hard gelatin capsule size no. 3, with grey opaque body, imprinted with "Altace" and powder blue opaque cap, imprinted with "15", contains: ramipril 15 mg. Nonmedicinal ingredients: pregelatinized starch; capsule: black iron oxide, D&C red No. 28, FD&C blue No. 1, gelatin and titanium dioxide. Cartons of 30 (2×15 blister-packed capsules). White, high-density polyethylene (HDPE) bottles of 100 and 500.

(Shown in Product Identification Section)

> The reader is invited to consult CPhA's monograph **ACE Inhibitors**.

Altace® HCT Pr

ramipril—hydrochlorothiazide

Angiotensin Converting Enzyme Inhibitor—Diuretic

sanofi-aventis

Date of Preparation: July 11, 2006

SUMMARY PRODUCT INFORMATION:

Route of Administration	Dosage Form/Strength	Clinically Relevant Nonmedicinal Ingredients
Oral	Tablets: 2.5 mg ramipril/12.5 mg hydrochlorothiazide 5 mg ramipril/12.5 mg hydrochlorothiazide 10 mg ramipril/12.5 mg hydrochlorothiazide 5 mg ramipril/25 mg hydrochlorothiazide 10 mg ramipril/25 mg hydrochlorothiazide	N/A For a complete listing see Dosage Forms, Composition and Packaging.

INDICATIONS AND CLINICAL USE: ALTACE HCT (ramipril/hydrochlorothiazide) is indicated for the treatment of essential hypertension in patients for whom this combination therapy is appropriate.

ALTACE HCT is not indicated for initial therapy (see Dosage and Administration). Patients in whom ramipril and diuretic are initiated simultaneously can develop symptomatic hypotension.

Patients should be titrated on individual drugs. If the fixed combination represents the dose and dosing frequency determined by this titration, the use of ALTACE HCT may be more convenient in the management of patients. If during maintenance therapy dosage adjustment is necessary it is advisable to use the individual drugs.

In using ALTACE HCT consideration should be given to the risk of angioedema (see Contraindications and Warnings and Precautions, Immune, Angioedema).

Geriatrics: There is limited clinical experience with ALTACE HCT in the elderly (>65 years) (see Warnings and Precautions, Special Populations, Geriatrics).

Pediatrics: The safety and effectiveness of ALTACE HCT in children have not been established; therefore use in this age group is not recommended (see Warnings and Precautions, Special Populations, Pediatrics).

CONTRAINDICATIONS: ALTACE HCT (ramipril/hydrochlorothiazide) is contraindicated in:

- patients who are hypersensitive to this drug, to any other angiotensin converting enzyme (ACE) inhibitor, or to any ingredient in the formulation (see Dosage Forms, Composition and Packaging).

Because of the ACE inhibitor component, ramipril, ALTACE HCT is contraindicated in:

- patients who have a history of angioedema (see Warnings and Precautions, Angioedema).
- during pregnancy and in breast feeding-women (see Warnings and Precautions, Special Populations, Pregnant Women, Nursing Women).

Because of the hydrochlorothiazide component, ALTACE HCT is contraindicated in:

- patients with anuria or hypersensitivity to thiazides and other sulfonamide-derived drugs (see Warnings and Precautions, Immune and Adverse Reactions, Post-Market Adverse Drug Reactions, Immune).

WARNINGS AND PRECAUTIONS:

> **Serious Warnings and Precautions**
> When used in pregnancy, angiotensin converting enzyme (ACE) inhibitors can cause injury or even death of the developing fetus (see Warnings and Precautions, Special Populations, Pregnant Women). When pregnancy is detected ALTACE HCT (ramipril/hydrochlorothiazide) should be discontinued as soon as possible.

General: Angioedema: Angioedema has been reported in patients treated with ACE inhibitors including ramipril. Angioedema associated with laryngeal involvement may be fatal. If laryngeal stridor or angioedema of the face, extremities, lips, tongue, or glottis occurs, ALTACE HCT should be discontinued immediately, the patient treated appropriately in accordance with accepted medical care, and carefully observed until the swelling disappears. In instances where swelling is confined to the face and lips, the condition generally resolves without treatment, although antihistamines may be useful in relieving symptoms. Where there is involvement of tongue, glottis, or larynx, likely to cause airway obstruction, appropriate therapy (including, but not limited to 0.3 to 0.5 mL of subcutaneous epinephrine solution 1:1000) should be administered promptly.

Angioedema, including laryngeal edema, may occur especially following the first dose of ALTACE HCT. Patients should be so advised and told to report immediately any signs or symptoms suggesting angioedema, such as swelling of face, extremities, eyes, lips, tongue, difficulty in swallowing or breathing. They should immediately stop taking ALTACE HCT and consult with their physician.

Intestinal angioedema has been reported in patients treated with ACE inhibitors. These patients presented with abdominal pain (with or without nausea or vomiting); in some cases facial angioedema also occurred. The intestinal angioedema symptoms resolved after stopping the ACE inhibitor (see Adverse Reactions, Post-Market Adverse Drug Reactions, Immune).

The incidence of angioedema during ACE inhibitor therapy has been reported to be higher in black than in non-black patients.

Patients with a history of angioedema unrelated to ACE inhibitor therapy may be at increased risk of angioedema while receiving an ACE inhibitor (see Contraindications).

Cough: A dry, persistent cough, which usually disappears only after withdrawal of ALTACE HCT, has been reported. This is likely related to ramipril, the ACE inhibitor component of ALTACE HCT. Such a possibility should be considered as part of the differential diagnosis of cough (see Adverse Reactions, Clinical Trial Adverse Drug Reactions).

Cardiovascular: Aortic Stenosis: There is concern, on theoretical grounds, that patients with aortic stenosis might be at particular risk of decreased coronary perfusion when treated with vasodilators because they do not develop as much afterload reduction.

Hypotension: Symptomatic hypotension has occurred after administration of ramipril, usually after the first or second dose or when the dose was increased. It is more likely to occur in patients who are volume depleted by diuretic therapy, dietary salt restriction, dialysis, diarrhea, or vomiting. In patients with ischemic heart disease or cerebrovascular disease, an excessive fall in blood pressure could result in a myocardial infarction or cerebrovascular accident (see Adverse Reactions, Cardiovascular, Hypotension). Because of the potential fall in blood pressure in these patients, therapy with ALTACE HCT should be started under close medical supervision. Such patients should be followed closely for the first weeks of treatment and whenever the dose of ALTACE HCT is increased. In patients with severe congestive heart failure, with or without associated renal insufficiency, ACE inhibitor therapy may cause excessive hypotension and has been associated with oliguria, and/or progressive azotemia, and rarely, with acute renal failure and/or death.

If hypotension occurs, the patient should be placed in a supine position and, if necessary, receive an intravenous infusion of 0.9% sodium chloride. A transient hypotensive response may not be a contraindication to further doses which usually can be given without difficulty once the blood pressure has increased after volume expansion in hypertensive patients. However, lower doses of ALTACE HCT should be considered. In patients receiving treatment following acute myocardial infarction, consideration should be given to discontinuation of ALTACE HCT (see Adverse Reactions, Cardiovascular, Hypotension).

ALTACE HCT may lower the state of patient alertness and/or reactivity, particularly at the start of treatment. Patients should be cautioned to report lightheadedness, especially during the first few days of ALTACE HCT therapy. If actual syncope occurs, the patients should be told to discontinue the drug and consult with their physician.

All patients should be cautioned that excessive perspiration and dehydration may lead to an excessive fall in blood pressure because of reduction in fluid volume. Other causes of volume depletion such as vomiting or diarrhea may also lead to a fall in blood pressure, patients should be advised to consult with their physician.

Hematologic: Neutropenia/Agranulocytosis: Agranulocytosis and bone marrow depression have been caused by ACE inhibitors. Several cases of agranulocytosis, neutropenia or leukopenia have been reported in which a causal relationship to ramipril cannot be excluded (see Adverse Reactions, Post-Market Adverse Drug Reactions). Current experience with the drug shows the incidence to be rare. Periodic monitoring of white blood cell counts should be considered especially in patients with collagen vascular disease and/or renal disease (see Warnings and Precautions, Monitoring and Laboratory Tests, Hematology).

Patients should be told to report promptly to their physician any indication of infection (e.g. sore throat, fever) as this may be a sign of neutropenia (see Adverse Reactions, Post-Market Adverse Drug Reactions).

Hepatic/Biliary/Pancreatic: Hepatitis (hepatocellular and/or cholestatic), elevations of liver enzymes and/or serum bilirubin have occurred during therapy with ACE inhibitors in patients with or without pre-existing liver abnormalities (see Adverse Reactions, Post-Market Adverse Drug Reactions). In most cases the changes were reversed on discontinuation of the drug.

Rarely, ACE inhibitors, including ramipril, have been associated with a syndrome that starts with cholestatic jaundice and progresses to fulminant hepatic necrosis and (sometimes) death. The mechanism of this syndrome is not understood. Patients receiving ACE inhibitors who develop jaundice or marked elevations of hepatic enzymes should discontinue the ACE inhibitor and receive appropriate medical follow-up.

Patients should be advised to return to their physician if they experience any symptoms possibly related to liver dysfunction. This would include "viral-like symptoms" in the first weeks to months of therapy (such as fever, malaise, muscle pain, rash or adenopathy which are possible indicators of hypersensitivity reactions), or if abdominal pain, nausea or vomiting, loss of appetite, jaundice, itching or any other unexplained symptoms occur during therapy (see Adverse Reactions, Post-Market Adverse Drug Reactions).

Should the patient receiving ALTACE HCT experience any unexplained symptoms particularly during the first weeks or months of treatment, it is recommended that a full set of liver function tests and any other necessary investigations be carried out. Discontinuation of ALTACE HCT should be considered when appropriate.

Thiazides should be used with caution in patients with impaired hepatic function or progressive liver disease, since minor alterations of fluid and electrolyte balance may precipitate hepatic coma. There are no adequate studies in patients with cirrhosis and/or liver dysfunction. ALTACE HCT should be used with particular caution in patients with pre-existing liver abnormalities. In such patients baseline liver function tests should be obtained before administration of the drug and close monitoring of response and metabolic effects should apply.

Immune: Anaphylactoid Reactions to ACE Inhibitors: Anaphylactoid reactions have been reported in patients dialyzed with high-flux membranes [e.g. polyacrylonitrile (PAN)] and treated concomitantly with an ACE inhibitor. Dialysis should be stopped immediately if symptoms such as nausea, abdominal cramps, burning, angioedema, shortness of breath and severe hypotension occur. Symptoms are not relieved by antihistamines. In these patients consideration should be given to using a different type of dialysis membrane or a different class of antihypertensive agents.

Rarely, patients receiving ACE inhibitors during low density lipoprotein apheresis with dextran sulfate have experienced life-threatening anaphylactoid reactions. These reactions were avoided by temporarily withholding the ACE inhibitor therapy prior to each apheresis.

There have been isolated reports of patients experiencing sustained life threatening anaphylactoid reactions while receiving ACE inhibitors during desensitization treatment with hymenoptera (e.g. bees, wasps) venoma. In the same patients, these reactions have been avoided when ACE inhibitors were temporarily withheld for at least 24 hours, but they have reappeared upon inadvertent rechallenge.

Hypersensitivity to Thiazide Diuretics: Sensitivity reactions to hydrochlorothiazide may occur in patients with or without a history of allergy or bronchial asthma.

The possibility of exacerbation or activation of systemic lupus erythematosus has been reported in patients treated with hydrochlorothiazide.

Metabolism: Thiazides, including HCT, can cause fluid or electrolyte imbalance (hypokalemia, hyponatremia, and hypochloremic alkalosis).

Hyperuricemia may occur, or acute gout may be precipitated, in certain patients receiving thiazide therapy.

Thiazides may decrease serum PBI (protein-bound iodine) levels without signs of thyroid disturbance.

Thiazides have been shown to increase excretion of magnesium; this may result in hypomagnesemia.

Thiazides may decrease urinary calcium excretion. Thiazides may cause intermittent and slight elevation of serum calcium in the absence of known disorders of calcium metabolism. Marked hypercalcemia may be evidence of hidden hyperparathyroidism. Thiazides should be discontinued before carrying out tests of parathyroid function.

Increases in cholesterol, triglyceride and glucose levels may be associated with thiazide diuretic therapy.

Dosage adjustments of insulin or oral hypoglycemic agents may be required. Latent diabetes mellitus may become manifest during thiazide therapy.

Administration of ACE inhibitors in patients with diabetes may potentiate the blood glucose lowering effect of oral hypoglycemic agents or insulin (see Drug Interactions, Drug-Drug Interactions).

Elevated serum potassium (greater than 5.7 mEq/L) was observed in approximately 1% of hypertensive patients in clinical trials treated with the ACE inhibitor ramipril. In most cases these were isolated values which resolved despite continued therapy. Risk factors for the development of hyperkalemia may include renal insufficiency, diabetes mellitus, and the concomitant use of agents to treat hypokalemia or other drugs associated with increases in serum potassium (see Drug Interactions, Drug-Drug Interactions, Agents increasing serum potassium).

Patients should be told not to use salt substitutes containing potassium without consulting their physician.

Peri-Operative Considerations: Surgery/Anesthesia: In patients undergoing surgery or anesthesia with agents producing hypotension, ALTACE HCT may block angiotensin II formation secondary to compensatory renin release. If hypotension occurs and is considered to be due to this mechanism, it may be corrected by volume repletion.

Thiazides may increase the responsiveness to tubocurarine.

Patients planning to undergo surgery and/or anesthesia should be told to inform their physician that they are taking an ACE inhibitor.

Renal: As a consequence of inhibiting the renin-angiotensin-aldosterone system, changes in renal function have been seen in susceptible individuals. In patients whose renal function may depend on the activity of the renin-angiotensin-aldosterone system, such as patients with bilateral renal artery stenosis, unilateral renal artery stenosis to a solitary kidney, or severe congestive heart failure, treatment with agents that inhibit this system has been associated with oliguria, progressive azotemia, and rarely, acute renal failure and/or death. In susceptible patients, concomitant diuretic use may further increase risk.

Use of ALTACE HCT should include appropriate assessment of renal function.

ALTACE HCT should be used with caution in patients with renal insufficiency as they may require reduced or less frequent doses (see Dosage and Administration). Close monitoring of renal function during therapy should be performed as deemed appropriate in patients with renal insufficiency (see Warnings and Precautions, Monitoring and Laboratory Tests, Renal Function).

Thiazides may not be appropriate diuretics for use in patients with renal impairment and are ineffective at creatinine clearance values of 30 mL/min or below (i.e., moderate or severe renal insufficiency).

Azotemia may be precipitated or increased by hydrochlorothiazide. Cumulative effects of the drug may develop in patients with impaired renal function. If increasing azotemia and oliguria occur during treatment of severe progressive renal disease the diuretic should be discontinued.

Special Populations: Pregnant Women: ACE inhibitors can cause fetal and neonatal morbidity and mortality when administered to pregnant women. Several dozen cases have been reported in the world literature. When pregnancy is detected, ALTACE HCT should be discontinued as soon as possible.

In rare cases (probably less than one in every thousand pregnancies) in which no alternative to ACE inhibitor therapy will be found, the mother(s) should be apprised of the potential hazard(s) to their fetus(es). Serial ultrasound examinations should be performed to assess fetal development and well-being and the volume of amniotic fluid.

If oligohydramnios is observed, ALTACE HCT should be discontinued unless it is considered life-saving for the mother. A non-stress test (NST), and/or a biophysical profiling (BPP) may be appropriate, depending upon the week of pregnancy. If concerns regarding fetal well-being still persist, a contraction stress testing (CST) should be considered. Patients and physicians should be aware, however, that oligohydramnios may not appear until the fetus has sustained irreversible injury.

Infants with a history of in utero exposure to ACE inhibitors should be closely observed for hypotension, oliguria, and hyperkalemia. If oliguria occurs, attention should be directed toward support of blood pressure and renal perfusion. Exchange transfusion or dialysis may be required as a means of reversing hypotension and/or substituting for impaired renal function; however, limited experience with those procedures has not been associated with significant clinical benefit. It is not known if ramipril or ramiprilat can be removed from the body by hemodialysis.

Since the use of ALTACE HCT during pregnancy can cause injury and even death of the developing fetus, patients should be advised to report promptly to their physician if they become pregnant.

Human Data: It is not known whether exposure limited to the first trimester of pregnancy can adversely affect fetal outcome. The use of ACE inhibitors during the second and third trimesters of pregnancy has been associated with fetal and neonatal injury including hypotension, neonatal skull hypoplasia, anuria, reversible or irreversible renal failure, and death. Oligohydramnios has also been reported, presumably resulting from decreased fetal renal function; oligohydramnios in this setting has been associated with fetal limb contractures, craniofacial deformation, and hypoplastic lung development. Prematurity and patent ductus arteriosus have also been reported, although it is not clear whether these occurrences were due to the ACE-inhibitor exposure.

Animal Data: No teratogenic effects of ramipril were seen in studies of pregnant rats, rabbits, and cynomolgus monkeys. The doses used were: 10, 100, or 1000 mg/kg in rats (2500 times maximum human dose), 0.4, 1.0, or 2.5 mg/kg in rabbits (6.25 times maximum human dose), and 5, 50, or 500 mg/kg in cynomolgus monkeys (1250 times maximum human dose). In rats, the highest dose caused reduced food intake in the dams, with consequent reduced birth weights of the pups and weight development during the lactation period. In rabbits, maternal effects were mortalities (high and middle dose) and reduced body weight. In monkeys, maternal effects were mortalities (high and middle dose), vomiting, and reduced weight gain.

Nursing Women: Ingestion of a single 10 mg oral dose of ramipril resulted in undetectable amounts of ramipril and its metabolites in breast milk. However, because multiple doses may produce low milk concentrations that are not predictable from single doses and because thiazides do appear in human milk, ALTACE HCT should not be administered to nursing mothers (see Action and Clinical Pharmacology, Pharmacokinetics, Special Populations and Conditions, Nursing Women).

Pediatrics: The safety and effectiveness of ALTACE HCT in children have not been established; therefore use in this age group is not recommended.

Geriatrics: Because of decreased cardiac reserve, greater sensitivity in older patients (>65 years) may be expected.

Monitoring and Laboratory Tests: Hematology: Periodic monitoring of white blood cell counts should be considered to permit detection of a possible leukopenia due to ACE inhibitor component of ALTACE HCT, ramipril. More frequent monitoring is advised in the initial phase of treatment and in patients with impaired renal function, those with concomitant collagen disease (e.g. lupus erythematosus or scleroderma) or those treated with other drugs that can cause changes in the blood picture (see Warnings and Precautions, Hematologic, Neutropenia/Agranulocytosis).

Metabolism: Appropriate monitoring of electrolytes and blood sugar is required.

Renal Function: Use of ALTACE HCT should include appropriate assessment of renal function. Close monitoring of renal function during therapy should be performed as deemed appropriate in patients with renal insufficiency (see Warnings and Precautions, Renal).

ADVERSE REACTIONS: Adverse Drug Reaction Overview: The most frequent adverse drug reactions observed with ALTACE HCT (ramipril/hydrochlorothiazide) were: headache (3.9%), dizziness (2.2%) and bronchitis (2.1%). The common serious adverse event pooled from the different clinical trials was tachycardia (0.2%). See Table 1.

Clinical Trial Adverse Drug Reactions: Because clinical trials are conducted under very specific conditions the adverse drug reaction rates observed in the clinical trials may not reflect the rates observed in practice and should not be compared to the rates in the clinical trials of another drug. Adverse drug reaction information from clinical trials is useful for identifying drug-related adverse events and for approximating rates.

Table 1: ALTACE HCT

Adverse Events Occurring ≥1% in Patients Taking Ramipril+HCT in Controlled Clinical Trials

Adverse Events	Ramipril+HCT[a] n=967 (%)	Ramipril n=1058 (%)	HCT n=515 (%)	Placebo n=44 (%)
Headache	3.9	1.7	6.0	4.5
Dizziness	2.2	1.5	1.0	4.5
Bronchitis	2.1	0.5	0.4	0.0
Neuralgia	1.9	0.4	0.4	2.3
Infection	1.8	0.4	1.2	2.3
Upper respiratory infection	1.4	0.4	0.8	2.3
Asthenia	1.3	1.3	1.6	2.3
Cough increased	1.3	1.2	1.0	0.0
Back pain	1.0	0.6	0.6	0.0

[a] Patients taking ALTACE HCT or ramipril+hydrochlorothiazide in combination.

Less Common Clinical Trial Adverse Drug Reactions (<1%): Body as a Whole: allergic reactions, fever, shock.

Cardiovascular System: angina pectoris, hypotension, palpitation, postural hypotension, syncope, tachycardia.

Digestive System: constipation, gastroenteritis, gastrointestinal pain, nausea.

Metabolic and Nutritional Disorders: excessive thirst, gout, hyperglycemia, hyperuricemia, hypokalemia and peripheral edema.

Musculoskeletal System: arthralgia, myalgia.

Nervous System: anxiety, apathy, depression, dry mouth, hot flushes, nervousness, paresthesia, sleep disorder, somnolence, sweating and tremor.
Respiratory System: dyspnea, and sinusitis.
Skin and Appendages: alopecia, angioedema, maculopapular rash, pruritus, psoriasis, rash.
Special Senses: conjunctivitis, taste loss, and tinnitus.
Urogenital System: impotence, renal failure, kidney function abnormal.
Abnormal Hematologic and Clinical Chemistry Findings: Hydrochlorothiazide: Renal Function Test: increased serum concentrations of uric acid.
Cholesterol: increase in serum cholesterol and triglycerides.
Glucose: lower tolerance to glucose. In patients with diabetes mellitus, this may lead to a deterioration of the metabolic control.
Post-Market Adverse Drug Reactions: Cardiovascular: tachycardia, palpitations, disturbed orthostatic regulation, hypotension, asthenia, angina pectoris, cardiac arrhythmias, syncope, myocardial infarction, ischaemic stroke and peripheral oedema.
Central Nervous System: headache, disorders of balance, weakness and light-headedness, dizziness, tinnitus, paraesthesiae, nervousness, depressed mood, tremor, restlessness, confusion, feeling of anxiety, transient erectile impotence, sweating and somnolence.
Dermatologic: cutaneous or mucosal reactions such as rash, pruritus or urticaria, maculopapular rash, erythema multiforme, Stevens-Johnson syndrome, toxic epidermal necrolysis, alopecia or photosensitivity, pemphigus, exacerbation of psoriasis, psoriasiform or pemphigoid exanthema and enanthema, or onycholysis.
Endocrine and Metabolism: decline in serum sodium concentration, hypochloraemia, hypomagnesaemia, hypercalcaemia, development or aggravation of a metabolic alkalosis, increase in the concentration of serum potassium due to ramipril, decrease in potassium concentration due to hydrochlorothiazide. General signs of disturbances in the electrolyte balance: headache, drowsiness, confusion and muscle cramps. Increased fluid excretion.
Gastrointestinal: vasculitis, nausea, increases in serum levels of hepatic enzymes and/or bilirubin, cholestatic and jaundice, dryness of the mouth, glossitis, inflammatory reactions of the oral cavity and gastrointestinal tract, abdominal discomfort, gastric pain (including gastritic-like gastric pain), digestive disturbances, smell and taste disturbances, constipation, diarrhea, vomiting, increased levels of pancreatic enzymes, pancreatitis, liver damage (including acute liver failure).
Genitourinary: increase in serum urea and serum creatinine and impairment of renal function, progression to acute renal failure, interstitial nephritis and pre-existing proteinuria may deteriorate (though ACE inhibitors usually reduce proteinuria), reduced libido, transient erectile impotence.
Hematologic: Hematological reactions to ACE inhibitors are more likely to occur in patients with impaired renal function and in those with concomitant collagen disease (e.g., lupus erythematosus or scleroderma) or in those treated with other drugs that may cause changes of the blood picture (see Warnings and Precautions, Hematologic and Drug Interactions). Haemolytic anaemia, reduction in the white blood cell or blood platelet count, agranulocytosis, pancytopenia and bone marrow depression.
Immune: Fever, eosinophilia, angioedema and other, not pharmacologically mediated anaphylactic or anaphylactoid reactions to ramipril or any of the other ingredients are rare (see Warnings and Precautions, Immune). Anaphylactic reactions to hydrochlorothiazide are possible. The likelihood and the severity of anaphylactoid reactions to insect venoma are increased under ACE inhibition.
Musculoskeletal: myalgia, arthralgia, muscle cramps develop.
Respiratory: dry (non-productive) tickling cough, nasal congestion, sinusitis, bronchitis, bronchospasm and dyspnoea.
Special Senses: visual disturbances, disturbed hearing.
DRUG INTERACTIONS: Overview: Drug-Drug Interactions: See Table 2.

Table 2: ALTACE HCT
Established or Potential Drug-Drug Interactions

Proper Name	Ref	Effect	Clinical Comment
Concomitant Diuretic Therapy	CT	Hypotensive effects	Patients concomitantly taking ACE inhibitors and diuretics, and especially those in whom diuretic therapy was recently instituted, may occasionally experience an excessive reduction of blood pressure after initiation of therapy. The patient should be closely observed for several hours following the initial dose and until blood pressure has stabilized (see Warnings and Precautions and Dosage and Administration).
Agents Increasing Serum Potassium	CT	Elevation of serum potassium	Since ramipril decreases aldosterone production, elevation of serum potassium may occur. Potassium sparing diuretics such as spironolactone, triamterene or amiloride, or potassium supplements should be given only for documented hypokalemia and with caution and frequent monitoring of serum potassium, since they may lead to a significant increase in serum potassium. Salt substitutes which contain potassium should also be used with caution (see also Non-steroidal anti-inflammatory agents).
Agents Causing Renin Release	T	Antihypertensive effect augmented	The antihypertensive effect of ramipril is augmented by antihypertensive agents that cause renin release.
Lithium	CT	Increased serum lithium levels and symptoms of lithium toxicity	Increased serum lithium levels and symptoms of lithium toxicity have been reported in patients receiving ACE inhibitors and thiazides during therapy with lithium. If these drugs must be used together, decrease lithium dose by 50% with close monitoring of lithium concentration, serum electrolytes and fluid intake. These drugs should be administered with caution, and frequent monitoring of serum lithium levels is recommended. If a diuretic is also used, the risk of lithium toxicity may be further increased.
Antacids	CT	No effect	In one open-label, randomized, cross-over single dose study in 24 male subjects, it was determined that the bioavailability of ramipril and the pharmacokinetic profile of ramiprilat were not affected by concomitant administration of the antacid, magnesium and aluminum hydroxides.
Digoxin	CT	No changes in serum levels of ramipril, ramiprilat, and digoxin with ramipril intake. Thiazide-induced electrolyte disturbances (mainly hypokalemia and hypomagnesemia) increase risk of digoxin toxicity.	In one open-label study in 12 subjects, administered multiple doses of both ramipril and digoxin, no changes were found in serum levels of ramipril, ramiprilat, and digoxin. Clinical significance of digoxin toxicity with thiazides is high. Monitor serum electrolytes, particularly potassium and magnesium levels. Administer potassium and/or magnesium supplements as required.
Warfarin		No alteration of the anticoagulant effects with ramipril.	The coadministration of ramipril with warfarin did not alter the anticoagulant effects.

(cont'd)

Table 2: ALTACE HCT *(cont'd)*
Established or Potential Drug-Drug Interactions

Proper Name	Ref	Effect	Clinical Comment
Acenocoumarol	CT	No significant change in blood pressure, thrombotest time and coagulation factors with ramipril.	In a multi-dose double-blind, placebo-controlled, pharmacodynamic interaction study with 14 patients with mild hypertension administered both ramipril and therapeutic doses of acenocoumarol, blood pressure, thrombotest time and coagulation factors were not significantly changed.
Non-steroidal anti-inflammatory agents	CT	Increased risk of worsening of renal function and an increase in serum potassium. Possible attenuation of the diuretic, natriuretic, and antihypertensive effects.	The antihypertensive effects of ACE inhibitors may be reduced with concomitant administration of non-steroidal anti-inflammatory agents (e.g. indomethacin). Concomitant treatment with Non-Steroidal Anti-Inflammatory drugs may lead to an increased risk of worsening of renal function and an increase in serum potassium (see also Agents Increasing Serum Potassium). Avoid if possible. If not possible, close monitoring of serum creatinine, potassium and patient's weight is recommended if using NSAIDs with ALTACE HCT (ramipril/hydrochlorothiazide). Observe the patient to ensure diuretic effects are obtained. Monitor blood pressure and diuretic effect and increase dose if necessary or discontinue NSAID. Also monitor renal function.
Antidiabetic agents (e.g. insulin and sulfonylurea derivates)	CT	Hypoglycemic reactions with ACE inhibitors. Hyperglycemic reactions with thiazides.	ACE inhibitors drugs may reduce insulin resistance. In isolated cases, such reduction may lead to hypoglycaemic reactions in patients concomitantly treated with antidiabetics. Particularly close blood glucose monitoring is, therefore, recommended in the initial phase of co-administration. Clinical significance is minimal to moderate but likely. Effect may occur after several days to several months of therapy. Monitor for changes in glycemic control and ensure adequate potassium levels are maintained. Supplement potassium and/or adjust dose of antidiabetic medications if required.
Skeletal muscle relaxants (Curare type)	T	Thiazide drugs may enhance the effects of nondepolarizing skeletal muscle relaxants	Thiazides may enhance the effects of nondepolarizing skeletal muscle relaxants potentially leading to prolonged respiratory depression. Thiazide-induced hypokalemia increases resistance to depolarization by hyperpolarizing the end plate resulting in enhanced myoneural blockade. Monitor and correct thiazide-induced hypokalemia. Consider decreasing dose of nondepolarizing skeletal muscle relaxant if hypokalemia cannot be corrected before administration of muscle relaxants is required. Clinical significance is unknown.
Sympathomimetics	T	Reduce the antihypertensive effect.	May decrease antihypertensive effect. May decrease arterial responsiveness to norepinephrine but this diminution is not sufficient to preclude effectiveness of the pressor agent for therapeutic use. Clinical significance is unknown.
Alcohol, barbiturates, narcotics	T	Orthostatic hypotension	Orthostatic hypotension may occur. Alcohol, barbiturates and narcotics may potentiate the antihypertensive effects. Avoid alcohol, especially with initiation of therapy (see Warnings and Precautions).
Corticosteroids	T	Possible hypokalemia. Possible reversal of thiazide antihypertensive response via corticosteroid-induced salt and water retention.	Monitor serum potassium levels and replace potassium if required. Monitor blood pressure and adjust medications as required.

Legend:
T=Theoretical, CT=Clinical Trial.

Drug-Food Interactions: No substantial drug-food interaction has been detected with ramipril or hydrochlorothiazide.
Drug-Laboratory Test Interactions: Tests for Parathyroid Function: Hydrochlorothiazide stimulates renal calcium reabsorption and may cause hypercalcemia. This must be considered when carrying out tests for parathyroid function.
Drug-Lifestyle Interactions: No information available.

DOSAGE AND ADMINISTRATION: Dosing Considerations:
- Dosage should be individualized.
- ALTACE HCT (ramipril/hydrochlorothiazide) is not for initial therapy.
- The dose of ALTACE HCT should be determined by the titration of the individual components.
- Special attention for dialysis patients.

Recommended Dose and Dosage Adjustment: Once the patient has been successfully titrated with the individual components as described below, ALTACE HCT may be substituted if the titrated dose and dosing schedule can be achieved by the fixed combination (see Indications and Clinical Use and Warnings and Precautions).
Usual dosage: 2.5 mg ramipril and 12.5 mg hydrochlorothiazide (corresponding to 1 tablet ALTACE HCT 2.5/12.5) daily. Generally it is recommended that the daily dose be administered in the morning as a single dose.
Titration will be based on physician's judgement according to severity of hypertension and other associated risk factors.
Maximum daily dose: 10 mg ramipril and 50 mg hydrochlorothiazide (corresponding to 4 tablets ALTACE HCT 2.5/12.5 or 2 tablets ALTACE HCT 5/25).
Dosage in Patients with Impaired Renal Function: Creatinine clearance 30 to 60 mL/min per 1.73 m^2 body surface area: the maximum recommended daily dose for renally impaired patients is 5 mg ramipril/25 mg hydrochlorothiazide (corresponding to 2 tablets ALTACE HCT 2.5/12.5 or 1 tablet ALTACE HCT 5/25).
Missed Dose: If a dose of this medication has been missed, it should be taken as soon as possible. However, if it is almost time for the next dose, skip the missed dose and go back to the regular dosing schedule. Do not double doses.
Administration: ALTACE HCT tablets should be swallowed with sufficient amounts of liquid (approximately ½ glass). The tablets must not be chewed or crushed.
Generally, it is recommended that the daily dose be administered in the morning as a single dose. No substantial food effects is to be expected with ALTACE HCT.

OVERDOSAGE:
Overdosage may cause persistent diuresis, excessive peripheral vasodilatation (with marked hypotension, electrolyte disturbances, cardiac arrhythmias, impairment of consciousness up to and including coma and cerebral convulsions).
Management: Treatment is symptomatic and supportive. Primary detoxification by, for example, administration of adsorbants may be considered. In the event of hypotension, administration of α_1-adrenergic agonists (e.g. norepinephrine, dopamine) or angiotensin II (angiotensinamide), must be considered in addition to volume and salt substitution.

In attempting to eliminate ramipril, or ramiprilat, limited/no experience is available concerning the efficacy of forced diuresis, altering urine pH, haemofiltration or dialysis. If dialysis or haemofiltration is nevertheless contemplated, consider risks of anaphylactoid reactions with high flux membrane (see Warnings and Precautions, Immune, Anaphylactoid Reactions to ACE Inhibitors).

Removal of thiazide diuretics by dialysis is negligible.

For management of a suspected drug overdose, CPhA recommends that you contact your **regional Poison Control Centre**. See the *CPS* Directory section for a list of Poison Control Centres.

ACTION AND CLINICAL PHARMACOLOGY: Mechanism of Action: ALTACE HCT (ramipril/hydrochlorothiazide) has antihypertensive and diuretic effects. Ramipril and hydrochlorothiazide are used singly or together for antihypertensive therapy. The antihypertensive effects of both substances are complementary.

The blood-pressure-lowering effects of both components together are greater than the effect of either monotherapy. In patients treated with ramipril and a thiazide diuretic there was essentially no change in serum potassium (see Warnings and Precautions, Metabolism).

Pharmacodynamics: Ramipril: Administration of ramipril causes a marked reduction in peripheral arterial resistance. Administration of ramipril to patients with hypertension leads to a reduction in supine and standing blood pressure without a compensatory rise in heart rate.

In most patients the onset of the antihypertensive effect of a single dose becomes apparent 1 to 2 hours after oral administration. The peak effect of a single dose is usually reached 3 to 6 hours after oral administration. The antihypertensive effect of a single dose usually lasts for 24 hours.

Abrupt discontinuation of ramipril does not produce a rapid and excessive rebound increase in blood pressure.

Hydrochlorothiazide: Electrolyte and water excretion starts approximately 2 hours after administration, reaches its peak after 3 to 6 hours and lasts from 6 to 12 hours.

The onset of the antihypertensive effect requires several days and administration for 2 to 4 weeks is necessary for optimal therapeutic effect.

Pharmacokinetics: See Table 3.

Table 3: ALTACE HCT

Summary of Pharmacokinetic Parameters After Single Doses of 5/25 mg ALTACE HCT, 5 mg Ramipril, 25 mg HCT or 5 mg Ramipril+25 mg HCT From Study HOE9829/1502

	Arithmetic Mean (CV%) (Geometric LS Mean)			
Substrate	**C_{max} [ng/mL]**	**t_{max} [h]**	**AUC_T [ng·h/mL]**	**$AUC_{(0-72)}$ [ng·h/mL]**
ALTACE HCT 5/25 mg tablet				
ramipril	19.348±37.7 (17.896)	0.50±26.8	25.256±63.3 (21.646)	—
ramiprilat	6.576±47.4 (6.061)	2.50±33.3	—	119.102±25.3 116.192
HCT	140.95±23.8 (137.08)	2.00±44.2	993.53±18.5 (980.65)	—
Ramipril 5 mg tablet				
ramipril	21.712±42.2 (19.649)	0.50±70.0	26.546±70.9 (22.500)	—
ramiprilat	6.588±62.7 (5.703)	2.57±51.3	—	116.693±29.0 110.362
HCT 25 mg tablet				
HCT	140.52±24.2 (136.21)	2.00±47.3	1048.70±24.8 (1021.52)	—
5 mg ramipril tablet+25 mg HCT tablet				
ramipril	21.035±33.1 (19.896)	0.53±35.3	25.317±65.1 (22.024)	—
ramiprilat	5.941±51.6 (5.328)	3.00±38.0	—	108.716±21.1 105.633
HCT	144.85±30.3 (138.38)	2.00±36.5	969.92±21.5 (953.41)	—

No significant pharmacokinetic interaction has been observed between ramipril and hydrochlorothiazide administered as a fixed combination formulation of ramipril/hydrochlorothiazide tablets (ramipril/hydrochlorothiazide 5 mg/25 mg tablet sanofi-aventis Canada Inc.) under fasting conditions, on the basis of ramipril and hydrochlorothiazide parameters (C_{max} and AUC).

Ramipril: Absorption: Ramipril is rapidly absorbed after oral administration. As measured by the recovery of radioactivity in the urine, which represents only one of the elimination routes, absorption of ramipril is at least 56%. Administration of ramipril at the same time as food has no relevant effect on absorption.

Distribution: As a result of this activation/metabolization of the prodrug, approximately 20% of orally administered ramipril is bioavailable.

The bioavailability of ramiprilat after oral administration of 2.5 and 5 mg ramipril is approximately 45% compared with its availability after intravenous administration of the same doses.

Peak plasma concentrations of ramipril are reached within 1 hour after oral administration. Peak plasma concentrations of ramiprilat are reached 2 to 4 hours after oral administration of ramipril.

The protein-binding of ramipril and ramiprilat is approximately 73% and approximately 56% respectively.

Metabolism: The prodrug ramipril undergoes an extensive hepatic first pass metabolism, which is essential for the formation of the sole active metabolite ramiprilat (hydrolysis, which occurs principally in the liver). In addition to this activation into ramiprilat, ramipril is glucuronized and transformed into ramipril diketopiperazine (ester). Ramiprilat is glucuronized as well and transformed into ramiprilat diketopiperazine (acid).

When high doses (10 mg) of ramipril are administered, impairment of hepatic function retards the activation of ramipril into ramiprilat, resulting in increased ramipril plasma levels.

Excretion: Following oral administration of 10 mg of radioactive labelled ramipril, approximately 40% of total radioactivity is excreted in faeces and approximately 60% in urine. The elimination half-life of ramipril is approximately 1 hour.

Approximately 80 to 90% of the metabolites in urine and bile have been identified as ramiprilat or ramiprilat metabolites. Ramipril glucuronide and ramipril diketopiperazine represented approximately 10 to 20% of the total amount, whereas unmetabolized ramipril accounted for approximately 2%.

Plasma concentrations of ramiprilat decline in a polyphasic manner. The initial distribution and elimination phase has a half-life of approximately 3 hours. It is followed by an intermediate phase (half-life approximately 15 hours) and a terminal phase with very low plasma ramiprilat concentrations and a half-life of approximately 4 to 5 days.

Despite this long terminal phase, a single daily dose of 2.5 mg ramipril or more yields steady state plasma concentrations of ramiprilat after approximately 4 days. The "effective" half-life, which is relevant for dosage, is 13 to 17 hours under multiple-dose conditions.

Renal excretion of ramiprilat is reduced in patients with impaired renal function, and renal ramiprilat clearance is proportionally related to creatinine clearance. This results in elevated plasma concentrations of ramiprilat, which decrease more slowly than in persons with normal renal function (see Warnings and Precautions, Renal).

Hydrochlorothiazide: Absorption: Approximately 70% of hydrochlorothiazide is absorbed after oral administration; the bioavailability of hydrochlorothiazide after oral administration is approximately 70%.

Distribution: Approximately 40% of hydrochlorothiazide is bound to plasma proteins.

Metabolism: Hydrochlorothiazide undergoes negligible hepatic metabolism and has not been shown to induce or inhibit any CYP450 isoenzymes.

Excretion: Hydrochlorothiazide is excreted almost entirely (more than 95%) by renal route in unchanged form. After oral administration of a single dose, 50 to 70% is excreted within 24 hours.

The elimination half-life is 5 to 6 hours. In renal insufficiency excretion is reduced and the half-life prolonged. Renal clearance of hydrochlorothiazide correlates closely with creatinine clearance.

Special Populations and Conditions: Pediatrics: No data available.

Geriatrics: In healthy subjects aged between 65 and 76 years ramipril and ramiprilat kinetics are similar to those in healthy young subjects.

Gender: No data available.

Race: The average response to ACE inhibitor monotherapy was lower in black hypertensive patients (usually a low-renin hypertensive population) than in non-black patients.

Cardiovascular Insufficiency: The clearance of hydrochlorothiazide may be decreased in patients with congestive heart failure.

Nursing Women: Hydrochlorothiazide passes into breast milk in small quantities. Studies in lactating animals have shown that ramipril passes into the milk. (Warnings and Precautions, Nursing Women.)

Hepatic Insufficiency: No relevant changes in the pharmacokinetics of hydrochlorothiazide have been noted in liver cirrhosis.

In patients with impaired liver function, plasma ramipril levels increased about 3-fold, although peak concentrations of ramiprilat in these patients were not different from those seen in patients with normal hepatic function.

Hepatic metabolism does not play a significant role in the elimination of hydrochlorothiazide.

Hydrochlorothiazide should not be administered in hepatic coma or pre-coma. It should be used only with caution in patients with progressive hepatic disease (see Warnings and Precautions, Hepatic/Biliary/Pancreatic).

Renal Insufficiency: Renal excretion of ramipril, ramiprilat, and its metabolite is reduced in patients with impaired renal function, and renal ramiprilat clearance is proportionally related to creatinine clearance. This results in elevated plasma concentrations of ramiprilat, which decreases more slowly than in persons with normal renal function.

In patients with creatinine clearance less than 40 mL/min/1.73 m², increases in C_{max} and AUC of ramipril and ramiprilat compared to normal subjects were observed following multiple dosing with 5 mg ramipril (see Dosage and Administration, Dosage in Patients with Impaired Renal Function).

The clearance of hydrochlorothiazide is decreased in renal failure.

Hydrochlorothiazide must be present at the site of action in the renal tubule in sufficient concentration in order to achieve its therapeutic effect. Hydrochlorothiazide reaches its site of action almost exclusively by secretion into the tubular fluid via the organic acid cotransporter. In mild renal insufficiency, higher doses are required to achieve sufficient concentrations of drug at the site of action due to decreased tubular secretion in renal failure. However, hydrochlorothiazide becomes ineffective once creatinine clearance drops below 30 to 50 mL/min.

Genetic Polymorphism: No information available.

STORAGE AND STABILITY: Store ALTACE HCT (ramipril/hydrochlorothiazide) in original container at room temperature, between 15 and 30°C and not beyond the date indicated on the container.

INFORMATION FOR THE PATIENT: Published in e-CPS, available by subscription at www.e-cps.ca.

DOSAGE FORMS, COMPOSITION AND PACKAGING: ALTACE HCT 2.5/12.5: Each white to almost white oblong tablet, with score line on both sides, upper stamp: HNV/HNV, lower stamp: no lower stamp, contains: ramipril 2.5 mg/ hydrochlorothiazide 12.5 mg. Nonmedicinal ingredients: hydroxypropylmethylcellulose, microcrystalline cellulose, pregelatinized maize starch and sodium stearyl fumarate. Cartons of 28 (2×14 blister-packed) aluminum/PVC blisters.

ALTACE HCT 5/12.5: Each pink oblong tablet, with score line on both sides, upper stamp: 41/AV, lower stamp: no lower stamp, contains: ramipril 5 mg/hydrochlorothiazide 12.5 mg. Nonmedicinal ingredients: hydroxypropylmethylcellulose, microcrystalline cellulose, pregelatinized maize starch, red ferric oxide and sodium stearyl fumarate. Cartons of 28 (2×14 blister-packed) aluminum/PVC blisters.

ALTACE HCT 5/25: Each white to almost white oblong tablet, with score line on both sides, upper stamp: HNW/HNW, lower stamp: no lower stamp, contains: ramipril 5 mg/hydrochlorothiazide 25 mg. Nonmedicinal ingredients: hydroxypropylmethylcellulose, microcrystalline cellulose, pregelatinized maize starch and sodium stearyl fumarate. Cartons of 28 (2×14 blister-packed) aluminum/PVC blisters.

ALTACE HCT 10/12.5: Each orange oblong tablet, with score line on both sides, upper stamp: 42/AV, lower stamp: no lower stamp, contains: ramipril 10 mg/hydrochlorothiazide 12.5 mg. Nonmedicinal ingredients: hydroxypropylmethylcellulose, microcrystalline cellulose, pregelatinized maize starch, red ferric oxide, yellow ferric oxide and sodium stearyl fumarate. Cartons of 28 (2×14 blister-packed) aluminum/PVC blisters.

ALTACE HCT 10/25: Each pink oblong tablet, with score line on both sides, upper stamp: 39/AV, lower stamp: no lower stamp, contains: ramipril 10 mg/hydrochlorothiazide 25 mg. Nonmedicinal ingredients: hydroxypropylmethylcellulose, microcrystalline cellulose, pregelatinized maize starch, red ferric oxide and sodium stearyl fumarate. Cartons of 28 (2×14 blister-packed) aluminum/PVC blisters.

(Shown in Product Identification Section)

The reader is invited to consult CPhA's monograph **Corticosteroids: Inhaled.**

Alvesco® ℞

ciclesonide

Corticosteroid for Oral Inhalation

Nycomed

Date of Preparation: September 8, 2006
Date of Revision: December 24, 2009

SUMMARY PRODUCT INFORMATION:

Route of Administration	Dosage Form/ Strength	All Nonmedicinal Ingredients
Oral Inhalation	Metered Dose Inhaler 100 µg, 200 µg per actuation (ex-valve)	Propellant HFA-134a (norflurane) and ethanol

Note: All doses given in this monograph are ex-valve unless specified otherwise.

INDICATIONS AND CLINICAL USE: Alvesco (ciclesonide) is indicated for:

- prophylactic management of steroid-responsive bronchial asthma in adults, adolescents and children 6 years of age and older.

Pediatrics: At present, there is limited data regarding the use of Alvesco in patients <6 years of age and therefore Alvesco is not recommended for patients younger than 6 years.

Geriatrics (>65 years of age): Based on the pharmacokinetic characteristics obtained in patients older than 65 years of age, dose adjustment is not necessary in elderly patients.

CONTRAINDICATIONS:

- Alvesco is contraindicated in patients with known hypersensitivity to any of the ingredients. For a complete listing, see Dosage Forms, Composition and Packaging.
- Alvesco is contraindicated in patients with untreated fungal, bacterial or tuberculosis infections of the respiratory tract.
- Alvesco is not to be used in the primary treatment of status asthmaticus or other acute episodes of asthma, or in patients with moderate to severe bronchiectasis.

WARNINGS AND PRECAUTIONS: General: It is essential that patients be instructed that Alvesco is a preventative agent which must be taken daily at the intervals recommended by their doctors and is not to be used as acute treatment for an asthmatic attack. Patients should be advised to inform subsequent physicians of the prior use of corticosteroids. Treatment with Alvesco should not be stopped abruptly, but tapered off gradually.

Monitoring Asthma Control: Patients with severe asthma are at risk of acute attacks and should have regular assessments of their asthma control including pulmonary function tests. Increasing use of short-acting bronchodilators to relieve asthma symptoms indicate deterioration of asthma control. If patients find that short-acting relief bronchodilator treatment becomes less effective, or they need more inhalations than usual, medical attention should be sought. In this situation, patients should be reassessed and consideration given to the need for increased anti-inflammatory treatment therapy (either higher doses of Alvesco or a course of oral corticosteroids). Severe asthma exacerbations should be managed according to standard medical practice.

Endocrine and Metabolism: Hypothyroidism: There is an enhanced effect of corticosteroids on patients with hypothyroidism.

Hematologic: Eosinophilic Conditions: In rare cases, patients on inhaled corticosteroid therapy may present with systemic eosinophilic conditions, with some patients presenting with clinical features of vasculitis consistent with Churg-Strauss syndrome, a condition that is often treated with systemic corticosteroid therapy. These events usually, but not always, have been associated with the reduction and/or withdrawal of oral corticosteroid therapy following the introduction of inhaled corticosteroids, and cases of serious eosinophilic conditions have been reported in this clinical setting.

Physicians should be alert to eosinophilia, vasculitic rash, worsening pulmonary symptoms, cardiac complications, and/or neuropathy presenting in their patients. A causal relationship between ciclesonide and these underlying conditions has not been established.

Hypoprothrombinemia: Acetylsalicylic acid should be used cautiously in conjunction with corticosteroids in hypoprothrombinemia.

Hepatic/Biliary/Pancreatic: Cirrhosis: There is an enhanced effect of corticosteroids on patients with cirrhosis.

Hepatic Insufficiency: Based on the pharmacokinetic characteristics obtained in patients with hepatic insufficiency, dose adjustment is not necessary in this population. There is limited data available in patients with severe hepatic impairment. An increased exposure in patients with severe hepatic impairment is expected and these patients should therefore be monitored for potential systemic effects.

Immune: Patients who are on drugs that suppress the immune system are more susceptible to infections than healthy individuals. Chickenpox and measles, for example, can have a more serious or even fatal course in susceptible children or adults on corticosteroids. In such children or adults who have not had these diseases, particular care should be taken to avoid exposure. How the dose, route, and duration of corticosteroid administration affect the risk of developing a disseminated infection is not known. The contribution of the underlying disease and/or prior corticosteroid treatment to the risk is also not known. If exposed to chickenpox, prophylaxis with varicella zoster immune globulin (VZIG) may be indicated. If exposed to measles, prophylaxis with intramuscular pooled immunoglobulin (IG) may be indicated. If chickenpox develops, treatment with antiviral agents may be considered.

Corticosteroids may mask some signs of infections and new infections may appear. A decreased resistance to localised infections has been observed during corticosteroid therapy. This may require treatment with appropriate therapy or stopping the administration of ciclesonide until the infection is eradicated.

Infection: Candidiasis and Oral Hygiene: Therapeutic dosages of inhaled corticosteroids may cause the appearance of *C. albicans* (thrush) in the mouth and throat. The rate reported of candidiasis in clinical trials with Alvesco was low (0.6%, see Adverse Reactions). The development of pharyngeal and laryngeal candidiasis is a cause for concern because the extent of its penetration into the respiratory tract is unknown. Adequate oral hygiene is of primary importance in minimizing overgrowth of micro-organisms such as *C. albicans*. Patients may find it helpful to rinse and gargle with water after using Alvesco. Symptomatic candidiasis can be treated with topical anti-fungal therapy while still continuing to use Alvesco.

Renal: Renal Insufficiency: Due to the lack of renal excretion of the active metabolite, dose adjustment should not be necessary in renally impaired patients, however, specific studies in this patient group have not been performed.

Respiratory: Paradoxical Bronchospasm: As with other inhalation therapy, paradoxical bronchospasm may occur which is characterized by an immediate increase in wheezing after dosing. This should be treated immediately with a fast-acting inhaled bronchodilator to relieve acute asthmatic symptoms. Alvesco should be discontinued immediately, the patient assessed, and if necessary, alternative therapy instituted.

Systemic Steroid Replacement by Inhaled Steroid: Particular care is needed in asthmatic patients who are transferred from systemically active corticosteroids to inhaled corticosteroids because deaths due to adrenal insufficiency have occurred during and after transfer. For the transfer of patients being treated with oral corticosteroids, Alvesco inhalation aerosol should first be added to the existing oral steroid therapy, which is then gradually withdrawn. Patients with adrenocortical suppression should be monitored regularly and the oral steroid reduced cautiously. Some patients transferred from other inhaled steroids or oral steroids remain at risk of impaired adrenal reserve for a considerable time after transferring to inhaled ciclesonide.

After withdrawal from systemic corticosteroids, a number of months are required for recovery of hypothalamic-pituitary-adrenal (HPA) function. During this period of HPA suppression, patients may exhibit signs and symptoms of adrenal insufficiency when exposed to trauma, surgery or infections, particularly gastroenteritis. Although Alvesco inhalation aerosol may provide control of asthmatic symptoms during these episodes, it does not provide the systemic steroid which is necessary for coping with these emergencies. The physician may consider supplying oral steroids for use in times of stress (e.g. worsening asthma attacks, chest infections, surgery). During periods of stress or a severe asthmatic attack, patients who have been withdrawn from systemic corticosteroids should be instructed to resume systemic steroids immediately and to contact their physician for further instruction. These patients should also be instructed to carry a warning card indicating that they may need supplementary systemic steroids during periods of stress or a severe asthma attack. To assess the risk of adrenal insufficiency in emergency situations, routine tests of adrenal cortical function, including measurement of early morning and evening cortisol levels, should be performed periodically in all patients. An early morning resting cortisol level may be accepted as normal only if it falls at or near the normal mean level.

Transfer of patients from systemic steroid therapy to Alvesco inhalation aerosol may unmask allergic conditions outside the pulmonary tract that were previously suppressed by the systemic steroid therapy, e.g., rhinitis, conjunctivitis, and eczema. These allergies should be symptomatically treated with anti-histamine and/or topical preparations, including topical steroids.

Systemic Effects: Systemic effects of inhaled corticosteroids may occur, particularly at high doses prescribed for prolonged periods. These effects are much less likely to occur than with oral corticosteroids. Possible systemic effects include adrenal suppression, growth retardation in children and adolescents, decrease in bone mineral density, cataract and increased intraocular pressure, with or without glaucoma. Therefore, it is important that the dose of inhaled corticosteroid is titrated to the lowest dose at which effective control of asthma is maintained.

Long-Term Effects: The long-term effects of ciclesonide in human subjects are still unknown. In particular, the local effects of the drug on developmental or immunologic processes in the mouth, pharynx, trachea, and lungs are unknown. There is also no information about the possible long-term systemic effects of the agent (see Monitoring and Laboratory Tests).

Special Populations: Pregnant Women: There are no adequate and well controlled studies in pregnant women. However, serum concentrations of ciclesonide are generally very low following inhaled administration; thus, fetal exposure is expected to be negligible and the potential for reproductive toxicity low. As with other inhaled corticosteroids, ciclesonide should only be used during pregnancy when the potential benefit to the mother justifies the potential risk to the mother, fetus or infant. Infants born to mothers who received corticosteroids during pregnancy should be observed carefully for hypoadrenalism.

The extent of exposure in pregnancy during clinical trials: Very Limited; individual cases only.

Nursing Women: It is unknown if ciclesonide and/or its active metabolite is excreted in human milk. In rats, however, very low levels of ciclesonide and/or its metabolites (<0.05% of dose) were found to be excreted into the milk following intravenous or oral administration. As with other inhaled corticosteroids, Alvesco should only be used in nursing women when the potential benefit to the mother justifies the potential risk to the mother and/or infant.

Pediatrics (<6 years of age): At present, there is limited data regarding the use of Alvesco in patients <6 years of age and therefore Alvesco is not recommended for patients younger than 6 years.

Geriatrics (>65 years of age): Based on the pharmacokinetic characteristics obtained in patients older than 65 years of age, dose adjustment is not necessary in this population.

Monitoring and Laboratory Tests: As with all inhaled corticosteroids, during long-term therapy, HPA axis function (e.g. blood cortisol levels) and effects on the eye (examination for cataracts, increased intraocular pressure and glaucoma) should be assessed periodically by a specialist. See Systemic Effects.

ADVERSE REACTIONS: Adverse Drug Reaction Overview: Inhaled corticosteroid therapy may be associated with dose dependent increases in incidence of ocular complications, reduced bone density, suppression of HPA axis responsiveness to stress, and inhibition of growth velocity in children. Although such events have been associated with inhaled corticosteroid therapy, no significant difference was detected between inhaled Alvesco and placebo on HPA function and serum cortisol levels.

Glaucoma may be exacerbated by inhaled corticosteroid treatment for asthma or rhinitis. In patients with established glaucoma who require long-term inhaled corticosteroid treatment, it is prudent to measure intraocular pressure before commencing the inhaled corticosteroid and to monitor it subsequently. In patients without established glaucoma, but with a potential for developing intraocular hypertension, intraocular pressure should be monitored at appropriate intervals. In all patients who are receiving long-term inhaled corticosteroid therapy, intraocular pressure should be monitored at appropriate intervals (see Warnings and Precautions, Monitoring and Laboratory Tests).

In elderly patients treated with inhaled corticosteroids, the prevalence of posterior subcapsular and nuclear cataracts is probably low but increases in relation to the daily and cumulative lifetime dose. Cofactors such as smoking, ultraviolet B exposure, or diabetes may increase the risk.

A reduction of growth velocity in children or teenagers may occur as a result of inadequate control of chronic diseases such as asthma or from use of corticosteroids for treatment. Physicians should closely follow growth of all children taking corticosteroids by any route and weigh the benefits of corticosteroid therapy and asthma control against the possibility of growth suppression if any child's or adolescent's growth appears slowed. In a one-year study, Alvesco was shown to have no effect on growth rates compared to placebo when administered to pediatric patients at doses of up to 200 µg per day.

Osteoporosis and bone fracture are complications of long term asthma treatment with parenteral or oral steroids. Inhaled corticosteroid therapy has also been associated with dose dependent bone loss, although the risk is much less with inhaled therapy than with oral and parenteral therapy.

Clinical Trial Adverse Drug Reactions: Because clinical trials are conducted under very specific conditions the adverse drug reaction rates observed in the clinical trials may not reflect the rates observed in practice and should not be compared to the rates in the clinical trials of another drug. Adverse drug reaction information from clinical trials is useful for identifying drug-related adverse events and for approximating rates.

Use in Adolescents and Adults: The clinical trial safety database for Alvesco consists of a total of 9162 patients (740 adolescents and 8422 adults) treated with Alvesco, 100 to 1600 µg per day, in clinical studies ranging in duration from 2 weeks to 1 year. The majority of short-term trials had a randomized, blinded design. Three long-term studies were of open-label design.

Approximately 6.6% of patients in placebo-controlled clinical trials experienced adverse events assessed as possibly related to treatment with Alvesco by the investigator and/or sponsor (vs. 6.5% of patients treated with placebo). In the majority of cases (56.4%), these were mild and did not require discontinuation of treatment with Alvesco. Approximately 6.2% of patients treated with Alvesco discontinued clinical trial participation due to an adverse event vs. 16.4% of patients in the placebo group. The primary adverse event leading to discontinuation was asthma in both treatment groups (Alvesco, 4.4% vs. placebo, 13.8%).

The following adverse reactions (see Table 1) were reported during placebo-controlled clinical trials in ≥1% of patients.

Table 1: Alvesco

Common Adverse Reactions[a] (≥1-<10%) in Placebo-Controlled Clinical Trials

	Alvesco n=1850 (%)	Placebo n=934 (%)
Respiratory		
Paradoxical bronchospasm[b]	1.8	1.9

[a] Assessed as possibly related to the treatment by investigator and/or sponsor.
[b] Paradoxical bronchospasm refers to a known adverse drug reaction of all inhaled drugs, which may be related to the active drug substance, excipients, or in the case of metered dose inhalers, to the cooling caused by the propellant or evaporation. Suspected paradoxical bronchospasm includes the preferred terms: chest discomfort, chest pain, asthma, bronchospasm, cough, dyspnea, obstructive airways disorder, wheezing.

Dose Response Information: The incidence of possibly treatment-related adverse events was generally comparable among the Alvesco dose groups, with the exception of respiratory, thoracic and mediastinal disorders which showed a trend towards dose dependency. This could be due to the fact that the higher dose groups tended to include patients with more severe asthma.

Special Populations: No safety signals specific for gender or for age were found in clinical trials.

The following adverse reactions (assessed as possibly related to treatment by the investigator and/or sponsor) were reported in clinical trials with Alvesco (placebo-controlled, active-controlled and open label studies):

Common Clinical Trial Adverse Drug Reactions (≥1%-<10%): Respiratory: paradoxical bronchospasm (1.6%), dysphonia (1.0%).

Uncommon Clinical Trial Adverse Drug Reactions (≥0.1% to <1%): Cardiovascular: palpitations (0.1%).

Eye: cataract subcapsular (0.1%).

Gastrointestinal: nausea (0.2%), dry mouth (0.1%), dyspepsia (0.1%).

Infections: oral candidiasis (0.6%), candidiasis (0.1%), oral fungal infection (0.1%), pharyngitis (0.1%).

Injury: contusion (0.1%).

Investigations: ALT increased (0.1%), gamma-glutamyltransferase increased (0.1%), weight increased (0.1%).

Nervous System: headache (0.4%), dysgeusia (0.3%), dizziness (0.1%).

Respiratory, Thoracic and Mediastinal Disorders: pharyngolaryngeal pain (0.4%), throat irritation (0.3%), dry throat (0.1%).

Skin: rash (0.1%).

The incidence of local oropharyngeal adverse reactions in Alvesco-treated patients was low and comparable to placebo, see Table 2.

Table 2: Alvesco

Local Adverse Reactions[a] in Placebo-Controlled Clinical Studies

	Alvesco n=1850 (%)	Placebo n=934 (%)
Gastrointestinal		
Dry Mouth	0.2	0.1
Local Infections		
Oral Candidiasis	0.5	0.4
Oral Fungal Infection NOS	0.1	0.0
Nervous System		
Dysgeusia	0.4	0.1
Respiratory		
Dysphonia/Hoarseness	0.9	0.4
Dry Throat	0.2	0.0
Pharyngitis	0.1	0.0

(cont'd)

Table 2: Alvesco *(cont'd)*

Local Adverse Reactions[a] in Placebo-Controlled Clinical Studies

	Alvesco n=1850 (%)	Placebo n=934 (%)
Throat Irritation	0.1	0.0

[a] Adverse events considered to be possibly related to treatment by investigator and/or sponsor.

Use in Children: The clinical trial safety database for Alvesco in pediatric patients consists of a total of 3754 children 4-11 years of age treated with Alvesco, 50 to 200 µg per day, in clinical studies ranging in duration from 2 weeks to 1 year. The incidence of possibly treatment related adverse events was similar in frequency and nature to that seen in adults and adolescents. The most commonly reported adverse drug reaction was headache (0.5%).

Abnormal Hematologic and Clinical Chemistry Findings: Examination of the percentage of patients with normal values at baseline and values above or below the normal range at the end of treatment did not demonstrate any trends with respect to changes in hematology and biochemistry values. See Uncommon Clinical Trial Adverse Drug Reactions (≥0.1% to <1%).

Post-Market Adverse Drug Reactions: Spontaneous adverse events reported during postmarketing use of ciclesonide are described below. As the events were reported spontaneously, no exact incidences can be provided. The following events were reported in postmarketing use, and causal relation to ciclesonide treatment could not be ruled out:

There have been rare reports of immediate or delayed hypersensitivity reactions such as angioedema with swelling of lips, tongue and pharynx as well as increased intraocular pressure in susceptible patients.

Post-Market Clinical Trial Adverse Drug Reactions: There have been uncommon reports of vomiting, bad taste; cough after inhalation, and eczema, and rare reports of abdominal pain and hypertension in the ongoing clinical trial database.

DRUG INTERACTIONS: Overview: In vitro data indicate that CYP3A4 is the major enzyme involved in the metabolism of the active metabolite of ciclesonide (M1) in man.

The serum levels of ciclesonide and its active metabolite M1, are low. However, co-administration with a potent inhibitor of the cytochrome P 450 3A4 system (e.g. itraconazole, ritonavir or nelfinavir) should be considered with caution because there might be an increase in ciclesonide/active metabolite serum levels, as was observed when orally inhaled ciclesonide was concomitantly administered with ketoconazole (see Drug-Drug Interactions). The risk of clinical adverse effect (e.g. cushingoid syndrome) cannot be excluded.

Drug-Drug Interactions: The drugs listed in Table 3 are based on drug-drug interaction clinical studies:

Table 3: Alvesco

Summary of Drug-Drug Interaction Clinical Trials Conducted with Ciclesonide

Ciclesonide	Effect	Clinical Comment
Ketoconazole	The exposure of the ciclesonide active metabolite (M1) increased approximately 3.5 fold.	Co-administration should be considered with caution. The risk of clinical adverse effect cannot be excluded.
Erythromycin	No pharmacokinetic interaction was observed in this study.	No special precautions are necessary.

Ciclesonide is not expected to influence the metabolism of other drugs.

Drug-Food Interactions: Interactions with food have not been established. Drug-food interactions are unlikely for inhaled corticosteroids.

Drug-Herb Interactions: Interactions with herbal products have not been established.

Drug-Laboratory Test Interactions: Interactions with laboratory tests have not been established. Drug-laboratory interactions are unlikely for inhaled corticosteroids.

DOSAGE AND ADMINISTRATION: Recommended Dose and Dosage Adjustment: Adults and Adolescents 12 Years of Age and Older:

- The recommended starting dose of Alvesco therapy for most patients, whether previously maintained on either bronchodilators alone or inhaled corticosteroids, is 400 µg once daily.
- The recommended dose range is 100 to 800 µg per day.
- Alvesco can be administered as 1 or 2 puffs once daily either in the morning or evening.
- Some patients with more severe asthma may be more adequately controlled on 800 µg daily (administered as 400 µg twice daily).
- As with all inhaled corticosteroids, the dose of Alvesco should be adjusted according to individual response.

Children 6-11 Years of Age :

- The recommended starting dose of Alvesco therapy for most patients, whether previously maintained on either bronchodilators alone or inhaled corticosteroids, is 100 to 200 µg once daily.
- The recommended dose range is 100 to 200 µg per day, administered as 1 or 2 puffs once daily either in the morning or evening.
- As with all inhaled corticosteroids, the dose of Alvesco should be adjusted according to individual response.

At present there is limited efficacy data regarding the use of Alvesco in patients <6 years of age and therefore Alvesco is not recommended for patients younger than 6 years.

Symptoms can start to improve with Alvesco within 24 hours of treatment. Clinically, Alvesco has been shown to improve lung function as measured by FEV_1, peak expiratory flow, improved asthma symptom control, reduced exacerbations, and decreased need for inhaled beta-2 agonists.

It is important to gain control of asthma symptoms and optimize pulmonary function as soon as possible. If there has been no improvement within one to two weeks, the patient should consult with their physician. Due to its prophylactic nature, Alvesco should be taken regularly even when patients are asymptomatic. The patient should be aware that the benefit of Alvesco depends on regular use even when they are experiencing no symptoms. When patient symptoms remain under satisfactory control, the dose of Alvesco should be titrated to the lowest dose at which effective control of asthma is maintained. Patients should be instructed to seek medical attention if their asthma symptoms worsen, or if their need for rescue medication increases.

Dose adjustments are not necessary in elderly patients, patients with liver impairment and patients with renal impairment.

Missed Dose: It is very important that ciclesonide is used regularly. If a dose is missed, the next dose should be taken when it is due.

Administration: Alvesco is for oral inhalation use only. To ensure the proper dosage and administration of the drug, the patient must be instructed by a physician or other health professional in the use of the inhalation aerosol (see Information for the Patient). Inhaler technique of patients should be checked regularly to make sure that correct method is used and inhaler actuation is synchronized with inhalation to ensure optimum delivery to the lungs.

In patients who find co-ordination of a pressurized metered dose inhaler difficult, a spacer device (AeroChamber Plus) may be used with Alvesco.

If the inhaler is new or has not been used for one week or more, three puffs should be released into the air. No shaking is necessary as Alvesco is a solution aerosol. The mouthpiece should be cleaned with a dry tissue or cloth weekly. No part of the inhaler should be washed or put into water.

Patients should be instructed to use the following technique to administer their medication:

- Instruct the patient to remove the mouthpiece cover, place the inhaler in their mouth, close their lips around the mouthpiece, and breathe in slowly and deeply.
- After starting to breathe in through the mouth, the top of the inhaler should be pressed down.
- Then, patients should move the inhaler away from their mouth, and hold their breath for about 10 seconds, or as long as is comfortable.
- The patient should not breathe out into the inhaler.
- Finally, patients should breathe out slowly, and replace the mouthpiece cover.

Transferring a Patient From an Oral Steroid to Alvesco: The patient should be in a relatively stable phase. A high dose of Alvesco should be given in combination with the oral steroid for about 10 days. Then the oral steroid should be gradually reduced to the lowest possible level. The gradual withdrawal of the systemic steroid is started by reducing the daily dose by 1.0 mg of prednisone (or equivalent of another corticosteroid) at seven day intervals if the patient is under close observation. If close observation is not feasible, the withdrawal of the systemic steroid should be more gradual at approximately 1.0 mg of the daily dose of prednisone (or equivalent) every ten days. If withdrawal symptoms appear, the previous dose of the systemic drug should be resumed for a week before any further decrease is attempted.

OVERDOSAGE:

Single doses of up to 3200 µg inhaled Alvesco were administered to healthy volunteers and were well tolerated.

The potential for acute toxic effects following overdose of inhaled ciclesonide is low. The only effect that follows inhalation of large amounts of the drug over a short period of time may be temporary suppression of adrenal function, symptoms of which may include: weakness, nausea, and hypotension. In such cases, treatment with Alvesco should be continued at a dose sufficient to control asthma. Recovery of adrenal function can be verified by measuring plasma cortisol.

If higher than recommended doses are administered continuously over prolonged periods, some degree of adrenal suppression may occur, therefore monitoring of adrenal reserve should be considered. Gradual reduction of the inhaled dose may be required. Treatment with Alvesco should be continued at a dose sufficient to control asthma.

> For management of a suspected drug overdose, contact your **regional Poison Control Centre**. See the *CPS* Directory section for a list of Poison Control Centres.

ACTION AND CLINICAL PHARMACOLOGY: Mechanism of Action: Ciclesonide exhibits low binding affinity to the glucocorticoid receptor and is pharmacologically inactive. Once inhaled, ciclesonide is converted by esterases in the lungs to its active metabolite, 21 des-methylpropionyl-ciclesonide (M1), which is a potent glucocorticoid that binds to glucocorticoid receptors in the lung resulting in local pronounced anti-inflammatory activity.

Pharmacodynamics: The active metabolite of ciclesonide (M1) exhibits high receptor affinity. Ciclesonide possesses a unique combination of properties that limits systemic exposure to the active drug including: the conversion to the active metabolite predominantly in the lung, high lung deposition, reversible formation of fatty acid conjugates of M1 in lung tissue slices, high clearance, low oral bioavailability, high protein binding, and low receptor affinity of metabolites other than M1. The clinical effects of ciclesonide on the HPA function and serum cortisol levels were investigated and, at therapeutic doses, no significant difference was detected between inhaled ciclesonide and placebo.

Pharmacokinetics: Ciclesonide is presented in HFA-134a propellant and ethanol as a solution aerosol, delivering 50 µg, 100 µg or 200 µg ciclesonide ex-valve. The doses are proportionally formulated with respect to dose and puff strength and exhibit bioequivalent systemic exposure when the same dose is inhaled by the three different formulation strengths. Across the recommended dose range, ciclesonide demonstrates linear pharmacokinetics with increases in systemic exposure proportional to dose. When a single dose of 3200 µg of ciclesonide was administered, a greater than proportional increase in systemic exposure was observed.

The pharmacokinetic characterization of ciclesonide focused on the active metabolite (M1) of ciclesonide, as it is the active moiety. While systemic drug levels of M1 are relevant for the systemic effect profile, a close relationship between systemic exposure and efficacy response is not assumed for asthma treatment with inhaled corticosteroids due to their topical mode of action. Since ciclesonide is poorly absorbed via the gastrointestinal tract and shows an extensive first pass metabolism, systemic exposure will depend on the drug fraction that is absorbed via the lung. Table 4 describes the pharmacokinetic characteristics of the active metabolite M1 in healthy patients between 22 and 43 years of age following single and repeated inhalation of 400 µg ciclesonide once daily. Pharmacokinetic data of healthy subjects and asthma patients were also shown to be similar.

Table 4: Alvesco

Summary of the Pharmacokinetic Parameters of Ciclesonide Active Metabolite (M1) in Healthy Subjects Following Inhalation of 400 µg Ciclesonide (n=18), Mean Values (Standard Deviation)

	Active Metabolite (M1)			
	C_{max} (µg/L)	AUC[a] (µg·h/L)	t_{max} (h)	$t_{½}$ (h)
Single Dose	0.30 (0.13)	1.72 (0.73)	1.08 (0.62)	5.23 (1.28)
Steady State	0.37 (0.06)	2.18 (0.42)	0.94 (0.44)	6.72 (1.04)

[a] Single Dose=$AUC_{(0,inf)}$; Steady State=$AUC_{(0,24h)}$.

Absorption: Studies with oral and intravenous dosing of radiolabelled drug have shown low oral absorption (24.5%). When inhaled the oral bioavailability of both ciclesonide and the active metabolite is negligible (<0.5% for ciclesonide, <1% for the active metabolite). Based on a γ-scintigraphy experiment, lung deposition in healthy subjects is 52%. The systemic bioavailability for the active metabolite is >50% when using the ciclesonide metered-dose inhaler. As the oral bioavailability for the active metabolite is <1%, the swallowed portion of the inhaled drug effectively does not contribute to the systemic absorption. Ciclesonide undergoes extensive first pass metabolism. See Table 4 for information regarding the pharmacokinetic characteristics (AUC, T_{max} and C_{max}) of ciclesonide following single and repeated dose administration.

Distribution: Following intravenous administration to healthy subjects, the volume of distribution averaged 2.9 L/kg. The total serum clearance of ciclesonide is high (average 2.0 L/h/kg) indicating a high hepatic extraction. The percentage of ciclesonide bound to human plasma proteins is 99% and that of the active metabolite is greater than 98%. Only the unbound drug in the systemic circulation (approximately 1-2%) is available for further systemic pharmacodynamic effect. The active metabolite showed no accumulation in red blood cells, as could be concluded from high plasma/whole blood ratio of 1.5-1.6 at 0.5-6 hours post-dosing.

Metabolism: Ciclesonide is a prodrug and is hydrolysed to its pharmacologically active metabolite by esterase enzymes primarily in the lungs. Investigation of the enzymology of further metabolism by human liver microsomes showed that this compound is mainly metabolized to hydroxylated inactive metabolites by CYP3A4 catalysis. Lipophilic fatty acid ester conjugates of the active metabolite in the lung were detected using in vitro techniques.

Excretion: After oral and intravenous administration, ciclesonide is predominantly excreted via the faeces (78 and 68%, respectively), indicating that excretion via the bile is the major route of elimination. After intravenous administration, the clearance of ciclesonide was 152±37 L/h and that of the active metabolite, M1 (assuming full conversion from ciclesonide) was 228±65 L/h. The half-life estimated from the terminal elimination phase after inhaled administration of ciclesonide was approximately 6 h.

Special Populations and Conditions: Geriatrics: In a comparison between one study in elderly subjects and another study in young healthy subjects, there was an approximately 2-fold increase in the rate and extent of exposure to the active metabolite in elderly patients. However, in a population pharmacokinetic analysis of 9 studies, age did not impact the clearance or volume of distribution of the active metabolite.

Pediatrics: In two 12 week clinical studies investigating the safety and efficacy of Alvesco in asthmatic patients between 4-11 years of age, serum samples were taken from 53 patients for pharmacokinetic analysis. The pharmacokinetics of the active metabolite M1 were found to be similar to adults.

Hepatic Insufficiency: Reduced liver function may affect the elimination of corticosteroids. In a study including patients with hepatic impairment suffering from liver cirrhosis, a higher systemic exposure (1.8 to 2.8 times) to the active metabolite was observed.

Renal Insufficiency: Due to the low rate of renal excretion of ciclesonide metabolites, studies on renally impaired patients have not been performed.

STORAGE AND STABILITY: The container contains a pressurized liquid and should not be pierced. It is recommended that Alvesco be stored at room temperature between 15-30°C. Do not freeze.

INFORMATION FOR THE PATIENT: Published in e-CPS, available by subscription at www.e-cps.ca.

DOSAGE FORMS, COMPOSITION AND PACKAGING: Alvesco is a solution aerosol. Additional ingredients are propellant HFA-134a (Norflurane) and ethanol. The inhaler is comprised of an aluminum canister sealed with a metering valve, actuator and cap.

Alvesco is available in two strengths: 100 µg per actuation (ex-valve) and 200 µg per actuation (ex-valve). Alvesco is available in canisters containing 30 or 120 actuations.

(Shown in Product Identification Section)

Amantadine 🄿
Antiviral—Antiparkinsonian Agent

CPhA Monograph

Date of Preparation: August 2009
Date of Revision: October 2009

This monograph has been compiled by CPhA and reviewed by experts. It may contain information different from that found in Health Canada-approved Product Monographs. The reader is referred to the *CPS* Editorial Policy for more information.

SUMMARY PRODUCT INFORMATION:

Route of Administration	Dosage Form	Strength
Oral	Capsule	100 mg
	Syrup	10 mg/mL

INDICATIONS AND CLINICAL USE:
- Amantadine is indicated for the prevention and treatment of influenza A infections. Due to a high incidence of resistance, current guidelines and recommendations should be consulted to determine susceptibility prior to the use of amantadine. Immunization with trivalent inactivated influenza vaccine remains the primary tool for the prevention of influenza infection and illness.
- Amantadine is indicated for the treatment of early stage Parkinson's disease as monotherapy.
- Amantadine is indicated for the treatment of drug-induced extrapyramidal symptoms, including levodopa-induced dyskinesia.

CONTRAINDICATIONS:
- Patients who are hypersensitive to amantadine hydrochloride or to any ingredient in the formulation or component of the container.

WARNINGS AND PRECAUTIONS:

Serious Warnings and Precautions
- Neuroleptic malignant syndrome (NMS): Cases of possible neuroleptic malignant syndrome have been reported in association with dose reduction or withdrawal of amantadine therapy. Neuroleptic malignant syndrome (NMS) is potentially fatal and is characterized by hyperpyrexia, muscle rigidity, altered mental status and autonomic instability (irregular pulse and blood pressure, tachycardia, diaphoresis and cardiac dysrhythmia).
- Abrupt discontinuation of amantadine has led to parkinsonian crisis in patients with Parkinson's syndrome. There is a risk of marked clinical deterioration.
- Suicide attempts and suicidal ideation, including fatalities, have been reported rarely in patients with and without prior history of psychiatric illness.

General: Avoid simultaneous use of amantadine for prophylaxis and treatment of amantadine-sensitive influenza A within a health care facility as this may increase the development of amantadine resistance.
Cardiovascular: Patients with a history of heart failure or peripheral edema should be followed closely as heart failure has been reported in patients receiving amantadine.
Dermatologic: Eczematoid rash has been reported and is more likely in those with a history of the condition. Use with caution in patients with recurrent eczematoid dermatitis.
Hepatic/Biliary/Pancreatic: Use with caution in patients with liver disease.
Neurologic: Use with caution in patients with history of epilepsy or other seizures. Monitor patients for increased seizure activity.
Ophthalmologic: Increased risk of mydriasis; should not be used in patients with angle-closure glaucoma.
Psychiatric: Use with caution in patients with a history of psychiatric disorders as symptoms may be exacerbated.
Renal: Dosage adjustment in renal impairment is recommended (see Dosage and Administration).
Sensitivity/Resistance: The prevalence of amantadine resistance among strains of influenza A virus varies on a yearly basis depending on the season's circulating strains. Resistance seems to result from alterations in the transmembrane domain of the viral M2 protein, and can occur spontaneously or emerge rapidly within 2-3 days of initiating therapy. Susceptibility testing is conducted by the National Microbiology Laboratory each year, and current guidelines and recommendations should be consulted prior to the use of amantadine [www.phac-aspc.gc.ca/naci-ccni/index-eng.php].
Special Populations: Pregnant Women: There are no adequate and well controlled studies on the effects of amantadine in pregnancy. Although a small number of birth defects have been reported in women using amantadine during the first trimester, a causal relationship has not been established. No specific data is available, but it is expected that amantadine would pass to the placenta based on its small molecular size. Amantadine should be used only when the potential benefits outweigh the possible risks to the fetus.
Nursing Women: Amantadine is excreted into breast milk. Use is not recommended in nursing mothers.
Pediatrics (birth to <1 year old): Safety and efficacy of amantadine in neonates and infants less than 1 year old have not been established.
Geriatrics: Careful attention is required when used in the elderly as they may be more susceptible to CNS effects. Dosage adjustment may be necessary (see Dosage and Administration).
Occupational Hazards: Patients should be cautioned about performing tasks which require mental alertness, such as driving or operating heavy machinery, as amantadine can cause decreased alertness and blurred vision.

ADVERSE REACTIONS: More Common Adverse Drug Reactions (≥1%): Table 1 lists the more common adverse effects of amantadine.

Table 1: Amantadine
More Common Adverse Drug Reactions (≥1%)

Body System	Effect	Approximate Incidence (%)
CNS	Dizziness	5–10
	Insomnia	5–10
	Agitation	1–5
	Anxiety and irritability	1–5
	Ataxia	1–5
	Confusion	1–5
	Delirium	1–5
	Depression	1–5
	Dream abnormality	1–5
	Hallucinations	1–5
	Headache	1–5
	Nervousness	1–5
	Somnolence	1–5
Gastrointestinal	Nausea	5–10
	Anorexia	1–5
	Constipation	1–5
	Diarrhea	1–5
	Xerostomia	1–5
Dermatologic	Livedo reticularis	1–5
Cardiovascular	Orthostatic hypotension	1–5
	Peripheral edema	1–5
Respiratory	Dry nose	1–5

Less Common Adverse Drug Reactions (<1%): Cardiovascular: heart failure, hypertension
Central Nervous System: amnesia, euphoria, hyperkinesia, psychosis, seizures, slurred speech, suicidal ideation, suicide, abnormal thinking, weakness, aggressive behaviour, paresthesia, impulsive/compulsive behaviour.
Dermatologic/Hypersensitivity: Allergic reactions including anaphylaxis, pruritus, eczematoid dermatitis, skin rash, photosensitization and diaphoresis have occurred rarely.
Gastrointestinal: vomiting, dysphagia.
Genitourinary: Urinary retention, which can be an early sign of toxicity.
Hematologic: leukopenia, neutropenia.
Hepatic/Biliary/Pancreatic: elevations of alkaline phosphatase, ALT, AST and bilirubin.
Ophthalmologic: visual disturbance including punctate subepithelial or other corneal opacity, corneal edema, decreased visual acuity, sensitivity to light and optic nerve palsy; oculogyric episodes, mydriasis.
Renal: elevation of blood urea nitrogen, creatinine.
Respiratory: dyspnea, pulmonary edema, respiratory failure.
Sexual Function/Reproduction: decreased libido.
DRUG INTERACTIONS: Drug-Drug Interactions: Drug-drug interactions involving amantadine are listed in Table 2.

Table 2: Amantadine
Drug-Drug Interactions

Interacting Drug	Effect	Clinical Comment
Antipsychotics (first or second-generation)	May antagonize the antiparkinson effect of amantadine.	Use with caution. Consider therapy modification.
Anticholinergic agents	May potentiate anticholinergic side effects.	Dosage adjustment of both drugs may be needed.
CNS stimulants	Concurrent use of CNS stimulants and amantadine may potentiate CNS stimulant effects.	Use with caution.
Ethanol	Concurrent use of ethanol and amantadine may result in increased CNS effects.	Avoid excessive use of ethanol.
Metoclopramide	May antagonize antiparkinson effect of amantadine.	Monitor therapy.
Potassium chloride	Concurrent use of amantadine and solid oral dosage forms of potassium chloride may result in increased risk of gastrointestinal lesions.	Use with caution. Consider liquid dosage form of potassium.
Trimethoprim	Concurrent use of amantadine and trimethoprim may cause increased serum levels of each drug possibly through competitive inhibition of renal tubule secretion.	Monitor for CNS side effects of amantadine.

DOSAGE AND ADMINISTRATION: Dosing Considerations:
- **Due to the high incidence of resistance, consult current guidelines and recommendations prior to the use of amantadine for prophylaxis or treatment of influenza A.**
- The usual dosage of amantadine may need to be reduced in patients with heart failure, peripheral edema, orthostatic hypotension or impaired renal function.
- If insomnia occurs after amantadine administration, the last daily dose should be taken several hours before bedtime.
- There are no known interactions between amantadine and food.
- Dividing the daily dosage may reduce CNS adverse effects.

Recommended Dose and Dosage Adjustment: Adults: See Table 3.

Table 3: Amantadine
Dose in Adult Patients

Indication	Usual Dose	Clinical Comment
Influenza A (treatment)	100 mg po twice daily or 200 mg po once daily	Initiate within 24–48 hours after onset of symptoms; continue for 24–48 hours after symptoms disappear or up to 5 days.

(cont'd)

Table 3: Amantadine *(cont'd)*
Dose in Adult Patients

Indication	Usual Dose	Clinical Comment
Influenza A (prophylaxis)	100 mg po twice daily or 200 mg po once daily	Continue for at least 10 days following a known exposure. Prophylaxis may be discontinued 2 weeks after vaccination. For patients who cannot be vaccinated, continue prophylaxis for the duration of influenza activity in the community.
Parkinsonism (monotherapy)	100 mg po twice daily	May initiate at 100 mg daily and increase after 1–2 weeks to minimize side effects. Maximum: 400 mg/day in divided doses.
Drug-induced extrapyramidal effects	100 mg po twice daily	Maximum dose of 300 mg/day in divided doses.

Geriatrics: Usual dose for all indications is 100 mg/day. Further adjust dose based on renal function. See Table 5.
Pediatrics: See Table 4.

Table 4: Amantadine
Dose in Pediatric Patients

Indication	Age/Weight	Usual Dose	Maximum Dose	Clinical Comment
Influenza A (treatment)	1–9 years	5 mg/kg/day	150 mg/day	In 2 divided doses. Initiate within 24–48 hours after onset of symptoms; continue for 24–48 hours after symptoms disappear or up to 5 days.
	≥10 years and <40 kg	5 mg/kg/day	200 mg/day	
	≥10 years and ≥40 kg	Refer to adult dosing	200 mg/day	
Influenza A (prophylaxis)	1–9 years	5 mg/kg/day	150 mg/day	Continue for at least 10 days following a known exposure. Prophylaxis may be discontinued 2 weeks after vaccination. For children <9 years old who are vaccinated for the first time, continue prophylaxis until 2 weeks after the 2nd dose. For patients who cannot be vaccinated, continue prophylaxis for the duration of influenza activity in the community.
	≥10 years and <40 kg	5 mg/kg/day	200 mg/day	
	≥10 years and ≥40 kg	Refer to adult dosing	200 mg/day	

Renal Impairment: See Table 5.

Table 5: Amantadine
Dose in Adult Patients with Renal Impairment

Creatinine Clearance (mL/min/1.73m²)	Dosage Adjustment (<65 y)	Dosage Adjustment (≥65 y)[a]
30–50	200 mg on day 1, then 100 mg/day	100 mg/day
15–29	200 mg on day 1, then 100 mg on alternate days	100 mg on alternate days
<15	200 mg every 7 days	100 mg every 7 days

[a] Dose reduced further in those ≥65 years because dose-related side-effects are reported more frequently in the elderly.

Dosage in Dialysis: Prophylaxis and Treatment: 200 mg every 7 days.

OVERDOSAGE:
Signs and Symptoms: Acute toxic psychosis (disorientation, confusion, visual hallucinations and aggressive behaviour), urinary retention/renal failure, a mixed acid-base disturbance, seizures, arrhythmia (e.g., QT prolongation and torsades de pointes), cardiac arrest and death. Death has been in reported in doses as low as 1 g.
Recommended Management: There is no specific antidote for amantadine overdosage. General supportive measures should be instituted and cardiovascular status (ECG/telemetry), blood pressure, pulse, respiration, temperature, serum electrolytes, urinary output and urine pH should be monitored.

For management of a suspected drug overdose, CPhA recommends that you contact your **regional Poison Control Centre**. See the *CPS* Directory section for a list of Poison Control Centres.

ACTION AND CLINICAL PHARMACOLOGY: Mechanism of Action: Amantadine acts as an antiviral by inhibiting viral uncoating through interference of M2 ion-channel function. In certain influenza strains, the irreversible conversion of hemagglutinin and subsequent prevention of virus release may also contribute to antiviral effects. Amantadine has no appreciable activity against Influenza B virus.

The exact mechanism of amantadine in the treatment of parkinsonian syndrome and drug-induced extrapyramidal reactions is not known. Amantadine is a non-competitive N-methyl-D-Aspartic acid (NMDA) receptor antagonist. There is some evidence that amantadine may exert its antiparkinsonian activity through inhibition of the NMDA receptor as well as by augmenting the release of dopamine from nerve terminals and delaying dopamine re-uptake.
Pharmacokinetics: Adults: Absorption: Amantadine is well absorbed after oral administration. Peak serum concentrations occur within about 2 to 4 hours after administration.
Distribution: The volume of distribution of amantadine ranges from 3 to 8 L/kg. Amantadine is distributed into tissues and fluids including saliva, tear film and nasal secretions and crosses the blood brain barrier. Amantadine is 67% protein bound.
Metabolism: The metabolism of amantadine is minimal though small amounts of N-acetylated metabolites may be identified.
Excretion: Principally, amantadine is excreted unchanged in the urine (80-90%). The elimination half-life ranges from 10 to 25 hours. In patients with renal insufficiency (creatinine clearance less than 40 mL/min/ 1.73 m²), the elimination half-life is prolonged by two- to three-fold or greater. Amantadine is minimally removed by hemodialysis. The average elimination half life in patients on chronic maintenance hemodialysis is 8 days.
Special Populations: Geriatrics: The elimination half-life in elderly males is prolonged and ranges from 20 to 41 hours.
STORAGE AND STABILITY: Store at controlled room temperature (15 to 30°C) in a tightly closed container.

The reader is invited to consult CPhA's monograph **Sulfonylureas**.

Amaryl®
glimepiride
Oral Hypoglycemic Agent (Sulfonylurea)
sanofi-aventis

Date of Revision: August 7, 2008
SUMMARY PRODUCT INFORMATION:

Route of Administration	Dosage Form/Strength	Clinically Relevant Nonmedicinal Ingredients
Oral	Tablet 1, 2, and 4 mg	Lactose For a complete listing see Dosage Forms, Composition and Packaging.

INDICATIONS AND CLINICAL USE: AMARYL (glimepiride) is indicated for:
- AMARYL (glimepiride) is indicated as an adjunct to proper dietary management, exercise and weight reduction to lower the blood glucose in patients with type 2 diabetes whose hyperglycemia cannot be controlled by diet and exercise alone.
- AMARYL may be used in combination with metformin when diet and exercise, and AMARYL or metformin alone do not result in adequate glycemic control.
- AMARYL is also indicated for use in combination with insulin to lower blood glucose in patients with type 2 diabetes whose hyperglycemia cannot be controlled by diet and exercise in conjunction with an oral hypoglycemic agent alone.

CONTRAINDICATIONS: AMARYL (glimepiride) is contraindicated in patients with:
- Type 1 diabetes (formerly known as insulin-dependent diabetes mellitus or IDDM).
- Known hypersensitivity or allergy to any sulfonylurea or sulfonamides or any other component of the formulation. For a complete listing, see Dosage Forms, Composition and Packaging.
- Diabetic ketoacidosis, with or without coma. This condition should be treated with insulin.
- Pregnant or breast-feeding women.

No experience has been gained concerning the use of AMARYL in patients with severe impairment of liver function and in dialysis patients. In patients with severe impairment of renal or hepatic function, change-over to insulin is indicated, to achieve optimal metabolic control.
WARNINGS AND PRECAUTIONS: General: Use of AMARYL (glimepiride) must be considered as treatment in addition to a proper dietary regimen and not as a substitute for diet.

Over a period of time, patients may become progressively less responsive to therapy with oral hypoglycemic agents because of deterioration of their diabetic state. Patients should therefore be monitored with regular clinical and laboratory evaluations, including blood glucose and glycosylated hemoglobin (HbA_{1C}) determinations, to determine the minimum effective dosage and to detect primary failure (inadequate lowering of blood glucose concentrations at the maximum recommended dosage) or secondary failure (progressive deterioration in blood sugar control following an initial period of effectiveness). The rate of primary failure will vary greatly depending upon patient selection and adherence to diet and exercise. The etiology of secondary failure is multifactorial and may involve progressive β-cell failure as well as exogenous diabetogenic factors such as obesity, illness, drugs, or tachyphylaxis to the sulfonylurea. If a loss of adequate blood glucose lowering response to a sulfonylurea is detected, the addition of a different type of oral antidiabetic may be considered, although insulin is often required. Certain patients who demonstrate an inadequate response or true primary or secondary failure to one sulfonylurea may benefit from a switch to another sulfonylurea.

In initiating treatment for type 2 diabetes, non-pharmacologic therapy (proper dietary management, exercise and weight reduction) should be emphasized as the initial form of treatment. Caloric restriction, weight loss and exercise are essential in the obese diabetic patient. Proper dietary management and exercise alone may be effective in controlling the blood glucose and symptoms of hyperglycemia. In addition to regular physical activity, cardiovascular risk factors should be identified and corrective measures taken when possible.
Patient Selection and Follow-up: Careful selection of patients is important. Patients most likely to respond to sulfonylurea therapy are: obese or normal body weight; duration of diabetes less than 5 to 10 years before initiation of therapy; and, absence of ketoacidosis. It is imperative that there be careful attention to diet, careful adjustment of dosage, instruction of the patient on hypoglycemic reactions and their treatment, as well as regular, thorough follow-up examinations.

If non-pharmacologic therapy fails to reduce symptoms and/or blood glucose, the use of an oral sulfonylurea should be considered. Use of AMARYL (glimepiride) must be viewed by both the physician and patient as a treatment in addition to diet and exercise and not as a substitute for proper dietary management, exercise and weight reduction or as a convenient mechanism for avoiding dietary restraint. Furthermore, loss of blood glucose control on diet and exercise alone may be transient, thus requiring only short-term administration of AMARYL.
Loss of Control of Blood Glucose: When a patient stabilized on any diabetic regimen is exposed to stress such as illness during therapy, fever, trauma, infection, or surgery, a loss of glycemic control may occur. At such times, it may be necessary to adjust the dosage of AMARYL, add insulin in combination with AMARYL or even use insulin monotherapy. The effectiveness of any oral hypoglycemic drug, including AMARYL, in lowering blood glucose to a desired level decreases in many patients over a period of time, which may be due to progression of the severity of the diabetes or to diminished responsiveness to the drug. This phenomenon, known as secondary failure, is distinctive of primary failure in which the drug is ineffective in an individual patient when given for the first time. Should secondary failure occur or if target blood glucose levels are not attainable with AMARYL monotherapy, metformin may be added until the maximum dose of both agents is reached. Should secondary failure occur with AMARYL-metformin combination therapy, AMARYL-insulin combination therapy may be instituted.
Hypoglycemia: All sulfonylurea drugs are capable of producing severe hypoglycemia. In the initial weeks of treatment, the risk of hypoglycemia seen with glimepiride may be even further increased and necessitates closer and more frequent monitoring.

Signs of severe hypoglycemia can include disorientation, loss of consciousness, and seizures. Proper patient selection, dosage, and instructions are important to avoid hypoglycemic episodes. Elderly, debilitated or malnourished patients, and those with adrenal, pituitary, or hepatic insufficiency are particularly susceptible to the hypoglycemic action of glucose-lowering drugs. Patients with impaired renal function may be more sensitive to the glucose-lowering effect of AMARYL. A starting dose of 1 mg once daily followed by appropriate dose titration is also recommended in those patients. Hypoglycemia may be difficult to recognize in the elderly and in people who are taking beta-adrenergic blocking drugs or other sympatholytic agents. Hypoglycemia is more likely to occur when caloric intake is deficient, after severe or prolonged exercise, when alcohol is ingested, or when other drugs causing lowering of blood glucose are used concomitantly with AMARYL (see Drug Interactions, Drug-Drug Interactions). In clinical trials, patients receiving AMARYL in combination with insulin reported more incidence of hypoglycemia than patients on monotherapy.
Cardiovascular: It has been suggested, based on a study conducted by the University Group Diabetes Program (UGDP), that certain sulfonylurea antidiabetic agents increase cardiovascular mortality in diabetic patients, a population at greater risk of cardiovascular disease. This finding was not confirmed by a more recent trial, the United Kingdom Prospective Diabetes Study (UKPDS) which showed that intensive glycemic control with either sulfonylureas or insulin did not have an adverse effect on cardiovascular outcomes. Despite questions regarding the design of these studies and interpretation of the results, the results of these studies provide a basis for caution, especially high risk patients with cardiovascular disease.

In clinical trials more patients receiving AMARYL and insulin reported an increase in peripheral edema compared to patients receiving insulin alone. Patients receiving this combination therapy should be asked to report any edema or weight gain.
Hematologic: Treatment of patients with G6PD-deficiency with sulfonylurea agents can lead to hemolytic anemia. Since AMARYL belongs to the class of sulfonylurea agents, caution should be used in patients with G6PD-deficiency and a nonsulfonylurea alternative should be considered.
Renal: In patients with renal insufficiency, the initial dosing, dose increments, and maintenance dosage should be conservative to avoid hypoglycemic reactions.

Special Populations: Pregnant Women: There are no adequate and well-controlled studies in pregnant women. On the basis of results from animal studies, AMARYL (glimepiride) should not be used during pregnancy. Recent information suggests that abnormal blood glucose levels during pregnancy are associated with a higher incidence of congenital abnormalities. Experts, including the Canadian Diabetes Association and the Canadian Medical Association recommend that insulin be used during pregnancy to maintain blood glucose levels as close to normal as possible.

Teratogenic Effects: Glimepiride did not produce teratogenic effects in rats exposed orally up to 4000 mg/kg body weight (approximately 4000 times the maximum recommended human dose based on surface area) or in rabbits exposed up to 32 mg/kg body weight (approximately 60 times the maximum recommended human dose based on surface area). Glimepiride has been shown to be associated with intrauterine fetal death in rats when given in doses as low as 50 times the human dose based on surface area and in rabbits when given in doses as low as 0.1 times the human dose based on surface area. This fetotoxicity, observed only at doses inducing maternal hypoglycemia, has been similarly noted with other sulfonylureas, and is believed to be directly related to the pharmacologic (hypoglycemic) action of glimepiride.

Nonteratogenic Effects: In some studies in rats, offspring of dams exposed to high levels of glimepiride during pregnancy and lactation developed skeletal deformations consisting of shortening, thickening, and bending of the humerus during the postnatal period. Significant concentrations of glimepiride were observed in the serum and breast milk of the dams as well as in the serum of the pups. These skeletal deformations were determined to be the result of nursing from mothers exposed to glimepiride.

Prolonged severe hypoglycemia (4 to 10 days) has been reported in neonates born to mothers who were receiving a sulfonylurea drug at the time of delivery. This has been reported more frequently with the use of agents with prolonged half-lives. Patients who are planning a pregnancy should consult their physician, and it is recommended that they change over to insulin for the entire course of pregnancy and lactation.

Nursing Women: In rat reproduction studies, significant concentrations of glimepiride were observed in the serum and breast milk of the dams, as well as in the serum of the pups. Although it is not known whether AMARYL is excreted in human milk, other sulfonylureas are excreted in human milk. Since the potential for hypoglycemia in nursing infants may exist, and because of the effects on nursing animals, AMARYL should be discontinued in nursing mothers. If AMARYL is discontinued, and if diet and exercise alone are inadequate for controlling blood glucose, insulin therapy should be considered (see Pregnant Women, Nonteratogenic Effects).

Pediatrics: Safety and efficacy in pediatric type 2 diabetes patients have not been established.

Monitoring and Laboratory Tests: Fasting blood glucose should be monitored periodically to determine therapeutic response. Glycosylated hemoglobin (HbA_{1C}) should also be monitored, usually every 3 to 6 months, to more precisely assess long-term glycemic control.

Occupational Hazards: Driving a vehicle or operating machinery: Alertness and reactions may be impaired due to hypo- or hyperglycemia, especially when beginning or after altering treatment or when AMARYL (glimepiride) is not taken regularly. This may, for example, affect the ability to drive or to operate machinery.

ADVERSE REACTIONS: Adverse Drug Reaction Overview: The safety profile of Amaryl (glimepiride) has been evaluated in clinical trials and further assessed during post-marketing experience. A total of 2013 patients were exposed to AMARYL in US controlled trials, 1489 patients in European trials and 783 patients in Japanese trials. More than 1800 of these patients were treated for at least 1 year.

The overall incidence of hypoglycemia with AMARYL (glimepiride) was approximately 14% in placebo controlled trials, the incidence of hypoglycemia ranged from 2.1 to 3.1% in two long-term, well-controlled studies, and hypoglycemic episodes occurred in 22 and 51% in clinical trials involving patients treated with AMARYL in combination with metformin or insulin, respectively.

The most frequent adverse events occurring in US placebo-controlled trials were: dizziness (1.7%); asthenia (1.6%); headache (1.5%); nausea (1.1%).

Clinical Trial Adverse Drug Reactions: Because clinical trials are conducted under very specific conditions the adverse drug reaction rates observed in the clinical trials may not reflect the rates observed in practice and should not be compared to the rates in the clinical trials of another drug. Adverse drug reaction information from clinical trials is useful for identifying drug-related adverse events and for approximating rates.

The overall incidence of hypoglycemia with AMARYL (glimepiride) in placebo controlled trials was approximately 14% versus 2% for placebo. In two long-term (2-2.5 years) and well-controlled studies, the incidence of hypoglycemic reaction ranged from 2.1 to 3.1%. In clinical trials involving patients treated with AMARYL in combination with metformin or insulin, hypoglycemic episodes occurred in 22 and 51% of the patients, respectively.

Adverse events, other than hypoglycemia, considered to be possibly or probably related to study drug that occurred in US placebo-controlled trials in more than 1% of patients treated with AMARYL (see Table 1).

Table 1: AMARYL

Adverse Events Occurring in >1% AMARYL Patients

	AMARYL		Placebo	
	No. patients (n=746)	%	No. patients (n=294)	%
Dizziness	13	1.7	1	0.3
Asthenia	12	1.6	3	1.0
Headache	11	1.5	4	1.4
Nausea	8	1.1	0	0.0

Endocrine and Metabolism: Hepatic porphyria reactions and disulfiram-like reactions have been reported with sulfonylureas; however, no cases have yet been reported with AMARYL (glimepiride). Cases of hyponatremia have been reported with glimepiride and all other sulfonylureas, most often in patients who are on other medications or have medical conditions known to cause hyponatremia or increased release of antidiuretic hormones. Although there have been no reports for AMARYL, the syndrome of inappropriate antidiuretic hormone (SIADH) secretion has been reported with certain other sulfonylureas, and it has been suggested that these sulfonylureas may augment the peripheral (antidiuretic) action of ADH and/or increased release of ADH.

Gastrointestinal: Gastrointestinal (GI) disturbances e.g. nausea, GI fullness, occur occasionally. Vomiting, gastrointestinal pain, and diarrhea have been reported, but the incidence in placebo-controlled trials was similar to that of placebo. In rare cases, there may be elevation of liver enzyme levels. Sulfonylureas, including AMARYL (glimepiride), may also—in isolated instances—cause impairment of liver function (e.g. with cholestasis and jaundice), as well as hepatitis which may also lead to liver failure.

Skin: Allergic or pseudoallergic skin reactions, e.g., pruritus, erythema, urticaria, vasculitis, and morbilliform or maculopapular eruptions, occur in less than 1% of treated patients. Such mild reactions may develop into serious reactions with dyspnoea and hypotension, sometimes progressing to shock. These may be transient and may disappear despite continued use of AMARYL; if skin reactions persist, the drug should be discontinued. Although there have been no reports for AMARYL, porphyria cutanea tarda has been reported with sulfonylureas.

Other Adverse Reactions: Changes in accommodation and/or blurred vision may occur with the use of AMARYL. This is thought to be due to changes in blood glucose, and may be more pronounced when treatment is initiated. This condition is also seen in untreated diabetic patients, and may actually be reduced by treatment. In placebo-controlled trials of AMARYL, the incidence of blurred vision was placebo, 3.4%, and AMARYL, 1.7%.

Less Common Clinical Trial Adverse Drug Reactions (<1%): Clinical adverse events occurring in less than 1% of patients treated with AMARYL in all US clinical trials are listed below by body system:

Body as a Whole: abdominal pain, laboratory test abnormal, and pain in extremity.

Cardiovascular: palpitation and vasodilation.

Digestive: diarrhea, increased appetite, dyspepsia, anorexia, and gastrointestinal pain.

Metabolic and Nutritional Disorders: hypoglycemic reaction and hyperglycemia.

Nervous System: tremor, insomnia, sweating increased, nervousness, dry mouth, hot flashes, and paresthesia.

Skin and Appendages: pruritus and urticaria.

Special Senses: blurred vision.

Urogenital System: increased urinary frequency and nocturia.

Post-Market Adverse Drug Reactions: The following adverse events, not seen in clinical trials, have been reported during post-marketing surveillance:

Hematologic: Changes in the blood picture may occur. Rarely (≥1/10 000 and <1/1000), thrombopenia and, in isolated cases (<1/10 000), leukopenia, hemolytic anemia, erythrocytopenia, granulocytopenia, agranulocytosis or pancytopenia may develop.

Skin: In isolated cases (<1/10 000), allergic vasculitis or hypersensitivity of the skin to light may occur.

Other: In isolated cases (<1/10 000), a decrease in serum sodium concentration may occur.

DRUG INTERACTIONS: Overview: Glimepiride is metabolized by cytochrome P450 2C9 (CYP2C9). This should be taken into account when glimepiride is coadministered with inducers (e.g. rifampicin) or inhibitors (e.g. fluconazole) of CYP 2C9. Both acute and chronic alcohol intake may potentiate or weaken the blood-glucose-lowering action of AMARYL in an unpredictable fashion.

Drug-Drug Interactions: The drugs listed in Table 2 are based on either drug interaction case reports or studies, or potential interactions due to the expected magnitude and seriousness of the interaction (i.e., those identified as contraindicated).

Table 2: AMARYL

Established or Predicted Drug-Drug Interactions

Proper Name	Ref	Effect	Clinical Comments
Acetylsalicylic acid (ASA)	CT	↓ 34% mean glimepiride AUC ↑ 34% mean glimepiride Cl/F ↓ 4% mean glimepiride C_{max}	Blood glucose and serum C-peptide concentrations were unaffected and no hypoglycemic symptoms were reported. Pooled data from clinical trials showed no evidence of clinically significant adverse interactions with uncontrolled concurrent administration of acetylsalicylic acid and other salicylates.
Cimetidine or ranitidine	CT	No clinically significant effect	Coadministration of either cimetidine (800 mg once daily) or ranitidine (150 mg bid) with a single 4-mg oral dose of AMARYL did not significantly alter the absorption and disposition of glimepiride, and no differences were seen in hypoglycemic symptomatology. Pooled data from clinical trials showed no evidence of clinically significant adverse interactions with uncontrolled concurrent administration of H2-receptor antagonists.
Propranolol	CT	↑ glimepiride C_{max} by 23% ↑ glimepiride AUC by 22% ↑ glimepiride $T_{1/2}$ by 15% ↓ glimepiride Cl/F by 18%	The recovery of M1 and M2 metabolites from urine did not change. The pharmacodynamic responses to glimepiride were nearly identical in normal subjects receiving propranolol and placebo. Pooled data from clinical trials in patients with type 2 diabetes showed no evidence of clinically significant adverse interactions with uncontrolled concurrent administration of beta-blockers. However, if beta-blockers are used, caution should be exercised and patients should be warned about the potential for hypoglycemia.
Warfarin	CT	No clinically significant effect	Concomitant administration of AMARYL (glimepiride) (4 mg once daily) did not alter the pharmacokinetic characteristics of R- and S-warfarin enantiomers following administration of a single dose (25 mg) of racemic warfarin to healthy subjects. No changes were observed in warfarin plasma protein binding. AMARYL treatment did result in a slight, but statistically significant, decrease in the pharmacodynamic response to warfarin. The reductions in mean area under the prothrombin time (PT) curve and maximum PT values during AMARYL treatment were very small (3.3% and 9.9%, respectively) and are unlikely to be clinically important.
Ramipril	CT	No clinically significant effect	The responses of serum glucose, insulin, C-peptide, and plasma glucagon to 2 mg AMARYL were unaffected by coadministration of ramipril 5 mg once daily in normal subjects. No hypoglycemic symptoms were reported. Pooled data from clinical trials in patients with type 2 diabetes showed no evidence of clinically significant adverse interactions with uncontrolled concurrent administration of ACE inhibitors.
Drugs metabolized by cytochrome P450 2C9	T	Potential interactions	Potential interactions of glimepiride with other drugs metabolized by cytochrome P450 2C9 also include phenytoin, diclofenac, ibuprofen, naproxen, and mefenamic acid.

Legend: CT=clinical trial; T=theoretical.

Although no specific interaction studies were performed, pooled data from clinical trials showed no evidence of clinically significant adverse interactions with uncontrolled concurrent administration of calcium-channel blockers, estrogens, fibrates, NSAIDS, HMG CoA reductase inhibitors, sulfonamides, or thyroid hormone.

The hypoglycemic action of sulfonylureas may be potentiated by certain drugs, including anabolic steroids and male sex hormones, ACE inhibitors, insulin and other oral antidiabetics, nonsteroidal anti-inflammatory drugs and other drugs that are highly protein bound, such as azapropazone, sulfonamides (e.g. sulphaphenazole), chloramphenicol, clarithromycin, coumarins, cyclophosphamide, disopyramide, fenyramidol, fenfluramine, fibrates, fluconazole, fluoxetine, guanethidine, ifosfamide, miconazole, monoamine oxidase inhibitors, oxyphenbutazone, para-aminosalicylic acid, pentoxifylline (high dose parenteral), phenylbutazone, probenecid, propranolol, quinolones, salicylates, sulfonamide antibiotics, sulfinpyrazone, and tetracycline.

When these drugs are administered to a patient receiving AMARYL, the patient should be observed closely for hypoglycemia. When these drugs are withdrawn from a patient receiving AMARYL, the patient should be observed closely for loss of glycemic control.

Certain drugs tend to produce hyperglycemia and may lead to loss of glycemic control. These drugs include the thiazides and other diuretics, acetazolamide, barbiturates, corticosteroids, diazoxide, epinephrine and other sympathomimetic agents, glucagon, isoniazid, laxatives (after protracted use), nicotinic acid (in high dose), estrogens and progestogens, phenothiazines, phenytoin, rifampicin and thyroid products. When these drugs are administered to a patient receiving AMARYL, the patient should be closely observed for loss of glycemic control. When these drugs are withdrawn from a patient receiving AMARYL, the patient should be observed closely for hypoglycemia.

Concurrent use of H_2 receptor antagonists, beta-blockers, clonidine or reserpine may lead to either potentiation or weakening of the blood-glucose-lowering effect.

Under the influence of sympatholytic drugs such as beta-blockers, clonidine, guanethidine and reserpine, the signs of adrenergic counter-regulation to hypoglycaemia may be reduced or absent.

The effect of coumarin derivatives may be potentiated or weakened.

Drug-Food Interactions: Interactions with food have not been established.

Drug-Herb Interactions: Interactions with herbal products have not been established.

Drug-Laboratory Interactions: Interactions with laboratory tests have not been established.

DOSAGE AND ADMINISTRATION: **Dosing Considerations:** The patient's fasting blood glucose and HbA_{1C} must be measured periodically to determine the minimum effective dose for the patient; to detect primary failure, i.e., inadequate lowering of blood glucose at the maximum recommended dose of medication; and to detect secondary failure, i.e., loss of adequate blood glucose lowering response after an initial period of effectiveness. Glycosylated hemoglobin levels (HbA_{1C}) should be performed to monitor the patient's response to therapy.

Short-term administration of AMARYL (glimepiride) may be sufficient during periods of transient loss of glycemic control in patients usually controlled well on diet and exercise.

Recommended Dose and Dosage Adjustment: Usual Starting Dose: The usual starting dose of AMARYL as initial therapy is 1 mg once daily, administered with breakfast or the first main meal. Those patients who may be more sensitive to hypoglycemic drugs should be titrated carefully (see Warnings and Precautions). Failure to follow an appropriate dosage regimen may precipitate hypoglycemia. Patients who do not adhere to their prescribed dietary, exercise, weight loss and drug regimen are more prone to exhibit unsatisfactory response to therapy.

Adjustment of dosage must also be considered, whenever:

- The patient's weight changes,
- The patient's life-style changes, other factors arise which cause an increased susceptibility to hypoglycemia or hyperglycemia (see Warnings and Precautions).

Usual Maintenance Dose: The usual maintenance dose is 1 to 4 mg once daily. The maximum recommended dose is 8 mg once daily. After reaching a dose of 2 mg, dosage increases should be made in increments of no more than 1 mg at 1-2 week intervals based upon the patient's blood glucose response. Long-term efficacy should be monitored by measurement of HbA_{1C} levels, for example every 3 to 6 months.

AMARYL-Metformin Combination Therapy: Combination therapy with AMARYL and metformin may be used in patients who do not respond adequately to the maximal dose of AMARYL or in secondary failure patients. With concomitant AMARYL and metformin therapy, the desired control of blood glucose may be obtained by adjusting the dose of each drug. Attempts should be made to identify the minimum effective dose of each drug to achieve this goal. With combination AMARYL and metformin therapy, the risk of hypoglycemia may increase. Appropriate precautions should be taken.

AMARYL-Insulin Combination Therapy: Combination therapy with AMARYL and insulin may be used in secondary failure patients. The recommended AMARYL dose is 8 mg once daily administered with the first main meal. After starting with low-dose insulin, upward adjustments of insulin can be done approximately weekly as guided by frequent measurements of fasting blood glucose. Once stable, combination-therapy patients should monitor their capillary blood glucose on an ongoing basis, preferably daily. Periodic adjustments of insulin may also be necessary during maintenance as guided by glucose and HbA_{1C} levels.

Specific Patient Populations: AMARYL is not recommended for use in pregnancy, nursing mothers, or children. In elderly, debilitated, or malnourished patients, or in patients with renal or hepatic insufficiency, the initial dosing, dose increments, and maintenance dosage should be conservative to avoid hypoglycemic reactions (see Action and Clinical Pharmacology, Special Populations and Conditions and Warnings and Precautions, General).

Changeover from Other Oral Hypoglycemic Agents: No exact dosage relationship exists between AMARYL and the other oral hypoglycemic agents. When substituting AMARYL for other oral hypoglycemic agents, it is recommended that the procedure be the same as for initial dosage starting with daily doses of 1 mg. Consideration must be given to the potency and duration of the previous antidiabetic agent. Patients should be observed carefully (1-2 weeks) for hypoglycemia when being transferred from longer half-life sulfonylureas (e.g., chlorpropamide) to AMARYL due to potential overlapping of drug effect.

A break from medication may be required to avoid any summation of effects entailing a risk of hypoglycemia.

Missed Dose: The missed dose should be taken as soon as possible, unless it is almost time for the next dose. The patient should be advised not to take two doses at the same time.

OVERDOSAGE:

Overdosage of sulfonylureas, including AMARYL (glimepiride), can produce hypoglycemia. Mild hypoglycemic symptoms without loss of consciousness or neurologic findings should be treated with oral glucose and adjustments in drug dosage and/or meal patterns. Close monitoring should continue until the physician is assured that the patient is out of danger. Severe hypoglycemic reactions with coma, seizure, or other neurological impairment occur infrequently, but constitute medical emergencies requiring immediate hospitalization. In case of overdosage, current medical intervention for the treatment of hypoglycemia should be followed according to the condition of the patient. Patients should be closely monitored for a minimum of 24 to 48 hours, because hypoglycemia may recur after apparent clinical recovery.

For management of a suspected drug overdose, CPhA recommends that you contact your **regional Poison Control Centre**. See the *CPS* Directory section for a list of Poison Control Centres.

ACTION AND CLINICAL PHARMACOLOGY: **Mechanism of Action:** The primary mechanism of action of glimepiride in lowering blood glucose appears to be dependent on stimulating the release of insulin from functioning pancreatic beta cells. In addition, extra-pancreatic effects may also play a role in the activity of glimepiride. This is supported by both preclinical and clinical studies demonstrating that glimepiride administration can lead to increased sensitivity of peripheral tissues to insulin. These findings are consistent with the results of a long-term, randomized, placebo-controlled trial in which AMARYL (glimepiride) therapy improved postprandial insulin/C-peptide responses and overall glycemic control without producing clinically meaningful increases in fasting insulin/C-peptide levels. However, the mechanism by which glimepiride lowers blood glucose during long-term administration has not been clearly established.

Pharmacodynamics: A mild glucose-lowering effect first appeared following single oral doses as low as 0.5-0.6 mg in healthy subjects. The time required to reach the maximum effect (i.e., minimum blood glucose level [T_{min}]) was about 2 to 3 hours. In type 2 diabetes (formerly known as non-insulin-dependent diabetes mellitus or NIDDM) patients, both fasting and 2-hour postprandial glucose levels were significantly lower with glimepiride (1, 2, 4, and 8 mg once daily) than with placebo after 14 days of oral dosing. The glucose-lowering effect in all active treatment groups was maintained over 24 hours.

In larger dose-ranging studies, blood glucose and glycosylated hemoglobin (HbA_{1C}) were found to respond in a dose-dependent manner over the range of 1 to 4 mg of AMARYL once daily. Some patients, particularly those with higher fasting plasma glucose (FPG) levels, may benefit from doses of AMARYL up to 8 mg once daily. No difference in the decrease in blood glucose and HbA_{1C} concentrations were found when AMARYL was administered once or twice daily.

In two 14-week, placebo-controlled studies in 720 subjects, the average net reduction in HbA_{1C} for AMARYL (glimepiride) patients treated with 8 mg once daily was 2.0% (0.02) in absolute units compared with placebo-treated patients. Efficacy results were not affected by age, gender, weight, or race.

In a 22-week, randomized, placebo-controlled study of Type 2 diabetic patients unresponsive to dietary management, AMARYL therapy improved postprandial insulin/C-peptide responses, and 75% of patients achieved and maintained control of blood glucose and HbA_{1C}. The results of three long-term studies demonstrated that AMARYL, when administered over a prolonged treatment period of one-year (n=986), was effective in maintaining metabolic control in type 2 diabetic patients who were responders to sulfonylurea therapy. In an extension of long-term trials with patients previously treated with AMARYL, no meaningful deterioration in mean fasting blood glucose (FBG) or HbA_{1C} levels was seen after up to 2.5 years of AMARYL therapy (n=445).

Combination therapy with AMARYL and metformin was compared with glimepiride and metformin monotherapy in Type 2 diabetic patients. The results of the study indicated that the combination of metformin and glimepiride was more effective than either treatment alone, with regards to improving HbA_{1C}, fasting blood glucose and postprandial blood glucose levels.

Combination therapy with AMARYL and insulin (70% NPH/30% regular) was compared to placebo/insulin in secondary failure patients whose body weight was >130% of their ideal body weight. Initially, 5-10 units of insulin were administered with the main evening meal and titrated upward weekly to achieve predefined FPG values. Both groups in this double-blind study achieved similar reductions in FPG levels but the AMARYL/insulin therapy group showed an insulin sparing effect with a use of 38% less insulin.

AMARYL therapy is effective in controlling blood glucose without deleterious changes in the plasma lipoprotein profiles of patients treated for Type 2 diabetes.

Pharmacokinetics: Absorption: After oral administration, glimepiride is completely (100%) absorbed from the GI tract. Studies with single oral doses in normal subjects and with multiple oral doses in patients with type 2 diabetes have shown significant absorption of glimepiride within 1 hour after administration and peak drug levels (C_{max}) at 2 to 3 hours. When glimepiride was given with meals, the mean T_{max} (time to reach C_{max}) was slightly increased (12%) and the mean C_{max} and AUC (area under the curve) were slightly decreased (8% and 9%, respectively). In normal healthy volunteers, the intra-individual variabilities of C_{max}, AUC, and total body clearance after oral dosing (Cl/F) for glimepiride were 23%, 17%, and 15%, respectively, and the inter-individual variabilities were 25%, 29%, and 24%, respectively.

The pharmacokinetics of glimepiride obtained from a single-dose, crossover, dose-proportionality (1, 2, 4, and 8 mg) study in normal subjects and from a single- and multiple-dose, parallel, dose-proportionality (4 and 8 mg) study in patients with type 2 diabetes are summarized in Table 3.

Table 3: AMARYL
Pharmacokinetics of AMARYL in Healthy Volunteers and Type 2 Diabetic Patients

	Volunteers	Patients with Type 2 Diabetes	
	Single Dose Mean±SD (n)	Single Dose (Day 1) Mean±SD (n)	Multiple Dose (Day 10) Mean±SD (n)
C_{max} (ng/mL)			
1 mg	103±34 (12)	—	—
2 mg	177±44 (12)	—	—
4 mg	308±69 (12)	352±222 (12)	309±134 (12)
8 mg	551±152 (12)	591±232 (14)	578±265 (11)
T_{max} (h)			
1 mg	2.3±0.5 (12)	—	—
2 mg	2.4±0.5 (12)	—	—
4 mg	2.1±0.6 (12)	2.08±0.51 (12)	2.22±1.21 (12)
8 mg	2.8±1.2 (12)	2.80±1.46 (14)	3.46±2.82 (11)
Cl/F (mL/min)			
1 mg	55.3±16.3 (12)	—	—
2 mg	53.5±15.5 (12)	—	—
4 mg	53.6±10.6 (12)	54.2±41.1 (12)	63.4±53.5 (12)
8 mg	56.5±21.1 (12)	43.6±13.0 (14)	41.0±11.2 (11)
Vd/f (L)			
1 mg	10.6±1.8 (12)	—	—
2 mg	12.6±2.9 (12)	—	—
4 mg	15.7±5.4 (12)	20.8±11.3 (12)	40.2±22.3 (12)
8 mg	20.9±6.9 (12)	18.9±14.1 (14)	33.8±12.6 (11)
$t_{1/2}$ (h)			
1 mg	1.2±0.5 (12)	—	—
2 mg	1.3±0.4 (12)	—	—
4 mg	1.5±0.5 (12)	5.30±2.54 (12)	8.82±4.36 (12)
8 mg	1.5±0.4 (12)	4.69±2.61 (14)	9.63±2.63 (11)

Legend: (n)=number of subjects; Vd/f=volume of distribution calculated after oral dosing.

These data indicate that glimepiride did not accumulate in serum, and the pharmacokinetics of glimepiride were not different in healthy volunteers and in type 2 diabetic patients. Oral clearance of glimepiride did not change over the 1-8-mg dose range, indicating linear pharmacokinetics.

Distribution: After intravenous dosing in normal subjects, the volume of distribution (Vd) was 8.8 L (113 mL/kg), and the total body clearance (CL) was 47.8 mL/min. Protein binding was greater than 99.5%.

Metabolism: Glimepiride is completely metabolized by oxidative biotransformation after either IV or oral administration. The major metabolites are the cyclohexyl hydroxy methyl derivative (M1) and the carboxyl derivative (M2). Cytochrome P450 2 C9 has been shown to be involved in the biotransformation of glimepiride to M1. M1 is further metabolized to M2 by one or several cytosolic enzymes. M1, but not M2, possesses about 1/3 of the pharmacological activity as compared to its parent in an animal model; however, whether the glucose-lowering effect of M1 is clinically meaningful in humans is not clear.

Excretion: When ^{14}C-glimepiride was given as a single dose orally, approximately 60% of the total radioactivity was recovered in the urine in 7 days and metabolites M1 (predominant) and M2 accounted for 80-90% of that recovered in the urine. Approximately 40% of the total radioactivity was recovered in feces and metabolites M1 and M2 (predominant) accounted for about 70% of that recovered in feces. After IV dosing in patients, no significant biliary excretion of glimepiride or its M1 metabolite has been observed.

Special Populations and Conditions: **Pediatrics:** No studies were performed in pediatric patients.

Geriatrics: Comparison of glimepiride pharmacokinetics in type 2 diabetic patients ≤65 years and those >65 years was performed in a study using a dosing regimen of 6 mg daily. There were no significant differences in glimepiride pharmacokinetics between the two age groups. The mean AUC at steady state for the older patients was about 13% lower than that for the younger patients; the mean weight-adjusted clearance for the older patients was about 11% higher than that for the younger patients (see Warnings and Precautions, General).

Gender: There were no differences between males and females in the pharmacokinetics of glimepiride when adjusting for differences in body weight.

Race: No pharmacokinetic studies to assess the effects of race have been performed, but in placebo-controlled studies of AMARYL (glimepiride) in patients with type 2 diabetes, the hypoglycemic effect was comparable in whites (n=536), blacks (n=63), and Hispanics (n=63).

Hepatic Insufficiency: No studies were performed in patients with hepatic insufficiency.

Renal Insufficiency: A single-dose, open-label study was conducted in 15 patients with renal impairment. AMARYL (3 mg) was administered to 3 groups of patients with different levels of mean creatinine clearance (CL_{cr}): Group I, CL_{cr}=77.7 mL/min (1.30 mL/sec), n=5; Group II, CL_{cr}=27.7 mL/min (0.462 mL/sec), n=3; and Group III, CL_{cr}=9.4 mL/min (0.16 mL/sec), n=7. AMARYL was found to be well tolerated in all 3 groups. The results showed that M1 and M2 metabolites serum levels (mean AUC values) increased 2.2 and 6.1 times from Group I to Group III as renal function decreased. The apparent terminal half-life ($T_{1/2}$) for glimepiride did not change, while the half-lives for metabolites M1 and M2 increased as renal function decreased. Mean urinary excretion of metabolites M1 plus M2 as percent of dose, however, decreased (44.4%, 21.9%, and 9.3% for Groups I to III).

A multiple-dose titration study was also conducted in 16 type 2 diabetic patients with renal impairment using doses ranging from 1-8 mg daily for 3 months. The results were consistent with those observed after single doses. All patients with a CL_{cr} less than 22 mL/min (0.37 mL/sec) had adequate control of their glucose levels with a dosage regimen of only 1 mg daily. The results from this study suggested that a starting dose of 1 mg AMARYL may be given to type 2 diabetic patients with kidney disease, and the dose may be titrated based on fasting blood glucose levels (see Warnings and Precautions, Renal).

Other Populations: There were no important differences in glimepiride metabolism in subjects identified as phenotypically different drug-metabolizers by their metabolism of sparteine.

The pharmacokinetics of glimepiride in morbidly obese patients were similar to those in the normal weight group, except for a lower C_{max} and AUC. However, since neither C_{max} nor AUC values were normalized for body surface area, the lower values of C_{max} and AUC for the obese patients were likely the result of their excess weight and not due to a difference in the kinetics of glimepiride.

STORAGE AND STABILITY: Store between 15 and 30°C. Dispense in well-closed container.

INFORMATION FOR THE PATIENT: Published in e-CPS, available by subscription at www.e-cps.ca.

DOSAGE FORMS, COMPOSITION AND PACKAGING: 1 mg: Each pink, flat-faced, oblong tablet with notched sides at the bisect, imprinted with "AMARYL" on one side and plain with bisect on the other, contains: glimepiride 1 mg. Nonmedicinal ingredients: ferric oxide, lactose, magnesium stearate, microcrystalline cellulose, povidone and sodium starch glycolate. Plastic bottles of 30.
2 mg: Each green, flat-faced, oblong tablet with notched sides at the bisect, imprinted with "AMARYL" on one side and plain with bisect on the other, contains: glimepiride 2 mg. Nonmedicinal ingredients: FD&C Blue #2 Aluminum Lake, ferric oxide, lactose, magnesium stearate, microcrystalline cellulose, povidone and sodium starch glycolate. Plastic bottles of 30.
4 mg: Each blue, flat-faced, oblong tablet with notched sides at the bisect, imprinted with "AMARYL" on one side and plain with bisect on the other, contains: glimepiride 4 mg. Nonmedicinal ingredients: FD&C Blue #2 Aluminum Lake, lactose, magnesium stearate, microcrystalline cellulose, povidone and sodium starch glycolate. Plastic bottles of 30.

(Shown in Product Identification Section)

AmBisome® Ⓟ

liposomal amphotericin B

Antifungal

Astellas

PHARMACOLOGY: The active component of AmBisome is amphotericin B which acts by binding to the ergosterol component in the cell membrane of susceptible fungi. This results in a change in membrane permeability allowing leakage of cell components. While amphotericin B has a higher affinity for the ergosterol component of the fungal cell membrane, it can also bind to the cholesterol component of the mammalian cell membrane and the damage to human cells and fungal cells may share a common mechanism.

AmBisome is a true single bilayer liposomal drug delivery system. Liposomes are closed, spherical vesicles created by mixing specific proportions of amphiphilic substances such as phospholipids and cholesterol so that they arrange themselves into multiple concentric bilayer membranes when hydrated in aqueous solutions. AmBisome consists of these unilamellar bilayer liposomes with amphotericin B intercalated within the membrane, forming a charge transfer complex with the distearoylphosphatidylglycerol. Due to the nature and quantity of amphiphilic substances used, and the lipophilic moiety in the amphotericin B molecule, the drug is an integral part of the overall structure of the AmBisome liposomes. AmBisome contains true liposomes that are less than 100 nm in diameter. The unique size of the liposomes results in therapeutic levels at diverse sites of fungal infections within the body.

Studies have shown that AmBisome can remain as an intact liposome and stay in circulation for prolonged periods of time. It is taken up and retained in tissues rich in reticuloendothelial cells where fungal infection may occur. Preclinical studies have shown that liposomes with and without amphotericin B bind to the fungal cell wall. Liposomal amphotericin B acts by liposomal binding to the outer cell wall of fungi followed by drug release. On release the drug is thought to transfer to the ergosterol-rich fungal cell wall for which it has high affinity. Interaction with fungi occurs both within and outside macrophages. Liposomal and various lipid-complexed amphotericin B preparations differ significantly in their pharmacokinetic profile and tissue distribution.
Pharmacokinetics: The pharmacokinetic profile of amphotericin B after administration of liposomal amphotericin B is different from that of conventional amphotericin B (amphotericin B desoxycholate). In Phase I pharmacokinetic studies, liposomal amphotericin B produced higher peak serum concentrations between daily doses of 1 to 5 mg/kg/day (6- to 10-fold greater) and area under the serum concentration curve (AUC, approximately 13-fold higher) than those reported for conventional amphotericin B. The apparent volume of distribution ranged from 18.9 to 49.1 L. The total body clearance of liposomal amphotericin B ranged from 0.5 to 1.3 L/h. Data are shown in Table 1. Detailed comparative studies with conventional amphotericin B are lacking. Some variability of the data in patients has been observed.

Amphotericin B concentrations were measured in autopsy material from 3 patients who died within 24 hours of receiving their last dose of liposomal amphotericin B. Drug concentrations were highest in the liver and spleen (tissues rich in reticuloendothelial cells) confirming data obtained from animal studies. Concentrations in lungs, kidneys, brain and heart were comparatively low. Detailed human tissue distribution have not been established for liposomal amphotericin B.

Table 1: AmBisome

Pharmacokinetic Parameters of AmBisome

Dose (mg/kg/day)	1.0		2.5		5.0	
Day	1 n=8	Last n=7	1 n=7	Last n=7	1 n=12	Last n=9
Parameters						
C_{max} (µg/mL)	7.3 ± 3.8	12.2 ± 4.9	17.2 ± 7.1	31.4 ± 17.8	57.6 ± 21.0	83.0 ± 35.2
AUC_{0-24} (µg·h/mL)	27 ± 14	60 ± 20	65 ± 33	197 ± 183	269 ± 96	555 ± 311
$t_{1/2}$ (h)	10.7 ± 6.4	7.0 ± 2.1	8.1 ± 2.3	6.3 ± 2.0	6.4 ± 2.1	6.8 ± 2.1
V (L/kg)	0.58 ± 0.40	0.16 ± 0.04	0.69 ± 0.85	0.18 ± 0.13	0.22 ± 0.17	0.11 ± 0.08
Vss (L/kg)	0.44 ± 0.27	0.14 ± 0.05	0.40 ± 0.37	0.16 ± 0.09	0.16 ± 0.10	0.10 ± 0.07
Cl (mL/h/kg)	39 ± 22	17 ± 6	51 ± 44	22 ± 15	21 ± 14	11 ± 6

INDICATIONS: For empirical therapy for presumed fungal infection in febrile, neutropenic patients and for treatment of cryptococcal meningitis in HIV-infected patients. Liposomal amphotericin B is also indicated for the treatment of systemic or disseminated infections due to Candida, Aspergillus or Cryptococcus in patients who are refractory to or intolerant to conventional amphotericin B therapy or renally impaired patients.

In a randomized, double-blind study of 687 febrile, neutropenic patients treated with either liposomal amphotericin B or conventional amphotericin B following at least 96 hours of broad spectrum antibiotic therapy, overall therapeutic success rates for liposomal amphotericin B and conventional amphotericin B were equivalent (49.9% vs 49.1%, respectively). In a randomized, double-blind study of 267 HIV positive patients with cryptococcal meningitis, treated with either liposomal amphotericin B or conventional amphotericin B mycological success rates at week 2 for liposomal amphotericin B and conventional amphotericin B were equivalent (53% vs 48%, respectively).

Liposomal amphotericin B was used in a compassionate study of 133 patients who had failed conventional amphotericin B therapy or who had nephrotoxicity from previous therapy or had renal insufficiency. Overall mycological eradication rate was 62% (33/53 patients) and the overall clinical success rate was 82% (75/91 patients). Patients who entered this trial with high creatinine values due to nephrotoxicity returned to or toward normal values during liposomal amphotericin B therapy.

CONTRAINDICATIONS: In patients who have demonstrated or have known hypersensitivity to conventional amphotericin B or any other constituents of AmBisome unless, in the opinion of the treating physician, the benefit of therapy outweighs the risk.

WARNINGS: Anaphylaxis has been reported with conventional amphotericin B and other amphotericin-containing drugs. Anaphylactoid type reactions have been reported with liposomal amphotericin B. If a severe reaction occurs, the infusion should be immediately discontinued. The patient should not receive further infusions of liposomal amphotericin B.

Liposomal amphotericin B should be administered primarily to patients with progressive, potentially fatal infections. This drug should not be used to treat the common apparent forms of fungal diseases which show only positive skin or serologic tests.

PRECAUTIONS: General: As with any amphotericin B-containing product, the drug should be administered by medically trained personnel. During the initial dosing period, patients should be under close clinical observation. Liposomal amphotericin B has been shown to be significantly less toxic than traditional amphotericin B; however, adverse events may still occur. In general, patients should be monitored for any of the adverse events associated with the use of amphotericin B. In particular, caution should be exercised when prolonged therapy is required.
Geriatrics: Experience with liposomal amphotericin B in the elderly (≥65 years) is comprised of 71 patients. It has not been necessary to alter the dose of liposomal amphotericin B for this population. As with most other drugs, elderly patients receiving liposomal amphotericin B should be carefully monitored. The pharmacokinetics of amphotericin B after administration of liposomal amphotericin B in elderly patients has not been studied.
Children: Pediatric patients age 1 month to 16 years with presumed fungal infections (empirical therapy), confirmed systemic fungal infections or with visceral leishmaniasis have been treated with liposomal amphotericin B. In studies which included 302 pediatric patients administered liposomal amphotericin B there was no evidence of any differences in efficacy or safety of liposomal amphotericin B compared to adults. Since pediatric patients have received liposomal amphotericin B at doses comparable to those used in adults on a per kilogram body weight basis, no dosage adjustment is required in this population. Safety and effectiveness in pediatric patients below the age of 1 month has not been established. The pharmacokinetics of amphotericin B after administration of liposomal amphotericin B in pediatric patients has not been studied.
Pregnancy: Reproduction studies in animals have revealed no evidence of teratogenicity at human therapeutic doses. There have been no adequate and well-controlled studies of liposomal amphotericin B in pregnant women. Systemic fungal infections have been successfully treated in pregnant women with conventional amphotericin B without obvious effects to the fetus, but the number of case reports has been small. Because animal reproduction studies are not always predictive of human response, and adequate and well controlled studies have not been conducted in pregnant women, this drug should be administered during pregnancy with caution and only if the potential benefit to the mother outweighs the potential risk to the fetus.
Lactation: Many drugs are excreted in human milk. However, it is not known whether liposomal amphotericin B is excreted in human milk. Due to the potential for serious adverse reactions in breast-fed infants, a decision should be made whether to discontinue nursing or whether to discontinue the drug, taking into account the importance of the drug to the mother.
Carcinogenicity/Mutagenicity: Liposomal amphotericin B has not undergone testing for mutagenic or carcinogenic potential.
Special Diseases or Conditions: Hepatic Impairment: The effect of hepatic impairment on the disposition of liposomal amphotericin B is not known.
Renal Impairment: The effect of renal impairment on the disposition of liposomal amphotericin B has not been studied. However, liposomal amphotericin B has been successfully administered to patients with pre-existing renal impairment.
Diabetic Patients: It should be noted that liposomal amphotericin B contains approximately 900 mg of sucrose in each vial.
Renal Dialysis Patients: The administration of liposomal amphotericin B should be initiated after dialysis is completed.
Laboratory Tests: Patient management should include laboratory evaluation of renal, hepatic and hematopoietic function, complete blood counts and serum electrolytes (particularly magnesium and potassium).
Drug Interactions: No formal clinical studies of drug interactions have been conducted with liposomal amphotericin B. However, the following drugs are known to interact with amphotericin B and may interact with liposomal amphotericin B:
Antineoplastic Agents: Concurrent use of antineoplastic agents may enhance the potential for renal toxicity, bronchospasm and hypotension. Antineoplastic agents should be given concomitantly with caution.
Corticosteroids and Corticotrophin (ACTH): Concurrent use of corticosteroids and corticotropin (ACTH) may potentiate hypokalemia which could predispose the patient to cardiac dysfunction. If used concomitantly, serum electrolytes and cardiac function should be closely monitored.
Digitalis Glycosides: Concurrent use may induce hypokalemia and may potentiate digitalis toxicity. When administered concomitantly, serum potassium levels should be closely monitored.
Flucytosine: Concurrent use of flucytosine with amphotericin B-containing preparations may increase the toxicity of flucytosine by possibly increasing its cellular uptake and/or impairing its renal excretion. Flucytosine should be given concomitantly with liposomal amphotericin B with caution.
Azoles (e.g., ketoconazole, miconazole, clotrimazole, fluconazole, etc.): In vitro and in vivo animal studies of the combination of amphotericin B and imidazoles suggest that imidazoles may induce fungal resistance to amphotericin B. Combination therapy should be administered with caution, especially in immunocompromised patients.
Leukocyte Transfusions: Acute pulmonary toxicity has been reported in patients simultaneously receiving i.v. amphotericin B and leukocyte transfusions. Leukocyte transfusions should not be given concurrently.
Other Nephrotoxic Agents: Concurrent use of amphotericin B and agents such as aminoglycosides and pentamidine may enhance the potential for drug-induced renal toxicity and should be used only with caution. Intensive monitoring of renal function is recommended in patients requiring any combination of nephrotoxic medications.
Skeletal Muscle Relaxants: Amphotericin B-induced hypokalemia may enhance the curariform effect of skeletal muscle relaxants (e.g., tubocurarine) due to hypokalemia. When administered concomitantly, serum potassium levels should be closely monitored.

ADVERSE EFFECTS: The following adverse events are based on the experience of 592 adult patients (295 treated with liposomal amphotericin B and 297 treated with amphotericin B desoxycholate) and 95 pediatric patients (48 treated with liposomal amphotericin B and 47 treated with amphotericin B desoxycholate) in Study 94-0-002, a randomized, double-blind, multicentre study for the empiric treatment of febrile, neutropenic patients. Liposomal amphotericin B and amphotericin B were infused over 2 to 4 hours.

The incidence of common adverse events occurring with either liposomal amphotericin B or amphotericin B desoxycholate, regardless of relationship to study drug, is shown in Table 2.

Table 2: AmBisome

Empirical Therapy Study 94-0-002 Common (≥10% incidence) Adverse Events

Adverse Event by Body System	AmBisome n=343 %	Amphotericin B n=344 %
Body as a Whole		
Abdominal Pain	19.8	21.8
Asthenia	13.1	10.8
Back Pain	12.0	7.3
Blood Product Transfusion Reaction	18.4	18.6
Chills	47.5	75.9
Fever	89.5	91.0
Infection	11.1	9.3
Pain	14.0	12.8
Procedural Complication	19.8	19.8
Sepsis	14.0	11.3
Cardiovascular System		
Chest Pain	12.0	11.6
Hypertension	7.9	16.3
Hypotension	14.3	21.5

(cont'd)

Table 2: AmBisome *(cont'd)*

Empirical Therapy Study 94-0-002 Common (≥10% incidence) Adverse Events

Adverse Event by Body System	AmBisome n=343 %	Amphotericin B n=344 %
Tachycardia	13.4	20.9
Digestive System		
Diarrhea	30.3	27.3
Gastrointestinal Hemorrhage	9.9	11.3
Nausea	39.7	38.7
Vomiting	31.8	43.9
Metabolic and Nutritional Disorders		
Alkaline Phosphatase Increased	22.2	19.2
ALT Increased	14.6	14.0
AST Increased	12.8	12.8
Bilirubinemia	18.1	19.2
BUN Increased	21.0	31.1
Creatinine Increased	22.4	42.2
Edema	14.3	14.8
Hyperglycemia	23.0	27.9
Hypernatremia	4.1	11.0
Hypervolemia	12.2	15.4
Hypocalcemia	18.4	20.9
Hypokalemia	42.9	50.6
Hypomagnesemia	20.4	25.6
Peripheral Edema	14.6	17.2
Nervous System		
Anxiety	13.7	11.0
Confusion	11.4	13.4
Headache	19.8	20.9
Insomnia	17.2	14.2
Respiratory System		
Cough Increased	17.8	21.8
Dyspnea	23.0	29.1
Epistaxis	14.9	20.1
Hypoxia	7.6	14.8
Lung Disorder	17.8	17.4
Pleural Effusion	12.5	9.6
Rhinitis	11.1	11.0
Skin and Appendages		
Pruritus	10.8	10.2
Rash	24.8	24.4
Sweating	7.0	10.8
Urogenital System		
Hematuria	14	14

Liposomal amphotericin B was well tolerated. Liposomal amphotericin B had a lower incidence of chills, hypotension, hypertension, tachycardia, hypoxia, hypokalemia, and various events related to decreased kidney function as compared to amphotericin B desoxycholate.

In pediatric patients (16 years of age or less) in this double-blind study, liposomal amphotericin B compared to amphotericin B desoxycholate had a lower incidence of hypokalemia (37% vs 55%), chills (29% vs 68%), vomiting (27% vs 55%), and hypertension (10% vs 21%). Similar trends, although with a somewhat lower incidence, were observed in open-label, randomized Study 104-14 involving 205 febrile neutropenic pediatric patients (141 treated with liposomal amphotericin B and 64 treated with amphotericin B desoxycholate). Pediatric patients appear to have more tolerance than older individuals for the nephrotoxic effects of amphotericin B desoxycholate.

The following adverse events are based on the experience of 244 patients (202 adult and 42 pediatric patients) of whom 85 patients were treated with liposomal amphotericin B 3 mg/kg, 81 patients were treated with liposomal amphotericin B 5 mg/kg and 78 patients treated with amphotericin B lipid complex 5 mg/kg in Study 97-0-034, a randomized, double-blind, multicentre study in febrile, neutropenic patients. Liposomal amphotericin B and amphotericin B lipid complex were infused over 2 hours.

Patients administered liposomal amphotericin B (3 mg/kg/day and/or 5 mg/kg/day) had a statistically lower incidence of chills, hypertension, hypotension, tachycardia, increased creatinine, hypoxia, hyperventilation and asthma than those administered amphotericin B lipid complex. These adverse events were 2.5 to 13 times more frequent for patients in the amphotericin B lipid complex group compared with those administered liposomal amphotericin B. However, confusion was more common (nearly 4 times more frequent) with 3 mg/kg/day liposomal amphotericin B than with amphotericin B lipid complex.

The incidence of adverse events with statistically significant differences between liposomal amphotericin B (3 mg/kg and/or 5 mg/kg) and amphotericin B lipid complex treatment groups regardless of relationship to study drug are summarized in Table 3.

Table 3: AmBisome

Empirical Therapy Study 97-0-034

	Incidence and p-value[a] (Fisher's Exact Test)		
	AmBisome 3 mg/kg	**AmBisome 5 mg/kg**	**Amphotericin B lipid complex**
Total number of patients	85	81	78
Chills/Rigors	40.0% p<0.001	48.1% p<0.001	89.7%
Hypertension	10.6% p=0.037	19.8% p=0.700	23.1%
Hypotension	10.6% p=0.129	7.4% p=0.035	19.2%
Tachycardia	9.4% p=0.020	18.5% p=0.559	23.1%
Creatinine Increased	20.0% p<0.001	18.5% p<0.001	48.7%
Confusion	12.9% p=0.050	8.6% p=0.329	3.8%
Hypoxia	7.1% p=0.020	6.2% p=0.009	20.5%
Hyperventilation	3.5% p=0.197	1.2% p=0.032	9.0%
Asthma	0 p=0.050	1.2% p=0.204	5.1%

[a] p-values vs amphotericin B lipid complex.

In a double-blind, placebo-controlled study of patients undergoing bone marrow transplantation or chemotherapy, there were no significant differences between liposomal amphotericin B and placebo in the incidence of adverse events.

Study 94-0-013, was a randomized, double-blind, multicentre comparative trial of 2 doses of liposomal amphotericin B versus amphotericin B, for a target 14 day induction period. Treatment was followed by fluconazole as consolidation therapy to complete a total of 10 weeks of therapy for the treatment of acute cryptococcal meningitis in AIDS patients. The following adverse events are based on the experience of 267 patients (266 adult and 1 pediatric patient) of whom 86 patients were treated with liposomal amphotericin B 3 mg/kg/day, 94 patients were treated with liposomal amphotericin B 6 mg/kg/day and 87 patients were treated with amphotericin B desoxycholate 0.7 mg/kg/day. Liposomal amphotericin B and amphotericin B were infused over 2 to 4 hours.

The incidence of adverse events occurring in more than 10% of subjects in 1 or more treatment arms is provided in Table 4.

Table 4: AmBisome

Incidence of Common (≥10% incidence) Non-infusion-Related Adverse Events (Weeks 1-4) Study 94-0-013

Adverse Event by Body System	AmBisome 3 mg/kg n=86 %	AmBisome 6 mg/kg n=94 %	Ampho B 0.7 mg/kg n=87 %
Body as a Whole			
Abdominal Pain	7.0	7.4	10.3
Infection	12.8	11.7	6.9
Procedural Complication	8.1	9.6	10.3
Cardiovascular System			
Phlebitis	9.3	10.6	25.3
Digestive System			
Anorexia	14.0	9.6	11.5
Constipation	15.1	14.9	20.7
Diarrhea	10.5	16.0	10.3
Nausea	16.3	21.3	25.3
Vomiting	10.5	21.3	20.7
Hemic and Lymphatic System			
Anemia	26.7	47.9	43.7
Leukopenia	15.1	17.0	17.2
Thrombocytopenia	5.8	12.8	6.9
Metabolic and Nutritional Disorders			
Bilirubinemia	0	8.5	12.6

(cont'd)

Table 4: AmBisome *(cont'd)*

Incidence of Common (≥10% incidence) Non-infusion-Related Adverse Events (Weeks 1-4) Study 94-0-013

Adverse Event by Body System	AmBisome 3 mg/kg n=86 %	AmBisome 6 mg/kg n=94 %	Ampho B 0.7 mg/kg n=87 %
BUN Increased	9.3	7.4	10.3
Creatinine Increased	18.6	39.4	43.7
Hyperglycemia	9.3	12.8	17.2
Hypocalcemia	12.8	17.0	13.8
Hypokalemia	31.4	51.1	48.3
Hypomagnesemia	29.1	48.9	40.2
Hyponatremia	11.6	8.5	9.2
Liver Function Tests Abnormal	12.8	4.3	9.2
Nervous System			
Dizziness	7.0	8.5	10.3
Insomnia	22.1	17.0	20.7
Respiratory			
Cough Increased	8.1	2.1	10.3
Skin and Appendages			
Rash	4.7	11.7	4.6

Among non-infusion-related adverse events, overall cardiovascular adverse events and phlebitis were lower in both liposomal amphotericin B groups as shown in Table 5.

Table 5: AmBisome

Cardiovascular Adverse Events Study 94-0-013

	AmBisome 3 mg/kg	AmBisome 6 mg/kg	Amphotericin B
Total number of patients receiving at least 1 dose of study drug	86	94	87
Cardiovascular system any adverse event	23 (27%)	27 (29%)	39 (45%)
Phlebitis	8 (9%)	10 (11%)	22 (25%)

The following adverse events occurred at a significantly higher rate with the 6 mg/kg/day liposomal amphotericin B dose compared to the 3 mg/kg/day liposomal amphotericin B dose: overall incidence of hemic and lymphatic system adverse events, anemia, hypokalemia, hypomagnesemia, creatinine increased and bilirubinemia.

Infusion Related Reactions: In Study 94-0-002, the large, double-blind study of pediatric and adult febrile neutropenic patients, no premedication to prevent infusion related reaction was administered prior to the first dose of study drug (Day 1). Liposomal amphotericin B-treated patients had a lower incidence of infusion related fever (17% vs 44%), chills/rigors (18% vs 54%) and vomiting (6% vs 8%) on Day 1 as compared to amphotericin B desoxycholate-treated patients.

The incidence of infusion-related reactions on Day 1 in pediatric and adult patients is summarized in Table 6.

Table 6: AmBisome

Incidence of Day 1 Infusion-Related Reactions (IRR) By Patient Age

	Pediatric Patients (≤16 years of age)		Adult Patients (>16 years of age)	
	AmBisome	Amphotericin B	AmBisome	Amphotericin B
Total number of patients receiving at least 1 dose of study drug	48	47	295	297
Patients with fever[a] increase ≥1°C	6 (13%)	22 (47%)	52 (18%)	128 (43%)
Patients with chills/rigors	4 (8%)	22 (47%)	59 (20%)	165 (56%)
Patients with nausea	4 (8%)	4 (9%)	38 (13%)	31 (10%)
Patients with vomiting	2 (4%)	7 (15%)	19 (6%)	21 (7%)
Patients with other reactions	10 (21%)	13 (28%)	47 (16%)	69 (23%)

[a] Day 1 body temperature increased above the temperature taken within 1 hour prior to infusion (preinfusion temperature) or above the lowest infusion value (no preinfusion temperature recorded).

Cardiorespiratory events, except for vasodilatation (flushing), during all study drug infusions were more frequent in amphotericin B-treated patients as summarized in Table 7.

The percentage of patients who received drugs either for the treatment or prevention of infusion related reactions (e.g., acetaminophen, diphenhydramine, meperidine and hydrocortisone) was lower in liposomal amphotericin B-treated patients compared with amphotericin B desoxycholate-treated patients.

In the empirical therapy study 97-0-034, on Day 1, where no premedication was administered, the overall incidence of infusion related events of chills/rigors was significantly lower for patients administered liposomal amphotericin B compared with amphotericin B lipid complex. In addition, a lower incidence of chills/rigors on Day 1 was evident regardless of age, sex, receipt of bone marrow transplant or transplant type, or the use of immunosuppressants. Fever, chills/rigors and hypoxia were significantly lower for each liposomal amphotericin B group compared with the amphotericin B lipid complex group. The infusion-related event hypoxia was reported for 11.5% of amphotericin B lipid complex-treated patients compared with 0% of patients administered 3 mg/kg/day liposomal amphotericin B and 1.2% of patients treated with 5 mg/kg/day liposomal amphotericin B. See Table 8.

Table 7: AmBisome

Incidence of Infusion-Related Cardiorespiratory Events

Event	AmBisome n=343	Amphotericin B n=344
Hypotension	12 (3.5%)	28 (8.1%)
Tachycardia	8 (2.3%)	43 (12.5%)
Hypertension	8 (2.3%)	39 (11.3%)
Vasodilatation	18 (5.2%)	2 (0.6%)
Dyspnea	16 (4.7%)	25 (7.3%)
Hyperventilation	4 (1.2%)	17 (4.9%)
Hypoxia	1 (0.3%)	22 (6.4%)

Table 8: AmBisome

Incidence of Day 1 Infusion-Related Reactions (IRR) Chills/Rigors Empirical Therapy Study 97-0-034

	AmBisome 3 mg/kg/day	AmBisome 5 mg/kg/day	AmBisome Both	Amphotericin B lipid complex 5 mg/kg/day
Total number of patients	85	81	166	78
Patients with chills/rigors	16 (18.8%)	19 (23.5%)	35 (21.1%)	62 (79.5%)
Total number with IRR	44 (51.8%)	39 (48.1%)	83 (50.0%)	69 (88.5%)
Patients with fever[a] ≥1°C increase in temperature	20 (23.5%)	16 (19.8%)	36 (21.7%)	45 (57.7%)
Patients with nausea	9 (10.6%)	7 (8.6%)	16 (9.6%)	9 (11.5%)
Patients with vomiting	5 (5.9%)	5 (6.2%)	10 (6.0%)	11 (14.1%)
Patients with other significant reactions	16 (18.8%)	21 (25.9%)	37 (22.3%)	32 (41.0%)
Hypertension	4 (4.7%)	7 (8.6%)	11 (6.6%)	12 (15.4%)
Tachycardia	2 (2.4%)	8 (9.9%)	10 (6.0%)	14 (17.9%)
Dyspnea	4 (4.7%)	8 (9.9%)	12 (7.2%)	8 (10.3%)
Hypoxia	0	1 (1.2%)	1 (<1%)	9 (11.5%)

[a] Day 1 body temperature increased above the temperature taken within 1 hour prior to infusion (preinfusion temperature) or above the lowest infusion value (no preinfusion temperature recorded). Patients were not administered premedications to prevent infusion related reactions prior to the Day 1 study drug infusion.

In Study 94-0-013, a randomized, double-blind, multicentre trial comparing liposomal amphotericin B and amphotericin B desoxycholate as initial therapy for cryptococcal meningitis, in 266 adult and 1 pediatric HIV positive patients, premedications to prevent infusion related reactions were permitted. The proportion of patients in the amphotericin B group who required medication for the treatment of infusion related reactions was >2X that in the liposomal amphotericin B group. Liposomal amphotericin B-treated patients again had a lower incidence of fever, chills/rigors and respiratory adverse events as summarized in Table 9.

Table 9: AmBisome

Incidence of Infusion-Related Reactions Study 94-0-013

	AmBisome 3 mg/kg	AmBisome 6 mg/kg	Amphotericin B
Total number of patients receiving at least 1 dose of study drug	86	94	87
Patients with fever increase of >1°C	6 (7%)	8 (9%)	24 (28%)
Patients with chills/rigors	5 (6%)	8 (9%)	42 (48%)
Patients with nausea	11 (13%)	13 (14%)	18 (20%)
Patients with vomiting	14 (16%)	13 (14%)	16 (18%)
Respiratory adverse events	0	1 (1%)	8 (9%)

There have been a few reports of flushing, back pain with or without chest tightness, and chest pain associated with liposomal amphotericin B administration; on occasion this has been severe. Where these symptoms were noted, the reaction developed within a few minutes after the start of infusion and disappeared rapidly when the infusion was stopped. The symptoms do not occur with every dose and usually do not recur on subsequent administrations when the infusion rate is slowed.

Toxicity and Discontinuation of Dosing: In Study 94-0-002, a significantly lower incidence of grade 3 or 4 toxicity was observed in the liposomal amphotericin B group compared with the amphotericin B group. In addition, nearly 3 times as many patients administered amphotericin B required a reduction in dose due to toxicity or discontinuation of study drug due to an infusion related reaction compared with those administered liposomal amphotericin B.

In empirical therapy study 97-0-034, a significantly higher percentage of patients in the amphotericin B lipid complex group discontinued the study drug due to an adverse event than in the liposomal amphotericin B groups (32% vs 13%, respectively). The incidence of discontinuations due to increased creatinine was significantly higher in the amphotericin B lipid complex group than in the liposomal amphotericin B 5 mg/kg/day group (10% vs 1%, respectively) or the liposomal amphotericin B 3 mg/kg/day group (10% vs 2%, respectively). In addition, the incidence of discontinuation was significantly higher in the amphotericin B lipid complex group than in the liposomal amphotericin B 3 mg/kg/day group due to fever (6% vs 0%, respectively) and in the liposomal amphotericin B 5 mg/kg/day group due to hypoxia (8% vs 0%, respectively).

Less Common Adverse Events: The following adverse events also have been reported in 2% to 10% of liposomal amphotericin B-treated patients receiving chemotherapy or bone marrow transplantation or had HIV disease in 6 comparative, clinical trials:

Body as a Whole: abdomen enlarged, allergic reaction, cellulitis, cell mediated immunological reaction, face edema, graft versus host disease, malaise, neck pain, and procedural complication.

Cardiovascular System: arrhythmia, atrial fibrillation, bradycardia, cardiac arrest, cardiomegaly, hemorrhage, postural hypotension, valvular heart disease, vascular disorder, and vasodilatation (flushing).

Digestive System: anorexia, constipation, dry mouth/nose, dyspepsia, dysphagia, eructation, fecal incontinence, flatulence, hemorrhoids, gum/oral hemorrhage, hematemesis, hepatocellular damage, hepatomegaly, ileus, liver function test abnormal, mucositis, rectal disorder, stomatitis, ulcerative stomatitis, and veno-occlusive liver disease.

Hemic and Lymphatic Systems: anemia, coagulation disorder, ecchymosis, fluid overload, petechia, prothrombin decreased, prothrombin increased, and thrombocytopenia.

Metabolic and Nutritional Disorders: acidosis, amylase increased, hyperchloremia, hyperkalemia, hypermagnesemia, hyperphosphatemia, hyponatremia, hypophosphatemia, hypoproteinemia, lactate dehydrogenase increased, nonprotein nitrogen (NPN) increased, and respiratory alkalosis.

Musculoskeletal System: arthralgia, bone pain, dystonia, myalgia, and rigors.

Nervous System: agitation, coma, convulsion, depression, dysesthesia, dizziness, hallucinations, nervousness, paresthesia, somnolence, thinking abnormality, and tremor.

Respiratory System: asthma, atelectasis, hemoptysis, hiccup, hyperventilation, influenza-like symptoms, lung edema, pharyngitis, pneumonia, respiratory insufficiency, respiratory failure, and sinusitis.

Skin and Appendages: alopecia, dry skin, Herpes simplex, injection site reactions involving pain and inflammation, maculopapular rash, purpura, skin discoloration, skin disorder, skin ulcer, urticaria, and vesiculobullous rash.

Special Senses: conjunctivitis, dry eyes, and eye hemorrhage.

Urogenital System: abnormal renal function, acute kidney failure, acute renal failure, dysuria, kidney failure, toxic nephropathy, urinary incontinence, and vaginal hemorrhage.

The following adverse experiences have been reported infrequently in postmarketing surveillance, in addition to those mentioned above: agranulocytosis, anaphylactic reaction, angioedema, bronchospasm/wheezing, cholestasis, cyanosis/hypoventilation, erythema, epilepsy, fever, generalized edema, headache, hemorrhagic cystitis, hyperbilirubinemia, hypocalcemia, jaundice, increased liver enzymes, leukopenia, multiorgan failure, myocardial infarction, pelvic bleeding, pulmonary edema, renal impairment, retrosternal pain, stomach pain, sweating, swelling (face, lips, eyes), tachycardia, urea increase, urticaria.

Clinical Laboratory Values: The effect of liposomal amphotericin B on renal and hepatic function and on serum electrolytes was assessed from laboratory values measured repeatedly in randomized clinical trials. The laboratory data from the controlled clinical trials previously discussed were used in this analysis. Nephrotoxicity was defined as creatinine values increasing 100% or more over pretreatment levels in pediatric patients and creatinine values increasing 100% or more over pretreatment levels in adult patients provided the peak creatinine concentration was >1.2 mg/dL. Hypokalemia was defined as potassium levels ≤2.5 mmol/L any time during treatment.

The incidence of hepatotoxicity appeared similar in the liposomal amphotericin B and amphotericin B treatment groups. Hepatotoxicity was defined as significant changes from baseline in serum concentrations of AST or ALT. Significant changes were an increase to a value >5× baseline in cases where baseline is <2× the upper limit of normal, an increase to a value >3× baseline in cases where baseline is 2 to 5× the upper limit of normal, and an increase to a value >2× baseline in cases where baseline is >5× the upper limit of normal.

In study 94-0-002 for liposomal amphotericin B, 18.7% of patients had nephrotoxicity compared with 33.7% for patients treated with conventional amphotericin B. For hypokalemia, 6.7% of liposomal amphotericin B-treated patients had decreased serum potassium levels compared with 11.6% of patients who received the traditional amphotericin B formulation. For the empirical study 97-0-034, the incidence of nephrotoxicity by all measures was significantly lower, at 14.5%, for patients administered liposomal amphotericin B compared with 42.5% in patients administered amphotericin B lipid complex.

The incidence of nephrotoxicity in the comparative trial for cryptococcal meningitis, Study 94-0-013, was lower in the combined liposomal amphotericin B group (3 and 6 mg/kg/day), at 17.8%, compared to those treated with amphotericin B (0.7 mg/kg/day), for which 33.3% of the patients experienced nephrotoxicity.

OVERDOSE:

The toxicity of liposomal amphotericin B due to overdose has not been defined. A maximum tolerated dose was not observed with repeated daily doses up to 10 mg/kg in pediatric patients and 15 mg/kg in adult patients.

Treatment: If an overdose is suspected, discontinue therapy, monitor the patient's clinical status and administer supportive therapy as required. Particular attention should be given to monitoring renal function.

For management of a suspected drug overdose, CPhA recommends that you contact your **regional Poison Control Centre**. See the *CPS* Directory section for a list of Poison Control Centres.

DOSAGE: Liposomal amphotericin B should be administered by i.v. infusion over a period of approximately 120 minutes. Infusion time may be reduced to approximately 60 minutes in patients in whom the treatment is well-tolerated. If the patient experiences discomfort during infusion, the duration of infusion may be increased. The recommended concentration for i.v. infusion is 0.5 to 2 mg/mL of liposomal amphotericin B.

The daily dose and duration of therapy of liposomal amphotericin B should be based on the infecting organism, the patient's condition and the response to therapy. Treatment should be continued until clinical parameters and laboratory tests indicate that an active fungal infection has been cured or subsided. An inadequate period of treatment may lead to recurrence of active infection. Dose, rate of infusion and duration of treatment may have to be individualized for the needs of specific patients. The recommended initial dosage of liposomal amphotericin B for each indication for adult, pediatric and special population groups is outlined below.

Systemic Mycoses: Patients with a proven systemic infection with Aspergillus, Candida and/or Cryptococcus species who are refractory to or intolerant to conventional amphotericin B therapy or are renally impaired usually have therapy instituted at 3 mg/kg/day which is increased up to 5 mg/kg/day, as required.

Cryptococcal Meningitis in HIV-infected Patients: HIV-infected patients with cryptococcal meningitis were treated with a dose of 3 mg/kg/day or 6 mg/kg/day for an average of 14 days. Due to an increased incidence of adverse events with the 6 mg/kg/day dose, it is recommended patients be started with a dose of 3 mg/kg/day and increase to 6 mg/kg/day as required. Because of the high frequency of relapses, chronic suppressive therapy with another agent may be necessary after completion of a treatment course with liposomal amphotericin B.

Empirical Treatment: For empirical therapy liposomal amphotericin B was administered at an initial dose of 3 mg/kg/day, and increased or decreased as needed (dose range of 1.5 to 6 mg/kg/day) for 1 to 53 days at a cumulative dose of 33.4±30.8 mg/kg.

Maximum Dose: In maximum tolerated dose studies in patients with empirical or proven fungal infections, treatment has been administered an average of 9 to 29 days in adults at doses of 7.5 to 15 mg/kg/day and 8 to 15 days in children at 2.5 to 10 mg/kg/day without any dose-limiting toxicity detected.

Special Patient Groups: Renal Impairment: The effect of renal impairment on the disposition of liposomal amphotericin B has not been studied. Liposomal amphotericin B has been successfully administered to patients with pre-existing renal impairment. For renal dialysis patients, liposomal amphotericin B administration should be initiated after dialysis is completed.

Hepatic Impairment: The effect of hepatic impairment on the disposition of liposomal amphotericin B is unknown.

Stability and Storage: Unopened vials of lyophilized material are to be stored between temperatures of 2 to 25°C.

Reconstituted Product Concentrate: The reconstituted product concentrate may be stored for up to 24 hours at 2 to 8°C following reconstitution with Sterile Water for Injection USP. Do not freeze.

Reconstituted Product Diluted With 5% Dextrose: Do not freeze. Injection of liposomal amphotericin B should commence within 6 hours of dilution with 5% Dextrose.

Caution: Discard partially used vials.

Directions for Reconstitution and Dilution: **Read this entire section carefully before beginning reconstitution.**

Liposomal amphotericin B must be reconstituted using Sterile Water for Injection USP (without a bacteriostatic agent). Vials of liposomal amphotericin B containing 50 mg of amphotericin B are prepared as follows:

Reconstitution: 1) Aseptically add 12 mL of Sterile Water for Injection USP to each vial to yield a preparation containing 4 mg of amphotericin B/mL (50 mg/12.9 mL).

Caution: Do not reconstitute with saline or add saline to the reconstituted concentration, or mix with other drugs.

The use of any solution other than those recommended, or the presence of a bacteriostatic agent (e.g., benzyl alcohol) in the solution, may cause precipitation of liposomal amphotericin B.

2) **Shake the vials vigorously** for 30 seconds to completely disperse the liposomal amphotericin B. Liposomal amphotericin B forms a yellow, translucent suspension.

Dilution: 3) Calculate the amount of reconstituted (4 mg/mL) liposomal amphotericin B to be further diluted. Liposomal amphotericin B must be diluted with 5% dextrose injection to a final concentration between 0.5 and 2 mg/mL prior to administration.

Filtration: 4) Withdraw this amount of reconstituted liposomal amphotericin B into a sterile syringe.

5) Attach the 5-micron filter, provided, to the syringe. Inject the syringe contents through the filter, into the appropriate amount of 5% dextrose injection. (Use only one filter per vial of liposomal amphotericin B).

As with all parenteral drug products, the reconstituted liposomal amphotericin B should be inspected visually for particulate matter and discoloration prior to administration, whenever solution and container permit. Do not use material if there is any evidence of precipitation or foreign matter. Aseptic technique must be strictly observed in all handling since no preservative or bacteriostatic agent is present in AmBisome or in the materials specified for reconstitution and dilution.

An in-line membrane filter may be used for i.v. infusion of liposomal amphotericin B. However, **the mean pore diameter of the filter should not be less than 1 micron.**

Note: An existing i.v. line must be flushed with 5% Dextrose Injection prior to infusion of liposomal amphotericin B. If this is not feasible, liposomal amphotericin B should be administered through a separate line.

SUPPLIED: Each vial of sterile, nonpyrogenic lyophilized powder for i.v. infusion contains amphotericin B, USP 50 mg, intercalated into a liposomal membrane consisting of hydrogenated soy phosphatidylcholine, cholesterol, distearoylphosphtidylglycerol, α-tocopherol, together with sucrose, and disodium succinate hexahydrate (as buffer). Following reconstitution with Sterile Water for Injection, the resulting pH of the suspension is 5.0 to 6.0. Single unit vials, packs of 10 in individual cartons. Each carton contains 1 prepackaged, disposable sterile 5 micron filter. Unopened vials of lyophilized material are to be stored between temperatures of 2 to 25°C.

Amcinonide Ⓟ

CPhA Monograph

see *Corticosteroids: Topical*

Amerge® Ⓟ

naratriptan HCl

5-HT1 Receptor Agonist—Migraine Therapy

GlaxoSmithKline

Date of Revision: October 24, 2007

PHARMACOLOGY: Naratriptan has been demonstrated to be a selective agonist for a vascular 5-hydroxytryptamine$_1$ receptor subtype (probably a member of the 5-$HT_{1B/1D}$ family) with little or no binding affinity for 5-$HT_{2/3}$ receptor subtypes; alpha$_1$-, alpha$_2$-, or beta-adrenergic; dopamine$_1$; dopamine$_2$; muscarinic; or benzodiazepine receptors. Naratriptan did not exhibit agonist or antagonist activity in ex vivo assays of 5-HT_4 and 5-HT_7 receptor-mediated activities.

The therapeutic activity of naratriptan in migraine is generally attributed to its agonist activity at 5-HT_{1B}/5-HT_{1D} receptors. Two current theories have been proposed to explain the efficacy of 5-HT_1 receptor agonists in migraine. One theory suggests that activation of 5-HT_1 receptors located on intracranial blood vessels, including those on the arteriovenous anastomoses, leads to vasoconstriction, which is believed to be correlated with the relief of migraine headache. The other hypothesis suggests that activation of 5-HT_1 receptors on perivascular fibers of the trigeminal system results in the inhibition of pro-inflammatory neuropeptide release. These theories are not mutually exclusive.

Pharmacokinetics: Absorption: Naratriptan is well absorbed, with 74% oral bioavailability in females and 63% in males. After oral administration, the absorption is rapid and peak concentrations are obtained in 2 to 5 hours. A 2-period crossover study was performed in 15 female migraine patients who received naratriptan as a single 2.5 mg tablet during a migraine attack, followed 3 to 7 days later by another 2.5 mg treatment during a non-migraine period. During a migraine attack, absorption is slower, although exposure (AUC) and elimination half-life are not significantly affected. See Table 1.

Plasma levels of naratriptan increase in a dose-proportional manner consistent with linear pharmacokinetics over a 1 to 10 mg dose range. The absorption and elimination are independent of the dose. Administration with food does not appreciably influence the pharmacokinetics of naratriptan. Repeat administration (up to 10 mg once daily for 5 days) does not result in drug accumulation.

Table 1: Amerge

Pharmacokinetic Parameters in Female Migraine Patients After Receiving 2.5 mg Amerge Tablets[a]

Parameter	Migraine Attack (N=15)	Non-Migraine Period (N=15)
C_{max} (ng/mL)	7.66 (3.07)	9.50 (3.63)
t_{max} (h)	3.8 (2.1)	2.0 (1.0)
AUC (ng/mL·h)	86.7 (32.5)	92.0 (33.7)
Cl/F (mL/min)	467.5 (126.4)	520.7 (222.6)
$t_{1/2}$ (h)	6.75 (1.44)	7.02 (2.39)

[a] Values quoted are arithmetic mean (standard deviation).

Legend:

C_{max}=maximum concentrations.

Cl/F=apparent clearance.

AUC=area under the curve of concentration vs time extrapolated to infinity.

t_{max}=time to maximum concentration.

$t_{1/2}$=elimination half-life.

Metabolism and Distribution: In vitro, naratriptan is metabolized by a wide range of cytochrome P_{450} isoenzymes into a number of inactive metabolites. Naratriptan is a poor inhibitor of cytochrome P_{450} isoenzymes, and does not inhibit monoamine oxidase (MAO) enzymes; metabolic interactions between naratriptan and drugs metabolized by P_{450} or MAO are, therefore, unlikely. According to a population pharmacokinetic estimate, naratriptan is distributed into a volume of approximately 261 L.

Protein Binding: Plasma protein binding is low (29%).

Elimination: The elimination half-life generally ranges from 5 to 8 hours. Oral clearance is 509 mL/min in females and 770 mL/min in males. The renal clearance (220 mL/min) exceeds the glomerular filtration rate, suggesting that the drug undergoes active tubular secretion. Naratriptan is predominantly eliminated in urine, with 50% of the dose recovered unchanged and 30% as metabolites.

Special Populations: Age Effects: A study was performed to compare the pharmacokinetics of naratriptan in young (6 female/6 male, 24 to 44 years) and elderly (6 female/6 male, 65 to 77 years) subjects. The subjects received 2 doses each of placebo, 1 mg naratriptan, and 2.5 mg naratriptan separated by 4-hour intervals. A minimum 96-hour period intervened between consecutive treatment days.

Elderly subjects experienced a higher degree of exposure to naratriptan than did younger subjects. Mean C_{max} and area under the plasma concentration time curve values were 28% and 38% higher, respectively, for the 1 mg treatment group and 15% and 32% higher, respectively, for the 2.5 mg group. Total and renal clearance were decreased by about 30%, while the elimination half-life was increased by about 1 hour.

Elevations in systolic blood pressure at the 2.5 mg dose were more pronounced in the elderly subjects than in the young subjects (mean peak increases of 12 mmHg in elderly versus 2 mmHg in young subjects).

Renal Impairment: Renal excretion is the major route for elimination of naratriptan. A study to compare male and female subjects with mild to moderate renal impairment (n=15, 31 to 58 years; screening creatinine clearance: median 41.2 mL/min, range 18 to 115 mL/min) to gender-matched healthy subjects (n=8, 21 to 47 years) showed a decrease in oral clearance (mean decreased by 50%), resulting in a longer mean half-life (approximately 11 hours, range 7 to 20 hours) and an increase in the mean C_{max} (approximately 40%). In this study, blood pressure measurements suggested that increased exposure in renally-impaired subjects may be associated with increases in blood pressure which are larger than those seen in healthy subjects receiving the same dose (5 mg) (see Dosage).

Hepatic Impairment: Liver metabolism plays a limited role in the clearance of naratriptan. The pharmacokinetics of a single 2.5 mg dose of naratriptan were determined in subjects with moderate hepatic impairment (Child-Pugh grade A or B, n=8) and gender- and age-matched healthy subjects (n=8). Subjects with hepatic impairment showed a moderate decrease in clearance (approximately 30%) resulting in increases of approximately 40% in the half-life (range 8 to 16 hours) and the area under the plasma concentration time curve (see Dosage).

Clinical Studies: Therapeutic Clinical Trials: Four double-blind, placebo-controlled, dose-ranging clinical trials evaluated the safety and efficacy of naratriptan at oral doses ranging from 0.1 to 10 mg in a total of 3160 adult patients with migraine attacks characterized by moderate or severe pain. The minimal effective dose was 1.0 mg. In 3 of the 4 clinical trials, a higher overall rate of headache relief was achieved with a 2.5 mg dose. Single doses of 5 mg and higher are not recommended, due to an increased incidence of adverse events. Onset of significant headache relief (defined as no or mild pain) became apparent at 60 to 120 minutes after these doses. Naratriptan also relieved the nausea, phonophobia, and photophobia associated with migraine attacks.

Table 2 shows the 4-hour efficacy results obtained for the recommended doses of naratriptan in 2 of the 4 dose-ranging efficacy studies. In study 1, patients were randomised to receive placebo or a particular dose of naratriptan for the treatment of a single migraine attack according to a parallel group design, whereas, in study 2, patients were randomised to receive each of the treatments for separate migraine attacks according to a crossover design. In both studies, patients who achieved headache relief at 240 minutes post-dose, but experienced a worsening of severity between 4 and 24 hours post-dosing were permitted to take a second dose of double-blind medication identical to the first.

Table 2: Amerge

Results at 240 Minutes Post First Dose

Parameter	Study 1			Study 2		
	Placebo (n=107) %	Amerge 1 mg (n=219) %	Amerge 2.5 mg (n=209) %	Placebo (n=602) %	Amerge 1 mg (n=595) %	Amerge 2.5 mg (n=586) %
Pain Relief (0/1)[a]	27	52[e]	66[e,f]	33	57[e]	68[e,f]
Pain Free (0)[b]	10	26[e]	43[e,f]	15	33[e]	45[e]
Nausea Free	56	71[g]	77[g]	54	69[e]	75[e]
Photophobia Free	34	57[g]	67[g]	33	53[e]	61[e]
Phonophobia Free	[d]	[d]	[d]	36	55[e]	65[e]
Clinical Disability[c] (0/1)	49	62[g]	72[g]	50	70[e]	76[e]

[a] Pain relief is defined as a reduction in headache severity from grade 3 or 2 (severe or moderate) to grade 1 or 0 (mild or no pain).
[b] Pain free is defined as a headache severity score of 0 (no pain).
[c] Clinical disability is measured on a 4-point scale (0=able to function normally, 1=ability mildly impaired, 2=ability severely impaired, 3=bed rest required).
[d] Photophobia and phonophobia collected as one measure.
[e] p<0.01 vs placebo.
[f] p<0.01 vs Amerge 1 mg. Note comparisons were not performed for any parameter other than pain relief and pain free in study 1 and for pain relief in study 2.
[g] Statistical comparisons not performed.

Significant headache relief was sustained over 24 hours. Data from four placebo controlled studies (n=3160) showed that of the patients who achieved headache relief with naratriptan 2.5 mg, 72% to 83% did not experience recurrence of headache between 4 and 24 hours post-dosing.

Subgroup analyses of the overall population of patients participating in the placebo-controlled trials indicate that the efficacy of naratriptan was unaffected by migraine type (with/without aura), gender, oral contraceptive use, or concomitant use of common migraine prophylactic drugs (e.g., beta-blockers, calcium channel blockers, tricyclic antidepressants).

In a long-term, repeat dose, open study of 417 patients (all were initiated on a 2.5 mg dose of naratriptan but were given the option to titrate down to a 1 mg dose if 2.5 mg was not well tolerated) a total of 15 301 attacks were treated (mean number of treated attacks/patient=36 for the 2.5 mg dose and 8 for the 1 mg dose) over a period of up to 12 months. Headache response was sustained (as judged by the proportion of attacks treated with naratriptan resulting in headache relief). The median percentage of attacks per patient requiring a second dose for headache recurrence was 8%. Of the 417 patients treating attacks, 10 patients opted for a dosage reduction.

INDICATIONS: For the acute treatment of migraine attacks with or without aura.

Naratriptan is not intended for the prophylactic therapy of migraine or for use in the management of hemiplegic, basilar, or ophthalmoplegic migraine (see Contraindications). Safety and efficacy have not been established for cluster headache, which is present in an older, predominantly male population.

CONTRAINDICATIONS: Naratriptan is contraindicated in patients with history, symptoms, or signs of ischemic cardiac, cerebrovascular or peripheral vascular syndromes, valvular heart disease or cardiac arrhythmias (especially tachycardias). In addition, patients with other significant underlying cardiovascular diseases (e.g., atherosclerotic disease, congenital heart disease) should not receive naratriptan. Ischemic cardiac syndromes include, but are not limited to, angina pectoris of any type (e.g., stable angina of effort and vasospastic forms of angina such as the Prinzmetal's variant), all forms of myocardial infarction, and silent myocardial ischemia. Cerebrovascular syndromes include, but are not limited to, strokes of any type as well as transient ischemic attacks (TIAs). Peripheral vascular disease includes, but is not limited to, ischemic bowel disease, or Raynaud's syndrome (see Warnings).

Because naratriptan can give rise to increases in blood pressure, it is contraindicated in patients with uncontrolled or severe hypertension (see Warnings).

Ergot-containing drugs have been reported to cause prolonged vasospastic reactions. Because naratriptan may also cause coronary vasospasm and these effects may be additive, the use of naratriptan within 24 hours before or after treatment with other 5-HT$_1$ receptor agonists, or ergotamine-containing drugs or their derivatives (e.g., dihydroergotamine, methysergide) is contraindicated.

Naratriptan is contraindicated in patients with hemiplegic, basilar, or ophthalmoplegic migraine.

Naratriptan is contraindicated in patients with severe renal impairment (creatinine clearance <15 mL/min) (see Pharmacology and Dosage).

Naratriptan is contraindicated in patients with severe hepatic impairment (Child-Pugh grade C) (see Pharmacology and Dosage).

Naratriptan is contraindicated in patients with hypersensitivity to naratriptan or any component of the formulation.

WARNINGS: Naratriptan should only be used where a clear diagnosis of migraine has been established.

Risk of Myocardial Ischemia and/or Infarction and Other Adverse Cardiac Events: Naratriptan has been associated with transient chest and/or neck pain and tightness which may resemble angina pectoris. In rare cases, the symptoms have been identified as being the likely result of coronary vasospasm or myocardial ischemia. Rare cases of serious coronary events or arrhythmia have occurred following use of another 5-HT$_1$ agonist. Naratriptan should not be given to patients who have documented ischemic or vasospastic coronary artery disease (see Contraindications). It is strongly recommended that naratriptan not be given to patients in whom unrecognized coronary artery disease (CAD) is predicted by the presence of risk factors (e.g., hypertension, hypercholesterolemia, smoking, obesity, diabetes, strong family history of CAD, female who is surgically or physiologically postmenopausal, or male who is over 40 years of age) unless a cardiovascular evaluation provides satisfactory clinical evidence that the patient is reasonably free of coronary artery and ischemic myocardial disease or other significant underlying cardiovascular disease. The sensitivity of cardiac diagnostic procedures to detect cardiovascular disease or predisposition to coronary artery vasospasm is unknown. If, during the cardiovascular evaluation, the patient's medical history or electrocardiographic investigations reveal findings indicative of or consistent with coronary artery vasospasm or myocardial ischemia, naratriptan should not be administered (see Contraindications).

For patients with risk factors predictive of CAD who are considered to have a satisfactory cardiovascular evaluation, the first dose of naratriptan should be administered in the setting of a physician's office or similar medically staffed and equipped facility. Because cardiac ischemia can occur in the absence of clinical symptoms, consideration should be given to obtaining ECGs in patients with risk factors during the interval immediately following naratriptan administration on the first occasion of use. However, an absence of drug-induced cardiovascular effects on the occasion of the initial dose does not preclude the possibility of such effects occurring with subsequent administrations.

Intermittent long-term users of naratriptan who have or acquire risk factors predictive of CAD, as described above, should receive periodic interval cardiovascular evaluations over the course of treatment.

If symptoms consistent with angina occur after the use of naratriptan, ECG evaluation should be carried out to look for ischemic changes.

The systematic approach described above is intended to reduce the likelihood that patients with unrecognized cardiovascular disease will be inadvertently exposed to naratriptan.

Cardiac Events and Fatalities Associated with 5-HT$_1$ Agonists: Naratriptan can cause coronary artery vasospasm. Serious adverse cardiac events, including acute myocardial infarction, life-threatening disturbances of cardiac rhythm, and death have been reported within a few hours following the administration of 5-HT$_1$ agonists. Considering the extent of use of 5-HT$_1$ agonists in patients with migraine, the incidence of these events is extremely low.

Premarketing Experience with Naratriptan: Among approximately 3500 patients with migraine who participated in premarketing clinical trials of naratriptan, 4 patients treated with single oral doses of naratriptan ranging from 1 to 10 mg experienced asymptomatic ischemic ECG changes with at least 1, who took 7.5 mg, likely due to coronary vasospasm.

Cerebrovascular Events and Fatalities with 5-HT$_1$ Agonists: Cerebral hemorrhage, subarachnoid hemorrhage, stroke, and other cerebrovascular events have been reported in patients treated with 5-HT$_1$ agonists, and some have resulted in fatalities. In a number of cases, it appears possible that the cerebrovascular events were primary, the agonist having been administered in the incorrect belief that the symptoms experienced were a consequence of migraine, when they were not. Before treating migraine headaches with naratriptan in patients not previously diagnosed as migraineurs, and in migraineurs who present with atypical symptoms, care should be taken to exclude other potentially serious neurological conditions. If a patient does not respond to the first dose, the opportunity should be taken to review the diagnosis before a second dose is given. It should be noted that patients with migraine may be at increased risk of certain cerebrovascular events (e.g., stroke, hemorrhage, TIA).

Special Cardiovascular Pharmacology Studies: In subjects (n=10) with suspected coronary artery disease undergoing angiography, naratriptan at a s.c. dose of 1.5 mg produced an 8% increase in aortic blood pressure, an 18% increase in pulmonary artery blood pressure, and an 8% increase in systemic vascular resistance. In addition, mild chest pain or tightness was reported by 4 subjects. Clinically significant increases in blood pressure were experienced by 3 of the subjects (2 of whom also had chest pain/discomfort). Diagnostic angiogram results revealed that 9 subjects had normal coronary arteries and 1 had insignificant coronary artery disease.

Migraine patients (n=35) free of cardiovascular disease were subjected to assessments of myocardial perfusion by positron emission tomography while receiving s.c. naratriptan 1.5 mg in the absence of a migraine attack. Naratriptan was associated with a reduced coronary vasodilatory reserve (approximately 10%), increased coronary resistance (approximately 20%), and decreased hyperemic myocardial blood flow (approximately 10%). The relevance of these findings to the use of recommended oral doses of naratriptan is not known.

Hypersensitivity: Rare hypersensitivity (anaphylaxis/anaphylactoid) reactions may occur in patients receiving 5-HT$_1$ agonists such as naratriptan. Such reactions can be life-threatening or fatal. In general, hypersensitivity reactions to drugs are more likely to occur in individuals with a history of sensitivity to multiple allergens (see Contraindications). Owing to the possibility of cross-reactive hypersensitivity reactions, naratriptan should not be used in patients having a history of hypersensitivity to sumatriptan or chemically-related 5-HT$_1$ receptor agonists. As naratriptan contains a sulfonamide component, there is a theoretical risk of hypersensitivity reactions in patients with known hypersensitivity to sulfonamides.

Other Vasospasm-Related Events: 5-HT$_1$ agonists may cause vasospastic reactions other than coronary artery vasospasm. Extensive postmarket experience has shown the use of naratriptan to be associated with very rare occurrences of peripheral vascular ischemia and colonic ischemia with abdominal pain and bloody diarrhea.

Increases in Blood Pressure: Elevations in blood pressure have been reported following use of naratriptan. At the recommended oral doses, the elevations are generally small (population average maximum increases of <5 mmHg systolic and <3 mmHg diastolic at the 2.5 mg dose). The effects may be more pronounced in the elderly and hypertensive patients. In a pharmacodynamic study conducted in normotensive patients (n=12) and in hypertensive patients controlled by antihypertensive treatment (n=12), the pressor effects of naratriptan were greater in hypertensive patients (weighted mean increases in systolic and diastolic blood pressure of 6 and 4 mm Hg in hypertensive subjects vs 3 and 2 mmHg in normotensive patients receiving two 2.5 mg doses separated by a 2-hour time interval). Two hypertensive patients experienced 3 events of chest discomfort while receiving naratriptan. Significant elevation in blood pressure, including hypertensive crisis, has been reported on rare occasions in patients receiving 5-HT$_1$ agonists with and without a history of hypertension. Naratriptan is contraindicated in patients with uncontrolled or severe hypertension (see Contraindications).

In patients with controlled hypertension, naratriptan should be administered with caution, as transient increases in blood pressure and peripheral vascular resistance have been observed in a small portion of patients.

Selective Serotonin Reuptake Inhibitors/Serotonin Norepinephrine Reuptake Inhibitors and Serotonin Syndrome: Cases of life-threatening serotonin syndrome have been reported during combined use of selective serotonin reuptake inhibitors (SSRIs)/serotonin norepinephrine reuptake inhibitors (SNRIs) and triptans. If concomitant treatment with naratriptan and SSRIs (e.g., fluoxetine, paroxetine, sertraline) or SNRIs (e.g., venlafaxine) is clinically warranted, careful observation of the patient is advised, particularly during treatment initiation and dose increases. Serotonin syndrome symptoms may include mental status changes (e.g., agitation, hallucinations, coma), autonomic instability (e.g., tachycardia, labile blood pressure, hyperthermia), neuromuscular aberrations (e.g., hyperreflexia, incoordination) and/or gastrointestinal symptoms (e.g., nausea, vomiting, diarrhea) (see Precautions, Drug Interactions).

PRECAUTIONS: Cardiovascular: Discomfort in the chest, neck, throat, and jaw (including pain, pressure, heaviness, tightness, dyspnea) has been reported after administration of naratriptan. Because 5-HT$_1$ agonists may cause coronary artery vasospasm, patients who experience signs or symptoms suggestive of angina following naratriptan should be evaluated for the presence of CAD or a predisposition to variant angina before receiving additional doses, and should be monitored electrocardiographically if dosing is resumed and similar symptoms recur. Similarly, patients who experience other symptoms or signs suggestive of decreased arterial flow, such as ischemic bowel syndrome or Raynaud's syndrome following naratriptan administration should be evaluated for atherosclerosis or predisposition to vasospasm (see Contraindications and Warnings).

Neurologic Conditions: Care should be taken to exclude other potentially serious neurologic conditions before treating headache in patients not previously diagnosed with migraine or who experience a headache that is atypical for them. There have been rare reports where patients received 5-HT$_1$ agonists for severe headaches that were subsequently shown to have been secondary to an evolving neurologic lesion. For newly diagnosed patients or patients presenting with atypical symptoms, the diagnosis of migraine should be reconsidered if no response is seen after the first dose of naratriptan.

Seizures: Caution should be observed if naratriptan is to be used in patients with a history of epilepsy or structural brain lesions which lower the convulsion threshold.

Renal or Hepatic Impairment: Naratriptan should be administered with caution to patients with impaired renal or hepatic function (see Pharmacology, Contraindications and Dosage).

Occupational Hazards: Psychomotor Impairment: In a study of psychomotor function in healthy volunteers, single oral 5 and 10 mg doses of naratriptan were associated with sedation and decreased alertness. Although these doses are higher than those recommended for the treatment of migraine, patients should be cautioned that drowsiness may occur following treatment with naratriptan. They should be advised not to perform skilled tasks (e.g., driving or operating machinery) if drowsiness occurs.

Medication Overuse Headache: Overuse of acute migraine treatments has been associated with the exacerbation of headache (medication overuse headache, MOH) in susceptible patients. Withdrawal of the treatment may be necessary.

Drug Interactions: The limited metabolism of naratriptan and the wide range of cytochrome P_{450} isoenzymes involved, as determined by in vitro studies, suggest that significant drug interactions with naratriptan are unlikely. Naratriptan did not inhibit MAO enzymes (MAO-A or MAO-B) in vitro. The possibility of pharmacodynamic in vivo interactions between naratriptan and MAO inhibitors has not been investigated.

Ergot-Containing Drugs: Ergot-containing drugs have been reported to cause prolonged vasospastic reactions. Because there is a theoretical basis for these effects being additive, ergot-containing or ergot-type medications (like dihydroergotamine or methysergide) are contraindicated within 24 hours of naratriptan administration (see Contraindications).

Other 5-HT$_1$ agonists: The administration of naratriptan with other 5-HT$_1$ agonists has not been evaluated in migraine patients. As an increased risk of coronary vasospasm is a theoretical possibility with coadministration of 5-HT$_1$ agonists, use of these drugs within 24 hours of each other is contraindicated.

Selective Serotonin Reuptake Inhibitors/Serotonin Norepinephrine Reuptake Inhibitors: Cases of life-threatening serotonin syndrome have been reported during combined use of selective serotonin reuptake inhibitors (SSRIs) or serotonin norepinephrine reuptake inhibitors (SNRIs) and triptans (see Warnings).

Hormonal Contraceptives: In a population pharmacokinetic study in migraine patients, hormonal contraceptive use was associated with a 32% decrease in naratriptan clearance.

Tobacco: In a population pharmacokinetic study in migraine patients, tobacco use was associated with a 29% increase in naratriptan clearance.

Alcohol and Food: Clinical studies did not reveal any pharmacokinetic interaction when naratriptan was administered together with alcohol or food.

Pregnancy: The safety of naratriptan for use during human pregnancy has not been established. Naratriptan should be used during pregnancy only if the potential benefit justifies the potential risk to the fetus. To monitor fetal outcomes of pregnant women exposed to naratriptan, GlaxoSmithKline Inc. maintains a Naratriptan Pregnancy Registry. Health care providers are encouraged to register patients by calling 1-800-336-2176.

Lactation: Naratriptan and/or its metabolites are distributed into the milk of lactating rats (at 2 hours post oral gavage dosing, levels in milk were 3.5 times higher than maternal plasma levels). Therefore, caution should be exercised when considering the administration of naratriptan to nursing women.

Children: Safety and effectiveness of naratriptan have not been studied in children under 12 years of age. Use of the drug in this age group is, therefore, not recommended.

Adolescents: The efficacy of naratriptan at single doses of 0.25, 1.0 and 2.5 mg was not demonstrated to be greater than placebo in adolescents (12 to 17 years). Therefore, the use of the drug in adolescents is not recommended.

Geriatrics: The safety and effectiveness of naratriptan have not been adequately studied in individuals over 65 years of age. Naratriptan is known to be substantially excreted by the kidney, and the risk of adverse reactions to this drug may be greater in elderly patients who have reduced renal function. In addition, elderly patients are more likely to have decreased hepatic function; they are at higher risk for CAD; and blood pressure increases may be more pronounced in the elderly. Clinical studies of naratriptan did not include patients over 65 years of age. Its use in this age group is, therefore, not recommended.

Drug/Laboratory Test Interactions: Naratriptan is not known to interfere with commonly employed clinical laboratory tests.

Dependence Liability: In 1 clinical study enrolling 12 subjects, all of whom had experience using oral opiates and other psychoactive drugs, subjective responses typically associated with many drugs of abuse were produced with less intensity during treatment with naratriptan (1 to 5 mg) than with codeine (30 to 90 mg). Long-term studies (12 months) in migraine patients using naratriptan revealed no evidence of increased drug utilization.

Melanin Binding: In pigmented rats treated with a single oral dose (10 mg/kg) of radiolabeled naratriptan, radioactivity was detected in the eyes at 3 months postadministration, a finding which suggests that the drug or its metabolites may bind to the melanin of the eye. The possible clinical significance of this finding is unknown. No systematic monitoring of ophthalmologic function was undertaken in clinical trials. Prescribers should consider the possibility of long-term ophthalmologic effects due to accumulation of naratriptan in melanin-rich tissues.

ADVERSE EFFECTS: Serious cardiac events, including some that have been fatal, have occurred following the use of 5-HT$_1$ agonists. These events are extremely rare and most have been reported in patients with risk factors predictive of CAD. Events reported have included coronary artery vasospasm, transient myocardial ischemia, myocardial infarction, ventricular tachycardia, and ventricular fibrillation (see Contraindications, Warnings and Precautions).

Experience in Controlled Clinical Trials with Naratriptan: Typical 5-HT$_1$ Agonist Adverse Reactions: As with other 5-HT$_1$ agonists, naratriptan has been associated with sensations of heaviness, pressure, tightness or pain which may be intense. These may occur in any part of the body including the chest, throat, neck, jaw and upper limb.

Acute Safety: The safety and efficacy of the 1 and 2.5 mg doses of naratriptan were investigated in 4 placebo-controlled clinical trials in adult migraine patients. Two of these trials were of parallel group design and involved the treatment of a single migraine attack. A third study was of crossover design and involved the treatment of one migraine attack per dose group. The fourth study was a parallel group trial in which patients treated up to 3 migraine attacks. In all studies, patients who achieved headache relief at 240 minutes postdose, but experienced a worsening of severity between 4 and 24 hours postdosing, were permitted to take a second dose of double-blind medication identical to the first.

The overall incidence of adverse events following doses of naratriptan 1 mg or 2.5 mg (1 or 2 doses) were similar to placebo (28.5 and 30.2% vs 28.9% with placebo). Naratriptan is generally well tolerated and most adverse reactions were mild, transient and self-limiting. The most common adverse events to occur at a higher rate than in the corresponding placebo group were malaise/fatigue (2.4% vs 0.8% with placebo) and neck/throat/jaw sensations (2.1% vs 0.3% with placebo). Table 3 lists the most common adverse events that occurred in the 4 large placebo-controlled clinical trials. Only events that occurred at a frequency of 1% or more in the naratriptan 2.5 mg or 1 mg group and were more frequent in that group than in the placebo group are included in Table 3. From this table, it appears that many of these adverse events are dose-related.

Table 3: Amerge

Treatment-Emergent Adverse Events in Placebo-Controlled Clinical Trials Reported by at Least 1% of Patients with Migraine[a]

	Placebo	Amerge 1 mg	Amerge 2.5 mg
Number of Patients	922	1024	1016
Number of Migraine Attacks Treated	1059	1387	1368
Symptoms of Potentially Cardiac Origin			
Neck/Throat/Jaw Sensations[a]	0.3%	1.7%	2.1%
Chest Sensations[a]	1.1%	0.8%	1.2%
Upper Limb Sensations[a]	0.3%	0.5%	1.4%
Neurological			
Dizziness	1.5%	1.0%	2.2%
Drowsiness/Sleepiness	0.8%	0.9%	1.7%
Paresthesia	0.8%	1.6%	1.5%
Head/Face sensations[a]	0.5%	0.5%	1.3%
Headache	0.2%	0.4%	1.0%
Gastrointestinal			
Nausea	6.2%	5.9%	6.3%
Hyposalivation	0.3%	0.5%	1.0%
Non-Site Specific			
Malaise and fatigue	0.8%	1.6%	2.4%

[a] The term "sensations" encompasses adverse events described as pain and discomfort, pressure, heaviness, constriction, tightness, heat/burning sensation, paresthesia, numbness, tingling, and strange sensations.

Long-Term Safety: In a long-term open study, 417 patients treated 15 301 migraine attacks with naratriptan over a period of up to 1 year. The most common adverse events in descending order of frequency were as follows: nausea (16%); malaise/fatigue (11%); drowsiness (10%); chest sensations* (8%); neck/throat/jaw sensations* (8%); paresthesia (7%); head/face sensations* (6%); vomiting (6%); and dizziness (5%). Due to the lack of a placebo arm in this study, the role of naratriptan in causation cannot be reliably determined.

Other Adverse Events Observed in Association with Naratriptan: In the paragraphs that follow, the frequencies of less commonly reported adverse clinical events are presented. Because some events were observed in open and uncontrolled studies, the role of naratriptan in their causation cannot be reliably determined. All reported events are included except those already listed in Table 3, those too general to be informative, and those not reasonably associated with the use of the drug. Event frequencies are calculated as the number of patients reporting an event divided by the total number of patients (n=2790) exposed to naratriptan. Events are further classified within body system categories and enumerated in order of decreasing frequency using the following definitions: frequent adverse events are defined as those occurring in at least 1/100 patients; infrequent adverse events are those occurring in 1/100 to 1/1000 patients; rare adverse events are those occurring in fewer than 1/1000 patients.

Cardiovascular: Infrequent: palpitations, increased blood pressure, tachyarrhythmias and abnormal ECGs. Rare: bradycardia, hypotension, varicosities and heart murmur.

Ear, Nose and Throat: Frequent: ear, nose and throat infections. Infrequent: phonophobia, sinusitis, and upper respiratory inflammation. Rare: allergic rhinitis, labyrinthitis, tinnitus, ear, nose and throat hemorrhage and hearing difficulty.

Endocrine and Metabolic: Infrequent: thirst and polydipsia, dehydration and fluid retention. Rare: hyperlipidemia, hypercholesterolemia, hypothyroidism, hyperglycemia, glycosuria and ketonuria and parathyroid neoplasm.

Eye: Infrequent: photophobia. Rare: eye hemorrhage, dry eyes and difficulty focusing.

Gastrointestinal: Frequent: vomiting. Infrequent: dyspeptic symptoms, diarrhea, hyposalivation, gastrointestinal discomfort and pain, gastroenteritis and constipation. Rare: abnormal liver function tests, abnormal bilirubin levels, salivary gland swelling, hemorrhoids, gastritis, esophagitis, oral itching and irritation, regurgitation and reflux and gastic ulcers.

Musculoskeletal: Infrequent: musculoskeletal/muscle pain, muscle cramps and spasms, arthralgia and articular rheumatism. Rare: joint and muscle stiffness, tightness and rigidity.

Neurology: Frequent: migraine. Infrequent: vertigo, tremors, sleep disorders, cognitive function disorders and hyperesthesia. Rare: disorders of equilibrium, decreased consciousness, confusion, sedation, coordination disorders, neuritis, dreams, altered sense of taste, motor retardation, muscle twitching and fasciculation.

Non-Site Specific: Frequent: paresthesia and heat sensations. Infrequent: chills and/or fever, descriptions of odor or taste and feelings of pressure/tightness/heaviness. Rare: allergies and allergic reactions, mobility disorders and faintness.

Psychiatry: Infrequent: anxiety and depressive disorders. Rare: aggression, agitation and detachment.

Reproduction: Rare: lumps of female reproductive tract and inflammation of the fallopian tube.

Skin: Infrequent: skin photosensitivity, skin rashes, pruritus, sweating and urticaria. Rare: skin erythema, dermatitis and dermatosis, and pruritic skin rash.

Urology: Infrequent: urinary infections. Rare: urinary tract hemorrhage, urinary urgency and pyelitis.

Post-Marketing Experience: The following section enumerates potentially important adverse events that have occurred in clinical practice and that have been reported spontaneously to various surveillance systems. The events enumerated represent reports arising from both domestic and nondomestic use of naratriptan. These events do not include those already listed in the Adverse Effects section above. Because the reports cite events reported spontaneously from worldwide postmarketing experience, frequency of events and the role of naratriptan in their causation cannot be reliably determined.

Cardiovascular: angina, myocardial infarction (see Precautions and Warnings).

Gastrointestinal: colonic ischemia (see Warnings).

Lower Respiratory: dyspnea (see Precautions).

Neurologic: cerebral vascular accident, including transient ischemic attack, subarachnoid hemorrhage, and cerebral infarction (see Warnings).

General: hypersensitivity, including anaphylaxis/anaphylactoid reactions, in some cases severe (e.g., circulatory collapse) (see Warnings).

OVERDOSE:

Symptoms: In clinical studies, numerous patients (n=222) and healthy subjects (n=196) have received naratriptan at doses of 5 to 25 mg. In the majority of cases, no serious adverse events were reported. One patient treated with a 7.5 mg dose experienced ischemic ECG changes which were likely due to coronary vasospasm. This event was not associated with a serious clinical outcome. A patient who was mildly hypertensive experienced a significant increase in blood pressure (baseline value of 150/98 to 204/144 mmHg at 225 minutes) beginning 30 minutes after the administration of a 10 mg dose (4 times the maximum recommended single dose). The event resolved with antihypertensive treatment. Administration of 25 mg (10 times the maximum recommended single dose) in 1 healthy male subject increased blood pressure from 120/67 mmHg pretreatment up to 191/113 mmHg at approximately 6 hours postdose and resulted in adverse events including lightheadedness, tension in the neck, tiredness, and loss of coordination. Blood pressure returned to near baseline by 8 hours after dosing without any pharmacological intervention.

Treatment: The elimination half-life of naratriptan is about 5 to 8 hours (see Pharmacology), and therefore monitoring of patients after overdose with naratriptan should continue for at least 24 hours or longer if symptoms or signs persist. Standard supportive treatment should be applied as required. If the patient presents with chest pain or other symptoms consistent with angina pectoris, ECG monitoring should be performed for evidence of ischemia. Appropriate treatment (e.g., nitroglycerin or other coronary artery vasodilators) should be administered as required.

It is unknown what effect hemodialysis or peritoneal dialysis has on the serum concentrations of naratriptan.

For management of a suspected drug overdose, CPhA recommends that you contact your **regional Poison Control Centre**. See the *CPS* Directory section for a list of Poison Control Centres.

DOSAGE: Naratriptan is recommended only for the acute treatment of migraine attacks. Naratriptan should not be used prophylactically.

Adults: The minimal effective single adult dose of naratriptan is 1 mg. The maximum recommended single dose is 2.5 mg (see Clinical Studies in Table 4).

Table 4: Amerge

Percentage of Patients with Headache Relief at 4 Hours Postdosing[a]

	Placebo		Amerge 1 mg		Amerge 2.5 mg	
	%	(N)	%	(N)	%	(N)
Study 1	39	(91)	64	(85)	63[b]	(87)
Study 2	34	(122)	50[c]	(117)	60[b,c]	(127)
Study 3	27	(107)	52[c]	(219)	66[c,d]	(209)
Study 4	33	(602)	57[c]	(595)	68[c,d]	(586)

[a] Pain relief is defined as a reduction in headache severity from grade 3 or 2 (severe or moderate) to grade 1 or 0 (mild or no pain).
[b] Comparison between 1 and 2.5 mg Amerge doses was not performed.
[c] $p<0.05$ vs placebo.
[d] $p<0.01$ vs Amerge 1 mg.

In 3 of the 4 studies, optimal rates of headache relief were achieved with a 2.5 mg dose. As patients may vary in their dose-responsiveness, the choice of dose should be made on an individual basis, weighing the possible benefit of the 2.5 mg dose with the potential for a greater risk of adverse events.

If the migraine headache returns, or if a patient has a partial response, the initial dose may be repeated once after 4 hours, for a maximum dose of 5 mg in a 24-hour period.

* The term "sensations" encompasses adverse events described as pain and discomfort, pressure, heaviness, constriction, tightness, heat/burning sensation, paresthesia, numbness, tingling, and strange sensations.

The safety of treating, on average, more than 4 headaches in a 30-day period has not been established.

Naratriptan tablets should be swallowed whole with fluids. Naratriptan tablets should be taken as early as possible after the onset of a migraine headache, but are effective if taken at a later stage.

If a patient does not respond to the first dose of naratriptan, a second dose should not be taken for the same attack, as it is unlikely to be of benefit.

Renal disease/functional impairment causes prolongation of the half-life of orally administered naratriptan. Consequently, if treatment is deemed advisable in the presence of renal impairment, a maximum single dose of 1 mg should be administered. No more than a total of 2 mg should be taken in any 24-hour period. Repeated dosing in renally impaired patients has not been evaluated (see Pharmacology). Administration of naratriptan in patients with severe renal impairment (creatinine clearance <15 mL/min) is contraindicated (see Contraindications).

Hepatic disease/functional impairment causes prolongation of the half-life of orally administered naratriptan. Consequently, if treatment is deemed advisable in the presence of hepatic impairment, a maximum single dose of 1 mg should be administered. No more than a total of 2 mg should be taken in any 24-hour period (see Pharmacology). Administration of naratriptan in patients with severe hepatic impairment (Child-Pugh grade C) is contraindicated (see Contraindications).

Hypertension: Naratriptan should not be used in patients with uncontrolled or severe hypertension. Patients with mild to moderate controlled hypertension should be treated cautiously at the lowest effective dose.

INFORMATION FOR THE PATIENT: Published in e-CPS, available by subscription at www.e-cps.ca.

SUPPLIED: 1 mg: Each white film-coated, D-shaped tablet, embossed GXCE3 on one side, contains: naratriptan (base) 1 mg as the HCl salt. Nonmedicinal ingredients: croscarmellose sodium, hydroxypropyl methylcellulose, lactose, magnesium stearate, microcrystalline cellulose, titanium dioxide and triacetin. Blister packs of 2, cartons of 4 blisters. Store below 30°C.

2.5 mg: Each green film-coated, D-shaped tablet, embossed GXCE5 on one side, contains: naratriptan (base) 2.5 mg as the HCl salt. Nonmedicinal ingredients: croscarmellose sodium, hydroxypropyl methylcellulose, indigo carmine aluminium lake (FD&C Blue No. 2), iron oxide yellow, lactose, magnesium stearate, microcrystalline cellulose, titanium dioxide and triacetin. Blister packs of 2 and 6, cartons of 4 blisters. Store below 30°C.

(Shown in Product Identification Section)

Amevive® Ⓟ

alefacept

Selective Immunomodulating Antipsoriatic Agent

Astellas

Date of Revision: June 1, 2006

SUMMARY PRODUCT INFORMATION:

Route of Administration	Dosage Form/ Strength	Clinically Relevant Nonmedicinal Ingredients
Intramuscular Injection	Lyophilized powder for reconstitution/ 15 mg per 0.5 mL	None For a complete listing see Dosage Forms, Composition and Packaging.

DESCRIPTION: AMEVIVE (alefacept) is a recombinant dimeric fusion protein that consists of the extracellular CD2-binding portion of the human leukocyte function antigen-3 (LFA-3) linked to the Fc (hinge, C_H2 and C_H3 domains) portion of human IgG_1. Alefacept is produced by recombinant DNA technology in a Chinese Hamster Ovary (CHO) mammalian cell expression system. The molecular weight of alefacept is 91.4 kilodaltons.

INDICATIONS AND CLINICAL USE: AMEVIVE (alefacept) is indicated for:

- treatment of patients with moderate to severe chronic plaque psoriasis who are candidates for phototherapy or systemic therapy.

Summary of Clinical Studies: The safety and efficacy of AMEVIVE (alefacept) in psoriasis were evaluated in two randomized, double-blind, placebo-controlled phase III studies in 1060 adults. In both studies, patients had chronic plaque psoriasis for more than one year and a minimum body surface area involvement of 10% prior to study entry. The patients' ages ranged from 16 to 84 years. Patients received a treatment consisting of weekly doses of either AMEVIVE or placebo over 12 weeks and were followed for an additional 12 weeks without treatment after dosing. The use of low-potency topical steroids was allowed, but concomitant phototherapy or systemic therapy was not allowed. Study 1 evaluated the efficacy and safety of one versus two 12-week courses of AMEVIVE 7.5 mg administered by intravenous (IV) bolus. A total of 553 patients received either two courses of AMEVIVE, one course of AMEVIVE followed by one course of placebo, or one course of placebo followed by one course of AMEVIVE.

In Study 2, which examined the safety and efficacy of two different doses of AMEVIVE, patients received either 10 mg, 15 mg, or placebo, administered weekly for 12 weeks by intramuscular injection. Results are presented below for the 15 mg dose versus placebo only since 15 mg IM once weekly is the recommended dose.

In both studies, one course was defined as a 12-week treatment of once weekly injection followed by a 12-week observation period.

Efficacy Results: In Study 1, a greater proportion of patients (14%) treated with AMEVIVE (alefacept) compared with 4% of patients receiving placebo (p<0.001), achieved PASI 75 or greater response two weeks after the last dose of Course 1. The proportion of patients who achieved PASI 50 or greater response was 38% of patients treated with AMEVIVE, compared to 10% who received placebo (p<0.001). A PGA assessment of almost clear or clear was achieved in 11% of patients treated with AMEVIVE compared with 4% who received placebo (p=0.004).

In Study 2, the proportion of patients achieving PASI 75 or greater response two weeks after the last dose in the AMEVIVE and placebo groups were 21% and 5% (p<0.001), respectively. The proportion of patients achieving PASI 50 or greater was 42% and 18% in the AMEVIVE and placebo groups, respectively (p<0.001). The response rates for PGA almost clear or clear were 14% and 5% in the AMEVIVE and placebo groups (p=0.006), respectively.

Assessment of clinical response at any time during the course of treatment and follow-up in Study 1 demonstrated that 28% of patients treated with AMEVIVE achieved PASI 75 or greater compared with 8% for placebo (p<0.001) and 56% of patients treated with AMEVIVE achieved PASI 50 at any time compared to 24% for placebo (p<0.001). Also 23% of patients treated with AMEVIVE achieved PGA almost clear or clear at any time compared to 6% for placebo (p<0.001).

Similarly in Study 2, 33% of patients treated with AMEVIVE achieved PASI 75 or greater at any time during treatment and follow-up compared to 13% for placebo (p<0.001) and 57% of patients treated with AMEVIVE achieved PASI 50 or greater at any time compared to 35% for placebo (p<0.001). Also 24% of patients treated with AMEVIVE achieved PGA almost clear or clear at any time compared to 8% for placebo (p<0.001).

Assessment of clinical response with a second course of AMEVIVE is based upon the comparison between the 154 patients in Cohort 1 and the 142 patients in Cohort 2 of Study 1. Patients in Cohort 1 received AMEVIVE during both courses of treatment (AMEVIVE/AMEVIVE) while patients in Cohort 2 received AMEVIVE during the first course and placebo during the second course (AMEVIVE/placebo). At two weeks after the last dose of course 2, 23% of patients treated with AMEVIVE/AMEVIVE achieved PASI 75 or greater compared to 7% of patients who received AMEVIVE/placebo (p<0.001), 48% of patients treated with AMEVIVE/AMEVIVE achieved PASI 50 or greater compared to 25% of patients who received AMEVIVE/placebo (p<0.001) and 20% of patients treated with AMEVIVE/AMEVIVE achieved PGA almost clear or clear compared to 6% of patients who received AMEVIVE/placebo (p=0.006). At any time during treatment and follow-up 37% of patients treated with AMEVIVE/AMEVIVE achieved PASI 75 or greater compared to 19% who received AMEVIVE/placebo (p<0.001), 64% of patients treated with AMEVIVE/AMEVIVE achieved PASI 50 or greater compared to 49% who received AMEVIVE/placebo (p=0.002) and 30% of patients treated with AMEVIVE/AMEVIVE achieved PGA almost clear or clear compared to 18% who received AMEVIVE/placebo (p=0.011).

In patients in Study 1 who were randomized to receive two courses of AMEVIVE, 71% achieved a reduction in PASI score of at least 50% from baseline and 40% achieved a reduction in PASI score of at least 75% from baseline at any time after the start of dosing.

Clinical responses were initially evident within six weeks after the first dose in both studies. Maximal clinical responses may be seen up to six weeks post-dosing. Return of disease activity following cessation of treatment was generally slow. A second course of therapy provided additional benefit.

In general, clinical responses to AMEVIVE were durable. Patients were followed for up to 36 weeks following the completion of dosing patients with AMEVIVE (Study 1, cohort 2). Patients achieving a 75% reduction in PASI following a single 12-week treatment of AMEVIVE maintained at least a 50% reduction in PASI for a median of over seven months (216 days).

Following repeat courses of therapy, median duration of response was generally longer than following a single course. Intermittent treatment with additional 12-week courses of AMEVIVE therapy has been demonstrated to be safe and effective. Courses were separated by at least a 12-week monitoring period (see Dosage and Administration).

Following cessation of treatment, no disease rebound or flaring occurred at any time in either study.

Beneficial effects on Quality of Life (QOL), as measured by the Dermatology Life Quality Index (DLQI), were evident in both phase III studies.

Geriatrics (>60 years of age): During clinical studies, no overall differences in safety or effectiveness were observed between patients aged >60 years and younger patients.

Pediatrics (<16 years of age): The safety and effectiveness of AMEVIVE (alefacept) in children below the age of 16 years has not been studied. AMEVIVE should not be administered in these patients.

CONTRAINDICATIONS:

- Patients who are hypersensitive to this drug or to any ingredient in the formulation or component of the container. For a complete listing, see Dosage Forms, Composition and Packaging.
- AMEVIVE (alefacept) should not be administered to patients infected with HIV. AMEVIVE reduces CD4+ T lymphocyte counts, which might accelerate disease progression or increase complications of disease in these patients (see Warnings and Precautions, General and Immune).

WARNINGS AND PRECAUTIONS: General: AMEVIVE (alefacept) induces dose-dependent reductions in circulating CD4+ and CD8+ T lymphocyte counts. AMEVIVE should not be administered to patients with a baseline total lymphocyte or CD4+ T cell count below normal. Beginning two weeks after the first dose, the CD4+ T lymphocyte counts should be monitored every two weeks during dosing and continuing throughout the course of the 12-week dosing regimen to guide subsequent dosing. If the CD4+ T cell count falls below 250 cells/μL, subsequent doses of AMEVIVE should be withheld until the CD4+ T cell count increases to 250 cells/μL or more. AMEVIVE should be permanently discontinued in patients if CD4+ T lymphocyte counts remain below 250 cells/μL for one month. Prior to initiating another course of therapy, it is recommended that patients have total lymphocyte and CD4+ T cell counts within the normal range (see Dosage and Administration). Patients who develop a new clinically significant infection while undergoing treatment with AMEVIVE should be clinically monitored closely. If a patient develops a severe infection, dosing should be discontinued until the infection is completely resolved (see Warnings and Precautions, Immune).

Patients should be informed that:

- AMEVIVE (alefacept) needs to be administered under the guidance and supervision of a qualified health care professional.
- There is a need for regular monitoring of white blood cell (lymphoctye) counts during therapy and that results of this biweekly blood test should be confirmed **before** administration of subsequent injections.
- AMEVIVE reduces lymphocyte counts, which may increase their chances of developing an infection or malignancy. Patients should be advised to inform their physician if they develop an infection or malignancy while undergoing a course of therapy with AMEVIVE.

When a physician determines that AMEVIVE can be used outside of the physician's office, persons who will be administering AMEVIVE 15 mg IM should receive instruction in reconstitution and injection, including a review of the injection procedures. If a patient is to self-administer, the physical ability of the patient to self-inject IM should be assessed. If home use is chosen, the first IM injection should be performed under the supervision of a qualified healthcare professional. Patients should be instructed in the technique and importance of proper syringe and needle disposal and be cautioned against reuse of these items. A puncture resistant container for disposal of needles should be used (see Information for the Patient).

Carcinogenesis and Mutagenesis: AMEVIVE (alefacept) may increase the risk of malignancies. Some patients who received AMEVIVE in clinical studies developed malignancies. The observed rates and incidences were similar to those expected for the population studied (see Adverse Reactions, Malignancies). In non-clinical studies, animals developed B cell hyperplasia and one animal developed a lymphoma. AMEVIVE should not be administered to patients with a history of systemic malignancy. Caution should be exercised when considering the use of AMEVIVE in patients at high risk for malignancy. If a patient develops a malignancy, AMEVIVE should be discontinued.

No carcinogenicity or fertility studies were conducted.

Mutagenicity studies were conducted in vitro and in vivo; no evidence of mutagenicity was observed.

Hepatic/Biliary/Pancreas: During post-marketing surveillance there have been reports of liver injury, including hepatitis, decompensation of cirrhosis and acute liver failure. Some cases were reported with concomitant alcohol use. The role of AMEVIVE (alefacept) in these events has not been established. AMEVIVE should be discontinued in patients who develop clinical signs of liver injury.

Immune: AMEVIVE (alefacept) has the potential to increase the risk of infection and may reactivate latent, chronic infections. AMEVIVE should not be administered to patients with a clinically important infection. Caution should be exercised when considering the use of AMEVIVE in patients with chronic infections or a history of recurrent infection. Patients should be monitored for signs and symptoms of infection during or after a course of AMEVIVE. New infections should be monitored closely. If a patient develops a serious infection, AMEVIVE should be discontinued (see Adverse Reactions, Infections).

During the clinical development of AMEVIVE, no generalised immunosuppressive effects were observed in psoriasis patients. In a controlled study (n=46), there was no evidence to suggest impaired antibody (IgM and IgG) responses either during or after alefacept therapy. The data from this study suggest that patients treated with AMEVIVE mounted a normal antibody response to the tetanus toxoid (recall antigen) and to an experimental neo-antigen. The safety and efficacy of live or live-attenuated vaccines administered to patients being treated with AMEVIVE is unknown.

Patients were tested at multiple time points for antibodies to AMEVIVE. Low titers of antibodies to AMEVIVE were detected in sera of less than 3% of psoriasis patients receiving AMEVIVE. No apparent correlation between antibody development and clinical response or adverse events was observed. The long-term immunogenicity of AMEVIVE is unknown.

The data reflect the percentage of patients whose test results were considered positive for antibodies to alefacept in an ELISA assay, and are highly dependent on the sensitivity and specificity of the assay. Additionally, the observed incidence of antibody positivity in an assay may be influenced by several factors including sample handling, timing of sample collection, concomitant medications and underlying disease.

Sensitivity/Resistance: Hypersensitivity reactions (urticaria, angioedema) were associated with the administration of alefacept. If an anaphylactic reaction or other serious allergic reaction occurs, administration of AMEVIVE (alefacept) should be discontinued immediately and appropriate therapy initiated.

Special Populations: Pregnant Women: There were no abortifacient or teratogenic effects in pregnant non-human primates. No evidence of fetal toxicity, malformations, or adverse effects on growth or development was observed in any of these animals. Trans-placental passage was observed.

No studies were conducted in pregnant women. Patients planning to become pregnant should not be treated with AMEVIVE (alefacept). If pregnancy inadvertently occurs during treatment, discontinuation of AMEVIVE is recommended. Women of child-bearing potential receiving AMEVIVE should be advised to take adequate contraceptive measures. It is not known if AMEVIVE alters the efficacy of oral contraceptives.

Data on a limited number (2) of exposed pregnancies indicate no adverse effect of AMEVIVE on pregnancy or on the health of the fetus or newborn child.

Nursing Women: It is not known whether AMEVIVE is excreted in human milk. Treatment with AMEVIVE should be avoided while nursing.

Pediatrics (<16 years of age): The safety and effectiveness of AMEVIVE (alefacept) in children below the age of 16 years have not been studied. AMEVIVE should not be administered to these patients.

Geriatrics (>60 years of age): Of the 1357 patients who received AMEVIVE (alefacept) in clinical studies, a total of 135 psoriasis patients aged 60-69 years and a total of 30 patients age >69 years have been treated with AMEVIVE. No overall differences in safety or effectiveness were observed between these patients and younger patients.

Monitoring and Laboratory Tests: CD4+ T lymphocyte counts should be monitored every two weeks during the 12-week dosing period and used to guide dosing. Patients should have normal CD4+ T lymphocyte counts prior to an initial or a subsequent course of treatment with AMEVIVE (alefacept). Dosing should be withheld if CD4+ T lymphocyte counts are below 250 cells/μL. AMEVIVE should be discontinued if CD4+ T lymphocyte counts remain below 250 cells/μL for one month.

ADVERSE REACTIONS: Adverse Drug Reaction Overview: Events Leading to Discontinuation of Treatment: The proportion of patients who discontinued treatment due to adverse events was approximately 2% of patients treated with AMEVIVE (alefacept) and 1% of placebo-treated patients. The most frequent adverse events leading to discontinuation in patients treated with AMEVIVE included headache and nausea. Infections leading to discontinuation included isolated cases of pneumonia and herpes zoster.

In Study 1, 10% of patients temporarily discontinued treatment and 2% permanently discontinued treatment due to CD4+ T cell counts below the specified threshold of 250 cells/µL. In Study 2, 4% temporarily discontinued treatment and none permanently discontinued treatment due to CD4+ counts below the specified threshold of 250 cells/µL.

Effects on Liver Function: In placebo-controlled studies, elevations of liver function tests were observed at a similar rate of incidence in placebo and patients treated with AMEVIVE (alefacept) following single or repeated courses of treatment. Rare cases of elevations of transaminases to 5-10 times the upper limit of normal without associated hyperbilirubinemia were observed in both patients treated with AMEVIVE and placebo.

During post-marketing surveillance rare hepatic events, including a case of hepatitis associated with transient coagulopathy and hyperbilirubinemia, have been reported.

Injection Site Reactions: In Study 2, 16% of patients treated with AMEVIVE (alefacept) and 8% of placebo-treated patients reported injection site reactions. Reactions at the site of injection were generally mild, typically occurred on single occasions, and included either pain (7%), inflammation (4%), bleeding (4%), edema (2%), non-specific reaction (2%), mass (1%), or skin hypersensitivity (<1%). During clinical trials, there was only one case of injection site reaction leading to the discontinuation of AMEVIVE.

Effect on Lymphocyte Levels: Overall in the first course of Studies 1 and 2, the mean total lymphocyte, CD4+ and CD8+ T cell counts remained above the lower limit of normal (LLN) throughout the 12 weeks of dosing and 12 weeks of follow-up. The maximal effects on lymphocytes were observed within 6 to 8 weeks of initiation of treatment with a rise in mean counts on cessation of treatment. Recovery rates varied between individuals with the majority of recovery occurring immediately in the 12 weeks following cessation of dosing. Table 1 provides the proportion of patients who experienced a maximal reduction in lymphocytes below the LLN and those who, within the period of observation (12 weeks post dosing), had lymphocyte counts below the LLN. In both studies 1 and 2, there was no evidence of predisposition to infections in patients with a low total lymphocyte count (see Warnings and Precautions, Immune).

Table 1: AMEVIVE

Lymphocyte, CD4+ and CD8+ Counts in Patients Treated with AMEVIVE

Lymphocyte parameters	Study 1	Study 2
Total Lymphocytes		
Mean count at baseline	2089	2159
Patients <LLN at time of maximum reduction	18%	9%
Mean count at time of maximum reduction	1236	1384
Patients <LLN at 12 weeks post dosing	4%	2%
Mean count at 12 weeks post dosing (cells/µL)	1724	1841
CD4+ T cells		
Mean count at baseline	901	909
Patients <LLN at time of maximum reduction	46%	31%
Mean count at time of maximum reduction	459	542
Patients <LLN at 12 weeks post dosing	19%	7%
Mean count at 12 weeks post dosing (cells/µL)	634	745
CD8+ T cells		
Mean count at baseline	495	508
Patients <LLN at time of maximum reduction	58%	46%
Mean count at time of maximum reduction	231	269
Patients <LLN at 12 weeks post dosing	36%	22%
Mean count at 12 weeks post dosing (cells/µL)	336	396

Legend: LLN=total lymphocytes 910 cells/µL; CD4+ 404 cells/µL; CD8+ 220 cells/µL.

Infections: In the first course of placebo-controlled studies, adverse events considered as infections were reported in a total of 176 patients (43%) following placebo and 393 patients (45%) following AMEVIVE (alefacept). Infections reported at an incidence of 5% or greater in the first course of therapy were pharyngitis, flu syndrome, nasopharyngitis (common cold), and viral infection. The incidence of infection did not increase with subsequent courses of therapy.

In the first course of placebo-controlled studies, infections requiring hospitalization were seen at a rate of less than 1%, similar to that of the placebo group. The nature of infections reported was similar to the nature of infections reported in the placebo-treated patients. In patients receiving repeated courses of therapy, the rates were 1% and 2% in the second and third course of therapy respectively. Infections requiring hospitalization included cellulitis, abscess, post-operative and burn wound infection, appendicitis, cholecystitis, gastroenteritis, toxic shock, and pneumonia. In general these infections occurred in patients with pre-existing risk factors. No opportunistic infections were reported.

Malignancies: In the 24-week period constituting the first course of placebo-controlled studies, 13 malignancies were diagnosed in 11 patients treated with AMEVIVE (alefacept). The incidence of malignancies was 1.3% (11/876) for patients treated with AMEVIVE compared to 0.5% (2/413) in the placebo group.

During clinical development the most common malignancy in patients treated with AMEVIVE was squamous cell and basal cell cancers of the skin. Most of the patients had pre-existing risk factors such as PUVA/UVB exposure. In placebo-controlled clinical studies skin carcinoma was observed in 0.7% (6/876) of patients treated with AMEVIVE and 0.2% (1/413) of placebo-treated patients. Uncommon cases of lymphoma (non-Hodgkin's follicular cell lymphoma and Hodgkin's disease) have also been observed. The incidence of lymphoid malignancies was consistent with that expected in the moderate to severe psoriasis population. The role of AMEVIVE in the development of lymphoid malignancies is unknown.

The observed rates and incidences were similar to those expected for the population studied (see Warnings and Precautions).

Hypersensitivity Reactions: In clinical studies, two patients were reported to experience angioedema, one of whom was hospitalized. In the 24-week period constituting the first course of placebo-controlled studies, urticaria was reported in <1% (6/876) patients treated with AMEVIVE (alefacept) vs. 1 of 413 patients in the control group. Urticaria resulted in discontinuation of therapy in one of the patients treated with AMEVIVE.

Clinical Trial Adverse Drug Reactions: Because clinical trials are conducted under very specific conditions the adverse reaction rates observed in the clinical trials may not reflect the rates observed in practice and should not be compared to the rates in the clinical trials of another drug. Adverse drug reaction information from clinical trials is useful for identifying drug-related adverse events and for approximating rates.

AMEVIVE (alefacept) has been studied in 1357 psoriasis patients who received at least one course of AMEVIVE, of whom 876 patients received their first course in placebo-controlled studies. Ages ranged from 16 to 84 years with a mean age of 45 years; 69% were males and 31% were females.

Table 2 shows the incidence of adverse events experienced in at least 5% of patients in the first course of treatment in placebo-controlled studies. Adverse events overall were similar to placebo. Chills was the only event seen at an incidence of 5% or greater in AMEVIVE versus placebo-treated patients. Chills were most frequently observed within 24 hours of dosing when AMEVIVE was administered intravenously. Chills were mild to moderate severity and were not dose limiting.

Table 2: AMEVIVE

Incidence of Adverse Events Experienced in at Least 5% of Patients in the First Course of AMEVIVE (alefacept) in Placebo-controlled Studies

	AMEVIVE n=876 %	Placebo n=413 %
No. patients with an event	730 (83%)	327 (79%)
Headache	17	18
Accidental injury	15	13
Pharyngitis	15	13
Infection	11	11
Pruritus	11	8
Rhinitis	11	10
Flu syndrome	9	9
Viral infection	6	7
Asthenia	6	7
Chills	6	1
Pain	6	5
Diarrhea	5	5
Dizziness	5	3
Arthralgia	5	6
Nausea	5	3

Multiple Course Experience: In clinical studies, 346 patients received at least two courses, 125 patients received at least three courses, and 56 patients received at least four courses of AMEVIVE (alefacept) administered intravenously over a period of up to two years. The safety experience in those patients that received multiple courses of therapy was similar to that observed in patients that received a single course.

The incidence of adverse events experienced in at least 5% of patients receiving multiple courses of AMEVIVE include headache, pharyngitis, accidental injury, rhinitis, infection, flu-syndrome, pruritus, chills, asthenia, pain, diarrhea, nausea, viral infection, dizziness, and sinusitis.

Less Common Clinical Trial Adverse Drug Reactions (<1%): In the first course of placebo-controlled studies, adverse events requiring hospitalization were observed at a rate of 5% in both patients treated with AMEVIVE (alefacept) and placebo-treated patients. The rate of occurrence of these events did not increase with subsequent courses of treatment. The most commonly reported adverse events requiring hospitalization in patients treated with AMEVIVE were cardiovascular events including coronary artery disease, myocardial infarction, chest pain, atrial fibrillation, complete atrio-ventricular block, and congestive heart failure. These events were infrequent and were generally observed in patients with pre-existing risk factors.

Other less common events (incidence of at least 1%) that were observed at a higher rate in patients treated with AMEVIVE in comparison with placebo are listed below by body system.

Body as a Whole: back pain, abdominal pain, fever, malaise, chest pain.
Cardiovascular: hypertension.
Digestive: tooth disorder, periodontal abscess, vomiting.
Musculoskeletal: myalgia, arthritis.
Nervous System: anxiety, hypertonia, paresthesis, somnolence.
Respiratory: increased cough, asthma.
Skin and Appendages: rash, herpes simplex, acne, benign skin neoplasm, contact dermititis.
Special Senses: conjunctivitis.
Urogenital: vaginal moniliasis.

Use with Other Psoriasis Therapies: The safety profile of AMEVIVE (alefacept) was evaluated when used in combination with other psoriasis treatments. In two studies involving 261 patients AMEVIVE 15 mg once weekly for 12 weeks was used both alone (n=116) or in combination with either UVB (n=49) or cyclosporine (n=16) or methotrexate (n=21) or systemic retinoids (n=10), or mid- to high- potency topical treatments (n=48). The incidence of adverse events was similar in all the patient groups that received combination therapies. The safety profile was demonstrated to be similar to that observed in the phase III clinical trials in terms of the types and frequencies of adverse events, indicating that AMEVIVE, in combination with other psoriasis treatments, was well tolerated. The most common adverse events were headache (12%) and nasopharyngitis(8%).

In both studies, there were no reports of opportunistic infection nor was there an increased risk of infection or malignancy observed. Three patients had non-serious skin malignancies diagnosed. One patient receiving AMEVIVE alone had both a squamous cell and a basal cell carcinoma, one patient receiving AMEVIVE with 12 weeks UVB experienced a basal cell carcinoma and one patient receiving AMEVIVE with cyclosporine experienced a squamous cell carcinoma. During the dosing period at the time of maximal reduction in circulating CD4 T-cell counts no significant differences were observed between those patients receiving AMEVIVE alone or those patients receiving AMEVIVE in combination with the other psoriasis treatments. The clinical correlation and significance of these results require further assessment.

DRUG INTERACTIONS: Overview: No formal drug interaction studies have been conducted with AMEVIVE (alefacept). Topical medications such as topical steroids and emollients can be used concomitantly with AMEVIVE.

DOSAGE AND ADMINISTRATION: Dosing Considerations:

- AMEVIVE (alefacept) is intended for use under the guidance and supervision of a health care professional.
- Patients may self-inject the intramuscular injection only if their physician determines that it is appropriate and with medical follow-up, as necessary, after proper training in IM injection technique.
- Total lymphocyte and CD4+ T lymphocyte counts should be normal prior to initiating treatment with AMEVIVE. CD4+ T lymphocyte counts should be monitored every two weeks during the 12-week dosing regimen. Dosing should be withheld if CD4+ T lymphocyte counts are below 250 cells/µL. AMEVIVE should be discontinued if the counts remain below 250 cells/µL for one month (see Warnings and Precautions, Monitoring and Laboratory Tests).

Recommended Dose and Dosage Adjustment:

- 15 mg given once weekly as an intramuscular injection

The recommended regimen is a course of up to 12 injections over a 12-week period. Intermittent re-treatment with subsequent courses may be initiated as needed provided that total lymphocyte and CD4+ T cell counts are within the normal range and a minimum of a 12-week interval has passed between courses of treatment.

Missed Dose: If you forget to take a dose on the day it is scheduled, you should contact your doctor.

Administration: AMEVIVE (alefacept) must be reconstituted with supplied sterile Water for Injection using aseptic technique prior to intramuscular administration.

Reconstitution: Parenteral Products:

Vial Size	Volume of Water for Injection to be used for reconstitution	Available Volume	Nominal Concentration per 0.5 mL
15 mg for intramuscular administration	0.6 mL	0.5 mL	15 mg

During reconstitution of AMEVIVE, inject the sterile Water for Injection very slowly into the vial, keeping the needle pointed at the sidewall of the vial. Some foaming will occur, which is normal. To avoid excessive foaming, do not shake or vigorously agitate. The contents should be swirled gently during dissolution. Generally, dissolution of AMEVIVE takes less than two minutes.

The reconstituted solution should be clear and colourless to slightly yellow and used as soon as possible after reconstitution. Visually inspect the solution for particulate matter and discolouration prior to administration. The solution should not be used if discoloured or cloudy, or if particulate matter remains.

Remove the needle used for reconstitution and attach the other supplied needle. Withdraw the solution into the syringe, removing only 0.5 mL from the vial. Some foam or bubbles may remain in the vial.

Do not add other medications to solutions containing AMEVIVE. Do not reconstitute AMEVIVE with other diluents. Do not filter reconstituted solution during preparation or administration.

Once reconstituted, the solution should be used immediately.

For intramuscular use, inject the full 0.5 mL of solution. Rotate injection sites so that a different site is used for each new injection. New injections should be given at least 1 inch from an old site and never into areas where the skin is tender, bruised, red or hard.

OVERDOSE:

Symptoms: The highest doses tested in humans (up to 0.75 mg/kg IV) were associated with chills, headache, arthralgia, and sinusitis.

Treatment: Patients inadvertently administered an excess of the recommended dose should be monitored for effects on total lymphocyte count and CD4+ T cell count.

> For management of a suspected drug overdose, CPhA recommends that you contact your **regional Poison Control Centre**. See the *CPS* Directory section for a list of Poison Control Centres.

ACTION AND CLINICAL PHARMACOLOGY: Mechanism of Action: AMEVIVE (alefacept) exerts its effect via a dual mechanism of action. Chronic plaque psoriasis is a T cell mediated disorder that is characterized by the presence of memory-effector T cells (CD45RO+) in skin lesions. The majority of T cells express activation markers (CD2, CD25, CD69) and release inflammatory cytokines (IFNγ). T lymphocyte activation includes an interaction between LFA-3 on antigen presenting cells (APC) and CD2 on T lymphocytes. AMEVIVE prevents T cell activation by specifically binding to CD2 on the T-cell thereby inhibiting the interaction between CD2 on the T-cell and LFA-3 on the Antigen Presenting Cell. In addition, the Fc portion of AMEVIVE binds to Fc gamma receptors on cytotoxic cells, such as natural killer cells, leading to apoptosis of CD2+ target T cells. AMEVIVE selectively targets T cells that express high levels of CD2, such as activated and memory-effector T cells.

In vivo, exposure to AMEVIVE is associated with reductions in the number of circulating activated CD25+, CD4+CD45RO+, and CD8+CD45RO+ memory-effector T cells, detectable as a reduced total lymphocyte, CD4+, or CD8+ T cell count. Repeat courses of alefacept induce effects that are similar on circulating total lymphocytes as those seen following one course of therapy.

CD4+ and CD8+ T cells are the predominant phenotype within the psoriatic lesions. The reduction of CD4+CD45RO+ and CD8+CD45RO+ memory T cells is correlated with clinical outcome after the administration of AMEVIVE to psoriatic patients. Patients with a >50% reduction in Psoriasis Area Severity Index (PASI) score had a significant reduction in intra-lesional lymphocytes, particularly IFNγ-secreting T cells.

Pharmacodynamics: Therapy with AMEVIVE (alefacept) results in dose-dependent decreases in circulating total lymphocyte, CD4+, and CD8+ T cell counts. AMEVIVE does not cause general immunosuppresion. Rather, AMEVIVE exhibits specificity against CD4+CD45RO+ and CD8+CD45RO+ memory-effector T cells (see Figure 1). Naïve T cells (CD4+CD45RA+ and CD8+CD45RA+), B cells, and natural killer cells do not demonstrate significant changes in circulating levels during single or multiple courses of AMEVIVE therapy. Reductions in lymphocyte counts could occur in the first six weeks of therapy.

Figure 1: AMEVIVE

Effect of AMEVIVE on Naïve and Memory-Effector T Cells

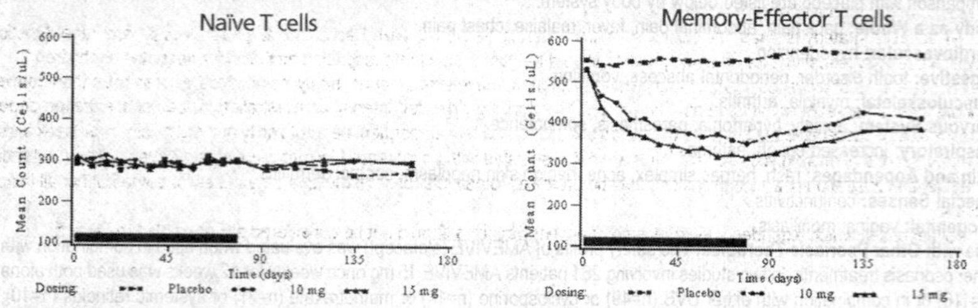

Legend: Solid bar indicates dosing interval.

Pharmacokinetics: The pharmacokinetics of AMEVIVE (alefacept) have been evaluated following both single and repeat dosing by intravenous (IV) and intramuscular (IM) routes of administration. Following repeat dosing to psoriasis patients, the disposition of AMEVIVE was consistent following IV and IM dosing. The bioavailability of AMEVIVE following IM administration in healthy volunteer studies was approximately 63%.

Table 3: AMEVIVE

Pharmacokinetic parameters of AMEVIVE following repeat-dosing to psoriasis patients

	Mean elimination $t_{1/2}$ (h)	Mean clearance (mL/h/kg)	Mean volume of distribution (mL/kg)
15 mg IM injection n=166	270	0.46[a]	167[a]
7.5 mg IV injection n=520	267	0.25	94

[a] Unadjusted for bioavailability

Special Populations and Conditions: Pediatrics and Geriatrics: The pharmacokinetics of AMEVIVE (alefacept) in children and the elderly have not been studied.

Gender or Race: No differences in pharmacokinetics have been observed as a function of gender or ethnicity.

Hepatic or Renal Insufficiency: Effects on the pharmacokinetics of AMEVIVE have not been studied.

Duration of Effect: Duration of effect represents the maximum period of response. In general, clinical responses to AMEVIVE (alefacept) were durable. Patients were followed for up to 36 weeks following the completion of dosing patients with AMEVIVE (Study 1, cohort 2). Patients achieving a 75% reduction in PASI following a single 12-week treatment of AMEVIVE maintained at least a 50% reduction in PASI for a median of over seven months (216 days).

This remittive and sustained effectiveness was also observed with patients who reached a PGA of "almost clear" or "clear". A prolonged effect of at least a 50% reduction in PASI for a median of eight months (241 days) was maintained in these patients.

Following repeat courses of therapy, median duration of response was generally longer than following a single course. Intermittent treatment with additional 12-week courses of AMEVIVE therapy has been demonstrated to be safe and effective. Courses were separated by at least a 12-week monitoring period (see Dosage and Administration).

Following cessation of treatment, no disease rebound or flaring occurred at any time in either study.

STORAGE AND STABILITY: Do not use a dose administration pack beyond the expiry date stamped on the carton, dose tray label, vial label, or diluent container label. The dose administration pack containing AMEVIVE (alefacept) lyophilized powder must be stored in the refrigerator (2 to 8°C).

If refrigeration is unavailable, AMEVIVE can be stored at temperatures up to 30°C for up to 48 hours.

Once reconstituted, the solution should be used immediately. If not administered immediately after reconstitution, AMEVIVE may be stored in the vial for up to 4 hours if refrigerated at 2 to 8°C. **Any AMEVIVE not used within 4 hours of reconstitution should be discarded.**

INFORMATION FOR THE PATIENT: Published in e-CPS, available by subscription at www.e-cps.ca.

DOSAGE FORMS, COMPOSITION AND PACKAGING: Each single-use vial of sterile, white to off-white, preservative-free, lyophilized powder for parenteral administration contains: alefacept 15 mg. Nonmedicinal ingredients: citric acid monohydrate, glycine, sodium citrate dihydrate and sucrose. Each dose pack contains one 15 mg single-use vial of AMEVIVE, one single-use 10 mL sterile Water for Injection vial, one syringe, two needles, two alcohol prep pads, one gauze pad, and one bandage. Cartons containing 1 and 4 administration dose packs.

Amikacin 🄿

Antibacterial

CPhA Monograph

Date of Preparation: November 2007

> This monograph has been compiled by CPhA and reviewed by experts. It may contain information different from that found in Health Canada-approved Product Monographs. The reader is referred to the *CPS* Editorial Policy for more information.

SUMMARY PRODUCT INFORMATION:

Route of Administration	Dosage Form	Strength
Injectable (IV, IM)	Solution	250 mg/mL (2 mL)

INDICATIONS AND CLINICAL USE: Amikacin is an aminoglycoside antibacterial agent. The spectrum of activity of amikacin includes primarily aerobic gram-negative bacteria including nosocomial pathogens.

Amikacin is indicated for:

- treatment of nosocomial infections due to susceptible aerobic gram-negative bacteria
- use in synergistic antibacterial combination regimens for empiric treatment of hospital-acquired pneumonia, ventilator-associated pneumonia in patients with late-onset disease or risk factors for multidrug-resistant pathogens
- empiric treatment of infections in febrile neutropenic patients in combination with another agent
- treatment of active *M. tuberculosis* infection, when used as a second-line agent in combination with other antitubercular agents
- treatment of nontubercular mycobacterial infections when used in combination with other agents

Aminoglycosides are active against *P. aeruginosa*. Among aerobic gram-negative bacteria, *S. maltophilia* and *B. cepacia* are unusual in that they are not considered to be susceptible to aminoglycosides. Amikacin is active against *M. tuberculosis* and a wide range of nontuberculous mycobacteria including *M. avium* complex, *M. kansasii*, *M. abscessus*, *M. chelonae*, *M. fortuitum*, *M. haemophilum*, *M. immunogenum* and *M. smegmatis*. Amikacin has less activity against *M. chelonae* than tobramycin.

Anaerobic bacteria are not susceptible to aminoglycosides.

Acquired resistance to aminoglycosides is mediated via numerous aminoglycoside-modifying enzymes produced by bacteria that alter specific amino or hydroxyl functions on the drug. Acquired resistance to one aminoglycoside does not necessarily confer resistance to other agents in the class.

Amikacin is eliminated almost exclusively by renal excretion and is associated with nephrotoxicity. For this reason the drug must be used with caution and the dose must be individualized in patients with renal impairment. Monitoring of renal function (i.e., BUN and serum creatinine) is recommended during treatment.

Amikacin is also associated with ototoxicity, which is usually not reversible. Some individuals are predisposed to aminoglycoside-associated ototoxicity because of a maternally inherited mutation in mitochondrial DNA that makes the human mitochondrial ribosome more closely resemble the bacterial ribosome, which is the site of action for these drugs [BMJ 2007;335:784-5].

Geriatrics: Elderly patients may be more susceptible to aminoglycoside-associated nephrotoxicity due to the age-related decline in renal function. The dosage regimen of amikacin must be tailored to renal function.

Pediatrics: Aminoglycoside antibiotics have been used extensively in pediatric patients including neonates. Changes in renal function during the neonatal period (see Warnings and Precautions, Special Populations, Pediatrics) must be considered when selecting a dosing regimen for amikacin or another aminoglycoside antibiotic.

CONTRAINDICATIONS:

- Patients who are hypersensitive to amikacin, or other aminoglycoside antibiotics, or to any ingredient in the formulation.

WARNINGS AND PRECAUTIONS:

> **Serious Warnings and Precautions**
> - Nephrotoxicity and ototoxicity are serious adverse effects associated with amikacin and other aminoglycosides. These effects may be seen in any patient treated with these drugs, but are more likely to occur in the following settings: pre-existing renal, vestibular or auditory impairment, older individuals, dehydration, concomitant therapy with other nephrotoxic or ototoxic agents, or prolonged therapy.
> - Neuromuscular blockade has been associated with aminoglycoside antibiotics.

Neurologic: Aminoglycosides are associated with eighth cranial nerve toxicity, which may affect the vestibular and the auditory senses. Symptoms of vestibular toxicity include nausea, vomiting, dizziness, nystagmus, vertigo and ataxia. Symptoms of cochlear (auditory) toxicity include tinnitus, roaring in the ears and hearing impairment. Loss of high frequency auditory perception, which may be detected by audiometric testing, usually precedes clinically detectable hearing loss. Some individuals have a genetic predisposition to aminoglycoside-induced ototoxicity. Ototoxicity has occurred within the recommended target serum concentration range. Patients receiving high cumulative doses of amikacin or therapy for protracted periods are at increased risk of developing ototoxicity. In patients receiving protracted therapy, consideration should be given to performing regular audiograms (e.g., weekly) to detect signs of ototoxicity before it becomes clinically significant.

Neuromuscular blockade associated with aminoglycosides is dose-related and generally self-limiting, but may rarely lead to respiratory muscle paralysis. Clinical manifestations include flaccid paralysis, dilated pupils and weakness of the respiratory musculature. Neuromuscular effects occur more commonly after application to serosal surfaces (e.g., after intrapleural injection or peritoneal instillation), after administration to patients with neuromuscular disease (e.g., myasthenia gravis), hypocalcemia or hypomagnesemia, or after concomitant administration with neuromuscular blocking agents. Rapid injection of aminoglycoside antibiotics is a risk factor for neuromuscular blockade; therefore, these drugs should be infused over at least 30 minutes.

Perioperative Considerations: Aminoglycosides may produce neuromuscular blockade when used in combination with neuromuscular blocking agents (e.g., succinylcholine, tubocurarine).

Renal: Aminoglycosides are associated with renal tubular necrosis, which decreases the glomerular filtration rate and is reflected in increased concentrations of BUN and serum creatinine. Aminoglycoside-associated nephrotoxicity is most often evident as nonoliguric azotemia; oliguria is rare. Changes in renal function are usually reversible when the drug is discontinued.

Patient-related factors associated with an increased risk of aminoglycoside-associated nephrotoxicity include older age, pre-existing renal disease, volume depletion, hypotension, hepatic dysfunction and recent treatment with an aminoglycoside antibiotic. Concomitant administration of nephrotoxic drugs may increase the clinical risk of aminoglycoside-associated nephrotoxicity.

Factors that decrease the risk of aminoglycoside-associated nephrotoxicity include younger age, normal renal and hepatic function, use of smaller cumulative doses and treatment for less than 3 days, and use of extended interval dosing ("once daily") regimens (see Dosage and Administration).

Nephrotoxicity has occurred within the recommended target serum concentration range. Peak serum aminoglycoside levels are not a clinical risk factor for aminoglycoside-associated nephrotoxicity. In contrast, nephrotoxicity is associated with persistently elevated trough serum concentrations.

Special Populations: Pregnant Women: Amikacin crosses the placenta and is distributed into the fetal circulation and amniotic fluid; it is not considered to be teratogenic and has been used to treat serious infections in pregnancy.

Nursing Women: Amikacin is excreted in breast milk, but is considered to be compatible with breast-feeding because it is minimally absorbed from the gastrointestinal tract.

Pediatrics: Amikacin is used in children and for the treatment of suspected or confirmed infections in neonates. The pharmacokinetics of amikacin differs in neonates compared with older children in that renal clearance of the drug is prolonged in neonates. Specialized references for neonates and children should be consulted.

Geriatrics: Elimination of amikacin is prolonged in elderly patients because of the age-related decline in glomerular filtration rate. Renal function should be determined at baseline and monitored during therapy with amikacin. Specific dosage guidelines should be consulted and the dosage regimen should be adjusted according to renal function.

Monitoring and Laboratory Tests: Renal function (BUN and serum creatinine) should be monitored before and during therapy with amikacin.

When extended interval dosing (Table 6) of amikacin is employed it is not necessary to monitor peak serum drug levels. Some extended interval dosing protocols require measurement of the serum concentration.

It is necessary to measure serum drug concentrations and individualize the dose of amikacin if achievement of specific peak and trough serum concentrations is desired. Some authors have argued that dose individualization is preferred to the use of dosing nomograms because of the wide interindividual variation in aminoglycoside pharmacokinetics [see Clin Pharmacokinet 1999;36(2):89-98 and Pharmacotherapy 2002;22(9):1077-1083].

If amikacin is dosed in the conventional manner (Table 7), monitoring of peak and trough amikacin levels is recommended in patients receiving prolonged courses of therapy, and in those with renal dysfunction or serious infections. Calculation of pharmacokinetic parameters is done with steady state versions of one-compartment equations. Serum concentrations should be measured at steady state, which is achieved after 3 to 5 half-lives have elapsed. If no loading dose is administered, steady state will usually be achieved after the third or fourth dose (this is also the case after each dose adjustment). Peak concentrations should be measured after the distribution phase is complete; ideally 30 to 60 minutes after the end of the infusion. Trough concentrations may be measured 30 minutes before infusion of the next dose. Specific target peak and trough concentrations are provided in Table 7. If a higher peak concentration is desired, the dose of amikacin should be increased. If a lower trough concentration is desired, prolonging the dosing interval is preferred. Determination of peak and trough levels should be repeated after dosage adjustments to ensure the desired results have been obtained.

ADVERSE REACTIONS: More Common Adverse Drug Reactions (> 1%): See Table 1.

Table 1: Amikacin

More Common Adverse Drug Reactions (≥ 1%)

Body System	Effect	Clinical Comment
Renal	Nephrotoxicity. Damage to proximal tubule marked by elevated BUN, elevated serum creatinine and decreased urine specific gravity. May involve proteinuria, nonoliguric azotemia, aminoaciduria and metabolic acidosis, electrolyte wasting and renal failure.	Monitor renal function at baseline and during treatment. Individualize dose based on renal function and adjust the dose based on changes in renal function and or serum drug levels. Consider alternative antibiotics in patients at risk.

Less Common Adverse Drug Reactions (< 1%): Overview: Cardiovascular: tachycardia, hypotension, hypertension.

Central Nervous System: headache, dizziness, nystagmus, vertigo, ataxia, tinnitus, roaring in the ears, hearing impairment, loss of high frequency hearing perception.

Allergic/Dermatologic: local irritation, phlebitis, rash, urticaria, stomatitis, pruritus, fever, toxic epidermal necrolysis, erythema multiforme, Stevens-Johnson syndrome. Hypersensitivity reactions are rare with aminoglycosides. Cross-allergenicity with aminoglycosides has been reported.

Gastrointestinal: anorexia, weight loss, nausea and vomiting.

Hematologic: anemia, leukopenia, granulocytopenia, thrombocytopenia.

Hepatic/Biliary/Pancreatic: hepatic necrosis, hepatomegaly, splenomegaly, transient increase in serum transaminase, alkaline phosphatase and bilirubin levels.

Neurologic: peripheral neuropathy, numbness, tingling, muscle twitching, seizures, myasthenia gravis-like syndrome, tremor.

Abnormal Hematologic and Clinical Chemistry Findings: See Table 2.

DRUG INTERACTIONS:

Serious Drug Interactions

- Concomitant administration of nephrotoxic drugs may increase the clinical risk of aminoglycoside-associated nephrotoxicity.
- Concomitant administration of amikacin with neuromuscular blocking agents may result in an increased risk of neuromuscular blockade.

Overview: Because potential drug interactions involving amikacin generally involve combinations that result in additive nephrotoxicity or ototoxicity, it is best to avoid combined use of amikacin with any agent that is known to be nephrotoxic or ototoxic. If combined use cannot be avoided, monitoring of renal function and serum amikacin levels and adjustment of the dosage of amikacin are recommended. Amikacin does not alter the pharmacokinetics of other drugs.

Drug-Drug Interactions: See Table 3.

Table 2: Amikacin

Abnormal Hematologic and Clinical Chemistry Findings

Test	Effect	Clinical Comment
BUN	Increased	An increase in BUN and serum creatinine over baseline is an indication of nephrotoxicity. In patients with a serum creatinine in the normal range before therapy, an increase to > 133 µmol/L or an absolute increase of > 35 µmol/L may indicate nephrotoxicity. In patients with a baseline serum creatinine concentration > 133 µmol/L, an increase of > 44 µmol/L is indicative of nephrotoxicity; in those with a baseline serum creatinine concentration > 265 µmol/L, an increase of > 88 µmol/L is indicative of nephrotoxicity. If nephrotoxicity occurs during treatment with amikacin, the preferred strategy is discontinuation of the drug and substitution with an alternative non-nephrotoxic agent. If discontinuation is not possible, then the dosage should be adjusted accordingly and renal function monitored.
Serum creatinine	Increased	

Table 3: Amikacin

Drug-Drug Interactions

Interacting Drug	Effect	Clinical Comment
Amphotericin B	Additive nephrotoxicity	Monitor renal function and adjust the dose of amikacin if BUN or SCr increases.
Cisplatin	Additive nephrotoxicity	Monitor renal function and adjust the dose of amikacin if BUN or SCr increases.
Cyclosporine	Additive nephrotoxicity	Monitor renal function and adjust the dose of amikacin if BUN or SCr increases.
Vancomycin	Additive nephrotoxicity	Monitor renal function and adjust the dose of amikacin if BUN or SCr increases.
Ethacrynic acid	Additive ototoxicity	Avoid combination use. Monitor for signs and symptoms of ototoxicity.
Furosemide or bumetanide	Increased risk of nephrotoxicity or ototoxicity	Monitor renal function and adjust the dose of amikacin if BUN or SCr increases Monitor for signs of ototoxicity.
Indomethacin	Increased amikacin serum levels in infants	Monitor renal function and serum levels of amikacin and adjust the dose of amikacin accordingly.
Neuromuscular blocking agents	Additive neuromuscular blockade	Monitor respiratory function. Provide supportive care if an interaction occurs. May respond to neostigmine.
Botulinum toxin	Additive neuromuscular blockade	Avoid concurrent use. If given together, monitor respiratory function.

DOSAGE AND ADMINISTRATION: Dosing Considerations: Amikacin may be administered by iv or im injection.

In contemporary clinical practice there are two broad strategies used to dose amikacin. Extended interval ("once daily") administration involves administration of single large iv doses of amikacin at prolonged intervals (i.e., 24 hours or longer). The alternative (conventional) approach involves administering lower doses of the drug at more frequent intervals (e.g., q8h) with monitoring of peak and trough serum concentrations.

Whichever strategy is used, the dose of amikacin should be individualized according to patient weight and renal function. Specific recommendations for pediatric patients should be consulted when prescribing amikacin for neonates or children.

Several lines of evidence suggest that extended interval administration of aminoglycosides may be less toxic than conventional three-times-daily administration. The principles underlying extended interval administration include concentration-dependent killing of susceptible bacteria, the post-antibiotic effect, and time-dependent nephrotoxicity and ototoxicity. High peak serum concentrations of aminoglycoside antibiotics are not associated with an increased incidence of adverse events. Thus, extended interval administration of aminoglycosides may be preferred to administration of multiple daily doses for some but not all indications.

Situations in which extended interval dosing of aminoglycosides should not be considered are presented in Table 5.

Table 4: Amikacin

Indications and Recommended Regimens

Indication	Route	Recommended Regimen (see also Table 5, Table 6, Table 7, Table 8)	Duration of Treatment	Clinical Comment
Treatment of serious infections in adults	IV/IM	Extended interval ("once daily") iv dosing. Alternative: conventional divided daily dosing.	Dependent upon susceptibility of organisms and response to therapy.	Usually used in combination with other agents. Switch to a suitable oral antibiotic as soon as feasible.
Empiric treatment of febrile neutropenic adult patients	IV/IM	Extended interval ("once daily") iv dosing. Alternative: conventional divided daily dosing.	Dependent upon susceptibility of organisms and response to therapy.	Administer in combination with a broad spectrum antipseudomonal agent (i.e., cephalosporin, antipseudomonal penicillin, carbapenem). Monitor renal function and adjust dosage (as per Table 8 recommendations).
M. tuberculosis	IV/IM	Usual adult dose: 15 mg/kg once daily (max 1000 mg) Patients aged > 50 years: 10 mg/kg once daily (max 750 mg) Children: 15–30 mg/kg once daily (max 1000 mg)	Administer on 5 to 7 days per week during the first 2 to 4 months of therapy, then 2 or 3 times per week after culture conversion depending on the sensitivity of the isolate.	Given only in combination with other agents. Amikacin is a second-line agent.
M. avium complex lung disease in adults	IV/IM	25 mg/kg/day three times weekly	Give during the first 2 to 3 months of therapy.	Given only in combination with other agents for treatment of patients with cavitary disease, severe disease or previously-treated disease.
M. avium complex infection in patients with AIDS	IV/IM	Adults: 10–15 mg/kg once daily Children: 15–30 mg/kg/day in one or two divided doses (max 1500 mg)	Treatment of MAC is lifelong unless immune restoration is achieved with antiretroviral therapy.	Given only in combination with other agents. Amikacin is considered an alternative agent for use in patients with severe or disseminated disease.
M. abscessus infection in adults	IV/IM	10–15 mg/kg once daily Or 25 mg/kg three times weekly	Treat serious skin and soft tissue infections for a minimum of 4 months and bone infections for 6 months. Periodic administration of amikacin plus other agents over several months may help control symptoms and retard progression of lung infections, which are more difficult to treat than skin, soft tissue and bone infections.	Given only in combination with other agents.

There are several protocols for extended interval dosing of aminoglycosides. One approach is presented in Table 6. The Hartford method is an alternative in which the dose of amikacin is 15 mg/kg. The serum concentration is determined 6 to 14 hours after the start of an infusion and the measured serum level is divided by 2 and plotted on the nomogram to determine the dosage interval [Antimicrob Agent Chemother 1995;39:650-55]. The Hartford nomogram and more information on this method is available online at www.bugsanddrugs.ca.

Recommended Dose and Dosage Adjustment: See Table 4 Table 5, Table 6, Table 7, Table 8, Table 9 and Table 10.

Table 5: Amikacin

Situations in Which Extended Interval ("Once Daily") Dosing of Amikacin is not Recommended in Adults

Extensive burns (> 20% body surface area)
Ascites (altered volume of distribution)
Pregnancy/postpartum (altered volume of distribution)
Patients with gram-positive infections for which gentamicin is used for synergy (exception: endocarditis due to viridans group streptococci)
Surgical prophylaxis

Table 6: Amikacin

Extended Interval ("Once Daily") Administration in Adults[a]

Estimated ClCr[b] (mL/min)	Dosage interval (h)	Dose (mg/kg IBW[c])
90	24	15
70	24	12
50	24	7.5
30	24	4
20	48	7.5
10	48	4
Hemodialysis	48 (give after dialysis)	3

[a] Measure the trough level prior to the third dose.

[b] ClCr=creatinine clearance (estimate using the Cockcroft-Gault equation)

$$\text{ClCr (mL/min)} = \frac{1.2\ (140 - \text{age})\ (\text{wt in kg})}{\text{serum creatinine } (\mu\text{mol/L})}$$

For females, multiply the result by 0.85.

[c] IBW = ideal body weight.
IBW (kg; males) = 50 + (2.3 × height in inches over 5 feet).
IBW (kg; females) = 45.5 + (2.3 × height in inches over 5 feet).
Adjusted body weight (ABW) has been recommended for dosing aminoglycosides in obese individuals (i.e. if total body weight is >25% above the IBW [see Br J Clin Pharmacol 2004;58(2):119-33 and Antimicrob Agents Chemother 1995;39(2):545-8].
ABW = IBW + 0.4 × (total body weight−IBW).

Table 7: Amikacin

Conventional Dosing in Adults with ClCr >90 mL/min (as an alternative to extended interval dosing)

Route	Loading Dose	Maintenance Dose	Desired Serum Concentration	
			Peak	Trough
IV/IM	7.5 mg/kg (IBW[a])	5 mg/kg (IBW) q8h	20–30 μg/mL	< 8 μg/mL

[a] IBW = ideal body weight.
IBW (kg; males) = 50 + (2.3 × height in inches over 5 feet).
IBW (kg; females) = 45.5 + (2.3 × height in inches over 5 feet).
Adjusted body weight (ABW) has been recommended for dosing aminoglycosides in obese individuals (i.e. if total body weight is > 25% above the IBW [see Br J Clin Pharmacol 2004;58(2):119-33 and Antimicrob Agents Chemother 1995;39(2):545-8].
ABW = IBW + 0.4 × (total body weight−IBW).

Table 8: Amikacin

Conventional Dose in Adults with Renal Dysfunction (as an alternative to extended interval dosing)

Route	ClCr[a] (mL/min)	Dose	Clinical comment
IV/IM	> 50–90	60–90% of recommended dose q12h (see Table 7)	Monitor serum concentration and adjust dosage regimen to achieve desired peak and trough serum levels.
IV/IM	10–50	30–70% of recommended dose q12–18h (see Table 7)	
IV/IM	< 10	20–30% of recommended dose q24–48h (see Table 7)	
IV/IM	Hemodialysis	Dose as for ClCr < 10 mL/min; give supplemental ½ dose after dialysis	

[a] ClCr=creatinine clearance (estimate using the Cockcroft-Gault equation)

$$\text{ClCr (mL/min)} = \frac{1.2\ (140 - \text{age})\ (\text{wt in kg})}{\text{serum creatinine } (\mu\text{mol/L})}$$

For females, multiply the result by 0.85.

Dosage in Continuous Ambulatory Peritoneal Dialysis: In adult patients receiving continuous ambulatory peritoneal dialysis it is estimated that 15 to 20 mg of amikacin will be lost per litre of dialysate each day. Thus in a patient receiving 8 L of dialysate per day a total of 120 to 160 mg will be lost daily and may be replaced intravenously.

In patients receiving hemodialysis a supplemental dose of 50% may be given after each dialysis session.

Hepatic Impairment: Amikacin is not eliminated by hepatic metabolism; hence no dosage adjustments are required in patients with hepatic dysfunction. However, patients with severe hepatic dysfunction are at increased risk of nephrotoxicity, so careful monitoring of renal function is advised in these individuals.

Pediatrics: Regimens recommended in the SickKids Drug Handbook and Formulary 2007–2008 are presented in Table 9 for neonates and in Table 10 for older infants and children.

There have been numerous studies of extended interval dosing of aminoglycosides in children. A meta-analysis of 24 studies concluded that this approach simplifies administration and provides similar or better efficacy and safety compared with conventional multiple daily dose regimens [Pediatrics 2004;114(1):111-8]. Amikacin was administered at dosages ranging from 15 to 20 mg/kg once daily in the studies that were considered in the analysis.

Table 9: Amikacin

Dose in Neonates

Route	Age and Weight	Dose
IV	Neonates ≤ 7 days and < 2 kg[a]	15 mg/kg/day divided q12h
IV	Neonates ≤ 7 days and ≥ 2 kg[a]	20 mg/kg/day divided q12h
IV	Neonates > 7 days and < 2 kg[a]	20 mg/kg/day divided q8h
IV	Neonates > 7 days and ≥ 2 kg[a]	30 mg/kg/day divided q8h (maximum 500 mg/dose prior to measuring serum levels)
The peak concentration is measured 30 to 60 minutes after infusion to allow for distribution. If given q8h the trough concentration is measured 30 minutes prior to infusion of the next dose. The desired trough level is 2.5–10 μg/mL and the desired peak concentration is 15–35 μg/mL.		

[a] Applies to neonates until a postconceptual age of > 38 weeks and a postnatal age of 28 days is achieved [SickKids Drug Handbook and Formulary 2007-2008].

Table 10: Amikacin

Dose in Pediatric Patients

Route	Age and Weight	Dose
IM/IV	Infants > 28 days and children	15–30 mg/kg/day divided q8h
IV	Infants and children > 28 days[a]	20 mg/kg/day q24h (no dose limit)
If given q8h the peak concentration is measured 30 to 60 minutes after infusion to allow for distribution. If given q8h the trough concentration is measured 30 minutes prior to infusion of the next dose. The desired trough level is 2.5–10 μg/mL and the desired peak concentration is 15–35 μg/mL.		

[a] This regimen is used in hematology and oncology patients and in recipients of hematopoietic progenitor cell transplants with fever and neutropenia [SickKids Drug Handbook and Formulary 2007-2008].

Administration: Amikacin may be administered by iv or im injection. It is impractical to administer large injection volumes, such as those required in extended interval regimens, by im injection. When large doses are given by iv infusion the drug should be infused over at least 30 minutes to minimize the possibility of neuromuscular blockade.

OVERDOSAGE:

For management of a suspected drug overdose, CPhA recommends that you contact your **regional Poison Control Centre**. See the *CPS* Directory section for a list of Poison Control Centres.

ACTION AND CLINICAL PHARMACOLOGY: Mechanism of Action: Amikacin is highly water soluble, a property that limits its ability to cross lipid-rich cellular membranes. The drug is also positively charged, such that activity is enhanced at alkaline pH and decreased at acidic pH. Transport of aminoglycosides across bacterial cytoplasmic membranes is an energy-dependent process. Amikacin binds to the 30S subunit of prokaryotic ribosomes. This results in a conformational change in the structure of the ribosomal subunit and impairs messenger RNA translation and translocation. The drug also binds electrostatically to the lipopolysaccharide layer of gram-negative bacteria, an effect that ultimately disrupts the permeability of the bacterial cell wall.

Aminoglycosides are bactericidal antibiotics that are characterized by concentration-dependent killing of susceptible bacteria. As the rate of killing increases in proportion to the serum concentration, achievement of higher serum concentrations may enhance efficacy. This phenomenon forms part of the rationale for extended interval dosing regimens.

Aminoglycosides are associated with a significant post-antibiotic effect. This phenomenon results in persistent suppression of bacterial growth after exposure to the antibiotic. The duration of the post-antibiotic effect is prolonged after exposure to high drug concentrations and persists after the concentration falls below the minimal inhibitory concentration of the organism. The post-antibiotic effect forms part of the rationale for extended interval dosing of aminoglycosides.

The uptake of aminoglycosides by gram-positive cocci is enhanced by concomitant exposure to cell-wall active agents, a phenomenon which forms the basis for the clinical use of aminoglycosides and penicillins as a synergistic combination against certain pathogens.

The antibacterial efficacy of aminoglycosides is not affected by the size of the inoculum.

Pharmacokinetics: Adults: Absorption: Aminoglycosides are minimally absorbed from the gastrointestinal tract and thus must be administered intravenously or intramuscularly in order to treat systemic infections. Absorption may be delayed in patients with hypotension or poor tissue perfusion.

Distribution: Aminoglycoside antibiotics are minimally bound to plasma proteins (~10%) and, given their high water solubility, are distributed in the vascular space and interstices of most tissues. Drug concentrations in interstitial fluids at steady state approximate those of plasma. The volume of distribution of aminoglycosides is typically on the order of 0.2 to 0.3 L/kg. However, the volume of distribution increases in certain clinical situations including extensive burns, ascites, pregnancy and the postpartum state.

Aminoglycosides accumulate in the cells of the proximal convoluted tubule to concentrations that exceed those in plasma. Nephrotoxicity is probably due to time-dependent accumulation of drug within cells of the proximal convoluted tubule. Thus, minimizing exposure to the drug, as with extended interval administration, may minimize the risk of nephrotoxicity. This reasoning supports the concept of extended interval administration of aminoglycosides.

Concentrations of aminoglycosides in vitreous humour are approximately 40% of serum levels. Aminoglycosides have poor penetration across the blood-brain barrier and into bronchial secretions, the biliary tract and abscesses.

Amikacin crosses the placenta and is distributed into fetal circulation and amniotic fluid. Amikacin is excreted in breast milk, but the drug is poorly absorbed orally so is unlikely to result in significant plasma levels in infants.

Excretion: Amikacin is not metabolized, but rather is eliminated almost exclusively by glomerular filtration. In adults over the age of 6 months with normal renal function, the elimination half-life of amikacin typically ranges from 2 to 3 hours. In adults with normal renal function, > 90% of an administered dose is recoverable in urine within 24 hours.

The elimination half-life may be shortened in patients with febrile conditions and is prolonged in elderly patients and in those with renal dysfunction in proportion to the extent of the impairment in glomerular filtration rate.

Special Populations: Pediatrics: The elimination half-life of aminoglycoside antibiotics is prolonged in neonates. Specific dosing guidelines should be consulted when prescribing amikacin for newborns.

Geriatrics: Due to the age-related decline in glomerular filtration rate, the terminal elimination half-life of amikacin is prolonged in elderly patients. The dose must be individualized according to renal function.

Amikacin Sulfate Injection USP

amikacin sulfate

Antibiotic

Sandoz

SUPPLIED: Each mL of sterile aqueous solution contains: amikacin sulfate equivalent to 250 mg of amikacin, sodium bisulfite, sodium citrate, sulfuric acid to adjust pH and water for injection. Single-use vials of 2 mL, boxes of 10. Store between 15 and 30°C. Protect from light. Discard unused portion.

Aminophylline

CPhA Monograph

see *Theophyllines*

Aminophylline

aminophylline

Bronchodilator

Hospira

SUPPLIED: Each mL contains: aminophylline 25 mg. Nonmedicinal ingredients: ethylenediamine and water for injection. Ampuls of 10 and 20 mL, boxes of 5. Protect from light.

Amiodarone Hydrochloride for Injection Sandoz Standard

amiodarone HCl

Antiarrhythmic

Sandoz

PHARMACOLOGY: Amiodarone hydrochloride is generally considered a Class III antiarrhythmic drug, but it possesses electrophysiologic characteristics of all four Vaughan Williams classes. Like Class I drugs, amiodarone blocks sodium channels at rapid pacing frequencies, and like Class II drugs, it exerts antisympathetic activity. One of its main effects, with prolonged administration, is to lengthen the cardiac action potential, a Class III effect. The negative chronotropic effect of amiodarone in nodal tissues is similar to the effect of Class IV drugs. In addition to blocking sodium channels, amiodarone blocks myocardial potassium channels, which contributes to the slowing of conduction and prolongation of refractoriness. The antisympathetic action and block of calcium and potassium channels are responsible for the negative dromotropic effects on the sinus node and for the slowing of conduction and prolongation of refractoriness in the atrioventricular (AV) node.

Additionally, amiodarone has vasodilatory action that can decrease cardiac workload and consequently myocardial oxygen consumption.

A comparison of the electrophysiologic effects of oral and IV amiodarone is shown in Table 1.

Table 1: Amiodarone Hydrochloride for Injection Sandoz Standard

Effects of Oral and IV Amiodarone HCl on Electrophysiologic Parameters

Formulation	SCL	QRS	QTc	AH	HV	ERP RA	ERP RV	ERP AVN
Oral	↑	←→	↑	↑	←→	↑	↑	↑
I.V.	←→	←→	←→	↑	←→	←→	←→	↑

←→ No change.

Legend: SCL=sinus cycle length; QRS=a measure of intraventricular conduction; QTc=corrected QT, a measure of repolarization; AH=atrial HIS, a measure of intranodal conduction; HV=HIS ventricular, a measure of intranodal conduction; ERP=effective refractory period; RA=right atrium; RV=right ventricle; AVN=atrioventricular node.

At higher doses (>10 mg/kg) of intravenous amiodarone, prolongation of the ERP RV and modest prolongation of the QRS have been seen. These differences between oral and intravenous administration suggest that the initial acute effects of intravenous amiodarone may be predominantly focused on the AV node, causing an intranodal conduction delay and increased nodal refractoriness due to calcium channel blockade (Class IV activity) and β-adrenoreceptor antagonism (Class II activity).

Pharmacodynamics: Amiodarone has been reported to produce negative inotropic and vasodilating effects in animals and humans. After long-term treatment with oral amiodarone in a dose range of 200 to 600 mg/day, patients with decreased left ventricular ejection fraction (LVEF) show no significant change in mean LVEF. Hypotension is uncommon (<1%) during chronic oral amiodarone therapy. In clinical studies of patients with refractory ventricular fibrillation (VF) or hemodynamically unstable ventricular tachycardia (VT), drug-related hypotension occurred in 15.6% of 1836 patients treated with intravenous amiodarone. No correlations have been seen between the baseline ejection fraction and the occurrence of clinically significant hypotension during intravenous infusion of amiodarone.

Rapid onset of antiarrhythmic activity, well before significant blood levels of DEA (Desethylamiodarone) are present, has been shown in both a placebo-controlled study of intravenous amiodarone in patients with supraventricular arrhythmias and 2- to 3-consecutive beat ventricular arrhythmias, and in a pharmacokinetic/pharmacodynamic study evaluating rapid intravenous loading in patients with recurrent, refractory VT/VF. Approximately 1500 mg/day of intravenous amiodarone were administered using 2- and 3-stage infusion regimens. In the patients with complex ventricular arrhythmias, including sustained and nonsustained VT, amiodarone therapy reduced episodes of VT by 85%.

The acute effectiveness of intravenous amiodarone in suppressing recurrent VF or hemodynamically unstable VT has been supported by two randomized, parallel, dose-response studies of approximately 300 patients each. In these studies, patients with at least 2 episodes of VF or hemodynamically unstable VT in the preceding 24 hours were randomly assigned to receive doses of approximately 125 or 1000 mg over the first 24 hours, an 8-fold difference. In one study, a middle dose of approximately 500 mg was evaluated. The dose regimen consisted of an initial rapid loading infusion, followed by a slower 6-hour loading infusion, and then an 18-hour maintenance infusion. The maintenance infusion was continued up to hour 48. Additional supplemental infusions of 150 mg were given for "breakthrough" VT/VF more frequently to the 125-mg dose group, thereby considerably reducing the planned 8-fold differences in total dose to 1.8- and 2.6-fold, respectively, in the two studies.

The prospectively defined primary efficacy end point was the rate of VT/VF episodes per hour. For both studies, the median rate was 0.02 episodes per hour in patients receiving the high dose and 0.07 episodes per hour in patients receiving the low dose, or approximately 0.5 versus 1.7 episodes per day (p=0.07, 2-sided, in both studies). In one study, the time to first episode of VT/VF was significantly prolonged (approximately 10 hours in patients receiving the low dose and 14 hours in patients receiving the high dose). In both studies, significantly fewer supplemental infusions were given to patients in the high-dose group. Mortality was not affected in these studies.

Pharmacokinetics: The absorption of oral amiodarone is slow and variable, with peak serum amiodarone concentrations being attained at 3 to 12 hours after administration. Absorption may continue for up to 15 hours after oral ingestion. There is extensive intersubject variation: mean oral bioavailability is approximately 50% (mean range, 33 to 65%). First-pass metabolism in the gut wall and liver appears to be an important factor in determining the systemic availability of the drug. The mean terminal half-life after steady-state administration is approximately 50 days and has been found in one study (n=8) to range from 26 to 107 days. Since at least 3 to 4 half-lives are needed to approach steady-state concentrations, loading doses must be administered at the onset of oral amiodarone therapy.

Amiodarone has a very high apparent volume of distribution (approximately 5000 L) with an extensive accumulation in tissues, especially adipose tissues, and in highly perfused organs such as liver, lung, spleen, heart and kidney. One major metabolite of amiodarone, desethylamiodarone, has been identified, but the pharmacological activity of this metabolite is not known. During chronic treatment, the plasma ratio of metabolite to parent compound is approximately 1.

In patients on long-term oral therapy, amiodarone has a biphasic elimination pattern, with an initial decline in plasma levels observed from 2.5 to 10 days after discontinuation of therapy. This initial phase is followed by a marked rebound in plasma levels at 12 to 20 days post-dosing, before settling into a slower terminal elimination phase. In one study (n=8), the plasma elimination half-life of the parent compound ranged from 26 to 107 days (mean: 53 days).

Amiodarone exhibits complex disposition characteristics after intravenous administration. Peak serum concentrations after single 5 mg/kg 15-minute intravenous infusions in healthy subjects range between 5 and 41 mg/L. Peak concentrations after 150 mg supplemental infusions in patients with VF or hemodynamically unstable VT range between 7 and 26 mg/L. Due to rapid disposition, serum concentrations decline to 10% of peak values within 30 to 45 minutes after the end of the infusion. In clinical trials, after 48 hours of continued infusions (125, 500, or 1000 mg/day) plus supplemental (150 mg) infusions (for recurrent arrhythmias), amiodarone mean serum concentrations between 0.7 to 1.4 mg/L were observed (n=260).

Amiodarone is eliminated primarily by hepatic metabolism and biliary excretion. Desethylamiodarone (DEA) is the major active metabolite of amiodarone. At the usual amiodarone hydrochloride daily maintenance dose of 400 mg, mean steady-state DEA/amiodarone ratios ranged from 0.61 to 0.93. High-dose oral amiodarone loading in patients yielded 24-hour DEA/amiodarone ratios of 0.083 to 0.19. High-dose intravenous loading yielded a mean 24-hour DEA/amiodarone ratio of 0.041. No data are presently available on the activity of DEA in humans, but animal studies have shown that it has significant electrophysiologic and antiarrhythmic properties. The major enzyme responsible for the N-deethylation to DEA is believed to be cytochrome P450 3A4. Large interindividual variability in CYP-450 3A4 activity may explain the variable systemic availability of amiodarone. DEA is highly lipophilic and has a very large apparent volume of distribution, showing a higher concentration than amiodarone in all tissue except fat at steady state. Myocardial concentrations of DEA are approximately 3- to 4.5-fold greater than those of amiodarone during long-term oral amiodarone therapy. However, after either acute oral or acute intravenous administration, both mean serum and mean myocardial DEA concentrations are quite low compared to those of amiodarone.

There is negligible excretion of amiodarone or DEA in urine and neither is dialyzable. Amiodarone and DEA cross the placenta and both appear in breast milk.

Table 2 summarizes the mean ranges of pharmacokinetic parameters of amiodarone reported in single dose IV (5 mg/kg over 15 min) and oral (400 or 600 mg) studies of healthy subjects and in in vitro studies. Pharmacokinetics were similar in males and females.

Table 2: Amiodarone Hydrochloride for Injection Sandoz Standard

Amiodarone Pharmacokinetic Profile

Drug	Clearance (mL/h/kg)	V_C (L/kg)	V_{SS} (L/kg)	$t_{1/2}$ (days)	Protein Binding	F_{oral} (%)
Amiodarone	90–158	0.2	40–84	20–47	>0.96	33–65
Desethylamiodarone	197–290	—	68–168	≥AMI $t_{1/2}$	—	—

Notes: V_C and V_{SS} denote=the central and steady-state volumes of distribution from IV studies; F_{oral} is=systemic availability of oral amiodarone; "—" denotes=not available; AMI is=amiodarone; $t_{1/2}$=terminal phase elimination half-life.
Desethylamiodarone clearance and volume involve an unknown biotransformation factor.

During chronic treatment with oral amiodarone, close monitoring may be prudent for elderly patients and those with severe left ventricular dysfunction. However, during short-term intravenous use, age, sex, renal disease, and hepatic disease (cirrhosis) do not have clinically significant effects on the disposition of amiodarone and DEA. No dosage adjustment is necessary for patients in any of these populations.

There is no well-established relationship between drug concentration and therapeutic response for long-term oral or short-term intravenous use. Steady-state amiodarone concentrations of 1 to 2.5 mg/L, however, have been effective with minimal toxicity following chronic oral amiodarone.

INDICATIONS:

No antiarrhythmic drug has been shown to reduce the incidence of sudden death in patients with asymptomatic ventricular arrhythmias. Most antiarrhythmic drugs have the potential to cause dangerous arrhythmias; some have been shown to be associated with an increased incidence of sudden death. In light of the above, physicians should carefully consider the risks and benefits of antiarrhythmic therapy for all patients with ventricular arrhythmias.

Amiodarone HCl therapy should be initiated in hospital and continued in a monitored environment until adequate control of the arrhythmia has occurred.

Patients treated with amiodarone should be under the supervision of a cardiologist or a physician with equivalent experience in cardiology.

Amiodarone Hydrochloride for Injection is indicated for initiation of treatment of documented, life-threatening, frequently recurring ventricular fibrillation and hemodynamically unstable ventricular tachycardia in patients refractory to all other treatment. Additionally, intravenous amiodarone can be used to treat patients with VT/VF for whom oral amiodarone is indicated, but who are unable to take oral medication. During or after treatment with intravenous amiodarone patients may be transferred to oral amiodarone therapy.

Amiodarone Hydrochloride for Injection should be used for acute treatment until the patient's ventricular arrhythmias are stabilized. Most patients will require this therapy for 48 to 96 hours, but intravenous amiodarone may be administered for longer periods, if necessary.

CONTRAINDICATIONS: In patients with known hypersensitivity to any of the components of Amiodarone Hydrochloride for Injection, and in patients with cardiogenic shock, marked sinus bradycardia, and second- or third-degree AV block unless a functioning pacemaker is available.

WARNINGS: Pulmonary Toxicity: One of the most serious complications resulting from oral amiodarone HCl therapy is pulmonary toxicity, characterized by pneumonitis. Clinical symptoms include cough, dyspnea, weight loss, and weakness.

On chest X-ray, there is a diffuse interstitial pattern of lung involvement frequently with patchy alveolar infiltrates, particularly in the upper lobe. Predicting which patient will develop pulmonary toxicity has been difficult (see Contraindications). Pulmonary toxicity can appear abruptly either early or late during therapy and it commonly mimics viral or bacterial infection or worsening congestive heart failure. The relationship of pulmonary toxicity to duration of therapy, maintenance dose, and total dose is unclear. Besides an immediate cessation of amiodarone administration, steroid therapy may be beneficial. The majority of patients have recovered with this management, although some fatalities have occurred. Chest X-rays and pulmonary function tests are recommended prior to, and periodically during, the chronic administration of oral amiodarone.

Only 1 of more than 1000 patients treated with intravenous amiodarone in clinical studies developed pulmonary fibrosis. The condition was diagnosed 3 months after treatment with intravenous amiodarone, during which time the patient had received oral amiodarone. Intravenous amiodarone therapy should be discontinued if a diagnosis of pulmonary fibrosis is made.

During clinical studies using intravenous amiodarone, 2% of patients were reported to have adult respiratory distress syndrome (ARDS). ARDS is a disorder characterized by bilateral, diffuse pulmonary infiltrates with pulmonary edema and varying degrees of respiratory insufficiency. The clinical and radiographic picture can arise after a variety of lung injuries, such as those resulting from trauma, shock, prolonged cardiopulmonary resuscitation, and aspiration pneumonia, conditions present in many of the patients enrolled in the clinical studies. It is not possible to determine what role, if any, intravenous amiodarone played in causing or exacerbating the pulmonary disorder in those patients.

Proarrhythmia/QT Interval Prolongation: Amiodarone may cause a worsening of the existing arrhythmias or precipitate a new arrhythmia. Amiodarone causes prolongation of the QT interval. Proarrhythmia, primarily torsades de pointes, has been associated with prolongation of the QTc interval to 500 ms or greater. Proarrhythmia has been reported (2 to 5%) with oral amiodarone, especially in the presence of concomitant antiarrhythmic therapy and has included new-onset VF, incessant VT, increased resistance to cardioversion, and paroxysmal polymorphic VT associated with QT prolongation (torsades de pointes). Although QTc prolongation occurred frequently in patients receiving intravenous amiodarone, torsades de pointes or new-onset VF occurred infrequently (less than 2% of all patients treated with intravenous amiodarone in controlled clinical trials). Patients should be monitored carefully for QTc prolongation during amiodarone therapy.

Bradycardia and AV Block: Bradycardia was reported as an adverse drug reaction in 4.9% of patients receiving intravenous amiodarone for life-threatening VT/VF in clinical trials. AV block was reported as an adverse drug reaction in 1.4% of patients receiving intravenous amiodarone. There was no dose-related increase in bradycardia or AV block in these studies.

During intravenous amiodarone therapy, bradycardia should be treated by slowing the infusion rate or discontinuing therapy. In some patients inserting a pacemaker is required. Despite such measures, bradycardia was progressive and terminal in 1 (<1%) patient during controlled clinical trials. Patients with a known predisposition to bradycardia or AV block should be treated with intravenous amiodarone in a setting where a temporary pacemaker is available.

Hypotension: Hypotension is the most common adverse event seen with intravenous amiodarone therapy. In double-blind controlled clinical trials, hypotension was reported as an adverse event in 316 (39%) of 814 patients treated with intravenous amiodarone. Clinically significant hypotension during infusions was seen most often in the first several hours of treatment and was not dose related, but appeared to be related to the rate of infusion. Hypotension necessitating temporary discontinuation of intravenous amiodarone therapy was reported in 3% of the 814 patients, with permanent discontinuation required in an additional 2% of the 814 patients. Hypotension should be treated initially by slowing the infusion: additionally standard therapy may be needed including vasopressor drugs, positive inotropic agents and volume expansion. **The initial rate of infusion should be monitored closely and should not exceed that recommended in the Dosage section.**

PRECAUTIONS: General: Patients with life-threatening arrhythmias may experience serious adverse events during their treatment and therefore should be properly monitored. Amiodarone hydrochloride should be administered only by physicians who are experienced in the treatment of life-threatening arrhythmias, who are thoroughly familiar with the risks and benefits of amiodarone therapy, and who have access to facilities adequate for monitoring the effectiveness and adverse events of treatment (see Indications).

Liver Enzyme Elevations: In patients with life-threatening arrhythmias, the potential risk of hepatic injury should be weighed against the potential benefit of amiodarone therapy. However, patients receiving oral or intravenous amiodarone should be monitored carefully for evidence of progressive hepatic injury.

Elevations of blood hepatic enzyme values-alanine aminotransferase (ALT), aspartate aminotransferase (AST) and gamma-glutamyl transferase (GGT)-are seen commonly in patients with immediately life-threatening VT/VF. Interpreting elevated AST activity can be difficult because the values may be elevated in patients with recent myocardial infarction, congestive heart failure, and in those who have received multiple electrical defibrillations.

Approximately 54% of patients receiving intravenous amiodarone in clinical studies had baseline elevations in liver enzyme values, and 13% had clinically significant elevations. In 81% of patients with baseline and on-therapy data available, the liver enzyme elevations either improved during therapy or remained at baseline levels. Baseline abnormalities in hepatic enzymes are not a contraindication to treatment.

Two cases of fatal hepatocellular necrosis after treatment with intravenous amiodarone have been reported. The patients, one 28 years of age and the other 60 years of age, were treated for atrial arrhythmias with an initial infusion of 1500 mg over 5 hours, a rate much higher than recommended. Both patients developed hepatic and renal failure within 24 hours after the start of intravenous amiodarone treatment and died on day 14 and day 4, respectively. Because these episodes of hepatic necrosis may have been due to the rapid rate of infusion and hypotension is related to the rate of infusion, **the initial rate of infusion should be monitored closely and should not exceed that recommended in the Dosage section.**

Electrolyte Disturbances: Patients with hypokalemia or hypomagnesemia should have the condition corrected whenever possible before being treated with amiodarone, since these disorders can exaggerate the degree of QTc prolongation and increase the potential for torsades de pointes. Special attention should be given to electrolyte and acid-base balance in patients experiencing severe or prolonged diarrhea and receiving concomitant diuretics.

Children: The safety and efficacy of amiodarone in children have not been established; therefore, its use in children is not recommended. Experience with the use of oral or intravenous amiodarone has been reported in the medical literature but is limited.

Amiodarone Hydrochloride for Injection contains the preservative benzyl alcohol. There have been reports of fatal "gasping syndrome" in neonates (children less than one month of age) following the administration of intravenous solutions containing the preservative benzyl alcohol. Manifestations of the disease included: metabolic acidosis, respiratory distress, gasping respirations, central-nervous system dysfunction, convulsions, intracranial hemorrhages, hypoactivity, hypotonia, cardiovascular collapse and death.

Amiodarone Hydrochloride for Injection has been found to leach out **plasticizers**, such as DEHP (di-[2-ethylhexyl] phthalate) from intravenous tubing (including PVC tubing). The degree of leaching increases when infusing Amiodarone Hydrochloride for Injection at higher concentrations and at lower flow rates than provided in Dosage. DEHP is used in various plastic medical devices, generally to increase flexibility.

Based on data from animal studies, there was concern that exposure to DEHP may adversely affect male reproductive tract development during fetal, infant and toddler stages of development if the exposure in these immature stages is several fold higher than in adults, a situation that might be associated with intensive medical procedures such as those used in critically ill infants. Although a no-observable-adverse-effect level (NOAEL), by the oral route was identified for sexually mature rats (3.7-14 mg/kg per day), a NOAEL was not identified for rats in the postnatal stage. The maximum anticipated exposure to DEHP following Amiodarone IV administration under conditions of pediatric administration was calculated to be about 1.9 mg/kg per day for a 3 kg infant, which produces a safety margin of between twofold and sevenfold.

Pregnancy: Amiodarone has been shown to be embryotoxic in some animal species. In 3 different human case reports, both the parent drug and its DEA metabolite have been shown to pass through the placenta, quantitatively ranging between 10 and 50% of human maternal serum concentrations. Although amiodarone use during pregnancy is uncommon, there have been a small number of published reports of congenital goiter/hypothyroidism and hyperthyroidism. Therefore, amiodarone should be used during pregnancy only if the potential benefit to the mother justifies the risk to the fetus.

Use During Labor and Delivery: It is not known whether the use of amiodarone during labour or delivery has any immediate or delayed adverse effects. Preclinical studies in rodents have not shown any effect on the duration of gestation or on parturition.

Lactation: Amiodarone and its DEA metabolite are excreted in human milk, suggesting that breast-feeding could expose the nursing infant to a significant dose of the drug. Nursing offspring of lactating rats administered amiodarone have demonstrated reduced viability and reduced body weight gains. The risk of exposing the infant to amiodarone should be weighed against the potential benefit of arrhythmia suppression in the mother. The mother should be advised to discontinue nursing.

Drug Interactions: Amiodarone can inhibit the metabolism mediated by cytochrome P450 enzymes, probably accounting for the significant effects of oral amiodarone (and presumably intravenous amiodarone) on the pharmacokinetics of various therapeutic agents including digoxin, quinidine, procainamide, warfarin, dextromethorphan, and cyclosporine. Hemodynamic and electrophysiologic interactions have also been observed after concomitant administration with propranolol, diltiazem, and verapamil. Conversely, agents producing a significant effect on amiodarone pharmacokinetics include phenytoin, cimetidine, and cholestyramine. The potential for drug interactions may persist long after discontinuation of amiodarone administration because of its long half-life. Few data are available on drug interactions with intravenous amiodarone.

Beta-Blockers: Since amiodarone has weak beta-blocking activity, use with beta-blocking agents could increase risk of hypotension and bradycardia.

Calcium Channel Blockers: Amiodarone may have additive effects on atrioventricular conduction or myocardial contractility, increasing the risk of hypotension.

In addition to the interactions noted above, chronic (>2 weeks) oral amiodarone administration impairs metabolism of phenytoin, dextromethorphan, and methotrexate.

ADVERSE EFFECTS: Intravenous Amiodarone: In a total of 1836 patients in controlled and uncontrolled clinical trials, 14% of patients received intravenous amiodarone for up to 1 week, 5% received it for up to 2 weeks, 2% received it for up to 3 weeks, and 1% received it for more than 3 weeks, without an increased incidence of serious adverse events. The mean duration of therapy in these studies was 5.6 days.

Overall, treatment was discontinued in 9% of the patients because of adverse events. The most common serious adverse events leading to discontinuation of intravenous amiodarone therapy were ventricular tachycardia (2%), hypotension (2%), cardiac arrest (asystole/cardiac arrest/electromechanical dissociation) (1%), and cardiogenic shock (1%).

Table 3 lists the most common (incidence ≥1%) adverse drug reactions during i.v. amiodarone therapy that were collected from controlled and open-label clinical trials involving 1836 patients with hemodynamically unstable VT or VF.

Table 3: Amiodarone Hydrochloride for Injection Sandoz Standard

Adverse Drug Reactions in Patients Receiving IV Amiodarone in Controlled and Open-label Studies (≥1% incidence)

Study Event	Controlled Trials (N=814)	Open-label Trials (N=1022)	Total Incidence (N=1836)
Any Adverse Reaction	412 (50.6%)	384 (37.5%)	796 (43.3%)
Body as a Whole	54 (6.6%)	32 (3.1%)	86 (4.6%)
Fever	24 (2.9%)	13 (1.2%)	37 (2%)
Cardiovascular System	308 (37.8%)	264 (25.8%)	572 (31.1%)
Atrial Fibrillation	15 (1.8%)	9 (<1%)	24 (1.3%)
AV Block	14 (1.5%)	12 (1.2%)	26 (1.4%)
Bradycardia	49 (6.0%)	41 (4.0%)	90 (4.9%)
Congestive Heart Failure	18 (2.2%)	21 (2.0%)	39 (2.1%)
Heart Arrest	29 (3.5%)	26 (2.5%)	55 (2.9%)
Hypotension	165 (20.2%)	123 (12%)	288 (15.6%)
Nodal Arrhythmia	15 (1.8%)	15 (1.4%)	30 (1.6%)
QT Interval Prolonged	15 (1.8%)	4 (<1%)	19 (1.0%)
Shock	13 (1.5%)	12 (1.1%)	25 (1.3%)
Ventricular Fibrillation	12 (1.4%)	13 (1.2%)	25 (1.3%)
Ventricular Tachycardia	15 (1.8%)	30 (2.9%)	45 (2.4%)
Digestive System	102 (12.5%)	97 (9.4%)	199 (10.8%)
Diarrhea	8 (<1%)	12 (1.1%)	20 (1.0%)
Abnormal Liver Function Tests	35 (4.2%)	29 (2.8%)	64 (3.4%)
Nausea	29 (3.5%)	43 (4.2%)	72 (3.9%)
Vomiting	16 (1.9%)	17 (1.6%)	33 (1.7%)
Hemic and Lymphatic System	34 (4.1%)	34 (3.3%)	68 (3.7%)
Thrombocytopenia	14 (1.7%)	16 (1.5%)	30 (1.6%)
Metabolic and Nutritional	56 (6.8%)	49 (4.7%)	105 (5.7%)
AST Increased	14 (1.7%)	6 (<1%)	20 (1.0%)
ALT Increased	14 (1.7%)	5 (<1%)	19 (1.0%)
Nervous System	46 (5.6%)	38 (3.7%)	84 (4.5%)
Respiratory System	54 (6.6%)	61 (5.9%)	115 (6.2%)
Lung Edema	6 (<1%)	15 (1.4%)	21 (1.1%)
Respiratory Disorder	11 (1.3%)	8 (<1%)	19 (1.0%)
Urogenital System	27 (3.3%)	30 (2.9%)	57 (3.1%)
Kidney Function Abnormal	8 (<1%)	16 (1.5%)	24 (1.3%)

OVERDOSE:

Symptoms: Intravenous Overdose: The most likely effects of an inadvertent overdose of intravenous amiodarone are hypotension, cardiogenic shock, bradycardia, AV block, and hepatotoxicity.

Treatment: Hypotension and cardiogenic shock should be treated by slowing the infusion rate or with standard therapy: vasopressor drugs, positive inotropic agents and volume expansion. Bradycardia and AV block may require temporary pacing. Hepatic enzyme concentrations should be monitored closely.

Neither amiodarone nor DEA is dialyzable.

For management of a suspected drug overdose, CPhA recommends that you contact your **regional Poison Control Centre**. See the *CPS* Directory section for a list of Poison Control Centres.

DOSAGE: Amiodarone Hydrochloride for Injection must be diluted prior to use and is for intravenous infusion only.

Amiodarone Hydrochloride for Injection has been found to leach out plasticizers, such as DEHP [di-(2-ethylhexyl) phthalate] from intravenous tubing (including PVC tubing). The degree of leaching increases when infusing Amiodarone Hydrochloride for Injection at higher concentrations and lower flow rates than provided in Dosage (see Precautions, Children).

Amiodarone Hydrochloride for Injection must be delivered by a volumetric infusion pump. The surface properties of solutions containing injectable amiodarone are altered such that the drop size may be reduced. This reduction may lead to underdosage of the patient by up to 30% if drop counter infusion sets are used.

Amiodarone Hydrochloride for Injection should, whenever possible, be administered through a central venous catheter dedicated to that purpose. An in-line filter should be used during administration.

Amiodarone hydrochloride concentrations greater than 3 mg/mL in Dextrose 5% Injection have been associated with a high incidence of peripheral vein phlebitis; however, concentrations of 2.5 mg/mL or less appear to be less irritating. Therefore, for infusions longer than 1 hour, Amiodarone Hydrochloride for Injection concentrations should not exceed 2 mg/mL unless a central venous catheter is used.

Amiodarone Hydrochloride for Injection should be diluted in Dextrose 5% Injection (in PVC bags, glass or polyolefin bottles), at a concentration ranging from 1 mg/mL to 6 mg/mL. Amiodarone losses of approximately 10-12% were observed after 2 hours when Amiodarone Hydrochloride for Injection was diluted in Dextrose 5% Injection in PVC bags. Those losses may be attributed to adsorption of amiodarone to the PVC. However, when diluted in polyolefin or glass containers, no apparent losses were observed within 24 hours.

Infusions of Amiodarone Hydrochloride for Injection exceeding 2 hours must be administered in glass or polyolefin bottles containing Dextrose 5% for Injection.

It is well known that amiodarone adsorbs to polyvinyl chloride (PVC) tubing and the clinical trial dose administration schedule was designed to account for this adsorption. All of the clinical trials were conducted using PVC tubing and its use is therefore recommended. The concentrations and rates of infusion provided in Dosage reflect doses identified in these studies.

Amiodarone Hydrochloride for Injection does not need to be protected from light during administration.

Preparation of IV Solution: Amiodarone Hydrochloride for Injection must be diluted prior to use and is for intravenous infusion only.

IV Stability: See Table 4.

Table 4: Amiodarone Hydrochloride for Injection Sandoz Standard

Stability of Diluted Amiodarone Hydrochloride for Injection in Dextrose 5%

Solution	Concentration (mg/mL)	Container	Comments
5% Dextrose in Water	1–6	PVC	Physically compatible, with amiodarone loss of approximately 10–12% at 2 hours at room temperature
5% Dextrose in Water	1–6	Polyolefin, Glass	Physically compatible, with no amiodarone loss at 24 hours at room temperature

As with all parenteral drug products, intravenous admixtures should be inspected visually for clarity, particulate matter, precipitation, discolouration and leakage prior to administration whenever solution and container permit. Unused portions should be discarded.

Admixture Incompatibility: Amiodarone Hydrochloride for Injection in Dextrose 5% Injection (D_5W) is physically incompatible with the drugs shown in Table 5.

Table 5: Amiodarone Hydrochloride for Injection Sandoz Standard

Y-site Injection Incompatibility

Drug	Vehicle	Amiodarone Concentration mg/mL	Comments
Aminophylline	D_5W	4	Precipitate
Cefamandole Nafate	D_5W	4	Precipitate
Cefazolin Sodium	D_5W	4	Precipitate
Mezlocillin Sodium	D_5W	4	Precipitate
Heparin Sodium	D_5W	—	Precipitate
Sodium Bicarbonate	D_5W	3	Precipitate

Amiodarone shows considerable interindividual variation in response. Thus, although a starting dose adequate to suppress life-threatening arrhythmias is needed, close monitoring with adjustment of dose is essential. The recommended starting dose of Amiodarone Hydrochloride for Injection is about 1000 mg over the first 24 hours of therapy, delivered by the infusion regimen in Table 6. It is important that the recommended infusion regimen be followed closely.

Table 6: Amiodarone Hydrochloride for Injection Sandoz Standard

Intravenous Dose Recommendations—First 24 Hours

Loading Infusions	**Rapid: 150 mg over 10 minutes (15 mg/min).** Add 3 mL of Amiodarone Hydrochloride for Injection (150 mg) to 100 mL Dextrose 5% Injection (concentration=1.5 mg/mL). Infuse 100 mL over 10 minutes.
	Slow: 360 mg over 6 hours (1 mg/min). Add 18 mL of Amiodarone Hydrochloride for Injection (900 mg) to 500 mL Dextrose 5% Injection (concentration=1.8 mg/mL).
Maintenance Infusion	**540 mg over 18 hours (0.5 mg/min).** Decrease the rate of the slow loading infusion to 0.5 mg/min.

After the first 24 hours, the maintenance infusion rate of 0.5 mg/min (720 mg/24 hours) should be continued utilizing a concentration of 1 to 6 mg/mL (Amiodarone Hydrochloride for Injection concentrations greater than 2 mg/mL should be administered via a central venous catheter). In the event of breakthrough episodes of VF or hemodynamically unstable VT, 150 mg supplemental infusions of Amiodarone Hydrochloride for Injection mixed in 100 mL of Dextrose 5% Injection may be administered. Such infusions should be administered over 10 minutes to minimize the potential for hypotension. The rate of the maintenance infusion may be increased to achieve effective arrhythmia suppression.

The first 24-hour dose may be individualized for each patient; however, in controlled clinical trials, mean daily doses above 2100 mg were associated with an increased risk of hypotension. The initial rate of infusion should not exceed 30 mg/min.

Based on the experience from clinical studies of intravenous amiodarone, a maintenance infusion of up to 0.5 mg/min can be cautiously continued for 2 to 3 weeks regardless of the patient's age, renal function, or left ventricular function. There has been limited experience in patients receiving intravenous amiodarone for longer than 3 weeks.

Intravenous to Oral Transition: Patients whose arrhythmias have been suppressed by Amiodarone Hydrochloride for Injection may be switched to oral amiodarone. The optimal dose for changing from intravenous to oral administration of amiodarone will depend on the dose of Amiodarone Hydrochloride for Injection already administered as well as the bioavailability of oral amiodarone. When changing to oral amiodarone therapy, clinical monitoring is recommended, particularly for elderly patients.

Table 7 provides suggested doses of oral formulation amiodarone to be initiated after varying durations of Amiodarone Hydrochloride for Injection administration. These recommendations are made on the basis of a comparable total body amount of amiodarone delivered by the intravenous and oral routes, based on a 50% bioavailability of oral amiodarone. **Please refer to the Product Monograph of amiodarone oral formulations for detailed information on dosing and administration of oral amiodarone.**

Table 7: Amiodarone Hydrochloride for Injection Sandoz Standard

Recommendations for Oral Dosage After IV Infusion

Duration of Amiodarone HCl for Injection Infusion[a]	Initial Daily Dose of Oral Amiodarone (mg)
<1 week	800–1600
1–3 weeks	600–800
>3 weeks[b]	400

[a] Assuming a 720 mg/day infusion (0.5 mg/min).
[b] Amiodarone HCl for injection is not intended for maintenance treatment.

Preparation of IV Solution: **Amiodarone Hydrochloride for Injection must be diluted prior to use and is for intravenous infusion only.**

Amiodarone Hydrochloride for Injection should be diluted in Dextrose 5% Injection (in PVC bags, glass or polyolefin bottles), at a concentration ranging from 1 mg/mL to 6 mg/mL. Amiodarone losses of approximately 10-12% were observed after 2 hours when Amiodarone Hydrochloride for Injection was diluted in Dextrose 5% Injection in PVC bags. These losses may be attributed to adsorption of amiodarone to the PVC. However, when diluted in polyolefin or glass container, no apparent losses were observed within 24 hours.

Infusions of Amiodarone Hydrochloride for Injection exceeding 2 hours must be administered in glass or polyolefin bottles containing Dextrose for Injection.

Parenteral Products: As with all parenteral drug products, intravenous admixtures should be inspected visually for clarity, particulate matter, precipitation, discolouration and leakage prior to administration whenever solution and container permit. Discard unused portion.

SUPPLIED: Each mL of clear, pale yellow, sterile aqueous solution contains: amiodarone HCl 50 mg. Nonmedicinal ingredients: benzyl alcohol 20.2 mg, polysorbate 80 100 mg, sodium hydroxide and/or hydrochloric acid (to adjust pH) and water for injection. Amber glass single use vials of 3 mL fill in 5 mL vials (boxes of 10), 6 mL fill in 10 mL vials (boxes of 5), 9 mL fill in 10 mL vials (boxes of 1), and 18 mL fill in 20 mL vials (boxes of 1). Store between 15 and 30°C. Protect from light and excessive heat. Discard unused portion.

Amitriptyline

Antidepressant—Analgesic

CPhA Monograph

Date of Revision: November 2009

> This monograph has been compiled by CPhA and reviewed by experts. It may contain information different from that found in Health Canada-approved Product Monographs. The reader is referred to the *CPS* Editorial Policy for more information.

PHARMACOLOGY: Amitriptyline is a tertiary amine tricyclic antidepressant (TCA). The mechanism of action of TCAs believed to be related to their inhibition of the presynaptic reuptake of neurotransmitters, including serotonin and norepinephrine, which potentiates the effects of the neurotransmitters.

Amitriptyline exhibits strong anticholinergic activity, cardiovascular effects including orthostatic hypotension, changes in heart rhythm and conduction, and a lowering of the seizure threshold. As with other antidepressants, several weeks of therapy may be required to achieve the full antidepressant effect of amitriptyline; however, analgesic effects may become apparent within 1 to 2 weeks.

Pharmacokinetics: Amitriptyline is well absorbed from the gastrointestinal tract with peak plasma concentrations occurring between 2 and 12 hours after administration. Bioavailability of the drug is between 30 and 60% due to extensive first-pass metabolism of the drug in the liver. Amitriptyline is demethylated in the liver to its primary active metabolite, nortriptyline, and is a substrate for numerous isozymes of CYP450, including CYP1A2, CYP2C9, CYP2C19, CYP2D6 and CYP3A4.

Amitriptyline is over 90% protein bound. Its elimination half-life varies from 10 to 50 hours, with an average of 15 hours. Within 24 hours, approximately 25 to 50% of a dose of amitriptyline is excreted in the urine as inactive metabolites; small amounts are excreted in the bile.

Routine serum drug concentration monitoring is not warranted but may be useful to assess compliance or suspected toxicity. Recommended therapeutic trough levels, i.e., the sum of both amitriptyline and its metabolite nortriptyline, vary widely and range from 250 to 900 nmol/L (60 to 250 ng/mL). Ideally, the trough level should be taken 12 hours following administration of the last dose.

INDICATIONS: In the pharmacologic management of depressive illness.

The use of amitriptyline in patients with bipolar disorder may precipitate a hypomanic or manic state.

Patients with transient mood disturbances or normal grief reaction are not expected to benefit from TCAs.

Although not a labelled indication, amitriptyline is widely used as an atypical analgesic in the management of several conditions including fibromyalgia, migraine prophylaxis, rheumatoid arthritis and various neuropathies (e.g., post-herpetic neuralgia, diabetic peripheral neuropathy).

Though amitriptyline can be sedating, it is not recommended for use purely as a sedative-hypnotic, as other agents with greater efficacy and fewer adverse effects are available.

CONTRAINDICATIONS: Amitriptyline is contraindicated in patients who have shown hypersensitivity to the drug. Cross-sensitivity between amitriptyline and related TCAs is possible.

Hypertension, tachycardia, confusion, hyperpyretic crisis, severe convulsions and death have occurred in patients receiving TCAs and MAO inhibiting drugs simultaneously. Normally, when amitriptyline must be substituted for an MAO inhibitor or vice versa, a minimum of 14 days should elapse after the initial drug is discontinued before the new drug is cautiously started; however, patients with refractory depression have received combination therapy without significant adverse effects, under certain strict conditions and under the supervision of prescribers experienced with such therapy.

Amitriptyline is not recommended during the acute recovery phase following myocardial infarction or in the presence of congestive heart failure (see Warnings).

WARNINGS: Anticholinergic Effects: Because of its strong anticholinergic properties, amitriptyline must be used with caution in patients with urinary retention, benign prostatic hyperplasia, angle-closure glaucoma or increased intraocular pressure.

Cardiovascular: Orthostatic hypotension, arrhythmias and conduction abnormalities have occurred during therapy with amitriptyline. An increased incidence of sudden death has been reported in cardiac patients receiving therapeutic doses of tricyclic antidepressants. Caution is advised if TCAs are used in patients with pre-existing cardiovascular disease.

Sedation: Patients should be warned about the possible sedation and mental or motor impairment associated with amitriptyline therapy and advised of the potential danger of operating machinery or driving a motor vehicle if this occurs.

Suicide: The potential for attempted suicide must always be considered in depressed patients. Concern has been raised about potential worsening of depression or suicidality during therapy with antidepressants including amitriptyline, in both adults and children. Patients should be closely monitored during therapy. It is considered prudent to provide a limited supply of amitriptyline to patients thought to be at risk of suicide.

PRECAUTIONS: Bipolar Illness: The use of antidepressants during the depressed phase of bipolar illness may precipitate a hypomanic or manic state.

Cardiovascular: TCAs may have significant effects on the cardiovascular system (see Adverse Effects). Patients with a history of cardiovascular disease who require treatment with amitriptyline should be started on a low dose which may be cautiously increased over time. These patients also require close monitoring, including periodic ECG. In addition, all patients receiving higher than usual dosage should have periodic ECG, regardless of the presence or absence of cardiac abnormalities prior to treatment.

Central Nervous System: Sedation is the most common CNS effect of tricyclic antidepressants. Other reactions have occurred such as agitation, confusion, nightmares, restlessness, hostility, exacerbation of psychosis and extrapyramidal symptoms. Elderly patients may be more susceptible to some of these effects, especially those with pre-existing cognitive impairment or dementia.

Elective surgery: Temporary discontinuation of amitriptyline should be considered prior to elective surgery. Patients receiving amitriptyline in the perioperative period may be predisposed to intraoperative dysrhythmias. Risks of temporary discontinuation must be weighed against those of continued therapy throughout the perioperative period. If therapy is to be interrupted, amitriptyline should be stopped approximately 10 days prior to surgery. If the patient is at risk of experiencing withdrawal symptoms, consideration should be given to tapering the dose (see Adverse Effects).

Endocrine: TCAs should be used with caution in patients who are hyperthyroid or receiving thyroid medication, because of the possibility of cardiac arrhythmias.

Hematologic: Rarely, blood dyscrasias have occurred in patients taking TCAs. A leukocyte and differential count should be performed in patients who develop symptoms such as sore throat and fever while taking these drugs.

Hypersensitivity: Allergic reactions have included rash, edema, drug fever and photosensitivity. The possibility of cross-sensitivity among the tricyclic agents must be considered.

Seizures: TCAs can lower the seizure threshold and should be used with caution in patients with a history of seizures or those who may be predisposed to seizures.

Drug Interactions: Anticholinergics: Concurrent use of TCAs and other drugs with anticholinergic activity may necessitate dosage adjustments to minimize the additive effects. Hyperpyrexia has been reported when TCAs are administered with other anticholinergic agents, particularly during hot weather. Elderly patients may be particularly susceptible to excessive anticholinergic effects.

Antihypertensives: TCAs may antagonize the antihypertensive effects of clonidine.

CNS Depressants: The concomitant use of TCAs and other CNS depressants may result in additive depressant effects.

Inducers of cytochrome P450 enzymes (e.g., barbiturates, carbamazepine, phenytoin, rifampin): decreased serum concentrations of amitriptyline may result. Monitor for therapeutic failure of amitriptyline and adjust dose as indicated.

Inhibitors of cytochrome P450 enzymes (e.g., cimetidine, fluconazole, isoniazid, itraconazole, ketoconazole, quinidine, ritonavir, SSRIs): Increased amitriptyline concentrations can result. Consider alternative therapy when possible. Monitor for increased adverse effects/toxicity of amitriptyline; adjust dose as indicated. Dose reductions of up to 75% may be necessary when amitriptyline is used concurrently with potent enzyme inhibitors.

Lithium: There is some evidence that concurrent use of lithium and TCAs may increase the risk of neurotoxicity, particularly in the elderly. It has been suggested that reducing the dose of lithium in elderly patients may reduce the risk of neurotoxicity without compromising its clinical effect. Elderly patients should be monitored carefully for signs of neurotoxicity (e.g., tremor, ataxia, seizures) when on combined therapy.

MAO Inhibitors: Because of the additive serotonergic effects, combination therapy with TCAs and MAO inhibitors is not recommended, except under certain conditions (see Contraindications).

Serotonergic Drugs: Rarely, serotonin syndrome (characterized by symptoms such as confusion, agitation, hyperthermia, diaphoresis, hyperreflexia, shivering, ataxia) has occurred when amitriptyline was used concurrently with other serotonergic drugs such as trazodone, sibutramine, St. John's wort or SSRIs. Concurrent use should be avoided when possible.

Sympathomimetics: TCAs can significantly enhance the pressor response to norepinephrine and may potentiate the cardiovascular effects (e.g., arrhythmia) of sympathomimetics in general.

Thyroid Hormones: Concomitant use of amitriptyline and levothyroxine may potentiate the cardiovascular effects (e.g., arrhythmias) of both drugs.

Pregnancy: Amitriptyline has not been proven to be without risk to the developing fetus; however, it is sometimes continued during pregnancy when the need to treat an underlying depression justifies the potential risk to the fetus.

Lactation: Amitriptyline and its metabolite are excreted into breast milk, although levels have not been detected in infants' serum. Amitriptyline's effect in breastfeeding is unknown.

Children: Amitriptyline should be used cautiously and with close monitoring (e.g., serum concentration monitoring) in children and adolescents. The manufacturer recommends against its use for treatment of depression in children under 12 years of age.

Geriatrics: Elderly patients may be more susceptible to the anticholinergic, cardiovascular and CNS effects of TCAs. For this reason, many clinicians prefer to avoid the use of amitriptyline in elderly patients when a suitable alternative is available. When amitriptyline is prescribed to an older patient, lower initial dosages with more gradual increases are recommended.

ADVERSE EFFECTS: The more common adverse reactions involve anticholinergic effects such as dry mouth, disturbances of visual accommodation, constipation and urinary retention. Also commonly seen are light-headedness, drowsiness, decreased perspiration and mild tremors, as well as insomnia. Adverse reactions of the cardiovascular system may be much more serious; however, these occur less frequently.

Note: Some of the following adverse reactions have been reported with other TCAs and not specifically with amitriptyline. Pharmacologic similarities among the TCA drugs require that each reaction be considered when amitriptyline is administered.

Anticholinergic: Frequently: dry mouth and rarely associated sublingual adenitis, blurred vision, disturbances of accommodation, constipation, perspiration, flushing. Occasionally: delayed micturition, dilation of the urinary tract. In isolated cases: mydriasis, glaucoma, paralytic ileus, urinary frequency.

Behavioral: Occasionally: confusional states (especially in the elderly) with hallucinations, disorientation, delusions, anxiety, agitation, insomnia, restlessness, nightmares, hypomania, mania, exacerbation of psychosis, decrease in memory, feeling of unreality. In isolated cases: feeling of weakness, aggressiveness.

Cardiovascular: Frequently: hypotension, particularly orthostatic hypotension with associated vertigo, tachycardia, ECG changes (including flattening or inversion of T waves). Occasionally: arrhythmia, disturbances in cardiac conduction, palpitation, syncope. In isolated cases: hypertension, congestive heart failure, myocardial infarction, heart block, asystole, stroke, peripheral vasospastic reactions.

Central Nervous System: Frequently: drowsiness, fatigue, tremors. Occasionally: insomnia, dizziness, headache, paresthesia (numbness, tingling sensation, symptoms suggestive of peripheral neuropathy). Rarely: seizures. In isolated cases: tinnitus, incoordination, ataxia, alterations in EEG patterns, extrapyramidal symptoms, myoclonus, speech disorders.

Endocrine: Frequently: weight gain. Occasionally: increased or decreased libido, impotence. In isolated cases: gynecomastia in the male, breast enlargement and galactorrhea in the female, testicular swelling, elevation or depression of blood sugar levels, weight loss, syndrome of inappropriate antidiuretic hormone secretion (SIADH).

Hematologic: In isolated cases: agranulocytosis, eosinophilia, leukopenia, purpura and thrombocytopenia may occur as an idiosyncratic response.

Hypersensitivity: Occasionally: skin rash, urticaria. In isolated cases: petechiae, itching, photosensitization (avoid excessive exposure to sunlight), edema (general or of face and tongue), drug fever, obstructive jaundice, nasal congestion, alopecia, allergic alveolitis (pneumonia) with or without eosinophilia.

Gastrointestinal : Occasionally: nausea, vomiting, anorexia. Rarely: elevated transaminases. In isolated cases: diarrhea, bitter taste, stomatitis, epigastric distress, abdominal cramps, black tongue, dysphagia, increased salivation, hepatitis with or without jaundice.

Withdrawal: If prolonged treatment is abruptly terminated, withdrawal symptoms may occur. These may include sleep disturbances, gastrointestinal discomfort, flu-like symptoms, anxiety, depression, hypomania, mania, panic and depersonalization, delirium, dizziness, tremor, muscle twitching and, rarely, dyskinesia. These usually occur within 1 to 3 days of discontinuation, are mild and self-limiting and resolve within 2 weeks. Very rarely, cardiac disturbances may also occur.

OVERDOSE:

Symptoms: Amitriptyline and other TCAs are extremely toxic in overdose. Consultation with a Poison Control Centre is recommended. See the *CPS* Directory section for contact numbers.

Cardiac arrhythmias and CNS involvement pose the greatest threat and may occur suddenly even when initial symptoms appear to be mild. The toxic dose is variable but, in general, acute ingestion of 10 to 20 mg/kg may result in serious toxicity and may be lethal. TCA overdose has one of the highest mortality rates of any type of ingestion. Toxicity most commonly begins within two hours of ingestion. The onset of symptoms is frequently precipitous, with patients progressing from a wakeful, interactive state to having severe CNS and cardiac involvement within a matter of minutes.

Peripheral anticholinergic symptoms may include urinary retention, dry mucous membranes, mydriasis, constipation, and occasionally adynamic ileus. Patients may also be hyperpyrexic. CNS signs and symptoms can be highly variable and may range from somnolence to agitation, irritability, confusion, delirium, and hallucinations . In severe cases, patients may display extreme drowsiness, areflexia, respiratory depression, and coma. Patients may occasionally become hypothermic. Seizures are common and may precipitate cardiac toxicity.

Cardiac irregularities are frequent. Sinus tachycardia is common. Its presence is not a reliable predictor of serious toxicity, and its absence does not ensure a benign clinical course. An effect on cardiac conduction similar to that of quinidine may be seen with slowing of conduction, widening of the QRS complex, rightward shift in the axis of the terminal 40 milliseconds of the QRS complex, prolongation of the PR and QT intervals, right bundle branch and AV block, ventricular tachyarrhythmias (including torsades de pointes and fibrillation), and death. Prolongation of the QRS duration to more than 0.1 seconds is generally associated with more severe toxicity. Bradycardia may be seen in severely poisoned patients. Hypotension is common and may be severe, resulting from vasodilation, central and peripheral alpha-adrenergic blockade, and myocardial depression. Metabolic and/or respiratory acidosis may occur secondary to seizures, poor tissue perfusion, respiratory depression or poor gas exchange. In an otherwise healthy young person, prolonged resuscitation may be required.

Treatment: All cases of accidental pediatric exposure or adult overdose should be monitored at a health care facility. Asymptomatic cases without ECG abnormalities should be monitored for a minimum of 6 hours. Plasma concentrations of amitriptyline are of little use and should not guide management of the patient. In managing overdose, consider the possibility of multiple drug overdose, interactions among drugs and altered pharmacokinetics, including delayed absorption. Protect the patient's airway and support ventilation and perfusion. Closely monitor and maintain the patient's vital signs, ECG, blood gases, serum electrolytes, and acid-base balance. Minimize external stimulation to reduce the risk of seizures.

Consultation with a regional poison centre is advisable in all patients with TCA overdose. Activated charcoal (1 gram per kilogram) may reduce absorption of drug from the gastrointestinal tract, and should be considered in patients who present within 2 hours of ingestion. This can be given through a nasogastric tube if necessary. Although it should not be routinely performed, gastric lavage may be considered in the unusual case where a patient presents within 30 to 60 minutes of a massive TCA overdose, but only on the advice of a Poison Control Centre. If performed, gastric lavage should be followed by administration of activated charcoal. If the patient has a decreased level of consciousness, consideration should be given to placement of an endotracheal tube with cuff inflated before beginning the lavage procedure, to lessen the likelihood of aspiration of gastric contents.

Hypotension should be promptly corrected. If hypotension does not respond to a rapid isotonic fluid bolus and the patient has a widened QRS interval (> 0.1 seconds), sodium bicarbonate boluses should be administered at a dose of 1 to 2 mmol/kg (an average adult would typically receive 1 to 3 ampoules of 50 mmol/50 mL). If hypotension still hasn't responded, vasopressors should be employed, with a direct-acting agonist such as norepinephrine being the drug of choice.

Widened QRS intervals (> 0.14 seconds) and ventricular dysrhythmias should be treated with iv sodium bicarbonate. An i.v. bolus of 1 to 2 mmol/kg (typically 1 to 3 ampoules of 50 mmol/50 mL) should be administered and repeated if necessary to achieve a serum pH of 7.45 to 7.55. Maintain the pH between 7.45 and 7.55. Do not exceed pH 7.6. Monitor for hypokalemia and fluid overload. Hyperventilation may also be used to maintain alkalemia.

Ventricular arrhythmias refractory to sodium bicarbonate may respond to lidocaine. Quinidine, procainamide and other type IA or IC antiarrhythmics should not be used because they may exacerbate arrhythmias and conduction slowing due to the overdosage. Overdrive pacing should be considered in patients whose arrhythmias are not responsive to drug therapy.

In patients with severe/refractory toxicity, consideration should be given to the use of intravenous lipid emulsion. Consult a toxicologist.

Seizures should be aggressively treated with iv benzodiazepines such as lorazepam or diazepam. If this is unsuccessful, barbiturates and other measures should be employed as for status epilepticus. However, phenytoin is no longer recommended for the treatment of TCA-induced seizures.

Diuresis, hemoperfusion and dialysis are not helpful in TCA overdose.

Flumazenil is contraindicated in any patient with an altered level of consciousness who has or may have taken a TCA or any drug that can cause seizures or arrhythmias, as it may precipitate seizures or even cardiac arrest. This is true even in cases of mixed overdose where the patient is known to have coingested benzodiazepines.

For management of a suspected drug overdose, CPhA recommends that you contact your **regional Poison Control Centre**. See the *CPS* Directory section for a list of Poison Control Centres.

DOSAGE: Dosage should be initiated at a low level and increased gradually, noting carefully the clinical response and any evidence of adverse effects.

Depression: Initial dose for adults: 25 to 50 mg/day. The dose may be gradually increased, if necessary, to the level providing maximal clinical benefit with minimal adverse effects. The usual effective dose is 75 to 200 mg/day. Some patients may require high-dose therapy to a maximum of 300 mg daily.

It is generally recommended that therapy for depression be continued for a year for first episodes and for at least two years for subsequent episodes. Some experts recommend lifelong therapy for patients who have had more than two episodes. Hospitalized patients may require higher initial or overall dosage.

Adolescents: An initial dose of 10 mg 3 times daily with 20 mg at bedtime is recommended. The dose may be increased to a maximum of 100 mg daily, either in divided doses or as a single bedtime dose.

Geriatrics: Recommended initial dose is 10 to 25 mg at bedtime. May be increased by 10 to 25 mg daily, at weekly intervals, up to 150 mg daily.

Maintenance: When satisfactory improvement has been achieved, dosage should be reduced to the lowest amount that will maintain relief of symptoms. In suitable patients, the total daily dosage may be given in a single dose, preferably at bedtime. Once remission is achieved, therapy should continue for one year for first episode depression and at least two years for subsequent episodes.

Neuropathic Pain: Usual starting dose is 10 to 25 mg at bedtime or 2 to 3 hours before bedtime. Geriatric or debilitated patients should start with 10 mg at bedtime. Dosage should then be increased weekly by 10 to 25 mg/day until reasonable pain relief is obtained or side effects occur, or to a maximum of 150 mg/day.

Fibromyalgia: 10 to 25 mg at bedtime or 2 to 3 hours before bedtime.

Migraine Prophylaxis: 10 mg at bedtime initially. Increase gradually if necessary; range 10 to 150 mg at bedtime.

Rheumatoid Arthritis: see Neuropathic Pain.

Amlodipine Ⓟ

CPhA Monograph

see *Calcium Channel Blockers*

Amoxicillin Ⓟ

Antibiotic

CPhA Monograph

Date of Revision: March 2008

This monograph has been compiled by CPhA and reviewed by experts. It may contain information different from that found in Health Canada-approved Product Monographs. The reader is referred to the *CPS* Editorial Policy for more information.

SUMMARY PRODUCT INFORMATION:

Route of Administration	Dosage Form	Strength
Oral	Capsule	250 mg, 500 mg
	Chewable tablet	125 mg, 250 mg
	Powder for oral suspension[a]	125 mg/5 mL, 250 mg/5 mL

[a] Also available in sugar-free formulation.

INDICATIONS AND CLINICAL USE: Amoxicillin is used in the following clinical settings to treat or prevent infections caused by susceptible organisms:

- Treatment of upper respiratory tract infections such as pharyngitis and sinusitis.
- Treatment of lower respiratory tract infections such as community-acquired pneumonia and acute exacerbations of chronic obstructive pulmonary disease.
- Treatment of acute otitis media caused by susceptible bacteria (*S. pneumoniae*, *H. influenza* and *M. catarrhalis*).
- Treatment of hematogenous osteomyelitis in children following initial iv therapy.
- Treatment of uncomplicated urinary tract infections. Not used as first-line treatment because of the incidence of resistance, and may be less effective than agents such as trimethoprim/sulfamethoxazole even when the causative bacteria are susceptible [Guidelines for antimicrobial treatment of uncomplicated acute bacterial cystitis and acute pyelonephritis in women. Infectious Diseases Society of America (IDSA).*Clin Infect Dis* 1999;29(4):745-58]. It may be used as first-line therapy in pregnant women with acute cystitis, due to the relatively small number of available agents which are considered safe in all stages of pregnancy. However, culture should always be done to ensure susceptibility, and treatment may need modification [Rosser WW et al. *Anti-infective guidelines for community-acquired infections*; 2005. p. 56,60,61; Guidelines for antimicrobial treatment of uncomplicated acute bacterial cystitis and acute pyelonephritis in women. *Clin Infect Dis* 1999;29(4):745-58].
- Treatment of asymptomatic bacteriuria in pregnancy [Rosser WW et al. *Anti-infective guidelines for community-acquired infections*; 2005. p. 59; Infectious Diseases Society of America guidelines for the diagnosis and treatment of asymptomatic bacteriuria in adults. *Clin Infect Dis* 2005;40(5):643-54].
- Treatment of *H. pylori* infection.
- Treatment of urethral, endocervical or rectal chlamydia infections in pregnant and nursing women [Canadian STI guidelines on chlamydia at http://www.phac-aspc.gc.ca/std-mts/sti_2006/pdf/05sti2006b_e.pdf].
- Treatment of lyme disease (*B. burgdorferi*) [The clinical assessment, treatment, and prevention of lyme disease, human granulocytic anaplasmosis, and babesiosis: clinical practice guidelines by the Infectious Diseases Society of America. *Clin Infect Dis* 2006;43(9):1089-134].

- Treatment of typhoid fever in children with fully susceptible *S. enterica* serotype typhi [Management of typhoid fever in children. *Pediatr Infect Dis J* 2002;21(2):157-8].
- Prevention of infective endocarditis in susceptible patients.

Amoxicillin is used for prophylaxis against infective endocarditis in patients undergoing certain dental or surgical procedures who have any of the following conditions: prosthetic heart valves or prosthetic material used for cardiac valve region, previous infective endocarditis, heart transplantation recipients who develop cardiac valvulopathy, congenital heart disease, i.e., unrepaired cyanotic congenital heart disease, including palliative shunts and conduits; repaired congenital heart disease with residual defects at the site or adjacent to the site of a prosthetic patch or prosthetic device which inhibits endothelialization; completely repaired congenital heart defect with prosthetic material or device, whether placed by surgery or by catheter intervention, during the first six months after the procedure [Prevention of infective endocarditis: guidelines from the American Heart Association. *Circulation* 2007;116(15):1736-54]. These procedures are dental procedures that involve manipulation of gingival tissue or the periapical region of teeth or perforation of the oral mucosa, procedures on respiratory tract involving incision or biopsy of respiratory mucosa and procedures in patients with infected skin, skin structures or musculoskeletal tissue.

Antibiotic prophylaxis against infective endocarditis is not recommended for genitourinary or gastrointestinal tract procedures [Prevention of infective endocarditis: guidelines from the American Heart Association. *Circulation* 2007;116(15):1736-54].

CONTRAINDICATIONS:

- Patients who are hypersensitive to amoxicillin or to any ingredient in the formulation.
- Patients who are hypersensitive to penicillins or other β-lactam antibiotics.

WARNINGS AND PRECAUTIONS:

Serious Warnings and Precautions

- Serious and occasionally fatal hypersensitivity reactions have been reported in patients on penicillin therapy. Prior to prescribing or administering amoxicillin, a careful inquiry should be made concerning previous reactions to penicillins, other β-lactam antibiotics or other allergen, including type and severity of the reaction.
- Patients with a history of immediate-sensitivity reaction to penicillin (e.g., anaphylaxis, bronchospasms and/or hypotension) are considered to be at increased risk of similar reactions to cephalosporins. Administration of cephalosporins to patients with a history of severe allergic reactions to penicillin antibiotics should only be considered in situations where the benefit outweighs the potential risks, and in consultation with an expert. If an allergic reaction occurs, discontinue amoxicillin and institute appropriate therapy.
- *C. difficile*-associated diarrhea or colitis has been reported with amoxicillin and should be considered in the differential diagnosis of patients who develop diarrhea during or following amoxicillin therapy.

General: The use of anti-infective agents may alter the flora of the gastrointestinal tract and other non-sterile sites, sometimes leading to overgrowth of nonsusceptible organisms such as *C. albicans*.

Amoxicillin is renally excreted. An interval adjustment may be required depending on kidney function (see Table 4).

Amoxicillin should be used with caution if infectious mononucleosis, acute lymphocytic leukemia or cytomegalovirus infection is suspected, due to an increased incidence of maculopapular rash when it is used in these settings.

Special Populations: Pregnant Women: Pregnancy Category B_M. Amoxicillin readily crosses the placenta and is generally considered to pose no significant teratogenic risk. Amoxicillin has been used to treat urinary tract and chlamydial infections during pregnancy with no evidence of adverse effects on the fetus.

Nursing Women: Amoxicillin appears in breast milk in low concentrations. Potential risks to the infant include altered bowel flora, diarrhea and hypersensitivity reactions. According to the American Academy of Pediatrics, amoxicillin is considered compatible with breastfeeding.

ADVERSE REACTIONS: Dermatologic: A morbilliform, erythematous, urticarial rash, similar to those reported with other penicillins, may occur. In addition, aminopenicillins may cause an erythematous, maculopapular rash which may or may not be immunologically mediated.

Amoxicillin should be used with caution if infectious mononucleosis is suspected; an increased incidence of maculopapular rash occurs when used in this setting.

Gastrointestinal: nausea or vomiting, diarrhea, anorexia, epigastric distress and gastritis. Black hairy tongue, glossitis and stomatitis have also been noted. Diarrhea is generally less frequent than with ampicillin. Amoxicillin-associated hemorrhagic colitis and *C. difficile*-associated diarrhea has been reported.

Hematologic: anemia (rare), thrombocytopenia, thrombocytopenic purpura, eosinophilia, leukopenia, neutropenia, agranulocytosis. These reactions are usually reversible on discontinuation of therapy.

Hepatic: Moderate rise in serum aspartate transferase, alkaline phosphatase and lactic dehydrogenase has been noted, but the significance of these findings is unknown.

Hypersensitivity: rash, serum sickness-like reactions, anaphylaxis.

Neurologic : aseptic meningitis (rare).

Renal: acute interstitial nephritis resulting in acute renal failure (rare), tubulitis.

Miscellaneous: A Jarisch-Herxheimer type of reaction may occur when Lyme disease is treated with amoxicillin (case report).

DRUG INTERACTIONS: Drug-Drug Interactions: See Table 1.

DOSAGE AND ADMINISTRATION: Recommended Dose and Dosage Adjustment: Amoxicillin is given orally and because it is stable in the presence of gastric acid, it may be given without regard to meals. The duration of therapy depends on the type and severity of the infection, and can vary from 7 to 10 days to several weeks. See Table 2 and Table 3.

Adults: See Table 2.

Table 1: Amoxicillin

Drug-Drug Interactions

Interacting Drug	Effect	Clinical Comment
Methotrexate	Penicillins compete with renal tubular secretion of methotrexate resulting in ↓ clearance of methotrexate. Concomitant use may ↑ methotrexate serum concentrations, ↑ the risk of toxicity (e.g., neutropenia).	If concomitant treatment is necessary, monitor patients for signs and symptoms of methotrexate toxicity, e.g., hematologic, gastrointestinal.
Contraceptives, oral	Antibacterials may destroy intestinal bacteria that provide hydrolytic enzymes essential for enterohepatic recirculation of ethinyl estradiol resulting in ↓ plasma concentration of ethinyl estradiol. Effectiveness of oral contraceptives may be ↓.	Possible contraceptive failure. Consider use of additional method of contraception, e.g., barrier, for duration of cycle to avoid ↑ risk of pregnancy.
Probenecid	Probenecid inhibits renal tubular excretion of amoxicillin, thereby ↓ elimination of amoxicillin.	This interaction has been exploited to increase serum levels of penicillins.
Tetracyclines (doxycycline, minocycline, tetracycline)	Bacteriostatic action of tetracyclines may inhibit bactericidal activity of penicillins.	The combination of penicillins and tetracyclines is avoided in pneumococcal meningitis and scarlet fever because tetracycline reduces the effectiveness of penicillin. The clinical significance of the interaction in other infections is unknown.

Pediatrics: See Table 3.

Renal Impairment: See Table 4.

Dialysis: Adults: 250 to 500 mg orally every 24 hours. An additional 250 mg may be given after each dialysis period.

Table 2: Amoxicillin

Dose in Adult Patients

Indications	Route	Usual Dose	Duration of Treatment	Clinical Comment
Respiratory tract infection, upper	PO	500 mg Q8H	Continue for 48–72h after patient is asymptomatic or evidence of eradication of infection is obtained. Treatment duration ranges from 7 to 10 days. Severe or persistent infections may require several weeks of therapy.	
Respiratory tract infection, lower	PO	500–1000 mg Q8H For community-acquired pneumonia: 1 g po TID **plus** a macrolide [*Clin Infect Dis* 2007;44(Suppl 2):S27-72]. See comments.		For community-acquired pneumonia, current IDSA guidelines recommend combination treatment with a macrolide in patients with comorbidities[a] [*Clin Infect Dis* 2007;44(Suppl 2):S27-72].
Urinary tract infection, acute	PO	250–500 mg Q8H	7 days	
Bacteriuria, asymptomatic in pregnancy	PO	250–500 mg Q8H	3 days	Perform follow-up culture and repeat culture monthly. Repeat culture if necessary.
Otitis media, acute	PO	500 mg Q8H	7–10 days	
Chlamydia, urethral, endocervical or rectal in pregnant and nursing women	PO	500 mg Q8H	7 days	A test to confirm cure is recommended 3–4 weeks after completion of treatment. Patients should abstain from sexual intercourse during and for 7 days after therapy until all sexual partners are treated.
H. pylori -positive peptic ulcer disease, treatment	PO	1 g BID in combination with a proton-pump inhibitor and clarithromycin	7 days	Consider local resistance patterns for choice of antibiotic. Duration of treatment lengthens if treatment failure is suspected.
Infective endocarditis, prevention	PO	2 g	Single dose	Give 30 to 60 minutes prior to procedure.
Lyme disease, early localized or Lyme disease, early disseminated with erythema migrans	PO	500 mg TID	14–21 days, 28 days for Lyme arthritis	Longer duration and parenteral therapy should be considered in patients with: acute neurological disease, 3rd degree heart-block, CNS or peripheral nervous system disease in late Lyme disease and persistent recurrent arthritis after usage of oral regimen [*Clin Infect Dis* 2006;43(9):1089-134].

[a] Examples of comorbidities include diabetes mellitus, alcoholism, use of antibiotics within previous 3 months, chronic heart, lung or kidney disease or immunosuppressive conditions, e.g., malignancies, HIV infection, chronic use of oral corticosteroids.

Table 3: Amoxicillin

Dose in Pediatrics[a] (Infants >3 Months and Children)

Indication	Route	Usual Dose	Duration of Treatment	Clinical Comment
Respiratory tract infection, upper	PO	40–50 mg/kg daily divided Q8H. For known or drug-resistant *S. pneumoniae*: 80–90 mg/kg daily (high-dose)[b] divided BID or TID. Maximum 4 g/day.	Continue for 48–72h after patient is asymptomatic or evidence of eradication of infection is obtained. Duration of therapy is usually 10 days. Severe or persistent infections may require several weeks of therapy.	
Respiratory tract infection, lower	PO	40–50 mg/kg daily divided Q8H. For known or drug-resistant *S. pneumoniae*: 80–90 mg/kg daily (high-dose)[b] divided BID or TID Maximum 4 g/day.		
Urinary tract infection, acute	PO	40 mg/kg daily divided Q8H		Prior to prescribing amoxicillin, check local resistance patterns for *E. coli*.
Otitis media, acute	PO	40 mg/kg daily divided Q8H; for known or suspected drug resistant *S. pneumoniae* 80–90 mg/kg (high-dose)[b] daily divided BID or TID	For children >2 years, 5 days of treatment is as effective as 10 days of treatment. For children ≤2 years, treatment duration is 10 days.	Reassess patients who fail to respond to therapy within 48–72 hours.

(cont'd)

Table 3: Amoxicillin *(cont'd)*

Dose in Pediatrics[a] (Infants >3 Months and Children)

Indication	Route	Usual Dose	Duration of Treatment	Clinical Comment
Osteomyelitis, hematogenous	PO	100 mg/kg daily divided TID; maximum 3 g/day	Minimum 4 weeks of antibiotics including iv therapy. Some clinicians recommend 6 weeks if initial presentation is more severe, there is extensive bone involvement and slow resolution of systemic and local signs [*Can J Infect Dis* 1994;4:10-2]	May be given as step-down therapy after initial iv therapy.
Infective endocarditis, prevention	PO	50 mg/kg per dose	Single dose	Give 30 to 60 minutes prior to procedure.
Lyme disease, early localized or Lyme disease, early disseminated with erythema migrans	PO	50 mg/kg daily divided Q8H; max 500 mg/dose	14–21 days, 28 days for Lyme arthritis	One of the recommended treatments in children <8 years. Longer duration and parenteral therapy should be considered in patients with: acute neurological disease, 3rd degree heart-block, CNS or peripheral nervous system disease in late Lyme disease and persistent recurrent arthritis after usage of oral regimen [*Clin Infect Dis* 2006;43(9):1089-134].
Typhoid fever	PO	100 mg/kg daily divided Q8H, maximum 4 g/day	14 days	For fully susceptible *S. enterica* serotype typhi.

a Dose in neonates is 20-30 mg/kg daily divided q12h depending on type and severity of infection.
b Recommended if recent (<3 months) exposure to antibiotics and/or attends day care.

Table 4: Amoxicillin

Dose in Adult Patients with Renal Impairment

Creatinine Clearance	Interval Adjustment
>50 mL/min	Q8H
10–50 mL/min	Q8–12H
<10 mL/min	Q24H

OVERDOSAGE:

Signs and Symptoms: Serious toxicity is unlikely following large doses of amoxicillin. Acute ingestion of large doses of amoxicillin may cause nausea, vomiting, diarrhea and abdominal pain. Acute oliguric renal failure and hematuria may occur following large doses.

Recommended Management: Activated charcoal is recommended only for very large recent ingestions. For amoxicillin ingestions of less than 250 mg/kg, treatment is not usually required in patients with normal renal function. Monitor fluid and electrolyte status and renal function in patients with severe vomiting and/or diarrhea. Hemodialysis may be useful following severe overdose with renal impairment.

For management of a suspected drug overdose, CPhA recommends that you contact your **regional Poison Control Centre**. See the *CPS* Directory section for a list of Poison Control Centres.

ACTION AND CLINICAL PHARMACOLOGY: Amoxicillin, a semisynthetic penicillin of the aminopenicillin group, is bactericidal against sensitive organisms. It acts through the inhibition of peptidoglycan synthesis in the bacterial cell wall. This leads to the formation of a defective cell wall with eventual lysis and death to the cell.

The spectrum of activity of amoxicillin includes gram-negative susceptible bacteria such as *H. influenzae, E. coli, P. mirabilis, S. enterica* serotype typhi, as well as penicillin-sensitive gram-positive bacteria such as *S. pneumoniae*, enterococci, nonpenicillinase-producing staphylococci and Listeria (see Penicillin G/Penicillin V, CPhA Monograph). Some isolates of *H. influenza*, Enterobacteriaceae, Salmonella and Shigella species are resistant due to β-lactamase production or other mechanisms. The proportion of strains which are sensitive varies widely among different populations.

Pharmacokinetics: Amoxicillin is rapidly absorbed after oral administration and is stable in the presence of gastric acid. Peak serum concentrations are usually attained within 1 to 2 hours following oral administration and are generally 2 to 2.5 times greater than those obtained with an equivalent dose of oral ampicillin. The peak plasma concentration ranged from 2.65 to 5.75 μg/mL after administration of a single dose of 250 mg of reconstituted amoxicillin granules suspension. Oral amoxicillin has better bioavailability than oral ampicillin. Amoxicillin diffuses readily into most body tissues and fluids, e.g., middle ear fluid, synovial fluid. Amoxicillin is not highly protein bound. Its elimination half-life ranges from 0.7 to 1.4 hours in patients with normal renal function and 7 to 10 hours in patients with impaired renal function. Amoxicillin is partially metabolized to inactive metabolites and then rapidly excreted in urine. Small amounts of the compounds are excreted in feces and bile.

Ampicillin Pr

ampicillin sodium
ampicillin trihydrate

Antibiotic

CPhA Monograph

Date of Preparation: November 2004
Date of Revision: March 2008

This monograph has been compiled by CPhA and reviewed by experts. It may contain information different from that found in Health Canada-approved Product Monographs. The reader is referred to the *CPS* Editorial Policy for more information.

SUMMARY PRODUCT INFORMATION:

Drug	Route of Administration	Dosage Form	Product Strength
Ampicillin trihydrate	Oral	Capsule	250 mg, 500 mg
		Powder for suspension	125 mg/5 mL, 250 mg/5 mL
Ampicillin sodium	Parenteral	Dry powder vial for reconstitution	250 mg, 500 mg, 1000 mg, 2000 mg

INDICATIONS AND CLINICAL USE: Ampicillin is used in the following clinical settings to treat or prevent infections caused by susceptible organisms:

- Treatment of pyelonephritis and complicated urinary tract infections (UTIs). Given in combination with an aminoglycoside in the treatment of complicated UTIs. Empirically, ampicillin can be added to gentamicin in the treatment of pyelonephritis, especially in patients with diabetes or pregnant women; these patient groups are more susceptible to Group B Streptococcus [Rosser WW et al. *Anti-infective guidelines for community-acquired infections*; 2005. p. 62-4].
- Recommended treatment for bacterial meningitis caused by *L. monocytogenes* and *S. agalactiae* (group B streptococci) in adults and neonates. Recommended empiric treatment in combination with third-generation cephalosporin when *S. agalactiae* and *L. monocytogenes* have not been ruled out. Infection with either of these microorganisms may require the addition of gentamicin [Practice guidelines for the management of bacterial meningitis. *Clin Infect Dis* 2004;39(9):1267-84].
- Empiric treatment of septicemia, especially if enterococcus is a concern.
- Alternative agent for the prophylaxis of intrapartum streptococcus group B infection of the infant. Penicillin is the preferred agent [Prevention of perinatal group B streptococcal disease. Revised guidelines from CDC. *MMWR Recomm Rep* 2002;51[RR-11]:1-22].
- Treatment of native or prosthetic valve enterococcal endocarditis. Given in combination with gentamicin, streptomycin, ceftriaxone or imipenem-cilastatin depending on susceptibility of strains [Infective endocarditis: diagnosis, antimicrobial therapy, and management of complications. *Circulation* 2005;111(23):e394-434]. For enterococcal endocarditis, the combination therapy with a cephalosporin or imipenem has been used experimentally to treat vancomycin-resistant enterococcus, but there is little clinical data to support this.
- Prevention of infective endocarditis in susceptible patients. Oral amoxicillin is preferred; however, parenteral ampicillin is recommended in patients who are unable to take oral medications [Prevention of infective endocarditis: guidelines from the American Heart Association. *Circulation* 2007;116(15):1736-54].

Parenteral ampicillin is used for prophylaxis against infective endocarditis in patients undergoing certain dental or surgical procedures who have any of the following conditions: prosthetic heart valves or prosthetic material used for the cardiac valve region, previous infective endocarditis, heart transplantation recipients who develop cardiac valvulopathy, congenital heart disease, i.e., unrepaired cyanotic congenital heart disease, including palliative shunts and conduits; repaired congenital heart disease with residual defects at the site or adjacent to the site of a prosthetic patch or prosthetic device which inhibits endothelialization; completely repaired congenital heart defect with prosthetic material or device, whether placed by surgery or by catheter intervention, during the first six months after the procedure [Prevention of infective endocarditis: guidelines from the American Heart Association. *Circulation* 2007;116(15):1736-54]. These procedures are dental procedures that involve manipulation of gingival tissue or the periapical region of teeth or perforation of the oral mucosa, procedures on respiratory tract involving incision or biopsy of respiratory mucosa and procedures in patients with infected skin, skin structures or musculoskeletal tissue.

Antibiotic prophylaxis against infective endocarditis is not recommended for genitourinary or gastrointestinal tract procedures [Prevention of infective endocarditis: guidelines from the American Heart Association. *Circulation* 2007;116(15):1736-54].

CONTRAINDICATIONS:

- Patients who are hypersensitive to ampicillin or to any ingredient in the formulation.
- Patients who are hypersensitive to penicillin or other β-lactam antibiotics.

WARNINGS AND PRECAUTIONS:

Serious Warnings and Precautions

- Serious and occasionally fatal hypersensitivity reactions have been reported in patients on penicillin therapy. Prior to prescribing or administering ampicillin, a careful inquiry should be made concerning previous reactions to penicillins, other β-lactam antibiotics or other allergen, including type and severity of the reaction.
- Patients with a history of immediate-sensitivity reaction to penicillin (e.g., anaphylaxis, bronchospasms and/or hypotension) are considered to be at increased risk of similar reactions to cephalosporins. Administration of cephalosporins to patients with a history of severe allergic reactions to penicillin antibiotics should only be considered in situations where the benefit outweighs the potential risks, and in consultation with an expert. If an allergic reaction occurs, discontinue ampicillin and institute appropriate therapy.
- *C. difficile*-associated diarrhea or colitis has been reported with ampicillin and should be considered in the differential diagnosis of patients who develop diarrhea during or following ampicillin therapy.

Hematologic: Monitor hematologic systems periodically while on prolonged therapy of ampicillin since hematologic adverse effects have been reported (see Adverse Reactions).

Hepatic: Monitor liver enzymes periodically while on prolonged therapy of ampicillin since transient increases in aminotransferases and hepatic dysfunction have been reported (see Adverse Reactions).

Immune: Serious and occasionally fatal hypersensitivity reactions have been reported in patients on penicillin therapy. Although anaphylaxis is more frequent following parenteral therapy, it has occurred in patients taking oral penicillins. These reactions are more likely to occur in individuals with a history of sensitivity to multiple allergens.

Renal: Ampicillin is renally excreted. An interval adjustment may be required depending on kidney function (see Dosage and Administration). Monitor kidney function periodically while on prolonged therapy of ampicillin since interstitial nephritis has been reported.

Skin: Ampicillin should be used with caution if infectious mononucleosis, acute lymphocytic leukemia or cytomegalovirus infection is suspected, due to an increased incidence of maculopapular rash when it is used in this setting.

Special Populations: Pregnant Women: Pregnancy Category B. Ampicillin readily crosses the placenta and is generally considered to pose no significant teratogenic risk to the fetus. Ampicillin has been used in pregnant women (e.g., urinary tract infections) without adverse effects to the fetus.

Nursing Women: Ampicillin appears in breast milk in low concentrations. Potential risks to the infant include altered bowel flora, diarrhea, obscured diagnosis of fever specifically interpretation of culture results and hypersensitivity reactions.

Pediatrics (birth to 16 years old): Renal, hepatic and hematologic systems should be evaluated periodically during treatment, especially in premature babies, neonates and other infants.

Geriatrics: There are no specific precautions for use in the elderly.

ADVERSE REACTIONS: More Common Adverse Drug Reactions: See Table 1.

Table 1: Ampicillin

More Common Adverse Drug Reactions

Body System	Ampicillin (%)
Dermatologic	
Rash	1–10
Gastrointestinal	
Abdominal cramps	1–10
Diarrhea	9–17 (oral); 3 (iv)

(cont'd)

Table 1: Ampicillin *(cont'd)*

More Common Adverse Drug Reactions

Body System	Ampicillin (%)
Nausea	2–2.9 (oral); 3 (iv)
Oral candidiasis	1–10
Vomiting	2–2.9 (oral); 3 (iv)
Miscellaneous	
Allergic reaction	1–10
Pain at injection site	10

Less Common Adverse Drug Reactions (<1%): CNS: dizziness, headache, penicillin encephalopathy, seizures (with large iv doses, especially in patients with renal failure).
Hematologic: decreased lymphocytes, eosinophilia, granulocytopenia, hemolytic anemia, leukopenia, neutropenia, thrombocytopenia, thrombocytopenia purpura.
Hepatic: hepatic dysfunction, increase in AST and/or ALT.
Renal: interstitial nephritis.

DRUG INTERACTIONS: Drug-Drug Interactions: See Table 2.

Table 2: Ampicillin

Established or Predicted Drug-Drug Interactions

Interacting Drug	Effect	Clinical Comment
Allopurinol	Increased rate of ampicillin-induced skin rash with concurrent allopurinol use.	Monitor for rashes. If a skin rash develops, consider ↓ dose of allopurinol or using alternative therapy.
Aminoglycosides	Concurrent administration of penicillins and aminoglycosideshas resulted in the inactivation of aminoglycosides.	Do not mix parenteral aminoglycosides and penicillins in the same solution.
Atenolol	Ampicillin may ↓ GI absorption of atenolol, resulting in blood pressure elevation and reduced antianginal effects.	Monitor blood pressure when initiating, during and discontinuing ampicillin therapy.
Methotrexate	Penicillins compete with renal tubular secretion of methotrexate, resulting in a ↓ methotrexate clearance. Concomitant use may ↑ methotrexate serum concentrations, thereby ↑ the risk of toxicity (e.g., neutropenia).	If concomitant treatment is necessary, monitor patients for signs and symptoms of methotrexate toxicity, e.g., hematologic, gastrointestinal.
Oral contraceptives	Antibacterial agents may destroy intestinal flora that provide hydrolytic enzymes essential for enterohepatic recirculation of ethinyl estradiol resulting in ↓ plasma concentration of ethinyl estradiol. Effectiveness of oral contraceptives may be ↓.	Possible contraceptive failure. Consider use of additional method of contraception (e.g., barrier) for duration of cycle to avoid ↑ risk of pregnancy.
Probenecid	Probenecid inhibits renal tubular excretion of ampicillin, thereby ↓ elimination of ampicillin.	This interaction has been exploited to increase serum levels of penicillins.
Tetracyclines (doxycycline, minocycline, tetracycline)	Bacteriostatic action of tetracyclines may inhibit the bactericidal activity of penicillins.	The combination of penicillins and tetracyclines is avoided in pneumococcal meningitis and scarlet fever because tetracycline reduces the effectiveness of penicillin. The clinical significance of this interaction in other infections is unknown.
Warfarin	Effects of warfarin may be increased, resulting in ↑ risk of bleeding (mostly associated with large iv doses of penicillins).	Monitor INR upon addition and withdrawal of ampicillin. INR should be periodically reassessed for at least 3 weeks after ampicillin discontinuation, since adjustment in the warfarin dose may be necessary to maintain an effective level of anticoagulation.

Drug-Food Interactions: Food decreases the absorption of orally administered ampicillin. Oral ampicillin should be taken 1 hour before or 2 hours after meals.

DOSAGE AND ADMINISTRATION: Dosing Considerations: Parenteral ampicillin should be reserved for moderately severe to severe infections and for patients who are unable to take oral medication. Change to oral therapy as soon as it is appropriate.
Recommended Dose and Dosage Adjustment: (See Table 3, Table 4, Table 5.)

Table 3: Ampicillin

Dose in Adult Patients

Indication	Route	Usual Dose	Duration of Treatment	Detailed Information
Urinary tract infections, complicated[a] and pyelonephritis	IV	500–1000 mg Q6H	Modify treatment according to culture results. Continue for 48–72 hours after patient is asymptomatic or evidence of eradication of infection is obtained. Severe infections may require several weeks of therapy.	For severe infections, larger doses may be required. Given in combination with an aminoglycoside in complicated UTIs (see Indications and Clinical Use).
Meningitis or septicemia	IV	12 g daily divided Q4H		iv should be used initially for at least 3 days
Infective endocarditis, prevention	IM or IV	2 g	Single dose	For patients who are unable to take oral medications. Give 30–60 minutes prior to procedure
Infective endocarditis, treatment	IV	12 g per 24 h	4–6 weeks	Give as continuous infusion or in 6 equally divided doses
Prevention of intrapartum streptococcus group B infection of the infant	IV	2 g as initial dose, then 1 g Q4H until delivery	Until delivery	Penicillin is the preferred agent for Group B Streptococcus prophylaxis

[a] Complicated UTIs in men and structural abnormalities, e.g., obstruction, spinal cord injury.

Table 4: Ampicillin

Dose in Pediatric Patients other than Neonates

Indication	Route	Usual Dose	Duration of Treatment	Detailed Information
Genitourinary tract infection	IV	100–200 mg/kg daily divided Q6H	Continue for 48–72 hours after patient is asymptomatic or evidence of eradication of infection is obtained. Severe infections may require several weeks of therapy.	
Meningitis	IV (should be given iv for at least the first 3 days)	200–400 mg/kg daily divided Q6H		Maximum daily dose is 12 g
Septicemia	IM or IV	100–200 mg/kg daily divided Q6H		Maximum daily dose is 12 g
Infective endocarditis, prevention	IM or IV	50 mg/kg	Single dose	For patients who are unable to take oral medications. Give 30 to 60 minutes prior to procedure

Table 5: Ampicillin

Dose in Neonates (≤1 month)

Indication	Age	Weight	Usual Dose[b]/Route	Duration of Treatment
Meningitis, Group B Streptococcus[a]	≤7 days	Regardless of weight	200 mg/kg daily iv divided Q8H	Continue for 48–72 hours after patient is asymptomatic or evidence of eradication of infection is obtained. Severe infections may require several weeks of therapy.
	>7 days	Regardless of weight	300 mg/kg daily iv divided Q6H	
Meningitis	≤7 days	<2 kg	100 mg/kg daily iv divided Q12H	
		≥2 kg	150 mg/kg daily iv divided Q8H	
	>7 days	<2 kg	150 mg/kg daily iv divided Q8H	
		≥2 kg	200 mg/kg daily iv divided Q6H	
Other infections	≤7 days	<2 kg	50 mg/kg daily iv divided Q12H	
		≥2 kg	75 mg/kg daily iv divided Q8H	
	>7 days	<2 kg	75 mg/kg daily iv divided Q8H	
		≥2 kg	100 mg/kg daily iv divided Q6H	
Urinary tract infection, prophylaxis	Regardless of age	Regardless of weight	50 mg/kg daily iv divided Q12H	

[a] Group B streptococci is also known as *S. agalactiae*.
[b] The maximum recommended dose should not exceed the adult dose.

Table 6: Ampicillin

Dose in Adult Patients with Renal Impairment

Creatinine Clearance	Interval Adjustment
>50 mL/min	Q6H
10–50 mL/min	Q6–12H
<10 mL/min	Q12–24H

Dosage in Dialysis: Ampicillin is dialyzable. An extra dose of ampicillin is recommended after hemodialysis. The recommended dose of ampicillin for patients on peritoneal dialysis is 250 mg q12h. For patients receiving continuous arterio-venous hemofiltration (CAVH) or continuous veno-venous hemofiltration (CVVH), dose according to creatinine clearance of 10-50 mL/min (see Table 6).
Administration: Oral ampicillin should be taken 1 hour before or 2 hours after meals.

Ampicillin may be administered by iv infusion at a concentration of ≤30 mg/mL over 30 minutes or by iv direct at a concentration of ≤100 mg/mL at a maximum rate of 100 mg/min.

OVERDOSAGE:

For management of a suspected drug overdose, CPhA recommends that you contact your **regional Poison Control Centre**. See the *CPS* Directory section for a list of Poison Control Centres.

ACTION AND CLINICAL PHARMACOLOGY: Ampicillin, an aminopenicillin, is bactericidal against sensitive organisms. It acts through the inhibition of peptidoglycan synthesis in the bacterial cell wall. This leads to the formation of a defective cell wall with eventual lysis and death to the cell.

The spectrum of activity includes susceptible gram-negative bacteria such as *H. influenzae*, *E. coli*, *P. mirabilis*, *S. epidermidis*, as well as penicillin-sensitive gram-positive bacteria such as *S. pneumoniae*, enterococci, nonpenicillinase-producing staphylococci and Listeria (see Penicillin G/Penicillin V, CPhA monograph). Some isolates of *H. influenza*, Enterobacteriaceae, Salmonella and Shigella species are resistant due to β-lactamase production or other mechanisms. The proportion of strains which are sensitive varies widely among different patient populations. Ampicillin is slightly more active against enterococcus than penicillin G or penicillin V, but resistance to penicillin implies resistance to ampicillin. For severe infections, since ampicillin alone is only bacteriostatic, the addition of an aminoglycoside (usually gentamicin) is often indicated.

Pharmacokinetics: Ampicillin is well absorbed after oral administration. Ampicillin is taken on an empty stomach. A decrease and delay in the peak levels of ampicillin occur if taken with food. Peak blood levels are usually attained within 1 to 2 hours following oral administration. Amoxicillin is the preferred oral agent over ampicillin as it has better bioavailability. Ampicillin diffuses readily into most body tissues and fluids especially in the presence of inflammation. Ampicillin is not highly protein bound (20%). Its elimination half-life ranges from 0.8 to 1.5 hours in patients with normal renal function. Significant levels are achieved in the bile and stool as ampicillin undergoes enterohepatic circulation. Ampicillin is renally excreted.

Anafranil® Ⓟ

clomipramine HCl

Antidepressant—Antiobsessional

Sepracor

Date of Preparation: August 4, 2009

PHARMACOLOGY: Clomipramine is a tricyclic agent with both antidepressant and antiobsessional properties. Like other tricyclics, clomipramine inhibits norepinephrine and serotonin uptake into central nerve terminals, possibly by blocking the membrane-pump of neurons, thereby increasing the concentration of transmitter monoamines at receptor sites. Clomipramine is presumed to influence depression and obsessive and compulsive behavior through its effects on serotonergic neurotransmission. The actual neurochemical mechanism is unknown, but clomipramine's capacity to inhibit serotonin reuptake is thought to be important. Clomipramine appears to have a mild sedative effect which may be helpful in alleviating the anxiety component often accompanying depression.

As with other tricyclic compounds, clomipramine possesses anticholinergic properties which are responsible for certain side effects. It also has weak antihistamine and antiserotonin properties, lowers the convulsive threshold, potentiates the effect of norepinephrine and other drugs acting on the CNS, has a quinidine-like effect on the heart and may impair cardiac conduction.

The action of clomipramine on the human EEG is one of desynchronization. Clomipramine causes a persistent increase in the frequency of shifts into stage I sleep and produces marked reduction or suppression of rapid eye movement sleep (REM or paradoxical sleep). Partial recovery occurs within 3 to 4 weeks as does a rebound after drug withdrawal which appears to last approximately the same time. In normal human volunteers tricyclic antidepressants tend to produce a sedative effect accompanied by atropine-like symptoms and may produce some difficulty in concentrating and thinking.

Pharmacokinetics: Clomipramine is rapidly and completely absorbed after oral administration in humans. Peak plasma levels are usually reached 2 hours after dosage but much individual variation occurs. The plasma half-life after a single oral dose is approximately 21 hours. After 28 days of oral administration to patients in a daily dosage of 75 mg, plasma concentrations of clomipramine ranged from 17 to 70 ng/mL (mean=35.7 ng/mL). The concentration of the active metabolite, desmethylclomipramine, was about twice as high. The binding of clomipramine to serum proteins is very high at 96 to 97% and is practically concentration-independent within the therapeutic range. Clomipramine has a volume of distribution of approximately 12 L/kg.

Clomipramine is extensively metabolized in the body with hydroxylation, demethylation and N-oxidation being the quantitatively more important routes of metabolism.

Owing to the lower clearance of clomipramine in plasma, elderly patients require lower doses of clomipramine than patients in younger age groups.

As expected, the metabolites of clomipramine are quite similar to those of imipramine, all retaining the benzazepine structure. Two-thirds of clomipramine is excreted as water-soluble conjugates in the urine and approximately one-third in the feces. After a 25 mg radiolabeled dose of clomipramine in 2 subjects, the urinary recoveries of clomipramine and desmethylclomipramine were about 2% and 0.5% of the total radioactivity, respectively.

INDICATIONS: For the treatment of depression. Clomipramine also appears to have a mild sedative effect which may be helpful in alleviating the anxiety component often accompanying depression.

For the treatment of obsessions and compulsions in patients with obsessive compulsive disorder (OCD). The obsessions and compulsions must cause marked distress, be time-consuming, or significantly interfere with social or occupational functioning.

The effectiveness of clomipramine for long-term use (e.g., for more than 10 weeks) has not been systematically evaluated in placebo-controlled trials. The physician who elects to use clomipramine for extended periods should periodically re-evaluate the long-term usefulness of the drug for the individual patient.

CONTRAINDICATIONS: Patients who have known or suspected hypersensitivity to the drug or its excipients, or have known or suspected hypersensitivity to tricyclic antidepressants belonging to the dibenzazepine group.

Clomipramine should not be given in conjunction with or within 14 days before or after treatment with a MAO inhibitor (see Drug Interactions). The concomitant treatment with selective, reversible MAO A inhibitors, such as moclobemide, is also contraindicated. Hypertensive crises, hyperactivity, hyperpyrexia, spasticity, severe convulsions or coma, and death have been reported in patients receiving such combinations.

It is contraindicated during the acute recovery phase following myocardial infarction and in the presence of acute congestive heart failure.

Clomipramine is contraindicated in patients with existing liver or kidney damage and should not be administered to patients with a history of blood dyscrasias.

Clomipramine is contraindicated in patients with glaucoma, as the condition may be aggravated due to the atropine-like effects of the drug.

WARNINGS: Seizures: Tricyclic agents are known to lower the convulsive threshold and clomipramine should, therefore, be used with extreme caution in patients with a history of convulsive disorders and other predisposing factors, e.g., brain damage of varying etiology, concomitant use of neuroleptics, alcoholism and withdrawal from alcohol, and concomitant use with other drugs that lower the seizure threshold. It appears that the occurrence of seizures is dose dependent. Therefore, the recommended total daily doses should not be exceeded (see Dosage).

Concurrent administration of ECT and clomipramine may be hazardous and such treatment should be limited to patients for whom it is essential. Physicians should discuss with patients the risk of taking clomipramine while engaging in activities in which a sudden loss of consciousness could result in serious injury to the patient or others, e.g., the operation of complex machinery, driving, swimming, or climbing.

Cardiovascular: Tricyclic antidepressants, particularly in high doses, have been reported to produce sinus tachycardia, changes in conduction time and arrhythmias. A few instances of unexpected death have been reported in patients with cardiovascular disorders. Myocardial infarction and stroke have also been reported with drugs of this class. Therefore, clomipramine should be administered with extreme caution to patients with a history of cardiovascular disorders, especially those with cardiovascular insufficiency, conduction disorders (e.g., atrioventricular block grades I to III) or other arrhythmias, those with circulatory lability and elderly patients. Clomipramine also has a hypotensive action which may be detrimental in these circumstances. In such cases, treatment should be initiated at low doses with progressive increases only if required and tolerated, and the patients should be under close surveillance at all dosage levels. Monitoring of cardiac function and the ECG is indicated in such patients as well as in the elderly.

There may be a risk of QTc prolongation at supra-therapeutic doses or supra-therapeutic plasma concentrations of clomipramine, as occur in the case of co-medication with selective serotonin reuptake inhibitors (SSRIs) (see Precautions). It is established that hypokalemia is a risk factor of QTc prolongation and torsades de pointes. Therefore, hypokalemia should be treated before initiating treatment with clomipramine and clomipramine should be used with caution when combined with SSRIs or diuretics (see Precautions).

Use in Concomitant Illness: Caution should be observed in prescribing clomipramine in hyperthyroid patients or for patients receiving thyroid medication. Transient cardiac arrhythmias have occurred in rare instances in patients who have been receiving other tricyclic compounds concomitantly with thyroid medication.

Because of its anticholinergic properties, clomipramine should be used with caution in patients with increased intraocular pressure, narrow angle glaucoma or urinary retention, particularly in the presence of prostatic hypertrophy.

Tricyclic antidepressants may give rise to paralytic ileus, particularly in the elderly and in hospitalized patients. Therefore, appropriate measures should be taken if constipation occurs.

Caution is called for when employing clomipramine in patients with tumors of the adrenal medulla (e.g., pheochromocytoma, neuroblastoma) in whom the drug may provoke hypertensive crisis.

Clomipramine should be kept in a safe place, well out of the reach of children.

Pregnancy: The safety of use in pregnant women has not been established. Therefore, clomipramine should not be administered to women of childbearing potential, or during pregnancy, unless, in the opinion of the physician, the expected benefit to the patient outweighs the potential risk to the fetus. Withdrawal symptoms including tremors, dyspnea, lethargy, colic, irritability, hypotonia/hypertonia, convulsions, and respiratory depression have been reported in neonates whose mothers received tricyclic antidepressants during the third trimester of pregnancy. To avoid such symptoms, clomipramine should, if possible, be gradually withdrawn at least 7 weeks before the calculated date of confinement.

Lactation: Since clomipramine passes into breast milk, the drug should be gradually withdrawn or the infant weaned if the patient is breast-feeding.

PRECAUTIONS: Suicide: The possibility of a suicide attempt is inherent in depression with or without obsessive compulsive disorder. These patients should be carefully supervised during treatment with clomipramine, and hospitalization or concomitant ECT may be required. To minimize the risk of an intentional overdose by a depressed patient, prescriptions for clomipramine should be written for the smallest possible quantity of the drug consistent with good patient management.

Psychosis, Mania-Hypomania And Other Neuropsychiatric Phenomena: In patients treated with tricyclic antidepressants, activation of latent schizophrenia or aggravation of existing psychotic manifestations in schizophrenic patients may occur. Patients with manic-depressive tendencies may experience hypomanic or manic shifts. Hyperactive or agitated patients may become over-stimulated. A reduction in dose or discontinuation of clomipramine should be considered under these circumstances.

In predisposed and elderly patients, tricyclic antidepressants may, particularly at night, provoke pharmacogenic (delirious) psychoses that disappear within a few days of withdrawing the drug.

Occupational Hazards: Since clomipramine may produce sedation, particularly during the initial phase of therapy, patients should be cautioned about the danger of engaging in activities requiring mental alertness, judgement and physical coordination.

Cardiovascular: Before initiating treatment, it is advisable to check the patient's blood pressure, because individuals with hypotension or a labile circulation may react to the drug with a fall in blood pressure. Regular measurements of blood pressure should be performed in susceptible patients. Postural hypotension may be controlled by reducing the dosage or administering circulatory stimulants.

ECG abnormalities have been observed in patients treated with clomipramine. The most common ECG changes were premature ventricular contractions (PVCs), ST-T wave changes, and abnormalities in intraventricular conduction. These changes were rarely associated with significant clinical symptoms. Nevertheless, caution is necessary when treating patients with heart disease, as well as elderly subjects. In these patients cardiac function should be monitored and ECG examinations performed during long-term therapy. Gradual dose titration is also recommended.

Hepatic Changes: Clomipramine has occasionally been associated with elevations in AST and ALT of potential clinical significance (e.g., values greater than 3 times the upper limit of normal). In the majority of cases, these enzyme elevations were not associated with other clinical findings suggestive of hepatic injury.

Isolated cases of obstructive jaundice have been reported. Caution is indicated in treating patients with known liver disease, and periodic monitoring of hepatic function is recommended in such patients.

Hematologic Changes: Isolated cases of bone marrow depression with agranulocytosis have been reported. Leukocyte and differential blood cell counts are recommended in patients receiving treatment with clomipramine over prolonged periods, and should be performed for patients who develop fever, an influenzal infection, or sore throat. In the event of an allergic skin reaction, clomipramine should be withdrawn.

Central Nervous System: More than 30 cases of hyperthermia have been recorded by nondomestic post-marketing surveillance systems. Most cases occurred when clomipramine was used in combination with other drugs. When clomipramine and a neuroleptic were used concomitantly, the cases were sometimes considered to be examples of a neuroleptic malignant syndrome.

Withdrawal Symptoms: A variety of withdrawal symptoms has been reported in association with abrupt discontinuation of clomipramine, including dizziness, nausea, vomiting, headache, malaise, sleep disturbance, hyperthermia and irritability. In addition, such patients may experience a worsening of psychiatric status. While the withdrawal effects of clomipramine have not been systematically evaluated in controlled trials, they are well known with closely related tricyclic antidepressants. It is recommended that the dosage be tapered gradually and the patient monitored carefully during discontinuation.

Metabolic Effects: Tricyclic antidepressants have been associated with porphyrinogenicity in susceptible patients.

Renal Function: It is advisable to monitor renal function during long-term therapy with tricyclic antidepressants.

Dental Effects: Lengthy treatment with tricyclic antidepressants can lead to an increased incidence of dental caries.

Lacrimation: Decreased lacrimation and accumulation of mucoid secretions, due to the anticholinergic properties of tricyclic antidepressants, may cause damage to the corneal epithelium in patients with contact lenses.

Endocrine Effects: As with certain other psychotherapeutic drugs, clomipramine elevates prolactin levels. Tissue culture experiments indicate that approximately one-third of human breast cancers are prolactin dependent in vitro, a factor of potential importance if the prescription of clomipramine is contemplated in a patient with a previously detected breast cancer. Although disturbances such as galactorrhea, amenorrhea, gynecomastia, and impotence have been reported, the clinical significance of elevated serum prolactin levels is unknown for most patients. An increase in mammary neoplasms has been found in rodents after chronic administration of neuroleptic drugs. Neither clinical studies nor epidemiologic studies conducted to date, however, have shown an association between chronic administration of these drugs and mammary tumorigenesis: the available evidence is considered too limited to be conclusive at this time.

Children: As clomipramine has not been studied in patients under 10 years of age, specific recommendations for use in this age group cannot be provided. The long-term effects of clomipramine on childhood growth and development have not been determined.

Drug Interactions: Patients should be warned that, while taking clomipramine, their responses to alcoholic beverages, other CNS depressants (e.g., barbiturates, benzodiazepines or general anesthetics) or anticholinergic agents (e.g., atropine, antihistamines, biperiden, levodopa) may be exaggerated.

When tricyclic antidepressants are given in combination with anticholinergics or neuroleptics with an anticholinergic action, hyperexcitation states or delirium may occur, as well as attacks of glaucoma.

Tricyclic antidepressants should not be employed in combination with antiarrhythmic agents of the quinidine type (see Warnings, Cardiovascular).

Since clomipramine may diminish or abolish the antihypertensive effects of guanethidine, bethanidine, clonidine, reserpine, or alpha-methyldopa, patients requiring concomitant treatment for hypertension should be given antihypertensives of a different type (e.g., vasodilators, beta-blockers).

Co-medication with diuretics may lead to hypokalemia, which should be treated prior to administration of clomipramine.

Clomipramine may potentiate the cardiovascular effects of norepinephrine or epinephrine, amphetamine, as well as nasal drops and local anesthetics containing sympathomimetics (e.g., isoprenaline, ephedrine, phenylephrine).

Fluoxetine, fluvoxamine and other selective serotonin reuptake inhibitors (SSRIs) may increase the activity and plasma concentrations of tricyclic antidepressants, such as clomipramine, with corresponding adverse effects. Co-medication with SSRIs may lead to additive effects on the serotoninergic system.

Caution should be exercised if clomipramine is administered together with cimetidine or methylphenidate since these drugs have been shown to inhibit the metabolism of several tricyclic antidepressants. Clinically significant increases in plasma levels of clomipramine may occur, necessitating a dosage reduction.

Substances which activate the hepatic mono-oxygenase enzyme system (e.g., barbiturates, carbamazepine, phenytoin, nicotine and oral contraceptives) may lower plasma concentrations of tricyclic antidepressants and so reduce their antidepressive effects. In addition, clomipramine may increase plasma levels of phenytoin and carbamazepine, therefore, it may be necessary to adjust the dosage of these drugs.

Clomipramine should not be administered for a period of at least 14 days after the discontinuation of treatment with MAO inhibitors due to the potential for severe interactions (see Contraindications). The same caution should also be observed when administering an MAO inhibitor after previous treatment with clomipramine.

Clomipramine should be discontinued prior to elective surgery for as long as is clinically feasible, since little is known about the interaction with general anesthetics.

Concomitant treatment with neuroleptic agents (e.g., phenothiazines and butyrophenones) may result in increased plasma concentrations of clomipramine, a lowered convulsion threshold and seizures. Combination with thioridazine may produce cardiac arrhythmias. No such effects are known to occur in combination with diazepam but it might be necessary to lower the dosage of clomipramine if administered concomitantly with alprazolam or disulfiram.

Tricyclic antidepressants may potentiate the anticoagulant effect of coumarin drugs by inhibiting hepatic metabolism of these drugs. Careful monitoring of plasma prothrombin is therefore advised.

If administered concomitantly with estrogens, the dose of clomipramine should be reduced since steroid hormones inhibit the metabolism of clomipramine.

Teratology: No teratogenic effects were observed in rats and mice at doses up to 20 times the maximum daily human dose. Slight nonspecific fetotoxic effects were seen in the offspring of pregnant mice given doses 10 times the maximum daily human dose. Slight nonspecific embryotoxicity was observed in rats given doses 5 to 10 times the maximum daily human dose.
Animal Toxicology: As with tricyclic compounds, clomipramine has been associated with changes in testicular and lung tissue in long-term animal toxicology studies. In 1- and 2 year studies in rats, a dose 4 times the maximum daily human dose was associated with phospholipidosis in the lungs and changes in the testes (atrophy, aspermatogenesis, and calcification). In a 1 year toxicity study in dogs, testicular atrophy was detected in animals receiving 10 times the maximum recommended daily human dose.

ADVERSE EFFECTS: The most commonly observed adverse events associated with the use of clomipramine and not seen at an equivalent incidence among placebo-treated patients were gastrointestinal complaints, including dry mouth, constipation, nausea, dyspepsia, and anorexia; nervous system complaints, including somnolence, tremor, dizziness, nervousness and myoclonus; genitourinary complaints including changed libido, ejaculatory failure, impotence and micturition disorder; and other miscellaneous complaints, including fatigue, sweating, increased appetite, weight gain, and visual changes.

If severe neurological or psychiatric reactions occur, clomipramine should be withdrawn.

Elderly patients are particularly susceptible to anticholinergic, psychiatric, neurological and cardiovascular effects.

The following adverse reactions have also been reported with clomipramine or other tricyclic antidepressants. (Frequency estimates: Frequent: >10%; Occasional: >1 to 10%; Rare: >0.01 to 1%; Isolated cases: <0.01%).
Neurological: Occasional: headache, paresthesia (numbness, tingling sensation, symptoms suggestive of peripheral neuropathy), delirium, muscle hypertonia, muscle weakness. Rare: epileptic seizures. Isolated cases: tinnitus, incoordination, ataxia, alterations in EEG patterns, extrapyramidal symptoms, speech disorders, weakness, hyperpyrexia.
Behavioral: Occasional: drowsiness, insomnia, confusional states with hallucinations (particularly in geriatric patients and patients suffering from Parkinson's disease), anxiety, agitation, restlessness, sleep disturbances, nightmares, aggravated depression, hypomania, mania, decrease in memory, feeling of unreality, depersonalization, yawning, disorientation. Rare: activation of latent psychosis. Isolated cases: aggressiveness.
Anticholinergic: Frequent: dry mouth and rarely associated sublingual adenitis, disturbances of visual accommodation, hot flushes. Occasional: dilation of the urinary tract. Isolated cases: mydriasis, glaucoma, paralytic ileus.
Cardiovascular: Frequent: hypotension, particularly orthostatic hypotension with associated vertigo, sinus tachycardia, ECG changes (including flattening or inversion of T wave, depressed S-T segments) in patients of normal cardiac status. Occasional: arrhythmia, palpitation, syncope. Isolated cases: hypertension, congestive heart failure, myocardial infarction, heart block, asystole, stroke, peripheral vasospastic reactions, disturbances in cardiac conduction (e.g. widening of QRS complex, PQ changes, bundle-branch block, prolonged QT interval, torsades de pointes in hypokalemia).
Hematologic: Isolated cases: agranulocytosis, eosinophilia, leukopenia, purpura and thrombocytopenia may occur as an idiosyncratic response. One case of pancytopenia has been reported.
Gastrointestinal: Occasional: vomiting, abdominal cramps. Rare: diarrhea, elevated transaminases. Isolated cases: bitter taste, stomatitis, epigastric distress, black tongue, dysphagia, increased salivation, hepatitis with or without jaundice.
Respiratory: Isolated cases: bronchospasm.
Endocrine: Isolated cases: gynecomastia in the male, breast enlargement and galactorrhea in the female, testicular swelling, elevation or depression of blood sugar levels, weight loss, inappropriate antidiuretic hormone (SIADH) secretion syndrome, increase in prolactin levels, menstrual irregularity.
Allergic or Toxic: Occasional: skin rash, urticaria. Isolated cases: petechiae, itching, photosensitization (avoid excessive exposure to sunlight), edema (general or of face and tongue), drug fever, obstructive jaundice, nasal congestion, alopecia, allergic alveolitis (pneumonia) with or without eosinophilia, systemic analphylactic/anaphylactoid reactions including hypotension.
Withdrawal Symptoms: Abrupt cessation of treatment with tricyclic antidepressants after prolonged administration may occasionally produce nausea, vomiting, abdominal pain, diarrhea, insomnia, nervousness, anxiety, headache and malaise. These symptoms are not indicative of addiction.

OVERDOSE:
Since children may be more sensitive than adults to acute overdosage with tricyclic antidepressants, and since fatalities in children have been reported, effort should be made to avoid potential overdose particularly in this age group.

Symptoms: These may vary in severity depending on various factors such as the amount of drug absorbed, the interval between drug ingestion and start of treatment, and the age of the patient. Accidental ingestion in children should be regarded as serious and potentially fatal.

Symptoms generally appear within 4 hours of ingestion and reach maximum severity after 24 hours. Owing to delayed absorption (increased anticholinergic effect due to overdose), long half-life and enterohepatic recycling of the drug, the patient may be at risk for up to 4 to 6 days.

Symptoms may include drowsiness, stupor, ataxia, vomiting, cyanosis, restlessness, agitation, delirium, severe perspiration, hyperactive reflexes, muscle rigidity, athetoid and choreiform movements, and convulsions. Hyperpyrexia, mydriasis, bowel and bladder paralysis, and respiratory depression may occur.

Hypotension and initial hypertension may occur. However, the usual finding is increasing hypotension which may lead eventually to shock. Serious cardiovascular disturbances are frequently present, including tachycardia, cardiac arrhythmias (flutter, atriofibrillation, premature ventricular beats and ventricular tachycardia) as well as impaired myocardial conduction, atrioventricular and intraventricular block, ECG abnormalities (such as widened QRS complexes, marked S-T shifts and QTc prolongation), signs of congestive heart failure and cardiac arrest. Coma may ensue.

Treatment: Patients in whom overdosage is suspected should be admitted to hospital without delay. No specific antidote is available and treatment is essentially symptomatic and supportive.

Gastric lavage or aspiration should be performed promptly and is recommended up to 12 hours or even more after the overdose, since the anticholinergic effect of the drug may delay gastric emptying. Administration of activated charcoal may help to reduce absorption of the drug. As clomipramine is largely protein bound, forced diuresis, peritoneal dialysis and hemodialysis are unlikely to be of value.

Treatment should be designed to insure maintenance of the vital functions. An open airway should be maintained in comatose patients and assisted ventilation instituted, if necessary, but respiratory stimulants should not be used. Hyperpyrexia should be controlled by external measures, such as ice packs and cooling sponge baths. Acidosis may be treated by cautious administration of sodium bicarbonate. Adequate renal function should be maintained.

ECG monitoring in an intensive care unit is recommended in all patients, particularly in the presence of ECG abnormalities, and should be maintained for several days after the cardiac rhythm has returned to normal. Unexpected deaths attributed to cardiac arrhythmias have been reported several days following an apparent recovery from tricyclic antidepressant overdose. Correction of hypoxia and acidosis, if present, may be beneficial. Correction of metabolic acidosis and low potassium concentrations by means of bicarbonate i.v. and potassium substitution may also be effective for treatment of arrhythmias. If bradyarrhythmia or AV-block occur, consider temporary insertion of a cardiac pacemaker. Because of its effect on cardiac conduction, digitalis should be used only with caution. If rapid digitalization is required for the treatment of congestive heart failure, special care should be exercised in using the drug.

External stimulation should be minimized to reduce the tendency to convulsions. If convulsions occur, anticonvulsants (preferably i.v. diazepam) should be administered. Barbiturates may intensify respiratory depression, particularly in children, and aggravate hypotension and coma. Paraldehyde may be used in some children to counteract muscular hypertonus and convulsions with less likelihood of causing respiratory depression. If the patient fails to respond rapidly to anticonvulsants, artificial ventilation should be instituted. Prompt control of convulsions is essential since they aggravate hypoxia and acidosis and may thereby precipitate cardiac arrhythmias and arrest.

Shock should be treated with supportive measures, such as i.v. fluids, plasma expanders and oxygen. The use of corticosteroids in shock is controversial and may be contraindicated in tricyclic antidepressant overdose. Hypotension usually responds to elevation of the foot of the bed. Pressor agents (but **not** epinephrine) should be given cautiously, if indicated. In the event of reduced myocardial function, consider recourse to treatment with dopamine or dobutamine by i.v. drip.

Since it has been reported that physostigmine may cause severe bradycardia, asystole and seizures, its use is not recommended in cases of overdosage with clomipramine.

Deaths by deliberate or accidental overdosage have occurred with this class of drugs. Since the propensity for suicide is high in depressed patients, a suicide attempt by other means may occur during the recovery phase. The possibility of simultaneous ingestion of other drugs should also be considered.

For management of a suspected drug overdose, CPhA recommends that you contact your **regional Poison Control Centre**. See the *CPS* Directory section for a list of Poison Control Centres.

DOSAGE: Dosage should be individualized according to the requirements of each patient. Treatment should be initiated at the lowest recommended dose and increased gradually, noting carefully the clinical response and any evidence of intolerance. During the initial dose titration phase, the total daily dose of clomipramine should be divided and administered with meals to reduce gastrointestinal side effects.

Owing to the long elimination half-lives of clomipramine and its active metabolite, desmethylclomipramine, steady-state plasma levels may not be achieved until 2 to 3 weeks after a dosage adjustment. It may thus be advisable to wait 2 to 3 weeks after the initial dose titration phase, before attempting further dosage adjustments. It should be kept in mind that a lag in therapeutic response usually occurs at the onset of therapy, lasting from several days to a few weeks. Increasing the dosage does not normally shorten this latent period and may increase the incidence of side effects.
Depression: Initial Dosage: Adults: Clomipramine therapy should be initiated at daily doses of 25 mg. Dosage may be increased by 25 mg increments, as tolerated, at 3 to 4 day intervals up to a total daily dose of 150 mg by the end of 2 weeks. Thereafter, the dose may be gradually increased over a period of several weeks to 200 mg. Doses in excess of 200 mg daily are not recommended for outpatients. Occasionally, in more severely depressed hospitalized patients, dosages up to 300 mg daily may be required.
Elderly and Debilitated Patients: In general, lower dosages are recommended for these patients. Initially, 20 to 30 mg daily in divided doses is suggested, with very gradual increments, depending on tolerance and response. Blood pressure and cardiac rhythm should be checked frequently, particularly in patients who have unstable cardiovascular function.
Maintenance Dosage: Dosage during maintenance therapy should be kept at the lowest effective level. To minimize daytime sedation during maintenance treatment, the total daily dosage may be given as a single dose at bedtime. Medication should be continued for the expected duration of the depressive episode in order to minimize the possibility of relapse following clinical improvement.
Obsessive Compulsive Disorders: Initial Dosage: Adults: Clomipramine therapy in adult obsessive compulsive patients should be initiated at daily doses of 25 mg. Dosage may be increased by 25 mg increments, as tolerated, at 3 to 4 day intervals up to a total daily dose of 100 or 150 mg by the end of 2 weeks. Thereafter, the dose may be gradually increased over a period of several weeks to 200 mg. Doses in excess of 200 mg/day are not generally recommended for outpatients. However, in the treatment of severe cases of Obsessive Compulsive Disorder, daily doses of up to 250 mg may be required.
Children and Adolescents: In children aged 10 to 17 years, an initial dose of 25 mg/day is recommended. Dosage may be increased by 25 mg increments, as tolerated, at 3 to 4 day intervals. By the end of 2 weeks, patients may be titrated up to 100 to 150 mg/day or 3 mg/kg, whichever is lower. Thereafter, the dose may be gradually increased to 200 mg or 3 mg/kg whichever is lower. A total daily dose above 200 mg should not be used in children or adolescents.
Elderly and Debilitated Patients: In general, lower dosages are recommended for these patients. Initially, 20 to 30 mg daily in divided doses is suggested, with very gradual increments, depending on tolerance and response. Blood pressure and cardiac rhythm should be checked frequently, particularly in patients who have unstable cardiovascular function.
Maintenance Dosage (Adults, Children, and Adolescents): Double-blind extension phase studies of clomipramine therapy in patients with Obsessive Compulsive Disorder have followed patients for up to 52 weeks. Although placebo enrollment in these studies was inadequate to permit a controlled comparison, data suggest that clomipramine therapy can be continued for up to a year without loss of efficacy.

Dosage adjustments may be made during maintenance therapy with the objective of maintaining the patient at the lowest effective dose. To minimize daytime sedation during maintenance treatment, the total daily dosage may be given as a single dose at bedtime. If symptoms recur, the dosage should be increased until the symptoms are controlled. Patients should be reassessed periodically to determine the need for continued treatment. To avoid withdrawal symptoms upon discontinuation of therapy, a gradual decrease in dosage and careful patient monitoring are recommended.

SUPPLIED: 10 mg: Each cream-colored, triangular, sugar-coated tablet, contains: clomipramine HCl 10 mg. Nonmedicinal ingredients: cellulose compounds, cornstarch, gelatin, glycerin, iron oxide, lactose, magnesium stearate, polyethylene glycol, polyvinylpyrrolidone, sucrose, talc and titanium dioxide. Bottles of 100. Protect from heat. Store between 2 and 30°C. Keep out of reach of children.
25 mg: Each cream-colored, round, biconvex, sugar-coated tablet, branded GEIGY on one side and FH on the other side in black, contains: clomipramine HCl 25 mg. Nonmedicinal ingredients: cellulose compounds, colloidal silicon dioxide, cornstarch, glycerin, iron oxide, lactose, magnesium stearate, polyethylene glycol, polyvinylpyrrolidone, stearic acid, sucrose, talc and titanium dioxide. Bottles of 100. Protect from heat. Store between 2 and 30°C. Keep out of reach of children.
50 mg: Each white, round, beveled edge, film-coated tablet, engraved GEIGY on one side and LP on the other side, contains: clomipramine HCl 50 mg. Nonmedicinal ingredients: cellulose compounds, colloidal silicon dioxide, lactose, magnesium stearate, polysorbates, talc and titanium dioxide. Bottles of 100. Protect from heat. Store between 2 and 30°C. Keep out of reach of children.

Anandron® Pr
nilutamide
Nonsteroidal Antiandrogen

sanofi-aventis

Date of Revision: May 15, 2008

PHARMACOLOGY: Nilutamide is a pure, nonsteroidal antiandrogen which blocks androgens binding at receptor target cells. Nilutamide is specific and does not bind to any other steroidal receptors; therefore, it does not have any other hormonal or antihormonal activity.

Nilutamide demonstrates potent antiandrogenic effects by inhibiting androgen uptake and/or inhibiting nuclear binding of androgen in target tissues. In adult male rats, ventral prostate and seminal vesicle weights were markedly reduced by daily administration of nilutamide.

Androgen-sensitive prostatic carcinoma cells respond to treatment that counteracts the effect of androgen and/or removes the source of androgen e.g., castration. Combined with castration, nilutamide exerts a total peripheral antiandrogenic activity by antagonizing the action of androgens of adrenal origin which otherwise may maintain the proliferation of prostatic cancer cells.

Nilutamide also inhibits the consequences of the initial rise of testosterone plasma levels observed after treatment with LHRH agonists.

Clinical studies with nilutamide have demonstrated improvement in metastatic bone pain, diminished consumption of analgesics, regression of the cancer together with reduced rate of objective progression and higher survival actuarial rate of patients with metastatic prostate cancer.

Nilutamide is rapidly and completely absorbed as indicated by the low level of fecal radioactivity measured after administration of radiolabeled nilutamide. Unchanged nilutamide represents the major active compound. In patients, nilutamide has a long half-life of 56 hours (range from 23 to 87 hours). Nilutamide is 84% bound to plasma proteins. The plasma concentrations are dose-related and steady-state levels are reached approximately 2 weeks after initiation of treatment. No evidence of accumulation has been demonstrated.

Nilutamide is mainly excreted in the urine as metabolites. Using radiolabeled nilutamide, unchanged drug accounts for only 3% of recovered urinary radioactivity. Fecal excretion accounts for 1.4 to 7% of the total administered dose after 4 to 5 days. The major metabolic pathway is by reduction of the nitro group and the amino derivative of nilutamide represents the major metabolite. Among the metabolites of nilutamide only the hydroxymethylnitro derivative shows some androgen receptor binding affinity.

INDICATIONS: In the treatment of metastatic prostatic carcinoma (Stage D_2) in conjunction with surgical castration.

CONTRAINDICATIONS: Patients with known hypersensitivity to the drug or to any constituents of the drug product and in patients with severe hepatic dysfunction or with severe respiratory insufficiency.

Nilutamide is contraindicated in women and children.

WARNINGS: The hepatic and respiratory state of the patient should be evaluated and the necessity to report any respiratory symptoms as soon as they appear should be emphasized.

Cases of interstitial lung disease have been reported with the use of nilutamide. If dyspnea or worsening of dyspnea occurs, treatment should be interrupted and a chest x ray performed immediately. If interstitial pneumopathy is diagnosed, nilutamide must be discontinued and corticosteroid treatment may be considered.

Cases of hepatic dysfunction have been reported with the use of nilutamide. If clinical symptoms give rise to a suspicion of liver dysfunction, transaminases should be measured. If an increase in serum transaminases above 3 times the upper limit of normal laboratory range is shown, treatment must be interrupted.

Antiandrogen Withdrawal Syndrome: In some patients with metastatic prostate cancer, antiandrogens (steroidal or non-steroidal), may promote, rather than inhibit, the growth of prostate cancer. A decrease in PSA and/or clinical improvement following the discontinuation of antiandrogens have been reported. It is recommended that patients prescribed an antiandrogen, who have PSA progression, should have the antiandrogen discontinued immediately and be monitored for 6 to 8 weeks for a withdrawal response prior to any decision to proceed with other prostate cancer therapy.

PRECAUTIONS: Information to Be Provided to the Patient: Patients should be informed that they should not interrupt their dosing or stop taking nilutamide without consulting their physician(s).

Occupational Hazards: Where patients are participating in activities such as driving an automobile or operating machinery, attention should be drawn to possible visual disturbances mainly due to an increase in adaptation time when passing from a well lit area to a more dimly lit area. These disturbances, should they occur, can decrease even if treatment is continued and can be ameliorated with the use of sunglasses.

Patients should be informed about signs/symptoms suggestive of liver dysfunction (e.g., right upper quadrant tenderness, dark urine, persistent anorexia, nausea, vomiting, jaundice, pruritus or unexplained flu-like symptoms) and be advised to contact their physician should these occur.

Patients administered nilutamide should be warned against consuming alcohol because of a possible disulfiram-like reaction.

Drug Interactions: Nilutamide, apparently through an effect on certain oxidative microsomal enzymes, may reduce the hepatic metabolism of warfarin-type anticoagulants, phenytoin, propranolol, chlordiazepoxide, lidocaine, diazepam and theophylline, thereby delaying elimination and increasing blood levels of these drugs. Benzodiazepines that are not oxidized by the hepatic system do not exhibit this effect.

Dosage of the drugs mentioned above, and other similarly metabolized drugs, may require adjustment when starting or stopping concomitantly administered nilutamide, to maintain safe optimum therapeutic blood levels.

In case of associated treatment with warfarin-type anticoagulants, close monitoring of prothrombin time is recommended and adjustment of the anticoagulant dose may be necessary.

Alcohol intolerance (disulfiram-like reaction) may occur if alcohol is consumed during treatment with nilutamide.

Specific Patient Populations: In an uncontrolled pilot study conducted in a Japanese population, interstitial pneumonitis was reported and was considered possibly or probably related to nilutamide in 6 out of 47 patients (12.8%). This incidence figure is higher than the incidence of interstitial pneumonitis available from the international database of placebo-controlled trials in orchiectomized patients (1.1%; see Adverse Effects). In concurrent pharmacokinetics/metabolism investigations in Japanese vs Caucasian patients, no differences in the results could account for the higher incidence of this event in this race. The incidence rate of raised transaminases in the Japanese study was 19%. Special care should be observed when treating Asian patients.

ADVERSE EFFECTS: Clinical Trials: Adverse Drug Reactions: Table 1 lists the possibly or probably drug-related adverse events (adverse reactions) most frequently reported during placebo-controlled clinical trials of nilutamide in conjunction with surgical castration. Hot flushes, decreased libido, impotence and body hair loss are known to occur with surgical castration.

Table 1: Anandron
Adverse Effects

Adverse Reaction	Percentage of Patients: Nilutamide (n=560)	Placebo (n=558)
Hot flushes	13.8	9.7
Impaired adaptation to darkness	10.5	0.7
Nausea	4.3	1.1
Alcohol intolerance	4.1	0.2
Dizziness	2.9	0.5
Chromatopsia	2.5	0
ALT increased	2.0	0.7
Abnormal vision	1.8	0.5
AST increased	1.4	0.4
Photophobia	1.4	0
Hyperglycemia	1.3	1.6
Impotence	1.3	0.5
Dyspnea	1.1	0.2
Gynecomastia	1.1	1.3
Impaired light adaptation	1.1	0
Interstitial lung disease	1.1	0
Eye disorder	0.9	0.4
Libido decreased	0.9	0
Sweating increased	0.9	0.5
Vomiting	0.9	0
Anorexia	0.7	0
Blurred vision	0.7	0
Hepatitis	0.7	0
Hypertension	0.7	0.2
Anemia	0.5	0.2
Asthenia	0.5	0.4
Gastrointestinal pain	0.5	0.2
Lung disorder	0.5	0
Malaise	0.5	0

Adverse Events Irrespective of Relationship with Nilutamide: Other adverse events reported overall in clinical trials (of which most occurred with similar frequencies in patients receiving placebo), others known to commonly occur in elderly patients or expected in patients with metastatic prostate cancer included:
Cardiovascular: cerebrovascular accident (1.4%), heart failure (1.0%). Rare cases of tachycardia.
Digestive: constipation (2.6%), gastrointestinal disorder (2.0%). Rare cases of diarrhea.
Metabolic and Nutritional: peripheral edema (1.5%).
Nervous System: headache (2.6%), depression (1.1%), insomnia (1.1%). Rare cases of drowsiness and anxiety.
Skin and Appendages: pruritus (1.1%). Rare cases of maculopapular rash and hirsutism.
Special Senses: rare cases of dazzle and dry mouth.
Urogenital: urinary tract infection (1.3%).
No causal relationship of these experiences with drug treatment has been established.

Post-Marketing Surveillance: The adverse events which have been spontaneously reported worldwide further to marketing of nilutamide and which are considered possibly or probably related to the drug (adverse reactions) include the following: interstitial pneumonitis (most of the cases showed a favorable outcome after treatment discontinuation, however, there have been reports of fatality), hepatocellular or mixed liver injury, fulminant hepatitis, and unspecified vision disorders. Isolated cases of angina pectoris, anxiety dyspnea palpitation, cold extremities, dizziness, headache, gynecomastia, maculopapular rash, urticaria, vomiting and weight increase have been reported.

Aplastic anemia (including 1 fatality) has been reported rarely in patients treated with nilutamide but no specific relationship to the drug product has been ascertained.

OVERDOSE:

Symptoms: At the dose of 900 mg (3 to 6 times the recommended daily dose), nilutamide caused malaise, dizziness, nausea and vomiting which disappeared upon discontinuation of treatment.

The effects of ingestion of a very high dose of nilutamide have been described in 1 case report. A 79-year-old man was admitted 2 hours after the ingestion of 13 g of nilutamide (170 mg/kg or 43 times the therapeutic dose). He had been receiving nilutamide 300 mg/day for 2 weeks. On admission, he underwent gastric lavage immediately, followed by administration of a 20 g oral dose of activated charcoal. Clinical and biological parameters were monitored. There were no changes in the biological parameters as compared to the pre-treatment values either early post ingestion or upon control on days 4, 9 and 30. The clinical manifestations were limited to moderate vomiting and diarrhea during the first 12 hours post ingestion and the patient recovered. Plasma and serum concentrations were measured. The initial level reached 6 times the usual therapeutic range of 4.4 to 8.5 mg/L. Levels 3.5 times greater than the normal range were measured 72 hours post-ingestion.

The ingested dose (170 mg/kg) is close to the lethal dose in animals, the oral LD_{50} being 215 mg/kg (180 to 240) in mice and 195 mg/kg (160 to 230) in rats. However, the extent of absorption was probably limited by early therapeutic intervention. The lethal dose in man has not been established.

For management of a suspected drug overdose, CPhA recommends that you contact your **regional Poison Control Centre**. See the *CPS* Directory section for a list of Poison Control Centres.

DOSAGE: Treatment with nilutamide should be initiated immediately after surgical castration.
Initial Dosage: 300 mg once daily for the first month of treatment. Maintenance treatment may be started earlier should intolerance occur.
Maintenance Dosage: 150 mg once daily.

Nilutamide should be taken before breakfast, until more information is available.

Discontinuation of nilutamide should be considered once objective evidence of disease progression is noted.

INFORMATION FOR THE PATIENT: Published in e-CPS, available by subscription at www.e-cps.ca.

SUPPLIED: Each white, round, biconvex tablet, debossed with "168" over "A" on one side and with the Roussel logo on the other side contains: nilutamide 50 mg. Nonmedicinal ingredients: cornstarch, lactose, magnesium stearate, povidone, sodium docusate and talc. Blister packs of 90. Store between 15 and 30°C. Protect from light, heat and humidity.

(Shown in Product Identification Section)

Anbesol® Gel
benzocaine
Topical Anesthetic

Paladin

Anbesol® Gel Extra Strength
benzocaine
Topical Anesthetic

Paladin

Anbesol® Liquid Extra Strength
benzocaine
Topical Anesthetic

Paladin

Anbesol® Baby Grape Gel
benzocaine
Topical Anesthetic

Paladin

SUPPLIED: Anbesol Gel: Each plastic tube contains: benzocaine 10%. Nonmedicinal ingredients: benzyl alcohol, carbomer, D&C Red No. 33, D&C Yellow No. 10, FD&C Blue No. 1, FD&C Yellow No. 6, flavour, glycerin, methylparaben, polyethylene glycol, propylene glycol and saccharin. Tubes of 7 g.
Anbesol Gel Extra Strength: Each plastic tube contains: benzocaine 20%. Nonmedicinal ingredients: benzyl alcohol, carbomer, D&C Yellow No. 10, FD&C Blue No. 1, FD&C Red No. 40, flavour, glycerin, methylparaben, polyethylene glycol, propylene glycol and saccharin. Tubes of 7 g.
Anbesol Liquid Extra Strength: Each glass bottle contains: benzocaine 20%. Nonmedicinal ingredients: benzyl alcohol, D&C Yellow No. 10, FD&C Blue No. 1, FD&C Red No. 40, flavour, methylparaben, polyethylene glycol, propylene glycol and saccharin. Bottles of 13 mL.
Anbesol Baby Grape Gel: Each plastic tube contains: benzocaine 7.5%. Nonmedicinal ingredients: benzoic acid, carbomer, D&C Red No. 33, disodium edetate, FD&C Blue No. 1, flavour, glycerin, parabens, polyethylene glycol, saccharin and water. Tubes of 7 g.

Andriol®
testosterone undecanoate
Androgen

Schering-Plough

Date of Revision: December 15, 2008

SUMMARY PRODUCT INFORMATION:

Route of Administration	Dosage Form/ Strength	Clinically Relevant Nonmedicinal Ingredients
Oral	Capsule 40 mg	Castor oil, gelatin For a complete listing see Dosage Forms, Composition and Packaging.

INDICATIONS AND CLINICAL USE: Andriol (testosterone undecanoate capsules) is indicated for testosterone replacement therapy in adult males for conditions associated with a deficiency or absence of endogenous testosterone.

Andriol should not be used to treat non-specific symptoms suggestive of hypogonadism if testosterone deficiency has not been demonstrated and if other etiologies responsible for the symptoms have not been excluded. Testosterone deficiency should be clearly demonstrated by clinical features and confirmed by two separate validated biochemical assays (morning testosterone) before initiating therapy with any testosterone replacement, including Andriol treatment.

Geriatrics (>65 years of age): There is limited Andriol use in the geriatric population.

Pediatrics (<18 years of age): Andriol is not indicated for use in children <18 years of age since safety and efficacy have not been established in this patient population (see Warnings and Precautions).

CONTRAINDICATIONS:
- Andriol (testosterone undecanoate capsules) should not be used in patients with known hypersensitivity to any of its ingredients. For a complete listing of ingredients see Dosage Forms, Composition and Packaging.
- Testosterone replacement therapies are contraindicated in men with known or suspected carcinoma of the prostate or breast.
- Andriol is not indicated for use in women.
- Contraindicated drug-drug interactions appear in the Drug Interactions section (see Drug Interactions).

WARNINGS AND PRECAUTIONS: General: There is very limited data from clinical trials with Andriol (testosterone undecanoate capsules) in the geriatric male (>65 years of age) to support the efficacy and safety of prolonged use. Impacts to prostate and cardiovascular event rates and patient important outcomes are unknown.

Patients with clinical or demographic characteristics that are recognized to be associated with an increased risk of prostate cancer should be evaluated for the presence of prostate cancer prior to initiation of testosterone replacement therapy.

Testosterone replacement therapy should not be used to attempt to improve body composition, bone and muscle mass, increase lean body mass and decrease total fat mass. Efficacy and safety have not been established. Serious long term deleterious health issues may arise. Testosterone replacement therapy has not been shown to be safe and effective for the enhancement of athletic performance. Because of the potential risk of serious adverse health effects, this drug should not be used for such purpose.

If testosterone deficiency has not been established, testosterone replacement therapy should not be used for the treatment of sexual dysfunction.

Clinical studies have not established testosterone replacement therapy as a treatment for male infertility.

Carcinogenesis and Mutagenesis: Prostatic: Geriatric patients treated with testosterone products may be at an increased risk for the development of prostatic hyperplasia and prostatic carcinoma but their role in the initiation of either disease is unknown.

Breast: Patients using long-term parenteral testosterone replacement therapy may be at an increased risk for the development of breast cancer.

Skeletal: Patients with skeletal metastases are at a risk of exacerbating hypercalcemia/ hypercalciuria with concomitant testosterone replacement therapy.

Cardiovascular: Testosterone may increase blood pressure and should be used with caution in patients with hypertension.

Edema, with or without congestive heart failure, may be a serious complication in patients with pre-existing cardiac, renal, or hepatic disease. Diuretic therapy may be required, in addition to discontinuation of the drug.

Dependence/Tolerance: Andriol contains testosterone, a Schedule G controlled substance as defined by the Food and Drugs Act.

Endocrine and Metabolism: Testosterone products have been shown to alter glucose tolerance tests. Diabetics should be followed carefully and the insulin or oral hypoglycemic dosage adjusted accordingly (see Drug Interactions, Drug-Drug Interactions).

Hypercalciuria/hypercalcemia (caused by malignant tumors) may be exacerbated by androgen treatment. Androgens should be used with caution in cancer patients at risk of hypercalcemia (and associated hypercalciuria). Regular monitoring of serum calcium concentrations is recommended in patients at risk of hypercalciuria/hypercalcemia. Hypercalcemia may occur in immobilized patients. If any hypercalcemia occurs, the drug should be discontinued.

Genitourinary: Patients with benign prostatic hyperplasia may develop acute urethral obstruction.

Hematologic: Hemoglobin and hematocrit levels should be checked periodically (to detect polycythemia) in patients on long-term testosterone replacement therapy (see Monitoring and Laboratory Tests).

Respiratory: The treatment of hypogonadal men with testosterone products may potentiate sleep apnea, particularly for those with risk factors such as obesity or chronic lung diseases.

Sexual Function/Reproduction: Gynecomastia may develop and occasionally persist in patients being treated for hypogonadism. Priapism or excessive sexual stimulation may develop.

Oligospermia may occur after prolonged administration or excessive dosage.

Special Populations: Pregnant Women and Nursing Women: Andriol should not be used in pregnant or nursing women. Testosterone may cause fetal harm. Testosterone exposure during pregnancy has been reported to be associated with fetal abnormalities (see Contraindications).

Pediatrics (<18 years of age): Testosterone replacement therapy should be used cautiously in males with hypogonadism causing delayed puberty. Androgens can accelerate bone maturation without producing compensatory gain in linear growth. This adverse effect may result in compromised adult stature. The younger the child is the greater risk of compromising final mature height. The effect of androgens on bone maturation should be monitored closely by assessing bone age of the wrist and hand on a regular basis.

Geriatrics (>65 years of age): There are very limited controlled clinical study data supporting the use of testosterone in the geriatric population and virtually no controlled clinical studies on subjects 75 years and over.

Geriatric patients treated with testosterone products may be at an increased risk for the development of prostatic hyperplasia and prostatic carcinoma but their role in the initiation of either disease is unknown.

In men receiving testosterone replacement therapy, surveillance for prostate cancer should be consistent with current practices for eugonadal men.

Monitoring and Laboratory Tests: The patient should be monitored (including serum testosterone levels) on a regular basis to ensure adequate response to treatment. Good clinical judgment must be employed using serum bioavailable testosterone levels or if this is unavailable Calculated Free Testosterone Fractions since the levels have daily fluctuations with use of Andriol. Serum Bioavailable Testosterone (Bio-T) level or Calculated Free Testosterone Fractions must be obtained about 5 hours after Andriol Capsule intake, at Cmax, and in a non-fasted subject.

Currently there is no consensus about age specific testosterone levels. The normal serum testosterone level for young eugonadal men is generally accepted to be approximately 10.4-34.6 nmol/L (300-1000 ng/dL). It should be taken into account that physiological testosterone levels (mean and range) decrease with increasing age.

The following laboratory tests, performed routinely, are recommended to ensure that adverse experience possibly caused by or related to testosterone replacement therapy is detected and addressed:
- hemoglobin and hematocrit levels should be checked periodically (to detect polycythemia);
- liver function tests;
- prostate specific antigen (PSA), digital rectal examination (DRE), especially if the patient presents with progressive difficulty with urination or a change in voiding habits;
- lipid profile, total cholesterol, LDL, HDL, and triglycerides; serum cholesterol levels may increase and/or decrease during androgen therapy;
- diabetics should be followed carefully and the insulin or oral hypoglycemic dosage adjusted accordingly (see Drug Interactions, Drug-Drug Interactions).

ADVERSE REACTIONS: Clinical Trial Adverse Drug Reactions: Because clinical trials are conducted under very specific conditions the adverse reaction rates observed in the clinical trials may not reflect the rates observed in practice and should not be compared to the rates in the clinical trials of another drug. Adverse drug reaction information from clinical trials is useful for identifying drug-related adverse events and for approximating rates.

The following adverse reactions have occurred with androgen therapy in general: fluid retention, nervousness, mood disturbance, myalgia, hypertension, pruritus, priapism, prostatic cancer, prostatic disorder, abnormal hepatic function , lipid abnormality, increased PSA, inhibition of testicular function, testicular atrophy and oligospermia, impotence, gynecomastia, epididymitis and bladder irritability, nausea, cholestatic jaundice, peliosis hepatis, polycythemia, headache, anxiety, depression, generalized paresthesia and rarely anaphylactoid reaction. In addition, the following reactions are known to occur with anabolic steroids: increased or decreased libido, flushing of the skin, acne, habituation, excitation and sleeplessness, chills, leukopenia, and bleeding in patients on concomitant anticoagulant therapy.

Post-Market Adverse Drug Reactions: In addition to those adverse events reported during clinical trials, the following adverse reactions have been identified during post-marketing use of Andriol (testosterone undecanoate capsules) (see Table 1) and known reactions of other testosterone preparations in general (see Table 2). Because these reactions are reported voluntarily from a population of uncertain size, it is not always possible to reliably estimate their frequency or establish a causal relationship to drug exposure.

Table 1: Andriol
Adverse Drug Reactions from Post-Marketing Experience of Andriol

MedDRA System Organ Class (SOC)	Adverse Drug Reaction
Blood and The Lymphatic System Disorders	Polycythemia
Endocrine Disorders	Abnormal accelerated growth
Gastrointestinal Disorders	Nausea, vomiting, diarrhea, abdominal pain, gastrointestinal bleeding
General Disorders and Administration Site Conditions	Edema, malaise, fatigue
Hepatobiliary Disorders	Hepatic neoplasms
Immune System Disorders	Allergic reaction/hypersensitivity reaction
Investigations	Weight increase, fluctuating testosterone levels, testosterone decreased, abnormal liver function tests (e.g. elevated GGTP), lipid abnormalities
Metabolism and Nutrition Disorders	Increased appetite, electrolyte changes (nitrogen, potassium, phosphorus, sodium), glucose tolerance impaired, elevated cholesterol
Musculoskeletal and Connective Tissue Disorders	Myalgia, arthralgia
Nervous System Disorders	Headache, dizziness
Psychiatric Disorders	Personality disorder, confusion, aggression, depression, anxiety, decreased libido, cognitive disturbance
Renal and Urinary Disorders	Renal disorders
Reproductive System and Breast Disorders	Prostate carcinoma, enlarged prostate (benign), free prostate-specific antigen increased, epididymitis, oligospermia, priapism, impotence, precocious puberty, gynecomastia
Skin and Subcutaneous Tissue Disorders	Pruritus, rash, urticaria, vesiculo-bullous rash, acne, alopecia, hirsutism
Vascular Disorders	Hypertension

Table 2: Andriol
Adverse Drug Reactions from Other Testosterone Preparations

MedDRA System Organ Class (SOC)	Adverse Drug Reaction
Blood and The Lymphatic System Disorders	Erythropoiesis abnormal
General Disorders and Administration Site Conditions	Application site burning, application site induration, application site rash, application site dermatitis, application site blister, application site erythema
Hepatobiliary Disorders	Peliosis hepatis
Metabolism and Nutrition Disorders	Urine calcium decrease
Nervous System Disorders	Insomnia
Psychiatric Disorders	Anger
Renal and Urinary Disorders	Dysuria, hematuria, incontinence, bladder irritability
Reproductive System and Breast Disorders	Testicular atrophy, mastodynia
Respiratory, Thoracic and Mediastinal Disorders	Dyspnea, sleep apnea
Skin and Subcutaneous Tissue Disorders	Seborrhea, male pattern baldness, hirsutism

DRUG INTERACTIONS: Drug-Drug Interactions: Insulin: In diabetic patients, the metabolic effects of Androgens may decrease blood glucose and, therefore, insulin requirements.

Propranolol: In a published pharmacokinetic study of an injectable testosterone product, administration of testosterone cypionate led to an increased clearance of propranolol in the majority of men tested. It is unknown if this would apply to Andriol (testosterone undecanoate capsules).

Corticosteroids: The concurrent administration of testosterone with ACTH or corticosteroids may enhance edema formation; thus these drugs should be administered cautiously particularly in patients with cardiac, renal or hepatic disease.

Anticoagulants: Androgens may increase sensitivity to oral anticoagulants. Dosage of the anticoagulant may require reduction in order to maintain satisfactory therapeutic hypoprothrombinemia.

Cyclosporine: Testosterone replacement therapy may potentiate cyclosporine and increase risk of nephrotoxicity.

Drug-Food Interactions: Andriol must be taken with meal since fat enhances its absorption.

Drug-Herb Interactions: It was found that some herbal products (e.g. St. John's Wort) which are available as over-the-counter (OTC) products might interfere with steroid metabolism and therefore may decrease plasma testosterone levels.

Drug-Laboratory Test Interactions: Testosterone products may decrease levels of thyroxine-binding globulin, resulting in decreased total T_4 serum levels and increased resin uptake of T_3 and T_4. Free thyroid hormone levels remain unchanged, however, and there is no clinical evidence of thyroid dysfunction.

DOSAGE AND ADMINISTRATION: Recommended Dose and Dosage Adjustment: Usually, a daily dosage of 120-160 mg divided in two doses, taken once in the morning and once in the evening for 2-3 weeks is adequate. Subsequent dosage (40-120 mg daily) should be based on the subsequent testosterone levels and/or clinical effect obtained during therapy.

Missed Dose: Should you forget a dose, take your dose at the next scheduled time. Do not take a double dose of this medicine.

Administration: To ensure adequate absorption, Andriol (testosterone undecanoate capsules) must be taken with a meal and swallowed without chewing.

OVERDOSAGE:
No experience with overdosage has been reported. No specific antidote is available.

For management of a suspected drug overdose, CPhA recommends that you contact your **regional Poison Control Centre**. See the *CPS* Directory section for a list of Poison Control Centres.

ACTION AND CLINICAL PHARMACOLOGY: Mechanism of Action: Testosterone undecanoate, an orally active testosterone preparation, is a fatty acid ester of the natural androgen testosterone. Unlike other oral testosterone preparations, testosterone undecanoate is able to by-pass the liver via the lymphatic system and is therefore orally bioavailable.

Therapy with testosterone undecanoate increases plasma levels of testosterone and its active metabolites, leading to a regular therapeutic effect. In eugonadal men, peak testosterone levels are reached approximately 4-5 hours after ingestion, returning to basal levels after about 10 hours. In volunteers and hypogonadal men, 77-93% of an orally administered dose of testosterone undecanoate was excreted in the urine and faeces within 3 to 4 days.

Andriol (testosterone undecanoate dissolved in a mixture of castor oil and propylene glycol monolaurate) has been found to exhibit comparable testosterone bioavailability to Andriol (testosterone undecanoate in oleic acid).

Andriol delivers physiologic amounts of testosterone, producing circulating testosterone levels that approximate normal levels (e.g. 10.4-34.6 nmol/L [300-1000 ng/dL]) seen in young healthy men.

Pharmacodynamics: Testosterone and Hypogonadism: Testosterone and dihydrotestosterone (DHT), endogenous androgens, are responsible for normal growth and development of the male sex organs and for maintenance of secondary sex characteristics. These effects include the growth and maturation of the prostate, seminal vesicles, penis, and scrotum; the development of male hair distribution, such as facial, pubic, chest, and axillary hair; laryngeal enlargement; vocal cord thickening; alterations in body musculature; and fat distribution.

Male hypogonadism results from insufficient secretion of testosterone and is characterized by low serum testosterone concentrations. Symptoms associated with male hypogonadism include decreased sexual desire with or without impotence, fatigue and loss of energy, mood depression, regression of secondary sexual characteristics, and osteoporosis. Hypogonadism is a risk factor for osteoporosis in men.

General Androgen Effects: Drugs in the androgen class also promote retention of nitrogen, sodium, potassium, phosphorus, and decreased urinary excretion of calcium.

Androgens have been reported to increase protein anabolism and decrease protein catabolism. Nitrogen balance is improved only when there is sufficient intake of calories and protein.

Androgens have been reported to stimulate the production of red blood cells by enhancing erythropoietin production.

Androgens are responsible for the growth spurt of adolescence and for the eventual termination of linear growth brought about by fusion of the epiphyseal growth centers. In children, exogenous androgens accelerate linear growth rates but may cause a disproportionate advancement in bone maturation. Use over long periods may result in fusion of the epiphyseal growth centers and termination of the growth process.

During exogenous administration of androgens, endogenous testosterone release may be inhibited through feedback inhibition of pituitary luteinizing hormone (LH). At large doses of exogenous androgens, spermatogenesis may also be suppressed through feedback inhibition of pituitary follicle-stimulating hormone (FSH).

In hypogonadal men treatment with Andriol results in improvement of testosterone deficiency symptoms. Testosterone treatment has been reported to increase bone mineral density and lean body mass and decrease body fat with no clinical relevance. Serum cholesterol, LDL, HDL, and triglycerides levels may increase and/or decrease during androgen therapy. Hemoglobin and hematocrit increase during testosterone therapy in a dose dependant manner. In small clinical studies reported in the literature Andriol has not been associated with increases in serum liver enzyme activities. In short term (up to 2 years) studies involving small numbers of patients Andriol has not been shown to be associated with significant increases in PSA levels. In other trials testosterone therapy has a variable effect on PSA measurements. Clinical studies report that testosterone treatment including Andriol may result in an increase in prostate size but this has not been associated with symptoms of prostatism. In hypogonadal diabetic patients the metabolic effects of Androgens may decrease blood glucose, and therefore insulin requirements.

Pharmacokinetics: Absorption: The active substance of Andriol is well absorbed from the gastrointestinal tract. Both testosterone undecanoate and the newly formed 5-alpha-dihydrotestosterone undecanoate are partly absorbed via the lymphatic system, circumventing first passage through the liver. Following oral administration of Andriol, an important part of the active substance testosterone undecanoate is co-absorbed with the lipophilic solvent from the intestine into the lymphatic system, thus partially circumventing the first-pass inactivation by the liver. Andriol must be taken with a normal meal or breakfast to ensure absorption. The bioavailability is about 7%.

Distribution: Administration of radioactively labelled testosterone undecanoate (^{3}H-TU) to men resulted in radioactivity in the lymph associated with unmetabolized testosterone undecanoate and 5-alpha-dihydrotestosterone undecanoate. Peak levels of radioactivity appeared in the lymph and plasma 2.5-5 hours after administration.

Metabolism: It is metabolized partly in the intestinal wall into 5-alpha-dihydrotestosterone undecanoate (DHTU) and in plasma and tissues TU is hydrolyzed to free testosterone and DHTU to DHT. Free testosterone is rapidly converted to 5-alpha-dihydrotestosterone, androstenedione and estradiol.

Excretion: The highest concentration of radioactivity in urine was found 2 hours later. During the first 24 hours approximately 40% of the administered dose was found in urine and the total recovery of the dose in urine during the first week was 45-48%.

Special Populations and Conditions: Pediatrics: Andriol may be used to stimulate puberty in carefully selected males with clearly delayed puberty not secondary to a pathological disorder. Androgens can accelerate bone maturation without producing compensatory gain in linear growth. The effect on bone maturation should be monitored by assessing bone age of the wrist and hand every six months. These adverse effects may result in compromised adult stature. The younger the child the greater the risk of compromising final mature height.

Geriatrics: Geriatric patients treated with androgens may be at an increased risk of developing prostatic hypertrophy and prostatic carcinoma although conclusive evidence to support this concept is lacking.

STORAGE AND STABILITY: Store between 15-30°C. Protect from light and moisture. Do not refrigerate. Keep blister in the outer carton.

SPECIAL HANDLING INSTRUCTIONS: Not applicable.

INFORMATION FOR THE PATIENT: Published in e-CPS, available by subscription at www.e-cps.ca.

DOSAGE FORMS, COMPOSITION AND PACKAGING: Each oval, orange, soft gelatin capsule, coded in white ORG DV3, contains: testosterone undecanoate 40 mg. Nonmedicinal ingredients: castor oil and propylene glycol monolaurate; capsule shell: FD&C Yellow #6, gelatin and glycerin. Blister packs of 10 capsules (boxes of 12 blister packs).

(Shown in Product Identification Section)

Androcur® Ⓟ
cyproterone acetate
Antiandrogen

Bayer

Androcur® Depot Ⓟ
cyproterone acetate
Antiandrogen

Bayer

Date of Revision: May 28, 2009

PHARMACOLOGY: Cyproterone is a steroid which clinically demonstrates 2 distinct properties: antiandrogenic: cyproterone blocks the binding of dihydrotestosterone—the active metabolite of testosterone—to the specific receptors in the prostatic carcinoma cell. Progestogenic/antigonadotrophic: Cyproterone exerts a negative feed-back on the hypothalamo-pituitary axis, by inhibiting the secretion of LH leading to diminished production of testicular testosterone.

The absorption of cyproterone following oral administration is complete. Peak plasma levels are reached 3 to 4 hours after administration. Plasma levels fall rapidly during the first 24 hours as a result of tissue distribution and excretion, and plasma half-life was 38±5 hours.

Most of the cyproterone is excreted unchanged in the feces (60%) or urine (33%) within 72 hours.

Cyproterone is eliminated in the urine mainly in the form of unconjugated metabolites and in the bile via feces in the form of glucuronidized metabolites.

The principal metabolite identified was 15 β-hydroxy-cyproterone acetate.

Androcur Depot: Following i.m. administration, mean maximum blood levels are attained 3.4 days after injection. The mean elimination half-life was found to be 4 days.

INDICATIONS: For the palliative treatment of patients with advanced prostatic carcinoma.

CONTRAINDICATIONS: Known hypersensitivity to the drug. Active liver disease and hepatic dysfunction. Renal insufficiency.

WARNINGS: Liver Function: Direct hepatic toxicity, including jaundice, hepatitis and hepatic failure, which has been fatal in some cases, has been reported in patients treated with 200 to 300 mg cyproterone. Most reported cases are in men with prostatic cancer. Toxicity is dose-related and develops usually, several months after treatment has begun. Liver function tests should be performed before treatment and whenever any symptoms or signs suggestive of hepatotoxicity occur. If hepatotoxicity is confirmed, cyproterone should normally be withdrawn, unless the hepatotoxicity can be explained by another cause, e.g., metastatic disease, in which case cyproterone should be continued only if the perceived benefit outweighs the risk.

Inhibition of Spermatogenesis: The sperm count and the volume of ejaculate are reduced at oral doses of 50 to 300 mg/day. Infertility is usual, and there may be azoospermia after 8 weeks of therapy, which is associated with atrophy of seminiferous tubules.

Follow-up examinations on discontinuation of therapy have shown these changes to be reversible.

Spermatogenesis usually reverts to its previous level about 3 to 5 months after stopping cyproterone, or in some patients, after up to 20 months. Production of abnormal spermatozoa during cyproterone therapy has been observed; their relationship to abnormal fertilization or malformed embryos is not known.

Gynecomastia: Benign nodules (hyperplasia) of the breast have been reported, these generally subside 1 to 3 months after discontinuation of therapy and/or after a reduction of dosage. The reduction of dosage should be weighed against the risk of inadequate tumor control.

Depression: Cyproterone therapy has occasionally been associated with an increased incidence of depressive mood changes, especially during the first 6 to 8 weeks of therapy. Similar mood changes have also been seen following surgical castration and are considered to be due to androgen deprivation. Patients with tendencies to depressive reaction should be carefully observed.

Antiandrogen Withdrawal Syndrome: In some patients with metastatic prostate cancer, antiandrogens (steroidal or nonsteroidal), may promote, rather than inhibit, the growth of prostate cancer. A decrease in PSA and/or clinical improvement following the discontinuation of antiandrogens have been reported. It is recommended that patients prescribed an antiandrogen, who have PSA progression, should have the antiandrogen discontinued immediately and be monitored for 6-8 weeks for a withdrawal response prior to any decision to proceed with other prostate cancer therapy.

PRECAUTIONS: Thromboembolism: Clinical investigations have shown that when cyproterone is used alone it has a minor effect on blood clotting factors. However, when cyproterone was combined with ethinyl estradiol, changes were found in increased coagulation capability. There is an inherent risk for those patients with a history of thrombophlebitis or thromboembolism for recurrence of the disease. Cyproterone should be discontinued at the first sign of thrombophlebitis or thromboembolism. And, the patient should be carefully re-evaluated if manifestations of thrombotic disorders (thrombophlebitis, cerebrovascular complications, retinal thrombosis or pulmonary embolism) occur.

Adrenocortical Function: Suppression of adrenocortical function tests have occurred in patients receiving high doses (100 mg/m^2) of cyproterone.

Reduced response to endogenous ACTH was noted by metyrapone test; furthermore, reduced ACTH and cortisol blood levels determined by the Mattingly method were also found.

It is therefore recommended that adrenocortical function tests should be monitored periodically by serum cortisol assay.

Diabetes: Cyproterone may impair carbohydrate metabolism. Parameters of carbohydrate metabolism, fasting blood glucose and glucose tolerance test, should be examined carefully in all patients and particularly in all diabetics before and regularly during therapy with cyproterone.

Hematology: Hypochromic anemia has been observed rarely during therapy with cyproterone. Regular hematological assessment is recommended.

Nitrogen Balance: A negative nitrogen balance is usual at the start of therapy, but does generally correct itself within 3 months of continued therapy.

Metabolic Effects: Fluid retention, hypercalcemia and changes in plasma lipid profile may occur. Accordingly, cyproterone should be used with caution in patients with cardiac disease.

Skin: Cyproterone therapy may cause a reduction of sebum production leading to dryness of the skin, and transient patchy loss of body hair.

Concomitant Alcohol: Alcohol may reduce the antiandrogenic effect of cyproterone in hypersexuality. The relevance of this in prostatic carcinoma is not known, however, it would be prudent to inform the patients that the use of alcohol during cyproterone therapy is not advisable.

Physical Performance: Patients should be informed that fatigue and lassitude are common in the first few weeks of therapy, but usually becomes much less pronounced from the third month on.

Marked lassitude and asthenia necessitate special care when driving or operating machinery.

ADVERSE EFFECTS: The adverse events associated most frequently with the use of cyproterone are those related to the hormonal effects of the drug. These reactions usually disappear upon discontinuation of therapy or reduction of dose: decreased libido, breast enlargement, breast tenderness, benign nodular hyperplasia of the breast, galactorrhea, gynecomastia, abnormal spermatozoa, impotence and inhibition of spermatogenesis.

Other adverse events which have been reported are listed below:

Cardiovascular: hypotension, tachycardia, heart failure, syncope, myocardial infarct, hemorrhage, cerebrovascular accident, cardiovascular disorder, retinal vascular disorder, embolus, pulmonary embolism, superficial and deep thrombophlebitis, thrombosis, retinal vein thrombosis, phlebitis, vascular headache and shock.

Gastrointestinal System: constipation, diarrhea, indigestion, anorexia, nausea, vomiting, cholestatic jaundice, cirrhosis of liver, hepatic coma, hepatitis, hepatoma, hepatomegaly, jaundice, liver carcinoma, liver failure, abnormal liver function test, liver necrosis, pancreatitis and glossitis.

Hematology: increased fibrinogen, decreased prothrombin, thrombocytopenia, anemia, hemolytic anemia, hypochromic anemia, normocytic anemia, leukopenia and leukocytosis.

Metabolism: negative nitrogen balance, decreased response to ACTH, hyperglycemia, lowered cortisol, hypercalcemia, increased AST, increased ALT, increased creatinine, hypernatremia, edema, weight gain, weight loss and diabetes mellitus.

Musculoskeletal: myasthenia, osteoporosis.

Central Nervous System: fatigue, lassitude, weakness, hot flashes, increased sweating, aphasia, coma, depression, dizziness, encephalopathy, hemiplegia, personality disorder, psychotic depression, abnormal gait and headache.

Cerebral meningiomas (single and multiple) have been reported in association with long-term use (several years) of ANDROCUR.

Respiratory System: asthma, increased cough, dyspnea, hyperventilation, respiratory disorder, shortness of breath on effort, lung fibrosis.

Skin: eczema, urticaria, erythema nodosum, exfoliative dermatitis, rash, maculopapular rash, dryness of the skin, pruritus, alopecia, hirsutism, skin discolouration, photosensitivity reactions and scleroderma.

Sensory System: ear disorder, optic atrophy, optic neuritis, abnormality of accommodation, abnormal vision, blindness and retinal disorder.

Urogenital: enlarged uterine fibroids, uterine hemorrhage, increased urinary frequency, bladder carcinoma, kidney failure, hematuria, urate crystalluria, urine abnormality.

Other: ascites, allergic reaction, asthenia, chills, fetal chromosome abnormality, death, fever, hernia, malaise and injection site reaction.

Adverse reactions are rarely of sufficient severity to require dosage reduction or discontinuation of treatment.

If reactions are severe, it may be beneficial to reduce the dosage.

OVERDOSAGE:

Treatment: There have been no reports of fatal overdosage in man with cyproterone. There are no specific antidotes and treatment should be symptomatic. If oral overdosage is discovered within 2 to 3 hours, gastric lavage can safely be used if indicated.

For management of a suspected drug overdose, CPhA recommends that you contact your **regional Poison Control Centre**. See the *CPS* Directory section for a list of Poison Control Centres.

DOSAGE: Oral Tablets: The usual daily initial and maintenance dose is 4 to 6 tablets (200 to 300 mg) divided into 2 to 3 doses and taken after meals.

After orchiectomy a lower daily dose of 2 to 4 tablets (100 to 200 mg) is recommended.

Injectable: The usual initial and maintenance dose is one weekly i.m. injection of 3 mL (300 mg). For orchiectomized patients, the recommended dose is one i.m. injection of 3 mL (300 mg) every 2 weeks.

Oral or i.m depot therapy should not be discontinued when remission or improvement occurs.

Because of their pharmacokinetic properties, the oral and i.m. depot can be interchanged in the course of long-term treatment. The dosage may be reduced if side effects are intolerable but should be kept within the oral range of 100 to 300 mg daily (2 to 6 tablets) or i.m. injections of 300 mg (3 mL) at weekly intervals, or every 2 weeks.

SUPPLIED: Androcur: Each white, round, flat-sided tablet with beveled edges, imprinted one side "BV" in a regular hexagon, other side scored, contains: cyproterone acetate 50 mg. Nonmedicinal ingredients: aerosil (colloidal silicic acid), cornstarch, lactose, magnesium stearate and polyvinylpyrrolidone. Gluten- and tartrazine-free. Blisters of 10 tablets, cartons of 6 blisters. Bottles of 60.

Androcur Depot: Each ampul contains: cyproterone acetate 100 mg/mL in a castor oil solution. Nonmedicinal ingredients: benzyl benzoate and castor oil. Ampuls of 3 mL, boxes of 4.

(Shown in Product Identification Section)

Androderm® Ⓒ

testosterone

Testosterone Replacement Therapy

Paladin

SUPPLIED: 12.2 mg: Each patch has a 7.5 cm^2 central drug delivery reservoir surrounded by a peripheral adhesive area. The total contact surface area is 37 cm^2. Each patch contains: testosterone 12.2 mg, dissolved in an alcohol-based gel, and delivers 2.5 mg/24 hours/patch. Nonmedicinal ingredients: alcohol, carbomer, glycerin, glycerol monooleate, methyl laurate, purified water and sodium hydroxide. Cartons of 60.

24.3 mg: Each patch has a 15 cm^2 central drug delivery reservoir surrounded by a peripheral adhesive area. The total contact surface area is 44 cm^2. Each patch contains: testosterone USP 24.3 mg, dissolved in an alcohol-based gel, and delivers 5 mg/24 hours/patch. Nonmedicinal ingredients: alcohol, carbomer, glycerin, glycerol monooleate, methyl laurate, purified water and sodium hydroxide. Cartons of 30.

Store at room temperature, 15 to 30°C. Do not store outside the pouch provided. Apply immediately upon removal from the protective pouch. Damaged patches should not be used. Keep out of the reach of children both before and after use. The drug reservoir may be burst by excessive pressure or heat. May be discarded with household waste in a manner that avoids accidental contact by others.

AndroGel® Ⓒ

testosterone

Androgens

Abbott Products

Date of Revision: April 15, 2010

SUMMARY PRODUCT INFORMATION:

Route of Administration	Dosage Form/ Strength	Clinically Relevant Nonmedicinal Ingredients
Topical	1% gel	Alcohol For a complete listing see Dosage Forms, Composition and Packaging.

INDICATIONS AND CLINICAL USE: ANDROGEL is indicated for testosterone replacement therapy in adult males for conditions associated with a deficiency or absence of endogenous testosterone (hypogonadism).

ANDROGEL should not be used to treat non-specific symptoms suggestive of hypogonadism if testosterone deficiency has not been demonstrated and if other etiologies responsible for the symptoms have not been excluded. Testosterone deficiency should be clearly demonstrated by clinical features and confirmed by biochemical assays (Endocrine Society Guidelines recommend two separate tests preferably in the morning) before initiating therapy with any testosterone replacement, including ANDROGEL treatment.

Geriatrics (>65 years of age): There are limited controlled clinical study data supporting the use of ANDROGEL in the geriatric population (see Warnings and Precautions).

Pediatrics (<18 years of age): ANDROGEL is not indicated for use in children <18 years of age since safety and efficacy have not been established in this patient population (see Warnings and Precautions, Special Populations).

CONTRAINDICATIONS:

- **ANDROGEL is not indicated for use in women.**
- **Pregnant and nursing women should avoid skin contact with ANDROGEL application sites on men. Testosterone may cause fetal harm. Testosterone exposure during pregnancy has been reported to be associated with fetal abnormalities (see Warnings and Precautions, Potential for Secondary Exposure to Testosterone and Special Populations).** In the event that unwashed or unclothed skin to which ANDROGEL has been applied or clothing exposed to ANDROGEL comes in direct contact with the skin of a pregnant or nursing woman, the general area of contact on the woman should be immediately washed with soap and water.
- Androgens are contraindicated in men with known or suspected carcinoma of the prostate or breast.
- ANDROGEL should not be used in patients with known hypersensitivity to any of its ingredients, including testosterone USP that is chemically synthesized from soy. For a complete listing, see Dosage Forms, Composition and Packaging.

WARNINGS AND PRECAUTIONS:

> **Serious Warnings and Precautions**
> **SECONDARY EXPOSURE TO TESTOSTERONE**
> - **Virilization has been reported in children who were secondarily exposed to testosterone gel, including ANDROGEL.**
> - **Children should avoid contact with unwashed or unclothed application sites in men using ANDROGEL.**
> - **Healthcare providers should advise patients to strictly adhere to recommended instructions for use.**
>
> **(See Warnings and Precautions, Potential for Secondary Exposure to Testosterone, Strict adherence to the following precautions is advised in order to minimize the potential for secondary exposure to testosterone from ANDROGEL-treated skin.)**

Potential for Secondary Exposure to Testosterone: Secondary exposure to testosterone in children and women can occur with testosterone gel use in men. Cases of secondary exposure resulting in virilization of children have been reported in postmarketing surveillance. Signs and symptoms have included enlargement of the penis or clitoris, development of pubic hair, increased erections and libido, aggressive behavior, and advanced bone age. In most cases, these signs and symptoms regressed with removal of the exposure to testosterone gel. In a few cases, however, enlarged genitalia did not fully return to age-appropriate normal size, and bone age remained modestly greater than chronological age. The risk of transfer was increased in some of these cases by not adhering to precautions for the appropriate use of testosterone gel.

Inappropriate changes in genital size or development of pubic hair or libido in children, or changes in body hair distribution, significant increase in acne, or other signs of virilization in adult women should be brought to the attention of a physician and the possibility of secondary exposure to testosterone gel should also be brought to the attention of a physician. Testosterone gel should be promptly discontinued until the cause of virilization has been identified.

Strict adherence to the following precautions is advised in order to minimize the potential for secondary exposure to testosterone from ANDROGEL-treated skin:

- Children and women should avoid contact with unwashed or unclothed application site(s) of men using testosterone gel.
- ANDROGEL should only be applied to the shoulders, upper arms, and/or abdomen (area of application should be limited to the area that will be covered by the patient's short sleeve t-shirt); when a shirt is used to cover the application site(s), the transfer of ANDROGEL from the male to the female partner can be completely prevented.
- Patients should wash their hands immediately with soap and water after applying ANDROGEL.
- Patients should cover the application site(s) with clothing (e.g., a shirt) after the gel has dried.
- Prior to any situation in which skin-to-skin contact with the application site is anticipated, patients should wash the application site(s) thoroughly with soap and water to remove any testosterone residue.
- In the events that unwashed or unclothed skin to which ANDROGEL has been applied and/or that the testosterone gel user's unwashed shirts and/or other fabrics (such as towels and sheets) come in direct contact with the skin of another person, the general area of contact on the other person should be washed with soap and water as soon as possible. Studies show that residual testosterone is removed from the skin surface by washing with soap and water.

General: There is very limited data from clinical trials with ANDROGEL in the geriatric male (>65 years of age) to support the efficacy and safety of prolonged use. Impacts to prostate and cardiovascular event rates and patient important outcomes are unknown.

ANDROGEL should not be used to improve body composition, bone and muscle mass, increase lean body mass and decrease total fat mass. Efficacy and safety have not been established. Serious long term deleterious health issues may arise.

ANDROGEL has not been shown to be safe and effective for the enhancement of athletic performance. Because of the potential risk of serious adverse health effects, this drug should not be used for such purpose.

If testosterone deficiency has not been established, testosterone replacement therapy should not be used for the treatment of sexual dysfunction.

Testosterone replacement therapy is not a treatment for male infertility.

Gels are flammable. Following application of ANDROGEL (testosterone gel), allow gel to dry completely before smoking or going near an open flame.

Carcinogenesis: Prostatic: Geriatric patients treated with androgens may be at an increased risk for the development of prostatic hyperplasia and prostatic carcinoma (see Special Populations, Geriatrics (>65 years of age)).

Breast: Patients using long-term androgen therapy may be at an increased risk for the development of breast cancer.

Hepatic: Prolonged use of high doses of orally active 17-alpha-alkyl androgens (e.g., methyltestosterone) has been associated with serious hepatic adverse effects (peliosis hepatis, hepatic neoplasms, cholestatic hepatitis, and jaundice). Peliosis hepatis can be a life-threatening or fatal complication. Long-term therapy with testosterone enanthate, which elevates blood levels for prolonged periods, has produced multiple hepatic adenomas. ANDROGEL is not known to produce these adverse effects.

Skeletal: Patients with skeletal metastases are at a risk of exacerbating hypercalcemia/hypercalciuria with concomitant androgen therapy.

Cardiovascular: Testosterone may increase blood pressure and should be used with caution in patients with hypertension.

Edema, with or without congestive heart failure, may be a serious complication in patients with pre-existing cardiac, renal, or hepatic disease. Diuretic therapy may be required, in addition to discontinuation of the drug.

Dependence/Tolerance: ANDROGEL contains testosterone, a Schedule G controlled substance as defined by the Food and Drugs Act.

Endocrine and Metabolism: Androgens have been shown to alter glucose tolerance tests. Diabetics should be followed carefully and the insulin or oral hypoglycemic dosage adjusted accordingly (see Drug Interactions, Drug-Drug Interactions).

Hypercalciuria/hypercalcemia (caused by malignant tumors) may be exacerbated by androgen treatment. Androgens should be used with caution in cancer patients at risk of hypercalcemia (and associated hypercalciuria). Regular monitoring of serum calcium concentrations is recommended in patients at risk of hypercalciuria/hypercalcemia.

Hypercalcemia may occur in immobilized patients. If this occurs, the drug should be discontinued.

Hematologic: Hemoglobin and hematocrit levels should be checked periodically (to detect polycythemia) in patients on long-term androgen therapy (see Monitoring and Laboratory Tests).

Oral alkylated derivatives of testosterone such as methandrostenolone, have been reported to decrease the anticoagulant requirement of patients receiving oral anticoagulants (e.g. warfarin). Patients receiving oral anticoagulants therapy require close monitoring, especially when androgens are started or stopped (see Drug Interactions, Drug-Drug Interactions).

Respiratory: The treatment of hypogonadal men with testosterone may potentiate sleep apnea, particularly for those with risk factors such as obesity or chronic lung diseases.

Sexual Function/Reproduction: Gynecomastia may frequently develop and occasionally persist in patients being treated for hypogonadism.

Priapism or excessive sexual stimulation may develop.

Oligospermia may occur after prolonged administration or excessive dosage.

Skin: Changes in body hair distribution, significant increase in acne, or other signs of virilization of the female partner or in any person (including children) exposed to skin-to skin contact, should be brought to the attention of a physician.

Application site reactions associated with the use of transdermal testosterone may manifest as skin irritation (including erythema, induration or burning).

Special Populations: Pregnant Women: Pregnant and nursing women should avoid skin contact with ANDROGEL application sites on men. Testosterone may cause fetal harm. Testosterone exposure during pregnancy has been reported to be associated with fetal abnormalities. In the event that unwashed or unclothed skin to which ANDROGEL has been applied or clothing exposed to ANDROGEL comes in direct contact with the skin of a pregnant or nursing woman, the general area of contact on the woman should be immediately washed with soap and water (see Contraindications).

Nursing Women: See Pregnant Women.

Pediatrics (<18 years of age): ANDROGEL is not indicated for use in children <18 years of age since safety and efficacy have not been established in this patient population.

Androgen therapy should be used cautiously in males with hypogonadism causing delayed puberty. Androgens can accelerate bone maturation without producing compensatory gain in linear growth. This adverse effect may result in compromised adult stature. The younger the child is the greater risk of compromising final mature height. The effect of androgens on bone maturation should be monitored closely by assessing bone age of the wrist and hand on a regular basis.

Geriatrics (>65 years of age): There are very limited controlled clinical study data supporting the use of testosterone in the geriatric population and virtually no controlled clinical studies on subjects 75 years and over.

Geriatric patients treated with androgens may be at an increased risk for the development of prostatic hyperplasia and prostatic carcinoma.

Geriatric patients and other patients with clinical or demographic characteristics that are recognized to be associated with an increased risk of prostate cancer should be evaluated for the presence of prostate cancer prior to initiation of testosterone replacement therapy.

Monitoring and Laboratory Tests: The patient should be monitored (including serum testosterone levels) on a regular basis to ensure adequate response to treatment.

Currently there is no consensus about age specific testosterone levels. The normal serum testosterone level for young eugonadal men is generally accepted to be approximately 10.4-34.6 nmol/L (300-1000 ng/dL). However, it should be taken into account that physiologically testosterone levels (mean and range) decrease with increasing age. Men with levels below their laboratory's reference range and who are experiencing symptoms are candidates for testosterone replacement therapy and should be evaluated as such.

The following laboratory tests, performed routinely, are recommended to ensure that adverse experience is detected and addressed:

- hemoglobin and hematocrit levels should be checked periodically (to detect polycythemia);
- liver function tests, to detect hepatotoxicity associated with the use of androgens;
- prostate specific antigen (PSA), Digital Rectal Examination (DRE), especially if the patient presents with progressive difficulty with urination or a change in voiding habits;
- lipid profile, total cholesterol, LDL, HDL, and triglycerides;
- diabetics should be followed carefully and the insulin or oral hypoglycemic dosage adjusted accordingly (see Drug Interactions, Drug-Drug Interactions).

Table 1: ANDROGEL

Adverse Events Possibly, Probably or Definitely Related to Use of ANDROGEL in the 180-Day Controlled Clinical Trial

Adverse Event	5 g n=77	7.5 g n=40	10 g n=78
Acne	1%	3%	8%
Alopecia	1%	0%	1%
Application Site Reaction	5%	3%	4%
Asthenia	0%	3%	1%
Depression	1%	0%	1%
Emotional Lability	0%	3%	3%
Gynecomastia	1%	0%	3%
Headache	4%	3%	0%
Hypertension	3%	0%	3%
Lab Test Abnormal[a]	6%	5%	3%
Libido Decreased	0%	3%	1%
Nervousness	0%	3%	1%
Pain Breast	1%	3%	1%
Prostate Disorders[b]	3%	3%	5%
Testis Disorder[c]	3%	0%	0%

[a] **Lab test abnormal** occurred in 9 patients with 1 or more of the following events: elevated hemoglobin or hematocrit, hyperlipidemia, elevated triglycerides, hypokalemia, decreased HDL, elevated glucose, elevated creatinine, or elevated total bilirubin.

[b] **Prostate disorders** included 5 patients with enlarged prostate, 1 patient with BPH (Benign Prostatic Hypertrophy), and 1 patient with elevated PSA (Prostatic Specific Antigen) results.

[c] **Testis disorders** were reported from two patients: one patient with left varicocele and one patient with slight sensitivity of left testis.

ADVERSE REACTIONS: Clinical Trial Adverse Drug Reactions: Because clinical trials are conducted under very specific conditions the adverse reaction rates observed in the clinical trials may not reflect the rates observed in practice and should not be compared to the rates in the clinical trials of another drug. Adverse drug reaction information from clinical trials is useful for identifying drug-related adverse events and for approximating rates.

In a controlled clinical study, 154 patients were treated with ANDROGEL (testosterone gel) for up to 6 months. Adverse Events possibly, probably or definitely related to the use of ANDROGEL and reported by ≥1% of the patients are listed in Table 1. The four most reported adverse events are: acne (1-8%), lab test abnormal* (3-6%), application site reaction (3-5%), and prostate disorders† (3-5%).

Less Common Clinical Trial Adverse Drug Reactions (<1%): Endocrine Disorders: hirsutism.
General Disorders and Administration: peripheral edema.
Genitourinary Disorders: impaired urination.
Nervous System Disorders: dizziness.
Psychiatric Disorders: anxiety, hostility, amnesia.
Reproductive System and Breast Disorders: penis disorder.

* **Lab test abnormal** occurred in nine patients with one or more of the following events: elevated hemoglobin or hematocrit, hyperlipidemia, elevated triglycerides, hypokalemia, decreased HDL, elevated glucose, elevated creatinine, or elevated total bilirubin.

† **Prostate disorders** included five patients with enlarged prostate, one patient with BPH, and one patient with elevated PSA (Prostatic Specific Antigen) results.

Skin and Subcutaneous Tissue Disorders: dry skin, discolored hair, sweating, paresthesia.
Vascular Disorders: vasodilation.

The following adverse events possibly related to the use of ANDROGEL occurred in fewer than 1% of patients: amnesia, anxiety, discolored hair, dizziness, dry skin, hirsutism, hostility, impaired urination, paresthesia, penis disorder, peripheral edema, sweating, and vasodilation.

In this clinical trial of ANDROGEL, skin reactions at the site of application were occasionally reported with ANDROGEL, but none was severe enough to require treatment or discontinuation of drug. Six (4%) patients in this trial had adverse events that led to discontinuation of ANDROGEL. These events included the following: cerebral hemorrhage, convulsion (neither of which were considered related to ANDROGEL administration), depression, sadness, memory loss, elevated prostate specific antigen and hypertension. No ANDROGEL patients discontinued due to skin reactions.

In an uncontrolled pharmacokinetic study of 10 patients, two had adverse events associated with ANDROGEL; these were asthenia and depression in one patient and increased libido and hyperkinesia in the other. In further studies in 17 patients, there was one instance each of acne, erythema at the thoracic level and benign prostate adenoma associated with a 2.5% testosterone gel formulation applied dermally.

One hundred and sixty-two (162) patients have received ANDROGEL for up to 3 years in a long-term follow-up study for patients who completed the controlled clinical trial. Table 2 summarizes those adverse events possibly, probably or definitely related to the use of ANDROGEL and reported by 2 or more subjects in at least one treatment group during longterm exposure to ANDROGEL.

Table 2: ANDROGEL

Incidence of Treatment-Emergent Adverse Events Possibly, Probably or Definitely Related to the Use of ANDROGEL in the 3 Year Open-Label Extension Clinical Trial

Adverse Event Category/Classification	Treatment Group n=162 (%)
Lab Test Abnormal[a]	15 (9.3)
Skin Dry	3 (1.9)
Application Site Reaction	9 (5.6)
Acne	5 (3.1)
Pruritus	3 (1.9)
Enlarged Prostate	19 (11.7)
Carcinoma of Prostate	2 (1.2)
Urinary symptoms[b]	6 (3.7)
Gynecomastia	4 (2.5)
Testis Disorder[c]	3 (1.9)
Anemia	4 (2.5)

[a] **Lab test abnormal** occurred in fifteen patients with one or more of the following events: elevated AST, elevated ALT, elevated testosterone, elevated hemoglobin or hematocrit, elevated cholesterol, elevated cholesterol/LDL ratio, elevated triglycerides, elevated HDL, or elevated serum creatinine.

[b] **Urinary symptoms** included nocturia, urinary hesitancy, urinary incontinence, urinary retention, urinary urgency and weak urinary stream.

[c] **Testis disorder** included three patients. There were two patients with a non-palpable testis and one patient with slight right testicular tenderness.

Two patients reported serious adverse events considered possibly related to treatment: deep vein thrombosis (DVT) and prostate disorder requiring a transurethral resection of the prostate (TURP). Nine patients discontinued treatment due to adverse events possibly related to treatment with ANDROGEL, including two patients with application site reactions, one with kidney failure, and five with prostate disorders (including increase in serum PSA in 4 patients and increase in PSA with prostate enlargement in a fifth patient). All patients who discontinued due to an increase in serum PSA did so by Day 357.

Table 3: ANDROGEL

Laboratory Test Results of Clinical Concern Appearing at Day 90 or Final Visit but Not Baseline

		Day 90						Final Visit							
		Very low values			Very high values			Very low values				Very high values			
Lab source/ Test	Criteria for Very Low and Very High Lab Test Results	T-Gel 50	T-Gel 100	T-patch	T-Gel 50	T-Gel 100	T-patch	T-Gel 50	T-Gel 75	T-Gel 100	T-patch	T-Gel 50	T-Gel 75	T-Gel 100	T-patch
CHEM															
Glucose	VL: <=40; VH: >=175	0 (0%)	0 (0%)	0 (0%)	2 (3%)	0 (0%)	1 (1%)	0 (0%)	0 (0%)	0 (0%)	0 (0%)	2 (3%)	1 (3%)	0 (0%)	0 (0%)
Potassium (K)	VL: <=3; VH: >=6	0 (0%)	0 (0%)	0 (0%)	1 (1%)	1 (1%)	1 (1%)	0 (0%)	0 (0%)	0 (0%)	0 (0%)	0 (0%)	1 (3%)	0 (0%)	0 (0%)
Calcium (CA)	VL: <=8.2; VH: >=12	1 (1%)	1 (1%)	1 (1%)	0 (0%)	0 (0%)	0 (0%)	0 (0%)	2 (5%)	0 (0%)	1 (1%)	0 (0%)	0 (0%)	0 (0%)	0 (0%)
Inorganic phosphorus	VL: <=1.7; VH: >=9	1 (1%)	0 (0%)	0 (0%)	0 (0%)	0 (0%)	0 (0%)	0 (0%)	0 (0%)	0 (0%)	0 (0%)	0 (0%)	0 (0%)	0 (0%)	0 (0%)
AST	VH: >=2.6 ULN	0 (0%)	0 (0%)	0 (0%)	0 (0%)	0 (0%)	0 (0%)	0 (0%)	0 (0%)	0 (0%)	0 (0%)	1 (1%)	0 (0%)	0 (0%)	0 (0%)
Triglycerides	VH: >=450	0 (0%)	0 (0%)	0 (0%)	2 (3%)	0 (0%)	0 (0%)	0 (0%)	0 (0%)	0 (0%)	0 (0%)	0 (0%)	0 (0%)	1 (1%)	1 (1%)
HEMA															
WBC	VL: <2.5; VH: >16	0 (0%)	1 (1%)	0 (0%)	0 (0%)	0 (0%)	0 (0%)	1 (1%)	1 (3%)	0 (0%)	0 (0%)	0 (0%)	0 (0%)	0 (0%)	0 (0%)
Hemoglobin	VL: <9.4; VH: >18	0 (0%)	0 (0%)	0 (0%)	1 (1%)	3 (4%)	0 (0%)	1 (1%)	0 (0%)	0 (0%)	0 (0%)	1 (1%)	1 (3%)	1 (1%)	1 (1%)
Hematocrit	VL: <37; VH: >56	1 (1%)	1 (1%)	1 (1%)	0 (0%)	1 (1%)	0 (0%)	0 (0%)	0 (0%)	0 (0%)	3 (4%)	0 (0%)	0 (0%)	1 (1%)	0 (0%)
IMMU															
Prostate specific antigen	VH: >5.5	0 (0%)	0 (0%)	0 (0%)	0 (0%)	0 (0%)	0 (0%)	0 (0%)	0 (0%)	0 (0%)	0 (0%)	0 (0%)	1 (3%)	0 (0%)	0 (0%)

Only patients with lab test results meeting the criteria for Clinical Concern for the first time at Day 90 or Final visit are included in this table.
Legend: VL=Very Low lab test result; VH=Very High lab test result; ULN=Upper Limit of Normal.

During the initial 6-month study, the mean change in PSA values had a statistically significant increase of 0.26 ng/mL. Serum PSA was measured every 6 months thereafter. While there were no statistically significant increases in mean PSA from 6 months through 36 months of ANDROGEL treatment for the overall group of 162 patients enrolled in the long-term extension study, there were increases in serum PSA seen in approximately 18% of individual patients. In the long-term extension study, the overall mean change from baseline in serum PSA values for the entire group was 0.11 ng/mL.

Twenty-nine (29) (18%) patients met the per-protocol criterion for increase in serum PSA value, defined as a value ≥2× the baseline value or any single absolute value ≥6 ng/mL. Twenty-five of these patients met this criterion by virtue of a post-baseline value at least twice the baseline value. In most of these cases (22/25), the maximum serum PSA value attained was ≤2 ng/mL. The first occurrence of a pre-specified, post-baseline increase in serum PSA was seen at or prior to Month 12 in most of the patients who met this criterion (23 of 29; 79%).

Four patients met this criterion by having a serum PSA ≥6 ng/mL and in these, maximum serum PSA values were 6.2 ng/mL, 6.6 ng/mL, 6.7 ng/mL, and 10.7 ng/mL (in ANDROGEL-treated patients). In two of these ANDROGEL-treated patients, prostate cancer was detected on biopsy. The first patient's PSA levels were 4.7 ng/mL and 6.2 ng/mL at baseline and at Month 6/Final, respectively. The second patient's PSA levels were 4.2 ng/mL, 5.2 ng/mL, 5.8 ng/mL, and 6.6 ng/mL at baseline, Month 6, Month 12, and Final, respectively.

Abnormal Hematologic and Clinical Chemistry Findings: See Table 3.

Post-Market Adverse Drug Reactions: Secondary Exposure to Testosterone in Children: Cases of secondary exposure to testosterone resulting in virilization of children have been reported in postmarket surveillance. Signs and symptoms of these reported cases have included enlargement of the clitoris (with surgical intervention) or of the penis, premature development of pubic hair, increased erections and libido, aggressive behavior, and advanced bone age. In most cases with a reported outcome, these signs and symptoms were reported to have regressed with removal of the testosterone gel exposure. In a few cases, however, enlarged genitalia did not fully return to age appropriate normal size, and bone age remained modestly greater than chronological age. In some of the cases, direct contact with the sites of application on the skin of men using testosterone gel was reported. In at least one reported case, the reporter considered the possibility of secondary exposure from items such as the testosterone gel user's shirts and/ or other fabric, such as towels and sheets (see Warnings and Precautions).

In addition to those adverse events reported during clinical trials, the following adverse reactions have been identified during post-marketing use of ANDROGEL. Because these reactions are reported voluntarily from a population of uncertain size, it is not always possible to reliably estimate their frequency or establish a causal relationship to drug exposure: see Table 4.

Table 4: ANDROGEL

Adverse Drug Reactions from Post-Marketing Experience of ANDROGEL and Known Reactions of General Testosterone Treatment

MedDRA System Organ Class (SOC)	Adverse Drug Reaction
Blood and the Lymphatic System Disorders	Polycythemia, erythropoiesis abnormal
Endocrine Disorders	Abnormal accelerated growth Male pattern baldness, hirsuitism
Gastrointestinal Disorders	Nausea, vomiting, diarrhea, abdominal pain, gastrointestinal bleeding
General Disorders and Administration Site Conditions	Edema, malaise, fatigue, application site burning, application site induration, application site rash, application site dermatitis, application site blister, application site erythema
Genitourinary Disorders	Dysuria, hematuria, incontinence, bladder irritability
Hepatobiliary Disorders	Hepatic neoplasms, peliosis hepatis
Immune System Disorders	Allergic reaction, hypersensitivity reaction
Investigations	Weight increase, fluctuating testosterone levels, testosterone decreased, abnormal liver function tests (e.g. elevated GGTP), lipid abnormalities
Metabolism and Nutrition Disorders	Increased appetite, electrolyte changes (nitrogen, potassium, phosphorus, sodium), urine calcium decrease, glucose tolerance impaired, elevated cholesterol
Musculoskeletal and Connective Tissue Disorders	Myalgia, arthralgia
Nervous System Disorders	Insomnia, headache, dizziness, sleep apnea
Psychiatric Disorders	Personality disorder, confusion, anger, aggression, depression, anxiety, decreased libido, cognitive disturbance
Reproductive System and Breast Disorders	Prostate carcinoma, enlarged prostate (benign), free prostate-specific antigen increased, testicular atrophy, epididymitis, oligospermia, priapism, impotence, precocious puberty, gynecomastia, mastodynia
Respiratory, Thoracic and Mediastinal Disorders	Dyspnea
Skin and Subcutaneous Tissue Disorders	Pruritus, rash, urticaria, vesiculo-bullous rash, seborrhea, acne, alopecia
Vascular Disorders	Hypertension

In addition, one patient reported experiencing serum sickness and another patient reported experiencing both a hepatoma and polycystic kidneys.

DRUG INTERACTIONS: Drug-Drug Interactions: Insulin: In diabetic patients, the metabolic effects of androgens may decrease blood glucose and, therefore, insulin requirements.

Propranolol: In a published pharmacokinetic study of an injectable testosterone product, administration of testosterone cypionate led to an increased clearance of propranolol in the majority of men tested. It is unknown if this would apply to ANDROGEL.

Corticosteroids: The concurrent administration of testosterone with ACTH or corticosteroids may enhance edema formation; thus these drugs should be administered cautiously particularly in patients with cardiac, renal or hepatic disease.

Anticoagulants: Androgens may increase sensitivity to oral anticoagulants. Dosage of the anticoagulant may require reduction in order to maintain satisfactory therapeutic hypoprothrombinemia.

Drug-Food Interactions: Interactions with food have not been established.

Drug-Herb Interactions: Literature reports indicate that some herbal products (e.g. St John's wort) which are available as over-the-counter (OTC) products might interfere with steroid metabolism and therefore may decrease plasma testosterone levels.

Drug-Laboratory Test Interactions: Androgens may decrease levels of thyroxine-binding globulin, resulting in decreased total T_4 serum levels and increased resin uptake of T_3 and T_4. Free thyroid hormone levels remain unchanged, however, and there is no clinical evidence of thyroid dysfunction.

DOSAGE AND ADMINISTRATION: ANDROGEL is a clear, colorless, fragrance free, hydroalcoholic gel containing 1% testosterone. ANDROGEL provides continuous transdermal delivery of testosterone, the primary circulating endogenous androgen, for 24 hours following a single application to intact, clean, dry skin of the shoulders, upper arms and/or abdomen.

A daily application of ANDROGEL (testosterone gel) 5 g, 7.5 g, or 10 g delivers 50 mg, 75 mg, or 100 mg of testosterone, respectively, per day, to the skin's surface. Approximately 10% of the applied testosterone dose is absorbed across skin of average permeability during a 24-hour period. ANDROGEL delivers physiologic amounts of testosterone, producing circulating testosterone concentrations that approximate normal levels (10.3-36.2 nmol/L or 300-1000 ng/dL) seen in healthy men.

Recommended Dose and Dosage Adjustment: The recommended starting and usual dose of ANDROGEL is 5 g (to deliver 50 mg of testosterone) applied once daily (preferably in the morning) to clean, dry, intact skin of the shoulders and upper arms and/or abdomen.

As some patients may benefit from higher doses, serum testosterone levels should be measured after initiation of therapy to assist in proper dosing. If the desired clinical response is not achieved or if the serum testosterone concentration is below the lower limit of the normal range (10.3 nmol/L or 300 ng/dL), the daily ANDROGEL 1% dose may be increased from 5 g to 7.5 g and from 7.5 g to 10 g.

ANDROGEL is available in either 2.5 g or 5.0 g gel unit-dose packets or a 60 actuation metered-dose pump. The pump delivers 1.25 g of gel for each time the pump mechanism is fully depressed (actuation).

Administration: If using the metered-dose ANDROGEL pump, patients should be instructed to prime the new pump prior to using it for the first time. Up to five depressions may be needed before all of the air is removed from the pump and gel is discharged. The first two actuations which deliver gel, should be discarded to assure precise dose delivery. Discard this portion of gel in household trash in a manner that prevents accidental application or ingestion by household members, especially nursing/pregnant women and children. After priming, patients should completely depress the pump once (1 actuation) for every 1.25 g of gel required to achieve the daily prescribed dosage. The gel should be delivered directly into the palm of the hand and then applied to the desired application sites, either one actuation at a time or upon completion of all actuations, required for the daily dose. Alternatively, the product can be applied directly to the application sites. Application directly to the sites may prevent loss of product that may occur during transfer from the palm of the hand onto the application sites.

For specific dosing guidelines when using the ANDROGEL pump, refer to the chart below:

Prescribed Daily Dose	Number of Full Pump Actuations
5.0 g	4
7.5 g	6
10.0 g	8

If using the unit-dose ANDROGEL packet, one half (½) of the contents of the packet should be squeezed into the palm of the hand and immediately applied to the application sites. Once the first half of the packet has been applied, the second half of the packet should be applied in the same manner. Application sites should be allowed to dry for a few minutes prior to dressing. Hands should be washed with soap and water immediately after ANDROGEL has been applied.

Special Notes on Administration: The physician or health care professional should advise patients of the following:

- ANDROGEL should not be applied to the scrotum.
- ANDROGEL should be applied daily to clean, dry, healthy, intact skin.
- Currently it is unknown how long showering or swimming should be delayed after application of ANDROGEL. For optimal absorption of testosterone, it appears reasonable to wait at least 5-6 hours after application prior to showering or swimming. Nevertheless, showering or swimming after just 1 hour should have a minimal effect on the amount of ANDROGEL absorbed if done very infrequently.

Transference of ANDROGEL to another person can be completely prevented when application site is covered with a long-sleeved shirt (cotton-polyester blend).

Potential for Secondary Exposure to Testosterone and Steps to Prevent Secondary Exposure: Secondary exposure to testosterone in children and women can occur with the use of testosterone gel in men. Cases of secondary exposure to testosterone have been reported in children with signs and symptoms including enlargement of the penis or clitoris, premature development of pubic hair, increased erections, and aggressive behavior.

- Physicians should advise patients of the reported signs and symptoms of secondary exposure which may include the following:
  - In children; unexpected sexual development including inappropriate enlargement of the penis or clitoris, premature development of pubic hair, increased erections, and aggressive behavior.
  - In women; changes in hair distribution, increase in acne, or other signs of testosterone effects.
- The possibility of secondary exposure to testosterone gel should be brought to the attention of a healthcare provider.
- Testosterone gel should be promptly discontinued until the cause of virilization is identified.

Strict adherence to the following precautions is advised to minimize the potential for secondary exposure to testosterone from testosterone gel in men:

- **Children and women should avoid contact with unwashed or unclothed application site(s)** of men using testosterone gel.
- **To minimize the potential for transfer** to others, patients using ANDROGEL should apply the product as directed and strictly adhere to the following:
  - **Wash hands** with soap and water after application.
  - **Cover the application site(s)** with clothing after the gel has dried.
  - **Wash the application site(s) thoroughly** with soap and water prior to any situation where skin-to-skin contact of the application site with another person is anticipated.
  - In the events that unwashed or unclothed skin to which ANDROGEL has been applied and/or that the testosterone gel user's unwashed shirts and/ or other fabrics (such as towels and sheets) come in direct contact with the skin of another person, the general area of contact on the other person should be washed with soap and water as soon as possible. Studies show that residual testosterone is removed from the skin surface by washing with soap and water.

OVERDOSAGE:

Symptoms of a testosterone overdose are not known. No specific antidote is available. Symptomatic and supportive treatment should be given.

> For management of a suspected drug overdose, CPhA recommends that you contact your **regional Poison Control Centre**. See the *CPS* Directory section for a list of Poison Control Centres.

ACTION AND CLINICAL PHARMACOLOGY: ANDROGEL (testosterone gel) contains 1% testosterone and provides continuous transdermal delivery of testosterone, the primary circulating endogenous androgen.

Pharmacodynamics: Testosterone and Hypogonadism: Testosterone and dihydrotestosterone (DHT), endogenous androgens, are responsible for the normal growth and development of the male sex organs and for maintenance of secondary sex characteristics. These effects include the growth and maturation of prostate, seminal vesicles, penis, and scrotum; the development of male hair distribution, such as facial, pubic, chest, and axillary hair; laryngeal enlargement; vocal chord thickening; alterations in body musculature; and fat distribution.

Male hypogonadism results from insufficient secretion of testosterone and is characterized by low serum testosterone concentrations. Symptoms associated with male hypogonadism include decreased sexual desire with or without erectile dysfunction, fatigue and loss of energy, mood depression/ disorder and depressive symptoms, regression of some secondary sexual characteristics, osteoporosis, weakness, irritability and decreased motivation. Although causality has not been established, there are associations between hypogonadism and depression, osteoporosis, metabolic syndrome, type 2 diabetes, cardiovascular disease and increased mortality in men. Hypogonadism is a risk factor for osteoporosis in men.

General Androgen Effects: Drugs in the androgen class also promote retention of nitrogen, sodium, potassium, phosphorus, and decreased urinary excretion of calcium.

Androgens have been reported to increase protein anabolism and decrease protein catabolism. Nitrogen balance is improved only when there is sufficient intake of calories and protein. Androgens have been reported to stimulate the production of red blood cells by enhancing erythropoietin production.

Androgens are responsible for the growth spurt of adolescence and for the eventual termination of linear growth brought about by fusion of the epiphyseal growth centers. In children, exogenous androgens accelerate linear growth rates but may cause a disproportionate advancement in bone maturation. Use over long periods may result in fusion of the epiphyseal growth centers and termination of the growth process.

During exogenous administration of androgens, endogenous testosterone release may be inhibited through feedback inhibition of pituitary luteinizing hormone (LH). At large doses of exogenous androgens, spermatogenesis may also be suppressed through feedback inhibition of pituitary follicle-stimulating hormone (FSH).

Pharmacokinetics: Absorption: ANDROGEL (testosterone gel) is a hydroalcoholic formulation that dries quickly when applied to the skin surface. The skin serves as a reservoir for the sustained release of testosterone into the systemic circulation. In a study with the 10 g dose (to deliver 100 mg testosterone), all patients showed an increase in serum testosterone within 30 minutes, and eight of nine patients had a serum testosterone concentration within normal range by 4 hours after the initial application. Absorption of testosterone into the blood continues for the entire 24-hour dosing interval. Serum concentrations approximate the steady state level by the end of the first 24 hours and are at steady state by the second or third day of dosing.

Approximately 10% of testosterone from the applied ANDROGEL dose is absorbed across the skin during 24 hours, resulting in about 9-14% bioavailability of testosterone from the T-gel formulation. Nearly 1% of absorbed testosterone appears in the systemic circulation as dihydrotestosterone (DHT). There is no accumulation of testosterone or its metabolites such as estradiol and DHT, during continuous treatment.

With single daily applications of ANDROGEL, follow-up measurements 30, 90 and 180 days after starting treatment have confirmed that serum testosterone concentrations are generally maintained within the eugonadal range. Similar trends were observed in patients followed up to 3 years. Figure 1 summarizes the 24-hour pharmacokinetic profiles of testosterone for hypogonadal men (<300 ng/dL) maintained on 5 g or 10 g of ANDROGEL (to deliver 50 or 100 mg of testosterone, respectively) for 30 days. The average (±SD) daily testosterone concentration produced by ANDROGEL 10 g on Day 30 was 27.5 (±10.2) nmol/L and by ANDROGEL 5 g, 19.6 (±9.1) nmol/L.

Figure 1: ANDROGEL

Mean (SD) Steady-State Serum Testosterone Concentrations on Day 30 in Patients Applying ANDROGEL Once Daily

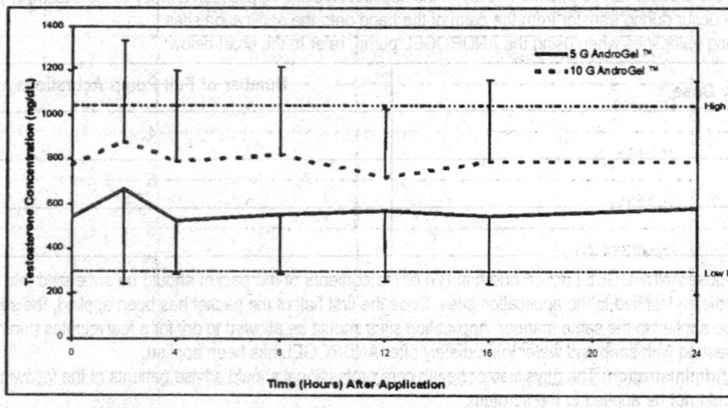

Distribution: Circulating testosterone is chiefly bound in the serum to sex hormone-binding globulin (SHBG) and albumin. The albumin-bound fraction of testosterone easily dissociates from albumin and is presumed to be bioactive. The portion of testosterone bound to SHBG is not considered biologically active. Approximately 40% of testosterone in plasma is bound to SHBG, 2% remains unbound (free) and the rest is bound to albumin and other proteins. The amount of SHBG in the serum and the total testosterone level will determine the distribution of bioactive and nonbioactive androgen.

Metabolism: There is considerable variation in the half-life of testosterone as reported in the literature, ranging from ten to 100 minutes.

When ANDROGEL treatment is discontinued after achieving steady state, serum testosterone levels remain in the normal range for 24 to 48 hours but return to their pretreatment levels by the fifth day after the last application.

Testosterone is metabolized to various 17-keto steroids through two different pathways. The major active metabolites of testosterone are estradiol and dihydrotestosterone (DHT). Testosterone is metabolized to DHT by steroid 5α reductase located in the skin, liver, and the urogenital tract of the male. Estradiol is formed by an aromatase enzyme complex in the brain, fat, and testes. DHT binds with greater affinity to SHBG than does testosterone. In many tissues the activity of testosterone depends on its reduction to DHT, which binds to cytosol receptor proteins. The steroid-receptor complex is transported to the nucleus where it initiates transcription and cellular changes related to androgen action. In reproductive tissues, DHT is further metabolized to 3-α and 3-β androstanediol.

DHT concentrations increased in parallel with testosterone concentrations during testosterone gel treatment. After 90 days of treatment, mean DHT concentrations remained generally within the normal range for testosterone gel-treated subjects.

Excretion: About 90% of a dose of testosterone given intramuscularly is excreted in the urine as glucuronic and sulfuric acid conjugates of testosterone and its metabolites; about 6% of a dose is excreted in the feces, mostly in the unconjugated form. Inactivation of testosterone occurs primarily in the liver.

Special Populations and Conditions: In patients treated with ANDROGEL, there are no observed differences in the average daily serum testosterone concentration at steady-state based on age, cause of hypogonadism or body mass index. Since no formal studies were conducted involving patients with renal or hepatic insufficiencies, the use of ANDROGEL is not recommended in men with serious liver or kidney disorders.

STORAGE AND STABILITY: Store at controlled room temperature (15-30°C).

SPECIAL HANDLING INSTRUCTIONS: None.

INFORMATION FOR THE PATIENT: Published in e-CPS, available by subscription at www.e-cps.ca.

DOSAGE FORMS, COMPOSITION AND PACKAGING: Each g of clear, colorless, fragrance-free, hydroalcoholic gel contains: testosterone USP 1%. Nonmedicinal ingredients: alcohol, Carbopol 980, isopropyl myristate, purified water and sodium hydroxide. Non-aerosol, metered-dose pump composed of plastic and stainless steel and a LDPE/aluminum foil inner liner encased in rigid plastic with a polypropylene cap. Cartons of 2 pumps. Each pump is capable of dispensing sixty 1.25 g doses. Unit-dose aluminum foil packets of 2.5 g (25 mg of testosterone) and 5 g (50 mg of testosterone), cartons of 30.

ANDROGEL is supplied as follows:

Strength	Package Size
1% (25 mg testosterone)	30 packets: 2.5 g gel per packet
1% (50 mg testosterone)	30 packets: 5.0 g gel per packet
1%	Two 60-actuation metered-dose pumps: 1.25 g gel per actuation

Disposal: Used ANDROGEL pumps or used ANDROGEL packets should be discarded in household trash in a manner that prevents accidental application or ingestion by household members, especially nursing/pregnant women and children.

(Shown in Product Identification Section)

Anexate®

flumazenil

Benzodiazepine Antagonist

Roche

Date of Preparation: September 8, 1993
Date of Revision: June 3, 2008

PHARMACOLOGY: ANEXATE (flumazenil), an imidazobenzodiazepine, is a benzodiazepine antagonist which blocks the central effects of agents that act via the benzodiazepine receptor, by competitive inhibition. The antagonism is specific, since in animal experiments the effects of compounds which have no affinity for the benzodiazepine receptor (e.g., barbiturates, meprobamate, ethanol, GABA-mimetics, and adenosine receptor agonists) were not affected by flumazenil. Flumazenil does not reverse the central effects of opioids.

Following the intravenous administration of radiolabelled ANEXATE to human volunteers, the distribution of radioactivity corresponded closely to the distribution of benzodiazepine receptors as determined by positron emission tomography.

The hypnotic-sedative effects of benzodiazepines are rapidly reversed by ANEXATE. However, the residual effects may reappear gradually within a few hours, depending on the dose and plasma concentrations of ANEXATE, the time elapsed since the benzodiazepine agonist was given, and the dose and elimination half-life of the previously administered benzodiazepine agonist. ANEXATE has shown some weak intrinsic agonistic (e.g., anticonvulsant) activity without therapeutic relevance.

Pharmacokinetics: In young male volunteers, the pharmacokinetics of intravenous flumazenil were linear over a dose range of 2-100 mg. Increasing doses of flumazenil were accompanied by a corresponding increase in the area under the plasma concentration-time curve (AUC: 37 ng/mL·h at 2 mg and 1906 ng/mL·h at 100 mg), and maximum plasma concentration (C_{max}: 55 ng/mL at 2 mg and 3332 ng/mL at 100 mg). However, elimination half-life, volume of distribution at steady-state, and plasma clearance were independent of dose over the entire range studied. The mean elimination half-life of flumazenil following the administration of single intravenous doses to healthy subjects was approximately one hour.

Plasma protein binding is low. Over a concentration range of 24 to 570 ng/mL, flumazenil was found to be 50% bound to human plasma proteins. Albumin accounts for approximately two-thirds of the plasma protein binding. The binding of flumazenil was not affected by a high concentration of diazepam (10 µg/mL), and flumazenil did not interfere with the binding of diazepam.

Flumazenil undergoes rapid and extensive hepatic metabolism; less than 0.2% of the administered dose is eliminated unchanged in the urine. The major metabolites of flumazenil identified in the urine are the free acid and its glucuronide conjugate.

In healthy volunteers, approximately 70% of an intravenous dose of flumazenil was excreted within the first two hours after dosing and another 16% during the next two hours. Elimination was essentially complete within 72 hours, with 90 to 95% of the total radioactivity appearing in the urine and 5 to 10% in the feces. Ingestion of food during an intravenous infusion of flumazenil results in a 50% increase in clearance, most likely due to the increased hepatic blood flow that accompanies a meal.

Table 1 summarizes the ranges of mean pharmacokinetic parameters reported in a series of studies, after single intravenous doses of flumazenil.

Table 1: ANEXATE

Pharmacokinetics

Subjects	Dose (mg)	Elimination Half-life ($t_{1/2\beta}$) (min)	Volume of Distribution at Steady-state (Vd_{ss}) (L/kg)	Plasma Clearance (Cl_p) (L/h)
Male volunteers 23–26 years	2–100	48–55	0.83–0.86	55–57
Male volunteers 28–42 years	2.5	42–72	0.63	41
Volunteers 39 years	2	46	0.62	74
Cirrhosis				
– moderate 45 years	2	76	0.68	29
– severe 45 years	2	142	0.85	19
Volunteers 37 years	1	51	0.91	60
Chronic Renal Failure				
– without dialysis 36 years	1	38	0.94	75
– with dialysis 55 years	1	43	1.07	75
Age Volunteers				
Male				
20–28 years	2	54	0.87	56
65–77 years	2	66	0.93	56
Female				
24–30 years	2	48	0.96	66
63–67 years	2	54	0.78	44

There were no statistically significant differences between the distribution and elimination parameters of 12 elderly (8 males and 4 females) and 6 young (4 males and 2 females) healthy volunteers, following the administration of a 2 mg intravenous dose.

When administered together with the benzodiazepines midazolam, flunitrazepam or lormetazepam, the pharmacokinetic parameters of flumazenil were not affected. Similarly, the pharmacokinetics of benzodiazepines remained unaltered in the presence of the antagonist flumazenil.

Hepatic Impairment: In patients with cirrhosis, the pharmacokinetics of flumazenil were altered, particularly in patients with severely impaired liver function. Elimination half-life was prolonged and plasma clearance markedly decreased. Since plasma protein binding is lower in cirrhotic patients than in healthy subjects, the levels of free drug are substantially increased, namely from 55% in controls to 64% and 79% in patients with moderate and severe liver dysfunction, respectively. Caution should be exercised with initial and/or repeated dosing to patients with liver disease.

Renal Impairment: In patients with chronic stabilized renal failure (creatinine clearance <10 mL/min) in the absence and presence of dialysis, the pharmacokinetics of flumazenil remained essentially unaltered.

INDICATIONS: ANEXATE (flumazenil) is indicated for the complete or partial reversal of the central sedative effects of benzodiazepines. It may therefore be used in anaesthesia and intensive care in the following situations: Termination of general anaesthesia induced and/or maintained with benzodiazepines. Reversal of benzodiazepine sedation in short diagnostic and therapeutic procedures. For the diagnosis and/or as an adjunct to supportive measures used for the management of deliberate or accidental benzodiazepine overdosage.

Geriatrics (>65 years of age): Elderly patients may be more sensitive to the effects of ANEXATE. For a brief description, see Precautions, Geriatrics.

Pediatrics (<18 years of age): The safety and effectiveness of ANEXATE in children below the age of 18 has not been established.

CONTRAINDICATIONS: ANEXATE (flumazenil) is contraindicated: In patients with known hypersensitivity to ANEXATE or to benzodiazepines. In epileptic patients who have been receiving benzodiazepine treatment for a prolonged period. The abrupt suppression of the protective effect of benzodiazepines may induce convulsions in epileptic patients. In patients who are showing signs of serious cyclic antidepressant overdose (see Precautions). In patient who have been given a benzodiazepine for a potentially life-threatening conditions (e.g. intracranial pressure).

WARNINGS:

In view of the short duration of action of ANEXATE and the possible need for repeat doses, the patient should remain closely monitored until all possible central benzodiazepine effects have subsided.

The immediate availability of oxygen, resuscitative equipment and skilled personnel for the maintenance of airway, ventilation and cardiac function should be ensured before the administration of any benzodiazepine or ANEXATE.

Resedation: ANEXATE is a competitive inhibitor of benzodiazepines at the receptor site and does not affect the pharmacokinetics of benzodiazepines. Thus, when the effect of ANEXATE wears off, the patient returns to the point of residual sedation that would have been present at that time had ANEXATE not been given. In patients administered large doses of long-acting benzodiazepines or in critically ill patients, this could be deep sedation. In a U.S. clinical study in patients with benzodiazepine intoxication, 90/133 (67.7%) patients became resedated. **Therefore, ANEXATE should be administered only when the continued observation of patients for recurrence of sedation, respiratory depression or residual benzodiazepine effects can be assured.**

Respiration: When used in anaesthesiology at the end of surgery, ANEXATE should not be given until the effects of neuromuscular blockade have been completely antagonized and careful monitoring of the respiratory depressant effect of opiate analgesics has been assured. After the benzodiazepine has been antagonized with ANEXATE, any residual respiratory depressant effect of benzodiazepines and other agents, such as opiates, may require interventions such as establishing an airway and assisted ventilation.

The ability of ANEXATE to reverse benzodiazepine-induced respiratory depression is equivocal; in some studies residual effects of benzodiazepines on respiration were still present despite reversal of sedation.

Seizures: Rapid intravenous injections should be avoided in patients treated for long periods of time and/or with high doses of benzodiazepines, as ANEXATE may trigger withdrawal symptoms (e.g., convulsions, agitation, anxiety, emotional lability as well as mild confusion and sensory distortions). Seizures have been reported in patients known to suffer from epilepsy, or severe hepatic impairment, particularly after long-term treatment with benzodiazepines or in cases of mixed-drug overdose. Most convulsions associated with flumazenil administration require treatment and have been successfully managed with benzodiazepines, phenytoin or barbiturates.

PRECAUTIONS: General: In high-risk patients (e.g., patients treated with benzodiazepines for long periods of time, overdose with signs of cyclic antidepressant overdosage), the advantages of counteracting benzodiazepine-related sedation should be weighed against the drawbacks of rapid awakening.

Postoperative pain must be taken into account. Following a major intervention, it may be preferable to maintain a moderate degree of sedation.

ANEXATE is not recommended either as a treatment for benzodiazepine dependence or for the management of protracted benzodiazepine abstinence syndromes.

Anxiety and Panic Disorder: The dosage of ANEXATE (flumazenil) should be adjusted carefully in patients suffering from preoperative anxiety or having a history of chronic or episodic anxiety. In anxious patients, particularly those with coronary heart disease, it is preferable to maintain a degree of sedation throughout the early postoperative period rather than bring about complete arousal.

ANEXATE has been reported to provoke panic attacks in patients with a history of panic disorders.

Instruction to Patients Upon Discharge: Occupational Hazards: Patients who have received ANEXATE to reverse the effects of benzodiazepine sedation should be instructed, if possible in writing, not to drive, to operate machinery or to engage in any other physically or mentally demanding activity for 24 hours or until the effects of the benzodiazepine have subsided, since the effect of the benzodiazepine may return. Patients should also be warned not to take alcohol, or drugs not prescribed by their physician, until the effects of the benzodiazepines have subsided.

Children: The safety and effectiveness of ANEXATE in children below the age of 18 has not been established.

Geriatrics: In the absence of data on the use of ANEXATE in elderly patients, it should be borne in mind that this population is generally more sensitive to the effects of drugs and should be treated with due caution.

Pregnancy: Although studies in animals have not shown evidence of embryotoxicity or teratogenicity, ANEXATE should be used during pregnancy only, if in the opinion of the treating physician, the possible benefit to the patient outweighs the potential risks to the fetus.

Lactation: It is not known whether ANEXATE is excreted in human milk. For this reason, breast-feeding should be interrupted for 24 hours when ANEXATE is used during lactation.

Hepatic Impairment: In patients with liver insufficiency, the elimination of ANEXATE can be delayed. Caution should be exercised with initial and/or repeated dosing to patients with liver disease (see Pharmacology, Pharmacokinetics, Hepatic Impairment and Dosage).

Seizures have been reported in patients known to suffer from severe hepatic impairment, particularly after long-term treatment with benzodiazepines or in cases of mixed-drug overdose.

Renal Impairment: No dosage adjustments are necessary in patients with renal impairment.

Use in Respiratory Disease: The primary treatment of patients with serious lung disease who experience serious respiratory depression due to benzodiazepines should be given appropriate ventilatory support, rather than administration of ANEXATE.

Use in Acute Myocardial Infarction or Cardiac Arrhythmias: Flumazenil abruptly terminates the effects of benzodiazepines. As a result, sympathetic tone may be increased and thus, cardiac electrical instability enhanced. Consequently, caution is advised when administering ANEXATE to patients with myocardial infarction or cardiac arrhythmias.

Use in Patients with Increased Intracranial Pressure Receiving Benzodiazepines (e.g., head injury, brain tumor, intracranial hemorrhage): In patients with increased intracranial pressure, ANEXATE may further increase intracranial pressure cerebral perfusion pressure, or precipitate convulsions. In such patients, ANEXATE should be used with extreme caution and only by practitioners prepared to manage such complications, should they occur.

Multiple Drug Overdosage: Particular caution is necessary when using ANEXATE in cases of multiple drug overdosage, since the toxic effects (cardiac arrhythmias and/or convulsions) of other psychotropic drugs, especially cyclic antidepressants, may increase as the effects of benzodiazepines subside.

Patients should be evaluated for the signs and symptoms (autonomic, neurological or cardiovascular) of a cyclic antidepressant overdose. A diagnostic ECG can be used to confirm the presence of these agents; a QRS duration of 0.1 seconds or greater indicates a serious overdosage with cyclic antidepressants, which should be treated with appropriate measures. Depending on the extent of involvement of benzodiazepines in the multiple drug overdose, this may or may not include ANEXATE.

Use in the ICU: ANEXATE should be used with caution in the Intensive Care Unit because of the increased risk of unrecognized benzodiazepine dependence in such settings. ANEXATE may produce convulsions in patients physically dependent on benzodiazepine (see Warnings, Seizures).

<u>Drug Interactions:</u> Interactions with central nervous system depressants other than benzodiazepines have not been studied specifically.

ANEXATE blocks the central effects of benzodiazepines by competitive interaction at the receptor level; the effects of non-benzodiazepines which act via the benzodiazepine receptor, such as zopiclone, triazolopyridazines and others, are also blocked. However, ANEXATE does not reverse the effects of drugs that do not act via this route, such as opioids.

The pharmacokinetics of ANEXATE are unaltered in the presence of benzodiazepines, and similarly, ANEXATE does not affect the kinetics of benzodiazepines.

There is no pharmacokinetic interaction between ethanol and flumazenil.

ADVERSE EFFECTS: ANEXATE (flumazenil) is generally well tolerated. In postoperative use, nausea and/or vomiting are observed, particularly if opiates have also been employed. Flushing has also been noted. If patients are awakened too rapidly, they may become agitated, anxious or fearful. Transient increases in blood pressure and heart rate may also occur.

Excessively and/or rapidly injected doses of ANEXATE may induce benzodiazepine withdrawal symptoms such as anxiety attacks, tachycardia, dizziness and sweating in patients on long-term benzodiazepine treatment.

Although clinical experience with ANEXATE is limited, seizures and/or cardiac arrhythmias have been observed in patients who are physically dependent on benzodiazepines, and in multiple drug overdose, particularly in the presence of tricyclic antidepressants.

ANEXATE has been reported to provoke panic attacks in patients with a history of panic disorders.

Table 2 summarizes the adverse reactions which occurred with an incidence of >1%.

Other clinical adverse events which occurred with an incidence of <1% are as follows:

Cardiovascular: ventricular premature beats, arrhythmia, palpitations, bradycardia, flush, hypotension, chest pain.

Respiratory: dyspnea, hypopnea, nasal congestion, cough, subjective suffocation.

CNS/Neuromuscular: startle reaction, fear, nervousness, restlessness, excitation, aggressiveness, anger; euphoria, hallucinations, vertigo, confusion, tiredness/drowsiness, depression, involuntary/spontaneous movement, tremor, mouth movement, tetany, speech disorder.

Gastrointestinal: salivation, dry mouth, hiccoughs.

Dermatological: urticaria, pruritus.

Miscellaneous: pain, allergic reaction, strabismus, sweating.

Local Tolerance: Slight to moderate pain at the site of injection occurred in 2.5% of patients and redness was observed in 1.3% of patients in clinical trials, one hour after the administration of ANEXATE.

OVERDOSE:

Symptoms: ANEXATE (flumazenil), administered intravenously to healthy volunteers at a dosage of 100 mg, did not produce symptoms of overdosage. Reversal of sedation or general anesthesia with excessively high doses of flumazenil may produce symptoms of benzodiazepine withdrawal, such as anxiety, agitation, increased muscle tone, hyperesthesia, and possible convulsions.

Table 2: ANEXATE

Clinical Adverse Events >1%

Organ System	Adverse Event	Frequency (%) General Anaesthesia/ Sedation n=7365	Frequency (%) Known or Suspected Benzodiazepine Overdose n=764
CNS	Agitation	0.2	5.8
	Crying/Tears	0.5	3.5
	Headache	0.5	1.6
	Anxiety/Anxious Feeling	0.3	1.4
	Seizures/Convulsions	—	1.3
	Dizziness	1.4	1.2
Gastrointestinal	Nausea	4.3	2.2
	Vomiting	2.6	2.0
Cardiovascular	Hypertension	0.1	1.4
	Tachycardia	0.1	1.2
Miscellaneous	Shivering/Cold Sensation/Chills	0.5	1.2

There is very limited experience of acute overdose in humans with ANEXATE. There is no specific antidote for overdose with ANEXATE. Treatment of an overdose with ANEXATE should consist of general supportive measures including monitoring of vital signs and observation of the clinical status of the patient. Convulsions associated with the ANEXATE (flumazenil) administration have been successfully managed with benzodiazepines, phenytoin or barbiturates (see Warnings, Seizures).

Treatment: See Symptoms.

For management of a suspected drug overdose, CPhA recommends that you contact your **regional Poison Control Centre**. See the *CPS* Directory section for a list of Poison Control Centres.

<u>DOSAGE</u>: ANEXATE (flumazenil) should be administered intravenously by a physician with experience in anaesthesiology.

ANEXATE is not indicated for epileptic patients who have been treated with benzodiazepines for a prolonged period. The abrupt cessation of the protective effect of benzodiazepines may induce convulsions in epileptic patients.

Caution should be exercised with initial and repeated dosing to patients with hepatic insufficiency as elimination of ANEXATE (flumazenil) can be delayed in these patients (see Pharmacology, Pharmacokinetics, Hepatic Impairment).

The dose of ANEXATE should always be individually titrated to the desired response to avoid abrupt awakening. Particular care is needed with patients who are physically dependent on benzodiazepines, patients who have ingested multiple drugs, and patients who are prone to anxiety. In the intensive care unit, in patients treated with high doses of benzodiazepines and/or for long periods of time, the individually titrated injections of ANEXATE, slowly administered, should not produce withdrawal syndromes (see Precautions). If unexpected symptoms occur, diazepam or midazolam could be carefully titrated intravenously according to patient's response.

ANEXATE may be used concurrently with other resuscitative procedures (see Known or Suspected Benzodiazepine Overdose).

ANEXATE is compatible with 5% dextrose in water, lactated Ringer's, and normal saline solutions. If ANEXATE is drawn into a syringe or mixed with any of these solutions, it should be discarded after 24 hours.

Reversal of General Anaesthesia/Sedation: The recommended initial dose is 0.2 mg administered intravenously over 15 seconds. If the desired level of consciousness is not obtained within 60 seconds, a further dose of 0.1 mg can be injected and repeated at 60 second intervals, up to a maximum total dose of 1 mg. The usual dose is between 0.3 and 0.6 mg.

Known or Suspected Benzodiazepine Overdose: Necessary measures should be taken to monitor the patient's vital signs and institute supportive treatment as indicated by the patient's clinical state. In particular, patients may require symptomatic treatment for cardiorespiratory effects or central nervous system effects. ANEXATE (flumazenil) is intended as an adjunct to, not as a substitute for, supportive measures used to manage overdose (e.g., proper management of airway, assisted breathing, circulatory access and support, internal decontamination by charcoal and possibly lavage, and adequate clinical evaluation).

For the reversal of excessive sedative effects of benzodiazepines in overdose cases, titrate ANEXATE as described below, until the patient clearly responds or until the maximum recommended dose has been reached.

The recommended initial dose is 0.3 mg administered intravenously over 30 seconds, followed by a series of 0.3 mg injections, each administered over a 30-second period, at 60-second intervals. The maximum recommended dose is 2 mg.

If a significant improvement in the level of consciousness and respiratory function is not achieved after repeated injections of ANEXATE, a non-benzodiazepine aetiology must be assumed.

If drowsiness recurs, an intravenous infusion of 0.1-0.4 mg/hr may be useful. The rate of the infusion should be individually adjusted to the desired level of arousal.

INFORMATION FOR THE PATIENT: Published in e-CPS, available by subscription at <u>www.e-cps.ca</u>.

SUPPLIED: Each mL of the colorless aqueous solution contains: flumazenil 0.1 mg. Nonmedicinal ingredients: acetic acid, disodium edetate, methylparaben, propylparaben and sodium chloride. Sodium hydroxide and hydrochloric acid added to adjust pH to approximately 4. Multidose vials of 5 mL, packs of 10. Store at 15 to 30°C.

Angeliq® Ⓟ

drospirenone—estradiol-17β

Progestin—Estrogen

Bayer

Date of Revision: May 26, 2009

SUMMARY PRODUCT INFORMATION:

Route of Administration	Dosage Form/ Strength	Clinically Relevant Nonmedicinal Ingredients
Oral	Film-coated tablet, 1 mg drospirenone/1 mg estradiol-17β	None For a complete listing see Dosage Forms, Composition and Packaging.

INDICATIONS AND CLINICAL USE: ANGELIQ (drospirenone and estradiol-17β) is indicated for:

- treatment of the climacteric syndrome (vasomotor symptoms) in postmenopausal women. This may include the treatment of the symptoms of vulvar and vaginal dryness associated with menopause. When prescribing solely for the treatment of symptoms of vulvar and vaginal dryness, topical vaginal products should be considered. ANGELIQ is recommended for use only in patients with an intact uterus since the regimen includes a progestin whose role is to assist in the prevention of endometrial hyperplasia.

CONTRAINDICATIONS:

- active hepatic dysfunction or disease, especially of the obstructive type
- personal history of known or suspected estrogen-dependent or progestin-dependent malignant neoplasia (eg, breast cancer or endometrial cancer)
- presence or history of liver tumors (benign or malignant)
- presence or history of severe renal disease as long as renal function values have not returned to normal
- severe hypertriglyceridemia
- endometrial hyperplasia
- undiagnosed abnormal genital bleeding
- known or suspected pregnancy
- lactation
- active or past history of arterial thromboembolic disease (e.g., stroke, myocardial infarction, coronary heart disease)
- classical migraine
- active or past history of confirmed venous thromboembolism (such as deep vein thrombosis or pulmonary embolism) or active thrombophlebitis
- partial or complete loss of vision due to ophthalmic vascular disease
- hypersensitivity to this drug or to any ingredient in the formulation or component of the container. For a complete listing, see Dosage Forms, Composition and Packaging.

WARNINGS AND PRECAUTIONS:

Serious Warnings and Precautions

The Women's Health Initiative (WHI) trial examined the health benefits and risks of oral combined estrogen plus progestin therapy (n=16 608) and oral estrogen-alone therapy (n=10 739) in postmenopausal women aged 50 to 79 years.

The estrogen plus progestin arm of the WHI trial (mean age 63.3 years) indicated an increase risk of myocardial infarction (MI), stroke, invasive breast cancer, pulmonary emboli and deep vein thrombosis in postmenopausal women receiving treatment with combined conjugated equine estrogens (CEE, 0.625 mg/day) and medroxyprogesterone acetate (MPA, 2.5 mg/day) for 5.2 years compared to those receiving placebo.

The estrogen-alone arm of the WHI trial (mean age 63.6 years) indicated an increased risk of stroke and deep vein thrombosis in hysterectomized women treated with CEE-alone (0.625 mg/day) for 6.8 years compared to those receiving placebo.

Therefore, the following should be given serious consideration at the time of prescribing:

- Estrogens with or without progestins **should not** be prescribed for primary or secondary prevention of cardiovascular diseases.
- Estrogens with or without progestins should be prescribed at **the lowest effective dose** for the approved indication.
- Estrogens with or without progestins should be prescribed for **the shortest period** possible for the approved indication.

Carcinogenesis and Mutagenesis: Breast Cancer: Available epidemiological data indicate that the use of combined estrogen plus progestin by postmenopausal women is associated with an increased risk of invasive breast cancer.

In the estrogen plus progestin arm of the WHI trial, among 10 000 women over a one-year period, there were:

- 8 more cases of invasive breast cancer (38 on combined HRT versus 30 on placebo).

The WHI study also reported that the invasive breast cancers diagnosed in the estrogen plus progestin group were similar in histology but were larger (mean (SD) 1.7 cm (1.1) vs 1.5 cm (0.9), respectively; P=0.04) and were at a more advanced stage compared with those diagnosed in the placebo group. The percentage of women with abnormal mammograms (recommendations for short-interval follow-up, a suspicious abnormality, or highly suggestive of malignancy) was significantly higher in the estrogen plus progestin group versus the placebo group. This difference appeared at year one and persisted in each year thereafter.

In the estrogen-alone arm of the WHI trial, there was no statistically significant difference in the rate of invasive breast cancer in hysterectomized women treated with conjugated equine estrogens versus women treated with placebo.

It is recommended that estrogens with or without progestins not be given to women with existing breast cancer or those with a previous history of the disease. There is a need for caution in prescribing estrogens with or without progestins for women with known risk factors associated with the development of breast cancer, such as strong family history of breast cancer (first degree relative) or who present a breast condition with an increased risk (abnormal mammograms and/or atypical hyperplasia at breast biopsy). Other known risk factors for the development of breast cancer such as nulliparity, obesity, early menarche, late age at first full term pregnancy and at menopause should also be evaluated.

It is recommended that women undergo mammography prior to the start of HRT treatment and at regular intervals during treatment, as deemed appropriate by the treating physician and according to the perceived risks for each patient.

The overall benefits and possible risks of hormone replacement therapy should be fully considered and discussed with patients. It is important that the modest increased risk of being diagnosed with breast cancer after 4 years of treatment with combined estrogen plus progestin HRT (as reported in the results of the WHI trial) be discussed with the patient and weighed against its known benefits.

Instructions for regular self-examination of the breasts should be included in this counselling.

Liver Tumors: In rare cases, benign and even more rarely, malignant liver tumors have been observed after the use of hormonal substances such as those contained in HRT products. In isolated cases, these tumors led to life-threatening intra-abdominal hemorrhage. A hepatic tumor should be considered in the differential diagnosis if upper abdominal pain, enlarged liver, or signs of intra-abdominal hemorrhage occur.

Endometrial Hyperplasia and Endometrial Carcinoma: The use of unopposed estrogens in women with intact uteri has been associated with an increased risk of endometrial cancer.

Clinical surveillance of all women taking estrogen/progestin combinations is important. Adequate diagnostic measures, including endometrial sampling when indicated, should be undertaken to rule out malignancy in all cases of undiagnosed persistent or recurring abnormal vaginal bleeding. Adding a progestin to estrogen therapy has been shown to reduce the risk of endometrial hyperplasia, which may be a precursor to endometrial cancer.

Pituitary Tumors: Any suspicion of prolactinoma should be ruled out before starting treatment.

Cardiovascular: The results of the Heart and Estrogen/progestin Replacement Studies (HERS and HERS II) and the Women's Health Initiative (WHI) trial indicate that the use of estrogen plus progestin is associated with an increased risk of coronary heart disease (CHD) in postmenopausal women. The results of the WHI trial indicate that the use of estrogen-alone and estrogen plus progestin is associated with an increased risk of stroke in postmenopausal women.

WHI Trial Findings: In the combined estrogen plus progestin arm of the WHI trial, among 10 000 women over a one-year period, there were:

- 8 more cases of stroke (29 on combined HRT versus 21 on placebo)
- 7 more cases of CHD (37 on combined HRT versus 30 on placebo).

In the estrogen-alone arm of the WHI trial of women with prior hysterectomy, among 10 000 women over a one-year period, there were/was:

- 12 more cases of stroke (44 on estrogen-alone therapy versus 32 on placebo)
- no statistically significant difference in the rate of CHD.

HERS and HERS II Findings: In the Heart and Estrogen/progestin Replacement Study (HERS) of postmenopausal women with documented heart disease (n=2763, average age 66.7 years), a randomized placebo-controlled clinical trial of secondary prevention of coronary heart disease (CHD), treatment with 0.625 mg/day oral conjugated equine estrogen (CEE) plus 2.5 mg medroxyprogesterone acetate (MPA) demonstrated no cardiovascular benefit. Specifically, during an average follow-up of 4.1 years, treatment with CEE plus MPA did not reduce the overall rate of CHD events in postmenopausal women with established coronary heart disease. There were more CHD events in the hormone-treated group than in the placebo group in year 1, but not during the subsequent years.

From the original HERS trial, 2321 women consented to participate in an open label extension of HERS, known as HERS II. Average follow-up in HERS II was an additional 2.7 years, for a total of 6.8 years overall. After 6.8 years, hormone therapy did not reduce the risk of cardiovascular events in women with CHD.

Blood Pressure: Women using hormone replacement therapy sometimes experience increased blood pressure. Blood pressure should be monitored with HRT use. Elevation of blood pressure in previously normotensive or hypertensive patients should be investigated and HRT may have to be discontinued.

Endocrine and Metabolism: Glucose and Lipid Metabolism: A worsening of glucose tolerance and lipid metabolism has been observed in a significant percentage of peri- and postmenopausal patients. Therefore, diabetic patients or those with a predisposition to diabetes should be observed closely to detect any alterations in carbohydrate or lipid metabolism, especially in triglyceride blood levels.

Women with moderately elevated levels of triglycerides need special surveillance. HRT in these women may be associated with a further increase in triglyceride levels bearing the risk of acute pancreatitis.

Women with familial hyperlipidemias or porphyria need special surveillance. Lipid-lowering measures are recommended additionally, before treatment is started.

Calcium and Phosphorus Metabolism: Because the prolonged use of estrogens with or without progestins influences the metabolism of calcium and phosphorus, estrogens with or without progestins should be used with caution in patients with metabolic and malignant bone diseases associated with hypercalcemia and in patients with renal insufficiency.

Hypothyroidism: Patients who require thyroid hormone replacement therapy and who are also taking estrogen should have their thyroid function monitored regularly to ensure that thyroid hormone levels remain in an acceptable range (see Drug-Laboratory Test Interactions).

Genitourinary: Vaginal Bleeding: Abnormal vaginal bleeding, due to its prolongation, irregularity or heaviness, occurring during therapy should prompt diagnostic measures like hysteroscopy, endometrial biopsy, or curettage to rule out the possibility of uterine malignancy and the treatment should be re-evaluated.

Uterine Leiomyomata: Pre-existing uterine leiomyoma may increase in size during estrogen use. Growth, pain, or tenderness of uterine leiomyoma requires discontinuation of medication and appropriate investigation.

Endometriosis: Symptoms and physical findings associated with a previous diagnosis of endometriosis may reappear or become aggravated with estrogen use. Should endometriosis be reactivated under treatment, discontinuation of therapy is recommended.

Hematologic: Venous Thromboembolism: Available epidemiological data indicate that use of estrogen with or without progestin by postmenopausal women is associated with an increased risk of developing venous thromboembolism (VTE).

In the estrogen plus progestin arm of the WHI trial, among 10 000 women on combined HRT over a one-year period, there were 18 more cases of venous thromboembolism, including 8 more cases of pulmonary embolism.

In the estrogen-alone arm of the WHI trial, among 10 000 women on estrogen therapy over a one-year period, there were 7 more cases of venous thromboembolism, although there was no statistically significant difference in the rate of pulmonary embolism.

Generally recognized risk factors for VTE include a personal history, a family history (the occurrence of VTE in a direct relative at a relatively early age may indicate genetic predisposition), and severe obesity (body mass index >30 kg/m²). The risk of VTE also increases with age and smoking.

The risk of VTE may be temporarily increased with prolonged immobilization, major surgery, or trauma. In women on HRT, attention should be given to prophylactic measures to prevent VTE following surgery. Also, patients with varicose veins should be closely supervised. The physician should be alert to the earliest manifestations of thrombotic disorders (thrombophlebitis, retinal thrombosis, cerebral embolism and pulmonary embolism). If these occur or are suspected, hormone therapy should be discontinued immediately, given the risks of long-term disability or fatality.

If feasible, estrogens with or without progestins should be discontinued at least 4 weeks before major surgery which may be associated with an increased risk of thromboembolism, or during periods of prolonged immobilization.

Hepatic/Biliary/Pancreatic: Gallbladder Diseases: A 2- to 4-fold increase in the risk of gallbladder disease requiring surgery in women receiving postmenopausal estrogens has been reported.

Jaundice: Caution is advised in patients with a history of liver and/or biliary disorders. If cholestatic jaundice develops during treatment, the treatment should be discontinued and appropriate investigations carried out.

Liver Function Tests: Liver function tests should be done periodically in subjects who are suspected of having hepatic disease. For information on endocrine and liver function tests, see the section under Monitoring and Laboratory Tests.

Immune: Angioedema: Exogenous estrogens may induce or exacerbate symptoms of angioedema, in particular in women with hereditary angioedema. Discontinuation of this medication should be considered.

Neurologic: Cerebrovascular Insufficiency: Patients who develop visual disturbances, classical migraine, transient aphasia, paralysis, or loss of consciousness should discontinue medication.

Patients with a previous history of classical migraine and who develop a recurrence or worsening of migraine symptoms should be re-evaluated.

Dementia: Available epidemiological data indicate that the use of combined estrogen plus progestin in women age 65 and over may increase the risk of developing probable dementia.

The Women's Health Initiative Memory Study (WHIMS), a clinical substudy of the WHI, was designed to assess whether postmenopausal hormone replacement therapy (estrogen plus progestin or estrogen-alone) reduces the risk of dementia in women aged 65 and over and free of dementia at baseline.

In the estrogen plus progestin arm of the WHIMS (n=4532), women with an intact uterus were treated with daily 0.625 mg conjugated equine estrogens (CEE) plus 2.5 mg medroxyprogesterone acetate (MPA) or placebo for an average of 4.05 years. The results, when extrapolated to 10 000 women treated over a one-year period showed:

- 23 more cases of probable dementia (45 on combined HRT versus 22 on placebo).

In the estrogen-alone arm of the WHIMS (n=2947), women with prior hysterectomy were treated with daily 0.625 mg CEE or placebo for an average of 5.21 years. The results, when extrapolated to 10 000 women treated over a one-year period showed:

- 12 more cases of probable dementia (37 on estrogen-alone versus 25 on placebo), although this difference did not reach statistical significance.

When data from the estrogen plus progestin arm of the WHIMS and the estrogen-alone arm of the WHIMS were combined, as per the original WHIMS protocol, in 10 000 women over a one-year period, there were:

- 18 more cases of probable dementia (41 on estrogen plus progestin or estrogen-alone versus 23 on placebo).

Renal: Fluid Retention: Estrogens with or without progestins may cause fluid retention. Therefore, particular caution is indicated in cardiac or renal dysfunction, epilepsy or asthma. Treatment should be stopped if there is an increase in epileptic seizures. If, in any of the above-mentioned conditions, a worsening of the underlying disease is diagnosed or suspected during treatment, the benefits and risks of treatment should be reassessed based on the individual case.

Nonsevere disturbances of liver function, including hyperbilirubinemias such as Dubin-Johnson syndrome or Rotor syndrome, require close supervision. In case of deterioration of markers of liver function, the use of HRT should be discontinued.

Skin: Chloasma may occasionally occur, especially in women with a history of chloasma gravidarum. Women with a tendency to chloasma should avoid exposure to the sun or ultraviolet radiation while taking HRT.

Special Populations: Pregnant Women: ANGELIQ must not be used during pregnancy and lactation (see Contraindications). If pregnancy occurs during medication with ANGELIQ, treatment must be discontinued immediately.

Monitoring and Laboratory Tests: Before ANGELIQ (drospirenone and estradiol-17β) is administered, the patient should have a complete physical examination, including a blood pressure determination. Breasts and pelvic organs should be appropriately examined and a Papanicolaou smear should be performed. Endometrial biopsy should be done when indicated. Baseline tests should include mammography, measurement of blood glucose, calcium, triglycerides and cholesterol, and liver function tests.

The first follow-up examination should be done within 3 to 6 months after initiation of treatment to assess response to treatment. Thereafter, examinations should be made at intervals of at least once a year. Appropriate investigations should be arranged at regular intervals as determined by the physician. **It is important that patients are encouraged to practice frequent self examination of the breasts.**

ADVERSE REACTIONS: Adverse Drug Reaction Overview: See Warnings and Precautions regarding potential induction of malignant neoplasms and adverse effects similar to those of oral contraceptives.

The following adverse reactions have been reported with estrogen/progestin combinations in general:

Blood and Lymphatic System Disorders: altered coagulation tests (see Drug Interactions, Drug-Laboratory Test Interactions).

Cardiac Disorders: palpitations; increase in blood pressure (see Warnings and Precautions); coronary thrombosis.

Endocrine Disorders: increased blood sugar levels; decreased glucose tolerance.

Eye Disorders: neuro-ocular lesions (e.g., retinal thrombosis, optic neuritis); visual disturbances; steepening of the corneal curvature; intolerance to contact lenses.

Gastrointestinal Disorders: nausea; vomiting; abdominal discomfort (cramps, pressure, pain, bloating).

General Disorders and Administration Site Conditions: fatigue; changes in appetite; changes in body weight; change in libido.

Hepatobiliary Disorders: gallbladder disorder; asymptomatic impaired liver function; cholestatic jaundice.

Musculoskeletal and Connective Tissue Disorders: musculoskeletal pain including leg pain not related to thromboembolic disease (usually transient, lasting 3 to 6 weeks) may occur.

Nervous System Disorders: aggravation of migraine episodes; headaches, dizziness; neuritis.

Psychiatric Disorders: mental depression; nervousness; irritability.

Renal and Urinary Disorders: cystitis; dysuria; sodium retention; edema.

Reproductive System and Breast Disorders: breakthrough bleeding; spotting; change in menstrual flow; dysmenorrheal; vaginal itching/discharge; dyspareunia; endometrial hyperplasia; premenstrual-like syndrome; reactivation of endometriosis; changes in cervical erosion and amount of cervical secretion; breast swelling and tenderness.
Skin and Subcutaneous Tissue Disorders: chloasma or melasma, which may persist when drug is discontinued; erythema multiforme; erythema nodosum; hemorrhagic eruption; loss of scalp hair; hirsutism and acne.
Vascular Disorders: isolated cases of: thrombophlebitis; thromboembolic disorders.

Exogenous estrogens may induce or exacerbate symptoms of angioedema, in particular in women with hereditary angioedema (see Warnings and Precautions).

Clinical Trial Adverse Drug Reactions: Because clinical trials are conducted under very specific conditions the adverse reaction rates observed in the clinical trials may not reflect the rates observed in practice and should not be compared to the rates in the clinical trials of another drug. Adverse drug reaction information from clinical trials is useful for identifying drug-related adverse events and for approximating rates.

A clinical trial dataset of 1532 patients was used to generate the adverse drug reaction profile of ANGELIQ to support market authorization in Canada (market authorization clinical trials dataset). Subsequent to market introduction, additional adverse drug reaction data from clinical trials (n=892) has become available for a total database of 2424 patients.

Market Authorization Clinical Trials Dataset: The most commonly reported adverse reaction to ANGELIQ (drospirenone and estradiol-17β) in the clinical trials upon which market authorization is based (n=1532) were breast pain, vaginal bleeding, abdominal pain, headache, enlarged abdomen, breast neoplasm, asthenia, depression, hot flashes, emotional lability, nausea, enlarged uterine fibroids, cervix neoplasm, leukorrhea, fibrocystic breast, pain in extremity, nervousness, breast enlargement, peripheral edema, and vaginitis.

The following are adverse events reported with ANGELIQ treatment in these clinical trials, including strengths of drospirenone in combination with estradiol that are not approved (i.e., containing 1, 2, or 3 mg DRSP): see Table 1.

Table 1: ANGELIQ

Adverse Events Considered at Least Possibly Related to ANGELIQ in Four Phase III Clinical Trials (n=1532)

	Adverse Event	
Organ System	**Common (≥1/100, <1/10)**	**Uncommon (≥1/1000, <1/100)**
Body as a Whole	Abdominal pain Asthenia Pain in extremity	Pain in back or pelvis Chills Malaise Laboratory test abnormal
Cardiovascular System		Migraine Hypertension Chest pain Palpitation Varicose veins Venous thrombosis Superficial thrombophlebitis Vasodilation
Digestive	Nausea	Gastrointestinal disorder Increased appetite Liver function test abnormal
Metabolic and Nutritional Disorders		Generalized or localized edema Weight gain Hyperlipemia
Musculoskeletal System		Muscle cramps Arthralgia
Nervous System	Headache Mood swings Hot flushes Nervousness	Insomnia Dizziness Libido decreased Concentration ability impaired Paresthesia Sweating increased Anxiety Dry mouth Vertigo
Respiratory System		Dyspnea
Skin and Appendages	Benign breast neoplasms Breast enlargement	Alopecia Skin or hair disorder Hirsutism Breast carcinoma Breast engorgement
Special Senses		Taste disturbance
Urogenital	Uterine fibroids enlarged Cervix neoplasm Leukorrhea	Vulvovaginitis Endometrial or cervical disorder Bleeding Dysmenorrhea Ovarian cyst Urinary tract infections Incontinence

Additional Related Adverse Drug Reactions: The following **additional** adverse drug reactions were observed in clinical trials (n=2424), including strengths of drospirenone in combination with estradiol that are not approved in Canada (i.e., containing 0.5, 1, 2, or 3 mg DRSP), and are considered at least possibly related to ANGELIQ by the investigator:
Uncommon (≥1/1000, <1/100): Digestive System: anorexia, constipation, diarrhea, flatulence, vomiting.
Skin and Appendages: acne, pruritus, rash.
Special Senses: abnormal vision.
Rare (<1/1000): Digestive System: cholelithiasis.
Hematic and Lymphatic: anemia.
Skin and Appendages: tinnitus.
Urogenital System: salpingitis.

The following adverse reactions, considered at least possibly related to ANGELIQ were recorded in 2 clinical trials in hypertensive women: hyperkalemia, cardiac failure, atrial flutter, QT interval prolonged, cardiomegaly, blood aldosterone increased.

DRUG INTERACTIONS: Overview: Estrogens may diminish the effectiveness of anticoagulants, antidiabetics, and antihypertensive agents.

Preparations inducing liver enzymes (eg, barbiturates, hydantoins, carbamazepine, meprobamate, phenylbutazone, or rifampicin) may interfere with the activity of orally administered estrogens.

Acute alcohol ingestion during use of HRT may lead to elevations of circulating estradiol levels.

Drug-Drug Interactions: Clinical pharmacokinetic studies have not demonstrated any consistent effect of antibiotics (other than rifampin) on plasma concentrations of synthetic steroids.

Effects of Drospirenone on Other Drugs: Metabolic Interactions: Metabolism of DRSP and potential effects of DRSP on hepatic cytochrome P450 (CYP) enzymes have been investigated in in vitro and in vivo studies (see Action and Clinical Pharmacology, Pharmacokinetics). In in vitro studies, DRSP did not affect turnover of model substrates of CYP1A2 and CYP2D6, but had an inhibitory influence on the turnover of model substrates of CYP1A1, CYP2C9, CYP2C19, and CYP3A4, with CYP2C19 being the most sensitive enzyme. The potential effect of DRSP on CYP2C19 activity was investigated in a clinical pharmacokinetic study using omeprazole as a marker substrate. In the study with 24 postmenopausal women (including 12 women with homozygous (wild type) CYP2C19 genotype and 12 women with heterozygous CYP2C19 genotype), the daily oral administration of 3 mg DRSP for 14 days did not affect the oral clearance of omeprazole (40 mg, single oral dose). Based on the available results of in vivo and in vitro studies, it can be concluded that, at clinical dose level, DRSP is unlikely to interact significantly with cytochrome P450 enzymes.

In vitro and in vivo studies have shown that estrogens are metabolized partially by cytochrome P450 3A4 (CYP3A4). Therefore, inducers or inhibitors of CYP3A4 may affect estrogen drug metabolism. Inducers of CYP3A4 such as St. John's Wort preparations (Hypericum perforatum), phenobarbital, carbamazepine, and rifampin may reduce plasma concentrations of estrogens, possibly resulting in a decrease in therapeutic effects and/or changes in the uterine bleeding profile. Inhibitors of CYP3A4 such as erythromycin, clarithromycin, ketoconazole, itraconazole, ritonavir, and grapefruit juice may increase plasma concentrations of estrogens and may result in side effects.

Coadministration with Drugs that Have the Potential to Increase Serum Potassium: Nonsteroidal Anti-inflammatory Drugs (NSAIDs): The interaction of DRSP 3 mg/E2 1 mg and indomethacin was studied in 32 postmenopausal women who were coadministered 150 mg indomethacin daily for 17 days. No subject developed hyperkalemia during the study. A complete 24-hour serum potassium profile showed no clinically or statistically significant difference between serum potassium concentrations in subjects on indomethacin alone or the combination of DRSP/E2 + indomethacin. The combined intake of a potent NSAID, indomethacin and DRSP 3 mg/E2 1 mg did not cause hyperkalemia in healthy postmenopausal women.

ACE Inhibitors or Angiotensin Receptor Blockers (ARB) + Nonsteroidal Anti-inflammatory Drugs (NSAIDs): Combined effects of an ACEI or ARB with an NSAID were studied in 230 postmenopausal women with hypertension and/or diabetes mellitus requiring an ACE inhibitor or angiotensin receptor blocker (ARB). Of these, 26 patients had a creatinine clearance >50 mL/min to <80 mL/min. Patients were given DRSP 3 mg/E2 1 mg or placebo over 28 days. Nondiabetic patients also received ibuprofen 1200 mg/day for 5 days during the study. The range of mean serum potassium values during the treatment phase was similar in both groups, 4.35 to 4.42 mEq/L for the DRSP/E2 group and 4.27 to 4.34 mEq/L for the placebo group. After 28 days of exposure the mean change from baseline for the DRSP/E2 group was 0.11 mEq/L and 0.08 mEq/L for the placebo group.

Serum potassium levels ≥5.5 mEq/L were observed in 8 (7.3%) DRSP/E2-treated subjects (3 diabetic and 5 nondiabetic) and 3 (2.6%) placebo-treated subjects (2 diabetic and 1 nondiabetic). None of the subjects with serum potassium levels ≥5.5 mEq/L had cardiovascular adverse events. The elevated levels returned to normal even with continuous treatment. The addition of ibuprofen resulted in a slight increase in the number of subjects with potassium values greater than 5.5 mEq/mL. The addition of an NSAID can increase the risk of elevated potassium in both diabetics and nondiabetics receiving ACEI and ARBs. DRSP/E2 administered concomitantly slightly increases the probability of elevated potassium, although the results were not statistically significant.

ACE Inhibitors: A 2-week study in 24 mildly hypertensive postmenopausal women taking enalapril maleate 10 mg twice daily with placebo or DRSP 3 mg/E2 1 mg was performed to assess the effect on serum potassium. Of them, 8 had mild renal insufficiency. Potassium levels were obtained every other day. Mean serum potassium levels in the DRSP/E2 treatment group relative to baseline were 0.22 mEq/L higher that those in the placebo group. Serum potassium concentrations also were measured at multiple timepoints over 24 hours at baseline and on Day 14. The ratios for serum potassium C_{max} and AUC in the DRSP/E2 group to those in the placebo group were 0.955 (90% CI: 0.914, 0.999) and 1.010 (90% CI: 0.944, 1.080), respectively. No patient in either treatment group experienced serum potassium above the upper limit of normal.

Physicians and other health care providers should be aware of other nonprescription products concomitantly used by the patient, including herbal and natural products obtained from the widely spread health stores.

Coadministration with Drugs that Have the Potential to Decrease Serum Potassium: Hydrochlorothiazide: A 4-week study in 36 mildly hypertensive postmenopausal women taking hydrochlorothiazide (HCTZ) 25 mg once daily with placebo or DRSP 3 mg/E2 1 mg was performed to assess potential interactions with HCTZ. The pharmacokinetics of HCTZ was not affected by coadministration with DRSP 3 mg/E2 1 mg. Therefore, no dosage adjustment is required when administering ANGELIQ with HCTZ.

Drug-Food Interactions: The effect of food on the absorption and bioavailability of DRSP and E2 have not been investigated following the administration of ANGELIQ. However, clinical studies with formulations containing DRSP or E2 have shown that the bioavailability of both drugs is not affected by concomitant food intake.

Drug-Herb Interactions: It was found that some herbal products (e.g., St. John's wort) which are available as over-the-counter (OTC) products might interfere with steroid metabolism and therefore alter the efficacy and safety of estrogen/progestin products.

Physicians and other health care providers should be made aware of the other nonprescription products concomitantly used by the patient, including herbal and natural products obtained from the widely spread health stores.

Drug-Laboratory Test Interactions: The results of certain endocrine and liver function tests may be affected by estrogen-containing products:

- increased prothrombin time and partial thromboplastin time; increased levels of fibrinogen and fibrinogen activity; increased coagulation factors VII, VIII, IX, X; increased norepinephrine-induced platelet aggregability; decreased antithrombin III
- increased thyroxine-binding globulin (TBG), leading to increased circulating total thyroid hormone (T_4) as measured by column or radioimmunoassay; free T_3 resin uptake is decreased, reflecting the elevated TBG; free T_4 concentration is unaltered
- other binding proteins may be elevated in serum, i.e., corticosteroid binding globulin (CBG), sex hormone-binding globulin (SHBG), leading to increased circulating corticosteroids and sex steroids, respectively; free or biologically active hormone concentrations are unchanged (see Action and Clinical Pharmacology, Pharmacokinetics).
- impaired glucose tolerance
- reduced serum folate concentration
- increased serum triglyceride and phospholipid concentration

In Study 96097 on endometrial safety, additional metabolic variables were investigated as safety variables in a subgroup of 210 patients. No relevant changes in insulin and glucose levels in the oral glucose tolerance tests performed after one year of treatment with the E2/DRSP combinations were observed. Overall, none of the E2/DRSP combinations impaired glucose tolerance. In addition, a number of coagulation parameters including activated partial thromboplastin time, fibrinogen level, and plasminogen activator inhibitor level were tested. These coagulation parameters generally decreased during treatment with E2 alone, as well as with the combinations of 1 mg E2 with 0.5 to 3 mg DRSP. The decreases of the activated partial thromboplastin time were statistically significant for all E2/DRSP combinations, the decrease in plasminogen activator inhibitor levels was only significant for the combination of 1 mg E2 with 3 mg DRSP, and the decrease in the fibrinogen levels was significant only for E2 alone. This hormone-associated reduction of plasminogen activator inhibitor was observed despite increased levels of triglycerides, which are known to induce the levels of plasminogen activator inhibitor.

The magnitude of the observed changes was small. It should also be noted that a predictive value of these changes for the risk of VTEs is not established.

The results of the above laboratory tests should not be considered reliable unless therapy has been discontinued for two to four weeks. The pathologist should be informed that the patient is receiving estrogen/progestin therapy when relevant specimens are submitted.

DOSAGE AND ADMINISTRATION: Dosing Considerations: ANGELIQ tablets are a combination of estradiol-17β (estrogen) and drospirenone (progestin) intended for continuous administration as hormone replacement therapy. Women who do not take estrogens or women who change from a continuous combination product may start treatment at any time. Patients changing from a sequential combined HRT regimen should be started at the end of the scheduled bleeding.

Recommended Dose and Dosage Adjustment: One tablet is taken daily. Each blister pack is for 28 days of treatment. The tablets are to be swallowed whole with some liquid, irrespective of food intake. There is no need for the patient to count days between cycles because there are no "pill-free days". The tablets should be taken at the same time every day.

Missed Dose: In the case of a missed tablet, it should be taken as soon as possible. If more than 24 hours have elapsed, no extra tablet needs to be taken. If several tablets are forgotten, bleeding may occur. Irregular uterine bleeding may occur, particularly in the first 6 months, but generally decreases with time, and eventually may lead to an amenorrheic state. Patients should be re-evaluated after the first three months of therapy, then at regular (ie, three to six months) intervals or if significant bleeding occurs after three months.

OVERDOSAGE:
Symptoms of Overdose: Numerous reports of ingestion of large doses of estrogen products and estrogen-containing oral contraceptives by young children have not revealed acute serious ill effects. Overdosage with estrogen may cause nausea, breast discomfort, fluid retention, bloating or vaginal bleeding in women.

Progestin (eg, norethindrone acetate) overdosage has been characterized by depressed mood, tiredness, acne, and hirsutism.
Treatment of Overdose: In the event of a possible overdose, the physician should observe the patient closely and symptomatic treatment should be given.

For management of a suspected drug overdose, CPhA recommends that you contact your **regional Poison Control Centre**. See the *CPS* Directory section for a list of Poison Control Centres.

ACTION AND CLINICAL PHARMACOLOGY: Mechanism of Action: ANGELIQ is a continuous dosage regimen of an estrogen-progestin combination for oral administration as hormone replacement therapy (HRT). ANGELIQ contains 17β-estradiol, which is chemically and biologically identical to endogenous human estradiol, and the synthetic progestin, drospirenone. 17β-estradiol provides hormone replacement during and after the climacteric. The addition of drospirenone opposes the development of endometrial hyperplasia thought to be caused by estrogens.

Pharmacodynamics: Clinical Pharmacology of Estrogens: Endogenous estrogens are largely responsible for the development and maintenance of the female reproductive system and secondary sexual characteristics. Although circulating estrogens exist in a dynamic equilibrium of metabolic interconversions, estradiol-17β (E2) is the principal intracellular human estrogen and is substantially more potent than its metabolites, estrone and estriol, at the receptor level.

The primary source of estrogen in normally cycling adult women is the ovarian follicle, which secretes 70 to 500 µg of estradiol daily, depending on the phase of the menstrual cycle. After menopause, most endogenous estrogen is produced by conversion of androstenedione, secreted by the adrenal cortex, to estrone by peripheral tissues. Thus, estrone and the sulphate conjugated form, estrone sulphate, are the most abundant circulating estrogens in postmenopausal women.

Estrogens act through binding to nuclear receptors in estrogen-responsive tissues. To date, two estrogen receptors have been identified. These vary in proportion from tissue to tissue.

Circulating estrogens modulate the pituitary secretion of the gonadotropins, luteinizing hormone (LH), and follicle-stimulating hormone (FSH) through a negative feedback mechanism. Estrogen replacement therapy acts to reduce the elevated levels of these hormones seen in postmenopausal women.

Loss of ovarian estradiol-17β production after menopause can result in instability of thermoregulation, causing hot flushes associated with sleep disturbance and excessive sweating. Estrogen replacement therapy is effective in reducing the number and intensity of hot flushes associated with menopause.

Clinical Pharmacology of Progestins: Drospirenone (DRSP), a spironolactone analogue, is a progestogen with antimineralocorticoid activity. Similar to spironolactone and endogenous progesterone, drospirenone affects the renin-angiotensin-aldosterone system (RAAS) by competitive binding to the aldosterone receptor. As an aldosterone antagonist, drospirenone may retain potassium and cause excess amounts of sodium to be excreted.

In animals, drospirenone has no glucocorticoid or antiglucocorticoid activity. Drospirenone is devoid of estrogenic and androgenic activity but is antiandrogenic in animal and in vitro models.

Drospirenone has no effect on glucose tolerance and insulin resistance. In women, glucose tolerance is not compromised by the use of ANGELIQ.

Progestins exert their effects in target cells by binding to specific progesterone receptors that interact with progesterone response elements in target genes. Progesterone receptors have been identified in the female reproductive tract, breast, pituitary, hypothalamus, and central nervous system. Progestins produce similar endometrial changes to those of the naturally occurring hormone progesterone.

Progestin compounds enhance cellular differentiation and generally oppose the actions of estrogens by decreasing estrogen receptor levels, increasing local metabolism of estrogens to less active metabolites, or inducing gene products that blunt cellular responses to estrogen.

The use of unopposed estrogen therapy has been associated with an increased risk of endometrial hyperplasia, a possible precursor of endometrial adenocarcinoma. The addition of a progestin, in adequate doses and appropriate duration, to an estrogen replacement regimen reduces the incidence of endometrial hyperplasia, and the attendant risk of carcinoma in women with an intact uterus.

Pharmacokinetics: This section makes reference to strengths of DRSP in combination with E2 that are not approved (ie, strengths other than 1 mg DRSP/1 mg E2).

Absorption: DRSP is rapidly and almost completely absorbed following oral administration. Its absolute bioavailability ranges between 76% to 85%. Serum concentrations of DRSP reached peak levels within approximately 1 hour after administration of ANGELIQ. Estradiol is well absorbed through the gastrointestinal tract. Following oral administration of ANGELIQ, peak serum estradiol concentrations are typically reached 6 to 8 hours after dosing. The oral relative bioavailability of estradiol and DRSP following administration of ANGELIQ is 107% and 102%, respectively, when compared to a combination oral microcrystalline suspension.

Figure 1: ANGELIQ

Mean Steady-State Serum Drospirenone Concentrations Following Repeated Daily Oral Administration of 1 mg DRSP/1 mg Estradiol (n=18)

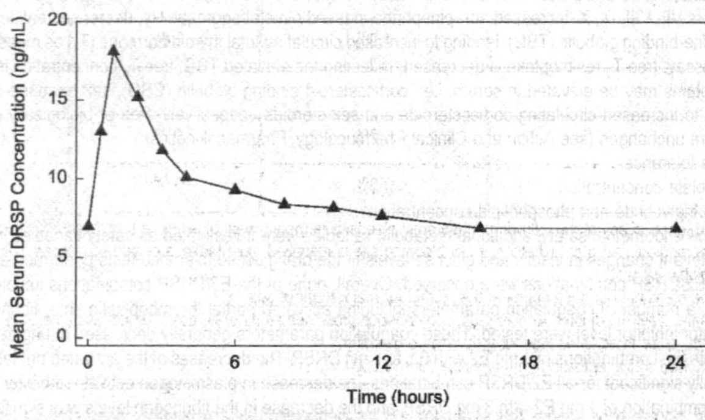

Figure 2: ANGELIQ

Mean Steady-State Serum Estradiol Concentrations Following Repeated Daily Oral Administration of 1 mg DRSP/1 mg Estradiol (n=18)

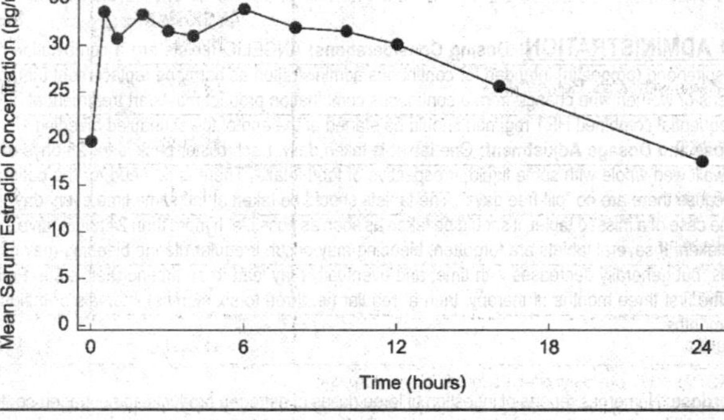

The pharmacokinetics of DRSP are dose proportional within the dose range of 1 to 4 mg. Following daily dosing of ANGELIQ, steady-state DRSP concentrations were observed after 10 days. Mean accumulation ratios for estradiol and DRSP were 1.9 and 2.4, respectively. Mean steady-state serum concentrations are shown in Figure 1 and Figure 2 and a summary of primary pharmacokinetic parameters following the administration of ANGELIQ for 28 days is presented in Table 2.

Table 2: ANGELIQ

Mean Steady-State Pharmacokinetic Parameters of ANGELIQ Tablets (Drospirenone and Estradiol)

Dose	No. of Subjects	C_{max} (ng/mL)	t_{max} (h)	$AUC_{(0-24h)}$ (ng· h/mL)	$t_{½}$ (h)
Drospirenone (Mean[a]±SD)					
1 mg E2/1 mg DRSP	14	18.3±5.55	1.07±0.27	208±83	42.3±21.3
1 mg E2/4 mg DRSP	16	74.2±16.3	1.34±0.89	865±258	35.6±6.30
Estradiol (Mean±SD)					
Dose	**No. of Subjects**	**C_{max} (ng/mL)**	**t_{max} (h)**	**$AUC_{(0-24h)}$ (ng· h/mL)**	**$t_{½}$ (h)**
1 mg E2/1 mg DRSP	14	43.8±10.0	4.8±4.4	665±178	NA
1 mg E2/4 mg DRSP	16	44.6±18.4	3.8±2.6	683±330	NA
Estrone (Mean±SD)					
Dose	**No. of Subjects**	**C_{max} (ng/mL)**	**t_{max} (h)**	**$AUC_{(0-24h)}$ (ng· h/mL)**	**$t_{½}$ (h)**
1 mg E2/1 mg DRSP	14	245±50.6	4.2±1.3	3814±1159	23±6.2
1 mg E2/4 mg DRSP	16	283±143	4.1±1.6	4254±2121	22.4±4.5

[a] Arithmetic mean, NA=not available; C_{max}=maximum serum concentration; AUC=area under the curve; t_{max}=time of maximum serum concentration; $t_{½}$=half-life; SD=standard deviation.

Effect of Food: The effect of food on the absorption and bioavailability of DRSP and E2 have not been investigated following the administration of ANGELIQ. However, clinical studies with formulations containing DRSP or E2 have shown that the bioavailability of both drugs is not affected by concomitant food intake.

Distribution: DRSP does not bind to sex hormone-binding globulin (SHBG) or corticosteroid-binding globulin (CBG) but binds about 97% to serum protein, thought to be albumin. The distribution of exogenous estrogens is similar to that of endogenous estrogens. Estrogens are widely distributed in the body and are generally found in higher concentrations in the sex hormone target organs. Estradiol circulates in the blood bound to SHBG (37%) and to albumin (61%), while only approximately 1% to 2% is unbound.

Metabolism: DRSP is extensively metabolized after oral administration. The two main metabolites of DRSP found in human plasma were identified to be the acid form of DRSP generated by opening of the lactone ring and the 4,5-dihydrodrospirenone-3-sulfate, both of which are formed without the involvement of the cytochrome P450 system. These metabolites were shown not to be pharmacologically active. In in vitro studies with human liver microsomes, DRSP was metabolized only to a minor extent mainly by cytochrome P450 3A4 (CYP3A4).

Exogenous estrogens are metabolized in the same manner as endogenous estrogens. Circulating estrogens exist in a dynamic equilibrium of metabolic interconversions. These transformations take place mainly in the liver. Estradiol is converted reversibly to estrone, and both can be converted to estriol, which is the major urinary metabolite. Estrogens also undergo enterohepatic recirculation via sulphate and glucuronide conjugation in the liver, biliary secretion of conjugates into the intestine, and hydrolysis in the gut followed by reabsorption. In postmenopausal women, a significant proportion of the circulating estrogens exist as sulphate conjugates, especially estrone sulphate, which serves as a circulating reservoir for the formation of more active estrogens.

Excretion: DRSP serum levels are characterized by a terminal elimination half-life of approximately 36 to 42 hours. Excretion of DRSP was nearly complete after ten days and amounts excreted were slightly higher in feces compared to urine. DRSP was extensively metabolized and only trace amounts of unchanged DRSP were excreted in urine and feces. At least 20 different metabolites were observed in urine and feces. About 38% to 47% of the metabolites in urine were glucuronide and sulphate conjugates. In feces, about 17% to 20% of the metabolites were excreted as glucuronides and sulphates. Estradiol, estrone, and estriol are excreted in the urine along with glucuronide and sulphate conjugates.

Special Populations and Conditions: Geriatrics (>65 years of age): ANGELIQ should not be used in geriatric patients (>65 years of age) as there are no studies showing benefits to geriatric patients.

Pediatrics: No pharmacokinetic study for ANGELIQ has been conducted in a pediatric population. ANGELIQ is not indicated in the pediatric population.

Gender: ANGELIQ is indicated for use in women only.

Race: No studies were done to determine the effect of race on the pharmacokinetics of ANGELIQ.

Hepatic Insufficiency: ANGELIQ is contraindicated in patients with active hepatic dysfunction or disease (see Contraindications and Warnings and Precautions).

The safety and the pharmacokinetics of a single dose of DRSP 3 mg/E2 1 mg was evaluated in 10 female patients with moderate hepatic impairment and 10 healthy female subjects matched for age, weight, and smoking history. Small changes (not statistically significant) in serum potassium were observed, although clinical significance cannot be determined. DRSP was rapidly absorbed reaching equal peak serum DRSP for both groups of subjects. However, the total exposure of DRSP in the patients with moderate hepatic impairment was almost doubled compared to that of the normal volunteers due to prolongation of the DRSP half-life.

Renal Insufficiency: ANGELIQ is contraindicated in patients with severe renal insufficiency (see Contraindications and Warnings and Precautions).

The effects of severe renal insufficiency on the pharmacokinetics of DRSP (3 mg daily for 14 days) and the effects of DRSP on serum potassium levels were investigated in female subjects (n=28, age 30-65) with normal (11 patients) renal function and mild (10 patients) and moderate (7 patients) renal impairment. All subjects were on a low potassium diet. During the study, 7 subjects continued the use of potassium-sparing drugs for the treatment of the underlying illness. On the 14th day (steady-state) of DRSP treatment, serum DRSP levels in the group with mild renal impairment (creatinine clearance CLcr, 50-80 mL/min) were comparable to those in the group with normal renal function (CLcr, >80 mL/min). The serum DRSP levels were on average 37% higher in the group with moderate renal impairment (CLcr, 30-50 mL/min) compared to those in the group with normal renal function. DRSP treatment was well tolerated by all groups. DRSP treatment did not show any clinically significant effect on serum potassium concentration. Hyperkalemia was not observed in the study, in five of the seven subjects who continued use of potassium-sparing drugs during the study, individual mean serum potassium levels increased by up to 0.33 mEq/L (to 4.67 mEq/L), which is well within the normal serum potassium range.

STORAGE AND STABILITY: Store in original packaging between 15°C and 30°C. Do not refrigerate or freeze. **Keep out of the reach of children and pets.**

INFORMATION FOR THE PATIENT: Published in e-CPS, available by subscription at www.e-cps.ca.

DOSAGE FORMS, COMPOSITION AND PACKAGING: Each round, biconvex, dark pink, film-coated tablet, embossed on one side with the letters "DU" inside a regular hexagon contains: 1 mg of drospirenone and 1 mg of estradiol. Nonmedicinal ingredients: corn starch, ferric oxide pigment, hydroxypropylmethyl cellulose, lactose monohydrate, macrogol 6000, magnesium stearate, modified starch, povidone 25 000, talc, and titanium dioxide. Blister packs of 28 tablets, cartons of 1.

(Shown in Product Identification Section)

Angiomax® Ⓟ

bivalirudin

Direct Thrombin Inhibitor

Sepracor

Date of Revision: July 29, 2010

SUMMARY PRODUCT INFORMATION:

Route of Administration	Dosage Form/Strength	Nonmedicinal Ingredients
Intravenous injection	250 mg/vial	Mannitol, sodium hydroxide and trifluoroacetate

INDICATIONS AND CLINICAL USE: ANGIOMAX (bivalirudin) is indicated for use as an anticoagulant in patients undergoing percutaneous coronary intervention and in the treatment of patients with moderate to high risk acute coronary syndromes due to unstable angina or non-ST-segment elevation in whom early percutaneous coronary intervention is planned [see also Dosage and Administration, Use Subsequent to Unfractionated Heparin (UFH) or Low Molecular Weight Heparin (LMWH)].

ANGIOMAX is intended for use with acetylsalicylic acid (ASA) and has been studied only in patients receiving concomitant ASA. Clopidogrel can also be administered.

ANGIOMAX is also indicated in patients with or at risk of heparin induced thrombocytopenia or heparin induced thrombocytopenia thrombosis syndrome (HIT/TS) undergoing PCI or cardiac surgery. ANGIOMAX may be administered with or without ASA in patients undergoing cardiac surgery.

The safety and effectiveness of ANGIOMAX have not been established in patients with acute coronary syndromes who are not undergoing PCI.

Pediatrics (<18 years of age): No studies in patients under 18 years of age have been conducted with ANGIOMAX.

CONTRAINDICATIONS: ANGIOMAX (bivalirudin) is contraindicated in patients with:

- Hypersensitivity to this drug or to any ingredient in the formulation or component of the container. For a complete listing, see Dosage Forms, Composition and Packaging.
- Uncontrollable active bleeding
- Major blood clotting disorders
- Acute gastric or duodenal ulcer
- Cerebral hemorrhage
- Severe cerebro-spinal trauma
- Bacterial endocarditis
- Severe uncontrolled hypertension
- Diabetic or hemorrhagic retinopathy
- Proximal use of spinal/epidural anesthesia

WARNINGS AND PRECAUTIONS: General: ANGIOMAX (bivalirudin) should not be administered intramuscularly.

There is no known antidote to ANGIOMAX. ANGIOMAX is hemodialysable (see Action and Clinical Pharmacology, Pharmacokinetics).

Brachytherapy: To date, no formal clinical trials have been conducted with ANGIOMAX as the principal anticoagulant when performing catheter-based brachytherapy (beta or gamma) to reduce the risk of in-stent restenosis. Therefore, ANGIOMAX is not recommended for use in brachytherapy procedures.

An increased risk of thrombus formation has been associated with the use of ANGIOMAX in gamma brachytherapy, including fatal outcomes.

Cardiac Surgery: When ANGIOMAX is used in cardiac surgery, techniques that allow blood or blood-based solutions to lie stagnant should be avoided. Local bivalirudin levels may decrease due to metabolism by proteases from blood exposed to wound or foreign surfaces, potentially leading to local clot formation. During surgery, blood should not be allowed to stand in grafts, and grafts should preferably be stored and tested for flow and leakage with saline, instead of blood. Care should be taken to avoid stasis in the internal mammary artery after harvest. Circulation throughout the cardiopulmonary bypass (CPB) circuit must be ensured with particular attention paid to bypass lines that are blood-filled and then clamped off, or lines that are intermittently used for perfusion.

Hematologic: Hemorrhage: Bleeding may occur in conjunction with use of any anticoagulant drug. As with other anticoagulants, ANGIOMAX should be used with extreme caution in patients at increased risk of hemorrhage. Bleeding can occur at any site during therapy with ANGIOMAX. An unexpected drop in hematocrit or blood pressure should lead to a search for a bleeding site (see Drug Interactions and Adverse Reactions, Bleeding).

Immune: Immunogenicity/Re-exposure: In in vitro studies, ANGIOMAX exhibited no platelet aggregation response against sera from patients with a history of HIT/TS.

Among 494 patients who received ANGIOMAX in clinical trials and were tested for antibodies, two had treatment-emergent positive bivalirudin antibody tests. Neither patient demonstrated clinical evidence of allergic or anaphylactic reactions, and repeat testing was not performed. Nine other patients who had initial positive tests were negative on repeat testing. Of fifteen healthy volunteers who were exposed to ANGIOMAX twice, none developed antibodies.

Special Populations: Pregnant Women: There are no studies available evaluating ANGIOMAX in pregnant women.

Studies in rats and rabbits have demonstrated no evidence of impaired fertility or harm to the fetus attributable to bivalirudin at clinically relevant doses. Because animal reproduction studies are not always predictive of human response, ANGIOMAX should be used during pregnancy only if clearly indicated.

In PCI, ANGIOMAX is intended for use with ASA (see Indications and Clinical Use). Because of possible adverse effects on the neonate and the potential for increased maternal bleeding, particularly during the third trimester, ANGIOMAX and ASA should be used together during pregnancy only with caution and if benefit is thought to outweigh risk.

Nursing Women: It is not known whether ANGIOMAX is excreted in human milk. Because many drugs are excreted in human milk, caution should be exercised when ANGIOMAX is administered to a nursing woman.

Pediatrics (<18 years of age): The safety and efficacy of ANGIOMAX in children have not been established.

Geriatrics (>65 years of age): Across studies approximately 45% of patients were ≥65 years of age and 18% of patients were ≥75 years old. Elderly patients experienced more bleeding events than younger patients.

ADVERSE REACTIONS: Adverse Drug Reaction Overview: As with any antithrombotic treatment, hemorrhagic manifestations can occur. Risk factors for bleeding identified with the use of ANGIOMAX (bivalirudin) include elderly status, female gender, and the concomitant use of drugs known to cause bleeding, such as heparin, warfarin and thrombolytics. These risks are comparable to those seen in heparin-treated patients. Petechiae or easy bruising may precede frank hemorrhage. The early signs of bleeding may include epistaxis, hematuria, or melena. Bleeding may occur at any site and be difficult to detect, for example, retroperitoneal bleeding. Bleeding may also occur at surgical sites. Major hemorrhage, including retroperitoneal or intracranial bleeding, has been associated with ANGIOMAX use, in some cases leading to a fatal outcome.

ACUITY (UA/NSTEMI): The type and severity of adverse events observed in the ACS trials were similar between the ANGIOMAX and other treatment groups, and were typical of ACS trials. Few patients discontinued due to an adverse event, and the overall incidence and types of events that led to discontinuation were balanced between treatment groups. Very few of these events were associated with bleeding.

REPLACE-2 (PCI): Adverse events observed in clinical trials are similar between the ANGIOMAX-treated patients and the control groups. Adverse events seen are those typical of PCI trials. In clinical trials, adverse events leading to discontinuation occurred in 2% of ANGIOMAX patients and 7% of heparin patients.

CHOOSE and EVOLUTION (Cardiac Surgery): Pleural effusion, atelectasis and atrial fibrillation were the most frequent adverse events observed in the clinical trials in both the bivalirudin group and the control group; these events are common following cardiac surgery.

Clinical Trial Adverse Drug Reactions: Because clinical trials are conducted under very specific conditions the adverse reaction rates observed in the clinical trials may not reflect the rates observed in practice and should not be compared to the rates in the clinical trials of another drug. Adverse drug reaction information from clinical trials is useful for identifying drug-related adverse events and for approximating rates.

Bleeding: ACUITY (UA/NSTEMI): In 13 819 patients with ACS treated in the ACUITY trial, patients administered ANGIOMAX monotherapy exhibited statistically significantly lower rates of bleeding, and transfusions when compared to those patients who received heparin+GPI. There was no statistical difference in bleeding rates when ANGIOMAX+GPI was compared to heparin+GPI (Table 1).

Table 1: ANGIOMAX

Bleeding Rates ACUITY Study

	ANGIOMAX[a] Alone (N=4612)	ANGIOMAX + GPI (N=4606)	Heparin[e] + GPI[e] (UFH or Enoxaparin) (N=4603)
ACUITY-defined Bleeding			
Major[b]	3.0%	5.3%	5.7%
Minor[c]	12.9%	21.8%	21.6%
TIMI-defined Bleeding[d]			
Major	0.9%	1.6%	1.9%
Minor	3.7%	6.1%	6.4%
Transfusions	1.6%	2.6%	2.7%

[a] GPIs were administered to <7% of patients in the ANGIOMAX group for procedural complications.

[b] Defined as the occurrence of any of the following: intracranial bleeding, retroperitoneal bleeding, intraocular bleeding, a transfusion of any units of blood/blood products, a fall in haemoglobin (Hgb) ≥4 g/dL, whether or not bleeding site is identified, spontaneous or non-spontaneous blood loss with a decrease in Hgb ≥3 g/dL, reoperation for bleeding, access site bleeding requiring surgical or radiological intervention, or a hematoma ≥5 cm at puncture site.

[c] Defined as observed bleeding that does not meet the criteria for major bleeding.

[d] Thrombolysis in Myocardial Infarction (TIMI) major bleeding is defined as: intracranial, or a fall in adjusted Hgb >5 g/dL or hematocrit (Hct) of >15%; TIMI minor bleeding is defined as a fall in adjusted Hgb of 3 to <5 g/dL or a fall in adjusted Hct of 9 to <15%, with a bleeding site such as hematuria, hematemesis, hematomas, retroperitoneal bleeding or a decrease in Hgb of >4 g/dL with no bleeding site.

[e] Heparin was either unfractioned heparin (UFH) or enoxaparin.

REPLACE-2 (PCI) and BAT (PTCA): In 6010 patients undergoing PCI treatment in a double-blind trial, ANGIOMAX patients plus provisional GPI (7.2%) exhibited statistically significant lower rates of bleeding, transfusions, and thrombocytopenia than patients receiving heparin plus a glycoprotein IIb/IIIa (GPIIb/IIIa) inhibitor, as noted in Table 2. Major bleeding was seen in 2.4% of patients treated with ANGIOMAX+GPI compared to 4.1% in the patients treated with heparin+GPI.

Table 2: ANGIOMAX

Major Hematologic Outcomes REPLACE-2 Study (Safety Population)

	ANGIOMAX N=2914	Heparin+GPIIb/IIIa N=2987	P Value
% Patients with Major Hemorrhage[a]	2.3%	4.0%	<0.001
Non-Access Site Bleeding			
Retroperitoneal Bleeding	0.2%	0.5%	0.069
Intracranial Bleeding	<0.1%	0.1%	1
Required Transfusion (any)	1.5%	2.5%	0.009
Access Site Bleeding			
Sheath Site Bleeding	0.9%	2.4%	<0.001
% Patients with Minor Hemorrhage[b]	13.6%	25.8%	<0.001
TIMI-Definition Bleeding[c]			
Major and Minor	1.9%	3.8%	<0.001
Thrombocytopenia[d]			
<100 000 mm³	0.7%	1.7%	<0.001
<50 000 mm³	0.3%	0.6%	0.039

[a] Defined as the occurrence of any of the following: intracranial bleeding, retroperitoneal bleeding, a transfusion ≥2 units of blood/blood products, a fall in hemoglobin >4 g/dL, whether or not bleeding site is identified, spontaneous or non-spontaneous blood loss with a decrease in hemoglobin ≥3 g/dL.

[b] Defined as observed bleeding that does not meet the criteria for major hemorrhage.

[c] Defined as: intracranial, a fall in adjusted Hgb >5 g/dL, spontaneous gross hematuria or hematemesis, bleeding associated with a fall in adjusted Hgb >3 g/dL, a fall in adjusted Hgb >4 g/dL with no bleeding.

[d] If platelets <100 000 **and** >25% reduction from baseline, or <50 000.

In two randomised, double-blind studies that evaluated 4312 patients with unstable angina undergoing percutaneous transluminal coronary angioplasty (PTCA), ANGIOMAX patients exhibited lower rates of major bleeding and lower requirements for blood transfusions than patients treated with heparin (Table 3). It should be noted that the comparator dose of heparin used in these studies was 175 IU/kg, a dose significantly higher than generally used currently.

Table 3: ANGIOMAX

Major Bleeding and Transfusions in BAT Trial: All Patients[a] During Hospitalization Period

	ANGIOMAX N=2161	Heparin N=2151
Number (%) of Patients with Major Hemorrhage[b]	79 (3.7)	199 (9.3)
-with ≥3g/dL fall in Hgb	41 (1.9)	124 (5.8)
-with ≥5g/dL fall in Hgb	14 (<1)	47 (2.2)
-Retroperitoneal Bleeding	5 (<1)	15 (<1)
-Intracranial Bleeding	1 (<1)	2 (<1)
-Required Transfusion	43 (2.0)	123 (5.7)

[a] No monitoring of ACT (or PTT) was done after a target ACT was achieved.

[b] Major hemorrhage was defined as the occurrence of any of the following: intracranial bleeding, retroperitoneal bleeding, clinically overt bleeding with a decrease in hemoglobin ≥3 g/dL or leading to a transfusion of ≥2 units of blood. This table includes data from entire hospital period.

Table 4: ANGIOMAX

Summary of Bleeding Related Safety Data at Day 7/Discharge in the CHOOSE Studies and in Pooled On- and Off-pump Studies in Cardiac Surgery (Safety Population)

	CHOOSE Studies (HIT/TS)[a]				Pooled Studies (HIT/TS and Non-HIT/TS)[a]			
	On-pump		Off-pump		On-pump		Off-pump	
Parameter	Angiomax N=49 n (%)	Historical control N=75 n (%)	Angiomax N=51 n (%)	Historical control N=36 n (%)	Angiomax N=147 n (%)	Heparin/ protamine N=121 n (%)	Angiomax N=152 n (%)	Heparin/ protamine N=88 n (%)
Incidence of transfusions	41 (83.7)	69 (92.0)	27 (52.9)	32 (88.9)	98 (66.7)	94 (77.7)	73 (48.0)	61 (69.3)
Patients with major bleeding events	2 (4.1)	6 (8.0)	2 (3.9)	3 (8.3)	8 (5.4)	6 (5.0)	11 (7.2)	5 (5.7)
Patients with persistent hemorrhage requiring repeat operation	2 (4.1)	4 (5.3)	2 (3.9)	3 (8.3)	8 (5.4)	5 (4.1)	10 (6.6)	5 (5.7)
Median total postoperative blood loss (mL) up to 24 hours	N=47 880.0	N=62 797.5	N=51 780.0	N=35 990.0	N=143 815.0	N=106 750.0	N=131 713.0	N=75 750.0

[a] 10 historical patients from the CHOOSE studies were administered an anticoagulant other than heparin/protamine and are excluded from this analysis.

CHOOSE and EVOLUTION (Cardiac Surgery): In the CHOOSE and EVOLUTION studies the incidence of blood product transfusions was lower in the bivalirudin treatment group (Table 4). The incidence of major bleeding and median total postoperative blood loss volumes were similar.

Other Adverse Reactions: ACUITY (UA/NSTEMI): In 13 819 patients with UA/NSTEMI in the ACUITY study, those treated with ANGIOMAX had similar rates of non-bleeding adverse events compared to the patients who received heparin plus GPI. No individual adverse reaction occurred with a frequency higher than 0.1% in the ANGIOMAX population.

REPLACE-2 (PCI) and BAT (PTCA): In the REPLACE-2 trial similar non-bleeding adverse events were reported in the two treatment groups as shown below in Table 5.

Table 5: ANGIOMAX

Adverse Events Other than Bleeding Occurring in ≥2% of Patients in Either Treatment Group in REPLACE-2

	Treatment Group	
	ANGIOMAX (n=2914)	Heparin+GP IIb/IIIa (n=2987)
Event	Number of Patients (%)	
Cardiovascular		
Hypotension	91 (3.1)	120 (4.0)
Angina Pectoris	155 (5.3)	156 (5.2)
Gastrointestinal		
Nausea	86 (3.0)	96 (3.2)
Miscellaneous		
Back pain	268 (9.2)	263 (8.8)
Pain	98 (3.4)	72 (2.4)
Chest Pain	68 (2.3)	69 (2.3)
Headache	75 (2.6)	83 (2.8)
Injection site pain	80 (2.7)	80 (2.7)

All adverse events other than bleeding reported for ≥5% of patients in either treatment group in the BAT trial are shown below in Table 6.

Table 6: ANGIOMAX

Adverse Events Other than Bleeding Occurring in ≥5% of Patients in Either Treatment Group in BAT Trial

	Treatment Group	
	ANGIOMAX (n=2161)	Heparin (n=2151)
Event	Number of Patients (%)	
Cardiovascular		
Hypotension	262 (12)	371 (17)
Hypertension	135 (6)	115 (5)
Bradycardia	118 (5)	164 (8)
Gastrointestinal		
Nausea	318 (15)	347 (16)
Vomiting	138 (6)	169 (8)
Dyspepsia	100 (5)	111 (5)
Genitourinary		
Urinary retention	89 (4)	98 (5)

(cont'd)

Table 6: ANGIOMAX *(cont'd)*

Adverse Events Other than Bleeding Occurring in ≥5% of Patients in Either Treatment Group in BAT Trial

	Treatment Group	
	ANGIOMAX (n=2161)	Heparin (n=2151)
Event	Number of Patients (%)	
Miscellaneous		
Back pain	916 (42)	944 (44)
Pain	330 (15)	358 (17)
Headache	264 (12)	225 (10)
Injection site pain	174 (8)	274 (13)
Insomnia	142 (7)	139 (6)
Pelvic pain	130 (6)	169 (8)
Anxiety	127 (6)	140 (7)
Abdominal pain	103 (5)	104 (5)
Fever	103 (5)	108 (5)
Nervousness	102 (5)	87 (4)

CHOOSE and EVOLUTION (Cardiac Surgery): All adverse events other than bleeding reported for ≥5% of patients in either treatment group are shown below in Table 7. Adverse events were not collected for the historical cohort in the CHOOSE studies. Prolongations of activated partial thromboplastin time (aPTT) and prothrombin time (PT) were reported more frequently in the bivalirudin group. This is expected with ANGIOMAX due to absence of a reversal agent, and was reported as an adverse event by a single site. All other differences in adverse event rates that were statistically significant occurred in the heparin/protamine group.

Table 7: ANGIOMAX

Adverse Events Other Than Bleeding Occurring in ≥5% of Patients in Either Treatment Group in the Pooled Cardiac Surgery Studies

Adverse Event	Bivalirudin N=379	Heparin/protamine[a] N=158
Number of patients with any common adverse event	256 (67.5)	115 (72.8)
Pleural effusion	94 (24.8)	55 (34.8)
Atrial fibrillation	59 (15.6)	28 (17.7)
Atelectasis	49 (12.9)	37 (23.4)
Nausea	44 (11.6)	29 (18.4)
Anaemia NOS	41 (10.8)	15 (9.5)
Hypotension NOS	34 (9.0)	12 (7.6)
Activated partial thromboplastin time	26 (6.9)	0 (0.0)
Pain NOS	26 (6.9)	23 (14.6)
Oedema peripheral	26 (6.9)	12 (7.6)
Prothrombin time prolonged	24 (6.3)	0 (0.0)
Pericardial effusion	23 (6.1)	12 (7.6)
Constipation	21 (5.5)	13 (8.2)
Wound secretion	20 (5.3)	19 (12.0)

(cont'd)

Table 7: ANGIOMAX *(cont'd)*

Adverse Events Other Than Bleeding Occurring in ≥5% of Patients in Either Treatment Group in the Pooled Cardiac Surgery Studies

Adverse Event	Bivalirudin N=379	Heparin/protamine[a] N=158
Oliguria	20 (5.3)	12 (7.6)
Vomiting NOS	18 (4.7)	13 (8.2)
Anxiety	15 (4.0)	14 (8.9)
Hypertension NOS	13 (3.4)	8 (5.1)
Chest pain	12 (3.2)	10 (6.3)

[a] Does not include data from the historical cohort of the CHOOSE studies.

Less Common Clinical Trial Adverse Drug Reactions: Rarely, the following have been reported with ANGIOMAX use, without attribution to cause: thrombocytopenia, urticaria, rash.

Post-Market Adverse Drug Reactions: The following events have been reported: fatal bleeding; hypersensitivity and allergic reactions including very rare reports of anaphylaxis; thrombus formation during PCI with and without intracoronary brachytherapy, including reports of fatal outcomes.

DRUG INTERACTIONS: Overview: In clinical trials in patients undergoing PCI, coadministration of ANGIOMAX (bivalirudin) with heparin, warfarin or thrombolytics was associated with increased risk of major bleeding events compared to patients not receiving these concomitant medications.

The safety and effectiveness of ANGIOMAX have not been formally established when used in conjunction with GPIIb/IIIa inhibitors. In two clinical trials, however, it was noted that the apparent bleeding advantage of ANGIOMAX over heparin plus planned GPIIb/IIIa inhibitor (Table 1 and Table 2; see also Adverse Reactions, Bleeding) was practically nullified when a GPIIb/IIIa inhibitor was added to ANGIOMAX therapy.

No formal drug interaction studies have been carried out with bivalirudin. Clinical studies evaluating pharmacodynamic effects and providing preliminary safety information of various products when used in combination with ANGIOMAX have been carried out, including the adenosine diphosphate antagonist, ticlopidine, and the GPIIb/IIIa inhibitors, abciximab, tirofiban and eptifibatide. Although data are limited, precluding conclusions regarding efficacy and safety in combination with these agents, the results do not suggest interaction between ANGIOMAX and the individual drugs studied in respect of their pharmacodynamic activities. These results are not sufficient to conclude definitively that no interaction exists.

DOSAGE AND ADMINISTRATION: Dosing Considerations:

- ANGIOMAX should be administered with ASA. Clopidogrel can also be administered.
- Patients can be started with ANGIOMAX 30 minutes after discontinuation of UFH given intravenously, or 8 hours after discontinuation of LMWH given subcutaneously.

UA/NSTEMI: In patients presenting with unstable angina (UA)/non-ST-segment elevation myocardial infarction (NSTEMI), the recommended dose of ANGIOMAX is an initial intravenous bolus of 0.1 mg/kg bivalirudin followed by an infusion of 0.25 mg/kg/h prior to angiography and continued through angiography and as long as needed. The dose should be administered before assignment to a procedure (PCI, CABG, or drug therapy management).

Patients who are to be medically managed may continue the infusion of 0.25 mg/kg/h for up to 72 hours. No dosage adjustment is needed for these patients.

If the patient proceeds to PCI, an additional bolus of 0.5 mg/kg should be administered and the infusion increased to 1.75 mg/kg/h for the duration of the procedure. Following PCI, the reduced infusion dose of 0.25 mg/kg/h may be resumed for 4 to 12 hours as clinically necessary.

For patients who proceed to CABG surgery off-pump, the i.v. infusion of ANGIOMAX should be continued until the time of surgery. Just prior to surgery, a 0.5 mg/kg bolus dose should be administered followed by a 1.75 mg/kg/h infusion for the duration of the surgery.

For patients who proceed to CABG surgery on-pump, the i.v. infusion of ANGIOMAX should be continued until 1 hour prior to surgery after which the infusion should be discontinued and the patient treated with unfractionated heparin.

PCI: The recommended dosage of ANGIOMAX is an i.v. bolus of 0.75 mg/kg. This should be followed by an infusion of 1.75 mg/kg/hr for the duration of the PCI procedure (see also Table 8). Five (5) minutes after the bolus dose has been administered, an ACT should be performed and an additional bolus of 0.3 mg/kg should be given if needed. GPI administration should be considered in the event that any of the conditions listed in "CLINICAL TRIALS Replace-2" is present.

Continuation of the infusion following PCI for up to 4 hours post-procedure is optional, at the discretion of the treating physician. After 4 hours, an additional IV infusion of ANGIOMAX may be initiated at a rate of 0.2 mg/kg/h for up to 20 hours, if needed. ANGIOMAX is intended for use with aspirin (300-325 mg daily) and has only been studied in patients receiving concomitant aspirin.

Cardiac Surgery (see also Table 8): On-pump Cardiac Surgery: The recommended dosage of ANGIOMAX is an i.v. bolus of 1 mg/kg immediately followed by a 2.5 mg/kg/hr i.v. infusion. ANGIOMAX infusion may be terminated approximately 15 minutes prior to the anticipated end of cardiopulmonary bypass (CPB). The ACT may be used to check that the patient is anticoagulated following administration of ANGIOMAX. Infusion dose adjustment should not be necessary. For patients in whom hemofiltration is required during bypass, periodic ACT monitoring may be used (see Dosing Pre- and Post-cardiac Surgery, Medical Management Guidelines for Cardiac Surgery). If CPB is not terminated within 20 minutes or in patients who need to go back on bypass, a bivalirudin i.v. bolus of 0.5 mg/kg should be administered and a 2.5 mg/kg/hr i.v. infusion restarted and continued until 15 minutes prior to the anticipated end of CPB (see Dosage and Administration, Dosing Pre- and Post-cardiac Surgery, Medical Management Guidelines for Cardiac Surgery for dosing of the CPB pump with ANGIOMAX).

Off-pump Cardiac Surgery: The recommended dosage of ANGIOMAX is an i.v. bolus of 0.75 mg/kg immediately followed by a 1.75 mg/kg/hr i.v. infusion for the duration of the procedure. The ACT may be used to check that the patient is anticoagulated following administration of ANGIOMAX. In clinical trials, investigators had the option to administer additional boluses of 0.1-0.5 mg/kg or make adjustments to the infusion rate in 0.25 mg/kg/hr increments if a higher level of anticoagulation was desired. The data suggest that infusion dose adjustments should not be necessary.

For patients who may need to go on-pump, an additional ANGIOMAX i.v. bolus dose of 0.25 mg/kg should be administered to the systemic circulation and the infusion rate should be increased to 2.5 mg/kg/hr. In addition, see Dosing Pre- and Post-cardiac Surgery, Medical Management Guidelines for Cardiac Surgery for dosing of the pump.

Dosing Pre- and Post-cardiac Surgery: ANGIOMAX may be used for anticoagulation up to 48 hours prior to surgery or in the postoperative phase up to 14 days after the procedure. An ANGIOMAX i.v. bolus of 0.1 mg/kg followed by an i.v. infusion of 0.2 mg/kg/hr may be administered, with aPTT monitoring to attain the clinically desired range of 1.5-2.5 times the baseline value.

Medical Management Guidelines for Cardiac Surgery: CPB: Use of ANGIOMAX for anticoagulation during CPB requires little modification to the conventional bypass circuit setup. Before initiation of CPB, a bolus dose of 50 mg ANGIOMAX should be added to the circuit regardless of patient weight or volume of the prime. Either an open system or a closed system may be used for venous drainage. A closed system with venous reservoir bags generally has better flow characteristics with more internal mixing than a hardshell open venous reservoir. After completion of CPB, once it is clear that return to bypass support will not be needed, processing of the remaining circuit volume with a cell saver prior to a readministration to the patient is recommended. Provision to allow recirculation of the circuit following termination from CPB may be provided by administration of 50 mg of ANGIOMAX to the circuit followed by a continuous infusion of 50 mg/hr.

Cardioplegia: Crystalloid or blood-based cardioplegia may be used. If blood-based cardioplegia is used, blood should be obtained directly from the circuit and, after mixing with cardioplegia solution, should be immediately infused into the coronary system. If there are non-circulating portions of line between the pump and the patient, these lines should be flushed prior to cardioplegia administration. The cardioplegia setup can be circulated continuously by use of a connector. The volume of the cardioplegia circuit is typically 250 mL; for this volume, a continuous infusion of ANGIOMAX of 6.25 mg/hr will maintain anticoagulation within the circuit.

Hemofiltration: It is recommended that the ACT be measured frequently during hemofiltration to ensure the adequacy of anticoagulation.

Cell Saver: If a cell saver is used, an anticoagulant is necessary. A citrate-based solution (citrate phosphate dextrose [CPD], acid citrate dextrose [ACD], sodium citrate) is recommended.

Dosage Adjustment for Patients with Renal Impairment: No reduction in the bolus dose of ANGIOMAX is needed regardless of the patient's baseline renal function.

No infusion dose adjustment is required for patients with mild or moderate renal impairment undergoing either PCI or cardiac surgery. In PCI patients, reduction of the infusion rate to 1 mg/kg/hr should be considered if the creatinine clearance is less than 30 mL/min. If a PCI patient is dependent on hemodialysis, the infusion rate should be reduced to 0.25 mg/kg/hr. Patients with creatinine clearance below 30 mL/min have not been studied in cardiac surgery. See "Action and Clinical Pharmacology, Pharmacokinetics" for details regarding bivalirudin pharmacokinetics in patients with renal impairment.

In patients with renal impairment, the ACT should be monitored with any dose alterations. ACT should be checked at 5 and 45 minutes. If the ACT is ≤250 seconds for renally-impaired patients, administer a second bolus (0.3 mg/kg) and double the infusion rate to maintain the ACT at approximately 350 seconds. If the ACT is 250-300 seconds in renally-impaired patients, re-bolus (0.3 mg/kg) to maintain the ACT approximately 350 seconds. ANGIOMAX is hemodialysable (see Action And Clinical Pharmacology, Pharmacokinetics).

Use Subsequent to Unfractionated Heparin (UFH) or Low Molecular Weight Heparin (LMWH): Patients can be started with ANGIOMAX 30 minutes after discontinuation of UFH given intravenously, or 8 hours after discontinuation of LMWH given subcutaneously.

Administration: ANGIOMAX is intended for i.v. injection and infusion after dilution (see Reconstitution). The dose to be administered is adjusted according to the patient's weight (see Table 8).

Table 8: ANGIOMAX

ANGIOMAX Weight Based Dosing Table for Patients Undergoing PCI or Cardiac Surgery[a]

	Using 5 mg/mL Concentration				Using 0.5 mg/mL Concentration
	PCI and Off-Pump Cardiac Surgery		On-Pump Cardiac Surgery		
Weight (kg)	Bolus (0.75 mg/kg) (mL)	Infusion (1.75 mg/kg/hr) (mL/hr)	Bolus (1 mg/kg) (mL)	Infusion (2.5 mg/kg/hr) (mL/hr)	Subsequent Low-Rate Infusion (0.2 mg/kg/hr) (mL/hr)
43–47	7	16	9	23	18
48–52	7.5	17.5	10	25	20
53–57	8	19	11	28	22
58–62	9	21	12	30	24
63–67	10	23	13	33	26
68–72	10.5	24.5	14	35	28
73–77	11	26	15	38	30
78–82	12	28	16	40	32
83–87	13	30	17	43	34
88–92	13.5	31.5	18	45	36
93–97	14	33	19	48	38
98–102	15	35	20	50	40
103–107	16	37	21	53	42
108–112	16.5	38.5	22	55	44
113–117	17	40	23	58	46
118–122	18	42	24	60	48
123–127	19	44	25	63	50
128–132	19.5	45.5	26	65	52
133–137	20	47	27	68	54
138–142	21	49	28	70	56
143–147	22	51	29	73	58
148–152	22.5	52.5	30	75	60

[a] If patients have undergone treatment with ANGIOMAX for ACS prior to PCI and/or CABG, see above for dosing recommendations.

ANGIOMAX should be administered via an intravenous line. No incompatibilities have been observed with glass bottles or polyvinyl chloride bags and administration sets. The following nine drugs should **not** be administered in the same intravenous line with ANGIOMAX, since they resulted in haze formation, microparticulate formation, or gross precipitation when mixed with ANGIOMAX: alteplase, amiodarone HCl, amphotericin B, chlorpromazine HCl, diazepam, prochlorperazine edisylate, reteplase, streptokinase, and vancomycin HCl.

The following six drugs show dose-concentration physical incompatibilities with bivalirudin (i.e. gross precipitation, turbidity changes visible in normal diffuse room light with the unaided eye, increases in measured turbidity, and microprecipitation) during Y-site coadministration at room temperature (23°C): dobutamine HCl, famotidine, haloperidol lactate, labetalol HCl, lorazepam, promethazine HCl. Therefore, the administration of these medicinal products in the same intravenous line as bivalirudin is not recommended.

As with all parenteral drug products, i.v. mixtures should be inspected visually for clarity, particulate matter, precipitate, discolouration and leakage prior to administration whenever solution and container permit. Solutions showing haziness, particulate matter, precipitate, discolouration or leakage should not be used. Discard unused portion.

Reconstitution: ANGIOMAX is to be reconstituted with Water for Injection, USP as summarized below.

Vial Size	Volume of Diluent to be Added to Vial	Approximate Available Volume	Nominal Concentration per mL
250 mg	5 mL	5.5 mL	50 mg/mL

To each 250 mg vial add 5 mL of Sterile Water for Injection, USP. Gently swirl until all material is dissolved. Each reconstituted vial should be further diluted in 50 mL of 5% Dextrose in Water or 0.9% Sodium Chloride for Injection to yield a final concentration of 5 mg/mL (e.g., 1 vial in 50 mL; 2 vials in 100 mL; 5 vials in 250 mL). The dose to be administered is adjusted according to the patient's weight, see Table 8.

If the low-rate infusion is to be used after the initial infusion, a lower concentration bag should be prepared. In order to prepare this bag, reconstitute the 250 mg vial with 5 mL of Sterile Water for Injection, USP. Gently swirl until all material is dissolved. Each reconstituted vial should be further diluted in 500 mL of 5% Dextrose in Water or 0.9% Sodium Chloride for Injection to yield a final concentration of 0.5 mg/mL. The infusion rate to be administered should be selected from the right-hand column in Table 8.

Do not freeze reconstituted or diluted ANGIOMAX. Reconstituted material may be stored at 2-8°C for up to 24 hours. Diluted ANGIOMAX with a concentration of between 0.5 mg/mL and 5 mg/mL is stable at room temperature for up to 24 hours.

OVERDOSAGE:
Bleeding has been reported in some cases of overdose with single bolus doses of ANGIOMAX (bivalirudin) up to 7.5 mg/kg. Discontinuation of ANGIOMAX leads to a gradual reduction in anticoagulant effects due to metabolism of the drug. There has been no experience of overdosage in human clinical trials. In case of overdosage, ANGIOMAX should be discontinued and the patient should be closely monitored for signs of bleeding. Supportive therapy should be instituted, as necessary. There is no known antidote to ANGIOMAX. ANGIOMAX is hemodialysable (see Action and Clinical Pharmacology, Pharmacokinetics).

> For management of a suspected drug overdose, contact your regional Poison Control Centre. See the *CPS* Directory section for a list of Poison Control Centres.

ACTION AND CLINICAL PHARMACOLOGY: Mechanism of Action: ANGIOMAX (bivalirudin) is a specific and reversible direct thrombin inhibitor. The active substance is a synthetic peptide composed of twenty amino acids. ANGIOMAX directly inhibits thrombin by specifically binding both to the catalytic site and to the anion-binding exosite of circulating and clot-bound thrombin. Thrombin is a serine proteinase that plays a central role in the thrombotic process, acting to cleave fibrinogen into fibrin monomers and to activate Factor XIII to Factor XIIIa, which allows fibrin to develop a covalently cross-linked framework, thus stabilising formed thrombus. Thrombin also activates Factors V and VIII, promoting further thrombin generation; and activates platelets, stimulating aggregation and granule release. The binding of ANGIOMAX to thrombin is reversible as thrombin slowly cleaves the bivalirudin-Arg_3-Pro_4 bond, resulting in recovery of thrombin active site functions.

In in vitro studies, bivalirudin inhibited both soluble (free) and clot-bound thrombin, and was not neutralized by products of the platelet release reaction. The clinical relevance of these findings is unknown. It also prolonged the aPTT, thrombin time (TT), and PT of normal human plasma in a concentration-dependent manner.

Pharmacodynamics: In healthy volunteers and patients undergoing routine angioplasty, bivalirudin exhibits linear dose-dependent and concentration-dependent anticoagulant activity as evidenced by prolongation of the ACT, aPTT, PT, and TT. Intravenous administration of ANGIOMAX produces a prompt anticoagulant effect. Coagulation times return to the normal range approximately 1-2 hours following cessation of ANGIOMAX administration in patients with normal renal function.

In 291 patients undergoing routine angioplasty, a positive correlation was observed between the dose of ANGIOMAX and the proportion of patients achieving ACT values of 300 or 350 seconds. In the subset of patients receiving ANGIOMAX at a dose of 1 mg/kg i.v. bolus plus 2.5 mg/kg/hr i.v. infusion for 4 hours, then followed by 0.2 mg/kg/hr, all patients reached maximal ACT values >300 seconds.

The correlation of various clotting tests with bivalirudin plasma concentration was studied in patients undergoing cardiac surgery. The data confirmed that, as during PCI, the activated clotting times were prolonged in a concentration-dependent manner during cardiac surgery.

Pharmacokinetics: Absorption: Bivalirudin exhibits linear pharmacokinetics following i.v. administration to patients undergoing PTCA. In these patients, a mean steady state bivalirudin concentration of 12.3±1.7 μg/mL is achieved after administration of an i.v. bolus of 1 mg/kg followed by a 2.5 mg/kg/hr i.v. infusion given for 4 hours.

Distribution: Bivalirudin does not bind to plasma proteins other than thrombin, or to red blood cells.

Excretion: Bivalirudin is cleared from plasma by a combination of renal mechanisms and proteolytic cleavage, with a half-life in patients with normal renal function of about 25 minutes. Bivalirudin is hemodialysable, with approximately 25% cleared by hemodialysis.

Special Populations and Conditions: Renal Insufficiency: The disposition of bivalirudin was also studied in PTCA patients with mild and moderate renal impairment and in patients with severe renal impairment. Drug elimination was related to glomerular filtration rate (GFR), see Table 9.

Table 9: ANGIOMAX

Pharmacokinetics in Patients with Renal Impairment[a]

Renal Function (GFR, mL/min)	Clearance (mL/min/kg)	Half-life (minutes)
Normal renal function (≥90 mL/min)	3.4	25
Mild renal impairment (60-89 mL/min)	3.4	22
Moderate renal impairment (30-59 mL/min)	2.7	34
Severe renal impairment (10–29 mL/min)	2.8	57
Dialysis-dependent patients (off dialysis)	1.0	3.5 hours

[a] The ACT should be monitored in renally-impaired patients.

For patients with renal impairment, the ACT should be monitored. In patients with renal impairment, the initial bolus dose should not be adjusted, however a reduction of the infusion dose to be administered may be required (see Dosage and Administration, Dosage Adjustment for Patients with Renal Impairment).

Cardiac Surgery: In a population of patients undergoing cardiac surgery utilizing CPB with normal renal function or mild/moderate renal dysfunction at baseline, the mean plasma bivalirudin concentration 5 minutes after administration of an i.v. bolus dose of 1 mg/kg followed by a 2.5 mg/kg/hr i.v. infusion was 13.3±2.4 μg/mL. Bivalirudin levels were maintained at or above this concentration for the duration of infusion. Bivalirudin was eliminated with a clearance of 198 mL/min (2.34 mL/min/kg). Following termination of infusion, plasma bivalirudin concentrations declined biexponentially with an initial half-life of 27 minutes and a terminal half-life of 77 minutes. Temperature had no detectable effect on bivalirudin clearance. The clearance of bivalirudin was reduced by 20-30% in patients with mild or moderate renal impairment. The pharmacokinetics of bivalirudin in off-pump cardiac surgery patients was similar to that in on-pump surgery patients.

STORAGE AND STABILITY: ANGIOMAX dosage units are to be shipped and stored at controlled room temperature (15-25°C). Do not freeze. Discard any unused portion of reconstituted solution remaining in the vial.

Do not freeze reconstituted or diluted ANGIOMAX. Reconstituted material may be stored at 2-8°C for up to 24 hours. Diluted ANGIOMAX with a concentration of between 0.5 mg/mL and 5 mg/mL is stable at room temperature for up to 24 hours.

INFORMATION FOR THE PATIENT: Published in e-CPS, available by subscription at www.e-cps.ca.

DOSAGE FORMS, COMPOSITION AND PACKAGING: Each vial of sterile, lyophilized product contains: bivalirudin 250 mg. Single-use glass vials. Reconstitution of ANGIOMAX with 5 mL Water for Injection, USP yields a solution of pH 5.0-6.0 with the following composition: bivalirudin, 50 mg/mL; mannitol, 25 mg/mL; bound trifluoroacetate, 4-6 mg/mL; and sodium hydroxide to adjust pH to 5.0-6.0. Reconstituted material will be a clear to slightly opalescent, colourless to slightly yellow solution. Discard any unused portion of reconstituted solution remaining in the vial.

Anodan™-HC Pr
hydrocortisone acetate—zinc sulfate monohydrate
Anorectal Therapy

Odan

SUPPLIED: Ointment: Each g contains: hydrocortisone acetate 0.5% and zinc sulfate monohydrate 0.5% in a petrolatum ointment base. Nonmedicinal ingredients: Germaben II and petrolatum. Tubes of 15 and 30 g with rectal applicator.

Suppositories: Each suppository contains: zinc sulfate monohydrate 10 mg, hydrocortisone acetate 10 mg in a triglyceride base. Nonmedicinal ingredients: methylparaben, propylparaben and triglyceride. Boxes of 12 and 24. Store between 15 and 30°C. Avoid freezing.

Ansaid® Pr
flurbiprofen
Nonsteroidal Anti-inflammatory Drug (NSAID)

Pfizer

Date of Revision: February 3, 2010

SUMMARY PRODUCT INFORMATION:

Route of Administration	Dosage Form/ Strength	Clinically Relevant Nonmedicinal Ingredients
Oral	Tablet/50 mg, 100 mg	Lactose For a complete listing see Dosage Forms, Composition and Packaging.

INDICATIONS AND CLINICAL USE: Ansaid (flurbiprofen) is indicated for the following:

- Relief of signs and symptoms of rheumatoid arthritis, osteoarthritis and ankylosing spondylitis.
- Relief of pain associated with dysmenorrhoea.
- Relief of mild to moderate pain accompanied by inflammation (e.g. bursitis, tendinitis, soft tissue trauma).

For patients with an increased risk of developing CV and/or GI adverse events, other management strategies that do not include the use of NSAIDs should be considered first (see Contraindications and Warnings and Precautions). Use of Ansaid should be limited to the lowest effective dose for the shortest possible duration of treatment in order to minimize the potential risk for cardiovascular or gastrointestinal adverse events (see Contraindications and Warnings and Precautions).

Ansaid, as a NSAID, does **not** treat clinical disease or prevent its progression.

Ansaid, as a NSAID, only relieves symptoms and decreases inflammation for as long as the patient continues to take it.

Geriatrics (>65 years of age): Evidence from clinical studies and postmarket experience suggests that use in the geriatric population is associated with differences in safety (see Warnings and Precautions, Special Populations).

Pediatrics (<18 years of age): Safety and efficacy have not been established in the pediatric population (see Contraindications).

CONTRAINDICATIONS: Ansaid (flurbiprofen) is contraindicated in:

- The peri-operative setting of coronary artery bypass graft surgery (CABG). Although Ansaid has **not** been studied in this patient population, a selective COX-2 inhibitor NSAID studied in such a setting has led to an increased incidence of cardiovascular/thromboembolic events, deep surgical infections and sternal wound complications.
- The third trimester of pregnancy, because of risk of premature closure of the ductus arteriosus and prolonged parturition.
- Women who are breastfeeding, because of the potential for serious adverse reactions in nursing infants.
- Severe uncontrolled heart failure.
- Known or suspected hypersensitivity to flurbiprofen or to any of the components/excipients, or other nonsteroidal anti-inflammatory drugs (NSAIDs).
- History of asthma, urticaria, or allergic-type reactions after taking ASA or other NSAIDs (i.e. complete or partial syndrome of ASA-intolerance—rhinosinusitis, urticaria/angioedema, nasal polyps, asthma). Fatal asthmatic and anaphylactoid reactions have occurred in such individuals. As well, individuals with the above medical problems are at risk of a severe reaction even if they have taken NSAIDs in the past without any adverse effects. The potential for cross-reactivity between different NSAIDs must be kept in mind (see Warnings and Precautions, Hypersensitivity Reactions, Anaphylactoid Reactions).
- Active gastric/duodenal/peptic ulcer, active GI bleeding, a history of recurrent ulceration or active inflammatory disease of the gastrointestinal system.
- Cerebrovascular bleeding or other bleeding disorders.
- Inflammatory bowel disease.
- Severe liver impairment or active liver disease.
- Severe renal impairment (creatinine clearance <30 mL/min or 0.5 mL/sec) or deteriorating renal disease (individuals with lesser degrees of renal impairment are at risk of deterioration of their renal function when prescribed NSAIDs and must be monitored) (see Warnings and Precautions, Renal).
- Known hyperkalemia (see Warnings and Precautions, Renal, Fluid and Electrolyte Balance).
- Children and adolescents less than 18 years of age.

WARNINGS AND PRECAUTIONS:

> **Serious Warnings and Precautions**
> **Risk of Cardiovascular (CV) Adverse Events: Ischemic Heart Disease, Cerebrovascular Disease, Congestive Heart Failure (NYHA II-IV) (see Warnings and Precautions, Cardiovascular).**
> **Ansaid is a non-steroidal anti-inflammatory drug (NSAID). Use of some NSAIDs is associated with an increased incidence of cardiovascular adverse events (such as myocardial infarction, stroke or thrombotic events) which can be fatal. The risk may increase with duration of use. Patients with cardiovascular disease or risk factors for cardiovascular disease may be at greater risk.**
> **Caution should be exercised in prescribing Ansaid to any patient with ischemic heart disease (including but not limited to acute myocardial infarction, history of myocardial infarction and/or angina), cerebrovascular disease (including but not limited to stroke, cerebrovascular accident, transient ischemic attacks and/or amaurosis fugax) and/or congestive heart failure (NYHA II-IV).**
> **Use of NSAIDs, such as Ansaid, can promote sodium retention in a dose-dependent manner, through a renal mechanism, which can result in increased blood pressure and/or exacerbation of congestive heart failure (see also Warnings and Precautions, Renal, Fluid and Electrolyte Balance).**
> **Randomized clinical trials with Ansaid have not been designed to detect differences in cardiovascular events in a chronic setting. Therefore, caution should be exercised when prescribing Ansaid.**
> **Risk of Gastrointestinal (GI) Adverse Events (see Warnings and Precautions, Gastrointestinal (GI)).**
> **Use of NSAIDs, such as Ansaid, is associated with an increased incidence of gastrointestinal adverse events (such as peptic/duodenal ulceration, perforation, obstruction and gastrointestinal bleeding).**

General: Frail or debilitated patients may tolerate side effects less well and therefore special care should be taken in treating this population. **To minimize the potential risk for an adverse event, the lowest effective dose should be used for the shortest possible duration.** As with other NSAIDs, caution should be used in the treatment of elderly patients who are more likely to be suffering from impaired renal, hepatic or cardiac function. For high risk patients, alternate therapies that do not involve NSAIDs should be considered.

Ansaid is **not** recommended for use with other NSAIDs, with the exception of low-dose ASA for cardiovascular prophylaxis, because of the absence of any evidence demonstrating synergistic benefits and the potential for additive adverse reactions (see Drug Interactions, Drug/Drug Interactions, Acetylsalicylic Acid (ASA) or other NSAIDs). In common with other anti-inflammatory drugs, Ansaid may mask the usual signs of infection.

Cardiovascular: Ansaid is a non-steroidal anti-inflammatory drug (NSAID). Use of some NSAIDs is associated with an increased incidence of cardiovascular adverse events (such as myocardial infarction, stroke or thrombotic events) which can be fatal. The risk may increase with duration of use. Patients with cardiovascular disease or risk factors for cardiovascular disease may be at greater risk.

Caution should be exercised in prescribing Ansaid to patients with risk factors for cardiovascular disease, cerebrovascular disease or renal disease, such as any of the following (not an exhaustive list): hypertension, dyslipidemia/hyperlipidemia, diabetes mellitus, congestive heart failure (NYHA I), coronary artery disease (atherosclerosis), peripheral arterial disease, smoking, creatinine clearance <60 mL/min or 1 mL/sec.

For patients with a high risk of developing an adverse CV event, other management strategies that do **not** include the use of NSAIDs should be considered first. **To minimize the potential risk for an adverse CV event, the lowest effective dose should be used for the shortest possible duration.**

Cardiovascular Thrombotic Events: Physicians and patients should remain alert for the development of such events, even in the absence of previous CV symptoms. Patients should be informed about the signs and/or symptoms of serious CV events and the steps to take if they occur.

There is no consistent evidence that concurrent use of ASA mitigates the increased risk of serious CV thrombotic events associated with NSAID use. The concurrent use of ASA and an NSAID does increase the risk of serious GI events (see Warnings and Precautions, Gastrointestinal (GI)).

Hypertension: NSAIDs including Ansaid, can lead to onset of new hypertension or worsening of pre-existing hypertension, either of which may contribute to the increased incidence of CV events. Patients taking thiazides or loop diuretics may have impaired response to these therapies when taking NSAIDs. NSAIDs, including Ansaid, should be used with caution in patients with hypertension. Blood pressure (BP) should be monitored closely during the initiation of NSAID treatment and throughout the course of therapy.

Congestive Heart Failure and Edema: Fluid retention and edema have been observed in patients treated with Ansaid. Therefore, as with many other NSAIDs, the possibility of precipitating congestive heart failure in elderly patients or those with compromised cardiac function should be borne in mind. Ansaid should be used with caution in patients with heart failure, hypertension or other conditions predisposing to fluid retention (see Warnings and Precautions, Renal, Fluid and Electrolyte Balance).

Endocrine and Metabolism: With nonsteroidal anti-inflammatory treatment there is a potential risk of hyperkalemia, particularly in patients with conditions such as diabetes mellitus or renal failure; elderly patients; or in patients receiving concomitant therapy with beta-adrenergic blockers, angiotensin converting enzyme inhibitors or some diuretics. Serum electrolytes should be monitored periodically during long-term therapy, especially in those patients who are at risk.

Corticosteroids: Ansaid (flurbiprofen) is **not** a substitute for corticosteroids. It does **not** treat corticosteroid insufficiency. Abrupt discontinuation of corticosteroids may lead to exacerbation of corticosteroid-responsive illness. Patients on prolonged corticosteroid therapy should have their therapy tapered slowly if a decision is made to discontinue corticosteroids (see Drug Interactions, Drug-Drug Interactions, Glucocorticoids).

Gastrointestinal (GI): Serious GI toxicity (sometimes fatal), such as peptic/duodenal ulceration, inflammation, perforation, obstruction and gastrointestinal bleeding, can occur at any time, with or without warning symptoms, in patients treated with NSAIDs, such as Ansaid. Minor upper GI problems, such as dyspepsia, commonly occur at any time. Health care providers should remain alert for ulceration and bleeding in patients treated with Ansaid, even in the absence of previous GI tract symptoms. Most spontaneous reports of fatal GI events are in elderly or debilitated patients and therefore special care should be taken in treating this population. **To minimize the potential risk for an adverse GI event, the lowest effective dose should be used for the shortest possible duration.** For high risk patients, alternate therapies that do not involve NSAIDs should be considered (see Warnings and Precautions, Special Populations, Geriatrics (>65 years of age)).

Patients should be informed about the signs and/or symptoms of serious GI toxicity and instructed to discontinue using Ansaid and seek emergency medical attention if they experience any such symptoms. The utility of periodic laboratory monitoring has **not** been demonstrated, nor has it been adequately assessed. Most patients who develop a serious upper GI adverse event on NSAID therapy have no symptoms. Upper GI ulcers, gross bleeding or perforation, caused by NSAIDs, appear to occur in approximately 1% of patients treated for 3-6 months, and in about 2-4% of patients treated for one year. These trends continue, thus increasing the likelihood of developing a serious GI event at some time during the course of therapy. Even short-term therapy has its risks.

The incidence of these complications increases with increasing dose.

Caution should be taken if prescribing Ansaid to patients with a prior history of peptic/duodenal ulcer disease or gastrointestinal bleeding as these individuals have a greater than 10-fold higher risk for developing a GI bleed when taking a NSAID than patients with neither of these risk factors. In these cases the physician must weigh the benefits of treatment against the possible hazards. Other risk factors for GI ulceration and bleeding include the following: *H. pylori* infection, increased age, prolonged use of NSAID therapy, excess alcohol intake, smoking, female gender, poor general health status or concomitant therapy with any of the following: Anti-coagulants (e.g. warfarin); Anti-platelet agents (e.g. ASA, clopidogrel); Oral corticosteroids (e.g. prednisone); Selective Serotonin Reuptake Inhibitors (SSRIs) (e.g. citalopram, fluoxetine, paroxetine, sertraline).

Ansaid should be given under close medical supervision to patients prone to gastrointestinal tract irritation particularly those with a history of peptic ulcer, diverticulosis or other inflammatory disease of the gastrointestinal tract such as ulcerative colitis and Crohn's disease. In these cases the physician must weigh the benefits of treatment against the possible hazards.

If ulceration is suspected or confirmed, or if GI bleeding occurs, Ansaid should be discontinued immediately, appropriate treatment instituted and the patient monitored closely.

No studies to date have identified any group of patients not at risk of developing ulceration and bleeding. Studies to date show that all NSAIDs can cause GI tract adverse events as existing data do not clearly identify differences in risk between various NSAIDs.

There is no definitive evidence that the concomitant administration of histamine H_2-receptor antagonists and/or antacids will either prevent the occurrence of gastrointestinal side effects or allow the continuation of Ansaid therapy when and if these adverse reactions appear.

Genitourinary: Some NSAIDs are associated with persistent urinary symptoms (bladder pain, dysuria, urinary frequency), hematuria or cystitis. The onset of these symptoms may occur at any time after the initiation of therapy with an NSAID. Some cases have become severe on continued treatment. Should urinary symptoms occur, in the absence of an alternate explanation, treatment with Ansaid should be stopped to ascertain if symptoms disappear. This should be done before any urological investigations or treatments are carried out.

Hematologic: NSAIDs inhibiting prostaglandin biosynthesis interfere with platelet function to varying degrees; patients who may be adversely affected by such an action, such as those on anti-coagulants or suffering from haemophilia or platelet disorders, should be carefully observed when Ansaid is administered.

Anti-coagulants: Numerous studies have shown that the concomitant use of NSAIDs and anti-coagulants increases the risk of bleeding. Concurrent therapy of Ansaid with warfarin requires close monitoring of the international normalized ratio (INR).

Even with therapeutic INR monitoring, increased bleeding may occur.

Anti-platelet Effects: NSAIDs inhibit platelet aggregation and have been shown to prolong bleeding time in some patients. Unlike acetylsalicylic acid (ASA), their effect on platelet function is quantitatively less, or of shorter duration, and is reversible.

Ansaid and other NSAIDs have no proven efficacy as anti-platelet agents and should **not** be used as a substitute for ASA or other anti-platelet agents for prophylaxis of cardiovascular thromboembolic diseases. Anti-platelet therapies (e.g. ASA) should **not** be discontinued. There is some evidence that use of NSAIDs with ASA can markedly attenuate the cardioprotective effects of ASA (see Drug Interactions, Drug-Drug Interactions, Acetylsalicylic Acid (ASA) or other NSAIDs).

Concomitant administration of Ansaid with low dose ASA increases the risk of GI ulceration and associated complications.

Blood Dyscrasias: Blood dyscrasias (such as neutropenia, leukopenia, thrombocytopenia, aplastic anemia and agranulocytosis) associated with the use of NSAIDs are rare, but could occur with severe consequences.

Anemia is sometimes seen in patients receiving NSAIDs, including Ansaid. This may be due to fluid retention, GI blood loss, or an incompletely described effect upon erythropoiesis. Patients on long-term treatment with NSAIDs, including Ansaid, should have their hemoglobin or hematocrit checked if they exhibit any signs or symptoms of anemia or blood loss.

Hepatic/Biliary/Pancreatic: As with other NSAIDs, borderline elevations of one or more liver enzyme tests (AST, ALT, alkaline phosphatase) may occur in up to 15% of patients. These abnormalities may progress, may remain essentially unchanged, or may be transient with continued therapy.

A patient with symptoms and/or signs suggesting liver dysfunction, or in whom an abnormal liver function test has occurred, should be evaluated for evidence of the development of a more severe hepatic reaction while on therapy with Ansaid. The ALT test is probably the most sensitive indicator of liver injury. Meaningful (3 times the upper limit of normal) elevations of ALT or AST have been reported in controlled clinical trials in less than 1% of patients.

Severe hepatic reactions including jaundice and cases of fatal hepatitis, liver necrosis and hepatic failure, some of them with fatal outcomes, have been reported with NSAIDs.

Although such reactions are rare, if abnormal liver tests persist or worsen, if clinical signs and symptoms consistent with liver disease develop (e.g. jaundice), or if systemic manifestations occur (e.g. eosinophilia, rash, etc.), this drug should be discontinued.

During long-term therapy, liver function tests should be monitored periodically. If there is a need to prescribe this drug in the presence of impaired liver function, it must be done under strict observation.

Hypersensitivity Reactions: Anaphylactoid Reactions: As with NSAIDs in general, anaphylactoid reactions have occurred in patients without known prior exposure to Ansaid. In post-marketing experience, rare cases of anaphylactic anaphylactoid reactions and angioedema have been reported in patients receiving Ansaid. Ansaid should **not** be given to patients with the ASA-triad. This symptom complex typically occurs in asthmatic patients who experience rhinitis with or without nasal polyps, or who exhibit severe, potentially fatal bronchospasm after taking ASA or other NSAIDs (see Contraindications).

ASA-Intolerance: Ansaid should **not** be given to patients with complete or partial syndrome of ASA-intolerance (rhinosinusitis, urticaria/angioedema, nasal polyps, asthma) in whom asthma, anaphylaxis, urticaria/angioedema, rhinitis or other allergic manifestations are precipitated by ASA or other NSAIDs. Fatal anaphylactoid reactions have occurred in such individuals. As well, individuals with the above medical problems are at risk of a severe reaction even if they have taken NSAIDs in the past without any adverse reaction (see Contraindications).

Cross-sensitivity: Patients sensitive to one NSAID may be sensitive to any of the other NSAIDs as well.

Serious Skin Reactions: (See Warnings and Precautions, Skin.)

Immune: (See Warnings and Precautions, Infection, Aseptic Meningitis.)

Infection: Ansaid, in common with other NSAIDs, may mask signs and symptoms of an underlying infectious disease.

Aseptic Meningitis: Rarely, with some NSAIDs, the symptoms of aseptic meningitis (stiff neck, severe headaches, nausea and vomiting, fever or clouding of consciousness) have been observed. Patients with autoimmune disorders (systemic lupus erythematosus, mixed connective tissue diseases, etc.) seem to be pre-disposed. Therefore, in such patients, the health care provider must be vigilant to the development of this complication.

Neurologic: Some patients may experience drowsiness, dizziness, blurred vision, vertigo, tinnitus, hearing loss, insomnia or depression with the use of NSAIDs, such as Ansaid. In clinical trials, 1-3% of patients experienced drowsiness, dizziness, vertigo, insomnia or depression with the use of Ansaid. If patients experience these side effects, they should exercise caution in carrying out activities that require alertness.

Ophthalmologic: Blurred and/or diminished vision has been reported with the use of NSAIDs, including Ansaid. If such symptoms develop, Ansaid should be discontinued and an ophthalmologic examination performed. Ophthalmologic examination should be carried out at periodic intervals in any patient receiving Ansaid for an extended period of time.

Peri-Operative Considerations: (See Contraindications, Coronary Artery Bypass Graft Surgery.)

Psychiatric: Some patients may experience depression with the use of Ansaid (see Warnings and Precautions, Neurologic).

Renal: Long-term administration of NSAIDs to animals has resulted in renal papillary necrosis and other abnormal renal pathology. In humans, there have been reports of acute interstitial nephritis with hematuria, low-grade proteinuria, and occasionally nephrotic syndrome.

Renal insufficiency due to NSAID use is seen in patients with pre-renal conditions leading to reduction in renal blood flow or blood volume. Under these circumstances, renal prostaglandins have a supportive role in the maintenance of renal perfusion and glomerular filtration rate (GFR). In these patients, administration of a NSAID may cause a dose-dependent reduction in prostaglandin synthesis leading to impaired renal function. Patients at greatest risk of this reaction are those with pre-existing insufficiency (GFR <60 mL/min or 1 mL/s), dehydrated patients, patients on salt restricted diets, those with congestive heart failure, cirrhosis, liver dysfunction, taking angiotensin-converting enzyme inhibitors, angiotensin-II receptor blockers, cyclosporin, diuretics, and the elderly. Serious or life-threatening renal failure has been reported in patients with normal or impaired renal function after short term therapy with NSAIDs. Even patients at risk who demonstrate the ability to tolerate a NSAID under stable conditions may decompensate during periods of added stress (e.g. dehydration due to gastroenteritis). Discontinuation of NSAIDs is usually followed by recovery to the pre-treatment state.

Caution should be used when initiating treatment with NSAIDs, such as Ansaid, in patients with considerable dehydration. It is advisable to rehydrate patients first prior to initiation of therapy. Caution is also recommended in patients with pre-existing kidney disease. Ansaid and its metabolites are eliminated primarily by the kidneys, therefore the drug should be used with great caution in patients with impaired renal function. In these cases, utilization of lower doses of Ansaid should be considered and patients carefully monitored.

During long-term therapy, kidney function should be monitored periodically.

Advanced Renal Disease: (See Contraindications.)

Fluid and Electrolyte Balance: Use of NSAIDs, such as Ansaid, can promote sodium retention in a dose-dependent manner, which can lead to fluid retention and edema, and consequences of increased blood pressure and exacerbation of congestive heart failure. Thus, caution should be exercised in prescribing Ansaid in patients with a history of congestive heart failure, compromised cardiac function, hypertension, increased age or other conditions predisposing to fluid retention (see Warnings and Precautions, Cardiovascular).

Use of NSAIDs, such as Ansaid, can increase the risk of hyperkalemia, especially in patients with diabetes mellitus, renal failure, increased age, or those receiving concomitant therapy with adrenergic blockers, angiotensin-converting enzyme inhibitors, angiotensin-II receptor antagonists, cyclosporin, or some diuretics.

Electrolytes should be monitored periodically (see Contraindications).

Respiratory: ASA-induced asthma is an uncommon but very important indication of ASA and NSAID sensitivity. It occurs more frequently in patients with asthma who have nasal polyps.

Sexual Function/Reproduction: The use of Ansaid, as with any drug known to inhibit cyclooxygenase/prostaglandin synthesis, may impair fertility and is not recommended in women attempting to conceive. Therefore, in women who have difficulties conceiving, or who are undergoing investigation of infertility, withdrawal of Ansaid should be considered.

Skin: In rare cases, serious skin reactions such as Stevens-Johnson syndrome, toxic epidermal necrolysis, exfoliative dermatitis and erythema multiforme have been associated with the use of some NSAIDs. Because the rate of these reactions is low, they have usually been noted during post-marketing surveillance in patients taking other medications also associated with the potential development of these serious skin reactions. Thus, causality is **not** clear. These reactions are potentially life threatening but may be reversible if the causative agent is discontinued and appropriate treatment instituted. Patients should be advised that if they experience a skin rash they should discontinue their NSAID and contact their physician for assessment and advice, including which additional therapies to discontinue.

Special Populations: Pregnant Women: Ansaid is contraindicated for use during the third trimester of pregnancy because of risk of premature closure of the ductus arteriosus and the potential to prolong parturition.

Caution should be exercised in prescribing Ansaid during the first and second trimesters of pregnancy.

Inhibition of prostaglandin synthesis may adversely affect pregnancy and/or the embryo-fetal development. Data from epidemiological studies suggest an increased risk of miscarriage and of cardiac malformation after use of a prostaglandin synthesis inhibitor in early pregnancy.

In animals, administration of a prostaglandin synthesis inhibitor has been shown to result in increased pre- and post-implantation loss and embryo-fetal lethality. In addition, increased incidences of various malformations, including cardiovascular, have been reported in animals given a prostaglandin synthesis inhibitor during the organogenetic period. Although no teratogenic effects were seen in animal studies, parturition was delayed and prolonged, and there was an increase in the number of stillbirths. Flurbiprofen has been found to cross the placental barrier.

Nursing Women: The safe use of flurbiprofen during lactation has not been established. Flurbiprofen is secreted in breast milk. The use of this drug is not recommended during lactation (see Contraindications).

Pediatrics (<18 years of age): (See Contraindications.)

Geriatrics (>65 years of age): As with all NSAIDs, Ansaid (flurbiprofen) should be used with caution in the elderly, particularly women (see Action and Clinical Pharmacology, Pharmacokinetics).

Patients older than 65 years (referred to in this document as older or elderly) and frail or debilitated patients are more susceptible to a variety of adverse reactions from NSAIDs. The incidence of these adverse reactions increases with dose and duration of treatment. In addition, these patients are less tolerant to ulceration and bleeding. Most reports of fatal GI events are in this population. Older patients are also at risk of lower esophageal ulceration and bleeding. For such patients, consideration should be given to a starting dose lower than the one usually recommended, with individual adjustment when necessary, and under close supervision. See information in this section under Endocrine and Metabolism, and Renal for further advice. See also information under Drug Interactions, Glucocorticoids.

Monitoring and Laboratory Tests: Cardiovascular: (Hypertension): Blood pressure should be monitored regularly during therapy with Ansaid (see Warnings and Precautions, Cardiovascular, Hypertension).

Renal: Renal function (serum creatinine, and serum urea, etc.) should be monitored in high-risk populations, such as the elderly, patients with advanced renal disease, patients with cardiovascular disease and diabetes mellitus, as well as in the setting of concomitant use of diuretics, ACE inhibitors, and methotrexate (see Contraindications; Drug Interactions, Anti-hypertensives and Methotrexate; Warnings and Precautions, Fluid and Electrolyte Balance). If abnormal renal tests persist or worsen, Ansaid should be discontinued.

Patients on long term treatment with NSAIDs, including Ansaid, should have their electrolytes such as serum potassium checked regularly if they exhibit any signs or symptoms of renal disease (see Warnings and Precautions, Fluid and Electrolyte Balance).

Hepatic: Patient with symptoms and/or signs of liver dysfunction, or in whom an abnormal liver function test has occurred, should be monitored carefully for evidence of the development of a more severe hepatic reaction while on therapy with Ansaid. If abnormal liver tests persist or worsen, Ansaid should be discontinued (see Warnings and Precautions, Hepatic/Biliary/Pancreatic).

Hematologic: Anemia is commonly observed in rheumatoid arthritis and is sometimes aggravated by NSAIDs, which may produce fluid retention or minor gastrointestinal blood loss in some patients. Therefore, patients who have initial hemoglobin values of 10 g/dL or less, and who are to receive long-term therapy, should have hemoglobin values determined periodically (see Warnings and Precautions, Hematologic, Blood Dyscrasias).

Concurrent therapy of Ansaid with warfarin requires close monitoring of the international normalized ratio (INR) (see Warnings and Precautions, Hematologic, Anti-coagulants).

Plasma Lithium: When lithium and flurbiprofen are concurrently administered, a reduction in lithium dose is recommended and plasma concentrations of lithium should be monitored. Plasma concentrations of lithium should also be monitored when stopping or starting an NSAID (see Drug Interactions, Lithium).

Vision Changes: Blurred and/or diminished vision has been reported with the use of Ansaid and other NSAIDs. Patients experiencing eye complaints should have ophthalmologic examinations (see Warnings and Precautions, Ophthalmologic).

ADVERSE REACTIONS: Adverse Drug Reaction Overview: The most common adverse reactions encountered with NSAIDs are gastrointestinal, of which peptic ulcer, with or without bleeding, is the most severe. Fatalities have occurred, particularly in the elderly.

Clinical Trial Adverse Drug Reactions: Because clinical trials are conducted under very specific conditions, the adverse reaction rates observed in the clinical trials may not reflect the rates observed in practice and should not be compared to the rates in the clinical trials of another drug. Adverse drug reaction information from clinical trials is useful for identifying drug-related adverse events and for approximating rates.

In company-sponsored clinical trials of Ansaid (flurbiprofen) in which a total of 2820 patients were treated, gastrointestinal adverse reactions were those most commonly seen, the most severe of which were gastrointestinal bleeding and ulceration. See Table 1.

Table 1: Ansaid

Events Occurring in ≥1% with Ansaid Patients from Clinical Trials

Central Nervous System	
Headache	2.6%
Asthenia	1.0%
Gastrointestinal	
Abdominal pain	6.8%
Dyspepsia	6.0%
Diarrhea	5.7%
Nausea	4.5%
Constipation	2.6%
Gastrointestinal bleeding	1.7%
Flatulence	1.4%
Emesis	1.2%
Elevated liver enzymes	1.4%
Dermatologic	
Rash	1.9%
General Body	
Edema	2.6%
Pain	1.9%
Flu syndrome	2.0%
Hematologic	
Decrease in hemoglobin and hematocrit	4.6%
Respiratory	
Pharyngitis	6.1%
Infection	1.2%
Rhinitis	1.3%
Sinusitis	1.6%
Special Senses	
Dizziness	1.5%
Tinnitus	1.2%
Urogenital	
Urinary tract infections	1.5%

Less Common Clinical Trial Adverse Drug Reactions (<1%): Cardiovascular: Incidence 0.1 to 1.0%: hypertension, arrhythmias, inotropic problems, palpitations, vasodilatation, angina, phlebitis, vascular distress, extrasystoles, right heart failure, myocardial infarction, vasculitis. Incidence less than 0.1%: tachycardia, syncope.

Central Nervous System: Incidence 0.1% to 1.0%: somnolence, hypertonia, insomnia, nervousness, paresthesia, depression, mood changes, tremors, anxiety, amnesia, migraine, ataxia, cerebrovascular accident, confusion, cerebral ischemia, malaise, increased reflex. Incidence less than 0.1%: EEG abnormalities, neuralgia, convulsions, meningitis, speech disorder, twitch, euphoria, decreased libido.

Dermatologic: Incidence 0.1 to 1.0%: herpetic infections, alopecia, dry skin, eczema, nail discoloration, pruritus, sweating, skin ulcerations, urticaria. Incidence less than 0.1%: seborrhea, angioedema, exfoliation.

Gastrointestinal: Incidence 0.1 to 1.0%: increased appetite, stomatitis, gastrointestinal distress, gastritis, gastroenteritis, ulcer (peptic, gastric or duodenal), melena (includes rectal bleed, bloody diarrhea), oral inflammation, eructation, dry mouth, esophagitis, hematemesis, colitis, hepatitis, rectal discomfort, periodontal abscess, gingivitis, glossitis, anorexia, vomiting. Incidence less than 0.1%: gums bleeding, cholecystitis.

General Body: Incidence 0.1% to 1.0%: fever, abdominal enlargement, chills, infection, allergic reaction, death. Incidence less than 0.1%: injury.

Hematologic: Incidence 0.1% to 1.0%: iron deficiency anemia, ecchymosis, eosinophilia, leukopenia, lymphadenopathy, neutropenia. Incidence less than 0.1%: anemia, leukocytosis, petechia, thrombocytopenia, WBC abnormality.

Metabolic: Incidence 0.1 to 1.0%: weight changes, hyperuricemia. Incidence less than 0.1%: electrolyte changes (Ca++, K+), increased CPK, thirst.

Musculoskeletal: Incidence 0.1 to 1.0%: arthritis, injury, myalgia. Incidence less than 0.1%: myasthenia, tenosynovitis, joint disease.

Respiratory: Incidence 0.1 to 1.0%: bronchitis, epistaxis, increase in cough, dyspnea, laryngitis, lung disorder, asthma, voice alterations. Incidence less than 0.1%: hyperventilation, pleural distress, pulmonary infarct, pulmonary embolism, pneumonia.

Special Senses: Ear: vertigo 0.6%; pain 0.3%; disorder 0.2%. Incidence less than 0.1%: vestibular disturbances.
Eye: ocular inflammations 0.3%; amblyopia 0.6%; vision disturbances 0.4%; blepharitis 0.1%; conjunctivitis 0.5%; keratoconjunctivitis 0.1%; photophobia 0.1%. Incidence less than 0.1%: diplopia, visual field problems, corneal opacity, lacrimal distress, glaucoma, pain, scleritis.
Others: taste changes 0.2%; parosmia <0.1%.

Urogenital: Incidence 0.1 to 1.0%: urine abnormalities, hematuria, cystitis, frequency, vaginitis, breast pain, kidney function abnormalities. Incidence less than 0.1%: dysuria, albuminuria, pyuria, pain, kidney stones, kidney failure, incontinence, ejaculatory abnormality, leukorrhea, urethritis, retention, dysmenorrhea, menstrual distress, impotence.

Post-Market Adverse Drug Reactions: Additional reports of serious adverse events temporally associated with Ansaid during worldwide post-marketing experience are included below. Because these events are reported voluntarily from a population of uncertain size, it is not always possible to reliably estimate their frequency or clearly establish a causal relationship to Ansaid exposure. These include the following: Aseptic meningitis, cholestatic and non-cholestatic jaundice, exacerbation of inflammatory bowel disease, small intestine inflammation with loss of blood and protein, photosensitivity, toxic epidermal necrolysis, interstitial nephritis anaphylaxis, Stevens-Johnson syndrome.

Abnormal Hematologic and Clinical Chemistry Findings: Decrease in hemoglobin and hematocrit was observed in clinical trials at an incidence of 4.6 %. Iron deficiency anemia, ecchymosis, eosinophilia, leukopenia, lymphadenopathy, neutropenia were reported in clinical trials at an incidence of 0.1% to 1.0% (see Adverse Reactions, Clinical Trial Adverse Drug Reactions).

DRUG INTERACTIONS: Overview: Factors such as excess alcohol intake, smoking, age, female gender and concomitant NSAID and oral steroid or anticoagulant use have been associated with increased risk of GI adverse events such as ulceration and bleeding.

Ansaid is extensively protein bound (99%) to human serum albumin. Less than 10% of the primary binding sites were estimated to be occupied at therapeutic drug concentrations. In vitro studies suggest that Ansaid binds to a different primary site on albumin (Type II) than drugs such as anticoagulants, sulfonamides and phenytoin (Type I). However, patients with such combination therapy should be monitored.

Flurbiprofen metabolism is predominantly mediated via cytochrome P450 CYP 2C9 in the liver. Patients who are known or suspected to be poor CYP2C9 metabolizers based on previous history/experience with other CYP2C9 substrates should be administered flurbiprofen with caution as they may have abnormally high plasma levels due to reduced metabolic clearance.

Drug-Drug Interactions: Acetylsalicylic Acid (ASA) or other NSAIDs: The use of Ansaid in addition to any other NSAID, including over-the-counter ones (such as ASA and ibuprofen) for analgesic and/or anti-inflammatory effects is **not** recommended because of the absence of any evidence demonstrating synergistic benefits and the potential for additive adverse reactions.

The exception is the use of low dose ASA for cardiovascular protection, when another NSAID is being used for its analgesic/anti-inflammatory effect, keeping in mind that combination NSAID therapy is associated with additive adverse reactions. The concurrent administration of Ansaid and ASA may result in significantly lowering flurbiprofen concentrations.

Some NSAIDs (e.g. ibuprofen) may interfere with the anti-platelet effects of low dose ASA, possibly by competing with ASA for access to the active site of cyclooxygenase-1.

Antacids: In geriatric subjects, antacid suspensions caused a reduction in the rate but not the extent of flurbiprofen absorption.

Anticoagulants: Numerous studies have shown that the concomitant use of NSAIDs and anticoagulants increases the risk of GI adverse events such as ulceration and bleeding (see Warnings and Precautions, Hematologic, Anti-coagulants).

Because prostaglandins play an important role in hemostasis, and NSAIDs affect platelet function, concurrent therapy of Ansaid with warfarin requires close monitoring to be certain that no change in anticoagulant dosage is necessary.

Anti-hypertensives: NSAIDs may diminish the anti-hypertensive effect of Angiotensin Converting Enzyme (ACE) inhibitors.

Combinations of ACE inhibitors, angiotensin-II antagonists, or diuretics with NSAIDs might have an increased risk for acute renal failure and hyperkalemia. Blood pressure and renal function (including electrolytes) should be monitored more closely in this situation, as occasionally there can be a substantial increase in blood pressure.

Anti-platelet Agents (including ASA): There is an increased risk of bleeding, via inhibition of platelet function, when anti-platelet agents are combined with NSAIDs, such as Ansaid (see Warnings and Precautions, Hematologic, Anti-platelet Effects).

β-adrenergic Blocking Agents: Ansaid pretreatment attenuated the hypotensive effect of propranolol but did not appear to affect the ß-blocker mediated reduction in heart rate.

Cimetidine/Ranitidine: A small but statistically significant increase in flurbiprofen serum concentration may result with administration of these agents.

Cyclosporin and Tacrolimus: Although this interaction has not been studied with flurbiprofen, co-administration of cyclosporin or tacrolimus and any NSAID may increase the nephrotoxic effect of cyclosporin or tacrolimus due to the NSAID's effect on renal prostaglandins. Renal function should be monitored when flurbiprofen and either of these drugs are used in combination.

CYP2C9 Substrates: Flurbiprofen metabolism is predominantly mediated via cytochrome P450 CYP 2C9 in the liver. Patients who are known or suspected to be poor CYP2C9 metabolizers based on previous history/experience with other CYP2C9 substrates should be administered flurbiprofen with caution as they may have abnormally high plasma levels due to reduced metabolic clearance.

Digoxin: Concurrent administration with flurbiprofen did not reveal a change in steady state serum levels of either drug.

Diuretics: Clinical studies as well as post-marketing observations have shown that NSAIDs can reduce the effect of diuretics.

Ansaid can interfere with the effects of furosemide. NSAIDs have been shown to interfere with the action of thiazide diuretics and potassium-sparing diuretics.

Glucocorticoids: Numerous studies have shown that the concomitant use of NSAIDs and oral glucocorticoids increases the risk of GI side effects such as ulceration and bleeding. This is especially the case in older (>65 years of age) individuals.

Lithium: Combined use of lithium and flurbiprofen resulted in significant elevation of lithium trough plasma concentration and area under the curve. When lithium and flurbiprofen are concurrently administered, a reduction in lithium dose is recommended. Plasma concentrations of lithium should also be monitored when stopping or starting a NSAID.

Methotrexate: Although a pharmacokinetic interaction has not been reported between low dose methotrexate and flurbiprofen, in rheumatoid arthritis patients with normal renal function, monitoring of toxic signs and symptoms and renal function is recommended. The dose of methotrexate should be reduced if toxicity or impairment of renal function is observed. The interaction of intermediate and high dose methotrexate and flurbiprofen has not been studied. Since significant toxicity has been reported with coadministration of intermediate or high dose methotrexate and other NSAIDs, the concomitant use of intermediate or high dose methotrexate and flurbiprofen should be avoided.

Oral Contraceptives: No drug interaction data are available for Ansaid and the co-administration of oral contraceptives.

Oral Hypoglycemics: Concomitant administration of flurbiprofen and hypoglycemic agents revealed a slight reduction in blood sugar concentrations but no signs or symptoms of hypoglycemia.

Selective Serotonin Reuptake Inhibitors (SSRIs): Concomitant administration of NSAIDs and SSRIs may increase the risk of gastrointestinal ulceration and bleeding (see Warnings and Precautions, Gastrointestinal (GI)).

Drug-Food Interactions: Interactions with food have not been established.

Drug-Herb Interactions: Interactions with herbal products have not been established.

Drug-Laboratory Test Interactions: Interactions with laboratory tests have not been established.

DOSAGE AND ADMINISTRATION: Dosing Considerations: Consideration should be given to reducing the starting dose in elderly patients.

Flurbiprofen metabolism is predominantly mediated via cytochrome P450 CYP 2C9 in the liver. Patients who are known or suspected to be poor CYP2C9 metabolizers based on previous history/experience with other CYP2C9 substrates should be administered flurbiprofen with caution as they may have abnormally high plasma levels due to reduced metabolic clearance.

Recommended Dose and Dosage Adjustment: Rheumatoid Arthritis, Osteoarthritis, Ankylosing Spondylitis: The recommended dose is 200 mg per day given in divided doses. Some patients may require up to 300 mg per day. The dose should be adjusted until the minimum effective maintenance dose is established. During the course of treatment, the maximum daily dose of 300 mg should be used only during symptom exacerbations and not for maintenance therapy (see Adverse Reactions).

Dysmenorrhoea: The recommended dosage is 50 mg given four times daily.

Mild to Moderately Severe Pain: The usual recommended dose is 50 mg given every four to six hours as needed.

Missed Dose: The missed dose should be taken as soon as remembered. If the next dose is due within 2 hours, a single dose should be taken and the next dose skipped.

Administration: Ansaid (flurbiprofen) should be taken immediately after a meal, or with food or milk.

OVERDOSAGE:

Information on Ansaid (flurbiprofen) overdosage is available for 13 children and 12 adults; all persons receiving only a flurbiprofen overdose and all but one person exposed to more than one drug recovered. Manifestations of flurbiprofen overdose have included decreased mental status, coma, diminished muscle tone, headache, diplopia, elevated liver enzymes, respiratory depression, nausea, and epigastric pain.

Patients should be managed by symptomatic and supportive care following overdose with a nonsteroidal anti-inflammatory drug. There are no specific antidotes. Emesis and/or activated charcoal (60 to 100 g in adults, 1 to 2 g/kg in children) and/or osmotic cathartic may be indicated in patients seen within 4 hours of ingestion with symptoms, or following a large overdose (5 to 10 times the usual dose). Forced diuresis, alkalization of urine, hemodialysis, or hemoperfusion may not be useful due to high protein binding.

For management of a suspected drug overdose, CPhA recommends that you contact your **regional Poison Control Centre**. See the *CPS* Directory section for a list of Poison Control Centres.

ACTION AND CLINICAL PHARMACOLOGY: Mechanism of Action: The mode of action of flurbiprofen, like that of other NSAID agents, is not known. However, its therapeutic action is not due to pituitary-adrenal stimulation. Flurbiprofen is an inhibitor of prostaglandin synthesis. The resulting decrease in prostaglandin synthesis may partially explain the drug's anti-inflammatory effect at the cellular level.

Pharmacodynamics: Ansaid (flurbiprofen), a phenylalkanoic acid derivative, is a NSAID which also possesses analgesic and antipyretic activities.

Pharmacokinetics: See Table 2.

Table 2: Ansaid

Summary of Mean (SD) Flurbiprofen Pharmacokinetic Parameters

	Peak Conc. (μg/mL)	Time of Peak Conc. (h)	Area Under the Curve (AUC[a]) (μg h/mL)	Apparent Volume of Distribution (Vz/F, L)	Terminal Disposition Half-life ($t_{1/2}$, h)
100 mg single-dose Normal Healthy Adults (18 to 40 years) N=15	14 (4)	1.9 (1.5)	83 (20)	14 (3)	7.5 (0.8)
Steady-state (100 mg every 12 hours) Geriatric Arthritis Patients (65 to 83 years) N=13	16 (5)	2.2 (3)	77 (24)	12 (5)	5.8 (1.9)

[a] AUC from 0 to infinity for single doses and from 0 to the end of the dosing interval for multiple-doses.

Absorption: In bioavailability studies in normal volunteers, Ansaid reached peak blood levels in approximately 2 hours (range of 0.5 to 4 hours). Administration of Ansaid with food does not alter total drug availability but delays absorption.

Distribution: Ansaid is extensively bound (99%) to human plasma protein such as albumin, but less than 10% of the primary albumin binding sites would be occupied by the drug. Flurbiprofen binds to a different primary site on albumin than do anticoagulants, sulfonamides and phenytoin. Mean peak serum concentrations of flurbiprofen were higher in the elderly female patients.

Metabolism: Flurbiprofen metabolism is predominantly mediated via cytochrome P450 CYP 2C9 in the liver. Ansaid is rapidly metabolized and excreted in the urine as free and unaltered intact drug (20%) and hydroxylated metabolites (50%). About 90% of the flurbiprofen in urine is present as conjugates. In animal models of inflammation the metabolites showed little activity.

Excretion: The elimination half life of flurbiprofen is approximately 7 hours with a range of 3 to 9 hours. Excretion of Ansaid is 88-98% complete within 24 hours after the last dose.

Special Populations and Conditions: Geriatrics: With the exception of elderly females, flurbiprofen pharmacokinetics were similar in geriatric arthritis patients, younger arthritis patients, and young healthy volunteers receiving Ansaid Tablets 100 mg as either single or multiple doses. Mean peak serum concentrations of flurbiprofen were higher in the elderly female patients, therefore dosage adjustment may be necessary.

Poor CYP2C9 metabolizers: Flurbiprofen metabolism is predominantly mediated via cytochrome P450 CYP 2C9 in the liver. Patients who are known or suspected to be poor CYP2C9 metabolizers based on previous history/experience with other CYP2C9 substrates should be administered flurbiprofen with caution as they may have abnormally high plasma levels due to reduced metabolic clearance.

Hepatic Insufficiency: Hepatic metabolism may account for >90% of flurbiprofen elimination, so patients with hepatic disease may require reduced doses of Ansaid Tablets compared to patients with normal hepatic function. The pharmacokinetics of R- and S-flurbiprofen were similar, however, in alcoholic cirrhosis patients (N=8) and young healthy volunteers (N=8) following administration of a single 200 mg dose of Ansaid tablets. Flurbiprofen plasma protein binding may be decreased in patients with liver disease and serum albumin concentrations below 3.1 g/dL (see Warnings and Precautions, Hepatic/Biliary/Pancreatic).

Renal Insufficiency: Renal clearance is an important route of elimination for flurbiprofen metabolites, but a minor route of elimination for unchanged flurbiprofen (≈3% of total clearance). The unbound clearances of R- and S-flurbiprofen did not differ significantly between normal healthy volunteers (N=6, 50 mg single dose) and patients with renal impairment (N=8, inulin clearances ranging from 11 to 43 mL/min, 50 mg multiple doses). Flurbiprofen plasma protein binding may be decreased in patients with renal impairment and serum albumin concentrations below 3.9 g/dL. Elimination of flurbiprofen metabolites may be reduced in patients with renal impairment (Warnings and Precautions, Renal).

Flurbiprofen is not significantly removed from the blood into dialysate in patients undergoing continuous ambulatory peritoneal dialysis.

STORAGE AND STABILITY: Store at controlled room temperature (15 to 30°C).

INFORMATION FOR THE PATIENT: Published in e-CPS, available by subscription at www.e-cps.ca.

DOSAGE FORMS, COMPOSITION AND PACKAGING: 50 mg: Each white, elliptical, film-coated tablet imprinted with Ansaid logo contains: flurbiprofen 50 mg. Nonmedicinal ingredients: carnauba wax, colloidal silicon dioxide, croscarmellose sodium, hypromellose, lactose, magnesium stearate, microcrystalline cellulose, propylene glycol and titanium dioxide. Bottles of 100.

100 mg: Each blue, elliptical, film-coated tablet imprinted with Ansaid logo contains: flurbiprofen 100 mg. Nonmedicinal ingredients: carnauba wax, colloidal silicon dioxide, croscarmellose sodium, FD&C Blue No. 2, hypromellose, lactose, magnesium stearate, microcrystalline cellulose, propylene glycol and titanium dioxide. Bottles of 100.

(Shown in Product Identification Section)

Antizol® Pr

fomepizole

Synthetic Alcohol Dehydrogenase Inhibitor

Paladin

Date of Revision: November 20, 2006

PHARMACOLOGY: Mechanism of Action: Fomepizole is a competitive inhibitor of alcohol dehydrogenase. Alcohol dehydrogenase catalyzes the oxidation of ethanol to acetaldehyde. Alcohol dehydrogenase also catalyzes the initial steps in the metabolism of ethylene glycol and methanol to their toxic metabolites.

Ethylene glycol, the main component of most antifreezes and coolants, is metabolized to glycoaldehyde, which undergoes subsequent sequential oxidations to yield glycolate, glyoxylate, and oxalate. Glycolate and oxalate are the metabolic by-products primarily responsible for the metabolic acidosis and renal damage seen in ethylene glycol toxicosis which presents with the following morbidities: nausea/vomiting, seizures, cardiac arrhythmias, stupor, coma, calcium oxaluria, acute tubular necrosis and death, depending on the amount of ethylene glycol ingested and the time elapsing from ingestion. The lethal dose of ethylene glycol in humans is approximately 1.4 mL/kg.

Methanol, the main component of windshield wiper fluid, is slowly metabolized via alcohol dehydrogenase to formaldehyde with subsequent oxidation via formaldehyde dehydrogenase to yield formic acid. Formic acid is primarily responsible for the metabolic acidosis and visual disturbances (e.g., decreased visual acuity and potential blindness) associated with methanol poisoning. A lethal dose of methanol in humans is approximately is 1 to 2 mL/kg.

Fomepizole has been shown in vitro and in vivo to block alcohol dehydrogenase enzyme activity in dog, monkey, and human liver. The relative affinity of fomepizole for human ADH is 80 000 times greater than that of methanol and ethylene glycol, and 8 000 times greater than that of ethanol. The concentration of fomepizole at which alcohol dehydrogenase is inhibited by 50% in vitro is approximately 0.1 μmol/L. The plasma concentrations achieved in humans with the proposed dosage regimen are well above this, with peak concentrations of fomepizole between 100 to 300 μmol/L (8.6 to 24.6 mg/L). These levels are achieved with oral or i.v. fomepizole doses of 10 to 20 mg/kg. Fomepizole is most effective when given in close proximity to the ethylene glycol or methanol ingestion before significant target organ damage occurs.

Pharmacokinetics: The plasma half-life of fomepizole varies with dose, even in patients with normal renal function, and has not been calculated.

Distribution: After i.v. infusion, fomepizole rapidly distributes to total body water. The volume of distribution is between 0.6 L/kg and 1.02 L/kg.

Metabolism: In healthy volunteers, only 1 to 3.5% of the administered dose of fomepizole (7 to 20 mg/kg oral and i.v.) was excreted unchanged in the urine, indicating that metabolism is the major route of elimination. In humans, the primary metabolite of fomepizole is 4-carboxypyrazole (approximately 80 to 85% of administered dose), which is excreted in the urine. Other metabolites of fomepizole observed in the urine are 4-hydroxymethylpyrazole and the N-glucuronide conjugates of 4-carboxypyrazole and 4-hydroxymethylpyrazole.

Excretion: After a single dose, the elimination of fomepizole is best characterized by Michaelis-Menten kinetics with saturable elimination occurring at plasma concentrations of 100 to 300 μmol/L, 8.2 to 24.6 mg/L.

With multiple doses, fomepizole rapidly induces its own metabolism via the cytochrome P450 mixed-function oxidase system, which produces a significant increase in the elimination rate after about 30 to 40 hours. After enzyme induction, elimination follows first-order kinetics.

Special Populations: Fomepizole has not been studied sufficiently to determine whether the pharmacokinetics differ for geriatric or pediatric populations, between genders, or for patients with renal or hepatic impairment.

INDICATIONS: As an antidote for ethylene glycol (such as antifreeze) or methanol poisoning (such as windshield washer fluid), or for use in suspected ethylene glycol or methanol ingestion, either alone or in combination with hemodialysis (see Dosage).

CONTRAINDICATIONS: Fomepizole should not be administered to patients with a documented serious hypersensitivity reaction to fomepizole or other pyrazoles.

WARNINGS: No data supplied by the manufacturer.

PRECAUTIONS: General: **Fomepizole injection should not be given undiluted or by bolus injection.** Venous irritation and phlebosclerosis were noted in 2 of 6 normal volunteers given bolus injections (over 5 minutes) of fomepizole at a concentration of 25 mg/mL.

Minor allergic reactions (mild rash, eosinophilia) have been reported in a few patients receiving fomepizole (see Adverse Effects). Therefore, patients should be monitored for signs of allergic reactions.

Drug Interactions: Oral doses of fomepizole (10 to 20 mg/kg), via alcohol dehydrogenase inhibition, significantly reduced the rate of elimination of ethanol (by approximately 40%) given to healthy volunteers in moderate doses. Similarly, ethanol decreased the rate of elimination of fomepizole (by approximately 50%) by the same mechanism.

Reciprocal interactions may occur with concomitant use of fomepizole and drugs that increase or inhibit the cytochrome P450 system (e.g., phenytoin, carbamazepine, cimetidine, ketoconazole), though this has not been studied.

Pregnancy: Animal reproduction studies have not been conducted with fomepizole. It is also not known whether fomepizole can cause fetal harm when administered to pregnant women or can affect reproduction capacity. Antizol should be given to pregnant women only if clearly needed.

Lactation: It is not known whether fomepizole is excreted in human milk. Because many drugs are excreted in human milk, caution should be exercised when fomepizole is administered to a nursing woman.

Children: Safety and effectiveness in pediatric patients have not been established.

Geriatrics: Fomepizole is metabolized by the liver and excreted by the kidney. The functions of both organs are generally lower in elderly patients; therefore, care should be taken when selecting the dose of fomepizole for elderly patients.

ADVERSE EFFECTS: The most frequent adverse events reported as drug-related or unknown relationship to study drug in the 78 patients and 63 normal volunteers who received fomepizole injection were headache (14%), nausea (11%), and dizziness, increased drowsiness, and bad taste/metallic taste (6% each). All other adverse events in this population were reported in approximately 3% or fewer of those receiving fomepizole and were as follows:

Body as a Whole: abdominal pain, fever, pain during fomepizole injection, inflammation at injection site, lumbalgia/backache, hangover.

Cardiovascular: phlebosclerosis, phlebitis, hypotension.

Gastrointestinal: vomiting, diarrhea, dyspepsia, heartburn, decreased appetite, transient increase in liver function tests.

Hemic/Lymphatic: Eosinophilia/hypereosinophilia, lymphangitis, anemia.

Nervous: lightheadedness, agitation, feeling drunk, facial flush, vertigo, nystagmus, anxiety, "felt strange", decreased environmental awareness.

Respiratory: hiccups, pharyngitis.

Skin/Appendages: application site reaction, rash.

Special Senses: abnormal smell, speech/visual disturbances, transient blurred vision, roar in ear.

OVERDOSE:

Symptoms: Nausea, dizziness, and vertigo were noted in healthy volunteers receiving 50 and 100 mg/kg doses of fomepizole injection (at plasma concentrations of 290 to 520 μmol/L, 23.8 to 42.6 mg/L). These doses are 3 to 6 times the recommended dose. This dose-dependent CNS effect was short-lived in most subjects and lasted up to 30 hours in 1 subject.

Treatment: Fomepizole is dialyzable, and hemodialysis may be useful in treating cases of overdosage.

For management of a suspected drug overdose, CPhA recommends that you contact your **regional Poison Control Centre**. See the *CPS* Directory section for a list of Poison Control Centres.

DOSAGE: Treatment Guidelines: Treatment of ethylene glycol and methanol poisonings consists of blocking the formation of toxic metabolites using inhibitors of alcohol dehydrogenase, such as fomepizole injection, and correction of metabolic abnormalities. In patients with high ethylene glycol or methanol concentrations (≥50 mg/dL), significant metabolic acidosis, or renal failure, hemodialysis should be considered in addition to treatment with fomepizole to remove ethylene glycol or methanol and the respective toxic metabolites of these alcohols.

Treatment with Fomepizole: Begin fomepizole treatment immediately upon suspicion of ethylene glycol or methanol ingestion based on patient history and/or anion gap metabolic acidosis, increased osmolar gap, visual disturbances, or oxalate crystals in the urine, **or** a documented serum ethylene glycol or methanol concentration greater than 20 mg/dL.

In addition to specific antidote treatment with fomepizole, patients intoxicated with ethylene glycol or methanol should be managed as appropriate for metabolic acidosis, acute renal failure (ethylene glycol), adult respiratory distress syndrome, visual disturbances (methanol) and hypocalcemia. At frequent intervals throughout the treatment, patients poisoned with ethylene glycol should be monitored for ethylene glycol concentrations in serum and urine, and the presence of urinary oxalate crystals. Similarly, serum methanol concentrations should be monitored in patients poisoned with methanol. Hepatic enzymes and white blood cell counts should be monitored during treatment, as transient increases in serum transaminase concentrations and eosinophilia have been noted with repeated fomepizole dosing.

Dosing of Fomepizole: A loading dose of 15 mg/kg should be administered, followed by doses of 10 mg/kg every 12 hours for 4 doses, then 15 mg/kg every 12 hours thereafter until ethylene glycol or methanol concentrations are undetectable or have been reduced below 20 mg/dL, and the patient is asymptomatic with normal pH. All doses should be administered as a slow i.v. infusion over 30 minutes (see Preparation for I.V. Administration).

Dosage with Hemodialysis: Hemodialysis should be considered in addition to fomepizole in the case of renal failure, significant or worsening metabolic acidosis, or a measured ethylene glycol or methanol concentration if greater than or equal to 50 mg/dL. Patients should be dialyzed to correct metabolic abnormalities and to lower the ethylene glycol concentrations below 50 mg/dL.

The following guidelines for administering fomepizole during hemodialysis should be used: Before dialysis: Administer next scheduled dose if >6 hours since the last dose. During dialysis: Administer doses every 4 hours. Postdialysis: If time since last dose is <1 hour, then give the next scheduled dose 12 hours from the last dose administered, and then follow the normal dosing schedule (see Dosing of Fomepizole).

If time since last dose is ≥1 hour but <3 hours, then immediately administer 50% of the next scheduled dose, and then follow the normal dosing schedule. If time since last dose is ≥3 hours, then immediately administer 100% of the next scheduled dose, and then follow the normal dosing schedule.

Discontinuation of Fomepizole Treatment: Treatment with fomepizole may be discontinued when ethylene glycol or methanol concentrations are undetectable or have been reduced below 20 mg/dL, and the patient is asymptomatic with normal pH.

Preparation for I.V. Administration: When preparing fomepizole solution avoid ocular, dermal, or inhalation exposures. In case of eye or skin exposure, flush immediately with copious amounts of water. Seek medical attention if irritation persists. Prepare solution in well-ventilated area. If accidental inhalation occurs, move to fresh air.

Fomepizole solidifies at temperatures less than 25°C. If the fomepizole solution has become solid in the vial, the solution should be liquefied by running the vial under warm water or by holding in the hand. Solidification does not affect the efficacy, safety, or stability of fomepizole. Using sterile technique, the appropriate dose of fomepizole should be drawn from the vial with a syringe and injected into **at least 100 mL of sterile 0.9% Sodium Chloride Injection or Dextrose 5% Injection.** Mix well. The entire contents of the resulting solution should be infused over 30 minutes. Fomepizole, like all parenteral products, should be inspected visually for particulate matter prior to administration.

Parenteral Products: Stability: Antizol diluted in 0.9% Sodium Chloride Injection or Dextrose 5% Injection remains stable and sterile for at least 24 hours when stored refrigerated or at room temperature. Antizol does not contain preservatives. Therefore, maintain sterile conditions, and after dilution do not use beyond 24 hours. Solutions showing haziness, particulate matter, precipitate, discoloration or leakage should not be used.

SUPPLIED: Each mL of clear to yellow, sterile solution for i.v. injection, contains: fomepizole 1 g. Nonmedicinal ingredients: none. Preservative-free. Single-use vials of 1.5 mL, packages of 4. Store at controlled room temperature (20 to 25°C). Discard any unused portion.

Anugesic-HC™ Ⓟ

pramoxine HCl—hydrocortisone acetate—zinc sulfate monohydrate

Anorectal Therapy

McNeil Consumer Healthcare

PHARMACOLOGY: Anugesic-HC combines the antiseptic, emollient and astringent effects of Anusol with the anti-inflammatory action of hydrocortisone and topical analgesic effect of pramoxine. Pramoxine provides the surface analgesia within 2 to 3 minutes which lasts up to 4 hours and is less toxic and less sensitizing than benzocaine, cocaine, procaine and dibucaine (cinchocaine).

INDICATIONS: For the relief of the pain and discomfort following anorectal surgery of all types and that which is associated with the acute phase of common anorectal disorders. These include hemorrhoids, internal and external (including those accompanying pregnancy) whether or not complicated by thrombosis and prolapse; pruritis ani; proctitis, cryptitis, fissures, and incomplete fistulas; and other congestive allergic or inflammatory conditions. May also be used prior to rectal examination to anesthetize the area where it is too tender or where there is too much spasm to admit the examining finger. To be followed by maintenance management with regular Anusol preparations as required.

CONTRAINDICATIONS: In patients with a sensitivity to any of the components. Not to be used in the presence of existing tuberculous, fungal and viral lesions of the skin.

WARNINGS: No data supplied by the manufacturer.

PRECAUTIONS: Until an adequate proctological examination is completed and a diagnosis made, Anugesic-HC or any preparation containing hydrocortisone should not be used. In addition, specific measures against infection, allergy and other causal factors must not be neglected. Prolonged use of this medication could produce systemic corticosteroid effects, although none have been noted to date. As with all medication that is applied locally, if idiosyncratic reactions occur, medication should be discontinued. (Do not use on infected lesions unless accompanied by appropriate anti-infective agents. Discontinue use if sensitivity develops.)

Pregnancy: The safe use of topical corticosteroids during pregnancy and lactation has not been fully established. Therefore, during pregnancy, Anugesic-HC should not be used unnecessarily on extended areas (ointment), in large amounts, or for prolonged periods of time.

Lactation: See Pregnancy.

ADVERSE EFFECTS: Occasionally, patients may experience burning upon application of Anugesic-HC especially if the anoderm is not intact. Local sensitivity reactions have been rare.

OVERDOSE:

Symptoms: No toxic effects have been reported with Anugesic-HC.

Treatment: In case of accidental ingestion, perform gastric lavage.

> For management of a suspected drug overdose, CPhA recommends that you contact your **regional Poison Control Centre**. See the *CPS* Directory section for a list of Poison Control Centres.

DOSAGE: Suppositories: Administer Anugesic-HC suppositories in the morning and again at bedtime, and after each evacuation. Continue this treatment until the acute phase of pain and discomfort passes and the inflammation subsides. Thereafter, maintain patient comfort and continue treatment with 1 daily application after the morning stool. Bathe and dry the affected anal area. Then insert 1 suppository into the rectum. Suppositories are most easily administered in a stooped or squatting position, or while lying on the side with knees flexed. The exertion of a slight bearing down pressure relaxes the anal sphincter which permits painless insertion of the suppository.

Ointment: Administer Anugesic-HC ointment in the morning and again at bedtime, and after each evacuation. Continue this treatment until the acute phase of pain and discomfort passes and the inflammation subsides. Thereafter, maintain patient comfort and continue treatment with 1 daily application after the morning stool. Bathe and dry the affected anal area. Attach the plastic applicator to the tube and insert it into the rectum to its full extent. Then, slowly withdraw while gently squeezing the tube. Regardless of whether the ointment form is used for internal medication, the ointment may also be applied to the exterior surface of the anus for relief of any external anorectal discomfort often associated with the former conditions.

SUPPLIED: Ointment: Each tube contains: pramoxine HCl 1%, hydrocortisone acetate 0.5%, zinc sulfate monohydrate 0.5% in a petroleum ointment base. Nonmedicinal ingredients: calcium phosphate, methylparaben, mineral oil, petrolatum, poloxyl-2-oleyl ether and propylparaben. Tubes of 30 g with plastic applicator and guard. Store between 15 and 30°C.

Suppositories: Each white-colored suppository contains: pramoxine HCl 20 mg, hydrocortisone acetate 10 mg, zinc sulfate monohydrate 10 mg, in a base of triglycerides. Nonmedicinal ingredients: calcium phosphate, magnesium stearate, methylparaben, propylparaben and triglyceride base. Boxes of 12. Store between 15 and 30°C.

Anusol®

zinc sulfate monohydrate

Anorectal Therapy

McNeil Consumer Healthcare

Anusol® Plus

pramoxine HCl—zinc sulfate monohydrate

Anorectal Therapy

McNeil Consumer Healthcare

INDICATIONS: Symptomatic relief of pain and discomfort as in: external and internal hemorrhoids, proctitis, papillitis, cryptitis, fissures, incomplete fistulas and relief of local pain following anorectal surgery.

CONTRAINDICATIONS: History of sensitivity to any component.

WARNINGS: No data supplied by the manufacturer.

PRECAUTIONS: In case of rectal bleeding, consult physician promptly.

ADVERSE EFFECTS: An occasional patient may experience burning upon application, especially if the anoderm is not intact. Discontinue medication if irritation or sensitivity is suspected.

OVERDOSE:

No data supplied by the manufacturer.

> For management of a suspected drug overdose, CPhA recommends that you contact your **regional Poison Control Centre**. See the *CPS* Directory section for a list of Poison Control Centres.

DOSAGE: Ointment: Bathe and dry the affected anal area. Apply ointment freely to the affected area every 4 hours or as needed and after each bowel movement.

Suppositories: Bathe and dry the affected anal area. Insert 1 suppository in the morning, at bedtime and after each bowel movement.

SUPPLIED: Anusol: Ointment: A smooth, colorless, translucent ointment contains: zinc sulfate monohydrate 0.5% w/w. Nonmedicinal ingredients: calcium phosphate, mineral oil, oleth-2, parabens and petrolatum. Tubes of 30 g with applicator.

Suppositories: Each white, opaque suppository contains: zinc sulfate monohydrate 10 mg. Nonmedicinal ingredients: calcium phosphate, magnesium stearate, parabens and vegetable oil. Boxes of 24.

Anusol Plus: Ointment: Each tube of smooth, colorless, translucent ointment contains: pramoxine HCl 1% w/w and zinc sulfate monohydrate 0.5% w/w. Nonmedicinal ingredients: calcium phosphate, mineral oil, oleth-2, parabens and petrolatum. Tubes of 30 g with applicator.

Suppositories: Each white, opaque suppository contains: pramoxine HCl 20 mg and zinc sulfate monohydrate 10 mg. Nonmedicinal ingredients: calcium phosphate, magnesium stearate, parabens and vegetable oil. Boxes of 12 and 24.

Store between 15 and 30°C.

Anusol-HC™ Ⓟ

hydrocortisone acetate—zinc sulfate monohydrate

Anorectal Therapy

McNeil Consumer Healthcare

INDICATIONS: For the relief of the pain and discomfort following anorectal surgery of all types and that which is associated with the acute phase of common anorectal disorders. These include hemorrhoids, internal and external (including those accompanying pregnancy) whether or not complicated by thrombosis and prolapse; pruritis ani; proctitis, cryptitis, fissures, and incomplete fistulas; and other congestive allergic or inflammatory conditions.

CONTRAINDICATIONS: In patients with a sensitivity to any of the components. Not to be used in the presence of existing tuberculous, fungal and viral lesions of the skin.

WARNINGS: No data supplied by the manufacturer.

PRECAUTIONS: Until an adequate proctological examination is completed and a diagnosis made, Anusol-HC or any preparation containing hydrocortisone should not be used. In addition, specific measures against infection, allergy and other causal factors must not be neglected. Prolonged use of this medication could produce systemic corticosteroid effects, although none have been noted to date. As with all medication that is applied locally, if idiosyncratic reactions occur, medication should be discontinued.

Pregnancy: The safe use of topical corticosteroids during pregnancy and lactation has not been fully established. Therefore, during pregnancy, Anusol-HC should not be used unnecessarily on extended areas (ointment), in large amounts, or for prolonged periods of time.

Lactation: See Pregnancy.

ADVERSE EFFECTS: Occasionally, patients may experience burning upon application of Anusol-HC especially if the anoderm is not intact. Local sensitivity reactions have been rare.

OVERDOSE:

Symptoms: The chances of overdosage are very rare, and no toxic reactions or side effects have been reported with Anusol-HC.

Treatment: In case of accidental ingestion, perform gastric lavage followed by a purgative dose of magnesium sulfate.

> For management of a suspected drug overdose, CPhA recommends that you contact your **regional Poison Control Centre**. See the *CPS* Directory section for a list of Poison Control Centres.

DOSAGE: Ointment: Apply Anusol-HC ointment internally and on the exterior surface of the anus in the morning and at bedtime, and after each bowel movement, or as directed by a physician.

Suppositories: Remove wrapper from suppository and apply Anusol-HC suppository internally in the anus in the morning and at bedtime, and after each bowel movement, or as directed by a physician.

SUPPLIED: Ointment: Each tube contains: zinc sulfate monohydrate 0.5% and hydrocortisone acetate 0.5% in a petroleum ointment base. Nonmedicinal ingredients: calcium phosphate, methylparaben, mineral oil, petrolatum, poloxyl-2-oleyl ether and propylparaben. Tube of 30 g with a plastic applicator. Store between 15 and 30°C.

Suppositories: Each suppository contains: zinc sulfate monohydrate 10 mg, hydrocortisone acetate 10 mg in a triglyceride base. Nonmedicinal ingredients: calcium phosphate, magnesium stearate, methylparaben, propylparaben and triglyceride base. Boxes of 12 and 24. Store in a cool place between 15 and 30°C.

Anzemet® Ⓟ

dolasetron mesylate

Antiemetic

sanofi-aventis

Date of Revision: October 12, 2006

PHARMACOLOGY: Dolasetron and its active metabolite, hydrodolasetron (MDL 74156), are selective 5-HT_3 receptor antagonists shown not to have activity at other known serotonin receptors and with low affinity for dopamine receptors. The serotonin 5-HT_3 receptors are located on the nerve terminals of the vagus in the periphery and centrally in the chemoreceptor trigger zone of the area postrema. It is thought that chemotherapeutic agents produce nausea and vomiting by releasing serotonin from the enterochromaffin cells of the small intestine, and that serotonin then activates the 5-HT_3 receptors located on vagal afferents to initiate the vomiting reflex.

Acute, reversible, ECG changes (PR and QTc; QRS widening), caused by dolasetron, have been observed in controlled clinical trials. Dolasetron appears to prolong both depolarization and, to a lesser extent, repolarization time. Although QTc prolongation is primarily due to QRS widening, JT prolongation has also been observed. The magnitude and frequency of the ECG changes increased with dose (related to the peak plasma concentration of hydrodolasetron but not the parent compound). These ECG changes usually returned to baseline within 6 to 8 hours, but in some patients have lasted 24 hours or longer. Dolasetron administration has little or no effect on blood pressure.

In healthy volunteers (N=4), dolasetron in single i.v. doses up to 5 mg/kg produced no effect on pupil size or meaningful changes in EEG tracings. Results from neuropsychiatric tests revealed that dolasetron does not alter mood or concentration. Multiple daily doses of dolasetron have no effect on colonic transit in humans. Dolasetron has no effect on plasma prolactin concentrations.

Pharmacokinetics: Pharmacokinetics in Humans (I.V. Administration): I.V. dolasetron is rapidly eliminated ($t_{1/2}$ <10 min) and completely metabolized to the most clinically relevant species, hydrodolasetron. Hydrodolasetron appears rapidly in plasma, with a maximum concentration occurring approximately 0.6 hours after the end of i.v. treatment, and is eliminated with a mean half-life of 7.3 hours (CV=24%, n=30) in adult cancer patients. Hydrodolasetron is eliminated by multiple routes, including renal excretion, after metabolism mainly by glucuronidation and hydroxylation. Hydrodolasetron exhibits linear pharmacokinetics over the i.v. dose range of 50 to 200 mg and they are independent of infusion rate. Doses lower than 50 mg have not been studied. Two-thirds of the administered dose is recovered in the urine and one-third in the feces. Hydrodolasetron is widely distributed in the body with a mean apparent volume of distribution of 5.8 L/kg (CV=25%; n=24) in adults.

Sixty-nine to 77% of hydrodolasetron is bound to plasma proteins. In a study with ^{14}C-labeled dolasetron, the distribution of radioactivity to blood cells was not extensive. The binding of hydrodolasetron to α1-acid glycoprotein is approximately 51%. The pharmacokinetics are similar in men and women. The pharmacokinetics of hydrodolasetron, in special and targeted patient populations following i.v. administration of dolasetron, are summarized in Table 1. The pharmacokinetics of hydrodolasetron are similar in adult healthy volunteers and adult cancer patients receiving chemotherapeutic agents. The apparent clearance of hydrodolasetron is not affected by age in adult cancer patients. Following i.v. administration, the apparent clearance of hydrodolasetron remains unchanged with severe hepatic impairment and decreases 47% with severe renal impairment.

Table 1: Anzemet

Pharmacokinetic Values for Hydrodolasetron Following I.V. Administration of Dolasetron Mesylate (1.8 mg/kg)

	Age (years)	Cl_{app} (mL/min/kg)	$t_{1/2}$ (h)	AUC_{∞} (ng/mL×h)	C_{max} (ng/mL)
Young healthy volunteers (n=24)	19–40	9.4 (28%)	7.3 (24%)	2567[a]	457[a]
Elderly healthy volunteers (n=15)	65–75	8.3 (30%)	6.9 (22%)	3021[a]	465[a]
Cancer patients (n=273)	19–87	10.2 (34%)	7.5 (43%)	3640 (32%)	505 (26%)

a Results dose-normalized to the recommended dose assuming linear kinetics.

Legend:
Cl_{app}=apparent clearance.
C_{max}=maximal serum concentration.
$t_{1/2}$=terminal elimination half-life.
Values in brackets ( ) represent the coefficient of variation in %.

Pharmacokinetics in Humans (Oral Administration): Oral dolasetron is well absorbed, although the parent drug is rarely detected in plasma due to rapid and complete metabolism to the most clinically relevant species, hydrodolasetron. Hydrodolasetron appears rapidly in plasma, with a maximum concentration occurring approximately 1 hour after dosing, and is eliminated with a mean half-life of 8.1 hours (CV=18%; n=30). The apparent absolute bioavailability of oral dolasetron, determined by the major active metabolite hydrodolasetron, is about 75%. Food does not affect the apparent bioavailability of dolasetron taken by mouth. Hydrodolasetron is eliminated by multiple routes, including renal excretion, after metabolism, mainly glucuronidation and hydroxylation. Two-thirds of the administered dose is recovered in the urine and one-third in the feces. Hydrodolasetron is widely distributed in the body with a mean apparent volume of distribution of 5.8 L/kg (CV=25%; n=24). Sixty-nine to 77% of hydrodolasetron is bound to plasma proteins. The binding of hydrodolasetron to α1-acid glycoprotein is approximately 51%. In a study with ^{14}C-labeled dolasetron, the distribution of radioactivity to blood cells was not extensive. The pharmacokinetics of hydrodolasetron are linear and similar in men and women.

The pharmacokinetics of hydrodolasetron following oral administration, in special and targeted patient populations, are summarized in Table 2. The pharmacokinetics of hydrodolasetron are similar between adult healthy volunteers and cancer patients receiving chemotherapeutic agents. The apparent clearance of hydrodolasetron following oral administration of dolasetron is not affected by age in adult cancer patients. The apparent clearance of hydrodolasetron decreases 42% with severe hepatic impairment and 44% with severe renal impairment.

Table 2: Anzemet

Pharmacokinetic Values for Hydrodolasetron Following Oral Administration of Dolasetron Mesylate (100 mg)

	Age (years)	Cl_{app} (mL/min/kg)	$t_{1/2}$ (h)	AUC_{∞} (ng/mL×h)	C_{max} (ng/mL)
Young healthy volunteers (n=24)	19–45	10.5 (32%)	8.2 (21%)	1605[a]	299[a]
Elderly healthy volunteers (n=14)	65–75	9.5 (36%)	7.2 (32%)	2106[a]	402[a]
Cancer patients (n=17)	30–84	11.5 (47%)	7.9 (33%)	—[b]	—[b]

a Results dose-normalized to the recommended dose assuming linear kinetics.
b Sampling times did not allow for determination.

Legend:
Cl_{app}=apparent oral clearance.
C_{max}=maximal serum concentration.
$t_{1/2}$=terminal elimination half-life.
Values in brackets ( ) represent the coefficient of variation in %.

Clinical Trials: I.V. Administration: One thousand nine hundred and seventeen patients receiving emetogenic chemotherapy (including high dose cisplatin ≥70 mg/m²) were studied in 5 randomized, double blind trials in which 597 patients were treated with the recommended dose of 1.8 mg/kg dolasetron injection (see Table 3). Efficacy was based on complete response rates (no emetic episodes and no rescue medication). Dolasetron administered i.v. at a dose of 1.8 mg/kg gave similar results in preventing nausea and vomiting as the other selective 5-HT_3 receptor antagonists studied as active comparators. Dolasetron injection was more effective than metoclopramide.

Table 3: Anzemet

Prevention of Chemotherapy-induced Nausea and Emesis in Cisplatin[a] Chemotherapy with Anzemet Injection (1.8 mg/kg)

Response over 24 hours	Patients Responding (%) (n=597)
Complete Response[b]	313 (52.4%)
Nausea Score[c]	10.5
Total Response[d]	223 (37.4%)

a Cisplatin was used at moderately and highly emetogenic doses; cyclophosphamide, doxorubicin, fluorouracil, epirubicin and vincristine were used at moderately emetogenic doses and were the most commonly used chemotherapeutic agents in these trials.
b No emetic episodes and no rescue medication.
c Median 24-hour change from baseline nausea score using visual analog scale (VAS); score range 0="none" to 100="nausea as bad as it could be".
d Complete response plus no nausea (VAS <5 mm).

Oral Administration: One thousand and twenty-six patients receiving emetogenic chemotherapy were studied in 3 randomized, double blind trials in which 227 patients were treated with 100 mg oral dolasetron (see Table 4). Efficacy was based on complete response rates (no emetic episodes and no rescue medication). Dolasetron administered at an oral dose of 100 mg gave similar results in preventing nausea and vomiting as the other selective 5-HT_3 receptor antagonists studied as active comparators.

INDICATIONS: Adults: For the prevention of nausea and vomiting associated with initial and repeat courses of emetogenic cancer chemotherapy, including high dose cisplatin.
Pediatrics (<18 years of age): See Contraindications.

CONTRAINDICATIONS: In patients with known hypersensitivity to the drug or any components of its formulations (see Supplied).
Any therapeutic use in children and adolescents under 18 years of age.
The prevention and treatment of post-operative nausea and vomiting in adults.
These contraindications apply to **both** intravenous (IV) and oral formulations.

Table 4: Anzemet

Prevention of Chemotherapy-induced Nausea and Vomiting in Moderately Emetogenic Chemotherapy with Anzemet Tablets (100 mg)[a]

Response over 24 hours	Patients Responding (%) (n=227)
Complete Response[b]	147 (64.8%)
Nausea Score[c]	2.5
Total Response[d]	111 (48.9%)

a Cisplatin, carboplatin, doxorubicin and cyclophosphamide were used at moderately emetogenic doses.
b No emetic episodes and no rescue medication.
c Median 24-hour change from baseline nausea score using visual analog scale (VAS); score range 0="none" to 100="nausea as bad as it could be".
d Complete response and no nausea (VAS <5 mm).

WARNINGS: ECG changes and cardiovascular events: **Dolasetron can cause ECG interval changes (PR and QTc prolongations and QRS widening) in healthy volunteers and patients. In patients receiving chemotherapy or undergoing surgery, JT prolongations have also been observed following dolasetron, active comparator or placebo. JT prolongations have not been observed in healthy volunteers receiving dolasetron. ECG interval changes are related in magnitude and frequency to blood levels of the active metabolite, hydrodolasetron. These changes are self-limiting with declining blood levels. Some patients have interval prolongations for 24 hours or longer. Interval prolongations could lead to cardiovascular consequences, including heart block or cardiac arrhythmias. These have been rarely reported n patients receiving dolasetron.**

Complete heart block was observed interoperatively in a 61 year-old woman who received 200 mg dolasetron oral tablet for the prevention of postoperative nausea and vomiting. This patient was also taking verapamil. A 66 year-old man receiving chemotherapy was found dead 6 hours after receiving 1.8 mg/kg (119 mg) i.v. dolasetron injection and concomitant anthracycline therapy. Vital signs taken at 1 and 4.5 hours after dolasetron injection indicated an adequate blood pressure and increasing heart rate. This patient had other potential risk factors including substantial exposure to doxorubicin and concomitant cyclophosphamide.

The use of dolasetron mesylate is contraindicated in children and adolescents under 18 years of age and in adults for the prevention and treatment of post-operative nausea and vomiting (see Contraindications) as:

- acute electrocardiographic changes have occurred very commonly in pediatrics aged 2 to 18 years;
- individual cases of sustained supraventricular and ventricular arrhythmias, myocardial infarction and one case of fatal cardiac arrest have been reported in association with dolasetron in pediatrics. A causal relationship with dolasetron was suspected based on temporal association in all cases. Most of the cases of cardiovascular events occurred in adolescents. In all cases dolasetron was indicated for postoperative nausea and vomiting. They concerned mainly the I.V. route, and in one case oral administration.

Dolasetron (5-HT_3 receptor antagonist) should be administered with caution in patients who have or may develop prolongation of cardiac conduction intervals, particularly QTc, due to potential for additive effects. These include, also patients with AV block II-III, bundle branch block, patients receiving concomitant class I and III antiarrhythmics and patients with hypokalemia or hypomagnesemia, patients taking diuretics with potential for inducing electrolyte abnormalities, patients with congenital QT syndrome, patients taking anti-arrhythmic drugs or other drugs which lead to QT prolongation, and cumulative high dose anthracycline therapy. Interval prolongation could lead to cardiovascular consequences, including heart block or cardiac arrhythmias.

Because dolasetron affects cardiac conductivity, the recommended doses should not be exceeded.

Allergic Reactions: Cross hypersensitivity reactions have been reported in patients who have received other selective 5HT_3 receptor antagonists. It has not been seen with dolasetron.

PRECAUTIONS: Cardiovascular: **Dolasetron (5-HT_3 receptor antagonist) should be administered with caution in patients who have or may develop prolongation of cardiac conduction intervals, particularly QTc, due to potential for additive effects (see Warnings, ECG changes and cardiovascular events).**

Children (<18 years of age): See Contraindications.

Renal Impairment: Dosage adjustment is not necessary in mild to moderate renal impairment. However, dolasetron is not recommended in patients with severe renal impairment because of the possibility of prolonged QTc intervals and other cardiac conduction abnormalities from elevated hydrodolasetron levels.

Hepatic Impairment: Dosage adjustment is not necessary in mild to moderate hepatic impairment. The oral formulation of dolasetron is not recommended in patients with severe hepatic impairment because of the possibility of prolonged QTc intervals and other cardiac conduction abnormalities from elevated hydrodolasetron levels.

Pregnancy: There are no adequate and well-controlled studies in pregnant women. This drug is not recommended for use during pregnancy. Animal reproduction studies have shown no evidence of teratogenicity when dolasetron was administered throughout organogenesis.

Lactation: It is not known whether dolasetron is excreted in human milk. Dolasetron should not be administered to a nursing woman.

Geriatrics: Dosage adjustment is not needed in patients over 65.

Carcinogenicity: In a 24-month carcinogenicity study in CD-1 mice, there was a statistically significant (p=0.001) increase in the incidence of combined hepatocellular adenomas and carcinomas in male mice treated orally with 150 mg/kg/day dolasetron and above. No increase in liver tumors was observed at a dose of 75 mg/kg/day in male mice and at doses up to 300 mg/kg/day in female mice.

In a 24-month carcinogenicity study in Sprague-Dawley rats, oral dolasetron mesylate was not tumorigenic at doses up to 150 mg/kg/day in males and 300 mg/kg/day in females.

Drug Interactions: The potential for clinically significant drug-drug interactions posed by dolasetron and hydrodolasetron appears to be low for drugs commonly used in chemotherapy or surgery (see Warnings for information about potential interaction with other drugs that prolong QTc intervals). Blood levels of hydrodolasetron increased 24% when dolasetron was coadministered with cimetidine (nonselective inhibitor of cytochrome P450) for 7 days, and decreased 28% with coadministration of rifampin (potent inducer of cytochrome P450) for 7 days. Dolasetron injection has been safely coadministered with drugs used in chemotherapy and surgery. In patients taking furosemide, nifedipine, diltiazem, ACE inhibitors, verapamil, glyburide, propranolol, and various chemotherapy agents, no effect was shown on the clearance of hydrodolasetron. Clearance of hydrodolasetron decreased by about 27% when dolasetron was administered concomitantly with atenolol. Dolasetron does not influence anesthesia recovery time in patients. Dolasetron did not inhibit the antitumor activity of 4 chemotherapeutic agents (cisplatin, 5-fluorouracil, doxorubicin, cyclophosphamide) in 4 murine models.

ADVERSE EFFECTS: The safety of dolasetron has been evaluated in over 7000 patients in North American and European clinical trials. Dolasetron was well tolerated, with headache being the most frequently reported adverse event. The incidence of adverse events from pivotal controlled clinical trials is presented in Table 5 and Table 6.

Injection: In controlled and uncontrolled clinical trials, 2265 adult patients received dolasetron injection of which 731 patients were treated at the recommended therapeutic dose (1.8 mg/kg). The most frequently reported adverse events (≥2%) in patients receiving dolasetron injection are presented in Table 5. Patients were receiving chemotherapy (primarily cisplatin) and i.v. fluids. Adverse events were recorded for at least 24 hours following dolasetron injection administration.

Oral Administration: In controlled clinical trials, 943 patients received oral dolasetron of which 227 patients were treated at the recommended therapeutic dose (100 mg). These patients were receiving concurrent chemotherapy, predominantly cyclophosphamide and doxorubicin regimens. Table 6 lists adverse events occurring in ≥2% of patients in comparative clinical trials.

Table 5: Anzemet

Anzemet I.V. Adverse Events ≥2% in Chemotherapy-Induced Nausea and Vomiting

Event	Anzemet Injection 1.8 mg/kg (n=731)
Headache	188 (25.7%)
Diarrhea	93 (12.7%)
Fever	36 (4.9%)
Hepatic Function Abnormal[a]	28 (3.8%)
Fatigue	25 (3.4%)
Abdominal Pain	23 (3.1%)
Tachycardia	21 (2.9%)
Chills/Shivering	20 (2.7%)
Hypertension	20 (2.7%)
Extrasystoles	19 (2.6%)
Pain	18 (2.5%)
Dizziness	15 (2.1%)

[a] Includes events coded as AST- or ALT-increased.

Table 6: Anzemet

Oral Anzemet Adverse Events Occurring ≥ 2% in Chemotherapy-Induced Nausea and Vomiting Patients

	Anzemet 100 mg (n=227)
Headache	52 (22.9%)
Diarrhea	12 (5.3%)
Fatigue	13 (5.7%)
Bradycardia	9 (4.0%)
Pain	7 (3.1%)
Dizziness	7 (3.1%)
Tachycardia	6 (2.6%)
T Wave Change	6 (2.6%)
ST-T Wave Change	6 (2.6%)
Chills/Shivering	5 (2.2%)
Dyspepsia	5 (2.2%)

Less frequently occurring adverse events: Injection: In controlled and uncontrolled clinical trials the following adverse events occurred at a frequency of 0.3 to 2.0% in patients treated with dolasetron injection at the recommended dose (1.8 mg/kg):
Application Site: injection site pain.
Autonomic Nervous System: dry mouth, flushing.
Body as a Whole: malaise.
Cardiovascular (general): chest pain, edema, edema peripheral, fluid overload, hypotension.
Central and Peripheral Nervous Systems: drowsiness, paresthesia, tremor, vertigo.
Gastrointestinal: abdominal distention, anorexia, appetite increased, constipation, dyspepsia, flatulence, hiccup, nausea, stomatitis.
Hearing, Taste, and Vision: taste perversion.
Heart Rate and Rhythm: atrial arrhythmia, sinus arrhythmia, atrial flutter/fibrillation, first degree AV block, bradycardia, cardiac arrest, ECG abnormal specific, QT/QTc prolonged, ST-T wave change, T wave change.
Hematologic: bone marrow aplasia, epistaxis.
Musculoskeletal: myalgia.
Psychiatric: agitation, anxiety, confusion, sleep disorder.
Resistance Mechanism: sepsis.
Respiratory System: abnormal breath sounds, bronchospasm, cough, dyspnea, pneumonia, pulmonary congestion, throat irritation, upper respiratory congestion.
Skin and Appendages: facial edema, increased sweating.
Urinary System: urinary retention.
Oral Administration: In controlled clinical trials the following adverse events occurred at a frequency of 0.9 to 2.0% in patients treated with oral dolasetron at the recommended dose (100 mg):
Autonomic Nervous System: dry mouth, flushing.
Body as a Whole: fever.
Cardiovascular (general): dependent edema, hypotension.
Central and Peripheral Nervous Systems: drowsiness.
Gastrointestinal: abdominal pain, anorexia, increased appetite, constipation, eructation, flatulence, nausea.
Hearing, Taste, and Vision: taste perversion.
Heart Rate and Rhythm: atrial arrhythmia, sinus arrhythmia, extrasystoles.
Liver and Biliary System: AST increased.
Metabolic and Nutritional: dehydration.
Resistance Mechanism: influenza-like symptoms.
Respiratory System: dyspnea, nasal irritation, sneezing, throat irritation.
Postmarket Surveillance Injection: Cases of local pain and burning on i.v. administration have been observed. In very rare cases, severe hypotension, bradycardia and possibly loss of consciousness may occur immediately or closely following i.v. bolus administration of dolasetron. These events have occurred in patients receiving dolasetron for the prevention of cancer chemotherapy-induced nausea and vomiting.

Dolasetron has been shown to cause ECG prolongations, including QTc, PR and QRS intervals. These changes are related in magnitude and frequency to blood levels of the active metabolite; the changes are self-limiting with declining blood levels. Some patients have interval prolongation for 24 hours or longer. Interval prolongation could lead to cardiovascular consequences including heart block or cardiac arrhythmias. There are very rare reports of wide complex tachycardia or ventricular tachycardia and of ventricular fibrillation/cardiac arrest following intravenous administration.

Individual cases of sustained supraventricular and ventricular arrhythmias, myocardial infarction and one case of fatal cardiac arrest have been reported in association with dolasetron in pediatrics. A causal relationship with dolasetron was suspected based on temporal association in all cases. Most of the cases of cardiovascular events occurred in adolescents. In all cases dolasetron was indicated for postoperative nausea and vomiting. They concerned mainly the I.V. route, and in one case oral administration.

There are rare reports of anaphylactic/anaphylactoid reactions including skin reactions such as rash, puritus, and urticaria, respiratory reactions such as bronchospasm, very rare reports of facial edema/angioedema and shock.

OVERDOSE:

Symptoms: There have been reports of overdose. Severe hypotension, dizziness and prolongation of the PR, QRS and QTc intervals were reported after overdose intravenous infusion.

Single i.v. doses of dolasetron at 160 mg/kg in male mice and 140 mg/kg in female mice and rats of both sexes were lethal. Symptoms of acute toxicity were tremors, depression and convulsions.

Treatment: It is not known if dolasetron is removed by hemodialysis or peritoneal dialysis.

Following a suspected overdose of dolasetron, a patient found to have second-degree or higher AV conduction block should undergo cardiac telemetry monitoring.

There is no known specific antidote for dolasetron, and patients with suspected overdose should be managed with supportive therapy. Individual doses as large as 5 mg/kg i.v. or 400 mg orally have been safely given to healthy volunteers or cancer patients.

For management of a suspected drug overdose, CPhA recommends that you contact your **regional Poison Control Centre**. See the *CPS* Directory section for a list of Poison Control Centres.

DOSAGE: The following recommended doses should not be exceeded due to the effects on cardiac conductivity (see Warnings and Precautions).

Adults: Dolasetron is contraindicated for the prevention and treatment of post-operative nausea and vomiting in adults (see Contraindications).

I.V. Administration: The recommended i.v. dosage is 1.8 mg/kg given as a single dose approximately 30 minutes before chemotherapy. Most patients can be adequately treated with 100 mg. For light patients (<56 kg) or heavy patients (>90 kg), 1.8 mg/kg should be used.

The injection solution can be infused as rapidly as 100 mg over 30 seconds, or it can be diluted in a compatible i.v. solution such as normal saline or 5% dextrose to 50 mL and infused over 15 minutes. More rapid i.v. administration should be avoided (see Adverse Effects). Dolasetron should not be mixed with other drugs. Flush the infusion line before and after administration of dolasetron.

Oral Administration: The recommended oral dosage is one 100 mg tablet given within 1 hour prior to chemotherapy.
Children: Dolasetron is contraindicated for any therapeutic use in children and adolescents under 18 years of age (see Contraindications).
Geriatrics: It is not necessary to adjust the dose of dolasetron in elderly patients.
Hepatic Impairment: No dosage adjustment is necessary in mild to moderate hepatic impairment. However, oral dolasetron is not recommended in patients with severe hepatic impairment because of the possibility of prolonged QTc intervals and other cardiac conduction abnormalities from elevated hydrodolasetron levels.
Renal Impairment: No dosage adjustment is necessary in mild to moderate renal impairment. However, dolasetron is not recommended in patients with severe renal impairment because of the possibility of prolonged QTc intervals and other cardiac conduction abnormalities from elevated hydrodolasetron levels.
Parenteral Products: Administration of I.V. Infusion Solutions: Compatibility with I.V. Solutions: Dolasetron injection should only be admixed with the following recommended infusion fluids: 0.9% w/v Sodium Chloride Injection, 5% w/v Glucose Injection, 10% w/v Mannitol Injection, 0.45% w/v Sodium Chloride and 5% w/v Glucose Injection, Lactated Ringer's Injection, 5% w/v Glucose Injection and Lactated Ringer's Injection.

Dolasetron is compatible with polypropylene syringes, i.v. bags, and associated tubing.

Compatibility with Other Drugs: Dolasetron should not be mixed with other drugs. Flush the infusion line before and after administration of dolasetron.

Anzemet injection at a 4 mg/mL concentration has been determined to be physically incompatible with the following drugs when administered through the same i.v. line: carmustine, 5-fluorouracil, acyclovir sodium, ampicillin sodium, cefazolin sodium, chloramphenicol sodium succinate, clindamycin phosphate, dexamethasone sodium phosphate, methylprednisolone sodium succinate, trimethoprim with sulfamethoxazole, aminophylline, amphotericin B, heparin sodium, potassium phosphate and sodium bicarbonate. Anzemet injection at a concentration of 20 mg/mL is physically incompatible with thiopental sodium.

Note: As with all parenteral drug products, i.v. admixtures should be inspected visually for clarity, particulate matter, precipitate, discoloration and leakage prior to administration, whenever solution and container permit. Solutions showing haziness, particulate matter, precipitate, discoloration or leakage should not be used.

Dilution: To prepare dolasetron injection for i.v. infusion, aseptically transfer the appropriate amount of dolasetron injection to the desired volume of infusion fluid. See Table 7.

Table 7: Anzemet

Dilution

Diluent Volume	Quantity of Anzemet Injection	Final Concentration	Administration[a]	
			Dose	Infusion Rate
50 mL	50 mg (2.5 mL)	0.95 mg/mL	50 mg/15 min	53 mL/15 min
50 mL	100 mg (5 mL)	1.82 mg/mL	100 mg/15 min	55 mL/15 min

[a] Anzemet Injection can also be injected over 30 seconds.

Stability and Storage of Diluted Solutions: Dilutions of i.v. fluids should be used immediately after preparation or stored for no more than 24 hours at 2 to 8°C.

INFORMATION FOR THE PATIENT: Published in e-CPS, available by subscription at www.e-cps.ca.

SUPPLIED: Injection: Each mL of clear, colorless, sterile, nonpyrogenic solution for i.v. injection contains: dolasetron mesylate monohydrate 20 mg. Nonmedicinal ingredients: glacial acetic acid, mannitol and sodium acetate trihydrate. pH: 3.2 to 3.8. Clear glass vials of 5 mL.

Tablets: 50 mg: Each pale pink, round, film-coated tablet, printed "50" in the center of the tablet and "A" on the other side, contains: dolasetron mesylate monohydrate 50 mg. Nonmedicinal ingredients: carnauba wax, croscarmellose sodium, hydroxypropyl methylcellulose, lactose, magnesium stearate, polyethylene glycol, polysorbate 80, pregelatinized starch, iron oxide, titanium dioxide and white wax. Bottles of 15.

100 mg: Each pink, oval, film-coated tablet, printed with "ANZEMET" on one side and "100" on the other, contains: dolasetron mesylate monohydrate 100 mg. Nonmedicinal ingredients: carnauba wax, croscarmellose sodium, hydroxypropyl methylcellulose, lactose, magnesium stearate, polyethylene glycol, polysorbate 80, pregelatinized starch, iron oxide, titanium dioxide and white wax. Bottles of 15.

Store at 15 to 30°C and protect from light.

(Shown in Product Identification Section)

Apidra®

insulin glulisine (rDNA origin)

Antidiabetic—Short-acting Recombinant Human Insulin Analogue

sanofi-aventis

Date of Revision: June 8, 2010

SUMMARY PRODUCT INFORMATION:

Route of Administration	Dosage Form/ Strength	Clinically Relevant Nonmedicinal Ingredients
Subcutaneous	Solution for injection 100 U/mL	m-cresol, trometamol, sodium chloride, polysorbate 20, water for injection, hydrochloric acid and sodium hydroxide (for pH adjustment) For a complete listing see Dosage Forms, Composition and Packaging.

DESCRIPTION: APIDRA [insulin glulisine (rDNA origin)] is a recombinant human insulin analogue that is a rapid-acting, parenteral blood glucose-lowering agent. Insulin glulisine is produced by recombinant DNA technology utilizing a non-pathogenic laboratory strain of *E. coli* (K12).

Insulin glulisine differs from human insulin* in that the amino acid asparagine at position B3 is replaced by lysine and the lysine in position B29 is replaced by glutamic acid.

INDICATIONS AND CLINICAL USE: APIDRA [insulin glulisine (rDNA origin)] is a recombinant human insulin analogue indicated for:

- the treatment of adult patients with diabetes mellitus where treatment with insulin is required.
- the treatment of pediatric patients with type 1 diabetes mellitus who require a short acting insulin. There is insufficient clinical data on the use of APIDRA in children below the age of 6 years (see Warnings and Precautions, Special Populations, Pediatrics).

APIDRA has a more rapid onset of action and a shorter duration of action than regular human insulin. APIDRA should normally be used in regimens that include a longer-acting insulin or basal insulin analogue to maintain adequate glucose control (see Dosage and Administration). APIDRA can be used with oral hypoglycemic agents.

CONTRAINDICATIONS:

- Patients who are hypersensitive to this drug or to any ingredient in the formulation or component of the container. For a complete listing, see Dosage Forms, Composition and Packaging.

WARNINGS AND PRECAUTIONS: General: APIDRA differs from regular human insulin by its rapid onset of action and shorter duration of action. When used as a meal time insulin, the dose of APIDRA should be given within 15 minutes before or within 20 minutes after starting a meal.

Because of the short duration of action of APIDRA, patients with diabetes also require a longer-acting insulin or insulin infusion pump therapy to maintain adequate glucose control.

Hypoglycemia may occur if the insulin dose is too high in relation to the insulin requirement (see Hypoglycemia). The use of too low insulin dosages or discontinuation of treatment, especially in Type 1 diabetes, may lead to hyperglycemia and diabetic ketoacidosis. Uncorrected hypoglycemic or hyperglycemic reactions can cause loss of consciousness, coma, or death.

Any change of insulin should be made cautiously and only under medical supervision. As with other insulins, additional caution should be exercised in patients with a long history of diabetes on insulin who might be prone to develop hypoglycemia and in patients with a previous history of cardiac ischemic disorders who might be prone to develop cardiac adverse events. Changes in insulin strength, manufacturer, type (e.g. regular, NPH, or insulin analogues), or species (animal, human), or method of manufacture (recombinant DNA versus animal-source insulin) may result in the need for a change in dosage. Concomitant oral antidiabetic treatment may need to be adjusted.

As with all insulin preparations, the time course of APIDRA action may vary in different individuals or at different times in the same individual and is dependent on site of injection, blood supply, temperature, and physical activity. Adjustment of dosage of any insulin may be necessary if patients change their physical activity or their usual meal plan.

Glucose monitoring is recommended for all patients with diabetes.

Thiazolidinediones (TZDs), alone or in combination with other antidiabetic agents (including insulin), can cause heart failure and edema. The combination of TZD with insulin is not indicated for the treatment of Type 2 Diabetes Mellitus. Please refer to the respective TZD product monograph Warnings and Precautions information when the use of these drugs in combination with any insulin, including APIDRA, is contemplated.

Hepatic/Biliary/Pancreatic: Studies have not been performed in patients with hepatic impairment. APIDRA requirements may be diminished due to reduced capacity for gluconeogenesis and reduced insulin metabolism, similar to observations found with other insulins (see Action and Clinical Pharmacology).

Hypoglycemia: As with all insulin preparations, hypoglycemic reactions may be associated with the administration of APIDRA. Use caution in patients with hypoglycemia unawareness and in patients who may be predisposed to hypoglycemia (e.g., the pediatric population and patients who fast or have erratic food intake). Early warning symptoms of hypoglycemia may be different, be less pronounced or absent, under certain conditions, as for example if glycemic control is markedly improved, if hypoglycemia is developing gradually, in elderly patients, in patients with a long history of diabetes, in patients with diabetic nerve disease, in patients using some medications such as beta-blockers, or intensified diabetes control (see Drug Interactions). Such situations may result in severe hypoglycemia (and possibly, loss of consciousness) prior to patients' awareness of hypoglycemia.

Severe hypoglycemia may require the assistance of another person. Patients who are unable to take sugar orally or who are unconscious may require an intramuscular/subcutaneous injection of glucagon or should be treated with intravenous administration of glucose by medical personnel. Without immediate medical help, serious reactions or even death could occur.

Hypoglycemia is the most common adverse effect of insulin therapy, including APIDRA. As with all insulins, the timing of hypoglycemia may differ among various insulin formulations.

The time of occurrence of hypoglycemia depends on the action profile of the insulins used and may, therefore, change when treatment regimen is changed.

Intercurrent Conditions: Insulin requirements may be altered during illness, emotional disturbances or stress.

Insulin Pumps: When used in an external insulin pump for subcutaneous infusion, APIDRA SHOULD NOT be mixed with any other insulin or diluted with any other solution. Patients using external pump infusion therapy should be trained appropriately. Physicians and patients should carefully evaluate information on pump use in the APIDRA product monograph, package insert, and the pump manufacturer's manual.

APIDRA specific information should be followed for period of use, frequency of changing infusion sets, or other details specific to APIDRA usage, because APIDRA specific information may differ from general or other insulin's pump manual instructions. Pump or infusion set malfunctions or insulin degradation can lead to hyperglycemia and ketosis in a short time. This is especially pertinent for rapid-acting insulin analogues that are more rapidly absorbed and have a shorter duration of action. Prompt identification and correction of the cause of hyperglycemia or ketosis is necessary. Interim therapy with subcutaneous injection may be required (see Dosage and Administration, Continuous Subcutaneous Insulin Infusion Pump, Information for the Patient, Vials, Continuous Subcutaneous Insulin Infusion Pump, Storage and Stability).

Renal: The pharmacokinetic properties of APIDRA were generally maintained in subjects with renal impairment. However, as with all insulins, the requirements for APIDRA may be reduced in patients with renal impairment (see Action and Clinical Pharmacology).

Special Populations: Pregnant Women: There are no well-controlled clinical studies of the use of APIDRA in pregnant women. Animal reproduction studies have not revealed any differences between APIDRA and human insulin regarding pregnancy, embryonal/foetal development, parturition or postnatal development.

It is essential for patients with pre-existing or gestational diabetes to maintain good metabolic control before conception and during pregnancy. Insulin requirements may decrease during the first trimester and generally increase during the second and third trimesters. Immediately after delivery, insulin requirements decline rapidly.

Careful monitoring of glucose control is essential.

* In some studies regular human insulin refers to short acting insulin marketed internationally.

Patients with diabetes must inform their doctor if they are pregnant or are contemplating pregnancy.

Nursing Women: It is unknown whether APIDRA is excreted in human milk. Many drugs including human insulin, are excreted in human milk. For this reason, caution should be exercised when APIDRA is administered to a nursing woman. Lactating women may require adjustments in insulin dose and diet.

Pediatrics: The safety and effectiveness of APIDRA have been investigated in pediatric patients (age 4 to 17 years) with Type 1 diabetes [9(1.6%) <6 years, 32 (5.6%) between 6 and 8 years, 149 (26%) between 8 and 12 years, and 382 (67%) above 12 years old]. APIDRA has not been studied in pediatric patients younger than 4 years of age. There is insufficient clinical data on the use of APIDRA in children below the age of 6 years.

As in adults, the dosage of APIDRA must be individualized in pediatric patients based on metabolic needs and frequent monitoring of blood glucose.

Geriatrics (≥65 years of age): Hypoglycemia may be difficult to recognize in the elderly. In Phase III clinical trials (n=2408), APIDRA was administered to 147 patients ≥65 years of age and 27 patients ≥75 years of age. The majority of these were patients with Type 2 diabetes. The change in glycated hemoglobin (A1c) values and hypoglycemia frequencies did not differ by age, but greater sensitivity of some older individuals cannot be ruled out.

Occupational Hazards: The patient's ability to concentrate and react may be impaired as a result of hypoglycemia or hyperglycemia or, for example, as a result of visual impairment. This may constitute a risk in situations where these abilities are of special importance (e.g. driving a car or operating machinery).

Patients should be advised to take precautions to avoid hypoglycemia whilst driving. This is particularly important in those who have reduced or absent awareness of the warning symptoms of hypoglycemia or have frequent episodes of hypoglycemia. It should be considered whether it is advisable to drive or operate machinery in these circumstances.

ADVERSE REACTIONS: Adverse Drug Reaction Overview: Overall, clinical studies comparing APIDRA with short-acting insulins did not demonstrate a difference in frequency of adverse events.

Adverse events commonly associated with human insulin therapy include the following:

Body as a Whole: Local Allergy: As with other insulin therapy, local allergy in patient may occur as redness, itching, swelling, or hemorrhage. These minor reactions usually resolve in a few days to a few weeks. In some instances, these reactions may be related to factors other than insulin, such as irritants in a skin cleansing agent or poor injection technique.

Systemic Allergy: Less common, but potentially more serious, is generalized allergy to insulin, which may cause rash (including pruritus) over the whole body, shortness of breath, wheezing, reduction in blood pressure, rapid pulse, or sweating. Severe cases of generalized allergy, including anaphylactic reactions, may be life threatening.

Localized reactions and generalized myalgias have been reported with the use of m-cresol as an injectable excipient.

Hypoglycemia: Hypoglycemia, a frequent adverse reaction to insulin therapy, may occur if the insulin dose is too high in relation to the insulin requirement.

As with all insulins, prolonged or severe hypoglycemic attacks, especially if recurrent, may lead to neurological damage, loss of consciousness, coma or death.

The risk of all categories of symptomatic hypoglycemia did not differ between APIDRA and short-acting insulin comparators in subjects with type 1 or type 2 diabetes (see Warnings and Precautions and Table 1).

Table 1: APIDRA

Number of Subjects with at Least One Episode of Symptomatic Hypoglycemia in Studies in Adults with Type 1 and Type 2 Diabetes

	Type 1 Diabetes				Type 2 Diabetes			
	Glulisine		Comparator[a]		Glulisine		Comparator[b]	
	n/N	%	n/N	%	n/N	%	n/N	%
Subcutaneous Injection	783/921	85.0	516/611	84.5	562/883	63.6	578/833	65.5
Continuous[c] Subcutaneous Infusion	26/29	89.7	24/30	80.0	—	—	—	—

a Insulin lispro, regular human insulin.
b Regular human insulin.
c Insulin aspart.
Legend: n=number of subjects with at least 1 episode of hypoglycemia; N=total number of evaluable ITT subjects.

Table 2: APIDRA

Number (percentage) of Pediatric Subjects with Type 1 Diabetes with All Symptomatic Hypoglycemia

	Glulisine			Lispro		
	n/N	(%)	Number of Episodes	n/N	(%)	Number of Episodes
Screening/run-in phase	198/277	(71.5)	1269	213/295	(72.2)	1144
Month 1	195/277	(70.4)	1212	184/295	(62.4)	973
Month 2	125/274	(45.6)	781	125/295	(42.4)	756
Month 3	158/270	(58.5)	864	168/292	(57.5)	870
Month 4—treatment end	199/268	(74.3)	2686	199/291	(68.4)	2747
Entire treatment phase	230/277	(83.0)	5543	238/295	(80.7)	5346

Legend: n=number of subjects reporting at least one episode of symptomatic hypoglycemia; N=number of randomized and treated subjects evaluable.

In pediatric subjects with type 1 diabetes, the overall incidence of symptomatic hypoglycaemia was comparable between the treatment groups (83% for insulin glulisine vs. 81% for insulin lispro). However, there was a significant difference between treatment groups during the first month of treatment in the frequency (70.4% in the insulin glulisine group, 62.4% in the insulin lispro group, p=0.0330) and in the monthly rate (4.77 vs. 3.59 respectively, p=0.0094) of symptomatic hypoglycemia. For nocturnal symptomatic hypoglycemia, a difference was noted between the two treatment groups in the frequency and monthly rate per subject, with a higher frequency (39.7% vs. 30.5%) and more events (0.25 vs. 0.19) reported in the insulin glulisine group. The difference was especially notable in the first month of treatment (frequency (19.9% vs. 11.2%) and events (0.41 vs 0.23)), when all subjects had been randomized following a 4-week of run-in period with individualized dose adjustment of insulin lispro. The incidence of severe symptomatic hypoglycemia and the incidence of severe nocturnal symptomatic hypoglycemia were comparable between the treatment groups.

Skin and Appendages: As with other insulin therapy, lipodystrophy may occur at the injection site and delay insulin absorption. Continuous rotation of the injection site within a given area may help to reduce or prevent these reactions.

Weight Gain: Weight gain can occur with insulin therapy, including APIDRA, and has been attributed to the anabolic effects of insulin and the decrease in glucosuria.

Clinical Trial Adverse Drug Reactions: Because clinical trials are conducted under very specific conditions the adverse reaction rates observed in the clinical trials may not reflect the rates observed in practice and should not be compared to the rates in the clinical trials of another drug. Adverse drug reaction information from clinical trials is useful for identifying drug-related adverse events and for approximating rates. See Table 3.

Table 3: APIDRA
Common (≥1%) Adverse Drug Reactions in Pooled Adult Type 1 and 2 Studies

Adverse Event System Organ Class/Preferred Term	Insulin Glulisine (all studies) n=1833 (% of subjects)	Lispro n=333 (% of subjects)	Regular Insulin n=1161 (% of subjects)	Aspart n=30 (% of subjects)
General Disorders and Administration Site Condition				
Injection site hypertrophy	9 (0.5)	7 (2.1)	— (—)	— (—)
Metabolism and Nutrition Disorders				
Hypoglycemia NOS[a]	83 (4.5)	22 (6.6)	33 (2.8)	2 (6.7)
Hypoglycemic seizure	16 (0.9)	7 (2.1)	9 (0.8)	— (—)
Hypoglycemic unawareness	1 (0.1)	4 (1.2)	— (—)	2 (6.7)
Nervous System Disorders				
Hypoglycemic coma	49 (2.7)	13 (3.9)	19 (1.6)	— (—)

[a] Not otherwise specified.

Table 4 summarizes the adverse reactions occurring with frequency higher than 1% in a clinical study in children and adolescents with type 1 diabetes treated with insulin glulisine (n=277) or insulin lispro.

Table 4: APIDRA
Common (≥1%) Adverse Drug Reactions in Children and Adolescents with Type 1 Diabetes

Adverse Event System Organ Class/Preferred Term	Insulin Glulisine n=277 (% of subjects)	Lispro n=295 (% of subjects)
General Disorders and Administration Site Condition		
Injection site hypertrophy	3 (1.1)	1 (0.3)
Metabolism and Nutrition Disorders		
Hypoglycemia NOS[a]	6 (2.2)	7 (2.4)
Hypoglycemic seizure	17 (6.1)	14 (4.7)
Nervous System Disorders		
Hypoglycemic coma	1 (0.4)	3 (1.0)

[a] Not otherwise specified.

During clinical studies, there were no clinically noteworthy differences between insulin glulisine and comparator short-acting insulins in the overall incidences of adverse events. The adverse events observed were those known in this pharmacological class and consequently common to insulins.

Less Common Clinical Trial Adverse Drug Reactions (<1%): Gastrointestinal Disorders: nausea.
General Disorders Administration Site Conditions: fatigue, injection site reaction NOS†, peripheral oedema, asthenia, increased fat tissue, injection site stinging.
Infections and Infestations: cellulitis.
Injury, Poisoning and Procedural (complications): overdose NOS.†
Metabolism and Nutrition Disorders: hyperglycemia NOS.†
Nervous System Disorders: paraesthesia.
Skin and Subcutaneous Tissue Disorders: acquired lipodystrophy.
Post-Market Adverse Drug Reactions: Other: Medication errors have been reported in which other insulins, particularly long-acting insulins, have been accidentally administered instead of insulin glulisine.
DRUG INTERACTIONS: Overview: Drug-Drug Interactions: The following are examples of potential drug-drug interactions that may occur with APIDRA treatment: see Table 5.
Drug-Food Interactions: Interactions with food have not been established.
Drug-Herb Interactions: Interactions with herbal products have not been established.
Drug-Laboratory Test Interactions: Interactions with laboratory tests have not been established.

DOSAGE AND ADMINISTRATION: Dosing Considerations: The dosage of APIDRA should be individualized and determined based on the physician's advice in accordance with the needs of the patient.

APIDRA [insulin glulisine (rDNA origin)] is a recombinant human insulin analogue that has been shown to be equipotent to human insulin. One unit of APIDRA has the same glucose-lowering effect as one unit of regular human insulin. After subcutaneous administration it has a more rapid onset and a shorter duration of action (see Action and Clinical Pharmacology).

APIDRA should be given by injection within 15 minutes before or within 20 minutes after starting a meal. APIDRA should normally be used in regimens that include a longer-acting insulin or basal insulin analogue.

APIDRA is intended for subcutaneous administration by injection and for use as a continuous subcutaneous insulin infusion (CSII) in pump systems suitable for insulin infusion.

APIDRA should be administered by subcutaneous injection in the abdominal wall, the thigh, the buttock or the deltoid or by continuous subcutaneous infusion (CSII) in the abdominal wall. As with all insulins, injection sites and infusion sites within an injection area (abdomen, thigh, buttock or deltoid) should be rotated from one injection to the next.

As for all insulins, the rate of absorption, and consequently the onset and duration of action, may be affected by injection site, exercise and other variables. Blood glucose monitoring is recommended for all patients with diabetes.

Administration: Preparation and Handling: APIDRA must only be used if the solution is clear, colourless, with no solid particles visible, and if it is of a water-like consistency. To minimize local irritation at the injection site, it is recommended to allow the insulin to reach room temperature before injection.

The instructions for using the APIDRA in a pump or with an injection pen must be followed carefully.

An empty vial, cartridge, or SoloSTAR must never be reused and must be properly discarded.

Vials: Before withdrawing insulin from the vial for the first time, remove the plastic protective cap.

Do not shake the vial vigorously as this may cause frothing. Froth may interfere with the correct measurement of the dose.

Mixing of Insulins: APIDRA can be mixed with NPH human insulin (except when administered with pump (see Dosage and Administration, Continuous Subcutaneous Insulin Infusion Pump)).

If APIDRA is mixed with NPH human insulin, APIDRA should be drawn into the syringe first. Injection should be made immediately after mixing.

† Not otherwise specified.

No data are available on mixing APIDRA with insulin preparations other than NPH human insulin.

Mixtures should not be administered intravenously.

Cartridges or SoloSTAR: APIDRA cartridges or APIDRA SoloSTAR are not designed to allow any other insulin to be mixed in the cartridge.

If the injection pen malfunctions, the solution may be drawn from the cartridge into a syringe (suitable for an insulin with U-100) and injected.

Table 5: APIDRA
Established or Potential Drug-Drug Interactions

Proper Name	Ref	Effect	Clinical Comment
Oral antidiabetic agents ACE inhibitors Disopyramide Fibrates Fluoxetine MAO inhibitors Pentoxifylline Propoxyphene Salicylates Sulfonamide antibiotics	Theoretical	May enhance the blood-glucose-lowering effect and increase susceptibility to hypoglycemia	May require close monitoring of blood glucose level and dose adjustment (reduction) of APIDRA
Corticosteroids Danazol Diazoxide Diuretics Glucagon Isoniazid Estrogens and progestogens (e.g. in oral contraceptives) Phenothiazine derivatives Somatropin Sympathomimetic agents (e.g. epinephrine, salbutamol, terbutaline) Protease inhibitors Atypical antipsychotic medications (e.g. olanzapine and clozapine)	Theoretical	May reduce the blood-glucose-lowering effect. May enhance or decrease the insulin requirements	May require close monitoring of blood glucose level and dose adjustment (increase or decrease) of APIDRA
Thyroid hormones	Theoretical	May enhance or decrease the insulin requirements	May require close monitoring of blood glucose level and dose adjustment (increase or decrease) of APIDRA
Alcohol Beta-blockers Clonidine Lithium salts	Theoretical	May either potentiate or weaken the blood-glucose-lowering effect of insulin	May require close monitoring of blood glucose level and dose adjustment (increase or decrease) of APIDRA
Pentamidine	Theoretical	May cause hypoglycemia, which may sometimes be followed by hyperglycemia	May require close monitoring of blood glucose level and dose adjustment (increase or decrease) of APIDRA
Sympatholytic medicinal products such as beta-blockers, clonidine, guanethidine and reserpine	Theoretical	The signs of hypoglycemia may be reduced or absent	May require close monitoring of blood glucose level and dosage adjustment (increase or decrease) of APIDRA

Continuous Subcutaneous Insulin Infusion Pump: APIDRA may be used for Continuous Subcutaneous Insulin Infusion (CSII) in pump systems suitable for insulin infusion.

When used with an insulin infusion pump, APIDRA should not be mixed with any other insulin or diluted with any other solution.

Patients using CSII should be comprehensively instructed on the use of the system pump. The infusion set and reservoir should be changed every 48 hours using aseptic technique.

Patients administering APIDRA by CSII must have an alternative insulin delivery system available in case of pump system failure.

OVERDOSAGE:
Hypoglycemia may occur as a result of an excess of insulin relative to food intake, energy exposure or both.

Mild/moderate episodes of hypoglycemia can usually be treated with oral carbohydrates. Adjustments in dosage of the medicinal product, meal patterns, or physical activity may be needed.

Severe episodes with coma, seizure, or neurologic impairment may be treated with intramuscular/subcutaneous glucagon or concentrated intravenous glucose.

Sustained carbohydrate intake and observation may be necessary because hypoglycemia may recur after apparent clinical recovery.

> For management of a suspected drug overdose, contact your regional Poison Control Centre. See the *CPS* Directory section for a list of Poison Control Centres.

ACTION AND CLINICAL PHARMACOLOGY: Pharmacodynamics: The primary activity of insulins and insulin analogues, including insulin glulisine, is regulation of glucose metabolism. Insulins lower blood glucose levels by stimulating peripheral glucose uptake by skeletal muscle and fat, and by inhibiting hepatic glucose production. Insulins inhibit lipolysis in the adipocyte, inhibit proteolysis, and enhance protein synthesis.

The glucose lowering activities of APIDRA and of regular human insulin are equipotent when administered by the intravenous route.

After subcutaneous administration the effect of APIDRA is more rapid in onset and of shorter duration compared to regular human insulin. This has been demonstrated in studies in healthy volunteers and patients with diabetes.

In a study in patients with Type 1 diabetes (n=20), the glucose-lowering profiles of APIDRA and regular human insulin were assessed at various times in relation to a standard meal at a dose of 0.15 U/kg (see Figure 1).

Glucose-lowering Effect Over 6 Hours: See Figure 1.

APIDRA given 2 minutes (glulisine-pre) before the start of a meal compared to regular human insulin given 30 minutes (Regular-30 min) before start of the meal (Figure 1) and compared to regular human insulin (Regular-pre) given 2 minutes before a meal (Figure 2). APIDRA given 15 minutes (glulisine-post) after start of a meal compared to regular human insulin (Regular-pre) given 2 minutes before a meal (Figure 3). On the x-axis zero (0) is the start of a 15-minute meal.

Figure 1: APIDRA

Glucose-lowering Effect Over 6 Hours

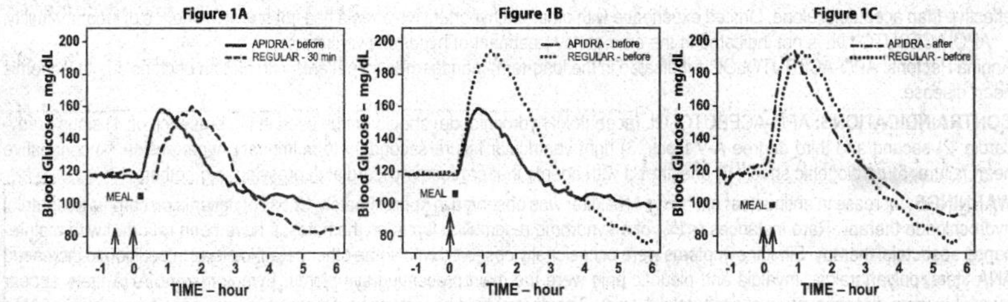

Legend: ↑=Injection time Regular Human Insulin; ↑=Injection time APIDRA.

Pharmacokinetics: APIDRA exhibits dose-proportionality in insulin exposure and less than dose-proportional increases in effect, as common to short and rapid acting insulins. See Table 6.

Table 6: APIDRA

Pharmacokinetic and Pharmacodynamic Results in Type 1 Diabetes Mellitus Subjects Treated with S.C. Insulin Glulisine

	Pharmacokinetic Parameters		
Dose	0.075 U/kg	0.15 U/kg	0.3 U/kg
$AUC_{0\text{-}2h}$ (μU.min.mL⁻¹)	**3792** 3855±677	**6676** 6832±1461	**12 992** 13 237±2599
$AUC_{0\text{-}end}$ (μU.min.mL⁻¹)	**5341** 5372±589	**11 196** 11 284±1456	**24 891** 25 076±3209
C_{max} (μU.mL⁻¹)	**42** 43±9	**72** 73±16	**140** 142±25
MRT (min)	**115** 122±50	**121** 125±34	**134** 136±28
T_{max} Min (*)	47 34–99	57 44–93	72 50–112
$T_{10\%\text{-}AUC}$ Min (*)	26 18–53	31 24–52	39 28–64
$T_{90\%\text{-}AUC}$ Min (*)	149 116–260	205 141–295	242 169–345
$T_{½}$ (min)	64±33	55±17	56±17
Volume of Distribution (mL/kg)	1075±362	986±274	930±216
	Glucose Infusion Rate—Pharmacodynamic Parameters		
$GIR\text{-}AUC_{(0\text{-}2h)}$ (mg/kg)	314±156	491±167	536±153
$GIR\text{-}AUC_{(0\text{-}end)}$ (mg/kg)	499±233	1090±271	1476±300

Values in bold font represent the geometric means, all others are based on the mean & standard deviation, unless denoted with (*) to indicate the median, minimum & maximum range.

Table 7 compares pharmacokinetic and pharmacodynamic parameters for APIDRA (s.c.) from a study in patients with Type I diabetes (n=18) with historical data for Huminsulin Normal 100 (s.c.) from a study in healthy adult subjects (n=24; see Table 7).

Table 7: APIDRA

Pharmacokinetic and Pharmacodynamic Results for S.C. APIDRA and Huminsulin Normal 100

	APIDRA (N=18)[b]	Huminsulin Normal 100[a] (N=24)[c]
Dose	0.3 U/kg	0.3 IU/kg
	Pharmacokinetic Parameters	
$AUC_{0\text{-}end}$ (μU.min.mL⁻¹)	25 076±3209	17 417±2348
C_{max} (μU.mL⁻¹)	142±25	56±16
MRT (min)	136±28	229±41
T_{max} Min (*)	72 50–112	120 60–240
$T_{10\%\text{-}AUC}$ Min (*)	39 28–64	58 45–81
$T_{90\%\text{-}AUC}$ Min (*)	242 169–345	448 321–590
$T_{1/2}$ (min)	56±17	64±28[d]
Volume of Distribution (mL/kg)	930±216	2375±963
	Glucose Infusion Rate—Pharmacodynamic Parameter	

(cont'd)

Table 7: APIDRA *(cont'd)*

Pharmacokinetic and Pharmacodynamic Results for S.C. APIDRA and Huminsulin Normal 100

	APIDRA (N=18)[b]	Huminsulin Normal 100[a] (N=24)[c]
$GIR\text{-}AUC_{(0\text{-}end)}$ (mg/kg)	1476±300	3032±743

[a] Historical data and different radioimmunoassay from APIDRA study.
[b] Type 1 Diabetes patients.
[c] Healthy adult subjects.
[d] N=23.
Values represent mean and standard deviation, unless denoted with (*) to indicate the median, minimum & maximum range.

Absorption and Bioavailability: Pharmacokinetic profiles in healthy volunteers and diabetes patients (Type 1 or 2) demonstrated that absorption of insulin glulisine was up to twice as fast with a peak concentration approximately up to twice as high compared to regular human insulin.

In a study in patients with type 1 diabetes (n=20) after subcutaneous administration of 0.15 U/kg, the median time to maximum concentration (T_{max}) was 55 minutes (range 34 to 91 minutes) and the peak concentration (C_{max}) was 82 μU/mL (range 42 to 134 μU/mL) for insulin glulisine compared to a median T_{max} of 82 minutes (range 52 to 308 minutes) and a C_{max} of 46 μIU/mL (range 32 to 70 μIU/mL) for regular human insulin. The mean residence time of insulin glulisine was shorter (median: 98 minutes, range 55 to 149 minutes) than for regular human insulin (median: 161 minutes, range 133 to 193 minutes). (See Figure 2.)

Figure 2: APIDRA

Pharmacokinetic Profile of Insulin Glulisine and Regular Human Insulin in Patients with Type 1 Diabetes After a Dose of 0.15 U/kg

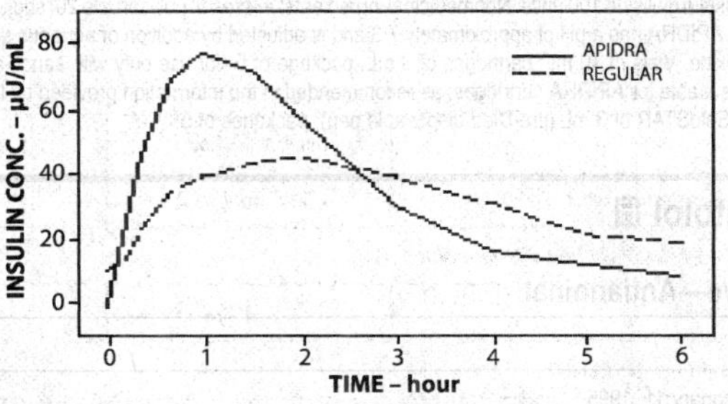

When APIDRA was injected subcutaneously into different areas of the body, the time-concentration profiles were similar with a slightly faster absorption when administered in the abdomen compared to the deltoid or thigh. (See Dosage and Administration.) The absolute bioavailability of insulin glulisine after subcutaneous administration is about 70%, regardless of injection area (abdomen 73%, deltoid 71%, thigh 68%). The T_{max} for the abdomen was 44 min (range 27-69 min); 58 min for the deltoid (range 30-85 min), and 66 min for the thigh (range 35-108 min).

Distribution and Excretion: The distribution and elimination of insulin glulisine and regular human insulin after intravenous administration are similar with volumes of distribution of 13 L and 21 L and half lives of 13 and 17 minutes, respectively. After subcutaneous administration, insulin glulisine is eliminated more rapidly than regular human insulin with an apparent half life of 42 minutes compared to 86 minutes.

Special Populations and Conditions: Pediatrics: The pharmacokinetic and pharmacodynamic properties of insulin glulisine and regular human insulin were assessed in a study conducted in pediatric patients with Type 1 diabetes (children [7-11 years, n=10] and adolescents [12-16 years, n=10]). The relative differences in pharmacokinetics and pharmacodynamics between insulin glulisine and regular human insulin in pediatric patients with Type 1 diabetes were similar to those in healthy adult subjects and adults with Type 1 diabetes.

Gender: Information on the effect of gender on the pharmacokinetics of insulin glulisine is not available. However, in Phase III clinical trials in adults (n=2408), subgroup analyses based on gender did not show differences in safety and efficacy between insulin glulisine and other short-acting insulin formulations.

Race: Information on the effect of race on the pharmacokinetics of insulin glulisine is not available.

Hepatic Insufficiency: The effect of hepatic impairment on the pharmacokinetics of insulin glulisine has not been studied. However, some studies with human insulin have shown increased circulating levels of insulin in patients with liver failure (see Warnings and Precautions).

Renal Insufficiency: Studies with human insulin have shown increased circulating levels of insulin in patients with renal failure. In a study performed in 24 non-diabetic subjects covering a wide range of renal function (CrCl >80 mL/min; 30-50 mL/min; <30 mL/min), the pharmacokinetic properties of insulin glulisine were generally maintained (see Warnings and Precautions).

Pregnancy: The effect of pregnancy on the pharmacokinetics and pharmacodynamics of insulin glulisine has not been studied.

Lactation: It is unknown whether APIDRA is excreted in human milk.

Obesity: The more rapid onset of action and shorter duration of activity of insulin glulisine and insulin lispro compared to regular human insulin were maintained in an obese non-diabetic population. The rapid onset of action was better maintained with insulin glulisine than with insulin lispro (see Figure 3).

Figure 3: APIDRA

Glucose Infusion Rates (GIR) After Subcutaneous Injection of 0.3 U/kg of APIDRA (Glulisine), Insulin Lispro or Regular Human Insulin in an Obese Population

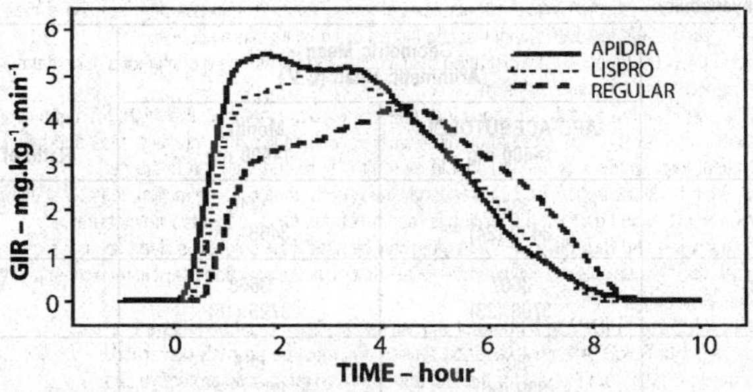

STORAGE AND STABILITY: Vials: Unopened Vial: Unopened APIDRA vials should be stored in a refrigerator, between 2-8°C. Keep APIDRA away from direct heat and light. APIDRA should not be stored in the freezer and it should not be allowed to freeze. If APIDRA freezes or overheats, discard it.

Opened (In Use) Vial: The opened vial can be kept refrigerated or unrefrigerated (15-25°C) for up to 28 days away from direct heat and light, as long as the temperature is not greater than 25°C. Opened APIDRA vials, whether or not refrigerated, must be discarded after 28 days even if they contain insulin.

Opened APIDRA vials should not be stored in the freezer and should not be allowed to freeze. If a vial freezes or overheats, discard it.

Cartridges: Unopened Cartridge: Unopened APIDRA cartridges should be stored in a refrigerator, between 2-8°C. Keep APIDRA away from direct heat and light. APIDRA should not be stored in the freezer and it should not be allowed to freeze. If APIDRA freezes or overheats, discard it.
Opened (In Use) Cartridge: The opened cartridge in use must be kept unrefrigerated (15-25°C) for up to 28 days away from direct heat and light, as long as the temperature is not greater than 25°C. If the cartridge overheats or if there is any remaining insulin after 28 days, discard it. The opened cartridge in use must never be removed from and reinserted into the injection pen.
SoloSTAR: Unopened SoloSTAR: Unopened APIDRA SoloSTAR should be stored in a refrigerator, between 2-8°C. Keep APIDRA away from direct heat and light. APIDRA should not be stored in the freezer and it should not be allowed to freeze. If APIDRA freezes or overheats, discard it.
Opened (In Use) SoloSTAR: Opened APIDRA SoloSTAR in use must be kept unrefrigerated (15-25°C) for up to 28 days away from direct heat and light, as long as the temperature is not greater than 25°C. If the APIDRA SoloSTAR overheats or if there is any remaining insulin after 28 days, discard it.

Opened APIDRA SoloSTAR should not be stored in the freezer and should not be allowed to freeze. If APIDRA SoloSTAR freezes discard it.

As with all medications and devices, keep out of reach of children.
Infusion Sets: Infusion sets (reservoirs, tubing, and catheters) and the APIDRA in the reservoir should be discarded after no more than 2 days of use or after exposure to temperatures that exceed 37°C.

SPECIAL HANDLING INSTRUCTIONS: See also Information for the Patient, and refer patients to the APIDRA Information for the Patient circular for APIDRA Vial, APIDRA Cartridge, and APIDRA SoloSTAR for additional information. Refer patients to the User Manual for sanofi-aventis insulin injection pens or injection pens suitable for APIDRA cartridges **as recommended in the information provided by the injection pen manufacturer** and User Manual for the APIDRA SoloSTAR for additional information on use of the pens.

INFORMATION FOR THE PATIENT: Published in e-CPS, available by subscription at www.e-cps.ca.

DOSAGE FORMS, COMPOSITION AND PACKAGING: The vials, cartridges, and SoloSTAR contain a sterile solution of insulin glulisine for use as an injection. APIDRA [insulin glulisine (rDNA origin)] consists of insulin glulisine dissolved in a clear aqueous solution.

Each mL contains: insulin glulisine 100 units. Nonmedicinal ingredients: m-cresol, polysorbate 20, sodium chloride, trometamol and water for injection. APIDRA has a pH of approximately 7.3 and is adjusted by addition of aqueous solutions of hydrochloric acid and sodium hydroxide. Vials of 10 mL; cartridges of 3 mL, package of 5 (for use only with sanofi-aventis insulin injection pens or injection pens suitable for APIDRA cartridges, as recommended in the information provided by the injection pen manufacturer) and APIDRA SoloSTAR of 3 mL (pre-filled disposable pen), packages of 5.

Apo®-Acebutolol Ⓟ

acebutolol HCl

Antihypertensive—Antianginal

Apotex

Date of Preparation: January 11, 1995
Date of Revision: August 16, 1995

PHARMACOLOGY: Acebutolol is a beta-adrenergic receptor blocking agent. In vitro and in vivo animal studies have shown that it has a preferential effect on $beta_1$ adrenoreceptors, chiefly located in cardiac muscle. This preferential effect is not absolute, however, and at higher doses acebutolol also inhibits $beta_2$ adrenoreceptors, chiefly located in the bronchial and vascular musculature. It possesses some partial agonist activity (or intrinsic sympathomimetic activity—ISA). It is used in the treatment of hypertension and/or prophylaxis of angina pectoris.

The mechanism of the antihypertensive effect has not been established. Among the factors that may be involved are: a) competitive ability to antagonize catecholamine-induced tachycardia at the beta-receptor sites in the heart, thus decreasing cardiac output; b) inhibition of renin release by the kidneys; c) inhibition of the vasomotor centres.

The mechanism of the anti-anginal effect is also uncertain. An important factor may be the reduction of myocardial oxygen requirements by blocking catecholamine-induced increases in heart rate, systolic blood pressure, and the velocity and extent of myocardial contraction.

Acebutolol hydrochloride is well absorbed from the gastrointestinal tract. It undergoes extensive first-pass hepatic biotransformation, with an absolute bioavailability of approximately 40% for the parent compound. The major metabolite, an N-acetyl derivative (diacetolol), is pharmacologically active. This metabolite is equipotent to acebutolol and, in cats, is more cardioselective than acebutolol; therefore, this first-pass phenomenon does not attenuate the therapeutic effect of acebutolol. Food intake does not have a significant effect on the area under the plasma concentration time curve [AUC] of acebutolol although the rate of absorption and peak concentration decreased slightly.

The plasma elimination half-life of acebutolol is approximately 3 to 4 hours, while that of its metabolite, diacetolol, is 8 to 13 hours. The time to reach peak concentration for acebutolol is 2.5 hours and for diacetolol, after oral administration of acebutolol, 3.5 hours.

Within the single oral dose range of 200 to 400 mg, the kinetics are dose proportional. However, this linearity is not seen at higher doses, probably due to saturation of hepatic biotransformation sites. In addition, after multiple dosing the lack of linearity is also seen by AUC increases of approximately 100% as compared to single oral dosing. Elimination via renal excretion is approximately 30% to 40% and by non-renal mechanisms 50% to 60%, which includes excretion into the bile and direct passage through the intestinal wall.

Acebutolol has a low binding affinity for plasma proteins (about 26%). Acebutolol and its metabolite, diacetolol, are relatively hydrophilic and therefore only minimal quantities have been detected in the cerebrospinal fluid (CSF).
Comparative Bioavailability: A comparative bioavailability study was performed using healthy human volunteers. The rate and extent of absorption of acebutolol were measured and compared after a single oral 400 mg dose of APO-ACEBUTOLOL (one 400 mg tablet) and Monitan (one 400 mg tablet). The results are summarized in Table 1.

Table 1: APO-ACEBUTOLOL

Comparative Bioavailability

	Geometric Mean Arithmetic Mean (C.V.)		
Parameter	**APO-ACEBUTOLOL 1×400 mg**	**Monitan 1×400 mg**	**Ratio of Means (%)**
AUC_T (ng·hr/mL)	3340 3439 (24)	3413 3468 (18)	98.0
AUC_I (ng·hr/mL)	3607 3708 (23)	3668 3725 (18)	98.5
C_{max} (ng/mL)	802 839 (30)	847 882 (33)	94.7
T_{max}[a] (hr)	2.26 (0.71)	2.32 (0.93)	—
$t_{½}$[a] (hr)	2.91 (0.36)	2.92 (0.49)	—

[a] For the T_{max} and $t_{½}$ parameters, these are the arithmetic means (standard deviations).

INDICATIONS: Hypertension: APO-ACEBUTOLOL (acebutolol hydrochloride) is indicated in patients with mild to moderate hypertension. It is usually used in combination with other drugs, particularly a thiazide diuretic. However, it may be tried alone as an initial agent in those patients in whom, in the judgement of the physician, treatment should be started with a beta-blocker rather than a diuretic.

In patients with severe hypertension, a beta-adrenergic blocking agent may be used as part of a multiple drug regimen which would normally include a diuretic and a vasodilator.

The combination of acebutolol with a diuretic or peripheral vasodilator has been found to be compatible and generally more effective than acebutolol alone. Limited experience with other antihypertensive agents has not shown evidence of incompatibility.

APO-ACEBUTOLOL is not indicated in the emergency treatment of hypertensive crises.
Angina Pectoris: APO-ACEBUTOLOL is indicated in the long-term management of patients with angina pectoris due to ischemic heart disease.

CONTRAINDICATIONS: APO-ACEBUTOLOL (acebutolol hydrochloride) should not be used in the presence of: 1) sinus bradycardia; 2) second and third degree A-V block; 3) right ventricular failure secondary to pulmonary hypertension; 4) congestive heart failure; 5) cardiogenic shock; 6) anesthesia with agents that produce myocardial depression, e.g., ether.

WARNINGS: Increase in antinuclear antibody (ANA) titer was observed in approximately 12.5% of patients on chronic acebutolol hydrochloride therapy. Rare instances (<1%) of a syndrome resembling lupus erythematosus have been reported with maintenance acebutolol therapy. Similar symptoms were occasionally observed with some other beta-blockers. In addition to increased ANA titers, polyarthralgia, myalgia and pleuritic pain were the main presenting symptoms. Symptoms and ANA titers appear reversible upon discontinuation of acebutolol therapy. The drug should be withdrawn if symptoms appear or if the results of ANA testing are significantly positive. Patients should be followed up both clinically and serologically until resolution of symptoms.
Cardiac Failure: Special caution should be exercised when administering APO-ACEBUTOLOL (acebutolol hydrochloride) to patients with a history of heart failure. Sympathetic stimulation is a vital component supporting circulatory function in congestive heart failure, and inhibition with beta-blockade always carries the potential hazard of further depressing myocardial contractility and precipitating cardiac failure. APO-ACEBUTOLOL acts selectively without abolishing the inotropic action of digitalis on the heart muscle. However, the positive inotropic action of digitalis may be reduced by the negative inotropic effect of acebutolol hydrochloride when the two drugs are used concomitantly.

The effects of beta-blockers and digitalis are additive in depressing A-V conduction.

In patients without a history of cardiac failure, continued depression of myocardium over a period of time can, in some cases, lead to cardiac failure. Therefore, at the first sign or symptom of impending cardiac failure, patients should be fully digitalized and/or given a diuretic and the response observed closely. If cardiac failure continues despite adequate digitalization and diuretic therapy, APO-ACEBUTOLOL therapy should be immediately withdrawn.
Abrupt Cessation of Therapy with APO-ACEBUTOLOL: Patients with angina should be warned against abrupt discontinuation of APO-ACEBUTOLOL. There have been reports of severe exacerbation of angina, and of myocardial infarction or ventricular arrhythmias occurring in patients with angina pectoris, following abrupt discontinuation of beta-blocker therapy. The last two complications may occur with or without preceding exacerbation of angina pectoris. Therefore, when discontinuation of APO-ACEBUTOLOL is planned in patients with angina pectoris, the dosage should be gradually reduced over a period of about two weeks and the patient should be carefully observed. The same frequency of administration should be maintained. In situations of greater urgency, acebutolol hydrochloride therapy should be discontinued stepwise and under conditions of closer observation. If angina markedly worsens or acute coronary insufficiency develops, it is recommended that treatment with APO-ACEBUTOLOL be reinstituted promptly, at least temporarily.

Various skin rashes and conjunctival xerosis have been reported with beta-blockers, including acebutolol. A severe syndrome (oculo-muco-cutaneous syndrome) whose signs include conjunctivitis sicca and psoriasiform rashes, otitis, and sclerosing serositis has occurred with the chronic use of one beta-adrenergic blocking agent (practolol). This syndrome has not been observed with acebutolol or any other such agent. However, physicians should be alert to the possibility of such reactions and should discontinue treatment in the event that they occur.

Severe sinus bradycardia may occur with the use of acebutolol from unopposed vagal activity remaining after blockade of $beta_1$-adrenergic receptors; in such cases, dosage should be reduced.

In patients with thyrotoxicosis, the possible deleterious effects from long-term use of acebutolol have not been adequately appraised. APO-ACEBUTOLOL may give a false impression of improvement by masking the clinical signs of continuing hyperthyroidism or its complications. Therefore, abrupt withdrawal of APO-ACEBUTOLOL may be followed by an exacerbation of the symptoms of hyperthyroidism, including thyroid storm.
Pregnancy: Reproduction studies have been performed with acebutolol in rats and rabbits at doses of up to 60 mg/kg/day by the oral route and 18 mg/kg/day by the I.V. route. In one rabbit study where acebutolol was administered by the I.V. route, the following malformations were observed: rib defects, gastroschisis, ventricular septal defect, dysplasia of urogenital system and umbilical hernia. These results could not be confirmed in a repeat intravenous study and were not seen in a study using the oral route.

Studies have also been performed with diacetolol (the major metabolite of acebutolol in man) at doses of up to 450 mg/kg/day p.o. in rabbits and 1800 mg/kg/day p.o. in rats. There was a significant elevation of postimplantation loss in rabbit dams receiving 450 mg/kg/day, a level at which food consumption and body weight gain were reduced; a non-statistically significant increase in incidence of bilateral cataracts was also noticed in rat fetuses from dams treated with 1800 mg/kg/day.

There has been no experience with the use of acebutolol in pregnant women; however, studies have shown that both acebutolol and diacetolol cross the placenta. APO-ACEBUTOLOL should not be given to pregnant patients. Its use in women with child bearing potential requires that the anticipated benefit be cautiously weighed against possible hazards.
Lactation: Acebutolol and diacetolol appear in breast milk with a milk: plasma ratio of 7.1 and 12.2 respectively. Use in nursing mothers is not recommended.

PRECAUTIONS: Patients with bronchospastic disease should, in general, not receive a beta-blocker. Because of its relative $beta_1$ selectivity, however, low doses of APO-ACEBUTOLOL (acebutolol hydrochloride) may be used with caution in patients with bronchospastic disease who do not respond to, or who cannot tolerate, alternative treatment. Since $beta_1$ selectivity is not absolute and is dose-dependent, a $beta_2$ stimulating agent should be administered concomitantly and the lowest possible dose of acebutolol should be used initially, preferably in divided doses to avoid the higher plasma levels associated with the longer dose interval.

There may be increased difficulty in treating an allergic type reaction in patients on beta-blockers. In these patients, the reaction may be more severe due to pharmacological effects of beta-blockers and problems with fluid changes. Epinephrine should be administered with caution since it may not have its usual effects in the treatment of anaphylaxis. On the one hand, larger doses of epinephrine may be needed to overcome the bronchospasm, while on the other, these doses can be associated with excessive alpha-adrenergic stimulation with consequent hypertension, reflex bradycardia and heart-block and possible potentiation of bronchospasm. Alternatives to the use of large doses of epinephrine include vigorous supportive care such as fluids and the use of beta-agonists including parenteral salbutamol or isoproterenol to overcome bronchospasm, and norepinephrine to overcome hypotension.

APO-ACEBUTOLOL should be administered with caution to patients subject to spontaneous hypoglycemia, or to diabetic patients (especially those with labile diabetes) who are receiving insulin or oral hypoglycemic agents. Beta-adrenergic blockers may mask the premonitory signs and symptoms of acute hypoglycemia.

APO-ACEBUTOLOL should be administered with caution to patients with impaired renal function. Acebutolol hydrochloride is excreted through the G.I. tract, but the active metabolite diacetolol, is eliminated predominantly by the kidney. There is a linear relationship between renal clearance of diacetolol and creatinine clearance. The daily dose of APO-ACEBUTOLOL should be reduced in patients with a creatinine clearance less than 50 mL/min.
Geriatrics: Acebutolol has been used in the elderly without specific adjustment of dosage. However, this patient population may require lower maintenance doses because the bioavailability of both acebutolol hydrochloride and its metabolite are approximately doubled in this age group. This increased bioavailability is probably due to decreases in first-pass metabolism and renal function in the elderly.

APO-ACEBUTOLOL dosage should be individually adjusted when used concomitantly with other antihypertensive agents (see Dosage).

Liver function tests should be performed at regular intervals during long-term treatment.
In Patients Undergoing Elective or Emergency Surgery: The management of patients being treated with beta-blockers and undergoing elective or emergency surgery is controversial. Although beta-adrenergic receptor blockade impairs the ability of the heart to respond to beta-adrenergically-mediated reflex stimuli, abrupt discontinuation of therapy with APO-ACEBUTOLOL may be followed by severe complications (see Warnings). Some patients receiving beta-adrenergic blocking agents have been subject to protracted severe hypotension during anesthesia. Difficulty in restarting and maintaining the heartbeat has also been reported. For these reasons, in patients with angina undergoing elective surgery, APO-ACEBUTOLOL should be withdrawn gradually following the recommendation given under Warnings, Abrupt Cessation of Therapy with APO-ACEBUTOLOL. According to available evidence, all clinical and physiological effects of beta-blockade are no longer present 72 hours after cessation of medication.

In emergency surgery, since APO-ACEBUTOLOL is a competitive inhibitor of beta-adrenergic receptor agonists, its effects may be reversed, if necessary, by sufficient doses of such agonists as isoproterenol.
Children: There is no experience with APO-ACEBUTOLOL in the treatment of pediatric age groups and therefore use in children is not recommended.

Drug Interactions: Catecholamine-depleting drugs, such as reserpine, may have an additive effect when given with β-blocking agents. Patients treated with APO-ACEBUTOLOL plus catecholamine depletors should, therefore be observed closely for evidence of marked bradycardia or hypotension which may present as vertigo, syncope/pre-syncope, or orthostatic changes in blood pressure without compensatory tachycardia.

Exaggerated hypertensive responses have been reported from the combined use of β-adrenergic antagonists and α-adrenergic stimulants, including those contained in proprietary cold remedies and vasoconstrictive nasal drops. Patients receiving β-blockers should be warned of this potential hazard.

No significant interactions of acebutolol with digoxin, hydrochlorothiazide, hydralazine, sulfinpyrazone, oral contraceptives, tolbutamide or warfarin have been observed. Should it be decided to discontinue therapy in patients receiving beta-blockers and clonidine concurrently, the beta-blocker should be discontinued several days before the gradual withdrawal of clonidine. It has been suggested that withdrawal of clonidine in the presence of beta-blockade may exaggerate the clonidine withdrawal syndrome (see also prescribing information for clonidine).

ADVERSE EFFECTS: The incidence of treatment-related side effects is derived from clinical trials in 3090 patients with hypertension, angina pectoris or arrhythmia.

The most serious adverse reactions encountered with acebutolol hydrochloride are congestive heart failure, severe bradycardia and bronchospasm occurring in less than 1% of patients.

The most common adverse reactions reported are fatigue (4%), dyspnea (2.5%), nausea (2%), dizziness (2%), hypotension (1%) and rashes (1%).

Adverse reactions grouped by systems are as follows:

Cardiovascular: congestive heart failure (see Warnings); secondary effects of decreased cardiac output which include: syncope, vertigo, lightheadedness and postural hypotension; severe bradycardia, lengthening of PR interval, second and third degree A-V block, sinus arrest, palpitation, chest pain, cold extremities, Raynaud's phenomenon, hot flushes, pain in legs, edema.

Central Nervous System: headache, dizziness, mental depression, tiredness, drowsiness or somnolence, lightheadedness, anxiety, tinnitus, weakness, confusion, vivid dreams, paresthesia, insomnia.

Gastrointestinal: nausea and vomiting, heartburn, indigestion, flatulence, abdominal pain, diarrhea, constipation.

Respiratory: dyspnea, cough, shortness of breath, wheezing, bronchospasm.

Allergic/Dermatological: (See Warnings): urticaria, pruritus, sweating, exfoliative dermatitis, psoriasiform rash; Lupus-like syndrome with arthralgia, myalgia, dyspnea and pleuritic pain, reversible upon cessation of the drug.

EENT: blurred vision and non-specific visual disturbances, itching eyes, conjunctivitis.

Miscellaneous: weight gain, loss of appetite, decrease in libido, shivering, micturition (frequency), nocturia.

Laboratory Tests: occasional reports of increased transaminase, alkaline phosphatase and lactic dehydrogenase values; positive antinuclear antibodies (see Warnings).

OVERDOSE:

Symptoms: The most common signs to be expected with a beta-adrenergic blocking agent are bradycardia, congestive heart failure, hypotension, bronchospasm and hypoglycemia.

Treatment: If overdosage occurs, in all cases therapy with APO-ACEBUTOLOL (acebutolol hydrochloride) should be discontinued and the patient observed closely. In addition, if required, the following therapeutic measures are suggested:

Bradycardia: atropine or another anticholinergic drug.

Heart block (second or third degree): isoproterenol or transvenous cardiac pacemaker.

Congestive heart failure: conventional therapy.

Hypotension (depending on associated factors): Epinephrine rather than isoproterenol or norepinephrine may be useful in addition to atropine and digitalis. [See Precautions concerning the use of epinephrine in β-blocked patients.]

Bronchospasm: aminophylline or isoproterenol.

Hypoglycemia: intravenous glucose.

APO-ACEBUTOLOL and its major metabolite are dialyzable.

It should be remembered that APO-ACEBUTOLOL is a competitive antagonist of isoproterenol and hence large doses of isoproterenol can be expected to reverse many of the effects of excessive doses of APO-ACEBUTOLOL. However, the complications of excess isoproterenol should not be overlooked.

For management of a suspected drug overdose, CPhA recommends that you contact your **regional Poison Control Centre**. See the *CPS* Directory section for a list of Poison Control Centres.

DOSAGE: The dose of APO-ACEBUTOLOL (acebutolol hydrochloride) must always be adjusted to the individual requirements of the patient in accordance with the following guidelines:

Hypertension: APO-ACEBUTOLOL is usually used in conjunction with other antihypertensive agents, particularly thiazide diuretics but may be used alone (see Indications).

APO-ACEBUTOLOL treatment should be initiated with doses of 100 mg b.i.d. If an adequate response is not seen after one week, the dosage should be increased to 200 mg b.i.d. In some cases, the daily dosage may need further increments of 100 mg b.i.d. at intervals of not less than two weeks, up to the maximum of 400 mg b.i.d.

The maintenance dose is within the range of 400 to 800 mg daily. Patients who show a satisfactory response at a daily dose of 400 mg or less may be given the total dose once daily in the morning. Daily doses above this should be divided into two equal doses.

Angina Pectoris: The initial dose is 200 mg b.i.d. If after two weeks a satisfactory response has not been obtained, the dosage should be increased to a maximum of 300 mg b.i.d.

The usual maintenance dose of APO-ACEBUTOLOL in angina pectoris is in the range of 200 to 600 mg daily administered in two divided doses. In patients adequately controlled on 400 mg daily, a lower maintenance dose of 100 mg twice a day may be tried.

Geriatrics: Older patients have an approximately 2-fold increase in bioavailability and are likely to require lower maintenance doses.

Use in Patients with Impaired Renal Function: The daily dose of acebutolol hydrochloride should be reduced by 50% when creatinine clearance is less than 50 mL/min and by 75% when it is less than 25 mL/min (see Precautions).

APO-ACEBUTOLOL and its metabolite are dialyzable.

SUPPLIED: 100 mg: Each white, round, biconvex, film-coated tablet, scored and engraved "APO" over "100" on one side, contains: acebutolol HCl equivalent to acebutolol 100 mg. Nonmedicinal ingredients: carnauba wax, colloidal silicon dioxide, dextrates, hydroxypropyl methylcellulose, magnesium stearate, polyethylene glycol and titanium dioxide. Bottles of 100 and 500.
200 mg: Each white, oval, biconvex, film-coated tablet, scored and engraved "APO 200" on one side, contains: acebutolol HCl equivalent to acebutolol 200 mg. Nonmedicinal ingredients: carnauba wax, colloidal silicon dioxide, dextrates, hydroxypropyl methylcellulose, magnesium stearate, polyethylene glycol and titanium dioxide. Bottles of 100 and 500.
400 mg: Each white, capsule-shaped, biconvex, film-coated tablet, scored and engraved "APO 400" on one side, contains: acebutolol HCl equivalent to acebutolol 400 mg. Nonmedicinal ingredients: carnauba wax, colloidal silicon dioxide, dextrates, hydroxypropyl methylcellulose, magnesium stearate, polyethylene glycol and titanium dioxide. Bottles of 100 and 500.

Store at 15 to 30°C. Protect from light.

The reader is invited to consult CPhA's monograph **ACE Inhibitors**.

Apo®-Amiloride

amiloride HCl

Antikaliuretic Agent—Diuretic

Apotex

Date of Preparation: June 11, 2004

PHARMACOLOGY: Amiloride hydrochloride is an antikaliuretic drug with mild natriuretic diuretic and antihypertensive activity. These activities may be additive to the effects of thiazides or other saluretic-diuretic agents. The principal use of amiloride hydrochloride is to conserve potassium in selected patients receiving kaliuretic-diuretic agents. Amiloride hydrochloride interferes with the mechanism involved in the exchange of sodium for potassium in the distal convoluted tubule and collecting duct of the nephron. An increase in sodium and a decrease in potassium and hydrogen ion excretion are induced in the presence or absence of aldosterone, thereby suggesting a direct tubular action of the drug. Chloride excretion may remain unchanged or increase slowly with continued therapy.

Amiloride hydrochloride when administered with hydrochlorothiazide has been shown to result in less excretion of magnesium than thiazide or loop diuretics used alone.

Approximately 50% of an oral dose is absorbed. Amiloride hydrochloride usually begins to act within 2 hours after an oral dose. Its effect on electrolyte excretion reaches a peak between 6 and 10 hours and lasts about 24 hours. Peak plasma levels are obtained in 3 to 4 hours and plasma half-life varies from 6 to 9 hours.

Amiloride hydrochloride is not metabolized by the liver. About 50% of a 20 mg dose of amiloride hydrochloride is excreted unchanged in the urine and 40% is excreted in the stool within 72 hours. In clinical studies of amiloride hydrochloride was found to have little effect on glomerular filtration rate or renal blood flow.

Comparative Bioavailability: A comparative bioavailability study was performed using healthy human volunteers. The rate and extent of absorption of amiloride hydrochloride was measured and compared following oral administration of APO-AMILORIDE (1×5 mg) tablets or Midamor (1×5 mg) tablets. The results from measured data are summarized as follows (see Table 1).

Table 1: APO-AMILORIDE

Summary Table of the Comparative Bioavailability Data (Dose: 1×5 mg) From Measured Data

Parameter	Geometric Mean Arithmetic Mean (CV%)		Ratio of Geometric Means (%)[b]
	APO-AMILORIDE	Midamor[c]	
AUC_T (ng·hr/mL)	85.8 88.2 (23)	86.9 89.3 (21)	98.7
AUC_{0-72} (ng·hr/mL)	91.6 92.9 (17)	91.7 93.1 (17)	99.8
AUC_I (ng·hr/mL)	92.9 95.7 (23)	92.6 95.3 (22)	100.3
C_{max} (ng/mL)	5.45 5.57 (20)	5.46 5.56 (19)	99.9
T_{max} (hr)[a]	3.92 (25)	3.86 (27)	—
$t_{1/2}$ (hr)[a]	20.4 (47)	17.4 (25)	—

[a] Arithmetic means (CV%).
[b] Based on the least squares estimate.
[c] Midamor is marketed by Merck Frosst, and was purchased in Canada.

INDICATIONS: APO-AMILORIDE (amiloride hydrochloride) is indicated for use alone or concomitantly with thiazide diuretics or other kaliuretic-diuretic agents in the treatment of patients with cirrhosis of the liver with ascites and edema.

APO-AMILORIDE is indicated as an adjunct to the treatment with thiazide diuretics or other kaliuretic-diuretic agents in those patients with edema of cardiac origin or hypertension who: a) have hypokalemia, or b) in whom maintenance of normal serum potassium levels is considered to be clinically important, e.g., digitalized patients, patients in whom adequate dietary intake of potassium is not feasible or patients with cardiac arrhythmias.

Use in Hepatic Cirrhosis with Ascites and Edema: APO-AMILORIDE used alone may provide satisfactory diuresis with diminished potassium loss and with a reduced risk of metabolic alkalosis. In resistant cases APO-AMILORIDE may be used with kaliuretic-diuretic agents to help produce satisfactory diuresis, while maintaining a more balanced serum electrolyte pattern. As with all therapy for the ascites of hepatic cirrhosis, gradual weight loss and avoidance of electrolyte imbalance are the chief objectives (see Precautions).

CONTRAINDICATIONS: Hyperkalemia: APO-AMILORIDE (amiloride hydrochloride) should not be used in the presence of elevated serum potassium levels (see Warnings).

Antikaliuretic Therapy or Potassium Salts: Other antikaliuretic agents and potassium supplements are contraindicated in patients receiving amiloride hydrochloride (such combination therapy is commonly associated with rapid increases in plasma potassium levels).

Impaired Renal Function: Anuria, acute renal failure, severe or progressive renal disease, and diabetic nephropathy are contraindications to the use of APO-AMILORIDE (see Warnings).

Hypersensitivity: APO-AMILORIDE is contraindicated in patients who are hypersensitive to any component of this product.

WARNINGS: Hyperkalemia: Hyperkalemia (i.e., serum potassium levels over 5.5 mEq/L), has been observed in patients who received amiloride hydrochloride tablets either alone or with diuretics. This has been noted particularly in elderly patients, in diabetic patients, and in hospitalized patients with hepatic cirrhosis or cardiac edema who had known renal impairment, were seriously ill, or were receiving vigorous diuretic therapy. Since fatalities have occurred, patients should be monitored carefully for clinical, laboratory, and electrocardiographic (ECG) evidence of hyperkalemia and for acidosis. Monitoring of the serum potassium level is important because hyperkalemia is not always associated with an abnormal ECG.

Warning signs or symptoms of hyperkalemia include paresthesias, muscular weakness, fatigue, flaccid paralysis of the extremities, bradycardia, shock, and ECG abnormalities.

When abnormal, the ECG in hyperkalemia is characterized primarily by tall, peaked T waves or elevations from previous tracings. There may also be lowering of the R wave and increased depth of the S wave, widening and even disappearance of the P wave, progressive widening of the QRS complex, prolongation of the PR interval, and ST depression.

If hyperkalemia occurs in patients taking APO-AMILORIDE (amiloride hydrochloride), the drug should be discontinued immediately. If the serum potassium level exceeds 6.5 mEq per liter, active measures should be taken to reduce it. Such measures include the intravenous administration of sodium bicarbonate solution or oral or parenteral glucose with a rapid-acting insulin preparation. If needed, a cation exchange resin such as sodium polystyrene sulfonate may be given orally or by enema. Patients with persistent hyperkalemia may require dialysis.

Diabetes Mellitus: In diabetic patients, hyperkalemia has been commonly reported with the use of amiloride hydrochloride, particularly if they have chronic renal disease or prerenal azotemia. Some deaths occurred in this last group of patients. Therefore, if therapy with APO-AMILORIDE is considered essential, the drug should be used with caution in diabetic or suspected diabetic patients and only after first determining the status of renal function.

Careful monitoring of serum potassium levels is required throughout the therapy.

One patient with poorly controlled diabetes mellitus who became severely hyperkalemic while on amiloride hydrochloride died following two repeated intravenous glucose tolerance tests. Therefore, APO-AMILORIDE should be discontinued at least 3 days before glucose tolerance testing.

Metabolic or Respiratory Acidosis: Antikaliuretic therapy should be instituted only with caution in patients in whom respiratory or metabolic acidosis may occur, such as patients with cardiopulmonary disease or diabetes. If APO-AMILORIDE is given to these patients, frequent monitoring of acid-base balance is necessary. Shifts in acid-base balance alter the ratio of extracellular/intracellular potassium, and the development of acidosis may be associated with rapid increases in serum potassium levels.

Impaired Renal Function: Patients with impaired renal function other than those listed under Contraindications and who have BUN levels over 30 mg per 100 mL, serum creatinine levels over 1.5 mg per 100 mL, or with whole blood urea values over 60 mg per 100 mL or with diabetes mellitus, should not receive the drug without careful, frequent monitoring of serum electrolytes, creatinine, and BUN levels. Potassium retention associated with the use of amiloride hydrochloride is accentuated in the presence of renal impairment and may result in the rapid development of hyperkalemia. Prolongation of amiloride hydrochloride excretion was observed in patients with renal impairment.

PRECAUTIONS: Electrolyte Imbalance and BUN Increases: Hyponatremia and hypochloremia may occur when APO-AMILORIDE (amiloride hydrochloride) is used with other diuretics. Increases in BUN levels have been reported. These increases usually have accompanied vigorous fluid elimination, especially when diuretic therapy was used in seriously ill patients, such as those who had hepatic cirrhosis with ascites and metabolic alkalosis, or those with resistant edema. Therefore, careful monitoring of serum electrolytes and BUN levels is important when using APO-AMILORIDE.

Effects Related to Diuresis in Cirrhotic Patients: Patients with hepatic cirrhosis and ascites are intolerant of acute shifts in electrolyte balance and often have pre-existing hypokalemia as a result of associated secondary hyperaldosteronism. When oral diuretic therapy is used, these patients should be carefully monitored and diuresis should be gradual.

Hepatic encephalopathy, manifested by tremors, confusion, and coma, has been reported in association with amiloride hydrochloride therapy.

In a few cirrhotic patients, pre-existing jaundice increased, but the relationship to drug is uncertain.

Pregnancy: Teratologic studies with amiloride hydrochloride in rabbits and mice revealed no evidence of harm to the fetus. Reproduction studies in rats showed no evidence of impaired fertility. At approximately 5 or more times the expected maximum daily dose for humans, some toxicity was seen in adult rats and rabbits and a decrease in rat pup growth and survival occurred.

In rats a trace of drug crossed the placental barrier.

Because clinical experience is limited, APO-AMILORIDE is not recommended for use during pregnancy. The potential benefits of the drug must be weighed against possible hazards to the fetus if it is administered to a woman of childbearing age.

Lactation: It is not known whether amiloride hydrochloride is excreted in human milk. In rats secretion of amiloride hydrochloride in milk has been demonstrated. Because many drugs are excreted in human milk and because of the potential for serious adverse reactions, a decision should be made whether to discontinue nursing or to discontinue the drug taking into account the importance of the drug to the mother.

Children: The use of amiloride hydrochloride in children has not been established; therefore APO-AMILORIDE is not recommended in the pediatric age group.

Drug Interactions: Lithium should generally not be given with diuretics because they reduce the renal clearance of lithium and add a high risk of lithium toxicity.

When amiloride HCl is administered concomitantly with an angiotensin-converting enzyme inhibitor, cyclosporine or tacrolimus, the risk of hyperkalemia may be increased. Therefore, if concomitant use of these agents is indicated because of demonstrated hypokalemia, they should be used with caution and with frequent monitoring of serum potassium.

Concomitant administration of non-steroidal anti-inflammatory drugs (NSAIDs) and potassium-sparing agents, including amiloride hydrochloride, may cause hyperkalemia and renal failure, particularly in elderly patients. Therefore, when amiloride hydrochloride is used concomitantly with NSAIDs, renal function and serum potassium levels should be carefully monitored.

ADVERSE EFFECTS: While rare, the most serious adverse effect of amiloride hydrochloride is symptomatic hyperkalemia (symptoms of hyperkalemia may include paresthesias, muscular weakness, fatigue, flaccid paralysis of the extremities, bradycardia, shock and ECG abnormalities) (see Contraindications and Warnings).

The following incidence of adverse reactions was determined from clinical trials (837 patients treated with amiloride hydrochloride). See Table 2.

Table 2: APO-AMILORIDE

Adverse Reactions

	Incidence ≥3%	Incidence >1%–<3%	Incidence ≤1%
Gastrointestinal (in 12.1% of patients)	Nausea/anorexia (6.1%) Diarrhea (3.8%) Vomiting (3.3%)	Abdominal pain Gas pain Appetite changes Constipation	Jaundice GI bleeding Abdominal fullness GI disturbance Thirst Heartburn Flatulence Dyspepsia Dryness of the mouth
Central Nervous System (In 9.6% of patients)	Headache (7.6%)	Dizziness Encephalopathy	Paresthesia Tremors Vertigo Nervousness Mental confusion Insomnia Decreased libido Depression Somnolence
Metabolic (In 8.0% of patients)	Asymptomatic hyperkalemia (8.0%)		Symptomatic hyperkalemia Hyponatremia
Musculoskeletal (In 6.1% of patients)		Muscle cramps Weakness Fatigability	Joint pain Leg ache Back pain Chest pain Neck/shoulder ache Pain extremities
Respiratory (in 2.0% of patients)		Cough Dyspnea	Shortness of breath
Urogenital (in 3.8% of patients)		Impotence	Polyuria Dysuria Urinary frequency Bladder spasms
Cardiovascular (In 1.5% of patients)			Angina pectoris Orthostatic hypotension Arrhythmia Palpitation One patient with a partial heart block developed complete heart block
Dermatologic (In 1.9% of patients)			Skin rash Pruritus Alopecia
Special Senses (In 2.9% of patients)			Visual disturbances Nasal congestion Increased intraocular pressure Tinnitus

Causal Relationship Unknown: A causal relationship could not be established with other reactions reported rarely. However, the possibility could not be excluded. These reactions were: activation of probable pre-existing peptic ulcer; aplastic anemia; neutropenia; abnormalities of liver function tests; hyperuricemia.

In cirrhotic patients, jaundice associated with the underlying disease process has deepened in a few instances, but the relationship to drug is uncertain.

In patients with pre-existing severe liver disease, hepatic encephalopathy, manifested by tremors, confusion, and coma, and increased jaundice, have been reported in association with diuretics, including amiloride hydrochloride.

OVERDOSE:

Symptoms: No data are available in regard to overdosage in humans.

It is not known whether the drug is dialyzable.

If hyperkalemia occurs, active measures should be taken to reduce the serum potassium levels (see Warnings).

The most likely signs and symptoms to be expected with overdosage are dehydration and electrolyte imbalance. These can be treated by established procedures. Therapy with APO-AMILORIDE (amiloride hydrochloride) should be discontinued and the patient observed closely.

There is no specific antidote. Emesis should be induced or gastric lavage performed. Treatment is symptomatic and supportive.

Treatment: See Symptoms.

> For management of a suspected drug overdose, CPhA recommends that you contact your **regional Poison Control Centre**. See the *CPS* Directory section for a list of Poison Control Centres.

DOSAGE: The incidence of hyperkalemia is dose-related and this should be considered especially when daily doses over 10 mg are used.

Hepatic Cirrhosis with Ascites and Edema: Treatment should be started with a small dose of APO-AMILORIDE (amiloride hydrochloride), i.e., one 5 mg tablet daily, plus a small dose of a diuretic agent (other than antikaliuretics). If necessary, dosages of both drugs may be increased gradually until effective diuresis is obtained. The dosage of APO-AMILORIDE should not exceed four tablets (20 mg) a day. Maintenance doses may be lower than those required to initiate diuresis; therefore, reduction in the daily dosage should be attempted when the patient's weight is stabilized. In cirrhotic patients, gradual weight reduction is especially desirable to reduce the likelihood ofuntoward reactions associated with diuretic therapy.

In those instances where APO-AMILORIDE is used alone, the initial daily dosage should be two 5 mg tablets (as a single dose or one tablet twice a day). Dosage may be increased depending on the need. The total daily dosage should not exceed four tablets (20 mg). After diuresis has been achieved the dosage may be reduced by decrements of one tablet to the least amount required.

Edema of Cardiac Origin: APO-AMILORIDE, one or two 5 mg tablets daily, may be given with the usual doses of a diuretic agent (other than antikaliuretics). This dose is sufficient in most cases. If potassium levels remain low, the dosage of APO-AMILORIDE may be increased gradually. The dosage of APO-AMILORIDE should not exceed four tablets (20 mg) a day.

The optimal dosage is determined by the serum potassium level. Reduction in dosage should be attempted for maintenance therapy. Maintenance therapy may be on an intermittent basis.

Hypertension: APO-AMILORIDE, one or two 5 mg tablets daily, is given with the usual antihypertensive dosage of a diuretic agent (other than antikaliuretics). The dosage may be adjusted if necessary. More than two 5 mg tablets of APO-AMILORIDE daily usually is not needed; in any event, the maximum dosage is four tablets (20 mg) a day.

SUPPLIED: Each yellow, diamond-shaped, biconvex tablet, engraved "APO" over "5" on one side and plain on the other, contains: amiloride HCl 5 mg. Nonmedicinal ingredients: croscarmellose sodium, lactose monohydrate, magnesium stearate, microcrystalline cellulose and yellow ferric oxide. Bottles of 100. Store at room temperature (15-30°C).

Apo®-Benzydamine Ⓟ

benzydamine HCl

Local Analgesic

Apotex

Date of Preparation: November 5, 1998

PHARMACOLOGY: Animal studies using parenteral route have shown that benzydamine hydrochloride possesses properties of an analgesic/anti-inflammatory agent. This effect is not mediated through the pituitary-adrenal axis. Studies using the topical route have demonstrated local anesthetic properties of benzydamine hydrochloride. In controlled studies in humans with oro–pharyngeal mucosity due to radiation therapy, benzydamine hydrochloride oral rinse use has provided relief through reduction of pain and edema. Similar studies in patients with acute sore throat demonstrated relief from pain.

Benzydamine hydrochloride has been detected in blood and urine after gargling four times for 20 seconds, in rapid succession, each time with a volume equivalent to 25.5 mg benzydamine per 70 kg body weight (approximately 17 mL per gargle). The average maximum plasma level of 59 ng/mL (range 17 to 173) was obtained 2 hours after gargling. For comparison, one dose of 17 mL, when swallowed, yielded an average maximum plasma level of 180 ng/mL (range 102 to 324), also at 2 hours after ingestion. Benzydamine was still detectable 24 hours later in 7 out of 10 subjects after the gargling (average plasma level of 7 ng/mL) and in 9 out of 10 subjects after the ingestion (average 32 ng/mL).

The urinary excretion was completed within 3-4 days after the single dose in both groups; about 46% of the dose was recovered in garglers, about 26% in ingestors. Repeated administration for 7 days did not result in a significant accumulation of benzydamine hydrochloride in plasma.

INDICATIONS: APO-BENZYDAMINE (benzydamine hydrochloride) Oral Rinse is indicated for relief of pain in acute sore throat and for the symptomatic relief of oro-pharyngeal mucositis caused by radiation therapy.

CONTRAINDICATIONS: APO-BENZYDAMINE (benzydamine hydrochloride) Oral Rinse is contraindicated in subjects with a history of hypersensitivity to any of its components.

WARNINGS: No data supplied by the manufacturer.

PRECAUTIONS: The use of undiluted APO-BENZYDAMINE (benzydamine hydrochloride) may produce local irritation manifested by burning sensation in patients with mucosal defects. If necessary, it may be diluted (1:1) with lukewarm water.

Since APO-BENZYDAMINE is absorbed from oral mucosa and then excreted mostly unchanged in the urine, a possibility of its systemic action has to be considered in patients with renal impairment.

Pregnancy: The safety of benzydamine hydrochloride has not been established in pregnant patients. Risk to benefit ratio should be established if APO-BENZYDAMINE Oral Rinse is to be used in these patients.

Children: Safety and dose directions have not been established for children five years of age and younger.

ADVERSE EFFECTS: The most frequent adverse reactions reported are: local numbness (9.7%), local burning or stinging sensation (8.2%), nausea and/or vomiting (2.1%).

The least frequent were reports of throat irritation, cough, dryness of the mouth associated with thirst, drowsiness and headache.

OVERDOSE:

There are no known cases of overdosage with benzydamine hydrochloride oral rinse formulations. Since no specific antidote for benzydamine is available, cases of excessive ingestion of the liquid should receive supportive symptomatic treatment aimed at rapid elimination of the drug.

> For management of a suspected drug overdose, CPhA recommends that you contact your **regional Poison Control Centre**. See the *CPS* Directory section for a list of Poison Control Centres.

DOSAGE: Not less than 15 mL of the liquid should be used for each gargle or rinse and repeated three or four times a day, depending on the severity of the treated condition. The liquid should be kept in contact with the inflamed mucosa for at least 30 seconds and then expelled from the mouth. Administration should begin the day prior to commencement of radiation therapy and continue daily during the treatment period as well as after cessation of radiation applications until desired improvement is obtained.

In acute sore throat, gargle with 15 mL every 1.5 to 3 hours. The solution should be expelled from the mouth after use.

SUPPLIED: Each bottle of clear yellow-green liquid with a distinctive mint-like odor contains: benzydamine HCl 0.15% w/v. Nonmedicinal ingredients: artificial freshmint flavour, D&C Yellow No. 10, ethanol, FD&C Blue No. 1, glycerin, methylparaben, polysorbate 80, propylparaben and purified water. PET bottles of 100 and 250 mL. Store at room temperature (15 to 30°C). Protect from freezing.

Apo®-Bromazepam

bromazepam

Anxiolytic—Sedative

Apotex

Date of Preparation: July 14, 1995
Date of Revision: February 6, 2001

PHARMACOLOGY: APO-BROMAZEPAM (bromazepam) is a benzodiazepine with anxiolytic and sedative properties which are of value in the symptomatic relief of pathological anxiety in psychoneurotic patients.

Orally administered bromazepam is completely absorbed with peak blood levels achieved 1 to 4 hours after administration. Bromazepam has a mean serum half-life of 12 hours (8 to 19 hours). Over a 72-hour interval, 69% of a 12 mg oral dose was recovered in the urine in the form of conjugated 3-hydroxybromazepam and conjugated 2-(2-amino-5-bromo-3-hydroxybenzoyl)-pyridine.

Comparative Bioavailability: A controlled, three-way crossover bioavailability was conducted in 18 volunteers to compare the drug plasma levels produced by a single 6 mg oral dose of bromazepam. The products compared were APO-BROMAZEPAM 1.5 and 6 mg tablets manufactured by Apotex Inc. and Lectopam 6 mg tablets manufactured by Hoffman-La Roche Ltd. The following mean pharmacokinetic values were reported: see Table 1 and Table 2.

Table 1: APO-BROMAZEPAM

APO-BROMAZEPAM 6 mg Tablets versus Lectopam 6 mg Tablets

Parameter	Geometric Mean Arithmetic Mean (C.V.) APO-BROMAZEPAM 6 mg	 Lectopam 6 mg	Ratio of Means (%)
AUC_T (ng·hr/mL)	1575.0 1646.9 (33)	1614.9 1716.0 (38)	97.5
AUC_I (ng·hr/mL)	1797.2 1870.7 (31)	1839.0 1965.5 (42)	97.7
C_{max} (ng/mL)	71.5 73.8 (28)	73.4 75.4 (23)	97.4
T_{max} (hours)[a]	1.72 (57)	1.42 (35)	—
$t_{1/2}$ (hours)[a]	20.6 (27)	20.2 (24)	

[a] Arithmetic means only (C.V.).

Table 2: APO-BROMAZEPAM

APO-BROMAZEPAM 1.5 mg Tablets versus Lectopam 6 mg Tablets

Parameter	Geometric Mean Arithmetic Mean (C.V.) APO-BROMAZEPAM 1.5 mg	 Lectopam 6 mg	Ratio of Means (%)
AUC_T (ng·hr/mL)	1680.8 1801.7 (35)	1614.9 1716.0 (38)	104
AUC_I (ng·hr/mL)	1933.3 2078.5 (37)	1839.0 1965.5 (42)	105.1
C_{max} (ng/mL)	75.5 78.4 (28)	73.4 75.4 (23)	102.8
T_{max} (hours)[a]	1.67 (54)	1.42 (35)	—
$t_{1/2}$ (hours)[a]	22.0 (26)	20.2 (24)	

[a] Arithmetic means only (C.V.).

INDICATIONS: APO-BROMAZEPAM (bromazepam) is useful for the short-term, symptomatic relief of manifestations of excessive anxiety in patients with anxiety neurosis.

CONTRAINDICATIONS: APO-BROMAZEPAM (bromazepam) is contraindicated in patients with known hypersensitivity to benzodiazepines and in patients with myasthenia gravis.

WARNINGS: APO-BROMAZEPAM (bromazepam) is not recommended for use in patients with depressive disorders or psychosis. Patients should be advised against the concurrent use of alcohol and other CNS depressant drugs.

Children: Because of the lack of sufficient clinical experience, bromazepam is not recommended for use in patients less than 18 years of age.

Occupational Hazards: Driving and Hazardous Activities: Since bromazepam has a central nervous system depressant effect, patients should be warned against driving, operating dangerous machinery, or engaging in other hazardous activities requiring mental alertness and physical coordination and should be cautioned that the effects of alcohol on such activities may be increased.

Pregnancy: The safety of use of bromazepam in pregnancy has not been established. Therefore, bromazepam should not be used during pregnancy. Several studies have suggested an increased risk of congenital malformations with the use of the benzodiazepines, chlordiazepoxide and diazepam, and meprobamate during the first trimester of pregnancies. Since bromazepam is also a benzodiazepine derivative, its administration is rarely justified in women of child-bearing potential. If the drug is prescribed to a woman of child-bearing potential, she should be warned to consult her physician regarding discontinuation of the drug if she plans to become or suspects that she is pregnant.

Lactation: Bromazepam and its metabolites are probably excreted in human milk. Therefore, this drug should not be given to nursing mothers.

PRECAUTIONS: Geriatrics: Elderly and debilitated patients, or those with organic brain syndrome, have been found to be prone to CNS depression after even low doses of benzodiazepines. Therefore, medication should be initiated in these patients with very low initial doses and increments should be made gradually, depending on the response of the patient, in order to avoid oversedation or neurological impairment. The initial dose for the elderly or debilitated patients should not exceed 3 mg.

Dependence Liability: APO-BROMAZEPAM (bromazepam) should not be administered to individuals prone to drug abuse.

Caution should be observed with all patients who are considered to have potential for psychological dependence.

Withdrawal symptoms similar to those occurring with other drugs of this class, including alcohol, have been observed after abrupt discontinuation of the drug. These include irritability, nervousness, insomnia, agitation, tremors, convulsions, diarrhea, abdominal cramps, vomiting and memory impairment. Since these symptoms are similar to those for which the patient is being treated, it may appear that the patient has suffered a relapse upon discontinuation of the drug. It is suggested that the drug should be withdrawn gradually, if the individual is suspected of being dependent, or the drug perhaps has been used in prolonged high doses.

Mental and Emotional Disorders: It should be recognized that suicidal tendencies may be present in patients with emotional disorders and that protective measures and appropriate treatment may be necessary and should be instituted without delay.

Since excitement and other paradoxical reactions can result from the use of anxiolytic sedatives in psychotic patients, bromazepam should not be used in ambulatory patients suspected of having psychotic tendencies.

As with other benzodiazepines, bromazepam should not be used in individuals with physiological anxiety or normal stresses of daily living, but only in the presence of disabling manifestations of an appropriate pathological anxiety disorder. These drugs are not effective in patients with characterological and personality disorders or those with obsessive-compulsive disorders. Bromazepam is also not recommended for management of depressive or psychotic disorders.

Impaired Hepatic or Renal Function: In patients with impaired hepatic or renal function, it is recommended to initiate therapy, if necessary, at a very low dose and to increase the dosage only to the extent that such an increase is compatible with the degree of residual function of these organs. Such patients should be followed closely and have periodic laboratory assessments.

Laboratory Tests: If bromazepam should be administered for repeated cycles of therapy, periodic blood counts and liver function tests are advisable.

Drug Interactions: Bromazepam may potentiate or interact with the effects of other CNS-acting drugs such as alcohol, narcotics, barbiturates, non-barbiturate hypnotics, antihistamines, phenothiazines, thioxanthenes, butyrophenones, monoamine oxidase inhibitors, tricyclic antidepressants and anticonvulsants. Therefore, if bromazepam is to be combined with other drugs acting on the CNS, careful consideration should be given to the pharmacology of the agent involved because of the possible additive or potentiation of drug effects. Patients should also be advised against the simultaneous use of other CNS depressant drugs and should be cautioned not to take alcohol during the administration of bromazepam because of the potentiation of effects that might occur.

ADVERSE EFFECTS: The most frequently reported adverse reactions with bromazepam have been drowsiness, ataxia and dizziness. Release of hostility and other paradoxical effects such as irritability and excitability are known to occur with the use of benzodiazepines.

Other side effects less frequently reported, listed by body systems, include the following:
Neurologic: blurred vision, headache, seizures, slurred speech, difficulty in depth perception.
Psychiatric: agitation, mental confusion, depression, irritability, nervousness, sleep disorders, euphoria, lethargy, stupor.
Gastrointestinal: dry mouth, nausea, non-specific gastrointestinal disturbances, vomiting.
Musculoskeletal: muscle spasm, muscle weakness.
Cardiovascular: hypotension, palpitations, tachycardia.
Dermatologic: pruritus, rash.
Genitourinary: incontinence, change in libido.
Hematologic: decreased hemoglobin and hematocrit, increased and decreased WBC.
Hepatic: elevations of alkaline phosphatase, bilirubin, AST and ALT.
Miscellaneous Blood Chemistry: increased and decreased blood sugar levels.

OVERDOSE:

Symptoms: Overdosage manifestations include drowsiness, somnolence, ataxia, impaired vision, depressed reflexes and finally coma. Hypotension and respiratory depression may occur with large overdoses.

Treatment: Vital signs should be monitored and general supportive measures should be employed as indicated. Gastric lavage should be instituted as soon as possible. Vomiting may be induced if the patient is fully awake. The value of dialysis has not been determined.

As is frequently the case in intentional overdosage, the probability of multiple agents having been ingested should be considered.

For management of a suspected drug overdose, CPhA recommends that you contact your **regional Poison Control Centre**. See the *CPS* Directory section for a list of Poison Control Centres.

DOSAGE: The dosage of APO-BROMAZEPAM (bromazepam) must be individualized and carefully titrated in order to avoid excessive sedation or mental and motor impairment. Short course of treatment should usually be the rule for the symptomatic relief of excessive anxiety and the initial course of treatment should not last longer than one week without reassessment of the need for a limited extension. If necessary, drug dosage can be adjusted after one week of treatment. Initially, not more than one week's supply of the drug should be provided and automatic prescription renewals should not be allowed. Subsequent prescriptions, when required, should be limited to a short course of therapy.

Usual Adult Dosage: The recommended initial adult daily dosage is 6 to 18 mg in equally divided doses, depending on the severity of symptoms and response of the patient. Treatment should be initiated by lower doses and adjusted as necessary. The optimal dosage may range from 6 to 30 mg daily in individual patients, in divided doses. Doses up to 60 mg daily may be used in exceptional cases.

Elderly and Debilitated Patients: The initial daily dose in these patients should not exceed 3 mg in divided doses. This dosage can be carefully adjusted, depending on tolerance and response of the patient.

SUPPLIED: 1.5 mg: Each white, round, flat-faced, beveled-edge, scored tablet, engraved "APO" over "B-1.5" on one side, contains: bromazepam 1.5 mg. Nonmedicinal ingredients: cornstarch, lactose, magnesium stearate and microcrystalline cellulose. Bottles of 100.

3 mg: Each pink, round, flat-faced, beveled-edge, scored tablet, engraved "APO" over "B-3" on one side, contains: bromazepam 3 mg. Nonmedicinal ingredients: cornstarch, D&C Red #7 Calcium Lake, D&C Red #30 Aluminum Lake, lactose, magnesium stearate and microcrystalline cellulose. Bottles of 100 and 500.

6 mg: Each green, round, flat-faced, beveled-edge, scored tablet, engraved "APO" over "B-6" on one side, contains: bromazepam 6 mg. Nonmedicinal ingredients: Blue #1 Aluminum Lake, cornstarch, D&C yellow #10 Lake, ferric ferrous oxide, lactose, magnesium stearate and microcrystalline cellulose. Bottles of 100 and 500.

Store at controlled room temperature (15 and 30°C).

Apo®-Bromocriptine

bromocriptine mesylate

Prolactin Inhibitor—Growth Hormone Suppressant in Acromegaly—Adjunctive Medication in Parkinson's Disease

Apotex

Date of Preparation: May 13, 1994
Date of Revision: December 31, 1996

PHARMACOLOGY: APO-BROMOCRIPTINE (bromocriptine mesylate) is a dopaminomimetic ergot derivative with D_2 type dopamine receptor agonist activity, and has also D_1 dopamine receptor antagonist properties.

Bromocriptine inhibits the release and synthesis of prolactin by acting directly on the prolactin secreting cells of the anterior pituitary. In patients with acromegaly, apart from lowering prolactin and elevated levels of growth hormone, bromocriptine has a beneficial effect on clinical symptoms and on glucose tolerance.

The dopaminomimetic activity of bromocriptine in nigro-striatal pathway is considered responsible for the clinical benefits seen in patients with Parkinson's disease.

The metabolism of dopamine, from exogenous and endogenous origin, is known to involve the formation of peroxides and free radicals. It has been postulated that these agents may in fact contribute to the progression of Parkinson's disease by accelerating the rate at which neuronal cells are lost. Bromocriptine's metabolic pathway does not involve the formation of such peroxides and free radicals. It has been suggested that because bromocriptine attenuates the timing and rate of levodopa dosage increase, early use of the drug may reduce risk of formation of potentially toxic peroxides and free radicals.

In man, bromocriptine is rapidly absorbed after oral administration with an absorption half-life of approximately 0.3 hours. The amount absorbed is about 65-95% of the oral dose. About 7% of the dose reaches the systemic circulation unchanged, due to a high hepatic extraction rate and first pass metabolism. The plasma protein binding amounts to 96%. Bromocriptine is extensively metabolized by the liver. Only traces of the unchanged compound are found in urine, together with 2 major metabolites. Unchanged drug represents about 10-15% of peak levels of radioactivity in plasma measured after a single dose of labelled drug. The active parent drug and the metabolites are primarily excreted via the liver, with only 6% being eliminated via the kidney. In plasma, the elimination half-life was between 2 to 8 hours for the parent drug and 50 to 70 hours for the metabolites after single oral doses.

The extreme variability in GI tract absorption and the extensive and individually variable first-pass metabolism are responsible for the broad variability in plasma concentrations of bromocriptine and, in part, for the variability in dose response.

Comparative Bioavailability: A comparative bioavailability study was performed using normal healthy human volunteers. The rate and extent of absorption after a single 7.5 mg dose of APO-BROMOCRIPTINE 2.5 mg tablets and Parlodel 2.5 mg tablets was measured and compared. The results are summarized in Table 1.

Table 1: APO-BROMOCRIPTINE

Rate and Extent of Absorption After a Single 7.5 mg Dose of APO-BROMOCRIPTINE 2.5 mg Tablets and Parlodel 2.5 mg Tablets

	APO-BROMOCRIPTINE	Parlodel[c]	Percentage of Parlodel
AUC_T[a] (ng·hr/mL)	5.66 (16)	5.46 (23)	103.7
AUC_I[a] (ng·hr/mL)	7.00 (15)	6.72 (22)	104.2
C_{max}[a] (ng/mL)	0.99 (14)	0.99 (16)	100
T_{max}[b] (hr)	1.18 (0.33)	1.18 (0.35)	—
$t_{½}$[b] (hr)	6.09 (1.00)	5.95 (1.44)	—

[a] Geometric means (CV).
[b] Arithmetic means (SD).
[c] Parlodel (Sandoz) from a Canadian pharmacy.

A second bioavailability study was performed using normal healthy human volunteers. The rate and extent of absorption after a single 10 mg dose of APO-BROMOCRIPTINE 5 mg capsules and Parlodel 5 mg capsules was measured and compared. The potency corrected results are summarized as follows (see Table 2).

Table 2: APO-BROMOCRIPTINE

Rate and Extent of Absorption After a Single 10 mg Dose of APO-BROMOCRIPTINE 5 mg Capsules and Parlodel 5 mg Capsules

	APO-BROMOCRIPTINE	Parlodel[c]	Ratio of Geometric Means (%)
AUC_T (pg·hr/mL)	511[a] 586 (51)[b]	514[a] 582 (47)[b]	99
AUC_I (pg·hr/mL)	618[a] 696 (48)[b]	610[a] 672 (43)[b]	101
C_{max} (pg/mL)	208[a] 224 (39)[b]	207[a] 227 (46)[b]	100
T_{max} (hr)	1.39 (34)[b]	1.29 (43)[b]	—
$t_{½}$ (hr)	2.44 (65)[b]	2.21 (53)[b]	—

[a] Geometric means.
[b] Arithmetic means (CV).
[c] Parlodel (Sandoz) from a Canadian pharmacy.

Note: The two summary tables simply serve as a convenient way of comparing the bioavailability of APO-BROMOCRIPTINE and Parlodel within each study, not between studies. Due to advancement of analytical technology, the radioimmunoassay used in the capsule study for measuring plasma drug concentrations is evidently more selective and sensitive than the one used in the tablet study. This results in differences in observed pharmacokinetic parameter values between the two studies. Therefore, the results from these two studies should not be used as a basis for dose adjustment when switching between tablets and capsules.

INDICATIONS: Galactorrhea with or without amenorrhea due to hyperprolactinemia.

Prolactin-dependent menstrual disorders and infertility: e.g. secondary amenorrhea, ovulatory insufficiency and short luteal phase.

Prolactin-secreting adenomas: as a treatment for inoperable macroadenomas or prior to surgery in order to facilitate removal, and as an alternative to surgery in patients with microadenomas.

Prolactin-dependent male hypogonadism.

Acromegaly: The first-line treatment of this condition is by surgery or radiotherapy. APO-BROMOCRIPTINE (bromocriptine mesylate) may be a useful adjunct to such treatment, and can be used as monotherapy in special cases.

Parkinson's Disease: APO-BROMOCRIPTINE is effective when used as adjunct therapy to levodopa in the symptomatic management of Parkinson's Disease. Used concomitantly with levodopa, bromocriptine facilitates the use of lower doses of levodopa in early disease and attenuates the rate of increase in the levodopa dosages on long-term usage. In this way the risk of long-term complications such as prominent dyskinesias and/or end-of-dose failure can be reduced.

CONTRAINDICATIONS: Uncontrolled hypertension of pregnancy, a history of toxemia of pregnancy, sensitivity to ergot alkaloids. For procedure during pregnancy see Pregnancy under Precautions.

WARNINGS: In women with non-puerperal galactorrhea, reduction of prolactin levels may lead to resumption of normal menses. Following discontinuation of medication, galactorrhea returns in some patients and leads to suspicion of pituitary adenomas; a complete investigation at specialized units to identify these patients is advisable.

Treatment with APO-BROMOCRIPTINE (bromocriptine mesylate) may effectively lower prolactin levels in patients with pituitary tumors but does not obviate the necessity for radiotherapy or surgical intervention where appropriate.

Long-term treatment (6-36 months) with bromocriptine in doses ranging from 20-100 mg/day has been associated with pulmonary infiltrates, pleural effusion and thickening of the pleura in a few patients. In those instances in which bromocriptine treatment was terminated, the changes slowly reverted towards normal.

To date, there have been seven (7) reported cases of retroperitoneal fibrosis occurring in parkinsonian patients on long-term treatment (15 months-10 years) with bromocriptine at daily doses higher than 30 mg. To recognize retroperitoneal fibrosis at an early, reversible stage it is recommended to look for its manifestations (e.g. back pain, edema of the lower limbs, impaired kidney function) in this category of patients. APO-BROMOCRIPTINE medication should be withdrawn immediately if fibrotic changes in the retroperitoneum are diagnosed or suspected.

Although there is no conclusive evidence which demonstrates the interaction between bromocriptine and other ergot alkaloids, the concomitant use of these medications is not recommended.

Particular attention should be paid to patients who have recently received other drugs that can alter the blood pressure.

PRECAUTIONS: APO-BROMOCRIPTINE (bromocriptine mesylate) may cause hypotension, primarily postural; periodic monitoring of the blood pressure, particularly during the first days of therapy, is advisable. In some patients, dizziness (vertigo) may occur with bromocriptine; patients should therefore be cautioned against activities requiring rapid and precise responses such as driving an automobile or operating dangerous machinery until their response has been determined.

Care should be exercised when administering APO-BROMOCRIPTINE concomitantly with phenothiazines or with other medications known to lower blood pressure. Dosage should be adjusted accordingly.

Alcohol should be avoided during treatment with bromocriptine. In some patients the concomitant use of bromocriptine and alcohol has given rise to alcohol intolerance and an increase in the severity and incidence of bromocriptine's possible adverse reactions.

Although there is no conclusive evidence demonstrating interactions between bromocriptine and other ergot derivatives, it is not recommended to administer concomitantly APO-BROMOCRIPTINE and any drug with potential vasoconstrictor activity.

In patients being treated with APO-BROMOCRIPTINE for galactorrhea, prolactin induced amenorrhea, menstrual disorders or acromegaly, infertility might be reversed by restoration of normal menses and ovulation. Women who do not wish to conceive should, therefore, use a reliable method of contraception. Since pregnancy may occur prior to initiation of menses it is recommended that a pregnancy test be conducted at least every four weeks during the amenorrheic period, and, once menses are reinitiated, every time a patient misses a menstrual period.

There have been occasional reports of gastrointestinal bleeding in acromegalic patients, both in those treated with bromocriptine and in those given a different or no medication. Until further data are available, therefore, acromegalic patients with a history or evidence of peptic ulceration should preferably be given alternative treatment. If bromocriptine must be used in such patients they should be instructed to report promptly any gastrointestinal reactions.

The use of APO-BROMOCRIPTINE is not recommended for patients with uncontrolled hypertension or toxemia of pregnancy.

In postpartum women treated with bromocriptine mesylate, some rare serious adverse events (about 1 in 100 000) have been reported. These include hypertension, visual disturbances, myocardial infarction, seizures and strokes, or psychic disorders. In some patients the occurrence of seizures or strokes was preceded by severe headache and/or visual disturbances. Causal relationship of these events to the drug is uncertain.

Safety and efficacy of bromocriptine has not been established in patients with severe renal or hepatic disease.

Bromocriptine therapy has been demonstrated to be effective in the short term management of amenorrhea/galactorrhea. Data are not available on the safety or effectiveness of its use in long-term continuous dosage in this indication or in patients given repeated courses of treatment following recurrence of amenorrhea/galactorrhea after initial treatment. Recurrence rates are reportedly very high, ranging from 70 to 80%.

Bromocriptine should always be taken with food. In cases where adverse effects, such as nausea, vomiting and vertigo are severe or persisting, the therapeutic dosage of APO-BROMOCRIPTINE should be reduced to half of one tablet daily (1.25 mg) and increased gradually to the recommended dose. The dopamine antagonist domperidone may be useful in the control of severe gastrointestinal side effects in Parkinsonian patients receiving bromocriptine (see Drug Interactions).

As with all medication, APO-BROMOCRIPTINE should be kept safely out of the reach of children.

Pregnancy: In patients receiving APO-BROMOCRIPTINE, immunological confirmation of suspected conception should be performed as soon as possible and treatment stopped unless, in the opinion of the treating physician, the possible benefit to the patient outweighs the potential risk to the fetus. In any event, the patient must be monitored closely throughout pregnancy for signs and symptoms which may develop if a previously undetected prolactin-secreting tumor enlarges.

In human studies with bromocriptine, there were 1410 reported pregnancies, which yielded 1236 live and 5 stillborn infants from women who took bromocriptine during early pregnancy.

Among the 1241 infants, 43 cases (31 minor and 12 major) of congenital anomalies were reported. The incidence (3.46%) and type of congenital malformations and the incidence of spontaneous abortions (11.13%) in this group of pregnancies do not exceed those generally reported for such occurrences in the population at large.

Patients with pronounced enlargement of the sella turcica or a visual field defect should, in the first instance, be treated by surgery and/or radiotherapy. If pregnancy occurs in the presence of a pituitary microadenoma, close supervision throughout pregnancy is essential. This includes regular checking of the visual fields.

Small prolactin-secreting adenomas not detected previously may rapidly increase in size during pregnancy. Optic nerve compression may occur and emergency pituitary surgery or other appropriate measures may be necessary.

Use in Parkinson's Disease: Use of APO-BROMOCRIPTINE, particularly in high doses, may be associated with mental confusion and mental disturbances. Since patients with Parkinson's Disease may manifest varying degrees of dementia, caution should be exercised when treating such patients with bromocriptine.

APO-BROMOCRIPTINE administered alone or concomitantly with levodopa may cause visual or auditory hallucinations. These usually resolve with dosage reduction, but discontinuation of bromocriptine may be required in some cases. Rarely, after high doses, hallucinations have persisted for several weeks following discontinuation of bromocriptine. Caution should be exercised when administering APO-BROMOCRIPTINE to patients with a history of myocardial infarction, particularly if they have a residual atrial, nodal or ventricular arrhythmia.

Symptomatic hypotension can occur and, therefore, caution should be exercised when administering APO-BROMOCRIPTINE, particularly in patients receiving antihypertensive medication. Periodic evaluation of hepatic, hematopoietic, cardiovascular and renal function is recommended.

Drug Interactions: The concomitant use of erythromycin may increase bromocriptine plasma levels.

Domperidone, a peripheral dopamine antagonist, may cause increases in serum prolactin. In so doing, domperidone may antagonize the therapeutically-relevant prolactin lowering effect of bromocriptine. It is possible that the anti-tumorigenic effect of bromocriptine in patients with prolactinomas may be partially blocked by domperidone administration.

ADVERSE EFFECTS: The most frequently observed adverse reactions are nausea, vomiting, headache and gastrointestinal side effects such as abdominal pain, diarrhea and constipation. All these effects may be minimized or even prevented by giving small initial doses of bromocriptine and by taking it with food.

Postural hypotension can, on rare occasions, lead to fainting, and shock-like syndromes have been reported in sensitive patients. This is most likely to occur during the first few days of APO-BROMOCRIPTINE (bromocriptine mesylate) treatment.

In clinical studies to date, the following adverse reactions were noted:

In postpartum women treated with bromocriptine mesylate, some rare serious adverse events (about 1 in 100 000) have been reported. These include hypertension, visual disturbances, myocardial infarction, seizures and strokes, or psychic disorders. In some patients, the occurrence of seizures or strokes was preceded by severe headache and/or visual disturbances. Causal relationship of these events to the drug is uncertain.

Amenorrhea/Galactorrhea/Female Infertility/Acromegaly: The incidence of side effects in these indications is higher (68%), reflecting the larger doses required, but they are generally mild to moderate in degree. Therapy was discontinued in approximately 6% of patients because of adverse effects. In decreasing order of frequency these are: nausea 51%, headache 18%, dizziness 16%, fatigue 8%, abdominal cramps 7%, lightheadedness 6%, vomiting 5%, nasal congestion 5%, constipation 3%, and diarrhea 3%.

Parkinson's Disease: When bromocriptine is added to levodopa therapy, the incidence of adverse reactions may increase. The most common newly appearing adverse reactions in combination therapy with levodopa are: nausea, abnormal involuntary movements, hallucinations, confusion, "on-off" phenomenon, dizziness, drowsiness, faintness, fainting, vomiting, asthenia, abdominal discomfort, visual disturbance, ataxia, insomnia, depression, hypotension, shortness of breath, constipation and vertigo.

General: Less common adverse reactions include, anorexia, anxiety, blepharospasm, dry mouth, dysphagia, edema of the feet and ankles, erythromelalgia, epileptiform seizures, fatigue, headache, lethargia, mottling of skin, nasal stuffiness, nervousness, nightmares, paresthesia, skin rash, changes in urinary frequency, urinary incontinence, urinary retention and rarely signs and symptoms of ergotism such as tingling of fingers, cold feet, numbness, muscle cramps of feet and legs or exacerbation of Raynaud's syndrome.

Abnormalities in laboratory tests may include elevation of blood urea nitrogen, AST, ALT, GGPT, CPK, alkaline phosphatase and uric acid, which are usually transient and not of clinical significance.

The occurrence of adverse reactions may be lessened by temporarily reducing the dosage to 1.25 mg two or three times daily.

OVERDOSE:

Symptoms: There have been several reports of acute overdosage with bromocriptine in children and adults. No life threatening reactions have occurred. Symptoms reported could have resulted from over-stimulation of dopaminergic receptors: they included nausea, vomiting, dizziness, drowsiness, hypotension, sweating and hallucinations.

Treatment: The management of acute intoxication is largely symptomatic. The cardiovascular system should be monitored. Metoclopramide can be used to antagonize the emesis and hallucinations in patients who have taken high doses.

For management of a suspected drug overdose, CPhA recommends that you contact your **regional Poison Control Centre**. See the *CPS* Directory section for a list of Poison Control Centres.

DOSAGE: APO-BROMOCRIPTINE (bromocriptine mesylate) should always be taken with food. In order to establish tolerance, the first dose of 1.25-2.5 mg (½-1 tablet), depending on the indication should be given at bedtime with food. Please consult the detailed dosage recommendations for each indication.

Galactorrhea with or Without Amenorrhea Due to Hyperprolactinemia: 1.25-2.5 mg (½ to 1 tablet) at bedtime with food to establish tolerance; gradually increase after 2-3 days to 2.5 mg (1 tablet) twice daily with meals. If required the dose may be increased to 2.5 mg three times daily. Continue treatment until milk secretion has ceased completely or, in the case of menstrual dysfunction, until the menstrual cycle has returned to normal.

Prolactin-dependent Menstrual Disorders and Infertility: 1.25-2.5 mg (½ to 1 tablet) at bedtime with food to establish tolerance. Gradually increase after 2-3 days to one tablet twice daily with meals. If required the dose may be increased to 2.5 mg three times daily.

Prolactin Secreting Adenomas: 1.25 mg (½ tablet) 2 or 3 times daily, increasing gradually (average maintenance dose: 5-7.5 mg daily). If necessary to keep plasma prolactin adequately suppressed, dosage may be increased gradually over a period of several weeks to 10-20 mg (4 to 8 tablets or 2 to 4 capsules) daily with meals.

Prolactin Dependent Male Hypogonadism: 1.25-2.5 mg (½ to 1 tablet) at bedtime to establish tolerance. Gradually increase after 2 to 3 days to 2.5 mg twice daily with meals or more, as required to 2.5 mg three times per day with meals.

Acromegaly: 1.25-2.5 mg (½ to 1 tablet) at bedtime with food to establish tolerance, increasing gradually over a period of 2 to 4 weeks to 10-20 mg (4 to 8 tablets or 2 to 4 capsules) daily with meals, depending on clinical response. Daily requirements of 20 mg should be taken in four equally divided doses.

For convenience and after initial titration, some patients may use the 5 mg capsules for maintenance therapy.

The maximum recommended daily dose is 20 mg (eight 2.5 mg tablets or four 5 mg capsules).

In the event of serious or persistent adverse effects, the dosage should be reduced to 1.25 mg (½ tablet) and increased again gradually to the recommended dose. If reactions such as nausea, vomiting, vertigo or headaches continue to be severe, APO-BROMOCRIPTINE should be discontinued.

Parkinson's Disease: APO-BROMOCRIPTINE should be added to levodopa therapy. It is desirable to combine a slow increase of bromocriptine with a concomitant, limited and gradual reduction of levodopa. APO-BROMOCRIPTINE dosage should be individualized. The initial dose is 1.25 mg (½ tablet) at bedtime to establish tolerance. Thereafter, the recommended dosage is 2.5 mg daily in two divided doses, with meals.

The dosage may be increased, if necessary, by adding an additional 2.5 mg per day, once every 2 to 4 weeks, taken in 2 or 3 divided doses with meals. The maximum recommended daily dosage is 40 mg. Clinical assessments are recommended during dosage titration to ensure that the lowest effective dose is employed. Where dose levels permit, use of the 5 mg capsule may be found more convenient by many patients.

SUPPLIED: 2.5 mg: Each white, oval-shaped tablet, scored and engraved APO 2.5, contains: bromocriptine 2.5 mg (as mesylate). Nonmedicinal ingredients: croscarmellose sodium, lactose, magnesium stearate and microcrystalline cellulose. Bottles of 100. Store between 15 and 30°C. Protect from light and moisture.

5 mg: Each white and caramel No. 4 opaque capsule, imprinted APO 5, contains: bromocriptine 5 mg (as mesylate). Nonmedicinal ingredients: cornstarch, lactose, stearic acid and talc; capsule shell: gelatin, sodium lauryl sulfate, silicon dioxide, titanium dioxide, red iron oxide and yellow iron oxide; edible black ink: synthetic black iron oxide, D&C Yellow #10 aluminum lake, FD&C Blue #1 aluminum lake, FD&C Blue #2 aluminum lake, FD&C Red #40 aluminum lake, pharmaceutical glaze, n-butyl alcohol, propylene glycol and SDA-3A alcohol. Bottles of 100. Store between 15 and 30°C. Protect from light.

Apo®-Butorphanol Ⓒ

butorphanol tartrate

Analgesic

Apotex

Date of Preparation: October 22, 2003

PHARMACOLOGY: Butorphanol acts as an agonist at kappa-opioid receptors and a mixed agonist-antagonist at mu-opioid receptors in the central nervous system to alter the perception of pain. The drug is believed to act at sites in the periventricular and periaqueductal grey matter, and at sites in the spinal cord.

In an animal model, the dose of butorphanol tartrate required to antagonize morphine analgesia by 50% was similar to that for nalorphine, less than that for pentazocine and more than that for naloxone.

The analgesic activity of 2 mg of butorphanol tartrate administered parenterally is approximately equivalent to 10 mg morphine sulfate, 80 mg meperidine hydrochloride or 40 mg pentazocine. In normal volunteers, the same doses of these drugs produced nearly equivalent respiratory depression. Butorphanol, in contrast to morphine or meperidine, produces respiratory depression in a limited dose range, reaching a plateau at approximately 4 mg. The magnitude of respiratory depression with butorphanol is not appreciably increased at a dose of 4 mg; however, the duration of respiratory depression appears to be dose-related. Respiratory rates were monitored in controlled clinical studies with therapeutic doses of butorphanol tartrate nasal spray and no untowards effects were observed. Respiratory depression noted after administration of butorphanol by any route is reversed by treatment with naloxone, a specific opioid antagonist (see Overdose, Symptoms and Treatment).

Butorphanol tartrate has a marked sedative effect that is dose related and this property should be considered in its clinical application (see Precautions).

The hemodynamic changes after the intravenous administration of butorphanol are similar to those produced by pentazocine. These include increased pulmonary artery pressure, pulmonary wedge pressure, left ventricular end diastolic pressure, systemic arterial pressure, and pulmonary vascular resistance. Although smaller than those associated with pentazocine, these changes are nevertheless in a direction that increases the work of the heart, especially in the pulmonary circuit.

Butorphanol, like other mixed agonist-antagonists with a high affinity for the kappa receptor, produced unpleasant psychotomimetic effects in some individuals.

Pharmacokinetics: The pharmacokinetics (including absorption times and peak blood levels) of a nasal spray dose and an intramuscular dose of butorphanol tartrate are similar. In addition, after an initial absorption phase, the pharmacokinetics of a nasal spray dose are also similar to those of an intravenous dose.

Table 1: APO-BUTORPHANOL

Mean Pharmacokinetic Parameters of Butorphanol Tartrate Nasal Spray in Young and Elderly Subjects[a]

Parameter	Young	Elderly
T_{max}[b] (hr)	0.62 (0.50–2.00)[e]	0.75 (0.25–3.00)
C_{max}[c] (ng/mL)	1.04 (0.35–1.97)	0.90 (1.10–2.68)
$AUC_{(inf)}$[d] (hr·ng/mL)	4.93 (2.16–7.27)	5.24 (0.30–10.34)
Half-life (hr)	4.7 (2.89–8.79)	6.6 (3.75–9.17)
Absolute Bioavailability (%)	69 (44–113)	62 (3–121)
Volume of Distribution[f] (L)	487 (305–901)	552 (305–737)
Clearance[f] (L/hr)	98 (70–154)	82 (52–143)

[a] Young subjects (n=24) are from 20 to 40 years old (mean M/F, 25/30 years) and elderly subjects (n=24) are from 65 to 83 years old (mean M/F, 71 years).
[b] Time to peak plasma concentration, median values.
[c] Peak plasma concentration normalized to 1 mg dose.
[d] Area under the plasma concentration time curve after a 1 mg dose.
[e] (Range of observed values).
[f] Derived from IV data.

Butorphanol tartrate is rapidly absorbed without significant biotransformation following nasal administration. In both young and elderly normal volunteers, peak blood levels occur around one-half hour following nasal administration. Peak plasma concentrations after a 1 mg dose vary from a mean of 0.9 to 1.04 ng/mL (see Table 1). Elderly subjects may have a somewhat decreased ability to eliminate butorphanol, with an apparent elimination half-life of 6.6 hours as opposed to 4.7 hours for younger subjects. The mean absolute bioavailability may be somewhat less for elderly women (48%) than for elderly men or younger subjects (75% and 69% respectively).

The mean plasma half-life of butorphanol is 5.1 hours after a 2 mg intranasal administration.

Serum protein binding is independent of concentration over the range achieved in clinical practice (up to 7 ng/mL) with a bound fraction of approximately 80%. Butorphanol crosses the blood brain and placental barriers and is found in human milk (see Precautions).

The volume of distribution of butorphanol varies from 305-901 litres and total body clearance from 52-154 litres/hour.

Intranasal butorphanol pharmacokinetic studies determined that steady state plasma levels of butorphanol were dose proportional (in doses up to 4 mg every 6 hours). Steady state is achieved within 2 days, and plasma concentrations are approximately 1.8 times those following a single dose.

Butorphanol is extensively metabolized in the liver and is eliminated as oxidized and conjugated metabolites. Metabolism is qualitatively and quantitatively similar with nasal, intravenous, or intramuscular administration. Less than 5% of an intravenous dose is recovered in the urine as unchanged drug. Because of extensive first-pass metabolism, the bioavailability of oral butorphanol is less than 10%.

Hydroxybutorphanol is the main urinary metabolite of butorphanol (49% of dose); small amounts of norbutorphanol (<5%) are also excreted in urine. The analgesic activity of these two metabolites has not been determined in humans.

In Patients with Renal Insufficiency: Eighteen female volunteers (age 30-65 years) with normal or varying degrees of renal impairment were given single 1 mg intranasal doses of butorphanol. As shown below, the elimination half-life of butorphanol was prolonged, and the AUC increased, in patients with reduced creatinine clearance (CrCl). No effect, however, was observed on C_{max} or T_{max}.

	CrCl (mL/min)	$t_{½}$ (h)	AUC (h·ng/mL)
Normal	>70	5.75	4.32 (1.63)[a]
Moderately impaired	30–60	8.55	6.49 (1.32)
Severely impaired	<30	10.48	7.41 (2.64)

[a] Standard Deviation.

In Patients with Hepatic Disease: The pharmacokinetics and absolute bioavailability of a 1 mg dose of transnasal butorphanol tartrate was studied in 12 (8M, 4F) subjects with hepatic impairment, and 12 normal subjects matched for sex, age and weight. Compared to normal subjects, patients with hepatic impairment had on average a 3-fold increase in $t_{½}$ and a 2 to 3-fold increase in AUC. Absolute bioavailability was 99% in the subjects with hepatic impairment compared to 73% in controls. C_{max} and T_{max}, however, remained unaltered regardless of the liver conditions.

Pharmacodynamics: Following intranasal administration of butorphanol tartrate nasal spray, onset of analgesia is within 15-30 minutes, and peak analgesic activity generally occurs within 1-2 hours. The duration of analgesia varies depending on the pain model but is generally 3-6 hours with intranasal doses of 1-2 mg.

Clinical Studies: Migraine Headache Pain: The analgesic efficacy of two 1 mg doses one hour apart of butorphanol tartrate nasal spray in migraine headache pain was compared with a single dose of 10 mg intramuscular methadone or placebo (32 patients per treatment group). Significant onset of analgesia occurred within 15 minutes for both butorphanol tartrate nasal spray and intramuscular methadone. Peak analgesic effect occurred at 2 hours for butorphanol tartrate nasal spray and 1.5 hours for methadone. The median duration of pain relief was 6 hours with butorphanol tartrate nasal spray and 4 hours with methadone as judged by the time when approximately half of the patients remedicated.

In the two other trials in patients with migraine headache pain, a 2 mg initial dose of butorphanol tartrate nasal spray followed by an additional 1 mg dose 1 hour later (76 patients) was compared with either 75 mg intramuscular meperidine (24 patients) or placebo (72 patients). Onset peak activity and duration were similar with both active treatments; however, the incidence of adverse experiences (nausea, vomiting, dizziness) was higher in these two trials with the 2 mg initial dose of butorphanol tartrate nasal spray than in the trial with the 1 mg initial dose.

Postoperative Analgesia: The analgesic efficacy of butorphanol tartrate nasal spray was investigated in placebo-controlled studies in postoperative surgical pain (abdominal, orthopedic, gynecologic) and in postoperative caesarian section pain. Patients had moderate to severe pain at baseline.

In the general surgery study, a single 1 or 2 mg dose of butorphanol tartrate nasal spray (33 to 36 patients per treatment group) was compared to a single dose of 37.5 or 75 mg intramuscular meperidine. In this blinded study, the effects of the lower doses of each drug could be distinguished from those of the higher doses. Analgesia provided by the 1 and 2 mg doses of butorphanol was equivalent to that of 37.5 and 75 mg of meperidine respectively. The duration of pain relief was 2 to 3 hours with 1 mg butorphanol tartrate nasal spray and 3 to 4 hours with 2 mg butorphanol tartrate nasal spray, as judged by the time when approximately half of the patients required a repeat dose.

In the caesarian section study, a single dose of 2 mg butorphanol tartrate nasal spray (37 patients) or two 1 mg doses of butorphanol tartrate nasal spray given 1 hour apart (35 patients), were compared to a single dose of 2 mg intravenous butorphanol (37 patients) or placebo (37 patients).

Significant pain relief began within 5 minutes for intravenous butorphanol, 15 minutes for 2 mg butorphanol tartrate nasal spray, and 30 minutes for the two 1 mg doses of butorphanol tartrate nasal spray. Peak analgesic effects were similar for the three butorphanol treatments. The duration of pain relief, as judged by this time when approximately half of the patients required a repeat dose, was 2 to 3 hours for 2 mg i.v. butorphanol and 4 to 5 hours for 2 mg butorphanol tartrate nasal spray administered either as a single dose or two 1 mg doses given 1 hour apart.

INDICATIONS: APO-BUTORPHANOL (butorphanol tartrate) Nasal Spray is indicated for the relief of moderate to severe acute pain. The efficacy of APO-BUTORPHANOL Nasal Spray for periods longer than 3 days has not been established.

CONTRAINDICATIONS: APO-BUTORPHANOL (butorphanol tartrate) Nasal Spray is contraindicated in patients hypersensitive to butorphanol tartrate or to any component of the preparation.

WARNINGS: Patients Dependent on Narcotics: Because of the opioid antagonist properties of butorphanol tartrate, patients who are physically dependent on narcotics should not be given butorphanol tartrate as they may experience withdrawal symptoms. Such patients should have an adequate period of withdrawal from opioid drugs prior to beginning butorphanol tartrate nasal spray therapy.

Butorphanol tartrate nasal spray has precipitated opioid withdrawal symptoms in patients taking opioid analgesics chronically. Adverse experiences include those of the central nervous system (anxiety, agitation, mood changes, hallucinations, and dysphoria) more frequently than typical somatic opioid withdrawal symptoms. Because of the difficulty in assessing opioid tolerance in patients who have recently received repeated doses of narcotic analgesic medication, caution should be used in the administration of butorphanol tartrate nasal spray to such patients.

PRECAUTIONS: General: Hypotension associated with syncope during the first hour of dosing with butorphanol tartrate nasal spray has been reported rarely, particularly in patients with past history of similar reactions to opioid analgesics. Therefore, patients should be advised to avoid activities with potential risks.

The sedative property should be considered in the clinical use of butorphanol tartrate nasal spray. In addition, patients receiving recommended therapeutic doses may experience severe dizziness, nausea, vomiting and confusion. Infrequently, hallucinations have also occurred at 2 mg. The patient should be advised accordingly (see Adverse Effects).

Limited clinical experience appears to suggest that patients with migraine headache may be more susceptible to certain adverse reactions associated with butorphanol tartrate nasal spray (see Adverse Effects).

Head Injury and Increased Intracranial Pressure: As with other opioids, butorphanol used in patients with head injury may be associated with carbon dioxide retention and secondary elevation of cerebrospinal fluid pressure, miosis, and alterations in mental state that would obscure the interpretation of the clinical course of head injuries. In such patients, butorphanol should be used only if the benefits of use outweigh the risks.

Respiratory Depression: As a class, the mixed agonist-antagonist opioid drugs are less likely than morphine to produce significant respiratory depression. Nevertheless, drugs of this class may produce respiratory depression in susceptible individuals, especially patients receiving other CNS active agents or suffering from CNS diseases or respiratory impairment.

Hepatic Disease: Butorphanol tartrate nasal spray should be administered with caution to patients with liver disease (see Pharmacology, Pharmacokinetics, and Dosage, Dosage Adjustments).

Renal Disease: Impaired renal function necessitates alterations in dosing schedule (see Pharmacology, Pharmacokinetics, and Dosage, Dosage Adjustments).

Cardiovascular Effects: Because butorphanol tartrate nasal spray increases the work of the heart, especially the pulmonary circuit, the use of this drug in acute myocardial infarction or in cardiac patients with ventricular dysfunction or coronary insufficiency should be limited to those patients for whom the benefits clearly outweigh the risk.

Severe hypertension has been reported rarely during parenteral administration of butorphanol. Because of the similarity in pharmacokinetics (see Pharmacology), this adverse event could potentially occur during use of butorphanol tartrate nasal spray. In such cases, butorphanol should be discontinued and the hypertension treated with antihypertensive drugs. In patients who are not opioid dependent, naloxone has also been reported to be effective.

Use in Anesthesia: Butorphanol tartrate nasal spray has not been evaluated for use in anesthesia.

Occupational Hazards: Use in Ambulatory Patients: Drowsiness and dizziness related to the use of butorphanol tartrate nasal spray may impair mental and/or physical abilities required for the performance of potentially hazardous tasks (e.g., driving, operating machinery, etc.). Patients should be told to use caution in such activities until their individual response to butorphanol has been well characterized.

Pregnancy: There are no adequate and well-controlled studies of butorphanol in pregnant women before 37 weeks of gestation. The use of butorphanol tartrate in women of childbearing potential requires that the expected benefit of the drug be weighed against the potential risk to the mother and fetus.

Reproduction studies in mice, rats and rabbits during organogenesis did not reveal any teratogenic potential of butorphanol. Pregnant rats treated subcutaneously with butorphanol at 1 mg/kg (5.9 mg/m²) had a higher frequency of stillbirths than controls. Butorphanol administered orally at 30 mg/kg (5.1 mg/m²) and 60 mg/kg (10.2 mg/m²) also showed higher incidences of post-implantation loss in rabbits.

Use in Labour and Delivery: Butorphanol tartrate nasal spray is not recommended during labour or delivery because there is no clinical experience with its use in this setting. Butorphanol tartrate injection has been used during labour, and there have been rare reports of neonatal respiratory depression of the newborn occurring after delivery.

Lactation: There is no clinical experience with the use of butorphanol tartrate nasal spray in nursing mothers. If butorphanol tartrate is administered to a nursing mother, consideration should be given to the possibility that pharmacologically active drug could be available to a nursing infant. Butorphanol tartrate administered intravenously or intramuscularly is secreted in low concentrations in human milk; however, the clinical significance of this finding has not been systematically evaluated.

Children: Safety and efficacy of butorphanol tartrate nasal spray in patients under 18 years of age have not been established.

Geriatrics: The mean half-life of butorphanol tartrate is increased to 6 hours in patients over the age of 65 (see Pharmacology). In addition to having a somewhat reduced ability to eliminate butorphanol, elderly patients may be more sensitive to its side effects, particularly dizziness (see Dosage).

Dependence Liability: Although, as a class, the mixed agonist-antagonist opioid analgesics have a much lower abuse potential than morphine, all such drugs have been reported to be abused.

Among 161 patients who used butorphanol tartrate nasal spray for 2 months or longer, during a controlled clinical trial, there were 5 reports suggestive of possible abuse, including 3 reports of clinically significant overuse. Post-treatment symptoms such as anxiety, agitation, and diarrhea were observed in 6 patients. Symptoms suggestive of opioid withdrawal occurred in 2 patients who stopped the drug abruptly after using 16 mg a day or more for longer than 3 months.

Neither withdrawal nor symptoms suggestive of withdrawal occurred when the drug was used for less than a week or when the dose was tapered if use exceeded 1-2 weeks. Special care should be exercised in administering butorphanol to emotionally unstable patients and to those with a history of drug abuse.

Drug Interactions: Concurrent use of butorphanol tartrate with central nervous system depressants (e.g., alcohol, barbiturates, tranquillizers, and antihistamines) may result in additive central nervous system depressant effects. The dose of butorphanol tartrate nasal spray should be minimized and the frequency of dosing reduced when it is administered concomitantly with drugs that potentiate the action of opioids.

It is not known if the effects of butorphanol are altered by concomitant medications that affect hepatic metabolism of drugs (erythromycin, theophylline, etc.), but physicians should be alert to the possibility that longer intervals between doses may be needed.

Caution should be exercised in using butorphanol concomitantly with MAO inhibitors, as the latter have been associated with severe and sometimes fatal adverse reactions in certain susceptible individuals when used with meperidine and other narcotic analgesics.

Administration of a single 2 mg dose of butorphanol tartrate nasal spray to 18 subjects with allergic rhinitis resulted in a higher C_{max} and shorter T_{max} compared to healthy subjects, although bioavailabilities were similar. When these 18 subjects were pre-treated with the nasal vasoconstrictor, oxymetazoline, bioavailability of butorphanol was not affected, however, C_{max} was reduced and T_{max} was increased to values similar to those observed in healthy subjects.

No significant pharmacokinetic interactions between butorphanol tartrate nasal spray (1 mg) and sumatriptan (6 mg s.c.) were observed in a single dose clinical trial involving 24 healthy volunteers. However, the safety and efficacy of butorphanol tartrate nasal spray in the treatment of migraine headache pain refractory to sumatriptan has not been established.

In another study among 16 healthy male volunteers, the plasma concentrations of a 1 mg dose of butorphanol tartrate nasal spray (q.i.d. for 4 days) were not affected when cimetidine was coadministered (300 mg q.i.d. for 4 days). Conversely, the pharmacokinetics of cimetidine (300 mg q.i.d. for 4 days) were not altered when butorphanol tartrate nasal spray (1 mg q.i.d.) was coadministered for 4 days.

ADVERSE EFFECTS: Commonly Observed: Across all controlled and uncontrolled acute treatment clinical trials (799 patients exposed to butorphanol tartrate nasal spray) the most commonly observed adverse experiences (with incidence of least 10%) regardless of relationship to butorphanol tartrate nasal spray were; drowsiness (35%), somnolence (17%), dizziness (25%), and nausea and vomiting (11%). These adverse events appeared dose-related. They also occurred more frequently in patients given butorphanol tartrate nasal spray for migraine. In nearly all cases, the type and incidence of side effects were those expected of a potent opioid analgesic, and no unforeseen or unusual toxicity was reported.

Severe Adverse Reactions: During controlled and uncontrolled acute clinical trials involving 799 patients exposed to butorphanol tartrate nasal spray, the following adverse events regardless of relationship (incidence in parentheses) were rated as severe in greater than 1% of patients: drowsiness and somnolence (7.7%), dizziness (4.4%), nausea and vomiting (3.4%), and confusion (1%).

Controlled Clinical Studies: The incidences of adverse reactions (>3%) to butorphanol tartrate nasal spray in Table 2 are derived from placebo-controlled trials (N=662) in a variety of post-operative pain models at doses of 1 or 2 mg, and from two placebo-controlled trials involving the treatment of migraine pain at doses of 2-3 mg.

Table 2: APO-BUTORPHANOL

Summary of Adverse Events in Patients Receiving Butorphanol Tartrate Nasal Spray or Placebo in Post Operative Pain and Migraine Trials. Only Adverse Events Reported by >3% of Patients Treated with Butorphanol Tartrate Nasal Spray at the Specified Dose Are Included

	Migraine Pain Trials (% of Patients)				Post Operative Pain (% of Patients)			
	Butorphanol Tartrate Nasal Spray			Placebo	Butorphanol Tartrate Nasal Spray			Placebo
	1+1 mg N=32	2 mg N=33	2+1 mg N=16	N=78	1 mg N=128	1+1 mg N=70	2 mg N=149	N=156
Body as a Whole								
Asthenia	9	18	6	3				
Chills	—	6	—	3				
Headache					4	4	—	3
Pain	—	6	—	1				
Sensation of Heat	6	12	6	3	—	—	5	1
Cardiovascular								
Chest Pain	—	6	—	—				
Palpitation	6	—	—	—				
Syncope	—	9	—	—				
Vasodilation	6	—	6	1				
Digestive								
Dry Mouth	6	21	12	—				
Increased Appetite	—	6	—	—				
Nausea/Vomiting	22	61	37	4				
Thirst	—	—	6	—	—	—	8	1
Nervous System								
Abnormal Feelings	6	12	6	—				
Abnormal Thinking	—	6	—	—				
Anxiety	—	6	—	—				
Confusion	9	24	6	—	—	6	—	—
Dizziness	50	85	75	10	23	6	25	1
Drowsiness	41	51	50	5	26	33	40	16
Euphoria	—	3	6	—				
Incoordination	—	6	—	—				
Nervousness	16	9	6	—				
Paresis	—	15	6	—				
Paresthesia	6	21	—	—				
Somnolence					23	36	39	12
Vertigo	9	6	—	1				
Respiratory								
Epistaxis	—	—	6	—				
Nasal Irritation	—	6	6	1				
Dermatological								
Pruritus	6	12	6	—				
Sweating	6	30	19	—	—	4	—	1
Special Senses								
Blurred Vision	12	9	12	1	—	—	—	—
Diplopia	6	—	—	—	—	—	—	—
Ear Disorder	—	6	—	—	—	—	—	—
Hearing Loss	—	—	6	—	—	—	—	—
Unpleasant Taste	12	9	6	—	—	—	—	—

(cont'd)

Table 2: APO-BUTORPHANOL *(cont'd)*

Summary of Adverse Events in Patients Receiving Butorphanol Tartrate Nasal Spray or Placebo in Post Operative Pain and Migraine Trials. Only Adverse Events Reported by >3% of Patients Treated with Butorphanol Tartrate Nasal Spray at the Specified Dose Are Included

Other adverse reactions (≤3%) that were reported with butorphanol tartrate nasal spray in all acute (controlled and non-controlled) clinical trials (N=799) are listed below.

These adverse events, regardless of relationship to butorphanol tartrate nasal spray, are listed in order of decreasing frequency according to the following definitions: Frequent events were reported on one or more occasions by at least 1/100 individuals; Infrequent events by 1/100 to 1/1000 individuals. (**All events except those already listed in Table 2 are included**.)

Body as a Whole: Infrequent: sensation of cold, fever, edema, accidental injury, back pain.

Gastrointestinal: Infrequent: pharyngitis, stomach pain, abdominal pain, dysphagia, flatulence.

Cardiovascular: Frequent: hypotension. Infrequent: blood pressure elevated, hypertension, tachycardia, pallor, arrythmia.

Musculoskeletal: Infrequent: muscle relaxation, leg pain.

Nervous System: Infrequent: hallucinations, feel calm, insomnia, abnormal dreams, agitation, abnormal gait, dysarthria, ataxia, tremor, derealization, intoxication, spasms, stupor, hyperesthesia, motor retardation, vivid imagination, abnormal involuntary movement, slowed movement.

Respiratory: Infrequent: dyspnea, cough, hypoventilation, respiratory disorder, sinus congestion, nasal congestion.

Dermatological: Infrequent: rash, erythema.

Genitourinary: Infrequent: impaired urination, libido increased.

Nasal Experiences: Infrequent: nasal symptoms, nose pain.

Special Senses: Infrequent: visual disturbance, photophobia, hyperacusia, eye pain, ear pain, tinnitus, eye disorder, taste loss.

Hemic and Lymphatic: Infrequent: petechiae.

Postmarketing Experience: The following adverse events also have occurred in less than 1% of patients in short-term butorphanol trials and postmarketing experience.

Body as a Whole: Excessive drug effect associated with transient difficulty speaking and/or executing purposeful movements.
Cardiovascular: chest pain, hypertension, tachycardia.
Nervous System: convulsions, drug dependence.

OVERDOSE:

Symptoms: Based on its pharmacology, butorphanol tartrate overdosage could produce signs of respiratory depression, cardiovascular failure (especially in predisposed patients), or central nervous system depression. There have been no clinical reports of fatal overdosage of butorphanol as a single drug in healthy individuals, but the injectable product has been reported in a fatal overdose in combination with other drugs or alcohol.

Treatment: The specific treatment of suspected butorphanol tartrate overdosage is immediate establishment of adequate airway and ventilation, followed (if necessary) by an opioid antagonist such as intravenous naloxone. Physicians are reminded that the duration of butorphanol action exceeds the duration of action of naloxone, and repeated dosing of naloxone may be required. The patient should be carefully monitored, especially the respiratory and cardiac status, and appropriate supportive measures, such as oxygen, intravenous fluids and/or vasopressors, should be instituted if necessary.

For management of a suspected drug overdose, CPhA recommends that you contact your **regional Poison Control Centre**. See the *CPS* Directory section for a list of Poison Control Centres.

DOSAGE: APO-BUTORPHANOL (butorphanol tartrate) Nasal Spray has an onset of effect within 15-30 minutes, and requires individualization of dosage based on clinical response.

Adults: The usual recommended dose for initial nasal administration is one (1) spray in one (1) nostril (1 mg). Adherence to this dose may reduce the likelihood of drowsiness, dizziness, and nausea and vomiting. If adequate pain relief is not achieved within 60 to 90 minutes, an additional 1 mg dose may be given.

The initial dose sequence of APO-BUTORPHANOL Nasal Spray may be repeated in 3-4 hours as needed. Due to limited clinical experience with higher doses, total daily doses of more than 16 mg are not recommended.

Depending on the severity of the pain, an initial dose of 2 mg (1 spray in each nostril) may be used in patients who will be able to remain recumbent in the event drowsiness or dizziness occur. In such patients, additional doses should not be given for 3-4 hours.

Dosage Adjustments: Patients with Hepatic Impairment: The elimination half-life of APO-BUTORPHANOL Nasal Spray is prolonged in patients with impaired hepatic function (see Pharmacology, Pharmacokinetics). APO-BUTORPHANOL Nasal Spray should thus be used with caution in this population. The initial dosage interval should be increased to 6-12 hours until the response is well characterized. Subsequent dosings should be determined by patient response rather than being scheduled at fixed intervals.

Patients with Renal Impairment: The elimination half-life of APO-BUTORPHANOL Nasal Spray is prolonged in patients with impaired renal function (see Pharmacology, Pharmacokinetics). Dosage adjustments may thus be necessary. In patients with severe renal disease (i.e., creatinine clearance <30 mL/min), the initial dosage interval should be increased to 6-8 hours until the response has been well characterized. Subsequent dosings of APO-BUTORPHANOL Nasal Spray should be determined by patient response rather than being scheduled at fixed intervals.

Geriatrics: Because elderly patients may have a somewhat decreased ability to eliminate butorphanol (see Pharmacology, Pharmacokinetics) and may be more sensitive to butorphanol's side effects, the effects of the initial dose should be carefully assessed, and it may be appropriate to modify the frequency of subsequent dosing.

Initially a 1 mg dose of APO-BUTORPHANOL Nasal Spray should generally be used in elderly patients, and 90-120 minutes should elapse before deciding whether a second 1 mg dose is needed. The repeat dose sequence should be determined by the patient's response rather than at fixed times, but will generally be no less than at 6 hour intervals (see Precautions).

INFORMATION FOR THE PATIENT: Published in e-CPS, available by subscription at www.e-cps.ca.

SUPPLIED: Each mL of clear, colourless aqueous solution contains: butorphanol tartrate 10 mg. Nonmedicinal ingredients: 0.2 mg/mL benzethonium chloride as a preservative, citric acid, purified water with hydrochloric acid and sodium hydroxide. Bottles of 2.5 mL with a metered-dose spray pump with protective clip and dust cover and a patient instruction leaflet. The 2.5 mL bottle wil deliver on average 14 to 15 metered doses, if no repriming is necessary. Store at room temperature (15 to 30°C).

Special Instructions: APO-BUTORPHANOL Nasal Spray is an open delivery system that has a risk of accidental exposure to health care workers. In the priming process, a certain amount of butorphanol may be aerosolized; therefore, the pump sprayer should be aimed away from the patient or animals.

Significant absorption from accidental dermal exposure is unlikely, and the contents of a spilled system should be washed from the skin by rinsing with cool water.

The best way to dispose of the unit safely is to unscrew the cap, rinse the bottle and spray assembly under the water faucet, then dispose of the parts in a waste can where children cannot get to them easily.

Information for the Pharmacist: Instructions for Assembly of Nasal Spray Unit: Assemble APO-BUTORPHANOL prior to dispensing to the patient, according to the following instructions.

1. Open the container and remove the spray pump and solution bottle.
2. Assemble APO-BUTORPHANOL Nasal Spray by first unscrewing the white cap from the solution bottle and screwing the pump unit tightly onto the bottle. Make sure the clear cover is on the pump unit.
3. Return APO-BUTORPHANOL Nasal Spray bottle to the container for dispensing to the patient. Patients should be instructed in the proper use of APO-BUTORPHANOL Nasal Spray.

Apo®-Carvedilol ℞

carvedilol

Congestive Heart Failure Agent

Apotex

Date of Preparation: July 25, 2003

PHARMACOLOGY: Carvedilol is a cardiovascular agent for the treatment of congestive heart failure that combines beta-adrenoceptor blockade and vasodilation in a single racemic mixture. Nonselective beta-adrenoceptor blocking activity is present in the S(−) enantiomer and alpha_1-adrenoceptor blocking activity is present at equal potency in both the R(+) and S(−) enantiomers. Carvedilol has no intrinsic sympathomimetic activity. Its action on beta-receptors is 10 times stronger than on alpha_1-receptors.

Carvedilol reduces peripheral vascular resistance by vasodilation, thereby causing a fall in systemic blood pressure after acute administration, predominantly mediated through selective alpha_1-antagonism. Beta blockade prevents reflex tachycardia with the net result that heart rate is unchanged or decreased. Carvedilol reduces renin release through beta blockade.

In two studies that compared the acute hemodynamic effects of carvedilol to baseline measurements in patients with congestive heart failure, there were significant reductions in systemic blood pressure, pulmonary artery pressure, pulmonary capillary wedge pressure, and heart rate. Initial effects on cardiac output, stroke volume index and systemic vascular resistance were small and variable.

In terms of chronic hemodynamic effects (12 to 14 weeks), carvedilol significantly reduced systemic blood pressure, pulmonary artery pressure, right atrial pressure, systemic vascular resistance and heart rate while stroke volume index was increased.

The mechanism for the beneficial effects of carvedilol in congestive heart failure has not been established.

In a US multicentre program, 1197 patients with stable symptomatic congestive heart failure, NYHA class II to IV, were challenged with a low dose of carvedilol (3.125 or 6.25 mg twice daily) for 2 to 4 weeks to determine tolerability. Of these patients, 1094 were then randomized to double-blind treatment with carvedilol (n=696) or placebo (n=398) and stratified to one of four studies based on baseline exercise performance, with the prestated objective to evaluate total mortality. The average duration of therapy on carvedilol was 6.5 months in this program. Patients entering the program had symptomatic congestive heart failure due to ischemic or non-ischemic cardiomyopathy with an ejection fraction ≤35%. All patients received conventional therapy, i.e. diuretics, angiotensin-converting enzyme (ACE) inhibitors, if tolerated, with or without digoxin.

On an intent-to-treat basis, total mortality in this program was 3.2% in the carvedilol group and 7.8% in the placebo group. Thus a relative risk reduction of 65% (95% confidence limits 39 and 80%, p=0.001) was observed. Treatment with carvedilol was associated with a significant decrease in the relative risk of death from progressive pump failure (81%, p=0.001) and the relative risk of sudden death (56%, p=0.033). The incidence of cardiovascular hospitalizations was 13% in the carvedilol group and 21% in the placebo group, with a relative risk reduction of 36% (95% confidence limits: 14% and 53%, p=0.004).

Improved patient well-being was observed with carvedilol treatment in the US multicentre program, as indicated by a change in the NYHA class from baseline to endpoint for the four US phase III placebo-controlled studies. The overall between-group difference in distributions, stratified by protocol and baseline classification, was significant (p<0.001) and as also indicated by patient and physician global assessments during US Phase III trials, 78% of patients in the carvedilol group rated their condition as improved compared to 63% in the placebo group (p values over four studies from 0.001 to 0.032). However, exercise tolerance was not improved.

In a large multicentre trial of carvedilol, performed in Australia and New Zealand, 443 patients with stable symptomatic congestive heart failure NYHA Class I to III, were challenged with a low dose of carvedilol (3.125 mg or 6.25 mg twice daily) for 2-4 weeks to determine tolerability. Of these patients 415 were then randomized to double-blind treatment with carvedilol (n=207) or placebo (n=208). The average duration of therapy on carvedilol was 16.1 months in this study. Patients entering the program had symptomatic congestive heart failure due to ischemic cardiomyopathy with an ejection fraction ≤45%. All patients received conventional therapy, i.e., diuretics, angiotensin-converting enzyme (ACE) inhibitors, if tolerated, with or without digoxin.

On an intent-to-treat basis, total mortality in this Australia and New Zealand trial was 10.1% in the carvedilol group and 13.9% in the placebo group, a non-statistically significant relative risk reduction of 29% (confidence limits −24% and 59%, p=0.231). Cardiovascular hospitalizations were 31% in the carvedilol group and 40% in the placebo group, a relative risk reduction of 28% (95% confidence limits: 1% and 48%, p=0.044). Patient well-being as judged by NYHA class or Specific Activity Scale rating, as well as exercise tolerance were no different in the carvedilol group compared to the placebo group.

In the COPERNICUS trial, 2289 patients with severe heart failure were randomly assigned to treatment with placebo or carvedilol for up to 29 months. Patients had symptoms at rest or on minimal exertion and had a left ventricular ejection fraction <25% (mean 20%), despite treatment with diuretics (99%), an ACE inhibitor (89%), and digitalis (66% worldwide, 85% within Canada) for more than 2 months. Patients with cardiac impairment not related to left ventricular dysfunction were excluded as were patients with prior cardiac transplant, cardioplasty, unstable angina, myocardial infarction, destabilizing cardiac arrhythmias, or treatment within 1 month with an α-adrenoceptor antagonist (except for prostatism), a calcium channel blocker or a class I antiarrhythmic agent. The trial was followed by a data safety monitoring committee, which stopped the trial early after a median follow-up of 10.4 months because of an observed reduction in total mortality, the primary endpoint, from 19.7% per patient-year on placebo to 12.8% per patient-year on carvedilol, (a relative risk reduction of 35%; hazard ratio 0.65, 95% CI 0.52 and 0.81, and a P value adjusted for interim analyses of 0.0014). The results are summarized as follows: see Table 1.

Table 1: APO-CARVEDILOL

Results of the COPERNICUS trial

End Point	Placebo N=1133	Carvedilol N=1156	Hazard Ratio (95% CI)	% Reduction	Nominal P value
Mortality	190	130	0.65 (0.52–0.81)	35	0.00013
Mortality + all hospitalization	507	425	0.76 (0.67–0.87)	24	0.00004
Martality + CV hospitalization	395	314	0.73 (0.63–0.84)	27	0.00002
Mortality + CHF hospitalization	357	271	0.69 (0.59–0.81)	31	0.00004

Pharmacokinetics: Carvedilol is rapidly absorbed following oral administration, with peak plasma concentrations of carvedilol observed at 1 hour post-dose in fasting subjects. Despite being well absorbed, absolute bioavailability is approximately 25% to 35% due to a significant degree of first-pass metabolism.

Plasma concentrations achieved are proportional to the oral dose administered. When administered with food, the rate of absorption is slowed, as evidenced by a delay in time to reach peak plasma concentrations (about 2.3 hours post-dose), with no significant difference in extent of bioavailability.

Carvedilol is highly bound to plasma proteins, (greater than 98%) primarily to albumin. The plasma-protein binding is independent of concentration over the therapeutic range. Carvedilol is a basic, lipophilic compound with a steady-state volume of distribution of approximately 115 L.

Following oral administration, the apparent mean terminal elimination half-life of carvedilol ranges from 7 to 10 hours. Plasma clearance ranges from 500 to 700 mL/min. Carvedilol is extensively metabolized with less than 2% of the dose excreted unchanged in the urine. Carvedilol is metabolized mainly by glucuronidation and aromatic ring oxidation by the cytochrome P450 system (primarily CYP2D6 and CYP2C9 isozymes). The metabolites of carvedilol are excreted mainly via the bile into the feces. Elimination is mainly biliary. The primary route of excretion is via the feces. A minor part is eliminated via the kidneys in the form of various metabolites.

Carvedilol undergoes stereo selective first-pass metabolism with plasma levels of R(+)-carvedilol approximately 2- to 3-fold higher than S(−)-carvedilol following oral administration in healthy subjects. The mean apparent terminal elimination half-life for R(+)-carvedilol ranges from 5 to 9 hours compared with 7 to 11 hours for the S(−) enantiomer.

Carvedilol is subject to genetic polymorphism with poor metabolizers of debrisoquin (deficient in CYP2D6) exhibiting 2- to 3-fold higher plasma concentrations of the R(+)-carvedilol compared to extensive metabolizers. In contrast, plasma levels of S(−)-carvedilol are increased only about 20% to 25% in poor metabolizers, indicating that the metabolism of this enantiomer is affected to a lesser extent by CYP2D6 than R(+)-carvedilol. The Pharmacokinetics of carvedilol enantiomers do not appear to be different in poor metabolizers of 5-mephenytoin, i.e. deficient in CYP 2C19.

There are at least 5 pharmacologically active metabolites of carvedilol: desmethyl, 4'-hydroxyphenyl, 5'-hydroxyphenyl, 1-hydroxycarbazolyl and 8-hydroxycarbazolyl metabolites. Each of these metabolites has two enantiomeric forms and each metabolite possesses different relative potencies with regard to alpha-and beta-receptor blocking activities. Plasma concentrations of these metabolites are 10 to 50-fold lower than those observed for the parent compound. Therefore, even for metabolites that are more active, or at least as active as carvedilol itself, they are present at such low concentrations that they would produce effects less than, or at least not greater than, the parent compound.

In patients with cirrhotic liver disease, the absolute bioavailability of carvedilol was 4 times greater as compared to healthy subjects with median C_{max} and AUC values for carvedilol 4 to 7 times higher in patients with liver disease following oral administration (see Contraindications, Warnings and Precautions).

Although carvedilol is metabolized primarily by the liver, plasma concentrations of carvedilol have been reported to be increased in patients with renal impairment. Based on AUC data, approximately 40% to 50% higher plasma concentrations of carvedilol were observed in hypertensive patients with moderate to severe renal impairment compared to a control group of hypertensive patients with normal renal function. However, the ranges of AUC values were similar for both groups. Changes in C_{max} data were less pronounced, approximately 12% to 26% higher in patients with impaired renal function.

The pharmacokinetics of carvedilol are not altered by hemodialysis.

Steady-state plasma concentrations of carvedilol and its enantiomers increased proportionally over the 6.25 to 50 mg b.i.d. dose range in patients with congestive heart failure. Compared to healthy subjects, patients with Class IV congestive heart failure had increased mean AUC and C_{max} values for carvedilol and its enantiomers with up to 50% to 100% higher values than normal volunteers. The mean apparent terminal elimination half-life for carvedilol was similar to that observed in healthy subjects.

Compared to young subjects (18-43 years old), AUC values for carvedilol were, on average, 38% higher in elderly (65-76 years old) subjects. Moreover, AUC values were 50% higher for S(−)-carvedilol and 23% for R(+)-carvedilol in the elderly compared to the young subjects. Changes in C_{max} values for carvedilol and its enantiomers were less pronounced, approximately 8% to 17% higher in elderly subjects with no apparent change in T_{max}. Although the terminal elimination half-lives of carvedilol were similar in both young and elderly subjects, the initial decline in plasma concentrations in the elderly appeared to be slower than in the young subjects, suggesting a decrease in systemic clearance of carvedilol in the elderly (see Precautions and Dosage).

Comparative Bioavailability: A comparative bioavailability study was performed on healthy volunteers. The rate and extent of absorption of carvedilol was measured and compared following oral administration of 1×25 mg of either APO-CARVEDILOL 25 mg tablets or Coreg 25 mg tablets. The results from measured data are summarized in Table 2.

Table 2: APO-CARVEDILOL

Summary Table of the Comparative Bioavailability Data. Carvedilol (Dose: 1×25 mg) from Measured Data—Under Fed Conditions

Parameter	Geometric Mean Arithmetic Mean (CV%)		Ratio of Geometric Means (%)[b]
	APO-CARVEDILOL	Coreg[c]	
AUC_T (ng·hr/mL)	329 362 (46)	306 344 (51)	107.5
AUC_I (ng·hr/mL)	336 370 (47)	321 359 (50)	109.3
C_{max} (ng/mL)	65.0 73.5 (55)	70.2 82.3 (61)	92.6
T_{max} (hr)[a]	2.62 (52.9)	1.84 (60.1)	
$t_{1/2}$ (hr)[a]	9.99 (34)	10.0 (43)	

a Arithmetic means (CV%).
b Based on the least squares estimate.
c Coreg is manufactured by Hoffmann-La Roche Limited, marketed by SmithKlineBeecham and was purchased in Canada.

INDICATIONS: APO-CARVEDILOL (carvedilol) is indicated for treatment of mild, moderate or severe heart failure of ischemic or non-ischemic origin to increase survival and also, to reduce the combined risk of all-cause mortality and cardiovascular or non-cardiovascular hospitalizations.

In general, APO-CARVEDILOL is used in conjunction with diuretics and an ACE inhibitor, with or without digitalis.

APO-CARVEDILOL should be prescribed by a physician experienced in the treatment of heart failure.

> Beta blockers can cause worsening heart failure (see Precautions). Since carvedilol has beta-blocking properties, care must be taken during initiation and up-titration of the drug in heart failure patients, since worsening heart failure has been observed during this phase of treatment. In order to minimize the risk of these events, it is critical to carefully follow the recommended dosing for carvedilol in patients with congestive heart failure (see Dosage).

CONTRAINDICATIONS: APO-CARVEDILOL (carvedilol) is contraindicated in patients with: decompensated cardiac failure requiring intravenous inotropic therapy with sympathomimetic agents; bronchial asthma or related bronchospastic conditions (see Precautions); second- or third- degree AV block, or sick sinus syndrome (unless a permanent pacemaker is in place); cardiogenic shock; severe hypotension (see Warnings); severe bradycardia (see Warnings); primary obstructive valvular heart disease; clinically manifest hepatic impairment (jaundice, ascites, spider angiomata, esophageal varices, etc.); mental incapacity (eg. severe Alzheimer's, alcoholism, drug abuse), unless closely supervised by an appropriate caregiver; hypersensitivity to carvedilol or any component of APO-CARVEDILOL.

WARNINGS: Hypotension: Hypotension and postural hypotension in congestive heart failure patients occurred with a higher incidence in carvedilol-treated than in placebo-treated patients (see Adverse Effects). The risk of these events was highest during initiation of therapy and during the first 30 days of dosing corresponding to the up-titration period. Therefore, it is of critical importance that the dosing recommendation be followed (see Dosage).

Sinus Bradycardia: Severe sinus bradycardia may occur with the use of carvedilol. In such cases, dosage should be discontinued.

In clinical trials, patients with a resting heart rate of less than or equal to 68 beats/minute prior to initiation of carvedilol were not studied.

Hepatic Injury: Hepatocellular injury, confirmed by rechallenge, has occurred rarely with carvedilol therapy.

Hepatic injury has been reversible and has occurred after short-and/or long-term therapy with minimal clinical symptomatology. No deaths due to liver function abnormalities have been reported in association with the use of carvedilol.

At the first symptom/sign of liver dysfunction (e.g. pruritus, dark urine, persistent anorexia, jaundice, right upper quadrant tenderness or unexplained "flu-like" symptoms) laboratory testing should be performed. If the patient has laboratory evidence of liver injury or jaundice, APO-CARVEDILOL (carvedilol) should be stopped and not restarted.

Abrupt Cessation of Therapy: In patients with heart failure treated chronically with carvedilol, abrupt cessation of therapy may lead to deterioration. Therefore discontinuation of carvedilol should be done gradually, if possible.

Patients with ischemic heart disease should be warned against abrupt discontinuation of beta-adrenergic blocking agents. There have been reports of severe exacerbation of angina, and of myocardial infarction or ventricular arrhythmias occurring in patients with angina pectoris, following abrupt discontinuation of beta-blocker therapy.

The last two complications may occur with or without preceding exacerbation of angina pectoris. Therefore, when discontinuing APO-CARVEDILOL in patients with angina pectoris, the dosage should be gradually reduced over a period of about 2 weeks and the patient should be carefully observed. The same frequency of administration should be maintained. In situations of greater urgency, carvedilol therapy should be discontinued stepwise and under conditions of closer observation. If angina markedly worsens or acute coronary insufficiency develops, it is recommended that treatment with the drug be re-instituted promptly, at least temporarily.

Oculomucocutaneous Syndrome: Various skin rashes and conjunctival xerosis have been reported with beta-blockers. A severe syndrome (oculomucocutaneous syndrome) whose signs include conjunctivitis sicca and psoriasiform rashes, otitis, and sclerosing serositis has occurred with the chronic use of one beta-adrenergic blocking agent (practolol). This syndrome has not been observed in association with carvedilol or any other such agent. However, physicians should be alert to the possibility of such reactions and should discontinue treatment in the event that they occur.

Uveal Binding: Animal studies have shown that carvedilol binds to the melanin of the uveal tract. The significance of this in humans is not known but periodic ophthalmic examinations are advisable while the patient is taking APO-CARVEDILOL.

Hyperthyroidism: In patients with thyrotoxicosis, possible deleterious effects from long-term use of carvedilol have not been appraised. Beta-blockade, in general, may mask the clinical signs of continuing hyperthyroidism or complications, and give a false impression of improvement. Therefore, abrupt withdrawal of carvedilol may be followed by an exacerbation of the symptoms of hyperthyroidism, including thyroid storm.

Pheochromocytoma: The effect of carvedilol in patients with pheochromocytoma has not been studied. Since paradoxical hypertensive responses have been reported in a few patients with this tumor when treated with beta-blockers, physicians should use caution when administering carvedilol to patients with pheochromocytoma.

PRECAUTIONS: Cardiac Failure: Worsening cardiac failure may occur during initiation and up-titration of APO-CARVEDILOL (carvedilol). Sympathetic stimulation is a vital component supporting circulatory function in congestive heart failure, and inhibition with beta blockade may further depress myocardial contractility.

Cardiac failure should be controlled for at least 4 weeks before APO-CARVEDILOL treatment is initiated. In clinical trials of mild to moderate heart failure, patients were required to be on stable doses of diuretics and ACE inhibitors (if tolerated) prior to the initiation of carvedilol. Despite these steps to ensure stability, a small number of patients developed worsening heart failure. During the initiation of therapy (doses of 3.125-6.25 mg b.i.d over 2-4 weeks) 6.0 % of patients developed worsening congestive heart failure. During up-titration (12.5-50 mg b.i.d over 2-6 weeks), worsening heart failure was reported in 5.1% of patients treated with carvedilol and in 4.1% of placebo patients.

In a placebo-controlled trial of patients with severe heart failure (COPERNICUS trial), worsening heart failure occurred during up-titration although the frequency reported during the first 3 months was similar with carvedilol (15.4%) and with placebo (14.8%). When treatment was maintained beyond 3 months, worsening heart failure was reported less frequently in patients treated with carvedilol than with placebo. Worsening heart failure observed during long-term therapy is more likely to be related to the patients' underlying disease than to treatment with carvedilol.

Administration of APO-CARVEDILOL to patients with controlled heart failure must be carried out under careful supervision. If symptoms occur, diuretics should be increased and the carvedilol dose not advanced or even lowered until clinical stability resumes (see Dosage). However, it may be necessary to discontinue APO-CARVEDILOL. Such episodes may not preclude subsequent successful titration of the drug or a favourable response to carvedilol.

Renal Function: Rarely, use of APO-CARVEDILOL in patients with congestive heart failure has resulted in acute renal failure and deterioration of renal function, likely on a pre-renal basis. Patients at risk appear to be those with low blood pressure (systolic BP<100 mm Hg), ischemic heart disease and diffuse vascular disease, and/or underlying renal insufficiency. Renal function has returned to baseline when carvedilol was stopped. In patients with these risk factors it is recommended that renal function be monitored during up-titration of APO-CARVEDILOL and the drug discontinued or dosage reduced if worsening of renal function occurs (see Dosage).

Hepatic Impairment: Since carvedilol undergoes first-pass metabolism in the liver, reduced hepatic metabolism could lead to greater systemic bioavailability of carvedilol in patients with hepatic impairment. Care should be taken in selecting an appropriate dosage regimen for these patients (see Contraindications and Dosage). Physicians should be aware of the potential for increased manifestations of vasodilation (dizziness, postural hypotension, hypotension, syncope) or beta-blockade (bradycardia, AV block) in patients with mild hepatic impairment receiving APO-CARVEDILOL (see Dosage).

Bronchospasm (e.g. chronic bronchitis and emphysema): Patients with bronchospastic disease should, in general, not receive beta-blockers (see Contraindications).

In clinical trials of patients with congestive heart failure, patients with bronchospastic disease were enrolled if they did not require oral or inhaled medication to treat their bronchospastic disease. In such patients, it is recommended that carvedilol be used with caution. The dosing recommendations should be followed closely and the dose should be lowered if any evidence of bronchospasm is observed during up-titration.

Allergic Reaction: There may be increased difficulty in treating an allergic-type reaction in patients on beta-blockers. In these patients, the reaction may be more severe due to pharmacological effects of beta-blockers and problems with fluid changes. Epinephrine should be administered with caution since it may not have its usual effects in the treatment of anaphylaxis.

On the one hand, larger doses of epinephrine may be needed to overcome the bronchospasm, while on the other, these doses can be associated with excessive alpha-adrenergic stimulation with consequent hypertension, reflex bradycardia and heart block and possible potentiation of bronchospasm. Alternatives to the use of large doses of epinephrine include vigorous supportive care such as fluids and the use of beta agonists including parenteral salbutamol or isoproterenol to overcome bronchospasm and norepinephrine to overcome hypotension.

Prinzmetal's Angina: Beta-blocking agents may provoke chest pain in patients with Prinzmetal's angina. There has been no clinical experience with carvedilol in these patients. Caution should be taken in the administration of APO-CARVEDILOL to patients suspected of having Prinzmetal's variant angina.

Primary Regurgitative Valvular Heart Disease: APO-CARVEDILOL should be used with caution in patients with primary regurgitative valvular disease as experienced in this patient population is limited.

Patients with Diabetes: APO-CARVEDILOL should be administered with caution to patients subject to spontaneous hypoglycemia, or to diabetic patients (especially those with labile diabetes) who are receiving insulin or oral hypoglycemic agents. Beta-adrenergic blocking drugs may enhance hypoglycemia in patients prone to this condition. Also, diabetics on insulin or oral hypoglycemic medication may have an increased tendency towards hypoglycemia when treated with these drugs. It may also be necessary to adjust the dosage of oral hypoglycemics or insulin. Early signs of acute hypoglycemia, especially tachycardia, may be masked or attenuated. Regular monitoring of blood glucose is therefore recommended when carvedilol is initiated, adjusted or discontinued.

Thyrotoxicosis: β-adrenergic blockade may mask clinical signs of hyperthyroidism, such as tachycardia. Abrupt withdrawal of β-blockade may be followed by an exacerbation of the symptoms of hyperthyroidism or may precipitate thyroid storm.

Peripheral Vascular Disease: Beta-blockers can precipitate or aggravate symptoms of arterial insufficiency in patients with peripheral vascular disease. Caution should be exercised in such individuals.

Patients and General Surgery: Because of the synergistic negative inotropic and vasodilating effects of carvedilol and anaesthetic drugs, the potential for pronounced hypotension during anesthesia exists. If treatment with APO-CARVEDILOL is to be continued perioperatively, particular care should be taken when anesthetic agents which depress myocardial function are used.

Contact Lens Use: Wearers of contact lenses should bear in mind the possibility of reduced lacrimation.

Geriatrics: Pharmacokinetic studies indicate that AUC and T_{max} values are increased in elderly patients. Plasma levels of carvedilol averaged about 38% higher in elderly compared to young subjects. Therefore, dosage adjustments should be made with particular caution (see Dosage).

Pregnancy: There have been no clinical studies carried out to specifically examine the use of carvedilol in pregnant women. Beta-blockers reduce placental perfusion, which may result in intrauterine fetal death, immature and premature deliveries. In addition, adverse effects (especially hypoglycemia and bradycardia) may occur in the fetus and neonate. There is an increased risk of cardiac and pulmonary complications in the neonate in the postnatal period.

Animal reproduction studies have revealed no teratogenic potential for carvedilol. Embryotoxicity was observed only after large doses in rabbits. The relevance of these findings for humans is uncertain.

APO-CARVEDILOL should be used during pregnancy only if the potential benefit justifies the potential risk to the fetus.

Lactation: Carvedilol and/or its metabolites are excreted in breast milk. Therefore, breast feeding is not recommended during administration of APO-CARVEDILOL.

Children: Safety and efficacy in children have not been established.

Drug Interactions: Antihypertensive Agents: When administered concomitantly with other drugs that are antihypertensive in action or have hypotension as part of their adverse effect profile, carvedilol may have additive effects to excessively lower blood pressure.

Catecholamine-depleting agents: Patients taking both agents with beta-blocking properties and a drug that can deplete catecholamines (e.g., reserpine and monoamine oxidase inhibitors) should be observed closely for evidence of hypotension and/or marked bradycardia.

Antiarrhythmics and Calcium Channel Blockers: Isolated cases of conduction disturbance (rarely with hemodynamic compromise) have been observed when carvedilol is co-administered with anti-arrhythmic agents or calcium channel blockers such as diltiazem and verapamil that can slow cardiac conduction. As with other agents with beta-blocking properties, if APO-CARVEDILOL is to be administered orally with antiarrhythmics that slow conduction or calcium channel blockers of the verapamil or diltiazem type, it is recommended that ECG and blood pressure be monitored.

Digoxin: Following concomitant administration of carvedilol and digoxin, peak concentration of digoxin increased by approximately 30% and steady-state trough concentrations of digoxin were increased by about 15%. Both digoxin and carvedilol slow AV conduction. Therefore, increased monitoring of digoxin levels is recommended when initiating, adjusting or discontinuing APO-CARVEDILOL.

Clonidine: Concomitant administration of clonidine with agents with beta-blocking properties may potentiate blood pressure and heart rate lowering effects. When concomitant treatment with agents with beta-blocking properties and clonidine is to be terminated, the beta-blocking agent should be discontinued first. Clonidine therapy can then be discontinued several days later by gradually decreasing the dosage.

Cyclosporine: Modest increases in mean trough cyclosporine concentrations were observed following initiation of carvedilol treatment in 21 renal transplant patients suffering from chronic vascular rejection. In about 30% of patients, the dose of cyclosporine had to be reduced in order to maintain cyclosporine concentrations within the therapeutic range, while in the remainder no adjustment was needed. On the average for the group, the dose of cyclosporine was reduced about 20% in these patients. Due to wide inter-individual variability in the dose adjustment required, it is recommended that cyclosporine concentrations be monitored closely after initiation of carvedilol therapy and that the dose of cyclosporine be adjusted as appropriate.

Inducers and Inhibitors of Cytochrome P450: Since carvedilol undergoes substantial oxidative metabolism, care may be required in patients receiving inducers or inhibitors of cytochrome P450, as plasma concentrations may be altered. Pre-treatment with rifampin (600 mg daily for 12 days) decreased the AUC and C_{max} for carvedilol approximately 70% following a single oral dose of carvedilol. Co-administration of carvedilol and cimetidine (1000 mg/day) resulted in a 30% increase in median AUC for carvedilol. Despite the reduction in oral clearance, peak plasma concentrations of carvedilol were unchanged due to an apparent decrease in rate of absorption.

Grapefruit Juice: Following simultaneous administration of a single dose of 25 mg of carvedilol with 300 mL of grapefruit juice (an inhibitor of CYP3A4 and CYP1A2), AUC for carvedilol was approximately 16% higher than following administration of carvedilol with 300 mL of water.

Nitroglycerin: The effect of carvedilol co-administration with nitroglycerin has not been studied. Carvedilol could blunt the reflex tachycardia produced by nitroglycerin through its beta-adrenergic blocking activity. When it is used with nitroglycerin in patients with angina pectoris, additional decreases in blood pressure may occur.

Insulin or Oral Hypoglycemics: Agents with beta-blocking properties may enhance the blood-sugar reducing effect of insulin and oral hypoglycemics. Therefore, in patients taking insulin or oral hypoglycemics, regular monitoring of blood glucose is recommended.

Tricyclic Antidepressants: The effect of carvedilol co-administration with tricyclic antidepressants has not been studied. As an increased incidence of tremor has been observed with other drugs of this class upon co-administration of tricyclic antidepressants, the possibility of a drug interaction cannot be excluded.

Warfarin: Carvedilol (12.5 mg twice daily for 7 days) did not have an effect on warfarin-induced increase in steady-state prothrombin time ratios and did not alter the pharmacokinetics of both enantiomers of warfarin following concomitant administration with warfarin in healthy volunteers.

ADVERSE EFFECTS: Mild to Moderate Heart Failure—Controlled Trials: In six US placebo controlled trials, 1313 patients were challenged with carvedilol over a 2-4 week period. Of these patients, 1202 were randomized to double blind treatment with carvedilol (n=765) or placebo (n=437). 92.5% of those treated with carvedilol reported at least one adverse experience.

During the double-blind phase of these trials, adverse experiences rated as serious were reported in 22.4% of patients treated with carvedilol and 31.8% in the placebo group. The most serious adverse experiences reported with carvedilol were cardiac failure (5.6%), syncope (1.8%), bradycardia (1.6%), hypotension (1.3%), myocardial infarction (0.9%), acute renal failure (0.8%), and AV block (0.7%).

Adverse experiences rated as severe in intensity during the double-blind phase of these trials were reported in 24.3% of patients treated with carvedilol. The most frequent severe adverse experiences were cardiac failure (2.9%), fatigue (2.2%), dizziness (2.0%), dyspnea (1.8%), and syncope (1.7%).

The most common adverse experiences reported in the double-blind phase of the US clinical trial experience (see Table 3) with carvedilol were dizziness (32.4%), fatigue (23.9%), dyspnea (21.3%), upper respiratory infection (18.3%) cardiac failure (15.3%) and chest pain (14.4%).

Of the 1202 patients who received randomized treatment in these trials, 5.4% of patients treated with carvedilol withdrew because of adverse experiences compared with 8.0% of placebo patients. Bradycardia, fatigue, hypotension, dizziness and dyspnea were the most commonly reported adverse experiences leading to discontinuation in patients treated with carvedilol (see Table 3).

Six deaths occurred in 1319 patients enrolled in the screening phase (3-4 weeks), eleven deaths occurred in 1313 patients challenged with carvedilol (2-4 weeks). There were 8 deaths (3/765 carvedilol; 5/437 placebo) during up titration phase (2-6 weeks) and 47 deaths (20/765 carvedilol; 27/437 placebo) during the maintenance phase (up to 12 months) of the studies.

Withdrawals due to worsening heart failure in U.S. placebo controlled trials were as follows: during challenge 1.4% of patients (18/1313 for 24 weeks); during up-titration 0.9% (7/765) of patients treated with carvedilol and 0% (0/437) of placebo patients (2-6 weeks); during the maintenance phase 0.7% (5/765) of patients treated with carvedilol and 2.3% (10/437) of placebo patients (up to 12 months).

Worsening renal function, including acute renal failure (see Table 3), has been seen in some patients (carvedilol 9.5% and placebo 7.6%). Patients at greatest risk include those with pre-existing renal insufficiency, hypotension and ischemic cardiomyopathy, previous renal insufficiency due to ACE inhibitors, diffuse vascular disease, or evidence of renal artery stenosis.

Table 3 shows adverse events reported in patients with mild to moderate heart failure enrolled in U.S. placebo-controlled clinical trials. Shown are adverse events that occurred more frequently in carvedilol-treated patients than placebo-treated patients with an incidence >1% regardless of causality. Median study medication exposure was 6.3 months for carvedilol and placebo patients.

Table 3: APO-CARVEDILOL

Adverse Events in (% Occurrence and % Withdrawal) Occurring More Frequently with Carvedilol than with Placebo in Patients with Mild to Moderate Heart Failure Enrolled in U.S. Heart Failure Trials (Incidence >1%, Regardless of Causality; Withdrawal Rates due to Adverse Events)

	Adverse Reactions		Withdrawals	
	Carvedilol (n=765) % occurrence	**Placebo (n=437) % occurrence**	**Carvedilol (n=765) % withdrawals**	**Placebo (n=437) % withdrawals**
Autonomic Nervous System				
Sweating increased	2.9	2.1		
Body as a Whole				
Fatigue	23.9	22.4	0.7	0.7
Chest Pain	14.4	14.2	0.1	
Pain	8.6	7.6		0.2
Injury	5.9	5.5		
Drug level increased	5.1	3.7		0.2
Edema generalized	5.1	2.5		
Edema dependent	3.7	1.8		
Fever	3.1	2.3		
Edema legs	2.2	0.2	0.1	0.2
Edema peripheral	1.6	0.7		
Allergy	1.4	0.2		
Sudden death	1.3	1.1		
Malaise	1.3	0.7		
Hypovolemia	1.2	0.2		
Cardiovascular				
Bradycardia	8.8	0.9	0.8	
Hypotension	8.5	3.4	0.4	0.2
Syncope	3.4	2.5	0.3	0.2
Hypertension	2.9	2.5	0.1	
AV block	2.9	0.5		
Angina pectoris aggravated	2.0	1.1		
Fluid overload	1.7	1.6		
Postural hypotension	1.2	0.2		
Central Nervous System				

(cont'd)

Table 3: APO-CARVEDILOL *(cont'd)*

Adverse Events in (% Occurrence and % Withdrawal) Occurring More Frequently with Carvedilol than with Placebo in Patients with Mild to Moderate Heart Failure Enrolled in U.S. Heart Failure Trials (Incidence >1%, Regardless of Causality; Withdrawal Rates due to Adverse Events)

	Adverse Reactions		Withdrawals	
	Carvedilol (n=765) % occurrence	**Placebo (n=437) % occurrence**	**Carvedilol (n=765) % withdrawals**	**Placebo (n=437) % withdrawals**
Dizziness	32.4	19.2	0.4	
Headache	8.1	7.1	0.3	
Paresthesia	2.0	1.8	0.1	
Hypesthesia	1.7	1.1		
Vertigo	1.4	1.1		
Confusion	1.3	0.9		
Somnolence	1.2	0.9		0.2
Gastrointestinal				
Diarrhea	11.8	5.9	0.3	
Nausea	8.5	4.8		
Abdominal pain	7.2	7.1	0.3	
Vomiting	6.3	4.3	0.1	
Melena	1.4	1.1		
Periodontitis	1.3	0.7		
Hematologic				
Thrombocytopenia	2.0	0.5	0.1	
Prothrombin decreased	1.3	1.1		
Purpura	1.3	0.2		
Metabolic				
Hyperglycemia	12.2	7.8	0.1	
Weight increase	9.7	6.9	0.1	0.5
Gout	6.3	6.2		
BUN increased	6.0	4.6	0.3	0.2
NPN increased	5.8	4.6	0.3	0.2
Hypocholesterolemia	4.1	2.5		
Dehydration	2.1	1.6		
Hypervolemia	2.0	0.9		
Hyperuricemia	1.8	1.6		
Hypoglycemia	1.6	1.4	0.1	
ALT increased	1.4	0.9		
Hyponatremia	1.3	1.1		
Phosphatase alkaline increase	1.2	1.1		
AST increased	1.2	0.9		
Glycosuria	1.2	0.7		
Musculoskeletal				
Back pain	6.9	6.6		
Arthralgia	6.4	4.8	0.1	0.2
Myalgia	3.4	2.7		
Resistance Mechanism				
Upper respiratory tract infection	18.3	17.6		
Infection	2.2	0.9		
Reproductive Male				
Impotence	1.7	0.9		
Respiratory				
Sinusitis	5.4	4.3		

(cont'd)

Table 3: APO-CARVEDILOL *(cont'd)*

Adverse Events in (% Occurrence and % Withdrawal) Occurring More Frequently with Carvedilol than with Placebo in Patients with Mild to Moderate Heart Failure Enrolled in U.S. Heart Failure Trials (Incidence >1%, Regardless of Causality; Withdrawal Rates due to Adverse Events)

	Adverse Reactions		Withdrawals	
	Carvedilol (n=765) % occurrence	Placebo (n=437) % occurrence	Carvedilol (n=765) % withdrawals	Placebo (n=437) % withdrawals
Bronchitis	5.4	3.4		0.2
Pharyngitis	3.1	2.7		
Urinary/Renal				
Urinary tract infection	3.1	2.7		
Hematuria	2.9	2.1		
Renal function abnormal	1.7	1.4	0.3	
Albuminuria	1.6	1.1		
Acute renal failure	1.2	0.5	0.3	
Vision				
Vision abnormal	5.0	1.8	0.1	

In addition to the events in Table 3, the following events occurred in more than 1% of carvedilol-treated patients but rates were equal to, or more common in, placebo-treated patients: asthenia, cardiac failure, flatulence, anorexia, dyspepsia, palpitation, ventricular tachycardia, atrial fibrillation, extrasystoles, bilirubinemia, hyperkalemia, arthritis, angina pectoris, insomnia, depression, amnesia, anemia, viral infection, dyspnea, coughing, respiratory disorder, pneumonia, rhinitis, rash, pruritus, and leg cramps.

Adverse experiences related to laboratory parameters reported in greater than 1% of patients are in Table 3. Adverse experiences related to laboratory parameters reported in ≤1% but more than 0.1% of patients included increased hepatic enzymes (0.4% of congestive heart failure patients were discontinued from therapy because of increases in hepatic enzymes; see Precautions, Hepatic Impairment), hypokalemia, hypertriglyceridemia, anemia, leukopenia.

Severe Heart Failure—Controlled Trial: In a clinical trial in severe heart failure that compared carvedilol in daily doses of 50 mg (n=1156) with placebo (n=1133), 9.4% of patients treated with carvedilol discontinued treatment for adverse experiences versus 11.2% of placebo patients.

The most common adverse experiences reported with carvedilol were dizziness (24.1%), hypotension (13.9%) and upper respiratory infection (see Table 4). Median study exposure was 10.4 months for both carvedilol and placebo patients.

Table 4 shows adverse events reported in patients with severe heart failure enrolled in multinational placebo-controlled clinical trial. Shown are adverse events that occurred more frequently in carvedilol-treated patients than placebo-treated patients with an incidence >1% regardless of causality.

Table 4: APO-CARVEDILOL

Adverse Events in (% Occurrence and % Withdrawal) Occurring More Frequently with Carvedilol than with Placebo in Patients with Severe Heart Failure (Incidence >1%, Regardless of Causality)

	Adverse Reactions		Withdrawals	
	Carvedilol (n=1156) % occurrence	Placebo (n=1133) % occurrence	Carvedilol (n=1156) % withdrawals	Placebo (n=1133) % withdrawals
Body as a Whole				
Asthenia	10.9	9.4	0.4	0.7
Infection	2.5	2.4		
Back pain	2.9	1.4		
Cardiovascular				
Hypotension	13.9	8.2	0.6	0.4
Bradycardia	10.3	2.7	0.6	
Syncope	7.6	5	0.4	0.4
Angina pectoris	5.5	4.1	0.1	0.1
Hypertension	2.6	2.2		0.1
Postural hypotension	1.8	1	0.1	0.1
Sinus bradycardia	1.7	0.4		
Palpitation	1.6	1.5		0.1
Gastrointestinal				
Diarrhea	4.8	3.1	0.3	
Nausea	3.8	3.3		0.1
Gastrointestinal disorder	1.6	1.1	0.1	0.1
Hematologic				
Anemia	2.4	2		
Metabolic and Nutritional				
Weight gain	11.7	10.7	0.1	0.1
Peripheral edema	7.0	6.4	0.2	0.1
Generalized edema	6.0	4.9	0.2	0.2
Hyperglycemia	4.5	3.3	0.0	0.1
Gout	3.5	2.7		
Hyperkalemia	3.3	1.9	0.2	0.1
Creatinine increased	2.9	1.4		0.1
Diabetes mellitus	2.0	1.7		
Weight loss	1.4	1.1		
GGT increased	1.3	1.1		
Nervous System				
Dizziness	24.1	16.8	1.3	0.6
Headache	4.8	3.0		0.1
Paresthesia	1.7	1.4		
Respiratory				
Upper respiratory tract infection	13.6	12.6	0.1	
Dyspnea	11.2	11.0	0.5	0.3
Bronchitis	5.2	4.5	0.1	
Cough increased	4.5	4.2	0.1	0.2
Lung disorder	4.0	3.2	0.1	
Sinusitis	1.6	1.1		
Special Senses				
Blurred vision	2.8	2.2	0.2	0.1
Urogenital				
Kidney failure	1.6	1.3	0.1	

In addition to the events in Table 4, when compared with placebo, carvedilol-treated patients had fewer of the following adverse events related to the cardiovascular system and occurring in or equal to 2% of patients: sudden death, atrial fibrillation, chest pain, congestive heart failure, heart failure, peripheral vascular disorder, unstable angina pectoris and ventricular tachycardia. Other adverse experiences occurring in greater or equal to 2% but reported less frequently in carvedilol-treated patients include: abdominal pain, pain in the extremity, hypokalemia, lung edema, pneumonia, abnormal kidney function and urinary tract infection.

Hypertension and Heart Failure—Open and Controlled Trials: The following adverse events were reported as possibly or probably related in worldwide open or controlled trials with carvedilol in patients with hypertension or congestive heart failure at an incidence of >0.1% to ≤1%:

Cardiovascular: peripheral ischemia, tachycardia.
Central and Peripheral Nervous Systems: hypokinesia.
General: substernal chest pain, edema.
Psychiatric: sleep disorder, aggravated depression, impaired concentration, abnormal thinking, paroniria, emotional lability.
Respiratory System: asthma.
Reproductive, Male: decreased libido.
Skin and Appendages: pruritus, rash erythematous, rash maculopapular, rash psoriaform, photosensitivity reaction.
Special Senses: tinnitus.
Urinary System: micturition frequency.
Autonomic Nervous System: dry mouth, sweating increased.
Metabolic and Nutritional: diabetes mellitus.

The following adverse events were reported as possibly or probably related in worldwide open or controlled trials with carvedilol in patients with hypertension or congestive heart failure at an incidence of ≤0.1%, and are potentially important: complete AV block, bundle branch block, myocardial ischemia, cerebrovascular disorder, convulsions, migraine, neuralgia, paresis, anaphylactoid reaction, alopecia, exfoliative dermatitis, amnesia, GI hemorrhage, bronchospasm, pulmonary edema, decreased hearing, respiratory alkalosis, decreased HDL, pancytopenia, and atypical lymphocytes.

Post-Marketing Experience: The following adverse reaction has been reported in post-marketing experience: reports of aplastic anemia have been rare and received only when carvedilol was administered concomitantly with other medications associated with the event.

OVERDOSE:

Symptoms: Cases of overdosage with carvedilol alone or in combination with other drugs have been reported. Quantities ingested in some cases exceeded 1000 mg. Clinical signs experienced included low blood pressure and heart rate. Standard supportive treatment was provided and individuals recovered.

In the event of inadvertent or intentional overdosage with carvedilol, there may be severe hypotension, excessive bradycardia, heart failure, cardiogenic shock, and cardiac arrest due to its pharmacologic activities. There may also be respiratory distress, bronchospasm, vomiting, disturbed consciousness, and generalized seizures.

Treatment: Patients who have taken an overdose of carvedilol should be placed supine, with their legs raised. For removal of the drug shortly after ingestion, gastric lavage or pharmacologically induced emesis may be useful. Carvedilol is not removed by hemodialysis. In addition to these general procedures, the patient's vital signs should be monitored under intensive care conditions with continuous monitoring, if necessary.

The following additional supportive therapies can be used:

If excessive hypotension occurs, vasopressors, norepinephrine or noradrenaline should be administered with continuous monitoring of the circulatory system. Digitalis, diuretics, and if necessary, dopamine or dobutamine should be administered if cardiac failure occurs.

(cont'd)

For excessive bradycardia, atropine 0.5 to 2 mg should be given intravenously. In addition, glucagon 1 to 10 mg given intravenously over 30 seconds initially, followed by a continuous infusion of 2 to 2.5 mg/h, has been shown to be effective when severe overdosage of beta blockers causes hypotension and or bradycardia. For therapy-resistant bradycardia, pacemaker therapy may be necessary.

For bronchospasm, beta-sympathomimetics (as aerosol or intravenously) or intravenous aminophylline should be given.

In the event of seizures, slow intravenous injection of diazepam or clonazepam is recommended.

Note: In the event of severe intoxication where there are symptoms of shock, treatment must be continued for a sufficiently long period of time consistent with the 7-10 hour elimination half-life of carvedilol.

> For management of a suspected drug overdose, CPhA recommends that you contact your **regional Poison Control Centre**. See the *CPS* Directory section for a list of Poison Control Centres.

DOSAGE: Dosage must be individualized and patients closely monitored during initiation and up-titration by a physician experienced in the treatment of heart failure.

All patients in whom APO-CARVEDILOL (carvedilol) therapy is to be considered must be clinically stable for 4 weeks prior to initiation of APO-CARVEDILOL.

Prior to initiation of therapy with APO-CARVEDILOL, patients should be on stable doses of diuretics and angiotensin converting enzyme inhibitors, with or without digitalis. In clinical trials, patients were on the above regimen unless they were intolerant to an ACE inhibitor.

The recommended starting dose of APO-CARVEDILOL is 3.125 mg twice daily for two weeks. If this dose is tolerated, it can then be increased to 6.25, 12.5 and 25 mg twice daily over successive intervals of at least 2 weeks. Patients should be maintained on the highest tolerated dose. The maximum recommended dose is 25 mg twice daily. The dose of APO-CARVEDILOL should not be increased until symptoms of worsening heart failure or vasodilation have stabilized.

Patients should be advised that initiation of treatment and, to a lesser extent, dosage increases may be associated with transient symptoms of dizziness or lightheadedness, and rarely syncope, within the first 2 hours after dosing. During these periods, they should avoid situations such as driving or dangerous tasks where symptoms could result in injury. In addition, APO-CARVEDILOL should be taken with food to slow the rate of absorption and reduce the incidence of orthostatic effects, especially during up-titration. Symptoms of hypotension do not often require treatment, but it may be useful to separate the time of dosing of APO-CARVEDILOL from that of the ACE inhibitor, or to reduce temporarily the dose of the ACE inhibitor.

The risk/benefit of carvedilol therapy in clinically stable heart failure patients with a heart rate lower than 68 beats per minute should be carefully considered prior to initiation of carvedilol since carvedilol has not been studied in these patients (see Warnings).

Before each dose increase the patient should be seen in the office and evaluated for symptoms of worsening heart failure, vasodilation (dizziness, lightheadedness, symptomatic hypotension) or bradycardia, in order to determine tolerability of APO-CARVEDILOL. Transient worsening of heart failure may be treated with increased doses of diuretics, lowering the dose of APO-CARVEDILOL or, if necessary, discontinuation of APO-CARVEDILOL. Symptoms of vasodilation such as dizziness, lightheadedness or decreasing blood pressure may respond to a reduction in the dose of diuretics. If these changes do not relieve symptoms, the dose of APO-CARVEDILOL should be decreased. If the dose of APO-CARVEDILOL was decreased, it should not be increased again until symptoms of worsening heart failure or vasodilation have been stabilized for 2 weeks. Initial difficulty with titration may not preclude later attempts to re-introduce or resume titration of APO-CARVEDILOL, however caution is required in these circumstances. If congestive heart failure patients experience bradycardia (pulse rate below 55 beats/min.), the dose of APO-CARVEDILOL should be reduced, or may require discontinuation.

Geriatrics: The frequency and pattern of adverse reactions in patients ≥65 years was similar to that in younger patients. However, plasma levels of carvedilol are higher in older patients compared to younger patients (see Precautions). Therefore, after initiating APO-CARVEDILOL at the same dose in the elderly as in younger patients, up-titration should be done more cautiously in the elderly. A lower total daily dose may be reached at the end of up-titration in such patients compared to younger patients.

Hepatic Impairment: APO-CARVEDILOL is contraindicated in patients with clinically manifest liver disease (see Contraindications). In patients with milder hepatic impairment, there is a potential for increased manifestations of vasodilation and beta-blockade (see Pharmacology, Pharmacokinetics, and Precautions). Therefore, after initiating APO-CARVEDILOL at the same dose in patients with hepatic impairment as in other patients, up-titration should be done more cautiously in patients with hepatic impairment. A lower total daily dose may be reached at the end of up-titration in such patients compared to other patients.

Renal Impairment: Acute, reversible renal failure has been seen in some patients treated with APO-CARVEDILOL, particularly those with underlying renal impairment (see Precautions). Therefore, after initiating APO-CARVEDILOL at the same dose in patients with renal impairment as in other patients, up-titration should be done more cautiously in patients with renal impairment. Renal function (BUN and creatinine) should be checked in such patients as appropriate. If renal function has deteriorated, the dose of APO-CARVEDILOL may need to be reduced or discontinued.

Discontinuation: APO-CARVEDILOL should be gradually reduced over a period of about 2 weeks, if possible, and the patient should be carefully observed (see Warnings, Abrupt Cessation of Therapy).

INFORMATION FOR THE PATIENT: Published in e-CPS, available by subscription at www.e-cps.ca.

SUPPLIED: 3.125 mg: Each oval, white, film-coated tablet, engraved "APO" on one side and "C3" on the other, contains: carvedilol 3.125 mg. Nonmedicinal ingredients: croscarmellose sodium, hydroxyethyl cellulose, lactose monohydrate, magnesium stearate, microcrystalline cellulose, polyethylene glycol and titanium dioxide. Bottles of 100. Store at room temperature between (15 and 30°C). Protect from heat and moisture. Dispense in a tight, light-resistant container.

6.25 mg: Each oval, white, film-coated tablet, engraved "APO" on one side and "6.25" on the other, contains: carvedilol 6.25 mg. Nonmedicinal ingredients: croscarmellose sodium, hydroxyethyl cellulose, lactose monohydrate, magnesium stearate, microcrystalline cellulose, polyethylene glycol and titanium dioxide. Bottles of 100. Store at room temperature between (15 and 30°C). Protect from heat and moisture. Dispense in a tight, light-resistant container.

12.5 mg: Each oval, white, film-coated tablet engraved "APO" on one side and "12.5" on the other, contains: carvedilol 12.5 mg. Nonmedicinal ingredients: croscarmellose sodium, hydroxyethyl cellulose, lactose monohydrate, magnesium stearate, microcrystalline cellulose, polyethylene glycol and titanium dioxide. Bottles of 100. Store at room temperature between (15 and 30°C). Protect from heat and moisture. Dispense in a tight, light-resistant container.

25 mg: Each oval, white, film-coated tablet engraved "APO" on one side and "C25" on the other, contains: carvedilol 25 mg. Nonmedicinal ingredients: croscarmellose sodium, hydroxyethyl cellulose, lactose monohydrate, magnesium stearate, microcrystalline cellulose, polyethylene glycol and titanium dioxide. Bottles of 100. Store at room temperature between (15 and 30°C). Protect from heat and moisture. Dispense in a tight, light-resistant container.

Apo®-Doxepin 🄿

doxepin HCl

Antidepressant—Anxiolytic

Apotex

Date of Preparation: October 12, 1993
Date of Revision: October 30, 2001

PHARMACOLOGY: Doxepin is a tricyclic antidepressant closely related in structure to other tricyclic antidepressant drugs, such as amitriptyline and imipramine. It also has sedative and anticholinergic effects, and, in the higher dosage range, it produces peripheral adrenergic blocking effects.

Electroencephalographic (EEG) studies in humans have shown decreases in amplitude and amplitude variability, and also increases in delta, theta, and 24-35 CPS activities.

After single oral doses peak plasma concentrations of doxepin were reached between 1 and 4 hours, and peak concentrations of the active metabolite, desmethyldoxepin, between 2 and 10 hours. As with other tricyclic antidepressants, there is extensive first-pass metabolism and large inter-subject variability in plasma levels. The mean elimination half-life of doxepin was 16 to 18 hours, and of desmethyldoxepin between 28 and 51 hours. With repeated administration of doxepin 75 mg daily in two subjects, steady-state was reached by the ninth day in both subjects.

A bioavailability study was performed using normal human volunteers. The rate and extent of absorption of doxepin and desmethyldoxepin were measured and compared after a single 150 mg dose of Apo-Doxepin 150 mg capsules and Sinequan 150 mg capsules. The results are summarized in Table 1 and Table 2.

Table 1: Apo-Doxepin

Rate and Extent of Absorption of Doxepin and Desmethyldoxepin Measured and Compared After a Single 150 mg Dose of Apo-Doxepin 150 mg Capsules and Sinequan 150 mg Capsules—Doxepin

Parameter	Geometric Mean Arithmetic Mean (CV%)		Ratio of Means (%)
	Apo-Doxepin	Sinequan	
AUC_T (ng·hr/mL)	380 485 (62)	392 495 (66)	97
AUC_I (ng·hr/mL)	441 539 (59)	450 564 (69)	98
C_{max} (ng/mL)	39.3 46.7 (53)	43.4 53.9 (71)	91
T_{max}[a] (hr)	2.32 (0.92)	2.19 (0.99)	—
$t_{½}$[a] (hr)	12.6 (6.6)	11.9 (6.1)	—

[a] For the T_{max} and $t_{½}$ parameters, these are the arithmetic means (standard deviation).

Table 2: Apo-Doxepin

Rate and Extent of Absorption of Doxepin and Desmethyldoxepin Measured and Compared After a Single 150 mg Dose of Apo-Doxepin 150 mg Capsules and Sinequan 150 mg Capsules—Desmethyldoxepin

Parameter	Geometric Mean Arithmetic Mean (CV%)		Ratio of Means (%)
	Apo-Doxepin	Sinequan	
AUC_T (ng·hr/mL)	196 357 (108)	215 357 (107)	91.3
C_{max} (ng/mL)	8.72 9.97 (52)	8.96 10.0 (49)	97.4
T_{max}[a] (hr)	9.4 (16.5)	7.2 (7.8)	—

[a] For the T_{max} parameter, these are the arithmetic means (standard deviation).

INDICATIONS: The antidepressant and anxiolytic properties of Apo-Doxepin (doxepin hydrochloride) have been found to be of value in the drug treatment of: 1) Psychoneurotic patients with anxiety and/or depressive reactions; anxiety neurosis associated with somatic disorders; alcoholic patients with anxiety and/or depression. 2) Psychotic depression, including manic-depressive illness (depressed type) and involutional melancholia.

CONTRAINDICATIONS: Apo-Doxepin (doxepin hydrochloride) is contraindicated in individuals who have shown hypersensitivity to the drug or to other dibenzoxepine compounds.

It is not recommended for children under 12 years of age, since sufficient data on its use in this age group is not yet available.

Because of its anticholinergic activity, doxepin should not be administered to patients with glaucoma, increased intraocular pressure or a tendency to urinary retention.

Tricyclic agents are generally contraindicated during the acute recovery phase following myocardial infarction and in the presence of acute congestive heart failure, as well as in patients with a history of blood dyscrasias and severe liver disease. Doxepin should not be administered concomitantly with MAO inhibitors, since such a combination may cause a syndrome of intensive sympathetic stimulation. Drugs of this type should be discontinued at least two weeks before instituting doxepin therapy.

WARNINGS: Tricyclic antidepressant drugs, particularly when given in high doses, can induce sinus tachycardia, changes in conduction time and arrhythmias. A few instances of unexpected death have been reported in patients with cardiovascular disorders. Myocardial infarction and stroke have also been reported with drugs of this class. Therefore, Apo-Doxepin (doxepin hydrochloride) should be administered with extreme caution to patients with a history of cardiovascular disease, those with circulatory lability and elderly patients. In such cases, treatment should be initiated with low doses, with progressive increases only if required and tolerated, and the patient should be under close surveillance at all dosage levels.

Close supervision is required when doxepin is given to hyperthyroid patients or those receiving thyroid medication because of the possibility of cardiovascular toxicity. At doses above 150 mg daily doxepin may block the antihypertensive effect of guanethidine and related compounds.

Since tricyclic agents are known to lower the seizure threshold, doxepin should be used with caution in patients with a history of convulsive disorders. Concurrent administration of ECT and doxepin may be hazardous, and therefore, such treatment should be limited to patients for whom it is essential.

Pregnancy: The safety of doxepin during pregnancy and lactation has not been established.

Therefore, it should not be used in women of childbearing potential or nursing mothers, unless, in the opinion of the physician, the potential benefits to the patient outweigh the possible hazards to the fetus, or child.

Lactation: See Pregnancy.

PRECAUTIONS: Since drowsiness may occur with the use of doxepin, patients should be cautioned against driving a motor vehicle, operating hazardous machinery, or engaging in activities requiring mental alertness and physical coordination while taking the drug.

Combined use with other drugs acting on the central nervous system should be undertaken with due recognition of the possibility of potentiation. The response to alcohol, barbiturates, and other CNS depressants may be modified by doxepin.

Tricyclic antidepressants may precipitate or aggravate psychotic manifestations in schizophrenic patients, and hypomanic or manic episodes in manic-depressive patients. This may require a reduction in dosage, discontinuation of the drug, and/or administration of an antipsychotic agent.

The possibility of suicide in seriously depressed patients may remain until significant remission occurs. Such patients should be closely supervised throughout therapy and consideration should be given to the possible need for hospitalization. This type of patient should not have easy access to large quantities of doxepin.

Tricyclic antidepressants may also give rise to paralytic ileus, particularly in the elderly and in hospitalized patients. Therefore, appropriate measures should be taken if constipation occurs.

Close supervision and careful adjustment of dosages are required when doxepin is given concomitantly with anticholinergic or sympathomimetic drugs, due to the possibility of additive effects.

Caution should be exercised if Apo-Doxepin (doxepin hydrochloride) is administered together with cimetidine, since the latter has been shown to inhibit the metabolism of several tricyclic antidepressants, including doxepin, and clinically significant increases in plasma levels of doxepin may occur.

Doxepin should be discontinued prior to elective surgery for as long as clinically feasible, since little is known about the interaction between doxepin and general anesthetics.

The use of Apo-Doxepin on a once-a-day dosage regimen in geriatric patients, patients with intercurrent illnesses, or patients taking other medications should be adjusted carefully, based on the patient's condition. This is especially important if the patient is receiving other medications with anticholinergic effects.

Doxepin should be used with caution in patients with impaired liver function, or with a history of hepatic damage or blood dyscrasias. Leukocyte and differential blood counts and liver function studies should be performed when patients receive doxepin in large doses or over prolonged periods.

ADVERSE EFFECTS: Although some of the adverse reactions included in the following list have not been reported with doxepin, pharmacological similarities among the tricyclic antidepressants require that each of the reactions be considered when prescribing Apo-Doxepin (doxepin hydrochloride).

Behavioural: drowsiness, fatigue, excitement, agitation, restlessness, insomnia, nightmares, hypomania, anxiety, confusion, disorientation, disturbed concentration, delusions, hallucinations, activation of latent pyschosis.
Neurological: seizures, alteration in EEG patterns, dizziness, tremors, extrapyramidal symptoms, numbness, tingling, paresthesias of the extremities, peripheral neuropathy, tinnitus, syndrome of inappropriate ADH (antidiuretic hormone) secretion.
Cardiovascular: hypotension, hypertension, tachycardia, palpitations. A quinidine-like effect and other reversible ECG changes such as flattening or inversion of T-waves, bundle branch block, depressed S-T segments, prolonged conduction time and asystole, arrhythmias, heart block, fibrillation, myocardial infarction, stroke and unexpected death in patients with cardiovascular disorders have been reported with other tricyclic antidepressants.
Autonomic: dry mouth, blurred vision, disturbances of accommodation, mydriasis, constipation, nasal stuffiness, delayed micturition, sublingual adenitis, paralytic ileus, urinary retention, dilation of the urinary tract, precipitation of latent and aggravation of existing glaucoma, vertigo.
Endocrine: increased or decreased libido, impotence, menstrual irregularity, testicular swelling, breast enlargement and galactorrhea in the female, gynecomastia in the male, elevation and lowering of blood sugar levels.
Allergic or Toxic: pruritus, skin rash, photosensitization, edema, drug fever, leukopenia, urticaria, petechiae, obstructive jaundice and bone marrow depression, including agranulocytosis, eosinophilia, purpura and thrombocytopenia.
Gastrointestinal: nausea, epigastric distress, vomiting, flatulence, abdominal pain, diarrhea, peculiar taste, stomatitis.
Miscellaneous: weakness, headache, weight gain or loss, excessive appetite, anorexia, increased perspiration, urinary frequency, lacrimation, alopecia, parotid swelling, black tongue, hepatitis.
Withdrawal Symptoms: Abrupt cessation of treatment with tricyclic antidepressants after prolonged administration may produce nausea, headache and malaise. These symptoms are not indicative of addiction.

OVERDOSE:

Symptoms: Excessive drowsiness leading to minor alterations of consciousness and even unresponsiveness could be an early indication of excessive dosage.

However, overdosage with Apo-Doxepin (doxepin hydrochloride) is more likely to be manifested by increased psychomotor agitation and convulsions leading to apnoea and coma. The ECG changes (broadening of QRS and T wave abnormalities) tend to be a late finding and are not always accompanied by cardiovascular hemodynamic changes.

Treatment: In general, treatment of overdosage should be symptomatic and supportive. Cardiac arrhythmias and CNS involvement pose the greatest threat with tricyclic anti-depressant overdosage and may occur suddenly even when initial symptoms appear to be mild. Therefore, patients who may have ingested an overdosage of doxepin, particularly children, should be hospitalized and kept under close surveillance.

If the patient is conscious, induced emesis followed by gastric lavage, with appropriate precautions to prevent pulmonary aspiration, should be accomplished as soon as possible. Following lavage, activated charcoal may be administered to reduce absorption. An adequate airway should be established in comatose patients and assisted ventilation instituted, if necessary. The possibility of occurrence of seizures should be kept in mind. External stimulation should be minimized to reduce the tendency to convulsions. Convulsions, should they occur, may respond to standard anticonvulsant therapy; however, barbiturates should be avoided since they may potentiate respiratory depression, particularly in children, and aggravate hypotension and coma.

ECG monitoring in an intensive care unit is recommended in all patients, particularly in the presence of ECG abnormalities, and should be maintained for several days after the cardiac rhythm has returned to normal. A patient who has ingested a toxic overdose of a tricyclic antidepressant may remain medically and psychiatrically unstable for several days due to sustained excessive drug levels. Unexpected cardiac deaths have occurred up to 6 days after overdose with other antidepressants. The QRS interval of the electrocardiogram appears to be a reliable correlate of the severity of overdosage. If the QRS interval exceeds 100 milliseconds any time during the first 24 hours after overdosage, cardiac function should be continuously monitored for 5 or 6 days. Because of its effect on cardiac conduction, digitalis should be used only with caution. If rapid digitalization is required for the treatment of congestive heart failure, special care should be exercised in using the drug.

Shock should be treated with supportive measures such as intravenous fluids, oxygen and corticosteroids. Pressor agents, such as noradrenaline (but **not** adrenaline), are rarely indicated and should be given only after careful consideration and under continuous monitoring.

The slow intravenous administration of physostigmine salicylate has been reported to reverse most of the cardiovascular and CNS anticholinergic manifestations of tricyclic overdosage. The recommended dosage in adults has been 1 to 2 mg in **very slow** intravenous injection. In children, the initial dosage should not exceed 0.5 mg and should be adjusted to age and response. Since physostigmine has a short duration of action, administration may have to be repeated at 30 to 60 minute intervals.

Deaths by deliberate or accidental overdosage have occurred with this class of drugs. Since the propensity for suicide is high in depressed patients, a suicide attempt by other means may occur during the recovery phase. The possibility of simultaneous ingestion of other drugs should also be considered.

> For management of a suspected drug overdose, CPhA recommends that you contact your **regional Poison Control Centre**. See the *CPS* Directory section for a list of Poison Control Centres.

DOSAGE: An optimum daily dosage of Apo-Doxepin (doxepin hydrochloride) depends on the condition which is being treated and the response of the individual.

Some patients respond promptly: others may not respond for 2 weeks or longer. An initial dosage of 25 mg t.i.d. is recommended in most patients. This dosage should be increased as required by 25 mg increments at appropriate intervals until a therapeutic response is obtained. The usual optimum dosage range is 100-150 mg per day. In some patients, up to 300 mg per day may be required, but there is rarely any benefit to be obtained by increasing this dosage.
Geriatrics: In elderly patients it is advisable to proceed more cautiously with dosage increments and to initiate treatment with a lower dosage.

Once a satisfactory therapeutic response has been obtained, it is generally possible to reduce the dosage and still maintain this effect.

For maintenance therapy in depressed patients, the total daily dosage, up to 150 mg, may be given on a once-a-day schedule. This dosage should be established as described above and should preferably be given at bedtime.

SUPPLIED: 10 mg: Each pink and scarlet hard gelatin capsule, imprinted "APO 10", contains: doxepin HCl equivalent to doxepin base 10 mg. Nonmedicinal ingredients: colloidal silicon dioxide, croscarmellose sodium, lactose, microcrystalline cellulose, stearic acid and talc; capsule shell: D&C Red # 28, D&C Red # 33, D&C Yellow # 10, FD&C Blue # 1, FD&C Red # 40, gelatin and titanium dioxide, edible black ink (pharmaceutical glaze, synthetic black iron oxide, FD&C Blue # 2 aluminum lake, FD&C Red # 40 aluminum lake, FD&C Blue # 1 aluminum lake, D&C Yellow # 10 aluminum lake; may contain: n-butyl alcohol, propylene glycol, SDA-3A alcohol). Bottles of 100.
25 mg: Each pink and blue hard gelatin capsule, imprinted "APO 25", contains: doxepin HCl equivalent to doxepin base 25 mg. Nonmedicinal ingredients: colloidal silicon dioxide, croscarmellose sodium, lactose, microcrystalline cellulose, stearic acid and talc; capsule shell: D&C Red # 28, FD&C Blue #1, FD&C Red # 40, titanium dioxide and gelatin, edible black ink (pharmaceutical glaze, synthetic black iron oxide, FD&C Blue # 2 aluminum lake, FD&C Red # 40 aluminum lake, FD&C Blue # 1 aluminum lake, D&C Yellow # 10 aluminum lake; may contain: n-butyl alcohol, propylene glycol, SDA-3A alcohol). Bottles of 100.
50 mg: Each flesh and pink hard gelatin capsule, imprinted "APO 50", contains: doxepin HCl equivalent to doxepin base 50 mg. Nonmedicinal ingredients: colloidal silicon dioxide, croscarmellose sodium, lactose, microcrystalline cellulose, stearic acid and talc; capsule shell: D&C Red # 28, D&C Yellow # 10, FD&C Blue # 1, FD&C Red # 40, titanium dioxide and gelatin, edible black ink (pharmaceutical glaze, synthetic black iron oxide, FD&C Blue # 2 aluminum lake, FD&C Red # 40 aluminum lake, FD&C Blue # 1 aluminum lake, D&C Yellow # 10 aluminum lake; may contain: n-butyl alcohol, propylene glycol, SDA-3A alcohol). Bottles of 100.
75 mg: Each flesh and flesh hard gelatin capsule, imprinted "APO 75", contains: doxepin HCl equivalent to doxepin base 75 mg. Nonmedicinal ingredients: colloidal silicon dioxide, croscarmellose sodium, lactose, microcrystalline cellulose, stearic acid and talc; capsule shell: D&C Red # 28, D&C Yellow # 10, FD&C Blue # 1, titanium dioxide and gelatin, edible black ink (pharmaceutical glaze, synthetic black iron oxide, FD&C Blue # 2 aluminum lake, FD&C Red # 40 aluminum lake, FD&C Blue # 1 aluminum lake, D&C Yellow # 10 aluminum lake; may contain: n-butyl alcohol, propylene glycol, SDA-3A alcohol). Bottles of 100.
100 mg: Each flesh and blue hard gelatin capsule, imprinted "APO 100", contains: doxepin HCl equivalent to doxepin base 100 mg. Nonmedicinal ingredients: colloidal silicon dioxide, croscarmellose sodium, lactose, microcrystalline cellulose, stearic acid and talc; capsule shell: D&C Red # 28, D&C Yellow # 10, FD&C Blue # 1, titanium dioxide and gelatin, edible black ink (pharmaceutical glaze, synthetic black iron oxide, FD&C Blue # 2 aluminum lake, FD&C Red # 40 aluminum lake, FD&C Blue # 1 aluminum lake, D&C Yellow # 10 aluminum lake; may contain: n-butyl alcohol, propylene glycol, SDA-3A alcohol). Bottles of 100.

Store at room temperature 15 to 30°C.

Apo®-Etodolac Ⓟ

etodolac

Anti-inflammatory

Apotex

Date of Preparation: August 13, 1997

PHARMACOLOGY: Etodolac is a nonsteroidal anti-inflammatory drug (NSAID) that exhibits anti-inflammatory, analgesic and antipyretic properties in animal models. The pharmacological actions of etodolac are thought to be related to inhibition of prostaglandin biosynthesis at the site of inflammation.

APO-ETODOLAC (etodolac) is a racemic mixture of R- and S-etodolac. As with other NSAIDs, it has been demonstrated in animals that the S-form is biologically active and the R- form is not. Both enantiomers are stable and there is no R-to-S conversion in vivo.

According to in vitro studies of human chondrocytes, etodolac may preserve collagen phenotype while still inhibiting prostaglandin (PGE_2) biosynthesis. The results demonstrated that normal chondrocyte function remained unaffected by etodolac, as assessed by the rate of DNA synthesis, proteoglycan synthesis, type II collagen production, and collagenase production. Etodolac maintained type II collagen synthesis and partially blocked the effects of interleukin-1 (IL-1). Nevertheless, PGE_2 synthesis was significantly decreased in the presence of etodolac. These results need to be verified through in vivo testing.

Pharmacokinetics: Etodolac is well absorbed following oral administration. The systemic availability of etodolac is at least 80%, and the drug does not undergo significant first-pass metabolism. The dose-proportionality based on AUC (the area under the plasma concentration-time curve) is linear following doses up to 600 mg every 12 hours. Etodolac is more than 99% bound to plasma proteins.

Table 1: APO-ETODOLAC

Etodolac Steady-State Pharmacokinetic Parameters (n=267)

Kinetic Parameters	Scientific Notation (Units)	Mean±SD
Extent of Oral Absorption (Bioavailability)	F (%)	≥80
Peak Concentration Time	t_{max} (hr)	1.7±1.3
Oral-Dose Clearance	CL/F (mL/hr/kg)	47±6
Central Compartment Volume	V_c/F (mL/kg)	132±47
Steady-State Volume	V_{ss}/F (mL/kg)	362±29
Distribution Half-Life	$t_{½}$ α (hr)	0.71±0.50
Terminal Half-Life	$t_{½}$ β (hr)	7.3±4.0

Mean peak plasma concentrations range from approximately 14±4 to 37±9 µg/mL after 200 to 600 mg single doses and are reached in 80±30 minutes. The mean plasma clearance of etodolac is 47 (±16) mL/hr/kg, and terminal disposition half-life is 7.3 (±4.0) hours.

Etodolac is extensively metabolized in the liver, with renal elimination of etodolac and its metabolites being the primary route of excretion. Approximately 72% of the administered dose is recovered in the urine as the following, indicated as % of the administered dose:

Etodolac, unchanged	1%
Etodolac glucuronide	13%
Hydroxylated metabolites (6-, 7- and 8-OH)	5%
Hydroxylated metabolite glucuronides	20%
Unidentified metabolites	33%

Fecal excretion accounted for 16% of the dose. Therefore, enterohepatic circulation, if present, is not extensive.

The extent of absorption of etodolac is not affected when it is administered after a meal or with an antacid. Food intake, however, reduces the peak concentration reached by approximately one-half, and increases the time-to-peak concentration by 1.4 to 3.8 hours. Coadministration with an antacid decreases the peak concentration reached by about 15-20%, with no measurable effect on time-to-peak.

In studies in the elderly, age was found to have no effect on etodolac half-life or protein binding, and there was no drug accumulation. Etodolac clearance was reduced by about 15%. Because the reduction in clearance is small, no dosage adjustment is generally necessary in the elderly on the basis of pharmacokinetics. The elderly may need dosage adjustment, however, on the basis of body size, and they may be more sensitive to antiprostaglandin effects than younger patients.

In studies of the effects of mild to moderate renal impairment, no significant differences in the disposition of total and free etodolac were observed. In patients undergoing hemodialysis, there was a 50% greater apparent clearance of total etodolac, due to a 50% greater unbound fraction. Free etodolac clearance was not altered, indicating the importance of protein binding in etodolac's disposition. Nevertheless, etodolac is not dialyzable. No adjustment of etodolac is generally required in patients with mild to moderate renal impairment; however, etodolac should be used with caution in such patients because, as with other NSAIDs, it may further decrease renal function in some patients with impaired renal function.

In patients with compensated hepatic cirrhosis, the disposition of total and free etodolac is not altered. Although no dosage adjustment is generally required in this patient population, etodolac clearance is dependent on hepatic function and could be reduced in patients with severe hepatic failure.

Comparative Bioavailability: A standard, randomized, two-way crossover study was conducted in 24 healthy, adult, male volunteers to evaluate the relative bioavailability of single oral doses (300 mg) of APO-ETODOLAC capsules manufactured by Apotex Inc. and Ultradol capsules manufactured by Procter & Gamble Pharmaceuticals Canada, Inc. The mean pharmacokinetic parameters of the 23 subjects completing the study are listed below: see Table 2.

Table 2: APO-ETODOLAC

Summary Table of the Comparative Bioavailability Data. Etodolac (Dose: 300 mg) from Measured Data

Parameter	Geometric Mean Arithmetic Mean (CV%)		Ratio of Means (%)
	APO-ETODOLAC	Ultradol[b]	
AUC_T (µg·hr/mL)	93.60 97.25 (30)	97.03 100.99 (31)	96.6
AUC_I (µg·hr/mL)	96.45 100.88 (34)	100.18 105.20 (36)	96.5

(cont'd)

Table 2: APO-ETODOLAC *(cont'd)*

Summary Table of the Comparative Bioavailability Data. Etodolac (Dose: 300 mg) from Measured Data

Parameter	Geometric Mean Arithmetic Mean (CV%)		Ratio of Means (%)
	APO-ETODOLAC	Ultradol[b]	
C_{max} (µg/mL)	17.53 17.80 (18)	19.99 20.76 (28)	88.1
T_{max} (hr)[a]	1.60 (42)	1.71 (61)	—
$t_{1/2}$ (hr)[a]	7.03 (25)	7.12 (30)	—

[a] The T_{max} and $t_{½}$ parameters are expressed as the arithmetic means (CV%).
[b] Ultradol is manufactured by Procter & Gamble Pharmaceuticals Canada Inc. and was purchased in Canada.

INDICATIONS: APO-ETODOLAC (etodolac) is indicated for acute or long-term use in the relief of signs and symptoms of rheumatoid arthritis and osteoarthritis (degenerative joint disease).

CONTRAINDICATIONS: APO-ETODOLAC (etodolac) should not be used in patients who have previously shown hypersensitivity to etodolac. Due to possible cross-reactivity, APO-ETODOLAC should not be administered to patients who experience asthma, rhinitis, urticaria or other allergic reactions during therapy with ASA or other NSAIDs. Fatal anaphylactoid reactions have occurred in such individuals.

APO-ETODOLAC should not be used in patients with an active peptic ulcer or inflammatory diseases of the gastrointestinal tract.

WARNINGS: Peptic ulceration, perforation and gastrointestinal bleeding, sometimes severe and occasionally fatal have been reported during therapy with nonsteroidal anti-inflammatory drugs (NSAIDs) including etodolac.

APO-ETODOLAC (etodolac) should be given under close medical supervision to patients prone to gastrointestinal tract irritation, particularly those with a history of peptic ulcer, melena, diverticulosis or other inflammatory disease of the gastrointestinal tract (such as ulcerative colitis or Crohn's disease). In these cases the physician must weigh the benefits of treatment against the possible hazards (see Contraindications and Adverse Effects).

Patients taking any NSAID including this drug should be instructed to contact a physician immediately if they experience symptoms or signs suggestive of peptic ulceration or gastrointestinal bleeding. These reactions can occur at any time during treatment, without warning symptoms or signs.

Elderly, frail and debilitated patients appear to be at higher risk from a variety of adverse reactions from NSAIDs. As with other NSAIDs, APO-ETODOLAC should be used with special caution and under close supervision in these patients and consideration should be given to a starting dose lower than usual, with individual adjustment when necessary.

Pregnancy and Lactation: The safety of APO-ETODOLAC during pregnancy and lactation has not been established and therefore its use during pregnancy and lactation is not recommended.

In teratology studies, isolated occurrences of alterations in limb development were found and included polydactyly, oligodactyly, syndactyly, and unossified phalanges in rats and oligodactyly and synostosis of metatarsal in rabbits. These were observed at dose levels (2-14 mg/kg/day) close to human clinical doses. However, the frequency and the dosage group distribution of these findings in initial or repeated studies did not establish a clear drug- or dose-response relationship.

In rat studies with etodolac, as with other drugs known to inhibit prostaglandin synthesis, an increased incidence of dystocia, delayed parturition, and decreased pup survival occurred. The effects of APO-ETODOLAC on labour and delivery in pregnant women are unknown.

It is not known whether etodolac is excreted in human milk. Caution should be exercised if APO-ETODOLAC is administered to a nursing woman because many drugs are excreted in human milk.

Children: The safety and effectiveness of APO-ETODOLAC in children have not been established and therefore, the drug is not recommended in this age group.

PRECAUTIONS: Gastrointestinal: If peptic ulceration is suspected or confirmed or if gastrointestinal bleeding or perforation occurs in patients under treatment with APO-ETODOLAC (etodolac), the drug should be immediately withdrawn, an appropriate treatment initiated and the patient closely monitored.

There is no definitive evidence that the concomitant administration of histamine H_2-receptor antagonists and/or antacids will either prevent the occurrence of gastrointestinal side effects or allow continuation of APO-ETODOLAC therapy when and if the adverse reactions appear.

Renal Function: As with other NSAIDs, long-term administration of etodolac to animals has resulted in renal papillary necrosis and other abnormal renal pathology. In humans there have been reports of acute interstitial nephritis with hematuria, proteinuria, and occasionally nephrotic syndrome.

In patients with prerenal conditions leading to reduction in renal blood flow or blood volume, where renal prostaglandins have a supportive role in the maintenance of renal perfusion, administration of nonsteroidal anti-inflammatory agents may precipitate overt renal decompensation due to a dose-dependent reduction in prostaglandin formation. Patients at greatest risk are those with impaired renal function, heart failure, liver dysfunction, those taking diuretics, and the elderly.

Discontinuation of NSAID therapy is usually followed by recovery to the pretreatment state.

Etodolac and its metabolites are eliminated primarily by the kidneys; therefore, the drug should be used with great caution in patients with impaired renal function. In these cases, lower doses of APO-ETODOLAC should be considered and patients carefully monitored. During long-term therapy, kidney function should be monitored periodically.

Hepatic Function: As with other NSAIDs, borderline elevations of one or more liver tests may occur in up to 15% of patients. These abnormalities may progress, may remain essentially unchanged, or may be transient with continued therapy. Meaningful (3 times the upper limit of normal) elevations of ALT or AST occurred in controlled clinical trials with etodolac in approximately 1% of patients. A patient with symptoms and/or signs suggesting liver dysfunction, or in whom an abnormal liver test has occurred, should be evaluated for evidence of the development of more severe hepatic reaction while on therapy with this drug. Severe hepatic reactions including jaundice and cases of fatal hepatitis have been reported with this drug as with other nonsteroidal anti-inflammatory drugs. Although such reactions are rare, if abnormal liver tests persist or worsen, if clinical signs and symptoms consistent with liver disease develop, or if systemic manifestations occur (e.g. eosinophilia, rash, etc.), this drug should be discontinued.

During long-term therapy, liver function tests should be monitored periodically. If this drug is to be used in the presence of impaired liver function, it must be done under strict observation.

Fluid and Electrolyte Balance: Fluid retention and edema have been reported; therefore, as with many other NSAIDs, the possibility of precipitating congestive heart failure in elderly patients or those with compromised cardiac function should be borne in mind. APO-ETODOLAC should be used with caution in patients with heart failure, hypertension and renal diseases and in those recovering from surgical operations under general anesthesia and other conditions predisposing to fluid retention. With NSAID treatment, there is a potential risk of hyperkalemia, particularly in patients with conditions such as diabetes mellitus or renal failure, elderly patients or in patients receiving concomitant therapy with beta-adrenergic blockers, angiotensin converting enzyme inhibitors or some diuretics.

Serum electrolytes should be monitored periodically during long-term therapy, especially in those patients at risk.

Hematology: Drugs inhibiting prostaglandin biosynthesis do interfere with platelet function and vascular response to bleeding to some degree; therefore, patients who may be adversely affected by such an action should be carefully observed when APO-ETODOLAC is administered.

Blood dyscrasias associated with the use of NSAIDs are rare, but could be with severe consequences.

Anemia is commonly observed in rheumatoid arthritis and is sometimes aggravated by NSAIDs, which may produce fluid retention or minor gastrointestinal blood loss in some patients. Therefore, patients with initial hemoglobin values of 10 g/dL or less who are to receive long-term therapy, should have hemoglobin values determined frequently.

Infection: In common with other anti-inflammatory drugs, etodolac may mask the usual signs of infection.

Ophthalmology: Blurred and/or diminished vision has been reported with the use of etodolac and other NSAIDs. If such symptoms develop, this drug should be discontinued and an ophthalmologic examination performed; ophthalmic examination should be carried out at periodic intervals in any patient receiving this drug for an extended period of time.

Hypersensitivity: As with other nonsteroidal anti-inflammatory drugs, allergic reactions, including anaphylactic/anaphylactoid reactions, can occur without prior exposure to drug; therefore, careful questioning of patients for a history of asthma, nasal polyps, urticaria, and hypotension associated with NSAIDs before starting therapy is important.

Drug Interactions: Antacids: The concomitant administration of antacids has no apparent effect on the extent of absorption of etodolac. However, antacids can decrease the peak concentration reached by 15-20% but have no detectable effect on the time-to-peak.

Acetylsalicylic Acid (ASA): When etodolac is administered with ASA, its protein binding is reduced although the clearance of free etodolac is not altered. The clinical significance of this interaction is not known; however, as with other NSAIDs, concomitant administration of APO-ETODOLAC and ASA is not generally recommended because of potential of increased adverse effects.

Warfarin: Concomitant administration of warfarin and etodolac results in reduced protein binding of warfarin, but there is no change in the clearance of free warfarin. There is no significant difference in the pharmacodynamic effect of warfarin administered alone and warfarin administered with etodolac as measured by prothrombin time. Thus, concomitant therapy with warfarin and APO-ETODOLAC should not require dosage adjustment of either drug. Caution should be exercised, nevertheless, because interactions have been seen with other NSAIDs.

Phenytoin: Etodolac has no apparent pharmacokinetic interaction when administered with phenytoin.

Glyburide: Etodolac has no apparent pharmacokinetic or pharmacodynamic interaction when administered with glyburide.

Diuretics: Etodolac has no apparent pharmacokinetic interaction when administered with furosemide or hydrochlorothiazide, nor does etodolac attenuate the diuretic response of either of these drugs in normal volunteers. APO-ETODOLAC, and other NSAIDs nevertheless, should be used with caution in patients receiving diuretics or who have cardiac, renal or hepatic failure (see Renal Function).

Antihypertensive Agents: NSAIDs can reduce the anti-hypertensive effect of propranolol and other beta-blockers as well as other antihypertensive agents.

Cyclosporine, Digoxin, Lithium, Methotrexate: Etodolac, like other NSAIDs, through effects on renal prostaglandins may cause changes in the elimination of these drugs leading to elevated serum levels of digoxin, lithium, and methotrexate and increased toxicity. Nephrotoxicity associated with cyclosporine may also be enhanced. Patients receiving these drugs who are given etodolac, or any other NSAID, and particularly those patients with altered renal function, should be observed for the development of the specific toxicities of these drugs (monitoring of plasma drug levels).

Protein Binding: Data from in vitro studies using peak serum concentrations at reported therapeutic doses in humans show that the etodolac free fraction is not significantly altered by ibuprofen, acetaminophen, phenytoin, probenecid, indomethacin, chlorpropamide, glyburide, naproxen, glipizide or piroxicam.

In contrast, phenylbutazone causes an increase (by about 80%) in the free fraction of etodolac. Although in vivo studies have not been done to see if etodolac clearance is changed by coadministration of phenylbutazone, it is not recommended that they be coadministered.

Laboratory Test Interactions: The urine of patients who take etodolac can give a false-positive reaction for urinary bilirubin (urorubin) due to the presence of phenolic metabolites of etodolac.

Diagnostic dip-stick methodology, used to detect ketone bodies in urine, has resulted in false-positive findings in some patients treated with etodolac. Generally, this phenomenon has not been associated with other clinically significant events. No dose-relationship has been observed.

Etodolac treatment is associated with a small decrease in serum uric acid levels. In clinical trials, mean decreases of 1-2 mg% were observed in arthritic patients receiving etodolac (600 mg to 1000 mg/day) after 4 weeks of therapy. These levels then remained stable for up to one year of therapy.

ADVERSE EFFECTS: The most common adverse reactions encountered with nonsteroidal anti-inflammatory drugs are gastrointestinal, of which peptic ulcer, with or without bleeding, is the most severe. Fatalities have occurred on occasion, particularly in the elderly.

Adverse reaction information for etodolac was derived from 2629 arthritic patients treated with etodolac in double-blind and open-label clinical trials of 4 to 320 weeks in duration and worldwide post-marketing surveillance studies in approximately 60 000 patients.

In clinical studies, etodolac was generally well tolerated. Most adverse reactions were mild and transient. The discontinuation rate in controlled clinical trials because of adverse events, was 9% for patients treated with etodolac.

Listed below are the patient complaints with an incidence of greater than, equal to, or less than 1% which occurred in clinical trials and post-marketing experience with etodolac at doses up to 1000 mg per day.

Incidence ≥1%: Gastrointestinal: nausea; diarrhea; epigastric pain; heartburn; indigestion; flatulence; abdominal pain; gastrointestinal cramps; abdominal distention; constipation; vomiting; dyspepsia; gastritis; melena.

Central Nervous System: headache; dizziness; drowsiness; insomnia; nervousness/anxiety; depression.

Dermatologic: dermatitis manifested as skin rash (erythematous, vesicular, maculopapular, morbilliform, petechial, or eczematous), or pruritus.

General Illness: fatigue; weakness/malaise.

Genitourinary: urinary frequency; dysuria.

Metabolic System: fluid retention/edema.

Eye, Ear, Nose and Throat: tinnitus; blurred vision.

Incidence <1%: Gastrointestinal: peptic ulcer with/without gastrointestinal hemorrhage and/or perforation; hematemesis; rectal bleeding; stool changes (loose, with mucus, or increase in number and/or frequency); taste abnormalities including loss of taste; eructation; stomatitis; hepatitis; cholestasis; jaundice; esophagitis with or without erosions or stricture or cardiospasm; colitis; pancreatitis.

Central Nervous System: restlessness; confusion; vertigo; syncope; nightmares; listlessness; inability to concentrate, somnolence.

Dermatologic: urticaria; angioedema; alopecia; sore, dry, inflamed or swollen mucous membranes including mouth, tongue, and lips; photosensitivity; peeling; easy bruising; brittle nails; exfoliative dermatitis; Stevens-Johnson syndrome, cutaneous vasculitis with purpura; erythema multiforme.

Eye, Ear, Nose and Throat: hearing loss, visual disturbances including teichopsia; epistaxis; ear ache; pressure/throbbing in ears; burning sensation of eyes/nose; twinging behind eyes; photophobia; conjunctivitis.

Extremities: paresthesias; muscle cramps; muscular fatigue; involuntary muscle movement; pain in arms/hands/shoulders; hand tremor; tenderness; subcutaneous nodule/first metatarsophalangeal joint.

General Illness: pyrexia; chills; lethargy; vasculitis; general deterioration; breast tenderness.

Genitourinary: dysuria; urinary urgency; hematuria; nocturia; vaginal bleeding; difficulty maintaining erection; recto-pubic pain; cystitis; leukorrhea; renal calculus; interstitial nephritis; papillary necrosis; renal failure; uterine bleeding irregularities.

Metabolic System: change in weight; change in appetite; flushing; anorexia; excessive thirst; hot flashes; diaphoresis.

Cardiovascular: hypertension; congestive heart failure; palpitations; tachycardia; chest pain (costal, costochondral, or retrosternal); arrhythmias; myocardial infarction; and chest tightness or fullness.

Respiratory: dyspnea; asthma; bronchospasm; hyperventilation; sneezing and sighing; bronchitis; pharyngitis; rhinitis; sinusitis.

Hypersensitivity: anaphylactic/anaphylactoid reaction; laryngeal edema.

Hematology: agranulocytosis; pancytopenia; decreased hemoglobin; decreased hematocrit; anemia; hemolytic anemia; thrombocytopenia; leukopenia; neutropenia; eosinophilia; atypical lymphocytes; increased bleeding time.

Laboratory: elevated hepatic enzymes; increased serum creatinine.

OVERDOSE:

Symptoms: Symptoms following acute NSAID overdose are usually limited to lethargy, drowsiness, nausea, vomiting and epigastric pain which are generally reversible with supportive care. Gastrointestinal bleeding can occur and coma has occurred following massive ibuprofen or mefenamic acid overdose. Hypertension, acute renal failure, and respiratory depression may occur, but are rare. Anaphylactoid reactions have been reported with therapeutic ingestion of NSAIDs, and may occur following overdose.

Treatment: Patients should be managed by symptomatic and supportive care following an NSAID overdose. There are no specific antidotes. Gut decontamination may be indicated in patients seen within 4 hours with symptoms or following a large overdose (5-10 times the usual dose). This should be accomplished via emesis and/or activated charcoal (60 to 100 g in adults, 1 to 2 g/kg in children) with an osmotic cathartic. Forced diuresis, alkalinization of the urine, hemodialysis or hemoperfusion would probably not be useful due to etodolac's high protein binding.

One case of intentional etodolac overdosage has been reported (*Human Toxicol* 1988;7:203-204). This 53-year-old female ingested from 15 to 46 two hundred mg etodolac capsules (3 to 8.6 g). Plasma etodolac concentrations were measured frequently over the next 4 days. At 5 hours after ingestion (3 hours after gastric lavage) the plasma etodolac level was 22 µg/mL. These plasma levels and her subsequent recovery with no signs or symptoms of etodolac toxicity were consistent with systemic absorption of 600 to 800 mg. Her laboratory tests on admission showed a prolonged prothrombin time and a false-positive urine bilirubin (attributed to the phenolic etodolac metabolites).

For management of a suspected drug overdose, CPhA recommends that you contact your **regional Poison Control Centre**. See the *CPS* Directory section for a list of Poison Control Centres.

DOSAGE: Adults: The recommended dosage of APO-ETODOLAC (etodolac) in the treatment of rheumatoid arthritis and osteoarthritis is 200 to 300 mg twice daily. Patients may also respond to a single daily (400 mg or 600 mg) dose administered in the evening.

The safety of doses in excess of 1000 mg per day for extended periods has not been established. In order to maximize the effectiveness of therapy, the dosage must be individualized for each patient.

Geriatrics: As with any NSAID, caution should be exercised in treating the elderly, and when individualizing their dosage, extra care should be taken when increasing the dose because the elderly seem to tolerate NSAID side effects less well than younger patients. In otherwise healthy patients 65 years and older, no substantial differences in the side-effects profile of etodolac were seen.

INFORMATION FOR THE PATIENT: Published in e-CPS, available by subscription at www.e-cps.ca.

SUPPLIED: 200 mg: Each hard gelatin, light grey/dark grey, size #1 capsule, imprinted "APO 200", contains: etodolac 200 mg. Nonmedicinal ingredients: colloidal silicon dioxide, croscarmellose sodium, lactose monohydrate, stearic acid and talc; capsule shell: black iron oxide, titanium dioxide, yellow iron oxide, gelatin; edible red ink (shellac glaze-45% in SDA-3A alcohol, FD&C Red # 3, n-butyl alcohol, propylene glycol, iron oxide yellow and titanium dioxide). Bottles of 100.

300 mg: Each hard gelatin, light grey/light grey, size #0 capsule, imprinted "APO 300", contains: etodolac 300 mg. Nonmedicinal ingredients: colloidal silicon dioxide, croscarmellose sodium, lactose monohydrate, stearic acid and talc; capsule shell: black iron oxide, titanium dioxide, yellow iron oxide, gelatin; edible red ink (shellac glaze-45% in SDA-3A alcohol, FD&C Red # 3, n-butyl alcohol, propylene glycol, iron oxide yellow and titanium dioxide). Bottles of 100.

Store at room temperature (15 to 30°C) and protect from moisture.

Apo®-Fenofibrate ℞
fenofibrate
Lipid Metabolism Regulator

Apotex

Apo®-Feno-Micro ℞
fenofibrate
Lipid Metabolism Regulator

Apotex

Date of Preparation: June 20, 1996
Date of Revision: January 5, 2001

PHARMACOLOGY: Fenofibrate lowers elevated serum lipids by decreasing the low-density lipoprotein (LDL) fraction rich in cholesterol and the very low-density lipoprotein (VLDL) fraction rich in triglycerides. In addition, fenofibrate increases the high-density lipoprotein (HDL) cholesterol fraction.

Fenofibrate appears to have a greater depressant effect on the very low density lipoproteins (VLDL) than on the low density lipoproteins (LDL). Therapeutic doses of fenofibrate produce variable elevations of HDL cholesterol, a reduction in the content of the total low density lipoproteins cholesterol, and a substantial reduction in the triglyceride content of very low density lipoproteins.

The mechanism of action of fenofibrate has not been definitively established. Work carried out to date suggests that fenofibrate: enhances the liver elimination of cholesterol as bile salts; inhibits the biosynthesis of triglycerides and enhances the catabolism of VLDL by increasing the activity of lipoprotein lipase; has an inhibitory effect on the biosynthesis of cholesterol by modulating the activity of HMG-CoA reductase.

After oral administration with food, fenofibrate is rapidly hydrolyzed into fenofibric acid, the active metabolite.

Fenofibrate's absorption is low and variable when the product is administered under fasting conditions. Fenofibrate's absorption is increased when the compound is given with food. In man, it is mainly excreted through the kidney. Half-life is about 20 hours. In patients with severe renal failure, significant accumulation was observed with a large increase in half-life. Therefore, the dose of fenofibrate may need to be reduced, depending on the rate of creatinine clearance.

The APO-FENO-MICRO formulation of fenofibrate offers in the order of 33% greater bioavailability than the APO-FENOFIBRATE formulation of fenofibrate. Thus, a 200 mg capsule of the APO-FENO-MICRO formulation of fenofibrate achieves equivalent plasma levels to a single dose of three 100 mg capsules of the APO-FENOFIBRATE formulation and a 67 mg capsule of the APO-FENO-MICRO formulation of fenofibrate achieves equivalent plasma levels to a 100 mg capsule of APO-FENOFIBRATE. In comparison with the APO-FENOFIBRATE formulation, the absorption of APO-FENO-MICRO is less influenced by fat content of the diet.

Comparative Bioavailability: A randomized, two-way crossover, single dose bioavailability study was conducted in fed, healthy, adult male subjects. The bioavailability of APO-FENO-MICRO Capsules, 200 mg, relative to Lipidil Micro Capsules, 200 mg, was determined following a single dose of 200 mg (1×200 mg capsule). The average values of the pharmacokinetic parameters determined for each of the formulations are listed in the following Table 1 for the 16 subjects completing the study.

Table 1: APO-FENO-MICRO

Summary Table of the Comparative Bioavailability Data. Fenofibrate (Dose: 1×200 mg capsule) (from measured data)

Parameter	Geometric Mean Arithmetic Mean (C.V.)		Ratio of Geometric Means (%)
	APO-FENO-MICRO	**Lipidil Micro[a]**	
AUC_{0-72} (μg·hr/mL)	133.6 139.2 (29)	140.7 146.2 (27)	95
AUC_I (μg·hr/mL)	140.6 147.1 (30)	147.8 154.1 (28)	95
C_{max} (μg/mL)	8.866 9.102 (24)	10.014 10.248 (23)	89
T_{max}[b] (hr)	6.66 (45)	6.31 (41)	—
$t_{1/2}$[b] (hr)	14.98 (34)	14.93 (29)	—

[a] Lipidil Micro is manufactured by Laboratoires Fournier S.C.A., France and distributed by Jouveinal Inc., and was purchased in Canada.
[b] The arithmetic means (CV) are presented for T_{max} and $t_{1/2}$.

INDICATIONS: APO-FENOFIBRATE (fenofibrate) and APO-FENO-MICRO (fenofibrate) are indicated as adjuncts to diet and other therapeutic measures for: 1) Treatment of patients with hypercholesterolemia, Fredrickson classification Types IIa and IIb mixed hyperlipidemias, to regulate lipid levels (reduce serum triglycerides and LDL cholesterol levels and increase HDL cholesterol). 2) Treatment of adult patients with very high serum triglyceride levels, Fredrickson classification Type IV and Type V hyperlipidemias, who are at a high risk of sequelae and complications (i.e., pancreatitis) from their hyperlipidemia.

APO-FENOFIBRATE and APO-FENO-MICRO alone may not be adequate therapy in some patients with familial combined hyperlipidemia with Type IIb and Type IV hyperlipoproteinemia.

Initial therapy for hyperlipidemia should include a specific diet (at least an equivalent to the American Heart Association [AHA] Step I diet), weight reduction, and an exercise program; and for patients with diabetes mellitus, good diabetic control.

CONTRAINDICATIONS: 1) Hepatic or severe renal dysfunction (creatinine clearance <20 mL/min), including primary biliary cirrhosis. 2) Pre-existing gallbladder disease (see Warnings). 3) Hypersensitivity to fenofibrate, or other drugs of the fibrate class. 4) The drug should not be used in pregnant or lactating patients. 5) APO-FENOFIBRATE (fenofibrate) and APO-FENO-MICRO (fenofibrate) are not indicated for the treatment of Type I hyperlipoproteinemia.

WARNINGS: *Drug Interactions:* Concomitant Oral Anticoagulants: Caution should be exercised when oral anticoagulants are given in conjunction with APO-FENOFIBRATE (fenofibrate) or APO-FENO-MICRO (fenofibrate). The dosage of oral anticoagulant should be reduced to maintain the prothrombin time at the desired level to prevent bleeding complications. Careful monitoring of prothrombin time is therefore recommended until it has been definitely determined that the prothrombin level has been stabilized.

Statins and Cyclosporine: Severe myositis and rhabdomyolysis have occurred when a statin or cyclosporine was administered in combined therapy with a fibrate. Therefore, the benefits and risks of using fenofibrate concomitantly with these drugs should be carefully considered.

MAO-Inhibitors: MAO-inhibitors with hepatotoxic potential must not be administered together with fibrates such as fenofibrate as they may increase the risk of hepatotoxicity.

Sulphonylureas and Insulin: It has been previously reported that the fibrates may potentiate the effects of these classes of drug. This effect has not yet been documented in the case of fenofibrate. No case of hypoglycemia or hypoglycemic reaction has been reported to date.

Children: Limited experience is available in children and adolescents, at the dose of 5 mg/kg/day, non-micronized formulation. However, safety and effectiveness has not been established in this sub-population.

Pregnancy: Strict birth control procedures must be exercised by women of childbearing potential. If pregnancy occurs despite birth control procedures, APO-FENOFIBRATE or APO-FENO-MICRO should be discontinued. Women who are planning pregnancy should discontinue fenofibrate products several months prior to conception.

Lactation: In the absence of information concerning the presence of fenofibrate in human breast milk, APO-FENOFIBRATE or APO-FENO-MICRO should not be used by nursing mothers.

Cholelithiasis: Fenofibrate may increase cholesterol excretion into the bile, and may lead to cholelithiasis. If cholelithiasis is suspected, gallbladder studies are indicated. APO-FENOFIBRATE or APO-FENO-MICRO should be discontinued if gallstones are found.

Other: Fenofibrate clinically and pharmacologically shows similarities with clofibrate. Physicians prescribing fenofibrate products should also be familiar with the risks and benefits of clofibrate.

In long-term, animal toxicity and carcinogenicity studies fenofibrate has been shown to be tumorigenic for the liver in male rats at 12 times the human dose. At this dose level in male rats there was also an increase in benign Leydig cell tumours. Pancreatic acinar cell tumours were increased in male rats at 9 and 40 times the human dose. However, mice and female rats were unaffected at similar doses. Florid hepatocellular peroxisome proliferation has been observed following fenofibrate administration to rats. Such changes have not been found in the human liver after up to 3.5 years of fenofibrate administration.

Since a relationship between reduction of mortality from coronary artery disease and total mortality has not been established, APO-FENOFIBRATE and APO-FENO-MICRO should be administered only to those patients described in Indications. If a significant serum lipid response is not obtained in three months, fenofibrate products should be discontinued. If APO-FENOFIBRATE or APO-FENO-MICRO is chosen for treatment, the prescribing physician should discuss the proposed therapy and inform the patient of the expected benefits and potential risks which may be associated with long-term administration (see Precautions).

PRECAUTIONS: Initial Therapy: Before instituting fenofibrate therapy, attempts should be made to control serum lipids with appropriate diet, exercise and weight loss in obese patients. Other medical problems, such as diabetes mellitus and hypothyroidism, should also be controlled. In patients at high risk, consideration should be given to the control of other risk factors such as smoking, excessive alcohol intake, hormonal contraceptive use, and inadequately controlled hypertension.

Long-term Therapy: Because long-term administration of fenofibrate is recommended, the potential risks and benefits should be carefully weighed. Adequate pretreatment laboratory studies should be performed to ensure that patients have elevated serum cholesterol and/or triglycerides or low HDL-cholesterol levels. Periodic determination of serum lipids, fasting glucose, creatinine and ALT should be considered during fenofibrate treatment, particularly during the first months of therapy.

Reproduction Studies: Standard tests for teratology, fertility and peri- and post-natal effects in animals have shown a relative absence of risk; however, embryotoxicity has occurred in animals at maternally toxic doses.

Hematologic Changes: Mild hemoglobin, hematocrit and white blood cell decreases have been observed occasionally in patients following initiation of fenofibrate therapy. However, these levels stabilize during long-term administration. Periodic blood counts are recommended during the first 12 months of fenofibrate administration.

Liver Function: Abnormal liver function tests have been observed occasionally during fenofibrate administration, including elevations of transaminases, and decreases or, rarely, increases in alkaline phosphatase. However, these abnormalities disappear when therapy with fenofibrate is discontinued. Therefore, periodic liver function tests (AST, ALT] and GGT [if originally elevated]) in addition to other baseline tests are recommended after 3 to 6 months and at least yearly thereafter. APO-FENOFIBRATE (fenofibrate) and APO-FENO-MICRO (fenofibrate) therapy should be terminated if abnormalities persist. Fenofibrate may increase cholesterol excretion into the bile, and may lead to cholelithiasis.

Hepatobiliary Disease: In patients with a past history of jaundice or hepatic disorder, fenofibrate should be used with caution.

Skeletal Muscle: Treatment with drugs of the fibrate class has been associated on rare occasions with rhabdomyolysis or myositis, usually in patients with impaired renal function. Myopathy should be considered in any patient with diffuse myalgias, muscle tenderness or weakness, and/or marked elevation of creatinine phosphokinase levels.

Patients should be advised to promptly report unexplained muscle pain, tenderness or weakness, particularly if accompanied by malaise or fever. CPK levels should be assessed in patients reporting these symptoms, and fenofibrate therapy should be discontinued if markedly elevated CPK levels (10 times the upper limit of normal) occur or myopathy is diagnosed.

Drug Interactions: (See also Warnings.)

Resins: When a fibrate is used concurrently with cholestyramine or any other resin, an interval of at least 2 hours should be maintained between the administration of the two drugs, since the absorption of fibrates are impaired by cholestyramine.

Estrogens: Since estrogens may lead to a rise in lipid levels, the prescribing of fibrates in patients taking estrogens or estrogen-containing contraceptives must be critically considered on an individual basis.

Renal Function: In patients with hypoalbuminemia, e.g., nephrotic syndrome, and in patients with renal insufficiency, the dosage of fibrates must be reduced and renal function should be monitored regularly (see Precautions, Skeletal Muscle and Dosage). Fenofibrate is not removed by hemodialysis and should not be used in dialysis patients.

ADVERSE EFFECTS: Clinical adverse effects of fenofibrate therapy have been reported at an incidence between 2 and 15% with a mean of 6.3% in European trials of less than 12 months duration. In longer term studies, the incidence was between 7 and 14% with a mean of 11.3%. The most frequently reported adverse events include:

Gastrointestinal: epigastric distress, flatulence, abdominal pain, nausea, diarrhea, constipation.
Dermatologic: erythema, pruritus, urticaria.
Musculoskeletal: muscle pain and weakness, arthralgia.
Central Nervous System: headache, dizziness, insomnia.
Miscellaneous: decreased libido, hair loss, weight loss.

In two separate controlled clinical studies conducted in the U.S., a total of 191 patients on non-micronized fenofibrate (116 Type II and 75 Type IV/V patients) were evaluated for adverse effects versus 183 patients on placebo (111 Type II and 72 Type IV/V patients). Listed in Table 2 are the adverse reactions considered by the investigators to be possibly or probably related to treatment, and reported by more than 1% of the patients receiving fenofibrate in these trials.

Table 2: APO-FENOFIBRATE/APO-FENO-MICRO

Number (%) of Patients Reporting Adverse Reactions

	U.S. Multicentre Studies Type II study (6-month treatment) Type IV/V study (2-month treatment)	
Adverse Reactions	**Fenofibrate (n=191)**	**Placebo (n=183)**
Gastrointestinal		
Dyspepsia	6 (3.1)	8 (4.4)
Flatulence	6 (3.1)	5 (2.7)
Nausea	4 (2.1)	3 (1.6)

(cont'd)

Table 2: APO-FENOFIBRATE/APO-FENO-MICRO *(cont'd)*

Number (%) of Patients Reporting Adverse Reactions

U.S. Multicentre Studies Type II study (6-month treatment) Type IV/V study (2-month treatment)		
Adverse Reactions	**Fenofibrate (n=191)**	**Placebo (n=183)**
Abdominal pain	4 (2.1)[a]	2 (1.1)
Constipation	3 (1.6)	1 (0.5)
Skin and Appendages		
Pruritus	6 (3.1)[a]	1 (0.5)
Rash	6 (3.1)	1 (0.5)
Hives	3 (1.6)	—
Body as a Whole		
Fatigue	4 (2.1)	2 (1.1)
Musculoskeletal		
Arthralgia	3 (1.6)[a]	—

[a] One patient reported multiple adverse effects.

In these studies, the difference between the numbers of fenofibrate and placebo patients reporting these adverse reactions was not statistically significant (p>0.05). While the nature of the reported adverse reactions was similar in both studies, these reactions were observed in most cases at a higher frequency in the longer term, six-month trial in Type II patients.

Adverse reactions for the APO-FENO-MICRO formulation of fenofibrate at recommended therapeutic doses in clinical trials have shown a comparable profile with those described for the APO-FENOFIBRATE formulation of fenofibrate.

Surveillance in countries in which fenofibrate has been marketed for up to 20 years such as France, Germany and the United Kingdom, indicates that clinical adverse effects reported include gastrointestinal complaints, painful muscles, skin disorders typically classified as pruritus, urticaria or erythema, loss of weight, impotence, diverse nervous complaints, hair loss, gallstones, pancreatitis and hepatitis.

Laboratory Tests: In most trials, sporadic and transient increases in aminotransferase levels have been associated with the use of fenofibrate. The reported frequency of AST and ALT elevations was variable; in the U.S. clinical trials, elevations above twice the upper limit of normal were observed in 6.8% of the patients treated with fenofibrate, versus 1.6% of the patients on placebo. Values usually return to normal without interruption of treatment. On some occasions, more severe elevations of transaminases (above twice the upper limit of normal values) were noted; such rises subside when fenofibrate therapy is discontinued (see Precautions). Reductions in alkaline phosphatase levels have also been observed.

Mild decreases in hemoglobin, hematocrit and white blood cell counts have been observed occasionally in patients following initiation of fenofibrate therapy. However, these levels stabilize during long-term administration. In addition, a decrease in haptoglobin concentration has been observed in some patients with Type IV hyperlipidemia during long-term use of fenofibrate. However, this decrease in haptoglobin was not associated with any other sign of blood dyscrasia and/or hemolysis.

The mean plasma levels of urea and creatinine showed increases, particularly during long-term fenofibrate treatment, most of them remaining within the limits of normal values.

Fenofibrate also has the potential to provoke CPK elevations and changes in hematologic parameters which generally subside when the drug is discontinued (see Precautions).

OVERDOSE:

Treatment: While there has been no reported case of overdosage, symptomatic and supportive measures should be taken. Because fenofibric acid (the main metabolite of fenofibrate) is highly bound to plasma proteins, hemodialysis should not be considered.

For management of a suspected drug overdose, CPhA recommends that you contact your **regional Poison Control Centre**. See the *CPS* Directory section for a list of Poison Control Centres.

DOSAGE: The recommended dose for APO-FENO-MICRO (fenofibrate) in adults is 200 mg daily administered as one 200 mg capsule taken with the main meal or, three 67 mg capsules in two or three divided doses taken with meals. The maximum recommended total daily dose is 267 mg.

The recommended dose of APO-FENOFIBRATE (fenofibrate) is 300 mg daily administered in three divided doses (three 100 mg capsules) to be taken with meals. The maximum recommended total daily dose is 400 mg.

In patients with renal insufficiency (creatinine clearance between 20 and 100 mL/min), APO-FENO-MICRO treatment should be initiated at the dose of 67 mg/day and increased progressively after evaluation of the tolerance and effects on the lipid parameters. Fenofibrate is not removed by hemodialysis and should not be used when the creatinine clearance is lower than 20 mL/min.

INFORMATION FOR THE PATIENT: Published in e-CPS, available by subscription at www.e-cps.ca.

SUPPLIED: APO-FENOFIBRATE: Each opaque, white, No. 2 hard gelatin capsule, imprinted "APO 100", contains: fenofibrate 100 mg. Nonmedicinal ingredients: lactose monohydrate spray-dried, starch (corn), stearic acid and talc; capsule shell: edible black ink (synthetic black iron oxide, FD&C Blue #1 aluminum lake, FD&C Blue No. 2 aluminum lake, FD&C Red No. 40 aluminum lake, D&C Yellow No. 10 aluminum lake, n-butyl alcohol, propylene glycol, pharmaceutical glaze (modified) in SD-45), gelatin, sodium lauryl sulphate and titanium dioxide. Bottles of 100. Store at controlled room temperature (15 to 25°C). Avoid excessive humidity.

APO-FENO-MICRO: 67 mg: Each yellow, No. 4 hard gelatin capsule, imprinted "APO 67" contains: fenofibrate 67 mg. Nonmedicinal ingredients: colloidal silicon dioxide, croscarmellose sodium, lactose monohydrate (spray-dried), stearic acid and talc; capsule shell: colloidal silicon dioxide, D&C Yellow No. 10, edible black ink (shellac, dehydrated alcohol, isopropyl alcohol, butyl alcohol, propylene glycol, purified water, strong ammonia solution, black iron oxide), FD&C Red No. 40, FD&C Yellow No. 6, gelatin, sodium lauryl sulfate and titanium dioxide. Bottles of 100. Store at controlled room temperature (15 to 25°C). Avoid excessive humidity.

200 mg: Each orange, No. 1 hard gelatin capsule, imprinted "APO 200" contains: fenofibrate 200 mg. Nonmedicinal ingredients: colloidal silicon dioxide, croscarmellose sodium, lactose monohydrate (spray-dried), stearic acid and talc; capsule shell: colloidal silicon dioxide, D&C Red No. 28, edible black ink (shellac, dehydrated alcohol, isopropyl alcohol, butyl alcohol, propylene glycol, purified water, strong ammonia solution, black iron oxide), FD&C Blue No. 1, FD&C Red No. 40, FD&C Yellow No. 6, gelatin and titanium dioxide. Bottles of 100. Blister packages of 30. Store at controlled room temperature (15 to 25°C). Avoid excessive humidity.

Apo-Flavoxate Ⓟ

flavoxate HCl

Urinary Tract Antispasmodic

Apotex

Date of Preparation: October 23, 2001
Date of Revision: July 4, 2002

PHARMACOLOGY: The basic action of flavoxate hydrochloride (HCl) is the relaxation of smooth muscle fibers of the urinary tract through a mechanism not yet defined.

By counteracting smooth muscle spasms of the urinary tract, it relieves the pain and discomfort accompanying a variety of urological disorders, e.g., frequency, dysuria, urgency, nocturia, and incontinence.

In addition, flavoxate HCl has been shown to have analgesic and local anaesthetic properties in laboratory animals (mouse).

Flavoxate hydrochloride is a spasmolytic drug directly counteracting smooth muscle spasms of the bladder and urinary tract. It was synthesized in 1960 by a team of chemists and pharmacologists in the Research Laboratories of Recordati, Milano, Italy.

Clinical Use: In human volunteers administered 800-1200 mg of flavoxate HCl daily for 90 days hemoglobin, hematocrit, white blood cell counts, blood urea nitrogen, blood glucose, bilirubin, alkaline phosphatase, ALT, prothrombin time, and body weight remained normal as did urine analyses performed routinely throughout the test period.

Following oral administration of 200 and 400 mg doses of flavoxate HCl to human volunteers, small concentrations only (0.3-0.7 µg/mL) were detected in plasma 1 hour after dosing. Concentrations of its major metabolite, 3-methyl flavone-8-carboxylic acid (MFCA), ranged from 5-10 µg/mL during this time interval, increasing to 9-15 µg/mL within 2 hours.

The author observed that 'flavoxate was very well tolerated by all subjects. There was a low incidence of side effects, in particular those usually observed with anticholinergic or related agents'.

Cystometric studies in 50 patients with normal as well as neurogenic bladders showed therapeutic effects, decreased resting bladder pressure and increased bladder capacity, within two hours. Comparing clinical responses observed after flavoxate HCl and propantheline administration, the authors concluded that the anticholinergic 'caused dryness in the oropharynx in about two thirds of the patients whereas none reported this or any other complaint after flavoxate HCl therapy'.

Studies have involved over 1000 patients (adults and children, male and female) ranging in age from 7 to 90 years. Collectively, these studies documented the safety and efficacy of flavoxate HCl for the indications described.

Clinical trials have shown that flavoxate HCl is well tolerated in both short and long-term therapy. Significant urine retention frequently observed in patients treated with anticholinergics was not seen in patients undergoing flavoxate HCl therapy.

Zaffiri et al. first reported the beneficial effects (alleviation of discomfort and pain) of flavoxate HCl administration in patients being prepared for prostate surgery.

In 1973 Stanton conducted a double-blind, crossover clinical trial comparing flavoxate HCl and emepronium bromide (dosages administered: 200 mg tablets three times a day) in 38 patients (32 women and 6 men) with urinary frequency, urgency, and incontinence.

Flavoxate HCl reduced intravesical bladder pressure to a greater extent than emepronium bromide (p almost 0.05). Both drugs delayed the onset of first sensation and increased overall bladder capacity, but flavoxaote HCl more so than emepronium bromide (p<0.02). Flavoxate HCl also improved to a greater extent stress incontinence associated with detrusor instability (75%) or sphincter dysfunction (50%) than emepronium bromide (25% and 36%, respectively) (p=0.003).

Flavoxate HCl provided, likewise, greater symptomatic relief of urgency associated with detrusor instability (83%) or sphincter dysfunction (50%) than emepronium bromide (66% and 36%, respectively) (p=0.145). Both drugs reduced diurnal frequency but flavoxate HCl was significantly more effective (p=0.038). Also patients undergoing flavoxate HCl therapy experienced fewer side effects (8%) than those undergoing emepronium bromide therapy (24%) (p=0.07).

In 1975, Gould reported a study comprising 9 separate clinical trials based on identical protocols. It involved 392 patients having urinary frequency, dysuria, nocturia, urgency, incontinence, and/or suprapubic pain associated with acute cystitis, prostatitis, urethritis, and/or trigonitis. They were randomly assigned to treatment with flavoxate HCl (two 100 mg tablets four times a day) or phenazopyridine (two 100 mg tablets three times a day). Altogether 289 women and 103 men, ranging in age from 7 to 90 years, participated in the study. Overall response was evaluated in 384 patients after five days of therapy.

In patients having prostatitis, response was satisfactory in 66% treated with flavoxate HCl, and in 31% treated with phenazopyridine.

In patients having acute cystitis, urethritis, and/or trigonitis overall response was satisfactory in 80% of patients receiving flavoxate HCl, compared with 56% of patients receiving phenazopyridine.

Adverse effects were reported in 8% of patients receiving flavoxate HCl, compared to 13% of patients receiving phenazopyridine.

In 1977, Delaere completed a study in which 42 patients ranging in age from 8 to 70 years, participated. They suffered from urodynamically proven detrusor instability treated previously without success by means of bladder distension, propantheline bromide and/or emepronium bromide therapy. The author noted that following administration of flavoxate HCl (400-1200 mg/day), and continued observation of all patients over a period of 2-18 months, 'five patients were completely relieved of all their complaints, and in 11 the symptoms improved (16%)'. Urgency and frequency showed the most favorable reaction to the treatment, nocturnal enuresis the least.

In 1979, Jonas et al. concluded a study during which 37 patients, 'ranging in age from 7 to 75 years, were administered flavoxate HCl (300-600 mg/day) because of a variety of urological disorders due to hyperactive detrusor muscle. Overall therapeutic response was as follows: subjective improvement 61.3%, daily frequency normalized or improved 47.8%, nocturia normalized or improved 50.0%, daily enuresis normalized or improved 67.8%, and nocturnal enuresis normalized or improved 41.2%.

Bladder volume at which uninhibited contractions were first seen was increased by 80.5% (from a mean of 74.5 mL to 134.5 mL), the amplitude of uninhibited detrusor contractions decreased by 49.5% (from a mean of 52.3 cm H_2O to 26.4 cm H_2O), and bladder capacity increased by 18.7% (from a mean of 231 mL to 284 mL).

In 1978 and 1980, Gaudenz and Weil, reported on studies comparing the safety and efficacy of flavoxate HCl (3×200 mg/day), emepronium bromide (3×200 mg/day), and propantheline (3×30 mg/day) following administration over a period of 12 weeks to 70 patients (17 to 79 years old) having urological disorders. They found that incontinence was improved in 87% of patients treated with flavoxate HCl, in 66% of patients treated with emepronium bromide, and in 50% of patients treated with propantheline.

Urinary frequency, nocturia and urgency were improved in 81% of patients undergoing flavoxate therapy, in 78% of patients undergoing emepronium bromide therapy, and in 48% of patients undergoing propantheline therapy. Bladder capacity increased in 50% of patients receiving either flavoxate HCl or emepronium bromide, and in 44% of patients receiving propantheline, mean increases being 83 mL for flavoxate HCl, 39 mL for emepronium bromide, and 28 mL for propantheline.

Subjectively, 50% of patients on flavoxate HCl, 34% of patients on emepronium bromide, and 15% of patients on propantheline were very satisfied. No improvement was experienced by 17% of patients receiving flavoxate HCl, 34% of patients receiving emepronium bromide, and 57% of patients receiving propantheline.

Fewer side effects were observed in patients treated with flavoxate HCl. Drug tolerance was judged to be excellent in 42% of patients on emepronium bromide, in 56% of patients on propantheline, and in 75% of patients on flavoxate HCl. Also, whereas 8% of patients treated with emepronium bromide and 11% of patients treated with propantheline withdrew from the study, no patient treated with flavoxate HCl discontinued the clinical trial.

Comparative Bioavailability: A comparative bioavailability study was performed using healthy volunteers. The rate and extent of absorption of flavoxate HCl was measured and compared following oral administration of a single 1×200 mg dose of APO-FLAVOXATE (flavoxate HCl) tablets, or Urispas (flavoxate HCl) tablets, under fed conditions. The results from measured data are summarized in Table 1.

INDICATIONS: APO-FLAVOXATE (flavoxate HCl) is indicated for the symptomatic relief of dysuria, urgency, nocturia, suprapubic pain, frequency and incontinence, as may occur in cystitis, prostatitis, urethritis, urethrocystitis, and urethrotrigonitis.

It is not indicated for the definitive treatment of urinary tract infections, but is compatible with drugs used for their management. Where evidence of such infection is present, appropriate anti-infective therapy should be instituted concomitantly. In non-infectious cases of bladder inflammation or irritation, APO-FLAVOXATE alone can provide symptomatic relief.

APO-FLAVOXATE is also indicated for the relief of vesicourethral spasms due to catheterization, cystoscopy or indwelling catheters, prior to cystoscopy or catheterization, and sequelae of surgical intervention of the lower urinary tract.

CONTRAINDICATIONS: APO-FLAVOXATE (flavoxate HCl) is contraindicated in patients who have any of the following conditions: pyloric or duodenal obstruction, obstructive intestinal lesions or ileus, achalasia, gastrointestinal hemorrhage and obstructive uropathies of the lower urinary tract. It is not yet recommended for infants and children under 12 years of age since safety and efficacy studies in this age group are not completed.

WARNINGS: APO-FLAVOXATE (flavoxate HCl) should be given cautiously to patients with suspected glaucoma. Although studies in sensitive animals have not shown any potential for teratogenic effects, the drug should only be used during pregnancy if, in the opinion of the physician, the anticipated benefits outweigh any risks.

PRECAUTIONS: In the event of drowsiness or blurred vision, the patient should not operate a motor vehicle or any machinery, and refrain from participating in activities requiring alertness.

ADVERSE EFFECTS: Adverse reactions reported include nausea and vomiting, dry mouth, nervousness, vertigo, headache, drowsiness, blurred vision, increased ocular tension, disturbance in eye accommodation, urticaria and other dermatoses, mental confusion, especially in the elderly patient, dysuria, tachycardia and palpitation, hyperpyrexia, eosinophilia and leukopenia (one case which was reversible upon discontinuation of the drug).

Table 1: APO-FLAVOXATE

Summary Table of the Comparative Bioavailability Data Flavoxate HCl Tablets (Dose: 1×200 mg) From Measured Data

Parameter	Geometric Mean Arithmetic Mean (CV%) APO-FLAVOXATE	Urispas[c]	Ratio of Geometric Means (%)[b]
AUC_T (μg·hr/mL)	15.5 16.0 (24)	15.9 16.4 (26)	97.5
AUC_I (μg·hr/mL)	15.9 16.3 (24)	16.4 16.9 (26)	97.2
C_{max} (μg/mL)	7.60 8.09 (36)	9.00 9.82 (43)	84.8
T_{max} (hr)[a]	1.50 (63)	1.74 (48)	
$t_{1/2}$ (hr)[a]	1.16 (27)	1.30 (30)	

[a] Arithmetic means (CV%).
[b] Based on the least squares estimate.
[c] Urispas is manufactured by Pharmascience Inc, and was purchased in Canada.

OVERDOSE:

Symptoms: Although no such experience has been reported to date, it is considered likely that the following symptoms may be observed: nausea, vomiting, dryness of the mouth, blurred vision, disturbance in visual accommodation, tachycardia, tachypnea, mental confusion, excitement, convulsions, respiratory failure, and coma.

Treatment: There is no known specific antidote. Treatment is, essentially, symptomatic with close monitoring of vital functions imperative

In a conscious, alert patient prompt evacuation of the stomach should be performed. When evacuation is complete, observation and further treatment should be made according to the attending physician's assessment of the patient.

If overdosage is extreme, or there is delay in removing the drug from the stomach, administration of a parasympathomimetic drug should be considered.

In the presence of severe anticholinergic reactions, slow intravenous injection of 1-4 mg of physostigmine is indicated, and in case of favorable response, repeated doses may be administered. If marked excitement is observed, diazepam may be given for sedation and control of convulsions. In a comatosed patient, a clear airway must be established immediately and artificial respiration instituted.

For management of a suspected drug overdose, CPhA recommends that you contact your **regional Poison Control Centre**. See the *CPS* Directory section for a list of Poison Control Centres.

DOSAGE: The recommended dosage for adults and children over 12 years of age is one tablet 3 or 4 times a day.

APO-FLAVOXATE (flavoxate HCl) is rapidly absorbed. Clinical response will vary depending on the nature and severity of symptoms diagnosed and the patient's overall condition. Therapeutic effects on bladder musculature may be observed within 2 to 3 hours.

In patients with infection, treatment is usually continued for as long as antibacterial or anti-infective medications are administered (i.e., a week or so). In patients with chronic bladder symptoms, maintenance therapy for prolonged periods may be required for optimum results. With improvement of symptoms, the dose may be reduced.

It is recommended that tablets be taken after meals.

SUPPLIED: Each white, round, biconvex, film-coated tablet, engraved "APO" on one side and "FLA" over "200" on the other contains: flavoxate HCl 200 mg. Nonmedicinal ingredients: colloidal silicon dioxide, hydroxypropyl cellulose, hydroxypropyl methylcellulose, magnesium stearate, microcrystalline cellulose, polyethylene glycol and titanium dioxide. HDPE bottles of 100. Store at room temperature (15 to 30°C), in tightly closed containers.

Apo-Floctafenine ℞

floctafenine

Anti-inflammatory—Analgesic

Apotex

Date of Preparation: October 22, 2001

PHARMACOLOGY: Floctafenine, an anthranilic acid derivative, is a non-steroidal anti-inflammatory agent with analgesic and anti-inflammatory properties. The analgesic activity is comparable to that of other mild analgesics in the relief of acute pain. Floctafenine has been shown to inhibit in vitro biosynthesis of prostaglandins PGE_2 and $PGF_{2\alpha}$. Gastrointestinal bleeding determined by daily fecal blood loss, was shown in one clinical trial to be approximately 1.2 mL after 1600 mg/day of floctafenine compared to 10.4 mL after 2400 mg/day of acetylsalicylic acid.

In normal volunteers, floctafenine was well absorbed after oral administration and peak plasma levels of floctafenic acid, the active metabolite, were attained 1-2 hours after administration and declined in a biphasic manner, with an initial (α phase) half-life of approximately 1 hour and a later (β phase) half-life of approximately 8 hours. Floctafenine and its metabolites do not accumulate following oral administration of multiple doses.

After oral and intravenous administration of ^{14}C labelled floctafenine, urinary excretion accounted for 40% and fecal and biliary excretion accounted for 60% of the recovered radioactivity. The main urinary metabolites are floctafenic acid and its conjugate with minimal amounts of free floctafenine.

Comparative Bioavailability: A comparative bioavailability study was performed on healthy human volunteers. The rate and extent of absorption of floctafenine was measured and compared following oral administration of 2×400 mg of either APO-FLOCTAFENINE 400 mg tablets or Idarac 400 mg tablets. The results from measured data are summarized as follows: see Table 1.

Table 1: APO-FLOCTAFENINE

Summary Table of the Comparative Bioavailability Data. Floctafenine (Dose: 2×400 mg) from Measured Data—Under Fasting Conditions

Parameter	Geometric Mean Arithmetic Mean (CV%) APO-FLOCTAFENINE	Idarac[c]	Ratio of Geometric Means (%)[b]
AUC_T (μg·hr/mL)	27.5 29.6 (37)	27.2 28.9 (39)	100.6
AUC_I (μg·hr/mL)	32.6 35.2 (39)	34.4 36.7 (38)	94.4
C_{max} (μg/mL)	7.81 8.66 (38)	6.72 7.79 (74)	116.0
T_{max} (hr)[a]	1.35 (47)	1.28 (50)	
$t_{1/2}$ (hr)[a]	22.1 (89)	22.3 (61)	

[a] Arithmetic means (CV%).
[b] Based on the least squares estimate.
[c] Idarac is manufactured by Sanofi Canada Inc., formerly Sanofi Winthrop, and was purchased in Canada.

INDICATIONS: APO-FLOCTAFENINE (floctafenine) is indicated for short-term use in acute pain of mild and moderate severity.

CONTRAINDICATIONS: The following are contraindications to the use of APO-FLOCTAFENINE (floctafenine):

1. Active peptic ulcer, a history of recurrent ulceration or active inflammatory disease of the gastrointestinal system.
2. Known or suspected hypersensitivity to the drug or other non-steroidal anti-inflammatory drugs. The potential for cross-reactivity between different NSAIDs must be kept in mind.
   APO-FLOCTAFENINE should not be used in patients with the complete or partial syndrome of nasal polyps, or in whom asthma, anaphylaxis, urticaria, rhinitis or other allergic manifestations are precipitated by ASA or other non-steroidal anti-inflammatory agents. Fatal anaphylactoid reactions have occurred in such individuals. As well, individuals with the above medical problems are at risk of a severe reaction even if they have taken NSAIDs in the past without any adverse effects.
3. On occasion, it has been observed that intermittent use may have resulted in increased sensitivity. Since severe cases of hypersensitivity reactions have been reported with floctafenine, its use in severe cardiac insufficiency and ischemic cardiomyopathy is contraindicated.
4. Significant hepatic impairment or active liver disease.
5. Severely impaired or deteriorating renal function (creatinine clearance <30 mL/min). Individuals with lesser degrees of renal impairment are at risk of deterioration of their renal function when prescribed NSAIDs and must be monitored.
6. APO-FLOCTAFENINE is not recommended for use with other NSAIDs because of the absence of any evidence demonstrating synergistic benefits and the potential for additive side effects.
7. Severe heart failure.
8. Coronary heart disease.
9. Associated treatment with beta-blocking agents (see Precautions, Drug Interactions).

WARNINGS: Gastrointestinal System (GI): Serious GI toxicity, such as peptic ulceration, perforation and gastrointestinal bleeding, sometimes severe and occasionally fatal can occur at any time, with or without symptoms in patients treated with non-steroidal anti-inflammatory drugs (NSAIDs) including floctafenine.

Minor upper GI problems, such as dyspepsia, are common, usually developing early in therapy. Physicians should remain alert for ulceration and bleeding in patients treated with non-steroidal anti-inflammatory drugs, even in the absence of previous GI tract symptoms.

In patients observed in clinical trials of such agents, symptomatic upper GI ulcers, gross bleeding, or perforation appear to occur in approximately 1% of patients treated for 3-6 months and in about 2-4% of patients treated for one year. The risk continues beyond one year and possibly increases. APO-FLOCTAFENINE (floctafenine), however, is only recommended for short-term use.

The incidence of these complications increases with increasing dose.

APO-FLOCTAFENINE (floctafenine) should be given under close medical supervision to patients prone to gastrointestinal tract irritation particularly those with a history of peptic ulcer, diverticulosis or other inflammatory disease of the gastrointestinal tract such as ulcerative colitis and Crohn's disease. In these cases the physician must weigh the benefits of treatment against the possible hazards.

Physicians should inform patients about the signs and/or symptoms of serious GI toxicity and instruct them to contact a physician immediately if they experience persistent dyspepsia or other symptoms or signs suggestive of gastrointestinal ulceration or bleeding.

If ulceration is suspected or confirmed, or if GI bleeding occurs, APO-FLOCTAFENINE should be discontinued immediately, appropriate treatment instituted and the patient monitored closely.

No studies to date, have identified any group of patients **not** at risk of developing ulceration and bleeding. A prior history of serious GI events and other factors such as excess alcohol intake, smoking, age, female gender and concomitant oral steroid and anti-coagulant use have been associated with increased risk.

Studies to date show that all NSAIDs can cause GI tract adverse events. Although existing data does not clearly identify differences in risk between various NSAIDs, this may be shown in the future.

Use in the Elderly: Patients older than 65 years and frail or debilitated patients are most susceptible to a variety of adverse events from non-steroidal anti-inflammatory drugs (NSAIDs): the incidence of these adverse reactions increases with dose and duration of treatment. In addition, these patients are less tolerant to ulceration and bleeding. Most reports of fatal GI events are in this population. Older patients are also at risk of lower esophageal ulceration and bleeding.

For such patients, consideration should be given to a starting dose lower than the one usually recommended, with individual adjustment when necessary and under close supervision. See Precautions for further advice.

Sensitivity and Cross-Sensitivity: Avoid occasional repeated dosing which may cause sensitization (notably for some acute pain states). Generalized and mucocutaneous allergic reactions possibly culminating in shock, may occur. These may often be preceded by the appearance of minor allergic symptoms: formication of the palms and soles, sudden reddening of the face and neck, rash, laryngeal tickling sensation and malaise. This type of previous history should be systematically evaluated before each new prescription. It is a contraindication to continuing or resuming treatment with floctafenine either alone or in combination with compounds having a similar chemical structure because of possible cross-sensitivity.

Aseptic Meningitis: In occasional cases, with some NSAIDs, the symptoms of aseptic meningitis (stiff neck, severe headaches, nausea and vomiting, fever or clouding of consciousness) have been observed. Patients with autoimmune disorders (systemic lupus erythematosus, mixed connective tissue diseases, etc.) seem to be pre-disposed. Therefore, in such patients, the physician must be vigilant to the development of this complication.

Pregnancy: As floctafenic acid crosses the placental barrier, the use of APO-FLOCTAFENINE in women of childbearing potential requires that the likely benefit of the drug be weighed against the possible risk to the mother and fetus.

Use in Labour: See Pregnancy.

Lactation: It has been shown that floctafenic acid is slightly secreted in breast milk. Therefore, use of APO-FLOCTAFENINE in women who are nursing is not recommended.

Children: The safety and efficacy of APO-FLOCTAFENINE in children have not been established and therefore its use in this age group is not recommended.

The safety and efficacy of long-term use of APO-FLOCTAFENINE have not been clearly established.

PRECAUTIONS: Gastrointestinal System: There is no definitive evidence that the concomitant administration of histamine H_2-receptor antagonists and/or antacids will either prevent the occurrence of gastrointestinal side effects or allow the continuation of APO-FLOCTAFENINE (floctafenine) therapy when and if these adverse reactions appear.

Renal Function: Long-term administration of non-steroidal anti-inflammatory drugs to animals has resulted in renal papillary necrosis and other abnormal renal pathology. In humans, there have been reports of acute interstitial nephritis with hematuria, proteinuria, and occasionally nephrotic syndrome.

A second form of renal toxicity has been seen in patients with prerenal conditions leading to the reduction in renal blood flow or blood volume, where the renal prostaglandins have a supportive role in the maintenance of renal perfusion. In these patients, administration of a non-steroidal anti-inflammatory drug may cause a dose-dependent reduction in prostaglandin formation and may precipitate overt renal decompensation. Patients at greatest risk of this reaction are those with impaired renal function, heart failure, liver dysfunction, those taking diuretics, and the elderly. Discontinuation of non-steroidal anti-inflammatory therapy is usually followed by recovery to the pre-treatment state.

Floctafenine and its metabolites are eliminated primarily by the kidneys, therefore the drug should be used with great caution in patients with impaired renal function. In these cases, utilization of lower doses of APO-FLOCTAFENINE should be considered and patients monitored.

In clinical trials with floctafenine, dysuria, without apparent changes in renal function, was reported. The incidence of dysuria was greater in males than in females and occurred primarily in the first morning voiding. It has not been established whether dysuria is related to dose and/or duration of drug administration.

Genitourinary Tract: Some NSAIDs are known to cause persistent urinary symptoms (bladder pain, dysuria, urinary frequency), hematuria or cystitis. The onset of these symptoms may occur at any time after the initiation of therapy with an NSAID. Some cases have become severe on continued treatment. Should urinary symptoms occur, treatment with APO-FLOCTAFENINE **must be stopped immediately** to obtain recovery. This should be done before any urological investigations or treatments are carried out.

Hepatic Function: As with other non-steroidal anti-inflammatory drugs, borderline elevations of one or more liver function tests may occur in up to 15% of patients. These abnormalities may progress, may remain essentially unchanged, or may be transient with continued therapy. A patient with symptoms and/or signs suggesting liver dysfunction, or in whom an abnormal liver test has occurred, should be evaluated for evidence of the development of more severe hepatic reaction while on therapy with this drug. Severe hepatic reactions including jaundice and cases of fatal hepatitis have been reported with non-steroidal anti-inflammatory drugs. Although such reactions are rare, if abnormal liver tests persist or worsen, if clinical signs and symptoms consistent with liver disease develop, or if systemic manifestations occur (e.g. eosinophilia, rash, etc.) this drug should be discontinued.

If there is a need to prescribe this drug in the presence of impaired liver function, it must be done under strict observation.

Fluid and Electrolyte Balance: Fluid retention and edema have been observed in patients treated with floctafenine. Therefore, as with many other non-steroidal anti-inflammatory drugs, the possibility of precipitating congestive heart failure in elderly patients or those with compromised cardiac function should be borne in mind. APO-FLOCTAFENINE should be used with caution in patients with heart failure, hypertension or other conditions predisposing to fluid retention.

With non-steroidal anti-inflammatory treatment, there is a potential risk of hyperkalemia, particularly in patients with conditions such as diabetes mellitus or renal failure; elderly patients; or in patients receiving concomitant therapy with β-adrenergic blockers, angiotensin converting enzyme inhibitors or some diuretics.

Hematology: Drugs inhibiting prostaglandin biosynthesis do interfere with platelet function to varying degrees; therefore, patients who may be adversely affected by such an action should be carefully observed when APO-FLOCTAFENINE is administered.

Blood dyscrasias (such as neutropenia, leukopenia, thrombocytopenia, aplastic anemia and agranulocytosis) associated with the use of non-steroidal anti-inflammatory drugs are rare, but could occur with severe consequences.

Infection: In common with other anti-inflammatory drugs, APO-FLOCTAFENINE may mask the usual signs of infection.

Ophthalmology: Blurred and/or diminished vision has been reported with the use of floctafenine and other non-steroidal anti-inflammatory drugs. If such symptoms develop, this drug should be discontinued and an ophthalmologic examination performed.

Central Nervous System: Some patients may experience drowsiness, dizziness, vertigo, insomnia or depression with the use of floctafenine. If patients experience these side effects, they should exercise caution in carrying out activities that require alertness.

Hypersensitivity Reactions: Floctafenine should not be used in patients with the complete or partial syndrome of nasal polyps, or in whom asthma, anaphylaxis, urticaria, rhinitis or other allergic manifestations are precipitated by ASA or other non-steroidal anti-inflammatory agents. Fatal anaphylactoid reactions have occurred in such individuals. As well, individuals with the above medical problems are at risk of a severe reaction even if they have taken NSAIDs in the past without any adverse effects. On occasion, it has been observed that intermittent use may have resulted in increased sensitivity.

Cardiovascular Function: Since severe cases of hypersensitivity reactions have been reported with floctafenine, its use in severe cardiac insufficiency and ischemic cardiomyopathy is contraindicated.

Geriatrics: As with other non-steroidal anti-inflammatory drugs, APO-FLOCTAFENINE should be used with caution in the elderly and consideration given to administration of a lower starting dose. (See Warnings.)

Drug Interactions: Acetylsalicylic Acid (ASA) or Other NSAIDs: The use of floctafenine in addition to any other NSAID, including those over the counter ones (such as ASA and ibuprofen) is not recommended due to the possibility of additive side effects.

Concomitant administration of acetylsalicylic acid results in decreased peak serum concentration of non-steroidal anti-inflammatory drugs and slight increases in both clearance and apparent half-life. The clinical significance of these changes is unknown.

Beta-Blocking Drugs: Associated treatment with beta-blocking drugs is contraindicated; in the event of an anaphylactic-type reaction, such treatment may lead to or aggravate hypotension or shock. These compounds decrease cardiovascular compensatory mechanisms.

Anticoagulants: Numerous studies have shown that the concomitant use of NSAIDs and anticoagulants increases the risk of GI adverse events such as ulceration and bleeding.

Because prostaglandins play an important role in hemostasis, and NSAIDs affect platelet function, concurrent therapy of floctafenine with warfarin requires close monitoring to be certain that no change in anticoagulant dosage is necessary.

Oral Hypoglycemics: NSAIDs are known to be extensively bound to serum albumin. This may lead to interaction with hypoglycemic agents; therefore, caution should be observed when these drugs are used concomitantly.

Diuretics: Floctafenine may cause water retention and therefore could interfere with diuretics in the treatment of hypertension.

Vitamin K Antagonists: Changes in prothrombin time have been noted in patients undergoing long-term treatment with vitamin K antagonists and floctafenine. The prothrombin time or INR should be monitored during long-term treatment with floctafenine.

Glucocorticoids: Numerous studies have shown that the concomitant use of NSAIDs and oral glucocorticoids increases the risk of GI side effects such as ulceration and bleeding. This is especially the case in older (>65 years of age) individuals.

Antacids: No pharmacokinetic interaction has been noted with concomitant administration of antacids.

Methotrexate: See Other Drug Interactions below.

Lithium: See Other Drug Interactions below.

Other Drug Interactions: Non-steroidal anti-inflammatory drugs are known to be extensively bound to serum albumin. This may lead to interaction with anticoagulants, sulfonylureas, hypoglycemic agents, sulfonamides, phenytoin, lithium and certain chemotherapeutic agents such as methotrexate. Therefore, caution should be observed regarding possible interaction between floctafenine and any of these drugs should they be used concurrently.

In patients receiving concomitant steroid therapy, any reduction in steroid dosage should be gradual to avoid the possible complications of sudden steroid withdrawal.

Clinical Laboratory Tests: The administration of floctafenine is not known to interfere with laboratory and diagnostic tests.

ADVERSE EFFECTS: The most common adverse reactions encountered with non-steroidal anti-inflammatory drugs are gastrointestinal, of which peptic ulcer, with or without bleeding, is the most severe. Fatalities have occurred, particularly in the elderly.

The most commonly occurring side effects reported during floctafenine therapy were:

Gastrointestinal System: nausea, diarrhea, vomiting, abdominal pain or discomfort, heartburn, constipation, abnormal liver function, gastrointestinal bleeding.

Allergic-Type Reactions: maculopapular skin rash, pruritus, urticaria, redness and itching of the face and neck. Cases of anaphylactic shock and angioedema have been reported in clinical use (see Warnings). Sensation of burning of the face and extremities, asthmatic type dyspnea, sensation of malaise.

Central Nervous System: drowsiness, dizziness, headache, insomnia, nervousness, irritability.

Urogenital System: dysuria, burning micturition, polyuria, strong smelling urine, urethritis and cystitis. Reversible acute renal insufficiency with or without oliguria/anuria.

Other less frequently occurring side effects were: tinnitus, blurred vision, dry mouth, thirst, bitter taste, anorexia, stomach cramps, flatulence, hot flushes and sweating, tachycardia, weakness and tiredness. Very rarely: thrombocytopenia.

OVERDOSE:

A few cases of overdose have been reported with floctafenine. No common symptoms resulting from overdosing could be distinguished among these patients. In all cases the outcome was favourable and the patients recovered well. Standard procedures to evacuate gastric contents, maintain urinary output and provide general supportive care should be employed in cases of overdose.

For management of a suspected drug overdose, CPhA recommends that you contact your **regional Poison Control Centre**. See the *CPS* Directory section for a list of Poison Control Centres.

DOSAGE: Adults: The usual adult dose of APO-FLOCTAFENINE (floctafenine) is 200 to 400 mg every 6 to 8 hours as required. The maximum recommended daily dose is 1200 mg. APO-FLOCTAFENINE is recommended for short-term management of acute pain.

The tablets should be taken after a meal or food with a glass of water.

Elderly and Debilitated: Elderly and debilitated individuals are most susceptible to adverse events from non-steroidal anti-inflammatory drugs, the incidence of which increases with dose and duration of treatment. For such patients, consideration should be given to a starting dose lower than usual, with individual adjustment when necessary and under close supervision.

Children: APO-FLOCTAFENINE is not recommended for use in children.

Other Special Precautions: Adults with renal insufficiency—serum levels are slightly elevated and the dose may therefore be reduced.

INFORMATION FOR THE PATIENT: Published in e-CPS, available by subscription at www.e-cps.ca.

SUPPLIED: 200 mg: Each creamy white, round, biconvex tablet, engraved "APO" on one side and "FLO" over "200" on the other, contains: floctafenine 200 mg. Nonmedicinal ingredients: colloidal silicon dioxide, croscarmellose sodium, magnesium stearate, microcrystalline cellulose and stearic acid. Bottles of 100.

400 mg: Each creamy white, round, biconvex tablet, engraved "APO" on one side and "FLO" over "400" on the other, contains: floctafenine 400 mg. Nonmedicinal ingredients: colloidal silicon dioxide, croscarmellose sodium, magnesium stearate, microcrystalline cellulose and stearic acid. Bottles of 100.

Store at room temperature (15 to 30°C). Protect from light.

Apo-Granisetron Ⓟ

granisetron HCl

Antiemetic—5-HT3 Receptor Antagonist

Apotex

Date of Preparation: April 11, 2008

SUMMARY PRODUCT INFORMATION:

Route of Administration	Dosage Form/ Strength	Clinically Relevant Nonmedicinal Ingredients
Oral	Tablet/1 mg	Lactose monohydrate For a complete listing see Dosage Forms, Composition and Packaging.

INDICATIONS AND CLINICAL USE: Indications: APO-GRANISETRON (granisetron hydrochloride) is indicated for:

Adults:

- The prevention of nausea and vomiting associated with emetogenic cancer chemotherapy, including high dose cisplatin.
- The prevention of nausea and vomiting associated with radiation, including total body irradiation and fractionated abdominal radiation.

Geriatrics (>65 years of age): Chemotherapy-induced and Radiation-induced Nausea and Vomiting: Safety and efficacy of granisetron appear to be similar to that observed in younger adults (see Warnings and Precautions and Dosage and Administration).

Pediatrics: Safety and efficacy of APO-GRANISETRON has not been adequately studied in children or adolescents under 18 years of age and it is not indicated for use in this population (see Warnings and Precautions and Dosage and Administration).

CONTRAINDICATIONS: APO-GRANISETRON (granisetron hydrochloride) is contraindicated in patients with a known hypersensitivity to the drug or to any component of its formulations.

WARNINGS AND PRECAUTIONS: Carcinogenesis and Mutagenesis: Granisetron hydrochloride has been associated with an increased occurrence of hepatocellular tumours in carcinogenicity studies performed in rodents at doses in excess of the recommended human dose. Although the clinical significance of these findings has not been determined, the use of this drug should be restricted to the treatment of nausea and vomiting in patients undergoing emetogenic cancer chemotherapy. The recommended dosage of granisetron hydrochloride should not be exceeded.

Granisetron was administered to rats in the diet in a 24 month carcinogenicity study. The incidence of hepatocellular carcinomas and adenomas was significantly increased in male rats treated at doses of 5 mg/kg/day and in rats of both sexes treated with 25 mg/kg/day. No increase in the rate of occurrence of liver tumours was observed in the 1 mg/kg/day treatment group (100 times the recommended human dose given intravenously).

In another 24 month carcinogenicity study, mice were administered granisetron in the diet at doses of 1, 5, and 50 mg/kg/day. There was a statistically significant increase in the incidence of hepatocellular carcinomas in males and hepatocellular adenomas in females dosed with 50 mg/kg/day. No statistically significant increase in liver tumours was observed in mice at a dose of 5 mg/kg/day (500 times the recommended human dose given intravenously).

Gastrointestinal: Granisetron hydrochloride is not a drug that stimulates gastric or intestinal peristalsis. It should not be used instead of nasogastric suction. The use of granisetron hydrochloride in patients with chemotherapy-induced nausea and vomiting may mask a progressive ileus and/or gastric distention. Patients with signs of sub-acute intestinal obstruction should be monitored following administration of granisetron hydrochloride.

Sensitivity/Resistance: Hypersensitivity reactions may occur in patients who have exhibited hypersensitivity to other selective 5-HT3 receptor antagonists.

Special Populations: Pregnant Women: The use of granisetron hydrochloride in pregnant women has not been studied and is not recommended. Reproduction studies performed in pregnant rats given granisetron at intravenous dosages up to 9 mg/kg/day and pregnant rabbits at intravenous dosage up to 3 mg/kg/day revealed no evidence of impaired fertility or harm to the fetus due to granisetron.

Nursing Women: It is not known whether granisetron is excreted in human milk. Nursing is not recommended during treatment with granisetron hydrochloride.

Pediatrics: The safety and efficacy of granisetron hydrochloride has not been adequately studied in children or adolescents under 18 years of age (see Indications and Clinical Use and Dosage and Administration).

Geriatrics (>65 years of age): During clinical trials of 325 patients 65 years of age or older who received oral granisetron hydrochloride, 298 were 65 to 74 years of age and 27 were 75 years of age or older. The efficacy and safety of granisetron hydrochloride did not appear to be age dependent (see Indications and Clinical Use and Dosage and Administration).

Information to Be Provided to the Patient: Effect on Ability to Drive and Use Machinery: There are no data on the effect of granisetron hydrochloride on the ability to drive. As there have been occasional reports of somnolence in clinical studies, patients should be advised to avoid driving a car or operating hazardous machinery until they are reasonably certain that the drug treatment does not affect them adversely.

ADVERSE REACTIONS: Because clinical trials are conducted under very specific conditions the adverse reaction rates observed in the clinical trials may not reflect the rates observed in practice and should not be compared to the rates in the clinical trials of another drug. Adverse drug reaction information from clinical trials is useful for identifying drug-related adverse events and for approximating rates.

Adverse Drug Reaction Overview: The most common adverse events reported by patients receiving oral granisetron hydrochloride in single-day chemotherapy trials are: headache, asthenia, somnolence, diarrhea, constipation, and abdominal pain (see Table 1 for the percentages of patients with these events). The only two common adverse experiences recognized to be causally related to granisetron hydrochloride are constipation and headache.

Clinical Trial Adverse Drug Reactions: Chemotherapy-induced Nausea and Vomiting: Oral granisetron hydrochloride was given either as a single dose or divided dose for 1, 7, or 14 days. Patients received cancer chemotherapy which consisted primarily of cisplatin or cyclophosphamide regimens. Adverse events were recorded over seven days when granisetron hydrochloride was given on a single day and up to 28 days when granisetron hydrochloride was administered for 7 or 14 days. In the absence of a placebo group, the relationship of observed adverse events to treatment with granisetron hydrochloride is difficult to judge.

Table 1 gives the frequencies of the six adverse events most commonly reported by patients receiving oral granisetron hydrochloride in single-day chemotherapy trials. This table does not include those events that are commonly associated with chemotherapy or the underlying malignant disease.

The only two common adverse experiences recognized to be causally related to granisetron hydrochloride are constipation and headache. As with other drugs of this class, rare cases of hypersensitivity reactions, sometimes severe (e.g. anaphylaxis, shortness of breath, hypotension, urticaria) have been reported.

Radiation-induced Nausea and Vomiting: In controlled clinical trials, the adverse events reported by patients receiving granisetron hydrochloride tablets and concurrent radiation were similar to those reported by patients receiving granisetron hydrochloride tablets prior to chemotherapy. The most frequently reported adverse events were diarrhea (25.6%), asthenia (22.0%) and constipation (15.5%). Headache (7.7%), however, was less prevalent in this patient population. Table 2 lists the adverse experiences (>5%) in patients who received granisetron hydrochloride tablets or placebo.

Table 1: APO-GRANISETRON

Principal Adverse Events in Clinical Trials of Single-Day Chemotherapy

	Percentage of Patients with Event Oral Granisetron Hydrochloride (1.0 mg b.i.d. or 2.0 mg u.i.d.), (n=1322)
Headache	22%
Asthenia	15%
Somnolence	2%
Diarrhea	8%
Constipation	17%
Abdominal Pain	6%

Table 2: APO-GRANISETRON

Principal Adverse Events in Clinical Trials—RINV

	Percentage of Patients with Event Oral Granisetron Hydrochloride (1.0 mg b.i.d.), (n=134)	Percentage of Patients with Event Placebo (n=128)
Diarrhea	28%	34%
Asthenia	25%	20%
Constipation	19%	5%
Abdominal Pain	11%	9%
Nausea (after 20 radiation fractions)	11%	9%
Decreased appetite	10%	7%
Pain	8%	4%
Headache	5%	11%

Less Common Clinical Trial Adverse Drug Reactions (≤1%): Chemotherapy-induced Nausea and Vomiting: The safety profile of granisetron hydrochloride has been evaluated in 3269 patients receiving intravenous granisetron hydrochloride (2 to 160 μg/kg) and 2600 patients receiving oral granisetron hydrochloride (0.25-20 mg) in single day and multiple-day clinical trials with emetogenic cancer therapies. In the listings which follow, a COSTART-based dictionary terminology has been used to classify reported adverse experiences. The frequencies presented, therefore, represent the proportion of the patients who experienced an event of the type cited on at least one occasion while receiving granisetron hydrochloride.

Experiences are further classified within body system categories and enumerated in order of decreasing frequency using the following definitions: frequent adverse experiences are defined as: those occurring on one or more occasion in at least 1/100 patients; infrequent adverse experiences as: those occurring in less than 1/100 but at least 1/1000 patients; rare experiences as: those occurring in less than 1/1000 patients.

Many adverse experiences are observed in cancer chemotherapy patients. All adverse experiences are included except those for which the drug cause was remote, those reported in terms so general as to be uninformative and those already listed in Table 1.

Body as a Whole: Frequent: abdominal pain. Infrequent: abdomen enlarged, chills, fever, malaise. Rare: allergic reaction, chest pain.

Cardiovascular System: Infrequent: hypertension, hypotension, migraine, syncope, vasodilatation. Rare: arrhythmia, bradycardia, palpitation, postural hypotension, tachycardia, ventricular arrhythmia, angina pectoris, and atrial fibrillation.

Gastrointestinal System: Frequent: decreased appetite. Infrequent: dry mouth, dyspepsia, flatulence, jaundice, liver function tests abnormal [elevation of AST and ALT (>2 times the upper limit of normal)], nausea. Rare: gastrointestinal haemorrhage, hepatic coma, ileus, liver damage, melena, vomiting.

Hemic and Lymphatic System: Rare: coagulation time increased, eosinophilia, leukopenia, anemia, thrombocytopenia.

Metabolic and Nutritional: Infrequent: hypokalemia. Rare: bilirubinemia, edema, hyperphosphatemia, hyponatremia.

Nervous System: Infrequent: agitation, anxiety, dizziness, drugged feeling, insomnia, nervousness, paresthesia, tremor. Rare: coma, depersonalisation, grand mal convulsion, vertigo.

Respiratory System: Infrequent: dyspnea, hiccup. Rare: epistaxis, rhinitis, sinusitis.

Skin and Appendages: Infrequent: pruritus, rash, sweating. Rare: photosensitivity.

Special Searches: Rare: puncture site pain.

Special Senses: Infrequent: taste perversion. Rare: abnormal vision.

Urogenital System: Infrequent: dysuria. Rare: urinary incontinence.

DRUG INTERACTIONS: Overview: Granisetron does not induce or inhibit the cytochrome P450 drug metabolizing enzyme system.

DOSAGE AND ADMINISTRATION:

Recommended Dose, Dosage Adjustment and Administration: Emetogenic Chemotherapy: Adults: The recommended dosage of oral granisetron hydrochloride is 2 mg on the day of chemotherapy. This may be administered either as a single dose (2×1 mg) one hour before chemotherapy or as a divided dose of 1 mg one hour before chemotherapy followed by a second 1 mg dose 12 hours post-chemotherapy. The need for additional doses beyond 24 hours post-chemotherapy has not been investigated.

Geriatrics: Available clinical data suggest that dosage reductions may not be necessary in this patient population (see Indications and Clinical Use and Warnings and Precautions).

Pediatrics: See Indications and Clinical Use and Warnings and Precautions.

Renally Impaired Patients: Available clinical data suggest that dosage reductions may not be necessary in this patient population.

Hepatically Impaired Patients: The clearance of granisetron hydrochloride is reduced by half in patients with hepatic impairment. The dose response of granisetron hydrochloride in patients with hepatic impairment has not been determined.

Radiation (either Total Irradiation or Fractionated Abdominal Radiation): Adults: The recommended adult dosage of oral granisetron hydrochloride is 2 mg once daily. 2×1 mg tablets are taken one hour before radiation.

Geriatrics: Available clinical data suggest that dosage reductions may not be necessary in this patient population (see Indications and Clinical Use and Warnings and Precautions).

Pediatrics: See Indications and Clinical Use and Warnings and Precautions.

OVERDOSAGE:

There is no specific antidote for granisetron hydrochloride overdosage. In the case of overdosage, symptomatic treatment should be given. Overdose has been reported with both the intravenous and oral formulations. Overdosage of up to 38.5 mg of granisetron hydrochloride injection has been reported without symptoms or with the occurrence of a slight headache.

For management of a suspected drug overdose, contact your regional Poison Control Centre. See the *CPS Directory* section for a list of Poison Control Centres.

ACTION AND CLINICAL PHARMACOLOGY: Mechanism of Action: Granisetron hydrochloride is a selective antagonist of 5-hydroxytryptamine (5-HT3) receptors. Following exposure to emetogenic cancer chemotherapy, mucosal enterochromaffin cells release serotonin which stimulates 5-HT3 receptors located peripherally on vagal nerve terminals and centrally in the nucleus tractus solitarus. The antiemetic effect of granisetron appears to involve antagonism of the serotonin-induced stimulation of vagal afferent activity.

Radioligand binding studies have demonstrated that granisetron hydrochloride has negligible affinity for other 5-HT receptors or for dopamine D2 receptor binding sites.

Pharmacodynamics: In healthy subjects, granisetron hydrochloride produced no consistent or clinically significant changes in pulse rate, blood pressure or ECG. Following single and multiple oral doses, granisetron hydrochloride slowed colonic transit in normal volunteers.

Pharmacokinetics: Chemotherapy-Induced Nausea and Vomiting: Injection: In adult cancer patients undergoing chemotherapy and in healthy volunteers, infusion of a single 40 μg/kg dose of granisetron hydrochloride produced the following pharmacokinetic data: See Table 3.

Table 3: APO-GRANISETRON

Pharmacokinetic Parameters in Adult Cancer Patients Undergoing Chemotherapy and in Volunteers, Following a Single Intravenous 40 μg/kg Dose of Granisetron Hydrochloride.

	Peak Plasma Concentration (ng·mL)	Terminal Plasma Half-Life (h)	AUC (ng·h/mL)	Total Clearance (L/h)
Cancer Patients (n=14)				
Mean	63.8[a]	8.95[a]	167[a]	25.8[a]
Range	18.0 to 176	0.90 to 31.1	26.0 to 294	8.92 to 95.2
Young Adult Volunteers 21 to 42 years (n=20)				
Mean	64.3[b]	4.91[b]	89.7[b]	51.8[b]
Range	11.2 to 182	0.88 to 15.2	15.6 to 201	11.3 to 176
Elderly Volunteers 65 to 81 years (n=20)				
Mean	57.0[b]	7.69[b]	115[b]	27.1[b]
Range	14.6 to 153	2.65 to 17.7	37.7 to 240	10.9 to 58.4

[a] Infusion over 5 minutes.
[b] Infusion over 3 minutes.

Oral: In healthy volunteers and adult cancer patients undergoing chemotherapy, administration of oral granisetron hydrochloride produced the following mean pharmacokinetic data (Table 4):

Table 4: APO-GRANISETRON

Pharmacokinetic Parameters (Mean [range]) In Adult Cancer Patients Undergoing Chemotherapy and in Volunteers Following Oral Granisetron Hydrochloride

	Peak Plasma Concentation (ng·mL)	Terminal Plasma Half-Life (h)	Area under Curve (ng· h/mL)	Total Clearance (L/h)
Cancer Patients				
1.0 mg, b.i.d., 7 days (n=24)	8.19 [1.97 to 18.4]	N.D.[a]	54.2 [10.2 to 126]	34.1 [7.94 to 98.0]
Volunteers single dose (n=25)				
1.0 mg	4.10 [0.58 to 7.37]	8.74 [2.40 to 19.9]	43.7 [2.85 to 142]	53.3 [7.04 to 351]
2.5 mg	9.44 [1.68 to 19.5]	7.24 [2.54 to 17.0]	105 [7.75 to 319]	67.2 [7.84 to 323]

[a] Not determined after oral administration.

Distribution: Granisetron hydrochloride is extensively distributed between plasma and red blood cells with a mean volume of distribution of approximately 3 L/kg. Plasma protein binding is approximately 65%.

Metabolism: The clearance of granisetron occurs predominantly through hepatic metabolism. Biotransformation pathways involve N-demethylation and aromatic ring oxidation followed by conjugation.

Excretion: In normal volunteers, the urinary excretion of unchanged granisetron hydrochloride averages 12% of the administered dose over a period of 48 hours, while the remainder of the dose is excreted as metabolites, 47% in the urine and 34% in the feces. The metabolism of granisetron involves N-demethylation and aromatic ring oxidation followed by conjugation.

Special Populations and Conditions: Pediatrics: The safety and efficacy of granisetron hydrochloride has not been adequately studied in children or adolescents under 18 years of age.

Geriatrics: In geriatric (mean age 71 yrs) subjects after single intravenous doses of 40 μg/kg, pharmacokinetic parameters were within the range found for young subjects (mean age 29 yrs). Although the elimination half-life was prolonged and the total plasma clearance reduced in the geriatric relative to the young subject group, no significant differences were determined between the two groups with regard to maximum plasma concentration or area under the plasma concentration time curve values (see Table 3).

Gender/Race: There were too few male and Black patients to adequately assess differences in effect in either population.

Hepatic Insufficiency: A pharmacokinetic study in patients with hepatic impairment due to neoplastic liver involvement showed that total clearance was approximately halved and mean area under the plasma concentration time curve (AUC) values were approximately doubled compared to patients without hepatic impairment.

Renal Insufficiency: Renal Insufficiency: Although renal clearance was decreased in subjects with severe renal impairment (N=11) relative to normal volunteers (N=12), total plasma clearance was numerically higher in this renally impaired group (43 L/h) than in the normal volunteers (32 L/h). Mean area under the plasma concentration time curve values were similar for the two subject groups.

Cancer Patients: Following intravenous administration, mean terminal elimination half-life values are approximately twice as long in cancer patients as they are in healthy adult volunteers, while clearance values are decreased by approximately 50% (see Table 3). Available data do not allow a formal comparison of elimination half-life or clearance between volunteers and cancer patients receiving oral granisetron hydrochloride.

STORAGE AND STABILITY: Store tablets at room temperature 15-30°C.

INFORMATION FOR THE PATIENT: Published in e-CPS, available by subscription at www.e-cps.ca.

DOSAGE FORMS, COMPOSITION AND PACKAGING: Each white to off-white, triangular biconvex film-coated tablet, engraved "APO" on one side, "GR" over "1" on the other side, contains: granisetron 1 mg as granisetron hydrochloride. Nonmedicinal ingredients: colloidal silicon dioxide, hydroxypropyl cellulose, hydroxypropyl methylcellulose, lactose monohydrate, magnesium stearate, microcrystalline cellulose, polyethylene glycol, sodium starch glycolate and titanium dioxide. Unit dose blister packs of 10.

Apo®-Hydralazine ℞

hydralazine HCl

Antihypertensive

Apotex

Date of Preparation: August 28, 1990
Date of Revision: July 6, 1998

PHARMACOLOGY: Although the precise mechanism of action of hydralazine hydrochloride is not fully understood, the major effects are on the cardiovascular system. Hydralazine apparently lowers blood pressure by exerting a peripheral vasodilating effect through a direct relaxation of vascular smooth muscle. Hydralazine, by altering cellular calcium metabolism, interferes with the calcium movements within the vascular smooth muscle that are responsible for initiating or maintaining the contractile state.

The peripheral vasodilating effect of hydralazine results in decreased arterial blood pressure (diastolic more than systolic); decreased peripheral vascular resistance; and an increased heart rate, stroke volume, and cardiac output. The vasodilating effect is much greater on arterioles than on veins, and vascular resistance decreases more in the coronary, cerebral, splanchnic and renal circulations than in skin and muscle.

Hydralazine usually increases renin activity in plasma, presumably as a result of increased secretion of renin by the renal juxtaglomerular cells in response to reflex sympathetic discharge. This increase in renin activity leads to the production of angiotensin II, which then causes stimulation of aldosterone and consequent sodium reabsorption and fluid retention.

Sodium retention and excessive sympathetic stimulation of the heart caused by hydralazine may be precluded by co-administration of a thiazide diuretic and a beta-blocker. Beta-adrenergic blocking drugs and hydralazine are complementary in their pharmacologic effects, a beta-adrenergic blocking agent minimizes hydralazine-induced increases in cardiac rate and output, and hydralazine prevents the reflex increase in peripheral resistance induced by beta-blockers.

Pharmacokinetics: Hydralazine is rapidly and fairly completely absorbed after oral administration. In the plasma only small amounts of the free drug can be traced, the bulk circulating in conjugated form, i.e. pyruvic acid hydrazone. Peak serum concentrations are reached within one to two hours after a dose. Plasma levels of hydralazine vary widely among individuals. Orally administered hydralazine undergoes extensive, saturable first-pass metabolism (systemic availability: 26-55%), this first-pass effect being dependent on the individual's acetylator status. In response to the same oral dose, slow-acetylators show higher "apparent" plasma hydralazine levels than rapid acetylators and require lower doses to maintain control of blood pressure.

After intravenous administration of hydralazine no first-pass effect occurs; acetylator status therefore has no influence on the plasma levels.

Hydralazine is widely distributed in the body. The apparent volume of distribution of hydralazine is approximately 50% body weight. Binding to plasma proteins (chiefly albumin) is 85-90%.

Hydralazine crosses the placental barrier and is excreted in the breast milk.

The pattern of the metabolites depends on the subject's acetylator and presumably hydroxylator status. The main metabolite, NAc-HPZ (N-acetyl-hydrazine-phthalazinone), was found to be the relevant indicator for the drug-related phenotype.

The plasma half-life generally ranges between 1.7 and 3.0 hours in most subjects, but in rapid acetylators it is shorter, averaging 45 minutes.

Hydralazine and its metabolites are rapidly excreted by the kidney and 80% of the oral dose appears in the urine within 48 hours. The bulk of the hydralazine excreted is in the form of acetylated and hydroxylated metabolites, some of which are conjugated with glucuronic acid; 2-14% is excreted as "apparent" hydralazine.

Comparative Bioavailability: A comparative bioavailability study was performed using normal human volunteers. The rate and extent of absorption after a 50 mg single dose of APO-HYDRALAZINE (5×10 mg tablets) and Apresoline (5×10 mg tablets) were measured and compared. Plasma levels of free and total hydralazine were measured. The results can be summarized as follows: see Table 1.

Table 1: APO-HYDRALAZINE
Rate and Extent of Absorption After a 50 mg Single Dose of APO-HYDRALAZINE (5×10 mg tablets) and Apresoline (5×10 mg tablets)

Parameter	APO-HYDRALAZINE	Apresoline
Free Hydralazine		
AUC_{0-24} (ng·hr/mL)	42.45±29.57	42.30±27.15
C_{max} (ng/mL)	40.58±37.51	39.51±36.34
T_{max} (hr)	0.47±0.23	0.63±0.36
$t_{1/2}$ (hr)	2.23±1.08	2.10±1.03
Total Hydralazine		
AUC_{0-24} (ng·hr/mL)	1915.33±783.56	1841.29±782.41
C_{max} (ng/mL)	775.81±260.06	754.67±247.49
T_{max} (hr)	0.52±0.23	0.68±0.38
$t_{1/2}$ (hr)	3.11±0.73	3.02±0.61

The rate and extent of absorption after a 50 mg single dose of APO-HYDRALAZINE (1×50 mg tablet) and Apresoline (1×50 mg tablet) were measured and compared in two studies. The first study on 23 healthy male volunteers measured free and total hydralazine. The second study on 24 healthy male volunteers measured free hydralazine and was combined with the first study. The results can be summarized in arithmetic means and standard deviation as follows: see Table 2.

Table 2: APO-HYDRALAZINE
Rate and Extent of Absorption After a 50 mg Single Dose of APO-HYDRALAZINE (1×50 mg tablet) and Apresoline (1×50 mg tablet)

Parameter	APO-HYDRALAZINE	Apresoline
Free Hydralazine		
AUC_{0-24} (ng·hr/mL)	40.38±20.90	37.09±20.82
C_{max} (ng/mL)	44.38±32.44	40.60±28.90
T_{max} (hr)	0.59±0.34	0.73±0.24
$t_{1/2}$ (hr)	2.41±1.56	2.45±1.39
Total Hydralazine		
AUC_{0-24} (ng·hr/mL)	1915.11±644.81	1928.48±801.80
C_{max} (ng/mL)	730.96±178.39	727.78±224.22
T_{max} (hr)	0.62±0.21	0.80±0.24
$t_{1/2}$ (hr)	3.05±0.56	2.92±0.57

(cont'd)

Table 2: APO-HYDRALAZINE (cont'd)

INDICATIONS: APO-HYDRALAZINE (hydralazine hydrochloride) is indicated in the treatment of essential hypertension. It is used in conjunction with other antihypertensives such as beta-blockers and diuretics.

CONTRAINDICATIONS: Hypersensitivity to hydralazine or other hydrazinophthalazine derivatives.

Idiopathic systemic lupus erythematosus (SLE) and related diseases.

Severe tachycardia and heart failure with a high cardiac output (e.g. in thyrotoxicosis).

Myocardial insufficiency due to mechanical obstruction (e.g. in the presence of aortic or mitral stenosis or constrictive pericarditis).

Isolated right-ventricular heart failure due to pulmonary hypertension (cor pulmonale).

Acute dissecting aneurysm of the aorta.

Coronary artery disease.

WARNINGS: Hydralazine may provoke in a few patients a clinical picture simulating systemic lupus erythematosus (SLE) including glomerulonephritis. In its mild form this syndrome is reminiscent of rheumatoid arthritis (arthralgia, sometimes associated with fever and skin rash). When fully developed a syndrome resembling disseminated lupus erythematosus occurs.

Should this SLE-like syndrome develop, treatment should be discontinued immediately. Symptoms and signs usually regress when the drug is discontinued but residua have been detected many years later. Long-term treatment with adrenocorticosteroids may be necessary.

The frequency of these untoward effects increases with dosage and duration of exposure to the drug and is higher in slow than in fast acetylators. When treated with the same dosage, slow acetylators have higher serum concentrations than fast acetylators. The lowest effective dosage should therefore be used for maintenance therapy. If 100 mg daily fails to elicit an adequate clinical effect, the patient's acetylator status should be evaluated.

Slow acetylators and women run a greater risk of developing this SLE-like syndrome. In such cases dosage should be kept below 100 mg daily and the patients carefully monitored for clinical signs and symptoms suggestive of this syndrome.

Complete blood counts, examination of lupus erythematosus cell preparations, antinuclear antibody titer determinations and urine analysis are indicated before and periodically (e.g. every 6 months) during prolonged therapy with hydralazine even though the patient is asymptomatic. These tests are also indicated if the patient develops arthralgia, fever, chest pain, continued malaise or other unexplained signs or symptoms. If the results of these tests are abnormal, treatment should be discontinued.

Antinuclear antibody may be found in the blood of as many as 50 percent of patients receiving hydralazine who remain asymptomatic. A positive antinuclear antibody titer requires that the physician carefully weigh the implications of the test results against the benefits to be derived from antihypertensive therapy with hydralazine.

Microhematuria and/or proteinuria, in particular together with positive titres of antinuclear antibodies, may be initial signs of immune-complex glomerulonephritis associated with the SLE-like syndrome.

The chronotropic and inotropic effects of hydralazine increase myocardial oxygen requirements. It can cause electrocardiographic changes of myocardial ischemia, and in patients with coronary artery disease may precipitate angina pectoris or congestive heart failure. Hydralazine has been implicated in the production of myocardial infarction. APO-HYDRALAZINE must therefore be used with caution in patients with suspected coronary artery disease. It should be given only in combination with a beta-blocker or other suitable sympatholytic agents. The beta-blocker medication should be commenced a few days before the start of treatment with APO-HYDRALAZINE.

Patients who have survived a myocardial infarction should not receive APO-HYDRALAZINE until post-infarction stabilization has been achieved.

The "hyperdynamic" circulation caused by hydralazine may accentuate specific cardiovascular inadequacies (e.g. hydralazine may increase pulmonary artery pressure in patients with mitral valvular disease).

Pregnancy: Animal studies indicate that high doses of hydralazine are teratogenic in mice, possibly in rabbits, but not in rats). Teratogenic effects observed were cleft palate and malformation of facial and cranial bones. There are no adequate and well-controlled studies in pregnant women. Although clinical experience does not include any positive evidence of adverse effects on the human fetus, hydralazine should be used during pregnancy only if the benefit clearly justifies the potential risk to the fetus.

PRECAUTIONS: Postural hypotension may result from hydralazine, but is less common than with ganglionic blocking agents. The drug should be used with caution in patients with cerebral vascular disease since abrupt decreases in blood pressure should be avoided in these patients.

A pronounced lowering of the blood pressure may adversely affect the patient's reactions (e.g. as in driving or operating machinery).

In hypertensive patients with normal kidneys who are treated with hydralazine, there is evidence of increased renal blood flow and a maintenance of glomerular filtration rate. In some instances improved renal function has been noted where control values were below normal prior to hydralazine administration. However, as with any antihypertensive agent, APO-HYDRALAZINE should be used with caution in patients with advanced renal damage.

In patients with renal impairment, serum levels of hydralazine increased as compared to those in patients with normal renal function, therefore the dose or the dosing interval has to be adapted according to the clinical response, in order to avoid accumulation of the "apparent" active substance.

In patients with hepatic dysfunction, serum levels of hydralazine increased as compared to those in patients with normal hepatic function, therefore the dose or the dosing interval has to be adapted according to the clinical response, in order to avoid accumulation of the "apparent" active substance.

Peripheral neuritis, evidenced by paresthesias, numbness and tingling in the extremities has been observed. Published evidence suggests an antipyridoxine effect and the addition of pyridoxine to the regimen if symptoms develop.

Blood dyscrasias consisting of reduction in hemoglobin and red cell count, leukopenia, agranulocytosis and purpura have been reported. Periodic blood counts are advised during therapy. If such abnormalities develop, therapy should be discontinued.

Tumorigenicity and Mutagenicity: Hydralazine hydrochloride in chronic toxicity studies has been shown to increase the incidence of some tumors in aging rodents. A mutagenic potential was observed in some but not all mutagenicity tests. The extent to which these findings indicate a risk to man is uncertain. While long-term clinical observations have not suggested that human cancer is associated with hydralazine use, epidemiologic studies have so far been insufficient to arrive at any conclusion.

Lactation: Hydralazine passes into breast milk. Alternatives to hydralazine should be considered in nursing mothers.

Geriatrics: The elderly may be more sensitive to the hypotensive effects. In addition the risk of hydralazine-induced hypothermia may be increased in elderly patients.

Children: Although there is some experience with the use of hydralazine hydrochloride in children, controlled clinical trials to establish safety and effectiveness in this age group have not been conducted.

Drug Interactions: Concomitant treatment with other vasodilators, calcium antagonists, ACE inhibitors, diuretics, antihypertensives, tricyclic antidepressants and major tranquilizers, as well as the consumption of alcohol, may potentiate the hypotensive effect of hydralazine.

Administration of hydralazine shortly before or after diazoxide may lead to marked hypotension. When potent antihypertensive drugs, such as diazoxide, are used in combination with APO-HYDRALAZINE, patients should be continuously observed for several hours for any excessive fall in blood pressure.

Concurrent administration of hydralazine with beta-blockers subject to a strong first-pass effect (e.g. propranolol) may increase their bioavailability. Downward dosage adjustment of these drugs may be required when they are given concomitantly.

Monoamine oxidase (MAO) inhibitors should be used with caution in patients receiving hydralazine. Hydralazine may reduce the pressor responses to epinephrine.

ADVERSE EFFECTS: The most common adverse reactions are tachycardia, palpitation, anginal symptoms, flushing, headache and gastro-intestinal disturbances. These are more frequent at the start of treatment, especially if the dosage is raised rapidly. However, such reactions generally subside in the further course of treatment or following a reduction of dosage.

The most severe adverse reactions are neuropathy, blood dyscrasias, and an acute rheumatoid state resulting in a syndrome resembling disseminated lupus erythematosus (see Warnings and Precautions).

Cardiovascular System: tachycardia, palpitation, flushing, hypotension, anginal symptoms, edema, heart failure, paradoxical pressor responses.

Central and Peripheral Nervous Systems: headache, dizziness, peripheral neuritis evidenced by paresthesia, numbness and tingling, polyneuritis, tremor, agitation, anorexia, anxiety, depression, hallucinations, disorientation, sleep disturbances.

Musculo-Skeletal System: arthralgia, joint swelling, myalgia, muscle cramps.

Skin and Appendages: rash.

Urogenital System: proteinuria, increased plasma creatinine, hematuria sometimes in association with glomerulonephritis, acute renal failure, urinary retention, difficulty in micturition.

Gastrointestinal Tract: gastrointestinal disturbances, diarrhea, constipation, nausea, vomiting, jaundice, liver enlargement, abnormal liver function sometimes in association with hepatitis, paralytic ileus.

Blood: anemia, leukopenia, neutropenia, thrombocytopenia with or without purpura, hemolytic anemia, leucocytosis, lymphadenopathy, pancytopenia, splenomegaly, agranulocytosis, antinuclear antibodies.

Sense Organs: increased lacrimation, conjunctivitis, nasal congestion, blurred vision.

Hypersensitivity Reactions: SLE-like syndrome (see Warnings), chills, eosinophilia, hypersensitivity reactions such as pruritus, urticaria, vasculitis, hepatitis.

Respiratory Tract: dyspnea, pleural pain.

Miscellaneous: fever, weight decrease, malaise, exophthalmos, decreased libido, pancreatitis. Hyperuricemia, hyperglycemia and hypokalemia have been reported.

OVERDOSE:

Symptoms: Hypotension, tachycardia, headache, generalized skin flushing, sweating, nausea and dizziness. Myocardial ischemia with angina pectoris, cardiac arrhythmia and profound shock can develop.

Further signs may include impairment of consciousness, vomiting, tremor, convulsions, oliguria and hypothermia.

Treatment: There is no known specific antidote.

Evacuate gastric contents by induction of emesis or gastric lavage, taking adequate precautions against aspiration and for protection of the airway. If general conditions permit, administer activated charcoal slurry and possibly an osmotic cathartic. These procedures may have to be omitted or carried out after cardiovascular status has been stabilized, since they might precipitate cardiac arrhythmias or increase the depth of shock.

Support of the cardiovascular system is of primary importance. Shock should be treated with volume expanders without resorting to use of vasopressors. The use of dopamine to elevate systolic blood pressure to 90 mmHg may be considered in an emergency. If a vasopressor drug is required, a type that is least likely to precipitate or aggravate cardiac arrhythmia should be used, and the ECG should be monitored while it is being administered. Digitalization may be necessary. Renal function must be monitored and supported as required.

No experience has been reported with extracorporeal or peritoneal dialysis.

> For management of a suspected drug overdose, CPhA recommends that you contact your **regional Poison Control Centre**. See the *CPS* Directory section for a list of Poison Control Centres.

DOSAGE: The dose of APO-HYDRALAZINE (hydralazine hydrochloride) must always be individualized and adjusted according to the patient's blood pressure response.

Initially, one 10 mg tablet 4 times daily for the first 2 to 4 days. The dose is increased to 25 mg 4 times daily for the remainder of the first week. Dosage is then increased to 50 mg 4 times daily for the second and subsequent weeks of treatment.

For maintenance, adjust dosage to lowest effective levels. The incidence of toxic reactions, particularly the lupus erythematosus syndrome, is highest in the group of patients receiving large doses of hydralazine.

The usual effective maintenance daily dose ranges from 50 to 200 mg. However, the dose should not be increased above 100 mg per day without determining the acetylator phenotype.

After the titration period, some patients may be maintained on a twice daily schedule.

The influence of food on the bioavailability of hydralazine is uncertain. Contradictory results have been obtained.

Note: Geriatric patients may be more sensitive to the effects of the usual adult dose. Response should be monitored and the dosage adjusted accordingly to lowest effective levels.

In patients with renal impairment the dose or the dosing interval should be adapted according to the clinical response, in order to avoid accumulation of the "apparent" active substance. In patients with hepatic dysfunction the dose or the dosing interval should be adapted according to the clinical response, in order to avoid accumulation of the "apparent" active substance.

SUPPLIED: 10 mg: Each round, yellow, biconvex tablet, scored and engraved "APO" over "H10" on one side, contains: hydralazine HCl 10 mg. Nonmedicinal ingredients: cornstarch, D&C Yellow #10 Aluminum Lake, FD&C Yellow #6 Aluminum Lake, magnesium stearate and microcrystalline cellulose. Bottles of 100.

25 mg: Each round, blue, biconvex, film-coated tablet, engraved "25" on one side, contains: hydralazine HCl 25 mg. Nonmedicinal ingredients: carnauba wax, croscarmellose sodium, D&C Yellow #10 Aluminum Lake, FD&C Blue #1 Aluminum Lake, hydroxypropyl methylcellulose, magnesium stearate, microcrystalline cellulose, polyethylene glycol and titanium dioxide. Bottles of 100 and 500.

50 mg: Each round, pink, biconvex, film-coated tablet, engraved "50" on one side, contains: hydralazine HCl 50 mg. Nonmedicinal ingredients: carnauba wax, colloidal silicon dioxide, croscarmellose sodium, FD&C Red #3 Aluminum Lake, hydroxypropyl methylcellulose, magnesium stearate, microcrystalline cellulose, polyethylene glycol and titanium dioxide. Bottles of 100.

Store at room temperature (15-30°C).

> The reader is invited to consult CPhA's monograph **Thiazide Diuretics**.

Apo®-Hydro Ⓟ

hydrochlorothiazide

Diuretic—Antihypertensive

Apotex

Date of Preparation: July 6, 1995

PHARMACOLOGY: Hydrochlorothiazide inhibits reabsorption of sodium and chloride in the distal tubule thus promoting water loss. The higher urine volume increases potassium loss; this loss can often be decreased by restricting sodium intake. Oral doses are well absorbed and reach peak effect in about 4 hours, with a 6 to 12 hour duration. It is excreted unchanged in the urine with a half-life of 3 to 5 hours.

The mild blood pressure reducing effects are initially due to volume reduction but the persisting effect includes other undetermined mechanisms that reduce peripheral resistance. A high salt intake reverses its antihypertensive effect.

INDICATIONS: Adjunctive therapy in edema associated with congestive heart failure, hepatic cirrhosis, in drug induced edema (corticosteroid and estrogen therapy) and in edema of renal origin (i.e. nephrotic syndrome, acute glomerulonephritis, chronic renal disease).

In the management of hypertension, hydrochlorothiazide may be used alone or as an adjunct to other antihypertensive drugs. Since it enhances the action of these agents, their dosage must be reduced to avoid an excessive drop in blood pressure and other adverse effects.

CONTRAINDICATIONS: Anuria; discontinue if increasing azotemia and oliguria occur during treatment of severe progressive renal disease. Do not use in patients known to be sensitive to thiazides or other sulfonamide derived drugs.

WARNINGS: No data supplied by the manufacturer.

PRECAUTIONS: May precipitate or increase azotemia; cumulative effects may develop in presence of impaired renal function; discontinue if increasing azotemia and oliguria occur during treatment of severe progressive renal disease. Use with caution in impaired hepatic function or progressive liver disease since minor alterations of fluid and electrolyte balance or of serum ammonia may precipitate hepatic coma.

The possibility of sensitivity reactions should be considered in patients with or without a history of allergy or bronchial asthma.

The possibility of exacerbation or activation of systemic lupus erythematosus has been reported.

Check carefully for signs of fluid and electrolyte imbalance, namely hyponatremia, hypochloremic alkalosis and hypokalemia. Serum and urine electrolyte determinations are particularly important when the patient has other disorders that predispose to fluid and electrolyte imbalance such as vomiting, diarrhea, heart failure, liver or renal disease, is on a salt-restricted diet, or is receiving parenteral fluids. The elderly may be at greater risk for developing electrolyte abnormalities, including hypomagnesemia, due to age-related changes in renal function. Warning signs, irrespective of cause, are: dryness of mouth, thirst, weakness, lethargy, drowsiness, restlessness, muscle pains or cramps, muscular fatigue, hypotension, oliguria, tachycardia, and gastrointestinal disturbances.

Prevent or treat hypokalemia with foods high in potassium, or, if necessary, with supplemental potassium chloride.

Dilutional hyponatremia may occur in edematous patients in hot weather; appropriate therapy is water restriction, rather than administration of salt except in rare instances when the hyponatremia is life-threatening.

Although any chloride deficit is generally mild and usually does not require specific treatment except under extraordinary circumstances (as in liver disease or renal disease), chloride replacement may be required in the treatment of metabolic or hypochloremic alkalosis.

Should hypochloremic alkalosis or hyponatremia occur, withdrawal of the diuretic, fluid restriction and other appropriate therapy should be considered.

Pathological changes in the parathyroid glands with hypercalcemia and hypophosphatemia have been observed in a few patients on prolonged thiazide therapy. The common complications of hyperparathyroidism such as renal lithiasis, bone resorption, and peptic ulceration have not been seen. Discontinue thiazides before carrying out parathyroid function tests.

Caution is necessary in patients with hyperuricemia or a history of gout since gout may be precipitated.

Drug Interactions: Hypokalemia may develop (especially with brisk diuresis) in severe cirrhosis; with concomitant steroid or ACTH therapy; or with inadequate electrolyte intake. Hypokalemia can sensitize or exaggerate the response of the heart to toxic effects of digitalis.

Thiazides may increase responsiveness to tubocurarine. The antihypertensive effect of the drug may be enhanced in the post sympathectomy patient.

Insulin or oral hypoglycemic dosage requirements may be altered by thiazides. Latent diabetes mellitus may become manifest.

Hydrochlorothiazide may add to or potentiate the action of other antihypertensive drugs, and decrease responsiveness to norepinephrine.

Diuretics enhance the cardiotoxic (e.g. ECG changes) and neurotoxic (e.g. ataxia, confusion and mental disorientation) effects of lithium and these drugs should ordinarily not be administered concurrently. In those rare instances when these drugs must be given together, patients should be observed closely for signs and symptoms of lithium toxicity. Close monitoring of serum electrolytes and lithium concentrations and maintenance of adequate fluid, potassium and sodium intake also are necessary.

Pregnancy: The routine use of thiazide diuretics in an otherwise healthy pregnant woman with or without edema is not appropriate. Edema in pregnancy, resulting from restriction of venous return by the expanded uterus, is treated though elevation of the lower extremities and use of support hose. A short course of diuretics may be appropriate in patients with severe hypervolemia not relieved by rest or these measures. Pathological edema such as cardiac, nephrotic or hepatic edema may be an indication for use of thiazide diuretics. Thiazides do not prevent toxemia of pregnancy, nor are they useful in its treatment.

Thiazides cross the placental barrier. Possible risks include fetal or neonatal jaundice, thrombocytopenia, and possibly other adverse reactions that have occurred in the adult.

Lactation: Thiazides are excreted into the milk of nursing women, although apparently not in significant amounts. The potential for idiosyncratic or allergic reaction in the infant should be considered. It should be noted that diuretics may partially inhibit lactation.

ADVERSE EFFECTS: Gastrointestinal: anorexia, gastric irritation, nausea, vomiting, cramping, diarrhea, constipation, jaundice (intrahepatic cholestatic), pancreatitis, sialadenitis.

CNS: dizziness, vertigo, paresthesias, headache, xanthopsia.

Hypersensitivity: purpura, photosensitivity, rash, urticaria, necrotizing angiitis, fever, respiratory distress including pneumonitis, anaphylactic reactions.

Hematologic: leukopenia, thrombocytopenia, agranulocytosis, aplastic anemia, hemolytic anemia.

Cardiovascular: orthostatic hypotension may occur, especially in elderly patients with reduced plasma volume and may be potentiated by alcohol, barbiturates or narcotics.

Miscellaneous: muscle spasm, weakness, restlessness, hyperglycemia, glycosuria, hyperuricemia, transient blurred vision. Whenever adverse reactions are moderate or severe, thiazide dosage should be reduced or therapy withdrawn.

OVERDOSE:

Symptoms: Overdosage may lead to excessive diuresis with electrolyte depletion (hypokalemia, hypochloremia, hyponatremia) and dehydration. If digitalis has also been administered, hypokalemia may accentuate myocardial abnormalities (e.g. cardiac arrhythmias).

Signs are dry mouth, thirst, weakness, lethargy, drowsiness, restlessness, muscle pains or cramps, muscular fatigue, hypotension, oliguria, tachycardia, gastrointestinal disturbances, mental confusion, delirium, convulsions, shock, coma.

Treatment: There is no specific antidote. If ingestion is recent, gastric lavage or emesis may reduce absorption; activated charcoal may be given. Otherwise, management includes symptomatic treatment with special attention to cardiac rate and output, blood volume, electrolyte balance, dehydration, paralytic ileus, urinary function, hepatic coma, and cerebral activity. Administration of sympathomimetic drugs (e.g. dopamine) may be indicated. Administer oxygen or artificial respiration for respiratory impairment.

> For management of a suspected drug overdose, CPhA recommends that you contact your **regional Poison Control Centre**. See the *CPS* Directory section for a list of Poison Control Centres.

DOSAGE: Diuresis: The usual adult dose is 25 to 200 mg per day; the maintenance dose is 25 to 100 mg per day, depending on patient response. Some patients may respond to intermittent therapy (alternate days or 3 to 5 days per week). The usual oral dosage for children is 2 mg/kg per day, given in 2 divided doses. Infants under 6 months of age may require up to 3 mg/kg per day, in 2 divided doses.

Hypertension: Doses as low as 12.5 mg daily may be effective, especially in the elderly. Usual adult dose is 25 to 50 mg daily. Doses above this level may increase effectiveness very little but cause more side effects such as hypokalemia. In hypertension associated with renal failure volume overload, more potent diuretics, such as loop diuretics may have to be used.

SUPPLIED: 25 mg: Each round, pale pink, flat-faced, beveled edge tablet, scored and identified APO over 25, contains: hydrochlorothiazide 25 mg. Nonmedicinal ingredients: colloidal silicon dioxide, cornstarch, FD&C Yellow #6 aluminum lake, lactose, magnesium stearate and microcrystalline cellulose. Bottles of 100 and 1000. Unit dose packages of 100.

50 mg: Each round, pale pink, flat-faced, beveled edge tablet, scored and identified APO over 50, contains: hydrochlorothiazide 50 mg. Nonmedicinal ingredients: colloidal silicon dioxide, cornstarch, lactose, FD&C Yellow #6 aluminum lake, magnesium stearate and microcrystalline cellulose. Bottles of 100 and 1000.

100 mg: Each round, pale pink, flat-faced, beveled edge tablet, scored and identified APO over 100, contains: hydrochlorothiazide 100 mg. Nonmedicinal ingredients: colloidal silicon dioxide, cornstarch, FD&C Yellow #6 aluminum lake, lactose, magnesium stearate and microcrystalline cellulose. Bottles of 100.

The reader is invited to consult CPhA's monograph **Thiazide Diuretics**.

Apo®-Hydro (12.5 mg)
hydrochlorothiazide
Diuretic—Antihypertensive

Apotex

Date of Preparation: June 25, 2009

SUMMARY PRODUCT INFORMATION:

Route of Administration	Dosage Form/ Strength	Clinically Relevant Nonmedicinal Ingredients
Oral	Tablet 12.5 mg	Lactose monohydrate For a complete listing see Dosage Forms, Composition and Packaging.

INDICATIONS AND CLINICAL USE: Apo-Hydro (hydrochlorothiazide) tablets are indicated for the treatment of:
- Edema
- Hypertension
- Toxemia of Pregnancy

Edema: Apo-Hydro (hydrochlorothiazide) is indicated in edema associated with congestive heart failure, hepatic cirrhosis, corticosteroid and estrogen therapy, premenstrual tension with edema and in edema of renal origin (i.e. nephritic syndrome, acute glomerulonephrities and chronic renal disease). In obese patients in whom fluid retention is a complicating factor, it may help to initiate a loss of fluid and, thus of weight.
Hypertension: Apo-Hydro may be used alone or as an adjunct to other antihypertensive drugs. Since it enhances the action of these agents, their dosage must be reduced to avoid an excessive drop in pressure and other unwanted side effects.
Toxemia of Pregnancy: Apo-Hydro may be effective in the treatment of toxemia of pregnancy (including eclampsia).
Geriatrics (>65 years of age): No data available.
Pediatrics (0 to 16 years of age): No data available.

CONTRAINDICATIONS:
- Apo-Hydro (hydrochlorothiazide), as all diuretics, is contraindicated in anuria.
- Apo-Hydro should be discontinued if increasing azotemia and oliguria occur during treatment of severe progressive renal disease.
- Apo-Hydro is contraindicated in persons known to be sensitive to hydrochlorothiazide or to other sulfonamide-derived drugs.
- Patients who are hypersensitive to any ingredient in the formulation of Apo-Hydro or component of the container. For a complete listing, see Dosage Forms, Composition and Packaging.

WARNINGS AND PRECAUTIONS: General: Patients on long therapy with hydrochlorothiazide are required to be on potassium rich diet. Periodic determinations of serum electrolytes to detect possible electrolyte imbalance should be performed.

The antihypertensive effects of the drug may be enhanced in the postsympathectomy patient.

Carcinogenesis and Mutagenesis: No data available.
Cardiovascular: No data available.
Ear/Nose/Throat: No data available.
Endocrine and Metabolism: Calcium: Calcium excretion is decreased by thiazides.
Chloride: Chloride deficiency is generally mild and does not require specific treatment except under special conditions such as renal or/and hepatic disease.
Dilutional Hyponatremia: Dilutional hyponatremia may occur in edematous patients in hot weather; appropriate therapy is water restriction rather than administration of salt except when hyponatremia is life threatening. In actual salt depletion, appropriate replacement is the therapy of choice.
Fluid and Electrolyte Imbalance: All patients receiving thiazide should be observed for clinical signs of fluid or electrolyte imbalance: namely hyponatremia, hypochloremic alkalosis, and hypokalemia. Serum and urine electrolyte determinations are particularly important when the patient is vomiting excessively, or receiving parenteral fluids. Warning signs of serum electrolyte imbalance, irrespective of cause are: dryness of mouth, thirst, weakness, lethargy, drowsiness, restlessness, muscle pains or cramps, muscular fatigue, hypotension, oliguria, tachycardia, and gastrointestinal disturbances such as nausea and vomiting. Serum electrolytes may also be influenced by medication such as digitalis.
Hyperuricemia: Hyperuricemia may occur or frank gout may be precipitated in certain patients receiving thiazide therapy.
Hypokalemia: Hypokalemia may develop, especially with rapid diuresis, when severe cirrhosis is present or during concomitant use of corticosteroids or ACTH. Deficient oral electrolyte intake will also contribute to hypokalemia. Hypokalemia may sensitize or exaggerate the response of the heart to the toxic effects of digitalis (e.g. increased ventricular irritability). Hypokalemia may be avoided or treated by the use of potassium supplements.
Insulin: Insulin requirements in diabetic patients may be increased, decreased, or remain unchanged. Latent diabetes mellitus may become manifest during thiazide therapy. Concomitant therapy with lithium is not recommended with diuretics because of the reduction of renal clearance of lithium and therefore an added risk of lithium toxicity.
Parathyroid Gland: Pathological changes in the parathyroid gland with hypercalcemia and hypophosphatemia have been observed in a few patients on prolonged thiazide therapy. The common complications of hyperparathyroidism such as renal lithiasis, bone resorption, and peptic ulceration have not been reported. Use of thiazides should be discontinued before carrying out tests for parathyroid function.
Protein Bound Iodine (PBI): Thiazides may decrease serum PBI levels without signs of thyroid disturbance.
Gastrointestinal: Non-specific small bowel lesions consisting of stenosis with or without ulceration, may occur in association with the administration of enteric coated potassium salts, alone or with oral diuretics. These small bowel lesions have caused obstruction, hemorrhage and perforation. Surgery was frequently required and deaths have occurred. Available information tends to implicate enteric coated potassium salts, although lesions of this type also occur spontaneously. Such preparations should be used only when adequate dietary supplementation is not practical, and should be discontinued immediately if abdominal pain, distension, nausea, vomiting or gastrointestinal bleeding occur.
Genitourinary: No data available.
Hematologic: No data available.
Hepatic/Biliary/Pancreatic: Hydrochlorothiazide should be used with caution in patients with impaired hepatic function or progressive liver disease, since minor alterations of fluid and electrolyte balance or of serum ammonia may precipitate hepatic coma.
Immune: The possibility of exacerbation or activation of systemic lupus erythematosus has been reported.

Sensitivity reactions may occur in patients with or without a history of allergy or bronchial asthma.

Neurologic: No data available.
Ophthalmologic: No data available.
Peri-Operative Considerations: No data available.
Psychiatric: No data available.
Renal: In progressive renal impairment, therapy with hydrochlorothiazide should be withheld or discontinued.

Hydrochlorothiazide may commence or precipitate azotemia. It should be used with caution in patients with severely impaired renal function to avoid toxic or cumulative effect. If azotemia becomes more severe and oliguria occurs during treatment of patients with severe renal disease, administration of the diuretic must be stopped.

Respiratory: No data available.
Sensitivity/Resistance: No data available.
Sexual Function/Reproduction: No data available.
Skin: No data available.
Special Populations: Pregnant Women: Thiazides cross the placental barrier and appear in cord blood. When hydrochlorothiazide is used in pregnancy or in women of child-bearing age, the potential benefits of the drug should be weighed against the possible hazards to the fetus. These hazards include fetal or neonatal jaundice, thrombocytopenia, and possibly other adverse reactions which have occurred in the adult.

The routine use of diuretics in otherwise healthy pregnant women with or without mild edema is not indicated.
Nursing Women: Since thiazides appear in breast milk, hydrochlorothiazide is contraindicated in nursing mothers. If use of the drug is deemed essential, the patient should stop nursing.
Pediatrics (0 to 18 years of age): Safety and effectiveness in children under 18 years of age have not been established.
Geriatrics: Safety and effectiveness in adults over 65 years of age have not been established.

ADVERSE REACTIONS: Adverse Drug Reaction Overview: Whenever adverse reactions are moderate or severe, thiazide dosage should be reduced or therapy withdrawn.
Cardiovascular: orthostatic hypotension (may be aggravated by alcohol, barbiturates, or narcotics).
Central Nervous System: dizziness, vertigo, paresthesias, headache, xanthopsia.
Gastrointestinal System: anorexia, gastric irritation, nausea, vomiting, cramps, diarrhea, constipation, jaundice (intrahepatic cholestatic jaundice), pancreatitis, sialadenitis.
Hematologic: leukopenia, agranulocytosis, thrombocytopenia, aplastic anemia.
Hypersensitivity: pupura, photosensitivity, rash, urticaria, necrotizing angitis (vasculitis), fever, respiratory distress including pneumonitis, anaphylactic reactions.
Other: hyperglycemia, glycosuria, hyperuricemia, muscle spasm, weakness, restlessness, transient blurred vision.

DRUG INTERACTIONS: Hydrochlorothiazide adds to or potentiates the action of other antihypertensive drugs. Potentiation occurs especially with ganglionic or peripheral adrenergic blocking drugs.
Drug-Drug Interactions: Alcohol, Barbiturates or Narcotics: Orthostatic hypotension may occur and may be potentiated by alcohol, barbiturates, or narcotics.
Lithium: Concomitant therapy with lithium is not recommended with diuretics because of the reduction of renal clearance of lithium and therefore an added risk of lithium toxicity.
Norepinephrine: Thiazides may decrease arterial responsiveness to norepinephrine. This diminution is not sufficient to preclude effectiveness of the pressor agent for therapeutic use.
Probenecid: The rate of elimination of hydrochlorothiazide is decreased some what by the coadministration of probenecid without, however, an accompanying reduction in diuresis.
Tubocurarine: Thiazide drugs may increase the responsiveness to tubocurarine.
Drug-Food Interactions: Interactions with food have not been established.
Drug-Herb Interactions: Interactions with herbal products have not been established.
Drug-Laboratory Test Interactions: There are no known interactions of Hydrochlorothiazide with commonly used laboratory tests.

DOSAGE AND ADMINISTRATION: Therapy should be individualized according to the patients requirement. Use the smallest dosage necessary to achieve the required response.
Dosing Considerations: Adult Patients:
- Diuresis
- Toxemia of pregnancy
- Premenstrual tension with edema
- Control of hypertension

Infants and Children: Adult Patients: Diuresis: The recommended adult dosage is 50 to 100 mg once or twice a day. Many patients respond to intermittent therapy, i.e. administration on alternate days or on three to five days each week.

With an intermittent schedule, excessive response and the resulting undesirable electrolyte imbalance are less likely to occur.
Toxemia of Pregnancy: The recommended dosage is 100 mg daily, or in severe cases and for brief periods, 200 mg daily (in divided doses). Frequency of administration may range from once every four days to daily.
Premenstrual Tension with Edema: The recommended dosage is 25 to 50 mg once or twice a day from the first appearance of symptoms until onset of the menses.
Control of Hypertension: The usual recommended starting dosage is 50 or 100 mg a day as a single or divided dose. Dosage is increased or decreased according to the blood pressure response of the patient. Some patients may require doses of 200 mg a day in divided doses.

Careful observation for changes in blood pressure must be made when Apo-Hydro (hydrochlorothiazide) is used with other anti-hypertensive drugs, especially during initial therapy. The dosage of other agents must be reduced by at least 50%, as soon as it is added to the regimen, to prevent excessive drop in blood pressure. As the blood pressure falls under the potentiating effect of this agent, a further reduction in dosage, or discontinuation of other antihypertensive drugs may be necessary. A single daily dose as low as 12.5 mg of Hydrochlorothiazide could be used in combination with another antihypertensive.

In the case of hypertension monotherapy, doses as low as a single daily dose 12.5 mg may be effective (especially in the elderly or as a starting dose), as well as a daily dose of 25 mg given in two divided doses.
Infants and Children: The usual recommended pediatric dosage is based on 1.0 mg of Apo-Hydro per pound of body weight per day in two doses. Infants under 6 months of age may require up to 1.5 mg per pound per day in two doses.

On this basis, infants up to 2 years of age may be given 12.5 to 37.5 mg daily in two doses. Children from 2 to 12 years of age may be given 37.5 to 100 mg daily in two doses. Dosage in both age groups should be based on body weight.

OVERDOSAGE:
Symptoms: Overdosage of hydrochlorothiazide may produce diuresis accompanied with electrolyte imbalance (hypokalemia, hyponatremia and hypochloremic alkalosis) and dehydration.

The symptoms are as follows: dryness of mouth, thirst, weakness, lethargy, drowsiness, restlessness, muscle pains or cramps, muscular fatigue, hypotension, oliguria, tachycardia, gastrointestinal disturbances, mental confusion, delirium, convulsions, shock, coma.

Hypokalemia can sensitize or exaggerate the response of the heart to the toxic effects of digitalis (e.g. increased ventricular irritability).

Hydrochlorothiazide may precipitate hepatic coma in patients with cirrhosis; increase the effect of other antihypertensive agents and decrease arterial responsiveness to norepinephrine.
Treatment: No specific antidote is available.

Treatment is symptomatic and supportive. Induce emesis or perform gastric lavage. Correct dehydration, electrolyte imbalance, hepatic coma, and hypotension by established procedures. Administer oxygen or artificial respiration for respiratory impairment.

For management of a suspected drug overdose, contact your regional Poison Control Centre. See the *CPS* Directory section for a list of Poison Control Centres.

ACTION AND CLINICAL PHARMACOLOGY: Mechanism of Action: Hydrochlorothiazide is a diuretic and an antihypertensive agent. The exact mechanism of the antihypertensive effect is unknown. Hydrochlorothiazide has no effect on normal blood pressure.

Hydrochlorothiazide affects the renal tubular mechanism of electrolyte reabsorption. It increases excretion of sodium and chloride in approximately equivalent amounts and reduces the rate of formation of solute-free water. Natriuresis causes a secondary loss of potassium and bicarbonate.
Pharmacokinetics: Absorption: Hydrochlorothiazide is rapidly absorbed from the gastrointestinal tract. Onset of action after oral administration occurs in 2 hours and the peak effect at approximately 4 hours. Duration of action persists for approximately 6 to 12 hours.
Distribution: The drug is distributed throughout the extracellular space and does not accumulate in tissues other than the kidney. It passes readily through the placental barrier to the fetus.
Metabolism: Hydrochlorothiazide is not metabolized.
Excretion: Hydrochlorothiazide is eliminated rapidly by the kidney.

STORAGE AND STABILITY: Apo-Hydro (hydrochlorothiazide) tablets should be stored at controlled room temperature (15 to 30°C).

INFORMATION FOR THE PATIENT: Published in e-CPS, available by subscription at www.e-cps.ca.

DOSAGE FORMS, COMPOSITION AND PACKAGING: Each pale pink, round, flat-faced bevelled-edge, tablet, engraved "APO" over "12.5" on one side, plain on the other side contains: hydrochlorothiazide, USP 12.5 mg. Nonmedicinal ingredients: colloidal silicon dioxide, lactose monohydrate (spray dried), magnesium stearate, microcrystalline cellulose, starch (corn) and sunset yellow aluminum lake 40%. HDPE bottles of 100, 500 and 1000. Blisters of 100.

Apo®-Keto Pr
ketoprofen
Anti-inflammatory—Analgesic

Apotex

Apo®-Keto-E Pr
ketoprofen
Anti-inflammatory—Analgesic

Apotex

Apo®-Keto SR Pr
ketoprofen
Anti-inflammatory—Analgesic

Apotex

Date of Preparation: October 11, 1989
Date of Revision: July 7, 2000

PHARMACOLOGY: Animal pharmacological studies have shown that ketoprofen is a NSAID that possesses anti-inflammatory, analgesic, and antipyretic properties. The anti-inflammatory action is not mediated through the pituitary-adrenal axis.

Its therapeutic effectiveness has been demonstrated by a reduction in joint swelling, pain and duration of morning stiffness, and by increased grip strength and an improvement in functional capacity.

Clinical trials in rheumatoid arthritis have shown that the anti-arthritic activity of ketoprofen 200 mg/day was similar to that of acetylsalicylic acid 3.6 g/day.

Ketoprofen 200 mg daily induced less gastrointestinal bleeding than acetylsalicylic acid 3.6 g daily.

The effectiveness of ketoprofen as a general purpose analgesic has been studied in standard pain models which have shown the effectiveness of doses of 25 to 150 mg. Doses of 25 mg were superior to placebo. Larger doses than 25 mg generally could not be shown significantly more effective but there was a tendency toward faster onset and greater duration of action with 50 mg and, in the case of dysmenorrhea, a significantly greater effect overall with 75 mg. Doses greater than 50 to 75 mg did not have increased analgesic effect.

Pharmacokinetics: In man, ketoprofen is rapidly and almost completely absorbed from the gastrointestinal tract. Maximum plasma levels are reached within 1/2 to 2 hours after administration of capsules; however, peak plasma levels are delayed by a further 1 to 2 hours with enteric-coated tablets and by 5 to 6 hours with sustained-release tablets. The biotransformation of ketoprofen is characterized by two main processes: hydroxylation and conjugation, the latter being the main metabolic pathway in man.

The drug is 99% bound to plasma proteins, mainly to the albumin fraction. Metabolites as well as the unchanged drug are excreted mainly in the urine. Fecal excretion is negligible.

Following the administration of capsules or enteric-coated tablets in man, 25% to 90% of the drug is excreted in the urine within 24 hours, with the major portion being excreted during the first 6 hours. The elimination half-life is approximately 2 hours. Following administration of slow release ketoprofen, absorption is gradual, reaching a plateau during which plasma levels remain steady from the fifth to the twelfth hour after ingestion and decrease with an apparent half-life of 3 to 4 hours. No accumulation of ketoprofen was found following repeated once-daily administration of ketoprofen sustained-release tablets. Repeated administration of the drug, in both animals and man, caused no induction of liver enzymes.

When ketoprofen capsules are administered with food, the total bioavailability (AUC) is not altered; however, the rate of absorption is slowed resulting in delayed and reduced peak concentrations (C_{max}). Following a single 50 mg dose of ketoprofen while fasting, the mean C_{max} was 4.1 mg/L (at 1.1 hours); when administered after food, it decreased to 2.4 mg/L (at 2.0 hours).

The composition of the diet slightly but significantly alters the extent of absorption of ketoprofen from sustained-release tablets: a high-fat/high-calorie meal (3000 calories/day) was associated with lower ketoprofen bioavailability values (about 20%) than a low-fat/low-calorie content (1200 calories/day). Mean trough ketoprofen plasma concentrations were similar after high or low fat meals.

To date, studies of the effects of age and renal function impairment have been small, generally involving 5 to 8 subjects per group, but they indicate modest decrease in clearance in the elderly and in patients with impaired renal function. In normal elderly volunteers (mean age 73 years), the plasma and renal clearance and protein binding were reduced while the V_d increased when compared to a younger normal population (mean age 27 years). (Plasma clearance and V_d were 0.05 L/kg/hr and 0.4 L/kg in elderly and 0.06 L/kg/hr and 0.3 L/kg in young subjects, respectively). The mean half-life of ketoprofen in this normal geriatric population, as well as in a rheumatoid elderly population (mean age 64 years), was about 5 hours as compared to 3 hours in the younger population.

Patients with impaired renal function (mean age 44 years) also demonstrate decreases in plasma clearance (0.04 L/kg/hr) of drug, with the mean half-life increasing to about 3.5 hours.

Comparative Bioavailability: Bioavailability studies were performed using normal human volunteers. The rate and extent of absorption of ketoprofen after a single oral 50 mg dose of ORUDIS 50 mg and APO-KETO 50 mg capsules were measured and compared. The results are summarized as follows: see Table 1.

Table 1: APO-KETO

Rate and Extent of Absorption of Ketoprofen After a Single Oral 50 mg Dose of ORUDIS 50 mg and APO-KETO 50 mg Capsules

	ORUDIS 50 mg	APO-KETO 50 mg	% Diffr.
AUC_{0-12} (µg·hr/mL)	9.93	9.49	−4.4
C_{max} (µg/mL)	5.31	4.39	−17.3
T_{max} (hr)	1.12	1.35	+20.4
$t_{1/2}$ (hr)	1.7	1.6	−5.9

The rate and extent of absorption of ketoprofen after a single oral 50 mg dose of ORUDIS E 50 mg and APO-KETO-E 50 mg enteric-coated tablets were measured and compared. The results are summarized as follows: see Table 2.

Table 2: APO-KETO-E

Rate and Extent of Absorption of Ketoprofen After a Single Oral 50 mg Dose of ORUDIS E 50 mg and APO-KETO-E 50 mg Enteric-coated Tablets

	ORUDIS E 50 mg	APO-KETO-E 50 mg	% Diffr.
AUC_{0-12} (µg·hr/mL)	9.59	9.72	+1.4
C_{max} (µg/mL)	6.09	4.41	−27.7
T_{max} (hr)	1.5	1.6	+10.6
$t_{1/2}$ (hr)	1.8	1.8	0.0

Two additional bioavailability studies were performed using sustained-release tablets, one with food and one without food. The rate and extent of absorption of ketoprofen after a single oral 200 mg dose of ORUDIS SR 200 mg and APO-KETO SR 200 mg tablets were measured and compared. The results from measured data are summarized as follows: see Table 3 and Table 4.

Table 3: APO-KETO SR
Study 1 (Without Food)

	Geometric Mean Arithmetic Mean (CV%)		
Parameter	**APO-KETO SR**	**ORUDIS SR[a]**	**Ratio of Means (%)**
AUC_T (µg·hr/mL)	30.3 31.0 (19)	31.2 31.7 (19)	96.9[b]
AUC_I (µg·hr/mL)	34.5 35.1 (19)	35.5 36.1 (21)	97.1[b]
AUC_x(µg·hr/mL)	30.3 31.9 (19)	31.2 31.6 (19)	97.2[b]
C_{max} (µg/mL)	3.32 3.45 (32)	3.29 3.39 (28)	99.7[b]
T_{max} (hr)	10.2 (37)	7.08 (45)	—
$t_{1/2}$ (hr)	2.93 (23)	3.87 (53)	—

[a] ORUDIS SR (Rhône-Poulenc Rorer) was purchased at a Canadian retail pharmacy.
[b] Based on the least squares estimate of the geometric means.
The T_{max} and $t_{1/2}$ parameters are expressed as the arithmetic means.

Table 4: APO-KETO SR
Study 2 (With Food)

	Geometric Mean Arithmetic Mean (CV%)		
Parameter	**APO-KETO SR**	**ORUDIS SR[a]**	**Ratio of Means (%)**
AUC_T (µg·hr/mL)	26.6 29.5 (44)	26.0 28.7 (45)	98.4[b]
AUC_I (µg·hr/mL)	30.6 33.5 (39)	29.4 32.2 (42)	97.6[b]
AUC_x(µg·hr/mL)	25.3 27.9 (43)	24.3 26.3 (39)	101.8[b]
C_{max} (µg/mL)	3.46 3.53 (20)	3.94 4.14 (29)	82.2[b]
T_{max} (hr)	11.9 (39)	9.69 (61)	—
$t_{1/2}$ (hr)	3.13 (53)	2.15 (41)	—

[a] ORUDIS SR (Rhône-Poulenc Rorer) was purchased at a Canadian retail pharmacy.
[b] Based on the least squares estimate of the geometric means.
The T_{max} and $t_{1/2}$ parameters are expressed as the arithmetic means.

INDICATIONS: APO-KETO (ketoprofen) is indicated in the treatment of rheumatoid arthritis, ankylosing spondylitis and osteoarthritis.

APO-KETO is also indicated for the treatment of primary dysmenorrhea as well as for the relief of mild to moderate acute pain associated with musculotendinous trauma (sprains and strains), postoperative (including dental surgery) or postpartum pain.

CONTRAINDICATIONS: APO-KETO (ketoprofen) is contraindicated in patients with active peptic ulcers or active inflammatory diseases of the gastrointestinal tract.

Known or suspected hypersensitivity to the drug. APO-KETO should not be used in patients in whom acute asthmatic attacks, urticaria, rhinitis or other allergic manifestations are precipitated by ASA or other nonsteroidal anti-inflammatory agents. Fatal anaphylactoid reactions have occurred in such individuals.

WARNINGS: Peptic ulceration, perforation and gastrointestinal bleeding, sometimes severe and occasionally fatal have been reported during therapy with nonsteroidal anti-inflammatory drugs (NSAIDs) including ketoprofen. Unlike most adverse reactions, which usually manifest themselves in the first month if they are going to occur in an individual, new peptic ulcers keep appearing in patients under treatment with ketoprofen at a rate of greater than 1% per year.

APO-KETO (ketoprofen) should be given under close medical supervision to patients prone to gastrointestinal tract irritation particularly those with a history of peptic ulcer, diverticulosis or other inflammatory disease of the gastrointestinal tract. In these cases the physician must weigh the benefits of treatment against the possible hazards.

Patients taking any NSAID including this drug should be instructed to contact a physician immediately if they experience symptoms or signs suggestive of peptic ulceration or gastrointestinal bleeding. These reactions can occur without warning symptoms or signs and at any time during the treatment.

Elderly, frail and debilitated patients appear to be at higher risk from a variety of adverse reactions from nonsteroidal anti-inflammatory drugs (NSAIDs). For such patients, consideration should be given to a starting dose lower than usual, with individual adjustment when necessary and under close supervision. See Precautions for further advice.

Pregnancy: The safety of APO-KETO when administered to pregnant or nursing women has not been determined and therefore such use is not recommended. Pregnant rats who received ketoprofen 6 and 9 mg/kg/day p.o. from day 15 of gestation, showed dystocia and increased pup mortality.

Lactation: In rats, ketoprofen at doses of 9 mg/kg (approximately 1.5 times the maximum human therapeutic dose) did not affect perinatal development. Upon administration to lactating dogs, the milk concentration of ketoprofen was found to be 4 to 5% of the plasma drug level. Data on secretion in human milk after ingestion of ketoprofen do not exist. As with other drugs that are excreted in milk, APO-KETO is not recommended for use in nursing mothers.

Children: The conditions for safe and effective use of APO-KETO in children under 12 years of age have not been established and the drug is therefore not recommended in this age group.

PRECAUTIONS: Gastrointestinal System: If peptic ulceration is suspected or confirmed, or if gastrointestinal bleeding or perforation occurs, APO-KETO (ketoprofen) should be discontinued, an appropriate treatment instituted and the patient closely monitored.

There is no definitive evidence that the concomitant administration of histamine H_2-receptor antagonists and/or antacids will either prevent the occurrence of gastrointestinal side effects or allow continuation of ketoprofen therapy when and if these adverse reactions appear.

Renal Function: As with other nonsteroidal anti-inflammatory drugs, long-term administration of ketoprofen to animals has resulted in renal papillary necrosis and other abnormal renal pathology. In humans, there have been reports of acute interstitial nephritis with hematuria, proteinuria, and occasionally nephrotic syndrome.

A second form of renal toxicity has been seen in patients with prerenal conditions leading to the reduction in renal blood flow or blood volume, where the renal prostaglandins have a supportive role in the maintenance of renal perfusion. In these patients, administration of a nonsteroidal anti-inflammatory drug may cause a dose dependent reduction in prostaglandin formation and may precipitate overt renal decompensation. Patients at greatest risk of this reaction are those with impaired renal function, heart failure, liver dysfunction, those taking diuretics, and the elderly. Discontinuation of nonsteroidal anti-inflammatory therapy is usually followed by recovery to the pre-treatment state.

Ketoprofen and its metabolites are eliminated primarily by the kidneys, therefore the drug should be used with great caution in patients with impaired renal function. In these cases lower doses of APO-KETO should be anticipated and patients carefully monitored.

During long-term therapy kidney function should be monitored periodically.

Hepatic Function: As with other nonsteroidal anti-inflammatory drugs, borderline elevations of one or more liver tests may occur in up to 15% of patients. These abnormalities may progress, may remain essentially unchanged, or may be transient with continued therapy. Meaningful (3 times the upper limit of normal) elevations of ALT or AST occurred in controlled clinical trials in less than 1% of patients. A patient with symptoms and/or signs suggesting liver dysfunction, or in whom an abnormal liver test has occurred, should be evaluated for evidence of the development of more severe hepatic reaction while on therapy with this drug. Severe hepatic reactions including jaundice and cases of fatal hepatitis have been reported with this drug as with other nonsteroidal anti-inflammatory drugs. Although such reactions are rare, if abnormal liver tests persist or worsen, if clinical signs and symptoms consistent with liver disease develop, or if systemic manifestations occur (e.g. eosinophilia, rash, etc.), this drug should be discontinued.

During long-term therapy, liver function tests should be monitored periodically. If this drug is to be used in the presence of impaired liver function, it must be done under strict observation.

Fluid and Electrolyte Balance: Fluid retention and edema have been observed in approximately 2% of patients treated with ketoprofen. Therefore, as with many other nonsteroidal anti-inflammatory drugs, the possibility of precipitating congestive heart failure in elderly patients or those with compromised cardiac function should be borne in mind. APO-KETO should be used with caution in patients with heart failure, hypertension or other conditions predisposing to fluid retention.

Serum electrolytes should be monitored periodically during long-term therapy, especially in those patients at risk.

Hematology: Drugs inhibiting prostaglandin biosynthesis do interfere with platelet function to some degree; therefore, patients who may be adversely affected by such an action should be carefully observed when APO-KETO is administered.

Blood dyscrasias associated with the use of nonsteroidal anti-inflammatory drugs are rare, but could be with severe consequences.

Anemia is commonly observed in rheumatoid arthritis and is sometimes aggravated by nonsteroidal anti-inflammatory drugs, which may produce fluid retention or minor gastrointestinal blood loss in some patients. Therefore, patients with initial hemoglobin values of 10 g/dL or less who are to receive long-term therapy should have hemoglobin values determined frequently.

Infection: In common with other anti-inflammatory drugs, APO-KETO may mask the usual signs of infection.

Ophthalmology: Blurred and/or diminished vision has been reported with the use of ketoprofen and other NSAIDs. If such symptoms develop APO-KETO should be discontinued and an ophthalmological examination performed. Ophthalmic examination should be carried out at periodic intervals in any patients receiving this drug for an extended period of time.

Drug Interactions: Methotrexate: The concomitant administration of ketoprofen and high dose methotrexate has been associated with prolonged and marked enhancement of serum methotrexate levels resulting in severe methotrexate toxicity. This may also apply to some other nonsteroidal anti-inflammatory drugs. There were no abnormalities in methotrexate kinetics or evidence of toxicity when ketoprofen was given at least 12 hours after completion of high-dose methotrexate infusion. APO-KETO should not be used in patients receiving high-dose methotrexate.

The potential for severe toxicity should be kept in mind when prescribing ketoprofen and low-dose methotrexate concurrently. APO-KETO should not be administered within 12 hours of methotrexate infusion.

Acetylsalicylic Acid: Concurrent administration of acetylsalicylic acid (ASA) decreased ketoprofen protein binding and increased its plasma clearance. The overall result was a 40% reduction in the AUC of ketoprofen. APO-KETO does not alter ASA absorption.

Oral Anticoagulants: Ketoprofen has been shown to depress platelet aggregation and it can prolong bleeding time by approximately 3 to 4 minutes from baseline values. However, a study conducted in 20 patients undergoing therapy with Coumadin and simultaneously receiving ketoprofen, failed to demonstrate potentiation of anticoagulant effect. Nevertheless, close monitoring of patients is recommended when APO-KETO is given concomitantly with anticoagulants.

Diuretics: Hydrochlorothiazide, given concomitantly with ketoprofen produces a reduction in urinary potassium and chloride excretion compared to hydrochlorothiazide alone. Patients taking diuretics are at greater risk of developing renal failure secondary to a decrease in renal blood flow caused by prostaglandin inhibition.

Antacids: Concomitant administration of magnesium hydroxide and aluminum hydroxide does not interfere with the rate or extent of the absorption of ketoprofen.

Lithium: Nonsteroidal anti-inflammatory agents have been reported to increase steady-state plasma lithium levels. It is recommended that plasma lithium levels be monitored when APO-KETO is coadministered with lithium.

Probenecid: Concurrent administration of probenecid increases both free and bound ketoprofen through reducing the plasma clearance of ketoprofen to about one-third as well as decreasing its protein binding. APO-KETO is not recommended in association with probenecid.

Ketoprofen is extensively (99%) protein bound to human serum albumin and may compete for binding sites with drugs such as sulfonamides, oral hypoglycemic agents, phenytoin or lithium. Although no significant interaction has been documented, patients with such combination therapy should be monitored.

Clinical Laboratory Tests: The presence of ketoprofen and its metabolites in urine has been shown to interfere with certain tests which are used to detect albumin, bile salts, 17-ketosteroids or 17-hydroxycorticosteroids in urine and which rely upon acid precipitation as an end point or upon color reactions for carbonyl groups. No interference was seen in the tests for proteinuria using Albustix, Hema-Combistix or Labstix Reagent Strips.

Ketoprofen decreases platelet adhesion and aggregation. Therefore, it can prolong bleeding time by approximately 3 to 4 minutes from baseline values. There is no significant change in platelet count, prothrombin time, partial thromboplastin time, or thrombin time.

ADVERSE EFFECTS: The most common adverse reactions encountered with nonsteroidal anti-inflammatory drugs are gastrointestinal, of which peptic ulcer, with or without bleeding, is the most severe. Fatalities have occurred on occasion, particularly in the elderly.

In clinical trials of ketoprofen involving 1542 patients, the most common side effects reported were gastrointestinal (22%). The most severe were peptic ulcer or GI bleeding which occurred in controlled clinical trials in less than 1% of 1076 patients; however, in open label continuation studies in 1292 patients the rate was greater than 2%.

The detailed breakdown of side effects with their corresponding frequencies (not indicated when <1%) is given herewithin. That includes rare adverse reactions collected from foreign reports to manufacturers and regulatory agencies, publications and U.S. clinical trials:

Gastrointestinal (22%): dyspepsia (12.8%), nausea (4.0%), indigestion and flatulence (2.8%), vomiting (2.0%), constipation (2.0%), diarrhea (1.4%), anorexia, ulcer, GI bleeding and perforation, melena, hematemesis, stomatitis.

Central Nervous System (3-5%): headache (1.7%), fatigue (1%), dizziness, tension, anxiety, depression, drowsiness, impotence, vertigo, migraine, paresthesia.

Body as a Whole: angioedema, asthma, life threatening bronchospasm, anaphylaxis.

Dermatological (<3%): rashes (1.7%), pruritus, flushing, excessive perspiration, alopecia, bullous rash, exfoliative dermatitis, photosensitivity, purpuric rash, urticaria, onycholysis.

Cardiovascular: peripheral edema (2%), palpitation, congestive heart failure, hypertension.

Special Senses: tinnitus, visual disturbance, conjunctivitis, taste perversion, conjunctivitis sicca, hearing impairment.

Hematological: hypocoagulability, agranulocytosis, anemia, hemolysis, purpura, thrombocytopenia.

Renal: interstitial nephritis, hematuria, nephrotic syndrome, impairment of renal function, acute renal failure.

Hepatic: hepatic dysfunction, jaundice.

Laboratory Tests: Abnormal alkaline phosphatase, lactic dehydrogenase, glutamic oxaloacetic transaminase and blood urea nitrogen values were found in some patients receiving ketoprofen therapy. The abnormalities did not lead to discontinuation of treatment and, in some cases, returned to normal while the drug was continued. There have been sporadic reports of decreased hematocrit and hemoglobin values without progressive deterioration on prolonged administration of the drug.

OVERDOSE:

Symptoms: Of 20 cases of overdosage (doses up to 5000 mg) reported in Great Britain (5 children, 14 adolescents or young adults, and 1 elderly), only 4 had mild symptoms (vomiting in 3, drowsiness in 1 child).

Treatment: Administer gastric lavage or an emetic and treat symptomatically: compensate for dehydration, monitor urinary excretion and correct acidosis if present.

The drug is dialyzable; therefore, hemodialysis may be useful to remove circulating drug and to assist in case of renal failure.

> For management of a suspected drug overdose, CPhA recommends that you contact your **regional Poison Control Centre**. See the *CPS* Directory section for a list of Poison Control Centres.

DOSAGE: Adults: Rheumatoid Arthritis and Osteoarthritis: The usual dosage for APO-KETO (ketoprofen) capsules or enteric-coated tablets is 150 to 200 mg per day in 3 or 4 divided doses.

Once the maintenance dosage has been established, patients may be tried on a twice daily dosing regimen. Clinical trials, however, show that some rheumatoid arthritis patients respond better to more frequent dosing. The usual maintenance dose is 100 mg twice daily.

Patients with rheumatoid arthritis or osteoarthritis on a maintenance dose of 200 mg/day may be changed to a once daily dose of APO-KETO SR 200 mg tablets administered in the morning or evening. APO-KETO SR tablets should be swallowed whole.

APO-KETO E and APO-KETO SR tablets provide alternative presentations for those who may prefer these dosage forms. No difference in toxicity profile was documented.

The total daily dose of APO-KETO capsules or tablets should not exceed 200 mg per day. When the patient's response warrants it, the dose may be decreased to the minimum effective level.

In severe cases during a flare-up of rheumatic activity or if a satisfactory response cannot be obtained with the lower dose, a daily dosage in excess of 200 mg may be used, but a dose of 300 mg/day should not be exceeded.

Primary Dysmenorrhea and Mild to Moderate Pain: The usual dose for APO-KETO (ketoprofen) is 25 to 50 mg 3 or 4 times daily as necessary.

A larger dose may be tried if the patient's response to a previous dose was less than satisfactory, but individual doses above 50 mg have not been shown to give added analgesia. The total daily dose should not exceed 300 mg. In most types of acute pain, a course of 3 to 7 days has been shown to be sufficient.

Elderly and Debilitated Patients: Initial dosage should be reduced by 1/2 to 1/3 in patients with impaired renal function and the elderly.

Children: APO-KETO (ketoprofen) is not indicated in children under 12 years of age because clinical experience in this age group is insufficient.

INFORMATION FOR THE PATIENT: Published in e-CPS, available by subscription at www.e-cps.ca.

SUPPLIED: APO-KETO: Each dark green and ivory, hard gelatin no. 2 capsule, identified APO 50, contains: ketoprofen 50 mg. Nonmedicinal ingredients: colloidal silicon dioxide, croscarmellose sodium, dextrates (hydrous), lactose monohydrate, magnesium stearate and talc; capsules shell: D&C Yellow #10, FD&C Yellow #6, FD&C Green #3, gelatin, and titanium dioxide. The capsule is imprinted with edible red ink (pharmaceutical shellac, SDA-3A alcohol, FD&C Yellow #6 aluminum lake, n-butyl alcohol, D&C Red #7 calcium lake, 2-ethoxyethanol and titanium oxide). Bottles of 100.

APO-KETO-E: 50 mg: Each round, biconvex, yellow, enteric-coated tablet, engraved "50" on one side, contains: ketoprofen 50 mg. Nonmedicinal ingredients: colloidal silicon dioxide, croscarmellose sodium, D&C Yellow #10, dextrates, FD&C Yellow #6, guar gum, hydroxypropyl cellulose, hydroxypropyl methylcellulose, magnesium stearate, methacrylic acid copolymer, methylcellulose, polyethylene glycol, talc, titanium dioxide and triethyl citrate. Bottles of 100 and 500.

100 mg: Each round, biconvex, yellow, enteric-coated tablet, engraved "APO" over "100" on one side, contains: ketoprofen 100 mg. Nonmedicinal ingredients: colloidal silicon dioxide, croscarmellose sodium, D&C Yellow #10, dextrates, FD&C Yellow #6, guar gum, hydroxypropyl cellulose, hydroxypropyl methylcellulose, magnesium stearate, methacrylic acid copolymer, methylcellulose, polyethylene glycol, titanium dioxide and triethyl citrate. Bottles of 100 and 500.

APO-KETO SR: Each round, biconvex, white, enteric-coated, sustained release tablet, engraved "APO" on one side and "200" on the other, contains: ketoprofen 200 mg. Nonmedicinal ingredients: colloidal silicon dioxide, dextrates, hydroxypropyl cellulose, hydroxypropyl methylcellulose, magnesium stearate, methanol, polyethylene glycol, polyvinyl acetate phthalate, stearic acid, titanium dioxide and triethyl citrate. Bottles of 100.

Store at a controlled room temperature 15-30°C.

Apo®-Lactulose

lactulose

Laxative

Apotex

Date of Preparation: August 29, 2000
Date of Revision: May 10, 2004

PHARMACOLOGY: Lactulose is poorly absorbed from the gastrointestinal tract and no enzyme capable of hydrolysis of this disaccharide is present in human gastrointestinal tissue. As a result, oral doses of lactulose reach the colon virtually unchanged. In the colon, lactulose is broken down to lactic acid (and other short-chain carboxylic acids) by the action of colonic bacteria. The resulting increase in osmotic pressure and acidification of portions of the colonic contents are believed to be responsible for the increase in stool volume and frequency observed during lactulose administration.

INDICATIONS: The alleviation of constipation in chronically constipated patients.

CONTRAINDICATIONS: Since lactulose solution contains galactose (less than 107 mg/mL), it is contraindicated in patients who require a low galactose diet.

WARNINGS: Lactulose should not be taken for more than one week, unless ordered by a physician. Overuse or extended use may cause dependence for bowel function. Lactulose should not be taken within two hours of another medicine because the desired effect of the other medication may be reduced. Lactulose should not be used in the presence of abdominal pain, nausea, fever or vomiting.

PRECAUTIONS: *Pregnancy:* Animal studies have not revealed significant adverse effects. However, the use of lactulose by women who are pregnant or may become pregnant requires that the potential benefits be weighed against the potential risks.

Lactulose solution contains galactose (less than 107 mg/mL) and lactose (less than 80 mg/mL) and it should be used with caution in diabetics.

ADVERSE EFFECTS: Initial dosing may produce flatulence and intestinal cramps, which are usually transient. Excessive dosage can lead to diarrhea. Nausea has been reported.

OVERDOSE:

Symptoms and Treatment: Diarrhea and abdominal cramps may be controlled by a reduction of the dosage.

> For management of a suspected drug overdose, CPhA recommends that you contact your **regional Poison Control Centre**. See the *CPS* Directory section for a list of Poison Control Centres.

DOSAGE: Usual dose is 1 to 4 tablespoonfuls (15 to 60 mL) daily as required.

SUPPLIED: Each mL of clear, yellow to golden yellow solution contains: lactulose 667 mg. Nonmedicinal ingredients: D&C Yellow No. 10, FD&C Yellow No. 6, galactose, lactose, other sugars and purified water. Bottles of 500 mL and 1 L. Store at room temperature 15-30°C. Protect from freezing. Prolonged exposure to high temperature or direct light may cause some darkening of solution or a cloudy appearance, but no loss of therapeutic effect. Freezing will change the solution to semisolid state, which returns to normal when warmed to room temperature. Dilution and subsequent storage is not recommended.

Apo-Methazolamide Ⓟ

methazolamide

Carbonic Anhydrase Inhibitor—Ocular Pressure Lowering Therapy

Apotex

Date of Preparation: May 7, 2002
Date of Revision: January 21, 2004

PHARMACOLOGY: Methazolamide is a potent inhibitor of the enzyme carbonic anhydrase. The oral administration of the drug inhibits ocular carbonic anhydrase therefore decreasing formation of aqueous humor and intraocular pressure. The time of onset of intraocular pressure fall occurs within 2 to 4 hours, with a peak effect in 6 to 8 hours. The effect lasts for 10 to 18 hours.

Methazolamide is absorbed more slowly from the gastrointestinal tract and disappears more slowly from the plasma than does acetazolamide. Methazolamide is distributed throughout the body and can be assayed in the blood plasma, the cerebrospinal fluid, the aqueous humor of the eye, the red blood cell, in the bile and the extracellular fluid.

At present, the metabolism of methazolamide is not well characterized.

Methazolamide is a sulfonamide derivative, however, it does not have any clinically significant antimicrobial properties. Although concentration in the cerebrospinal fluid is high, it is not considered an effective anticonvulsant.

Methazolamide does have a weak transient diuretic effect. The drug should not be used as a diuretic. Serum changes in sodium, potassium and chloride are minimal and return to pretreatment levels after daily administration for 3 to 4 days. Inhibition of renal bicarbonate reabsorption produces an alkaline urine. Plasma bicarbonate decreases temporarily and a relative and transient metabolic acidosis may occur due to a disequilibrium in CO_2 transport in the red cell. This is quickly restored to balance by the initiation of compensatory mechanisms. The excretion of urinary citrate and uric acid is decreased by up to 40%. The effect on citrate excretion is less than that attributed to acetazolamide and varies according to urinary output.

Comparative Bioavailability Study—APO-METHAZOLAMIDE (Methazolamide) vs Neptazane: A comparative bioavailability study was performed using healthy human volunteers. The rate and extent of absorption of methazolamide was measured and compared following oral administration of a single 1×50 mg dose of APO-METHAZOLAMIDE (methazolamide) or Neptazane (methazolamide) tablets, under fasting conditions. The results from measured data are summarized in Table 1.

Table 1: APO-METHAZOLAMIDE

Summary Table of the Comparative Bioavailability Data. Methazolamide (Dose: 1×50 mg under fasting conditions) From Measured Data

Parameter	Geometric Mean Arithmetic Mean (CV%) APO-METHAZOLAMIDE	Neptazane[c]	Ratio of Geometric Means (%)[b]
AUC_{0-72} (µg·hr/mL)	577 584 (15)	598 602 (11)	96.5
AUC_I[a] (µg·hr/mL)	— —	— —	—
C_{max} (µg/mL)	11.1 11.4 (23)	11.1 11.2 (14)	100
T_{max} (hr)	— 4.79 (93)	— 4.28 (160)	—
$t_{1/2}$ (hr)[a]	— —	— —	—

[a] The determination of AUC_I and $t_{1/2}$ is not necessary because methazolamide is a drug with a long half-life (>24 hours).
[b] Based on the least squares estimate.
[c] Neptazane is manufactured by Wyeth-Ayerst Canada Inc., and was purchased in Canada.

INDICATIONS: Adjunctive treatment of chronic simple (open-angle) glaucoma, secondary glaucoma and preoperatively in acute angle closure glaucoma, where delay of surgery is desired in order to lower intraocular pressure.

CONTRAINDICATIONS: Severe or absolute glaucoma and chronic noncongestive angle-closure glaucoma. It is of doubtful use in glaucoma due to severe peripheral anterior synechiae or haemorrhagic glaucoma.

Methazolamide is contraindicated in patients with adrenocortical insufficiency, hepatic insufficiency, renal insufficiency, or an electrolyte imbalance state such as hyperchloremic acidosis, and sodium and potassium depletion states.

WARNINGS: *Pregnancy:* Studies in rats have demonstrated teratogenic effects (skeletal anomalies) at high doses. There is no evidence of these effects in human beings and no fetal defects have been reported. However, methazolamide should not be used in women of childbearing potential or in pregnancy, especially in the first trimester, unless the benefits to be gained in the control of glaucoma outweigh potential adverse effects.

PRECAUTIONS: Potassium excretion is increased initially, upon administration of methazolamide, and in patients with cirrhosis or hepatic insufficiency could precipitate a hepatic coma. It should be used with caution in patients on steroid therapy because of the potentiality of a hypokalemic state.

Adequate and balanced electrolyte intake is essential in all patients whose concomitant clinical condition may bring about electrolyte imbalance.

The potential for drug accumulation and toxic manifestations exists in patients with renal insufficiency.

In patients with pulmonary obstruction or emphysema where alveolar ventilation may be impaired, methazolamide, which may precipitate or aggravate acidosis, should be used with caution.

Since systemically administered carbonic anhydrase inhibitors may cause hyperglycemia and glycosuria in patients with diabetes mellitus, the drug should be used with caution in these patients.

ADVERSE EFFECTS: Most adverse reactions to methazolamide have been relatively mild in character and disappear upon withdrawal of the drug or adjustment of dosage. They are as follows: anorexia, nausea, vomiting, malaise, fatigue or drowsiness, headache, vertigo, mental confusion, depression. Paresthesias of fingers, toes, hands or feet and, occasionally, at the mucocutaneous junction of the lips, mouth and anus can be experienced. Dose reduction may be required in patients who experience paresthesia following the use of methazolamide. Rarely photosensitivity has been reported.

Adverse reactions common to all sulfonamide derivatives may occur: anaphylaxis, fever, rash (including erythema multiforme, Stevens-Johnson syndrome, toxic necrolysis), crystalluria, renal calculus.

Bone marrow depression, thrombocytopenic purpura, hemolytic anemia, leukopenia, pancytopenia, and agranulocytosis can occur. Baseline and periodic hematological determinations thereafter should be performed for early detection of blood dyscrasias. If significant changes are detected in laboratory parameters, the drug should be discontinued and appropriate therapy instituted.

OVERDOSE:

For management of a suspected drug overdose, CPhA recommends that you contact your **regional Poison Control Centre**. See the *CPS* Directory section for a list of Poison Control Centres.

DOSAGE: The dosage of methazolamide must be adjusted to the patient's requirements and response. The effective therapeutic dose administered in tablet form varies from 50 to 100 mg 2 to 3 times daily. The drug may be used concomitantly with miotic and osmotic agents.

SUPPLIED: Each white, round, biconvex, straight edge tablet, engraved "APO" on one side, scored and engraved "MZ" over "50" on the other, contains: methazolamide 50 mg. Nonmedicinal ingredients: colloidal silicon dioxide, magnesium stearate and methylcellulose. Bottles of 100. Store at room temperature (15 to 30°C), in well closed containers.

Apo®-Misoprostol ℞

misoprostol

Mucosal Protective Agent

Apotex

Date of Preparation: May 28, 2001
Date of Revision: June 14, 2001

PHARMACOLOGY: Misoprostol is a synthetic analogue of prostaglandin E_1. In animals and man, orally administered misoprostol has both gastric antisecretory and mucosal protective effects. Its antisecretory activity is mediated by misoprostol acid binding to specific prostaglandin receptors on gastric parietal cells. The mechanism of the gastrointestinal mucosal protective effect of misoprostol is not as well understood, but is thought to involve the replacement of prostaglandins following their depletion or inhibition of production, the increasing of mucus production, the increasing of bicarbonate secretion in the duodenum, increased mucosal blood flow, decreased vascular permeability, increased cellular proliferation and migration, and the restoration of the gastric potential difference. Studies conducted in animals and clinical trials in humans have demonstrated that misoprostol can protect the gastric mucosa against various irritants such as alcohol, acetylsalicylic acid, naproxen, tolmetin and sodium taurocholate.

Misoprostol is a prodrug for the active de-esterified misoprostol acid. Conversion to misoprostol acid occurs rapidly in the stomach. The misoprostol acid then binds locally to receptors (e.g. on the parietal cells), undergoes additional hydrolysis, is taken up and metabolized by cells lining the stomach or in the liver, or is passed on to the small intestine along with stomach contents.

In a recent cross-over study (1995), a single 200 µg oral dose of misoprostol administered to sixteen fasting, healthy male subjects produced mean C_{max}, AUC (0-24), T_{max} and elimination half-life of misoprostol acid of: 206.5 pg/mL, 141.8 pg·hr/mL, 0.42 hours, and 0.48 hours respectively. The values of these pharmacokinetic parameters differ from those which were obtained from a pilot study conducted in 1984 (as previously reported). Despite the low systemic bioavailability of misoprostol (~7%), misoprostol acid is very potent and even these sub-nanomolar systemic concentrations may elicit prostaglandin-like effects in other tissues. These effects have been associated with diarrhea uterine contractions and menstrual irregularities.

Misoprostol has both local and systemic activity. Although misoprostol systemic $t_{1/2}$ is very short with plasma levels not typically detectable beyond 2 hours, the duration of its activities, e.g. antisecretory properties, in the gastric tissues are greater than 3 but less than 6 hours.

Pharmacokinetic studies in patients with varying degrees of renal impairment showed an approximate doubling of $t_{1/2}$, C_{max}, and AUC compared to normals, but no clear correlation between the degree of impairment and AUC. In subjects over 64 years of age, the AUC for misoprostol acid is increased. No routine dosage adjustment is recommended in older patients or patients with renal impairment, but dosage may need to be reduced if the usual dose is not tolerated.

Comparative Bioavailability: A comparative bioavailability study was performed using healthy human volunteers. The rate and extent of absorption of misoprostol was measured and compared following oral administration of 400 µg (two APO-MISOPROSTOL 200 µg tablets or two Cytotec 200 µg tablets). The results from measured data are summarized in Table 1.

Table 1: APO-MISOPROSTOL

Summary Table of the Comparative Bioavailability Data. Misoprostol (Dose: 400 µg) From Measured Data

Parameter	Geometric Mean Arithmetic Mean (CV%) APO-MISOPROSTOL	Cytotec[c]	Ratio of Geometric Means (%)[b]
AUC_T (pg·hr/mL)	561 585 (33)	588 615 (31)	95.4
AUC_I (pg·hr/mL)	588 610 (31)	614 638 (29)	95.8
C_{max} (pg/mL)	242 267 (48)	251 273 (47)	95.2
T_{max} (hr)[a]	0.97 (120)	0.66 (72)	—
$t_{1/2}$ (hr)[a]	0.88 (49)	0.77 (51)	—

[a] Arithmetic means (CV%).
[b] Based on the least squares estimate.
[c] Cytotec (Searle Canada) was purchased at a Canadian retail pharmacy.

INDICATIONS: APO-MISOPROSTOL (misoprostol) is indicated for the treatment and prevention of NSAID-induced gastroduodenal ulcers. APO-MISOPROSTOL is also indicated for the treatment of duodenal ulcers caused by Peptic Ulcer Disease (PUD).

Patients at high risk of developing NSAID-induced complications and who may require protection include: Patients with a previous history of ulcer disease or a significant gastrointestinal event. Patients over 60 years of age. Patient judged to be at risk because of general poor health, severe concomitant medical disease, or patients who are poor surgical risks. Patients disabled by joint symptoms (e.g. HAQ Disability Index Score >1.5) or those with severe systemic manifestations of arthritis. Patients taking other drugs known to damage or exacerbate damage to the gastrointestinal tract such as corticosteroids or anticoagulants. Patients taking a high dosage or multiple NSAIDs, including those available Over-The-Counter.

The risk of NSAID-induced complications may be highest in the first three months of NSAID therapy.

CONTRAINDICATIONS: Known sensitivity to prostaglandins, prostaglandin analogues, or excipients.

APO-MISOPROSTOL (misoprostol), or misoprostol in any form, should not be used in pregnant women because it induces uterine contractions and therefore has abortifacient potential. Anecdotal reports, primarily from Brazil, of congenital anomalies and reports of fetal death subsequent to misuse of misoprostol as an abortifacient have been received. Uterine perforation has been reported with misuse of misoprostol for cervical ripening or labor induction.

Women of childbearing potential should not be started on APO-MISOPROSTOL until pregnancy is excluded, and should be fully counseled on the importance of adequate contraception while undergoing treatment. If pregnancy is suspected, use of the product should be discontinued.

WARNINGS: Women of childbearing potential should employ adequate contraception (i.e., oral contraceptives or intrauterine devices) while receiving APO-MISOPROSTOL (misoprostol) (see Contraindications).

Lactation: It is unlikely that misoprostol is excreted in human milk since it is rapidly metabolized throughout the body. However, it is not known if the active metabolite (misoprostol acid) is excreted in human milk. Therefore, APO-MISOPROSTOL should not be administered to nursing mothers because the potential excretion of misoprostol acid could cause significant diarrhea in nursing infants.

Children: Safety and effectiveness in patients below the age of 18 have not been established.

PRECAUTIONS: Selection of Patients: Caution should be used when using symptomatology as the sole diagnosis and follow-up procedure, since misoprostol has not been shown to have an effect on gastrointestinal pain or discomfort.

When misoprostol is used for the treatment of ulcers, a positive diagnosis of duodenal ulcer or NSAID-induced gastroduodenal ulcer should be made. The general health of the patient should be considered. Misoprostol is rapidly metabolized by most body tissues to inactive metabolites. Nevertheless, caution should be exercised when patients have impairment of renal or hepatic function.

Diarrhea: Rare instances of profound diarrhea leading to severe dehydration have been reported. Patients with an underlying condition such as irritable bowel disease, or those in whom dehydration, were it to occur, would be dangerous, should be monitored carefully if APO-MISOPROSTOL (misoprostol) is prescribed.

Use in Elderly or Renally Impaired: Considerations for Dosage Adjustment: In subjects over 64 years of age or those who are renally impaired the pharmacokinetics may be affected, but not to a clinically significant degree (see Dosage). No routine dosage adjustment is recommended in older patients or those patients with renal impairment. Dosage may need to be reduced if the usual dose is not tolerated. In patients with renal failure, a starting dose in the low range (100 µg QID) is recommended.

Drug Interactions: No clinically significant drug interactions attributable to misoprostol have been observed to date.

The serum protein binding of misoprostol acid (the active metabolite of misoprostol) was not affected by: indomethacin, ranitidine, digoxin, phenylbutazone, warfarin, diazepam, methyldopa, propranolol, triamterene, cimetidine, acetaminophen, ibuprofen, chlorpropamide, and hydrochlorothiazide.

Salicylic acid (300 µg/mL) lowered the protein binding of misoprostol from 84% to 52%; this is not considered clinically significant since the binding of misoprostol acid is not extensive and its elimination half-life is very short.

In laboratory studies, misoprostol has shown no significant effect on the cytochrome P450 linked hepatic mixed function oxidase system, and therefore should not affect the metabolism of theophylline, warfarin, benzodiazepines or other drugs normally metabolized by this system.

Misoprostol does not interfere with the beneficial effects of NSAIDS on the signs and symptoms of rheumatoid arthritis and osteoarthritis.

Magnesium containing antacids may increase the likelihood of diarrhea.

Some prostaglandins and prostaglandin analogues have the capacity to produce hypotension through peripheral vasodilation. APO-MISOPROSTOL should be used with caution in the presence of disease states where hypotension might precipitate severe complications, e.g., cerebral vascular disease or coronary artery disease.

Epileptic seizures have been reported with prostaglandins and prostaglandin analogues administered by routes other than oral. Therefore, misoprostol tablets should be used in known epileptics only when their epilepsy is adequately controlled and then only when expected benefits outweigh potential risks.

Gastrointestinal bleeding, ulceration and perforation have occurred in NSAID-treated patients receiving misoprostol. Physicians and patients should remain alert for ulceration, even in the absence of gastrointestinal symptoms.

Symptomatic responses to misoprostol do not preclude the presence of gastric malignancy.

Keep APO-MISOPROSTOL out of the reach of children.

ADVERSE EFFECTS: Gastrointestinal: In subjects and patients receiving at least one dose of misoprostol in clinical trials, the most frequent gastrointestinal adverse events were diarrhea (14.6%), abdominal pain (12.7%), nausea (7.3%), flatulence (6.8%), dyspepsia (6.3%), vomiting (2.3%) and constipation (1.7%). The events were usually transient and mild to moderate in severity.

Diarrhea and abdominal pain, when they occurred, usually developed early in the course of therapy, were self limiting and required discontinuation of misoprostol in less than 5% of the patients. Diarrhea is dose related. The incidence of diarrhea can be minimized by reducing the dose of misoprostol, by administering immediately after a meal or with food or milk, and by avoiding co-administration of misoprostol with magnesium-containing antacids.

Gynecological: Women who received misoprostol during clinical trials reported the following gynecological disorders: spotting, uterine cramps, menorrhagia, menstrual disorder, dysmenorrhea and vaginal hemorrhage (including postmenopausal bleeding). The incidence of each of these adverse events in women was <1%. The overall incidence of gynecological disorders was lower in women over 50 years of age.

Elderly: In clinical trials, there were no significant differences in the safety profile of misoprostol in approximately 500 ulcer patients who were 65 years of age or older, compared with younger patients.

Confusion has been reported in a small number of patients in post-marketing surveillance of misoprostol.

Incidence greater than 1%: In clinical trials, the following adverse reactions were reported by more than 1% of the subjects receiving misoprostol: headache and dizziness. However, there were no clinically significant differences between the incidences of these events for misoprostol and placebo.

The profile for adverse reactions with ≥1% incidence was similar for short-term (four to twelve weeks duration) and long-term (up to one year) clinical trials. Therefore, misoprostol may be administered for up to one year without expecting an increase in adverse events. This includes no adverse or unusual change in the morphology of gastric mucosa, as determined by gastric biopsy.

Adverse reactions reported from post-marketing experience are consistent with those reported from clinical trials.

OVERDOSE:

Symptoms: The toxic dose of misoprostol in human beings has not been determined. Cumulative total daily doses of 1600 µg have been tolerated with only symptoms of gastrointestinal discomfort being reported. In animals, the acute toxic effects are similar to those reported for other prostaglandins and prostaglandin analogues: relaxation of smooth muscle, respiratory difficulties, and depression of the central nervous system. Possible clinical signs that may indicate an overdose may include: sedation, tremor, fever, convulsions, dyspnea, abdominal pain and cramping, severe or profound diarrhea, palpitations, hypotension, or bradycardia.

Treatment: Treatment should be symptomatic and supportive.

It is not known if misoprostol acid is dialyzable. However, because misoprostol has a large volume of distribution and is metabolized like a fatty acid, it is unlikely that dialysis would be appropriate treatment for overdosage.

For management of a suspected drug overdose, CPhA recommends that you contact your **regional Poison Control Centre**. See the *CPS* Directory section for a list of Poison Control Centres.

DOSAGE: APO-MISOPROSTOL (misoprostol) should be taken with food or milk. To minimize the risk of diarrhea, magnesium-containing antacids should be avoided. Aluminum-based antacids may be used as needed for relief of heartburn/epigastric pain.

Treatment and Prevention of NSAID-Induced Gastroduodenal Ulcers: The recommended adult oral dose of APO-MISOPROSTOL for the prevention and treatment of NSAID-induced gastroduodenal ulcer is 400 to 800 µg a day in divided doses. NSAIDs should be taken according to the schedule prescribed by the physician. When appropriate, APO-MISOPROSTOL and NSAIDs are to be taken simultaneously. APO-MISOPROSTOL should be taken after a meal or with food or milk.

Treatment of Duodenal Ulcer: The recommended adult oral dose of APO-MISOPROSTOL for duodenal ulcer is 800 µg per day for 4 weeks in two or four equally divided doses (i.e., 200 µg QID or 400 µg BID). The last dose should be taken at bedtime with food. Treatment should be continued for a total of 4 weeks unless healing in less time had been documented by endoscopic examination. In the small number of patients who may not have fully healed after 4 weeks, therapy with APO-MISOPROSTOL may be continued for a further 4 weeks.

Use in Elderly and Renally Impaired: Consideration for Dosage Adjustment: Pharmacokinetic studies in patients with varying degrees of renal impairment showed an approximate doubling of $t_{1/2}$, C_{max} and AUC compared to normals. There was no clear correlation between degree of impairment and AUC. In subjects over 64 years of age, the pharmacokinetics may be affected. In both patient groups, the pharmacokinetic changes are not clinically significant. No routine dosage adjustment is recommended in older patients or those patients with renal impairment. Dosage may need to be reduced if the usual dose is not tolerated. In patients with renal failure, a starting dose in the low range (100 µg QID) is recommended.

INFORMATION FOR THE PATIENT: Published in e-CPS, available by subscription at www.e-cps.ca.

SUPPLIED: 100 µg: Each round, white, flat-faced, beveled-edged tablet, engraved "APO" on one side and "MIS" over "100" on the other side, contains: misoprostol 100 µg. Nonmedicinal ingredients: croscarmellose sodium, hydroxypropyl methylcellulose, magnesium stearate and microcrystalline cellulose. Bottles of 100.

200 µg: Each hexagonal, white, flat-faced, beveled-edged tablet, scored and engraved "MIS" over "200" on one side and "APO" on the other side, contains: misoprostol 200 µg. Nonmedicinal ingredients: croscarmellose sodium, hydroxypropyl methylcellulose, magnesium stearate and microcrystalline cellulose. Bottles of 100.

Store between 15 and 30 °C, protect from humidity. Keep container closed when not in use.

Apo®-Moclobemide Ⓟ

moclobemide

Antidepressant

Apotex

Date of Preparation: August 8, 1997
Date of Revision: March 10, 2009

ACTIONS AND CLINICAL PHARMACOLOGY: Moclobemide is a short-acting, reversible inhibitor of monoamine oxidase type A (RIMA). It is a benzamide derivative which inhibits the deamination of serotonin, noradrenaline and dopamine. This action leads to increased concentrations of these neurotransmitters, which may account for the antidepressant activity of moclobemide.

Monoamine oxidases are currently subclassified into two types, A and B, which differ in their substrate specificity. Moclobemide preferentially inhibits MAO-A; at a 300 mg dose, the inhibition of MAO-A is approximately 80%, while that of MAO-B is approximately 20-30%. The estimated MAO-A inhibition is short-lasting (maximum 24 hours) and reversible.

Pharmacokinetics: Volunteers: General: Following oral administration, moclobemide is 98% absorbed from the gastrointestinal tract. Due to hepatic first pass effect, absolute bioavailability is approximately 55% after single doses, but 90% after multiple doses. The apparent volume of distribution is approximately 1.2 L/kg, indicating extensive tissue distribution.

Moclobemide is extensively metabolized, largely via oxidative reactions on the morpholine moiety of the molecule. While 95% of the administered dose is excreted in the urine, less than 1% of this is in the unchanged form. Active metabolites recovered in vitro or in animal experiments are present only at very low concentrations in the systemic circulation in man. Moclobemide is 50% bound to plasma proteins, mainly to albumin.

The presence of food reduces the rate, but not the extent of moclobemide absorption.

Single Dose: Following the administration of a 100 mg single oral dose of moclobemide to healthy subjects, peak plasma concentrations ranged from 488 ng/mL to 1450 ng/mL (mean C_{max}: 849 ng/mL) and were reached in 0.5 to 3.5 hours (mean T_{max}: 49 min). The elimination half-life is 1.5 hours. Up to 200 mg, the pharmacokinetics of moclobemide are linear. At higher doses, non-linear pharmacokinetics are observed. In a dose range of 400 mg to 1200 mg, maximum plasma concentrations increased and clearance decreased in a non dose-proportional manner. With increasing doses, the elimination half-life also becomes prolonged.

Multiple Dose: During the second week of a 100 mg t.i.d. dosing regimen in healthy subjects, the steady-state trough concentrations of moclobemide ranged between 114 ng/mL and 517 ng/mL. An increase in the dose to 150 mg t.i.d. resulted in a greater than proportional increase in moclobemide steady-state trough concentrations, namely to concentrations ranging between 346 ng/mL and 1828 ng/mL.

Patients: Hepatic Impairment, Single Dose: In patients with liver cirrhosis, the administration of a single 100 mg dose of moclobemide resulted in approximately a three-fold increase in peak plasma concentrations (C_{max}: 1607 ng/mL) and elimination half-life ($t_{½β}$: 4.0 hr), while clearance decreased about four-fold (Cl: 337 mL/min).

Renal Impairment, Single Dose: In patients with renal insufficiency, the administration of a single 100 mg dose of moclobemide did not appreciably alter the pharmacokinetics of the drug, except for an increase in absorption time.

Elderly Patients, Single and Multiple Dose: Following a 100 mg t.i.d. dosing regimen in elderly subjects (65 to 77 years old), C_{max} and AUC values were somewhat higher than in young subjects (21 to 34 years old), namely 1498 versus 950 ng/mL and 5,571 versus 3,102 ng·h/mL, respectively. Clearance in the elderly was reduced (19.7 versus 32.3 L/h).

Slow Metabolisers: Because moclobemide is partially metabolized by polymorphic isozymes (CYP2C19 and CYP2D6), blood levels of the drug can be affected in patients with genetically or drug-induced poor metabolism. Approximately 2% of the Caucasian population and 15% of the Asian population can be genetically phenotyped as slow metabolisers with respect to oxidative hepatic metabolism. It was found that the area under the curve (AUC) measurement in slow metaboliser subjects was approximately 1.5 times greater than in extensive metaboliser subjects for the same dose of moclobemide. This increase is within the normal range of variation (up to two-fold) typically seen in patients.

Comparative Bioavailability: Two comparative bioavailability studies were performed using healthy human volunteers. The rate and extent of absorption of moclobemide was measured and compared after administration of a single oral dose of 1) Apo-Moclobemide or Manerix 150 mg tablets after a 10 hour fast, and 2) Apo-Moclobemide or Manerix 300 mg tablets after a standardized meal. The results are summarized in Table 1 and Table 2.

Table 1: APO-MOCLOBEMIDE

Fasting Study: Summary Table of the Comparative Bioavailability Data. Moclobemide (Dose: 1×150 mg) from Measured Data

Parameter	Geometric Mean Arithmetic Mean (CV%) APO-MOCLOBEMIDE	Manerix[c]	Ratio of Geometric Means (%)[b]	90% CI[b]
AUC_T (ng·hr/mL)	2592 2920 (46)	2671 3053 (49)	97.7	94.2-101.3
AUC_I (ng·hr/mL)	2760 3133 (48)	2840 3275 (52)	97.8	94.2-101.5
C_{max} (ng/mL)	773 836 (39)	748 823 (39)	103.3	93.6-114.1
T_{max} (hr)[a]	2.09 (63)	1.78 (40)	—	—
$t_{½}$ (hr)[a]	1.84 (31)	1.83 (30)	—	—

[a] Arithmetic means (CV%).
[b] Based on the least square estimate of the geometric means.
[c] Manerix (Hoffmann-La Roche Ltd.) was purchased at a Canadian retail pharmacy.

Table 2: APO-MOCLOBEMIDE

Fed Study: Summary Table of the Comparative Bioavailability Data. Moclobemide (Dose: 1×300 mg) from Measured Data

Parameter	Geometric Mean Arithmetic Mean (CV%) APO-MOCLOBEMIDE	Manerix[c]	Ratio of Geometric Means (%)[b]	90% CI[b]
AUC_T (ng·hr/mL)	8144 9189 (50)	7801 8782 (54)	104.3	97.9-111.2
AUC_I (ng·hr/mL)	8708 10121 (59)	8350 9712 (62)	104.2	—
C_{max} (ng/mL)	2065 2179 (32)	1861 1958 (33)	111.0	100.5-122.50
T_{max} (hr)[a]	1.92 (53)	2.25 (44)	—	—
$t_{½}$ (hr)[a]	2.34 (45)	2.35 (45)	—	—

[a] Arithmetic means (CV%).
[b] Based on the least square estimate of the geometric means.
[c] Manerix (Hoffmann-La Roche Ltd.) was purchased at a Canadian retail pharmacy.

INDICATIONS AND CLINICAL USE: APO-MOCLOBEMIDE (moclobemide) is indicated for the symptomatic relief of depressive illness.

CONTRAINDICATIONS: APO-MOCLOBEMIDE (moclobemide) is contraindicated in patients with a known hypersensitivity to moclobemide or any component of the product. As with any other exogenous compound the possibility of hypersensitivity reaction should be considered in susceptible patients. Symptoms of hypersensitivity may include rash and edema. APO-MOCLOBEMIDE is also contraindicated in patients in an acute confusional state.

In a clinical study designed to test the interaction between moclobemide and a tricyclic antidepressant (clomipramine), severe adverse reactions emerged and the study was terminated. Data involving other tricyclic antidepressants are limited. Consequently, the concomitant use of APO-MOCLOBEMIDE and tricyclic antidepressants is contraindicated.

Clinical data are not available on the concomitant use of moclobemide and selective serotonin reuptake inhibitors or conventional MAO inhibitors. Therefore, until such data become available, APO-MOCLOBEMIDE should not be administered in combination with these agents.

Although there is limited experience with the concomitant use of moclobemide and narcotics, death has occurred in patients receiving a conventional MAO inhibitor and meperidine (pethidine) given concomitantly. Moclobemide should not be used in combination with meperidine.

The concomitant use of APO-MOCLOBEMIDE and Mellaril (thioridizine) is contraindicated (see Precautions).

As safety and effectiveness of APO-MOCLOBEMIDE in children below the age of 18 have not been established, pediatric use is not recommended.

PRECAUTIONS: General: The possibility of suicide in depressed patients is inherent in their illness and may persist until remission occurs. Therefore, patients must be carefully supervised during all phases of treatment with APO-MOCLOBEMIDE (moclobemide). Prescriptions in potentially suicidal patients should be written for a limited supply only.

In patients with thyrotoxicosis or pheochromocytoma, conventional MAO-inhibitors may precipitate a hypertensive reaction. Because there are no data available on the use of moclobemide in such patients, caution is advised when prescribing APO-MOCLOBEMIDE to these subjects.
Occupational Hazards: Patients should be cautioned against driving an automobile or performing hazardous tasks until they are certain of the effect that APO-MOCLOBEMIDE has on them.
Pregnancy: Safety of use in pregnancy has not been established. Therefore, APO-MOCLOBEMIDE is not recommended in women who may be pregnant, unless, in the opinion of the physician, the expected benefits to the patient markedly outweigh the possible risk to the fetus.
Lactation: Clinical data suggest that small quantities of moclobemide are excreted in human milk. Therefore, APO-MOCLOBEMIDE is not recommended in nursing mothers unless the anticipated benefits outweigh the potential harm to the infant.
Hepatic Dysfunction: In patients with severe liver dysfunction, the daily dose of APO-MOCLOBEMIDE should be substantially reduced to one-third or one-half of the standard dose (see Actions and Clinical Pharmacology, Pharmacokinetics).
Renal Dysfunction: Single dose pharmacokinetic data suggest that no dosage adjustment may be required in patients with impaired renal function (see Actions and Clinical Pharmacology, Pharmacokinetics). However, multiple dose studies with moclobemide have not been performed in patients with renal dysfunction, therefore, APO-MOCLOBEMIDE should be used with caution in this patient population. In normal volunteers, the absolute bioavailability almost doubles following multiple dosing as compared to a single dose.
Dextromethorphan: Co-administration of moclobemide and dextromethorphan which may be contained in cough and cold medicines is not recommended (see Drug Interactions).
Thioridazine: A study to evaluate the potential of moclobemide to inhibit the cytochrome P-450 isoenzyme CYP2D6 concluded that moclobemide can affect the pharmakokinetics of drugs (such as thioridazine) that are mainly metabolized by CYP2D6. Thioridazine administration results in a dose-dependent prolongation of the QTc interval, which may cause serious ventricular arrhythmias including torsades de pointes-type arrhythmias and sudden death. This risk is expected to increase with moclobemide-induced inhibition of thioridazine metabolism (see Contraindications).
Drug Interactions: Cimetidine: Cimetidine doubles the AUC (area under the plasma concentration-time curve) of moclobemide and is expected to approximately double moclobemide steady-state concentrations.

In patients receiving APO-MOCLOBEMIDE concomitantly with cimetidine, a 50% reduction in the dosage of APO-MOCLOBEMIDE may be necessary.
Tyramine: During studies conducted at the maximum recommended moclobemide dose of 600 mg/day, the mean dose of tyramine required to produce a 30 mm Hg increase in systolic blood pressure was 148+50 mg (76-200 mg) when moclobemide was administered immediately after tyramine. The threshold dose of tyramine was reduced to 84+23 mg (54-112 mg) when the sequence of administration was reversed so that moclobemide was administered one hour before tyramine. These findings indicate that the potentiation of tyramine may be minimized by administering moclobemide after, instead of prior to, a tyramine-enriched meal. There is limited experience in patients who took moclobemide before meals. Most clinical trial protocols specified that the drug be taken immediately after meals. Therefore, patients should be instructed to take APO-MOCLOBEMIDE immediately after meals.

Treatment with APO-MOCLOBEMIDE does not necessitate special dietary restrictions. In clinical studies, it was demonstrated that up to 100 mg tyramine can be safely ingested during treatment with moclobemide 600 mg/day when moclobemide was given after meals. This amount of tyramine, 100 mg, corresponds to 1000 g to 2000 g mild or 200 g strong cheese, or to 70 g Marmite yeast extract.

As a safety measure, patients should be urged to report immediately the abrupt occurrence of any of the following symptoms; occipital headache, palpitations, neck stiffness, tachycardia or bradycardia or other atypical or unusual symptoms not previously experienced.
Other Antidepressants: Concomitant Use: Clinical interaction studies between moclobemide and a tricyclic antidepressant (clomipramine) resulted in severe adverse reactions (see Contraindications). Data involving other tricyclic antidepressants are limited. Therefore, the concomitant use of APO-MOCLOBEMIDE and tricyclic antidepressants is contraindicated.

Clinical data are not available on the concomitant use of moclobemide and selective serotonin re-uptake inhibitors, or conventional monoamine oxidase inhibitors. Therefore, until clinical data becomes available, APO-MOCLOBEMIDE should not be administered in combination with these agents.
Sequential Use: Treatment with a tricyclic antidepressant may be initiated following the discontinuation of moclobemide with a short washout period of no less than two days.

When switching patients from serotonergic antidepressants to a conventional MAO-inhibitor, it is standard practice to allow for a washout period equivalent to at least 4-5 half-lives of the previously administered drug or any active metabolites. This recommendation also applies to APO-MOCLOBEMIDE.
Fluoxetine: An exception is fluoxetine; at least five weeks should elapse between its discontinuation and initiation of treatment with moclobemide.
Buspirone: To date, there is no experience regarding the co-administration of moclobemide and buspirone. Therefore, patients should be carefully monitored should concomitant administration be implemented.
Antipsychotics: In depressed patients with schizophrenic or schizoaffective disorder, psychotic symptoms may be exacerbated during treatment with APO-MOCLOBEMIDE. There is little experience regarding the concomitant use of moclobemide and antipsychotic drugs. Therefore, patients should be carefully monitored should concomitant treatment be undertaken.
Thioridazine: A study to evaluate the potential of moclobemide to inhibit the cytochrome P-450 isoenzyme CYP2D6 concluded that moclobemide can affect the pharmakokinetics of drugs (such as thioridazine) that are mainly metabolized by CYP2D6. Thioridazine administration results in a dose dependent prolongation of the QTc interval, which may cause serious ventricular arrhythmias including torsades de pointes-type arrhythmias and sudden death. This risk is expected to increase with moclobemide-induced inhibition of thioridazine metabolism (see Contraindications).
Alcohol: Excessive alcohol consumption should be avoided. Alcohol interaction studies were performed at blood alcohol concentrations of 0.05%. However, no studies were conducted at blood alcohol concentrations recognized as legally intoxicating.
Anesthetic Agents: While specific data on the use of moclobemide in patients undergoing anesthesia are not available, based on its reversible action and short elimination half-life (see Actions and Clinical Pharmacology), APO-MOCLOBEMIDE should be discontinued no less than two days before the administration of anesthetic agents, especially spinal or local anesthetic agents that contain epinephrine.

In animals, moclobemide has been shown to potentiate the effects of opiates. The combination of moclobemide and meperidine (pethidine) is not recommended (see Contraindications). Other opioid analgesics should be used with extreme caution, if at all, and a dosage adjustment may be necessary for these drugs.
Sympathomimetics: Following multiple oral doses of moclobemide (total dose: 600 mg/day), a phenylephrine-induced increase in systolic blood pressure was potentiated (1.6 times) after intravenous administration. Patients should be advised to avoid the concomitant use of sympathomimetic amines (e.g., amphetamine and ephedrine like compounds contained in many proprietary cold, hay fever or weight-reducing preparations), until further studies have been conducted.
Dextromethorphan: In isolated cases, the co-administration of moclobemide and dextromethorphan resulted in adverse events, including vertigo, tremor, nausea and vomiting. Since cough and cold medicines may contain dextromethorphan, they should not be taken without prior consultation with the physician, such that non-dextromethorphan containing alternatives may be given (see Precautions).
Antihypertensive Agents: Clinical trials with moclobemide have shown inconsistent effects on the blood pressure of hypertensive patients. Therefore, careful monitoring is recommended during initial treatment.

ADVERSE EFFECTS: Table 3 lists the adverse events reported during clinical trials in which 1922 patients were treated with 50-600 mg/day moclobemide for depressive illness. Limited experience in 60 patients treated with 601 to 750 mg/day of moclobemide suggests that the incidence of adverse reactions may increase at higher doses.

Other clinical adverse events with an incidence of <1% in clinical trials, or reported in postmarketing surveillance, are as follows:
Psychiatric: difficulties falling asleep, nightmares/dreams, hallucinations, memory disturbances, confusion, disorientation, delusions, increased depression, excitation/irritability, hypomanic symptoms, aggressive behavior, apathy, tension.
Central and Peripheral Nervous Systems: migraine, extrapyramidal effects, tinnitus, paresthesia, dysarthria.
Gastrointestinal: heartburn, gastritis, meteorism, indigestion.
Cardiovascular: hypertension, bradycardia, extrasystoles, angina/chest pain, phlebitic symptoms, flushing.
Dermatological/Mucocutaneous: exanthema/rash, allergic skin reaction, itching, gingivitis, stomatitis, dry skin, conjunctivitis, pruritus, urticaria.
Genitourinary: disturbances of micturition (dysuria, polyuria, tenesmus) metrorrhagia, prolonged menstruation.
Miscellaneous: general malaise, skeletal/muscular pain, altered taste sensations, hot flushes/cold sensation, photopsia, dyspnea, visual disturbances.

Laboratory Abnormalities: Laboratory examinations were performed in a total of 1401 patients during clinical trials with moclobemide. Reductions were observed in leucocyte, AST and ALT values, however, these reductions were attributed to raised baseline values returning to normal, and were not considered clinically relevant. No other laboratory abnormalities were noted during clinical trials.

In post-market surveillance, there appeared to be a low incidence of raised liver enzymes, without associated clinical sequelae.

Table 3: APO-MOCLOBEMIDE
Clinical Adverse Events >1%

Organ System	Adverse Event	% Moclobemide (n=1922)	% Placebo (n=271)
Central Nervous System	headache, pressure in head	8.0	11.1
	insomnia, sleep disturbances	7.3	4.8
	dizziness	5.1	8.1
	tremor	5.0	3.0
	increased agitation	4.5	2.6
	restlessness, nervousness	4.1	2.6
	sleepiness, somnolence	3.7	5.5
	tiredness, sedation	3.0	4.1
	increased anxiety, acute anxiety state	2.8	2.2
	weakness or faintness	1.2	1.8
Gastrointestinal	nausea	5.2	4.8
	constipation	3.9	3.3
	gastrointestinal pain, epigastric discomfort	2.3	2.6
	sickness	1.9	1.1
	diarrhea	1.8	1.1
	abdominal fullness, abdominal pain	1.6	1.5
	vomiting	1.6	0.4
Cardiovascular	tachycardia, palpitations	3.8	3.3
	hypotension	3.0	0.4
	orthostatic, reactive hypotension	2.3	3.3
Anticholinergic	dry mouth	9.2	10.7
Miscellaneous	sweating	2.4	2.2
	blurred vision	1.8	1.1
	increase/loss of appetite	1.3	1.8

OVERDOSE:
Symptoms: Signs and symptoms of overdosage with moclobemide include nausea, vomiting, drowsiness, disorientation, slurred speech, amnesia, reduced reflexes, agitation, hypertension and convulsions. One patient remained stuporous for 36 hours following an overdose of 1550 mg moclobemide. All abnormal laboratory values and vital signs returned to within normal range 1 to 5 days after overdosage. No organ toxicity was reported.
Treatment: The treatment of overdosage should consist of general supportive measures. Gastric lavage or induction of emesis, activated charcoal and fluid control may be of benefit.

As with other antidepressants, mixed overdoses of moclobemide with other drugs (e.g., agents active on the CNS), could be life-threatening. Serotonergic syndrome and death have been reported after combined overdose of moclobemide and other antidepressants. Therefore, such patients should be closely monitored so that appropriate care and treatment may be given.

For management of a suspected drug overdose, contact your regional Poison Control Centre. See the *CPS* Directory section for a list of Poison Control Centres.

DOSAGE: Note: APO-MOCLOBEMIDE (moclobemide) should always be taken after meals (see Precautions, Drug Interactions).
Usual Adult Dosage: The administration of APO-MOCLOBEMIDE should be initiated at 300 mg daily dose (in 2 divided doses), and increased gradually to a maximum of 600 mg/day if needed, noting carefully the clinical response and any evidence of intolerance. Individual patient response may allow for a reduction of the daily dose. As with other antidepressants, it should be kept in mind that there may be a lag time in therapeutic response. There is no evidence that increasing the dosage rapidly shortens this latent period and may, in fact, increase the incidence of side-effects. Furthermore, because bioavailability of moclobemide has been shown to increase over the first week of dosing (see Actions and Clinical Pharmacology, Pharmacokinetics), the initial daily dose of 300 mg should not be increased until after this first week of therapy.
Liver Dysfunction: When hepatic metabolism is severely impaired by hepatic disease or inhibited by a drug that affects microsomal mixed function oxidase activity (e.g., cimetidine), the daily dose of APO-MOCLOBEMIDE should be reduced to one-third or one-half of the standard dose.
Renal Dysfunction: Single dose pharmacokinetic data suggest that no dosage adjustment may be required in patients with impaired renal function. However, multiple dose studies with moclobemide have not been performed in patients with renal dysfunction, therefore, APO-MOCLOBEMIDE should be used with caution in this patient population. In normal volunteers, the absolute bioavailability almost doubles following multiple dosing as compared to a single dose.
Geriatrics: No dosage adjustments are necessary in elderly patients.
Cimetidine: Cimetidine doubles the AUC (area under the plasma concentration-time curve) of APO-MOCLOBEMIDE and is expected to approximately double moclobemide steady-state concentrations (see Precautions, Drug Interactions).

In patients receiving moclobemide concomitantly with cimetidine, a 50% reduction in the dosage of moclobemide may be necessary.

INFORMATION FOR THE PATIENT: Published in e-CPS, available by subscription at www.e-cps.ca.

SUPPLIED: 100 mg: Each orange, oval, biconvex, film-coated tablet, scored on one side and engraved APO over 100 on the other, contains: moclobemide 100 mg. Nonmedicinal ingredients: carnauba wax, colloidal silicon dioxide, croscarmellose sodium, dextrates, hydroxypropyl methylcellulose, magnesium stearate, polydextrose, polyethylene glycol 3350 (carbowax), red ferric oxide, titanium dioxide and yellow ferric oxide. Bottles of 100. Stable for 24 months. Store at room temperature 15-30°C.
150 mg: Each pale yellow, oval, biconvex, film-coated tablet, scored on one side and engraved APO over 150 on the other, contains: moclobemide 150 mg. Nonmedicinal ingredients: carnauba wax, colloidal silicon dioxide, croscarmellose sodium, dextrates, hydroxypropyl methylcellulose, magnesium stearate, polydextrose, polyethylene glycol 3350 (carbowax), titanium dioxide and yellow ferric oxide. Bottles of 100 and 500. Stable for 24 months. Store at room temperature 15-30°C.
300 mg: Each white, oval, biconvex, film-coated tablet, scored on one side and engraved APO over 300 on the other, contains: moclobemide 300 mg. Nonmedicinal ingredients: colloidal silicon dioxide, croscarmellose sodium, hydroxypropyl cellulose, hydroxypropyl methylcellulose, magnesium stearate, methylcellulose, microcrystalline cellulose, polyethylene glycol and titanium dioxide. Bottles of 100. Stable for 24 months. Store at room temperature 15-30°C.

Apo®-Orciprenaline ℞

orciprenaline sulfate

β2-adrenergic Stimulant—Bronchodilator

Apotex

Date of Preparation: October 31, 1997
Date of Revision: October 26, 2004

PHARMACOLOGY: Orciprenaline sulphate is a bronchodilating agent. The bronchospasm associated with various pulmonary diseases—chronic bronchitis, pulmonary emphysema, bronchial asthma, silicosis, tuberculosis, sarcoidosis and carcinoma of the lung, has been successfully reversed by therapy with orciprenaline sulphate.
Orciprenaline sulphate has the following major characteristics:

1. Pharmacologically, the action of orciprenaline sulphate is one of beta stimulation. Receptor sites in the bronchi and bronchioles are more sensitive to the drug than those in the heart and blood vessels, so that the ratio of bronchodilating to cardiovascular effects is favourable. Consequently, it is usually possible clinically to produce good bronchodilation at dosage levels which are unlikely to cause cardiovascular side effects.
2. The efficacy of the bronchodilator after both oral and inhalation administration has been demonstrated by pulmonary function studies (spirometry, and by measurement of airways resistance by body plethysmography).
3. Rapid onset of action follows administration of orciprenaline sulphate inhalants, and the effect is usually noted immediately. Following oral administration, the effect is usually noted within 30 minutes.
4. The peak effect of bronchodilator activity following orciprenaline sulphate generally occurs within 60 to 90 minutes, and this activity lasts for 3 to 6 hours.
5. Orciprenaline sulphate taken orally potentiates the action of a bronchodilator inhalant administered 90 minutes later, whereas no additive effect occurs when the drugs are given in reverse order.
6. Patients have not developed tolerance to the drug during prolonged therapy.
7. No toxic effects on the liver, kidneys or hematologic system have been reported in the long-term use of orciprenaline sulphate in man.

INDICATIONS: Orciprenaline sulphate has been found useful in the following conditions:

- bronchial asthma
- chronic bronchitis
- pulmonary emphysema

Orciprenaline sulphate is also useful in sarcoidosis, silicosis, carcinoma of the lung and tuberculosis when bronchospasm contributes to the disability.

The efficacy of orciprenaline sulphate has been demonstrated by improvement of flow rates (FEV_1, MMFR, MEFR) and airways resistance measurements (body plethysmography). Repeated measurements of pulmonary function made over a 4-hour period show that orciprenaline sulphate 20 mg orally gives a generally better result regarding duration of action and magnitude of response than placebo, 100 mg methoxyphenamine, 30 mg ephedrine by mouth, or 10 mg isoproterenol sublingually.

The effect of an inhalant bronchodilator may be potentiated by oral administration of 20 mg of orciprenaline sulphate 90 minutes prior to use of the inhalant. No additive effect occurs when the drugs are given in reverse order. The probable reason for this is that a bronchodilator delivered to the lungs via the vascular system (intravenous or oral medication) acts upon bronchioles whether or not they are occluded. Such an effect causes a wider distribution in the lungs of a subsequently given drug, and consequently the bronchodilation is more intense. Knowledge of this interaction is of value when instructing patients in the combined use of oral and inhalant forms of orciprenaline sulphate.

Orciprenaline sulphate may be given orally in dosages ranging from 60 mg to 120 mg daily. **An effective clinical response in adults and children above 12 years can be achieved by 20 mg orciprenaline sulphate 3 times daily, and at this dosage side effects are not significantly different from those following placebo. Orciprenaline sulphate at a dosage of 20 mg 4 times daily is well tolerated and side effects are usually mild.** Only at dosages of 100 mg daily and above, do palpitations and tremulousness become troublesome. If high doses of orciprenaline sulphate are necessary, it may be possible to eliminate the side effects whilst continuing the same total daily dose, by administering 10 mg single doses at more frequent intervals.

The low incidence of side effects together with effective bronchodilation make orciprenaline sulphate acceptable to patients with chronic **bronchial asthma** for continuous use either alone or concurrently with corticosteroids. Some of these patients may be controlled with orciprenaline sulphate as the sole medication, and it may be possible to avoid the use of steroid therapy. In a proportion of individuals who are already taking corticosteroids, it may be possible to withdraw this medication and continue with orciprenaline sulphate alone. However, caution should be observed in this regard as many patients, particularly those with severe bronchial asthma, can be managed satisfactorily only if steroids and bronchodilators are given together.

Prolonged studies have shown that patients with bronchitis and emphysema respond to continuous therapy with orciprenaline sulphate. The frequency and severity of acute attacks decrease, and patients experience relief of wheezing, chest congestion and shortness of breath. A close association is apparent between objective measurements of pulmonary function and the subjective response.

CONTRAINDICATIONS: Known sensitivity to the drug or other sympathomimetic amines. The use of APO-ORCIPRENALINE (orciprenaline sulphate) and other beta stimulators is generally considered to be contraindicated in patients with hypertrophic obstructive cardiomyopathy and cardiac arrhythmias associated with tachycardia.

Beta-blocking agents, e.g., propranolol, effectively antagonize the action of APO-ORCIPRENALINE. Their concomitant use, except in the treatment of accidental overdosage, is therefore contraindicated.

APO-ORCIPRENALINE should not be taken in patients with a history of hypersensitivity to the active ingredient or other components of the product.

WARNINGS: Like other β_2-agonists, APO-ORCIPRENALINE (orciprenaline sulphate) should not be used on a regular daily basis without appropriate concomitant anti-inflammatory therapy (see Dosage).

APO-ORCIPRENALINE should not be administered to pregnant women or to women of childbearing potential unless in the opinion of the physician the expected benefits outweigh the possible risks to the fetus. In rabbits, high oral doses (100 mg/kg) and low subcutaneous doses (0.2 mg/kg) have resulted in malformed offspring in some experiments, but not in others. Studies in the rat, mouse and rhesus monkey have shown no adverse effects on the developing fetus. Other sympathomimetic drugs tested, viz., ephedrine and phenylephrine, produced teratogenic effects in the rabbit when given orally at high doses as did isoproterenol given subcutaneously at low doses. The significance of these findings is not known.

However, clinical evidence presently available from the use of APO-ORCIPRENALINE in pregnancy is limited. β_2-agonists should be used with caution before childbirth in view of their inhibiting effect on uterine contractions.

Care should be taken in patients suffering from myocardial insufficiency, cardiac arrhythmias, recent myocardial infarction, severe organic heart and/or other vascular disorders, hypertension, hyperthyroidism phaeochromocytoma or diabetes mellitus.

Occasional patients have been reported to have developed severe paradoxical airways resistance with repeated excessive use of sympathomimetic inhalation preparations. The cause of this refractory state is unknown. It is advisable that in such instances the use of the preparation be discontinued immediately and alternate therapy instituted since, in the reported cases, the patients did not respond to other forms of therapy until the drug was withdrawn. **Fatalities have been reported following excessive use of isoproterenol inhalation preparations and the exact cause is unknown. Cardiac arrest was noted in several instances.**

Patients should be advised to seek medical aid in the event that they do not respond to their **usual dose** of a sympathomimetic amine aerosol. The failure to respond may be due to retention of viscid bronchial secretions, associated with an allergic or infective exacerbation of the patient's condition. Increased airways resistance on the basis of bronchospasm alone is reversed promptly by bronchodilators and, if this does not occur, a more serious condition should be suspected. Admission to hospital for intensive support of the cardiovascular and respiratory systems may be necessary.

Potentially serious hypokalemia may result from β_2-agonist therapy, mainly from parenteral and nebulized administration. Particular caution is advised in acute severe asthma as this may be potentiated by concomitant treatment with xanthine derivatives, steroids and diuretics; the adverse effects of hypokalemia on cardiac rhythm may be exacerbated by hypoxia. It is recommended that serum potassium levels be monitored in such situations. Hypokalemia will increase the susceptibility of digitalis-treated patients to cardiac arrhythmias.

PRECAUTIONS: If therapy does not produce a significant improvement or if the patient's condition gets worse, medical advice must be sought in order to determine a new plan of treatment. In the case of acute or rapidly worsening dyspnea, a doctor should be consulted immediately.

Increasing use of β_2-agonists to control symptoms of bronchial obstruction, especially administration on a regular basis or in high amounts, indicates deterioration of asthma control. Under these conditions, the patient's therapy plan has to be revised. It is inadequate simply to increase the use of bronchodilators under these circumstances, in particular over extended periods of time (see Dosage).

In acute tests, orciprenaline sulphate has been shown to have minimal effect on blood pressure and pulse. The drug should be used with care, however, in asthmatic or emphysematous patients who also have systemic hypertension, coronary artery disease, acute and recurring congestive heart failure, diabetes mellitus, glaucoma or hyperthyroidism or in patients sensitive to sympathomimetic amines.

Drug Interactions: Concomitant use of orciprenaline sulphate with other sympathomimetic agents is not recommended since the combined use may lead to deleterious cardiovascular effects. If concomitant use is necessary, this should take place only under strict medical supervision.

Extreme care must also be exercised in the concomitant use of orciprenaline sulphate with epinephrine, monoamine oxidase inhibitors or tricyclic antidepressants since the action of beta adrenergic agonists may be enhanced.

Inhalation of halogenated hydrocarbon anaesthetics such as halothane, trichloroethylene and enflurane may increase the susceptibility to the cardiovascular effects of beta-agonists.

Pregnancy: There is no well documented experience in pregnant women. Orciprenaline sulphate should only be used during pregnancy if the potential benefit outweighs the potential risk to the fetus.

Lactation: It is not known whether orciprenaline sulphate is excreted in human milk; therefore, orciprenaline sulphate should be used during nursing only if the potential benefit justifies the possible risk to the newborn.

ADVERSE EFFECTS: In the recommended dosage, the most frequently observed adverse reactions to orciprenaline sulphate include, fine tremor of skeletal muscles, nervousness, headache, dizziness, tachycardia, and palpitations.

As with other beta-mimetics, nausea, vomiting, sweating, weakness and myalgia/muscle cramps may occur. In rare cases decrease in diastolic blood pressure, increase in systolic blood pressure, arrhythmia, particularly after higher doses, may occur.

In rare cases skin reactions or allergic reactions have been reported, especially in hypersensitive patients. There have been isolated cases of anaphylactic or anaphylactoid reactions.

In individual cases psychological alterations have been reported under inhalational therapy with beta-mimetics.

Potentially serious hypokalemia may result from β_2-agonist therapy.

As with use of other inhalation therapy, cough, local irritation, and less common, paradoxical bronchoconstriction have been reported.

OVERDOSE:

Symptoms: The symptoms of overdosage are those of excess beta stimulation including exaggeration of the known pharmacological effects, i.e. any of the symptoms listed under Adverse Effects, the most prominent being tachycardia, palpitation, tremor, hypertension, hypotension, widening of the pulse pressure, anginal pain, arrhythmias, and flushing.

Treatment: Therapy may include administration of sedative, tranquilizers or in severe cases, intensive therapy.

Beta-receptor blockers, preferably $beta_1$-selective, are suitable as specific antidotes; however, a possible increase in bronchial obstruction must be taken into account and the dose should be adjusted carefully in patients suffering from asthma. It has been shown that the beta-blocker propranolol effectively antagonizes the action of orciprenaline sulphate and the use of this agent should be considered under these circumstances.

For management of a suspected drug overdose, CPhA recommends that you contact your **regional Poison Control Centre**. See the *CPS* Directory section for a list of Poison Control Centres.

DOSAGE: Dosage should be individualized, and patient response should be monitored by the prescribing physician on an ongoing basis.

If a previous effective dosage regimen fails to provide the usual relief, medical advice should be sought immediately as this is a sign of seriously worsening asthma that requires reassessment of therapy.

In accordance with the present practice for asthma treatment, concomitant anti-inflammatory therapy should be part of the regimen when a β_2-agonist needs to be used on a regular daily basis.

The following recommended dosages represent general guidelines that are suitable for the majority of patients.

Syrup: Adults: 20 mg (10 mL) t.i.d. or q.i.d.
Children: Ages 4-12: 10 mg (5 mL) t.i.d.
Above 12: 20 mg (10 mL) t.i.d.

INFORMATION FOR THE PATIENT: Published in e-CPS, available by subscription at www.e-cps.ca.

SUPPLIED: Each mL of clear, grape-flavoured syrup contains: orciprenaline sulfate 2 mg. Nonmedicinal ingredients: artificial grape flavour, edetate disodium dihydrate, glycerin, hydroxyethyl cellulose, methylparaben, propylparaben, purified water, sorbitol and sulfuric acid. Amber-coloured bottles of 250 mL. Store at room temperature (15 to 30°C). Protect from light.

Apo®-Pimozide ℞

pimozide

Antipsychotic

Apotex

Date of Preparation: February 14, 2002

PHARMACOLOGY: Pimozide is a diphenylbutylpiperidine derivative with neuroleptic properties that has been found to be useful in the management of chronic schizophrenic patients. It is relatively non-sedating and can be administered in a single daily dosage.

It is assumed that the basic mechanism of action of pimozide is related to its action on central aminergic receptors. It appears to have a selective ability to block central dopaminergic receptors, although it affects noradrenaline turnover at higher doses. The extrapyramidal effects typical of other neuroleptic agents are seen also with pimozide, but it appears to have fewer autonomic effects. As with other neuroleptics, endocrine effects and ECG changes have also been reported with pimozide.

Pharmacokinetics: The peak plasma level of pimozide in man occurs between 3 and 8 hours after administration and plasma levels decrease slowly to about 50% of the peak level at 48 to 72 hours after dosing. In a single-dose study involving healthy volunteers, the mean plasma half-life of tritiated pimozide (total radioactivity) was found to be 29±10 (S.D.) hours. In a repeat-dose study of short duration involving chronic schizophrenics, the mean plasma half-life was 55±20 (S.D.) hours. There was a 13-fold interindividual difference in the area under the serum pimozide concentration-time curve and an equivalent degree of variation in peak serum levels among patients studied. The significance of this is unclear since there are few correlations between plasma levels and clinical findings. In the single-dose study, 19% (range 8 to 32%) of the radioactivity was excreted in urine in 24 hours. Approximately 40 to 50% was excreted in urine and 20% in feces within a week. Negligible amounts were excreted after the 7th day, although labelled material was detected up to 14 days after administration. The main metabolite in both urine and feces is 4-bis (p-fluorophenyl) butyric acid. Unchanged pimozide constitutes at least 50% of the fecal radioactivity but only a very small fraction of the plasma and urinary radioactivity.

Comparative Bioavailability: A comparative bioavailability study was performed using healthy human volunteers. The rate and extent of absorption of pimozide was measured and compared following oral administration of a 4 mg dose of APO-PIMOZIDE (pimozide) 4 mg tablets or ORAP (pimozide) 4 mg tablets, under fasted conditions. The results from measured data are summarized in Table 1.

Table 1: APO-PIMOZIDE

Summary Table of the Comparative Bioavailability Data. Pimozide (Dose: 4 mg) from Measured Data

Parameter	Geometric Mean Arithmetic Mean (CV%)		Ratio of Geometric Means (%)[b]
	APO-PIMOZIDE	Orap[c]	
AUC_{0-72h} (ng·hr/mL)	62.1 70.6 (64)	58.7 66.7 (61)	105.9
AUC_I (ng·hr/mL)	73.1 84.8 (68)	68.9 80.1 (67)	106.2
C_{max} (ng/mL)	2.29 2.50 (49)	2.11 2.31 (49)	108.1
T_{max} (hr)[a]	6.41 (22)	6.96 (38)	—
$t_{½}$ (hr)[a]	25.4 (21)	25.2 (19)	—

[a] Arithmetic means (CV%).
[b] Based on the least squares estimate.
[c] Orap was manufactured by Janssen-Ortho Inc., and was purchased in Canada.

INDICATIONS: APO-PIMOZIDE (pimozide) is indicated in the management of the manifestations of chronic schizophrenia in which the main manifestations do not include excitement, agitation or hyperactivity. Pimozide has relatively little sedative action and can be used as a once-daily medication.

CONTRAINDICATIONS: APO-PIMOZIDE (pimozide) is contraindicated in central nervous system depression, comatose states, liver disorders, renal insufficiency, and blood dyscrasias, and in individuals who have previously displayed hypersensitivity to the drug. It should not be used in depressive disorders or Parkinson's syndrome.

APO-PIMOZIDE therapy is contraindicated in patients with congenital long QT syndrome or with a family history of this syndrome and in patients with a history of cardiac arrhythmias. A pre-treatment ECG is thus recommended to exclude these conditions. In the case of acquired long QT interval, such as associated with concomitant use of drugs known to prolong the QT interval (see Drug Interactions), known hypokalemia or hypomagnesemia, or clinically significant bradycardia, APO-PIMOZIDE tablets should not be used.

The concomitant use of CYP 3A4-inhibiting drugs such as azole antimycotics, antiviral protease inhibitors, macrolide antibiotics and nefazodone is contraindicated. The concomitant use of CYP 2D6-inhibiting drugs such as quinidine is also contraindicated. The inhibition of either or both cytochrome P450 systems may result in the elevation of pimozide blood concentration and increase the possibility of QT-prolongation.

WARNINGS: Increased Psychomotor Activity: Clinical trials with pimozide indicate that it is not effective in, and therefore should not be used in the management of manifestations of chronic schizophrenia in which the main symptoms include agitation, excitement and anxiety.

Cardiac Monitoring: As with other neuroleptics, cases of sudden, unexpected deaths have occurred with pimozide, mainly at doses above 20 mg/day. ECG changes have been reported in association with the use of pimozide (see Adverse Effects), and one possible mechanism for the deaths is prolongation of the QT interval, predisposing patients to ventricular arrhythmia. Periodic assessment of cardiac function, primarily ECG, should be undertaken in those patients receiving pimozide in excess of 16 mg daily. Any indication of repolarization changes, such as prolongation of QT intervals beyond 0.52 seconds in adults, or more than 25% above the patient's original baseline, or T-wave or U-wave changes should be considered a basis for stopping further increases, possibly lowering the dose, and reviewing the need for pimozide. Caution should be exercised if it is necessary to use pimozide in patients with cardiovascular disorders. Electrolyte imbalance, particularly hypokalemia, should be considered a risk factor.

Liver Disease: Caution is advised in patients with liver disease because pimozide is metabolized in the liver.

Tardive Dyskinesia: As with all antipsychotic agents, tardive dyskinesia may appear in some patients on long-term therapy or after drug discontinuation. The syndrome is mainly characterized by rhythmical involuntary movements of the tongue, face, mouth or jaw. The manifestations may be permanent in some patients. The syndrome may be masked when treatment is reinstituted, when the dosage is increased or when a switch is made to a different antipsychotic drug. Treatment should be discontinued as soon as possible.

Neuroleptic Malignant Syndrome: In common with other antipsychotic drugs, pimozide has been associated with neuroleptic malignant syndrome: an idiosyncratic response characterized by hyperthermia, generalised muscle rigidity, autonomic instability, altered consciousness. Hyperthermia is often an early sign of this syndrome. Antipsychotic treatment should be withdrawn immediately and appropriate supportive therapy and careful monitoring instituted.

Hyperpyrexia, not associated with the above symptom complex, has been reported with other antipsychotic drugs.

Withdrawal Emergent Neurological Signs: Generally, patients receiving short-term therapy experience no problems with abrupt discontinuation of antipsychotic drugs. However, some patients on maintenance treatment experience transient dyskinetic signs after abrupt withdrawal. In certain of these cases the dyskinetic movements are indistinguishable from the syndrome described above under "Tardive Dyskinesia" except for duration. It is not known whether gradual withdrawal of antipsychotic drugs will reduce the rate of occurrence of withdrawal emergent neurological signs but, until further evidence becomes available, it seems reasonable to gradually withdraw use of antipsychotic drugs.

In schizophrenia, the response to antipsychotic drug treatment may be delayed. If drugs are withdrawn, recurrence of symptoms may not become apparent for several weeks or months. Acute withdrawal symptoms, including nausea, vomiting, transient dyskinetic signs, and insomnia, have very rarely been described after abrupt cessation of high doses of antipsychotic drugs. Gradual withdrawal is advisable.

Potential for Hypotension: Patients receiving pimozide should be observed for evidence of hypotension. Some individuals, especially the elderly or debilitated, have demonstrated transient hypotension for several hours following drug administration.

PRECAUTIONS: Blood Dyscrasia: Leukopenia, granulocytopenia, agranulocytosis and anemia have been reported occasionally following antipsychotic therapy, notably with phenothiazines. Therefore, the possibility of blood dyscrasias cannot be ruled out in patients receiving treatment with pimozide, and they should be observed for any signs or symptoms of blood dyscrasia.

Anticonvulsants: Since pimozide may lower the convulsive threshold, it should be used with caution in epileptic patients and adequate anticonvulsive medication should be maintained.

Antiemetic Effects: As with other antipsychotics, pimozide has a substantial antiemetic effect. Thus, caution should be exercised in cases where the suppression of nausea and vomiting might hinder the diagnosis of an underlying physical disorder.

Pregnancy: The safety of use of pimozide in pregnancy has not been established. Therefore, it should not be administered to women of child-bearing potential, particularly during the first trimester of pregnancy, unless, in the opinion of the physician, the expected benefits of the drug to the patient outweigh the potential risk to the fetus or child.

Lactation: Pimozide may be excreted in breast milk. If the use of pimozide tablets is considered essential, breast feeding should be discontinued.

Children: Safety and effectiveness in children have not been established, therefore, this drug is not recommended for use in the pediatric age group.

Geriatrics: For recommendations for use in elderly see Dosage.

Occupational Hazards: Effects On Driving Ability And Use Of Machinery: Pimozide may impair alertness, especially at the start of treatment. These effects may be potentiated by alcohol. Patients should be warned of the risks of sedation and advised not to drive or operate machinery during treatment until their susceptibility is known.

Drug Interactions: CNS: Potentiation of the effects of drugs acting on the central nervous system (anesthetics, opiates, alcohol, etc.) as well as atropine and organophosphorous insecticides may occur with the use of pimozide. Both animal and human data indicate that pimozide may block the action of amphetamines. Therefore, concomitant use of the two medications is not recommended.

Levodopa: Pimozide may, in a dose-related way, impair the antiparkinson effect of levodopa.

Antihypertensives: Concomitant administration of antihypertensive agents should be undertaken with caution in view of the fact that other antipsychotics, notably the phenothiazines, have blocked the action of these agents.

Drugs That Inhibit Cytochrome P450: Pimozide is metabolized mainly via the cytochrome P450 subtype 3A4 (CYP 3A4) enzyme system and more discreetly via the CYP 2D6 subtype. In vitro data indicate that especially potent inhibitors of CYP 3A4 enzyme system, such as azole antimycotics, antiviral protease inhibitors, macrolide antibiotics and nefazodone will inhibit the metabolism of pimozide, resulting in markedly elevated plasma levels of pimozide. In vitro data also indicate that quinidine diminishes the CYP 2D6 dependent metabolism of pimozide. Elevated pimozide levels may enhance the risk of QT prolongation.

As CYP 1A2 may also contribute to the metabolism of pimozide tablets, prescribers should be aware of the theoretical potential for drug interactions with inhibitors of this enzymatic system.

Drugs That Prolong QT Interval: Drugs known to prolong the QT interval are also contraindicated. Examples include certain antiarrhythmics, such as those of Class IA (such as quinidine, disopyramide and procainamide) and Class III (such as amiodarone and sotalol), tricyclic antidepressants (such as amitriptyline), certain tetracyclic antidepressants (such as maprotiline), certain other antipsychotic medications (such as phenothiazines, and sertindole), certain antihistamines (such as astemizole and terfenadine), cisapride, bepridil, halofantrine and sparfloxacin.

Particular care should be taken to avoid toxic plasma levels of lithium when this agent is administered together with pimozide, since such toxic levels have also been associated with QT prolongation.

Grapefruit Juice: As grapefruit juice is known to inhibit the metabolism of CYP 3A4 metabolized drugs, concomitant use of grapefruit juice with pimozide tablets should be avoided.

ADVERSE EFFECTS: The following adverse reactions have been reported with pimozide or with other antipsychotic agents:

Extrapyramidal Symptoms: In common with all neuroleptics, extrapyramidal symptoms may occur, i.e. tremor, rigidity, hypersalivation, bradykinesia, akathisia, and acute dystonia. Antiparkinson drugs of the anticholinergic type may be prescribed as required, but should not be prescribed routinely as a preventive measure.

Tardive Dyskinesia: As with all antipsychotic agents, tardive dyskinesia may appear in some patients on long-term therapy or may appear after drug therapy has been discontinued (see Warnings).

Neuroleptic Malignant Syndrome: In common with other antipsychotic drugs, pimozide has been associated with neuroleptic malignant syndrome (see Warnings).

Other CNS Effects: These are occasionally reported and include: insomnia, restlessness, agitation, drowsiness, decreased attention, fatigue and depression, which have been most commonly observed with pimozide. Irritability, tension, jitteriness, excitement, aggressiveness, anxiety, confusion, nightmares and hallucinations have also been recorded. In some instances, aggravation of the patient's psychotic symptoms has occurred. Toxic confusional states and euphoria have been reported with other antipsychotic therapy.

The most commonly reported neurological adverse reactions are extrapyramidal, including parkinsonism. As with most neuroleptics, reports of parkinsonian side effects, such as tremor, rigidity and sialorrhea, are not uncommon. Akathisia occurs relatively frequently, but can usually be managed by reducing the dosage of pimozide or by the concomitant administration of an antiparkinsonian agent.

Dystonic reactions have been reported, the most common being torticollis, which is generally accom-panied by oro-facial symptoms, and in some instances, oculogyric crises, as well as spasms of the face, tongue and jaw. Mouth and throat area dyskinesias, trismus, dysarthria, muscle cramps and athetoid movements have also been observed occasionally. In addition, dizziness or vertigo, weakness, excessive sweating, body temperature disregulation, headache, EEG changes, and an increased incidence of epileptic seizures have been reported, and in association with other antipsychotics, opisthotonus, hyperreflexia and grand mal convulsions.

Autonomic Effects: Autonomic adverse reactions that have occurred with pimozide are dry mouth, blurred vision, difficulty with accommodation, urinary retention, and urinary and fecal incontinence. Nasal congestion, paralytic ileus and reversed epinephrine effect have been reported with the use of other antipsychotics.

Cardiovascular Effects: Hypotension, tachycardia and fluctuations in blood pressure have been noted with pimozide. Hypertension has occasionally occurred. QT interval prolongation and/or ventricular arrhythmias have very rarely been reported, and predominantly with high doses and in predisposed patients.

Gastrointestinal Effects: anorexia, nausea and/or vomiting, constipation, diarrhea, and abdominal cramps or pain have been observed in some patients receiving pimozide.

Endocrine Effects: Hormonal effects of antipsychotic neuroleptic drugs include hyperprolactinemia, which may cause galactorrhea, gynecomastia, oligomenorrhea or amenorrhea and impotence. Very rarely, cases of hyponatremia due to either Syndrome of Inappropriate Antidiuretic Hormone (SIADH) secretion or psychogenic polydipsia, have been reported.

Miscellaneous: Cases of urticaria and erythematous rash have been reported with pimozide, as well as instances of severe edema, generally limited to the facial area.

Fever, laryngeal edema, angioneurotic edema, asthma, anaphylactoid reactions, hyperpyrexis, obstructive jaundice, biliary stasis, photosensitivity, eczema, exfoliative dermatitis, maculopapular and acneiform reactions, and alopecia have been reported in association with the use of other antipsychotics. Blood dyscrasias (agranulocytosis, leukopenia, granulocytopenia, pancytopenia, thrombocytopenic purpura, eosinophilia, anemia, and aplastic anemia) have also occurred.

Cerebral edema, peripheral edema and altered cerebrospinal fluid proteins have been observed with other antipsychotic agents.

Since a peculiar skin-eye syndrome has been recognized as a side effect following long-term treatment with certain phenothiazines, the possibility of this side effect occurring with pimozide cannot be excluded. This reaction is marked by progressive pigmentation of areas of skin or conjunctivae and may be accompanied by discolouration of the exposed sclera and cornea. Opacities of the anterior lens and cornea described as irregular or stellate in shape have also been reported.

Hyperpyrexia: Hyperpyrexia has been reported with other antipsychotic drugs.

OVERDOSE:

Symptoms: In general, the signs and symptoms of overdosage with pimozide would be an exaggeration of known pharmacologic effects and adverse reactions, the most prominent of which would be extrapyramidal symptoms. The risk of cardiac arrhythmias, possibly associated with QT prolongation should be considered. If these arrhythmias are severe, they can be associated with hypotension and circulatory collapse.

Treatment: There is no specific antidote for pimozide. In the event of overdosage, gastric lavage, establishment of a patent airway and, if necessary, mechanically-assisted respiration are advised. Electrocardiographic monitoring should commence immediately and continue until the ECG parameters are within the normal range. Hypotension and circulatory collapse may be counteracted by use of intravenous fluids, plasma, or concentrated albumin, and vasopressor agents such as metaraminol, phenylephrine and norepinephrine. **Epinephrine should not be used.** In case of severe extrapyramidal reactions, antiparkinson medication should be administered. Because of the long half-life of pimozide, patients who take an overdose should be observed for at least 4 days. As with all drugs, the physician should consider contacting a poison control center for additional information on the treatment of overdose.

For management of a suspected drug overdose, CPhA recommends that you contact your **regional Poison Control Centre**. See the *CPS* Directory section for a list of Poison Control Centres.

DOSAGE: A single morning dose is recommended for all patients.

Adults: The initial recommended dose in patients with chronic schizophrenia for whom pimozide might be indicated is 2 to 4 mg once daily, with weekly increments of 2 to 4 mg until a satisfactory level of therapeutic effect is attained or excessive adverse effects occur. The average maintenance dose is 6 mg daily with the usual range of 2 to 12 mg per day. Daily doses above 20 mg are not recommended.

Geriatrics: The maintenance dose is the same as in adults but it is recommended to start with half of the adult starting dose.

SUPPLIED: 2 mg: Each round, white, flat-faced, bevelled-edge tablet, engraved "APO" on one side and scored and engraved "PIM" over "2" on the other side, contains: pimozide 2 mg. Nonmedicinal ingredients: anhydrous lactose, croscarmellose sodium, and magnesium stearate. Bottles of 100. Store at controlled room temperature (15 to 30°C) in tight containers.

4 mg: Each round, light green, flat-faced, bevelled-edge tablet, engraved "APO" on one side and scored and engraved "PIM" over "4" on the other side, contains: pimozide 4 mg. Nonmedicinal ingredients: anhydrous lactose, croscarmellose sodium, D&C Yellow #10 aluminum lake, FD&C Blue #2 aluminum lake, and magnesium stearate. Bottles of 100. Store at controlled room temperature (15 to 30°C) in tight containers.

Apo®-Prazo ℞
prazosin HCl
Antihypertensive

Apotex

Date of Preparation: April 30, 1990
Date of Revision: December 8, 1997

PHARMACOLOGY: Prazosin causes a decrease in total peripheral resistance. Animal studies suggest that the vasodilator effect of prazosin is related to selective blockade of postsynaptic alpha$_1$-adrenoceptors. The results of dog forelimb experiments demonstrate that the peripheral vasodilator effect is confined mainly to the level of the resistance vessels (arterioles). Hemodynamic studies have been carried out in man following acute single dose administration and during the course of long term maintenance therapy. The results confirm that the therapeutic effect is a fall in blood pressure unaccompanied by a clinically significant change in heart rate, renal blood flow and glomerular filtration rate. In patients with hypertension, there is little change in cardiac output. In addition, clinical pharmacology studies have shown that prazosin antagonizes the vasopressor effect of intravenous phenylephrine, an alpha$_1$-agonist.

In man, blood pressure is lowered in both the supine and standing positions. The hypotensive effect of prazosin hydrochloride is greater when the patient is standing, and a mild reflex tachycardia can result. Tolerance has not been observed to develop in long term hypertensive therapy. Rebound elevation of blood pressure does not seem to occur following abrupt cessation of therapy with prazosin.

Following oral administration of prazosin in normal volunteers and hypertensive patients, plasma concentrations reach a peak at about 3 hours with a plasma half-life of 2-3 hours. The drug is highly bound to plasma protein (97 percent). After chronic administration, no apparent drug accumulation was observed nor were any obvious decreases in plasma concentrations noted. Secondary plasma drug peaks and shoulders suggested probable enterohepatic circulation. Animal studies indicate that prazosin hydrochloride is extensively metabolized, primarily by demethylation and conjugation and excreted (primarily as glucuronide conjugates) mainly via bile and feces. Similar metabolism and excretion has been documented in human studies.

Most clinical studies indicate that chronic therapy with prazosin has little effect on plasma renin activity. However, one report suggests a transient increase in plasma renin activity following the initial dose, as well as attenuated transient increase with subsequent doses.

Comparative Bioavailability: Comparative bioavailability studies were performed using healthy human volunteers. The rate and extent of absorption after a single 2 mg dose of APO-PRAZO 1 mg and MINIPRESS 1 mg tablets was measured and compared. The results are summarized as follows: see Table 1.

Table 1: APO-PRAZO

APO-PRAZO 1 mg Tablets versus MINIPRESS 1 mg Tablets

Parameter	APO-PRAZO (SD) 1 mg	MINIPRESS (SD[a]) 1 mg
AUC_{0-24} (ng·hr/mL)	109 (34.9)	99.8 (32.4)
AUC_{0-Inf} (ng·hr/mL)	111 (36.1)	102 (33.4)
C_{max} (ng/mL)	25.4 (7.5)	21.6 (6.4)
T_{max} (hr)	0.95 (0.40)	1.05 (0.55)
$t_{1/2}$ (hr)	3.95 (0.92)	3.88 (0.96)

[a] SD=Standard Deviation.

The rate and extent of absorption after a single 2 mg dose of APO-PRAZO 2 mg and MINIPRESS 2 mg tablets was measured and compared. The results are summarized as follows: see Table 2.

Table 2: APO-PRAZO

APO-PRAZO 2 mg Tablets versus MINIPRESS 2 mg Tablets

Parameter	APO-PRAZO (SD) 2 mg	MINIPRESS (SD[a]) 2 mg
AUC_{0-24} (ng·hr/mL)	84.7 (27.5)	85.4 (20.0)
AUC_{0-Inf} (ng·hr/mL)	85.9 (27.6)	86.4 (20.3)
C_{max} (ng/mL)	17.7 (7.9)	18.2 (5.1)
T_{max} (hr)	1.59 (1.53)	1.21 (0.77)
$t_{1/2}$ (hr)	3.69 (0.98)	3.59 (0.89)

[a] SD=Standard Deviation.

INDICATIONS: APO-PRAZO (prazosin hydrochloride) is indicated in the treatment of mild to moderate essential hypertension. It is employed in a general treatment program in association with a thiazide diuretic and/or other antihypertensive agents as needed for proper patient response. It may be tried as a sole therapy in those patients in whom treatment with other agents causes adverse effects or is inappropriate.

CONTRAINDICATIONS: APO-PRAZO (prazosin hydrochloride) is contraindicated in patients with a known sensitivity to quinazolines.

WARNINGS: APO-PRAZO (prazosin hydrochloride) may cause syncope and/or excessive hypotension with sudden loss of consciousness. In most cases this is believed to be due to an excessive postural hypotensive effect, although occasionally the syncopal episode has been associated with a bout of severe tachycardia with heart rates of 120-160 beats per minute. The incidence of syncopal episodes is approximately 0.8% when the gradual dose build up described under Dosage is followed. The incidence is higher if the initial dose exceeds 0.5 mg. Syncopal episodes have occurred within 30 to 90 minutes of the initial dose of the drug. They have also been reported in association with dosage increases or the introduction of APO-PRAZO into the regimen of a patient taking another antihypertensive agent or a diuretic. Physicians are therefore advised to limit the initial dose of the drug to 0.5 mg b.i.d. or t.i.d., to subsequently increase the dosage slowly, and to introduce any additional antihypertensive drugs into the patient's regimen with caution.

Patients whose blood pressure is not adequately controlled by high doses of a beta-adrenergic blocking agent such as propranolol may develop acute hypotension when prazosin is added. To minimize the incidence of acute hypotension in such patients, the dose of beta adrenergic blocking agent should be reduced before APO-PRAZO is administered. A low initial dose of APO-PRAZO is also strongly recommended (see Dosage).

If syncope occurs, the patient should be placed in the recumbent position and supportive measures instituted. This adverse effect is self limiting and in most cases does not recur once a steady maintenance level is initiated. Patients should be cautioned to avoid situations where injury could result should syncope occur during APO-PRAZO therapy especially in the initial dose adjustment period.

More common than loss of consciousness are the symptoms often associated with lowering of the blood pressure, namely, dizziness and lightheadedness. The patient should be cautioned about these possible adverse effects and advised what measures to take should they develop.

Pregnancy: Although no teratogenic effects were seen in animal testing, there are no adequate and well controlled studies which establish the safety of APO-PRAZO in pregnant women. Limited uncontrolled use in the management of hypertension in the later stages of pregnancy suggests that prazosin hydrochloride in combination with a beta-blocker can lower blood pressure in pregnant patients. The drug appears to be less effective in patients with proteinuria in whom the addition of i.v. hydralazine was usually required. Accordingly APO-PRAZO should be used during pregnancy only if in the opinion of the physician the potential benefit outweighs potential risk to mother and child.

Lactation: Prazosin has been shown to be excreted in small amounts in human milk. Caution should be exercised when APO-PRAZO is administered to nursing mothers.

Children: APO-PRAZO is not recommended for the treatment of children under the age of twelve years since safe conditions for its use have not been established in this group.

PRECAUTIONS: Use in Patients with Moderate to Severe Grades of Renal Impairment: Because some patients with moderate to severe grades of renal impairment have responded to smaller than usual doses of prazosin hydrochloride, it is recommended that therapy with APO-PRAZO (prazosin hydrochloride) be initiated at 0.5 mg daily and that dose increases be instituted cautiously.

Drug Interactions: Prazosin has been administered without any adverse drug interaction in limited clinical experience to date with the following: (1) cardiac glycosides—digitalis and digoxin; (2) hypoglycemics—insulin, chlorpropamide, tolazamide, and tolbutamide; (3) tranquilizers and sedatives—chlordiazepoxide, diazepam, and phenobarbital; (4) antigout—allopurinol, colchicine, and probenecid; (5) antiarrhythmics—procainamide, propranolol (see Warnings however), and quinidine; and (6) analgesics, antipyretics, and anti-inflammatories—propoxyphene, ASA, indomethacin, and phenylbutazone.

Addition of a diuretic or other antihypertensive agent to prazosin hydrochloride has been shown to cause an additive hypotensive effect (see Warnings and Dosage). An exaggerated hypotensive response has also been observed.

Drug/Laboratory Test Interactions: False positive results may occur in screening tests for pheochromocytoma (urinary vanillylmandelic acid [VMA] and methoxyhydroxyphenyl glysol [MHPG] urinary metabolites of norepinephrine) in patients who are being treated with prazosin. If an elevated VMA is found, APO-PRAZO should be discontinued and the patient retested after a month.

ADVERSE EFFECTS: The most common reactions associated with prazosin therapy are postural dizziness (11%), nausea (9.5%), drowsiness (8.7%), headache (8.4%), palpitations (6.6%), dry mouth (5.6%), weakness (4.6%), and fatigue/malaise (4.5%). In most instances side effects have disappeared with continued therapy or have been tolerated with no decrease in dose of drug. The following reactions have also been observed during prazosin administration.

Gastrointestinal: vomiting, diarrhea, constipation, abdominal discomfort and/or pain.
Cardiovascular: syncope (see Warnings), edema, dyspnea, orthostatic hypotension, tachycardia, faintness.
Central Nervous System: nervousness, vertigo, depression, paresthesia, hallucinations.
Dermatologic: rash, pruritus, alopecia, lichen planus.
Genitourinary: urinary frequency, incontinence, impotence, priapism.
EENT: blurred vision, reddened sclera, epistaxis, tinnitus, nasal congestion.
Hepatic: liver function abnormalities, pancreatitis.
Hematologic: decreased hematocrit/hemoglobin.
Other: diaphoresis, fever, positive ANA titer, arthralgia.

Single reports of pigmentary mottling and serous retinopathy have been reported. In these instances, the exact causal relationship has not been established because the baseline observations were frequently inadequate.

In more specific slit-lamp and funduscopic studies which included adequate baseline examinations, no drug-related abnormal ophthalmological findings have been reported.

Literature reports exist associating prazosin hydrochloride therapy with a worsening of pre-existing narcolepsy. A causal relationship is uncertain in these cases.

OVERDOSE:

Symptoms: A few reports of prazosin hydrochloride overdose have been documented. The most frequently observed symptoms of overdose include hypotension and somnolence.

Accidental ingestion of at least 50 mg of prazosin in a two-year-old child resulted in profound drowsiness and depressed reflexes. No decrease in blood pressure was noted. Recovery was uneventful.

Treatment: Should overdosage lead to hypotension, support of the cardiovascular system is of first importance. Restoration of blood pressure and normalization of heart rate may be accomplished by keeping the patient in the supine position. If necessary, vasopressors should be used. If this measure is inadequate, shock should then be treated with volume expanders. Renal function should be monitored and supported as needed. Laboratory data indicate that prazosin is not dialysable because it is protein bound.

For management of a suspected drug overdose, CPhA recommends that you contact your **regional Poison Control Centre**. See the *CPS* Directory section for a list of Poison Control Centres.

DOSAGE: Note: When titration is to be undertaken using the tablet formulation it will be necessary to split the 1 mg scored tablet to obtain the 0.5 mg starting dose.

It is recommended that the starting dose of 0.5 mg be given with food preferably with the evening meal, at least two or three hours before retiring. The dose should be built up gradually with 0.5 mg being given b.i.d. or t.i.d. for at least three days. Unless adverse effects occur and subject to the blood pressure lowering effect, this dose should be increased to 1 mg given b.i.d. or t.i.d. for at least a further three days.

Thereafter, as determined by the patient's response to the blood pressure lowering effect, the dose should be increased gradually. Response to APO-PRAZO (prazosin hydrochloride) is usually seen within one to fourteen days if it is to occur at any particular dose. When a response is seen, therapy should be continued at that dose until the degree of response has reached the optimum before the next dose increment is added. Incremental increases should be continued until a desired effect is achieved or a maximum daily dose of 20 mg is reached.

The maintenance dose of APO-PRAZO may be given as a twice or three times daily dosage regimen.

In patients with moderate to severe grades of renal impairment, it is recommended that therapy be initiated at 0.5 mg daily and that dose increases be instituted gradually.

Use with Other Drugs: Patients Receiving Diuretic Therapy: The diuretic should be reduced to a maintenance dose level for the particular agent and APO-PRAZO initiated at 0.5 mg h.s. then proceeding to 0.5 mg b.i.d. or t.i.d. After the initial period of observation, the dose of APO-PRAZO should be gradually increased as determined by the patient's response.

Patients Receiving Other Antihypertensive Agents: Because some additive effect is anticipated, the other agent (e.g. propranolol* or other beta-adrenergic blocking agents*, alpha methyldopa, reserpine, clonidine*, etc.) should be reduced and APO-PRAZO initiated at 0.5 mg h.s. then proceeding to 0.5 mg b.i.d. or t.i.d. Subsequent dosage increase should be made depending upon the patient's response.

Patients on APO-PRAZO to Whom Other Antihypertensive Agents Are Added: When adding a diuretic or other antihypertensive agent, the dose of APO-PRAZO should be reduced to 1 mg or 2 mg b.i.d. or t.i.d. and retitration then carried out.

SUPPLIED: 1 mg: Each capsule-shaped, peach, flat-faced with bevelled edge tablet, scored and engraved APO P1 on one side, contains: prazosin HCl equivalent to prazosin 1 mg. Nonmedicinal ingredients: croscarmellose sodium, D&C Yellow #10, FD&C Yellow #6, lactose, magnesium stearate, microcrystalline cellulose and polysorbate 80. Bottles of 100 and 500.

2 mg: Each round, white, biconvex tablet, scored and engraved APO over P2 on one side, contains: prazosin HCl equivalent to prazosin 2 mg. Nonmedicinal ingredients: croscarmellose sodium, lactose, magnesium stearate, microcrystalline cellulose and polysorbate 80. Bottles of 100.

5 mg: Each diamond-shaped, white, biconvex tablet, scored and engraved APO over P5 on one side, contains: prazosin HCl equivalent to prazosin 5 mg. Nonmedicinal ingredients: croscarmellose sodium, lactose, magnesium stearate, microcrystalline cellulose and polysorbate 80. Bottles of 100.

Store at room temperature (15 to 30°C).

* Appropriate precautions should be observed when the dosage of these other antihypertensive agents is reduced.

Apo®-Prochlorazine 🅿

prochlorperazine maleate

Antipsychotic—Antiemetic

Apotex

Date of Preparation: November 11, 1999
Date of Revision: February 13, 2001

PHARMACOLOGY: Prochlorperazine is a piperazine phenothiazine derivative with antipsychotic, antiemetic and weak sedative activity.

Prochlorperazine has actions similar to those of other phenothiazine derivatives but appears to be less sedating and to have a weak propensity for causing hypotension or potentiating the effects of CNS depressants and anesthetics. However, it produces a high incidence of extrapyramidal reactions.

Prochlorperazine is well absorbed from the gastrointestinal tract. Onset of action following oral administration is 30 to 40 minutes; 60 minutes for suppositories and 10 to 20 minutes after i.m. administration. Duration of action for all routes is 3 to 4 hours. Prochlorperazine distributes to most body tissues with high concentrations being distributed into liver and spleen. Prochlorperazine enters the enterohepatic circulation and is excreted chiefly in the feces.

INDICATIONS: In the management of manifestations of psychotic disorders such as agitation, confusion, delusion, tension and anxiety.

It is also effective in controlling nausea and vomiting due to stimulation of the chemoreceptor trigger zone.

In selected patients, prochlorperazine may be of value for the relief of excessive anxiety, accompanied by severe tension and agitation, associated with psychoneurotic or somatic conditions.

CONTRAINDICATIONS: Should not be administered in the presence of circulatory collapse, altered states of consciousness or comatose states, particularly when these are due to intoxication with central depressant drugs (alcohol, hypnotics, narcotics). It is contraindicated in severely depressed patients, in the presence of blood dyscrasias, liver disease, renal insufficiency, pheochromocytoma, or in patients with severe cardiovascular disorders or a history of hypersensitivity to phenothiazine derivatives.

As with other phenothiazines, prochlorperazine is contraindicated in patients with suspected or established subcortical brain damage, with or without hypothalamic damage, since a hyperthermic reaction with temperatures above 40°C may occur, sometimes not until 14 to 16 hours after drug administration.

Phenothiazine compounds should not be used in patients receiving large doses of hypnotics, due to the possibility of potentiation.

Prochlorperazine is contraindicated in children undergoing surgery.

WARNINGS: The antiemetic action of prochlorperazine may mask the signs and symptoms of overdosage of other drugs and may obscure the diagnosis and treatment of other conditions such as brain tumour or intestinal obstruction. Therefore the etiology of nausea and vomiting should be established before using the drug.

Occupational Hazards: The use of this drug may impair the mental and physical abilities required for the performance of potentially hazardous tasks, such as driving a car or operating machinery.

Potentiation of the effects of alcohol may also occur.

Pregnancy: Safety during pregnancy has not been established. Therefore, it is recommended that the drug be given to pregnant patients only when, in the judgement of the physician, the potential benefit to the patient outweighs the possible risk to the fetus.

Children: The drug should not be used in children under 2 years unless potentially life-saving.

The extrapyramidal symptoms which can occur secondary to prochlorperazine may be confused with the CNS signs of an undiagnosed primary disease responsible for the vomiting, e.g. Reye's syndrome or other encephalopathy. The use of prochlorperazine should be avoided in children and adolescents whose signs and symptoms suggest Reye's syndrome.

PRECAUTIONS: The increased incidence of seizures, which occasionally occur in epileptics started on antipsychotic medication, may be controlled by increasing the dosage of their anticonvulsant. Patients with a familial history of seizures or febrile convulsions are more likely to develop seizures than those who have no such history.

Phenothiazines may increase the effects of general anesthetics, opiates, barbiturates, and other CNS depressants and the doses of these drugs should be reduced if administered concomitantly with prochlorperazine.

On long-term therapy, particularly during the first 2 or 3 months, it is advisable to perform periodic liver function tests and blood counts as cholestatic jaundice and blood dyscrasias may occur, necessitating discontinuation of treatment. Renal function should be monitored and, if BUN becomes abnormal, treatment should be discontinued.

To lessen the likelihood of adverse reactions related to drug accumulation, patients on long-term therapy, particularly on high doses, should be evaluated periodically to decide whether the maintenance dosage could be lowered or drug therapy discontinued.

Because of its anticholinergic action, prochlorperazine should be used with great caution in patients with glaucoma or prostatic hypertrophy.

The effects of anticholinergic drugs may be potentiated by prochlorperazine. Paralytic ileus, even resulting in death, may occur, especially in the elderly. Caution should be observed if constipation develops.

Retinal changes, lenticular and corneal deposits and abnormal skin pigmentation have been observed with other phenothiazines and may occur after prolonged therapy. The possibility of persistent tardive dyskinesia should also be borne in mind when patients are under long-term treatment.

Patients receiving prochlorperazine should be cautioned against exposure to extreme heat or organophosphorous insecticides.

Hypotension and ECG changes, particularly non-specific and usually reversible Q and T wave distortions, have been associated with the administration of phenothiazines. Therefore, prochlorperazine should be used with caution in patients with compensated cardiovascular and cerebrovascular disorders.

Unexpected, sudden deaths have occurred in hospitalized patients treated with phenothiazines. Previous brain damage or seizures may predispose. High doses should be avoided in known seizure patients. Sudden exacerbations of psychotic behaviour patterns occurred in several patients shortly before death. Acute fulminating pneumonia or pneumonitis and aspiration of gastric contents were also observed. Therefore, the physician also should keep in mind the possible development of silent pneumonias.

Neuroleptic drugs elevate prolactin levels; the elevation persists during chronic administration. Tissue culture experiments indicate that approximately one-third of human breast cancers are prolactin-dependent in vitro, a factor of potential importance if the prescription of these drugs is contemplated in a patient with a previously detected breast cancer. Although disturbances such as galactorrhea, amenorrhea, gynecomastia and impotence have been reported, the clinical significance of elevated serum prolactin levels is unknown for most patients. An increase in mammary neoplasms has been found in rodents after chronic administration of neuroleptic drugs. Neither clinical studies, nor epidemiologic studies conducted to date, however, have shown an association between chronic administration of these drugs and mammary tumorigenesis; the available evidence is considered too limited to be conclusive at this time.

Withdrawal Emergent Neurological Signs: Abrupt withdrawal after short-term administration of antipsychotic drugs does not generally pose problems. However, transient dyskinetic signs are experienced by some patients on maintenance therapy after abrupt withdrawal. The signs are very similar to those described under Tardive Dyskinesia, except for duration. Although it is not known whether gradual withdrawal of antipsychotic drugs will decrease the incidence of withdrawal emergent neurological signs, gradual withdrawal would appear to be advisable.

Geriatrics: The incidence of adverse reactions may be greater in patients over 55 years of age, since the half-lives of antipsychotic drugs are often prolonged. To minimize this possibility, the maintenance dosage should be reduced to the lowest effective level as soon as possible after initial titration and periodically reviewed.

Since psychiatric syndromes in the elderly can be caused by drugs or organic disease, withdrawal of the precipitating drug or treatment of the medical condition should supersede initiation of antipsychotic medication. These agents should not be used for non-psychiatric conditions for which other drugs are available, since the elderly are especially prone to develop adverse effects from antipsychotic drugs.

Children: Children with an acute febrile illness or suffering from dehydration seem to be much more susceptible than adults to neuromuscular reactions, particularly dystonias. In such patients, the drug should be used under close supervision and at low doses.

ADVERSE EFFECTS: Adverse reactions with different phenothiazines vary in type, frequency, and mechanism of occurrence, i.e., some are dose-related, while others involve individual patient sensitivity. Some adverse reactions may be more likely to occur with greater intensity, in patients with special medical problems.

Not all of the following adverse reactions have been observed with every phenothiazine derivative, but they have been reported with one or more and should be borne in mind when drugs of this class are administered.

Neurological: extrapyramidal reactions including tremor, rigidity, akathisia, dystonia, dyskinesia, oculogyric crises, opisthotonos, hyperreflexia and sialorrhea. EEG changes, disturbed temperature regulation and seizures have also been encountered.

Persistent Tardive Dyskinesia: As with other antipsychotic agents, tardive dyskinesia may occur in patients on long-term therapy or may be observed after drug therapy has been discontinued. The risk seems to be greater in elderly patients on high doses, especially females. The symptoms are persistent and in some patients appear to be irreversible. The syndrome is characterized by rhythmical involuntary movements of the tongue, face, mouth or jaw (e.g., protrusion of tongue, puffing of cheeks, puckering of mouth, chewing movements). Sometimes, these may be accompanied by involuntary movements of the extremities.

There is no known effective treatment for tardive dyskinesia; antiparkinsonian agents usually do not alleviate the symptoms of this syndrome. It is suggested that all antipsychotic agents be discontinued if these symptoms appear. Should it be necessary to reinstitute treatment, or increase the dosage of the agent, or switch to a different antipsychotic agent, the syndrome may be masked. It has been reported that the fine vermicular movements of the tongue may be an early sign of the syndrome and if the medication is stopped at that time, the syndrome may not develop. The physician may be able to reduce the risk of this syndrome by minimizing the unnecessary use of neuroleptic drugs and reducing the dose or discontinuing the drug, if possible, when manifestations of this syndrome are recognized, particularly in patients over the age of 50.

Behavioral: Sleep disturbances, drowsiness, fatigue, insomnia, and depression have been reported and may, in severe cases, necessitate reduction in dosage. As with other phenothiazine derivatives, reactivation or aggravation of psychotic processes may be encountered. Paradoxical effects such as agitation, anxiety, restlessness, excitement and bizarre dreams, have been observed.

Autonomic Nervous System: Dry mouth, nasal congestion, headache, nausea, constipation, tachycardia, hypotension, syncope, dizziness, blurred vision, vomiting, sweating and urinary incontinence have been observed.

Patients with pheochromocytoma, cerebral vascular or renal insufficiency, or a severe cardiac reserve deficiency such as mitral insufficiency appear to be particularly prone to hypotensive reactions with phenothiazine compounds, and should therefore be observed closely when the drug is administered. Should hypotension occur in patients receiving prochlorperazine and a vasopressor agent be required, i.v. levarterenol or phenylephrine should be used, and **not** epinephrine, since phenothiazine derivatives can reverse the pressor effect of the latter drug.

Other autonomic reactions which have occurred with phenothiazines are salivation, polyuria, glaucoma, bladder paralysis, adynamic ileus, and fecal compaction.

Metabolic and Endocrine: Anorexia, menstrual irregularities, impotence, and increased thirst, weight changes, increased appetite, peripheral edema, galactorrhea, gynecomastia, false positive pregnancy tests, and changes in libido have also occurred in patients receiving phenothiazine therapy.

Allergic or Toxic: pruritus, dermatitis, rash, erythema, urticaria, seborrhea, eczema, exfoliative dermatitis, and photosensitivity. The possibility of an anaphylactoid reaction should be borne in mind.

Blood dyscrasias including leukopenia, agranulocytosis, pancytopenia, thrombocytopenic or non-thrombocytopenic purpura, eosinophilia, and anemia, have been associated with phenothiazine therapy. Routine blood counts are therefore advisable during prolonged therapy. If any soreness of the mouth, gums or throat or any symptoms of upper respiratory infection occur and confirmatory leukocyte count indicates cellular depression, therapy should be discontinued and other appropriate measures instituted immediately.

Cholestatic jaundice and biliary stasis may be encountered, particularly during the first months of therapy, and require immediate discontinuation of treatment.

Miscellaneous: The following adverse reactions have been reported in patients receiving phenothiazine derivatives: headache, asthma, laryngeal, cerebral and angioneurotic edema, altered cerebrospinal fluid proteins, systemic lupus erythematosus-like syndrome, hyperpyrexia, ECG and EEG changes and hypotension severe enough to cause fatal cardiac arrest. Skin pigmentation, epithelial keratopathy, lenticular and corneal deposits have been associated with long-term administration.

Sudden, unexpected and unexplained deaths have been reported in hospitalized psychotic patients receiving phenothiazines. Previous brain damage or seizures may be predisposing factors; high doses should be avoided in known seizure patients. Several patients have shown flare-ups of psychotic behaviour patterns shortly before deaths. Autopsy findings have usually revealed acute fulminating pneumonia or pneumonitis, aspiration of gastric contents or intramyocardial lesions.

Potentiation of CNS depressants (barbiturates, narcotics, analgesics, alcohol, antihistamines) may occur.

Neuroleptic Malignant Syndrome: As with other neuroleptic drugs, a symptom complex sometimes referred to as neuroleptic malignant syndrome (NMS) may occur. Cardinal features of NMS are hyperpyrexia, muscle rigidity, altered mental status (including catatonic signs), and evidence of autonomic instability (irregular pulse or blood pressure). Additional signs may include elevated CPK, myoglobinuria (rhabdomyolysis), and acute renal failure. NMS is potentially fatal and requires symptomatic treatment and immediate discontinuation of neuroleptic treatment.

OVERDOSE:

Symptoms: Primarily extrapyramidal reactions, CNS depression which may vary from simple lethargy to coma. Agitation and restlessness may also occur. Other possible manifestations include convulsions, fever and autonomic reactions such as hypotension, dry mouth and ileus.

Treatment: Essentially symptomatic and supportive. Early gastric lavage may be helpful.

Maintain an open airway. If hypotension occurs, the standard measures for managing circulatory shock should be initiated; if a pressor agent is required give levarterenol or phenylephrine and **not** epinephrine as it may further depress the blood pressure. Extrapyramidal reactions should be treated with an antiparkinsonian agent.

Centrally-acting emetics will be ineffective because of prochlorperazine's antiemetic action. Limited experience indicates that phenothiazines are not dialyzable.

For management of a suspected drug overdose, CPhA recommends that you contact your **regional Poison Control Centre**. See the *CPS* Directory section for a list of Poison Control Centres.

DOSAGE: Begin with the lowest recommended dosage. Adjust to response of the individual.

Adults: To control nausea, vomiting or excessive anxiety: usually 5 to 10 mg, 3 or 4 times daily; in mild cases, a single dose of 5 to 10 mg is often adequate. In psychiatry for moderate to severe conditions, the usual starting dosage is 10 mg 3 or 4 times a day; increase dosage gradually by 5 to 10 mg every 2 or 3 days until symptoms are controlled or adverse reactions intervene. Some patients respond satisfactorily on 50 to 75 mg per day. In more severe disturbances it may reach 100 to 150 mg a day. For maintenance therapy, the dosage should be reduced to the minimum effective dose.

Children: Daily dosage, administered in divided doses, should be based on body weight rather than on age, and should not be exceeded. Do not administer to children under 2 years of age or 9 kg of body weight. Occasionally the patient may react to the drug with signs of restlessness and excitement; if this occurs, treatment should be discontinued.

From 9 to 14 kg: 2.5 mg, 1 or 2 times a day, maximum 7.5 mg/day. From 14 to 18 kg: 2.5 mg, 2 or 3 times a day, maximum 10 mg/day. From 18 to 39 kg: 2.5 mg, 3 times a day, or 5 mg 2 times a day, maximum 15 mg/day. Vomiting usually subsides after a single day of treatment. In psychiatry: on the first day of treatment a dosage of 10 mg, in divided doses, should not be exceeded. The maximum total daily dosage reached by gradual increments should not exceed 20 mg for children of 2 to 5 years, and 25 mg for children of 6 to 12 years.

SUPPLIED: 5 mg: Each orange, round, biconvex, film-coated tablet, engraved APO over 5 on one side, contains: prochlorperazine maleate equivalent to prochlorperazine 5 mg. Nonmedicinal ingredients: carnauba wax, croscarmellose sodium, dextrates and magnesium stearate; film coat: D&C Yellow No. 10 Lake, FD&C Yellow No. 6 Lake, hydroxypropyl methylcellulose, polyethylene glycol and titanium dioxide. Bottles of 100.

10 mg: Each orange, round, biconvex, film-coated tablet, engraved APO over 10 on one side, contains: prochlorperazine maleate equivalent to prochlorperazine 10 mg. Nonmedicinal ingredients: carnauba wax, croscarmellose sodium, dextrates and magnesium stearate; film coat: D&C Yellow No. 10 Lake, FD&C Yellow No. 6 Lake, hydroxypropyl methylcellulose, polyethylene glycol and titanium dioxide. Bottles of 100.

Store at room temperature (15 to 30°C). Protect from light.

Apo®-Sotalol 🅿

sotalol HCl

Antiarrhythmic

Apotex

Date of Preparation: January 25, 1996

PHARMACOLOGY: Sotalol hydrochloride has both beta-adrenoreceptor blocking (Vaughan Williams Class II) and cardiac action potential duration prolongation (Vaughan Williams Class III) antiarrhythmic properties. Sotalol hydrochloride is a racemic mixture of d- and l-sotalol. Both isomers have similar Class III antiarrhythmic effects, while the l-isomer is responsible for virtually all of the beta-blocking activity. Sotalol is non-cardioselective and is not associated with partial agonist or membrane stabilizing activity. Whereas significant beta-blockade may occur at oral doses as low as 25 mg, Class III effects are seen at daily doses of 160 mg and above. The antiarrhythmic activity of sotalol appears to be primarily due to the drug's Class III property, based on animal models.

Pharmacologically, in addition to its antiarrhythmic properties, sotalol hydrochloride also has antihypertensive and antianginal properties.

Electrophysiology: Sotalol hydrochloride prolongs the plateau phase of the cardiac action potential in the isolated myocyte, as well as in isolated tissue preparations of ventricular and atrial muscle (Class III activity). In intact animals it slows heart rate, decreases A-V nodal conduction and increases the refractory periods of atrial and ventricular muscle and conduction tissue.

In man, the Class II (beta-blockade) electrophysiological effects of sotalol are manifested by increased sinus cycle length, decreased AV nodal conduction and increased AV nodal refractoriness. The Class III electrophysiological effects in man include prolongation of the atrial and ventricular monophasic action potentials, and effective refractory period prolongation of atrial muscle, ventricular muscle, and atrioventricular accessory pathways (where present) in both the anterograde and retrograde directions. With oral doses of 160 to 640 mg/day, the surface ECG shows dose-related mean increases of 40-100 msec in QT and 10-40 msec in QT_c. No significant alteration in QRS interval is observed.

In a small study (n=25) of patients with implanted defibrillators treated concurrently with sotalol hydrochloride, the average defibrillatory threshold was 6 joules (range 2-15 joules) compared to a mean of 16 joules for a non-randomized comparative group primarily receiving amiodarone.

In a randomized clinical trial [Electrophysiologic Study Versus Electrocardiographic Monitoring (ESVEM) Trial] comparing choice of antiarrhythmic therapy by PES suppression versus Holter monitor selection (in each case followed by treadmill exercise testing) in patients with a history of sustained VT/VF who were also inducible by PES, the effectiveness acutely and chronically of sotalol hydrochloride was compared with 6 other drugs (procainamide, quinidine, mexiletine, propafenone, imipramine and pirmenol). Overall response, limited to first randomized drug, was 39% for sotalol and 30% for the pooled other drugs. Acute response rate for first drug randomized using suppression of PES induction was 36% for sotalol hydrochloride versus a mean of 13% for the other drugs. Using the Holter monitoring endpoint (complete suppression of sustained VT, 90% suppression of NSVT, 80% suppression of VPC pairs, and at least 70% suppression of VPC's), sotalol hydrochloride yielded 41% response versus 45% for the other drugs combined. Among responders placed on long-term therapy identified acutely as effective (by either PES or Holter), sotalol hydrochloride, when compared to the pool of other drugs, had the lowest two-year mortality (13% versus 22%), the lowest two-year VT recurrence rate (30% versus 60%), and the lowest withdrawal rate (38% versus about 75-80%). The most commonly used doses of sotalol hydrochloride in this trial were 320-480 mg/day (66% of patients), with 16% receiving 240 mg/day or less and 18% receiving 640 mg or more.

It cannot be determined, however, in the absence of a controlled comparison of sotalol hydrochloride versus no pharmacologic treatment (e.g., in patients with implanted defibrillators) whether sotalol response causes improved survival or identifies a population with a good prognosis.

Hemodynamics: In a study of systemic hemodynamic function measured invasively in 12 patients with a mean left ventricular (LV) ejection fraction of 37% and ventricular tachycardia (9 sustained and 3 non-sustained), a median dose of 160 mg twice daily of sotalol hydrochloride produced a 28% reduction in heart rate and a 24% decrease in cardiac index at 2 hours post-dosing at steady-state. Concurrently, systemic vascular resistance and stroke volume showed non-significant increases of 25% and 8%, respectively. Pulmonary capillary wedge pressure increased significantly from 6.4 mmHg to 11.8 mmHg in the 11 patients who completed the study. One patient was discontinued because of worsening congestive heart failure. Mean arterial pressure, mean pulmonary artery pressure and stroke work index did not significantly change. Exercise and isoproterenol induced tachycardia are antagonized by sotalol hydrochloride and total peripheral resistance increases by a small amount.

In hypertensive patients, sotalol hydrochloride produces significant reductions in both systolic and diastolic blood pressures. Although sotalol is usually well tolerated hemodynamically, caution should be exercised in patients with marginal cardiac compensation as deterioration in cardiac performance may occur (see Warnings, Congestive Heart Failure).

Pharmacokinetics: In Healthy Subjects: The oral bioavailability of sotalol hydrochloride is 90-100%. After oral administration, peak plasma concentrations are reached in 2.5 to 4 hours, and steady-state plasma concentrations are attained within 2-3 days. Over the dosage range of 160-640 mg/day, sotalol hydrochloride displays dose proportionality with respect to plasma concentrations. Distribution occurs to a central (plasma) and to a peripheral compartment, with a mean elimination half-life of 7-15 hours.

Sotalol hydrochloride does not bind to plasma proteins and is not metabolized. The pharmacokinetics of the d and l enantiomers of sotalol are essentially identical. Sotalol crosses the blood brain barrier poorly. In one study, mean cerebrospinal fluid concentrations following a single oral dose ranged from 5% to 28% of those observed in plasma.

In Renally-Impaired Patients: Excretion is predominantly via the kidney in the unchanged form, and therefore lower doses are necessary in renal impairment (see Dosage and Precautions).

In Hepatically-Impaired Patients: Since sotalol hydrochloride is not subject to first-pass metabolism, patients with hepatic impairment show no alteration in clearance of sotalol hydrochloride.

Geriatrics: Age per se does not significantly alter the pharmacokinetics of sotalol hydrochloride, but impaired renal function in elderly patients can increase the terminal elimination half-life, resulting in increased drug accumulation.

Effect of Food: When sotalol hydrochloride was administered with a standard meal, the absorption was reduced by approximately 20% compared to that in the fasting state.

A blinded, randomized, cross-over, single-dose bioavailability study was conducted in 18 healthy male volunteers to compare the bioavailability of APO-SOTALOL (160 mg) tablets to Sotacor (160 mg) tablets. The pharmacokinetic results are listed in Table 1.

Table 1: APO-SOTALOL

Summary Table of the Sotalol HCl 160 mg Tablet Comparative Bioavailability Data (Dose: 160 mg) (from measured data)

	Geometric Mean[a] Arithmetic Mean[b] (CV%)		
Parameter	**APO-SOTALOL**	**Sotacor**	**Ratio of Means**
AUC_T (ng·hr/mL)	16 237 16 729 (22)	16 523 16 786 (19)	98.3
AUC_I (ng·hr/mL)	16 703 17 186 (22)	16 989 17 241 (18)	98.3
C_{max}(ng/mL)	1414 1459 (24)	1420 1450 (21)	99.5
T_{max} (hr)	3.0 (0.74)	3.4 (0.61)	—
$t_{1/2}$ (hr)	10.8 (1.59)	10.7 (1.67)	—

[a] The geometric means are presented for AUC_T, AUC_I and C_{max} parameters.
[b] For T_{max} and $t_{1/2}$ parameters, the arithmetic means (SD) are presented.

These results demonstrate the bioequivalence of these two formulations.

INDICATIONS:

No antiarrhythmic drug has been shown to reduce the incidence of sudden death in patients with **asymptomatic** ventricular arrhythmias. Most antiarrhythmic drugs have the potential to cause dangerous arrhythmias; some have been shown to be associated with an increased incidence of sudden death. In light of the above, physicians should carefully consider the risks and benefits of antiarrhythmic therapy for all patients with ventricular arrhythmias.

APO-SOTALOL (sotalol hydrochloride) is indicated for the treatment of documented life-threatening ventricular arrhythmias such as sustained ventricular tachycardia. APO-SOTALOL may also be used for the treatment of patients with documented symptomatic ventricular arrhythmias when the symptoms are of sufficient severity to require treatment. Because of the proarrhythmic effects of APO-SOTALOL, its use should be reserved for patients in whom, in the opinion of the physician, the benefit of treatment clearly outweighs the risks.

For patients with sustained ventricular tachycardia, APO-SOTALOL therapy should be initiated in the hospital. Hospitalization may also be required for certain other patients depending on their cardiac status and underlying cardiac disease.

In view of the proarrhythmic effects of APO-SOTALOL, its use in patients with hypertension or angina pectoris is not recommended unless they also require APO-SOTALOL for the treatment of ventricular arrhythmias.

CONTRAINDICATIONS: APO-SOTALOL (sotalol hydrochloride) is contraindicated in patients with bronchial asthma, allergic rhinitis, severe sinus node dysfunction, sinus bradycardia, second and third degree AV block (unless a functioning pacemaker is present), congenital or acquired long QT syndrome, cardiogenic shock, severe or uncontrolled congestive heart failure, hypokalemia, anesthesia with agents that produce myocardial depression and previous evidence of hypersensitivity to sotalol.

WARNINGS: Mortality: The results of the Cardiac Arrhythmia Suppression Trial (CAST) in post-myocardial infarction patients with asymptomatic ventricular arrhythmias showed a significant increase in mortality and in non-fatal cardiac arrest rate in patients treated with encainide or flecainide compared with a matched placebo-treated group. CAST was continued using a revised protocol with the moricizine and placebo arms only. The trial was prematurely terminated because of a trend towards an increase in mortality in the moricizine treated group. The applicability of these results to other populations or other antiarrhythmic agents is uncertain, but at present it is prudent to consider these results when using any antiarrhythmic agent.

Proarrhythmia: APO-SOTALOL (sotalol hydrochloride) may cause new or worsen existing arrhythmias. Such proarrhythmic effects range from an increase in frequency of premature ventricular contractions to the development of more severe ventricular tachycardia, ventricular fibrillation or torsade de pointes. It is therefore essential that each patient administered APO-SOTALOL be evaluated clinically and electrocardiographically prior to, and during therapy to determine whether the response to APO-SOTALOL supports continued treatment. Sotalol hydrochloride, like some antiarrhythmic agents, has been associated with a specific form of arrhythmia, torsade de pointes, which is defined as a polymorphic ventricular tachycardia with prolongation of the QT interval and QRS complexes of changing amplitude that appear to twist around the isoelectric axis. Torsades have been observed more frequently in patients with an elevated baseline QT (>430 msec), on-therapy QT of >500 msec, bradycardia (heart rate <50 bpm), hypokalemia and hypomagnesemia (see Warnings, Electrolyte Disturbances) and congestive heart failure. Because of the variable temporal recurrence of arrhythmias, it is not always possible to distinguish between a new or aggravated arrhythmic event and lack of efficacy. Thus, the incidence of drug-related events cannot be precisely determined and the rates of occurrence provided below must be considered approximations. It should be noted that drug-induced arrhythmias may often not be identified until late after starting the drug because of infrequent monitoring. Due to the possibility of proarrhythmic effects, APO-SOTALOL is not recommended for the treatment of patients with asymptomatic premature contractions (see Indications).

Overall in clinical trials with sotalol, 4.3% of 3257 patients experienced a new or worsened ventricular arrhythmia. Of this 4.3%, new or worsened sustained ventricular tachycardia was reported in approximately 1% of patients, and torsade de pointes in 2.4%. Additionally, in approximately 1% of patients, deaths were considered possibly drug-related; such cases, although difficult to evaluate, may have been associated with proarrhythmic events. In patients with a history of sustained ventricular tachycardia, the incidence of torsade de pointes was 4%, and worsened VT was approximately 1%; in patients with other, less serious, ventricular arrhythmias and supraventricular arrhythmias, the incidence of torsade de pointes was 1% and 1.4%, respectively.

As shown in Table 2, torsade de pointes arrhythmias as well as the prolongation of QT (QT_c) interval were dose related.

Table 2: APO-SOTALOL

Percent Incidence of Torsade de Pointes and Mean QT_c Interval by Dose for Patients with Sustained VT/VF

Daily Dose (mg)	Incidence of Torsade de Pointes	Mean QT_c[a](msec)
80	0 (69)	463 (17)
160	0.5 (832)	467 (181)
320	1.6 (835)	473 (344)
480	4.4 (459)	483 (234)
640	3.7 (324)	490 (185)
>640	5.8 (103)	512 (62)

[a] Highest on-therapy value.
Legend: ( ) Number of patients assessed.

In addition to dose and presence of sustained VT, other risk factors for torsade de pointes were gender (females had a higher incidence), excessive prolongation of the QT_c interval (see Table 3) and history of cardiomegaly or congestive heart failure. Patients with sustained ventricular tachycardia and a history of congestive heart failure appear to have the highest risk for serious proarrhythmia (7%). Of the patients experiencing torsade de pointes, approximately two-thirds spontaneously reverted to their baseline rhythm. The others were either converted electrically (D/C cardioversion or overdrive pacing) or treated with other drugs (see Overdose, Symptoms and Treatment). It is not possible to determine whether some sudden deaths represented episodes of torsade de pointes, but in some instances sudden death did follow a documented episode of torsade de pointes. Although sotalol therapy was discontinued in most patients experiencing torsade de pointes, 17% were continued on a lower dose. Nonetheless, APO-SOTALOL should be used with particular caution if the QT_c is greater than 500 msec on-therapy and serious consideration should be given to reducing the dose or discontinuing therapy when the QT_c exceeds 550 msec. Due to the multiple risk-factors associated with torsade de pointes, however, caution should be exercised regardless of the QT_c interval. Table 3 relates the incidence of torsade de pointes to on-therapy QT_c and change in QT_c from baseline. It should be noted, however, that the highest on-therapy QT_c was in many cases the one obtained at the time of the torsade de pointes event, so that the table overstates the predictive value of a high QT_c.

Table 3: APO-SOTALOL

Relationship Between QT_C Interval Prolongation and Torsade de Pointes

On-Therapy QT_C Interval (msec)	Incidence of Torsade de Pointes	Change in QT_C Interval from Baseline (msec)	Incidence of Torsade de Pointes
<500	1.3% (1787)	<65	1.6% (1516)
500–525	3.4% (236)	65–80	3.2% (158)
525–550	5.6% (125)	80–100	4.1% (146)
>550	10.8% (157)	100–130	5.2% (115)
		>130	7.1% (99)

Legend: ( ) Number of patients assessed.

Proarrhythmic events must be anticipated not only on initiating therapy, but with every upward dose adjustment. Proarrhythmic events most often occur within 7 days of initiating therapy or of an increase in dose; 75% of serious proarrhythmias (torsade de pointes and worsened VT) occurred within 7 days of initiating sotalol therapy, while 60% of such events occurred within 3 days of initiation or a dosage change. Initiating therapy at 80 mg b.i.d. with gradual upward dose titration and appropriate evaluations for efficacy (e.g., PES or Holter) and safety (e.g., QT interval, heart rate and electrolytes) prior to dose escalation should reduce the risk of proarrhythmia. Avoiding excessive accumulation of sotalol in patients with diminished renal function, by appropriate dose reduction, should also reduce the risk of proarrhythmia (see Dosage).

Electrolyte Disturbances: APO-SOTALOL should not be used in patients with hypokalemia or hypomagnesemia prior to correction of such imbalance, as these conditions can exaggerate the degree of QT prolongation and increase the potential for torsade de pointes. The serum electrolytes must be monitored regularly and more frequently if diuretics are used concomitantly. Special attention should be given to electrolyte and acid-base balance in patients experiencing severe or prolonged diarrhea or patients receiving concomitant diuretics.

Congestive Heart Failure: Sympathetic stimulation is a vital component supporting circulatory function in congestive heart failure (CHF), and beta-blockade carries the potential hazard of further depressing myocardial contractility and precipitating more severe failure. Moreover, patients with CHF have a higher risk of torsade de pointes (see Warnings, Proarrhythmia).

In patients with controlled CHF, APO-SOTALOL should be administered cautiously. The positive inotropic action of digitalis may be reduced when the two drugs are used concomitantly. Both digitalis and sotalol slow AV conduction. If cardiac failure continues despite adequate digitalization, APO-SOTALOL should be discontinued.

In patients without a history of heart failure, continued depression of the myocardium over a period of time can, in some cases, lead to cardiac failure. At the first sign of impending heart failure, appropriate therapy must be established and consideration should be given to discontinuation of treatment with APO-SOTALOL.

In clinical trials, new or worsened congestive heart failure (CHF) occurred in 3.3% (n=3257) of patients and led to discontinuation in approximately 1% of patients receiving APO-SOTALOL. The incidence was higher in patients presenting with sustained ventricular tachycardia/fibrillation (4.6%, n=1363), or a prior history of heart failure (7.3%, n=696). Based on a life-table analysis, the one-year incidence of new or worsened CHF was 3% in patients without a prior history and 10% in patients with a prior history of CHF. NYHA Classification was also closely associated to the incidence of new or worsened heart failure in patients receiving sotalol (1.8% in 1395 Class I patients, 4.9% in 1254 Class II patients and 6.1% in 278 Class III or IV patients).

Conduction Disturbances: Excessive prolongation of the QT interval (>550 msec) can promote serious arrhythmias and should be avoided (see Proarrhythmia). Sinus bradycardia (heart rate less than 50 bpm) occurred in 13% of patients receiving sotalol hydrochloride in clinical trials, and led to discontinuation in about 3% of patients. Bradycardia itself increases the risk of torsade de pointes. Sinus pause, sinus arrest and sinus node dysfunction occur in less than 1% of patients. The incidence of 2nd- or 3rd-degree AV block is approximately 1%.

Recent Myocardial Infarction: Caution should be exercised when APO-SOTALOL is given to patients with recent myocardial infarction. Experience in the use of sotalol hydrochloride in the early stage of recovery from acute myocardial infarction is limited and, at least at high initial doses, not reassuring. In the first 2 weeks following acute myocardial infarction, particular caution is advised. Careful dose titration is especially important, particularly in patients with impaired ventricular function.

In a double-blind, placebo-controlled secondary prevention trial in 1456 post-infarction patients who did not necessarily have ventricular arrhythmias, sotalol hydrochloride was given as a non-titrated dose of 320 mg once daily. The results did not suggest an adverse effect on survival; however, there was a suggestion of excess mortality (3% on sotalol hydrochloride versus 2% on placebo) during the first ten days of the trial. In another trial, where high doses of sotalol hydrochloride (320 mg twice daily) were given to a small number of high-risk post-infarction patients (n=17 randomized to sotalol), there were four fatalities and three serious hemodynamic/electrical adverse events within two weeks of initiating sotalol hydrochloride.

Abrupt Cessation of Therapy: Patients should be warned against abrupt interruption or discontinuation of APO-SOTALOL. Hypersensitivity to catecholamines has been observed in patients withdrawn from beta blocker therapy. There have been occasional reports of severe exacerbation of angina pectoris, ventricular arrhythmias and in some cases myocardial infarction following abrupt discontinuation of beta blocker therapy. The last two complications may occur with or without preceding exacerbation of angina pectoris. Therefore, it is prudent when discontinuing chronically administered APO-SOTALOL, particularly in patients with ischemic heart disease, to carefully monitor the patient and to discontinue APO-SOTALOL in a stepwise manner or consider the temporary use of an alternate beta-blocker if appropriate. If possible, the dosage should be gradually reduced over a period of one to two weeks and the patient should be carefully observed. The same frequency of administration should be maintained. If angina markedly worsens or acute coronary insufficiency develops, appropriate therapy should be instituted promptly. Because coronary artery disease is common and may be unrecognized in patients receiving APO-SOTALOL, abrupt discontinuation in patients with arrhythmias may unmask latent coronary insufficiency.

Anaphylaxis: While taking beta blockers, patients with a history of anaphylactic reactions to a variety of allergens may have a more severe reaction on repeated challenge, either accidental, diagnostic or therapeutic.

There may be increased difficulty in treating an allergic type reaction in patients on beta-blockers. In these patients, the reaction may be more severe due to pharmacologic effects of the beta-blockers and problems with fluid changes. Epinephrine should be administered with caution since it may not have its usual effects in the treatment of anaphylaxis. On the one hand, larger doses of epinephrine may be needed to overcome the bronchospasm, while on the other hand, these doses can be associated with excessive alpha adrenergic stimulation with consequent hypertension, reflex bradycardia and heart block and possible potentiation of bronchospasm. Alternatives to the use of large doses of epinephrine include vigorous supportive care such as fluids and the use of beta agonists including parenteral salbutamol or isoproterenol to overcome bronchospasm and norepinephrine to overcome hypotension.

Non-Allergic Bronchospasm (e.g. Chronic Bronchitis and Emphysema): **Patients with bronchospastic diseases should in general not receive beta-blockers.** It is prudent, if APO-SOTALOL is to be administered, to use the smallest effective dose, so that inhibition of bronchodilation produced by endogenous or exogenous catecholamine stimulation of $beta_2$ receptors may be minimized.

Sick Sinus Syndrome: APO-SOTALOL should be used only with extreme caution in patients with sick sinus syndrome associated with symptomatic arrhythmias, because it may cause sinus bradycardia, sinus pauses or sinus arrest.

Skin Rashes and Oculomucocutaneous Syndrome: Various skin rashes and conjunctival xerosis have been reported with beta blockers, including sotalol hydrochloride. A severe syndrome (oculomucocutaneous syndrome) whose signs include conjunctivitis sicca and psoriasiform rashes, otitis, and sclerosing serositis has occurred with the chronic use of one beta-adrenergic-blocking agent (practolol). This syndrome has not been observed with sotalol hydrochloride. Physicians, however, should be alert to the possibility of such reactions and should discontinue treatment in the event that they occur.

Thyrotoxicosis: In patients with thyrotoxicosis, APO-SOTALOL may mask the clinical signs of hyperthyroidism or its complications and give a false impression of improvement. Patients suspected of developing thyrotoxicosis should be managed carefully to avoid abrupt withdrawal of APO-SOTALOL which might be followed by an exacerbation of the symptoms of hyperthyroidism, including thyroid storm.

PRECAUTIONS: Renal Impairment: Renal function tests should be carried out at appropriate intervals. Caution should be observed in patients with impaired renal function since APO-SOTALOL (sotalol hydrochloride) is eliminated mainly via the kidneys through glomerular filtration and to a small degree by tubular secretion. There is a direct relationship between renal function, as measured by serum creatinine or creatinine clearance, and the elimination rate of sotalol. Guidance for dosing in conditions of renal impairment can be found under Dosage.

Diabetes: APO-SOTALOL should be administered with caution to patients with history of spontaneous hypoglycemia or to patients with diabetes (especially labile diabetes) receiving insulin or oral hypoglycemic agents. Beta-adrenergic blockers may mask the premonitory signs and symptoms of acute hypoglycemia; e.g. tachycardia.

Anesthesia: It is not advisable to withdraw beta-adrenoceptor blocking drugs prior to surgery in the majority of patients. However, care should be taken when using APO-SOTALOL with anesthetic agents such as those which may depress the myocardium. Vagal dominance, if it occurs, may be corrected with atropine (1 to 2 mg i.v.).

Some patients receiving beta-adrenoceptor blocking agents have been subject to protracted severe hypotension during anesthesia. Difficulty in restarting the heart and maintaining the heart beat has also been reported.

In emergency surgery, since sotalol is a competitive antagonist at beta-adrenoceptor sites, its effects may be reversed, if required, by sufficient doses of such agonists as isoproterenol or noradrenaline.

Pregnancy: There are no studies in pregnant women. Sotalol hydrochloride has been shown to cross the placenta, and is found in amniotic fluid. There has been a report of subnormal birth weight with sotalol hydrochloride. Therefore, APO-SOTALOL should be used during pregnancy only if the potential benefit outweighs the potential risk.

Lactation: Sotalol has been reported to be present in human milk. Because of the potential for adverse reactions from APO-SOTALOL in nursing infants, a decision should be made whether to discontinue nursing or to discontinue the drug, taking into account the importance of the drug to the mother.

Children: The safety and effectiveness of APO-SOTALOL in children have not been established.

Drug Interactions: Antiarrhythmics: Class Ia antiarrhythmic drugs, such as disopyramide, quinidine and procainamide, and Class III drugs (e.g. amiodarone) are not recommended as concomitant therapy with APO-SOTALOL because of their potential to prolong refractoriness (see Warnings). There is only limited experience with the concomitant use of Class Ib or Ic antiarrhythmics. Additive Class II effects would also be anticipated with the use of other beta-blocking agents concomitantly with APO-SOTALOL.

Drugs Prolonging the QT Interval: APO-SOTALOL should also be given with extreme caution in conjunction with other drugs known to prolong the QT interval, such as Class I and Class III antiarrhythmics, phenothiazines, tricyclic antidepressants, terfenadine, astemizole, erythromycin, lithium and liquid protein diets.

Digoxin: Single and multiple doses of sotalol hydrochloride do not significantly affect serum digoxin levels. Proarrhythmic events were more common in sotalol hydrochloride treated patients also receiving digoxin. It is not clear whether this represents an interaction or is related to the presence of CHF, a known risk factor for proarrhythmia, in the patients receiving digoxin.

Calcium Blocking Drugs: APO-SOTALOL should be administered with caution in conjunction with calcium blocking drugs because of possible synergistic impairment of atrioventricular conduction and of ventricular function. Additionally, concomitant use of these drugs may have additive effects on blood pressure, possibly leading to hypotension.

Catecholamine-Depleting Agents: Concomitant use of catecholamine-depleting drugs, such as reserpine and guanethidine, with a beta-blocker may produce an excessive reduction of resting sympathetic nervous tone. Patients treated with APO-SOTALOL plus a catecholamine-depletor should therefore be closely monitored for evidence of hypotension and/or marked bradycardia, which may produce syncope.

Insulin and Oral Hypoglycemics: Hypoglycemia and hyperglycemia may occur and the dosage of antidiabetic drugs should be adjusted accordingly (see Precautions, Diabetes).

Clonidine: Beta-blocking drugs may potentiate the rebound hypertension sometimes observed after discontinuation of clonidine; therefore, the beta-blocker should be discontinued several days before the gradual withdrawal of clonidine.

Beta-2-Receptor Stimulants: Beta-agonists such as salbutamol, terbutaline and isoprenaline may have to be administered in increased dosages when used concomitantly with APO-SOTALOL.

ADVERSE EFFECTS: During premarketing trials, 3186 patients with cardiac arrhythmias (1363 with sustained ventricular tachycardia) received oral sotalol hydrochloride, of whom 2451 received the drug for at least two weeks. The most important adverse effects are torsade de pointes and other serious new ventricular arrhythmias (see Warnings), occurring at rates of almost 4% and 1%, respectively, in the VT/VF population. Overall, discontinuation because of unacceptable side effects was necessary in 17% of all patients in clinical trials, and in 13% of patients treated for at least two weeks. The most common adverse reactions leading to discontinuation of sotalol hydrochloride are as follows: fatigue 4%, bradycardia (<50 bpm) 3%, dyspnea 3%, proarrhythmia 3%, asthenia 2% and dizziness 2%.

Occasional reports of elevated serum liver enzymes have occurred with sotalol therapy but no cause and effect relationship has been established.

One case of peripheral neuropathy which resolved on discontinuation of sotalol and recurred when the patient was rechallenged with the drug was reported in an early dose tolerance study. Elevated blood glucose levels and increased insulin requirements can occur in diabetic patients.

Table 4 lists as a function of dosage the most common (incidence of 2% or greater) adverse effects, regardless of relationship to therapy and the percent of patients discontinued due to the event, as collected from clinical trials involving 1292 patients with sustained VT/VF.

Table 4: APO-SOTALOL

Incidence (%) of Adverse Events and Discontinuations

	Daily Dose						
Body System	**160 mg (n=832)**	**240 mg (n=263)**	**320 mg (n=835)**	**480 mg (n=459)**	**640 mg (n=324)**	**Any Dose[a] (n=1292)**	**% Patients Discont. (n=1292)**
Body as a Whole							
Infection	1	2	2	2	3	4	<1
Fever	1	2	3	2	2	4	<1
Localized pain	1	1	2	2	2	3	<1
Cardiovascular							
Dyspnea	5	8	11	15	15	21	2
Bradycardia	8	8	9	7	5	16	2
Chest pain	4	3	10	10	14	16	<1
Palpitation	3	3	8	9	12	14	<1
Edema	2	2	5	3	5	8	1
ECG abnormal	4	2	4	2	2	7	1
Hypotension	3	4	3	2	3	6	2
Proarrhythmia	<1	<1	2	4	5	5	3
Syncope	1	1	3	2	5	5	1
Heart failure	2	3	2	2	2	5	1
Presyncope	1	2	2	4	3	4	<1
Peripheral vascular disorder	1	2	1	1	2	3	<1
Cardiovascular disorder	1	<1	2	2	2	3	<1
Vasodilation	1	<1	1	2	1	3	<1
AICD discharge	<1	2	2	2	2	3	<1
Hypertension	<1	1	1	1	2	2	<1
Nervous							
Fatigue	5	8	12	12	13	20	2
Dizziness	7	6	11	11	14	20	1
Asthenia	4	5	7	8	10	13	1
Lightheaded	4	3	6	6	9	12	1
Headache	3	2	4	4	4	8	<1
Sleep problem	1	1	5	5	6	8	<1
Perspiration	1	2	3	4	5	6	<1

(cont'd)

Table 4: APO-SOTALOL *(cont'd)*

Incidence (%) of Adverse Events and Discontinuations

Body System	Daily Dose						
	160 mg (n=832)	240 mg (n=263)	320 mg (n=835)	480 mg (n=459)	640 mg (n=324)	Any Dose[a] (n=1292)	% Patients Discont. (n=1292)
Altered consciousness	2	3	1	2	3	4	<1
Depression	1	2	2	2	3	4	<1
Paresthesia	1	1	2	3	2	4	<1
Anxiety	2	2	2	3	2	4	<1
Mood change	<1	<1	1	3	2	3	<1
Appetite disorder	1	2	2	1	3	3	<1
Stroke	<1	<1	1	1	<1	1	<1
Digestive							
Nausea/vomiting	5	4	4	6	6	10	1
Diarrhea	2	3	3	3	5	7	<1
Dyspepsia	2	3	3	3	3	6	<1
Abdominal pain	<1	<1	2	2	2	3	<1
Colon problem	2	1	1	<1	2	3	<1
Flatulence	1	<1	1	1	2	2	<1
Respiratory							
Pulmonary problem	3	3	5	3	4	8	<1
Upper respiratory tract problem	1	1	3	4	3	5	<1
Asthma	1	<1	1	1	1	2	<1
Urogenital							
Genitourinary disorder	1	0	1	1	2	3	<1
Sexual dysfunction	<1	1	1	1	3	2	<1
Metabolic							
Abnormal lab value	1	2	3	2	1	4	<1
Weight change	1	1	1	<1	2	2	<1
Musculoskeletal							
Extremity pain	2	2	4	5	3	7	<1
Back pain	1	<1	2	2	2	3	<1
Skin and Appendages							
Rash	2	3	2	3	4	5	<1
Hematologic							
Bleeding	1	<1	1	<1	2	2	<1
Special Senses							
Visual problem	1	1	2	4	5	5	<1

[a] Because patients are counted at each dose level tested, the "Any Dose" column cannot be determined by adding across the doses.

Potential Adverse Effects: Marketing experience with sotalol hydrochloride showed an adverse experience profile similar to that described above from clinical trials. Voluntary reports since introduction include rare reports (less than one report per 10 000 patients) of: emotional lability, slightly clouded sensorium, incoordination, vertigo, paralysis, thrombocytopenia, eosinophilia, leukopenia, photosensitivity reaction, fever, pulmonary edema, hyperlipidemia, myalgia, pruritus, reversible alopecia.

Additional adverse effects have been reported with other beta-adrenergic blocking agents.

Central Nervous System: reversible mental depression progressing to catatonia; and acute reversible syndrome characterized by disorientation for time and place, short-term memory loss and decreased performance on neuropsychometrics.

Allergic: fever, combined with aching and sore throat, laryngospasm; respiratory distress.

Hematologic: agranulocytosis; thrombocytopenic or nonthrombocytopenia purpura.

Gastrointestinal: mesenteric arterial thrombosis; ischemic colitis.

Other: Peyronie's disease, Raynaud's phenomenon.

OVERDOSE:

Intentional or accidental overdosage with sotalol hydrochloride has rarely resulted in death.

Symptoms: The most common signs to be expected are bradycardia, congestive heart failure, hypotension, bronchospasm and hypoglycemia. In cases of massive intentional overdosage (2-16 g) with sotalol hydrochloride, the following clinical findings were seen: hypotension, bradycardia, prolongation of QT interval, torsade de pointes, ventricular tachycardia, and premature ventricular complexes.

Treatment: If overdosage occurs, therapy with sotalol hydrochloride should be discontinued. Close monitoring of the electrocardiogram in patients with suspected sotalol intoxication is essential. Because of the lack of protein binding, hemodialysis is useful for reducing sotalol plasma concentrations. Patients should be carefully observed until QT_c intervals are normalized.

Every effort should be made to correct promptly metabolic and electrolyte imbalances which might contribute to the initiation of ventricular arrhythmias (see Warnings).

If required, the following therapeutic measures are suggested:

Bradycardia: atropine, another anticholinergic drug, a beta-adrenergic agonist or transvenous cardiac pacing.

Heart Block (second and third degree): isoproterenol or transvenous cardiac pacemaker.

Congestive Heart Failure: conventional therapy.

Hypotension: (Depending on associated factors) epinephrine rather than isoproterenol or norepinephrine may be useful in addition to atropine and digitalis (see Precautions).

Bronchospasm: aerosolized beta-2-receptor stimulant or aminophylline.

Hypoglycemia: intravenous glucose.

Torsade de pointes: epinephrine, magnesium sulphate, transvenous cardiac pacing, DC cardioversion.

It should be remembered that sotalol hydrochloride is a competitive antagonist of isoproterenol and, hence, large doses of isoproterenol can be expected to reverse many of the effects of excessive doses of APO-SOTALOL. However, the complications of excess isoproterenol should not be overlooked.

For management of a suspected drug overdose, CPhA recommends that you contact your **regional Poison Control Centre**. See the *CPS* Directory section for a list of Poison Control Centres.

DOSAGE: APO-SOTALOL (sotalol hydrochloride), when used for the treatment of documented life-threatening ventricular arrhythmias, should be initiated and dose increased in a hospital with facilities for cardiac rhythm monitoring and assessment (see Indications). APO-SOTALOL should be administered only after appropriate clinical assessment and the dosage of APO-SOTALOL must be individualized on the basis of therapeutic response and tolerance. The usefulness of monitoring plasma level for optimization of therapy has not been established. Proarrhythmic events can occur not only at the initiation of therapy, but also with each upward dosage adjustment.

Dosage of APO-SOTALOL should be adjusted gradually, allowing 2-3 days between dosing increments in order to attain steady-state plasma concentrations and to allow monitoring of QT intervals. Graded dose adjustment will help prevent the use of doses which are higher than necessary to control the arrhythmia. The recommended initial dose is 80 mg twice daily. If needed, this dose may be increased, after appropriate evaluation, to 240 or 320 mg/day. In most patients, a therapeutic response is obtained at a total daily dose of 160 to 320 mg/day, given in two divided doses. Some patients with life-threatening refractory arrhythmias may require doses as high as 480-640 mg/day; however, these doses should only be prescribed when the potential benefit outweighs the increased risk of adverse events, in particular proarrhythmias. Because of the long elimination half-life of sotalol hydrochloride, dosing on more than a twice daily regimen is not usually necessary.

Patients experiencing bradycardia or hypotension on initial administration of APO-SOTALOL should be removed from therapy; APO-SOTALOL may be later reintroduced at a lower dose. A dose reduction may also be advisable to alleviate symptoms of weakness and dizziness in cases where blood pressure remains low after more than a month of therapy.

Renal Impairment: Because sotalol is excreted predominantly in urine and its elimination half-life is prolonged in conditions of renal impairment, a longer duration of dosing is required to reach steady state. The dosing interval of APO-SOTALOL should then be modified, when creatinine clearance is <60 mL/min., as shown in the following table:

Creatinine Clearance (mL/min)	Dosing Interval (hours)
>60	12
30–60	24
10–30	36–48
<10	Dose should be individualized

Dose increases in renal impairment should only be done after administration of at least 5 or 6 doses at appropriate intervals.

Transfer to and from APO-SOTALOL: Based on theoretical considerations rather than experimental data, the following suggestion is made: when transferring patients from another antiarrhythmic drug to APO-SOTALOL or from APO-SOTALOL to another antiarrhythmic agent, allow at least 3 to 4 half-lives to elapse for the drug being discontinued before starting the alternative drug at the usual dosage. In patients where withdrawal of a previous antiarrhythmic agent is likely to produce life-threatening arrhythmias, the physician should consider hospitalizing the patient.

SUPPLIED: 80 mg: Each blue, capsule-shaped, biconvex tablet, identified "APO-80" on one side and scored on the other, contains: sotalol HCl 80 mg. Nonmedicinal ingredients: colloidal silicon dioxide, dextrates, FD&C Blue # 2 aluminum lake, magnesium stearate and methylcellulose. Bottles of 100 and 500. Store at room temperature (15 to 30°C).

160 mg: Each blue, capsule-shaped, biconvex tablet, identified "APO-160" on one side and scored on the other, contains: sotalol HCl 160 mg. Nonmedicinal ingredients: colloidal silicon dioxide, dextrates, FD&C Blue # 2 aluminum lake, magnesium stearate and methylcellulose. Bottles of 100 and 500.

Store at room temperature (15 to 30°C). Protect from light.

Apo®-Tenoxicam

tenoxicam

Anti-inflammatory—Analgesic

Apotex

Date of Preparation: February 14, 1997
Date of Revision: November 8, 2001

PHARMACOLOGY: Tenoxicam is a nonsteroidal anti-inflammatory agent with analgesic and antipyretic properties. Its mechanism of action, as with other nonsteroidal anti-inflammatory agents, is not yet completely known. Tenoxicam is an inhibitor of prostaglandin biosynthesis both in vitro and in vivo (protects mice against arachidonic acid induced toxicity). In vitro tests of leukocyte peroxidase also suggest that tenoxicam may act as a scavenger for active oxygen at the site of inflammation. These effects probably explain in part, the activity of tenoxicam in the treatment of painful inflammatory and degenerative diseases of the musculoskeletal system. Tenoxicam does not act by pituitary-adrenal stimulation.

After 4, 7, 10 or 14 days of culture with tenoxicam (2.4, 12, 48 µg/mL), there was no significant effect on the amount of cartilage proteoglycans synthesized and released into the culture medium of human chondrocytes, as compared to untreated cultures.

In vitro studies have also shown that tenoxicam inhibits the activity of both proteoglycanase and collagenase enzymes obtained from human osteoarthritic cartilage. These in vitro results suggest a positive effect of tenoxicam on the joint cartilage under experimental conditions by slowing down the enhanced catabolism of the osteoarthritic cartilage matrix. The clinical significance of these findings is not yet known and is being investigated.

Pharmacokinetics: Tenoxicam is extensively absorbed following oral administration with an absolute bioavailability of approximately 100%. Following a single oral dose of a 20 mg tablet, peak plasma concentrations (1.46 to 3.31 µg/mL) were reached within one-half hour to six hours (median: 1.25 hours), and the mean half-life was 72±28 hours (range: 32-110 hours) in eight fasted healthy males. When taken with a meal, tenoxicam is absorbed to the same extent but at a slower rate (peak plasma concentration is attained after four hours).

Approximately two-thirds of a single 40 mg oral dose of tenoxicam is excreted in the urine, mainly as inactive 5'hydroxy-tenoxicam (20-30%). Only small amounts of the unchanged drug (0.5%) were found in the urine.

Following multiple doses of 20 mg once daily, steady-state conditions are reached within 10-15 days. Maximum steady-state plasma concentrations fall within the range of 10-15 µg/mL.

An average of 17% (4.8-45.3%) of a 20 mg oral dose is found in the bile as the C-7 or C-8 0-glucuronide of tenoxicam.

In 14 elderly patients suffering from osteoarthritis or rheumatoid arthritis, the mean peak plasma concentration after a single 20 mg dose of tenoxicam was 2.6 µg/mL, and the mean maximum steady-state plasma concentration after multiple dosing was 12.4 µg/mL.

In eight male and four female patients with renal insufficiency (creatinine clearance 6-57 mL/min), peak plasma concentrations were in the range of 1.2-5.2 mg/mL and the half-life of elimination ranged from 30-110 hours after a single 20 mg dose of tenoxicam. Pharmacokinetic parameters in patients with renal insufficiency were not significantly different from those in healthy volunteers.

In four male and two female patients with liver cirrhosis, the mean peak plasma concentration was 2.6 µg/mL and the half-life of elimination ranged between 26-84 hours after a single 20 mg dose of tenoxicam.

Tenoxicam is highly bound to the albumin component of plasma proteins (98-99%).

The sex-dependent difference in the disposition of tenoxicam was investigated. There was no difference in the maximum plasma concentrations, whereas a difference, at the 0.10 level of significance, was seen for the time to reach maximum drug concentrations (3.6 hours for males, 1.52 hours for females), and for the half-life of elimination (72.4 hours for males and 61.8 hours for females).

Total tenoxicam concentrations in synovial fluid were determined in six patients (three male, three female) after receiving a single 40 mg oral dose of tenoxicam. Peak synovial concentrations (1.82 µg/mL) were reached after 10 hours. The area under the synovial fluid tenoxicam concentration-time curve was 40-50% of the area under the plasma tenoxicam concentration-time curve.

Over a 2-week period of observation, six healthy volunteers taking tenoxicam 20 mg daily in a single dose, showed significantly less mean daily fecal blood loss (5.71 mL/week) than they did when taking 1.2-3.0 g of acetylsalicylic acid daily (9.41 mL/week).

Comparative Bioavailability: A standard, randomized, two-way crossover study was conducted in 19 healthy, fasted, adult, male volunteers to evaluate the relative bioavailability of single oral doses (2×20 mg) of APO-TENOXICAM 20 mg tablets manufactured by Apotex Inc. and Mobiflex tablets manufactured by Hoffman-La Roche Limited. The mean pharmacokinetic parameters, corrected for potency, are listed in Table 1.

Table 1: APO-TENOXICAM

APO-TENOXICAM 20 mg Tablets versus Mobiflex Tablets

Parameter	Geometric Mean Arithmetic Mean (CV%)		Ratio of Means (%)
	APO-TENOXICAM	Mobiflex	
AUC_{0-72} (µg·hr/mL)	241 245 (16.9)	233 237 (17.5)	103
AUC_I (µg·hr/mL)	517 565 (44.5)	507 541 (39.5)	102
C_{max} (µg/mL)	5.85 5.91 (15.5)	6.1 6.18 (16.2)	96
T_{max} (hrs)[a]	1.75 (64.9)	1.21 (47.8)	—
$t_{½}$ (hrs)[a]	84.3 (47.7)	83.5 (33.2)	—

[a] The $t_{½}$ and T_{max} parameters are expressed as arithmetic means (CV).

INDICATIONS: APO-TENOXICAM (tenoxicam) is indicated for the symptomatic treatment of rheumatoid arthritis, osteoarthritis, ankylosing spondylitis and extra-articular inflammations such as tendinitis, bursitis and periarthritis of the shoulders or hips.

CONTRAINDICATIONS: APO-TENOXICAM (tenoxicam) should not be administered to patients with active peptic ulcer or active inflammatory diseases of the gastrointestinal tract. APO-TENOXICAM is contraindicated in patients who have shown hypersensitivity to the drug. It should not be used in patients in whom acute asthmatic attacks, urticaria, rhinitis or other allergic manifestations are precipitated by ASA or other nonsteroidal anti-inflammatory agents. Fatal anaphylactoid reactions have occurred in such individuals.

Before anesthesia or surgery, APO-TENOXICAM should not be given to elderly patients, to patients at risk of renal failure, or to patients with increased risk of bleeding, because of an increased risk of acute renal failure and possibility of impaired hemostasis.

WARNINGS: Peptic ulcerations, perforation and gastrointestinal bleeding, sometimes severe and occasionally fatal have been reported during therapy with nonsteroidal anti-inflammatory drugs (NSAIDs) including tenoxicam.

Caution should be exercised when a NSAID such as tenoxicam is used in patients with a history suggestive of peptic ulcer, melena or any gastrointestinal disease. In these cases, the physician must weigh the benefits of treatment against the possible hazards.

Patients taking any NSAID including this drug should be instructed to contact a physician immediately if they experience symptoms or signs suggestive of peptic ulceration or gastrointestinal bleeding. These reactions can occur without warning symptoms or signs and at any time during the treatment.

Elderly, frail and debilitated patients appear to be at higher risk from a variety of adverse reactions from nonsteroidal anti-inflammatory drugs (NSAIDs). As with other nonsteroidal anti-inflammatory drugs, APO-TENOXICAM (tenoxicam) should be used with special caution in these patients.

Pregnancy: The safety of APO-TENOXICAM during pregnancy has not been established and therefore its use during pregnancy is not recommended.

No teratogenic effects were observed in animal reproductive studies. Rats receiving tenoxicam during pregnancy showed delayed delivery.

Lactation: The safety of APO-TENOXICAM during lactation has not been established and therefore its use during lactation is not recommended.

Tenoxicam readily passes into the milk of lactating rats.

Children: APO-TENOXICAM is not recommended for use in patients under 16 years of age, as the dose and indications in this population have not been established.

PRECAUTIONS: Gastrointestinal System: If peptic ulceration or gastrointestinal bleeding occur in patients under treatment with APO-TENOXICAM (tenoxicam), the drug should be immediately withdrawn.

There is no definitive evidence that the concomitant administration of histamine H_2-receptor antagonists and/or antacids will either prevent the occurrence of gastrointestinal side effects or allow continuation of APO-TENOXICAM therapy when and if these adverse reactions appear.

Renal Function: As with other nonsteroidal anti-inflammatory drugs, long-term administration of tenoxicam to animals has resulted in renal papillary necrosis and other abnormal renal pathology. In humans, there have been reports of acute interstitial nephritis with hematuria, proteinuria, and occasionally nephrotic syndrome.

A second form of renal toxicity has been seen in patients with prerenal conditions leading to the reduction in renal blood flow or blood volume, where the renal prostaglandins have a supportive role in the maintenance of renal perfusion. In these patients, administration of a nonsteroidal anti-inflammatory drug may cause a dose-dependent reduction in prostaglandin formation and may precipitate overt renal decompensation. Patients at greatest risk of this reaction are those with impaired renal function, heart failure, liver dysfunction, those taking diuretics, and the elderly. Discontinuation of nonsteroidal anti-inflammatory therapy is usually followed by recovery to the pre-treatment state.

Reversible elevation of BUN and serum creatinine have been reported with tenoxicam. The effect is thought to result from inhibition of renal prostaglandin synthesis resulting in changes in medullary and deep cortical blood flow with an attendant effect on renal function. Patients with impaired renal function or on diuretics, as well as elderly patients and those with congestive heart failure or liver ascites, are more at risk.

During long-term therapy, kidney function should be monitored periodically.

Hepatic Function: As with other nonsteroidal anti-inflammatory drugs, borderline elevations of one or more liver tests may occur. These abnormalities may progress, may remain essentially unchanged, or may be transient with continued therapy. A patient with symptoms and/or signs suggesting liver dysfunction, or in whom an abnormal liver test has occurred, should be evaluated for evidence of the development of more severe hepatic reactions while on therapy with this drug. Severe hepatic reactions including jaundice and cases of fatal hepatitis have been reported with this drug as with other nonsteroidal anti-inflammatory drugs. Although such reactions are rare, if abnormal liver tests persist or worsen, if clinical signs and symptoms consistent with liver disease develop, or if systemic manifestations occur (e.g. eosinophilia, rash, etc.), this drug should be discontinued.

During long-term therapy, liver function tests should be monitored periodically.

Fluid and Electrolyte Balance: Fluid retention and edema have been observed in patients treated with tenoxicam. Therefore, as with many other nonsteroidal anti-inflammatory drugs, the possibility of precipitating congestive heart failure in elderly patients or those with compromised cardiac function should be borne in mind. APO-TENOXICAM should be used in caution in patients with heart failure, hypertension or other conditions predisposing to fluid retention.

With NSAID treatment, there is a potential risk of hyperkalemia particularly in patients with conditions such as diabetes mellitus or renal failure; elderly patients; and patients receiving concomitant therapy with β-adrenergic blockers, angiotensin-converting enzyme inhibitors or some diuretics. Serum electrolytes should be monitored periodically during long-term therapy, especially in those patients at risk.

Hematology: Drugs inhibiting prostaglandin biosynthesis do interfere with platelet function to some degree; therefore, patients who may be adversely affected by such an action should be carefully observed when APO-TENOXICAM is administered.

Blood dyscrasias associated with the use of nonsteroidal anti-inflammatory drugs are rare, but could be with severe consequences.

Infection: In common with other anti-inflammatory drugs, APO-TENOXICAM may mask the usual signs of infection.

Ophthalmology: Blurred and/or diminished vision has been reported with the use of tenoxicam and other nonsteroidal anti-inflammatory drugs. If such symptoms develop, this drug should be discontinued and an ophthalmologic examination performed; ophthalmic examination should be carried out at periodic intervals in any patient receiving this drug for an extended period of time.

Hypersensitivity Reactions: As with other NSAIDs, allergic reactions may occur. Manifestation of allergic reactions include urticaria, bronchospasm and anaphylaxis, and in rare instances, severe skin reactions such as Stevens-Johnson syndrome and Lyell Syndrome.

Drug Interactions: Acetylsalicylic Acid or Other NSAIDs: Plasma concentrations of tenoxicam are reduced to approximately 80% of their normal concentrations when single doses of tenoxicam are administered in conjunction with acetylsalicylic acid (2600 to 3900 mg/day). At steady state, simultaneous administration of ASA does not appear to have a significant effect on the plasma concentration of tenoxicam. The use of APO-TENOXICAM in conjunction with acetylsalicylic acid or other nonsteroidal anti-inflammatory agents is not recommended since data are not available demonstrating that the combination produces greater improvement than that achieved with either drug alone, and the potential for adverse reactions is increased.

Protein-Bound Drugs: As with other NSAIDs, APO-TENOXICAM is highly protein-bound, and therefore, might be expected to displace other protein-bound drugs, such as anticoagulants, oral hypoglycemics (sulfonylureas), phenytoin and sulfonamides.

Short-term pharmacodynamic studies have demonstrated that tenoxicam does not potentiate the anticoagulant effect of coumarin-type anticoagulants nor the hypoglycemic effect of sulfonylurea drugs. However, when a NSAID such as APO-TENOXICAM is administered concomitantly with anticoagulants, oral hypoglycemics, or other highly protein-bound drugs, the patient should be monitored and dosage adjustments made, if necessary.

Diuretics/Antihypertensives: As with other nonsteroidal anti-inflammatory drugs, APO-TENOXICAM can attenuate the blood pressure lowering effect of hydrochlorothiazide and the peak excretion rates of Na^+ and Cl^- in patients with hypertension. Therefore, close monitoring of patients on this drug combination is advisable. The excretion of electrolytes was not significantly affected when tenoxicam (two-day loading dose of 40 mg daily, followed by 20 mg daily) was administered to normotensive patients receiving furosemide therapy (40 mg daily).

Some NSAIDs have been reported to reduce the antihypertensive effects of certain β-blockers. The interaction between APO-TENOXICAM and β-blockers has not been studied.

Digoxin: In elderly patients with normal plasma creatinine levels, plasma digoxin levels were not altered by the concomitant administration of tenoxicam (30 mg daily).

Antacids: The administration of 15 mL of an aluminum hydroxide or an aluminum and magnesium hydroxide antacid just prior to a single 20 mg oral dose of tenoxicam did not affect the bioavailability of tenoxicam.

Cholestyramine: The average half-life of tenoxicam, after a single 20 mg intravenous dose, was reduced from 67.4 hours to 31.9 hours following the administration of cholestyramine (4 g in 200 mL water p.o. t.i.d.). The apparent drug clearance of tenoxicam increased by 105%.

Lithium: Nonsteroidal anti-inflammatory agents have been reported to increase steady state plasma lithium concentrations. It is recommended that these concentrations be monitored when initiating, adjusting and discontinuing APO-TENOXICAM treatment.

Methotrexate: The co-administration of some NSAIDs and methotrexate has been associated with reduced renal tubular secretion of methotrexate, higher plasma concentrations, and severe methotrexate toxicity. Therefore, caution should be exercised when NSAIDs, such as APO-TENOXICAM, are administered concurrently with methotrexate. The interaction between tenoxicam and methotrexate has not been studied.

ADVERSE EFFECTS: The most common adverse reactions encountered with nonsteroidal anti-inflammatory drugs are gastrointestinal, of which peptic ulcer, with or without bleeding, is the most severe. Fatalities have occurred on occasion, particularly in the elderly.

In approximately 12 000 patients administered tenoxicam 10-40 mg/day (approximately four-fifths receiving 20 mg/day), the incidence of peptic ulceration and the incidence of gastrointestinal bleeding (including hematemesis and melena) was 0.1-0.6%.

The approximate incidences of other adverse effects listed by systems are summarized below:

Gastrointestinal (10.4-23.0%): dyspepsia (0.1-9.7%), nausea (2.0-6.7%), constipation (0.5-2.9%), abdominal pain (0.7-3.3%), diarrhea (0.5-2.3%), flatulence (0.04-1.9%), vomiting (0.2-1.1%), ulcerative stomatitis (0.1-0.7%), gastritis (0.1-0.8%), esophagitis (0.2%), abdominal discomfort (1.4-2.2%), pyrosis (1.3-1.9%), epigastric discomfort (0.2-0.4%), epigastric pain (1.8-2.5%), hyperacidity (0.02-0.4%), anorexia (0.05-0.4%), indigestion (0.1-0.2%), meteorism (0.2-0.4%), gastric pressure (0.5-1.0%), mouth dryness (0.1-0.3%). Glossitis, stomatitis, dysphagia and reflux esophagitis were each reported in less than 0.1% of the patients.

Dermatologic (1.6-3.9%): rash (0.2-1.4%), pruritus (0.3-1.3%), sweating (0.06-0.3%), exanthema (0.2-0.3%), itching (0.05-0.4%). Photosensitivity reaction, seborrhea, urticaria, eczema and nail disorder were each reported in 0.1% or less of the patients. One case of angioedema was also reported.

Central Nervous System (2.0-9.1%): headache (0.9-4.3%), dizziness (0.8-3.3%), malaise (0.04-0.8%), paresthesia (0.02-0.5%), somnolence (0.1-0.7%), vertigo (0.2-0.4%), confusion (0.2%), fatigue (0.1-0.9%), depression (0.6%), insomnia (0.1-0.2%). Leg cramps, nervousness, fever and paresis were each reported in 0.1% of the patients.

Cardiovascular: hypertension (0.02-0.3%), palpitations (0.02-0.2%), flushing (0.02-0.03%), purpura (0.02-0.2%). Tachycardia was reported in less than 0.1% of the patients.

Hematologic: anemia (0.04-0.3%), leukopenia (0.04-0.4%). Thrombocytopenia was reported in 0.1% or less of the patients.

Renal: hematuria (0.02-0.2%), edema (0.2-1.3%), micturition frequency (0.02-0.3%), polyuria (0.03-0.1%). Dysuria, cystitis, increased BUN, increased creatinine, and albuminuria were each reported in less than 0.1% of the patients. Isolated cases of abnormal renal function and one case of renal failure were reported.

Hepatic (0.06-0.4%): abnormal hepatic function (0.3%). Jaundice, increased AST, ALT, gamma GT and bilirubin were each reported in less than 0.1% of the patients. Hepatitis, hepatic coma and hepatic failure were each reported once.

Respiratory (0.02-0.65%): dyspnea (0.2%), bronchospasm (0.1%).

Eyes, Ears, Nose, Throat: vision abnormal (0.02-0.3%). Diplopia, conjunctivitis, tinnitus, deafness, epistaxis, abnormal lacrimation were each reported in 0.1% or less of the patients.

OVERDOSE:

Cases of overdose with tenoxicam have not been reported. In the event of overdosage with APO-TENOXICAM (tenoxicam), supportive and symptomatic therapy is indicated.

For management of a suspected drug overdose, CPhA recommends that you contact your **regional Poison Control Centre**. See the *CPS* Directory section for a list of Poison Control Centres.

DOSAGE: A single daily dose of 20 mg APO-TENOXICAM (tenoxicam) should be taken orally at the same time each day. Higher doses should be avoided as they do not usually achieve a significantly greater therapeutic effect, but may be associated with a higher risk of adverse events.

In some patients, a 10 mg (½ tablet) daily dose may be sufficient. The smallest effective dose should be prescribed.

Geriatrics: As with other NSAIDs, APO-TENOXICAM should be used with special caution in elderly patients since they may be less able to tolerate side effects than younger patients. They are also more likely to be receiving concomitant medication or to have impaired hepatic, renal or cardiovascular function.

INFORMATION FOR THE PATIENT: Published in e-CPS, available by subscription at www.e-cps.ca.

SUPPLIED: Each yellow, oval, biconvex, film-coated tablet, engraved "APO" on one side and "20" and partially bisected on the other side, contains: tenoxicam 20 mg. Nonmedicinal ingredients: carnauba wax, colloidal silicon dioxide, croscarmellose sodium, hydroxypropyl methylcellulose, lactose hydrous, magnesium stearate, microcrystalline cellulose, polydextrose, polyethylene glycol, titanium dioxide and yellow ferric oxide. Bottles of 100. Store at 15 to 30°C.

Apo®-Timol
timolol maleate
Antihypertensive—Antianginal

Apotex

Date of Revision: August 14, 2002

PHARMACOLOGY: Timolol is a beta-adrenergic receptor blocking agent. The mechanism of the antihypertensive effect of beta-adrenergic receptor blocking agents has not yet been established. Among the factors that may be involved are; competitive ability to antagonize catecholamine-induced tachycardia at the beta receptor sites in the heart, thus decreasing cardiac output; inhibition of renin release by the kidneys; inhibition of the vasomotor centres.

The exact mechanism by which timolol exercises its antianginal effect is not certain but it may reduce the oxygen requirements of the heart by blocking catecholamine-induced increases in heart rate, systolic blood pressures and the velocity and extent of myocardial contraction. However oxygen requirements may be increased by such actions as increases in left ventricular fibre length, end diastolic pressure and the systolic ejection period. When the net physiological effect is advantageous in anginal patients it manifests itself during exercise or stress by delaying the onset of pain and reducing the incidence and severity of anginal attacks. Timolol can therefore increase the capacity for work and exercise in such patients. In a multi-clinic study, two-thirds of the patients treated with timolol maleate benefited to some degree.

Timolol has been found effective in prophylactic use for secondary prevention in patients with ischemic heart disease who have survived the acute phase of a myocardial infarction. At the present time, the mechanism of this protective effect of timolol is unknown.

Comparative Bioavailability: The bioavailability of a single oral dose of Apo-Timol 10 mg was compared with that of Blocadren 10 mg in normal human volunteers, with results as follows: See Table 1.

Table 1: Apo-Timol
Summary Table of the Comparative Bioavailability Data Apo-Timol (Dose: 10 mg) Tablet from Measured Data

	Geometric Mean Arithmetic Mean (CV %)		
Parameter	**Blocadren[b] 10 mg**	**Timolol[a] 10 mg**	**Percent Difference**
AUC 0-24 (ng·hr/mL)	123.5	124.9	+1.1
C_{max} (ng/mL)	24.08	26.42	+9.7
T_{max} (hr)[a]	1.6	1.5	−6.6
$t_{1/2}$ (hr)[a]	3.4	3.2	−5.9

[a] Timolol maleate 10 mg tablet.
[b] Blocadren is manufactured by Frosst, and was purchased in Canada.

INDICATIONS: For patients with mild or moderate hypertension. Timolol is usually used in combination with other drugs, particularly a thiazide diuretic. However, timolol may be tried alone, as an initial agent in those patients in whom, in the judgement of the physician, treatment should be started with a beta-blocker rather than a diuretic.

The combination of timolol maleate with a diuretic or peripheral vasodilator has been found to be compatible and generally more effective than timolol alone. Limited experience with other antihypertensive agents has not shown evidence of incompatibility with timolol.

Timolol is not indicated in the treatment of hypertensive emergencies.

Angina pectoris due to ischemic heart disease.

Patients who have survived the acute phase of a myocardial infarction, and are clinically stable, to reduce cardiovascular mortality and the risk of re-infarction. In the study, which showed these benefits, treatment with timolol was begun 7 to 28 days after the acute phase. Data are not available as to whether benefit would ensue if the treatment is initiated later.

Prophylactic treatment of migraine. Timolol is not indicated in the management of acute migraine attacks.

CONTRAINDICATIONS: Congestive heart failure (see Warnings); right ventricular failure secondary to pulmonary hypertension; significant cardiomegaly; sinus bradycardia; AV block; cardiogenic shock; allergic rhinitis, bronchospasm (including asthma), or a history of bronchospasm or severe chronic obstructive pulmonary disease (including severe chronic bronchitis and emphysema) (see Warnings); anesthesia with agents that produce myocardial depression, e.g., ether; hypersensitivity to any component of this product.

WARNINGS: Cardiac Failure: Special caution should be exercised when administering timolol to patients with a history of heart failure. Sympathetic stimulation is a vital component supporting circulatory function in congestive heart failure, and inhibition with beta blockade always carries a potential hazard of further depressing myocardial contractility and precipitating cardiac failure.

In patients without a history of cardiac failure, continued depression of the myocardium over a period of time can, in some cases, lead to cardiac failure. In rare instances this has been observed during therapy with timolol.

Therefore, at the first sign or symptom of impending cardiac failure occurring during drug therapy, patients should be fully digitalized and/or given a diuretic, and the response observed closely. Timolol acts selectively without blocking the inotropic action of digitalis on the heart muscle. However, the positive inotropic action of digitalis may be reduced by the negative inotropic effect of timolol when the 2 drugs are used concomitantly. The effects of timolol and digitalis are additive in depressing AV conduction. If cardiac failure persists, therapy with timolol should be discontinued (see below).

Abrupt Cessation of Therapy: Patients with ischemic heart disease should be warned against stopping timolol abruptly. Hypersensitivity to catecholamines has been observed in patients withdrawn from beta-blocker therapy. Myocardial infarction, ventricular arrhythmias, or sudden death has been reported in such patients following abrupt discontinuation of therapy with beta-adrenergic receptor blocking agents, with or without preceding exacerbation of angina pectoris. Therefore, in angina and postmyocardial infarction, the dosage of timolol should be gradually reduced over about 2 weeks (maintaining the same frequency of administration) and the patient should be carefully observed. In patients with angina pectoris, if the angina still markedly worsens, or in any patient if acute coronary insufficiency develops, it is recommended that timolol be reinstated, at least temporarily.

Since ischemic heart disease may be unrecognized, the above advice should be followed in patients considered to be at risk of having asymptomatic ischemic heart disease.

Patients with chronic obstructive pulmonary disease (e.g., chronic bronchitis, emphysema) of mild to moderate severity should in general not receive beta-blockers, particularly the nonselective beta-blockers such as timolol (see Contraindications). If timolol must be given to such patients, it should be given with caution and under careful medical supervision since it may block bronchodilation produced by endogenous catecholamine stimulation of beta receptors (see Precautions).

Various skin rashes and conjunctival xerosis have been reported with beta-blockers including timolol. A severe syndrome (oculomucocutaneous syndrome) whose signs include conjunctivitis sicca and psoriasiform rashes, otitis and sclerosing serositis have occurred with the chronic use of one beta-adrenergic blocking agent. This syndrome has not been observed with timolol. However, physicians should be alert to the possibility of such reactions and should discontinue treatment in the event that they occur.

Severe sinus bradycardia due to unopposed vagal activity may result from the administration of timolol; in such cases, consider the use of i.v. atropine, and, if no improvement is seen, i.v. isoproterenol.

In patients with thyrotoxicosis, timolol may give a false impression of improvement by diminishing peripheral manifestations of hyperthyroidism without improving thyroid function. Special considerations should be given to the potential of timolol to aggravate congestive heart failure. Timolol does not alter thyroid function tests. Patients suspected of developing thyrotoxicosis should be managed carefully to avoid abrupt withdrawal of beta blockade which might precipitate a thyroid storm.

PRECAUTIONS: There may be increased difficulty in treating an allergic-type reaction in patients on beta-blockers. In these patients, the reaction may be more severe due to pharmacologic effects of the beta-blocker and problems with fluid changes. Epinephrine should be administered with caution since it may not have its usual effects in the treatment of anaphylaxis. On the one hand, larger doses of epinephrine may be needed to overcome the bronchospasm, while on the other, these doses can be associated with excessive alpha-adrenergic stimulation with consequent hypertension, reflex bradycardia, heart block and possible potentiation of bronchospasm. Alternatives to the use of large doses of epinephrine include vigorous supportive care such as fluids and the use of beta-agonists including parenteral salbutamol or isoproterenol to overcome bronchospasm and norepinephrine to overcome hypotension.

Timolol should be administered with caution to patients subject to spontaneous hypoglycemia, or to diabetic patients (especially those with labile diabetes) who are receiving insulin or oral hypoglycemic agents. Beta-adrenergic blocker may mask the premonitory signs and symptoms of acute hypoglycemia.

Timolol dosage should be individually adjusted when used concomitantly with other antihypertensive agents (see Dosage).

Suitable laboratory tests should be carried out at appropriate intervals and caution should be observed in patients with impaired renal or hepatic function. Since timolol is partially metabolized in the liver and excreted mainly by the kidneys, dosage reduction may be necessary when hepatic or renal insufficiency is present. Marked hypotension has been observed in patients with severe renal insufficiency undergoing renal hemodialysis following oral administration of 20 mg of timolol.

Beta-adrenergic blockade has been reported to potentiate muscle weakness consistent with certain myasthenic symptoms (e.g., diplopia, ptosis and generalized weakness). Timolol has been reported rarely to increase muscle weakness in some patients with myasthenic symptoms.

Because of potential effects of beta-adrenergic blocking agents relative to blood pressure and pulse, these agents should be used with caution in patients with cerebrovascular insufficiency. If signs or symptoms suggesting reduced cerebral blood flow are observed, consideration should be given to discontinuing these agents.

Patients Undergoing Elective or Emergency Surgery: The management of patients with angina, being treated with beta-blockers and undergoing elective or emergency surgery, is controversial because beta-adrenergic receptor blockade impairs the ability of the heart to respond to beta-adrenergically mediated reflex stimuli, but abrupt discontinuation of therapy may be followed by severe complications (see Warnings). Some patients receiving beta-adrenergic blocking agents have been subject to protracted severe hypotension during anesthesia. Difficulty in restarting and maintaining the heartbeat has also been reported.

For these reasons, in patients with angina undergoing elective surgery, timolol should be withdrawn gradually following the recommendation given under Abrupt Cessation of Therapy (see Warnings). According to available evidence, all clinical and physiologic effects of beta blockade are no longer present 48 hours after cessation of medication.

In emergency surgery, since timolol is a competitive Inhibitor of beta-adrenergic receptor agonists, its effcts may be reversed, if necessary, by sufficient doses of such agonists as isoproterenol, levarterenol, dopamine or dobutamine.

Pregnancy: Since timolol has not been studied in human pregnancy, the drug should not be given to pregnant women. The use of any drug in patients of childbearing potential requires that the anticipated benefit be weighed against possible hazards.

Lactation: Timolol is detectable in human milk. Because of the potential for serious adverse reactions from timolol in infants, a decision should be made whether to discontinue nursing or to discontinue the drug, taking into account the importance of the drug to the mother.

Children: Safety and effectiveness in children have not been established.

Risk of Anaphylactic Reaction: While taking beta-blockers, patients with a history of atopy or a history of severe anaphylactic reaction to a variety of allergens may be more reactive to repeated challenge with such allergens, either accidental, diagnostic or therapeutic. Such patients may be unresponsive to the usual doses of epinephrine used to treat anaphylactic reactions.

Drug Interactions: Close observation of the patient is recommended when timolol is administered to patients receiving catecholamine-depleting drugs such as reserpine or guanethidine, because of possible additive effects and the production of hypotension and/or marked bradycardia, which may produce vertigo, syncope, or postural hypotension.

Attenuation of the antihypertensive effect of beta-adrenoceptor blocking agents by NSAIDs has been reported. When using these agents concomitantly, patients should be observed carefully to confirm that the desired therapeutic effect has been obtained.

The potential exists for hypotension, AV conduction disturbances and left ventricular failure to occur in patients receiving a beta-blocking agent and an oral calcium entry blocker concurrently. The nature of any cardiovascular adverse effect tends to depend on the type of calcium entry blocker used. The dihydropyridine derivatives such as nifedipine are more likely to lead to hypotension whereas verapamil and diltiazem have a greater propensity to lead to AV conduction disturbances or left ventricular failure when used with a beta-blocker. Oral calcium antagonists may be used with caution in combination with beta-adrenergic blocking agents when cardiac function is normal, but should be avoided in patients with impaired cardiac function. However in exceptional cases, when in the opinion of the physician, concomitant use is considered essential in patients with impaired cardiac function, such use should be instituted gradually, in a hospital setting, under careful supervision.

I.V. calcium entry blockers should not be used in patients receiving beta-adrenoceptor blocking agents.

The concomitant use of beta-adrenergic blocking agents and digitalis with either diltiazem or verapamil may have additive effects in prolonging cardiac AV conduction time.

ADVERSE EFFECTS: Trials:

Cardiovascular: Congestive heart failure in 3 to 4% of patients (see Warnings). Secondary effects of decreased cardiac output, about 4%, which could include: syncope, vertigo, lightheadedness, postural hypotension; decreased renal perfusion. Severe bradycardia in about 1% of patients, lengthening of the PR interval, 2nd-and 3rd-degree A-V block, sinus arrest (if SA node previously diseased), cold extremities, Raynaud's phenomenon, claudication or paresthesia, hypotension.

Respiratory: dyspnea has occurred in about 10% of patients, bronchospasm in about 1% of patients, laryngospasm occurs rarely.

CNS: Most frequently reported: headache, tinnitus. Less frequently: drowsiness, anxiety, vertigo, dizziness, weakness, insomnia, sedation, and mental depression. Rarely: vivid dreams.

Integumentary: (See Warnings): Occasionally rashes, including one case of psoriasiform rash reported to date, and pruritus. Rarely: exfoliative dermatitis (one case).

Gastrointestinal: vomiting in about 4% of patients, diarrhea in about 5% of patients, constipation, epigastric distress, nausea.

Special Senses: dry eyes.

Adverse Reactions Reported Since the Drug Was Marketed:

Cardiovascular: cardiac arrest, cerebral vascular accident, palpitation, arrhythmia, edema, pulmonary edema, worsening of arterial insufficiency, worsening of angina pectoris, vasodilatation.

Hematologic: nonthrombocytopenic purpura.

Respiratory: rales, cough.

CNS: Rarely: nightmares, nervousness, diminished concentration, hallucinations, increased dreaming, decreased libido.

Integumentary: (See Warnings): skin irritation, increased pigmentation, sweating.

Gastrointestinal: dyspepsia, hepatomegaly.

Special Senses: visual disturbances, diplopia, ptosis, and eye irritation.

Urogenital: impotence, micturition difficulties.

Body as a Whole: asthenia, fatigue, chest pain, extremity pain, decreased exercise tolerance, weight loss.

Musculoskeletal: arthralgia.

Endocrine: hypoglycemia, hyperglycemia.

Clinical Laboratory: Slight increases in blood urea nitrogen, serum potassium, serum uric acid and triglycerides, and slight decreases in hemoglobin, hematocrit, and HDL-cholesterol have occurred, but were not progressive or associated with clinical manifestations. Slight increases in ALT have also occurred.

OVERDOSE:

Symptoms: The most common signs expected are bradycardia, hypotension, bronchospasm, or acute cardiac failure.

If overdosage occurs, in all cases therapy with timolol should be discontinued and the patient observed closely. In addition, the following therapeutic measures are suggested:

Treatment: Gastric lavage.

Bradycardia:
Use atropine sulfate i.v. 0.25 mg to 2 mg to induce vagal blockade. If bradycardia persists, i.v. isoproterenol HCl should be administered cautiously. In refractory cases the use of a cardiac pacemaker may be considered.

Heart Block (second degree or complete):
isoproterenol HCl or a cardiac pacemaker.

Acute Cardiac Failure:
Conventional therapy with digitalis, diuretics, and oxygen should be instituted immediately. In refractory cases the use of i.v. aminophylline is suggested. This may be followed, if necessary, by glucagon HCl which has been reported to be useful.

Hypotension:
Use sympathomimetic pressor drug therapy, such as levarterenol, epinephrine, dopamine or dobutamine. The response to epinephrine in such patients may be altered (see Precautions). In refractory cases the use of glucagon HCl has been reported to be useful.
Bronchospasm:
Use isoproterenol HCl. Additional therapy with aminophylline may be considered.
Hypoglycemia:
I.V. glucose and/or i.m. glucagon.
An in vitro hemodialysis study, using C^{14} timolol added to human plasma or whole blood, showed that timolol was readily dialyzed from these fluids; however, a study of patients with renal failure showed that timolol did not dialyze readily.

It should be remembered that timolol is a competitive antagonist of isoproterenol and hence large doses of isoproterenol can be expected to reverse many of the effects of excessive doses of timolol. However, the complications of excess isoproterenol, such as tachycardia, headache, flushing of the skin, arrhythmia, nausea, weakness, tremor and sweating, should not be overlooked.

For management of a suspected drug overdose, CPhA recommends that you contact your **regional Poison Control Centre.** See the *CPS* Directory section for a list of Poison Control Centres.

DOSAGE: Hypertension: Timolol is usually used in conjunction with other antihypertensive agents, particularly a thiazide diuretic, but may be used alone (see Indications).

The dose must always be adjusted to the individual requirements of the patient, in accordance with the following guidelines.

When timolol is given to patients already receiving other antihypertensive agents, the initial dose should be 5 to 10 mg twice a day. If after 1 to 2 weeks an adequate response is not observed, dosage may be increased by increments of 5 mg twice daily, at intervals of 2 weeks. A 60 mg daily dose should not be exceeded.

When timolol is used alone the initial dose should be 10 mg twice a day and dosage increased if required, following the regimen described above.

In those patients who are found to be adequately controlled on daily doses of 20 mg or less, the administration of the total dose in the morning should be tried, as studies show adequate response to this dose regimen.

Angina: The recommended dosage range is 15 to 45 mg/day. The majority of patients respond to a daily dosage of 35 to 45 mg. Therapy should be initiated with 5 mg 2 or 3 times a day. Depending on response, increases in dosage may be necessary. The first increase should not exceed 10 mg/day in divided doses. Subsequent increases should not exceed 15 mg/day in divided doses. A total daily dose of 45 mg should not be exceeded. There should be an interval of at least 3 days between increases in dosage.

After the titration period, some patients may be maintained on a twice-daily schedule.

Preventive Use in Ischemic Heart Disease: For long-term preventive use in patients who have survived the acute phase of myocardial infarction, the maintenance dose is 10 mg twice daily. Therapy should be initiated with 5 mg twice daily and the patient observed carefully. If no adverse reaction occurs, the dosage should then be increased after 2 days to 10 mg twice daily. In the studies evaluating timolol following myocardial infarction, treatment was begun 7 to 28 days after the acute phase.

Migraine: Dosage must be individualized. The recommended dosage for prevention of migraine headache is 10 mg twice daily. The dosage range is 10 to 30 mg/day. If a satisfactory response is not obtained after 6 to 8 weeks of the maximum suggested dosage, therapy with timolol should be discontinued.

SUPPLIED: 5 mg: Each white, round, flat faced, bevelled-edge tablet, scored and engraved with 'APO' over 'T5' on one side, contains: timolol maleate equivalent to 5 mg. Nonmedicinal ingredients: croscarmellose sodium, lactose monohydrate, magnesium stearate and microcrystalline cellulose. Bottles of 100.

10 mg: Each light blue, round, flat faced, bevelled-edge tablet, scored and engraved with 'APO' over 'T10' on one side, contains timolol maleate equivalent to 10 mg. Nonmedicinal ingredients: croscarmellose sodium, FD&C Blue #1 aluminum lake, FD&C Blue #2 aluminum lake, lactose monohydrate, magnesium stearate and microcrystalline cellulose. Bottles of 100.

20 mg: Each light blue, capsule-shaped, scored tablet, engraved with 'APO T20' on one side, contains: timolol maleate equivalent to 20 mg. Nonmedicinal ingredients: FD&C Blue # 1 aluminum lake, FD&C Blue # 2 aluminum lake, croscarmellose sodium, lactose monohydrate, magnesium stearate and microcrystalline cellulose. Bottles of 100.

Store at temperatures between 15 and 30°C. Preserve in well closed containers.

Apresoline® Pr

hydralazine HCl

Antihypertensive

SteriMax

SUPPLIED: Each ampoule of sterile, lyophilized powder contains: 20 mg of hydralazine hydrochloride, for reconstitution to 20 mg/mL. Alcohol-, bisulfite-, gluten-, lactose-, sodium-, parabens- and tartrazine-free. Cartons of 10. Store below 30°C. Protect from heat and light.

Apri 21 Pr

desogestrel—ethinyl estradiol

Oral Contraceptive

Apotex

Apri 28 Pr

desogestrel—ethinyl estradiol

Oral Contraceptive

Apotex

Date of Preparation: September 22, 2008

PHARMACOLOGY: Combination oral contraceptives act by suppression of gonadotropins. Although the primary mechanism of this action is inhibition of ovulation, other alterations include changes in the cervical mucus (which increase the difficulty of sperm entry into the uterus) and the endometrium (which reduces the likelihood of implantation).

Desogestrel, the progestogen component of desogestrel/ethinyl estradiol (150 μg/30 μg) tablets, displays low androgenic activity in relation to its progestogenic effects and may increase the HDL/LDL ratio and apoprotein A-1/B ratio without affecting HDL_2. Like other oral contraceptives, these changes in lipid profile can be associated with an increase in triglycerides.

INDICATIONS: Conception control.

CONTRAINDICATIONS: History of/or actual thrombophlebitis or thromboembolic disorders. History of/or actual cerebrovascular disorders. History of/or actual myocardial infarction or coronary arterial disease. Active liver disease or history of/or actual benign or malignant liver tumours. Known or suspected carcinoma of the breast. Known or suspected estrogen-dependent neoplasia. Undiagnosed abnormal vaginal bleeding. Any ocular lesion arising from ophthalmic vascular disease, such as partial or complete loss of vision or defect in visual fields. When pregnancy is suspected or diagnosed.

WARNINGS: Predisposing Factors for Coronary Artery Disease: Cigarette smoking increases the risk of serious cardiovascular side effects and mortality. Birth control pills increase this risk, especially with increasing age. Convincing data are available to support an upper age limit of 35 years for oral contraceptive use in women who smoke.

Other women who are independently at high risk for cardiovascular disease include those with diabetes, hypertension, abnormal lipid profile, or a family history of these. Whether oral contraceptives accentuate this risk is unclear.

In low risk, non-smoking women of any age, the benefits of oral contraceptive use outweigh the possible cardiovascular risks associated with low dose formulations. Consequently, oral contraceptives may be prescribed for these women up to the age of menopause.

Cigarette smoking increases the risk of serious adverse effects on the heart and blood vessels. This risk increases with age and becomes significant in oral contraceptive-users over 35 years of age. Women should be counselled not to smoke.

Epidemiological studies have suggested an association between the use of COCs and an increased risk of venous thrombotic and thromboembolic diseases.

Venous thromboembolism (VTE) manifesting as deep vein thrombosis and/or pulmonary embolism, may occur during the use of all COCs. The approximate incidence of VTE in users of low estrogen dose (<0.05 mg EE) OCs is up to 4 per 10 000 woman years compared to 0.5-3 per 10 000 woman years in non-OC users. The incidence of VTE associated with pregnancy is 6 per 10 000 woman years.

Several epidemiological studies indicate that third generation oral contraceptives, including those containing desogestrel, are associated with a higher risk of venous thromboembolism than certain second generation oral contraceptives. These studies indicate an approximate 2-fold difference in risk, which corresponds to 1-2 cases of venous thromboembolism per 10 000 women-years of use. However, data from additional studies have not shown this difference in risk.

Discontinue medication at the earliest manifestation of:
A. Thromboembolic and cardiovascular disorders such as thrombophlebitis, pulmonary embolism, cerebrovascular disorders, myocardial ischemia, mesenteric thrombosis, and retinal thrombosis.
B. Conditions which predispose to venous stasis and to vascular thrombosis e.g. immobilization after accidents or confinement to bed during long-term illness. Other non-hormonal methods of contraception should be used until regular activities are resumed. For use of oral contraceptives when surgery is contemplated, see Precautions.
C. Visual defects, partial or complete.
D. Papilledema, or ophthalmic vascular lesions.
E. Severe headache of unknown etiology or worsening of pre-existing migraine headache.

PRECAUTIONS: Physical Examination and Follow-up: Before oral contraceptives are used, a thorough history and physical examination should be performed, including a blood pressure determination. Breasts, liver, extremities and pelvic organs should be examined. A Papanicolaou smear should be taken if the patient has been sexually active.

The first follow-up visit should be done three months after oral contraceptives are prescribed. Thereafter, examinations should be performed at least once a year or more frequently if indicated. At each annual visit, examination should include those procedures that were done at the initial visit as outlined above or per recommendations of the Canadian Task Force on the Periodic Health Examination.

Pregnancy: Oral contraceptives should not be taken by pregnant women. However, if conception accidentally occurs while taking the pill, there is no conclusive evidence that the estrogen and progestin contained in the oral contraceptive will damage the developing child.

Lactation: In breast-feeding women, the use of oral contraceptives results in the hormonal components being excreted in breast milk and may reduce its quantity and quality. If the use of oral contraceptives is initiated after the establishment of lactation, there does not appear to be any effect on the quantity and quality of the milk. There is no evidence that low dose oral contraceptives are harmful to the nursing infant.

Hepatic Function: Patients who have had jaundice including a history of cholestatic jaundice during pregnancy should be given oral contraceptives with great care and under close observation.

The development of severe generalized pruritus or icterus requires that the medication be withdrawn until the problem is resolved.

If the jaundice should prove to be cholestatic in type, the use of oral contraceptives should not be resumed. In patients taking oral contraceptives, changes in the composition of the bile may occur and an increased incidence of gallstones has been reported.

Hepatic nodules (adenoma and focal nodular hyperplasia) have been reported, particularly in long-term users of oral contraceptives. Although these lesions are extremely rare, they have caused fatal intra-abdominal hemorrhage and should be considered in women presenting with an abdominal mass, acute abdominal pain, or evidence of intra-abdominal bleeding.

Hypertension: Patients with essential hypertension whose blood pressure is well-controlled may be given oral contraceptives but only under close supervision. If a significant elevation of blood pressure in previously normotensive or hypertensive subjects occurs at any time during the administration of the drug, cessation of medication is necessary.

Migraine and Headache: The onset or exacerbation of migraine or the development of headache of a new pattern which is recurrent, persistent or severe, requires discontinuation of oral contraceptives and evaluation of the cause.

Diabetes: Current low dose oral contraceptives exert minimal impact on glucose metabolism. Diabetic patients, or those with a family history of diabetes, should be observed closely to detect any worsening of carbohydrate metabolism. Patients predisposed to diabetes who can be kept under close supervision may be given oral contraceptives. Young diabetic patients whose disease is of recent origin, well-controlled, and not associated with hypertension or other signs of vascular disease such as ocular fundal changes, should be monitored more frequently while using oral contraceptives.

Ocular Disease: Patients who are pregnant or are taking oral contraceptives, may experience corneal edema that may cause visual disturbances and changes in tolerance to contact lenses, especially of the rigid type. Soft contact lenses usually do not cause disturbances. If visual changes or alterations in tolerance to contact lenses occur, temporary or permanent cessation of wear may be advised.

Breasts: Increasing age and a strong family history are the most significant risk factors for the development of breast cancer. Other established risk factors include obesity, nulliparity and late age at first full-term pregnancy. The identified groups of women that may be at increased risk of developing breast cancer before menopause are long-term users of oral contraceptives (more than 8 years) and starters at early age. In a few women, the use of oral contraceptives may accelerate the growth of an existing but undiagnosed breast cancer. Since any potential increased risk related to oral contraceptive use is small, there is no reason to change prescribing habits at present.

Women receiving oral contraceptives should be instructed in self-examination of their breasts. Their physicians should be notified whenever any masses are detected. A yearly clinical breast examination is also recommended because, if a breast cancer should develop, estrogen-containing drugs may cause a rapid progression.

Vaginal Bleeding: Persistent irregular vaginal bleeding requires assessment to exclude underlying pathology.

Fibroids: Patients with fibroids (leiomyomata) should be carefully observed. Sudden enlargement, pain, or tenderness require discontinuation of the use of oral contraceptives.

Emotional Disorders: Patients with a history of emotional disturbances, especially the depressive type, may be more prone to have a recurrence of depression while taking oral contraceptives. In cases of a serious recurrence, a trial of an alternate method of contraception should be made which may help to clarify the possible relationship. Women with premenstrual syndrome (PMS) may have a varied response to oral contraceptives, ranging from symptomatic improvement to worsening of the condition.

Laboratory Tests: Results of laboratory tests should be interpreted in the light that the patient is on oral contraceptives. The following laboratory tests are modified.
A. Liver function tests: Aspartate serum transaminase (AST)—variously reported elevations. Alkaline phosphatase and gamma glutamine transaminase (GGT)—slightly elevated.
B. Coagulation tests: Minimal elevation of test values reported for such parameters as prothrombin and Factors VII, VIII, IX and X.
C. Thyroid function tests: Protein binding of thyroxine is increased as indicated by increased total serum thyroxine concentrations and decreased T_3 resin uptake.
D. Lipoproteins: Small changes of unproven clinical significance may occur in lipoprotein cholesterol fractions.
E. Gonadotropins: LH and FSH levels are suppressed by the use of oral contraceptives. Wait two weeks after discontinuing the use of oral contraceptives before measurements are made.

Tissue Specimens: Pathologists should be advised of oral contraceptive therapy when specimens obtained from surgical procedures and Pap smears are submitted for examination.

Return to Fertility: After discontinuing oral contraceptive therapy, the patient should delay pregnancy until at least one normal spontaneous cycle has occurred in order to date the pregnancy. An alternate contraceptive method should be used during this time.

Amenorrhea: Women having a history of oligomenorrhea, secondary amenorrhea, or irregular cycles may remain anovulatory or become amenorrheic following discontinuation of estrogen-progestin combination therapy.

Amenorrhea, especially if associated with breast secretion, that continues for six months or more after withdrawal, warrants a careful assessment of hypothalamic-pituitary function.

Thromboembolic Complications—Post-surgery: There is an increased risk of post-surgery thromboembolic complications in oral contraceptive users, after major surgery. If feasible, oral contraceptives should be discontinued and an alternative method substituted at least one month prior to **major** elective surgery. Oral contraceptives should not be resumed until the first menstrual period after hospital discharge following surgery.

Drug Interactions: The concurrent administration of oral contraceptives with other drugs may result in an altered response to either agent (Table 1 and Table 2). Reduced effectiveness of the oral contraceptive, should it occur, is more likely with the low dose formulations. It is important to ascertain all drugs that a patient is taking, both prescription and non-prescription, before oral contraceptives are prescribed.

Table 1: Apri

Drugs Which May Decrease the Efficacy of Oral Contraceptives

Class of Compound	Drug	Proposed Mechanism	Suggested Management
Anticonvulsants	Carbamazepine Ethosuximide Phenobarbital Phenytoin Primidone	Induction of hepatic microsomal enzymes: Rapid metabolism of estrogen and increased binding of progestin and ethinyl estradiol to SHBG.	Use higher dose OCs (50 µg ethinyl estradiol) another drug or another method.
Antibiotics	Ampicillin Cotrimoxazole Penicillin	Enterohepatic circulation disturbance, intestinal hurry.	For short course, use additional method or use another drug. For long course, use another method.
	Rifampicin	Increased metabolism of progestins. Suspected acceleration of estrogen metabolism.	Use another method.
	Chloramphenicol Metronidazole Neomycin Nitrofurantoin Sulfonamides Tetracyclines	Induction of hepatic microsomal enzymes. Also disturbance of enterohepatic circulation.	For short course, use additional method or use another drug. For long course, use another method.
	Troleandomycin	May retard metabolism of OCs increasing the risk of cholestatic jaundice.	
Antifungals	Griseofulvin	Stimulation of hepatic metabolism of contraceptive steroids may occur.	Use another method.
Sedatives and Hypnotics	Benzodiazepines Barbiturates Chloral hydrate Glutethimide Meprobamate	Induction of hepatic microsomal enzymes.	For short course, use additional method or another drug. For long course, use another method or higher dose OCs.
Antacids		Decreased intestinal absorption of progestins.	
Other Drugs	Phenylbutazone Antihistamines Analgesics Antimigraine Preparations Vitamin E	Reduced OC efficacy has been reported. Remains to be confirmed.	

Table 2: Apri

Modification of Other Drug Action by Oral Contraceptives

Class of Compound	Drug	Modification of Drug Action	Suggested Management
Alcohol		Possible increased levels of ethanol or acetaldehyde.	Use with caution.
Alpha-II Adrenoreceptor Agents	Clonidine	Sedation effect increased.	Use with caution.
Anticoagulants	All	OC's increase clotting factors, decrease efficacy. However OCs may potentiate action in some patients.	Use another method.
Anticonvulsants	All	Fluid retention may increase risk of seizures.	Use another method.
Antidiabetic drugs	Oral hypoglycemics and insulin	OCs may impair glucose tolerance and increase blood glucose.	Use low dose estrogen and progestin OC or another method. Monitor blood glucose.
Antihypertensive agents	Guanethidine and methyldopa	Estrogen component causes sodium retention, progestin has no effect.	Use low dose estrogen OC or use another method.
	Beta blockers	Increased drug effect (decreased metabolism)	Adjust dose of drug if necessary. Monitor cardiovascular status.
Antipyretics	Acetaminophen	Increased renal clearance.	Dose of drug may have to be increased.
	Antipyrine	Impaired metabolism	Decrease dose of drug.
	ASA	Effects of ASA may be decreased by the short-term use of OCs.	Patients on chronic ASA therapy may require an increase in ASA dosage.

(cont'd)

Table 2: Apri *(cont'd)*

Modification of Other Drug Action by Oral Contraceptives

Class of Compound	Drug	Modification of Drug Action	Suggested Management
Aminocaproic Acid		Theoretically, a hypercoagulable state may occur because OCs augment clotting factors.	Avoid concomitant use.
Betamimetic Agents	Isoproterenol	Estrogen causes decreased response to these drugs.	Adjust dose of drug as necessary. Discontinuing OCs can result in excessive drug activity.
Caffeine		The actions of caffeine may be enhanced as OCs may impair the hepatic metabolism of caffeine.	Use with caution.
Cholesterol Lowering Agents	Clofibrate	OCs may increase the clearance of clofibrate leading to decreased level of clofibrate.	Use with caution.
Corticosteroids	Prednisone	Markedly increased serum levels.	Possible need for decrease in dose.
Cyclosporine		May lead to an increase in cyclosporine levels and hepatotoxicity.	Monitor hepatic function. The cyclosporine dose may have to be decreased.
Folic Acid		OCs have been reported to impair folate metabolism.	
Meperidine		Possible increased analgesia and CNS depression due to decreased metabolism of meperidine.	Use combination with caution.
Phenothiazine Tranquilizers	All phenothiazines, reserpine and similar drugs	Estrogen potentiates the hyperprolactinemia effect of these drugs.	Use other drugs or lower dose OCs. If galactorrhea or hyperprolactinemia occurs, use other method.
Sedatives and Hypnotics	Chlordiazepoxide Lorazepam Oxazepam Diazepam	Increased effect (increased metabolism)	Use with caution
Theophylline	All	Decreased oxidation, leading to possible toxicity.	Use with caution. Monitor theophylline levels.
Tricyclic Antidepressants	Clomipramine (possibly others)	Increased side effects; i.e., depression.	Use with caution
Vitamin B_{12}		OCs have been reported to reduce serum levels of Vitamin B_{12}.	

Non-Contraceptive Benefits of Oral Contraceptives: Several health advantages other than contraception have been reported.

1. Combination oral contraceptives reduce the incidence of cancer of the endometrium and ovaries.
2. Oral Contraceptives reduce the likelihood of developing benign breast disease and as a result decrease the incidence of breast biopsies.
3. Oral contraceptives reduce the likelihood of development of functional ovarian cysts.
4. Pill-users have less menstrual blood loss and have more regular cycles, thereby reducing the chance of developing iron-deficiency anemia.
5. The use of oral contraceptives may decrease the severity of dysmenorrhea and premenstrual syndrome and may improve acne vulgaris, hirsutism and other androgen-mediated disorders.
6. Oral contraceptives decrease the incidence of acute pelvic inflammatory disease and thereby reduce as well the incidence of ectopic pregnancy.
7. Oral contraceptives have potential beneficial effects on endometriosis.

Oral Contraceptives **do not protect** against sexually transmitted diseases (STDs), including HIV/AIDS. For protection against STDs, it is advisable to use latex condoms **in combination with** oral contraceptives.

ADVERSE EFFECTS: An increased risk of the following serious adverse reactions has been associated with the use of oral contraceptives: thrombophlebitis, pulmonary embolism, mesenteric thrombosis, neuro-ocular lesions, e.g., retinal thrombosis, myocardial infarction, cerebral thrombosis, cerebral hemorrhage, hypertension, benign hepatic tumours, gallbladder disease, congenital anomalies.

The following adverse reactions also have been reported in patients receiving oral contraceptives: Nausea and vomiting, usually the most common adverse reaction, occurs in approximately 10% or less of patients during the first cycle.

Other reactions, as a general rule, are seen less frequently or only occasionally, as follows: gastrointestinal symptoms (such as abdominal cramps and bloating), breakthrough bleeding, spotting, change in menstrual flow, dysmenorrhea, amenorrhea during and after treatment, temporary infertility after discontinuance of treatment, edema, chloasma or melasma which may persist, breast changes: tenderness, enlargement, and secretion, change in weight (increase or decrease), endocervical hyperplasias, possible diminution in lactation when given immediately post-partum, cholestatic jaundice, migraine, increase in size of uterine leiomyomata, rash (allergic), mental depression, reduced tolerance to carbohydrates, vaginal candidiasis, premenstrual-like syndrome, intolerance to contact lenses, change in corneal curvature (steepening), cataracts, optic neuritis, retinal thrombosis, changes in libido, chorea, changes in appetite, cystitis-like syndrome, rhinitis, headache, nervousness, dizziness, hirsutism, loss of scalp hair, erythema multiforme, erythema nodosum, hemorrhagic eruption, vaginitis, porphyria, impaired renal function, Raynaud's phenomenon, auditory disturbances, hemolytic uremic syndrome, pancreatitis.

OVERDOSE:

Symptoms: Serious ill effects have not been reported following acute ingestion of large doses of oral contraceptives by young children. Overdosage may cause nausea, and withdrawal bleeding may occur in females.

For management of a suspected drug overdose, contact your **regional Poison Control Centre**. See the *CPS* Directory section for a list of Poison Control Centres.

DOSAGE: Information to Patients on How to Take the Birth Control Pill:

1. **Read these directions:**

- before you start taking your pills, and
- any time you are not sure what to do.

2. **Look at your pill pack** to see if it has 21 or 28 pills:
   - 21-pill pack: 21 active pills (with hormones) taken daily for three weeks, and then take no pills for one week

   or
   - 28-pill pack: 21 active pills (with hormones) taken daily for three weeks, and then seven "reminder" pills (no hormones) taken daily for one week.

   Also check the pill pack for instructions on 1) where to start and 2) direction to take pills.
3. You may wish to use a second method of birth control (e.g. latex condoms and spermicidal foam or gel) for the first seven days of the first cycle of pill use. This will provide a back-up in case pills are forgotten while you are getting used to taking them.
4. When receiving any medical treatment, be sure to tell your doctor that you are using birth control pills.
5. **Many women have spotting or light bleeding, or may feel sick to their stomach during the first three months on the pill.** If you do feel sick, do not stop taking the pill. The problem will usually go away. If it does not go away, check with your doctor or clinic.
6. **Missing pills also can cause some spotting or light bleeding**, even if you make up the missed pills. You also could feel a little sick to your stomach on the days you take two pills to make up for missed pills.
7. **If you miss pills at any time, you could get pregnant. The greatest risks for pregnancy are:**
   - when you start a pack late
   - when you miss pills at the beginning or at the very end of the pack.
8. **Always be sure you have ready:**
   - **Another kind of birth control** (such as latex condoms and spermicidal foam or gel) to use as a back-up in case you miss pills, and
   - **An extra, full pack of pills.**
9. **If you have vomiting or diarrhea, or if you take some medicines**, such as antibiotics, your pills may not work as well. Use a back-up method, such as latex condoms and spermicidal foam or gel, until you can check with your doctor or clinic.
10. **If you forget more than one pill two months in a row**, talk to your doctor or clinic about how to make pill-taking easier or about using another method of birth control.
11. **If your questions are not answered here, call your doctor or clinic.**

When to start the first pack of pills: Be sure to read these instructions:

- before you start taking your pills, and
- any time you are not sure what to do.

Decide with your doctor or clinic what is the best day for you to start taking your first pack of pills. Your pills may be either a 21-day or a 28-day type.

A. **Apri 21-Day Combination:** With this type of birth control pill, you are 21 days on pills with seven days off pills. You must not be off the pills for more than seven days in a row.
   1. **The first day of your menstrual period (bleeding) is day 1 of your cycle.** Your doctor may advise you to start taking the pills on Day 1 or on the first Sunday after your period begins. If your period starts on Sunday, start that same day.
   2. Take one pill at approximately the same time every day for 21 days; **then take no pills for seven days**. Start a new pack on the eighth day. You will probably have a period during the seven days off the pill. (This bleeding may be lighter and shorter than your usual period.)

B. **Apri 28-Day Combination:** With this type of birth control pill, you take 21 pills which contain hormones and seven pills which contain no hormones.
   1. **The first day of your menstrual period (bleeding) is day 1 of your cycle.** Your doctor may advise you to start taking the pills on Day 1 or on the first Sunday after your period begins. If your period starts on Sunday, start that same day.
   For Day 1 start: Label the dispenser by selecting the appropriate day label strip that starts with Day 1 of your menstrual period (first day of menstruation is Day 1).
   or
   For Sunday start: Label the dispenser by selecting the day label strip that starts with Sunday.
   Place the day label strip in the space where you see the words "Place Day Label Here". Having the dispenser labeled with the days of the week will help remind you to take your pill every day.
   2. Take one pill at approximately the same time every day for 28 days. Begin a new pack the next day, **not missing any days on the pills**. Your period should occur during the last seven days of using that pill pack.

What to do during the month:

1. **Take a pill at approximately the same time every day until the pack is empty.**
   - Try to associate taking your pill with some regular activity like eating a meal or going to bed.
   - Do not skip pills even if you have bleeding between monthly periods or feel sick to your stomach (nausea).
   - Do not skip pills even if you do not have sex very often.
2. **When you finish a pack:**
   - **21 pills: Wait seven days** to start the next pack. You will have your period during that week.
   - **28 pills:** Start the next pack **on the next day**. Take one pill every day. Do not wait any days between packs.

What to do if you miss pills: Table 3 outlines the actions you should take if you miss one or more birth control pills. Match the number of pills missed with the appropriate starting time for the type of pill pack.

Table 3: Apri

What to Do if You Miss Pills

Sunday Start	Day 1 Start
Miss 1 pill	**Miss 1 pill**
Take it as soon as you remember, and take the next pill at the usual time. This means that you might take 2 pills in one day.	Take it as soon as you remember, and take the next pill at the usual time. This means that you might take 2 pills in one day.
Miss 2 pills in a row	**Miss 2 pills in a row**
First 2 Weeks: 1. Take 2 pills the day you remember and 2 pills the next day. 2. Then take 1 pill a day until you finish the pack. 3. Use a back-up method of birth control if you have sex in the 7 days after you miss the pills. **Third Week:** 1. Keep taking 1 pill a day until Sunday. 2. On Sunday, safely discard the rest of the pack and start a new pack that day. 3. Use a back-up method of birth control if you have sex in the 7 days after you miss the pills. 4. You may not have a period this month. **If You Miss 2 Periods In a Row, Call Your Doctor, Pharmacist or Clinic.**	**First 2 Weeks:** 1. Take 2 pills the day you remember and 2 pills the next day. 2. Then take 1 pill a day until you finish the pack. 3. Use a back-up method of birth control if you have sex in the 7 days after you miss the pills. **Third Week:** 1. Safely dispose of the rest of the pill pack and start a new pack that same day. 2. Use a back-up method of birth control if you have sex in the 7 days after you miss the pills. 3. You may not have a period this month. **If You Miss 2 Periods In a Row, Call Your Doctor, Pharmacist or Clinic.**
Miss 3 or More Pills in a Row	**Miss 3 or More Pills in a Row**

(cont'd)

Table 3: Apri *(cont'd)*

What to Do if You Miss Pills

Sunday Start	Day 1 Start
Anytime in the Cycle: 1. Keep taking 1 pill a day until Sunday. 2. On Sunday, safely discard the rest of the pack and start a new pack that day. 3. Use a back-up method of birth control if you have sex in the 7 days after you miss the pills. 4. You may not have a period this month. **If You Miss 2 Periods In a Row, Call Your Doctor, Pharmacist or Clinic.**	**Anytime in the Cycle:** 1. Safely dispose of the rest of the pill pack and start a new pack that same day. 2. Use a back-up method of birth control if you have sex in the 7 days after you miss the pills. 3. You may not have a period this month. **If You Miss 2 Periods In a Row, Call Your Doctor, Pharmacist or Clinic.**

Note: 28-Day Pack: If you forget any of the seven "reminder" pills (without hormones) in Week 4, just safely dispose of the pills you missed. Then keep taking one pill each day until the pack is empty. You do not need to use a back-up method.

Always be sure you have on hand:

- a back-up method of birth control (such as latex condoms and spermicidal foam or gel) in case you miss pills, and
- an extra, full pack of pills.

If you forget more than one pill two months in a row, talk to your doctor or clinic. Talk about ways to make pill-taking easier or about using another method of birth control.

INFORMATION FOR THE PATIENT: Published in e-CPS, available by subscription at www.e-cps.ca.

SUPPLIED: Apri 21: Each round, rose tablet, debossed with "dp" on one side and "575" on the other side, contains: desogestrel 0.15 mg and ethinyl estradiol 0.03 mg. Nonmedicinal ingredients: colloidal silicon dioxide, FD&C Blue no. 2 aluminum lake, FD&C Red no. 40 aluminum lake, lactose monohydrate, Opadry Clear YS-1-7472 (hydroxypropyl methylcellulose and polyethylene glycol), Opadry Maroon YS-1-16002 (hydroxypropyl methylcellulose, polyethylene glycol and titanium dioxide), polysorbate 80, povidone, pregelatinized starch, stearic acid and vitamin E. Sachets containing an Aclar blister dispenser with 21 rose active tablets. Store between 15-30°C. Protect from light once opened using the protective covering provided. Keep out of reach of children.

Apri 28: Each round, rose tablet, debossed with "dp" on one side and "575" on the other side, contains: desogestrel 0.15 mg and ethinyl estradiol 0.03 mg. Each round, white tablet, debossed with "dp" on one side and "570" on the other side, contains: inert ingredients. Nonmedicinal ingredients: rose tablet: colloidal silicon dioxide, FD&C Blue no. 2 aluminum lake, FD&C Red no. 40 aluminum lake, lactose monohydrate, Opadry Clear YS-1-7472 (hydroxypropyl methylcellulose and polyethylene glycol), Opadry Maroon YS-1-16002 (hydroxypropyl methylcellulose, polyethylene glycol and titanium dioxide), polysorbate 80, povidone, pregelatinized starch, stearic acid and vitamin E; white tablet: anhydrous lactose; magnesium stearate, microcrystalline cellulose and pregelatinized starch. Sachets containing an Aclar blister dispenser with 21 rose active tablets and 7 white inert tablets. Store between 15-30°C. Protect from light once opened using the protective covering provided. Keep out of reach of children.

Aptivus® ℞

tipranavir

Non-Peptidic Protease Inhibitor (NPPI)

Boehringer Ingelheim

Date of Revision: May 14, 2009

SUMMARY PRODUCT INFORMATION:

Route of Administration	Dosage Form/ Strength	Clinically Relevant Nonmedicinal Ingredients
Oral	Capsules 250 mg	Sorbitol, ethanol and Cremophor EL For a complete listing see Dosage Forms, Composition and Packaging.

INDICATIONS AND CLINICAL USE: APTIVUS (tipranavir) co-administered with 200 mg ritonavir, is indicated for combination antiretroviral treatment of HIV-1 infected adults, who are treatment experienced and infected with HIV-1 strains resistant to more than one protease inhibitor.

In deciding on a new regimen for patients who have failed an antiretroviral regimen, careful consideration should be given to the treatment history of the individual patient and the patterns of mutations associated with different drugs.

Geriatrics (>65 years): Clinical studies of APTIVUS did not include sufficient number of subjects aged 65 and over to determine whether they respond differently from younger subjects. In general, caution should be exercised in the administration and monitoring of APTIVUS in elderly patients reflecting the greater frequency of decreased hepatic, renal, or cardiac function, and of concomitant disease or other drug therapy. See Action and Clinical Pharmacology, Warnings and Precautions, Adverse Reactions, and Dosage and Administration.

Pediatrics (2-18 years of age): The safety and efficacy of APTIVUS in this population has not yet been fully established. Treatment of children with APTIVUS is therefore not recommended. See Action and Clinical Pharmacology, Warnings and Precautions, Adverse Reactions, and Dosage and Administration.

CONTRAINDICATIONS: APTIVUS (tipranavir) is contraindicated in patients with known hypersensitivity to the active substance or to any of the ingredients of the product. For a complete listing, see Dosage Forms, Composition and Packaging.

In case of rare hereditary conditions that may be incompatible with an excipient of the product (please refer to Warnings and Precautions) the use of the product is contraindicated.

APTIVUS is contraindicated in patients with moderate or severe (Child-Pugh Class B or C respectively) hepatic insufficiency.

Combination of rifampicin (rifampin) with APTIVUS with concomitant 200 mg ritonavir is contraindicated (see also Drug Interactions).

Herbal preparations containing St. John's wort (hypericum perforatum) must not be used while taking APTIVUS, co-administered with 200 mg ritonavir, due to the risk of decreased plasma concentrations and reduced clinical effects of tipranavir (see also Drug Interactions).

APTIVUS contains Cremophor EL. Caution should be used when administering medicines containing Cremophor EL (e.g. cyclosporine i.v. and paclitaxel i.v.) to patients with a prior hypersensitivity reaction to Cremophor EL.

Co-administration of APTIVUS with 200 mg ritonavir, with drugs that are highly dependent on CYP3A for clearance and for which elevated plasma concentrations are associated with serious and/or life-threatening events is contraindicated. These drugs are listed in Table 1.

Table 1: APTIVUS

Drugs that are Contraindicated with APTIVUS, Co-Administered with Ritonavir

Drug Class	Drugs within Class that are Contraindicated with APTIVUS, Co-administered with Ritonavir
Antiarrhythmics	Amiodarone, bepridil, flecainide, propafenone, quinidine
Antihistamines	Astemizole[a], terfenadine[a]
Ergot derivatives	Dihydroergotamine, ergonovine, ergotamine, methylergonovine

(cont'd)

Table 1: APTIVUS *(cont'd)*

Drugs that are Contraindicated with APTIVUS, Co-Administered with Ritonavir

Drug Class	Drugs within Class that are Contraindicated with APTIVUS, Co-administered with Ritonavir
GI motility agent	Cisapride[a]
HMG-CoA reductase inhibitors	Lovastatin, simvastatin
Neuroleptic	Pimozide
Sedatives/hypnotics	Midazolam, triazolam
PDE5 Inhibitors	Levitra (vardenafil)

[a] Cisapride, astemizole and terfenadine are not marketed in Canada.

Due to the need for co-administration of APTIVUS with low-dose ritonavir (RTV), please refer to ritonavir product monograph for a description of ritonavir contraindications.

WARNINGS AND PRECAUTIONS:

APTIVUS co-administered with 200 mg ritonavir has been associated with reports of both fatal and non-fatal intracranial hemorrhage.

APTIVUS co-administered with 200 mg ritonavir has been associated with reports of clinical hepatitis and hepatic decompensation including some fatalities. Extra vigilance including increased clinical and laboratory monitoring is warranted in patients with chronic hepatitis B or hepatitis C co-infection, as these patients have an increased risk of hepatotoxicity (see Hepatic Impairment).

General: APTIVUS (tipranavir) must be administered with 200 mg ritonavir to ensure its therapeutic effect (see Dosage and Administration). Failure to correctly co-administer APTIVUS with ritonavir will result in reduced plasma levels of tipranavir that may be insufficient to achieve the desired antiviral effect. Patients should be instructed accordingly. Please refer to ritonavir product monograph for additional information on precautionary measures.

APTIVUS contains up to 50.4 mg sorbitol per maximum recommended daily dose. Patients with the rare hereditary condition of fructose intolerance should not take this medicine.

Intracranial Hemorrhage: APTIVUS, co-administered with 200 mg of ritonavir, has been associated with reports of both fatal and non-fatal intracranial hemorrhage (ICH). Many of these patients had other medical conditions or were receiving concomitant medications that may have caused or contributed to these events. No pattern of abnormal coagulation parameters has been observed in patients in general, or preceding the development of ICH. Therefore, routine measurement of coagulation parameters is not currently indicated in the management of patients on APTIVUS.

Effects on Platelet Aggregation and Coagulation: APTIVUS co-administered with ritonavir, should be used with caution in patients who may be at risk of increased bleeding from trauma, surgery or other medical conditions, or who are receiving medications known to increase the risk of bleeding such as antiplatelet agents and anticoagulants, or who supplement high doses of vitamin E.

In in vitro experiments, tipranavir was observed to inhibit human platelet aggregation at levels consistent with exposures observed in patients receiving APTIVUS, co-administered with ritonavir.

In rats, co-administration of a Vitamin E derivative increased the bleeding effects of tipranavir. However, analyses of stored plasma from adults treated with APTIVUS capsules plus low-dose ritonavir, and from paediatric patients treated with APTIVUS capsules or tipranavir oral solution (which contains a vitamin E derivative) plus low-dose ritonavir have demonstrated that with or without the vitamin E-containing oral solution there was no effect of tipranavir on vitamin K-dependent coagulation factors (Factor II and Factor VII), Factor V, or on prothrombin or activated partial thromboplastin times.

Carcinogenesis and Mutagenesis: Long-term carcinogenicity studies in mice and rats have been conducted with tipranavir. Mice were administered 30, 150 or 300 mg/kg/day tipranavir, 150/40 mg/kg/day tipranavir/ritonavir in combination, or 40 mg/kg/day ritonavir. The incidences of benign hepatocellular adenomas and combined adenomas/carcinomas were increased in females of all groups except the low dose of tipranavir. These tumors were also increased in male mice at the high-dose of tipranavir and the tipranavir/ritonavir combination group. Hepatocellular carcinoma incidence was increased in female mice given the high dose of tipranavir and both sexes receiving tipranavir/ritonavir. The combination of tipranavir and ritonavir caused an exposure-related increase in this same tumor type in both sexes. The clinical relevance of the carcinogenic findings in mice is unknown. Systemic exposures in mice (based on AUC or C_{max}) at all dose levels tested were below those in humans receiving the recommended dose level. Rats were administered 30, 100 or 300 mg/kg/day tipranavir, 100/26.7 mg/kg/day tipranavir/ritonavir in combination, or 10 mg/kg/day ritonavir. No drug-related findings in male rats were observed. At the highest dose of tipranavir, an increased incidence of benign follicular cell adenomas of the thyroid gland was observed in female rats. Based on AUC measurements, exposure to tipranavir at this dose level in rats is approximately equivalent to exposure in humans at the recommended therapeutic dose. This finding is probably not relevant to humans, because thyroid follicular cell adenomas are considered a rodent-specific effect secondary to enzyme induction.

Tipranavir showed no evidence of genetic toxicity in a battery of five in vitro and in vivo tests assessing mutagenicity and clastogenicity.

In a study conducted in rats with tipranavir at systemic exposure levels (AUC) of 1670 μM·h, equivalent to human exposure at the adult human clinical dose, no adverse effects on mating or fertility were observed. Tipranavir did not produce teratogenic effects at maternal doses producing systemic drug exposure levels of 1310 μM·h in rats or 120 μM·h in rabbits-equivalent to or below the exposure at the adult human clinical dose (APTIVUS/ritonavir 500 mg/200 mg bid), respectively.

At tipranavir exposures of 1310 μM·h in rats (0.8-fold human exposure at the clinical dose), fetal toxicity (decreased sternebrae ossification and body weights) was observed. In pre- and post-natal development studies with tipranavir in rats, no adverse effects were noted at 340 μM·h (0.2-fold human exposure), but growth inhibition of pups was observed at maternally toxic doses of 1310 μM·h (0.8-fold human exposure). Calculated exposure in animal studies were equivalent to or below human therapeutic exposure levels. For the animal studies reported above, exposures were three to five fold lower at the end of the dosing period compared to the start of the dosing period.

Cardiovascular: QT Prolongation: A specific study was conducted using the therapeutic and supratherapeutic doses of APTIVUS co-administered with RTV (TPV/r 500/200 mg and TPV/r 750/200 mg) on the QTc interval in healthy male and female volunteers using moxifloxacin (400 mg) as a positive control. There was no clinically relevant prolongation of the QT interval or other electrocardiac abnormalities compared to the baseline with either dose.

Endocrine and Metabolism: Diabetes Mellitus/Hypergylcemia: New onset diabetes mellitus, exacerbation of pre-existing diabetes mellitus and hyperglycemia have been reported during post-marketing surveillance in HIV-infected patients receiving protease inhibitor therapy. Some patients required either initiation or dose adjustments of insulin or oral hypoglycemic agents for treatment of these events. In some cases, diabetic ketoacidosis occurred. In those patients who discontinued protease inhibitor therapy, hyperglycemia persisted in some cases. Because these events have been reported voluntarily during clinical practice, estimates of frequency cannot be made. The causal relationship between protease inhibitor therapy and these events has not been established.

Lipid Elevation: Treatment with APTIVUS co-administered with ritonavir, and other antiretroviral agents, has resulted in increased plasma total triglycerides and cholesterol. Triglyceride and cholesterol testing should be performed prior to initiating APTIVUS therapy and during therapy. Treatment-related lipid elevations should be managed as clinically appropriate.

Fat Redistribution: Redistribution/accumulation of body fat including central obesity, dorsocervical fat enlargement (buffalo hump), peripheral wasting, facial wasting, breast enlargement, and "cushingoid appearance" have been observed in patients receiving antiretroviral therapy. The mechanism and long-term consequences of these events are currently unknown. A causal relationship has not been established.

Hematologic: Hemophilia: There have been reports of increased bleeding, including spontaneous skin haematomas and haemarthrosis in patients with haemophilia type A and B treated with protease inhibitors. In some patients additional Factor VIII was given. In more than half of the reported cases, treatment with protease inhibitors was continued or reintroduced if treatment had been discontinued. A causal relationship between protease inhibitors and these events has not been established.

Hepatic/Biliary/Pancreatic: Hepatic Impairment: APTIVUS is contraindicated in patients with moderate or severe hepatic insufficiency (Child-Pugh Class B or C, respectively) (see Contraindications). Limited data are currently available for the use of APTIVUS, co-administered with ritonavir, in patients co-infected with hepatitis B or C. Patients with chronic hepatitis B or C and treated with antiretroviral agents are at an increased risk for severe and potentially fatal hepatic adverse events. APTIVUS should be used in this patient population only if the potential benefit outweighs the potential risk, and with increased clinical and laboratory monitoring.

Patients with mild hepatic impairment (Child-Pugh Class A) should be closely monitored.

Caution should be exercised when administering APTIVUS/ritonavir to patients with liver enzyme abnormalities or history of hepatitis. Appropriate laboratory testing should be conducted prior to initiating therapy with APTIVUS and ritonavir, and frequently during treatment. Increased monitoring should be considered when APTIVUS and ritonavir are administered to patients with elevated baseline transaminase levels, or active hepatitis B or C, as patients with underlying hepatitis B or C and marked elevations in transaminases prior to treatment may be at increased risk for developing further transaminase elevations or hepatic decompensation. APTIVUS/ritonavir should be discontinued once signs of worsening liver function occur in patients with pre-existing liver disease.

APTIVUS co-administered with ritonavir, has been associated with reports of clinical hepatitis and hepatic decompensation, including some fatalities. These have generally occurred in patients with advanced HIV disease taking multiple concomitant medications. A causal relationship to APTIVUS co-administered with ritonavir could not be established. Physicians and patients should be vigilant for the appearance of signs or symptoms of hepatitis, such as fatigue, malaise, anorexia, nausea, jaundice, liver tenderness or hepatomegaly. Patients with signs or symptoms of hepatitis should discontinue APTIVUS/ritonavir treatment and seek medical evaluation.

Tipranavir is principally metabolised by the liver. Therefore caution should be exercised when administering this drug to patients with hepatic impairment because tipranavir concentrations may be increased.

For information on the multi-dose pharmacokinetics of tipranavir in hepatically impaired patients, see Action and Clinical Pharmacology.

Immune: Immune Reconstitution Syndrome: During the initial phase of treatment, patients responding to antiretroviral therapy may develop an inflammatory response to indolent or residual opportunistic infections (such as MAC, CMV, PCP, and TB), which may necessitate further evaluation and treatment.

Renal: Renal Impairment: Since the renal clearance of tipranavir is negligible, increased plasma concentrations are not expected in patients with renal impairment.

Sensitivity/Resistance: Sulfonamide Allergy: APTIVUS (tipranavir) should be used with caution in patients with a known sulfonamide allergy. Tipranavir contains a sulfonamide moiety. The potential for cross-sensitivity between drugs in the sulfonamide class and tipranavir is unknown.

Sexual Function/Reproduction: Teratogenic Effects: No observable teratogenicity was detected in reproductive studies performed in pregnant rats and rabbits.

Investigation of fertility and early embryonic development with tipranavir disodium was performed in rats, teratogenicity studies were performed in rats and rabbits, and pre- and post-natal development were explored in rats.

No teratogenicity was detected in reproductive studies performed in pregnant rats and rabbits up to dose levels of 1000 mg/kg/day and 150 mg/kg/day tipranavir, respectively. At 400 mg/kg/day and above in rats, fetal toxicity (decreased sternebrae ossification and body weights) was observed, corresponding to an AUC of 1310 μM·h or 1.4 fold human exposure at the recommended dose. In rats and rabbits, fetal toxicity was not noted at 40 mg/kg/day and 150 mg/kg/day, respectively, corresponding accordingly to $C_{max}/AUC_{0\text{-}24}$ levels of 30.4 μM/340 μM·h/mL and 8.4 μM/120 μM·h/mL. These exposure levels (AUC) are 0.4 fold and 0.1 fold the exposure in humans at the recommended dose.

In pre- and post-development studies in rats, tipranavir showed no adverse effects at 40 mg/kg/day, but caused growth inhibition in pups and maternal toxicity at dose levels of 400 mg/kg/day and above. No post-weaning functions were affected at any dose level.

Skin: Rash: Urticarial rash, maculopapular rash, and possible photosensitivity have been reported in subjects receiving APTIVUS/ritonavir. In Phase 2 and 3 trials, rash was observed in 14% of females and in 8-10% of males receiving APTIVUS/ritonavir. Additionally, in one drug interaction trial in healthy female volunteers administered a single dose of ethinyl estradiol followed by APTIVUS/ritonavir, 33% of subjects developed a rash. Rash accompanied by joint pain or stiffness, throat tightness, or generalized pruritus has been reported in both men and women receiving APTIVUS/ritonavir. The risk of rash increases in patients with lower CD4 cell counts.

Special Populations: Pregnant Women: There are no adequate and well-controlled studies in pregnant women for the treatment of HIV-1 infection. APTIVUS should be used during pregnancy only if the potential benefit justifies the potential risk to the fetus.

Nursing Women: APTIVUS was shown to be excreted in breast milk in rats/mice. It is unknown if the drug is excreted in human milk. Because many drugs are excreted in human milk, precaution should be exercised. Consistent with the recommendation that HIV-infected mothers not breast-feed their infants to avoid risking postnatal transmission of HIV, mothers should discontinue breast-feeding if they are receiving APTIVUS.

Antiretroviral Pregnancy Registry: To monitor maternal-fetal outcomes of pregnant women exposed to APTIVUS, an Anti-retroviral Pregnancy Registry has been established. Physicians are encouraged to register patients by calling toll-free 1-800-258-4263.

Pediatrics (2-18 years of age): Safety and efficacy of APTIVUS in this population has not yet been fully established. Treatment of children with APTIVUS is therefore not recommended.

There are no data available in children younger than 2 years of age.

Geriatrics (>65 years of age): Clinical studies of APTIVUS did not include sufficient numbers of subjects aged 65 and over to determine whether they respond differently from younger subjects. In general, caution should be exercised in the administration and monitoring of APTIVUS in elderly patients reflecting the greater frequency of decreased hepatic, renal, or cardiac function, and of concomitant disease or other drug therapy.

Monitoring and Laboratory Tests: Appropriate laboratory testing should be conducted prior to initiating therapy with APTIVUS and low-dose ritonavir, and during treatment. Increased monitoring should be considered when APTIVUS and low dose ritonavir are administered to patients with elevated AST and ALT levels, or chronic hepatitis-B or -C.

Triglyceride and cholesterol testing should be performed prior to initiating tipranavir therapy and during therapy.

ADVERSE REACTIONS: Clinical Trial Adverse Drug Reactions: Because clinical trials are conducted under very specific conditions the adverse reaction rates observed in the clinical trials may not reflect the rates observed in practice and should not be compared to the rates in the clinical trials of another drug. Adverse drug reaction information from clinical trials is useful for identifying drug-related adverse events and for approximating rates.

APTIVUS (tipranavir) co-administered with low-dose ritonavir has been studied in a total of 6308 HIV-positive adults as combination therapy in clinical trials. Of these, 1299 treatment-experienced patients received the dose of 500 mg/200 mg bid in formal clinical trials. Nine hundred and nine (909) and 552 adults, including 541 and 381 in the RESIST-1 and RESIST-2 Phase III pivotal trials, have been treated for at least 48 and 96 weeks, respectively. Table 2, Table 3, Table 4 and Table 5 contain adverse events observed within the RESIST trials with no assigned causality.

Due to the need for co-administration of APTIVUS with low-dose ritonavir, please refer to ritonavir product monograph for ritonavir-associated adverse reactions.

Table 2: APTIVUS

Serious Adverse Events (SAE) Occurring in ≥0.5% of RESIST Trial Patients

	TPV/r[a]		CPI/r[b]	
Preferred Term	**No. (%) of Patients**	**Events/100 PEY**	**No. (%) of Patients**	**Events/100 PEY**
Total treated	749 (100.0)	1159.6	737 (100.0)	659.3
Total of any SAE	217 (29.0)	22.4	156 (21.2)	27.0
Blood and Lymphatic System Disorders	15 (2.0)	1.3	15 (2.0)	2.3
Anemia	7 (0.9)	0.6	8 (1.1)	1.2
Gastrointestinal Disorders	49 (6.5)	4.3	25 (3.4)	3.8

(cont'd)

Table 2: APTIVUS *(cont'd)*

Serious Adverse Events (SAE) Occurring in ≥0.5% of RESIST Trial Patients

	TPV/r[a]		CPI/r[b]	
Preferred Term	**No. (%) of Patients**	**Events/100 PEY**	**No. (%) of Patients**	**Events/100 PEY**
Diarrhea	13 (1.7)	1.1	7 (1.0)	1.1
Pancreatitis	8 (1.1)	0.7	2 (0.3)	0.3
Abdominal pain	7 (0.9)	0.6	3 (0.4)	0.5
Vomiting	5 (0.7)	0.4	3 (0.4)	0.5
Dysphagia	4 (0.5)	0.3	2 (0.3)	0.3
General Disorders and Administration Site Conditions	44 (5.9)	3.9	25 (3.4)	3.9
Pyrexia	24 (3.2)	2.1	11 (1.5)	1.7
Chills	4 (0.5)	0.3	1 (0.1)	0.2
Asthenia	4 (0.5)	0.3	3 (0.4)	0.5
Chest pain	5 (0.7)	0.4	3 (0.4)	0.5
Hepatobiliary Disorders	12 (1.6)	1.0	3 (0.4)	0.5
Hepatic failure	4 (0.5)	0.3	0 (0.0)	0.0
Infections and Infestations	104 (13.9)	9.6	72 (9.8)	11.5
Pneumonia	23 (3.1)	2.0	5 (0.7)	0.8
Gastroenteritis	5 (0.7)	0.4	4 (0.5)	0.6
Cytomegalovirus chorioretinitis	4 (0.5)	0.3	4 (0.5)	0.6
P. jiroveci pneumonia	10 (1.3)	0.9	8 (1.1)	1.2
Esophageal candidiasis	8 (1.1)	0.7	7 (1.0)	1.1
Bronchitis	4 (0.5)	0.3	1 (0.1)	0.2
Condyloma acuminatum	5 (0.7)	0.4	1 (0.1)	0.2
Sepsis	5 (0.7)	0.4	0 (0.0)	0.0
Appendicitis	4 (0.5)	0.3	1 (0.1)	0.2
HIV infection	4 (0.5)	0.3	0 (0.0)	0.0
Sinusitis	4 (0.5)	0.3	2 (0.3)	0.3
Injury, Poisoning and Procedural Complications	14 (1.9)	1.2	9 (1.2)	1.4
Hip fracture	4 (0.5)	0.3	0 (0.0)	0.0
Road traffic accident	4 (0.5)	0.3	2 (0.3)	0.3
Investigations	17 (2.3)	1.5	11 (1.5)	1.7
ALT increased	6 (0.8)	0.5	1 (0.1)	0.2
AST increased	5 (0.7)	0.4	1 (0.1)	0.2
Weight decreased	4 (0.5)	0.3	3 (0.4)	0.5
Metabolism and Nutrition Disorders	20 (2.7)	1.7	10 (1.4)	1.5
Dehydration	11 (1.5)	1.0	4 (0.5)	0.6
Neoplasms Benign, Malignant and Unspecified (including cysts and polyps)	39 (5.2)	3.4	23 (3.1)	3.6
Basal cell carcinoma	4 (0.5)	0.3	1 (0.1)	0.2
Hodgkin's disease	5 (0.7)	0.4	0 (0.0)	0.0
Nervous System Disorders	31 (4.1)	2.7	22 (3.0)	3.4
Headache	6 (0.8)	0.5	4 (0.5)	0.6
Convulsions	4 (0.5)	0.3	4 (0.5)	0.6
Psychiatric Disorders	5 (0.7)	0.4	12 (1.6)	1.8
Depression	1 (0.1)	0.1	5 (0.7)	0.8
Renal and Urinary Disorders	24 (3.2)	2.1	9 (1.2)	1.4
Acute renal failure	11 (1.5)	1.0	2 (0.3)	0.3
Renal failure	7 (0.9)	0.6	3 (0.4)	0.5

(cont'd)

Table 2: APTIVUS *(cont'd)*

Serious Adverse Events (SAE) Occurring in ≥0.5% of RESIST Trial Patients

	TPV/r[a]		CPI/r[b]	
Preferred Term	**No. (%) of Patients**	**Events/100 PEY**	**No. (%) of Patients**	**Events/100 PEY**
Respiratory, Thoracic and Mediastinal Disorders	23 (3.1)	2.0	11 (1.5)	1.7
Dyspnea	5 (0.7)	0.4	4 (0.5)	0.6
Respiratory failure	4 (0.5)	0.3	0 (0.0)	0.0

a Dose is TPV/r 500 mg/200 mg BID.

b Doses are BID and in mg: LPV/r 400/100, IDV/r 800/100, SQV/r 1000/100 or SQV/r 800/200, APV/r 600/100.

In RESIST-1 and RESIST-2 in the APTIVUS/ritonavir arm, the most frequent adverse events were diarrhoea, nausea, headache, pyrexia, vomiting, fatigue and abdominal pain. The 48 Week Kaplan-Meier rates of adverse events leading to discontinuation were 13.3 % for APTIVUS/ritonavir-treated patients and 10.8% for the comparator arm patients.

The following clinical safety features (intracranial hemorrhage, hepatotoxicity, hyperlipidemia) were seen at higher frequency among APTIVUS/ritonavir treated patients when compared with the comparator arm treated patients in the RESIST trials.

Intracranial Hemorrhage (ICH): Five cases of ICH in 4 patients (1246 patient exposure years) were observed in patients receiving APTIVUS/ritonavir compared to no cases in the comparator arm (660 patient exposure years). Fourteen intracranial hemorrhage events (ICH), including 8 fatalities, occurred in 13 out of 6840 HIV-1 infected individuals receiving APTIVUS (tipranavir) capsules, as part of combination antiretroviral therapy, in clinical trials. Many of these patients had other medical conditions or were receiving concomitant medications that may have caused or contributed to these events. An increased risk of ICH has previously been observed in patients with advanced HIV disease/AIDS. No pattern of abnormal coagulation parameters has been observed in patients in general, or preceding the development of ICH. The median time to onset of an ICH event was 525.5 days on treatment.

Hepatotoxicity: The frequency of Grade 3 or 4 ALT and/or AST abnormalities was higher in APTIVUS/ritonavir patients compared with comparator arm patients. Multivariate analyses showed that baseline ALT or AST above DAIDS Grade 1 and co-infection with hepatitis B or C were risk factors for these elevations.

Hyperlipidaemia: Grade 3 or 4 elevations of triglycerides and cholesterol occurred more frequently in the APTIVUS/ritonavir arm compared with the comparator arm. The clinical significance of these observations has not been fully established.

Table 3: APTIVUS

Percentage of Patients with Treatment Emergent Adverse Events of at Least Moderate Intensity (Grades 2-4) in ≥2% of Patients in Either Treatment Group[a] in the RESIST Trials at the 48-Week Time Point

	Phase 3 Studies 1182.12 and 1182.48 (48-weeks)	
	Percentage of Patients (rate per 100 patient-exposure years)	
	APTIVUS/Ritonavir (500/200 mg BID)+OBR (n=749; 757.4 patient-exposure years)	Comparator PI/Ritonavir[b]+OBR (n=737; 503.9 patient-exposure years)
Blood and Lymphatic Disorders		
Anemia	3.3% (3.4)	2.3% (3.4)
Neutropenia	2.0% (2.0)	1.0% (1.4)
Gastrointestinal Disorders		
Diarrhea	15.0% (16.5)	13.4% (21.6)
Nausea	8.5% (9.0)	6.4% (9.7)
Vomiting	5.9% (6.0)	4.1% (6.1)
Abdominal pain	4.4% (4.5)	3.4% (5.1)
Abdominal pain upper	1.5% (1.5)	2.3% (3.4)
General Disorders		
Pyrexia	7.5% (7.7)	5.4% (8.2)
Fatigue	5.7% (5.9)	5.6% (8.4)
Investigations		
Weight decreased	3.1% (3.1)	2.2% (3.2)
ALT increased	2.0% (2.0)	0.5% (0.8)
GGT increased	2.0% (2.0)	0.4% (0.6)
Metabolism and Nutrition Disorders		
Hypertriglyceridemia	3.9% (4.0)	2.0% (3.0)
Hyperlipidemia	2.5% (2.6)	0.8% (1.2)
Dehydration	2.1% (2.1)	1.1% (1.6)
Musculoskeletal and Connective Tissue Disorders		
Myalgia	2.3% (2.3)	1.8% (2.6)
Nervous System Disorders		
Headache	5.2% (5.3)	4.2% (6.3)
Peripheral neuropathy	1.5% (1.5)	2.0% (3.0)

(cont'd)

Table 3: APTIVUS *(cont'd)*

Percentage of Patients with Treatment Emergent Adverse Events of at Least Moderate Intensity (Grades 2-4) in ≥2% of Patients in Either Treatment Group[a] in the RESIST Trials at the 48-Week Time Point

	Phase 3 Studies 1182.12 and 1182.48 (48-weeks)	
	Percentage of Patients (rate per 100 patient-exposure years)	
	APTIVUS/Ritonavir (500/200 mg BID)+OBR (n=749; 757.4 patient-exposure years)	Comparator PI/Ritonavir[b]+OBR (n=737; 503.9 patient-exposure years)
Psychiatric Disorders		
Insomnia	1.7% (1.7)	3.7% (5.5)
Respiratory, Thoracic and Mediastinal Disorders		
Dyspnea	2.1% (2.1)	1.0% (1.4)
Skin and Subcutaneous Tissue Disorders		
Rash	3.1% (3.1)	3.8% (5.7)

[a] Excludes laboratory abnormalities that were Adverse Events.
[b] Comparator PI/RTV: lopinavir/ritonavir 400/100 mg BID, indinavir/ritonavir 800/100 mg BID, saquinavir/ritonavir 1000/100 mg BID, amprenavir/ritonavir 600/100 mg BID.

Table 4: APTIVUS

Adverse Events Resulting in Clinical Intervention (Discontinuation) in the RESIST Trials 1182.12 and 1182.14

System Organ Class/Preferred Term	Treatment Group TPV/r N (%)	TPV/r Events/100 PEY	CPI/r N (%)	CPI/r Events/100 PEY
Total Treated	749 (100.0)	1159.6	737 (100.0)	659.3
Total With Any AE Leading to Discontinuation	117 (15.6)	10.3	69 (9.4)	10.7
Gastrointestinal Disorders	41 (5.5)	3.6	28 (3.8)	4.3
Nausea	13 (1.7)	1.1	11 (1.5)	1.7
Vomiting	12 (1.6)	1.0	9 (1.2)	1.4
Diarrhea	14 (1.9)	1.2	10 (1.4)	1.5
Abdominal pain	2 (0.3)	0.2	6 (0.8)	0.9
Abdominal pain upper	2 (0.3)	0.2	1 (0.1)	0.2
Pancreatitis	3 (0.4)	0.3	0 (0.0)	0.0
Gastrointestinal disorder	2 (0.3)	0.2	1 (0.1)	0.2
General Disorders and Administration Site Conditions	15 (2.0)	1.3	10 (1.4)	1.5
Asthenia	2 (0.3)	0.2	0 (0.0)	0.0
Fatigue	4 (0.5)	0.3	4 (0.5)	0.6
Malaise	2 (0.3)	0.2	0 (0.0)	0.0
Pyrexia	4 (0.5)	0.3	2 (0.3)	0.3
Hepatobiliary Disorders	8 (1.1)	0.7	2 (0.3)	0.3
Cytolytic Hepatitis	2 (0.3)	0.2	1 (0.1)	0.2
Infections and Infestations	17 (2.3)	1.5	10 (1.4)	1.5
Retroviral infections	2 (0.3)	0.2	2 (0.3)	0.3
P. jiroveci pneumonia	2 (0.3)	0.2	0 (0.0)	0.0
Investigations	26 (3.5)	2.3	3 (0.4)	0.5
ALT Increased	7 (0.9)	0.6	1 (0.1)	0.2
AST Increased	3 (0.4)	0.3	1 (0.1)	0.2
GGT Increased	5 (0.7)	0.4	0 (0.0)	0.0
Hepatic Enzyme Increased	4 (0.5)	0.3	1 (0.1)	0.2
Liver Function Test Abnormal	3 (0.4)	0.3	0 (0.0)	0.0
Transaminases Increased	3 (0.4)	0.3	0 (0.0)	0.0
Weight decreased	3 (0.4)	0.3	0 (0.0)	0.0
Blood Triglycerides Increased	2 (0.3)	0.2	0 (0.0)	0.0

(cont'd)

Table 4: APTIVUS *(cont'd)*

Adverse Events Resulting in Clinical Intervention (Discontinuation) in the RESIST Trials 1182.12 and 1182.14

System Organ Class/Preferred Term	Treatment Group TPV/r N (%)	TPV/r Events/100 PEY	CPI/r N (%)	CPI/r Events/100 PEY
Metabolism and Nutrition Disorders	14 (1.9)	1.2	6 (0.8)	0.9
Anorexia	4 (0.5)	0.3	1 (0.1)	0.2
Cachexia	2 (0.3)	0.2	0 (0.0)	0.0
Hypertriglyceridemia	2 (0.3)	0.2	1 (0.1)	0.2
Dehydration	3 (0.4)	0.3	0 (0.0)	0.0
Hyperlipidaemia	2 (0.3)	0.2	0 (0.0)	0.0
Musculoskeletal and Connective Tissue Disorders	5 (0.7)	0.4	3 (0.4)	0.5
Arthralgia	1 (0.1)	0.1	2 (0.3)	0.3
Back pain	0 (0.0)	0.0	2 (0.3)	0.3
Myalgia	2 (0.3)	0.2	0 (0.0)	0.0
Neoplasms Benign, Malignant and Unspecified (including cysts and polyps)	3 (0.4)	0.3	9 (1.2)	1.4
Lymphoma	0 (0.0)	0.0	3 (0.4)	0.5
Nervous System Disorders	13 (1.7)	1.1	4 (0.5)	0.6
Headache	3 (0.4)	0.3	2 (0.3)	0.3
Dizziness	2 (0.3)	0.2	0 (0.0)	0.0
Psychiatric Disorders	2 (0.3)	0.2	0 (0.0)	0.0
Renal and Urinary Disorders	4 (0.5)	0.3	3 (0.4)	0.5
Renal failure acute	2 (0.3)	0.2	0 (0.0)	0.0
Nephrolithiasis	0 (0.0)	0.0	2 (0.3)	0.3
Respiratory, Thoracic and Mediastinal Disorders	6 (0.8)	0.5	1 (0.1)	0.2
Skin and Subcutaneous Tissue Disorders	7 (0.9)	0.6	8 (1.1)	1.2
Rash	5 (0.7)	0.4	4 (0.5)	0.6
Vascular Disorders	2 (0.3)	0.2	0 (0.0)	0.0

Table 5: APTIVUS

Study-Drug-Related Adverse Events Occurring in 1% or More of Patients in Either Treatment Group in the RESIST Trials

System Organ Class/ Preferred Term	Treatment Group/Number (%) of Patients and Events/100 PEY TPV/r[a]	Events/100 PEY	CPI/r[a]	Events/100 PEY
Total treated	749 (100.0)	1159.6	737 (100.0)	659.3
Total with any study drug-related adverse event	412 (55.0)	65.9	300 (40.7)	67.3
Gastrointestinal Disorders	268 (35.8)	33.4	226 (30.7)	45.3
Diarrhea	144 (19.2)	14.9	138 (18.7)	24.4
Nausea	105 (14.0)	10.2	87 (11.8)	14.5
Vomiting	41 (5.5)	3.7	28 (3.8)	4.4
Flatulence	26 (3.5)	2.3	25 (3.4)	3.9
Abdominal distension	22 (2.9)	2.0	19 (2.6)	2.9
Abdominal pain	22 (2.9)	1.9	29 (3.9)	4.6
Abdominal pain upper	10 (1.3)	0.9	11 (1.5)	1.7
Dyspepsia	9 (1.2)	0.8	9 (1.2)	1.4
Dry mouth	4 (0.5)	0.3	7 (1.0)	1.1
Gastritis	2 (0.3)	0.2	7 (1.0)	1.1
General Disorders and Administration Site Conditions	58 (7.7)	5.3	53 (7.2)	8.5
Fatigue	39 (5.2)	3.5	29 (3.9)	4.5

(cont'd)

Table 5: APTIVUS *(cont'd)*

Study-Drug-Related Adverse Events Occurring in 1% or More of Patients in Either Treatment Group in the RESIST Trials

System Organ Class/ Preferred Term	Treatment Group/Number (%) of Patients and Events/100 PEY			
	TPV/r[a]	Events/100 PEY	CPI/r[a]	Events/100 PEY
Asthenia	4 (0.5)	0.3	13 (1.8)	2.0
Investigations	64 (8.5)	5.8	19 (2.6)	2.9
ALT increased	18 (2.4)	1.6	4 (0.5)	0.6
GGT increased	16 (2.1)	1.4	1 (0.1)	0.2
Blood triglycerides increased	15 (2.0)	1.3	6 (0.8)	0.9
AST increased	12 (1.6)	1.0	3 (0.4)	0.5
Transaminases increased	8 (1.1)	0.7	0 (0.0)	0.0
Metabolism and Nutrition Disorders	83 (11.1)	7.8	48 (6.5)	7.7
Hypertriglyceridemia	33 (4.4)	2.9	17 (2.3)	2.6
Hyperlipidemia	23 (3.1)	2.0	7 (1.0)	1.1
Anorexia	10 (1.3)	0.9	8 (1.1)	1.2
Nervous System Disorders	59 (7.9)	5.4	56 (7.6)	9.0
Headache	29 (3.9)	2.6	15 (2.0)	2.3
Dizziness	12 (1.6)	1.1	11 (1.5)	1.7
Somnolence	5 (0.7)	0.4	7 (1.0)	1.1
Neuropathy peripheral	3 (0.4)	0.3	7 (1.0)	1.1
Psychiatric Disorders	19 (2.5)	1.7	20 (2.7)	3.1
Insomnia	5 (0.7)	0.4	7 (1.0)	1.1
Skin and Subcutaneous Tissue Disorders	58 (7.7)	5.3	40 (5.4)	6.2
Rash	16 (2.1)	1.4	12 (1.6)	1.8
Lipodystrophy acquired	9 (1.2)	0.8	3 (0.4)	0.5
Pruritus	12 (1.6)	1.1	3 (0.4)	0.5

[a] Doses are BID and in mg. TPV/r doses are 500/200; CPI/r doses are LPV/r 400/100, IDV/r 800/100, SQV/r 1000/100 or SQV/r 800/200, APV/r 600/100.

Less Common Clinical Trial Adverse Drug Reactions (<1%): Clinically meaningful adverse reactions of moderate to severe intensity occurring in less than 1% (<1/100) of adult patients in all Phase II and III trials treated with the 500 mg/200 mg APTIVUS/ritonavir dose (n=1397) are listed below by system organ class and frequency according to the following catergories:
Blood and Lymphatic System Disorders: anaemia, neutropenia, thrombocytopenia.
Gastrointestinal Disorders: gastrooesophageal reflux disease, pancreatitis.
General Disorders: influenza like illness, malaise, pyrexia.
Hepatobiliary Disorders: hepatitis, cytolytic hepatitis, toxic hepatitis, hepatic steatosis, hepatic failure (including fatal outcome), hyperbilirubinemia.
Immune System Disorders: hypersensitivity.
Investigations: hepatic enzymes increased, liver function test abnormal, weight decreased, lipase increased.
Metabolism and Nutrition Disorders: decreased appetite, diabetes mellitus, hyperamylasaemia, hypercholesterolaemia, dehydration, facial wasting, hyperglycaemia.
Musculoskeletal and Connective Tissue Disorders: muscle cramp, myalgia.
Nervous System Disorders: dizziness, neuropathy peripheral, somnolence, intracranial hemorrhage.
Psychiatric Disorders: insomnia, sleep disorder.
Renal and Urinary Disorders: renal insufficiency.
Respiratory, Thoracic and Mediastinal Disorders: dyspnoea.
Skin and Subcutaneous System Disorders: exanthem, lipoatrophy, lipodystrophy acquired, lipohypertrophy.

Reactivation of herpes simplex and varicella zoster virus infections were observed in the RESIST trials.

Abnormal Hematologic and Clinical Chemistry Findings: Frequencies of marked clinical laboratory abnormalities (Grade 3 or 4) reported in at least 2 % of patients in the APTIVUS/ritonavir (TPV/r) arms in the Phase III clinical studies (RESIST-1 and RESIST-2) after 48-weeks were increased AST (6.1 %), increased ALT (9.6 %), increased ALT and/or AST (6.2 %), increased amylase (6.0 %), increased cholesterol (4.2%), increased triglycerides (24.9 %) and decreased white blood cell counts (5.7 %).

In clinical trials RESIST-1 and RESIST-2 extending up to 96-weeks, the proportion of patients who developed Grade 2-4 ALT and/or AST elevations increased from 26% at week 48 to 29.3% at week 96 with APTIVUS/ritonavir and from 13.7% at week 48 to 14.6% at week 96 with Comparator PI/ritonavir, showing that the risk of developing transaminase elevations during the second year of therapy is lower than during the first year. Grade 3/4 ALT and/or AST elevations with APTIVUS coadministered with low dose ritonavir continued to increase from 10.0% at week 48 to 14.7% at week 96, and for comparator PI/ritonavir from 3.4% to 4.5% at weeks 48 and 96, respectively.

Marked clinical laboratory abnormalities (Grade 3 or 4) reported in phase III clinical studies (RESIST-1 and RESIST-2) in adults are summarized in Table 6.

Post-Market Adverse Drug Reactions: In addition to adverse events identified in clinical trials, the following events have been reported since market introduction of APTIVUS. Because they are reported spontaneously from a population of unknown size, estimates of frequency cannot be made. The following events have been chosen for inclusion due to their seriousness, frequency of reporting, potential causal connection to APTIVUS, or a combination of these factors.
Blood and Lymphatic System Disorders: thrombocytopenia.
Gastrointestinal Disorders: diarrhoea, nausea, pancreatitis, vomiting.
Hepatobiliary Disorders: hepatitis, hepatotoxicity, hyperbilirubinaemia, jaundice.
Immune System Disorders: hypersensitivity.
Investigations: alanine aminotransferase increased, aspartate aminotransferase increased, blood bilirubin increased, blood triglycerides increased, gamma glutamyl transferase increased, hepatic enzyme increased, liver function test abnormal, transaminases increased.
Metabolism and Nutrition Disorders: anorexia, hypertriglyceridaemia.
Musculoskeletal, Connective Tissue and Bone Disorders: haemarthrosis, muscle haemorrhage.
Nervous System Disorders: dizziness, haemorrhage intracranial, headache, somnolence.
Psychiatric Disorders: insomnia.
Renal and Urinary Disorders: renal failure.
Skin and Subcutaneous Disorders: rash, subcutaneous haemorrhage.

Table 6: APTIVUS

Grade 3-4 Laboratory Abnormalities Reported in ≥2% of Adult Patients

	RESIST-1/RESIST-2 (48-weeks) Percentage of Patients (events per 100 patient-exposure years)	
	APTIVUS/RTV (500 mg/200 mg BID)+OBR (n=738) %	Comparator PI/RTV+OBR[a] (n=724) %
Hematology		
WBC count decrease	5.7 (5.8)	5.9 (9.5)
Chemistry		
ALT	9.6 (10.1)	2.1 (3.3)
AST	6.1 (6.3)	1.8 (2.8)
ALT and/or AST	10.3 (10.9)	2.9 (4.6)
Amylase	6.0 (6.2)	7.0 (11.6)
Lipase	2.8 (2.9)	2.6 (4.2)
Total cholesterol	4.2 (4.3)	0.4 (0.7)
Triglycerides	24.9 (30.8)	13.0 (22.9)
Glucose (increase)	1.9 (1.9)	1.8 (2.8)

[a] OBR—optimized background regimen—Comparator PI/r: LPV/r 400/100 mg BID, IDV/r 800/100 mg BID, SQV/r 1000/100 mg BID, APV/r 600/100 mg BID.

DRUG INTERACTIONS:

Tipranavir is a substrate, an inducer and an inhibitor of cytochrome P450 CYP3A. However, when co-administered with ritonavir at the recommended dosage, there is a net inhibition of P450 CYP3A. Co-administration of APTIVUS and ritonavir with agents primarily metabolised by CYP3A may result in changed plasma concentrations of tipranavir or the other agents, which could alter their therapeutic and adverse effects. Agents that are contraindicated specifically due to the expected magnitude of interaction and potential for serious adverse events are listed in Contraindications and in Drug Interactions, Table 7, Drugs that Should Not Be Co-Administered with APTIVUS/Ritonavir.

Tipranavir is metabolised by CYP3A and is a Pgp substrate. Co-administration of tipranavir and agents that induce CYP3A and/or Pgp may decrease tipranavir concentrations and reduce its therapeutic effect. Co-administration of APTIVUS and medicinal products that inhibit Pgp may increase tipranavir plasma concentrations. Interaction with other drugs and other potentially significant drug interactions are discussed in greater detail in this section.

Overview: APTIVUS co-administered with ritonavir at the recommended dose is a net inhibitor of CYP3A and may increase plasma concentrations of agents that are primarily metabolized by CYP3A. Thus, co-administration of APTIVUS/ritonavir with drugs highly dependent on CYP3A for clearance and for which elevated plasma concentrations are associated with serious and/or life-threatening events is contraindicated (see Contraindications). Co-administration with other CYP3A substrates may require a dose adjustment or additional monitoring (see Drug Interactions).

A phenotypic cocktail study was conducted with 16 healthy volunteers to quantify the influence of 10 days of APTIVUS/ritonavir administration on the activity of hepatic CYP 1A2 (caffeine), 2C9 (warfarin), 2C19 (omeprazole), 2D6 (dextromethorphan) and the activity of intestinal and hepatic CYP3A4/5 (midazolam) and P-glycoprotein (P-gp) (digoxin). This study determined the first-dose and steady-state effects of 500 mg of APTIVUS, co-administered with 200 mg of ritonavir twice-daily in capsule form.

There was no net effect on CYP2C9 or hepatic P-gp at first dose or steady state. There was no net effect after first dose on CYP1A2, but there was moderate induction at steady state. There was slight inhibition after first dose on CYP2C19 and moderate induction at steady state. Potent inhibition of CYP2D6 and both hepatic and intestinal CYP3A4/5 activities were observed after first dose and steady state.

Intestinal and hepatic P-gp activity was assessed by administering oral and intravenous digoxin, respectively. The digoxin results indicate that P-gp was inhibited after the first dose of APTIVUS/ritonavir followed by induction of P-gp over time. Thus, it is difficult to predict the net effect of APTIVUS administered with ritonavir on oral bioavailability and plasma concentrations of drugs that are dual substrates of CYP3A and P-gp. The net effect will vary depending on the relative affinity of the co-administered drugs for CYP3A and P-gp, and the extent of intestinal first-pass metabolism/efflux. An in vitro induction study in human hepatocytes showed an increase in UGT1A1 by tipranavir similar to that evoked by rifampin. The clinical consequences of this finding have not been established.

Table 7: APTIVUS

Drugs That Should not be Co-Administered with APTIVUS/Ritonavir

Drug Class: Drug Name	Clinical Comment
Antiarrhythmics: amiodarone, bepridil, flecainide, propafenone, quinidine	**Contraindicated.** Concentrations of amiodarone, bepridil, flecainide, propafenone, quinidine may be increased when co-administered with APTIVUS/ritonavir.
Antihistamines: astemizole[a], terfenadine[a]	**Contraindicated** due to potential for serious and/or life-threatening reactions such as cardiac arrhythmias.
Ergot Derivatives: dihydroergotamine, ergonovine, ergotamine, methylergonovine	**Contraindicated** due to potential for serious and/or life-threatening reactions such as acute ergot toxicity characterized by peripheral vasospasm and ischemia of the extremities and other tissues.

(cont'd)

Table 7: APTIVUS *(cont'd)*

Drugs That Should not be Co-Administered with APTIVUS/Ritonavir

Drug Class: Drug Name	Clinical Comment
Fluticasone Propionate	A drug interaction study in healthy subjects has shown that ritonavir significantly increases plasma fluticasone propionate exposures, resulting in significantly decreased serum cortisol concentrations. Concomitant use of APTIVUS, co-administered with ritonavir, and fluticasone propionate may produce the same effects. Systemic corticosteroid effects including Cushing's syndrome and adrenal suppression have been reported during post-marketing use in patients receiving ritonavir and inhaled or intranasally administered fluticasone propionate. Therefore, co-administration of fluticasone propionate and APTIVUS/ritonavir is not recommended unless the potential benefit to the patient outweighs the risk of systemic corticosteroid side effects.
GI Motility Agent: cisapride[a]	**Contraindicated** due to potential for serious and/or life-threatening reactions such as cardiac arrhythmias.
HMG-CoA Reductase Inhibitors: lovastatin, simvastatin	**Contraindicated** due to an increased risk of myopathy, including rhabdomyolysis.
HMG-CoA Reductase Inhibitors: atorvastatin	The concomitant use of APTIVUS, co-administered with low-dose ritonavir with atorvastatin is not recommended due to an increased risk of myopathy, including rhabdomyolysis.
Neuroleptic: pimozide	**Contraindicated** due to the potential for serious and/or life-threatening reactions such as cardiac arrhythmias.
Phosphodiesterase (PDE5) Inhibitors: vardenafil	**Contraindicated** as co-administration of APTIVUS and ritonavir with PDE5 inhibitors is expected to substantially increase PDE5 inhibitors concentrations and may result in an increase in PDE5 inhibitor-associated adverse events including hypotension, visual changes and priapism (see Drug Interactions, Table 8, and complete prescribing information for PDE5 inhibitors).
Proton Pump Inhibitors/ H_2 Antagonists: omeprazole, esomeprazole	A drug interaction study in healthy subjects has shown that APTIVUS/ritonavir significantly decreased plasma omeprazole exposures (AUC and C_{max} by 71% and 73%, respectively). Therefore, co-administration of omeprazole or esomeprazole with APTIVUS/ritonavir is not recommended. If unavoidable, upward dose adjustments for either omeprazole or esomeprazole should be considered based on clinical response to therapy. Recommendations for maximal doses of omeprazole or esomeprazole are found in their corresponding product monographs.
Protease Inhibitors: atazanavir, fosamprenavir, lopinavir, saquinavir	In a clinical study of dual-boosted protease inhibitor combination therapy in multiple-treatment experienced HIV-positive adults, APTIVUS, co-administered with 200 mg ritonavir, caused a 55%, 70% and 78% reduction in the C_{min} of amprenavir, lopinavir and saquinavir, respectively. An 81% reduction in the C_{min} of atazanavir was similarly observed in a healthy volunteer interaction study. Concomitant use of APTIVUS, co-administered with 200 mg ritonavir, with the protease inhibitors fosamprenavir, atazanavir, lopinavir or saquinavir (each co-administered with low-dose ritonavir) results in significant decreases in plasma concentrations of these protease inhibitors (see Drug Interactions, Table 10). Combining a protease inhibitor with APTIVUS/ritonavir is not recommended.
Rifampicin (Rifampin):	Concomitant use of APTIVUS and rifampicin (rifampin) is contraindicated. Co-administration of protease inhibitors, including APTIVUS, with rifampicin (rifampin) is expected to substantially decrease protease inhibitor concentrations and may result in sub-optimal levels of tipranavir and lead to loss of virologic response and possible resistance to APTIVUS or to the class of protease inhibitors.
Sedatives/Hypnotics: midazolam, triazolam	**Contraindicated** due to the potential for serious and/or life-threatening reactions such as prolonged or increased sedation or respiratory depression. Ritonavir is a potent inhibitor of CYP 3A, and therefore will affect drugs metabolized by this enzyme. Concentrations of intravenously administered single dose midazolam were increased 2.8-fold (AUC_{0-24h}) and concentrations of orally administered midazolam were increased 10-fold when co-administered with APTIVUS/ritonavir at steady state.

[a] Cisapride, astemizole and terfenadine are no longer marketed in Canada.

The drugs listed in Table 8 are based on either drug interaction case reports or studies, or potential interactions due to the expected magnitude and seriousness of the interaction (i.e. those identified as contraindicated).

Table 8: APTIVUS

Established and Other Potentially Significant Drug Interactions: Alterations in Dose or Regimen May be Recommended Based on Drug Interaction Studies or Predicted Interaction

Concomitant Drug Class: Drug Name	Effect on Concentration of APTIVUS, Co-Administered with Ritonavir or Concomitant Drug	Clinical Comment
HIV-Antiviral Agents		
Nucleoside Reverse Transcriptase Inhibitors:		
Abacavir	↓ Abacavir AUC by approximately 40%	Clinical relevance of reduction in abacavir levels not established. Dose adjustment of abacavir cannot be recommended at this time.
Didanosine (EC)	↓ Didanosine	Clinical relevance of reduction in didanosine levels not established. For optimal absorption, didanosine should be separated from APTIVUS co-administered with ritonavir dosing by at least 2 hours to avoid formulation incompatibility.
Zidovudine	↓ Zidovudine AUC by approximately 35%. ZDV glucuronide concentrations were unaltered.	Clinical relevance of reduction in zidovudine levels not established. Dose adjustment of zidovudine cannot be recommended at this time.
Lamivudine and stavudine	No significant change in the AUC of lamivudine or stavudine	No dosage adjustment of lamivudine or stavudine is recommended.
Tenofovir	No significant change in the plasma concentrations of tenofovir.	No dosage adjustment of tenofovir is recommended.
Non-nucleoside Reverse Transcriptase Inhibitors:		

(cont'd)

Table 8: APTIVUS *(cont'd)*

Established and Other Potentially Significant Drug Interactions: Alterations in Dose or Regimen May be Recommended Based on Drug Interaction Studies or Predicted Interaction

Concomitant Drug Class: Drug Name	Effect on Concentration of APTIVUS, Co-Administered with Ritonavir or Concomitant Drug	Clinical Comment
Efavirenz	No significant impact on the AUC and C_{min} of efavirenz.	Steady-state efavirenz 600 mg qd co-administered with steady-state APTIVUS and ritonavir (500/200 mg BID) had no significant impact on tipranavir AUC and C_{max} (2.9% and 8.3% decreases, respectively) and resulted in a clinically unimportant increase in Cp_{12h} (19.2%). Therefore no dose adjustment is necessary.
Nevirapine	No significant interaction with nevirapine was observed.	Therefore no dose adjustments are necessary.
Fusion Inhibitors:		
Enfurvitide	No formal drug interaction data are currently available on interactions of APTIVUS, co-administered with 200 mg ritonavir, with fusion inhibitors.	The co-administration of enfurvitide with APTIVUS, co-administered with ritonavir, is associated with an increase in steady-state plasma tipranavir trough concentration for the study population by approximately 45%. Similar increases also have been observed for lopinavir (23%) and saquinavir (63%) plasma trough concentrations after combination with enfuvirtide. The mechanism for this interaction is not known. Tipranavir or ritonavir dose adjustment is not recommended.
Other Agents for Opportunistic Infections		
Antifungals:		
Fluconazole Itraconazole Ketoconazole Voriconazole	↑ Tipranavir, ↔ Fluconazole ↑ Itraconazole (not studied) ↑ Ketoconazole (not studied) ↑↓ Voriconazole (not studied)	Fluconazole increases TPV concentrations but dose adjustments are not needed. Fluconazole doses >200 mg/day are not recommended. Based on theoretical considerations itraconazole and ketoconazole should be used with caution. High doses (200 mg/day) are not recommended. Due to multiple CYP isoenzymes systems involved with voriconazole metabolism, it is difficult to predict the interaction with APTIVUS, co-administered with ritonavir.
Antimycobacterials:		
Clarithromycin	↑ Tipranavir, ↑ Clarithromycin, ↓ 14-hydroxy-clarithromycin metabolite	No dose adjustment of APTIVUS or clarithromycin for patients with normal renal function is necessary. For patients with renal impairment the following dosage adjustments should be considered: • For patients with CL_{CR} 30 to 60 mL/min the dose of clarithromycin should be reduced by 50%. • For patients with CL_{CR} <30 mL/min the dose of clarithromycin should be decreased by 75%.
Rifabutin	Tipranavir not changed, ↑ Rifabutin ↑ Desacetyl-rifabutin	Single dose study. Dosage reductions of rifabutin by 75% are recommended (e.g. 150 mg every other day). Increased monitoring for adverse events in patients receiving the combination is warranted. Further dosage reduction may be necessary.
Other Agents Commonly Used		
Antacids	↓ Tipranavir	When APTIVUS/ritonavir, was co-administered with 20 mL of aluminum and magnesium-based liquid antacid, tipranavir AUC_{12h}, C_{max} and C_{12h} were reduced by 27, 25, and 29%, respectively. Consideration should be given to separating APTIVUS/ritonavir dosing from antacid administration to prevent reduced absorption of tipranavir.
Anticonvulsants:		
Carbamazepine Phenobarbital Phenytoin	↓ Tipranavir ↑ Carbamazepine	Carbamazepine, phenobarbital and phenytoin should be used with caution in combination with APTIVUS/ritonavir. APTIVUS may be less effective due to decreased tipranavir plasma concentration in patients taking these agents concomitantly. Concomitant use of carbamazepine at a dose of 200 mg BID resulted in increased carbamazepine plasma concentrations (by approximately 23 % in geometric mean C_{min} for the total of carbamazepine and carbamazepine-10,11 -epoxide; both are pharmacologically active moieties), and a decrease in tipranavir C_{min} (by approximately 61% compared to historical controls), which may result in decreased effectiveness. Higher doses of carbamazepine may result in even larger decreases in tipranavir plasma concentrations.
Valproic Acid	↓ Valproic Acid	Caution should be used when prescribing valproic acid. Valproic acid may be less effective due to decreased valproic acid plasma concentration in patients taking Aptivus concomitantly.
Antidepressants:		

(cont'd)

Table 8: APTIVUS *(cont'd)*

Established and Other Potentially Significant Drug Interactions: Alterations in Dose or Regimen May be Recommended Based on Drug Interaction Studies or Predicted Interaction

Concomitant Drug Class: Drug Name	Effect on Concentration of APTIVUS, Co-Administered with Ritonavir or Concomitant Drug	Clinical Comment
Trazodone	↑ Trazodone	Adverse events of nausea, dizziness, hypotension, and syncope have been observed following co-administration of trazodone and ritonavir. If trazodone is used with APTIVUS/ritonavir, the combination should be used with caution and a lower dose of trazodone should be considered.
Calcium Channel Blockers:		
Diltiazem Felodipine Nicardipine Nisoldipine Verapamil	Combination with APTIVUS/ritonavir not studied. Cannot predict effect of APTIVUS/ritonavir on calcium channel blockers that are dual substrates of CYP 3A and P-gp due to conflicting effect of APTIVUS/ritonavir on CYP 3A and P-gp. ↑↓ Diltiazem ↑ Felodipine (CYP 3A substrate but not P-gp substrate) ↑↓ Nicardipine ↑↓ Nisoldipine (CYP 3A substrate but not clear whether it is a P-gp substrate) ↑↓ Verapamil	Caution is warranted and clinical monitoring of patients is recommended.
Despiramine	Combination with APTIVUS/ritonavir not studied ↑ Despiramine	Dosage reduction and concentration monitoring of despiramine is recommended.
Disulfiram/ Metronidazole	Combination with APTIVUS/ritonavir not studied	APTIVUS capsules contain alcohol that can produce disulfiram-like reactions when co-administered with disulfiram or other drugs which produce this reaction (e.g. metronidazole).
HMG-CoA Reductase Inhibitors:		
Rosuvastatin Pravastatin Fluvastatin	↑ Tipranavir ↑ Rosuvastatin	APTIVUS, co-administered with ritonavir, increases the AUC (37%) and C_{max} (123%) of rosuvastatin. Co-administration of APTIVUS/r and rosuvastatin should be initiated with the lowest dose (5mg/day) of rosuvastatin, titrated to treatment response, and accompanied with careful clinical monitoring for rosuvastatin associated symptoms as described in the label of rosuvastatin. Based on similarities in the elimination of pravastatin and rosuvastatin it is also recommended to initiate pravastatin on the lowest possible dose (10 gm/day) with careful monitoring for pravastatin associated symptoms as described in the label of pravastatin.
Hypoglycemics:		
Glimepiride Glyburide Pioglitazone Repaglinide Tolbutamide	Combination with APTIVUS/ritonavir not studied. ↔ Glimepiride (CYP 2C9) ↔ Glyburide (CYP 2C9) ↑↓ Pioglitazone (CYP 2C8 and CYP 3A4) ↑↓ Repaglinide (CYP 2C8 and CYP 3A4) ↔ Tolbutamide (CYP 2C9) The effect of APTIVUS/ritonavir on CYP 2C8 and CYP 2C9 substrates is not known.	Careful glucose monitoring is warranted.
Immunosuppressants:		
Cyclosporine Sirolimus Tacrolimus	Combination with APTIVUS/ritonavir not studied. Cannot predict effect of TPV/ritonavir on immunosuppressants due to conflicting effect of TPV/ritonavir on CYP 3A and P-gp. ↑↓ Cyclosporine ↑↓ Sirolimus ↑↓ Tacrolimus The effect of co-administration of APTIVUS with ritonavir on a substrate for CYP3A4/5 showed potent inhibition at both first-dose and steady-state APTIVUS/ritonavir. When APTIVUS with ritonavir was co-administered with a substrate for P-gp moderate inhibition of P-gp occurred with first-dose APTIVUS/ritonavir, however no effect on P-gp occurred with steady-state APTIVUS/ritonavir. It is anticipated that similar effects will be seen with these immunosuppressants.	More frequent concentration monitoring of these medicinal products is recommended until blood levels have been stabilized.

(cont'd)

Table 8: APTIVUS *(cont'd)*

Established and Other Potentially Significant Drug Interactions: Alterations in Dose or Regimen May be Recommended Based on Drug Interaction Studies or Predicted Interaction

Concomitant Drug Class: Drug Name	Effect on Concentration of APTIVUS, Co-Administered with Ritonavir or Concomitant Drug	Clinical Comment
Loperamide	A pharmacodynamic interaction study in healthy volunteers demonstrated that administration of loperamide and APTIVUS, co-administered with low-dose ritonavir, does not cause any clinically relevant change in the respiratory response to carbon dioxide. The pharmacokinetic analysis showed that the AUC and C_{max} of loperamide are reduced by 51% and 61%, respectively, and the C_{min} of tipranavir by 26%.	The clinical relevance of these changes is unknown.
Narcotic Analgesics:		
Meperidine	Combinations with APTIVUS/ritonavir not studied ↓ Meperidine, ↑ Normeperidine	Dosage increase and long-term use of meperidine are not recommended due to increased concentrations of the metabolite normeperidine which has both analgesic activity and CNS stimulant activity (e.g. seizures).
Methadone	↓ Methadone AUC and C_{max} by 50%	Because APTIVUS/ritonavir decreases methadone AUC and C_{max} patients should be monitored for opiate withdrawal syndrome. Dosage of methadone may need to be increased when co-administered with tipranavir and 200 mg of ritonavir.
Oral Contraceptives/Estrogens:		
Ethinyl estradiol	↓ Ethinyl estradiol concentrations by 50%	Alternative methods of nonhormonal contraception should be used when estrogen based oral contraceptives are co-administered with APTIVUS and ritonavir. Patients using estrogens as hormone replacement therapy should be clinically monitored for signs of estrogen deficiency. Women using estrogens may have an increased risk of rash.
PDE5 Inhibitors:		
Sildenafil Tadalafil Vardenafil	Only the combination of tadalafil with APTIVUS/ritonavir has been studied ↑ Sildenafil (not studied) ↑ Tadalafil with first dose APTIVUS/ritonavir ↔ Tadalafil at APTIVUS/ritonavir steady-state	Concomitant use of APTIVUS, co-administered with 200 mg ritonavir, and tadalafil resulted in a 2.3-fold increase in tadalafil exposure with first-dose APTIVUS/ritonavir and no change in tadalafil exposure with steady-state tipranavir/ritonavir. If tadalafil is used within the first days of APTIVUS/ritonavir treatment, then the lowest dose should be administered. However, after 7-10 days of APTIVUS/ritonavir dosing, steady-state for tipranavir and ritonavir is achieved and the dose of tadalafil may be increased, as clinically necessary. Concomitant use of PDE5 inhibitors with APTIVUS and ritonavir should be used with caution and in no case should the starting dose of: • sildenafil exceed 25 mg within 48 hours • tadalafil exceed 10 mg every 72 hours • vardenafil is contraindicated
Selective Serotonin-Reuptake Inhibitors:		
Fluoxetine Paroxetine Sertraline	Combination with APTIVUS/ritonavir not studied ↑ Fluoxetine ↑ Paroxetine ↑ Sertraline	Antidepressants have a wide therapeutic index, but doses may need to be adjusted upon initiation of APTIVUS/ritonavir therapy.
Theophylline	APTIVUS, co-administered with low-dose ritonavir, is expected to decrease theophylline concentrations.	Increased dosage of theophylline may be required and therapeutic monitoring should be considered.
Warfarin and other oral anticoagulants	↔ S-Warfarin	Clinical and biological (INR measurement) monitoring is recommended when these medicinal products are combined.
Buprenor- phine/naloxone	↔ Buprenorphine/naloxone ↓ Tipranavir	A pharmacokinetic study (n=10) indicated that buprenorphine AUC and Cp24h were not significantly affected by co-administered TPV/rtv. Compared to historical controls the C_{min} of tipranavir was decreased by 39% with this combination.
Bupropion	↓ Bupropion	APTIVUS, co-administered with ritonavir at steady-state resulted in approximately a 50% decrease in bupropion C_{max} and AUC. Careful clinical monitoring should be recommended when combining these three drugs.

Drug-Food Interactions: APTIVUS capsules, administered under high fat meal conditions or with a light snack of toast and skimmed milk, were tested in a multiple dose study. Food enhanced the extent of bioavailability (AUC point estimate 1.31, confidence interval 1.23-1.39), but had minimal effect on peak tipranavir concentrations (C_{max} point estimate 1.16, confidence interval 1.09-1.24).

APTIVUS may be safely taken with standard or high-fat meals. APTIVUS capsules, co-administered with ritonavir, should be taken with food.

Drug-Herb Interactions: Herbal preparations containing St. John's wort should not be combined with APTIVUS, co-administered with low dose ritonavir. Co-administration of protease inhibitors, including APTIVUS, with St. John's wort is expected to substantially decrease protease inhibitor concentrations and may result in sub-optimal levels of tipranavir and lead to loss of virologic response and possible resistance to APTIVUS or to the class of protease inhibitors.

Drug-Laboratory Test Interactions: Interactions with laboratory tests have not been established.

Drug-Lifestyle Interactions: Driving and Using Machines: There are no specific studies about the ability to drive vehicles and use machinery.

Other Medications: The following medications were discouraged in the pivotal trials: amitriptyline, benazepril, buspirone, carbamazepine, cimetidine, clonazepam, desiryl, encainide erythromycin, fentanyl, loratadine, milk thistle, mirtazapine, nortriptyline, phenobarbital, phenytoin, quetiapine fumarate, risperidone, sublimaze, sulfinpyrazone, systemic cytotoxic chemotherapy, temazepam, troleandomycin, venlafaxine, verapamil, zaleplon, and zolpidem tartrate. Clinicians should monitor patients taking any of these medications concomitantly with APTIVUS/r.

Table 9: APTIVUS

Drug Interactions: Pharmacokinetic Parameters for Tipranavir in the Presence of Co-Administered Drugs

Co-Administered Drug	Co-Administered Drug Dose (Schedule)	APTIVUS/Ritonavir Drug Dose (Schedule)	n	PK	Ratio (90% Confidence Interval) of Tipranavir Pharmacokinetic Parameters with/without Co-Administered Drug		
					C_{max}	AUC	C_{min}
Atorvastatin	10 mg (1 dose)	500/200 mg BID (14 doses)	22	↔	0.96 (0.86, 1.07)	1.08 (1.00, 1.15)	1.04 (0.89, 1.22)
Clarithromycin	500 mg BID (25 doses)	500/200 mg BID[a]	24 (68)	↑	1.40 (1.24, 1.47)	1.66 (1.43, 1.73)	2.00 (1.58, 2.47)
Didanosine	400 mg (1 dose)	500/100 mg BID (27 doses)	5	↓	1.32 (1.09, 1.60)	1.08 (0.82, 1.42)	0.66 (0.31, 1.43)
Efavirenz	600 mg QD (8 doses)	500/100 mg BID[a]	21 (89)	↓	0.79 (0.69, 0.89)	0.69 (0.57, 0.83)	0.58 (0.36, 0.86)
		750/200 mg BID[a]	25 (100)	↔	0.97 (0.85, 1.09)	1.01 (0.85, 1.18)	0.97 (0.69, 1.28)
Ethinyl estradiol/ Norethindrone	0.035/1.0 mg (1 dose)	500/100 mg BID (21 doses)	21	↓	1.10 (0.98, 1.24)	0.98 (0.88, 1.11)	0.73 (0.59, 0.90)
		750/200 mg BID (21 doses)	13	↔	1.01 (0.96, 1.06)	0.98 (0.90, 1.07)	0.91 (0.69, 1.20)
Fluconazole	100 mg QD (12 doses)	500/200 mg BID[a]	20 (68)	↑	1.32 (1.18, 1.47)	1.50 (1.29, 1.73)	1.69 (1.33, 2.09)
Loperamide	16 mg (1 dose)	750/200 mg BID (21 doses)	24	↓	1.03 (0.92, 1.17)	0.98 (0.86, 1.12)	0.74 (0.62, 0.88)
Rifabutin	150 mg (1 dose)	500/200 mg BID (15 doses)	21	↔	0.99 (0.93, 1.07)	1.00 (0.96, 1.04)	1.16 (1.07, 1.27)
Tenofovir	300 mg (1 dose)	500/100 mg BID	22	↓	0.83 (0.74, 0.94)	0.82 (0.75, 0.91)	0.79 (0.70, 0.90)
		750/200 mg BID (23 doses)	20	↔	0.89 (0.84, 0.96)	0.91 (0.85, 0.97)	0.88 (0.78, 1.00)
Zidovudine	300 mg (1 dose)	500/100 mg BID	29	↓	0.87 (0.80, 0.94)	0.82 (0.76, 0.89)	0.77 (0.68, 0.87)
		750/200 mg BID (23 doses)	25	↔	1.02 (0.94, 1.10)	1.02 (0.92, 1.13)	1.07 (0.86, 1.34)

[a] Steady state comparison to historical data (n).

Table 10: APTIVUS

Drug Interactions: Pharmacokinetic Parameters for Co-Administered Drug in the Presence of APTIVUS/Ritonavir

Co-Administered Drug	Co-Administered Drug Dose (Schedule)	APTIVUS/Ritonavir Drug Dose (Schedule)	n	PK	Ratio (90% Confidence Interval) of Co-Administered Drug Pharmacokinetic Parameters with/without APTIVUS/Ritonavir; No Effect=1.00		
					C_{max}	AUC	C_{min}
Amprenavir/RTV[a]	600/100 mg BID (27 doses)	500/200 mg BID (28 doses)	16	↓	0.61 (0.51, 0.73)[d]	0.56 (0.49, 0.64)[d]	0.45 (0.38, 0.53)[d]
			74	↓	—	—	0.44 (0.39, 0.49)[e]
Abacavir[a]	300 mg BID (43 doses)	250/200 mg BID	28	↓	0.56 (0.48, 0.66)	0.56 (0.49, 0.63)	—
		750/100 mg BID	14	↓	0.54 (0.47, 0.63)	0.64 (0.55, 0.74)	—
		1250/100 mg BID (42 doses)	11	↓	0.48 (0.42, 0.53)	0.65 (0.55, 0.76)	—
Atorvastatin	10 mg (1 dose)	500/200 mg BID (17 doses)	22	↑	8.61 (7.25, 10.21)	9.36 (8.02, 10.94)	5.19 (4.21, 6.40)
Orthohydroxy-atorvastatin			21, 12, 17	↓	0.02 (0.02, 0.03)	0.11 (0.08, 0.17)	0.07 (0.06, 0.08)
Parahydroxy-atorvastatin			13, 22, 1	↓	1.04 (0.87, 1.25)	0.18 (0.14, 0.24)	0.33 (NA)
Clarithromycin	500 mg BID (25 doses)	500/200 mg BID (15 doses)	21	↑	0.95 (0.83, 1.09)	1.19 (1.04, 1.37)	1.68 (1.42, 1.98)
14-OH-clarithromycin			21	↓	0.03 (0.02, 0.04)	0.03 (0.02, 0.04)	0.05 (0.04, 0.07)
Didanosine[b]	200 mg BID, ≥60 kg 125 mg BID, <60 kg (43 doses)	250/200 mg BID	10	↓	0.57 (0.42, 0.79)	0.67 (0.51, 0.88)	—
		750/100 mg BID	8	↔	0.76 (0.49, 1.17)	0.97 (0.64, 1.47)	—
		1250/100 mg BID (42 doses)	9	↔	0.77 (0.47, 1.26)	0.87 (0.47, 1.65)	—
	400 mg (1 dose)	500/100 mg BID (27 doses)	5	↔	0.80 (0.63, 1.02)	0.90 (0.72, 1.11)	1.17 (0.62, 2.20)
Efavirenz[b]	600 mg QD (15 doses)	500/100 mg BID	24	↔	1.09 (0.99, 1.19)	1.04 (0.97, 1.12)	1.02 (0.92, 1.12)
		750/200 mg BID (15 doses)	22	↔	1.12 (0.98, 1.28)	1.00 (0.93, 1.09)	0.94 (0.84, 1.04)
Ethinyl estradiol	0.035 mg (1 dose)	500/100 mg BID	21	↓	0.52 (0.47, 0.57)	0.52 (0.48, 0.56)	—
		750/200 mg BID (21 doses)	13	↓	0.48 (0.42, 0.57)	0.57 (0.54, 0.60)	—
Fluconazole	200 mg (Day 1) then 100 mg QD (6 or 12 doses)	500/200 mg BID (2 or 14 doses)	19	↔	0.97 (0.94, 1.01)	0.99 (0.97, 1.02)	0.98 (0.94, 1.02)
			19	↔	0.94 (0.91, 0.98)	0.92 (0.88, 0.95)	0.89 (0.85, 0.92)
Lopinavir/RTV[a]	400/100 mg BID (27 doses)	500/200 mg BID (28 doses)	21	↓	0.53 (0.40, 0.69)[d]	0.45 (0.32, 0.63)[d]	0.30 (0.17, 0.51)[d]
			69	↓	—	—	0.48 (0.40, 0.58)[e]

(cont'd)

Table 10: APTIVUS *(cont'd)*

Drug Interactions: Pharmacokinetic Parameters for Co-Administered Drug in the Presence of APTIVUS/Ritonavir

Co-Administered Drug	Co-Administered Drug Dose (Schedule)	APTIVUS/Ritonavir Drug Dose (Schedule)	n	PK	Ratio (90% Confidence Interval) of Co-Administered Drug Pharmacokinetic Parameters with/without APTIVUS/Ritonavir; No Effect=1.00		
					C_{max}	AUC	C_{min}
Loperamide	16 mg (1 dose)	750/200 mg BID (21 doses)	24	↓	0.39 (0.31, 0.48)	0.49 (0.40, 0.61)	—
N-Demethyl-Loperamide			24	↓	0.21 (0.17, 0.25)	0.23 (0.19, 0.27)	—
Lamivudine[a]	150 mg BID (43 doses)	250/200 mg BID	64	↔	0.96 (0.89, 1.03)	0.95 (0.89, 1.02)	—
		750/100 mg BID	46	↔	0.86 (0.78, 0.94)	0.96 (0.90, 1.03)	—
		1250/100 mg BID (42 doses)	35	↔	0.71 (0.62, 0.81)	0.82 (0.66, 1.00)	—
Nevirapine[a]	200 mg BID (43 doses)	250/200 mg BID	26	↔	0.97 (0.90, 1.04)	0.97 (0.91, 1.04)	0.96 (0.87, 1.05)
		750/100 mg BID	22	↔	0.86 (0.76, 0.97)	0.89 (0.78, 1.01)	0.93 (0.80, 1.08)
		1250/100 mg BID (42 doses)	17	↔	0.71 (0.62, 0.82)	0.76 (0.63, 0.91)	0.77 (0.64, 0.92)
Norethindrone	1.0 mg (1 dose)	500/100 mg BID	21	↔	1.03 (0.94, 1.13)	1.14 (1.06, 1.22)	—
		750/200 mg BID (21 doses)	13	↔	1.08 (0.97, 1.20)	1.27 (1.13, 1.43)	—
Rifabutin	150 mg (1 dose)	500/200 mg BID (15 doses)	20	↑	1.70 (1.49, 1.94)	2.90 (2.59, 3.26)	2.14 (1.90, 2.41)
25-O-desacetyl-rifabutin			20	↑	3.20 (2.78, 3.68)	20.71 (17.66, 24.28)	7.83 (6.70, 9.14)
Rifabutin + 25-O-desacetyl-rifabutin[c]			20	↑	1.86 (1.63, 2.12)	4.33 (3.86, 4.86)	2.76 (2.44, 3.12)
Saquinavir/RTV[a]	600/100 mg BID (27 doses)	500/200 mg BID (28 doses)	20	↓	0.30 (0.23, 0.40)[d]	0.24 (0.19, 0.32)[d]	0.18 (0.13, 0.26)[d]
			68	↓	—	—	0.20 (0.16, 0.25)[e]
Stavudine[a]	40 mg BID, ≥60 kg 30 mg BID, <60 kg (43 doses)	250/200 mg BID	26	↔	0.90 (0.81, 1.02)	1.00 (0.91, 1.11)	—
		750/100 mg BID	22	↔	0.76 (0.66, 0.89)	0.84 (0.74, 0.96)	—
		1250/100 mg BID (42 doses)	19	↔	0.74 (0.69, 0.80)	0.93 (0.83, 1.05)	—
Tenofovir	300 mg (1 dose)	500/100 mg BID	22	↓	0.77 (0.68, 0.87)	0.98 (0.91, 1.05)	1.07 (0.98, 1.17)
		750/200 mg BID (23 doses)	20	↓	0.62 (0.54, 0.71)	1.02 (0.94, 1.10)	1.14 (1.01, 1.27)
Zidovudine[b]	300 mg BID	250/200 mg BID	48	↓	0.54 (0.47, 0.62)	0.58 (0.51, 0.66)	—
	300 mg BID	750/100 mg BID	31	↓	0.51 (0.44, 0.60)	0.64 (0.55, 0.75)	—
	300 mg BID (43 doses)	1250/100 mg BID (42 doses)	23	↓	0.49 (0.40, 0.59)	0.69 (0.49, 0.97)	—
	300 mg (1 dose)	500/100 mg BID	29	↓	0.39 (0.33, 0.45)	0.57 (0.52, 0.63)	0.89 (0.81, 0.99)
		750/200 mg BID (23 doses)	25	↑	0.44 (0.36, 0.54)	0.67 (0.62, 0.73)	1.25 (1.08, 1.44)
Zidovudine glucuronide		500/100 mg BID	29	↑	0.82 (0.74, 0.90)	1.02 (0.97, 1.06)	1.52 (1.34, 1.71)
		750/200 mg BID (23 doses)	25	↑	0.82 (0.73, 0.92)	1.09 (1.05, 1.14)	1.94 (1.62, 2.31)

[a] HIV+ patients.
[b] HIV+ patients (APTIVUS/ritonavir 250 mg/200 mg, 750 mg/200 mg and 1250 mg/100 mg) and healthy volunteers (APTIVUS/ritonavir 500 mg/100 mg and 750 mg/200 mg).
[c] Normalized sum of parent drug (rifabutin) and active metabolite (25-O-desacetyl-rifabutin).
[d] Intensive PK analysis.
[e] Drug levels obtained at 8-16 hrs post-dose.

DOSAGE AND ADMINISTRATION:

Dosing Considerations: APTIVUS must be administered with 200 mg ritonavir to ensure its therapeutic effect. Patients should be instructed accordingly.

Please also refer to the ritonavir product monograph for contraindications, warnings, precautions, side effects and potential drug interactions.

Triglyceride and cholesterol testing should be performed prior to initiating tipranavir therapy and during therapy.

Dosage for Elderly Patients: In general, caution should be exercised in the administration and monitoring of APTIVUS in elderly patients reflecting the greater frequency of decreased hepatic, renal or cardiac function, and of concomitant disease or other drug therapy. See Action and Clinical Pharmacology, Warnings and Precautions, and Adverse Reactions.

Dosage for Pediatric Patients: The safety and efficacy of APTIVUS in this population has not been established. Treatment of children with APTIVUS is therefore not recommended. See Action and Clinical Pharmacology, Warnings and Precautions, Special Populations, and Adverse Reactions.

Dosage for Hepatically Impaired Patients: APTIVUS is contraindicated in patients with moderate or severe hepatic insufficiency (Child-Pugh Class B or C, respectively) (see Contraindications). APTIVUS co-administered with 200 mg ritonavir should be used with caution in patients with mild hepatic insufficiency (Child-Pugh Class A); these patients should be monitored closely.

Recommended Dose and Dosage Adjustment: The recommended dose of APTIVUS (tipranavir) Capsules is 500 mg (two 250 mg capsules), co-administered with 200 mg ritonavir (low-dose ritonavir), twice daily.

APTIVUS, co-administered with 200 mg ritonavir, should be administered with food.

APTIVUS, co-administered with 200 mg ritonavir, should be taken with at least two additional antiretroviral agents. The manufacturers' product monograph of the antiretroviral agents should be followed.

APTIVUS, co-administered with 200 mg ritonavir, causes a reduction in the AUC of didanosine. Dosing of enteric-coated didanosine and tipranavir, co-administered with 200 mg ritonavir, should be separated by at least 2 hours to avoid formulation incompatibility.

Missed Dose: Patients should be advised of the need to take APTIVUS every day as prescribed. If a dose is missed the patient should not double the next dose but should take the next dose as soon as possible.

OVERDOSAGE:

There is no known antidote for APTIVUS overdose. Treatment of overdose should consist of general supportive measures, including monitoring of vital signs and observation of the patient's clinical status. Administration of activated charcoal may also be used to aid in removal of unabsorbed drug. Since tipranavir is highly protein bound, dialysis is unlikely to be beneficial in significant removal of this medicine.

For management of a suspected drug overdose, contact your **regional Poison Control Centre**. See the *CPS* Directory section for a list of Poison Control Centres.

ACTION AND CLINICAL PHARMACOLOGY:

Microbiology: Mechanism of Action: The human immunodeficiency virus (HIV-1) encodes an aspartyl protease that is essential for the cleavage and maturation of viral protein precursors. Tipranavir is a non-peptidic inhibitor of the HIV-1 protease that inhibits viral replication by preventing the maturation of viral particles.

Pharmacokinetics: In order to achieve effective tipranavir plasma concentrations and a BID dosing regimen, co-administration of APTIVUS with 200 mg ritonavir twice daily is essential (see Dosage and Administration). Ritonavir acts by inhibiting hepatic cytochrome P450 CYP3A, the intestinal P-glycoprotein (Pgp) efflux pump and possibly intestinal cytochrome P450 CYP3A as well. As demonstrated in a dose-ranging evaluation in 113 HIV-negative healthy male and female volunteers, ritonavir increases $AUC_{0\text{-}12h}$, C_{max} and C_{min} and decreases the clearance of tipranavir. APTIVUS co-administered with ritonavir (500 mg/200 mg twice daily) was associated with a 29-fold increase in the geometric mean morning steady-state trough plasma concentrations compared to APTIVUS 500 mg twice daily without ritonavir.

Dosing APTIVUS 500 mg with 200 mg ritonavir twice-daily for greater than 2 weeks and without meal restriction produced the pharmacokinetic parameters for male and female HIV-positive patients presented in Table 11.

A trial of HIV infected patients assessed the pharmacokinetics and safety of APTIVUS/ritonavir 500/200 mg administered with and without lopinavir, amprenavir, or saquinavir compared to ritonavir 100 mg administered with lopinavir, amprenavir, or saquinavir. The mean systemic ritonavir concentration when 200 mg of ritonavir was given with APTIVUS was similar to the concentrations observed when 100 mg was given with the other protease inhibitors.

Table 11: APTIVUS

Pharmacokinetic Parameters[a] of Tipranavir/Ritonavir 500/200 mg for HIV+Patients by Gender

	Females (n=14)	Males (n=106)
Cp_{trough} (μM)	41.6±24.3	35.6±16.7
C_{max} (μM)	94.8±22.8	77.6±16.6
T_{max} (h)	2.9	3.0
$AUC_{0\text{-}12h}$ (μM·h)	851±309	710±207
CL (L/h)	1.15	1.27
V (L)	7.7	10.2
$t_{½}$ (h)	5.5	6.0

[a] Population pharmacokinetic parameters reported as mean±standard deviation.

Absorption: Absorption of tipranavir in humans is limited, although no absolute quantification of absorption is available. Tipranavir is a P-gp substrate, a weak P-gp inhibitor, and appears to be a potent P-gp inducer as well. In vivo data suggest that tipranavir/ritonavir, at the dose of 500/200 mg, is a P-gp inhibitor after the first dose and induction of P-gp occurs over time. Tipranavir trough concentrations at steady-state are about 70% lower than those on Day 1, presumably due to intestinal P-gp induction. Steady state is attained in most subjects after 7-10 days of dosing.

Peak plasma concentrations are reached within 1 to 5 hours after dose administration depending upon the dosage used. With repeated dosing, tipranavir plasma concentrations are lower than predicted from single dose data, presumably due to hepatic and transporter enzyme induction. Steady state is attained in most subjects after 7 days of dosing. APTIVUS, co-administered with 200 mg ritonavir, exhibits linear pharmacokinetics at steady-state.

Dosing with APTIVUS 500 mg concomitant with 200 mg ritonavir twice daily for 2 to 4 weeks and without meal restriction produced a mean tipranavir peak plasma concentration (C_{max}) of 94.8±22.8 μM for female patients (n=14) and 77.6±16.6 μM for male patients (n=106), occurring approximately 3 hours after administration.

The mean steady-state trough concentration prior to the morning dose was 41.6±24.3 μM for female patients and 35.6±16.7 μM for male patients. Tipranavir AUC over a 12 hour dosing interval averaged 851±309 μM·h (CL=1.15 L/h) for female patients and 710±207 μM·h (CL=1.27 L/h) for male patients. The mean half-life was 5.5 (females) or 6.0 hours (males).

Effects of Food on Oral Absorption: For APTIVUS capsules co-administered with ritonavir at steady-state, no clinically significant changes in C_{max}, Cp_{12h}, and AUC were observed under fed conditions (500-682 Kcal, 23-25% calories from fat) compared to fasted conditions. In view of the better tolerability of ritonavir when taken with food and the importance of taking APTIVUS and ritonavir together, APTIVUS/ritonavir should be taken with food (see Dosage and Administration).

When APTIVUS, co-administered with 200 mg ritonavir, was co-administered with 20 mL of aluminium and magnesium-based liquid antacid, tipranavir AUC_{12h}, C_{max} and C_{12h} were reduced by 25-29 %. Consideration should be given to separating APTIVUS/ritonavir dosing from antacid administration to prevent reduced absorption of tipranavir.

Distribution: Tipranavir is extensively bound to plasma proteins (>99.9%). From clinical samples of healthy volunteers and HIV-positive subjects who received APTIVUS without ritonavir the mean fraction of tipranavir unbound in plasma was similar in both populations (healthy volunteers 0.015%±0.006%; HIV positive subjects 0.019%±0.076%). Total plasma tipranavir concentrations for these samples ranged from 9 to 82 μM. The unbound fraction of tipranavir appeared to be independent of total drug concentration over this concentration range.

No studies have been conducted to determine the distribution of tipranavir into human cerebrospinal fluid or semen.

Metabolism: In vitro metabolism studies with human liver microsomes indicated that CYP3A4 is the predominant CYP isoform involved in tipranavir metabolism.

The oral clearance of tipranavir decreased after the addition of ritonavir which may represent diminished first-pass clearance of the drug at the gastrointestinal tract as well as the liver.

The metabolism of tipranavir in the presence of low-dose ritonavir is minimal. In a ^{14}C-tipranavir human study (^{14}C-tipranavir/ritonavir, 500 mg/200 mg bid), unchanged tipranavir was predominant and accounted for 98.4% or greater of the total plasma radioactivity circulating at 3, 8, or 12 hours after dosing. Only a few metabolites were found in plasma, and all were at trace levels (0.2% or less of the plasma radioactivity). In feces, unchanged tipranavir represented the majority of fecal radioactivity (79.9% of fecal radioactivity). The most abundant fecal metabolite, at 4.9% of fecal radioactivity (3.2% of dose), was a hydroxyl metabolite of tipranavir. In urine, unchanged tipranavir was found in trace amounts (0.5% of urine radioactivity). The most abundant urinary metabolite, at 11.0% of urine radioactivity (0.5% of dose) was a glucuronide conjugate of tipranavir.

Excretion: Administration of ^{14}C-tipranavir to subjects (n=8) that received APTIVUS/ritonavir 500 mg/200 mg BID dosed to steady-state demonstrated that most radioactivity (median 82.3%) was excreted in faeces, while only a median of 4.4% of the radioactive dose administered was recovered in urine. In addition, most radioactivity (56.3 %) was excreted between 24 and 96 hours after dosing. The effective mean elimination half-life of tipranavir/ritonavir in healthy volunteers (n=67) and HIV-infected adult patients (n=120) was 4.8 and 6.0 hours, respectively, at steady state following a dose of 500/200 mg BID daily with a light meal.

Special Populations and Conditions: Geriatrics: Evaluation of steady-state plasma tipranavir trough concentrations at 10-14 h after dosing from the RESIST-1 and RESIST-2 studies demonstrated that there was no change in median trough tipranavir concentrations as age increased for either gender through 65 years of age. There were an insufficient number of women greater than age 65 years in the two trials to evaluate the elderly, but the trend of consistent trough tipranavir concentrations with increasing age through 80 years for men was supported.

Gender: Evaluation of steady-state plasma tipranavir trough concentrations at 10-14 h after dosing from the RESIST-1 and RESIST-2 studies demonstrated that females generally had higher tipranavir concentrations than males. After 4 weeks of APTIVUS/ritonavir 500 mg/200 mg BID, the median plasma trough concentration of tipranavir was 43.9 μM for females and 31.1 μM for males. This difference in concentrations does not warrant a dose adjustment.

Race: Evaluation of steady-state plasma tipranavir trough concentrations at 10-14 h after dosing from the RESIST-1 and RESIST-2 studies demonstrated that white males generally had more variability in tipranavir concentrations than black males, but the median concentration and the range making up the majority of the data are comparable between the races. Females of either race generally had higher trough tipranavir concentrations than males.

Renal Insufficiency: Tipranavir pharmacokinetics have not been studied in patients with renal dysfunction. However, since the renal clearance of tipranavir is negligible, a decrease in total body clearance is not expected in patients with renal insufficiency.

Hepatic Insufficiency: In a study comparing 9 patients with mild (Child-Pugh A) hepatic impairment to 9 controls, the single and multiple dose pharmacokinetic profiles of tipranavir and ritonavir were increased in patients with hepatic impairment but still within the range observed in the clinical studies. No dosing adjustment is required in patients with mild hepatic impairment; however, patients should be closely monitored.

The influence of moderate hepatic impairment (Child Pugh B) on the multiple-dose pharmacokinetics of either tipranavir or ritonavir has not been evaluated. APTIVUS is contraindicated in patients with moderate or severe hepatic impairment.

STORAGE AND STABILITY: APTIVUS capsules should be stored under refrigeration (2 to 8°C). Once opened, the bottle can be stored at 25°C, excursions permitted to 15 to 30°C for up to 60 days.

INFORMATION FOR THE PATIENT: Published in e-CPS, available by subscription at www.e-cps.ca.

DOSAGE FORMS, COMPOSITION AND PACKAGING: Each pink, oblong soft gelatin capsule, imprinted in black with "TPV 250", contains: tipranavir 250 mg. Nonmedicinal ingredients: Cremophor EL, ethanol, mono/diglycerides of caprylic/capric acid, propyl gallate, propylene glycol, purified water and trometamol; shell: gelatin, iron oxide red, propylene glycol, purified water, 'sorbitol special glycerin blend' (d-sorbitol, 1,4-sorbitan, mannitol and glycerin) and titanium dioxide; black printing ink: ammonium hydroxide, ethylacetate, iron oxide black, isopropyl alcohol, Macrogol, polyvinyl acetate phthalate, propylene glycol, purified water and SDA 35 alcohol. HDPE unit-of-use bottles with a child resistant closure and 120 capsules.

(Shown in Product Identification Section)

Aranesp® 🅿

darbepoetin alfa

Erythropoiesis Regulating Hormone

Amgen

Date of Revision: July 12, 2010

SUMMARY PRODUCT INFORMATION:

Route of Administration	Dosage Form/ Strength	Clinically Relevant Nonmedicinal Ingredients
Chronic Kidney Disease (CKD): subcutaneous (SC) or intravenous (IV) **Cancer:** subcutaneous (SC)	**Pre-filled Syringes:** 10, 20, 30, 40, 50, 60, 80, 100, 130, 150, 200, 300, 500 μg/syringe	Not applicable For a complete listing see Dosage Forms, Composition and Packaging.

DESCRIPTION: Aranesp (darbepoetin alfa) is an erythropoiesis-stimulating agent produced in Chinese hamster ovary (CHO) cells by recombinant DNA technology. The final processed form is a 165-amino acid protein containing 5 N-linked oligosaccharide chains and 1 O-linked oligosaccharide chain. Aranesp has a molecular weight of 37.1 kd (based on known amino acid and carbohydrate structure).

INDICATIONS AND CLINICAL USE: Treatment of Anemia in Chronic Kidney Disease: Aranesp (darbepoetin alfa) is indicated for the treatment of anemia associated with chronic kidney disease (CKD), including patients on dialysis and patients not on dialysis.

Aranesp is not intended for patients who require immediate correction of severe anemia or emergency transfusions.

Blood pressure should be adequately controlled prior to initiation of Aranesp therapy and must be closely monitored and controlled during treatment.

Aranesp is not indicated for other causes of anemia such as iron or folate deficiencies, hemolysis, or gastrointestinal bleeding which should be managed appropriately.

Treatment of Anemia due to Chemotherapy in Patients with Non-Myeloid Malignancies: Aranesp is indicated for the treatment of anemia due to the effect of concomitantly administered chemotherapy based on studies that have shown a reduction in the need for red blood cell (RBC) transfusions in patients with advanced or metastatic, non-myeloid malignancies. Studies to determine whether Aranesp increases mortality or decreases progression-free/recurrence-free survival are ongoing.

- In patients with a long life expectancy, the decision to administer erythropoiesis-stimulating agents (ESAs) should be based on a benefit-risk assessment with the participation of the individual patient. This should take into account the specific clinical context such as (but not limited to) the type of tumor and its stage, the degree of anemia, life expectancy, the environment in which the patient is being treated and known risks of transfusions and ESAs.
- If appropriate, red blood cell transfusion should be the preferred treatment for the management of anemia in patients with a long life expectancy and who are receiving myelosuppressive chemotherapy.
- Aranesp is not indicated for use in patients receiving hormonal agents, therapeutic biologic products, or radiotherapy unless receiving concomitant myelosuppressive chemotherapy.

CONTRAINDICATIONS: Aranesp (darbepoetin alfa) is contraindicated in patients:

- with uncontrolled hypertension
- who develop Pure Red Cell Aplasia (PRCA) following treatment with any ESAs
- with known hypersensitivity to the active substance or any of the excipients
- with sensitivity to mammalian cell-derived products
- with sensitivity to albumin (where applicable with the albumin formulation)*

WARNINGS AND PRECAUTIONS:

Serious Warnings and Precautions

All Patients

- To minimize the risks for death, serious cardiovascular events, and stroke, follow the recommended dosage for each indication for Aranesp and other erythropoiesis-stimulating agents (ESAs) (see Warnings and Precautions, Increased Mortality, Serious Cardiovascular Events, Thromboembolic Events and Stroke, and Dosage and Administration).
- Patients with uncontrolled hypertension should not be treated with Aranesp; blood pressure should be adequately controlled before initiation of therapy with Aranesp.
- Aranesp should be used with caution in patients with a history of seizures.
- Antibody-mediated Pure Red Cell Aplasia (PRCA) has been reported after months to years of treatment with ESAs.

Chronic Kidney Disease Patients

- In clinical studies, patients experienced greater risks for death, serious cardiovascular events, and stroke when administered ESAs to target hemoglobin levels of 130 g/L and above. Individualize dosing to achieve and maintain hemoglobin levels within the range of 100 to 120 g/L.

Cancer Patients

- ESAs increased the risks for death, serious cardiovascular and thromboembolic events in some controlled clinical trials.
- ESAs shortened overall survival and/or increased the risk of tumor progression or recurrence in some clinical studies in patients with breast, head and neck, lymphoid, cervical and non-small cell lung cancers when dosed to target a hemoglobin level of ≥120 g/L.
- To minimize the above risks, use the lowest dose needed to avoid red blood cell (RBC) transfusions.
- Use ESAs only for treatment of anemia due to concomitant myelosuppressive chemotherapy.
- If appropriate, red blood cell transfusion should be the preferred treatment for the management of anemia in patients with a long life expectancy and who are receiving myelosuppressive chemotherapy.
- Discontinue Aranesp following the completion of a chemotherapy course.

General: Albumin (Human)*: Aranesp (darbepoetin alfa) is supplied in 2 formulations with different excipients, one containing polysorbate 80 and another containing albumin (human), a derivative of human blood. Based on effective donor screening and product manufacturing processes, Aranesp formulated with albumin carries an extremely remote risk for transmission of viral diseases. A theoretical risk for transmission of Creutzfeldt-Jakob disease (CJD) also is considered extremely remote. No cases of transmission of viral diseases or CJD have ever been identified for albumin.

Cardiovascular: Hypertension: Patients with uncontrolled hypertension should not be treated with Aranesp; blood pressure should be controlled adequately before initiation of therapy. Blood pressure may rise during treatment of anemia with Aranesp or rHuEPO. In Aranesp CKD clinical trials, approximately 40% of patients required initiation or intensification of antihypertensive therapy during the early phase of treatment when the hemoglobin was increasing. Hypertensive encephalopathy and seizures have been observed in patients with CKD treated with Aranesp or rHuEPO.

Special care should be taken to closely monitor and control blood pressure in patients treated with Aranesp During Aranesp therapy, patients should be advised of the importance of compliance with antihypertensive therapy and dietary restrictions. If blood pressure is difficult to control by pharmacologic or dietary measures, the dose of Aranesp should be reduced or withheld (see Dosage and Administration, Dose Adjustment for CKD Patients). A clinically significant decrease in hemoglobin may not be observed for several weeks.

Increased Mortality, Serious Cardiovascular Events, Thromboembolic Events and Stroke: Patients with chronic kidney disease experienced greater risks for death, serious cardiovascular events, and stroke when administered ESAs to target hemoglobin levels of 130 g/L and above in clinical studies. Patients with chronic kidney disease and an insufficient hemoglobin response to ESA therapy may be at even greater risk for cardiovascular events and mortality than other patients. Serious cardiovascular events included myocardial infarction, stroke, congestive heart failure, and an increased risk of serious arterial and venous thromboembolic events including hemodialysis vascular access thrombosis. A rate of hemoglobin rise of >10 g/L over 2 weeks may contribute to these risks.

Aranesp and other ESAs increased the risks for death, serious cardiovascular and thromboembolic events and stoke in some controlled clinical trials of patients with cancer. A rate of hemoglobin rise of >10 g/L over 2 weeks may contribute to these risks.

* Note: Albumin formulation not currently available in Canada.

CKD patients with hypo-responsiveness to ESAs may be at an increased risk for mortality and cardiovascular events. These patients should be evaluated for treatable conditions (see Warnings and Precautions, Lack or Loss of Response to Aranesp and Dosage and Administration, Dose Adjustment for CKD Patients). These risks should be carefully weighed against the benefit to be derived from treatment with ESAs, particularly in cancer patients with increased risk factors of thrombotic events, such as patients with a prior history of TVEs (e.g. deep venous thrombosis or pulmonary embolism) (see Dosage and Administration, Chronic Kidney Disease Patients; Cancer Patients Receiving Chemotherapy).

To minimize the risks for death and serious cardiovascular events, follow the recommended dosage for each indication for Aranesp and other ESAs. For CKD patients, individualize dosing to achieve and maintain hemoglobin levels within the recommended range of 100-120 g/L. For patients with cancer, use the lowest dose sufficient to avoid blood transfusions. The rate of hemoglobin increase should not exceed 10 g/L in any 2 week period (see Dosage and Administration).

An increased incidence of thromboembolic events has been observed in patients treated with erythropoietic agents. The anticipated benefits of Aranesp must be weighed against the potential for increased risks associated with therapy in the following populations: patients at risk for thrombosis; patients with pre-existing vascular disease; and in those patients with a known intolerance to antithrombotic agents.

An increased incidence of deep vein thrombosis (DVT) in patients receiving ESAs and undergoing surgical orthopedic procedures has been observed. Increased mortality was observed in patients receiving ESAs who were undergoing coronary artery bypass surgery. Aranesp is not authorized for reduction in allogeneic RBC transfusions in patients scheduled for surgical procedures.

Hematologic: The safety and efficacy of Aranesp (darbepoetin alfa) therapy has not been established in patients with underlying hematologic diseases (e.g., hemolytic anemia, sickle cell anemia, thalassemia, porphyria).

In order to ensure effective erythropoiesis, iron status should be evaluated for all patients before and during treatment as the majority of patients will eventually require supplemental iron therapy. Supplemental iron therapy is recommended for all patients whose serum ferritin is below 100 µg/L or serum transferrin saturation is below 20%.

Neurologic: Seizures: Use with caution in patients with a history of seizures. Seizures have occurred in patients participating in clinical trials of Aranesp and rHuEPO. During the first several months of therapy, blood pressure and the presence of premonitory neurologic symptoms should be monitored closely. Patients should be cautioned to avoid potentially hazardous activities such as driving heavy machinery during this period. While the relationship between seizures and the rate of rise of hemoglobin is uncertain, it is recommended that the dose of Aranesp be decreased if the hemoglobin increase exceeds 10 g/L in any 2-week period in CKD patients or 15 g/L in any 3-week period in cancer patients.

Sensitivity/Resistance: There have been reports of serious allergic reactions including anaphylactic reaction, angioedema, skin rash, urticaria and allergic bronchospasm associated with Aranesp. Symptoms have recurred with rechallenge, suggesting a causal relationship exists in some instances. If a serious allergic or an anaphylactic reaction occurs, appropriate therapy should be administered and Aranesp should be immediately and permanently discontinued.

Lack or Loss of Response to Aranesp: A lack of response or failure to maintain a hemoglobin response with Aranesp (darbepoetin alfa) doses within the recommended dosing range should prompt a search for causative factors. Deficiencies of iron, folic acid, or vitamin B_{12} should be excluded or corrected. Depending on the clinical setting, intercurrent infections, inflammatory or malignant processes, osteofibrosis cystica, occult blood loss, severe aluminum toxicity, bone marrow fibrosis, insufficient dialysis and malnutrition may compromise an erythropoietic response.

If patients are hyporesponsive, or fail to respond to other erythropoietic agents, Pure Red Cell Aplasia (PRCA) or anti-erythropoietin antibody formation should be excluded. Patients with confirmed antibody-mediated PRCA should not be switched to Aranesp. See Dosage and Administration, Dose Adjustment for CKD Patients for the management of patients with an insufficient hemoglobin response to Aranesp therapy.

Pure Red Cell Aplasia: Cases of pure red cell aplasia (PRCA) and of severe anemia, with or without other cytopenias, associated with neutralizing antibodies to erythropoietin have been reported in patients treated with Aranesp. This has been reported predominantly in CKD patients receiving Aranesp by subcutaneous administration. For additional information on the use of ESAs and PRCA reactions in non-CKD patients, see Adverse Reactions, Post-Market Adverse Drug Reactions.

Any patient who develops a sudden loss of response to Aranesp, accompanied by severe anemia and low reticulocyte count should be evaluated for the etiology of loss of effect, including the presence of neutralizing antibodies to erythropoietin. If anti-erythropoietin antibody-associated anemia is suspected, withhold Aranesp and other ESAs. Contact Amgen Canada (1-866-502-6436) to perform assays for binding and neutralizing antibodies. Aranesp should be permanently discontinued in patients with antibody-mediated anemia. Patients should not be switched to other ESAs as antibodies may cross react (see Adverse Reactions, Immunogenicity).

Suspected cases of PRCA in association with Aranesp should be reported to Amgen who may assist in this evaluation.

Sexual Function/Reproduction: No data are available from human studies with regard to impairment of fertility.

Special Populations: Chronic Kidney Disease Patients: Patients with CKD Not Requiring Dialysis: Patients with CKD not yet requiring dialysis (pre-dialysis patients) may require lower maintenance doses of Aranesp than patients receiving dialysis. Though CKD patients not receiving dialysis generally receive less frequent monitoring of blood pressure and laboratory parameters than dialysis patients, CKD patients not receiving dialysis may be more responsive to the effects of Aranesp, and require judicious monitoring of blood pressure and hemoglobin. Renal function and fluid and electrolyte balance should also be closely monitored.

Dialysis Management: Therapy with Aranesp results in an increase in the number of red blood cells (RBCs) and a decrease in plasma volume, which could reduce dialysis efficiency; patients who are marginally dialyzed may require adjustments in their dialysis prescription.

The importance of compliance with a prescribed diet should be reinforced. Notably hyperkalemia is not uncommon in this patient population.

Cancer Patients: Increased Mortality and/or Increased Risk of Tumor Progression or Recurrence: Erythropoiesis-stimulating agents (ESAs), when administered to target a hemoglobin level of >120 g/L, shortened the time to tumor progression in patients with advanced head and neck cancer receiving radiation therapy. ESAs also shortened survival in patients with metastatic breast cancer and in patients with lymphoid malignancy receiving chemotherapy when administered to target a hemoglobin level ≥120 g/L.

In addition, ESAs shortened survival in patients with non-small cell lung cancer and in a study enrolling patients with various malignancies who were not receiving chemotherapy or radiotherapy; in these two studies, ESAs were administered to target a hemoglobin level of ≥120 g/L.

An increased risk of death was observed in a clinical study when ESAs were administered to target hemoglobin of 120 g/L in patients with active malignant disease who were not being treated with either chemotherapy or radiation therapy. Aranesp is not indicated for use in patients with cancer who have anemia that is not associated with chemotherapy.

In view of the above, where appropriate red blood cell transfusion should be the preferred treatment for the management of anemia in patients with cancer. The decision to administer ESAs should be based on a benefit-risk assessment with the participation of the individual patient. This should take into account the specific clinical context such as (but not limited to) the type of tumor and its stage, the degree of anemia, life-expectancy, the environment in which the patient is being treated, and known risks of transfusions and ESAs.

Pregnant Women: There are no adequate and well-controlled studies in pregnant women. Aranesp should be used during pregnancy only if the potential benefit justifies the potential risk to the fetus.

Reproductive studies in rats showed no significant placental transfer of Aranesp. Studies in rats and rabbits, in which Aranesp was administered during gestation, showed no evidence of direct embryotoxic, fetotoxic, or teratogenic properties at doses up to 40 times the human dose. The only adverse effect observed was a slight reduction in fetal weight, which was seen at doses causing exaggerated pharmacological effects in the dams. No treatment effects on uterine implantation were seen in either species.

Nursing Women: It is not known whether Aranesp is excreted in human milk. Because many drugs are excreted in human milk, caution should be exercised when Aranesp is administered to a nursing woman.

Pediatrics: The safety and efficacy of Aranesp in pediatric patients has not been established.

Geriatrics: Chronic Kidney Disease Patients: The results of clinical trials with Aranesp suggest no increased safety risk with increasing age. Of more than 1500 patients with CKD treated with Aranesp, 43% were 65 years of age or older. Of these geriatric patients, 35% were 75 years of age or older. Regardless of age, the administration of Aranesp, either IV or SC, resulted in a dose-dependent and sustained increase in hemoglobin. No differences in dose requirements between geriatric and younger adults were observed. No overall differences in safety or efficacy were observed between these subjects and younger subjects. A greater sensitivity in older patients cannot be ruled out.

Cancer Patients: Of the 873 cancer patients in clinical studies receiving Aranesp and concomitant chemotherapy, 45% were age 65 and over, while 14% were 75 and over. No overall differences in safety or efficacy were observed between these patients and younger patients.

Monitoring and Laboratory Tests: Chronic Kidney Disease Patients: In order to avoid an excessive rate of rise or exceeding the recommended hemoglobin range of 100-120 g/L, the guidelines for dose and frequency of dose adjustments should be followed. After initiation of Aranesp therapy, the hemoglobin should be determined weekly until it has stabilized and the maintenance dose has been established (see Dosage and Administration, Chronic Kidney Disease Patients). After a dose adjustment, the hemoglobin should be determined weekly for at least 4 weeks until it has been determined that the hemoglobin has stabilized in response to the dose change. The hemoglobin should then be monitored at regular intervals.

In order to ensure effective erythropoiesis, iron status should be evaluated for all patients before and during treatment, as the majority of patients will eventually require supplemental iron therapy. Supplemental iron therapy is recommended for all patients whose serum ferritin is below 100 µg/L or whose serum transferrin saturation is below 20%.

Cancer Patients: The hemoglobin concentration after initiation of Aranesp therapy should be monitored at regular intervals to assess the need to modify dose based on the individual patient's response (see Dosage and Administration, Cancer Patients Receiving Chemotherapy).

ADVERSE REACTIONS: All Patients: Thrombotic/Vascular Events: The following thrombotic/vascular events have been reported in patients receiving ESAs (some with fatal outcomes): venous and arterial thromboses and embolism (such as deep venous thrombosis, arterial thrombosis, pulmonary emboli, aneurysms, retinal thrombosis, clotting of vascular access), cerebrovascular accidents (including cerebral infarction and cerebral hemorrhage) and transient ischemic attacks.

Chronic Kidney Disease Patients: In all studies with CKD patients, the most frequently reported serious adverse reactions with Aranesp were vascular access thrombosis, congestive heart failure, sepsis, and cardiac arrhythmia. The most commonly reported adverse reactions were infection, hypertension, hypotension, myalgia, headache, and diarrhea (see Warnings and Precautions, Increased Mortality, Serious Cardiovascular Events, Thromboembolic Events and Stroke). The most frequently reported adverse reactions resulting in clinical intervention (eg, discontinuation of Aranesp, adjustment in dosage, or the need for concomitant medication to treat an adverse reaction symptom) were hypotension, hypertension, fever, myalgia, nausea, and chest pain.

The data described below reflect exposure to Aranesp in 1598 CKD patients, including 675 exposed for at least 6 months, of whom 185 were exposed for greater than 1 year. Aranesp was evaluated in active-controlled (n=823) and uncontrolled studies (n=775).

The rates of adverse events and association with Aranesp are best assessed in the results from studies in which Aranesp was used to stimulate erythropoiesis in patients anemic at study baseline (n=348), and, in particular, the subset of these patients in randomized controlled trials (n=276). Because there were no substantive differences in the rates of adverse reactions between these subpopulations, or between these subpopulations and the entire population of patients treated with Aranesp, data from all 1598 patients were pooled.

The population encompassed an age range from 18 to 91 years. Fifty-seven percent of the patients were male. The percentages of Caucasian, Black, Asian, and Hispanic patients were 83%, 11%, 3%, and 1%, respectively. The median weekly dose of Aranesp was 0.45 µg/kg (25th, 75th percentiles: 0.29, 0.66 µg/kg).

Some of the adverse events reported are typically associated with CKD, or recognized complications of dialysis, and may not necessarily be attributable to Aranesp therapy. No important differences in adverse event rates between treatment groups were observed in controlled studies in which patients received Aranesp or other ESAs.

The data in Table 1 reflect those adverse events occurring in at least 5% of CKD patients treated with Aranesp.

Table 1: Aranesp

Adverse Events Occurring in ≥5% of CKD Patients

Event	CKD Patients Treated with Aranesp (n=1598) %
Application Site	
Injection Site Pain	7
Body as a Whole	
Peripheral Edema	11
Fatigue	9
Fever	9
Death	7
Chest Pain, Unspecified	6
Fluid Overload	6
Access Infection	6
Influenza-like Symptoms	6
Access Hemorrhage	6
Asthenia	5
Cardiovascular	
Hypertension	23
Hypotension	22
Cardiac Arrhythmias/Cardiac Arrest	10
Angina Pectoris/Cardiac Chest Pain	8
Thrombosis Vascular Access	8
Congestive Heart Failure	6
CNS/PNS	
Headache	16
Dizziness	8
Gastrointestinal	
Diarrhea	16
Vomiting	15
Nausea	14

(cont'd)

Table 1: Aranesp *(cont'd)*
Adverse Events Occurring in ≥5% of CKD Patients

Event	CKD Patients Treated with Aranesp (n=1598) %
Abdominal Pain	12
Constipation	5
Musculoskeletal	
Myalgia	21
Arthralgia	11
Limb Pain	10
Back Pain	8
Resistance Mechanism	
Infection[a]	27
Respiratory	
Upper Respiratory Infection	14
Dyspnea	12
Cough	10
Bronchitis	6
Skin and Appendages	
Pruritus	8

[a] Infection includes sepsis, bacteremia, pneumonia, peritonitis, and abscess.

The incidence rates for other clinically significant events are shown in Table 2.

Table 2: Aranesp
Percent Incidence of Other Clinically Significant Events in CKD Patients

Event	CKD Patients Treated with Aranesp (n=1598) %
Acute Myocardial Infarction	2
Seizure	1
Stroke	1
Transient Ischemic Attack	1

Vascular access thrombosis occurred in CKD clinical trials at an annualized rate of 0.22 events per patient year of Aranesp therapy. Rates of thrombotic events (e.g., vascular access thrombosis, venous thrombosis, and pulmonary emboli) with Aranesp therapy were similar to those observed with rHuEPO therapy in these trials.

Cancer Patients Receiving Chemotherapy: The data described below reflect the exposure to Aranesp in 873 cancer patients. Aranesp was evaluated in seven studies that were active-controlled and/or placebo-controlled studies of up to 6 months duration. The Aranesp-treated patient demographics were as follows: median age of 63 years (range of 20 to 91 years); 40% male; 88% Caucasian, 5% Hispanic, 4% Black, and 3% Asian. Over 90% of patients had locally advanced or metastatic cancer, with the remainder having early stage disease. Patients with solid tumors (e.g., lung, breast, colon, ovarian cancers), and lymphoproliferative malignancies (e.g., lymphoma, multiple myeloma) were enrolled in the clinical studies. All of the 873 Aranesp-treated subjects also received concomitant cyclic chemotherapy.

The most frequently reported serious adverse events included death (10%), fever (4%), pneumonia (3%), dehydration (3%), vomiting (2%), and dyspnea (2%). The most commonly reported adverse events were fatigue, edema, nausea, vomiting, diarrhea, fever, and dyspnea (see Table 3). The most commonly reported adverse reaction was injection site pain (see Table 4).

Except for those events listed in Table 3, the incidence of adverse events in clinical studies occurred at a similar rate compared with patients who received placebo and were generally consistent with the underlying disease and its treatment with chemotherapy. The most frequently reported events leading to discontinuation of Aranesp were progressive disease, death, discontinuation of the chemotherapy, asthenia, dyspnea, pneumonia, and gastrointestinal hemorrhage. No important differences in adverse event rates between treatment groups were observed in controlled studies in which patients received Aranesp or other ESAs.

Table 3: Aranesp
Adverse Events[a] Occurring in ≥5% of Cancer Patients Receiving Chemotherapy

Event	Aranesp (n=873) %	Placebo (n=221) %
Body as a Whole		
Fatigue	33	30
Edema	21	10
Fever	19	16
CNS/PNS		
Dizziness	14	8
Headache	12	9
Gastrointestinal		
Diarrhea	22	12
Constipation	18	17
Metabolic/Nutrition		
Dehydration	5	3
Musculoskeletal		
Arthralgia	13	6
Myalgia	8	5
Skin and Appendages		
Rash	7	3

[a] An adverse event is defined as an event that presents during treatment but does not necessarily have a causal relationship to Aranesp.

Table 4: Aranesp
Adverse Reactions Occurring in ≥1% of Cancer Patients Receiving Chemotherapy

Event	Aranesp (n=873) n (%)	Placebo (n=221) n (%)
Number of Patients with an Adverse Reaction[a]	98 (11)	14 (6)
Injection Site Pain	36 (4)	6 (3)

[a] An adverse reaction is defined as an event determined to be causally related to treatment with Aranesp.

Adverse reactions occurring in less than 1% of cancer patients treated with Aranesp include the following events:
Application Site: injection site ecchymosis, injection site edema, injection site paresthesia, injection site rash, injection site reaction.
Body as a Whole: fever, pain, peripheral edema, rigors, allergic reaction, fatigue, malaise, chest pain.
CNS/PNS: headache, dizziness, insomnia, cerebrovascular disorder, hypertonia, hypoesthesia, peripheral neuropathy, paresthesia.
Cardiovascular: hypertension, hypotension.
Gastrointestinal: diarrhea, nausea, vomiting, constipation, abdominal pain, anorexia, dry mouth, dyspepsia, tongue edema, GI hemorrhage, oral moniliasis, mucositis.
Hematologic: ecchymosis, hematoma, thrombocytopenia.
Metabolic/Nutrition: hypomagnesemia.
Musculoskeletal: involuntary muscular contraction, skeletal pain, myalgia, limb pain, arthralgia, back pain, joint stiffness, muscle weakness.
Resistance Mechanism: Herpes Zoster, sepsis.
Respiratory: dyspnea, cough, pulmonary embolism, hemoptysis, rhinitis, sore throat.
Skin and Appendages: increased sweating, erythema, skin lesion, rash, pruritus, maculo-papular rash, dry skin, skin ulceration.
Special Senses: parosmia, taste perversion.
Urinary Disorders: nocturia.
Vascular Disorders: deep venous thrombosis, thrombosis.
Vision Disorders: abnormal lacrimation, abnormal vision.

Table 5: Aranesp
Incidence of Other Clinically Significant Adverse Events in Patients Receiving Chemotherapy

Event	All Aranesp (n=873) %	Placebo (n=221) %
Hypertension	3.7	3.2
Seizures/Convulsions[a]	0.6	0.5
Thrombotic Events	6.2	4.1
Pulmonary Embolism	1.3	0.0
Thrombosis[b]	5.6	4.1

[a] Seizures/Convulsions include the preferred terms: convulsions, convulsions grand mal, and convulsions local.
[b] Thrombosis includes: thrombophlebitis, thrombophlebitis deep, thrombosis venous, thrombosis venous deep, thromboembolism, and thrombosis.

Once-every-3-week dosing in chemotherapy-treated patients was assessed in a 705 patient active-controlled, double-blind study with 4 months of Aranesp treatment. The incidence of adverse reactions was similar between subjects treated with Aranesp at the starting dose of 500 µg once every 3 weeks and Aranesp at the starting dose of 2.25 µg/kg/week.

Thrombotic and Cardiovascular Events: Overall, the incidence of thrombotic events was 6.2% for Aranesp and 4.1% for placebo. The following events were reported more frequently in Aranesp-treated patients than in placebo controls: pulmonary embolism, thromboembolism, thrombosis, and thrombophlebitis (deep and/or superficial). In addition, edema of any type was more frequently reported in Aranesp-treated (21%) patients than in patients who received placebo (10%). (See Table 3.)

Immunogenicity: As with all therapeutic proteins, there is a potential for immunogenicity. Radioimmunoprecipitation assays were performed on sera from 1534 CKD patients and 833 cancer patients treated with Aranesp. High-titer antibodies were not detected, but assay sensitivity may be inadequate to reliably detect lower titers. Since the incidence of antibody formation is highly dependent on the sensitivity and specificity of the assay, and the observed incidence of antibody positivity in an assay may additionally be influenced by several factors including sample handling, concomitant medications, and underlying disease, comparison of the incidence of antibodies to Aranesp with the incidence of antibodies to other products may be misleading.

Post-Market Adverse Drug Reactions: In the post-marketing experience, the following have been reported in patients treated with Aranesp:

- Very rare cases of PRCA associated with neutralizing anti-erythropoietin antibodies (see Warnings and Precautions, Pure Red Cell Aplasia).
- Convulsions/seizures
- Serious allergic reactions including anaphylactic reaction, angioedema, allergic bronchospasm, skin rash and urticaria

Cases of PRCA have been rarely reported in patients with hepatitis C treated with interferon and ribavirin, when ESAs are used concomitantly. ESAs are not approved for the management of anemia associated with hepatitis C.

(cont'd)

DRUG INTERACTIONS: No formal drug interaction studies of Aranesp with other medications commonly used in CKD or cancer patients have been performed.

DOSAGE AND ADMINISTRATION: Dosing Considerations: Important: See Warnings and Precautions, Boxed Serious Warnings and Precautions, and Increased Mortality, Serious Cardiovascular Events, Thromboembolic Events and Stroke. Aranesp dosing regimens are different for each of the indications described in the Indications and Clinical Use of this product monograph. Aranesp should be administered under the supervision of a healthcare professional. Due to the longer serum half-life, Aranesp should be administered less frequently than Epoetin alfa (for example, where Epoetin alfa is administered three times a week, Aranesp should be administered weekly). When changing the route of administration, the same dose should be used and the hemoglobin monitored so that the appropriate dose adjustments can be made to keep the hemoglobin at the desired concentration.

Chronic Kidney Disease Patients: Aranesp is administered either IV or SC as a single injection administered weekly or once every two weeks. The dose should be started and slowly adjusted as described below based on hemoglobin levels. If a patient fails to respond or maintain a response, other etiologies should be considered and evaluated (see Warnings and Precautions, Monitoring and Laboratory Tests, Lack or Loss of Response to Aranesp, Pure Red Cell Aplasia). When Aranesp therapy is initiated or adjusted, the hemoglobin should be followed weekly until stabilized and monitored at least monthly thereafter.

For patients who respond to Aranesp with a rapid increase in hemoglobin (e.g., more than 10 g/L in any 2-week period), the dose of Aranesp should be reduced (see Dosage and Administration, Dose Adjustment for CKD Patients) because of the association of excessive rate of rise of hemoglobin with adverse events (see Warnings and Precautions, Increased Mortality, Serious Cardiovascular Events, Thromboembolic Events and Stroke).

It should be recognized that subcutaneous administration of recombinant human proteins may increase the risk of immunogenicity. In patients on hemodialysis, the IV route is recommended.

Correction of Anemia in Chronic Kidney Disease Patients: The recommended starting dose of Aranesp for the correction of anemia in CKD patients is 0.45 μg/kg body weight, administered as a single IV or SC injection once weekly. Doses should be titrated to achieve and maintain the hemoglobin within the recommended range of 100-120 g/L. If hemoglobin excursions outside the recommended range occur Aranesp dose should be adjusted using the dosing recommendations below (see Dosage and Administration, Dose Adjustment for CKD Patients). For many patients, the appropriate maintenance dose will be lower than this starting dose. CKD patients not receiving dialysis, in particular, may require lower maintenance doses. Also, some patients have been treated successfully with a SC dose of Aranesp administered once every 2 weeks.

Conversion to Aranesp from Recombinant Human Erythropoietin in CKD Patients: The clinical studies demonstrated that the relationship between baseline rHuEPO and maintenance Aranesp is nonlinear across the dosing spectrum. Consequently, the starting weekly dose of Aranesp should be estimated on the basis of the weekly Epoetin alfa dose at the time of substitution (see Table 6). Due to the longer serum half-life, Aranesp should be administered less frequently than rHuEPO. Patients receiving rHuEPO 2 or 3 times weekly should change to once weekly Aranesp at a dose equivalent to their total weekly dose of rHuEPO. Patients receiving rHuEPO once per week should change to Aranesp once every 2 weeks at a dose that is equivalent to the sum of 2 weekly doses of rHuEPO. The same route of administration should be used. For patients prescribed prefilled syringes the calculated dose should be rounded upward to the next available syringe strength.

Table 6: Aranesp

Estimated Aranesp Starting Dose (μg/week) Based on Previous Epoetin alfa Dose (Units/week) for CKD Patients

Previous Weekly Epoetin alfa Dose (CKD Patients) (Units/week)	Weekly Aranesp Dose (CKD Patients) (μg/week)
<2500	6.25
2500 to 4999	12.5
5000 to 10 999	25
11 000 to 17 999	40
18 000 to 33 999	60
34 000 to 89 999	100
≥90 000	200

Patients should be carefully monitored to ensure appropriate dose adjustments in order to maintain appropriate hemoglobin levels (see Dosage and Administration, Dose Adjustment for CKD Patients).

Data from approximately 800 patients receiving Aranesp in clinical studies were analysed to assess the dose required to maintain hemoglobin; no difference was observed between the average weekly dose administered by the IV or SC routes of administration.

Because of intersubject variability, titration to the optimal therapeutic Aranesp dose is required for individual patients. When a patient's hemoglobin is stabilized within the recommended range it should be monitored monthly and adjustments made as described below (see Dosage and Administration, Dose Adjustment for CKD Patients).

Dose Adjustment for CKD Patients: The dose of Aranesp should be individualized to achieve and maintain the hemoglobin within the recommended range of 100-120 g/L. If hemoglobin excursions outside the recommended range occur Aranesp dose should be adjusted using the dosing recommendations below.

Because of the time required for erythropoiesis and the red cell half-life, an interval of 2 to 6 weeks may occur between the time of a dose adjustment and a significant change in hemoglobin. Increases in dose should not be made more frequently than once a month. If the hemoglobin is increasing and approaching 120 g/L, the dose should be reduced by approximately 25%. If after a dose reduction, the hemoglobin continues to increase, the dose should be temporarily withheld until the hemoglobin begins to decrease, at which point therapy should be reinitiated at a dose approximately 25% below the previous dose. If the hemoglobin increases by more than 10 g/L in a 2-week period, the dose should be decreased by approximately 25%.

After Aranesp initiation or dose increase, if the increase in hemoglobin is less than 10 g/L over 4 weeks and iron stores are adequate (see Warnings and Precautions, Hematologic), the dose of Aranesp may be increased by approximately 25% of the previous dose. Further increases may be made at 4-week intervals until the desired response is attained.

For patients whose hemoglobin does not attain a level within the range of 100 to 120 g/L despite the use of appropriate Aranesp dose titrations over a 12-week period:

- do not administer higher Aranesp doses and use the lowest dose that will maintain a hemoglobin level sufficient to avoid the need for recurrent RBC transfusions,
- evaluate and treat for other causes of anemia (see Warnings and Precautions, Increased Mortality, Serious Cardiovascular Events, Thromboembolic Events and Stroke), and
- thereafter, hemoglobin should continue to be monitored and if responsiveness improves, Aranesp dose adjustments should be made as described above; discontinue Aranesp if responsiveness does not improve and the patient needs recurrent RBC transfusions.

Maintenance Dose for CKD Patients: Aranesp dosage should be individualized to maintain the hemoglobin within the recommended range of 100-120 g/L. If hemoglobin excursions outside the recommended range occur Aranesp dose should be adjusted using the dosing recommendations above. If the hemoglobin exceeds 120 g/L, the dose may be adjusted as described above. Doses must be individualized to ensure that hemoglobin is maintained at an appropriate level for each patient.

Cancer Patients Receiving Chemotherapy: Aranesp should not be initiated at hemoglobin levels ≥100 g/L. Two dosing regimens may be used in adults; 500 μg SC once every 3 weeks or 2.25 μg/kg SC once weekly. Aranesp administration should be discontinued following the completion of a chemotherapy course.

Discontinue Aranesp if after 8 weeks of therapy there is no response as measured by increased hemoglobin levels or decreased need for RBC transfusions.

Once-Every-Three-Week (Q3W) Dosing: The recommended starting dose for Aranesp administered once every 3 weeks is 500 μg as a SC injection.

The dose should be adjusted for each patient to maintain the lowest hemoglobin level sufficient to avoid the need for RBC transfusion and not to exceed 120 g/L. Hemoglobin levels should be monitored, prior to dosing, at least every 3 weeks until the lowest level sufficient to avoid the need for RBC transfusion is reached and thereafter.

Doses of Aranesp should be decreased by approximately 40% (e.g., 300 μg once every 3 weeks) when the hemoglobin reaches a level needed to avoid red blood cell transfusion or increases by more than 10 g/L in a 2-week period or 15 g/L in any 3-week period. If the hemoglobin exceeds a level needed to avoid transfusion, Aranesp should be temporarily withheld until the hemoglobin approaches a level where RBC transfusions may be required. At this point, therapy should be reinitiated at a dose 40% below the previous dose (e.g., 300 μg once every 3 weeks).

Once-Weekly Dosing: The recommended starting dose of Aranesp administered weekly is 2.25 μg/kg as a SC injection. The dose should be adjusted for each patient to maintain the lowest hemoglobin level sufficient to avoid the need for RBC transfusion and not to exceed 120 g/L.

If the increase in hemoglobin is inadequate (≤10 g/L) or if the response is not satisfactory in terms of reducing RBC transfusion requirements after approximately 6 weeks of therapy, the dose of Aranesp should be increased up to 4.5 μg/kg/week. For patients prescribed prefilled syringes the calculated dose should be rounded upward to the next available syringe strength.

Hemoglobin levels should be monitored, prior to dosing, on a weekly basis until the lowest level sufficient to avoid the need for RBC transfusion is reached, and every 3 weeks thereafter. Doses of Aranesp should be decreased by 40% as the hemoglobin reaches a level needed to avoid RBC transfusion or the rate of hemoglobin increase is more than 10 g/L in a 2-week period or 15 g/L in a 3-week period. If the hemoglobin exceeds a level needed to avoid RBC transfusion, doses should be temporarily withheld until the hemoglobin approaches a level where RBC transfusions may be required. At this point, therapy should be reinitiated at a dose 40% below the previous dose.

Administration: Information to Be Provided to the Patient: In those situations in which the physician determines that a patient can safely and effectively self-administer Aranesp, the patient should be instructed as to the proper dosage and administration technique. Patients should be referred to Information for the Patient. This is intended as a guide for patients; however, it is not a disclosure of all possible side effects. Patients should be informed of the signs and symptoms of allergic drug reactions and advised of appropriate actions.

Following administration of Aranesp from the prefilled syringe, the patient should activate the UltraSafe Needle Guard by placing their hands behind the needle, grasping the guard with one hand, and sliding the guard forward until the needle is completely covered and the guard clicks into place. **Note:** If an audible click is not heard, the needle guard may not be completely activated.

If home use is prescribed for a patient, the patient should be thoroughly instructed in the importance of proper disposal of syringes and cautioned against the reuse of needles, syringes, or drug product. A puncture-resistant container for the disposal of used syringes and needles should be available to the patient. The full container should be disposed of according to the directions provided by the physician, pharmacist or nurse.

OVERDOSAGE:

If overdosage occurs, the patient's hemoglobin, blood pressure, and any premonitionary neurologic symptoms should be carefully monitored.

The maximum amount of Aranesp (darbepoetin alfa) that can be safely administered in single or multiple doses has not been determined. Therapy with Aranesp can result in polycythemia if the hemoglobin is not carefully monitored and the dose appropriately adjusted. If the recommended hemoglobin range is exceeded, Aranesp should be temporarily withheld until the hemoglobin returns to the recommended range; Aranesp therapy may then be resumed using a lower dose (see Dosage and Administration). If clinically indicated, phlebotomy may be performed.

> For management of a suspected drug overdose, contact your regional Poison Control Centre. See the *CPS* Directory section for a list of Poison Control Centres.

ACTION AND CLINICAL PHARMACOLOGY: Mechanism of Action: Aranesp (darbepoetin alfa) is an erythropoiesis-stimulating agent produced in Chinese hamster ovary (CHO) cells by recombinant DNA technology. The final processed form is a 165-amino acid protein containing 5 N-linked oligosaccharide chains, whereas endogenous erythropoietin (EPO) or recombinant human erythropoietin (rHuEPO) contain only 3. Erythropoietin is a glycoprotein that is the primary regulator of erythropoiesis through specific interaction with the erythropoietin receptor on the erythroid progenitor cells in the bone marrow. The production of erythropoietin primarily occurs in and is regulated by the kidney in response to changes in tissue oxygenation. Hypoxia and anemia generally result in an increase in endogenous erythropoietin production, which in turn stimulates erythropoiesis. Aranesp stimulates erythropoiesis by the same mechanism as endogenous erythropoietin.

Endogenous erythropoietin production is impaired in patients with chronic kidney disease (CKD) and EPO deficiency is the primary cause of their anemia. Aranesp has been shown to stimulate erythropoiesis in anemic CKD patients resulting in the correction of anemia and maintenance of hemoglobin levels within a defined target range in patients not previously receiving rHuEPO. In patients previously maintained on rHuEPO who were switched to Aranesp, hemoglobin levels were maintained within a defined target range.

The etiology of anemia in cancer patients is multifactorial. Erythropoietin deficiency and a blunted response of erythroid progenitor cells to endogenous erythropoietin contribute significantly towards anemia in these patients. Aranesp has been shown to stimulate erythropoiesis, resulting in increased hemoglobin levels and a reduced need for red blood cell (RBC) transfusions in cancer patients. Increased hemoglobin levels have been shown to result in improved quality of life.

Pharmacokinetics: Due to its increased sialic acid containing carbohydrate content, Aranesp has an approximately 3-fold longer terminal half-life than rHuEPO and consequently a greater in vivo activity when administered by either the subcutaneous (SC) or intravenous (IV) route. Receptor-binding studies indicate that Aranesp has a reduced binding affinity to the EPO receptor compared with rHuEPO, explained by the addition of sialic acids; however, the relationship between the increased amount of sialic acid-containing carbohydrate on the molecule and an increase in serum half-life accounts for the observed greater biological effect with Aranesp. The pharmacokinetics of Aranesp were studied in adults with chronic kidney disease and adult cancer patients receiving chemotherapy.

Chronic Kidney Disease Patients: Following IV administration to adult CKD patients, Aranesp serum concentration-time profiles are biphasic, with a distribution half-life of approximately 1.4 hours and mean terminal half-life of approximately 21 hours.

Following SC administration, the absorption is slow and rate-limiting, and the terminal half-life is 49 hours (range: 27 to 89 hours), which reflects the absorption half-life. The peak concentration occurs at 34 hours (range: 24 to 72 hours) post-SC administration in adult CKD patients, and bioavailability is approximately 37% (range: 30% to 50%).

The distribution of Aranesp in adult CKD patients is predominantly confined to the vascular space (approximately 60 mL/kg). The pharmacokinetic parameters indicate dose-linearity over the therapeutic dose range. With once weekly dosing, steady-state serum levels are achieved within 4 weeks with <2-fold increase in peak concentration when compared to the initial dose. Accumulation was negligible following both IV and SC dosing over 1 year of treatment.

Cancer Patients: Following SC administration of 2.25 μg/kg/week to adult cancer patients (n=26), a mean peak concentration of 10.6 ng/mL (range: 1.23 to 25.2 ng/mL) was achieved at a mean time of 90.5 hours (range: 70.8 to 123 hours). The data were consistent with dose-linear pharmacokinetics over a wide dose range (0.5 to 8.0 μg/kg weekly and 3.0 to 9.0 μg/kg every 2 weeks). Upon multiple dosing over 12 weeks (dosing every week or every 2 weeks), the pharmacokinetic properties did not change. The expected moderate increases (<2-fold) in Aranesp serum concentrations upon multiple dosing were observed as steady state was approached. Accumulation was negligible across a wide range of doses at once weekly and once every 2 weeks dosing schedules. Although the accumulation potential of Aranesp is unknown for longer-term (i.e. >12 weeks) treatment in cancer patients, the extent (<2-fold) accumulation observed at 12 weeks was the same as that observed at 4 weeks.

Over the dose range of 4.5 to 15 μg/kg administered on a once-every-3-week (Q3W) schedule to cancer patients receiving chemotherapy, Aranesp pharmacokinetics were approximately linear with respect to dose, and no evidence of accumulation was observed.

Following SC administration of 6.75 μg/kg (equivalent to 500 μg for a 74-kg patient) on a Q3W schedule to cancer patients, peak concentrations occurred at 71 hours (range: 28 to 120 hours), and a terminal half-life of 74 hours (range: 24 to 144 hours) was observed. No evidence of marked (>2-fold) accumulation was observed upon Q3W SC dosing of 6.75 μg/kg. Exposure to Aranesp when administered on a Q3W schedule (6.75 μg/kg), either on the same day of chemotherapy or mid cycle was comparable, with mean AUC values differing by less than 28% between groups. Although approximately 30-70% differences in mean terminal half-life or peak concentration values were observed between groups, no clinically significant differences in efficacy or safety between groups was observed, suggesting limited clinical significance of the findings. Following IV or SC administration of 4.5 μg/kg on a Q3W schedule, mean trough or 1- to 2-week postdose Aranesp serum levels were comparable between the IV and SC groups after multiple dosing.

STORAGE AND STABILITY: Store at 2 to 8°C. Do not freeze or shake. Protect from light. Do not use Aranesp beyond the expiry date shown on the label.

INFORMATION FOR THE PATIENT: Published in e-CPS, available by subscription at www.e-cps.ca.

DOSAGE FORMS, COMPOSITION AND PACKAGING: Each SingleJect, prefilled syringe, contains: darbepoetin alfa as 10, 20, 30, 40, 50, 60, 80, 100, 130, 150, 200, 300 or 500 µg per syringe in the following concentrations and fill volumes: 25 µg/mL in 0.4 mL; 40 µg/mL in 0.5 mL; 100 µg/mL in 0.3 mL, 0.4 mL and 0.5 mL; 200 µg/mL in 0.3 mL, 0.4 mL, 0.5 mL and 0.65 mL; 500 µg/mL in 0.3 mL, 0.4 mL, 0.6 mL and 1 mL. Nonmedicinal ingredients: polysorbate 80, sodium chloride, sodium phosphate dibasic anhydrous, sodium phosphate monobasic monohydrate and sterile water for injection, USP. Preservative-free. pH of polysorbate solution is 6.2±0.2. The needle cover of the pre-filled syringe contains dry natural rubber (a derivative of latex).

To reduce the risk of accidental needle sticks to users, each prefilled syringe is equipped with an UltraSafe Needle Guard that is manually activated to cover the needle during disposal.

Arava® Ⓟ

leflunomide

Antirheumatic—Immunomodulator Agent

sanofi-aventis

Date of Revision: July 19, 2010

SUMMARY PRODUCT INFORMATION:

Route of Administration	Dosage Form/Strength	Clinically Relevant Nonmedicinal Ingredients
Oral	Film-coated tablets 10, 20, 100 mg	Lactose monohydrate For a complete listing see Dosage Forms, Composition and Packaging.

INDICATIONS AND CLINICAL USE: ARAVA (leflunomide) should be used only by physicians who have fully familiarized themselves with the efficacy and safety profile of ARAVA and who are experienced in the therapy of rheumatoid diseases.

ARAVA is indicated in adults for the treatment of active rheumatoid arthritis.

Geriatrics (>65 years of age): No dosage adjustment is needed in patients over 65 years of age.

Pediatrics (<18 years of age): The use in patients less than 18 years of age is contraindicated.

CONTRAINDICATIONS: ARAVA is contraindicated in:

1. Patients with known hypersensitivity to ARAVA (especially previous Stevens-Johnson syndrome, toxic epidermal necrolysis or erythema multiforme) or to any of ARAVA excipients.
2. Due to the lack of clinical experience in the following three patient populations, ARAVA is not to be administered to these patients due to its potential for immunosuppression:
   i. Patients with immunodeficiency states (e.g. AIDS), due to causes other than rheumatoid arthritis (see Warnings and Precautions, Immune).
   ii. Patients with impaired bone marrow function or significant anaemia, leucopenia, neutropenia or thrombocytopenia due to causes other than rheumatoid arthritis.
   iii. Patients with serious infections.
3. Patients with moderate to severe renal insufficiency because the kidney plays a role in the elimination of ARAVA.
4. Patients with impairment of liver function (ARAVA in monotherapy or in combination with other hepatotoxic drugs e.g. Disease Modifying Antirheumatic Drugs [DMARDs] such as methotrexate) given the possible risk of increased hepatotoxicity and the role of the liver in activation, elimination and recycling of ARAVA (see Drug Interactions).

   While the mechanism of action of ARAVA and methotrexate are different, their pharmacodynamic action of interfering with cell division is similar. Concomitant treatment with methotrexate and/or other liver and bone marrow toxic medications is associated with an increased risk of serious hepatic or marrow reactions and requires strict vigilance in monitoring (see Warnings and Precautions, Monitoring and Laboratory Tests).

   If a switch in treatment from ARAVA to another hepatotoxic DMARD is required the washout and monitoring must be adhered to as mentioned in the Warnings and Precautions, Monitoring and Laboratory Tests and General, Washout Procedures).
5. Patients with severe hypoproteinemia (e.g. in nephrotic syndrome). Since the active metabolite of ARAVA, A771726, is highly protein-bound and cleared via hepatic metabolism and biliary secretion.
6. Pregnant women, or women of childbearing potential who are not using reliable contraception before, during, and for a period of two years after treatment with ARAVA (or as long as the plasma levels of the active metabolite are above 0.02 mg/L). Pregnancy must be excluded before start of treatment with ARAVA (see Warnings and Precautions, Special Populations, Pregnant Women).
7. Women who are breast feeding (see Warnings and Precautions, Special Population, Nursing Women).
8. Patients less than 18 years of age.

Male patients should be aware of the possible male-mediated foetal toxicity. Reliable contraception during treatment with ARAVA should also be guaranteed (see Warnings and Precautions, Sexual Function/Reproduction and Special Population, Pregnant Women).

WARNINGS AND PRECAUTIONS: General: The active metabolite of ARAVA, A771726, has a long half-life. Serious undesirable effects might occur (e.g. hepatotoxicity, haematotoxicity or allergic reactions, see below), even if the treatment with ARAVA has been stopped. For the management of the above-mentioned toxicities a washout procedure should be performed.

If a severe adverse reaction to ARAVA occurs, or if for any other reason A771726 needs to be cleared rapidly from the body, cholestyramine or activated charcoal has to be initiated and continued/repeated as clinically necessary (see Overdosage). For suspected severe immunologic/allergic reactions, more prolonged cholestyramine or activated charcoal administration may be necessary to achieve rapid and sufficient clearance (see below the Washout Procedures).

Similarly, when switching to another DMARD (e.g. methotrexate) after treatment with ARAVA a washout procedure should be performed since there exist a possibility of additive risks of adverse events for a long time after the switching (see Washout Procedures and see also Contraindications and Drug Interactions).

Recent treatment with hepatotoxic DMARDs may result in increased side effects; therefore, the initiation of ARAVA treatment has to be carefully considered regarding these benefit/risk aspects. Caution and careful monitoring of liver and bone marrow function is necessary if these drugs are used concomitantly (see Contraindications and Drug Interactions).

Washout Procedures: One of the following is recommended to achieve a fast decrease in plasma levels after stopping treatment with ARAVA:

1. 8 g cholestyramine 3 times daily for 11 days **or**
2. 50 g activated charcoal 4 times daily for 11 days

The duration may be modified depending on clinical or laboratory variables.

Similarly low A771726 plasma levels may be expected 2 years after stopping ARAVA without one of the above washout methods. Due to individual variation in drug clearance, some patients may decrease to below this plasma level in less time (e.g. 6 months).

For information regarding measurements of A771726, please contact sanofi-aventis Canada Inc.

Carcinogenesis and Mutagenesis: Malignancy: The risk of malignancy, particularly lymphoproliferative disorders, is increased with the use of some immunosuppressive medications. There is a potential for immunosuppression with ARAVA. No apparent increase in the incidence of malignancies and lymphoproliferative disorders was reported in the clinical trials of ARAVA, but larger and longer-term studies would be needed to determine whether there is an increased risk of malignancies or lymphoproliferative disorders with ARAVA.

Carcinogenesis, and Mutagenesis: No evidence of carcinogenicity was observed in a 2-year bioassay in rats at oral doses of ARAVA up to the maximally tolerated dose of 6 mg/kg (approximately 1/40 the maximum human A771726 systemic exposure based on the area under the curve [AUC]). However, male mice in a 2-year bioassay exhibited an increased incidence in lymphoma at an oral dose of 15 mg/kg, the highest dose studied (1.7 times the human A771726 exposure based on AUC). Female mice in the same study exhibited a dose-related increased incidence of bronchoalveolar adenomas and carcinomas combined beginning at 1.5 mg/kg (approximately 1/10 the human A771726 exposure based on AUC). The significance of the findings in mice relative to the clinical use of ARAVA is not known.

ARAVA was not mutagenic in the Ames Assay, the Unscheduled DNA Synthesis Assay, or in the HGPRT Gene Mutation Assay. In addition, ARAVA was not clastogenic in the in vivo Mouse Micronucleus Assay nor in the in vivo Cytogenetic Test in Chinese Hamster Bone Marrow Cells. However, 4-trifluoromethylanaline (TFMA), a minor metabolite of ARAVA, was mutagenic in the Ames Assay and in the HGPRT Gene Mutation Assay and was clastogenic in the in vitro Assay for Chromosome Aberrations in the Chinese Hamster Cells. TFMA was not clastogenic in the in vivo Mouse Micronucleus Assay nor in the in vivo Cytogenetic Test in Chinese Hamster Bone Marrow Cells.

Dependence/Tolerance: ARAVA should have no potential for abuse or dependence.

Hematologic: Monitoring for hematologic toxicity must be adhered to (see Warnings and Precautions, Monitoring and Laboratory Tests).

ARAVA is contraindicated in patients with impaired bone marrow function or significant anaemia, leucopenia, neutropenia or thrombocytopenia due to causes other than rheumatoid arthritis (see Contraindications). In patients with a lesser degree of pre-existing anemia, leucopenia, and/or thrombocytopenia as well as in patients with impaired bone marrow function or those at risk of bone marrow suppression, the risk of hematological disorders is increased. The same effects also occur in patients on concomitant myelosuppressive medications, for example methotrexate, therefore strict vigilance in monitoring is recommended for all patients on ARAVA on concomitant myelosuppressive medication. If such effects occur, a washout procedure to reduce plasma levels of A771726 should be considered.

In case of severe hematological reactions, including pancytopenia, ARAVA and any concomitant myelosuppressive medication must be discontinued and a washout procedure initiated (see Warnings and Precautions, General, Washout Procedures).

Hepatic/Biliary/Pancreatic: Monitoring for hepatotoxicity must be adhered to (see Warnings and Precautions, Monitoring and Laboratory Tests).

ARAVA is contraindicated in patients with impairment of liver function (see Contraindications). Given the possible risk of increased hepatotoxicity and the role of the liver in drug activation, elimination and recycling, the use of ARAVA is not recommended in patients with positive Hepatitis B or C serologies or pre-existing hepatic disease.

Rare cases (defined by Regulatory definition as events occurring at a frequency ranging from 0.01 to 0.1%) of serious liver injury, including liver failure some with a fatal outcome, have been reported during treatment with ARAVA. Most of the cases occurred within the first 6 months of treatment. While confounding factors were seen in many cases such as other hepatotoxic drugs such as methotrexate and/or Non-Steroidal Anti-inflammatory Drugs (NSAIDs), a causal relationship to ARAVA cannot be excluded. It is essential that the monitoring recommendations be adhered to and washout procedure performed in appropriate cases (see Warnings and Precautions, Monitoring and Laboratory Tests).

Due to a potential for additive hepatotoxic effects, it is recommended that alcohol consumption be avoided during treatment with ARAVA.

In clinical trials, ARAVA treatment was associated with elevations of liver function tests, primarily ALT and AST in a significant number of patients; these effects were generally reversible. Most transaminase elevations were mild (≤2×ULN) (upper limit of normal) and usually resolved while continuing treatment. Clinically significant elevations (>2 and ≤3×ULN) were less common and were generally asymptomatic and reversible with dose reduction or, if persistent, by discontinuing ARAVA. More marked elevations (>3×ULN) occurred infrequently and usually reversed with dose reduction; persistent elevations resolved after discontinuation of ARAVA. Some patients received cholestyramine to enhance clearance. Overall, persistent elevations after dose reduction were uncommon and were usually associated with concomitant NSAIDs use. Limited biopsy data did not suggest that ARAVA was associated with the development of cirrhosis or hepatic fibrosis.

Table 1 shows liver enzyme elevations seen with monthly monitoring in clinical trials US301, MN301 and MN302. It was notable that the absence of folate use in MN302 was associated with a considerably greater incidence of liver enzyme elevation on methotrexate.

Table 1: ARAVA

Liver Enzyme Elevations >3-fold Upper Limit of Normal (ULN)

	US301			MN301			MN302	
	No. of Patients (% patients)			No. of Patients (% patients)			No. of Patients (% patients)	
	LEF	PBO	MTX	LEF	PBO	SSZ	LEF	MTX
ALT >3-fold ULN (%)	8 (4.4)	3 (2.5)	5 (2.7)	2 (1.5)	1 (1.1)	2 (1.5)	13 (2.6)	83 (16.7)
Reversed to ≤2-fold ULN	8	3	5	2	1	2	12	82
Timing of Elevation								
0-3 Months	6	1	1	2	1	2	7	27
4-6 Months	1	1	3	—	—	—	1	34
7-9 Months	1	1	1	—	—	—	—	16
10-12 Months	—	—	—	—	—	—	5	6
AST >3-fold ULN (%)	4 (2.2)	2 (1.7)	1 (0.6)	2 (1.5)	0	5 (3.6)	7 (1.4)	29 (5.8)
Reversed to ≤2-fold ULN	4	2	1	2	0	4	5	29
Timing of Elevation								
0-3 Months	2	1	—	2	—	4	3	10
4-6 Months	1	1	1	—	—	1	1	11
7-9 Months	1	—	—	—	—	—	—	8
10-12 Months	—	—	—	—	—	—	1	—

Legend: LEF=leflunomide; PBO=placebo; MTX=methotrexate; SSZ=sulfasalazine.

Guidelines for dose adjustment or discontinuation based on the severity and persistence of ALT elevation are recommended as follows: If ALT elevations between 2- and 3-fold the upper limit of normal persist or if ALT elevations of more than 3-fold the upper limit of normal are present, ARAVA should be discontinued. Cholestyramine or activated charcoal should be administered to more rapidly lower A771726 level (see Warnings and Precautions, General, Washout Procedures and Monitoring and Laboratory Tests).

Rare elevations of alkaline phosphatase and bilirubin have been observed. Trial US301 used ACR Methotrexate Liver Biopsy Guidelines for monitoring therapy. One of 182 patients receiving ARAVA and 1 of 182 patients receiving methotrexate underwent liver biopsy at 106 and 50 weeks, respectively. The biopsy for the leflunomide subject was Roegnik Grade IIIA and for the methotrexate subject Roegnik Grade I.

Immune: ARAVA is not recommended for patients with bone marrow dysplasia, or severe, uncontrolled infections or immunodeficiency due to causes other than rheumatoid arthritis (see Contraindications).

Medications like ARAVA that have immunosuppression potential may cause patients to be more susceptible to infections, including opportunistic infections (see Adverse Reactions). Infections may be more severe in nature.

It is known that patients with rheumatoid arthritis have an increased risk of severe infections, which may lead to sepsis and death. Rare cases of severe infection (including *P. jiroveci* and cytomegalovirus infections) and sepsis (with fatal outcome in isolated cases) were reported in patients treated with ARAVA. Although in most cases a causal relationship to leflunomide has not been established and multiple confounding factors were present, infections developing in patients receiving ARAVA may require early and vigorous treatment.

In the event that a severe or uncontrolled infection occurs, it may be necessary to interrupt ARAVA treatment and administer a washout procedure (see Warnings and Precautions, General, Washout Procedures).

Patients should be questioned about history of tuberculosis or tuberculin reactivity and, if positive, they should be carefully monitored for tuberculosis reactivation.

Renal: ARAVA is contraindicated in patients with moderate to severe renal impairment. Because the kidney plays a role in the elimination of ARAVA, and without sufficient studies of the use of ARAVA in patients with renal insufficiency, caution should be used when considering the administration of ARAVA to patients with mild renal insufficiency.

Respiratory: Rare (<0.1%) spontaneous reports of interstitial lung disease occurring during treatment with ARAVA have been received worldwide (see Adverse Reactions, Respiratory, Thoracic and Mediastinal Disorders). Several of these cases had a fatal outcome. In a Japanese postmarketing surveillance program of 3658 patients with rheumatoid arthritis, the rate of interstitial lung disease was estimated at 0.8%, regardless of causality. Twenty-nine (29) cases of interstitial pneumonitis were reported, 11 with a fatal outcome. Assessment of the causality between ARAVA use and the reported interstitial lung disease is frequently confounded by pre-existing pulmonary disease (e.g. interstitial pneumonitis), and/or previous or concomitant use of other DMARDs known to induce interstitial lung disease (including methotrexate).

In patients with a current or previous history of pulmonary disease or who have been recently treated with drugs known to induce interstitial lung disease, it is recommended that pulmonary status be evaluated prior to initiation of ARAVA therapy and that patients be closely monitored during treatment.

Interstitial lung disease is a potentially fatal disorder, which may occur acutely at any time during therapy and has a variable clinical presentation. New onset or worsening pulmonary symptoms, such as cough and dyspnea, with or without associated fever, may be a reason for discontinuation of the therapy and for further investigation, as appropriate. If discontinuation of the drug is needed, the long half-life of the active metabolite of ARAVA may necessitate the initiation of washout procedures (see Warnings and Precautions, General, Washout Procedures).

Patients should be informed about the early warning signs of interstitial lung disease and asked to contact their physician as soon as possible if these symptoms appear or worsen during therapy.

Sexual Function/Reproduction: Procreation: Pregnancy must be avoided if either partner is receiving ARAVA.

Females: There are no adequate and well-controlled studies evaluating ARAVA in pregnant women. However, based on animal studies, ARAVA may cause fetal death or teratogenic effects when administered to a pregnant woman. Women of childbearing potential must not be started on ARAVA until pregnancy is excluded and it has been confirmed that they are using reliable contraception.

Before starting treatment with ARAVA, patients must be fully counselled on the potential for serious risk to the fetus. Patient must be advised that if there is any delay in onset of menses or any other reason to suspect pregnancy, they must notify the physician immediately for pregnancy testing. Should pregnancy occur, the physician and patient should discuss the risk of continuing the pregnancy (see Information for the Patient). It is possible that rapidly lowering the blood level of the active metabolite, by instituting the drug elimination procedure described below, at the first delay of menses may decrease the risk to the fetus from ARAVA.

For women who have received ARAVA treatment and wish to become pregnant, one of the following procedures is recommended:

- After stopping treatment with ARAVA, cholestyramine 8 g is administered 3 times daily for a period of 11 days **or**
- After stopping treatment with ARAVA, 50 g of activated charcoal is administered 4 times daily for a period of 11 days.

The plasma levels of the active metabolite (A771726) must be less than 0.02 mg/L (0.02 µg/mL). Below this plasma level (to be verified by 2 separate tests at an interval of at least 14 days), the teratogenic risk is considered very low (see Contraindications and Warnings and Precautions, General, Washout Procedures).

Without the drug elimination procedure, it may take up to 2 years to reach A771726 levels <0.02 mg/L. However, also after such a waiting period, verification of A771726 levels less than 0.02 mg/L (0.02 µg/mL) by 2 separate tests at an interval of a least 14 days is required.

If a waiting period of up to approximately 2 years under reliable contraception is considered unpractical, prophylactic institution of a washout procedure may be advisable (see Warnings and Precautions, General, Washout Procedures).

Reliable contraception with oral contraceptive may not be guaranteed during the washout procedure with cholestyramine or activated charcoal. Use of alternative contraceptive methods is recommended.

Males: ARAVA must not be used by men who could potentially father a child and are not using reliable contraception during and for a total of 2 years after treatment with ARAVA, if no elimination procedure is used.

There are no specific data on the risk of male-mediated foetal toxicity. However, animal studies to evaluate this specific risk have not been conducted. To minimize any possible risk, men wishing to father a child should consider discontinuing use of ARAVA and use elimination procedure or wait 2 years after treatment cessation.

For men having received ARAVA treatment and wishing to father a child, plasma levels of the active metabolite (A771726) must be less than 0.02 mg/L (0.02µg/mL) to be verified by two separate tests at an interval of at least 14 days. **After the second test confirming that the plasma concentration is below 0.02 mg/L an additional waiting period of 3 months is required.** After that period, the risk of male-mediated foetal toxicity is considered very low (see Contraindications and Warnings and Precautions, General, Washout Procedures).

Impairment of Fertility: ARAVA had no effect on fertility in either male or female rats at oral doses up to 0.4 mg/kg (approximately 1/30 the human A771726 exposure based on AUC).

Skin: In case of ulcerative stomatitis, ARAVA administration should be discontinued.

Very rare cases of Stevens-Johnson syndrome or toxic epidermal necrolysis have been reported in patients treated with ARAVA. As soon as skin and/or mucosal reactions are observed which raise the suspicion of such severe reactions, ARAVA and any other possibly associated medication must be discontinued, and a washout procedure initiated immediately. A complete washout is essential in such cases. In such cases re-exposure to ARAVA is contraindicated (see Contraindications and Warnings and Precautions, General, Washout Procedures).

Special Populations: Pregnant Women: ARAVA must not be administered to pregnant women or women of child bearing potential. ARAVA must not be administered to male subjects who wish to father a child (see Contraindications and Warnings and Precautions, Sexual Function/Reproduction).

Nursing Women: Animal studies indicate that ARAVA or its metabolites pass into breast milk. Therefore, ARAVA must not be administered to nursing mothers (see Contraindications).

Pediatrics (<18 years of age): The safety and efficacy of ARAVA in the pediatric population have not been fully evaluated, and its use in patients less than 18 years of age is contraindicated.

Geriatrics (>65 years of age): No dosage adjustment is needed in patients over 65 years of age.

Monitoring and Laboratory Tests: ARAVA should be administered to patients only under careful medical supervision.

AST and ALT must be checked before initiation of the treatment and at monthly or more frequent intervals during the first 6 months, and every 8 weeks thereafter (See Warnings and Precautions, Hepatic/Biliary/Pancreatic).

ALT values are elevated more frequently than AST.

For confirmed ALT elevations between 2- and 3-times the upper limit of normal, dose may be reduced from 20 to 10 mg/day and monitoring should be performed weekly. If ALT elevations of more than 2- times the upper limit of normal persist, or, if confirmed ALT increases to more than 3- times the upper limit of normal, ARAVA must be discontinued and washout procedures initiated.

If a severe undesirable effect of ARAVA occurs, or if for any other reason the active metabolite needs to be cleared rapidly from the body (e.g.: desired or unintended pregnancy, switching to another DMARD such as methotrexate), the washout procedures should be initiated. Cholestyramine or activated charcoal should be administered to more rapidly lower A771726 levels (see Contraindications, Warnings and Precautions, General, Washout Procedures).

A complete blood cell count, including differential white blood cell count and platelets, must be performed before start of ARAVA treatment as well as every 2 weeks for the first 6 months of treatment and every 8 weeks thereafter (see Warnings and Precautions, Hematologic).

In addition to hypertension noted in Clinical Trials, isolated reports of difficulty with blood pressure control including cases of malignant hypertension and hypertensive crisis have been submitted. Although a causal relationship to ARAVA has not been established and confounding factors were present in most cases, it is considered essential that monitoring recommendations are closely followed. Therefore, blood pressure must be checked before the start of ARAVA treatment and periodically thereafter (see Adverse Reactions, Clinical Trial Adverse Drug Reactions).

In patients with a current or previous history of pulmonary disease or who have been recently treated with drugs known to induce interstitial lung disease, it is recommended that pulmonary status be evaluated prior to initiation of ARAVA therapy and that patients be closely monitored during treatment.

Other Laboratory Tests Changes: Due to an uricosuric effect presumably at the brush border of the proximal renal tubule, uric acid levels usually decrease. Phosphaturia and hypokalemia may also occur.

ADVERSE REACTIONS: Adverse Drug Reaction Overview: Hypertension, gastrointestinal disturbances, weight loss, headache, dizziness, paresthesia, asthenia, musculoskeletal and skin disorder are considered as some common adverse reactions seen with ARAVA.

Leucopenia and hypersensitivity reactions may occur and very rarely, cases of Stevens-Johnson syndrome or toxic epidermal necrolysis have been reported.

Hepatotoxicity has occurred. It is usually mild and reversible but cases of severe, sometimes fatal, liver disease, including acute hepatic necrosis, have been observed. There have been reports of pancreatitis, interstitial lung disease, and infections, including fatal sepsis (see Clinical Trial Adverse Drug Reactions and Less Common Clinical Trial Adverse Drug Reactions/Post-Market Adverse Drug Reactions).

Clinical Trial Adverse Drug Reactions: Because clinical trials are conducted under very specific conditions the adverse reaction rates observed in the clinical trials may not reflect the rates observed in practice and should not be compared to the rates in the clinical trials of another drug. Adverse drug reaction information from clinical trials is useful for identifying drug-related adverse events and for approximating rates.

There were a total of 5419 adverse events reported in 1339 subjects treated with ARAVA. Four percent (4%) of the subjects in controlled studies of ARAVA had a dose reduction as a result of an adverse event and 15.5% discontinued study treatment due to adverse events. There was a total of 377 serious adverse events which occurred in 294 (22%) ARAVA treated subjects. The percent of ARAVA treated patients experiencing an adverse event was similar to methotrexate, the next largest treatment population.

The most common adverse events, in the controlled clinical trials, considered related to ARAVA administration were of gastrointestinal origin and consisted predominantly of diarrhea (26.7% ARAVA, 11.9% placebo, 9.8% sulfasalazine, 12.5% methotrexate), LFT (liver function test) abnormalities (10.2% ARAVA, 2.4% placebo, 3.8% sulfasalazine, 15.1% methotrexate), abdominal pain (5.7% ARAVA, 4.3% placebo, 6.8% sulfasalazine, 7.5% methotrexate), and nausea and/or vomiting (17.8% ARAVA, 14.3% placebo, 22.6% sulfasalazine, 19.9% methotrexate). These disorders may as well be associated with concomitant NSAID administration, common in all treatment groups. The occurrences of hypertension and hypokalemia observed in patients treated with ARAVA may have been influenced by concomitant NSAID and/or steroid use. Monitoring blood pressure in patients on ARAVA should be considered as addition to the recommended Monitoring of hematologic and hepatic function (see Warnings and Precautions, Monitoring and Laboratory Tests).

Adverse reactions associated with the use of ARAVA in rheumatoid arthritis include diarrhea, elevated liver transaminases (ALT and AST, alopecia, rash, and hypertension. In the controlled studies, the following adverse events were reported regardless of causality (see Table 2).

Table 2: ARAVA

Percentage of Patients with Adverse Events ≥3% in any ARAVA-treated Group

	All RA Studies	Placebo-controlled Trials				Active-controlled Trials	
		MN 301 and US 301				MN 302[a]	
	LEF (N=1339) (%)	LEF (N=315) (%)	PBO (N=210) (%)	SSZ (N=133) (%)	MTX (N=182) (%)	LEF (N=501) (%)	MTX (N=498) (%)
General Disorder							
Allergic Reaction	—	5	2	0	6	—	2
Worsening RA	8	5	11	20	4	17	19
Asthenia	3	6	4	5	6	3	3
Flu Syndrome	—	4	2	0	7	—	0
Infection	4	—	0	0	0	—	0
Injury Accident	5	7	5	3	11	6	7
Pain	—	4	2	2	5	—	<1
Abdominal Pain	6	5	4	4	8	6	4
Back Pain	5	6	3	4	9	8	7
Cardiovascular Disorders							
Hypertension	10	9	4	4	3	10	4
Chest Pain	—	4	2	2	4	—	2
Gastrointestinal Disorders							
Anorexia	3	3	2	5	2	3	3
Diarrhea	17	27	12	10	20	22	10
Dyspepsia	5	10	10	9	13	6	7
Gastroenteritis	3	—	1	0	6	3	3
Abnormal Liver Function Tests	5	10	2	4	10	6	17
Nausea	9	13	11	19	18	13	18
Gastrointestinal/Abdominal Pain	5	6	4	7	8	8	8
Mouth Ulcer	3	5	4	3	10	3	6
Vomiting	3	5	4	4	3	3	3
Blood and Lymphatic Disorders							

(cont'd)

Table 2: ARAVA *(cont'd)*

Percentage of Patients with Adverse Events ≥3% in any ARAVA-treated Group

	All RA Studies	Placebo-controlled Trials				Active-controlled Trials	
		MN 301 and US 301				MN 302[a]	
	LEF (N=1339) (%)	LEF (N=315) (%)	PBO (N=210) (%)	SSZ (N=133) (%)	MTX (N=182) (%)	LEF (N=501) (%)	MTX (N=498) (%)
Leucopenia (>2.0 G/L)	3	—	0	2	1	4	3
Metabolic and Nutritional Disorders							
Hypokalemia	—	3	1	1	1	—	<1
Weight Decrease	4	—	1	2	0	—	2
Musculoskeletal System and Connective Tissue Disorders							
Leg Cramps	—	4	2	2	6	—	0
Joint Disorder	4	—	2	2	2	8	6
Synovitis	—	—	1	0	2	4	2
Tenosynovitis	3	—	0	1	2	5	1
Nervous System Disorders							
Dizziness	4	5	3	6	5	7	6
Headache	7	13	11	12	21	10	8
Paresthesia	—	3	1	1	2	4	3
Respiratory, Thoracic and Mediastinal Disorders							
Bronchitis	7	5	2	4	7	8	7
Increased Cough	3	4	5	3	6	5	7
Respiratory Infection	15	21	21	20	32	27	25
Pharyngitis	3	—	1	2	1	3	3
Pneumonia	—	3	0	0	1	—	2
Rhinitis	—	5	2	4	3	—	2
Sinusitis	—	5	5	0	10	—	1
Skin and Subcutaneous Tissue Disorders							
Alopecia	10	9	1	6	6	17	10
Eczema	—	—	1	1	1	3	2
Pruritus	4	5	2	3	2	6	2
Rash	10	12	7	11	9	11	10
Dry Skin	—	3	2	2	0	3	1
Renal and Urinary Disorders							
Urinary Tract Infection	5	5	7	4	2	5	6

[a] Study MN 302, an active-controlled study, treated a total of 999 subjects using 1:1 randomization to (1) ARAVA 20 mg/day after a loading dose of 100 mg/day for 3 days, or (2) methotrexate 10 mg/week or escalation to 15 mg/week. Treatment duration was 52 weeks.

Legend: LEF=leflunomide; SSZ=sulfasalazine; PBO=placebo; MTX=methotrexate; RA=rheumatoid arthritis.

Less Common Clinical Trial Adverse Drug Reactions/Post-Market Adverse Drug Reactions: The following adverse events have been reported in 1% to <3%, less than 1%, less than 0.1% or less than 0.01% of the rheumatoid arthritis patients in the ARAVA treatment group in controlled clinical trials or during post-marketing surveillance:

Blood and Lymphatic System Disorders: 1% to <3%: anemia (including iron deficiency anemia), ecchymosis, leucopenia (leucocytes >2×10⁹/L [2 g/L]). Less than 1%: eosinophilia, leucopenia (leucocytes <2 g /L), lymphadenopathy, pancytopenia, thrombocytopenia. Less than 0.01%: agranulocytosis.

Cardiovascular Disorders: 1% to <3%: angina pectoris, palpitation, tachycardia, vasodilatation, varicose vein.

Endocrine Disorders: 1% to <3%: diabetes mellitus, hyperthyroidism.

Eye Disorders: 1% to <3%: amblyopia, cataract, conjunctivitis, eye disorders.

Gastrointestinal Disorders: 1% to <3%: colitis, constipation, esophagitis, flatulence, gastritis, gingivitis, melena, oral moniliasis, pharyngitis, salivary gland enlarged, stomatitis (or aphthous stomatitis), tooth disorder, taste perversion.

General Disorders: 1% to <3%: abscess, cyst, fever, hernia, malaise, pain, neck pain, pelvic pain, migraine.

The risk of malignancy, particularly lymphoproliferative disorders, is also known to be increased with use of some immunosuppressive drugs (see Warnings and Precautions, Carcinogenesis and Mutagenesis).

Hepatobiliary Disorders: 1% to <3%: cholelithiasis. Less than 1%: hepatitis, jaundice/cholestasis, severe disturbances in liver function; increase in alkaline phosphatase and lactate dehydrogenase (LDH). Less than 0.01%: severe liver injury such as hepatic failure and acute hepatic necrosis that may be fatal, pancreatitis.

Infection and Infestations: Less than 0.1%: Severe infections including opportunistic infections and sepsis, which may be fatal.

Metabolism and Nutrition Disorders: 1% to <3%: creatine phosphokinase increased, peripheral edema, hyperglycemia, hyperlipidemia. Less than 1%: hypokalemia, hypophosphatemia.

Uric acid levels usually decrease, due to an uricosyric effect.

Musculoskeletal System and Connective Tissue Disorders: 1% to <3%: arthrosis, bursitis, muscle cramps, myalgia, bone necrosis, bone pain, tendon rupture.

Nervous System Disorders: 1% to <3%: anxiety, asthenia, depression, dry mouth, insomnia, neuralgia, neuritis, sleep disorder, sweat, vertigo. Less than 0.01%: peripheral neuropathy.

Respiratory, Thoracic and Mediastinal Disorders: 1% to <3%: asthma, dyspnea, epistaxis, lung disorder. Less than 0.1%: interstitial lung disease (including interstitial pneumonitis and pulmonary fibrosis), sometimes fatal.

Skin and Subcutaneous Tissue Disorders and Allergic Reactions: 1% to <3%: acne, contact dermatitis, fungal dermatitis, hair discoloration, hematoma, herpes simplex, herpes zoster, nail disorder, skin nodule, subcutaneous nodule, maculopapular rash, skin disorder, skin discolour, skin ulcer. Less than 1%: urticaria, anaphylactoid reactions, severe anaphylactic reaction. Less than 0.01%: erythema multiforme, Stevens-Johnson syndrome, toxic epidermal necrolysis, vasculitis, including cutaneous necrotizing vasculitis.

Renal and Urinary Disorders: 1% to <3%: albuminuria, cystitis, dysuria, hematuria, prostate disorder, urinary frequency.

Reproductive System and Breast Disorders: 1% to <3%: menstrual disorder, vaginal moniliasis.

Causal relationship of these events to ARAVA has not been established.

Adverse events during a second year of treatment with ARAVA in clinical trials were consistent with those observed during the first year of treatment and occurred at a similar or lower incidence.

DRUG INTERACTIONS: Overview: Increased side effects may occur when ARAVA is given concomitantly with hepatotoxic, hematotoxic or immunosuppressive substances. This is also to be considered when ARAVA treatment is followed by such drugs without a washout period (see Contraindications and Warnings and Precautions, General, Washout Procedures). Strict vigilance in monitoring of hepatic and hematologic functions is recommended for all patients prescribed ARAVA with other medications associated with increased risk of hepatotoxicity or hematotoxicity.

Due to a potential for additive hepatotoxic effects, it is recommended that alcohol consumption be avoided during treatment with ARAVA.

In vitro studies indicate that A771726 inhibits cytochrome P4502C9 (CYP2C9) activity. In clinical trials no safety problems were observed when ARAVA and NSAIDs metabolised by CYP2C9 were coadministered. Caution is advised when ARAVA is given together with drugs, other than NSAIDs, that are metabolised by CYP2C9 such as phenytoin, warfarin, and tolbutamide (see Drug-Drug Interactions).

Drug-Drug Interactions: Aspirin, NSAIDs, Corticosteroids: In clinical trials of over 1339 rheumatoid arthritis patients there were no apparent interactions between ARAVA and concomitantly administered aspirin (acetylsalicylic acid), NSAIDs, and/or low dose corticosteroids. It has been shown that corticosteroid doses may be reduced gradually in patients who respond to ARAVA.

In vitro studies indicate that A771726 inhibits cytochrome P4502C9 (CYP2C9) activity. In clinical trials no safety problems were observed when ARAVA and NSAIDs metabolised by CYP2C9 were coadministered.

Based on protein binding measured in vitro using therapeutic concentrations, there was no effect of ibuprofen, or diclofenac on the protein binding of A771726. A771726 lead to a 13% to 50% increase in the unbound fractions of diclofenac and ibuprofen, which would not be expected to be clinically significant.

Aspirin (acetylsalicylic acid), NSAIDs, and/or low dose corticosteroids may be continued during treatment with ARAVA. These combined used of ARAVA with NSAIDs and/or corticosteroids may be associated with hypertension.

Cholestyramine or Activated Charcoal: Concomitant administration of ARAVA with cholestyramine or activated charcoal will lead to a rapid and significant decrease in plasma A771726 (the active metabolite of ARAVA) concentration.

Cimetidine: When coadministered with cimetidine (nonspecific Cytochrome P450 inhibitor), there were no changes in the pharmacokinetics of A771726 or TFMA, and slight increases in ARAVA concentrations were observed in some subjects.

Methotrexate: Concomitant administration of ARAVA with methotrexate has not been approved in Canada.

In an open label study, 30 patients with active rheumatoid arthritis despite methotrexate therapy (17±4 mg/week (mean±S.D.) for at least six months were administered ARAVA 10-20 mg/day. Twenty-three patients completed one year of treatment. No pharmacokinetic interaction between the methotrexate and ARAVA was noted. A 2- to 3-fold elevation in liver enzymes was seen in 5 of 30 patients. All elevations resolved, 2 with continuation of both drugs and 3 after discontinuation of ARAVA. A more than 3-fold increase was seen in another 5 patients. All of these also resolved, 2 with continuation of both drugs and 3 after discontinuation of leflunomide. Sixteen patients met ACR 20% criteria for clinical response. In the two patients that underwent liver biopsies there was no evidence of significant fibrosis.

Changing from ARAVA to methotrexate without a washout period may raise the possibility of additive risks even for a long time after the switching (i.e. kinetic interaction, organ toxicity) (see Warnings and Precautions, General). In addition, if ARAVA and methotrexate are given concomitantly, ACR guidelines for monitoring methotrexate liver toxicity must be followed with ALT, AST, and serum albumin testing monthly (see Warnings and Precautions, Hepatic/Biliary/Pancreatic).

Other DMARDs: The combined use of ARAVA with antimalarials, intramuscular or oral gold, D penicillamine or azathioprine has not been adequately studied. The risk associated with combination therapy, in particular in long-term treatment, is unknown. Since such therapy can lead to additive or even synergistic toxicity (e.g. hepato- or hematotoxicity), combination with another DMARD is not advisable.

Phenytoin: In vitro studies indicate that A771726 inhibits cytochrome P4502C9 (CYP2C9) activity. Caution is advised when ARAVA is given together with drugs, other than NSAIDs that are metabolised by CYP2C9 such as phenytoin.

Warfarin: In vitro studies indicate that A771726 inhibits cytochrome P4502C9 (CYP2C9) activity. Caution is advised when ARAVA is given together with drugs, other than NSAIDs that are metabolised by CYP2C9 such as warfarin.

Based on protein binding measured in vitro using therapeutic concentrations, there was no effect of warfarin on the protein binding of A771726. A771726 had no effect on the binding of warfarin.

There have been case reports of increased prothrombin time when ARAVA and warfarin were coadministered.

Tolbutamide: In vitro studies indicate that A771726 inhibits cytochrome P4502C9 (CYP2C9) activity. Caution is advised when ARAVA is given together with drugs, other than NSAIDs that are metabolised by CYP2C9 such as tolbutamide.

In vitro, A771726 lead to a 13% to 50% increase in the unbound fractions of tolbutamide, which would not be expected to be clinically significant. Tolbutamide led to an increase in the percent of unbound A771726, which was dependent upon the concentration of tolbutamide but independent of the concentration of A771726.

Oral Contraceptives: In a study in which ARAVA was given concomitantly with a triphasic oral contraceptive pill containing 30 µg ethinyloestradiol to healthy female volunteers, there was no reduction in contraceptive activity and A771726 pharmacokinetic parameters were within predicted ranges.

Rifampin: Following concomitant administration of a single dose of ARAVA to subjects receiving multiple doses of rifampin, A771726 levels were increased approximately 40% over those seen when ARAVA was administered alone. Because of the potential for ARAVA levels to continue to increase with multiple dosing, caution should be used if patients are to be receiving both ARAVA and rifampin.

Vaccination: No clinical data are available on the efficacy and safety of vaccination during ARAVA treatment. Vaccination with live vaccines is, however, not recommended. A live vaccine should only be given after a period of at least 6 months has elapsed after stopping ARAVA.

Drug-Food Interactions: ARAVA can be taken during meals or at any time between meals.

Drug-Herb Interactions: Interactions with herbal products have not been established.

Drug-Laboratory Test Interactions: Interactions with laboratory tests have not been established.

DOSAGE AND ADMINISTRATION: Recommended Dose and Dosage Adjustment: Loading Dose: Due to the long half-life in patients with rheumatoid arthritis and recommended dosing interval (24 hr), a loading dose is needed to yield steady-state concentrations more rapidly. It is recommended that ARAVA therapy be initiated with a loading dose of one 100 mg tablet per day for 3 days.

Maintenance Therapy: Daily dosing of 20 mg is recommended for treatment of patients with rheumatoid arthritis. A small cohort of patients (n=104) treated with 25 mg/day experienced a greater incidence of side effects: alopecia, weight loss, liver enzyme elevations. Doses higher than 20 mg/day are not recommended. If dosing at 20 mg/day is not well tolerated clinically, the dose may be decreased to 10 mg daily. Due to the prolonged half-life of the active metabolite of ARAVA, patients should be carefully observed after dose reduction since it may take several weeks for metabolite levels to decline (see Warnings and Precautions, Monitoring and Laboratory Tests).

ARAVA can be taken with or without food, without regard to meals, at the same time everyday.

A treatment effect may be evident after 4 weeks and may further improve up to 4 to 6 months after start of treatment.

Geriatric Use: No dosage adjustment is needed in patients over 65 years of age.

Impaired Renal Function: Because the kidney plays a role in the elimination of ARAVA, and without sufficient studies of the use of ARAVA in patients with renal insufficiency, caution should be used when considering the administration of ARAVA to patients with mild renal insufficiency (see Contraindications).

Missed Dose: If the patient forgot to take a tablet of ARAVA they should be advised to take it as soon as they remember, unless it is nearly time for their next dose. The patient should be advised not to double-up on the next dose to make up for the missed dose.

Administration: ARAVA tablets should be swallowed whole, with sufficient liquid.

OVERDOSAGE:
There have been reports of chronic overdose in patients taking ARAVA at daily doses up to five times the recommended daily dose and reports of acute overdose in adults or children. The majority of the reported overdoses were without adverse events. In cases where adverse events were reported, they were consistent with the safety profile for ARAVA (see Adverse Reactions). The most frequent adverse events observed were diarrhea, abdominal pain, leucopenia, anemia and elevated liver function tests.

In the event of relevant overdose or toxicity, cholestyramine or activated charcoal administration is recommended.

Cholestyramine given orally at a dose of 8 g three times a day for 24 hours to three healthy volunteers decreased plasma levels of A771726 by approximately 40% in 24 hours and by 49-65% in 48 hours (see Warnings and Precautions, General, Washout Procedures).

Administration of activated charcoal (powder made into a suspension) orally or via nasogastric tube (50 g every 6 hours for 24 hours) has been shown to reduce plasma concentrations of the active metabolite, A771726, by 37% in 24 hours and by 48% in 48 hours.

These washout procedures may be repeated if clinically necessary.

Studies with both hemodialysis and CAPD (chronic ambulatory peritoneal dialysis) indicate that A771726, the primary metabolite of ARAVA, is not dialyzable.

> For management of a suspected drug overdose, CPhA recommends that you contact your **regional Poison Control Centre**. See the *CPS* Directory section for a list of Poison Control Centres.

ACTION AND CLINICAL PHARMACOLOGY: Mechanism of Action: Leflunomide is an isoxazole immunomodulatory agent which inhibits de novo pyrimidine synthesis and has antiproliferative activity. Following oral administration, it is rapidly metabolized to A771726, which is active in vitro and is presumed to be the active drug in vivo. Leflunomide has demonstrated prophylactic and therapeutic effects in animal models of autoimmune disease. In addition, leflunomide has exhibited antiinflammatory and weak analgesic and antipyretic activity. In a model of experimental septicemia, leflunomide did not alter the resistance of mice to bacterial pathogens.

In vitro, after mitogen stimulation, A771726 inhibits T-cell proliferation, DNA synthesis, and expression of certain cell surface and nuclear antigens directly involved in T-cell activation and proliferation. It inhibits antigen-stimulated proliferation of human peripheral blood mononuclear cells (PBMCs) and proliferation in transformed murine and human cell lines, in a dose-dependent fashion. The antiproliferative activity is reversed by the addition of uridine to the cell culture, indicating that A771726 acts at the level of the de novo pyrimidine biosynthesis.

Leflunomide inhibition of GvHD in vivo is also reversed by feeding uridine, further indicating that A771726 acts at the level of the de novo pyrimidine biosynthesis pathway.

It has been demonstrated that A771726 binds to and is a potent inhibitor of dihydroorotate dehydrogenase (DHODH), an enzyme in the de novo pyrimidine synthesis pathway important for DNA synthesis. In the heterotopic cardiac transplant model, DHODH activity is decreased in lymphocytes infiltrating heart allograft tissue in leflunomide-treated animals. In vitro, incubation of PHA/IL 2 stimulated human peripheral T cells with A771726 triggered cell cycle arrest at the GI phase or, in those cells undergoing DNA synthesis, at S phase. Exogenous uridine reversed this effect, and no increase in apoptotic cell numbers was observed. Increased levels of the tumor suppressor protein p53 with subsequent expression of the cyclin-dependent kinase (CDK) inhibitor p21 appear to mediate this reversible cell cycle arrest.

In vitro incubation of A771726 with rat, mouse, and human DHODH demonstrated inhibition of enzyme activity at concentrations lower than those, which exert antiproliferative effects upon rapidly dividing cells (10-367 mM). Rat and mouse enzymes are more sensitive to the inhibitory effect of A771726 (IC_{50} 0.14±0.08 and 16±11 μM, respectively) than the human enzyme (IC_{50} 46±6 μM).

Together, these data suggest that, in vivo at concentrations achievable in patients, leflunomide inhibits de novo pyrimidine synthesis in activated lymphocytes and other rapidly dividing cell populations resulting in reversible cell cycle arrest.

The inhibition of tyrosine kinase activities has also been reported for both in vitro and in vivo situations. These effects are observed at A771726 concentrations much higher than those needed for DHODH inhibition and could be secondary to the effect on DHODH. In addition, leflunomide orally and A771726 in vitro have been demonstrated to modulate the cell adhesion process in rheumatoid arthritis patients.

Pharmacokinetics: The pharmacokinetics of leflunomide, based upon plasma concentrations of the active metabolite, A771726, have been studied in healthy subjects and in patients with rheumatoid arthritis.

Absorption: After oral administration of a 100 mg dose of ^{14}C-leflunomide to healthy volunteers, leflunomide was not detectable (<25 ng/mL) in plasma over the plasma sampling period (0.5 hrs to 37 days). Plasma concentrations of total radioactivity and A771726 were superimposable, demonstrating extensive conversion to the active metabolite A771726 during the absorption process. The minor metabolite 4-trifluoromethylaniline (TFMA) has been detected in the plasma of animals and man, but at concentrations (ng/mL) much less than those of A771726 (μg/mL). The slow but nearly complete recovery of radioactivity as metabolites indicated near complete absorption of leflunomide in man.

In a 24-week study in patients with rheumatoid arthritis, steady-state was reached between 7 and 8 weeks. Mean plasma A771726 concentrations 24 hours after a 100 mg loading dose (8.5 μg/mL) were twice those after a 50 mg loading dose (4.0 μg/mL). Pre-dose plasma concentrations after 24 weeks of dosing were linearly related to the maintenance dose (9, 18, and 63 μg/mL after 5, 10 or 25 mg/day, respectively). The pharmacokinetics of A771726 are, therefore, linear over the range of loading and maintenance doses to be used clinically.

After single doses of ARAVA to healthy subjects, peak plasma concentrations of A771726 were approached between 6 and 12 hours. Based on determination of A771726, the bioavailability of leflunomide from a tablet formulation relative to an oral solution was 80%. ARAVA administered with a high fat/high carbohydrate meal was bioequivalent to administration under fasted conditions.

Distribution: In studies with plasma samples obtained from healthy subjects, A771726 was extensively bound to protein (>99%) (albumin). The unbound fraction of A771726 was 0.62%. Binding of A771726 was linear up to 573 μg/mL. Compared to healthy subjects, the unbound fraction was slightly increased (0.80%) in plasma from patients with rheumatoid arthritis and was approximately doubled in patients with chronic renal insufficiency. The extensive protein binding of A771726 is consistent with its low volume of distribution. After independent intravenous administration of A771726, steady-state volume of distribution averaged 11 L.

Metabolism: Following oral administration, leflunomide is rapidly converted to the active metabolite, A771726. Animal studies suggest that conversion takes place during passage through both the gut wall and the liver.

The metabolic biotransformation of A771726 is not controlled by a single enzyme and has been shown to occur in microsomal and cytosolic cellular fractions.

The urinary metabolites were primarily glucuronide conjugates of leflunomide and an oxanilic acid derivative of A771726, while A771726 was the primary metabolite in the feces.

Excretion: After oral administration of a 100 mg dose of ^{14}C-leflunomide to healthy volunteers, urinary and fecal recovery of ^{14}C-leflunomide over 28 days accounted for 43% and 48% of total radioactivity, respectively. Unchanged leflunomide was not detected in urine or feces. A771726 is cleared by slow excretion in feces, probably by biliary elimination and slow metabolism to the oxanilic acid metabolite excreted in urine.

After independent intravenous administration of A771726, clearance averaged 31 mL/hr and elimination half-life 10 days. A similar clearance estimate (29±17 mL/h) was obtained from population pharmacokinetics analysis of rheumatoid arthritis patients enrolled in pivotal safety and efficacy studies.

After single doses of ARAVA to healthy subjects, plasma concentrations of A771726 declined monoexponentially, with a half-life of approximately 8 days. After 24 weeks, the elimination half-life averaged 14-18 days.

The elimination half-life in patients is approximately 2 weeks. Oral administration of activated charcoal or cholestyramine is effective in enhancing the elimination of A771726. During oral administration of activated charcoal (50 g four times a day) or cholestyramine (8 g three times a day), the half-life of A771726 decreased to approximately 24 hours. Although the mechanism for the enhanced elimination is unknown, it may be related to interruption of enterohepatic recycling and/or dialysis across the gastrointestinal mucosa.

Special Populations and Conditions: Renal Insufficiency: When subjects with end-stage renal disease were administered a single 100 mg dose of leflunomide orally, plasma concentrations of A771726 both prior to and after dialysis (chronic ambulatory peritoneal dialysis [CAPD] or hemodialysis) were comparable to those of healthy volunteers administered the same dose. With hemodialysis, A771726 was cleared somewhat more rapidly and with a shorter half-life. The pharmacokinetic parameters for the CAPD patients were consistent with the values for healthy volunteers.

STORAGE AND STABILITY: Store at room temperature (15 to 30°C), in a dry place. Protect from exposure to light. Keep in a safe place out of the reach of children.

INFORMATION FOR THE PATIENT: Published in e-CPS, available by subscription at www.e-cps.ca.

DOSAGE FORMS, COMPOSITION AND PACKAGING: 10 mg: Each film-coated, white, round tablet, with 'ZBN' code on one side, contains: leflunomide 10 mg. Nonmedicinal ingredients: colloidal silicon dioxide, crospovidone, hydroxypropyl methylcellulose, lactose monohydrate, magnesium stearate, polyethylene glycol, povidone, starch, talc and titanium dioxide. HDPE bottles of 30.

20 mg: Each film-coated, light yellow, triangular tablet, with 'ZBO' code on one side, contains: leflunomide 20 mg. Nonmedicinal ingredients: colloidal silicon dioxide, crospovidone, hydroxypropyl methylcellulose, lactose monohydrate, magnesium stearate, polyethylene glycol, povidone, starch, talc, titanium dioxide and yellow ferric oxide. HDPE bottles of 30.

100 mg: Each film-coated, white, round tablet, with 'ZBP' code on one side, contains: leflunomide 100 mg. Nonmedicinal ingredients: colloidal silicon dioxide, crospovidone, hydroxypropyl methylcellulose, lactose monohydrate, magnesium stearate, polyethylene glycol, povidone, starch, talc and titanium dioxide. Aluminium/aluminium blister packs of 3.

(Shown in Product Identification Section)

Aredia® Ⓟ

pamidronate disodium

Bone Metabolism Regulator

Novartis Pharmaceuticals

Date of Preparation: February 24, 1993
Date of Revision: May 4, 2010

SUMMARY PRODUCT INFORMATION:

Route of Administration	Dosage Form/ Strength	Clinically Relevant Nonmedicinal Ingredients
I.V. infusion	Sterile lyophilized powder: • 30 mg/vial • 90 mg/vial	• mannitol • phosphoric acid

INDICATIONS AND CLINICAL USE:
- **Tumour-induced hypercalcemia following adequate saline rehydration.**
  Prior to treatment with AREDIA (pamidronate disodium), renal excretion of excess calcium should be promoted by restoring and maintaining adequate fluid balance and urine output.
- **Conditions associated with increased osteoclast activity: predominantly lytic bone metastases and multiple myeloma.**
- **Symptomatic Paget's disease of bone.**

CONTRAINDICATIONS: AREDIA is contraindicated:
- in patients with known or suspected hypersensitivity to AREDIA (pamidronate disodium), to any of its excipients (see Dosage Forms, Composition and Packaging), or to other bisphosphonates.
- in pregnancy.
- in breast-feeding women.

WARNINGS AND PRECAUTIONS:

> **Serious Warnings and Precautions**
> - The following are serious adverse events:
>   - Osteonecrosis of the jaw (ONJ) (see Warnings and Precautions, General)
>   - Deterioration in renal function (see Warnings and Precautions, Renal)
> - AREDIA should not be administered to patients with severe renal impairment except in cases of life-threatening tumour-induced hypercalcemia (see Warnings and Precautions, Special Populations, Renal Impairment and Dosage and Administration)
> - Single doses of AREDIA should not exceed 90 mg and the recommended infusion time should be observed (see Warnings and Precautions, Renal and Dosage and Administration)

General: AREDIA (pamidronate disodium) must never be given as a bolus injection since severe local reactions and thrombophlebitis may result from high local concentrations.

AREDIA should always be diluted and administered as a slow intravenous infusion (see Dosage and Administration). Regardless of the volume of solution in which AREDIA is diluted, slow intravenous infusion is absolutely necessary for safety.

AREDIA should not be given together with other bisphosphonates to treat hypercalcemia since the combined effects of these agents are unknown.

AREDIA should not be mixed with calcium-containing intravenous infusions.

Patients must be assessed prior to and during administration of AREDIA to assure that they are appropriately hydrated. This is especially important for patients receiving diuretic therapy.

It is essential in the initial treatment of tumour-induced hypercalcemia that intravenous rehydration be instituted to restore urine output. Patients should be hydrated adequately throughout treatment but overhydration must be avoided.

Cardiovascular: In patients with cardiac disease, especially in the elderly, additional saline overload may precipitate cardiac failure (left ventricular failure or congestive heart failure). Fever (influenza-like symptoms) may also contribute to this deterioration.

Atrial Fibrillation: When the effects of zoledronic acid (4 mg) and pamidronate (90 mg) were compared in one clinical trial, the number of atrial fibrillation adverse events was higher in the pamidronate group (12/556, 2.2%) than in the zoledronic acid group (3/563, 0.5%). Previously, it has been observed in a clinical trial investigating patients with postmenopausal osteoporosis, that zoledronic acid treated patients (5 mg) had an increased rate of atrial fibrillation serious adverse events compared to placebo (1.3% compared to 0.6%). The mechanism of this increased incidence of atrial fibrillation in isolated studies with some bisphosphonates, including AREDIA, is unknown.

Effects on Ability to Drive or Use Machines: Somnolence and/or dizziness may occur following AREDIA infusion, in which case the patient should not drive, operate potentially dangerous machinery or engage in other activities that may be hazardous because of decreased alertness.

Endocrine and Metabolism: Paget's Disease: Pre-existing hypocalcemia must be treated by adequate intake of calcium and Vitamin D before initiating AREDIA. Other disturbances of mineral metabolism (e.g., parathyroidectomy resulting in partial or complete hypoparathyroidism) must also be effectively managed. It is recommended that patients with Paget's disease of bone have their serum calcium levels assessed before and during treatment with AREDIA (e.g., as part of their annual examination). All patients should be counselled regarding the importance of calcium and vitamin D supplementation in maintaining serum calcium levels and on the symptoms of hypocalcemia.

Lytic Bone Metastases or Multiple Myeloma: In the absence of hypercalcemia, patients who are at risk of calcium or vitamin D deficiency, should be given oral calcium and Vitamin D supplementation in order to minimize the risk of hypocalcemia. In the event that hypercalcemia develops, calcium and Vitamin D supplements should be discontinued immediately.

Hepatic/Biliary/Pancreatic: There are no clinical data available in patients with severe hepatic insufficiency.

Musculoskeletal Pain: In post-marketing experience, severe and occasionally incapacitating bone, joint, and/or muscle pain has been reported in patients taking bisphosphonates. However, such reports occur rarely. This category of drugs includes AREDIA (pamidronate disodium for injection). The time to onset of symptoms varied from one day to several months after starting the drug. Most patients had relief of symptoms after stopping treatment. A subset of patients had recurrence of symptoms when re-challenged with the same drug or another bisphosphonate.

Ophthalmologic: Ocular disturbances (conjunctivitis, uveitis, episcleritis and orbital inflammation) have been reported with bisphosphonate therapy, including AREDIA. Patients with ocular events other than uncomplicated conjunctivitis should be referred to an ophthalmologist for evaluation. Treatment with AREDIA may need to be discontinued.

Osteonecrosis of the Jaw: Osteonecrosis of the jaw (ONJ) has been reported in cancer patients treated with bisphosphonates, including AREDIA. Although no causal relationship has been established, there is an association between bisphosphonate use and the development of ONJ. Post-marketing experience suggests a greater frequency of reports of ONJ based on tumour type (advanced breast cancer, multiple myeloma) and dental status (dental extractions, periodontal disease and local trauma including poorly fitting dentures); these are associated with a greater risk of developing ONJ. Cancer patients also receive other treatments that may play a role in the development of ONJ, such as chemotherapy and glucocorticosteroids. Many patients had signs of local infection including osteomyelitis.

Presentation of ONJ may include altered local sensation (hyperaesthesia or numbness), maxillofacial pain, "toothaches", denture sore spots, loose teeth, exposed bone in the oral cavity, impaired healing, recurrent or persistent soft tissue infection in the oral cavity and marked oral odour. The onset can be from months to years after commencing bisphosphonate therapy. Cancer patients should maintain good oral hygiene; it is recommended that advanced cancer patients be encouraged to have an oral examination of both hard and soft tissues, with preventive dentistry prior to treatment with bisphosphonates, and that such assessments continue at regularly scheduled intervals after bisphosphonate therapy is initiated. While on bisphosphonate treatment, these patients should avoid invasive dental procedures if possible. Biopsies are not recommended unless metastasis to the jaw is suspected. For patients who develop ONJ while on bisphosphonate therapy, dental surgery may exacerbate the condition. For patients requiring dental procedures, there is no data available to suggest whether discontinuation of bisphosphonate treatment reduces the risk of ONJ. Clinical judgment of the treating physician should guide the management plan of each patient based on individual benefit/risk assessment.

Renal: Bisphosphonates, including AREDIA, have been associated with renal toxicity manifested as deterioration of renal function and potential renal failure. Renal deterioration, progression to renal failure (some with fatal outcome) have been reported very rarely in patients after the initial dose or a single dose of AREDIA. Deterioration of renal function (including renal failure) has also been reported following long-term treatment with AREDIA in patients with multiple myeloma.

Due to the risk of clinically significant deterioration in renal function which may progress to renal failure, single doses of AREDIA should not exceed 90 mg and the recommended infusion time should be observed (see Dosage and Administration).

Special Populations: Pregnant Women: It has been shown that AREDIA can cross the placenta in rats and has produced marked maternal and embryo/fetal adverse effects in rats and rabbits.

There are no adequate and well-controlled studies in pregnant women and no clinical evidence to support the use of AREDIA in pregnant women. Therefore, AREDIA should not be used during pregnancy (see Contraindications).

Bisphosphonates are incorporated into the bone matrix, from where they are gradually released over periods of weeks to years. The extent of bisphosphonate incorporation into adult bone, and hence, the amount available for release back into the systemic circulation, is directly related to the total dose and duration of bisphosphonate use. Although there are very limited data on fetal risk in humans, bisphosphonates do cause fetal harm in animals, and animal data suggest that uptake of bisphosphonates into fetal bone is greater than into maternal bone. Therefore, there is a theoretical risk of fetal harm (e.g., skeletal and other abnormalities) if a woman becomes pregnant after completing a course of bisphosphonate therapy. The impact of variables such as time between cessation of bisphosphonate therapy to conception, the particular bisphosphonate used, and the route of administration (intravenous versus oral) on this risk has not been established.

Nursing Women: There is no clinical experience with AREDIA in lactating women. A study in lactating rats has shown that pamidronate passes into the milk. Mothers treated with AREDIA should therefore not breast feed their infants.

Pediatrics: The safety and efficacy of AREDIA in children has not been established. Until further experience is gained, AREDIA is only recommended for use in adult patients.

Renal Impairment: AREDIA is excreted intact primarily via the kidney (see Action and Clinical Pharmacology, Pharmacokinetics), thus the risk of adverse reactions may be greater in patients with impaired renal function. Single doses of AREDIA should not exceed 90 mg and the recommended infusion time should be observed (see Dosage and Administration).

As with other i.v. bisphosphonates renal monitoring is recommended, for instance, measurement of serum creatinine prior to each dose of AREDIA. Experience with AREDIA in patients with severe renal impairment (serum creatinine >440 μmol/L in TIH patients; >180 μmol/L in multiple myeloma patients) is limited. If clinical judgment determines that the potential benefits outweigh the risk in such cases, AREDIA should be used cautiously and renal function carefully monitored. Patients treated with AREDIA for bone metastases or multiple myeloma should have their dose withheld if renal function has deteriorated (see Dosage and Administration, Renal Impairment).

Monitoring and Laboratory Tests: Patients should have standard serum creatinine and clinical renal function parameters periodically evaluated. Patients receiving frequent AREDIA infusions over a prolonged period of time, and those with pre-existing renal disease or a predisposition to renal impairment (e.g., patients with multiple myeloma and/or tumour-induced hypercalcemia) should have evaluations of standard laboratory and clinical parameters of renal function prior to each dose of AREDIA. Fluid balance (urine output, daily weights) should also be followed carefully. If there is deterioration of renal function during AREDIA therapy, the infusion must be stopped (see Warnings and Precautions).

AREDIA is excreted intact primarily via the kidney, thus the risk of renal adverse reactions may be greater in patients with impaired renal function.

Serum electrolytes, calcium and phosphate should be monitored following initiation of therapy with AREDIA. Patients with anemia, leukopenia or thrombocytopenia should have regular hematology assessments. Occasional cases of mild, transient hypocalcemia, usually asymptomatic, have been reported. Symptomatic hypocalcemia occurs rarely and can be reversed with calcium gluconate. Patients who have undergone thyroid surgery may be particularly susceptible to develop hypocalcemia due to relative hypoparathyroidism.

In tumour-induced hypercalcemia, either ionized calcium or total serum calcium corrected (adjusted) for albumin should be monitored during treatment with AREDIA. Serum calcium levels in patients who have hypercalcemia of malignancy may not reflect the severity of hypercalcemia, since hypoalbuminemia is commonly present. Corrected serum calcium values should be calculated using established algorithms, such as:

$$cCa = tCa + (0.02 \times [40 - ALB])$$

where:

cCa=adjusted calcium concentration (mmol/L)
tCa=measured total calcium concentration (mmol/L)
ALB=measured albumin concentration (g/L)

Although mild hypercalcemia may be asymptomatic, moderate to severe hypercalcemia is usually associated with a variety of signs and symptoms, and can be life-threatening if not promptly recognized and treated. Individuals at risk and their caregivers should be made aware that signs and symptoms of hypercalcemia include: lethargy, fatigue, confusion, loss of appetite, nausea and vomiting, constipation, excessive thirst and urination. Measures such as maintaining mobility and ensuring adequate hydration could diminish the symptoms of hypercalcemia. However, when symptoms of hypercalcemia are detected, it is important to seek medical assistance promptly.

ADVERSE REACTIONS: Adverse Drug Reaction Overview: Adverse reactions with AREDIA (pamidronate disodium) are usually mild and transient. The most common adverse reactions are influenza-like symptoms and mild fever (an increase in body temperature of >1°C, which may last up to 48 hours). Fever usually resolves spontaneously and does not require treatment. Acute "influenza-like" reactions usually occur only with the first AREDIA infusion. Table 1 and Table 2 show the incidence of the more commonly observed adverse effects overall and by indication.

Clinical Trial Adverse Drug Reactions: Frequency estimates: Very common (≥1/10), common (≥1/100, <1/10), uncommon (≥1/1000, <1/100), rare (≥1/10 000, <1/1000), very rare (<1/10 000), including isolated reports.

Infections and Infestations: Very rare: reactivation of Herpes simplex and Herpes zoster.

Blood and Lymphatic System Disorders: Common: anemia, thrombocytopenia, lymphocytopenia. Very rare: leukopenia. One case of acute lymphoblastic leukemia has been reported in a patient with Paget's disease. The causal relationship to the treatment or the underlying disease is unknown.

Immune System Disorders: Uncommon: allergic reactions including anaphylactoid reactions, bronchospasm, dyspnea, Quincke's (angioneurotic) oedema. Very rare: anaphylactic shock.

Metabolism and Nutrition Disorders: Very common: hypocalcemia, hypophosphatemia. Common: hypokalemia, hypomagnesemia, increase in serum creatinine. Uncommon: abnormal liver function tests, increase in serum urea. Very rare: hyperkalemia, hypernatremia.

Nervous System Disorders: Common: symptomatic hypocalcemia (paresthesia, tetany), headache, insomnia, somnolence. Uncommon: seizures, agitation, dizziness, lethargy. Very rare: confusion, visual hallucinations.

Eye Disorders: Common: conjunctivitis. Uncommon: uveitis (iritis, iridocyclitis). Very rare: scleritis, episcleritis, xanthopsia.

Cardiac Disorders: Atrial fibrillation: When the effects of zoledronic acid (4 mg) and pamidronate (90 mg) were compared in one clinical trial, the number of atrial fibrillation adverse events was higher in the pamidronate group (12/556, 2.2%) than in the zoledronic acid group (3/563, 0.5%). Previously, it has been observed in a clinical trial investigating patients with postmenopausal osteoporosis, that zoledronic acid treated patients (5 mg) had an increased rate of atrial fibrillation serious adverse events compared to placebo (1.3% compared to 0.6%). The mechanism of this increased incidence of atrial fibrillation in isolated studies with some bisphosphonates, including AREDIA, is unknown.

Very rare: left ventricular failure (dyspnea, pulmonary edema), congestive heart failure (edema) due to fluid overload.

Vascular Disorders: Common: hypertension. Uncommon: hypotension.

Gastrointestinal Disorders: Common: nausea, vomiting, anorexia, abdominal pain, diarrhea, constipation, gastritis. Uncommon: dyspepsia.

Skin and Subcutaneous Disorders: Common: rash. Uncommon: pruritus.

Musculoskeletal and Connective Tissue Disorders: Common: transient bone pain, arthralgia, myalgia, generalized pain. Uncommon: osteonecrosis of the jaw (ONJ), muscle cramps.

Renal and Urinary Disorders: Uncommon: acute renal failure. Rare: focal segmental glomerulosclerosis including the collapsing variant, nephrotic syndrome. Very rare: hematuria, deterioration of pre-existing renal disease.

General Disorders and Administration Site Conditions: Very common: fever and influenza-like symptoms sometimes accompanied by malaise, rigor, fatigue and flushes. Common: reactions at the infusion site: pain, redness, swelling, induration, phlebitis, thrombophlebitis).

Many of these adverse events may have been related to the underlying disease.

Tumour-Induced Hypercalcemia and Paget's Disease: Adverse events considered to be related to AREDIA occurring in ≥1% patients in the specified indication (see Table 1).

Table 1: AREDIA

Adverse Events Considered to be Related to Pamidronate Occurring in ≥1% Patients in the Specified Indication

Adverse Events	Tumor-Induced Hypercalcemia	Paget's Disease
No. of Patients	**n=910**	**n=395**
Fever	6.9%	8.9%
Headache	0.0%	4.8%
Hypocalcemia	3.2%	0.8%
Influenza-like symptoms	0.0%	11.9%
Infusion site reaction	1.7%	1.8%
Malaise	0.0%	5.8%
Myalgia	0.0%	2.0%
Nausea	0.9%	2.0%
Pain (bone)	0.0%	8.9%
Pain (unspecified)	0.0%	7.9%
Rigors	0.0%	2.8%

Bisphosphonates, including AREDIA, have been associated with renal toxicity manifested as deterioration of renal function and potential renal failure (see Warnings and Precautions). Since many patients with tumour-induced hypercalcemia have compromised renal function prior to receiving antihypercalcemia therapy (see Warnings and Precautions), it is difficult to estimate the role of individual bisphosphonates in subsequent changes in renal function. Deterioration of renal function (elevation of serum creatinine of >20% above baseline) which could not be readily explained in terms of pre-existing renal disease, prior nephrotoxic chemotherapies or compromised intravascular volume status has been noted in 7 cases of 404 patients treated with AREDIA where these data have been reported. As with other i.v. bisphosphonates, renal monitoring is recommended (see Warnings and Precautions, Monitoring and Laboratory Tests).

Bone Metastases and Multiple Myeloma: The most commonly reported adverse events regardless of relationship to therapy are shown in Table 2.

Deterioration of renal function (including renal failure) has been associated with bisphosphonates including AREDIA. Renal monitoring is recommended (see Warnings and Precautions, Monitoring and Laboratory Tests).

Table 2: AREDIA

Commonly Reported Adverse Events in Three Controlled Trials (regardless of causality)

Bone Metastases and Multiple Myeloma Patients		
Adverse Event	**AREDIA 90 mg n=572**	**Placebo n=573**
General		
Asthenia	16.4	15.4
Fatigue	30.4	35.5
Fever	35.5	30.5
Metastases	14.0	13.6
Digestive System		
Anorexia	20.8	18.0
Constipation	27.6	30.9
Diarrhea	24.3	26.2
Dyspepsia	13.6	12.4
Nausea	48.4	46.4
Pain abdominal	17.3	14.0
Vomiting	30.9	28.1
Hemic and Lymphatic Systems		
Anemia	35.1	32.6
Granulocytopenia	16.8	17.3
Thrombocytopenia	11.0	13.1

(cont'd)

Table 2: AREDIA *(cont'd)*

Commonly Reported Adverse Events in Three Controlled Trials (regardless of causality)

	Bone Metastases and Multiple Myeloma Patients	
Adverse Event	**AREDIA 90 mg n=572**	**Placebo n=573**
Musculoskeletal System		
Myalgias	22.6	16.9
Skeletal pain	59.4	69.1
CNS		
Headache	24.0	19.7
Insomnia	18.2	17.3
Respiratory System		
Coughing	21.2	18.8
Dyspnea	23.3	18.7
Upper respiratory infection	19.8	20.9
Urogenital System		
Urinary tract infection	14.5	10.8

Post-Market Adverse Drug Reactions: Cases of osteonecrosis of the jaw (ONJ) are uncommon, although data suggest a higher number of reported cases in certain cancers, such as advanced breast cancer and multiple myeloma. The majority of reported cases of ONJ are associated with invasive dental procedures (such as tooth extraction or dental surgery and local trauma including poorly fitting dentures) or periodontal disease. Many patients had signs of local infection including osteomyelitis.

The following adverse reactions have been reported in post-marketing use:

General: reactivation of Herpes simplex and Herpes zoster, influenza-like symptoms.

CNS: confusion and visual hallucinations, sometimes in the presence of electrolyte imbalance.

Skin: rash, pruritus.

Special Senses: conjunctivitis, scleritis, orbital inflammation.

Renal: focal segmental glomerulosclerosis including the collapsing variant, nephrotic syndrome.

Laboratory Abnormalities: hyperkalemia, hypernatremia, hematuria. Instances of allergic manifestations have been reported, including hypotension, dyspnea, or angioedema, and anaphylactic shock.

DRUG INTERACTIONS: Drug interaction studies with AREDIA in humans have not been conducted.

Caution is warranted when AREDIA is used with other potentially nephrotoxic drugs.

In multiple myeloma patients, the risk of renal dysfunction may be increased when AREDIA is used in combination with thalidomide.

AREDIA should not be used in combination with other bisphosphonates.

DOSAGE AND ADMINISTRATION: Dosing Considerations: Dosing recommendations differ for tumour-induced hypercalcemia, lytic bone metastases and multiple myeloma, and Paget's disease. For patients suffering from TIH and multiple myeloma, see the TIH dosage guidelines.

AREDIA (pamidronate disodium) must never be given as a bolus injection (see Warnings and Precautions). AREDIA should be administered in a compatible calcium-free intravenous solution (e.g., sterile normal saline or dextrose 5% in water). AREDIA should be infused slowly.

To minimize local reactions the cannula should be carefully inserted in a relatively large vein.

The infusion rate should never exceed 60 mg/h (1 mg/min) and the concentration of AREDIA in the infusion solution should not exceed 90 mg/250 mL. A dose of 90 mg should normally be administered as a 2-hour infusion in 250 mL infusion solution. **However, in patients with multiple myeloma and in patients with tumour-induced hypercalcemia it is recommended not to exceed 90 mg in 500 mL over 4 hours (i.e., an infusion rate of 22.5 mg/h).**

Renal Impairment: AREDIA should not be administered to patients with severe renal impairment (creatinine clearance <30 mL/min) unless in cases of life-threatening tumour-induced hypercalcemia where the benefit outweighs the potential risk.

As with other i.v. bisphosphonates, renal monitoring is recommended, for instance, measurement of serum creatinine prior to each dose of AREDIA. In patients receiving AREDIA for bone metastases or multiple myeloma who show evidence of deterioration in renal function, AREDIA treatment should be withheld until renal function returns to within 10% of the baseline value. This recommendation is based on a clinical study, in which renal deterioration was defined as follows: For patients with normal baseline creatinine, increase of 0.5 mg/dL. For patients with abnormal baseline creatinine, increase of 1.0 mg/dL.

A pharmacokinetic study conducted in patients with cancer and normal or impaired renal function indicates that the dose adjustment is not necessary in mild (creatinine clearance 61 to 90 mL/min) to moderate renal impairment (creatinine clearance 30 to 60 mL/min). In such patients, the infusion rate should not exceed 90 mg/4h (approximately 20 to 22 mg/h).

Hepatic Impairment: A pharmacokinetic study indicates that no dose adjustment is necessary in patients with mild to moderate abnormal hepatic function. AREDIA has not been studied in patients with severe hepatic impairment (see Warnings and Precautions).

Recommended Dose and Dosage Adjustment: Dosing Guidelines for Tumour-Induced Hypercalcemia: Patients must be adequately rehydrated prior to and during administration of AREDIA.

In tumour-induced hypercalcemia, either ionized calcium or total serum calcium corrected (adjusted) for albumin should be monitored during treatment with AREDIA. Serum calcium levels in patients who have hypercalcemia of malignancy may not reflect the severity of hypercalcemia, since hypoalbuminemia is commonly present. Corrected serum calcium values should be calculated using established algorithms, such as:

cCa= tCa+(0.02×[40–ALB])

where:

cCa=adjusted calcium concentration (mmol/L)

tCa=measured total calcium concentration (mmol/L)

ALB=measured albumin concentration (g/L)

Although mild hypercalcemia may be asymptomatic, moderate to severe hypercalcemia usually associated with a variety of signs and symptoms, and can be life-threatening if not promptly recognized and treated. Individuals at risk and their caregivers should be made aware that signs and symptoms of hypercalcemia include: lethargy, fatigue, confusion, loss of appetite, nausea and vomiting, constipation, excessive thirst and urination. Measures such as maintaining mobility and ensuring adequate hydration could diminish the symptoms of hypercalcemia. However, when symptoms of hypercalcemia are detected, it is important to seek medical assistance promptly.

The recommended total dose of AREDIA for a treatment course depends upon initial plasma calcium levels. Doses should be adapted to the degree of severity of hypercalcemia to ensure normalization of plasma calcium and to optimize the duration of response. **A dose of 90 mg should be administered in 500 mL of infusion solution. The infusion rate should not exceed 22.5 mg/hour.**

The total dose for a treatment course may be given as a single infusion, or in multiple infusions spread over 2 to 4 consecutive days. The **maximum dose** of AREDIA per treatment course is 90 mg whether for initial or repeat treatment courses. Higher doses have not been associated with increased clinical effect.

Table 3 presents dosing guidelines for AREDIA derived from clinical data on uncorrected calcium values. These dose ranges also apply for calcium corrected for serum protein.

Table 3: AREDIA

Tumour-Induced Hypercalcemia

Initial Serum Calcium				
(mmol/L)	**(mg %)**	**Total Dose (mg)**	**Concentration of Infusate (mg/mL)**	**Maximum Infusion Rate (mg/h)**
Up to 3.0	Up to 12.0	30	30 mg/125 mL	22.5 mg/h
3.0–3.5	12.0–14.0	30 or 60[a]	30 mg/125 mL 60 mg/250 mL	22.5 mg/h 22.5 mg/h
3.5–4.0	14.0–16.0	60[a] or 90	60 mg/250 mL 90 mg/500 mL	22.5 mg/h 22.5 mg/h
>4.0	>16.0	90	90 mg/500 mL	22.5 mg/h

[a] Two vials of 30 mg each may be used.

Decreases in serum calcium levels are generally observed within 24 to 48 hours after drug administration, with maximum lowering occurring by 3 to 7 days. If hypercalcemia recurs, or if plasma calcium does not decrease within 2 days, repeat infusions of AREDIA may be given, according to the dosing guidelines. The limited clinical experience available to date has suggested the possibility that AREDIA may produce a weaker therapeutic response with repeat treatment in patients with advanced cancer.

Dosing Guidelines for Bone Metastases and Multiple Myeloma: The recommended dose of AREDIA for the treatment of predominantly lytic bone metastases and multiple myeloma is 90 mg administered as a single infusion every 4 weeks. In patients with bone metastases who receive chemotherapy at 3-weekly intervals, AREDIA 90 mg may also be given every 3 weeks. A dose of 90 mg should normally be administered as a 2-hour infusion in 250 mL of infusion solution. However, in patients with multiple myeloma it is recommended not to exceed 90 mg in 500 mL over 4 hours.

Radiotherapy is the treatment of choice for patients with solitary lesions in weight bearing bones (see Table 4).

Table 4: AREDIA

Dosing Guidelines for Bone Metastases and Multiple Myeloma

Disease State	Dosing Schedule	Concentration of Infusate (mg/mL)
Bone metastases	90 mg/2 hours every 3[a] –4 weeks	90 mg/250 mL
Multiple myeloma	90 mg/4 hours every 4 weeks	90 mg/500 mL

[a] For patients receiving chemotherapy every 3 weeks.

Dosing Guidelines for Paget's Disease of Bone: The recommended total dose of AREDIA for a treatment course is 180 to 210 mg. This may be administered as 6 doses of 30 mg once a week (total dose 180 mg). Alternatively, 3 doses of 60 mg may be administered every second week, but treatment should be initiated with a 30 mg dose (total dose 210 mg) as influenza-like reactions are common only with the first infusion. Each dose of 30 mg or 60 mg should be diluted in at least 250 mL or 500 mL, respectively, of normal saline or D5W. An infusion rate of 15 mg per hour is recommended. This regimen, omitting the initial dose, can be repeated after 6 months until remission of disease is achieved, and when relapse occurs (see Table 5).

Table 5: AREDIA

Recommended Treatment Regimens for Paget's Disease

	Recommended total dose/treatment course: 180–210 mg		
Regimen	**Dosing Schedule**	**Concentration of Infusate (mg/mL)**	**Infusion Rate (mg/h)**
Regimen 1 Total dose 180 mg	30 mg once weekly for 6 weeks	30 mg in 250–500 mL	15 mg/h
Regimen 2 Total Dose 210 mg	Infusions administered every 2 weeks. Initial dose (week 1)=30 mg; Subsequent doses (weeks 3, 5 & 7)=60 mg	30/60 mg[a] in 250–500 mL	15 mg/h
Re-treatment Regimen Total dose 180 mg	60 mg every 2 weeks for a total of 3 infusions	60 mg[a] in 500 mL	15 mg/h

[a] Two vials of 30 mg each may be used.

Administration: Reconstitution: Each vial of sterile lyophilized powder should be reconstituted with Sterile Water for Injection prior to dilution as given in Table 6.

Table 6: AREDIA

Reconstitution Table

Vial Size	Volume of Diluent to be Added to the Vial	Approximate Available Volume	Nominal Concentration
30 mg/10 mL vial	10 mL	10 mL	3 mg/mL
90 mg/10 mL vial	10 mL	10 mL	9 mg/mL

Dilution of Reconstituted Solution for I.V. Infusion: Reconstituted solutions that have been prepared with Sterile Water for Injection should be further diluted with either 0.9% w/v sodium chloride or 5% w/v glucose solution prior to intravenous infusion administration. The reconstituted solution is chemically and physically stable for 24 hours at room temperature. However, from a microbiological point of view, it is preferable to use the product immediately after aseptic reconstitution and dilution.

If not used immediately, the duration and conditions of storage prior to use are the care provider's responsibility. The total time between reconstitution, dilution and end of administration must not exceed 24 hours.

All parenteral products should be visually inspected for particulate matter and discoloration prior to administration. Any solution found to have particulate matter or discoloration should be discarded.

Incompatibilities: Pamidronate forms complexes with divalent cations. For this reason, AREDIA reconstituted solution must not be mixed with calcium-containing intravenous solutions such as Ringer's solution. AREDIA reconstituted solution should be diluted with 0.9% w/v sodium chloride solution of 5% w/v glucose solution. Studies with containers and infusion sets/devices for infusion made of glass, polyethylene and polyvinylchloride have been shown to be compatible with diluted AREDIA solution.

OVERDOSAGE:
Patients who have received doses higher than those recommended should be carefully monitored. Clinically significant hypocalcemia with paresthesia, tetany and hypotension, may be reversed by an infusion of calcium gluconate. Acute hypocalcemia is not expected to occur with AREDIA (pamidronate disodium) since plasma calcium levels fall progressively for several days after treatment.

For management of a suspected drug overdose, contact your regional Poison Control Centre. See the *CPS* Directory section for a list of Poison Control Centres.

ACTION AND CLINICAL PHARMACOLOGY: Mechanism of Action: AREDIA (pamidronate disodium) belongs to a class of bisphosphonates (previously termed diphosphonate), which inhibit bone resorption. The therapeutic activity of AREDIA is attributable to its potent anti-osteoclastic activity on bone. In animal studies, at therapeutic doses, pamidronate disodium inhibits bone resorption apparently without inhibiting bone formation and mineralization.

The predominant means by which AREDIA reduces bone turnover both in vitro and in vivo appears to be through the local, direct antiresorptive effect of bone-bound bisphosphonate. Pamidronate disodium binds to calcium phosphate (hydroxyapatite) crystals and directly inhibits the formation and dissolution of this bone mineral component in vitro. In vitro studies indicate that pamidronate disodium is a potent inhibitor of osteoclastic bone resorption. Pamidronate disodium also suppresses the migration of osteoclast precursors onto the bone and their subsequent transformation into the mature resorbing osteoclast.

Tumour-Induced Hypercalcemia: In tumour-induced hypercalcemia, AREDIA normalizes plasma calcium between 3 and 7 days following the initiation of treatment irrespective of the type of malignancy or presence of detectable metastases. This effect is dependent on initial calcium levels.

AREDIA improves symptoms associated with hypercalcemia, e.g. anorexia, nausea, vomiting and diminished mental status.

The kidneys play a prominent role in calcium homeostasis. In addition to skeletal osteolysis, renal dysfunction contributes to the pathogenesis of tumour-induced hypercalcemia. When diagnosed, most hypercalcemic patients are significantly dehydrated. Elevated plasma calcium antagonizes antidiuretic hormone-induced renal concentration, and thus results in polyuria and excessive fluid loss. Hydration status is further compromised by reduced fluid intake due to nausea, vomiting and diminished mental status. Furthermore, dehydration often leads to a fall in glomerular filtration rate (GFR).

Before AREDIA therapy is initiated, patients should be adequately rehydrated with isotonic saline (0.9%) (see Warnings and Precautions, General). Normalization of plasma calcium levels by AREDIA in adequately hydrated patients may also normalize plasma parathyroid hormone (PTH) which is suppressed by hypercalcemia.

The duration of normocalcemia following AREDIA treatment varies in patients with tumour-induced hypercalcemia because of early mortality, and the heterogeneity of diseases and cancer therapies. In general, recurrences tend to occur preferentially after treatment with lower doses: at doses of 30 mg or less, plasma calcium levels tend to increase after approximately 1 week, while at high doses (total treatment doses of 45 to 90 mg) plasma calcium levels remained normal for at least 2 weeks and up to several months. One study has shown a clear relationship between recurrence rates and AREDIA dose: in patients treated with single i.v. infusions of 30, 45, 60 and 90 mg AREDIA, recurrence rates were lower for the higher dose group 9 months after initial treatment. In patients in whom the underlying disease is well controlled by cancer therapy, the duration of response tends to be more prolonged.

Clinical experience with AREDIA in relapsed tumour-induced hypercalcemia is limited. In general, with re-treatment, the response is similar to that with the first AREDIA treatment, unless the cancer has progressed significantly. Therefore, AREDIA treatment appears effective for recurrent hypercalcemia at doses established for the initial treatment course (see Dosage and Administration). The mechanisms underlying possible decreased effects of repeat treatment with AREDIA in advanced cancer are unknown.

In severe forms of hypercalcemia the dose of AREDIA may be increased, or eventually, a combination drug therapy should be considered (see Warnings and Precautions).

Bone Metastases and Multiple Myeloma: Lytic bone metastases in cancer patients are caused by increased osteoclast activity. Metastatic tumour cells secrete paracrine factors which stimulate neighboring osteoclasts to resorb bone. By inhibiting osteoclast function, bisphosphonates interrupt the cascade of events which lead to tumour-induced osteolysis. Lytic bone destruction causes significant complications and associated morbidity.

Clinical trials in patients with predominantly lytic bone metastases or multiple myeloma showed that AREDIA prevented or delayed skeletal-related events, (SREs: hypercalcemia, pathologic fractures, radiation therapy to bone, orthopedic surgery, spinal cord compression) and decreased bone pain. When used in combination with standard anticancer treatment, AREDIA led to a delay in progression of bone metastases. In addition, osteolytic bone metastases which have proved refractory to cytotoxic and hormonal therapy may show radiological evidence of disease stabilization or sclerosis.

A significant reduction in bone pain was also demonstrated, which in some patients led to decreased analgesic intake and increased mobility. Greater deteriorations in ECOG performance status and Spitzer quality of life scores were seen in the placebo patients compared to AREDIA-treated patients.

Paget's Disease: Paget's disease of bone, which is characterized by local areas of increased bone resorption and formation with qualitative changes in remodelling, responds well to treatment with AREDIA. Repeated infusions of pamidronate disodium do not lead to reduced efficacy. In addition, patients resistant to etidronate and calcitonin respond well to AREDIA infusions. In long-term follow-up to clinical trials, bone fracture rate does not appear to be increased following treatment with pamidronate disodium relative to the normally occurring rate in patients with Paget's disease.

Clinical and biochemical remission of Paget's disease has been demonstrated by bone scintigraphy, by decreases in urinary hydroxyproline and serum alkaline phosphatase, and by symptomatic improvement. Bone scans show that AREDIA reduces the number of bones and the percent of the skeleton affected and that bone scintigraphy significantly improves. Bone biopsies consistently show histological and histomorphometric improvement indicating the reversal of the disease process. Symptoms improve even in those with severe disease.

Pharmacokinetics: Plasma concentrations of pamidronate rise rapidly after infusion is started and fall rapidly when the infusion is stopped. The apparent plasma half-life is about 0.8 hours. Apparent steady state is therefore achieved with infusions of more than about 2 to 3 hours' duration. When infused i.v. at 60 mg over 1 hour, the peak plasma concentration is about 10 nmol/mL and the apparent total plasma clearance is about 180 mL/min.

As pamidronate has a strong affinity for calcified tissues, total elimination is not observed within the time frame of experimental studies.

After an i.v. infusion, about 20 to 55% of the dose is recovered in the urine within 72 hours as unchanged pamidronate, the majority being excreted within the first 24 hours. Pamidronate does not appear to be metabolized, and the remaining fraction of the dose is retained in the body (within the time frame of the studies). The percentage of the dose retained is independent of both the dose (range 15 to 180 mg) and the infusion rate (range 1.25 to 60 mg/h).

Retention is similar after each dose of pamidronate disodium. Thus, accumulation in bone is not capacity limited and is dependent solely on the cumulative dose.

Urinary elimination is biphasic ($t_{½α}$=1.6 h; $t_{½β}$=27.2 h). The apparent renal clearance is about 54 mL/min, and there is a tendency for renal clearance to correlate with creatinine clearance.

Pamidronate disodium binding to human serum proteins is relatively low (about 54%) but increases to approximately 5 mmol when exogenous 95% calcium is added to human plasma.

Special Populations and Conditions: Hepatic Insufficiency: The pharmacokinetics of pamidronate were studied in male cancer patients at risk for bone metastases with normal hepatic function (n=6) and mild to moderate hepatic dysfunction (n=9). Each patient received a single 90 mg dose of AREDIA infused over 4 hours. Although there was a statistically significant difference in the pharmacokinetics between patients with normal and impaired hepatic function, the difference was not considered clinically relevant. Patients with hepatic impairment exhibited higher mean AUC (39.7%) and Cmax (28.6%) values. Nevertheless, pamidronate was still rapidly cleared from the plasma. Drug levels were not detectable in patients by 12 to 36 hours after drug infusion. Because AREDIA is administered on a monthly basis, drug accumulation is not expected. No changes in AREDIA dosing regimen are recommended for patients with mild to moderate abnormal hepatic function (see Dosage and Administration).

Hepatic and metabolic clearance of AREDIA are insignificant. AREDIA thus displays little potential for drug interactions at either the metabolic or protein binding level.

Renal Insufficiency: A pharmacokinetic study conducted in patients with cancer showed no differences in plasma AUC of pamidronate between patients with normal renal function and patients with mild to moderate renal impairment. In patients with severe renal impairment (creatinine clearance <30 mL/min), the AUC of pamidronate was approximately 3 times higher than in patients with normal renal function (creatinine clearance >90 mL/min) (see Dosage and Administration).

STORAGE AND STABILITY: Protect vials from heat (i.e., store below 30°C).

AREDIA must be kept out of the reach and sight of children and pets.

INFORMATION FOR THE PATIENT: Published in e-CPS, available by subscription at www.e-cps.ca.

DOSAGE FORMS, COMPOSITION AND PACKAGING: 30 mg: Each vial of sterile, white to practically white lyophilized powder contains: pamidronate disodium (anhydrous) 30 mg and mannitol 470 mg. Phosphoric acid is employed to adjust the pH to 6.3. Preservative-free. Vials of 10 mL, cartons of 1.

90 mg: Each vial of sterile, white to practically white lyophilized powder contains: pamidronate disodium (anhydrous) 90 mg and mannitol 375 mg. Phosphoric acid is employed to adjust the pH to 6.3. Preservative-free. Vials of 10 mL, cartons of 1.

(Shown in Product Identification Section)

Aricept® Ⓟ
donepezil HCl
Cholinesterase Inhibitor

Pfizer

Aricept RDT™ Ⓟ
donepezil HCl
Cholinesterase Inhibitor

Pfizer

Date of Revision: June 25, 2007

SUMMARY PRODUCT INFORMATION:

Route of Administration	Dosage Form/ Strength	Clinically Relevant Nonmedicinal Ingredients
Oral	Tablets 5 mg and 10 mg	Lactose monohydrate For a complete listing see Dosage Forms, Composition and Packaging.
Oral	Rapidly Disintegrating Tablets 5 mg and 10 mg	No known clinically relevant nonmedicinal ingredients For a complete listing see Dosage Forms, Composition and Packaging.

INDICATIONS AND CLINICAL USE: ARICEPT (donepezil hydrochloride) is indicated for: symptomatic treatment of patients with mild, moderate and severe dementia of the Alzheimer's type.

Efficacy of ARICEPT in patients with mild to moderate Alzheimer's disease was established in two 24 week and one 54-week placebo-controlled trials. Efficacy in patients with severe Alzheimer's disease was established in two 24-week/6 month placebo-controlled trials.

ARICEPT tablets should only be prescribed by (or following consultation with) clinicians who are experienced in the diagnosis and management of Alzheimer's disease.

CONTRAINDICATIONS: ARICEPT (donepezil hydrochloride) is contraindicated in patients with known hypersensitivity to donepezil hydrochloride or to piperidine derivatives.

WARNINGS AND PRECAUTIONS: Cardiovascular: Because of their pharmacological action, cholinesterase inhibitors may have vagotonic effects on heart rate (eg, bradycardia). The potential for this action may be particularly important to patients with "sick sinus syndrome" or other supraventricular cardiac conduction conditions.

In clinical trials in Alzheimer's disease, most patients with serious cardiovascular conditions were excluded. Patients such as those with controlled hypertension (DBP<95 mmHg), right bundle branch blockage, and pacemakers were included. Therefore, caution should be taken in treating patients with active coronary artery disease and congestive heart failure. Syncopal episodes have been reported in association with the use of ARICEPT. It is recommended that ARICEPT should not be used in patients with cardiac conduction abnormalities (except for right bundle branch block) including "sick sinus syndrome" and those with unexplained syncopal episodes.

Gastrointestinal: Through their primary action, cholinesterase inhibitors may be expected to increase gastric acid secretion due to increased cholinergic activity. Therefore, patients at increased risk for developing ulcers, eg, those with a history of ulcer disease or those receiving concurrent nonsteroidal anti-inflammatory drugs (NSAIDS) including high doses of acetylsalicylic acid (ASA), should be monitored for symptoms of active or occult gastrointestinal bleeding. Clinical studies of ARICEPT have shown no increase, relative to placebo in the incidence of either peptic ulcer disease or gastrointestinal bleeding (see Adverse Reactions).

ARICEPT, as a predictable consequence of its pharmacological properties, has been shown to produce, in controlled clinical trials in patients with Alzheimer's disease, diarrhea, nausea and vomiting. These effects, when they occur, appear more frequently with the 10 mg dose than with the 5 mg dose. In most cases, these effects have usually been mild and transient, sometimes lasting 1 to 3 weeks and have resolved during continued use of ARICEPT (see Adverse Reactions). Treatment with the 5 mg/day dose for 4-6 weeks prior to increasing the dose to 10 mg/day is associated with a lower incidence of gastrointestinal intolerance.

Genitourinary: Although not observed in clinical trials of ARICEPT, cholinomimetics may cause bladder outflow obstruction.

Hepatic/Biliary/Pancreatic: There is limited information regarding the pharmacokinetics of ARICEPT in hepatically impaired Alzheimer disease patients (see Action and Clinical Pharmacology, Pharmacokinetics).

Close monitoring for adverse effects in patients with hepatic disease being treated with ARICEPT is therefore recommended.

Neurologic: Seizures: Some cases of seizures have been reported with the use of ARICEPT in clinical trials and from spontaneous Adverse Reaction reporting. Cholinomimetics can cause a reduction of seizure threshold, increasing the risk of seizures. However, seizure activity may also be a manifestation of Alzheimer's disease. The risk/benefit of ARICEPT treatment for patients with a history of seizure disorder must therefore be carefully evaluated.

ARICEPT has not been studied in patients with Parkinsonian features. The efficacy and safety of ARICEPT in these patients are unknown.

Peri-Operative Considerations: Anesthesia: ARICEPT, as a cholinesterase inhibitor, is likely to exaggerate succinylcholine-type muscle relaxation during anesthesia.

Renal: There is limited information regarding the pharmacokinetics of ARICEPT in renally impaired Alzheimer disease patients (see Action and Clinical Pharmacology, Pharmacokinetics).

Close monitoring for adverse effects in patients with renal disease being treated with ARICEPT is therefore recommended.

Respiratory: Because of their cholinomimetic action, cholinesterase inhibitors should be prescribed with care to patients with a history of asthma or obstructive pulmonary disease. ARICEPT has not been studied in patients under treatment for these conditions and should therefore be used with particular caution in such patients.

Special Populations: Pregnant Women and Nursing Women: The safety of ARICEPT during pregnancy and lactation has not been established and therefore, it should not be used in women of childbearing potential or in nursing mothers unless, in the opinion of the physician, the potential benefits to the patient outweigh the possible hazards to the fetus or the infant.

Teratology studies conducted in pregnant rats at doses of up to 16 mg/kg/day and in pregnant rabbits at doses of up to 10 mg/kg/day did not disclose any evidence for a teratogenic potential of ARICEPT.

Pediatrics: There are no adequate and well-controlled trials to document the safety and efficacy of ARICEPT in any illness occurring in children. Therefore, ARICEPT is not recommended for use in children.

Geriatrics (≥65 years of age): In controlled clinical studies with 5 and 10 mg ARICEPT in patients with mild to moderate Alzheimer's disease, there were 536 patients between the ages of 65 to 84, and 37 patients aged 85 years or older treated with ARICEPT. In controlled clinical trials of patients with severe Alzheimer's disease there were 158 patients who were 74 years of age or less, 276 patients between the ages of 75 and 84, and 139 patients aged 85 years or older treated with ARICEPT. In Alzheimer's disease patients, nausea, diarrhea, vomiting, insomnia, fatigue and anorexia increased with dose and age and the incidence appeared to be greater in female patients. Since cholinesterase inhibitors as well as Alzheimer's disease can be associated with significant weight loss, caution is advised regarding the use of ARICEPT in low body weight elderly patients, especially in those ≥85 years old.

Use in Elderly Patients with Comorbid Disease: There is limited safety information for ARICEPT in patients with mild to moderate or severe Alzheimer's disease and significant comorbidity. The use of ARICEPT in Alzheimer's disease patients with chronic illnesses common among the geriatric population, should be considered only after careful risk/benefit assessment and include close monitoring for adverse events. Caution is advised regarding the use of ARICEPT doses above 5 mg in this patient population.

In severe Alzheimer's disease, the possibility of comorbid vascular disease and risk factors for vascular adverse events and mortality should be considered.

Patients with Vascular Dementia: Three clinical trials, each of 6 months duration, were conducted to evaluate the safety and efficacy of ARICEPT for the symptomatic treatment of individuals meeting the NINDS-AIREN criteria for probable or possible vascular dementia. The NINDS-AIREN criteria are designed to identify patients with dementia that appears to be due solely to vascular causes, and to exclude patients with Alzheimer's disease. ARICEPT was not shown to be an effective treatment for patients with vascular dementia in two of these clinical trials.

The safety profile from these controlled clinical trials in vascular dementia patients indicates that the rate of occurrence of treatment emergent adverse events overall was higher in vascular dementia patients (86%) than in Alzheimer's disease patients (75%). This was seen in both ARICEPT-treated subjects and placebo-treated subjects and may relate to the greater number of co-morbid medical conditions in the vascular dementia population.

In two of the clinical trials there was a higher rate of mortality among patients treated with ARICEPT, during double-blind treatment; this result was statistically significant for one of these two trials. For the three vascular dementia studies combined, the mortality rate in the ARICEPT group (1.7%, 25/1475) was numerically higher than in the placebo group (1.1%, 8/718), but this difference was not statistically significant.

These results are summarized as follows: (see Table 1).

Table 1: ARICEPT

Mortality Rates in ARICEPT Vascular Dementia Clinical Trials

Study	Placebo	ARICEPT 5 mg	p-value[b]	ARICEPT 10 mg	p-value[b]
307	3.5% (7/199)	1.0% (2/198)	0.17	2.4% (5/206)	0.57
308	0.5% (1/193)	1.9% (4/208)	0.37	1.4% (3/215)	0.62
319	0% (0/326)	1.7% (11/648)	0.02	[a]	NA
Combined	1.1% (8/718)	1.7% (25/1475)			0.35

[a] No 10 mg ARICEPT treatment arm in Study 319.

[b] p-values are for 5 mg donepezil vs placebo and 10 mg donepezil vs placebo.

The majority of deaths in patients taking either ARICEPT or placebo appear to have resulted from various vascular related causes, which may be expected in this elderly, fragile, population with co-morbid vascular disease. In the three combined vascular dementia trials there were similar proportions of patients with serious AEs in both treatment groups (approximately 15%), and similar proportions of patients with serious cardiovascular or cerebrovascular adverse events (non-fatal and fatal, approximately 8%). The proportion of patients who had a fatal cardiovascular or cerebrovascular adverse event was numerically higher in the ARICEPT group than in the placebo group, but this difference was not statistically significant across the three trials.

There is no evidence of an increase risk of mortality when ARICEPT is used in patients with mild to moderate Alzheimer's disease.

ADVERSE REACTIONS: Adverse Drug Reaction Overview: Alzheimer's Disease: Mild to Moderate Alzheimer's Disease: A total of 747 patients with mild to moderate Alzheimer's disease were treated in controlled clinical studies with ARICEPT (donepezil hydrochloride). Of these patients, 613 (82%) completed the studies. The mean duration of treatment for all ARICEPT groups was 132 days (range 1-356 days).

Adverse Events Leading to Discontinuation: The rates of discontinuation from controlled clinical trials of ARICEPT due to adverse events for the ARICEPT 5 mg/day treatment groups were comparable to those of placebo-treatment groups at approximately 5%. The rate of discontinuation of patients who received the 10 mg/day dose after only a 1 week initial treatment with 5 mg/day ARICEPT was higher at 13%.

The most common adverse events leading to discontinuation, defined as those occurring in at least 2% of patients and at twice the incidence seen in placebo patients, are shown in Table 2.

Table 2: ARICEPT

Most Frequent Adverse Events in Patients with Mild to Moderate Alzheimer's Disease Leading to Withdrawal from Controlled Clinical Trials by Dose Group

Dose Group	Placebo	5 mg/day ARICEPT	10 mg/day ARICEPT
Number of Patients Randomized	355	350	315
Events/% Discontinuing			
Nausea	1%	1%	3%
Diarrhea	0%	<1%	3%
Vomiting	<1%	<1%	2%

Most Frequent Adverse Clinical Events Seen in Association with the Use of ARICEPT: The most common adverse events, defined as those occurring at a frequency of at least 5% in patients receiving 10 mg/day and twice the placebo rate, are largely predicted by ARICEPT's cholinomimetic effects. These include nausea, diarrhea, insomnia, vomiting, muscle cramp, fatigue and anorexia.

These adverse events were often of mild intensity and transient, resolving during continued ARICEPT treatment without the need for dose modification.

There is evidence to suggest that the frequency of these common adverse events may be affected by the duration of treatment with an initial 5 mg daily dose prior to increasing the dose to 10 mg/day. An open label study was conducted with 269 patients who received placebo in the 15- and 30-week studies. These patients received a 5 mg/day dose for 6 weeks prior to initiating treatment with 10 mg/day. The rates of common adverse events were lower than those seen in controlled clinical trial patients who received 10 mg/day after only a 1 week initial treatment period with a 5 mg daily dose, and were comparable to the rates noted in patients treated only with 5 mg/day.

See Table 3 for a comparison of the most common adverse events following 1- and 6-week initial treatment periods with 5 mg/day ARICEPT.

Clinical Trial Adverse Drug Reactions: The events cited reflect experience gained under closely monitored conditions of clinical trials in a highly selected patient population. In actual clinical practice or in other clinical trials, these frequency estimates may not apply, as the conditions of use, reporting behavior, and the kinds of patients treated may differ.

Table 4 lists treatment-emergent signs and symptoms (TESS) that were reported in at least 2% of patients from placebo-controlled clinical trials who received ARICEPT and for which the rate of occurrence was greater for ARICEPT than placebo-assigned patients. In general, adverse events occurred more frequently in female patients and with advancing age.

Other Adverse Events Observed During Clinical Trials in Mild to Moderate Alzheimer's Disease: During the premarketing phase, ARICEPT has been administered to over 1700 individuals with mild to moderate Alzheimer's disease for various lengths of time during clinical trials worldwide. Approximately 1200 patients have been treated for at least 3 months, and more than 1000 patients have been treated for at least 6 months. Controlled and uncontrolled trials in the United States included approximately 900 patients. In regards to the highest dose of 10 mg/day, this population includes 650 patients treated for 3 months, 475 patients treated for 6 months and 115 patients treated for over 1 year. The range of patient exposure is from 1 to 1214 days.

Table 3: ARICEPT

Comparison of Rates of Adverse Events in Patients with Mild to Moderate Alzheimer's Disease Treated with 10 mg/day after 1 and 6 weeks of Initial Treatment with 5 mg/day

	No Initial Treatment		1-Week Initial Treatment with 5 mg/day	6-Week Initial Treatment with 5 mg/day
Adverse Event	**Placebo (N=315) %**	**5 mg/day (N=311) %**	**10 mg/day (N=315) %**	**10 mg/day (N=269) %**
Nausea	6	5	19	6
Diarrhea	5	8	15	9
Insomnia	6	6	14	6
Fatigue	3	4	8	3
Vomiting	3	3	8	5
Muscle cramps	2	6	8	3
Anorexia	2	3	7	3

Table 4: ARICEPT

Mild to Moderate Alzheimer's Disease: Adverse Events Reported in Controlled Clinical Trials in at Least 2% of Patients Receiving ARICEPT and at a Higher Frequency than Placebo-treated Patients

Body System/Adverse Events	Placebo n=355	ARICEPT n=747
Percent of Patients with any Adverse Event	72	74
Body as a Whole		
Headache	9	10
Pain, various locations	8	9
Accident	6	7
Fatigue	3	5
Cardiovascular System		
Syncope	1	2
Digestive System		
Nausea	6	11
Diarrhea	5	10
Vomiting	3	5
Anorexia	2	4
Hemic and Lymphatic System		
Ecchymosis	3	4
Metabolic and Nutritional		
Weight Decrease	1	3
Musculoskeletal System		
Muscle Cramps	2	6
Arthritis	1	2
Nervous System		
Insomnia	6	9
Dizziness	6	8
Depression	<1	3
Abnormal Dreams	0	3
Somnolence	<1	2
Urogenital		
Frequent Urination	1	2

Treatment-emergent signs and symptoms that occurred during 3 placebo-controlled clinical trials and 2 open-label trials of patients with mild to moderate Alzheimer's disease were recorded as adverse events by the clinical investigators using terminology of their own choosing. To provide an overall estimate of the proportion of individuals having similar types of events, the studies were integrated and the events were grouped into a smaller number of standardized categories using a modified COSTART dictionary and event frequencies were calculated across all studies. These categories are used in the listing below. The frequencies represent the proportion of 900 patients from these trials who experienced that event while receiving ARICEPT. All adverse events occurring at least twice are included. Adverse events already listed in Table 3 and Table 4 are not repeated here (ie, events occurring at an incidence >2%). Also excluded are COSTART terms too general to be informative, or events less likely to be drug-caused. Events are classified by body system and listed as occurring in ≥1% and <2% of patients (ie, in 1/100 to 2/100 patients: frequent) or in <1% of patients (ie, in 1/100 to 1/1000 patients: infrequent). These adverse events are not necessarily related to ARICEPT treatment and in most cases were observed at a similar frequency in placebo-treated patients in the controlled studies.

Adverse Events Occurring in ≥1% and <2% or <1% of Patients Receiving ARICEPT: Body as a Whole: (≥1% and <2%) influenza, chest pain, toothache; (<1%) fever, edema face, periorbital edema, hernia hiatal, abscess, cellulitis, chills, generalized coldness, head fullness, head pressure, listlessness.
Cardiovascular System: (≥1% and <2%) hypertension, vasodilation, atrial fibrillation, hot flashes, hypotension; (<1%) angina pectoris, postural hypotension, myocardial infarction, premature ventricular contraction, arrhythmia, AV Block (first degree), congestive heart failure, arteritis, bradycardia, peripheral vascular disease, supraventricular tachycardia, deep vein thromboses.
Digestive System: (≥1% and <2%) fecal incontinence, gastrointestinal bleeding, bloating, epigastric pain; (<1%) eructation, gingivitis, increased appetite, flatulence, periodontal abscess, cholelithiasis, diverticulitis, drooling, dry mouth, fever sore, gastritis, irritable colon, tongue edema, epigastric distress, gastroenteritis, increased transaminases, hemorrhoids, ileus, increased thirst, jaundice, melena, polydipsia, duodenal ulcer, stomach ulcer.
Endocrine System: (<1%) diabetes mellitus, goiter.
Hemic & Lymphatic System: (<1%) anemia, thrombocythemia, thrombocytopenia, eosinophilia, erythrocytopenia.
Nutritional Disorders: (≥1% and <2%) dehydration; (<1%) gout, hypokalemia, increased creatine kinase, hyperglycemia, weight increase, increased lactate dehydrogenase.
Musculoskeletal System: (≥1% and <2%) bone fracture; (<1%) muscle weakness, muscle fasciculation.
Nervous System: (≥1% and <2%) delusions, tremor, irritability, paresthesia, aggression, vertigo, ataxia, libido increased, restlessness, abnormal crying, nervousness, aphasia; (<1%) cerebrovascular accident, intracranial hemorrhage, transient ischemic attack, emotional lability, neuralgia, coldness (localized), muscle spasm, dysphoria, gait abnormality, hypertonia, hypokinesia, neurodermatitis, numbness (localized), paranoia, dysarthria, dysphasia, hostility, decreased libido, melancholia, emotional withdrawal, nystagmus, pacing, seizures.
Respiratory System: (≥1% and <2%) dyspnea, sore throat, bronchitis; (<1%) epistaxis, postnasal drip, pneumonia, hyperventilation, pulmonary congestion, wheezing, hypoxia, pharyngitis, pleurisy, pulmonary collapse, sleep apnea, snoring.
Skin and Appendages: (≥1% and <2%) abrasion, pruritus, diaphoresis, urticaria; (<1%) dermatitis, erythema, skin discoloration, hyperkeratosis, alopecia, fungal dermatitis, herpes zoster, hirsutism, skin striae, night sweats, skin ulcer.
Special Senses: (≥1% and <2%) cataract, eye irritation, blurred vision; (<1%) dry eyes, glaucoma, earache, tinnitus, blepharitis, decreased hearing, retinal hemorrhage, otitis externa, otitis media, bad taste, conjunctival hemorrhage, ear buzzing, motion sickness, spots before eyes.
Urogenital System: (≥1% and <2%) urinary incontinence, nocturia; (< 1%) dysuria, hematuria, urinary urgency, metrorrhagia, cystitis, enuresis, prostate hypertrophy, pyelonephritis, inability to empty bladder, breast fibroadenosis, fibrocystic breast, mastitis, pyuria, renal failure, vaginitis.
Long-Term Safety: Patients were exposed to ARICEPT in 2 open-label extension mild to moderate Alzheimer's disease studies (n=885) of over 2 years. In 1 of the studies, 763 patients who previously completed 1 of 2 placebo-controlled studies of 15 or 30 weeks duration continued to receive ARICEPT and were evaluated for safety and neuropsychological evaluations for up to 152 weeks; the safety profile of ARICEPT in this extension study remained consistent with that observed in placebo-controlled trials. Following 1 and 2 years of treatment, 76% (n=580) and 49% (n=374) of these patients, respectively, were still receiving therapy (cumulative Weeks 48 and 108).
Severe Alzheimer's Disease: A total of 573 patients with severe Alzheimer's disease were treated in controlled clinical studies with ARICEPT. Of these patients, 441 (77%) completed the studies. The duration of double blind treatment in all studies was 24 weeks. The mean duration of treatment for all ARICEPT groups was 148.4 days (range 1-231 days). The mean daily dose of ARICEPT was 7.5 mg/day.

In clinical trials of patients with severe Alzheimer's disease, most patients with significant comorbid conditions were excluded. The use of ARICEPT in Alzheimer's disease patients with chronic illnesses common among the geriatric population, should be considered only after careful risk/benefit assessment and should include close monitoring for adverse events.
Adverse Events Leading to Discontinuation: In controlled clinical trials in severe Alzheimer's disease, the rate of discontinuation due to adverse events was 11.3% in patients treated with ARICEPT compared to 6.7% in the placebo group. The most common adverse events that led to discontinuation, more often in patients treated with ARICEPT than placebo, were diarrhea, nausea, vomiting, urinary tract infection, decreased appetite, and aggression. Each of these adverse events led to discontinuation of less than 2% of patients treated with ARICEPT.
Most Frequent Adverse Clinical Events Seen in Association with the Use of ARICEPT: The incidence profile for adverse events for severe Alzheimer's disease was similar to that of mild to moderate Alzheimer's disease (see Table 5).

The most common adverse events, defined as those occurring at a frequency of at least 5% in patients and twice the placebo rate, were vomiting, diarrhea, nausea, and aggression. Overall, the majority of adverse events were judged by the investigators to be mild or moderate in intensity.

Table 5 lists treatment-emergent signs and symptoms (TESS) that were reported in at least 2% of patients from placebo-controlled clinical trials who received ARICEPT and for which the rate of occurrence was greater for ARICEPT than placebo-assigned patients.

Table 5: ARICEPT

Severe Alzheimer's Disease: Adverse Events Reported in Controlled Clinical Trials in at Least 2% of Patients Receiving ARICEPT and at a Higher Frequency than Placebo-treated Patients

Body System/Adverse Events	Placebo n=465	ARICEPT N=573
Percent of Patients with Any Adverse Event	**74**	**81**
Gastrointestinal		
Diarrhea	4	10
Vomiting	4	8
Nausea	3	6
Fecal incontinence	1	2
General		
Pyrexia	1	2
Chest pain	0	2
Infections and Infestations		
Urinary tract infection	7	8
Nasopharyngitis	6	8
Pneumonia	3	4
Injury, Poisoning, Procedural Complications		
Fall	9	10
Contusion	2	4
Skin laceration	1	2
Investigations		

(cont'd)

Table 5: ARICEPT *(cont'd)*

Severe Alzheimer's Disease: Adverse Events Reported in Controlled Clinical Trials in at Least 2% of Patients Receiving ARICEPT and at a Higher Frequency than Placebo-treated Patients

Body System/Adverse Events	Placebo n=465	ARICEPT N=573
Blood creatine phosphokinase increased	1	2
Metabolism and Nutrition		
Anorexia	2	4
Decreased appetite	1	3
Dehydration	1	2
Musculoskeletal and Connective Tissue		
Back pain	2	3
Osteoarthritis	1	2
Nervous System		
Headache	3	5
Somnolence	0	2
Psychiatric		
Aggression	2	5
Insomnia	3	4
Restlessness	2	3
Hallucination	1	2
Confusional state	1	2
Renal and Urinary		
Urinary incontinence	2	3
Respiratory		
Cough	1	2
Skin		
Eczema	1	2
Vascular		
Hypertension	1	2

A frequency of 0 has been used when frequencies were <0.5%.

Results from the controlled clinical trials indicate that the incidence of adverse events such as vomiting, urinary tract infection, urinary incontinence, pneumonia, falls, decreased appetite, aggression, restlessness, hallucination and confusion may be higher in ARICEPT and placebo-treated patients with severe Alzheimer's disease than in patients with mild to moderate Alzheimer's disease.

Other adverse events that occurred with an incidence of at least 2% in ARICEPT treated patients and at an equal or lower rate than in placebo treated patients included: abdominal pain, fatigue, gastroenteritis, excoriation, dizziness, anxiety and depression.
Long-term Safety for Severe Alzheimer's Disease: In Study 315, which was a 24 week, randomized, placebo controlled study in severe Alzheimer's patients, at the end of double-blind treatment 229 patients entered open label ARICEPT treatment for up to an additional 12 weeks. Therefore, at the end of the open label phase, 111 patients had received up to 36 weeks of ARICEPT treatment and 118 patients had received up to 12 weeks of ARICEPT treatment.

The most commonly affected body systems, types and frequencies of adverse events reported during 12 weeks of open label ARICEPT treatment were similar to what was observed during 24 weeks of double-blind treatment.

Gastrointestinal adverse events (diarrhea, nausea, vomiting, anorexia) were reported at a higher frequency in patients who received up to12 weeks of ARICEPT treatment. Other adverse events reported at higher frequencies in the patients treated with ARICEPT for up to 12 weeks included infection, insomnia, pneumonia, fever, dizziness, hypertension, asthenia, tremor, pharyngitis, hallucinations, convulsions and cysts.

In patients treated with ARICEPT for up to 36 weeks, accidental injury, urinary incontinence and urinary tract infections were reported at higher frequencies.
Post-Market Adverse Drug Reactions: Voluntary reports of adverse events temporally associated with ARICEPT that have been received since market introduction that are not listed above, and that there is inadequate data to determine the causal relationship with the drug include the following: abdominal pain, cholecystitis, convulsions, heart block (all types), hemolytic anemia, hepatitis, hyponatremia, pancreatitis, and rash.
DRUG INTERACTIONS: Concomitant Use with Other Drugs: Use with Anticholinergics: Because of their mechanism of action, cholinesterase inhibitors have the potential to interfere with the activity of anticholinergic medications.
Use with Cholinomimetics and Other Cholinesterase Inhibitors: A synergistic effect may be expected when cholinesterase inhibitors are given concurrently with succinylcholine, similar neuromuscular blocking agents or cholinergic agonists such as bethanechol.
Use with Other Psychoactive Drugs: Few patients in controlled clinical trials received neuroleptics, antidepressants or anticonvulsants. There is thus limited information concerning the interaction of ARICEPT with these drugs.
Drug-Drug Interactions: Pharmacokinetic studies, limited to short-term, single-dose studies in young subjects evaluated the potential of ARICEPT for interaction with theophylline, cimetidine, warfarin and digoxin administration. No significant effects on the pharmacokinetics of these drugs were observed. Similar studies in elderly patients were not done.
Drugs Highly Bound to Plasma Proteins: Drug displacement studies have been performed in vitro between donepezil, a highly bound drug (96%) and other drugs such as furosemide, digoxin, and warfarin. Donepezil at concentrations of 0.3-10 μg/mL did not affect the binding of furosemide (5 μg/mL), digoxin (2 ng/mL) and warfarin (3 μg/mL) to human albumin. Similarly, the binding of donepezil to human albumin was not affected by furosemide, digoxin and warfarin.
Effect of ARICEPT on the Metabolism of Other Drugs: In vitro studies show a low rate of donepezil binding to CYP 3A4 and CYP 2D6 isoenzymes (mean Ki about 50-130 μM), which, given the therapeutic plasma concentrations of donepezil (164 nM), indicates little likelihood of interferences. In a pharmacokinetic study involving 18 healthy volunteers, the administration of ARICEPT at a dose of 5 mg/day for 7 days had no clinically significant effect on the pharmacokinetics of ketoconazole. No other clinical trials have been conducted to investigate the effect of ARICEPT on the clearance of drugs metabolized by CYP 3A4 (eg, cisapride, terfenadine) or by CYP 2D6 (e.g., imipramine).

It is not known whether ARICEPT has any potential for enzyme induction.

Effect of Other Drugs on the Metabolism of ARICEPT: Ketoconazole and quinidine, inhibitors of CYP450, 3A4 and 2D6, respectively, inhibit donepezil metabolism in vitro. In a pharmacokinetic study, 18 healthy volunteers received 5 mg/day ARICEPT together with 200 mg/day ketoconazole for 7 days. In these volunteers, mean donepezil plasma concentrations were increased by about 30%-36%.

Inducers of CYP 2D6 and CYP 3A4 (eg, phenytoin, carbamazepine, dexamethasone, rifampin and phenobarbital) could increase the rate of elimination of ARICEPT.

Pharmacokinetic studies demonstrated that the metabolism of ARICEPT is not significantly affected by concurrent administration of digoxin or cimetidine.

Drug-Food Interactions: Food does not have an influence on the rate and extent of donepezil hydrochloride absorption.

Drug-Herb Interactions: Interactions with herbal products have not been established.

Drug-Laboratory Test Interactions: Interactions with laboratory tests have not been established.

DOSAGE AND ADMINISTRATION: Dosing Considerations: ARICEPT (donepezil hydrochloride) or ARICEPT RDT should only be prescribed by (or following consultation with) clinicians who are experienced in the diagnosis and management of Alzheimer's disease.

Special Populations: The use of ARICEPT in Alzheimer's disease patients with chronic illnesses common among the geriatric population, should be considered only after careful risk/benefit assessment and include close monitoring for adverse events. It is recommended that ARICEPT be used with caution in these patient populations. Adverse events are more common in individuals of low body weight, in patients ≥85 years old and in females.

Recommended Dose and Dosage Adjustment: Adults: The recommended initial dose of ARICEPT or ARICEPT RDT is 5 mg taken once daily. Therapy with the 5 mg dose should be maintained for 4-6 weeks before considering a dose increase, in order to avoid or decrease the incidence of the most common adverse reactions to the drug (see Adverse Reactions) and to allow plasma levels to reach steady state. Based on clinical judgement, the 10 mg daily dose may be considered following 4-6 weeks of treatment at 5 mg/day. The maximum recommended dose is 10 mg taken once daily.

Following initiation of therapy or any dosage increase, patients should be closely monitored for adverse effects.

Special Populations: Adverse events are more common in individuals of low body weight, in patients ≥85 years old and in females. It is recommended that ARICEPT be used with caution in these patient populations. In elderly women of low body weight, the dose should not exceed 5 mg/day.

In a population of cognitively-impaired individuals, safe use of this and all other medications may require supervision.

ARICEPT should be taken once daily in the morning or evening. It may be taken with or without food.

Administration: ARICEPT tablets should be swallowed whole with water.

ARICEPT RDT should be placed on the tongue and allowed to disintegrate before swallowing with water.

OVERDOSAGE:

Symptoms: Overdosage with cholinesterase inhibitors can result in cholinergic crisis characterized by severe nausea, vomiting, salivation, sweating, bradycardia, hypotension, respiratory depression, collapse and convulsions. Increasing muscle weakness is a possibility and may result in death if respiratory muscles are involved.

Treatment: The elimination half-life of ARICEPT (donepezil hydrochloride) at recommended doses is approximately 70 hours, thus, in the case of overdose, it is anticipated that prolonged treatment and monitoring of adverse and toxic reactions will be necessary. As in any case of overdose, general supportive measures should be utilized.

Tertiary anticholinergics such as atropine may be used as an antidote for ARICEPT overdosage. Intravenous atropine sulfate titrated to effect is recommended: an initial dose of 1.0 to 2.0 mg IV with subsequent doses based upon clinical response. Atypical responses in blood pressure and heart rate have been reported with other cholinomimetics when co-administered with quaternary anticholinergics such as glycopyrrolate. It is not known whether ARICEPT and/or its metabolites can be removed by dialysis (hemodialysis, peritoneal dialysis, or hemofiltration).

Dose-related signs of toxicity observed in animals included reduced spontaneous movement, prone position, staggering gait, lacrimation, clonic convulsions, depressed respiration, salivation, miosis, fasciculation, and lower body surface temperature.

> For management of a suspected drug overdose, CPhA recommends that you contact your **regional Poison Control Centre**. See the *CPS* Directory section for a list of Poison Control Centres.

ACTION AND CLINICAL PHARMACOLOGY: Mechanism of Action: ARICEPT (donepezil hydrochloride) is a piperidine-based, reversible inhibitor of the enzyme acetylcholinesterase (AChE).

A consistent pathological change in Alzheimer's disease is the degeneration of cholinergic neuronal pathways that project from the basal forebrain to the cerebral cortex and hippocampus. The resulting hypofunction of the cholinergic systems is thought to account for some of the clinical manifestations of dementia. Donepezil is postulated to exert its therapeutic effect by enhancing cholinergic function. This is accomplished by increasing the concentration of acetylcholine (ACh) through reversible inhibition of its hydrolysis by AChE.

There is no evidence that donepezil alters the course of the underlying dementing process.

Pharmacokinetics: Absorption: Donepezil is well absorbed with a relative oral bioavailability of 100% and reaches peak plasma concentrations (C_{max}) approximately 3 to 4 hours after dose administration. Plasma concentrations and area under the curve (AUC) were found to rise in proportion to the dose administered within the 1 to 10 mg dose range studied. The terminal disposition half-life ($t_{1/2}$) is approximately 70 hours and the mean apparent plasma clearance (Cl/F) is 0.13 L/hr/kg. Following multiple dose administration, donepezil accumulates in plasma by 4-7 fold and steady state is reached within 15 days. The minimum, maximum and steady-state plasma concentrations (C) and pharmacodynamic effect (E, percent inhibition of AChE in erythrocyte membranes) of donepezil in healthy adult male and female volunteers are given in Table 6.

Table 6: ARICEPT

Plasma Concentrations and Pharmacodynamic Effect of Donepezil Hydrochloride at Steady-state (Mean±S.D.)

Dose (mg/day)	C_{min} (ng/mL)	C_{max} (ng/mL)	C_{ss}[a] (ng/mL)	E_{min} %	E_{max} %	E_{ss}[b] %
5	21.4±3.8	34.1±7.3	26.5±3.9	62.2±5.8	71.8±4.3	65.3±5.2
10	38.5±8.6	60.5±10.0	47.0±8.2	74.7±4.4	83.6±1.9	77.8±3.0

[a] C_{ss}: Plasma concentration at steady-state.
[b] E_{ss}: Inhibition of erythrocyte membrane acetylcholinesterase at steady-state.

The range of inhibition of erythrocyte membrane AChE noted in Alzheimer's disease patients in controlled clinical trials was 40 to 80% and 60 to 90% for the 5 mg/day and 10 mg/day doses, respectively.

Pharmacokinetic parameters from healthy adult male and female volunteers participating in a multiple-dose study where single daily doses of 5 mg or 10 mg of donepezil hydrochloride were administered each evening are summarized in Table 7. Treatment duration was 1 month. However, volunteers randomized to the 10 mg/day dose group initially received 5 mg daily doses of donepezil for 1 week before receiving the 10 mg daily dose for the next 3 weeks in order to avoid acute cholinergic effects.

Neither food nor time of dose administration (ie, morning versus evening dose) have an influence on the rate and extent of donepezil hydrochloride absorption.

The effect of achlorhydria on the absorption of donepezil hydrochloride is unknown.

Distribution: Donepezil hydrochloride is about 96% bound to human plasma proteins, mainly to albumins (~75%) and α_1-acid glycoprotein (~21%) over the concentration range of 2 to 1000 ng/mL.

Metabolism/Excretion: Donepezil hydrochloride is extensively metabolized and is also excreted in the urine as parent drug. The rate of metabolism of donepezil hydrochloride is slow and does not appear to be saturable. There are 4 major metabolites—2 of which are known to be active—and a number of minor metabolites, not all of which have been identified. Donepezil is metabolized by CYP 450 isoenzymes 2D6 and 3A4 and undergoes glucuronidation. Following administration of a single 5 mg dose of ^{14}C-labelled donepezil hydrochloride, plasma radioactivity, expressed as a percent of the administered dose, was present primarily as unchanged donepezil hydrochloride (53%), and as 6-O-desmethyl donepezil (11%) which has been reported to inhibit AChE to the same extent as donepezil in vitro and was found in plasma at concentrations equal to about 20% of donepezil. Approximately 57% of the total administered radioactivity was recovered from the urine and 15% was recovered from the feces (total recovery of 72%) over a period of 10 days. Approximately 28% of the labelled donepezil remained uncovered, with about 17% of the donepezil dose recovered in the urine as parent drug.

Table 7: ARICEPT

Pharmacokinetic Parameters of Donepezil Hydrochloride at Steady-state (Mean±S.D.)

Dose (mg/day)	t_{max} (h)	AUC_{0-24} (ng·h/mL)	Cl_T/F (L/h/kg)	V_z/F (L/kg)	$t_{1/2}$ (h)
5	3.0±1.4	634.8±92.2	0.110±0.02	11.8±1.7	72.7±10.6
10	3.9±1.0	1127.8±195.9	0.110±0.02	11.6±1.9	73.5±11.8

Legend:
t_{max}: Time to maximal plasma concentration.
AUC_{0-24}: Area under the plasma concentration vs. time curve from 0 to 24 hours.
Cl_T/F: Mean apparent plasma clearance.
V_z/F: Apparent volume of distribution.
$t_{1/2}$: Elimination half-life.

Special Populations and Conditions: Gender/Age: No formal pharmacokinetic study was conducted to examine age and gender related differences in the pharmacokinetic profile of donepezil. However, mean plasma donepezil concentrations measured during therapeutic drug monitoring of elderly male and female patients with Alzheimer's disease are comparable to those observed in young healthy volunteers.

Race: No specific pharmacokinetic study was conducted to investigate the effects of race on the disposition of donepezil. However, retrospective pharmacokinetic analysis indicates that gender and race (Japanese and Caucasians) did not affect the clearance of donepezil.

Hepatic Insufficiency: In a study of 10 patients with stable alcoholic cirrhosis, the clearance of donepezil was decreased by 20% relative to 10 healthy age and sex matched subjects.

Renal Insufficiency: In a study of 4 patients with moderate to severe renal impairment (Cl_{cr} <22 mL/min/1.73 m²) the clearance of donepezil did not differ from that of 4 age and sex matched healthy subjects.

STORAGE AND STABILITY: ARICEPT tablets and ARICEPT RDT should be stored at controlled room temperature, 15 to 30°C and away from moisture.

ARICEPT RDT should not be removed from blisters until immediately prior to administration. Protect from light.

INFORMATION FOR THE PATIENT: Published in e-CPS, available by subscription at www.e-cps.ca.

DOSAGE FORMS, COMPOSITION AND PACKAGING: ARICEPT: 5 mg: Each white, film-coated tablet, embossed with the name "ARICEPT" and the strength, contains: donepezil HCl 5 mg equivalent to donepezil free base 4.56 mg. Nonmedicinal ingredients: cornstarch, hydroxypropylcellulose, lactose monohydrate, magnesium stearate and microcrystalline cellulose; film-coating: hypromellose, polyethylene glycol, talc and titanium dioxide. HDPE bottles of 30. Boxed blister strips of 7, 14 and 28 (combination of 2 strips of 14).

10 mg: Each yellow, film-coated tablet, embossed with the name "ARICEPT" and the strength, contains: donepezil HCl 10 mg equivalent to donepezil free base 9.12 mg. Nonmedicinal ingredients: cornstarch, hydroxypropylcellulose, lactose monohydrate, magnesium stearate and microcrystalline cellulose; film-coating: hypromellose, iron oxide, polyethylene glycol, talc and titanium dioxide. HDPE bottles of 30. Boxed blister strips of 7, 14 and 28 (combination of 2 strips of 14).

ARICEPT RDT: 5 mg: Each white, uncoated, rapidly disintegrating tablet, embossed with the name "ARICEPT" and the strength, contains: donepezil HCl 5 mg equivalent to donepezil free base 4.56 mg. Nonmedicinal ingredients: κ-carrageenan, mannitol, polyvinyl alcohol and silica colloidal anhydrous. Boxed blister strips of 7, 28 and 30.

10 mg: Each yellow, uncoated, rapidly disintegrating tablet, embossed with the name "ARICEPT" and the strength, contains: donepezil HCl 10 mg equivalent to donepezil free base 9.12 mg. Nonmedicinal ingredients: κ-carrageenan, iron oxide, mannitol, polyvinyl alcohol and silica colloidal anhydrous. Boxed blister strips of 7, 28 and 30.

(Shown in Product Identification Section)

Arimidex® 🅿

anastrozole

Nonsteroidal Aromatase Inhibitor

AstraZeneca

Date of Revision: December 4, 2009

SUMMARY PRODUCT INFORMATION:

Route of Administration	Dosage Form/ Strength	Clinically Relevant Nonmedicinal Ingredients
Oral	Tablet/1 mg	Lactose monohydrate, macrogol 300, magnesium stearate, hypromellose, povidone, sodium starch glycolate and titanium dioxide For a complete listing see Dosage Forms, Composition and Packaging.

INDICATIONS AND CLINICAL USE: ARIMIDEX (anastrozole) is indicated for the adjuvant treatment of postmenopausal women with hormone receptor positive early breast cancer.

Approval is based on superior disease-free survival for ARIMIDEX in comparison to tamoxifen. However, overall survival was not significantly different between the two treatments.

ARIMIDEX (anastrozole) is indicated for hormonal treatment of advanced breast cancer in postmenopausal women.

Geriatrics: No changes in dose are necessary for elderly patients.

Pediatrics: ARIMIDEX is not recommended for use in pediatric patients as safety and efficacy have not been established in this group of patients.

CONTRAINDICATIONS:

- Patients who are hypersensitive to ARIMIDEX (anastrozole) or to any ingredient in the formulation. For a complete listing, see Dosage Forms, Composition and Packaging.
- Pregnant or lactating women.

WARNINGS AND PRECAUTIONS:

> **Serious Warnings and Precautions**
> - Not recommended for use in pre-menopausal women as safety and efficacy have not been established in these patients (see Action and Clinical Pharmacology).
> - Not recommended for use in pediatric patients as safety and efficacy have not been established in these patients (see Special Populations, Pediatrics).
> - Potential risk/benefit should be carefully assessed in patients with severe hepatic and severe renal impairment (see Hepatic/Biliary and Renal).
> - Potential risk/benefit should be carefully assessed in patients with osteoporosis or risk factors for osteoporosis (see Musculoskeletal).
> - Should be administered under the supervision of a qualified physician experienced in the use of anti-cancer agents (see Dosage and Administration).

Body as a Whole: ARIMIDEX is unlikely to impair the ability of patients to drive and operate machinery. However, asthenia and somnolence have been reported with the use of ARIMIDEX and caution should be observed when driving or operating machinery while such symptoms persist.

Cardiovascular: In the ATAC trial, ischemic cardiovascular events were reported more frequently in patients treated with ARIMIDEX compared to those treated with tamoxifen, although the difference was not statistically significant. A retrospective evaluation has shown that this numerical difference was associated with a sub-group of patients with pre-existing ischemic heart disease. A statistical analysis could not be performed on this subgroup evaluation. Serious adverse events continued to be collected during the off-treatment follow-up and the incidence of cardiovascular events reported was similar in the ARIMIDEX and tamoxifen arms (3.9% vs. 3.7%, respectively).

Hepatic/Biliary: Anastrozole pharmacokinetics have been investigated in subjects with stable hepatic cirrhosis related to alcohol abuse. The apparent oral clearance of anastrozole was approximately 30% lower in subjects with hepatic cirrhosis than in control subjects with normal liver function. However, plasma anastrozole concentrations in the subjects with hepatic cirrhosis are within the range of concentrations seen in normal subjects across all clinical trials. Dosage adjustment in patients with mild-to-moderate hepatic dysfunction is not necessary.

ARIMIDEX has not been investigated in patients with severe hepatic impairment. The potential risk/benefit to such patients should be carefully considered before administration of ARIMIDEX.

Musculoskeletal: The use of estrogen lowering agents, including ARIMIDEX, may cause a reduction in bone mineral density with a possible consequent increased risk of fracture. Data available from a phase III/IV study [SABRE (Study of Anastrozole with the Bisphosphonate RisedronatE)] showed that in postmenopausal women with hormone receptor positive early breast cancer with existing moderate (T-score <−1.0 in either lumbar spine or total hip, provided neither of these was less than −2.0, and with no personal history of a fragility fracture) or high risk (T-score <−2.0 in either the lumbar spine, or hip, or a personal history of fragility fracture) of fragility fracture, bone mineral density (BMD) loss could be inhibited by using ARIMIDEX together with a bisphosphonate (risedronate). All patients in the study received vitamin D and calcium supplementation. Patients at existing low risk (T-score in both the lumbar spine, and total hip, of −1.0 or higher, and no personal history of fragility fracture) of fragility fracture in the study were treated with ARIMIDEX only and did not have a loss of lumbar spine BMD following 12 months of treatment although statistically significant changes were seen following 24 months of treatment (estimated percentage change −2.07%; 95% CI: −3.60, −0.53; p=0.0109). No change in total hip BMD was seen at 12 and 24 months in the low-risk group. Women should have their osteoporosis risk assessed and managed according to local clinical practice and guidelines.

Other: ARIMIDEX has not been investigated in patients with any degree of brain or leptomeningeal involvement or with pulmonary lymphangitic disseminated disease.

Renal: Anastrozole pharmacokinetics have been investigated in subjects with renal insufficiency. Anastrozole renal clearance decreased proportionately with creatinine clearance and was approximately 50% lower in subjects with severe renal impairment (creatinine clearance less than 30 mL/min/1.73 m^2 or 0.5 mL/sec/1.73 m^2) compared to controls. Because renal clearance is not a significant pathway of elimination, the apparent oral clearance of anastrozole is unchanged even in severe renal impairment. Dosage adjustment in patients with renal dysfunction is not necessary.

ARIMIDEX has not been investigated in patients with breast cancer and severe renal impairment. The potential risk/benefit to patients with severe renal impairment should be carefully considered prior to the administration of ARIMIDEX.

Special Populations: Pregnant Women: ARIMIDEX is contraindicated in pregnant women.

The extent of exposure in pregnancy to ARIMIDEX during clinical trials and postmarketing is very limited to individual cases only. If a patient becomes pregnant while receiving this drug, the patient should be apprised of the potential hazard to the fetus or potential risk for loss of the pregnancy.

Anastrozole has been found to cross the placenta following oral administration of 0.1 mg/kg in rats and rabbits. Studies in both rats and rabbits at doses equal to or greater than 0.1 and 0.02 mg/kg/day, respectively (about 1 and 1/3, respectively, the recommended human dose on a mg/m^2 basis), administered during the period of organogenesis showed that anastrozole increased pregnancy loss (increased pre- and/or post-implantation loss, increased resorption and decreased numbers of live fetuses). Effects were dose related in rats. Placental weights were significantly increased in rats at doses of 0.1 mg/kg/day or more.

Evidence of fetotoxicity, including delayed fetal development (i.e. incomplete ossification and depressed fetal body weights), was observed in rats administered doses of 1 mg/kg/day (about 8 times the recommended human dose on a mg/m^2 basis). There was no evidence of teratogenicity in rats administered doses up to 1 mg/kg/day. In rabbits, anastrozole caused pregnancy failure at doses equal to or greater than 1 mg/kg/day (about 16 times the recommended human dose on a mg/m^2 basis). There was no evidence of teratogenicity in rabbits administered 0.2 mg/kg/day (about 3 times the recommended human dose on a mg/m^2 basis).

Nursing Women: ARIMIDEX is contraindicated in lactating women.

Pediatrics: ARIMIDEX is not recommended for use in pediatric patients as safety and efficacy have not been established.

Geriatrics: Anastrozole pharmacokinetics have been investigated in postmenopausal female volunteers and patients with breast cancer. The pharmacokinetics were similar in volunteers and in patients, and no age related effects were seen.

Monitoring and Laboratory Tests: ARIMIDEX has not been observed to interfere with routine clinical laboratory test results.

During the ATAC trial, more patients receiving ARIMIDEX were reported to have elevated serum cholesterol compared to patients receiving tamoxifen (9.0% versus 3.5%, respectively). Lipid profile was assessed as part of the SABRE trial. In this study, treatment for 12 months with ARIMIDEX alone had a neutral effect on lipid profile.

ADVERSE REACTIONS: Adverse Drug Reaction Overview: ARIMIDEX (anastrozole) has generally been well tolerated. Adverse events have usually been mild to moderate with few withdrawals from treatment due to undesirable events.

The pharmacological action of ARIMIDEX may give rise to certain expected effects. Hot flushes were reported very commonly (≥10%). Common adverse reactions (≥1%-10%) are: asthenia, joint pain/stiffness, bone pain, carpal tunnel syndrome, vaginal dryness, hair thinning (alopecia), rash, nausea, diarrhea, headache and increases in alkaline phosphatase, alanine aminotransferase and aspartate aminotransferase. Uncommonly reported adverse reactions (≥0.1%-1%) are: vaginal bleeding, trigger finger, anorexia, hypercholesterolaemia, vomiting, and somnolence, hepatitis and increases in gamma-GT and bilirubin. Very rare cases (<0.01%) of erythema multiforme, Stevens-Johnson syndrome and allergic reactions including angioedema, urticaria and anaphylaxis have also been reported. These reported frequencies are generated from a number of ARIMIDEX studies as well as post-marketing reports.

In the ATAC trial, ischemic cardiovascular events were reported more frequently in patients treated with ARIMIDEX compared to those treated with tamoxifen, although the difference was not statistically significant. A retrospective evaluation has shown that this numerical difference was associated with a sub-group of patients with pre-existing ischemic heart disease. A statistical analysis could not be performed on this subgroup evaluation. Serious adverse events continued to be collected during the off-treatment follow-up and the incidence of cardiovascular events reported was similar in the ARIMIDEX and tamoxifen arms (3.9% vs. 3.7%, respectively).

Events of carpal tunnel syndrome have been reported in patients receiving ARIMIDEX treatment in clinical trials in greater numbers than those receiving treatment with tamoxifen. The majority of these events occurred in patients with identifiable risk factors for the development of the condition. In the ATAC adjuvant trial, 83 events of carpal tunnel syndrome occurred in 78 patients in the ARIMIDEX monotherapy arm, and 22 events occurred in 22 patients in the tamoxifen arm.

Vaginal bleeding has been reported infrequently, mainly in patients during the first few weeks after changing from existing hormonal therapy to treatment with ARIMIDEX. If bleeding persists, further evaluation should be considered.

Clinical Trial Adverse Drug Reactions: Adjuvant Treatment of Early Breast Cancer in Postmenopausal Women: ARIMIDEX was generally well tolerated in the ATAC trial. At the time of the 5-year treatment completion analysis, the median duration of adjuvant treatment was 59.8 months and 59.6 months for patients receiving ARIMIDEX 1 mg and tamoxifen 20 mg, respectively. The combination of ARIMIDEX and tamoxifen did not demonstrate any safety benefits in comparison to tamoxifen alone after the results from the first analysis (median duration of treatment was approximately 33 months).

ARIMIDEX was associated with statistically significant fewer discontinuations from treatment as a result of an adverse event compared to tamoxifen (11.1% vs. 14.3%) and fewer adverse drug reactions leading to discontinuation (6.5% vs. 8.9%). The incidence of on-treatment serious adverse events is significantly lower in patients receiving ARIMIDEX 1 mg relative to tamoxifen 20 mg (33.3% versus 36.0%).

Adverse events occurring with an incidence of at least 5% in either treatment group during treatment or within 14 days of the end of treatment are presented in Table 1.

Certain adverse events (irrespective of drug causality) and combinations of adverse events were prospectively specified for analysis, based on the known pharmacological properties and side effect profiles of ARIMIDEX and tamoxifen. Tamoxifen was statistically superior to ARIMIDEX for the adverse events of joint disorders and fractures (including fractures of spine, hip and wrist) while ARIMIDEX was statistically superior to tamoxifen for the adverse events of hot flushes, vaginal bleeding, vaginal discharge, endometrial cancer, venous thromboembolic events (including deep thromboembolic events) and ischemic cerebrovascular events.

A fracture rate of 22 per 1000 patient years was observed on ARIMIDEX and 15 per 1000 patient years with the tamoxifen group with a median follow-up of 68 months. The rate of hip fractures was similar for ARIMIDEX and tamoxifen in the ATAC trial. After a median follow-up of 100 months, fractures were reported more frequently in patients treated with ARIMIDEX in comparison to tamoxifen, both during and off-treatment (13.7% vs 10.1%; see Table 2), but the rate of fracture remained stable between the two groups. During the post-treatment follow-up period, the annual fracture rates were similar in the ARIMIDEX and tamoxifen arms and the increased fracture episode rate seen during treatment was not observed following treatment completion as shown in Figure 1.

Table 1: ARIMIDEX

Adverse Events Occurring with an Incidence of at Least 5% in any Treatment Group During or Within 14 Days of the End of Treatment from the ATAC Trial

Body System and Adverse Event by COSTART-preferred Term	Number (%) of Patients[a]			
	33-month Analysis (data cut-off 29 June 2001)		5-year Treatment Completion Analysis (data cut-off 31 March 2004)	
	Anastrozole 1 mg (N=3092)	Tamoxifen 20 mg (N=3094)	Anastrozole 1 mg (N=3092)	Tamoxifen 20 mg (N=3094)
Body as a Whole				
Asthenia	483 (15.6)	466 (15.1)	575 (18.6)	544 (17.6)
Pain	432 (14.0)	413 (13.3)	533 (17.2)	485 (15.7)
Back pain	238 (7.7)	234 (7.6)	321 (10.4)	309 (10.0)
Headache	253 (8.2)	197 (6.4)	314 (10.2)	249 (8.0)
Accidental injury	195 (6.3)	189 (6.1)	311 (10.1)	303 (9.8)
Infection	197 (6.4)	205 (6.6)	285 (9.2)	276 (8.9)
Abdominal pain	202 (6.5)	211 (6.8)	271 (8.8)	276 (8.9)
Chest pain	145 (4.7)	115 (3.7)	200 (6.5)	150 (4.8)
Flu syndrome	146 (4.7)	164 (5.3)	175 (5.7)	195 (6.3)
Neoplasm	101 (3.3)	99 (3.2)	162 (5.2)	144 (4.7)
Cyst	96 (3.1)	110 (3.6)	138 (4.5)	162 (5.2)
Cardiovascular				
Vasodilation	1060 (34.3)	1229 (39.7)	1104 (35.7)	1264 (40.9)
Hypertension	255 (8.2)	218 (7.0)	402 (13.0)	349 (11.3)
Digestive				
Nausea	287 (9.3)	281 (9.1)	343 (11.1)	335 (10.8)
Diarrhea	206 (6.7)	168 (5.4)	265 (8.6)	216 (7.0)
Constipation	183 (5.9)	203 (6.6)	249 (8.1)	252 (8.1)
Gastrointestinal disorder	126 (4.1)	104 (3.4)	210 (6.8)	158 (5.1)
Dyspepsia	150 (4.9)	124 (4.0)	206 (6.7)	169 (5.5)
Haemic and Lymphatic				
Lymphoedema	247 (8.0)	277 (9.0)	304 (9.8)	341 (11.0)
Anemia	73 (2.4)	102 (3.3)	113 (3.7)	159 (5.1)
Metabolic and Nutritional				
Peripheral edema	236 (7.6)	246 (8.0)	311 (10.1)	343 (11.1)
Weight gain	234 (7.6)	236 (7.6)	285 (9.2)	274 (8.9)
Hypercholesterolemia	186 (6.0)	68 (2.2)	278 (9.0)	108 (3.5)
Musculoskeletal Disorders				
Arthritis	380 (12.3)	296 (9.6)	512 (16.6)	445 (14.4)
Arthralgia	386 (12.5)	252 (8.1)	467 (15.1)	344 (11.1)
Osteoporosis	192 (6.2)	134 (4.3)	325 (10.5)	226 (7.3)
Fracture	183 (5.9)	115 (3.7)	315 (10.2)	209 (6.8)
Arthrosis	161 (5.2)	112 (3.6)	207 (6.7)	156 (5.0)
Bone pain	158 (5.1)	139 (4.5)	201 (6.5)	185 (6.0)
Joint disorder	102 (3.3)	95 (3.1)	184 (6.0)	160 (5.2)
Myalgia	114 (3.7)	103 (3.3)	179 (5.8)	160 (5.2)
Nervous System				
Depression	323 (10.4)	315 (10.2)	413 (13.4)	382 (12.3)
Insomnia	253 (8.2)	226 (7.3)	309 (10.0)	281 (9.1)
Dizziness	180 (5.8)	191 (6.2)	236 (7.6)	234 (7.6)
Paraesthesia	181 (5.9)	106 (3.4)	215 (7.0)	145 (4.7)
Anxiety	147 (4.8)	147 (4.8)	195 (6.3)	180 (5.8)
Respiratory				

(cont'd)

Table 1: ARIMIDEX *(cont'd)*

Adverse Events Occurring with an Incidence of at Least 5% in any Treatment Group During or Within 14 Days of the End of Treatment from the ATAC Trial

Body System and Adverse Event by COSTART-preferred Term	Number (%) of Patients[a]			
	33-month Analysis (data cut-off 29 June 2001)		5-year Treatment Completion Analysis (data cut-off 31 March 2004)	
	Anastrozole 1 mg (N=3092)	Tamoxifen 20 mg (N=3094)	Anastrozole 1 mg (N=3092)	Tamoxifen 20 mg (N=3094)
Pharyngitis	335 (10.8)	327 (10.6)	443 (14.3)	422 (13.6)
Cough increased	194 (6.3)	216 (7.0)	261 (8.4)	287 (9.3)
Dyspnea	173 (5.6)	164 (5.3)	234 (7.6)	237 (7.7)
Sinusitis	137 (4.4)	118 (3.8)	184 (6.0)	159 (5.1)
Bronchitis	126 (4.1)	107 (3.5)	167 (5.4)	153 (4.9)
Skin and Appendages				
Rash	281 (9.1)	314 (10.1)	333 (10.8)	387 (12.5)
Sweating	112 (3.6)	158 (5.1)	145 (4.7)	177 (5.7)
Special Senses				
Cataract specified	107 (3.5)	116 (3.7)	182 (5.9)	213 (6.9)
Urogenital				
Breast pain	176 (5.7)	121 (3.9)	251 (8.1)	169 (5.5)
Urinary tract infection	169 (5.5)	224 (7.2)	244 (7.9)	313 (10.1)
Vulvovaginitis	169 (5.5)	119 (3.8)	194 (6.3)	150 (4.8)
Breast neoplasm	94 (3.0)	89 (2.9)	164 (5.3)	139 (4.5)
Vaginitis	79 (2.6)	122 (3.9)	125 (4.0)	158 (5.1)
Vaginal hemorrhage[b]	100 (3.2)	151 (4.9)	122 (3.9)	180 (5.8)
Leucorrhea	68 (2.2)	264 (8.5)	86 (2.8)	286 (9.2)

[a] Patients with multiple events in the same category are counted only once in that category. Patients with events in more than 1 category are counted once in each of those categories.
[b] Vaginal hemorrhage without further diagnosis.
Legend: COSTART=Coding Symbols for Thesaurus of Adverse Reaction Terms; N=Number of patients treated.

Table 2: ARIMIDEX

Incidence of Fractures (during or off-trial treatment)

Category	Number (%) of Patients[a]	
	2007 Update Analysis (data cut-off 31 March 2007)	
	Anastrozole 1 mg (N=3092)	Tamoxifen 20 mg (N=3094)
Non-serious or Serious		
All Fractures	425 (13.7)	313 (10.1)
Wrist/Colles	95 (3.1)	84 (2.7)
Spine	61 (2.0)	38 (1.2)
Hip	49 (1.6)	42 (1.4)
Serious		
All fractures	212 (6.9)	170 (5.5)
Wrist/Colles	49 (1.6)	45 (1.5)
Spine	23 (0.7)	18 (0.6)
Hip	46 (1.5)	40 (1.3)

[a] Patients with multiple events in the same category are counted only once in that category. Patients with events in more than 1 category are counted once in each of those categories.
Note: Off-trial treatment AEs were SAEs and any fracture event reported as being serious or non-serious that occurred more than 14 days after stopping study treatment (but within 10 years of starting study treatment). AEs starting after the patients first recurrence visit were not reported.
Note: Off-trial treatment AEs included all off-treatment reports regardless of whether a patient had had a similar report on treatment.
Legend: N=Number of patients treated.

In the ATAC trial, ischemic cardiovascular events were reported more frequently in patients treated with ARIMIDEX compared to those treated with tamoxifen, although the difference was not statistically significant (see Table 3). A retrospective evaluation has shown that this numerical difference was associated with a sub-group of patients with pre-existing ischemic heart disease. A statistical analysis could not be performed on this subgroup evaluation. From the 33 month analysis to the 68 month analysis, the incidence of cardiovascular events also remains stable over time between the two treatment groups. The incidence of myocardial infarctions increased by 0.1% in the ARIMIDEX treatment group and 0.2% in the tamoxifen treatment group; the incidence of cerebrovascular accidents increased by 0.3% in each treatment group. During the off-treatment follow-up, when serious adverse events continued to be collected, the incidence of myocardial infarctions and cerebrovascular accidents was similar in both treatment groups.

Table 3 provides a summary of the pre-specified adverse events that occurred in either treatment group during treatment and after cessation of trial therapy.

Figure 1: ARIMIDEX

Annual First Event Rates of All Fractures On or Off Study Therapy

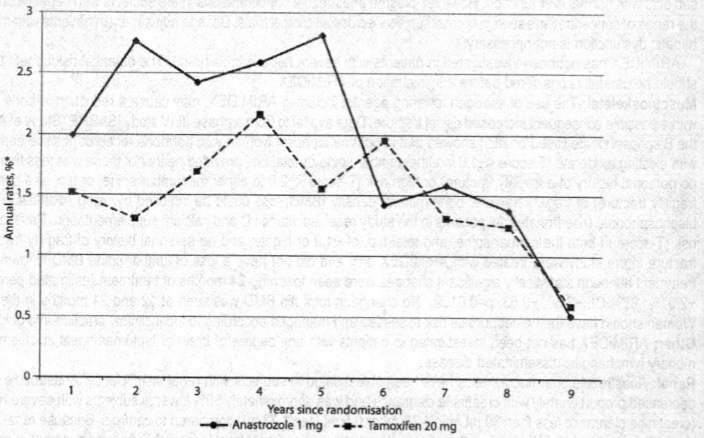

Table 3: ARIMIDEX

Incidence of Pre-specified Adverse Events Occurring in Either Treatment Group During Treatment and After Cessation of Trial Therapy From the ATAC Trial[a]

Adverse Event	Number (%) of Patients[b]			
	5-year Treatment Completion Analysis (data cut-off 31 March 2004)			
	Anastrozole 1 mg (N=3092)	Tamoxifen 20 mg (N=3094)	Odds Ratio[c]	p-value
Hot flushes	1104 (35.7)	1264 (40.9)	0.80	<0.0001
Mood disturbances	600 (19.4)	557 (18.0)	1.10	0.2
Fatigue/asthenia	577 (18.7)	544 (17.6)	1.08	0.3
Nausea and vomiting	396 (12.8)	385 (12.4)	1.03	0.7
Vaginal discharge	111 (3.6)	407 (13.2)	0.25	<0.0001
Vaginal bleeding	171 (5.5)	323 (10.4)	0.50	<0.0001
Joint pain/stiffness	1111 (35.9)	922 (29.8)	1.32	<0.0001
Fractures	340 (11.0)	238 (7.7)	1.48	<0.0001
Fractures of the spine, hip, or wrist/colles	148 (4.8)	112 (3.6)	1.34	0.02
Hip[d]	37 (1.2)	31 (1.0)	NC	NC
Spine[d]	45 (1.5)	27 (0.9)	NC	NC
Wrist/colles[d]	72 (2.3)	63 (2.0)	NC	NC
Cataracts	191 (6.2)	219 (7.1)	0.86	0.2
Ischemic cardiovascular disease	137 (4.4)	119 (3.8)	1.16	0.2
Angina pectoris[d]	75 (2.4)	56 (1.8)	NC	NC
Myocardial infarct[d]	42 (1.4)	40 (1.3)	NC	NC
Coronary artery disorder[d]	26 (0.7)	27 (0.9)	NC	NC
Myocardial ischemia[d]	24 (0.8)	16 (0.5)	NC	NC
Venous thromboembolic events	95 (3.1)	151 (4.9)	0.62	0.0003
Deep venous thromboembolic events	57 (1.8)	83 (2.7)	0.68	0.03
Ischemic cerebrovascular events	67 (2.2)	94 (3.0)	0.71	0.03
Endometrial cancer[e]	5 (0.2)	17 (0.8)	0.29	0.02

[a] All adverse events occurring during treatment or within 14 days of the end of treatment; all serious adverse events and all non-serious fractures occurring after 14 days from the end of treatment and prior to the confirmation of recurrence of breast cancer.
[b] Patients with multiple events in the same category are counted only once in that category. Patients with events in more than 1 category are counted once in each of those categories.
[c] Odds ratios of <1.00 indicate that treatment with anastrozole 1 mg is associated with a lower incidence of a specific event than tamoxifen 20 mg.
[d] Individual COSTART-preferred terms for a particular category of event—the broader category was the "pre-specified adverse event".
[e] Percentages calculated based upon the numbers of patients with an intact uterus at baseline (N=2229 for anastrozole and N=2236 for tamoxifen).
Legend: N=Number of patients treated; NC=Not calculated.

Patients with Advanced Breast Cancer: Two controlled clinical trials involving postmenopausal women with advanced breast cancer, compared treatment with tamoxifen (20 mg daily) versus treatment with anastrozole (1 mg daily). Table 4 presents adverse events reported in these trials with an incidence of greater than 5% in either treatment group, regardless of causality.

Table 4: ARIMIDEX

Number (%) of Patients with Adverse Events from Trials 0027 and 0030[a]

Adverse Event by Body System	ARIMIDEX 1 mg (n=506)	Tamoxifen 20 mg (n=511)
Body as a Whole		
Asthenia	83 (16.4)	81 (15.9)
Pain	70 (13.8)	73 (14.3)
Back pain	60 (11.9)	68 (13.3)
Headache	47 (9.3)	40 (7.8)
Chest pain	37 (7.3)	37 (7.2)
Flu syndrome	35 (6.9)	30 (5.9)
Pelvic pain	23 (4.5)	30 (5.9)
Cardiovascular		
Vasodilation	128 (25.3)	106 (20.7)
Hypertension	25 (4.9)	36 (7.0)
Digestive		
Nausea	94 (18.6)	106 (20.7)
Constipation	47 (9.3)	66 (12.9)
Abdominal pain	40 (7.9)	38 (7.4)
Diarrhea	40 (7.9)	33 (6.5)
Vomiting	38 (7.5)	36 (7.0)
Anorexia	26 (5.1)	46 (9.0)
Metabolic and Nutritional		
Peripheral edema	51 (10.1)	41 (8.0)
Musculoskeletal Disorders		
Bone pain	54 (10.7)	52 (10.2)
Nervous System		
Insomnia	30 (5.9)	28 (5.5)
Dizziness	30 (5.9)	22 (4.3)
Depression	23 (4.5)	32 (6.3)
Hypertonia	16 (3.2)	26 (5.1)
Respiratory		
Cough increased	55 (10.9)	52 (10.2)
Dyspnea	51 (10.1)	47 (9.2)
Pharyngitis	49 (9.7)	68 (13.3)
Skin and Appendages		
Rash	38 (7.5)	34 (6.7)
Urogenital		
Leucorrhea	9 (1.8)	31 (6.1)

[a] A patient may have more than one adverse event.

Based on results from the established safety profiles of ARIMIDEX and tamoxifen, the incidences of nine pre-specified adverse event categories, potentially causally related to one or both therapies because of their pharmacology, were statistically analyzed. No statistically significant differences were seen between treatment groups. The results are shown in Table 5.

Table 5: ARIMIDEX

Number (%) of Patients from Trials 0027 and 0030[a]

Adverse Event by Body System	ARIMIDEX 1 mg n=506 (%)	Tamoxifen 20 mg n=511 (%)
Body as a Whole		
Tumour flare	15 (3.0)	18 (3.5)
Cardiovascular		
Hot flushes	134 (26.5)	118 (23.1)
Thromboembolic disease	23 (4.5)	39 (7.6)
Digestive		
Gastrointestinal disturbances	170 (33.6)	196 (38.4)
Metabolic and Nutritional		
Weight gain	11 (2.2)	8 (1.6)
Nervous System		
Depression	23 (4.5)	32 (6.3)
Lethargy	6 (1.2)	15 (2.9)
Urogenital		
Vaginal dryness	15 (3.0)	13 (2.5)
Vaginal bleeding	5 (1.0)	11 (2.2)

[a] Patients may appear in more than one row.

The low incidence of vaginal bleeding and vaginal discharge was consistent with the known pharmacology of ARIMIDEX, which would be predicted to have no estrogenic effect, and no effect on the endometrium. Despite the lack of estrogenic activity, there was no increase in myocardial infarction or pathological fracture when compared with tamoxifen. There was a low incidence of thromboembolic disease.

Patients with Advanced Breast Cancer who had Disease Progression Following Tamoxifen Therapy: For two controlled clinical trials comparing ARIMIDEX (1 mg and 10 mg) versus megestrol acetate (160 mg), adverse events reported in greater than 5% of the patients in any of the treatment groups, regardless of causality, are presented in Table 6.

Table 6: ARIMIDEX

Number (n) and Percentage of Patients with Adverse Events from Trials 0004 and 0005[a]

Adverse Event by Body System	ARIMIDEX 1 mg (n=262) n (%)	ARIMIDEX 10 mg (n=246) n (%)	Megestrol Acetate (160 mg) n=253
Body as a Whole			
Asthenia	42 (16.0)	33 (13.4)	47 (18.6)
Headache	34 (13.0)	44 (17.9)	24 (9.5)
Pain	28 (10.7)	38 (15.4)	29 (11.5)
Back pain	28 (10.7)	26 (10.6)	19 (7.5)
Pelvic pain	14 (5.3)	17 (6.9)	13 (5.1)
Chest pain	13 (5.0)	18 (7.3)	13 (5.1)
Cardiovascular			
Hot flushes	32 (12.2)	29 (10.6)	21 (8.3)
Digestive			
Nausea	41 (15.6)	48 (19.5)	28 (11.1)
Vomiting	24 (9.2)	26 (10.6)	16 (6.3)
Diarrhea	22 (8.4)	18 (7.3)	7 (2.8)
Constipation	18 (6.9)	18 (7.3)	21 (8.3)
Abdominal pain	18 (6.9)	14 (5.7)	18 (7.1)
Anorexia	18 (6.9)	19 (7.7)	11 (4.3)
Dry mouth	15 (5.7)	11 (4.5)	13 (5.1)
Metabolic and Nutritional			
Peripheral edema	14 (5.3)	21 (8.5)	28 (11.1)
Weight gain	4 (1.5)	9 (3.7)	30 (11.9)
Increased appetite	0 (0)	1 (0.4)	13 (5.1)
Musculoskeletal Disorders			
Bone pain	17 (6.5)	26 (11.8)	19 (7.5)
Nervous System			
Dizziness	16 (6.1)	12 (4.9)	15 (5.9)
Depression	14 (5.3)	6 (2.4)	5 (2.0)
Paresthesia	12 (4.6)	15 (6.1)	9 (3.6)
Respiratory			
Dyspnea	24 (9.2)	27 (11.0)	53 (20.9)
Cough increased	22 (8.4)	18 (7.3)	19 (7.5)

(cont'd)

Table 6: ARIMIDEX *(cont'd)*

Number (n) and Percentage of Patients with Adverse Events from Trials 0004 and 0005[a]

Adverse Event by Body System	ARIMIDEX 1 mg (n=262) n (%)	ARIMIDEX 10 mg (n=246) n (%)	Megestrol Acetate (160 mg) n=253
Pharyngitis	16 (6.1)	23 (9.3)	15 (5.9)
Skin and Appendages			
Rash	15 (5.7)	15 (6.1)	19 (7.5)
Sweating	4 (1.5)	3 (1.2)	16 (6.3)
Urogenital			
Vaginal hemorrhage	6 (2.3)	4 (1.6)	13 (5.1)

[a] A patient may have more than one adverse event.

Other less frequent (2% to 5%) adverse experiences reported in patients receiving ARIMIDEX 1 mg in the two pivotal clinical trials are listed below. These adverse experiences are listed by body system and are in order of decreasing frequency within each body system regardless of assessed causality.

Body as a Whole: flu syndrome; fever; neck pain; malaise; accidental injury; infection.
Cardiovascular: hypertension; thrombophlebitis.
Hepatic: gamma GT increased; AST increased; ALT increased.
Hematologic: anemia; leukopenia.
Metabolic and Nutritional: alkaline phosphatase increased; weight loss.

Mean serum total cholesterol levels increased by 0.5 mmol/L among patients receiving ARIMIDEX. Increases in LDL cholesterol have been shown to contribute to these changes.

Musculoskeletal: myalgia; arthralgia; pathological fracture.
Nervous: somnolence; confusion; insomnia; anxiety; nervousness.
Respiratory: sinusitis; bronchitis; rhinitis.
Skin and Appendages: hair thinning; pruritus.
Urogenital: urinary tract infection; breast pain.

The incidence of the following adverse event groups, potentially causally related to one or both of the therapies because of their pharmacology, were statistically analyzed: weight gain, edema, thromboembolic disease, gastrointestinal disturbance, hot flushes, and vaginal dryness. These six groups, and the adverse events captured in the groups, were prospectively defined. The results are shown in Table 7.

Table 7: ARIMIDEX

Number (n) and Percentage of Patients from Trials 0004 and 0005

Adverse Event by Body System	ARIMIDEX 1 mg (n=262) n (%)	ARIMIDEX 10 mg (n=246) n (%)	Megestrol Acetate 160 mg n=253 n (%)
Cardiovascular			
Hot flushes	33 (12.6)	29 (11.8)	35 (13.8)
Thromboembolic disease	9 (3.4)	4 (1.6)	12 (4.7)
Digestive			
Gastrointestinal disturbance	77 (29.4)	81 (32.9)	54 (21.3)
Metabolic and Nutritional			
Edema	19 (7.3)	28 (11.4)	35 (13.8)
Weight gain	4 (1.5)	10 (4.1)	30 (11.9)
Urogenital			
Vaginal dryness	5 (1.9)	3 (1.2)	2 (0.8)

More patients treated with megestrol acetate reported weight gain as an adverse event compared to patients treated with ARIMIDEX 1 mg (p<0.0001). Other differences were not statistically significant.

An examination of the magnitude of change in weight in all patients was also conducted. Thirty-four percent (87/253) of the patients treated with megestrol acetate experienced weight gain of 5% or more and 11% (27/253) of the patients treated with megestrol acetate experienced weight gain of 10% or more. Among patients treated with ARIMIDEX 1 mg, 13% (33/262) experienced weight gain of 5% or more and 3% (6/262) experienced weight gain of 10% or more. On average, this 5 to 10% weight gain represented between 6 and 12 pounds.

No patients receiving ARIMIDEX or megestrol acetate discontinued treatment due to drug-related weight gain.

Abnormal Hematologic and Clinical Chemistry Findings: Systematic collection of laboratory results (including total cholesterol) was not performed as specific endpoints in the ATAC trial. Abnormal laboratory results in ATAC are reported as an adverse event. During the ATAC trial, more patients receiving ARIMIDEX were reported to have elevated serum cholesterol levels compared to patients receiving tamoxifen (9% versus 3.5%, respectively). In the SABRE trial, which was designed to specifically evaluate lipid levels in patients on ARIMIDEX, no difference was observed in levels of low density lipoprotein-cholesterol (LDL-C), total cholesterol or triglycerides in patients taking ARIMIDEX for 12 months compared to levels prior to commencing ARIMIDEX treatment. There was a statistically significant increase in high density lipoprotein-cholesterol (HDL-C) in patients taking ARIMIDEX for 12 months compared to levels prior to commencing ARIMIDEX treatment. On the basis of the SABRE data, no specific requirements for lipid monitoring due to ARIMIDEX therapy are recommended.

Post-Market Adverse Drug Reactions: A case of severe acute hepatitis has been reported. Although late onset hepatotoxicity due to previous chemotherapy could not be ruled out, the temporal evidence suggested ARIMIDEX as a possible cause. Rare cases of toxic hepatitis have been reported in association with ARIMIDEX administration.

DRUG INTERACTIONS: Overview: Anastrozole inhibits reactions catalyzed by cytochrome P450 1A2, 2C8/9, and 3A4 in vitro with Ki values which are approximately 30 times higher than the mean plasma steady-state C_{max} values observed following a 1 mg daily dose. Anastrozole has no inhibitory effect on reactions catalyzed by cytochrome P450 2A6 or 2D6 in vitro. Administration of a single 30 mg or multiple 10 mg doses of anastrozole to subjects had no effect on the clearance of antipyrine or urinary recovery of antipyrine metabolites. Based on these in vitro and in vivo results, it is unlikely that the administration of ARIMIDEX 1 mg will result in clinically significant inhibition of cytochrome P450-mediated metabolism of coadministered drugs.

Antipyrine, cimetidine, tamoxifen and warfarin clinical interaction studies indicate that the coadministration of ARIMIDEX (anastrozole) with other drugs is unlikely to result in clinically significant drug interactions mediated by cytochrome P450.

A review of AstraZeneca's global clinical trial safety database did not reveal evidence of clinically significant interactions in patients treated with ARIMIDEX who also received other commonly prescribed drugs.

Estrogen-containing therapies should not be used with ARIMIDEX as they may counteract the goal of achieving estrogen suppression.

Drug-Drug Interactions: Warfarin: The pharmacokinetics and anticoagulant activity of warfarin (25 mg) coadministered with anastrozole (1 mg daily) have been studied in healthy male volunteers. The mean plasma concentrations of anastrozole achieved throughout the warfarin dosing and sampling period were within the range seen in postmenopausal women with advanced breast cancer taking the clinically recommended dose of the drug. Overall, there was no evidence to suggest that anastrozole has any clinically relevant effects on the pharmacokinetics or anti-coagulant activity of warfarin.

Bisphosphonates: A review of AstraZeneca's global clinical trial safety database showed that there are no clinically significant interactions with bisphosphonates. Results from the SABRE trial demonstrate that anastrozole in combination with the bisphosphonate, risedronate, was well tolerated.

Tamoxifen: The effect of anastrozole on tamoxifen (20 mg daily) pharmacokinetics has been studied in postmenopausal women with early breast cancer, who were already receiving tamoxifen as adjuvant therapy. There was no evidence of anastrozole having any significant effect on blood levels of tamoxifen compared to placebo (p=0.919).

Coadministration of ARIMIDEX and tamoxifen did not affect tamoxifen or N-desmethyltamoxifen plasma concentrations, however, ARIMIDEX plasma concentrations were reduced by 27% compared to those achieved with ARIMIDEX alone. Combination treatment of ARIMIDEX with tamoxifen has shown that ARIMIDEX does not have a significant effect on blood levels of tamoxifen; estradiol suppression is consistent with that seen in patients treated with ARIMIDEX alone.

Results from the ATAC trial (median follow-up of 33 months) suggest that tamoxifen should not be coadministered with ARIMIDEX. The combination did not demonstrate any efficacy or safety benefit when compared to ARIMIDEX or tamoxifen treatment alone, subsequently resulting in the discontinuation of the combination arm from the ATAC trial. See Table 8.

Table 8: ARIMIDEX

Established or Potential Drug-drug Interactions

Anastrozole	Ref	Effect	Clinical Comment
Tamoxifen	CT	Tamoxifen and metabolite N-desmethyltamoxifen concentrations not affected. Anastrozole concentrations are decreased.	ATAC results indicate that the anastrozole-tamoxifen combination does not demonstrate any efficacy or safety benefits compared to tamoxifen monotherapy.

Legend: C=case study; CT=clinical trial; T=theoretical.

Drug-Food Interactions: Interactions with particular food has not been established.
Drug-Herb Interactions: Interactions with herbal products have not been established. Estrogen-containing herb therapies should not be used with ARIMIDEX as they may counteract the goal of achieving estrogen suppression.
Drug-Laboratory Test Interactions: ARIMIDEX has not been observed to interfere with routine clinical laboratory tests results.

DOSAGE AND ADMINISTRATION:

Dosing Considerations: Age: Patients should be postmenopausal.
Recommended Dose and Dosage Adjustment: ARIMIDEX (anastrozole) should be administered 1 mg orally, once a day.

In the adjuvant setting, it is currently recommended that treatment be given for 5 years.

Elderly: No changes in dose are necessary for elderly patients.
Hepatic Impairment: Although the apparent oral clearance of anastrozole was decreased in subjects with cirrhosis due to alcohol abuse, plasma anastrozole concentrations remained within the range seen across all clinical trials in subjects without liver disease. Therefore, no changes in dose are recommended for patients with mild-to-moderate hepatic impairment, although patients should be monitored for side effects. ARIMIDEX has not been studied in patients with severe hepatic impairment. The potential risk/benefit to such patients should be carefully considered before administration of ARIMIDEX.
Renal Impairment: No changes in dose are necessary for patients with renal impairment. The potential risk/benefit to patients with severe renal impairment should still be considered prior to the administration of ARIMIDEX in these patients.
Missed Dose: A missed dose should be taken as soon as possible, as long as it is taken at least 12 hours before the next dose is due. A missed dose should not be taken within 12 hours of the next dose.
Administration: Patients should swallow ARIMIDEX with fluids.

Patients should try to take ARIMIDEX at the same time each day.

OVERDOSAGE:

There is limited clinical experience of accidental overdosage. Acute toxicity was seen in animals at a dose greater than 45 mg/kg (equivalent to 2.7 g). Clinical trials have been conducted with various dosages of ARIMIDEX (anastrozole), up to 60 mg in a single dose given to healthy male volunteers and up to 10 mg daily given to post-menopausal women with advanced breast cancer; these dosages were well tolerated. A single dose of ARIMIDEX that results in life-threatening symptoms has not been established.

There is no specific antidote to overdosage and treatment must be symptomatic. In the management of an overdose, consideration should be given to the possibility that multiple agents may have been taken. Vomiting may be induced if the patient is alert. Dialysis may be helpful because ARIMIDEX is not highly protein bound. General supportive care, including frequent monitoring of vital signs and close observation of the patient, is indicated.

For management of a suspected drug overdose, contact your **regional Poison Control Centre**. See the *CPS* Directory section for a list of Poison Control Centres.

ACTION AND CLINICAL PHARMACOLOGY: Mechanism of Action: Many breast cancers have estrogen receptors and growth of these tumours can be stimulated by estrogens. In post-menopausal women, the principal source of circulating estrogen (primarily estrone) is conversion of adrenally-generated androstenedione to estrone by aromatase in peripheral tissues, such as adipose tissue, with further conversion of estrone to estradiol. Many breast cancers also contain aromatase; the importance of tumour-generated estrogens is uncertain.

Treatment of breast cancer has included efforts to decrease estrogen levels by ovariectomy pre-menopausally and by use of anti-estrogens and progestational agents both pre- and post-menopausally, and these interventions lead to decreased tumour mass or delayed progression of tumour growth in some women.

ARIMIDEX (anastrozole) is a potent and selective non-steroidal aromatase inhibitor. It significantly lowers serum estradiol concentrations and has no detectable effect on formation of adrenal corticosteroids or aldosterone.

Pharmacodynamics: Inhibition of aromatase activity is primarily due to anastrozole, the parent drug.

The relationship between dose and response, measured as suppression of serum estradiol, was studied in postmenopausal women. Daily doses of ARIMIDEX at 1 mg for 14 days produced estradiol suppression of greater than 80%. Suppression of serum estradiol was maintained for up to 6 days after cessation of daily dosing with 1 mg ARIMIDEX.

In a study of 14 postmenopausal women diagnosed with locally advanced (Stage T3-T4) breast cancer with non-inflammatory, estrogen-receptor positive tumours, anastrozole was shown to be a potent suppressor of intra-tumoural estrogen levels. Following use as a 15-week primary systemic treatment (prior to any local surgery and/or radiotherapy), anastrozole suppressed intra-tumoural concentrations of estradiol (E_2), estrone (E_1) and estrone sulfate (E_1S) to mean values of 11.1%, 16.7% and 26.6%, respectively, of baseline levels. Three patients had intra-tumoural levels of E_2, E_1 and E_1S suppressed below assay detection limits.

The selectivity of ARIMIDEX to the aromatase enzyme, rather than other cytochrome P450 enzymes controlling glucocorticoid and mineralocorticoid synthesis in the adrenal gland, has been established. Furthermore, provocative stimulation of the adrenal glands by ACTH in subjects under treatment with ARIMIDEX up to 10 mg, produced a normal response in terms of cortisol and aldosterone secretion. Therefore, patients treated with ARIMIDEX do not require glucocorticoid or mineralocorticoid replacement therapy.

ARIMIDEX does not possess direct progestogenic, androgenic or estrogenic activity and does not interfere with secretion of thyroid stimulating hormone (TSH).

Because of its pharmacological action, patients with estrogen and/or progesterone receptor-positive disease are the most appropriate population for ARIMIDEX therapy.

Pharmacokinetics: Absorption: Absorption of anastrozole is rapid and maximum plasma concentrations typically occur within 2 hours of dosing under fasted conditions. Studies with radiolabeled drug have demonstrated that orally administered anastrozole is well absorbed into the systemic circulation. Food reduces the rate, but not the overall extent of anastrozole absorption.

Distribution: The pharmacokinetics of anastrozole are linear over the dose range of 1 to 20 mg and do not change with repeated dosing. Consistent with the 50-hour plasma elimination half-life, plasma concentrations of anastrozole approach steady-state concentrations after 7 days of once daily dosing and are approximately three- to four-fold higher than the concentrations observed after a single dose of anastrozole. The protein binding of anastrozole to plasma proteins is about 40% and independent of concentration over a range, which includes therapeutic concentrations.

Metabolism: Metabolism of anastrozole occurs by N-dealkylation, hydroxylation and glucuronidation. Three metabolites of anastrozole (triazole, a glucuronide conjugate of hydroxy-anastrozole, and a glucuronide conjugate of anastrozole itself) have been identified in human plasma or urine. Several minor (less than 5% of the radioactive dose) metabolites excreted in the urine have not been identified. The major metabolite of anastrozole in the circulation, triazole, lacks pharmacologic activity.

Excretion: Studies in postmenopausal women with radiolabeled anastrozole demonstrated that elimination occurs primarily via metabolism (approximately 85%) and to a lesser extent renal excretion of unchanged anastrozole (approximately 11%). Anastrozole is eliminated slowly with a plasma elimination half-life of approximately 50 hours in postmenopausal women.

Special Populations and Conditions: Geriatrics: Anastrozole pharmacokinetics have been investigated in post-menopausal female volunteers and patients with breast cancer. The pharmacokinetics were similar in volunteers and in patients and no age related effects were seen.

Race: Anastrozole pharmacodynamics and pharmacokinetics have been studied in healthy, postmenopausal women in Japan, dosed for 16 days. The pharmacodynamic effect and pharmacokinetics of anastrozole 1 mg daily were similar in Japanese and Caucasian volunteers, and there was no indication that there would be any clinically significant differences in therapeutic responses to anastrozole between Japanese and Caucasian patients with breast cancer.

Hepatic Insufficiency: Anastrozole pharmacokinetics have been investigated in subjects with stable hepatic cirrhosis related to alcohol abuse. The apparent oral clearance of anastrozole was approximately 30% lower in subjects with hepatic cirrhosis than in control subjects with normal liver function. However, plasma anastrozole concentrations in the subjects with hepatic cirrhosis are within the range of concentrations seen in normal subjects across all clinical trials. Dosage adjustment in patients with mild to moderate hepatic impairment is not necessary. ARIMIDEX has not been studied in patients with severe hepatic impairment. The potential risk/benefit to such patients should be carefully considered before administration of ARIMIDEX.

Renal Insufficiency: Anastrozole pharmacokinetics have been investigated in subjects with renal insufficiency. Anastrozole renal clearance decreased proportionately with creatinine clearance and was approximately 50% lower in volunteers with severe renal impairment (creatinine clearance less than 30 mL/min/1.73 m^2 or 0.5 mL/sec/1.73 m^2) compared to controls. Because renal clearance is not a significant pathway of elimination, the apparent oral clearance of anastrozole is unchanged even in severe renal impairment. Dosage adjustment in patients with renal dysfunction is not necessary. The potential risk/benefit to patients with severe renal impairment should still be considered prior to the administration of ARIMIDEX in these patients.

STORAGE AND STABILITY: ARIMIDEX should be stored at room temperature (15 to 30°C).

SPECIAL HANDLING INSTRUCTIONS: No special instructions for handling are required.

INFORMATION FOR THE PATIENT: Published in e-CPS, available by subscription at www.e-cps.ca.

DOSAGE FORMS, COMPOSITION AND PACKAGING: Each white, biconvex, film-coated tablet, intagliated with "Adx 1" on one side and a logo on the other side ("A" for ARIMIDEX), contains: anastrozole 1 mg. Nonmedicinal ingredients: hypromellose, lactose monohydrate, macrogol 300, magnesium stearate, povidone, sodium starch glycolate and titanium dioxide. Blister-packs of 30.

(Shown in Product Identification Section)

The reader is invited to consult CPhA's monograph **Corticosteroids: Topical.**

Aristocort®, Creams and Ointments Ⓟ

triamcinolone acetonide

Topical Corticosteroid

Valeo Pharma

Date of Revision: February 22, 2005

PHARMACOLOGY: Topical steroid products are effective because of their anti-inflammatory, antipruritic and vasoconstrictive properties.

INDICATIONS: Indicated for topical therapy of corticosteroid responsive acute and chronic dermatoses, where an anti-inflammatory, anti-allergenic and antipruritic activity in topical management is required.

ARISTOCORT triamcinolone acetonide topical preparations have been demonstrated to be effective in the adjunctive treatment of the following dermatoses: atopic dermatitis, pruritus vulvae and ani, generalized erythrodermia, external otitis, seborrheic dermatitis, eczematized psoriasis, neurodermatitis.

The concentrated 0.5 % ARISTOCORT C triamcinolone acetonide preparation has been of greatest usefulness in the initial suppression of the acute manifestations of difficult to manage dermatologic conditions. The regular 0.1% ARISTOCORT R topical preparations are indicated for the control of dermatoses, once difficult conditions are suppressed.

ARISTOCORT Ointment is preferable to creams when one is dealing with a dry lesion, whereas the cream base formulations are preferable on weeping lesions.

It must be remembered that steroid therapy, although responsible for remissions of dermatoses, especially of allergic origin, cannot be expected to prevent recurrence. In the case of contact or allergic dermatitis, it is important to investigate causal factors and to remove the offending material or allergen.

CONTRAINDICATIONS: Topical steroids are contraindicated in: 1) Untreated bacterial, tubercular and fungal infections involving the skin, and in certain viral diseases such as herpes simplex, chicken pox, and vaccinia. 2) Hypersensitivity to any of the components.

WARNINGS: *Pregnancy:* The safety of topical corticosteroids during pregnancy and lactation has not been established. The potential benefit of topical corticosteroids, if used during pregnancy and lactation, should be weighed against possible hazard to the foetus or the nursing infant.

Lactation: See Pregnancy.

If used under an occlusive dressing, particularly over extensive areas, sufficient absorption may take place to give rise to adrenal suppression and other systemic effects.

Topical corticosteroids are not for ophthalmic use.

PRECAUTIONS: Should not be used on lesions close to the eye. Although hypersensitivity reactions have been rare with topically applied steroid products, the drug should be discontinued and appropriate therapy initiated if there are signs of reaction.

Prolonged use of topical corticosteroid products may produce atrophy of the skin and of subcutaneous tissues, particularly on flexor surfaces and on the face. If this is noted, discontinue the use of this product.

In cases of bacterial infections of the skin, appropriate antibacterial agents should be used as primary therapy. If it is considered necessary, the topical corticosteroid product may be used as an adjunct to control inflammation, erythema and itching.

The product should be used with caution in patients with stasis dermatitis and other skin diseases associated with impaired circulation.

If symptomatic response is not noted within a few days to a week, the local applications of corticosteroid should be discontinued and the patient re-evaluated. During the use of topical corticosteroids secondary infections may occur.

Significant systemic absorption may result when steroids are applied over large areas of the body. To minimize this possibility, when long-term therapy is anticipated, interrupt treatment periodically or treat one area of the body at a time.

Patients should be advised to inform subsequent physicians of the prior use of corticosteroids. Occlusive dressings should not be applied if there is an elevation of body temperature.

ADVERSE EFFECTS: When occlusive dressings are used, pustules, miliaria, folloculitis and pyoderma may occur. The following adverse skin reactions have been reported with the use of topical steroids: dryness, itching, burning, local irritation, striae, skin atrophy, hypertrichosis, change in pigmentation and secondary infection. Adrenal suppression has also been reported following topical corticosteroid therapy. Posterior subcapsular cataracts have been reported following systemic use of corticosteroids.

OVERDOSE:

For management of a suspected drug overdose, CPhA recommends that you contact your **regional Poison Control Centre**. See the *CPS* Directory section for a list of Poison Control Centres.

DOSAGE AND ADMINISTRATION: Apply in small quantities to the affected areas 3 or 4 times daily.

SUPPLIED: Cream: Aristocort "C" (0.5%), concentrate, 15 g tubes and 50 g tubes; Aristocort "R" (0.1%), regular, 30 g tubes and 500 g jars. Nonmedicinal ingredients: benzyl alcohol, emulsifying wax, glycerin, isopropyl palmitate, lactic acid, purified water and sorbitol solution.

Ointment: Aristocort "R" (0.1%) regular, 30 g tubes. Nonmedicinal ingredient: white petrolatum. No preservative.

Arixtra® Ⓟ

fondaparinux sodium

Synthetic Antithrombotic

GlaxoSmithKline

Date of Revision: May 26, 2010

SUMMARY PRODUCT INFORMATION:

Route of Administration	Dosage Form/Strength	Nonmedicinal Ingredients
Subcutaneous	Injection/ 2.5 mg/0.5 mL 7.5 mg/0.6 mL	Isotonic solution of sodium chloride, water for injection and if necessary, sodium hydroxide or hydrochloric acid for pH adjustment (pH 5-8).
Intravenous	2.5 mg/0.5 mL	

INDICATIONS AND CLINICAL USE: ARIXTRA (fondaparinux sodium) is indicated for:

- Prophylaxis of venous thromboembolic events (VTE) for up to one month post-surgery in patients undergoing orthopedic surgeries of the lower limbs such as hip fracture, knee surgery or hip replacement surgery.
- Prophylaxis of venous thromboembolic events (VTE) in patients undergoing abdominal surgery who are at high risk of thromboembolic complications, such as patients undergoing abdominal cancer surgery.
- Treatment of Acute Deep Vein Thrombosis (DVT) and treatment of Acute Pulmonary Embolism (PE).
- Management of unstable angina or non-ST segment elevation myocardial infarction (UA/NSTEMI) for the prevention of death and subsequent myocardial infarction.
- Management of ST segment elevation myocardial infarction (STEMI) for the prevention of death and myocardial reinfarction in patients who are managed with thrombolytics or who initially are to receive no form of reperfusion therapy.

Geriatrics (>65 years of age): ARIXTRA should be used with caution in elderly patients due to the risk of hemorrhage.

Pediatrics (<17 years of age): The safety and effectiveness of ARIXTRA in children has not been established.

CONTRAINDICATIONS:

- Patients who are hypersensitive to this drug or to any ingredient in the formulation.
- Thrombocytopenia associated with a positive in vitro test for anti-platelet antibody in the presence of fondaparinux sodium.
- Active clinically significant bleeding.
- Acute bacterial endocarditis.

WARNINGS AND PRECAUTIONS: General: ARIXTRA (fondaparinux sodium) must be administered only by the subcutaneous (SC) or intravenous (IV) route. **ARIXTRA must not be administered intramuscularly.**

Latex Allergy: The needle guard of the pre-filled syringe contains dry natural latex rubber that has the potential to cause allergic reactions in latex sensitive individuals.

Cardiovascular: Risk of catheter thrombosis during PCI: In patients undergoing any percutaneous coronary intervention (PCI), the use of ARIXTRA as the sole anticoagulant during PCI is not recommended because of an increased risk of guiding catheter thrombosis. An effective anti-thrombin regimen such as unfractionated heparin (UFH) should be used as an adjunct to PCI, according to standard practice (see Dosage and Administration).

In STEMI patients undergoing primary PCI for reperfusion, the use of ARIXTRA prior to and during PCI is not recommended (see Adverse Reactions, Risk of Catheter Thrombosis During PCI, and Dosage and Administration).

Clinical trials have shown a low but increased risk of guiding catheter thrombosis in patients treated solely with ARIXTRA for anticoagulation during PCI compared to control. Incidences during PCI in UA/NSTEMI were 1.00% with ARIXTRA, 0.32% with enoxaparin alone, and 0.16% with enoxaparin with adjunctive UFH (see Adverse Reactions, Risk of Catheter Thrombosis During PCI). In patients with STEMI undergoing primary PCI, incidences were 1.18% with ARIXTRA and 0% with UFH. Use of ARIXTRA during primary PCI is not recommended.

It is to be expected that the risk of peri-procedural myocardial infarction (MI) may be increased in patients who develop guiding catheter thrombosis, irrespective of anticoagulant used (see Adverse Reactions, Risk of Catheter Thrombosis During PCI).

Hematologic: Hemorrhage: ARIXTRA, like other antithrombotic drugs, should be used with caution in patients who have an increased risk of hemorrhage, such as those with congenital or acquired bleeding disorders, active ulcerative gastrointestinal disease and recent intracranial hemorrhage or shortly after brain, spinal, or ophthalmological surgery.

Risk of hemorrhage is expected to increase with decreasing renal function (see Adverse Reactions). Appropriate caution should be exercised in patients with moderate to severe renal impairment (see Warnings and Precautions, Renal).

Prophylaxis and Treatment of VTE: Agents that may enhance the risk of hemorrhage, with the exception of vitamin K antagonists used concomitantly for treatment of VTE, should be discontinued prior to initiation of ARIXTRA therapy. If co-administration is necessary, close monitoring may be appropriate (see Drug Interactions).

Prophylaxis of VTE Following Orthopedic or Abdominal Surgery (timing of first fondaparinux injection): The timing of the first dose of ARIXTRA following surgery requires strict adherence. The first dose should be given no earlier than 6 hours following surgical closure, and only after hemostasis has been established. Administration before 6 hours has been associated with an increased risk of major bleeding (see Dosage and Administration). Patient groups at particular risk are those older than 75 years of age, body weight of less than 50 kg or renal impairment with creatinine clearance less than 50 mL/min.

Management of UA/NSTEMI, STEMI: ARIXTRA should be used with caution in patients who are being treated concomitantly with other therapies that increase the risk of hemorrhage (such as GPIIb/IIIa inhibitors or thrombolytics).

Thrombocytopenia: Thrombocytopenia of any degree should be monitored closely. If the platelet count falls below 50 000/mm^3, ARIXTRA should be discontinued. ARIXTRA is contraindicated in patients with thrombocytopenia associated with a positive in vitro test for anti-platelet antibody in the presence of fondaparinux.

Rare spontaneous reports of heparin-induced thrombocytopenia (HIT) in patients treated with fondaparinux have been received.

Prophylaxis of VTE Following Orthopedic or Abdominal Surgery: Thrombocytopenia can occur with the administration of ARIXTRA as well as any major surgical procedure. Moderate thrombocytopenia (platelet counts between 100 000/mm^3 and 50 000/mm^3) occurred at a rate of 3.0% in patients given ARIXTRA 2.5 mg in the peri-operative orthopedic and abdominal surgery clinical trials. Severe thrombocytopenia (platelet counts less than 50 000/ mm^3) occurred at a rate of 0.2% in patients given 2.5 mg in peri-operative clinical trials. During extended prophylaxis no cases of moderate or severe thrombocytopenia were reported (0/327).

Treatment of DVT and PE: Moderate thrombocytopenia occurred at a rate of 0.5% in patients given the ARIXTRA treatment regimen in the DVT and PE treatment clinical trials. Severe thrombocytopenia occurred at a rate of 0.04% in patients given the ARIXTRA treatment regimen.

Hepatic/Biliary/Pancreatic: There is no evidence that fondaparinux is metabolized or eliminated hepatically. Following a single subcutaneous dose of 7.5 mg of ARIXTRA in patients with moderate hepatic impairment (Child-Pugh Category B) compared to subjects with normal liver function, changes from baseline in aPTT, PT/INR, and antithrombin III were similar in the two groups (see Action and Clinical Pharmacology, Special Populations and Conditions, Hepatic Insufficiency). However, a higher incidence of hemorrhage was observed in subjects with moderate hepatic impairment than in normal subjects, especially mild hematomas at the blood sampling or injection site. The pharmacokinetics of fondaparinux have not been studied in patients with severe hepatic impairment. The use of ARIXTRA should be considered with caution because of an increased risk of bleeding due to a deficiency of coagulation factors in patients with severe hepatic insufficiency. Thus, in patients with severe hepatic insufficiency, ARIXTRA should be used only with care.

Peri-operative Considerations: There have been cases of intra-spinal hematomas with the concurrent use of antithrombotics (i.e. low molecular weight heparins) and spinal/epidural anaesthesia resulting in long-term or permanent paralysis. The risk of these events may be higher with the use of post-operative indwelling epidural catheters or by the concomitant use of drugs affecting hemostasis: nonsteroidal anti-inflammatory drugs (NSAIDS), platelet inhibitors, or other drugs affecting coagulation. The risk also appears to be increased by traumatic or repeated epidural or spinal procedure. **ARIXTRA should only be used concurrently with spinal/epidural anaesthesia when the therapeutic benefits to the patients outweigh the possible risks.** Careful vigilance for neurological signs is recommended with rapid diagnosis and treatment, if signs occur.

Renal: The plasma clearance of fondaparinux decreases with the severity of renal impairment, and is associated with an increased risk of hemorrhage (see Action and Clinical Pharmacology, Renal Insufficiency). This has also been observed with all low molecular weight heparins (LMWH).

Prophylaxis of VTE Following Orthopedic or Abdominal Surgery: Occurrences of major bleeding in patients receiving prophylactic therapy following orthopedic surgery with normal renal function, mild renal insufficiency, moderate renal insufficiency and severe renal insufficiency have been found to be 1.6% (25/1565), 2.4% (31/1288), 3.8% (19/504) and 4.8% (4/83) respectively.

Major bleeding in patients receiving prophylactic therapy in abdominal surgery in an active-controlled trial with dalteparin sodium, occurred in 2.1% (13/606) of patients with normal renal function, in 3.6% (22/613) with mild renal impairment, in 6.7% (12/179) with moderate renal impairment, and in 7.1% (1/14) with severe renal impairment.

Therefore, ARIXTRA prophylactic therapy following orthopedic or abdominal surgery is not recommended in patients with severe renal insufficiency (creatinine clearance <30 mL/min) and should be used with caution in patients with moderate renal insufficiency (creatinine clearance 30-50 mL/min) (see Action and Clinical Pharmacology, Renal Insufficiency).

Renal function should be assessed periodically in orthopedic and abdominal surgery patients receiving prophylactic therapy. Consideration of immediate discontinuation of ARIXTRA should be undertaken for patients who develop severe renal insufficiency or labile renal function while on prophylactic therapy. After discontinuation of ARIXTRA prophylactic therapy, its anticoagulant effects may persist for 2-4 days in patients with normal renal function (ie. at least 3-5 half-lives). The anticoagulant effects of ARIXTRA prophylactic therapy may persist even longer in patients with renal insufficiency.

Treatment of DVT and PE: No dosing adjustment is generally necessary in patients with mild to moderate renal insufficiency, however, close monitoring of these patients is recommended. In patients with severe renal impairment (creatinine clearance ≤30 mL/min) use is not recommended due to risk of hemorrhage.

Management of UA/NSTEMI, STEMI: There are limited clinical data available on the use of fondaparinux 2.5 mg once daily in patients with creatinine clearance ≤30 mL/min (see Dosage and Administration and Action and Clinical Pharmacology, Renal Insufficiency).

Special Populations: Low Body Weight: Prophylaxis of VTE Following Orthopedic or Abdominal Surgery: Patients with body weight <50 kg are at increased risk of bleeding. ARIXTRA prophylactic therapy should be used only with caution in patients with body weight <50 kg undergoing orthopedic surgery.

Treatment of DVT and PE: For DVT and PE treatment, patients with body weight <50 kg a daily dose of 5 mg is recommended. In patients with body weight >100 kg a daily dose of 10 mg is recommended (see Dosage and Administration).

Management of UA/NSTEMI, STEMI: Patients with body weight less than 50 kg may be at increased risk of bleeding due to reduced clearance of ARIXTRA. ARIXTRA should be used with caution in patients weighing <50 kg.

Pregnant Women: There are very limited clinical data available on the use of ARIXTRA in pregnant women. Caution should be exercised when prescribing ARIXTRA to pregnant women. ARIXTRA should not be prescribed to pregnant women unless the potential benefit outweighs the risk. Animal studies do not indicate either direct or indirect harmful effects with respect to pregnancy, embryonal/fetal development, parturition or post-natal development.

Nursing Women: Although it is not known whether fondaparinux is excreted in human milk, it has been shown to be excreted in the milk of lactating rat dams. Because many drugs may be excreted in human milk, breast feeding is not recommended during treatment with ARIXTRA.

Pediatrics: The safety and effectiveness of ARIXTRA in children under the age of 17 years has not been established.

Geriatrics (>65 years of age): ARIXTRA should be used with caution in elderly patients because of increased risk of hemorrhage (see Adverse Reactions). Since fondaparinux sodium is substantially excreted by the kidney, risks associated with its use may be expected to be greater in patients with impaired renal function (see Adverse Reactions, and Dosage and Administration). Because elderly patients are more likely to have decreased renal function, it may be useful to monitor renal function (see Warnings and Precautions, Renal).

Monitoring, Laboratory and Coagulation Tests: Since the international standards of heparin or low molecular weight heparins (LMWH) are not appropriate calibrators, the activity of fondaparinux sodium is expressed in milligrams (mg) of the fondaparinux and cannot be compared with activities of heparin or LMWH.

At the 2.5 mg dose, ARIXTRA does not have a clinically relevant effect on routine coagulation tests such as activated partial thromboplastin time (aPTT), activated clotting time (ACT) or prothrombin time (PT)/International Normalized Ratio (INR) tests in plasma. When administered at the recommended prophylactic dose, routine coagulation tests such as PT and aPTT are relatively insensitive measures of ARIXTRA activity, and therefore unsuitable for monitoring. Although monitoring of ARIXTRA is generally not required, the anti-factor Xa assay is the preferred test to measure the anti-coagulant activity of ARIXTRA. Only fondaparinux can be used to calibrate the anti-Xa assay (see Action and Clinical Pharmacology, Mechanism of Action).

If during ARIXTRA therapy, unexpected changes in coagulation parameters or major bleeding occurs, ARIXTRA should be discontinued and a search for other causes such as concomitant medications that could interfere with coagulation, should be undertaken.

ADVERSE REACTIONS: Clinical Trial Adverse Drug Reactions: Because clinical trials are conducted under very specific conditions the adverse reaction rates observed in the clinical trials may not reflect the rates observed in practice and should not be compared to the rates in the clinical trials of another drug. Adverse drug reaction information from clinical trials is useful for identifying drug-related adverse events and for approximating rates.

The data described below reflect experience in over 25 000 patients randomized to ARIXTRA (fondaparinux sodium) Injection in controlled trials of hip fracture, hip replacement, major knee, or abdominal surgeries, treatment of DVT and PE, and the management of UA/NSTEMI and STEMI. Patients received ARIXTRA primarily in two large peri-operative dose-response trials (n=989), four active-controlled peri-operative VTE prophylaxis trials with enoxaparin sodium (n=3616), an extended VTE prophylaxis trial (n=327), an active-controlled VTE prophylaxis trial with dalteparin sodium (n=1425) in abdominal surgery, a dose-response trial (n=111) and an active-controlled trial with enoxaparin sodium in DVT treatment (n=1091); an active-controlled trial with heparin in PE treatment (n=1092), OASIS 5, an active-controlled trial with enoxaparin in the treatment of UA/NSTEMI (n=9979), and OASIS 6, an active and placebo-controlled trial with standard of care in the treatment of STEMI (n=5954).

Hemorrhage: As with any antithrombotic treatment, hemorrhagic manifestations can occur. The incidence of major hemorrhagic complications during ARIXTRA treatment has been low and generally did not differ from that observed with other antithrombotics. In clinical trials or in post-marketing experience, rare cases of intracranial/intracerebral or retroperitoneal bleedings have been reported.

Prophylaxis of VTE Following Orthopedic Surgery: The rates of major bleeding events reported during the orthopedic surgery clinical trials with ARIXTRA 2.5 mg injection are provided in Table 1, Table 2 and Table 3.

Major bleeding from the first active ARIXTRA dose decreased by 26% if the first dose was given 6 hours after surgical closure: major bleeding with ARIXTRA started <6 hours after surgical closure was 2.6% (n=1337) versus major bleeding with ARIXTRA started 6 hours after surgical closure which was 1.9% (n=2230).

Geriatrics: Over 2300 patients, 65 years and older, have received ARIXTRA 2.5 mg in randomized clinical trials in the orthopedic surgery program. In the peri-operative, orthopedic surgery, clinical trials with patients receiving ARIXTRA 2.5 mg, the risk of ARIXTRA-associated non-fatal major bleeding increased with age: 1.8% (23/1253) in patients <65 years, 2.2% (24/1111) in those 65-74 years, and 2.7% (33/1227) in those ≥75 years. Serious adverse events increased with age for patients receiving ARIXTRA. In patients undergoing extended prophylaxis following the first week of therapy, the incidence of ARIXTRA-associated non-fatal major bleeding was: 1.9% (1/52) in patients <65 years, 1.4% (1/71) in those 65-74 years, and 2.9% (6/204) in those ≥75 years.

Prophylaxis of VTE Following Abdominal Surgery: The rates of major bleeding reported during an abdominal surgery clinical trial with ARIXTRA 2.5 mg are provided in Table 4.

Geriatrics: In the abdominal surgery active-controlled clinical trial with dalteparin sodium, the risk of major bleeding associated with use of ARIXTRA increased with age: 3.0% (19/644) in patients <65 years, 3.2% (16/507) in those 65-74 years, and 5.0% (14/282) in those ≥75 years.

Treatment of DVT and PE: The rates of major bleeding events reported during the DVT and PE clinical trials with the ARIXTRA injection treatment regimen are provided in Table 5.

Geriatrics: Over 1200 patients, 65 years and older, have received the ARIXTRA treatment regimen in the DVT and PE treatment clinical trials. In the DVT and PE treatment clinical trials with patients receiving the ARIXTRA treatment regimen, the risk of ARIXTRA-associated non-fatal major bleeding increased with age: 0.6% (7/1151) in patients <65 years, 1.6% (9/560) in those 65-74 years, and 2.1% (12/583) in those ≥75 years. Careful attention to dosing directions and concomitant medications (especially antiplatelet medication) is advised (see Drug Interactions).

Management of UA/NSTEMI: The rates of major bleeding events reported during the management of UA/NSTEMI clinical trials with ARIXTRA 2.5 mg injection are provided in Table 6 and Table 7.

Table 1: ARIXTRA

Summary of Bleeding Results From First Injection up to Day 11–(%) of Patients

Surgery Type		Bleeding	ARIXTRA 2.5 mg Daily (%)	Enoxaparin (%)
Hip Fracture		Major bleeding[a]	18/831 (2.2)	19/842 (2.3)
		Minor bleeding[b]	34 /831 (4.1)	18/842 (2.1)
Knee Replacement		Major bleeding	11 /517 (2.1[e])	1/517 (0.2)
		Minor bleeding	14/517 (2.7)	19/517 (3.7)
Hip Replacement	Study 1[d]	Major bleeding	20/1128 (1.8)	11/1129 (1.0)
		Minor bleeding	17/1128 (1.5)	24/1129 (2.1)
	Study 2[c]	Major bleeding	47/1140 (4.1)	32/1133 (2.8)
		Minor bleeding	44/1140 (3.9)	38/1133 (3.4)

[a] Major bleeding was defined as clinically overt bleeding that was (1) fatal, (2) at a critical site (e.g. Intracranial, retroperitoneal, intra-ocular, pericardial, spinal or into adrenal gland), (3) associated with re-operation or (4) Bleeding Index (BI) ≥2 i.e. BI=drop in hemoglobin (Hb) pre-bleed minus post-bleed + number of units transfused. There were no fatal bleeds or bleeds at a critical site in the ARIXTRA group, and one fatal bleed and one bleed into a critical site in the enoxaparin group.

[b] Minor bleeding was clinically overt bleeding that was not major.

[c] Comparator was Enoxaparin 40 mg o.d.

[d] Comparator was Enoxaparin 30 mg bid.

[e] p value versus enoxaparin is 0.0081.

Table 2: ARIXTRA

Bleeding Across Hip Fracture, Hip Replacement, and Knee Replacement Surgery Studies

	ARIXTRA 2.5 mg SC Once Daily N=3616	Comparator: Enoxaparin Sodium[a] N=3956
Major bleeding[b]	96 (2.7%)	75 (1.9%)
Fatal bleeding	0 (0.0%)	1 (<0.1%)
Non-fatal bleeding at critical site	0 (0.0%)	1 (<0.1%)
Re-operation due to bleeding	12 (0.3%)	10 (0.3%)
Bleeding Index (BI) ≥2[c,e]	84 (2.3%)	63 (1.6%)
Minor bleeding[d]	109 (3.0%)	116 (2.9%)

[a] Enoxaparin Sodium dosing regimen: 30 mg every 12 hours or 40 mg once daily.

[b] Major bleeding was defined as clinically overt bleeding that was (1) fatal (2) bleeding at critical site (e.g. intracranial, retroperitoneal, intra-ocular, pericardial, spinal or into adrenal gland) (3) associated with reoperation at operative site, or (4) with a bleeding index (BI) ≥2.

[c] BI ≥2: overt bleeding associated only with a bleeding index ≥2 [calculated as number of whole blood or packed red blood cells units transfused + [(pre-bleeding) − (post-bleeding)] hemoglobin (g/dL) values].

[d] Minor bleeding was defined as clinically overt bleeding that was not major.

[e] Incidence of BI ≥2 with ARIXTRA across the 4 phase III studies decreased when the first dose was given ≥6 hours after surgical closure.

Table 3: ARIXTRA

Number (Percentage) of Patients with Adjudicated Bleeding Events in Hip Fracture Surgery

	Pre-randomization Open-Label Period (Day 1 to Day 7±1 post-surgery)	Randomized Double-Blind Extended Prophylaxis Period (Day 8 to Day 28±2 post-surgery)	
	ARIXTRA N=737	ARIXTRA N=327	Placebo N=329
Any bleeding	37 (5.0%)	13 (4.0%)	4 (1.2%)
Minor bleeding only[a]	15 (2.0%)	5 (1.5%)	2 (0.6%)
Any major bleeding[b]	22 (3.0%)	8 (2.4%)	2 (0.6%)
Fatal bleeding	2 (0.3%)	0 (0.0%)	0 (0.0%)
Non-fatal bleeding	1 (0.1%)	0 (0.0%)	0 (0.0%)
Other non-fatal major bleeding:	19 (2.6%)	8 (2.4%)	2 (0.6%)
At surgical site leading to Re-operation	3 (0.4%)	2 (0.6%)	2 (0.6%)
Only Bleeding Index (BI) ≥2[c]	16 (2.2%)	6 (1.8%)	0 (0.0%)

[a] Minor bleeding was defined as clinically overt bleeding that was not major.

[b] Major bleeding was defined as clinically overt bleeding that was (1) fatal (2) bleeding at critical site (e.g. intracranial, retroperitoneal, intra-ocular, pericardial, spinal or into adrenal gland) (3) associated with reoperation at operative site, or (4) with a bleeding index (BI) ≥2.

[c] Adjudicated as major and with BI ≥2 and/or decrease of hemoglobin ≥2 g/dL and/or number of units transfused ≥2.

Risk of Catheter Thrombosis During PCI: Clinical trials have shown an increased risk of guiding catheter thrombosis in patients treated solely with ARIXTRA for anticoagulation during percutaneous coronary intervention (PCI) compared to control (see Warnings and Precautions, Cardiovascular). The incidence of catheter thrombosis in UA/NSTEMI patients undergoing PCI were 1.00% (29/2888) with ARIXTRA, 0.32% (6/1883) with enoxaparin alone, and 0.16% (2/1286) with enoxaparin with adjunctive UFH. In OASIS 5, patients randomized to ARIXTRA received ARIXTRA as the sole adjunctive therapy during PCI whereas enoxaparin subjects received enoxaparin with or without UFH during PCI based on the timing since the last subcutaneous injection of enoxaparin.

ARIXTRA should not be used as the sole anticoagulant during PCI because of an increased risk of guiding catheter thrombosis. An effective anti-thrombin regimen such as unfractionated heparin (UFH) should be administered as an adjunct to PCI according to standard practice.

Geriatrics: Over 6000 UA/NSTEMI patients, 65 years or older, received treatment with ARIXTRA. In the UA/NSTEMI clinical trials with patients receiving ARIXTRA, the risk of major bleeding was: 1.3% (50/3885) in patients <65 years, 2.4% (89/3644) in those 65-74 years, and 2.9% (71/2450) in those ≥75 years.

Management of STEMI: The rates of major bleeding events reported during the management of STEMI clinical trials with ARIXTRA 2.5 mg injection are provided in Table 8.

Table 4: ARIXTRA

Major and Non-major Bleeding Episodes[a] in a Randomized, Controlled, Abdominal Surgery Study

	Study 1	
	ARIXTRA 2.5 mg SC Once Daily N=1433	**Dalteparin Sodium 5000 IU SC Once Daily N=1425**
Major bleeding[a]	49 (3.4%)	34 (2.4%)
Fatal bleeding	2 (0.1%)	2 (0.1%)
Non-fatal bleeding at critical site	0 (0.0%)	0 (0.0%)
Other non-fatal major bleeding		
Surgical site	38 (2.7%)	26 (1.8%)
Non-surgical site	9 (0.6%)	6 (0.4%)
Minor bleeding[b]	31 (2.2%)	23 (1.6%)

[a] Major bleeding was defined as bleeding that was (1) fatal, (2) bleeding at the surgical site leading to intervention, (3) non-surgical bleeding at a critical site (eg. intracranial, retroperitoneal, intra-ocular, pericardial, spinal, or into adrenal gland), or leading to an intervention, and/or with a bleeding index (BI ≥2 calculated as [number of whole blood or packed red blood cell unites transfused + [(pre-bleeding) – (post-bleeding)] hemoglobin (g/dL) values]).

[b] Minor bleeding was defined as clinically overt bleeding that was not major.

Table 5: ARIXTRA

Major Bleeding Episodes[a,b] in DVT and PE Treatment Studies

Indications	ARIXTRA Treatment Regimen N=2294	Enoxaparin Sodium[a] mg/kg SC q 12h N=1101	Heparin IV aPTT Adjusted N=1092
DVT and PE Treatment	28 (1.2%)	13 (1.2%)	12 (1.1%)

[a] Major bleeding was defined as clinically overt—and/or contributing to death—and/or in a critical organ including intracranial, retroperitoneal, intraocular, spinal, pericardial or adrenal gland—and/or associated with a fall in hemoglobin level = 2 g/dL—and/or leading to a transfusion ≥2 units of packed red blood cells or whole blood.

[b] Bleeding rates are during the study drug treatment period (approximately 7 days). Patients were also treated with vitamin K antagonists initiated within 72 hours after the first study drug administration.

Table 6: ARIXTRA

Bleeding Episodes in OASIS 5, a Randomized, Controlled Study in UA/NSTEMI[e]

	Up to 9 Days After Presenting with UA/NSTEMI	
	ARIXTRA[e] N=9979	**Enoxaparin[f] N=9969**
Investigator Reported Major Bleeding[a]	205 (2.1%)	410 (4.1%)
Fatal bleeding	7 (<0.1%)	22 (0.2%)
Intracranial	7 (<0.1%)	7 (<0.1%)
Retroperitoneal	9 (<0.1%)	36 (0.4%)
Requiring surgical intervention	39 (0.4%)	78 (0.8%)
Drop in hemoglobin ≥3 g/dL	189 (1.9%)	385 (3.9%)
Blood transfusion ≥2 units	156 (1.6%)	280 (2.8%)
Modified TIMI Severe Hemorrhage[b]	148 (1.5%)	260 (2.6%)
Minor Bleeding[c]	115 (1.2%)	320 (3.2%)
PCI-related bleed[d]	82 (0.8%)	183 (1.8%)
CABG-related bleed[d]	86 (0.9%)	72 (0.7%)

[a] Major bleeding was defined as clinically overt bleeding with at least one of the following criteria: fatal, symptomatic intracranial hemorrhage, retroperitoneal hemorrhage, intraocular hemorrhage leading to significant vision loss, bleeding requiring surgical intervention, decrease in Hb of ≥3 g/dL, or blood transfusion ≥2 units.

[b] Modified TIMI severe hemorrhage was defined as fatal hemorrhage, intracranial hemorrhage, cardiac tamponade, or a clinically significant hemorrhage with a decrease in Hb of >5 g/dL.

[c] Minor bleeding was defined as clinically overt bleeding that was not major and that led to interruption of study drug for at least 24 hours, or transfusion of one unit of blood.

[d] The number of patients undergoing PCI was 3422 for ARIXTRA and 3410 for enoxaparin and the number of patients undergoing CABG was 956 for ARIXTRA and 886 for enoxaparin.

[e] Patients randomized to ARIXTRA received 2.5 mg fondaparinux SC once daily for up to 8 days or discharge.

[f] Patients randomized to enoxaparin sodium received 1 mg/kg enoxaparin SC twice daily (once daily if creatinine clearance was between 20 mL/min and 30 mL/min) for 2-8 days or until clinically stable.

In those patients who underwent non-primary PCI <6 hours after the last dose of fondaparinux, the median dose of UFH used was 5000 IU and the incidence of major bleeding was 4.1% (2/49). In those patients who underwent non-primary PCI 6-24 hours after the last dose of fondaparinux, the median dose of UFH was 8000 IU and the incidence of major bleeding was 2% (2/98).

The relative effects of ARIXTRA compared to control on severe hemorrhage or any hemorrhage up to Day 9 by clopidogrel use were consistent with that observed for the overall population.

Table 7: ARIXTRA

Incidence of Adjudicated Major Bleeding in OASIS 5 at Day 9 in UA/NSTEMI Patients Treated with ARIXTRA by Renal Function Status at Baseline

Covariate Endpoint/ Timepoint	Number Events/Number Analyzed		OR/HR[a] (95% CI)	Interaction p-value[d]
	ARIXTRA[b]	**Enoxaparin[c]**		
On therapy	183/9943 (1.8%)	388/9928 (3.9%)	0.46 (0.38, 0.55)	0.343
<20 mL/min	1/40 (2.5%)	5/43 (11.6%)	0.19 (0.02, 1.75)	
≥20–<30 mL/min	4/240 (1.7%)	19/239 (7.9%)	0.20 (0.07, 0.59)	
≥30–<50 mL/min	47/1649 (2.9%)	104/1715 (6.1%)	0.45 (0.32, 0.65)	
≥50–<80 mL/min	93/4257 (2.2%)	185/4188 (4.4%)	0.48 (0.38, 0.62)	
≥80 mL/min	38/3757 (1.0%)	75/3743 (2.0%)	0.50 (0.34, 0.74)	
Creatinine clearance not recorded	0/36	1/41 (2.4%)		
Day 9	209/9979 (2.1%)	405/9969 (4.1%)	0.51 (0.43, 0.60)	0.248
<20 mL/min	2/40 (5.0%)	5/43 (11.6%)	0.41 (0.08, 2.11)	
≥20–<30 mL/min	4/240 (1.7%)	21/239 (8.8%)	0.19 (0.06, 0.54)	
≥30–<50 mL/min	54/1649 (3.3%)	107/1715 (6.2%)	0.52 (0.37, 0.71)	
≥50–<80 mL/min	103/4257 (2.4%)	193/4188 (4.6%)	0.52 (0.41, 0.66)	
≥80 mL/min	46/3757 (1.2%)	79/3743 (2.1%)	0.58 (0.40, 0.83)	
Creatinine clearance not recorded	0/36	1/41 (2.4%)		

[a] Odds ratio for the on-therapy analysis; hazard ratio for the Day 9 analysis.

[b] Patients randomized to ARIXTRA received 2.5 mg fondaparinux SC once daily for up to 8 days or discharge.

[c] Patients randomized to enoxaparin sodium received 1 mg/kg enoxaparin SC twice daily (once daily if creatinine clearance was between 20 mL/min and 30 mL/min) for 2–8 days or until clinically stable.

[d] Treatment by Covariate Interaction (test for homogeneity of treatment effect).

Note: Creatinine clearance was included as a continuous variable in the estimate of the overall hazard/odds ratio and covariate p-value.

Risk of Catheter Thrombosis During PCI: Clinical trials have shown an increased risk of guiding catheter thrombosis in patients treated solely with ARIXTRA for anticoagulation during percutaneous coronary intervention (PCI) compared to control (see Warnings and Precautions, Cardiovascular). The incidence of catheter thrombus in STEMI patients undergoing primary PCI were 1.18% (22/1862) for ARIXTRA, when ARIXTRA was used as the sole adjunctive therapy, compared to 0% for UFH (0/1853). In STEMI patients treated with ARIXTRA undergoing non-primary PCI (234 patients, 238 procedures) who received UFH as an adjunct to the procedure, no cases of guiding catheter thrombus occurred.

In STEMI patients undergoing primary percutaneous coronary intervention (PCI) for reperfusion, the use of ARIXTRA prior to and during PCI is not recommended (see Adverse Reactions, Risk of catheter thrombosis during PCI, and Dosage and Administration).

Geriatrics: Over 2300 STEMI patients, 65 years or older, received treatment with ARIXTRA. In the STEMI clinical trials with patients receiving ARIXTRA, the risk of severe hemorrhage was: 0.6% (22/3565) in patients <65 years, 1.5% (23/1518) in those 65-74 years, and 2.2% (19/871) in those ≥75 years.

Other, Non-hemorrhagic Events: Other adverse events that occurred during treatment with ARIXTRA or enoxaparin sodium in clinical trials with patients undergoing hip fracture surgery, hip replacement surgery, or knee replacement surgery and that occurred at a rate of at least 2% in either treatment group, are provided in Table 9 and Table 10.

Other adverse events that occurred during treatment with ARIXTRA or dalteparin sodium in a clinical trial with patients undergoing abdominal surgery that occurred at a rate of at least 2% in either treatment group are provided in Table 11.

Other adverse events that occurred during treatment with ARIXTRA, enoxaparin sodium or heparin in the DVT and PE treatment clinical trials and that occurred at a rate of at least 2% in any treatment group are provided in Table 12.

Adverse events that occurred during treatment with ARIXTRA in acute coronary syndromes are described in Table 13.

Thrombocytopenia: See Warnings and Precautions, Hematologic.

Liver Function Tests: Prophylaxis of VTE Following Orthopedic Surgery: Transient elevation of liver transaminases (AST and ALT) to >3 times the upper limit of laboratory range have been observed with the peri-operative prophylactic use of ARIXTRA as have been seen with other antithrombotics such as low molecular weight heparins. Such elevations are fully reversible and are rarely associated with increases in bilirubin. Transient transaminase increases >3 times upper limit of laboratory range during the extended prophylaxis clinical trial were as follows: ALT–4 /272 (1.5%) ARIXTRA vs. 2 /274 (0.7%) placebo; AST–2 /268 (0.7%) ARIXTRA vs. 1/ 271 (0.4%) placebo. However, these increases were reversible and there was no significant difference in the change in the hepatic enzymes between the two treatment groups from the baseline post-randomization period to the last value on double blind treatment.

Treatment of DVT and PE: In the DVT and PE treatment clinical trials asymptomatic increases in AST and ALT levels >3 times the upper limit of normal of the laboratory reference range have been reported in 0.7% and 1.3% of patients, respectively, during the ARIXTRA injection treatment regimen.

In comparison, these increases have been reported in 4.8% and 12.3% of patients, respectively, in the DVT treatment trial during treatment with enoxaparin sodium 1 mg/kg every 12 hours, and in 2.9% and 8.7% of patients, respectively, in the PE treatment trial during treatment with aPTT adjusted heparin.

Allergic Reaction: Skin rash and allergic reactions are rare but occur with many antithrombotics. As with any subcutaneous injection, mild local irritation (injection site bleeding, rash and pruritus) may occur following subcutaneous injection of ARIXTRA.

Post-Market Adverse Drug Reactions: The following adverse reactions have been identified during post-approval use of ARIXTRA.

Rare spontaneous reports of elevated aPTT have been received at the 2.5 mg dose. A causal association between treatment with fondaparinux and the occurrence of elevated aPTT has not been established.

DRUG INTERACTIONS: Drug-Drug Interactions: In clinical studies performed with ARIXTRA (fondaparinux sodium), the concomitant use of oral anticoagulants (warfarin), platelet inhibitors (acetylsalicylic acid), NSAIDs (piroxicam) and digoxin did not interact with the pharmacokinetics/pharmacodynamics of ARIXTRA. In addition, ARIXTRA neither influenced the pharmacodynamics of warfarin, acetylsalicylic acid, piroxicam and digoxin, nor the pharmacokinetics of digoxin at steady state.

Agents that may enhance the risk of hemorrhage should be discontinued prior to initiation of ARIXTRA therapy unless indicated for the management of the underlying condition, such as vitamin K antagonists for the treatment of venous thromboembolism (VTE). If co-administration is necessary, close monitoring may be appropriate.

Since fondaparinux does not inhibit CYP450s (CYP1A2, CYP2A6, CYP2C9, CYP2C19, CYP2D6, CYP2E1 or CYP3A4) in vitro, ARIXTRA is not expected to interact with other drugs metabolized in vivo via these isoenzymes.

ARIXTRA does not bind significantly to plasma proteins other than ATIII, therefore, drug interactions by protein binding displacement are not expected.

Drug-Food Interactions: Interactions with food have not been established.

Drug-Herb Interactions: Interactions with herbal products have not been established.

Drug-Laboratory Interactions: See Warnings and Precautions, Monitoring, Laboratory and Coagulation Tests.

Table 8: ARIXTRA

Bleeding Episodes[a,b] in OASIS 6, Randomized, Controlled Study in STEMI[c]

	Up to 9 Days After Presenting with STEMI (Number (%) Subjects)					
	Overall		Stratum 1		Stratum 2	
Investigator Reported Bleeding Events	ARIXTRA[c] N=5954	Control (UFH/placebo) N=5947	ARIXTRA[c] N=2808	Placebo N=2818	ARIXTRA[c] N=3146	UFH N=3129
Modified TIMI Severe Hemorrhage[a]	78 (1.3%)	94 (1.6%)	34 (1.2%)	48 (1.7%)	44 (1.4%)	46 (1.5%)
Fatal	35 (0.6%)	48 (0.8%)	19 (0.7%)	32 (1.1%)	16 (0.5%)	16 (0.5%)
Intracranial	12 (0.2%)	12 (0.2%)	6 (0.2%)	7 (0.2%)	6 (0.2%)	5 (0.2%)
Cardiac tamponade	26 (0.4%)	47 (0.8%)	15 (0.5%)	30 (1.1%)	11 (0.3%)	17 (0.5%)
Drop in Hgb ≥5 g/dL	37 (0.6%)	34 (0.6%)	12 (0.4%)	10 (0.4%)	25 (0.8%)	24 (0.8%)
By Reperfusion strategy						
No reperfusion	13/1415 (0.9%)	20/1367 (1.5%)	3/620 (0.5%)	5/599 (0.8%)	10/795 (1.3%)	15/768 (2.0%)
Thrombolytic group	34/2676 (1.3%)	55/2711 (2.0%)	25/2182 (1.1%)	41/2214 (1.9%)	9/494 (1.8%)	14/497 (2.8%)
Primary PCI	17/1863 (0.9%)	8/1869 (0.4%)	0/6	0/5	17/1857 (0.9%)	8/1864 (0.4%)
Major Bleeding[b]	104 (1.7%)	131 (2.2%)	40 (1.4%)	61 (2.2%)	64 (2.0%)	70 (2.2%)
Minor Bleeding	37 (0.6%)	23 (0.4%)	19 (0.7%)	6 (0.2%)	18 (0.6%)	17 (0.5%)
PCI related bleeding	45 (0.8%)	47 (0.8%)	7 (0.2%)	3 (0.1%)	38 (1.2%)	44 (1.4%)
CABG related bleeding	3 (<0.1%)	6 (0.1%)	1 (<0.1%)	3 (0.1%)	2 (<0.1%)	3 (<0.1%)

[a] Severe hemorrhage was defined according to a modified TIMI criteria as: fatal hemorrhage, intracranial hemorrhage, cardiac tamponade, or a clinically significant hemorrhage with a decrease in Hb of >5 g/dL.
[b] Major bleeding was defined as clinically overt bleeding with at least one of the following criteria: fatal, symptomatic intracranial hemorrhage, retroperitoneal hemorrhage, intraocular hemorrhage leading to significant vision loss, bleeding requiring surgical intervention, decrease in Hb of >3.0 g/dL, or blood transfusion ≥2 units.
[c] Patients randomized to ARIXTRA received an IV bolus injection of 2.5 mg followed by 2.5 mg by SC injection daily for up to 8 days or discharge.

Table 9: ARIXTRA

Adverse Events Occurring in ≥2% of ARIXTRA or Enoxaparin Sodium Treated Patients Regardless of Relationship to Study Drug Across Hip Fracture, Hip Replacement Surgery, or Knee Replacement Surgery Studies

Adverse Events	ARIXTRA 2.5 mg SC Once Daily N=3616 %	Comparator: Low Molecular Weight Heparin or Enoxaparin Sodium[a] N=3956 %
Anemia	19.6	16.9
Fever	13.6	15.4
Nausea	11.3	12.2
Edema	8.7	8.8
Constipation	8.5	10.5
Rash	7.5	8.3
Vomiting	5.9	6.0
Insomnia	5.0	5.4
Wound drainage increased	4.5	4.7
Hypokalemia	4.2	4.1
Urinary tract infection	3.8	3.4
Dizziness	3.6	4.2
Purpura	3.5	3.5
Hypotension	3.5	3.2
Confusion	3.1	3.3
Bullous eruption	3.1	2.6
Urinary retention	2.9	3.0
Hematoma	2.8	2.8
Diarrhea	2.5	2.6
Dyspepsia	2.4	2.6
Post-operative hemorrhage	2.4	1.7
Headache	2.0	2.5
Pain	1.7	2.6

[a] Enoxaparin Sodium dosing regimen: 30 mg every 12 hours or 40 mg once daily.

Table 10: ARIXTRA

Adverse Events Occurring in ≥2% of ARIXTRA or Placebo Treated Patients Regardless of Relationship to Study Drug During Pre-randomization Open Label Period and Extended Prophylaxis Period After Hip Fracture Surgery

	Pre-randomization Open-Label Period (Day 1 to Day 7±1 post-surgery)	Randomized Double-Blind Extended Prophylaxis Period (Day 8 to Day 28±2 post-surgery)	
Adverse Events	ARIXTRA N=737 %	ARIXTRA N=327 %	Placebo SC N=329 %
Constipation	7.1	1.8	2.1
Anemia	5.8	1.5	1.2
Nausea	4.6	0.3	1.2
Confusion	4.1	1.2	0.3
Fever	4.1	0.3	1.2
Urinary tract infection	3.1	4.0	4.0
Vomiting	2.7	0.6	1.2
Post-operative hemorrhage	2.4	0.6	0.6
Hematoma	1.2	2.1	0.3
Surgical site reaction	0.7	1.5	2.4
Diarrhea	0.5	1.8	2.4

Table 11: ARIXTRA

Adverse Events Occurring in ≥2% of Patients Treated with ARIXTRA or Dalteparin Sodium Undergoing Abdominal Surgery Regardless of Relationship to Study Drug

Adverse Events	ARIXTRA 2.5 mg SC Once Daily N=1433	Dalteparin Sodium 5000 IU SC Once Daily N=1425
Post-operative wound infection	4.9%	4.8%
Post-operative haemorrhage	4.3%	2.9%
Fever	3.7%	3.8%
Surgical site reaction	3.2%	2.8%
Anaemia	2.4%	1.8%
Hypertension	2.4%	2.9%
Pneumonia	2.3%	1.6%

(cont'd)

Table 11: ARIXTRA *(cont'd)*

Adverse Events Occurring in ≥2% of Patients Treated with ARIXTRA or Dalteparin Sodium Undergoing Abdominal Surgery Regardless of Relationship to Study Drug

Adverse Events	ARIXTRA 2.5 mg SC Once Daily N=1433	Dalteparin Sodium 5000 IU SC Once Daily N=1425
Vomiting	2.2%	1.8%

Table 12: ARIXTRA

Adverse Events Occurring in ≥2% of ARIXTRA or Enoxaparin Sodium or Heparin Treated Patients Regardless of Relationship to Study Drug Across VTE Treatment Studies

Adverse Events	ARIXTRA Treatment Regimen N=2294	Enoxaparin Sodium 1 mg/kg SC q 12h N=1101	Heparin IV aPTT Adjusted N=1092
Constipation	106 (4.6%)	32 (2.9%)	93 (8.5%)
Headache	104 (4.5%)	37 (3.4%)	65 (6.0%)
Insomnia	86 (3.7%)	19 (1.7%)	75 (6.9%)
Fever	81 (3.5%)	32 (2.9%)	47 (4.3%)
Nausea	76 (3.3%)	29 (2.6%)	53 (4.9%)
Urinary Tract Infection	53 (2.3%)	20 (1.8%)	24 (2.2%)
Coughing	48 (2.1%)	7 (0.6%)	26 (2.4%)
Diarrhea	43 (1.9%)	22 (2.0%)	27 (2.5%)
Abdominal Pain	33 (1.4%)	14 (1.3%)	28 (2.6%)
Chest Pain	33 (1.4%)	8 (0.7%)	26 (2.4%)
Leg Pain	31 (1.4%)	10 (0.9%)	22 (2.0%)
Back Pain	30 (1.3%)	11 (1.0%)	34 (3.1%)
Epistaxis	30 (1.3%)	12 (1.1%)	41 (3.8%)
Prothrombin decreased	30 (1.3%)	3 (0.3%)	34 (3.1%)
Anemia	28 (1.2%)	3 (0.3%)	23 (2.1%)
Vomiting	26 (1.1%)	14 (1.3%)	27 (2.5%)
Hypokalemia	25 (1.1%)	2 (0.2%)	23 (2.1%)
Bruise	24 (1.0%)	24 (2.2%)	14 (1.3%)
Anxiety	18 (0.8%)	8 (0.7%)	22 (2.0%)
Hepatic Function abnormal	10 (0.4%)	14 (1.3%)	24 (2.2%)
Hepatic Enzymes increased	7 (0.3%)	52 (4.7%)	30 (2.7%)
ALT increased	7 (0.3%)	47 (4.3%)	8 (0.7%)
AST increased	4 (0.2%)	31 (2.8%)	3 (0.3%)

DOSAGE AND ADMINISTRATION: Recommended Dose and Dosage Adjustment: Prophylaxis of VTE following Orthopaedic Surgery: The recommended dose of ARIXTRA (fondaparinux sodium) is 2.5 mg once daily administered post-operatively by subcutaneous injection.

After hemostasis has been established, the initial dose should be given no earlier than 6 hours after surgical closure. In clinical studies, 99% of the patients had received the initial dose of ARIXTRA by 18 hours after surgical closure. **Administration before 6 hours after orthopedic surgery has been associated with an increased risk of major bleeding.** The timing of the first dose of ARIXTRA following surgery requires strict adherence (see Warning and Precautions, Hemorrhage, and Peri-operative Considerations; Action and Clinical Pharmacology).

The usual duration of prophylactic therapy with ARIXTRA is 7±2 days. Treatment should be continued for as long as the risk of VTE persists. In patients for whom extended prophylaxis is indicated, administration of ARIXTRA in or out of the hospital up to an additional 24 days is recommended. In clinical trials of extended prophylaxis, a total of 32 days (peri-operative and extended prophylaxis) has been tolerated.

Prophylaxis of VTE Following Abdominal Surgery: The recommended dose of ARIXTRA is 2.5 mg once daily administered post-operatively by subcutaneous injection after hemostasis has been established.

The initial dose should be given 6 to 8 hours after surgery. **Administration before 6 hours after abdominal surgery has been associated with an increased risk of major bleeding.** The timing of the first dose of ARIXTRA following surgery requires strict adherence (see Warnings and Precautions, Hemorrhage, and Peri-operative Considerations; Action and Clinical Pharmacology).

The usual duration of administration is 5 to 9 days, and up to 10 days of ARIXTRA injection has been administered.

Treatment of DVT and PE: The recommended dose of ARIXTRA is 5 mg (body weight <50 kg), 7.5 mg (body weight 50-100 kg) or 10 mg (body weight >100 kg) by subcutaneous injection once daily.

Concomitant oral anticoagulation treatment should be initiated as soon as possible, usually within 72 hours. ARIXTRA injection treatment should be continued for at least 5 days and until a therapeutic oral anticoagulant effect is established (INR 2.0 to 3.0).

The average duration of administration is 7 days. In controlled clinical trials administration of ARIXTRA injection for up to 26 days to a small number of patients has been well tolerated.

Management of Unstable Angina/Non-ST Segment Elevation Myocardial Infarction (UA/NSTEMI): The recommended dose of ARIXTRA is 2.5 mg once daily, administered by subcutaneous injection. Treatment should be initiated as soon as possible following diagnosis and may be continued for up to 8 days or until hospital discharge.

If a patient is to undergo percutaneous coronary intervention (PCI) while being treated with ARIXTRA, an effective anti-thrombin regimen such as unfractionated heparin (UFH) should be administered as an adjunct to PCI, as per standard practice, taking into account the patient's potential risk of bleeding, including the time since the last dose of ARIXTRA (see Warnings and Precautions, Risk of catheter thrombosis during PCI, and Hemorrhage).

The timing of restarting subcutaneous ARIXTRA after sheath removal should be based on clinical judgment. In the UA/NSTEMI clinical trials treatment with ARIXTRA was restarted no earlier than 2 hours after sheath removal.

In patients who are to undergo coronary artery bypass graft (CABG) surgery, ARIXTRA where possible, should not be given during the 24 hours before surgery and may be restarted 48 hours post-operatively.

Management of ST Segment Elevation Myocardial Infarction (STEMI): The recommended dose of ARIXTRA is 2.5 mg once daily. The first dose of ARIXTRA is administered intravenously and subsequent doses are administered by subcutaneous injection. Treatment should be initiated as soon as possible following diagnosis and continued for up to 8 days or until hospital discharge.

ARIXTRA should not be used if primary PCI is the planned reperfusion therapy (see Indications and Clinical Use, and Warnings and Precautions, Risk of catheter thrombosis during PCI). ARIXTRA is indicated for use in patients who are managed with thrombolytics or who initially are to receive no form of reperfusion therapy.

If a patient is to undergo subsequent PCI while being treated with ARIXTRA, an effective anti-thrombin regimen such as unfractionated heparin (UFH) should be administered as an adjunct to PCI as per standard practice, taking into account the patient's potential risk of bleeding, including the time since the last dose of ARIXTRA (see Warnings and Precautions, Risk of catheter thrombosis during PCI, and Hemorrhage).

There are limited data on the use of UFH during non-primary PCI in patients treated with fondaparinux. In those patients with STEMI who underwent non-primary PCI in OASIS-6 less than 6 hours after the last dose of fondaparinux, the median dose of UFH was 5000 IU and the incidence of major bleeding was 4.1% (2/49). In those patients who underwent non-primary PCI 6-24 hours after the last dose of fondaparinux, the median dose of UFH was 8000 IU and the incidence of major bleeding was 2% (2/98).

The timing of restarting subcutaneous fondaparinux after sheath removal should be based on clinical judgment. In the STEMI clinical trials treatment with fondaparinux was restarted no earlier than 3 hours after sheath removal.

In patients who are to undergo coronary artery bypass graft (CABG) surgery, fondaparinux where possible, should not be given during the 24 hours before surgery and may be restarted 48 hours post-operatively.

General Dosing Considerations: Use in Patients with Renal Insufficiency: The risk of hemorrhage increases with increasing renal insufficiency. ARIXTRA should be used with caution in patients with moderate renal insufficiency (creatinine clearance 30-50 mL/min) (see Action and Clinical Pharmacology, Renal Insufficiency). In severe renal impairment, the use of ARIXTRA should be avoided or, if the physician determines that the benefit outweighs the risk, ARIXTRA should only be used with caution.

Renal function should be assessed periodically in patients receiving the drug. For prophylactic use following orthopedic surgery, ARIXTRA should be discontinued immediately in patients who develop severe renal insufficiency or labile renal function while on therapy. After discontinuation of ARIXTRA, its anticoagulant effects may persist for 2-4 days in patients with normal renal function (i.e., at least 3-5 half-lives). The anticoagulant effects of ARIXTRA may persist even longer in patients with renal insufficiency.

Use in Patients with Hepatic Insufficiency: No dose adjustment is recommended in patients with mild to moderate hepatic impairment, based upon single-dose pharmacokinetic data. Pharmacokinetic data are not available for patients with severe hepatic impairment. Patients with hepatic impairment may be particularly vulnerable to bleeding during ARIXTRA therapy. Observe these patients closely for signs and symptoms of bleeding (see Warnings and Precautions).

Use in Geriatric Patients: Use with caution in elderly patients (see Warnings and Precautions, Geriatrics (>65 years of age), and Adverse Reactions, Geriatrics).

Use in Patients with Low Body Weight: For patients of body weight <50 kg, ARIXTRA should be used with caution (see Warnings and Precautions, Low Body Weight).

Administration: Subcutaneous Administration: Administration is by subcutaneous injection only. **Do not inject ARIXTRA intramuscularly.**

Table 13: ARIXTRA

Adverse Events Occurring in ≥2% of ARIXTRA or Control[a] Treated Patients Regardless of Relationship to Study Drug Across Studies of UA/NSTEMI and STEMI

	Number (%) Subjects									
	OASIS 5		OASIS 6							
			Overall		Stratum 1		Stratum 2			
	ARIXTRA N=9979	Enoxaparin N=9969	ARIXTRA N=5954	Control[a] N=5947	ARIXTRA N=2808	Placebo N=2818	ARIXTRA N=3146	UFH N=3129		
Any AE[b]	2426 (24)	2785 (28)	1933 (32)	1959 (33)	922 (33)	954 (34)	1011 (32)	1005 (32)		
Headache	227 (2)	226 (2)	105 (2)	118 (2)	60 (2)	63 (2)	45 (1)	55 (2)		
Atrial fibrillation	103 (1)	124 (1)	164 (3)	126 (2)	69 (2)	57 (2)	95 (3)	69 (2)		
Pyrexia	96 (<1)	110 (1)	189 (3)	200 (3)	119 (4)	125 (4)	70 (2)	75 (2)		
Chest pain	148 (1)	147 (1)	108 (2)	79 (1)	50 (2)	42 (1)	58 (2)	37 (1)		
Vomiting	50 (<1)	62 (<1)	74 (1)	74 (1)	47 (2)	42 (1)	27 (1)	32 (1)		
Ventricular tachycardia	35 (<1)	28 (<1)	76 (1)	81 (1)	26 (<1)	29 (1)	50 (2)	52 (2)		

[a] OASIS 5 is a study in UA/NSTEMI and OASIS 6 is a study in STEMI. Control for the OASIS 5 study was enoxaparin and for the OASIS 6 study was placebo or UFH.
[b] Includes any efficacy outcomes (except hemorrhagic stroke), non-fatal cardiac arrest and heart failure reported as AEs by the investigator in contravention of the protocol.

To avoid the loss of medicinal product when using the pre-filled syringe do not expel the air bubble from the syringe before the injection. For step-by-step instructions for use, please see Information for the Patient.

Intravenous Administration: For STEMI patients treated with ARIXTRA, the initial dose is to be administered intravenously. Administration should be through an existing intravenous line either directly or using a small volume (25 mL or 50 mL) 0.9% saline minibag as the first dose in the treatment of STEMI.

To avoid the loss of medicinal product when using the pre-filled syringe, do not expel the air bubble from the syringe before the injection. The intravenous tubing should be well flushed with saline after the administration of ARIXTRA injection to ensure that all of the medicinal product is administered. If administered via a minibag, the infusion should be given over 1 to 2 minutes.

If ARIXTRA is added to a 0.9% saline minibag it should be infused immediately, but can be stored between 15-30°C for up to 24 hours. Minibags are typically composed of a variety of polymers including PVC, polyethylene, polypropylene, or styrene-ethylene-butadiene, individually or in combination.

In the absence of compatibility studies, ARIXTRA must not be mixed with other medicinal products.

OVERDOSAGE:

For management of a suspected drug overdose, contact your regional Poison Control Centre. See the *CPS* Directory section for a list of Poison Control Centres.

Hemorrhage is the major clinical sign of overdosage. Minor bleeding rarely requires specific therapy, and reducing or delaying subsequent doses of ARIXTRA (fondaparinux sodium) is usually sufficient.

Overdosage associated with bleeding complications should lead to treatment discontinuation, search for the primary cause of bleeding and initiation of appropriate therapy.

ACTION AND CLINICAL PHARMACOLOGY: Mechanism of Action: ARIXTRA (fondaparinux sodium) Injection is a synthetic and specific inhibitor of activated Factor X (Xa). As ARIXTRA has no animal-sourced components, there is no risk of animal contamination such as transmissable spongiform encephalitis (TSE).

The mechanism of action of ARIXTRA is the potentiation of antithrombin III (ATIII) which selectively inhibits Factor Xa. By selectively binding to ATIII, ARIXTRA potentiates approximately 300 times the neutralization of Factor Xa. Neutralization of Factor Xa interrupts the blood coagulation cascade and thus inhibits thrombin formation and thrombus development.

ARIXTRA does not inactivate thrombin (activated Factor II) and has no effect on platelets. At the recommended dose, ARIXTRA does not affect fibrinolytic activity or bleeding time.

At equivalent antithrombotic concentrations, experimental bleeding models demonstrate that ARIXTRA induces less bleeding than unfractionated heparin.

ARIXTRA does not bind to Human Platelet Factor 4 (unlike heparin) and does not cross-react with sera from patients with heparin-induced thrombocytopenia. No thrombocytopenia with suspected immuno-allergic pathophysiology was documented in the overall clinical development program.

Anti-Xa Activity: The pharmacodynamics/pharmacokinetics of fondaparinux sodium are derived from fondaparinux plasma concentrations quantified via anti-Factor Xa activity. Only fondaparinux can be used to calibrate the anti-Xa assay. (The international standards of heparin or Low Molecular Weight Heparin [LMWH] are not appropriate for this use). As a result, the activity of fondaparinux sodium is expressed as milligram (mg) of the fondaparinux calibrator. The anti-Xa activity of the drug increases with increasing drug concentration, reaching maximum values in approximately 3 hours.

Pharmacokinetics: Absorption: Following a single 4 mg i.v. bolus administration to normal healthy subjects, mean peak fondaparinux plasma concentration is approximately 0.81 mg/L at the first sampling time point of 5 minutes. After subcutaneous dosing, fondaparinux is completely and rapidly absorbed, with an absolute bioavailability of 100%. Following a single subcutaneous injection of 2.5 mg, peak plasma concentration (C_{max}=0.34 mg/L) is obtained 2 hours post-dosing. Plasma concentrations of half the mean C_{max} values are reached 25 minutes post-dosing.

Pharmacokinetics of fondaparinux are linear in the range of 2 to 8 mg by the subcutaneous route. At steady state, mean plasma concentrations 2 hours post dosing ranged between 0.32 and 0.47 mg/L in patients undergoing orthopedic surgeries receiving ARIXTRA 2.5 mg.

In patients with symptomatic deep vein thrombosis and pulmonary embolism undergoing treatment with fondaparinux sodium injection 5 mg (body weight <50 kg), 7.5 mg (body weight 50-100 kg) and 10 mg (body weight >100 kg) once daily, the body-weight-adjusted doses provide similar exposure across all body weight categories. The peak steady-state plasma concentration is, on average, 1.20-1.26 mg/L. In these patients, the minimum steady-state plasma concentration is 0.46-0.62 mg/L.

Distribution: In healthy adults, intravenously or subcutaneously administered fondaparinux distributes mainly in blood as evidenced by steady state and non-steady state apparent volume of distribution of 7 to 11 L.

In vitro fondaparinux is highly (at least 94% in the concentration range from 0.5 to 2 mg/L) and specifically bound to ATIII and does not bind significantly to other plasma proteins, including Platelet Factor 4 (PF4).

Metabolism: There is no evidence that fondaparinux is metabolized since most of the administered dose is eliminated unchanged in urine.

Excretion: The elimination half-life ($T_{1/2}$) is 17 to 21 hours in healthy subjects.

Up to 77% of a single subcutaneous dose of fondaparinux is excreted in urine as unchanged compound in 72 hours in healthy individuals up to 75 years of age.

Special Populations and Conditions: Geriatrics: Fondaparinux elimination is prolonged in patients over 75 years old. In studies evaluating fondaparinux sodium 2.5 mg prophylaxis in hip fracture surgery or elective hip surgery, the total clearance of fondaparinux was approximately 25% lower in patients over 75 years old as compared to patients less than 65 years old. A similar pattern is observed in DVT and PE treatment patients.

Following a single intravenous dose of fondaparinux 4 mg in healthy elderly subjects, a mean C_{max} of 0.86 mg/L was observed at the first sampling timepoint of 5 minutes. Other pharmacokinetic parameters following intravenous administration were similar to those observed for subcutaneous administration.

Renal Insufficiency: Fondaparinux elimination is prolonged in patients with renal insufficiency since the major route of elimination is urinary excretion of unchanged drug. In patients undergoing prophylaxis following elective hip surgery or hip fracture surgery, the total clearance of fondaparinux is approximately 25% lower in patients with mild renal insufficiency (creatinine clearance 50 to 80 mL/min), approximately 40% lower in patients with moderate renal insufficiency (creatinine clearance 30 to 50 mL/min) and approximately 55% lower in patients with severe renal insufficiency (<30 mL/min) compared to patients with normal renal function. The associated terminal half-life values were 29 hours in moderate and 72 hours in patients with severe renal insufficiency. A similar pattern is observed in DVT and PE treatment patients (see Warnings and Precautions, Renal.)

Patients Weighing Less Than 50 kg: Total clearance of fondaparinux sodium is decreased by approximately 30% in patients weighing less than 50 kg (see Dosage and Administration).

Hepatic Insufficiency: Unbound concentrations of fondaparinux are expected to be unchanged in patients with mild to moderate hepatic insufficiency, and therefore, no dose adjustment is necessary based on pharmacokinetics. Following a single, subcutaneous dose of fondaparinux in subjects with moderate hepatic insufficiency (Child-Pugh Category B), C_{max} and AUC were decreased by 22% and 39%, respectively, as compared to subjects with normal liver function. The lower plasma concentrations of fondaparinux were attributed to reduced binding to ATIII secondary to the lower ATIII plasma concentrations in subjects with hepatic insufficiency thereby resulting in increased renal clearance of fondaparinux. There were no clinically relevant differences in the pharmacodynamic measures as assessed by aPTT, PT and ATIII concentrations, indicating that the effect of fondaparinux in subjects with hepatic impairment was similar to that in individuals with normal liver function.

The pharmacokinetics of fondaparinux have not been studied in patients with severe hepatic insufficiency (see Dosage and Administration, Use in Patients with Hepatic Insufficiency and Warnings and Precautions).

Patients Weighing Less Than 50 kg: Total clearance of fondaparinux sodium is decreased by approximately 30% in patients weighing less than 50 kg (see Dosage and Administration).

Pediatrics: The pharmacokinetics of fondaparinux have not been investigated in pediatric patients.

STORAGE AND STABILITY: ARIXTRA (fondaparinux sodium) injection should be stored between 15-30°C. Do not freeze.

If ARIXTRA is added to a 0.9% saline minibag it should be infused immediately, but can be stored between 15-30°C for up to 24 hours. Minibags are typically composed of a variety of polymers including PVC, polyethylene, polypropylene, or styrene-ethylene-butadiene, individually or in combination.

SPECIAL HANDLING INSTRUCTIONS: Keep out of reach of children. Single dose syringes. Discard unused portion.

INFORMATION FOR THE PATIENT: Published in e-CPS, available by subscription at www.e-cps.ca.

DOSAGE FORMS, COMPOSITION AND PACKAGING: 2.5 mg/0.5 mL: Each pre-filled 0.5 mL single use syringe, affixed with a 27 gauge x ½ inch needle with a blue plunger within a built-in automatic needle protection, contains: fondaparinux sodium 2.5 mg. Packages of 10.

7.5 mg/0.6 mL: Each 0.6 mL single use pre-filled syringe, affixed with a 27-gauge x ½ inch needle with a magenta plunger within a built-in automatic needle protection, contains: fondaparinux sodium 7.5 mg. Packages of 10.

As with all parenteral drug products, syringes should be inspected visually for clarity, particulate matter, precipitate, discolouration and leakage prior to administration. Solutions showing haziness, particulate matter, precipitate, discolouration or leakage should not be used.

Aromasin™ Pr

exemestane

Aromatase Inactivator—Antitumor Agent

Pfizer

Date of Revision: January 7, 2009

SUMMARY PRODUCT INFORMATION:

Route of Administration	Dosage Form/ Strength	Clinically Relevant Nonmedicinal Ingredients
Oral	Tablet 25 mg	Not applicable. For a complete listing see Dosage Forms, Composition and Packaging.

INDICATIONS AND CLINICAL USE: AROMASIN (exemestane) is indicated for the sequential adjuvant treatment of postmenopausal women with estrogen receptor-positive early breast cancer who have received 2-3 years of initial adjuvant tamoxifen therapy.

Approval is based on improved disease-free survival for sequential AROMASIN in comparison to continuous tamoxifen. However, overall survival was not significantly different between the two treatments.

AROMASIN (exemestane) is also indicated for hormonal treatment of advanced breast cancer in women with natural or artificially induced postmenopausal status whose disease has progressed following antiestrogen therapy.

CONTRAINDICATIONS: AROMASIN (exemestane) Tablets are contraindicated in patients with a known hypersensitivity to the drug or to any of the excipients.

WARNINGS AND PRECAUTIONS:

Serious Warnings and Precautions

Aromasin should be administered under the supervision of a qualified physician experienced in the use of anti-cancer agents.

- Not recommended for use in pre-menopausal women (see General)
- Osteoporosis (see Musculoskeletal).

General: AROMASIN should not be administered to women with premenopausal endocrine status as safety and efficacy have not been established in these patients. AROMASIN should not be coadministered with estrogen-containing agents as these could interfere with its pharmacologic action.

Carcinogenesis and Mutagenesis: In a carcinogenicity study conducted in rats, exemestane was administered by gavage at doses of 30, 100 and 315 mg/kg/day for 92 weeks in males and 104 weeks in females. No evidence of carcinogenic activity was observed in female rats. The male rat study was inconclusive since it was terminated prematurely at Week 92.

In a 2-year carcinogenicity study in mice, exemestane, dosed at 50, 150 and 450 mg/kg/day, induced an increased incidence of hepatocellular adenomas and carcinomas at the high dose in both sexes. An increased incidence of renal tubular adenomas was also observed in male mice at the high dose. Plasma levels in male and female mice at the high dose were approximately 34 and 75-fold higher than the AUC in postmenopausal patients at the therapeutic dose. Since the doses tested in mice did not achieve an MTD, neoplastic findings in organs other than liver and kidneys remain unknown.

Cardiovascular: The use of aromatase inhibitors, including AROMASIN, may increase the risk of ischemic cardiovascular diseases. During the Intergroup Exemestane Study (IES), more patients receiving exemestane were reported to have ischemic cardiac events (myocardial infarction, angina, and myocardial ischemia) compared to patients receiving tamoxifen (treatment-emergent cases: 2.0% versus 1.3%; all-cases [either on treatment or during follow up]: 5.8% versus 3.8%). In addition, a larger number of events were reported for exemestane in comparison to tamoxifen for some individual treatment-emergent cardiovascular events including hypertension (9.9% versus 8.4%), myocardial infarction (0.6% versus 0.2%) and cardiac failure (1.1% versus 0.7%). Women with significant cardiac disorders were excluded from the clinical studies of exemestane in early breast cancer.

Gastrointestinal: The use of AROMASIN may increase the risk of gastric ulcer. In the early breast cancer IES trial, gastric ulcer was observed at a slightly higher frequency in the exemestane arm compared to tamoxifen (0.7% versus <0.1%). The majority of patients on exemestane with gastric ulcer received concomitant treatment with non-steroidal anti-inflammatory agents and/or had a prior history.

Hepatic/Biliary/Pancreatic: Use in Patients with Hepatic Dysfunction: Following a single 25-mg oral dose, the AUC of exemestane was approximately 3 times higher than that observed in healthy volunteers. However, no dosage adjustment is required for patients with liver impairment since exemestane was well tolerated in patients with breast cancer at doses 8 to 24 times higher than the recommended 25 mg daily dose (see Action and Clinical Pharmacology). AROMASIN should be used with caution in patients with hepatic impairment (see Adverse Reactions, Post-Market Adverse Drug Reactions).

Musculoskeletal: The use of estrogen lowering agents, including AROMASIN, may cause a reduction in bone mineral density (BMD) with a possible consequent increased risk of fracture. Women should have their osteoporosis risk assessed and managed according to local clinical practice and guidelines. Women with clinical evidence of severe osteoporosis or a history of osteoporotic fracture were excluded from the clinical studies of exemestane in early breast cancer. Reductions in BMD over time were seen with exemestane use in these clinical trials; Table 1 describes changes in BMD from baseline to 24 months in patients receiving exemestane compared to patients receiving tamoxifen (IES) or placebo (027).

Table 1: AROMASIN

Percent Change in BMD from Baseline to 24 Months, Exemestane vs. Control

	IES		027	
BMD	Exemestane	Tamoxifen	Exemestane N=59	Placebo N=65
Lumbar spine (%)	−3.68 (N=82)	−0.19 (N=94)	−3.51	−2.39
Femoral neck (%)	−3.96 (N=77)	−0.69 (N=87)	−4.57	−2.59

The use of aromatase inhibitors, including AROMASIN, may cause arthralgias and/or myalgias, which may impact on treatment compliance and quality of life. In the IES study, 17.6% of patients in exemestane arm reported arthralgia as an adverse event versus 10.8% of patients in tamoxifen arm. Arthralgia-related disorders such as arthralgia, back pain, and pain in limb led to study drug discontinuation more often in AROMASIN-treated patients than tamoxifen-treated patients (1.3% versus 0.3% of total patients treated, respectively).

Renal: Use in Patients with Renal Dysfunction: The AUC of exemestane after a single 25-mg dose was approximately 3 times higher in subjects with severe renal insufficiency (creatinine clearance <30 mL/min/1.73 m²) compared with the AUC in healthy volunteers. However, no dosage adjustment is required for patients with renal impairment since exemestane was well tolerated in patients with breast cancer at doses 8 to 24 times higher than the recommended dose (see Action and Clinical Pharmacology).

Special Populations: Pregnant Women: AROMASIN (exemestane) Tablets might cause fetal harm when administered to a pregnant woman. Exemestane caused placental enlargement, dystocia, and prolonged gestation when given to pregnant rats at doses greater than 4 mg/kg/day (24 mg/m²/day), approximately 1.5 times the recommended human daily dose (16 mg/m²/day) on a mg/m² basis. There are no adequate and well-controlled studies in pregnant women using exemestane. If this drug is used during pregnancy, or if the patient becomes pregnant while taking this drug, the patient should be apprised of the potential hazard to the fetus or the potential risk for loss of the pregnancy.

Increased resorption, reduced number of live fetuses, decreased fetal weight, and retarded ossification were also observed at these doses. The administration of exemestane to pregnant rats at doses of 50 mg/kg/day during the organogenesis period caused an increase in fetal resorption, but there was no evidence of teratogenicity up to the dose of 810 mg/kg/day (4860 mg/m²/day).

Daily doses of exemestane 270 mg/kg/day (4320 mg/m²/day), which is greater than 200 times the recommended human daily dose, given to rabbits during organogenesis caused abortions, an increase in resorptions, and a reduction in fetal body weight; there was no increase in the incidence of malformations.

Nursing Women: Although it is not known whether exemestane is excreted in human milk, the drug was shown to be excreted in the milk of lactating rats. Because there is a potential for serious adverse reactions in nursing infants, nursing should be discontinued when receiving therapy with AROMASIN.

Pediatrics: The safety and effectiveness of AROMASIN in pediatric patients have not been established.

Geriatrics: Healthy postmenopausal women aged 43 to 68 years were studied in the pharmacokinetic trials. Age-related alterations in exemestane pharmacokinetics were not seen over this age range (see Action and Clinical Pharmacology).

Monitoring and Laboratory Tests: The use of aromatase inhibitors, including AROMASIN, may increase the occurrence of hypercholesterolemia. During the IES study, more patients receiving exemestane were reported to have treatment-emergent hypercholesterolemia compared to patients receiving tamoxifen (3.7% vs. 2.1%, respectively). Physicians should continue their routine practice of checking lipid levels on a regular basis.

In patients receiving tamoxifen and warfarin concurrently, re-titration of the warfarin dose may be required following the switch from tamoxifen to exemestane. Possible interaction between tamoxifen and warfarin that required dose adjustments have been described. As a result, patients on warfarin treatment were excluded from the IES trial because the risk of experiencing a coagulation problem in switching from previous tamoxifen to exemestane could not be excluded. Although a potential interaction between warfarin and exemestane has not been studied clinically, in vitro studies have demonstrated that exemestane does not inhibit the activity of CYP2C9 (enzyme responsible for the metabolism of s-warfarin) and exemestane is not anticipated to alter the pharmacokinetics of warfarin. Therefore, the dosage of warfarin should be controlled by periodic determinations of prothrombin times (PT) ratio/International Normalized Ratio (INR) or other suitable coagulation tests at the time of switch from tamoxifen to exemestane as per recommendations in the warfarin Product Monograph.

In a study in postmenopausal women with early breast cancer at low risk treated with exemestane (n=73) or placebo (n=73) (Study 027), there was no change in the coagulation parameters activated partial thromboplastin time [APTT], prothrombin time [PT] and fibrinogen. Plasma HDL cholesterol was decreased 6-9% in exemestane-treated patients; total cholesterol, LDL-cholesterol, triglycerides, apolipoprotein-A1, apolipoprotein-B, and lipoprotein-a were unchanged. An 18% increase in homocysteine levels was observed in exemestane-treated patients compared with a 12% increase seen with placebo. Exemestane induced a significant increase in both bone formation and bone resorption markers [bone-specific alkaline phosphatase (BAP), serum procollagen type I N propeptide (PINP) and serum osteocalcin; serum and urinary C-terminal cross-linked telopeptide of type 1 collagen (CTX-I), and urinary N-terminal cross-linked telopeptide of type I collagen (NTX-I)].

In patients with early breast cancer (IES Study) the incidence of hematological abnormalities of Common Toxicity Criteria (CTC) grade ≥1 was lower in the exemestane treatment group, compared with tamoxifen. Incidence of CTC grade 3 or 4 abnormalities was low (approximately 0.1%) in both treatment groups. Approximately 20% of patients receiving AROMASIN in clinical studies in advanced breast cancer, particularly those with pre-existing lymphocytopenia, experienced a moderate transient decrease in lymphocytes. However, mean lymphocyte values in these patients did not change significantly over time. Patients did not have a significant increase in viral infections, and no opportunistic infections were observed.

In patients with early breast cancer, elevations in bilirubin, alkaline phosphatase, and creatinine were more common in those receiving exemestane than either tamoxifen or placebo. Treatment emergent bilirubin elevations occurred in 5.9% of exemestane-treated patients compared to 0.9% of tamoxifen-treated patients on the IES, and in 6.9% of exemestane-treated patients versus 0% of placebo-treated patients on the 027 study; CTC grade 3-4 increases in bilirubin occurred in 0.9% of exemestane-treated patients compared to 0.1% of tamoxifen-treated patients on the IES. Alkaline phosphatase elevations occurred in 15.9% of exemestane-treated patients compared to 3.1% of tamoxifen-treated patients on the IES, and in 13.7% of exemestane-treated patients compared to 6.9% of placebo-treated patients on Study 027. Creatinine elevations occurred in 6.4% of exemestane-treated patients versus 5.0% of tamoxifen-treated patients on the IES and in 5.5% of exemestane-treated patients versus 0% of placebo-treated patients on Study 027.

In patients treated for advanced breast cancer, elevation of the serum levels of AST, ALT, alkaline phosphatase and gamma glutamyl transferase >5 times the upper value of the normal range have been reported rarely. These changes were mostly attributable to the underlying presence of liver and/or bone metastases. In the Phase III study in advanced breast cancer patients, elevation of the gamma glutamyl transferase without documented evidence of liver metastasis was reported in 2.7% of patients treated with AROMASIN and in 1.8% of patients treated with megestrol acetate.

Potential Effect on Antithrombin III: To date, there is no indication that exemestane affects antithrombin III. Some steroidal compounds are known to affect antithrombin III, increasing the risk of thromboembolic events. Preclinical data evaluating exemestane's potential to affect antithrombin III is not available; however, studies in humans are ongoing.

ADVERSE REACTIONS: Adjuvant Treatment of Early Breast Cancer: Adverse Drug Reaction Overview: AROMASIN (exemestane) Tablets tolerability in postmenopausal women with early breast cancer was evaluated in two well-controlled trials: the Intergroup Exemestane Study 031 (IES) and the 027 study (a randomized, placebo-controlled, double-blind, parallel group, phase II study specifically designed to assess the effects of exemestane on bone metabolism, hormones, lipids and coagulation factors over 2 years of treatment).

Certain adverse events, expected based on the known pharmacological properties and side effect profiles of test drugs, were actively sought through a positive checklist. Signs and symptoms were graded for severity using CTC in both studies. Within the IES study, the presence of some illnesses/conditions was monitored through a positive checklist without assessment of severity. These included myocardial infarction, other cardiovascular disorders, gynecological disorders, osteoporosis, osteoporotic fractures, other primary cancer, and hospitalizations.

The median duration of adjuvant treatment was 30.0 months and 29.9 months for patients receiving AROMASIN or tamoxifen, respectively, within the IES study, and 23.9 months for patients receiving AROMASIN or placebo within the 027 study. Median duration of observation after randomization at the time of primary analysis, for AROMASIN was 40.4 months and for tamoxifen 39.1 months; and at the time of the updated analysis for AROMASIN was 53.6 months and for tamoxifen 51.6 months. Median duration of observation was 30 months for both groups in the 027 study.

AROMASIN was generally well tolerated, and adverse events were usually mild to moderate. Within the IES study discontinuations due to adverse events occurred in 7.4% and 6.2% of patients receiving AROMASIN and tamoxifen, respectively, and in 12.3% and 4.1% of patients receiving exemestane or placebo within Study 027. Within the IES study, the most commonly reported adverse reactions were hot flushes (AROMASIN 22%; tamoxifen 20%), arthralgias (AROMASIN 18%; tamoxifen 11%), and fatigue (AROMASIN 16%; tamoxifen 15%). On-treatment deaths due to any cause were reported for 1.5% of the exemestane-treated patients, and 1.5% of the tamoxifen-treated patients within the IES study. There were 6 on-treatment deaths due to stroke and 3 due to cardiac failure in the AROMASIN-treated patients compared with 2 deaths due to stroke and 1 due to cardiac failure in the tamoxifen-treated patients. There were no deaths in Study 027.

Clinical Trial Adverse Drug Reactions: Treatment-emergent adverse events and illnesses including all causalities and occurring with an incidence of ≥5% in either treatment group of the IES study during or within one month of the end of treatment are shown in Table 2.

Table 2: AROMASIN

Incidence (%) of Adverse Events of all Grades[a] and Illnesses Occurring in ≥5% of Patients in Any Treatment Group in Study IES in Postmenopausal Women with Early Breast Cancer

Body System and Adverse Event by MedDRA Dictionary	% of patients	
	AROMASIN 25 mg daily (N=2249)	Tamoxifen 20 mg daily[b] (N=2279)
Gastrointestinal		
Nausea[c]	8.9	9.1
General Disorders		
Fatigue[c]	16.3	15.1
Investigations		
Weight increased	5.7	6.1
Musculoskeletal		
Arthralgia	17.6	10.8
Pain in limb	6.4	4.7
Back pain	9.3	7.7
Osteoarthritis	6.1	4.7
Osteoporosis	5.2	2.9
Nervous		
Headache[c]	13.6	11.2
Dizziness[c]	10.0	8.8
Psychiatric		
Insomnia[c]	12.9	9.0
Depression	6.2	5.6
Reproductive System		
Vaginal hemorrhage	4.0	5.3
Skin & Subcutaneous Tissue		
Increased sweating[c]	12.0	10.6
Vascular		
Hot flushes[c]	21.8	20.1
Hypertension[c]	9.9	8.4

[a] Graded according to Common Toxicity Criteria.
[b] 75 patients received tamoxifen 30 mg daily.
[c] Event actively sought.

In the IES study, more patients receiving exemestane were reported to have ischemic cardiac events (myocardial infarction, angina, and myocardial ischemia) compared to patients receiving tamoxifen (treatment-emergent cases: 2.0% versus 1.3%; all-cases [either on treatment or during follow up]: 5.8% versus 3.8%). No significant difference was noted for any individual treatment-emergent cardiovascular event including hypertension (9.9% versus 8.4%), myocardial infarction (0.6% versus 0.2%) and cardiac failure (1.1% versus 0.7%). The proportion of patients reporting hypercholesterolemia was 3.7% in the AROMASIN-treated group versus 2.1% in the tamoxifen-treated group.

In the IES study, as compared to tamoxifen, AROMASIN was associated with a higher incidence of events in the musculoskeletal disorders and in the nervous system disorders, including the following events occurring with frequency lower than 5%: paraesthesia (2.8% vs. 1.0%), carpal tunnel syndrome (2.8% vs. 0.2%) and neuropathy (0.5% vs. <0.1%).

AROMASIN was associated with a significantly higher incidence of gastric ulcer events in comparison to tamoxifen (0.7% vs. <0.1%). In addition, diarrhea was also more frequent in the AROMASIN group (4.2% vs. 2.2%). The majority of patients on AROMASIN with gastric ulcer received concomitant treatment with non-steroidal anti-inflammatory agents and/or had a prior history.

Clinical fractures were reported in 101 patients receiving exemestane (4.5%) and 75 patients receiving tamoxifen (3.3%).

Tamoxifen was associated with a greater incidence of muscle cramps (3.2% vs. 1.4%), uterine polyps (1.8% vs. 0.4%), venous thromboembolic disease (1.8% vs. 0.7%), endometrial hyperplasia (0.9% vs. <0.1%) and uterine polypectomy (0.8% vs. 0.2%).

A lower incidence of other second (non-breast) primary cancers was observed in the AROMASIN-treated patients versus tamoxifen-treated patients (3.6% vs. 5.3%) in the IES study.

Based on reports of adverse events in 73 postmenopausal women in each treatment group in the 027 study, Table 3 shows treatment-emergent adverse events including all causalities and occurring with an incidence of ≥5% in either treatment group.

Table 3: AROMASIN

Incidence (%) of Adverse Events of all Grades[a] Occurring in ≥5% of Patients in either Treatment Group in Study 027

Body System and Adverse Event by MedDRA Dictionary	% of Patients	
	AROMASIN	Placebo
Gastrointestinal		
Nausea	12.3	16.4
Abdominal pain	11.0	13.7
Diarrhea	9.6	1.4
General Disorders		
Fatigue	11.0	19.2

(cont'd)

Table 3: AROMASIN *(cont'd)*

Incidence (%) of Adverse Events of all Grades[a] Occurring in ≥5% of Patients in either Treatment Group in Study 027

Body System and Adverse Event by MedDRA Dictionary	% of Patients	
	AROMASIN	**Placebo**
Musculoskeletal		
Arthralgia	28.8	28.8
Pain in limb	8.2	6.9
Myalgia	5.5	4.1
Tendonitis	5.5	5.5
Nervous		
Dizziness	9.6	9.6
Headache	6.9	4.1
Psychiatric		
Insomnia	13.7	15.1
Depression	9.6	6.9
Anxiety	4.1	5.5
Reproductive System		
Urinary tract infection	8.2	8.2
Skin & Subcutaneous Tissue		
Increased sweating	17.8	20.6
Alopecia	15.1	4.1
Dermatitis	6.9	1.4
Vascular		
Hot flushes	32.9	24.7
Hypertension	15.1	6.9

[a] Graded according to Common Toxicity Criteria.

Events were mostly grade 1 or 2 in severity for both AROMASIN and placebo treated patients.

Treatment of Advanced Breast Cancer: Adverse Drug Reaction Overview: A total of 1058 patients were treated with AROMASIN (exemestane) Tablets 25 mg once daily in the clinical trials program. AROMASIN was generally well tolerated and adverse events were usually mild to moderate. Only one death was potentially related to treatment with AROMASIN; an 80-year-old woman with known coronary artery disease had a myocardial infarction with multiple organ failure after 9 weeks on study treatment. In the clinical trials program, only 2.8% of the patients discontinued treatment with AROMASIN because of adverse events, mainly within the first 10 weeks of treatment; late discontinuations due to adverse events were uncommon (0.3%).

Clinical Trial Adverse Drug Reactions: In the Phase III study, 358 patients were treated with AROMASIN and 400 patients were treated with megestrol acetate. Fewer patients receiving exemestane discontinued treatment because of adverse events than those treated with megestrol acetate (1.7% versus 5%). Adverse events in the Phase III study that were considered drug related or of indeterminate cause included hot flashes (12.6%), nausea (9.2%), fatigue (7.5%), increased sweating (4.5%), and increased appetite (2.8%). The proportion of patients experiencing an excessive weight gain (>10% of their baseline weight) was significantly higher with megestrol acetate than with exemestane (17.1% versus 7.6%, p=0.001). Table 4 shows the adverse events of all National Cancer Institute (NCI) Common Toxicity grades regardless of causality reported in 5% or greater of patients in the Phase III study treated either with AROMASIN or megestrol acetate.

Table 4: AROMASIN

Incidence (%) of Adverse Events of all NCI[a] Common Toxicity Grades and Causes Occurring in >5% of Patients in the Phase III Study

Event	AROMASIN 25 mg Once Daily (N=358)	Megestrol Acetate 40 mg QID (N=400)
Any Adverse Event	79.3	80
Autonomic Nervous		
Increased sweating	6.1	9.0
Body as a Whole		
Fatigue	21.8	29.3
Hot flushes	13.4	5.5
Pain	13.1	12.5
Influenza-like symptoms	5.9	5.3
Cardiovascular		
Hypertension	4.7	5.8
Nervous		
Depression	12.8	8.8
Insomnia	10.9	9.0
Anxiety	10.1	10.8
Dizziness	8.1	5.8
Headache	8.1	6.5
Gastrointestinal		
Nausea	18.4	11.5
Vomiting	7.3	3.8
Abdominal pain	6.1	10.5
Anorexia	6.1	4.8
Constipation	4.7	8.0
Diarrhea	3.6	5.0
Increased appetite	2.8	5.8
Respiratory		
Dyspnea	9.8	15.0
Coughing	5.9	7.0

(cont'd)

Table 4: AROMASIN *(cont'd)*

Incidence (%) of Adverse Events of all NCI[a] Common Toxicity Grades and Causes Occurring in >5% of Patients in the Phase III Study

[a] NCI = National Cancer Institute.

In the overall clinical trials program (N=1058), adverse events reported in 5% or greater of patients treated with AROMASIN 25 mg once daily included pain at tumor site (8%), asthenia 5.8%) and fever (5%). Less frequent adverse events (2% to 5%) reported in all patients receiving AROMASIN 25 mg once daily were arthralgia, peripheral edema, back pain, dyspepsia, paresthesia, bronchitis, rash, chest pain, edema, hypertension, upper respiratory tract infection, pruritus, urinary tract infection, pathological fracture, alopecia, leg edema, sinusitis, skeletal pain, infection, pharyngitis, rhinitis, hypoesthesia, confusion, and lymphedema.

Post-Market Adverse Drug Reactions: Among the most frequently reported serious post-market adverse events/illnesses in clinical trial and non-clinical trial cases were cerebrovascular accident, pulmonary embolus, cardiac failure, deep vein thrombosis, and myocardial infarction. Because these events are reported voluntarily from a population of uncertain size, it is not always possible to reliably estimate their frequency or clearly establish a casual relationship to AROMASIN exposure. Carpal tunnel syndrome has also been frequently reported as a post-marketing adverse drug reaction. Rare cases of hepatitis including cholestatic hepatitis have been observed in clinical trials and reported through post-marketing surveillance. Also, elevation of the serum levels of AST, ALT, alkaline phosphatase and gamma glutamyl transferase >5 times the upper value of the normal range have been reported. Increase in liver enzymes was not due to liver or bone metastases and normalization of liver enzyme values post discontinuation of drug has been observed. Severe cutaneous reactions erythema multiforme and acute generalized exanthematus pustulosis have also been reported in association with AROMASIN.

DRUG INTERACTIONS: Drug-Drug Interactions: In vitro evidence showed that AROMASIN (exemestane) is metabolized by cytochrome P450 (CYP) 3A4 and aldoketoreductases, and does not inhibit any of the major CYP isoenzymes, including CYP 1A2, 2C9, 2D6, 2E1, and 3A. In a clinical pharmacokinetic study, the specific inhibition of CYP3A4 by ketoconazole administration showed no significant influence on the pharmacokinetics of exemestane. Although pharmacokinetic effects were observed in a pharmacokinetic interaction study with rifampin, a potent CYP3A4 inducer, the suppression of plasma estrogen concentrations (estrone sulfate) produced by exemestane was not affected and a dosage adjustment is not required.

In patients receiving tamoxifen and warfarin concurrently, re-titration of the warfarin dose may be required following the switch from tamoxifen to exemestane. Possible interaction between tamoxifen and warfarin that required dose adjustments have been described. As a result, patients on warfarin treatment were excluded from the IES trial because the risk of experiencing a coagulation problem in switching from previous tamoxifen to exemestane could not be excluded. Although a potential interaction between warfarin and exemestane has not been studied clinically, in vitro studies have demonstrated that exemestane does not inhibit the activity of CYP2C9 (enzyme responsible for the metabolism of s-warfarin) and exemestane is not anticipated to alter the pharmacokinetics of warfarin. Therefore, the dosage of warfarin should be controlled by periodic determinations of prothrombin times (PT) ratio/International Normalized Ratio (INR) or other suitable coagulation tests at the time of switch from tamoxifen to exemestane as per recommendations in the warfarin Product Monograph.

Drug-Laboratory Test Interactions: No clinically relevant changes in the results of clinical laboratory tests have been observed.

DOSAGE AND ADMINISTRATION: Recommended Dose and Dosage Adjustment: The recommended dose of AROMASIN (exemestane) Tablets in early and advanced breast cancer is 25 mg once daily after a meal.

In postmenopausal women with early breast cancer, treatment with AROMASIN should continue until completion of five years of adjuvant endocrine therapy, or until local or distant recurrence or new contralateral breast cancer.

In patients with advanced breast cancer, treatment with AROMASIN should continue until tumor progression is evident.

No dose adjustments are required for patients with hepatic or renal insufficiency.

OVERDOSAGE:
Clinical trials have been conducted with AROMASIN (exemestane) Tablets given up to 800 mg as a single dose to healthy female volunteers and up to 600 mg daily for 12 weeks to postmenopausal women with advanced breast cancer. These dosages were well tolerated. There is no specific antidote to overdosage and treatment must be symptomatic. General supportive care, including frequent monitoring of vital signs and close observation of the patient, is indicated.

A male child (age unknown) accidentally ingested a 25-mg tablet of exemestane. The initial physical examination was normal, but blood tests performed 1 hour after ingestion indicated leucocytosis (WBC:25 000/mm^3 with 90% neutrophils). Blood tests were repeated 4 days after the incident and were normal. No treatment was given.

In rats and dogs, mortality was observed after single oral doses of 5000 mg/kg (about 2000 times the recommended human dose on a mg/m^2 basis) and of 3000 mg/kg (about 4000 times the recommended human dose on a mg/m^2 basis), respectively.

> For management of a suspected drug overdose, CPhA recommends that you contact your **regional Poison Control Centre**. See the *CPS* Directory section for a list of Poison Control Centres.

ACTION AND CLINICAL PHARMACOLOGY: Mechanism of Action: Breast cancer cell growth is often estrogen-dependent and anti-tumour activity is expected following effective and continuous estrogen suppression in patients with hormone-sensitive breast cancer. Aromatase is the key enzyme that converts androgens to estrogens both in pre- and postmenopausal women. While the main source of estrogen (primarily estradiol) is the ovary in premenopausal women, the principal source of circulating estrogens in postmenopausal women is from conversion of adrenal and ovarian androgens (mainly androstenedione) to estrogens (primarily estrone) by the aromatase enzyme in peripheral tissues. This occurs mainly in the adipose tissue, but also in the liver, muscle, hair follicles, and breast tissue. Estrogen deprivation through aromatase inhibition is an effective and selective treatment for postmenopausal patients with hormone-dependent breast cancer.

AROMASIN (exemestane) is a potent aromatase inactivator, causing estrogen suppression and inhibition of peripheral aromatisation. It is a steroidal irreversible Type I aromatase inhibitor, structurally related to the natural substrate androstenedione. Exemestane is a specific competitive inactivator of human placental aromatase, which has been shown to be more potent than the irreversible aromatase inhibitor formestane or the reversible inhibitor aminoglutethimide in vitro.

In vivo studies of aromatase inactivation indicate that exemestane, by the oral route, is several times more potent than formestane. It acts as a false substrate for the aromatase enzyme, and is processed to an intermediate that binds irreversibly to the active site of the enzyme causing its inactivation, an effect also known as "suicide inhibition". De novo aromatase enzyme synthesis is required for recovery of enzyme activity. Exemestane significantly lowers circulating estrogen concentrations in postmenopausal women, but has no detectable effect on adrenal biosynthesis of corticosteroids or aldosterone. Exemestane has no effect on other enzymes involved in the steroidogenic pathway up to a concentration at least 600 times higher than that inhibiting the aromatase enzyme.

Pharmacokinetics: Absorption: Following oral administration of radiolabeled exemestane, at least 42% of radioactivity was absorbed from the gastrointestinal tract. Maximum exemestane plasma concentration (C_{max}) was observed within 2 hours of receiving exemestane. Exemestane plasma levels increased by approximately 40% after a high-fat breakfast; however, no further effect on estrogen suppression was observed since maximum activity was already achieved under fasting conditions. Exemestane appears to be more rapidly absorbed in women with breast cancer than in healthy women. After repeated doses, mean T_{max} was 1.2 hours in the women with breast cancer and 2.9 hours in the healthy women. Mean AUC values following repeated doses were approximately 2-fold higher in women with breast cancer (75.4 ng·h/mL) compared with healthy women (41.4 ng·h/mL). However, there was considerable overlap between the range of pharmacokinetic parameters observed in these two populations.

Distribution: Exemestane is distributed extensively into tissues. Exemestane is 90% bound to plasma proteins and the fraction bound is independent of the total concentration. Albumin and α_1-acid glycoprotein contribute equally to the binding. The distribution of exemestane and its metabolites into blood cells is negligible.

Metabolism and Excretion: After reaching maximum plasma concentration, exemestane levels declined polyexponentially with a mean terminal half-life of about 24 hours. Following administration of a single oral dose of radiolabeled exemestane, the elimination of drug-related products was essentially complete within 1 week. Approximately equal proportions of the dose were eliminated in urine and feces. The amount of drug excreted unchanged in urine was less than 1% of the dose, indicating that renal excretion is a limited elimination pathway. Exemestane was extensively metabolized, with levels of the unchanged drug in plasma accounting for less than 10% of the total radioactivity. The initial steps in the metabolism of exemestane are oxidation of the methylene group in position 6 and reduction of the 17-keto group with subsequent formation of many secondary metabolites. Each metabolite accounts only for a limited amount of drug-related material. The metabolites are inactive or demonstrate minimal ability to inhibit aromatase compared with the parent drug. Studies using human liver preparations indicate that cytochrome P-450 3A4 (CYP 3A4) is the principal isoenzyme involved in the oxidation of exemestane. Additional studies in humans demonstrated that exemestane does not affect the activity of CYP3A4 to any great extent. No significant inhibition of any of the CYP isoenzymes (including CYP3A4) involved in xenobiotic metabolism was observed in human liver preparations. This would suggest that possible drug-drug interactions involving inhibition of CYP by co-administration with exemestane are unlikely.

Special Populations and Conditions: Pediatrics: The pharmacokinetics of exemestane have not been studied in pediatric patients.

Geriatrics: Although women ranging in age up to 99 years were enrolled in the clinical studies (see Warnings and Precautions), healthy postmenopausal women aged 43 to 68 years were enrolled in the pharmacokinetic trials. Age-related alterations in exemestane pharmacokinetics were not seen over this age range.

Gender: The pharmacokinetics of exemestane following administration of a single, 25 mg tablet to fasted healthy males (mean age 32 years; range 19 to 51 years) or to fasted healthy postmenopausal women (mean age 55 years; range 45 to 68 years) have been compared. Mean C_{max} and AUC values in healthy males (12.3±5.8 ng/mL and 28.4±17.3 ng·h/mL, respectively) were similar to those determined in healthy postmenopausal women (11.1±4.4 ng/mL and 29.7±7.8 ng·h/mL, respectively). Thus, the pharmacokinetics of exemestane does not appear to be influenced by gender.

Race: The influence of race on exemestane pharmacokinetics has not been formally evaluated.

Hepatic Insufficiency: The pharmacokinetics of exemestane have been investigated in subjects with moderate and severe hepatic insufficiency. Following a single 25-mg oral dose, the AUC of exemestane was approximately 3 times higher than that observed in healthy volunteers. However no dosage adjustment is required for patients with liver impairment since exemestane was well tolerated in patients with breast cancer at doses 8 to 24 times higher than the recommended 25-mg daily dose (see Warnings and Precautions).

Renal Insufficiency: The AUC of exemestane after a single 25-mg dose was approximately 3 times higher in subjects with severe renal insufficiency (creatinine clearance <30 mL/min/1.73 m²) compared with the AUC in healthy volunteers. However, no dosage adjustment is required for patients with renal impairment since exemestane was well tolerated in patients with breast cancer at doses 8 to 24 times higher than the recommended dose (see Warnings and Precautions).

STORAGE AND STABILITY: Store between 15 to 30°C.

SPECIAL HANDLING INSTRUCTIONS: Not applicable.

INFORMATION FOR THE PATIENT: Published in e-CPS, available by subscription at www.e-cps.ca.

DOSAGE FORMS, COMPOSITION AND PACKAGING: Each round, biconvex, off-white to slightly gray tablet, printed on one side with the number "7663" in black contains: exemestane 25 mg. Nonmedicinal ingredients: carnauba wax, cetyl esters wax, crospovidone, hypromellose, iron oxides, magnesium carbonate, magnesium stearate, mannitol, methyl-p-hydroxybenzoate, microcrystalline cellulose, polyethyleneglycol 6000, polysorbate 80, polyvinyl alcohol, shellac, silicon dioxide, simethicone, sodium starch glycolate, sucrose, talc and titanium dioxide. Aluminium-PVDC/PVC-PVDC opaque white blisters of 30.

(Shown in Product Identification Section)

Arthrotec® Ⓟ

diclofenac sodium—misoprostol

NSAID—Mucosal Protective Agent

Pfizer

Date of Revision: February 3, 2010

SUMMARY PRODUCT INFORMATION:

Route of Administration	Dosage Form/ Strength	Clinically Relevant Nonmedicinal Ingredients
Oral	Enteric coated tablets: 50 mg diclofenac/200 µg misoprostol 75 mg diclofenac/200 µg misoprostol	Lactose For a complete listing see Dosage Forms, Composition and Packaging.

INDICATIONS AND CLINICAL USE: Arthrotec (diclofenac sodium plus misoprostol) is indicated for acute and chronic use in the relief of the signs and symptoms of rheumatoid arthritis and osteoarthritis.

For patients with an increased risk of developing CV and/or GI adverse events, other management strategies that do not include the use of NSAIDs should be considered first.

Use of Arthrotec should be limited to the lowest effective dose for the shortest possible duration of treatment in order to minimize the potential risk for cardiovascular or gastrointestinal adverse events. (See Contraindications and Warnings and Precautions.)

Arthrotec, as a NSAID, does **not** treat clinical disease or prevent its progression.

Arthrotec, as a NSAID, only relieves symptoms and decreases inflammation for as long as the patient continues to take it.

Geriatrics (>65 years of age): Evidence from clinical studies and experience suggests that use in geriatric patients is associated with differences in safety or effectiveness (see Warnings and Precautions, Special Populations).

Pediatrics (<18 years of age): Not recommended for pediatric use (see Contraindications).

CONTRAINDICATIONS: Arthrotec (diclofenac sodium plus misoprostol) is contraindicated in:

- The peri-operative setting of coronary artery bypass graft surgery (CABG). Although Arthrotec has **not** been studied in this patient population, a selective COX-2 inhibitor NSAID studied in such a setting has led to an increased incidence of cardiovascular/thromboembolic events, deep surgical infections and sternal wound complications.
- The women who are **pregnant**, or in whom **pregnancy has not been excluded**. Women of childbearing potential should be fully counseled about misoprostol's abortifacient potential and the importance of effective contraception (oral contraceptive or intrauterine device) and prevention of pregnancy while undergoing treatment (see Warnings and Precautions, Special Populations, Pregnant Women).
- Women who are breastfeeding, because of the potential for serious adverse reactions in nursing infants.
- Severe uncontrolled heart failure.
- Known or suspected hypersensitivity to diclofenac sodium, misoprostol, or any other ingredient of the product, other NSAIDs including aspirin, or other prostaglandins. The potential for cross-reactivity between different NSAIDs must be kept in mind.
- History of asthma, urticaria, or allergic-type reactions after taking ASA or other NSAIDs (i.e. complete or partial syndrome of ASA-intolerance—rhinosinusitis, urticaria/angioedema, nasal polyps, asthma) (see Warnings and Precautions, Anaphylactoid Reactions). Fatal anaphylactoid reactions have occurred in such individuals. As well, individuals with the above medical problems are at risk of a severe reaction even if they have taken NSAIDs in the past without any adverse effects.
- Patients with active gastric/duodenal/peptic ulcer active gastrointestinal bleeding, a history of recurrent ulceration or active inflammatory disease of the gastrointestinal system.
- Cerebrovascular bleeding or other bleeding disorders.
- Inflammatory bowel disease.
- Significant hepatic impairment or active liver disease.
- Severely impaired or deteriorating renal function (creatinine clearance <30 mL/min or 0.5 mL/sec). Individuals with lesser degrees of renal impairment are at risk of deterioration of their renal function when prescribed NSAIDs and must be monitored (see Warnings and Precautions, Renal).
- Known hyperkalemia (see Warnings and Precautions, Renal, Fluid and Electrolyte Balance).
- Children and adolescents less than (18) years of age.
- Diclofenac is not recommended for use with other NSAIDs because of the absence of any evidence demonstrating synergistic benefits and the potential for additive side effects (see Drug Interactions).

WARNINGS AND PRECAUTIONS:

> **Serious Warnings and Precautions**
>
> **Risk of Cardiovascular (CV) Adverse Events: ischemic heart disease cerebrovascular disease, congestive heart failure (NYHA II-IV) (see Warnings and Precautions, Cardiovascular).**
>
> **Arthrotec is a non-steroidal anti-inflammatory drug (NSAID). Use of some NSAIDs is associated with an increased incidence of cardiovascular adverse events (such as myocardial infarction, stroke or thrombotic events) which can be fatal. The risk may increase with duration of use. Patients with cardiovascular disease or risk factors for cardiovascular disease may be at greater risk.**
>
> **Caution should be exercised in prescribing Arthrotec to any patient with ischemic heart disease (including but not limited to acute myocardial infarction, history of myocardial infarction and/or angina), cerebrovascular disease (including but not limited to stroke, cerebrovascular accident, transient ischemic attacks and/or amaurosis fugax) and/or congestive heart failure (NYHA II-IV).**
>
> **Use of NSAIDs, such as Arthrotec, can promote sodium retention in a dose-dependent manner, through a renal mechanism, which can result in increased blood pressure and/or exacerbation of congestive heart failure (see also Warnings and Precautions, Renal, Fluid and Electrolyte Balance).**
>
> **Randomized clinical trials with Arthrotec have not been designed to detect differences in cardiovascular events in a chronic setting. Therefore, caution should be exercised when prescribing Arthrotec.**
>
> **Risk of Gastrointestinal (GI) Adverse Events (see Warnings and Precautions, Gastrointestinal).**
>
> **Patients should not give Arthrotec to anyone else. Arthrotec has been prescribed for the patient's specific condition, may not be the correct treatment for another person and may be dangerous to that person if she were to become pregnant.**

General: Frail or debilitated patients may tolerate side effects less well and therefore special care should be taken in treating this population. **To minimize the potential risk for an adverse event, the lowest effective dose should be used for the shortest possible duration.** As with other NSAIDs, caution should be used in the treatment of elderly patients who are more likely to be suffering from impaired renal, hepatic or cardiac function. For high risk patients, alternate therapies that do not involve NSAIDs should be considered.

Arthrotec is **not** recommended for use with other NSAIDs, with the exception of low-dose ASA for cardiovascular prophylaxis, because of the absence of any evidence demonstrating synergistic benefits and the potential for additive adverse reactions (see Drug Interactions, Drug-Drug Interactions, Acetylsalicylic Acid (ASA) or other NSAIDs).

In common with other anti-inflammatory drugs, Arthrotec may mask the usual signs of infection, such as fever.

Cardiovascular: Arthrotec is a non-steroidal anti-inflammatory drug (NSAID). Use of some NSAIDs is associated with an increased incidence of cardiovascular adverse events (such as myocardial infarction, stroke or thrombotic events) which can be fatal. Large population-based observational studies, meta-analyses and systematic reviews suggest an increased risk of myocardial infarction and stroke in association with the use of diclofenac. The risk may increase with the dose and duration of use. Patients with cardiovascular disease or risk factors for cardiovascular disease may be at greater risk.

Caution should be exercised in prescribing Arthrotec to patients with risk factors for cardiovascular disease, cerebrovascular disease or renal disease, such as any of the following (not an exhaustive list):

- **Hypertension**
- **Dyslipidemia/Hyperlipidemia**
- **Diabetes Mellitus**
- **Congestive Heart Failure (NYHA I)**
- **Coronary Artery Disease (Atherosclerosis)**
- **Peripheral Arterial Disease**
- **Smoking**
- **Creatinine Clearance <60 mL/min or 1 mL/sec**

Use of NSAIDs, such as Arthrotec, can lead to new hypertension or can worsen pre-existing hypertension, either which may increase the risk of cardiovascular events as described above. Thus blood pressure should be monitored regularly. Consideration should be given to discontinuing Arthrotec should hypertension either develop or worsen with its use.

For patients with a high risk of developing an adverse CV event, other management strategies that do **not** include the use of NSAIDs should be considered first. **To minimize the potential risk for an adverse CV event, the lowest effective dose should be used for the shortest possible duration.**

Congestive Heart Failure and Edema: Fluid retention and edema have been observed in patients treated with Arthrotec. Therefore, as with many other nonsteroidal anti-inflammatory drugs, the possibility of precipitating congestive heart failure in elderly patients or those with compromised cardiac function should be borne in mind. Arthrotec should be used with caution in patients with heart failure, hypertension or other conditions predisposing to fluid retention. (See Warnings and Precautions, Renal, Fluid and Electrolyte Balance.)

Endocrine and Metabolism: With nonsteroidal anti-inflammatory treatment there is a potential risk of hyperkalemia, particularly in patients with conditions such as diabetes mellitus or renal failure; elderly patients; or in patients receiving concomitant therapy with beta-adrenergic blockers, angiotensin converting enzyme inhibitors or some diuretics. Serum electrolytes should be monitored periodically during long-term therapy, especially in those patients who are at risk.

Corticosteroids: Arthrotec (diclofenac sodium plus misoprostol) is **not** a substitute for corticosteroids. It does **not** treat corticosteroid insufficiency. Abrupt discontinuation of corticosteroids may lead to exacerbation of corticosteroidresponsive illness. Patients on prolonged corticosteroid therapy should have their therapy tapered slowly if a decision is made to discontinue corticosteroids (see Drug Interactions, Drug-Drug Interactions, Glucocorticoids).

Gastrointestinal: The presence of misoprostol in the product may protect against the mucosal damaging effects of the other component, diclofenac.

However, serious GI toxicity, such as peptic/duodenal ulceration, inflammation, perforation, obstruction and gastrointestinal bleeding, **sometimes severe and occasionally fatal** can occur at any time, with or without symptoms in patients treated with nonsteroidal anti-inflammatory drugs (NSAIDs) including Arthrotec (diclofenac sodium plus misoprostol). NSAIDs, including Arthrotec, should be used with caution in patients with a history of, or active, GI disease, such as ulceration, bleeding, or inflammatory conditions. Most spontaneous reports of fatal GI events are in elderly or debilitated patients and therefore special care should be taken in treating this population. **To minimize the potential risk for an adverse GI event, the lowest effective dose should be used for the shortest possible duration.** For high risk patients, alternate therapies that do not involve NSAIDs should be considered (see Warnings and Precautions, Special Populations, Geriatrics (>65 years of age)).

Minor upper GI problems, such as dyspepsia, commonly occur at any time. Physicians should remain alert for ulceration and bleeding in patients treated with nonsteroidal anti-inflammatory drugs, even in the absence of previous GI tract symptoms.

Physicians should inform patients about the signs and/or symptoms of serious GI toxicity and instruct them to discontinue using Arthrotec and seek emergency medical attention if they experience any such symptoms.

Because serious GI tract ulceration and bleeding can occur without warning symptoms, physicians should follow chronically treated patients by checking their hemoglobin periodically and by being vigilant for the signs and symptoms of ulceration and bleeding and should inform the patients of the importance of this follow-up.

The utility of periodic laboratory monitoring has **not** been demonstrated, nor has it been adequately assessed. Most patients who develop a serious upper GI adverse event on NSAID therapy have no symptoms. Upper GI ulcers, gross bleeding or perforation, caused by NSAIDs, appear to occur in approximately 1% of patients treated for 3-6 months, and in about 2-4% of patients treated for one year. These trends continue, thus increasing the likelihood of developing a serious GI event at some time during the course of therapy. Even short-term therapy has its risks.

Caution should be taken if prescribing Arthrotec to patients with a prior history of peptic/duodenal ulcer disease or gastrointestinal bleeding as these individuals have a greater than 10-fold higher risk for developing a GI bleed when taking a NSAID than patients with neither of these risk factors. Other risk factor for GI ulceration and bleeding include the following: *H. pylori* infection, increased age, prolonged use of NSAID therapy, excess alcohol intake, smoking, female gender, poor general health status or concomitant therapy with any of the following:

- Anti-coagulants (e.g. warfarin)
- Anti-platelet agents (e.g. ASA, clopidogrel)
- Oral corticosteroids (e.g. prednisone)
- Selective Serotonin Reuptake Inhibitors (SSRIs) (e.g. citalopram, fluoxetine, paroxetine, sertraline)

If ulceration is suspected or confirmed, or if GI bleeding occurs, Arthrotec should be discontinued immediately, appropriate treatment instituted and the patient monitored closely. No studies, to date, have identified any group of patients not at risk of developing ulceration and bleeding. Studies to date show that all NSAIDs can cause GI tract adverse events. Although existing data do not clearly identify differences in risk between various NSAIDs, this may be shown in the future.

Genitourinary: Some NSAIDs are associated with persistent urinary symptoms (bladder pain, dysuria, urinary frequency), hematuria or cystitis. The onset of these symptoms may occur at any time after the initiation of therapy with an NSAID. Some cases have become severe on continued treatment. Should urinary symptoms occur, in the absence of an alternate explanation, treatment with Arthrotec (diclofenac sodium plus misoprostol) must be stopped to ascertain if symptoms disappear. This should be done before any urological investigations or treatments are carried out.

Post-menopausal vaginal bleeding may be related to Arthrotec administration. If this occurs, diagnostic workup should be undertaken to rule out gynecological pathology (see Adverse Reactions).

Hematologic: NSAIDs inhibiting prostaglandin biosynthesis interfere with platelet function to varying degrees; patients who may be adversely affected by such an action, such as those on anti-coagulants or suffering from haemophilia or platelet disorders should be carefully monitored when diclofenac is administered (see Drug Interactions, Drug-Laboratory Test Interactions).

Anti-Coagulants: Numerous studies have shown that the concomitant use of NSAIDs and anti-coagulants increases the risk of bleeding. Concurrent therapy of Arthrotec with warfarin requires close monitoring of the international normalized ratio (INR).

Even with therapeutic INR monitoring, increased bleeding may occur.

Anti-Platelet Effects: NSAIDs inhibit platelet aggregation and have been shown to prolong bleeding time in some patients. Unlike acetylsalicylic acid (ASA), their effect on platelet function is quantitatively less, or of shorter duration, and is reversible. Misoprostol does not exacerbate the effects of diclofenac on platelet activity.

In clinical trials, there has been no evidence that Arthrotec affects hemostasis.

Arthrotec and other NSAIDs have no proven efficacy as anti-platelet agents and should **not** be used as a substitute for ASA or other anti-platelet agents for prophylaxis of cardiovascular thromboembolic diseases. Anti-platelet therapies (e.g. ASA) should **not** be discontinued. There is some evidence that use of NSAIDs with ASA can markedly attenuate the cardioprotective effects of ASA (see Drug Interactions, Drug-Drug Interactions, Acetylsalicylic Acid (ASA) or other NSAIDs).

Concomitant administration of Arthrotec with low dose ASA increases the risk of GI ulceration and associated complications.

Blood Dyscrasias: Blood dyscrasias (such as neutropenia, leucopenia, thrombocytopenia, aplastic anemia and agranulocytosis) associated with the use of NSAIDs are rare, but could occur with severe consequences.

Anemia is sometimes seen in patients receiving NSAIDs, including Arthrotec. This may be due to fluid retention, GI blood loss, or an incompletely described effect upon erythropoiesis. Patients on long-term treatment with NSAIDs, including Arthrotec, should have their haemoglobin or hematocrit checked if they exhibit any signs or symptoms of anemia or blood loss.

Hepatic/Biliary/Pancreatic: As with other NSAIDs, borderline elevations of one or more liver function tests (AST, ALT, alkaline phosphatase) may occur in up to 15% of patients. These abnormalities may progress, may remain essentially unchanged, or may be transient with continued therapy. In clinical trials of 4 to 12 weeks duration, clinically significant (>3 times the upper limit of normal) elevations of ALT and/or AST, were observed in 2.5% or less of patients who received diclofenac/misoprostol or diclofenac/placebo.

A patient with symptoms and/or signs suggesting liver dysfunction, or in whom an abnormal liver test has occurred, should be evaluated for evidence of the development of more severe hepatic reaction while on therapy with this drug. Severe hepatic reactions including jaundice and cases of fatal hepatitis, liver necrosis and hepatic failure have been reported with nonsteroidal anti-inflammatory drugs.

Although such reactions are rare, if abnormal liver tests persist or worsen, if clinical signs and symptoms consistent with liver disease develop (e.g. jaundice), or if systemic manifestations occur (e.g. eosinophilia, rash, etc.), this drug should be discontinued.

During long-term therapy, liver function tests should be monitored periodically. If there is a need to prescribe this drug in the presence of impaired liver function, it must be done under strict observation.

Hypersensitivity Reactions: Anaphylactoid Reactions: As with NSAIDs in general, anaphylactoid reactions have occurred in patients without known prior exposure to Arthrotec. In post-marketing experience, rare cases of anaphylactic/anaphylactoid reactions and angioedema have been reported in patients receiving Arthrotec. Arthrotec should **not** be given to patients with the ASA-triad. This symptom complex typically occurs in asthmatic patients who experience rhinitis with or without nasal polyps, or who exhibit severe, potentially fatal bronchospasm after taking ASA or other NSAIDs (see Contraindications).

ASA-Intolerance: Arthrotec should **not** be given to patients with complete or partial syndrome of ASA-intolerance (rhinosinusitis, urticaria/angioedema, nasal polyps, asthma) in whom asthma, anaphylaxis, urticaria/angioedema, rhinitis or other allergic manifestations are precipitated by ASA or other NSAIDs. Fatal anaphylactoid reactions have occurred in such individuals. As well, individuals with the above medical problems are at risk of a severe reaction even if they have taken NSAIDs in the past without any adverse reaction (see Contraindications).

Cross-Sensitivity: Patients sensitive to one NSAID may be sensitive to any of the other NSAIDs as well.

Serious Skin Reactions: (See Warnings and Precautions, Skin).

Immune: (See Warnings and Precautions, Infection, Aseptic Meningitis).

Infection: Arthrotec, in common with other NSAIDs, may mask signs and symptoms of an underlying infectious disease.

Aseptic Meningitis: Rarely, with some NSAIDs, the symptoms of aseptic meningitis (stiff neck, severe headaches, nausea and vomiting, fever or clouding of consciousness) have been observed. Patients with autoimmune disorders (systemic lupus erythematosus, mixed connective tissue diseases, etc.) seem to be pre-disposed. Therefore, in such patients, the health care provider must be vigilant to the development of this complication.

Neurologic: Some patients may experience drowsiness, dizziness, blurred vision, vertigo, tinnitus, hearing loss, insomnia or depression with the use of NSAIDs such as Arthrotec. If patients experience these side effects, they should exercise caution in carrying out activities that require alertness.

Ophthalmologic: Blurred, diminished vision, and/or sensitivity to light have been reported with the use of NSAIDs. If such symptoms develop this drug should be discontinued and an ophthalmologic examination performed; ophthalmologic examination should be carried out at periodic intervals in any patient receiving Arthrotec for an extended period of time.

Peri-Operative Considerations: See Contraindications, Coronary Artery Bypass Graft Surgery).

Psychiatric: Some patients may experience depression with the use of diclofenac. (See Warnings and Precautions, Neurologic.)

Renal: Long-term administration of nonsteroidal anti-inflammatory drugs to animals has resulted in renal papillary necrosis and other abnormal renal pathology. In humans, there have been reports of acute interstitial, nephritis, hematuria, low grade proteinuria, and occasionally nephrotic syndrome.

Renal insufficiency due to NSAID use is seen in patients with prerenal conditions leading to the reduction in renal blood flow or blood volume. Under these circumstances, renal prostaglandins help maintain renal perfusion and glomerular filtration rate (GFR). In these patients, administration of a NSAID may cause a reduction in prostaglandin formation and may precipitate overt renal decompensation. Patients at greatest risk of this reaction are those with pre-existing renal insufficiency (GFR <60 mL/min or 1 mL/s), dehydrated patients, patients on salt-restricted diets, heart failure, cirrhosis, liver dysfunction, those taking angiotensin-converting enzyme inhibitors, angiotensin-II receptor blockers, cyclosporin, diuretics, and the elderly. Serious or life-threatening renal failure has been reported in patients with normal or impaired renal function after short term therapy with NSAIDs. Even patients at risk who demonstrated the ability to tolerate a NSAID under stable conditions may decompensate during periods of added stress (e.g. dehydration due to gastroenteritis). Discontinuation of NSAIDs is usually followed by recovery to the pre-treatment state.

Diclofenac and its metabolites are eliminated primarily by the kidneys, therefore the drug should be used with great caution in patients with impaired renal function. In these cases, utilization of lower doses of diclofenac should be considered and patients carefully monitored. Caution should be used when initiating treatment in patients with dehydration. **It is advisable to rehydrate patients first and then start therapy.** The dose should be kept as low as possible and renal function should be monitored.

During long-term therapy kidney function should be monitored periodically.

Advanced Renal Disease: (See Contraindications.)

Fluid and Electrolyte Balance: Use of NSAIDs, such as Arthrotec, can promote sodium retention in a dose-dependent manner, which can lead to fluid retention and edema, and consequences of increased blood pressure and exacerbation of congestive heart failure. Thus, caution should be exercised in prescribing Arthrotec in patients with a history of congestive heart failure, compromised cardiac function, hypertension, increased age or other conditions predisposing to fluid retention (see Warnings and Precautions, Cardiovascular).

Use of NSAIDs, such as Arthrotec, can increase the risk of hyperkalemia, especially in patients with diabetes mellitus, renal failure, increased age, or those receiving concomitant therapy with adrenergic blockers, angiotensin-converting enzyme inhibitors, angiotensin-II receptor antagonists, cyclosporin, or some diuretics.

Electrolytes should be monitored periodically (see Contraindications).

Respiratory: ASA-induced asthma is an uncommon but very important indication of ASA and NSAID sensitivity. It occurs more frequently in patients with asthma who have nasal polyps.

Sexual Function/Reproduction: The use of Arthrotec, as with any drug known to inhibit cyclooxygenase/prostaglandin synthesis, may impair fertility and is not recommended in women attempting to conceive. Therefore, in women who have difficulties conceiving, or who are undergoing investigation of infertility, withdrawal of Arthrotec should be considered.

Skin: In rare cases, serious skin reactions such as Stevens-Johnson syndrome, toxic epidermal necrolysis, exfoliative dermatitis and erythema multiforme have been associated with the use of some NSAIDs. Because the rate of these reactions is low, they have usually been noted during post-marketing surveillance in patients taking other medications also associated with the potential development of these serious skin reactions. Thus, causality is **not** clear. These reactions are potentially life-threatening but may be reversible if the causative agent is discontinued and appropriate treatment instituted. Patients should be advised that if they experience a skin rash they should discontinue their NSAID and contact their physician for assessment and advice, including which additional therapies to discontinue.

Arthrotec may cause sensitivity to sunlight. Any exposure to sunlight or sunlamps may cause sunburn, skin blisters, skin rash, redness, itching or discoloration. Patients should be advised that if they experience any of these symptoms, they should discontinue their NSAID and contact their physician for assessment and advice, including which additional therapies to discontinue.

Special Populations: Pregnant Women: Arthrotec is contraindicated for use in women who are **pregnant**, or in whom **pregnancy has not been excluded** (see Contraindications, Boxed Serious Warnings and Precautions, Adverse Reactions and Post-Market Adverse Drug Reactions). Misoprostol administration to pregnant women induces uterine contractions and is associated with abortion, premature birth, birth defects and fetal death. Misoprostol can cause uterine tetany and uterine rupture if administered to pregnant women beyond the eighth week of pregnancy. (See Contraindications and Adverse Reactions, Post-Market Adverse Drug Reactions.)

Nursing Women: Misoprostol is rapidly metabolised in the mother to misoprostol acid, which is biologically active and is excreted in breast milk. Diclofenac/misoprostol is contraindicated in nursing mothers because the excretion of misoprostol acid could cause undesirable effects such as diarrhea in nursing infants (see Contraindications).

Pediatrics (<18 years of age): (See Contraindications.)

Geriatrics (>65 years of age): Patients older than 65 years and frail or debilitated patients are most susceptible to a variety of adverse reactions from NSAIDs. The incidence of these adverse reactions increases with dose and duration of treatment. In addition, these patients are less tolerant to ulceration and bleeding. Most reports of fatal GI events are in this population. Older patients are also at risk of lower esophageal ulceration and bleeding (see Action and Clinical Pharmacology). For such patients, consideration should be given to a starting dose lower than the one usually recommended, with individual adjustment when necessary and under close supervision.

As with any NSAID, the elderly are likely to tolerate adverse events less well than younger patients.

Diclofenac is known to be substantially excreted by the kidney, and the risk of toxic reactions to Arthrotec may be greater in patients with impaired renal function. Because elderly patients are more likely to have decreased renal function, care should be taken in dose selection, and it may be useful to monitor renal function (see Warnings and Precautions, Renal).

Monitoring and Laboratory Tests: Cardiovascular: (Hypertension): Blood pressure should be monitored regularly during therapy with Arthrotec.

Hematologic: Patients on long-term treatment with NSAIDs, including Arthrotec, should have their hemoglobin or hematocrit checked if they exhibit any signs or symptoms of anemia or blood loss. Concurrent therapy of Arthrotec with warfarin requires close monitoring of the international normalized ratio (INR).

Hepatic: Patient with symptoms and/or signs of liver dysfunction, or in whom an abnormal liver function test has occurred, should be monitored carefully for evidence of the development of a more severe hepatic reaction while on therapy with Arthrotec. If abnormal liver tests persist or worsen, Arthrotec should be discontinued.

Renal: Renal function should be monitored in high-risk populations, such as the elderly, patients with advanced renal disease, patients with cardiovascular disease and diabetes mellitus, as well as in the setting of concomitant use of diuretics and ACE inhibitors (see Contraindications). If abnormal renal tests persist or worsen, Arthrotec should be discontinued.

Laboratory abnormalities included increased alkaline phosphatase, decreased hematocrit and elevated ALT.

Persistently abnormal or worsening renal, hepatic or hematological test values should be followed up carefully since they may be related to therapy.

ADVERSE REACTIONS: Adverse Drug Reaction Overview: The most common adverse reactions encountered with nonsteroidal anti-inflammatory drugs are gastrointestinal, of which peptic ulcer, with or without bleeding, is the most severe. Fatalities have occurred, particularly in the elderly.

Most fatal gastrointestinal events occur in the elderly or debilitated patients. Gastrointestinal adverse events can develop at any time in the course of the therapy.

Clinical Trial Adverse Drug Reactions: Because clinical trials are conducted under very specific conditions the adverse reaction rates observed in the clinical trials may not reflect the rates observed in practice and should not be compared to the rates in the clinical trials of another drug. Adverse drug reaction information from clinical trials is useful for identifying drug-related adverse events and for approximating rates.

In clinical trials, 3549 arthritic patients have been treated with Arthrotec (diclofenac sodium plus misoprostol), 506 of whom received Arthrotec for more than one year. A total of 285 patients have been treated with Arthrotec 75 in clinical trials for a duration of up to 12 weeks.

The following adverse reactions occurred with an incidence of 1% or greater with at least one of the Arthrotec or Diclofenac dosing regimens presented in Table 1.

Table 1: Arthrotec

Adverse Reactions Reported in ≥1% of Patients

	A50[a] BID N=391	A50[a] TID N=692	A50[a] BID/TID N=750	D50[b] BID/TID N=754	A75[c] BID[e] N=285	D75[d] BID[e] N=260
Body as a Whole						
Influenza-Like Symptoms	1.0	0.6	2.0	1.5	1.1	2.3
Pain	0.5	1.0	0.7	0.8	4.2	1.9
Back Pain	0.8	0.6	1.2	1.1	3.2	3.5
Chest Pain	1.0	0.3	1.1	0.5	0.7	3.1
Fever	0.0	0.6	0.7	1.1	1.4	0.0

(cont'd)

Table 1: Arthrotec *(cont'd)*
Adverse Reactions Reported in ≥1% of Patients

	A50[a] BID N=391	A50[a] TID N=692	A50[a] BID/TID N=750	D50[b] BID/TID N=754	A75[c] BID[e] N=285	D75[d] BID[e] N=260
Asthenia	0.0	0.1	0.1	0.7	1.1	0.4
Myalgia	0.8	0.7	0.8	0.3	1.1	0.4
Arthralgia	0.0	0.7	0.3	0.3	2.8	3.5
Arthrosis	0.0	0.1	0.3	0.0	1.4	1.2
Cardiovascular						
Hypertension	0.0	0.5	0.0	0.1	1.1	2.3
Edema	0.8	0.7	0.0	0.3	1.1	1.2
Dependent Edema	0.0	0.3	0.4	0.5	1.1	0.4
Leg Edema	0.0	0.1	0.0	0.1	1.1	0.8
Central Nervous System						
Headache	9.2	6.4	7.3	9.2	12.3	15.8
Dizziness	2.6	2.0	3.5	5.3	3.9	4.2
Migraine	1.3	0.6	0.4	0.9	1.4	0.8
Paresthesia	0.3	0.3	0.7	0.7	1.1	0.4
Dermatologic						
Rash	0.8	1.4	1.5	1.1	2.1	3.5
Pruritus	1.0	0.4	1.2	0.9	2.1	1.9
Skin Ulceration	0.0	0.0	0.1	0.0	1.1	0.4
Gastrointestinal						
Abdominal Pain	19.4	19.4	23.2	19.5	24.6	24.2
Diarrhea	15.9	17.8	19.9	11.3	20.4	16.2
Dyspepsia	7.2	14.5	11.3	7.8	33.3	34.6
Nausea	10.2	10.0	11.7	6.5	14.0	9.2
Flatulence	6.1	8.7	8.0	3.1	18.2	9.2
Gastritis	2.8	2.3	3.6	6.8	7.4	13.1
Vomiting	2.6	3.3	3.1	1.3	3.9	5.4
Constipation	1.8	2.6	2.1	2.9	4.9	6.9
Eructation	2.6	0.3	2.0	0.8	2.1	0.4
Esophagitis	0.8	1.7	1.1	0.8	3.9	1.9
Duodenitis	2.3	0.9	0.9	2.3	3.5	5.0
Gastroesophageal Reflux	0.0	1.0	0.4	1.7	1.1	1.2
Duodenal Ulcer	0.0	1.2	0.1	0.4	0.7	2.7
Gastric Ulcer	0.8	0.6	0.7	1.7	3.2	6.9
Tooth Disorder	0.3	0.6	0.0	0.0	1.1	0.8
Hepatic						
ALT Increased	0.5	0.6	0.1	0.7	2.5	2.3
AST Increased	0.5	0.4	0.0	0.5	1.1	2.3
Psychiatric						
Insomnia	1.3	0.4	0.9	1.2	2.5	1.9
Somnolence	0.8	0.6	0.7	0.9	1.1	0.8
Respiratory						
Upper Respiratory Tract Infection	1.0	2.7	1.1	2.1	2.8	3.8
Pharyngitis	0.5	1.9	1.1	1.9	3.5	1.5
Rhinitis	0.8	2.6	0.3	0.9	3.2	4.2
Sinusitis	0.0	0.9	0.1	0.1	6.0	2.7
Coughing	0.3	1.2	0.4	1.2	1.8	3.5

(cont'd)

Table 1: Arthrotec *(cont'd)*
Adverse Reactions Reported in ≥1% of Patients

	A50[a] BID N=391	A50[a] TID N=692	A50[a] BID/TID N=750	D50[b] BID/TID N=754	A75[c] BID[e] N=285	D75[d] BID[e] N=260
Bronchitis	0.0	0.4	0.7	1.1	2.1	1.5
Dyspnea	0.3	0.4	0.4	0.7	1.4	0.4
Urogenital						
Menorrhagia	0.9	0.6	1.3	0.0	0.0	0.5
Vaginitis	0.0	0.9	0.0	0.0	1.0	1.1
Perineal Pain, Male	0.6	0.0	0.0	0.0	1.1	0.0

[a] A50=Arthrotec 50.
[b] D50=Diclofenac 50 mg.
[c] A75=Arthrotec 75.
[d] D75=Diclofenac 75 mg.
[e] Patients must have experienced ulceration in order to enter study. This represents an extremely high risk cohort.

Abdominal pain and diarrhea were generally transient and mild to moderate in severity, occurring early in the course of therapy and lasting several days. The abdominal pain and diarrhea usually resolved spontaneously while continuing Arthrotec.

Less Common Clinical Trial Adverse Drug Reactions (<1%) : The following adverse events were reported by 1% or less of the subjects receiving Arthrotec. Causal relationships between Arthrotec and these events have not been established but cannot be excluded.

Body as a Whole: hot flushes, malaise, rigors.
Cardiovascular: palpitation and syncope.
Central Nervous System/Psychiatric: anorexia, anxiety, concentration impaired, depression, hypoesthesia, mouth dry, speech disorder and vertigo.
Dermatologic: angioedema, erythematous rash, sweating increased, urticaria and purpura.
Gastrointestinal: abdomen enlarged, esophageal ulceration, gall bladder disorder, glossitis, hematemesis, hiccup and melena.
Gynecological: menstrual disorder, intermenstrual bleeding, dysmenorrhea, leukorrhea, vaginal bleeding, breast pain and uterine cramping. (Post-menopausal vaginal bleeding may be related to Arthrotec administration. If this occurs, diagnostic workup should be undertaken to rule out gynecological pathology.)
Hematologic: leukopenia and thrombocytopenia.
Hepatic: bilirubinemia, abnormal hepatic function, LDH increased, and alkaline phosphatase increased.
Metabolic: BUN increased and glycosuria.
Respiratory: hyperventilation and sputum increased.
Special Senses: earache, eye pain, taste loss, taste abnormalities, tinnitus and vision abnormal.
Urinary: dysuria and urine abnormal.

Abnormal Hematologic and Clinical Chemistry Findings: See Drug Interactions, Drug-Laboratory Test Interactions.

Post-Market Adverse Drug Reactions: Additional reports of serious adverse events temporally associated with Arthrotec during worldwide post-marketing experience are included below. Because these events are reported voluntary from a population of uncertain size, it is not always possible to reliably estimate their frequency or establish a causal relationship to Arthrotec exposure.

Allergic: reactions including anaphylaxis and angioedema.
Cardiovascular: myocardial infarction, stroke, transient ischemic attack, cerebral hemorrhage.
Central Nervous System/Psychiatric: changes in mood, nightmares.
Dermatologic: cutaneous reactions (including rash, pruritus and bullous eruption), rare cases of mucocutaneous reactions, edema, urticaria.
Gastrointestinal: dyspnea, hepatitis, interstitial nephritis, pancreatitis, stomatitis.
Gynecological: abnormal uterine contractions, uterine hemorrhage, uterine rupture/perforation, retained placenta, amniotic fluid embolism, incomplete abortion, premature birth, fetal death, and birth defects.
Hematology: thrombocytopenia.
Special Senses: blurred vision.
Urogenital: renal failure.

DRUG INTERACTIONS: Overview: Factors such as excess alcohol intake, smoking, and concomitant NSAID and oral steroid or anticoagulant use have been associated with increased risk of GI adverse events such as ulceration and bleeding. In laboratory studies, misoprostol has shown no significant effect on the cytochrome P450-linked hepatic mixed function oxidase system, and therefore should not affect the metabolism of theophylline, warfarin, benzodiazepines or other drugs normally metabolized by this system.

Diclofenac metabolism is predominantly mediated via cytochrome P450 CYP 2C9 in the liver. Patients who are known or suspected to be poor CYP2C9 metabolizers based on previous history/experience with other CYP2C9 substrates should be administered diclofenac with caution as they may have abnormally high plasma levels due to reduced metabolic clearance.

Drug-Drug Interactions: Misoprostol has been used concomitantly with at least 44 different classes of drugs, including more than 150 drugs. There were no reports of any clinically significant drug interactions.

Acetylsalicylic Acid (ASA) or other NSAIDs: When diclofenac and ASA are taken simultaneously, the bioavailability of each is reduced. Concomitant administration of Arthrotec and ASA is not recommended because diclofenac is displaced from its binding sites by ASA, resulting in lower plasma concentrations, peak plasma levels and AUC values. Misoprostol does not affect the kinetics of other NSAIDs (e.g., ibuprofen, indomethacin and piroxicam). The use of Arthrotec in addition to any other NSAID, including those over the counter ones (such as ASA and ibuprofen) for analgesic and/or anti-inflammatory effects is **not** recommended because of the absence of any evidence demonstrating synergistic benefits and the possibility of additive side effects.

The exception is the use of low dose ASA for cardiovascular protection, when another NSAID is being used for its analgesic/anti-inflammatory effect, keeping in mind that combination NSAID therapy is associated with additive adverse reactions.

Some NSAIDs (e.g. ibuprofen) may interfere with the anti-platelet effects of low dose ASA, possibly by competing with ASA for access to the active site of cyclooxygenase-I.

Antacids: Only aluminum-based antacids should be used with Arthrotec as magnesium-based antacids may increase the potential for diarrhea (see Adverse Reactions). The concomitant administration of aluminum hydroxide or magnesium hydroxide antacids may delay the absorption of diclofenac but does not affect the total amount of the drug absorbed. The total availability of misoprostol acid is reduced by antacids in large doses.

Anticoagulants: Numerous studies have shown that the concomitant use of NSAIDs and anticoagulants increases the risk of GI adverse events such as ulceration and bleeding. Pharmacodynamic studies have shown no potentiation of anticoagulant drugs due to concurrent administration with diclofenac. However, other NSAIDs have been shown to interact with anticoagulant agents. Although clinical investigations would appear to indicate that diclofenac has no influence on the effect of anticoagulants, there are isolated reports of an increased risk of hemorrhage with the combined use of diclofenac and nicoumalone anticoagulant therapy. Special caution is therefore recommended and frequent laboratory tests should be performed to check that the desired response to the anticoagulant is being maintained. Because prostaglandins play an important role in hemostasis and NSAIDs affect platelet function as well, concurrent therapy of Arthrotec with warfarin requires close monitoring to be certain no change in anticoagulant dosage is necessary (see Warnings and Precautions, Hematologic, Anti-Coagulants).

Anti-Hypertensives: NSAIDs may diminish the anti-hypertensive effect of Angiotensin Converting Enzyme (ACE) inhibitors.

Combinations of ACE inhibitors, angiotensin-II antagonists, or diuretics with NSAIDs might have an increased risk for acute renal failure and hyperkalemia. Blood pressure and renal function (including electrolytes) should be monitored more closely in this situation, as occasionally there can be a substantial increase in blood pressure.

Anti-Platelet Agents (including ASA): There is an increased risk of bleeding, via inhibition of platelet function, when anti-platelet agents are combined with NSAIDs, such as Arthrotec (see Warnings and Precautions, Hematologic, Anti-Platelet Effects).

Cyclosporin or Tacrolimus: Although this interaction has not been studied with Arthrotec, co-administration of cyclosporin or tacrolimus and any NSAID may increase the nephrotoxic effect of cyclosporin or tacrolimus due to the NSAID's effect on renal prostaglandins. Renal function should be monitored when Arthrotec and either of these drugs is used in combination.

CYP2C9 Substrates: Diclofenac metabolism is predominantly mediated via cytochrome P450 CYP 2C9 in the liver. Patients who are known or suspected to be poor CYP2C9 metabolizers based on previous history/experience with other CYP2C9 substrates should be administered diclofenac with caution as they may have abnormally high plasma levels due to reduced metabolic clearance.
Digoxin: Diclofenac may increase the plasma concentration of digoxin. Dosage adjustment of the digoxin may be required with Arthrotec. Serum digoxin levels should be monitored for possible digoxin toxicity.
Diuretics/Antihypertensives: Clinical studies as well as post-marketing observations have shown that NSAIDs can reduce the effect of diuretics. Concomitant treatment of Arthrotec with potassium-sparing diuretics may be associated with increased serum potassium levels, thus making it necessary to monitor the latter. The antihypertensive effect of hydrochlorothiazide and ACE inhibitors may be decreased by diclofenac in patients with essential hypertension. Coadministration of Arthrotec with ACE inhibitors may result in an impairment of renal function.
Glucocorticoids: Some studies have shown that the concomitant use of NSAIDs and oral glucocorticoids increases the risk of GI side effects such as ulceration and bleeding. This is especially the case in older (>65 years of age) individuals.
Lithium: Diclofenac, when administered concomitantly with lithium, increases the lithium plasma concentration through an effect on lithium renal clearance. Lithium toxicity may develop in these patients. Dosage adjustment of lithium may be required with Arthrotec.
Methotrexate: Concurrent administration of methotrexate and diclofenac may result in increased plasma levels of methotrexate and rare cases of fatal renal toxicity have been reported. Thus, caution should be taken when administering Arthrotec and methotrexate.
Oral Hypoglycemic Agents: Diclofenac does not alter glucose metabolism in normal subjects, and pharmacodynamic studies have shown no potentiation of oral hypoglycemic drugs due to concurrent administration with diclofenac. However, other NSAIDs have been shown to interact with oral hypoglycemic agents. Therefore, Arthrotec should be administered with caution in patients receiving insulin or oral hypoglycemic agents.
Selective Serotonin Reuptake Inhibitors (SSRIs): Concomitant administration of NSAIDs and SSRIs may increase the risk of gastrointestinal ulceration and bleeding (see Warnings and Precautions, Gastrointestinal).
Voriconazole: Voriconazole increased C_{max} and AUC of diclofenac (50 mg single dose) by 114% and 78%, respectively.
Drug-Food Interactions: Interactions with food have not been established.
Drug-Herb Interactions: Interactions with herbal products have not been established.
Drug-Laboratory Test Interactions: Diclofenac increases platelet aggregation time but does not affect bleeding time, plasma prothrombin clotting time, plasma fibrinogens, or factors V and VII to XII. Statistically significant changes in prothrombin and partial thromboplastin times have been reported in normal volunteers. The mean changes were observed to be less than 1 second in both instances, and are unlikely to be clinically important.
Drug-Lifestyle Interactions: Smoking and alcohol intake should be discouraged while taking Arthrotec as they constitute risk factors for increased cardiovascular and gastrointestinal problems respectively.

DOSAGE AND ADMINISTRATION: Dosing Considerations: In Elderly Patients: The dosage should be reduced to the lowest dose that will provide control of symptoms, adjusted when necessary, and closely supervised.
Renal Insufficiency: In patients with mild to moderate renal insufficiency, the lowest dose of Arthrotec should be considered, and patients should be monitored closely (see Action and Clinical Pharmacology, Pharmacokinetics, Special Populations and Conditions, Renal Insufficiency). Arthrotec is contraindicated in patients with severe renal impairment (estimated creatinine clearance <30 mL/min or 0.5 mL/sec) (see Contraindications).
Hepatic Insufficiency: If Arthrotec must be used in patients with mild to moderate hepatic impairment, these patients must be closely monitored. ARTHROTEC is contraindicated in patients with significant hepatic impairment or active liver disease (see Contraindications).

Diclofenac metabolism is predominantly mediated via cytochrome P450 CYP 2C9 in the liver. Patients who are known or suspected to be poor CYP2C9 metabolizers based on previous history/experience with other CYP2C9 substrates should be administered diclofenac with caution as they may have abnormally high plasma levels due to reduced metabolic clearance.
Recommended Dose and Dosage Adjustment—18 years of age and older: Use of Arthrotec should be limited to the lowest effective dose in every patient (see Warnings and Precautions).

The recommended daily oral dose of Arthrotec (diclofenac sodium plus misoprostol) for treating the signs and symptoms of rheumatoid arthritis and osteoarthritis is 100 mg administered as two divided doses (50 mg twice per day). For patients experiencing an inflammatory flare, who do not achieve control of symptoms with 100 mg of diclofenac, the dosage may be increased to a maximum of 150 mg per day in divided doses (50 mg TID or 75 mg BID) for the shortest duration possible and under close monitoring (see Warnings and Precautions, Cardiovascular).

In elderly patients, patients with renal insufficiency, hepatic impairment and patients with a cardiovascular risk, the maximum daily dose is 100 mg of diclofenac (Arthrotec 50 BID) (see Dosing Considerations).

Arthrotec should be taken **immediately after a meal or with food or milk**.
Missed Dose: If a dose of Arthrotec is missed, the next dose should be taken at the regular time. The dose should not be doubled.
Administration: Arthrotec should be swallowed whole.

OVERDOSAGE:
Diclofenac Sodium: Worldwide reports on overdosage with diclofenac cover 27 cases. In 10 of these 27 cases, diclofenac was the only drug taken; all of these patients recovered. The highest dose of diclofenac was 2.5 g in a 20-year-old male who suffered acute renal failure as a consequence, and who was treated with dialysis sessions and recovered in 2 days. The next highest dose was 2.35 g in a 17-year-old female who experienced vomiting and drowsiness. A dose of 2.0 g of diclofenac was taken by a woman of unspecified age who remained asymptomatic.

There is no specific antidote for diclofenac. In cases of overdosage, absorption should be prevented as soon as possible by means of induction of vomiting, gastric lavage or treatment with activated charcoal.

Supportive and symptomatic treatment should be given for complications such as drowsiness, confusion, general hypotonia, hypotension, renal failure, convulsions, gastrointestinal irritation and respiratory depression. Measures to accelerate elimination (forced diuresis, hemoperfusion, dialysis) may be considered, but may be of limited use because of the high protein-binding and extensive metabolism (diclofenac 99% protein bound and misoprostol acid less than 90% protein bound).
Misoprostol: The toxic dose of misoprostol in humans has not been determined. Cumulative total daily doses of 1600 µg have been tolerated with only symptoms of gastrointestinal discomfort being reported.

Clinical signs that may indicate an overdose are sedation, tremor, convulsions, dyspnea, abdominal pain, diarrhea, fever, palpitations, hypotension, or bradycardia. Symptoms should be treated with supportive therapy.

It is not known if misoprostol acid is dialyzable. However, because misoprostol is metabolized like a fatty acid, it is unlikely that dialysis would be appropriate treatment for overdosage.

The use of oral activated charcoal may help to reduce the absorption of diclofenac and misoprostol.

> For management of a suspected drug overdose, CPhA recommends that you contact your **regional Poison Control Centre**. See the *CPS* Directory section for a list of Poison Control Centres.

ACTION AND CLINICAL PHARMACOLOGY: Mechanism of Action: Arthrotec (diclofenac sodium plus misoprostol) is a combination of a nonsteroidal anti-inflammatory drug (NSAID) with a mucosal protective synthetic analog of prostaglandin E_1.

Diclofenac inhibits prostaglandin synthesis by interfering with the action of prostaglandin synthetase. This inhibitory effect may partially explain its actions, both therapeutic and adverse.

Misoprostol has been shown to inhibit both basal and stimulated gastric acid secretion. In addition, increases in gastric mucosal blood flow, duodenal bicarbonate secretion and gastric mucus secretion have all been observed following treatment with misoprostol. It is not known whether the ability of misoprostol to prevent gastric and duodenal ulcers is the result of its antisecretory effect, its mucosal protective effect, or both.
Pharmacokinetics: The pharmacokinetic profiles of diclofenac and misoprostol administered alone are similar to the profiles when they are coadministered as separate tablets, or given as Arthrotec (diclofenac sodium plus misoprostol). No pharmacokinetic interaction between the two drugs has been observed following either single or multiple doses.

There was no accumulation of diclofenac or misoprostol acid in plasma following repeated doses of Arthrotec.
Absorption: Orally administered diclofenac is rapidly and almost completely absorbed.

Orally administered misoprostol is also rapidly and extensively absorbed.

With Arthrotec the effect of food on the bioavailability of the diclofenac and misoprostol components is similar to that reported for the individual drugs. The times of peak concentration (T_{max}) for diclofenac and misoprostol are prolonged by approximately 50% and 100% respectively, while the peak concentrations (C_{max}) are decreased by about 25% for diclofenac and 50% for misoprostol: the AUC for diclofenac is decreased by approximately 60%, while that of misoprostol is increased by about 25%.
Distribution: Diclofenac is highly but reversibly bound in the plasma. Following administration of enteric-coated tablets there is high between- and within-subject variability in the plasma concentrations of diclofenac, particularly if the tablets are taken with food. However, the plasma concentrations show a linear relationship to the amount of drug administered and no accumulation occurs provided that the recommended dosage intervals are observed.

There is high variability in plasma levels of misoprostol acid, but mean values after single doses show a linear relationship with dose over the range of 200 to 400 µg. No accumulation has been found in multiple dose studies and plasma steady state was achieved within two days.
Metabolism: Diclofenac metabolism is predominantly mediated via cytochrome P450 CYP 2C9 in the liver. Diclofenac undergoes single and multiple hydroxylation and methoxylation, producing 3'-, 4'-, 5-hydroxy, 4'-5-hydroxy and 3'-hydroxy-4'-methoxy derivatives of diclofenac. These phenolic metabolites are largely inactive, and (along with the parent compound) are mostly converted to glucuronide conjugates.

Misoprostol undergoes rapid metabolism to misoprostol acid.

Table 2: Arthrotec

Summary of Mean Arthrotec Pharmacokinetic Parameters

	C_{max}		AUC		T_{max}	
	D[a] (µg/mL)	M[a] (pg/mL)	D (µg·h/mL)	M (pg·h/mL)	D (h)	M (h)
Single dose of Arthrotec 50 Healthy Male Subjects N=36	1.13	136	1.63 ($AUC_{(0–24)}$)	238 ($AUC_{(0–4)}$)	3.9	0.87
Single dose of Arthrotec 75 Healthy Male and Female Subjects N=35	2.03	304	2.77 ($AUC_{(0-12)}$)	177 ($AUC_{(0-4)}$)	1.96	0.26

[a] D=diclofenac; M=misoprostol acid.

Excretion: The half-life of diclofenac is 1 to 2 hours. Forty to 60% of the drug and its metabolites are eliminated in the urine and the balance in the bile.

Misoprostol acid is quickly eliminated (elimination half-life of approximately 30 minutes). Approximately 70% of the dose of misoprostol is excreted in the urine, mainly as biologically inactive metabolites.
Special Populations and Conditions: Geriatrics: The kinetics and metabolism of diclofenac do not appear to be affected by age. In the elderly, the AUC of misoprostol acid is increased by roughly 40%.
Poor CYP2C9 Metabolizers: Diclofenac metabolism is predominantly mediated via cytochrome P450 CYP 2C9 in the liver. Patients who are known or suspected to be poor CYP2C9 metabolizers based on previous history/experience with other CYP2C9 substrates should be administered diclofenac with caution as they may have abnormally high plasma levels due to reduced metabolic clearance.
Hepatic Insufficiency: The kinetics and metabolism of diclofenac do not appear to be affected by hepatic impairment.

Misoprostol does not affect the hepatic mixed function oxidase (cytochrome P-450) enzyme system in animals. In a study of people with mild to moderate hepatic impairment, mean misoprostol acid AUC and C_{max} showed approximately double the mean values obtained in healthy people. Three people who had the lowest antipyrine and lowest indocyanine green clearance values had the highest misoprostol acid AUC and C_{max} values.
Renal Insufficiency: Differences in the pharmacokinetics of diclofenac (50 mg intravenously) have not been detected in studies of patients with renal impairment (N=5, creatinine clearance 3 to 42 mL/min). In these patients, AUC values and elimination rates were comparable to those in healthy people.

Following oral administration of misoprostol in patients with mild-to-moderate renal impairment, there was no significant effect on the pharmacokinetic profile compared to normal subjects. However, in anuric patients, an approximate doubling of C_{max}, AUC and $t_{½}$ of misoprostol acid has been observed compared to normal subjects.
STORAGE AND STABILITY: Store at 15 to 25°C and protect from heat and humidity.
INFORMATION FOR THE PATIENT: Published in e-CPS, available by subscription at www.e-cps.ca.
DOSAGE FORMS, COMPOSITION AND PACKAGING: Arthrotec 50: Each white to off-white, round and biconvex tablet, engraved "SEARLE" over "1411" on one side, 4×"A" around the circumference of the reverse side with "50" in the middle, contains: an enteric-coated core of diclofenac sodium 50 mg, surrounded by an outer mantle containing misoprostol 200 µg. Nonmedicinal ingredients: colloidal silicon dioxide, cornstarch, crospovidone, hydrogenated castor oil, hypromellose, lactose, magnesium stearate, methacrylic acid copolymer, microcrystalline cellulose, povidone K-30, sodium hydroxide, talc and triethyl citrate. Bottles of 250. **Pharmacist:** Dispense with Patient Insert.
Arthrotec 75: Each white to off-white, round and biconvex tablet, engraved "SEARLE" over "1421" on one side, 4×"A" around the circumference of the reverse side with a "75" in the middle, contains: an enteric-coated core of diclofenac sodium 75 mg, surrounded by an outer mantle containing misoprostol 200 µg. Nonmedicinal ingredients: colloidal silicon dioxide, cornstarch, crospovidone, hydrogenated castor oil, hypromellose, lactose, magnesium stearate, methacrylic acid copolymer, microcrystalline cellulose, povidone K-30, sodium hydroxide, talc and triethyl citrate. Bottles of 250. **Pharmacist:** Dispense with Patient Insert.

(Shown in Product Identification Section)

ASA

Analgesic—Antipyretic—Anti-inflammatory—Platelet Aggregation Inhibitor

CPhA Monograph

Date of Revision: November 2007

> This monograph has been compiled by CPhA and reviewed by experts. It may contain information different from that found in Health Canada-approved Product Monographs. The reader is referred to the CPS Editorial Policy for more information.

SUMMARY PRODUCT INFORMATION:

Route of Administration[a]	Dosage Form[a]	Strength[a]
Oral	Immediate-release tablet	80 mg, 325 mg, 500 mg
	Enteric-coated tablet	80 mg, 81 mg, 325 mg, 650 mg, 975 mg
	Chewable tablet	80 mg, 81 mg
Rectal	Suppository	150 mg, 650 mg

[a] ASA is also available in several combination products. Consult Health Canada's Drug Product Database, available at http://www.hc-sc.gc.ca/dhp-mps/prodpharma/databasdon/index_e.html

PHARMACOLOGY: ASA (acetylsalicylic acid) interferes with the production of prostaglandins in various organs and tissues through acetylation and inactivation of cyclooxygenase. The main action of the drug is thought to be peripheral; however, it may have similar activity in the CNS. The reduction in tissue levels of prostaglandins may be responsible for ASA's analgesic and anti-inflammatory effects. ASA is most effective in the management of pain of low to moderate intensity associated with inflammation.

ASA is also a potent antipyretic and lowers body temperature in patients with fever, mainly through inhibition of prostaglandin E_1 synthesis in the brain. Heat production is not affected but dissipation of heat is enhanced via increased blood flow through the skin and sweating.

ASA has antiplatelet activity through inhibition of thromboxane A_2 synthesis. Thromboxane A_2 plays an essential role in platelet aggregation. ASA prevents thromboxane A_2 formation by acetylating cyclooxygenase, a catalytic enzyme involved in the early stages of the inflammatory cascade. ASA's effect on the platelet is irreversible and persists for the life of the platelet (7 to 10 days).

Pharmacokinetics: Following oral administration, ASA is rapidly absorbed from the stomach and proximal small intestine, although there is some evidence that absorption may be substantially impaired in children during the febrile phase of Kawasaki syndrome (mucocutaneous lymph node syndrome).

Following oral administration, ASA is partially hydrolyzed to salicylate by esterases in the gastrointestinal mucosa. Once absorbed, further hydrolysis by esterases takes place, mainly in the liver but also in plasma, erythrocytes and synovial fluid.

Optimum absorption of salicylate occurs in the pH range of 2.15 to 4.1. Enteric-coated tablets resist disintegration at a pH less than 3.5 for a period of at least 2 hours, but can disintegrate in 10 to 30 minutes at a pH of greater than 5.5. Absorption of enteric-coated tablets takes place primarily in the duodenum.

Rectal absorption of ASA is slow, variable and usually incomplete and may be associated with rectal mucosal irritation.

Peak blood levels occur approximately 2 hours after ingestion of regular tablets and 6 to 8 hours after the ingestion of enteric-coated tablets.

ASA is widely distributed in most body tissues and fluids. The protein binding of salicylate is concentration dependent. The bound fraction decreases as the plasma concentration of salicylate increases; at low concentrations of less than 0.75 mmol/L about 90% of the drug is bound and at concentrations between 0.76 and 2.9 mmol/L, approximately 70 to 85% is bound.

The elimination half-life of ASA is 14 to 20 minutes. The half-life of salicylate is 2 to 3 hours after low doses of ASA and up to 15 to 30 hours after anti-inflammatory doses of ASA. Salicylate undergoes hepatic metabolism. Salicylate and its metabolites are rapidly and almost completely excreted in the urine. Only about 1% of ASA is excreted in the urine unchanged. This proportion is extremely variable and depends on dose and urinary pH.

Because of capacity-limited metabolism, serum concentrations of salicylate increase more than proportionally with an increase in dose.

INDICATIONS: ASA is used in the treatment of fever and mild to moderate pain. It is also used to relieve pain and inflammation associated with osteoarthritis, rheumatoid arthritis, juvenile arthritis and other musculoskeletal disorders.

As an antiplatelet agent, ASA is used to prevent thrombosis and reduce the risk of nonfatal MI, nonfatal stroke and death in the following clinical situations: ST segment elevation myocardial infarction (STEMI); non-ST segment elevation myocardial infarction (NSTEMI); unstable angina; primary prevention of ischemic stroke; primary prevention of coronary events in patients at high coronary risk, except in patients with a history of ASA intolerance or at increased risk of GI bleeding or hemorrhagic stroke; secondary prevention following myocardial infarction; chronic angina; secondary prevention following single or multiple transient ischemic attacks (TIAs) or ischemic stroke. It is unclear whether the potential benefit of ASA for primary prevention of coronary events in *low-risk* patients outweighs the potentially increased risk of GI bleeding or hemorrhagic stroke.

ASA is not recommended for prevention of a first stroke in otherwise healthy men. ASA can be useful in preventing a first stroke in women, particularly those over 65 years of age, but the decision should be individualized based on a benefit/risk analysis.

In general, ASA is more effective in men than women in preventing myocardial infarction.

Treatment with a proton pump inhibitor significantly reduces the rate of GI ulcer complications in patients receiving low-dose ASA who have a history of ASA-related ulcers [N Engl J Med 2002;346(26):2033-8]. Moreover, this combination is more effective than switching to clopidogrel in this population [N Engl J Med 2005;352(3):238-44].

ASA is used to prevent thrombotic complications in patients undergoing procedures such as coronary angioplasty, placement of intracoronary stents, coronary artery bypass or carotid endarterectomy and to prevent thrombosis in patients with atrial fibrillation who are at low risk of stroke (see Dosage) or in whom warfarin is contraindicated.

ASA is used in the treatment of acute pericarditis following MI and in the treatment of rheumatic fever, in conjunction with penicillin and other appropriate therapy. ASA is also used in the treatment of Kawasaki disease in conjunction with iv immune globulin.

CONTRAINDICATIONS: ASA is contraindicated in patients who have had a bronchospastic reaction, generalized urticaria, angioedema, severe rhinitis, laryngeal edema or shock precipitated by ASA or nonsteroidal anti-inflammatory drugs (see Precautions, Hypersensitivity).

ASA should not be used in patients with active peptic ulcer (see Warnings and Precautions).

WARNINGS: ASA is one of the most frequent causes of accidental poisoning in toddlers and infants. ASA-containing products should be kept well out of the reach of children.

ASA should not be used in children, teenagers or young adults with chickenpox, influenza or flu-like illness. A strong association has been made between development of Reye's syndrome and ingestion of salicylates (almost exclusively ASA) for these illnesses, although a causal relationship has not been established. Reye's syndrome is characterized by the onset of protracted vomiting 3 to 7 days following the onset of influenza, flu-like illness or chickenpox, with subsequent development of progressive CNS symptoms such as lethargy, drowsiness, combative behavior, confusion, delirium, seizures and coma. The liver is also affected, with fatty infiltrations and elevation of AST and ALT. Early recognition and treatment are crucial as this syndrome can be fatal or can result in permanent brain damage.

Most evidence to date, including a decline in the use of ASA in children and a continuing decline in reported cases of Reye's syndrome, supports an association between the two.

As with other nonsteroidal anti-inflammatory drugs, serious gastrointestinal toxicity, such as peptic ulceration, perforation and bleeding, sometimes severe and occasionally fatal, can occur at any time, with or without symptoms, in patients treated with ASA (see Precautions).

PRECAUTIONS: ASA should be used with extreme caution in patients with decreased renal function, bleeding tendencies, significant anemia, hypoprothrombinemia, thrombocytopenia, vitamin K deficiency or severe hepatic disease.

Gastrointestinal: Gastrointestinal toxicity may occur with the use of ASA (see Warnings). No studies, to date, have identified any group of patients not at risk of ulceration and bleeding. A history of serious gastrointestinal events and other factors such as ASA dosage, excessive alcohol intake, smoking, advanced age, female gender and concomitant corticosteroid or anticoagulant use have been associated with increased risk. Patients should be informed about the signs and symptoms of serious gastrointestinal toxicity and advised to contact their physician immediately if they occur. Because serious events can occur without warning symptoms, patients on long-term therapy should have periodic hemoglobin determinations in conjunction with vigilant follow-up.

Hypersensitivity: ASA sensitivity is rare, occurring in less than 1% of the general population. It usually involves bronchospasm, urticaria, angioedema and rarely, shock and death. ASA sensitivity occurs in a higher percentage (approximately 10%) of adults with asthma, more often in women than men, and rarely in children. The syndrome of ASA-induced asthma usually begins as chronic nasal congestion with subsequent development of nasal polyps. Asthma and ASA sensitivity follow, with disease progression despite avoidance of ASA and cross-reacting drugs. The mechanism is thought to involve inhibition of intracellular cyclooxygenase (COX) in respiratory cells. Patients with ASA-induced asthma should avoid other drugs that inhibit COX, such as NSAIDs, but the majority can safely take other salicylates that do not inhibit COX enzymes (e.g., bismuth subsalicylate). Dose-dependent cross-sensitivity with acetaminophen has been reported with frequencies of up to 34%. It is recommended that patients with ASA-induced asthma use low initial doses of acetaminophen (less than 1000 mg) with monitoring for 3 hours after initial doses.

Some patients with ASA-induced asthma have been desensitized with small incremental oral doses of ASA over the course of 2 to 3 days until 400 to 650 mg is tolerated, followed by maintenance doses of 80 to 325 mg daily. Cross-desensitization to other reacting drugs also occurs when patients are desensitized to ASA.

Salicylism: Chronic salicylate intoxication can occur when repeated large doses (> 100 mg/kg/day) are used for 2 or more days (see Overdose).

Surgery: ASA should be discontinued at least one week prior to elective surgery because of increased risk of bleeding.

Drug Interactions: Analgesics: Concurrent long-term use of ASA and other analgesic-antipyretic agents such as acetaminophen may be associated with analgesic nephropathy (papillary necrosis and tubulointerstitial inflammation).

Antacids: Chronic high-dose use of antacids may increase renal elimination of salicylates through alkalinization of the urine.

Anticoagulants: Concomitant use of ASA and anticoagulants increases the risk of bleeding. Large doses of ASA may enhance the hypoprothrombinemic response to warfarin; however, ASA is used in selected patients with prosthetic heart valves or coronary artery disease in conjunction with warfarin, with appropriate monitoring.

Antiepileptic Drugs: Large doses of ASA may increase phenytoin serum levels by inhibition of phenytoin metabolism. Valproic acid may cause hypoprothrombinemia and inhibit platelet aggregation. Concomitant use of ASA and valproic acid may cause increased valproic acid levels and may lead to an increased risk of bleeding.

Antihyperglycemic Agents: ASA increases the antihyperglycemic response to sulfonylureas, especially chlorpropamide. Large doses of ASA may cause a decrease in blood glucose, which may alter the insulin requirements of diabetic patients.

Corticosteroids: Corticosteroids may decrease the serum salicylate concentrations through increased excretion. Concomitant use may also increase the risk of gastrointestinal side effects.

Methotrexate: Concurrent use of ASA and methotrexate may lead to higher methotrexate serum levels, mainly through competition for renal excretion.

Nonsteroidal Anti-inflammatory Drugs (NSAIDs): Concomitant use of ASA and NSAIDs increases the risk of gastrointestinal side effects while providing no additional therapeutic benefit. It has also been suggested that ibuprofen and possibly other NSAIDs antagonize the antiplatelet effects of low-dose preventive ASA therapy, and that taking the daily ASA dose 2 hours before the other NSAID may help prevent this interaction.

Uricosuric Agents: ASA may decrease the uricosuric effects of sulfinpyrazone and probenecid.

Vancomycin: Use of vancomycin with ASA may increase the risk of ototoxicity.

Vitamin C: Large doses of vitamin C may decrease the excretion of ASA because of acidification of the urine.

Zidovudine: ASA may increase the risk of zidovudine toxicity by decreasing the hepatic metabolism of zidovudine.

Drug/Lab Test Interactions: Bleeding time: ASA may prolong bleeding time for 4 to 7 days due to its effects on platelet aggregation.

Copper Sulfate Urine Sugar Tests: Daily doses of ASA greater than 2.4 g may cause false positive results.

Thyroid Function Tests: Large doses of salicylates may increase T_3 resin uptake and decrease serum concentrations of T_3 and T_4 when determined by radioimmunoassay. Salicylates may also affect TRH-induced TSH release determinations.

Pregnancy: The use of full-dose ASA during pregnancy should generally be avoided, particularly in the 3rd trimester. ASA can affect hemostasis in both the mother and fetus, leading to higher risk of hemorrhage. Other possible effects include anemia and prolonged gestation and labor in the mother, and intrauterine growth retardation or premature closure of the ductus arteriosus in the fetus.

Low-dose ASA has been used therapeutically in very specific situations related to pregnancy, such as antiphospholipid syndrome and for prevention of pre-eclampsia; however more study is needed to establish the risk/benefit ratio of such therapy.

Lactation: ASA is excreted in breast milk in low concentrations. Because of the potential effects of ASA on nursing infants, caution is advised if ASA is used during lactation, particularly chronic high-dose therapy.

Geriatrics: Patients over 65 years of age and frail or debilitated patients are more susceptible to many adverse effects of ASA, including gastrointestinal toxicity. Consideration should be given to using lower initial dosages in this patient group.

ADVERSE EFFECTS: Cardiovascular: Pulmonary edema may occur with chronic or acute ingestion of large doses.

Dermatologic: Skin eruptions and lesions have been reported. Stevens-Johnson syndrome has rarely been associated with ASA.

Gastrointestinal: Ulcer, hemorrhage, dyspepsia, heartburn, epigastric distress, nausea, vomiting, diarrhea or abdominal pain may occur with increasing incidence at higher dosages (see Warnings and Precautions).

Hematologic: Leukopenia, thrombocytopenia, pancytopenia, agranulocytosis, aplastic anemia, purpura, eosinophilia associated with ASA-induced hepatoxicity have been reported rarely. Hematocrit and plasma iron concentration may be decreased with daily doses of 3 to 4 g.

Hepatic: Reversible hepatoxicity, particularly in patients with juvenile rheumatoid arthritis and systemic lupus erythematosus, has been reported rarely.

Hypersensitivity: See Precautions, Hypersensitivity.

Otic: Tinnitus and hearing loss, usually completely reversible, may occur in patients receiving large doses of ASA or with long-term use and are dose-related.

OVERDOSE:

Acute ASA intoxication can result from single ingestions of 150 mg/kg or more. Chronic ASA intoxication, also known as salicylism, can occur during high-dose therapy, e.g., > 100 mg/kg/day for 2 or more days. Salicylism most often occurs in an elderly patient being treated for a chronic condition such as rheumatoid arthritis, in whom a small increase in dose or a small decrease in clearance can result in a significant increase in serum salicylate concentration.

Symptoms: Acute: The severity of symptoms depends on the size of the dose ingested. Mild to moderate toxicity usually results from ingestion of 150 to 300 mg/kg; single doses of 300 to 500 mg/kg can lead to severe intoxication and over 500 mg/kg can be lethal.

Early signs and symptoms of an acute overdose of ASA include nausea, vomiting, diaphoresis and tinnitus (which often progresses to decreased auditory acuity or even deafness). Other CNS symptoms include hyperventilation, vertigo, agitation, delirium, hallucinations, convulsions, lethargy and stupor. Hyperthermia also occurs, and a marked temperature increase indicates severe toxicity. Acid-base disturbances are typical. A respiratory alkalosis secondary to hyperventilation usually predominates initially, but then gives way to a wide anion gap acidosis. Adults usually present with a mixed respiratory alkalosis and metabolic acidosis, while children often present with significant metabolic acidosis. Patients who have co-ingested a CNS depressant may present with respiratory acidosis, as may those with salicylate-induced pulmonary edema or severe fatigue from prolonged hyperventilation.

Chronic: Symptoms of chronic intoxication may include tinnitus, hearing loss, dizziness, confusion, drowsiness, hyperventilation, metabolic acidosis, respiratory alkalosis, tachycardia, hyperthermia, nausea and vomiting. The diagnosis of chronic salicylate intoxication is often delayed, possibly because symptoms have a slower onset and appear less severe than those of acute intoxication. Patients may initially be diagnosed as having delirium, sepsis, respiratory failure, cardiopulmonary disease (e.g., heart failure) or another disorder.

Treatment: Acute: Treatment of acute ASA overdose consists of intensive symptomatic and supportive therapy aimed at removal of unabsorbed ASA from the gut, prevention of further ASA absorption, enhancement of ASA elimination and correction of fluid, electrolyte and acid-base disturbances. Although specific recommendations regarding gut decontamination can vary considerably, at least one dose of activated charcoal (1 g/kg body weight) should be administered. A Poison Control Centre should be consulted regarding the potential need for additional decontamination, and for advice concerning other therapy. Other therapeutic measures may include: monitoring serum salicylate levels; correction of hypoglycemia, acidosis and hypokalemia with iv glucose, potassium and bicarbonate as required; management of seizures with iv diazepam; alkalinization of the urine; hemodialysis.

Chronic: Management of chronic ASA intoxication depends on the severity of the patient's clinical condition. Mild toxicity can usually be managed with reduction of the dose or discontinuation of ASA and symptomatic and supportive measures as required. Severe intoxication may require the same measures as for acute ingestions. Hemodialysis may be particularly beneficial, even in the absence of high serum salicylate levels.

> For management of a suspected drug overdose, CPhA recommends that you contact your **regional Poison Control Centre**. See the *CPS* Directory section for a list of Poison Control Centres.

DOSAGE: ASA should be taken with food or milk to minimize gastric irritation. Enteric-coated tablets may be used in patients with gastric intolerance to regular ASA tablets.

ASA should not be used for self-medication of high fever (greater than 39.5°C), fever persisting longer than 3 days, or recurrent fever, unless directed by a physician since such fevers may indicate serious illness requiring prompt medical attention.

ASA should not be used for self-medication of pain for longer than 10 days in adults or 5 days in children, unless directed by a physician, since pain of such intensity and duration may indicate a pathological condition requiring medical evaluation.

Enteric-coated preparations are not recommended for use in fever or in children under 2 years.

Analgesic/Antipyretic: Oral: Adults: 325 to 650 mg 4 to 6 times daily as necessary.

Children: **ASA should not be used in children, teenagers or young adults with chickenpox, influenza or flu-like symptoms** (see Warnings). 10 to 15 mg/kg every 4 to 6 hours as needed up to a maximum of 65 mg/kg/day. Alternatively, Table 1 gives dosage recommendation for children.

Table 1: ASA

Dosage Recommendations for Children[a,b]

Age (years)	Single Dose	Maximum Daily Dose
< 2	Recommendation of physician	
2 to < 4	160 mg	800 mg
4 to < 6	240 mg	1200 mg
6 to < 9	320 mg	1600 mg
9 to < 11	400 mg	2000 mg

(cont'd)

Table 1: ASA *(cont'd)*

Dosage Recommendations for Children[a,b]

Age (years)	Single Dose	Maximum Daily Dose
11 to < 12	480 mg	2400 mg

[a] The recommended dose may be given every 4 hours as necessary. Do not administer more than 5 doses to children in any 24-hour period.
[b] See Warnings, regarding possible association with Reye's syndrome.

Rectal: Adults: 650 mg 4 to 6 times a day as required. Children: As for oral analgesic/antipyretic dose outlined above.
Anti-inflammatory: Dosage must be individualized according to the patient's response, tolerance and serum salicylate levels. Serum salicylate concentration determinations are recommended if high dosage regimens are used, due to wide interindividual variations in pharmacokinetics. Usual serum salicylate concentrations for anti-inflammatory effect range from 1.1 to 2.2 mmol/L.
Adults: Usual initial anti-inflammatory dose is 2.4 to 3.6 g daily in divided doses. Dosage may be increased gradually if necessary. The usual maintenance dose is 3.6 to 5.4 g daily in divided doses, but higher doses may be required.
Children (see Warnings): Usual initial anti-inflammatory dose is 60 to 90 mg/kg daily in divided doses, up to 100 mg/kg daily. Adjust dosage slowly according to patient's tolerance to achieve optimal therapeutic response.
Platelet Antiaggregant: Adults: The following dosages represent recommended regimens based on current guidelines, and are expressed in accordance with marketed tablet strengths.
STEMI [*Circulation* 2004;110:588-636]: Initial dose of 162 to 325 mg, preferably nonenteric coated, chewed and swallowed, then 80 to 162 mg po daily, continued indefinitely.
Pericarditis following STEMI [*Circulation* 2004;110:588-636]: Up to 650 mg every 4 to 6 hours may be required.
Post coronary artery bypass graft [*Circulation* 2004;110:588-636]: 80 to 325 mg daily, started as soon as possible (within 24 hours) and continued indefinitely.
NSTEMI/Unstable angina [*Circulation* 2007;116:e148-304]: Initial dose of 162 to 325 mg, preferably nonenteric coated, chewed and swallowed. In patients receiving medical therapy without a stent: 80 to 162 mg daily, continued indefinitely, plus clopidogrel 75 mg daily for the first 1 to 12 months. Patients receiving bare metal stents: 162 to 325 mg daily for at least one month then 80 to 162 mg daily continued indefinitely, plus clopidogrel 75 mg daily for the first 1 to 12 months. Patients receiving drug-eluting stents: ASA 162 to 325 mg daily for at least 3 months for sirolimus-eluting stents and at least 6 months for paclitaxel–eluting stents, then 80 to 162 mg daily continued indefinitely, plus clopidogrel 75 mg daily for at least the first 12 months.

In this setting, it has been shown that maintenance doses of ASA as low as 75 mg daily yield outcomes similar to 325 mg daily, but with a lower risk of adverse effects [*Circulation* 2006;113:156–175].
Primary prevention of coronary events in patients with 10-year coronary risk ≥ 10% [*Circulation* 2002;106:388–91]: 80 to 325 mg daily continued indefinitely. In this patient group, ASA is not recommended in patients with a history of ASA intolerance or at increased risk of GI bleeding or hemorrhagic stroke.
Chronic angina [*Circulation* 2007 Nov 12;116:Epub ahead of print]: 80 to 325 mg daily continued indefinitely.
Secondary prevention of ischemic stroke (history of TIA or ischemic stroke) [*Stroke* 2006;37:577-617]: 80 to 325 mg daily. Patients who also have persistent or paroxysmal atrial fibrillation and who cannot take warfarin should take 325 mg daily.
Primary prevention of ischemic stroke in patients with atrial fibrillation [*Stroke* 2006; 37:1583-1633]: Preventive therapy can be determined using the $CHADS_2$ score, calculated as follows: 1 point each for presence of heart failure, hypertension, age ≥ 75 years or diabetes mellitus; 2 points for history of stroke or TIA; maximum score = 6.

For patients with a $CHADS_2$ score of 0: ASA 80 to 325 mg daily; those with a $CHADS_2$ score of 1 may receive ASA 80 to 325 mg daily or warfarin; patients with $CHADS_2$ scores of ≥ 2 should receive warfarin, but patients who cannot take warfarin may receive ASA 325 mg daily.
Vascular procedures: Recommendations vary according to procedure.
Kawasaki syndrome: Children: Initial (febrile phase): 80 to 100 mg/kg per day in 4 divided doses with serum level monitoring. Some patients may require higher doses to achieve therapeutic levels because of impaired absorption during the febrile phase of the disease. When fever subsides, the dose should be reduced to 3 to 5 mg/kg once daily until 6 to 10 weeks after initial onset of illness. In patients with coronary involvement, ASA is often continued due to the potential benefit of its antithrombotic effects.
Acute Rheumatic Fever: Usual adult dose is 5 to 8 g daily and for children, 60 to 100 mg/kg/day administered in 4 to 6 divided doses for 1 to 2 weeks; then decreased to 60 to 70 mg/kg/day for 1 to 6 weeks or until required; then gradually withdrawn over 1 to 2 weeks.

Asacol® Pr

5-ASA

Lower Gastrointestinal Anti-inflammatory

Warner Chilcott

SUPPLIED: Each brown-red, capsule-shaped, enteric-coated tablet, printed in black ink with "ASACOL NE", contains: 5-ASA (mesalamine) 400 mg. Each colon-targeted tablet is coated with a special acrylic-based resin, Eudragit S (methacrylic acid copolymer Type B [USP]), which delays release of the 5-ASA until the tablet reaches the terminal ileum. Nonmedicinal ingredients: colloidal silicon dioxide, dibutyl phthalate, edible black ink (ammonium hydroxide, n-butyl alcohol, propylene glycol, shellac glaze [modified] in SD-45 and synthetic black iron oxide), Eudragit S (methacrylic acid copolymer Type B [USP]), iron oxide red, iron oxide yellow, lactose, magnesium stearate, polyethylene glycol, polyvinylpyrrolidone, sodium starch glycolate and talc. Bottles of 180. Store at controlled room temperature (15-30°C).

(Shown in Product Identification Section)

Asacol® 800 Pr

5-ASA

Lower Gastrointestinal Anti-inflammatory

Warner Chilcott

Date of Revision: February 3, 2010

SUMMARY PRODUCT INFORMATION:

Route of Administration	Dosage Form/ Strength	Clinically Relevant Nonmedicinal Ingredients
Oral	Mesalamine Delayed Release Tablets, 800 mg	Lactose For a complete listing see Dosage Forms, Compositions and Packaging.

INDICATIONS AND CLINICAL USE: ASACOL 800 (800 mg tablet; mesalamine or 5-aminosalicylic acid) is indicated for:
- treatment of moderately active ulcerative colitis.

In the pivotal clinical trial with ASACOL 800 (800 mg tablet), moderately active ulcerative colitis was determined by a Physician Global Assessment (PGA) which included clinical and endoscopic evaluations scored as a 2 on a 0 (normal) to 3 (severe) scale.

Patients with ulcerative colitis should be made aware that ulcerative colitis rarely remits completely. Abrupt discontinuation of mesalamine therapy is not recommended, and may result in relapse. It is important for patients to comply with the dosage prescribed by their doctors; by doing so, the risk of relapse can be substantially reduced.
Relevant Clinical Information: Findings from the clinical studies for ASACOL 800 (800 mg tablet), that a higher dose of mesalamine shows greater efficacy in patients with moderately active disease, is consistent with previous findings seen with ASACOL (400 mg tablet). The demonstrated efficacy of ASACOL 800 (800 mg tablet) administered at 4.8 g/day in patients with moderately active disease offers this patient population convenient dosing over ASACOL (400 mg tablet) tablets by reducing the number of tablets by half. **Interchangeability between ASACOL (400 mg tablet) and ASACOL 800 (800 mg tablet) has not been established.** For information on the ASACOL (400 mg tablet), please refer to the current Product Monograph for the ASACOL (400 mg tablet) tablet.
Geriatrics: No data are available.
Pediatrics: Clinical trials of ASACOL 800 (800 mg tablet) did not include pediatric patients. ASACOL 800 (800 mg tablet) is contraindicated in patients unable to swallow an intact tablet and in patients less than 2 years of age.

CONTRAINDICATIONS: ASACOL 800 (800 mg tablet) is contraindicated in:
- patients who are hypersensitive to this drug or to any ingredient in the formulation or component of the container. For a complete listing, see Dosage Forms, Compositions and Packaging.
- patients with a history of sensitivity to salicylates
- patients with existing gastric or duodenal ulcer
- patients with urinary tract obstruction
- patients unable to swallow the intact tablet and
- infants under 2 years of age.

WARNINGS AND PRECAUTIONS:

Serious Warnings and Precautions
Hypersensitivity: If toxic or hypersensitivity reactions occur, the drug should be discontinued. In assessing liver and joint complications, it should be kept in mind that these are frequently associated with ulcerative colitis.
Renal: Renal impairment, including minimal change nephropathy and acute and chronic interstitial nephritis, and renal failure has been reported in patients taking mesalamine products. Caution should be exercised when using ASACOL 800 (800 mg tablet) (or other compounds that contain or are converted to mesalamine or its metabolites) in patients with a history of renal disease. ASACOL 800 (800 mg tablet) is not recommended for use in patients with renal impairment. It is recommended that all patients have an evaluation of renal function prior to initiation of ASACOL 800 (800 mg tablet) and periodically while on ASACOL 800 (800 mg tablet) therapy.

General: ASACOL 800 (800 mg tablet) and other mesalamine-containing products have differences in formulation and release characteristics that may lead to differences in concentrations of mesalamine delivered to the colon. If it is deemed necessary to switch from one mesalamine-containing product to another mesalamine-containing product, the prescriber should carefully assess the overall benefit-risk analysis based on the patient's clinical conditions and on all available information for the various mesalamine-containing products.
Gastrointestinal: Acute exacerbation of the symptoms of colitis, characterized by cramping, abdominal pain, bloody diarrhea, and occasionally by fever, headache, malaise, pruritus, rash, and conjunctivitis, has been reported in 3% of patients in controlled clinical trials of ASACOL (400 mg tablet) versus sulfasalazine. This reaction has been reported after initiation of other mesalamine-containing products, and was reported by 2% of patients receiving ASACOL 800 (800 mg tablet) in two controlled clinical trials. Symptoms usually abate when mesalamine therapy is discontinued.

Patients with pyloric stenosis may have prolonged gastric retention of ASACOL 800 (800 mg tablet) tablets that could delay release of mesalamine in the colon.

What appears to be intact or partially intact tablets may be observed in the stool.
Hepatic/Biliary/Pancreatic: Caution should be exercised when using ASACOL 800 (800 mg tablet) (or other compounds that contain or are converted to mesalamine or its metabolites) in patients with hepatic dysfunction.

In assessing liver complications, it should be kept in mind that these are frequently associated with ulcerative colitis.
Immune: Some patients who have experienced a hypersensitivity reaction to sulfasalazine may have a similar reaction to ASACOL 800 (800 mg tablet) tablets or to other compounds that contain, or are converted to, mesalamine. ASACOL 800 (800 mg tablet) does not contain a sulfa moiety, thus sulfa-related side effects are avoided.
Special Populations: Pregnant Women: In non-clinical reproduction studies, mesalamine administered orally at a dosage of 480 mg/kg/day to pregnant rats and rabbits showed no evidence of impaired female fertility or harm to the fetus. Mesalamine crosses the placenta, there are, however, no adequate and well-controlled studies in pregnant women. Because animal reproduction studies are not always predictive of human response, this drug should be used during pregnancy only if clearly needed.
Nursing Women: Literature reports indicate that, following oral or rectal administration of mesalamine-containing products to lactating women, small amounts of 5-ASA and higher concentrations of the metabolite N-acetyl-5-ASA are found in breast milk. While the clinical significance of this has not been determined, caution should be exercised when ASACOL 800 (800 mg tablet) tablets are administered to a nursing woman.
Pediatrics: Safety and effectiveness of ASACOL 800 (800 mg tablet) therapy in patients younger than 18 years of age has not been established.
Geriatrics: Less than 10% of patients in the ASACOL 800 (800 mg tablet) clinical trial were ≥65 years of age. Patients in this age range were not significantly different from the overall patient population with respect to safety and efficacy responses.
Monitoring and Laboratory Tests: It is recommended that all patients have an evaluation of renal function prior to initiation of ASACOL 800 (800 mg tablet) tablets and periodically while on ASACOL 800 (800 mg tablet) therapy.

ADVERSE REACTIONS: Adverse Drug Reaction Overview: ASACOL is generally well tolerated. The most commonly reported adverse reactions were nausea, diarrhea, abdominal pain and headache. Other common adverse reactions seen in clinical trials with ASACOL were acute exacerbation of ulcerative colitis symptoms, abnormal hepatic functions tests and rash. Adverse events seen in clinical trials with ASACOL tablets have generally been mild and reversible, and have seldom resulted in discontinuation of treatment.
Clinical Trial Adverse Drug Reactions: Because clinical trials are conducted under very specific conditions, the adverse reaction rates observed in the clinical trials may not reflect the rates observed in practice and should not be compared to the rates in the clinical trials of another drug. Adverse drug reaction information from clinical trials is useful for identifying drug-related adverse events and approximate rates of occurrence.

In two double-blind, randomized 6 week, parallel-group design clinical trials in patients with mildly to moderately active ulcerative colitis, the safety and efficacy of ASACOL 800 (800 mg tablet), dosed at 4.8 g/day, was compared to the safety and efficacy of ASACOL (400 mg tablet), dosed at 2.4 g/day. In these trials, the overall incidence of adverse events was comparable between the two treatment groups, and similar to that observed previously with ASACOL (400 mg tablet) therapy.

Table 1 presents adverse events assessed as possibly or probably related to the study drug in 1% ore more of patients in either treatment group.

Table 1: ASACOL 800

Assessed as Possibly or Probably Related to Study Drug Occuring in >=1% in Either Treatment Group by MedDRA PT

MedDRA Preferred Term	2.4 g/day ASACOL (400 mg tablet) (N=349) n (%)	4.8 g/day ASACOL (800 mg tablet) (N= 338) n (%)
Headache	13 (3.7%)	12 (3.6%)
Nausea	6 (1.7%)	8 (2.4%)
Vomiting	3 (0.9%)	4 (1.2%)
Abdominal pain	7 (2.0%)	3 (0.9%)
Ulcerative colitis	4 (1.1%)	3 (0.9%)
Abdominal distension	5 (1.4%)	1 (0.3%)

Post-Market Adverse Drug Reactions: In addition to the adverse events reported above in the two clinical trials involving ASACOL 800 (800 mg tablet), the following adverse events have been reported in controlled clinical trials, open-label studies, literature reports, or foreign and domestic marketing experience with ASACOL (400 mg tablet) or other products that contain or are metabolized to mesalamine. Because many of these events were reported voluntarily from a population of unknown size, estimates of frequency cannot be made. The relationship of the reported events to ASACOL is unclear in many cases, and some may be part of the clinical presentation of ulcerative colitis.

Body as a Whole: allergic reaction, facial edema, edema, peripheral edema, asthenia, drug fever (rare), chills, malaise, pain, neck pain, chest pain, back pain, abdominal enlargement, lupus-like syndrome, flu syndrome, infection.

Cardiovascular: pericarditis (rare), myocarditis (rare), palpitations, vasodilation, migraine.

Digestive: dry mouth, stomatitis, oral ulcers, anorexia, increased appetite, dyspepsia, eructation, flatulence, pancreatitis, gastritis, gastroenteritis, gastrointestinal bleeding, perforated peptic ulcer (rare), constipation, rectal hemorrhage, bloody diarrhea, tenesmus, rectal disorder, stool abnormality.

Hepatic: hepatitis (rare), cholecystitis. Asymptomatic elevations of liver function tests have occurred in patients taking ASACOL tablets. These elevations usually resolve during continued therapy or with discontinuation of ASACOL. When any elevations in liver enzymes are assessed, it should be kept in mind that hepatic complications are frequently associated with inflammatory bowel disease.

Hematologic: agranulocytosis (rare), aplastic anemia (rare), leukopenia, anemia, thrombocytopenia, eosinophilia, lymphadenopathy.

Musculoskeletal: gout, rheumatoid arthritis, arthritis, arthralgia, joint disorder, myalgia, hypertonia, leg cramps.

Nervous: anxiety, depression, somnolence, insomnia, nervousness, confusion, emotional lability, dizziness, vertigo, tremor, paresthesia, hyperesthesia, peripheral neuropathy (rare), Guillain-Barré syndrome (rare), and transverse myelitis (rare).

Respiratory/Pulmonary: epistaxis, rhinitis, sinusitis, pharyngitis, dyspnea, increased cough, asthma exacerbation, pleuritis, bronchitis, pneumonia, eosinophilic pneumonia, interstitial pneumonitis, lung disorder.

Skin: alopecia, psoriasis (rare), pyoderma gangrenosum (rare), erythema nodosum, acne, dry skin, sweating, pruritus, urticaria.

Special Senses: ear pain, tinnitus, deafness, ear congestion, ear disorder, conjunctivitis, eye pain, amblyopia, blurred vision, vision abnormality, lacrimation disorder, taste perversion.

Urogenital: interstitial nephritis (rare), minimal change nephropathy (rare), renal failure (rare) (see also Warnings and Precautions), cystitis, urinary tract infection, dysuria, urinary urgency, increased urination, hematuria, urine abnormality, epididymitis, prostate disorder, decreased libido, dysmenorrhea, menorrhagia, vaginitis, vaginal moniliasis.

Laboratory Abnormalities: elevated AST or ALT, elevated alkaline phosphatase, elevated serum creatinine and BUN.

DRUG INTERACTIONS: Overview: There are no known drug interactions with ASACOL (400 mg tablet). No drug interaction studies were performed with ASACOL 800 (800 mg tablet). In clinical trials of ASACOL 800 (800 mg tablet), there were no restrictions on the concomitant use of antacids, H_2-receptor antagonists, proton-pump inhibitors, or other preparations affecting gastrointestinal pH. In subgroup analyses, patients receiving H_2-receptor antagonists or proton-pump inhibitors were not significantly different from the overall patient population with respect to safety and efficacy response.

Drug-Food Interactions: Administration of the ASACOL 800 (800 mg tablet) tablet immediately following a high fat meal had no significant effect on the extent of exposure to 5-ASA and N-acetyl-5-ASA based on AUC and percent of dose excreted in urine (Ae%). A reduction of approximately 50% was observed in C_{max}, due to significantly delayed t_{max} when dosed following a high fat meal compared to dosing under fasting condition. However, no impact was observed on the safety profile or systemic exposure to 5-ASA and N-acetyl-5ASA in the clinical trials where doses were given without regards to meals. Therefore, ASACOL 800 (800 mg tablet) can be taken in a fasted or fed state.

Drug-Herb Interactions: Interactions with herbal products have not been established.

Drug-Laboratory Interactions: Interactions with laboratory tests have not been established.

DOSAGE AND ADMINISTRATION: Dosing Considerations: Patients with ulcerative colitis should be made aware that ulcerative colitis rarely remits completely. Abrupt discontinuation of ASACOL 800 (800 mg tablet) is not recommended, and may result in relapse. It is important for patients to comply with the dosage prescribed by their doctors; by doing so, the risk of relapse can be substantially reduced.

Recommended Dose and Dosage Adjustment: For the treatment of moderately active ulcerative colitis: Usual daily adult dose is 6 ASACOL 800 (800 mg tablet) tablets, taken orally in divided doses. ASACOL 800 (800 mg tablet) may be given without regards to meals.

For alternate dosing for moderately active ulcerative colitis, see the ASACOL (400 mg tablet) Product Monograph.

Missed Dose: If a dose of this medication has been missed, it should be taken as soon as possible. However, if it is almost time for the next dose, skip the missed dose and go back to the regular dosing schedule. Do not take double the dose.

Administration:

1. Swallow tablets whole, taking care not to break the outer coating. The outer coating is designed to remain intact, to protect the active ingredient until it reaches the terminal ileum, where the tablet coating dissolves and the contents of the tablet are released into the terminal ileum and colon.
2. Take ASACOL 800 (800 mg tablet) tablets only as prescribed. Do not change the number or frequency of tablets ingested without first consulting your physician.
3. What appears to be intact or partially intact tablets may infrequently appear in the stool. If this occurs repeatedly, consult your physician.

OVERDOSAGE:

There is no clinical experience with overdose of ASACOL 800 (800 mg tablet). Mesalamine is not metabolized to salicylate. There is no specific antidote for mesalamine overdose, and treatment is symptomatic and supportive.

> For management of a suspected drug overdose, contact your **regional Poison Control Centre**. See the *CPS* Directory section for a list of Poison Control Centres.

ACTION AND CLINICAL PHARMACOLOGY: Mechanism of Action: The active ingredient in ASACOL 800 (800 mg tablet) is mesalamine (5-aminosalicylic acid, also referred to as 5-ASA). The available evidence suggests that mesalamine has a topical anti-inflammatory effect on the colon, where it inhibits prostaglandin and leukotriene synthesis.

Pharmacodynamics: ASACOL 800 (800 mg tablet) tablets have a special acrylic-based resin coating, which does not allow the drug to be released below pH 7. The coating delays release of mesalamine until the tablets reach the terminal ileum and colon. ASACOL 800 (800 mg tablet) demonstrated expected enteric coating properties that were comparable to those of the ASACOL (400 mg tablet) tablet, as indicated by in-vitro dissolution data as well as prolonged t_{max} and t_{lag} following oral administration.

Pharmacokinetics: Once released in the colon, mesalamine is minimally absorbed and plasma levels are similar to those found in previous studies following oral administration of doses given as 400 mg tablets. The bioequivalence between ASACOL 800 (800 mg tablet) and ASACOL (400 mg tablet) tablets has not been established. Following oral administration of a single, 800 mg tablet under fasting conditions, the time to peak plasma concentration (t_{max}) is approximately 10 hours while the terminal elimination half-life ($t½_{elm}$) is 12 to 19 hours for both mesalamine and its metabolite, N-acetyl-5-ASA.

Approximately 20% of the administered dose is absorbed systemically; the remainder is available for therapeutic activity in the colon and excretion in the feces. The extent of systemic exposure to mesalamine is similar in fasted and fed subjects. The absorbed mesalamine is rapidly acetylated through the gut mucosal wall and by the liver. It is mainly excreted by the kidney, as N-acetyl-5-ASA.

Table 2 presents the mean pharmacokinetic parameters of 5-ASA and N-acetyl-5-ASA (N-Ac-5-ASA) following single and multiple dosing of ASACOL 800 (800 mg tablet) in healthy subjects.

Table 2: ASACOL 800

Summary of Mean Pharmacokinetic Parameters of 5-ASA and N-Ac-5-ASA Following Single and Multiple Dosing in Healthy Subjects

Mean Pharmacokinetic Parameters of 5-ASA		
Parameter	**Single Dose (1×800 mg)**	**Multiple Dose (4.8 g/day×6 Days)**
AUC_{tlast} (ng·h/mL)	3449.2	—
AUC (ng·h/mL)	3548.2	20 282.0[a]
C_{max} (ng/mL)	354.03	4972.1
t_{max} (h)	9.61	2.63
t_{lag} (h)	6.20	—
$t_{½,Z}$ (h)	13.41	11.89
$\%A_e$ (%)	0.21	9.28
Mean Pharmacokinetic Parameters of N-Ac-5-ASA		
Parameter	**Single Dose (1×800 mg)**	**Multiple Dose (4.8 g/day×6 Days)**
AUC_{tlast} (ng·h/mL)	19 900.8	—
AUC (ng·h/mL)	22 034.2	24 864.0[a]
C_{max} (ng/mL)	1028.68	4614.78
t_{max} (h)	11.13	3.13
t_{lag} (h)	5.39	—
$t_{½,Z}$ (h)	13.62	19.56
$\%A_e$ (%)	12.04	19.01

[a] AUC_τ is the area under the plasma concentration-time curve over a dosing interval.

Legend: AUC_{tlast} is the area under the plasma concentration-time curve from time zero to the last quantifiable concentration; AUC is the area under the plasma concentration-time curve from time zero to infinity; C_{max} is the maximum plasma concentration; t_{max} is the time at which C_{max} is observed; t_{lag} is the lag time before the onset of drug absorption; $t_{½,Z}$ is the terminal exponential half-life; $\%A_e$ is the percentage of dose excreted in urine.

STORAGE AND STABILITY: Store at controlled room temperature (15 to 30°C).

INFORMATION FOR THE PATIENT: Published in e-CPS, available by subscription at www.e-cps.ca.

DOSAGE FORMS, COMPOSITIONS AND PACKAGING: Each red-brown, capsule-shaped, enteric coated tablet, printed in black ink with "PG 800", available for oral administration, contains: mesalamine 800 mg. Nonmedicinal ingredients: colloidal silicon dioxide, dibutyl phthalate, edible black ink (ammonium hydroxide, n-butyl alcohol, shellac glaze [modified] in SD-45, propylene glycol, synthetic black iron oxide), iron oxide red, iron oxide yellow, lactose, magnesium stearate, Eudragit-L {methacrylic acid copolymer Type A (USP)}, Eudragit-S {methacrylic acid copolymer Type B (USP)}, polyethylene glycol, polyvinylpyrrolidone, sodium starch glycolate and talc. The colon-targeted tablets are coated with a special acrylic-based resin, Eudragit-S {methacrylic acid copolymer Type B (USP)}, which dissolves at pH 7 or greater, that delays release of the mesalamine until the tablets reach the terminal ileum. A second enteric coating which begins to dissolve earlier in the gastrointestinal tract is added after the Eudragit-S. The outer coating consists of a combination of Eudragit-S and another acrylic-based resin, Eudragit-L {methacrylic acid copolymer Type A (USP)}. Bottles of 180.

(Shown in Product Identification Section)

Asaphen

ASA

Platelet Aggregation Inhibitor

Pharmascience

Asaphen E.C.

ASA

Platelet Aggregation Inhibitor

Pharmascience

SUPPLIED: Asaphen: Each chewable, salmon, round, biconvex tablet, debossed with "ASA 80" on one side and scored on the other side contains: ASA 80 mg. Nonmedicinal ingredients: cornstarch, D&C Yellow No. 10 Aluminum Lake, FD&C Red No. 40 Aluminum Lake, mannitol, orange flavor, sodium saccharin and stearic acid. Bottles of 100 and 500. Store at room temperature (15-30°C).

Asaphen E.C.: Each round, white enteric-coated tablet contains: ASA 80 mg. Nonmedicinal ingredients: colloidal silicon dioxide, cornstarch, lactose, methacrylic acid copolymer, methylated silica, methylcellulose, polydimethylsiloxane, polyethylene glycol, sodium bicarbonate, sodium lauryl sulfate, sorbitan tristearate, stearic acid, talc, titanium dioxide and triethyl citrate. Bottles of 120, 500 and 1000. Store at room temperature (15-30°C).

Asatab™

ASA

Analgesic—Antipyretic

Odan

SUPPLIED: Each chewable, orange-coloured, round, biconvex tablet, embossed "ASATAB 80" on one side contains: ASA 80 mg. Nonmedicinal ingredients: FD&C yellow #6, lactose, mannitol, orange flavour, pregelatinized starch, sodium saccharin and stearic acid. Packages of 100 and 500.

Ascorbic Acid

CPhA Monograph

see *Vitamin C*

Aspirin®
ASA
Analgesic—Anti-inflammatory—Antipyretic—Platelet Aggregation Inhibitor

Bayer Consumer Care

PHARMACOLOGY: ASA interferes with the production of prostaglandins in various organs and tissues through acetylation of the enzyme cyclo-oxygenase. Prostaglandins are themselves powerful irritants and produce headaches and pain on injection in man. Prostaglandins also appear to sensitize pain receptors to other noxious substances such as histamine and bradykinin. By preventing the synthesis and release of prostaglandins in inflammation, ASA may avert the sensitization of pain receptors.

The antipyretic activity of ASA is due to its ability to interfere with the production of prostaglandin E_1 in the brain. Prostaglandin E_1 is one of the most powerful pyretic agents known.

The inhibition of platelet aggregation by ASA is due to its ability to interfere with the production of thromboxane A_2 within the platelet. Thromboxane A_2 is largely responsible for the aggregating properties of platelets.

When ASA is taken orally, it is rapidly absorbed from the stomach and proximal small intestine. The gastric mucosa is permeable to the nonionized form of ASA, which passes through the stomach wall by a passive diffusion process.

Optimum absorption of salicylate in the human stomach occurs in the pH range of 2.15 to 4.10. Absorption in the small intestine occurs at a significantly faster rate than in the stomach. After an oral dose of 650 mg ASPIRIN, the plasma acetylsalicylate concentration in man usually reaches a level between 0.6 and 1.0 mg% in 20 minutes after ingestion and drops to 0.2 mg% within an hour. Within the same period of time, half or more of the ingested dose is hydrolyzed to salicylic acid by esterases in the gastrointestinal mucosa and the liver, the total plasma salicylate concentration reaching a peak between 1 or 2 hours after ingestion, averaging between 3 and 7 mg%. Many factors influence the speed of absorption of ASA in a particular individual at a given time; tablet disintegration, solubility, particle size, gastric emptying time, psychological state, physical condition, nature and quantity of gastric contents, etc., all affect absorption.

Distribution of salicylate throughout most body fluids and tissues proceeds at a rapid rate after absorption. Aside from the plasma itself, fluids which have been found to contain substantial amounts of salicylate after oral ingestion include spinal, peritoneal and synovial fluids, saliva and milk. Tissues containing high concentrations of the drug are the kidney, liver, heart and lungs. Concentrations in the brain are usually low, and are minimal in feces, bile and sweat.

The drug readily crosses the placental barrier. At clinical concentrations, from 50% to 90% of the salicylate is bound to plasma proteins especially albumin, while ASA itself is bound to only a very limited extent. However, ASA has the capacity of acetylating various proteins, hormones, DNA, platelets and hemoglobin, which at least partly explains its wide-ranging pharmacological actions.

The liver appears to be the principal site for salicylate metabolism, although other tissues may also be involved. The three chief metabolic products of salicylic acid are salicyluric acid, the ether or phenolic glucuronide and the ester or acyl glucuronide. A small fraction is also converted to gentisic acid and other hydroxybenzoic acids. The half-life of ASA in the circulation is from 13 to 19 minutes so that the blood level drops quickly after absorption is complete. However, the half-life of the salicylate ranges between 3.5 and 4.5 hours, which means that 50% of the ingested dose leaves the circulation within that time.

Excretion of salicylates occurs principally via the kidney, through a combination of glomerular filtration and tubular excretion, in the form of free salicylic acid, salicyluric acid, as well as phenolic and acyl glucuronides. Salicylate can be detected in the urine shortly after its ingestion but the full dose requires up to 48 hours for complete elimination. The rate of excretion of free salicylate is extremely variable, reported recovery rates in human urine ranging from 10% to 85%, depending largely on urinary pH. In general, it can be stated that acid urine facilitates reabsorption of salicylate by renal tubules, while alkaline urine promotes excretion of the drug.

INDICATIONS: The relief of pain, fever and inflammation of a variety of conditions such as influenza, common cold, low back and neck pain, dysmenorrhea, headache, toothache, sprains and strains, myositis, neuralgia, synovitis, arthritis, bursitis, burns, injuries, following surgical and dental procedures.

ASPIRIN Extra Strength is also indicated for relief of migraines including pain and the associated symptoms of photophobia (sensitivity to light) and phonophobia (sensitivity to sound), and improves overall quality of life.

ASPIRIN 325 mg or ASPIRIN 81 mg is indicated for the following uses, based on its platelet aggregation inhibitory properties:

For reducing the risk of vascular mortality in patients with a suspected acute myocardial infarction.

For reducing the risk of a **first** non-fatal myocardial infarction in individuals deemed to be at sufficient risk of such an event by their physician. There is no evidence for a reduction in the risk of a **first** fatal myocardial infarction.

ASPIRIN does not reduce the risk of either cardiovascular mortality of **first** strokes, fatal or non-fatal.

The decrease in the risk of **first** non-fatal myocardial infarction must be assessed against a much smaller but not insignificant increase in risk of haemorrhagic stroke as well as gastrointestinal bleeding.

For reducing the risk of morbidity and death in patients with unstable angina and in those with previous myocardial infarction.

For reducing the risk of transient ischemic attacks (TIA) and for secondary prevention of atherothrombotic cerebral infarction.

Prophylaxis of venous thromboembolism after total hip replacement. (ASPIRIN 325 mg only).

Reduction of the adhesive properties of the platelets in patients following carotid endarterectomy to prevent recurrence of TIA and in hemodialysis patients with a silicone rubber arteriovenous cannula. (ASPIRIN 325 mg only).

CONTRAINDICATIONS: Patients who are hypersensitive to this drug or to any ingredient in the formulation or component of the container (see Supplied); patients with a history of asthma induced by the administration of salicylates or substances with a similar action, notably nonsteroidal anti-inflammatory drugs; combination with methotrexate at doses of 15 mg/week or more; last trimester of pregnancy; hemorrhagic diathesis; active peptic ulcer.

WARNINGS: ASA is one of the most frequent causes of accidental poisonings in toddlers and infants. Tablets should be kept well out of the reach of children.

Salicylates should be administered cautiously to patients with: hypersensitivity to anti-inflammatory or antirheumatic drugs or other allergens, impaired renal function or hepatic function, a history of chronic or recurrent gastrointestinal ulcerations and bleeds, a history of bleeding tendencies, significant anemia and/or hypothrombinemia.

ASPIRIN may precipitate bronchospasm and induce asthma attacks or other hypersensitivity reactions. Risk factors are present bronchial asthma, hay fever, nasal polyps, or chronic respiratory disease. This applies also for patients showing allergic reactions (e.g. cutaneous reactions, itching, urticaria) to other substances.

Due to effect on platelet aggregation, ASPIRIN may be associated with an increased risk of bleeding. Caution is necessary when salicylates and anticoagulants are prescribed concurrently, as salicylates can depress the concentration of prothrombin in the plasma.

Due to its inhibitory effect on platelet aggregation ASPIRIN may lead to an increased bleeding tendency during and after surgical operations (including minor surgeries, e.g. dental extractions).

Pregnancy: Use of salicylates in the first 3 months of pregnancy has been associated in several epidemiological studies with an elevated risk of malformations (cleft palate, heart malformations). After normal therapeutic doses this risk seems to be low: a prospective study with exposure of about 32 000 mother-child pairs has not yielded any association with the risk of malformations.

Salicylates should be taken during pregnancy only after strict risk-benefit evaluation.

In the last 3 months of pregnancy administration of salicylates in high doses (>300 mg/day) can lead to prolongation of the gestation period, premature closure of the arterial duct and inhibition of uterine contractions. An increased hemorrhagic tendency has been observed in both mother and child.

Administration of ASPIRIN in high doses (>300 mg/day) shortly before birth can lead to intracranial hemorrhages, particularly in premature babies.

Lactation: ASPIRIN and its metabolites pass into breast milk in small quantities. Since no adverse effects on the infant have been observed after occasional use, interruption of breast-feeding is usually unnecessary. However, on regular use or on intake of high doses, breast feeding should be discontinued early.

A possible association between Reye's syndrome and the use of salicylates has been suggested but not established. Reye's syndrome has also occurred in many patients not exposed to salicylates.

ASPIRIN should not be used in children and teenagers for viral infections with or without fever without consulting a physician.

In certain viral illnesses, especially influenza A, influenza B and varicella, there is a risk of Reye's syndrome, a very rare but possibly life-threatening illness requiring immediate medical action. The risk may be increased when ASPIRIN is given concomitantly; however, no causal relationship has been proven. Should persistent vomiting occur with such diseases; this may be a sign of Reye's syndrome.

At low doses, ASPIRIN reduces excretion of uric acid. This can trigger gout in patients who already tend to have low uric acid excretion.

Salicylates can produce changes in thyroid function tests.

Isolated cases of liver function disturbances (transaminases increase) have been described.

Drug Interactions: ASPIRIN should be used with caution with other products that have anticoagulation or antiplatelet effects, as these effects may be potentiated. Drugs that bind to protein binding sites should also be used cautiously since ASPIRIN may displace drugs from their protein binding site.

Methotrexate, used at 15 mg/week or less: Salicylates may retard the elimination of methotrexate by decreasing renal clearance of methotrexate, displacing methotrexate from protein binding sites, and thereby increasing its hematological toxicity.

Anticoagulants, e.g. warfarin, heparin: Caution is necessary when salicylates and anticoagulants are prescribed concurrently, as salicylates can depress the concentration of prothrombin in the plasma.

Oral hypoglycemics, e.g. insulin, sulfonylureas: Large doses of salicylates have a hypoglycemic action and may enhance the effect of oral hypoglycemic agents. Diabetics receiving concurrent salicylate and hypoglycemic therapy should be monitored closely: reduction of the sulfonylurea hypoglycemic drug dosage may be necessary.

Diuretics: Sodium excretion produced by spironolactone may be decreased by salicylate administration.

Uricosuric Agents: Salicylates in large doses are uricosuric agents; smaller amounts may depress uric acid clearance and thus decrease the uricosuric effects of other drugs.

Valproic Acid: Salicylates may alter valproic acid (VPA) metabolism and may displace VPA from protein binding sites, possibly intensifying the effects of VPA. Caution is recommended when VPA is administered concomitantly with salicylates.

Glucocorticoids (systemic), except hydrocortisone used as replacement therapy in Addison's disease: Decreased blood salicylate levels during corticosteroid treatment and risk of salicylate overdose after this treatment is stopped via increased elimination of salicylates by corticosteroids.

Angiotensin Converting Enzyme (ACE) Inhibitors: The hyponatremic and hypotensive effects of ACE inhibitors may be diminished by the concomitant administration of ASPIRIN due to its indirect effect on the renin-angiotensin conversion pathway. The potential interaction may be related to the dose of ASPIRIN (3 g/day or more).

Digoxin: Plasma concentrations of digoxin are increased due to a decrease in renal excretion.

ASPIRIN and other NSAIDs: The use of other nonsteroidal anti-inflammatory drugs with salicylates at high doses (equal to/more than 3 g/day) may increase the risk of ulcers and gastrointestinal bleeding due to a synergistic effect.

Ibuprofen: Ibuprofen may interfere with the cardioprotective effects and platelet aggregation inhibitory properties of ASPIRIN. Patients should talk to their doctor if they are on an ASPIRIN regimen and take ibuprofen for pain. Studies have shown that single doses and multiple doses of ibuprofen may interfere with the anti-platelet effects of low dose ASPIRIN.

PRECAUTIONS: See Warnings.

ADVERSE EFFECTS: Many adverse reactions due to ASPIRIN ingestion are dose-related. The following is a list of adverse reactions that have been reported in the literature and from both clinical and post-marketing experience.

Gastrointestinal: (the frequency and severity of these adverse effects are dose-related): nausea, vomiting, diarrhea, gastrointestinal bleeding and/or ulceration, dyspepsia, heartburn, hematemesis, melena.

Ear: tinnitus, vertigo, hearing loss.

Hematologic: leukopenia, thrombocytopenia, purpura, anemia.

Dermatologic and Hypersensitivity: urticaria, angioedema, pruritus, skin eruptions, asthma, anaphylaxis, Quincke edema.

Miscellaneous: mental confusion, drowsiness, sweating, thirst.

OVERDOSE:

Symptoms: Mild Overdose or Early Poisoning: Burning in the mouth, lethargy, nausea, vomiting, tinnitus, sweating, thirst, tachycardia or dizziness.

Moderate Overdose: All of the symptoms from mild overdose plus tachypnea, hyperpyrexia, sweating, dehydration, loss of coordination, restlessness, mental confusion.

Severe Overdose: All of the symptoms from moderate overdose plus hypotension, hallucinations, stupor, hypoglycemia, convulsions, cerebral edema, oliguria, renal failure, cardiovascular failure, coma, hemorrhage, metabolic acidosis, respiratory alkalosis and/or failure.

Treatment: Emergency Management: Immediate transfer to hospital and maintain cardiovascular and respiratory support. Gastric lavage, administration of activated charcoal. Check of acid-base balance and correct if necessary. Alkaline diuresis so as to obtain urine pH between 7.5 and 8 should be considered when plasma salicylate concentration is greater than 500 mg/L (3.6 mmol/L) in adults or 300 mg/L (2.2 mmol/L) in children. Hemodialysis should be considered in severe poisoning 800 mg/L (5.8 mmol/L) in adults and 700 mg/L (5.0 mmol/L) in children, as renal elimination of salicylates may be slow due to the presence of acidic urine and renal failure. Hemodialysis should also be considered if the patient is experiencing severe systemic metabolic acidosis (arterial pH <7.2), acute renal failure, pulmonary edema or CNS symptoms such as: drowsiness, agitation, coma or convulsions. Fluid losses should be replaced with hypotonic solution (e.g. half saline) and supplemented with glucose 50 to 100 g/L. Symptomatic treatment. Fatal Dose: varies from 10 to 30 g of ASA. However, (in one case) 130 g of ASA was ingested without fatal outcome.

> For management of a suspected drug overdose, CPhA recommends that you contact your **regional Poison Control Centre**. See the *CPS* Directory section for a list of Poison Control Centres.

DOSAGE: Analgesic and Antipyretic: Adults: 1 to 2 tablets (325 to 650 mg) orally every 4 hours. Children under 12: 10 to 15 mg/kg every 6 hours, not to exceed total daily dose of 2.4 g.

Migraine Pain and Associated Symptoms: Adults: 1000 mg (2×500 mg tablets) at onset of pain or symptoms. Children: Clinical studies to support migraine relief in children have not been conducted with acetylsalicylic acid.

Anti-inflammatory: Adults: 3 tablets (975 mg) 4 to 6 times a day, up to 30 tablets daily, may be required for optimal anti-inflammatory effect. A blood level between 15 and 30 mg/100 mL is in the desirable therapeutic range.

Children: 60 to 125 mg/kg daily in 4 to 6 divided doses.

Platelet Aggregation Inhibitor: Suspected Acute Myocardial Infarction: An initial dose of at least 160-162.5 mg chewed or crushed to ensure rapid absorption as soon as a myocardial infarction is suspected. The same dose should be given as maintenance over the next 30 days. After 30 days, consider further therapy based on dosage and administration for prevention of recurrent MI (see Prior Myocardial Infarction below).

Prevention of a First Non-fatal Myocardial Infarction: 80-325 mg once daily, according to the individual needs of the patient, as determined by the physician.

Prior Myocardial Infarction or Unstable Angina Pectoris: 80-325 mg daily according to the individual needs of the patient, as determined by the physician.

Transient Ischemic Attack (TIA) and Secondary Prevention of Atherothrombotic Cerebral Infarction: 80-325 mg daily according to the individual needs of the patient, as determined by the physician.

Prophylaxis of Venous Thromboembolism after Total Hip Replacement: 650 mg twice a day (1300 mg daily), started 1 day before surgery and continued for 14 days.

SUPPLIED: ASPIRIN Tablets, 325 mg: Each white tablet, with the Bayer Cross on both sides, contains: ASA 325 mg. Nonmedicinal ingredients: corn starch, hypromellose, powdered cellulose and triacetin. Blister packages of 8 and bottles of 24, 50, 100, 200 and 400.

ASPIRIN Caplets, 325 mg: Each white, capsule-shaped tablet (caplet), with BAYER on one side and a score on the other, contains: ASA 325 mg. Nonmedicinal ingredients: corn starch, hypromellose, powdered cellulose and triacetin. Packages of 50 and 100.

ASPIRIN Extra Strength Tablets, 500 mg: Each white tablet, with the Bayer Cross in red ink on one side, contains: ASA 500 mg. Nonmedicinal ingredients: carnauba wax, corn starch, D&C Red #7, FD&C Blue #2, FD&C Red #40, hypromellose, powdered cellulose, propylene glycol, shellac, titanium dioxide and triacetin. Packages of 50 and 100.

ASPIRIN Stomach Guard with Calcium Carbonate: Each white, film-coated tablet, with BAYER PLUS in blue ink on one side, contains: ASA 325 mg. Nonmedicinal ingredients: calcium carbonate, carnauba wax, colloidal silicon dioxide, corn starch, FD&C Blue #2, hypromellose, propylene glycol, shellac, sodium starch glycolate, titanium dioxide, microcrystalline cellulose and zinc stearate. Packages of 36.

ASPIRIN Extra Strength Stomach Guard with Calcium Carbonate: Each white, film-coated caplet, with BAYER PLUS 500 on one side in blue ink, contains: ASA 500 mg. Nonmedicinal ingredients: calcium carbonate, carnauba wax, colloidal silicon dioxide, corn starch, FD&C Blue #2, hypromellose, propylene glycol, shellac, sodium starch glycolate, titanium dioxide, microcrystalline cellulose and zinc stearate. Packages of 60.

ASPIRIN Arthritis Pain Relief Caplets, 325 mg: Each pale yellow, enteric coated caplet, with BAYER 325 in brown ink on one side, contains: ASA 325 mg. Nonmedicinal ingredients: black and brown iron oxides, carnauba wax, corn starch, D&C Yellow #10, D&C Yellow #7, hypromellose, methacrylic acid copolymer, polysorbate 80, powdered cellulose, sodium lauryl sulphate, talc, titanium dioxide, triacetin and triethyl citrate. Bottles of 50, 100 and 200.

ASPIRIN Arthritis Pain Relief Extra Strength Caplets, 500 mg: Each pale yellow, enteric coated caplet, with BAYER 500 in brown ink on one side, contains: ASA 500 mg. Nonmedicinal ingredients: black and brown iron oxides, carnauba wax, corn starch, D&C Yellow #10, D&C Yellow #7, hypromellose, methacrylic acid copolymer, polysorbate 80, powdered cellulose, sodium lauryl sulphate, talc, titanium dioxide, triacetin and triethyl citrate. Bottles of 100.
ASPIRIN 81 mg: Each pale blue, enteric coated tablet, with 81 in dark blue ink on one side, contains: ASA 81 mg. Nonmedicinal ingredients: carnauba wax, corn starch, croscarmellose sodium, FD&C Blue #1, FD&C Blue #2, hypromellose, lactose monohydrate, methacrylic acid copolymer, microcrystalline cellulose, polysorbate 80, powdered cellulose, propylene glycol, shellac, sodium lauryl sulphate, starch, titanium dioxide and triacetin. Bottles of 30, 120 and 180.
ASPIRIN 81 mg Quick Chews: Each peach-coloured tablet, with the Bayer Cross on one side, contains: ASA 81 mg. Nonmedicinal ingredients: corn starch, dextrose, FD&C Yellow #6, orange flavour and sodium cyclamate. Bottles of 30 and 100.

(Shown in Product Identification Section)

Atacand® Ⓟ

candesartan cilexetil

Angiotensin II AT1 Receptor Blocker

AstraZeneca

Date of Revision: December 29, 2008

SUMMARY PRODUCT INFORMATION:

Route of Administration	Dosage Form/ Strength	All Nonmedicinal Ingredients
Oral	Tablets: 4 mg, 8 mg, 16 mg and 32 mg	Calcium carboxymethylcellulose, maize starch, hydroxypropyl cellulose, iron oxide (except 4 mg tablets), lactose, magnesium stearate, polyethylene glycol

INDICATIONS AND CLINICAL USE: ATACAND (candesartan cilexetil) is indicated for:
- Hypertension:
  - The treatment of mild to moderate essential hypertension.
  - ATACAND may be used alone or concomitantly with thiazide diuretics.
  - The safety and efficacy of concurrent use with calcium channel blockers and angiotensin converting enzyme inhibitors have not been established.
- Heart Failure:
  - The treatment of NYHA Class II and III heart failure with ejection fraction ≤40% in addition to standard therapy, with or without an ACE inhibitor.

Geriatrics (>65 years of age): No overall differences in safety or effectiveness were observed between these subjects and younger subjects, and other reported clinical experience has not identified differences in responses between the elderly and younger patients, but greater sensitivity of some older individuals cannot be ruled out.
Pediatrics (<18 years of age): The safety and efficacy of ATACAND have not been established in children.
CONTRAINDICATIONS: ATACAND (candesartan cilexetil) is contraindicated in:
- Patients who are hypersensitive to any component of this product (see Dosage Forms, Composition and Packaging).

WARNINGS AND PRECAUTIONS:

> **Serious Warnings and Precautions**
> When used in pregnancy, angiotensin receptor (AT_1) blockers (ARBs) can cause injury or even death of the developing fetus. When pregnancy is detected, ATACAND should be discontinued as soon as possible (see Warnings and Precautions, Special Populations, Pregnant Women).

Cardiovascular: Hypotension: Occasionally, symptomatic hypotension has occurred after administration of candesartan cilexetil. It is more likely to occur in patients who are volume-depleted by diuretic therapy, dietary salt restriction, dialysis, diarrhea or vomiting, or undergoing surgery with anaesthesia. In these patients, because of the potential fall in blood pressure, therapy should be started under close medical supervision. Similar considerations apply to patients with ischemic heart or cerebrovascular disease, in whom an excessive fall in blood pressure could result in myocardial infarction or cerebrovascular accident.

Patients with heart failure given candesartan cilexetil commonly have some reduction in blood pressure. Caution should be observed when initiating therapy.

The effect of ATACAND (candesartan cilexetil) on the ability to drive and use machines has not been studied, but based on its pharmacodynamic properties ATACAND is unlikely to affect this ability. When driving vehicles or operating machines, it should be taken into account that dizziness or weariness may occur during treatment.
Valvular Stenosis: There is concern on theoretical grounds that patients with aortic stenosis might be at particular risk of decreased coronary perfusion when treated with vasodilators because they do not develop as much afterload reduction.
Endocrine and Metabolism: Hyperkalemia: In heart failure patients treated with ATACAND, hyperkalemia may occur. During treatment with ATACAND in patients with heart failure, periodic monitoring of serum potassium is recommended, especially when taken concomitantly with ACE inhibitors and potassium-sparing diuretics such as spironolactone.
Renal: Renal Impairment: As a consequence of inhibiting the renin-angiotensin-aldosterone system, changes in renal function have been seen in susceptible individuals. In patients whose renal function may depend on the activity of the renin-angiotensin-aldosterone system, such as patients with bilateral renal artery stenosis, unilateral renal artery stenosis to a solitary kidney, or severe congestive heart failure, treatment with agents that inhibit this system has been associated with oliguria, progressive azotemia, and rarely, acute renal failure and/or death. In susceptible patients, concomitant diuretic use may further increase risk.

Use of ATACAND should include appropriate assessment of renal function.

In heart failure patients, increases in serum creatinine may occur. Dosage reduction, and/or discontinuation of the diuretic, and/or ATACAND, and/or volume repletion may be required. Monitoring of serum creatinine is recommended during dose escalation and periodically thereafter.
Special Populations: Pregnant Women: Drugs that act directly on the renin-angiotensin-aldosterone-system (RAAS) can cause fetal and neonatal morbidity and death when administered to pregnant women. When pregnancy is detected, ATACAND should be discontinued as soon as possible.

The use of ARBs is not recommended during pregnancy. Epidemiological evidence regarding the risk of teratogenicity following exposure to angiotensin converting enzyme inhibitors (another class of therapeutic products interfering with the RAAS) during the first trimester of pregnancy has not been conclusive; however a small increase in risk cannot be excluded. Given the current evidence available on the risk with ARBs, similar risks may exist for this class of drugs. Patients planning pregnancy should be changed to alternative anti-hypertensive treatments which have an established safety profile for use in pregnancy. When pregnancy is diagnosed, treatment with angiotensin receptor (AT_1) blockers should be stopped immediately, and, if appropriate, alternative therapy should be started.

The use of ARBs during the second and third trimesters is known to induce human fetotoxicity (decreased renal function, oligohydramnios, skull ossification retardation) and neonatal toxicity (renal failure, hypotension, hyperkalaemia).

Infants with a history of in utero exposure to ARBs should be closely observed for hypotension, oliguria, and hyperkalemia. If oliguria occurs, attention should be directed toward support of blood pressure and renal perfusion. Exchange transfusion or dialysis may be required as a means of reversing hypotension and/or substituting for impaired renal function; however, limited experience with those procedures has not been associated with significant clinical benefit. Candesartan cilexetil is not removed from plasma by dialysis.
Animal Data: Oral doses ≥10 mg candesartan cilexetil/kg/day administered to pregnant rats during late gestation and continued through lactation were associated with reduced survival and an increased incidence of hydronephrosis in the offspring. Candesartan cilexetil given to pregnant rabbits at an oral dose of 3 mg/kg/day caused maternal toxicity (decreased body weight and death) but, in surviving dams, had no adverse effects on fetal survival, fetal weight, or external, visceral, or skeletal development. No maternal toxicity or adverse effects on fetal development were observed when oral doses up to 1000 mg candesartan cilexetil/kg/day were administered to pregnant mice.

Nursing Women: It is not known whether candesartan is excreted in human milk, but significant levels have been found in the milk of lactating rats. Because many drugs are excreted in human milk, and because of their potential for affecting the nursing infant adversely, a decision should be made whether to discontinue nursing or to discontinue the drug, taking into account the importance of the drug to the mother.
Pediatrics (<18 years of age): The safety and efficacy of ATACAND have not been established in children.
Geriatrics (>65 years of age): No overall differences in safety or effectiveness were observed between these subjects and younger subjects, and other reported clinical experience has not identified differences in responses between the elderly and younger patients, but greater sensitivity of some older individuals cannot be ruled out.
ADVERSE REACTIONS: Adverse Drug Reaction Overview: Hypertension: ATACAND (candesartan cilexetil) has been evaluated for safety in more than 8700 patients treated for hypertension, including 677 treated for six months or more, and 626 for about one year or more. Of these, 8694 were treated with candesartan cilexetil monotherapy in controlled clinical trials.

In placebo-controlled clinical trials, discontinuation due to adverse events occurred in 2.9% and 2.7% of patients treated with ATACAND monotherapy and placebo, respectively.

The following potentially serious adverse reactions have been reported rarely with candesartan cilexetil in controlled clinical trials: syncope, hypotension.
Heart Failure: The adverse event profile of ATACAND in heart failure patients was consistent with the pharmacology of the drug and the health status of the patients. In the CHARM Alternative and CHARM-Added studies comparing ATACAND in total daily doses up to 32 mg once daily to placebo, 23.2 % of ATACAND and 18.4% of placebo patients discontinued the treatment due to adverse events.

Severe adverse reactions most commonly seen in CHARM-Alternative and CHARM Added were hypotension, hyperkalemia and renal impairment.
Clinical Trial Adverse Drug Reactions: Because clinical trials are conducted under very specific conditions the adverse reaction rates observed in the clinical trials may not reflect the rates observed in practice and should not be compared to the rates in the clinical trials of another drug. Adverse drug reaction information from clinical trials is useful for identifying drug-related adverse events and for approximating rates.
Hypertension: In the double blind, placebo-controlled trials, the overall incidence of adverse events showed no association with dose, age or gender. In these trials, the following adverse events reported with ATACAND occurred in ≥1% of patients, regardless of drug relationship (see Table 1).

Table 1: ATACAND
Adverse Events that Occurred in ≥1% of Patients, Regardless of Drug Relationship

	ATACAND n=1388 (%)	Placebo n=573 (%)
Body as a Whole		
Back Pain	3.2	0.9
Fatigue	1.5	1.6
Abdominal Pain	1.5	1.3
Peripheral Edema	1.0	0.7
Digestive		
Nausea	1.9	1.3
Diarrhea	1.5	1.9
Vomiting	1.0	1.2
Nervous/Psychiatric		
Headache	10.4	10.3
Dizziness	2.5	2.3
Respiratory		
Upper Respiratory Infection	5.1	3.8
Coughing	1.6	1.1
Influenza-like Symptoms	1.5	0.8
Pharyngitis	1.1	0.4
Bronchitis	1.0	2.2
Rhinitis	1.0	0.4

Clinical trials in which doses up to 32 mg were administered did not result in a significant increase in any of the adverse events listed above.
Heart Failure: In these trials, the following adverse events reported with ATACAND occurred in ≥1% of patients and with higher frequency than placebo, regardless of drug relationship (see Table 2).

Table 2: ATACAND
Adverse Events Reported in CHARM-Alternative and CHARM-Added and Occurring with Frequency of ≥1% Regardless of Drug Relationship

	ATACAND n=2289 (%)	Placebo n=2287 (%)
Body as a Whole		
Fatigue	1.4	0.9
Cardiovascular Disorders		
Hypotension	20.9	11.0
Syncope	3.3	3.2
Coronary Artery Disorder	4.2	3.5

(cont'd)

Table 2: ATACAND *(cont'd)*

Adverse Events Reported in CHARM-Alternative and CHARM-Added and Occurring with Frequency of ≥1% Regardless of Drug Relationship

	ATACAND n=2289 (%)	Placebo n=2287 (%)
Cardiac Arrest	1.3	1.1
Blood Disorders		
Anemia	2.8	2.3
Gastrointestinal System Disorders		
Diarrhea	2.4	1.1
Gastroenteritis	1.1	0.7
Liver and Biliary System Disorders		
Cholelithiasis	1.1	0.9
Metabolic and Nutritional Disorders		
Hyperkalemia	7.6	2.6
Dehydration	2.5	1.3
Nonprotein Nitrogen Increased	1.3	0.3
Uremia	1.1	0.5
Gout	1.0	0.9
Musculoskeletal System Disorders		
Arthrosis	1.2	1.0
Nervous System Disorders		
Dizziness	3.4	2.1
Headache	1.0	0.7
Urinary System Disorders		
Renal Function Abnormal	14.3	7.2
Renal Failure Acute	3.0	1.8

Less Common Clinical Trial Adverse Drug Reactions: Hypertension: The following adverse events were reported at an incidence of <1% in controlled clinical trials (in more than one patient, with higher frequency than placebo):
Body as a Whole: allergy, asthenia, pain, syncope.
Cardiovascular: angina pectoris, circulatory failure, flushing, hypotension, myocardial infarction, peripheral ischemia, thrombophlebitis.
Central and Peripheral Nervous System: hypertonia, hypoesthesia, paresthesia, vertigo.
Gastrointestinal: constipation, dyspepsia, dry mouth, toothache.
Hearing: tinnitus.
Metabolic and Nutritional: diabetes mellitus, hyperkalemia, hyponatremia.
Musculoskeletal: arthritis, arthropathy, myalgia, myopathy, skeletal pain, tendon disorder.
Blood: anemia, epistaxis.
Psychiatric: depression, impotence, neurosis.
Reproductive: menopausal symptoms.
Resistance Mechanism: otitis.
Respiratory: laryngitis.
Skin: eczema, pruritus, rash, skin disorder, sweating, (rarely) urticaria.
Urinary: abnormal urine, cystitis.
Vision: conjunctivitis.

In studies using daily doses greater than 16 mg, the following adverse events were reported at a rate greater than 1% but at about the same or greater incidence in patients receiving placebo: chest pain, sinusitis, arthralgia and albuminuria. Other adverse events reported at an incidence of 0.5% or greater from more than 3200 patients treated worldwide include fever, gastroenteritis, tachycardia, palpitation, increased creatinine phosphokinase, hyperglycemia, hypertriglyceridemia, hyperuricemia, anxiety, somnolence, dyspnea, and hematuria.

Heart Failure: The following listed adverse events occurred in less than 1% of ATACAND treated patients but in at least 2 patients and with more frequent occurrence in the ATACAND group than in the placebo group (CHARM-Alternative and CHARM-Added).
Skin and Appendages Disorders: rash, pruritus, angioedema.
Liver and Biliary System Disorders: hepatic function abnormal.
White Cell and Resistance Disorders: granulocytopenia, leukopenia.

Abnormal Hematologic and Clinical Chemistry Findings: Laboratory Test Findings: Hypertension: In controlled clinical trials, clinically important changes in standard laboratory parameters were rarely associated with administration of ATACAND.
Liver Function Tests: In controlled clinical trials, elevations of AST and ALT (>3 times the upper limit of normal) occurred in 0.3% and 0.5% of patients treated with ATACAND monotherapy compared to 0.2% and 0.4% of patients receiving placebo.
Serum Potassium: A small increase (mean increase of 0.1 mEq/L) was observed in hypertensive patients treated with ATACAND alone but was rarely of clinical importance.
Creatinine, Blood Urea Nitrogen, and Sodium: Minor increases in blood urea nitrogen (BUN) and serum creatinine were observed infrequently, as were decreases in sodium.
Hemoglobin and Hematocrit: Small decreases in hemoglobin and hematocrit (mean decreases of approximately 0.2 g/dL and 0.5 volume %, respectively) were observed in patients treated with ATACAND alone but were rarely of clinical importance. Anemia, leukopenia and thrombocytopenia were associated with withdrawal of one patient each from clinical trials.
Hyperuricemia: Hyperuricemia was rarely found (0.6% of patients treated with ATACAND and 0.5% of patients treated with placebo).
Heart Failure: Increases in serum creatinine, potassium and urea, and decreases in hemoglobin and hematocrit were observed.
Post-Market Adverse Drug Reactions: Angioedema, (involving swelling of the face, lips and/or tongue), has been reported rarely in patients treated with ATACAND.

In other post-marketing experience, renal impairment, including renal failure in elderly susceptible patients, has been observed (see Warnings and Precautions, Renal, Renal Impairment for definition of susceptible patients).

Very rare cases of abnormal hepatic function or hepatitis have also been reported.

Other adverse events reported for ATACAND where a causal relationship could not be established include very rare cases of leukopenia, neutropenia and agranulocytosis.

Cases of muscle pain, muscle weakness, myositis and rhabdomyolysis have been reported in patients receiving angiotensin II receptor blockers.

DRUG INTERACTIONS: Overview: Warfarin: When candesartan cilexetil was administered at 16 mg once daily under steady state conditions, no pharmacodynamic effect on prothrombin time was demonstrated in subjects stabilized on warfarin.
Digoxin: Combination treatment with candesartan cilexetil and digoxin in healthy volunteers had no effect on AUC or C_{max} values for digoxin compared to digoxin alone. Similarly, combination treatment had no effect on AUC or C_{max} values for candesartan compared to candesartan cilexetil alone.
Other: No significant drug interactions have been reported with glyburide, nifedipine or oral contraceptives co-administered with candesartan cilexetil to healthy volunteers. While there is no clinically relevant interaction between candesartan and enalapril, patients with renal impairment showed a higher exposure to both drugs. This is consistent with known pharmacokinetics of these two compounds.
Drug-Drug Interactions: The drugs listed in Table 3 are based on either drug interaction case reports or studies or potential interactions due to the expected magnitude and seriousness of the interaction (i.e. those identified as contraindicated).

Table 3: ATACAND

Established or Potential Drug-Drug Interactions

Candesartan Cilexetil	Effect	Clinical Comment
Diuretics	Patients on diuretics, and especially those in whom diuretic therapy was recently instituted, may occasionally experience an excessive reduction of blood pressure after initiation of therapy with ATACAND (candesartan cilexetil).	The possibility of symptomatic hypotension with the use of ATACAND can be minimized by discontinuing the diuretic prior to initiation of treatment and/or lowering the initial dose of candesartan cilexetil (see Warnings and Precautions, Cardiovascular, Hypotension and Dosage and Administration). No drug interaction of clinical significance has been identified with thiazide diuretics in patients treated with up to 25 mg hydrochlorothiazide with 16 mg ATACAND for 8 weeks.
Agents Increasing Serum Potassium	ATACAND decreases the production of aldosterone.	Potassium-sparing diuretics or potassium supplements should be given only for documented hypokalemia and with frequent monitoring of serum potassium. Potassium-containing salt substitutes should also be used with caution.
Lithium Salts	As with other drugs which eliminate sodium, lithium clearance may be reduced.	Serum lithium levels should be monitored carefully if lithium salts are to be administered.

Drug-Food Interactions: ATACAND may be taken with or without food (see Dosage and Administration).

DOSAGE AND ADMINISTRATION: Dosing Considerations: The dosage of ATACAND (candesartan cilexetil) must be individualized.
Recommended Dose and Dosage Adjustment: ATACAND should be taken once daily, at approximately the same time each day, with or without food.
Hypertension: Initiation of therapy requires consideration of recent antihypertensive treatment, the extent of blood pressure elevation, salt restriction, and other pertinent clinical factors. The dosage of other antihypertensive agents used with ATACAND may need to be adjusted. Blood pressure response is dose related over the range of 4 to 32 mg.

The recommended initial dose of ATACAND is 16 mg, once daily when used as monotherapy. Total daily doses of ATACAND should range from 8 to 32 mg. Doses higher than 32 mg do not appear to have a greater effect on blood pressure reduction, and there is relatively little experience with such doses. Most of the antihypertensive effect is present within 2 weeks and the maximal blood pressure reduction is generally obtained within 4 weeks. For patients with possible depletion of intravascular volume (e.g. patients treated with diuretics, particularly those with impaired renal function) consideration should be given to administration of a lower dose. If blood pressure is not controlled by ATACAND alone, candesartan cilexetil may be used together with a thiazide diuretic (see Drug Interactions, Drug-Drug Interactions, Table 3: Diuretics).
Concomitant Diuretic Therapy: In patients receiving diuretics, ATACAND therapy should be initiated with caution, since these patients may be volume-depleted and thus more likely to experience hypotension following initiation of additional antihypertensive therapy.

Whenever possible, all diuretics should be discontinued two to three days prior to the administration of ATACAND, to reduce the likelihood of hypotension (see Warnings and Precautions, Cardiovascular, Hypotension). If this is not possible because of the patient's condition, ATACAND should be administered with caution and the blood pressure monitored closely. Thereafter, the dosage should be adjusted according to the individual response of the patient.
Hepatic Impairment: No dosage adjustment is necessary in patients with mild to moderate chronic liver disease.

There is only limited experience available in patients with severe hepatic impairment and/or cholestasis. In patients with severely impaired hepatic function, a lower initial dose of 4 mg should be considered.
Renal Impairment: No dosage adjustment is necessary in patients with mildly impaired renal function.

In patients with moderately or severely impaired renal function, or in patients undergoing dialysis, a lower initial dose of 4 mg should be considered.
Geriatrics (>65 years of age): No dosage adjustment is necessary for elderly patients. As greater sensitivity of some older patients cannot be ruled out, appropriate caution is recommended (see Warnings and Precautions, Special Populations, Geriatrics (>65 years of age)).
Pediatrics (<18 years of age): The safety and efficacy of ATACAND have not been established in children.
Heart Failure: The usual recommended initial dose for treating heart failure is 4 mg once daily. The target dose is 32 mg once daily which is achieved by doubling the dose at approximately 2 week intervals, as tolerated by the patient. ATACAND can be administered with other heart failure treatments including ACE inhibitors, beta-blockers, diuretics, digoxin, and/or spironolactone.

No initial dose adjustment is necessary for elderly patients or in patients with renal or hepatic impairment.
Missed Dose: If a patient misses a dose of ATACAND and remembers within 12 hours, the patient should take the dose as soon as possible and then go back to the regular schedule. If it is more than 12 hours after the patient remembers, they should not take the missed dose; the next dose should be taken on time.

A double dose of ATACAND should never be taken to make up for a missed dose.

OVERDOSAGE:
Limited data are available in regard to overdosage in humans. The most likely manifestations of overdosage would be hypotension, dizziness and tachycardia; bradycardia could occur from reflex parasympathetic (vagal) stimulation. In case reports detailing overdosage (up to 672 mg ATACAND (candesartan cilexetil) patient recovery was uneventful.

If symptomatic hypotension should occur, supportive treatment should be instituted and vital signs monitored. The patient should be placed supine with the legs elevated. If this is not sufficient, plasma volume should be increased by infusion of, for example, isotonic saline solution. Sympathomimetic drugs may also be administered if the above-mentioned measures are not sufficient. Candesartan cilexetil is not removed from the plasma by hemodialysis.

For management of a suspected drug overdose, CPhA recommends that you contact your **regional Poison Control Centre**. See the *CPS* Directory section for a list of Poison Control Centres.

ACTION AND CLINICAL PHARMACOLOGY: Mechanism of Action: ATACAND (candesartan cilexetil) antagonizes angiotensin II by blocking the angiotensin type one (AT_1) receptor. Angiotensin II is the primary vasoactive hormone of the renin-angiotensin-aldosterone system with effects that include vasoconstriction, stimulation of aldosterone secretion and renal reabsorption of sodium.

Candesartan cilexetil, a prodrug, is rapidly converted to the active drug, candesartan, during absorption from the gastrointestinal tract.

Candesartan blocks the vasoconstrictor and aldosterone secreting effects of angiotensin II by selectively blocking the binding of angiotensin II to the AT_1 receptor in many tissues, such as vascular smooth muscle and the adrenal gland. Its action is therefore independent of the pathways for angiotensin II synthesis. There is also an AT_2 receptor found in many tissues, but it plays no known role in cardiovascular homeostasis to date. Candesartan has a much greater affinity (>10 000 fold) for the AT_1 receptor than for the AT_2 receptor. The strong bond between candesartan and the AT_1 receptor is a result of tight binding to and slow dissociation from the receptor.

Candesartan does not inhibit angiotensin converting enzyme (ACE), also known as kininase II, the enzyme that converts angiotensin I to angiotensin II and degrades bradykinin, nor does it bind to or block other hormone receptors or ion channels known to be important in cardiovascular regulation.

Pharmacodynamics: Candesartan inhibits the pressor effects of angiotensin II infusion in a dose dependent manner. After 1 week of once-daily dosing of 8 mg candesartan cilexetil, the pressor effect was inhibited by approximately 90% at peak (4-8 hours after dosing) with approximately 50% inhibition persisting at 24 hours.

Plasma concentrations of angiotensin I, angiotensin II, and plasma renin activity, increased in a dose-dependent manner after single and repeated administration of candesartan cilexetil to healthy subjects, hypertensive, and heart failure patients. A decrease in the plasma concentration of aldosterone was observed when 32 mg of candesartan cilexetil was administered to hypertensive patients.

Pharmacokinetics: Absorption: Following oral administration of candesartan cilexetil as a tablet, the absolute bioavailability of candesartan was estimated to be approximately 15%. After tablet ingestion, the peak serum concentration (C_{max}) is reached after 3-4 hours. Food does not affect the bioavailability of candesartan after candesartan cilexetil administration.

Distribution: The volume of distribution of candesartan is 0.13 L/kg. Candesartan is highly bound to plasma proteins (>99%) and does not penetrate red blood cells. The protein binding is constant at candesartan plasma concentrations well above the range achieved with recommended doses. In rats, it has been demonstrated that candesartan does cross the blood-brain barrier. It has also been demonstrated in rats that candesartan passes across the placental barrier and is distributed in the fetus.

Metabolism: Candesartan cilexetil is rapidly and completely bioactivated by ester hydrolysis during absorption from the gastrointestinal tract to candesartan. It undergoes minor hepatic metabolism by O-deethylation to an inactive metabolite. In vitro studies indicate that cytochrome P450 isoenzyme CYP 2C9 is involved in the biotransformation of candesartan to its inactive metabolite. Based on in vitro data, no interaction would be expected to occur in vivo with drugs whose metabolism is dependent upon cytochrome P450 isoenzymes CYP1A2, CYP2A6, CYP2C9, CYP2C19, CYP2D6, CYP2E1 or CYP3A4.

Excretion: Total plasma clearance of candesartan is 0.37 mL/min/kg, with a renal clearance of 0.19 mL/min/kg. Candesartan is mainly excreted unchanged in urine and feces (via bile). When candesartan cilexetil is administered orally, about 26% of the dose is excreted as candesartan in urine. Following an oral dose of 14C-labeled candesartan cilexetil, approximately 33% of radioactivity is recovered in urine and approximately 67% in feces. Following an intravenous dose of 14C-labeled candesartan, approximately 59% of radioactivity is recovered in urine and approximately 36% in feces. Biliary excretion contributes to the elimination of candesartan. The elimination half-life of candesartan is approximately 9 hours. After single and repeated administration, the pharmacokinetics of candesartan are linear for oral doses up to 32 mg. Candesartan and its inactive metabolite do not accumulate in serum upon repeated once-daily dosing.

Special Populations and Conditions: Geriatrics: The plasma concentration of candesartan was higher in the elderly (≥65 years) (C_{max} was approximately 50% higher, and AUC was approximately 80% higher) compared to younger subjects administered the same dose. The pharmacokinetics of candesartan were linear in the elderly, and candesartan and its inactive metabolite did not accumulate in the serum of these subjects upon repeated, once-daily administration.

Gender: No gender-related differences in the pharmacokinetics of candesartan have been observed.

Hepatic Insufficiency: In patients with mild to moderate hepatic impairment, there was an increase in the AUC of candesartan of approximately 20%. There was no drug accumulation in plasma in these patients. In patients with moderate to severe hepatic impairment, the C_{max} and AUC increased up to five times in a very small group administered a single dose of 16 mg candesartan (see Dosage and Administration, Hepatic Impairment).

Renal Insufficiency: In patients with mild to moderate renal impairment (Cl_{creat} 31-60 mL/min/1.73m²), C_{max} and AUC of candesartan increased by 40-60% and 50-90%, respectively, but t½ was not altered, compared to patients with normal renal function (Cl_{creat} >60 mL/min/1.73m²) during repeated dosing. There was no drug accumulation in plasma in patients with mild to moderate renal impairment. The increases in C_{max} and AUC in patients with severe renal impairment (Cl_{creat} 15-30 mL/min/1.73m²) were 40-60% and 110%, respectively. The terminal t½ of candesartan was approximately doubled in patients with severe renal impairment, and these changes resulted in some accumulation in plasma. The pharmacokinetics of candesartan in patients undergoing hemodialysis were similar to those in patients with severe renal impairment (see Dosage and Administration, Renal Impairment).

STORAGE AND STABILITY: Store at 15-30°C.

INFORMATION FOR THE PATIENT: Published in e-CPS, available by subscription at www.e-cps.ca.

DOSAGE FORMS, COMPOSITION AND PACKAGING: 4 mg: Each circular, biconvex, white tablet, with a score and marked A/CF on one side and marked 004 on the other side, contains: candesartan cilexetil 4 mg. Nonmedicinal ingredients: calcium carboxymethylcellulose, cornstarch, hydroxypropyl cellulose, lactose, magnesium stearate and polyethylene glycol. Blister packs of 30.

8 mg: Each circular, biconvex, light pink tablet, with a score and marked A/CG on one side and marked 008 on the other side, contains: candesartan cilexetil 8 mg. Nonmedicinal ingredients: calcium carboxymethylcellulose, cornstarch, hydroxypropyl cellulose, iron oxide, lactose, magnesium stearate and polyethylene glycol. Blister packs of 30. Bottles of 100.

16 mg: Each circular, biconvex, pink tablet, with a score and marked A/CH on one side and marked 016 on the other side, contains: candesartan cilexetil 16 mg. Nonmedicinal ingredients: calcium carboxymethylcellulose, cornstarch, hydroxypropyl cellulose, iron oxide, lactose, magnesium stearate and polyethylene glycol. Blister packs of 30. Bottles of 100.

32 mg : Each circular, biconvex, pink tablet, with a score and marked A/CL on one side and marked 032 on the other side, contains: candesartan cilexetil 32 mg. Nonmedicinal ingredients: calcium carboxymethylcellulose, cornstarch, hydroxypropyl cellulose, iron oxide, lactose, magnesium stearate and polyethylene glycol. Blister packs of 30.

(Shown in Product Identification Section)

Atacand® Plus 🅿

candesartan cilexetil—hydrochlorothiazide

Angiotensin II AT1 Receptor Blocker—Diuretic

AstraZeneca

Date of Preparation: May 29, 2001
Date of Revision: August 28, 2009

SUMMARY PRODUCT INFORMATION:

Route of Administration	Dosage Form/ Strength	All Nonmedicinal Ingredients
Oral	Tablet: 16 mg/12.5 mg, 32 mg/12.5 mg and 32 mg/25 mg	Calcium carboxymethylcellulose, hydroxypropyl cellulose, iron oxide, lactose, magnesium stearate, maize starch, polyethylene glycol

INDICATIONS AND CLINICAL USE: ATACAND PLUS (candesartan cilexetil/hydrochlorothiazide) is indicated for the treatment of essential hypertension in patients for whom combination therapy is appropriate.

ATACAND PLUS is not indicated for initial therapy (see Dosage and Administration).

The dosage of ATACAND PLUS must be individualized. The dose of ATACAND PLUS should be determined by titration of the individual components.

Geriatrics (>65 years of age): No overall differences in safety or effectiveness were observed between the younger and elderly patients but greater sensitivity of some older patients cannot be ruled out and appropriate caution is recommended.

Pediatrics (<18 years of age): The safety and efficacy of ATACAND PLUS have not been established in children.

CONTRAINDICATIONS: ATACAND PLUS (candesartan cilexetil/hydrochlorothiazide) is contraindicated in:

- Patients who are hypersensitive to any component of this product (see Dosage Forms, Composition and Packaging).
- Patients with anuria and patients who are hypersensitive to other sulfonamide-derived drugs, because of the hydrochlorothiazide component (see Warnings and Precautions, Immune and Adverse Reactions, Post-Market Adverse Drug Reactions).

WARNINGS AND PRECAUTIONS:

> **Serious Warnings and Precautions**
> When used in pregnancy, angiotensin receptor (AT_1) blockers (ARBs) can cause injury or even death of the developing fetus. When pregnancy is detected, ATACAND PLUS should be discontinued as soon as possible (see Warnings and Precautions, Special Populations, Pregnant Women).

Cardiovascular: Hypotension: Occasionally, symptomatic hypotension has occurred after administration of candesartan cilexetil. It is more likely to occur in patients who are volume-depleted by diuretic therapy, dietary salt restriction, dialysis, diarrhea or vomiting, or undergoing surgery with anaesthesia. In these patients, because of the potential fall in blood pressure, therapy should be started under close medical supervision. Similar considerations apply to patients with ischemic heart or cerebrovascular disease, in whom an excessive fall in blood pressure could result in myocardial infarction or cerebrovascular accident.

The effect of ATACAND PLUS on the ability to drive and use machines has not been studied, but based on its pharmacodynamic properties ATACAND PLUS is unlikely to affect this ability. When driving vehicles or operating machines, it should be taken into account that occasionally dizziness or weariness may occur during treatment of hypertension.

Valvular Stenosis: There is concern on theoretical grounds that patients with aortic stenosis might be at particular risk of decreased coronary perfusion when treated with vasodilators because they do not develop as much afterload reduction.

Endocrine and Metabolism: Metabolism: Patients receiving thiazides, including hydrochlorothiazide (HCTZ), should be carefully observed for clinical signs of fluid and electrolyte imbalance (hyponatremia, hypochloremic alkalosis and hypokalemia).

Periodic determinations of serum electrolytes, to detect possible electrolyte disturbance, should be performed at appropriate intervals. Warning signs or symptoms of fluid and electrolyte imbalance include dryness of the mouth, thirst, weakness, lethargy, drowsiness, restlessness, muscle pain or cramps, muscle fatigue, hypotension, oliguria, tachycardia and gastrointestinal disturbances such as nausea and vomiting.

Hypokalemia may develop, especially with brisk diuresis, when severe cirrhosis is present, or after prolonged therapy.

Interference with adequate oral electrolyte intake will also contribute to hypokalemia. Hypokalemia can sensitize or exaggerate the response of the heart to the toxic effects of digitalis (e.g. increased ventricular irritability).

Any chloride deficit during thiazide therapy is generally mild and usually does not require specific treatment except under extraordinary circumstances (as in liver disease or renal disease). Dilutional hyponatremia may occur in edematous patients in hot weather. Appropriate therapy is water restriction rather than administration of salt, except in rare instances, when the hyponatremia is life threatening. In actual salt depletion, appropriate replacement is the therapy of choice.

Hyperuricemia may occur or acute gout may be precipitated in certain patients receiving thiazide therapy.

Thiazides may decrease serum PBI (protein bound iodine) levels without signs of thyroid disturbance.

Thiazides have been shown to increase excretion of magnesium; this may result in hypomagnesemia.

Thiazides may decrease urinary calcium excretion and may cause intermittent and slight elevation of serum calcium in the absence of known disorders of calcium metabolism. Marked hypercalcemia may be evidence of hidden hyperparathyroidism. Thiazides should be discontinued before carrying out tests for parathyroid function.

Treatment with a thiazide diuretic may impair glucose tolerance. Increases in cholesterol and triglyceride levels may be associated with thiazide diuretic therapy. However, at the doses contained in ATACAND PLUS (candesartan cilexetil/hydrochlorothiazide), minimal effects were observed.

Hepatic/Biliary/Pancreatic: Hepatic Impairment: Thiazides should be used with caution in patients with impaired hepatic function or progressive liver disease, since minor alterations of fluid or electrolyte balance may precipitate hepatic coma (see Dosage and Administration, Hepatic Impairment).

No studies were carried out with candesartan cilexetil/hydrochlorothiazide fixed combination in patients with impaired hepatic function.

Immune: Hypersensitivity Reactions: Sensitivity reactions to hydrochlorothiazide may occur in patients with or without a history of allergy or bronchial asthma.

The possibility of exacerbation or activation of systemic lupus erythematosus has been reported in patients treated with hydrochlorothiazide.

Peri-Operative Considerations: Thiazides may increase the responsiveness to tubocurarine.

Renal: Renal Impairment: As a consequence of inhibiting the renin-angiotensin-aldosterone system, changes in renal function have been seen in susceptible individuals. In patients whose renal function may depend on the activity of the renin-angiotensin-aldosterone system, such as patients with bilateral renal artery stenosis, unilateral renal artery stenosis to a solitary kidney, or severe congestive heart failure, treatment with agents that inhibit this system has been associated with oliguria, progressive azotemia, and rarely, acute renal failure and/or death. In susceptible patients, concomitant diuretic use may further increase risk.

Use of candesartan cilexetil should include appropriate assessment of renal function. Thiazides should be used with caution.

Because of the hydrochlorothiazide component, ATACAND PLUS is not recommended in patients with severe renal impairment (creatinine clearance <30 mL/min/1.73 m² BSA).

Azotemia: Azotemia may be precipitated or increased by hydrochlorothiazide. Cumulative effects of the drug may develop in patients with impaired renal function. If increasing azotemia and oliguria occur during treatment of severe progressive renal disease the diuretic should be discontinued.

Special Populations: Pregnant Women: Drugs that act directly on the renin-angiotensin-aldosterone-system (RAAS) can cause fetal and neonatal morbidity and death when administered to pregnant women. When pregnancy is detected, ATACAND PLUS should be discontinued as soon as possible.

The use of ARBs is not recommended during pregnancy. Epidemiological evidence regarding the risk of teratogenicity following exposure to angiotensin converting enzyme inhibitors (another class of therapeutic products interfering with the RAAS) during the first trimester of pregnancy has not been conclusive; however a small increase in risk cannot be excluded. Given the current evidence available on the risk with ARBs, similar risks may exist for this class of drugs. Patients planning pregnancy should be changed to alternative anti-hypertensive treatments which have an established safety profile for use in pregnancy. When pregnancy is diagnosed, treatment with angiotensin receptor (AT_1) blockers should be stopped immediately, and, if appropriate, alternative therapy should be started.

The use of ARBs during the second and third trimesters is known to induce human fetotoxicity (decreased renal function, oligohydramnios, skull ossification retardation) and neonatal toxicity (renal failure, hypotension, hyperkalaemia).

Infants with a history of in utero exposure to ARBs should be closely observed for hypotension, oliguria, and hyperkalemia. If oliguria occurs, attention should be directed toward support of blood pressure and renal perfusion. Exchange transfusion or dialysis may be required as a means of reversing hypotension and/or substituting for impaired renal function; however, limited experience with those procedures has not been associated with significant clinical benefit. Candesartan cilexetil is not removed from plasma by dialysis.

Thiazides cross the placental barrier and appear in cord blood. The routine use of diuretics in otherwise healthy pregnant women is not recommended and exposes mother and fetus to unnecessary hazard including fetal or neonatal jaundice, thrombocytopenia and possibly other adverse experiences which have occurred in the adult. Diuretics do not prevent development of toxemia of pregnancy and there is no satisfactory evidence that they are useful in the treatment of toxemia.

Animal Data: Oral doses ≥10 mg candesartan cilexetil/kg/day administered to pregnant rats during late gestation and continued through lactation were associated with reduced survival and an increased incidence of hydronephrosis in the offspring. Candesartan cilexetil given to pregnant rabbits at an oral dose of 3 mg/kg/day caused maternal toxicity (decreased body weight and death) but, in surviving dams, had no adverse effects on fetal survival, fetal weight, or external, visceral, or skeletal development. No maternal toxicity or adverse effects on fetal development were observed when oral doses up to 1000 mg candesartan cilexetil/kg/day were administered to pregnant mice.

Nursing Women: It is not known whether candesartan is excreted in human milk, but significant levels have been found in the milk of lactating rats. Thiazides appear in human milk. Because many drugs are excreted in human milk, and because of their potential for affecting the nursing infant adversely, a decision should be made whether to discontinue nursing or to discontinue the drug, taking into account the importance of the drug to the mother.

Pediatrics (<18 years of age): The safety and efficacy of ATACAND PLUS have not been established in children.

Geriatrics (>65 years of age): No overall differences in safety or effectiveness were observed between the younger and elderly patients but greater sensitivity of some older patients cannot be ruled out and appropriate caution is recommended.

ADVERSE REACTIONS: Adverse Drug Reaction Overview: ATACAND PLUS (candesartan cilexetil/hydrochlorothiazide) has been evaluated for safety in over 2500 patients treated for hypertension, including more than 700 treated for six months or more, and 500 for about one year or more. In placebo controlled double blind studies to support ATACAND PLUS 16 mg/12.5 mg, candesartan cilexetil/hydrochlorothiazide combination was administered to 1025 hypertensive patients. Approximately 600 patients received ATACAND PLUS 16 mg/12.5 mg. The overall exposure amounts to 977 patient-years. Safety of the higher strength combinations of ATACAND PLUS, 32 mg/12.5 mg and 32 mg/25 mg, has also been evaluated. In controlled clinical studies 718 patients were treated with candesartan/hydrochlorothiazide 32 mg/12.5 mg and 1155 patients were treated with 32 mg/25 mg; the total exposure in patient years in these studies was 107.8 and 175.3 years, respectively.

In general, adverse events were mild and transient in controlled clinical studies with various doses of candesartan cilexetil/hydrochlorothiazide (candesartan cilexetil up to 32 mg and hydrochlorothiazide up to 25 mg). The overall incidence of adverse events showed no association with age or gender.

In controlled clinical studies, discontinuation due to adverse events occurred in 2.3-3.3% and 2.7-4.3% of patients treated with ATACAND PLUS and placebo, respectively. In studies to support the 16 mg/12.5 mg strength, the incidence of serious adverse events observed with candesartan cilexetil/hydrochlorothiazide was 2.7% (71 out of 2582 patients). The incidence of serious adverse events was lower in the candesartan cilexetil/hydrochlorothiazide 32 mg/12.5 mg and 32 mg/25 mg dosage groups with the highest frequency of 0.8% (5 out of 664 patients) observed in the 32 mg/25 mg group.

Clinical Trial Adverse Drug Reactions: Because clinical trials are conducted under very specific conditions the adverse reaction rates observed in the clinical trials may not reflect the rates observed in practice and should not be compared to the rates in the clinical trials of another drug. Adverse drug reaction information from clinical trials is useful for identifying drug-related adverse events and for approximating rates.

In the double blind placebo controlled studies to support candesartan cilexetil/hydrochlorothiazide 16 mg/12.5 mg, the overall incidence of adverse events showed no association with age or gender. In these studies the following adverse events reported with candesartan cilexetil/hydrochlorothiazide occurred in ≥1% of patients, regardless of drug relationship (see Table 1).

Table 1: ATACAND PLUS

Adverse Events Reported with Candesartan Cilexetil/Hydrochlorothiazide in ≥1% of Patients Regardless of Causality in Studies Supporting the 16 mg/12.5 mg Strength

	Candesartan Cilexetil/ Hydrochlorothiazide (n=1025) (%)	Candesartan Cilexetil (n=749) (%)	Hydrochlorothiazide (n=603) (%)	Placebo (n=526) (%)
Body as a Whole				
Back Pain	3.8	5.5	5.1	3.0
Arthralgia	1.5	1.3	1.3	0.8
Fatigue	1.4	1.2	1.7	1.0
Abdominal Pain	1.3	1.7	0.7	1.1
Urinary				
Urinary Tract Infection	1.6	1.3	1.8	1.0
Digestive				
Nausea	1.5	0.9	1.2	0.6
Diarrhea	1.1	0.7	0.5	1.3
Gastroenteritis	1.0	0.5	1.0	0.4
Cardiovascular				
Tachycardia	1.3	0.9	1.2	0.8
ECG Abnormal	1.2	1.2	0.3	0.8
Edema Peripheral	1.1	1.6	2.2	1.3
Chest Pain	1.0	0.7	1.0	0.6
Metabolic Disorders				
Hyperuricemia	1.1	0.7	0.8	0.4
Hyperglycemia	1.0	0.9	0.5	0.2
Nervous/Psychiatric				
Headache	4.3	7.6	7.6	7.0
Dizziness	3.1	3.9	2.0	1.5
Inflicted Injury	2.0	2.0	3.0	1.9
Respiratory				
Upper Respiratory Tract Infection	3.7	5.1	5.6	1.9
Influenza-like Symptoms	2.8	2.3	3.0	2.9
Sinusitis	2.3	2.9	3.5	1.9
Bronchitis	2.1	2.8	2.5	2.5
Pharyngitis	1.4	0.9	1.0	1.7
Cough	0.9	2.3	1.7	1.0
Rhinitis	1.2	1.5	1.2	0.4

In double blind, controlled studies with candesartan cilexetil/hydrochlorothiazide 32 mg/12.5 mg, and 32 mg/25 mg the following adverse events reported with candesartan cilexetil/hydrochlorothiazide occurred in ≥1% of patients, regardless of drug relationship (see Table 2).

Table 2: ATACAND PLUS

Adverse Events Reported with Candesartan Cilexetil/Hydrochlorothiazide 32 mg/12.5 mg and 32 mg/25 mg in ≥1% of Patients Regardless of Causality

	Candesartan Cilexetil/ Hydrochlorothiazide (n=1873)				
	32 mg/12.5 mg (n=718) %	32 mg/25 mg (n=1155) %	Candesartan Cilexetil (n=1188) %	Hydrochlorothiazide (n=540) %	Placebo (n=163) %
Body as a Whole					
Back pain	2.4	1.6	1.1	0.6	2.5
Fatigue	1.1	0.9	0.8	0.4	2.5
Arthralgia	0.6	1.1	0.6	1.1	1.8
Digestive					
Diarrhea	1.1	0.4	0.7	0.4	1.8
Metabolic Disorders					
Dyslipidaemia	3.3	2.5	1.9	0.4	0
Nervous/Psychiatric					
Dizziness	2.5	2.9	1.3	2.4	0.6
Headache	2.4	2.0	5.1	7.6	7.4
Respiratory					
Cough	1.4	0.7	0.6	1.3	1.2
Nasopharyngitis	1.3	1.4	1.0	0.6	0
Upper respiratory tract infection	1.3	0.3	1.7	3.5	5.5
Bronchitis	1.1	0.9	1.0	1.3	1.2

Less Common Clinical Trial Adverse Drug Reactions (<1%): Candesartan Cilexetil: The following adverse events were reported at an incidence of <1% in controlled clinical trials (in more than one patient, with higher frequency than placebo):

Body as a Whole: allergy, asthenia, pain, syncope.
Cardiovascular: angina pectoris, circulatory failure, flushing, hypotension, myocardial infarction, peripheral ischemia, thrombophlebitis.
Central and Peripheral Nervous System: hypertonia, hypoesthesia, paresthesia, vertigo.
Gastrointestinal: constipation, dyspepsia, dry mouth, toothache.
Hearing: tinnitus.
Metabolic and Nutritional: diabetes mellitus, hyperkalaemia, hyponatraemia.
Musculoskeletal: arthritis, arthropathy, myalgia, myopathy, skeletal pain, tendon disorder.
Blood: anemia, epistaxis.
Psychiatric: depression, impotence, neurosis.
Reproductive: menopausal symptoms.
Resistance Mechanism: otitis.
Respiratory: laryngitis.
Skin: eczema, pruritus, rash, skin disorder, sweating, (rarely) urticaria.
Urinary: abnormal urine, cystitis.
Vision: conjunctivitis.

There was no clear indication of dose-response relationship for any of the most common adverse events.

Abnormal Hematologic and Clinical Chemistry Findings: Laboratory Test Findings: In controlled clinical trials, clinically important changes in standard laboratory parameters were rarely associated with administration of ATACAND PLUS.

Liver Function Tests: In controlled clinical trials, elevations of ALT (>3 times the upper limit of normal) occurred in 0.9% of patients treated with ATACAND PLUS compared to 0% of patients receiving placebo. Minor increases in serum AST have been observed in single patients receiving candesartan cilexetil/hydrochlorothiazide.

Serum Potassium, Sodium: A small decrease (mean decrease of 0.1 mmol/L) in serum potassium was observed in patients treated with ATACAND PLUS but was rarely of clinical importance. Values of serum potassium below the predefined lower critical limit were recorded in 0.6% of patients in controlled clinical trials with ATACAND PLUS. An increase in serum potassium has rarely been observed with ATACAND PLUS. A decrease in sodium has been observed with ATACAND PLUS.

Hemoglobin and Hematocrit: Small decreases in hemoglobin were observed in patients treated with ATACAND PLUS but were rarely of clinical importance. Values of hemoglobin below the predefined critical limit were recorded in 0.9% of patients in controlled clinical trials with ATACAND PLUS.

Blood Glucose: In controlled clinical trials, elevations of blood glucose occurred in 1.0% of patients treated with ATACAND PLUS compared to 0.2% of patients receiving placebo.

Hyperuricemia: Increases in serum uric acid were found in 1.1% of patients treated with ATACAND PLUS and 0.4% of patients treated with placebo.

Creatinine, Urea: An increase in creatinine and urea has been observed with ATACAND PLUS.

Post-Market Adverse Drug Reactions: Candesartan cilexetil: Angioedema, (involving swelling of the face, lips and/or tongue) has been reported rarely in patients treated with candesartan cilexetil.

In other post-marketing experience, renal impairment, including renal failure in susceptible patients, has been observed (see Warnings and Precautions, Renal, Renal Impairment for definition of susceptible patients).

Very rare cases of abnormal hepatic function or hepatitis have also been reported.

Other adverse events reported for candesartan cilexetil where a causal relationship could not be established include very rare cases of leukopenia, neutropenia and agranulocytosis.

Cases of muscle pain, muscle weakness, myositis and rhabdomyolysis have been reported in patients receiving angiotensin II receptor blockers.

Hydrochlorothiazide: Potentially serious clinical adverse events have been reported to occur with hydrochlorothiazide, such as: jaundice (intrahepatic cholestatic jaundice), pancreatitis, leukopenia, neutropenia/agranulocytosis, thrombocytopenia, aplastic anemia, haemolytic anemia, photosensitivity reactions, necrotising angitis (vasculitis), toxic epidermal necrolysis, anaphylactic reactions, respiratory distress (including pneumonitis and pulmonary edema), hypokalemia, renal dysfunction and interstitial nephritis.

DRUG INTERACTIONS: Overview: Warfarin: When candesartan cilexetil was administered at 16 mg once daily under steady state conditions, no pharmacodynamic effect on prothrombin time was demonstrated in subjects stabilized on warfarin.

Digoxin: Combination treatment with candesartan cilexetil and digoxin in healthy volunteers had no effect on AUC or C_{max} values for digoxin compared to digoxin alone. Similarly, combination treatment had no effect on AUC or C_{max} values for candesartan compared to candesartan cilexetil alone.

Thiazide-induced electrolyte disturbances may predispose to digitalis-induced arrhythmias.

d-Tubocurarine: Thiazide drugs may increase the responsiveness to tubocurarine.

Insulin: Insulin requirements in diabetic patients treated with diuretics may be increased, decreased or unchanged. Diabetes mellitus which has been latent may become manifest during thiazide administration.

Alcohol, Barbiturates or Narcotics: Thiazide diuretic potentiation of orthostatic hypotension may occur.

Corticosteroids, ACTH: Intensified electrolyte depletion, particularly hypokalemia, may occur when given concomitantly with thiazide diuretics.

Pressor Amines (e.g., norepinephrine): In the presence of thiazide diuretics possible decreased response to pressor amines may be seen but not sufficient to preclude their use.

Other: No significant drug interactions have been reported with glyburide, nifedipine or oral contraceptives co-administered with candesartan cilexetil to healthy volunteers. Co-administration of thiazide diuretics may increase the incidence of hypersensitivity reactions to allopurinol, may increase the risk of adverse effects caused by amantadine, may enhance the hyperglycemic effect of diazoxide, and may reduce the renal excretion of cytotoxic drugs (e.g. cyclophosphamide, methotrexate) and potentiate their myelosuppressive effects.

The bioavailability of thiazide diuretics may be increased by anticholinergic agents (e.g. atropine, biperiden), apparently due to a decrease in gastrointestinal motility and the stomach emptying rate.

There have been reports in the literature of hemolytic anemia occurring with concomitant use of hydrochlorothiazide and methyldopa.

Absorption of thiazide diuretics is decreased by cholestyramine.

Administration of thiazide diuretics with vitamin D or with calcium salts may potentiate the rise in serum calcium.

Concomitant treatment with cyclosporin may increase the risk of hyperuricemia and gout type complications.

Drug-Drug Interactions: The drugs listed in Table 3 are based on either drug interaction case reports or studies or potential interactions due to the expected magnitude and seriousness of the interaction (i.e. those identified as contraindicated).

Table 3: ATACAND PLUS

Established or Potential Drug-Drug Interactions

Candesartan cilexetil	Effect	Clinical Comment
Diuretics	Patients on diuretics, and especially those in whom diuretic therapy was recently instituted, may occasionally experience an excessive reduction of blood pressure after initiation of therapy with candesartan cilexetil.	The possibility of symptomatic hypotension with the use of ATACAND (candesartan cilexetil) can be minimized by discontinuing the diuretic prior to initiation of treatment and/or lowering the initial dose of candesartan cilexetil (see Warnings and Precautions, Cardiovascular, Hypotension and Dosage and Administration). No drug interaction of clinical significance has been identified with thiazide diuretics.
Agents Increasing Serum Potassium	ATACAND decreases the production of aldosterone.	Potassium-sparing diuretics or potassium supplements should be given only for documented hypokalemia and with frequent monitoring of serum potassium. Potassium-containing salt substitutes should also be used with caution. Concomitant thiazide diuretic use may attenuate any effect that candesartan cilexetil may have on serum potassium.
Lithium Salts	As with other drugs which eliminate sodium, lithium clearance may be reduced. Lithium generally should not be given with diuretics. Diuretic agents reduce the renal clearance of lithium and add a high risk of lithium toxicity.	Serum lithium levels should be monitored carefully if lithium salts are to be administered.
NSAIDS	In some patients, the administration of a nonsteroidal anti-inflammatory agent/drug (NSAID) can reduce the diuretic, natriuretic, and antihypertensive effects of loop, potassium-sparing and thiazide diuretics.	When ATACAND PLUS (candesartan cilexetil/hydrochlorothiazide) and NSAIDs are used concomitantly, the patient should be observed closely to determine if the desired effect of the diuretic is obtained.

Drug-Food Interactions: ATACAND PLUS may be taken with or without food (see Dosage and Administration).

DOSAGE AND ADMINISTRATION:

Dosing Considerations: The dosage of ATACAND PLUS (candesartan cilexetil/hydrochlorothiazide) must be individualized. The fixed combination is not for initial therapy. The dose of ATACAND PLUS should be determined by titration of the individual components.

Recommended Dose and Dosage Adjustment: Once the patient has been stabilized on the individual components, one ATACAND PLUS 16 mg/12.5 mg, 32 mg/12.5 mg or 32 mg/25 mg tablet once daily may be taken if the doses on which the patient was stabilized are the same as those in the fixed combination (see Indications and Clinical Use).

Initiation of therapy requires consideration of recent antihypertensive treatment, the extent of blood pressure elevation, salt restriction, and other pertinent clinical factors.

ATACAND PLUS should be taken once daily, at approximately the same time each day, with or without food.

Candesartan Cilexetil Monotherapy: The recommended initial dose of candesartan cilexetil is 16 mg, once daily. Total daily doses of candesartan cilexetil should range from 8 to 32 mg. Doses higher than 32 mg do not appear to have a greater effect on blood pressure reduction, and there is relatively little experience with such doses. Most of the antihypertensive effect is present within 2 weeks and the maximal blood pressure reduction is generally obtained within 4 weeks. For patients with possible depletion of intravascular volume (e.g. patients treated with diuretics, particularly those with impaired renal function) consideration should be given to administration of a lower dose. If blood pressure is not controlled by ATACAND alone, a thiazide diuretic may be added (see Drug Interactions, Drug-Drug Interaction, Table 3: Diuretics).

Concomitant Diuretic Therapy: In patients receiving diuretics, candesartan cilexetil therapy should be initiated with caution, since these patients may be volume-depleted and thus more likely to experience hypotension following initiation of additional antihypertensive therapy.

Whenever possible, all diuretics should be discontinued two to three days prior to the administration of candesartan cilexetil, to reduce the likelihood of hypotension (see Warnings and Precautions, Cardiovascular, Hypotension). If this is not possible because of the patient's condition, candesartan cilexetil should be administered with caution and the blood pressure monitored closely. Thereafter, the dosage should be adjusted according to the individual response of the patient.

Dosing Considerations in Special Populations: Hepatic Impairment: No dosage adjustment of ATACAND PLUS is necessary in patients with mild to moderate chronic liver disease.

Since dosage adjustment of candesartan cilexetil is necessary in patients with severely impaired hepatic function and/or cholestasis, and thiazide diuretics may precipitate hepatic coma, use of ATACAND PLUS is not recommended in these patients (see Warnings and Precautions, Hepatic Impairment).

Renal Impairment: No dosage adjustment of candesartan cilexetil is necessary in patients with mildly impaired renal function.

In patients with moderately or severely impaired renal function, or in patients undergoing dialysis, a lower initial dose of 4 mg should be considered.

The usual regimens of therapy with ATACAND PLUS may be followed as long as the patient's creatinine clearance is >30 mL/min/1.73 m² BSA. In patients with more severe renal impairment, loop diuretics are preferred to thiazides, so ATACAND PLUS is not recommended.

Geriatrics (>65 years of age): No dose adjustment of ATACAND PLUS is necessary for elderly patients. As greater sensitivity of some older patients cannot be ruled out, appropriate caution is recommended (see Warnings and Precautions, Geriatrics (>65 years of age)).

Pediatrics (<18 years of age): The safety and efficacy of ATACAND PLUS have not been established in children.

Missed Dose: If a patient misses a dose of ATACAND PLUS and remembers within 12 hours, the patient should take the dose as soon as possible and then go back to the regular schedule. If it is more than 12 hours after the patient remembers, they should not take the missed dose; the next dose should be taken on time.

A double dose of ATACAND PLUS should never be taken to make up for a missed dose.

OVERDOSAGE:

No specific information is available on the treatment of overdosage with ATACAND PLUS (candesartan cilexetil/hydrochlorothiazide). Treatment is symptomatic and supportive.

Candesartan Cilexetil: Limited data are available in regard to overdosage of candesartan cilexetil in humans. The most likely manifestations of overdosage would be hypotension, dizziness and tachycardia; bradycardia could occur from reflex parasympathetic (vagal) stimulation. If symptomatic hypotension should occur, supportive treatment should be instituted and vital signs monitored. The patient should be placed supine with the legs elevated. If this is not sufficient, plasma volume should be increased by infusion of, for example, isotonic saline solution. Sympathomimetic drugs may also be administered if the above-mentioned measures are not sufficient. In case reports detailing overdosage (up to 672 mg candesartan cilexetil) patient recovery was uneventful.

Candesartan cilexetil is not removed from the plasma by hemodialysis.

Hydrochlorothiazide: The most common symptoms observed from overdosage of hydrochlorothiazide are those caused by electrolyte depletion (hypokalemia, hypochloremia, hyponatremia) and dehydration resulting from excessive diuresis. If digitalis has also been administered, hypokalemia may accentuate cardiac arrhythmias. The degree to which hydrochlorothiazide is removed by hemodialysis has not been established.

For management of a suspected drug overdose, contact your **regional Poison Control Centre**. See the *CPS* Directory section for a list of Poison Control Centres.

ACTION AND CLINICAL PHARMACOLOGY: Mechanism of Action: ATACAND PLUS (candesartan cilexetil/hydrochlorothiazide) combines the actions of candesartan cilexetil, an angiotensin II AT_1 receptor blocker, and that of a thiazide diuretic, hydrochlorothiazide.

Candesartan Cilexetil: Candesartan cilexetil antagonizes the action of angiotensin II by blocking the angiotensin type one (AT_1) receptor. Angiotensin II is the primary vasoactive hormone of the renin-angiotensin-aldosterone system with effects that include vasoconstriction, stimulation of aldosterone secretion, and renal reabsorption of sodium.

Candesartan cilexetil, a prodrug, is rapidly converted to the active drug, candesartan, during absorption from the gastrointestinal tract.

Candesartan blocks the vasoconstrictor and aldosterone secreting effects of angiotensin II by selectively blocking the binding of angiotensin II to the AT_1 receptor in many tissues, such as vascular smooth muscle and the adrenal gland. Its action is therefore independent of the pathways for angiotensin II synthesis. There are also AT_2 receptors found in many tissues, but they play no known role in cardiovascular homeostasis to date. Candesartan has a much greater affinity (>10 000-fold) for the AT_1 receptor than for the AT_2 receptor. The strong bond between candesartan and the AT_1 receptor is a result of tight binding to and slow dissociation from the receptor.

Candesartan does not inhibit angiotensin converting enzyme (ACE), also known as kininase II, the enzyme that converts angiotensin I to angiotensin II and degrades bradykinin, nor does it bind to or block other hormone receptors or ion channels known to be important in cardiovascular regulation.

Hydrochlorothiazide: Hydrochlorothiazide is a diuretic and antihypertensive which interferes with the renal tubular mechanism of electrolyte reabsorption. It inhibits the active reabsorption of sodium, mainly in the distal kidney tubules, and promotes the excretion of sodium, chloride and water. The renal excretion of potassium and magnesium increases dose-dependently, while calcium is reabsorbed to a greater extent. While this compound is predominantly a saluretic agent, in vitro studies have shown that it has a carbonic anhydrase inhibitory action which seems to be relatively specific for the renal tubular mechanism. It does not appear to be concentrated in erythrocytes or the brain in sufficient amounts to influence the activity of carbonic anhydrase in those tissues.

Hydrochlorothiazide is useful in the treatment of hypertension. It may be used alone or as an adjunct to other antihypertensive drugs. Hydrochlorothiazide does not affect normal blood pressure.

Pharmacodynamics: Candesartan cilexetil: Candesartan inhibits the pressor effects of angiotensin II infusion in a dose-dependent manner. After 1 week of once-daily dosing of 8 mg candesartan cilexetil, the pressor effect was inhibited by approximately 90% at peak (4-8 hours after dosing) with approximately 50% inhibition persisting at 24 hours. Plasma concentrations of angiotensin I, angiotensin II, and plasma renin activity, increased in a dose-dependent manner after single and repeated administration of candesartan cilexetil to healthy subjects and hypertensive patients. A decrease in the plasma concentration of aldosterone was observed when 32 mg of candesartan cilexetil was administered to hypertensive patients.

Hydrochlorothiazide: Onset of the diuretic action following oral administration occurs in 2 hours and the peak action in about 4 hours. Diuretic activity lasts about 6 to 12 hours.

Pharmacokinetics: Concomitant administration of candesartan cilexetil and hydrochlorothiazide has no clinically significant effect on the pharmacokinetics of either medicinal product.

Candesartan Cilexetil: Absorption: Following oral administration of candesartan cilexetil as a tablet, the absolute bioavailability of candesartan was estimated to be approximately 15%. After tablet ingestion, the peak serum concentration (C_{max}) is reached after 3-4 hours. Food does not affect the bioavailability of candesartan after candesartan cilexetil administration.

Distribution: The volume of distribution of candesartan is 0.13 L/kg. Candesartan is highly bound to plasma proteins (>99%) and does not penetrate red blood cells. The protein binding is constant at candesartan plasma concentrations well above the range achieved with recommended doses. In rats, it has been demonstrated that candesartan does cross the blood-brain barrier. It has also been demonstrated in rats that candesartan passes across the placental barrier and is distributed in the fetus.

Metabolism: Candesartan cilexetil is rapidly and completely bioactivated by ester hydrolysis during absorption from the gastrointestinal tract to candesartan. It undergoes minor hepatic metabolism by O-deethylation to an inactive metabolite. In vitro studies indicate that cytochrome P450 isoenzyme CYP 2C9 is involved in the biotransformation of candesartan to its inactive metabolite. Based on in vitro data, no interaction would be expected to occur in vivo with drugs whose metabolism is dependent upon cytochrome P450 isoenzymes CYP1A2, CYP2A6, CYP2C9, CYP2C19, CYP2D6, CYP2E1 or CYP3A4.

Excretion: Total plasma clearance of candesartan is 0.37 mL/min/kg, with a renal clearance of 0.19 mL/min/kg. Candesartan is mainly excreted unchanged in urine and feces (via bile). When candesartan cilexetil is administered orally, about 26% of the dose is excreted as candesartan in urine. Following an oral dose of ^{14}C-labeled candesartan cilexetil, approximately 33% of radioactivity is recovered in urine and approximately 67% in feces. Following an intravenous dose of ^{14}C-labeled candesartan, approximately 59% of radioactivity is recovered in urine and approximately 36% in feces. Biliary excretion contributes to the elimination of candesartan. The elimination half-life of candesartan is approximately 9 hours. After single and repeated administration, the pharmacokinetics of candesartan are linear, for oral doses up to 32 mg. Candesartan and its inactive metabolite do not accumulate in serum upon repeated once-daily dosing.

Hydrochlorothiazide: Absorption: hydrochlorothiazide is rapidly absorbed from the gastrointestinal tract with an absolute bioavailability of approximately 70%. Concomitant food intake increases the absorption by approximately 15%.

Distribution: The bioavailability may decrease in patients with cardiac failure and pronounced edema. The plasma protein binding of hydrochlorothiazide is approximately 60%. The apparent volume of distribution is approximately 0.8 L/kg.

Excretion: Hydrochlorothiazide is not metabolized and is excreted almost entirely as unchanged drug by glomerular filtration and active tubular secretion. The terminal $t_{½}$ of hydrochlorothiazide is approximately 8 hours. Approximately 70% of an oral dose is eliminated in the urine within 48 hours. The half-life of hydrochlorothiazide remains unchanged (8 hours) after administration of hydrochlorothiazide in combination with candesartan cilexetil. No accumulation of hydrochlorothiazide occurs after repeated doses of the combination compared to monotherapy.

The terminal $t_{½}$ of hydrochlorothiazide is prolonged in the elderly and in patients with renal failure or chronic heart failure.

Hydrochlorothiazide crosses the placental but not the blood-brain barrier and is excreted in breast milk.

Special Populations and Conditions: Geriatrics: The plasma concentration of candesartan was higher in the elderly (≥65 years) (C_{max} was approximately 50% higher, and AUC was approximately 80% higher) compared to younger subjects administered the same dose. The pharmacokinetics of candesartan were linear in the elderly, and candesartan and its inactive metabolite did not accumulate in the serum of these subjects upon repeated, once-daily administration.

Gender: No gender-related differences in the pharmacokinetics of candesartan have been observed.

Hepatic Insufficiency: In patients with mild to moderate hepatic impairment, there was an increase in the AUC of candesartan of approximately 20%. There was no drug accumulation in plasma in these patients. In patients with moderate to severe hepatic impairment, the C_{max} and AUC increased up to five times in a very small group administered a single dose of 16 mg candesartan (see Dosage and Administration, Hepatic Impairment).

Renal Insufficiency: In patients with mild to moderate renal impairment (Cl_{creat} 31-60 mL/min/1.73 m²), C_{max} and AUC of candesartan increased by 40-60% and 50-90%, respectively, but $t_{½}$ was not altered, compared to patients with normal renal function (Cl_{creat} >60 mL/min/1.73 m²) during repeated dosing. There was no drug accumulation in plasma in patients with mild to moderate renal impairment. The increases in C_{max} and AUC in patients with severe renal impairment (Cl_{creat} 15-30 mL/min/1.73 m²) were 40-60% and 110%, respectively. The terminal $t_{½}$ of candesartan was approximately doubled in patients with severe renal impairment, and these changes resulted in some accumulation in plasma. The pharmacokinetics of candesartan in patients undergoing hemodialysis were similar to those in patients with severe renal impairment (see Dosage and Administration, Renal Impairment).

STORAGE AND STABILITY: Store at 15-30°C.

INFORMATION FOR THE PATIENT: Published in e-CPS, available by subscription at www.e-cps.ca.

DOSAGE FORMS, COMPOSITION AND PACKAGING: 16 mg/12.5 mg: Each oval, biconvex, peach tablet, with a score and marked ĉs on one side, contains: candesartan cilexetil 16 mg and hydrochlorothiazide 12.5 mg. Nonmedicinal ingredients: calcium carboxymethylcellulose, hydroxypropyl cellulose, iron oxide, lactose, magnesium stearate, maize starch and polyethylene glycol. Blister packs of 30.

32 mg/12.5 mg: Each oval, biconvex, yellow tablet, with a score and marked ĉs on one side, contains: candesartan cilexetil 32 mg and hydrochlorothiazide 12.5 mg. Nonmedicinal ingredients: calcium carboxymethylcellulose, hydroxypropyl cellulose, iron oxide, lactose, magnesium stearate, maize starch and polyethylene glycol. Blister packs of 30.

32 mg/25 mg: Each oval, biconvex, pink tablet, with a score and marked ĉs on one side, contains: candesartan cilexetil 32 mg and hydrochlorothiazide 25 mg. Nonmedicinal ingredients: calcium carboxymethylcellulose, hydroxypropyl cellulose, iron oxide, lactose, magnesium stearate, maize starch and polyethylene glycol. Blister packs of 30.

(Shown in Product Identification Section)

Atasol®-8, -15, -30 Ⓝ

acetaminophen—codeine phosphate—caffeine citrate

Analgesic—Antipyretic

Church & Dwight

INDICATIONS: The relief of mild to moderate pain of various causes as in headache, migraine, dental pain, dysmenorrhea, myalgias and neuralgias. As an antipyretic when fever accompanies painful conditions.

CONTRAINDICATIONS: Acetaminophen and/or codeine hypersensitivity.

WARNINGS: No data supplied by the manufacturer.

PRECAUTIONS: See Atasol Preparations.

ADVERSE EFFECTS: Codeine: Adverse reactions due to codeine phosphate may include drowsiness, nausea, vomiting and constipation. Infrequent adverse effects include palpitation, pruritus and, rarely, hyperhidrosis and agitation have been reported. Respiratory depression is seen in higher dosage and the potential for habituation may occur.

For acetaminophen see Atasol Preparations.

OVERDOSE:

Symptoms: See Atasol Preparations. Codeine overdosage is manifested by marked respiratory depression, significant miosis (pinpoint pupils), sweating, itching, lightheadedness, headache, nausea, vomiting, insensibility to pain. In severe cases: deep coma and significant CNS depression. Death is usually produced by respiratory failure.

Treatment: See Atasol Preparations.

Codeine: Gastric lavage, intubation measures aimed at supporting respiration and the administration of a narcotic antagonist, e.g., naloxone.

For management of a suspected drug overdose, CPhA recommends that you contact your **regional Poison Control Centre**. See the *CPS* Directory section for a list of Poison Control Centres.

DOSAGE: Atasol-8: Adults: 1 to 2 tablets every 4 hours (maximum: 2 tablets 6 times daily). Children: 12 to 14 years: only when recommended by a physician or dentist: 1 tablet 3 times daily (maximum: 1 tablet 4 times daily).

Atasol-15 and Atasol-30: Adults: 2 to 4 tablets daily or as prescribed by a physician or dentist.

SUPPLIED: Atasol-8: Each light peach, round, biconvex tablet bisected on one side, imprinted ATASOL on one section, and 8 on the other, plain on other side, contains: acetaminophen 325 mg, codeine phosphate 8 mg, caffeine citrate 30 mg (equivalent to 15 mg caffeine). Nonmedicinal ingredients: alumina, cellulose, D&C Yellow No. 10, FD&C Yellow 6, magnesium stearate, silicon dioxide and starch (corn). Energy: 0.4 kJ (0.1 kcal). Gluten- and tartrazine-free. Bottles of 30 and 100.

Atasol-15: Each light yellow, round, biconvex tablet bisected on one side, imprinted ATASOL on one section, and 15 on the other, plain on the other side, contains: acetaminophen 325 mg, codeine phosphate 15 mg, caffeine citrate 30 mg (equivalent to 15 mg caffeine). Nonmedicinal ingredients: alumina, cellulose, D&C Yellow No. 10, FD&C Yellow No. 6, magnesium stearate, silicon dioxide and starch (corn). Energy: 0.4 kJ (0.1 kcal). Gluten- and tartrazine-free. Bottles of 100. Hospital Control Packs of 800.

Atasol-30: Each pale green, round, biconvex tablet bisected on one side, imprinted ATASOL on one section, and 30 on the other section, plain on the other side, contains: acetaminophen 325 mg, codeine phosphate 30 mg, caffeine citrate 30 mg (equivalent to 15 mg caffeine). Nonmedicinal ingredients: alumina, cellulose, FD&C Blue No. 1, FD&C Yellow No. 5, magnesium stearate, silicon dioxide and starch (corn). Energy: 0.4 kJ (0.1 kcal). Also contains tartrazine. Gluten-free. Bottles of 100 and 500. Hospital Control Packs of 800.

(Shown in Product Identification Section)

Atasol® Preparations

acetaminophen

Analgesic—Antipyretic

Church & Dwight

INDICATIONS: As an analgesic for the relief of pain in headache, dysmenorrhea, myalgias and neuralgias; arthritis, sprains, toothache, and fever caused by cold or flu. As an antipyretic when fever accompanies painful conditions.

CONTRAINDICATIONS: Acetaminophen hypersensitivity.

WARNINGS: No data supplied by the manufacturer.

PRECAUTIONS: The incidence of gastrointestinal upset is less than after salicylate administration. If a rare sensitivity reaction occurs, discontinue the drug. Hypersensitivity to acetaminophen is usually manifested by a rash or urticaria.

Regular use of acetaminophen has been shown to produce a slight increase in prothrombin time in patients receiving oral anticoagulants. Chronic, high-dose administration of acetaminophen may potentiate the anticoagulant effect of warfarin. Patients stabilized on oral anticoagulants should be advised to limit their intake of acetaminophen to not more than 2 g daily for no more than a few days at a time.

Acetaminophen poisoning can result in severe hepatic damage. Phenobarbital increases the activity of microsomal enzymes which produce a toxic metabolite and therefore acetaminophen's hepatotoxicity may be enhanced. Thus, concomitant ingestion of phenobarbital may increase the likelihood of liver necrosis in acetaminophen overdose. The chronic ingestion of alcohol may be implicated in the increasing potential for hepatic toxicity.

Lactation: Acetaminophen is excreted in human breast milk, but may be used without danger, in therapeutic dosages, for short-term treatment. Peak concentrations in breast milk occur 1 to 2 hours after a dose.

Pregnancy: Acetaminophen crosses the placenta and is apparently safe for short-term use when therapeutic doses are used.

ADVERSE EFFECTS: In therapeutic doses, acetaminophen is relatively nontoxic. Chronic use of large doses of acetaminophen may produce more significant toxicity.

Hepatic: Hepatic toxicity has been associated with acetaminophen in overdose. Chronic use of high doses, e.g., ≥5 g daily for several weeks in adults or 150 mg/kg/day for 2 to 4 days in children, has also been associated with hepatotoxicity. Alcoholics, patients with liver disease, the malnourished and patients taking drugs that induce hepatic microsomal enzymes, may be at increased risk for hepatic toxicity.

Renal: Nephropathy, including papillary renal failure has been reported following consumption of large amounts of acetaminophen. Renal tubular necrosis has been associated occasionally with hepatic injury produced by acetaminophen overdose.

Hematologic: Neutropenia and thrombocytopenia purpura have been reported and rarely agranulocytosis.

Hypersensitivity: Laryngeal edema, angioedema and anaphylactoid reactions may occur rarely.

OVERDOSE:

In adults, hepatotoxicity may occur after ingestion of a single dose of more than 7.5 g (adults) or 150 mg/kg (children) of acetaminophen; a dose of 10 g or more is potentially fatal. However, reports have indicated hepatic necrosis with a single dose of 6 g and death occurring with a single dose of 13 g. Nonfatal overdoses of 12.5 to 31.5 g have also been reported.

Symptoms: Symptoms during the first 2 days of acute poisoning by acetaminophen do not reflect the potential seriousness of the intoxication. Nausea, vomiting, anorexia and abdominal pain occur during the initial 24 hours and may persist for a week or more. Liver injury may become manifest the second day, initially by elevation of serum transaminase and lactic dehydrogenase activity, increased serum bilirubin concentration and prolongation of prothrombin time. Alkaline phosphatase activity and serum albumin concentration may remain normal. The hepatotoxicity may progress to encephalopathy, coma and death. Liver biopsy reveals centrilobular necrosis with sparing of the periportal area. In nonfatal cases, the hepatic lesions are reversible over a period of weeks or months. Transient azotemia is apparent in most patients and acute renal failure occurs in some. Hypoglycemia may occur, but glycosuria and impaired glucose tolerance have also been reported. Both metabolic acidosis and metabolic alkalosis have been noted; cerebral edema and nonspecific myocardial depression have also occurred.

In addition to hepatic damage, clotting defects, and myocardial damage with ST segment abnormalities, T wave flattening and pericarditis have been reported.

Since acetaminophen is metabolized primarily by the liver, in cases of acute poisoning, prolongation of the plasma half-life beyond 3 hours may be indicative of liver injury. Hepatic necrosis should be anticipated if the half-life exceeds 4 hours, and hepatic coma is likely if the half-life is greater than 12 hours. A single determination of serum acetaminophen concentration is a less reliable predictor of hepatic injury. However, only minimal liver damage has developed when the serum concentration was below 120 µg/mL at 4 hours or less than 50 µg/mL at 12 hours after ingestion of the drug. Encephalopathy should also be anticipated if serum bilirubin concentration exceeds 4 mg/100 mL during the first 5 days.

Treatment: Treatment of acute acetaminophen overdosage is symptomatic; vigorous supportive therapy is essential in severe intoxication. Since the hepatic injury is dose dependent and occurs early in the course of intoxication, procedures to limit continuing absorption of the drug must be initiated promptly. Gastric lavage or emesis can be used if the drug has been recently ingested. Persistent vomiting induced by ipecac may interfere with acetylcysteine administration. If activated charcoal has been administered prior to initiation of acetylcysteine therapy, gastric lavage should be performed before the first dose of oral acetylcysteine is given, as charcoal may interfere with acetylcysteine absorption and reduces its effectiveness.

Although appropriate i.v. administration of cysteine or cysteamine may decrease the risk of acetaminophen-induced hepatic necrosis, these drugs are not readily available in Canada at this time. Current evidence suggests that oral N-acetylcysteine may exert a protective effect against hepatic necrosis. Call the nearest Poison Control Centre for the most recent information on treatment.

For management of a suspected drug overdose, CPhA recommends that you contact your **regional Poison Control Centre**. See the *CPS* Directory section for a list of Poison Control Centres.

DOSAGE: Adults: 325 to 650 mg every 4 to 6 hours, not to exceed 4000 mg/24 hours.

Children: 10 to 15 mg/kg every 4 to 6 hours, not to exceed 65 mg/kg/24 hours. Alternatively, see Table 1.

Table 1: Atasol Preparations

Dosage in Children

Age	Single Dose (mg)	Max. Daily Dose (mg)
0 to under 4 months	40	200
4 months to under 1 year	80	400
1 year to under 2	120	600
2 to under 4	160	800
4 to under 6	240	1200
6 to under 9	320	1600
9 to under 11	400	2000
11 to under 12	480	2400

SUPPLIED: Atasol Regular Tablets: Each white, round, biconvex tablet, bisected on one side and imprinted ATASOL on one section and plain on the other side, contains: acetaminophen 325 mg. Nonmedicinal ingredients: cellulose, cornstarch, povidone and stearic acid. Alcohol-, sucrose- and tartrazine-free. Energy: 1.3 kJ (0.3 kcal). Sodium: <1 mmol (0.1 mg). Bottles of 30 and 100.

Atasol Forte Tablets: Each white, shield-shaped tablet, biconvex, diagonally scored on one side, imprinted ATASOL FORTE and plain on the other side, contains: acetaminophen 500 mg (Atasol Forte). Nonmedicinal ingredients: cellulose, cornstarch, povidone and stearic acid. Alcohol-, sucrose- and tartrazine-free. Energy: 1.3 kJ (0.3 kcal). Sodium: <1 mmol (0.1 mg). Bottles of 30, 100 and 120.

Atasol Forte Caplets: Each white, film-coated, biconvex caplet, imprinted ATASOL on one side and FORTE on the other, contains: acetaminophen 500 mg. Nonmedicinal ingredients: alumina, cellulose, cornstarch, FD&C Blue No. 2, magnesium stearate, polyethylene glycol, povidone, stearic acid and titanium dioxide. Alcohol-, sucrose- and tartrazine-free. Bottles of 30 and 100.

Atasol Drops: Each mL of red, fruit-flavored solution contains: acetaminophen 80 mg. Nonmedicinal ingredients: citric acid, dibasic sodium phosphate, FD&C Red No. 2 and No. 40, flavor, glycerin, parabens, polyethylene glycol, sodium cyclamate, sorbitol and sucrose. Alcohol- and tartrazine-free. Energy: 10 kJ (2.4 kcal). Sodium: <1 mmol (0.9 mg). Plastic bottles of 24 mL with graduated dropper.

(Shown in Product Identification Section)

Atgam®

lymphocyte immune globulin—anti-thymocyte globulin (equine)

Immunosuppressant

Pfizer

PHARMACOLOGY: Atgam is the purified, concentrated, and sterile gamma globulin, primarily monomeric IgG, from hyperimmune plasma of horses immunized with human thymus lymphocytes.

Atgam is a lymphocyte-selective immunosuppressant as is demonstrated by its ability to reduce the number of circulating, thymus-dependent lymphocytes that form rosettes with sheep erythrocytes. This antilymphocyte effect is believed to reflect an alteration of the function of the T-lymphocytes, which are responsible in part for cell-mediated immunity and are involved in humoral immunity. In addition to its antilymphocyte activity, Atgam contains low concentrations of antibodies against other formed elements of the blood. In rhesus and cynomolgus monkeys, Atgam reduces lymphocytes in the thymus-dependent areas of the spleen and lymph nodes. It also decreases the circulating sheep-erythrocyte-rosetting lymphocytes that can be detected, but Atgam does not cause severe lymphopenia.

In general, when Atgam is given with other immunosuppressive therapy, such as antimetabolites and corticosteroids, the patient's own antibody response to horse gamma globulin is minimal. In a small clinical study, Atgam administered with other immunosuppressive therapy and measured as horse IgG had a serum half-life of 5.7±3 days.

INDICATIONS: For any patient in whom reduction of peripheral T-lymphocyte function as measured by rosette-forming cell assay could be desirable.

During controlled clinical trials, this immunosuppression has been demonstrated in renal allograft recipients treated with Atgam. When administered with conventional therapy at the time of rejection, it increases the frequency of resolution of the acute rejection episode. The drug has also been administered as an adjunct to other immunosuppresssive therapy to delay the onset of the first rejection episode.

In noncontrolled clinical studies, Atgam has been administered to other patients in whom reduction of T-cell function could be desirable. They had aplastic anemia, T-cell malignancies, or graft-versus-host disease, or had received skin, cardiac, liver, or bone marrow transplants. Anecdotal reports of benefit have been published, but to date controlled studies to establish safety and efficacy in circumstances other than renal transplantation have not been completed.

CONTRAINDICATIONS: Should not be administered to a patient who has had a severe systemic reaction during prior administration of the drug or any other equine gamma globulin preparation.

WARNINGS: Only physicians experienced in immunosuppressive therapy and management of renal transplant patients should use Atgam.

Patients receiving Atgam should be managed in facilities equipped and staffed with adequate laboratory and supportive medical resources.

Treatment with Atgam should be discontinued if any of the following occurs: anaphylaxis (see Adverse Effects); severe and unremitting thrombocytopenia; severe and unremitting leukopenia.

This product is manufactured using components of human blood which may contain the causative agent of hepatitis and other viral diseases. Prescribed manufacturing procedures utilized in blood collection centres and the plasma testing laboratories are designed to reduce the risk of transmitting viral infection. However, the risk of viral infectivity from this product cannot be totally excluded.

PRECAUTIONS: Because Atgam is an immunosuppressive agent ordinarily given with corticosteroids and antimetabolites, patients should be monitored carefully for signs of leukopenia, thrombocytopenia or concurrent infection. If infection occurs, appropriate adjunctive therapy should be instituted promptly. The physician should decide whether or not to continue therapy with Atgam depending on clinical circumstances.

Some studies have suggested an increase in the incidence of cytomegalovirus infection in patients receiving Atgam. Some physicians have found that it may be possible to reduce this by decreasing the dosage of other immunosuppressive agents which might be administered concomitantly with Atgam.

Dilution of Atgam in dextrose infusion solutions is not recommended, as low salt concentration may result in precipitation. The use of highly acidic infusion solutions is also not recommended because of possible physical instability over time.

Drug Interactions: When the dose of corticosteroids and other immunosuppressants is being reduced, some previously masked reactions to Atgam may appear. Under these circumstances, observe patients especially carefully during therapy with Atgam.

Pregnancy: Atgam has not been evaluated in pregnant women.

Lactation: Atgam has not been evaluated in lactating women.

Children: Experience with children has been limited. Atgam has been administered safely to a small number of pediatric renal, liver and bone marrow allograft recipients and aplastic anemia patients at dosage levels comparable to those in adults.

ADVERSE EFFECTS: The primary clinical experience with Atgam has been in renal allograft patients, who were also receiving concurrent standard immunosuppressive therapy (azathioprine, corticosteroids).

In controlled clinical trials, the following adverse reactions have been reported:

Incidence greater than 5%: fever (33%), chills (14%), leukopenia (14%), thrombocytopenia (11%) and dermatological reactions such as rash, pruritus, urticaria, wheal and flare (12.5%).

Incidence of 1 to 5%: arthralgia, chest and/or back pain, clotted A/V fistula, diarrhea, dyspnea, headache, hypotension, nausea and/or vomiting, night sweats, pain at the infusion site, peripheral thrombophlebitis and stomatitis.

The incidence of adverse reactions has been higher in patients being treated for aplastic anemia. Frequently reported adverse reactions among patients enrolled in aplastic anemia studies were arthralgia, chills, fever, skin rashes and thrombocytopenia. The high incidence of skin rashes and arthralgia was believed by investigators to represent serum sickness. In patients with aplastic anemia and other hematologic abnormalities who have received Atgam, abnormal tests of liver function (AST, ALT, alkaline phosphatase) and renal function (serum creatinine) have been observed. In some trials, clinical and laboratory findings of serum sickness have been seen in a majority of patients.

Other reactions reported in renal allograft or aplastic anemia patients receiving therapy have included: back pain, chest pain, clotted A/V fistula, diarrhea, dyspnea, headache, hypotension, nausea, night sweats, pain at the infusion site, peripheral thrombophlebitis, stomatitis and vomiting.

Reactions reported **rarely** have been: agitation, anaphylaxis, dizziness, edema, epigastric pain or hiccups, herpes simplex reactivation, hyperglycemia, hypertension, iliac vein obstruction, infection, laryngospasm, lymphadenopathy, malaise, paresthesia, periorbital edema, pleural effusions, possible encephalitis, proteinuria, pulmonary edema, renal artery thrombosis, seizure, tachycardia, toxic epidermal necrosis, weakness or faintness, and wound dehiscence.

Postmarketing Experience: During approximately 5 years of postapproval marketing experience, the frequency of adverse reactions in voluntarily reported cases is as follows: chills (16%), fever (51%), leukopenia (14%), rashes (27%), systemic infection (13%), thrombocytopenia (30%).

Events reported with a frequency of 5 to 10% include: abnormal renal function tests, arthralgia, chest, back or flank pain, diarrhea, dyspnea/apnea, nausea and/or vomiting and serum sickness-like symptoms.

Events reported with a frequency of <5% include: abnormal involuntary movement or tremor, abnormal liver function tests, abdominal pain, acute renal failure, anaphylaxis, anemia, aplasia or pancytopenia, confusion or disorientation, cough, deep vein thrombosis, dizziness, edema, enlarged or ruptured kidney, eosinophilia, epigastric or stomach pain, faintness, gastrointestinal bleeding or perforation, hemolysis or hemolytic anemia, headache, herpes simplex infection, hyperglycemia, hypertension, hypotension, localized infection, lymphadenopathy, malaise, myalgias or leg pains, neutropenia or granulocytopenia, nosebleed, pain, swelling or redness at infusion site, paresthesias, pulmonary edema or congestive heart failure, renal artery thrombosis, rigidity, seizures, sore mouth-throat, sweating, laryngospasm/edema, tachycardia, thrombophlebitis, vasculitis, and viral hepatitis.

The recommended management for some of the adverse reactions that could occur during treatment with Atgam follows: Anaphylaxis is uncommon but serious and may occur during therapy with Atgam. If this condition does occur, infusion of Atgam should be discontinued immediately; 0.3 mL aqueous epinephrine (1:1 000 dilution) should be administered i.m. along with steroids. Respiration should be assisted and other resuscitative measures provided. Do not resume therapy with Atgam.

Hemolysis can usually be detected only in the laboratory. Fulminant hemolysis has been reported rarely. Appropriate treatment of hemolysis often includes transfusion of erythrocytes; if necessary, administer i.v. mannitol, furosemide, sodium bicarbonate, and fluids. Severe and unremitting hemolysis may necessitate discontinuation of therapy with Atgam.

Thrombocytopenia and leukopenia are usually transient. Platelet and white cell counts generally return to adequate levels without interrupting therapy and without transfusions. If thrombocytopenia and leukopenia become severe, it may be helpful to decrease the dose of concomitant immunosuppressant (particularly azathioprine). If after 1 or 2 days the situation does not improve, the dose of Atgam may also be reduced (see Warnings).

Respiratory distress may indicate an anaphylactoid reaction. Infusion of Atgam should be discontinued. If distress persists, antihistamine, epinephrine, corticosteroid, or some combination of the three should be administered.

Pain in chest, flank or back may indicate anaphylaxis or hemolysis. Treatment is the same as for respiratory distress or, if hemolysis has occurred, the same as listed for hemolysis.

Hypotension may indicate anaphylaxis. Infusion of Atgam should be discontinued and blood pressure stabilized with pressor agents if necessary.

Chills and fever occur frequently in patients receiving Atgam. Atgam may release endogenous leukocyte pyrogens. Prophylactic and/or therapeutic administration of antihistamines or corticosteroids generally controls this reaction.

Chemical phlebitis can be caused by infusion of Atgam through peripheral veins. This often can be avoided by administering the infusion solution into a high-flow vein. A s.c. arterialized vein produced by a Brescia fistula is also a useful administration site.

Itching and erythema probably result from the effect of Atgam on blood elements. Antihistamines generally control the symptoms.

Serum sickness-like symptoms in aplastic anemia patients that have been treated with oral and i.v. corticosteroids. Resolution of symptoms has generally been prompt and long-term sequelae have not been observed. Prophylactic administration of corticosteroids may decrease the frequency of this reaction.

OVERDOSE:

Symptoms: Because of its mode of action and because it is a biologic substance, the maximum tolerated dose of Atgam would be expected to vary from patient to patient. To date, the largest single daily dose administered to a patient (renal transplant recipient) was 7 000 mg administered at a concentration of approximately 10 mg/mL of saline, 7 times the recommended total dose and infusion concentration. In this patient, the administration of Atgam was not associated with any signs of acute intoxication or late sequelae.

The greatest number of doses (10 to 20 mg/kg/dose) that can be administered to a single patient has not yet been determined. Some renal transplant patients have received up to 50 doses in 4 months, and others have received 28 day courses of 21 doses followed by as many as 3 more courses for the treatment of acute rejection. The incidence of toxicologic manifestations did not increase with any of these regimens.

For management of a suspected drug overdose, CPhA recommends that you contact your **regional Poison Control Centre**. See the *CPS* Directory section for a list of Poison Control Centres.

DOSAGE: Renal-Allograft Recipients: Adult renal allograft patients have received Atgam at the dose of 10 to 30 mg/kg of body weight daily. The few children studied received 5 to 25 mg/kg daily. Atgam has been used to delay the onset of the first rejection episode and at the time of the first rejection episode. Most patients who received Atgam for the treatment of acute rejection had not received it starting at the time of transplantation.

Usually, Atgam is used concomitantly with azathioprine and corticosteroids, which are commonly used to suppress the immune response. Exercise caution during repeat courses of Atgam; carefully observe patients for signs of allergic reactions.

Delaying the Onset of Allograft Rejection: The recommended dose is 15 mg/kg daily for 14 days, then every other day for 14 days for a total of 21 doses in 28 days. The first dose should be administered within 24 hours before or after the transplant.

Treatment of Rejection: The first Atgam dose can be delayed until the diagnosis of the first rejection episode. The recommended dose is 10 to 15 mg/kg daily for 14 days. Additional alternate-day therapy up to a total of 21 doses can be given.

Other Allograft Recipients: Atgam has been used in liver transplant recipients at daily doses of 8 to 15 mg/kg. The duration of therapy averaged 13 days. In heart transplant patients, intermittent daily doses averaged 8 mg/kg (range: 5 to 11 mg/kg), duration of therapy averaged 4 months, and the number of doses averaged 29 (range: 7 to 49). In burn patients who had received temporary skin allografts, Atgam dosage ranged from 10 to 15 mg/kg for up to 24 doses. All patients received the first Atgam dose in the 24 hour period immediately before or after the surgical procedure.

Bone Marrow Transplantation: Several different Atgam dosage regimens have been used in patients receiving bone marrow transplants. Generally patients received Atgam 7 to 20 mg/kg for 3 to 14 doses. The first dose was given 9 days before transplant for pre-conditioning, 7 to 30 days after transplant for prophylaxis of graft-versus-host disease or when graft-versus-host disease was diagnosed.

Aplastic Anemia: Patients with aplastic anemia have received Atgam in several regimens, generally 10 to 20 mg/kg for 8 to 21 doses.

Other Indications: Atgam has also been used in patients with Sezary syndrome, T-cell leukemia, and nephrotic syndrome. Although some patients have received multiple high doses intermittently over long periods, a standard dosage regimen has not been established.

Preparation and Administration: Skin Testing: Before the first i.v. infusion of Atgam, it is **strongly** recommended that skin testing potential recipients take place before commencing treatment. First the patient should receive an epicutaneous (prick) testing with undiluted Atgam. If a wheal does not develop 10 minutes after pricking, then proceed to intradermal testing with 0.02 mL of a 1:1000 v/v saline dilution of Atgam with a separate saline control injection of similar volume. After 10 minutes read the results. A wheal at the Atgam site of 3 mm or larger in diameter compared to the saline control site suggests clinical sensitivity and an increased possibility of a systemic allergic reaction. Where an Atgam skin test causes a locally positive reaction, serious consideration should be given to alternative forms of therapy. The risk to benefit ratio must be carefully weighed. If therapy with Atgam is deemed appropriate following a locally positive skin test, treatment should be administered in a setting where intensive life support facilities are immediately available and a physician familar with the treatment of potentially life-threatening allergic reactions is in attendance.

A systemic reaction such as generalized rash, tachycardia, dyspnea, hypotension, or anaphylaxis precludes additional administration of Atgam.

Note: The predictive value of this test has not been clinically proven. Allergic reactions to Atgam can occur in the presence of a negative skin test. Also, skin testing will not predict for later development of serum sickness (see Warnings, Precautions and Adverse Effects).

Infusion Instruction: Parenteral drug products should be inspected visually for particulate matter and discoloration prior to administration whenever solution and container permit. Because Atgam is a gamma globulin product, it can be transparent to slightly opalescent, colorless to faintly pink or brown, and may develop a slight granular or flaky deposit during storage. Atgam (diluted or undiluted) should not be shaken because excessive foaming and/or denaturation of the protein may occur.

Atgam should be diluted for i.v. infusion in an inverted bottle of sterile vehicle, so that the undiluted Atgam does not contact the air inside. Add the total daily dose of Atgam to the sterile vehicle, with a concentration not exceeding 4 mg of Atgam Sterile Solution per mL. The diluted solution should be gently rotated or swirled to effect complete mixing. Once diluted, Atgam has been shown to be physically and chemically stable for up to 24 hours at concentrations of up to 4 mg/mL in the following diluents: 0.9% Sodium Chloride Injection, 5% Dextrose and 0.225% Sodium Chloride Injection, 5% Dextrose and 0.45% Sodium Chloride Injection.

Adding Atgam to dextrose injection is not recommended, as low salt concentrations can cause precipitation. Highly acidic infusion solutions can also contribute to physical instability over time.

Atgam should not be kept in a diluted form for more than 24 hours (including actual infusion time). It is recommended that diluted Atgam be stored in a refrigerator if it is prepared prior to time of infusion. The diluted Atgam solution should be allowed to reach room temperature before infusion.

During the clinical trials, most investigators chose to infuse Atgam into a vascular shunt, arterial venous fistula, or a high-flow central vein through an in-line filter with a pore size of 0.2 to 1.0 micron. The in-line filter should be used with all i.v. infusions to prevent the inadvertent administration of any insoluble material that may develop in the product during storage.

Using high-flow veins will minimize the occurrence of phlebitis and thrombosis.

Do not infuse a dose of Atgam in less than 4 hours.

Always keep a tray containing epinephrine, antihistamines, corticosteroids, syringes, and an airway at the patient's bedside while Atgam is being administered.

Observe the patient continuously for possible allergic reactions throughout the infusion (see Adverse Effects).

SUPPLIED: Each mL contains: horse gamma globulin 50 mg stabilized in 0.3 molar glycine to a pH of approximately 6.8. Cartons of 5 ampuls of 5 mL. Store in refrigerator at 2 to 8°C. **Do not freeze.** Protect from light; store ampuls in carton.

Ativan®

lorazepam

Anxiolytic—Sedative

Pfizer

SUPPLIED: Oral Tablets: 0.5 mg: Each white, round, flat tablet, engraved with W on one side and 0.5 on the other side, contains: lorazepam 0.5 mg. Nonmedicinal ingredients: lactose, magnesium stearate, microcrystalline cellulose and polacrilin potassium. Energy: 0.84 kJ (0.20 kcal). Gluten- and tartrazine-free. Bottles of 100 and 500. Store at controlled room temperature (15 to 30°C).

1 mg: Each white, scored, oblong tablet, engraved with Ativan on one side and 1 on the other side, contains: lorazepam 1 mg. Nonmedicinal ingredients: lactose, magnesium stearate, microcrystalline cellulose and polacrilin potassium. Energy: 1.63 kJ (0.39 kcal). Gluten- and tartrazine-free. Bottles 100 and 1000. Store at controlled room temperature (15 to 30°C).

2 mg: Each white, scored, ovoid tablet, engraved with Ativan on one side and 2 on the other side, contains: lorazepam 2 mg. Nonmedicinal ingredients: lactose, magnesium stearate, microcrystalline cellulose and polacrilin potassium. Energy: 2.05 kJ (0.49 kcal). Gluten- and tartrazine-free. Bottles of 100 and 1000. Store at controlled room temperature (15 to 30°C).
Sublingual Tablets: 0.5 mg: Each pale green, round, flat tablet, engraved with W on one side and 0.5 on the other side contains: lorazepam 0.5 mg. Nonmedicinal ingredients: cornstarch, dye D&C Yellow 10 Aluminum Lake, dye FD&C Blue 1 Aluminum Lake, dye FD&C Yellow 6 Aluminum Lake, lactose, magnesium stearate and microcrystalline cellulose. Energy: 0.59 kJ (0.14 kcal). Gluten- and tartrazine-free. Bottles of 100. Protect from light. Store at controlled room temperature (15 to 30°C).
1 mg: Each white, round, flat tablet, engraved with W on one side and 1 on the other side, contains: lorazepam 1 mg. Nonmedicinal ingredients: cornstarch, lactose, magnesium stearate and microcrystalline cellulose. Energy: 0.59 kJ (0.14 kcal). Gluten- and tartrazine-free. Bottles of 100. Store at controlled room temperature (15 to 30°C).
2 mg: Each blue, round, flat tablet, engraved with W on one side and 2 on the other side, contains: lorazepam 2 mg. Nonmedicinal ingredients: cornstarch, dye FD&C Blue 2 Aluminum Lake, lactose, magnesium stearate and microcrystalline cellulose. Energy: 0.80 kJ (0.19 kcal). Gluten- and tartrazine-free. Bottles of 100. Protect from light. Store at controlled room temperature (15 to 30°C).

(Shown in Product Identification Section)

Atorvastatin Ⓟ

CPhA Monograph

see *HMG-CoA Reductase Inhibitors*

Atracurium Besylate Injection Ⓟ

atracurium besylate

Skeletal Neuromuscular Blocking Agent

Sandoz

SUPPLIED: Each mL of sterile solution contains: atracurium besylate 10 mg. Nonmedicinal ingredients: benzenesulfonic acid (to adjust pH), benzyl alcohol 0.9% v/v (as preservative) and water for injection. Amber multidose vials of 10 mL, boxes of 10. Refrigerate between 2 and 8°C. Protect from freezing. Protect from light.

Atriance™ Ⓟ

nelarabine

Antineoplastic Agent

GlaxoSmithKline

Date of Revision: March 5, 2009

ATRIANCE (nelarabine), indicated for the treatment of patients with T-cell acute lymphoblastic leukemia and T-cell lymphoblastic lymphoma whose disease has not responded to or has relapsed following treatment with at least two chemotherapy regimens, has been issued marketing authorization with conditions, pending the results of studies to verify its clinical benefit. Patients should be advised of the nature of the authorization.

SUMMARY PRODUCT INFORMATION:

Route of Administration	Dosage Form/ Strength	Clinically Relevant Nonmedicinal Ingredients
Intravenous infusion	Injection 5 mg/mL	Not applicable For a complete listing see Dosage Forms, Composition and Packaging.

INDICATIONS AND CLINICAL USE: ATRIANCE (nelarabine) is indicated for the treatment of patients with T-cell acute lymphoblastic leukemia and T-cell lymphoblastic lymphoma whose disease has not responded to or has relapsed following treatment with at least two chemotherapy regimens.

Approval is based on the unconfirmed surrogate endpoint of clinical response only.

CONTRAINDICATIONS: ATRIANCE (nelarabine) is contraindicated in patients who have a history of hypersensitivity to nelarabine or any other component of ATRIANCE.

WARNINGS AND PRECAUTIONS:

Serious Warnings and Precautions
ATRIANCE (nelarabine) Injection should be administered under the supervision of a physician experienced in the use of cancer chemotherapeutic agents. This product is for intravenous use only.
Severe Neurologic Events: These events included:
- Altered mental states including severe somnolence
- Central nervous system effects including convulsions
- Peripheral neuropathy including numbness, paresthesias, motor weakness, paralysis, craniospinal demyelination, and ascending peripheral neuropathies similar to Guillain-Barré syndrome

Some of these neurologic adverse events are irreversible.
ATRIANCE should be discontinued at the first sign of neurologic events of NCI Common Toxicity Criteria grade 2 or greater.
Close monitoring for neurological events is strongly recommended.

General: Patients receiving ATRIANCE should receive intravenous hydration according to standard medical practice for the management of hyperuricemia in patients at risk for tumour lysis syndrome. Consideration should be given to the use of allopurinol in patients at risk of hyperuricemia (see Dosage and Administration).

Administration of live vaccines to immunocompromised patients should be avoided.
Carcinogenesis and Mutagenesis: Carcinogenicity testing of nelarabine has not been performed. Nelarabine, however, is known to be genotoxic to mammalian cells.
Cardiovascular: The effect of nelarabine on QT interval prolongation has not been investigated.
Hematologic: Leukopenia, thrombocytopenia, anemia, and neutropenia, including febrile neutropenia have been associated with nelarabine therapy. Complete blood counts including platelets should be monitored regularly (see Adverse Reactions and Dosage and Administration).
Neurologic: Neurotoxicity is the dose-limiting toxicity of nelarabine. Patients undergoing therapy with ATRIANCE should be closely observed for signs and symptoms of neurologic toxicity.

Patients treated previously or concurrently with intrathecal chemotherapy or previously with craniospinal irradiation may be at increased risk for neurologic adverse events (see Dosage and Administration). Patients with CNS disease at baseline may have an increased risk of experiencing more severe (grade ≥3) neurological events.

Common signs and symptoms of nelarabine-related neurotoxicity include somnolence, confusion, convulsions, ataxia, paraesthesias and hypoesthesia. Severe neurologic toxicity can manifest as coma, status epilepticus, craniospinal demyelination, or ascending neuropathy similar in presentation to Guillain-Barré syndrome.
Sexual Function/Reproduction: The effects of nelarabine on human fertility have not been investigated.
Special Populations: Pregnant Women: ATRIANCE may cause fetal harm when administered to a pregnant woman. There are no studies of ATRIANCE in pregnant women.

If this drug is used during pregnancy, or if the patient becomes pregnant while taking this drug, the patient should be warned of the potential hazard to the fetus. Women of childbearing potential should be advised to avoid becoming pregnant while receiving treatment with ATRIANCE.
Nursing Women: Nelarabine is a pro-drug of the deoxyguanosine analogue 9-β-D-arabinofuranosylguanine (ara-G) (see Action and Clinical Pharmacology). It is not known whether nelarabine or ara-G is excreted in human milk. Because many drugs are excreted in human milk and because of the potential for serious adverse reactions in nursing infants from ATRIANCE, it is recommended that nursing be discontinued in women who are receiving therapy with ATRIANCE.
Geriatrics: Clinical studies of ATRIANCE did not include sufficient numbers of patients aged 65 and over to determine whether they respond differently than younger patients. In an exploratory analysis, increasing age, especially aged 65 years and older, appeared to be associated with increased rates of neurologic adverse events.
Renally Impaired Patients: Nelarabine has not been studied in individuals with renal impairment. Nelarabine and ara-G are partially renally excreted. Because the risk of adverse reactions to this drug may be greater in patients with decreased renal function (CrCl <50 mL/min), these patients should be closely monitored for toxicities when treated with ATRIANCE (see Dosage and Administration).
Hepatically Impaired Patients: The influence of hepatic impairment on the pharmacokinetics of nelarabine has not been evaluated. Because the risk of adverse reactions to this drug may be greater in patients with severe hepatic impairment, these patients should be closely monitored for toxicities when treated with ATRIANCE.

ADVERSE REACTIONS: Clinical Trial Adverse Drug Reactions: ATRIANCE (nelarabine) was studied in 459 patients in Phase I and Phase II clinical trials. The safety profile for the recommended dosages of ATRIANCE is based on data from 103 adult patients enrolled and treated in the CALGB19801 Study and an adult chronic lymphocytic leukemia study (PGAA2003) who were treated with the recommended dose and schedule. The safety profile for children is based on data from 84 pediatric patients enrolled and treated in the COGP9673 study who were treated with the recommended dose and schedule.

The most common adverse events in pediatric patients, regardless of causality, were hematologic disorders (anemia, leukopenia, neutropenia and thrombocytopenia). Of the non-hematologic adverse events in pediatric patients, the most frequent events reported were headache, increased transaminase levels, decreased blood potassium, decreased blood albumin, increased blood bilirubin and vomiting.

Table 1: ATRIANCE

Most Commonly Reported (≥5% Overall) Adverse Events Regardless of Causality in Pediatric Patients Treated with 650 mg/m² of ATRIANCE Administered Intravenously Over 1 Hour Daily for 5 Consecutive Days Repeated Every 21 Days

	Percentage of Patients: 650 mg/m²; N=84		
		Toxicity Grade	
System Organ Class Preferred Term	**Grade 3 %**	**Grade 4+ %**	**All Grades %**
Blood and Lymphatic System Disorders			
Anemia	45	10	95
Neutropenia	17	62	94
Thrombocytopenia	27	32	88
Leukopenia	14	7	38
Hepatobiliary Disorders			
Transaminases increased	4	0	12
Blood albumin decreased	5	1	10
Blood bilirubin increased	7	2	10
Metabolic/Laboratory			
Blood potassium decreased	4	2	11
Blood calcium decreased	1	1	8
Blood creatinine increased	0	0	6
Blood glucose decreased	4	0	6
Blood magnesium decreased	2	0	6
Nervous System Disorders (see Table 3)			
Gastrointestinal Disorders			
Vomiting	0	0	10
General Disorders and Administration Site Conditions			
Asthenia	1	0	6
Infections & Infestations			
Infection	2	1	5

Grade 4+ = Grade 4 and Grade 5.
Three (3) patients had a fatal event. Fatal events included neutropenia and pyrexia (n=1), status epilepticus/seizure (n=1), and fungal pneumonia (n=1). The status epilepticus was thought to be related to treatment with ATRIANCE. All other fatal events were unrelated to treatment with ATRIANCE.

The most common adverse events in adults, regardless of causality, were fatigue; gastrointestinal (GI) disorders (nausea, diarrhea, vomiting, and constipation); hematologic disorders (anemia, leukopenia, neutropenia and thrombocytopenia); respiratory disorders (cough and dyspnea); nervous system disorders (somnolence and dizziness); and pyrexia.

The most common adverse events by System Organ Class, regardless of causality, including severe or life threatening events (NCI Common Toxicity Criteria grade 3 or grade 4) and fatal events (grade 5) are shown in Table 1 for pediatric patients and Table 2 for adult patients.

Table 2: ATRIANCE

Most Commonly Reported (≥5% Overall) Adverse Events Regardless of Causality in ADULT Patients Treated with 1500 mg/m² of ATRIANCE Administered Intravenously Over 2 Hours on Days 1, 3, and 5 Repeated Every 21 Days

System Organ Class Preferred Term	Percentage of Patients; N=103 Toxicity Grade Grade 3 %	 Grade 4+ %	 All Grades %
Blood and Lymphatic System Disorders			
Anemia	20	14	99
Thrombocytopenia	37	22	86
Neutropenia	14	49	81
Febrile neutropenia	9	1	12
Cardiac Disorders			
Sinus tachycardia	1	0	8
Gastrointestinal Disorders			
Nausea	0	0	41
Diarrhea	1	0	22
Vomiting	1	0	22
Constipation	1	0	21
Abdominal pain	1	0	9
Stomatitis	1	0	8
Abdominal distension	0	0	6
General Disorders and Administration Site Conditions			
Fatigue	10	2	50
Pyrexia	5	0	23
Asthenia	0	1	17
Edema, peripheral	0	0	15
Edema	0	0	11
Pain	3	0	11
Rigors	0	0	8
Gait, abnormal	0	0	6
Chest pain	0	0	5
Non-cardiac chest pain	0	1	5
Infections			
Infection	2	1	9
Pneumonia	4	1	8
Hepatobiliary Disorders			
AST increased	1	1	6
Metabolism and Nutrition Disorders			
Anorexia	0	0	9
Dehydration	3	1	7
Hyperglycemia	1	0	6
Musculoskeletal and Connective Tissue Disorders			
Myalgia	1	0	13
Arthralgia	1	0	9
Back pain	0	0	8
Muscular weakness	5	0	8
Pain in extremity	1	0	7
Nervous System Disorders (see Table 4)			
Psychiatric Disorders			
Confusional state	2	0	8

(cont'd)

Table 2: ATRIANCE *(cont'd)*

Most Commonly Reported (≥5% Overall) Adverse Events Regardless of Causality in ADULT Patients Treated with 1500 mg/m² of ATRIANCE Administered Intravenously Over 2 Hours on Days 1, 3, and 5 Repeated Every 21 Days

System Organ Class Preferred Term	Percentage of Patients; N=103 Toxicity Grade Grade 3 %	 Grade 4+ %	 All Grades %
Insomnia	0	0	7
Depression	1	0	6
Respiratory, Thoracic, and Mediastinal Disorders			
Cough	0	0	25
Dyspnea	4	2	20
Pleural effusion	5	1	10
Epistaxis	0	0	8
Dyspnea, exertional	0	0	7
Wheezing	0	0	5
Vascular Disorders			
Petechiae	2	0	12
Hypotension	1	1	8

Grade 4+=Grade 4 and Grade 5.
Five (5) patients had a fatal event. Fatal events included hypotension (n=1), respiratory arrest (n=1), pleural effusion/pneumothorax (n=1), pneumonia (n=1), and cerebral hemorrhage/coma/ leukoencephalopathy (n=1). The cerebral hemorrhage/coma/leukoencephalopathy was thought to be related to treatment with ATRIANCE. All other fatal events were unrelated to treatment with ATRIANCE.

Other Adverse Events: Blurred vision was also reported in 4% of adult patients. There was a single report of biopsy confirmed progressive multifocal leukoencephalopathy in the adult patient population. In addition to the safety data from the pivotal clinical trials, tumour lysis syndrome has been observed (see Warnings and Precautions, General).

Neurologic Adverse Events: Nervous system events, regardless of drug relationship, were reported for 64% of patients across the Phase I and Phase II studies.

Most patients in clinical studies with ATRIANCE had no apparent CNS involvement of their disease at the time of therapy initiation with ATRIANCE. However, in an exploratory analysis of 459 nelarabine treated patients across multiple dose levels and regimens, the presence of CNS involvement with malignancy at baseline was associated with an increased risk (odds ratio 3.35 in regression analysis, p=0.0002) of grade ≥3 neurologic toxicity during therapy with ATRIANCE.

Pediatric: The most common neurologic adverse events regardless of causality, including all grades (NCI Common Toxicity Criteria) are shown in Table 3 for pediatric patients.

Table 3: ATRIANCE

Neurologic Adverse Events (≥1%) Regardless of Causality in Pediatric Patients Treated with 650 mg/m² of ATRIANCE Administered Intravenously Over 1 Hour Daily for 5 Consecutive Days Repeated Every 21 Days

Nervous System Disorders Preferred Term	Percentage of Patients; N=84 Grade 1 %	 Grade 2 %	 Grade 3 %	 Grade 4+ %	 All Grades %
Headache	8	2	4	2	17
Peripheral neurologic disorders, any event	1	4	6	0	12
Peripheral neuropathy	0	4	2	0	6
Peripheral motor neuropathy	1	0	2	0	4
Peripheral sensory neuropathy	0	0	6	0	6
Somnolence	1	4	1	1	7
Hypoesthesia	1	1	4	0	6
Seizures	0	0	0	6	6
Convulsions	0	0	0	3	4
Grand mal convulsions	0	0	0	1	1
Status epilepticus	0	0	0	1	1
Motor dysfunction	1	1	1	0	4
Nervous system disorder	1	2	1	0	4
Paresthesia	0	2	1	0	4
Tremor	1	2	0	0	4
Ataxia	1	0	1	0	2

Grade 4+=Grade 4 and Grade 5.
One (1) patient had a fatal neurologic event, status epilepticus. This event was thought to be related to treatment with ATRIANCE.

The other grade 3 event in pediatric patients, regardless of causality, was hypertonia reported in 1 patient (1%). The additional grade 4+ events, regardless of causality, were 3rd nerve paralysis, and 6th nerve paralysis, each reported in 1 patient (1%).

The other neurologic adverse events, regardless of causality, reported as grade 1, 2, or unknown in pediatric patients were dysarthria, encephalopathy, hydrocephalus, hyporeflexia, lethargy, mental impairment, paralysis, and sensory loss, each reported in 1 patient (1%).

Adults: The most common neurologic adverse events, regardless of causality, including all grades (NCI Common Toxicity Criteria) are shown in Table 4 for adult patients.

Table 4: ATRIANCE

Neurologic Adverse Events (≥1%) Regardless of Causality in Adult Patients Treated with 1500 mg/m² of ATRIANCE Administered Intravenously Over 2 Hours on Days 1, 3, and 5 Repeated Every 21 Days

	Percentage of Patients; N=103				
System Organ Class Preferred Term	**Grade 1 %**	**Grade 2 %**	**Grade 3 %**	**Grade 4 %**	**All Grades %**
Somnolence	20	3	0	0	23
Dizziness	14	8	0	0	21
Peripheral neurologic disorders, any event	8	12	2	0	21
Neuropathy	0	4	0	0	4
Peripheral neuropathy	2	2	1	0	5
Peripheral motor neuropathy	3	3	1	0	7
Peripheral sensory neuropathy	7	6	0	0	13
Hypoesthesia	5	10	2	0	17
Headache	11	3	1	0	15
Paresthesia	11	4	0	0	15
Ataxia	1	6	2	0	9
Depressed level of consciousness	4	1	0	1	6
Tremor	2	3	0	0	5
Amnesia	2	1	0	0	3
Dysgeusia	2	1	0	0	3
Balance disorder	1	1	0	0	2
Sensory loss	0	2	0	0	2

One (1) patient had a fatal neurologic event, cerebral hemorrhage/coma/leukoencephalopathy. This event was thought to be related to treatment with ATRIANCE.

Most nervous system events in the adult patients were evaluated as grade 1 or 2. The additional grade 3 events in adult patients, regardless of causality, were aphasia, convulsion, hemiparesis, and loss of consciousness, each reported in 1 patient (1%). The additional grade 4 events, regardless of causality, were cerebral hemorrhage, coma, intracranial hemorrhage, leukoencephalopathy, and metabolic encephalopathy, each reported in one patient (1%).

The other neurologic adverse events, regardless of causality, reported as grade 1, 2, or unknown in adult patients were abnormal coordination, burning sensation, disturbance in attention, dysarthria, hyporeflexia, neuropathic pain, nystagmus, peroneal nerve palsy, sciatica, sensory disturbance, sinus headache, and speech disorder, each reported in one patient (1%).

Other Neurologic Events: There have also been reports of events associated with demyelination and ascending peripheral neuropathies similar in appearance to Guillain-Barré syndrome.

Post-Market Adverse Drug Reactions: Several cases of serious spinal cord disorders including spinal cord ischaemia and myelitis transverse have been reported. These events presented with symptoms including leg weakness, numbness, quadriplegia, fecal incontinence and urinary incontinence. Causality assessment with regard to the contributory role of nelarabine is uncertain due to a number of confounding factors; however, a contribution by nelarabine cannot be excluded.

In addition, there have been two reports* of leukoencephalopathy in the pediatric population.

DRUG INTERACTIONS: No formal drug interaction studies have been carried out with nelarabine.

In one pharmacokinetic study, fludarabine administered prior to nelarabine did not affect the plasma pharmacokinetics of nelarabine and ara-G or ara-GTP.

The involvement of cytochrome P450 enzymes in the metabolism of nelarabine has not been investigated.

There is in vitro evidence that pentostatin is a strong inhibitor of adenosine deaminase. This may result in a reduction in the conversion of the prodrug nelarabine to its active moiety and consequently in a reduction in efficacy of nelarabine and/or change in the adverse event profile of either drug. Therefore administration of nelarabine in combination with adenosine deaminase inhibitors, such as pentostatin, is not recommended.

DOSAGE AND ADMINISTRATION: Dosing Considerations: Appropriate measures (e.g. hydration, urine alkalinization, and prophylaxis with allopurinol) must be taken to prevent hyperuricemia associated with tumour lysis syndrome.

Supportive measures (e.g. antiemetic agents) and medical care (e.g. antibiotics, blood and platelet transfusions) are recommended, as clinically indicated.

Recommended Dose and Dosage Adjustment: Adults: The recommended adult dose of ATRIANCE is 1500 mg/m²/day administered intravenously over 2 hours on days 1, 3, and 5, repeated every 21 days.

Children: The recommended pediatric dose of ATRIANCE is 650 mg/m²/day administered intravenously over 1 hour on days 1 to 5, repeated every 21 days.

The optimal dosing regimen for patients between the ages of 16 and 21 years of age has not been determined.

The recommended duration of treatment has not been clearly established. In clinical trials, treatment was generally continued until there was evidence of disease progression, the patient experienced unacceptable toxicity, the patient became a candidate for bone marrow transplant, or the patient no longer continued to benefit from treatment.

ATRIANCE has not been studied in patients with hepatic or renal dysfunction. No dose adjustment is recommended for CrCl ≥50 mL/min. There are insufficient data to support a dose recommendation for CrCl <50 mL/min (see Action and Clinical Pharmacology, Renal Insufficiency).

ATRIANCE (nelarabine) should be discontinued at the first sign of neurologic events of NCI Common Toxicity Criteria grade 2 or greater. Administration of the next treatment cycle may be delayed for other toxicity including hematologic toxicity.

Administration: Nelarabine Injection is intended to be used without further dilution.

Nelarabine Injection is stable in polyvinylchloride (PVC) infusion bags and glass containers for up to 8 hours at up to 30°C.

OVERDOSAGE:

There is no known antidote for overdoses of ATRIANCE (nelarabine). It is anticipated that overdosage would result in severe neurotoxicity (possibly including paralysis, coma), myelosuppression, and potentially death. In the event of overdose, supportive care consistent with good clinical practice should be provided.

* One case was received from a non-GlaxoSmithKline Inc (GSK) study prior to launch and approval of nelarabine. A second case was received during post marketing surveillance as part of a non-GSK study.

Nelarabine has been administered in clinical trials up to a dose of 75 mg/kg (approximately 2250 mg/m²) daily for 5 days to 1 pediatric subject and up to a dose of 60 mg/kg (approximately 2400 mg/m²) daily for 5 days to 5 adult patients.

Nelarabine has been administered in clinical trials up to a dose of 2900 mg/m² on days 1, 3, and 5 to 2 adult patients. At a dose of 2200 mg/m² given on days 1, 3, and 5 every 21 days, 2 patients developed a significant grade 3 ascending sensory neuropathy. MRI evaluations of the 2 patients demonstrated findings consistent with a demyelinating process in the cervical spine.

Because strategies for the management of overdose are continually evolving, it is advisable to contact a poison control center to determine the latest recommendations for the management of an overdose of any drug.

For management of a suspected drug overdose, CPhA recommends that you contact your **regional Poison Control Centre**. See the *CPS* Directory section for a list of Poison Control Centres.

ACTION AND CLINICAL PHARMACOLOGY: Mechanism of Action: Nelarabine is a pro-drug of the deoxyguanosine analogue antimetabolite, 9-β-D-arabinofuranosylguanine (ara-G). Nelarabine is rapidly demethylated by adenosine deaminase (ADA) to ara-G and then phosphorylated intracellularly by deoxyguanosine kinase and deoxycytidine kinase to its 5′-monophosphate. The monophosphate is subsequently converted intracellularly to the active 5′-triphosphate, ara-GTP. Accumulation of ara-GTP in leukemic cells allows for incorporation of ara-GTP into deoxyribonucleic acid (DNA) leading to inhibition of DNA synthesis which results in cell death. Other mechanisms may contribute to the cytotoxic effects of nelarabine. In vitro, T-cells are more sensitive than B-cells to the cytotoxic effects of nelarabine.

In a cross-study analysis using data from four Phase I studies, the pharmacokinetics of nelarabine and ara-G were characterized in patients aged less than 18 years and adult patients with refractory leukemia or lymphoma.

Pharmacokinetics: Absorption: Plasma ara-G C_{max} values generally occurred at the end of the nelarabine infusion and were generally higher than nelarabine C_{max} values, suggesting rapid and extensive conversion of nelarabine to ara-G. After infusion of 1500 mg/m² nelarabine over two hours in adult patients, mean plasma nelarabine and ara-G C_{max} values were 13.9 μM and 115 μM), respectively. Mean plasma nelarabine and ara-G AUC values were 13.5 μM.h and 571 μM.h, respectively, after infusion of 1500 mg/m². Intracellular C_{max} for ara-GTP appeared within 3 to 25 hours on Day 1. Mean intracellular ara-GTP C_{max} and AUC values were 95.6 μM and 2214 μM.h at this dose. No pharmacokinetic data are available in pediatric patients at the once daily 650 mg/m² nelarabine dose.

Distribution: Nelarabine and ara-G are extensively distributed throughout the body based on combined Phase I pharmacokinetic data at nelarabine doses of 104 to 2900 mg/m² in 135 patients with refractory leukemia or lymphoma in four Phase I studies. Specifically, for nelarabine, V_{ss} values were 115 L/m² and 89.4 L/m² in adult and pediatric patients, respectively. For ara-G, V_{ss}/F values were 44.8 L/m² and 32.1 L/m² in adult and pediatric patients, respectively. Nelarabine volume of distribution (V_{ss}) and ara-G V_{ss}/F were influenced by body surface area (BSA), which supports dosing based on BSA.

Nelarabine and ara-G are not substantially bound to human plasma proteins (less than 25%) in vitro, and binding is independent of nelarabine or ara-G concentrations up to 600 μM.

Metabolism: The principal route of metabolism for nelarabine is O-demethylation by adenosine deaminase to form ara-G, which undergoes hydrolysis to form guanine. In addition, some nelarabine is hydrolyzed to form methylguanine, which is O-demethylated to form guanine. Guanine is N-deaminated to form xanthine, which is further oxidized to yield uric acid.

Excretion: Pharmacokinetic studies in adult patients with refractory leukemia or lymphoma have demonstrated that nelarabine is rapidly eliminated from plasma with a half-life of approximately 30 minutes. Ara-G is eliminated from plasma at a slower rate than nelarabine, with a half-life of 2.0 and 3.2 hours for pediatric and adult patients, respectively.

Combined Phase 1 pharmacokinetic data at nelarabine doses of 104 to 2900 mg/m² on Day 1 indicate that geometric mean clearance (CL) values for nelarabine are 138 L/h/m² and 125 L/h/m² in adult and pediatric patients, respectively, on Day 1 (n=65 adults, n=1 pediatric patients). The apparent clearance of ara-G (CL/F) is comparable between the two groups (9.5 L/h/m² in adult patients and 10.8 L/h/m² in pediatric patients) on Day 1. Ara-G CL/F was influenced by body surface area (BSA), which supports dosing based on BSA.

Nelarabine and ara-G are partially eliminated by the kidneys. Mean urinary excretion of nelarabine and ara-G was 5.3% and 23.2% of the administered dose, respectively, in 28 adult patients over the 24 hours after nelarabine infusion on Day 1. Renal clearance averaged 16.4 L/h for nelarabine and 4.9 L/h for ara-G in 21 adult patients. Ara-G clearance (CL/F) was influenced by baseline calculated creatinine clearance (CLcr). No accumulation of nelarabine or ara-G was observed in plasma after nelarabine administration on either a daily or a day 1, 3, 5 schedule.

Intracellular ara-GTP concentrations in leukemic blasts were quantifiable for a prolonged period after nelarabine administration, and the elimination half-life could not be accurately estimated. Intracellular ara-GTP accumulated with repeated administration of nelarabine; on the Day 1, 3, and 5 schedule, C_{max} and $AUC_{(0-t)}$ values on Day 3 were approximately 50% and 30%, respectively, greater than C_{max} and $AUC_{(0-t)}$ values on Day 1. There is substantial intersubject variability in nelarabine, ara-G, and intracellular ara-GTP pharmacokinetics. Intracellular ara-GTP AUC and C_{max} values were higher in patients who responded to treatment with nelarabine than in patients who did not respond. Nelarabine and ara-G exposure were not associated with response.

Special Populations and Conditions: Pediatrics: No pharmacokinetic data are available in pediatric patients at the once daily 650 mg/m² nelarabine dosage. Combined Phase 1 pharmacokinetic data at nelarabine doses of 104 to 2900 mg/m² on Day 1 indicate that the geometric mean clearance (CL) values for nelarabine are 138 L/h/m² and 125 L/h/m² in adult and pediatric patients, respectively, on Day 1 (n=65 adults, n=21 pediatric patients). The apparent clearance of ara-G (CL/F) is comparable between the two groups (9.5 L/h/m² in adult patients and 10.8 L/h/m² in pediatric patients) on Day 1.

Nelarabine and ara-G are extensively distributed throughout the body. Specifically, for nelarabine, V_{ss} values were 115 L/m² and 89.4 L/m² in adult and pediatric patients, respectively. The volume of distribution of ara-G (V_{ss}/F) is 44.8 L/m² and 32.1 L/m² in adult and pediatric patients, respectively.

Geriatrics: Nelarabine and ara-G pharmacokinetics have not been specifically studied in an elderly population. Age has no effect on the pharmacokinetics of nelarabine or ara-G. Decreased renal function, which is more common in the elderly, may reduce ara-G clearance (see Warnings and Precautions).

Gender: The effect of gender on nelarabine and ara-G pharmacokinetics has not been specifically studied. In a pharmacokinetic/pharmacodynamic cross-study analysis, nelarabine and ara-G pharmacokinetics were not different between adult male and female patients; however, intracellular ara-GTP C_{max} and $AUC_{(0-t)}$ values at the same dose level were 2- to 3- fold greater on average in adult female than in adult male patients. There was no apparent difference in safety or efficacy parameters were observed by gender in clinical trials.

Race: The effect of race on nelarabine and ara-G pharmacokinetics has not been specifically studied. In a pharmacokinetic/pharmacodynamic cross-study analysis, race (Caucasian/other) had no apparent effect on nelarabine, ara-G, or intracellular ara-GTP pharmacokinetics.

Hepatic Insufficiency: The influence of hepatic impairment on the pharmacokinetics of nelarabine has not been evaluated.

Renal Insufficiency: The pharmacokinetics of nelarabine and ara-G have not been specifically studied in renally impaired or hemodialyzed patients. Nelarabine is excreted by the kidney to a small extent (5 to 10% of the administered dose). Ara-G is excreted by the kidney to a greater extent (20 to 30% of the administered nelarabine dose). In a pharmacokinetic/pharmacodynamic cross-study analysis with a limited number of renally impaired patients (n=2 with CLcr <50 mL/min), baseline calculated creatinine clearance (CLcr) was a significant predictor of ara-G apparent clearance (CL/F). The mean apparent clearance (CL/F) of ara-G was about 7% lower in patients with mild renal impairment (CLcr 50 to 80 mL/min) than in patients with normal renal function (>80 mL/min). Because the risk of adverse reactions to this drug may be greater in patients with decreased renal function (CLcr <50 mL/min), these patients should be closely monitored for toxicities when treated with ATRIANCE (see Dosage and Administration).

STORAGE AND STABILITY: Store at 25°C; excursions permitted to 15 to 30°C.

SPECIAL HANDLING INSTRUCTIONS: Caution should be used during handling, preparation and disposal of nelarabine. Use of gloves and other protective clothing to prevent skin contact is recommended. Proper aseptic technique should be used.

Guidelines on the proper handling and disposal of anticancer drugs should be consulted.

INFORMATION FOR THE PATIENT: Published in e-CPS, available by subscription at www.e-cps.ca.

DOSAGE FORMS, COMPOSITION AND PACKAGING: Each mL of clear, colorless solution contains: 5 mg nelarabine and 4.5 mg sodium chloride in Water for Injection, USP. Hydrochloric acid and sodium hydroxide may have been used to adjust the pH. The solution pH ranges from 5.0 to 7.0. Type I, clear glass, single use vials with a gray butyl rubber (latex-free) stopper and a red snap-off aluminum seal containing 250 mg nelarabine in 50 mL Water for Injection, USP. Cartons of 6 single use vials.

Atripla® 🅿

efavirenz—emtricitabine—tenofovir disoproxil fumarate

Antiretroviral Agent

Gilead Sciences

Date of Revision: July 19, 2010

SUMMARY PRODUCT INFORMATION:

Route of Administration	Dosage Form/ Strength	Clinically Relevant Nonmedicinal Ingredients
Oral	Tablet Efavirenz 600 mg/ Emtricitabine 200 mg/ Tenofovir Disoproxil Fumarate 300 mg	None For a complete listing, see Dosage Forms, Composition and Packaging.

INDICATIONS AND CLINICAL USE: ATRIPLA is indicated for use alone as a complete regimen or in combination with other antiretroviral agents for the treatment of HIV-1 infection in adults (see Adverse Reactions).

Geriatrics (>65 years of age): Clinical studies of the components of ATRIPLA did not include sufficient numbers of subjects aged 65 and over to determine whether they respond differently from younger subjects.

Pediatrics (<18 years of age): Safety and effectiveness in pediatric patients have not been established. ATRIPLA is not recommended for pediatric administration.

CONTRAINDICATIONS: ATRIPLA is contraindicated in patients with previously demonstrated hypersensitivity to any of the components of the product. For a complete listing, see Dosage Forms, Composition and Packaging.

Competition for CYP3A4 by efavirenz could result in inhibition of metabolism of some drugs and create the potential for serious and/or life-threatening adverse events. Drugs that are contraindicated with ATRIPLA are listed in Table 1. See also Drug Interactions, Drug-Drug Interactions.

Table 1: ATRIPLA

Drugs That Should Not Be Coadministered with ATRIPLA

Drug Class: Drug Name	Clinical Comment
Antifungal: voriconazole	**Contraindicated** because efavirenz significantly decreases voriconazole plasma concentrations, and coadministration may decrease the therapeutic effectiveness of voriconazole. Also, voriconazole significantly increases efavirenz plasma concentrations, which may increase the risk of efavirenz-associated side effects. Because ATRIPLA is a fixed dose combination product, the dose of efavirenz cannot be altered; therefore, voriconazole and ATRIPLA cannot be coadministered.
Antimigraine: ergot derivatives (dihydroergotamine, ergonovine, ergotamine, methylergonovine)	**Contraindicated** due to potential for serious and/or life-threatening reactions such as acute ergot toxicity characterized by peripheral vasospasm and ischemia of the extremities and other tissues.
Benzodiazepines: midazolam, triazolam	**Contraindicated** due to potential for serious and/or life-threatening reactions such as prolonged or increased sedation or respiratory depression.
Neuroleptic: pimozide	**Contraindicated** due to potential for serious and/or life-threatening reactions such as cardiac arrhythmias.
GI motility agent: cisapride[a]	**Contraindicated** due to potential for serious and/or life-threatening reactions such as cardiac arrhythmias.

[a] Cisapride is not marketed in Canada.

WARNINGS AND PRECAUTIONS:

> Lactic acidosis and severe hepatomegaly with steatosis, including fatal cases, have been reported with the use of nucleoside analogs including VIREAD, a component of ATRIPLA, alone or in combination with other antiretrovirals (see Warnings and Precautions, Hepatic/Biliary/Pancreatic).
>
> ATRIPLA is not approved for the treatment of chronic hepatitis B virus (HBV) infection and the safety and efficacy of ATRIPLA have not been established in patients coinfected with HBV and HIV. Severe acute exacerbations of hepatitis B have been reported in patients who are coinfected with HBV and HIV after the discontinuation of EMTRIVA or VIREAD, two of the components of ATRIPLA. In some patients infected with HBV and treated with EMTRIVA, the exacerbations of hepatitis B were associated with liver decompensation and liver failure. Hepatic function should be closely monitored with both clinical and laboratory follow up for at least several months in patients who discontinue ATRIPLA and are coinfected with HIV and HBV. If appropriate, initiation of anti-hepatitis B therapy may be warranted (see Warnings and Precautions, Special Populations).
>
> Renal failure, renal insufficiency, elevated creatinine, hypophosphatemia, and Fanconi syndrome have been reported with the use of tenofovir DF during clinical practice (see Warnings and Precautions).

General: As a fixed-dose combination of efavirenz, emtricitabine and tenofovir DF, ATRIPLA should not be administered with SUSTIVA, EMTRIVA, VIREAD, OR TRUVADA. Due to similarities between emtricitabine and lamivudine, ATRIPLA should not be administered with drugs containing lamivudine including Combivir, 3TC, Heptovir, Kivexa, and Trizivir.

ATRIPLA should not be administered with HEPSERA (adefovir dipivoxil).

Clinical trial data of patients who were switched to ATRIPLA from a prior PI-containing regimen suggest that they may have lower response rates than patients who remain on their baseline regimens. Therefore, patients who are switched to ATRIPLA from a prior PI-containing regimen should be monitored for both treatment-emergent adverse events and rises in viral load.

Concomitant use of St. John's Wort (Hypericum perforatum) or St. John's Wort-containing products with ATRIPLA is not recommended. Coadministration of non-nucleoside reverse transcriptase inhibitors (NNRTIs), including efavirenz, with St. John's Wort is expected to substantially decrease NNRTI concentrations. Decreased concentrations may result in suboptimal levels of efavirenz and lead to loss of virologic response and possible resistance to efavirenz or to the class of NNRTIs.

Efavirenz may cause dizziness, impaired concentration, and/or drowsiness. Patients should be instructed that, if they experience these symptoms, they should avoid potentially hazardous tasks such as driving or operating machinery. (See Warnings and Precautions, Neurologic.)

Carcinogenesis, Mutagenesis, Impairment of Fertility: Efavirenz: Oral carcinogenicity studies in mice and rats were carried out with efavirenz. Mice were dosed with 0, 25, 75, 150, or 300 mg/kg/day for 2 years. Incidences of hepatocellular adenomas and carcinomas and pulmonary alveolar/bronchiolar adenomas at all doses were increased above background in females. No increases in tumor incidence above background were seen in males. The systemic exposure (based on AUCs) in mice was approximately 1.7-fold that in humans receiving the 600 mg/day dose. Rats were administered efavirenz at doses of 0, 25, 50, or 100 mg/kg/day for 2 years; no increases in tumor incidence above background were observed. The exposure in rats was lower than that in humans.

The mechanism of the carcinogenic potential is unknown. However, in genetic toxicology assays, efavirenz showed no evidence of mutagenic or clastogenic activity in a battery of in vitro and in vivo studies. These included bacterial mutation assays in *S. typhimurium* and *E. coli*, mammalian mutation assays in Chinese hamster ovary cells, chromosome aberration assays in human peripheral blood lymphocytes or Chinese hamster ovary cells, and an in vivo mouse bone marrow micronucleus assay. Given the lack of genotoxic activity of efavirenz, the relevance to humans of neoplasms in efavirenz-treated mice is not known.

Efavirenz did not impair mating or fertility of male or female rats, and did not affect sperm of treated male rats. The reproductive performance of offspring born to female rats given efavirenz was not affected. As a result of the rapid clearance of efavirenz in rats, systemic drug exposures achieved in these studies were equivalent to or below those achieved in humans given therapeutic doses of efavirenz.

Emtricitabine: In long-term oral carcinogenicity studies of emtricitabine, no drug-related increase in tumor incidence was found in mice at doses up to 750 mg/kg/day (26 times the human systemic exposure at the therapeutic dose of 200 mg/day) or in rats at doses up to 600 mg/kg/day (31 times the human systemic exposure at the therapeutic dose).

Emtricitabine was not genotoxic in the in vitro reverse mutation bacterial test (Ames test), or in vivo mouse lymphoma or mouse micronucleus assays.

Emtricitabine did not affect fertility in male rats at approximately 140 fold or in male and female mice at approximately 60-fold higher exposures (AUC) than in humans given the recommended 200 mg daily dose. Fertility was normal in the offspring of mice exposed daily from before birth (in utero) through sexual maturity at daily exposures (AUC) of approximately 60-fold higher than human exposures at the recommended 200 mg daily dose.

Tenofovir Disoproxil Fumarate: Tenofovir disoproxil fumarate (tenofovir DF) did not show any carcinogenic potential in a long-term oral carcinogenicity study in rats. A long-term oral carcinogenicity study in mice showed a low incidence of duodenal tumors, considered likely related to high local concentrations in the gastrointestinal tract at the high dose of 600 mg/kg/day. The mechanism of tumor formation in mice and potential relevance for humans is uncertain.

Tenofovir DF was mutagenic in the in vitro mouse lymphoma assay and negative in an in vitro bacterial mutagenicity test (Ames test). In an in vivo mouse micronucleus assay, tenofovir DF was negative at doses up to 2000 mg/kg when administered orally to male mice.

There were no effects on fertility, mating performance or early embryonic development when tenofovir disoproxil fumarate was administered at 600 mg/kg/day to male rats for 28 days prior to mating and to female rats for 15 days prior to mating through day seven of gestation. There was, however, an alteration of the estrous cycle in female rats. A dose of 600 mg/kg/day is equivalent to 19 times the human dose based on body surface area comparisons.

Endocrine and Metabolism: Fat Redistribution: Redistribution/accumulation of body fat (lipodystrophy) including central obesity, dorsocervical fat enlargement (buffalo hump), peripheral wasting, facial wasting, breast enlargement, and "cushingoid appearance" have been observed in patients receiving antiretroviral therapy. The mechanism and long-term consequences of these events are currently unknown. A causal relationship has not been established.

Hepatic/Biliary/Pancreatic: Lactic Acidosis/Severe Hepatomegaly with Steatosis: Lactic acidosis and severe hepatomegaly with steatosis, including fatal cases, have been reported with the use of antiretroviral nucleoside analogs including the tenofovir DF component of ATRIPLA, alone or in combination with other antiretrovirals in the treatment of HIV infection. A majority of these cases have been in women. Obesity and prolonged nucleoside exposure may be risk factors. Particular caution should be exercised when administering nucleoside analogs to any patient with known risk factors for liver disease; however, cases have also been reported in patients with no known risk factors. Treatment with ATRIPLA should be suspended in any patient who develops clinical or laboratory findings suggestive of lactic acidosis or pronounced hepatotoxicity (which may include hepatomegaly and steatosis even in the absence of marked transaminase elevations).

Hepatic Impairment: The pharmacokinetics of efavirenz has not been adequately studied in patients with hepatic impairment and its use is not recommended in patients with severe hepatic impairment (Child-Pugh Class C). Because of the extensive cytochrome P450-mediated metabolism of efavirenz and limited clinical experience in patients with mild or moderate hepatic impairment, caution should be exercised in administering ATRIPLA to these patients. Patients should be monitored carefully for adverse events, and laboratory tests to evaluate the liver disease should be performed at periodic intervals.

Tenofovir and tenofovir disoproxil are not metabolized by liver enzymes. Clinically relevant pharmacokinetic changes in patients with hepatic impairment are not observed. Emtricitabine has not been evaluated in patients with hepatic impairment; however, emtricitabine has not been shown to be metabolized by liver enzymes, so the impact of liver impairment is likely to be limited.

The safety and efficacy of ATRIPLA have not been established or specifically studied in patients with underlying liver disorders. Patients with chronic hepatitis B or C and treated with antiretroviral therapy are at increased risk for severe and potentially fatal hepatic adverse events. In case of concomitant antiviral therapy for hepatitis B or C, please refer also to the relevant product information for these medicinal products (see Warnings and Precautions, Special Populations).

Pancreatitis: Pancreatitis has occurred during therapy with combination regimens that included tenofovir DF. Caution should be used when administering nucleoside analogues (including ATRIPLA) to patients with a history of pancreatitis or risk factors for the development of pancreatitis. Therapy should be suspended in patients with suspected pancreatitis.

In controlled clinical studies the rate of clinical pancreatitis was similar in patients receiving [1/1008 (0.1%)] and not receiving [2/635 (0.3%)] efavirenz. Asymptomatic increases in serum amylase levels were observed in a significantly higher number of patients treated with efavirenz 600 mg than in control patients.

Elevated triglycerides have been reported in patients receiving efavirenz, in some cases to levels which can predispose a patient to pancreatitis. Among patients with elevated triglycerides, there have been no cases of pancreatitis. Because these triglyceride levels were not obtained in a fasting state, the exact clinical relevance of these measurements is not known.

Immune: Hypersensitivity Reactions: In clinical trials, hypersensitivity reactions were uncommon (<1%) in patients treated with efavirenz.

Immune Reconstitution: Immune reconstitution syndrome has been reported in patients treated with combination antiretroviral therapy, including the components of ATRIPLA. During the initial phase of treatment, patients responding to antiretroviral therapy may develop an inflammatory response to indolent or residual opportunistic infections (such as *M. avium* infections, cytomegalovirus, *P. jiroveci* pneumonia (PCP), and tuberculosis), which may necessitate further evaluation and treatment.

Musculoskeletal: Bone Effects: Bone monitoring should be considered for HIV infected patients who have a history of pathologic bone fracture or are at risk for osteopenia. Although the effect of supplementation with calcium and vitamin D was not studied, such supplementation may be beneficial for all patients. If bone abnormalities are suspected then appropriate consultation should be obtained.

In a 144 week study of treatment-naïve patients, decreases from baseline in bone mineral density (BMD) were seen at the lumbar spine and hip in both arms of the study. At Week 144, there was a significantly greater mean percentage decrease from baseline in BMD at the lumbar spine in patients in the tenofovir DF + lamivudine + efavirenz group compared with patients in the stavudine + lamivudine + efavirenz group. Changes in BMD at the hip were similar in the two treatment groups. In both groups, the majority of the reduction in BMD occurred in the first 24-48 weeks of the study and this reduction was sustained through Week 144. Twenty-eight percent of tenofovir DF-treated patients vs. 21% of the stavudine-treated patients lost at least 5% of BMD at the spine or 7% of BMD at the hip. Clinically relevant fractures (excluding fingers and toes) were reported in 4 patients in the tenofovir DF group and 6 patients in the stavudine group. In addition, there were significant increases in biochemical markers of bone metabolism (serum bone-specific alkaline phosphatase, serum osteocalcin, serum C-telopeptide, and urinary N-telopeptide) in the tenofovir DF group relative to the stavudine group, suggesting increased bone turnover. Serum parathyroid hormone levels and 1,25 Vitamin D levels were also higher in the tenofovir DF group. Except for bone specific alkaline phosphatase, these changes resulted in values that remained within the normal range. The effects of tenofovir DF-associated changes in BMD and biochemical markers on long-term bone health and future fracture risk are unknown.

Cases of osteomalacia (associated with proximal renal tubulopathy and infrequently contributing to fractures) have been reported in association with the use of tenofovir DF (see Adverse Reactions, Post-Market Adverse Drug Reactions, Tenofovir DF).

For additional information, please consult the VIREAD Product Monograph.

Neurologic: Nervous System Symptoms: Fifty-three percent (531/1008) of patients receiving efavirenz in controlled clinical trials reported central nervous system symptoms (any grade, regardless of causality) compared to 25% (156/635) of patients receiving control regimens. These symptoms included, but were not limited to, dizziness (28.1% of the 1008 patients), insomnia (16.3%), impaired concentration (8.3%), somnolence (7.0%), abnormal dreams (6.2%), and hallucinations (1.2%). Other reported symptoms were euphoria, confusion, agitation, amnesia, stupor, abnormal thinking, and depersonalization. The majority of these symptoms were mild-moderate (50.7%); symptoms were severe in 2.0% of patients. Overall, 2.1% of patients discontinued therapy as a result. These symptoms usually begin during the first or second day of therapy and generally resolve after the first 2-4 weeks. After 4 weeks of therapy the prevalence of nervous system symptoms of at least moderate severity ranged from 5-9% in patients treated with regimens containing efavirenz and from 3-5% in patients treated with a control regimen. Patients should be informed that these symptoms are likely to improve with continued therapy. Dosing at bedtime improves tolerability of these symptoms.

Analysis of long-term data from a clinical study, (median follow-up 180 weeks, 102 weeks, and 76 weeks for patients treated with efavirenz + zidovudine + lamivudine, efavirenz + indinavir, and indinavir + zidovudine + lamivudine, respectively) showed that, beyond 24 weeks of therapy, the incidences of new-onset nervous system symptoms among efavirenz-treated patients were generally similar to those in the indinavir-containing control arm.

Patients receiving ATRIPLA should be alerted to the potential for additive central nervous system effects when ATRIPLA is used concomitantly with alcohol or psychoactive drugs. Patients should be informed that ATRIPLA may cause dizziness, impaired concentration, and/or drowsiness. Patients should be instructed that if they experience these symptoms they should avoid potentially hazardous tasks such as driving or operating machinery. (See Warnings and Precautions, General.)

Seizures: Caution should be taken in any patient with any history of seizures. Convulsions have been observed infrequently in patients receiving efavirenz, generally in the presence of known medical history of seizures. Overall, the rate of seizure in controlled clinical trials has been 0.89% in efavirenz treated patients and 0.63% in the control patients. Patients who are receiving concomitant anticonvulsant medications primarily metabolized by the liver such as phenytoin, carbamazepine, and phenobarbital, may require periodic monitoring of plasma levels (see Drug Interactions).

Psychiatric: Serious psychiatric adverse reactions have been reported in patients treated with efavirenz. In controlled trials of 1008 patients treated with regimens containing efavirenz for an average of 2.1 years and 635 patients treated with control regimens for an average of 1.5 years, the frequency (regardless of causality) of specific serious psychiatric events among patients who received efavirenz or control regimens respectively, were: severe depression (2.4%, 0.9%), suicidal ideation (0.7%, 0.3%), non-fatal suicide attempts (0.5%, 0%), aggressive behavior (0.4%, 0.5%), paranoid reactions (0.4%, 0.3%), and manic reactions (0.2%, 0.3%). When psychiatric symptoms similar to those noted above were combined and evaluated as a group in a multifactorial analysis of data from a clinical study, treatment with efavirenz was associated with an increase in the occurrence of these selected psychiatric symptoms. Other factors associated with an increase in the occurrence of these psychiatric symptoms were history of injection drug use, psychiatric history, and receipt of psychiatric medication at study entry; similar associations were observed in both the efavirenz and control treatment groups. In Study 006, onset of new serious psychiatric symptoms occurred throughout the study for both efavirenz-treated and control-treated patients. One percent of efavirenz-treated patients discontinued or interrupted treatment because of one or more of these selected psychiatric symptoms. There have also been occasional postmarketing reports of death by suicide, delusions, and psychosis-like behavior, although a causal relationship to the use of efavirenz cannot be determined from these reports. Patients with serious psychiatric adverse experiences should seek immediate medical evaluation to assess the probability that the symptoms may be related to the use of ATRIPLA, and if so, to determine whether the risks of continued therapy outweigh the benefits.

Renal: Nephrotoxicity: Emtricitabine and tenofovir are principally eliminated by the kidney, however efavirenz is not. Since ATRIPLA is a combination product and the dose of the individual components cannot be altered, patients with creatinine clearance <50 mL/min should not receive ATRIPLA.

Renal impairment, including cases of acute renal failure and Fanconi syndrome (renal tubular injury with severe hypophosphatemia), has been reported in association with the use of tenofovir DF (see Adverse Reactions, Post-Market Adverse Drug Reactions). The majority of these cases occurred in patients with underlying systemic or renal disease, or in patients taking nephrotoxic agents, however, some cases occurred in patients without identified risk factors.

It is recommended that creatine clearance be calculated in all patients prior to initiating therapy and as clinically appropriate during therapy with ATRIPLA. Routine monitoring of calculated creatine clearance and serum phosphorus should be performed in patients at risk for renal impairment, including patients who have previously experienced renal events while receiving HEPSERA.

ATRIPLA should be avoided with concurrent or recent use of a nephrotoxic agent. Examples of nephrotoxic agents include but are not limited to aminoglycosides, amphotericin B, foscarnet, ganciclovir, pentamidine, vancomycin, cidofovir, or interleukin-2. Particular caution should be exercised when administering ATRIPLA to patients with known risk factors for renal disease and a history of renal dysfunction; however, cases of renal failure have also been reported in patients with no known risk factors.

Skin: Rash: In controlled clinical trials, 26% (266/1008) of patients treated with 600 mg efavirenz experienced new onset skin rash compared with 17% (111/635) of patients treated in control groups. Rash associated with blistering, moist desquamation or ulceration occurred in 0.9% (9/1008) of patients treated with efavirenz. Rashes are usually mild-to-moderate maculopapular skin eruptions that occur within the first 2 weeks of initiating therapy with efavirenz (median time to onset of rash in adults was 11 days) and in most patients continuing therapy with efavirenz, rash resolves within 1 month (median duration, 16 days). The discontinuation rate for rash in clinical trials was 6.4% (17/266) among patients with rash and 1.7% (17/1008) overall.

Grade 4 rash (including erythema multiforme, Stevens-Johnson syndrome, toxic epidermal necrolysis, and exfoliative dermatitis) was uncommon (<1%) in patients treated with efavirenz in clinical studies.

Experience with efavirenz in patients who discontinued other antiretroviral agents of the NNRTI class is limited. Nineteen patients who discontinued nevirapine because of rash have been treated with efavirenz. Nine of these patients developed mild-to-moderate rash while receiving therapy with efavirenz, and two of these patients discontinued because of rash.

ATRIPLA can be reinitiated in patients interrupting therapy because of Grades 1 and 2 rash. ATRIPLA should be discontinued in patients developing severe rash associated with blistering, desquamation, mucosal involvement or fever. Appropriate antihistamines and/or corticosteroids may improve the tolerability and hasten the resolution of rash.

Special Populations: Patients with HIV and Hepatitis B Virus Coinfection: It is recommended that all patients with HIV be tested for the presence of HBV before initiating antiretroviral therapy. ATRIPLA is not approved for the treatment of chronic HBV infection and the safety and efficacy of ATRIPLA have not been established in patients coinfected with HBV and HIV. Severe acute exacerbations of hepatitis B have been reported in patients who are coinfected with HBV and HIV after the discontinuation of EMTRIVA and VIREAD, two of the components of ATRIPLA. In some patients infected with HBV and treated with EMTRIVA, the exacerbations of hepatitis B were associated with liver decompensation and liver failure. Hepatic function should be closely monitored with both clinical and laboratory follow-up for at least several months in patients who discontinue ATRIPLA and are coinfected with HIV and HBV. If appropriate, initiation of anti-hepatitis B therapy may be warranted. In patients with advanced liver disease or cirrhosis, post-treatment exacerbation of hepatitis may lead to hepatic decompensation. Therefore, in these patients, discontinuation of treatment without initiation of alternative anti-hepatitis B therapy is not recommended.

Pregnant Women: Efavirenz may cause fetal harm when administered during the first trimester to a pregnant woman. Pregnancy should be avoided in women receiving ATRIPLA and for 12 weeks after discontinuation. Barrier contraception must always be used in combination with other methods of contraception (e.g., oral or other hormonal contraceptives) (see Drug Interactions). Because of the long half-life of efavirenz, use of adequate contraceptive measures for 12 weeks after discontinuation of ATRIPLA is recommended. Women of childbearing potential should undergo pregnancy testing prior to initiation of ATRIPLA.

There are no adequate and well-controlled studies in pregnant women. ATRIPLA should be used in pregnant women only if the potential benefits outweigh the potential risks to the fetus, such as in pregnant women without other therapeutic options.

Efavirenz: As of July 2009, the Antiretroviral Pregnancy Registry has received prospective reports of 661 pregnancies exposed to efavirenz-containing regimens, nearly all of which were first-trimester exposures (606 pregnancies). Birth defects occurred in 14 of 501 live births (first-trimester exposure) and 2 of 55 live births (second-/third-trimester exposure). One of these prospectively reported defects with first-trimester exposure was a neural tube defect. A single case of anophthalmia with first-trimester exposure to efavirenz has also been prospectively reported; however, this case included severe oblique facial clefts and amniotic banding, a known association with anophthalmia. There have been six retrospective reports of findings consistent with neural tube defects, including meningomyelocele. All mothers were exposed to efavirenz-containing regimens in the first trimester. A causal relationship of these events to the use of efavirenz cannot be established.

Malformations have been observed in 3 of 20 fetuses/infants from efavirenz-treated cynomolgus monkeys (versus 0 of 20 concomitant controls) in a developmental toxicity study. The pregnant monkeys were dosed throughout pregnancy (postcoital days 20-150) with efavirenz 60 mg/kg daily, a dose which resulted in plasma drug concentrations similar to those in humans given 600 mg/day of efavirenz. Anencephaly and unilateral anophthalmia were observed in one fetus, microophthalmia was observed in another fetus, and cleft palate was observed in a third fetus. Efavirenz crosses the placenta in cynomolgus monkeys and produces fetal blood concentrations similar to maternal blood concentrations. Efavirenz has been shown to cross the placenta in rats and rabbits and produces fetal blood concentrations of efavirenz similar to maternal concentrations. An increase in fetal resorptions was observed in rats at efavirenz doses that produced peak plasma concentrations and AUC values in female rats equivalent to or lower than those achieved in humans given 600 mg once daily of efavirenz. Efavirenz produced no reproductive toxicities when given to pregnant rabbits at dose that produced peak plasma concentrations similar to and AUC values approximately half of those achieved in humans given 600 mg once daily of efavirenz.

Emtricitabine: The incidence of fetal variations and malformations was not increased in embryo-fetal toxicity studies performed with emtricitabine in mice at exposures (AUC) approximately 60-fold higher and in rabbits at approximately 120-fold higher than human exposures at the recommended daily dose.

Tenofovir DF: Reproduction studies have been performed in rats and rabbits at doses up to 14 and 19 times the human dose based on body surface area comparisons and revealed no evidence of impaired fertility or harm to the fetus due to tenofovir. Reduced pup body weights, survival and delay in sexual maturation was observed in a peri- and postnatal toxicity study in rats at the maternally toxic doses of 450 and 600 mg/kg (approximately 14 and 19 times the human dose based on body surface area comparisons).

Antiretroviral Pregnancy Registry: To monitor fetal outcomes of pregnant women exposed to ART (antiretroviral therapy) including ATRIPLA, an Antiretroviral Pregnancy Registry has been established. Healthcare providers are encouraged to register patients, http://www.apregistry.com. Telephone: (800) 258-4263. Fax: (800) 800-1052.

Nursing Women: HIV-1 infected mothers should not breast-feed their infants to avoid risking postnatal transmission of HIV. Studies in rats and rhesus monkeys have demonstrated that tenofovir is secreted in milk. Studies in rats have demonstrated that efavirenz is excreted in milk. It is not known whether efavirenz, emtricitabine or tenofovir is excreted in human milk. Because of both the potential for HIV transmission and the potential for serious adverse reactions in nursing infants, **mothers should be instructed not to breast-feed if they are receiving ATRIPLA.**

Pediatrics (<18 years of age): Safety and effectiveness in pediatric patients have not been established. ATRIPLA is not recommended for pediatric administration.

Geriatrics (>65 years of age): Clinical studies of efavirenz, emtricitabine or tenofovir DF did not include sufficient numbers of subjects aged 65 and over to determine whether they respond differently than younger subjects. In general, dose selection for the elderly patient should be cautious, keeping in mind the greater frequency of decreased hepatic, renal, or cardiac function, and of concomitant disease or other drug therapy.

Monitoring and Laboratory Tests: Liver Enzymes: In patients with known or suspected history of Hepatitis B or C infection and in patients treated with other medications associated with liver toxicity, monitoring of liver enzymes is recommended. Postmarketing reports of hepatic failure have occurred including some cases in patients with no pre-existing hepatic disease or other identifiable risk factors (see Post-Market Adverse Drug Reactions). Liver enzyme monitoring should also be considered for patients without pre-existing hepatic dysfunction or other risk factors. In patients with persistent elevations of serum transaminases to greater than five times the upper limit of the normal range, the benefit of continued therapy with ATRIPLA needs to be weighed against the potential risks of significant liver toxicity. (See Adverse Reactions, Laboratory Abnormalities and Warnings and Precautions, Renal.)

ADVERSE REACTIONS: Clinical Trial Adverse Drug Reactions: Because clinical trials are conducted under very specific conditions the adverse reaction rates observed in the clinical trials may not reflect the rates observed in practice and should not be compared to the rates in the clinical trials of another drug. Adverse drug reaction information from clinical trials is useful for identifying drug related adverse events and for approximating rates.

Adverse Drug Reaction Overview: The combination of efavirenz + emtricitabine + tenofovir DF has been studied in 460 patients either as the fixed-dose dose combination tablet ATRIPLA (Study 073) or as the component products (Study 934). Adverse reactions observed in Study 934 (Phase III) and Study 073 (Phase IV) were generally consistent with those seen in previous studies of the individual components.

The most common adverse events reported in Study 934 associated with study regimen of efavirenz + emtricitabine + tenofovir DF through Week 144 were dizziness (25%), nausea (18%), and abnormal dreams (17%). Study regimen was discontinued due to an adverse event for 5% of subjects (13/257) in the efavirenz + emtricitabine + tenofovir DF group and 11% of subjects (29/254) in the lamivudine/zidovudine + efavirenz group.

In study 073, the most frequently reported adverse events associated with ATRIPLA among patients treated up to 48 weeks were psychiatric disorders (16%); nervous system disorders (13%); and gastrointestinal disorders (7%). The majority of adverse events associated with ATRIPLA were mild in severity with dizziness (11%) and abnormal dreams (7%) being the most common specific adverse events reported. Adverse events that led to study drug discontinuation were experienced by 5% of subjects in the ATRIPLA group and 1% of subjects who stayed on their baseline regimen (SBR group); the majority of subjects who discontinued study drug due to adverse events had switched to ATRIPLA from a prior protease inhibitor-based regimen and the events that led to discontinuation were expected events consistent with the known safety profile of efavirenz e.g. nervous system symptoms.

Study 934: Study 934—Treatment-Emergent Adverse Events: Assessment of adverse reactions is based on data from Study 934 in which 511 antiretroviral-naïve patients received either emtricitabine + tenofovir DF administered in combination with efavirenz (N=257) or lamivudine/zidovudine administered in combination with efavirenz (N=254). Adverse events observed in this study were generally consistent with those seen in other studies in treatment experienced or treatment-naïve patients (Table 2). The most common adverse events that occurred in patients receiving efavirenz + emtricitabine + tenofovir DF were mild to moderate dizziness, nausea or diarrhea.

Table 2: ATRIPLA

Selected Treatment-Emergent Adverse Events (Grades 2-4) Reported in ≥3% in Any Treatment Group in Study 934 (0-48 Weeks)

	FTC+TDF+EFV N=257 %	AZT/3TC+EFV N=254 %
Blood and Lymphatic System Disorders		
Anemia	<1	5
Gastrointestinal Disorders		
Diarrhea	7	4
Nausea	8	6
Vomiting	1	4
General Disorders and Administration Site Conditions		
Fatigue	7	6
Infections and Infestations		
Sinusitis	4	2
Upper Respiratory Tract Infections	3	3
Nasopharyngitis	3	1
Nervous System Disorders		
Somnolence	3	2
Headache	5	4
Dizziness	8	7
Psychiatric Disorders		
Depression	4	7
Insomnia	4	5
Abnormal Dreams	4	3
Skin and Subcutaneous Tissue Disorders		

(cont'd)

Table 2: ATRIPLA *(cont'd)*

Selected Treatment-Emergent Adverse Events (Grades 2-4) Reported in ≥3% in Any Treatment Group in Study 934 (0-48 Weeks)

	FTC+TDF+EFV N=257 %	AZT/3TC+EFV N=254 %
Rash	5	4

Patients who received efavirenz + emtricitabine + tenofovir DF up to 144 weeks in Study 934 reported adverse events similar in nature and severity to those reported in the first 48 weeks of treatment.

Laboratory Abnormalities: Laboratory abnormalities observed in this study were generally consistent with those seen in other studies (Table 3).

Table 3: ATRIPLA

Significant Laboratory Abnormalities Reported in ≥1% in Any Treatment Group in Study 934 (0-48 Weeks)

	FTC+TDF+EFV N=257 %	AZT/3TC+EFV N=254 %
Any ≥Grade 3 Laboratory Abnormality	25	22
Fasting Cholesterol (>240 mg/dL)	15	17
Creatine Kinase (M: >990 U/L) (F: >845 U/L)	7	6
Serum Amylase (>175 U/L)	7	3
Alkaline Phosphatase (>550 U/L)	1	0
AST (M: >180 U/L) (F: >170 U/L)	3	2
ALT (M: >215 U/L) (F: >170 U/L)	2	2
Hemoglobin (<8.0 mg/dL)	0	3
Hyperglycemia (>250 mg/dL)	1	1
Hematuria (>75 RBC/HPF)	2	2
Neutrophil (<750/mm³)	3	4
Fasting Triglycerides (>750 mg/dL)	4	2

Laboratory abnormalities in patients who received treatment up to 144 weeks in Study 934 were consistent with those observed in the first 48 weeks of treatment.

Through 48 weeks, 7 patients in the efavirenz + emtricitabine + tenofovir DF group and 5 patients in the efavirenz + lamivudine/zidovudine group experienced a new CDC Class C event (10 and 6 patients, respectively, through 144 weeks). Renal safety assessed by laboratory abnormalities was similar in the two groups and no patient discontinued study drug due to renal events. At Weeks 48 and 144, total limb fat (as measured by dual-energy x-ray absorptiometry) was significantly less in a subgroup of patients in the efavirenz + lamivudine/zidovudine group compared to the efavirenz + emtricitabine + tenofovir DF subgroup (see Table 4).

Table 4: ATRIPLA

Study 934 Total Limb Fat at Week 144[a] (Dual-Energy X-Ray Absorptiometry)

	FTC+TDF+EFV	AZT/3TC+EFV
Week 48[b]	**N=51**	**N=49**
Total Limb Fat (kg) Mean±S.D (Median)	8.9±5.4 (7.4)	6.9±3.9 (6.0)
Week 144[c]	**N=145**	**N=124**
Total Limb Fat (kg) Mean±S.D (Median)	9.2±5.4 (7.9)	6.5±4.4 (5.4)
Change from Week 48 to Week 144[d]	**N=48**	**N=38**
Total Limb Fat (kg) Mean±S.D (Median)	1.1±1.9 (0.9)	−1.1±1.7 (−0.8)

a Baseline data are not available.
b P=0.03 for the comparison between arms.
c P<0.001 for the comparison between arms.
d P<0.001 for the comparison between arms; P<0.001 for the comparison within arms.

Lipids: In Study 934 at Week 144, the mean increase from baseline fasting triglyceride concentrations was 4 mg/dL for the tenofovir DF, emtricitabine and efavirenz group and 36 mg/dL for the zidovudine/lamivudine and efavirenz group. For fasting total, LDL, and HDL cholesterol concentrations, the mean increases from baseline were 24 mg/dL, 13 mg/dL, and 10 mg/dL, respectively, for the tenofovir DF group and 36 mg/dL, 16 mg/dL, and 12 mg/dL, respectively, for the zidovudine/lamivudine group. The differences between treatment groups reached statistical significance for fasting triglycerides (p=0.047) and fasting total serum cholesterol (p=0.005).

Hepatic Events: In Study 934, 10 patients treated with efavirenz, emtricitabine, and tenofovir DF and 16 patients treated with efavirenz and fixed-dose zidovudine/lamivudine were Hepatitis C antibody positive. Among these HCV coinfected patients, one patient (1/10) in the efavirenz, emtricitabine and tenofovir DF arm had elevations in ALT and AST to greater than five times ULN through 144 weeks. One patient (1/16) in the fixed-dose zidovudine/lamivudine arm had elevations in ALT to greater than five times ULN through 144 weeks, and one patient (1/16) in the fixed-dose zidovudine/lamivudine arm had elevations in AST to greater than five times ULN through 144 weeks. Nine patients treated with efavirenz, emtricitabine and tenofovir DF and 4 patients treated with efavirenz and fixed-dose zidovudine/lamivudine were Hepatitis B surface antigen positive. None of these patients had treatment-emergent elevations in ALT and AST to greater than five times ULN through 144 weeks. No HBV and/or HCV coinfected patient discontinued from the study due to hepatobiliary disorders (see Warnings and Precautions, Hepatic/Biliary/Pancreatic and Monitoring and Laboratory Tests).

Study 073: In study 073, patients with stable virologic suppression on antiretroviral therapy and no history of virologic failure were randomized to receive ATRIPLA or to stay on their baseline regimen. The adverse reactions observed in Study 073 were generally consistent with those seen in Study 934 and those seen with individual components of ATRIPLA when each was administered in combination with other antiretroviral agents.

In such an open label switch study, subjects may experience an adverse event or laboratory abnormality when they switch to a new treatment compared to subjects who remain on their baseline regimen.

Treatment-emergent AEs such as nervous system symptoms were more frequent in subjects who switched to ATRIPLA than those who stayed on their baseline regimen (SBR group). Such events can be expected in subjects receiving an efavirenz based regimen for the first time, and are consistent with the known safety profile of efavirenz.

Table 5: ATRIPLA

Selected Treatment-Emergent Adverse Events Reported for ≥3% of Subjects in Any Treatment Group in Study 073 (0-48 Weeks)

	FTC+TDF+EFV N=203 %	SBR N=97 %
Gastrointestinal Disorders		
Diarrhea	3	0
Nausea	3	2
Nervous System Disorders		
Somnolence	3	0
Dizziness	11	1
Psychiatric Disorders		
Insomnia	4	0
Abnormal Dreams	7	0

Laboratory abnormalities observed in the ATRIPLA group in Study 073 (Table 6) were generally consistent with those in Study 934.

Table 6: ATRIPLA

Laboratory Abnormalities (≥Grade 3) Reported in ≥1% of Subjects in Any Treatment Group in Study 073 (0-48 Weeks)

	FTC+TDF+EFV N=203 %	SBR N=97 %
Any ≥Grade 3 Laboratory Abnormality	9	15
Fasting Cholesterol (>300 mg/dL)	<1	2
Serum Amylase (>200 U/L)	3	2
AST (M: >180 U/L) (F: >170 U/L)	1	1
ALT (M: >215 U/L) (F: >170 U/L)	2	0
Hemoglobin (<7.5 g/dL)	0	1
Hyperglycemia (>250 mg/dL)	1	1
Neutrophil (<750/mm³)	0	1
Fasting Triglycerides (>750 mg/dL)	2	2
Total Bilirubin (>3 mg/dL)	0	7

In addition to the adverse events in Study 934 (Table 2) and Study 073 (Table 5), the following adverse events were reported in clinical studies of efavirenz, emtricitabine, or tenofovir DF in combination with other antiretroviral agents. This list is not all inclusive. For additional safety information about SUSTIVA (efavirenz), EMTRIVA (emtricitabine) or VIREAD (tenofovir DF), consult the Product Monographs for these products.

Efavirenz: The most significant adverse events observed in patients treated with efavirenz are nervous system symptoms, psychiatric symptoms, and rash (see Warnings and Precautions). Selected clinical adverse events of moderate or severe intensity reported in ≥2% of efavirenz-treated patients in three controlled clinical trials included abdominal pain, dyspepsia, anorexia, nausea, vomiting, diarrhea, anxiety, insomnia, dizziness, impaired concentration, nervousness, fatigue, pain, abnormal dreams, headache, depression, rash, somnolence, lipodystrophy, and pruritus.

Other adverse events of moderate or severe intensity reported in <2% of patients in all Phase II/III studies as well as post-marketing spontaneous reports included:

Body as a Whole: alcohol intolerance, allergic reaction, asthenia, fever, hot flushes, influenza-like symptoms, malaise, pain, peripheral edema, syncope, dysregulated body temperature, flank pain, hypersensitivity reactions. Redistribution/accumulation of body fat (see Warnings and Precautions, Endocrine and Metabolism, Fat Redistribution).

Cardiovascular: arrhythmia, flushing, palpitations, tachycardia, thrombophlebitis, hypertension, congestive heart failure, chest pain.

Central and Peripheral Nervous System: ataxia, confusion, convulsions, impaired coordination, migraine headaches, neuralgia, parasthesia, hypoesthesia, peripheral neuropathy, speech disorder, stupor, tremor, neuromuscular paresis, paranoid reaction.

Gastrointestinal: dry mouth, pancreatitis, constipation, malabsorption.

Liver and Biliary System: hepatic enzymes increased (including ALT, AST and GGT), hepatitis, jaundice, hepatomegaly (see Post-Market Adverse Drug Reactions).

Metabolic and Nutritional: hypercholesterolemia, hypertriglyceridemia.

Miscellaneous: thrombocytopenia, proteinuria, anemia, pancytopenia, increased sweating.

Psychiatric: aggressive reactions, abnormal thinking, aggravated depression, agitation, delusions, amnesia, anxiety, apathy, delirium, depersonalization, emotional lability, euphoria, hallucination, manic reaction, psychosis, neurosis, paranoia, suicide, suicidal ideation, non-fatal suicide attempts.

Respiratory: asthma, apnea, dyspnea.

Skin and Appendages: acne, alopecia, eczema, folliculitis, skin defoliation, urticaria, erythema nodosum, erythema multiforme, Stevens-Johnson syndrome, verruca, nail disorders, skin disorders, photosensitivity reaction.

Special Senses: abnormal vision, diplopia, glaucoma, iritis, parosmia, taste perversion, tinnitus.

Urinary System: polyuria.
For more information, please consult the SUSTIVA Product Monograph.
Emtricitabine and Tenofovir: Adverse events that occurred in at least 3-5% of patients receiving emtricitabine or tenofovir DF with other antiretroviral agents in clinical trials include: anorexia, anxiety, arthralgia, asthenia, increased cough, depressive disorders, dyspepsia, fever, flatulence, myalgia, pain, abdominal pain, back pain, chest pain, paresthesia, peripheral neuropathy (including peripheral neuritis and neuropathy), pneumonia, rhinitis, rash event (including rash, pruritus, maculopapular rash, urticaria, vesiculobullous rash, pustular rash and allergic reaction), sweating and weight loss. Skin discoloration has been reported with higher frequency among emtricitabine treated patients. Skin discoloration, manifested by hyperpigmentation on the palms and/or soles was generally mild and asymptomatic and of little clinical significance. The mechanism is unknown. In addition to the laboratory abnormalities described for Study 934 (Table 3), Grade 3/4 elevations of bilirubin (>2.5×ULN), pancreatic amylase (>2.0×ULN), serum glucose (<40 or >250 mg/dL), serum lipase (>2.0×ULN), and urine glucose (≥3+) occurred in up to 3% of patients treated with emtricitabine or tenofovir DF with other antiretroviral agents in clinical trials. For more information, please consult the VIREAD and EMTRIVA Product Monographs.
Post-Market Adverse Drug Reactions: In addition to the adverse reaction reports from clinical trials, the following possible adverse reactions have been identified during post-approval use of efavirenz, emtricitabine, or tenofovir DF. Because these events have been reported voluntarily from a population of unknown size, estimates of frequency cannot be made. These events have been considered possible adverse reactions due to a combination of their seriousness, frequency of reporting or potential causal relationship with treatment.
Efavirenz: Additional adverse experiences* reported in postmarketing surveillance include:
Endocrine: gynecomastia.
Eye Disorders: blurred vision.
Immune System Disorders: immune reconstitution syndrome.
Musculoskeletal: rhabdomyolysis.
Nervous System Disorders: cerebellar coordination and balance disturbances.
Psychiatric: neurosis.
Renal and Urinary Disorders: increased CPK.
Skin and Subcutaneous Tissue Disorders: photoallergic dermatitis.
Hepatic failure has been reported post-marketing, including some cases in patients with no pre-existing hepatic disease or other identifiable risk factors and also some cases characterized by a fulminant course, sometimes progressing to transplantation or death.
Additional cases of pancreatitis have been reported in post-marketing surveillance. Please see Warnings and Precautions, Hepatic/Biliary/Pancreatic.
Emtricitabine: The following adverse experiences have been reported in post-marketing experience without regard to causality; some events represent a single report.
Blood and Lymphatic System Disorders: thrombocytopenia.
Gastrointestinal Disorders: pancreatitis.
General Disorders and Administrative Site Conditions: pyrexia.
Metabolism and Nutrition Disorders: lactic acidosis.
Tenofovir DF: Immune System Disorders: allergic reaction (including angioedema).
Metabolism and Nutrition Disorders: lactic acidosis, hypokalemia, hypophosphatemia.
Respiratory, Thoracic and Mediastinal Disorders: dyspnea.
Gastrointestinal Disorders: pancreatitis, increased amylase, abdominal pain.
Hemic and Lymphatic System Disorders: thrombocytopenia.
Hepatobiliary Disorders: hepatic steatosis, hepatitis, increased liver enzymes (most commonly AST, ALT, GGT).
Skin and Subcutaneous Tissue Disorders: rash.
Musculoskeletal and Connective Tissue Disorders: rhabdomyolysis, osteomalacia (manifested as bone pain and infrequently contributing to fractures), muscular weakness, myopathy.
Renal and Urinary Disorders: acute renal failure, renal failure, acute tubular necrosis, Fanconi syndrome, proximal renal tubulopathy, interstitial nephritis (including acute cases), nephrogenic diabetes insipidus, renal insufficiency, increased creatinine, proteinuria, polyuria.
General Disorders and Administrative Site Conditions: asthenia.
The following adverse reactions, listed under the body system headings above, sometimes appeared to be concurrent with proximal renal tubulopathy: rhabdomyolysis, osteomalacia (manifested as bone pain and infrequently contributing to fractures), hypokalemia, muscular weakness, myopathy, hypophosphatemia.
There have been three post marketing reports of acute renal failure in patients on concomitant NSAIDs therapy where a relationship to tenofovir DF could not be excluded. These events mostly occurred in medically complex patients, where underlying disease processes confound interpretation.
Immune Reconstitution Syndrome: In HIV-infected patients with severe immune deficiency at the time of initiation of antiretroviral therapy an inflammatory reaction to infectious pathogens (active or inactive) may arise (see Warnings and Precautions).
Exacerbations of Hepatitis After Discontinuation of Treatment: Tenofovir DF and Emtricitabine-Containing Products: In HIV infected patients coinfected with HBV, clinical and laboratory evidence of exacerbations of hepatitis have occurred after discontinuation of treatment (see Warnings and Precautions, Special Populations, Patients with HIV and Hepatitis B Virus Coinfection).
DRUG INTERACTIONS: Drug-Drug Interactions: No drug interaction studies have been conducted with ATRIPLA tablets. The drug interactions described in Table 7 and Table 8 are based on studies conducted with efavirenz, emtricitabine or tenofovir DF as individual agents or are potential drug interactions. The tables include potentially significant interactions, but may not be inclusive of all potential interactions.

Table 7: ATRIPLA

Drugs That Are Not Recommended for Use with ATRIPLA

Drug Class: Drug Name	Clinical Comment
Antiretrovirals (related drugs): EMTRIVA (emtricitabine), VIREAD (tenofovir DF), TRUVADA (emtricitabine/tenofovir DF), SUSTIVA (efavirenz), HEPSERA (adefovir dipivoxil)	Not for use with ATRIPLA because the active ingredients of EMTRIVA (emtricitabine), VIREAD (tenofovir DF), TRUVADA (emtricitabine/tenofovir DF) and SUSTIVA (efavirenz) are components of ATRIPLA. Coadministration of ATRIPLA with HEPSERA is not recommended due to the possible risk of renal toxicity.
Antiretrovirals (similar drugs): 3TC (lamivudine), Combivir (lamivudine/zidovudine), Heptovir (lamivudine-HBV), Kivexa (abacavir sulfate/lamivudine), Trizivir (abacavir sulfate/lamivudine/zidovudine)l	Lamivudine (3TC), which is similar to emtricitabine, is a component of Combivir, Heptovir, Kivexa, and Trizivir.
Protease inhibitor: Atazanavir	**Not recommended:** Sufficient data are not available to make a dosing recommendation for atazanavir or atazanavir/ritonavir with ATRIPLA. Plasma concentrations of atazanavir were decreased by both efavirenz and tenofovir DF. Atazanavir has been shown to increase tenofovir concentrations.
St. John's Wort (Hypericum perforatum)	**Not recommended:** Expected to substantially decrease plasma levels of efavirenz; has not been studied in combination with efavirenz.

* Those adverse events not already included under Clinical Trial Adverse Drug Reactions, Efavirenz.

Table 8: ATRIPLA

Established[a] and Other Potentially Significant[b] Drug Interactions: Alteration in Dose or Regimen May Be Recommended Based on Drug Interaction Studies or Predicted Interaction

Concomitant Drug Class: Drug Name	Effect[c]	Clinical Comment
Antiretroviral Agents		
Protease Inhibitor: Fosamprenavir calcium	↓ amprenavir concentration	Fosamprenavir (unboosted): Appropriate doses of fosamprenavir and ATRIPLA with respect to safety and efficacy have not been established. Fosamprenavir/ritonavir: An additional 100 mg/day (300 mg total) of ritonavir is recommended when ATRIPLA is administered with fosamprenavir/ritonavir once daily. No change in the ritonavir dose is required when ATRIPLA is administered with fosamprenavir plus ritonavir twice daily.
Protease Inhibitor: Indinavir	↓ indinavir concentration	The optimal dose of indinavir, when given in combination with efavirenz, is not known. Increasing the indinavir dose to 1000 mg every 8 hours does not compensate for the increased indinavir metabolism due to efavirenz.
Protease Inhibitor: Lopinavir/ritonavir	↓ lopinavir concentration ↑ tenofovir concentration	For lopinavir/ritonavir capsules or oral solution, a dose increase to 533/133 mg (4 capsules or 6.5 mL) twice daily taken with food is recommended when used in combination with efavirenz in patients for whom reduced susceptibility to lopinavir is clinically suspected (by treatment history or laboratory evidence). A dose increase of lopinavir/ritonavir tablets to 600/150 mg (3 tablets) twice daily may be considered when used in combination with efavirenz in treatment-experienced patients where decreased susceptibility to lopinavir is clinically suspected (by treatment history or laboratory evidence). **Patients should be monitored for tenofovir-associated adverse events. ATRIPLA should be discontinued in patients who develop tenofovir-associated adverse events.**
CCR5 Co-receptor Antagonist : Maraviroc	↓ maraviroc	Refer to the full prescribing information for maraviroc for guidance on coadministration with ATRIPLA.
Protease Inhibitor: Ritonavir	↑ ritonavir concentration ↑ efavirenz concentration	When ritonavir 500 mg every 12 hours was coadministered with efavirenz 600 mg once daily, the combination was associated with a higher frequency of adverse clinical experiences (eg, dizziness, nausea, paresthesia) and laboratory abnormalities (elevated liver enzymes). Monitoring of liver enzymes is recommended when ATRIPLA is used in combination with ritonavir.
Protease Inhibitor: Saquinavir	↓ saquinavir concentration	Should not be used as sole protease inhibitor in combination with ATRIPLA.
NRTI: Didanosine	↑ didanosine concentration	Higher didanosine concentrations could potentiate didanosine-associated adverse events, including pancreatitis, and neuropathy. **In adults weighing ≥60 kg, the didanosine EC dose should be reduced to 250 mg if coadministered with ATRIPLA. For patients with body weight <60 kg, and creatinine clearance ≥60 mL/min, the recommended dose of ddI-EC is 200 mg. Data are not available to recommend a dose adjustment of didanosine for patients with creatinine clearance <60 mL/min. Coadministration of ATRIPLA and didanosine EC should be undertaken with caution and patients receiving this combination should be monitored closely for didanosine-associated adverse events. For additional information, please consult the Videx/Videx EC (didanosine) prescribing information.**
Other Agents		
Anticoagulant: Warfarin	↑ or ↓ warfarin concentration	Plasma concentrations and effects potentially increased or decreased by efavirenz.
Anticonvulsants: Carbamazepine	↓ carbamazepine concentration ↓ efavirenz concentration	Periodic monitoring of carbamazepine plasma levels should be conducted. There are insufficient data to make a dose recommendation for ATRIPLA. Alternative anticonvulsant treatment should be considered.
Phenytoin Phenobarbital	↓ anticonvulsant concentration ↓ efavirenz concentration	Potential for reduction in anticonvulsant and/or efavirenz plasma levels; periodic monitoring of anticonvulsant plasma levels should be conducted.
Antidepressant: Sertraline	↓ sertraline concentration	It may be necessary to retitrate the sertraline dose to achieve the desired clinical effect. In a drug interaction study in healthy subjects, an increased incidence of impaired concentration was seen in subjects receiving sertraline concomitantly with efavirenz.
Antifungals:		See Contraindications for other antifungals.
Itraconazole	↓ itraconazole concentration ↓ hydroxy-itraconazole concentration	Since no dose recommendation for itraconazole can be made, alternative antifungal treatment should be considered.
Posaconazole	↓ posaconazole	Avoid concomitant use of posaconazole and ATRIPLA unless the benefit to the patient outweighs the risk.
Ketoconazole	↓ ketoconazole concentration	Drug interaction studies with ATRIPLA and ketoconazole have not been conducted. Efavirenz has the potential to decrease plasma concentrations of ketoconazole.

(cont'd)

Table 8: ATRIPLA *(cont'd)*

Established[a] and Other Potentially Significant[b] Drug Interactions: Alteration in Dose or Regimen May Be Recommended Based on Drug Interaction Studies or Predicted Interaction

Concomitant Drug Class: Drug Name	Effect[c]	Clinical Comment
Anti-infective: Clarithromycin	↓ clarithromycin concentration ↑ 14-OH metabolite concentration	Clinical significance unknown. In uninfected volunteers, 46% developed rash while receiving efavirenz and clarithromycin. No dose adjustment of ATRIPLA is recommended when given with clarithromycin. Alternatives to clarithromycin, such as azithromycin, should be considered. Not all macrolide antibiotics have been studied in combination with efavirenz.
Antimycobacterials: Rifabutin	↓ rifabutin concentration	Increase daily dose of rifabutin by 50%. Consider doubling the rifabutin dose in regimens where rifabutin is given 2 or 3 times a week.
Rifampin	↓ efavirenz concentration	An additional 200 mg/day (800 mg total) of efavirenz is recommended when ATRIPLA is administered with rifampin.
Calcium Channel Blockers: Diltiazem	↓ diltiazem ↓ desacetyl diltiazem ↓ N-mono desmethyl diltiazem	Diltiazem levels are markedly decreased when coadministered with efavirenz. Efavirenz levels decreased to a lesser extent (see Table 9 and Table 10). Patients should be closely monitored for possible decreased diltiazem effects and increased adverse events and laboratory abnormalities associated with efavirenz. Refer to the prescribing information for diltiazem for guidance on dose adjustment.
Others (e.g. felodipine, nifedipine, verapamil)	↓ calcium channel blocker	No data are available on the potential interactions of efavirenz with other calcium channel blockers that are substrates of the CYP3A4 enzyme. The potential exists for reduction in plasma concentrations of the calcium channel blocker. Dose adjustments should be guided by clinical response (refer to the prescribing information for the calcium channel blocker).
Immunosuppressants: Cyclosporine, tacrolimus, sirolimus	↓ cyclosporine, tacrolimus, sirolimus concentration	When an immunosuppressant metabolized by CYP3A4 is administered with efavirenz, decreased exposure of the immunosuppressant may be expected due to CYP3A4 induction. Immunosuppressants metabolized by CYP3A4 are not anticipated to affect exposure of efavirenz. There were no clinically significant pharmacokinetic interactions when emtricitabine/tenofovir DF was coadministered with tacrolimus. Dose adjustments of the immunosuppressant may be required when used with ATRIPLA. Close monitoring of immunosuppressant concentrations for at least 2 weeks (until stable concentrations are reached) is recommended when starting or stopping treatment with ATRIPLA.
HMG-CoA Reductase Inhibitors:		Plasma concentrations of atorvastatin, pravastatin, and simvastatin decreased with efavirenz. Consult the complete prescribing information for the HMG-CoA reductase inhibitor for guidance on individualizing the dose.
Atorvastatin	↓ atorvastatin concentration	
Pravastatin	↓ pravastatin concentration	
Simvastatin	↓ simvastatin concentration	
Hormonal Contraceptive:		A reliable method of barrier contraception must be used in addition to hormonal contraceptives.
Oral: Ethinyl estradiol/ Norgestimate	↓ active metabolites of norgestimate	Efavirenz had no effect on ethinyl estradiol concentrations, but progestin levels (norelgestromin and levonorgestrel) were markedly decreased. The clinical significance of these effects is not known. No effect of ethinyl estradiol/norgestimate on efavirenz plasma concentrations was observed.
Implant: Etonogestrel	↓ etonogestrel	The interaction between etonogestrel and efavirenz has not been studied. Decreased exposure of etonogestrel may be expected (CYP3A4 induction), and there have been occasional postmarketing reports of contraceptive failure with etonogestrel in efavirenz-exposed patients.
Narcotic Analgesic: Methadone	↓ methadone concentration	Coadministration of efavirenz in HIV-infected individuals with a history of injection drug use resulted in decreased plasma levels of methadone and signs of opiate withdrawal. Patients should be monitored for signs of withdrawal and their methadone dose increased as required to alleviate withdrawal symptoms.

[a] See Table 9, Table 10, Table 11, Table 12.
[b] This table is not all inclusive.
[c] Increase=↑; Decrease=↓.

Efavirenz: Efavirenz has been shown in vivo to cause hepatic enzyme induction, thus increasing the biotransformation of some drugs metabolized by CYP3A4. In vitro studies have demonstrated that efavirenz inhibits 2C9, 2C19 and 3A4 isozymes in the range of observed efavirenz plasma concentrations. Coadministration of efavirenz with drugs primarily metabolized by these isozymes may result in altered plasma concentrations of the coadministered drug. Therefore, appropriate dose adjustments may be necessary for these drugs.

Drugs which induce CYP3A4 activity (e.g., phenobarbital, rifampin, rifabutin) would be expected to increase the clearance of efavirenz resulting in lowered plasma concentrations.

Drug interaction studies were performed with efavirenz and other drugs likely to be coadministered or drugs commonly used as probes for pharmacokinetic interaction. There was no clinically significant interaction observed between efavirenz and zidovudine, lamivudine, azithromycin, fluconazole, lorazepam, cetirizine, or paroxetine. Single doses of famotidine or an aluminum and magnesium antacid with simethicone had no effects on efavirenz exposures. The effects of coadministration of efavirenz on C_{max} and AUC are summarized in Table 9 (effect of other drugs on efavirenz) and Table 10 (effect of efavirenz on other drugs). (See Contraindications.)

Specific drug interaction studies have not been performed with efavirenz and NRTIs other than lamivudine, zidovudine and tenofovir DF. The steady-state pharmacokinetics of efavirenz and tenofovir were unaffected when efavirenz and tenofovir DF were administered together versus each agent dosed alone. Clinically significant interactions would not be expected since the NRTIs are metabolized via a different route than efavirenz and would be unlikely to compete for the same metabolic enzymes and elimination pathways.

Emtricitabine and Tenofovir DF: The steady state pharmacokinetics of emtricitabine and tenofovir were unaffected when emtricitabine and tenofovir DF were administered together versus each agent dosed alone.

In vitro and clinical pharmacokinetic drug-drug interaction studies have shown that the potential for CYP450 mediated interactions involving emtricitabine and tenofovir with other medicinal products is low.

Emtricitabine and tenofovir are primarily excreted by the kidneys by a combination of glomerular filtration and active tubular secretion. No drug-drug interactions due to competition for renal excretion have been observed. Since emtricitabine and tenofovir are primarily eliminated by the kidneys, coadministration of ATRIPLA with drugs that reduce renal function (see Warnings and Precautions, Renal) or compete for active tubular secretion may increase serum concentrations of emtricitabine, tenofovir, and/or other renally eliminated drugs. Some examples of drugs that compete for active tubular secretion include, but are not limited to cidofovir, acyclovir, valacyclovir, ganciclovir, and valganciclovir.

ATRIPLA should not be administered with HEPSERA (adefovir dipivoxil).

No clinically significant drug interactions have been observed between emtricitabine and famciclovir, indinavir, zidovudine, stavudine, and tenofovir DF. Similarly, no clinically significant drug interactions have been observed between tenofovir DF and abacavir, ribavirin, efavirenz, emtricitabine, entecavir, indinavir, lamivudine, lopinavir/ritonavir, methadone, oral contraceptives, nelfinavir or saquinavir/ritonavir in studies conducted in healthy volunteers.

Atazanavir and lopinavir/ritonavir have been shown to increase tenofovir concentrations (see Table 7 and Table 8). The mechanism of this interaction is unknown. The effects of coadministration of tenofovir on C_{max}, C_{min} and AUC are summarized in Table 11 (effect of other drugs on tenofovir) and Table 12 (effect of tenofovir on other drugs).

Table 9: ATRIPLA

Drug Interactions: Changes in Pharmacokinetic Parameters for Efavirenz in the Presence of the Coadministered Drug

Coadministered Drug	Dose of Coadministered Drug (mg)	Efavirenz Dose (mg)	N	Mean % Change of Efavirenz Pharmacokinetic Parameters[a] C_{max}	AUC	C_{min}
Atazanavir[d]	400 mg qd×20 days	600 mg qd d 7–20	—	↔	↔	NA
Indinavir	800 mg q8h×14 days	200 mg×14 days	11	↔	↔	↔
Lopinavir/Ritonavir	400/100 mg q12h×9 days	600 mg×9 days	11, 12[b]	↔	↓ 16	↓ 16
Nelfinavir	750 mg q8h×7 days	600 mg×7 days	10	↓ 12	↓ 12	↓ 21
Ritonavir	500 mg q12h×8 days	600 mg×10 days	9	↑ 14	↑ 21	↑ 25
Saquinavir SGC[c]	1200 mg q8h×10 days	600 mg×10 days	13	↓ 13	↓ 12	↓ 14
Tenofovir disoproxil fumarate	300 mg qd	600 mg×14 days	30	↔	↔	↔
Clarithromycin	500 mg q12h×7 days	400 mg×7 days	12	↑ 11	↔	↔
Azithromycin	600 mg single dose	400 mg×7 days	14	↔	↔	↔
Rifabutin	300 mg qd×14 days	600 mg×14 days	11	↔	↔	↓ 12
Rifampin	600 mg×7 days	600 mg×7 days	12	↓ 20	↓ 26	↓ 32
Antacid: Aluminiumhydroxide 400 mg Magnesium hydroxide 400 mg + simethicone 30 mg	30 mL single dose	400 mg single dose	17	↔	↔	NA
Carbamazepine	200 mg qd×3 days, 200 mg bid×3 days, then 400 mg qd×15 days	600 mg×35 days	14	↓ 21	↓ 36	↓ 47
Paroxetine	20 mg qd×14 days	600 mg×14 days	12	↔	↔	↔
Sertraline	50 mg qd×14 days	600 mg×14 days	13	↑ 11	↔	↔
Fluconazole	200 mg×7 days	400 mg×7 days	10	↔	↑ 16	↑ 22
Itraconazole	200 mg q 12h×14 days	600 mg×28 days	16	↔	↔	↔
Voriconazole	400 mg po q12h×1 day then 200 mg po q12h×8 days	400 mg×9 days	—	↑ 38	↑ 44	NA
	300 mg po q12h days 2–7	300 mg×7 days	—	↓ 14[e]	↔[e]	NA
	400 mg po q12h days 2–7	300 mg×7 days	—	↔[e]	↑ 17[e]	NA
Diltiazem	240 mg×14 days	600 mg×28 days	12	↑ 16	↑ 11	↑ 13
Cetirizine	10 mg single dose	600 mg×10 days	11	↔	↔	↔
Famotidine	40 mg single dose	400 mg single dose	17	↔	↔	NA
Atorvastatin	10 mg qd×4 days	600 mg×15 days	14	↔	↔	↔
Pravastatin	40 mg qd×4 days	600 mg×15 days	11	↔	↔	↔
Simvastatin	40 mg qd×4 days	600 mg×15 days	14	↓ 12	↔	↓ 12

[a] Increase=↑; Decrease=↓; No Effect=↔.
[b] Parallel-group design; N for efavirenz + lopinavir/ritonavir, N for efavirenz alone.
[c] Soft Gelatin Capsule.
[d] Comparison with historical data suggests that Atazanavir does not affect Efavirenz PK.
[e] Relative to steady-state administration of efavirenz (600 mg once daily for 9 days).

Table 10: ATRIPLA

Drug Interactions: Changes in Pharmacokinetic Parameters for Coadministered Drug in the Presence of Efavirenz

Coadministered Drug	Dose of Coadministered Drug (mg)	Efavirenz Dose (mg)	N	Mean % Change of Coadministered Drug Pharmacokinetic Parameters[a]		
				C_{max}	AUC	C_{min}
Atazanavir	400 mg qd with a light meal d 1–20	600 mg qd with a light meal d 7–20	27	↓ 59	↓ 74	↓ 93
	400 mg qd d 1–6, then 300 mg qd d 7–20 with ritonavir 100 mg qd and a light meal	600 mg qd 2 h after atazanavir and ritonavir d 7–20	13	↑ 14[c]	↑ 39[c]	↓ 48[c]
	300 mg qd/ritonavir 100 mg qd d 1–10 (pm), then 400 mg qd/ritonavir 100 mg qd d 11–24 (pm) (simultaneous with efavirenz)	600 mg qd d 11–24 (pm)	14	↑ 17%	↔	↑ 42
Indinavir	1000 mg q8h×10 days	600 mg×10 days	20			
	After morning dose			↔[d]	↓ 33[d]	↓ 39[d]
	After afternoon dose			↔[d]	↓ 37[d]	↓ 52[d]
	After evening dose			↓ 29[d]	↓ 46[d]	↓ 57[d]
Indinavir/Ritonavir	Indinavir 800 mg + ritonavir 100 mg q12h d 1–29	600 mg d 15–29		↓ 17[e]	↓ 25[e]	↓ 50[e]
Lopinavir/Ritonavir	400/100 mg (capsule) q12h×9 days	600 mg×9 days	11, 7[f]	↔[g]	↓ 19[g]	↓ 39[g]
	600/150 mg (tablet) q12h×10 days with efavirenz compared to 400/100 mg q12h alone	600 mg×9 days	23	↑ 36	↑ 36	↑ 32
Nelfinavir	750 mg q8h×7 days	600 mg×7 days	10	↑ 21	↑ 20	↔
Metabolite AG-1402				↓ 40	↓ 37	↓ 43
Ritonavir	500 mg q12h×8 days	600 mg×10 days	11			
	After AM dose			↑ 24	↑ 18	↑ 42
	After PM dose			↔	↔	↑ 24
Saquinavir SGC[i]	1200 mg q8h×10 days	600 mg×10 days	12	↓ 50	↓ 62	↓ 56
Lamivudine	150 mg q 12 h×14 days	600 mg×14 days	9	↔	↔	↑ 265
Zidovudine	300 mg q 12 h×14 days	600 mg×14 days	9	↔	↔	↑ 225
Tenofovir disoproxil fumarate	300 mg qd	600 mg×14 days	29	↔	↔	↔
Maraviroc	100 mg bid	600 mg qd	12	↓ 51	↓ 45	↓ 45
Clarithromycin	500 mg q12h×7 days	400 mg×7 days	11	↓ 26	↓ 39	↓ 53
14-OH Metabolite				↑ 49	↑ 34	↑ 26
Azithromycin	600 mg single dose	400 mg×7 days	14	↑ 22	↔	NA
Rifabutin 25-0-desacetylrifabutin	300 mg qd×14 days	600 mg×14 days	9	↓ 32 ↓ 49[b]	↓ 38 ↓ 74[b]	↓ 45 NA
Carbamazepine	200 mg qd×3 days, 200 mg bid×3 days, then 400 mg qd×29 days	600 mg×14 days	12	↓ 20	↓ 27	↓ 35
Epoxide Metabolite				↔	↔	↓ 13
Paroxetine	20 mg daily×14 days	600 mg×14 days	16	↔	↔	↔
Oral contraceptive:						
Ethinyl estradiol/	0.035 mg/ 0.25 mg×14 days	600 mg×14 days				
Ethinyl estradiol			21	↔	↔	↔
Norelgestromin			21	↓ 46	↓ 64	↓ 82
Levonorgestrel			6	↓ 80	↓ 83	↓ 86
Methadone	Stable maintenance 35–100 mg daily	600 mg 14–21 days	11	↓ 45	↓ 52	NA
Sertraline	50 mg qd×14 days	600 mg×14 days	13	↓ 29	↓ 39	↓ 46

(cont'd)

Table 10: ATRIPLA *(cont'd)*

Drug Interactions: Changes in Pharmacokinetic Parameters for Coadministered Drug in the Presence of Efavirenz

Coadministered Drug	Dose of Coadministered Drug (mg)	Efavirenz Dose (mg)	N	Mean % Change of Coadministered Drug Pharmacokinetic Parameters[a]		
				C_{max}	AUC	C_{min}
N desmethyl sertraline				↓ 17	↓ 20	↓ 20
Fluconazole	200 mg×7 days	400 mg×7 days	10	↔	↔	↔
Itraconazole Hydro-intraconazole	200 mg q12h×28 days	600 mg×14 days	18	↓ 37 ↓ 35	↓ 39 ↓ 37	↓ 44 ↓ 43
Posaconazole	400 mg (oral suspension) bid×10 and 20 days	400 mg×10 and 20 days		↓ 45	↓ 50	NA
Voriconazole	400 mg po q12h×1 day then 200 mg po q12h×8 days	400 mg×9 days	—	↓ 61	↓ 77	NA
	300 mg po q12h days 2–7	300 mg×7 days	—	↓ 36[h]	↓ 55[h]	NA
	400 mg po q12h days 2–7	300 mg×7 days	—	↑ 23[h]	↔[h]	NA
Lorazepam	2 mg single dose	600 mg×10 days	12	↑ 16	↔	NA
Diltiazem	240 mg×21 days	600 mg×14 days	13	↓ 60	↓ 69	↓ 63
Desacetyl diltiazem				↓ 64	↓ 75	↓ 62
N-monodesmethyl diltiazem				↓ 28	↓ 37	↓ 37
Cetirizine	10 mg single dose	600 mg×10 days	11	↓ 24	↔	NA
Atorvastatin	10 mg qd×4 days	600 mg×15 days	14	↓ 14	↓ 43	↓ 69
Total active (including metabolites)				↓ 15	↓ 32	↓ 48
Pravastatin	40 mg qd×4 days	600 mg×15 days	13	↓ 32	↓ 44	↓ 19
Simvastatin	40 mg qd×4 days	600 mg×15 days	14	↓ 72	↓ 68	↓ 45
Total active (including metabolites)				↓ 68	↓ 60	NA

a Increase=↑; Decrease=↓; No Effect=↔.
b Based on arithmetic means.
c Compared with atazanavir 400 mg qd alone.
d Comparator dose of indinavir was 800 mg q8h×10 days.
e Compared to indinavir 800 twice daily given with ritonavir 100 mg twice daily without efavirenz. The geometric C_{min} for indinavir (0.33 mg/L) when given with ritonavir and efavirenz was higher than the mean historical C_{min} (0.15 mg/L) when indinavir was given alone at 800 mg every 8 hours. When efavirenz 600 mg once daily was given with indinavir/ritonavir 800/100 mg twice daily in HIV-1-infected patients (n=6), the pharmacokinetics of indinavir and efavirenz were generally comparable to these data from uninfected volunteers.
f Parallel-group design; N for efavirenz + lopinavir/ritonavir, N for lopinavir/ritonavir alone.
g Values are for lopinavir. The pharmacokinetics of ritonavir 100 mg q12h are unaffected by concurrent efavirenz.
h Relative to steady-state administration of voriconazole (400 mg for 1 day, then 200 mg po q12h for 2 days).
i Soft Gelatin Capsule.

Table 11: ATRIPLA

Drug Interactions: Changes in Pharmacokinetic Parameters for Tenofovir in the Presence of the Coadministered Drug[a,b]

Coadministered Drug	Dose of Coadministered Drug (mg)	N	Mean % Change of Tenofovir Pharmacokinetic Parameters[c] (90% CI)		
			C_{max}	AUC	C_{min}
Atazanavir[d]	400 once daily×14 days	33	↑ 14 (↑ 8 to ↑ 20)	↑ 24 (↑ 21 to ↑ 28)	↑ 22 (↑ 15 to ↑ 30)
Didanosine (enteric-coated)	400 once	25	↔	↔	↔
Didanosine (buffered)	250 or 400 once daily ×7 days	14	↔	↔	↔
Entecavir	1 mg once daily×10 days	28	↔	↔	↔
Lopinavir/ Ritonavir	400/100 twice daily ×14 days	24	↔	↑ 32 (↑ 25 to ↑ 38)	↑ 51 (↑ 37 to ↑ 66)

a All interaction studies conducted in healthy volunteers.
b Patients received tenofovir DF 300 mg once daily.
c Increase=↑; Decrease=↓; No Effect=↔.
d Reyataz prescribing information.

Table 12: ATRIPLA

Drug Interactions: Changes in Pharmacokinetic Parameters for Coadministered Drug in the Presence of Tenofovir[a,b]

Coadministered Drug	Dose of Coadministered Drug (mg)	N	Mean % Change of Coadministered Drug Pharmacokinetic Parameters[c] (90% CI) C_{max}	AUC	C_{min}
Atazanavir[d]	400 once daily×14 days	34	↓ 21 (↓ 27 to ↓ 14)	↓ 25 (↓ 30 to ↓ 19)	↓ 40 (↓ 48 to ↓ 32)
	Atazanavir/ritonavir 300/100 once daily×42 days	10	↓ 28 (↓ 50 to ↑ 5)	↓ 25[e] (↓ 42 to ↓ 3)	↓ 23[e] (↓ 46 to ↑ 10)
Entecavir	1 mg once daily×10 days	28	↔	↑ 13 (↑ 11 to ↑ 15)	↔
Lopinavir	Lopinavir/ritonavir 400/100 twice daily×14 days	24	↔	↔	↔
Ritonavir	Lopinavir/ritonavir 400/100 twice daily×14 days	24	↔	↔	↔

a All interaction studies conducted in healthy volunteers.
b Patients received tenofovir DF 300 mg once daily.
c Increase=↑; Decrease=↓; No Effect=↔.
d Reyataz prescribing information.
e In HIV-infected patients, addition of tenofovir DF to atazanavir 300 mg plus ritonavir 100 mg, resulted in AUC and C_{min} values of atazanavir that were 2.3- and 4-fold higher than the respective values observed for atazanavir 400 mg when given alone.

Coadministration of tenofovir DF with didanosine results in changes in the pharmacokinetics of didanosine that may be of clinical significance. Table 13 summarizes the effects of tenofovir DF on the pharmacokinetics of didanosine. Concomitant dosing of tenofovir DF with didanosine buffered tablets or enteric-coated capsules significantly increased the C_{max} and AUC of didanosine. When didanosine 250 mg enteric-coated capsules were administered with tenofovir DF, systemic exposures of didanosine were similar to those seen with the 400 mg enteric-coated capsules alone under fasted conditions. The mechanism of this interaction is unknown. **Increases in didanosine concentrations of this magnitude could potentiate didanosine-associated adverse events, including pancreatitis, lactic acidosis, and neuropathy.** In addition, suppression of CD4 counts has been observed in patients receiving tenofovir DF with didanosine at a dose of 400 mg daily.

Therefore, the recommended dose of didanosine EC is 250 mg for HIV infected adults with body weight ≥60 kg and creatinine clearance ≥60 mL/min when coadministered with ATRIPLA. For patients with body weight <60 kg, and creatinine clearance ≥60 mL/min, the recommended dose of ddI-EC is 200 mg. Data are not available to recommend a dose adjustment of didanosine for patients with creatinine clearance <60 mL/min (for didanosine EC dosing adjustment recommendations, see Table 8). **Coadministration of ATRIPLA and didanosine should be undertaken with caution and patients receiving this combination should be monitored closely for didanosine-associated adverse events.**

Caution should be used when coadministering reduced-dose didanosine, tenofovir, and an NNRTI in treatment-naïve patients with high viral loads at baseline since such use has been associated with reports of a high rate of virologic failure and emergence of resistance at an early stage. All patients receiving tenofovir disoproxil fumarate and didanosine concomitantly should be closely monitored for didanosine-related adverse events and clinical response.

Table 13: ATRIPLA

Drug Interactions: Changes in Pharmacokinetic Parameters for Didanosine in the Presence of Tenofovir Disoproxil Fumarate[a,b]

Didanosine Dose (mg)/ Method of Administration[d]	Tenofovir DF Method of Administration[b,d]	N	Mean % Change (90% CI) vs. Didanosine 400 mg Alone, Fasted[c] C_{max}	AUC
Buffered Tablets				
400 once daily[e]×7 days	Fasted 1 hour after didanosine	14	↑ 28 (↑ 11 to ↑ 48)	↑ 44 (↑ 31 to ↑ 59)
Enteric Coated Capsules				
400 Once, Fasted	With food, 2 h after didanosine	26	↑ 48 (↑ 25 to ↑ 76)	↑ 48 (↑ 31 to ↑ 67)
400 Once, with Food	Simultaneously with didanosine	26	↑ 64 (↑ 41 to ↑ 89)	↑ 60 (↑ 44 to ↑ 79)
250 Once, Fasted	With food, 2 h after didanosine	28	↓ 10 (↓ 22 to ↑ 3)	↔
250 Once, Fasted	Simultaneously with didanosine	28	↔	↑ 14 (0 to ↑ 31)
250 Once, with Food	Simultaneously with didanosine	28	↓ 29 (↓ 39 to ↓18)	↓ 11 (↓ 23 to ↑ 2)

a All interaction studies conducted in healthy volunteers.
b Patients received tenofovir DF 300 mg once daily.
c Increase=↑; Decrease=↓; No Effect=↔.
d Administration with food was with a light meal (~373 kcal, 20% fat).
e Includes 4 subjects weighing <60 kg receiving ddI 250 mg.

Drug-Food Interactions: Interactions of ATRIPLA with food have not been established. In studies of the individual components of ATRIPLA, increased efavirenz and tenofovir concentrations were observed following administration with food (see Action and Clinical Pharmacology, Effect of Food on Oral Absorption).

Drug-Herb Interactions: Interactions of ATRIPLA with herbs have not been established. St. John's Wort is expected to substantially decrease plasma levels of efavirenz but has not been studied in combination with efavirenz. ATRIPLA should not be coadministered with St. John's Wort.

Drug-Laboratory Test Interactions: Interactions of ATRIPLA with laboratory tests have not been established.

Efavirenz Assay Interference: Cannabinoid Test Interaction: Efavirenz does not bind to cannabinoid receptors. False-positive urine cannabinoid test results have been observed in non-HIV-infected volunteers receiving efavirenz when the Microgenics Cedia DAU Multi-Level THC assay was used for screening. Negative results were obtained when more specific confirmatory testing was performed with gas chromatography/mass spectrometry. For more information, please consult the SUSTIVA Product Monograph.

DOSAGE AND ADMINISTRATION: The dose of ATRIPLA is one tablet (containing 600 mg of efavirenz, 200 mg of emtricitabine and 300 mg of tenofovir disoproxil fumarate) once daily taken orally on an empty stomach. Dosing at bedtime may improve the tolerability of nervous system symptoms (see Warnings and Precautions, Neurologic and Information for the Patient).

Dose Adjustment for Renal Impairment: Because ATRIPLA is a fixed-dose combination, it should not be prescribed for patients requiring dosage adjustment such as those with moderate to severe renal impairment (creatinine clearance <50 mL/min).

Missed Dose: If a patient misses a dose at the regularly scheduled time, but then remembers it that same day, the patient should take the missed dose immediately. The patient should **not** take more than 1 dose of ATRIPLA in a day.

OVERDOSAGE:

If overdose occurs the patient must be monitored for evidence of toxicity, and standard supportive treatment applied as necessary including monitoring of vital signs and observation of the patient's clinical status. Administration of activated charcoal may be used to aid removal of efavirenz. Hemodialysis can remove both emtricitabine and tenofovir DF (refer to information below), but, since efavirenz is highly protein bound, dialysis is unlikely to significantly remove the drug from blood. There is no specific antidote for overdose with efavirenz.

Efavirenz: Some patients accidentally taking 600 mg twice daily have reported increased nervous system symptoms. One patient experienced involuntary muscle contractions and a second patient experienced vomiting after taking twice the recommended dose.

Emtricitabine: Limited clinical experience is available at doses higher than the therapeutic dose of EMTRIVA. In one clinical pharmacology study single doses of emtricitabine 1200 mg were administered to 11 patients. No severe adverse reactions were reported. The effects of higher doses are not known.

Hemodialysis treatment removes approximately 30% of the emtricitabine dose over a 3 hour dialysis period starting within 1.5 hours of emtricitabine dosing (blood flow rate of 400 mL/min and a dialysate flow rate of 600 mL/min), however, a single treatment does not significantly affect emtricitabine C_{max} or AUC. It is not known whether emtricitabine can be removed by peritoneal dialysis.

Tenofovir DF: Limited clinical experience is available at doses higher than the therapeutic dose of tenofovir DF 300 mg. In one study, 600 mg tenofovir DF was administered to 8 patients orally for 28 days. No severe adverse reactions were reported. The effects of higher doses are not known.

Tenofovir is efficiently removed by hemodialysis with an extraction coefficient of approximately 54%. Following a single 300 mg dose of tenofovir DF, a four-hour hemodialysis session removed approximately 10% of the administered tenofovir dose.

For management of a suspected drug overdose, contact your regional Poison Control Centre. See the *CPS* Directory section for a list of Poison Control Centres.

ACTION AND CLINICAL PHARMACOLOGY: Mechanism of Action: Efavirenz: Efavirenz is a non-nucleoside reverse transcriptase (RT) inhibitor of human immunodeficiency virus type 1 (HIV-1). Efavirenz is predominantly a non-competitive inhibitor of HIV-1 RT. HIV-2 RT and human cellular DNA polymerases α, β, γ, and δ are not inhibited by efavirenz.

Emtricitabine: Emtricitabine, a synthetic nucleoside analog of cytidine, is phosphorylated by cellular enzymes to form emtricitabine 5'-triphosphate. Emtricitabine 5'-triphosphate inhibits the activity of the HIV-1 RT by competing with the natural substrate deoxycytidine 5'-triphosphate and by being incorporated into nascent viral DNA which results in chain termination. Emtricitabine 5'-triphosphate is a weak inhibitor of mammalian DNA polymerases α, β, ε, and mitochondrial DNA polymerase γ.

Tenofovir DF: Tenofovir DF is an acyclic nucleoside phosphonate diester analog of adenosine monophosphate. Tenofovir DF requires initial diester hydrolysis for conversion to tenofovir and subsequent phosphorylations by cellular enzymes to form tenofovir diphosphate. Tenofovir diphosphate inhibits the activity of HIV-1 RT by competing with the natural substrate deoxyadenosine 5'-triphosphate and, after incorporation into DNA, by DNA chain termination. Tenofovir diphosphate is a weak inhibitor of mammalian DNA polymerases α, β, and mitochondrial DNA polymerase γ.

Pharmacodynamics: Antiviral Activity In Vitro: Efavirenz, Emtricitabine and Tenofovir DF: In combination studies evaluating the in vitro antiviral activity of efavirenz and emtricitabine together, efavirenz and tenofovir together and emtricitabine and tenofovir together, additive to synergistic antiviral effects were observed.

Efavirenz: The concentration of efavirenz inhibiting replication of wild-type laboratory adapted strains and clinical isolates in cell culture by 90-95% (EC_{90-95}) ranged from 1.7-25 nM in lymphoblastoid cell lines, peripheral blood mononuclear cells, and macrophage/monocyte cultures. Efavirenz demonstrated antiviral activity against most non-clade B isolates (subtypes A, AE, AG, C, D, F, G, J, and N), but had reduced antiviral activity against group O viruses.

Emtricitabine: The in vitro antiviral activity of emtricitabine against laboratory and clinical isolates of HIV was assessed in lymphoblastoid cell lines, the MAGI-CCR5 cell line, and peripheral blood mononuclear cells. The EC_{50} (50% effective concentration) values for emtricitabine were in the range of 0.0013-0.64 μM (0.0003-0.158 μg/mL). Emtricitabine displayed antiviral activity in vitro against HIV-1 clades A, B, C, D, E, F, and G (EC_{50} values ranged from 0.007-0.075 μM) and showed strain specific activity against HIV-2 (EC_{50} values ranged from 0.007-1.5 μM).

Tenofovir DF: The antiviral activity in cell culture of tenofovir against laboratory and clinical isolates of HIV-1 was assessed in lymphoblastoid cell lines, primary monocyte/macrophage cells and peripheral blood lymphocytes. The EC_{50} values for tenofovir were in the range of 0.04-8.5 μM. Tenofovir displayed antiviral activity in vitro against HIV-1 clades A, B, C, D, E, F, G, and O (EC_{50} values ranged from 0.5-2.2 μM) and showed strain specific activity against HIV-2 (EC_{50} values ranged from 1.6 μM to 4.9 μM).

Pharmacokinetics: ATRIPLA: One ATRIPLA Tablet was bioequivalent to one SUSTIVA tablet (600 mg) plus one EMTRIVA Capsule (200 mg) plus one VIREAD Tablet (300 mg) following single-dose administration to fasting healthy subjects (N=45).

Efavirenz: In HIV-infected patients time-to-peak plasma concentrations were approximately 3-5 hours and steady-state plasma concentrations were reached in 6-10 days. In 35 patients receiving efavirenz 600 mg once daily, steady-state C_{max} was 12.9 μM, C_{min} was 5.6 μM, and AUC was 184 μM/h. Efavirenz is highly bound (approximately 99.5-99.75%) to human plasma proteins, predominantly albumin. Following administration of ^{14}C-labeled efavirenz, 14-34% of the dose was recovered in the urine (mostly as metabolites) and 16-61% was recovered in feces (mostly as parent drug).

In vitro studies suggest CYP3A4 and CYP2B6 are the major isozymes responsible for efavirenz metabolism. Efavirenz has been shown to induce P450 enzymes, resulting in induction of its own metabolism.

Efavirenz has been shown in vivo to cause hepatic enzyme induction, thus increasing the biotransformation of some drugs metabolized by CYP3A4. In vitro studies have demonstrated that efavirenz inhibits 2C9, 2C19 and 3A4 isozymes with K_i values (8.5-17 μM) in the range of observed efavirenz plasma concentrations. In in vitro studies, efavirenz did not inhibit CYP2E1 and inhibited CYP2D6 and CYP1A2 (K_i values 82-160 μM) only at concentrations well above those achieved clinically. Coadministration of efavirenz with drugs primarily metabolized by 2C9, 2C19, and 3A4 isozymes may result in altered plasma concentrations of the coadministered drug. Drugs which induce CYP3A4 activity would be expected to increase the clearance of efavirenz resulting in lowered plasma concentrations.

Efavirenz plasma exposure may be increased in patients with the homozygous G156T genetic variant of the CYP2B6 isozyme. The clinical implications of such an association are unknown; however, the potential for an increased frequency and severity of efavirenz-associated adverse events cannot be excluded.

Efavirenz has a terminal half-life of 52-76 hours after single doses and 40-55 hours after multiple doses.

Emtricitabine: Following oral administration, emtricitabine is rapidly absorbed with peak plasma concentrations occurring at 1-2 hours post-dose. In vitro binding of emtricitabine to human plasma proteins is <4% and is independent of concentration over the range of 0.02-200 μg/mL. Following administration of radiolabelled emtricitabine, approximately 86% is recovered in the urine and 13% is recovered as metabolites. The metabolites of emtricitabine include 3'-sulfoxide diastereomers and their glucuronic acid conjugate. Emtricitabine is eliminated by a combination of glomerular filtration and active tubular secretion. Following a single oral dose, the plasma emtricitabine half-life is approximately 10 hours.

Tenofovir DF: Following oral administration of tenofovir DF, maximum tenofovir serum concentrations are achieved in 1.0±0.4 hour. In vitro binding of tenofovir to human plasma proteins is <0.7% and is independent of concentration over the range of 0.01-25 μg/mL. Approximately 70-80% of the intravenous dose of tenofovir is recovered as unchanged drug in the urine. Tenofovir is eliminated by a combination of glomerular filtration and active tubular secretion. Following a single oral dose of tenofovir DF, the terminal elimination half-life of tenofovir is approximately 17 hours.

Effect of Food on Oral Absorption: ATRIPLA has not been evaluated in the presence of food. Administration of efavirenz tablets with a high fat meal increased the mean AUC and C_{max} of efavirenz by 28% and 79%, respectively, compared to administration in the fasted state. Compared to fasted administration, dosing of tenofovir DF/emtricitabine in combination with either a high fat meal or a light meal increased the mean AUC and C_{max} of tenofovir by 35% and 15%, respectively, without affecting emtricitabine exposures.

Special Populations and Conditions: Pediatrics and Geriatrics: Pharmacokinetics of tenofovir have not been evaluated in children (<18 years). Efavirenz has not been studied in children below 3 years of age or who weigh less than 13 kg. Emtricitabine has been studied in pediatric patients from 3 months to 17 years of age. ATRIPLA is not recommended for pediatric administration. Pharmacokinetics of efavirenz, emtricitabine, and tenofovir have not been fully evaluated in the elderly (>65 years).

Race: Efavirenz: The pharmacokinetics of efavirenz in patients appear to be similar among the ethnic groups studied.
Emtricitabine: No pharmacokinetic differences due to race have been identified following the administration of emtricitabine.
Tenofovir DF: There were insufficient numbers from racial and ethnic groups other than Caucasian to adequately determine potential pharmacokinetic differences among these populations following administration of tenofovir DF.
Gender: Efavirenz, emtricitabine and tenofovir pharmacokinetics are similar in male and female patients.
Hepatic Insufficiency: The pharmacokinetics of tenofovir following a 300 mg single dose of tenofovir DF have been studied in non-HIV infected subjects with moderate to severe hepatic impairment. There were no substantial alterations in tenofovir pharmacokinetics in subjects with hepatic impairment compared with unimpaired subjects. The pharmacokinetics of efavirenz or emtricitabine have not been studied in patients with hepatic impairment; however, emtricitabine has not been shown to be significantly metabolized by liver enzymes, so the impact of liver impairment should be limited (see Warnings and Precautions, Hepatic/Biliary/Pancreatic).
Renal Insufficiency: The pharmacokinetics of efavirenz have not been studied in patients with renal insufficiency; however, less than 1% of efavirenz is excreted unchanged in the urine, so the impact of renal impairment on efavirenz elimination should be minimal. The pharmacokinetics of emtricitabine and tenofovir are altered in patients with renal insufficiency (see Warnings and Precautions, Renal, Nephrotoxicity). In patients with creatinine clearance <50 mL/min, C_{max} and $AUC_{0-\infty}$ of emtricitabine and tenofovir were increased. Because ATRIPLA is a fixed dose combination, it should not be prescribed for patients requiring dosage adjustment such as those with moderate to severe renal impairment (creatinine clearance <50 mL/min).

STORAGE AND STABILITY: Store at 15-30°C. Keep container tightly closed. Dispense only in original container. Do not use if seal over bottle opening is broken or missing.

SPECIAL HANDLING INSTRUCTIONS: There are no special handling instructions.

INFORMATION FOR THE PATIENT: Published in e-CPS, available by subscription at www.e-cps.ca.

DOSAGE FORMS, COMPOSITION AND PACKAGING: Each pink, capsule-shaped, film-coated tablet, debossed with "123" on one side and plain-faced on the other side contains: efavirenz 600 mg, emtricitabine 200 mg and tenofovir disoproxil fumarate 300 mg (which is equivalent to 245 mg of tenofovir disoproxil). Nonmedicinal ingredients: croscarmellose sodium, hydroxypropyl cellulose, magnesium stearate, microcrystalline cellulose and sodium lauryl sulfate; Opadry II Pink 85F94172 coating: iron oxide black, iron oxide red, polyethylene glycol, polyvinyl alcohol, talc, and titanium dioxide. Bottles of 30 with a silica gel desiccant, closed with a child-resistant closure.

Atropine Sulfate Injection, USP

atropine sulfate

Anticholinergic

Hospira

SUPPLIED: Each mL contains: atropine sulfate monohydrate 0.1 mg (100 µg). Nonmedicinal ingredients: sodium chloride, sulfuric acid and/or sodium hydroxide and water for injection. Syringes of 5 and 10 mL, boxes of 10.

Atropine Sulfate Injection USP

atropine sulfate

Anticholinergic

Sandoz

SUPPLIED: 0.4 mg/mL, Preservative-free formulation: Each mL contains: atropine sulfate 0.4 mg, sodium chloride for isotonicity, sulfuric acid to adjust pH and water for injection. Ampoules of 1 mL, boxes of 10. Store between 15 and 30°C.
0.4 mg/mL, multidose formulation: Each mL contains: atropine sulfate 0.4 mg, chlorobutanol 0.5% (as preservative), ethanol, sodium chloride for tonicity, sulfuric acid to adjust pH and water for injection. Multidose vials of 10 mL, boxes of 10. Store between 15 and 30°C. Protect from light. Discard 28 days after initial use.
0.6 mg/mL, Preservative-free formulation: Each mL contains: atropine sulfate 0.6 mg, sodium chloride, sulfuric acid to adjust pH and water for injection. Ampoules of 1 mL, boxes of 10. Store between 15 and 30°C.

Atropine: Systemic

Anticholinergic

CPhA Monograph

Date of Revision: June 2009

> This monograph has been compiled by CPhA and reviewed by experts. It may contain information different from that found in Health Canada-approved Product Monographs. The reader is referred to the *CPS* Editorial Policy for more information.

SUMMARY PRODUCT INFORMATION:

Route of Administration	Dosage Form	Product Strength
Parenteral (im, iv, sc)	Solution	0.1 mg/mL
Parenteral (im, iv, sc)	Solution	0.4 mg/mL
Parenteral (im, iv, sc)	Solution	0.6 mg/mL

INDICATIONS AND CLINICAL USE: Atropine is used during cardiopulmonary resuscitation for its anticholinergic positive chronotropic effect. It is recommended for symptomatic sinus bradycardia, asystole, slow pulseless electrical activity or symptomatic heart block at nodal level or above. See the Advanced Cardiac Life Support (ACLS) guidelines for the role of atropine in cardiac arrest. Generally, atropine may reverse sinus bradycardia when it is secondary to extracardiac causes. Atropine has little effect when bradycardia is caused by intrinsic disease of the SA node.

Atropine can reverse decreased heart rate, blood pressure and systemic vascular resistance that is cholinergically mediated. It is indicated in the management of acute myocardial infarction (AMI) in the following situations (from early onset to 6 to 8 hours afterwards): patients with sinus bradycardia with low cardiac output and peripheral hypoperfusion or frequent premature ventricular complexes (PVC) at onset of symptoms of AMI; acute inferior infarction with type I second- or third-degree AV block associated with symptoms of hypotension, ventricular arrhythmias or ischemic discomfort; in myocardial infarction patients receiving nitroglycerin who are experiencing hypotension and sustained bradycardia or those receiving morphine who have nausea and vomiting; ventricular asystole. It is also used for symptomatic inferior infarcts and type I second or third-degree heart block at the AV node (i.e., with narrow QRS complex or with known existing bundle-branch block).

There is less evidence supporting the use of atropine for: second- or third-degree AV block of uncertain mechanism when pacing is not an option; asymptomatic patients with inferior infarction and type I second-degree heart block or third-degree heart block at the AV node; concomitant administration with morphine in the presence of sinus bradycardia.

Atropine could be harmful or ineffective for: type II AV block and third-degree AV block and third-degree AV block with new wide QRS complex (presumed acute myocardial infarction); sinus bradycardia that is greater than 40 bpm without hypoperfusion or frequent PVC.

Diagnostically, atropine is used for myocardial infarction in patients with Wolff-Parkinson-White syndrome. It is also used to assess sinus node dysfunction and during atrial pacing in the evaluation of coronary artery disease. It is used to treat sinus bradycardia caused by drugs or toxic substances that have cholinergic effects such as pilocarpine, organophosphate pesticides or Amanita muscaria mushrooms.

During hypotonic radiography atropine may be used to relax the upper GI tract and colon although glucagon is often preferred.

Although not needed as commonly with newer anesthetics, atropine can be given preoperatively as an antisialogogue to reduce salivation and excessive respiratory secretions. It is also used to prevent cholinergic effects which result from vagal stimulation during surgery (e.g., bradycardia, hypotension, cardiac arrhythmias). It is used with anticholinesterase agents (e.g., neostigmine, physostigmine, pyridostigmine) after surgery to terminate curarization.

In conjunction with a cholinesterase reactivator (e.g., pralidoxime), atropine is used in the treatment of organophosphate insecticide poisoning and nerve agent poisoning in terrorism or chemical warfare.

Pediatrics: Because hypoxia commonly causes bradycardia in children, atropine should not be used until the child has received adequate oxygenation and ventilation. See pediatric ACLS guidelines for the place of atropine in cardiac arrest.

CONTRAINDICATIONS: Atropine as an injection is contraindicated in patients with pyloric stenosis, thyrotoxicosis, obstructive gastrointestinal disease, paralytic ileus or prostatic hypertrophy (which may lead to bladder neck obstruction). It should not be used in patients with tachycardia or during acute hemorrhage in patients with unstable cardiovascular status or in those with severe ulcerative colitis or toxic megacolon. It is contraindicated in patients with myasthenia gravis unless it is being used to treat adverse effects caused by acetylcholinesterase inhibitors (e.g., neostigmine). Atropine is also contraindicated in patients with narrow-angle glaucoma. It is contraindicated in patients who are hypersensitive to any ingredient in the formulation or component of the container.

WARNINGS AND PRECAUTIONS:

> Atropine is a highly potent drug and due care is essential to avoid overdosage, especially with iv administration. Children are more susceptible than adults to the toxic effects of anticholinergic agents (e.g., agitation, confusion, drowsiness). Atropine may cause increased intraocular pressure leading to acute glaucoma and blindness, especially if the increase in pressure is maintained for an extended period. Use cautiously in patients with Down syndrome.

General: Especially in patients exposed to high environmental temperatures, atropine use may result in heat prostration characterized by fever and heat stroke due to decreased sweating. This risk may be increased in patients who are already febrile.

In patients with ileostomy or colostomy, diarrhea may be an early symptom of incomplete intestinal obstruction. Therefore treatment of diarrhea with atropine is not appropriate and could be harmful.

Cardiovascular: Investigate any tachycardia before giving atropine, as its administration may increase the heart rate. Parenteral atropine should be used with caution in patients with coronary heart disease, congestive heart failure, cardiac arrhythmias, tachycardia or hypertension.

Endocrine and Metabolism: Use parenteral atropine with caution in patients with hyperthyroidism as they may be tachycardic secondary to thyrotoxicosis.

Gastrointestinal: Anticholinergic drugs may produce a delay in gastric emptying time and may complicate oral treatment regimens or gastric ulcer. Atropine should also not be used in patients with GI infections (e.g., antibiotic-associated pseudomembranous colitis) as it may result in the causative organism/toxin being retained as a result of its effect on gastric motility.

Use parenteral atropine with caution in older individuals and in all patients with diarrhea. Large doses of atropine may suppress intestinal motility to the point of producing a paralytic ileus, which may precipitate or aggravate toxic megacolon especially in those with ulcerative colitis.

Atropine should be used with caution in patients with hiatal hernia associated with reflux esophagitis.

Conventional systemic doses may convert partial pyloric stenosis into complete obstruction.

Genitourinary: Conventional systemic doses may lead to complete urinary retention in patients with prostatic hypertrophy.

Hepatic/Biliary/Pancreatic: Use parenteral atropine with caution in patients with hepatic disease.

Neurologic: Use parenteral atropine with caution in patients with autonomic neuropathy as these patients are already at risk of urinary retention and constipation.

Ophthalmologic: Conventional systemic doses may precipitate acute glaucoma in susceptible patients, therefore an estimation of the depth of the angle of the anterior chamber should precede the use of atropine.

Renal: Parenteral atropine should be used with caution in patients with renal disease. Half-life may be prolonged in patients with renal dysfunction.

Respiratory: Conventional systemic doses may cause drying of bronchial secretions leading to formation of dangerous viscid plugs in the presence of chronic lung disease. To produce bronchodilation, administer atropine via oral inhalation.

Special Populations: Pregnancy: Use atropine with caution in pregnant women. Atropine crosses the placenta. Atropine as a premedication prior to cesarean section has not been associated with adverse fetal or neonatal effects. As a class, anticholinergics may be associated with minor malformations; however, there appears to be no specific link between gestational use of atropine and congenital malformations.

Lactation: The American Academy of Pediatrics considers use of atropine compatible with breastfeeding. The drug is possibly excreted in small amounts in breast milk and may decrease milk flow. However documentation is scant or conflicting. Infants of nursing mothers should be monitored for anticholinergic side effects.

Pediatrics: Children are more susceptible than adults to the toxic effects of anticholinergic agents. Atropine should be used with caution in children with spastic paralysis or brain damage.

Geriatrics: Atropine should be used with caution in the elderly (use with caution in all individuals over 40 years of age). Antimuscarinic agents, including atropine, may cause an increase in intraocular pressure leading to acute glaucoma and blindness, particularly if the increase in pressure is maintained for an extended period.

The elderly are at an increased risk for developing side effects such as delirium, confusion and hallucinations. Even small doses of atropine may result in excitement, agitation or drowsiness.

Occupational Hazards: Atropine may produce drowsiness, dizziness or blurred vision; caution patients who will be driving or performing other tasks requiring alertness.

ADVERSE REACTIONS: Adverse Drug Reaction Overview: Adverse effects of atropine are most often the result of excessive dosage. Most of the side effects of atropine are directly related to its antimuscarinic action.

Common Adverse Drug Reactions (1 to >10%): CNS: headache, restlessness, insomnia or dizziness.
Cardiovascular: tachycardia.
Dermatologic: dry, hot skin; light sensitivity.
Ophthalmologic: blurred vision, mydriasis.
Gastrointestinal: dry mouth, dysphagia, impaired GI motility and constipation.
Local: irritation at site of injection.
Less Common Adverse Drug Reactions (<1%): Autonomic: urinary retention.
Cardiovascular: palpitations and bradycardia following low-dose atropine (as low doses may be parasympathomimetic); arrhythmias, heart block, hypertension, increased myocardial ischemia or angina.
CNS: ataxia, disorientation, confusion, excitation, somnolence, headache, seizures, psychosis; delirium, hallucinations, respiratory depression and coma have been reported, mainly with administration of toxic doses.
Dermatologic: dry skin, flushing.
Gastrointestinal: vomiting, bloating, adynamic ileus.
Genitourinary: urinary hesitancy or retention, impotence.
Hematologic: leukocytosis.
Immune: severe allergic reactions, including anaphylaxis.
Ophthalmologic: photophobia, increased intraocular pressure, cycloplegia.
Psychiatric: hallucinations, delirium, excitement, agitation, confusion, especially in geriatric patients.
Miscellaneous: anaphylaxis (rare).

DRUG INTERACTIONS: Because atropine may slow GI motility, the bioavailability of nitrofurantoin and thiazide-diuretics may be increased. Atropine antagonizes the effects of metoclopramide on GI motility.

Table 1: Atropine

Drug-Drug Interactions

Interacting Drug	Effect	Clinical Comment
Amantadine	Increased anticholinergic activity (additive effect); confusion and hallucinations have been reported	Be alert for CNS effects when amantadine is combined with atropine. Consider decreasing dose of atropine.

(cont'd)

Table 1: Atropine *(cont'd)*

Drug-Drug Interactions

Interacting Drug	Effect	Clinical Comment
Anticholinergic agents	Increased effect of atropine	Be alert for excessive anticholinergic adverse effects (e.g., xerostomia, blurred vision, constipation).
Antihistamines (with anticholinergic activity)	Possible additive anticholinergic activity	Consider using an antihistamine with less anticholinergic activity. Monitor patient for troublesome anticholinergic effects (e.g., xerostomia, blurred vision, constipation).
Atenolol	Anticholinergics can increase heart rate (causing decreased bradycardic effects of atenolol) and may increase atenolol bioavailability, probably by slowing GI motility. Metoprolol and propranolol do not appear to be affected	No specific action is required, but be alert for evidence of the interaction.
Digoxin	Increased digoxin levels	Use with caution; monitor patient for signs of digitalis toxicity.
Disopyramide	Possible additive anticholinergic effects	Consider using an alternate antiarrhythmic with less anticholinergic activity; monitor patient for troublesome anticholinergic effects (e.g., xerostomia, blurred vision, constipation).
Levodopa	Decreased effect of levodopa	Monitor closely, increasing levodopa dose if necessary.
Meperidine	Possible additive anticholinergic effects	Consider using an alternate analgesic with less anticholinergic activity; monitor patient for troublesome anticholinergic effects (e.g., xerostomia, blurred vision, constipation).
Phenothiazines	Effects are variable: may worsen schizophrenic symptoms and decrease phenothiazine serum concentrations. Additive anticholinergic effects may result in paralytic ileus or heat stroke (both potentially fatal)	Routinely monitor patient for evidence of decreased phenothiazine effects and for symptoms of onset of adynamic ileus (e.g., constipation, abdominal pain, distention). Patient should take precautions to avoid heat stroke.
Tricyclic antidepressants (TCAs)	Additive anticholinergic effects	Use an antidepressant with less anticholinergic effect (e.g., trazodone, desipramine). Pyridoxine may prevent some anticholinergic side effects due to TCAs. Monitor patient for excessive anticholinergic effects (e.g., xerostomia, blurred vision, constipation).

Table 2: Atropine

Drug-Herb Interactions

Interacting Herb	Effect	Clinical Comment
Belladonna	Possible additive anticholinergic effects	Theoretical interaction resulting from belladonna's noted anticholinergic activity.
Henbane leaf	Possible additive anticholinergic effects	Theoretical interaction resulting from henbane leaf's noted anticholinergic activity.
Scopolia root	Possible additive anticholinergic effects	Theoretical interaction resulting from scopolia root's noted anticholinergic activity.
Yohimbe	Atropine may lower increased blood pressure caused by yohimbe. Atropine in moderate to high doses may increase yohimbe toxicity	Consider avoiding combination to decrease risk of toxicity.

DOSAGE AND ADMINISTRATION: Dosing Considerations:

Table 3: Atropine

Dose in Adult Patients[a]

Indication	Route	Usual Dose
Antimuscarinic	im, iv, sc	0.4–0.6 mg repeated after 4 to 6 h if necessary
Cardiopulmonary resuscitation Bradycardia	iv[b]	0.5 mg every 3 to 5 minutes to a total dose of 3 mg. Avoid doses less than 0.5 mg in adults as low doses may cause bradycardia.
Cardiopulmonary resuscitation Ventricular asystole and slow pulseless electrical activity (PEA)	iv[b]	1 mg; may repeat every 3 to 5 minutes to a total dose of 3 mg. 3 mg (0.04 mg/kg) will produce full vagal blockade; reserve this dose for asystolic cardiac arrest.
Hypotonic gastrointestinal radiography	im	1 mg
Preanesthesia (antisialagogue)	im, sc	0.2–0.6 mg 30 to 60 minutes before surgery
Cholinergic adjunct (curariform block)	iv	0.6–1.2 mg a few minutes before 0.5–2.5 mg of neostigmine or 10–20 mg of pyridostigmine. Administer in a syringe separate from the anticholinesterase agent.

(cont'd)

Table 3: Atropine *(cont'd)*

Dose in Adult Patients[a]

Indication	Route	Usual Dose
Antidote (to organophosphate poisoning)	im, iv	1–2 mg; repeat every 5 to 60 minutes until disappearance of muscarinic symptoms. 2–6 mg may be given initially in severe cases with doses repeated every 5 to 60 minutes. Continue dosage until definite improvement occurs and is maintained, sometimes for 2 days or more
Bronchospasm	inhalation	0.025 mg/kg diluted in 3–5 mL NS given TID-QID. Maximum dose required in adults usually 2.5 mg

[a] Adverse effects become more common in adults over 40 years of age; dosage adjustment may be necessary.
[b] Endotracheal tube can be used if iv route is not available. Dose is 2 to 2.5 times usual iv dose diluted in 10 mL NS; absorption may be unreliable. Intraosseus infusion can also be used if iv route not available. Administer usual iv dose.

Table 4: Atropine

Dose in Pediatric Patients[a]

Indication	Route	Usual Dose
Antimuscarinic	sc	0.01 mg/kg (not to exceed a 0.4 mg dose or 0.3 mg/m^2) every 4 to 6 h
Resuscitation[b]	iv/endotracheal tube	For bradycardia in neonates, reserve atropine for use in patients unresponsive to improved oxygenation and epinephrine. Neonates: 0.01–0.02 mg/kg/dose every 20 min as needed Infants and older children: 0.02 mg/kg/dose;minimum dose: 0.1 mg Maximum single dose: 0.5 mg in children and 1 mg in adolescents. May repeat in 5 minutes to a maximum cumulative dose of 1 mg in children or 2 mg in adolescents
Preanesthesia (antisialagogue)	im, sc	Infants and children: 0.01–0.02 mg/kg/dose 30–60 min preop. Minimum: 0.1 mg/dose; maximum: 0.6 mg/dose
Antidote (to organophosphate poisoning)	iv	0.02–0.05 mg/kg every 10 to 20 minutes until atropine effect seen (e.g., tachycardia, mydriasis, fever) then every 1 to 4 h for at least 24 h
Bronchospasm	inhalation	0.03–0.05 mg/kg/dose diluted in 3–5 mL NS given tid-qid. Maximum: 2.5 mg/dose

[a] Unless specified, neonatal dosing not included.
[b] Endotracheal tube can be used if iv route is not available. Doses 2-10 times the usual iv dose are diluted with normal saline to a total volume of 3-5 mL and followed with several positive-pressure ventilations; absorption may be unreliable. Intraosseus infusion can also be used if iv route not available. Dose is usual iv dose.

Administration: Although at least one manufacturer has recommended that atropine be given iv slowly and with caution, the drug is generally given iv rapidly since slow injection of the drug may cause a paradoxical slowing of the heart rate. Also administered im or sc. Atropine can also be given by endotracheal or intraosseous administration or by oral inhalation.

OVERDOSAGE:
Signs and Symptoms of Overdose: Gastrointestinal: dry mouth, dysphagia, nausea, abdominal distention, diminished or absent bowel sounds.
CNS: CNS stimulation, delirium, drowsiness, stupor, dizziness, headache, restlessness, seizures, tremor, hallucinations, ataxia, coma, psychotic behaviour.
Cardiovascular: circulatory failure, rapid pulse and respiration, tachycardia with weak pulse, palpitations, hypertension.
Genitourinary: urinary urgency with difficulty in micturition.
Ophthalmologic: blurred vision, photophobia, dilated pupils.
Miscellaneous: flushed, hot, dry skin (common), leukocytosis, respiratory failure.
Recommended Management of Overdose: Administer supportive and symptomatic therapy as indicated including ECG monitoring and maintenance of an adequate airway. Benzodiazepines may control excitement, but worsen confusion. Do not administer phenothiazines or other anticholinergic drugs. Hemodialysis is ineffective for atropine poisoning. Hyperpyrexia may be treated with physical cooling measures. If photophobia occurs, the patient may be kept in a dark room. Catheterization may be necessary for urinary retention. Pilocarpine may be administered to treat mydriasis.

If patients have severe CNS symptoms physostigmine use may be considered. Physostigmine is not currently marketed in Canada but is available through the Special Access Programme; see Appendix 2. Consult a toxicology specialist.
Human Lethal Dose: The fatal adult dose of atropine is not known.

In children, 10 mg or less may be fatal and symptoms of overdosage may occur with a dose as low as 0.5 mg.

For management of a suspected drug overdose, CPhA recommends that you contact your **regional Poison Control Centre**. See the *CPS* Directory section for a list of Poison Control Centres.

ACTION AND CLINICAL PHARMACOLOGY: Atropine (dl-hyoscyamine), a belladonna alkaloid, is commonly classified as an anticholinergic or antiparasympathetic drug. Atropine acts at muscarinic receptors as a competitive antagonist of acetylcholine. It acts on smooth muscles and secretory glands innervated by postganglionic cholinergic nerves (e.g., smooth and cardiac muscle) resulting in increased heart rate, decreased atrioventricular conduction time, decreased salivary, bronchial and gastric secretions, dilatation of bronchioles, decreased gastrointestinal smooth muscle tone and peristalsis and relaxation of the lower esophageal sphincter. Atropine facilitates relaxation of genitourinary, biliary and gastrointestinal tracts. Its direct vagolytic action enhances sinus node automaticity and AV conduction. Large doses of atropine can block nicotinic receptors at the autonomic ganglia and neuromuscular junction.
Pharmacokinetics: Absorption: Atropine is well absorbed following im administration, with peak plasma concentrations reached within 30 minutes. It is well absorbed after endotracheal administration appearing in serum within 30 seconds of administration.
Distribution: Atropine disappears rapidly from the blood following injection.

Atropine distributes throughout the body, including the CNS. Atropine is 18% bound to plasma proteins.

The heart rate increases 5 to 40 minutes after im administration and peaks within 20 to 60 minutes. The increase in heart rate peaks 2 to 4 minutes after iv administration and 2 to 10 minutes after endotracheal administration. Salivation is inhibited within 30 minutes of im administration and peaks at 1 to 1.6 hours.
Metabolism: Atropine is metabolized in the liver to several metabolites.
Excretion: From 30 to 50% of an atropine dose is excreted unchanged in the urine. Small amounts are excreted in feces and expired air. Based on im dosing, atropine half-life has 2 phases: an initial rate of 2 to 3 hours and a slower terminal rate of 12.5 hours or longer. Half-life is longer in older individuals, children less than 2 years of age and possibly in patients with hepatic or renal dysfunction.

Atrovent® HFA Inhalation Aerosol Ⓟ

ipratropium bromide

Bronchodilator

Boehringer Ingelheim

Date of Preparation: June 19, 2003
Date of Revision: June 9, 2009

SUMMARY PRODUCT INFORMATION:

Route of Administration	Dosage Form/ Strength	Clinically Relevant Nonmedicinal Ingredients
Oral	Inhalation Aerosol 20 µg/ metered dose	Citric acid, ethanol, propellant HFA 134a (1,1,1,2-tetrafluorethane) For a complete listing see Dosage Forms, Composition and Packaging.

INDICATIONS AND CLINICAL USE: ATROVENT HFA (ipratropium bromide) inhalation aerosol is indicated as:

- a bronchodilator for maintenance treatment of bronchospasm associated with chronic obstructive pulmonary disease, including chronic bronchitis and emphysema.

Pediatrics: ATROVENT HFA is recommended for the use in patients 18 years and older.

CONTRAINDICATIONS:

- ATROVENT HFA (ipratropium bromide) inhalation aerosol should not be taken by patients hypersensitive to ipratropium bromide, atropinics or any other aerosol components.

WARNINGS AND PRECAUTIONS: General: ATROVENT (ipratropium bromide) inhalation aerosol should not be used for the abatement of the acute episodes of bronchospasm where rapid response is required, since the drug has a slower onset of effect than that of an adrenergic β_2 agonist aerosol.

Care should be taken to ensure that ATROVENT inhalation aerosol does not reach the eye. There have been isolated reports of ocular complications (i.e., mydriasis, increased intraocular pressure, glaucoma and eye pain) when aerosolized ipratropium bromide, either alone or in combination with an adrenergic $beta_2$ agonist, has been released into the eyes.

Eye pain or discomfort, blurred vision, visual halos or coloured images in association with red eyes from conjunctival congestion and corneal oedema may be signs of acute narrow-angle glaucoma. Should any of these symptoms develop, treatment with miotic drops should be initiated and specialist advice sought immediately. In the event that glaucoma is precipitated or worsened, treatment should include standard measures for this condition.

Immediate hypersensitivity reactions may occur after administration of ATROVENT metered dose aerosol, as demonstrated by rare cases of urticaria, angio-oedema, rash, bronchospasm, oropharyngeal oedema and anaphylaxis.

To ensure optimal delivery of ATROVENT (ipratropium bromide) inhalation aerosol to the bronchial tree, the patient should be properly instructed by the physician or other health professional in the use of the inhaler.

When using the new formulation of ATROVENT inhalation aerosol (HFA) for the first time, some patients may notice that the taste is slightly different from that of the CFC-containing formulation. Patients should be made aware of this when changing from one formulation to the other. They should also be told that the formulations have been shown to be interchangeable and that the difference in taste has no consequences in terms of the safety or the efficacy of the new formulation.

Caution is advised against the release of the aerosol into the eyes.

In patients with narrow-angle glaucoma, prostatic hyperplasia, urinary retention or bladder neck obstruction, ATROVENT should be used with caution.

If a reduced response to ATROVENT becomes apparent, the patient should seek medical advice.

Gastrointestinal: Patients with cystic fibrosis may be more prone to gastrointestinal motility disturbances.

Special Populations: Pregnant Women: The safety of ATROVENT inhalation aerosol in pregnancy has not been established. The benefits of using ATROVENT when pregnancy is present or suspected must be weighed against possible hazards caused to the fetus. Studies in rats, mice and rabbits showed no embryotoxic nor teratogenic effects.

Nursing Women: No specific studies have been conducted on excretion of this drug in breast milk. Benefits of ATROVENT inhalation aerosol use during lactation should therefore be weighed against possible effects on the infant.

Pediatrics: ATROVENT HFA is recommended for the use in patients 18 years and older.

ADVERSE REACTIONS: Adverse Drug Reaction Overview: The adverse event profile was examined in a total of 3250 patients that were treated in clinical trials with formulations of ATROVENT other than HFA (e.g. CFC, unit dose vials, capsules and solution for inhalation). The nature and frequency of adverse events in this extended population were similar to ATROVENT HFA with the exception that gastrointestinal motility disorders (constipation, diarrhoea and vomiting) were common adverse events while nausea was rare.

Clinical Trial Adverse Drug Reactions: Because clinical trials are conducted under very specific conditions the adverse reaction rates observed in the clinical trials may not reflect the rates observed in practice and should not be compared to the rates in the clinical trials of another drug. Adverse drug reaction information from clinical trials is useful for identifying drug-related adverse events and for approximating rates.

Table 1 summarizes the adverse events reported with a frequency of at least 1% in the ATROVENT HFA clinical trial safety data set, which includes a total of 1231 patients, of which 787 were treated with ATROVENT HFA at total daily doses of 20 µg to 320 µg for up to 4 months. Figures for ATROVENT CFC from the same data set are given for comparison. The adverse events reported are on the whole those that might be expected in a population of patients with COPD or asthma that is being treated with an inhaled anticholinergic. The only significant difference between the two placebo formulations is in the reporting frequency for "taste perversion", which was higher for placebo HFA than placebo CFC.

Table 1: ATROVENT HFA Inhalation Aerosol

Commonly Reported[a] Adverse Events

	ATROVENT				Placebo			
Formulation	**CFC**		**HFA**		**CFC**		**HFA**	
No. of patients exposed	**N=431**		**N=787**		**N=106**		**N=126**	
	n	**%**	**n**	**%**	**n**	**%**	**n**	**%**
Respiratory System Disorders								
Any AE Within the Body System	165	38	305	39	34	32	38	30
Rhinitis	40	9	59	7	7	7	5	4
Bronchitis	33	8	67	9	5	5	32	
Dyspnoea	34	8	57	7	5	5	4	3
Coughing	25	6	46	6	4	4	7	6
Chronic obstructive airways disease	26	6	37	5	9	8	8	6
Upper Resp Tract Infection	17	4	44	6	8	8	8	6
Pharyngitis	23	5	38	5	1	<1	4	3
Asthma	14	3	36	5	0	0	0	0
Sinusitis	8	2	10	1	2	2	3	2
Body as a Whole—General Disorders								
Any AE Within the Body System	62	14	134	17	11	10	16	13
Headache	32	7	59	7	7	7	7	6
Pain	8	2	24	3	0	0	4	3
Influenza-like symptoms	6	1	24	3	0	0	3	2
Back pain	7	2	8	1	1	<1	1	<1
Chest pain	6	1	10	1	0	0	0	0
Fatigue	3	<1	9	1	1	<1	1	<1
Gastrointestinal System Disorders								
Any AE Within the Body System	47	11	97	12	6	6	6	5
Nausea	7	2	23	3	2	2	1	<1
Mouth dry	7	2	18	2	0	0	2	2
Diarrhoea	6	1	15	2	0	0	0	0
Abdominal pain	7	2	13	2	1	<1	0	0
Vomiting	5	1	15	2	0	0	0	0
Constipation	6	1	7	<1	1	<1	1	<1
Dyspepsia	6	1	7	<1	1	<1	0	0
Central and Peripheral Nervous Systems Disorders								
Any AE Within the Body System	24	6	34	4	4	4	5	4
Dizziness	6	1	15	2	1	<1	2	2
Dysphonia	8	2	7	<1	0	0	1	<1
Special Senses Other, Disorders								
Any AE Within the Body System	18	4	28	4	0	0	8	6
Taste Perversion	18	4	28	4	0	0	8	6
Urinary System Disorders								
Any AE Within the Body System	10	2	15	2	5	5	4	3
Urinary tract infection	8	2	7	<1	2	2	1	<1
Musculo-skeletal System Disorders								
Any AE Within the Body System	14	3	13	2	2	2	2	2
Myalgia	7	2	4	<1	2	2	1	<1
Vision Disorders								
Any AE Within the Body System	6	1	20	3	3	3	0	0
Conjunctivitis	3	<1	11	1	0	0	0	0

[a] Commonly reported adverse events are those that were reported with a frequency of at least 1% in the global safety data set regardless of relationship to treatment.

Legend: AE: adverse event; n=no. of patients reporting AE; %=percentage of patients reporting AE; CFC: chlorofluorocarbon formulation; HFA: Alternative Propellant, hydrofluoroalkane formulation.

Adverse events occurring prior to the first intake of test treatment are not included.

Treatment was the last treatment the patient received prior to the onset or worsening of the adverse event.

The most frequent non-respiratory adverse events reported in clinical trials were headache, gastrointestinal motility disorders (constipation, diarrhea, vomiting), dizziness and dryness of the mouth/throat.

As with other inhaled therapy including bronchodilators, cough, local irritation, paradoxical bronchospasm and in very rare instances, exacerbation of symptoms have been observed.

Less Common Clinical Trial Adverse Drug Reactions (<1%): Anticholinergic side effects such as tachycardia and palpitations, supraventricular tachycardia and atrial fibrillation, ocular accommodation disturbances, nausea and urinary retention have been reversible, although the risk of urinary retention may be increased in patients with pre-existing outflow tract obstruction.

There have been isolated reports of ocular events such as mydriasis, increased intraocular pressure, glaucoma and eye pain associated with the release of aerosolized ATROVENT (ipratropium bromide) into the eyes.

Ocular side effects have been reported (see Warnings and Precautions).

Post-Market Adverse Drug Reactions: World-wide safety data, which includes post-marketing data, spontaneous reports and literature reports indicates that the most frequent non-respiratory side effects of ATROVENT are headache and dryness of mouth/throat.

Allergic-type reactions such as skin rash, pruritus, angioedema of the tongue, lips and face, urticaria (including giant urticaria), laryngospasm, oropharyngeal edema, bronchospasm and anaphylactic reactions may occur.

Dizziness has been reported.

DRUG INTERACTIONS: Drug-Drug Interactions: In patients receiving other anticholinergic drugs, ATROVENT should be used with caution because of possible additive effects.

Xanthine derivatives and $beta_2$ adrenergic agents may enhance the effect of ATROVENT inhalation aerosol.

DOSAGE AND ADMINISTRATION: Recommended Dose and Dosage Adjustment: The optimal maintenance dosage must be individually determined. The recommended dosage is 2 metered doses (actuations) (40 µg) 3 or 4 times daily. Some patients may need up to 4 metered doses (actuations) (80 µg) at a time to obtain maximum benefit during early treatment. The maximum daily dose should not exceed 12 metered doses (actuations) (240 µg) and the minimum interval between doses should not be less than 4 hours.

There are no clinical studies in COPD patients to support a recommendation to use a spacer device with ATROVENT HFA.

ATROVENT HFA is recommended for the use in patients 18 years and older.

Missed Dose: If a dose is missed, the next scheduled dose should be taken. An extra dose must not be taken.

OVERDOSAGE:

Doses of ATROVENT (ipratropium bromide) up to 1.2 mg (60 puffs) have been administered by inhalation without the appearance of serious systemic anticholinergic effects. Minor systemic manifestations of anticholinergic action, including dry mouth, visual accomodation disturbances and increase of heart rate may occur.

Should signs of serious anticholinergic toxicity appear, cholinesterase inhibitors may be considered.

For management of a suspected drug overdose, CPhA recommends that you contact your **regional Poison Control Centre**. See the *CPS* Directory section for a list of Poison Control Centres.

ACTION AND CLINICAL PHARMACOLOGY: Mechanism of Action: ATROVENT (ipratropium bromide), a quaternary ammonium derivative of atropine is an anticholinergic drug having bronchodilator properties. On inhalation the onset of action is noted within 5 to 15 minutes with a peak response between 1 and 2 hours, lasting about 2 additional hours with subsequent decline. An inhaled dose of 40 µg induces bronchodilator effect lasting for some 6 hours.

Significant alterations on airway mucous secretion, mucociliary clearance of sputum, or gas exchange have not been observed. Systemic absorption of ATROVENT is poor and the blood levels reached are very low. Metabolic studies with ATROVENT in healthy volunteers show an average elimination half-life of 3.5 hours (range 1.5-4). The drug is transformed to some 8 metabolites with little or no anticholinergic activity.

In controlled 90 day studies in patients with bronchospasm associated with chronic obstructive pulmonary disease (COPD, chronic bronchitis and emphysema) significant improvements in pulmonary function (FEV_1 and $FEF_{25-75\%}$ increases of 15% or more) occurred within 15 minutes, reached a peak in 1-2 hours, and persisted for periods of 3 to 4 hours in the majority of patients and up to 6 hours in some patients.

ATROVENT HFA Inhalation Aerosol is a CFC-free formulation which uses hydrofluoroalkane 134a (HFA-134a) as propellant. It replaces the original formulation of ATROVENT Inhalation Aerosol which used chlorofluorocarbons (CFC) as propellant. Clinical trials with a treatment duration of up to one year in which the HFA and the CFC formulations have been compared have shown the two formulations to be therapeutically equivalent.

Pharmacodynamics: Large, single inhaled doses of ATROVENT have been given to man without any signs of toxicity. After the administration of 400 µg to 10 normal subjects no changes were detected in pulse rate, blood pressure, intraocular pressure, salivary secretion, visual accommodation or electrocardiograms. Likewise, in another study, no changes in pulse rate or salivary secretion were seen when cumulative doses up to 1.2 mg were administered by inhalation to 12 normal volunteers.

Special studies utilizing normal therapeutic doses in asthmatic and chronic bronchitic patients again have not revealed any systemic anticholinergic effects.

In one study, 14 patients were treated for 45 days with either ATROVENT 40 µg q.i.d. or ATROVENT 40 µg q.i.d. plus oral Berotec 5 mg q.i.d. No changes in visual acuity, intraocular pressure, pupil size or accommodation of vision occurred. Micturition function studies in 20 male patients showed no differences in urinary flow, total flow time and time until maximum flow between placebo and ATROVENT 40 µg t.i.d administered for 3 days.

A wide variety of challenge studies have been conducted utilizing ATROVENT as a protective agent. In pharmacologically induced bronchospasm, ATROVENT, in clinical doses, was very effective against methacholine and acetylcholine, moderately effective against propranolol but had little or no effect against histamine or serotonin. Studies in exercise induced bronchospasm have yielded variable results. Some investigations have indicated that ATROVENT has little or no effect but other studies have shown that some patients, at least, are protected against bronchospasm induced by exercise. Likewise, the protective effects of ATROVENT against cold air induced bronchospasm have been variable.

Antigen challenge studies have demonstrated that ATROVENT offers some protection against the "early" allergic asthma response, but has no effect on the "late" response.

Pharmacokinetics: Absorption: Ipratropium bromide is absorbed quickly after oral inhalation of a nominal dose of 40 µg administered from a pressurized metered dose inhaler. The peak plasma concentration (mean C_{max}=32 pg/mL) is reached within 5 minutes after inhalation. The therapeutic effect of ipratropium bromide is produced by a local action in the airways. Therefore time courses of bronchodilation and systemic pharmacokinetics do not run in parallel.

Following inhalation dose portions from 10 to 30% depending on the formulation and inhalation technique, are generally deposited in the lungs. The major part of the dose is swallowed and passes the gastrointestinal tract.

Due to the negligible gastrointestinal absorption of ipratropium bromide the bioavailability of the swallowed dose portion accounts for only ≈2% of the dose. This fraction of the dose does not make a relevant contribution to the plasma concentrations of the active ingredient. The portion of the dose deposited in the lungs reaches the circulation rapidly (within minutes) and has a nearly complete systemic availability.

From data of renal excretion (0-24 hrs) the total systemic bioavailability (pulmonary and gastrointestinal portions) of inhaled doses of ipratropium bromide was estimated to be in the range 7 to 28%.

Distribution: The basic pharmacokinetic parameters were calculated from the plasma level data after i.v. administration. A rapid biphasic decline in plasma is noted for ipratropium. The half-life of the terminal elimination phase was about 1.6 hours. The half-life for elimination of the drug and metabolites was 3.6 hours, as determined after radio-labeling. The main metabolites found in urine bind poorly to the muscarinic receptor. The total clearance of the active ingredient is 2.3 L/minute. Approximately 40% of the clearance is renal (0.9 L/min) and 60% non-renal, i.e. mainly hepato-metabolic. The volume of distribution (Vz) is 338 L (corresponding to approx. 4.6 L/kg).

Plasma concentrations after inhaled ipratropium bromide were about 1000 times lower than equipotent oral or i.v. doses (15 and 0.15 mg, respectively).

The drug is minimally (less then 20%) bound to plasma proteins. The ipratropium ion does not cross the blood-brain barrier, consistent with the quaternary amine structure of the molecule.

Metabolism: Up to 8 metabolites of ipratropium bromide have been detected in man, rat and dog. In man, about 70% of the drug is excreted unchanged after i.v. administration and only one metabolite exceeds 10% of the total radioactivity. The elimination occurs primarily via the kidney with less than 10% of the total intravenous dose excreted via the biliary or fecal route. After oral or inhaled doses, however, up to 90% of the dose is detectable in the feces, suggesting poor absorption.

Excretion: Thirty-nine percent of the active ingredient is excreted renally after intravenous administration, 4.4%-13.1% after inhalation from a metered dose inhaler is excreted as unchanged compound in urine [U86-0434, U95-0343, U96-0020].

Special Populations and Conditions: Pediatrics: ATROVENT HFA is recommended for the use in patients 18 years and older.

STORAGE AND STABILITY: The aerosol canister should be stored at room temperature (15-30°C); the contents are stable up to the expiration date stamped on the label.

SPECIAL HANDLING INSTRUCTIONS: The product should be dispensed in the original container. Caution: Contents under pressure. Container may explode if heated. Do not place in hot water or near radiators, stoves or other sources of heat. Do not puncture or incinerate container or store at temperatures over 30°C. Keep out of reach of children. The product should be kept from freezing.

INFORMATION FOR THE PATIENT: Published in e-CPS, available by subscription at www.e-cps.ca.

DOSAGE FORMS, COMPOSITION AND PACKAGING: Each metal canister with mouthpiece (oral adaptor) contains: 200 actuations of ipratropium bromide. Each valve depression actuation delivers 20 µg of ipratropium bromide. Nonmedicinal ingredients: citric acid, ethanol, propellant (1,1,1,2-Tetrafluoroethane (HFA 134a)) and water. This product does not contain chlorofluorocarbons (CFCs) or soya lecithin.

(Shown in Product Identification Section)

Atrovent® Inhalation Solution Ⓟ

ipratropium bromide

Bronchodilator

Boehringer Ingelheim

Date of Preparation: September 19, 2003
Date of Revision: May 16, 2006

SUMMARY PRODUCT INFORMATION:

Route of Administration	Dosage Form/ Strength	Clinically Relevant Nonmedicinal Ingredients
Oral	Inhalation Solution 20 mL bottle, 1 mL and 2 mL Unit Dose Vials	Sodium chloride For a complete listing see Dosage Forms, Composition and Packaging.

INDICATIONS AND CLINICAL USE: ATROVENT (ipratropium bromide) solution administered either alone or with a adrenergic stimulant solution is indicated:

- As a bronchodilator for the maintenance treatment of bronchospasm associated with, or for the therapy of, acute exacerbations of chronic obstructive pulmonary disease, including chronic bronchitis and emphysema. ATROVENT solution, when used in conjunction with a β_2 adrenergic stimulant solution such as fenoterol or salbutamol, is indicated for acute asthmatic attacks. It is to be administered by compressed air or oxygen driven nebulizers.

Pediatrics: The efficacy and safety of ATROVENT in children younger than 5 years has not been established.

CONTRAINDICATIONS:

- Known hypersensitivity to ATROVENT (ipratropium bromide), to any of the product ingredients, or to atropinics.

WARNINGS AND PRECAUTIONS: General: ATROVENT (ipratropium bromide) solution in the 20 mL multidose bottle contains preservatives (benzalkonium chloride and disodium ethylene diamine tetra acetic acid—EDTA-disodium). It has been reported that these preservatives may cause bronchoconstriction in some patients with hyper reactive airways.

The unit dose vials do not contain preservatives.

ATROVENT should not be used alone for the abatement of an acute asthmatic attack since the drug has a slower onset of effect than that of an adrenergic β_2 agonist.

Immediate hypersensitivity reactions may occur after administration of ATROVENT Inhalation Solution, as demonstrated by rare cases of utricaria, angioedema, rash, bronchospasm, oropharyngeal edema and anaphylaxis.

ATROVENT solution (Bottle and UDV's) is intended only for inhalation with suitable nebulizing devices and should not be taken orally or administered parenterally.

Patients should be instructed in the proper use of the nebulizer. Caution is advised against accidental release of the solution into the eyes.

In patients with glaucoma, prostatic hyperplasia, urinary retention and bladder neck obstruction, ATROVENT (ipratropium bromide) should be used with caution.

If a reduced response to ATROVENT becomes apparent, the patient should seek medical advice.

ATROVENT solution, when administered to patients with acute severe asthma, should be used with concomitant β_2 adrenergic stimulant therapy.

Ear/Nose/Throat: Glaucoma, angle-closure: Care should be taken to ensure that the nebulizer mask fits the patient's face properly and that nebulized solution does not escape into the eyes. In patients with glaucoma or narrow anterior chambers, the administration by nebulizer of a combined ATROVENT/β_2 agonist solution should be avoided unless measures (eg., use of swimming goggles or use of a nebulizer with a mouth piece) are taken to ensure that nebulized solution does not reach the eye. There have been isolated reports of ocular complications (i.e., mydriasis, increased intraocular pressure, angle closure glaucoma) when nebulized ipratropium bromide either alone or in combination with an adrenergic β_2 agonist solution has escaped into the eyes.

Eye pain or discomfort, blurred vision, visual halos or coloured images in association with red eyes from conjunctival congestion and corneal edema may be signs of acute narrow-angle glaucoma. In the event that glaucoma is precipitated or worsened, treatment should include standard measures for this condition.

Gastrointestinal: Patients with cystic fibrosis may be more prone to gastro-intestinal motility disturbances.

Special Populations: Pregnant Women: The safety of ATROVENT inhalation aerosol in pregnancy has not been established. The benefits of using ATROVENT when pregnancy is present or suspected must be weighed against possible hazards caused to the fetus. Studies in rats, mice and rabbits showed no embryotoxic nor teratogenic effects.

Nursing Women: No specific studies have been conducted on excretion of this drug in breast milk. Benefits of ATROVENT inhalation aerosol use during lactation should therefore be weighed against possible effects on the infant.

Pediatrics: The efficacy and safety of ATROVENT in children younger than 5 years has not been established.

ADVERSE REACTIONS: Adverse Drug Reaction Overview: Side effects noted as with the use of other inhalation therapy are cough, local irritation and inhalation induced bronchospasm, and in very rare instances exacerbation of symptoms has been observed.

The most frequent non-respiratory adverse events reported in clinical trials were headache, gastro-intestinal motility (constipation, diarrhoea and vomiting), dizziness and dryness of the mouth/throat.

The adverse event profile was examined in a total of 214 patients receiving ATROVENT solution, 94 patients receiving ATROVENT plus a β_2 agonist (either fenoterol or saluutmaol) solution and in 96 patients receiving a β_2 agonist alone. Furthermore the frequency of adverse reactions reported as possibly related to ATROVENT treatment was studied in a 12-week controlled clinical trial in 219 COPD patients.

Clinical Trial Adverse Drug Reactions: Because clinical trials are conducted under very specific conditions the adverse reaction rates observed in the clinical trials may not reflect the rates observed in practice and should not be compared to the rates in the clinical trials of another drug. Adverse drug reaction information from clinical trials is useful for identifying drug-related adverse events and for approximating rates.

Acute Administration: The frequency of adverse reactions recorded in 214 patients receiving ATROVENT (ipratropium bromide) solution was as follows: see Table 1.

Table 1: ATROVENT Inhalation Solution

Frequency of Adverse Reactions

Adverse Reaction	% of Patients
Dry mouth or throat	9.3
Bad taste	5.1
Tremor	4.2
Exacerbation of symptoms	4.2
Burning eyes	0.9
Nausea	0.9
Sweating	0.9
Cough	0.9

(cont'd)

Table 1: ATROVENT Inhalation Solution *(cont'd)*

Frequency of Adverse Reactions

Adverse Reaction	% of Patients
Headache	0.5
Palpitations	0.5

The adverse reaction judged to be most severe was exacerbation of bronchospasm. This occurred in 8 patients treated with ATROVENT solution alone, 6 of whom withdrew from the clinical studies.

Bronchospasm occurred in 3 patients with acute severe asthma who received ATROVENT solution alone. In two patients, this was reversed after therapy with a β_2 sympathomimetic solution. The third patient received no other therapy.

Table 2 compares the incidence of adverse reactions of the combination of ATROVENT and a β_2 agonist (either fenoterol or salbutamol) solution with that of the β_2 agonist alone.

Table 2: ATROVENT Inhalation Solution

Comparison of Adverse Reactions

Adverse Reaction	Atrovent+β_2 agonist (% of 94 Patients)	β_2 agonist (% of 96 Patients)
Tremor	31.9	26.0
Dry mouth	16.0	28.1
Bad taste	16.0	13.5
Vomiting	2.1	2.1
Palpitations	2.1	1.0
Headache	1.1	2.1
Cough	1.1	0.0
Flushing	1.1	0.0
Dizziness	0.0	1.0
Numbness in leg	0.0	1.0

Chronic Administration: The frequency of adverse reactions reported as possibly related to ATROVENT treatment in 219 COPD patients participating in long-term (12-week) controlled clinical trials was as follows: see Table 3.

Table 3: ATROVENT Inhalation Solution

Frequency of Adverse Reactions

Adverse Reactions	% of Patients
Dry mouth	2.7
Coughing	1.8
Dyspnea	1.8
Headache	1.8
Urinary retention	1.4
Tremor	0.9
Nausea	0.9
Palpitation	0.9
Eye pain	0.9

Observed adverse events occurring in at least 1% of subjects include rhinitis (0.9) and sputum increase (0.9%).

The following other adverse reactions were reported in one patient each: bronchospasm, tachycardia and urticaria.

In addition, the following adverse events were observed in one patient each: bronchitis, chest pain, depression, fatigue, flu-symptoms, hypoaesthesia, increased saliva, insomnia, nervousness, pain, paraesthesia, pharyngitis, somnolence.

The frequency of adverse reactions reported as possibly related to drug treatment in greater than 1% of COPD patients participating in long-term (12-week) controlled clinical trials that compared the efficacy and safety of ATROVENT+ β_2 agonists (metaproterenol or salbutamol) versus the β_2 agonist alone, was as follows: see Table 4.

Table 4: ATROVENT Inhalation Solution

Comparison of Adverse Reactions

Adverse Effect	% of Patients: Atrovent+β_2 agonist (n=208)	% of Patients: β_2 agonist (n=417)
Headache	4.3	1.7
Tremor	3.8	3.4
Nervousness	3.8	1.9
Dyspnea	2.4	3.4
Dry mouth	2.4	1.0
Bronchitis	2.9	2.9
Dizziness	1.4	1.9

(cont'd)

Table 4: ATROVENT Inhalation Solution *(cont'd)*

Comparison of Adverse Reactions

Adverse Effect	% of Patients: Atrovent+β_2 agonist (n=208)	% of Patients: β_2 agonist (n=417)
Coughing	1.4	1.0
Taste perversion	1.9	1.2
Insomnia	1.9	0.2
Dysuria	1.0	0.2
Nausea	1.0	1.7
Abnormal vision	0.5	1.2
Chest pain	1.4	0.7
Constipation	1.4	0.0
Dysphonia	1.0	0.2
Dyspepsia	1.0	0.0
Bronchospasm aggravated	1.0	0.7
Micturition frequency	1.0	0.2

Less Common Clinical Trial Adverse Drug Reactions (<1%): There have been isolated reports of ocular effects such as mydriasis, increased intraocular pressure, and acute glaucoma associated with the escape of nebulized ipratropium bromide, alone or in combination with a β_2 agonist solution into the eyes.

Side effects such as tachycardia and palpitations, supraventricular tachycardia and atrial fibrillation, ocular accommodation disturbances, nausea and urinary retention have been reversible, although the risk of urinary retention may be increased in patients with pre-existing outflow tract obstruction.

Ocular side effects have been reported (see Warnings and Precautions).

Post-Market Adverse Drug Reactions: World-wide safety data, which includes post-marketing data, spontaneous reports and literature reports indicates that the most frequent non-respiratory side effects of ATROVENT are headache and dryness of mouth/throat.

Immediate hypersensitivity reactions may occur after administration of ATROVENT. Allergic type reactions such as skin rash, pruritus, angioedema of the tongue, lips and face, urticaria (including giant uritcaria), laryngospasm, oropharyngeal edema, bronchospasm, and anaphylactic reactions, may occur.

Dizziness has been reported.

DRUG INTERACTIONS: Overview: In patients receiving other anticholinergic drugs, ATROVENT should be used with caution because of possible additive effects.

ATROVENT solution with preservatives (i.e. from the 20 mL multidose bottle) should not be mixed with sodium cromoglycate, as this produces a cloudy solution caused by complexation between the preservatives and sodium cromoglycate. If the patient's condition requires the administration of sodium cromoglycate, it should be given in combination with ATROVENT solution without preservatives (i.e., from the unit dose vial).

In acute and maintenance therapy of chronic reversible airways obstruction, ATROVENT has been shown to provide additive bronchodilating effects to theophylline and beta-adrenoceptor agonists (sympathomimetic amines). Repeated inhalation of ATROVENT has not been linked to tolerance towards bronchodilating effects.

DOSAGE AND ADMINISTRATION: Recommended Dose and Dosage Adjustment: Counselling by physicians on smoking cessation should be the first step in treating patients with chronic obstructive pulmonary disease (COPD), who smoke, independent of the clinical presentation i.e. chronic bronchitis (with or without airflow limitation) or emphysema. Cessation of smoking produces dramatic symptomatic benefits and has been shown to confer a survival advantage.

In adults, the average single dose of ATROVENT (ipratropium bromide) solution is 250-500 µg of ipratropium bromide. In children, aged 5-12 years, the recommended dose is 125-250 µg of ipratropium bromide. In most cases, dilution of the dose with sterile preservative-free saline is not necessary. However, volumes of ATROVENT solution less than 2 mLs are not appropriate for nebulization and must be diluted with saline or another suitable nebulizer solution to make up a total fill volume of 2-5 mL.

Nebulization should take place using a gas flow (oxygen or compressed air) of 6-10 L/minute and the solution nebulized to dryness over a 10-15 minute period. The Hudson Updraft, Bennett Twin Jet, DeVilbiss, Pari Compressors and Inspiron Mini-Neb nebulizers, with facemask or mouthpiece have been used. The manufacturers' instructions concerning cleaning and maintenance of the nebulizer should be strictly followed.

Treatment with ATROVENT solution may be repeated every 4-6 hours as necessary.

Daily doses exceeding 2 mg in adults should be given under medical supervision.

For the maintenance treatment of bronchospasm associated with chronic obstructive pulmonary disease, the recommended dose is 500 µg of ATROVENT (ipratropium bromide) solution given 3-4 times per day.

Missed Dose: If a dose is missed, the next scheduled dose should be taken. An extra dose must not be taken.

OVERDOSAGE:

Doses of ATROVENT (ipratropium bromide) up to 1.2 mg (60 puffs) have been administered by inhalation without the appearance of serious systemic anticholinergic effects. Minor systemic manifestations of anticholinergic action, including dry mouth, visual accomodation disturbances and increase of heart rate may occur.

Should signs of serious anticholinergic toxicity appear, cholinesterase inhibitors may be considered.

> For management of a suspected drug overdose, CPhA recommends that you contact your **regional Poison Control Centre**. See the *CPS* Directory section for a list of Poison Control Centres.

ACTION AND CLINICAL PHARMACOLOGY: Mechanism of Action: ATROVENT (ipratropium bromide), a quaternary ammonium derivative of atropine is an anticholinergic drug having bronchodilator properties. On inhalation the onset of action is noted within 5 to 15 minutes with a peak response between 1 and 2 hours, lasting about 2 additional hours with subsequent decline. Bronchodilation is still evident 8 hours after inhalation.

Pharmacodynamics: Large, single inhaled doses of ATROVENT have been given to man without any signs of toxicity. After the administration of 400 µg by inhaler (10 times the recommended single dose) to 10 normal subjects, no changes were detected in pulse rate, blood pressure, intraocular pressure, salivary secretion, visual accommodation or electrocardiograms. Likewise, in another study, no changes in pulse rate or salivary secretion were seen when cumulative doses up to 1.2 mg were administered by inhaler to 12 normal volunteers.

Special studies utilizing normal therapeutic doses in asthmatic and chronic bronchitic patients again have not revealed any systemic anticholinergic effects. In one study, 14 patients were treated for 45 days with either ATROVENT inhaler 40 µg q.i.d. or ATROVENT inhaler 40 µg q.i.d. plus oral Berotec 5 mg q.i.d. No changes in visual acuity intraocular pressure, pupil size or accommodation of vision occurred. Micturition function studies in 20 male patients showed no differences in urinary flow, total flow time and time until maximum flow between placebo and ATROVENT inhaler 40 µg t.i.d administered for 3 days.

Deterioration in pulmonary function in patients treated in all clinical trials with therapeutic doses of ATROVENT solution was examined. Table 5 shows the number of patients who showed a 15% or greater fall in FEV_1 at any time within 2 hours following the administration of the drug. Also shown are the figures for comparative agents used.

Table 5: ATROVENT Inhalation Solution

Number of patients who showed a 15% or greater fall in FEV_1

Treatment	Incidence
Normal saline	15/90 (16.7%)
ATROVENT Solution	14/214 (6.5%)
ATROVENT Inhaler	4/78 (5.1%)
Berotec Solution	4/83 (4.8%)
ATROVENT Solution+Berotec Solution	1/81 (1.2%)

Dose titration studies in stable asthmatic patients with ATROVENT solution have indicated that maximal improvement in pulmonary function occurs at approximately 250 µg for adults and 125 µg for children over 5 years.

A clinical pharmacology study comparing single doses of ATROVENT inhaler (80 mg) and ATROVENT solution (250 mg) in 16 stable adult asthmatics was performed. No difference between the regimens was found, based on an improvement in pulmonary function over a 2 hour period.

A wide variety of challenge studies have been conducted utilizing ATROVENT as a protective agent. In pharmacologically induced bronchospasm, ATROVENT, in clinical doses, was very effective against methacholine and acetylcholine, moderately effective against propranolol but had little or no effect against histamine or serotonin. Studies in exercise induced bronchospasm have yielded variable results. Some investigations have indicated that ATROVENT has little or no effect but other studies have shown that some patients are protected against bronchospasm induced by exercise. Likewise, the protective effects of ATROVENT against cold air induced bronchospasm have been variable.

Antigen challenge studies have demonstrated that ATROVENT offers some protection against the "early" allergic asthma response, but has no effect on the "late" response.

Pharmacokinetics: Absorption: In man, inhalation of 555 µg by inhaler of radiolabelled ipratropium bromide, about 14 times the recommended therapeutic dose, produced peak plasma levels (ipratropium and its metabolites) of 0.06 ng/mL after 3 hours. The time to reach peak plasma concentration was similar to that seen after oral administration, likely reflecting the large fraction of inhaled dose which is deposited on the pharyngeal mucosae and swallowed.

Direct (non-radioactive) determination of ipratropium bromide revealed that this active ingredient is absorbed very quickly after oral administration. The peak plasma concentrations are reached only minutes after inhalation. The systemic bioavailability after inhalation of 2 mg ipratropium bromide, via an ultrasonic Mizer inhaler, over 20 minutes is estimated to be 7% of the dose. The bioavailability of the swallowed portion of the dose is approximately 2%.

Distribution: Intravenous administration of 1.0 mg in man showed a rapid distribution into tissues (half-life of an alpha phase approximately 5 minutes), and a terminal half-life (beta phase) of 3-4 hours. Plasma concentrations after inhaled ipratropium bromide were about 1000 times lower than equipotent oral or intravenous doses (15 and 0.15 mg, respectively).

Parameters describing the disposition of ipratropium bromide were calculated from the plasma concentrations after i.v. administration. A rapid biphasic decline in plasma is noted for ipratropium. The half-life of the terminal elimination phase is about 1.6 hours. The total clearance of the active ingredient is 2.3 L/min. Approximately 40% of the clearance is renal (0.9 L/min) and 60% non-renal i.e. mainly hepato-metabolic. The volume of distribution is 338 L (corresponding to approximately 4.6 L/kg).

Radio-labelled technetium was administered with ATROVENT solution in an adult dose finding study. Table 6 outlines the doses reaching the patient. The figures for ATROVENT inhaler are published estimates.

Table 6: ATROVENT Inhalation Solution

Doses reaching the patient

Dose Available (µg)	Amount Reaching Patient (µg)	Lung Dose (µg)
500	53	17.0
250	27	8.5
125	13	4.3
40 (ATROVENT Inhaler)	40	4.4

The drug is minimally (less than 20%) bound to plasma proteins. The ipratropium ion does not cross the blood-brain barrier, consistent with the quaternary amine structure of the molecule.

Metabolism: Up to 8 metabolites of ipratropium bromide have been detected in man, rat and dog. However, the main metabolites bind poorly to the muscarinic receptor.

Excretion: In man, about 70% of the ^{14}C labelled drug is excreted unchanged after i.v. administration and only one metabolite exceeds 10% of the total radioactivity. The elimination of ipratropium and its metabolites occurs primarily via the kidney with less than 10% of the total intravenous dose excreted via the biliary or fecal route. After oral or inhaled doses, however, up to 90% of the radiolabelled dose is detectable in the feces, suggesting relatively low lung deposition and poor absorption of the swallowed portion.

Renal excretion of the active ingredient is 46% of the dose after intravenous administration and 3% of the dose after oral inhalation. Depending on the formulation and inhalation technique, renal excretion may increase up to 13% of the dose (40 or 80 µg dose), reflecting a higher deposition in the airways and a higher bioavailability.

Special Populations and Conditions: Pediatrics: The efficacy and safety of ATROVENT in children younger than 5 years has not been established.

STORAGE AND STABILITY: Unopened bottles of ATROVENT solution should be stored at controlled room temperature (between 15 and 30°C). Solutions diluted with preservative free sterile Sodium Chloride Inhalation Solution, USP 0.9% should be used within 24 hours from time of dilution when stored at room temperature and within 48 hours when stored in the refrigerator.

A controlled Preservative Challenge test, done in accordance with the current USP guideline for Preservative Efficacy Testing, indicated that bottles of ATROVENT Inhalation Solution, opened and closed several times, simulating patient use, were stable for up to 28 days when stored at room temperature (15-30°C).

Controlled laboratory experiments using mixtures of ATROVENT solution with Alupent (orciprenaline sulfate), Berotec (fenoterol hydrobromide) or salbutamol sulfate (6 mg/mL preserved with benzalkonium chloride) solutions and diluted with a sterile bacteriostatic sodium chloride solution 0.9% (i.e. normal saline), preserved with benzalkonium chloride, indicated that such mixtures were stable for 7 days at room temperature. For the preparation of such mixtures, it is recommended that only sterile solutions of bacteriostatic sodium chloride 0.9% preserved with 0.01% benzalkonium chloride be used to maintain the level of preservative in the mixture.

The safety of preservatives other than benzalkonium chloride has not been established.

SPECIAL HANDLING INSTRUCTIONS: Incompatibilities: ATROVENT solution with preservatives (i.e. from the 20 mL multi-dose bottle) should not be mixed with sodium cromoglycate solution, as this produces a cloudy solution caused by complexation between the preservatives and sodium cromoglycate. If the patient's condition requires the administration of sodium cromoglycate, it should be given in combination with ATROVENT solution without preservatives (i.e., from the unit dose vial).

1 mL or 2 mL Unit Dose Vials: Unopened unit dose vials of ATROVENT solution should be stored at controlled room temperature (between 15 and 30°C) and protected from light. If required, the solution should be diluted with a preservative free sterile sodium chloride solution 0.9% and used immediately. Any solution remaining in the vial must be discarded.

The solution is physically compatible with Alupent (orciprenaline sulfate), Berotec (fenoterol hydrobromide) or salbutamol sulfate (6 mg/mL) solutions. If such mixtures are prepared, they should be diluted with preservative free sterile sodium chloride solution 0.9% and used immediately. Any unused portion of such combined solutions must be discarded.

INFORMATION FOR THE PATIENT: Published in e-CPS, available by subscription at www.e-cps.ca.

DOSAGE FORMS, COMPOSITION AND PACKAGING: Bottles: Each mL of clear, colorless or almost colorless solution contains: ipratropium bromide 250 µg (0.025%). Nonmedicinal ingredients: benzalkonium chloride, EDTA-disodium, purified water and sodium chloride. pH 3.4. Amber glass bottles of 20 mL with screwcap.

Unit Dose Vials: 125 µg/mL: Each mL of clear, colorless solution contains: ipratropium bromide 125 µg (0.0125%). Nonmedicinal ingredients: hydrochloric acid, purified water and sodium chloride. Plastic single use vials of 2 mL.

250 µg/mL: Each mL of clear, colorless solution contains: ipratropium bromide 250 µg (0.025%). Nonmedicinal ingredients: hydrochloric acid, purified water and sodium chloride. Plastic single use vials of 1 and 2 mL.

Atrovent® Nasal Spray ℞

ipratropium bromide

Topical Anticholinergic

Boehringer Ingelheim

Date of Revision: June 9, 2009

PHARMACOLOGY: Ipratropium, a quaternary ammonium derivative of atropine, is an anticholinergic drug. Ipratropium administered intranasally has a localized parasympathetic blocking action which reduces watery hypersecretion from mucosal glands in the nose.

Two nasal provocation trials in perennial rhinitis patients (n=44) using ipratropium nasal spray showed a dose-dependent increase in inhibition of methacholine-induced nasal secretion with an onset of action within 15 minutes. The duration of action of ipratropium nasal spray was also dose-dependent.

Ipratropium administration via nasal aerosol had no marked effect on sense of smell, nasal mucociliary transport, ciliary beat frequency or the air-conditioning capacity of the nose.

Ipratropium is not readily absorbed into the systemic circulation from the nasal mucosa as confirmed by blood level measurements and renal excretion studies with ipratropium nasal spray 0.03%, 0.06% and 0.12%. The plasma half-life in man is less than 2 hours after i.v. administration of ipratropium. Serum protein binding is less than 20%. In placebo-controlled pharmacokinetic trials in a total of 17 volunteers, 0.03%, 0.06%, and 0.12% concentrations of ipratropium nasal spray exhibited linear kinetics up to a total dose of 336 µg. One clinical trial has shown that the rate of ipratropium absorption was accelerated in a limited number of perennial rhinitis patients (n=4) using ipratropium nasal spray 0.06% chronically versus normal patients (cross trial comparison). This is presumably due to an inflamed nasal mucosa which is, therefore, more permeable. However, the extent of absorption was the same for patients and normal volunteer groups. Since there was no increase in the frequency of systemic adverse events, the clinical significance of this increased rate of absorption is not known.

Studies in rats have shown that ipratropium does not cross the blood-brain barrier.

In double-blind, placebo-controlled, crossover, single dose pharmacokinetic trials (n=17), ipratropium nasal spray 0.03%, 0.06%, and 0.12% (84 µg, 168 µg and 336 µg total nasal dose, respectively) did not significantly affect pupillary diameter, or have any systemic anticholinergic physiologic effect (i.e., changes in heart rate or systolic/diastolic blood pressure) or adverse events (e.g., dry mouth, blurred vision, constipation, difficulty urinating, etc.).

INDICATIONS: Nasal Spray 0.03%: For the symptomatic relief of rhinorrhea associated with allergic or nonallergic perennial rhinitis.

Nasal Spray 0.06%: For the symptomatic relief of rhinorrhea associated with the common cold.

CONTRAINDICATIONS: Known hypersensitivity to ipratropium, atropinics or to any of the ingredients of the nasal spray (see Supplied).

WARNINGS: Care should be taken to ensure that ipratropium nasal spray does not reach the eye. There have been isolated reports of ocular complications (i.e., mydriasis, increased intraocular pressure, narrow angle glaucoma and eye pain) when aerosolized ipratropium has been released into the eyes.

Eye pain or discomfort, blurred vision, visual halos or colored images in association with red eyes from conjunctival and corneal congestion may be signs of acute angle-closure glaucoma. Should any combination of these symptoms develop, treatment with miotic drops should be initiated and specialist advice sought immediately.

Patients must be instructed in the correct administration of ipratropium nasal spray. Care must be taken not to allow the aqueous spray into the eyes. Patients who may be predisposed to glaucoma should be warned specifically to protect their eyes.

Patients with cystic fibrosis may be more prone to gastrointestinal motility disturbances.

PRECAUTIONS: Caution should be taken to avoid accidental release of the nasal spray into the eyes.

Patients with or predisposed to narrow-angle glaucoma, prostatic hyperplasia or bladder neck obstruction should use ipratropium nasal spray with caution.

Immediate hypersensitivity reactions may occur after administration of ipratropium nasal spray, as demonstrated by rare cases of urticaria, angioedema, rash, bronchospasm, oropharyngeal edema, and anaphylaxis.

Pregnancy: The safety of ipratropium nasal spray administration during pregnancy has not yet been established. The benefits of using ipratropium when pregnancy is confirmed or suspected must be weighed against possible hazards to the fetus. Studies in rats, mice and rabbits showed no embryotoxic effects nor teratogenic effects.

Lactation: No specific studies have been conducted on excretion of ipratropium in breast milk. Benefits of ipratropium nasal spray use during lactation should therefore be weighed against possible effects on the infant.

Children: There is insufficient evidence available at present to recommend ipratropium nasal spray for use in children under 12 years of age.

Drug Interactions: If patients are receiving other anticholinergic drugs, including ipratropium containing aerosols for oral inhalation, ipratropium nasal spray should be used with caution because of possible additive effects.

Although the open-label, long-term studies to date have not shown a drug-drug interaction, ipratropium nasal spray should be used with caution in patients concomitantly using intranasal steroids because of the possible adverse local effects, (e.g., epistaxis, etc.). Any patient who experiences the above adverse effect should contact their doctor and a reduction in dose or frequency of ipratropium nasal spray or the nasal steroid should be considered.

ADVERSE EFFECTS: Nasal Spray 0.03%: Adverse reaction information concerning Atrovent nasal spray 0.03% in patients with perennial rhinitis is derived from 5 multicentre, placebo-controlled clinical trials involving 854 patients (454 patients on Atrovent and 400 patients on placebo), and a 1-year open-label, follow-up trial. In 3 of the placebo-controlled trials, patients received Atrovent nasal spray, 42 µg per nostril, or placebo 3 times daily, for 8 weeks. In the other 2 placebo-controlled trials, Atrovent nasal spray, 21 or 42 µg per nostril, was administered to patients 2 or 3 times daily for 4 weeks. Of the 285 patients who entered the open-label, follow-up trial, 232 were treated for 3 months, 200 for 6 months, and 159 up to 1 year, with the majority (>86%) of patients going 1 year being maintained on 42 µg per nostril, 2 or 3 times daily, of Atrovent nasal spray.

Adverse reactions reported for patients who received Atrovent nasal spray 0.03%, 42 µg per nostril, or placebo 2 or 3 times daily where the prevalence in the Atrovent group is 2% or greater and exceeds the prevalence in placebo group appear in Table 1.

Adverse reactions were usually mild to moderate and transient in the 5 placebo-controlled trials, resulting in discontinuation of treatment for 5.3% of the Atrovent nasal spray 0.03% and 5.3% of the placebo-treated patients. There was no evidence of nasal rebound (i.e., a clinically significant increase in rhinorrhea, posterior nasal drip, sneezing or nasal congestion severity compared to baseline) upon discontinuation of double-blind therapy in these trials. There were no drug-related serious or anticholinergic adverse reactions (with the exception of dry mouth reported for 1% of the Atrovent and 0.5% of the placebo-treated patients) during the placebo-controlled trials or the 1-year, open-label, follow-up trial in patients on Atrovent nasal spray 0.03%.

Nasal adverse events and adverse reactions were reported for 84 (29.5%) of the 285 patients in the 1-year open-label, follow-up trial. The incidence for the most frequently reported nasal adverse reactions were nasal congestion (1.4%), nasal dryness (9.5%), and epistaxis (4.2%).

Drug-related and non-drug related nasal dryness and/or epistaxis occurred in 45 patients. It resolved with continued treatment or dose reduction in 40 of these patients (89%), and required discontinuation of treatment in 5 patients (11%).

Adverse reactions, which were found in less than 2% of perennial rhinitis patients receiving Atrovent nasal spray 0.03% in the 5 multicentre, placebo-controlled clinical trials and 1-year open-label follow-up trial were: rash, urticaria, and conjunctivitis.

Adverse events, observed in perennial rhinitis patients receiving Atrovent nasal spray 0.03% in the 5 multicentre, placebo-controlled clinical trials and 1-year open-label follow-up trials were: paresthesia, fatigue, dizziness, insomnia, dysphonia, migraine, vertigo, furunculosis, generalized edema, diarrhea, abdominal pain, taste perversion and xerophthalmia.

There have been isolated reports of ocular events such as mydriasis, increased intraocular pressure, glaucoma and eye pain associated with the release of aerosolized ipratropium into the eyes. These ocular events have not been reported with the use of Atrovent nasal spray.

Table 1: Atrovent Nasal Spray
Adverse Reactions Associated with 0.03% Spray

	% of Patients Reporting Reactions[a]			
	Atrovent Nasal Spray 0.03% (n=356)		Placebo Spray (n=347)	
	Incidence %	Discontinued %	Incidence %	Discontinued %
Headache	9.8	0.6	9.2	0
Upper Respiratory Tract Infection	9.8	1.4	7.2	1.4
Epistaxis	9.0	0.3	4.6	0.3
Rhinitis[b]				
Nasal Dryness	5.1	0	0.9	0.3
Nasal Irritation[c]	2.0	0	1.7	0.6
Other Nasal Symptoms[d]	3.1	1.1	1.7	0.3
Pharyngitis	8.1	0.3	4.6	0
Nausea	2.2	0.3	0.9	0

a This table includes only adverse reactions for which the prevalence in the Atrovent group was 2% or greater and exceeds the prevalence in the placebo group.
b All reactions are listed by their WHO term; rhinitis has been presented by descriptive terms for clarification.
c Nasal irritation includes reports of nasal itching, nasal burning, nasal irritation and rhinitis ulcerative.
d Other nasal symptoms include reports of nasal congestion, increased rhinorrhea, increased rhinitis, posterior nasal drip, sneezing, nasal polyps and nasal edema.

Nasal Spray 0.06%: Adverse reaction information concerning Atrovent nasal spray 0.06% in patients with the common cold is derived from 2 multicentre, placebo-controlled clinical trials involving 1276 patients (195 patients on Atrovent nasal spray 0.03%, 352 patients on Atrovent nasal spray 0.06%, 189 patients on Atrovent nasal spray 0.12%, 351 patients on placebo and 189 patients receiving no treatment). The adverse reactions reported for patients receiving Atrovent nasal spray 0.06% administered 3 or 4 times daily, where the incidence in the Atrovent group is 1% or greater and exceeds the prevalence in the placebo group, appear in Table 2.

Table 2: Atrovent Nasal Spray
Adverse Reactions Associated with 0.06% Spray

	% of Patients Reporting Reactions[a]	
	Atrovent Nasal Spray 0.06% (n=352)	Placebo (n=351)
Epistaxis or Nosebleed	5.4%	1.4%
Nasal Dryness	4.8%	2.8%
Blood-tinged Nasal Mucus	2.8%	0.9%
Dry Mouth/Throat	1.4%	0.3%
Nasal Congestion	1.1%	0.0%

a This table includes only those adverse reactions for which the frequency in the Atrovent group was 1% or greater and exceeds the frequency in the placebo group.

Adverse reactions reported in less than 1% of patients with the common cold receiving Atrovent nasal spray 0.06% in 2 multicentre, placebo-controlled clinical trials were: tachycardia, conjunctivitis and abnormal vision.

Adverse events seen in the same population include paresthesia, dizziness, dysphonia, and taste perversion.

Atrovent nasal spray 0.06% was well tolerated by the patients, with the most frequently reported adverse reactions being minor local nasal reactions. The majority of the adverse reactions were mild to moderate in nature, none were considered serious, none resulted in hospitalization and no patient receiving Atrovent nasal spray 0.06% was discontinued from the trial due to an adverse reaction. There was no evidence of rebound of nasal symptoms.

There have been isolated reports of ocular events such as mydriasis, increased intraocular pressure, glaucoma and eye pain associated with the release of aerosolized ipratropium into the eyes. These ocular events have not been reported with the use of Atrovent nasal spray.

Postmarketing Experience: Worldwide safety data, which includes postmarketing data, spontaneous reports, literature reports, and clinical trial reports, indicate that the most frequent local undesirable effects of Atrovent nasal spray are nasal reactions such as epistaxis, dryness of the nose and nasal irritation, nasal congestion, nasal burning sensation, headache and nausea.

Anticholinergic side effects such as tachycardia and palpitations, dryness of mouth/throat, ocular accommodation disturbances, gastrointestinal motility disturbances and urinary retention are rare and reversible.

After oral inhalation of ipratropium bromide in patients suffering from COPD or asthma, supraventricular tachycardia and atrial fibrillation have been reported.

Allergic-type reactions such as skin rash, angioedema of tongue, lips and face, urticaria, laryngospasm and anaphylactic reactions may occur.

OVERDOSE:

Symptoms: Acute overdosage by intranasal administration is unlikely since ipratropium is not well absorbed systemically after intranasal or oral administration. Minor systemic manifestation of anticholinergic action, including dry mouth, visual accommodation disturbances and increased heart rate may occur.

Treatment: Should signs of serious anticholinergic toxicity appear, cholinesterase inhibitors may be considered.

For management of a suspected drug overdose, CPhA recommends that you contact your **regional Poison Control Centre**. See the *CPS* Directory section for a list of Poison Control Centres.

DOSAGE: The dose of ipratropium nasal spray 0.03% for symptomatic relief of rhinorrhea associated with allergic or nonallergic perennial rhinitis is 2 sprays (42 µg) per nostril 2 or 3 times a day (total dose 168 to 252 µg/day). Optimum dosage varies with the response of the individual patient.

The dose of ipratropium nasal spray 0.06% is 2 sprays (84 µg) per nostril 3 or 4 times daily (total dose 504 to 672 µg/day) as required for symptomatic relief of rhinorrhea associated with the common cold.

Treatment in the common cold has only been studied up to 4 days. Efficacy and safety of treatment beyond 4 days have not been established, although there has been no evidence of adverse safety effects with longer treatment in perennial rhinitis patients.

Children: Not recommended for use in children under 12 years of age.

INFORMATION FOR THE PATIENT: Published in e-CPS, available by subscription at www.e-cps.ca.

SUPPLIED: 0.03%: Each spray is designed to deliver 0.07 mL which contains: ipratropium bromide 21 µg. Nonmedicinal ingredients: benzalkonium chloride, edetate disodium, hydrochloric acid, sodium chloride, sodium hydroxide and purified water. Bottles of 30 mL, fitted with a metered nasal spray pump, a safety clip to prevent accidental discharge of the spray and a clear plastic dust cap. The 30 mL bottle is designed to deliver 345 sprays of 0.07 mL each or 28 days of therapy at the maximum recommended dose (2 sprays per nostril 3 times a day). Store tightly closed between 15 and 30°C. The contents are stable up to the expiration date stamped on the label. Avoid excessive heat or freezing. Keep out of reach of children.

0.06%: Each spray is designed to deliver 0.07 mL which contains: ipratropium bromide 42 µg. Nonmedicinal ingredients: benzalkonium chloride, edetate disodium, hydrochloric acid, sodium chloride, sodium hydroxide and purified water. Bottles of 15 mL, fitted with a metered nasal spray pump, a safety clip to prevent accidental discharge of the spray and a clear plastic dust cap. The 15 mL bottle is designed to deliver 165 sprays of 0.07 mL each or 10 days of therapy at the maximum recommended dose (2 sprays per nostril 4 times a day). Store tightly closed between 15 and 30°C. The contents are stable up to the expiration date stamped on the label. Avoid excessive heat or freezing. Keep out of reach of children.

Auralgan®
antipyrine—benzocaine
Analgesic—Antiphlogistic
Paladin

SUPPLIED: Each mL of otic solution contains: benzocaine 14 mg, antipyrine 54 mg. Nonmedicinal ingredients: glycerin and oxyquinoline sulfate. Does not contain alcohols, gluten, parabens, sugars, sulfites or tartrazine. Plastic dropper bottles of 14 mL.

Avalide®
irbesartan—hydrochlorothiazide
Angiotensin II AT1 Receptor Blocker—Diuretic
Bristol-Myers Squibb/sanofi-aventis

Date of Preparation: February 25, 2000
Date of Revision: December 29, 2008

SUMMARY PRODUCT INFORMATION:

Route of Administration	Dosage Form/ Strength	Clinically Relevant Nonmedicinal Ingredients
Oral	Tablet/ 150/12.5 mg, 300/12.5 mg, 300/25 mg	Lactose monohydrate For a complete listing, see Dosage Forms, Composition and Packaging.

INDICATIONS AND CLINICAL USE: AVALIDE (irbesartan/hydrochlorothiazide) is indicated for the treatment of essential hypertension in patients for whom combination therapy is appropriate (see Dosage and Administration).

AVALIDE is also indicated as initial therapy in patients with severe essential hypertension (Sitting DBP ≥110 mmHg) for whom the benefit of a prompt blood pressure reduction exceeds the risk of initiating combination therapy in these patients (see Dosage and Administration).

AVALIDE is not indicated as initial therapy in patients with mild to moderate essential hypertension.

Geriatrics (>65 years of age): In clinical studies, no overall differences in safety or efficacy were observed between patients over 65 years of age and younger patients (see Warnings and Precautions, Special Populations).

Pediatrics (<18 years of age): The safety and efficacy of AVALIDE in patients <18 years of age have not been established (see Warnings and Precautions, Special Populations).

CONTRAINDICATIONS: AVALIDE (irbesartan/hydrochlorothiazide) is contraindicated in patients who are hypersensitive to any component of this product.

Because of the hydrochlorothiazide component, this product is contraindicated in patients with anuria, and in patients who are hypersensitive to other sulfonamide-derived drugs.

WARNINGS AND PRECAUTIONS:

Serious Warnings and Precautions
When used in pregnancy, angiotensin receptor (AT_1) blockers (ARB) can cause injury and even death of the developing fetus. When pregnancy is detected, AVALIDE should be discontinued as soon as possible (see Warnings and Precautions, Special Populations).

General: The effect of irbesartan on ability to drive and use machines has not been studied, but based on its pharmacodynamic properties, irbesartan is unlikely to affect this ability. When driving vehicles or operating machines, it should be taken into account that occasionally dizziness or weariness may occur during treatment of hypertension.

Cardiovascular: Hypotension: Occasionally, symptomatic hypotension has occurred after administration of irbesartan, in some cases after the first dose. It is more likely to occur in patients who are volume depleted by diuretic therapy, dietary salt restriction, dialysis, diarrhea, or vomiting. In these patients, because of the potential fall in blood pressure, therapy should be started under close medical supervision (see Dosage and Administration). Similar considerations apply to patients with ischemic heart or cerebrovascular disease, in whom an excessive fall in blood pressure could result in myocardial infarction or cerebrovascular accident.

Valvular Stenosis: There is concern on theoretical grounds that patients with aortic stenosis might be at particular risk of decreased coronary perfusion when treated with vasodilators because they do not develop as much afterload reduction.

Endocrine and Metabolism: Thiazides, including hydrochlorothiazide, can cause fluid or electrolyte imbalance (hypokalemia, hyponatremia and hypochloremic alkalosis).

Calcium excretion is decreased by thiazides which may cause intermittent and slight elevation of serum calcium. If calcium or a calcium sparing drug (e.g., vitamin D therapy) is prescribed, serum calcium levels should be monitored and calcium dosage adjusted accordingly. Marked hypercalcemia suggests the possibility of hyperparathyroidism. Thiazides should be discontinued before carrying out tests for parathyroid function.

Thiazides have been shown to increase the urinary excretion of magnesium, which may result in hypomagnesemia.

Hyperuricemia may occur, and an acute attack of gout may be precipitated in certain patients receiving thiazide therapy.

Insulin requirements in diabetic patients may be altered and latent diabetes mellitus may become manifest during thiazide diuretic therapy.

Increases in cholesterol and triglyceride levels may be associated with thiazide diuretic therapy.

Thiazides may decrease serum PBI levels without signs of thyroid disturbance.

Hepatic/Biliary/Pancreatic: Thiazides should be used with caution in patients with impaired hepatic function or progressive liver disease, since minor alterations in fluid and electrolyte balance may precipitate hepatic coma.

Immune: Hypersensitivity Reaction: Sensitivity reactions to hydrochlorothiazide may occur in patients with or without a history of allergy or bronchial asthma.

Systemic Lupus Erythematosus: Thiazide diuretics have been reported to cause exacerbation or activation of systemic lupus erythematosus.

Renal: Azotemia: Azotemia may be precipitated or increased by hydrochlorothiazide. Cumulative effects of the drug may develop in patients with impaired renal function.

If increasing azotemia and oliguria occur during treatment of severe progressive renal disease the diuretic should be discontinued.

Renal Impairment: As a consequence of inhibiting the renin-angiotensin-aldosterone system, changes in renal function have been seen in susceptible individuals. In patients whose renal function may depend on the activity of the renin-angiotensin-aldosterone system, such as patients with bilateral renal artery stenosis, unilateral renal artery stenosis to a solitary kidney, or severe congestive heart failure, treatment with agents that inhibit this system has been associated with oliguria, progressive azotemia, and rarely, acute renal failure and/or death. In susceptible patients, concomitant diuretic use may further increase risk.

Use of irbesartan should include appropriate assessment of renal function.

Thiazides should be used with caution.

Because of the hydrochlorothiazide component, AVALIDE (irbesartan/hydrochlorothiazide) is not recommended in patients with severe renal impairment (creatinine clearance ≤30 mL/min).

Special Populations: Pregnant Women: Drugs that act directly on the renin-angiotensin system (RAAS) can cause fetal and neonatal morbidity and death when administered to pregnant women. When pregnancy is detected, AVALIDE should be discontinued as soon as possible.

The use of ARB is not recommended during pregnancy. Epidemiological evidence regarding the risk of teratogenicity following exposure to angiotensin converting enzyme inhibitors (another class of therapeutic products interfering with the RAAS) during the first trimester of pregnancy has not been conclusive; however a small increase in risk cannot be excluded. Given the current evidence available on the risk with ARB, similar risks may exist for this class of drugs. Patients planning pregnancy should be changed to alternative antihypertensive treatments which have an established safety profile for use in pregnancy. When pregnancy is diagnosed, treatment with angiotensin II antagonists should be stopped immediately, and, if appropriate, alternative therapy should be started. The use of ARBs during the second and third trimesters is known to induce human fetotoxicity (decreased renal function, oligohydramnios, skull ossification, retardation) and neonatal toxicity (renal failure, hypotension, hyperkalaemia).

Infants with histories of in utero exposure to ARBs should be closely observed for hypotension, oliguria, and hyperkalemia. If oliguria occurs, attention should be directed toward support of blood pressure and renal perfusion. Exchange transfusion may be required as means of reversing hypotension and/or substituting for impaired renal function; however, limited experience with those procedures has not been associated with significant clinical benefit. Irbesartan is not removed by hemodialysis.

Thiazides cross the placental barrier and appear in cord blood. The routine use of diuretics in otherwise healthy pregnant women is not recommended and exposes mother and fetus to unnecessary hazard, including fetal or neonatal jaundice, thrombocytopenia, and possibly other adverse reactions that have occurred in adults. Diuretics do not prevent development of toxemia of pregnancy and there is no satisfactory evidence that they are useful in the treatment of toxemia.

Nursing Women: It is not known whether irbesartan is excreted in human milk, but significant levels of radioactivity have been found in the milk of lactating rats. Thiazides appear in human milk. Because many drugs are excreted in human milk and because of their potential for affecting the nursing infant adversely, a decision should be made whether to discontinue nursing or discontinue the drug, taking into account the importance of the drug to the mother.

Pediatrics: Safety and effectiveness have not been established.

Geriatrics: Of the 2650 hypertensive patients receiving irbesartan/hydrochlorothiazide in clinical studies, 618 patients were 65 years of age and over. No overall age-related differences were seen in the adverse effect profile but greater sensitivity in some older individuals cannot be ruled out.

ADVERSE REACTIONS: Adverse Drug Reaction Overview: AVALIDE (irbesartan/hydrochlorothiazide) has been evaluated for safety in 2746 patients with essential hypertension including 968 patients for 1 year or more.

The most commonly reported adverse events (occurring in ≥10% of patients treated with AVALIDE) was headache (11.0%), which occurred at a significantly higher incidence in the placebo group (16.1%).

The adverse events most frequently resulting in clinical intervention (discontinuation of AVALIDE) were due to dizziness (0.7%) and headache (0.7%). The adverse event of hypotension is more likely to occur in volume depleted patients (see Warnings and Precautions related to Cardiovascular under Hypotension).

The following potentially serious adverse reactions have been reported rarely with irbesartan in controlled clinical trials: syncope, hypotension.

Clinical Trial Adverse Drug Reactions: Because clinical trials are conducted under very specific conditions the adverse reaction rates observed in the clinical trials may not reflect the rates observed in practice and should not be compared to the rates in the clinical trials of another drug. Adverse drug reaction information from clinical trials is useful for identifying drug-related adverse events and for approximating rates.

Hypertension: In placebo-controlled clinical trials, therapy was discontinued due to a clinical or laboratory adverse event in 3.6 percent of patients treated with irbesartan/hydrochlorothiazide, versus 6.8 percent of patients given placebo.

Adverse events regardless of drug relationship, occurring in ≥1% of the irbesartan/ hydrochlorothiazide patients in placebo-controlled clinical trials include the following (see Table 1):

Table 1: AVALIDE

Adverse Events Regardless of Drug Relationship, Occurring in ≥1% of the Irbesartan/ Hydrochlorothiazide Patients in Placebo-controlled Clinical Trials

	Irbesartan/HCTZ n=898 (%)	Irbesartan n=400 (%)	HCTZ n=380 (%)	Placebo n=236 (%)
Cardiovascular				
Edema	3.1	1.5	1.6	2.5
Tachycardia	1.2	0.5	0.5	0.4
Dermatologic				
Rash	1.2	1.8	3.2	1.7
Gastrointestinal				
Nausea/Vomiting	3.2	1.5	2.4	0.4
Dyspepsia	2.1	0.3	1.6	0.8
Diarrhea	2.1	2.8	1.1	3.4
Abdominal Pain	1.7	1.5	1.6	0.8
General				
Fatigue	6.5	4.0	3.2	3.0
Influenza	2.8	2.0	1.8	1.3
Chest Pain	1.8	1.5	1.6	1.3
Immunology				
Allergy	1.1	0.5	0.5	0
Musculoskeletal				
Musculoskeletal Pain	6.5	6.0	9.7	4.7
Muscle Cramp	1.0	0.8	2.1	1.3

(cont'd)

Table 1: AVALIDE *(cont'd)*

Adverse Events Regardless of Drug Relationship, Occurring in ≥1% of the Irbesartan/ Hydrochlorothiazide Patients in Placebo-controlled Clinical Trials

	Irbesartan/HCTZ n=898 (%)	Irbesartan n=400 (%)	HCTZ n=380 (%)	Placebo n=236 (%)
Nervous System				
Headache	11.0	9.3	11.6	16.1
Dizziness	7.6	5.5	4.7	4.2
Orthostatic Dizziness	1.1	1.0	0.8	0.4
Anxiety/Nervousness	1.0	1.0	0.5	1.7
Renal/Genitourinary				
Urination Abnormal	1.9	0.5	2.1	0.8
Urinary Tract Infection	1.6	1.5	2.4	2.5
Respiratory				
URTI	5.6	8.3	7.1	5.5
Sinus Disorder	2.9	4.5	3.2	4.7
Cough	2.2	2.3	2.6	3.0
Pharyngitis	2.1	2.3	2.9	1.7
Rhinitis	1.9	2.0	1.6	2.5

Severe Hypertension: In a clinical study in patients with severe hypertension (SeDBP ≥110 mmHg), the overall pattern of adverse events reported through seven weeks of follow-up was similar in patients treated with AVALIDE as initial therapy and in patients treated with irbesartan as initial therapy. See Table 2.

Table 2: AVALIDE

Most Common Adverse Events Regardless of Drug Relationship, Occurring in ≥1% of the Irbesartan/Hydrochlorothiazide Patients with Severe Hypertension in Controlled Clinical Trial

	Number (%) of Subjects Irbesartan/HCTZ N=468	Number (%) of Subjects Irbesartan N=227
Headache	19 (4.1)	15 (6.6)
Dizziness	16 (3.4)	9 (4.0)
Nasopharyngitis	8 (1.7)	10 (4.4)
Bronchitis	6 (1.3)	6 (2.6)
Fatigue	6 (1.3)	1 (0.4)
Upper Respiratory Tract Infection	6 (1.3)	4 (1.8)
Erectile Dysfunction	5 (1.1)	0
Nausea	5 (1.1)	5 (2.2)
Diarrhoea	4 (0.9)	3 (1.3)
Sinusitis	4 (0.9)	3 (1.3)
Cough	3 (0.6)	4 (1.8)
Muscle Spasms	2 (0.4)	3 (1.3)

The incidence of the pre-specified adverse events was: 0% reported cases of syncope in either treatment group; 0.6% and 0% cases of hypotension, 3.6% and 4.0% cases of dizziness, 4.3% and 6.6% cases of headache, 0.2% and 0% cases of hyperkalemia, and 0.6% and 0.4% cases of hypokalemia reported in the group treated with AVALIDE and the group treated with irbesartan, respectively.

The rate of discontinuation due to adverse events was 1.9% and 2.2% in the group treated with AVALIDE and the group treated with irbesartan, respectively.

Irbesartan Alone: In addition, the following potentially important events occurred in less than 1% of patients receiving irbesartan, regardless of drug relationship:

Body as a Whole: fever.

Cardiovascular: flushing, hypertension, myocardial infarction, angina pectoris, arrhythmic/conduction disorder, cardio-respiratory arrest, heart failure, hypertensive crisis.

Dermatologic: pruritus, dermatitis, ecchymosis, erythema, urticaria, photosensitivity.

Endocrine: sexual dysfunction, libido disorder, gout.

Gastrointestinal: constipation, gastroenteritis, flatulence, abdominal distention, hepatitis.

Musculoskeletal: muscle cramp, arthritis, myalgia, muscular weakness.

Nervous System: sleep disturbance, numbness, somnolence, vertigo, depression, paresthesia, tremor, transient ischemic attack, cerebrovascular accident.

Renal/Genitourinary: abnormal urination.

Respiratory: epistaxis, tracheobronchitis, pulmonary congestion, dyspnea, wheezing.

Special Senses: visual disturbance, hearing impaired, conjunctivitis, taste disturbance.

Abnormal Hematologic and Clinical Chemistry Findings: AVALIDE: Liver Function Tests: Occasional elevations of liver enzymes and/or serum bilirubin have occurred. In patients with essential hypertension treated with AVALIDE alone, one patient was discontinued due to elevated liver enzymes.

Creatinine, Blood Urea Nitrogen: Minor increases in blood urea nitrogen (BUN) or serum creatinine were observed in 2.3% of patient. No patient was discontinued due to increased BUN. One patient was discontinued due to a minor increase in serum creatinine.

Irbesartan: Liver Function Tests: In placebo-controlled trials, elevations of AST and ALT ≥3× upper limit of normal occured in 0.1% and 0.2%, respectively, of irbesartan treated patients compared to 0.3% and 0.3%, respectively, of patients receiving placebo. The cumulative incidence of AST and/or ALT elevations ≥3× upper limit of normal was 0.4% in patients treated with irbesartan for a mean duration of over 1 year.

Hyperkalemia: In placebo-controlled trials, greater than a 10% increase in serum potassium was observed in 0.4% of irbesartan treated patients compared to 0.5% of patients receiving placebo.

Creatinine, Blood Urea Nitrogen: Minor increases in blood urea nitrogen (BUN) or serum creatinine were observed in less than 0.7% of patients with essential hypertension treated with irbesartan alone versus 0.9% on placebo.

Hemoglobin: Mean decreases in hemoglobin of 0.16 g/dL were observed in patients receiving irbesartan. No patients were discontinued due to anemia.

Neutropenia: Neutropenia (<1000 cells/mm^3) was observed in 0.3% of irbesartan treated patients compared to 0.5% of patients receiving placebo.

In clinical trials, the following were noted to occur with an incidence of <1%, regardless of drug relationship: anemia, thrombocytopenia, lymphocytopenia, and increased CPK.

Post-Market Adverse Drug Reactions: Angioedema (involving swelling of the face, lips, and/or tongue) has been reported rarely in post marketing use. The following adverse reactions, regardless of drug relationship, were reported very rarely in post-marketing use: syncope, asthenia, jaundice, myalgia, elevated liver function tests, and impaired renal function including occasional cases of renal failure in patients at risk (see Warnings and Precautions, Renal, Renal Impairment).

Cases of muscle pain, muscle weakness, myositis and rhabdomyolysis have been reported in patients receiving angiotensin II receptor blockers.

DRUG INTERACTIONS: Drug-Drug Interactions: Diuretics: Patients on diuretics, and especially those in whom diuretic therapy was recently instituted, may occasionally experience an excessive reduction of blood pressure after initiation of therapy with irbesartan. The possibility of symptomatic hypotension with the use of irbesartan can be minimized by discontinuing the diuretic prior to initiation of treatment and/or lowering the initial dose of irbesartan (see Warnings and Precautions, Cardiovascular, Hypotension, and Dosage and Administration). No drug interaction of clinical significance has been identified with thiazide diuretics.

Agents Increasing Serum Potassium: Since irbesartan decreases the production of aldosterone, potassium-sparing diuretics or potassium supplements should be given only for documented hypokalemia and with frequent monitoring of serum potassium. Potassium-containing salt substitutes should also be used with caution. Concomitant thiazide diuretic use may attenuate any effect that irbesartan may have on serum potassium.

Lithium Salts: As with other drugs which eliminate sodium, lithium clearance may be reduced in the presence of irbesartan. Therefore, serum lithium levels should be monitored carefully if lithium salts are to be administered with irbesartan.

Lithium generally should not be given with diuretics. Diuretic agents reduce the renal clearance of lithium and increase risk of lithium toxicity.

Warfarin: When irbesartan was administered as 300 mg once daily under steady-state conditions, no pharmacodynamic effect on PT was demonstrated in subjects stabilized on warfarin.

Digoxin: When irbesartan was administered as 150 mg once daily under steady-state conditions, no effect was seen on the pharmacokinetics of digoxin at steady-state. Thiazide induced electrolyte disturbances may predispose to digitalis induced arrhythmias.

Simvastatin: When irbesartan was administered in a small single-dose study with 12 young, healthy males aged 19 to 39, the single-dose pharmacokinetics of simvastatin were not affected by the concomitant administration of 300 mg irbesartan. Simvastatin values were highly variable whether simvastatin was administered alone or in combination with irbesartan.

Nifedipine: The pharmacokinetics of irbesartan were not affected by coadministration of nifedipine.

Alcohol, Barbiturates, or Narcotics: Diuretic potentiation of orthostatic hypotension may occur.

Antidiabetic Drugs (oral agents and insulin): In the presence of diuretics, dosage adjustment of the antidiabetic drug may be required.

Other Antihypertensive Drugs: Diuretic additive effect or potentiation may occur.

Cholestyramine and Colestipol Resins: Absorption of hydrochlorothiazide is impaired in the presence of anionic exchange resins. AVALIDE should be taken at least one hour before or four hours after these medications.

Corticosteroids, ACTH: Intensified electrolyte depletion, particularly hypokalemia may occur when given concomitantly with diuretics.

Pressor Amines (e.g., Norepinephrine): In the presence of diuretics, possible decreased response to pressor amines may be seen but not sufficient to preclude their use.

Skeletal Muscle Relaxants, Nondepolarizing (e.g., Tubocurarine): In the presence of diuretics, possible increased responsiveness to the muscle relaxant may occur.

Nonsteroidal Anti-inflammatory Drugs: In some patients, the administration of a nonsteroidal anti-inflammatory agent can reduce the diuretic, natriuretic, and antihypertensive effects of loop, potassium-sparing and thiazide diuretics. Therefore, when AVALIDE and nonsteroidal anti- inflammatory agents are used concomitantly, the patient should be observed closely to determine if the desired effect of the diuretic is obtained.

Drug-Food Interactions: No statistically significant effects of food were observed on the C_{max}, $AUC_{(inf)}$ or $T_{1/2}$ of irbesartan or on the $AUC_{(inf)}$ or $T_{1/2}$ of hydrochlorothiazide. In the fasted and fed states, T_{max} increased from 1 to 2 hours for irbesartan and from 1.5 to 3.5 hours for hydrochlorothiazide. The C_{max} for hydrochlorothiazide decreased 21% in the fed state relative to the fasted state. None of these changes were considered to be clinically significant.

Drug-Herb Interactions: There have been no clinical studies to assess the possible interaction of any herbal products and AVALIDE.

DOSAGE AND ADMINISTRATION: Dosing Considerations:

- Dosage must be individualized.
- The fixed combination is not for initial therapy except for severe hypertension.
- The dose of AVALIDE (irbesartan/hydrochlorothiazide) should be determined by the titration of the individual components.
- Use AVALIDE with patients with liver impairment is not advisable.
- Dosage adjustment may be required in hemodialysis patients (see Recommended Dose and Dosage Adjustment, Renal Insufficiency).

Recommended Dose and Dosage Adjustment: Once the patient has been stabilized on the individual components as described below, either one tablet of AVALIDE 150/12.5 mg, 300/12.5 mg or 300/25 mg once daily may be substituted if the doses on which the patient was stabilized are the same as those in the fixed combination.

AVALIDE may be administered with or without food, however it should be taken consistently with respect to food intake.

Irbesartan Monotherapy: The recommended dose of irbesartan is 150 mg once daily. In patients whose blood pressure is not adequately controlled, the daily dose may be increased to 300 mg.

Severe Hypertension (Sitting DBP ≥110 mmHg): The starting dose of AVALIDE for initial treatment of severe hypertension is one tablet of AVALIDE 150/12.5 mg once daily (see Indications and Clinical Use). The dosage may be increased after two to four weeks of therapy to a maximum of one 300/25 mg tablet once daily. AVALIDE is not recommended as initial therapy in patients with intravascular volume depletion (see Warnings and Precautions, Hypotension).

Dose Adjustment in Special Population: Diuretic Treated Patients: In patients receiving diuretics, irbesartan therapy should be initiated with caution, since these patients may be volume-depleted and thus more likely to experience hypotension following initiation of additional antihypertensive therapy. Whenever possible, all diuretics should be discontinued two to three days prior to the administration of irbesartan to reduce the likelihood of hypotension (see Warnings and Precautions, Cardiovascular, Hypotension, and Drug Interactions). If this is not possible because of the patient's condition, irbesartan should be administered with caution and the blood pressure monitored closely. The recommended starting dose of irbesartan is 75 mg once daily in hypovolemic patients (see Warnings and Precautions, Cardiovascular, Hypotension). Thereafter, the dosage should be adjusted according to the individual response of the patient.

Geriatrics: No initial dosage adjustment in irbesartan is necessary for most elderly patients. Appropriate caution should nevertheless be used when prescribing to the elderly, as increased vulnerability to drug effect is possible in this patient population. (See Warnings and Precautions, Geriatrics.)

Hepatic Insufficiency: No initial dosage adjustment in irbesartan is generally necessary in patients with mild to moderate hepatic impairment. Since thiazide diuretics may precipitate hepatic coma, the use of a fixed combination product such as AVALIDE is not advisable.

Renal Insufficiency: No initial dosage adjustment in irbesartan is generally necessary in patients with renal impairment, although due to the apparent greater sensitivity of hemodialysis patients, an initial dose of 75 mg is recommended in this group of patients.

The usual regimens of therapy with AVALIDE may be followed as long as the patient's creatinine clearance is >30 mL/min. In patients with more severe renal impairment, loop diuretics are preferred to thiazides so AVALIDE is not recommended.

Missed Dose: Patients should be instructed to take AVALIDE at the next scheduled dose and not take two doses at the same time if they miss a dose.

OVERDOSAGE:

No specific information is available on the treatment of overdosage with AVALIDE (irbesartan/hydrochlorothiazide). The patient should be closely monitored, and the treatment should be symptomatic and supportive, including fluid and electrolyte replacement.

Irbesartan: No data or very little data available in regard to overdosage in humans.

The most likely manifestations of overdosage would be hypotension and/or tachycardia; bradycardia might also occur in this setting. Irbesartan is not removed by hemodialysis.

Hydrochlorothiazide: The most common signs and symptoms observed are those caused by electrolyte depletion (hypokalemia, hypochloremia, hyponatremia) and dehydration resulting from excessive diuresis. If digitalis has also been administered, hypokalemia may accentuate cardiac arrhythmias.

The degree to which hydrochlorothiazide is removed by hemodialysis has not been established.

For management of a suspected drug overdose, contact your **regional Poison Control Centre**. See the *CPS* Directory section for a list of Poison Control Centres.

ACTION AND CLINICAL PHARMACOLOGY: Mechanism of Action: AVALIDE (irbesartan/hydrochlorothiazide) combines the actions of irbesartan, an angiotensin II AT_1 receptor blocker, and that of a thiazide diuretic, hydrochlorothiazide.

Irbesartan: Irbesartan antagonizes angiotensin II by blocking AT_1 receptors.

Angiotensin II is the primary vasoactive hormone in the renin-angiotensin system. Its effects include vasoconstriction and the stimulation of aldosterone secretion by the adrenal cortex.

Irbesartan blocks the vasoconstrictor and aldosterone-secreting effects of angiotensin II by selectively blocking in a non competitive manner the binding of angiotensin II to the AT_1 receptor found in many tissues. Irbesartan has no agonist activity at the AT_1 receptor. AT_2 receptors have been found in many tissues, but to date they have not been associated with cardiovascular homeostasis. Irbesartan has essentially no affinity for the AT_2 receptors.

Irbesartan does not inhibit angiotensin converting enzyme, also known as kininase II, the enzyme that converts angiotensin I to angiotensin II and degrades bradykinin, nor does it affect renin or other hormone receptors or ion channels involved in cardiovascular regulation of blood pressure and sodium homeostasis.

Hydrochlorothiazide: Hydrochlorothiazide is a thiazide diuretic. Thiazides affect the renal tubular mechanisms of electrolyte reabsorption, directly increasing excretion of sodium and chloride in approximately equivalent amounts. Indirectly, the diuretic action of hydrochlorothiazide reduces plasma volume, with consequent increases in plasma renin activity, increases in aldosterone secretion, increases in urinary potassium loss, and decreases in serum potassium. The renin-aldosterone link is mediated by angiotensin II, so coadministration of an angiotensin II AT_1 receptor blocker tends to reverse the potassium loss associated with these diuretics.

The mechanism of the antihypertensive effect of thiazides is not fully understood.

Pharmacodynamics: Irbesartan : In healthy subjects, single oral doses of irbesartan up to 300 mg produced dose-dependent inhibition of the pressor effect of angiotensin II infusions. The inhibition was complete (100%) 4 hours following oral doses of 150 mg or 300 mg. Partial inhibition of 40% and 60% was still present 24 hours post-dose with 150 mg and 300 mg irbesartan respectively.

In hypertensive patients, angiotensin II receptor inhibition following chronic administration of irbesartan causes a 1.5-2 fold rise in angiotensin II plasma concentration and a 2-3 fold increase in plasma renin levels. Aldosterone plasma concentrations generally decline following irbesartan administration, however serum potassium levels are not significantly affected at recommended doses.

During clinical trials, minimal incremental blood pressure response was observed at doses greater than 300 mg.

The blood pressure lowering effect of irbesartan is apparent after the first dose and substantially present within 1-2 weeks, with the maximal effect occurring by 4-6 weeks. In long-term studies, the effect of irbesartan appeared to be maintained for more than one year. There was essentially no change in average heart rate in patients treated with irbesartan in controlled trials.

There is no rebound effect after withdrawal of irbesartan.

Black hypertensive patients had a smaller blood pressure response to irbesartan monotherapy than Caucasians.

Hydrochlorothiazide: Onset of the diuretic action following oral administration occurs in 2 hours and the peak action in about 4 hours. Diuretic activity lasts about 6 to 12 hours.

Irbesartan/Hydrochlorothiazide: The components of AVALIDE have been shown to have an additive effect on blood pressure reduction, reducing blood pressure to a greater degree than either component alone.

Pharmacokinetics: SeeTable 3 and Table 4.

Table 3: AVALIDE

Pharmacokinetic Parameters for Irbersartan

Irbesartan	T_{max} (h)	$t_{½}$ (h)	Clearance (mL/minute)	Volume of distribution (L)
Single Dose Mean	1.5–2	11–15	Plasma 157–176 Renal 3.0–3.5	53–93

Table 4: AVALIDE

Pharmacokinetic Parameters for Hydrochlorothiazide

Hydrochlorothiazide	T_{max}	$t_{½}$	Clearance (mL/minute)	Volume of distribution (L/kg)
Single Dose Mean	1.5–2	5–15	Plasma 192–343 Predominantly Renal (unchanged)	1.5–4.2

Irbesartan: Absorption: Irbesartan is an orally active agent. The oral absorption of irbesartan is rapid and complete with an average absolute bioavailability of 60%-80%. Following oral administration, peak plasma concentrations are attained at 1.5-2 hours after dosing. Steady-state concentrations are achieved within 3 days.

Distribution: The average volume of distribution of irbesartan is 53-93 litres.

Irbesartan is approximately 96% protein-bound in the plasma, primarily to albumin and α_1-acid glycoprotein.

Metabolism: Irbesartan is metabolized via glucuronide conjugation, and oxidation by the cytochrome P-450 system.

Excretion: Irbesartan and its metabolites are excreted by both biliary and renal routes. Following either oral or intravenous administration of ^{14}C-labeled irbesartan, about 20% of radioactivity is recovered in the urine and the remainder in the feces. Less than 2% of the dose is excreted in urine as unchanged irbesartan. Irbesartan exhibits linear pharmacokinetics over the therapeutic dose range with an average terminal elimination half-life of 11-15 hours.

Total plasma and renal clearances are in the range of 157-176 and 3.0-3.5 mL/minute, respectively.

Hydrochlorothiazide: Absorption: Hydrochlorothiazide is rapidly absorbed from the gastrointestinal tract. The bioavailability is approximately 65 to 70%.

Distribution: Hydrochlorothiazide crosses the placental but not the blood-brain barrier and is excreted in breast milk.

Metabolism: Hydrochlorothiazide is not metabolized.

Excretion: Hydrochlorothiazide is eliminated rapidly by the kidney. At least 61% of the oral dose is eliminated unchanged within 24 hours. The plasma half life has been observed to vary from 5.6 and 14.8 hours.

Special Populations and Conditions: Geriatrics: In subjects over the age of 65 years, irbesartan elimination half-life was not significantly altered, but AUC and C_{max} values were about 20-50% greater than those of young subjects.

Renal Insufficiency: The mean AUC and C_{max} of irbesartan were not altered in patients with any degree of renal impairment, including patients on hemodialysis. However, a wide variance was seen in patients with severe renal impairment.

Hepatic Insufficiency: The pharmacokinetics of irbesartan following repeated oral administration were not significantly affected in patients with mild to moderate cirrhosis of the liver. No data is available in patients with severe liver disease.

STORAGE AND STABILITY: AVALIDE (irbesartan/hydrochlorothiazide) tablets can be stored between 15 and 30°C.

INFORMATION FOR THE PATIENT: Published in e-CPS, available by subscription at www.e-cps.ca.

DOSAGE FORMS, COMPOSITION AND PACKAGING: 150/12.5 mg: Each peach, biconvex, oval tablet, with a heart shape debossed on one side and the digits 2775 on the other, contains: irbesartan 150 mg and hydrochlorothiazide 12.5 mg. Nonmedicinal ingredients: croscarmellose sodium, ferric oxide red, ferric oxide yellow, lactose, magnesium stearate, microcrystalline cellulose, pregelatinized starch and silicon dioxide. Bottles of 90.

300/12.5 mg: Each peach, biconvex, oval tablet, with a heart shape debossed on one side and the digits 2776 on the other, contains: irbesartan 300 mg and hydrochlorothiazide 12.5 mg. Nonmedicinal ingredients: croscarmellose sodium, ferric oxide red, ferric oxide yellow, lactose, magnesium stearate, microcrystalline cellulose, pregelatinized starch and silicon dioxide. Bottles of 90.

300/25 mg: Each pink, film-coated, biconvex, oval tablet, with a heart shape debossed on one side and the digits 2788 on the other, contains: irbesartan 300 mg and hydrochlorothiazide 25 mg. Nonmedicinal ingredients: black iron oxides, carnauba wax, croscarmellose sodium, ferric oxide red, ferric oxide yellow, hypromellose, lactose monohydrate, magnesium stearate, microcrystalline cellulose, polyethylene glycol, pregelatinized starch, silicon dioxide and titanium dioxide. Bottles of 90.

(Shown in Product Identification Section)

The reader is invited to consult CPhA's monograph **Corticosteroids: Eye, Ear, Nose.**

Avamys®

fluticasone furoate

Corticosteroid for Nasal Use

GlaxoSmithKline

Date of Revision: April 20, 2010

SUMMARY PRODUCT INFORMATION:

Route of Administration	Dosage Form/Strength	All Nonmedicinal Ingredients
Intranasal	Nasal Spray/27.5 µg	0.015% w/w benzalkonium chloride, carboxymethylcellulose sodium, dextrose anhydrous, edetate disodium, microcrystalline cellulose, polysorbate 80 and purified water

INDICATIONS AND CLINICAL USE: AVAMYS (fluticasone furoate nasal spray) is indicated for:
- treatment of seasonal and perennial allergic rhinitis and its associated symptoms in patients 12 years of age and older.

Pediatrics (2 years to <12 years of age):
- treatment of seasonal and perennial allergic rhinitis.

CONTRAINDICATIONS:
- AVAMYS (fluticasone furoate nasal spray) is contraindicated in patients with a hypersensitivity to any of its ingredients. For a complete listing, see Dosage Forms, Composition and Packaging.

WARNINGS AND PRECAUTIONS: Systemic and/or local corticosteroid use has been associated with the following risks:

General: In patients previously on systemic steroids, either over prolonged periods or in high doses, the replacement with a topical corticosteroid can be accompanied by symptoms of withdrawal e.g. joint and/or muscular pain, lassitude and depression and, in severe cases, adrenal insufficiency may occur, necessitating the temporary resumption of systemic steroid therapy.

Ear/Nose/Throat: In clinical studies of 2 to 52 weeks duration, epistaxis and nasal ulcerations were observed more frequently and some epistaxis events were more severe in patients treated with AVAMYS (fluticasone furoate nasal spray) than those who received placebo. These observations were more prevalent in a longer duration chronic use study (52 weeks in adults and adolescents) conducted in a perennial allergic rhinitis population and therefore may not be indicative of event rates incurred with short-term intermittent use (see Adverse Reactions). In pediatric studies of up to 12 weeks duration, epistaxis events occurred at a similar rate between the active and placebo groups (see Adverse Reactions). A well-controlled, randomized, parallel-group, open-label, multi-centered clinical trial evaluated the effects of 52-weeks of once-daily treatment with AVAMYS 110 µg (N=56) or mometasone furoate nasal spray (MFNS) 200 µg (N=60) on the nasal mucosa of patients 18 years of age and older. An untreated non-rhinitic healthy control (HC) group (N=30) also underwent nasal biopsy at baseline and endpoint. Overall, nasal biopsies from patients treated with AVAMYS exhibited no evidence of mucosal atrophy. The effects of AVAMYS on mucosal atrophy in adolescents and children, or beyond 52 weeks has not been studied.

C. albicans Infection: Evidence of localized infections of the nose with *C. albicans* was seen on nasal exams in 7 of 2745 patients treated with AVAMYS (fluticasone furoate nasal spray) during clinical trials and was reported as an adverse event in 3 patients. When such an infection develops, it may require treatment with appropriate local therapy and discontinuation of AVAMYS (fluticasone furoate nasal spray). Therefore, patients using AVAMYS (fluticasone furoate nasal spray) over several months or longer should be examined periodically for evidence of Candida infection or other signs of adverse effects on the nasal mucosa.

Impaired Wound Healing: Monitor patients periodically for signs of adverse effects on the nasal mucosa. Avoid use in patients with recent nasal ulcers, nasal surgery, or nasal trauma, because of the inhibitory effect of corticosteroids on wound healing.

Endocrine and Metabolism: There is no evidence of HPA axis suppression following prolonged (12 months) treatment with AVAMYS (fluticasone furoate nasal spray). When intranasal steroids are used at higher than recommended dosages or in susceptible individuals at recommended dosages, systemic corticosteroid effects may occur, such as hypercorticism, suppression of HPA function, and/or reduction of growth velocity in children or teenagers. The results of a controlled, 2-week, cross-over study in children aged 6 to 11 years with allergic rhinitis demonstrated that knemometric assessment of short-term lower-leg growth was similar after treatment with AVAMYS (fluticasone furoate nasal spray) 110 µg once daily compared with placebo. A phase IV clinical trial (one year linear growth study) is being carried out to evaluate the effect of AVAMYS (fluticasone furoate nasal spray) on long term growth in pediatric patients.

Physicians should closely follow the growth of children and adolescents taking corticosteroids, by any route, and weigh the benefits of corticosteroid therapy against the possibility of growth suppression if growth appears slowed. If such changes occur, the dosage of all corticosteroids, including AVAMYS (fluticasone furoate nasal spray) should be discontinued slowly (see also Action and Clinical Pharmacology, Pharmacodynamics).

Hepatic/Biliary/Pancreatic: Fluticasone furoate undergoes extensive first-pass metabolism by the liver enzyme CYP3A4, therefore the pharmacokinetics of AVAMYS (fluticasone furoate nasal spray) in patients with severe liver disease may be altered (see Action and Clinical Pharmacology, Special Populations and Conditions).

Based on data with another glucocorticoid metabolized by CYP3A4, coadministration with ritonavir is not recommended because of the risk of systemic effects secondary to increased exposure to fluticasone furoate. However, a study confirming the effects of ritonavir coadministration with AVAMYS (fluticasone furoate nasal spray) has not been conducted (see Drug Interactions).

Immune: Potential worsening of existing tuberculosis; fungal, bacterial, viral, or parasitic infections; or ocular herpes simplex may occur.

Corticosteroids may mask some signs of infection and new infections may appear. A decreased resistance to localized infections has been observed during corticosteroid therapy; this may require treatment with appropriate therapy or stopping the administration of AVAMYS (fluticasone furoate) nasal spray.

Patients who are on drugs that suppress the immune system are more susceptible to infections than healthy individuals. Chickenpox and measles, for example, can have a more serious or even fatal course in non-immune children or adults on corticosteroids. In such children or adults who have not had these diseases, particular care should be taken to avoid exposure. How the dose, route, and duration of corticosteroid administration affect the risk of developing a disseminated infection is not known. The contribution of the underlying disease and/or prior corticosteroid treatment to the risk is also not known. If exposed to chickenpox, prophylaxis with varicella zoster immune globulin (VZIG) may be indicated. If exposed to measles, prophylaxis with pooled intramuscular immunoglobulin (IG), as appropriate, may be indicated. If chickenpox develops, treatment with antiviral agents may be considered.

Ophthalmologic: Nasal and inhaled corticosteroids may result in the development of glaucoma and/or cataracts. Therefore, close monitoring is warranted in patients with a change in vision or with a history of increased intraocular pressure, glaucoma, and/or cataracts.

Glaucoma and cataract formation was evaluated with intraocular pressure measurements and slit lamp examinations in one controlled 12-month study in 806 adolescent and adult patients aged 12 years and older and in one controlled 12-week study in 558 pediatric patients aged 2 to 11 years. The patients had perennial allergic rhinitis and were treated with either AVAMYS (fluticasone furoate nasal spray) (110 µg once daily in adult and adolescent patients and 55 or 110 µg once daily in pediatric patients) or placebo. Intraocular pressure remained within the sponsor-defined threshold (<21 mmHg) in ≥98% of the patients in both studies (see also Adverse Reactions, Ophthalmologic Safety).

In the 52 week adult and adolescent study (FFR102123) intraocular pressure measurements increased above the sponsor-defined threshold (≥21 mmHg) in <2% of patients. These increases were not persistent or sustained at more than one timepoint. In the adult/adolescent study, 6 (1%) patients treated with AVAMYS (fluticasone furoate nasal spray) 110 µg once daily and 1 (0.5%) patient treated with placebo had cataracts identified during the study that were not present at baseline (note: subjects were randomized in a 3:1 ratio for fluticasone furoate nasal spray versus placebo). In the 12 week pediatric study (FFR30008), intraocular pressure measurements increased above the sponsor-defined threshold (≥21 mmHg) in <2% of patients. One (<1%) patient in the fluticasone furoate group reported a cataract at week 12 in both eyes that was not present at baseline. No visual disturbances or glaucoma was detected in either study (see also Adverse Reactions, Ophthalmologic Safety).

Other Systemic Effects: Rarely, immediate and delayed hypersensitivity reactions (e.g. angioedema, rash, urticaria and anaphylaxis) may occur after administration of AVAMYS.

Special Populations: Pregnant Women: There are no adequate and well controlled studies in pregnant women. AVAMYS (fluticasone furoate nasal spray) should be used during pregnancy only if the potential benefit justifies the potential risk to the fetus.

Nursing Women: It is not known whether fluticasone furoate is excreted in human breast milk. However, other corticosteroids have been detected in human milk. Since there are no data from controlled trials on the use of AVAMYS (fluticasone furoate nasal spray) by nursing mothers, caution should be exercised when AVAMYS (fluticasone furoate nasal spray) is administered to a nursing woman. The use of fluticasone furoate in nursing mothers requires that the possible benefits of the drug be weighed against the potential hazards to the infant.

Pediatrics (less than 2 years of age): The safety and effectiveness of AVAMYS (fluticasone furoate nasal spray) in children below 2 years of age have not been evaluated.

Pediatrics (2-17 years of age): A total of 344 subjects aged 12 to 17 years were randomized in clinical trials, with 198 of these subjects treated with AVAMYS (fluticasone furoate nasal spray). The proportion of subjects 12-17 years of age reporting adverse events in these clinical trials was generally lower than in the adult population (18 to <65 year age group). In addition, other clinical trials of AVAMYS (fluticasone furoate nasal spray) have been conducted in 1224 patients aged 2 to 11 years treated with AVAMYS (fluticasone furoate nasal spray) 110 or 55 µg. Overall adverse events for subjects in this age group were reported with approximately the same frequency in patients treated with AVAMYS (fluticasone furoate nasal spray) versus placebo (see Adverse Reactions).

Geriatrics (≥65 years of age): Clinical studies of AVAMYS (fluticasone furoate nasal spray) did not include sufficient numbers of subjects aged 65 and over to determine whether they respond differently from younger subjects. Other reported clinical experience has not identified differences in responses between the elderly and younger patients. In general, dose selection for an elderly patient should be cautious, reflecting the greater frequency of decreased hepatic, renal, or cardiac function, and of concomitant disease or other drug therapy.

ADVERSE REACTIONS: Adverse Drug Reaction Overview: In general, in adults, adolescents and children, adverse reactions to AVAMYS (fluticasone furoate nasal spray) were similar to those seen with other intranasal corticosteroids and were primarily associated with irritation of the nasal mucous membranes. Overall adverse events were reported with approximately the same frequency by patients treated with AVAMYS (fluticasone furoate nasal spray) and those receiving placebo. Less than 3% of patients in clinical trials discontinued treatment because of adverse events.

Clinical Trial Adverse Drug Reactions: Because clinical trials are conducted under very specific conditions the adverse reaction rates observed in the clinical trials may not reflect the rates observed in practice and should not be compared to the rates in the clinical trials of another drug. Adverse drug reaction information from clinical trials is useful for identifying drug-related adverse events and for approximating rates.

Systemic and local corticosteroid use may result in the following:
- Epistaxis, ulcerations, *C. albicans* infection, impaired wound healing (see Warnings and Precautions)
- Cataracts and glaucoma (see Warnings and Precautions)
- Immunosuppression (see Warnings and Precautions)
- Hypothalamic-pituitary-adrenal (HPA) axis effects, including growth reduction (see Warnings and Precautions, Endocrine and Metabolism)

Adults and Adolescents (12 years of age and older): The data described below reflect exposure to AVAMYS (fluticasone furoate nasal spray) in 1079 adult and adolescent patients (661 females and 418 males aged 12 years and older) with seasonal or perennial allergic rhinitis in 8 controlled clinical trials. Patients were treated with AVAMYS (fluticasone furoate nasal spray) 110 µg once daily for 2 to 6 weeks. The rate of withdrawal among patients receiving AVAMYS (fluticasone furoate nasal spray) in these clinical trials was similar or lower than the rate among patients receiving placebo.

Table 1 displays the common adverse events (≥1%) that occurred in patients treated with AVAMYS (fluticasone furoate nasal spray) compared with placebo treated patients. These represent the absolute number of reported adverse events, regardless of whether or not a causal association was established.

Table 1: AVAMYS

Summary of Adverse Events with an Incidence ≥1% During Treatment (ITT population-studies FFR20001/FFR20002/FFR30002/FFR30003/FFR103184/FFR104861/FFR106080/FFU111439)

	Number of Subjects (%)	
Adverse Event	**Placebo N=1079**	**FF 110 µg QD N=1077**
Any event	327 (30)	369 (34)
Headache	88 (8)	99 (9)
Epistaxis	51 (5)	82 (8)
Pharyngolaryngeal pain	15 (1)	31 (3)
Nasal septum ulceration	3 (<1)	13 (1)
Nasopharyngitis	20 (2)	26 (2)
Back pain	10 (<1)	12 (1)
Upper Respiratory Tract Infection	14 (1)	11 (1)
Nausea	4 (<1)	11 (1)

In one controlled clinical trial, 605 patients (307 females and 298 males aged 12 years and older) were treated with AVAMYS (fluticasone furoate nasal spray) 110 µg once daily for 12 months. Adverse events were similar in type and rate between the treatment groups. However, epistaxis occurred more frequently in the group receiving AVAMYS (fluticasone furoate nasal spray) (123/605, 20%) than in the placebo group (17/201, 8%). The episodes of epistaxis were of mild intensity in the majority of patients (83/123 in the group receiving AVAMYS (fluticasone furoate nasal spray) and 17/17 in the placebo group). The episodes were of moderate intensity in 39 patients and of severe intensity in 1 patient receiving AVAMYS (fluticasone furoate nasal spray). This was a longer duration chronic use study conducted in a perennial allergic rhinitis population and therefore may not be indicative of event rates with short-term, intermittent use.

Systemic corticosteroid side effects were not reported during this clinical study.

Less Common Clinical Trial Adverse Drug Reactions (<1%): Table 2 displays the less common adverse events (<1%) that occurred in patients treated with AVAMYS (fluticasone furoate nasal spray) compared with placebo treated patients. All incidences are included. These represent the absolute number of reported adverse events, regardless of whether or not a causal association was established.

Table 2: AVAMYS

Summary of Less Common Adverse Events with an Incidence <1% During Treatment (ITT population-studies FFR20001/FFR20002/FFR30002/FFR30003/FFR103184/FFR104861/FFR106080/ FFU111439)

Body System	Less Common Adverse Events	Number of Subjects (%) Placebo N=1079	FF 110 µg QD N=1077
Nervous System Disorders	dizziness	7 (<1%)	9 (<1%)
	migraine	7 (<1%)	4 (<1%)
	tremor	0	2 (<1%)
	psychomotor hyperactivity	0	1 (<1%)
Respiratory, Thoracic and Mediastinal Disorders	cough	11 (1%)	10 (<1%)
	dry throat	2 (<1%)	7 (<1%)
	nasal discomfort	7 (<1%)	5 (<1%)
	dysphonia	1 (<1%)	2 (<1%)
	dyspnea	2 (<1%)	2 (<1%)
	sinus congestion	0	1 (<1%)
	throat irritation	0	2 (<1%)
Infection	herpes simplex	5 (<1%)	2 (<1%)
	vaginal candidiasis	0	1 (<1%)
Metabolic	aspartate aminotransferase increased	2 (<1%)	2 (<1%)
	alanine aminotransferase increased	2 (<1%)	1 (<1%)
	blood pressure increased	2 (<1%)	2 (<1%)
	blood glucose increased	4 (<1%)	3 (<1%)
Cardiovascular	palpitations	0	2 (<1%)
	atrioventricular block second degree	0	1 (<1%)

Pediatrics (2 to <12 years of age): The data from pediatric patients are based upon 3 clinical trials in which 795 children with seasonal or perennial rhinitis (352 females and 443 males 2 to <12 years of age) were treated with AVAMYS (fluticasone furoate nasal spray) 55 or 110 µg once daily for 2 to 12 weeks.

Table 3 displays the common adverse events (≥1%) that occurred in patients treated with AVAMYS (fluticasone furoate nasal spray) compared with placebo treated patients. These represent the absolute number of reported adverse events, regardless of whether or not a causal association was established. In children, the adverse event profile was similar to that seen for the adults and adolescents.

Table 3: AVAMYS

Adverse Events with ≥1% Incidence in Controlled Clinical Trials of 2 to 12 Weeks Duration with AVAMYS in Pediatric Patients 2 to <12 Years of Age with Seasonal or Perennial Allergic Rhinitis—Studies FFR100010, FFR30008, FFR100012

Adverse Event	Number (%) of Subjects Placebo (n=429)	FF 55 µg QD (n=369)	FF 110 µg QD (n=426)
Any Event	157 (37)	158 (43)	174 (41)
Headache	30 (7)	28 (8)	32 (8)
Nasopharyngitis	21 (5)	20 (5)	21 (5)
Epistaxis	19 (4)	17 (5)	17 (4)
Pyrexia	7 (2)	17 (5)	19 (4)
Pharyngolaryngeal pain	14 (3)	16 (4)	12 (3)
Cough	12 (3)	12 (3)	16 (4)
Bronchitis	11 (3)	11 (3)	8 (2)

Less Common Clinical Trial Adverse Drug Events (<1%): One of the less common clinical trial adverse events was nasal ulceration which occurred at a lower frequency in pediatric patients (2 to <12 years of age) than in adult and adolescent patients. Drug-related nasal ulceration was reported in 1 patient receiving placebo (<1%), 1 patient receiving 55 µg AVAMYS (fluticasone furoate nasal spray) (<1%) and 4 patients receiving 110 µg AVAMYS (fluticasone furoate nasal spray) (<1%) once daily. Another less common adverse event was increased intraocular pressure. Drug-related increased intraocular pressure was reported in 1 patient receiving placebo (<1%), 2 patients receiving 55 µg AVAMYS (fluticasone furoate nasal spray) once daily (<1%) and 1 patient receiving 110 µg AVAMYS (fluticasone furoate nasal spray) once daily (<1%). One patient treated with 55 µg AVAMYS (fluticasone furoate nasal spray) reported a cataract in both eyes at Week 12 that were not detected at baseline and was considered a drug-related adverse event (see also Adverse Reactions, Ophthalmologic Safety).

Ophthalmologic Safety: Glaucoma and cataract formation was evaluated in one controlled 12-month study in 806 adolescent and adult patients aged 12 years and older, and in one controlled 12-week study in 558 pediatric patients aged 2 to 11 years. Both studies were in the perennial allergic rhinitis patient population.

Patients in the adult/adolescent study were randomized in a 3:1 ratio to treatment with either fluticasone furoate 110 µg (n=605) or placebo (n=201), once daily. Ophthalmic evaluations were performed at Baseline and Weeks 12, 24 and 52. Intraocular pressure (IOP) remained within the sponsor-defined threshold (<21 mmHg) in ≥98% of the patients. Nine patients, 5 in the fluticasone furoate group (<1%) and 4 in the placebo group (2%), had IOP measurements ≥21 mmHg at baseline. Of these 5 patients in the fluticasone furoate group, 1 patient had no further IOP measurements, 1 patient had an IOP of 22 mmHg at a subsequent visit but values were lower than at baseline, and the remaining 3 patients had IOP measurements <21 mmHg at all subsequent treatment assessments. During the study 12 patients in the fluticasone furoate group had IOP measurements that increased above the sponsor-defined threshold (≥21 mmHg). However, no patient had an IOP >21 mmHg at more than one treatment assessment. Therefore, these changes in IOP measurements would not be considered persistent/sustained at more than one timepoint during the study. In addition, funduscopic cup to disc percentage values remained below the sponsor-defined threshold (66%) in all of these patients at all assessments and no cataracts were reported for them. No visual disturbances or glaucoma were seen in the study.

Further, 7 patients [6 (1%) in the fluticasone furoate group and 1 (0.5%) in the placebo group] had cataracts identified during the study that were not present at baseline. Posterior subcapsular cataracts were reported as adverse events in 2 patients (0.33%) receiving fluticasone furoate and 1 patient (0.5 %) receiving placebo. However, upon post-study evaluation in a patient in the fluticasone furoate group, the posterior subcapsular cataract was no longer detected.

Patients in the pediatric study were randomized to treatment with either fluticasone furoate 110 µg (n=185), fluticasone furoate 55 µg (n=185) or placebo (n=188) once daily for 12 weeks. Ophthalmic evaluations were performed at baseline and Week 12. Intraocular pressure (IOP) remained within the sponsor-defined threshold (<21 mmHg) in ≥98% of the patients. Two patients [1 in the fluticasone furoate 55 µg group (<1%) and 1 in the fluticasone furoate 110 µg group (<1%)] had IOP measurements ≥21 mmHg at baseline. However, these IOP measurements had decreased to below 21 mmHg at Week 12. Four adverse events of increased intraocular pressure were considered drug-related (see Pediatrics (2 to <12 years of age), Less Common Clinical Trial Adverse Drug Events (<1%)). However, funduscopic cup to disc percentage values remained below the sponsor-defined threshold (≥66%) in all of these subjects at all assessments and none of these patients reported a cataract.

In the same pediatric study, 4 patients in the fluticasone furoate 55 µg group (2%) reported a cataract in at least one eye compared with 2 patients in the placebo group (1%). Of these, the following three reports of cataracts were considered to be drug-related adverse events: one patient in the fluticasone furoate 55 µg group reported a cataract in both eyes at week 12 that was not detected at baseline; and in the placebo group, two patients also reported a cataract in both eyes at the end of the study that was not detected at baseline. No patient in the 110 µg fluticasone furoate group reported a cataract. No visual disturbances or glaucoma were seen in the study.

Post-Market Adverse Drug Reactions: The following adverse reactions have been identified during post-approval use of AVAMYS. Rare reports of hypersensitivity reactions, including anaphylaxis, angioedema, dyspnoea, rash and urticaria.

Because these reactions are reported voluntarily from a population of uncertain size, it is not always possible to reliably estimate their frequency or establish a causal relationship to drug exposure.

DRUG INTERACTIONS: Overview: Fluticasone furoate is cleared by extensive first-pass metabolism mediated by the cytochrome P450 isozyme CYP3A4. In a drug interaction study of intranasal fluticasone furoate and the CYP3A4 inhibitor ketoconazole given as a 200 mg once-daily dose for 7 days, 6 of 20 subjects receiving fluticasone furoate and ketoconazole had measurable but low levels of fluticasone furoate compared with 1 of 20 receiving fluticasone furoate and placebo. Based on this study and the low systemic exposure, there was a 5% reduction in 24-hour serum cortisol levels with ketoconazole compared to placebo. The data from this study should be carefully interpreted because the study was conducted with ketoconazole 200 mg once daily rather than 400 mg, which is the maximum recommended dosage. Therefore, caution is required with the coadministration of AVAMYS (fluticasone furoate nasal spray) and ketoconazole or other potent CYP3A4 inhibitors.

Based on data with another glucocorticoid, fluticasone propionate, metabolized by CYP3A4, coadministration of AVAMYS (fluticasone furoate nasal spray) with the potent CYP3A4 inhibitor ritonavir is not recommended because of the risk of systemic effects secondary to increased exposure to fluticasone furoate. High exposure to corticosteroids increases the potential for systemic side effects, such as cortisol suppression.

Enzyme induction and inhibition data suggest that fluticasone furoate is unlikely to significantly alter the cytochrome P450-mediated metabolism of other compounds at clinically relevant intranasal dosages.

Drug-Drug Interactions: See Table 4.

Table 4: AVAMYS

Established or Potential Drug-Drug Interactions

Proper Name	Ref	Effect	Clinical Comment
Ritonavir	CS	Systemic effects including Cushing's syndrome and adrenal suppression.	Concomitant use of fluticasone furoate and ritonavir should be avoided. (See Drug interactions, Overview.)
Other inhibitors of cytochrome P450 3A4	CT	Potential increased systemic exposure to fluticasone furoate.	Care is advised when coadministering potent cytochrome P450 3A4 inhibitors. (See Drug interactions, Overview.)

Legend: CS=Class Statement; CT=Clinical Trial.

DOSAGE AND ADMINISTRATION: Dosing Considerations: For full therapeutic benefit, regular scheduled usage is recommended. Onset of action has been observed as early as 8 hours after initial administration in SAR and as early as 24 hours after initial administration in PAR. It may take several days of treatment to achieve maximum benefit. An absence of an immediate effect should be explained to the patient. Similarly, when corticosteroids are discontinued, symptoms may not return for several days.

Recommended Dose and Dosage Adjustment: Adults and Adolescents 12 Years of Age and Older: The recommended dosage is two sprays (27.5 µg of fluticasone furoate per spray) in each nostril once daily (total daily dose, 110 µg).

Pediatrics (2 to <12 years of age): The recommended starting dosage is one spray (27.5 µg of fluticasone furoate per spray) in each nostril once daily (total daily dose, 55 µg). Patients not adequately responding to one spray in each nostril once daily (total daily dose, 55 µg) may use two sprays in each nostril once daily (total daily dose, 110 µg). Once adequate control of symptoms is achieved, dose reduction to one spray in each nostril once daily (total daily dose, 55 µg) is recommended.

Missed Dose: If a single dose is missed, instruct the patient to take the next dose when it is due. Do not instruct the patient to take an extra dose.

Administration: AVAMYS (fluticasone furoate nasal spray) should be administered only by the intranasal route. It is necessary to prime the pump with 6 actuations before first use or after 30 days of non-use or if the cap has been left off for more than 5 days. AVAMYS (fluticasone furoate nasal spray) may be administered at any time of day. Illustrated instructions for proper use appear in Information for the Patient.

OVERDOSAGE:

Chronic overdosage may result in signs/symptoms of hypercorticism (see Warnings and Precautions, Endocrine and Metabolism). There are no data on the effects of acute or chronic overdosage with AVAMYS (fluticasone furoate nasal spray). Because of low systemic bioavailability and an absence of acute drug related systemic findings in clinical studies (with dosages of up to 440 µg/day for 2 weeks [4 times the maximum recommended daily dose]), overdose is unlikely to require any therapy other than observation.

Intranasal administration of up to 2640 µg/day (24 times the recommended adult dose) of AVAMYS (fluticasone furoate nasal spray) to healthy human volunteers for 3 days was well tolerated. The oral median lethal dose in mice and rats was >2000 mg/kg compared with the maximum recommended clinical dose of 2.2 µg/kg based on a 50 kg bodyweight.

Acute overdosage with the intranasal dosage form is unlikely since one bottle of AVAMYS (fluticasone furoate nasal spray) contains approximately 3 mg of fluticasone furoate, and the bioavailability of fluticasone furoate is 0.50% for 2.6 mg/day given intranasally and 1.26% for a single 2 mg dose 2 mg/day given as an oral solution.

For management of a suspected drug overdose, contact your regional Poison Control Centre. See the *CPS* Directory section for a list of Poison Control Centres.

ACTION AND CLINICAL PHARMACOLOGY: Mechanism of Action: Fluticasone furoate is a synthetic trifluorinated corticosteroid with potent anti-inflammatory activity. The precise mechanism through which fluticasone furoate affects rhinitis symptoms is not known. Corticosteroids have been shown to have a wide range of actions on multiple cell types (e.g. mast cells, eosinophils, neutrophils, macrophages, and lymphocytes) and mediators (e.g. histamine, eicosanoids, leukotrienes, and cytokines) involved in inflammation. These anti-inflammatory actions of corticosteroids may contribute to their efficacy in rhinitis.

Specific effects of fluticasone furoate demonstrated in in vitro and in vivo models included activation of the glucocorticoid response element and inhibition of pro inflammatory transcription factors such as NFκB, potent protection of respiratory cells against physical and chemical damage and inhibition of antigen induced lung eosinophilia in sensitized rats. Human glucocorticoid receptor binding studies demonstrated that fluticasone furoate binds with significantly greater affinity than fluticasone propionate and other intranasal corticosteroids. Fluticasone furoate has been shown in vitro to exhibit a binding affinity for the human glucocorticoid receptor that is approximately 29.9 times that of dexamethasone and 1.7 times that of fluticasone propionate. In addition, it has been shown that fluticasone furoate binds more avidly to respiratory tissue than other corticosteroids. The clinical significance of these findings is unknown.

AVAMYS (fluticasone furoate nasal spray), like other corticosteroids, does not have an immediate effect on rhinitis symptoms. Onset of action has been observed as early as 8 hours after initial administration in SAR and as early as 24 hours after initial administration in PAR. It may take several days of treatment to achieve maximum benefit. An absence of an immediate effect should be explained to the patient. Similarly, when corticosteroids are discontinued, symptoms may not return for several days.

Pharmacodynamics: Adrenal Function: The effects of AVAMYS (fluticasone furoate nasal spray) on adrenal function have been evaluated in two controlled clinical trials with domiciled visits at the beginning and end of treatment. The first study was a randomized, double blind, parallel group clinical trial conducted in adult and adolescent patients aged 12 years and older with perennial allergic rhinitis. Patients were treated once daily with AVAMYS (fluticasone furoate nasal spray) 110 μg (n=48), prednisone 10 mg (n=13), or placebo (n=51) for 6 weeks. The 24 hour serum cortisol weighted mean was similar after treatment with AVAMYS (fluticasone furoate nasal spray) compared with placebo (AVAMYS (fluticasone furoate nasal spray):placebo ratio 0.98 [95% CI 0.89, 1.07]). In contrast, the 24 hour serum cortisol weighted mean was reduced by treatment with prednisone (prednisone:placebo ratio 0.49 [95% CI 0.43, 0.57]). The second study was of a similar design, but with no prednisone comparison, in pediatric patients aged 2 to 11 years with perennial allergic rhinitis. Patients were treated once daily with AVAMYS (fluticasone furoate nasal spray) 110 μg (n=57) or placebo (n=55) for 6 weeks. The 24 hour serum cortisol weighted mean was similar for the 2 treatment groups (AVAMYS (fluticasone furoate nasal spray): placebo ratio 0.97 [95% CI 0.88, 1.07]). Both studies also assessed 24 hour urinary cortisol excretion during the domiciled visits. There were no differences between the groups receiving AVAMYS (fluticasone furoate nasal spray) or placebo in 24 hour urinary cortisol.

No evidence of a decrease in 24 hour urinary free cortisol excretion was observed in two placebo-controlled non domiciled (outpatient) clinical studies that included a 12 week study in patients 2 to 11 years and a one year study in patients 12 years and older.

Pharmacokinetics: Absorption: The activity of AVAMYS (fluticasone furoate nasal spray) is due to the parent drug, fluticasone furoate. Following intranasal administration of fluticasone furoate most of the dose is eventually swallowed and undergoes incomplete absorption and extensive first-pass metabolism in the liver and gut, resulting in negligible systemic exposure. At the highest recommended intranasal dose of 110 μg once daily for up to 12 months in adults, plasma concentrations of fluticasone furoate are typically not quantifiable despite the use of a sensitive HPLC-MS/MS assay with a lower limit of quantification (LOQ) of 10 pg/mL.

The absolute bioavailability was evaluated in 16 male and female subjects following supratherapeutic dosages of fluticasone furoate (880 μg given intranasally at 8-hour intervals for 10 doses, or 2640 μg/day). The average absolute bioavailability was 0.50% (90% CI 0.34%, 0.74%).

Distribution: The plasma protein binding of fluticasone furoate is greater than 99%. Fluticasone furoate is widely distributed with volume of distribution at steady-state of, on average, 608 L.

Metabolism: In vivo studies have revealed no evidence of cleavage of the furoate moiety to form fluticasone. Fluticasone furoate is rapidly cleared (total plasma clearance of 58.7 L/h) from systemic circulation principally by hepatic metabolism via the cytochrome P450 isozyme CYP3A4. The principal route of metabolism is hydrolysis of the S-fluoromethyl carbothioate function to form the 17β-carboxylic acid metabolite.

Excretion: Elimination was primarily via the fecal route following oral and intravenous administration indicative of excretion of fluticasone furoate and its metabolites via the bile. Following intravenous administration, the elimination phase half-life averaged 15.1 hours. Urinary excretion accounted for approximately 1 and 2% of the orally and intravenously administered dose, respectively.

Special Populations and Conditions: Hepatic Insufficiency: Reduced liver function may affect the elimination of corticosteroids. Since fluticasone furoate undergoes extensive first-pass metabolism by the hepatic cytochrome P450 isozyme CYP3A4, the pharmacokinetics of fluticasone furoate may be altered in patients with hepatic impairment. A study of a single 400 μg dose of orally inhaled fluticasone furoate in patients with moderate hepatic impairment (Child-Pugh Class B) resulted in increased C_{max} (42%) and $AUC_{(0-t)}$ (172%), resulting in an approximately 20% reduction in serum cortisol level in patients with hepatic impairment compared to healthy subjects. The systemic exposure would be expected to be higher than that observed had the study been conducted after multiple doses and/or in patients with severe hepatic impairment. Therefore, use AVAMYS (fluticasone furoate nasal spray) with caution in patients with severe hepatic impairment. No dosage adjustment is needed for patients with mild or moderate hepatic impairment.

Renal Insufficiency: Fluticasone furoate is not detectable in urine from healthy subjects following intranasal dosing. Less than 1% of dose-related material is excreted in urine. No dosage adjustment is required in patients with renal impairment.

Allergen Chamber Study: A placebo controlled clinical study was carried out in 382 patients with seasonal allergic rhinitis, of which 80% were African American, to determine the onset of action of fluticasone furoate using an allergen challenge chamber (ACC). Patients with a confirmed diagnosis of ragweed allergy were exposed to controlled pollen concentration in an Allergen Challenge Chamber (ACC) and then treated with a single dose of either fluticasone furoate 110 μg aqueous nasal spray or vehicle placebo nasal spray, following which, the iTNSS was determined hourly for 12 hours. A statistically significant difference versus placebo was not shown during the entire 12-hour study duration; therefore no efficacy was demonstrated with fluticasone furoate by which an onset of action could be determined based on the results of this study.

STORAGE AND STABILITY: Store the device between 4 and 30°C, in the upright position with the cap in place. Do not refrigerate or freeze.

INFORMATION FOR THE PATIENT: Published in e-CPS, available by subscription at www.e-cps.ca.

DOSAGE FORMS, COMPOSITION AND PACKAGING: AVAMYS (fluticasone furoate nasal spray) 27.5 μg is supplied in an amber glass bottle enclosed in a nasal device with a small, short nozzle and a side-actuated mist-release button to actuate the spray. Each bottle contains a net fill weight of 4.5 g or 10 g and will provide 30 or 120 metered sprays, respectively, after the initial priming. Each spray delivers a fine mist containing 27.5 μg of fluticasone furoate in 50 μL of formulation through the nozzle. The contents of the bottle can be viewed through an indicator window. The nasal device should be discarded after the labelled amount of sprays has been used. Beyond this, the correct amount of medication in each spray cannot be assured, even though the bottle is not completely empty.

AVAMYS (fluticasone furoate nasal spray) is an unscented, taste free, alcohol free, preserved aqueous suspension of micronized fluticasone furoate for topical administration to the nasal mucosa by means of a metering (50 μL), atomizing spray pump. Nonmedicinal ingredients: 0.015% w/w benzalkonium chloride, carboxymethylcellulose sodium, dextrose anhydrous, edetate disodium, microcrystalline cellulose, polysorbate 80 and purified water.

(Shown in Product Identification Section)

Avandamet® Pr

rosiglitazone maleate—metformin HCl

Antidiabetic

GlaxoSmithKline

Date of Revision: March 24, 2009

SUMMARY PRODUCT INFORMATION:

Route of Administration	Dosage Form/ Strength	Clinically Relevant Nonmedicinal Ingredients
Oral	Tablet/1 mg/500 mg, 2 mg/500 mg, 4 mg/500 mg, 2 mg/1000 mg, 4 mg/1000 mg	Lactose monohydrate For a complete listing see Dosage Forms, Composition and Packaging.

INDICATIONS AND CLINICAL USE: AVANDAMET (rosiglitazone maleate/metformin hydrochloride) is indicated for:

- use as an adjunct to diet and exercise to reduce insulin resistance and improve glycemic control in patients with type 2 diabetes mellitus when diet and exercise plus metformin do not result in adequate glycemic control.

Caloric restriction, weight loss, and exercise improve insulin sensitivity and are essential for the proper treatment of a diabetic patient. These measures are important not only in the primary treatment of type 2 diabetes, but also in maintaining the efficacy of drug therapy. Prior to initiation of therapy with AVANDAMET, secondary causes of poor glycemic control (e.g., infection) should be investigated and treated.

Geriatrics (≥65 years of age): Results of the population pharmacokinetic analysis (n=716 <65 years; n=331 ≥65 years) showed that age does not significantly affect the pharmacokinetics of rosiglitazone.

However, limited data from controlled pharmacokinetic studies of metformin hydrochloride in healthy elderly subjects suggest that total plasma clearance of metformin is decreased, the half-life is prolonged and C_{max} is increased, compared to healthy young subjects. From these data, it appears that the change in metformin pharmacokinetics with aging is primarily accounted for by a change in renal function. Metformin treatment and therefore treatment with AVANDAMET should not be initiated in patients 80 years of age or older unless measurement of creatinine clearance demonstrates that renal function is not reduced (see Warnings and Precautions and Dosage and Administration).

Pediatrics (<18 years of age): The safety and effectiveness of rosiglitazone and metformin have not been established in patients younger than 18 years of age, therefore, AVANDAMET is not indicated in patients younger than 18 years of age.

CONTRAINDICATIONS: AVANDAMET is contraindicated in:

- Patients with New York Heart Association (NYHA) Class I to IV heart failure.
- Patients with renal impairment or for whom renal function is not known, in patients with serum creatinine levels above the upper limit of normal range, and in patients with renal disease or renal dysfunction (e.g., as suggested by serum creatinine levels ≥136 μmol/L (males), ≥124 μmol/L (females) or abnormal creatinine clearance) (<60 mL/min) which may result from conditions such as cardiovascular collapse (shock), acute myocardial infarction, and septicemia (see Warnings and Precautions).
- Patients with known hypersensitivity to this product (rosiglitazone maleate or metformin hydrochloride), or any of its ingredients.
- Patients with acute or chronic metabolic acidosis, including diabetic ketoacidosis, with or without coma, history of ketoacidosis with or without coma. Diabetic ketoacidosis should be treated with insulin.
- Patients with a history of lactic acidosis, irrespective of precipitating factors.
- Patients with serious hepatic impairment (see Warnings and Precautions).
- Patients with Type 1 diabetes mellitus.
- Pregnancy. Insulin is recommended during pregnancy to control blood glucose levels. Oral antidiabetic agents should not be given (see Warnings and Precautions, Special Populations, Pregnant Women).
- Breastfeeding.
- Excessive alcohol intake, acute or chronic.
- In cases of cardiovascular collapse and in disease states associated with hypoxemia such as cardiorespiratory insufficiency, which are often associated with hyperlactacidemia.
- During stress conditions, such as severe infections, trauma or surgery and the recovery phase thereafter.
- In patients suffering from severe dehydration.

AVANDAMET should be temporarily discontinued in patients undergoing radiologic studies involving intravascular administration of iodinated contrast materials, because use of such products may result in acute alteration of renal function (see Warnings and Precautions).

WARNINGS AND PRECAUTIONS: General: AVANDAMET: Administration with Other Drugs: For safety reasons, the use of AVANDAMET in combination with insulin is not indicated.

The use of AVANDAMET in combination with a sulfonylurea (triple therapy) is not indicated. An increase in reporting of fluid retention related events (including congestive heart failure) has been seen in patients receiving rosiglitazone in combination with metformin and a sulfonylurea.

Close monitoring of glycemic control and dose adjustment of the rosiglitazone or metformin components may be needed when AVANDAMET is coadministered with CYP2C8 inhibitors or inducers or cationic drugs that are eliminated by renal tubular excretion (see Drug Interactions).

Rosiglitazone maleate: Due to its mechanism of action, rosiglitazone is active only in the presence of endogenous insulin. Therefore, AVANDAMET should not be used in patients with type 1 diabetes.

Metformin hydrochloride: Radiologic studies involving the use of intravascular iodinated contrast materials (for example, intravenous urogram, intravenous cholangiography, angiography, and computed tomography (CT) scans with contrast materials): Intravascular contrast studies with iodinated materials can lead to acute alteration of renal function and have been associated with lactic acidosis in patients receiving metformin (see Contraindications). Therefore, in patients in whom any such study is planned, AVANDAMET should be temporarily discontinued at the time of or prior to the procedure, and withheld for 48 hours subsequent to the procedure and reinstituted only after renal function has been re-evaluated and found to be normal.

Change in Clinical Status of Previously Controlled Diabetic: A diabetic patient previously well controlled on AVANDAMET who develops laboratory abnormalities or clinical illness (especially vague and poorly defined illness) should be evaluated promptly for evidence of ketoacidosis or lactic acidosis. Evaluation should include serum electrolytes and ketones, blood glucose and, if indicated, blood pH, lactate, pyruvate and metformin levels. If acidosis of either form occurs, AVANDAMET must be stopped immediately and appropriate corrective measures initiated (see Warnings and Precautions, Lactic Acidosis).

Cardiovascular: Rosiglitazone maleate: Congestive Heart Failure: Thiazolidinediones, like rosiglitazone, alone or in combination with other antidiabetic agents, can cause fluid retention, which can exacerbate or lead to congestive heart failure. The fluid retention may very rarely present as rapid and excessive weight gain. All patients should be monitored for signs and symptoms of adverse reactions relating to fluid retention and heart failure (see Adverse Reactions). An increase in reporting of fluid retention related events including congestive heart failure has been seen in patients receiving rosiglitazone in combination with metformin and a sulfonylurea. This triple therapy regimen is not an approved indication.

Treatment with thiazolidinediones has been associated with cases of congestive heart failure, some of which were difficult to treat unless the medication was discontinued. AVANDAMET should be discontinued if any deterioration in cardiac status occurs.

AVANDAMET is contraindicated in patients with NYHA Class I, II, III and IV heart failure. Patients with severe heart failure (including NYHA Class III and IV cardiac status) were not studied during the clinical trials.

Patients experiencing acute coronary syndromes (ACS) have not been studied in rosiglitazone controlled clinical trials. Since patients experiencing ACS are at an increased risk of developing heart failure, and in view of the potential for rosiglitazone to cause or exacerbate heart failure, initiation of AVANDAMET in patients experiencing an acute coronary event is not recommended. Furthermore, discontinuation of AVANDAMET during the acute phase should be considered.

Ischemic Heart Disease: In a retrospective analysis of data from pooled clinical studies, which included patients on combination therapy with insulin as well as patients with NYHA Class I and II heart failure, the overall incidence of events typically associated with cardiac ischemia was higher for rosiglitazone containing regimens, 2.00% versus comparators, 1.53% [Hazard ratio 1.30 (95% confidence interval 1.004-1.69)]. In a subgroup analysis of this data, this risk was further increased in patients receiving nitrates with approximately twice as many events in patients receiving rosiglitazone versus comparators. **The use of AVANDAMET is therefore not recommended for patients being treated with nitrates.**

The completion of an adequately-designed cardiovascular outcome study is needed to further evaluate the risk of myocardial ischemic events associated with rosiglitazone.

In a large observational study where patients were well matched at baseline, the incidence of the composite endpoint of myocardial infarction and coronary revascularization was 1.75 events per 100 person years for rosiglitazone containing regimens and 1.76 events per 100 person years for other anti-diabetic agents [Hazard ratio 0.93 (95% confidence interval 0.80-1.10)].

Edema: AVANDAMET should be used with caution in patients with edema. In healthy volunteers who received rosiglitazone 8 mg once daily as monotherapy for 8 weeks, there was a statistically significant increase in median plasma volume (1.8 mL/kg) compared to placebo. In controlled clinical trials of patients with Type 2 diabetes, mild to moderate edema was observed at a greater frequency in patients treated with rosiglitazone, and may be dose related (see Adverse Reactions). For information on macular edema, see Warnings and Precautions, Ophthalmologic.

Metformin hydrochloride: Hypoxic States: Cardiovascular collapse (shock) from whatever cause, acute congestive heart failure, acute myocardial infarction and other conditions characterized by hypoxemia have been associated with lactic acidosis and may also cause prerenal azotemia. When such events occur in patients receiving AVANDAMET, the drug should be promptly discontinued.

Endocrine and Metabolism: AVANDAMET: Loss of Control of Blood Glucose: When a patient stabilized on any diabetic regimen is exposed to stress such as fever, trauma, infection, or surgery, a temporary loss of glycemic control may occur. At such times, it may be necessary to withhold AVANDAMET and temporarily administer insulin. AVANDAMET may be reinstituted after the acute episode is resolved.

Rosiglitazone maleate: Weight Gain: Dose-related weight gain was seen with rosiglitazone alone and in combination with other hypoglycemic agents. Treatment should be re-evaluated in patients with excessive weight gain (see Action and Clinical Pharmacology and Adverse Reactions).

Fractures: In a 4 to 6 year comparative study (ADOPT) of glycemic control with monotherapy in recently diagnosed patients with Type 2 diabetes mellitus, an increased incidence of bone fracture was noted in female patients taking rosiglitazone maleate (9.3%, 2.7 patients per 100 patient-years) versus glyburide (3.5%, 1.3 patients per 100 patient-years) or metformin (5.1%, 1.5 patients per 100 patient-years). The majoritiy of the fractures in the females who received rosiglitazone maleate were reported in the upper arm, hand, and foot (see Adverse Reactions). The risk of fracture should be considered in the care of patients, especially female patients, treated with rosiglitazone maleate, and attention should be given to assessing and maintaining bone health according to current standards of care.

Metformin hydrochloride: Lactic Acidosis: Lactic acidosis is a rare, but serious, metabolic complication that occurs due to metformin accumulation during treatment with AVANDAMET; when it occurs, it is fatal in approximately 50% of cases. Lactic acidosis may also occur in association with a number of pathophysiologic conditions, including diabetes mellitus, and whenever there is significant tissue hypoperfusion and hypoxemia. Lactic acidosis is characterized by elevated blood lactate levels (>5 mmol/L), decreased blood pH, electrolyte disturbances with an increased anion gap, and an increased lactate/pyruvate ratio. When metformin is implicated as the cause of lactic acidosis, metformin plasma levels >5 µg/mL are generally found.

The reported incidence of lactic acidosis in patients receiving metformin is very low (approximately 0.03 cases/1000 patient-years, with approximately 0.015 fatal cases/1000 patient-years). Reported cases have occurred primarily in diabetic patients with significant renal insufficiency, including both intrinsic renal disease and renal hypoperfusion, often in the setting of multiple concomitant medical/surgical problems and multiple concomitant medications. Patients with congestive heart failure requiring pharmacologic management, in particular those with unstable or acute congestive heart failure who are at risk of hypoperfusion and hypoxemia, are at increased risk of lactic acidosis. In particular, treatment of the elderly should be accompanied by careful monitoring of renal function. AVANDAMET treatment should not be initiated in patients 80 years of age or older, unless measurement of creatinine clearance demonstrates that renal function is not reduced, as these patients are more susceptible to developing lactic acidosis. The risk of lactic acidosis increases with the degree of renal dysfunction and the patient's age. The risk of lactic acidosis may, therefore, be significantly decreased by regular monitoring of renal function in patients taking AVANDAMET and by use of the minimum effective dose of AVANDAMET.

In addition, AVANDAMET should be promptly withheld in the presence of any condition associated with hypoxemia, dehydration or sepsis. Because impaired hepatic function may significantly limit the ability to clear lactate, AVANDAMET should generally be avoided in patients with clinical or laboratory evidence of hepatic disease.

Patients should be cautioned against excessive alcohol intake, either acute or chronic, when taking AVANDAMET, since alcohol potentiates the effects of metformin on lactate metabolism.

The onset of lactic acidosis often is subtle, and accompanied only by nonspecific symptoms such as malaise, myalgias, respiratory distress, increasing somnolence and nonspecific abdominal distress. There may be associated hypothermia, hypotension and resistant bradyarrhythmias with more marked acidosis. The patient and the patient's physician must be aware of the possible importance of such symptoms and the patient should be instructed to notify the physician immediately if they occur (see General). AVANDAMET should be withdrawn until the situation is clarified. Serum electrolytes, ketones, blood glucose and, if indicated, blood pH, lactate levels and even blood metformin levels may be useful. Once a patient is stabilized on any dose level of AVANDAMET, gastrointestinal symptoms, which are common during initiation of therapy, are unlikely to be drug related. Later occurrence of gastrointestinal symptoms could be due to lactic acidosis or other serious disease. Levels of fasting venous plasma lactate above the upper limit of normal but less than 5 mmol/L in patients taking AVANDAMET do not necessarily indicate impending lactic acidosis and may be explainable by other mechanisms, such as poorly controlled diabetes or obesity, vigorous physical activity or technical problems in sample handling. Lactic acidosis should be suspected in any diabetic patient with metabolic acidosis lacking evidence of ketoacidosis (ketonuria and ketonemia).

Lactic acidosis is a medical emergency that must be treated in a hospital setting. In a patient with lactic acidosis who is taking AVANDAMET, the drug should be discontinued immediately and general supportive measures promptly instituted. Because metformin hydrochloride is dialyzable (with a clearance of up to 170 mL/min under good hemodynamic conditions), prompt hemodialysis is recommended to correct the acidosis and remove the accumulated metformin. Such management often results in prompt reversal of symptoms and recovery (see Cardiovascular, Renal, Hepatic, and Contraindications).

If acidosis of any kind develops, AVANDAMET should be discontinued immediately.

Vitamin B_{12} Levels: Impairment of vitamin B_{12} and folic acid absorption has been reported in some patients on metformin. Therefore, measurements of serum vitamin B_{12} and folic acid are advisable at least every one to two years in patients on long-term treatment with AVANDAMET.

A decrease to subnormal levels of previously normal serum vitamin B_{12} levels, without clinical manifestations, is observed in approximately 7% of patients receiving metformin hydrochloride in controlled clinical trials of 28 weeks duration. Such a decrease, possibly due to interference with B_{12} absorption from the B_{12}-intrinsic factor complex, is, however, very rarely associated with anemia and appears to be rapidly reversible with discontinuation of metformin or vitamin B_{12} supplementation. Measurement of hematologic parameters on an annual basis is advised in patients on AVANDAMET and any apparent abnormalities should be appropriately investigated and managed (see Monitoring and Laboratory Tests). Certain individuals (those with inadequate vitamin B_{12} or calcium intake or absorption) appear to be predisposed to developing subnormal vitamin B_{12} levels.

Hypoglycemia: Hypoglycemia does not occur in patients receiving metformin alone under usual circumstances of use, but could occur when caloric intake is deficient, when strenuous exercise is not compensated by caloric supplementation, or during concomitant use with hypoglycemic agents (such as sulfonylureas) or ethanol. Elderly, debilitated or malnourished patients, and those with adrenal or pituitary insufficiency or alcohol intoxication are particularly susceptible to hypoglycemic effects. Hypoglycemia may be difficult to recognize in the elderly, and in people who are taking beta-adrenergic blocking drugs.

Hematologic: Rosiglitazone maleate: In controlled trials, there were dose-related decreases in hemoglobin and hematocrit. The magnitude of the decreases (≤11 g/L for hemoglobin and ≤0.034 for hematocrit) was small for rosiglitazone alone and rosiglitazone in combination with other hypoglycemic agents. The changes occurred primarily during the first 3 months of therapy or following an increase in rosiglitazone dose and remained relatively constant thereafter. Decreases may be related to increased plasma volume observed during treatment with rosiglitazone and have not been associated with any significant hematologic clinical effects (see Adverse Reactions, Abnormal Hematologic and Clinical Chemistry Findings). Patients with a hemoglobin value of <110 g/L for males and <100 g/L for females were excluded from the clinical trials.

Hepatic: Rosiglitazone maleate: Therapy with AVANDAMET should not be initiated in patients with increased baseline liver enzyme levels (ALT >2.5 times the upper limit of normal).

Rare cases of severe hepatocellular injury have been reported with thiazolidinediones.

In postmarketing experience with rosiglitazone, reports of hepatitis and of hepatic enzyme elevations to three or more times the upper limit of normal have been received. Very rarely, these reports have involved hepatic failure with and without fatal outcome, although causality has not been established (see Adverse Reactions, Post-Market Adverse Drug Reactions).

Liver enzymes should be checked prior to the initiation of therapy with AVANDAMET in all patients and periodically thereafter per the clinical judgement of the healthcare professional. Patients with mildly elevated liver enzymes (ALT levels ≤2.5 times the upper limit of normal) at baseline or during therapy with AVANDAMET should be evaluated to determine the cause of the liver enzyme elevation.

Initiation of, or continuation of, therapy with AVANDAMET in patients with mild liver enzyme elevations should proceed with caution and include appropriate close clinical follow-up, including more frequent liver enzyme monitoring, to determine if the liver enzyme elevations resolve or worsen. If at any time ALT levels increase to >3 times the upper limit of normal in patients on therapy with AVANDAMET, liver enzyme levels should be rechecked as soon as possible. If ALT levels remain >3 times the upper limit of normal, therapy with AVANDAMET should be discontinued (see Dosage and Administration).

If any patient develops symptoms suggesting hepatic dysfunction, which may include unexplained nausea, vomiting, abdominal pain, fatigue, anorexia and/or dark urine, liver enzymes should be checked. If jaundice is observed, drug therapy should be discontinued. In addition, if the presence of hepatic disease or hepatic dysfunction of sufficient magnitude to predispose to lactic acidosis is confirmed, therapy with AVANDAMET should be discontinued.

Metformin hydrochloride: Impaired Hepatic Function: Since impaired hepatic function has been associated with some cases of lactic acidosis, AVANDAMET should generally be avoided in patients with clinical or laboratory evidence of hepatic disease.

Ophthalmologic: Rosiglitazone maleate: New onset and/or worsening macular edema with decreased visual acuity has been reported rarely in postmarketing experience with AVANDAMET. In some cases, the visual events resolved or improved following discontinuation of AVANDAMET. Physicians should consider the possibility of macular edema if a patient reports disturbances in visual acuity (see Adverse Reactions, Post-Market Adverse Drug Reactions).

Peri-Operative Considerations: Metformin hydrochloride: Surgical Procedures: Use of AVANDAMET should be temporarily suspended for any surgical procedure (except minor procedures not associated with restricted intake of food and fluids). AVANDAMET should be discontinued 2 days before surgical intervention and should not be restarted until the patient's oral intake has resumed and renal function has been evaluated as normal.

Renal: Metformin hydrochloride: Use of concomitant medications that may affect renal function or metformin disposition: Concomitant medication(s) that may affect renal function or result in significant hemodynamic change or may interfere with the disposition of metformin, such as cationic drugs that are eliminated by renal tubular secretion (see Drug Interactions), should be used with caution.

Sexual Function/Reproduction: Rosiglitazone maleate: Ovulation: As with other thiazolidinediones, rosiglitazone may result in resumption of ovulation in premenopausal, anovulatory women with insulin resistance (e.g., patients with polycystic ovary syndrome). **As a consequence of their improved insulin sensitivity, these patients may be at risk of pregnancy if adequate contraception is not used.**

Although hormonal imbalance has been seen in preclinical studies, no significant adverse experiences associated with menstrual disorders have been reported in clinical trial participants, including premenopausal women. If unexpected menstrual dysfunction occurs, the benefits of continued therapy should be reviewed.

Special Populations: Pregnant Women: There are no controlled trials of AVANDAMET in pregnant women. Rosiglitazone has been reported to cross the human placenta and to be detectable in fetal tissues. AVANDAMET is contraindicated for use in pregnant women. Because current information strongly suggests that abnormal blood glucose levels during pregnancy are associated with a higher incidence of congenital anomalies as well as increased neonatal morbidity and mortality, most experts recommend that insulin be used during pregnancy to maintain blood glucose levels as close to normal as possible. In animal studies, rosiglitazone was not teratogenic but treatment during mid-late gestation caused fetal death and growth retardation in both rats and rabbits at 19- and 73-fold clinical systemic exposure, respectively.

Labour and Delivery: The effect of AVANDAMET or its components on labour and delivery in humans is unknown.

Nursing Women: No studies have been conducted with the combined components of AVANDAMET. In studies performed with the individual components, both rosiglitazone-related material and metformin were detectable in milk from lactating rats. It is not known whether rosiglitazone and/or metformin is excreted in human milk. Because many drugs are excreted in human milk, AVANDAMET should not be administered to a nursing woman. If AVANDAMET is discontinued, and if diet alone is inadequate for controlling blood glucose, insulin therapy should be considered.

Pediatrics (<18 years of age): There are no data on the use of AVANDAMET in patients under 18 years of age; therefore, AVANDAMET is not indicated for use in patients under 18 years of age. Thiazolidinediones promote the maturation of preadipocytes and have been associated with weight gain. Obesity is a major problem in adolescents with type 2 diabetes.

Geriatrics (≥65 years of age): Metformin is known to be substantially excreted by the kidney and because the risk of serious adverse reactions to the drug is greater in patients with impaired renal function, AVANDAMET should only be used in patients with normal renal function (see Contraindications and Warnings and Precautions). Because aging is associated with reduced renal function, AVANDAMET should be used with caution as age increases. Care should be taken in dose selection and should be based on careful and regular monitoring of renal function. Generally, elderly patients should not be titrated to the maximum dose of AVANDAMET (see Warnings and Precautions and Dosage and Administration).

Monitoring and Laboratory Tests: Periodic fasting blood glucose and A1C measurements should be performed to monitor therapeutic response.

Liver enzyme monitoring is recommended prior to initiation of therapy with AVANDAMET in all patients and periodically thereafter (see Warnings and Precautions, Hepatic).

Initial and periodic monitoring of hematologic parameters (e.g., hemoglobin/hematocrit and red blood cell indices) should be performed, at least on an annual basis. While megaloblastic anemia has rarely been seen with metformin therapy, if this is suspected, vitamin B_{12} deficiency should be excluded.

Monitoring of Renal Function: Metformin is known to be substantially excreted by the kidney, and the risk of metformin accumulation and lactic acidosis increases with the degree of impairment of renal function. Thus, patients with serum creatinine levels above the upper limit of normal for their age should not receive AVANDAMET (see Endocrine and Metabolism, Geriatrics (≥65 years of age); and Dosage and Administration).

Before initiation of therapy with AVANDAMET and every 6 months while on AVANDAMET therapy, renal function should be assessed and verified as being within normal range. In patients in whom development of renal dysfunction is anticipated, renal function should be assessed more frequently and AVANDAMET discontinued if evidence of renal impairment is present.

ADVERSE REACTIONS: Adverse Drug Reaction Overview: Rosiglitazone maleate: In clinical trials, anemia and edema were generally dose-related, mild to moderate in severity and usually did not require discontinuation of treatment with rosiglitazone.

In clinical trials, edema was reported in 4.8% of patients taking rosiglitazone compared to 1.3% on placebo, and 2.2% on metformin monotherapy and 4.4% on rosiglitazone in combination with maximum doses of metformin. Treatment was required for 1.2% of patients on rosiglitazone monotherapy with an adverse event of edema. These adverse experiences rarely led to withdrawal. In these clinical trials, few patients (1.0%) were enrolled with a presenting medical condition of congestive heart failure (NYHA Class I/II). Edema was more frequently observed when rosiglitazone was used in combination with insulin (see Warnings And Precautions, General).

In double blind studies where rosiglitazone was administered for up to one year, serious adverse experiences of ischemic heart disease were reported in 1.3% of patients taking rosiglitazone maleate compared to 0.5% on placebo, 1.3% on metformin and 1.2% on rosiglitazone in combination with maximum doses of metformin.

In a retrospective analysis of data from pooled clinical studies, which included patients on combination therapy with insulin as well as patients with NYHA Class I and II heart failure, the overall incidence of events typically associated with cardiac ischemia was higher for rosiglitazone containing regimens, 2.00% versus comparators, 1.53% [Hazard ratio 1.30 (95% confidence interval 1.004-1.69)]. In a subgroup analysis of this data, this risk was further increased in patients receiving nitrates with approximately twice as many events in patients receiving rosiglitazone versus comparators (see Warnings and Precautions, Cardiovascular, Rosiglitazone maleate, Ischemic Heart Disease). In a large observational study where patients were well matched at baseline, the incidence of the composite endpoint of myocardial infarction and coronary revascularization was 1.75 events per 100 person years for rosiglitazone containing regimens and 1.76 events per 100 person years for other antidiabetic agents [Hazard ratio 0.93 (95% confidence interval 0.80-1.10)].

In clinical trials, dose-related weight gain was seen with rosiglitazone alone and in combination with other hypoglycemic agents (see Action and Clinical Pharmacology and Warnings and Precautions).

Hypoglycemia was commonly observed and generally mild to moderate in nature and was dose-related when rosiglitazone was used in combination with metformin. Patients receiving rosiglitazone in combination with oral hypoglycemic agents may be at risk for hypoglycemia, and a reduction in the dose of rosiglitazone may be necessary.

In double blind studies, anemia was reported in 1.9% of patients taking rosiglitazone compared to 0.7% on placebo, and 2.2% on metformin and 7.1% on rosiglitazone in combination with maximum doses of metformin. Treatment was required for 0.3% of patients with an adverse event of anemia. These adverse experiences rarely led to withdrawal. Lower pre-treatment hemoglobin/hematocrit levels in patients enrolled in the metformin combination clinical trials may have contributed to the higher reporting rate of anemia in these studies (see Adverse Reactions, Abnormal Hematologic and Clinical Chemistry Findings).

Constipation was commonly observed and generally mild to moderate in nature in clinical trials of rosiglitazone with metformin.

A long-term study (ADOPT) compared the use of rosiglitazone maleate (n=1456), glyburide (n=1441), and metformin (n=1454) as monotherapy in type 2 diabetes patients followed up to 6 years. Fractures were reported in a greater number of females with rosiglitazone maleate (9.3%, 2.7/100 patient-years) compared to glyburide (3.5%, 1.3/100 patient-years) or metformin (5.1%, 1.5/100 patient years). The majority of the fractures in the females who received rosiglitazone maleate were reported in the upper arm, hand, and foot (see Warnings and Precautions, Endocrine and Metabolism, Rosiglitazone maleate, Fractures). The observed incidence of fractures for male patients was similar among the 3 treatment groups.

Metformin hydrochloride: Gastrointestinal Reactions: Gastrointestinal symptoms (diarrhea, nausea, vomiting, abdominal bloating, flatulence, and anorexia) are the most common reactions to metformin and are approximately 30% more frequent in patients on metformin monotherapy than in placebo-treated patients, particularly during initiation of metformin therapy. These symptoms are generally transient and resolve spontaneously during continued treatment. Occasionally, temporary dose reduction may be useful.

Because gastrointestinal symptoms during therapy initiation appear to be dose-related, they may be decreased by gradual dose escalation and by having patients take AVANDAMET with meals (see Dosage and Administration).

Special Senses: During initiation of AVANDAMET therapy, approximately 3% of patients may complain of an unpleasant or metallic taste, which usually resolves spontaneously.

Dermatologic Reactions: The incidence of rash/dermatitis in controlled clinical trials was comparable to placebo for metformin monotherapy.

Clinical Trial Adverse Drug Reactions: Because clinical trials are conducted under very specific conditions the adverse reaction rates observed in the clinical trials may not reflect the rates observed in practice and should not be compared to the rates in the clinical trials of another drug. Adverse drug reaction information from clinical trials is useful for identifying drug-related adverse events and for approximating rates.

Controlled Clinical Trials: The incidence and types of adverse events reported in clinical trials of rosiglitazone as monotherapy or in combination with maximum doses of metformin of 2500 mg/day are shown in Table 1.

Table 1: AVANDAMET

Adverse Events (≥5% in Any Treatment Group) Reported by Patients in Double-blind Clinical Trials with Rosiglitazone as Monotherapy or in Combination with Metformin

Preferred Term	Rosiglitazone N=2526 %	Placebo N=601 %	Metformin N=225 %	Rosiglitazone plus metformin N=338 %
Upper respiratory tract infection	9.9	8.7	8.9	16.0
Injury[a]	7.6	4.3	7.6	8.0
Headache	5.9	5.0	8.9	6.5
Back pain	4.0	3.8	4.0	5.0
Hyperglycemia	3.9	5.7	4.4	2.1
Fatigue	3.6	5.0	4.0	5.9
Sinusitis	3.2	4.5	5.3	6.2
Diarrhea	2.3	3.3	15.6	12.7
Viral infection	3.2	4.0	3.6	5.0
Arthralgia	3.0	4.0	2.2	5.0
Anemia	1.9	0.7	2.2	7.1

[a] Includes cuts, burns, sprains, fractures, falls, accidents and surgical procedure.

In clinical trials, reports of hypoglycemia in patients treated with rosiglitazone added to maximum metformin monotherapy were more frequent than in patients treated with rosiglitazone or metformin monotherapies. In double-blind studies, hypoglycemia was reported by 0.6% of patients receiving rosiglitazone as monotherapy compared to 0.2% on placebo and by 3.0% of patients receiving rosiglitazone in combination with maximum doses of metformin compared to 1.3% on metformin monotherapy.

Abnormal Hematologic and Clinical Chemistry Findings: Hematological: Small decreases in hematological parameters were more common in the patients treated with rosiglitazone than in placebo-treated patients. Leukopenia was reported in 0.4% of rosiglitazone patients compared to 0.2% of patients on placebo, 0% on metformin and 0.3% on rosiglitazone in combination with maximum doses of metformin. Decreases may be related to increased plasma volume observed with treatment with rosiglitazone. The mean decrease in hemoglobin in patients treated with rosiglitazone was approximately 10 to 12 g/L; the decrease in hematocrit was 0.03 to 0.04.

During controlled clinical trials of 29 weeks duration, approximately 9% of patients on metformin monotherapy developed asymptomatic subnormal serum vitamin B_{12} levels; serum folic acid levels did not decrease significantly. However, only five cases of megaloblastic anemia have been reported with metformin administration (none during U.S. clinical studies) and no increased incidence of neuropathy has been observed. Therefore, serum vitamin B_{12} levels should be appropriately monitored or periodic parenteral B_{12} supplementation considered (see Warnings and Precautions).

Lipids: Small increases in total cholesterol and LDL have been observed following treatment with rosiglitazone (see Action and Clinical Pharmacology, Pharmacodynamics and Clinical Effects).

Serum Transaminase Levels: In clinical studies in 4598 patients treated with rosiglitazone encompassing approximately 3600 patient years of exposure, there was no evidence of drug-induced hepatotoxicity or elevated ALT levels.

In the controlled trials (including patients with ALT/AST of up to 2.5 times the upper limit of the reference range at study entry), 0.2% of patients treated with rosiglitazone had reversible elevations in ALT >3 times the upper limit of the reference range compared to 0.2% on placebo and 0.5% on active comparators. Hyperbilirubinemia was found in 0.3% of patients treated with rosiglitazone compared with 0.9% treated with placebo and 1% in patients treated with active comparators. Overall, there was a decrease in mean values for ALT, AST, alkaline phosphatase and bilirubin over time in patients treated with rosiglitazone (see Warnings and Precautions, Hepatic).

In the clinical program including long-term, open-label experience, the rate per 100 patient years exposure of ALT increase to >3 times the upper limit of normal was 0.35 for patients treated with rosiglitazone, 0.59 for placebo-treated patients, and 0.78 for patients treated with active comparator agents.

In pre-approval clinical trials, there were no cases of idiosyncratic drug reactions leading to hepatic failure.

Post-Market Adverse Drug Reactions: In postmarketing experience with rosiglitazone, as monotherapy and in combination with other antidiabetic agents, adverse events potentially related to volume expansion (e.g., congestive heart failure, pulmonary edema, and pleural effusions) have been reported (see Warnings and Precautions, Cardiovascular).

Reports of events related to cardiovascular ischemia including myocardial infarction, and hypertension or hypertension accelerated have been received.

Reports of new onset and/or worsening macular edema with decreased visual acuity occurring with the use of rosiglitazone have been received rarely. These patients frequently reported concurrent peripheral edema. In some cases, symptoms improved following discontinuation of rosiglitazone (see Warnings and Precautions, Ophthalmologic).

Reports of anaphylactic reaction (such as angioedema and urticaria), rash and pruritus have been received very rarely.

Reports of hepatitis and of hepatic enzyme elevations to three or more times the upper limit of normal have been received. Very rarely, these reports have involved hepatic failure with and without fatal outcome, although causality has not been established.

Postmarketing reports of parotid gland enlargement have been associated with rosiglitazone and approximately one third of the reports resolved or improved following discontinuation of rosiglitazone.

DRUG INTERACTIONS: Overview: Rosiglitazone maleate: Drugs Metabolized by Cytochrome P450: It has been shown in vitro that rosiglitazone does not inhibit any of the major P450 enzymes at clinically relevant concentrations. In vitro studies demonstrate that rosiglitazone is predominantly metabolized by CYP2C8, with CYP2C9 as only a minor pathway. In vitro studies have shown that montelukast is an inhibitor of CYP2C8 and may inhibit the metabolism of drugs primarily metabolized by CYP2C8 (e.g. paclitaxel, rosiglitazone, repaglinide). No in vivo interaction studies have been performed with the CYP 2C8 inhibitor, montelukast; or, with CYP2C8 substrate paclitaxel. Although rosiglitazone is not anticipated to affect the pharmacokinetics of paclitaxel, concomitant use is likely to result in inhibition of the metabolism of rosiglitazone.

Coadministration of rosiglitazone with CYP2C8 inhibitors (e.g. gemfibrozil) resulted in increased rosiglitazone plasma concentrations. Since there is a potential for an increase in the risk of dose-related adverse reactions, a decrease in rosiglitazone may be needed when CYP2C8 inhibitors are coadministered.

Coadministration of rosiglitazone with a CYP2C8 inducer (e.g. rifampin) resulted in decreased rosiglitazone plasma concentrations. Therefore, close monitoring of glycemic control and changes in diabetic treatment should be considered when CYP2C8 inducers are coadministered. Clinically significant interactions with CYP2C9 substrates or inhibitors are not anticipated.

CYP3A4 Substrates: Rosiglitazone (8 mg once daily) was shown to have no clinically relevant effect on the pharmacokinetics of nifedipine and oral contraceptives (ethinylestradiol and norethindrone), which are predominantly metabolized by CYP3A4. The results of these two drug interaction studies suggest that rosiglitazone is unlikely to cause clinically important drug interactions with other drugs metabolized via CYP3A4.

Metformin hydrochloride: In healthy volunteers, the pharmacokinetics of propranolol and ibuprofen were not affected by metformin when coadministered in single-dose interaction studies. Metformin is negligibly bound to plasma proteins and is therefore, less likely to interact with highly protein-bound drugs such as salicylates, sulfonamides, chloramphenicol and probenecid.

Alcohol Intake: Alcohol is known to potentiate the effect of metformin on lactate metabolism. Patients, therefore, should be warned against excessive alcohol intake, acute or chronic, while receiving AVANDAMET.

Drug-Drug Interactions: AVANDAMET: Concurrent administration of rosiglitazone (2 mg twice daily) and metformin (500 mg twice daily) in healthy volunteers for 4 days had no effect on the steady-state pharmacokinetics of either metformin or rosiglitazone.

Rosiglitazone maleate: Oral Contraceptives: In 32 healthy women, rosiglitazone maleate (8 mg once daily) was shown to have no statistically significant effect on the pharmacokinetics of oral contraceptives (ethinylestradiol and norethindrone). Breakthrough bleeding occurred in 5 individuals when rosiglitazone was coadministered with an oral contraceptive. In one of these subjects a 40% decrease in ethinylestradiol exposure (AUC) was recorded. This was not correlated with a reduction in exposure to norethindrone, nor was there a consistent relationship between the occurrence of breakthrough bleeding and the pharmacokinetics of either ethinylestradiol or norethindrone in individual subjects.

Digoxin: Repeat oral dosing of rosiglitazone (8 mg once daily) for 14 days did not alter the steady-state pharmacokinetics of digoxin (0.375 mg once daily) in healthy volunteers. However, metformin has the potential for interaction with digoxin (see Drug Interactions, Cationic Drugs).

Warfarin: Coadministration of rosiglitazone (4 mg twice daily for 7 days) did not alter the anticoagulant response of steady-state warfarin in healthy volunteers with baseline values of INR of <2.75. Repeat dosing with rosiglitazone had no clinically relevant effect on the steady-state pharmacokinetics of warfarin.

Gemfibrozil: A study conducted in normal healthy volunteers showed that gemfibrozil (an inhibitor of CYP2C8) administered as 600 mg twice daily, increased rosiglitazone systemic exposure two-fold at steady state (see Warnings and Precautions, General).

Rifampin: A study conducted in normal healthy volunteers showed that rifampin (an inducer of CYP2C8) administered as 600 mg daily, decreased the rosiglitazone systemic exposure three-fold (see Warnings and Precautions, General).

Methotrexate: An interaction study of 22 adult patients with psoriasis examined the effect of repeat doses of rosiglitazone (8 mg daily as a single dose for 8 days) on the pharmacokinetics of oral methotrexate administered as single oral doses of 5 to 25 mg weekly. Following 8 days of rosiglitazone administration, the C_{max} and $AUC_{(0-inf)}$ of methotrexate increased by 18% (90% CI: 11% to 26%) and 15% (90% CI: 8% to 23%), respectively, when compared to the same doses of methotrexate administered in the absence of rosiglitazone.

Metformin hydrochloride: Furosemide: A single-dose, metformin-furosemide drug interaction study in healthy subjects demonstrated that pharmacokinetic parameters of both compounds were affected by coadministration. Furosemide increased the metformin plasma and blood C_{max} by 22% and blood AUC by 15%, without any significant change in metformin renal clearance. When administered with metformin, the C_{max} and AUC of furosemide were 31% and 12% smaller, respectively, than when administered alone, and the terminal half-life was decreased by 32%, without any significant change in furosemide renal clearance. No information is available about the interaction of metformin and furosemide when coadministered chronically.

Nifedipine: A single-dose, metformin-nifedipine drug interaction study in normal healthy volunteers demonstrated that coadministration of nifedipine increased plasma metformin C_{max} and AUC by 20% and 9%, respectively, and increased the amount excreted in the urine. T_{max} and half-life were unaffected. Nifedipine appears to enhance the absorption of metformin. Metformin had minimal effects on nifedipine.

Cationic Drugs: Cationic drugs (e.g., amiloride, digoxin, morphine, procainamide, quinidine, quinine, ranitidine, triamterene, trimethoprim, and vancomycin) that are eliminated by renal tubular secretion, theoretically have the potential for interaction with metformin by competing for common renal tubular transport systems. Such an interaction has been observed between metformin and oral cimetidine in normal healthy volunteers in both single- and multiple-dose, metformin-cimetidine drug interaction studies. These studies showed a 60% increase in peak metformin plasma and whole blood concentrations and a 40% increase in plasma and whole blood metformin AUC. There was no change in elimination half-life in the single-dose study. Metformin had no effect on cimetidine pharmacokinetics. Therefore, careful patient monitoring and dose adjustment of AVANDAMET or the interfering drug is recommended in patients who are taking cationic medications that are excreted via the proximal renal tubular secretory system.

Other: Other drugs tend to produce hyperglycemia and may lead to a loss of blood sugar control. These include thiazides and other diuretics, corticosteroids, phenothiazines, thyroid products, estrogens, estrogen plus progestogen, oral contraceptives, phenytoin, nicotinic acid, sympathomimetics, calcium channel blocking drugs, and isoniazid. When such drugs are administered to patients receiving AVANDAMET, the patient should be closely observed to maintain adequate glycemic control.

Drug-Food Interactions: Interactions with food have not been established.

Drug-Herb Interactions: Interactions with herbal products have not been established.

Drug-Laboratory Test Interactions: Interactions with laboratory tests have not been established.

DOSAGE AND ADMINISTRATION: Dosing Considerations: The management of antidiabetic therapy with AVANDAMET should be individualized on the basis of effectiveness and tolerability while not exceeding the maximum recommended daily dose of 8 mg rosiglitazone/2000 mg metformin.

Consistent with the dosing of metformin (i.e., in divided doses), AVANDAMET should be given in divided doses with meals, with gradual dose escalation. This reduces GI side effects (largely due to metformin) and permits determination of the minimum effective dose for the individual patient.

Sufficient time should be given after initiation of AVANDAMET therapy or any dose increase to assess adequacy of therapeutic response. Fasting plasma glucose (FPG) should be used to determine the therapeutic response to AVANDAMET. After an increase in metformin dosage, dose titration is recommended if patients are not adequately controlled after 1-2 weeks. After an increase in rosiglitazone dosage, dose titration is recommended if patients are not adequately controlled after 8-12 weeks.

Increases in the rosiglitazone component to 8 mg/day should be undertaken cautiously following appropriate clinical evaluation to assess the patient's risk of developing adverse reactions relating to fluid retention (see Warnings and Precautions and Adverse Reactions).

No studies have been performed specifically examining the safety and efficacy of AVANDAMET in patients previously treated with other oral hypoglycemic agents and switched to AVANDAMET. Any change in therapy of type 2 diabetes should be undertaken with care and appropriate monitoring as changes in glycemic control can occur.

Specific Patient Populations: AVANDAMET is not recommended for use in pregnancy or for use in pediatric patients.

The initial and maintenance dosing of AVANDAMET should be conservative in patients with advanced age, due to the potential for decreased renal function in this population. Any dosage adjustment should be based on a careful assessment of renal function. Generally, elderly, debilitated, and malnourished patients should not be titrated to the maximum dose of AVANDAMET. Monitoring of renal function is necessary to aid in prevention of metformin-associated lactic acidosis, particularly in the elderly (see Warnings and Precautions).

Therapy with AVANDAMET should not be initiated if the patient exhibits clinical evidence of active liver disease or increased serum transaminase levels (ALT >2.5 times the upper limit of normal at start of therapy) (see Warnings and Precautions, Hepatic and Action and Clinical Pharmacology, Special Populations and Conditions, Hepatic Insufficiency). Liver enzyme monitoring is recommended in all patients prior to initiation of therapy with AVANDAMET and periodically thereafter. AVANDAMET is contraindicated in patients with serious hepatic impairment (see Contraindications, Warnings and Precautions, Hepatic).

Recommended Dose and Dosage Adjustment: For patients inadequately controlled on metformin monotherapy: the usual starting dose of AVANDAMET is 4 mg rosiglitazone (total daily dose) plus the dose of metformin already being taken (see Table 2).

Table 2: AVANDAMET

AVANDAMET Starting Dose

Prior Therapy	Usual AVANDAMET Starting Dose	
Total Daily Dose	**Tablet Strength**	**Number of Tablets**
Metformin HCl[a]		
1000 mg/day	2 mg/500 mg	1 tablet b.i.d
2000 mg/day	2 mg/1000 mg	1 tablet b.i.d

[a] For patients on 1500, 1700 or 2550 mg/day of metformin, initiation of AVANDAMET requires individualization of therapy.

When switching from combination therapy of rosiglitazone plus metformin as separate tablets: the usual starting dose of AVANDAMET is the dose of rosiglitazone and metformin already being taken.

If additional glycemic control is needed: the daily dose of AVANDAMET may be increased by increments of 4 mg rosiglitazone and/or 500 mg metformin, up to the maximum recommended total daily dose of 8 mg/2000 mg.

Missed Dose: If a dose of AVANDAMET is missed, the patient should be advised to take one dose as soon as they remember and the next dose at the usual time. Three doses should never be taken in one day to make up for a missed dose the day before. If a whole day of AVANDAMET is missed, the usual dosing schedule should be followed the next day without making up for the missed doses.

OVERDOSAGE:
In the event of an overdose, appropriate supportive treatment should be initiated as dictated by the patient's clinical status.

No data are available with regard to overdosage of AVANDAMET. In clinical studies in volunteers, rosiglitazone has been administered at single oral doses of up to 20 mg and was well tolerated.

Hypoglycemia has not been seen even with ingestion of up to 85 g of metformin hydrochloride, although lactic acidosis has occurred in such circumstances (see Warnings and Precautions). Metformin is dialyzable with a clearance of up to 170 mL/min under good hemodynamic conditions. Therefore, hemodialysis may be useful for removal of accumulated drug from patients in whom metformin overdosage is suspected.

> For management of a suspected drug overdose, contact your **regional Poison Control Centre.** See the *CPS* Directory section for a list of Poison Control Centres.

ACTION AND CLINICAL PHARMACOLOGY: Mechanism of Action: AVANDAMET tablets combine two antidiabetic agents with different but complementary mechanisms of action to improve glycemic control while reducing circulating insulin levels in patients with type 2 diabetes: rosiglitazone maleate, a member of the thiazolidinedione class and metformin hydrochloride, a member of the biguanide class. Thiazolidinediones are insulin sensitizing agents that act primarily by enhancing peripheral glucose utilization, whereas biguanides act primarily by decreasing endogenous hepatic glucose production.

Rosiglitazone maleate is an oral antidiabetic agent which acts primarily by increasing insulin sensitivity in type 2 diabetes. Rosiglitazone, a member of the thiazolidinedione class of antidiabetic agents, improves glycemic control while reducing circulating insulin levels. It improves sensitivity to insulin in muscle and adipose tissue and inhibits hepatic gluconeogenesis. Rosiglitazone is not chemically or functionally related to the sulfonylureas, the biguanides or the alpha-glucosidase inhibitors. Rosiglitazone is a highly selective and potent agonist for the peroxisome proliferator-activated receptor-gamma (PPARγ). In humans, PPAR receptors are found in key target tissues for insulin action such as adipose tissue, skeletal muscle and liver. Activation of PPARγ nuclear receptors regulates the transcription of insulin-responsive genes involved in the control of glucose production, transport, and utilization. In addition, PPARγ-responsive genes also participate in the regulation of fatty acid metabolism and in the maturation of preadipocytes, predominantly of subcutaneous origin.

Insulin resistance is a primary feature characterizing the pathogenesis of type 2 diabetes. Rosiglitazone maleate results in increased responsiveness of insulin-dependent tissues and significantly improves hepatic and peripheral (muscle) tissue sensitivity to insulin in patients with type 2 diabetes. Clinical studies in patients with type 2 diabetes treated with rosiglitazone either as monotherapy or in combination with metformin showed improved beta-cell function and decreased fasting plasma glucose, insulin and C-peptide values following 26 weeks of treatment. A homeostasis model assessment (HOMA) was conducted using fasting plasma glucose and insulin or C-peptide levels as a measure of insulin sensitivity and beta-cell function. In these studies, reductions in mean plasma pro-insulin and pro-insulin split product concentrations were also observed.

Rosiglitazone significantly reduced hemoglobin A1C (A1C, a marker for long term glycemic control), and fasting blood glucose (FBG) in patients with type 2 diabetes. Inadequately controlled hyperglycemia is associated with an increased risk of diabetic complications, including cardiovascular disorders and diabetic nephropathy, retinopathy and neuropathy.

Studies between 8 and 26 weeks with rosiglitazone have shown a statistically significant reduction in markers of inflammation, C-reactive protein (CRP) and matrix metalloproteinase-9 (MMP-9). The clinical significance of these effects are still unknown. Further long term clinical trials are needed.

Estimates of LDL particle size can be determined by the LDL cholesterol (LDL) to apolipoprotein B (Apo B) ratio. In controlled clinical trials, rosiglitazone has been shown to increase the LDL cholesterol to Apo B ratio consistent with a beneficial change in LDL particle size from small dense LDL particles to larger more buoyant particles. This change has been confirmed by measuring LDL particle buoyancy (Rf) following 8 weeks treatment with rosiglitazone in an open-label study.

Metformin hydrochloride is an antihyperglycemic agent, which improves glucose tolerance in type 2 diabetes subjects, lowering both basal and postprandial plasma glucose. Metformin is not chemically or pharmacologically related to the oral sulfonylureas, thiazolidinediones, or alpha-glucosidase inhibitors. Metformin decreases hepatic glucose production, decreases intestinal absorption of glucose and improves insulin sensitivity by increasing peripheral glucose uptake and utilization. Unlike sulfonylureas, metformin does not produce hypoglycemia in either patients with type 2 diabetes or normal subjects (except in special circumstances, see Warnings and Precautions) and does not cause hyperinsulinemia. With metformin therapy, insulin secretion remains unchanged while fasting insulin levels and day-long plasma insulin response may actually decrease.

Pharmacodynamics and Clinical Effects: In clinical studies, treatment with rosiglitazone resulted in an improvement in glycemic control, as measured by fasting plasma glucose (FPG) and haemoglobin A1C, with a concurrent reduction in insulin and C-peptide. Postprandial glucose and insulin were also reduced. This is consistent with the mechanism of action of rosiglitazone as an insulin sensitizer. The improvement in glycemic control was durable. In open-labelled extension studies sustained improvements in glycemic control (as measured by A1C levels) were observed in patients receiving rosiglitazone monotherapy for 36 months.

Rosiglitazone is believed to act primarily on muscle and adipose tissue whereas metformin acts primarily on the liver to decrease hepatic glucose output. The coadministration of rosiglitazone with metformin resulted in significantly improved glycemic control compared to either of these agents alone. These results are consistent with a synergistic effect on glycemic control when rosiglitazone is used in combination with metformin. In patients whose type 2 diabetes was inadequately controlled with metformin monotherapy, the addition of rosiglitazone led to reductions in A1C levels that were sustained for over 30 months of treatment, in open-labelled studies.

Weight gain has been observed in clinical studies with rosiglitazone (see Table 3). In addition, rosiglitazone significantly decreased visceral (abdominal) fat stores while increasing subcutaneous abdominal fat. The reduction in visceral fat correlates with improved hepatic and peripheral tissue insulin sensitivity. Weight gain with thiazolidinediones can result from increases in subcutaneous adipose tissue and/or from fluid retention. Treatment should be re-evaluated in patients with excessive weight gain (see Warnings and Precautions and Adverse Reactions).

Table 3: AVANDAMET

Weight Changes (kg) from Baseline During Clinical Trials with Rosiglitazone

Treatment Group	Duration	Control Group	Control Group: median (25th, 75th percentile) (range)	Rosiglitazone 4 mg: median (25th, 75th percentile) (range)	Rosiglitazone 8 mg: median (25th, 75th percentile) (range)
Monotherapy					
Rosiglitazone	26 weeks	placebo	−0.9 (−2.8, 0.9) (−9.6 to 6.8) n=210	1.0 (−0.9, 3.6) (−11.6 to 12.7) n=436	3.1 (1.1, 5.8) (−6.8 to 13.9) n=439
Rosiglitazone	52 weeks	sulfonylurea	2.0 (0, 4.0) (−11.5 to 12.2) n=173	2.0 (−0.6, 4.0) (−7.0 to 16.0) n=150	2.6 (0, 5.3) (−11.0 to 22.0) n=157
Combination Therapy					
Rosiglitazone + sulfonylurea	26 weeks	sulfonylurea	0 (−1.3, 1.2) (−6.0 to 14.0) n=1043	1.8 (0, 3.1) (−5.0 to 11.5) n=392	—
Rosiglitazone + metformin	26 weeks	metformin	−1.4 (−3.2, 0.2) (−7.7 to 5.9) n=175	0.8 (−1.0, 2.6) (−6.8 to 9.8) n=100	2.1 (0, 4.3) (−5.4 to 13.1) n=184

Patients with lipid abnormalities were not excluded from clinical trials of rosiglitazone. In all 26-week controlled trials, across the recommended dose range, rosiglitazone as monotherapy was associated with increases in total cholesterol, LDL, and HDL and decreases in free fatty acids. These changes were statistically significantly different from controls.

Increases in LDL occurred primarily during the first 1 to 2 months of therapy with rosiglitazone and LDL levels remained stable, but elevated above baseline throughout the trials. In contrast, HDL continued to rise over time. As a result, the LDL/HDL ratio peaked after 2 months of therapy and then appeared to decrease over time. The pattern of LDL and HDL changes following therapy with rosiglitazone in combination with metformin was generally similar to those seen with rosiglitazone in monotherapy.

The changes in triglycerides during therapy with rosiglitazone were variable and were generally not statistically different from controls.

The long term significance of the lipid changes is not known.

Pharmacokinetics: Bioavailability: AVANDAMET: In a bioequivalence and dose proportionality study of AVANDAMET 4 mg/500 mg, both the rosiglitazone component and the metformin component were bioequivalent to coadministered 4 mg rosiglitazone maleate tablet and 500 mg metformin hydrochloride tablet under fasted conditions (see Table 4). In this study, dose proportionality of rosiglitazone in the combination formulations of 1 mg/500 mg and 4 mg/500 mg was demonstrated.

Table 4: AVANDAMET

Mean (SD) Pharmacokinetic Parameters for Rosiglitazone and Metformin

Regimen	N	AUC (0-inf) (ng·h/mL)	C_{max} (ng/mL)	T_{max}[a] (h)	$T_{½}$ (h)
Rosiglitazone					
A	25	1442 (324)	242 (70)	0.95 (0.48–2.47)	4.26 (1.18)
B	25	1398 (340)	254 (69)	0.57 (0.43–2.58)	3.95 (0.81)
C	24	349 (91)	63.0 (15.0)	0.57 (0.47–1.45)	3.87 (0.88)
Metformin					
A	25	7116 (2096)	1106 (329)	2.97 (1.02–4.02)	3.46 (0.96)
B	25	7413 (1838)	1135 (253)	2.50 (1.03–3.98)	3.36 (0.54)
C	24	6945 (2045)	1080 (327)	2.97 (1.00–5.98)	3.35 (0.59)

[a] Median and range presented for T_{max}.
Regimen Key: Regimen A=4 mg/500 mg AVANDAMET; Regimen B=4 mg rosiglitazone maleate tablet+500 mg metformin hydrochloride tablet; Regimen C=1 mg/500 mg AVANDAMET.

Administration of AVANDAMET 4 mg/500 mg with food resulted in no change in overall exposure (AUC) for either rosiglitazone or metformin. However, there were decreases in C_{max} of both components (22% for rosiglitazone and 15% for metformin, respectively) and a delay in T_{max} of both components (1.5 hrs for rosiglitazone and 0.5 hrs for metformin, respectively). These changes are not likely to be clinically significant. The pharmacokinetics of both the rosiglitazone component and the metformin component of AVANDAMET when taken with food were similar to the pharmacokinetics of rosiglitazone and metformin when administered concomitantly as separate tablets with food.

Absorption: Rosiglitazone maleate: Rosiglitazone is rapidly and completely absorbed after oral administration with negligible first-pass metabolism. The absolute bioavailability of rosiglitazone is 99%. Peak plasma concentrations are observed by 1 hour after dosing. Maximum plasma concentration (C_{max}) and the area under the curve ($AUC_{0\text{-}inf}$) of rosiglitazone increase in a dose-proportional manner over the therapeutic dose range. The elimination half-life is 3 to 4 hours and is independent of dose.

Metformin hydrochloride: Metformin absorption is relatively slow and may extend over about 6 hours. The absolute bioavailability of a 500 mg metformin hydrochloride tablet given under fasting conditions is approximately 50-60%. Studies using single oral doses of metformin tablets of 500 mg and 1500 mg, and 850 mg to 2550 mg, indicate that there is a lack of dose proportionality with increasing doses, which is due to decreased absorption rather than an alteration in elimination.

Distribution: Rosiglitazone maleate: The mean (SD) volume of distribution (Vss) of rosiglitazone after intravenous administration to healthy subjects is approximately 14.1 (3.1) L. Rosiglitazone is approximately 99.8% bound to plasma proteins, primarily albumin.

Metformin hydrochloride: The apparent volume of distribution (V/F) of metformin following single oral doses of 850 mg metformin hydrochloride averaged 654±358 L. Metformin is negligibly bound to plasma proteins. Metformin partitions into erythrocytes, most likely as a function of time. At usual clinical doses and dosing schedules of metformin, steady state plasma concentrations of metformin are reached within 24-48 hours and are generally <1 µg/mL. During controlled clinical trials, maximum metformin plasma levels did not exceed 5 µg/mL, even at maximum doses.

Metabolism: Rosiglitazone maleate: Rosiglitazone is extensively metabolized with no unchanged drug excreted in the urine. The major routes of metabolism were N-demethylation and hydroxylation, followed by conjugation with sulfate and glucuronic acid. All the circulating metabolites are considerably less potent than the parent drug and, therefore, are not expected to contribute to the insulin-sensitizing activity of rosiglitazone. In vitro data demonstrate that rosiglitazone is predominantly metabolized by cytochrome P450 isoenzyme CYP2C8, with CYP2C9 contributing as only a minor pathway.

Metformin hydrochloride: Intravenous single-dose studies in normal subjects demonstrate that metformin is excreted unchanged in the urine and does not undergo hepatic metabolism (no metabolites have been identified in humans) nor biliary excretion. Renal clearance is approximately 3.5 times greater than creatinine clearance which indicates that tubular secretion is the major route of metformin elimination.

Excretion: Rosiglitazone maleate: Following oral or intravenous administration of [^{14}C] rosiglitazone maleate, approximately 64% and 23% of the dose was eliminated in the urine and in the feces, respectively. The plasma half-life of [^{14}C] related material ranged from 103 to 158 hours.

Metformin hydrochloride: Following oral administration, approximately 90% of the absorbed drug is eliminated via the renal route within the first 24 hours, with a plasma elimination half-life of approximately 6.2 hours. In blood, the elimination half-life is approximately 17.6 hours, suggesting that the erythrocyte mass may be a compartment of distribution.

Special Populations and Conditions: Pediatrics: The safety and effectiveness of rosiglitazone and metformin have not been established in patients younger than 18 years of age, therefore, AVANDAMET is not indicated in patients younger than 18 years of age. Thiazolidinediones promote the maturation of preadipocytes and have been associated with weight gain. Obesity is a major problem in adolescents with type 2 diabetes.

Geriatrics: Results of the population pharmacokinetic analysis (n=716 <65 years; n=331 ≥65 years) showed that age does not significantly affect the pharmacokinetics of rosiglitazone.

However, limited data from controlled pharmacokinetic studies of metformin hydrochloride in healthy elderly subjects suggest that total plasma clearance of metformin is decreased, the half-life is prolonged and C_{max} is increased, compared to healthy young subjects. From these data, it appears that the change in metformin pharmacokinetics with aging is primarily accounted for by a change in renal function. Metformin treatment and therefore treatment with AVANDAMET should not be initiated in patients 80 years of age or older unless measurement of creatinine clearance demonstrates that renal function is not reduced (see Warnings and Precautions and Dosage and Administration).

Gender: Results of the population pharmacokinetic analysis showed that the mean oral clearance of rosiglitazone in female patients (n=405) was 15% lower compared to male patients (n=642), primarily related to lower body weight in females. In rosiglitazone and metformin combination studies, efficacy was demonstrated with no gender differences in glycemic response.

Metformin pharmacokinetic parameters did not differ significantly between normal subjects and patients with type 2 diabetes when analyzed according to gender (males=19, females=16). Similarly, in controlled clinical studies in patients with type 2 diabetes, the antihyperglycemic effect of metformin hydrochloride tablets was comparable in males and females.

Race: Results of a population pharmacokinetic analysis including subjects of white, black, and other ethnic origins indicate that race has no influence on the pharmacokinetics of rosiglitazone.

No studies of metformin hydrochloride pharmacokinetic parameters according to race have been performed. In controlled clinical studies of metformin in patients with type 2 diabetes, the antihyperglycemic effect was comparable in whites (n=249), blacks (n=51) and Hispanics (n=24).

Hepatic Insufficiency: Unbound oral clearance of rosiglitazone was significantly lower in patients with moderate to severe liver disease (Child-Pugh Class B/C) compared to healthy subjects. As a result, unbound C_{max} and AUC_{0-inf} were increased 2- and 3-fold, respectively. Elimination half-life for rosiglitazone was about 2 hours longer in patients with liver disease, compared to healthy subjects. Therapy with AVANDAMET should not be initiated if the patient exhibits clinical evidence of active liver disease or increased serum transaminase levels (ALT >2.5 times the upper limit of normal) at baseline (see Warnings and Precautions, Hepatic).

No pharmacokinetic studies have been conducted in subjects with hepatic insufficiency with metformin.

Renal Insufficiency: In subjects with decreased renal function (based on measured creatinine clearance), the plasma and blood half-life of metformin is prolonged and the renal clearance is decreased in proportion to the decrease in creatinine clearance (see Warnings and Precautions).

Since metformin is contraindicated in patients with renal impairment, administration of AVANDAMET is contraindicated in these patients.

STORAGE AND STABILITY: Store at controlled room temperature 15 to 30°C.

SPECIAL HANDLING INSTRUCTIONS: Dispense in a tight, light-resistant container.

INFORMATION FOR THE PATIENT: Published in e-CPS, available by subscription at www.e-cps.ca.

DOSAGE FORMS, COMPOSITION AND PACKAGING: 1 mg/500 mg: Each yellow, film-coated, oval tablet, debossed with gsk on one side and 1/500 on the other, contains: rosiglitazone maleate equivalent to rosiglitazone 1 mg and metformin HCl 500 mg. Nonmedicinal ingredients: hydroxypropyl methylcellulose, lactose monohydrate, magnesium stearate, microcrystalline cellulose, polyethylene glycol 400, povidone 29-32, sodium starch glycolate, titanium dioxide and one or more of the following: red and yellow iron oxides. Bottles of 100.

2 mg/500 mg: Each pale pink, film-coated, oval tablet, debossed with gsk on one side and 2/500 on the other, contains: rosiglitazone maleate equivalent to rosiglitazone 2 mg and metformin HCl 500 mg. Nonmedicinal ingredients: hydroxypropyl methylcellulose, lactose monohydrate, magnesium stearate, microcrystalline cellulose, polyethylene glycol 400, povidone 29-32, sodium starch glycolate, titanium dioxide and one or more of the following: red and yellow iron oxides. Bottles of 100.

4 mg/500 mg: Each orange, film-coated, oval tablet, debossed with gsk on one side and 4/500 on the other, contains: rosiglitazone maleate equivalent to rosiglitazone 4 mg and metformin HCl 500 mg. Nonmedicinal ingredients: hydroxypropyl methylcellulose, lactose monohydrate, magnesium stearate, microcrystalline cellulose, polyethylene glycol 400, povidone 29-32, sodium starch glycolate, titanium dioxide and one or more of the following: red and yellow iron oxides. Bottles of 100.

2 mg/1000 mg: Each yellow, film-coated, oval tablet, debossed with gsk on one side and 2/1000 on the other, contains: rosiglitazone maleate equivalent to rosiglitazone 2 mg and metformin HCl 1000 mg. Nonmedicinal ingredients: hydroxypropyl methylcellulose, lactose monohydrate, magnesium stearate, microcrystalline cellulose, polyethylene glycol 400, povidone 29-32, sodium starch glycolate, titanium dioxide and one or more of the following: red and yellow iron oxides. Bottles of 100.

4 mg/1000 mg: Each pink, film-coated, oval tablet, debossed with gsk on one side and 4/1000 on the other, contains: rosiglitazone maleate equivalent to rosiglitazone 4 mg and metformin HCl 1000 mg. Nonmedicinal ingredients: hydroxypropyl methylcellulose, lactose monohydrate, magnesium stearate, microcrystalline cellulose, polyethylene glycol 400, povidone 29-32, sodium starch glycolate, titanium dioxide and one or more of the following: red and yellow iron oxides. Bottles of 100.

(Shown in Product Identification Section)

The reader is invited to consult CPhA's monograph **Sulfonylureas**.

Avandaryl™ Ⓟ

rosiglitazone maleate—glimepiride

Antidiabetic

GlaxoSmithKline

Date of Revision: May 8, 2009

SUMMARY PRODUCT INFORMATION:

Route of Administration	Dosage Form/ Strength	Clinically Relevant Nonmedicinal Ingredients
Oral	Tablet 4 mg/1 mg, 4 mg/2 mg, 4 mg/4 mg	Lactose monohydrate For a complete listing see Dosage Forms, Composition and Packaging.

INDICATIONS AND CLINICAL USE: AVANDARYL (rosiglitazone maleate and glimepiride) is indicated for use as an adjunct to diet and exercise to reduce insulin resistance and improve glycemic control in patients with type 2 diabetes mellitus:

- who show intolerance to metformin or for whom metformin is contraindicated, when diet and exercise plus sulfonylurea or rosiglitazone monotherapy do not result in adequate glycemic control.

Caloric restriction, weight loss, and exercise improve insulin sensitivity and are essential for the proper treatment of a diabetic patient. These measures are important not only in the primary treatment of type 2 diabetes, but also in maintaining the efficacy of drug therapy. Prior to initiation of therapy with AVANDARYL, secondary causes of poor glycemic control (e.g., infection) should be investigated and treated.

The safety and efficacy of AVANDARYL as initial pharmacologic therapy for patients with type 2 diabetes after a trial of caloric restriction, weight loss, and exercise has not been established.

Geriatrics (≥65 years of age): Results of the population pharmacokinetic analysis (n=716 <65 years; n=331 ≥65 years) showed that age does not significantly affect the pharmacokinetics of rosiglitazone.

Comparison of glimepiride pharmacokinetics in type 2 diabetic patients ≤65 years and those ≥65 years was performed in a study using a dosing regimen of 6 mg daily. There were no significant differences in glimepiride pharmacokinetics between the two age groups. The mean AUC at steady state for the older patients was about 13% lower than that for the younger patients; the mean weight adjusted clearance for the older patients was about 11% higher than that for the younger patients (see Warnings and Precautions, Special Populations, Geriatrics (≥65 years of age)).

Pediatrics (<18 years of age): There are no data on the use of AVANDARYL in patients younger than 18 years; therefore, the use of AVANDARYL in pediatric patients is not recommended.

CONTRAINDICATIONS: AVANDARYL is contraindicated in:

- Patients with New York Heart Association (NYHA) Class I to IV heart failure.
- Type 1 diabetes (formerly known as insulin-dependent diabetes mellitus or IDDM)
- Patients with known hypersensitivity to rosiglitazone maleate, glimepiride, other sulfonylureas or sulfonamides, or any of the ingredients of AVANDARYL.
- Patients with serious hepatic impairment (see Warnings and Precautions).
- Patients with diabetic ketoacidosis, with or without coma. This condition should be treated with insulin.
- Pregnancy or breastfeeding women. Insulin is recommended during pregnancy to control blood glucose levels. Oral antidiabetic agents should not be given (see Warnings and Precautions, Special Populations, Pregnant Women).

WARNINGS AND PRECAUTIONS: General: AVANDARYL: Administration with Other Drugs: For safety reasons, the use of AVANDARYL in combination with insulin is not indicated.

The use of AVANDARYL in combination with metformin (triple therapy) is not indicated. An increase in reporting of fluid retention related events (including congestive heart failure) has been seen in patients receiving rosiglitazone in combination with metformin **and** a sulfonylurea.

Close monitoring of glycemic control and dose adjustment of the rosiglitazone maleate or glimepiride components may be needed when AVANDARYL is coadministered with CYP2C8 or CYP2C9 inhibitors or inducers (see Drug Interactions).

Rosiglitazone Maleate: Due to its mechanism of action, rosiglitazone is active only in the presence of endogenous insulin. Therefore, AVANDARYL should not be used in patients with type 1 diabetes or for the treatment of diabetic ketoacidosis.

Cardiovascular: Rosiglitazone Maleate: Congestive Heart Failure: Thiazolidinediones, like rosiglitazone maleate, alone or in combination with other antidiabetic agents, can cause fluid retention, which can exacerbate or lead to congestive heart failure. The fluid retention may very rarely present as rapid and excessive weight gain. All patients should be monitored for signs and symptoms of adverse reactions relating to fluid retention and heart failure. In particular, patients who are at risk for heart failure including those receiving concurrent therapy which increases insulin levels (i.e. sulfonylureas) should be closely monitored (see Adverse Reactions). An increase in reporting of fluid retention related events including congestive heart failure has been seen in patients receiving rosiglitazone in combination with metformin and a sulfonylurea. This triple therapy regimen is not an approved indication.

Treatment with thiazolidinediones has been associated with cases of congestive heart failure, some of which were difficult to treat unless the medication was discontinued. AVANDARYL should be discontinued if any deterioration in cardiac status occurs.

AVANDARYL is contraindicated in patients with NYHA Class I, II, III and IV heart failure. Patients with severe heart failure (including NYHA Class III and IV cardiac status) were not studied during the clinical trials.

Patients experiencing acute coronary syndromes (ACS) have not been studied in rosiglitazone controlled clinical trials. Since patients experiencing ACS are at an increased risk of developing heart failure, and in view of the potential for rosiglitazone to cause or exacerbate heart failure, initiation of AVANDARYL in patients experiencing an acute coronary event is not recommended. Furthermore, discontinuation of AVANDARYL during the acute phase should be considered.

Ischemic Heart Disease: In a retrospective analysis of data from pooled clinical studies, which included patients on combination therapy with insulin as well as patients with NYHA Class I and II heart failure, the overall incidence of events typically associated with cardiac ischemia was higher for rosiglitazone containing regimens, 2.00% versus comparators, 1.53% [hazard ratio 1.30 (95% confidence interval 1.004-1.69)]. In a subgroup analysis of this data, this risk was further increased in patients receiving nitrates with approximately twice as many events in patients receiving rosiglitazone versus comparators. **The use of AVANDARYL is therefore not recommended for patients being treated with nitrates.**

The completion of an adequately-designed cardiovascular outcome study is needed to further evaluate the risk of myocardial ischemic events associated with rosiglitazone.

In a large observational study where patients were well matched at baseline, the incidence of the composite endpoint of myocardial infarction and coronary revascularization was 1.75 events per 100 person years for rosiglitazone containing regimens and 1.76 events per 100 person years for other anti-diabetic agents [hazard ratio 0.93 (95% confidence interval 0.80-1.10)].

Edema: AVANDARYL should be used with caution in patients with edema. The maximum approved dose of rosiglitazone to be used in combination with a sulfonylurea is 4 mg. In healthy volunteers who received rosiglitazone maleate 8 mg once daily as monotherapy for 8 weeks, there was a statistically significant increase in median plasma volume (1.8 mL/kg) compared to placebo. In controlled clinical trials of patients with type 2 diabetes, mild to moderate edema was observed at a greater frequency in patients treated with rosiglitazone maleate and may be dose related (see Adverse Reactions). For information on macular edema, see Warnings and Precautions, Ophthalmologic.

Glimepiride: It has been suggested, based on a study conducted by the University Group Diabetes Program (UGDP), that certain sulfonylurea antidiabetic agents increase cardiovascular mortality in diabetic patients, a population at greater risk of cardiovascular disease. This finding was not confirmed by a more recent trial, the United Kingdom Prospective Diabetes Study (UKPDS) which showed that intensive glycemic control with either sulfonylureas or insulin did not have an adverse effect on cardiovascular outcomes. Despite questions regarding the design of these studies and interpretation of the results, the results of these studies provide a basis for caution, especially high risk patients with cardiovascular disease.

In clinical trials more patients receiving glimepiride and insulin reported an increase in peripheral edema compared to patients receiving insulin alone.

Endocrine and Metabolism: Hypoglycemia: AVANDARYL is a combination tablet containing rosiglitazone maleate and glimepiride, a sulfonylurea. All sulfonylurea drugs are capable of producing severe hypoglycemia. Proper patient selection, dosage, and instructions are important to avoid hypoglycemic episodes. Elderly, debilitated or malnourished patients, and those with adrenal, pituitary, or hepatic insufficiency are particularly susceptible to the hypoglycemic action of glucose-lowering drugs. Patients with impaired renal function may be more sensitive to the glucose-lowering effect of glimepiride. A starting dose of 1 mg glimepiride, as contained in AVANDARYL 4 mg/1 mg, followed by appropriate dose titration is also recommended in these patients (see Action and Clinical Pharmacology, Special Populations and Conditions, Renal Insufficiency).

Hypoglycemia may be difficult to recognize in the elderly and in people who are taking beta-adrenergic blocking drugs or other sympatholytic agents. Hypoglycemia is more likely to occur when caloric intake is deficient, after severe or prolonged exercise, when alcohol is ingested, or when other drugs with blood-glucose lowering potential are used.

Patients receiving rosiglitazone maleate in combination with a sulfonylurea may be at risk for hypoglycemia, and a reduction in the dose of either agent may be necessary (see Dosage and Administration, Specific Patient Populations).

Loss of Control of Blood Glucose: When a patient stabilized on any antidiabetic regimen is exposed to stress such as fever, trauma, infection, or surgery, a temporary loss of glycemic control may occur. At such times, it may be necessary to withhold AVANDARYL and temporarily administer insulin. AVANDARYL may be reinstituted after the acute episode is resolved.

If risk factors for hypoglycemia are present, including renal insufficiency, low body weight, malnourishment or coadministration of certain other drugs (see Warnings and Precautions, Hypoglycemia; Drug Interactions and Dosage and Administration), it may be necessary to adjust the dosage of glimepiride or the entire therapy during such situations. This also applies whenever illness occurs during therapy or the patient's life-style changes.

Rosiglitazone Maleate: Weight Gain: Dose-related weight gain was seen with rosiglitazone maleate alone and in combination with other hypoglycemic agents. Treatment should be re-evaluated in patients with excessive weight gain (see Action and Clinical Pharmacology and Adverse Reactions).

Fractures: In a 4 to 6 year comparative study (ADOPT) of glycemic control with monotherapy in recently diagnosed patients with Type 2 diabetes mellitus, an increased incidence of bone fracture was noted in female patients taking rosiglitazone (9.3%, 2.7 patients per 100 patient-years) versus glyburide (3.5%, 1.3 patients per 100 patient-years) or metformin (5.1%, 1.5 patients per 100 patient-years). The majority of the fractures in the females who received rosiglitazone were reported in the upper arm, hand, and foot (see Adverse Reactions). The risk of fracture should be considered in the care of patients, especially female patients, treated with rosiglitazone, and attention should be given to assessing and maintaining bone health according to current standards of care.

Hematologic: Rosiglitazone Maleate: In controlled trials, there were dose-related decreases in hemoglobin and hematocrit. The magnitude of the decreases (≤11 g/L for hemoglobin and ≤0.034 for hematocrit) was small for rosiglitazone maleate alone and rosiglitazone maleate in combination with other hypoglycemic agents. The changes occurred primarily during the first 3 months of therapy or following an increase in rosiglitazone maleate dose and remained relatively constant thereafter. Decreases may be related to increased plasma volume observed during treatment with rosiglitazone maleate and have not been associated with any significant hematologic clinical effects (see Adverse Reactions, Abnormal Hematologic and Clinical Chemistry Findings). Patients with a hemoglobin value of <110 g/L for males and <100 g/L for females were excluded from the clinical trials.

Glimepiride: Treatment of patients with glucose-6-phosphate dehydrogenase (G6PD)-deficiency with sulfonylurea agents can lead to hemolytic anemia. Since glimepiride belongs to the class of sulfonylurea agents, caution should be used in patients with G6PD-deficiency and a non-sulfonylurea alternative should be considered.

Hepatic: Rosiglitazone Maleate: Therapy with AVANDARYL should not be initiated in patients with increased baseline liver enzyme levels (ALT >2.5 times the upper limit of normal).

Rare cases of severe hepatocellular injury have been reported with thiazolidinediones.

In postmarketing experience with rosiglitazone, reports of hepatitis and of hepatic enzyme elevations to three or more times the upper limit of normal have been received. Very rarely, these reports have involved hepatic failure with and without fatal outcome, although causality has not been established (see Adverse Reactions, Post-Market Adverse Drug Reactions).

Liver enzymes should be checked prior to the initiation of therapy with AVANDARYL in all patients and periodically thereafter per the clinical judgement of the healthcare professional. Patients with mildly elevated liver enzymes (ALT levels ≤2.5 times the upper limit of normal) at baseline or during therapy with AVANDARYL should be evaluated to determine the cause of the liver enzyme elevation.

Initiation of, or continuation of, therapy with AVANDARYL in patients with mild liver enzyme elevations should proceed with caution and include appropriate close clinical follow-up, including more frequent liver enzyme monitoring, to determine if the liver enzyme elevations resolve or worsen. If at any time ALT levels increase to >3 times the upper limit of normal in patients on therapy with AVANDARYL, liver enzyme levels should be rechecked as soon as possible. If ALT levels remain >3 times the upper limit of normal, therapy with AVANDARYL should be discontinued (see Dosage and Administration).

If any patient develops symptoms suggesting hepatic dysfunction, which may include unexplained nausea, vomiting, abdominal pain, fatigue, anorexia and/or dark urine, liver enzymes should be checked. The decision whether to continue the patient on therapy with AVANDARYL should be guided by clinical judgment pending laboratory evaluations. If jaundice is observed, drug therapy should be discontinued.

Ophthalmologic: Rosiglitazone Maleate: New onset and/or worsening macular edema with decreased visual acuity has been reported rarely in postmarketing experience with AVANDARYL. In some cases, the visual events resolved or improved following discontinuation of AVANDARYL. Physicians should consider the possibility of macular edema if a patient reports disturbances in visual acuity (see Post-Market Adverse Drug Reactions).

Renal: Glimepiride: In patients with renal insufficiency, the initial dosing, dose increments, and maintenance dosage should be conservative to avoid hypoglycemic reactions (see Dosage and Administration).

There are no data from the use of glimepiride in patients on renal dialysis (see Action and Clinical Pharmacology).

Sexual Function/Reproduction: Rosiglitazone Maleate: Ovulation: As with other thiazolidinediones, rosiglitazone maleate may result in resumption of ovulation in premenopausal, anovulatory women with insulin resistance (e.g., patients with polycystic ovary syndrome). **As a consequence of their improved insulin sensitivity, these patients may be at risk of pregnancy if adequate contraception is not used.**

Although hormonal imbalance has been seen in preclinical studies, no significant adverse experiences associated with menstrual disorders have been reported in clinical trial participants, including premenopausal women. If unexpected menstrual dysfunction occurs, the benefits of continued therapy should be reviewed.

Special Populations: Pregnant Women: There are no controlled trials of AVANDARYL in pregnant women. Rosiglitazone has been reported to cross the human placenta and to be detectable in fetal tissues. AVANDARYL is contraindicated for use in pregnant women. Because current information strongly suggests that abnormal blood glucose levels during pregnancy are associated with a higher incidence of congenital anomalies as well as increased neonatal morbidity and mortality, most experts recommend that insulin be used during pregnancy to maintain blood glucose levels as close to normal as possible.

Teratogenic Effects: In animal studies rosiglitazone maleate was not teratogenic but treatment during mid-late gestation caused fetal death and growth retardation in both rats and rabbits at 19- and 73-fold clinical systemic exposure, respectively. In animal studies, glimepiride did not produce teratogenic effects but has been shown to be associated with intrauterine fetal death in rats when given in doses as low as 50 times the human dose based on surface area and in rabbits when given in doses as low as 0.1 times the human dose based on surface area. This fetotoxicity, observed only at doses inducing maternal hypoglycaemia, has been similarly noted with other sulfonylureas, and is believed to be directly related to the pharmacologic (hypoglycemic) action of glimepiride.

Nonteratogenic Effects: In some studies in rats, offspring of dams exposed to high levels of glimepiride during pregnancy and lactation developed skeletal deformations consisting of shortening, thickening and bending of the humerus during the postnatal period. Significant concentrations of glimepiride were observed in the serum and breast milk of the dams as well as in the serum of the pups. These skeletal deformations were determined to be the result of nursing from mothers exposed to glimepiride.

Prolonged severe hypoglycemia (4 to 10 days) has been reported in neonates born to mothers who were receiving a sulfonylurea drug. at the time of delivery. Patients who are planning a pregnancy should consult their physician.

Labour and Delivery: The effect of AVANDARYL or its components on labour and delivery in humans is not known.

Nursing Women: No studies have been conducted with AVANDARYL. Rosiglitazone and/or its metabolites have been detected in the milk of lactating rats. In rat reproduction studies, significant concentrations of glimepiride were observed in the serum and breast milk of the dame, as well as in the serum of the pups. Although it is not known whether rosiglitazone and/or glimepiride are excreted in human milk, many drugs, including other sulfonylureas, are excreted in human milk. Since the potential for hypoglycemia in nursing infants exist, and because of the effects on nursing animals (see Pregnant Women, Nonteratogenic Effects), AVANDARYL should not be administered to a nursing woman. If AVANDARYL is discontinued, and if diet alone is inadequate for controlling blood glucose, insulin therapy should be considered (see Pregnant Women).

Pediatrics (<18 years of age): There are no data on the use of AVANDARYL in patients under 18 years of age; therefore, AVANDARYL is not indicated for use in patients under 18 years of age.

Geriatrics (≥65 years of age): Glimepiride is known to be substantially excreted by the kidney, and the risk of toxic reactions to this drug may be greater in patients with impaired renal function. Because elderly patients are more likely to have decreased renal function, care should be taken in dose selection, and it may be useful to monitor renal function.

Elderly patients are particularly susceptible to the hypoglycemic action of glucose-lowering drugs. Therefore, the initial dosing, dose increments, and maintenance dosage should be conservative based upon blood glucose levels prior to and after initiation of treatment to avoid hypoglycemic reactions (see Warnings and Precautions, Hypoglycemia and Dosage and Administration, Specific Patient Populations).

Monitoring and Laboratory Tests: Periodic fasting blood glucose and A1C measurements should be performed to monitor therapeutic response.

Liver enzyme monitoring is recommended prior to initiation of therapy with AVANDARYL in all patients and periodically thereafter (see Warnings and Precautions, Hepatic).

ADVERSE REACTIONS: Adverse Drug Reaction Overview: In clinical trials, reports of hypoglycemia in patients treated with rosiglitazone maleate and sulfonylurea combination therapy were similar to reports in patients treated with sulfonylurea monotherapies. In double-blind studies, hypoglycemia was reported by 5.2% of patients receiving rosiglitazone maleate in combination with a sulfonylurea, by 5.9% receiving sulfonylurea monotherapy, by 0.6% receiving rosiglitazone maleate monotherapy, and by 0.2% receiving placebo.

Hypoglycemia was generally mild to moderate in nature and was dose-related when rosiglitazone maleate was used in combination with a sulfonylurea. Patients receiving rosiglitazone maleate in combination with oral hypoglycemic agents may be at risk for hypoglycemia, and a reduction in the dose of either agent may be necessary.

The overall incidence of hypoglycemia with glimepiride in placebo controlled trials was approximately 14%. In two long-term (2-2.5 years) and well-controlled studies, the incidence of hypoglycemic reaction ranged from 2.1 to 3.1%.

Rosiglitazone Maleate: In clinical trials, anemia and edema tended to be reported more frequently at higher doses, were generally mild to moderate in severity and usually did not require discontinuation of treatment with rosiglitazone maleate.

In clinical trials, edema was reported in 4.8% of patients taking rosiglitazone maleate as monotherapy compared to 1.3% on placebo, 1.0% on sulfonylureas and 4.0% on rosiglitazone maleate in combination with sulfonylureas. Treatment was required for 1.2% of patients on rosiglitazone maleate monotherapy with an adverse event of edema. In these clinical trials, few patients (1.0%) were enrolled with a presenting medical condition of congestive heart failure (NYHA Class I/II). Edema was more frequently observed when rosiglitazone maleate was used in combination with a sulfonylurea (see Warnings and Precautions, General and Cardiovascular).

In clinical trials, an increased incidence of heart failure has been observed when rosiglitazone maleate was added to a sulfonylurea (see Warnings and Precautions, Cardiovascular).

In double blind studies where rosiglitazone maleate was administered for up to one year, serious adverse experiences of ischemic heart disease were reported in 1.3% of patients taking rosiglitazone maleate compared to 0.5% on placebo, 0.8% on sulfonylureas and 1.2% on rosiglitazone maleate in combination with sulfonylureas.

In clinical trials, dose-related weight gain was seen with rosiglitazone maleate alone and in combination with other hypoglycemic agents (see Action and Clinical Pharmacology and Warnings and Precautions).

In a retrospective analysis of data from pooled clinical studies, which included patients on combination therapy with insulin as well as patients with NYHA Class I and II heart failure, the overall incidence of events typically associated with cardiac ischemia was higher for rosiglitazone containing regimens, 2.00% versus comparators, 1.53% [hazard ratio 1.30 (95% confidence interval 1.004-1.69)]. In a subgroup analysis of this data, this risk was further increased in patients receiving nitrates with approximately twice as many events in patients receiving rosiglitazone versus comparators (see Warnings and Precautions, Cardiovascular, Rosiglitazone Maleate, Ischemic Heart Disease). In a large observational study where patients were well matched at baseline, the incidence of the composite endpoint of myocardial infarction and coronary revascularization was 1.75 events per 100 person years for rosiglitazone containing regimens and 1.76 events per 100 person years for other anti-diabetic agents [hazard ratio 0.93 (95% confidence interval 0.80-1.10)].

A long-term study (ADOPT) compared the use of rosiglitazone (n=1456), glyburide (n=1441) and metformin (n=1454) as monotherapy in type 2 diabetes patients followed up to 6 years. Fractures were reported in a greater number of females with rosiglitazone (9.3%, 2.7/100 patient-years) compared to glyburide (3.5%, 1.3/100 patient-years) or metformin (5.1%, 1.5/100 patient-years). The majority of the fractures in the females who received rosiglitazone were reported in the upper arm, hand, and foot (see Warnings and Precautions, Fractures). The observed incidence of fractures for male patients was similar among the 3 treatment groups.

Anemia was reported in 1.9% of patients taking rosiglitazone maleate as monotherapy compared to 0.7% on placebo, 0.6% on sulfonylureas and 2.0% on rosiglitazone maleate in combination with a sulfonylurea.

Increased appetite was observed in clinical trials of rosiglitazone maleate as monotherapy or concomitantly with a sulfonylurea.

Constipation was observed to be generally mild to moderate in nature during clinical trials of rosiglitazone maleate as monotherapy, or concomitantly with a sulfonylurea.

Glimepiride: Adverse events, other than hypoglycemia, considered to be possibly or probably related to study drug that occurred in US placebo-controlled trials in more than 1% of patients treated with glimepiride included dizziness (1.7%), asthenia (1.6%), headache (1.5%), and nausea (1.1%).

Clinical Trial Adverse Drug Reactions: Because clinical trials are conducted under very specific conditions the adverse reaction rates observed in the clinical trials may not reflect the rates observed in practice and should not be compared to the rates in the clinical trials of another drug. Adverse drug reaction information from clinical trials is useful for identifying drug-related adverse events and for approximating rates.

Rosiglitazone Maleate: Controlled Clinical Trials: The incidence and types of adverse events reported in controlled, 26-week clinical trials in association with rosiglitazone maleate in combination with a sulfonylurea, in comparison to adverse events reported in association with rosiglitazone maleate and sulfonylurea monotherapies are shown in Table 1.

Table 1: AVANDARYL

Adverse Events (≥5% in Any Treatment Group) Reported by Patients in 26-week Double-blind Clinical Trials with Rosiglitazone Maleate as Monotherapy or in Combination with a Sulfonylurea

Preferred Term	Rosiglitazone Maleate N=2526 %	Placebo N=601 %	Sulfonylurea N=626 %	Rosiglitazone Maleate 4 mg plus Sulfonylurea N=405 %
Upper Respiratory Tract Infection	9.9	8.7	7.3	8.6
Injury[a]	7.6	4.3	6.1	6.7
Headache	5.9	5.0	5.4	4.9
Back Pain	4.0	3.8	5.0	2.0
Hyperglycemia	3.9	5.7	8.1	4.2
Fatigue	3.6	5.0	1.9	1.7
Hypoglycemia	0.6	0.2	5.9	5.2
Dizziness	2.5	1.7	3.0	5.4
Hypercholesterolemia	3.4	0.5	1.3	5.2

[a] Includes cuts, burns, sprains, fractures, falls, accidents and surgical procedures.

Overall, the types of adverse experiences reported when rosiglitazone maleate was used in combination with a sulfonylurea were similar to those during monotherapy with rosiglitazone maleate.

Glimepiride: Digestive Tract Reactions: Gastrointestinal (GI) disturbances e.g. nausea, GI fullness, occur occasionally. Vomiting, gastrointestinal pain, and diarrhea have been reported, but the incidence in placebo-controlled trials was similar to that of placebo. In rare cases, there may be elevation of liver enzyme levels. Sulfonylureas, including glimepiride, may also, in isolated instances, cause impairment of liver function (e.g. with cholestasis and jaundice), as well as hepatitis which may also lead to liver failure.

Dermatologic Reactions: Allergic skin reactions, e.g., pruritus, erythema, urticaria, and morbilliform or maculopapular eruptions, occur in less than 1% of treated patients. These may be transient and may disappear despite continued use of glimepiride. If those hypersensitivity reactions persist or worsen, the drug should be discontinued. Porphyria cutanea tarda, photosensitivity reactions, and allergic vasculitis, in some cases, progressing from mild to serious reactions (including anaphylactic shock) have been reported with sulfonylureas, including glimepiride.

Hematologic Reactions: Leukopenia, agranulocytosis, hemolytic anemia, thrombocytopenia, aplastic anemia, erythrocytopenia, granulocytopenia, and pancytopenia have been reported with sulfonylureas, including glimepiride.

Metabolic Reactions: Hepatic porphyria reactions and disulfiram-like reactions have been reported with sulfonylureas; however, no cases have yet been reported with glimepiride. Cases of hyponatremia have been reported with glimepiride and all other sulfonylureas, most often in patients who are on other medications or have medical conditions known to cause hyponatremia or increase release of antidiuretic hormone. Although there have been no reports for glimepiride, the syndrome of inappropriate antidiuretic hormone (SIADH) secretion has been reported with certain other sulfonylureas, and it has been suggested that these sulfonylureas may augment the peripheral (antidiuretic) action of ADH and/or increase release of ADH.

Other Adverse Reactions: Changes in accommodation and/or blurred vision may occur with the use of glimepiride. This is thought to be due to changes in blood glucose, and may be more pronounced when treatment is initiated. This condition is also seen in untreated diabetic patients, and may actually be reduced by treatment. In placebo-controlled trials of glimepiride, the incidence of blurred vision was placebo, 3.4%, and glimepiride, 1.7%.

Human Ophthalmology Data: Ophthalmic examinations were carried out in over 500 subjects during long-term studies of glimepiride using the methodology of Taylor and West and Laties et al. No significant differences were seen between glimepiride and glyburide in the number of subjects with clinically important changes in visual acuity, intra-ocular tension, or in any of the five lens-related variables examined. Ophthalmic examinations were carried out during long-term studies using the method of Chylack et al. No significant or clinically meaningful differences were seen between glimepiride and glipizide with respect to cataract progression by subjective LOCS II grading and objective image analysis systems, visual acuity, intraocular pressure, and general ophthalmic examination.

Abnormal Hematologic and Clinical Chemistry Findings: Hematological: Small decreases in hematological parameters were more common in the patients treated with rosiglitazone maleate than in placebo-treated patients. Leukopenia was reported in 0.4% of rosiglitazone maleate patients compared to 0.2% of patients on placebo, 0.6% on sulfonylureas and 1.1% on rosiglitazone maleate in combination with sulfonylureas. Decreases may be related to increased plasma volume observed with treatment with rosiglitazone maleate. The mean decrease in hemoglobin was approximately 10 to 12 g/L; the decrease in hematocrit was 0.03 to 0.04.

Lipids: Small increases in total cholesterol and LDL have been observed following treatment with rosiglitazone maleate (see Table 3, Action and Clinical Pharmacology, Pharmacodynamics and Clinical Effects).

Serum Transaminase Levels: In clinical studies in 4598 patients treated with rosiglitazone maleate encompassing approximately 3600 patient years of exposure, there was no evidence of drug-induced hepatotoxicity or elevated ALT levels.

In the controlled trials (including patients with ALT/AST of up to 2.5 times the upper limit of the reference range at study entry), 0.2% of patients treated with rosiglitazone maleate had reversible elevations in ALT >3 times the upper limit of the reference range compared to 0.2% on placebo and 0.5% on active comparators. Hyperbilirubinemia was found in 0.3% of patients treated with rosiglitazone maleate compared with 0.9% treated with placebo and 1% in patients treated with active comparators. Overall, there was a decrease in mean values for ALT, AST, alkaline phosphatase and bilirubin over time in patients treated with rosiglitazone maleate (see Warnings and Precautions, Hepatic).

In the clinical program including long-term, open-label experience, the rate per 100 patient years exposure of ALT increase to >3 times the upper limit of normal was 0.35 for patients treated with rosiglitazone maleate, 0.59 for placebo-treated patients, and 0.78 for patients treated with active comparator agents.

In pre-approval clinical trials, there were no cases of idiosyncratic drug reactions leading to hepatic failure.

Post-Market Adverse Drug Reactions: In postmarketing experience with rosiglitazone maleate as monotherapy and in combination with other oral antidiabetic agents, adverse events potentially related to volume expansion (e.g., congestive heart failure, pulmonary edema, and pleural effusions) have been reported. See Warnings and Precautions, Cardiovascular.

Reports of events related to cardiovascular ischemia including myocardial infarction, and hypertension or hypertension accelerated have been received.

Reports of new onset and/or worsening macular edema with decreased visual acuity occurring with the use of rosiglitazone maleate have been received rarely. These patients frequently reported concurrent peripheral edema. In some cases, symptoms improved following discontinuation of rosiglitazone maleate (see Warnings and Precautions, Ophthalmologic).

Reports of anaphylactic reaction, rash and pruritus have been received very rarely.

Reports of hepatitis and of hepatic enzyme elevations to three or more times the upper limit of normal have been received. Very rarely, these reports have involved hepatic failure with and without fatal outcome, although causality has not been established.

Postmarketing reports of parotid gland enlargement have been associated with rosiglitazone and approximately one third of the reports resolved or improved following discontinuation of rosiglitazone.

DRUG INTERACTIONS: Overview: Rosiglitazone Maleate: Drugs Metabolized by Cytochrome P450: It has been shown in vitro that rosiglitazone does not inhibit any of the major P450 enzymes at clinically relevant concentrations. In vitro studies demonstrate that rosiglitazone is predominantly metabolized by CYP2C8, with CYP2C9 as only a minor pathway. In vitro studies have shown that montelukast is an inhibitor of CYP 2C8 and may inhibit the metabolism of drugs primarily metabolized by CYP 2C8 (e.g. paclitaxel, rosiglitazone, repaglinide). No in vivo interaction studies have been performed with the CYP2C8 substrates cerivastatin and paclitaxel. The potential for a clinically relevant interaction with cerivastatin is considered to be low. Although rosiglitazone is not anticipated to affect the pharmacokinetics of paclitaxel, concomitant use is likely to result in inhibition of the metabolism of rosiglitazone.

Coadministration of rosiglitazone maleate with CYP2C8 inhibitors (e.g. gemfibrozil) resulted in increased rosiglitazone plasma concentrations. Since there is a potential for an increase in the risk of dose-related adverse reactions, a decrease in rosiglitazone maleate may be needed when CYP2C8 inhibitors are coadministered.

Coadministration of rosiglitazone maleate with a CYP2C8 inducer (e.g. rifampin) resulted in decreased rosiglitazone plasma concentrations. Therefore, close monitoring of glycemic control and changes in diabetic treatment should be considered when CYP2C8 inducers are coadministered.

Clinically significant interactions with CYP2C9 substrates or inhibitors are not anticipated.

CYP3A4 Substrates: Rosiglitazone maleate (8 mg once daily) was shown to have no clinically relevant effect on the pharmacokinetics of nifedipine and oral contraceptives (ethinylestradiol and norethindrone), which are predominantly metabolized by CYP3A4. The results of these two drug interaction studies suggest that rosiglitazone is unlikely to cause clinically important drug interactions with other drugs metabolized via CYP3A4.

Glimepiride: Glimepiride is metabolized by CYP2C9. This should be taken into account when glimepiride is coadministered with inducers or inhibitors of CYP2C9.

Coadministration of glimepiride with CYP2C9 inhibitors (e.g. fluconazole) resulted in increased glimepiride plasma concentrations. Since there is a potential for an increase in the risk of dose-related adverse reactions (e.g. hypoglycemia), a decrease in glimepiride dose may be needed when CYP2C9 inhibitors are coadministered.

Drug-Drug Interactions: AVANDARYL: Single oral doses of glimepiride in 14 healthy adult subjects had no clinically significant effect on the steady-state pharmacokinetics of rosiglitazone. No clinically significant reductions in glimepiride AUC and C_{max} were observed after repeat doses of rosiglitazone maleate for 8 days in healthy adult subjects.

Rosiglitazone Maleate: Oral Contraceptives: In 32 healthy women, rosiglitazone maleate (8 mg once daily) was shown to have no statistically significant effect on the pharmacokinetics of oral contraceptives (ethinylestradiol and norethindrone). Breakthrough bleeding occurred in 5 individuals when rosiglitazone maleate was coadministered with an oral contraceptive. In one of these subjects a 40% decrease in ethinylestradiol exposure (AUC) was recorded. This was not correlated with a reduction in exposure to norethindrone, nor was there a consistent relationship between the occurrence of breakthrough bleeding and the pharmacokinetics of either ethinylestradiol or norethindrone in individual subjects.

Digoxin: Repeat oral dosing of rosiglitazone maleate (8 mg once daily) for 14 days did not alter the steady-state pharmacokinetics of digoxin (0.375 mg once daily) in healthy volunteers.

Warfarin: Coadministration of rosiglitazone maleate (4 mg twice daily for 7 days) did not alter the anticoagulant response of steady-state warfarin in healthy volunteers with baseline values of INR of <2.75. Repeat dosing with rosiglitazone maleate had no clinically relevant effect on the steady-state pharmacokinetics of warfarin.

Gemfibrozil: A study conducted in normal healthy volunteers showed that gemfibrozil (an inhibitor of CYP2C8) administered as 600 mg twice daily, increased rosiglitazone systemic exposure two-fold at steady state (see Warnings and Precautions, General).

Rifampin: A study conducted in normal healthy volunteers showed that rifampin (an inducer of CYP2C8) administered as 600 mg daily, decreased the rosiglitazone systemic exposure three-fold (see Warnings and Precautions, General). Additional pharmacokinetic studies demonstrated no clinically relevant effect of acarbose, ranitidine, or metformin on the pharmacokinetics of rosiglitazone.

Methotrexate: An interaction study of 22 adult patients with psoriasis examined the effect of repeat doses of rosiglitazone maleate (8 mg daily as a single dose for 8 days) on the pharmacokinetics of oral methotrexate administered as single oral doses of 5 to 25 mg weekly. Following 8 days of rosiglitazone maleate administration, the C_{max} and $AUC_{(0-inf)}$ of methotrexate increased by 18% (90% CI: 11% to 26%) and 15% (90% CI: 8% to 23%), respectively, when compared to the same doses of methotrexate administered in the absence of rosiglitazone maleate.

Glimepiride: Coadministration of acetylsalicylic acid (1 g three times daily) and glimepiride led to a 34% decrease in the mean glimepiride AUC and, therefore, a 34% increase in the mean CL/f. The mean C_{max} had a decrease of 4%. Blood glucose and serum C-peptide concentrations were unaffected and no hypoglycemic symptoms were reported.

Coadministration of either cimetidine (800 mg once daily) or ranitidine (150 mg twice daily) with a single 4-mg oral dose of glimepiride did not significantly alter the absorption and disposition of glimepiride, and no differences were seen in hypoglycemic symptomatology.

Concomitant administration of propranolol (40 mg three times daily) and glimepiride significantly increased C_{max}, AUC, and $T_{½}$ of glimepiride by 23%, 22%, and 15%, respectively, and it decreased CL/f by 18%. The recovery of the major metabolites, cyclohexyl hydroxy methyl derivative (M1) and the carboxyl derivative (M2), from urine, however, did not change. The pharmacodynamic responses to glimepiride were nearly identical in normal subjects receiving propranolol and placebo. Pooled data from clinical trials in patients with type 2 diabetes showed no evidence of clinically significant adverse interactions with uncontrolled concurrent administration of beta-blockers. However, if beta-blockers are used, caution should be exercised and patients should be warned about the potential for hypoglycemia.

Concomitant administration of glimepiride tablets (4 mg once daily) did not alter the pharmacokinetic characteristics of R- and S-warfarin enantiomers following administration of a single dose (25 mg) of racemic warfarin to healthy subjects. No changes were observed in warfarin plasma protein binding. Glimepiride treatment did result in a slight, but statistically significant, decrease in the pharmacodynamic response to warfarin. The reductions in mean area under the prothrombin time (PT) curve and maximum PT values during glimepiride treatment were very small (3.3% and 9.9%, respectively) and are unlikely to be clinically important.

The responses of serum glucose, insulin, C-peptide, and plasma glucagon to 2 mg glimepiride were unaffected by coadministration of ramipril (an ACE inhibitor) 5 mg once daily in normal subjects. No hypoglycemic symptoms were reported.

A study conducted in twelve normal healthy volunteers showed that fluconazole (an inhibitor of CYP2C9) administered as 200 mg once daily, increased glimepiride systemic exposure approximately two and a half-fold (see Warnings and Precautions, General).

A study conducted in ten normal healthy volunteers showed that rifampin (an inducer of CYP2C9) administered as 600 mg once daily, decreased glimepiride systemic exposure by 34% (see Warnings and Precautions, General).

Potential interactions of glimepiride with other drugs metabolized by cytochrome P450 2C9 also include phenytoin, diclofenac, ibuprofen, naproxen, and mefenamic acid. Although no specific interaction studies were performed, pooled data from clinical trials showed no evidence of clinically significant adverse interactions with uncontrolled concurrent administration of calcium-channel blockers, estrogens, fibrates, NSAIDs, HMG-CoA reductase inhibitors, sulfonamides, or thyroid hormone.

The hypoglycemic action of sulfonylureas may be potentiated by certain drugs, including anabolic steroids and male sex hormones, ACE inhibitors, insulin and other oral antidiabetics nonsteroidal anti-inflammatory drugs and other drugs that are highly protein bound, such as azapropazone, sulfonamides (e.g. sulphaphenazole), chloramphenicol, clarithromycin, coumarins, cyclophosphamine, disopyramide, fenyramidol, fenfluramine, fibrates, fluconazole, fluoxetine, guanethidine, ifosfamide, miconazole, monoamine oxidase inhibitors, oxyphenbutazone, para-aminosalicylic acid, pentoxifylline (high dose parenteral), phenylbutazone, probenecid, propranolol, quinolones, salicylates, sulfonamide antibiotics, sulfinpyrazone and tetracyclines. When these drugs are administered to a patient receiving glimepiride, the patient should be observed closely for hypoglycemia. When these drugs are withdrawn from a patient receiving glimepiride, the patient should be observed closely for loss of glycemic control.

Certain drugs tend to produce hyperglycemia and may lead to loss of glycemic control. These drugs include the thiazides and other diuretics, acetazolamide, barbiturates, corticosteroids, diazoxide, epinephrine and other sympathomimetic agents, glucagon, isoniazid, laxatives (after protracted use), nicotinic acid (in high dose), estrogens and progestogens, phenothiazines, phenytoin, rifampin and thyroid products. When these drugs are administered to a patient receiving glimepiride, the patient should be closely observed for loss of glycemic control. When these drugs are withdrawn from a patient receiving glimepiride, the patient should be observed closely for hypoglycemia.

H_2 receptor antagonists, beta-blockers, clonidine and reserpine may lead to either potentiation or weakening of the blood-glucose-lowering effect.

Drug-Food Interactions: Interactions with food have not been established.

Drug-Herb Interactions: Interactions with herbal products have not been established.

Drug-Laboratory Test Interactions: Interactions with laboratory tests have not been established.

DOSAGE AND ADMINISTRATION:

Dosing Considerations: AVANDARYL should be given once daily with a meal. The dosage of antidiabetic therapy with AVANDARYL should be individualized on the basis of effectiveness and tolerability. No exact dosage relationship exists between AVANDARYL and other antidiabetic agents.

The safety and efficacy of AVANDARYL as initial therapy for patients with type 2 diabetes have not been established. No studies have been performed specifically examining the safety and efficacy of AVANDARYL in patients previously treated with other oral hypoglycemic agents and switched to AVANDARYL. Any change in therapy of type 2 diabetes should be undertaken with care and appropriate monitoring as changes in glycemic control can occur.

Specific Patient Populations: AVANDARYL should not be used in pregnancy or in nursing mothers. There are no data on the use of AVANDARYL in patients younger than 18 years; therefore, the use of AVANDARYL in pediatric patients is not recommended.

In elderly, debilitated, or malnourished patients, or in patients with renal insufficiency, the initial dosing, dose increments, and maintenance dosage of AVANDARYL should be conservative to avoid hypoglycemic reactions. (See Action and Clinical Pharmacology, Special Populations and Conditions and Warnings and Precautions, Hypoglycemia.)

Therapy with AVANDARYL should not be initiated if the patient exhibits clinical evidence of active liver disease or increased serum transaminase levels (ALT >2.5 times the upper limit of normal at start of therapy) (see Warnings and Precautions, Hepatic and Action and Clinical Pharmacology, Hepatic Insufficiency). Liver enzyme monitoring is recommended in all patients prior to initiation of therapy with AVANDARYL and periodically thereafter. AVANDARYL is contraindicated in patients with serious hepatic impairment (see Contraindications, Warnings and Precautions, Hepatic).

Recommended Dose and Dosage Adjustment: AVANDARYL is available for oral administration as tablets containing a fixed dose of 4 mg rosiglitazone maleate with variable doses of glimepiride (1, 2, or 4 mg) in a single tablet formulation.

For patients inadequately controlled on rosiglitazone or sulfonylurea monotherapy, the usual starting dose of AVANDARYL is 4 mg/1 mg or 4 mg/2 mg once daily. When switching from combination therapy of rosiglitazone maleate plus glimepiride as separate tablets, the usual starting dose of AVANDARYL is the dose of rosiglitazone maleate and glimepiride already being taken. The maximum recommended daily dose of AVANDARYL is 4 mg of rosiglitazone maleate and 4 mg of glimepiride.

Sufficient time should be given to assess adequacy of therapeutic response. Fasting glucose should be used to determine the therapeutic response to AVANDARYL:

- For patients previously treated with rosiglitazone monotherapy switched to AVANDARYL, dose titration is recommended if patients are not adequately controlled after 1 to 2 weeks. If additional glycemic control is needed, the daily dose of AVANDARYL may be increased by increasing the glimepiride component in no more than 2 mg increments at 1 to 2 week intervals up to the maximum recommended total daily dose of 4 mg rosiglitazone maleate/4 mg glimepiride.
- For patients previously treated with sulfonylurea monotherapy switched to AVANDARYL, it may take 2 weeks to see a reduction in blood glucose and 2 to 3 months to see the full effect of the rosiglitazone component. If additional glycemic control is needed, the dose of the glimepiride component may be increased. The dose of the rosiglitazone component should not exceed 4 mg. As with other sulfonylurea-containing antidiabetic agents, no transition period is necessary when transferring patients to AVANDARYL. Patients should be observed carefully (1 to 2 weeks) for hypoglycemia when being transferred from longer half-life sulfonylureas (e.g., chlorpropamide) to glimepiride due to potential overlapping of drug effect.
- If hypoglycemia occurs during up-titration of the dose or while maintained on therapy, a dosage reduction of the sulfonylurea component of AVANDARYL may be considered.

Missed Dose: If a dose of AVANDARYL is missed, the patient should be advised to take the dosage as soon as they remember anytime during the day. If a whole day is missed, the usual dose should be taken the next day. The patient should be advised not to take a double dose.

OVERDOSAGE:

In the event of an overdose, appropriate supportive treatment should be initiated as dictated by the patient's clinical status.

No data are available with regard to overdosage of AVANDARYL. Overdosage of glimepiride can produce hypoglycemia. Mild hypoglycemic symptoms without loss of consciousness or neurologic findings should be treated with oral glucose and adjustments in drug dosage and/or meal patterns. Close monitoring should continue until the physician is assured that the patient is out of danger. Severe hypoglycemic reactions with coma, seizure, or other neurological impairment occur infrequently, but constitute medical emergencies requiring immediate hospitalization. Patients should be closely monitored for a minimum of 24 to 48 hours, because hypoglycemia may recur after apparent clinical recovery.

> For management of a suspected drug overdose, contact your **regional Poison Control Centre**. See the *CPS* Directory section for a list of Poison Control Centres.

ACTION AND CLINICAL PHARMACOLOGY: Mechanism of Action: AVANDARYL tablets combines 2 antidiabetic agents with complementary mechanisms of action to improve glycemic control while reducing circulating insulin levels in patients with type 2 diabetes: Rosiglitazone, a member of the thiazolidinedione class, and glimepiride, a member of the sulfonylurea class. Thiazolidinediones are insulin sensitizing agents that act primarily by enhancing peripheral glucose utilization, whereas sulfonylureas act primarily by stimulating release of insulin from functioning pancreatic beta cells.

Rosiglitazone maleate is an oral antidiabetic agent which acts primarily by increasing insulin sensitivity in type 2 diabetes. Rosiglitazone, a member of the thiazolidinedione class of antidiabetic agents, improves glycemic control while reducing circulating insulin levels. It improves sensitivity to insulin in muscle and adipose tissue and inhibits hepatic gluconeogenesis. Rosiglitazone is not chemically or functionally related to the sulfonylureas, the biguanides or the alpha-glucosidase inhibitors. Rosiglitazone is a highly selective and potent agonist for the peroxisome proliferator-activated receptor-gamma (PPARγ). In humans, PPAR receptors are found in key target tissues for insulin action such as adipose tissue, skeletal muscle and liver. Activation of PPARγ nuclear receptors regulates the transcription of insulin-responsive genes involved in the control of glucose production, transport, and utilization. In addition, PPARγ-responsive genes also participate in the regulation of fatty acid metabolism and in the maturation of preadipocytes, predominantly of subcutaneous origin.

Insulin resistance is a primary feature characterizing the pathogenesis of type 2 diabetes. The use of rosiglitazone maleate results in increased responsiveness of insulin-dependent tissues and significantly improves hepatic and peripheral (muscle) tissue sensitivity to insulin in patients with type 2 diabetes. Clinical studies in patients with type 2 diabetes treated with rosiglitazone maleate either as monotherapy or in combination with sulfonylureas showed improved beta-cell function and decreased fasting plasma glucose, insulin and C-peptide values following 26 weeks of treatment. A homeostasis model assessment (HOMA) was conducted using fasting plasma glucose and insulin or C-peptide levels as a measure of insulin sensitivity and beta-cell function. In these studies, reductions in mean plasma pro-insulin and pro-insulin split product concentrations were also observed.

Rosiglitazone maleate significantly reduced hemoglobin A1C (A1C, a marker for long term glycemic control), and fasting blood glucose (FBG) in patients with type 2 diabetes. Inadequately controlled hyperglycemia is associated with an increased risk of diabetic complications, including cardiovascular disorders and diabetic nephropathy, retinopathy and neuropathy.

Studies between 8 and 26 weeks with rosiglitazone maleate have shown a statistically significant reduction in markers of inflammation, C-reactive protein (CRP) and matrix metalloproteinase-9 (MMP-9). The clinical significance of these effects are still unknown. Further long term clinical trials are needed.

Estimates of LDL particle size can be determined by the LDL cholesterol (LDL) to apolipoprotein B (Apo B) ratio. In controlled clinical trials, rosiglitazone maleate has been shown to increase the LDL cholesterol to Apo B ratio consistent with a beneficial change in LDL particle size from small dense LDL particles to larger more buoyant particles. This change has been confirmed by measuring LDL particle buoyancy (Rf) following 8 weeks treatment with rosiglitazone maleate in an open-label study.

The primary mechanism of action of glimepiride in lowering blood glucose appears to be dependent on stimulating the release of insulin from functioning pancreatic beta cells. In addition, extrapancreatic effects may also play a role in the activity of glimepiride. This is supported by both preclinical and clinical studies demonstrating that glimepiride administration can lead to increased sensitivity of peripheral tissues to insulin. These findings are consistent with the results of a long-term, randomized, placebo-controlled trial in which glimepiride therapy improved postprandial insulin/C-peptide responses and overall glycemic control without producing clinically meaningful increases in fasting insulin/C-peptide levels. However, the mechanism by which glimepiride lowers blood glucose during long-term administration has not been clearly established.

Pharmacodynamics and Clinical Effects: In clinical studies, treatment with rosiglitazone maleate resulted in an improvement in glycemic control, as measured by fasting plasma glucose (FPG) and hemoglobin A1c (A1C), with a concurrent reduction in insulin and C-peptide levels. Post-prandial glucose and insulin levels were also reduced. This is consistent with the mechanism of action of rosiglitazone as an insulin sensitizer. The improvement in glycemic control was durable with maintenance of effect for at least 52 weeks. In open-labelled extension studies sustained improvements in glycemic control (as measured by A1C levels) were observed in patients receiving rosiglitazone maleate monotherapy for 36 months.

Rosiglitazone is believed to act primarily on muscle and adipose tissue whereas sulfonylureas act primarily by stimulating the release of insulin from functioning pancreatic beta cells. The coadministration of rosiglitazone maleate with sulfonylureas resulted in significantly improved glycemic control compared to either of these agents alone. These results are consistent with a synergistic effect on glycemic control when rosiglitazone maleate is used in combination with sulfonylureas. In patients whose type 2 diabetes was inadequately controlled with sulfonylurea monotherapy, the addition of rosiglitazone maleate led to reductions in A1C levels that were sustained for over 30 months of treatment, in open-labelled studies.

Weight gain has been observed in clinical studies with rosiglitazone maleate (see Table 2). In addition, rosiglitazone maleate significantly decreased visceral (abdominal) fat stores while increasing subcutaneous abdominal fat. The reduction in visceral fat correlates with improved hepatic and peripheral tissue insulin sensitivity. Weight gain with thiazolidinediones can result from increases in subcutaneous adipose tissue and/or from fluid retention. Treatment should be re-evaluated in patients with excessive weight gain (see Warnings and Precautions and Adverse Reactions).

Table 2: AVANDARYL

Weight Changes (kg) from Baseline During Clinical Trials with Rosiglitazone Maleate

			Control Group	Rosiglitazone Maleate 4 mg	Rosiglitazone Maleate 8 mg
Treatment Group	**Duration**	**Control Group**	**Median (25th, 75th percentile) (range)**	**Median (25th, 75th percentile) (range)**	**Median (25th, 75th percentile) (range)**
Monotherapy					
Rosiglitazone maleate	26 weeks	placebo	−0.9 (−2.8, 0.9) (−9.6 to 6.8) n=210	1.0 (−0.9, 3.6) (−11.6 to 12.7) n=436	3.1 (1.1, 5.8) (−6.8 to 13.9) n=439
Rosiglitazone maleate	52 weeks	sulfonylurea	2.0 (0, 4.0) (−11.5 to 12.2) n=173	2.0 (−0.6, 4.0) (−7.0 to 16.0) n=150	2.6 (0, 5.3) (−11.0 to 22.0) n=157
Combination Therapy					
Rosiglitazone maleate + sulfonylurea	26 weeks	sulfonylurea	0 (−1.3, 1.2) (−6.0 to 14.0) n=1043	1.8 (0, 3.1) (−5.0 to 11.5) n=392	—
Rosiglitazone maleate + metformin	26 weeks	metformin	−1.4 (−3.2, 0.2) (−7.7 to 5.9) n=175	0.8 (−1.0, 2.6) (−6.8 to 9.8) n=100	2.1 (0, 4.3) (−5.4 to 13.1) n=184

Patients with lipid abnormalities were not excluded from clinical trials of rosiglitazone maleate. In all 26-week controlled trials, across the recommended dose range, rosiglitazone maleate as monotherapy was associated with increases in total cholesterol, LDL, and HDL and decreases in free fatty acids. These changes were statistically significantly different from placebo or glyburide controls (see Table 3).

Increases in LDL occurred primarily during the first 1 to 2 months of therapy with rosiglitazone maleate and LDL levels remained stable, but elevated above baseline throughout the trials. In contrast, HDL continued to rise over time. As a result, the LDL/HDL ratio peaked after 2 months of therapy and then appeared to decrease over time. Because of the temporal nature of lipid changes, the 52-week glyburide-controlled study is most pertinent to assess long-term effects on lipids. At baseline, week 26 and week 52, median LDL/HDL ratios were 3.0, 2.9 and 2.8, respectively for rosiglitazone maleate 4 mg twice daily and the median total cholesterol/HDL ratios were 4.76, 4.52 and 4.35, respectively. The corresponding values for glyburide were 3.2, 2.9 and 2.7 for the median LDL/HDL ratios and 4.90, 4.61 and 4.36 for the median total cholesterol/HDL ratios.

The pattern of LDL and HDL changes following therapy with rosiglitazone maleate in combination with sulfonylureas was generally similar to those seen with rosiglitazone maleate in monotherapy.

The changes in triglycerides during therapy with rosiglitazone maleate were variable and were generally not statistically different from placebo or glyburide controls.

Table 3: AVANDARYL

Summary of Lipid Changes in 26-week Placebo-controlled and 26-week/52-week Glyburide-controlled Monotherapy Studies

	Placebo-controlled Studies Week 26			Glyburide-controlled Study Week 26 and Week 52			
		Rosiglitazone Maleate		Glyburide Titration		Rosiglitazone Maleate 8 mg	
	Placebo	**4 mg daily**	**8 mg daily**	**wk 26**	**wk 52**	**wk 26**	**wk 52**
Free Fatty Acids (mmol/L)							
N	207	428	436	181	168	166	145
Baseline (median)	0.61	0.58	0.61	0.92	0.92	0.93	0.93
% change from baseline (median)	−4	−15.6	−23.5	−5.5	−9.7	−26.7	−24.7
LDL-cholesterol (mmol/L)							
N	190	400	374	175	160	161	133
Baseline (median)	3.15	3.26	3.19	3.68	3.55	3.62	3.62
% change from baseline (median)	+2.5	+10.3	+14.8	−3.7	−3.3	+7.1	+7.3
HDL-cholesterol (mmol/L)							
N	208	429	436	184	170	170	145
Baseline (median)	1.06	1.14	1.09	1.17	1.18	1.19	1.19
% change from baseline (median)	+8.2	+10.3	+11.3	+4.7	+8	+13.2	+17.4

(cont'd)

Table 3: AVANDARYL *(cont'd)*

Summary of Lipid Changes in 26-week Placebo-controlled and 26-week/52-week Glyburide-controlled Monotherapy Studies

The long term significance of the lipid changes is not known.

Pharmacokinetics: Bioavailability: AVANDARYL: In a bioequivalence study of AVANDARYL 4 mg/4 mg, the area under the curve (AUC) and maximum concentration (C_{max}) of rosiglitazone following a single dose of the combination tablet were bioequivalent to rosiglitazone maleate 4 mg concomitantly administered with glimepiride 4 mg under fasted conditions. The AUC and C_{max} of glimepiride following a single fasted 4 mg/4 mg dose was bioequivalent to glimepiride concomitantly administered with rosiglitazone maleate 4 mg (see Table 4 and Table 5—Comparative Bioavailability Data). The rate and extent of absorption of both the rosiglitazone component and glimepiride component of AVANDARYL when taken with food were equivalent to the rate and extent of absorption of rosiglitazone and glimepiride when administered concomitantly as separate tablets with food. A single dose, randomized 2-way crossover study was conducted in 30 healthy male and female volunteers under fasting conditions with AVANDARYL [1×(4 mg rosiglitazone maleate/4 mg glimepiride)] versus concomitant administration of AVANDIA (1×4 mg rosiglitazone maleate) and Amaryl (1×4 mg glimepiride).

Table 4: AVANDARYL

Table of the Comparative Bioavailability Data Rosiglitazone [1×4 mg administered as 1×(4 mg rosiglitazone maleate/4 mg glimepiride) and as 1×4 mg rosiglitazone maleate administered concomitantly with 1×4 mg glimepiride]

	From Measured Data Geometric Mean Arithmetic Mean (CV%)			
Parameter	**Test AVANDARYL**	**Reference AVANDIA[a]**	**Ratio of Geometric Means**	**90% Confidence Interval**
AUC_T (ng·h/mL)	1097 1269 (25.54)	1099 1245 (74.06)	100	96–104
AUC_I (ng·h/mL)	1134 1296 (24.88)	1136 1275 (67.52)	100	96–104
C_{max} (ng/mL)	231.4 263.8 (22.23)	226.1 257.0 (75.28)	102	92–114
T_{max}[b] (h)	1.11 (48.71)	1.14 (93.91)		
$T_{½}$[b] (h)	3.53 (13.66)	3.55 (18.78)		

a AVANDIA tablets, manufactured in the U.S. by GlaxoSmithKline Inc.
b Expressed as arithmetic mean (%CV) only.

Table 5: AVANDARYL

Table of the Comparative Bioavailability Data Glimepiride [1×4 mg administered as 1×(4 mg rosiglitazone maleate/4 mg glimepiride) and as 1×4 mg glimepiride administered concomitantly with 1×4 mg rosiglitazone maleate]

	From Measured Data Geometric Mean Arithmetic Mean (CV%)			
Parameter	**Test AVANDARYL**	**Reference Amaryl[a]**	**Ratio of Geometric Means**	**90% Confidence Interval**
AUC_T (ng·h/mL)	930 988 (35.55)	1022 1089 (33.16)	91	87–96
AUC_I (ng·h/mL)	1035 1093 (33.80)	1082 1157 (33.59)	96	91–100
C_{max} (ng/mL)	149 160.8 (40.01)	170 184.1 (40.46)	88	76–101
T_{max}[b] (h)	3.63 (45.23)	3.54 (61.57)		
$T_{½}$[b] (h)	7.48 (31.96)	5.10 (42.02)		

a Amaryl tablets, manufactured in the U.S. by Aventis Pharmaceuticals.
b Expressed as arithmetic mean (%CV) only.

The AUC and C_{max} of glimepiride increased in a dose-proportional manner following administration of AVANDARYL 4 mg/1 mg, 4 mg/2 mg, and 4 mg/4 mg. Administration of AVANDARYL with food decreased the rate, but not extent, of rosiglitazone absorption and increased both the rate and extent of absorption of glimepiride compared to the fasted state.

Absorption: Rosiglitazone Maleate: Rosiglitazone is rapidly and completely absorbed after oral administration with negligible first-pass metabolism. The absolute bioavailability of rosiglitazone is 99%. Peak plasma concentrations are observed by 1 hour after dosing. Maximum plasma concentration (C_{max}) and the area under the curve (AUC_{0-inf}) of rosiglitazone increase in a dose-proportional manner over the therapeutic dose range.

Glimepiride: After oral administration, glimepiride is completely (100%) absorbed from the GI tract. Studies with single oral doses in normal subjects and with multiple oral doses in patients with type 2 diabetes have shown significant absorption of glimepiride within 1 hour after administration and peak drug levels (C_{max}) at 2 to 3 hours.

Distribution: Rosiglitazone Maleate: The mean (SD) volume of distribution (Vss) of rosiglitazone after intravenous administration to healthy subjects is approximately 14.1 (3.1) L. Rosiglitazone is approximately 99.8% bound to plasma proteins, primarily albumin.

Glimepiride: After intravenous dosing in normal subjects, the volume of distribution (Vd) was 8.8 L (113 mL/kg), and the total body clearance (CL) was 47.8 mL/min. Protein binding was greater than 99.5%.

Metabolism: Rosiglitazone Maleate: Rosiglitazone is extensively metabolized with no unchanged drug excreted in the urine. The major routes of metabolism were N-demethylation and hydroxylation, followed by conjugation with sulfate and glucuronic acid. All the circulating metabolites are considerably less potent than the parent drug and, therefore, are not expected to contribute to the insulin-sensitizing activity of rosiglitazone. In vitro data demonstrate that rosiglitazone is predominantly metabolized by Cytochrome P450 (CYP) isoenzyme 2C8, with CYP 2C9 contributing as only a minor pathway.

Glimepiride: Glimepiride is completely metabolized by oxidative biotransformation after either IV or oral administration. The major metabolites are the cyclohexyl hydroxyl methyl derivative (M1) and the carboxyl derivative (M2). Cytochrome P450 2C9 has been shown to be involved in the biotransformation of glimepiride to M1. M1 is further metabolized to M2 by one or several cytosolic enzymes. M1, but not M2, possesses about 1/3 of the pharmacological activity as compared to its parent in an animal model; however, whether the glucose-lowering effect of M1 is clinically meaningful in humans is not clear.

Excretion: Rosiglitazone Maleate: Following oral or intravenous administration of [^{14}C] rosiglitazone maleate, approximately 64% and 23% of the dose was eliminated in the urine and feces, respectively. The plasma half-life of [^{14}C] related material ranged from 103 to 158 hours. The elimination half-life of rosiglitazone is 3 to 4 hours and is independent of dose.

Glimepiride: When ^{14}C-glimepiride was given as a single dose orally, approximately 60% of the total radioactivity was recovered in the urine in 7days and M1 (predominant) and M2 accounted for 80-90% of that recovered in the urine. Approximately 40% of the total radioactivity was recovered in feces and M1 and M2 (predominant) accounted for about 70% of that recovered in feces. After IV dosing in patients, no significant biliary excretion of glimepiride or its M1 metabolite has been observed.

Special Populations and Conditions: No pharmacokinetic data are available for AVANDARYL in the following special populations. Information is provided for the individual components of AVANDARYL.

Pediatrics: No pharmacokinetic data from studies in pediatric subjects are available for either rosiglitazone or glimepiride.

Geriatrics: Results of the population pharmacokinetic analysis (n=716 ≤65 years; n=331 ≥65 years) showed that age does not significantly affect the pharmacokinetics of rosiglitazone.

Comparison of glimepiride pharmacokinetics in type 2 diabetic patients ≤65 years and those >65 years was performed in a study using a dosing regimen of 6 mg daily. There were no significant differences in glimepiride pharmacokinetics between the two age groups. The mean AUC at steady state for the older patients was about 13% lower than that for the younger patients; the mean weight adjusted clearance for the older patients was about 11% higher than that for the younger patients (see Warnings and Precautions, Special Populations, Geriatrics (≥65 years of age)).

Gender: Results of the population pharmacokinetic analysis showed that the mean oral clearance of rosiglitazone in female patients (n=405) was 15% lower compared to male patients (n=642), primarily related to lower body weight in females. Combination therapy with rosiglitazone maleate and sulfonylureas improved glycemic control in both males and females. In rosiglitazone maleate and sulfonylurea combination studies, a greater therapeutic response was observed in females. For a given body mass index (BMI), females tend to have a greater fat mass than males. Since the molecular target of rosiglitazone, PPARγ, is expressed in adipose tissues, this differentiating characteristic may account, at least in part, for the greater response to rosiglitazone maleate in combination with sulfonylureas in females. Since therapy should be individualized, no dose adjustments are necessary based on gender alone.

There were no differences between males and females in the pharmacokinetics of glimepiride when adjusted for differences in body weight.

Race: Results of a population pharmacokinetic analysis including subjects of Caucasian, black and other ethnic origins indicate that race has no influence on the pharmacokinetics of rosiglitazone.

No pharmacokinetic studies to assess the effects of race have been performed, but in placebo-controlled studies of glimepiride in patients with type 2 diabetes, the hypoglycemic effect was comparable in whites (n=536), blacks (n=63), and Hispanics (n=63).

Hepatic Insufficiency: Unbound oral clearance of rosiglitazone was significantly lower in patients with moderate to severe liver disease (Child-Pugh Class B/C) compared to healthy subjects. As a result, unbound C_{max} and AUC_{0-inf} were increased 2- and 3-fold, respectively. Elimination half-life for rosiglitazone was about 2 hours longer in patients with liver disease, compared to healthy subjects. Therapy with AVANDARYL should not be initiated if the patient exhibits clinical evidence of active liver disease or increased serum transaminase levels (ALT >2.5 times the upper limit of normal at start of therapy). See Warnings and Precautions, Hepatic and Action and Clinical Pharmacology, Special Populations and Conditions, Hepatic Insufficiency.

No pharmacokinetic studies of glimepiride have been conducted in subjects with hepatic insufficiency.

Renal Insufficiency: There are no clinically relevant differences in the pharmacokinetics of rosiglitazone in patients with mild to severe renal impairment or in hemodialysis-dependent patients, compared to subjects with normal renal function.

There are no data from the use of glimepiride in patients on renal dialysis (see Warnings and Precautions).

A single-dose glimepiride, open-label study was conducted in 15 patients with renal impairment. Glimepiride (3 mg) was administered to 3 groups of patients with different levels of mean creatinine clearance (Clcr): Group I, Clcr=77.7 mL/min (1.30 mL/sec), n=5; Group II, Clcr=27.7 mL/min (0.462 mL/sec), n=3; and Group III, Clcr=9.4 mL/min (0.16 mL/sec), n=7. Glimepiride was found to be well tolerated in all 3 groups. The results showed that M1 and M2 serum levels (mean AUC values) increased 2.2 and 6.1 times from Group I to Group III as renal function decreased. The apparent terminal half life ($T_{½}$) for glimepiride did not change, while the half-lives for M1 and M2 increased as renal function decreased. Mean urinary excretion of M1 plus M2 as percent of dose, however, decreased (44.4%, 21.9%, and 9.3% for Groups I to III).

A multiple-dose glimepiride titration study was also conducted in 16 type 2 diabetic patients with renal impairment using doses ranging from 1-8 mg daily for 3 months. The results were consistent with those observed after single doses. All patients with a Clcr less than 22 mL/min (0.37 mL/sec) had adequate control of their glucose levels with a dosage regimen of only 1 mg daily. The results from this study suggested that a starting dose of 1 mg glimepiride, as in AVANDARYL 4 mg/1 mg, may be given to type 2 diabetic patients with kidney disease, and the dose may be titrated based on fasting blood glucose levels.

STORAGE AND STABILITY: Store at controlled room temperature 15 to 30°C.

SPECIAL HANDLING INSTRUCTIONS: Dispense in a tight, light-resistant container.

INFORMATION FOR THE PATIENT: Published in e-CPS, available by subscription at www.e-cps.ca.

DOSAGE FORMS, COMPOSITION AND PACKAGING: 4 mg/1 mg: Each yellow, rounded triangular tablet, debossed with gsk on one side and 4/1 on the other, contains: rosiglitazone maleate 4 mg and glimepiride 1 mg. Nonmedicinal ingredients: hypromellose 2910, lactose monohydrate, macrogol (polyethylene glycol), magnesium stearate, microcrystalline cellulose, sodium starch glycolate, titanium dioxide and one or more of the following: black, red or yellow iron oxides. Bottles of 100.

4 mg/2 mg: Each orange, rounded triangular tablet, debossed with gsk on one side and 4/2 on the other, contains: rosiglitazone maleate 4 mg and glimepiride 2 mg. Nonmedicinal ingredients: hypromellose 2910, lactose monohydrate, macrogol (polyethylene glycol), magnesium stearate, microcrystalline cellulose, sodium starch glycolate, titanium dioxide and one or more of the following: black, red or yellow iron oxides. Bottles of 100.

4 mg/4 mg: Each pink, rounded triangular tablet, debossed with gsk on one side and 4/4 on the other, contains: rosiglitazone maleate 4 mg and glimepiride 4 mg. Nonmedicinal ingredients: hypromellose 2910, lactose monohydrate, macrogol (polyethylene glycol), magnesium stearate, microcrystalline cellulose, sodium starch glycolate, titanium dioxide and one or more of the following: black, red or yellow iron oxides. Bottles of 100.

(Shown in Product Identification Section)

Avandia® P

rosiglitazone maleate

Antidiabetic—Insulin Resistance Reducing Agent

GlaxoSmithKline

Date of Revision: March 12, 2009

SUMMARY PRODUCT INFORMATION:

Route of Administration	Dosage Form/ Strength	Clinically Relevant Nonmedicinal Ingredients
Oral	Tablet/ 2 mg, 4 mg and 8 mg	Lactose monohydrate For a complete listing see Dosage Forms, Composition and Packaging.

INDICATIONS AND CLINICAL USE: AVANDIA (rosiglitazone maleate) is indicated for use as an adjunct to diet and exercise to reduce insulin resistance and improve glycemic control in patients with type 2 diabetes mellitus as follows:

Monotherapy:

- Use as monotherapy, in patients not controlled by diet and exercise alone and for whom metformin is inappropriate because of contraindications or intolerance.

Dual Therapy:

- Use in combination with metformin when diet and exercise plus metformin do not result in adequate glycemic control. For patients inadequately controlled on metformin, AVANDIA should be added to, not substituted for, metformin.
- Use in combination with a sulfonylurea in patients who show intolerance to metformin or for whom metformin is contraindicated, when diet and exercise plus sulfonylurea or AVANDIA monotherapy do not result in adequate glycemic control. For patients inadequately controlled on a sulfonylurea, AVANDIA should be added to, not substituted for, the sulfonylurea.

Caloric restriction, weight loss, and exercise improve insulin sensitivity and are essential for the proper treatment of a diabetic patient. These measures are important not only in the primary treatment of type 2 diabetes, but also in maintaining the efficacy of drug therapy. Prior to initiation of therapy with AVANDIA, secondary causes of poor glycemic control (e.g., infection) should be investigated and treated.

Geriatrics (≥65 years of age): Results of the population pharmacokinetic analysis (n=716 <65 years; n=331 ≥65 years) showed that age does not significantly affect the pharmacokinetics of rosiglitazone. Therefore, no dosage adjustments are required for the elderly.

Pediatrics (<18 years of age): The safety and effectiveness of rosiglitazone have not been established in patients younger than 18 years of age, therefore, AVANDIA is not indicated in patients younger than 18 years of age.

CONTRAINDICATIONS: AVANDIA is contraindicated in:

- Patients with New York Heart Association (NYHA) Class I to IV heart failure.
- Patients with known hypersensitivity to this product or any of its ingredients.
- Patients with serious hepatic impairment (see Warnings and Precautions).
- Pregnancy. Insulin is recommended during pregnancy to control blood glucose levels. Oral antidiabetic agents should not be given (see Warnings and Precautions, Special Populations, Pregnant Women).

WARNINGS AND PRECAUTIONS: General: AVANDIA is active only in the presence of insulin due to its mechanism of action. Therefore, AVANDIA should not be used in the treatment of type 1 diabetes or for the treatment of diabetic ketoacidosis.

For safety reasons, the use of AVANDIA in combination with insulin is not indicated.

The use of AVANDIA in combination with metformin **and** a sulfonylurea (triple therapy) is not indicated. An increase in reporting of fluid retention related events (including congestive heart failure) has been seen in patients receiving rosiglitazone in combination with metformin **and** a sulfonylurea.

Close monitoring of glycemic control and rosiglitazone dose adjustment may be needed when rosiglitazone is coadministered with CYP2C8 inhibitors or inducers (see Drug Interactions).

Cardiovascular: Congestive Heart Failure: Thiazolidinediones, like AVANDIA, alone or in combination with other antidiabetic agents, can cause fluid retention, which can exacerbate or lead to congestive heart failure. The fluid retention may very rarely present as rapid and excessive weight gain. All patients should be monitored for signs and symptoms of adverse reactions relating to fluid retention and heart failure. In particular, patients who are at risk for heart failure including those receiving concurrent therapy which increases insulin levels (i.e. sulfonylureas) should be closely monitored. (See Adverse Reactions.) An increase in reporting of fluid retention related events including congestive heart failure has been seen in patients receiving rosiglitazone in combination with metformin and a sulfonylurea. This triple therapy regimen is not an approved indication.

Treatment with thiazolidinediones has been associated with cases of congestive heart failure, some of which were difficult to treat unless the medication was discontinued. AVANDIA should be discontinued if any deterioration in cardiac status occurs.

AVANDIA is contraindicated in patients with NYHA Class I, II, III and IV heart failure. Patients with severe heart failure (including NYHA Class III and IV cardiac status) were not studied during the clinical trials.

Patients experiencing acute coronary syndromes (ACS) have not been studied in rosiglitazone controlled clinical trials. Since patients experiencing ACS are at an increased risk of developing heart failure, and in view of the potential for rosiglitazone to cause or exacerbate heart failure, initiation of AVANDIA in patients experiencing an acute coronary event is not recommended. Furthermore, discontinuation of AVANDIA during the acute phase should be considered.

Ischemic Heart Disease: In a retrospective analysis of data from pooled clinical studies, which included patients on combination therapy with insulin as well as patients with NYHA Class I and II heart failure, the overall incidence of events typically associated with cardiac ischemia was higher for AVANDIA containing regimens, 2.00% versus comparators, 1.53% [Hazard ratio 1.30 (95% confidence interval 1.004-1.69)]. In a subgroup analysis of this data, this risk was further increased in patients receiving nitrates with approximately twice as many events in patients receiving rosiglitazone versus comparators. **The use of AVANDIA is therefore not recommended for patients being treated with nitrates.**

The completion of an adequately-designed cardiovascular outcome study is needed to further evaluate the risk of myocardial ischemic events associated with AVANDIA.

In a large observational study where patients were well-matched at baseline, the incidence of the composite endpoint of myocardial infarction and coronary revascularization was 1.75 events per 100 person years for AVANDIA containing regimens and 1.76 events per 100 person years for other anti-diabetic agents [Hazard ratio 0.93 (95% confidence interval 0.80-1.10)].

Edema: AVANDIA should be used with caution in patients with edema. In healthy volunteers who received AVANDIA 8 mg once daily as monotherapy for 8 weeks, there was a statistically significant increase in median plasma volume (1.8 mL/kg) compared to placebo. In controlled clinical trials of patients with Type 2 diabetes, mild to moderate edema was observed at a greater frequency in patients treated with AVANDIA and may be dose related (see Adverse Reactions). For information on macular edema, see Warnings and Precautions, Ophthalmologic.

Endocrine and Metabolism: Loss of Control of Blood Glucose: When a patient stabilized on any antidiabetic regimen is exposed to stress such as fever, trauma, infection, or surgery, a temporary loss of glycemic control may occur. At such times, it may be necessary to withhold AVANDIA and temporarily administer insulin. AVANDIA may be reinstituted after the acute episode is resolved.

Hypoglycemia: Because AVANDIA does not stimulate insulin secretion, hypoglycemia is not expected to occur when AVANDIA is prescribed as monotherapy. Patients receiving AVANDIA in combination with other hypoglycemic agents (e.g. insulin secreting agents) may be at risk for hypoglycemia, and a reduction in the dose of either agent may be necessary.

Weight Gain: Dose-related weight gain was seen with AVANDIA alone and in combination with other hypoglycemic agents. Treatment should be re-evaluated in patients with excessive weight gain (see Action and Clinical Pharmacology and Adverse Reactions).

Fractures: In a 4 to 6 year comparative study (ADOPT) of glycemic control with monotherapy in recently diagnosed patients with Type 2 diabetes mellitus, an increased incidence of bone fracture was noted in female patients taking AVANDIA (9.3%, 2.7 patients per 100 patient-years) versus glyburide (3.5%, 1.3 patients per 100 patient-years) or metformin (5.1%, 1.5 patients per 100 patient-years). The majority of the fractures in the females who received AVANDIA were reported in the upper arm, hand, and foot (see Adverse Reactions). The risk of fracture should be considered in the care of patients, especially female patients, treated with AVANDIA, and attention should be given to assessing and maintaining bone health according to current standards of care.

Hematologic: In controlled trials, there were dose-related decreases in hemoglobin and hematocrit. The magnitude of the decreases (≤11 g/L for hemoglobin and ≤0.034 for hematocrit) was small for AVANDIA alone and AVANDIA in combination with metformin or in combination with sulfonylurea. The changes occurred primarily during the first 3 months of therapy or following an increase in AVANDIA dose and remained relatively constant thereafter. Decreases may be related to increased plasma volume observed during treatment with AVANDIA and have not been associated with any significant hematologic clinical effects (see Adverse Reactions, Abnormal Hematologic and Clinical Chemistry Findings). Patients with a hemoglobin value of <110 g/L for males and <100 g/L for females were excluded from the clinical trials.

Hepatic: Therapy with AVANDIA should not be initiated in patients with increased baseline liver enzyme levels (ALT >2.5 times the upper limit of normal).

Rare cases of severe hepatocellular injury have been reported with thiazolidinediones.

In postmarketing experience with AVANDIA, reports of hepatitis and of hepatic enzyme elevations to three or more times the upper limit of normal have been received. Very rarely, these reports have involved hepatic failure with and without fatal outcome, although causality has not been established (see Adverse Reactions, Post-Market Adverse Drug Reactions).

Liver enzymes should be checked prior to the initiation of therapy with AVANDIA in all patients and periodically thereafter per the clinical judgement of the healthcare professional.

Patients with mildly elevated liver enzymes (ALT levels ≤2.5 times the upper limit of normal) at baseline or during therapy with AVANDIA should be evaluated to determine the cause of the liver enzyme elevation.

Initiation of, or continuation of, therapy with AVANDIA in patients with mild liver enzyme elevations (ALT levels ≤2.5 times the upper limit of normal) should proceed with caution and include appropriate close clinical follow-up, including more frequent liver enzyme monitoring, to determine if the liver enzyme elevations resolve or worsen. If at any time ALT levels increase to >3 times the upper limit of normal in patients on therapy with AVANDIA, liver enzyme levels should be rechecked as soon as possible. If ALT levels remain >3 times the upper limit of normal, therapy with AVANDIA should be discontinued (see Dosage and Administration).

If any patient develops symptoms suggesting hepatic dysfunction, which may include unexplained nausea, vomiting, abdominal pain, fatigue, anorexia and/or dark urine, liver enzymes should be checked. The decision whether to continue the patient on therapy with AVANDIA should be guided by clinical judgment pending laboratory evaluations. If jaundice is observed, drug therapy should be discontinued.

Ophthalmologic: New onset and/or worsening macular edema with decreased visual acuity has been reported rarely in postmarketing experience with AVANDIA. In some cases, the visual events resolved or improved following discontinuation of AVANDIA. Physicians should consider the possibility of macular edema if a patient reports disturbances in visual acuity (see Adverse Reactions, Post-Market Adverse Drug Reactions).

Sexual Function/Reproduction: Ovulation: As with other thiazolidinediones, AVANDIA may result in resumption of ovulation in premenopausal, anovulatory women with insulin resistance (e.g., patients with polycystic ovary syndrome). **As a consequence of their improved insulin sensitivity, these patients may be at risk of pregnancy if adequate contraception is not used.**

Although hormonal imbalance has been seen in preclinical studies, no significant adverse experiences associated with menstrual disorders have been reported in clinical trial participants, including premenopausal women. If unexpected menstrual dysfunction occurs, the benefits of continued therapy should be reviewed.

Special Populations: Pregnant Women: There are no controlled trials of AVANDIA in pregnant women. Rosiglitazone has been reported to cross the human placenta and to be detectable in fetal tissues. AVANDIA is contraindicated for use in pregnant women. Because current information strongly suggests that abnormal blood glucose levels during pregnancy are associated with a higher incidence of congenital anomalies as well as increased neonatal morbidity and mortality, most experts recommend that insulin be used during pregnancy to maintain blood glucose levels as close to normal as possible. In animal studies AVANDIA was not teratogenic but treatment during mid-late gestation caused fetal death and growth retardation in both rats and rabbits at 19- and 73-fold clinical systemic exposure, respectively.

Labour and Delivery: The effect of rosiglitazone on labour and delivery in humans is not known.

Nursing Women: It is not known whether AVANDIA is excreted in human milk. Because many drugs are excreted in human milk, AVANDIA should not be administered to a nursing woman.

Pediatrics (<18 years of age): There are no data on the use of AVANDIA in patients under 18 years of age; therefore, AVANDIA is not indicated for use in patients under 18 years of age. Thiazolidinediones promote the maturation of preadipocytes and have been associated with weight gain. Obesity is a major problem in adolescents with type 2 diabetes.

Geriatrics (≥65 years of age): In the pooled population pharmacokinetic analysis, there were no marked differences in the pharmacokinetics of AVANDIA between elderly and non-elderly patients.

Monitoring and Laboratory Tests: Periodic fasting blood glucose and A1C measurements should be performed to monitor therapeutic response.

Liver enzyme monitoring is recommended prior to initiation of therapy with AVANDIA in all patients and periodically thereafter (see Warnings and Precautions, Hepatic).

ADVERSE REACTIONS: Adverse Drug Reaction Overview: In clinical trials, events of anemia and edema tended to be reported more frequently at higher doses, were generally mild to moderate in severity and usually did not require discontinuation of treatment with AVANDIA.

In clinical trials, edema was reported in 4.8% of patients taking AVANDIA as monotherapy compared to 1.3% on placebo, 1.0% on sulfonylureas and 2.2% on metformin. Treatment was required for 1.2% of patients on rosiglitazone monotherapy with an adverse event of edema. These adverse experiences rarely led to withdrawal. In these clinical trials, few patients (1.0%) were enrolled with a presenting medical condition of congestive heart failure (NYHA Class I/II). Edema was more frequently observed when AVANDIA was used in combination with a sulfonylurea or insulin (see Warnings and Precautions, General and Cardiovascular).

In clinical trials, an increased incidence of heart failure has also been observed when AVANDIA was added to a sulfonylurea (see Warnings and Precautions, Cardiovascular).

In double blind studies where AVANDIA was administered for up to one year, serious adverse experiences of ischemic heart disease were reported in 1.3% of patients taking AVANDIA compared to 0.5% on placebo, 0.8% on sulfonylureas and 1.3% on metformin.

In a retrospective analysis of data from pooled clinical studies, which included patients on combination therapy with insulin as well as patients with NYHA Class I and II heart failure, the overall incidence of events typically associated with cardiac ischemia was higher for AVANDIA containing regimens, 2.00% versus comparators, 1.53% [Hazard ratio 1.30 (95% confidence interval 1.004-1.69)]. In a subgroup analysis of this data, this risk was further increased in patients receiving nitrates with approximately twice as many events in patients receiving rosiglitazone versus comparators (see Warnings and Precautions, Cardiovascular, Ischemic Heart Disease). In a large observational study where patients were well-matched at baseline, the incidence of the composite endpoint of myocardial infarction and coronary revascularization was 1.75 events per 100 person years for AVANDIA containing regimens and 1.76 events per 100 person years for other anti-diabetic agents [Hazard ratio 0.93 (95% confidence interval 0.80-1.10)].

In clinical trials, dose-related weight gain was seen with AVANDIA alone and in combination with other hypoglycemic agents (see Action and Clinical Pharmacology and Warnings and Precautions). In a long-term monotherapy trial (ADOPT) in drug-naïve patients, median weight change (range) at 4 years was 3.5 kg (−31.0 to 41.3) for AVANDIA, 2.0 kg (−28.6 to 24.9) for glyburide, and −2.4 kg (−46.0 to 12.9) for metformin. This weight change with AVANDIA occurred consistently over the duration of the study.

A long-term study (ADOPT) compared the use of AVANDIA (n=1456), glyburide (n=1441), and metformin (n=1454) as monotherapy in type 2 diabetes patients followed up to 6 years. Fractures were reported in a greater number of females with AVANDIA (9.3%, 2.7/100 patient-years) compared to glyburide (3.5%, 1.3/100 patient-years) or metformin (5.1%, 1.5/100 patient-years). The majority of the fractures in the females who received AVANDIA were reported in the upper arm, hand, and foot (see Warnings and Precautions, Endocrine and Metabolism, Fractures). The observed incidence of fractures for male patients was similar among the 3 treatment groups.

Increased appetite was observed in clinical trials of rosiglitazone as monotherapy or concomitantly with a sulfonylurea.

Hypoglycemia was generally mild to moderate in nature and was dose-related when rosiglitazone was used in combination with metformin or a sulfonylurea. Patients receiving rosiglitazone in combination with oral hypoglycemic agents may be at risk for hypoglycemia, and a reduction in the dose of either agent may be necessary.

In double blind studies, anemia was reported in 1.9% of patients taking AVANDIA as monotherapy compared to 0.7% on placebo, 0.6% on sulfonylureas and 2.2% on metformin. Treatment was required for 0.3% of patients with an adverse event of anemia. These adverse experiences rarely led to withdrawal. Reports of anemia were greater in patients treated with a combination of AVANDIA and metformin (7.1%) compared to monotherapy with AVANDIA or AVANDIA in combination with a sulfonylurea (2.3%). Lower pre-treatment hemoglobin/hematocrit levels in patients enrolled in the metformin combination clinical trials may have contributed to the higher reporting rate of anemia in these studies.

Constipation was observed to be generally mild to moderate in nature during clinical trials of rosiglitazone as monotherapy, or concomitantly with metformin or a sulfonylurea.

Clinical Trial Adverse Drug Reactions: Because clinical trials are conducted under very specific conditions the adverse reaction rates observed in the clinical trials may not reflect the rates observed in practice and should not be compared to the rates in the clinical trials of another drug. Adverse drug reaction information from clinical trials is useful for identifying drug-related adverse events and for approximating rates.

Controlled Clinical Trials: The overall incidence and types of adverse experiences reported in clinical trials of rosiglitazone (16 weeks to 1 year) as monotherapy or in combination with metformin or sulfonylurea are shown in Table 1.

Table 1: AVANDIA

Adverse Experiences (≥5% in any treatment group) Reported by Patients in Double-blind Clinical Trials with AVANDIA as Monotherapy (16 weeks to 1 year)

	AVANDIA N=2526		Placebo N=601		Metformin N=225		Sulfonylureas N=626	
Preferred Term	n	%	n	%	n	%	n	%
Total Patients with Adverse Experiences	1742	**69.0**	374	**62.2**	172	**76.0**	438	**70.0**
Upper Respiratory Tract Infection	251	**9.9**	52	**8.7**	20	**8.9**	46	**7.3**
Injury[a]	192	**7.6**	26	**4.3**	17	**7.6**	38	**6.1**
Headache	148	**5.9**	30	**5.0**	20	**8.9**	34	**5.4**
Back Pain	102	**4.0**	23	**3.8**	9	**4.0**	31	**5.0**
Hyperglycemia	99	**3.9**	34	**5.7**	10	**4.4**	51	**8.1**
Fatigue	92	**3.6**	30	**5.0**	9	**4.0**	12	**1.9**
Sinusitis	82	**3.2**	27	**4.5**	12	**5.3**	19	**3.0**
Diarrhea	59	**2.3**	20	**3.3**	35	**16**	19	**3.0**
Hypoglycemia	16	**0.6**	1	**0.2**	3	**1.3**	37	**5.9**

[a] Includes cuts, burns, sprains, fractures, falls, accidents and surgical procedures.

Overall, the types of adverse experiences reported when AVANDIA was used in combination with a sulfonylurea or metformin were similar to those during monotherapy with AVANDIA.

Long-term Trial of AVANDIA as Monotherapy: In a 4 to 6 year monotherapy study (ADOPT), adverse reactions observed with AVANDIA were generally consistent to those observed in shorter-term trials as presented in Table 1, above). However, fractures were reported in a greater number of females with AVANDIA compared to glyburide or metformin (see Warnings and Precautions, Endocrine and Metabolism, Fractures and Adverse Reactions, Adverse Drug Reaction Overview).

Abnormal Hematologic and Clinical Chemistry Findings: Hematological: Small decreases in hematological parameters were more common in the patients treated with AVANDIA than in placebo-treated patients. Leukopenia was reported in 0.4% of AVANDIA patients compared to 0.2% of patients on placebo, 0.6% on sulfonylureas and 0% on metformin. Decreases may be related to increased plasma volume observed with treatment with AVANDIA. The mean decrease in hemoglobin was approximately 10 to 12 g/L; the decrease in hematocrit was 0.03 to 0.04.

Lipids: Small increases in total cholesterol and LDL have been observed following treatment with AVANDIA (see Table 3, Action and Clinical Pharmacology, Pharmacodynamics and Clinical Effects).

Serum Transaminase Levels: In clinical studies in 4598 patients treated with AVANDIA (rosiglitazone maleate) encompassing approximately 3600 patient years of exposure, there was no evidence of drug-induced hepatotoxicity or elevated ALT levels.

In the controlled trials (including patients with ALT/AST of up to 2.5 times the upper limit of the reference range at study entry), 0.2% of patients treated with AVANDIA had reversible elevations in ALT >3 times the upper limit of the reference range compared to 0.2% on placebo, 0.9% on metformin and 0.3% on sulfonylureas.

Hyperbilirubinemia was found in 0.3% of patients treated with AVANDIA compared with 0.9% treated with placebo. Overall, there was a decrease in mean values for ALT, AST, alkaline phosphatase and bilirubin over time in patients treated with AVANDIA (see Warnings and Precautions, Hepatic).

In the clinical program including long-term, open-label experience, the rate per 100 patient years exposure of ALT increase to >3 times the upper limit of normal was 0.35 for patients treated with AVANDIA, 0.59 for placebo-treated patients, and 0.78 for patients treated with active comparator agents.

In pre-approval clinical trials, there were no cases of idiosyncratic drug reactions leading to hepatic failure.

Post-Market Adverse Drug Reactions: In postmarketing experience with AVANDIA as monotherapy and in combination with other antidiabetic agents, adverse events potentially related to volume expansion (e.g., congestive heart failure, pulmonary edema, and pleural effusions) have been reported (see Warnings and Precautions, Cardiovascular).

Reports of events related to cardiovascular ischemia including myocardial infarction, and hypertension or hypertension accelerated have been received.

Reports of new onset and/or worsening macular edema with decreased visual acuity occurring with the use of AVANDIA have been received rarely. These patients frequently reported concurrent peripheral edema. In some cases, symptoms improved following discontinuation of AVANDIA (see Warnings and Precautions, Ophthalmologic).

Reports of anaphylactic reaction (such as angioedema and urticaria), rash and pruritus have been received very rarely.

Reports of hepatitis and of hepatic enzyme elevations to three or more times the upper limit of normal have been received. Very rarely, these reports have involved hepatic failure with and without fatal outcome, although causality has not been established.

Postmarketing reports of parotid gland enlargement have been associated with rosiglitazone and approximately one third of the reports resolved or improved following discontinuation of AVANDIA.

DRUG INTERACTIONS: Overview: Drugs Metabolized by Cytochrome P450: It has been shown in vitro that AVANDIA does not inhibit any of the major P450 enzymes at clinically relevant concentrations. In vitro studies demonstrate that rosiglitazone is predominantly metabolized by CYP2C8, with CYP2C9 as only a minor pathway. In vitro studies have shown that montelukast is an inhibitor of CYP2C8 and may inhibit the metabolism of drugs primarily metabolized by CYP2C8 (e.g. paclitaxel, rosiglitazone, repaglinide). No in vivo interaction studies have been performed with the CYP2C8 inhibitor, montelukast or with CYP2C8 substrates cerivastatin and paclitaxel. The potential for a clinically relevant interaction with cerivastatin is considered to be low. Although rosiglitazone is not anticipated to affect the pharmacokinetics of paclitaxel, concomitant use is likely to result in inhibition of the metabolism of rosiglitazone.

Coadministration of rosiglitazone with CYP2C8 inhibitors (e.g. gemfibrozil) resulted in increased rosiglitazone plasma concentrations. Since there is a potential for an increase in the risk of dose-related adverse reactions, a decrease in rosiglitazone may be needed when CYP2C8 inhibitors are coadministered.

Coadministration of rosiglitazone with a CYP2C8 inducer (e.g. rifampin) resulted in decreased rosiglitazone plasma concentrations. Therefore, close monitoring of glycemic control and changes in diabetic treatment should be considered when CYP2C8 inducers are coadministered.

Clinically significant interactions with CYP2C9 substrates or inhibitors are not anticipated.

CYP3A4 Substrates: AVANDIA (8 mg once daily) was shown to have no clinically relevant effect on the pharmacokinetics of nifedipine and oral contraceptives (ethinylestradiol and norethindrone), which are predominantly metabolized by CYP3A4. The results of these two drug interaction studies suggest that AVANDIA is unlikely to cause clinically important drug interactions with other drugs metabolized via CYP3A4.

Ethanol: A single administration of a moderate amount of alcohol did not increase the risk of acute hypoglycemia in type 2 diabetes mellitus patients treated with AVANDIA.

Drug-Drug Interactions: Oral Contraceptives: In 32 healthy women, AVANDIA (8 mg once daily) was shown to have no statistically significant effect on the pharmacokinetics of oral contraceptives (ethinylestradiol and norethindrone). Breakthrough bleeding occurred in 5 individuals when AVANDIA was coadministered with an oral contraceptive. In one of these subjects a 40% decrease in ethinylestradiol exposure (AUC) was recorded. This was not correlated with a reduction in exposure to norethindrone, nor was there a consistent relationship between the occurrence of breakthrough bleeding and the pharmacokinetics of either ethinylestradiol or norethindrone in individual subjects.

Glyburide: AVANDIA (2 mg twice daily) taken concomitantly with glyburide (3.75 to 10 mg/day) for 7 days did not alter the mean steady-state 24-hour plasma glucose concentrations in diabetic patients stabilized on glyburide therapy.

Glimepiride: Single oral doses of glimepiride in 14 healthy adult subjects had no clinically significant effect on the steady-state pharmacokinetics of AVANDIA. No clinically significant reductions in glimepiride AUC and C_{max} were observed after repeat doses of AVANDIA for 8 days in healthy adult subjects.

Metformin: Concurrent administration of AVANDIA (2 mg twice daily) and metformin (500 mg twice daily) in healthy volunteers for 4 days had no effect on the steady-state pharmacokinetics of either metformin or rosiglitazone.

Acarbose: Coadministration of acarbose (100 mg three times daily) for 7 days in healthy volunteers had no clinically relevant effect on the pharmacokinetics of a single oral dose of AVANDIA.

Digoxin: Repeat oral dosing of AVANDIA (8 mg once daily) for 14 days did not alter the steady-state pharmacokinetics of digoxin (0.375 mg once daily) in healthy volunteers.

Warfarin: Coadministration of AVANDIA (4 mg twice daily for 7 days) did not alter the anticoagulant response of steady-state warfarin in healthy volunteers with baseline values of INR of <2.75. Repeat dosing with AVANDIA had no clinically relevant effect on the steady-state pharmacokinetics of warfarin.

Ranitidine: Pretreatment with ranitidine (150 mg twice daily for 4 days) did not alter the pharmacokinetics of either single oral or intravenous doses of rosiglitazone in healthy volunteers. These results suggest that the absorption of oral rosiglitazone is not altered in conditions accompanied by increases in gastrointestinal pH.

Gemfibrozil: A study conducted in normal healthy volunteers showed that gemfibrozil (an inhibitor of CYP2C8) administered as 600 mg twice daily, increased rosiglitazone systemic exposure two-fold at steady state (see Warnings and Precautions, General).

Rifampin: A study conducted in normal healthy volunteers showed that rifampin (an inducer of CYP2C8) administered as 600 mg daily, decreased the rosiglitazone systemic exposure three-fold (see Warnings and Precautions, General).

Methotrexate: An interaction study of 22 adult patients with psoriasis examined the effect of repeat doses of rosiglitazone (8 mg daily as a single dose for 8 days) on the pharmacokinetics of oral methotrexate administered as single oral doses of 5 to 25 mg weekly. Following 8 days of rosiglitazone administration, the C_{max} and $AUC_{(0-inf)}$ of methotrexate increased by 18% (90% CI: 11% to 26%) and 15% (90% CI: 8% to 23%), respectively, when compared to the same doses of methotrexate administered in the absence of rosiglitazone.

Concomitant Medications in Phase III Clinical Trials: Results of the population pharmacokinetic analysis indicated that none of the following classes of concomitant medications (oral hypoglycemics, analgesics, calcium channel blockers, hypolipidemics, ACE inhibitors and steroid hormones) appear to alter the oral clearance or oral steady-state volume of distribution of AVANDIA.

Drug-Food Interactions: Interactions with food have not been established.

Drug-Herb Interactions: Interactions with herbal products have not been established.

Drug-Laboratory Test Interactions: Interactions with laboratory tests have not been established.

DOSAGE AND ADMINISTRATION:

Dosing Considerations: The management of antidiabetic therapy should be individualized.

Increases in rosiglitazone to 8 mg/day should be undertaken cautiously following appropriate clinical evaluation to assess the patient's risk of developing adverse reactions relating to fluid retention (see Warnings and Precautions and Adverse Reactions). The dose of AVANDIA used in combination with a sulfonylurea should not exceed 4 mg daily (see Recommended Dose and Dosage Adjustment, Combination Therapy with Sulfonylurea).

AVANDIA may be administered as a single daily dose in the morning, or divided and administered in the morning and evening. AVANDIA may be taken with or without food.

No dosage adjustments are required for the elderly, or in patients with renal impairment. Therapy with AVANDIA should not be initiated if the patient exhibits clinical evidence of active liver disease or increased serum transaminase levels (ALT >2.5 times the upper limit of normal at start of therapy). AVANDIA is contraindicated in patients with serious hepatic impairment. See Contraindications, Warnings and Precautions, Hepatic and Action and Clinical Pharmacology, Special Populations and Conditions, Hepatic Insufficiency.

Recommended Dose and Dosage Adjustment: Monotherapy: The usual starting dose of AVANDIA is 4 mg administered either as a single dose once daily or in divided doses twice daily. For patients who respond inadequately following 8 to 12 weeks of treatment as determined by reduction in fasting plasma glucose (FPG), the dose may be increased to 8 mg administered as a single dose once daily or in divided doses twice daily.

Combination Therapy with Metformin: The usual starting dose of AVANDIA in combination with metformin is 4 mg administered as either a single dose once daily or in divided doses twice daily. The dose of AVANDIA may be increased to 8 mg/day following 8 to 12 weeks of therapy if there is insufficient reduction in FPG.

Combination Therapy with Sulfonylurea: The recommended dose of AVANDIA when used in combination with sulfonylurea is 4 mg administered as either a single dose once daily or in divided doses twice daily. The dose of AVANDIA used in combination with a sulfonylurea should not exceed 4 mg daily. If patients report hypoglycemia, the dose of the sulfonylurea should be decreased (see Warnings and Precautions and Adverse Reactions).

Missed Dose: If a dose of AVANDIA is missed with once a day dosing, the patient should be advised to take the dose as soon as they remember anytime during the day. If a dose is missed with twice a day dosing, the patient should be advised to take the missed dose as soon as they remember and the next dose at the usual time. Three doses should never be taken in one day to make up for a missed dose the day before. If a whole day of AVANDIA is missed, the usual dosing schedule should be followed the next day without making up for the missed doses.

OVERDOSAGE:

In the event of an overdose, appropriate supportive treatment should be initiated as dictated by the patient's clinical status.

Limited data are available with regard to overdosage in humans. In clinical studies in volunteers, AVANDIA has been administered at single oral doses of up to 20 mg and was well tolerated.

> For management of a suspected drug overdose, contact your **regional Poison Control Centre**. See the *CPS* Directory section for a list of Poison Control Centres.

ACTION AND CLINICAL PHARMACOLOGY: Mechanism of Action: AVANDIA is an oral antidiabetic agent which acts primarily by increasing insulin sensitivity in type 2 diabetes. Rosiglitazone, a member of the thiazolidinedione class of antidiabetic agents, improves glycemic control while reducing circulating insulin levels. It improves sensitivity to insulin in muscle and adipose tissue and inhibits hepatic gluconeogenesis. Rosiglitazone is not chemically or functionally related to the sulfonylureas, the biguanides or the alpha-glucosidase inhibitors. Rosiglitazone is a highly selective and potent agonist for the peroxisome proliferator-activated receptor-gamma (PPARγ). In humans, PPAR receptors are found in key target tissues for insulin action such as adipose tissue, skeletal muscle and liver. Activation of PPARγ nuclear receptors regulates the transcription of insulin-responsive genes involved in the control of glucose production, transport, and utilization. In addition, PPARγ-responsive genes also participate in the regulation of fatty acid metabolism and in the maturation of preadipocytes, predominantly of subcutaneous origin.

Insulin resistance is a primary feature characterizing the pathogenesis of type 2 diabetes. AVANDIA results in increased responsiveness of insulin-dependent tissues and significantly improves hepatic and peripheral (muscle) tissue sensitivity to insulin in patients with type 2 diabetes. Clinical studies in patients with type 2 diabetes treated with AVANDIA either as monotherapy or in combination with metformin or sulfonylureas showed improved beta-cell function and decreased fasting plasma glucose, insulin and C-peptide values following 26 weeks of treatment. In a 4 to 6 year monotherapy study in drug-naïve patients, rosiglitazone treated patients showed an improvement in insulin sensitivity. The initial improvement in beta-cell function observed with AVANDIA was not sustained and gradually declined after one year for the duration of the study but continued to remain above baseline, as was the case for metformin and glyburide. A homeostasis model assessment (HOMA) was conducted using fasting plasma glucose and insulin or C-peptide levels as a measure of insulin sensitivity and beta-cell function. In these studies, reductions in mean plasma pro-insulin and pro-insulin split product concentrations were also observed.

AVANDIA significantly reduced hemoglobin A1C (A1C, a marker for long term glycemic control), and fasting blood glucose (FBG) in patients with type 2 diabetes. Inadequately controlled hyperglycemia is associated with an increased risk of diabetic complications, including cardiovascular disorders and diabetic nephropathy, retinopathy and neuropathy.

Studies between 8 and 26 weeks with AVANDIA have shown a statistically significant reduction in markers of inflammation, C-reactive protein (CRP) and matrix metalloproteinase-9 (MMP-9). The clinical significance of these effects are still unknown. Further long term clinical trials are needed.

Estimates of LDL particle size can be determined by the LDL cholesterol (LDL) to apolipoprotein B (Apo B) ratio. In controlled clinical trials, rosiglitazone has been shown to increase the LDL cholesterol to Apo B ratio consistent with a beneficial change in LDL particle size from small dense LDL particles to larger more buoyant particles. This change has been confirmed by measuring LDL particle buoyancy (Rf) following 8 weeks treatment with rosiglitazone in an open-label study.

Pharmacodynamics and Clinical Effects: In clinical studies, treatment with AVANDIA resulted in an improvement in glycemic control, as measured by fasting plasma glucose (FPG) and hemoglobin A1C (A1C), with a concurrent reduction in insulin and C-peptide. Post-prandial glucose and insulin levels were also reduced. This is consistent with the mechanism of action of AVANDIA as an insulin sensitizer. The improvement in glycemic control was durable, with maintenance of effect for at least 52 weeks. In open-labelled extension studies sustained improvements in glycemic control (as measured by A1C levels) were observed in patients receiving rosiglitazone monotherapy for 36 months. The maximum recommended daily dose of AVANDIA is 8 mg. Phase II studies indicated that no additional benefit was obtained with a total daily dose of 12 mg.

AVANDIA is believed to act primarily on muscle and adipose tissue whereas metformin acts primarily on the liver to decrease hepatic glucose output. The coadministration of AVANDIA with either metformin or sulfonylurea resulted in significantly improved glycemic control compared to any of these agents alone. These results are consistent with a synergistic effect on glycemic control when AVANDIA is used in combination therapy. In patients whose type 2 diabetes was inadequately controlled with metformin or sulfonylurea monotherapy, the addition of rosiglitazone led to reductions in A1C levels that were sustained for over 30 months of treatment, in open-labelled studies.

Weight gain has been observed in clinical studies with AVANDIA (see Table 2). In addition, AVANDIA significantly decreased visceral (abdominal) fat stores while increasing subcutaneous abdominal fat. The reduction in visceral fat correlates with improved hepatic and peripheral tissue insulin sensitivity. Weight gain with thiazolidinediones can result from increases in subcutaneous adipose tissue and/or from fluid retention. Treatment should be re-evaluated in patients with excessive weight gain (see Warnings and Precautions and Adverse Reactions).

Table 2: AVANDIA

Weight Changes (kg) from Baseline During Clinical Trials with AVANDIA

Treatment Group	Duration	Control Group		AVANDIA 4 mg	AVANDIA 8 mg
			median (25th, 75th percentile) (range)	median (25th, 75th percentile) (range)	median (25th, 75th percentile) (range)
Monotherapy					
AVANDIA	26 weeks	placebo	−0.9 (−2.8, 0.9) (−9.6 to 6.8) n=210	1.0 (−0.9, 3.6) (−11.6 to 12.7) n=436	3.1 (1.1, 5.8) (−6.8 to 13.9) n=439
AVANDIA	52 weeks	sulfonylurea	2.0 (0, 4.0) (−11.5 to 12.2) n=173	2.0 (−0.6, 4.0) (−7.0 to 16.0) n=150	2.6 (0, 5.3) (−11.0 to 22.0) n=157
Combination Therapy					
AVANDIA+ sulfonylurea	26 weeks	sulfonylurea	0 (−1.3, 1.2) (−6.0 to 14.0) n=1043	1.8 (0, 3.1) (−5.0 to 11.5) n=392	—
AVANDIA+ metformin	26 weeks	metformin	−1.4 (−3.2, 0.2) (−7.7 to 5.9) n=175	0.8 (−1.0, 2.6) (−6.8 to 9.8) n=100	2.1 (0, 4.3) (−5.4 to 13.1) n=184

In a long-term monotherapy trial (ADOPT) in drug-naïve patients, median weight change (range) at 4 years was 3.5 kg (−31.0 to 41.3) for AVANDIA, 2.0 kg (−28.6 to 24.9) for glyburide, and −2.4 kg (−46.0 to 12.9) for metformin.

Patients with lipid abnormalities were not excluded from clinical trials of AVANDIA. In all 26-week controlled trials, across the recommended dose range, AVANDIA as monotherapy was associated with increases in total cholesterol, LDL, and HDL and decreases in free fatty acids. These changes were statistically significantly different from placebo or glyburide controls (Table 3).

Increases in LDL occurred primarily during the first 1 to 2 months of therapy with AVANDIA and LDL levels remained stable, but elevated above baseline throughout the trials. In contrast, HDL continued to rise over time. As a result, the LDL/HDL ratio peaked after 2 months of therapy and then appeared to decrease over time. Because of the temporal nature of lipid changes, the 52-week glyburide-controlled study is most pertinent to assess long-term effects on lipids. At baseline, week 26, and week 52, median LDL/HDL ratios were 3.0, 2.9, and 2.8, respectively for AVANDIA 4 mg twice daily and the median total cholesterol/HDL ratios were 4.76, 4.52 and 4.35, respectively. The corresponding values for glyburide were 3.2, 2.9, and 2.7 for the median LDL/HDL ratios and 4.90, 4.61 and 4.36 for the median total cholesterol/HDL ratios.

The pattern of LDL and HDL changes following therapy with AVANDIA in combination with sulfonylurea or metformin were generally similar to those seen with AVANDIA in monotherapy.

The changes in triglycerides during therapy with AVANDIA were variable and were generally not statistically different from placebo or glyburide controls.

Table 3: AVANDIA

Summary of Lipid Changes in 26-Week Placebo-controlled and 26-Week/52-Week Glyburide-controlled Monotherapy Studies

	Placebo-controlled Studies Week 26			Glyburide-controlled Study Week 26 and Week 52			
		AVANDIA		Glyburide Titration		AVANDIA 8 mg	
	Placebo	4 mg daily	8 mg daily	wk 26	wk 52	wk 26	wk 52
Free Fatty Acids (mmol/L)							
N	207	428	436	181	168	166	145
Baseline (median)	0.61	0.58	0.61	0.92	0.92	0.93	0.93
% change from baseline (median)	−4.0	−15.6	−23.5	−5.5	−9.7	−26.7	−24.7
LDL-cholesterol (mmol/L)							
N	190	400	374	175	160	161	133
Baseline (median)	3.15	3.26	3.19	3.68	3.55	3.62	3.62
% change from baseline (median)	+2.5	+10.3	+14.8	−3.7	−3.3	+7.1	+7.3
HDL-cholesterol (mmol/L)							
N	208	429	436	184	170	170	145

(cont'd)

Table 3: AVANDIA *(cont'd)*

Summary of Lipid Changes in 26-Week Placebo-controlled and 26-Week/52-Week Glyburide-controlled Monotherapy Studies

	Placebo-controlled Studies Week 26			Glyburide-controlled Study Week 26 and Week 52			
		AVANDIA		Glyburide Titration		AVANDIA 8 mg	
	Placebo	4 mg daily	8 mg daily	wk 26	wk 52	wk 26	wk 52
Baseline (median)	1.06	1.14	1.09	1.17	1.18	1.19	1.19
% change from baseline (median)	+8.2	+10.3	+11.3	+4.7	+8.0	+13.2	+17.4

The long term significance of the lipid changes is not known.

Because AVANDIA does not stimulate insulin secretion, hypoglycemia is not expected to occur when AVANDIA is prescribed as monotherapy. Patients receiving AVANDIA in combination with other hypoglycemic agents (e.g. insulin secreting agents) may be at risk for hypoglycemia, and a reduction in the dose of the concomitant agent may be necessary. As insulin sensitizers can only work in the presence of insulin, AVANDIA should not be used in patients with type 1 diabetes.

Pharmacokinetics: Maximum plasma concentration (C_{max}) and the area under the curve ($AUC_{0\text{-}inf}$) of rosiglitazone increase in a dose-proportional manner over the therapeutic dose range (see Table 4). The elimination half-life is 3 to 4 hours and is independent of dose.

Table 4: AVANDIA

Mean (SD) Pharmacokinetic Parameters for Rosiglitazone Following Single Oral Doses (n=32)

Parameter	1 mg Fasting	2 mg Fasting	8 mg Fasting	8 mg Fed
$AUC_{0\text{-}inf}$ [ng·h/mL]	358 (112)	733 (184)	2971 (730)	2890 (795)
C_{max} [ng/mL]	76 (13)	156 (42)	598 (117)	432 (92)
T_{max} [h][a]	0.5 (0.5–1.5)	1.0 (0.5–2.0)	1.0 (0.5–1.5)	2.0 (1.0–5.0)
Half-life [h]	3.16 (0.72)	3.15 (0.39)	3.37 (0.63)	3.59 (0.70)
CL/F[b] [L/h]	3.03 (0.87)	2.89 (0.71)	2.85 (0.69)	2.97 (0.81)

[a] T_{max} presented as median (range).
[b] CL/F=Oral Clearance.

Absorption: Rosiglitazone is rapidly and completely absorbed after oral administration with negligible first-pass metabolism. The absolute bioavailability of rosiglitazone is 99%. Peak plasma concentrations are observed by 1 hour after dosing. Administration of rosiglitazone with food resulted in no change in overall exposure (AUC) but there was a decrease in the C_{max} (about 28%) and a delay in T_{max} of 1.75 hours. These changes are not likely to be clinically significant and AVANDIA may be administered with or without food.

Distribution: The mean (SD) volume of distribution (Vss) of rosiglitazone after intravenous administration to healthy subjects is approximately 14.1 (3.1) L. Rosiglitazone is approximately 99.8% bound to plasma proteins, primarily albumin.

Metabolism: Rosiglitazone is extensively metabolized with no unchanged drug excreted in the urine. The major routes of metabolism were N-demethylation and hydroxylation, followed by conjugation with sulfate and glucuronic acid. All the circulating metabolites are considerably less potent than the parent drug and, therefore, are not expected to contribute to the insulin-sensitizing activity of rosiglitazone. In vitro data demonstrate that rosiglitazone is predominantly metabolized by Cytochrome P450 (CYP) isoenzyme 2C8, with CYP2C9 contributing as only a minor pathway.

Excretion: Following oral or intravenous administration of [^{14}C] rosiglitazone maleate, approximately 64% and 23% of the dose was eliminated in the urine and in the feces, respectively. The plasma half-life of [^{14}C] related material ranged from 103 to 158 hours.

Special Populations and Conditions: Population pharmacokinetic analyses from three Phase III trials including 642 men and 405 women with type 2 diabetes (aged 35 to 80 years) showed that the pharmacokinetics of rosiglitazone are not influenced by age, race, smoking, or alcohol consumption. Both oral clearance (CL/F) and oral steady-state volume of distribution (Vss/F) were shown to increase with increases in body weight. Over the weight range observed in these analyses (50 to 150 kg), the range of predicted CL/F and Vss/F values varied by <1.7-fold and 2.3-fold, respectively. Additionally, rosiglitazone CL/F was shown to be lower (about 6%) in female patients compared to males of the same body weight. The population mean CL/F of rosiglitazone for a typical male weighing 84 kg was 2.48 L/h. The Vss/F in an 84 kg patient was 17.9L. The inter-patient variability in CL/F and Vss/F were 31% and 23%, respectively.

Pediatrics: The safety and effectiveness of rosiglitazone have not been established in patients younger than 18 years of age, therefore, AVANDIA is not indicated in patients younger than 18 years of age. Thiazolidinediones promote the maturation of preadipocytes and have been associated with weight gain. Obesity is a major problem in adolescents with type 2 diabetes.

Geriatrics: Results of the population pharmacokinetic analysis (n=716 <65 years; n=331 ≥65 years) showed that age does not significantly affect the pharmacokinetics of rosiglitazone.

Gender: Results of the population pharmacokinetic analysis showed that the mean oral clearance of rosiglitazone in female patients (n=405) was 15% lower compared to male patients (n=642), primarily related to lower body weight in females.

As monotherapy and in combination with metformin, AVANDIA improved glycemic control in both males and females. In metformin combination studies, efficacy was demonstrated with no gender differences in glycemic response.

In monotherapy studies, a greater therapeutic response was observed in females; however, in more obese patients, gender differences were less evident. For a given body mass index (BMI), females tend to have a greater fat mass than males. Since the molecular target PPARγ is expressed in adipose tissues, this differentiating characteristic may account, at least in part, for the greater response to AVANDIA in females. Since safety profiles were similar between male and female patients in clinical studies and, as therapy should be individualized, no dose adjustments are necessary based on gender.

Race: Results of a population pharmacokinetic analysis including subjects of Caucasian, black and other ethnic origins indicate that race has no influence on the pharmacokinetics of rosiglitazone.

Hepatic Insufficiency: Unbound oral clearance of rosiglitazone was significantly lower in patients with moderate to severe liver disease (Child-Pugh Class B/C) compared to healthy subjects. As a result, unbound C_{max} and $AUC_{0\text{-}inf}$ were increased 2- and 3-fold, respectively. Elimination half-life for rosiglitazone was about 2 hours longer in patients with liver disease, compared to healthy subjects. Therapy with AVANDIA should not be initiated if the patient exhibits clinical evidence of active liver disease or increased serum transaminase levels (ALT >2.5 times the upper limit of normal) at baseline (see Warnings and Precautions, Hepatic).

Renal Insufficiency: There are no clinically relevant differences in the pharmacokinetics of rosiglitazone in patients with mild to severe renal impairment or in hemodialysis-dependent patients, compared to subjects with normal renal function. No dosage adjustment is therefore required in such patients. Since metformin is contraindicated in patients with renal impairment, metformin in combination with AVANDIA is contraindicated in these patients.

STORAGE AND STABILITY: Store at controlled room temperature 15 to 30°C.

INFORMATION FOR THE PATIENT: Published in e-CPS, available by subscription at www.e-cps.ca.

DOSAGE FORMS, COMPOSITION AND PACKAGING: 2 mg: Each pink, pentagonal film-coated TILTAB tablet, debossed with SB or GSK on one side and "2" on the other, contains: rosiglitazone maleate equivalent to rosiglitazone 2 mg. Nonmedicinal ingredients: hydroxypropyl methylcellulose, lactose monohydrate, magnesium stearate, microcrystalline cellulose, polyethylene glycol 3000, sodium starch glycolate, titanium dioxide and triacetin; colorant: one or more of the following: synthetic red and yellow iron oxides and talc. Bottles of 60.

4 mg: Each orange, pentagonal film-coated TILTAB tablet, debossed with SB or GSK on one side and "4" on the other, contains: rosiglitazone maleate equivalent to rosiglitazone 4 mg. Nonmedicinal ingredients: hydroxypropyl methylcellulose, lactose monohydrate, magnesium stearate, microcrystalline cellulose, polyethylene glycol 3000, sodium starch glycolate, titanium dioxide and triacetin; colorant: one or more of the following: synthetic red and yellow iron oxides and talc. Bottles of 100.

8 mg: Each red-brown, pentagonal film-coated TILTAB tablet, debossed with SB or GSK on one side and "8" on the other, contains: rosiglitazone maleate equivalent to rosiglitazone 8 mg. Nonmedicinal ingredients: hydroxypropyl methylcellulose, lactose monohydrate, magnesium stearate, microcrystalline cellulose, polyethylene glycol 3000, sodium starch glycolate, titanium dioxide and triacetin; colorant: one or more of the following: synthetic red and yellow iron oxides and talc. Bottles of 60.

(Shown in Product Identification Section)

Avapro® Pr

irbesartan

Angiotensin II AT1 Receptor Blocker

Bristol-Myers Squibb/sanofi-aventis

Date of Preparation: May 27, 1998
Date of Revision: December 29, 2008

PHARMACOLOGY: Irbesartan antagonizes angiotensin II by blocking AT_1 receptors.

Angiotensin II is the primary vasoactive hormone in the renin-angiotensin system. Its effects include vasoconstriction and the stimulation of aldosterone secretion by the adrenal cortex.

Irbesartan blocks the vasoconstrictor and aldosterone-secreting effects of angiotensin II by selectively blocking in a noncompetitive manner the binding of angiotensin II to the AT_1 receptor found in many tissues. Irbesartan has no agonist activity at the AT_1 receptor. AT_2 receptors have been found in many tissues, but to date they have not been associated with cardiovascular homeostasis. Irbesartan has essentially no affinity for the AT_2 receptors.

Irbesartan does not inhibit angiotensin converting enzyme, also known as kininase II, the enzyme that converts angiotensin I to angiotensin II and degrades bradykinin, nor does it affect renin or other hormone receptors or ion channels involved in cardiovascular regulation of blood pressure and sodium homeostasis.

Pharmacokinetics: Irbesartan is an orally active agent. The oral absorption of irbesartan is rapid and complete with an average absolute bioavailability of 60 to 80%. Irbesartan exhibits linear pharmacokinetics over the therapeutic dose range with an average terminal elimination half-life of 11 to 15 hours. Following oral administration, peak plasma concentrations are attained at 1.5 to 2 hours after dosing. Steady-state concentrations are achieved within 3 days.

Irbesartan is approximately 96% protein-bound in the plasma, primarily to albumin and α_1-acid glycoprotein.

The average volume of distribution of irbesartan is 53 to 93 L. Total plasma and renal clearances are in the range of 157 to 176 and 3 to 3.5 mL/minute, respectively.

Irbesartan is metabolized via glucuronide conjugation, and oxidation by the cytochrome P450 system. Following either oral or i.v. administration of ^{14}C-labeled irbesartan, more than 80% of the circulating plasma radioactivity is attributable to unchanged irbesartan. The primary circulating metabolite is the inactive irbesartan glucuronide (approximately 6%). The remaining oxidative metabolites do not add appreciably to the pharmacologic activity.

Irbesartan and its metabolites are excreted by both biliary and renal routes. Following either oral or i.v. administration of ^{14}C-labeled irbesartan, about 20% of radioactivity is recovered in the urine and the remainder in the feces. Less than 2% of the dose is excreted in urine as unchanged irbesartan.

In vitro studies of irbesartan indicate that the oxidation of irbesartan is primarily by cytochrome P450 isoenzyme CYP2C9. Metabolism of irbesartan by CYP3A4 is negligible. Irbesartan is neither metabolized, nor does it substantially induce or inhibit the following isoenzymes: CYP1A1, 1A2, 2A6, 2B6, 2D6, 2E1. There was no induction or inhibition of CYP3A4.

In subjects over the age of 65 years, irbesartan elimination half-life was not significantly altered, but AUC and C_{max} values were about 20 to 50% greater than those of young subjects.

The mean AUC and C_{max} were not altered in patients with any degree of renal impairment, including patients on hemodialysis. However, a wide variance was seen in patients with severe renal impairment.

The pharmacokinetics of irbesartan following repeated oral administration were not significantly affected in patients with mild to moderate cirrhosis of the liver. No data are available in patients with severe liver disease.

Pharmacodynamics: In healthy subjects, single oral doses of irbesartan up to 300 mg produced dose-dependent inhibition of the pressor effect of angiotensin II infusions. The inhibition was complete (100%) 4 hours following oral doses of 150 mg or 300 mg. Partial inhibition of 40% and 60% was still present 24 hours post dose with 150 mg and 300 mg irbesartan respectively.

In hypertensive patients, angiotensin II receptor inhibition following chronic administration of irbesartan causes a 1.5- to 2-fold rise in angiotensin II plasma concentration and a 2- to 3-fold increase in plasma renin levels. Aldosterone plasma concentrations generally decline following irbesartan administration; however, serum potassium levels are not significantly affected at recommended doses.

During clinical trials, minimal incremental blood pressure response was observed at doses greater than 300 mg.

The blood pressure lowering effect of irbesartan is apparent after the first dose and substantially present within 1 to 2 weeks, with the maximal effect occurring by 4 to 6 weeks. In long-term studies, the effect of irbesartan appeared to be maintained for more than 1 year. There was essentially no change in average heart rate in patients treated with irbesartan in controlled trials.

There is no rebound effect after withdrawal of irbesartan.

Black hypertensive patients had a smaller blood pressure response to irbesartan monotherapy than Caucasians.

Clinical Trials: Two trials were done to investigate the effects of irbesartan in patients with hypertension and type 2 diabetic nephropathy, the IDNT and IRMA 2 trial.

IDNT: The Irbesartan Diabetic Nephropathy Trial (IDNT) was a multicenter, randomized, controlled, double-blind, morbidity and mortality trial comparing irbesartan, amlodipine and placebo. In 1715 hypertensive patients with type 2 diabetes (proteinuria ≥900 mg/day and serum creatinine 1.0-3.0 mg/dL) the long-term effects (mean 2.6 years) of irbesartan on the progression of renal disease and all-cause mortality were examined. In addition, a secondary endpoint, the effect of irbesartan on the risk of fatal or non-fatal cardiovascular events was assessed. Age of onset of Type II diabetes mellitus <20 years, renovascular occlusive disease affecting both kidneys or a solitary kidney and unstable angina pectoris were among the most important exclusion criteria.

Patients were randomized to receive irbesartan 75 mg (n=579), amlodipine 2.5 mg (n=567), or matching placebo (n=569) once-daily. Patients were then titrated to a maintenance dose of 300 mg irbesartan, 10 mg amlodipine, or placebo as tolerated. Additional antihypertensive agents for the three study arms (excluding ACE inhibitors, other angiotensin II receptor antagonists and calcium channel blockers) were added as needed to help achieve a blood pressure goal of 135/85 mmHg or less in all groups, or a 10 mmHg reduction in systolic pressure if baseline was >160 mmHg. Of the total of 579 patients randomized to irbesartan, 442 completed the double blind phase. All analyses were conducted on the intent to treat (ITT) patient population (see Figure 1 and Table 1).

Irbesartan demonstrated a 20% relative risk reduction (absolute risk reduction 6.4%) in the composite primary endpoint (first occurrence of any of the following: doubling of serum creatinine, end-stage renal disease (ESRD) or all-cause mortality) compared to placebo (p=0.023), and a 23% relative risk reduction (absolute risk reduction 8.5%) compared to amlodipine (p=0.006). When the individual components of the primary composite endpoint were analyzed, no effect in all-cause mortality and no significant effect on time to end stage renal disease were observed. However, a significant reduction was observed in doubling of serum creatinine. Irbesartan decreases the progression of renal disease in patients with chronic renal insufficiency and overt proteinuria. Irbesartan also produced significant reduction in the rate of urine excretion of protein and albumin relative to placebo or amlodipine (p<0.001 for both comparisons). Similar blood pressure was achieved in the irbesartan 300 mg and amlodipine 10 mg groups.

Treatment with irbesartan reduced the occurrence of sustained doubling of serum creatinine as a separate endpoint (33%) with an absolute risk reduction of 6.8%.

The risk of developing a doubling of serum creatinine or ESRD was reduced by 26% relative to placebo with an absolute risk reduction of 6.2% and 34% relative to amlodipine with an absolute risk reduction of 10.0% (pooled risk reduction 30%, p=0.0005). This renal protective effect of irbesartan appears to be independent of systemic blood pressure reduction.

There was no significant difference in the assessment of fatal or non-fatal cardiovascular events (cardiovascular death, non-fatal myocardial infarction, hospitalization for heart failure, permanent neurologic deficit attributed to stroke, or above-the-ankle amputation) among the three treatment groups.

Safety data from this trial has been reported in Adverse Effects.

Figure 1: Avapro

IDNT Primary Endpoint Time to Doubling of Serum Creatinine, ESRD, or Death

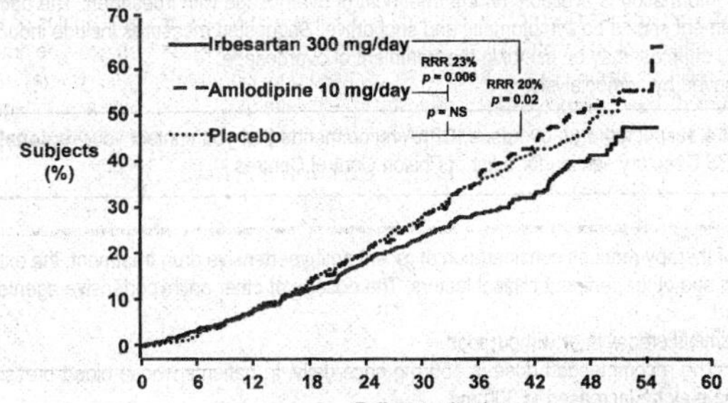

Table 1: Avapro

Primary Composite Endpoint Comparison (IDNT)

Event	Number (%) of Subjects			Relative Risk		
	Placebo N=569	Irbesartan N=579	Amlodipine N=567	Estimate (% Reduction)	95% Confidence Interval	p
Irbesartan vs Placebo						
Primary Composite Endpoint[a]	222 (39.0)	189 (32.6)	–	0.80 (20)	0.66–0.97	0.023
Irbesartan vs Amlodipine						
Primary Composite Endpoint[a]	–	189 (32.6)	233 (41.1)	0.77 (23)	0.63–0.93	0.006

[a] First occurrence of any of the following: doubling of serum creatinine, end-stage renal disease (ESRD) or all-cause mortality.

IRMA 2: The study of the Effects of Irbesartan on MicroAlbuminuria in Hypertensive Patients with Type 2 Diabetes Mellitus (IRMA 2) was a multicenter, randomized, placebo-controlled, double-blind morbidity study, conducted in 590 hypertensive patients with type 2 diabetes, microalbuminuria (20-200 µg/min; 30-300 mg/day) and normal renal function (serum creatinine ≤1.5 mg/dL in males and ≤1.1 mg/dL in females). Screening of urine for albumin has revealed that patients with microalbuminuria have a 10 to 20 fold higher risk of developing diabetic nephropathy than patients with normoalbuminuria. Of the 590 patients, 201 received placebo, 195 received irbesartan 150 mg and 194 patients received irbesartan 300 mg.

The study examined as a primary endpoint the long-term effects (2 years) of irbesartan on the progression to clinical (overt) proteinuria (urinary albumin excretion rate [AER] >200 µg/min [>300mg/day] and an increase in AER of at least 30% from baseline). In addition, after one and two years of treatment, the effect of irbesartan on the change in overnight AER and the change in 24-hour creatinine clearance was assessed. Age of onset of Type II diabetes mellitus <20 years, renovascular occlusive disease affecting both kidneys or a solitary kidney and unstable angina pectoris were among the most important exclusion criteria.

Irbesartan 300 mg demonstrated a 70% relative risk reduction (absolute risk reduction 9.8%) in the development of clinical (overt) proteinuria compared to placebo (p=0.0004). Relative risk reduction in the development of proteinuria with 150 mg irbesartan was not statistically significant. The slowing of progression to clinical (overt) proteinuria was evident as early as three months and continued over the 2 year period (see Figure 2 and Table 2).

Figure 2: Avapro

IRMA 2 Primary Endpoint Time to Overt Proteinuria

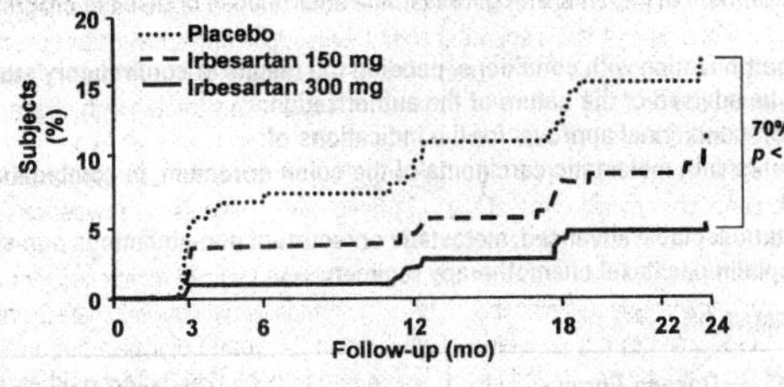

Table 2: Avapro

Time to Occurrence of Overt Proteinuria (Irbesartan 300 mg vs Placebo Comparison) (IRMA 2)

Event	Number (%) of Subjects		Relative Risk		
	Placebo N=201	Irbesartan N=195	Estimate (% Reduction)	95% Confidence Interval	p
Primary Endpoint	30 (14.9)	10 (5.2)	0.295 (70)	0.144 –0.606	0.0004

Regression to normoalbuminuria (<20 µg/min; <30 mg/day) was more frequent in the irbesartan 300 mg group (34%) than in the placebo group (21%). Irbesartan 300 mg reduced the level of urinary albumin excretion at 24 months by 43% (p=0.0001) (see Figure 3).

Safety data from this trial has been reported in Adverse Effects.

INDICATIONS: For the treatment of essential hypertension.

Irbesartan is also indicated for the treatment of hypertensive patients with type 2 diabetes mellitus and renal disease to reduce the rate of progression of nephropathy as measured by the reduction of microalbuminuria, and the occurrence of doubling of serum creatinine (see Pharmacology, Clinical Trials).

Irbesartan may be used alone or concomitantly with thiazide diuretics.

The safety and efficacy of concurrent use with angiotensin converting enzyme inhibitors have not been established.

Figure 3: Avapro

IRMA 2 Normalization of Urinary Excretion Rate

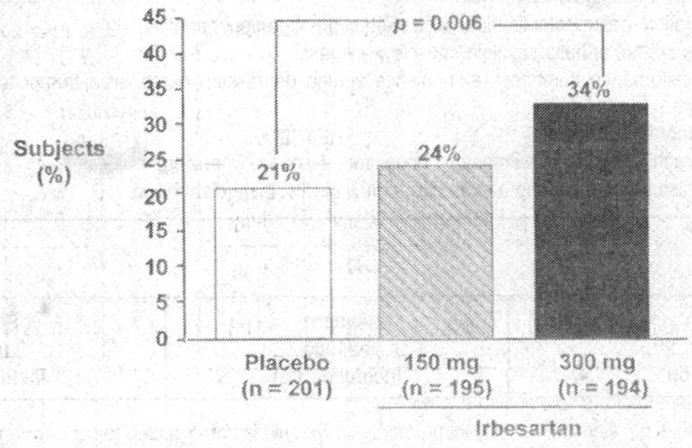

CONTRAINDICATIONS: In patients who are hypersensitive to any component of this product.

WARNINGS:

Serious Warnings and Precautions

When used in pregnancy, angiotensin receptor (AT_1) blockers (ARB) can cause injury or even death of the developing fetus. When pregnancy is detected, irbesartan should be discontinued as soon as possible (see Special Populations).

Special Populations: *Pregnancy:* Drugs that act directly on the renin-angiotensin system (RAAS) can cause fetal and neonatal morbidity and death when administered to pregnant women. When pregnancy is detected, irbesartan should be discontinued as soon as possible.

The use of ARB is not recommended during pregnancy. Epidemiological evidence regarding the risk of teratogenicity following exposure to angiotensin converting enzyme inhibitors (another class of therapeutic products interfering with the RAAS) during the first trimester of pregnancy has not been conclusive; however a small increase in risk cannot be excluded. Given the current evidence available on the risk with ARB, similar risks may exist for this class of drugs. Patients planning pregnancy should be changed to alternative anti-hypertensive treatments which have an established safety profile for use in pregnancy. When pregnancy is diagnosed, treatment with angiotensin II antagonists should be stopped immediately, and, if appropriate, alternative therapy should be started.

The use of ARBs during the second and third trimesters is known to induce human fetotoxicity (decreased renal function, oligohydramnios, skull ossification, retardation) and neonatal toxicity (renal failure, hypotension, hyperkalaemia).

Infants with histories of in utero exposure to an ARB should be closely observed for hypotension, oliguria, and hyperkalemia. If oliguria occurs, attention should be directed toward support of blood pressure and renal perfusion. Exchange transfusion may be required as means of reversing hypotension and/or substituting for impaired renal function; however, limited experience with those procedures has not been associated with significant clinical benefit. Irbesartan is not removed by hemodialysis.

Lactation: It is not known whether irbesartan is excreted in human milk, but significant levels have been found in the milk of lactating rats. Because many drugs are excreted in human milk, and because of their potential for affecting the nursing infant adversely, a decision should be made whether to discontinue nursing or discontinue the drug, taking into account the importance of the drug to the mother.

Hypotension: Volume Depleted Patients: Occasionally, symptomatic hypotension has occurred after administration of irbesartan, in some cases after the first dose. It is more likely to occur in patients who are volume depleted by diuretic therapy, dietary salt restriction, dialysis, diarrhea or vomiting. In these patients, because of the potential fall in blood pressure, therapy should be started under close medical supervision (see Dosage). Similar considerations apply to patients with ischemic heart or cerebrovascular disease, in whom an excessive fall in blood pressure could result in myocardial infarction or cerebrovascular accident.

PRECAUTIONS: Renal Impairment: As a consequence of inhibiting the renin-angiotensin-aldosterone system, changes in renal function have been seen in susceptible individuals. In patients whose renal function may depend on the activity of the renin-angiotensin-aldosterone system, such as patients with bilateral renal artery stenosis, unilateral renal artery stenosis to a solitary kidney, or severe congestive heart failure, treatment with agents that inhibit this system has been associated with oliguria, progressive azotemia, and rarely, acute renal failure and/or death. In susceptible patients, concomitant diuretic use may further increase risk.

Use of irbesartan should include appropriate assessment of renal function.

In hypertensive type 2 diabetic patients with proteinuria (≥900 mg/day), a population which has a high risk of renal artery stenosis, no patient treated with irbesartan in IDNT had an early acute rise in serum creatinine attributable to renal artery disease. (See Pharmacology, Clinical Trials, Hypertension and Type 2 Diabetic Renal Disease.)

Valvular Stenosis: There is concern on theoretical grounds that patients with aortic stenosis might be at particular risk of decreased coronary perfusion when treated with vasodilators because they do not develop as much afterload reduction.

Children: Safety and effectiveness have not been established.

Geriatrics: Of the 4140 hypertensive patients receiving irbesartan in clinical studies, 793 patients were 65 years of age and over. No overall age-related differences were seen in the adverse effect profile but greater sensitivity in some older individuals cannot be ruled out.

General: Occupational Hazards: The effect of irbesartan on the ability to drive and the use of machinery has not been studied, but based on its pharmacodynamic properties, irbesartan is unlikely to affect this ability. When driving vehicles or operating machinery, it should be taken into account that occasionally dizziness or weariness may occur during treatment of hypertension.

Drug Interactions: Diuretics: Patients on diuretics, and especially those in whom diuretic therapy was recently instituted, may occasionally experience an excessive reduction of blood pressure after initiation of therapy with irbesartan. The possibility of symptomatic hypotension with the use of irbesartan can be minimized by discontinuing the diuretic prior to initiation of treatment and/or lowering the initial dose of irbesartan (see Warnings, Hypotension and Dosage). No drug interaction of clinical significance has been identified with thiazide diuretics.

Agents Increasing Serum Potassium: Since irbesartan decreases the production of aldosterone, potassium-sparing diuretics or potassium supplements should be given only for documented hypokalemia and with frequent monitoring of serum potassium. Potassium-containing salt substitutes should also be used with caution.

Lithium Salts: As with other drugs which eliminate sodium, lithium clearance may be reduced. Therefore, serum lithium levels should be monitored carefully if lithium salts are to be administered.

Warfarin: When irbesartan was administered as 300 mg once daily under steady-state conditions, no pharmacodynamic effect on PT was demonstrated in subjects stabilized on warfarin.

Digoxin: When irbesartan was administered as 150 mg once daily under steady-state conditions, no effect was seen on the pharmacokinetics of digoxin at steady-state.

Simvastatin: When irbesartan was administered in a small single-dose study with 12 young, healthy males aged 19 to 39, the single-dose pharmacokinetics of simvastatin were not affected by the concomitant administration of 300 mg irbesartan. Simvastatin values were highly variable whether simvastatin was administered alone or in combination with irbesartan.

ADVERSE EFFECTS: Irbesartan has been evaluated for safety in more than 4100 patients with essential hypertension including approximately 1300 patients for over 6 months and 400 patients for 1 year or more.

In placebo-controlled clinical trials, therapy was discontinued due to a clinical adverse event in 3.3% of patients treated with irbesartan, versus 4.5% of patients given placebo.

The following potentially serious adverse reactions have been reported rarely with irbesartan in controlled clinical trials: syncope, hypotension.

Adverse events occurring in ≥1% or more of the 2606 hypertensive patients in placebo-controlled clinical trials include those shown in Table 3.

The incidence of hypotension or orthostatic hypotension occurred in 0.4% of irbesartan treated patients, unrelated to dosage, and in 0.2% of patients receiving placebo.

In addition, the following potentially important events occurred in less than 1% of patients receiving irbesartan, regardless of drug relationship:

Body as a Whole: fever.

Cardiovascular: flushing, hypertension, myocardial infarction, angina pectoris, arrhythmic/conduction disorder, cardiorespiratory arrest, heart failure, hypertensive crisis.
Dermatologic: pruritus, dermatitis, ecchymosis, erythema, urticaria, photosensitivity.
Endocrine: sexual dysfunction, libido change, gout.
Gastrointestinal: constipation, gastroenteritis, flatulence, distention abdomen, hepatitis.
Musculoskeletal: muscle cramp, arthritis, myalgia, muscle weakness.
Nervous System: sleep disturbance, numbness, somnolence, vertigo, depression, paresthesia, tremor, transient ischemic attack, cerebrovascular accident.
Renal/Genitourinary: abnormal urination.
Respiratory: epistaxis, tracheobronchitis, pulmonary congestion, dyspnea, wheezing.
Special Senses: visual disturbance, hearing abnormality, conjunctivitis, taste disturbance.

Table 3: Avapro
Adverse Events

Body System/Reaction	Avapro n=1965 Incidence (%)	Placebo n=641 Incidence (%)
General		
Abdominal Pain	1.4	2.0
Chest Pain	1.8	1.7
Edema	1.5	2.3
Fatigue	4.3	3.7
Cardiovascular		
Tachycardia	1.2	0.9
Dermatologic		
Rash	1.3	2.0
Gastrointestinal		
Diarrhea	3.1	2.2
Dyspepsia/Heartburn	1.7	1.1
Nausea/Vomiting	2.1	2.8
Musculoskeletal/Connective Tissue		
Musculoskeletal Pain	6.6	6.6
Nervous System		
Anxiety/Nervousness	1.1	0.9
Headache	12.3	16.7
Dizziness	4.9	5.0
Respiratory		
Cough	2.8	2.7
Urogenital System		
Urinary Tract Infection	1.1	1.4

Post-marketing Experience: Angioedema (involving swelling of the face, lips, and/or tongue) has been reported rarely in post-marketing use. The following adverse reactions, regardless of drug relationship, have been reported very rarely in post-marketing use, syncope, asthenia, myalgia, jaundice, elevated liver function tests and impaired renal function including isolated cases of renal failure in patients at risk (see Precautions, Renal Impairment).

Cases of muscle pain, muscle weakness, myositis and rhabdomyolysis have been reported in patients receiving angiotensin II receptor blockers.

Clinical Studies in Hypertension and Type 2 Diabetic Renal Disease: In clinical studies in patients with hypertension and type 2 diabetic renal disease (see Pharmacology, Clinical Trials, Hypertension and Type 2 Diabetic Renal Disease), the adverse drug experiences were similar to those in clinical trials of hypertensive patients with the exception of orthostatic symptoms (dizziness, orthostatic dizziness, and orthostatic hypotension) observed in IDNT (The Irbesartan Diabetic Nephropathy Trial) (proteinuria ≥900 mg/day, and serum creatinine from 1.0-3.0 mg/dL). In IDNT orthostatic symptoms occurred more frequently in the irbesartan group (dizziness 10.2%, orthostatic dizziness 5.4%, orthostatic hypotension 5.4%) than in the placebo group (dizziness 6.0%, orthostatic dizziness 2.7%, orthostatic hypotension 3.2%). The rates (percents) of discontinuations due to orthostatic symptoms for irbesartan versus placebo were: dizziness 0.3 vs 0.5; orthostatic dizziness 0.2 vs 0.0; and orthostatic hypotension, 0.0 vs 0.0.

Laboratory Test Findings: In controlled clinical trials, clinically important differences in laboratory tests were rarely associated with irbesartan.

Liver Function Tests: In placebo-controlled trials, elevations of AST and ALT ≥3 times upper limit of normal occurred in 0.1% and 0.2%, respectively, of irbesartan treated patients compared to 0.3% and 0.3%, respectively, of patients receiving placebo. The cumulative incidence of AST and/or ALT elevations ≥3 times upper limit of normal was 0.4% in patients treated with irbesartan for a mean duration of over 1 year.

Hyperkalemia: For hypertension with type 2 diabetes and renal disease in clinical trials conducted in patients with diabetic renal disease, the laboratory test parameter profile was similar to that of hypertension, with the exception of hyperkalemia. In a placebo-controlled trial in 590 patients with hypertension, type 2 diabetes, microalbuminuria, and normal renal function (IRMA 2), hyperkalemia ≥5.5 mEq/L occurred in 29.4% of the patients in the irbesartan 300 mg group and 22% of the patients in the placebo group. Discontinuation for hyperkalemia occurred in 0.5% of the patients in the irbesartan group.

In another placebo-controlled trial in 1715 patients with hypertension, type 2 diabetes, proteinuria ≥900 mg/day, and serum creatinine ranging from 1.0-3.0 mg/dL (IDNT), hyperkalemia ≥5.5 mEq/L occurred in 46.3% of the patients in the irbesartan group and 26.3% of the patients in the placebo group. Discontinuation for hyperkalemia occurred in 2.1% and 0.4% of the patients in the irbesartan and placebo groups, respectively.

Creatinine, Blood Urea Nitrogen: Minor increases in blood urea nitrogen (BUN) or serum creatinine were observed in less than 0.7% of patients with essential hypertension treated with irbesartan alone versus 0.9% on placebo.

Hemoglobin: Mean decreases in hemoglobin of 0.16 g/dL were observed in patients receiving irbesartan. No patients were discontinued due to anemia.

Neutropenia: Neutropenia (<1000 cells/mm³) was observed in 0.3% of irbesartan treated patients compared to 0.5% of patients receiving placebo.

In clinical trials, the following were noted to occur with an incidence of <1%, regardless of drug relationship: anemia, thrombocytopenia, lymphocytopenia and increased CPK.

OVERDOSE:

Symptoms: Few cases of overdosage with irbesartan have been reported, with no significant clinical sequelae. Reported overdoses ranged from 600-900 mg daily. Durations of overdosing ranged from 2-3 weeks up to 30 days and over. No complaints were associated with the overdoses and no clinical sequelae were observed. Experience in adults exposed to doses of up to 900 mg/day for 8 weeks revealed no toxicity.

The most likely manifestations of overdosage are expected to be hypotension and tachycardia; bradycardia might also occur from overdose.

Treatment: No specific information is available on the treatment of overdosage with irbesartan. The patient should be closely monitored, and the treatment should be symptomatic and supportive. Suggested measures include induction of emesis and/or gastric lavage. Activated charcoal may be useful in the treatment of overdosage.

Irbesartan is not removed by hemodialysis.

For management of a suspected drug overdose, CPhA recommends that you contact your **regional Poison Control Centre**. See the *CPS* Directory section for a list of Poison Control Centres.

DOSAGE: Initiation of therapy requires consideration of recent antihypertensive drug treatment, the extent of blood pressure elevation, salt restriction and other pertinent clinical factors. The dosage of other antihypertensive agents used with irbesartan may need to be adjusted.

Irbesartan may be administered with or without food.

Essential Hypertension: The recommended dose is 150 mg once daily. In patients whose blood pressure is not adequately controlled, the daily dose may be increased to 300 mg.

Essential Hypertension with Type 2 Diabetic Renal Disease: The recommended initial dose of irbesartan is 150 mg once daily. In patients whose blood pressure is not adequately controlled, the daily dose may be increased to 300 mg once daily, the preferred maintenance dose.

No initial dosage adjustment is required in the elderly or in patients with renal impairment (see Pharmacology, Pharmacokinetics and Precautions, Geriatrics). However, due to the apparent greater sensitivity of hemodialysis patients, an initial dose of 75 mg is recommended in this group of patients.

No initial dosage adjustment is required in patients with mild-to-moderate hepatic impairment (see Pharmacology, Pharmacokinetics).

Concomitant Diuretic Therapy: In patients receiving diuretics, irbesartan therapy should be initiated with caution, since these patients may be volume-depleted and thus more likely to experience hypotension following initiation of additional antihypertensive therapy. Whenever possible, all diuretics should be discontinued 2 to 3 days prior to the administration of irbesartan to reduce the likelihood of hypotension (see Warnings, Hypotension and Precautions, Drug Interactions). If this is not possible because of the patient's condition, irbesartan should be administered with caution and the blood pressure monitored closely. The recommended starting dose of irbesartan is 75 mg once daily in hypovolemic patients (see Warnings, Hypotension). Thereafter, the dosage should be adjusted according to the individual response of the patient.

INFORMATION FOR THE PATIENT: Published in e-CPS, available by subscription at www.e-cps.ca.

SUPPLIED: 75 mg: Each white to off-white biconvex, oval tablet, with a heart shape debossed on one side and the digits 2771 on the other, contains: irbesartan 75 mg. Nonmedicinal ingredients: croscarmellose sodium, lactose, magnesium stearate, microcrystalline cellulose, poloxamer 188, pregelatinized starch and silicon dioxide. Bottles of 90.
150 mg: Each white to off-white biconvex, oval tablet, with a heart shape debossed on one side and the digits 2772 on the other, contains: irbesartan 150 mg. Nonmedicinal ingredients: croscarmellose sodium, lactose, magnesium stearate, microcrystalline cellulose, poloxamer 188, pregelatinized starch and silicon dioxide. Bottles of 90.
300 mg: Each white to off-white biconvex, oval tablet, with a heart shape debossed on one side and the digits 2773 on the other, contains: irbesartan 300 mg. Nonmedicinal ingredients: croscarmellose sodium, lactose, magnesium stearate, microcrystalline cellulose, poloxamer 188, pregelatinized starch and silicon dioxide. Bottles of 90.

Store at room temperature (15 to 30°C).

(Shown in Product Identification Section)

Avastin® Ⓟ
bevacizumab
Antineoplastic

Roche

Date of Preparation: September 9, 2005
Date of Revision: March 24, 2010

AVASTIN, indicated

- **in combination with paclitaxel for the treatment of patients with metastatic HER2-negative breast cancer who are ECOG Class 0-1,**
- **as a single agent, for the treatment of patients with glioblastoma after relapse or disease progression, following prior therapy**

has been issued marketing authorization with conditions, pending the results of confirmatory studies to verify its clinical benefit. Patients should be advised of the nature of the authorization.

AVASTIN has been issued non-conditional approval for the indications of:

- **first-line treatment of patients with metastatic carcinoma of the colon or rectum, in combination with fluoropyrimidine-based chemotherapy**
- **treatment of patients with unresectable advanced, metastatic or recurrent non-squamous non-small cell lung cancer, in combination with carboplatin/paclitaxel chemotherapy regimen.**

SUMMARY PRODUCT INFORMATION:

Route of Administration	Dosage Form/ Strength	Clinically Relevant Nonmedicinal Ingredients
Intravenous	100 mg and 400 mg vials	None For a complete listing of nonmedicinal ingredients, see Dosage Forms, Composition and Packaging.

DESCRIPTION: AVASTIN (bevacizumab) is a recombinant humanised monoclonal antibody that selectively binds to and neutralises the biologic activity of human vascular endothelial growth factor (VEGF).

INDICATIONS AND CLINICAL USE: Metastatic Colorectal Cancer (mCRC): AVASTIN (bevacizumab) in combination with fluoropyrimidine-based chemotherapy is indicated for first-line treatment of patients with metastatic carcinoma of the colon or rectum.

So far AVASTIN has been shown in clinical trials to be effective and safe for the proposed indication in combination with irinotecan/intravenous 5-fluorouracil/leucovorin. Further data of AVASTIN in combination with intravenous 5-fluorouracil/leucovorin suggest superior objective response rates, progression free survival, and longer survival compared with 5-fluorouracil/leucovorin chemotherapy alone.

Consideration should be given to current standard of care guidelines for colorectal cancer.

Please refer to the Product Monographs for irinotecan, 5-fluorouracil and leucovorin for additional information on these products.

Metastatic Breast Cancer (mBC): AVASTIN (bevacizumab) in combination with paclitaxel is indicated for the treatment of patients with metastatic HER2-negative breast cancer who are ECOG Class 0-1.

The effectiveness of AVASTIN in metastatic breast cancer (mBC) is based on an improvement in progression-free survival. Currently, no data are available that demonstrate an improvement in disease-related symptoms or increased survival with AVASTIN in breast cancer.

Locally Advanced, Metastatic or Recurrent Non Small Cell Lung Cancer (NSCLC): AVASTIN, in combination with carboplatin/paclitaxel chemotherapy regimen, is indicated for treatment of patients with unresectable advanced, metastatic or recurrent non-squamous non-small cell lung cancer.

Malignant Glioma (WHO Grade IV)-Glioblastoma: AVASTIN, as a single agent, is indicated for the treatment of patients with glioblastoma after relapse or disease progression, following prior therapy.

The effectiveness of AVASTIN in glioblastoma is based on an improvement in objective response rate. There are no data demonstrating an improvement in disease-related symptoms or increased survival with AVASTIN.

Pediatrics: The safety and efficacy of AVASTIN in paediatric patients have not been assessed.

CONTRAINDICATIONS: AVASTIN (bevacizumab) is contraindicated in patients with known hypersensitivity to:

- Any components of the product (for a complete listing, see Dosage Forms, Composition and Packaging),
- Chinese hamster ovary cell products or other recombinant human or humanised antibodies.

AVASTIN is contraindicated in patients with untreated Central Nervous System (CNS) metastases (see Warnings and Precautions and Adverse Reactions).

WARNINGS AND PRECAUTIONS:

Serious Warnings and Precautions

Gastrointestinal Perforations/Wound Healing Complications: AVASTIN administration can result in the development of gastrointestinal perforation and wound dehiscence, in some instances resulting in fatality. Gastrointestinal perforation, sometimes associated with intra-abdominal abscess, occurred throughout treatment with AVASTIN (i.e. was not correlated to duration of exposure). The incidence of gastrointestinal perforation in patients receiving irinotecan/bolus 5-fluorouracil/leucovorin with AVASTIN was 2%. The typical presentation was reported as abdominal pain associated with symptoms such as constipation and vomiting. Gastrointestinal perforation should be included in the differential diagnosis of patients on AVASTIN presenting with abdominal pain. AVASTIN therapy should be permanently discontinued in patients with gastrointestinal perforation or wound dehiscence requiring medical intervention. AVASTIN therapy should not be initiated for at least 28 days following major surgery or until the surgical wound is fully healed (see Warnings and Precautions, Gastrointestinal and Peri-Operative Considerations).

Haemorrhage: Patients with non-small cell lung cancer treated with AVASTIN may be at risk for serious, and in some cases fatal, pulmonary haemorrhage/hemoptysis. Patients with recent pulmonary haemorrhage/hemoptysis (>1/2 teaspoon red blood) should not be treated with AVASTIN.

General: No studies on the effects on the ability to drive and use machines have been performed.

All patients discontinuing treatment with AVASTIN should be monitored according to medical practice.

Cardiovascular: The incidence of death from cardiovascular causes was higher in patients with mBC treated with AVASTIN + paclitaxel compared to patients treated with paclitaxel alone [8 (2.4 %) vs 4 (1.2 %) cases respectively].

Hypertension: An increased incidence of hypertension was observed in patients treated with AVASTIN (bevacizumab). Clinical safety data suggest that the incidence of hypertension is likely to be dose-dependent. Pre-existing hypertension should be adequately controlled before starting AVASTIN treatment. There is no information on the effect of AVASTIN in patients with uncontrolled hypertension at the time of initiating AVASTIN therapy. Frequent monitoring of blood pressure (e.g. 2-3 weeks) is recommended during AVASTIN therapy in order to detect certain potentially serious complications of therapy, including hypertensive encephalopathy and Reversible Posterior Leucoencephalopathy Syndrome (RPLS) (see Neurologic and Adverse Reactions).

In most cases hypertension was controlled adequately using standard antihypertensive treatment appropriate for the individual situation of the affected patient. AVASTIN treatment should be permanently discontinued if medically significant hypertension can not be adequately controlled with antihypertensive therapy, or, if the patient develops hypertensive crisis or hypertensive encephalopathy (see Adverse Reactions).

Arterial Thromboembolism: In five clinical trials, the incidence of arterial thromboembolic events including cerebrovascular accident, transient ischemic attack and myocardial infarction was higher in patients receiving AVASTIN in combination with chemotherapy compared to those who received chemotherapy alone.

AVASTIN should be permanently discontinued in patients who develop arterial thromboembolic events.

Patients receiving AVASTIN plus chemotherapy with a history of arterial thromboembolism or age greater than 65 years have an increased risk of developing arterial thromboembolic events during AVASTIN therapy. Caution should be used when treating such patients with AVASTIN (see Adverse Reactions). Regular clinical, and if necessary special radiological investigations should be performed to assess for signs of ATEs. Appropriate treatment, including permanent discontinuation of AVASTIN, should be carried out in case of identified ATE.

Venous Thromboembolism (see Adverse Reactions): Patients may be at risk of developing venous thromboembolic events, including pulmonary embolism under AVASTIN treatment. AVASTIN should be discontinued in patients with life-threatening (Grade 4) pulmonary embolism. Patients with ≤ grade 3 venous thromboembolism need to be monitored closely in accordance with local practice guidelines and receive appropriate treatment for VTEs including discontinuation of AVASTIN therapy if their condition deteriorates.

Congestive Heart Failure (CHF)/Cardiomyopathy: Events consistent with congestive heart failure (CHF) were reported in clinical trials. The symptoms ranged from asymptomatic declines in left ventricular ejection fraction to symptomatic CHF, requiring treatment or hospitalisation. Most of the patients who experienced CHF had metastatic breast cancer and had received previous treatment with anthracyclines, prior radiotherapy to the left chest wall or other risk factors for CHF, such as pre-existing coronary heart disease or concomitant cardiotoxic therapy (see Adverse Reactions). The signs and symptoms of CHF include unspecific symptoms like fatigue, weakness and fainting and depending on the side of heart affected, abdominal pain, nausea, orthopnea, pulmonary and/or peripheral oedema, shortness of breath, palpitations, irregular fast heartbeat.

Caution should be exercised when treating patients with clinically significant cardiovascular disease or pre-existing congestive heart failure with AVASTIN. If symptomatic cardiac failure develops during therapy with AVASTIN, it should be treated with the standard medications for this purpose. Discontinuation of AVASTIN should be strongly considered in patients who develop clinically significant congestive heart failure, taking into account a careful benefit-risk assessment.

Fistula (see Adverse Reactions): Patients may be at increased risk for the development of fistulae when treated with AVASTIN.

AVASTIN use has been associated with serious cases of fistulae including events resulting in death.

Permanently discontinue AVASTIN in patients with TE (tracheoesophageal) fistula or any grade 4 fistula. Limited information is available on the continued use of AVASTIN in patients with other fistulae. In cases of internal fistula not arising in the GI tract, discontinuation of AVASTIN should be considered.

In AVASTIN clinical trials, gastrointestinal fistulas have been reported with the highest incidence of around 2% in patients with metastatic colorectal cancer, but were also reported less commonly in patients with other types of cancers (e.g. breast cancer, lung cancer and others). Uncommon (≥0.1% to <1%) reports of other types of fistulas (e.g. bronchopleural, urogenital and biliary fistulas) were observed across various indications. Fistulas have also been reported in post-marketing experience. Although other risk factors (e.g. diagnosis of cancer, cancer progression, cancer treatments) are known to be associated with an increased risk of development of fistulas, a role for AVASTIN in increasing this risk cannot be excluded.

Tracheoesophageal (TE) Fistula: Cases of TE fistula have been reported in lung and esophageal cancer studies of AVASTIN in combination with chemotherapy alone or with concurrent radiation treatment. TE fistulas have not to date been reported in patients with metastatic colorectal cancer, but the possibility that this is a rare adverse drug reaction associated with AVASTIN in indications other than lung or esophageal cancer cannot be excluded.

Gastrointestinal: Gastrointestinal Perforations: Patients may be at increased risk for the development of gastrointestinal perforation and fistulas when treated with AVASTIN and chemotherapy (see Adverse Reactions). AVASTIN should be permanently discontinued in patients who develop gastrointestinal perforation.

Genitourinary: Patients with a history of hypertension are at increased risk for the development of proteinuria when treated with AVASTIN. There is evidence suggesting that ≥Grade 1 proteinuria may be related to AVASTIN dose. Monitoring of proteinuria by dipstick urinalysis is recommended prior to starting and during AVASTIN therapy. AVASTIN should be discontinued in patients who develop Grade 4 proteinuria (nephrotic syndrome) (see Adverse Reactions). Proteinuria may not completely resolve after discontinuation of AVASTIN.

Hematologic: Hemorrhage (see Adverse Reactions): Patients treated with AVASTIN have an increased risk of haemorrhage, especially tumour-associated haemorrhage. Patients should be monitored for bleeding events. AVASTIN should be permanently discontinued in patients who experienced Grade 3 or 4 bleeding (i.e. bleeding requiring medical intervention) during AVASTIN therapy, and aggressive medical management should be initiated. Routine assessment of this event should include serial complete blood counts and physical examination.

There is no information on the safety profile of AVASTIN in patients with congenital bleeding diathesis, acquired coagulopathy or in patients receiving full dose of anticoagulants for the treatment of thromboembolism prior to starting AVASTIN treatment, as such patients were excluded from clinical trials. Therefore, caution should be exercised before initiating AVASTIN therapy in these patients. However, patients who developed venous thrombosis while receiving AVASTIN therapy did not appear to have increased rate of Grade 3 or above bleeding when treated with full dose of warfarin and AVASTIN concomitantly.

CNS Hemorrhage: Cases of CNS hemorrhage, some with fatal outcome, have been observed with AVASTIN use. Patients should be monitored for signs and symptoms of CNS bleeding, and AVASTIN treatment discontinued in case of intracranial bleeding.

The risk of CNS hemorrhage in patients with CNS metastases receiving AVASTIN could not be fully evaluated, as these patients were excluded from clinical trials. A case of intracranial bleeding in a patient with occult, undiagnosed CNS metastasis was reported (see Contraindications).

Intracranial hemorrhage can occur in patients with relapsed glioblastoma. In study AVF3708g, CNS hemorrhage was reported in 2.4% (2/84) of patients in the AVASTIN-alone arm (Grade 1); and in 3.8% (3/79) of patients treated with AVASTIN and irinotecan (Grades 1, 2 and 4). CNS hemorrhage rates of 1.6-7.8% in patients with malignant glioma have been reported.

Neutropenia (see Adverse Reactions): Increased rates of severe neutropenia, febrile neutropenia, or infection with severe neutropenia (including some fatalities) have been observed in patients treated with some myelotoxic chemotherapy regimens plus AVASTIN in comparison to chemotherapy alone. Patients should be closely monitored for signs of febrile neutropenia, and white blood cell count carried out according to local oncology standards. Treatment of neutropenia and febrile neutropenia should follow established oncological standards.

Thrombocytopenia: The incidence of thrombocytopenia was higher in patients receiving AVASTIN in combination with chemotherapy (cisplatin/gemcitabine) compared to those who received chemotherapy alone. The incidence of Grade 3 thrombocytopenia was common in patients treated with AVASTIN. Patients >65 years of age appeared to be at higher risk for grade ≥3 thrombocytopenia compared with younger patients.

Hepatic/Biliary/Pancreatic: The safety and efficacy of AVASTIN has not been studied in patients with hepatic impairment.

Neurologic: Reversible Posterior Leukoencephalopathy Syndrome (RPLS): There have been rare reports of patients treated with AVASTIN developing signs and symptoms that are consistent with Reversible Posterior Leukoencephalopathy Syndrome (RPLS), a rare neurologic disorder, which can present with the following signs and symptoms among others: seizures, headache, altered mental status, visual disturbance, or cortical blindness, with or without associated hypertension. The symptoms of RPLS may be difficult to differentiate from those of uncontrolled hypertension, therefore neurological examination should be carried out in a patient presenting with the above signs and symptoms. Brain imaging, particularly MRI, confirms the diagnosis of RPLS. This syndrome may be reversible if recognised and treated promptly. The onset of symptoms has been reported to occur from 16 hours to 1 year after initiation of AVASTIN. In patients developing RPLS, treatment of specific symptoms including control of hypertension is recommended along with discontinuation of AVASTIN. Signs and symptoms of RPLS usually resolve within days, although neurologic sequelae may remain. The safety of reinitiating therapy with AVASTIN in patients previously experiencing RPLS is not known (see Adverse Reactions).

Proteinuria: In clinical trials, the incidence of proteinuria was higher in patients receiving AVASTIN in combination with chemotherapy compared to those who received chemotherapy alone. The incidence of Grade 3 proteinuria was common in patients treated with AVASTIN. Grade 4 proteinuria (nephrotic syndrome) was uncommon in patients with AVASTIN. The incidence of proteinuria (Grade 3-4) in metastatic breast cancer was 3% (Grade 4, 1.1%) in AVASTIN plus paclitaxel arm with no subjects with proteinuria Grade 3-4 in paclitaxel group. In the event of Grade 4 proteinuria AVASTIN treatment should be permanently discontinued (see Adverse Reactions).

Limited safety information is available for patients with proteinuria ≥0.5 g/24 hr urine collection as they were excluded from clinical trials.

Peri-Operative Considerations: Wound Healing: AVASTIN may adversely affect the wound healing process. AVASTIN therapy should not be initiated for at least 28 days following major surgery or until the surgical wound is fully healed. In patients who experience wound healing complications during AVASTIN treatment, AVASTIN should be withheld until the wound is fully healed. AVASTIN therapy should be withheld for elective surgery (see Adverse Reactions).

Pulmonary Haemorrhage/Hemoptysis: Patients with non-small cell lung cancer treated with AVASTIN may be at risk for serious, and in some cases fatal, pulmonary haemorrhage/hemoptysis. Patients with recent pulmonary haemorrhage/hemoptysis (>1/2 teaspoon red blood) should not be treated with AVASTIN (see Adverse Reactions, Hemorrhage (see Warnings and Precautions)).

Renal: The safety and efficacy of AVASTIN have not been studied in patients with renal Impairment (see Proteinuria and Genitourinary).

Hepatic: The safety and efficacy of AVASTIN have not been studied in patients with hepatic impairment.

Special Populations: Pregnant Women: There are no adequate and well controlled studies in pregnant women. IgGs are known to cross the placental barrier, and AVASTIN may inhibit angiogenesis in the fetus. Therefore, AVASTIN should not be used during pregnancy. In women with childbearing potential, appropriate contraceptive measures are recommended during AVASTIN therapy. Based on pharmacokinetic considerations, contraceptive measures are recommended for at least 6 months following the last dose of AVASTIN.

Angiogenesis has been shown to be critically important to fetal development. The inhibition of angiogenesis following administration of AVASTIN could result in an adverse outcome of pregnancy.

AVASTIN has been shown to be embryotoxic and teratogenic when administered to rabbits. Observed effects included decreases in maternal and fetal body weights, an increased number of fetal resorptions and an increased incidence of specific gross and skeletal fetal alterations. Adverse fetal outcomes were observed at all tested doses of 10-100 mg/kg.

Nursing Women: It is not known whether bevacizumab is excreted in human milk. As maternal IgG is excreted in milk and AVASTIN could harm infant growth and development, women should be advised to discontinue nursing during AVASTIN therapy and not to breast feed for at least 6 months following the last dose of AVASTIN.

Pediatrics: The safety and efficacy of AVASTIN in pediatric patients has not been studied.

Geriatrics (>65 years of age): Patients receiving AVASTIN plus chemotherapy with a history of arterial thromboembolism and age greater than 65 years have a higher risk of aterial thromboembolic events. Caution should be used when treating these patients with AVASTIN (see Adverse Reactions). In randomised clinical trials, age >65 years was associated with an increased risk of developing arterial thromboembolic events (including cerebrovascular accidents, transient ischemic attacks, myocardial infarction), grade 3-4 leucopenia, neutropenia, thrombocytopenia, proteinuria, diarrhea and fatigue as compared to those aged ≤65 years when treated with AVASTIN (see Warnings and Precautions and Adverse Reactions). The risk and benefit of AVASTIN administration in patients >65 should be carefully evaluated prior to initiating therapy.

More deaths were reported in patients with mBC >65 years of age treated with AVASTIN + paclitaxel compared to patients treated with paclitaxel alone (67/81 vs 57/83 deaths or 82.7% mortality vs 68.7%, respectively). Physicians are advised to assess risks and benefits in these patients.

ADVERSE REACTIONS: Adverse Drug Reaction Overview: Clinical trials have been conducted in patients with various malignancies treated with AVASTIN, predominantly in combination with chemotherapy. The safety profile from a clinical trial population of more than 3500 is presented in this section.

The most serious adverse events were:

- Gastrointestinal Perforations (see Warnings and Precautions)
- Hemorrhage including pulmonary haemorrhage/hemoptysis, which is more common in NSCLC patients (see Warnings and Precautions)
- Arterial Thromboembolism (see Warnings and Precautions)
- Non-gastrointestinal Fistula
- Hypertensive Crises
- Reversible Posterior Leukoencephalopathy Syndrome
- Neutropenia and Infections
- Nephrotic Syndrome
- Congestive Heart Failure

Analyses of the clinical safety data suggest that the occurrence of hypertension and proteinuria with AVASTIN therapy are likely to be dose-dependent.

The most frequently observed adverse drug reactions across all clinical trials in patients receiving AVASTIN were fatigue or asthenia, diarrhea, hypertension, and abdominal pain.

The most frequently observed adverse events (≥2% difference between treatment arms) across clinical trials in mBC patients receiving AVASTIN, with or without chemotherapy, were hypertension [very common], fatigue or asthenia, infection, neutrophil count abnormalities, nausea, vomiting, diarrhea, dehydration, headache, peripheral sensory neuropathy, proteinuria. Grades 1 and 2 AE were not captured.

Clinical Trial Adverse Drug Reactions: Because clinical trials are conducted under very specific conditions the adverse reaction rates observed in the clinical trials may not reflect the rates observed in practice and should not be compared to the rates in the clinical trials of another drug. Adverse drug reaction information from clinical trials is useful for identifying drug-related adverse events and for approximating rates.

Table 1 lists adverse drug reactions associated with the use of AVASTIN in combination with different chemotherapy regimens in multiple indications. These reactions had occurred either with at least a 2% difference compared to the control arm (NCI-CTC grade 3-5 reactions) or with at least a 10% difference compared to the control arm (NCI-CTC grade 1-5 reactions), in at least one of the major clinical trials. The adverse drug reactions listed in the table fall into the following categories (Very Common (≥10%) and Common (≥1%-<10%)). Adverse drug reactions are added to the appropriate category in the table according to the highest incidence seen in any of the major clinical trials. Within each frequency grouping adverse drug reactions are presented in order of decreasing seriousness. Some of the adverse reactions are reactions commonly seen with chemotherapy (e.g. palmar-plantar erythrodysaethesia syndrome with capecitabine and peripheral sensory neuropathy with paclitaxel or oxaliplatin) however an exacerbation by AVASTIN therapy can not be excluded.

Table 1: AVASTIN

Very Common and Common Adverse Drug Reactions

System Organ Class (SOC)	NCI-CTC Grade 3-5 Reactions (≥2% Difference Between the Study Arms in at Least one Clinical Trial): Very common (≥10%)	NCI-CTC Grade 3-5 Reactions: Common (≥1%-<10%)	All Grade Reactions (≥10% Difference Between the Study Arms in at Least one Clinical Trial): Very Common (≥10%)
Infections and Infestations		Sepsis Abscess Infection	
Blood and the Lymphatic Systems Disorders	Febrile neutropenia Leucopenia Neutropenia Thrombocytopenia	Anaemia	
Metabolism and Nutrition Disorders		Dehydration	Anorexia
Nervous System Disorders	Peripheral sensory neuropathy	Cerebrovascular accident Syncope Somnolence Headache	Dysgeusia Headache
Eye Disorders			Eye disorder Lacrimation increased
Cardiac Disorders		Cardiac failure congestive Supraventricular tachycardia	
Vascular Disorders	Hypertension	Thromboembolism (arterial) Deep vein thrombosis Haemorrhage	Hypertension
Respiratory, Thoracic and Mediastinal Disorders		Pulmonary embolism Dyspnoea Hypoxia Epistaxis	Dyspnoea Epistaxis Rhinitis
Gastrointestinal Disorders	Diarrhea Nausea Vomiting	Intestinal Perforation Ileus Intestinal obstruction Abdominal pain Gastrointestinal disorder Stomatitis	Constipation Stomatitis Rectal haemorrhage
Skin and Subcutaneous Tissue Disorders		Palmar-plantar erythrodysaesthesia syndrome	Exfoliative dermatitis Dry skin Skin discolouration
Musculoskeletal, Connective Tissue and Bone Disorders		Muscular weakness Myalgia	Arthralgia
Renal and Urinary Disorders		Proteinuria Urinary Tract infection	Proteinuria
General Disorders and Administration Site Conditions	Asthenia Fatigue	Pain Lethargy Mucosal Inflammation	Pyrexia Asthenia Pain Mucosal inflammation

Metastatic Breast Cancer:

Table 2: AVASTIN

AEs that Occured With At Least 1% Higher Incidence in the Bevacizumab Arm Compared To Control

Super Class Term	Preferred Term	PAC (n=348) No. (%)	PAC/BV (N=363) No. (%)
Gastrointestinal Disorders	Vomiting	8 (2.30)	20 (5.51)
	Diarrhea	5 (1.44)	17 (4.68)
	Nausea	5 (1.44)	15 (4.13)
	Abdominal pain	5 (1.44)	10 (2.75)
General Disorders And Administration Site Conditions, Infections And Infestations	Fatigue	18 (5.17)	39 (10.74)
	Neutropenic infection	5 (1.44)	9 (2.48)
	Infection	16 (4.60)	43 (11.85)
Investigations	Neutrophil count	11 (3.16)	23 (6.34)
	Aspartate aminotransferase	5 (1.44)	9 (2.48)
	Cardiac function test	1 (0.29)	5 (1.38)
Metabolism And Nutritional Disorders	Dehydration	3 (0.86)	12 (3.31)
	Hypokalaemia	2 (0.57)	6 (1.65)
	Hyponatraemia	0 (0.00)	5 (1.38)
Musculoskeletal And Connective Tissue Disorders	Muscular weakness	9 (2.59)	16 (4.41)
	Arthralgia	7 (2.01)	14 (3.86)
	Bone pain	6 (1.72)	13 (3.58)
	Myalgia	6 (1.72)	10 (2.75)
Nervous System Disorders	Headache	2 (0.57)	13 (3.58)
	Peripheral sensory	61 (17.53)	88 (24.24)
	Neuropathy syncope	2 (0.57)	8 (2.20)
	Cerebral ischaemia	0 (0.00)	7 (1.93)
	Peripheral motor neuropathy	6 (1.72)	11 (3.03)
Renal And Urinary Disorders	Proteinuria	0 (0.00)	10 (2.75)
Respiratory, Thoracic And Mediastinal Disorders	Dyspnoea	13 (3.74)	18 (4.96)
Skin And Subcutaneous Tissue Disorders	Exfoliative rash	1 (0.29)	7 (1.93)
Surgical And Medical Procedures	Packed red blood cell transfusion	1 (0.29)	5 (1.38)
Vascular Disorders	Hypertension	5 (1.44)	57 (15.70)
	Haemorrhage	0 (0.00)	4 (1.10)

Grades 3 and higher AEs only. Information from CRF toxicity form only.
AE and ADR Grades 1&2 were not captured, and Haematologic AE and ADR Grades 1-3 were not routinely captured.

Listing 1: AEs that Occured with Less Than 1% Incidence in the Bevacizumab Arm: Blood and Lymphatic System Disorders: febrile neutropenia, lymphatic disorder, lymphopenia.
Cardiac Disorders: cardiac disorder, myocardial ischaemia, arrhythmia, sinus bradycardia.
Ear and Labyrinth Disorders: vertigo, deafness.
Endocrine Disorders: hypothyroidism, cushingoid, virilism.
Eye Disorders: lacrimation increased, photophobia, vision blurred.
Gastrointestinal Disorders: constipation, ascites, colitis, gastrointestinal disorder, gastrointestinal haemorrhage, haematemesis, anal fistula, duodenal ulcer, gastric ulcer, gastritis, dyspepsia, dysphagia, ileus, proctitis.
General Disorders and Administration Site Conditions: chest pain, pyrexia, inevaluable event, death, sudden death.
Hepatobiliary Disorders: hepatic failure, hepatic pain, liver disorder.
Infections and Infestations: wound infection, catheter related infection.
Injury Poisoning and Procedural Complications: radiation associated pain.
Injury Poisoning and Procedural Complications, Investigations: wound, weight decreased, blood bilirubin, blood creatinine, haemoglobin, alanine aminotransferase, blood alkaline phosphatase, gamma-glutamyltransferase, platelet count, prothrombin time, weight increased, activated partial thromboplastin.
Metabolism and Nutrition Disorders: acidosis, alkalosis, hyperkalaemia, hypernatraemia, hypoalbuminaemia, hypocalcaemia, hypercalcaemia, hypertriglyceridaemia, metabolic disorder, hypoglycaemia.
Musculoskeletal and Connective Tissue Disorders: musculoskeletal disorder, arthritis, myositis.
Nervous System Disorders: ataxia, amnesia, convulsion, speech disorders, cranial neuropathy, extrapyramidal disorder.
Psychiatric Disorders: depression, hallucination, anxiety, insomnia.
Renal and Urinary Disorders: incontinence, urinary retention, renal failure.
Reproductive System and Breast Disorders: menstruation irregular.
Respiratory, Thoracic and Mediastinal Disorders: epistaxis, hypoxia, lung disorder, pleural effusion, pleuritic pain, pneumothorax.
Skin and Subcutaneous Tissue Disorders: skin disorder, photosensitivity reaction, pruritus, skin reaction, nail disorder.
Surgical and Medical Procedures: platelet transfusion.
Vascular Disorders: hot flush.

Grades 3 and higher AEs only. Information from CRF toxicity form only.

Locally Advanced, Metastatic or Recurrent Non Small Cell Lung Cancer (NSCLC) (Studies E4599 and AVF0757g): See Table 3.

Listing 2: Less Common NCI-CTC Grade 3-5 Non-Hematologic and Grade 4-5 Hematologic Clinical Trial Adverse Events (<1%) in Study E4599 Including Control Arms: Blood/Bone Marrow: hemoglobin.
Cardiovascular (Arrhythmia): vasovagal episode, sinus bradycardia, arrhythmia–other, conduction abnormality, dysrhythmia.
Cardiovascular (General): cardiac–left ventricular function, edema, cardiac troponin I, cardiac–other, pericardial effusion/pericarditis, cardiac troponin T.
Coagulation: any toxicity, PTT, PT.
Constitutional Symptoms: weight loss.
Dermatology/Skin: wound–infectious, alopecia, flushing, pruritus, radiation dermatitis, wound–non-infectious, dermatitis, skin–other, urticaria.
Endocrine: any toxicity, SIADH, hypothyroidism.
Gastrointestinal: dysphagia, GI–other, proctitis, colitis, ileus, dyspepsia, dysphagia–esophageal radiation, fistula–esophageal, fistula–rectal/anal, gastritis, pancreatitis.
Haemorrhage: CNS haemorrhage, epistaxis, hematemesis, haemorrhage–other, vaginal bleeding, haemorrhage with grade 3 or 4 platelets.
Hepatic: AST, alkaline phosphatase, bilirubin, GGT, hypoalbuminemia, hepatic–other, liver dysfunction/failure.
Infection/Febrile Neutropenia: infection w/unknown ANC, catheter-related infection.

Metabolic/Laboratory: hyperkalemia, amylase, hypoglycemia, hypercholesterolemia, hypocalcemia, hypercalcemia, hypermagnesemia, hypernatremia, hypertriglyceridemia, hyperuricemia, hypomagnesemia, lipase, metabolic–other, acidosis, alkalosis.
Musculoskeletal: osteonecrosis.
Neurology: depressed level of consciousness, ataxia, depression, neurologic–other, speech impairment, hallucinations, insomnia, seizure, memory loss, tremor, cognitive disturbance.
Ocular/Visual: any toxicity, double vision, cataract, blurred vision.
Pain: neuropathic pain, pleuritic pain, hepatic pain, pelvic pain, rigors/chills, weight gain.
Pulmonary: ARDS, pulmonary fibrosis, pneumothorax, apnea, voice changes/stridor.
Renal/Genitourinary: creatinine, incontinence, renal failure, renal/GU–other, urinary retention.
Syndromes: any toxicity, syndromes–other.

Table 3: AVASTIN

All NCI-CTC Grade 3-5 Non-Hematologic[a] and Grade 4-5 Hematologic[a] Adverse Events (i.e. regardless of drug relationship) Occurring in ≥1% of Patients in Study E4599 (NSCLC)

	Control Arm	Treatment Arm
	Carboplatin/Paclitaxel	Bevacizumab + Carboplatin/Paclitaxel
Toxicity Category and Term	**(n=441)**	**(n=427)**
Blood/Bone Marrow		
Neutrophils	76 (17.2%)	113 (26.5%)
Leukocytes	11 (2.5%)	19 (4.4%)
Platelets	1 (0.2%)	7 (1.6%)
Cardiovascular (Arrhythmia)		
Sinus Tachycardia	4 (0.9%)	7 (1.6%)
Supraventricular Arrhythmias	7 (1.6%)	2 (0.5%)
Cardiovascular (General)		
Hypertension	3 (0.7%)	33 (7.7%)
Thrombosis/Embolism	14 (3.2%)	24 (5.6%)
Hypotension	11 (2.5%)	14 (3.3%)
Cardiac-Ischemia	3 (0.7%)	7 (1.6%)
Constitutional Symptoms		
Fatigue	57 (12.9%)	67 (15.7%)
Constitutional	1 (0.2%)	19 (4.4%)
Fever	6 (1.4%)	7 (1.6%)
Dermatology/Skin		
Rash/Desquamation	4 (0.9%)	10 (2.3%)
Gastrointestinal		
Nausea	25 (5.7%)	27 (6.3%)
Vomiting	20 (4.5%)	25 (5.9%)
Anorexia	17 (3.9%)	24 (5.6%)
Dehydration	18 (4.1%)	23 (5.4%)
Constipation	15 (3.4%)	13 (3.0%)
Diarrhea	9 (2.0%)	15 (3.5%)
Stomatitis	5 (1.1%)	2 (0.5%)
Haemorrhage		
Hemoptysis	2 (0.5%)	9 (2.1%)
Melena/GI Bleeding	2 (0.5%)	5 (1.2%)
Hepatic		
ALT	3 (0.7%)	5 (1.2%)
Infection/Febrile Neutropenia		
Infection w/o Neutropenia	12 (2.7%)	30 (7.0%)
Febrile Neutropenia	8 (1.8%)	23 (5.4%)
Infection w/ Grade 3 or 4 Neutropenia	9 (2.0%)	19 (4.4%)
Infection-Other	1 (0.2%)	5 (1.2%)
Neurology		
Neuropathy-Sensory	48 (10.9%)	39 (9.1%)
Dizziness/Lightheadedness	8 (1.8%)	14 (3.3%)
Confusion	10 (2.3%)	11 (2.6%)
Syncope	9 (2.0%)	8 (1.9%)
Neuropathy-Motor	8 (1.8%)	7 (1.6%)
Cerebrovascular Ischemia	3 (0.7%)	6 (1.4%)
Anxiety/Agitation	6 (1.4%)	1 (0.2%)
Metabolic/Laboratory		
Hyperglycemia	17 (3.9%)	17 (4.0%)
Hyponatremia	5 (1.1%)	16 (3.7%)
Hypokalemia	5 (1.1%)	8 (1.9%)
Musculoskeletal		
Muscle Weakness	15 (3.4%)	17 (4.0%)
Musculoskeletal-Other	0 (0.0%)	6 (1.4%)
Allergy/Immunology		
Allergic Reaction	13 (2.9%)	17 (4.0%)
Pain		
Bone Pain	18 (4.1%)	18 (4.2%)
Myalgia	21 (4.8%)	17 (4.0%)
Arthralgia	16 (3.6%)	18 (4.2%)
Abdominal Pain	6 (1.4%)	14 (3.3%)
Headache	2 (0.5%)	13 (3.0%)
Chest Pain	4 (0.9%)	9 (2.1%)
Pain-Other	8 (1.8%)	6 (1.4%)
Tumor Pain	5 (1.1%)	5 (1.2%)
Pulmonary		
Dyspnea	66 (15.0%)	56 (13.1%)
Pneumonitis/Pulmonary Infiltrates	11 (2.5%)	21 (4.9%)
Hypoxia	15 (3.4%)	14 (3.3%)
Cough	8 (1.8%)	10 (2.3%)
Pulmonary-Other	5 (1.1%)	7 (1.6%)
Pleural Effusion	3 (0.7%)	5 (1.2%)
Renal/Genitourinary		
Proteinuria	0 (0.0%)	13 (3.0%)

[a] Grade 1-2 non-hematologic and grade 1-3 hematologic adverse events were not assessed in the clinical trial.
CP: Source: AE CRF Only; BC/CP: Source: AdEERS and AE CRF.

Table 4: AVASTIN

Adverse Events That Occurred with ≥2% Difference in Rates Between Treatment Arms: Treated Patients, Study E4599 (NSCLC)

	No. (%) of Patients	
	Control Arm	Treatment Arm
	Carboplatin Paclitaxel	Bevacizumab + Carboplatin Paclitaxel
NCI-CTC Category Term[a]	**(n=441)**	**(n=427)**
Any event	286 (64.9%)	327 (76.6%)
Blood/Bone Marrow		
Neutropenia	76 (17.2%)	112 (26.2%)
Constitutional Symptoms		

(cont'd)

Table 4: AVASTIN *(cont'd)*

Adverse Events That Occurred with ≥2% Difference in Rates Between Treatment Arms: Treated Patients, Study E4599 (NSCLC)

NCI-CTC Category Term[a]	No. (%) of Patients	
	Control Arm	Treatment Arm
	Carboplatin Paclitaxel	Bevacizumab + Carboplatin Paclitaxel
	(n=441)	(n=427)
Fatigue	57 (12.9%)	67 (15.7%)
Infection/Febrile Neutropenia		
Infection without neutropenia	12 (2.7%)	22 (5.2%)
Febrile neutropenia	8 (1.8%)	19 (4.4%)
Cardiovascular (general)		
Hypertension	3 (0.7%)	32 (7.5%)
Metabolic/Laboratory		
Hyponatremia	5 (1.1%)	15 (3.5%)
Pain		
Headache	2 (0.5%)	13 (3.0%)
Renal/Genitourinary		
Proteinuria	0 (0.0%)	13 (3.0%)

[a] Events were reported and graded according to NCI-CTC, Version 2.0. Per protocol, investigators were required to report only Grade 3-5 non-hematologic and Grade 4-5 hematologic events.
Legend: BV/CP=bevacizumab + carboplatin/paclitaxel; CP=carboplatin/paclitaxel.
Note: Events were sorted by highest relative frequency across all treatment groups combined.
Table 4 includes adverse events that occurred with ≥2% increased frequency in the AVASTIN group over the control arm.

Table 5: AVASTIN

Adverse Events (i.e. regardless of drug relationship) Occurring in ≥4%[a] of Patients in Study AVF0757g (NSCLC)

Body System/Preferred Term	Control Arm	Treatment Arm	Treatment Arm
	Carboplatin Paclitaxel	Bevacizumab 7.5 mg/kg + Carboplatin Paclitaxel	Bevacizumab 15 mg/kg + Carboplatin Paclitaxel
	(N=32)	(N=32)	(N=34)
Body as a Whole			
Asthenia	68.80%	75.00%	76.50%
Headache	9.40%	31.30%	47.10%
Pain	40.60%	40.60%	41.20%
Chest Pain	28.10%	18.80%	35.30%
Infection	25.00%	31.30%	35.30%
Fever	12.50%	34.40%	32.40%
Abdominal Pain	9.40%	12.50%	23.50%
Back Pain	6.30%	15.60%	11.80%
Chills	9.40%	12.50%	11.80%
Reaction Unevaluable	3.10%	12.50%	0.00%
Moniliasis	0.00%	0.00%	8.80%
Cellulitis	0.00%	6.30%	5.90%
Abscess	0.00%	0.00%	5.90%
Accidental Injury	3.10%	3.10%	5.90%
Mucous Membrane Disorder	6.30%	3.10%	5.90%
Allergic Reaction	6.30%	3.10%	0.00%
Cardiovascular			
Hypertension	3.10%	15.60%	17.60%
Haemorrhage	0.00%	12.50%	0.00%
Hypotension	3.10%	12.50%	8.80%

(cont'd)

Table 5: AVASTIN *(cont'd)*

Adverse Events (i.e. regardless of drug relationship) Occurring in ≥4%[a] of Patients in Study AVF0757g (NSCLC)

Body System/Preferred Term	Control Arm	Treatment Arm	Treatment Arm
	Carboplatin Paclitaxel	Bevacizumab 7.5 mg/kg + Carboplatin Paclitaxel	Bevacizumab 15 mg/kg + Carboplatin Paclitaxel
	(N=32)	(N=32)	(N=34)
Vasodilatation	9.40%	12.50%	11.80%
Syncope	6.30%	6.30%	11.80%
Cerebrovascular Accident	0.00%	0.00%	5.90%
Deep Thrombophlebitis	0.00%	3.10%	5.90%
Phlebitis	3.10%	0.00%	5.90%
Tachycardia	3.10%	3.10%	5.90%
Thrombosis	0.00%	0.00%	5.90%
Heart Arrest	6.30%	0.00%	0.00%
Digestive			
Nausea	46.90%	50.00%	50.00%
Anorexia	25.00%	28.10%	41.20%
Constipation	40.60%	40.60%	41.20%
Diarrhea	18.80%	28.10%	41.20%
Dyspepsia	21.90%	25.00%	17.60%
Stomatitis	9.40%	15.60%	23.50%
Vomiting	18.80%	18.80%	23.50%
Oral Moniliasis	0.00%	9.40%	2.90%
Dysphagia	6.30%	3.10%	8.80%
Flatulence	6.30%	3.10%	8.80%
Rectal Disorder	0.00%	0.00%	8.80%
Nausea And Vomiting	0.00%	6.30%	0.00%
Cheilitis	0.00%	0.00%	5.90%
Liver Function Tests Abnormal	3.10%	3.10%	5.90%
Rectal Haemorrhage	3.10%	3.10%	5.90%
Ulcerative Stomatitis	0.00%	0.00%	5.90%
Hemic and Lymphatic			
Leukopenia	31.30%	46.90%	55.90%
Anemia	21.90%	18.80%	29.40%
Thrombocytopenia	15.60%	6.30%	20.60%
Ecchymosis	0.00%	0.00%	11.80%
Hypochromic Anemia	3.10%	3.10%	5.90%
Metabolic/Nutrition			
Peripheral Edema	18.80%	21.90%	14.70%
Hyperglycemia	9.40%	12.50%	20.60%
Weight Loss	0.00%	6.30%	17.60%
Alkaline Phosphatase Increased	3.10%	0.00%	8.80%
Dehydration	6.30%	3.10%	8.80%
Hypocalcemia	3.10%	6.30%	2.90%
Edema	0.00%	3.10%	5.90%
AST Increased	3.10%	0.00%	5.90%
ALT Increased	6.30%	0.00%	5.90%
Musculoskeletal			
Arthralgia	50.00%	53.10%	41.20%
Myalgia	50.00%	28.10%	26.50%

(cont'd)

Table 5: AVASTIN *(cont'd)*

Adverse Events (i.e. regardless of drug relationship) Occurring in ≥4%[a] of Patients in Study AVF0757g (NSCLC)

	Control Arm	Treatment Arm	Treatment Arm
	Carboplatin Paclitaxel	Bevacizumab 7.5 mg/kg + Carboplatin Paclitaxel	Bevacizumab 15 mg/kg + Carboplatin Paclitaxel
Body System/Preferred Term	**(N=32)**	**(N=32)**	**(N=34)**
Arthritis	6.30%	12.50%	0.00%
Bone Pain	0.00%	9.40%	5.90%
Leg Cramps	3.10%	3.10%	8.80%
Myasthenia	6.30%	3.10%	8.80%
Nervous			
Peripheral Neuritis	28.10%	25.00%	38.20%
Paresthesia	21.90%	28.10%	35.30%
Insomnia	43.80%	25.00%	14.70%
Depression	6.30%	15.60%	23.50%
Anxiety	12.50%	9.40%	20.60%
Confusion	0.00%	6.30%	14.70%
Dizziness	12.50%	12.50%	14.70%
Neuropathy	28.10%	12.50%	14.70%
Somnolence	3.10%	0.00%	11.80%
Agitation	0.00%	6.30%	0.00%
Nervousness	6.30%	6.30%	5.90%
Amnesia	0.00%	0.00%	5.90%
Ataxia	3.10%	0.00%	5.90%
Emotional Lability	0.00%	3.10%	5.90%
Respiratory			
Cough Increased	25.00%	37.50%	50.00%
Epistaxis	6.30%	31.30%	44.10%
Dyspnea	34.40%	43.80%	41.20%
Hemoptysis	6.30%	28.10%	11.80%
Pharyngitis	9.40%	15.60%	26.50%
Rhinitis	0.00%	25.00%	20.60%
Voice Alteration	0.00%	15.60%	23.50%
Sinusitis	3.10%	9.40%	20.60%
Lung Disorder	9.40%	18.80%	17.60%
Bronchitis	3.10%	9.40%	11.80%
Hiccup	3.10%	6.30%	5.90%
Pleural Effusion	0.00%	6.30%	0.00%
Pneumonia	6.30%	6.30%	2.90%
Asthma	6.30%	3.10%	5.90%
Skin and Appendages			
Alopecia	53.10%	62.50%	64.70%
Rash	9.40%	34.40%	23.50%
Pruritus	0.00%	15.60%	5.90%
Sweating	9.40%	12.50%	11.80%
Acne	3.10%	0.00%	11.80%
Special Senses			
Taste Perversion	3.10%	9.40%	5.90%
Amblyopia	6.30%	0.00%	8.80%
Ear Pain	6.30%	3.10%	8.80%

(cont'd)

Table 5: AVASTIN *(cont'd)*

Adverse Events (i.e. regardless of drug relationship) Occurring in ≥4%[a] of Patients in Study AVF0757g (NSCLC)

	Control Arm	Treatment Arm	Treatment Arm
	Carboplatin Paclitaxel	Bevacizumab 7.5 mg/kg + Carboplatin Paclitaxel	Bevacizumab 15 mg/kg + Carboplatin Paclitaxel
Body System/Preferred Term	**(N=32)**	**(N=32)**	**(N=34)**
Tinnitus	3.10%	6.30%	2.90%
Urogenital			
Urinary Tract Infection	0.00%	3.10%	14.70%
Cystitis	0.00%	0.00%	8.80%
Urinary Incontinence	3.10%	0.00%	5.90%
Urinary Frequency	9.40%	0.00%	0.00%

[a] Due to the size of the trial and rates, the table of adverse events occurring in ≥1% patients was condensed to the table of adverse events occurring in ≥4 % of patients (1 patient per group equals <4%).

Listing 3: Clinical Trial Adverse Events (<4%*) in Study AVF0757g Including Control Arms: Body as a Whole: face edema, infection bacterial, injection site edema, injection site inflammation, injection site reaction, neoplasm, sepsis, abdomen enlarged, hernia, infection fungal, injection site pain, lab test abnormal, neck pain, neck rigidity, flank pain, flu syndrome.
Cardiovascular: arrhythmia, atrial fibrillation, bradycardia, cerebral ischemia, migraine, vascular anomaly, vascular disorder, endocarditis, palpitation, postural hypotension, angina pectoris, cardiovascular disorder, pericardial effusion, pulmonary embolus.
Digestive: gastrointestinal disorder, gastrointestinal haemorrhage, gingivitis, glossitis, hematemesis, hepatic failure, increased salivation, jaundice, melena, mouth ulceration, abnormal stools, eructation, gastroenteritis, intestinal obstruction, salivary gland enlargement, dry mouth, esophagitis.
Endocrine: diabetes mellitus, hypothyroidism.
Hemic and Lymphatic: prothrombin decreased, lymphadenopathy, lymphangitis, pancytopenia, thrombocythemia, leukocytosis, thromboplastin increased.
Metabolic/Nutrition: alkalosis, bilirubinemia, creatinine increased, hypercalcemia, hypoglycemia, hypokalemia, hypomagnesemia, hypophosphatemia, hypovolemia, respiratory alkalosis, amylase increased, hyperkalemia, calcium disorder, electrolyte depletion, weight gain.
Musculoskeletal: joint disorder, pathological fracture, tendon disorder, twitching.
Nervous: abnormal gait, hallucinations, hypertonia, incoordination, sleep disorder, speech disorder, thinking abnormal, tremor, vertigo, convulsion, hyperesthesia, myoclonus, neuralgia, nystagmus, reflexes increased, stupor, reflexes decreased, stupor, reflexes decreased.
Respiratory: emphysema, hypoxia, laryngitis, pleural disorder, pneumothorax, respiratory disorder.
Skin and Appendages: fungal dermatitis, pustular rash, vesiculobullous rash, dry skin, herpes simplex, hirsutism, maculopapular rash, skin discoloration, skin ulcer.
Special Senses: abnormal vision, dry eyes, otitis media, cataract nos, diplopia, ear disorder, keratitis.
Urogenital: albuminuria, nephrosis, nocturia, urination impaired, vaginal moniliasis, breast pain, hematuria, urinary retention, vaginal haemorrhage, dysuria.

Table 6: AVASTIN

Summary of Adverse Events that Occurred with ≥4%[a] Difference in Incidence Rate Between Treatment Arms in Study AVF0757g

	Control Arm	Treatment Arm	Treatment Arm
	Carboplatin Paclitaxel	Bevacizumab 7.5 mg/kg + Carboplatin Paclitaxel	Bevacizumab 15 mg/kg + Carboplatin Paclitaxel
Body System/Preferred Term	**(N=32)**	**(N=32)**	**(N=34)**
Body as a Whole			
Asthenia	68.80%	75.00%	76.50%
Headache	9.40%	31.30%	47.10%
Chest Pain	28.10%	18.80%	35.30%
Infection	25.00%	31.30%	35.30%
Fever	12.50%	34.40%	32.40%
Abdominal Pain	9.40%	12.50%	23.50%
Back Pain	6.30%	15.60%	11.80%
Reaction Unevaluable	3.10%	12.50%	0.00%
Moniliasis	0.00%	0.00%	8.80%
Cellulitis	0.00%	6.30%	5.90%
Abscess	0.00%	0.00%	5.90%
Cardiovascular			
Hypertension	3.10%	15.60%	17.60%
Haemorrhage	0.00%	12.50%	0.00%

* **Due to the size of the trial and rates (1 patient per group equals <4%), the listing of adverse events is presented as the listing of adverse events occurring in <4 % of patients.**

(cont'd)

Table 6: AVASTIN *(cont'd)*

Summary of Adverse Events that Occurred with ≥4%[a] Difference in Incidence Rate Between Treatment Arms in Study AVF0757g

	Control Arm	Treatment Arm	Treatment Arm
		Bevacizumab 7.5 mg/kg +	Bevacizumab 15 mg/kg +
	Carboplatin Paclitaxel	Carboplatin Paclitaxel	Carboplatin Paclitaxel
Body System/Preferred Term	**(N=32)**	**(N=32)**	**(N=34)**
Hypotension	3.10%	12.50%	8.80%
Syncope	6.30%	6.30%	11.80%
Cerebrovascular Accident	0.00%	0.00%	5.90%
Deep Thrombophlebitis	0.00%	3.10%	5.90%
Thrombosis	0.00%	0.00%	5.90%
Digestive			
Anorexia	25.00%	28.10%	41.20%
Diarrhea	18.80%	28.10%	41.20%
Stomatitis	9.40%	15.60%	23.50%
Vomiting	18.80%	18.80%	23.50%
Oral Moniliasis	0.00%	9.40%	2.90%
Rectal Disorder	0.00%	0.00%	8.80%
Nausea And Vomiting	0.00%	6.30%	0.00%
Cheilitis	0.00%	0.00%	5.90%
Ulcerative Stomatitis	0.00%	0.00%	5.90%
Endocrine			
Hemic and Lymphatic			
Leukopenia	31.30%	46.90%	55.90%
Anemia	21.90%	18.80%	29.40%
Thrombocytopenia	15.60%	6.30%	20.60%
Ecchymosis	0.00%	0.00%	11.80%
Metabolic/Nutrition			
Hyperglycemia	9.40%	12.50%	20.60%
Weight Loss	0.00%	6.30%	17.60%
Alkaline Phosphatase Increased	3.10%	0.00%	8.80%
Edema	0.00%	3.10%	5.90%
Musculoskeletal			
Arthritis	6.30%	12.50%	0.00%
Bone Pain	0.00%	9.40%	5.90%
Leg Cramps	3.10%	3.10%	8.80%
Nervous			
Peripheral Neuritis	28.10%	25.00%	38.20%
Paresthesia	21.90%	28.10%	35.30%
Depression	6.30%	15.60%	23.50%
Anxiety	12.50%	9.40%	20.60%
Confusion	0.00%	6.30%	14.70%
Somnolence	3.10%	0.00%	11.80%
Agitation	0.00%	6.30%	0.00%
Amnesia	0.00%	0.00%	5.90%
Emotional Lability	0.00%	3.10%	5.90%
Respiratory			
Cough Increased	25.00%	37.50%	50.00%
Epistaxis	6.30%	31.30%	44.10%

(cont'd)

Table 6: AVASTIN *(cont'd)*

Summary of Adverse Events that Occurred with ≥4%[a] Difference in Incidence Rate Between Treatment Arms in Study AVF0757g

	Control Arm	Treatment Arm	Treatment Arm
		Bevacizumab 7.5 mg/kg +	Bevacizumab 15 mg/kg +
	Carboplatin Paclitaxel	Carboplatin Paclitaxel	Carboplatin Paclitaxel
Body System/Preferred Term	**(N=32)**	**(N=32)**	**(N=34)**
Dyspnea	34.40%	43.80%	41.20%
Hemoptysis	6.30%	28.10%	11.80%
Pharyngitis	9.40%	15.60%	26.50%
Rhinitis	0.00%	25.00%	20.60%
Voice Alteration	0.00%	15.60%	23.50%
Sinusitis	3.10%	9.40%	20.60%
Lung Disorder	9.40%	18.80%	17.60%
Bronchitis	3.10%	9.40%	11.80%
Pleural Effusion	0.00%	6.30%	0.00%
Skin and Appendages			
Alopecia	53.10%	62.50%	64.70%
Rash	9.40%	34.40%	23.50%
Pruritus	0.00%	15.60%	5.90%
Acne	3.10%	0.00%	11.80%
Special Senses			
Taste Perversion	3.10%	9.40%	5.90%
Urogenital			
Urinary Tract Infection	0.00%	3.10%	14.70%
Cystitis	0.00%	0.00%	8.80%

[a] Due to the size of the trial and rates (1 patient per group equals <4%), the table is condensed to the table of adverse events occurring with ≥4% increased frequency in AVASTIN groups over the active control group.

Malignant Glioma (WHO Grade IV)—Glioblastoma:

Table 7: AVASTIN

Incidence of Adverse Events Occurring in ≥5% of Patients in Either Treatment Arm during the Planned Treatment Period in Study AVF3708g (All Grades)

System Organ Class/Preferred Term	Bevacizumab (N=84)	Bevacizumab + Irinotecan (N=79)
Blood and Lymphatic System Disorders		
Lymphopenia	7.1%	16.5%
Neutropenia	2.4%	15.2%
Anemia	1.2%	8.9%
Leukopenia	0.0%	8.9%
Thrombocytopenia	2.4%	6.3%
Endocrine Disorders		
Cushingoid	6.0%	6.3%
Eye Disorders		
Vision blurred	7.1%	6.3%
Gastrointestinal Disorders		
Diarrhea	21.4%	74.7%
Nausea	15.5%	67.1%
Constipation	14.3%	40.5%
Vomiting	6.0%	36.7%
Abdominal pain	3.6%	29.1%
Dyspepsia	1.2%	11.4%
Gingival bleeding	6.0%	5.1%
Hemorrhoids	4.8%	5.1%

(cont'd)

Table 7: AVASTIN *(cont'd)*

Incidence of Adverse Events Occurring in ≥5% of Patients in Either Treatment Arm during the Planned Treatment Period in Study AVF3708g (All Grades)

System Organ Class/Preferred Term	Bevacizumab (N=84)	Bevacizumab + Irinotecan (N=79)
Abdominal distension	2.4%	6.3%
Dysphagia	2.4%	5.1%
Rectal hemorrhage	2.4%	5.1%
Flatulence	1.2%	5.1%
Gastroesophageal reflux disease	1.2%	5.1%
Abdominal discomfort	0.0%	5.1%
General Disorders and Administration Conditions		
Fatigue	45.2%	75.9%
Edema peripheral	13.1%	17.7%
Gait disturbance	8.3%	13.9%
Asthenia	10.7%	8.9%
Pyrexia	8.3%	8.9%
Infections and Infestations		
Upper respiratory tract infection	11.9%	13.9%
Urinary tract infection	11.9%	8.9%
Candidiasis	3.6%	5.1%
Cellulitis	2.4%	6.3%
Nasopharyngitis	7.1%	1.3%
Pneumonia	1.2%	6.3%
Sinusitis	1.2%	5.1%
Oral herpes	0.0%	5.1%
Injury, Poisoning and Procedural Complications		
Contusion	9.5%	6.3%
Excoriation	3.6%	6.3%
Investigations		
Alanine aminotransferase increased	10.7%	10.1%
Weight decreased	6.0%	8.9%
White blood cell count decreased	3.6%	11.4%
Aspartate aminotransferase increased	7.1%	6.3%
Blood pressure increased	7.1%	6.3%
Tandem gait test abnormal	3.6%	6.3%
Weight increased	7.1%	2.5%
Blood calcium decreased	3.6%	5.1%
Hemoglobin decreased	0.0%	7.6%
Metabolism and Nutrition Disorders		
Hyperglycemia	16.7%	13.9%
Anorexia	13.1%	10.1%
Hypokalemia	8.3%	12.7%
Dehydration	8.3%	8.9%
Decreased appetite	6.0%	10.1%
Hyponatremia	3.6%	7.6%
Hypocalcemia	1.2%	6.3%
Musculoskeletal and Connective Tissue Disorders		
Pain in extremity	14.3%	13.9%
Arthralgia	14.3%	11.4%
Muscular weakness	9.5%	11.4%
Musculoskeletal pain	8.3%	8.9%

(cont'd)

Table 7: AVASTIN *(cont'd)*

Incidence of Adverse Events Occurring in ≥5% of Patients in Either Treatment Arm during the Planned Treatment Period in Study AVF3708g (All Grades)

System Organ Class/Preferred Term	Bevacizumab (N=84)	Bevacizumab + Irinotecan (N=79)
Back pain	8.3%	2.5%
Muscles spasms	0.0%	6.3%
Nervous System Disorders		
Headache	36.9%	32.9%
Convulsion	15.5%	19.0%
Aphasia	13.1%	17.7%
Cognitive disorder	13.1%	13.9%
Amnesia	13.1%	8.9%
Dizziness	7.1%	13.9%
Hemiparesis	10.7%	7.6%
Somnolence	9.5%	8.9%
Ataxia	10.7%	6.3%
Hypoesthesia	9.5%	6.3%
Tremor	6.0%	8.9%
Memory impairment	7.1%	6.3%
Speech disorder	4.8%	7.6%
Balance disorder	2.4%	7.6%
Paresthesia	4.8%	5.1%
Pyramidal tract syndrome	1.2%	6.3%
Coordination abnormal	1.2%	5.1%
Disturbance in attention	1.2%	5.1%
Cerebellar syndrome	0.0%	5.1%
Psychiatric Disorders		
Confusional state	14.3%	21.5%
Insomnia	14.3%	12.7%
Depression	7.1%	16.5%
Anxiety	6.0%	13.9%
Agitation	2.4%	6.3%
Respiratory, Thoracic and Mediastinal Disorders		
Epistaxis	19.0%	22.8%
Cough	14.3%	15.2%
Dyspnea	11.9%	12.7%
Dysphonia	10.7%	12.7%
Pharyngolaryngeal pain	7.1%	11.4%
Hemoptysis	2.4%	11.4%
Nasal congestion	3.6%	6.3%
Rhinorrhea	3.6%	6.3%
Hiccups	0.0%	8.9%
Sinus congestion	7.1%	1.3%
Postnasal drip	0.0%	5.1%
Skin and Subcutaneous Tissue Disorders		
Rash	13.1%	15.2%
Alopecia	1.2%	6.3%
Vascular Disorders		
Hypertension	29.8%	21.5%
Deep vein thrombosis	2.4%	7.6%

(cont'd)

Table 7: AVASTIN *(cont'd)*

Incidence of Adverse Events Occurring in ≥5% of Patients in Either Treatment Arm during the Planned Treatment Period in Study AVF3708g (All Grades)

System Organ Class/Preferred Term	Bevacizumab (N=84)	Bevacizumab + Irinotecan (N=79)
Flushing	1.2%	6.3%

Listing 4: Adverse Events (i.e. regardless of drug relationship) Occurring in <5%† of Patients in Either Treatment Arm during the Planned Treatment Period in Study AVF3708g (All Grades): Blood and Lymphatic System Disorders: hemoglobinemia, hemorrhagic diathesis, heparin-induced thrombocytopenia, splenomegaly.
Cardiac Disorders: tachycardia, bradycardia, sinus tachycardia, sinus bradycardia, aortic valve incompetence, cardiac flutter, myocardial infarction, myocardial ischemia, pericardial effusion.
Ear and Labyrinth Disorders: ear pain, hypoacusis, cerumen impaction, ear discomfort, deafness, tinnitus, vertigo.
Endocrine Disorders: Addison's disease.
Eye Disorders: visual acuity reduced, visual disturbance, conjunctivitis, diplopia, eye pain, eyelid ptosis, lacrimation increased, abnormal sensation in eye, blindness unilateral, dry eye, eye disorder, eye hemorrhage, keratitis, photopsia.
Gastrointestinal Disorders: fecal incontinence, abdominal pain upper, stomatitis, anal hemorrhage, mouth ulceration, oral pain, salivary hypersecretion, dental caries, dry mouth, hematochezia, abdominal pain lower, anal fissure, aphthous stomatitis, caecitis, cheilitis, epigastric discomfort, food poisoning, gastrointestinal perforation, glossitis, glossodynia, hypoaesthesia, inguinal hernia, intestinal perforation, lip ulceration, loose tooth, lumbar hernia, mucous stools, oral discomfort, periodontal disease, poor dental condition, proctalgia, sensitivity of teeth, stomach discomfort, swollen tongue, toothache.
General Disorders and Administration Site Conditions: chest pain, pain, chills, influenza like illness, impaired healing, irritability, chest discomfort, general physical health deterioration, injection site extravasation, catheter site edema, catheter site pain, cyst, extravasation, facial pain, feeling cold, feeling hot, generalised edema, induration , injection site bruising, injection site erythema, injection site hemorrhage, injection site nodule, injection site pain, injection site phlebitis, injection site reaction, malaise, mucosal inflammation, edema 1, peripheral coldness, pitting edema, secretion discharge, swelling, vessel puncture site hematoma.
Hepatobiliary Disorders: cholecystitis acute, cholelithiasis.
Immune System Disorders: seasonal allergy, contrast media allergy, iodine allergy.
Infections and Infestations: bronchitis, herpes zoster, infection, respiratory tract infection, ear infection, eye infection, fungal infection, gastroenteritis, gastroenteritis viral, localised infection, rhinitis, skin infection, tooth infection, acute sinusitis, anal candidiasis, catheter related infection, catheter site infection, cytomegalovirus colitis, eyelid infection, fungal skin infection, furuncle, genital herpes, gingival abscess, gingival infection, herpes simplex, influenza, laryngitis, metapneumovirus infection, neutropenic infection, onychomycosis, oral fungal infection, oral infection, otitis externa, otitis media, pharyngitis streptococcal, prostate infection, sepsis, staphylococcal infection, subcutaneous abscess, tinea pedis, tooth abscess, urinary tract infection fungal, vaginal candidiasis, viral infection, wound infection staphylococcal.
Injury, Poisoning and Procedural Complications: skin laceration, wound, arthropod bite, humerus fracture, incision site pain, procedural pain, rib fracture, tooth fracture, wound complication, ankle fracture, chest injury, concussion, facial bones fracture, fall, head injury, incision site complication, muscle strain, open wound, procedural headache, procedural nausea.
Investigations: blood glucose increased, blood sodium decreased, international normalised ratio increased, blood alkaline phosphatase increased, blood albumin decreased, blood potassium decreased, platelet count decreased, blood cholesterol increased, blood creatinine increased, blood sodium increased, blood urea increased, drug level increased, albumin urine present, blood albumin increased, blood bilirubin increased, blood chloride increased, blood glucose decreased, blood lactate dehydrogenase increased, blood magnesium decreased, blood potassium increased, blood testosterone decreased, blood thyroid stimulating hormone increased, blood uric acid increased, breath sounds abnormal, glucose urine, hematocrit decreased, heart rate increased, liver function test abnormal, lymphocyte count decreased, neutrophil count decreased, nuclear magnetic resonance imaging brain abnormal, past–pointing, positive Rombergism, protein total decreased, protein urine present, troponin I increased, urine ketone body present, urine output decreased.
Metabolism and Nutrition Disorders: hypercholesterolemia, hypoglycemia, hyperkalemia, hypernatremia, hypomagnesemia, hypophosphatemia, increased appetite, diabetes mellitus, hypercreatininemia, hyperlipidemia, hyperphagia, hypoalbuminemia, malnutrition, oral intake reduced, polydipsia.
Musculoskeletal and Connective Tissue Disorders: myopathy steroid, neck pain, arthritis, joint range of motion decreased, bone pain, groin pain, limb discomfort, muscle twitching, myopathy, arthropathy, coccydynia, intervertebral disc degeneration, joint stiffness, musculoskeletal chest pain, myositis, rhabdomyolysis, spinal osteoarthritis, tendonitis.
Neoplasms Benign, Malignant and Unspecified (incl cysts and polyps): lung neoplasm, adenocarcinoma, adrenal neoplasm, basal cell carcinoma, dysplastic naevus syndrome, hemangioma of liver, uterine leiomyoma.
Nervous System Disorders: facial paresis, upper motor neuron lesion, cerebral hemorrhage, dysgeusia, facial palsy, lethargy, neuropathy peripheral, peripheral sensory neuropathy, psychomotor skills impaired, syncope, visual field defect, complex partial seizures, nystagmus, burning sensation, dysarthria, grand mal convulsion, hemiplegia, hydrocephalus, hyperreflexia, hypertonia, intracranial hypotension, motor dysfunction, neurological symptom, sensory disturbance, akathisia, brain edema, carpal tunnel syndrome, cerebral ischemia, cerebral ventricle dilatation, cerebrovascular accident cholinergic syndrome, cranial neuropathy, depressed level of consciousness, drooling, dyskinesia, dysphasia, encephalopathy, hemicephalalgia, hyperesthesia, hypersomnia, hypogeusia, hypoglossal nerve disorder, intracranial pressure increased, mental impairment, neuralgia, neurologic neglect syndrome, pallanesthesia, parosmia, poor quality sleep, radiculopathy, reversible posterior leukoencephalopathy syndrome, sedation, sinus headache, status epilepticus, syncope vasovagal, VIIth nerve paralysis, VIth nerve paralysis, XIth nerve paralysis.
Psychiatric Disorders: disorientation, flat affect, personality change, abnormal behaviour, affective disorder, apathy, delirium, hallucination, libido decreased, mental status changes, abulia, affect lability, aggression, anger, anticipatory anxiety, confabulation, loss of libido, mood altered, panic attack, personality change due to a general medical condition, reading disorder, restlessness.
Renal and Urinary Disorders: urinary incontinence, pollakiuria, proteinuria, dysuria, micturition urgency, nocturia, urinary retention, hematuria, polyuria, renal cyst, renal failure, renal failure acute, stress urinary incontinence.
Reproductive System and Breast Disorders: erectile dysfunction, menorrhagia, amenorrhea, genital erythema, menstruation irregular, penile hemorrhage, pruritus genital, sexual dysfunction, testicular pain, vaginal hemorrhage, vulvovaginal pruritus.
Respiratory, Thoracic and Mediastinal Disorders: pulmonary embolism, dyspnea exertional, increased upper airway secretion, nasal dryness, allergic sinusitis, bronchitis chronic, dry throat, nasal discomfort, nasal mucosal discolouration, nasal mucosal disorder, pleural effusion, pneumonia aspiration, productive cough, pulmonary congestion, respiratory tract congestion, rhinalgia, rhinitis allergic, sneezing.
Skin and Subcutaneous Tissue Disorders: ecchymosis, dry skin, petechiae, skin disorder, erythema, blister, acne, decubitus ulcer, dermatitis contact, hyperhidrosis, ingrowing nail, night sweats, photosensitivity reaction, pruritus, rash maculo–papular, scab, skin discolouration, skin lesion, skin striae, actinic keratosis, dermatitis acneiform, eczema, hyperkeratosis, hypoesthesia facial, increased tendency to bruise, nail pitting, onychoclasis, pain of skin, palmar erythema, psoriasis, rash macular, skin exfoliation.
Vascular Disorders: hypotension, orthostatic hypotension, hot flush, bleeding varicose vein, embolism, hematoma, hemorrhage, lymphedema, varicose vein.
Further Information on Selected, Serious Adverse Drug Reactions: The following adverse drug reactions, reported using NCI-CTC (common toxicity criteria) for assessment of toxicity, have been observed in patients treated with AVASTIN:
Gastrointestinal Perforation (see Warnings and Precautions): AVASTIN has been associated with serious cases of gastrointestinal perforation or fistulae. Gastrointestinal perforations have been reported in clinical trials with an incidence of less than 1% in patients with metastatic breast cancer or non-squamous non-small cell lung cancer, and up to 2% in metastatic colorectal cancer patients. Fatal outcome was reported in approximately a third of serious cases of gastrointestinal perforations, which represents between 0.2%-1% of all AVASTIN treated patients.

† Due to the size of the trial and rates, the listing of adverse events is presented as the listing of adverse events occurring in <5% of patients.

‡ Of note: In the three Eastern Co-operative Oncology Group (ECOG) trials out of the ten mentioned trials, only grade 3 to 5 events were collected.

¶ Of note: In the three Eastern Co-operative Oncology Group (ECOG) trials out of the ten mentioned trials, only grade 3 to 5 events were collected.

Cases of GI perforations have also been observed in patients with relapsed glioblastoma.

The presentation of these events varied in type and severity, ranging from free air seen on the plain abdominal X-ray, which resolved without treatment, to an intestinal perforation with abdominal abscess and fatal outcome. In some cases, the underlying intra abdominal inflammation was present, either from gastric ulcer disease, tumour necrosis, diverticulitis or chemotherapy-associated colitis. A causal association of intra-abdominal inflammatory process and gastrointestinal perforation to AVASTIN has not been established.

Wound Healing (see Warnings and Precautions): As AVASTIN may adversely impact wound healing, patients who had major surgery within the last 28 days prior to starting AVASTIN treatment were excluded from participation in phase III trials.

Across metastatic colorectal cancer clinical trials there was no increased risk of post-operative bleeding or wound healing complications observed in patients who underwent major surgery between 28-60 days prior to starting AVASTIN therapy. An increased incidence of post-operative bleeding or wound healing complications occurring within 60 days of major surgery was observed, if the patient was being treated with AVASTIN at the time of surgery. The incidence varied between 10% (4/40) and 20% (3/15).

In the pivotal clinical trial in mBC, Grade 3-5 wound healing complications were observed in 1.1% of patients receiving AVASTIN + paclitaxel and in 0% of patients receiving paclitaxel alone. All wound healing complications were infective (no wound dehiscence or bleeding reported).

In the study of patients with relapsed glioblastoma (study AVF3708g), the incidence of post-operative wound healing complications (craniotomy site wound dehiscence and cerebrospinal fluid leak) was 3.6% in patients treated with single-agent AVASTIN and 1.3% in patients treated with AVASTIN plus irinotecan.

Hypertension (see Warnings and Precautions): An increased incidence of hypertension (all grades) of up to 34% has been observed in patients treated with AVASTIN compared with up to 14% in the comparator arm. In clinical trials across all indications the overall incidence of NCI-CTC Grade 3 and 4 hypertension in patients receiving AVASTIN ranged from 3.0% to 17.9%. Grade 4 hypertension (hypertensive crisis) occurred in up to 1.0% of patients treated with AVASTIN compared to up to 0.2% patients treated with the same chemotherapy alone.

Hypertension was generally adequately controlled with oral anti-hypertensives such as angiotensin converting enzyme inhibitors, diuretics and calcium-channel blockers. It rarely resulted in discontinuation of treatment with AVASTIN or hospitalisation. Very rare cases of hypertensive encephalopathy have been reported, some of which were fatal. The risk of hypertension associated with AVASTIN did not correlate with the patients' baseline characteristics, underlying disease or concomitant therapy. AVASTIN should be permanently discontinued in patients who develop hypertensive encephalopathy. Hypertensive encephalopathy is a complication of malignant hypertension. Signs and symptoms may include severe hypertension associated with headache, nausea, vomiting, convulsions, or confusion. Hypertensive encephalopathy may be reversible if treated by progressively reducing blood pressure to near normal ranges within several hours.

In the pivotal clinical trial in metastatic breast cancer, Grade 3-4 hypertension was observed in 15.5% of patients receiving AVASTIN + paclitaxel and in 1.4% of patients receiving paclitaxel alone. Grades 1 and 2 AEs were not captured.

Proteinuria (see Warnings and Precautions): In clinical trials proteinuria was very common and has been reported in up to 38% of patients receiving AVASTIN. Proteinuria ranged in severity from clinically asymptomatic, transient, trace proteinuria to nephrotic syndrome. Grade 3 proteinuria was reported in up to <3% of treated patients, and Grade 4 proteinuria (nephrotic syndrome) was seen in up to 1.4 % of treated patients.

The proteinuria seen in AVASTIN clinical trials was rarely associated with renal impairment (e.g., nephrotic syndrome, glomerulonephritis) which in some patients required permanent discontinuation.

The overall incidence of all grade adverse events suggestive of renal impairment was higher in the AVASTIN in combination with cisplatin/gemcitabine arms compared with chemotherapy arm.

Hemorrhage (see Warnings and Precautions): Eighteen patients (in studies in patients with non-small cell lung cancer (NSCLC)) prematurely discontinued at least one component of study treatment due to a bleeding adverse event. In clinical trials across all indications the overall incidence of NCI-CTC Grade 3-5 bleeding events ranged from 0.4% to 5% in patients treated with AVASTIN, compared to 0 to 2.9% of patients in the chemotherapy control group. The hemorrhagic events that have been observed in AVASTIN clinical studies were predominantly tumour-associated hemorrhage (see below) and minor mucocutaneous hemorrhage (e.g. epistaxis).

In the pivotal clinical trial in mBC, Grade 3-4 haemorrhage [i.e., requiring transfusion, endoscopic or surgical intervention] was observed in 1.7% of patients treated with AVASTIN + paclitaxel and in 0.3% patients receiving paclitaxel alone. No Grade 5 haemorrhage events were reported. Grades 1-3 Haematologic AEs were not routinely captured.

Tumour-associated Hemorrhage: Tumour associated hemorrhage was observed in AVASTIN studies. Major or massive pulmonary hemorrhage/hemoptysis has been observed primarily in studies in patients with non-small cell lung cancer and in studies that did not exclude patients with tumours of predominate squamous histology. These events can occur suddenly and can present as major or massive pulmonary hemorrhage/haemoptysis. Among the possible risk factors evaluated (including squamous cell histology, treatment with antirheumatic/anti-inflammatory drugs, treatment with anticoagulants, prior radiotherapy, AVASTIN therapy, previous medical history of atherosclerosis, central tumour location and cavitation of tumours during therapy) the only variables that showed statistically significant correlations with bleeding were AVASTIN therapy and squamous cell histology. Patients with NSCLC of known squamous cell histology or mixed cell type with predominant squamous cell histology were excluded from subsequent studies, while patients with unknown tumour histology were included.

In patients with NSCLC excluding predominant squamous histology, all grade pulmonary haemorrhage events were seen with a frequency of up to 9% when treated with AVASTIN plus chemotherapy compared with 5% in the patients treated with chemotherapy alone. Grade 3-5 pulmonary haemorrhage events have been observed in up to 2.3% of patients treated with AVASTIN plus chemotherapy as compared with <1% with chemotherapy alone. Grade 3-5 pulmonary haemorrhage/hemoptysis can occur suddenly and up to two thirds of these cases resulted in a fatal outcome.

There were four cases of cerebral haemorrhage; three cases were Grade 4 events and one case was a Grade 2 event. None of the patients with cerebral haemorrhage had brain metastasis at baseline.

Gastrointestinal hemorrhages, including rectal bleeding and melena have been reported in colorectal patients, and have been assessed as tumour-associated hemorrhages.

Tumour-associated hemorrhages were also seen rarely in other tumour types and locations and included a case of central nervous system (CNS) bleeding in a patient with hepatoma with occult CNS metastases and another patient who developed continuous oozing of blood from a thigh sarcoma with necrosis.

Within 10 randomized controlled Phase III trials across the tumour indications advanced or metastatic colorectal cancer, renal cell cancer, NSCLC, breast cancer and pancreatic cancer, representing a total of 8036 patients, the incidence of gastrointestinal bleeding (all Grades)‡ ranged between <1% and 9% in the control arms and between 1% and 10% in the bevacizumab arms. The incidence of Grade 5 events ranged between 0% and <1% in the control arms and between 0% and 1% in the bevacizumab arms.

CNS Hemorrhage: Cases of CNS hemorrhage, some with fatal outcome, have been observed in clinical trials of AVASTIN. Patients should be monitored for signs and symptoms of CNS bleeding, and Avastin treatment discontinued in case of intracranial bleeding.

Intracranial hemorrhage can occur in patients with relapsed glioblastoma. In study AVF3708g, CNS hemorrhage was reported in 2.4% (2/84) of patients in the AVASTIN-alone arm (Grade 1); and in 3.8% (3/79) of patients treated with AVASTIN and irinotecan (Grades 1, 2 and 4). CNS hemorrhage rates of 1.6-7.8% in patients with malignant glioma have been reported.

Within 10 randomized controlled Phase III trials across the tumour indications advanced or metastatic colorectal cancer, renal cell cancer, NSCLC, breast cancer and pancreatic cancer, representing a total of 8036 patients, the incidence of intracranial hemorrhage (all Grades)¶ ranged between 0% and <1% in both the control arms and in the bevacizumab arms, the incidence of Grade 5 events ranges between 0% and <1% in both the control arms and in the bevacizumab arms.

Mucocutaneous Hemorrhage: Across all AVASTIN clinical trials, mucocutaneous hemorrhage were seen in 20%-40% of patients treated with AVASTIN. These were most commonly NCI-CTC Grade 1 epistaxis that lasted less than 5 minutes, resolved without medical intervention and did not require any change in the AVASTIN treatment regimen. Clinical safety data suggest that the incidence of minor mucocutaneous haemorrhage (e.g. epistaxis) may be dose-dependant.

There have also been less common events of minor mucocutaneous hemorrhage in other locations, such as gingival bleeding or vaginal bleeding.

Arterial Thromboembolism (see Warnings and Precautions): An increased incidence of arterial thromboembolic events was observed in patients treated with AVASTIN across indications including cerebrovascular accidents, myocardial infarction, transient ischemic attacks, and other arterial thromboembolic events.

In clinical trials, the overall incidence ranged up to 3.8% in the AVASTIN containing arms compared up to 1.7% in the chemotherapy control arms. Fatal outcome was reported in 0.8% of patients receiving AVASTIN in combination with chemotherapy compared to 0.5% of patients receiving chemotherapy alone. Cerebrovascular accidents (including transient ischemic attacks) were reported in up to 2.3% of AVASTIN treated patients versus 0.5% of patients in the control group: myocardial infarction was reported in 1.4% of AVASTIN treated versus 0.7% of patients in the observed control group.

Patients with metastatic colorectal cancer who were not candidates for treatment with irinotecan, were included in clinical trial AVF2192g. In this trial arterial thromboembolic events were observed in 11% (11/100) of AVASTIN patients compared to 5.8% (6/104) in the chemotherapy control group.

Venous Thromboembolism: In clinical trials across indications the overall incidence of venous thromboembolic events ranged from 2.8% to 17.3% in the AVASTIN containing arms compared to 3.2% to 15.6% in the chemotherapy control arms. Venous thromboembolic events include deep venous thrombosis, pulmonary embolism.

Grade 3-5 venous thromboembolic events have been reported in up to 7.8% of patients treated with chemotherapy plus AVASTIN compared with up to 4.9% in patients with chemotherapy alone.

Patients who have experienced a venous thromboembolic event may be at higher risk for a recurrence if they receive AVASTIN in combination with chemotherapy versus chemotherapy alone.

Neutropenia (see Warnings and Precautions): An increased rate of severe neutropenia, febrile neutropenia, or infection with severe neutropenia, in some cases with a fatal outcome, was identified for patients treated with some but not all types of myelotoxic/myelosuppressive chemotherapy regimens in combination with bevacizumab compared to chemotherapy alone. These increases were seen in patients with non-small cell lung cancer, from ECOG4599 treated with carboplatin + paclitaxel in combination with bevacizumab (26.2% in the bevacizumab containing arm vs. 17.2% in the chemotherapy arm), and also in combination with myelosuppressive chemotherapy agents used to treat metastatic colorectal cancer (19.7% in the bevacizumab arm vs. 13.6% in the chemotherapy arm of AVF2107g) and metastatic breast cancer (5% in the bevacizumab containing arm vs. 3.2% in the chemotherapy arm of E2100).

Thrombocytopenia: The incidence of thrombocytopenia was higher in patients receiving AVASTIN in combination with cisplatin/gemcitabine chemotherapy compared to those who received chemotherapy alone. The incidence of Grade 3 thrombocytopenia was common in patients treated with AVASTIN. Patients >65 years of age appeared to at higher risk for grade ≥3 thrombocytopenia compared with younger patients.

Congestive Heart Failure (CHF) (see Warnings and Precautions): In clinical trials with AVASTIN, congestive heart failure (CHF) was observed in all cancer indications studied to date, but occurred predominantly in patients with metastatic breast cancer. In phase III studies (AVF2119g and E2100) in patients with metastatic breast cancer an increase of CHF Grade 3 or more with AVASTIN was seen. (Grades 1 and 2 AEs were not captured). The incidence of CHF in patients treated with AVASTIN ranged from 2.9% to 3.5% compared with 0 to 1.4% in the control arms.

Most of these patients showed improved symptoms and/or left ventricular function following appropriate medical therapy. In most clinical trials of AVASTIN, patients with pre-existing CHF of NYHA II-IV were excluded, therefore, no information is available on the risk of CHF in this population.

Prior anthracyclines exposure and/or prior radiation to the chest wall may be possible risk factors for the development of CHF.

Nasal Septum Perforations: Very rare cases of nasal septum perforations have been reported in patients treated with AVASTIN.

Fistula (see Warnings and Precautions): AVASTIN use has been associated with serious cases of fistulae including events resulting in death.

In AVASTIN clinical trials, gastrointestinal fistulae have been reported with an incidence of up to 2% in patients with metastatic colorectal cancer, but were also reported less commonly in patients with other types of cancers. Uncommon (≥0.1% to <1%) reports of other types of fistulae that involve areas of the body other than the gastrointestinal tract (e.g. bronchopleural, urogenital and biliary fistulae) were observed across various indications. Fistulae have also been reported in post-marketing experience.

Events were reported at various time points during treatment ranging from one week to greater than 1 year from initiation of AVASTIN, with most events occurring within the first 6 months of therapy.

Elderly Patients: In randomised clinical trials, age >65 years was associated with an increased risk of developing arterial thromboembolic events including cerebrovascular accidents, transient ischemic attacks, myocardial infarction, grade 3-4 leucopenia, neutropenia, diarrhea and fatigue as compared to those aged ≤65 years when treated with AVASTIN (see Warnings and Precautions and Adverse Reactions).

Other reactions with a higher frequency seen in patients over 65 were grade 3-4 leucopenia and thrombocytopenia; and all grade neutropenia, diarrhea, nausea, headache and fatigue.

No increase in the incidences of other reactions including gastrointestinal perforation, wound healing complications, hypertension and congestive heart failure was observed in elderly patients (>65 years) receiving AVASTIN as compared to those aged ≤65 years treated with AVASTIN.

Gender: In clinical trials in mNSCLC, female patients treated with AVASTIN had an increased risk of grade 3 adverse reactions of fatigue, abdominal pain and hypertension compared with males, and with females treated with chemotherapy. Grades 1 and 2 AEs were not captured.

Abnormal Hematologic and Clinical Chemistry Findings: Laboratory Abnormalities: Decreased neutrophil count, decreased white blood count and presence of urine protein may be associated with AVASTIN treatment.

Across clinical trials, the following Grade 3 and 4 laboratory abnormalities were seen with an increased (≥2%) incidence in patients treated with AVASTIN compared to those in the control groups: hyperglycaemia, decreased haemoglobin, hypokalemia, hyponatraemia, decreased white blood cell count, thrombocytopenia, increased PT prothrombin time and normalised ratio.

Post-Market Adverse Drug Reactions:

System Organ Class	Reactions (frequency)
Nervous System Disorders	Hypertensive encephalopathy (very rare) Reversible posterior leukoencephalopathy syndrome (rare) (see Warnings and Precautions)
Vascular Disorders	Renal thrombotic microangiopathy, clinically manifested as proteinuria (frequency not known). (See Warnings and Precautions, and Adverse Reactions)
Respiratory, Thoracic and Mediastinal Disorders	Nasal septum perforation (frequency not known) Pulmonary hypertension[a] (frequency not known) Dysphonia (common)

[a] Symptoms of pulmonary hypertension include dyspnea on exertion, fatigue, syncope, anginal chest pain, hemoptysis, and Raynaud's phenomenon).

Renal failure, sepsis, febrile neutropenia, non-gastrointestinal fistula and hypersensitivity reactions, including anaphylactic reaction were reported during postmarketing use of AVASTIN in combination with chemotherapy.

DRUG INTERACTIONS: Overview: No formal drug interaction studies with other antineoplastic agents have been conducted. However, the existing data suggest that bevacizumab does not affect the pharmacokinetics of 5-fluorouracil (5-FU), carboplatin, paclitaxel and doxorubicin.

Drug-Drug Interactions: In study AVF2107g, irinotecan concentrations were similar in patients receiving IFL (irinotecan/5-fluorouracil/leucovorin) alone and in combination with AVASTIN. Concentrations of SN38, the active metabolite of irinotecan, were analysed in a subset of patients, i.e. approximately 30 per treatment arms. Concentrations of SN38 were on average 33% higher in patients receiving IFL in combination with AVASTIN compared with IFL alone. Due to high inter-patient variability and limited sampling, it is unclear if the observed increase in SN38 levels was due to AVASTIN. There was a small increase in diarrhea and leukopenia adverse events (known adverse drug reactions of irinotecan), and also more dose reductions of irinotecan were reported in the patients treated with IFL + AVASTIN. Patients who develop severe diarrhea, leukopenia or neutropenia with AVASTIN and irinotecan combination therapy should have irinotecan dose modifications as specified in the irinotecan product information.

Sunitinib Malate: In two clinical studies of metastatic renal cell carcinoma, microangiopathic haemolytic anaemia (MAHA) was reported in 7 of 19 patients (37%) treated with bevacizumab (10 mg/kg every two weeks) and sunitinib malate (50 mg daily) combination.

MAHA is a haemolytic disorder which can present with red cell fragmentation, anaemia, and thrombocytopenia. In addition, hypertension (including hypertensive crisis), elevated creatinine, and neurological symptoms were observed in some of these patients. All of these findings were reversible upon discontinuation of bevacizumab and sunitinib malate (see Warnings and Precautions).

The safety and efficacy of AVASTIN in combination with sunitinib malate has not been established, therefore this combination is not recommended.

Radiotherapy: The safety and efficacy of concomitant administration of radiotherapy and AVASTIN has not been established.

DOSAGE AND ADMINISTRATION: Dosing Considerations: It is recommended that AVASTIN (bevacizumab) treatment be continued until progression of the underlying disease.

Recommended Dose and Dosage Adjustment: Metastatic Colorectal Cancer: The recommended dose of AVASTIN (bevacizumab) is 5 mg/kg of body weight given once every 14 days as an intravenous infusion.

Dose reduction of AVASTIN for adverse events is not recommended. If indicated, AVASTIN should either be permanently discontinued or temporarily suspended as described in the Warnings and Precautions.

Metastatic Breast Cancer: The recommended dose of AVASTIN (bevacizumab) for metastatic breast cancer treatment is 10 mg/kg of body weight given at weeks 1 and 3 of each 4-week cycle.

Locally Advanced, Metastatic or Recurrent Non Small Cell Lung Cancer (NSCLC): The recommended dose of AVASTIN, administered in addition to carboplatin + paclitaxel chemotherapy regimen, is 15 mg/kg of body weight given once every 3 weeks as an intravenous infusion.

In clinical trials, AVASTIN was administered in addition to carboplatin/paclitaxel chemotherapy for up to 6 cycles of treatment followed by AVASTIN as a single agent until disease progression.

Malignant Glioma (WHO Grade IV)-Glioblastoma: The recommended dose of AVASTIN is 10 mg/kg of body weight given once every 2 weeks as an intravenous infusion.

It is recommended that AVASTIN treatment be continued until progression of the underlying disease.

Administration: Do not administer as an intravenous push or bolus.

The initial AVASTIN dose should be delivered over 90 minutes as an intravenous infusion. If the first infusion is well tolerated, the second infusion may be administered over 60 minutes. If the 60-minute infusion is well tolerated, all subsequent infusions may be administered over 30 minutes.

AVASTIN infusions should not be administered or mixed with dextrose or glucose solutions. A concentration-dependent degradation profile of AVASTIN was observed when diluted with dextrose solutions (5%).

No incompatibilities between AVASTIN and polyvinyl chloride or polyolefin bags have been observed.

AVASTIN should be prepared by a healthcare professional using aseptic technique. Withdraw the necessary amount of bevacizumab and dilute to the required administration volume with 0.9% sodium chloride solution. The concentration of the final bevacizumab solution should be kept within the range of 1.4-16.5 mg/mL.

Discard any unused portion left in a vial, as the product contains no preservatives. Parenteral drug products should be inspected visually for particulate matter and discoloration prior to administration.

OVERDOSAGE:

In addition to the possible adverse reactions listed above, the highest dose of AVASTIN (bevacizumab) tested in humans (20 mg/kg of body weight, intravenous, multiple dose) was associated with severe migraine in several patients.

For management of a suspected drug overdose, CPhA recommends that you contact your **regional Poison Control Centre**. See the *CPS* Directory section for a list of Poison Control Centres.

ACTION AND CLINICAL PHARMACOLOGY: Mechanism of Action: AVASTIN (bevacizumab) is a recombinant humanised monoclonal antibody that selectively binds to and neutralises the biologic activity of human vascular endothelial growth factor (VEGF). Bevacizumab contains human framework regions with antigen binding regions of a humanised murine antibody that binds to VEGF. Bevacizumab is produced by recombinant DNA technology in a Chinese hamster ovary mammalian cell expression system in a nutrient medium containing the antibiotic gentamicin and is purified by a process that includes specific viral inactivation and removal steps. Gentamicin is detectable in the final product at ≤0.35 ppm. Bevacizumab consists of 214 amino acids and has a molecular weight of approximately 149 000 daltons.

AVASTIN inhibits the binding of VEGF to its receptors, Flt-1 and KDR, on the surface of endothelial cells. Neutralising the biologic activity of VEGF reduces the vascularisation of tumors, thereby inhibiting tumor growth. Administration of bevacizumab or its parental murine antibody to xenotransplant models of cancer in nude mice resulted in extensive anti-tumor activity in human tumor xenografts, including colon, breast, pancreas and prostate. Metastatic disease progression was inhibited and microvascular permeability was reduced.

Pharmacokinetics: The pharmacokinetic data for bevacizumab are available from eight clinical trials in patients with solid tumors. In all clinical trials, bevacizumab was administered as an intravenous infusion. The rate of infusion was based on tolerability, with an initial infusion duration of 90 minutes. In the first phase I study the pharmacokinetics of bevacizumab was linear at doses ranging from 1 to 10 mg/kg.

Distribution: Based on a population pharmacokinetic analysis of 491 subjects receiving AVASTIN weekly, every 2 weeks, or every 3 weeks, in doses ranging from 1 to 20 mg/kg, the volume of the central compartment (Vc) was 2.66 L and 3.25 L for female and male subjects, respectively. Results also indicated that, after correcting for body weight, male subjects had a larger Vc (+22%) than females.

Metabolism: Assessment of bevacizumab metabolism in rabbits following a single intravenous dose of ^{125}I-bevacizumab indicated that its metabolic profile was similar to that expected for a native IgG molecule which does not bind VEGF. The metabolism and elimination of bevacizumab is similar to endogenous IgG i.e. primarily via proteolytic catabolism throughout the body, including endothelial cells, and does not rely primarily on elimination through the kidneys and liver. Binding of the IgG to the FcRn receptor result in protection from cellular metabolism and the long terminal half-life.

Excretion: Bevacizumab clearance was 0.207 L/day for females and 0.262 L/day for males. The Vc and clearance correspond to an initial half life of 1.4 days and a terminal half life of 20 and 19 days for females and males, respectively. This half life is consistent with the terminal elimination half life for human endogenous IgG, which is 18 to 23 days. Results of the population pharmacokinetic analysis indicated that, after correcting for body weight, male subjects had a higher bevacizumab clearance (+26%) than females. However, no dose adjustment is required. There was no correlation between bevacizumab clearance and subject age. In patients with low albumin (≤29 g/dL) and high alkaline phosphatase (≥484 U/L) (both markers of disease severity), bevacizumab clearance was approximately 20% faster than in patients with median laboratory values.

Special Populations and Conditions: The population pharmacokinetics of bevacizumab were analysed to evaluate the effects of demographic characteristics. The results showed no significant difference in the pharmacokinetics of bevacizumab in relation to age.

Renal Insufficiency: No studies have been conducted to investigate the pharmacokinetics of bevacizumab in renally impaired patients since the kidneys are not a major organ for bevacizumab metabolism or excretion.

Hepatic Insufficiency: No studies have been conducted to investigate the pharmacokinetics of bevacizumab in patients with hepatic impairment since the liver is not a major organ for bevacizumab metabolism or excretion.

STORAGE AND STABILITY: Store vials in a refrigerator at 2-8°C. Keep vial in the outer carton in order to protect from light. **Do not freeze. Do not shake.**

AVASTIN (bevacizumab) does not contain any antimicrobial preservative; therefore, care must be taken to ensure the sterility of the prepared solution.

Chemical and physical in-use stability has been demonstrated for 48 hours at 2-30°C in 0.9% sodium chloride solution. From a microbiological point of view, the product should be used immediately. If not used immediately, in-use storage times and conditions are the responsibility of the user and would normally not be longer than 24 hours at 2 to 8°C, unless dilution has taken place in controlled and validated aseptic conditions.

INFORMATION FOR THE PATIENT: Published in e-CPS, available by subscription at www.e-cps.ca.

DOSAGE FORMS, COMPOSITION AND PACKAGING: Each vial contains: bevacizumab 25 mg/mL as either bevacizumab 100 mg in 4 mL or bevacizumab 400 mg in 16 mL. Nonmedicinal ingredients: α,α-trehalose dihydrate, polysorbate 20, sodium phosphate and water for injection. Preservative-free. Clear glass single-use vials with butyl rubber stopper, packs of 1.

Avaxim®
hepatitis A vaccine inactivated
Active Immunizing Agent

sanofi pasteur

Date of Revision: October 2005

PHARMACOLOGY: Hepatitis A, results from infection of the liver by hepatitis A virus (HAV), an RNA virus of a single serotype. Infection usually causes overt illness in adults and school-age children but is often asymptomatic in younger children. Humans are the principal reservoir for the virus. Typical symptoms of illness include anorexia, nausea, fatigue, fever and jaundice. Recovery often takes 4 to 6 weeks. About 25% of reported adult cases require hospitalization. Fulminant disease with liver necrosis is rare but can be fatal. The estimated mortality rate associated with hepatitis A is 0.1 - 0.3%, but this rises to 1.8% in persons over the age of 50. Individuals with pre-existing chronic liver disease are at increased risk of serious complications from hepatitis A infection.

Risk factors for infection in Canada include the following: residence in certain communities in rural or remote areas lacking adequate sanitation; residence in certain institutions, such as correctional facilities and those for developmentally challenged persons; oral or i.v. illicit drug use; sexual behaviours involving anal contact, particularly between men; travel to or residence in countries with inadequate sanitation.

Hepatitis A virus (HAV) infection in returned travellers and contacts of travellers including children account for a large proportion of cases reported in Canada; some cases have occurred in people who spent <2 weeks in an endemic area. The risk for susceptible travellers to developing countries has been estimated at 3 to 5 per 1000 per month and is up to six times higher for low-budget travellers eating in poorer hygienic conditions. In Canada, between 1990 and 1999, the annual number of cases of HAV infection reported to the National Notifiable Disease Registry varied from 890 to 3020, with corresponding rates from 3.0 to 10.8 per 100 000 population. Given under-reporting and asymptomatic infection, however, the actual number of cases is considerably higher. In 1999, the reported rate was 1.6 times higher among males than females. Age-specific incidence rates were highest among those 25 to 59 years of age and lowest among those <5 years or >59 years; 18% of all cases were <15 years old, an age group in which the disease is often asymptomatic. Although representative data are not available for the general Canadian population, studies indicate that immunity to HAV infection is evident in about 3% of Canadian-born preadolescents and in over 60% of those 60 years of age. The difference in levels of immunity reflects progressive accumulation of immunity over time and the greater likelihood of exposure in the past, when the infection was more common. Overall, the most commonly identified risk factor for HAV infection is household or sexual exposure to a recent case. In many infected persons no specific risk factor can be identified.

AVAXIM [Hepatitis A Vaccine Inactivated] confers immunity against hepatitis A virus (HAV) infection by inducing the production of specific anti-hepatitis A virus antibodies.

Clinical studies indicate that the vaccine confers immunity against hepatitis A virus by inducing antibody titres greater than those obtained after passive immunization with immunoglobulin. Immunity appears shortly after the first injection.

In clinical studies involving over 1000 volunteers, specific humoral antibodies against hepatitis A were elicited after the first injection and more than 90% of immunocompetent subjects were protected (titres above 20 mIU/mL) 14 days after vaccination. One month after the first injection, 100% of the subjects were protected. Immunity persisted for at least six months and was reinforced after a first booster dose.

In comparative trials with another hepatitis A vaccine, AVAXIM demonstrated a superior immunogenicity profile. Additionally, seroconversion rates at 14 days showed that the immune responses occur more rapidly with AVAXIM. This prompt immune response may be an important consideration when travellers must be vaccinated immediately prior to departure or when post-exposure prophylaxis cannot be done immediately after exposure.

INDICATIONS: AVAXIM [Hepatitis A Vaccine Inactivated] is indicated for active immunization against infection caused by hepatitis A virus (HAV) in persons 12 years of age and older. AVAXIM can be used for primary immunization or as a booster following primary immunization with AVAXIM or other similar hepatitis A vaccines.

AVAXIM is recommended for pre-exposure prophylaxis of individuals at increased risk of infection. Potential candidates for the vaccine are:

- travellers to countries where hepatitis A is endemic, especially when travel involves rural or primitive conditions;
- residents of communities with high endemic rates or recurrent outbreaks of HAV;
- members of the armed forces, emergency relief workers and others likely to be posted abroad at short notice to areas with high rates of HAV infection;
- residents and staff of institutions for the developmentally challenged where there is an ongoing problem with HAV transmission;
- inmates of correctional facilities in which there is an ongoing problem with HAV infection;
- people with life-style determined risks of infection, including those engaging in oral or intravenous illicit drug use in unsanitary conditions;
- men who have sex with men;
- people with chronic liver disease who may not be at increased risk of infection but are at increased risk of fulminant hepatitis A;
- patients with hemophilia A or B receiving plasma-derived replacement clotting factors;
- zoo-keepers, veterinarians and researchers who handle non-human primates;
- certain workers involved in research on hepatitis A virus or production of hepatitis A vaccine.

Outbreak Control: AVAXIM should be used as part of a coordinated public health response to hepatitis A outbreaks. Hepatitis A Vaccine has been used to arrest the transmission of the virus in communities.

Universal Immunization: WHO recommends targeted programs for countries with low endemicity, such as Canada.

CONTRAINDICATIONS: General: Immunization with AVAXIM [Hepatitis A Vaccine Inactivated] should be deferred in the presence of any acute illness, including febrile illness to avoid superimposing adverse effects from the vaccine on the underlying illness or mistakenly identifying a manifestation of the underlying illness as a complication of vaccine use. A minor afebrile illness such as mild upper respiratory infection is not usually reason to defer immunization.

Allergy to any component of AVAXIM (see components listed in Supplied) or an anaphylactic or other allergic reaction to a previous dose of AVAXIM are contraindications to vaccination.

The vaccine should not be administered intravenously or intradermally.

WARNINGS: AVAXIM [Hepatitis A Vaccine Inactivated] does not provide protection against infection caused by hepatitis B virus, hepatitis C virus, delta virus, hepatitis E virus, or by other liver pathogens, other than hepatitis A virus.

Seropositivity against hepatitis A virus is not a contraindication. AVAXIM is as well tolerated in seropositive as in seronegative subjects.

Because of the incubation period of hepatitis A, infection may be present at the time of vaccination; if so, the vaccine may be ineffective.

Intramuscular injections should be given with care in persons suffering from coagulation disorders or on anticoagulant therapy because of the risk of hemorrhage.

AVAXIM should not be administered into the buttocks due to the varying amount of fatty tissue in this region, nor by the intradermal route, since these methods of administration may induce a weaker immune response.

Immunocompromised persons (whether from disease or treatment) may not obtain the expected immune response. If possible, consideration should be given to delaying vaccination until after the completion of any immunosuppressive treatment. If AVAXIM is used in these persons, seroconversion should be confirmed by antibody testing.

As with any vaccine, immunization with AVAXIM may not protect 100% of susceptible individuals.

PRECAUTIONS: The possibility of allergic reactions in persons sensitive to components of the vaccine should be evaluated. Epinephrine Hydrochloride Solution (1:1000) and other appropriate agents should be available for immediate use in case an anaphylactic or acute hypersensitivity reaction occurs. Health-care providers should be familiar with current recommendations for the initial management of anaphylaxis in non-hospital settings, including proper airway management.

For instructions on recognition and treatment of anaphylactic reactions see the current edition of the Canadian Immunization Guide or visit the Health Canada website.

Before administration, take all appropriate precautions to prevent adverse reactions. This includes a review of the patient's history concerning possible hypersensitivity to the vaccine or similar vaccine, previous immunization history, the presence of any contraindications to immunization and current health status and a current knowledge of the literature concerning the use of the vaccine under consideration.

Before administration of AVAXIM [Hepatitis A Vaccine Inactivated], health-care providers should inform the parent or guardian or the patient to be immunized of the benefits and risks of immunization, inquire about the recent health status of the patient and comply with any local requirements with respect to information to be provided to the patient before immunization.

Do not inject into a blood vessel.

Use a separate sterile needle and syringe, or a sterile disposable unit, for each individual patient to prevent disease transmission.

There have been case reports of transmission of HIV and hepatitis by failure to scrupulously observe sterile technique.

Pregnancy: The effect of AVAXIM on the development of the embryo and fetus has not been assessed. Vaccination in pregnancy is not recommended unless there is a definite risk of acquiring hepatitis A. As the vaccine is inactivated, any risk to the embryo or the fetus is improbable. The benefits versus the risks of administering AVAXIM in pregnancy should carefully be evaluated.

Lactation: The effect of administration of AVAXIM during lactation has not been assessed. As AVAXIM is inactivated, any risk to the mother or the infant is improbable. The benefits versus the risks of administering AVAXIM during lactation should carefully be evaluated.

Drug Interactions: If indicated, AVAXIM may be administered simultaneously with immune globulin at separate sites with separate syringes. Seroconversion rates are not modified, but antibody titres could be lower than after vaccination with the vaccine alone.

As the vaccine is inactivated, concomitant administration of other vaccine(s) given at other injection sites is unlikely to interfere with immune responses. No interaction with other medication is currently known. AVAXIM has been shown to be safe and immunogenic when concomitantly administered with TYPHIM Vi using separate syringes at different sites.

Children: AVAXIM is indicated for persons 12 years of age and older. AVAXIM Pediatric, is used for children aged 12 months to 15 years of age. Either vaccine may be used for persons between 12 to 15 years of age.

ADVERSE EFFECTS: In six clinical trials conducted which involved over 2200 participants, adverse events were usually mild and confined to the first few days after vaccination with spontaneous recovery. The most common local reaction was mild pain (11.7%) at the injection site, occasionally associated with redness (0.5% over 3 cm). Mild fever (5.2%), weakness (13.5%), headache (9.7%), muscle or joint ache (10.3%) or gastro-intestinal tract disorders (6.1%) such as nausea, vomiting, diarrhea, or pain, were also reported.

Mild transient elevation of serum transaminases has been reported on rare occasions.

Adverse reactions were less frequently reported after the booster dose than after the first dose. In subjects seropositive to HAV, AVAXIM [Hepatitis A Vaccine Inactivated], was as well tolerated as in seronegative subjects.

In comparative trials with another hepatitis A vaccine, in a total of 423 adults, AVAXIM demonstrated significantly fewer local reactions after each injection.

Physicians, nurses, and pharmacists should report any adverse occurrences temporally related to the administration of the product in accordance with local requirements and to the Global Pharmacovigilance Department, Sanofi Pasteur Limited, 1755 Steeles Avenue West, Toronto, ON, M2R 3T4, Canada. 1-888-621-1146 (phone) or 416-667-2435 (fax).

DOSAGE: Primary immunization is achieved with one single dose of vaccine. In order to provide long term protection, a booster should be given six to twelve months later. Based on current data, a further booster dose may be required after 10 years.

The recommended dose is 0.5 mL administered intramuscularly.

Inspect for extraneous particulate matter and/or discolouration before use. If these conditions exist, the product should not be administered.

For information on vaccine administration see the current edition of the Canadian Immunization Guide or visit the Health Canada website.

Shake the prefilled syringe well to uniformly distribute the suspension before administration.

AVAXIM [Hepatitis A Vaccine Inactivated] may be packaged in one of two presentations: a pre-filled syringe with a choice of two needles; or a pre-filled syringe with attached needle.

If a choice of needles is present, select a needle of appropriate length to ensure that the vaccine will be delivered intramuscularly. Remove the tip cap from the syringe, take the chosen needle from the blister pack and fix to the tip of the prefilled syringe.

If a syringe with attached needle is present, the vaccine is ready to administer.

Aseptic technique must be used. Administer the vaccine **intramuscularly**. The preferred site is into the deltoid muscle or into the anterolateral aspect of the mid thigh (vastus lateralis muscle). Do not administer in the buttocks.

Do not inject intravenously.

In exceptional circumstances (e.g., in patients with thrombocytopenia or in patients at risk of hemorrhage) the vaccine may be injected by the subcutaneous route, however this may be associated with a higher risk of local reaction including injection site nodule.

Needles should not be recapped and should be disposed of properly.

Give the patient a permanent personal immunization record. In addition, it is essential that the physician or nurse record the immunization history in the permanent medical record of each patient. This permanent office record should contain the name of the vaccine, date given, dose, manufacturer and lot number.

SUPPLIED: The active ingredient is a purified and formaldehyde-inactivated hepatitis A virus. It is obtained from the GBM strain cultured on MRC-5 human diploid cells. Each human dose (0.5 mL) contains 160 antigen units (in the absence of an international standardized reference, the antigen content is expressed using an inhouse reference). Each (0.5 mL) dose contains: aluminum hydroxide (expressed as aluminum): 0.3 mg; 2-phenoxyethanol: 2.5 μL; formaldehyde: 12.5 μg; medium 199, water for injection up to 0.5 mL; neomycin: trace amounts. AVAXIM is a whitish, cloudy suspension. Packages of either one prefilled single dose syringe with a choice of two needles (1×25G×16 mm and 1×25G×25 mm), or one prefilled single dose syringe with attached needle. The plunger stoppers and needle shield for the syringes supplied with this product do not contain dry natural latex rubber.

Store at 2 to 8°C. **Do not freeze.** Discard product if exposed to freezing. Do not use after expiration date.

Avaxim®-Pediatric
hepatitis A vaccine inactivated
Active Immunizing Agent

sanofi pasteur

Date of Revision: November 2005

PHARMACOLOGY: Hepatitis A results from infection of the liver by hepatitis A virus (HAV), an RNA virus of a single serotype. Infection usually causes overt illness in adults and school-age children but is often asymptomatic in younger children. Humans are the principal reservoir for the virus. Typical symptoms of illness include anorexia, nausea, fatigue, fever and jaundice. Recovery often takes 4 to 6 weeks. About 25% of reported adult cases require hospitalization. Fulminant disease with liver necrosis is rare but can be fatal. The estimated mortality rate associated with hepatitis A is 0.1 - 0.3%, but this rises to 1.8% in persons over the age of 50. Individuals with pre-existing chronic liver disease are at increased risk of serious complications from hepatitis A infection.

Risk factors for infection in Canada include the following: residence in certain communities in rural or remote areas lacking adequate sanitation; residence in certain institutions, such as correctional facilities and those for developmentally challenged persons; oral or intravenous illicit drug use; sexual behaviours involving anal contact, particularly between men; travel to or residence in countries with inadequate sanitation.

Hepatitis A virus (HAV) infection in returned travellers and contacts of travellers including children account for a large proportion of cases reported in Canada; some cases have occurred in people who spent <2 weeks in an endemic area. The risk for susceptible travellers to developing countries has been estimated at 3 to 5 per 1000 per month and is up to six times higher for low-budget travellers eating in poorer hygienic conditions. In Canada, between 1990 and 1999, the annual number of cases of HAV infection reported to the National Notifiable Disease Registry varied from 890 to 3020 with corresponding rates from 3.0 to 10.8 per 100 000 population. Given under-reporting and asymptomatic infection; however, the actual number of cases is considerably higher. In 1999, the reported rate was 1.6 times higher among males than females. Age-specific incidence rates were highest among those 25 to 59 years of age and lowest among those <5 years or >59 years, 18% of all cases were <15 years old, an age group in which the disease is often asymptomatic. Although representative data are not available for the general Canadian population, studies indicate that immunity to HAV infection is evident in about 3% of Canadian-born preadolescents and in over 60% of those >60 years of age. The difference in levels of immunity reflects progressive accumulation of immunity over time and the greater likelihood of exposure in the past, when the infection was more common. Overall, the most commonly identified risk factor for HAV infection is household or sexual exposure to a recent case. In many infected persons no specific risk factor can be identified.

AVAXIM- Pediatric [Hepatitis A Vaccine Inactivated] confers immunity against hepatitis A virus (HAV) infection by inducing the production of specific anti-hepatitis A virus antibodies.

Clinical studies indicate that the vaccine confers immunity against hepatitis A virus by inducing antibody titres greater than those obtained after passive immunization with immunoglobulin. Immunity appears soon after the first injection.

In clinical studies involving over 1000 adult volunteers, specific humoral antibodies against hepatitis A were elicited after the first injection and more than 90% of immunocompetent subjects were protected (titres above 20 mIU/mL) 14 days after vaccination. One month after the first injection, 100% of the subjects were protected. Immunity persisted for at least six months and was reinforced after a first booster dose.

In comparative trials with another hepatitis A vaccine, AVAXIM [Hepatitis A Vaccine Inactivated] demonstrated a superior immunogenicity profile. Additionally, seroconversion rates at 14 days showed that the immune responses occur more rapidly with AVAXIM. This prompt immune response may be an important consideration when travellers must be vaccinated immediately prior to departure or when post-exposure prophylaxis cannot be done immediately after exposure.

In clinical studies for immunogenicity in 656 children aged 12 months to 15 years (inclusive), seroconversion rates 2 weeks following vaccination ranged from 95.4% to 99.1% depending on the study. One hundred percent of those tested at 24 and 28 weeks following vaccination had protective antibody levels. A second dose given 6 months following the initial dose resulted in a marked booster response (increase in antibody titres of 22.6-fold and 35.5-fold).

INDICATIONS: AVAXIM-Pediatric [Hepatitis A Vaccine Inactivated] is indicated for active immunization against infection caused by hepatitis A virus (HAV) in persons 12 months to 15 years of age inclusive.

AVAXIM-Pediatric can be used for primary immunization or as a booster following primary immunization with AVAXIM-Pediatric or other similar hepatitis A vaccines.

AVAXIM-Pediatric is recommended for pre-exposure prophylaxis of individuals at increased risk of infection. Potential candidates for the vaccine are:

- travellers to countries where hepatitis A is endemic, especially when travel involves rural or primitive conditions;
- residents of communities with high endemic rates or recurrent outbreaks of HAV;
- members of the armed forces, emergency relief workers and others likely to be posted abroad at short notice to areas with high rates of HAV infection;
- residents and staff of institutions for the developmentally challenged where there is an ongoing problem with HAV transmission;
- inmates of correctional facilities in which there is an ongoing problem with HAV infection;
- people with life-style determined risks of infection, including those engaging in oral or intravenous illicit drug use in unsanitary conditions;
- men who have sex with men;
- people with chronic liver disease who may not be at increased risk of infection but are at increased risk of fulminant hepatitis A;
- patients with hemophilia A or B receiving plasma-derived replacement clotting factors;
- zoo-keepers, veterinarians and researchers who handle non-human primates;
- certain workers involved in research on hepatitis A virus or production of hepatitis A vaccine.

Outbreak Control: AVAXIM-Pediatric should be used as part of a coordinated public health response to hepatitis A outbreaks. Hepatitis A Vaccine has been used to arrest the transmission of the virus in communities.

Universal Immunization: WHO recommends targeted programs for countries with low endemicity, such as Canada.

CONTRAINDICATIONS: General: Immunization with AVAXIM-Pediatric [Hepatitis A Vaccine Inactivated] should be deferred in the presence of any acute illness, including febrile illness to avoid superimposing adverse effects from the vaccine on the underlying illness or mistakenly identifying a manifestation of the underlying illness as a complication of vaccine use. A minor afebrile illness such as mild upper respiratory infection is not usually reason to defer immunization.

Allergy to any component of AVAXIM-Pediatric (see components listed in Supplied) or an anaphylactic or other allergic reaction to a previous dose of AVAXIM-Pediatric are contraindications to vaccination.

The vaccine should not be administered intravenously or intradermally.

WARNINGS: AVAXIM-Pediatric [Hepatitis A Vaccine Inactivated] does not provide protection against infection caused by hepatitis B virus, hepatitis C virus, delta virus, hepatitis E virus, or by other liver pathogens, other than hepatitis A virus.

Seropositivity against hepatitis A virus is not a contraindication. AVAXIM-Pediatric is as well tolerated in seropositive as in seronegative subjects.

Because of the incubation period of hepatitis A, infection may be present at the time of vaccination; if so, the vaccine may be ineffective.

AVAXIM-Pediatric should not be used for immunization of persons 16 years of age and older. AVAXIM [Hepatitis A Vaccine Inactivated] containing 160 antigen units should be used.

Intramuscular injections should be given with care in persons suffering from coagulation disorders or on anticoagulant therapy because of the risk of hemorrhage.

AVAXIM-Pediatric should not be administered into the buttocks due to the varying amount of fatty tissue in this region, nor by the intradermal route, since these methods of administration may induce a weaker immune response.

Immunocompromised persons (whether from disease or treatment) may not obtain the expected immune response. If possible, consideration should be given to delaying vaccination until after the completion of any immunosuppressive treatment. If AVAXIM-Pediatric is used in these persons, seroconversion should be confirmed by antibody testing.

As with any vaccine, immunization with AVAXIM-Pediatric may not protect 100% of susceptible individuals.

PRECAUTIONS: The possibility of allergic reactions in persons sensitive to components of the vaccine should be evaluated. Epinephrine Hydrochloride Solution (1:1000) and other appropriate agents should be available for immediate use in case an anaphylactic or acute hypersensitivity reaction occurs. Health-care providers should be familiar with current recommendations for the initial management of anaphylaxis in non-hospital settings, including proper airway management.

For instructions on recognition and treatment of anaphylactic reactions see the current edition of the Canadian Immunization Guide or visit the Health Canada website.

Before administration, take all appropriate precautions to prevent adverse reactions. This includes a review of the patient's history concerning possible hypersensitivity to the vaccine or similar vaccine, previous immunization history, the presence of any contraindications to immunization and current health status and a current knowledge of the literature concerning the use of the vaccine under consideration.

Before administration of AVAXIM-Pediatric [Hepatitis A Vaccine Inactivated], health-care providers should inform the parent or guardian or the patient to be immunized of the benefits and risks of immunization, inquire about the recent health status of the patient and comply with any local requirements with respect to information to be provided to the patient before immunization.

Do not inject into a blood vessel.

Use a separate sterile needle and syringe, or a sterile disposable unit, for each individual patient to prevent disease transmission.

There have been case reports of transmission of HIV and hepatitis by failure to scrupulously observe sterile technique.

Pregnancy: The effect of AVAXIM-Pediatric on the development of the embryo and fetus has not been assessed. Vaccination in pregnancy is not recommended unless there is a definite risk of acquiring hepatitis A. As the vaccine is inactivated, any risk to the embryo or the fetus is improbable. The benefits versus the risks of administering AVAXIM-Pediatric in pregnancy should carefully be evaluated.

Lactation: The effect of administration of AVAXIM-Pediatric during lactation has not been assessed. As AVAXIM-Pediatric is inactivated, any risk to the mother or the infant is improbable. The benefits versus the risks of administering AVAXIM-Pediatric during lactation should carefully be evaluated.

Drug Interactions: If indicated, AVAXIM-Pediatric may be administered simultaneously with immune globulin at separate sites using separate syringes. In adults seroconversion rates are not modified, but antibody titres could be lower than after vaccination with the vaccine alone.

As the vaccine is inactivated, concomitant administration of other vaccine(s) given at other injection sites is unlikely to interfere with immune responses. No interaction with other medication is currently known.

Adult Use: AVAXIM-Pediatric is indicated in children aged 12 months to 15 years of age. AVAXIM is indicated for persons 12 years of age and older. Either vaccine may be used for persons between 12 to 15 years of age.

ADVERSE EFFECTS: In three clinical trials in which over 2000 children received AVAXIM-Pediatric [Hepatitis A Vaccine Inactivated], adverse events were usually mild and confined to the first few days after vaccination with spontaneous recovery. Younger children experienced fewer reactions than older children. Reactions were reported less frequently after the booster dose than after the first dose (see Table 1).

Table 1: AVAXIM-Pediatric

Adverse Reactions within 7 Days Following AVAXIM-Pediatric

Reaction	First Dose (%) n=2363	Booster Dose (%) n=2294
Local	12.0	9.0
Pain	8.7	7.6
Redness	2.5	1.4
Hematoma	1.4	0.8
Induration/Edema	1.5	0.6
Pruritus	0.1	0
Systemic	11.3	6.5
Fever (>37.5°C axillary)	2.5	1.1
Asthenia/Drowsiness	1.9	1.0
Headache[a]	5.4	2.7
Myalgia/Arthralgia[a]	3.9	2.4
Gastrointestinal Disorders	4.0	2.0
Behavioral Changes	3.4	2.2
Skin Disorders	0.4	0.04

[a] Recorded only for age ≥4 years.

Mild transient elevation of serum transaminases has been reported on rare occasions.

In subjects seropositive to HAV, AVAXIM-Pediatric was as well tolerated as in seronegative subjects.

Reactions were less frequently reported after the booster dose than after the first dose.

Physicians, nurses, and pharmacists should report any adverse occurrences temporally related to the administration of the product in accordance with local requirements and to the Global Pharmacovigilance Department, Sanofi Pasteur Limited, 1755 Steeles Avenue West, Toronto, ON, M2R 3T4, Canada. 1-888-621-1146 (phone) or 416-667-2435 (fax).

DOSAGE: Primary immunization is achieved with one single dose of vaccine. In order to provide long term protection, a booster should be given six to twelve months later.

If the second dose is missed, it can be given at any time without repeat of the first dose.

The recommended dose is 0.5 mL administered intramuscularly.

Inspect for extraneous particulate matter and/or discolouration before use. If these conditions exist, the product should not be administered.

For information on vaccine administration see the current edition of the Canadian Immunization Guide or visit the Health Canada website.

AVAXIM-Pediatric may be packaged in one of three presentations: a pre-filled syringe with two needles; a pre-filled syringe with attached needle or a multidose vial. If two needles are present, select a needle of appropriate length to ensure that the vaccine will be delivered intramuscularly. **Shake the pre-filled syringe well** to uniformly distribute the suspension before administration. Remove the tip cap from the syringe, take the chosen needle from the blister pack and fix to the tip of the pre-filled syringe. If a syringe with attached needle is present, the vaccine is ready to administer.

Shake the vial to uniformly distribute the suspension before withdrawing each dose. When administering a dose from a stoppered vial, do not remove either the stopper or the metal seal holding it in place. Aseptic technique must be used for withdrawal of each dose (see Precautions).

Aseptic technique must be used. Administer the vaccine **intramuscularly**. The preferred site is into the deltoid muscle. Do not administer in the buttocks. Do not inject intravenously.

In exceptional circumstances (e.g., in patients with thrombocytopenia or in patients at risk of hemorrhage), the vaccine may be injected by the subcutaneous route; however, this may be associated with a higher risk of local reaction including injection site nodule.

Needles should not be recapped and should be disposed of properly.

Give the patient a permanent personal immunization record. In addition, it is essential that the physician or nurse record the immunization history in the permanent medical record of each patient. This permanent office record should contain the name of the vaccine, date given, dose, manufacturer and lot number.

SUPPLIED: The active ingredient is a purified and formaldehyde-inactivated hepatitis A virus. It is obtained from the GBM strain cultured on MRC-5 human diploid cells. Each dose (0.5 mL) contains 80 antigen units (in the absence of an international standardized reference, the antigen content is expressed using an in-house reference). Each dose contains: aluminum hydroxide (expressed as aluminum): 0.15 mg; 2-phenoxyethanol: 2.5 µL; formaldehyde: 12.5 µg; medium 199, water for injection up to: 0.5 mL; neomycin: trace amounts. AVAXIM-Pediatric is a whitish, cloudy suspension. Packages of either one prefilled single dose syringe with two needles (1×25G×16 mm and 1×25G×25 mm), one prefilled single dose syringe with attached needle or a multidose vial. The plunger stoppers and needle shields for the syringes supplied with this product do not contain dry natural latex rubber.

Store at 2 to 8°C. **Do not freeze.** Discard product if exposed to freezing. Do not use vaccine after expiration date.

The reader is invited to consult CPhA's monograph **Fluoroquinolones**.

Avelox® Ⓟ
moxifloxacin HCl
Antibacterial

Bayer

Avelox® I.V. Ⓟ
moxifloxacin HCl
Antibacterial

Bayer

Date of Revision: September 14, 2009

SUMMARY PRODUCT INFORMATION:

Route of Administration	Dosage Form/ Strength	Clinically Relevant Nonmedicinal Ingredients
Oral	Tablet, 400 mg moxifloxacin	Lactose monohydrate For a complete listing see Dosage Forms, Composition and Packaging.
Intravenous	Intravenous solution, 400 mg moxifloxacin/250 mL	For a complete listing see Dosage Forms, Composition and Packaging.

INDICATIONS AND CLINICAL USE: AVELOX (moxifloxacin hydrochloride) is indicated for the treatment of adults (≥18 years of age) with the following bacterial infections caused by susceptible strains of the designated microorganisms for which treatment is appropriate.

Oral Administration: Respiratory Tract Infections: Acute bacterial sinusitis caused by: *H. influenzae, M. catarrhalis, S. pneumoniae.*

Acute bacterial exacerbation of chronic bronchitis caused by: *H. influenzae, H. parainfluenzae, K. pneumoniae, M. catarrhalis, S. aureus, S. pneumoniae.*

Community acquired pneumonia of mild to moderate severity caused by: *C. pneumoniae, H. influenzae, M. catarrhalis, M. pneumoniae, S. pneumoniae* (including Multi-drug resistant strains).

Multi-Drug Resistant *S. pneumoniae* (MDRSP) are strains resistant to two or more of the following antibiotics: penicillin (MIC ≥2 μg/mL), 2nd generation cephalosporins (e.g., cefuroxime axetil), macrolides, tetracyclines, and trimethoprim/sulfamethoxazole.

Sequential Intravenous/Oral Administration: Intravenous administration is recommended when it offers a route of administration advantageous to the patient (e.g., severe infection or the patient cannot tolerate the oral dosage form, at the discretion of the physician).

Community acquired pneumonia in hospitalized patients caused by: *C. pneumoniae, H. influenzae, M. catarrhalis, M. pneumoniae, S. aureus, S. pneumoniae* (including Multi-drug resistant strains).

Multi-Drug Resistant *S. pneumoniae* (MDRSP) are strains resistant to two or more of the following antibiotics: penicillin (MIC ≥2 μg/mL), 2nd generation cephalosporins (e.g., cefuroxime axetil), macrolides, tetracyclines, and trimethoprim/sulfamethoxazole.

Complicated intra-abdominal infections due to polymicrobial and monomicrobial infections caused by: *B. fragilis**, *B. thetaiotaomicron, C. perfringens, E. faecalis* (Vancomycin sensitive strains only; many strains are only moderately susceptible), *E. coli, P. mirabilis, S. anginosus.*

Complicated skin and skin structure infections in hospitalized patients caused by: *E. cloacae, E. coli, K. pneumoniae, S. aureus* (methicillin-susceptible strains).

Appropriate culture and susceptibility tests should be performed before treatment with AVELOX in order to isolate and identify organisms causing the infection and to determine their susceptibility to moxifloxacin. Therapy with AVELOX may be initiated while awaiting the results of these tests; once results become available, appropriate therapy should be continued. Culture and susceptibility testing performed periodically during therapy will provide information not only on the therapeutic effect of the antimicrobial agent, but also on the possible emergence of bacterial resistance. The frequency of acquired resistance may vary geographically and with time for certain species. Local area information on resistance patterns is desirable, particularly when treating severe infections.

Pediatrics (<18 years of age): AVELOX is not recommended for children under the age of 18 years (see Warnings and Precautions).

Geriatrics (≥65 years of age): Clinical trial data demonstrate that there is no significant difference in the safety of AVELOX in patients aged 65 or older. Dosage adjustments based on age are not necessary (see Action and Clinical Pharmacology).

CONTRAINDICATIONS:
- Patients who are hypersensitive to AVELOX (moxifloxacin hydrochloride) or other quinolone antibacterial agents (see Warnings and Precautions and Adverse Reactions).
- Patients who are hypersensitive to any ingredient in the formulation or component of the container (see Dosage Forms, Composition and Packaging).

WARNINGS AND PRECAUTIONS:

Serious Warnings and Precautions
- AVELOX (moxifloxacin hydrochloride) has been shown to prolong the QT interval of the electrocardiogram in some patients (see Warnings and Precautions, Cardiovascular, QT Interval Prolongation).
- Serious hypersensitivity and/or anaphylactic reactions have been reported in patients receiving quinolone therapy, including AVELOX (see Warnings and Precautions, Hypersensitivity).
- Seizures may occur with quinolone therapy. AVELOX should be used with caution in patients with known or suspected CNS disorders which may predispose to seizures or lower the seizure threshold (see Warnings and Precautions, Neurologic).
- AVELOX should not be used in pregnant women unless the potential benefits outweigh the potential risk to the fetus (see Warnings and Precautions, Special Populations, Pregnant Women).
- For nursing mothers, a decision should be made to either discontinue nursing or discontinue the administration of AVELOX, taking into account the importance of AVELOX therapy to the mother and the possible risk to the infant (see Warnings and Precautions, Special Populations, Nursing Women).
- AVELOX is not recommended for children under the age of 18 years (see Warnings and Precautions, Special Populations, Pediatrics (<18 years of age)).
- Cases of fulminant hepatitis potentially leading to liver failure (including fatal case) have been reported with moxifloxacin (see Warnings and Precautions, Hepatic/Biliary/Pancreatic).

Carcinogenesis and Mutagenesis: From the results of animal studies, there is no evidence to suggest that AVELOX is carcinogenic or mutagenic.

Cardiovascular: QT Interval Prolongation: AVELOX has been shown to prolong the QT interval of the electrocardiogram in some patients. The drug should be avoided in patients with known prolongation of the QT interval, patients with hypokalemia and patients receiving Class IA (e.g., quinidine, procainamide) or Class III (e.g., amiodarone, sotalol) antiarrhythmic agents, due to the lack of clinical experience with the drug in these patient populations and the potential risk.

Sotalol, a Class III antiarrhythmic, has been shown to increase the QTc interval when combined with high doses of intravenous AVELOX in dogs.

Pharmacokinetic studies between moxifloxacin hydrochloride and other drugs that prolong the QT interval such as cisapride, erythromycin, antipsychotics and tricyclic antidepressants have not been performed. An additive effect of AVELOX and these drugs cannot be excluded, therefore AVELOX should be used with caution when given concurrently with these drugs.

The effect of AVELOX on patients with congenital prolongation of the QT interval has not been studied, but it is expected that these individuals may be more susceptible to drug-induced QT prolongation. AVELOX should be used with caution in patients with ongoing proarrhythmic conditions such as clinically significant bradycardia, acute myocardial ischemia, clinically relevant heart failure with reduced left-ventricular ejection fraction or previous history of symptomatic arrhythmias.

The magnitude of QT prolongation may increase with the infusion rate and with increasing plasma concentrations of the drug. Therefore, the recommended duration of infusion (60 minutes) should not be shortened and the recommended dose should not be exceeded (see Dosage and Administration).

QT prolongation may lead to an increased risk for ventricular arrhythmias including Torsades de Pointes. It has been observed with drugs that prolong the QT interval (including moxifloxacin) that females may be at greater risk compared to males for developing Torsades de Pointes because women tend to have a longer baseline QT interval compared to men. Elderly patients may also be more susceptible to drug-associated effects on the QT interval.

In 787 patients with paired valid ECGs in Phase III clinical trials, the mean±SD prolongation of the QTc interval after **oral** dosing with AVELOX 400 mg was 6±26 msec. In patients with paired valid ECGs in Phase III clinical trials, the mean±SD prolongation of the QTc interval within 0-4 hours after a one hour **infusion** of intravenous moxifloxacin hydrochloride 400 mg was 9±24 msec (Day 1; n=176) and 3±29 msec (Day 3; n=290) (see Action and Clinical Pharmacology).

No cardiovascular morbidity or mortality attributable to QTc prolongation occurred with AVELOX treatment in clinical trials involving over 4000 patients. However, certain predisposing conditions may increase the risk for ventricular arrhythmias.

When intravenous therapy is initiated, patients should be appropriately monitored. If signs of cardiac arrhythmia occur during treatment with AVELOX, treatment should be stopped and an ECG should be performed.

Moxifloxacin should be used with caution in patients with liver cirrhosis as pre-existing QT prolongation in these patients cannot be excluded.

To assure safe and effective use of AVELOX, patients should be advised of the following information and instructions when appropriate:
- that AVELOX may produce changes in the electrocardiogram (QTc interval prolongation)
- that AVELOX should be avoided if they are currently receiving Class IA (e.g., quinidine, procainamide) or Class III (e.g., amiodarone, sotalol) antiarrhythmic agents
- that AVELOX may add to the QTc prolonging effects of other drugs such as cisapride, erythromycin, antipsychotics and tricyclic antidepressants
- to inform their physician of any personal or family history of QTc prolongation or proarrhythmic conditions such as recent hypokalemia, significant bradycardia, acute myocardial ischemia, clinically relevant heart failure with reduced left-ventricular ejection fraction or previous history of symptomatic arrhythmias
- to contact their physician if they experience palpitations or fainting spells while taking AVELOX
- to inform their physician of any other medications being taken concurrently with AVELOX, including over-the-counter medications.

Atrial Fibrillation: Twenty-five patients from the moxifloxacin hydrochloride clinical datapool (7284 patients) had an episode of atrial fibrillation. In 4 of these patients the relationship between the event and moxifloxacin hydrochloride therapy was assessed as possible, though in each case it could also be explained by pre-existing cardiac disease. There was one episode of atrial fibrillation observed in patients who received a comparator agent (3994 patients).

Chondrotoxic Effects: As with other members of the quinolone class, moxifloxacin has caused arthropathy and/or chondrodysplasia in immature dogs. The significance of these findings to humans is unknown (see Action and Clinical Pharmacology).

Gastrointestinal: *C. difficile*-Associated Disease: *C. difficile*-associated disease (CDAD) has been reported with use of many antibacterial agents, including moxifloxacin (see Adverse Reactions). CDAD may range in severity from mild diarrhea to fatal colitis. It is important to consider this diagnosis in patients who present with diarrhea or symptoms of colitis, pseudomembranous colitis, toxic megacolon, or perforation of the colon subsequent to the administration of any antibacterial agent. CDAD has been reported to occur over 2 months after the administration of antibacterial agents.

Treatment with antibacterial agents may alter the normal flora of the colon and may permit overgrowth of *C. difficile. C. difficile* produces toxins A and B, which contribute to the development of CDAD. CDAD may cause significant morbidity and mortality. CDAD can be refractory to antimicrobial therapy.

If the diagnosis of CDAD is suspected or confirmed, appropriate therapeutic measures should be initiated. Mild cases of CDAD usually respond to discontinuation of antibacterial agents not directed against *C. difficile*. In moderate to severe cases, consideration should be given to management with fluids and electrolytes, protein supplementation, and treatment with an antibacterial agent clinically effective against *C. difficile*. Surgical evaluation should be instituted as clinically indicated since surgical intervention may be required in certain severe cases.

Hepatic/Biliary/Pancreatic: In 400 mg single dose studies in 6 patients with mild (Child Pugh Class A) and 10 patients with moderate (Child Pugh Class B) hepatic insufficiency, oral moxifloxacin mean systemic exposure (AUC) was 78% and 102%, respectively, of that in 18 healthy controls and mean peak concentration (C_{max}) was 79% and 84% of that in controls. The clinical significance of increased exposure to the sulfate and glucuronide conjugates has not been studied. No dosage adjustment is recommended for patients with mild or moderate hepatic insufficiency (Child Pugh Classes A and B). Due to limited clinical data, the use of moxifloxacin is not recommended for patients with severe hepatic insufficiency (Child Pugh Class C) (see Action and Clinical Pharmacology and Dosage and Administration).

Cases of fulminant hepatitis potentially leading to liver failure (including fatal cases) have been reported with moxifloxacin. Patients should be advised to discontinue treatment and contact their doctor immediately if they develop signs and symptoms of hepatitis (including abdominal pain, anorexia, jaundice, dark urine, pale stools, pruritus).

Hypersensitivity: Serious hypersensitivity and/or anaphylactic reactions have been reported in patients receiving quinolone therapy, including AVELOX.

There have been occasional reports of fatal hypersensitivity and/or anaphylactic reactions observed with quinolone therapy. These reactions may occur following the first dose. Some reactions have been accompanied by cardiovascular collapse, hypotension/shock, seizure, loss of consciousness, tingling, angioedema (including tongue, laryngeal, throat or facial edema/swelling), airway obstruction (including bronchospasm, shortness of breath and acute respiratory distress), dyspnea, urticaria, itching and other serious skin reactions.

AVELOX should be discontinued at the first appearance of a skin rash or any other sign of hypersensitivity. Serious acute hypersensitivity reactions may require treatment with epinephrine and other resuscitative measures, including oxygen, intravenous fluids, antihistamines, corticosteroids, pressor amines and airway management, as clinically indicated.

Serious and sometimes fatal events, some due to hypersensitivity and some due to uncertain etiology, have been reported in patients receiving therapy with all antibiotics, including moxifloxacin. These events may be severe and generally occur following the administration of multiple doses. Clinical manifestations may include one or more of the following: fever, rash or severe dermatologic reactions (e.g., toxic epidermal necrolysis, Stevens-Johnson Syndrome), vasculitis, arthralgia, myalgia, serum sickness, allergic pneumonitis, interstitial nephritis, acute renal insufficiency or failure, hepatitis, jaundice, acute hepatic necrosis or failure, anemia including hemolytic and aplastic, thrombocytopenia including thrombotic thrombocytopenic purpura, leukopenia, agranulocytosis, pancytopenia, and/or other hematologic abnormalities (see Contraindications and Adverse Reactions).

Musculoskeletal: Rupture of the shoulder, hand, and Achilles tendons that required surgical repair or resulted in prolonged disability have been reported in patients receiving quinolones, including AVELOX. AVELOX should be discontinued if the patient experiences pain, inflammation or rupture of a tendon. Patients should rest and refrain from exercise until the diagnosis of tendinitis or tendon rupture has been confidently excluded. The risk of developing fluoroquinolone-associated tendinitis and tendon rupture is further increased in older patients usually over 60 years of age, in patients taking corticosteroid drugs, and in patients with kidney, heart, or lung transplants. Factors, in addition to age and corticosteroid use, that may independently increase the risk of tendon rupture include strenuous physical activity, renal failure, and previous tendon disorders such as rheumatoid arthritis. Tendinitis and tendon rupture have also occurred in patients taking fluoroquinolones who do not have the above risk factors. Tendon rupture can occur during or after completion of therapy; cases occurring up to several months after completion of therapy have been reported. AVELOX should be discontinued if the patient experiences pain, swelling, inflammation, or rupture of a tendon. Patients should be advised to rest at the first sign of tendinitis or tendon rupture and to contact their healthcare provider regarding changing to a non quinolone antimicrobial drug.

Moxifloxacin should not be used in patients with a history of tendon disease/disorder related to previous quinolone treatment.

* Increasing resistance of *B. fragilis* to fluoroquinolones including moxifloxacin has been reported.

Neurologic: Convulsions, increased intracranial pressure and toxic psychosis have been reported in patients receiving quinolones. Quinolones, including moxifloxacin, may also cause central nervous system stimulation which may lead to abnormal dreams, agitation, anxiety, confusion, depression, dizziness, emotional lability, hallucinations, insomnia, lightheadedness, nervousness, nightmares, paranoia, restlessness and tremors. These reactions may occur after the first dose. If these reactions occur in patients receiving AVELOX, the drug should be discontinued and appropriate measures instituted.

As with all quinolones, AVELOX should be used with caution in patients with known or suspected CNS disorders, such as severe cerebral arteriosclerosis, epilepsy, and other factors that predispose to seizures or lower the seizure threshold (see Adverse Reactions).

AVELOX should be used with caution in patients with myasthenia gravis because the symptoms can be exacerbated.

Peripheral Neuropathy: Rare cases of sensory or sensorimotor axonal polyneuropathy affecting small and/or large axons resulting in paresthesias, hypoesthesias, dysesthesias and weakness have been reported in patients receiving quinolones.

Renal: The pharmacokinetic parameters of AVELOX are not significantly altered by mild, moderate, or severe renal impairment. No dosage adjustment is necessary in patients with renal impairment, including patients on chronic dialysis, i.e., hemodialysis or continuous ambulatory peritoneal dialysis. In clinical studies, as renal function decreased, mean exposure (AUC) to the glucuronide conjugate (M2) increased by a factor of 2.8 (Cl_{cr}<30 mL/min), 7.5 (hemodialysis) and 13.3 (continuous ambulatory peritoneal dialysis).

The sulfate and glucuronide conjugates are not microbiologically active, and the clinical implication of increased exposure to these metabolites in patients with renal impairment has not been studied (see Action and Clinical Pharmacology and Dosage and Administration).

Skin: Phototoxicity: Phototoxicity has been reported in patients receiving certain quinolones. In keeping with good medical practice, the patient should be advised to avoid excessive sunlight or artificial ultraviolet light (e.g., sunlamps) during treatment with AVELOX and for one day following completion of treatment. If a sunburn-like reaction or skin eruptions occur, the physician should be contacted. A study in human volunteers concluded that AVELOX has no measurable phototoxic potential.

Photocarcinogenicity: Some members of the fluoroquinolone class of drugs (of which AVELOX is a member) have been shown to produce skin tumours in the Hairless (Skh-1) mouse when concomitantly exposed to daily irradiations of UV-A light for 16 weeks. In this model, in the absence of exposure to UV-A light, mice treated with the fluoroquinolone did not develop skin tumours. The clinical significance of these findings, particularly for short term use, is not known. Photocarcinogenicity studies with AVELOX have not yet been carried out. During treatment with AVELOX and for one day following completion of treatment, exposure to excessive sunlight or artificial ultraviolet light (e.g., sunlamps) should be avoided.

Special Populations: The safety and efficacy of AVELOX (moxifloxacin hydrochloride) in children, pregnant women and nursing women have not been established.

Pregnant Women: Adequate and well-controlled studies have not been performed in pregnant women. The extent of exposure in pregnancy is very limited. AVELOX should not be used in pregnant women unless the potential benefits outweigh the potential risk to the fetus.

Moxifloxacin was not teratogenic when administered to pregnant rats during organogenesis at oral doses as high as 500 mg/kg/day or 0.24 times the maximum recommended human dose based on systemic exposure (AUC), but decreased fetal body weights and slightly delayed fetal skeletal development (indicative of fetotoxicity) were observed. Intravenous administration of 80 mg/kg to pregnant rats resulted in maternal toxicity and a marginal effect on fetal and placental weights and the appearance of the placenta. There was no evidence of teratogenicity at intravenous doses as high as 80 mg/kg/day. Intravenous administration of 20 mg/kg/day (approximately equal to the maximum recommended human oral dose based upon systemic exposure) to pregnant rabbits resulted in maternal toxicity, decreased fetal body weights and delayed fetal skeletal ossification. There was no evidence of teratogenicity when pregnant Cynomolgus monkeys were given oral doses as high as 100 mg/kg/day (12.5 times the maximum recommended human dose based upon systemic exposure). An increased incidence of smaller fetuses was observed at 100 mg/kg/day. In an oral pre- and postnatal development study conducted in rats, effects observed at 500 mg/kg/day included slight increases in duration of pregnancy and prenatal loss, reduced pup birth weight and decreased neonatal survival. Treatment-related maternal mortality occurred during gestation at 500 mg/kg/day in this study.

Nursing Women: The safety and efficacy of AVELOX (moxifloxacin hydrochloride) in nursing women have not been established.

AVELOX is excreted in the breast milk of rats and may also be excreted in human milk. Because of the potential for unknown effects from moxifloxacin in infants being nursed by mothers taking moxifloxacin, a decision should be made to either discontinue nursing or discontinue the administration of moxifloxacin, taking into account the importance of moxifloxacin therapy to the mother and the possible risk to the infant.

Pediatrics (<18 years of age): The safety and efficacy of AVELOX in pediatric populations less than 18 years of age have not been established. Quinolones, including AVELOX, cause arthropathy and osteochondrosis in juvenile animals of several species. The significance of these findings to humans is unknown.

Geriatrics (≥65 years of age): In controlled multiple-dose clinical trials with oral moxifloxacin, 23% of patients who received moxifloxacin were ≥65 years of age and 9% were ≥75 years of age. In intravenous multiple-dose trials, 45% of the patients who received intravenous moxifloxacin were ≥65 years of age, and 24% were ≥75 years of age. The clinical trial data demonstrate that there is no significant difference in the safety of moxifloxacin in patients aged 65 or older compared to younger adults (see Action and Clinical Pharmacology and Dosage and Administration).

In the pool of 248 moxifloxacin-treated and 243 comparator-treated elderly (≥65 years) patients enrolled in the two pivotal intravenous trials of community acquired pneumonia, the following ECG abnormalities were reported in moxifloxacin vs. comparator patients: QT prolongation (4 vs. 1), ventricular tachycardia (3 vs. 0), tachycardia (2 vs. 1), atrial fibrillation (1 vs. 0), supraventricular tachycardia (1 vs. 0), ventricular extrasystoles (1 vs. 0), and arrhythmia (0 vs. 1). A majority of these patients completed a full-course of therapy.

Monitoring and Laboratory Tests: There are no reported laboratory test interactions.

When intravenous therapy is initiated, patients should be appropriately monitored. If signs of cardiac arrhythmia occur during treatment with AVELOX, treatment should be stopped and an ECG should be performed (see Warnings and Precautions, Cardiovascular, QT Interval Prolongation).

ADVERSE REACTIONS: Adverse Drug Reaction Overview: Over 8600 courses of AVELOX (moxifloxacin hydrochloride tablets) and AVELOX I.V. (moxifloxacin hydrochloride injection) treatment have been evaluated for drug safety during clinical development. Of these, 8050 patients received the 400 mg dose. Most adverse events reported in trials were described as transient in nature, mild to moderate intensity, and required no additional treatment. AVELOX was discontinued due to adverse drug reactions (those judged by the investigators to be possibly or probably related to AVELOX) in 3.1% of patients (206 out of 6734) treated with moxifloxacin hydrochloride tablets and 7.0% of patients (131 out of 1872) treated with intravenous moxifloxacin hydrochloride.

Clinical Trial Adverse Drug Reactions: Because clinical trials are conducted under very specific conditions the adverse reaction rates observed in the clinical trials may not reflect the rates observed in practice and should not be compared to the rates in the clinical trials of another drug. Adverse drug reaction information from clinical trials is useful for identifying drug-related adverse events and for approximating rates.

The overall rate of adverse drug reactions during clinical trials was 26% (1734/6734) with AVELOX and 26% (483/1872) with AVELOX I.V. The major difference between the oral and intravenous treatment groups relates to local injection site reactions known to be associated with intravenous administration. The common adverse drug reactions seen in clinical trials (those judged by the investigators to be possibly or probably related to moxifloxacin) are summarized in Table 1.

Table 1: AVELOX

Most Common Clinical Trial Adverse Drug Reactions (≥1% to <10%)

	Moxifloxacin Hydrochloride n=8606 %
Body as a Whole	
Abdominal pain	2
Headache	2
Injection site reaction	1
Cardiovascular	
In patients with concomitant hypokalemia: QT interval prolongation	1
Digestive	
Nausea	7
Diarrhea	5
Dyspepsia	1
Vomiting	2
Metabolic	
Liver function test abnormal	1
Nervous	
Dizziness	3

(cont'd)

Less Common Clinical Trial Adverse Drug Reactions: Uncommon adverse drug reactions seen in clinical trials (those judged by the investigators to be possibly or probably related to moxifloxacin) are listed in Table 2 and Table 3.

Table 2: AVELOX

Uncommon Clinical Trial Adverse Drug Reactions (≥0.1% to <1%)

	Moxifloxacin Hydrochloride n=8606
Body as a Whole	asthenia, chest pain, fever, infection, malaise, moniliasis, pain
Cardiovascular	hypertension, palpitation, phlebitis, QT interval prolongation, tachycardia, vasodilatation
Digestive	anorexia, constipation, dry mouth, flatulence, gastrointestinal disorder, GGTP increased, glossitis, nausea and vomiting, oral moniliasis, stomatitis
Hemic and Lymphatic	anemia, eosinophilia, leukopenia, prothrombin/INR decreased, thrombocythemia
Metabolic and Nutritional	amylase increased, lactic dehydrogenase increased (in connection with abnormal liver function tests)
Musculoskeletal	arthralgia, myalgia
Nervous	anxiety, insomnia, nervousness, paresthesia, somnolence, tremor, vertigo
Respiratory	dyspnea, pharyngitis, pneumonia, rhinitis
Skin and Appendages	pruritus, rash, sweating, urticaria
Special Senses	taste perversion
Urogenital	kidney function abnormal, vaginal moniliasis, vaginitis

Table 3: AVELOX

Rare Clinical Trial Adverse Drug Reactions (<0.1%)

	Moxifloxacin Hydrochloride n=8606
Body as a Whole	abdomen enlarged, accidental overdose, aggravation reaction, allergic reaction, back pain, cachexia, cellulitis, chest pain substernal, chills, drug level increased, edema, face edema, hand pain, hernia, infection fungal, inflammation, injection site edema, injection site hypersensitivity, injection site inflammation, injection site pain, lab test abnormal, lack of drug effect, leg pain, multisystem organ failure, neoplasm, overdose, pelvic pain, peritonitis, photosensitivity reaction, reaction unevaluable, sepsis
Cardiovascular	AV block first degree, angina pectoris, atrial fibrillation, cardiovascular disorder, cerebrovascular accident, congestive heart failure, deep thrombophlebitis, electrocardiogram abnormal, heart failure, hemorrhage, hypotension, migraine, myocardial infarct, peripheral edema, peripheral vascular disorder, postural hypotension, shock, supraventricular tachycardia, syncope, thrombophlebitis, vascular headache, ventricular tachycardia, ventricular extrasystoles
Digestive	aphthous stomatitis, cheilitis, cholestatic jaundice, colitis, cholangitis, diarrhea (*C. difficile*), dysphagia, eructation, esophagitis, gastritis, gastroenteritis, gastrointestinal hemorrhage, gastrointestinal moniliasis, gingivitis, hepatic failure, hyperchlorhydria, increased appetite, jaundice (predominantly cholestatic), liver damage, melena, mouth ulceration, pancreatitis, pseudomembranous colitis, salivary gland enlargement, thirst, tongue discoloration, tongue disorder, tongue edema
Endocrine	diabetes mellitus, female lactation
Hemic and Lymphatic	abnormal platelets, coagulation disorder, hypochromic anemia, lymphocytosis, lymphangitis, monocytosis, pancytopenia, prothrombin/INR increased, sedimentation rate increased, thrombocytopenia, thromboplastin decreased
Hypersensitivity	allergic reaction, face edema, urticaria
Metabolic and Nutritional	bilirubinemia, dehydration, enzymatic abnormality, gamma globulins increased, gout, hypercholesteremia, hyperglycemia, hyperlipemia, hyperuricemia, hypoproteinemia, hypophosphatemia, lipase increased, NPN increased, weight gain

(cont'd)

Table 3: AVELOX *(cont'd)*

Rare Clinical Trial Adverse Drug Reactions (<0.1%)

	Moxifloxacin Hydrochloride n=8606
Musculoskeletal	arthritis, arthrosis, leg cramps, myasthenia, tendon disorder
Nervous	abnormal dreams, agitation, amnesia, aphasia, cerebral infarct, circumoral parasthesia, coma, confusion, convulsion, depersonalization, depression, emotional lability, euphoria, grand mal convulsion, hallucinations, hyperkinesia, hypertonia, hypesthesia, hypotonia, incoordination, parasthesia, personality disorder, sleep disorder, speech disorder, thinking abnormal, twitching, vestibular disorder
Respiratory	apnea, asthma, atrophic rhinitis, cough increased, dyspnea, epistaxis, hemoptysis, hiccup, hyperventilation, lung disorder, pleural effusion, respiratory disorder, sinusitis, surgery
Skin and Appendages	acne, dry skin, eczema, fungal dermatitis, herpes simplex, maculopapular rash, psoriasis, purpuric rash, pustular rash, skin disorder, skin ulcer, vesiculobullous rash, Stevens-Johnson syndrome
Special Senses	abnormal vision, amblyopia, blindness, deafness, diplopia, ear pain, eye disorder, hyperacusis, parosmia (including smell perversion, decreased smell and loss of smell), partial permanent deafness, photophobia, taste loss, tinnitus
Urogenital	acute kidney failure, albuminuria, balanitis, cystitis, dysuria, hematuria, hypomenorrhea, kidney function abnormal, kidney pain, leukorrhea, menstrual disorder, polyuria, pyuria, salpingitis, urinary frequency, urinary retention, urinary tract infection, urine abnormality, vulvovaginitis

Abnormal Hematologic and Clinical Chemistry Findings: Changes in laboratory parameters without regard to drug relationship that are not listed above as adverse drug reactions and which occurred in ≥2% of oral moxifloxacin-treated patients in controlled clinical trials (n=4301) are summarized in Table 4.

Table 4: AVELOX

Changes in Laboratory Parameters Seen in Clinical Trials

	Moxifloxacin Hydrochloride n=4301
Increases in:	albumin, alkaline phosphatase, amylase, basophils, bicarbonate, calcium, chloride, cholesterol, creatinine, eosinophils, globulin, glucose, hematocrit, hemoglobin, LDH, lymphocytes, monocytes, neutrophils, PCO_2, phosphorus, platelets, potassium, prothrombin time/INR, RBCs, serum transaminases, sodium, theophylline, total bilirubin, triglycerides, urea, uric acid, WBCs
Decreases in:	albumin, amylase, basophils, bicarbonate, calcium, chloride, creatinine, eosinophils, globulin, glucose, hematocrit, hemoglobin, LDH, lymphocytes, monocytes, neutrophils, phosphorus, platelets, PO_2, potassium, prothrombin time/INR, RBCs, serum transaminases, sodium, theophylline, total bilirubin, urea, uric acid, WBCs

Post-Market Adverse Drug Reactions: The safety of moxifloxacin has been studied in two prospective post-marketing surveillance studies involving nearly 33 000 patients.

Adverse reactions with moxifloxacin based on post-marketing reports (from more than eight million patient treatments) are summarized in Table 5.

Table 5: AVELOX

Adverse Reactions Identified in Post-Marketing Surveillance

Cardiovascular	ventricular tachyarrythmias including Torsades de Pointes and cardiac arrest have been reported especially in patients with severe underlying proarrhythmic conditions in very rare cases (see Warnings and Precautions; Incidence <0.01%)
Hepatic	hepatitis (predominantly cholestatic; Incidence <0.01%)
Hypersensitivity	anaphylactic reaction, shock (anaphylactic), angioedema (including laryngeal edema; potentially life-threatening; Incidence <0.01%)
Musculoskeletal	exacerbation of symptoms of myasthenia gravis, tendon rupture (Incidence <0.01%)
Nervous	psychotic reaction (Incidence <0.01%)

Additional serious adverse events reported with moxifloxacin regardless of drug relationship are listed in Table 6.

Table 6: AVELOX

Serious Adverse Events Reported Regardless of Drug Relationship

Cardiac	atrial arrhythmia, atrial flutter, bradycardia, myocardial infarct (death), tachyarrhythmia, ventricular fibrillation, ventricular tachycardia
Hepatic	cholestatic hepatitis, fulminant hepatitis potentially leading to life-threatening liver failure (including fatal cases), hepatic failure, hepatitis
Hypersensitivity	allergic vasculitis, anaphylactoid reaction, anaphylaxis, tongue edema
Renal	acute kidney failure
Skin and Appendages	toxic epidermal necrolysis (potentially life threatening)

DRUG INTERACTIONS: Overview: AVELOX (moxifloxacin hydrochloride) is metabolized via glucuronide and sulfate conjugation. The cytochrome P450 system is not involved in moxifloxacin metabolism, and is not affected by moxifloxacin. Moxifloxacin is unlikely to alter the pharmacokinetics of drugs metabolized by these enzymes. As with all other quinolones, iron and antacids significantly reduced bioavailability of moxifloxacin. (See Table 7.)

Drug-Drug Interactions: See Table 7.

Table 7: AVELOX

Established or Potential Drug-drug Interactions

Proper Name	Ref	Effect	Clinical Comment
Antacids, Sucralfate, Metal Cations, Multivitamins	CT/T	Quinolones form chelates with alkaline earth and transition metal cations. Administration of quinolones with antacids containing aluminum or magnesium, as well as sucralfate, metal cations such as iron, and multivitamins containing iron or zinc, and formulations containing divalent and trivalent cations such as didanosine chewable/buffered tablets or the pediatric powder for oral solution, may substantially interfere with the absorption of quinolones, resulting in systemic concentrations considerably lower than desired.	AVELOX should be taken at least 4 hours before or 8 hours after these agents (see Dosage and Administration).
Ranitidine	CT	Concomitant administration with ranitidine does not change the absorption characteristics of moxifloxacin. Absorption parameters (C_{max}, t_{max}, AUC) are comparable indicating absence of an influence of gastric pH on moxifloxacin uptake from the GI-tract.	No clinically relevant interactions.
Nonsteroidal anti-inflammatory drugs (NSAIDs)	T	Although not observed with moxifloxacin in preclinical and clinical trials, some quinolones have been reported to have proconvulsant activity that is exacerbated with concomitant use of non-steroidal anti-inflammatory drugs (NSAIDs).	Concomitant administration of a nonsteroidal anti-inflammatory drug with a quinolone may increase the risks of CNS stimulation and convulsions.
Calcium supplements	CT	When moxifloxacin is given with high dose calcium supplements, only a slightly reduced rate of absorption is observed while the extent of absorption remains unaffected.	No clinically relevant interactions.
Warfarin	CT	**Changes in INR:** Cases of increased anticoagulant activity have been reported in patients receiving oral anticoagulants concurrently with antibiotics, including moxifloxacin. The infectious disease (and its accompanying inflammatory process), age and general status of the patient are risk factors.	Although an interaction between moxifloxacin and warfarin was not demonstrated in clinical trials, INR monitoring should be performed, and if necessary, the oral anticoagulant dosage should be adjusted as appropriate.
Drugs metabolized by Cytochrome P450 enzymes (e.g., midazolam, cyclosporine, warfarin, theophylline)	CT/T	In vitro studies with cytochrome P450 isoenzymes (CYP) indicate that moxifloxacin does not inhibit CYP3A4, CYP2D6, CYP2C9, CYP2C19, or CYP1A2, suggesting that moxifloxacin is unlikely to alter the pharmacokinetics of drugs metabolized by these enzymes.	No clinically relevant interactions.
Antidiabetic agents	CT/T	Disturbances of blood glucose, including symptomatic hyper- and hypoglycemia, have been reported with quinolones, including moxifloxacin, usually in diabetic patients receiving concomitant treatment with an oral hypoglycemic agent (e.g., glyburide/glibenclamide, etc.) of with insulin.	In diabetic patients, careful monitoring of blood glucose is recommended. If a hypoglycemic reaction occurs in a patient receiving moxifloxacin, discontinue the drug immediately and an appropriate therapy should be instituted (see Adverse Reactions).
Oral contraceptives	CT	No interaction has occurred following concomitant oral administration of moxifloxacin with oral contraceptives.	No clinically relevant interactions.
Itraconazole	CT	Exposure (AUC) to itraconazole is only marginally altered under concomitant moxifloxacin treatment. Pharmacokinetics of moxifloxacin are not significantly altered by itraconazole.	No clinically relevant interactions.
Digoxin	CT	The pharmacokinetics of digoxin are not significantly influenced by moxifloxacin and vice versa. After repeated dosing in healthy volunteers, moxifloxacin increased C_{max} of digoxin by approximately 30% at steady state without affecting AUC or trough levels.	No clinically relevant interactions.
Morphine	CT	Parenteral administration of morphine does not reduce the oral availability of moxifloxacin and only slightly decreases C_{max} (17%).	No clinically relevant interactions.
Atenolol	CT	The pharmacokinetics of atenolol are not significantly altered by moxifloxacin. Following single dose administration in healthy subjects, AUC was marginally increased (by approximately 4%) and peak concentrations were decreased by 10%.	No clinically relevant interactions.
Probenecid	CT	No significant effect on apparent total body clearance and renal clearance of moxifloxacin was found in a clinical study investigating the impact of probenecid on renal excretion.	No clinically relevant interactions.

Legend: C=Case Study; CT=Clinical Trial; T=Theoretical.

Drug-Food Interactions: AVELOX may be taken with or without food.
Drug-Herb Interactions: Interactions with herbal products have not been established.
Drug-Laboratory Test Interactions: There are no reported laboratory test interactions.

DOSAGE AND ADMINISTRATION: Recommended Dose and Dosage Adjustment: The recommended dose for AVELOX (moxifloxacin hydrochloride tablets) and AVELOX I.V. (moxifloxacin hydrochloride injection) is 400 mg once daily for all indications. The duration of therapy and route of administration is dependent upon the type and severity of infection as described in Table 8.

Table 8: AVELOX

Dosage and Administration Information for Approved Indications

Infection[a]	Daily Dose	Route of Administration	Usual Duration
Acute Bacterial Sinusitis	400 mg	PO	7–10 days
Acute Bacterial Exacerbation of Chronic Bronchitis	400 mg	PO	5 days
Community Acquired Pneumonia (Mild/Moderate)	400 mg	PO	10 days
Community Acquired Pneumonia in Hospitalized Patients (Mild/Moderate/Severe)	400 mg	IV/PO	7–14 days
Complicated Intra-abdominal Infections	400 mg	IV/PO	5–14 days
Complicated Skin and Skin Structure Infections in Hospitalized Patients	400 mg	IV/PO	7–21 days

[a] Due to the designated pathogens (see Indications and Clinical Use).

Special Populations: Gender: Clinical trial data indicate that there are no significant differences in moxifloxacin pharmacokinetics between male and female subjects when differences in body weight are taken into consideration. Dosage adjustments based on gender are not necessary (see Action and Clinical Pharmacology).

Geriatrics (≥65 years of age): Clinical trial data demonstrate that there is no significant difference in the safety of moxifloxacin in patients aged 65 or older. Dosage adjustments based on age are not necessary (see Action and Clinical Pharmacology and Warnings and Precautions).

Hepatic Impairment: Based on the pharmacokinetic data, no dosage adjustment is required for patients with mild or moderate hepatic insufficiency (Child Pugh Classes A and B). Due to limited clinical data, the use of moxifloxacin is not recommended in patients with severe hepatic insufficiency (Child Pugh Class C) (see Action and Clinical Pharmacology and Warnings and Precautions).

Renal Impairment: Based on pharmacokinetic data, no dosage adjustment is necessary in renally impaired patients, including patients on chronic dialysis (i.e., hemodialysis or continuous ambulatory peritoneal dialysis). A study in 24 patients with renal impairment found no significant changes in the pharmacokinetic properties of oral moxifloxacin As renal function decreases, concentrations of the glucuronide conjugate (M2) increased by a factor of 2.8 (Cl_{cr}<30 mL/min), 7.5 (hemodialysis) and 13.3 (continuous ambulatory peritoneal dialysis) (see Action and Clinical Pharmacology and Warnings and Precautions).

The clinical implication of increased exposure to the sulfate (M1) and the glucuronide (M2) conjugates of moxifloxacin in renally impaired patients, including those undergoing hemodialysis and continuous ambulatory peritoneal dialysis (HD and CAPD), has not been studied. Clinical efficacy of moxifloxacin treatment in dialysis patients (HD and CAPD) has not been studied.

Administration: Oral Administration: AVELOX (moxifloxacin hydrochloride) is administered orally, independent of meals. The tablets are swallowed whole. Patients should be advised to drink fluids liberally and take moxifloxacin at least 4 hours before or 8 hours after antacids containing magnesium or aluminium, or multivitamins containing iron or zinc. Do not crush or chew the tablets. Swallow each tablet whole with a drink of water.

Intravenous Administration: AVELOX I.V. (moxifloxacin hydrochloride injection) should be administered over a period of 60 minutes by direct infusion or through a Y-type intravenous infusion set which may already be in place. Slow infusion into a large vein will minimize patient discomfort and reduce the risk of venous irritation. Rapid or bolus intravenous infusion must be avoided. It is not intended for intramuscular, intrathecal, intraperitoneal or subcutaneous administration. The recommended dose is 400 mg once daily for Community Acquired Pneumonia and Complicated Intra-abdominal Infections. The recommended duration of infusion should not be shortened and the recommended dose should not be exceeded (see Warnings and Precautions).

Sequential IV/PO Therapy: When switching from intravenous to oral dosage administration, no dosage adjustment is necessary. Patients whose therapy is initiated with AVELOX I.V. may be switched to AVELOX tablets when clinically indicated at the discretion of the physician.

As with all parenteral products, the intravenous mixture should be inspected visually for clarity, discolouration, particulate matter, precipitate and leakage prior to administration. Solutions showing haziness, particulate matter, precipitate, discolouration or leakage should not be used.

Since the premixed minibags are for single-use only, any unused portion should be discarded.

Since only limited data are available on the compatibility of moxifloxacin intravenous injection with other intravenous substances, additives or other medications should not be added to AVELOX I.V. or infused simultaneously through the same intravenous line. If the same intravenous line is used for sequential infusion of other drugs, the line should be flushed before and after infusion of AVELOX I.V. with an infusion solution compatible with AVELOX I.V. as well as with other drug(s) administered via this common line.

AVELOX I.V. is compatible with the following intravenous solutions at ratios from 1:10 to 10:1: 0.9% Sodium Chloride Injection, USP; 1M Sodium Chloride Injection; 5% Dextrose Injection, USP; Sterile Water for Injection, USP; 10% Dextrose for Injection, USP; Lactated Ringer's for Injection.

If the Y-type or "piggyback" method of administration is used, it is advisable to discontinue temporarily the administration of any other solutions during the infusion of AVELOX I.V.

Missed Dose: If a dose is missed, another should be taken as soon as possible. Continue with the next dose 24 hours later. Two doses should not be taken in any 24-hour period.

Reconstitution: Not applicable.

OVERDOSAGE:
In the event of acute overdosage of AVELOX (moxifloxacin hydrochloride), the stomach should be emptied. ECG monitoring is recommended due to the possible prolongation of the QT interval. The patient should be carefully observed and given supportive treatment. Adequate hydration must be maintained. Moxifloxacin and the glucuronide conjugate (M2) are removed from the body by hemodialysis (approximately 9% and 4%, respectively, 5 hour dialysis sessions) and by continuous ambulatory peritoneal dialysis (approximately 3% and 2%, respectively).

The administration of activated charcoal as soon as possible after oral overdose may prevent excessive increase of systemic moxifloxacin exposure.

Toxic signs after administration of a single high dose of moxifloxacin in animals included CNS and gastrointestinal effects (see Warnings and Precautions).

For management of a suspected drug overdose, contact your **regional Poison Control Centre**. See the *CPS* Directory section for a list of Poison Control Centres.

ACTION AND CLINICAL PHARMACOLOGY: Mechanism of Action: AVELOX (moxifloxacin hydrochloride) is a synthetic fluoroquinolone with a broad spectrum of activity and a bactericidal mode of action. The bactericidal action results from the interference of moxifloxacin with bacterial topoisomerases II (DNA gyrase) and IV. Topoisomerases are essential enzymes which control DNA topology and assist in DNA replication, repair and transcription.

Killing curves demonstrated that moxifloxacin exhibits a concentration dependent bactericidal effect. Minimum bactericidal concentrations are in the range of minimum inhibitory concentrations.

Fluoroquinolones, including moxifloxacin, differ in chemical structure and mechanism of action from macrolides, beta-lactams, aminoglycosides, or tetracyclines; therefore, microorganisms resistant to these classes of drugs may be susceptible to moxifloxacin. Conversely, microorganisms resistant to fluoroquinolones may be susceptible to other classes of antimicrobial agents. Although cross-resistance has been observed between moxifloxacin and other fluoroquinolones against Gram negative bacteria, Gram positive bacteria resistant to other fluoroquinolones may be susceptible to moxifloxacin. Conversely, Gram positive bacteria that are resistant to moxifloxacin may be susceptible to other fluoroquinolones.

Pharmacodynamics: Resistance: Resistance mechanisms which inactivate penicillins, cephalosporins, aminoglycosides, macrolides and tetracyclines do not interfere with the antibacterial activity of moxifloxacin. There is no cross-resistance between moxifloxacin and these agents. Plasmid-mediated resistance has not been observed to date.

It appears that the C8-methoxy moiety contributes to enhanced activity and lower selection of resistant mutants of Gram-positive bacteria compared to the C8-H moiety. The presence of the bulky bicycloamine substituent at the C-7 position prevents active efflux, a proposed mechanism of fluoroquinolone resistance.

In vitro resistance to moxifloxacin develops slowly via multiple-step mutations. Resistance to moxifloxacin occurs in vitro at a general frequency of between 1.8×10^{-9} to $<1\times10^{-11}$ in one strain of *S. aureus* and one strain of *S. pneumoniae*.

Effect on the Intestinal Flora: Treatment with antibacterial agents alters the normal flora of the colon and may permit overgrowth of clostridia.

Pharmacokinetics: Pharmacokinetics are linear in the range of 50-800 mg (single dose) and up to 600 mg (once daily oral dosing over 10 days).

The mean (±SD) C_{max} and AUC values at steady-state with a 400 mg oral once daily dosage regimen are 4.5±0.53 g/L and 48±2.7 mg·h/L, respectively. C_{max} is attained 1 to 3 hours after oral dosing. The mean (±SD) trough concentration is 0.95±0.10 mg/L. The mean (±SD) C_{max} and AUC values at steady-state with a once daily dosage regimen of 400 mg intravenous moxifloxacin hydrochloride infused over 60 minutes in healthy young males are 4.2±0.8 g/L and 38±4.7 mg·h/L, respectively. C_{max} is achieved at the end of a 60 minute infusion (see Dosage and Administration).

Plasma concentrations increase proportionately with dose up to the highest dose tested (1200 mg single oral dose). Moxifloxacin hydrochloride is eliminated from plasma by first-order process. The mean (±SD) elimination half-life from plasma is 12±1.3 hours; steady-state is achieved after at least three days with a 400 mg once daily regimen. The time course of plasma concentrations of moxifloxacin hydrochloride following steady-state oral and intravenous administration is illustrated in Figure 1, and pharmacokinetic parameters of moxifloxacin hydrochloride are presented in Table 9.

Figure 1: Avelox

Mean Steady-state Plasma Concentrations of Moxifloxacin Obtained with Once Daily Dosing of 400 mg Either Orally (n=10 males) or by I.V. Infusion (n=12 elderly males and females)

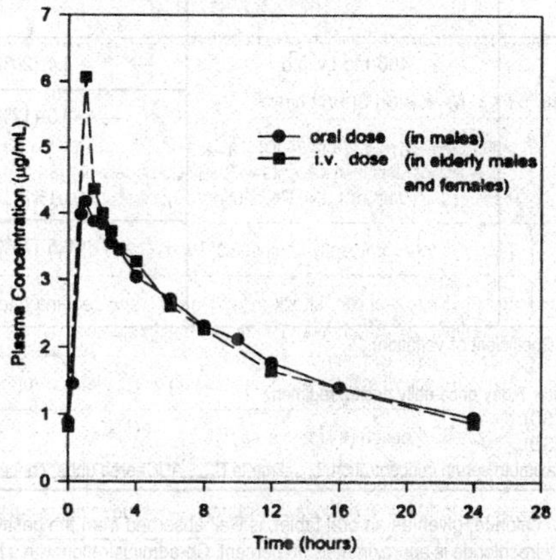

Table 9: AVELOX

Pharmacokinetic Parameters of Moxifloxacin After Oral and Intravenous Administration of 400 mg Single or Multiple Doses

Population Years (range)	Dose	C_{max} (CV)[a] mg/L	AUC (CV)[a] mg·h/L	t_{max}[b] (range) h	$t_{1/2}$ (CV)[a] h	Comment
Single Dose Studies—Oral Administration						
38 males (23–45)	400 mg	2.50 (27%)	26.9 (17%)	1.5 (0.5–2.6)	13.1 (6%)	
18 males (20–25)	400 mg	4.13 (27%)	51.5 (10%)	1.75 (0.5–2.5)	13.9 (10%)	
Single Dose Studies—Intravenous Administration						
6 males (19–43)	400 mg	4.6 (33%)	36.9 (19%)	N/A	13.4 (17%)	30 min. infusion
6 males (24–44)	400 mg	4.5 (25%)	34.0 (22%)	0.5	11.9 (10%)	30 min. infusion
12 males (20–44)	400 mg	4.3 (21%)	42.9 (11%)	0.5	13.5 (20%)	33 min. infusion
12 males (23–41)	400 mg	3.6 (28%)	34.6 (19%)	1.0 (1.0–1.25)	15.4 (16%)	60 min. infusion

(cont'd)

Table 9: AVELOX *(cont'd)*

Pharmacokinetic Parameters of Moxifloxacin After Oral and Intravenous Administration of 400 mg Single or Multiple Doses

Population Years (range)	Dose	C_{max} (CV)[a] mg/L	AUC (CV)[a] mg·h/L	t_{max}[b] (range) h	$t_{1/2}$ (CV)[a] h	Comment
9 males, 11 females (19–32)	400 mg	4.6 (18%)	46.3 (18%)	1.0 (0.5–1.3)	12.4 (10%)	60 min. infusion
13 males (24–36)	400 mg	3.6 (20%)	39.8 (14%)	1.0 (0.55–1.5)	14.1 (17%)	60 min. infusion
7 males (25–41)	400 mg	5.0 (22%)	44.7 (19%)	1.0 (0.5–1.0)	8.0 (18%)	60 min. infusion
Multiple Dose Studies						
8 males (22–43)	400 mg o.d./p.o.×5 days	3.10 (29%)	30.9 (11%)	0.5 (0.5–4.0)	9.6 (11%)	Day 1
		3.24 (17%)	33.9 (20%)	1.5 (0.5–3.0)	15.1 (5%)	Day 5
10 males 5 females (19–41)	400 mg o.d./ p.o.×10 days	3.4 (22%)	36.7 (13%)	1.8 (0.75–3.0)	9.3 (12%)	Day 1
		4.5 (12%)	48.0 (6%)	1.0 (0.75–2.5)	12.7 (15%)	Day 10
9 males (20–40)	400 mg o.d.	4.1 (39%)	40.9 (10%)	1.0 (0.5–2.5)	10.7 (16%)	Day 1
		4.1 (28%)	46.7 (15%)	1.8 (0.5–3.0)	14.0 (15%)	Day 7
9 males (23–38)	400 mg i.v.	6.6 (30%)	36.3 (11%)	0.25	9.3 (17%)	Day 1; 15 min. infusion
11 males, 7 females (65–75)	400 mg i.v.	6.6 (27%)	38.6 (21%)	0.26	8.6 (15%)	Day 1; 15 min. infusion
		5.9 (21%)	47.4 (20%)	1.0	10.1 (16%)	Day 5; 60 min. infusion
12 male (25–42); 8 active, 4 placebo	400 mg i.v.	3.6 (20%)	34.8 (11%)	1.0	9.9 (15%)	Day 1; 60 min. infusion
		4.1 (20%)	37.8 (11%)	1.0	14.7 (16%)	Day 10; 60 min. infusion
32 (23–74) 20 males and 12 females; varying degrees of renal function	400 mg p.o.	4.4 (34%)	43.4 (31%)	0.8 (0.5–1.5)	14.9 (38%)	Cl_{cr} >90 mL/min
		4.9 (30%)	40.1 (22%)	0.3 (0.3–2.5)	15.2 (15%)	Cl_{cr} >60–90 mL/min
		3.5 (41%)	35.8 (30%)	0.8 (0.5–2.5)	16.2 (15%)	Cl_{cr} >30–60 mL/min
		3.2 (14%)	43.9 (29%)	1.5 (0.5–2.5)	14.5 (19%)	Cl_{cr} <30 mL/min
16 (22–62) 12 males, 4 females; 8 HD, 8 CAPD	400 mg p.o.	3.2 (23%)[c]	40.4 (29%)[c,d]	3.0 (1.0–4.0)[c]	18.7 (25%)[c]	Cl_{cr} <20 mL/min and on HD
		4.0 (18%)[c]	49.6 (25%)[c,d]	2.5 (0.9–4.2)[c]	11.4 (23%)[c]	Cl_{cr} <20 mL/min and on CAPD
18 males (30–64) 10 healthy, 8 with hepatic disease	400 mg p.o.	3.0 (26%)	32.8 (26%)	0.8 (0.5–3.0)	13.4 (18%)	healthy volunteers
		2.5 (34%)	25.1 (26%)	0.5 (0.5–2.5)	11.7 (26%)	patients with hepatic disease, Child Pugh Class A and B
16 males (42–64) 8 healthy, 8 with hepatic disease	400 mg p.o.	3.3 (1.4)[e]	30.8 (1.3)[e]	1.5 (0.5–3.0)	11.6 (1.1)[e]	healthy volunteers
		2.6 (1.2)[e]	34.6 (1.2)[e]	1.25 (0.5–2.5)	13.6 (1.2)[e]	patients with hepatic disease, Child Pugh Class B
9 healthy males (23–45)	400 mg i.v./p.o.	3.4 (20%)	35.5 (14%)	1.0 (0.75–1.5)	11.6 (10%)	i.v. alone; 60 min. infusion
		3.0 (12%)	28.5 (12%)	1.0 (0.5–1.5)	11.8 (6%)	i.v. plus 5 g charcoal 5 minutes prior to infusion; immediately after infusion and 2, 4, 8 hours post-infusion; 60 min. infusion
		0.6 (73%)	5.4 (65%)	0.75 (0.5–1.25)	10.8 (11%)	p.o. plus 10 g charcoal 15 minutes before, 2, 4, 8 hours after dosing

[a] Values are geometric means (Coefficient of Variation).
[b] Median (range).
[c] Pharmacokinetic values are after 7 day once-daily dosing regimen.
[d] Values are geometric means (SD).
[e] Values are geometric means (SD).
Legend: o.d.=once daily; C_{max}=maximum serum concentration; t_{max}=time to C_{max}; AUC=area under concentration vs. time curve; $t_{1/2}$=serum half-life; Cl_{cr}=creatinine clearance; HD=hemodialysis; CAPD=Continuous Ambulatory Peritoneal Dialysis.

Absorption: Moxifloxacin hydrochloride, given as an oral tablet, is well absorbed from the gastrointestinal tract. The absolute bioavailability of moxifloxacin hydrochloride is approximately 90 percent. Co-administration with a high fat meal (i.e., 500 calories from fat) does not affect absorption of moxifloxacin hydrochloride.

Consumption of one cup of yogurt with moxifloxacin does not significantly affect the extent or rate of systemic absorption (AUC).

Distribution: Moxifloxacin hydrochloride is approximately 50% bound to serum proteins, independent of drug concentration. As shown in Table 10, the volume of distribution of moxifloxacin hydrochloride ranges from 1.7 to 2.7 L/kg. Moxifloxacin hydrochloride is widely distributed throughout the body, with tissue concentrations often exceeding plasma concentrations. Moxifloxacin has been detected in the saliva, nasal and bronchial secretions, mucosa of the sinuses, and abdominal tissues and fluids following oral or intravenous administration of 400 mg. Moxifloxacin concentrations measured post dose in various tissues and fluids following a 400 mg oral or I.V. dose are summarized in Table 10. The rates of elimination of moxifloxacin from tissues generally parallel the elimination from plasma.

In animal experiments, radiolabelled moxifloxacin hydrochloride was shown to cross the blood-brain barrier only to a small extent.

Metabolism: Moxifloxacin is metabolized via glucuronide and sulfate conjugation. The cytochrome P450 system is not involved in moxifloxacin metabolism, and is not affected by moxifloxacin. The sulfate conjugate (M1) accounts for approximately 38% of the dose, and is eliminated primarily in the feces. Approximately 14% of an oral dose is converted to a glucuronide conjugate (M2), which is found exclusively in the urine. Peak plasma concentrations of M2 are approximately 40% those of the parent drug, while plasma concentrations of M1 are generally less than 10% those of moxifloxacin. The sulfate (M1) and glucuronide (M2) conjugates are not microbiologically active.

Excretion: Approximately 45% of an oral dose of moxifloxacin is excreted as unchanged drug (~20% in urine and ~25% in feces). A total of 96%±4% of an oral dose is excreted as either unchanged drug or known metabolites. The mean (±SD) apparent total body clearance and renal clearance are 12±2.0 L/hr and 2.6±0.5 L/hr, respectively.

Special Populations and Conditions: Pediatrics (<18 years of age): The pharmacokinetics of moxifloxacin in pediatric subjects have not been studied.

Geriatrics (≥65 years of age): Following oral administration of 400 mg moxifloxacin for 10 days in 16 elderly (8 male; 8 female) and 16 young (8 male; 8 female) healthy volunteers, there were no age-related changes in moxifloxacin pharmacokinetics. In 16 healthy male volunteers (8 young; 8 elderly) given a single 200 mg oral dose of moxifloxacin, the extent of systemic exposure (AUC and C_{max}) was not statistically different between young and elderly males and elimination half-life was unchanged. No dosage adjustment is necessary based on age.

In Phase I studies, the pharmacokinetics in elderly patients following infusion of 400 mg were similar to those observed in young patients.

Gender: Following oral administration of 400 mg moxifloxacin daily for 10 days to 23 healthy males (19-75 years) and 24 healthy females (19-70 years), the mean AUC and C_{max} were 8% and 16% higher, respectively, in females compared to males. There are no significant differences in moxifloxacin pharmacokinetics between male and female subjects when differences in body weight are taken into consideration.

A 400 mg single dose study was conducted in 18 young males and females. The comparison of moxifloxacin pharmacokinetics in this study (9 young females and 9 young males) showed no differences in AUC or C_{max} due to gender. Dosage adjustments based on gender are not necessary.

Race: Steady state moxifloxacin pharmacokinetics in male Japanese subjects were similar to those determined in Caucasians, with a mean C_{max} of 4.1 mg/L, an AUC_{24} of 47 mg·h/mL, and an elimination half-life of 14 hours following 400 mg daily PO.

Hepatic Insufficiency: In 400 mg single oral dose studies in 6 patients with mild, (Child Pugh Class A) and 10 patients with moderate (Child Pugh Class B) hepatic insufficiency, moxifloxacin mean systemic exposure (AUC) was 78% and 102%, respectively, of that in 18 healthy controls. The mean peak concentration (C_{max}) was 79% and 84%, respectively, of control values.

The mean AUC of the sulfate conjugate of moxifloxacin (M1) increased by 3.9-fold (ranging up to 5.9-fold) and 5.7-fold (ranging up to 8.0-fold) in the mild and moderate groups, respectively. The mean C_{max} of M1 increased by approximately 3-fold in both groups (ranging up to 4.7- and 3.9-fold), respectively. The mean AUC of the glucuronide conjugate of moxifloxacin (M2) increased by 1.5-fold (ranging up to 2.5-fold) in both groups. The mean C_{max} of M2 increased by 1.6- and 1.3-fold (ranging up to 2.7- and 2.1-fold), respectively. The clinical significance of increased exposure to the sulfate and glucuronide conjugates has not been studied. No dosage adjustment is recommended for mild or moderate hepatic insufficiency (Child Pugh Classes A and B). Due to limited clinical data, the use of moxifloxacin is not recommended with severe hepatic insufficiency (Child Pugh Class C) (see Warnings and Precautions and Dosage and Administration).

Renal Insufficiency: The pharmacokinetic parameters of moxifloxacin are not significantly altered by mild, moderate, or severe renal impairment. No dosage adjustment is necessary in patients with renal impairment, including those patients on hemodialysis (HD) or continuous ambulatory peritoneal dialysis (CAPD).

In a single oral dose study of 24 patients with varying degrees of renal function from normal to severely impaired, the mean peak concentrations (C_{max}) of moxifloxacin were reduced by 22% and 21% in the patients with moderate (Cl_{cr}≥30 and ≤60 mL/min) and severe (Cl_{cr}<30 mL/min) renal impairment, respectively. The mean systemic exposure (AUC) in these patients was increased by 13%. In the moderate and severe renally impaired patients, the mean AUC for the sulfate conjugate (M1) increased by 1.7-fold (ranging up to 2.8-fold) and mean AUC and C_{max} for the glucuronide conjugate (M2) increased by 2.8-fold (ranging up to 4.8-fold) and 1.4-fold (ranging up to 2.5-fold), respectively. The sulfate and glucuronide conjugates are not microbiologically active, and the clinical implication of increased exposure to these metabolites in patients with renal impairment has not been studied.

The pharmacokinetics of single- and multiple-dose moxifloxacin were studied in patients with Cl_{cr}<20 mL/min on either hemodialysis or continuous ambulatory peritoneal dialysis (8 HD, 8 CAPD). Pharmacokinetic comparisons are to historical pharmacokinetic values from healthy volunteers (Cl_{cr}>90 mL/min; administered a single 400 mg oral dose of moxifloxacin). Following a single 400 mg oral dose, the AUC of moxifloxacin in these HD and CAPD patients did not vary significantly from the AUC generally found in healthy volunteers. C_{max} values of moxifloxacin were reduced by about 45% and 33% in HD and CAPD patients, respectively, compared to healthy subjects. The exposure (AUC) to the sulfate conjugate (M1) increased by 1.4- to 1.5-fold in these patients. The mean AUC of the glucuronide conjugate (M2) increased by a factor of 7.3 to 13.2, whereas the mean C_{max} values of the glucuronide conjugate (M2) increased by a factor of 2.5 to 3, compared to healthy subjects. The sulfate and the glucuronide conjugates of moxifloxacin are not microbiologically active, and the clinical implication of increased exposure to these metabolites in patients with renal disease including those undergoing HD and CAPD has not been studied.

Oral administration of 400 mg moxifloxacin once daily for 7 days to patients on HD or CAPD produced mean systemic exposure (AUC_{ss}) to moxifloxacin similar to that generally seen in healthy volunteers. Steady-state C_{max} values were about 28% lower in HD patients but were comparable between CAPD patients and healthy volunteers. Moxifloxacin and the glucuronide conjugate (M2) were removed from the body by HD (approximately 9% and 4%, respectively) and by CAPD (approximately 3% and 2%, respectively). Systemic exposure (AUC) to M2 was equal to or greater than moxifloxacin exposure in HD and CAPD subjects following single dosing and at steady state (see Warnings and Precautions and Dosage and Administration).

QT Prolongation: One pharmacokinetic study in 9 male and 9 female healthy volunteers showed that at the expected time of peak plasma concentrations and at a heart rate of 75 beats/minute, a 400 mg oral dose of moxifloxacin was associated with a mean QT prolongation (uncorrected for heart-rate) of 14±13 msec (3.8%±3.5%) compared to baseline. Exercise data indicated the absence of a reverse-rate dependence.

In clinical pharmacology studies (n=112 subjects), the aggregate mean prolongation of the QTc interval at the expected time of peak plasma concentrations after a single oral dose of 400 mg moxifloxacin was 7±23 msec (1.8%±5.6%). One patient had an increase in QTc greater than 60 msec.

In clinical pharmacology studies (n=29) with 400 mg intravenous moxifloxacin, the aggregate mean prolongation of the QTc interval at the end of a one hour infusion was 20.6±23 msec (5.5%±5.9%). Two patients had an increase in QTc greater than 60 msec (see Warnings and Precautions).

Table 10: AVELOX

Moxifloxacin Concentrations (mean±SD) in Plasma and Tissues After Oral or Intravenous Dosing with 400 mg[a]

Tissue or Fluid	N	Tissue or Fluid Concentration (mg/L or µg/g)	Tissue or Fluid: Plasma Ratio[b]
Respiratory			
Alveolar Macrophages	5	61.8±27.3	21.2±10.0
Bronchial Mucosa	8	5.5±1.3	1.7±0.3
Epithelial Lining Fluid	5	24.4±14.7	8.7±6.1
Sinus[c]			
Maxillary Sinus Mucosa	4	7.6±1.7	2.0±0.3
Anterior Ethmoid Mucosa	3	8.8±4.3	2.2±0.6
Nasal Polyps	4	9.8±4.5	2.6±0.6
Intra-Abdominal			
Abdominal Tissue[d]	8	7.6±2.0	2.7±0.8
Abdominal Exudate[d]	10	3.5±1.25	1.6±0.7
Abscess Fluid	6	2.3±1.5	0.8±0.4
Skin, Musculoskeletal			
Blister Fluid	5	2.6±0.9	0.9±0.2
Subcutaneous Tissue	6	0.9±0.3[e]	0.4±0.6
Skeletal Muscle	6	0.9±0.3[e]	0.4±0.1

[a] Moxifloxacin concentrations were measured 3 hours after a single oral or intravenous 400 mg dose, except as noted.
[b] Tissue or fluid: plasma ratio was determined on an individual patient basis and then averaged for each site of infection.
[c] Sinus concentrations were measured after 5 days of dosing.
[d] Measured 2 hours after dosing.
[e] Reflects only non-protein bound concentrations of drug.

STORAGE AND STABILITY: AVELOX tablets: Store at room temperature (15-30°C). Avoid freezing.
AVELOX I.V. minibags: Store at room temperature (15-30°C). **Do not refrigerate.** Protect from light.
Since the premixed minibags are for single-use only, any unused portion should be discarded.

SPECIAL HANDLING INSTRUCTIONS: Not applicable.

INFORMATION FOR THE PATIENT: Published in e-CPS, available by subscription at www.e-cps.ca.

DOSAGE FORMS, COMPOSITION AND PACKAGING: Injectable: Each premixed, ready-to-use 250 mL minibag contains: moxifloxacin HCl equivalent to 400 mg of moxifloxacin in 0.8% saline, with pH ranging from 4.1 to 4.6. The appearance of the intravenous solution is yellow and is not affected by, or indicative of, product stability. Nonmedicinal ingredients: sodium chloride, USP, and Water for Injection, USP. It may also contain hydrochloric acid and/or sodium hydroxide for pH adjustment. **No further dilution of this product is necessary.**

As with all parenteral products, the intravenous mixture should be inspected visually for clarity, discoloration, particulate matter, precipitate and leakage prior to administration. Solutions showing haziness, particulate matter, precipitate, discolouration or leakage should not be used.

Tablets: Each oblong, dull red film-coated tablet, engraved "BAYER" on one side and "M400" on the other, contains: moxifloxacin HCl equivalent to moxifloxacin 400 mg. Nonmedicinal ingredients: cellulose microcrystalline, croscarmellose sodium, hydroxypropyl methyl cellulose, lactose monohydrate, magnesium stearate, polyethylene glycol 4000, red ferric oxide and titanium dioxide. Bottles of 30.

(Shown in Product Identification Section)

Aviane™ 21 Pr
levonorgestrel—ethinyl estradiol
Oral Contraceptive

Apotex

Aviane™ 28 Pr
levonorgestrel—ethinyl estradiol
Oral Contraceptive

Apotex

Date of Preparation: August 15, 2007
Date of Revision: February 28, 2008

SUMMARY PRODUCT INFORMATION:

Route of Administration	Dosage Form/ Strength	Clinically Relevant Nonmedicinal Ingredients
Oral	Tablet 100 µg levonorgestrel, 20 µg ethinyl estradiol	Lactose For a complete listing see Dosage Forms, Composition and Packaging.

INDICATIONS AND CLINICAL USE: AVIANE 21 and AVIANE 28 (levonorgestrel and ethinyl estradiol) tablets are indicated for:
- conception control
- treatment of moderate acne vulgaris in women ≥14 years of age who have no known contraindications to oral contraceptive therapy, desire contraception, and have achieved menarche.

CONTRAINDICATIONS:
- Hypersensitivity to AVIANE 21 or AVIANE 28 (levonorgestrel/ethinyl estradiol tablets) or to any ingredient in the formulation or component of the container. For a complete listing, see Dosage Forms, Composition and Packaging.
- History of or actual thrombophlebitis or thromboembolic disorders.
- History of or actual cerebrovascular disorders.
- History of or actual myocardial infarction or coronary arterial disease.
- Deep vein thrombosis (current or history).
- Thrombogenic valvulopathies and thrombogenic rhythm disorders.
- Hereditary or acquired thrombophilias.
- Migraine with focal neurological symptoms such as aura (current or history).
- Active liver disease, or history of or actual benign or malignant liver tumors.
- Known or suspected carcinoma of the breast.
- Carcinoma of the endometrium or other known or suspected estrogen-dependent neoplasia.
- Undiagnosed abnormal vaginal bleeding.
- Any ocular lesion arising from ophthalmic vascular disease, such as partial or complete loss of vision or defect in visual fields.
- When pregnancy is suspected or diagnosed.
- Diabetes with vascular involvement.
- Uncontrolled hypertension.

WARNINGS AND PRECAUTIONS:

> **Serious Warnings and Precautions**
> Cigarette smoking increases the risk of serious adverse effects on the heart and blood vessels. This risk increases with age and becomes significant in oral contraceptive-users over 35 years of age. Women who use combination hormonal contraceptives including this product should be counselled not to smoke.
> Women using birth control pills should be counselled that this product (as with other combined hormonal contraceptives) **does not protect** against HIV infection (AIDS) and other sexually transmitted diseases (STDs). For protection against STDs, it is advisable to use latex condoms **in combination with** this product.

General: The following information is provided from studies of combination oral contraceptives (COCs). The use of combination hormonal contraceptives is associated with increased risks of several serious conditions including myocardial infarction, thromboembolism, stroke, hepatic neoplasia and gallbladder disease, although the risk of serious morbidity and mortality is small in healthy women without underlying risk factors. The risk of morbidity and mortality increases significantly if associated with the presence of other risk factors such as hypertension, hyperlipidemias, obesity and diabetes.

The information contained in this section is principally from studies carried out in women who used COCs with higher formulations of estrogens and progestogens than those in common use today. The effect of long-term use of combination hormonal contraceptives with lower doses of both estrogen and progestogen administered orally remains to be determined.

1. **Predisposing Factors for Coronary Artery Disease:** Cigarette smoking increases the risk of serious cardiovascular side effects and mortality from COC use. This risk increases with age and with the extent of smoking. Convincing data are available to support an upper age limit of 35 years for oral contraceptive use in women who smoke.
   Other women who are independently at high risk for cardiovascular disease include those with diabetes, hypertension, abnormal lipid profile, obesity or family history of these. Whether COCs accentuate this risk is unclear.
   In low risk, non-smoking women of any age, the benefits of oral contraceptive use outweigh the possible cardiovascular risks associated with low dose formulations. Consequently, oral contraceptives may be prescribed for these women up to the age of menopause.
2. **Discontinue Medication at the Earliest Manifestation of the Following:**
   a. **Venous and arterial thrombosis and thromboembolism:** Use of COCs is associated with an increased risk of venous and arterial thrombotic and thromboembolic events. For any particular estrogen/progestin combination, the dosage regimen prescribed should be one which contains the least amount of estrogen and progestin that is compatible with a low failure rate and the needs of the individual patient.
   New users of COCs should be started on preparations containing less than 50 µg of estrogen.
   Venous thrombosis and thromboembolism: Use of COCs increases the risk of venous thrombotic and thromboembolic events. Reported events include deep venous thrombosis, thrombophlebitis, pulmonary embolism and mesenteric thrombosis. For information on retinal vascular thrombosis see Ophthalmologic.
   The use of any COCs carries an increased risk of venous thrombotic and thromboembolic events compared with no use. The excess risk is highest during the first year a woman ever uses a COC. This increased risk is less than the risk of venous thrombotic and thromboembolic events associated with pregnancy which is estimated as 60 cases per 100 000 woman-years. Venous thromboembolism is fatal in 1-2% of cases.
   The risk of venous thrombotic and thromboembolic events is further increased in women with conditions predisposing for venous thrombosis and thromboembolism. Caution must be exercised when prescribing COCs for such women.
   Arterial thrombosis and thromboembolism: The use of COCs increases the risk of arterial thrombotic and thromboembolic events. Reported events include myocardial infarction and cerebrovascular events (ischemic and hemorrhagic stroke, transient ischemic attack). For information on retinal vascular thrombosis see Ophthalmologic .
   The risk of arterial thrombotic and thromboembolic event is further increased in women with underlying risk factors. Caution must be exercised when prescribing COCs for women with risk factors for arterial thrombotic and thromboembolic events.
   b. **Conditions that Predispose to Venous Thrombosis and Thromboembolism:** (e.g. obesity, surgery or trauma with increased risk of thrombosis, immobilization after accidents or confinement to bed during long-term illness, recent delivery or second-trimester abortion [see Dosing Considerations, Dosage and Administration]). Other nonhormonal methods of contraception should be used until regular activities are resumed. For use of oral contraceptives when surgery is contemplated, see Peri-Operative Considerations. Examples of risk factors for arterial thrombotic and thromboembolic events are smoking, hypertension, hyperlipidemias, obesity and increasing age.

c. **Visual Defects—Partial or Complete**
d. **Papilledema or Ophthalmic Vascular Lesions**
e. **Severe Headache of Unknown Etiology or Development of new Migraine** (particularly migraine with aura). Women with migraine who take COCs may be at increased risk of stroke.

Carcinogenesis and Mutagenesis: Breasts: A meta-analysis from 54 epidemiological studies reported that there is a slightly increased relative risk (RR=1.24) of having breast cancer diagnosed in women who are currently using COCs compared to never-users. The increased risk gradually disappears during the course of the 10 years after cessation of COC use. These studies do not provide evidence for causation. The observed pattern of increased risk of breast cancer diagnosis may be due to an earlier detection of breast cancer in COC users, the biological effects of COCs or a combination of both. Because breast cancer is rare in women under 40 years of age, the excess number of breast cancer diagnoses in current and recent COC users is small in relation to the lifetime risk of breast cancer. Breast cancers diagnosed in ever-users tend to be less advanced clinically than the cancers diagnosed in never-users.

Increasing age and a strong family history are the most significant risk factors for the development of breast cancer. Other established risk factors include obesity, nulliparity and late age for first full-term pregnancy. The identified groups of women that may be at increased risk of developing breast cancer before menopause are long-term users of COCs (more than eight years) and starters at early age. In a few women, the use of COCs may accelerate the growth of an existing but undiagnosed breast cancer. Since any potential increased risk related to COC use is small, there is no reason to change prescribing habits at present.

Women receiving COCs should be instructed in self-examination of their breasts. Their physicians should be notified whenever any masses are detected. A yearly clinical breast examination is also recommended because, if a breast cancer should develop, drugs that contain estrogen may cause a rapid progression.

Cervix: The most important risk factor for cervical cancer is persistent human papillomavirus infection. Some epidemiological studies suggest that long-term use of COCs may further contribute to this increased risk of cervical intraepithelial neoplasia or invasive cervical cancer. However, there continues to be controversy about the extent to which this finding is attributable to confounding effects, e.g. cervical screening and sexual behaviour including the use of barrier contraceptives. In cases of undiagnosed abnormal genital bleeding, adequate diagnostic measures are indicated.

Cardiovascular: Hypertension: Patients with essential hypertension whose blood pressure is well-controlled may be given oral COCs but only under close supervision. If a significant elevation of blood pressure in previously normotensive or hypertensive subjects occurs at any time during the administration of the drug, cessation of medication is necessary.

Increases in blood pressure have been reported in women taking COCs. Elevated blood pressure associated with COC use will generally return to baseline after stopping COCs, and there appears to be no difference in the occurrence of hypertension among ever- and never- users.

Endocrine and Metabolism: Diabetes: Glucose intolerance has been reported in combined oral contraceptive (COC) users. Current low-dose COCs exert minimal impact on glucose metabolism. Diabetic patients, or those with a family history of diabetes, should be observed closely to detect any worsening of carbohydrate metabolism. Patients predisposed to diabetes who can be kept under close supervision may be given combination hormonal contraceptives. Young diabetic patients whose disease is of recent origin, well-controlled, and not associated with hypertension or other signs of vascular disease such as ocular fundal changes, should be monitored more frequently while using combination hormonal contraceptives.

Lipid Effects: A small proportion of women will have adverse lipid changes while on COCs. Alternative contraception should be considered in women with uncontrolled dyslipidemias. Elevations of plasma triglycerides may lead to pancreatitis and other complications.

Women who are being treated for hyperlipidemias should be followed closely if they elect to use COCs.

Gastrointestinal: Diarrhea and/or vomiting may reduce hormone absorption resulting in decreased serum concentrations.

Genitourinary: Fibroids: Patients with fibroids (leiomyomata) should be carefully observed. Sudden enlargement, pain, or tenderness requires discontinuation of the use of combined oral contraceptives (COC).

Vaginal Bleeding: In some women withdrawal bleeding may not occur during the tablet-free interval. If the COC has not been taken according to directions prior to the first missed withdrawal bleed, or if two consecutive withdrawal bleeds are missed, tablet-taking should be discontinued and a nonhormonal back-up method of contraception should be used, and the possibility of pregnancy should be evaluated.

With all COC, irregular bleeding (breakthrough bleeding or spotting) may occur, especially during the first three months of use. Persistent irregular vaginal bleeding requires assessment to exclude underlying pathology.

Hematologic: See also Contraindications, Warnings and Precautions, General, Cardiovascular, and Peri-Operative Considerations.

Epidemiological studies have shown that the incidence of venous thromboembolism (VTE) in users of oral contraceptives with low estrogen content (<50 µg ethinyl estradiol) ranges from about 20 to 40 cases per 100 000 women-years, but this risk estimate varies according to the progestogen. This compares with 5 to 10 cases per 100 000 women-years for non-users.

The use of any combined oral contraceptive carries an increased risk of venous thromboembolism (VTE) compared with no use. The excess risk of VTE is highest during the first year a woman ever uses a combined oral contraceptive. The increased risk is less than the risk of venous thrombotic and thromboembolic events associated with pregnancy which is estimated as 60 cases per 100 000 women-years. VTE is fatal in 1-2% of cases.

Hepatic/Biliary/Pancreatic: Jaundice: Patients who have had jaundice, including a history of cholestatic jaundice during pregnancy, or a history of COC-related cholestasis, are more likely to have this condition with COC use and, they should be given COCs with great care and under close observation. If these patients receive a COC they should be carefully monitored and, if the condition recurs, the COC should be discontinued.

The development of severe generalized pruritus or icterus requires that the medication be withdrawn until the problem is resolved.

If a patient develops jaundice that proves to be cholestatic in type, the use of oral contraceptives should not be resumed. In patients taking oral contraceptives, changes in the composition of the bile may occur and an increased incidence of gallstones has been reported.

Liver Disorders: Hepatic nodules (adenoma and focal nodular hyperplasia) have been reported, particularly in long-term users of oral contraceptives. Although these lesions are extremely rare, they have caused fatal intra-abdominal hemorrhage and should be considered in women presenting with an abdominal mass, acute abdominal pain, or evidence of intra-abdominal bleeding.

Hepatocellular carcinoma may be associated with COC use. The risk appears to increase with duration of COC use. However, the attributable risk (the excess incidence) of liver cancer in OC users is extremely small.

Neurologic: The onset of a migraine or the development of headache of a new pattern that is recurrent, persistent or severe requires discontinuation of oral contraceptives and evaluation of the cause.

Ophthalmologic: Ocular Disease: Discontinue medication at the earliest manifestation of visual defects (partial or complete) and papilledema or ophthalmic vascular lesions.

Patients who are pregnant or are taking COCs, may experience corneal edema that may cause visual disturbances and changes in tolerance to contact lenses, especially of the rigid type. Soft contact lenses usually do not cause disturbances. If visual changes or alterations in tolerance to contact lenses occur, temporary or permanent cessation of wear may be advised.

With use of COCs, there have been reports of retinal vascular thrombosis which may lead to partial or complete loss of vision. If there are signs or symptoms such as visual changes, onset of proptosis or diplopia, papilledema, or retinal vascular lesions, the COC should be discontinued and the cause immediately evaluated.

Peri-Operative Considerations: Thromboembolic Complications—Post-surgery: There is an increased risk of thromboembolic complications in COC users after major surgery. If feasible, COCs should be discontinued and an alternative method substituted at least one month prior to **major** elective surgery and during periods of prolonged immobilization. OC use should not be resumed for at least two weeks after major elective surgery, and only after the first menstrual period after hospital discharge following surgery.

Psychiatric: Emotional Disorders: Patients with a history of emotional disturbances, especially the depressive type, may be more prone to have a recurrence of depression while taking oral contraceptives. In cases of a serious recurrence, a trial of an alternate method of contraception should be made, which may help to clarify the possible relationship. Women with premenstrual syndrome (PMS) may have a varied response to oral contraceptives, ranging from symptomatic improvement to worsening of the condition.

Renal: Fluid retention: Hormonal contraceptives may cause some degree of fluid retention. They should be prescribed with caution, and only with careful monitoring, in patients with conditions which might be aggravated by fluid retention.

Sexual Function/Reproduction: Amenorrhea: Women having a history of oligomenorrhea, secondary amenorrhea, or irregular cycles may remain anovulatory or become amenorrheic following discontinuation of estrogen-progestin combination therapy.

Amenorrhea, especially if associated with breast secretion, that continues for six months or more after withdrawal, warrants a careful assessment of hypothalamic-pituitary function.

Reduced Efficacy: The efficacy of COCs may be reduced in the event of missed tablets, gastro-intestinal disturbances or concomitant medication (see Drug Interactions).

Return to Fertility: After discontinuing oral contraceptive therapy, the patient should delay pregnancy until at least one normal spontaneous cycle has occurred in order to date the pregnancy. An alternate contraceptive method should be used during this time.

Special Populations: Pregnant Women: Oral contraceptives should not be taken by pregnant women. If conception accidentally occurs while taking the pill, there is no conclusive evidence that the estrogen and progestin contained in the oral contraceptive will damage the developing child. However, further intake of COCs should be stopped.

Nursing Women: In breast-feeding women, the use of oral contraceptives results in the hormonal components being excreted in breast milk and may reduce its quantity and quality. If the use of oral contraceptives is initiated after the establishment of lactation, there does not appear to be any effect on the quantity and quality of the milk. Some adverse effects on the child have been reported, including jaundice and breast enlargement.

The use of COCs is generally not recommended until the nursing mother has completely weaned her child.

Pediatrics: This medication should not be used before menarche.

Monitoring and Laboratory Tests: Physical Examination and Follow-up: Before oral contraceptives are used, a thorough history and physical examination should be performed, including a blood pressure determination. Breasts, liver, extremities and pelvic organs should be examined. A Papanicolaou smear should be taken if the patient has been sexually active.

The first follow-up visit should be three months after oral contraceptives are prescribed. Thereafter, examinations should be performed at least once a year, or more frequently if indicated. At each annual visit, examination should include those procedures that were done at the initial visit as outlined above or per recommendations of the Canadian Task Force on the Periodic Health examination.

ADVERSE REACTIONS: Adverse Drug Reaction Overview: An increased risk of the following serious adverse reactions has been associated with the use of COCs: thrombophlebitis; arterial thromboembolism; pulmonary embolism; mesenteric thrombosis; neuro-ocular lesions (e.g. retinal thrombosis); myocardial infarction; cerebral thrombosis; cerebral hemorrhage; hypertension; benign hepatic tumours; hepatic adenomas or benign liver tumours; gallbladder disease, including gallstones*; stroke; transient ischemic attack; venous thrombosis; cervical intraepithelial neoplasia; cervical cancer; being diagnosed with breast cancer.

The following adverse reactions also have been reported in patients receiving COCs: Nausea and vomiting, usually the most common adverse reaction, occurs in approximately 10 percent or fewer of patients during the first cycle. Other reactions, as a general rule, are seen less frequently or only occasionally.

Other Adverse Reactions: The following adverse reactions have been reported in patients receiving COC and are believed to be drug related: gastrointestinal symptoms (such as abdominal pain, cramps and bloating); breakthrough bleeding; spotting; change in menstrual flow; amenorrhea; dysmenorrhea; temporary infertility after discontinuance of treatment; fluid retention/edema; chloasma (melasma) which may persist; breast changes: pain, tenderness, enlargement, and secretion; change in weight (increase or decrease); change in cervical ectropion and secretion; diminution in lactation when given immediately postpartum; cholestatic jaundice; headache, including migraines; rash (allergic); mood changes, including depression; reduced tolerance to carbohydrates; vaginitis including candidiasis; change in corneal curvature (steepening); intolerance to contact lenses; retinal vascular thrombosis.

The following adverse reactions have been reported in users of COCs and the association has been neither confirmed nor refuted: congenital anomalies; premenstrual syndrome; cataracts; optic neuritis†; changes in appetite (increase or decrease); cystitis-like syndrome; nervousness; dizziness; hirsutism; loss of scalp hair; erythema multiforme; erythema nodosum; hemorrhagic eruption; vaginitis; exacerbation of porphyria; impaired renal function; hemolytic uremic syndrome; Budd-Chiari syndrome; acne; changes in libido; colitis; sickle-cell disease; cerebrovascular disease with mitral valve prolapse; lupus-like syndrome; anaphylactic (anaphylactoid reactions, including very rare cases of urticaria, angioedema, and severe reactions with respiratory and circulatory symptoms); exacerbation of systemic lupus erythematosus; exacerbation of chorea; aggravation of varicose veins; pancreatitis; hepatic adenomas; hepatocellular carcinomas; changes in serum lipid levels, including hypertriglyceridemia; decrease in serum folate levels.‡

Clinical Trial Adverse Drug Reactions: Because clinical trials are conducted under very specific conditions the adverse reactions rates observed in the clinical trials may not reflect the rates observed in practice and should not be compared to the rates in the clinical trials of another drug. Adverse drug reaction information from clinical trials is useful for identifying drug-related adverse events and for approximating rates.

Clinical Trials in Oral Contraception: A total of 1477 patients completed 7720 cycles with the combined oral contraceptive containing 0.10 mg levonorgesterol and 0.02 mg ethinyl estradiol during a 15 month period of use. The mean cycle length, excluding cycle 1, was 29.1 days, and 90% of the cycles ranged in duration from 26 to 30 days.

Breakthrough bleeding alone and spotting alone occurred during 4.3% and 12.1% of cycles, respectively. Breakthrough bleeding and spotting occurred during 11.0% of the cycles, while breakthrough bleeding and/or spotting occurred during 27.3% of the cycles. The medication should not be halted during intermenstrual bleeding. If the bleeding persists, the usual diagnostic procedures should be undertaken to determine the cause of the vaginal bleeding.

The incidence of amenorrhea was low with the use of 0.10 mg levonorgestrel and 0.02 mg ethinyl estradiol (Table 1). If one period is missed, however, appropriate diagnostic procedures should be undertaken to rule out pregnancy and medication should be discontinued during this time, and an alternate method of contraception employed.

Treatment-emergent study events (TESE) were analyzed for 1477 subjects exposed to the study drug for 7870 cycles. One or more TESE were reported for 1106 (75%) subjects. Table 1 lists the frequency of TESE that were reported by ≥2% of subjects.

Table 1: AVIANE

Frequency of TESE That Occurred in ≥2% of Subjects

Event	Number (%) of Subjects (n=1477)
Headache	400 (27)
Dysmenorrhea	210 (14)
Infection	200 (14)
Pharyngitis	146 (10)
Abdominal pain	134 (9)
Nausea	134 (9)
Metrorrhagia	123 (8)
Sinusitis	90 (6)
Flu syndrome	84 (6)
Vaginal moniliasis	71 (5)
Pain	71 (5)
Back pain	66 (4)
Breast pain	65 (4)
Accidental injury	64 (4)
Acne	62 (4)

(cont'd)

* COCs may worsen existing gallbladder disease and may accelerate the development of this disease in previously asymptomatic women.

† Optic neuritis may lead to partial or complete loss of vision.

‡ Serum folate levels may be depressed by COC therapy.

Table 1: AVIANE *(cont'd)*

Frequency of TESE That Occurred in ≥2% of Subjects

Event	Number (%) of Subjects (n=1477)
Rhinitis	54 (4)
Emotional lability	50 (3)
Vaginitis	48 (3)
Urinary tract infection	41 (3)
Dizziness	40 (3)
Diarrhea	40 (3)
Bronchitis	37 (3)
Depression	36 (2)
Asthenia	35 (2)
Vomiting	34 (2)
Allergic reaction other than to study drug	33 (2)
Amenorrhea	30 (2)

A total of 133 (9%) subjects stopped taking the study medication because of adverse events. Some of the study events that led to subject discontinuation were considered by the medical monitor to be potentially serious: headache (21), hypertension (7), migraine (3), phlebitis (1), palpitations (1), varicose veins (1), vascular disorder (1), hypercholesterolemia/hyperlipidemia (6), depression/emotional lability (16), hypesthesia (1), abnormal vision (2), visual field defect (1), amenorrhea (8), dysmenorrhea (4), menorrhagia (6), irregular bleeding (1), menstrual bloating (1), metrorrhagia (1), fibroid growth (1).

No deaths occurred during the multicentre study.

Clinical Trials in Acne: Two randomized, placebo-controlled, 6-cycle, multicenter clinical trials were conducted in 721 women with moderate acne. The measured weight change and the incidence of some adverse events commonly attributed to OC use (such as nausea, breast tenderness, headache) were similar in women treated with 0.10 mg levonorgestrel and 0.02 mg ethinyl estradiol, and with placebo (see Table 2). The safety profile of 0.10 mg levonorgestrel and 0.02 mg ethinyl estradiol was compared with that of placebo. Treatment-emergent adverse events that were reported by ≥2% of patients in either treatment group are presented in Table 2.

Table 2: AVIANE

Percentage of Patients (≥2%) Reporting Treatment-emergent Adverse Events in Either Treatment Group in Studies 0858A1-900,901

Adverse Event	Number (%) of Subjects (0.10 mg Levonorgestrel and 0.02 mg Ethinyl Estradiol) (n=349)	Placebo (n=355)
Headache	110 (31.5)	107 (30.1)
Metrorrhagia[a]	77 (21.8)	14 (3.9)
Nausea	49 (14.0)	40 (11.3)
Infection	48 (13.8)	49 (13.8)
Pharyngitis	46 (13.2)	58 (16.3)
Pain	31 (8.9)	36 (10.1)
Abdominal pain	27 (7.7)	24 (6.8)
Dysmenorrhea	27 (7.7)	39 (11.0)
Accidental injury	21 (6.0)	16 (4.5)
Menstrual disorder[a]	21 (6.0)	8 (2.3)
Flu syndrome	19 (5.4)	20 (5.6)
Allergic reaction[a]	16 (4.6)	6 (1.7)
Breast pain	16 (4.6)	11 (3.1)
Rhinitis	15 (4.0)	13 (3.7)
Sinusitis	14 (4.0)	2.0 (8)
Asthenia	13 (3.7)	5 (1.4)
Back pain	12 (3.4)	12 (3.4)
Dyspepsia	12 (3.4)	2.3 (8)
Weight gain	17 (3.4)	12 (2.3)
Emotional lability[a]	12 (3.4)	4 (1.1)
Acne	13 (3.4)	6 (1.4)
Migraine	11 (3.2)	8 (2.3)
Dizziness	11 (3.2)	10 (2.8)

(cont'd)

Table 2: AVIANE *(cont'd)*

Percentage of Patients (≥2%) Reporting Treatment-emergent Adverse Events in Either Treatment Group in Studies 0858A1-900,901

Adverse Event	Number (%) of Subjects (0.10 mg Levonorgestrel and 0.02 mg Ethinyl Estradiol) (n=349)	Placebo (n=355)
Cough increased	10 (2.9)	8 (2.3)
Vomiting	10 (2.6)	6 (1.7)
Depression	9 (2.6)	11 (2.5)
Moniliasis	7 (2.0)	8 (2.3)
Myalgia	7 (2.0)	5 (1.4)
Bronchitis	7 (2.0)	7 (2.0)
Rash	7 (2.0)	7 (2.0)
Urticaria[a]	7 (2.0)	0
Allergic reaction other than drug	7 (2.0)	7 (2.0)
Diarrhea	6 (1.7)	10 (2.8)
Unintended pregnancy[a]	2 (0.6)	12 (3.1)

[a] Statistically significantly different between treatment groups ($p<0.05$).

As expected, menstrual-related events were more frequent in women treated with 0.10 mg levonorgestrel and 0.02 mg ethinyl estradiol than with placebo. However, other adverse events often associated with oral contraceptive use, including nausea, vomiting, breast pain, headache, migraine and weight gain, occurred at similar rates in women treated with placebo or 0.10 mg levonorgestrel and 0.02 mg ethinyl estradiol.

DRUG INTERACTIONS: Overview: The concurrent administration of COCs with other substances may result in an altered response to either agent. Decreased ethinyl estradiol (EE) serum concentration may cause an increased incidence of breakthrough bleeding and menstrual irregularities and may possibly reduce efficacy of the COC. During concomitant use of EE containing products and substances that may lead to decreased EE serum concentration, it is recommended that a nonhormonal back-up method of birth control (such as condoms and spermicide) be used in addition to the regular intake of AVIANE 21 and AVIANE 28. In the case of prolonged use of such substances COCs should not be considered the primary contraceptive.

After discontinuation of substances that may lead to decreased EE serum concentrations, use of a nonhormonal back-up method is recommended for at least 7 days. Longer use of a back-up method is advisable after discontinuation of substances that have led to induction of hepatic microsomal enzymes, resulting in decreased EE serum concentrations. It may sometimes take several weeks until enzyme induction has completely subsided, depending on dosage, duration of use and rate of elimination of the inducing substance.

Reduced effectiveness of the COC, should it occur, is more likely with the low-dose formulations. It is important to ascertain all drugs that a patient is taking, both prescription and non-prescription, before COCs are prescribed.

Examples of substances that may decrease serum EE concentrations:

- Any substance that reduces gastrointestinal transit time
- Hypericum perforatum, also known as St. John's Wort, and ritonavir (possibly by induction of hepatic microsomal enzymes).
- Substances that induce hepatic microsomal enzymes, such as rifampicin, rifabutin, dexamethasone, modafinil, some protease inhibitors, topiramate.

Examples of substances that may increase serum EE concentrations:

- Atorvastatin
- Competitive inhibitors for sulfation in the gastrointestinal wall, such as ascorbic acid (vitamin C) and acetaminophen.
- Substances that inhibit cytochrome P 450 3A4 isoenzymes such as indinavir, fluconazole and troleandomycin.

Troleandomycin may increase the risk of intrahepatic cholestasis during coadministration with COCs.

Ethinyl estradiol may interfere with the metabolism of other drugs by inhibiting hepatic microsomal enzymes, or by inducing hepatic drug conjugation, particularly glucuronidation. Accordingly, plasma and tissue concentrations of some drugs may either be increased (eg. cyclosporine, theophylline, corticosteroids) or decreased (eg. lamotrigine) by ethinyl estradiol.

Drug-Drug Interactions: For possible drug interactions with COCs, see Table 3 and Table 4.

Table 3: AVIANE[a]

Drugs that May Decrease the Efficacy of Oral Contraceptives

Class of Compound	Drug	Proposed Mechanism	Suggested Management
Anticonvulsants	Carbamazepine Ethosuximide Phenobarbital Phenytoin Primidone	Induction of hepatic microsomal enzymes. Rapid metabolism of estrogen and increased binding of progestin and ethinyl estradiol to SHBG.	Use higher dose OCs (50 µg ethinyl estradiol), another drug or another method.
Antibiotics	Ampicillin Cotrimoxazole Penicillin	Enterohepatic circulation disturbance, intestinal hurry.	For short course, use additional method or use another drug. For long course, use another method.
	Rifampin	Increased metabolism of progestins. Suspected acceleration of estrogen metabolism.	Use another method.
	Chloramphenicol Metronidazole Neomycin Nitrofurantoin Sulfonamides Tetracyclines	Induction of hepatic microsomal enzymes. Also disturbance of enterohepatic circulation.	For short course, use additional method or use another drug. For long course, use another method.
	Troleandomycin	May retard metabolism of OCs, increasing the risk of cholestatic jaundice.	

(cont'd)

Table 3: AVIANE[a] *(cont'd)*

Drugs that May Decrease the Efficacy of Oral Contraceptives

Class of Compound	Drug	Proposed Mechanism	Suggested Management
Antifungals	Griseofulvin	Stimulation of hepatic metabolism of contraceptive steroids may occur.	Use another method.
Cholesterol Lowering Agents	Clofibrate	Reduces elevated serum triglycerides and cholesterol; this reduces OC efficacy.	Use another method.
Sedatives and Hypnotics	Benzodiazepines Barbiturates Chloral Hydrate Glutethimide Meprobamate	Induction of hepatic microsomal enzymes.	For short course, use additional method or another drug. For long course, use another method or higher dose OCs.
Antacids		Decreased intestinal absorption of progestins.	Dose two hours apart.
Other Drugs	Phenylbutazone[b] Antihistamines[b] Analgesics[b] Antimigraine Preparations[b] Vitamin E	Reduced OC efficacy has been reported. Remains to be confirmed.	

[a] Adapted from Dickey, RP, ed.: Managing Contraceptive Pill Patients, 5th edition Creative Informatics Inc., Durant, OK, 1987.
[b] Refer to *Oral Contraceptives* 1994, A Report by the Special Advisory Committee on Reproductive Physiology to the Drugs Directorate, Health Protection Branch, Health Canada.

Table 4: AVIANE[a]

Modification of Other Drug Action by Oral Contraceptives

Class of Compound	Drug	Modification of Drug Action	Suggested Management
Alcohol		Possible increased levels of ethanol or acetaldehyde.	Use with caution.
Alpha-II Adrenoreceptor Agents	Clonidine	Sedation effect increased.	Use with caution.
Anticoagulants	All	OCs increase clotting factors, decrease efficacy. However, OCs may potentiate action in some patients.	Use another method.
Anticonvulsants	All	Fluid retention may increase risk of seizures.	Use another method.
Antidiabetic Drugs	Oral Hypoglycemics and Insulin	OCs may impair glucose tolerance and increase blood glucose.	Use low-dose estrogen and progestin OC or another method. Monitor blood glucose.
Antihypertensive Agents	Guanethidine and Methyldopa	Estrogen component causes sodium retention, progestin has no effect.	Use low-dose estrogen OC or use another method.
	Beta Blockers	Increased drug effect (decreased metabolism).	Dose of drug may have to be increased.
Antipyretics	Acetaminophen	Increased metabolism and renal clearance.	Dose of drug may have to be increased.
	Antipyrine	Impaired metabolism.	Decrease dose of drug.
	ASA	Effects of ASA may be decreased by the short-term use of OCs.	Patients on chronic ASA therapy may require an increase in ASA dosage.
Aminocaproic Acid		Theoretically, a hypercoagulable state may occur because OCs augment clotting factors.	Avoid concomitant use.
Betamimetic Agents	Isoproterenol	Estrogen causes decreased response to these drugs.	Adjust dose of drug as necessary. Discontinuing OCs can result in excessive drug activity.
Caffeine		The actions of caffeine may be enhanced as OCs may impair the hepatic metabolism of caffeine.	Use with caution.
Cholesterol Lowering Agents	Clofibrate	Their action may be antagonized by OCs. OCs may also increase metabolism of clofibrate.	May need to increase dose of clofibrate.
Corticosteroids	Prednisone	Markedly increased serum levels.	Possible need for decrease in dose.
Cyclosporine		May lead to an increase in cyclosporine levels and hepatotoxicity.	Monitor hepatic function. The cyclosporine dose may have to be decreased.
Folic Acid		OCs have been reported to impair folate metabolism.	May need to increase dietary intake, or supplement.

(cont'd)

Table 4: AVIANE[a] *(cont'd)*

Modification of Other Drug Action by Oral Contraceptives

Class of Compound	Drug	Modification of Drug Action	Suggested Management
Meperidine		Possible increased analgesia and CNS depression due to decreased metabolism of meperidine.	Use combination with caution.
Phenothiazine Tranquilizers	All Phenothiazines, Reserpine and similar drugs	Estrogen potentiates the hyperprolactinemia effect of these drugs.	Use other drugs or lower dose OCs. If galactorrhea or hyperprolactinemia occurs, use other method.
Sedatives and Hypnotics	Chlordiazepoxide Lorazepam Oxazepam Diazepam	Increased effect (increased metabolism).	Use with caution.
Theophylline	All	Decreased oxidation, leading to possible toxicity.	Use with caution. Monitor theophylline levels.
Tricyclic Antidepressants	Clomipramine (possibly others)	Increased side effects: i.e., depression.	Use with caution.
Vitamin B_{12}		OCs have been reported to reduce serum levels of Vitamin B_{12}.	May need to increase dietary intake, or supplement.

[a] Adapted from Dickey, RP, ed.: Managing Contraceptive Pill Patients, 5th edition Creative Informatics Inc., Durant, OK, 1987.

Drug-Food Interactions: The actions of caffeine may be enhanced by concomitant use of oral contraceptives. Oral contraceptives may impair the hepatic metabolism of caffeine, therefore use with caution.

The use of alcohol with oral contraceptives may possibly result in increased levels of ethanol or acetaldehyde, therefore use with caution.

Drug-Herb Interactions: Herbal products containing St. John's Wort (hypericum perforatum) may induce hepatic enzymes (cytochrome P450) and p-glycoprotein transporter and may reduce the effectiveness of contraceptive steroids. This may also result in breakthrough bleeding. Physicians and other health care providers should be made aware of the non-prescription products concomitantly used by the patient, including herbal and natural products.

Drug-Laboratory Test Interactions: Results of laboratory tests should be interpreted in the light that the patient is on combined oral contraceptives. The following laboratory tests are modified:

Liver Function Tests	
Bromsulphthalein Retention Test (BSP)	Moderate increase
AST and GGT	Minor increase
Alkaline Phosphatase	Variable increase
Serum Bilirubin	Increased, particularly in conditions predisposing to or associated with hyperbilirubinemia
Coagulation Tests	
Factors II, VII, IX, X, XII and XIII	Increased
Factor VIII	Mild increase
Platelet aggregation and adhesiveness	Mild increase in response to common aggregating agents
Fibrinogen	Increased
Plasminogen	Mild increase
Antithrombin III	Mild decrease
Prothrombin Time	Increased
Thyroid Function Tests	
Protein-bound Iodine (PBI)	Increased
Total Serum Thyroxine (T_3 and T_4)	Increased
Thyroid Stimulating Hormone (TSH)	Unchanged
Free T3 Resin Uptake	Decreased
Adrenocortical Function Tests	
Plasma Cortisol	Increased
Cortisol Binding Globulin	Increased
Dehydroepiandrosterone sulfate (DHEAS)	Decreased
Renal Function	
Plasma Creatinine	Increased
Creatinine Clearance	Increased
Miscellaneous Tests	
Serum Folate	Occasionally decreased
Glucose Tolerance Test	Variable increase with return to normal after 6 to 12 months
Insulin Response	Mild to moderate increase
c-Peptide Response	Mild to moderate increase

Tissue Specimens: Pathologists should be advised of COC therapy when specimens obtained from surgical procedures and Pap smears are submitted for examination.

Non-Contraceptive Benefits of Oral Contraceptives: Several health advantages other than contraception have been reported.

1. Combination oral contraceptives reduce the incidence of cancer of the endometrium and ovaries.
2. Oral contraceptives reduce the likelihood of developing benign breast disease.
3. Oral contraceptives reduce the likelihood of development of functional ovarian cysts.
4. Pill users have less menstrual blood loss and have more regular cycles, thereby reducing the chance of developing iron-deficiency anemia.
5. The use of oral contraceptives may decrease the severity of dysmenorrhea and premenstrual syndrome, and may improve acne vulgaris, hirsutism, and other androgen-mediated disorders.
6. Other non-contraceptive benefits are outlined in *Oral Contraceptives* 1994 Health Canada.

DOSAGE AND ADMINISTRATION: Recommended Dose and Dosage Adjustment: Contraception: AVIANE 21 (21 Day Regimen): Each cycle consists of 21 days on medication and a 7-day interval without medication (three weeks on, one week off).

The dosage of AVIANE 21 is one tablet daily for 21 consecutive days per menstrual cycle, according to prescribed schedule. For the first cycle of medication, the patient is instructed to take one AVIANE tablet daily for 21 consecutive days beginning on Day 1 of her menstrual cycle, on Day 5, or on the first Sunday after her period begins. (For the first cycle only, the first day of menstrual flow is considered Day 1.) The tablets are then discontinued for seven days (one week). Withdrawal bleeding should usually occur within three days following discontinuation of AVIANE.

The patient begins her next and all subsequent 21-day courses of AVIANE tablets (following the same 21 days on, 7 days off) on the same day of the week that she began her first course. She begins taking her tablets seven days after discontinuation, regardless of whether or not withdrawal bleeding is still in progress.

AVIANE 28 (28 Day Regimen): Each cycle consists of 21 days of orange AVIANE tablets followed by 7 days of light green inert tablets (three weeks on AVIANE, one week on inert tablets).

The dosage of AVIANE 28 is one tablet daily for 21 consecutive days per menstrual cycle, according to prescribed schedule, followed by one inert tablet daily for 7 consecutive days according to prescribed schedule. For the first cycle of medication, the patient is instructed to take one orange tablet daily for 21 consecutive days beginning on Day 1 of her menstrual cycle, on Day 5, or on the first Sunday after her period begins. (For the first cycle only, the first day of menstrual flow is considered Day 1.) One light green tablet is taken daily for the following seven consecutive days. Withdrawal bleeding should usually occur within three days following the discontinuation orange AVIANE tablets, i.e., during the week the patient is taking the light green inert tablets.

The patient begins her next and all subsequent 28-day courses of tablets on the same day of the week that she began her first course. She continues her next course of 28 tablets immediately after the last course, regardless of whether or not a period of withdrawal bleeding is still in progress. There is no need for the patient to count days between cycles because there are no "off-tablet days".

Acne: The timing of initiation of AVIANE treatment for acne should follow the instructions for use of AVIANE for contraception (see above for dosing information for oral contraception).

Administration: It is recommended that AVIANE tablets be taken at the same time each day, preferably after the evening meal or at bedtime.

AVIANE is effective from the first day of therapy if the tablets are begun on the first day of the menstrual cycle.

If AVIANE tablets administration is initiated after Day 1 of the first menstrual cycle of medication or postpartum, contraceptive reliance should not be placed on AVIANE until after the first seven consecutive days of administration. The possibility of ovulation and conception prior to initiation of medication should be considered. Therefore, nonhormonal methods of contraception (such as condoms and spermicide) should be used for the first 7 days of tablet taking.

If spotting or breakthrough bleeding occurs, the patient is instructed to continue on the same regimen. This type of bleeding usually is transient and without significance; however, if the bleeding is persistent or prolonged, the patient is advised to consult her physician.

Special Notes on Administration: No preceding hormonal contraceptive use (in the past month): Tablet-taking should start on day 1 of the woman's natural cycle (i.e., the first day of her menstrual bleeding). Starting on days 2-7 (e.g. Sunday start) is allowed, but for the first 7 days of tablet-taking during the first cycle, a nonhormonal back-up method of birth control (such as condoms and spermicide) is recommended.

Changing from another combined oral contraceptive pill: The woman should start AVIANE preferably on the day after the last active tablet of her previous combined oral contraceptive (COC), but at the latest, on the day following the usual tablet-free or inactive tablet interval of her previous COC.

Changing from a progestin only method (progestin-only pill, injection, implant): The woman may switch any day from the progestin-only pill and should begin AVIANE the next day. She should start AVIANE on the day of an implant removal or, if using an injection, the day the next injection would be due. In all of these situations, the woman should be advised to use a nonhormonal back-up method for the first 7 days of tablet-taking.

Following first-trimester abortion: The woman may start AVIANE immediately. Additional contraceptive measures are not needed.

Following delivery or second-trimester abortion: Since the immediate post-partum period is associated with an increased risk of thromboembolism, oral contraceptives should be started no earlier than day 28 after delivery in the nonlactating mother or after second-trimester abortion. The woman should be advised to use a nonhormonal back-up method for the first 7 days of tablet-taking. However, if intercourse has already occurred, the possibility of pregnancy should be ruled out before the actual start of COC use or the woman must wait for her first menstrual period.

Advice in case of vomiting: If vomiting occurs within 3-4 hours after a tablet is taken, absorption may not be complete. In such event, advice concerning the management of missed tablet is outlined in Table 5. The woman must take the extra active tablet(s) needed from a backup pack.

Missed Dose: The patient should be instructed to use the following chart if she misses one or more of her birth control pills. She should be told to match the number of pills with the appropriate starting time for her type of pill. See Table 5.

Contraceptive reliability may be reduced if active tablets are missed and particularly if the missed tablets extend the tablet-free interval. If active tablets were missed and intercourse took place in the week before the tablets were missed, the possibility of pregnancy should be considered.

OVERDOSAGE:

Symptoms of COC overdosage in adults and children may include nausea, vomiting, breast tenderness, dizziness, abdominal pain, drowsiness/fatigue; withdrawal bleeding may occur in females. There is no specific antidote and further treatment of overdose, if necessary, is directed to the symptoms.

> For management of a suspected drug overdose, contact your **regional Poison Control Centre**. See the *CPS* Directory section for a list of Poison Control Centres.

ACTION AND CLINICAL PHARMACOLOGY: Mechanism of Action: Oral Contraception: Although the primary mechanism of action is inhibition of ovulation, the effectiveness of AVIANE may also result from other mechanisms of action, such as hostility of the cervical mucus to sperm penetration and migration.

Acne: Acne is a disease of the pilosebaceous apparatus characterized by abnormal keratinization, increased sebum production, and bacterial colonization. While the etiology of acne is multifactorial, there is evidence that androgenic action, including stimulation of sebaceous glands, is necessary for the development of acne. The suppression of gonadotropins by AVIANE leads to decreased ovarian production of the androgens, including androstenedione. AVIANE also significantly reduces bioavailable serum testosterone by preserving the estrogen-induced increases in sex hormone binding globulin (SHBG). In addition, AVIANE decreases serum levels of 3β-androstanediol glucuronide (a marker of peripheral 5 β-reductase activity). These biochemical changes produced by the coadministration of levonorgestrel and ethinyl estradiol are consistent with improvement of acne in otherwise healthy women.

Pharmacodynamics: Progestogens can have, in addition to progestational activity, estrogenic, anti-estrogenic and androgenic activity. When combined with estrogen, the progestogen will markedly affect the overall biological activity by producing a synergistic, summative or diminutional effect on activity.

Table 5: AVIANE

What to Do if You Miss Pills

Sunday Start	Other Than Sunday Start
Miss One Pill	**Miss One Pill**
Take it as soon as you remember, and take the next pill at the usual time. This means that you might take two pills in one day.	Take it as soon as you remember, and take the next pill at the usual time. This means that you might take two pills in one day.
Miss Two Pills in a Row	**Miss Two Pills in a Row**
First two weeks: 1. Take two pills the day you remember and two pills the next day. 2. Then take one pill a day until you finish the pack. 3. Use a nonhormonal back-up method of birth control if you have sex in the seven days after you miss the pills. **Third week:** 1. Keep taking one pill a day until Sunday. 2. On Sunday, safely discard the rest of the pack and start a new pack that day. 3. Use a nonhormonal back-up method of birth control if you have sex in the seven days after you miss the pills. 4. You may not have a period this month. **If You Miss Two Periods in a Row, Call Your Doctor, Pharmacist or Clinic.**	**First two weeks:** 1. Take two pills the day you remember and two pills the next day. 2. Then take one pill a day until you finish the pack. 3. Use a nonhormonal back-up method of birth control if you have sex in the seven days after you miss the pills. **Third week:** 1. Safely dispose of the rest of the pill pack and start a new pack that same day. 2. Use a nonhormonal back-up method of birth control if you have sex in the seven days after you miss the pills. 3. You may not have a period this month. **If You Miss Two Periods in a Row, Call Your Doctor, Pharmacist or Clinic.**
Miss Three or More Pills in a Row	**Miss Three or More Pills in a Row**
Anytime in the cycle: 1. Keep taking one pill a day until Sunday. 2. On Sunday, safely discard the rest of the pack and start a new pack that day. 3. Use a nonhormonal back-up method of birth control if you have sex in the seven days after you miss the pills. 4. You may not have a period this month. **If You Miss Two periods in a Row, Call Your Doctor, Pharmacist or Clinic.**	**Anytime in the cycle:** 1. Safely dispose of the rest of the pill pack and start a new pack that same day. 2. Use a nonhormonal back-up method of birth control if you have sex in the seven days after you miss the pills. 3. You may not have a period this month. **If You Miss Two periods in a Row, Call Your Doctor, Pharmacist or Clinic.**

Comparisons of progestogen potency are not considered scientifically valid because the effects of one progestogen cannot be directly compared with those of another.

A study of serum luteinizing hormone (LH), follicle stimulating hormone (FSH), progesterone and 17β-estradiol in patients taking low dose oral contraceptives indicated reduction or abolition of the mid-cycle ovulatory peak and post-ovulatory levels commonly associated with these hormones and gonadotrophins respectively.

Endometrial biopsies taken during the course of therapy with 250 µg d-norgestrel (as 500 µg of the dl-racemate) plus 50 µg ethinyl estradiol revealed a histological sequence in the menstrual cycle of early glandular epithelial stimulation followed by later inhibition after the first half of the menstrual cycle.

Cervical mucus studies with 250 µg d-norgestrel (as 500 µg of the dl-racemate) plus 50 µg ethinyl estradiol, and 37.5 µg d-norgestrel (as 75 µg of the dl-racemate) would suggest a similar action for AVIANE on the cervical mucus, viz., absence of ferning and decreased spinnbarkeit, indicative of poor conditions for sperm penetration and migration.

The results of assays for prolactin in a group of 11 normally ovulating women given 150 µg d-norgestrel (as 300 µg of the dl-racemate) plus 30 µg ethinyl estradiol over a continuous period of three months indicated no clinically or statistically significant elevation or depression of hormone levels during the course of active drug ingestion, nor in the first post-treatment cycle.

Pharmacokinetics: A human study of the metabolism of ^{14}C-labelled norgestrel, revealed that most of the urinary excretion of norgestrel occurred on the first day. There was no difference in the rate of excretion of norgestrel whether administered orally or intravenously. The amount of radioactivity in plasma fell rapidly within the first few hours and at the end of two days only small amounts were present. The foregoing and other studies with ^{14}C-labelled and unlabelled norgestrel have shown that saturation of the 4,5-double bond with and without concomitant reduction of the 3-carbonyl to a 3-hydroxyl group are important reactions during metabolism.

Special Populations and Conditions: Pediatrics: Pharmacokinetic differences in pediatrics in comparison to adults have not been studied. This medication should not be used before menarche.

Race: Pharmacokinetic differences based on race have not been studied.

Renal Insufficiency: No studies have been conducted in women with renal insufficiency.

Genetic Polymorphism: Pharmacokinetic differences based on genetic polymorphism have not been studied.

STORAGE AND STABILITY: Store at room temperature (15-30°C).

AVIANE 21 and AVIANE 28 should be protected from light once opened using the protective covering provided. Keep out of reach of children and pets.

INFORMATION FOR THE PATIENT: Published in e-CPS, available by subscription at www.e-cps.ca.

DOSAGE FORMS, COMPOSITION AND PACKAGING: AVIANE 21: Each orange, round tablet, debossed with 'dp' and '016', contains: levonorgestrel 100 µg and ethinyl estradiol 20 µg. Nonmedicial ingredients: FD&C yellow # 6 aluminum lake, hydroxypropyl methylcellulose, lactose monohydrate, magnesium stearate, microcrystalline cellulose, polyethylene glycol, pregelatinized starch, sodium starch glycolate and titanium dioxide. Packs of 21 active tablets.

AVIANE 28: Each orange, round tablet, debossed with 'dp' and '016', contains: levonorgestrel 100 µg and ethinyl estradiol 20 µg. The light green, round tablets, debossed with 'dp' and '519' are inert. Nonmedicial ingredients: Active tablets: FD&C yellow # 6 aluminum lake, hydroxypropyl methylcellulose, lactose monohydrate, magnesium stearate, microcrystalline cellulose, polyethylene glycol, pregelatinized starch, sodium starch glycolate and titanium dioxide. Inert tablets: D&C yellow #10 aluminum lake, FD&C yellow # 6 aluminum lake, FD&C blue # 1 aluminum lake, lactose monohydrate, magnesium stearate, microcrystalline cellulose and pregelatinized starch. Packs of 21 active tablets and 7 inert tablets.

Avodart® Ⓟ

dutasteride

Type I and II 5 Alpha-reductase Inhibitor

GlaxoSmithKline

Date of Revision: November 19, 2009

SUMMARY PRODUCT INFORMATION:

Route of Administration	Dosage Form/ Strength	Clinically Relevant Nonmedicinal Ingredients
Oral	Capsules, 0.5 mg	Gelatin For a complete listing see Dosage Forms, Composition and Packaging.

INDICATIONS AND CLINICAL USE: Monotherapy: AVODART (dutasteride) is indicated for the treatment of symptomatic Benign Prostatic Hyperplasia (BPH) in men with enlarged prostates.

Combination Therapy: AVODART (dutasteride) in combination with the alpha blocker tamsulosin is indicated for the treatment of moderate to severe symptomatic BPH in men with enlarged prostates.

AVODART administered as monotherapy has been shown to:

- reduce the risk of acute urinary retention (AUR)
- reduce the risk of the need for BPH related surgery

AVODART, administered alone or in combination with the alpha blocker tamsulosin, has been shown to:

- reduce prostate size, improve urinary flow and symptoms of BPH

CONTRAINDICATIONS: AVODART (dutasteride) is contraindicated for use in women and children (see Warnings and Precautions, Exposure of Women—Risk to Male Fetus).

AVODART is contraindicated in patients with known hypersensitivity to dutasteride, other 5 alpha-reductase inhibitors, or any component of the preparation.

WARNINGS AND PRECAUTIONS:

> **Serious Warnings and Precautions**
> **AVODART is for use for men only.**
> **Exposure of Women—Risk to Male Fetus:** Dutasteride is absorbed through the skin. Therefore, women who are pregnant or may be pregnant should not handle AVODART capsules.

General: Prior to treatment with AVODART, patients should be assessed thoroughly to rule out other urological diseases including prostate cancer.

Patients with a large residual urinary volume and/or severely diminished urinary flow may not be proper candidates for 5 alpha-reductase inhibitor therapy and should be carefully monitored for obstructive uropathy.

No study has been conducted to determine if AVODART can be used for the control of BPH in asymptomatic patients.

The long-term (>4 years) beneficial and adverse effects of AVODART have not been established.

Cardiovascular: In two 4-year clinical studies, the incidence of cardiac failure (a composite term of reported events, primarily cardiac failure and congestive cardiac failure) was higher among subjects taking the combination of AVODART and an alpha-blocker, primarily tamsulosin, than it was among subjects not taking the combination. The relative risk estimate for time to first cardiac failure event was 3.57 [95% CI: 1.17, 10.8] for combination treatment compared with AVODART monotherapy and 1.36 [95% CI: 0.61, 3.07] compared with tamsulosin monotherapy. In these 2 studies, the incidence of cardiac failure was low (≤1%) and variable between the studies. No imbalance was observed in the incidence of cardiovascular adverse events overall in either study. No causal relationship between AVODART (alone or in combination with an alpha-blocker) and cardiac failure has been established (see Adverse Reactions).

Endocrine and Metabolism: Hormone Levels: In healthy volunteers, 52 weeks of treatment with dutasteride 0.5 mg/day (n=26) resulted in no clinically significant change compared with placebo (n=23) in sex hormone binding globulin, estradiol, luteinizing hormone, follicle-stimulating hormone, thyroxine (free T4), and dehydroepiandrosterone. Statistically significant, baseline-adjusted mean increases compared with placebo were observed for total testosterone at 8 weeks (3.37 nmol/L, p<0.003) and thyroid-stimulating hormone (TSH) at 52 weeks (0.4 mcIU/mL, p<0.05). The median percentage changes from baseline within the dutasteride group were 17.9% for testosterone at 8 weeks and 12.4% for TSH at 52 weeks. After stopping dutasteride for 24 weeks, the mean levels of testosterone and TSH had returned to baseline in the group of subjects with available data at the visit. In patients with BPH treated with dutasteride 0.5 mg/day for 4 years, the median decrease in serum DHT was 94% at 1 year, 93% at 2 years, and 95% at both 3 and 4 years. The median increase in serum testosterone was 19% at both 1 and 2 years, 26% at 3 years, and 22% at 4 years, but the mean and median levels remained within the physiologic range. In patients with BPH treated with dutasteride in a large Phase III trial, there was a median percent increase in luteinizing hormone of 12% at 6 months and 19% at both 12 and 24 months.

Hematologic: Men treated with dutasteride should not donate blood until at least 6 months have passed following their last dose. The purpose of this deferred period is to prevent administration of dutasteride to a pregnant female transfusion recipient.

Hepatic: The effect of hepatic impairment on dutasteride pharmacokinetics has not been studied. Because dutasteride is extensively metabolized and has a half-life of 3 to 5 weeks, caution should be used in the administration of dutasteride to patients with liver disease.

Sexual Function/Reproduction: The effects of dutasteride 0.5 mg/day on semen characteristics were evaluated in normal volunteers aged 18 to 52 (n=27 dutasteride, n=23 placebo) throughout 52 weeks of treatment and 24 weeks of post treatment follow-up. At 52 weeks, the mean percent reduction from baseline in total sperm count, semen volume, and sperm motility were 23%, 26%, and 18%, respectively, in the dutasteride group when adjusted for changes from baseline in the placebo group. Sperm concentration and sperm morphology were unaffected. After 24 weeks of follow-up, the mean percent change in total sperm count in the dutasteride group remained 23% lower than baseline. While mean values for all semen parameters at all time points remained within the normal ranges and did not meet predefined criteria for a clinically significant change (30%), two subjects in the dutasteride group had decreases in sperm count of greater than 90% from baseline at 52-weeks, with partial recovery at the 24-week follow-up. The clinical significance of dutasteride's effect on semen characteristics for an individual patient's fertility is not known.

Exposure of Women—Risk to Male Fetus: Dutasteride is absorbed through the skin. Therefore, women who are pregnant or may be pregnant should not handle AVODART because of the possibility of absorption of dutasteride and the potential risk of a fetal anomaly to a male fetus. Pre-clinical data suggests that the suppression of circulating levels of dihydrotestosterone may inhibit the development of the external genital organs in a male foetus carried by a woman exposed to dutasteride. In addition, women should use caution whenever handling AVODART. If contact is made with leaking capsules, the contact area should be washed immediately with soap and water. It is not known whether dutasteride is excreted in human milk.

Special Populations: Nursing Women: It is not known whether dutasteride is excreted in human milk.

Pediatrics: BPH is not a disease of childhood. AVODART is not indicated for use in children. Safety and effectiveness in children have not been established. Dutasteride is absorbed through the skin and therefore contact with leaking capsules must be avoided. If contact is made with leaking capsules, the contact area should be washed immediately with soap and water.

Geriatrics: No dose adjustment is necessary in the elderly. The pharmacokinetics and pharmacodynamics of dutasteride were evaluated in 36 healthy male subjects between the ages of 24 and 87 years following administration of a single 5 mg dose of dutasteride. In this single dose study, dutasteride half life increased with age (approximately 170 hours in men aged 20 to 49 years, approximately 260 hours in men aged 50 to 69 years, and approximately 300 hours in men older than 70 years). Of 2167 men treated with dutasteride in the 3 pivotal studies, 60% were age 65 and over and 15% were age 75 and over. No overall differences in safety or efficacy were observed between these patients and younger patients.

Monitoring and Laboratory Tests: Effects on Prostate Specific Antigen (PSA) and Prostate Cancer Detection: Digital rectal examination, as well as other evaluations for prostate cancer, should be performed on patients with BPH prior to initiating therapy with AVODART (dutasteride) capsules and periodically thereafter.

Serum prostate-specific antigen (PSA) concentration is an important component of the screening process to detect prostate cancer. Generally, a total serum PSA concentration greater than 4 ng/mL (Hybritech) requires further evaluation and consideration of prostate biopsy. Physicians should be aware that a baseline PSA less than 4 ng/mL in patients taking AVODART does not exclude a diagnosis of prostate cancer. Dutasteride causes a decrease in serum PSA levels by approximately 50%, after 6 months, in patients with BPH, even in the presence of prostate cancer. Although there may be individual variation, the reduction in PSA by approximately 50% is predictable as it was observed over the entire range of baseline PSA values (1.5 to 10 ng/mL). Therefore, to interpret an isolated PSA value in a man treated with AVODART for six months or more, PSA values should be doubled (e.g.: multiplied by a factor of 2) for comparison with normal ranges in untreated men. This adjustment preserves the sensitivity and specificity of the PSA assay and maintains its ability to detect prostate cancer. Any sustained increases in PSA levels while on AVODART should be carefully evaluated to rule out prostate cancer.

Total serum PSA levels return to baseline within 6 months of discontinuing treatment with AVODART. The ratio of free to total PSA remains constant even under the influence of AVODART. If clinicians elect to use percent free PSA as an aid in the detection of prostate cancer in men undergoing AVODART therapy, no adjustment to its value appears necessary.

Co-administration of tamsulosin with dutasteride resulted in similar changes to total PSA as dutasteride monotherapy after 2 years.

ADVERSE REACTIONS: Adverse Drug Reaction Overview: Most adverse reactions were mild or moderate and generally resolved while on treatment in both the AVODART and placebo groups. The most common adverse events leading to withdrawal in both treatment groups were associated with the reproductive system.

Clinical Trial Adverse Drug Reactions: Because clinical trials are conducted under very specific conditions the adverse reaction rates observed in the clinical trials may not reflect the rates observed in practice and should not be compared to the rates in the clinical trials of another drug. Adverse drug reaction information from clinical trials is useful for identifying drug-related adverse events and for approximating rates.

Dutasteride Monotherapy: Over 4300 male subjects with BPH were randomly assigned to receive placebo or 0.5 mg daily doses of AVODART in 3 identical 2 year, placebo-controlled, double blind, Phase 3 treatment studies, each with 2 year open-label extensions. During the double blind treatment period, 2167 male subjects were exposed to AVODART, including 1772 exposed for 1 year and 1510 exposed for 2 years. When including the open label extensions, 1009 male subjects were exposed to AVODART for 3 years and 812 were exposed for 4 years.

The population was aged 47 to 94 years (mean age, 66 years) and greater than 90% Caucasian. Over the 2-year double-blind treatment period, 376 subjects (9% of each treatment group) were withdrawn from the studies due to adverse experiences, most commonly associated with the reproductive system, with similar findings during the 2-year open-label extensions. Withdrawals due to adverse events considered by the investigator to have a reasonable possibility of being caused by the study medication occurred in 4% of the subjects receiving AVODART and in 3% of the subjects receiving placebo. Table 1 summarizes clinical adverse reactions that were reported by the investigator as drug-related in at least 1% of subjects receiving AVODART and at a higher incidence than subjects receiving placebo.

Table 1: AVODART

Drug-Related Adverse Events[a] Reported in ≥1% Subjects Over a 48-Month Period and More Frequently in the Dutasteride Group Than the Placebo Group (Pivotal Studies Pooled)

	Adverse Event Onset					
	Double-Blind				Open-Label[c]	
Adverse Events	Month 0–6	Month 7–12	Month 13–18	Month 19–24	Month 25–36	Month 39–48
Dutasteride (n)	(n=2167)	(n=1901)	(n=1725)	(n=1605)	(n=1188)	(n=1041)
Placebo (n)	(n=2158)	(n=1922)	(n=1714)	(n=1555)	(n=1152)	(n=968)
Impotence						
Dutasteride	4.7%	1.4%	1.0%	0.8%	1.4%	0.4%
Placebo	1.7%	1.5%	0.5%	0.9%	2.8%	0.4%
Decreased Libido						
Dutasteride	3.0%	0.7%	0.3%	0.3%	0.4%	0.1%
Placebo	1.4%	0.6%	0.2%	0.1%	2.4%	0.2%
Ejaculation Disorder						
Dutasteride	1.4%	0.5%	0.5%	0.1%	0.3%	0.1%
Placebo	0.5%	0.3%	0.1%	0.0%	1.2%	0.3%
Breast Disorders[b]						
Dutasteride	0.5%	0.8%	1.1%	0.6%	1.8%	0.7%
Placebo	0.2%	0.3%	0.3%	0.1%	1.3%	0.9%

[a] A drug-related adverse event is one considered by the investigator to have a reasonable possibility of being caused by the study medication. In assessing causality, investigators were asked to select from 1 of 2 options: reasonably related to study medication or unrelated to study medication.

[b] Includes breast tenderness and breast enlargement.

[c] All subjects switched to open-label dutasteride for months 25 to 48.

The relationship between long-term use of Dutasteride and Leydig cell tumours of the testis, Hepatocellular adenomas, and the Gleason score (grade of malignancy) of prostate cancer in patients taking long term Alpha reductase inhibitors is currently unknown.

In postmarketing experience with AVODART, adverse events related to allergic reactions, including rash, pruritus, urticaria, localized edema and angioedema, have been reported very rarely.

Combination with Alpha-Blocker Therapy (CombAT) Study: The CombAT study is an ongoing 4-year multicenter, double-blind study in which 4844 male subjects with BPH are randomized to receive combination therapy (AVODART 0.5 mg/day plus tamsulosin 0.4 mg/day, n=1610), AVODART alone (n=1623) or tamsulosin alone (n=1611). During the first 2 years, 1623 subjects received monotherapy with Avodart; 1611 subjects received monotherapy with tamsulosin; and 1610 subjects received combination therapy. The population was aged 49 to 88 years (mean age 66 years) and 88% Caucasian.

The most common adverse reactions reported over the first 2 years in subjects receiving combination therapy (AVODART plus tamsulosin) were ejaculation disorders, impotence, decreased libido, breast disorders (including breast enlargement and tenderness) and dizziness. Over 2 years of treatment, drug-related ejaculation disorders occurred more frequently in subjects receiving combination therapy (9%) compared to AVODART monotherapy (2%) or tamsulosin monotherapy (3%).

Over the first 2 years of treatment, study withdrawal due to adverse reactions occurred in 5% of subjects receiving combination therapy (AVODART plus tamsulosin), 3% of subjects receiving AVODART monotherapy, and 3% of subjects receiving tamsulosin monotherapy. The most common adverse reaction leading to study withdrawal in subjects receiving combination therapy was impotence (1%). See Table 2.

Table 2: AVODART

Adverse Reactions Reported Over a 24-Month Period in ≥1% of Subjects in Any Treatment Group (CombAT)

	Adverse Reaction Onset			
Adverse Reactions	Month 0–6	Month 7–12	Month 13–18	Month 19–24
Combination[a]	(n=1610)	(n=1524)	(n=1424)	(n=1345)
AVODART	(n=1623)	(n=1547)	(n=1457)	(n=1378)
Tamsulosin	(n=1611)	(n=1542)	(n=1468)	(n=1363)
Impotence				
Combination	5.5%	1.2%	0.8%	0.3%
AVODART	3.9%	1.2%	0.6%	0.7%
Tamsulosin	2.7%	0.8%	0.4%	0.4%

(cont'd)

Table 2: AVODART *(cont'd)*

Adverse Reactions Reported Over a 24-Month Period in ≥1% of Subjects in Any Treatment Group (CombAT)

	Adverse Reaction Onset			
Adverse Reactions	**Month 0–6**	**Month 7–12**	**Month 13–18**	**Month 19–24**
Decreased Libido				
Combination	4.5%	0.9%	0.4%	<0.1%
AVODART	3.3%	0.6%	0.7%	0.2%
Tamsulosin	1.9%	0.6%	0.4%	0.2%
Ejaculation Disorders				
Combination	7.6%	1.6%	0.4%	<0.1%
AVODART	1.1%	0.6%	0.1%	0.1%
Tamsulosin	2.2%	0.5%	0.4%	0.1%
Breast Disorders[b]				
Combination	1.0%	1.1%	0.7%	0.3%
AVODART	0.9%	1.0%	0.8%	0.5%
Tamsulosin	0.4%	0.4%	0.2%	0.1%
Dizziness				
Combination	1.1%	0.4%	0.2%	0%
AVODART	0.4%	0.2%	<0.1%	<0.1%
Tamsulosin	0.9%	0.5%	0.3%	0.1%

[a] Combination=AVODART 0.5 mg once daily plus tamsulosin 0.4 mg once daily.
[b] Includes breast tenderness and breast enlargement.

Cardiovascular Disorders: In CombAT, after 4 years of treatment, the incidence of the composite term cardiac failure in the combination group (14/1,610, 0.9%) was higher than in either monotherapy group: AVODART, 4/1,623 (0.2%) and tamsulosin, 10/1,611 (0.6%). The relative risk estimate for time to first cardiac failure event was 3.57 [95% CI: 1.17, 10.8] for combination treatment compared with AVODART monotherapy and 1.36 [95% CI: 0.61, 3.07] compared with tamsulosin monotherapy, as shown in Table 3.

In a 4-year comparison of placebo and AVODART in men at risk of developing prostate cancer, there was a higher incidence of the composite term cardiac failure in subjects taking AVODART (30/4,105, 0.7%) versus placebo (15/4,126, 0.4%) for a relative risk estimate for time to first cardiac failure event of 2.04 [95% CI: 1.09, 3.78] (Table 3).

Table 3: AVODART

Number (%) of Subjects with Cardiac Failure Adverse Events in Study ARI40005 and Study ARI40006, Year 4

					Relative Risk Estimate[a] [95% CI]		
Study	**Dut + Tam (n/N (%))**	**Dutas-teride (n/N (%))**	**Tamsulosin (n/N (%))**	**Placebo (n/N (%))**	**Combina-tion vs. Dutasteride**	**Combina-tion vs. Tamsu-losin**	**Dutasteride vs. Placebo**
ARI40005	14/1610 (0.9)	4/1623 (0.2)	10/1611 (0.6)		3.57 (1.17, 10.8)	1.36 (0.61, 3.07)	
ARI40006		30/4105 (0.7)		15/4126 (0.4)			2.04 (1.09, 3.78)

[a] Relative risk (hazard ratio) based on Cox proportional hazards model.
ARI40005—CombAT study, a 4-year multicenter, double-blind study in which combination of dutasteride and tamsulosin administered randomly to male subjects with BPH.
ARI40006—4-year comparison of placebo and AVODART in men at risk of developing prostate cancer.

In a post-hoc analysis of concomitant alpha-blocker use, there was a higher incidence of the composite term cardiac failure in subjects taking AVODART and an alpha-blocker concomitantly (12/1,148, 1.0%), compared with subjects not taking AVODART and an alpha-blocker concomitantly: AVODART and no alpha-blocker (18/2,957, 0.6%), placebo and an alpha-blocker (1/1,387, <0.1%), placebo and no alpha-blocker (14/2,739, 0.5%).

No imbalance was observed in the incidence of overall cardiovascular adverse events in either study. No causal relationship between AVODART (alone or in combination with an alpha-blocker) and cardiac failure has been established (see Warnings and Precautions).

DRUG INTERACTIONS: Overview: Care should be taken when administering dutasteride to patients taking potent, chronic CYP3A4 inhibitors such as ritonavir, ketoconazole, verapamil, diltiazem, cimetidine, troleandomycin, and ciprofloxacin. Based on the in vitro data, blood concentrations of dutasteride may increase in the presence of CYP3A4 inhibitors.

Dutasteride does not inhibit the in vitro metabolism of model substrates for the major human cytochrome P450 isoenzymes (CYP1A2, CYP2C9, CYP2C19, CYP2D6, and CYP3A4) at a concentration of 1000 ng/mL, 25 times greater than steady-state serum concentrations in humans. In vitro studies demonstrate that dutasteride does not displace warfarin, diazepam, or phenytoin from plasma protein binding sites, nor do these model compounds displace dutasteride.

Drug-Drug Interactions: Digoxin: In a study of 20 healthy volunteers, AVODART did not alter the steady-state pharmacokinetics of digoxin when administered concomitantly at a dose of 0.5 mg/day for 3 weeks.

Warfarin: In a study of 23 healthy volunteers, 3 weeks of treatment with AVODART 0.5 mg/day did not alter the steady-state pharmacokinetics of the S- or R-warfarin isomers or alter the effect of warfarin on prothrombin time when administered with warfarin.

Alpha-Adrenergic Blocking Agents: In a single sequence, crossover study in healthy volunteers, the administration of tamsulosin or terazosin in combination with AVODART had no effect on the steady state pharmacokinetics of either alpha adrenergic blocker. The percent change in DHT concentrations was similar for AVODART alone compared with the combination treatment.

A clinical trial was conducted in which dutasteride and tamsulosin were administered in BPH patients concomitantly for 24 weeks followed by 12 weeks of treatment with either the dutasteride and tamsulosin combination or dutasteride monotherapy. Results from the second phase of the trial revealed no excess of serious adverse events or discontinuations due to adverse events in the combination group compared to the dutasteride monotherapy group.

If AVODART is administered in combination with the alpha-blocker tamsulosin, please refer to Warnings and Precautions and Adverse Reactions.

Calcium Channel Antagonists: In a population pharmacokinetics analysis, a decrease in clearance of dutasteride was noted when co-administered with the CYP3A4 inhibitors verapamil (−37%, n=6) and diltiazem (−44%, n=5). In contrast, no decrease in clearance was seen when amlodipine, another calcium channel antagonist that is not a CYP3A4 inhibitor, was co-administered with dutasteride (+7%, n=4).

The decrease in clearance and subsequent increase in exposure to dutasteride in the presence of verapamil and diltiazem is not considered to be clinically significant. No dose adjustment is recommended.

Cholestyramine: Administration of a single 5 mg dose of AVODART followed 1 hour later by 12 g cholestyramine did not affect the relative bioavailability of dutasteride in 12 normal volunteers.

Other Concomitant Therapy: Although specific interaction studies were not performed with other compounds, approximately 90% of the subjects in the 3 Phase III pivotal efficacy studies receiving AVODART were taking other medications concomitantly. No clinically significant adverse interactions could be attributed to the combination of AVODART and concurrent therapy when AVODART was co-administered with anti-hyperlipidemics, angiotensin converting enzyme (ACE) inhibitors, beta adrenergic blocking agents, calcium channel blockers, corticosteroids, diuretics, nonsteroidal anti-inflammatory drugs (NSAIDs), phosphodiesterase Type V inhibitors and quinolone antibiotics.

Drug-Food Interactions: Dutasteride absorption is not affected by food. The effects of CYP3A4 inhibitors found in foods on dutasteride pharmacokinetics have not been studied. Care should be taken when administering dutasteride to patients who chronically consume CYP3A4 inhibitors found in foods and beverages such as grapefruit juice.

Drug-Herb Interactions: The effects of herbal remedies on the pharmacokinetics of dutasteride have not been studied. Care should be taken when administering dutasteride to patients who chronically consume herbal remedies containing CYP3A4 inhibitors (e.g., milk thistle) or CYP3A4 inducers (e.g., St. John's wort).

Drug-Laboratory Test Interactions: Effects on Prostate Specific Antigen: PSA levels generally decrease in patients treated with AVODART as the prostate volume decreases. In approximately one-half of the subjects, a 20% decrease in PSA is seen within the first month of therapy. After 6 months of therapy, PSA levels stabilize to a new baseline that is approximately 50% of the pre-treatment value. Results of subjects treated with AVODART for up to 2 years indicate this 50% reduction in PSA is maintained. Therefore, a new baseline PSA concentration should be established after 3 to 6 months of treatment with AVODART (see Warnings and Precautions, Effects on PSA and Prostate Cancer Detection).

DOSAGE AND ADMINISTRATION: Recommended Dose and Dosage Adjustment: Adult Males (Including Elderly): Monotherapy: The recommended dose of AVODART (dutasteride) is, one 0.5 mg capsule taken orally once a day.

Combination Therapy: The recommended dose of AVODART in combination with alpha-blocker is 1 AVODART capsule (0.5 mg) taken once daily and tamsulosin 0.4 mg capsule taken once daily.

Administration: AVODART capsules should be swallowed whole and not chewed or opened, as contact with the capsule contents may result in irritation of the oropharyngeal mucosa. AVODART may be taken with or without food (see Warnings and Precautions, Exposure of Women—Risk to Male Fetus and Special Handling Instructions).

Renal Impairment: The effect of renal impairment on dutasteride pharmacokinetics has not been studied. However, less than 0.1% of a steady state 0.5 mg dose of dutasteride is recovered in human urine, and no adjustment in dose is anticipated for patients with renal impairment.

Hepatic Impairment: The effect of hepatic impairment on dutasteride pharmacokinetics has not been studied. Because dutasteride is extensively metabolized and has a half-life of 3 to 5 weeks, caution should be used in the administration of dutasteride to patients with liver disease.

Missed Dose: If a dose is missed the capsule can be taken at the next scheduled dose. Extra capsules taken for missed doses are not necessary.

OVERDOSAGE:

In volunteer studies of AVODART (dutasteride), single daily doses of dutasteride up to 40 mg/day (80 times the therapeutic dose) have been administered for 7 days without significant safety concerns. In clinical studies, doses of 5 mg daily have been administered to subjects for 6 months with no additional adverse effects to those seen at therapeutic doses of 0.5 mg.

There is no specific antidote for AVODART. Therefore, in cases of suspected overdosage, symptomatic and supportive treatment should be given as appropriate, taking the long half-life of dutasteride in consideration.

> For management of a suspected drug overdose, contact your regional Poison Control Centre. See the *CPS* Directory section for a list of Poison Control Centres.

ACTION AND CLINICAL PHARMACOLOGY: Mechanism of Action: Dutasteride, a synthetic 4-azasteriod compound, inhibits the conversion of testosterone to 5 α-dihydrotestosterone (DHT). DHT is the androgen primarily responsible for the initial development and subsequent enlargement of the prostate gland. Testosterone is converted to DHT by the enzyme 5 α-reductase, which exists as 2 isoforms, Type I and Type II. Both Type I and Type II isoenzymes are present in the prostate. The Type I isoenzyme is also responsible for testosterone conversion in the skin and liver. It has been observed that compared to normal tissue, the expression of both isoenzymes are increased in BPH tissue.

Dutasteride is a competitive and specific inhibitor of both Type I and Type II 5 α-reductase isoenzymes, with which it forms a stable enzyme complex. Dissociation from this complex has been evaluated under in vitro and in vivo conditions and is extremely slow. Dutasteride lowers DHT levels and leads to a reduction in prostatic volume. Dutasteride does not bind to the human androgen receptor.

Pharmacodynamics: The maximum effect of daily doses of dutasteride on the reduction on DHT is dose dependent and is observed within 1-2 weeks. After 1 week and 2 weeks of daily dosing of dutasteride 0.5 mg, median serum DHT concentrations were reduced by 85% and 90% respectively.

In patients with BPH treated with dutasteride 0.5 mg/day for 4 years, the median decrease in serum DHT was 94% at 1 year, 93% at 2 years, and 95% at both 3 and 4 years. The median increase in serum testosterone was 19% at both 1 and 2 years, 26% at 3 years, and 22% at 4 years. The testosterone concentrations remain within the physiological normal range.

In BPH patients treated with 5 mg/day of dutasteride or placebo for up to 12 weeks prior to transurethral resection of the prostate, mean DHT concentrations in prostatic tissue were significantly lower in the dutasteride group compared with placebo (784 and 5793 pg/g, respectively, p<0.001). Mean prostatic tissue concentrations of testosterone were significantly higher in the dutasteride group compared with placebo (2073 and 93 pg/g, respectively, p<0.001).

In BPH patients (N=43) treated with dutasteride 0.5 mg/day or placebo for 3 months prior to transurethral resection of the prostate (TURP), the adjusted mean intraprostatic DHT level was significantly lower in the dutasteride group compared to the placebo group (0.209 ng/g and 3.23 ng/g, respectively, p<0.001).

In another study, men with localized prostate cancer received a loading dose of dutasteride 10 mg/day for 7 days followed by dutasteride 5 mg/day for up to 10 weeks prior to radical prostatectomy. Mean DHT concentrations in prostatic tissue were substantially lower in the dutasteride group compared with placebo (177 and 6179 pg/g, respectively).

Pharmacokinetics: Absorption: Dutasteride is rapidly absorbed with peak concentrations occurring at 1 to 3 hours and absorption is not affected by food. Absolute bioavailability is approximate 60% relative to a 2-hour intravenous infusion.

Distribution: Dutasteride has a large volume of distribution (300-500 L) and is highly bound to proteins in plasma (>99.5%). The half-life of dutasteride is 3 to 5 weeks. Steady state serum concentrations (Css) of approximately 40 ng/mL are achieved after 6 months of dosing with dutasteride 0.5 mg once daily. Similarly, dutasteride concentrations in semen reached steady-state at 6 months. After 52 weeks of treatment, semen dutasteride concentrations averaged 3.4 ng/mL (range 0.4 to 14 ng/mL).

Metabolism: Dutasteride is extensively metabolized in humans. Studies showed that CYP3A4 isoenzymes are involved in metabolism of dutasteride.

Excretion: Dutasteride and its metabolites were excreted mainly in feces. Only trace amounts of unchanged dutasteride were found in urine (<1%).

Special Populations and Conditions: Geriatrics: No dose adjustment is necessary in the elderly. The pharmacokinetics and pharmacodynamics of dutasteride were evaluated in 36 healthy male subjects between the ages of 24 and 87 years following administration of a single 5 mg dose of dutasteride. In this single-dose study, dutasteride half-life increased with age (approximately 170 hours in men aged 20 to 49 years, approximately 260 hours in men aged 50 to 69 years, and approximately 300 hours in men older than 70 years). Of 2167 men treated with dutasteride in the 3 pivotal studies, 60% were age 65 and over and 15% were age 75 and over. No overall differences in safety or efficacy were observed between these patients and younger patients.

Gender: AVODART is not indicated for use in women (see Warnings and Precautions).

Race: The effect of race on dutasteride pharmacokinetics has not been studied.

Hepatic Insufficiency: The effect on the pharmacokinetics of dutasteride in hepatic impairment has not been studied.

Renal Insufficiency: The effect of renal impairment on dutasteride pharmacokinetics has not been studied. However, less than 0.1% of a steady-state 0.5 mg dose of dutasteride is recovered in human urine, so no adjustment in dosage is anticipated for patients with renal impairment.

STORAGE AND STABILITY: Store between 15 and 30°C.

SPECIAL HANDLING INSTRUCTIONS: Dutasteride is absorbed through the skin; therefore, women and children must avoid contact with leaking capsules. If contact is made with leaking capsules, the contact area should be washed immediately with soap and water (see Contraindications and Warnings and Precautions).

INFORMATION FOR THE PATIENT: Published in e-CPS, available by subscription at www.e-cps.ca.

DOSAGE FORMS, COMPOSITION AND PACKAGING: Each opaque, yellow, oblong-shaped, soft gelatin capsule, imprinted with GX CE2 in red ink on one side, contains: 0.5 mg of dutasteride dissolved in a mixture of mono-di-glycerides of caprylic/capric acid and butylated hydroxytoluene. Nonmedicinal ingredients: capsule shell: gelatin (from certified, BSE-free, nonporcine sources), glycerol, iron oxide yellow, lecithin, medium chain triglycerides and titanium dioxide. The capsules are printed with edible red ink containing iron oxide red as the colourant. Blister packages of 30.

(Shown in Product Identification Section)

Avonex® 🅿

interferon beta-1a

Immunomodulator

Biogen Idec

Avonex® PS 🅿

interferon beta-1a

Immunomodulator

Biogen Idec

Date of Revision: May 1, 2008

SUMMARY PRODUCT INFORMATION:

Route of Administration	Dosage Form/ Strength	Clinically Relevant Nonmedicinal Ingredients
Intramuscular injection	Lyophilized powder for reconstitution/30 or 60 µg per mL reconstituted solution	Human serum albumin For a complete listing see Dosage Forms, Composition and Packaging.
	Liquid for injection in prefilled syringe/30 µg per 0.5 mL	Not applicable For a complete listing see Dosage Forms, Composition and Packaging.

DESCRIPTION: AVONEX (interferon beta-1a) and AVONEX PS (interferon beta-1a) are produced by recombinant DNA technology. Interferon beta-1a is a 166 amino acid glycoprotein with a predicted molecular weight of approximately 22 500 daltons. It is produced by mammalian cells (Chinese Hamster Ovary cells) into which the human interferon beta gene has been introduced. The amino acid sequence of interferon beta-1a is identical to that of natural human interferon beta.

Using the World Health Organization (WHO) natural interferon beta standard, Second International Standard for Interferon, Human Fibroblast (Gb-23-902-531), AVONEX and AVONEX PS have a specific activity of approximately 200 million international units (IU) of antiviral activity per mg; 30 µg of AVONEX and AVONEX PS contains 6 million IU and 60 µg of AVONEX contains 12 million IU of antiviral activity.

INDICATIONS AND CLINICAL USE: AVONEX (interferon beta-1a) and AVONEX PS (interferon beta-1a) are indicated for:

- Treatment of relapsing forms of multiple sclerosis (MS):
  - To slow the progression of disability
  - To decrease the frequency of clinical exacerbations
  - To reduce the number and volume of active brain lesions identified on Magnetic Resonance Imaging (MRI) scans.
- A subgroup of relapsing MS includes secondary progressive MS (SPMS) patients who are still experiencing relapses, also known as relapsing progressive MS (RPMS). In a study of patients with relapsing progressive MS, AVONEX showed an improvement on relapse rates and MRI measures in those patients who had greater disability at baseline.
- Treatment of people who have experienced a single demyelinating event, accompanied by abnormal MRI scans, with lesions typical of MS:
  - To delay the onset of clinically definite MS (as determined by a second demyelinating event)
  - To decrease the number and volume of active brain lesions and overall disease burden (as identified by MRI scans). Before initiating treatment with AVONEX or AVONEX PS, alternate diagnoses should first be excluded.

Safety and efficacy have not been established in patients with primary progressive multiple sclerosis.

Clinical Effects in Relapsing Forms of MS: The clinical effects of AVONEX in MS were studied in a randomized, multicentre, double-blind, placebo-controlled study in patients with relapsing (stable or progressive) MS. In this study, 301 patients received either 6 million IU (30 µg) of AVONEX (n=158) or placebo (n=143) by IM injection once weekly over 2 years.

The primary outcome assessment was time to progression in disability, and the secondary outcomes included exacerbation frequency and results of MRI scans of the brain including gadolinium (Gd)-enhanced lesion number and volume and T2-weighted lesion volume.

Time to onset of sustained progression in disability was significantly longer in patients treated with AVONEX than in patients receiving placebo (p=0.02). The percentage of patients progressing by the end of two years was 34.9% for placebo-treated patients and 21.9% for AVONEX-treated patients, indicating a 37% reduction in the risk of disability progression in patients treated with AVONEX.

AVONEX treatment significantly decreased the frequency of exacerbations (relapses) in patients who were enrolled in the study for at least two years, from 0.90 in the placebo-treated group to 0.61 in the AVONEX-treated group (p=0.002). This represents a 32% reduction in the annual exacerbation rate. The percent of exacerbation-free patients was 38% (p=0.03) in the group treated with AVONEX.

Patients treated with AVONEX demonstrated significantly lower Gd-enhanced lesions number and volume (p=0.05). The percentage change in T2-weighted lesion volume (at year 1) was significantly lower in AVONEX-treated patients (p=0.02). A similar significant effect was seen in the number of active (new and enlarging) T2 lesions over two years (p=0.002).

Clinical Effects in Delaying Onset of Clinically Definite MS: A randomized, double-blind, multicentre study was conducted to determine whether AVONEX, when compared to placebo, could delay the onset of clinically definite MS (CDMS) in 383 patients who have experienced a single episode of optic neuritis, incomplete transverse myelitis, or brainstem/cerebellar syndrome, and who had at least two subclinical multiple sclerosis-like lesions on brain MRI. Patients received either 6 million IU (30 µg) AVONEX (n=193) or placebo (n=190) by IM injection once weekly. All patients were initially treated with corticosteroids.

The primary outcome measure was time to development of CDMS. Secondary outcomes were brain MRI measures of the cumulative increase in new pathologic events (number of new or enlarging T2 lesions), the change in overall burden of disease (change in T2 lesion volume compared to baseline), and inflammatory activity at the time of the scan (gadolinium-enhancing lesions).

Time to development of CDMS was significantly delayed in patients treated with AVONEX compared to placebo (p=0.002). The rate of developing CDMS as documented by a second event was 44% lower in the group treated with AVONEX than in the placebo-treated group.

Brain MRI showed a statistically significant reduced T2 lesion volume, fewer new or enlarging T2 lesions, and fewer new Gd-enhancing lesions in the AVONEX-treated group than in the placebo-treated group after 6, 12, and 18 months of treatment. At 18 months, the AVONEX-treated group compared to the placebo group showed 91% (p<0.001) less increase in the median T2 lesion volume, a 58% (p<0.001) decrease in the mean number of new or enlarging T2 lesions, and a 71% (p<0.001) decrease in the mean number of Gd-enhancing lesions.

The safety and immunogenicity of 30 µg AVONEX PS human serum albumin (HSA)-free liquid formulation given IM once-a-week was investigated in a multicentre, single-arm, open-label study. The results were consistent with previously reported results in clinical studies of patients with relapsing forms of MS given either 30 µg or 60 µg AVONEX lyophilized powder formulation. The incidence of serum neutralizing antibodies was low (4.0%) and comparable to that observed with the lyophilized formulation (see Warnings and Precautions, Immune). AVONEX PS was well tolerated and comparable to results reported in clinical studies of AVONEX (see Adverse Reactions).

In a bioequivalence comparison of AVONEX PS and AVONEX , the results of the ANOVA analysis demonstrate that the liquid formulation is more bioavailable compared to the lyophilized formulation. However, this does not translate into clinical and immunological differences between the two formulations (as measured by the presence of binding and neutralizing antibodies to human interferon beta-1a).

Other Studies: Secondary Progressive MS: The clinical effects of AVONEX were also investigated in a randomized, multicentre, double-blind, placebo-controlled, parallel-group study in male and female patients with secondary progressive MS. Patients received either AVONEX 60 µg (n=217) or placebo (n=219) by IM injection once weekly for 2 years. The study used a composite outcome measure, the Multiple Sclerosis Functional Composite (MSFC). The MSFC consists of the Timed 25-Foot Walk, Nine Hole Peg Test (9HPT), and Paced Auditory Serial Addition Test (PASAT). In both groups, the mean baseline EDSS score was 5.2 (range 3.5 to 6.5).

In the patients treated with AVONEX 60 µg, compared to the placebo group, disease progression was reduced by approximately 27% (based on mean MSFC score) or 40% (based on median MSFC score) (p=0.033). This result was mainly based on the 9HPT (upper extremity function measure) and the PASAT (cognitive function measure). For the Timed 25-foot walk, a difference between treatment arms was observed although this did not reach statistical significance. Sustained progression when measured by the Kurtze Expanded Disability Status Scale (EDSS) was similar (p=0.901) for patients receiving AVONEX 60 µg (32%) or placebo (37%). AVONEX 60 µg demonstrated statistically significant reductions of relapse rate (32%, p=0.008) and on all MRI outcome measures (p<0.0001) compared to placebo.

The treatment effect was strongest and approached clinical significance (p=0.074) in patients who had experienced relapse in the previous year. In this subgroup, active treatment reduced disease progression by 44% (based on mean MSFC score) or 59% (based on median MSFC score). In patients who had not had a clinical relapse in the previous year, however, active treatment reduced disease progression by 9.5% (based on mean MSFC score) or 27% (based on median MSFC score) that did not approach statistical significance (p=0.206). This suggests that patients with secondary progressive MS who have had recent relapses would achieve the most benefit from AVONEX 60 µg.

Dose-comparison Study: The clinical effects of AVONEX were investigated in another study comparing the safety and efficacy of 30 µg and 60 µg doses of AVONEX in relapsing MS patients, which included relapsing progressive MS (RPMS) patients similar to the patients with secondary progressive MS in the above study. The results of this dose-comparison study showed that patients meeting the definition of RPMS with a higher baseline EDSS demonstrated the benefit of the higher dose in an analysis of a number of EDSS milestones. For the overall RP group (n=120), no statistical difference between the two dose groups was found (p=0.902). However, statistical significance was reached for a small subgroup of subjects who had baseline EDSS >4.5 (n=25 each group, p=0.036). The advantage of 60 µg over 30 µg on time to reaching an EDSS of 6 or greater was most clear for RPMS patients with a high baseline EDSS. No evidence of an effect of 60 µg over 30 µg was observed for the same analysis in the RRMS patients in this study.

Geriatrics (>65 years of age): Clinical trials of AVONEX did not include sufficient numbers of patients aged 65 years and over to determine whether they respond differently than younger patients.

Pediatrics (<18 years of age): Safety and effectiveness have not been established in patients below the age of 18 years.

CONTRAINDICATIONS: AVONEX (interferon beta-1a) and AVONEX PS (interferon beta-1a) are contraindicated in:

- Persons with a history of hypersensitivity to natural or recombinant interferon beta.
- Persons with a history of hypersensitivity to any other component of the formulation or the container.
- For AVONEX (interferon beta-1a) only, a history of hypersensitivity to human serum albumin (HSA).
  For a complete listing, see Dosage Forms, Composition and Packaging.

WARNINGS AND PRECAUTIONS: General: AVONEX (interferon beta-1a) and AVONEX PS (interferon beta-1a) should be used under the supervision of a physician. The first injection should be performed under the supervision of an appropriately qualified health care professional (see Dosage and Administration).

Patients should be informed of the following information:

- The most common adverse events associated with interferon beta administration, including symptoms of the flu-like syndrome (see Adverse Reactions). These symptoms tend to be most prominent at the initiation of therapy and decrease in frequency and severity with continued treatment.
- To **not** stop or modify their treatment unless instructed by their physician.
- To report depression or suicidal ideation.
- The risk of decreased blood counts including white blood cells and platelet counts and of the requirement for periodic laboratory testing. Patients should be advised to report immediately any clinical symptoms associated with blood cell count abnormalities and laboratory testing should be performed according to standard medical practice. Patients with myelosuppression may require more intensive monitoring of complete blood cell counts, with differential and platelet counts.
- The potential risk of liver injury with AVONEX and AVONEX PS therapy, and of the requirement for frequent laboratory testing. Patients should be informed of the symptoms of suggestive liver dysfunction, such as loss of appetite accompanied by other symptoms such as nausea, vomiting, and jaundice, and advised to consult with their physician immediately should such symptoms arise.
- To report any symptoms of thyroid dysfunction (hypo or hyperthyroidism) and thyroid function tests should be performed according to standard medical practice.
- Female patients should be advised about the abortifacient potential of AVONEX and AVONEX PS and instructed to take adequate contraceptive measures.
- When a physician determines that AVONEX or AVONEX PS can be used outside the physician's office, persons who will be administering AVONEX or AVONEX PS should receive instruction in reconstitution and injection, including the review of the injection procedures (see Information for the Patient). If a patient is to self-administer, the physical ability of the patient to self-inject intramuscularly should be assessed. If home use is chosen, the first injection should be performed under the supervision of a qualified health care professional. Patients should be advised of the importance of rotating sites of injection with each dose, to minimize the likelihood of injection site reactions. A puncture-resistant container for disposal of needles and syringes should be used. Patients should be instructed in the technique and importance of proper syringe and needle disposal and be cautioned against reuse of these items.
- Patients receiving AVONEX 60 µg IM once a week in the relapsing MS population showed similar adverse event and tolerability patterns to the 30 µg dose. Adverse events known to be associated with interferon administration (e.g. flu syndrome, asthenia, depression, headache, myalgia, nausea, fever, diarrhea, dizziness and chills) generally occurred at similar frequencies between the two dose groups, with the exception of flu syndrome (AVONEX 30 µg vs AVONEX 60 µg: 85% vs 92%, respectively).

Carcinogenesis and Mutagenesis: No carcinogenicity data for interferon beta-1a are available in animals or humans.

Interferon beta-1a was not mutagenic when tested in the Ames bacterial test and in an in vitro cytogenetic assay in human lymphocytes in the presence and absence of metabolic activation. These assays are designed to detect agents that interact directly with and cause damage to cellular DNA. Interferon beta-1a is a glycosylated protein that does not directly bind to DNA.

Cardiovascular: Patients with cardiac disease, such as angina, congestive heart failure, or arrhythmia, should be closely monitored for worsening of their clinical condition during initiation and continued treatment with AVONEX or AVONEX PS. While AVONEX or AVONEX PS does not have any known direct-acting cardiac toxicity, during the post-marketing period infrequent cases of congestive heart failure, cardiomyopathy, and cardiomyopathy with congestive heart failure have been reported in patients without known predisposition to these events or other known etiologies. In rare cases, these events have been temporally related to the administration of AVONEX and have recurred upon re-challenge in patients with known predisposition.

Endocrine and Metabolism: Other interferons have been noted to reduce cytochrome P-450 oxidase-mediated drug metabolism. Formal hepatic drug metabolism studies with AVONEX or AVONEX PS in humans have not been conducted. Hepatic microsomes isolated from rhesus monkeys treated with AVONEX showed no influence of AVONEX on hepatic P-450 enzyme metabolism activity.

Hematologic: Decreased Peripheral Blood Counts: Decreased peripheral blood counts in all cell lines, including very rare pancytopenia and thrombocytopenia have been reported from post-marketing experience (see Adverse Reactions). Some cases of thrombocytopenia have had nadirs below 10 000/mL. Some cases reoccur with re-challenge. Patients should be monitored for signs of these disorders (see Monitoring and Laboratory Tests).

Hepatic/Biliary/Pancreatic: AVONEX and AVONEX PS, like other interferon beta products, have the potential for causing severe liver injury (see Adverse Reactions). Hepatic injury including elevated serum hepatic enzyme levels, hepatitis and autoimmune hepatitis (see Warnings and Precautions, Immune), some of which have been severe, has been reported post-marketing. In some patients a recurrence of elevated serum levels of hepatic enzymes have occurred upon AVONEX re-challenge. In some cases, these events have occurred in the presence of other drugs that have been associated with hepatic injury. The potential of additive effects from multiple drugs or other hepatotoxic agents (e.g., alcohol) has not been determined.

Cases of hepatic failure have been reported with interferon beta-1a in post-marketing, including very rare cases with AVONEX.

Patients should be monitored for signs of hepatic injury (see Monitoring and Laboratory Tests) and caution exercised when AVONEX or AVONEX PS is used concomitantly with other drugs associated with hepatic injury.

Immune: As with other interferon treatment, autoimmune disorders of multiple target organs have been reported post marketing including idiopathic thrombocytopenia, hyper and hypothyroidism, and rare cases of autoimmune hepatitis have also been reported. Patients should be monitored for signs of these disorders (see Monitoring and Laboratory Tests) and appropriate treatment implemented when observed.

Serum neutralizing antibodies were reported to develop in only 2% to 6% of patients treated with AVONEX and AVONEX PS. Although the exact clinical significance of antibodies has not been fully established, there are multiple literature reports indicating that the occurrence of neutralizing antibodies with beta interferon treatment impacts clinical efficacy, MRI measures and the induction of biological markers.

Neurologic: Seizures: Caution should be exercised when administering AVONEX or AVONEX PS to patients with pre-existing seizure disorder. In the two placebo-controlled studies of MS, four patients receiving AVONEX experienced seizures, while no seizures occurred in the placebo group. Of these four patients, three had no prior history of seizure. It is not known whether these events were related to the effects of MS alone, to AVONEX, or to a combination of both. For patients with no prior history of seizure who developed seizures during therapy with AVONEX and AVONEX PS, an etiologic basis should be established and appropriate anti-convulsant therapy instituted prior to considering resumption of treatment. The effect of AVONEX and AVONEX PS administration on the medical management of patients with seizure disorder is unknown.

Psychiatric: Depression and Suicide: AVONEX and AVONEX PS should be used with caution in patients with depression. Depression and suicide have been reported to occur in patients receiving other interferon compounds. Depression and suicidal ideation are known to occur at an increased frequency in the MS population. A relationship between the occurrence of depression and/or suicidal ideation and the use of AVONEX and AVONEX PS has not been established. An equal incidence of depression was seen in the placebo-treated and the patients treated with AVONEX in the placebo-controlled study of relapsing MS patients. In the study of patients with a single demyelinating event patients treated with AVONEX were more likely to experience depression than placebo-treated patients (p=0.05). Suicidal tendency occurred in one subject treated with placebo, and there were no reports of suicide attempts. Patients treated with AVONEX and AVONEX PS should be advised to report immediately any symptoms of depression and/or suicidal ideation to their prescribing physicians. If a patient develops depression, antidepressant therapy or cessation of AVONEX and AVONEX PS therapy should be considered.

Sensitivity/Resistance: Anaphylaxis has been reported as a rare complication of AVONEX and AVONEX PS use. Other allergic reactions have included dyspnea, orolingual edema, skin rash and urticaria (see Adverse Reactions).

Sexual Function/Reproduction: No studies were conducted to evaluate the effects of interferon beta on fertility in normal women or women with MS. It is not known whether AVONEX and AVONEX PS can affect human reproductive capacity. Menstrual irregularities were observed in monkeys administered interferon beta at a dose 100 times the recommended weekly human dose (based upon a body surface area comparison). Anovulation and decreased serum progesterone levels were also noted transiently in some animals. These effects were reversible after discontinuation of drug.

Treatment of monkeys with interferon beta at two times the recommended weekly human dose (based upon a body surface area comparison) had no effects on cycle duration or ovulation.

The accuracy of extrapolating animal doses to human doses is not known. In the placebo-controlled study, 6% of patients receiving placebo and 5% of patients receiving AVONEX experienced menstrual disorder. If menstrual irregularities occur in humans, it is not known how long they will persist following treatment.

Special Populations: Pregnant Women: The extent of exposure in pregnancy during clinical trials is: Limited: <1000 pregnancies.

AVONEX and AVONEX PS should not be administered in case of pregnancy. There are no adequate and well-controlled studies of AVONEX and AVONEX PS in pregnant women. Patients should be advised of the abortifacient potential of AVONEX and AVONEX PS. Fertile women receiving AVONEX and AVONEX PS should be advised to take adequate contraceptive measures. It is not known if interferons alter the efficacy of oral contraceptives.

If a woman becomes pregnant or plans to become pregnant while taking AVONEX or AVONEX PS, she should be informed of the potential hazards to the fetus, and it should be recommended that the woman discontinue therapy. The reproductive toxicity of AVONEX and AVONEX PS has not been studied in animals or humans. In pregnant monkeys given interferon beta at 100 times the recommended weekly human dose (based upon a body surface area comparison), no teratogenic or other adverse effects on fetal development were observed. Abortifacient activity was evident following 3 to 5 doses at this level. No abortifacient effects were observed in monkeys treated at two times the recommended weekly human dose (based upon a body surface area comparison). Although no teratogenic effects were seen in these studies, it is not known if teratogenic effects would be observed in humans. There are no adequate and well-controlled studies with interferons in pregnant women.

Nursing Women: AVONEX and AVONEX PS should not be administered in case of lactation. It is not known whether AVONEX or AVONEX PS is excreted in human milk. Because of the potential of serious adverse reactions in nursing infants, a decision should be made to either discontinue nursing or to discontinue AVONEX and AVONEX PS.

Pediatrics (<18 years of age): Safety and effectiveness have not been established.

Geriatrics (>65 years of age): Clinical studies with AVONEX did not include sufficient numbers of patients >65 years to determine whether they respond differently than younger patients.

Monitoring and Laboratory Tests: Laboratory abnormalities are associated with the use of interferons. During the placebo-controlled trials in multiple sclerosis, liver function tests were performed at least every 6 months. Liver function tests including serum ALT are recommended during AVONEX and AVONEX PS therapy and should be performed at baseline, monthly at months 1 through 6, and every 6 months thereafter. AVONEX and AVONEX PS should be initiated with caution in patients with a history of significant liver disease, clinical evidence of active liver disease, alcohol abuse, increased serum ALT (>2.5 times ULN), and in patients receiving concomitant medications associated with hepatic injury. These patients may require more frequent monitoring of serum hepatic enzymes. Discontinuation or interruption of AVONEX and AVONEX PS should be considered if ALT rises above 5 times the ULN. Treatment with AVONEX and AVONEX PS should be stopped if jaundice or other clinical symptoms of liver dysfunction appear. In addition to those laboratory tests normally required for monitoring patients with MS, and in addition to liver enzyme monitoring (see Warnings and Precaution, Hepatic/Biliary/Pancreatic) complete blood cell counts and white blood cell differential, platelet counts, and blood chemistries are recommended during AVONEX and AVONEX PS therapy (see Warnings and Precautions, Hematologic and Adverse Reactions). These tests should be performed at baseline, months 1, 3, 6, and every 6 months thereafter. Patients with myelosuppression may require more intensive monitoring of complete blood cell counts, with differential and platelet counts.

Patients being treated with interferon beta may occasionally develop new or worsening thyroid abnormalities. Thyroid testing should be performed at baseline and every 6 months. In case of abnormal results or in patients with a past history of thyroid dysfunction, any necessary treatment and more frequent testing should be performed as clinically indicated.

ADVERSE REACTIONS: Adverse Drug Reaction Overview: The five most common adverse events associated (at p<0.075) with AVONEX (interferon beta-1a) and AVONEX PS (interferon beta-1a) treatment were flu-like symptoms (otherwise unspecified), muscle ache, fever, chills, and asthenia. The incidence of all 5 adverse events diminished with continued treatment.

In the placebo-controlled study of patients with relapsing MS, one patient in the placebo group and no AVONEX-treated patients attempted suicide. The incidence of depression was equal in the two treatment groups. However, since depression and suicide have been reported with other interferon products, AVONEX or AVONEX PS should be used with caution in patients with depression (see Warnings and Precautions). Four patients receiving AVONEX experienced seizures, while no seizures occurred in the placebo group. Of these four patients, three had no prior history of seizure. It is not known whether these events were related to the effects of MS alone, to AVONEX, or to a combination of both (see Warnings and Precautions).

In the study of patients experiencing a single demyelinating event, the most common adverse events associated with AVONEX (p≤0.05) during the first six months of treatment were flu-like syndrome (AVONEX: 39%, placebo: 22%), fever (AVONEX: 17%, placebo: 6%) and chills (AVONEX: 17%, placebo: 3%). A higher proportion of patients treated with AVONEX (20%) experienced depression, as compared with placebo (13%) (p=0.05) (see Warnings and Precautions).

Patients receiving AVONEX 60 µg IM once a week in the relapsing MS population showed similar adverse event and tolerability patterns to the 30 µg dose. Adverse events known to be associated with interferon administration (e.g. flu syndrome, asthenia, depression, headache, myalgia, nausea, fever, diarrhea, dizziness and chills) generally occurred at similar frequencies between the two dose groups, with the exception of flu syndrome (AVONEX 30 µg vs AVONEX 60 µg: 85% vs 92%, respectively).

Serious adverse events occurred in 52% of patients in the 30 µg dose group and 45% of patients in the 60 µg dose group. The incidence of serious adverse events was similar between the two treatment groups, with the exception of accidental injury, which occurred more often in the 30 µg group (30 µg vs 60 µg: 4% vs 1% respectively). Overall the safety profile of AVONEX 60 µg appeared to be similar to that of AVONEX 30 µg in subjects with relapsing MS.

Clinical Trial Adverse Drug Reactions: Because clinical trials are conducted under very specific conditions the adverse reaction rates observed in the clinical trials may not reflect the rates observed in practice and should not be compared to the rates in the clinical trials of another drug. Adverse drug reaction information from clinical trials is useful for identifying drug-related adverse events and for approximating rates.

Relapsing Multiple Sclerosis: The safety data describing the use of AVONEX in MS patients are based on the placebo-controlled trial in which 158 patients with relapsing multiple sclerosis randomized to AVONEX were treated for up to 2 years.

Single Demyelinating Event: The adverse events observed in the placebo-controlled study of patients with a single demyelinating event were similar to those observed in the placebo-controlled study of relapsing MS patients. Patients in this trial (n=193) initiated treatment with AVONEX while on oral prednisone, which was used to treat the initial demyelinating event.

Table 1 enumerates adverse events and selected laboratory abnormalities that occurred at an incidence of 2% or more among the 158 patients with relapsing MS treated with 30 µg AVONEX once weekly by IM injection. Reported adverse events have been classified using standard COSTART terms. Terms so general as to be uninformative or more common in the placebo-treated patients have been excluded.

Table 1: AVONEX

Adverse Events and Selected Laboratory Abnormalities in the Placebo-controlled Study of Relapsing MS

	Placebo (%) n=143	AVONEX (%) n=158
Body as a Whole		
Headache	57	67
Flu-like Symptoms (otherwise unspecified)[a]	40	61
Pain	20	24
Fever[a]	13	23
Asthenia	13	21
Chills[a]	7	21
Infection	6	11
Abdominal Pain	6	9
Chest Pain	4	6
Injection Site Reaction	1	4
Malaise	3	4
Injection Site Inflammation	0	3
Hypersensitivity Reaction	0	3
Ovarian Cyst	0	3
Ecchymosis Injection Site	1	2
Cardiovascular System		
Syncope	2	4
Vasodilation	1	4
Digestive System		
Nausea	23	33
Diarrhea	10	16
Dyspepsia	7	11
Anorexia	6	7
Hemic and Lymphatic System		
Anemia[a]	3	8
Eosinophils ≥10%	4	5
HCT (%) ≤32 (females) or ≤37 (males)	1	3
Metabolic and Nutritional Disorders		
AST ≥3×ULN	1 %	3 %
Musculoskeletal System		
Muscle Ache[a]	15	34
Arthralgia	5	9
Nervous System		
Sleep Difficult	16	19
Dizziness	13	15
Muscle Spasm	6	7
Suicidal Tendency	1	4
Seizure	0	3
Speech Disorder	0	3
Ataxia	0	2
Respiratory System		

(cont'd)

Table 1: AVONEX *(cont'd)*

Adverse Events and Selected Laboratory Abnormalities in the Placebo-controlled Study of Relapsing MS

	Placebo (%) n=143	AVONEX (%) n=158
Upper Respiratory Tract Infection	28	31
Sinusitis	17	18
Dyspnea	3	6
Skin and Appendages		
Urticaria	2	5
Alopecia	1	4
Nevus	0	3
Herpes Zoster	2	3
Herpes Simplex	1	2
Special Senses		
Otitis Media	5	6
Hearing Decreased	0	3
Urogenital		
Vaginitis	2	4

[a] Significantly associated with AVONEX treatment (p≤0.05).

Other: AVONEX has also been evaluated in 290 patients with diseases other than MS. The majority of these patients were enrolled in studies to evaluate AVONEX treatment of chronic viral hepatitis B and C with AVONEX, in which the doses studied ranged from 15 µg to 75 µg, given subcutaneously (SC), 3 times a week, for up to 6 months. The incidence of common adverse events in these studies was generally seen at a frequency similar to that seen in the placebo-controlled MS study. In these non-MS studies, inflammation at the site of the SC injection was seen in 52% of treated patients. In contrast, injection site inflammation was seen in 3% of MS patients receiving AVONEX, 30 µg by IM injection. SC injections were also associated with the following local reactions: injection site necrosis, injection site atrophy, injection site edema, and injection site hemorrhage. None of the above was observed in the MS patients participating in the placebo-controlled study of relapsing MS.

AVONEX PS has been shown to have comparable safety and immunogenicity profiles compared to what has been reported with the use of AVONEX in previous clinical trials and in clinical practice. In the safety and immunogenicity study with AVONEX PS liquid formulation, three of the five adverse events in which the incidence was greater than 20% (flu syndrome: 134 (88%); headache: 69 (45%); asthenia: 40 (26%)), were attributable to the flu-like syndrome associated with interferon therapy. Paresthesia occurred in 33 (22%) patients, and MS exacerbation, an event inherent to the relapsing form of MS, was seen in 50 (33%) patients. Depression, which is known to be associated with MS and potentially with interferon therapy, was observed in 23 (15%) patients. There were no reported suicide attempts or suicidal tendency in this study. The incidence of depression in this study is similar to that observed in the group treated with AVONEX in the clinical studies (15%). Twenty-five percent of subjects (38/153) experienced an adverse event related to the injection site, the most frequent of which were injection site ecchymosis (12%) and injection site pain (11 %). These rates are similar to those seen with AVONEX in previous clinical studies. There were no unexpected laboratory abnormalities in this trial. Mild shifts outside of the normal range occurred with an incidence similar to that seen with AVONEX.

Post-Market Adverse Drug Reactions: Anaphylaxis and other allergic reactions and decreased peripheral blood counts have been reported in patients using AVONEX and AVONEX PS. Seizures, cardiovascular adverse events, and autoimmune disorders also have been reported in association with the use of AVONEX (see Warnings and Precautions).

Other events observed during premarket and postmarket evaluation of AVONEX, administered either SC or IM are listed below. Because most of the events were observed in open and uncontrolled studies, or in marketed use, the role of AVONEX and AVONEX PS in their causation cannot be reliably determined.

Body as a Whole: abscess, ascites, cellulitis, facial edema, hernia, injection site fibrosis, injection site hypersensitivity, injection site reaction (including pain, inflammation, and very rare cases of abscess or cellulitis) lipoma, neoplasm, photosensitivity reaction, rigors, sepsis, sinus headache, tachycardia, toothache.

Cardiovascular System: arrhythmia, arteritis, congestive heart failure, heart arrest, hemorrhage, hypotension, palpitation, pericarditis, peripheral ischemia, peripheral vascular disorder, postural hypotension, pulmonary embolus, spider angioma, tachycardia, telangiectasia, vascular disorder.

Digestive System: blood in stool, colitis, constipation, diverticulitis, dry mouth, gallbladder disorder, gastritis, gastrointestinal hemorrhage, gingivitis, gum hemorrhage, hepatitis, hepatoma, hepatomegaly, increased appetite, intestinal perforation, intestinal obstruction, liver function test abnormalities, periodontal abscess, periodontitis, proctitis, thirst, tongue disorder, vomiting.

Endocrine System: hyperthyroidism, hypothyroidism.

Hemic and Lymphatic System: coagulation time increased, ecchymosis, lymphadenopathy, petechia.

Metabolic and Nutritional Disorders: abnormal healing, dehydration, hypoglycemia, hypomagnesemia, hypokalemia.

Musculoskeletal System: arthritis, bone pain, myasthenia, osteonecrosis, synovitis.

Nervous System: abnormal gait, amnesia, anxiety, Bell's Palsy, clumsiness, confusion, depersonalization, drug dependence, emotional lability, facial paralysis, hyperesthesia, hypertonia, increased libido, neurosis, paresthesia, psychosis, transient severe weakness.

Respiratory System: emphysema, hemoptysis, hiccup, hyperventilation, laryngitis, pharyngeal edema, pneumonia.

Skin and Appendages: basal cell carcinoma, blisters, cold clammy skin, contact dermatitis, erythema, furunculosis, genital pruritus, nevus, pruritus, rash (including vesicular rash), seborrhea, skin ulcer, skin discoloration.

Special Senses: abnormal vision, conjunctivitis, earache, eye pain, labyrinthitis, vitreous floaters.

Urogenital: breast fibroadenosis, breast mass, dysuria, epididymitis, fibrocystic change of the breast, fibroids, gynecomastia, hematuria, kidney calculus, kidney pain, leukorrhea, menopause, nocturia, pelvic inflammatory disease, penis disorder, Peyronies Disease, polyuria, post menopausal hemorrhage, prostatic disorder, pyelonephritis, testis disorder, urethral pain, urinary urgency, urinary retention, urinary incontinence, vaginal hemorrhage.

DRUG INTERACTIONS: Overview: No formal drug interaction studies have been conducted with AVONEX (interferon beta-1a) and AVONEX PS (interferon beta-1a). In the placebo-controlled study, corticosteroids or ACTH were administered for treatment of exacerbations in some patients concurrently receiving AVONEX. In addition, some patients receiving AVONEX were also treated with anti-depressant therapy and/or oral contraceptive therapy. No unexpected adverse events were associated with these concomitant therapies.

Drug-Drug Interactions: As with all interferon products, proper monitoring of patients is required if AVONEX or AVONEX PS is given in combination with myelosuppressive agents.

DOSAGE AND ADMINISTRATION: Dosing Considerations:

- Intended for use under the guidance and supervision of a physician.
- Patients may self-inject only:
  - If their physician determines that it is appropriate
  - Appropriate medical follow-up is provided
  - After proper training in IM injection technique
- Injection sites (thigh or upper arm) should be rotated each week. Avoid injection into an area of skin that is sore, red, infected or otherwise damaged.
- Before initiating a patient on AVONEX (interferon beta-1a) or AVONEX PS (interferon beta-1a) therapy, note the following Contraindications:
  - In patients with a known hypersensitivity to natural or recombinant interferon beta, human serum albumin (AVONEX) or any other component of the formulation. Anaphylaxis has been observed with the use of AVONEX and AVONEX PS.
- Review the Warnings and Precautions section and ensure appropriate monitoring of patients with depression, hepatic dysfunction, a history of seizures, cardiac disease, thyroid dysfunction, myelosuppression, and female patients of child-bearing potential.
- Patients should be advised of the side-effects of AVONEX and AVONEX PS and instructed on the use of aseptic technique when administering AVONEX or AVONEX PS. Information for the Patient should be carefully reviewed with all patients, and patients should be educated on self-care and advised to continue to refer to Information for the Patient during treatment with AVONEX or AVONEX PS.
- A shorter thinner needle for intramuscular injection may be substituted by the prescribing physician, if deemed appropriate.

Recommended Dose and Dosage Adjustment: 30 µg injected intramuscularly once per week.

Patients with relapsing progressive MS or secondary progressive MS with recurrent attacks of neurological dysfunction could benefit from an increase of their dose of AVONEX up to 60 µg.

Missed Dose: If a dose is missed, the next dose should be taken as soon as possible. The regular schedule should be continued the following week. **Do not take AVONEX or AVONEX PS on two consecutive days.**

Administration: AVONEX lyophilized powder must be reconstituted by adding 1.1 mL of supplied sterile Water for Injection to the single-use vial of lyophilized powder prior to intramuscular injection. The 1.0 mL is withdrawn for administration (see Information for the Patient).

AVONEX PS in the prefilled syringe does not require reconstitution prior to injection.

Reconstitution: Parenteral Products:

Vial Size	Volume of Diluent to be Added to Vial	Approximate Available Volume	Nominal Concentration per mL
3 mL	1.1 mL	1.0 mL	30 µg or 60 µg

Use the reconstituted product as soon as possible, but within 6 hours if stored at 2 to 8°C. **Do not freeze** the reconstituted solution.

OVERDOSAGE:

In clinical studies, overdosage was not seen using interferon beta-1a at a dose of 75 µg given subcutaneously three times a week.

For management of a suspected drug overdose, CPhA recommends that you contact your **regional Poison Control Centre**. See the *CPS* Directory section for a list of Poison Control Centres.

ACTION AND CLINICAL PHARMACOLOGY: Mechanism of Action: Interferons are a family of naturally occurring proteins and glycoproteins that are produced by eukaryotic cells in response to viral infection and other biological inducers. Interferon beta, one member of this family, is produced by various cell types including fibroblasts and macrophages. Natural interferon beta and interferon beta-1a are similarly glycosylated. Glycosylation of other proteins is known to affect their stability, activity, biodistribution, and half-life in blood. Glycosylation of other proteins also decreases aggregation of proteins. Protein aggregates are thought to be involved in the immunogenicity of recombinant proteins. Aggregated forms of interferon beta are known to have lower levels of specific activity than monomeric (non-aggregated) forms of interferon beta.

Interferons are cytokines that mediate antiviral, antiproliferative, and immunomodulatory activities in response to viral infection and other biological inducers. Three major interferons have been distinguished: alpha, beta, and gamma. Interferons alpha and beta form the Type I class of interferons and interferon gamma is a Type II interferon. These interferons have overlapping but clearly distinct biological activities.

Interferon beta exerts its biological effects by binding to specific receptors on the surface of human cells. This binding initiates a complex cascade of intracellular events that lead to the expression of numerous interferon-induced gene products and markers. These include 2', 5'-oligoadenylate synthetase, β_2-microglobulin, and neopterin. These products have been measured in the serum and cellular fractions of blood collected from patients treated with AVONEX (interferon beta-1a).

The specific interferon-induced proteins and mechanisms by which AVONEX exerts its effects in MS have not been fully defined. To understand the mechanism(s) of action of AVONEX, studies were conducted to determine the effect of IM injection of AVONEX on levels of the immunosuppressive cytokine interleukin 10 (IL-10) in serum and cerebrospinal fluid (CSF) of treated patients. IL-10, or cytokine synthesis inhibitory factor, is a potent immunosuppressor of a number of pro-inflammatory cytokines such as interferon gamma (IFN-γ), tumor necrosis factor alpha (TNF-α), interleukin 1 (IL-1), tumor necrosis factor beta (TNF-β), and interleukin 6 (IL-6), which are secreted by T lymphocyte helper-1 (Th1) cells and macrophages. Elevated serum IL-10 levels were seen after IM injection of AVONEX, from 48 hours post-injection through at least 7 days. Similarly, in the Phase III study, IL-10 levels in CSF were significantly increased in patients treated with AVONEX compared to placebo. CSF IL-10 levels correlated with a favourable clinical treatment response to AVONEX.

Upregulation of IL-10 represents a possible mechanism of action of interferon beta in relapsing MS. IL-10 has been demonstrated to decrease relapses in acute and chronic relapsing experimental autoimmune encephalomyelitis (EAE), an animal model resembling MS. However, no relationship has been established between the absolute levels of IL-10 and the clinical outcome in MS.

STORAGE AND STABILITY: AVONEX: Vials of AVONEX (interferon beta-1a) should be stored in a refrigerator at 2 to 8°C. Should refrigeration be unavailable, vials of AVONEX can be stored at up to 25°C for a period of up to 30 days. If the product has been exposed to conditions other than those recommended, **discard the product and do not use.**

AVONEX PS: Prefilled syringes of AVONEX PS (interferon beta-1a) should be stored in a refrigerator at 2 to 8°C. Once removed from the refrigerator, the prefilled syringe should be allowed to warm to room temperature (approximately 30 minutes). Do not use external heat sources, such as hot water, to warm the prefilled syringe. AVONEX PS can be stored at room temperature (between 15-30°C) for up to one week. If the product has been exposed to conditions other than those recommended, **discard the product and do not use.**

Additional information for AVONEX vial and AVONEX PS prefilled syringe:

- Do not expose to high temperatures.
- Do not freeze.
- Do not use beyond the expiration date stamped on the vial.
- Protect from light.

SPECIAL HANDLING INSTRUCTIONS: The supplied diluent Sterile Water for Injection must be used for reconstitution of the lyophilized powder. No other diluent may be used.

INFORMATION FOR THE PATIENT: Published in e-CPS, available by subscription at www.e-cps.ca.

DOSAGE FORMS, COMPOSITION AND PACKAGING: AVONEX: Each single-use vial of sterile white to off-white lyophilized powder, contains: interferon beta-1a 33 µg (6.6 million IU) or 66 µg (13.2 million IU). Nonmedicinal ingredients: human serum albumin USP 16.5 mg, dibasic sodium phosphate USP 6.3 mg, monobasic sodium phosphate USP 1.3 mg and sodium chloride USP 6.4 mg. Preservative-free. Administration Dose Packs containing 1 vial of AVONEX (3 mL), 1 vial of sterile Water for Injection (10 mL), 2 alcohol wipes, 1 syringe (3 mL), 1 Micro Pin, 1 needle, 1 adhesive bandage, 1 gauze pad; packages of 4.

AVONEX PS: Each prefilled syringe of sterile liquid contains: interferon beta-1a 30 µg (6.0 million IU). Nonmedicinal ingredients: arginine hydrochloride USP 15.8 mg, glacial acetic acid USP 0.25 mg, polysorbate 20 0.025 mg, sodium acetate trihydrate USP 0.79 mg and Water for Injection USP 0.5 mL at a pH of 4.8. Administration Dose Packs containing 1 prefilled syringe of AVONEX PS liquid and 1 needle for injection and a reclosable accessory pouch containing 4 alcohol wipes, 4 gauze pads and 4 adhesive bandages; packages of 4.

Axert® Ⓟ

almotriptan malate

5-HT1 Receptor Agonist—Migraine Therapy

McNeil Consumer Healthcare

Date of Preparation: September 22, 2003
Date of Revision: March 4, 2009

PHARMACOLOGY: Mechanism of Action: AXERT (almotriptan malate) is a selective 5-hydroxytryptamine$_{1B/1D}$ (5-HT$_{1B/1D}$) receptor agonist. Almotriptan binds with high affinity to 5-HT$_{1D}$, 5-HT$_{1B}$ and 5-HT$_{1F}$ receptors. Almotriptan has a weak affinity for 5-HT$_{1A}$ and 5-HT$_7$ receptors, but has no significant affinity or pharmacological activity at 5-HT$_2$, 5-HT$_3$, 5-HT$_4$, 5-HT$_6$; alpha or beta adrenergic; adenosine (A$_1$, A$_2$); angiotensin (AT$_1$, AT$_2$); dopamine (D$_1$, D$_2$); endothelin (ET$_A$, ET$_B$); or tachykinin (NK$_1$, NK$_2$, NK$_3$) binding sites.

Current theories on the etiology of migraine headaches suggest that symptoms are due to local cranial vasodilatation and/or to the release of vasoactive and pro-inflammatory peptides from the sensory nerve endings in an activated trigeminal system. The therapeutic activity of almotriptan in migraine can most likely be attributed to agonist effects at 5-HT$_{1B/1D}$ receptors on the extracerebral, intracranial blood vessels that become dilated during a migraine attack, and on the nerve terminals in the trigeminal system. Activation of these receptors results in cranial vessel constriction, inhibition of the neuropeptide release, and reduced transmission in the trigeminal pain pathways.

Pharmacokinetics: Absorption: Almotriptan is well absorbed following oral administration. The mean oral absolute bioavailability is approximately 70%, and peak plasma concentrations of approximately 40 ng/mL are reached 1 to 3 hours after a single 12.5 mg dose. The rate and extent of absorption are not affected by food intake or by administration during a migraine attack. Almotriptan does not undergo substantial first-pass elimination.

Distribution: Almotriptan is extensively distributed. Almotriptan is minimally protein bound (approximately 35%), and the mean apparent volume of distribution is approximately 180 to 200 L.

Metabolism: Almotriptan is metabolized by one minor and two major pathways. Monoamine oxidase (MAO)-mediated oxidative deamination (approximately 27% of the dose) and cytochrome P450-mediated oxidation (approximately 12% of the dose) are the major routes of metabolism, while flavin mono-oxygenase is the minor route. MAO-A is responsible for the formation of the indoleacetic acid metabolite, whereas cytochrome P450 (3A4 and 2D6) catalyzes the hydroxylation of the pyrrolidine ring to an intermediate that is further oxidized by aldehyde dehydrogenase to the gamma-aminobutyric acid derivative. Both metabolites are inactive.

Excretion: The mean half-life of almotriptan is between 3 and 4 hours. The primary route of elimination is via renal clearance, accounting for 75% of the administered dose. Approximately 40% of an administered dose is excreted unchanged in urine. Renal clearance exceeds the glomerular filtration rate by approximately 3-fold, indicating an active mechanism. Approximately 13% of the administered dose is excreted via feces, both unchanged and metabolized.

Special Populations: Geriatric: Renal and total clearance, and amount of drug excreted in the urine (10 L/h, 33 L/h and 30% respectively) were lower in elderly non-migraineur volunteers (aged 65 to 76 years) than in younger non-migraineur volunteers (aged 19 to 34 years), resulting in longer terminal half-life (3.7 h vs 3.2 h) and higher area under the plasma concentration-time curve (405 ng·h/mL vs 325 ng·h/mL) in the elderly subjects. However, the differences do not appear to be clinically significant.

Pediatric: The pharmacokinetics of almotriptan have not been evaluated in pediatric patients.

Gender: No significant gender differences have been observed in pharmacokinetic parameters.

Race: No significant differences have been observed in the pharmacokinetic parameters between Caucasian and African-American volunteers.

Hepatic Impairment: The pharmacokinetics of almotriptan have not been assessed in this population. Based on the known mechanisms of the clearance of almotriptan, the maximum decrease in expected almotriptan clearance due to hepatic impairment would be 60% (see Dosage and Precautions, Hepatic Impairment).

Renal Impairment: The clearance of almotriptan was approximately 65% lower in patients with severe renal impairment (Cl/F=19.8 L/h; creatinine clearance between 10 and 30 mL/min) and approximately 40% lower in patients with moderate renal impairment (Cl/F=34.2 L/h; creatinine clearance between 31 and 71 mL/min) compared to healthy volunteers. Maximum plasma concentrations of almotriptan increased by approximately 80% in these patients (see Dosage and Precautions, Renal Impairment).

Clinical Studies: The pharmacological activity of almotriptan in the treatment of migraine has been assessed in Phase II and Phase III clinical trials.

The efficacy of AXERT (almotriptan malate) tablets was established in 3 multicentre, randomized, double-blind, placebo-controlled trials. Patients enrolled in these studies were primarily female (86%) and Caucasian (more than 98%), with a mean age of 41 years (range of 18 to 72). Patients were instructed to treat a moderate to severe migraine headache. Two hours after taking one dose of study medication, patients evaluated their headache pain. If the pain had not decreased in severity to mild or to no pain, the patient was allowed to take an escape medication. If the pain had decreased to mild or to no pain at 2 hours but subsequently increased in severity between 2 and 24 hours, it was considered a relapse and the patient was instructed to take a second dose of study medication. Associated symptoms of nausea, vomiting, photophobia, and phonophobia were also evaluated.

In these studies, the percentage of patients achieving a response (mild or no pain) 2 hours after treatment was significantly greater in patients who received either AXERT 6.25 mg or 12.5 mg, compared with those who received placebo. In study 1, Almotriptan 12.5 mg was superior to placebo as early as 30 minutes after drug administration (pairwise comparison, p=0.0485). A higher percentage of patients reported pain relief after treatment with the 12.5 mg dose than with the 6.25 mg dose. Doses greater than 12.5 mg did not lead to significantly better response. These results are summarized in Table 1.

Table 1: AXERT

Pain Relief Rates 2 Hours Following Treatment of Initial Headache

	Placebo	AXERT 6.25 mg	AXERT 12.5 mg
Study 1	32.5% (n=80)	56.3%[a] (n=167)	58.5%[b] (n=164)
Study 2	42.4% (n=98)		56.5%[c] (n=184)
Study 3	33.9% (n=176)	57.3% (n=360)	64.6%[b] (n=373)

[a] p value 0.002 in comparison to placebo.
[b] p value <0.001 in comparison to placebo.
[c] p value 0.008 in comparison to placebo.

These results cannot be validly compared with results of anti-migraine treatments in other studies. Because studies are conducted at different times, with different samples of patients, by different investigators, employing different criteria and/or different interpretations of the same criteria under different conditions (dose, dosing regimen, etc.), quantitative estimates of treatment responses and the timing of responses may be expected to vary considerably from study to study.

For patients with migraine-associated photophobia, phonophobia, nausea, and vomiting at baseline, there was a decreased incidence of these symptoms following administration of AXERT compared with placebo.

Two to 24 hours following the initial dose of study medication, patients were allowed to take an escape medication or a second dose of study medication for pain response. Escape medication was taken more frequently by patients in the placebo groups than by those in the active almotriptan treatment groups.

The efficacy of AXERT was unaffected by the presence of aura; by gender, weight, or age of the patient; or by concomitant use of common migraine prophylactic drugs (e.g. beta-blockers, calcium channel blockers, tricyclic antidepressants), or oral contraceptives. There were insufficient data to assess the effect of race on efficacy.

INDICATIONS: AXERT (almotriptan malate) tablets are indicated for the acute treatment of migraine with or without aura in adults.

AXERT is not intended for the prophylactic therapy of migraine or for use in the management of hemiplegic, ophthalmoplegic or basilar migraine (see Contraindications). Safety and effectiveness of AXERT have not been established for cluster headache, which presents in an older, predominantly male population.

CONTRAINDICATIONS: AXERT (almotriptan malate) is contraindicated in patients with history, symptoms, or signs of ischemic cardiac, cerebrovascular or peripheral vascular syndromes, valvular heart disease or cardiac arrhythmias (especially tachycardias). In addition, patients with other significant underlying cardiovascular diseases (e.g., atherosclerotic disease, congenital heart disease) should not receive AXERT. Ischemic cardiac syndromes include, but are not restricted to, angina pectoris of any type (e.g., stable angina of effort and vasospastic forms of angina such as the Prinzmetal's variant), all forms of myocardial infarction, and silent myocardial ischemia. Cerebrovascular syndromes include, but are not limited to, strokes of any type as well as transient ischemic attacks (TIAs). Peripheral vascular disease includes, but is not limited to, ischemic bowel disease, or Raynaud's syndrome (see Warnings).

Because AXERT may increase blood pressure, it should not be given to patients with uncontrolled hypertension (see Warnings).

AXERT should not be administered within 24 hours of treatment with another 5-HT$_1$ agonist, or an ergotamine-containing or ergot-type medication, such as dihydroergotamine or methylsergide.

AXERT should not be given to patients with hemiplegic, ophthalmoplegic or basilar migraine.

AXERT is contraindicated in patients who are hypersensitive to almotriptan or any other ingredients in AXERT.

WARNINGS: AXERT (almotriptan malate) tablets should only be used where a clear diagnosis of migraine has been established.

Risk of Myocardial Ischemia and/or Infarction and Other Adverse Cardiac Events: Because of the potential of this class of compounds (5-HT$_{1B/1D}$ agonists) to cause coronary vasospasm, AXERT should not be given to patients with documented ischemic or vasospastic coronary artery disease (see Contraindications). It is strongly recommended that 5-HT$_1$ agonists (including AXERT) not be given to patients in whom unrecognized coronary artery disease (CAD) is predicted by the presence of risk factors such as: hypertension, hypercholesterolemia, smoker, obesity, diabetes, strong family history of CAD, female with surgical or physiological menopause, or male over 40 years of age, unless a cardiovascular examination provides satisfactory clinical evidence that the patient is reasonably free of coronary artery and ischemic myocardial disease or other significant underlying cardiovascular disease. The sensitivity of cardiac diagnostic procedures to detect cardiovascular diseases or predisposition to coronary artery vasospasm is modest at best. If, during the cardiovascular evaluation, the patient's medical history, electrocardiogram (ECG) or other evaluations reveal findings indicative of, or consistent with, coronary artery vasospasm, or myocardial ischemia, AXERT should not be administered (see Contraindications).

These evaluations, however, may not identify every patient who has cardiac disease, and in very rare cases, serious cardiac events, such as myocardial infarction or coronary ischemia have occurred in patients without evidence of underlying cardiovascular disease.

For patients with risk factors predictive of CAD, who are determined to have a satisfactory cardiovascular evaluation, it is strongly recommended that administration of the first dose of AXERT take place in a clinical setting, such as the physician's office or a similarly staffed medical facility, unless the patient has previously received almotriptan. Because cardiac ischemia can occur in the absence of any clinical symptoms, consideration should be given to obtaining an ECG during the interval immediately following the first use of AXERT in a patient with risk factors. However, an absence of drug-induced cardiovascular effects on the occasion of the initial dose does not preclude the possibility of such effects occurring with subsequent administrations.

If symptoms consistent with angina occur after the use of AXERT, ECG evaluation should be carried out to look for ischemic changes.

It is recommended that patients who are intermittent long-term users of AXERT and who have or acquire risk factors predictive of CAD as described above undergo periodic interval cardiovascular evaluation as they continue to use AXERT.

The systematic approach described above is intended to reduce the likelihood that patients with unrecognized cardiovascular disease are inadvertently exposed to AXERT.

Cardiac Events and Fatalities Associated with 5-HT$_1$ Agonists: Serious adverse cardiac events, including acute myocardial infarction have been reported within a few hours following administration of almotriptan. Life-threatening disturbances of cardiac rhythm and death have been reported within a few hours following the administration of other 5-HT$_1$ agonists. Due to the common pharmacodynamic actions of 5-HT$_1$ agonists, the possibility of cardiovascular effects of the nature described below should be considered for all agents of this class. Considering the extent of use of 5-HT$_1$ agonists in patients with migraine, the incidence of these events is extremely low.

AXERT can cause coronary vasospasm; at least one of these events occurred in a patient with no cardiac history and with documented absence of coronary artery disease.

Patients with symptomatic Wolff-Parkinson-White syndrome or arrhythmias associated with other cardiac accessory conduction pathway disorders should not receive AXERT.

Premarketing Experience with Almotriptan: Among the 3865 subjects/patients who received AXERT in premarketing clinical trials, one patient was hospitalized for observation after a scheduled ECG was found to be abnormal (negative T-waves on the left leads) 48 hours after taking a single 6.25 mg dose of AXERT. The patient, a 48-year-old female, had previously taken 3 other doses for earlier migraine attacks. Myocardial enzymes at the time of the abnormal ECG were normal. The patient was diagnosed as having had myocardial ischemia, and it was also found that she had a family history of coronary disease. An ECG performed 2 days later was normal, as was a follow-up coronary angiography. The patient recovered without incident.

Postmarketing Experience with Almotriptan: Serious cardiovascular events have been reported in association with the use of AXERT. The uncontrolled nature of postmarketing surveillance, however, makes it impossible to definitely determine the proportion of the reported cases that were actually caused by almotriptan or to reliably assess causation in individual cases.

Cerebrovascular Events and Fatalities with 5-HT$_1$ Agonists: Cerebral hemorrhage, subarachnoid hemorrhage, stroke and other cerebrovascular events have been reported in patients treated with other 5-HT$_1$ agonists, and some have resulted in fatalities. In a number of cases, it appears possible that the cerebrovascular events were primary, the agonist having been administered in the belief that the symptoms experienced were a consequence of migraine, when they were not. Before treating migraine headaches with AXERT, in patients not previously diagnosed as migraineurs, and in migraineurs who present with atypical symptoms, care should be taken to exclude other potentially serious neurological conditions. If a patient does not respond to the first dose, the opportunity should be taken to review the diagnosis before a second dose is given. It should be noted, however, that patients who suffer from migraine may have an increased risk of certain cerebrovascular events such as stroke, hemorrhage or transient ischemic attack.

Other Vasospasm-Related Events: 5-HT$_1$ agonists may cause vasospastic reactions other than coronary artery vasospasm. Both peripheral vascular ischemia and colonic ischemia with abdominal pain and bloody diarrhea have been reported with 5-HT$_1$ agonists.

Increases in Blood Pressure: Significant elevations in systemic blood pressure, including hypertensive crisis, have been reported on rare occasions in patients with and without a history of hypertension treated with other 5-HT$_1$ agonists. AXERT is contraindicated in patients with uncontrolled hypertension (see Contraindications). In patients with controlled hypertension, AXERT should be administered with caution, as transient increases in blood pressure and peripheral vascular resistance have been observed in a small portion of patients. In volunteers, small increases in mean systolic and diastolic blood pressure relative to placebo were seen over the first 4 hours after administration of 12.5 mg of almotriptan (0.21 and 1.35 mm Hg, respectively). The effect of AXERT on blood pressure was also assessed in patients with hypertension controlled by medication. In this population, mean increases in systolic and diastolic blood pressure relative to placebo over the first 4 hours after administration of 12.5 mg of almotriptan were 4.87 and 0.26 mm Hg, respectively. The slight increases in blood pressure in both volunteers and controlled hypertensive patients were not considered clinically significant (see Adverse Effects and Precautions).

Special Cardiovascular Pharmacology Studies With Another 5-HT$_1$ Agonist: In subjects (n=10) with suspected coronary artery disease undergoing angiography, a 5-HT$_1$ agonist at a subcutaneous dose of 1.5 mg produced an 8% increase in aortic blood pressure, an 18% increase in pulmonary artery blood pressure, and an 8% increase in systemic vascular resistance. In addition, mild chest pain or tightness was reported by four subjects. Clinically significant increases in blood pressure were experienced by three of the subjects (two of whom also had chest pain/discomfort). Diagnostic angiogram results revealed that 9 subjects had normal coronary arteries and 1 had insignificant coronary artery disease.

In an additional study with this same drug, migraine patients (n=35) free of cardiovascular disease were subjected to assessments of myocardial perfusion by positron emission tomography while receiving a subcutaneous 1.5 mg dose in the absence of a migraine attack. Reduced coronary vasodilatory reserve (~10%), increased coronary resistance (~20%), and decreased hyperaemic myocardial blood flow (~10%) were noted. The relevance of these findings to the use of the recommended oral dose of this 5-HT$_1$ agonist is not known.

Similar studies have not been done with AXERT. However, owing to the common pharmacodynamic actions of 5-HT_1 agonists, the possibility of cardiovascular effects of the nature described above should be considered for any agent of this pharmacological class.

Hypersensitivity: Rare hypersensitivity (anaphylaxis/anaphylactoid) reactions have occurred in patients receiving other 5-HT_1 agonists. Such reactions can be life threatening or fatal. In general, hypersensitivity reactions to drugs are more likely to occur in individuals with a history of sensitivity to multiple allergens. Owing to the possibility of cross-reactive hypersensitivity reactions, AXERT should not be used in patients having a history of hypersensitivity to chemically-related 5-HT_1 receptor agonists (see Adverse Effects and Precautions).

Selective Serotonin Reuptake Inhibitors/Serotonin Norepinephrine Reuptake Inhibitors and Serotonin Syndrome: Cases of life-threatening serotonin syndrome have been reported during combined use of selective serotonin reuptake inhibitors (SSRIs)/serotonin norepinephrine reuptake inhibitors (SNRIs) and triptans. If concomitant treatment with AXERT and SSRIs (e.g., fluoxetine, paroxetine, sertraline) or SNRIs (e.g., venlafaxine) is clinically warranted, careful observation of the patient is advised, particularly during treatment initiation and dose increases. Serotonin syndrome symptoms may include mental status changes (e.g., agitation, hallucinations, coma), autonomic instability (e.g., tachycardia, labile blood pressure, hyperthermia), neuromuscular aberrations (e.g., hyperreflexia, incoordination) and/or gastrointestinal symptoms (e.g., nausea, vomiting, diarrhea) (see Precautions, Drug Interactions).

PRECAUTIONS: General: AXERT should be administered with caution to patients with diseases that may alter the absorption, metabolism or excretion of drugs, such as those with impaired hepatic or renal function (see Pharmacology, Special Populations and Dosage).

Caution should be exercised when prescribing almotriptan to patients with known hypersensitivity to sulfonamides.

Cardiovascular: As with other 5-HT_1 agonists, sensations of tightness, pain, pressure, and heaviness in the precordium, throat, neck and jaw have been reported after treatment with AXERT (almotriptan malate). These events have not been associated with arrhythmias or ischemic ECG changes in clinical trials. Because drugs in this class, including AXERT, may cause coronary artery vasospasm, patients who experience signs or symptoms suggestive of angina following dosing should be evaluated for the presence of CAD or a predisposition to Prinzmetal's variant angina before receiving additional doses of the medication, and should be monitored electrocardiographically if dosing is resumed and similar symptoms recur. Similarly, patients who experience other symptoms or signs suggestive of decreased arterial flow, such as ischemic bowel syndrome or Raynaud's syndrome following the use of any 5-HT_1 agonist, are candidates for further evaluation (see Contraindications and Warnings).

Neurologic Conditions: Care should be taken to exclude other potentially serious neurologic conditions before treating headache in patients not previously diagnosed with migraine or who experience a headache that is atypical for them. There have been rare reports where patients received 5-HT_1 agonists for severe headache that were subsequently shown to have been secondary to an evolving neurological lesion. For newly diagnosed patients or patients presenting with atypical symptoms, the diagnosis of migraine should be reconsidered if no response is seen after the first dose of AXERT.

Corneal Opacities: Three male dogs (out of a total of 14 treated) in a 52-week toxicity study of oral almotriptan developed slight corneal opacities that were noted after 51, but not after 25, weeks of treatment. The doses at which this occurred were 2, 5, and 12.5 mg/kg/day. The opacity reversed in the affected dog at 12.5 mg/kg/day after a 4-week drug-free period. Systemic exposure (plasma AUC) to parent drug at 2 mg/kg/day was approximately 2.5 times the exposure in humans receiving the maximum recommended daily dose of 25 mg. A no-effect dose was not established.

Binding to Melanin-Containing Tissues: When pigmented rats were given a single oral dose of 5 mg/kg of radiolabelled almotriptan, the elimination half-life of radioactivity from the eye was 22 days, suggesting that almotriptan and/or its metabolites may bind to the melanin of the eye. Because almotriptan could accumulate in the melanin-rich tissues over time, there is the possibility that it could cause toxicity in these tissues over extended use. However, no adverse ocular effects related to treatment with almotriptan were noted in any of the toxicity studies. Although no systemic monitoring of ophthalmic function was undertaken in clinical trials, and no specific recommendations for ophthalmic monitoring are offered, prescribers should be aware of the possibility of long-term ophthalmic effects.

Carcinogenesis: The carcinogenic potential of almotriptan was evaluated by oral gavage for up to 103 weeks in mice at doses of up to 250 mg/kg/day, and in rats for up to 104 weeks at doses up to 75 mg/kg/day. These doses were associated with plasma exposures (AUC) to parent drug that were approximately 40 and 78 times, in mice and rats respectively, the plasma AUC observed in humans receiving the MRDD of 25 mg. Because of high mortality rates in both studies, which reached statistical significance in high-dose female mice, all female rats, all male mice and high-dose female mice were terminated between weeks 96 and 98. There was no increase in tumors related to almotriptan administration.

Mutagenesis: Almotriptan was not mutagenic, with or without metabolic activation, when tested in two gene mutation assays, the Ames test and the in vitro thymidine locus mouse lymphoma assay. Almotriptan was not determined to be clastogenic in two in vitro cytogenetics assays in human lymphocytes and an in vivo mouse micronucleus assay. Almotriptan produced an equivocal weakly positive response in in vitro cytogenetics assays in human lymphocytes.

Impairment of Fertility: When female rats received almotriptan by oral gavage prior to and during mating and up to implantation at doses of 25, 100, and 400 mg/kg/day, prolongation of the estrous cycle was observed at a dose of 100 mg/kg/day (exposure, based on mg/m², was approximately 40 times exposure in humans receiving the maximum recommended daily dose (MRDD) of 25 mg). No effects on fertility were noted in female rats at 25 mg/kg/day (exposure approximately 10 times human exposure at MRDD). No adverse effects were noted in male rats at 400 mg/kg/day (160 times the human exposure based on mg/m²).

Pregnancy: When almotriptan was administered orally during organogenesis to pregnant rats at doses of 125, 250, 500 and 1000 mg/kg/day, an increase in embryolethality was seen at the 1000 mg/kg/day dose (maternal exposure [based on plasma AUC of parent drug] was approximately 958 times the human exposure at MRDD of 25 mg). Increased incidences of fetal skeletal variations (decreased ossification) were noted at doses greater than the no-observed-effect level in rats of 125 mg/kg/day (maternal exposure 80 times human exposure at MRDD). Similar studies in rabbits conducted with almotriptan at doses of 5, 20 and 60 mg/kg/day demonstrated increases in embryolethality at 60 mg/kg/day (maternal exposure, based on mg/m², 50 times human exposure at MRDD). When almotriptan was administered to rats throughout the periods of gestation and lactation at doses of 25, 100 and 400 mg/kg/day, gestation length was increased and litter size and offspring body weight were decreased at the high dose (maternal exposure, based on mg/m², 160 times human exposure at MRDD). The decrease in pup weight persisted throughout lactation. The no-observed-effect level in this study was 100 mg/kg/day (maternal exposure 40 times human exposure at MRDD).

There have been no adequate and well-controlled studies in pregnant women; therefore AXERT should only be used during pregnancy if the potential benefit justifies the risk to the fetus.

Hepatic Impairment: AXERT should be used with caution in patients with hepatic impairment. The maximum daily dose should not exceed 12.5 mg over a 24-hour period, and a starting dose of 6.25 mg is recommended (see Pharmacology, Special Populations and Dosage).

Renal Impairment: AXERT should be used with caution in patients with severe renal impairment. The maximum daily dose should not exceed 12.5 mg over a 24-hour period, and a starting dose of 6.25 mg should be used (see Pharmacology, Special Populations and Dosage).

Occupational Hazards: Patients should be advised to avoid driving a car or operating hazardous machinery until they are reasonably certain that AXERT does not affect them adversely.

Geriatrics: Clinical studies of AXERT did not include sufficient numbers of subjects over 65 years of age to determine whether they respond differently from younger subjects. Renal and total clearance, and amount of drug excreted in the urine were lower in elderly non-migraineur volunteers (age 65 to 76 years) than in younger non-migraineur volunteers (age 19 to 34 years), resulting in longer terminal half-life and higher area under the plasma concentration-time curve. Although clearance of almotriptan was lower in elderly volunteers, there were no differences in the safety and tolerability between the two populations (see Pharmacology, Special Populations). In general, dose selection for an elderly patient should be cautious, usually starting at the low end of the dosing range, reflecting the greater frequency of decreased renal, cardiac, and hepatic function, and of concomitant disease or other drug therapy.

Pediatrics: The safety and effectiveness of AXERT in pediatric patients has not been established; therefore, AXERT is not recommended for use in patients under 18 years of age.

Post-marketing experience with other triptans include a limited number of reports that describe pediatric (under 12 years of age) and adolescent (12-17 years of age) patients who have experienced clinically serious adverse events that are similar in nature to those reported as rare occurrences in adults.

Lactation: It is not known whether almotriptan is excreted in human milk. Since many drugs are excreted in human milk, caution should be exercised when AXERT is administered to a nursing woman.

Dependence Liability: Although the abuse potential of AXERT has not been specifically assessed, no abuse of, tolerance to, withdrawal from, or drug-seeking behaviour was observed in patients who received AXERT in clinical trials or their extensions. The 5-$HT_{1B/1D}$ agonists, as a class, have not been associated with drug abuse.

Drug Interactions: All drug interaction studies were performed in healthy volunteers using a single 12.5 mg dose of almotriptan and multiple doses of the other drug.

Ergot-Containing Drugs: These drugs have been reported to cause prolonged vasospastic reactions. As there is a theoretical basis that these effects may be additive, use of ergotamine-containing or ergot-type medications (dihydroergotamine or methylsergide) and AXERT within 24 hours of each other should be avoided (see Contraindications).

Monoamine Oxidase Inhibitors: Coadministration of almotriptan and moclobemide (150 mg b.i.d. for 8 days) resulted in a 27% decrease in almotriptan clearance and an increase in Cmax of approximately 6%. No dose adjustment is necessary.

Propranolol: Coadministration of almotriptan and propranolol (80 mg b.i.d. for 7 days) resulted in no significant changes in the pharmacokinetics of almotriptan.

Selective Serotonin Reuptake Inhibitors (SSRIs)/Serotonin Norepinephrine Reuptake Inhibitors (SNRIs): Cases of life-threatening serotonin syndrome have been reported during combined use of selective serotonin reuptake inhibitors (SSRIs) or serotonin norepinephrine reuptake inhibitors (SNRIs) and triptans (see Warnings).

Coadministration of almotriptan and fluoxetine (60 mg daily for 8 days), a potent inhibitor of CYP2D6, had no effect on almotriptan clearance, but maximal concentrations of almotriptan were increased by 18%. This difference is not clinically significant.

Verapamil: Coadministration of almotriptan and verapamil (120 mg sustained-release tablets b.i.d. for 7 days), an inhibitor of CYP4503A4, resulted in a 20% increase in the area under the plasma concentration-time curve, and in a 24% increase in maximal plasma concentrations of almotriptan. Neither of these changes is clinically significant.

Other 5-$HT_{1B/1D}$ Agonists: Concomitant use of other 5-$HT_{1B/1D}$ agonists within 24 hours of treatment with AXERT is contraindicated (see Contraindications).

Ketoconazole and Other Potent CYP3A4 Inhibitors: Coadministration of almotriptan and the potent CYP3A4 inhibitor ketoconazole (400 mg q.d. for 3 days) resulted in an approximately 60% increase in the area under the plasma concentration-time curve and maximal plasma concentrations of almotriptan. Although the interaction between almotriptan and other potent CYP3A4 inhibitors (e.g. itraconazole, ritonavir, and erythromycin) has not been studied, increased exposures to almotriptan may be expected when almotriptan is used concomitantly with these medications.

Laboratory Tests: Almotriptan is not known to interfere with any commonly employed clinical laboratory tests. No specific laboratory tests are recommended for monitoring patients.

ADVERSE EFFECTS: Serious cardiac events, including some that have been fatal, have occurred following use of other 5-HT_1 agonists. These events are extremely rare and most have been reported in patients with risk factors predictive of CAD. Events reported have included coronary artery vasospasms, transient myocardial ischemia, myocardial infarction, ventricular tachycardia, and ventricular fibrillation (see Contraindications, Warnings and Precautions).

Serious cardiac events, including myocardial infarction, coronary artery vasospasm and intermediate coronary syndrome, have occurred following the use of AXERT tablets. These events are extremely rare and have been reported mostly in patients with cardiovascular risk factors (see Warnings and Post-Marketing Adverse Reactions).

Experience in Controlled Clinical Trials with AXERT (almotriptan): Typical 5-HT_1 Agonist Adverse Reactions: As with other 5-HT_1 agonists, AXERT has been associated with sensations of heaviness, pressure, tightness or pain which may be intense. These may occur in any part of the body including the chest, throat, neck, jaw and upper limbs.

Increases in Blood Pressure: Significant elevations in systemic blood pressure, including hypertensive crisis, have been reported on rare occasions in patients with and without a history of hypertension treated with other 5-HT_1 agonists. AXERT is contraindicated in patients with uncontrolled hypertension (see Contraindications). In volunteers, small increases in mean systolic and diastolic blood pressure relative to placebo were seen over the first 4 hours after administration of 12.5 mg of almotriptan (0.21 and 1.35 mm Hg, respectively). The effect of AXERT on blood pressure was also assessed in patients with hypertension controlled by medication. In this population, mean increases in systolic and diastolic blood pressure relative to placebo over the first 4 hours after administration of 12.5 mg of almotriptan were 4.87 and 0.26 mm Hg, respectively. The slight increases in blood pressure in both volunteers and controlled hypertensive patients were not considered clinically significant (see also Contraindications and Warnings).

Acute Safety: Adverse events were assessed in controlled clinical trials that included 1840 patients who received one or two doses of AXERT (almotriptan malate) tablets and 386 patients who received placebo.

The most common adverse events during treatment with AXERT were nausea, somnolence, headache, paresthesia, and dry mouth. In long-term, open-label studies where patients were allowed to treat multiple attacks for up to one year, 5% (63 out of 1347 patients) withdrew due to adverse experiences.

Table 2 lists the adverse events that occurred in at least 1% of the patients treated with AXERT, and at an incidence greater than in patients treated with placebo, regardless of drug relationship. These events reflect experience gained under closely monitored conditions of clinical trials in a highly selected patient population. In actual clinical practice or in other clinical trials, these frequency estimates may not apply, as the conditions of use, reporting behaviour, and the kinds of patients treated may differ.

Table 2: AXERT

Incidence of Adverse Events in Controlled Clinical Trials (Reported in at Least 1% of Patients Treated with AXERT, and at an Incidence Greater than Placebo)

	Percentage of Patients Reporting the Event		
Adverse Event	**AXERT 6.25 mg (n=527)**	**AXERT 12.5 mg (n=1313)**	**Placebo (n=386)**
Digestive			
Nausea	1	2	1
Dry Mouth	1	1	0.5
Nervous			
Paresthesia	1	1	0.5

AXERT is generally well tolerated. Most adverse events were mild in intensity and were transient, and did not lead to long-lasting effects. The incidence of adverse events in controlled clinical trials was not affected by gender, weight, age, presence of aura, or use of prophylactic medications or oral contraceptives. There were insufficient data to assess the effect of race on the incidence of adverse events.

Other Events: The frequencies of less commonly reported adverse events are presented below. However, the role of AXERT in their causation cannot be reliably determined. Furthermore, variability associated with adverse event reporting, the terminology used to describe adverse events, etc., limit the value of the quantitative frequency estimates provided. Event frequencies are calculated as the number of patients who used AXERT in controlled clinical trials and reported an event, divided by the total number of patients exposed to AXERT in these studies. All reported events are included, except the ones already listed in Table 2, and those unlikely to be drug related. Events are further classified within body system categories and enumerated in order of decreasing frequency using the following definitions: frequent adverse events are those occurring in at least 1/100 patients; infrequent adverse events are those occurring in 1/100 to 1/1000 patients; and rare adverse events are those occurring in fewer than 1/1000 patients.

Total Body System: Frequent was headache. Infrequent were abdominal cramp or pain, asthenia, chills, back pain, chest pain, neck pain, fatigue, and rigid neck. Rare were fever and photosensitivity reaction.

Cardiovascular: Infrequent were vasodilation, palpitations, and tachycardia. Rare were intermediate coronary syndrome, abnormal cardiac rhythm, hypertension, and syncope.

Digestive: Infrequent were diarrhea, vomiting, and dyspepsia. Rare were decreased appetite, increased appetite, colitis, gastritis, gastroenteritis, esophageal reflux, increased thirst, and increased salivation.

Metabolic: Infrequent were hyperglycemia and increased serum creatine phosphokinase. Rare were increased gamma glutamyl transpeptidase and hypercholesteremia.

Musculoskeletal: Infrequent were myalgia and muscular weakness. Rare were arthralgia, arthritis, and myopathy.

Nervous System: Frequent were dizziness and somnolence. Infrequent were tremor, vertigo, anxiety, hypesthesia, restlessness, CNS stimulation, insomnia, and shakiness. Rare were change in dreams, impaired concentration, abnormal coordination, depressive symptoms, euphoria, hyperreflexia, hypertonia, nervousness, neuropathy, nightmares, and nystagmus.

Respiratory: Infrequent were pharyngitis, rhinitis, dyspnea, laryngismus, sinusitis, bronchitis, and epistaxis. Rare were hyperventilation, laryngitis, and sneezing.

Skin: Infrequent were diaphoresis, dermatitis, erythema, pruritus, and rash.

Special Senses: Infrequent were ear pain, conjunctivitis, eye irritation, hyperacusis, and taste alteration. Rare were diplopia, dry eyes, eye pain, otitis media, parosmia, scotoma, and tinnitus.
Urogenital: Dysmenorrhea was infrequent.
Long-Term Safety: In a long term open label study, 762 patients treated 13,751 migraine attacks with AXERT over a period of up to 1 year. Migraine headaches could be treated with either a single dose of 12.5 mg AXERT or an initial 12.5 mg dose followed by a second 12.5 mg dose if needed. In this study, 3% (24 of 762) of patients withdrew due to an adverse experience. The most common adverse events (defined as occurring in more than 3% of patients) in descending order frequency were as follows: back pain (8%), bronchitis (6.4%), influenza-like symptoms (5.8%), pharyngitis (4.6%), vomiting (4.2%), rhinitis (4.1%), skeletal pain (3.4%) and sinusitis (3.4%). Due to the lack of placebo control in this study, the role of AXERT in causation cannot be reliably determined.
Post-Marketing Adverse Reactions: In addition to the adverse experiences reported during clinical trials of AXERT, the following adverse events have been reported in patients receiving marketed AXERT from worldwide use since approval. Due to the uncontrolled nature of post-marketing surveillance, it is not possible to definitely determine the proportion of the reported cases that were actually caused by AXERT or to reliably assess causation.

Serious cardiovascular adverse events, including acute myocardial infarction, coronary vasospasm and angina pectoris have been reported within a few hours following administration of AXERT.

Although very rare, AXERT can cause coronary vasospasm; at least one of these events occurred in a patient with no cardiac history and with documented absence of coronary artery disease (see Contraindications, Warnings, Adverse Effects and Precautions).

OVERDOSE:

Symptoms: Patients and volunteers receiving single oral doses of 100 to 150 mg of AXERT did not experience significant adverse events. During the clinical trials, one patient ingested 62.5 mg in a five-hour period, and another patient ingested 100 mg in a 38-hour period. Neither patients experienced adverse reactions.

Based on the pharmacology of 5-HT_1 agonists, hypertension or other more serious cardiovascular symptoms could occur after overdosage.

Treatment: Gastrointestinal decontamination (i.e. gastric lavage followed by activated charcoal) should be considered in patients suspected of an overdose with AXERT. Clinical and electrocardiographic monitoring should be continued for at least 20 hours, even if clinical symptoms are not observed.

The effects of hemodialysis or peritoneal dialysis on plasma concentrations of almotriptan are unknown.

For management of a suspected drug overdose, CPhA recommends that you contact your **regional Poison Control Centre**. See the *CPS* Directory section for a list of Poison Control Centres.

DOSAGE: In controlled clinical trials, single doses of 6.25 mg and 12.5 mg of AXERT (almotriptan malate) were effective for the acute treatment of migraine in adults, with the 12.5 mg dose tending to be a more effective dose (see Pharmacology, Clinical Studies). Individuals may vary in response to doses of AXERT. The choice of dose should therefore be made on an individual basis.

If the headache returns, the dose may be repeated after 2 hours, but no more than two doses should be given within a 24-hour period. Controlled trials have not adequately established the effectiveness of a second dose if the initial dose is ineffective. The safety of treating an average of more than four headaches in a 30-day period has not been established.
Hepatic Impairment: The pharmacokinetics of almotriptan have not been assessed in this population. The maximum decrease expected in the clearance of almotriptan due to hepatic impairment is 60%. Therefore, the maximum daily dose should not exceed 12.5 mg over a 24-hour period, and a starting dose of 6.25 mg should be used (see Pharmacology, Special Populations and Precautions).
Renal Impairment: In patients with severe renal impairment, the clearance of almotriptan was decreased. Therefore, the maximum daily dose should not exceed 12.5 mg over a 24-hour period, and a starting dose of 6.25 mg should be used (see Pharmacology, Special Populations and Precautions).

INFORMATION FOR THE PATIENT: Published in e-CPS, available by subscription at www.e-cps.ca.

SUPPLIED: 6.25 mg: Each white, circular, biconvex tablet, printed in red with the code 2080, contains: almotriptan 6.25 mg. Nonmedicinal ingredients: carnauba wax, cellulose, hydroxypropyl methylcellulose, iron oxide, mannitol, polyethylene glycol, povidone, propylene glycol, sodium starch glycolate, sodium stearyl fumarate and titanium oxide. Unit dose (aluminum blister pack) of 6. Store between 15-30°C.
12.5 mg: Each white, circular, biconvex tablet, printed in blue with a stylized "A", contains: almotriptan 12.5 mg. Nonmedicinal ingredients: carnauba wax, cellulose, FD&C Blue No. 2, hydroxypropyl methylcellulose, mannitol, polyethylene glycol, povidone, propylene glycol, sodium starch glycolate, sodium stearyl fumarate and titanium oxide. Unit dose (aluminum blister pack) of 6. Store between 15-30°C.

(Shown in Product Identification Section)

Azarga® Ⓟ

brinzolamide—timolol maleate

Elevated Intraocular Pressure Therapy

Alcon

Date of Revision: August 7, 2009

SUMMARY PRODUCT INFORMATION:

Route of Administration	Dosage Form/ Strength	Clinically Relevant Nonmedicinal Ingredients
Ophthalmic (topical)	Suspension/brinzolamide 1.0% and timolol 0.5% (as timolol maleate)	Benzalkonium chloride For a complete listing see Dosage Forms, Composition and Packaging.

INDICATIONS AND CLINICAL USE: AZARGA (brinzolamide/timolol) ophthalmic suspension is indicated for the reduction of intraocular pressure (IOP) in patients with open-angle glaucoma or ocular hypertension for whom monotherapy provides insufficient IOP reduction and when the combination therapy is appropriate.
Geriatrics (>65 years of age): No overall differences in safety and effectiveness have been observed between elderly and other adult patients.
Pediatrics (<18 years of age): The safety and effectiveness of AZARGA suspension in pediatric patients have not been established. Its use is not recommended in these patients until further data become available.
CONTRAINDICATIONS:

- hypersensitivity to brinzolamide, timolol, or to any ingredient in the formulation or component of the container (for a complete listing, see Dosage Forms, Composition and Packaging)
- bronchial asthma, a history of bronchial asthma, or severe chronic obstructive pulmonary disease
- sinus bradycardia, second or third degree atrioventricular block, overt cardiac failure, or cardiogenic shock
- severe allergic rhinitis and bronchial hyper-reactivity; hypersensitivity to other beta-blockers
- hyperchloraemic acidosis
- severe renal impairment
- hypersensitivity to sulfonamides

No studies have been conducted with AZARGA (brinzolamide/timolol) ophthalmic suspension or timolol maleate ophthalmic solution in patients with hepatic or renal impairment, or in patients with hyperchloraemic acidosis. Since brinzolamide and its main metabolite are excreted predominantly by the kidney, AZARGA suspension is therefore contraindicated in patients with severe renal impairment.

WARNINGS AND PRECAUTIONS: General: Like other topically applied ophthalmic agents, brinzolamide and timolol are absorbed systemically.

Due to the beta-adrenergic component, timolol, the same types of cardiovascular and pulmonary adverse reactions as seen with systemic beta-adrenergic blocking agents may occur. Cardiac failure should be adequately controlled before beginning therapy with AZARGA (brinzolamide/timolol) ophthalmic suspension. Patients with a history of severe cardiac disease should be watched for signs of cardiac failure and have their pulse rates checked.

Respiratory reactions and cardiac reactions, including death due to bronchospasm in patients with asthma and rarely, death in association with cardiac failure, have been reported following administration of timolol maleate.

Beta adrenergic blocking agents should be administered with caution in patients subject to spontaneous hypoglycaemia or to patients with labile insulin-dependent diabetes as beta adrenergic blocking agents may mask the signs and symptoms of acute hypoglycaemia. They may also mask the signs of hyperthyroidism and cause worsening of Prinzmetal angina, severe peripheral and central circulatory disorders and hypotension.

Timolol may interact with other medicinal products.

The effect on intraocular pressure or the known effects of systemic beta blockade may be potentiated when AZARGA suspension is given to patients already receiving an oral beta-adrenergic blocking agent. The use of two local beta-adrenergic blocking agents or two local carbonic anhydrase inhibitors is not recommended.

AZARGA suspension contains brinzolamide, a sulphonamide. The same type of undesirable effects that are attributable to sulphonamides may occur with topical administration. Acid-base disturbances have been reported with oral carbonic anhydrase inhibitors. If signs of serious reactions or hypersensitivity occur, discontinue the use of this medicinal product.

There is potential for an additive effect on the known systemic effects of carbonic anhydrase inhibition in patients receiving an oral carbonic anhydrase inhibitor and AZARGA suspension. The concomitant administration of AZARGA suspension and oral carbonic anhydrase inhibitors has not been studied and is not recommended.
Hepatic/Biliary/Pancreatic: AZARGA suspension has not been studied in patients with hepatic impairment and therefore should be used with caution in such patients.
Immune: Anaphylactic Reactions: While taking beta adrenergic blocking agents, patients with a history of atopy of a history of severe anaphylactic reaction to a variety of allergens may be unresponsive to the usual doses of adrenaline used to treat anaphylactic reactions.
Ophthalmologic: There is limited experience with AZARGA suspension in the treatment of patients with pseudoexfoliative glaucoma or pigmentary glaucoma.

AZARGA suspension has not been studied in patients with narrow-angle glaucoma.

The possible role of brinzolamide on corneal endothelial function has not been investigated in patients with compromised corneas (particularly in patients with low endothelial count). Specifically, patients wearing contact lenses have not been studied and careful monitoring of these patients when using brinzolamide is recommended, since carbonic anhydrase inhibitors may affect corneal hydration and wearing contact lenses might increase the risk for the cornea. Likewise, in other cases of compromised corneas such as patients with diabetes mellitus, careful monitoring is recommended.

AZARGA suspension contains benzalkonium chloride which may cause eye irritation and is known to discolour soft contact lenses. Contact with soft contact lenses is to be avoided. Patients must be instructed to remove contact lenses prior to the application of AZARGA suspension and wait 15 minutes after instillation of the dose before reinsertion.

As with any eye drops, temporary blurred vision or other visual disturbances may affect the ability to drive or use machines. If blurred vision occurs at instillation, the patient must wait until the vision clears before driving or using machinery.
Special Populations: Pregnant Women: There are no adequate data from the use of brinzolamide in pregnant women. Studies in animals have shown reproductive toxicity. The potential risk for humans is unknown.

Well-controlled epidemiological studies with systemic use of beta adrenergic blocking agents did not indicate malformation effects, but some pharmacological effects such as bradycardia have been observed in fetuses or neonates. Data on a limited number of exposed pregnancies indicate no adverse effects of timolol in ophthalmic solutions on pregnancy or on the health of the fetus/newborn child but bradycardia and arrhythmia have been reported in one case in the fetus of a woman treated with timolol ophthalmic solution. To date, no other relevant epidemiological data are available.

AZARGA suspension should be used during pregnancy only if the potential benefit justifies the potential risk to the fetus.
Nursing Women: It is not known whether brinzolamide is excreted in human breast milk. Animal studies have shown excretion of brinzolamide in breast milk. Timolol does appear in breast milk. However, at therapeutic doses of timolol in ophthalmic solutions, the calculated dose of timolol for the nursing child would be too low to produce clinical beta-blockade.

Because of the potential for serious adverse reactions from AZARGA suspension in nursing infants, a decision should be made whether to discontinue nursing or to discontinue the drug, taking into account the importance of the drug to the mother.
Pediatrics (<18 years of age): Safety and effectiveness of AZARGA suspension in children have not been established.
Geriatrics (>65 years of age): Oral carbonic anhydrase inhibitors may impair the ability to perform tasks requiring mental alertness and/or physical coordination in elderly patients. AZARGA suspension is absorbed systemically and therefore this may occur with topical administration in elderly patients.
Monitoring and Laboratory Tests: No untoward safety issues were identified based upon a review of the laboratory data (haematology, blood chemistry, and urinalysis) from a single pharmacokinetic study.

ADVERSE REACTIONS: Adverse Drug Reaction Overview: In clinical studies involving over 500 patients treated with AZARGA (brinzolamide/timolol) ophthalmic suspension, the most frequently reported adverse drug reaction was temporary blurred vision (6%) upon instillation, lasting from a few seconds to a few minutes.

Dysgeusia (bitter or unusual taste in the mouth following topical ocular instillation) was the most frequently reported systemic adverse drug reaction. It is likely caused by passage of the eye drops in the nasopharynx via the nasolacrimal canal and is attributable to the brinzolamide component of this combination product. Nasolacrimal occlusion or gently closing the eyelid after instillation may help reduce the incidence of this effect.

AZARGA suspension contains brinzolamide which is a sulphonamide inhibitor of carbonic anhydrase with systemic absorption. Gastrointestinal, nervous system, haematological, renal and metabolic effects are generally associated with systemic carbonic anhydrase inhibitors. The same type of adverse drug reactions that are attributable to oral carbonic anhydrase inhibitors may occur with topical administration.
Clinical Trial Adverse Drug Reactions: Because clinical trials are conducted under very specific conditions the adverse reaction rates observed in the clinical trials may not reflect the rates observed in practice and should not be compared to the rates in the clinical trials of another drug. Adverse drug reaction information from clinical trials is useful for identifying drug-related adverse events and for approximating rates.

In 5 clinical studies, AZARGA suspension was administered to 501 patients at a dose of one drop two times daily for up to 1 year. The most frequent adverse drug reactions (≥1%) seen in clinical trials are presented in Table 1.

Table 1: AZARGA
Treatment-Related Adverse Drug Reactions ≥1%

MedDRA Preferred Term (Version 10.0)	AZARGA N=501 (%)	COSOPT N=264 (%)	AZOPT N=203 (%)	Timolol N=236 (%)
Eye Disorders				
Blurred vision	6%	1%	3%	1%
Eye irritation	4%	12%	2%	3%
Eye pain	3%	9%	0%	1%
Foreign body sensation in eyes	1%	0%	0%	0%
Nervous System Disorders				
Dysgeusia	2%	2%	5%	0%

Less Common Clinical Trial Adverse Drug Reactions (<1%): Eye Disorders: conjunctival hyperaemia, eye pruritus, intraocular pressure decreased, ocular hyperaemia, punctuate keratitis, dry eye, eye discharge, abnormal sensation in eye, anterior chamber flare, asthenopia, blepharitis, blepharitis allergic, conjunctivitis allergic, corneal disorder, corneal erosion, eyelid margin crusting, eyelids pruritus, erythema of eyelid, lacrimation increased, photophobia, scleral hyperaemia.
Psychiatric Disorders: insomnia.

Respiratory, Thoracic and Mediastinal Disorders: chronic obstructive pulmonary disease, cough, pharyngolaryngeal pain, rhinorrhoea.
Skin and Subcutaneous Tissue Disorders: hair disorder, lichen planus.
Vascular Disorders: blood pressure decreased.

Additional Adverse Reactions Observed with the Individual Components of AZARGA Suspension: AZARGA suspension contains brinzolamide and timolol (as timolol maleate). Additional adverse reactions associated with the use of the individual components observed in clinical studies that may potentially occur with AZARGA suspension include:

Brinzolamide 1.0% (Clinical trials): Blood and the Lymphatic System Disorders: blood chloride increased, red blood cell count decreased.
Cardiac Disorders: angina pectoris, arrhythmia, bradycardia, cardio-respiratory distress, heart rate increased, heart rate irregular, palpitation, tachycardia.
Ear and Labyrinth Disorders: tinnitus, vertigo.
Eye Disorders: conjunctivitis, corneal epithelium defect, corneal epithelium disorder, corneal staining, corneal oedema, deposit eye, diplopia, eye allergy, eye swelling, eyelid disorder, eyelid oedema, glare, hypoaesthesia eye, intraocular pressure increased, keratitis, keratoconjunctivitis sicca, keratopathy, madarosis, meibomianitis, ocular discomfort, optic nerve cup/disc ratio increased, photopsia, pterygium, scleral pigmentation, subconjunctival cyst, visual acuity reduced, visual disturbance.
Gastrointestinal Disorders: abdominal discomfort, diarrhea, dry mouth, dyspepsia, flatulence, frequent bowel movements, gastrointestinal disorder, hypoaesthesia oral, nausea, oesophagitis, paraesthesia oral, stomach discomfort, upper abdominal pain, vomiting.
General Disorders and Administration Site Conditions: asthenia, chest discomfort, chest pain, fatigue, feeling abnormal, feeling jittery, irritability, malaise, medication residue, pain, peripheral oedema.
Hepatobiliary Disorders: liver function test abnormal.
Immune System Disorders: hypersensitivity.
Infections and Infestations: nasopharyngitis, pharyngitis, rhinitis, sinusitis.
Injury, Poisoning and Procedural Complications: foreign body in eye.
Musculoskeletal and Connective Tissue Disorders: arthralgia, back pain, muscle spasms, myalgia, pain in extremity.
Nervous System Disorders: ageusia, amnesia, dizziness, headache, hypoaesthesia, motor dysfunction, memory impairment, paraesthesia, somnolence, tremor.
Psychiatric Disorders: apathy, depressed mood, depression, libido decreased, nervousness, nightmare.
Renal and Urinary Disorders: pollakiuria, renal pain.
Reproductive System and Breast Disorders: erectile dysfunction.
Respiratory, Thoracic and Mediastinal Disorders: asthma, bronchial hyperactivity, dyspnoea, epistaxis, nasal congestion, nasal dryness, postnasal drip, sneezing, throat irritation, upper respiratory tract congestion.
Skin and Subcutaneous Tissue Disorders: alopecia, dermatitis, erythema, pruritus generalized, rash, rash maculo-papular, skin tightness, urticaria.
Vascular Disorders: blood pressure increased, hypertension.

Timolol 0.5% (Clinical trials): Cardiac Disorders: arrhythmia, atrioventricular block, bradycardia, cardiac arrest, cardiac failure, palpitation.
Eye Disorders: conjunctivitis, diplopia, eyelid ptosis, keratitis, visual disturbance.
Gastrointestinal Disorders: diarrhoea, nausea.
General Disorders and Administration Site Conditions: asthenia, chest pain.
Metabolism and Nutrition Disorders: hypoglycemia.
Nervous System Disorders: cerebral ischaemia, cerebrovascular accident, dizziness, headache, myasthenia gravis, paresthesia, syncope.
Psychiatric Disorders: depression.
Respiratory, Thoracic and Mediastinal Disorders: bronchospasm, dyspnoea, nasal congestion, respiratory failure.
Skin and Subcutaneous Tissue Disorders: alopecia, rash.
Vascular Disorders: hypotension.

Abnormal Hematologic and Clinical Chemistry Findings: AZARGA suspension had no clinically relevant treatment-related effect on laboratory parameters.

Post-Market Adverse Drug Reactions: Adverse reactions identified from post-marketing experience with the individual components that have not been reported previously in clinical trials with AZARGA suspension, brinzolamide 1.0% or timolol 0.5% are listed below.

Brinzolamide 1.0% (Post-marketing): Blood and the Lymphatic System Disorders: agranulocytosis, thrombocytopenia.
Cardiac Disorders: cardiac disorder, supraventricular extrasystoles.
Congenital and Familial/Genetic Disorders: congenital anomaly.
Ear and Labyrinth Disorders: ear pain.
Eye Disorders: corneal opacity, iris disorder, periorbital disorder, accommodation disorder, anterior chamber fibrin, blepharospasm, choroidal detachment, conjunctival haemorrhage, conjunctival irritation, conjunctival oedema, conjunctival scar, corneal degeneration, dark circles under eyes, Descemet's membrane disorder, eye oedema, eyelid exfoliation, iritis, macular oedema, ocular vascular disorder, oculogyration, optic disc drusen, uveitis, visual brightness.
Gastrointestinal Disorders: abdominal pain, mouth haemorrhage, disphagia, pancreatitis acute.
General Disorders and Administration Site Conditions: drug intolerance, drug ineffective, condition aggravated, adverse drug reaction, face oedema, facial pain, feeling cold, pyrexia, sensation of foreign body.
Hepatobiliary Disorders: jaundice.
Immune System Disorders: anaphylactic shock.
Injury, Poisoning and Procedural Complications: injury, limb injury, drug exposure during pregnancy, periorbital haematoma, transplant failure.
Infections and Infestations: bronchitis, herpes ophthalmic, herpes virus infection, pneumonia.
Investigations: gamma-glutamyltransferase increased, hepatic enzyme increased, blood lactic acid increased, blood urea increased, body temperature decreased, electrocardiogram abnormal.
Metabolism and Nutrition Disorders: metabolic acidosis, anorexia.
Musculoskeletal and Connective Tissue Disorders: musculoskeletal discomfort.
Nervous System Disorders: hypogeusia, hyposmia, anosmia, aphonia, burning sensation, burning sensation mucosal, cerebral infarction, cerebrovascular accident, convulsion, disturbance in attention, facial palsy, hyperaesthesia, lethargy, loss of consciousness.
Psychiatric Disorders: anxiety, agitation, bradyphrenia, depressive symptom, fear, restlessness, thought blocking.
Renal and Urinary Disorders: micturition disorder, micturition urgency, renal failure acute.
Respiratory, Thoracic and Mediastinal Disorders: bronchospasm, dry throat, dysphonia, lung disorder, nasal discomfort, nasal turbinate abnormality, respiratory distress, respiratory failure.
Skin and Subcutaneous Tissue Disorders: pruritus, dermatitis contact, eczema, hyperhidrosis, dry skin, hair colour changes, hair texture abnormal, periorbital oedema, psoriasis, rash generalised, rash pruritic, rash vesicular, skin hyperpigmentation, skin reaction, swelling face, vascular purpura.
Surgical and Medical Procedures: sinus operation.
Vascular Disorders: angiopathy, haematoma, hot flush.

Timolol 0.5% (Post-marketing): Cardiac Disorders: atrioventricular block complete, accelerated idioventricular rhythm, cardiotoxicity, myocardial infarction, sinus bradycardia.
Congenital and Familial/Genetic Disorders: multiple congenital abnormalities.
Ear and Labyrinth Disorders: vertigo.
Endocrine Disorders: thyroid disorder.
Eye Disorders: visual acuity reduced, corneal deposits, conjunctival oedema, corneal oedema, corneal opacity, corneal scar, ectropion, eye allergy, eye disorder, keratopathy, miosis.
General Disorders and Administration Site Conditions: chest discomfort, drug ineffective, drug interaction, fatigue, peripheral coldness, tachyphylaxis.
Immune System Disorders: hypersensitivity.
Infections and Infestations: nasopharyngitis.
Injury, Poisoning and Procedural Complications: accidental exposure, drug exposure during pregnancy, fall, medication error, transplant failure.
Investigations: heart rate increased, blood phosphorus increased, pulse abnormal, respiratory rate increased, skin test positive.
Metabolism and Nutrition Disorders: metabolic acidosis.
Musculoskeletal and Connective Tissue Disorders: muscular weakness, myalgia.
Nervous System Disorders: amnesia, balance disorder, depressed level of consciousness, hypotonia, lethargy, nervous system disorder.
Psychiatric Disorders: confusional state, nervousness.
Reproductive System and Breast Disorders: menorrhagia.
Skin and Subcutaneous Tissue Disorders: pruritus, dermatitis, dermatitis contact, erythema, periorbital oedema, skin exfoliation, toxic epidermal necrolysis.

DRUG INTERACTIONS: Overview: Specific drug interaction studies were not conducted with AZARGA (brinzolamide/timolol) ophthalmic suspension. In clinical studies, AZARGA suspension was used concomitantly with the following systemic medications without evidence of adverse interactions: antihistamines, anti-infectives, cardiovascular medications, central nervous system medications, analgesic/antipyretic medications, non-steroidal anti-inflammatory drugs, psychotherapeutic agents, antidiabetic medications, and thyroid agents. However, the potential for interactions with any drug should be considered.

Drug-Drug Interactions: AZARGA suspension contains brinzolamide, a carbonic anhydrase inhibitor and, although administered topically, is absorbed systemically. Acid-base disturbances have been reported with oral carbonic anhydrase inhibitors. The potential for interactions must be considered in patients receiving AZARGA suspension.

The cytochrome P-450 isozymes responsible for metabolism of brinzolamide include CYP3A4 (main), CYP2A6, CYP2B6, CYP2C8 and CYP2C9. It is expected that inhibitors of CYP3A4 such as ketoconazole, itraconazole, clotrimazole, ritonavir and troleandomycin will inhibit the metabolism of brinzolamide by CYP3A4. Caution is advised if CYP3A4 inhibitors are given concomitantly. Brinzolamide is not an inhibitor of cytochrome P-450 isozymes.

There is a potential for additive effects resulting in hypotension and/or marked bradycardia when ophthalmic solutions with beta blockers such as timolol are administered concomitantly with oral calcium channel blockers, guanethidine other beta adrenergic blocking agents, antiarrhythmics, digitalis glycosides or parasympathomimetics.

The hypertensive reaction to sudden withdrawal of clonidine can be potentiated when taking beta adrenergic blocking agents.

Potentiated systemic beta-blockade (e.g. decreased heart rate) has been reported during combined treatment with CYP2D6 inhibitors (e.g. quinidine, cimetidine) and timolol.

Drug-Food Interactions: Interactions with food are not anticipated following topical ocular administration.
Drug-Herb Interactions: Interactions with herbal products are not anticipated following topical ocular administration.
Drug-Laboratory Test Interactions: Interactions with laboratory tests are not anticipated following topical ocular administration.

DOSAGE AND ADMINISTRATION: Dosing Considerations: When substituting another ophthalmic antiglaucoma agent with AZARGA (brinzolamide/timolol) ophthalmic suspension, the other agent should be discontinued and AZARGA suspension should be started the following day.

If more than one topical ophthalmic medicinal product is being used, the medicines must be administered at least 5 minutes apart.

Recommended Dose and Dosage Adjustment: The adult dose is one drop of AZARGA suspension in the conjunctival sac of the affected eye(s) twice daily.

Missed Dose: If a dose is missed, a single drop should be applied as soon as possible before reverting to regular routine. Do not use a double dose to make up for the one missed.

Administration: Nasolacrimal occlusion or gently closing the eyelid after instillation is recommended. This may reduce the systemic absorption of medications administered via the ocular route and result in a decrease in systemic adverse reactions.

Instruct patients to shake the bottle well before use.

To prevent contamination of the dropper tip and solution, care must be taken not to touch the eyelids, surrounding areas or other surfaces with the dropper tip of the bottle. Instruct patients to keep the bottle tightly closed when not in use.

OVERDOSAGE:
No data are available in humans with regards to overdosage by accidental or deliberate ingestion of AZARGA (brinzolamide/timolol) ophthalmic suspension.

If overdose with AZARGA suspension occurs, treatment should be symptomatic and supportive. Electrolyte imbalance, development of an acidotic state, and possibly central nervous system effects may occur. Serum electrolyte levels (particularly potassium) and blood pH levels should be monitored. Studies have shown that timolol does not dialyse readily.

> For management of a suspected drug overdose, contact your regional Poison Control Centre. See the *CPS* Directory section for a list of Poison Control Centres.

ACTION AND CLINICAL PHARMACOLOGY: Mechanism of Action: AZARGA (brinzolamide/timolol) ophthalmic suspension contains two active substances: brinzolamide and timolol maleate. These two components decrease elevated IOP primarily by reducing aqueous humour secretion, but do so by different mechanisms of action. The combined effect of these two agents results in additional IOP reduction compared to either compound alone.

Brinzolamide is a potent inhibitor of human CA-II, the predominant isozyme in the eye. Inhibition of carbonic anhydrase in the ciliary processes of the eye decreases aqueous humour secretion, presumably by slowing the formation of bicarbonate ions with subsequent reduction in sodium and fluid transport.

Timolol is a non-selective beta adrenergic blocking agent that has no intrinsic sympathomimetic, direct myocardial depressant or membrane-stabilising activity. Tonography and fluorophotometry studies in man suggest that its predominant action is related to reduced aqueous humour formation and a slight increase in outflow facility.

Pharmacodynamics: AZARGA suspension, when applied topically to the eye, has the action of reducing elevated as well as normal intraocular pressure, whether or not accompanied by glaucoma. Elevated intraocular pressure is a major risk factor in the pathogenesis of glaucomatous visual field loss. The higher the level of intraocular pressure, the greater the likelihood of glaucomatous visual field loss and optic nerve damage. The Advanced Glaucoma Intervention Study (AGIS) established elevated intraocular pressure as a positive risk factor for glaucomatous visual field loss. Eyes with intraocular pressures below 18 mmHg at all visits were found to have little to no visual field loss during the six-year monitoring period.

Clinical Effects: In a twelve-month, controlled clinical trial in patients with open-angle glaucoma or ocular hypertension who, in the investigator's opinion could benefit from a combination therapy, and who had baseline mean IOP of 25 to 27 mmHg, the mean IOP-lowering effect of AZARGA suspension dosed twice daily was 7 to 9 mmHg.

In a six-month, controlled clinical study in patients with open-angle glaucoma or ocular hypertension and baseline mean IOP of 25 to 27 mmHg, the mean IOP-lowering effect of AZARGA suspension dosed twice daily was 7 to 9 mmHg, and was up to 3 mmHg greater than that of brinzolamide 1.0% dosed twice daily and up to 2 mmHg greater than that of timolol 0.5% dosed twice daily. A statistically superior reduction in mean IOP was observed compared to both brinzolamide and timolol at all time-points and visits throughout the study.

In two controlled clinical trials, the ocular discomfort upon instillation of AZARGA suspension was significantly lower than that of COSOPT.

Pharmacokinetics: See Table 2 and Table 3.

Absorption: Following topical ocular administration of AZARGA suspension, brinzolamide and timolol are absorbed through the cornea and into the systemic circulation. In a pharmacokinetic study, healthy subjects received oral brinzolamide (1 mg) twice daily for 2 weeks to shorten the time to reach steady-state prior to the start of administering AZARGA suspension. Following twice daily dosing of AZARGA suspension in both eyes for 13 weeks, red blood cell (RBC) concentrations of brinzolamide averaged 18.8±3.29 μM, 18.1±2.68 μM and 18.4±3.01 μM at weeks 4, 10 and 15, respectively, indicating that steady-state RBC concentrations of brinzolamide were maintained (RBC saturation of CA-II at approximately 20 μM). The mean steady-state timolol plasma C_{max} was 0.824 ng/mL and T_{max} was 0.79 hours after dosing with AZARGA suspension.

Distribution: Plasma protein binding of brinzolamide is moderate (about 60%). Brinzolamide is sequestered in RBCs due to its high affinity binding to CA-II and to a lesser extent to CA-I. Its active N-desethyl metabolite also accumulates in RBCs where it binds primarily to CA-I. The affinity of brinzolamide and metabolite to RBC and tissue CA results in low plasma concentrations.

Timolol can be measured in human aqueous humour after administration of timolol ophthalmic solution and in plasma for up to 12 hours after administration of AZARGA suspension.

Metabolism: The metabolic pathways for the metabolism of brinzolamide involve N-dealkylations, O-dealkylations and oxidation of its N-propyl side chain. N-desethyl brinzolamide is a major metabolite of brinzolamide formed in humans, which also binds to CA-I in the presence of brinzolamide and accumulates in RBCs. In vitro cytochrome P450 isozyme studies show that the metabolism of brinzolamide mainly involves CYP3A4 as well as at least four other isozymes which include CYP2A6, CYP2B6, CYP2C8 and CYP2C9.

Timolol is metabolised by two pathways. One route yields an ethanolamine side chain on the thiadiazole ring and the other giving an ethanolic side chain on the morpholine nitrogen and a second similar side chain with a carbonyl group adjacent to the nitrogen. Timolol metabolism is mediated primarily by CYP2D6.

Excretion: Brinzolamide is eliminated primarily by renal excretion (approximately 60%). About 20% of the dose has been accounted for in urine as metabolite. Brinzolamide and N-desethyl-brinzolamide are the predominant components in the urine along with trace levels (<1%) of the N-desmethoxypropyl and O-desmethyl metabolites.

Timolol and its metabolites are primarily excreted by the kidneys. Approximately 20% of a timolol dose is excreted in the urine unchanged and the remainder excreted in urine as metabolites. The plasma $t_{½}$ of timolol is 4.8 hours after administration of AZARGA suspension.

Table 2: AZARGA

Steady State Red Blood Cell Concentrations of brinzolamide and N-desethyl Brinzolamide Following Administration of AZARGA Suspension in Healthy Subjects

	C_{107} (μM)	$AUC_{15-107\ day}$ (μM·day)
Brinzolamide	18.4±3.01	1681±225
N-desethyl-brinzolamide	1.57±1.13	118±61.8

Table 3: AZARGA

Steady State Plasma Concentrations of Timolol Following Administration of AZARGA Suspension in Healthy Subjects

	C_{max} (ng/mL)	T_{max} (h)	AUC_{0-12} (ng·h/mL)	$t_{½}$ (h)
Timolol	0.824±0.453	0.79±0.45	4.71±2.49	4.8±1.8 h

Special Populations and Conditions: Pediatrics: AZARGA suspension has not been evaluated in the pediatric population.
Geriatrics: No overall differences in safety and effectiveness have been observed between elderly and other adult patients.
Gender: Following topical ocular administration of AZARGA suspension, there were no clinically relevant differences in systemic exposure to brinzolamide, N-desethyl brinzolamide or timolol, when analyzed by gender.
Race: No efficacy and safety differences due to ethnicity are expected with AZARGA suspension.
Hepatic Insufficiency: AZARGA suspension has not been studied in patients with hepatic disease.
Renal Insufficiency: AZARGA suspension has not been studied in patients with renal impairment.

STORAGE AND STABILITY: Store at 2-30°C. Discard 60 days after opening.

SPECIAL HANDLING INSTRUCTIONS: None.

INFORMATION FOR THE PATIENT: Published in e-CPS, available by subscription at www.e-cps.ca.

DOSAGE FORMS, COMPOSITION AND PACKAGING: Each mL of ophthalmic suspension contains: brinzolamide 10 mg, timolol 5 mg as timolol maleate and the preservative benzalkonium chloride 0.01%. Nonmedicinal ingredients: carbomer 974P, edetate disodium, mannitol, purified water, sodium chloride, sodium hydroxide and/or hydrochloric acid (to adjust pH) and tyloxapol. AZARGA suspension is formulated at a pH of approximately 7.2 and is isotonic. Round low density polyethylene bottles of 8 mL with a low density polyethylene dispensing plug and white polypropylene cap. Tamper evidence is provided by a closure with an extended skirt that locks to the bottle finish on application and breaks away from the closure on opening. Net contents are 5 mL supplied in an 8 mL bottle.

Azilect® Pr

rasagiline mesylate

Antiparkinsonian Agent

Teva Canada Innovation

Date of Revision: June 7, 2010

PHARMACOLOGY: Mechanism of Action: AZILECT (rasagiline mesylate tablets) is an irreversible, monoamine oxidase inhibitor indicated for the treatment of idiopathic Parkinson's disease. AZILECT inhibits MAO type B, but adequate studies to establish whether rasagiline is selective for MAO type B (MAO-B) in humans have not yet been conducted. MAO, a flavin-containing enzyme, is classified into two major molecular species, A and B, and is localized in mitochondrial membranes throughout the body in nerve terminals, brain, liver and intestinal mucosa. MAO regulates the metabolic degradation of catecholamines and serotonin in the CNS and peripheral tissues. MAO-B is the major form in the human brain. In ex vivo animal studies in brain, liver and intestinal tissues rasagiline was shown to be a potent, irreversible monoamine oxidase type B (MAO-B) selective inhibitor. Rasagiline at the recommended therapeutic dose was also shown to be a potent and irreversible inhibitor of MAO-B in platelets. The dose at which rasagiline selectively inhibits only MAO-B (and not MAO-A) in humans and the sensitivity to tyramine during rasagiline treatment at doses higher than 1 mg have not been sufficiently characterized (see Precautions).

The precise mechanisms of action of rasagiline are unknown. One mechanism is believed to be related to its MAO-B inhibitory activity, which causes an increase in extracellular levels of dopamine in the striatum. The elevated dopamine level and subsequent increased dopaminergic activity are likely to mediate rasagiline's beneficial effects seen in models of dopaminergic motor dysfunction.

Pharmacodynamics: Platelet MAO Activity in Clinical Studies: Studies in healthy subjects and in Parkinson's disease patients have shown that rasagiline inhibits platelet MAO-B irreversibly. The inhibition lasts at least 1 week after last dose. Almost 25-35 % MAO-B inhibition was achieved after a single rasagiline dose of 1 mg/day and more than 55% of MAO-B inhibition was achieved after a single rasagiline dose of 2 mg/day. Over 90% inhibition was achieved 3 days after rasagiline daily dosing at 2 mg/day and this inhibition level was maintained 3 days post-dose. Multiple doses of rasagiline of 0.5, 1 and 2 mg per day resulted in complete MAO-B inhibition.

Pharmacokinetics: Rasagiline's pharmacokinetics are linear with doses over the range of 1-10 mg. Its mean steady-state half life is 3 hours but there is no correlation of pharmacokinetics with its pharmacological effect because of its irreversible inhibition of MAO-B.

Absorption: Rasagiline is rapidly absorbed, reaching peak plasma concentration (C_{max}) in approximately 1 hour. The absolute bioavailability of rasagiline is about 36%.

Food does not affect the T_{max} of rasagiline, although C_{max} and exposure (AUC) are decreased by approximately 60% and 20%, respectively, when the drug is taken with a high fat meal. Because AUC is not significantly affected, AZILECT can be administered with or without food (see Dosage).

Distribution: The mean volume of distribution at steady-state is 87 L indicating that the tissue binding of rasagiline is in excess of plasma protein binding. Plasma protein binding ranges from 88-94% with mean extent of binding of 61-63% to human albumin over the concentration range of 1-100 ng/mL.

Metabolism and Elimination: Rasagiline undergoes almost complete biotransformation in the liver prior to excretion. The metabolism of rasagiline proceeds through two main pathways: N-dealkylation and/or hydroxylation to yield: 1-aminoindan (AI), 3-hydroxy-N-propargyl-1-aminoindan (3-OH-PAI) and 3-hydroxy-1-aminoindan (3-OH-AI). In vitro experiments indicate that both routes of rasagiline metabolism are dependent on cytochrome P450 (CYP) system, with CYP 1A2 being the major iso-enzyme involved in rasagiline metabolism. Glucuronide conjugation of rasagiline and its metabolites, with subsequent urinary excretion, is the major elimination pathway.

After oral administration of ^{14}C-labeled rasagiline, elimination occurred primarily via urine and secondarily via feces (62% of total dose in urine and 7% of total dose in feces over 7 days), with a total recovery of 84% of the dose over a period of 38 days. Less than 1% of rasagiline was excreted as unchanged drug in urine.

Population Pharmacokinetics: Hepatic Insufficiency: Following repeat dose administration (7 days) of rasagiline (1 mg/day) in subjects with mild hepatic impairment (Child-Pugh score 5-6), AUC and C_{max} were increased by 2 fold and 1.4 fold, respectively, compared to healthy subjects. In subjects with moderate hepatic impairment (Child-Pugh score 7-9), AUC and C_{max} were increased by 7 fold and 2 fold, respectively, compared to healthy subjects. (See Warnings, Hepatic Insufficiency and Dosage, Patients with Hepatic Impairment.)

Renal Insufficiency: Conclusive data are not available for renally impaired patients. As unconjugated rasagiline is not excreted by the kidney, rasagiline can be given at usual doses in patients with mild renal impairment. Due to the absence of adequate safety data, rasagiline should not be administered to patients with moderate to severe renal impairment.

Geriatric: Since age has little influence on rasagiline pharmacokinetics, it can be administered at the recommended dose in the elderly.

Pediatric: AZILECT has not been investigated in patients below 18 years of age.

Gender: The pharmacokinetic profile of rasagiline is similar in men and women.

<u>*Drug Interactions:*</u> Tyramine Effect: (See Precautions; Overdose, Symptoms and Treatment; Dosage and Information for the Patient.)

Levodopa: Data from population pharmacokinetic studies comparing rasagiline clearance in the presence and absence of levodopa have given conflicting results. Although there may be some increase in rasagiline blood levels in the presence of levodopa, the effect is modest and rasagiline dosing need not be modified in the presence of levodopa.

Effect of Other Drugs on the Metabolism of AZILECT: In vitro metabolism studies showed that CYP 1A2 was the major enzyme responsible for the metabolism of rasagiline. There is the potential for inhibitors of this enzyme to alter AZILECT clearance when coadministered. (See Warnings, Ciprofloxacin and Other CYP1A2 Inhibitors and Dosage, Patients Taking Ciprofloxacin and Other CYP1A2 Inhibitors.)

Ciprofloxacin: When ciprofloxacin, an inhibitor of CYP 1A2, was administered to healthy volunteers (n=12) at 500 mg (BID) with 2 mg/day rasagiline, the AUC of rasagiline increased by 83% and there was no change in the elimination half life. (See Warnings, Ciprofloxacin and Other CYP1A2 Inhibitors and Dosage, Patients Taking Ciprofloxacin and Other CYP1A2 Inhibitors.)

Theophylline: Coadministration of rasagiline 1 mg/day and theophylline, a substrate of CYP 1A2, up to 500 mg twice daily to healthy subjects (n=24), did not affect the pharmacokinetics of either drug.

Antidepressants: Severe CNS toxicity associated with hyperpyrexia and death has been reported with the combination of tricyclic or tetracyclic antidepressants, selective serotonin reuptake inhibitors (SSRIs), or serotonin-norepinephrine reuptake inhibitors (SNRIs) and non-selective MAOIs or selective MAO-B inhibitors. Therefore, the coadministration of antidepressants with rasagiline is contraindicated (see Contraindications).

Effect of AZILECT on Other Drugs: No additional in vivo trials have investigated the effect of AZILECT on other drugs metabolized by the cytochrome P450 enzyme system. In vitro, studies showed that rasagiline at a concentration of 1 μg/ml (equivalent to a level that is 160 times the average C_{max} ~5.9-8.5 ng/mL in Parkinson's disease patients after 1 mg rasagiline multiple dosing, did not inhibit cytochrome P450 isoenzymes, CYP1A2, CYP2A6, CYP2C9, CYP2C19, CYP2D6, CYP2E1, CYP3A4 and CYP4A. These results indicate that rasagiline is unlikely to cause any clinically significant interference with substrates of these enzymes.

Clinical Trials: In phase II/III premarketing trials approximately 1361 patients received AZILECT with 771 being treated for at least one year, approximately 361 patients treated for at least two years, and 245 receiving AZILECT for more than 3 years.

The effectiveness of AZILECT for the treatment of Parkinson's disease was established in three 18- to 26-week, randomized, placebo-controlled trials. In one of these trials study TVP-1012/232 (TEMPO) AZILECT was given as initial monotherapy treatment and in the other two studies as adjunctive therapy to levodopa TVP-1012/133 (PRESTO) and TVP-1012/122 (LARGO).

Monotherapy Use of AZILECT: The monotherapy trial (TEMPO) was a double-blind, randomized, fixed-dose parallel group 26-week study in early Parkinson's disease patients not yet receiving any concomitant dopaminergic therapy at the start of the study. The majority of the patients were not treated with any anti-Parkinson's disease medication before receiving AZILECT treatment.

The first phase was placebo-controlled in which 404 patients were randomly assigned to receive placebo (138 patients), AZILECT 1 mg/day (134 patients) or AZILECT 2 mg/day (132 patients). Patients were not allowed to take levodopa, dopamine agonists, selegiline or amantadine, but if necessary, could take stable doses of anticholinergic medication. The average Parkinson's disease duration was approximately 1 year (range 0 to 11 years). Patients completing the first 26 weeks or patients requiring additional anti-PD therapy could start the second phase of double-blind treatment in which all patients received AZILECT, 1 or 2 mg once daily.

Three hundred eighty patients entered the second phase. Patients who received AZILECT in the first phase remained on their originally assigned dose. Patients who received placebo in the first phase were switched to AZILECT, 2 mg once daily.

The primary measure of effectiveness was the change from baseline in the total score of the Unified Parkinson's Disease Rating Scale (UPDRS), [mentation (Part I), + activities of daily living (ADL) (Part II) + motor function (Part III)]. The UPDRS is a multi-item rating scale that measures the ability of a patient to perform mental and motor tasks as well as activities of daily living. A reduction in the score represents improvement and a beneficial change from baseline appears as a negative number.

Rasagiline (1 or 2 mg once daily) had a significant beneficial effect relative to placebo on the primary measure of effectiveness in patients receiving six months of treatment and not on dopaminergic therapy. Patients who received rasagiline had significantly less worsening in the UPDRS score, compared to those who received placebo. The effectiveness of rasagiline 1 mg and 2 mg was comparable. Table 1 displays the results of the monotherapy trial.

Table 1: AZILECT

Parkinson's Disease Patients not on Dopaminergic Therapy (TEMPO)

	Primary Measure of Effectiveness: Change in Total UPDRS Score		
	Baseline Score	Change from Baseline to Termination Score	p-value vs. Placebo
Placebo	24.5	3.9	—
1.0 mg/day	24.7	0.1	0.0001
2.0 mg/day	25.9	0.7	0.0001

For the comparison between rasagiline 1 mg/day and placebo, no differences in effectiveness based on age or gender were detected.

In addition in the TEMPO study the following secondary measurements of effectiveness were statistically significant and the effects of AZILECT 1 mg tablets over placebo are presented below: UPDRS ADL (Activities of Daily Living) subscale score ($p=0.0003$); UPDRS Motor subscale score ($p<0.0001$).

Adjunctive Use of AZILECT: Two multicenter, randomized, multinational trials were conducted in more advanced Parkinson's disease patients treated chronically with levodopa and experiencing motor fluctuations (including but not limited to, end of dose "wearing off," sudden or random "off," etc.) Studies TVP-1012/133 (PRESTO) and TVP-1012/122 (LARGO). The first (PRESTO) was conducted in North America (U.S. and Canada) and compared two doses (0.5 mg and 1 mg daily) of rasagiline and placebo while the second (LARGO) was conducted outside of North America (several European countries, Argentina, Israel) and studied a single dose (1 mg daily) of rasagiline, a COMT inhibitor with each levodopa dose and placebo. Patients had had Parkinson's disease for an average of 9 years (range 5 months to 33 years), had been taking levodopa for an average of 8 years (range 5 months to 32 years), and had been experiencing motor fluctuations for approximately 3 to 4 years (range 1 month to 23 years). Patients kept home diaries just prior to baseline and at specified intervals during the trial. Diaries recorded one of the following four conditions for each half-hour interval over a 24-hour period: "ON" (period of relatively good function and mobility) as either "ON" with no dyskinesia or without troublesome dyskinesia, "ON" with troublesome dyskinesia, "OFF" (period of relatively poor function and mobility) or asleep. "Troublesome" dyskinesia is defined as that which interferes with the patient's daily activity. All patients had been inadequately controlled and were experiencing motor fluctuations typical of advanced stage disease despite receiving levodopa/decarboxylase inhibitor. The average dose of levodopa/decarboxylase inhibitor was approximately 700 to 800 mg (range 150 to 3000 mg/day). Patients were also allowed to take stable doses of additional anti-PD medications at entry into the trials. In both trials, approximately 65% of patients were on dopamine agonists and in the North American study (PRESTO) approximately 35% were on entacapone. The majority of patients taking entacapone were taking a dopamine agonist as well.

In both trials the primary measure of effectiveness was the change in the mean number of hours that were spent in the "OFF" state at baseline compared to the mean number of hours that were spent in the "OFF" state during the treatment period. Secondary measures of effectiveness included global assessments of improvement by the examiner, ADL subscale scores when Off and UPDRS motor while ON. A reduction in the UPDRS score represents improvement and a beneficial change from baseline appears as a negative number.

PRESTO was a double-blind, randomized, fixed-dose parallel group trial conducted in 472 levodopa-treated Parkinson's disease patients who were experiencing motor fluctuations. Patients were randomly assigned to receive placebo (159 patients), AZILECT 0.5 mg/day (164 patients), or AZILECT 1 mg/day (149 patients), and were treated for 26 weeks. Patients averaged approximately 6 hours daily in the "OFF" state at baseline, as confirmed by home diaries.

LARGO was a double-blind, randomized, parallel group trial conducted in 687 levodopa-treated Parkinson's disease patients who were experiencing motor fluctuations. Patients were randomly assigned to receive placebo (229 patients), AZILECT 1 mg/day (231 patients) or an active comparator, a COMT inhibitor taken along with scheduled doses of levodopa/decarboxylase inhibitor (227 patients). Patients were treated for 18 weeks. Patients averaged approximately 5.6 hours daily in the "OFF" state at baseline as confirmed by home diaries.

In both studies rasagiline 1 mg once daily reduced "OFF" time compared to placebo when added to levodopa in patients experiencing motor fluctuations (see Table 2 and Table 3). The lower dose (0.5 mg) of rasagiline also significantly reduced "OFF" time (see Table 2), but had a numerically smaller effect than the 1 mg dose of rasagiline. In LARGO, the active comparator also reduced "OFF" time when compared to placebo.

Table 2: AZILECT

Parkinson's Disease Patients Receiving AZILECT as Adjunct Therapy (PRESTO)

Primary Measure of Effectiveness: Change in Mean Total Daily "OFF" Time			
	Baseline (hours)	**Change from Baseline to Treatment Period (hours)**	**p-value vs. Placebo**
Placebo	6.0	−0.9	—
0.5 mg/day	6.0	−1.4	0.0199
1.0 mg/day	6.3	−1.9	<0.0001

Table 3: AZILECT

Parkinson's Disease Patients Receiving AZILECT as Adjunct Therapy (LARGO)

Primary Measure of Effectiveness: Change in Mean Total Daily "OFF" Time			
	Baseline (hours)	**Change from Baseline to Treatment Period (hours)**	**p-value vs. Placebo**
Placebo	5.5	−0.40	—
1.0 mg/day	5.6	−1.2	0.0001
COMT Inhibitor with Each Levodopa Dose	5.6	−1.2	<0.0001

In both studies, dosage reduction of levodopa was allowed within the first 6 weeks if dopaminergic side effects, including dyskinesia and hallucinations, emerged. In PRESTO, levodopa dosage reduction occurred in 8 % of patients in the placebo group and in 16 % and 17 % of patients in the 0.5 mg/day and 1 mg/day rasagiline groups, respectively. In those patients who had levodopa dosage reduced, the dose was reduced on average by about 7 %, 9%, and 13 % in the placebo, 0.5 mg/day, and 1 mg/day groups, respectively. In LARGO, levodopa dosage reduction occurred in 6 % of patients in the placebo group and in 9 % in the rasagiline 1 mg/day group. In patients who had their levodopa dosage reduced, the dose was reduced on average by about 13% and 11 % in the placebo and the rasagiline groups, respectively.

For the comparison between rasagiline 1 mg/day and placebo in both studies, no differences in effectiveness based on age or gender were detected.

Several secondary outcome assessments in the two studies showed statistically significant improvements with rasagiline. These included effects on the activities of daily living (ADL) subscale of the UPDRS performed during an "OFF" period, and the motor subscale of the UPDRS as performed during an "ON" period. In both scales, a negative response represents improvement. Table 4 and Table 5 show these results for PRESTO and LARGO.

Table 4: AZILECT

Secondary Measures of Effectiveness (PRESTO)

	Baseline (Score)	**Change from Baseline Last Value**	**p-value vs. Placebo**
Global Improvement Score, Rated by the Examiner			
Placebo	—	−0.02	—
0.5 mg/day	—	−0.40	0.0027
1.0 mg/day	—	−0.66	<0.0001
UPDRS ADL (Activities of Daily Living) Subscale Score While "OFF"			
Placebo	15.5	0.68	—
0.5 mg/day	15.8	−0.60	0.0069
1.0 mg/day	15.5	−0.68	0.0034
UPDRS Motor Subscale Score While "ON"			
Placebo	20.8	1.21	—
0.5 mg/day	21.5	−1.43	0.0010
1.0 mg/day	20.9	−1.3	0.0008

Table 5: AZILECT

Secondary Measures of Effectiveness (LARGO)

	Baseline (Score)	**Change from Baseline Last Value**	**p-value vs. Placebo**
Global Improvement Score, Rated by the Examiner			
Placebo	—	−0.44	—
1.0 mg/day	—	−0.93	<0.001
COMT Inhibitor with Each Levodopa Dose	—	−0.79	0.0002
UPDRS ADL (Activities of Daily Living) Subscale Score While "OFF"			
Placebo	18.7	−0.89	
1.0 mg/day	19.0	−2.61	<0.0001
COMT Inhibitor with Each Levodopa Dose	19.0	−2.3	0.0006
UPDRS Motor Subscale Score While "ON"			
Placebo	23.5	−0.82	
1.0 mg/day	23.8	−3.87	<0.0001
COMT Inhibitor with Each Levodopa Dose	23.0	−3.5	<0.0001

(cont'd)

Table 5: AZILECT *(cont'd)*

INDICATIONS: AZILECT (rasagiline mesylate tablets) is indicated for the treatment of the signs and symptoms of idiopathic Parkinson's disease as initial monotherapy and as adjunct therapy to levodopa.

The effectiveness of AZILECT was demonstrated in patients with early Parkinson's disease who were receiving AZILECT as monotherapy and who were not receiving any concomitant dopaminergic therapy. The effectiveness of AZILECT as adjunct therapy was demonstrated in patients with Parkinson's disease who were treated with levodopa.

CONTRAINDICATIONS: Meperidine and Other Analgesics: AZILECT is contraindicated for use with meperidine. Serious reactions have been precipitated with concomitant use of meperidine (e.g., Demerol and other tradenames) and MAO inhibitors including selective MAO-B inhibitors. These reactions have been characterized by coma, severe hypertension or hypotension, severe respiratory depression, convulsions, malignant hyperpyrexia, excitation, peripheral vascular collapse and death. At least 14 days should elapse between discontinuation of AZILECT and initiation of treatment with meperidine.

For similar reasons, AZILECT should not be administered with the analgesic agents tramadol, methadone, and propoxyphene.
Other Drugs: AZILECT should not be used with the antitussive agent dextromethorphan. The combination of MAO inhibitors and dextromethorphan has been reported to cause brief episodes of psychosis or bizarre behavior. AZILECT is also contraindicated for use with St. John's wort, and cyclobenzaprine (a tricyclic muscle relaxant).
Sympathomimetic Amines: Like other MAOIs, AZILECT is contraindicated for use with sympathomimetic amines, including amphetamines as well as cold products and weight-reducing preparations that contain vasoconstrictors (e.g., pseudoephedrine, phenylephrine and ephedrine). Severe hypertensive reactions have followed the administrations of sympathomimetics and non-selective MAO inhibitors. At least one case of hypertensive crisis has been reported in a patient taking the recommended doses of a selective MAO-B inhibitor and a sympathomimetic medication (ephedrine).
Antidepressants: AZILECT should not be administered concomitantly with antidepressants. Serotonin Syndrome has been observed following concomitant use of these medications both with selective and non-selective MAOI inhibitors. At least 14 days should elapse between discontinuation of AZILECT and initiation of treatment with a tricyclic, tetracyclic, SSRI, or SNRI antidepressant. Similarly, at least 14 days should elapse after discontinuing treatment with a tricyclic, tetracyclic, SSRI, or SNRI antidepressant before starting AZILECT. Because of the long half-lives of fluoxetine and its active metabolite, at least five weeks (perhaps longer, especially if fluoxetine has been prescribed chronically and/or at higher doses) should elapse between discontinuation of fluoxetine and initiation of AZILECT (see Warnings).
MAO Inhibitors: AZILECT should not be administered along with other MAO inhibitors because of the increased risk of non-selective MAO inhibition that may lead to a hypertensive crisis. At least 14 days should elapse between discontinuation of AZILECT and initiation of treatment with MAO inhibitors.
Surgery: As with other MAOIs, patients taking AZILECT should not undergo elective surgery requiring general anesthesia. Also, they should not be given local anesthesia containing cocaine or sympathomimetic vasoconstrictors. AZILECT should be discontinued at least 14 days prior to elective surgery. If surgery is necessary sooner, benzodiazepines, mivacurium, fentanyl, morphine, and codeine may be used cautiously.
Pheochromocytoma: As with other MAOIs, AZILECT is contraindicated in patients with pheochromocytoma.

WARNINGS: Serotonin Syndrome: Severe CNS toxicity associated with hyperpyrexia and death has been reported with the combination of tricyclic or tetracyclic antidepressants, non-selective MAOIs (NARDIL, PARNATE) including the reversible MAOI, moclobemide and a selective MAO-B inhibitor, selegiline. These adverse events have included behavioral and mental status changes, diaphoresis, muscular rigidity, hypertension, syncope and death.

Serious, sometimes fatal, reactions with signs and symptoms including hyperthermia, rigidity, myoclonus, autonomic instability with rapid vital sign fluctuations, and mental status changes progressing to extreme agitation, delirium, and coma have been reported in patients receiving a combination of selective serotonin reuptake inhibitors (SSRIs), including fluoxetine (PROZAC), fluvoxamine (LUVOX) sertraline (ZOLOFT), and paroxetine (PAXIL), non-selective MAOIs, including the reversible MAOI moclobemide, or the selective MAO-B inhibitor selegiline. Similar reactions have been reported with serotonin-norepinephrine reuptake inhibitors (SNRIs). In the post-marketing period, non-fatal cases of serotonin syndrome have been reported in patients treated with antidepressants concomitantly with AZILECT.

At least 14 days should elapse between discontinuation of AZILECT and initiation of treatment with a tricyclic, tetracyclic, SSRI, or SNRI antidepressant. Similarly, at least 14 days should elapse after discontinuing treatment with a tricyclic, tetracyclic, SSRI, or SNRI antidepressant before starting AZILECT. Because of the long half-lives of fluoxetine and its active metabolite, at least five weeks (perhaps longer, especially if fluoxetine has been prescribed chronically and/or at higher doses) should elapse between discontinuation of fluoxetine and initiation of AZILECT (see Contraindications).
Ciprofloxacin and Other CYP1A2 Inhibitors: Rasagiline plasma concentrations may increase up to 2 fold in patients using concomitant ciprofloxacin and other CYP1A2 inhibitors. (See Pharmacology, Drug Interactions and Dosage, Patients Taking Ciprofloxacin and Other CYP1A2 Inhibitors.)
Hepatic Insufficiency: AZILECT plasma concentration may increase in patients with mild (up to 2 fold, Child-Pugh score 5-6), moderate (up to 7 fold, Child-Pugh score 7-9), and severe hepatic Child-Pugh score 10-15) impairment. Patients with mild hepatic impairment should be given the dose of 0.5 mg/day. AZILECT should not be used in patients with moderate or severe hepatic impairment (see Pharmacology, Population Pharmacokinetics).

PRECAUTIONS: General: Tyramine/Rasagiline Interaction: Rasagiline should not be used at daily doses exceeding the maximum recommended (1 mg/day) because of the risks associated with nonselective inhibition of MAO. Adequate studies above this dose have not been conducted. Therefore, if rasagiline is to be used without restrictions being placed on diet and concomitant drug use, it is critical to adhere to this maximum dose.
Melanoma: Epidemiological studies have shown that patients with Parkinson's disease have a higher risk (2- to approximately 6-fold higher) of developing melanoma than the general population. Whether the increased risk observed was due to Parkinson's disease or other factors, such as drugs used to treat Parkinson's disease, is unclear.

For the reasons stated above, patients and providers are advised to monitor for melanomas frequently and on a regular basis when using AZILECT for **any** indication. Ideally periodic skin examinations should be performed by appropriately qualified individuals (e.g. dermatologists).
Dyskinesia Due to Levodopa Treatment: When used as an adjunct to levodopa AZILECT may potentiate dopaminergic side effects and exacerbate pre-existing dyskinesia (treatment-emergent dyskinesia occurred in about 18% of patients treated with 0.5 mg or 1 mg rasagiline as an adjunct to levodopa and 10% of patients who received placebo as an adjunct to levodopa). Decreasing the dose of levodopa may ameliorate this side effect.
Postural Hypotension: When used as monotherapy, postural hypotension was reported in approximately 3% of patients treated with 1 mg rasagiline and 5% of patients treated with placebo. In the monotherapy trial, postural hypotension did not lead to drug discontinuation and premature withdrawal in the rasagiline treated patients or the placebo treated patients.

When used as an adjunct to levodopa, postural hypotension was reported in approximately 6% of patients treated with 0.5 mg rasagiline, 9% of patients treated with 1 mg rasagiline and 3% of patients treated with placebo. Postural hypotension led to drug discontinuation and premature withdrawal from clinical trials in one (0.7%) patient treated with rasagiline 1 mg/day, no patients treated with rasagiline 0.5 mg/day and no placebo-treated patients.

Clinical trial data suggest that postural hypotension occurs most frequently in the first two months of rasagiline treatment and tends to decrease over time.

Hallucinations: In the monotherapy study, hallucinations were reported as an adverse event in 1.3% of patients treated with 1 mg rasagiline and in 0.7% of patients treated with placebo. In the monotherapy trial, hallucinations led to drug discontinuation and premature withdrawal from clinical trials in 1.3% of the 1 mg rasagiline treated patients and in none of the placebo treated patients.

When used as an adjunct to levodopa, hallucinations were reported as an adverse event in approximately 5% of patients treated with 0.5 mg/day, 4% of patients treated with 1 mg/day rasagiline and 3% of patients treated with placebo. Hallucinations led to drug discontinuation and premature withdrawal from clinical trials in about 1% of patients treated with 0.5 mg/day or 1 mg/day and none of the placebo treated patients.

Information to Be Provided to the Patient: Patients receiving Azilect should be given the following instructions by the physician:

The risk of exceeding the recommended daily dose (1 mg/day) should be explained. The explanation should describe the signs and symptoms associated with MAOI induced hypertensive reactions. Patients should be urged to immediately report any severe headache or other atypical or unusual symptoms not previously experienced.

Patients should be cautioned of the possibility of developing hallucinations and instructed to report them to their health care provider promptly should they develop.

Patients should be advised to inform their physician if they are taking, or planning to take, any prescription or over-the-counter drugs especially with antidepressants and over-the-counter cold medications since there is a potential for interaction with AZILECT. Patients should not use meperidine with AZILECT.

Patients taking AZILECT as adjunct to levodopa should be advised there is the possibility of increased dyskinesia and postural hypotension.

Patients are advised to monitor for melanomas frequently and on a regular basis. Ideally, periodic skin examinations should be performed by appropriately qualified individuals (e.g. dermatologists).

Patients should be instructed to take AZILECT as prescribed. If a dose is missed the next dose should be taken at the usual time on the following day. The patient should not double-up the dose of AZILECT.

Drug Interactions: Meperidine: Serious, sometimes fatal reactions have been precipitated with concomitant use of meperidine (e.g., Demerol and other tradenames) and MAO inhibitors including selective MAO-B inhibitors (see Contraindications).

Dextromethorphan: The concomitant use of AZILECT and dextromethorphan was not allowed in clinical studies. The combination of MAO inhibitors and dextromethorphan has been reported to cause brief episodes of psychosis or bizarre behavior. Therefore, in view of AZILECT's MAO inhibitory activity, dextromethorphan should not be used concomitantly with AZILECT (see Contraindications).

Sympathomimetic Medications: The concomitant use of AZILECT and sympathomimetic medications was not allowed in clinical studies. Severe hypertensive reactions have followed the administration of sympathomimetics and non-selective MAO inhibitors. One case of hypertensive crisis has been reported in a patient taking the recommended doses of a selective MAO-B inhibitor and a sympathomimetic medication (ephedrine). Therefore, in view of AZILECT's MAO inhibitory activity, AZILECT should not be used concomitantly with sympathomimetics including nasal and oral decongestants and cold remedies (see Contraindications).

MAO Inhibitors: AZILECT should not be administered along with other MAO inhibitors, including reversible MAOI (moclobemide) and selective MAO-B inhibitors (selegiline) because of the increased risk of non-selective MAO inhibition that may lead to a hypertensive crisis (see Contraindications).

Selective Serotonin Reuptake Inhibitors (SSRIs), Serotonin Norepinephrine Reuptake Inhibitors (SNRIs), Tricyclic and Tetracyclic Antidepressants: Concomitant use of SSRI, SNRI, tricyclic, and tetracyclic antidepressants with AZILECT is contraindicated (see Contraindications).

Levodopa/Carbidopa: (See Pharmacology, Drug Interactions and Precautions, General, Dyskinesia Due to Levodopa Treatment.)

Ciprofloxacin and Other CYP1A2 Inhibitors: Rasagiline plasma concentrations may increase up to 2-fold in patients using concomitant ciprofloxacin and other CYP1A2 inhibitors. This could result in increased adverse events. (See Pharmacology, Drug Interactions and Warnings, Ciprofloxacin and Other CYP1A2 Inhibitors.)

Theophylline: (See Pharmacology, Drug Interactions.)

Laboratory Tests: No specific laboratory tests are necessary for the management of patients on AZILECT.

Pregnancy: Reproductive studies conducted with rasagiline in animals did not reveal any negative effect at doses much higher than those used in the clinical studies. However, there are no adequate and well-controlled studies of rasagiline in pregnant women. Because animal reproduction studies are not always predictive of human response, AZILECT should be used during pregnancy only if clearly needed.

Lactation: Experimental data indicated that rasagiline inhibits prolactin secretion and, thus, may inhibit lactation. It is not known whether rasagiline is excreted in human milk. Because many drugs are excreted in human milk, caution should be exercised when AZILECT is administered to a nursing woman.

Children: The safety and effectiveness of AZILECT in patients below 18 years of age have not been established.

Geriatrics: Approximately half of patients in clinical trials were 65 years and over. There were no significant differences in the safety profile of the geriatric and non-geriatric patients.

Renal Insufficiency: Conclusive data are not available for renally impaired patients. As unconjugated rasagiline is not excreted by the kidney, rasagiline can be given at usual doses in patients with mild renal impairment. Due to the absence of adequate safety data, rasagiline should not be administered to patients with moderate to severe renal impairment.

ADVERSE EFFECTS: During the clinical development of AZILECT (rasagiline mesylate tablets), 1361 Parkinson's disease patients received AZILECT as initial monotherapy, or as adjunct therapy to levodopa. As these two populations differ, not only in the adjunct use of levodopa during AZILECT treatment, but also in the severity and duration of their disease, they may have differential risks for various adverse events. Therefore, most of the adverse events data in this section are presented separately for each population.

Monotherapy: Adverse Events Leading to Discontinuation in Controlled Clinical Studies: In the double-blind, placebo-controlled trials conducted in patients receiving AZILECT as monotherapy, approximately 5% of the 149 patients treated with rasagiline discontinued treatment due to adverse events compared to 2% of the 151 patients who received placebo.

The only adverse event that led to the discontinuation of more than one patient was hallucinations.

Adverse Event Incidence in Controlled Clinical Studies: The most commonly observed adverse events that occurred in ≥5% of patients receiving AZILECT 1 mg as monotherapy (n=149) participating in the double-blind, placebo-controlled trial and that were at least 1.5 times the incidence in the placebo group (n=151), were: flu syndrome, arthralgia, depression, dyspepsia and fall.

Table 6 lists treatment emergent adverse events that occurred in ≥2% of patients receiving AZILECT as monotherapy participating in the double-blind, placebo-controlled trial and were numerically more frequent than in the placebo group.

Table 6: AZILECT

Treatment Emergent[a] Adverse Events in AZILECT 1 mg-Treated Monotherapy Patients

Placebo-Controlled Studies Without Levodopa Treatment	AZILECT 1 mg (N=149) % of Patients	Placebo (N=151) % of Patients
Headache	14	12
Arthralgia	7	4
Dyspepsia	7	4
Depression	5	2
Fall	5	3
Flu Syndrome	5	1
Conjunctivitis	3	1

(cont'd)

Table 6: AZILECT *(cont'd)*

Treatment Emergent[a] Adverse Events in AZILECT 1 mg-Treated Monotherapy Patients

Placebo-Controlled Studies Without Levodopa Treatment	AZILECT 1 mg (N=149) % of Patients	Placebo (N=151) % of Patients
Fever	3	1
Gastroenteritis	3	1
Rhinitis	3	1
Arthritis	2	1
Ecchymosis	2	0
Malaise	2	0
Neck Pain	2	0
Paresthesia	2	1
Vertigo	2	1

[a] Incidence ≥2% in AZILECT 1 mg group and numerically more frequent than in placebo group.

Other events of potential clinical importance reported by 1% or more of Parkinson's disease patients receiving AZILECT as monotherapy, and at least as frequent as in the placebo group, in descending order of frequency include: dizziness, diarrhea, chest pain, albuminuria, allergic reaction, alopecia, angina pectoris, anorexia, asthma, hallucinations, impotence, leukopenia, libido decreased, liver function tests abnormal, skin carcinoma, syncope, vesiculobullous rash, vomiting.

There were no significant differences in the safety profile based on age or gender.

Adjunct Therapy: Adverse Events Leading to Discontinuation in Controlled Clinical Studies: In a double-blind, placebo-controlled trial (PRESTO) conducted in patients treated with AZILECT as adjunct to levodopa therapy, approximately 9% of the 164 patients treated with AZILECT 0.5 mg/day and 7% of the 149 patients treated with AZILECT 1 mg/day discontinued treatment due to adverse events compared to 6% of the 159 patients who received placebo. The AEs that led to discontinuation of more than one rasagiline treated patient were diarrhea, weight loss, hallucination, and rash. Adverse event reporting was considered more reliable for PRESTO than for the second controlled trial (LARGO); therefore only the adverse event data from PRESTO are presented in this section of labeling.

Adverse Event Incidence in Controlled Clinical Studies: The most commonly observed adverse events that occurred in ≥5% of patients receiving AZILECT 1 mg (n=149) as adjunct to levodopa therapy participating in the double-blind, placebo-controlled trial (PRESTO) and that were at least 1.5 times the incidence in the placebo group (n=159) in descending order of difference in incidence were dyskinesia, accidental injury , weight loss, postural hypotension, vomiting, anorexia, arthralgia, abdominal pain, nausea, constipation, dry mouth, rash, ecchymosis, somnolence and paresthesia.

Table 7 lists treatment emergent adverse events that occurred in ≥2% of patients treated with AZILECT 1 mg/day as adjunct to levodopa therapy participating in the double-blind, placebo-controlled trial (PRESTO) and that were numerically more frequent than the placebo group. The table also shows the rates for the 0.5 mg group in PRESTO.

Table 7: AZILECT

Incidence of Treatment Emergent[a] Adverse Events in Patients Receiving AZILECT as Adjunct to Levodopa Therapy in PRESTO

	AZILECT 1 mg + Levodopa (N=149) % of Patients	AZILECT 0.5 mg + Levodopa (N=164) % of Patients	Placebo + Levodopa (N=159) % of Patients
Dyskinesia	18	18	10
Accidental Injury	12	8	5
Nausea	12	10	8
Headache	11	8	10
Fall	11	12	8
Weight Loss	9	2	3
Constipation	9	4	5
Postural Hypotension	9	6	3
Arthralgia	8	6	4
Vomiting	7	4	1
Dry Mouth	6	2	3
Rash	6	3	3
Somnolence	6	4	4
Abdominal Pain	5	2	1
Anorexia	5	2	1
Diarrhea	5	7	4
Ecchymosis	5	2	3
Dyspepsia	5	4	4
Paresthesia	5	2	3
Abnormal Dreams	4	1	1
Hallucinations	4	5	3
Ataxia	3	6	1

(cont'd)

Table 7: AZILECT (*cont'd*)

Incidence of Treatment Emergent[a] Adverse Events in Patients Receiving AZILECT as Adjunct to Levodopa Therapy in PRESTO

	AZILECT 1 mg + Levodopa (N=149) % of Patients	AZILECT 0.5 mg + Levodopa (N=164) % of Patients	Placebo + Levodopa (N=159) % of Patients
Dyspnea	3	5	2
Infection	3	2	2
Neck Pain	3	1	1
Sweating	3	2	1
Tenosynovitis	3	1	0
Dystonia	3	2	1
Gingivitis	2	1	1
Hemorrhage	2	1	1
Hernia	2	1	1
Myasthenia	2	2	1

[a] Incidence ≥2% in AZILECT 1 mg group and numerically more frequent than in placebo group.

Several of the more common adverse events seemed dose-related, including weight loss, postural hypotension, and dry mouth.

Other events of potential clinical importance reported in PRESTO by 1% or more of patients treated with rasagiline 1 mg/day as adjunct to levodopa therapy and at least as frequent as in the placebo group, in descending order of frequency include: skin carcinoma, anemia, albuminuria, amnesia, arthritis, bursitis, cerebrovascular accident, confusion, dysphagia, epistaxis, leg cramps, pruritus, skin ulcer.

There were no significant differences in the safety profile based on age or gender.

Other Adverse Events Observed During All Phase II/III Clinical Trials: Rasagiline was administered to approximately 1361 patients during all PD phase II/III clinical trials. About 771 patients received rasagiline for at least one year, approximately 361 patients received rasagiline for at least two years and 245 patients received rasagiline for more than 3 years, with 138 patients treated for more than 5 years. The long-term safety profile was similar to that observed with shorter duration exposure.

The frequencies listed below represent the proportion of the 1361 individuals exposed to rasagiline who experienced events of the type cited.

All events that occurred at least twice (or once for serious or potentially serious events) except those already listed above, trivial events, terms too vague to be meaningful, adverse events with no plausible relation to treatment and events that would be expected in patients of the age studied were reported without regard to determination of a causal relationship to rasagiline.

Events are further classified within body system categories and enumerated in order of decreasing frequency using the following definitions: frequent adverse events are defined as those occurring in at least 1/100 patients, infrequent adverse events are defined as those occurring in less than 1/100 to at least 1/1000 patients and rare adverse events are defined as those occurring in fewer than 1/1000 patients.

Body as a Whole: Frequent: asthenia. Infrequent: chills, face edema, flank pain, photosensitivity reaction.

Cardiovascular System: Frequent: bundle branch block. Infrequent: deep thrombophlebitis, heart failure, migraine, myocardial infarct, phlebitis, ventricular tachycardia. Rare: arterial thrombosis, atrial arrhythmia, AV block complete, AV block second degree, bigeminy, cerebral hemorrhage, cerebral ischemia, ventricular fibrillation.

Digestive System: Frequent: gastrointestinal hemorrhage. Infrequent: colitis, esophageal ulcer, esophagitis, fecal incontinence, intestinal obstruction, mouth ulceration, stomach ulcer, stomatitis, tongue edema. Rare: hematemesis, hemorrhagic gastritis, intestinal perforation, intestinal stenosis, jaundice, large intestine perforation, megacolon, melena.

Hemic and Lymphatic Systems: Infrequent: macrocytic anemia. Rare: purpura, thrombocythemia.

Metabolic and Nutritional Disorders: Infrequent: hypocalcemia.

Musculoskeletal System: Infrequent: bone necrosis, muscle atrophy. Rare: arthrosis.

Nervous System: Frequent: abnormal gait, anxiety, hyperkinesia, hypertonia, neuropathy, tremor. Infrequent: agitation, aphasia, circumoral paresthesia, convulsion, delusions, dementia, dysarthria, dysautonomia, dysesthesia, emotional lability, facial paralysis, foot drop, hemiplegia, hypesthesia, incoordination, manic reaction, myoclonus, neuritis, neurosis, paranoid reaction, personality disorder, psychosis, wrist drop. Rare: apathy, delirium, hostility, manic depressive reaction, myelitis, neuralgia, psychotic depression, stupor.

Respiratory System: Frequent: cough increased. Infrequent: apnea, emphysema, laryngismus, pleural effusion, pneumothorax. Rare: interstitial pneumonia, larynx edema, lung fibrosis.

Skin and Appendages: Infrequent: eczema, urticaria. Rare: exfoliative dermatitis, leukoderma.

Special Senses: Infrequent: blepharitis, deafness, diplopia, eye hemorrhage, eye pain, glaucoma, keratitis, ptosis, retinal degeneration, taste perversion, visual field defect. Rare: blindness, parosmia, photophobia, retinal detachment, retinal hemorrhage, strabismus, taste loss, vestibular disorder.

Urogenital System: Frequent: hematuria, urinary incontinence. Infrequent: acute kidney failure, dysmenorrhea, dysuria, kidney calculus, nocturia, polyuria, scrotal edema, sexual function abnormal, urinary retention, urination impaired, vaginal hemorrhage, vaginal moniliasis, vaginitis. Rare: abnormal ejaculation, amenorrhea, anuria, epididymitis, gynecomastia, hydroureter, leukorrhea, priapism.

Postmarketing Experience: The following adverse events have been identified during postapproval use of AZILECT. Because these events are reported voluntarily from a population of uncertain size, it is not always possible to reliably estimate their frequency or establish a causal relationship to drug exposure.

Nervous System: Serotonin syndrome characterized by agitation, confusion, rigidity, pyrexia, and myoclonus has been reported by patients treated with antidepressants concomitantly with AZILECT.

Cardiovascular System: Cases of elevated blood pressure, including rare cases of hypertensive crisis, associated with ingestion of unknown amounts of tyramine-rich foods; one report of elevated blood pressure in a patient using the ophthalmic vasoconstrictor tetrahydrozoline hydrochloride.

OVERDOSE:

Symptoms: Symptoms reported following overdose of AZILECT in doses ranging from 3 mg to 100 mg include dysphoria, hypomania, hypertensive crisis, and serotonin syndrome.

The following description of presenting symptoms and clinical course is based upon overdose descriptions of non-selective MAO inhibitors.

Characteristically, signs and symptoms of non-selective MAOI overdose may not appear immediately. Delays of up to 12 hours between ingestion of drug and the appearance of signs may occur. Importantly, the peak intensity of the syndrome may not be reached for upwards of a day following the overdose. Death has been reported following overdosage. Therefore, immediate hospitalization, with continuous patient observation and monitoring for a period of at least two days following the ingestion of such drugs in overdose, is strongly recommended.

The clinical picture of MAOI overdose varies considerably; its severity may be a function of the amount of drug consumed. The central nervous and cardiovascular systems are prominently involved.

Signs and symptoms of overdosage may include, alone or in combination, any of the following: drowsiness, dizziness, faintness, irritability, hyperactivity, agitation, severe headache, hallucinations, trismus, opisthotonos, convulsions, and coma; rapid and irregular pulse, hypertension, hypotension and vascular collapse; precordial pain, respiratory depression and failure, hyperpyrexia, diaphoresis, and cool, clammy skin.

Treatment: There is no specific antidote for rasagiline overdose. The following suggestions are offered based upon the assumption that rasagiline overdose may be modeled after non-selective MAO inhibitor poisoning. Treatment of overdose with non-selective MAO inhibitors is symptomatic and supportive. Respiration should be supported by appropriate measures, including management of the airway, use of supplemental oxygen, and mechanical ventilatory assistance, as required. Body temperature should be monitored closely. Intensive management of hyperpyrexia may be required. Maintenance of fluid and electrolyte balance is essential.

For management of a suspected drug overdose, contact your regional Poison Control Centre. See the *CPS* Directory section for a list of Poison Control Centres.

DOSAGE: Dosing Considerations:

- The recommended and maximum dose in both monotherapy and adjunct therapy is 1 mg once daily.
- AZILECT can be taken with or without food.

There is no evidence that additional benefit will be obtained from the administration of doses higher than that recommended. Furthermore, higher doses will likely result in a loss of selectivity of rasagiline towards MAO-B with an increase in the inhibition of MAO-A. There is an increased risk of adverse reactions with higher doses as well as an increased risk of hypertensive episode ("cheese reaction").

Monotherapy: The recommended AZILECT dose for the treatment of Parkinson's disease patients is 1 mg administered once daily.

Adjunctive Therapy: The dosage of AZILECT shown to be effective in controlled clinical trials for adjunct therapy was 0.5-1 mg once daily. The recommended initial dose is 0.5 mg administered once daily. If a sufficient clinical response is not achieved, the dose may be increased to 1 mg administered once daily.

Change of Levodopa Dose in Adjunct Therapy: When AZILECT is used in combination with levodopa a reduction of the levodopa dosage may be considered based upon individual response. During the controlled trials of AZILECT as adjunct therapy to levodopa, levodopa dosage was reduced in some patients. In clinical studies, dosage reduction of levodopa was allowed within the first 6 weeks if dopaminergic side effects, including dyskinesia and hallucinations, emerged. In the PRESTO study levodopa dosage reduction occurred in 8 % of patients in the placebo group and in 16 % and 17 % of patients in the 0.5 mg/day and 1 mg/day rasagiline groups, respectively. In those patients who had levodopa dosage reduced, the dose was reduced on average by about 7 %, 9%, and 13 % in the placebo, 0.5 mg/day, and 1 mg/day groups, respectively. In the LARGO study levodopa dosage reduction occurred in 6 % of patients in the placebo group and in 9 % in the rasagiline 1 mg/day group. In patients who had their levodopa dosage reduced, the dose was reduced on average by about 13% and 11 % in the placebo and the rasagiline groups, respectively.

Patients with Hepatic Impairment: AZILECT plasma concentration will increase in patients with hepatic impairment. Patients with mild hepatic impairment AZILECT should use 0.5 mg daily of AZILECT. AZILECT should not be used in patients with moderate to severe hepatic impairment. (See Pharmacology, Population Pharmacokinetics, Hepatic Insufficiency and Warnings, Hepatic Insufficiency.)

Patients with Renal Impairment: Conclusive data are not available for renally impaired patients. As unconjugated rasagiline is not excreted by the kidney, rasagiline can be given at usual doses in patients with mild renal impairment. Due to the absence of adequate safety data, rasagiline should not be administered to patients with moderate to severe renal impairment.

Patients Taking Ciprofloxacin and Other CYP1A2 Inhibitors: Rasagiline plasma concentrations are expected to double in patients taking concomitant ciprofloxacin and other CYP1A2 inhibitors. Therefore, patients taking concomitant ciprofloxacin or other CYP1A2 inhibitors should use 0.5 mg daily of AZILECT (see Pharmacology, Drug Interactions, Ciprofloxacin and Effect of Other Drugs on the Metabolism of AZILECT and Warnings, Ciprofloxacin and Other CYP1A2 Inhibitors).

INFORMATION FOR THE PATIENT: Published in e-CPS, available by subscription at www.e-cps.ca.

SUPPLIED: 0.5 mg: Each white to off-white, round, flat, beveled tablet, debossed with "GIL" and "0.5" below on one side and plain on the other, contains: rasagiline 0.5 mg, as mesylate. Nonmedicinal ingredients: colloidal silicon dioxide, mannitol, pregelatinized starch, starch, stearic acid and talc. Bottles of 30. Store at 25°C with excursions permitted to 15-30°C.

1 mg: Each white to off-white, round, flat, beveled tablet, debossed with "GIL" and "1" below on one side and plain on the other, contains: rasagiline 1 mg, as mesylate. Nonmedicinal ingredients: colloidal silicon dioxide, mannitol, pregelatinized starch, starch, stearic acid and talc. Bottles of 30. Store at 25°C with excursions permitted to 15-30°C.

(*Shown in Product Identification Section*)

Azopt® Ⓟ

brinzolamide

Elevated Intraocular Pressure Therapy

Alcon

PHARMACOLOGY: Brinzolamide is a carbonic anhydrase inhibitor formulated for topical ophthalmic use.

Carbonic anhydrase (CA) is an enzyme found in many tissues of the body including the eye. It catalyzes the reversible reaction involving the hydration of carbon dioxide and the dehydration of carbonic acid. In humans, carbonic anhydrase exists as a number of isoenzymes, the most active being carbonic anhydrase II (CA-II), found primarily in red blood cells (RBC's), but also in other tissues. Inhibition of carbonic anhydrase in the ciliary processes of the eye decreases aqueous humor secretion, presumably by slowing the formation of bicarbonate ions with subsequent reduction in sodium and fluid transport. The result is a reduction in intraocular pressure (IOP).

Following topical ocular administration, brinzolamide is absorbed into the systemic circulation. Due to its high affinity for CA-II, brinzolamide distributes extensively into the RBCs and exhibits a long half-life in whole blood (approximately 111 days). In humans, the metabolite N-desethyl brinzolamide is formed, which also binds to CA and accumulates in RBCs. This metabolite binds mainly to CA-I in the presence of brinzolamide. In plasma, both parent brinzolamide and N-desethyl brinzolamide concentrations are low and generally below assay quantitation limits (<10 ng/mL). Binding to plasma proteins is not extensive (about 60%). Brinzolamide is eliminated predominantly in the urine as unchanged drug. N-Desethyl brinzolamide is also found in the urine along with trace concentrations (<1% of the dose) of the N-desmethoxypropyl and O-desmethyl metabolites.

INDICATIONS: In the treatment of elevated intraocular pressure in patients with ocular hypertension or open-angle glaucoma.

CONTRAINDICATIONS: Patients who are hypersensitive to any component of this product.

Brinzolamide has not been studied in patients with severe renal impairment (CrCl <30 mL/min). Because brinzolamide and its metabolite are excreted predominantly by the kidney, brinzolamide is not recommended in such patients.

There is a potential for an additive effect on the known systemic effects of carbonic anhydrase inhibition in patients receiving an oral carbonic anhydrase inhibitor and brinzolamide. The concomitant administration of brinzolamide and oral carbonic anhydrase inhibitors is not recommended.

WARNINGS: Brinzolamide is a sulfonamide and although administered topically, it is absorbed systemically. Therefore, the same types of adverse reactions that are attributable to sulfonamides may occur with topical administration of brinzolamide. Fatalities have occurred, although rarely, due to severe reactions to sulfonamides including Stevens-Johnson syndrome, toxic epidermal necrolysis, fulminant hepatic necrosis, agranulocytosis, aplastic anemia, and other blood dyscrasias. Sensitization may occur when a sulfonamide is readministered irrespective of the route of administration. If signs of serious reactions or hypersensitivity occur, discontinue the use of this preparation.

The management of patients with acute angle-closure glaucoma requires therapeutic interventions in addition to ocular hypotensive agents. Brinzolamide has not been studied in patients with acute angle-closure glaucoma.

Brinzolamide has not been studied in patients with hepatic impairment and should therefore be used with caution in such patients.

The preservative in AZOPT ophthalmic suspension, benzalkonium chloride, may be absorbed by soft contact lenses. Contact lenses should be removed during instillation of brinzolamide suspension but may be reinserted 15 minutes after instillation.

Children: Safety and effectiveness in pediatric patients have not been established.

Pregnancy: There are no adequate and well-controlled studies in pregnant women. Brinzolamide should be used during pregnancy only if the potential benefit justifies the potential risk to the fetus.

Lactation: It is not known whether this drug is excreted in human milk. Because many drugs are excreted in human milk and because of the potential for serious adverse reactions in nursing infants from brinzolamide suspension, a decision should be made whether to discontinue nursing or to discontinue the drug, taking into account the importance of the drug to the mother.

In a study of brinzolamide in lactating rats, decreases in body weight gain in offspring at an oral dose of 15 mg/kg/day (312 times the recommended human ophthalmic dose) were seen during lactation. No other effects were observed. However, following oral administration of ^{14}C-brinzolamide to lactating rats, radioactivity was found in milk at concentrations below those in the blood and plasma.

PRECAUTIONS: Carbonic anhydrase activity has been observed in both the cytoplasm and around the plasma membranes of the corneal endothelium. In a 12-month topical ocular primate study, continued administration of brinzolamide ophthalmic suspension resulted in no significant effect on the corneal endothelium as evaluated by specular microscopy.

Patients should be instructed to avoid allowing the tip of the dispensing container to contact the eye or surrounding structures or with other surfaces.

If more than 1 topical ophthalmic drug is being used, the drugs should be administered at least 10 minutes apart.

Occupational Hazards: Effects on Ability to Drive and to Use Machines: Brinzolamide may temporarily result in blurred vision following dosing. Care should be exercised in operating machinery or driving a motor vehicle.

Drug Interactions: Although acid-base and electrolyte alterations were not reported in the clinical trials with brinzolamide, these changes have been reported with oral carbonic anhydrase inhibitors and have, in some instances, resulted in drug interactions (e.g., toxicity associated with high-dose salicylate therapy). Therefore, the potential for such drug interactions should be considered in patients receiving brinzolamide suspension.

Geriatrics: In well-controlled clinical studies of brinzolamide, the probability of having an adverse reaction was independent of age. No difference in patients experiencing adverse reactions was noted in patients less than 65 years of age, between 65 and 75 years of age, and greater than 75 years of age.

ADVERSE EFFECTS: In well-controlled clinical studies of brinzolamide, adverse reactions related to brinzolamide were generally mild to moderate and usually did not lead to discontinuation of therapy. Table 1 lists for brinzolamide 1% and placebo reported adverse events possibly, probably or definitely related to therapy occurring at an incidence of 1% or greater.

Table 1: AZOPT

Adverse Events

	AZOPT 1% N=1173 % Incidence	Placebo N=101 % Incidence
Ocular		
Blurred Vision	5.0	2.0
Discomfort	2.6	3.0
Foreign Body sensation	1.8	0
Dry Eye	1.2	1.0
Hyperemia	1.1	1.0
Pain	1.0	1.0
Nonocular		
Body as a Whole		
Headache	1.5	1.0
Special Senses		
Taste Perversion	5.6	1.0

The following ocular-related adverse reactions to brinzolamide 1% suspension were reported at an incidence below 1%: pruritus, discharge, keratitis, blepharitis, tearing, conjunctivitis, lid margin crusting, sticky sensation, abnormal vision and eye fatigue.

The following nonocular related adverse reactions to brinzolamide 1% suspension were reported at an incidence below 1%: dry mouth, nausea, dyspepsia, depression, dizziness, paresthesia, rhinitis, pharyngitis, bronchitis, dyspnea, dermatitis and alopecia.

OVERDOSE:

Symptoms: Although no human data are available, electrolyte imbalance, development of an acidotic state, and possible nervous system effects may occur. Serum electrolyte levels (particularly potassium) and blood pH levels should be monitored. The oral LD_{50} of brinzolamide in rats was found to be between 1000 to 2000 mg/kg.

Treatment: The treatment should be symptomatic and supportive.

For management of a suspected drug overdose, CPhA recommends that you contact your **regional Poison Control Centre**. See the *CPS* Directory section for a list of Poison Control Centres.

DOSAGE: Shake well before use.

When used as a monotherapy, the recommended starting dose is 1 drop in the affected eye(s) 2 times daily. If the clinical response is not adequate after 4 weeks, the dosage may be increased to 1 drop 3 times daily.

Brinzolamide suspension may be used as adjunctive therapy with ophthalmic β-blockers.

When brinzolamide is used concomitantly with β-blockers, the recommended dosage is the same as when it is used as a monotherapy. The drugs should be administered at least 10 minutes apart.

INFORMATION FOR THE PATIENT: Published in e-CPS, available by subscription at www.e-cps.ca.

SUPPLIED: Each mL of sterile, aqueous suspension, formulated to be readily suspended and slow settling following shaking, contains: brinzolamide 10 mg. The pH has been adjusted to pH 7.5 (pH range 6.5 to 8.5) to match the physiologic pH of tears and the product has also been formulated to be iso-osmotic to optimize ocular comfort upon instillation. Nonmedicinal ingredients: carbomer 974P, edetate disodium, hydrochloric acid and/or sodium hydroxide (to adjust pH), mannitol, purified water, sodium chloride and tyloxapol. Benzalkonium chloride 0.01% is added as a preservative. Natural, plastic Drop-Tainer dispensers with a controlled dispensing-tip 5 mL. Store at 4 to 30°C. Shake well before use.

B

B

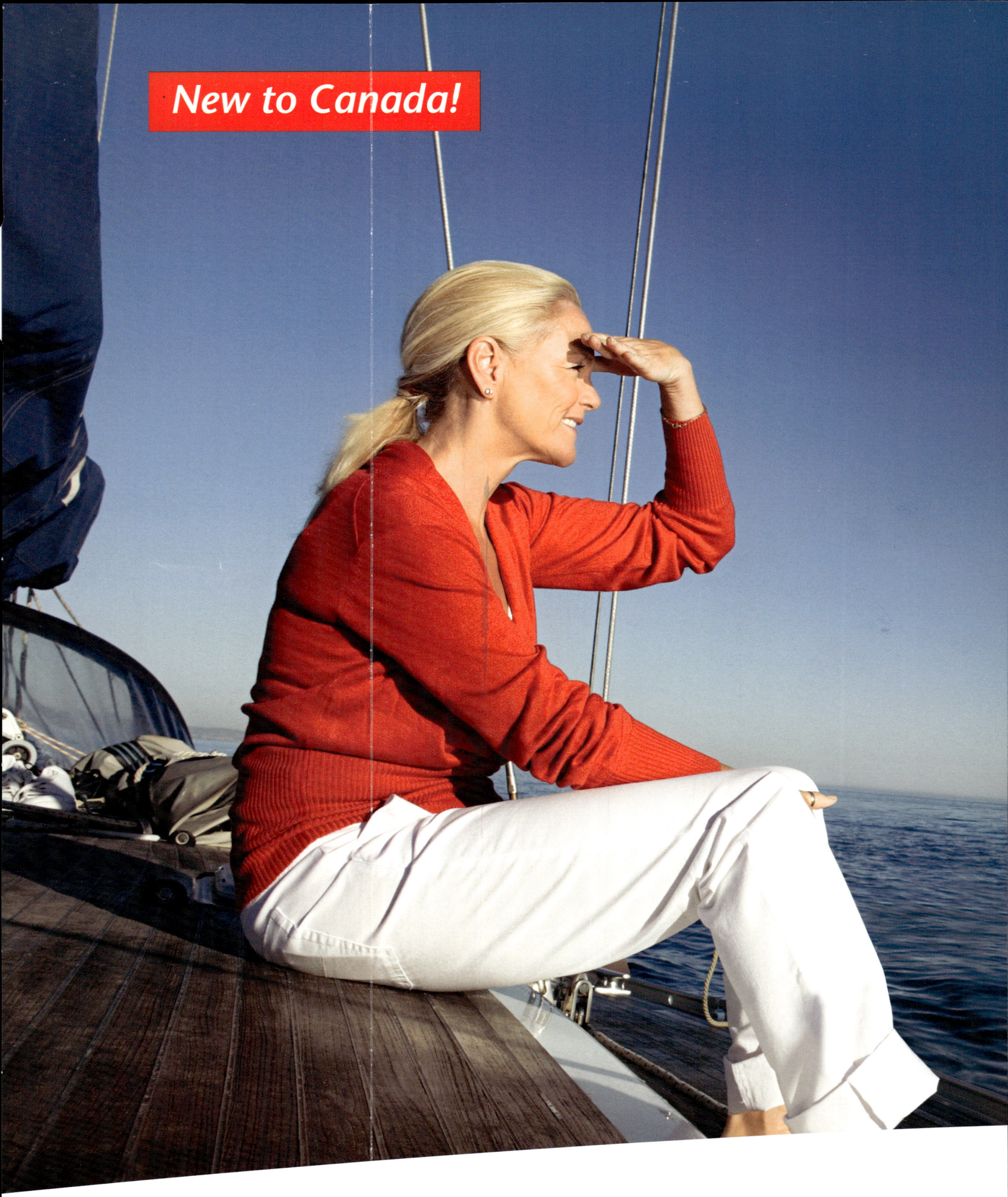

Help patients improve glycemic control with the efficacy of Onglyza

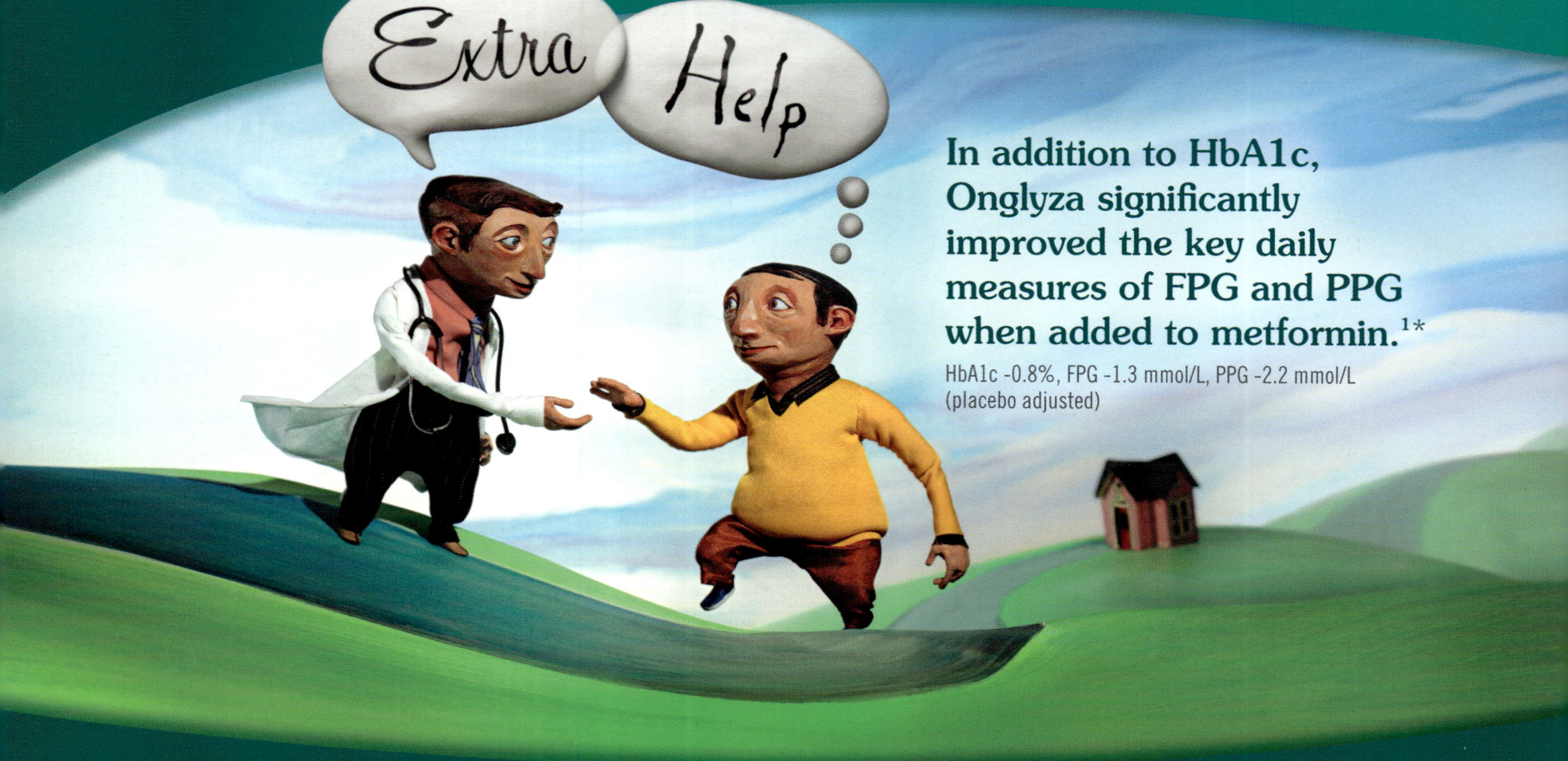

In addition to HbA1c, Onglyza significantly improved the key daily measures of FPG and PPG when added to metformin.[1*]

HbA1c -0.8%, FPG -1.3 mmol/L, PPG -2.2 mmol/L (placebo adjusted)

Add Onglyza for patients with type 2 diabetes when their HbA1c is above 7.0% on metformin alone

Onglyza is indicated in patients with type 2 diabetes mellitus to improve glycemic control in combination with metformin or a sulfonylurea, when metformin or the sulfonylurea used alone, with diet and exercise, does not provide adequate glycemic control.[1]

Onglyza is not recommended for the following: patients with moderate-to-severe renal impairment, including patients with end-stage renal disease requiring hemodialysis, patients with moderate-to-severe hepatic impairment, patients with congestive heart failure, or pregnant women. Onglyza should not be used by women who are nursing, pediatric patients (<18 years of age), patients with type 1 diabetes or for the treatment of diabetic ketoacidosis.[1]

Onglyza is contraindicated in patients who have had a history of any serious hypersensitivity to this drug or any ingredient in the formulation or to another DPP-4 inhibitor.[1]

In a clinical study that combined Onglyza with metformin, the most commonly reported adverse events, regardless of causality and more common with Onglyza than placebo, were nasopharyngitis (11.0% vs. 10.6%) and bronchitis (9.4% vs. 6.1%).[1]

In a clinical study that combined Onglyza with a sulfonylurea (glyburide), the most commonly reported adverse events, regardless of causality and more common with Onglyza than placebo, were hypoglycemia (19.8% vs. 18.4%) and urinary tract infection (13.8% vs. 10.9%).[1]

Please consult prescribing information for warnings, precautions and adverse events.

Reference: 1. AstraZeneca Canada Inc./Bristol-Myers Squibb Canada. Onglyza® Product Monograph, September 14, 2009.

* Randomized, double-blind placebo-controlled study of 24-week duration. Evaluated efficacy and safety of Onglyza in combination with metformin in patients with inadequate glycemic control (HbA1c ≥7.0% and ≤10.0%) on metformin alone. Placebo mean baseline HbA1c: 8.1%. Patients were required to be on a stable dose of metformin (1500–2550 mg daily) for at least 8 weeks to be enrolled in trial. Results demonstrated at trial's end were the following (placebo adjusted): -0.8% improvement in HbA1c, -1.3 mmol/L improvement in FPG and -2.2 mmol/L improvement in 2-hour PPG. Change in FPG and PPG from baseline was measured at 6 months. Onglyza baseline FPG was 9.9 mmol/L (n=187) and baseline PPG was 16.4 mmol/L (n=155). Placebo baseline FPG was 9.7 mmol/L (n=176) and baseline PPG was 16.4 mmol/L (n=135). P-values were p<0.0001 for HbA1c, FPG and 2-hour PPG when compared to placebo.

Bristol-Myers Squibb

PAAB 12/11

AstraZeneca

ONG073E

Member R&D

Pr onglyza®

(saxagliptin) 5 mg tablets

B

BaciJect
bacitracin
Antibiotic

SteriMax

SUPPLIED: Each vial of sterile, lyophilized powder for injection contains: bacitracin USP equivalent to 50 000 units. Reconstituted solution provides bacitracin equivalent to 5000 units per mL. Store BaciJect sterile dry powder in a refrigerator (2-8°C). Vials of 30 mL with latex free stoppers, cartons of 10.

Bacitracin
bacitracin
Antibiotic

Pfizer

PHARMACOLOGY: Bacitracin, an antibiotic substance derived from cultures of *B. subtilis* (Tracey), exerts pronounced antibacterial action in vitro against a variety of gram-positive and a few gram-negative organisms.

However, among systemic diseases, only staphylococcal infections qualify for consideration of bacitracin therapy. Bacitracin is assayed against a standard and its activity is expressed in units, 1 mg having a potency of not less than 50 units.

Susceptibility Plate Testing: If the Kirby-Bauer method of disc susceptibility is used, a 10-unit bacitracin disc should give a zone over 13 mm when tested against a bacitracin-susceptible strain of *S. aureus*. Absorption of bacitracin following i.m. injection is rapid and complete. A dose of 200 or 300 units/kg every 6 hours gives serum levels of 0.2 to 2 µg/mL in individuals with normal renal function. The drug is excreted slowly by glomerular filtration. It is widely distributed in all body organs and is demonstrable in ascitic and pleural fluids after i.m. injection.

INDICATIONS: The use of i.m. bacitracin is indicated in the treatment of infants with pneumonia and empyema caused by staphylococci shown to be susceptible to the drug.

Bacitracin solutions, applied locally in the form of compresses or instillations, may be used once or twice daily in secondarily infected wounds, ulcers, pyodermas and other superficial skin infections and in superficial infections of the eye caused by bacitracin-susceptible organisms. Bacitracin solutions may be instilled into the nasal cavities or administered by inhalation as an aerosol in the treatment of bacitracin-susceptible infections of the upper and lower respiratory tract. In severe or extensive infections, appropriate antibacterial therapy should be given in addition to local treatment with bacitracin.

CONTRAINDICATIONS: In those individuals with a history of previous hypersensitivity or toxic reaction to it.

WARNINGS: I.M.: Nephrotoxicity: Bacitracin in parenteral (i.m.) therapy may cause renal failure due to tubular and glomerular necrosis. Its use should be restricted to infants with staphylococcal pneumonia and empyema when due to organisms shown to be susceptible to bacitracin. It should be used only where adequate laboratory facilities are available and when constant supervision of the patient is possible.

Renal function should be carefully determined prior to and daily during therapy. The recommended daily dose should not be exceeded, and fluid intake and urinary output maintained at proper levels to avoid kidney toxicity. If renal toxicity occurs the drug should be discontinued. The concurrent use of other nephrotoxic drugs, particularly streptomycin, kanamycin, polymyxin B, polymyxin E (colistin), neomycin, and viomycin, should be avoided.

PRECAUTIONS: See Warnings for precautions in regard to kidney toxicity associated with i.m. use of bacitracin.

Adequate fluid intake should be maintained orally or, if necessary, by parenteral method.

As with other antibiotics, use of this drug may result in overgrowth of nonsusceptible organisms, including fungi. If superinfection occurs, appropriate therapy should be instituted.

ADVERSE EFFECTS: Nephrotoxic: albuminuria, cylindruria, azotemia, rising blood levels without any increase in dosage. Others: nausea and vomiting. Pain at site of injection. Skin rashes.

OVERDOSE:
No data supplied by the manufacturer.

> For management of a suspected drug overdose, CPhA recommends that you contact your **regional Poison Control Centre**. See the *CPS* Directory section for a list of Poison Control Centres.

DOSAGE: **To be administered i.m.**
Infants: For infants under 2500 g: 900 units/kg/24 hours in 2 or 3 divided doses. For infants over 2500 g: 1000 units/kg/24 hours in 2 or 3 divided doses. I.M. injections of the solution should be given in the upper outer quadrant of the buttocks, alternating right and left, and avoiding multiple injections in the same region because of the transient pain following injection.

Preparation of Solutions: Should be dissolved in sodium chloride injection containing 2% procaine HCl. The concentration of the antibiotic in the solution should not be less than 5000 units/mL nor more than 10 000 units/mL.

Diluents containing parabens should not be used to reconstitute bacitracin; cloudy solutions and precipitate formation have occurred. Reconstitution of the 50 000 unit vial with 9.8 mL of diluent will result in a concentration of 5000 units/mL.

To be administered topically.
Preparation of Solution: Solutions for topical application are prepared by dissolving bacitracin in Sterile Water for Injection or Sodium Chloride Injection in amounts to give the following concentrations: skin, 500 units/mL; ophthalmic solutions, 500 to 1000 units/mL; intranasal therapy, 250 units/mL; aerosol, 500 to 1000 units/mL.

SUPPLIED: Each vial contains: bacitracin 50 000 units. Cartons of 5. Store unreconstituted bacitracin in a refrigerator 2 to 8°C. Solutions are rapidly inactivated at room temperature but are stable for 1 week when stored in a refrigerator 2 to 8°C.

Bactine®
benzalkonium chloride—lidocaine HCl
Antiseptic—Anesthetic

Bayer Consumer Care

SUPPLIED: Each mL contains: benzalkonium chloride 0.13% w/w and lidocaine hydrochloride 2.5% w/w. Nonmedicinal ingredients: camphor, clove oil, edetate disodium, eucalyptus oil, marjoram oil, menthol, nonoxynol 9 and propylene glycol. Bottles of 120 mL. Pump spray bottles of 105 mL.

Bactroban® Ointment
mupirocin
Topical Antibiotic

GlaxoSmithKline

PHARMACOLOGY: Mupirocin exerts a bactericidal action against sensitive organisms by inhibiting bacterial protein synthesis. It reversibly and specifically binds to bacterial isoleucyl transfer-RNA synthetase.

INDICATIONS: For the topical treatment of the following, when caused by sensitive strains of staphylococcus and streptococcus species: impetigo, superficially infected dermatoses, lesions which are moist and weeping.

For abrasions, minor cuts and wounds, the use of mupirocin may prevent the development of infections by sensitive Gram-positive organisms.

No cross-resistance has been shown between mupirocin and other commonly used antibiotics.

CONTRAINDICATIONS: In patients with hypersensitivity to mupirocin or to other ointments containing polyethylene glycols.

WARNINGS: This mupirocin ointment formulation is not suitable for ophthalmic or intranasal use, or in conjunction with cannulae.

When mupirocin ointment is used on the face, care should be taken to avoid the eyes.

Polyethylene glycol (PEG) can be absorbed from open wounds and damaged skin. It is excreted by the kidneys. As with other PEG-based ointments, mupirocin ointment should not be used in conditions where absorption of large quantities of PEG is possible, especially if there is evidence of moderate or severe renal impairment.

In the rare event of a possible sensitization reaction or severe local irritation occurring with the use of mupirocin, treatment should be discontinued and appropriate alternative therapy for the infection instituted.

PRECAUTIONS: Use of topical antibiotics occasionally allows overgrowth of nonsusceptible organisms. If this occurs, or irritation or sensitization develop, treatment should be discontinued and appropriate therapy instituted.

Pregnancy: The safety of mupirocin ointment in the treatment of infections during pregnancy has not been established. If administration to pregnant patients is considered necessary, its potential benefits should be weighed against the possible hazards to the fetus.

Lactation: Caution should be exercised when mupirocin ointment is administered to nursing mothers. If a cracked nipple is to be treated, lactation from the affected breast should be maintained by manual expression until the end of treatment. During this time, milk from the affected breast should be discarded.

ADVERSE EFFECTS: The following local adverse reactions have been reported during therapy with mupirocin: itching, burning, erythema, stinging and dryness. It was not usually necessary to discontinue therapy due to these adverse reactions. Systemic allergic reactions have been reported with mupirocin ointment. Cutaneous sensitization reactions to mupirocin or the ointment base have been reported rarely.

OVERDOSE:
Overdosage has not been known to occur during topical therapy with mupirocin ointment.

> For management of a suspected drug overdose, CPhA recommends that you contact your **regional Poison Control Centre**. See the *CPS* Directory section for a list of Poison Control Centres.

DOSAGE: A small amount of the ointment should be applied to the affected area 3 times daily for up to 10 days, depending on the response. The area treated may be covered with a gauze dressing if desired.

SUPPLIED: Each g of ointment contains: mupirocin 20 mg (2%) in a bland water-soluble ointment base consisting of polyethylene glycol 400 and polyethylene glycol 3350 (polyethylene glycol ointment, USP). Tubes of 15 and 30 g. Store at room temperature.

Balminil Cough & Flu
dextromethorphan HBr—pseudoephedrine HCl—guaifenesin—acetaminophen
Antitussive—Decongestant—Expectorant—Analgesic—Antipyretic

Rougier Pharma

Balminil DM
dextromethorphan HBr
Antitussive

Rougier Pharma

Balminil DM Children
dextromethorphan HBr
Antitussive

Rougier Pharma

Balminil DM+Decongestant
dextromethorphan HBr—pseudoephedrine HCl
Antitussive—Decongestant

Rougier Pharma

Balminil DM+Decongestant+Expectorant
dextromethorphan HBr—pseudoephedrine HCl—guaifenesin
Antitussive—Decongestant—Expectorant

Rougier Pharma

Balminil DM+Expectorant
dextromethorphan HBr—guaifenesin
Antitussive—Expectorant

Rougier Pharma

Balminil Expectorant
guaifenesin
Expectorant

Rougier Pharma

Balminil Night-Time

dextromethorphan HBr—diphenhydramine HCl—ammonium chloride

Antitussive—Antihistamine—Expectorant

Rougier Pharma

SUPPLIED: Balminil Cough & Flu: Each 15 mL of clear, dark red, blackberry-flavored syrup contains: dextromethorphan HBr 15 mg, pseudoephedrine HCl 30 mg, guaifenesin 100 mg and acetaminophen 325 mg. Nonmedicinal ingredients: artificial coloring and flavoring, benzoic acid, caramel, citric acid, maltitol, polyethylene glycol, propylene glycol, purified water, sodium benzoate, sodium citrate and sodium cyclamate. Energy: 16.2 kcal/15 mL. Alcohol-, bisulfite-, gluten-, lactose-, parabens- and tartrazine-free. Bottles of 250 mL. Store between 15 and 30°C. Protect from freezing.

Balminil DM: Sucrose-free: Each 5 mL of orange, melon-flavored syrup contains: dextromethorphan HBr 15 mg. Nonmedicinal ingredients: artificial flavoring, citric acid, FD&C yellow #6, potassium sorbate, propylene glycol, purified water, sodium benzoate and sorbitol. Energy: 29.8 kJ (7 kcal)/5 mL. Alcohol-, gluten-, lactose-, parabens-, sucrose-, sulfite- and tartrazine-free. Bottles of 100 mL, 250 mL and 2 L. Store between 15 and 30°C. Protect from freezing.

Syrup: Each 5 mL of clear reddish-pink, cherry-flavored syrup contains: dextromethorphan HBr 15 mg. Nonmedicinal ingredients: artificial coloring and flavoring, citric acid, potassium sorbate, propylene glycol, purified water, sodium benzoate and sucrose. Energy: 51 kJ (12 kcal)/5 mL. Alcohol-, gluten-, lactose-, parabens-, sulfite- and tartrazine-free. Bottles of 100 mL and 250 mL. Store between 15 and 30°C. Protect from freezing.

Balminil DM Children: Sucrose-free: Each 5 mL of purple, grape-flavored syrup contains: dextromethorphan HBr 7.5 mg. Nonmedicinal ingredients: artificial coloring and flavoring, citric acid, FD&C blue #1, potassium sorbate, propylene glycol, purified water, sodium benzoate, sodium saccharin and sorbitol. Energy: 29.8 kJ (7 kcal)/5 mL. Alcohol-, gluten- lactose-, parabens-, sucrose-, sulfite- and tartrazine-free. Amber plastic bottles of 100 mL. Store between 15 and 30°C. Protect from freezing.

Balminil DM+Decongestant: Each 5 mL of reddish-pink colored syrup contains: dextromethorphan HBr 15 mg and pseudoephedrine HCl 30 mg. Nonmedicinal ingredients: artificial coloring and flavorings, citric acid, FD&C blue #1, potassium sorbate, propylene glycol, purified water, sodium benzoate, sorbitol and sucrose. Energy: 40 kJ (9.4 kcal)/5 mL. Alcohol-, gluten-, parabens-, sulfite- and tartrazine-free. Bottles of 100 and 250 mL. Store between 15 and 30°C. Protect from freezing.

Balminil DM+Decongestant+Expectorant: Extra-Strength: Each 5 mL of reddish-pink, minty-raspberry and menthol flavored syrup contains: dextromethorphan HBr 15 mg, pseudoephedrine HCl 30 mg and guaifenesin 200 mg. Nonmedicinal ingredients: artificial flavorings, citric acid, D&C red #33, FD&C red #40, glycerin, menthol, polyethylene glycol, propylene glycol, purified water, sodium benzoate, sodium carboxymethylcellulose, sodium citrate and sodium saccharin. Energy: 29.75 kJ (7 kcal)/5 mL. Alcohol-, gluten-, parabens-, sulfite- and tartrazine-free. Bottles of 100 and 250 mL. Store between 15 and 30°C. Protect from freezing.

Regular: Each 5 mL of reddish-pink, minty-raspberry and menthol flavored syrup contains: dextromethorphan HBr 15 mg, pseudoephedrine HCl 30 mg and guaifenesin 100 mg. Nonmedicinal ingredients: artificial flavorings, citric acid, D&C red #33, FD&C red #40, glycerin, menthol, polyethylene glycol, propylene glycol, purified water, sodium benzoate, sodium carboxymethylcellulose, sodium citrate and sodium saccharin. Energy: 29.75 kJ (7 kcal)/5 mL. Alcohol-, gluten-, parabens-, sucrose-, sulfite- and tartrazine-free. Bottles of 100 and 250 mL. Store between 15 and 30°C. Protect from freezing.

Balminil DM+Expectorant: Extra-Strength: Each 5 mL of reddish-pink, minty-grape and menthol flavored syrup contains: dextromethorphan HBr 15 mg and guaifenesin 200 mg. Nonmedicinal ingredients: artificial flavorings, citric acid, D&C red #33, FD&C red #40, glycerin, menthol, polyethylene glycol, propylene glycol, purified water, sodium benzoate, sodium carboxymethylcellulose, sodium citrate and sodium saccharin. Energy: 29.75 kJ (7 kcal)/5 mL. Alcohol-, gluten-, parabens-, sucrose-, sulfite- and tartrazine-free. Bottles of 100 and 250 mL. Store between 15 and 30°C. Protect from freezing.

Regular Strength: Each 5 mL of reddish-pink, wild-cherry- and menthol-flavored syrup contains: dextromethorphan HBr 15 mg and guaifenesin 100 mg. Nonmedicinal ingredients: artificial flavorings, citric acid, D&C red #33, FD&C red #40, menthol, potassium sorbate, propylene glycol, purified water, sodium benzoate, sodium carboxymethylcellulose, sodium saccharin and sorbitol. Energy: 27.6 kJ (6.5 kcal)/5 mL. Alcohol-, gluten-, parabens-, sucrose-, sulfite- and tartrazine-free. Bottles of 100 and 250 mL. Store between 15 and 30°C. Protect from freezing.

Balminil Expectorant: Sucrose-free: Each 5 mL of pink-reddish, wild-cherry-citrus-flavored syrup contains: guaifenesin 100 mg. Nonmedicinal ingredients: artificial coloring and flavoring, citric acid, D&C yellow #10, potassium sorbate, propylene glycol, purified water, sodium benzoate and sorbitol. Energy: 34.5 kJ (8.1 kcal)/5 mL. Alcohol-, gluten-, parabens-, sucrose-, sulfite- and tartrazine-free. Bottles of 100 mL, 250 mL and 2 L. Store between 15 and 30°C. Protect from freezing.

Syrup: Each 5 mL of pink-reddish, menthol-flavored syrup contains: guaifenesin 100 mg. Nonmedicinal ingredients: artificial coloring and flavoring, citric acid, FD&C yellow #6, menthol, potassium sorbate, propylene glycol, purified water, sodium benzoate and sucrose. Energy: 34.0 kJ (8.0 kcal)/5 mL. Alcohol-, gluten-, parabens-, sulfite- and tartrazine-free. Bottles of 100 mL and 250 mL. Store between 15 and 30°C. Protect from freezing.

Balminil Night-Time: Each 5 mL of clear reddish-pink, raspberry- and menthol-flavored syrup contains: dextromethorphan HBr 15 mg, diphenhydramine HCl 12.5 mg and ammonium chloride 125 mg. Nonmedicinal ingredients: alcohol, artificial coloring and flavoring, glycerin, menthol, methylparaben, propylparaben, purified water, simethicone, sorbitol and sucrose. Energy: 17.3 kcal/5 mL. Gluten-, sulfite- and tartrazine-free. Bottles of 250 mL. Store between 15 and 30°C. Protect from freezing.

Balminil Nasal Decongestant

xylometazoline HCl

Nasal Decongestant

Rougier Pharma

SUPPLIED: Each bottle contains: xylometazoline HCl 0.1%. Nonmedicinal ingredients: benzalkonium chloride, dibasic potassium phosphate, EDTA disodium, monobasic sodium phosphate, potassium chloride, purified water and sodium chloride. Plastic squeeze bottles of 20 mL. Keep this product and all medicine out of the reach of children. Protect from heat.

Baraclude™ Ⓟ

entecavir

Antiviral Agent

Bristol-Myers Squibb

Date of Preparation: June 16, 2006
Date of Revision: July 30, 2009

SUMMARY PRODUCT INFORMATION:

Route of Administration	Dosage Form/ Strength	Clinically Relevant Nonmedicinal Ingredients
Oral	Tablet 0.5 mg	Lactose monohydrate For a complete listing, see Dosage Forms, Composition and Packaging.
	Solution 0.05 mg/mL	Maltitol For a complete listing, see Dosage Forms, Composition and Packaging.

INDICATIONS AND CLINICAL USE: BARACLUDE (entecavir) is indicated for the treatment of chronic hepatitis B virus infection in adults with evidence of active viral replication and either evidence of persistent elevations in serum aminotransferases (ALT or AST) or histologically active disease.

This indication is based on efficacy and safety data in nucleoside-treatment-naive and in lamivudine-refractory adult patients with HBeAg-positive or HBeAg-negative chronic HBV infection with compensated liver disease and on more limited data in adult patients with HIV/HBV co-infection who have received prior lamivudine therapy.

CONTRAINDICATIONS: BARACLUDE is contraindicated in patients with previously demonstrated hypersensitivity to entecavir or any component of the product. (For a complete listing, see Dosage Forms, Composition and Packaging.)

WARNINGS AND PRECAUTIONS:

Serious Warnings and Precautions

Severe acute exacerbations of hepatitis B have been reported in patients who have discontinued anti-hepatitis B therapy, including entecavir. Hepatic function should be monitored closely with both clinical and laboratory follow-up for at least several months in patients who discontinue anti-hepatitis B therapy. If appropriate, re-initiation of anti-hepatitis B therapy may be warranted (see Adverse Reactions, Exacerbations of Hepatitis After Discontinuation of Treatment).

Lactic acidosis and severe hepatomegaly with steatosis, including fatal cases, have been reported with the use of nucleoside analogues alone or in combination with antiretrovirals.

Limited clinical experience suggests there is a potential for the development of resistance to HIV (human immunodeficiency virus) nucleoside reverse transcriptase inhibitors if BARACLUDE is used to treat chronic hepatitis B virus infection in patients with HIV infection that is not being treated. Therapy with BARACLUDE is not recommended for HIV/HBV co-infected patients who are not also receiving highly active antiretroviral therapy (HAART) (see Warnings and Precautions, Special Populations, Patients Co-Infected with HIV and HBV).

General: BARACLUDE tablets contain lactose and are not recommended for patients with rare hereditary problems of galactose intolerance, the Lapp lactase deficiency or glucose-galactose malabsorption. BARACLUDE Oral Solution is lactose-free and available as an alternative (see Dosage Forms, Composition and Packaging).

Carcinogenesis and Mutagenesis: Positive carcinogenic results were found in two-year carcinogenicity studies with entecavir conducted in mice and rats. In male mice, increases in the incidences of lung adenomas were observed at exposures ≥3 times the exposure in humans at 1 mg and lung carcinomas were observed in male and female mice at approximately 40 times the exposure in humans at 1 mg. Tumor development was preceded by pneumocyte proliferation in the lung, which was not observed in rats, dogs, or monkeys administered entecavir, indicating that a key event in lung tumor development observed in mice likely was species specific. Drug-related increased incidences of other types of tumors were seen at the highest entecavir exposures [in mice approximately 40 times and in rats 35 times (males) and 24 times (females) human exposure at 1 mg], including liver carcinomas in male mice, benign vascular tumors in female mice, brain microglial tumors in male and female rats, and liver adenomas and carcinomas in female rats. Skin fibromas were observed in female rats at both the high (0.4 mg/kg/day; equivalent to 4 times the exposure in humans at 1 mg) and highest (2.6 mg/kg/day; equivalent to 24 times the exposure in humans at 1 mg) doses.

It is not known how predictive the results of rodent carcinogenicity studies may be for humans.

Entecavir was clastogenic to human lymphocyte cultures and in mouse lymphoma cells in vitro. Entecavir was not mutagenic in the Ames bacterial reverse mutation assay, a mammalian-cell gene mutation assay, and a transformation assay with Syrian hamster embryo cells. Entecavir was also negative in an oral micronucleus study and an oral DNA repair study in rats. In reproductive toxicology studies in which rats were administered entecavir at up to 30 mg/kg for up to 4 weeks, no evidence of impaired fertility was seen in males or females at systemic exposures >90 times those in humans at 1 mg. In rodent and dog toxicology studies, seminiferous tubular degeneration was observed at ≥35 times the exposure in humans at 1 mg. No testicular changes were evident in monkeys administered entecavir for 1 year at 167 times the exposure in humans at 1 mg.

Liver Transplant Recipients: The safety and efficacy of BARACLUDE in liver transplant recipients are unknown. The potential for pharmacokinetic interaction between entecavir and the immunosuppressants cyclosporine A or tacrolimus was not formally evaluated. If BARACLUDE treatment is determined to be necessary for a liver transplant recipient who has received or is receiving cyclosporine or tacrolimus, renal function must be carefully monitored both before and during treatment with BARACLUDE (see Action and Clinical Pharmacology, Special Populations and Conditions and Dosage and Administration, Renal Impairment).

Renal Impairment: BARACLUDE is predominantly eliminated by the kidney. Dosage adjustment of BARACLUDE is recommended for patients with a creatinine clearance <50 mL/min, including patients on hemodialysis or CAPD [continuous ambulatory peritoneal dialysis] (see Dosage and Administration, Renal Impairment).

Special Populations: Patients Co-Infected with HIV and HBV: BARACLUDE has not been evaluated in patients who are co-infected with HIV and HBV and are not concurrently receiving effective HIV treatment. Limited clinical experience suggests there is a potential for the development of resistance to HIV nucleoside reverse transcriptase inhibitors if BARACLUDE is used to treat chronic hepatitis B virus infection in patients with HIV infection that is not being treated. Therefore therapy with BARACLUDE is not recommended for HIV/HBV co-infected patients who are not also receiving highly active antiretroviral therapy (HAART). BARACLUDE has not been studied as a treatment for HIV infection and is not recommended for this use (see Action and Clinical Pharmacology, Special Populations and Conditions, Patients Co-Infected with HIV and HBV).

Before initiating BARACLUDE therapy, HIV antibody testing should be offered to all patients.

Pregnant Women: There are no adequate and well-controlled studies in pregnant women. BARACLUDE should be used during pregnancy only if the potential benefit justifies the potential risk to the fetus.

Entecavir caused effects on embryo-fetal development in rats at doses that also produced maternal toxicity; at these doses, exposures to entecavir were 180 times those in humans at 1 mg. In rabbits, embryo-fetal toxicity was observed at exposures to entecavir 883 times those in humans at 1 mg. There were no adverse effects on growth, development, and reproductive performance in the progeny of rats administered entecavir at doses associated with exposures to entecavir >94 times those in humans at 1 mg.

Pregnancy Registry: To monitor maternal-fetal outcomes of pregnant women exposed to BARACLUDE a Pregnancy Registry has been established. To register patients, physicians must obtain prior consent. Physicians can register patients by calling 1-800-258-4263.

Labor and Delivery: There are no studies in pregnant women and no data on the effect of BARACLUDE on transmission of HBV from mother to infant. Therefore, appropriate interventions should be used to prevent neonatal acquisition of HBV.

Nursing Women: Entecavir is excreted in the milk of rats. It is not known whether this drug is excreted in human milk. Mothers should be instructed not to breast-feed if they are taking BARACLUDE.

Pediatrics (<16 years of age): Safety and effectiveness of BARACLUDE in pediatric patients below the age of 16 years have not been established.

Geriatrics (>65 years of age): Clinical studies of BARACLUDE did not include sufficient numbers of subjects aged 65 years and over to determine whether they respond differently from younger subjects. Entecavir is substantially excreted by the kidney, and the risk of toxic reactions to this drug may be greater in patients with impaired renal function. Because elderly patients are more likely to have decreased renal function, care should be taken in dose selection, and it may be useful to monitor renal function (see Dosage and Administration, Renal Impairment).

Use in Racial/Ethnic Groups: Clinical studies of BARACLUDE did not include sufficient numbers of subjects from some racial/ethnic minorities (black/African American, Hispanic) to determine whether they respond differently to treatment with the drug. There are no significant racial differences in entecavir pharmacokinetics.

ADVERSE REACTIONS: Adverse Drug Reaction Overview: Assessment of adverse reactions is based on four pivotal studies (AI463014, AI463022, AI463026, and AI463027) in which 1720 patients with chronic hepatitis B infection received double-blind treatment with BARACLUDE 0.5 mg/day (n=679), BARACLUDE 1 mg/day (n=183), or lamivudine (n=858) for up to two years (Studies AI463022, AI463027 for nucleoside-naïve patients and studies AI463014, AI463026 for lamivudine-refractory patients). The safety profiles of BARACLUDE and lamivudine were comparable in these studies.

The safety profile of BARACLUDE 1 mg (n=51) in HIV/HBV co-infected patients enrolled in Study AI463038 was similar to that of placebo (n=17) through 24 weeks of blinded treatment and similar to that seen in non-HIV infected patients (see Warnings and Precautions, Special Populations, Patients Co-Infected with HIV and HBV).

The most common (≥3%) adverse events of any severity with at least a possible relation to study drug for BARACLUDE-treated patients were headache, fatigue, dizziness, and nausea. The most common adverse events among lamivudine-treated patients were headache, fatigue, and dizziness. One percent of BARACLUDE-treated patients in these four studies compared with 4% of lamivudine-treated patients discontinued for adverse events or abnormal laboratory test results.

Clinical Trial Adverse Drug Reactions: Because clinical trials are conducted under very specific conditions the adverse reaction rates observed in the clinical trials may not reflect the rates observed in practice and should not be compared to the rates in the clinical trials of another drug. Adverse drug reaction information from clinical trials is useful for identifying drug-related adverse events and for approximating rates.

Clinical adverse reactions occurring in ≥3% of BARACLUDE-treated patients during therapy in four clinical studies in which BARACLUDE was compared with lamivudine, in addition to selected clinical adverse reactions that occurred in <3% of patients are presented in Table 1.

Table 1: BARACLUDE

Clinical Adverse Reactions Reported in ≥3% of BARACLUDE-treated Patients, Plus Selected Clinical Adverse Reactions in Four BARACLUDE Clinical Trials—Through 2 Years of Treatment

	Nucleoside-Naive[b]		Lamivudine-Refractory[c]	
Body System/ Adverse Event[a]	**BARACLUDE 0.5 mg n=679 %**	**Lamivudine 100 mg n=668 %**	**BARACLUDE 1 mg n=183 %**	**Lamivudine 100 mg n=190 %**
Gastrointestinal				
Nausea	3	2	4	3
Abdominal pain upper	3	2	2	5
Dyspepsia	2	2	3	<1
Diarrhea	1	<1	2	1
Vomiting	1	<1	1	<1
General				
Fatigue	5	5	9	6
Nervous System				
Headache	8	8	10	7
Dizziness	4	3	5	2
Somnolence	1	1	2	1
Psychiatric				
Insomnia	2	1	1	<1

[a] Includes events of possible, probable, certain, or unknown relationship to treatment regimen.
[b] Studies AI463022 and AI463027. Mean duration of therapy was 69 weeks for BARACLUDE-treated and 63 weeks for lamivudine-treated patients.
[c] Includes Study AI463026 and the BARACLUDE 1 mg and lamivudine treatment arms of Study AI463014, a Phase 2 multinational, randomized, double-blind study of three doses of BARACLUDE (0.1, 0.5, and 1 mg) once daily versus continued lamivudine 100 mg once daily for up to 52 weeks in patients who experienced recurrent viremia on lamivudine therapy. Mean duration of therapy was 73 weeks for BARACLUDE-treated and 51 weeks for lamivudine-treated patients.

Exacerbations of Hepatitis After Discontinuation of Treatment: In the Phase 3 studies, a subset of patients was allowed to discontinue treatment at or after 52 weeks if they achieved a protocol-defined response to therapy. An exacerbation of hepatitis or ALT flare was defined as ALT >10×ULN and >2× the patient's reference level (minimum of the baseline or last measurement at end of dosing). As demonstrated in Table 2, a proportion of patients experienced post-treatment ALT flares. If BARACLUDE is discontinued without regard to treatment response, the rate of post-treatment flares could be higher.

Table 2: BARACLUDE

Exacerbations of Hepatitis During Off-Treatment Follow-up, Patients in Studies AI463022, AI463027 and AI463026

	Patients with ALT Elevations >10×ULN and >2×Reference[a]	
	BARACLUDE	**Lamivudine**
Total Nucleoside-Naïve	28/476 (6%)	43/417 (10%)
HBeAg-positive	4/174 (2%)	13/147 (9%)
HBeAg-negative	24/302 (8%)	30/270 (11%)
Lamivudine-Refractory	6/52 (12%)	0/16

[a] Reference is the minimum of the baseline or last measurement at end of dosing. Median time to off-treatment exacerbation was 23 weeks for BARACLUDE-treated patients and 10 weeks for lamivudine-treated patients.

Abnormal Hematologic and Clinical Chemistry Findings: Frequencies of selected treatment-emergent laboratory abnormalities reported during therapy in four clinical trials of BARACLUDE compared with lamivudine are listed in Table 3.

Table 3: BARACLUDE

Selected Treatment-Emergent[a] Laboratory Abnormalities Reported in Four BARACLUDE Clinical Trials—Through 2 Years

	Nucleoside-Naive[b]		Lamivudine-Refractory[c]	
Test	**BARACLUDE 0.5 mg (n=679)**	**Lamivudine 100 mg (n=668)**	**BARACLUDE 1 mg (n=183)**	**Lamivudine 100 mg (n=190)**
ALT >10×ULN and >2× baseline	2%	4%	2%	11%
ALT >5.0×ULN	11%	16%	12%	24%
AST >5.0×ULN	5%	8%	5%	17%
Albumin <2.5 g/dL	<1%	<1%	0%	2%
Total bilirubin >2.5×ULN	2%	2%	3%	2%
Amylase >2.1×ULN	2%	2%	3%	3%
Lipase >2.1×ULN	7%	6%	7%	7%
Creatinine >3.0×ULN	0%	0%	0%	0%
Confirmed creatinine increase ≥44.2 mmol/L	1%	1%	2%	1%
Hyperglycemia fasting >13.8 mmol/L	2%	1%	3%	1%
Glycosuria[d]	4%	3%	4%	6%
Hematuria[e]	9%	10%	9%	6%
Platelets <50 000/mm³	<1%	<1%	<1%	<1%

(cont'd)

Table 3: BARACLUDE *(cont'd)*

Selected Treatment-Emergent[a] Laboratory Abnormalities Reported in Four BARACLUDE Clinical Trials—Through 2 Years

[a] On-treatment value worsened from baseline to Grade 3 or Grade 4 for all parameters except albumin (any on treatment value <2.5 g/dL), confirmed creatinine increase ≥44.2 mmol/L and ALT >10×ULN and >2×baseline.
[b] Studies AI463022 and AI463027. Mean duration of therapy was 69 weeks for BARACLUDE-treated and 63 weeks for lamivudine-treated patients.
[c] Includes Study AI463026 and the BARACLUDE 1 mg and lamivudine treatment arms of Study AI463014, a Phase 2 multinational, randomized, double-blind study of three doses of BARACLUDE (0.1, 0.5, and 1 mg) once daily versus continued lamivudine 100 mg once daily for up to 52 weeks in patients who experienced recurrent viremia on lamivudine therapy. Mean duration of therapy was 73 weeks for BARACLUDE-treated and 51 weeks for lamivudine-treated patients.
[d] Grade 3=3+, large, ≥500 mg/dL; Grade 4=4+, marked, severe.
[e] Grade 3=3+, large, Grade 4=≥4+, marked, severe, many.
Legend: ULN=upper limit of normal.

Among BARACLUDE-treated patients in these studies, on-treatment ALT elevations >10×ULN and >2×baseline generally resolved with continued treatment. A majority of these exacerbations were associated with a ≥2 log_{10}/mL reduction in viral load that preceded or coincided with the ALT elevation. Periodic monitoring of hepatic function is recommended during treatment.

Post-Market Adverse Drug Reactions: The following events have been identified during post-approval use of BARACLUDE. Because reports are voluntary from a population of unknown size, an estimate of frequency cannot be made, as well, the existence of underlying medical conditions confounds the assessment of causality.

Gastrointestinal Disorders: pancreatitis, upper abdominal pain.
Metabolism and Nutrition Disorders: lactose intolerance.
Skin and Subcutaneous Tissue Disorders: alopecia, rash.
Blood and Lymphatic System Disorders: leukopenia, neutropenia, platelet count decreased.
Immune System Disorders: hypersensitivity and drug hypersensitivity including anaphylactoid reaction.

DRUG INTERACTIONS: Overview: Since entecavir is primarily eliminated by the kidneys (see Action and Clinical Pharmacology, Metabolism and Excretion), coadministration of BARACLUDE with drugs that reduce renal function or compete for active tubular secretion may increase serum concentrations of either entecavir or the coadministered drug. In clinical trials, coadministration of BARACLUDE with lamivudine, adefovir dipivoxil, or tenofovir disoproxil fumarate did not result in significant drug interactions. The effects of coadministration of BARACLUDE with other drugs that are renally eliminated or are known to affect renal function have not been evaluated, and patients should be monitored closely for adverse events when BARACLUDE is coadministered with such drugs.

The metabolism of entecavir was evaluated in in vitro and in vivo studies. Entecavir is not a substrate, inhibitor, or inducer of the cytochrome P450 (CYP450) enzyme system. At concentrations up to approximately 10 000-fold higher than those obtained in humans, entecavir inhibited none of the major human CYP450 enzymes 1A2, 2C9, 2C19, 2D6, 3A4, 2B6, and 2E1. At concentrations up to approximately 340-fold higher than those observed in humans, entecavir did not induce the human CYP450 enzymes 1A2, 2C9, 2C19, 3A4, 3A5, and 2B6. (see Action and Clinical Pharmacology, Metabolism and Excretion). The pharmacokinetics of entecavir are unlikely to be affected by coadministration with agents that are either metabolized by, inhibit, or induce the CYP450 system. Likewise, the pharmacokinetics of known CYP substrates are unlikely to be affected by coadministration of BARACLUDE.

Drug-Drug Interactions: In clinical studies, the steady-state pharmacokinetics of BARACLUDE and coadministered drug were not altered in interaction studies of entecavir with lamivudine, adefovir dipivoxil, and tenofovir disoproxil fumarate.

Drug-Food Interactions: Oral administration of 0.5 mg of BARACLUDE with a standard high-fat meal (945 kcal, 54.6 g fat) or a light meal (379 kcal, 8.2 g fat) resulted in a minimal delay in absorption (1.0-1.5 hour fed vs 0.75 hours fasted), a decrease in C_{max} of 44%-46%, and a decrease in AUC of 18%-20%. Therefore, BARACLUDE should be administered on an empty stomach (at least 2 hours after a meal and 2 hours before the next meal).

DOSAGE AND ADMINISTRATION: Recommended Dose and Dosage Adjustment: The usual recommended dose of BARACLUDE for chronic hepatitis B virus infection in adults and adolescents 16 years of age or older is 0.5 mg once daily.

For adults and adolescents 16 years of age or older with a history of hepatitis B viremia while receiving lamivudine or with known lamivudine resistance mutations, the recommended dose of BARACLUDE is 1 mg (two 0.5 mg tablets) once daily.

BARACLUDE should be administered on an empty stomach (at least 2 hours after a meal and 2 hours before the next meal).

BARACLUDE Oral Solution contains 0.05 mg of entecavir per mL. Therefore, 10 mL of the oral solution provides a 0.5-mg dose and 20 mL provides a 1 mg dose of entecavir.

Renal Impairment: In patients with renal impairment, the apparent oral clearance of entecavir decreased as creatinine clearance decreased. Dosage adjustment is recommended for patients with creatinine clearance <50 mL/min, including patients on hemodialysis or CAPD (continuous ambulatory peritoneal dialysis), as shown in Table 4.

Table 4: BARACLUDE

Recommended Dosage of BARACLUDE in Patients with Renal Impairment

Creatinine Clearance (mL/min)	**Usual Dose (0.5 mg)**	**Lamivudine Refractory (1 mg)**
≥50	0.5 mg once daily	1 mg once daily
30 to <50	0.25 mg once daily[a] **or** 0.5 mg every 48 hours	0.5 mg once daily **or** 1 mg every 48 hours
10 to <30	0.15 mg once daily[a] **or** 0.5 mg every 72 hours	0.3 mg once daily[a] **or** 1 mg every 72 hours
<10, Hemodialysis[b] or CAPD	0.05 mg once daily[a] **or** 0.5 mg every 7 days	0.1 mg once daily[a] **or** 1 mg every 7 hours

[a] For doses less than 0.5 mg, BARACLUDE Oral Solution is recommended.
[b] On hemodialysis days, administer after hemodialysis.

Hepatic Impairment: No dosage adjustment is necessary for patients with hepatic impairment.

Duration of Therapy: The optimal duration of treatment with BARACLUDE for patients with chronic hepatitis B infection and the relationship between treatment and long-term outcomes such as cirrhosis and hepatocellular carcinoma are unknown.

OVERDOSAGE:
Activated charcoal may be administered to aid in the removal of unabsorbed drug. General supportive measures are recommended. Healthy subjects who received single entecavir doses up to 40 mg or multiple doses up to 20 mg/day for up to 14 days had no increase in, or unexpected, adverse events. If overdose occurs, the patient must be monitored for evidence of toxicity, and standard supportive treatment applied as necessary.

Following a single 1 mg dose of entecavir, a 4-hour hemodialysis session removed approximately 13% of the entecavir dose.

For management of a suspected drug overdose, contact your **regional Poison Control Centre**. See the *CPS* Directory section for a list of Poison Control Centres.

ACTION AND CLINICAL PHARMACOLOGY: Mechanism of Action: Entecavir is a guanosine nucleoside analogue that is efficiently phosphorylated to the active triphosphate form and exhibits selective activity against HBV polymerase, competes with the natural substrate deoxyguanosine triphosphate, and inhibits all three functional activities of the HBV polymerase (reverse transcriptase, rt): (1) base priming, (2) reverse transcription of the negative strand from the pregenomic messenger RNA, and (3) synthesis of the positive strand of HBV DNA. Entecavir triphosphate has an inhibition constant (Ki) for HBV DNA polymerase of 0.0012 μM and is a weak inhibitor of cellular DNA polymerases α, β, and δ and mitochondrial DNA polymerase γ with Ki values ranging from 18 to >160 μM.

Antiviral Activity: Entecavir inhibited HBV DNA synthesis (50% reduction, EC_{50}) at a concentration of 0.004 μM in human HepG2 cells transfected with wild-type HBV. The median EC_{50} value for entecavir against lamivudine-resistant HBV (rtL180M, rtM204V) was 0.026 μM (range 0.010-0.059 μM).

A comprehensive analysis of the inhibitory activity of entecavir against a panel of laboratory and clinical HIV-1 isolates using a variety of cells and assay conditions yielded EC50 values ranging from 0.026 to >10 μM: the lower EC_{50} values were observed when decreased levels of virus were used in the assay. In cell culture, entecavir selected for an M184I substitution in HIV reverse transcriptase at micromolar concentrations, confirming inhibitory pressure at high entecavir concentrations. HIV variants containing the M184I substitution showed loss of susceptibility to entecavir.

The coadministration of HIV nucleoside/nucleotide reverse transcriptase inhibitors (NRTIs) with BARACLUDE is unlikely to reduce the antiviral efficacy of BARACLUDE against HBV or of any of these agents against HIV. In HBV combination assays in vitro, abacavir, didanosine, lamivudine, stavudine, tenofovir, or zidovudine were not antagonistic to the anti-HBV activity of entecavir over a wide range of concentrations. In HIV antiviral assays, entecavir was not antagonistic to the in vitro anti-HIV activity of these six NRTIs or emtricitabine at concentrations greater than 100 times the C_{max} of entecavir using the 1 mg dose.

Drug Resistance: Clinical Studies: In nucleoside-naive studies (AI463022, AI463027, and rollover study AI463901) and in studies of lamivudine-refractory HBV (AI463026, AI463014, AI463015, and rollover study AI463901), patients initially treated with entecavir 0.5 mg (nucleoside-naïve) or 1.0 mg (lamivudine refractory) and with an on-therapy PCR HBV DNA measurement at or after Week 24 were monitored for resistance. Virologic breakthroughs due to resistance to entecavir are observed in viruses which harbour primary lamivudine resistance substitutions (M204I/V±L180M) along with additional substitutions at residues T184, S202 or M250 of the viral polymerase.

Nucleoside-Naïve patients: Through Year 5, genotypic evidence of entecavir resistance (ETVr) substitutions at residues T184, S202 or M250 was observed in 3 patients (<1%), 2 of whom experienced virologic breakthrough (see Table 5). The results reflect use of a 1 mg dose of entecavir in 147 patients in Year 3 and all patients in Years 4 and 5 and of entecavir-lamivudine combination therapy (followed by long-term entecavir monotherapy) for a median of 20 weeks for 130 patients in Year 3 and for 1 week for one patient in Year 4 in a rollover study.

Table 5: BARACLUDE

Genotypic Entecavir Resistance and Virologic Breakthrough with Resistance Through Year 5, Nucleoside-Naïve Studies

	Year 1	Year 2	Year 3[a]	Year 4[a]	Year 5[a]
Subjects treated and monitored for resistance[b]	663	278	149	121	108
Emerging genotypic ETV[c,d]	1	1	1	0	0
Genotypic ETVr[c,d] with virologic breakthrough[e]	1	0	1	0	0
Cumulative probability of emerging genotypic ETVr[c,d]	0.2%	0.5%	1.2%	1.2%	1.2%
Cumulative probability of genotypic ETVr[c,d] with virologic breakthrough[e]	0.2%	0.2%	0.8%	0.8%	0.8%

[a] Results reflect the use of a 1 mg dose of entecavir for 147 subjects in Year 3 and all subjects in Years 4 and 5 and of combination entecavir-lamivudine therapy (followed by long-term entecavir therapy) for a median of 20 weeks for 130 subjects in Year 3 and for 1 week for 1 subject in Year 4 in rollover study.
[b] Includes subjects with at least one on-therapy HBV DNA measurement by PCR at or after week 24 through week 58 (Year 1), after week 58 through week 102 (Year 2), after week 102 through week 156 (Year 3), after week 156 through week 204 (Year 4), or after week 204 through week 252 (Year 5).
[c] ETVr=entecavir resistance substitutions at residues T184, S202 or M250.
[d] Subjects also had lamivudine resistance substitutions (rtM204V and rtL180M).
[e] ≥1 log_{10} increase above nadir in HBV DNA by PCR, confirmed with successive measurements or at the end of the windowed point.

Emerging amino acid substitutions at M204I/V±L180M, L80I, or V173L, which conferred decreased phenotypic susceptibility to entecavir in the absence of S202, T184, or M250 changes, were detected in the HBV of 3 patients (3/663=<1%) who experienced virologic breakthrough by the end of Year 5.

Lamivudine-Refractory Patients: Through Year 5, genotypic evidence of entecavir resistance (ETVr) substitutions at residues T184, S202 or M250 was observed in 47 patients, 39 of whom experienced virologic breakthrough (see Table 6) The results reflect the use of entecavir-lamivudine combination therapy (followed by long-term entecavir monotherapy) for a median of 13 weeks for 48 patients in Year 3, for a median of 38 weeks for 10 patients in Year 4 and for 16 weeks for 1 patient in Year 5 in a rollover study.

The presence of ETVr substitutions at baseline in isolates from 10 (5%) of 187 lamivudine-refractory patients indicates that prior lamivudine treatment can select these resistance substitutions and they can exist at a low frequency before entecavir treatment. Through Year 5, 3 of the 10 patients experienced virologic breakthrough. Isolates from patients who experienced virologic breakthrough with the emergence of S202, T184 and/or M250 substitutions (n=39), had a median 285 fold-change in entecavir susceptibility as compared to wild type HBV. Three additional subjects experienced virologic breakthrough with the emergence of M204I/V±L180M, L80V or V173L/M alone.

Cross-resistance: Cross-resistance has been observed among HBV nucleoside analogues. In cell-based assays, HBV containing lamivudine resistance substitutions M204V/I±L180M was 8-fold less susceptible to entecavir than wild type virus. Further reductions (>70 fold) in entecavir phenotypic susceptibility required the presence of primary lamivudine resistance amino acid substitutions (M204V/I±L180M) along with additional substitutions at residues rtT184, rtS202, or rtM250, or a combination of these substitutions with or without an rtI169 substitution in the HBV polymerase.

Recombinant HBV genomes encoding adefovir resistance-associated substitutions at either rtN236T or rtA181V remained susceptible to entecavir. HBV isolates from lamivudine-refractory patients failing BARACLUDE therapy were susceptible in vitro to adefovir but retained resistance to lamivudine.

Pharmacokinetics: The single- and multiple-dose pharmacokinetics of entecavir were evaluated in healthy subjects and patients with chronic hepatitis B infection (including liver transplant recipients). Steady-state pharmacokinetics of entecavir are summarized in Table 7.

Absorption: Following oral administration in healthy subjects, entecavir was rapidly absorbed with peak plasma concentrations occurring between 0.5 and 1.5 hours. Following multiple daily doses ranging from 0.1 to 1.0 mg, C_{max} and area under the concentration-time curve (AUC) at steady state increased in proportion to dose. Steady state was achieved after 6-10 days of once-daily administration with approximately 2 fold accumulation. For a 0.5-mg oral dose, C_{max} at steady state was 4.2 ng/mL and trough plasma concentration (C_{trough}) was 0.3 ng/mL. For a 1 mg oral dose, C_{max} was 8.2 ng/mL and C_{trough} was 0.5 ng/mL.

A bioavailability study was performed on 24 healthy subjects under fasting conditions comparing the rate and extent of absorption of a 10 mL single oral dose of entecavir 0.05 mg/mL oral solution and a single oral dose of entecavir 0.5 mg tablet. Results showed that the bioavailability following administration of the 0.05 mg/mL oral solution was comparable to the bioavailability following administration of the 0.5 mg tablet.

Table 6: BARACLUDE

Genotypic Entecavir Resistance and Virologic Breakthrough with Resistance Through Year 5, Lamivudine-Refractory Studies

	Year 1	Year 2	Year 3[a]	Year 4[a]	Year 5[a]
Subjects treated and monitored for resistance[b]	187	146	80	52	33
Emerging genotypic ETV[c,d]	11	12	16	6	2
Genotypic ETVr[c,d] with virologic breakthrough[e]	2[f]	14[f]	13[f]	9[f]	1[f]
Cumulative probability of emerging genotypic ETVr[c,d]	6%	15%	36%	47%	51%
Cumulative probability of genotypic ETVr[c,d] with virologic breakthrough[e]	1%[f]	11%[f]	27%[f]	41%[f]	44%[f]

[a] Results reflect the use of combination entecavir-lamivudine therapy (followed by long-term entecavir therapy) for a median of 13 weeks for 48 subjects in Year 3, for a median of 38 weeks for 10 subjects in Year 4, and for 16 weeks for 1 patient in Year 5 in a rollover study.
[b] Includes subjects with at least one on-therapy HBV DNA measurement by PCR at or after week 24 through week 58 (Year 1), after week 58 through week 102 (Year 2), after week 102 through week 156 (Year 3), after week 156 through week 204 (Year 4), or after week 204 through week 252 (Year 5).
[c] ETVr=entecavir resistance substitutions at residues T184, S202 or M250.
[d] Subjects also had lamivudine resistance substitutions (rtM204V/I±rtL180M).
[e] ≥1 log_{10} increase above nadir in HBV DNA by PCR, confirmed with successive measurements or at the end of the windowed point.
[f] ETVr occuring in any year virologic breakthrough in a specified year.

Table 7: BARACLUDE

Summary of Entecavir Pharmacokinetic Parameters in Healthy Subjects

	C_{max}[a] (ng/mL)	$T_{½}$ (h)	AUC (TAU)[a] (ng·h/mL)	Clearance (CLT/F) (mL/min)	CLR (mL/min)
Steady-state mean (0.5 mg)	4.2	130	14.8	572	360
Steady-state mean (1.0 mg)	8.2	149	26.4	636	471

[a] Geometric mean.

Effects of Food on Oral Absorption: Oral administration of 0.5 mg of entecavir with a standard high-fat meal (945 kcal, 54.6 g fat) or a light meal (379 kcal, 8.2 g fat) resulted in a delay in absorption (1.0-1.5 hours fed vs. 0.75 hours fasted), a decrease in C_{max} of 44%-46%, and a decrease in AUC of 18%-20%. Therefore, BARACLUDE should be administered on an empty stomach (at least 2 hours after a meal and 2 hours before the next meal).

Distribution: Based on the pharmacokinetic profile of entecavir after oral dosing, the estimated apparent volume of distribution is in excess of total body water, suggesting that entecavir is extensively distributed into tissues. Protein binding to human serum protein in vitro was approximately 13%.

Metabolism: The metabolism of entecavir was evaluated in in vitro and in vivo studies. Entecavir is not a substrate, inhibitor, or inducer of the cytochrome P450 (CYP450) enzyme system. At concentrations approximately 10 000 fold higher than those obtained in humans, entecavir inhibited none of the major human CYP450 enzymes 1A2, 2C9, 2C19, 2D6, 3A4, 2B6, and 2E1. At concentrations approximately 340 fold higher than those observed in humans, entecavir did not induce the human CYP450 enzymes 1A2, 2C9, 2C19, 3A4, 3A5, and 2B6. Following administration of ^{14}C-entecavir in humans and rats, no oxidative or acetylated metabolites were observed. Minor amounts of the phase II metabolites glucuronide and sulfate conjugate were observed.

Excretion: After reaching peak concentration, entecavir plasma concentrations decreased in a bi-exponential manner with a terminal elimination half-life of approximately 128-149 hours.

The observed drug accumulation index is approximately 2 fold with once-daily dosing, indicating an effective accumulation half-life of approximately 24 hours.

Entecavir is predominantly eliminated by the kidney with urinary recovery of unchanged drug at steady state ranging from 62% to 73% of the administered dose. Renal clearance is independent of dose and ranges from 360 to 471 mL/min suggesting that entecavir undergoes both glomerular filtration and net tubular secretion (see Drug Interactions).

Special Populations and Conditions: Patients Co-Infected with HIV and HBV: Study AI463038 was a randomized, double-blind, placebo-controlled study of BARACLUDE versus placebo in 68 patients co-infected with HIV and HBV, who experienced recurrence of HBV viremia while receiving a lamivudine-containing highly active antiretroviral (HAART) regimen. Patients continued their lamivudine-containing HAART regimen (lamivudine dose 300 mg/day) and were assigned to add either BARACLUDE 1 mg once daily (51 patients) or placebo (17 patients) for 24 weeks followed by an open-label phase for an additional 24 weeks where all patients received BARACLUDE. At baseline, patients had a mean serum HBV DNA level by PCR of 9.13 log_{10} copies/mL. Ninety-nine percent of patients were HBeAg-positive at baseline, with a mean baseline ALT level of 71.5 U/L. Median HIV RNA level remained stable at approximately 2 log_{10} copies/mL through 24 weeks of blinded therapy. Virologic and biochemical endpoints at Week 24 are shown in Table 8. There are no data in patients with HIV/HBV co-infection who have not received prior lamivudine therapy. BARACLUDE has not been evaluated in HIV/HBV co-infected patients who were not simultaneously receiving effective HIV treatment (see Warnings and Precautions, Special Populations, Patients Co-Infected with HIV and HBV).

Table 8: BARACLUDE

Virologic and Biochemical Endpoints at Week 24, Study AI463038

	BARACLUDE 1 mg[a] N=51	Placebo[a] N=17
HBV DNA[b]		
Proportion undetectable (<300 copies/mL)	6%	0
Mean change from baseline (log_{10} copies/mL)	(−3.65[d])	(+0.11)
ALT normalization (≤1×ULN)	(34%[c])	(8%[c])

[a] All patients also received a lamivudine-containing HAART regimen.
[b] Roche COBAS Amplicor PCR assay (LLOQ=300 copies/mL).
[c] Percentage of patients with abnormal ALT (>1×ULN) at baseline who achieved ALT normalization (n=35 for BARACLUDE and n=12 for placebo).
[d] p<0.0001.

For patients originally assigned to BARACLUDE, at the end of the open-label phase (Week 48), 8% of patients had HBV DNA <300 copies/mL by PCR, the mean change from baseline HBV DNA by PCR was −4.20 log_{10} copies/mL, and 37% of patients with abnormal ALT at baseline had ALT normalization (≤1×ULN).

Pediatrics: Pharmacokinetic studies have not been conducted in children.

Geriatrics: The effect of age on the pharmacokinetics of entecavir was evaluated following administration of a single 1 mg oral dose in healthy young (20-40 years old) and elderly (65-83 years old) volunteers. Entecavir AUC was 29.3% greater in elderly subjects compared to young subjects. The disparity in exposure between elderly and young subjects was most likely attributable to differences in renal function. Dosage adjustment of BARACLUDE should be based on the renal function of the patient, rather than age (see Dosage and Administration, Renal Impairment).

Gender/Race: There are no significant gender/racial differences in entecavir pharmacokinetics.

Hepatic Insufficiency: No dosage adjustment of BARACLUDE is recommended for patients with hepatic impairment. The pharmacokinetics of entecavir following a single 1 mg dose were studied in patients (without chronic hepatitis B infection) with moderate and severe hepatic impairment. The pharmacokinetics of entecavir were similar between hepatically impaired patients and healthy control subjects.

Post-liver Transplant: The safety and efficacy of BARACLUDE in liver transplant recipients are unknown. However, in a small pilot study of entecavir use in HBV-infected liver transplant recipients on a stable dose of cyclosporine A (n=5) or tacrolimus (n=4), entecavir exposure was approximately 2 fold the exposure in healthy subjects with normal renal function. Altered renal function contributed to the increase in entecavir exposure in these patients. The potential for pharmacokinetic interactions between entecavir and cyclosporine A or tacrolimus was not formally evaluated. Renal function must be carefully monitored both before and during treatment with BARACLUDE in liver transplant recipients who have received or are receiving an immunosuppressant that may affect renal function, such as cyclosporine or tacrolimus (see Dosage and Administration, Renal Impairment).

Renal Insufficiency: The pharmacokinetics of entecavir following a single 1 mg dose were studied in patients (without chronic hepatitis B infection) with selected degrees of renal impairment, including patients whose renal impairment was managed by hemodialysis or continuous ambulatory peritoneal dialysis (CAPD). Results are shown in Table 9.

Table 9: BARACLUDE

Pharmacokinetic Parameters in Subjects with Selected Degrees of Renal Function

	Baseline Creatinine Clearance (mL/min)				Severe Managed with Hemodialysis[a] (n=6)	Severe Managed with CAPD (n=4)
	Unimpaired >80 (n=6)	Mild >50– ≤80 (n=6)	Moderate 30–50 (n=6)	Severe <30 (n=6)		
C_{max}(ng/mL) (CV%)	8.1 (30.7)	10.4 (37.2)	10.5 (22.7)	15.3 (33.8)	15.4 (56.4)	16.6 (29.7)
$AUC_{(0-T)}$ (ng·h/mL) (CV)	27.9 (25.6)	51.5 (22.8)	69.5 (22.7)	145.7 (31.5)	233.9 (28.4)	221.8 (11.6)
CLR (mL/min) (SD)	383.2 (101.8)	197.9 (78.1)	135.6 (31.6)	40.3 (10.1)	NA	NA
CLT/F (mL/min) (SD)	588.1 (153.7)	309.2 (62.6)	226.3 (60.1)	100.6 (29.1)	50.6 (16.5)	35.7 (19.6)

[a] Dosed immediately following hemodialysis.
Legend: CLR=renal clearance; CLT/F=apparent oral clearance.

Dosage adjustment is recommended for patients with a creatinine clearance <50 mL/min, including patients on hemodialysis or CAPD (see Dosage and Administration, Renal Impairment).

Following a single 1 mg dose of BARACLUDE, hemodialysis removed approximately 13% of the BARACLUDE dose over 4 hours and CAPD removed approximately 0.3% of the dose over 7 days. BARACLUDE should be administered after hemodialysis.

STORAGE AND STABILITY: BARACLUDE Tablets should be stored in a tightly closed container at 25°C; excursions permitted between 15-30°C.

BARACLUDE Oral Solution should be stored at 25°C; excursions permitted between 15-30°C. Protect from light. Store bottle in outer carton. After opening, the oral solution can be used up to the expiration date on the bottle. The bottle and its contents should be discarded after the expiration date.

INFORMATION FOR THE PATIENT: Published in e-CPS, available by subscription at www.e-cps.ca.

DOSAGE FORMS, COMPOSITION AND PACKAGING: Oral Solution: Each mL of ready-to-use orange-flavored, clear, colorless to pale yellow aqueous solution contains: entecavir 0.05 mg. Nonmedicinal ingredients: citric acid, maltitol, methylparaben, orange flavour, propylparaben and sodium citrate. Plastic bottles of 260 mL (quantity 210 mL) with child-resistant closures.

BARACLUDE Oral Solution is a ready-to-use product; dilution or mixing with water or any other solvent or liquid product is not recommended. Each bottle of the oral solution is accompanied by a dosing spoon that is calibrated in 1 mL increments up to 10 mL. Patients should be instructed to hold the spoon in a vertical position and fill it gradually to the mark corresponding to the prescribed dose. Rinsing of the dosing spoon with water is recommended after each daily dose.

Tablets: Each white to off-white, triangular-shaped, film-coated tablet, debossed with "BMS" on one side and "1611" on the other side, contains: entecavir 0.5 mg. Nonmedicinal ingredients: crospovidone, lactose monohydrate, magnesium stearate, microcrystalline cellulose and povidone; coating: hypromellose, polyethylene glycol 400, polysorbate 80 and titanium dioxide. Plastic bottles of 30 with child-resistant closures.

(Shown in Product Identification Section)

Barbiturates

butalbital
pentobarbital sodium
phenobarbital sodium
primidone
thiopental sodium

Antiepileptic—Sedative-Hypnotic

CPhA Monograph

Date of Revision: November 2007

This monograph has been compiled by CPhA and reviewed by experts. It may contain information different from that found in Health Canada-approved Product Monographs. The reader is referred to the *CPS* Editorial Policy for more information.

SUMMARY PRODUCT INFORMATION:

Drug	Route of Administration	Dosage Form	Strength
Butalbital ©	Oral	Tablet	50 mg (in combination with ASA 330 mg and caffeine 40 mg)
	Oral	Capsule	50 mg (in combination with ASA 300 mg, caffeine 40 mg ± codeine 15 or 30 mg)
Pentobarbital sodium ©	IM, IV	Solution	50 mg/mL, 2 mL amp (available through Special Access Programme, Health Canada)
Phenobarbital sodium ©	IM, IV	Solution	30 mg/mL, 120 mg/mL
	Oral	Tablet	15 mg, 30 mg, 60 mg, 100 mg
	Oral	Elixir	5 mg/mL
	Oral	Tablet	40 mg (in combination with belladonna 0.2 mg and ergotamine 0.6 mg
Primidone	Oral	Tablet	125 mg, 250 mg
Thiopental Sodium ©	IV	Sterile powder for reconstitution	250 mg syringe, 500 mg syringe, 1 g vial, 2.5 g vial, 5 g bottle

PHARMACOLOGY: Barbiturates are nonselective central nervous system (CNS) depressants, capable of producing all degrees of depression from mild sedation and hypnosis to general anesthesia, deep coma and death. The extent of CNS depression varies with the route of administration, dose and pharmacokinetic characteristics of the particular barbiturate. Patient-specific factors such as age, physical or emotional state and the concomitant use of other drugs will also affect response.

The mechanism of action of barbiturates is not completely known. They may act by enhancing and/or mimicking the synaptic action of gamma-aminobutyric acid (GABA), an inhibitory neurotransmitter. The sedative-hypnotic action of barbiturates may be due to an inhibition of conduction in the reticular formation resulting in a decrease in the number of impulses reaching the cerebral cortex.

Anticonvulsant activity may result from a reduction in CNS synaptic transmission and an increase in the threshold for electrical stimulation of the motor cortex. Phenobarbital is the only barbiturate with anticonvulsant activity at subhypnotic doses.

The therapeutic index of barbiturates is narrow. Therefore, the use of barbiturates is almost always accompanied by some degree of impairment of cognitive function. Supratherapeutic doses lead to marked mental and motor impairment. In some patients (especially children and the elderly), drowsiness may paradoxically be preceded by transient euphoria, elation, excitement and confusion.

Pharmacokinetics: See Table 1. After oral administration, absorption is usually rapid and relatively complete. The sodium salts undergo rapid dissolution and are absorbed more quickly than their corresponding free acids. The rate of absorption is increased when the barbiturate is formulated as a liquid, when the stomach is empty and when alcohol is ingested concurrently. The onset of action following rectal administration is similar to that following oral administration. After iv administration, the onset of action is immediate for pentobarbital and within 5 minutes for phenobarbital. The onset of action following im administration is slightly faster than when the drugs are administered orally or rectally.

Once absorbed, the barbiturates are rapidly distributed to all tissues and fluids. High concentrations appear in the brain, liver and kidneys. Phenobarbital is the least lipid soluble and has the slowest distribution. Barbiturates readily cross the placenta and are excreted into breast milk. Following iv administration, fetal blood concentrations are approximately equal to maternal serum concentration; with oral administration, fetal concentrations are less than maternal levels.

Barbiturates are slowly metabolized and/or conjugated in the liver and then excreted renally. Pentobarbital is almost completely metabolized. Due to its lower lipid solubility, phenobarbital is not metabolized as extensively and almost 25% is excreted unchanged in the urine. One of the metabolites of primidone is phenobarbital.

Metabolic elimination is influenced by age (slower in the elderly and infants), chronic liver disease and other drugs.

Table 1: Barbiturates

Pharmacokinetics

Drug	Onset of Action (minutes)	Half-life (hours)	Duration of Action
Butalbital[a]	15 to 60	35	4 to 6 h
Pentobarbital[b]	1	35–50	15 min
Phenobarbital[a]	60	80 to 120	10 to 12 h
Primidone	N/A	10 to 12	10 to 12 h
Thiopental[b]	1	8 to 10	10 to 30 min

[a] Following oral administration.
[b] Following intravenous administration.

INDICATIONS: The use of barbiturates as sedative/hypnotics has largely been replaced by less toxic agents such as benzodiazepines. Barbiturates have been used parenterally in the management of status epilepticus or acute seizure episodes that are secondary to meningitis or other causes.

Butalbital is used in combination with analgesics in the management of mild to moderate headache. Phenobarbital and primidone are used as second-line or adjunctive agents in the management of simple or complex partial seizures with or without secondary generalization. Phenobarbital is sometimes used in the management of acute alcohol withdrawal; it has also been used in combination with ergotamine and belladonna in the treatment of migraine. Pentobarbital is used as a sedative prior to surgery or other procedures. Thiopental is used as an anesthetic agent. Thiopental and pentobarbital are used in certain cases of increased intracranial pressure.

CONTRAINDICATIONS: Barbiturates should not to be administered to patients who are known to be hypersensitive to barbituric acid derivatives, or patients with porphyria, severe respiratory depression or pulmonary insufficiency.

WARNINGS: See Precautions.

PRECAUTIONS: Prolonged use of barbiturates, even in therapeutic dosages, may result in psychologic and physiologic dependence. Patients may escalate dosage without medical advice. Withdrawal symptoms may occur following abrupt termination of hypnotic doses causing nightmares, insomnia, sweating, irritability, tremor, weight loss or anorexia, or after chronic use of large doses resulting in delirium, seizures, or death. Withdrawal should be cautious and gradual.

Rarely, rickets and osteomalacia have been reported following prolonged usage of barbiturates due to increased metabolism of vitamin D.

Barbiturates should be used with caution in patients with impaired liver function or in patients with a history of drug dependence or abuse. Caution is essential when the drug is administered in the presence of any respiratory difficulty. Special care should be taken when barbiturates are administered to patients in whom the hypnotic effect may be prolonged or intensified, as in those suffering from shock, hepatic dysfunction, uremia, or after recent administration of other respiratory depressants.

Since barbiturates are potent CNS depressants, iv administration should not be attempted without adequate provisions for supporting respiration and circulation. Rapid injection can cause cardiovascular collapse. Slow administration will usually prevent this occurrence but may cause apnea, laryngospasm, coughing, or other respiratory difficulties.

With the exception of phenobarbital, barbiturates should be avoided in older individuals.

Barbiturates should be discontinued if cutaneous reactions occur, as they may herald the onset of a severe sensitivity reaction (see Adverse Effects, Hypersensitivity).

IM injection of pentobarbital should not exceed a volume of 5 mL (250 mg) at any one site because of possible tissue damage.

Barbiturate solutions are highly alkaline and should not be given sc. When they are administered iv, extreme care should be exercised to avoid extravasation or intra-arterial injection. Extravascular injection may cause local tissue damage with subsequent necrosis. The consequences of intra-arterial injection may vary from transient pain along the course of the artery to gangrene of the limb. Signs of accidental injection by this route include, in addition to pain, delayed onset of hypnosis, pallor and cyanosis of the extremity and patchy discoloration of the skin. Any complaint of pain in the limb warrants stopping the injection.

Hypotension may result from iv administration of the drug, particularly in patients with hypertension. Slow administration will usually prevent this occurrence.

Solutions that appear cloudy or in which a precipitate has formed should not be used.

Occupational Hazards: Barbiturates may impair the mental and/or physical abilities required for the performance of potentially hazardous tasks such as driving a vehicle or operating machinery. The concomitant use of alcohol or other CNS depressants may have an additive effect. Patients should be warned accordingly. The incidence of fractures due to falls may be increased, particularly in the elderly. Following use of barbiturates in office procedures, warn patients against operating motor vehicles for the remainder of the day.

Drug Interactions: Most of the following drug interactions have been documented with phenobarbital, however, they are likely applicable to other barbiturates as well. Barbiturates are inducers of cytochrome P450 isoenzymes CYP1A2, CYP2C9, CYP2C19 and CYP3A4, and are capable of increasing the clearance of many hepatically metabolized drugs. This can result in two concerns: i) decrease in or loss of effectiveness of other drug(s) during barbiturate use; ii) increase in effect or frank toxicity of the other drug(s) on discontinuation of the barbiturate.

When adding or deleting any barbiturate to or from a patient's therapeutic regimen, pharmacotherapy must be monitored closely as dosage adjustment of concurrent medications may be necessary.

Anticoagulants, Oral: Metabolism of coumarin anticoagulants (warfarin, nicoumalone/acenocoumarol) may be accelerated, resulting in decreased anticoagulant response. Correspondingly, if the barbiturate is discontinued from a stabilized regimen, the hypoprothrombinemic response may be greatly increased, potentially resulting in hemorrhagic complications. Prothrombin times should be monitored closely when barbiturates are added to or deleted from a regimen that includes oral anticoagulants.

Antidepressants, MAO Inhibitors: MAO inhibitors may inhibit barbiturate metabolism, resulting in increased CNS depressant effects. A reduction in barbiturate dosage may be required.

Antidepressants, Tricyclic: Barbiturates may increase metabolism of tricyclic antidepressants resulting in lack of effect. Plasma tricyclic concentrations should be monitored if possible, especially if the patient is not responding to standard dosages of antidepressant. The use of both drugs concomitantly may result in additive respiratory depressant effects.

Carbamazepine: When phenobarbital and carbamazepine are used together, the metabolism of carbamazepine is usually accelerated and plasma concentrations may be decreased. The clinical significance of this interaction is not known. Plasma concentrations of both drugs should be monitored when any change in the therapeutic regimen occurs.

CNS Depressants: Alcohol, benzodiazepines and other CNS depressants used concurrently with a barbiturate may result in excessive CNS depression.

Corticosteroids: Barbiturates may increase the metabolism of corticosteroids. There have been several reports of exacerbation of asthma and other conditions when barbiturates were added to regimens containing corticosteroids.

Contraceptives, Oral: Barbiturates may accelerate the metabolism of both the estrogenic and progestagenic components of the contraceptive, resulting in decreased effectiveness, which may or may not be signalled by breakthrough bleeding. There have been reports of pregnancy resulting from this combination. If the barbiturate is necessary, use of additional or alternative methods of contraception is recommended.

Doxycycline: Barbiturates have been reported to increase the metabolism and correspondingly reduce the effectiveness of doxycycline.

Ketamine: When ketamine is used for anesthesia following preoperative administration of a barbiturate, profound respiratory depression may result.

Phenytoin: When phenobarbital is used with phenytoin, concentrations of either or both drugs may be increased, decreased or unchanged. While phenobarbital may induce the metabolism of phenytoin, it may also decrease it because both drugs compete for the same metabolic pathway. Plasma concentrations of both drugs should be monitored when any change in the therapeutic regimen occurs.

Valproic Acid: Concomitant administration of valproic acid and phenobarbital usually results in increased levels of phenobarbital and resultant oversedation. There have been case reports of progression of CNS depression to coma. Plasma concentrations of both drugs should be monitored when any change in the therapeutic regimen occurs.

Pregnancy: Barbiturates readily cross the placental barrier.

Pentobarbital: There have been no reports of an increased risk of congenital defects associated with pentobarbital.

Phenobarbital and Primidone: The great majority of mothers on antiepileptic medication deliver normal infants. It is important to note that antiepileptic drugs should not be discontinued in patients in whom the drug is administered to prevent major seizures because of the strong possibility of precipitating status epilepticus with attendant hypoxia and threat to life. In individual cases where the severity and frequency of the seizure disorder are such that the removal of medication does not pose a serious threat to the patient, discontinuation of the drug may be considered prior to and during pregnancy, although it cannot be said with any confidence that even minor seizures do not pose some hazard to the developing embryo or fetus.

In addition to reports of increased incidence of congenital malformations such as cleft lip/palate and heart malformations in children of women receiving phenobarbital and other antiepileptic drugs, there have been rare reports of fetal hydantoin syndrome. This consists of prenatal growth deficiency, microcephaly and mental deficiency in children born to mothers who have received barbiturates, phenytoin, alcohol or trimethadione. However, these features are all inter-related and are frequently associated with intrauterine growth retardation from other causes.

The prescribing physician should weigh these considerations in treating or counseling women with epilepsy who are of child-bearing potential.

The serum level of antiepileptic drugs may decline during pregnancy, requiring adjustments in dosage. Postpartum restoration of the original dosage will probably be indicated.

Neonatal coagulation defects have been reported within the first 24 hours in babies born to mothers receiving phenobarbital, primidone and/or phenytoin for epilepsy. Vitamin K prevents or corrects this defect and can be given to the mother before delivery and to the neonate after birth.

Barbiturate withdrawal has occurred in newborns who were exposed to the drug in utero and may be characterized by hypotonia, irritability and vomiting.

Lactation: Breast milk concentrations of barbiturates are 35 to 50% of maternal serum concentrations. Barbiturates are eliminated slowly in neonates and may accumulate. Breast-fed infants should be observed for excessive drowsiness, feeding problems, rash or other adverse effects. If any of these occur, breast-feeding should be discontinued. When breast-feeding is discontinued there is a potential for withdrawal symptoms in infants.

ADVERSE EFFECTS: CNS: Drowsiness is frequent especially at initiation of therapy. Mild impairment of concentration, judgment, memory and fine motor skills may occur. Disturbances of sleep, dizziness, vertigo, headache and depression may occur. Patients with poorly controlled pain may experience paradoxical euphoria, elation or excitement as well as confusion, delirium or increased pain intensity. In children, hyperactivity is not uncommon; behavioral disturbances and cognitive impairment may occur. Geriatric patients may experience excitation, confusion or depression.

Cardiovascular: Hypotension may be observed with iv administration and is generally related to the rate of administration (see Precautions).

Gastrointestinal : nausea, vomiting, diarrhea and constipation.

Hematologic: megaloblastic anemia (responds to folic acid therapy). Agranulocytosis and thrombocytopenia are rare.

Hypersensitivity: Facial edema, skin rash (1 to 2%) may be purpuric, vesicular or erythematous. Exfoliative dermatitis and erythema multiforme are rare. Hypersensitivity reactions have a greater tendency to occur in patients with a history of asthma, urticaria or angioedema.

Metabolic: Barbiturates may increase vitamin D requirements, possibly by increasing vitamin D metabolism via enzyme induction. Rarely, rickets and osteomalacia have been reported following prolonged use of barbiturates.

Respiratory: respiratory depression (see Precautions).

Hepatic: Severe allergic reactions may result in jaundice due to degenerative changes in the liver. Toxic hepatitis is rare.

Miscellaneous: exacerbation of porphyria, pain at the injection site, withdrawal (see Precautions).

OVERDOSE:

Symptoms: Acute overdosage with barbiturates primarily affects the CNS and the cardiovascular system. Mild overdose resembles alcohol intoxication. Drowsiness, confusion, stupor, respiratory depression, ataxia, sluggish or absent reflexes, early hypothermia, late fever, cardiovascular depression with hypotension, renal failure, cardiac arrhythmias, pulmonary edema, aspiration pneumonia, bullae over pressure points and decreased gastrointestinal motility are all possible symptoms. Severe overdose may progress to shock, coma and death.

Doses that result in toxicity vary widely. A severe and potentially lethal overdose is about 10 times the usual hypnotic dose of pentobarbital (1 to 3 g). The lethal dose of phenobarbital is believed to be 5 g.

Chronic ingestion of barbiturates results in the development of tolerance and large doses can be ingested without overt toxicity. Serious toxicity can result at lower barbiturate levels if combined with alcohol or other CNS depressants.

Treatment: Patients who have ingested barbiturates in overdose often require respiratory and hemodynamic support. This may include intubation, ventilation, boluses of isotonic iv fluids, and inotrope infusions. Once a patient's airway is protected, activated charcoal should be administered to minimize absorption of orally administered barbiturates. Administering multiple doses of activated charcoal enhances the clearance of phenobarbital, though there is no evidence that this results in improved clinical outcomes (e.g., reduced duration of intubation). In patients with normal renal and cardiac function, urinary alkalinization also enhances phenobarbital clearance. Likewise, urinary alkalinization has not actually been shown to improve clinical outcomes.

For management of a suspected drug overdose, CPhA recommends that you contact your **regional Poison Control Centre**. See the *CPS* Directory section for a list of Poison Control Centres.

DOSAGE: The general use of barbiturates as sedatives or hypnotics has for the most part been supplanted by other less toxic drugs (i.e., benzodiazepines). Decreased dosage is recommended in older individuals and in patients with decreased renal or hepatic function. For more information on pediatric dosages, consult specialized pediatric references.

When used im, pentobarbital or phenobarbital should be given by deep im injection into a large muscle. For iv use, the rate of administration should not exceed 50 mg/min for pentobarbital and 60 mg/min for phenobarbital.

Butalbital: Oral: 50 to 100 mg, in combination with analgesics as per formulation, for acute headache; may be repeated in 4 hours. To prevent medication-overuse headache, combination analgesics should not be used on more than 10 days per month.

Pentobarbital: Adults: Preoperative sedation: 150-200 mg im.

Children: Procedural sedation: 2.5 mg/kg (max 50 mg) iv over 1 minute. Wait 1 minute. If necessary give 1.25 mg/kg (max 25 mg) iv over 30 seconds. Wait 1 minute. If necessary give 1.25 mg/kg (max 25 mg) iv over 30 seconds. Wait 1 minute. If necessary give 1 further dose of 1 mg/kg (max 20 mg) iv.

Note: Pentobarbital injection is available through the Special Access Programme, Health Canada.

Phenobarbital: Oral: Seizure Disorders: Adults: 90-120 mg po at bedtime. Children: 2-6 mg/kg/day po in 1 or 2 divided doses. Preoperative sedation: 100 to 200 mg im 60 to 90 minutes prior to surgery. Children: 1 to 3 mg/kg po or im 60 to 90 minutes prior to surgery.

Status Epilepticus: Adults: 20 mg/kg iv at a rate of 50-75 mg/min. Children: 20 mg/kg iv over 20 minutes.

Primidone: Adults: 125 mg po at bedtime for 3 days, then 125 mg po BID for 3 days then 125 mg po TID for 3 days; usual maintenance dose is 500 to 1000 mg/day in 3-4 divided doses. Children: 125 mg po at bedtime for 6 days, then 125 mg po BID for 7 days, then 125 mg po TID for 7 days, then 10-25 mg/kg/day in 3 to 4 divided doses (max 750-1500 mg/day).

Thiopental: Induction or maintenance of anesthesia, management of increased intracranial pressure: Dosage must be individualized; consult specialized references.

Barriere™
dimethylpolysiloxane
Skin Protectant

WellSpring

SUPPLIED: Each g of vanishing cream contains: dimethylpolysiloxane 20%. Also contains parabens. Tubes of 50 and 100 g; jars of 450 g.

BCG Vaccine (Freeze-Dried)
Bacillus Calmette-Guérin
Active Immunizing Agent

sanofi pasteur

Date of Revision: October 2005

DESCRIPTION: BCG Vaccine (Freeze-Dried) is a culture preparation of Bacillus Calmette-Guérin, Connaught substrain, an attenuated strain of *M. bovis* suspended in monosodium glutamate. BCG cultures are propagated on Sauton growth medium, then harvested, mixed with monosodium glutamate and lyophilized (freeze-dried). BCG cultures are viable upon reconstitution. BCG Vaccine is supplied in multi-dose vials with accompanying diluent, which consists of sterile phosphate-buffered saline containing 0.025% polysorbate 80. The concentration of the reconstituted vaccine is 8×10^5 to 32×10^5 colony forming units (CFU) per adult dose of 0.1 mL (=0.1 mg BCG), equivalent to 4×10^5 to 16×10^5 CFU per infant dose of 0.05 mL (=0.05 mg BCG).

Lyophilized vaccine for reconstitution with diluent	
Bacillus Calmette-Guérin	1.5 mg
Excipient	
Monosodium glutamate	1.5% w/v
Diluent	
Sodium chloride	0.85%
Disodium hydrogen phosphate	0.25%
Sodium dihydrogen phosphate	0.06%
Polysorbate 80	0.025%
Water for injection	q.s. 1.5 mL

PHARMACOLOGY: Tuberculosis (TB) is an infectious disease caused by *M. tuberculosis*. Mortality and morbidity from TB have declined significantly in Canada since the Second World War. After decades of continuous decline, however, the notification rate has essentially levelled off since 1987 to the current level. The incidence of TB varies from one geographic region to another. Groups at highest risk include Aboriginal populations and immigrants from areas with a high prevalence of the disease. Other persons at high risk include those infected with both HIV and tubercle bacilli, close contacts of persons with untreated TB, the elderly and the homeless.

BCG (Bacille Calmette-Guérin) is a live, attenuated vaccine derived from *M. bovis*. BCG has been used as a vaccine against TB since 1921. Its use in North America is confined to selected groups of people who still have high rates of tuberculosis.

Two meta-analyses have calculated summary estimates of BCG efficacy. Both studies concluded that there were very high rates of protection against meningeal and miliary tuberculosis, as high as 86% in one clinical trial. It was concluded from the clinical trials and case-control studies that BCG offered an overall protective effect of 51% and 50% against pulmonary tuberculosis. The protective effect is long lasting and has been demonstrated nearly 20 years after vaccination. The protective effect was greater among infants and children than among adults. An enhanced protective effect was also noted in studies in which BCG was given to newborns or infants. The protective effect of vaccination increases with increased distance from the equator.

Clinical Trials with BCG Vaccine (Freeze-Dried): Two retrospective case-control studies assessed the protective effect of BCG Vaccine (Freeze-Dried) in Aboriginal Canadian Indians. In one study, comparing the BCG vaccination status of 160 persons treated for tuberculosis between 1975 and 1979 with 232 controls, the protective effect of BCG vaccination was 57% (95% confidence interval (CI) 23-75%).

In the other study, the BCG vaccination history of 71 children, aged 15 years and under, newly diagnosed with TB (37 bacteriologically confirmed) between 1979 and 1983 was compared with 213 controls. A record of BCG vaccination was found in 49% of the tuberculosis cases compared to 77% of the controls. The protective effect for those who received BCG Vaccine (Freeze-Dried) at birth was 60%.

In a clinical trial in Chile in 1984, 148 neonates received 0.05 mg in 0.05 mL of BCG Vaccine (Freeze-Dried) and 105 neonates received the same dose of the WHO-reference BCG vaccine. By 6 months of age, PPD positivity (>10 mm induration to 5 TU of PPD) was demonstrated in 40 out of 97 (41.2%) of BCG Vaccine (Freeze-Dried) recipients and 38 out of 69 (55.0%) of WHO-reference BCG vaccine recipients.

In a clinical trial in Colombia in 1984, 445 PPD negative school children aged 5-14 years received 0.1 mg in 0.1 mL of BCG Vaccine (Freeze-Dried) and 138 received the same dose of the WHO-reference BCG vaccine. PPD positivity (>10 mm induration to 5 TU of PPD) was demonstrated among 305 out of 407 (74.9%) of BCG Vaccine (Freeze-Dried) recipients and 100 out of 130 (76.9%) of WHO-reference BCG vaccine recipients.

In a clinical trial of safety and immunogenicity of BCG Vaccine (Freeze-Dried) administered to PPD negative, healthy adult health-care workers aged 18-45 years in St. Louis, Missouri in 1994, PPD conversion (>5 mm induration to 5 or 10 TU of PPD) was demonstrated in 91% of 31 subjects.

INDICATIONS: BCG Vaccine (Freeze-Dried) is indicated for the prevention of tuberculosis in persons not previously infected with *M. tuberculosis* who are at high risk of exposure.

In accordance with the Canadian Tuberculosis Standards, BCG Vaccine may be considered for the following groups: newborn First Nations infants, particularly those living on reserve; individuals who are repeatedly exposed to persistently untreated or inadequately treated tuberculosis, particularly children from families in which there is a strong history of tuberculosis; communities or groups of persons in which high rates of new infection are demonstrated (annual infection rate >1%), for which other control measures have proved ineffective; health-care workers who may be at particular risk of exposure to unrecognized infectious forms of tuberculosis or who handle tubercle bacilli in laboratory cultures; newborn infants born to infectious mothers. Alternatively, BCG may be given 3 months after INH prophylaxis once the mother has ceased to be infectious, if the infant remains tuberculin negative; travellers visiting countries with a high prevalence of TB. A tuberculin skin test is recommended before departure except for those with known previous positive skin tests.

BCG Vaccine should be given only to persons who have not been infected with *M. tuberculosis* or who have a negative tuberculin skin test (Mantoux 5 TU). Infants <6 weeks of age do not need to be tuberculin tested before receiving BCG Vaccine since reactivity does not develop before this age.

BCG vaccination has NO value in the treatment of tuberculous disease.

In accordance with the recommendations of the National Advisory Committee on Immunization (NACI), BCG vaccination is recommended for the following persons: a) infants and children belonging to groups with high rates of new infections, i.e., in excess of 1% per year, when other control measures have proved ineffective; b) infants and children with negative tuberculin skin tests who are at high risk of intimate and prolonged exposure to persistently untreated or ineffectively treated patients (e.g., because of multidrug resistance) with infectious pulmonary TB, unless they can be removed from the source of exposure or given long-term preventive therapy; c) individuals repeatedly exposed to persons with untreated or inadequately treated active TB in conditions under which normal preventive measures are not possible or have been unsuccessful, e.g., when multidrug-resistant TB is involved. d) BCG vaccination may be considered for health-care workers (including medical laboratory workers) at considerable risk of exposure to tubercle bacilli, especially drug-resistant bacilli, when protective measures against infection are known to be ineffective or not feasible. Consultation with a regional TB and/or infectious disease expert is recommended before BCG Vaccine is administered. e) BCG vaccination may be considered for travellers planning extended stays in areas of high tuberculosis prevalence, particularly where a program of serial skin testing and appropriate chemotherapy may not be feasible or where primary isoniazid resistance of *M. tuberculosis* is high. Travellers are advised to consult a specialist in travel medicine or infectious disease when considering a decision for or against BCG immunization.

CONTRAINDICATIONS: Allergy to any component of BCG Vaccine (Freeze-Dried) including monosodium glutamate and polysorbate 80 or an anaphylactic or other allergic reaction to a previous dose of BCG vaccine are contraindications to vaccination.

BCG Vaccine (Freeze-Dried) should not be administered to persons with immune deficiency diseases, including HIV, congenital immunodeficiency such as chronic granulomatous disease or interferon gamma receptor deficiency, altered immune status due to malignant disease, or impaired immune function secondary to treatment with corticosteroids, chemotherapeutic agents, or radiation (see Adverse Effects).

Extensive skin disease or burns is also a contraindication to immunization with BCG Vaccine (Freeze-Dried).

BCG Vaccine (Freeze-Dried) is contraindicated for persons with a positive tuberculin skin test although vaccination of tuberculin reactors has frequently occurred without incident.

Immunization with BCG Vaccine (Freeze-Dried) should be deferred during the course of a moderate or severe febrile illness or acute infection (see Precautions) to avoid superimposing potential adverse effects of the vaccine on the underlying illness. A minor afebrile illness such as mild upper respiratory infection is not usually reason to defer immunization.

WARNINGS: As with any vaccine, immunization with BCG Vaccine (Freeze-Dried) may not protect 100% of persons.

BCG immunization will not prevent the development of active TB in persons who are already infected with *M. tuberculosis*.

BCG Vaccine (Freeze-Dried) is not a treatment for superficial cancer of the urinary bladder.

PRECAUTIONS: The stopper of the vial for this product contains dry natural latex rubber. Natural latex rubber has been associated with allergic reactions.

The possibility of allergic reactions in persons sensitive to components of the vaccine should be evaluated. Epinephrine Hydrochloride Solution (1:1000) should be available for immediate use in case an anaphylactic or acute hypersensitivity reaction occurs. Health-care providers should be familiar with current recommendations for the initial management of anaphylaxis in non-hospital settings, including proper airway management.

For instructions on recognition and treatment of anaphylactic reactions, see the current edition of the Canadian Immunization Guide, or visit the Health Canada website.

Before administration take all appropriate precautions to prevent adverse reactions. This includes a review of the patient's history concerning possible hypersensitivity to the vaccine or similar vaccine, previous immunization history, the presence of any contraindications to immunization and current health status.

BCG Vaccine (Freeze-Dried) should not be administered to persons receiving drugs with antituberculous activity, since these agents may be active against the vaccine strain.

Providers of BCG Vaccine should ascertain any family history suggestive of congenital immunodeficiency and any risk factors for HIV infection before administering BCG Vaccine. Infants who have potentially been exposed to HIV perinatally should not be given BCG Vaccine until they have been confirmed not to be infected with HIV.

Before administration of BCG Vaccine (Freeze-Dried) health-care providers should inform the patient, parent or guardian of the benefits and risks of immunization, inquire about the recent health status of the patient and comply with any local requirements regarding information to be provided to the patient before immunization.

Administer BCG Vaccine (Freeze-Dried) **intradermally**; do not inject subcutaneously, intramuscularly or intravenously.

Use a separate sterile needle and syringe, or a sterile disposable unit, for each individual patient to prevent disease transmission.

There have been case reports of transmission of HIV and hepatitis by failure to scrupulously observe sterile technique. In particular, the same needle and/or syringe must never be used to re-enter a multidose vial to withdraw vaccine even when it is to be used for inoculation of the same patient. This may lead to contamination of the vial contents and infection of patients who subsequently receive vaccine from the vial.

BCG Vaccine (Freeze-Dried) contains viable attenuated mycobacteria; it should be handled as an infectious agent at all times. See Dosage for recommended procedures for proper handling and disposal.

Pregnancy: Vaccination of pregnant women is usually delayed until after delivery, although no harmful effects on the fetus have been observed.

Animal reproduction studies have not been conducted with BCG Vaccine (Freeze-Dried). It is also not known whether BCG Vaccine (Freeze-Dried) can cause fetal harm when administered to a pregnant woman or can affect reproduction capacity.

Lactation: It is not known whether BCG Vaccine (Freeze-Dried) is excreted in human milk. Because live vaccines may be excreted in human milk, caution should be exercised when BCG Vaccine (Freeze-Dried) is administered to a nursing woman.

Simultaneous Use with Other Vaccines: Most inactivated and live vaccines may be given simultaneously at separate sites with separate syringes. Studies to examine the simultaneous administration of BCG Vaccine (Freeze-Dried) with hepatitis B immune globulin have not been conducted. A study which examined simultaneous administration of BCG Vaccine and hepatitis B vaccine at birth, showed that simultaneous administration impaired neither the immunogenicity nor the safety of either vaccine. One live vaccine may interfere with the effectiveness of another. BCG Vaccine should not be given within 4 weeks after administration of any live vaccine, since these vaccines are known to suppress the tuberculin response.

ADVERSE EFFECTS: The usual response to BCG vaccination is a red indurated area measuring 5-15 mm; the center is soft for 3 to 4 weeks and a crust is formed. When the crust falls off between the 6th and 10th week, a flat scar measuring 3-7 mm, usually with sharp punched-out edges which may be regular or irregular, remains.

Two studies of BCG Vaccine (Freeze-Dried) were conducted in Chile and in Colombia in 1984. In Chile, 148 neonates received 0.05 mg in 0.05 mL of BCG Vaccine (Freeze-Dried) and 105 neonates received the same dose of the WHO-reference BCG Vaccine. In Colombia, 445 PPD negative school children aged 5-14 years received 0.1 mg in 0.1 mL of BCG Vaccine (Freeze-Dried) and 138 received the same dose of the WHO-reference BCG vaccine. Table 1 outlines the reactions observed.

For these two studies, safety follow-up was not continued past 10 weeks. Systemic reactions were not monitored.

In a study of safety and immunogenicity of BCG Vaccine (Freeze-Dried) administered to 32 healthy PPD negative, HIV-negative adult health-care workers aged 18 - 45 years, in St. Louis, Missouri, in 1994, local and systemic reactions were monitored for 49 days, with any unresolved reactions being monitored up to 84 days. Local and systemic reactions were noted in Table 2.

Table 1: BCG Vaccine

Chile and Colombia Studies Reactions Observed in Chilean Neonates and Colombian School Children

Reaction Observed	Vaccine	Chile		Colombia	
		Post-vaccination		Post-vaccination	
		4 Weeks	8–10 Weeks	4 Weeks	8–10 Weeks
Induration ≥10 mm	BCG Vaccine (Freeze-Dried)	39.2%	7.4%	29.4%	16.2%
	WHO BCG vaccine	14.2%	15.2%	13.5%	14.0%
Ulceration 5–9 mm	BCG Vaccine (Freeze-Dried)	12.4%	56.1%	18.5%	34.7%
	WHO BCG vaccine	3.8%	59.0%	5.3%	21.5%
Ulceration 10–14 mm	BCG Vaccine (Freeze-Dried)	0%	2%	0%	0%
	WHO BCG vaccine	0%	2%	0%	0%
Regional Lymphadenopathy ≥10 mm; <20 mm	BCG Vaccine (Freeze-Dried)	34.6%	21.0%	9.5%	0.2%
	WHO BCG vaccine	41.5%	49.6%	0.8%	0%
Regional Lymphadenopathy ≥20 mm	BCG Vaccine (Freeze-Dried)	0%	0%	0%	0%
	WHO BCG vaccine	0.9%	6.7%	0%	0%

Table 2: BCG Vaccine

Local and Systemic Reactions to BCG Vaccine (Freeze-Dried), in Healthy US Adults

Days Post-BCG	0	1	3	14	28	49
	Number (%) of each reaction					
Any Reaction at Injection Site	24 (75)	31 (97)	32 (100)	32 (100)	31 (97)	25 (78)
>1" Erythema	2 (6.3)	1 (3.1)	5 (15.6)	2 (6.3)	0	0
Induration	1 (3.1)	3 (9.4)	12 (37.5)	12 (37.5)	4 (12.5)	0
Pain/Soreness	6 (19)	6 (19)	4 (13)	0	2 (6)	0
Ulceration	0	1 (3)	3 (9)	22 (69)	22 (69)	15 (47)
Fever >37.22°C	1 (3)	0	0	0	0	0
Regional Adenopathy[a]	1 (3)	1 (3)	1 (3)	1 (3)	1 (3)	1 (3)
Chills[b]	0	1 (3)	0			
Anorexia[b]	1 (3.1)	0	1 (3.1)			
Malaise[b]	6 (19)	5 (16)	4 (13)			

[a] Regional Adenopathy was observed in a single subject throughout the monitoring period.

[b] Except for fever and regional adenopathy, systemic reactions were not recorded after day 3 post-dose.

There were no episodes of nausea or vomiting. Ulceration had completely healed by 7 weeks in 18 of 32 subjects (56.3%), by 8 weeks in another 9 subjects (28.1%) and by 12 weeks in the remaining 5 (15.5%).

In studies of BCG Vaccine (Freeze-Dried) ulceration of >5 mm at the site of intradermal vaccination (the most common adverse reaction) occurred in approximately 50% (35-69%) of patients.

Regional (e.g., axillary) lymphadenopathy follows BCG vaccination (various strains from various manufacturers), with a frequency ranging from 1-10%. Suppurative lymphadenitis is much less common than lymphadenopathy, occurring in 0.03-0.5% of BCG Vaccine recipients. Multiple lymphadenitis, hepatomegaly, splenomegaly and other nonfatal disseminated lesions have occurred at rates of 0.31 to 0.39 per 1 million vaccinations.

One case of osteomyelitis associated with Sanofi Pasteur Limited's BCG Vaccine (Freeze-Dried) was reported in 1998. Osteitis has been observed mostly in Scandinavian countries, possibly related to the strain used. The risk for developing osteitis after BCG vaccination varies by country; in one review this risk ranged from 0.01 cases/million vaccinees in Japan to 43.4 cases/million vaccinees in Finland.

Disseminated *M. bovis*, var BCG, infection occurred in four Aboriginal Canadian infants who had been immunized with BCG Vaccine (Freeze-Dried) in the neonatal period. All cases were in infants with immunodeficiencies (including severe combined immunodeficiency, HIV/AIDS, defect in interferon gamma) which had not been detected before immunization.

Disseminated BCG infection, which may be fatal, occurs very rarely (about 1 in 1 million vaccinations), and is seen almost exclusively in persons with impaired immune responses.

HIV-infected Individuals: Several case reports of disseminated BCG in HIV-seropositive infants immunized during the first year of life and in adults with AIDS have raised concern that HIV infection may predispose to disease caused by BCG. In adults who have acquired AIDS, BCG adenitis has been reported up to 30 years after immunization with BCG.

Physicians, nurses and pharmacists should report any adverse occurrences temporally related to the administration of the product in accordance with local requirements and to the Global Pharmacovigilance Department, Sanofi Pasteur Limited, 1755 Steeles Avenue West, Toronto, ON, M2R 3T4, Canada 1-888-621-1146 (phone) or 416-667-2435 (fax).

OVERDOSE:

The recommended dosage for age should not be exceeded, as this may result in more extensive local reactions. Subcutaneous or intramuscular injection may result in an abscess at the injection site.

For management of a suspected drug overdose, CPhA recommends that you contact your **regional Poison Control Centre**. See the *CPS* Directory section for a list of Poison Control Centres.

DOSAGE: The recommended dose for newborns and infants ≤12 months of age is 0.05 mL (0.05 mg). Children over 12 months of age and adults should be given a 0.1 mL (0.1 mg) dose.

Reconstitution of Freeze-Dried Vaccine and Withdrawal from Stoppered Vial.

Do not remove the stopper from the vial.

Apply a **sterile** piece of cotton moistened with a suitable antiseptic to the surface of the stopper of the vial of vaccine. Withdraw the diluent into a syringe. Holding the plunger of the syringe containing the diluent steady, pierce the centre of the stopper in the vial and inject the required volume of sterile diluent into the freeze-dried vaccine. Do not try to force all of the diluent into the vial at once as this will create pressure. It is necessary gradually to allow air to escape into the syringe by intermittently aspirating air from the vial while injecting the diluent into the vial. Do not remove the needle from the stopper until the required volume of diluent has been injected. Shake the vial gently. **Avoid foaming** since this will prevent withdrawal of the proper dose. Withdraw the required dose of the reconstituted vaccine into a syringe. Aseptic technique must be used for withdrawal of each dose. (See Precautions.)

Inspect for extraneous particulate matter and/or discolouration before use. If these conditions exist, the product should not be administered.

Cleanse the outer surface of the upper arm with a suitable germicide and allow to dry. Using a 1.0 mL **sterile** syringe with a 26-gauge needle, inject 0.1 mL (0.05 mL for infants) of the reconstituted vaccine **intradermally** into the most superficial layers of the skin at one site. The bevelled side of the needle should face upwards.

The preferred site is over the area of the deltoid muscle of the arm.

Do not inject subcutaneously, intramuscularly or intravenously.

Needles should not be recapped and should be disposed of properly.

BCG Vaccine (Freeze-Dried) contains viable attenuated mycobacteria and should be **handled as an infectious agent at all times**. After use, any unused vaccine and all equipment, packaging and materials exposed to the product should be immediately placed in a container for biohazardous materials and disposed of as biohazardous waste.

Give the patient a permanent personal immunization record. In addition, it is essential that the physician or nurse record the immunization and PPD history (if applicable) in the permanent medical record of each patient. This permanent office record should contain the name of the vaccine, date given, dose, manufacturer and lot number.

Revaccination: Revaccination with BCG is not recommended and should be addressed in consultation with regional TB or infectious disease experts.

Storage: Store at 2 to 8°C. **Do not freeze.** Discard product if exposed to freezing. Do not use after expiration date. BCG Vaccine can be adversely affected by exposure to light. The product should be stored in the dark except when doses are actually being withdrawn from the vial. **The vaccine should be used immediately after reconstitution and any reconstituted vaccine not used within 8 hours must be discarded.** Any reconstituted product which exhibits flocculation or clumping that cannot be dispersed with gentle shaking should not be used. The reconstituted vaccine should be maintained at 2 to 8°C.

SUPPLIED: Package containing a multidose 1.5 mg vial of vaccine and accompanying 1.5 mL vial of diluent.

Beano®

alpha-D-galactosidase

Alpha Galactosidase Enzyme

GlaxoSmithKline Consumer Healthcare

PHARMACOLOGY: Hydrolysis converts raffinose, stachyose and verbascose into their digestible sugar components: glucose, galactose, sucrose and fructose. Raffinose yields sucrose+ galactose; stachyose yields sucrose+galactose; verbascose yields glucose+fructose+galactose.

INDICATIONS: Helps prevent gas. Beano enzyme has been shown to be effective in both clinical and anecdotal studies with humans when consuming foods with high alpha-linked sugar content. Use results in substantially reduced breath hydrogen emissions and marked reduction or elimination of symptoms, compared with identical challenges without Beano.

Flatulence and/or bloating as a result of eating a variety of grains, cereals, nuts, seeds and vegetables containing the sugars raffinose, stachyose and/or verbascose. This includes all or most legumes and all or most cruciferous vegetables. Examples of such foods are oats, wheat, beans of all kinds, chickpeas, peas, lentils, peanuts, soy-content foods, broccoli, brussels sprouts, cabbage, carrots, corn, leeks, onions, parsnips, squash.

Note: Beano has no effect on fibre. Most vegetables also contain fibre, which is gas productive in some people, but usually far less so than the alpha-linked sugars.

CONTRAINDICATIONS: Beano is made from a safe food-grade mold; however, if a rare sensitivity occurs, with allergic-type symptoms, discontinue use.

WARNINGS: No data supplied by the manufacturer.

PRECAUTIONS: Galactosemics should not use without their physicians' advice, since one of the breakdown sugars is galactose.

ADVERSE EFFECTS: Reports to date include gastroenterological symptoms, such as cramping and diarrhea as well as allergic-type reactions including rash and pruritus. Rare reports of more serious allergic reactions have been received.

OVERDOSE:

No data supplied by the manufacturer.

For management of a suspected drug overdose, CPhA recommends that you contact your **regional Poison Control Centre**. See the *CPS* Directory section for a list of Poison Control Centres.

DOSAGE: Tablets: 2 to 3, swallowed, chewed or crumbled with the first bite of food (1 tablet per ½ cup serving of gas producing food), should be enough for a meal of 1 to 3 servings of problem foods.

The optimum number of tablets required is a function of the quantity of food eaten, the levels of alpha-linked sugars in the food and the gas-producing propensity of the person.

Beano enzyme is inactivated at high temperatures. It should be added to foods at a temperature of less than 54°C. If the food is too hot to eat, it is too hot for the enzyme. Do not cook with Beano as the enzyme will be inactivated. Beano will hydrolyze the complex sugars (raffinose, stachyose and verbascose) into the simple sugars—glucose, galactose and fructose, and the easily digestible disaccharide, sucrose. This happens simultaneously with normal digestion.

SUPPLIED: Each tablet contains: not less than 150 GalU (galactose units) of alpha-D-galactosidase (following Food Chemical Codex (FCC) standards) derived from *A. niger* mold. Nonmedicinal ingredients: cellulose gel, colloidal silica, fish gelatin, invertase, magnesium stearate, mannitol and potato starch. Bottles of 30 and 60. Store at room temperature (avoid heat).

Beclomethasone Ⓟ

CPhA Monograph

see *Corticosteroids: Eye Ear Nose*

see *Corticosteroids: Inhaled*

Bellergal® Spacetabs ©

belladonna—ergotamine tartrate—phenobarbital

Anticholinergic—Antispasmodic—Sedative

Triton Pharma

SUPPLIED: Each compressed tablet contains: ergotamine tartrate USP 0.6 mg, levorotatory belladonna alkaloids 0.2 mg and phenobarbital USP 40 mg. Bottles of 100.

(Shown in Product Identification Section)

Benadryl® Allergy/Sinus/Headache

diphenhydramine HCl—pseudoephedrine HCl—acetaminophen

Antihistaminic—Decongestant—Analgesic

McNeil Consumer Healthcare

Benadryl® Total/Allergy/Regular Strength

diphenhydramine HCl—pseudoephedrine HCl—acetaminophen

Antihistaminic—Decongestant—Analgesic

McNeil Consumer Healthcare

Benadryl® Total/Allergy/Extra Strength

diphenhydramine HCl—pseudoephedrine HCl—acetaminophen

Antihistaminic—Decongestant—Analgesic

McNeil Consumer Healthcare

INDICATIONS: For relief of sneezing, runny nose, itchy watery eyes, sinus and nasal congestion, sinus pain and headache.

PRECAUTIONS: Benadryl Allergy/Sinus/Headache: Occupational Hazards: May cause drowsiness, use caution when driving a motor vehicle or operating machinery. Use only on the advice of a doctor. Avoid alcohol.

May cause excitability especially in children.

A physician should be consulted prior to using this product if patient has chronic alcoholism, serious kidney or liver disease, high blood pressure, heart or thyroid disease, diabetes, chronic lung disease, glaucoma or difficulty in urinating due to enlargement of the prostate gland, is elderly, pregnant, nursing or taking a drug for depression, including MAO inhibitor drugs, other antihistamines or sedating drugs.

If symptoms do not improve in 5 days or are accompanied by a fever, a physician should be consulted. Taking more than the recommended dose can cause serious liver damage, nervousness, dizziness or sleeplessness. In case of accidental overdose, contact a physician or Poison Control Centre immediately, even if there are no symptoms. **Keep out of reach of children.**

Benadryl Total/Allergy/Regular Strength: Occupational Hazards: May cause drowsiness, use caution when driving a motor vehicle or operating machinery. Use only on the advice of a doctor. Avoid alcohol.

A physician should be consulted prior to using this product if patient has chronic alcoholism, serious kidney or liver disease, high blood pressure, heart or thyroid disease, diabetes, chronic lung disease, glaucoma or difficulty in urinating due to enlargement of the prostate gland, is elderly, pregnant, nursing, or is taking other antihistamines, sedating drugs or drugs for depression, including MAO inhibitor drugs. If symptoms do not improve in 5 days or are accompanied by a fever, a physician should be consulted. Taking more than the recommended dose can cause serious liver damage, nervousness, dizziness or sleeplessness. In case of accidental overdose, contact a physician or Poison Control Centre immediately, even if there are no symptoms. **Keep out of reach of children.**

Benadryl Total/Allergy/Extra Strength: Occupational Hazards: May cause marked drowsiness; alcohol, sedatives and tranquilizers may increase the drowsiness effect. Use caution when driving a motor vehicle or operating machinery. Use only on the advice of a doctor. Avoid alcohol.

A physician should be consulted prior to using this product if patient has chronic alcoholism, serious kidney or liver disease, high blood pressure, heart or thyroid disease, diabetes, chronic lung disease, glaucoma or difficulty in urinating due to enlargement of the prostate gland, is elderly, pregnant, nursing, or is taking other antihistamines, sedating drugs or drugs for depression, including MAO inhibitor drugs. If symptoms do not improve in 5 days or are accompanied by a fever, a physician should be consulted. Taking more than the recommended dose can cause serious liver damage, nervousness, dizziness or sleeplessness. In case of accidental overdose, contact a physician or Poison Control Centre immediately, even if there are no symptoms. **Keep out of reach of children.**

OVERDOSE:

For management of a suspected drug overdose, CPhA recommends that you contact your **regional Poison Control Centre**. See the *CPS* Directory section for a list of Poison Control Centres.

DOSAGE: Benadryl Allergy/Sinus/Headache: Adults and children 12 years and over: 2 caplets every 6 hours. Do not exceed 8 caplets/day. Not recommended for children under 12 years.

Benadryl Total/Allergy/Regular Strength: Adults and children 12 years and over: 2 caplets every 6 hours. Do not exceed 8 caplets/day. Not recommended for children under 12 years.

Benadryl Total/Allergy/Extra Strength: Adults and children 12 years and over: 2 caplets every 6 hours while symptoms persist. Do not exceed 8 caplets/day. Not recommended for children under 12 years.

SUPPLIED: Benadryl Allergy/Sinus/Headache: Each light-green caplet, imprinted Benadryl on one side, contains: diphenhydramine HCl 12.5 mg, pseudoephedrine HCl 30 mg and acetaminophen 500 mg. Nonmedicinal ingredients: cellulose, D&C Yellow No. 10, FD&C Blue No. 1, FD&C Yellow No. 6, PEG, polysorbate, starches, stearic acid, titanium dioxide, wax and zinc stearate. Blister packages of 20. Store between 15 and 25°C.

Benadryl Total/Allergy/Regular Strength: Each light-green caplet, debossed with "WL 26" on one side and "B" on the other side, contains: diphenhydramine HCl 12.5 mg, pseudoephedrine HCl 30 mg and acetaminophen 500 mg. Nonmedicinal ingredients: celluloses, D&C Yellow No. 10, FD&C Blue No. 1, FD&C Yellow No. 6, PEG, polysorbate, starches, stearic acid, titanium dioxide, wax and zinc stearate. Blister packages of 20. Store between 15 and 25°C.

Benadryl Total/Allergy/Extra Strength: Each blue caplet, debossed with "WL 28" on one side and "B" on the other side, contains: diphenhydramine HCl 25 mg, pseudoephedrine HCl 30 mg and acetaminophen 500 mg. Nonmedicinal ingredients: cellulose, FD&C Blue No. 1 aluminum lake, magnesium stearate, PEG, polysorbate, starch, titanium dioxide and wax. Blister packages of 20. Store between 15 and 25°C.

Benadryl® Preparations

diphenhydramine HCl

Antihistaminic

McNeil Consumer Healthcare

Benadryl® Spray

diphenhydramine HCl—zinc acetate

Topical Analgesic—Skin Protectant

McNeil Consumer Healthcare

Benadryl® Stick

diphenhydramine HCl—zinc acetate

Topical Analgesic—Skin Protectant

McNeil Consumer Healthcare

Date of Revision: January 2008

INDICATIONS: Antihistamine, antiemetic and antispasmodic. Allergic diseases such as hay fever, allergic rhinitis, urticaria, angioedema, atopic dermatitis, contact dermatitis, gastrointestinal allergy, pruritus, physical allergies, reactions to injection of contrast media, reactions to therapeutic preparations, allergic transfusion reactions; postoperative nausea and vomiting and motion sickness.

Benadryl Itch Relief Cream is indicated for relief of itching due to insect bites, mild cases of sunburn, poison ivy or oak, and other minor skin irritations.

Benadryl Itch Relief Spray is indicated for temporary relief of pain and itching associated with rashes, oozing and weeping due to poison ivy, poison oak, sumac; minor burns, scrapes, sunburn, insect stings (bee, wasp), minor cuts, minor skin irritations and allergic itches.

Benadryl Itch Relief Stick is indicated for fast, effective relief of itch and pain from insect bites and stings.

CONTRAINDICATIONS: Cream, Stick and Spray should not be applied to extensively denuded or weeping skin areas.

WARNINGS: Antihistamines should be used with considerable caution in patients with narrow-angle glaucoma, stenosing peptic ulcer, pyloroduodenal obstruction, symptomatic prostatic hypertrophy, or bladder-neck obstruction. Not recommended for children with chronic lung disease or glaucoma.

Cream, Stick and Spray: For external use only. Do not apply to blistered, raw or oozing areas of the skin. Do not use on chickenpox, measles or extensive areas of the skin. If condition worsens or persists for more than 7 days, or recurs within a few days, discontinue use and consult a physician. Do not use other drugs containing diphenhydramine while using this product. Avoid contact with eyes or other mucous membranes; if this occurs rinse thoroughly with water. Keep out of reach of children. Keep Benadryl Stick and Spray away from fire or flame and store between 20 and 25°C. Use as Local Anesthetic: This drug should not be used as local anesthetic due to the risk of local tissue necrosis.

Children: In infants and children, especially, antihistamines in overdosage may cause hallucinations, convulsions, or death. As in adults, antihistamines may diminish mental alertness in children. In the young child, particularly, they may produce excitation.

Geriatrics (approximately 60 years or older): Antihistamines are more likely to cause dizziness, sedation and hypotension in elderly patients.

PRECAUTIONS: *Pregnancy:* Safety for use in pregnancy and lactation has not been established. Its use therefore in such patients should involve consideration of expected benefits and possible risks.

Lactation: Safety for use in pregnancy and lactation has not been established. Its use therefore in such patients should involve consideration of expected benefits and possible risks.

Occupational Hazards: Patients should be cautioned not to operate vehicles or hazardous machinery until their response to the drug has been determined.

Since the depressant effects of antihistamines are additive to those of other drugs affecting the CNS, patients should be cautioned against drinking alcoholic beverages or taking hypnotics, sedatives, psychotherapeutic agents or other drugs with CNS depressant effects during antihistaminic therapy.

Diphenhydramine has an atropine-like action and therefore should be used with caution in patients with a history of bronchial asthma, increased intraocular pressure, hyperthyroidism, cardiovascular disease or hypertension.

ADVERSE EFFECTS: Drowsiness, dizziness, dryness of mouth, nausea and nervousness may occur. Other infrequently reported effects are vertigo, palpitation, blurring of vision, headache, restlessness, insomnia and thickening of bronchial secretions. Allergic reactions, diarrhea, vomiting and excitation may also occur.

OVERDOSE:

> For management of a suspected drug overdose, CPhA recommends that you contact your **regional Poison Control Centre**. See the *CPS* Directory section for a list of Poison Control Centres.

DOSAGE: **Oral: Capsules or Caplets:** Adults and children 12 years and over: 25 to 50 mg 3 or 4 times daily. Maximum 4 doses/day. Capsules and caplets are not recommended for children under 12.

Extra Strength Nightime Caplets: Adults and children 12 years and over: 1 caplet at bedtime. Not recommended for children under 12 years. Do not take more than the recommended dosage.

Children's Benadryl Allergy Chewable Tablets: Adults and children 12 years and over: Use Adult BENADRYL. Children 6 to under 12 years: 1 to 2 tablets every 4 to 6 hours. Children 2 to under 6 years of age: Use BENADRYL Children's Liquid. Maximum 8 tablets/day. Chew tablets thoroughly before swallowing.

Elixir: Adults and children 12 years and over: 10 to 20 mL every 4 to 6 hours. Children, 6 to under 12 years: 5 to 10 mL every 4 to 6 hours. Maximum 4 doses/day.

Children's Liquid: Children under 2 years: 2.5 mL every 4 to 6 hours. Children 2 to 5 years: 5 mL every 4 to 6 hours. Children 6 to under 12 years: 10 to 20 mL every 4 to 6 hours. Maximum 4 doses/day.

Itch Relief Cream: Adults and children 2 years and over: Apply locally 3 or 4 times daily. Children under 2 years of age – Consult a doctor.

Itch Relief Spray: Adults and children 2 years of age and older: Shake well. Apply to affected area not more than 3 to 4 times daily. Children under 2 years of age – Consult a doctor.

Itch Relief Stick: Adults and children 2 years of age and older: Apply to affected area not more than 3 to 4 times daily. Children under 2 years of age – Consult a doctor. Shake well. Hold stick straight down over affected area and press tip of stick repeatedly until liquid flows, then dab sparingly.

SUPPLIED: Caplets: Each, pink, film-coated caplet, imprinted Benadryl on both sides contains: diphenhydramine HCl 25 mg. Nonmedicinal ingredients: celluloses, dicalcium phosphate, D&C Red No. 27, PEG, polysorbate, starch, stearic acid, titanium dioxide, wax and zinc stearate. Energy: 0.5 kJ (0.12 kcal). Gluten-, lactose-, paraben-, sodium-, sulfite- and tartrazine-free. Unit packages of 12 and 24. Bottles of 50 and 100.

Capsules: Each white capsule with pink cap contains: diphenhydramine HCl 50 mg. Nonmedicinal ingredients: lactose and talc; capsule shell: FD&C Blue No. 1, FD&C Red No. 3, gelatin, silicon dioxide, sodium lauryl sulfate and titanium dioxide. Energy: 2 kJ (0.47 kcal). Gluten-, paraben-, sodium-, sulfite- and tartrazine-free. Bottles of 100.

Children's Benadryl Allergy Chewable Tablets: Each purple, grape-flavored, round tablet, debossed "B" on one side and "FAST" over "MELT" on the other side contains: diphenhydramine HCl 12.5 mg. Nonmedicinal ingredients: artificial flavours, celluloses, corn starch, crospovidone, D&C Red No. 7 calcium lake, D&C Red No. 30 aluminum lake, dextrose, FD&C Blue No. 1 aluminum lake, gum arabic, magnesium stearate, maltodextrin, natural flavours, polymeric methacrylate, succinic acid, sucralose, tartaric acid and triacetin. Unit packages of 12.

Children's Liquid: Each 5 mL of colorless, bubble-gum flavored liquid contains: diphenhydramine HCl 6.25 mg. Nonmedicinal ingredients: artificial bubble gum flavor, carboxymethylcellulose, citric acid, glycerin, saccharin, sodium benzoate, sodium citrate, sorbitol, vanilla flavor and water. Energy: 43.68 kJ (10.4 kcal)/5 mL. Alcohol-, dye-, gluten-, lactose-, paraben-, sulfite- and tartrazine-free. Plastic bottles of 100 mL.

Cream: Each g of white emulsion for topical use contains: diphenhydramine 2% w/w. Nonmedicinal ingredients: alcohol, paraben, polyethylene glycol, propylene glycol and water. Tubes of 30 g.

Elixir: Each 5 mL of red elixir contains: diphenhydramine HCl 12.5 mg. Nonmedicinal ingredients: alcohol, FD&C Red No. 2, flavoring agents, sugar and water. Energy: 42.7 kJ (10.2 kcal)/5 mL. Gluten-, lactose-, paraben-, sodium-, sulfite- and tartrazine-free. Plastic bottles of 100 mL.

Extra Strength Nightime Caplets: Each white film-coated caplet, embossed "B" on one side and "50" on the other side contains: diphenhydramine HCl 50 mg. Nonmedicinal ingredients: calcium phosphate, cellulose, crospovidone, hydroxypropyl methylcellulose, magnesium stearate, polyethylene glycol, starch, stearic acid, titanium dioxide and wax. Gluten-, lactose-, paraben-, sodium-, sulfite- and tartrazine-free. Unit packages of 12. Child resistant package.

Spray: Each bottle contains: diphenhydramine HCl 2% w/v and zinc acetate 0.1% w/v. Nonmedicinal ingredients: alcohol, glycerin, povidone, tromethamine and water. Spray bottles of 59 mL.

Stick: Each stick contains: diphenhydramine HCl 2% w/v and zinc acetate 0.1% w/v. Nonmedicinal ingredients: alcohol, glycerin, povidone, tromethamine and water. Sticks of 14 mL.

Benazepril P

CPhA Monograph

see *ACE Inhibitors*

BeneFIX®

coagulation factor IX (recombinant) (nonacog alfa)

Antihemorrhagic Blood Coagulation Factor IX

Pfizer

Date of Preparation: March 21, 1997
Date of Revision: December 2, 2009

SUMMARY PRODUCT INFORMATION:

Route of Administration	Dosage Form/ Strength	Clinically Relevant Nonmedicinal Ingredients
Intravenous Injection	Lyophilized powder nominally containing 250, 500, 1000 and 2000 IU per vial The reconstituted product contains approximately: 50, 100, 200 and 400 IU/mL, respectively.	Glycine, sucrose, L-histidine, polysorbate 80

DESCRIPTION: BeneFIX is formulated as a sterile, nonpyrogenic, lyophilized powder preparation. It is a clear, colorless solution after reconstitution.

INDICATIONS AND CLINICAL USE: BeneFIX Coagulation Factor IX (Recombinant), is indicated for the control and prevention of hemorrhagic episodes in patients with hemophilia B (congenital factor IX deficiency or Christmas disease), including control and prevention of bleeding in surgical settings.

BeneFIX is not indicated for the treatment of other factor deficiencies (e.g., factors II, VII and X), nor for the treatment of hemophilia A patients with inhibitors to factor VIII, nor for the reversal of coumarin-induced anticoagulation, nor for the treatment of bleeding due to low levels of liver-dependent coagulation factors.

CONTRAINDICATIONS: Because BeneFIX Coagulation Factor IX (Recombinant), is produced in a Chinese Hamster ovary cell line, it may be contraindicated in patients with a known history of hypersensitivity to hamster protein.

WARNINGS AND PRECAUTIONS: General: Allergic-type hypersensitivity reactions, including anaphylaxis, have been reported for all factor IX products, including BeneFIX. Frequently, these events have occurred in close temporal association with the development of factor IX inhibitors. Patients should be informed of the early symptoms and signs of hypersensitivity reactions including hives, generalized urticaria, chills (rigors), flushing, angioedema, chest tightness, laryngospasm, bronchospasm, dyspnea, wheezing, faintness, hypotension, tachycardia, blurred vision and anaphylaxis. If allergic or anaphylactic reactions occur, administration of BeneFIX should be stopped immediately, and appropriate medical management should be given, which may include treatment for shock. Patients should be advised to discontinue use of the product and contact their physician and/or seek immediate emergency care, depending on the type/severity of the reaction, if any of these symptoms occur.

Nephrotic syndrome has been reported following immune tolerance induction with factor IX products in hemophilia B patients with factor IX inhibitors and a history of allergic reactions to factor IX. The safety and efficacy of using BeneFIX for immune tolerance induction has not been established.

Since the use of factor IX complex concentrates has historically been associated with the development of thromboembolic complications, the use of factor IX-containing products may be potentially hazardous in patients with signs of fibrinolysis and in patients with disseminated intravascular coagulation (DIC).

Historically, the administration of factor IX complex concentrates derived from human plasma, containing factors II, VII, IX and X, has been associated with the development of thromboembolic complications. Although BeneFIX, Coagulaton Factor IX (Recombinant), contains no Coagulation factor other than factor IX, the potential risk of thrombosis and DIC observed with other products containing factor IX should be recognized. Because of the potential risk of thromboembolic complications, caution should be exercised when administering this product to patients with liver disease, to patients post-operatively, to neonates, or to patients at risk of thromboembolic phenomena or DIC. In each of these situations, the benefit of treatment with BeneFIX should be weighed against the risk of these complications.

Twelve days after a dose of BeneFIX for a bleeding episode, one hepatitis C antibody positive patient developed a renal infarct. The relationship of the infarct to prior administration of BeneFIX is uncertain but was judged to be unlikely by the investigator. The patient continued to be treated with BeneFIX.

Dosing of BeneFIX may differ from that of plasma-derived factor IX products.

The safety and efficacy of BeneFIX administration by continuous infusion have not been established. There have been post-marketing reports of thrombotic events in patients receiving continuous-infusion BeneFIX through a central venous catheter, including life-threatening superior vena cava (SVC) syndrome in critically ill neonates.

Carcinogenesis and Mutagenesis: BeneFIX has been shown to be nonmutagenic in the Ames assay and nonclastogenic in a chromosomal aberrations assay. No investigations on carcinogenesis or impairment of fertility have been conducted.

Cardiovascular: Historically, the administration of factor IX complex concentrates derived from human plasma, containing factors II, VII, IX and X, has been associated with the development of thromboembolic complications. Although BeneFIX, Coagulaton Factor IX (Recombinant), contains no Coagulation factor other than factor IX, the potential risk of thrombosis and DIC observed with other products containing factor IX should be recognized. Because of the potential risk of thromboembolic complications, caution should be exercised when administering this product to patients with liver disease, to patients post-operatively, to neonates, or to patients at risk of thromboembolic phenomena or DIC. In each of these situations, the benefit of treatment with BeneFIX should be weighed against the risk of these complications.

Hematologic: See Cardiovascular.

Hepatic/Biliary/Pancreas: See Cardiovascular.

Immune: Activity-neutralizing antibodies (inhibitors) have been detected in patients receiving factor IX-containing products. As with all factor IX products, patients using BeneFIX should be monitored for the development of factor IX inhibitors. Patients with factor IX inhibitors may be at an increased risk of anaphylaxis upon subsequent challenge with factor IX. Patients experiencing allergic reactions should be evaluated for the presence of inhibitor. Preliminary information suggests a relationship may exist between the presence of major deletion mutations in a patient's factor IX gene and an increased risk of inhibitor formation and of acute hypersensitivity reactions. Patients known to have major deletion mutations of the factor IX gene should be observed closely for signs and symptoms of acute hypersensitivity reactions, particularly during the early phases of initial exposure to product. In view of the potential for allergic reactions with factor IX concentrates, the initial (approximately 10-20) administrations of factor IX should be performed under medical supervision where proper medical care for allergic reactions could be provided.

Peri-operative Considerations: See Cardiovascular.

Renal: Nephrotic syndrome has been reported following immune tolerance induction with factor IX products in hemophilia B patients with factor IX inhibitors and a history of allergic reactions to factor IX. The safety and efficacy of using BeneFIX for immune tolerance induction has not been established.

Twelve days after a dose of BeneFIX for a bleeding episode, one hepatitis C antibody positive patient developed a renal infarct. The relationship of the infarct to prior administration of BeneFIX is uncertain but was judged to be unlikely by the investigator. The patient continued to be treated with BeneFIX.

Respiratory: Patients should be informed of the early symptoms and signs of hypersensitivity reactions including hives, generalized urticaria, chills (rigors), flushing, angioedema, chest tightness, dyspnea, wheezing, faintness, hypotension, tachycardia, and anaphylaxis. Patients should be advised to discontinue use of the product and contact their physician and/or seek immediate emergency care, depending on the type/severity of the reaction, if any of these symptoms occur.

Sensitivity/Resistance: See General.

Sexual Function/Reproduction: See Special Populations.

Skin: See Sensitivity/Resistance.

Special Populations: Pregnant Women: Animal reproduction and lactation studies have not been conducted with BeneFIX Coagulation Factor IX (Recombinant). It is not known whether BeneFIX can affect reproductive capacity or cause fetal harm when given to pregnant women. BeneFIX should be administered to pregnant and lactating women only if clearly indicated.

Nursing Women: See Pregnant Women.

Pediatrics: Data from BeneFIX safety, efficacy, and pharmacokinetic studies have been evaluated in previously treated and previously untreated pediatric patients.

Nineteen (19) previously treated pediatric patients (range 4 to <15 years) underwent pharmacokinetic evaluations for up to 24 months. The mean increase in circulating factor IX activity was 0.7±0.2 IU/dL per IU/kg infused (range 0.3 to 1.1 IU/dL per IU/kg). The mean biological half-life was 20.2±4.0 hours (range 14 to 28 hours).

Fifty-eight previously untreated patients [PUPs] less than 15 years of age at baseline [3 neonates (0-<1 month), 45 infants (≥1 month-<2 years), 9 children (≥2 years-<12 years) and 1 adolescent >12 years)] underwent at least one recovery assessment within 30 minutes post-infusion in the presence or absence of hemorrhage during the study. The mean increase in circulating FIX activity was 0.7±0.3 IU/dL per IU/kg infused (range 0.2 to 2.1 IU/dL per IU/kg). In addition, there was no difference in the recoveries noted when data were evaluated by age group for infants (0.7±0.4 IU/dL per IU/kg; range 0.2 to 2.1 IU/dL per IU/kg) and children (0.7±0.2 IU/dL per IU/kg; range 0.2 to 1.5 IU/dL per IU/kg). The recoveries in these age groups were consistent with the recovery for the PUP study as a whole. There was insufficient sample size in the neonate and adolescent age groups to perform an analysis in these groups. Data from 57 patients who underwent repeat recovery testing for up to 60 months demonstrated that the average incremental FIX recovery was consistent over time. Additional safety and efficacy studies are ongoing in previously treated, minimally treated, and previously untreated pediatric patients.

Geriatrics: Clinical studies of BeneFIX did not include sufficient numbers of subjects aged 65 and over to determine whether they respond differently from younger subjects. As with any patient receiving BeneFIX, dose selection for an elderly patient should be individualized.

Monitoring and Laboratory Tests: Temporary correction of partial thromboplastin time (PTT) was observed. No effect on normal prothrombin time was seen. No significant increase in fibrinopeptide A or prothrombin fragment 1+2 was observed.

ADVERSE REACTIONS: Adverse Drug Reaction Overview: As with the intravenous administration of any protein product, the following reactions may be observed after administration: headache, fever, chills, flushing, nausea, vomiting, lethargy, or manifestations of allergic reactions. Should evidence of an acute hypersensitivity reaction be observed, the infusion should be stopped promptly and appropriate counter measures and supportive therapy should be administered.

Clinical Trial Adverse Drug Reactions: During uncontrolled open-label clinical studies with BeneFIX, Coagulation Factor IX (Recombinant), conducted in previously treated patients (PTPs), 131 adverse reactions with definite, probable, possible or unknown relation to BeneFIX therapy were reported among 27 of 65 patients (with some patients reporting more than one event) who received a total of 7573 infusions. These adverse reactions are summarized in Table 1.

Table 1: BeneFIX

Adverse Events Reported for PTPs[a]

Reaction	Total Number of Events with Definite, Probable, Possible or Unknown Relation to Therapy (n=129)	Number and (%) of Patients from Which the Reports Originated (n=65)	Number and (%) of Infusions Temporally Associated with the Reaction[b] (n=7573)
Nausea	27	4 (6.2%)	27 (0.36%)
Taste Perversion (Altered taste)	14	3 (4.6%)	19 (0.25%)
Hypoxia (Urge to cough with hypoxemia)	11	1 (1.5%)	11 (0.15%)
Injection Site Reaction	11	5 (7.7%)	12 (0.16%)
Injection Site Pain	10	4 (6.2%)	16 (0.21%)
Headache	10	7 (10.8%)	13 (0.17%)
Dizziness	7	5 (7.7%)	8 (0.11%)
Allergic Rhinitis	7	3 (4.6%)	9 (0.12%)
Pain (Burning sensation in the jaw and skull)	6	1 (1.5%)	7 (0.09%)
Rash	6	5 (7.7%)	7 (0.09%)
Hives	3	2 (3.1%)	3 (0.04%)
Flushing	3	2 (3.1%)	4 (0.05%)
Fever	2	2 (3.1%)	2 (0.03%)
Shaking	2	2 (3.1%)	1 (0.01%)
Factor IX Inhibitor[c]	1	1 (1.5%)	2 (0.03%)
Chest Tightness	1	1 (1.5 %)	4 (0.05 %)
Drowsiness	1	1 (1.5%)	1 (0.01%)
Visual Disturbance	1	1 (1.5%)	1 (0.01%)
Cellulitis at the IV site	1	1 (1.5%)	7 (0.09%)
Phlebitis at the IV Site	1	1 (1.5%)	7 (0.09%)
Dry Cough	1	1 (1.5%)	0 (0.00%)
Allergic Reaction	1	1 (1.5%)	1 (0.01%)
Diarrhea	1	1 (1.5%)	1 (0.01%)
Lung Disorder	1	1 (1.5%)	1 (0.01%)
Vomiting	1	1 (1.5 %)	1 (0.01 %)
Renal Infarct[d]	1	1 (1.5%)	1 (0.01%)
Total	131	27/65 (41.5%)	148/7573 (2.2%)

a More than one event in the table could have been associated with an infusion; however, the total represents the actual number of infusions given.
b Reaction occurring within 72 hours after infusion.
c Low titer transient inhibitor formation.
d The renal infarct developed in a hepatitis C antibody positive patient 12 days after a dose of BeneFIX for a bleeding episode. The relationship of the infarct to the prior administration of BeneFIX is uncertain (see Precautions, General).

One subject discontinued BeneFIX due to pulmonary allergic-type symptoms.

In the 63 treated PUPS, who received a total of 5538 infusions, 22 adverse reactions were reported as having definite, probable, possible or unknown relationship to BeneFIX. These events are summarized in Table 2.

Table 2: BeneFIX

Adverse Events Reported for PUPs[a]

Reaction	Total Number of Events with Definite, Probable, Possible or Unknown Relation to Therapy (n=22)	Number and (%) of Patients from Which the Reports Originated (n=63)	Number and (%) of Infusions Temporally Associated with the Reaction[b] (n=5538)
Diarrhea	5	1 (1.6 %)	11 (0.20%)
Urticaria (Hives)	3	3 (4.8 %)	3 (0.05%)
Factor IX Inhibitor[c]	2	2 (3.2%)	4 (0.07%)
Dyspnea (Respiratory distress)	2	2 (3.2 %)	2 (0.04%)
Increased Alkaline Phosphatase	1	1 (1.6 %)	3 (0.05%)
Elevated ALT	1	1 (1.6 %)	0 (0.00 %)
Rash (Body rash)	1	1 (1.6 %)	1 (0.02%)
Elevated AST	1	1 (1.6 %)	0 (0.00 %)
Chills (Rigors)	1	1 (1.6 %)	3 (0.05%)
Photosensitivity Reaction	1	1 (1.6 %)	0 (0.00 %)
Injection Site Reaction	1	1 (1.6 %)	2 (0.04%)
HAV Seroconversion[d]	1	1 (1.6 %)	2 (0.04%)
Parvovirus B19 Seroconversion[e]	1	1 (1.6 %)	1 (0.02%)
Asthma	1	1 (1.6 %)	1 (0.02%)
Total	22	11/63 (17.5%)	27/5538 (0.60%)

a More than one event in the table could have been assoc. with an infusion; however, the total represents the actual number of infusions given.
b Reaction occurring within 72 hours after infusion.
c Two subjects developed high titer inhibitor formation during treatment with BeneFIX.
d Relationship of HAV seroconversion to BeneFIX is unknown. HAV seroconversion was noted on 2 occasions in a single patient but was negative at final visit. The patient had no laboratory or clinical findings associated with active infection.
e Relationship of Parvovirus B19 seroconversion to BeneFIX is unknown. It was unlikely that seroconversion was related to BeneFIX due to the frequency of community acquired infection and viral safeguards built into the manufacturing process.

Less Common Clinical Trial Adverse Drug Reactions (<1%): In the section below the following frequency categories and terms are used: Uncommon: ≥0.1% and <1%. Rare: ≥0.01% and <0.1%. Very Rare: <0.01%.

Body as a Whole: Rare: hypersensitivity/allergic reactions (including, but not limited to hives, generalized urticaria, chills (rigors), flushing, angioedema, chest tightness, laryngospasm, bronchospasm, dyspnea, wheezing, faintness, hypotension, tachycardia, anaphylaxis), blurred vision.

Nervous System Disorders: Uncommon: dizziness, headache.

Cardiac Disorders: Rare: hypotension, tachycardia.

Vascular Disorders: Rare: phlebitis at the injection site.

Respiratory, Thoracic and Mediastinal Disorders: Rare: respiratory distress. Very Rare: dry cough.

Gastrointestinal Disorders: Uncommon: nausea. Rare: vomiting.

Skin: Rare: angioedema, cellulitis at the injection site, hives, rash.

Special Senses: Uncommon: altered taste.

General Disorder and Administration Site Conditions: Uncommon: injection site reaction. Rare: fever.

Abnormal Hematologic and Clinical Chemistry Findings: Temporary correction of partial thromboplastin time (PTT) was observed. No effect on normal prothrombin time was seen. No significant increase in fibrinopeptide A or prothrombin fragment 1+2 was observed.

Post-Market Adverse Drug Reactions: The following post-marketing adverse reactions have been reported for BeneFIX, as well as for plasma-derived factor IX products: inadequate factor IX recovery, inadequate therapeutic response, inhibitor development, anaphylaxis, laryngeal edema, angioedema, cyanosis, dyspnea, hypotension, and thrombosis.

There have been post-marketing reports of thrombotic events in patients receiving continuous-infusion BeneFIX through a central venous catheter, including life-threatening superior vena cava (SVC) syndrome in critically ill neonates. Cases of peripheral thrombophlebitis and deep vein thrombosis (DVT) have also been reported. In some, BeneFIX was administered via continuous infusion, which is not an approved method of administration.

If any adverse reaction takes place that is thought to be related to the administration of BeneFIX, the rate of infusion should be decreased or the infusion stopped.

DRUG INTERACTIONS: Overview: No interactions of recombinant coagulation factor IX products with other medicinal products are known.

Drug-Laboratory Interactions: No interactions of recombinant coagulation factor IX products with laboratory methods are known.

DOSAGE AND ADMINISTRATION: Dosage: Treatment should be initiated under the supervision of a physician experienced in the treatment of hemophilia B.

Treatment with all factor IX products, including BeneFIX, requires individualized dosage adjustment. The dosage and duration of treatment for all factor IX products depend on the severity of the factor IX deficiency, the location and extent of bleeding, and the patient's clinical condition. Dosing of BeneFIX may differ from that of plasma-derived factor IX products.

To ensure that the desired factor IX activity level has been achieved, precise monitoring using the factor IX activity assay is advised, in particular for surgical interventions. In order to adjust the dose as appropriate, doses should be titrated taking into consideration factor IX activity, pharmacokinetic parameters (such as half-life and recovery) as well as the clinical situation.

In an eleven patient, crossover, randomized PK evaluation of BeneFIX and a single lot of highpurity plasma-derived factor IX, the recovery was lower for BeneFIX. In the clinical efficacy studies, patients were initially administered the same dose previously used for plasma-derived factor IX. Even in the absence of factor IX inhibitor, approximately half of the patients increased their dose in these studies. Titrate the initial dose upward if necessary to achieve the desired clinical response. As with some plasma-derived factor IX products, patients at the low end of the observed factor IX recovery may require upward dosage adjustment to as much as two times (2X) the initial empirically calculated dose in order to achieve the intended rise in circulating factor IX activity.

Method of Calculating Dose: The method of calculating the factor IX dose is shown in the following equation:

$$\text{Number of factor IX IU required (IU)} = \text{Body weight (kg)} \times \text{Desired factor IX increase (\% or IU/dL)} \times \text{Reciprocal of observed recovery (IU/kg per IU/dL)}$$

In the presence of an inhibitor, higher doses may be required.

Adult Patients: In adult PTPs, on average, one international unit of BeneFIX per kilogram of body weight increased the circulating activity of factor IX by 0.8±0.2 (range 0.4 to 1.4) IU/dL. The method of dose estimation is illustrated in the following example. If you use 0.8 IU/dL average increase of factor IX per IU/kg body weight administered, then:

Number of factor IX IU required (IU)	=	Body weight (kg)	×	Desired factor IX increase (% or IU/dL)	×	1.2 (IU/kg per IU/dL)

Pediatric Patients (<15 years): In pediatric patients, on average, one international unit of BeneFIX per kilogram of body weight increased the circulating activity of factor IX by 0.7±0.3 (range 0.2 to 2.1) IU/dL. The method of dose estimation is illustrated in the following example. If you use 0.7 IU/dL average increase of factor IX per IU/kg body weight administered, then:

Number of factor IX IU required (IU)	=	Body weight (kg)	×	Desired factor IX increase (% or IU/dL)	×	1.4 (IU/kg per IU/dL)

Dosing for Bleeding Episodes and Surgery: Table 3 may be used to guide dosing in bleeding episodes and surgery:

Table 3: BeneFIX

Dosing in Bleeding Episodes and Surgery[a]

Type of Hemorrhage	Circulating Factor IX Activity Required (% or IU/dL)	Dosing Interval (h)	Duration of Therapy (days)
Minor Uncomplicated hemarthroses, superficial muscle, or soft tissue	20–30	12–24	1–2
Moderate Intramuscle or soft tissue with dissection, mucous membranes, dental extractions, or hematuria	25–50	12–24	Treat until bleeding stops and healing begins; about 2 to 7 days
Major Pharynx, retropharynx, retroperitoneum, CNS, surgery	50–100	12–24	7–10

[a] Adapted from: Roberts and Eberst.

Administration (Intravenous Injection): BeneFIX is administered by intravenous (IV) infusion after reconstitution with 0.234% sodium chloride solution.

BeneFIX should be administered using the infusion set provided in this kit, and the pre-filled diluent syringe provided or a single sterile disposable plastic syringe. In addition, the solution should be withdrawn from the vial using the vial adapter.

Detailed instructions for preparation and administration are contained in Part III: Consumer Information.

Reconstitute lyophilized BeneFIX powder for injection with the supplied diluent (0.234% sodium chloride solution) from the pre-filled syringe provided. Gently rotate the vial until all powder is dissolved.

After reconstitution, the solution is drawn back into the syringe. The solution should be clear and colorless. The solution should be discarded if visible particulate matter or discoloration is observed.

Note: Agglutination of red blood cells in the tubing/syringe has been reported with the administration of BeneFIX. No adverse events have been reported in association with this observation. To minimize the possibility of agglutination, it is important to limit the amount of blood entering the tubing. Blood should not enter the syringe. If red blood cell agglutination is observed in the tubing or syringe, discard all material (tubing, syringe and BeneFIX solution) and resume administration with a new package.

After reconstitution, BeneFIX should be injected intravenously over several minutes. The rate of administration should be determined by the patient's comfort level.

BeneFIX, when reconstituted, contains polysorbate-80, which is known to increase the rate of di-(2-ethylhexyl)phthalate (DEHP) extraction from polyvinyl chloride (PVC). This should be considered during the preparation and administration of BeneFIX, including storage time elapsed in a PVC container following reconstitution. It is important that the recommendations in Dosage and Administration be followed closely.

Dispose of all unused solution, empty vials, and used needles and syringes in an appropriate container for throwing away waste that might hurt others if not handled properly.

The administration of BeneFIX by continuous infusion has not been sufficiently evaluated in clinical trials to justify its use in this manner. BeneFIX should only be reconstituted with the diluent provided. BeneFIX should not be mixed with 5% dextrose or other parenteral infusion solutions.

OVERDOSAGE:

Symptoms: No symptoms of overdose are known.

For management of a suspected drug overdose, CPhA recommends that you contact your **regional Poison Control Centre**. See the *CPS* Directory section for a list of Poison Control Centres.

ACTION AND CLINICAL PHARMACOLOGY: Mechanism of Action: BeneFIX contains recombinant coagulation factor IX, (nonacog alfa). Recombinant coagulation factor IX is a single chain glycoprotein with an approximate molecular mass of 55 000 Daltons that is a member of the serine protease family of vitamin K-dependent coagulation factors. Recombinant coagulation factor IX is a recombinant DNA-based protein therapeutic, which has structural and functional characteristics comparable to endogenous factor IX. Factor IX is activated by factor VII/tissue factor complex in the extrinsic pathway as well as factor XIa in the intrinsic coagulation pathway. Activated factor IX, in combination with activated factor VIII, activates factor X. This results ultimately in the conversion of prothrombin to thrombin. Thrombin then converts fibrinogen into fibrin and a clot can be formed. Factor IX activity is absent or greatly reduced in patients with hemophilia B and substitution therapy may be required.

Hemophilia B is a sex-linked hereditary disorder of blood coagulation due to decreased levels of factor IX and results in profuse bleeding into joints, muscles or internal organs, either spontaneously or as a result of accidental or surgical trauma. By replacement therapy the plasma levels of factor IX are increased, thereby enabling a temporary correction of the factor deficiency and correction of the bleeding tendencies.

Pharmacodynamics: Factor IX is activated by factor VII/tissue factor complex in the extrinsic coagulation pathway as well as by factor XIa in the intrinsic coagulation pathway. Activated factor IX, in combination with activated factor VIII, activates factor X. This results ultimately in the conversion of prothrombin to thrombin. Thrombin then converts fibrinogen to fibrin, and a clot can be formed.

Factor IX is the specific clotting factor deficient in patients with hemophilia B and in patients with acquired factor IX deficiencies. The administration of BeneFIX Coagulation Factor IX (Recombinant), increases plasma levels of factor IX and can temporarily correct the coagulation defect in these patients.

Pharmacokinetics: After single intravenous (IV) doses of 50 IU/kg of BeneFIX, Coagulation Factor IX (Recombinant), in 37 previously treated adult patients (>15 years), each given as a 10-minute infusion, the mean increase from pre-infusion level in circulating factor IX activity was 0.8±0.2 IU/dL per IU/kg infused (range 0.4 to 1.4 IU/dL per IU/kg) and the mean biologic half-life was 18.8±5.4 hours (range 11 to 36 hours). In subsequent evaluations for up to 24 months, the pharmacokinetic parameters were similar to the initial results.

In the randomized, cross-over pharmacokinetic study in previously treated patients (PTPs), the in vivo recovery using BeneFIX was statistically significantly less (28% lower) than the recovery using a highly purified plasma-derived factor IX product. There was no significant difference in biological half-life. Structural differences of the rFIX molecule compared with pdFIX were shown to contribute to the lower recovery.

For specific information regarding pediatric pharmacology, see Warnings and Precautions, Special Populations.

Special Populations and Conditions: Pediatrics: See Warnings and Precautions, Special Populations.

Geriatrics: See Warnings and Precautions, Special Populations.

Hepatic Insufficiency: See Warnings and Precautions, Hepatic/Biliary/Pancreas.

Renal Insufficiency: See Warnings and Precautions, Hepatic/Biliary/Pancreas.

STORAGE AND STABILITY: Product as packaged for sale: BeneFIX, Coagulation Factor IX (Recombinant), should be stored under refrigeration at a temperature of 2 to 8°C. Prior to the expiration date, BeneFIX may also be stored at room temperature not to exceed 25°C for up to 6 months. The patient should make note of the date the product was placed at room temperature in the space provided on the outer carton. Freezing should be avoided to prevent damage to the diluent syringe.

Do not use BeneFIX after the expiry date on the label.

Product after reconstitution: The product does not contain a preservative and should be used within 3 hours.

SPECIAL HANDLING INSTRUCTIONS: Reconstituted Solutions: Detailed instructions for preparation and administration are contained in Part III: Information for the Patient. Patients should follow the specific reconstitution and administration procedures provided by their physicians.

Always wash your hands before performing the following procedures. Aseptic technique should be used during the reconstitution procedure.

BeneFIX, Coagulation Factor IX (Recombinant), will be administered by intravenous (IV) infusion after reconstitution with 0.234% sodium chloride solution (diluent).

BeneFIX should be administered within 3 hours after reconstitution. The reconstituted solution may be stored at room temperature prior to administration.

Table 4: BeneFIX

Parenteral Products (for reconstitution before use)

Vial Size	Volume of Diluent to Be Added to Vial	Nominal Concentration per mL
250 IU	5 mL	50 IU
500 IU	5 mL	100 IU
1000 IU	5 mL	200 IU
2000 IU	5 mL	400 IU

Reconstitute with 0.234% sodium chloride solution (USP).

INFORMATION FOR THE PATIENT: Published in e-CPS, available by subscription at www.e-cps.ca.

DOSAGE FORMS, COMPOSITION AND PACKAGING: Each single use vial of sterile, nonpyrogenic, lyophilized powder preparation for i.v. injection contains: coagulation factor IX (recombinant) nominally 250, 500, 1000 and 2000 IU. Nonmedicinal ingredients: glycine, L-histidine, polysorbate and sucrose. Includes one pre-filled syringe of solvent (5 mL sterile 0.234% sodium chloride solution for injection for reconstitution) with one plunger rod, one sterile vial adapter reconstitution device, one sterile infusion set, and two alcohol swabs, one plaster and one gauze pad. Actual factor IX activity in IU is stated on the label of each vial. Prior to use, the 250, 500, 1000 and 2000 IU per vial dosage forms are reconstituted in 5 mL of 0.234% sodium chloride solution. The reconstituted product contains approximately: 50, 100, 200 and 400 IU/mL Factor IX, respectively.

After reconstitution of the lyophilized drug product, the concentrations of the excipients are 0.234% sodium chloride, 8 mM L-histidine, 0.8% sucrose, 208 mM glycine and 0.004% polysorbate 80.

The container closure system for BeneFIX consists of a 10 mL USP Type I glass vial, a 20 mm grey rubber stopper, and a 20 mm diameter flip-off crimp seal.

Benoxyl® 5%

benzoyl peroxide

Keratolytic—Acne Therapy

Stiefel, a GSK company

Benoxyl® 10% and 20% Ⓟ

benzoyl peroxide

Keratolytic—Acne Therapy

Stiefel, a GSK company

SUPPLIED: Each mL of lotion contains: benzoyl peroxide 5%, 10% or 20% in a greaseless, washable lotion base. Nonmedicinal ingredients: glyceryl monostearate, imidurea, isopropyl palmitate, polyethylene glycol 20 monostearate, propylene glycol, purified water, stearic acid, xanthan gum and zinc stearate. Plastic bottles of 30 mL (5%) and 60 mL (5%, 10%, 20%) with dispenser top. Protect from heat.

Bentylol®

dicyclomine HCl

Antispasmodic

Axcan Pharma

PHARMACOLOGY: BENTYLOL (dicyclomine) relieves smooth muscle spasm of the gastrointestinal tract. Animal studies indicate that this action is achieved via a dual mechanism: 1) a specific anticholinergic effect (antimuscarinic) at the acetylcholine (ACh)-receptor sites with approximately 1/8 the milligram potency of atropine (in vitro guinea pig ileum); 2) a direct effect upon smooth muscle (musculotropic) as evidenced by dicyclomine's antagonism of bradykinin- and histamine-induced spasms of the isolated guinea pig ileum. Atropine did not affect responses to these 2 agonists. Animal studies showed dicyclomine to be equally potent against ACh- or barium chloride ($BaCl_2$)-induced intestinal spasm while atropine was at least 200 times more potent against the effects of ACh than against $BaCl_2$. Tests for mydriatic effects in mice showed that dicyclomine was approximately 1/500 as potent as atropine; antisialagogue tests in rabbits showed dicyclomine to be 1/300 as potent as atropine.

After a single oral 20 mg dose of dicyclomine in volunteers, peak plasma concentration reached a mean value of 58 ng/mL in 1 to 1.5 hours. The principal route of elimination is via the urine.

INDICATIONS: For the treatment of functional gastrointestinal tract conditions involving smooth muscle spasm such as irritable colon (mucous colitis, spastic colon, irritable bowel syndrome) and spastic constipation. It can also be used as adjunctive therapy in organic gastrointestinal conditions to relieve associated smooth muscle spasm such as in colitis, diverticulitis, regional enteritis, gastritis, and peptic ulcer.

CONTRAINDICATIONS: Known idiosyncrasy to BENTYLOL (dicyclomine). Infants less than 6 months of age (see Warnings) and in nursing mothers (see Precautions). Should not be used in patients with obstructive uropathy, obstructive disease of the gastrointestinal tract, paralytic ileus and intestinal atony, severe ulcerative colitis, myasthenia gravis, reflux esophagitis, glaucoma, unstable cardiovascular status in acute hemorrhage.

WARNINGS: Infants: There are reports of infants who, in their first 3 months of life, were given BENTYLOL (dicyclomine) syrup and evidenced respiratory symptoms (breathing difficulty, shortness of breath, breathlessness, respiratory collapse, apnea), as well as seizures, syncope, asphyxia, pulse rate fluctuations, muscular hypotonia, and coma. In some instances, these symptoms occurred within minutes of ingestion and lasted up to 20 to 30 minutes. The symptoms were reported in association with dicyclomine syrup therapy but a proven cause and effect relationship has not been established.

Worldwide, a few deaths have been reported in infants 3 months of age or less who had been given dicyclomine syrup. Two of these were reported to have been associated with excessively high dicyclomine blood levels.

Although no causal relationship between these effects, observed in infants, and dicyclomine administration has been established, dicyclomine is contraindicated in infants 6 months of age or less (see Contraindications).

Other: Diarrhea may be an early symptom of incomplete intestinal obstruction, especially in patients with ileostomy or colostomy. In this instance, treatment with this drug would be inappropriate and possibly harmful.
Occupational Hazards: Dicyclomine may produce drowsiness or blurred vision. The patient should be warned not to engage in activities requiring mental alertness, such as operating a motor vehicle or other machinery or performing hazardous work while taking this drug.

Psychosis has been reported in sensitive individuals given anticholinergic drugs. CNS signs and symptoms include confusion, disorientation, short-term memory loss, hallucinations, dysarthria, ataxia, coma, euphoria, decreased anxiety, fatigue, insomnia, agitation and mannerisms, and inappropriate affect. These CNS signs and symptoms usually resolve within 12 to 24 hours after discontinuation of the drug.

PRECAUTIONS: General: BENTYLOL (dicyclomine) should be used with caution in any patient with, or suspected of having: prostatic hypertrophy, hiatal hernia associated with reflux esophagitis because anticholinergic drugs may aggravate the condition, autonomic neuropathy, hepatic or renal disease, hyperthyroidism, hypertension, coronary heart disease, congestive heart failure, cardiac tachyarrhythmia.
Pregnancy: Epidemiologic studies in pregnant women with products containing dicyclomine (at doses up to 40 mg/day) have not shown that dicyclomine increases the risk of fetal abnormalities if administered during the first trimester of pregnancy. There are however no adequate and well-controlled studies in pregnant women at the recommended doses (80 to 160 mg/day). Animal reproduction studies have revealed no evidence of impaired fertility or harm to the fetus due to dicyclomine. Because animal reproduction studies are not always predictive of human response, BENTYLOL (dicyclomine) should be used during pregnancy only if required.
Lactation: Since dicyclomine has been reported to be excreted in human milk, BENTYLOL is contraindicated in nursing mothers (see Contraindications).
Drug Interactions: The following agents may increase certain actions or side effects of anticholinergic drugs: amantadine, antiarrhythmic agents of class I (e.g., quinidine), antihistamines, antipsychotic agents (e.g., phenothiazines), benzodiazepines, MAO inhibitors, narcotic analgesics (e.g., meperidine), nitrates and nitrites, sympathomimetic agents, tricyclic antidepressants, and other drugs having anticholinergic activity.

Anticholinergics antagonize the effects of antiglaucoma agents. Anticholinergic drugs in the presence of increased intraocular pressure may be hazardous when taken concurrently with agents such as corticosteroids.

Anticholinergic agents may affect gastrointestinal absorption of various drugs, such as slowly dissolving dosage forms of digoxin; increased serum digoxin concentrations may result. Anticholinergic drugs may antagonize the effects of drugs that alter gastrointestinal motility such as metoclopramide. Because antacids may interfere with the absorption of anticholinergic agents, simultaneous use of these drugs should be avoided.

The inhibiting effects of anticholinergic drugs on gastric hydrochloric acid secretion are antagonized by agents used to treat achlorhydria and those to test gastric secretion.

ADVERSE EFFECTS: Most adverse reactions reported in clinical trials conducted with dicyclomine were typically anticholinergic in nature and included, in decreasing order of frequency: dry mouth, dizziness, blurred vision, nausea, lightheadedness, drowsiness, weakness and nervousness.

Other adverse reactions reported with BENTYLOL (dicyclomine) and pharmacologically similar drugs, e.g., other anticholinergics and antispasmodics, were the following:
Gastrointestinal: vomiting, constipation, bloated feeling, abdominal pain, taste loss, anorexia.
Central Nervous System: tingling, headache, numbness, mental confusion and/or excitement (especially in elderly persons), dyskinesia, lethargy, syncope, speech disturbance, insomnia.
Ophthalmologic: diplopia, mydriasis, cycloplegia, increased ocular tension.
Dermatologic/Allergic: rash, urticaria, itching, and other dermal manifestations; severe allergic reaction or drug idiosyncrasies including anaphylaxis.
Genitourinary: urinary hesitancy, urinary retention.
Cardiovascular: tachycardia, palpitations.
Respiratory: dyspnea, apnea, asphyxia.
Other: decreased sweating, nasal stuffiness or congestion, sneezing, throat congestion, impotence, suppression of lactation (see Precautions).

OVERDOSE:
Symptoms: Signs and symptoms of BENTYLOL (dicyclomine) overdosage are headache; nausea; vomiting; blurred vision; dilated pupils; hot, dry skin; dizziness; dry mouth; difficulty in swallowing; and CNS stimulation. A curare-like action may occur (i.e., neuromuscular blockage leading to muscular weakness and possible paralysis).
Treatment: Treatment should consist of gastric lavage, emetics and activated charcoal. Sedatives (e.g., short-acting barbiturates, benzodiazepines) may be used for management of overt signs of excitement. If indicated, an appropriate parenteral cholinergic agent may be used as an antidote.
Dialysis: It is not known if dicyclomine is dialyzable.

> For management of a suspected drug overdose, CPhA recommends that you contact your **regional Poison Control Centre**. See the *CPS* Directory section for a list of Poison Control Centres.

DOSAGE: Dosage should be adjusted to individual patient needs.
Syrup and Tablets: Adults: 10 to 20 mg 3 to 4 times daily. Depending upon the patient's response during the first week of therapy, the dose should be increased to 160 mg/day unless side effects limit dose escalation. If efficacy is not achieved within 2 weeks or side effects require doses below 80 mg/day, the drug should be discontinued. Documented safety data are not available for doses above 80 mg daily for periods longer than 2 weeks.
Children (2 to 12 years): 10 mg 3 to 4 times daily.
Infants (6 months to 2 years): 5 to 10 mg 3 to 4 times daily, 15 minutes before feeding. Do not exceed 40 mg daily. Syrup should be diluted with equal volume of water.

SUPPLIED: Syrup: Each 5 mL of clear, red viscous syrup with a taste characteristic of raspberries, contains: dicyclomine HCl USP 10 mg. Nonmedicinal ingredients: amaranth color, blackcurrant artificial flavour, cherry natural/artificial flavour, citric acid, FD&C Yellow No. 6, glucose, methylparaben, propylene glycol, propylparaben, purified water, raspberry imitation fritzbro, sodium citrate, sodium cyclamate and vanilla flavour imitation. Bottles of 250 mL. Store at 15 to 30°C. Protect from excessive heat.
Tablets: 10 mg: Each white, round, flat-faced, beveled edged tablet, one side debossed with the letter "M" in a double circle, and the other with the number "10" contains: dicyclomine HCl USP 10 mg. Nonmedicinal ingredients: cornstarch, lactose monohydrate, magnesium stearate, microcrystalline cellulose and talc. Bottles of 100. Store at 15 to 30°C. Protect from excessive heat and moisture.
20 mg: Each white, round, flat-faced, beveled edged tablet, one side debossed with the letter "M" in a double circle, and the other side scored with the number "20" contains: dicyclomine HCl USP 20 mg. Nonmedicinal ingredients: cornstarch, lactose monohydrate, magnesium stearate, microcrystalline cellulose and talc. Bottles of 100. Store at 15 to 30°C. Protect from excessive heat and moisture.

(Shown in Product Identification Section)

Benuryl™ Ⓟ
probenecid
Uricosuric

Valeant

SUPPLIED: Each white, round, scored tablet, imprinted ICN B11, contains: probenecid, USP 500 mg. Nonmedicinal ingredients: colloidal silicon dioxide, lactose, magnesium stearate, microcrystalline cellulose, sodium starch glycolate, starch and talc. Bottles of 100 and 500.

Benylin® All-in-One® Cold and Flu Night PE
acetaminophen—phenylephrine HCl—diphenhydramine HCl
Analgesic—Decongestant—Antihistamine—Cough Suppressant

McNeil Consumer Healthcare

Benylin® 1 All-in-One® Cold and Flu
dextromethorphan HBr—pseudoephedrine HCl—guaifenesin—acetaminophen
Antitussive—Decongestant—Expectorant—Analgesic

McNeil Consumer Healthcare

Benylin® 1 All-in-One® Cold and Flu Nightime
dextromethorphan HBr—pseudoephedrine HCl—guaifenesin—acetaminophen—chlorpheniramine maleate
Antitussive—Decongestant—Expectorant—Analgesic—Antihistamine

McNeil Consumer Healthcare

Benylin® 2 All-in-One® Cold and Flu with Codeine (Non-prescription) Ⓝ
codeine phosphate—pseudoephedrine HCl—guaifenesin
Antitussive—Decongestant—Expectorant

McNeil Consumer Healthcare

Benylin® Cold and Sinus
phenylephrine HCl—acetaminophen
Decongestant—Analgesic

McNeil Consumer Healthcare

Benylin® Cold and Sinus Plus
phenylephrine HCl—acetaminophen—chlorpheniramine maleate
Decongestant—Analgesic—Antihistamine

McNeil Consumer Healthcare

Benylin® DM-D-E-A Cold and Sinus Rapid Gels
dextromethorphan HBr—pseudoephedrine HCl—guaifenesin—acetaminophen
Antitussive—Decongestant—Expectorant—Analgesic

McNeil Consumer Healthcare

Benylin® Night Cough
diphenhydramine HCl
Antitussive

McNeil Consumer Healthcare

Benylin® DM
dextromethorphan HBr
Antitussive

McNeil Consumer Healthcare

Benylin® DM 12 Hour (Nightime)
dextromethorphan polistirex
Antitussive

McNeil Consumer Healthcare

Benylin® DM for Children
dextromethorphan HBr
Antitussive

McNeil Consumer Healthcare

Benylin® DM for Children 12 Hour (Bedtime)
dextromethorphan polistirex
Antitussive

McNeil Consumer Healthcare

Benylin® DM-D (Adult)
dextromethorphan HBr—pseudoephedrine HCl
Antitussive—Decongestant

McNeil Consumer Healthcare

Benylin® DM-D for Children
dextromethorphan HBr—pseudoephedrine HCl
Antitussive—Decongestant

McNeil Consumer Healthcare

Benylin® DM-D-E Extra Strength with Menthactin®
dextromethorphan HBr—pseudoephedrine HCl—guaifenesin—menthol
Antitussive—Decongestant—Expectorant—Anesthetic—Analgesic

McNeil Consumer Healthcare

Benylin® DM-E
dextromethorphan HBr—guaifenesin
Antitussive—Expectorant

McNeil Consumer Healthcare

Benylin® DM-E Extra Strength with Menthactin®
dextromethorphan HBr—guaifenesin—menthol
Antitussive—Expectorant—Anesthetic—Analgesic

McNeil Consumer Healthcare

Benylin® E Extra Strength with Menthactin®
guaifenesin—menthol
Expectorant—Anesthetic—Analgesic

McNeil Consumer Healthcare

Date of Revision: August 2008

INDICATIONS: DM/Codeine: Antitussive Products (dextromethorphan)/(codeine): Suppression of dry hacking coughs.
E: Expectorant Products (guaifenesin): Loosens mucus/phlegm in chest coughs due to colds.
D: Decongestant Products (pseudoephedrine, phenylephrine): Relieves nasal congestion.
A: Analgesic/Antipyretic (acetaminophen): Relieves pain, fever, chills, headache, body aches, and sore throat pain.
AH (chlorpheniramine, diphenhydramine): Relieves runny nose, sneezing and itchy, watery eyes.
Benylin 1 Cold and Flu Caplets: For relief of: pain, fever, headache, stuffy nose, sore throat pain, dry cough, chest congestion, chills.
Benylin DM-D-E Extra Strength with Menthactin (dextromethorphan, pseudoephedrine, guaifenesin, menthol): For fast acting relief of cough, cold and sore throat.
Benylin DM-E Extra Strength with Menthactin (dextromethorphan, guaifenesin, menthol): For fast acting relief of chest cough and sore throat.
Benylin E Extra Strength with Menthactin (guaifenesin, menthol): For fast acting relief of chest congestion and sore throat.
Benylin Night Cough (diphenhydramine hydrochloride): For relief of dry cough.

CONTRAINDICATIONS: Sensitivity to any of the components.
DM or Codeine: Pre-existing respiratory depression.
DM or D (Decongestant): Patients receiving or having received MAO inhibitors in the preceding 3 weeks.

WARNINGS: Acetaminophen: Massive acetaminophen overdose can be toxic and potentially fatal. In adults, hepatotoxicity from acetaminophen is unlikely to occur with overdoses at less than 10 g ingested at one time and fatalities are unlikely to occur with overdoses of less than 15 g ingested at one time.
Benylin All-in-One Cold and Flu Night PE Caplets, Benylin 1 Cold and Flu Caplets, Benylin 1 Cold and Flu Syrup, Benylin Cold & Sinus, Benylin Night Cough: Do not use with other products containing any of these ingredients (see Supplied). Doing so may result in accidental overdose.

This package contains enough medicine to seriously harm a child. Keep out of reach of children. Avoid Alcohol. Use only on the advice of a doctor. Talk to a doctor before using this product if you have chronic alcoholism, serious liver or kidney disease, high blood pressure, heart or thyroid disease, diabetes, asthma, chronic lung disease/shortness of breath, persistent/chronic cough, glaucoma or difficulty urinating due to enlargement of prostate gland, or are elderly, pregnant, breast-feeding, or taking a drug for depression, including monoamine oxidase (MAO) inhibitor drugs. Check with a doctor if symptoms do not improve within 5 days or if cough worsens, lasts more than 7 days, or tends to recur or if you also have excessive secretions or fever for more than 3 days. Taking more than the recommended dose can cause serious liver damage, nervousness, dizziness or sleeplessness. In case of accidental overdose contact a doctor or Poison Control Centre immediately, even if there are no symptoms.
Benylin 1 Nightime Syrup: All warnings listed above apply. In addition, talk to a doctor before using this product if you are also taking other drugs such as antihistamines, sedatives and tranquilizers.

PRECAUTIONS: Before prescribing medication to suppress or modify cough, it is important to ascertain that the underlying cause of the cough is identified, that modification of the cough does not increase the risk of clinical or physiologic complications, and that appropriate therapy for the primary disease is provided.

If cough worsens, lasts for more than 1 week, tends to recur, or is accompanied by high fever, consult a physician. Do not exceed recommended dosage. Keep safely out of reach of children.

Caution should be exercised and dosage may need to be reduced when a codeine or dextromethorphan containing product is administered with other drugs which depress the CNS (including alcohol), phenothiazines or tricyclic antidepressants.
Codeine: May cause drowsiness, do not drive. In young children the respiratory centre is especially susceptible to the depressant action of narcotic cough suppressants. Benefit to risk ratio should be carefully considered especially in children with respiratory embarrassment, e.g., croup. Estimation of dosage relative to the child's age and weight is of great importance.
Dextromethorphan (DM) or Guaifenesin (E): Not recommended for patients with asthma, chronic lung disease, shortness of breath or persistent chronic cough unless directed by a physician.
Pseudoephedrine, Phenylephrine (D): This product should be used with caution in diabetics, hypertensive patients and patients with glaucoma, coronary artery disease, hyperthyroidism, urinary retention due to prostate enlargement.
Acetaminophen: This product should be used with caution in persons with chronic alcoholism, serious liver or kidney diseases. If symptoms do not improve in 5 days, consult a physician. Do not use with other products containing acetaminophen.
Chlorpheniramine, Diphenhydramine: Do not engage in activities requiring alertness.
Geriatrics: In elderly patients, consult a physician before using these products.
Pregnancy: In pregnant patients, consult a physician before using these products.
Lactation: In nursing patients, consult a physician before using these products.
Benylin DM for Children, Benylin DM-D for Children: In cases of overdose, the respiratory centre in young children is especially susceptible to depression. Estimation of dosage relative to the child's age and weight is of great importance.

Do not use in cases of high blood pressure, heart or thyroid disease, diabetes or asthma, except on the advice of a physician. Do not exceed recommended dosage. If cough worsens, lasts for more than 1 week, tends to recur, or is accompanied by high fever, consult a physician. Keep safely out of reach of children.

ADVERSE EFFECTS: Benylin DM (Adult and Children) or Benylin DM-E: Drowsiness, dizziness, constipation, nausea, vomiting and confusion have been encountered.
Benylin DM-D (Adult and Children), Benylin DM-D-E, Benylin 2 Cold and Flu with Codeine: Drowsiness, nausea, vomiting, constipation, palpitation, confusion, dizziness and tightness in the chest may be encountered.
Benylin E Extra Strength with Menthactin: Nausea, gastrointestinal upset and drowsiness occur infrequently.

OVERDOSE:

> For management of a suspected drug overdose, CPhA recommends that you contact your **regional Poison Control Centre**. See the *CPS* Directory section for a list of Poison Control Centres.

DOSAGE: Benylin All-in-One Cold and Flu Night PE (caplets): Adults and children 12 years and over: 2 caplets every 6 hours while symptoms persist. Do not exceed 8 caplets per day. Not recommended for children under 12 years.
Benylin 1 All-in-One Cold and Flu (caplets): Adults and children 12 years and over: 2 caplets every 6 hours. Maximum 8 caplets per day. Not recommended for children under 12 years.
Benylin 1 All-in-One Cold and Flu (syrup): Adults and children 12 years and over: 30 mL every 6 hours. Maximum 4 doses/day. Not recommended for children under 12 years.
Benylin 1 All-in-One Cold and Flu Nightime (syrup): Adults and children 12 years and over: 2 tablespoons (30 mL) every 6 hours. Maximum 4 doses/day. Not recommended for children under 12 years.
Benylin 2 All-in-One Cold and Flu with Codeine (Non-prescription): Adults: 10 mL every 6 hours. Up to a maximum of 4 doses/day.
Benylin Cold and Sinus: Adults: 1 to 2 caplets every 4-6 hours. Do not exceed 8 caplets per day.
Benylin Cold and Sinus Plus: Adults: 1 to 2 caplets every 4-6 hours. Do not exceed 8 caplets per day.
Benylin DM-D-E-A Cold and Sinus Rapid Gels: Adults/Children 12 years and older: 2 capsules every 4-6 hours. Do not exceed 8 capsules per day.
Benylin Night Cough: Adults and children 12 years and over: Take 1 capsule at night before bed.
Benylin DM: Adults and children 12 years and over: 10 mL every 6 hours. Children: 6 to 11 years: 5 mL every 6 hours; 2 to 5 years: 2.5 mL every 6 hours. Maximum 4 doses/day.
Benylin DM 12 Hour: Adults and children 12 years and over: 10 mL every 12 hours. Children 6 to 11 years: 5 mL every 12 hours. Children 2 to 5 years: 2.5 mL every 12 hours. Maximum 2 doses/day. Not recommended for children under 2 years of age except on the advice of a physician.
Benylin DM for Children: Children 6 to 11 years: 10 mL every 6 hours. 2 to 5 years: 5 mL every 6 hours. Maximum 4 doses/day. Not recommended for children under 2 years of age except on the advice of a physician.
Benylin DM for Children 12 Hour: Children 6 to 11 years (22 to 44 kg): 10 mL every 12 hours. Children 2 to 5 years (11 to 22 kg): 5 mL every 12 hours. Maximum 2 doses/day.
Benylin DM-D for Children: 6 to under 12 years: 10 mL every 6 hours. 2 to 5 years: 5 mL every 6 hours. Under 2 years: Consult a doctor.
Benylin DM-E, Benylin DM-D (Adult), Benylin DM-D-E: Adults and children 12 years and over: 10 mL every 6 hours. Children: 6 to 11 years: 5 mL every 6 hours; 2 to 5 years: 2.5 mL every 6 hours. Maximum 4 doses/day.
Benylin DM-D-E Extra Strength with Menthactin: Adults and children over 12 years: 10 mL every 6 hours. Maximum 4 doses/day. Not recommended for children under 12 years.
Benylin DM-E Extra Strength with Menthactin: Adults and children 12 years and over: 10 mL every 6 hours. Maximum 4 doses/day. Not recommended for children under 12 years.
Benylin E Extra Strength with Menthactin: Adults and Children 12 years and over: 5 to 10 mL every 6 hours. Maximum 40 mL/day. Not recommended for children under 12 years.

SUPPLIED: Benylin All-in-One Cold and Flu Night PE (Caplets): Each caplet contains: acetaminophen 325 mg, phenylephrine HCl 5 mg and diphenhydramine HCl 25 mg. Nonmedicinal ingredients: cellulose, corn starch, FD&C Blue No. 1 aluminum Lake, hypromellose, polyethylene glycol, polysorbate, povidone, silicon dioxide, starch, stearic acid, titanium dioxide and wax. Gluten-, lactose-, paraben-, sucrose- and tartrazine-free. Child resistant packages of 24. Store between 15 and 30°C. Protect from light. Keep dry.
Benylin 1 All-in-One Cold and Flu (Caplets): Each caplet contains: acetaminophen 500 mg, dextromethorphan HBr 15 mg, pseudoephedrine HCl 30 mg and guaifenesin 100 mg. Nonmedicinal ingredients: cellulose, D&C Yellow No. 10 aluminum Lake, FD&C Blue No. 1 aluminum Lake, hypromellose, polyethylene glycol, polysorbate, polyvinyl pyrrolidone, silica, starch, stearic acid, titanium dioxide, wax and zinc stearate. Gluten-, lactose-, paraben-, sucrose- and tartrazine-free. Child resistant packages of 12. Store between 15 and 30°C
Benylin 1 All-in-One Cold and Flu (Syrup): Each 15 mL of syrup contains: dextromethorphan HBr 15 mg, pseudoephedrine HCl 30 mg, guaifenesin 100 mg and acetaminophen 500 mg. Nonmedicinal ingredients: alcohol, artificial sweetness enhancer, citric acid, D&C Red No. 33, flavor, glycerin, menthol, monoammonium glycyrrhizinate, polyethylene glycol, propylene glycol, saccharin sodium, sodium benzoate, sodium carboxymethylcellulose, sodium citrate, sodium cyclamate, sorbitol and water. Energy: 82.44 kJ (19.7 kcal)/15 mL. Bottles of 180 mL.
Benylin 1 All-in-One Cold and Flu Nightime (Syrup): Each 15 mL of syrup contains: acetaminophen 500 mg, dextromethorphan HBr 15 mg, pseudoephedrine HCl 30 mg, guaifenesin 100 mg and chlorpheniramine maleate 2 mg. Nonmedicinal ingredients: alcohol, artificial sweetness enhancer, benzyl alcohol, citric acid, D&C Red No. 33, flavor, glycerin, menthol, monoammonium glycyrrhizinate, polyethylene glycol, propylene glycol, saccharin sodium, sodium benzoate, sodium carboxymethylcellulose, sodium citrate, sodium cyclamate, sorbitol and water. Energy: 19.7 kcal/15 mL. Corn-, gluten-, lactose-, paraben-, sucrose- and tartrazine-free. Bottles of 170 mL. Store between 15 and 30°C.
Benylin 2 All-in-One Cold and Flu with Codeine (Non-prescription) Syrup Ⓝ: Each 5 mL contains: codeine phosphate 3.3 mg, pseudoephedrine HCl 30 mg and guaifenesin 100 mg. Nonmedicinal ingredients: alcohol, citric acid, D&C Red No. 33, FD&C Red No. 2, flavor, glycerin, menthol, polyethylene glycol, propyl gallate, sodium benzoate, sodium carboxymethylcellulose, sodium citrate, sodium cyclamate, sorbitol and water. Energy: 42.7 kJ (10.2 kcal)/5 mL. Sodium: <1.1 mmol (25 mg)/5 mL. Gluten-, lactose-, paraben-, sucrose-, sulfite- and tartrazine-free. Bottles of 100 mL.
Benylin Cold and Sinus: Each caplet contains: acetaminophen 500 mg and phenylephrine HCl 5 mg. Nonmedicinal ingredients: celluloses, corn starch, FD&C Blue No. 2 aluminum Lake, FD&C Red 40 aluminum lake, FD&C Yellow No. 6, aluminum Lake, iron oxide yellow, polyethylene glycol, polyvinyl alcohol, povidone, silicon dioxide, stearic acid, talc and titanium dioxide. Gluten-, lactose-, paraben-, sucrose-, sulfite- and tartrazine-free. Child resistant packages of 24 and 48. Store between 15 and 30°C.
Benylin Cold and Sinus Plus: Each caplet contains: acetaminophen 500 mg, phenylephrine HCl 5 mg and chlorpheniramine maleate 2 mg. Nonmedicinal ingredients: celluloses, corn starch, FD&C Blue No. 1 aluminum Lake, FD&C Yellow No. 6 aluminum Lake, polyethylene glycol, polyvinyl alcohol, povidone, quinoline yellow aluminum lake, silicon dioxide, stearic acid, talc and titanium dioxide. Gluten-, lactose-, paraben-, sucrose-, sulfite- and tartrazine-free. Child resistant packages of 24 and 48. Store between 15 and 30°C.
Benylin DM-D-E-A Cold and Sinus Rapid Gels: Each soft gelatin capsule contains: dextromethorphan HBr 10 mg, pseudoephedrine HCl 30 mg, guaifenesin 100 mg and acetaminophen 250 mg. Nonmedicinal ingredients: D&C Yellow No. 10, FD&C Red No. 40, gelatin, polyethylene glycol, povidone, propylene glycol and water. Gluten-, lactose-, paraben-, sucrose-, sulfite- and tartrazine-free. Child resistant packages of 20. Store between 15 and 30°C. Protect from light. Keep dry.
Benylin Night Cough: Each soft gelatin capsule contains: diphenhydramine HCl 25 mg. Nonmedicinal ingredients: gelatin, glycerin, polyethylene glycol, sorbitol and titanium dioxide. Gluten-, lactose-, paraben-, sucrose-, sulfite- and tartrazine-free. Packages of 24. Store between 15 and 30°C. Protect from light. Keep dry.
Benylin DM: Each 5 mL of syrup contains: dextromethorphan HBr 15 mg. Nonmedicinal ingredients: artificial sweetness enhancer, citric acid, D&C Red No. 33, FD&C Red No. 40, flavor, glycerin, menthol, polyethylene glycol, sodium benzoate, sodium carboxymethylcellulose, sodium citrate, sodium cyclamate, sorbitol and water. Energy: 28 kJ (6.7 kcal)/5 mL. Sodium: <1 mmol (18.8 mg)/5 mL. Alcohol-, gluten-, lactose-, paraben-, sucrose-, sulfite- and tartrazine-free. Bottles of 100 and 250 mL.
Benylin DM 12 Hour: Each 5 mL of syrup contains: dextromethorphan polistirex in a controlled-release formula equivalent to dextromethorphan hydrobromide 30 mg. Nonmedicinal ingredients: D&C Red No. 33, disodium EDTA, flavor, menthol, parabens, polyethylene glycol, polysorbate, sorbitan monooleate, sorbitol, sucralose, tragacanth gum, water and xanthan gum. Energy: 12.6 kJ (3 kcal)/5 mL. Alcohol-, gluten-, lactose-, sucrose-, sulfite- and tartrazine-free. Bottles of 85 mL.
Benylin DM for Children: Each 5 mL of grape-flavored syrup contains: dextromethorphan HBr 7.5 mg. Nonmedicinal ingredients: citric acid, FD&C Blue No. 1, FD&C Red No. 2, flavor, glycerin, monoammonium glycyrrhizinate, sodium benzoate, sodium carboxymethylcellulose, sodium citrate, sodium cyclamate, sorbitol and water. Alcohol-, gluten-, lactose-, paraben-, sucrose-, sulfite- and tartrazine-free. Energy: 38.5 kJ (9.2 kcal)/5 mL. Bottles of 100 and 250 mL.
Benylin DM for Children 12 Hour: Each 5 mL of bubble gum flavored syrup contains: dextromethorphan polistirex in a controlled-release formula equivalent to dextromethorphan hydrobromide 15 mg. Nonmedicinal ingredients: D&C Red No. 33, disodium EDTA, flavor, maltol, parabens, polyethylene glycol, polysorbate, sorbitan monooleate, sorbitol, sucralose, tragacanth gum, water and xanthan gum. Energy: 12.6 kJ (3 kcal)/5 mL. Alcohol-, gluten-, lactose-, sucrose-, sulfite- and tartrazine-free. Bottles of 85 mL.
Benylin DM-D (Adult): Each 5 mL of syrup contains: dextromethorphan HBr 15 mg and pseudoephedrine HCl 30 mg. Nonmedicinal ingredients: artificial sweetness enhancer, citric acid, D&C Red No. 33, FD&C Red No. 40, flavor, glycerin, menthol, polyethylene glycol, sodium benzoate, sodium carboxymethylcellulose, sodium citrate, sodium cyclamate, sorbitol and water. Energy: 28 kJ (6.7 kcal)/5 mL. Sodium: <1 mmol (19 mg)/5 mL. Alcohol-, gluten-, lactose-, paraben-, sucrose-, sulfite- and tartrazine-free. Bottles of 100 mL.
Benylin DM-D for Children: Each 5 mL of grape-flavored syrup contains: dextromethorphan HBr 7.5 mg and pseudoephedrine HCl 15 mg. Nonmedicinal ingredients: cellulose, citric acid, FD&C Blue No. 1, FD&C Red No. 2, flavor, glycerin, monoammonium glycyrrhizinate, sodium benzoate, sodium citrate, sodium cyclamate, sorbitol and water. Energy: 38.6 kJ (9.2 kcal)/5 mL. Sodium: <1 mmol (11.04 mg)/5 mL. Alcohol-, gluten-, lactose-, paraben-, sucrose-, sulfite- and tartrazine-free. Bottles of 100 and 250 mL.

Benylin DM-D-E: Each 5 mL of syrup contains: dextromethorphan HBr 15 mg, pseudoephedrine HCl 30 mg and guaifenesin 100 mg. Nonmedicinal ingredients: alcohol, artificial sweetness enhancer, citric acid, D&C Red No. 33, FD&C Red No. 40, flavor, glycerin, menthol, polyethylene glycol, sodium benzoate, sodium carboxymethylcellulose, sodium citrate, sodium cyclamate, sorbitol and water. Energy: 34.7 kJ (8.3 kcal)/5 mL. Sodium: <1 mmol (20.6 mg)/5 mL. Gluten-, lactose-, paraben-, sucrose-, sulfite- and tartrazine-free. Bottles of 100 and 250 mL.

Benylin DM-D-E Extra Strength with Menthactin: Each 5 mL of syrup contains: dextromethorphan HBr 15 mg, pseudoephedrine HCl 30 mg, menthol 15 mg and guaifenesin 200 mg. Nonmedicinal ingredients: alcohol, citric acid, FD&C Blue No. 1, FD&C Red No. 40, flavor, glycerin, menthol, monoammonium glycyrrhizinate, polyethylene glycol, polyoxyl hydrogenated castor oil, propylene glycol, saccharin sodium, sodium benzoate, sodium chloride, sodium citrate, water and xanthan gum. Caloric content: 5.7 Kcal/5 mL. Gluten-, lactose-, paraben-, sucrose-, sulfite- and tartrazine-free. Bottles of 100 and 250 mL.

Benylin DM-E: Each 5 mL of syrup contains: dextromethorphan HBr 15 mg and guaifenesin 100 mg. Nonmedicinal ingredients: alcohol, artificial sweetness enhancer, citric acid, D&C Red No. 33, FD&C Red No. 40, flavor, glycerin, menthol, polyethylene glycol, sodium benzoate, sodium carboxymethylcellulose, sodium citrate, sodium cyclamate, sorbitol and water. Energy: 34.7 kJ (8.3 kcal)/5 mL. Sodium: <1 mmol (20.6 mg)/5 mL. Gluten-, lactose-, paraben-, sucrose-, sulfite- and tartrazine-free. Bottles of 100 and 250 mL.

Benylin DM-E Extra Strength with Menthactin: Each 5 mL of syrup contains: dextromethorphan HBr 15 mg, menthol 15 mg and guaifenesin 200 mg. Nonmedicinal ingredients: alcohol, citric acid, FD&C Blue No. 1, FD&C Red No. 40, flavor, glycerin, menthol, monoammonium glycyrrhizinate, polyethylene glycol, polyoxyl hydrogenated castor oil, propylene glycol, saccharin sodium, sodium benzoate, sodium chloride, sodium citrate, water and xanthan gum. Caloric content: 5.7 Kcal/5 mL. Gluten-, lactose-, paraben-, sucrose-, sulfite- and tartrazine-free. Bottles of 100 and 250 mL.

Benylin E Extra Strength with Menthactin: Each 5 mL of syrup contains: menthol 15 mg and guaifenesin 200 mg. Nonmedicinal ingredients: alcohol, citric acid, FD&C Blue No. 1, FD&C Red No. 40, flavor, glycerin, menthol, monoammonium glycyrrhizinate, polyethylene glycol, polyoxyl hydrogenated castor oil, propylene glycol, saccharin sodium, sodium benzoate, sodium chloride, sodium citrate, water, xanthan gum. Caloric content: 5.7 Kcal/5 mL. Gluten-, lactose-, paraben-, sucrose-, sulfite- and tartrazine-free. Bottles of 100 and 250 mL.

Benzac® AC 5
benzoyl peroxide
Acne Therapy

Galderma

Benzac® AC 10 ℞
benzoyl peroxide
Acne Therapy

Galderma

SUPPLIED: Each tube contains: benzoyl peroxide USP 5% or 10% in a water base gel. Nonmedicinal ingredients: acrylates copolymer, carbomer 940, docusate sodium, edetate disodium, glycerin, poloxamer 182, propylene glycol, purified water, silicon dioxide and sodium hydroxide. May contain citric acid to adjust pH. Plastic tubes of 60 g. Store at room temperature; avoid excessive heat.

BenzaClin® ℞
clindamycin phosphate—benzoyl peroxide
Acne Vulgaris Therapy

sanofi-aventis

Date of Revision: February 12, 2010

SUMMARY PRODUCT INFORMATION:

Route of Administration	Dosage Form/ Strength	Clinically Relevant Nonmedicinal Ingredients
Topical (dermal)	Topical Gel: 1% clindamycin, as phosphate and 5% benzoyl peroxide after reconstitution by the pharmacist	None For a complete listing of nonmedicinal ingredients, see Dosage Forms, Composition and Packaging.

INDICATIONS AND CLINICAL USE: BenzaClin Topical Gel (clindamycin, as phosphate, 1% and benzoyl peroxide 5%) is indicated for:

- The topical treatment of moderate acne vulgaris characterized by comedones, inflammatory papules/pustules, with or without an occasional cyst or nodule (Grade II to III)*.

  BenzaClin Topical Gel is not indicated for the treatment of cystic acne (Grade IV*).

CONTRAINDICATIONS:

- Patients who have a history of hypersensitivity to preparations containing clindamycin, lincomycin or any other component of the preparation. For a complete listing of the ingredients in the formulation, see Dosage Forms, Composition and Packaging.
- Patients with a history of regional enteritis, ulcerative colitis, or a history of antibiotic-associated colitis (see Warnings and Precautions).

WARNINGS AND PRECAUTIONS: General: For external (dermatological) use only. Not for ophthalmic use.

Concomitant topical acne therapy is not recommended because a possible cumulative irritancy effect may occur, especially with the use of peeling, desquamating, or abrasive agents.

Exposure to sunlight or unnecessary UV light should be minimized.

Gastrointestinal: Orally and parenterally administered clindamycin have been associated with severe colitis, which may result in patient death. Use of the topical formulation of clindamycin can result in absorption of the antibiotic from the skin surface. Diarrhea, bloody diarrhea, and colitis (including pseudomembranous colitis) have been reported with the use of topical and systemic clindamycin.

Studies indicate that a toxin produced by clostridia is a primary cause of antibiotic-associated colitis. The colitis is usually characterized by severe persistent diarrhea and severe abdominal cramps and may be associated with the passage of blood and mucus. Endoscopic examination may reveal pseudomembranous colitis. Stool culture for *C. difficile* and stool assay for *C. difficile* toxin may be helpful diagnostically. **When significant diarrhea occurs, the drug should be discontinued. Large bowel endoscopy should be considered to establish a definitive diagnosis in cases of severe diarrhea.**

Diarrhea, colitis, and pseudomembranous colitis have been observed to begin up to several weeks following cessation of oral and parenteral therapy with clindamycin.

Ophthalmologic/Mucosal/Skin: Avoid contact with eyes and mucous membranes. In the event of accidental contact with such sensitive surfaces (mucous membranes, eyes, abraded skin), rinse with large amounts of tepid tap water.

Special Populations: Pregnant Women: There are no well-controlled trials in pregnant women treated with BenzaClin Topical Gel (clindamycin, as phosphate, 1% and benzoyl peroxide 5%). It is not known whether BenzaClin Topical Gel can cause fetal harm when administered to a pregnant woman or can affect reproductive capacity. BenzaClin Topical Gel should not be given to a pregnant woman unless the benefits to the mother clearly outweigh the possible risks to the fetus.

Nursing Women: It is not known whether BenzaClin Topical Gel is excreted in human milk after topical application. However, orally and parenterally administered clindamycin has been reported to appear in breast milk. Because of the potential for serious adverse reactions in nursing infants, a decision should be made whether to discontinue nursing or to discontinue the drug, taking into account the importance of the drug to the mother.

* [Pillsbury DM., Heaton C. Manual of Dermatology 1980.]

Pediatrics (<12 years of age): The safety and effectiveness of this product in pediatric patients below the age of 12 have not been established.

Geriatrics (>65 years of age): The safety and effectiveness of this product in geriatric patients above the age of 65 years have not been established.

ADVERSE REACTIONS: Adverse Drug Reaction Overview: The most frequent adverse reactions that may occur with BenzaClin Topical Gel (clindamycin, as phosphate, 1% and benzoyl peroxide 5%) are mild to moderate adverse reactions of the skin; most commonly, dry skin.

Clinical Trial Adverse Drug Reactions: Because clinical trials are conducted under very specific conditions, the adverse reaction rates observed in the clinical trials may not reflect the rates observed in practice and should not be compared to the rates in the clinical trials of another drug. Adverse drug reaction information from clinical trials is useful for identifying drug-related adverse events and for approximating rates.

Table 1 presents a pooled summary of the most frequent (≥1%) adverse reactions reported during four randomized, double-blind, vehicle-controlled, multicentre trials conducted with BenzaClin Topical Gel in patients with moderate acne vulgaris. A total of 420 male and female patients with an average age of 19 years received BenzaClin Topical Gel in these studies; 168 patients received vehicle. The average duration of treatment with BenzaClin Topical Gel was 69 days.

Table 1: BenzaClin

Most Frequent Adverse Events (≥1%) Reported in the BenzaClin Topical Gel or Vehicle Groups Considered to be Possibly, Probably or Definitely Related to Product Administration

Body System: Skin and Appendages	BenzaClin Topical Gel n=420 %	Vehicle n=168 %
Very Common Adverse Reaction		
Dry Skin	12	6
Common Adverse Reactions		
Application Site Reaction	3	<1
Peeling	2	—
Pruritus	2	<1
Erythema	1	<1

Sunburn was observed in 1% of the BenzaClin Topical Gel group but considered related to the drug in less than 1% (2 patients). The use of a moisturizer in the studies may have reduced the incidence of dry skin.

Less Common Clinical Trial Adverse Drug Reactions (<1%): Body as a Whole: face edema, headache.

Nervous System: dizziness.

Skin and Appendages: rash, skin burning.

Post-Market Adverse Drug Reactions: The most frequently reported post-market adverse events are related to the application site, and are consistent with the type of events recorded in the controlled clinical trials. Typically, these application site reactions have included dry skin, erythema, burning sensation, rash, peeling and pruritus. Application site hypersensitivity (allergic reaction), colitis and diarrhea have also been reported.

DRUG INTERACTIONS: Drug-Drug Interactions: The interactions discussed in this section are based on either drug interaction case reports, or studies, or potential interactions due to the expected magnitude and seriousness of the interaction (i.e., those identified as contraindicated).

Clindamycin, erythromycin, lincomycin and chloramphenicol containing products should not be used concurrently. In vitro studies have shown antagonism among these antimicrobials. In vitro studies suggest that benzoyl peroxide contributes to the degradation of tretinoin especially when combined with exposure to UV light.

Drug-Food Interactions: Interactions with food have not been established.

Drug-Herb Interactions: Interactions with herbal products have not been established.

Drug-Laboratory Test Interactions: Interactions with laboratory tests have not been established.

DOSAGE AND ADMINISTRATION: Recommended Dose and Dosage Adjustment: BenzaClin Topical Gel (clindamycin, as phosphate, 1% and benzoyl peroxide 5%) should be applied twice daily, morning and evening, or as directed by a physician, to affected areas of the skin after it is gently washed with a mild non-medicated soap, rinsed with warm water and patted dry. Improvement has been seen as early as two weeks, although up to ten weeks of treatment may be required for best results.

Administration: Reconstitution: BenzaClin Topical Gel is supplied to the pharmacist as two components: 1) a jar of benzoyl peroxide gel; 2) a vial containing clindamycin phosphate powder, both of which are to be admixed by the pharmacist and dispensed to the patient in the jar as 1% clindamycin and 5% benzoyl peroxide. See Table 2.

Table 2: BenzaClin

How Supplied and Mixing Instructions for the Pharmacist

Size (Net Weight)	Benzoyl Peroxide Gel	Total Active Clindamycin Phosphate Powder	Purified Water to Be Added to Vial
50 g (pump)	41.4 g	0.6 g	10 mL

Prior to dispensing, tap the vial until powder flows freely. Add indicated amount of purified water to the vial (to the mark) and immediately shake to completely dissolve clindamycin. If needed, add additional purified water to bring level up to the mark. Add the solution in the vial to the gel and stir until homogenous in appearance (1 to 1½ minutes). Reassemble jar with pump dispenser. BenzaClin Topical Gel (as dispensed) can be stored between 15-25°C for 3 months. Place a 3-month expiration date on the label immediately following mixing.

OVERDOSAGE:

Acute overdosage with the topical use of BenzaClin Topical Gel (clindamycin, as phosphate, 1% and benzoyl peroxide 5%) is unlikely. If BenzaClin is applied excessively, marked dryness, peeling and redness might occur. The literature indicates that clindamycin could be absorbed topically (see Warnings and Precautions). In the event of accidental ingestion, treatment should be symptomatic.

For management of a suspected drug overdose, CPhA recommends that you contact your **regional Poison Control Centre**. See the *CPS* Directory section for a list of Poison Control Centres.

ACTION AND CLINICAL PHARMACOLOGY: BenzaClin Topical Gel (clindamycin, as phosphate, 1% and benzoyl peroxide 5%) contains 1% clindamycin (as phosphate) and 5% benzoyl peroxide. The use of a clindamycin and benzoyl peroxide combination product in acne is predicated upon the facts that both clindamycin and benzoyl peroxide are active against *P. acnes*, and benzoyl peroxide is an oxidizing agent exhibiting keratolytic and desquamative activity. Clindamycin phosphate is a water-soluble ester and semi-synthetic antibiotic which is derived from the parent antibiotic lincomycin. BenzaClin Topical Gel penetrates the skin and has greater clinical and *P. acnes* reducing effects than either of its components. BenzaClin Topical Gel inhibits clindamycin-resistant *P. acnes*. Topical clindamycin and benzoyl peroxide penetrate systemically to a minimal degree.

STORAGE AND STABILITY: Store BenzaClin Topical Gel and its individual components between 15 and 25°C (before and after reconstitution).

After reconstitution for dispensing to the patient, label BenzaClin Topical Gel with a 3-month expiration date.

Do not freeze. Keep tightly closed. Keep out of the reach of children.

INFORMATION FOR THE PATIENT: Published in e-CPS, available by subscription at www.e-cps.ca.

DOSAGE FORMS, COMPOSITION AND PACKAGING: BenzaClin Topical Gel (clindamycin, as phosphate, 1% and benzoyl peroxide 5%) is supplied as two components: a jar of benzoyl peroxide gel and a vial containing clindamycin phosphate powder. The pharmacist will dissolve the clindamycin phosphate powder in purified water, then add the solution to the jar of benzoyl peroxide gel and mix (see Dosage and Administration).

As dispensed to the patient after reconstitution by the pharmacist, BenzaClin Topical Gel contains 1% clindamycin (as clindamycin phosphate) and 5% benzoyl peroxide in an aqueous gel medium. It also contains the following nonmedicinal ingredients: carbomer, dioctyl sodium sulfosuccinate, purified water and sodium hydroxide. BenzaClin Topical Gel is dispensed in 50 g jars equipped with a hand actuated pump.

Benzac® W5

benzoyl peroxide

Acne Therapy

Galderma

SUPPLIED: Each tube contains: benzoyl peroxide USP 5% in a water base gel. Nonmedicinal ingredients: carbomer 940, docusate sodium, edetate disodium, poloxamer 182, propylene glycol, purified water, silicon dioxide and sodium hydroxide. May contain citric acid to adjust pH. Plastic tubes of 60 g. Store at room temperature; avoid excessive heat.

Benzac® W Wash 5

benzoyl peroxide

Acne Therapy

Galderma

Benzac® W Wash 10

benzoyl peroxide

Acne Therapy

Galderma

SUPPLIED: Each bottle contains: benzoyl peroxide USP 5% or 10% cleanser in a water base gel. Nonmedicinal ingredients: carbomer 940, citric acid, purified water and sodium C14-16 olefin sulfonate. Plastic bottles of 225 g. Store at room temperature; avoid excessive heat.

Benzamycin®

erythromycin—benzoyl peroxide

Acne Therapy

sanofi-aventis

Date of Revision: September 25, 2008

PHARMACOLOGY: Erythromycin is a bacteriostatic macrolide antibiotic, but may be bactericidal in high concentrations. Although the mechanism by which erythromycin acts in reducing inflammatory lesions of acne vulgaris is not fully elucidated, it is presumably due to its antibiotic action. It inhibits the growth of *P. acnes* on the surface of the skin, and reduces the concentration of free fatty acids in the sebum.

Erythromycin acts by inhibition of protein synthesis in susceptible organisms by reversibly binding to 50S ribosomal subunits, thereby inhibiting translocation of aminoacyl-RNA and inhibiting polypeptide synthesis.

Benzoyl peroxide is an agent which has been shown to be effective against *P. acnes*, an anaerobe found in sebaceous follicles and comedones. The antibacterial action of benzoyl peroxide is believed to be due to the release of active oxygen. Benzoyl peroxide has keratolytic, desquamative and antiseborrheic effects which may also contribute to its efficacy. Benzoyl peroxide has been shown to be absorbed by the skin where it is converted to benzoic acid. Approximately 5% of the metabolite is excreted unchanged in the urine.

INDICATIONS: For the topical treatment of moderate acne vulgaris characterized by comedones, inflammatory papules/pustules, with or without an occasional cyst or nodule (Grade II to III*). Benzamycin is not indicated for the treatment of cystic acne (Grade IV*).

CONTRAINDICATIONS: In those patients with a history of hypersensitivity to erythromycin, benzoyl peroxide or any of the ingredients in the preparation (see Supplied).

WARNINGS: For external use only.

Not for ophthalmic use. Avoid contact with eyes, nose, lips, mouth and other mucous membranes. If contact occurs, rinse thoroughly with water.

Benzamycin contains drying and peeling agents that are potential irritants. Therefore, reduction in frequency of application may be necessary to avoid excessive irritation. If severe irritation develops, discontinue use and institute appropriate therapy. Concomitant topical acne therapy should be used with caution because a possible cumulative irritancy effect may occur, especially with peeling, desquamating or abrasive agents.

PRECAUTIONS: General: The use of antibiotic agents may be associated with the overgrowth of nonsusceptible organisms including fungi. If this occurs, administration of Benzamycin should be discontinued, and appropriate measures taken.

Pregnancy: The safety of Benzamycin in pregnancy has not been established, nor have any animal reproduction studies been conducted with Benzamycin. It is also not known whether Benzamycin can cause fetal harm when administered to a pregnant woman or can affect reproductive capacity. Benzamycin should be given to a pregnant woman only if clearly needed.

Lactation: It is not known whether Benzamycin is excreted in human milk after topical application. However, erythromycin is excreted in human milk following oral and parenteral administration. Therefore, caution should be exercised when erythromycin is administered to a nursing woman.

Children: The safety and effectiveness of Benzamycin in children below the age of 12 years have not been established.

Drug Interactions: Antagonism has been demonstrated in vitro between erythromycin, lincomycin, chloramphenicol and clindamycin. Therefore erythromycin, lincomycin, chloramphenicol and clindamycin should not be used concomitantly with Benzamycin, although no studies have been conducted testing for antagonism of Benzamycin with these antibiotics.

ADVERSE EFFECTS: Local irritation reactions such as irritation of the skin including: peeling, itching, burning sensation, erythema, inflammation of the face, eyes and nose, irritation of the eyes, skin discoloration, oiliness, tenderness of the skin, pruritus and edema may occur while using Benzamycin.

In clinical trials conducted with Benzamycin, 5 of 155 patients experienced adverse reactions. Four of the adverse reactions were dryness, and 1 was an urticarial reaction which responded to symptomatic treatment.

OVERDOSE:
Acute overdosage with the topical use of Benzamycin is unlikely. In the event of accidental ingestion, appropriate intervention should be initiated.

For management of a suspected drug overdose, CPhA recommends that you contact your **regional Poison Control Centre.** See the *CPS* Directory section for a list of Poison Control Centres.

* [Pillsbury DM., Heaton C. Manual of Dermatology 1980.]

DOSAGE: Benzamycin should be applied as a thin layer to affected areas twice daily, morning and evening, or as directed by physician. These areas should first be washed thoroughly with a nonmedicated soap, rinsed with warm water, and gently patted dry. Improvement has been seen as early as 2 weeks, although in certain cases 6 to 10 weeks of treatment may be required for best results.

Compounding Directions: Benzamycin is supplied to the pharmacist in a package containing 40 g of benzoyl peroxide gel and 1.6 g of active erythromycin powder in a plastic vial (46.6 g net weight, as dispensed). **Prior to dispensing, tap the vial of erythromycin until all powder flows freely. For Benzamycin 46.6 g (net weight, as dispensed), add 6 mL of ethyl alcohol (70%) to the erythromycin vial (to the mark) and immediately shake to completely dissolve the powder.** Add this solution to the gel and stir until homogeneous in appearance (1-1½ minutes).

INFORMATION FOR THE PATIENT: Published in e-CPS, available by subscription at www.e-cps.ca.

SUPPLIED: Each g of topical gel contains: erythromycin 3% (30 mg/g) and benzoyl peroxide 5% (50 mg/g). Nonmedicinal ingredients: alcohol, carbomer, docusate sodium, lemon fragrance, methyl salicylate, purified water and sodium hydroxide.

Prior to dispensing, the package containing one jar of benzoyl peroxide gel (40 g) and one plastic vial of active erythromycin powder (1.6 g) should be stored at room temperature (15 to 25°C). Following compounding (see Dosage, Compounding Directions), Benzamycin should be stored under refrigeration (2 to 8°C). Do not freeze. A 3-month expiration date is to be placed on the label.

Benzodiazepines

alprazolam
bromazepam
chlordiazepoxide HCl
clobazam
clonazepam
clorazepate dipotassium
diazepam
flurazepam HCl
lorazepam
midazolam HCl
nitrazepam
oxazepam
temazepam
triazolam

Anticonvulsant—Anxiolytic—Hypnotic—Sedative

CPhA Monograph

Date of Revision: October 2009

This monograph has been compiled by CPhA and reviewed by experts. It may contain information different from that found in Health Canada-approved Product Monographs. The reader is referred to the *CPS* Editorial Policy for more information.

SUMMARY PRODUCT INFORMATION:

Drug	Route of Administration	Dosage Form	Strength
Alprazolam	Oral	Tablet	0.25 mg, 0.5 mg, 1 mg, 2 mg
Bromazepam	Oral	Tablet	1.5 mg, 3 mg, 6 mg
Chlordiazepoxide HCl	Oral	Capsule	5 mg, 10 mg, 25 mg
Clobazam	Oral	Tablet	10 mg
Clonazepam	Oral	Tablet	0.5 mg, 2 mg
Clorazepate dipotassium	Oral	Capsule	3.75 mg, 7.5 mg, 15 mg
Diazepam	Oral	Tablet	2 mg, 5 mg, 10 mg
	Rectal	Gel	5 mg/mL
	IM/IV	Injectable emulsion	5 mg/mL; 2 mL
	IM/IV	Injectable solution	5 mg/mL; 2 mL
Flurazepam HCl	Oral	Capsule	15 mg, 30 mg
Lorazepam	Oral	Tablet	0.5 mg, 1 mg, 2 mg
	Sublingual	Tablet	0.5 mg, 1 mg, 2 mg
	IM/IV	Injectable solution	4 mg/mL
Midazolam HCl	IM/IV	Injectable solution	1 mg/mL; 2, 5, or 10 mL
Nitrazepam	Oral	Tablet	5 mg, 10 mg
Oxazepam	Oral	Tablet	10 mg, 15 mg, 30 mg
Temazepam	Oral	Capsule	15 mg, 30 mg
Triazolam	Oral	Tablet	0.125 mg, 0.25 mg

PHARMACOLOGY: Benzodiazepines exhibit an affinity for benzodiazepine receptors which act as specific binding sites for gamma aminobutyric acid (GABA), the major inhibitory neurotransmitter in the CNS. Benzodiazepines are believed to produce their CNS effects by interacting with a macromolecular protein complex in the neuronal membrane which includes $GABA_A$ receptors, high-affinity benzodiazepine receptors and chloride channels.

Benzodiazepines with very similar chemical structures can differ in their potency, rate of absorption and other pharmacokinetic parameters. The potency of a benzodiazepine is correlated with its affinity for its binding site, the benzodiazepine receptor. In therapeutic use, the benzodiazepines, while differing in potency, have similar pharmacologic profiles.

Different types of benzodiazepine receptors in various areas of the CNS are thought to produce the different pharmacologic actions of the drugs. As the dose of benzodiazepine is increased, anxiolytic effects are first produced, followed by anticonvulsant effects, a reduction in muscle tonus, and finally sedation and hypnosis.

Pharmacokinetics: The primary differences among the benzodiazepines are in their pharmacokinetic properties, and these often are among the main factors considered in drug selection. Table 1 lists the major pharmacokinetic properties of these agents.

Benzodiazepines are widely distributed in the body and accumulate preferentially in lipid rich areas such as the CNS and adipose tissue. The more lipophilic agents have the fastest rates of absorption and onset of clinical effects. Benzodiazepines and their metabolites are highly bound to plasma proteins (80 to 99%).

Steady state plasma concentrations of benzodiazepines and their metabolites are reached after about 5 elimination half-lives, usually a few days to 2 weeks after initiation of therapy.

Benzodiazepines or active metabolites with very long elimination half-lives can accumulate with chronic dosing and produce prolonged effects, especially in elderly or obese patients, those with liver disease, or with concurrent use of other drugs that compete for hepatic oxidation. Benzodiazepines that undergo hepatic glucuronide conjugation and do not have active metabolites are unlikely to accumulate with chronic administration and require multiple daily dosing for sustained effects.

Most of the benzodiazepines are excreted almost entirely in the urine in the form of oxidized and glucuronide-conjugated metabolites. Benzodiazepines are not significantly removed by hemodialysis.

INDICATIONS: Benzodiazepines have similar pharmacologic actions; however, clinical uses of specific agents may reflect differences in their pharmacokinetic profiles, the availability of clinical evidence, or the labeled indications for a particular agent. Table 2 outlines the labeled indications of the benzodiazepines available in Canada.

Benzodiazepines are also used in the management of agitation, restless legs syndrome, skeletal muscle spasticity and alcohol withdrawal; they are also used adjunctively in the management of nausea and vomiting associated with cancer chemotherapy or prior to surgical or diagnostic procedures.

CONTRAINDICATIONS: Patients with known hypersensitivity to this class of drugs or to any component of the product in question. The manufacturers advise against the use of benzodiazepines in patients with myasthenia gravis and acute angle-closure glaucoma, but they may be used in patients receiving appropriate therapy for open-angle glaucoma. Specific product monographs should be consulted as individual products may have additional contraindications to their use.

WARNINGS: Benzodiazepines are not recommended for use in patients with a major depressive disorder or psychosis in which anxiety is not a prominent feature.

Benzodiazepines should be used with extreme caution in patients with severe pulmonary insufficiency or sleep apnea, especially the elderly or very ill patients, and those with limited pulmonary reserve.

Table 1: Benzodiazepines

Pharmacokinetic Properties[a]

Drug	Approximate Equivalent Oral Dose (mg)	Time to Peak Concentration (hours)	Onset of Action[b]	Active Metabolites	Pathway of Metabolism	Approximate Half-life (hours, parent compound and active metabolite)
Long-acting						
Chlordiazepoxide	10	0.5 to 4	I	Yes	Oxidation (CYP1A2)	100
Clorazepate	7.5	0.5 to 2	F	Yes	Oxidation	100
Diazepam	5	Oral: 0.5 to 2 h Rectal gel: 1.5 h Injectable emulsion: 15 min (iv); 2 h (im)	F	Yes	Oxidation (CYP1A2, 2C9, 2C19, 3A4)	100
Flurazepam	15	0.5 to 1	F	Yes	Oxidation	100
Intermediate-acting						
Alprazolam	0.5	1 to 2	I	Yes	Oxidation (CYP3A4)	12 to 15
Bromazepam	3	1 to 4	I	Yes	Conjugation	8 to 30
Clobazam	10	1 to 4	I	Yes	Oxidation	10 to 46
Clonazepam	0.25	1 to 2	I	No	Oxidation (CYP3A4); reduction	20 to 80
Lorazepam	1	2 to 4	I	No	Conjugation	10 to 20
Nitrazepam	5	2 to 3	I	No	Reduction	16 to 55
Oxazepam	15	2 to 4	S	No	Conjugation	5 to 15
Temazepam	15	2 to 3	I	No	Conjugation	10 to 20
Short-acting						
Midazolam[c]	Not applicable	See Onset of Action	IM: 5 to 15 min IV: 1.5 to 5 min[d]	Yes	Oxidation (CYP3A4)	1 to 4
Triazolam	0.25	1 to 2	F	No	Oxidation (CYP3A4)	1.5 to 5

[a] After oral administration, unless otherwise indicated.
[b] Legend: F = fast (< 1 h); I = intermediate (1–3 h); S = slow (> 3 h).
[c] Parenteral use only.
[d] Onset of action may be faster if opioid administered concurrently.

Table 2: Benzodiazepines

Labeled Indications[a]

Drug	Anxiety Disorders	Panic Disorder	Insomnia	Perioperative Medication	Seizure Disorders[b]	Skeletal Muscle Spasticity	Alcohol Withdrawal
Alprazolam	Yes	Yes	—	—	—	—	—
Bromazepam	Yes	—	—	—	—	—	—
Chlordiazepoxide	Yes	—	—	—	—	—	—
Clobazam	—	—	—	—	Yes	—	—
Clonazepam	—	—	—	—	Yes	—	—
Clorazepate	Yes	Yes	—	—	Yes	—	Yes
Diazepam	Yes	—	—	Yes	Yes	Yes	Yes
Flurazepam	—	—	Yes	—	—	—	—
Lorazepam	Yes	—	—	Yes	Yes	—	—
Midazolam	—	—	—	Yes	—	—	—
Nitrazepam	—	—	Yes	—	Yes	—	—
Oxazepam	Yes	—	—	—	—	—	Yes
Temazepam	—	—	Yes	—	—	—	—
Triazolam	—	—	Yes	—	—	—	—

[a] Refer to individual product monographs for more detailed information.
[b] Used in adults and children.

Resuscitative facilities and equipment should be available when benzodiazepines are administered parenterally, particularly iv. These agents should not be administered iv to patients in shock, coma, acute alcohol intoxication, or to patients who have recently received other respiratory depressant drugs.

Benzodiazepines should be used with caution in severely depressed patients or those in whom there is any sign of impending depression with an associated anxiety disorder, particularly in patients at risk of increased suicidal tendencies. Appropriate protective measures may be necessary during benzodiazepine therapy in these patients. Consideration should be given to the quantity of medication prescribed at any one time.

Patients should be informed about possible negative effects on memory and advised to report to their physician any mental or behavioral changes that develop during benzodiazepine therapy (see Precautions).

A Health Canada advisory was issued in October 2009 to make patients and clinicians aware of cases where patients took a sedative-hypnotic agent and subsequently engaged in activities such as driving, making phone calls or cooking/eating meals while not fully awake, and with no recall of the event(s). The concurrent use of alcohol or other CNS depressants or the use of higher than recommended sedative doses increases the risk of such events. The advisory applies to flurazepam, nitrazepam, temazepam and triazolam, which are the benzodiazepines officially indicated as hypnotics, as well as to the nonbenzodiazepine, zopiclone. If these events occur in a patient taking any benzodiazepine, consider discontinuing the drug in light of the safety implications of engaging in potentially hazardous activities such as driving while not fully awake. See also Precautions.

Occupational Hazards: Patients should be warned about the potential impairment of mental alertness or physical coordination which may decrease their ability to perform hazardous tasks such as driving or operating machinery. Elderly patients may be at particular risk for these CNS depressant effects, which may predispose them to falls or motor vehicle accidents.

Dependence and Withdrawal: Tolerance and the risk of psychological and physical dependence may occur following prolonged use of benzodiazepines at therapeutic doses. The possibility that such effects also may occur following short-term use of benzodiazepines, particularly at higher doses, should also be considered. Tolerance to the hypnotic and sedative effects develops rapidly. In contrast, clinically significant tolerance to the anxiolytic effect usually does not occur even after prolonged use.

Risk of benzodiazepine dependence can be minimized by titrating the dose, close observation and follow-up, proper screening for possible risk factors and education of the patient. Benzodiazepine use should be avoided in patients with a history of alcohol or substance abuse, except for the treatment of acute alcohol withdrawal.

Abrupt withdrawal of benzodiazepines may lead to symptoms such as anxiety, insomnia, psychomotor agitation, gastrointestinal discomfort, hand tremor, anorexia, diaphoresis, tachycardia, photophobia or phonophobia. More severe symptoms may occur such as confusion, depersonalization, myoclonus, delirium, psychosis or seizures. Rebound insomnia may occur, particularly following abrupt discontinuation of a benzodiazepine with a short elimination half-life.

Withdrawal can also be precipitated by dosage tapering or inadvertent withdrawal (e.g., forgotten doses or admission to hospital). Such effects can also emerge in the early morning following bedtime administration of a short-acting agent. In addition, an increase in daytime anxiety and/or restlessness may occur between doses of short-acting agents. Rebound or re-emergence of symptoms may occur after as little as 4 to 6 weeks' therapy. It is more likely if the drug is short-acting, taken regularly for >3 months and abruptly discontinued. Symptoms may be similar to those experienced by the patient prior to initiation of the benzodiazepine, but may be more intense.

Choice of withdrawal regimen may depend on the setting of detoxification, severity of dependence and concurrent drug or substance abuse. Patients should follow a structured discontinuation program. When discontinuing benzodiazepines in patients on prolonged therapy, dosage should be gradually decreased over about 6 to 12 weeks, especially in patients with a history of seizures or epilepsy, regardless of their concomitant antiepileptic drug therapy. If the patient had been taking a short-acting agent, a longer-acting benzodiazepine may be substituted, to provide a gradual decrease in drug concentration and reduce the possibility of withdrawal symptoms. Patients who were taking the equivalent of 60 mg or more of diazepam daily, or those with a history of serious withdrawal reactions, should be hospitalized during acute withdrawal, and dosage tapering should be more gradual than in those managed as outpatients.

PRECAUTIONS: CNS: Elderly or debilitated patients, children, and patients with liver disease or low serum albumin are most likely to experience CNS adverse effects. Generally it is recommended that therapy be initiated with low dosages and gradually titrated to the lowest effective dose, to minimize the possibility of ataxia, dizziness and oversedation. Benzodiazepines can produce prolonged CNS depression in neonates because of the inability to convert the benzodiazepine into inactive metabolites. Reversible dementia has also been reported in the elderly after prolonged administration of benzodiazepines.

Differences in the degree of residual and cumulative CNS depressant effects among the benzodiazepines may be particularly important in elderly patients, in patients with potentially impaired elimination of drugs and in individuals whose occupation or lifestyle requires unimpaired intellectual or psychomotor function. There is some evidence that ataxia and the risk of falling and associated hip fracture in elderly patients is greatest with the use of long-acting benzodiazepines as compared to short-acting agents. Long-acting benzodiazepines (chlordiazepoxide, clorazepate, diazepam and flurazepam) and triazolam should be avoided in elderly patients.

Benzodiazepine therapy should be individualized and closely monitored in elderly patients, and the need for continued therapy with these drugs should be re-evaluated frequently.

Anterograde amnesia has occurred following therapeutic doses of benzodiazepines. The degree of severity and duration of effects may vary depending on the drug, dosage, route of administration or individual patient (e.g., elderly patients may be at particular risk). Although amnesic effects have been more commonly associated with midazolam, triazolam and lorazepam, these effects have occurred with other benzodiazepines. Data suggest that anterograde amnesia and next day memory loss occur at a higher rate with triazolam, generally at a 0.5 mg dose. Cases of transient global amnesia and "traveler's amnesia" have also been associated with triazolam in patients taking the drug to induce sleep while traveling. These amnesic effects are unpredictable and not necessarily dose related. The manufacturers advise warning patients not to take triazolam under circumstances in which a full night's sleep and clearance of the drug from the body are not possible before they will need to resume full activity and alertness, e.g., an overnight flight of less than 7 to 8 hours. See also Warnings.

Paradoxical CNS stimulation has occurred in psychiatric patients and hyperactive, aggressive children. Such reactions include restlessness, anxiety, mania, insomnia, sleep disturbances, increased muscle spasticity, acute rage and hyperactivity, and have appeared early in therapy, usually in the first 2 weeks. Benzodiazepine therapy should be discontinued if CNS stimulation occurs.

Serious behavioral changes and abnormal thinking have occasionally been associated with benzodiazepine use. They may include hallucinations, depersonalization, agitation, bizarre behavior and decreased inhibition manifested as aggression or excessive extroversion, similar to that seen with alcohol and other CNS depressants.

Cardiovascular: Caution is advised during parenteral administration of benzodiazepines to elderly patients as they may be more likely to experience apnea, hypotension, bradycardia or cardiac arrest.

Dependence: Benzodiazepines may cause psychologic or physical dependence (see Warnings).

Other: Patients with compromised renal or hepatic function should be monitored and the dose carefully titrated to avoid accumulation of these agents.

Because of isolated reports of blood dyscrasias and abnormal liver function tests, periodic blood counts and liver function tests may be of benefit during long-term therapy.

Drug Interactions: Table 3 lists the more common interactions. Consult product monographs or specialized references for more detailed information.

Table 3: Benzodiazepines

Drug Interactions

Drug(s) Interacting with Benzodiazepines	Potential Effect
Alcohol and other CNS depressants	Additive CNS depressant effects. Tolerance may develop with chronic alcohol use. Increased risk of complex sleep-related behaviours such as sleep-driving (see Warnings)
Grapefruit juice	Increased serum levels of benzodiazepines metabolized by CYP3A4 (alprazolam, clonazepam, diazepam, midazolam, triazolam).
Hepatic enzyme inducers	Decreased serum concentrations and effects of benzodiazepines metabolized by the affected enzyme[a] (see Table 1).
Hepatic enzyme inhibitors	Increase in pharmacologic effects of benzodiazepines metabolized by the affected enzymes (see Table 1).

[a] Cigarette smoking may have a similar effect.

Children: Some benzodiazepines are used in children for many of the same indications as for adults. They share the same precautions as for adults, but can also cause paradoxical excitation in children. Specialized references should be consulted for detailed information.

Pregnancy: Benzodiazepines should generally be avoided during pregnancy. Benzodiazepines freely cross the placenta and accumulate in the fetal circulation, and may be associated with a lightly increased risk of congenital malformations following first-trimester exposure. Hypotonia, lethargy and sucking difficulties have been reported in infants whose mothers received benzodiazepines close to delivery. Chronic use of benzodiazepines during pregnancy has also been associated with neonatal withdrawal. The use of benzodiazepines solely as hypnotics is contraindicated during pregnancy. When a benzodiazepine is being used in the management of a seizure disorder, the risk of continued therapy must be weighed against the risk of discontinuation, and the lowest effective possible should be used. Abrupt discontinuation should be avoided.

Lactation: Benzodiazepines are excreted in breast milk. Because the ability of neonates to metabolize these drugs is limited, accumulation may occur. Benzodiazepine use is not recommended during lactation.

Occupational Hazards: Because of the CNS depressant effect of benzodiazepines, patients should be cautioned with regard to driving or performing other hazardous tasks that require mental alertness and physical coordination.

ADVERSE EFFECTS: The most common adverse effects reported with the use of benzodiazepines are dose-dependent CNS effects. Ataxia, dizziness, lightheadedness, drowsiness, including residual daytime drowsiness when used as a hypnotic, weakness, and fatigue usually occur in the first few days of therapy and may decrease with continued therapy. If these effects are persistent, a reduction in dosage may be necessary. Elderly or debilitated patients, children, and patients with liver disease or low serum albumin may be unusually sensitive to the CNS effects.

The more serious, occasionally reported adverse reactions are hypersensitivity reactions, mental depression, behavioral problems, paradoxical stimulant reactions, leukopenia, jaundice, hypotension, memory impairment, phlebitis or venous thrombosis, and seizures.

Other adverse effects less frequently reported include: abdominal or stomach cramps or pain, blurred vision or diplopia, sexual dysfunction, constipation, diarrhea, dry mouth or increased thirst, vertigo, syncope, confusion, vivid or disturbing dreams, slurred speech, euphoria, headache, increased bronchial secretions or watering of mouth, muscle spasm, nausea or vomiting, incontinence, urinary retention, tachycardia or palpitations, trembling and unusual tiredness or weakness.

OVERDOSE:

Symptoms: Symptoms of mild overdose include drowsiness, impaired coordination, diminished reflexes, confusion and lethargy. In more serious overdose, symptoms may include ataxia, hypotonia, hypotension, respiratory depression, seizures and coma. Although cardiac arrest has been reported, death from overdose of benzodiazepines in the absence of concurrent ingestion of alcohol or other CNS depressants is rare.

Treatment: Management consists of appropriate supportive and symptomatic therapy. The possibility of co-ingestion of other substances must be taken into consideration. In the case of a recent oral benzodiazepine overdose, activated charcoal (about 1 g/kg) may be administered, as long as the patient is sufficiently alert to adequately protect the airway. Vital signs and fluid balance should be monitored. An adequate airway should be maintained and respiration assisted as required. Hypotension is generally not problematic, and usually is adequately treated with boluses of isotonic iv fluids.

Flumazenil, a benzodiazepine antagonist, should be used cautiously, if at all, in patients with either a pure benzodiazepine or a mixed drug overdose (*except* those involving tricyclic antidepressants). Sudden reversal by flumazenil in patients who chronically take benzodiazepines can induce withdrawal and precipitate seizures. Furthermore, if patients have co-ingested a tricyclic antidepressant, sudden reversal with flumazenil can precipitate cardiac arrest. Consequently, flumazenil is *contraindicated* in any patient who might have co-ingested a tricyclic antidepressant or used benzodiazepines chronically.

The hypnotic-sedative effects of benzodiazepines are rapidly reversed. However, the residual effects may reappear gradually within a few hours, depending on the dose of flumazenil, the time elapsed since the benzodiazepine was administered, and elimination half-life of the benzodiazepine in question.

If flumazenil is used, it should be administered only when continuous monitoring for recurrence of sedation can be assured. Flumazenil is generally reserved for management of severely symptomatic pure benzodiazepine overdose. Flumazenil's effects on respiratory depression are inconsistent; in some studies residual respiratory depressant effects were still present despite reversal of sedation. Improved consciousness is expected within the first several minutes of flumazenil administration, but ventilatory support may be required for respiratory depression. Flumazenil does not consistently reverse benzodiazepine-associated amnesia. The flumazenil product monograph should be consulted for complete prescribing information.

Dialysis is of limited value in benzodiazepine overdose.

For management of a suspected drug overdose, CPhA recommends that you contact your **regional Poison Control Centre**. See the *CPS* Directory section for a list of Poison Control Centres.

DOSAGE: The dosage of benzodiazepines should be individualized and carefully titrated to avoid excessive sedation and mental or motor impairment. The lowest effective dose should be used and the need for continued therapy reassessed frequently. The risk of dependence may increase with the dose and duration of treatment. Individual product monographs may contain recommendations for maximum duration of use or maximum quantity per prescription, e.g., in the treatment of insomnia or anxiety. Oral dosages for the more common indications for each agent are included in Table 4.

Please refer to individual product monographs or other specialized references for dosage recommendations for specific patient groups such as children, elderly or debilitated patients, or those with hepatic or renal failure, or for indications not included in the table.

Table 4: Benzodiazepines

Dosage

Drug	Indication	Usual Oral Adult Dosage[a]
Alprazolam[a]	Anxiety	0.25 to 0.5 mg 3 times daily
	Panic disorder	0.5 mg 3 times daily
Bromazepam[a]	Anxiety	Initial: 6 to 18 mg/day in divided doses Usual maintenance range: 6 to 30 mg/day
Chlordiazepoxide[b]	Anxiety	5 to 25 mg 3 to 4 times daily
Clobazam[a]	Seizure disorders	Initial: 5 to 15 mg/day, preferably at bedtime Maintenance: 20 to 40 mg daily, in 1 or 2 divided doses
Clonazepam[a]	Anxiety, Panic disorder	0.25 to 0.5 mg twice daily
	Seizure disorders	Initial: 0.5 mg 3 times daily; increase by 0.5 to 1.0 mg daily every 3 days as needed and tolerated. Maximum: 20 mg/day
Clorazepate[a]	Anxiety	7.5 to 15 mg 2 to 4 times daily OR single dose of 15 to 22.5 mg at bedtime
	Seizure disorders	Initial: Up to 7.5 mg 2 to 3 times daily; increase by no more than 7.5 mg per week, to a maximum of 90 mg/day
Diazepam[b]	Anxiety/Seizure disorders	2 to 10 mg 2 to 4 times daily
Flurazepam[b]	Insomnia	15 to 30 mg at bedtime
Lorazepam[a]	Insomnia	0.5 to 1 mg at bedtime
Nitrazepam[a]	Insomnia	5 to 10 mg at bedtime

(cont'd)

Table 4: Benzodiazepines *(cont'd)*

Dosage

Drug	Indication	Usual Oral Adult Dosage[a]
Oxazepam[a]	Anxiety	10 to 30 mg 3 to 4 times daily
	Insomnia	15 mg 30 to 60 minutes before bedtime
Temazepam[a]	Insomnia	15 mg at bedtime
Triazolam[b]	Insomnia	0.125 to 0.25 mg at bedtime

[a] The dose is given for healthy younger adults. Elderly patients may be particularly sensitive to the CNS effects of benzodiazepines, and may have longer elimination half-lives due to decreased hepatic metabolism. In general, dosages of benzodiazepines for elderly patients tend to be approximately one-third to one-half of the recommended dose for younger adults.

[b] Not recommended in elderly patients.

Benztropine Mesylate

Antiparkinsonian Agent

CPhA Monograph

Date of Revision: November 2006

This monograph has been compiled by CPhA and reviewed by experts. It may contain information different from that found in Health Canada-approved Product Monographs. The reader is referred to the *CPS* Editorial Policy for more information.

PHARMACOLOGY: Benztropine is a synthetic tertiary amine with structural similarities to atropine and diphenhydramine. Benztropine exhibits anticholinergic, antihistaminic and local anesthetic properties. Its mechanism of action is not well understood, but it appears that by reducing cholinergic activity it helps to restore the functional balance between acetylcholine and dopamine in the basal ganglia of patients with parkinsonism. The proposed ability of benztropine to inhibit reuptake and storage of dopamine, thereby prolonging the action of dopamine, may also contribute to an effect on the equilibrium between acetylcholine and dopamine. The pharmacologic effects of the drug may not be apparent until 2 to 3 days after initiation of therapy and may persist for up to 24 hours after discontinuation of the drug.

Pharmacokinetics: When given orally, benztropine has an onset of action of between 1 and 2 hours. When given by im or iv injection, the onset of action is within minutes. Benztropine binds extensively, approximately 95%, with serum proteins. Benztropine crosses the blood-brain barrier.

INDICATIONS: The symptomatic treatment of all etiologic groups of parkinsonism and drug-induced extrapyramidal reactions.

CONTRAINDICATIONS: Benztropine is contraindicated in patients with a known hypersensitivity to benztropine or to any of its excipients, in patients with angle-closure glaucoma or severe ulcerative colitis. Because of its adverse anticholinergic effects, this drug is contraindicated in children under 3 years of age and should be used with caution in older children.

WARNINGS: Benztropine, alone or in combination with antipsychotics or anticholinergics, may cause anhidrosis and/or hyperthermia, which may be fatal. Patients should avoid becoming overheated from prolonged exposure to high environmental temperatures and/or from sustained heavy exercise. The elderly, the chronically ill, alcoholics and those with CNS disease may be particularly vulnerable. If there is evidence of anhidrosis, the dosage should be decreased so that the ability to maintain body temperature equilibrium by perspiration is not impaired. Benztropine should also be used with caution in patients with fever.

PRECAUTIONS: Because of its anticholinergic properties, benztropine should be used with caution in patients with cardiac arrhythmias, including sinus tachycardia, hypertension or hypotension, prostatic hypertrophy, liver or kidney disease or obstructive disease of the gastrointestinal or genitourinary tract.

Some experts recommend gonioscopic examination and monitoring of intraocular pressure (IOP) at regular intervals during prolonged therapy with benztropine. The drug may precipitate the onset of incipient angle-closure glaucoma and should not be used in predisposed patients (see Contraindications). Patients with primary open-angle glaucoma controlled with medication are at minimal risk of induction of an increase in IOP and many clinicians do not consider this condition a contraindication to therapy with benztropine.

Tardive dyskinesia may appear in some patients on long-term treatment with antipsychotics and related agents, or may occur after these drugs have been discontinued. Antiparkinsonian agents usually do not alleviate the symptoms of tardive dyskinesia and in some instances may aggravate or unmask such symptoms. Benztropine is not recommended in tardive dyskinesia.

When benztropine is used to treat extrapyramidal reactions caused by antipsychotic therapy in patients with a psychiatric illness, there may be an intensification of psychiatric illness. Although benztropine need not be discontinued when this occurs, its psychotogenic potential should be considered when planning the management of patients with psychiatric illness. When using benztropine in these patients, they should be carefully observed, especially at the beginning of treatment or if dosage is increased.

Use benztropine with extreme caution in patients with mild to moderate ulcerative colitis since antimuscarinic agents may suppress intestinal motility and produce paralytic ileus with resultant precipitation or aggravation of toxic megacolon. Use benztropine cautiously in those patients with known or suspected gastrointestinal infections since it may decrease gastrointestinal motility and prolong symptomatology by causing retention of the causative organism or toxin.

In patients with gastric ulcer, antimuscarinics in general may delay gastric emptying with possible antral stasis; therefore, benztropine should be used cautiously in these patients. Antimuscarinics may also relax the lower esophageal sphincter. This, combined with their effects on gastric emptying, may result in increased esophageal reflux in patients with gastroesophageal reflux disease or hiatus hernia associated with reflux esophagitis.

Due to its effects on bronchial secretions, benztropine should be used with caution in patients with chronic obstructive pulmonary disease. It should also be used with extreme caution in patients with autonomic neuropathy.

There have been occasional reports in the literature of benztropine abuse. Clinicians should remain aware of this possibility.

Drug Interactions: Amantadine: Benztropine and other anticholinergic drugs may potentiate CNS side effects of amantadine. Monitor patients for this effect and reduce the dose of one or both drugs as necessary.

Anticholinergics: Additive anticholinergic effects may occur when benztropine is used concurrently with drugs such as amantadine, atropine, MAO inhibitors, tricyclic antidepressants and phenothiazines. Paralytic ileus (sometimes fatal), hyperthermia and heat stroke may occur. Patients should be advised to report gastrointestinal problems, fever or heat intolerance promptly.

Cholinesterase Inhibitors: Benztropine and other anticholinergic drugs that readily penetrate the blood-brain barrier may, theoretically, interfere with the action of donepezil and other centrally-acting cholinesterase inhibitors. Conversely, cholinesterase inhibitors have the potential to interfere with the activity of anticholinergic medications.

CNS depressants: Benztropine may enhance the CNS depressant effects of drugs including alcohol, antiepileptics, barbiturates, MAO inhibitors, opioid analgesics, phenothiazines and tricyclic antidepressants.

Occupational Hazards: Benztropine may impair mental and/or physical abilities required for performance of hazardous tasks such as operating machinery or driving a motor vehicle.

Pregnancy: The safe use of this drug in pregnancy has not been established.

Lactation: It is not known if benztropine is excreted into breast milk.

Children: Benztropine is not recommended in children under 3 years of age (see Contraindications).

Geriatrics: Geriatric patients are frequently more sensitive to the adverse effects of anticholinergic medications, including benztropine. These patients may require lower doses, especially at the onset of therapy, and slower dose titration than younger adults.

ADVERSE EFFECTS: The adverse effects of benztropine are usually an extension of its pharmacologic action. They are usually dose related and may be reduced by lowering the dose.

Central Nervous System: nervousness, impaired memory, numbness of fingers, listlessness, depression. Mental confusion, excitement and visual hallucinations with high doses.

Gastrointestinal: dry mouth, constipation, nausea, vomiting, rarely paralytic ileus. Dry mouth may be relieved by the use of a saliva substitute or sugarless gum.

Ophthalmic: blurred vision, mydriasis.

Endocrine: hyperthermia, anhidrosis, heat stroke.

Genitourinary: urinary retention and/or dysuria.

Skeletomuscular: weakness and inability to move particular muscle groups.

Hypersensitivity: skin rash may occur occasionally.

Cardiovascular: tachycardia, arrhythmias.

OVERDOSE:

Symptoms: Symptoms of benztropine overdose are primarily extensions of its anticholinergic actions. Tachycardia, flushed/hot/dry skin, dry mucous membranes, mydriasis and blurred vision are common. Drowsiness, nervousness and lightheadedness may progress to, or alternate with, agitation, confusion, delirium and hallucinations, especially in children or the elderly. Urinary retention, hyperthermia, thirst and decreased gastrointestinal motility are also seen. Susceptible patients may experience angle-closure glaucoma. In severely poisoned patients coma or seizures may occur. Psychosis, rash, dystonic reactions, ataxia, weakness, respiratory depression, cardiac arrhythmia and rhabdomyolysis have been reported.

Treatment: Treatment is symptomatic and supportive. Consider administration of a single dose of activated charcoal to patients who present within 4 hours, since gastric emptying may be delayed. Monitor vital signs, urine output and ECG in severely poisoned patients. Maintain respiration and fluid and electrolyte balance. Hyperthermia can be managed with physical measures and control of agitation. Seizures may be treated with iv benzodiazepines. Physostigmine, a reversible cholinesterase inhibitor available through Health Canada's Special Access Programme, may be considered for management of delirium upon consultation with a regional poison control centre, and is preferable to benzodiazepines in many patients. Avoid antipsychotics and other anticholinergic drugs. If rhabdomyolysis does occur, hydration with crystalloid is the mainstay of treatment. Peritoneal dialysis and hemodialysis are of no value in the management of benztropine overdose.

For management of a suspected drug overdose, CPhA recommends that you contact your **regional Poison Control Centre**. See the *CPS* Directory section for a list of Poison Control Centres.

DOSAGE: Benztropine should be used orally in all cases when patients are able to take oral medication. When patients are unable to do so, or when more rapid response is desired, benztropine mesylate may be administered iv or im.

Since there is no significant difference in onset of effect after iv and im injection, there is usually no need to give benztropine iv. It is quickly effective by either route, with improvement sometimes noticeable a few minutes after injection.

Because benztropine has cumulative action, therapy should be initiated with a low dose, which is increased gradually by 0.5 mg increments at 5- or 6-day intervals, to the smallest amount necessary for optimal relief without excessive adverse effects. The maximum adult dose is 6 mg. Generally, older patients, thin patients and those with vascular parkinsonism cannot tolerate large doses. Most patients with postencephalitic parkinsonism need larger doses and tolerate them well. Patients with dementia or mental confusion are usually poor candidates for therapy.

Vascular (Arteriosclerotic), Idiopathic and Postencephalitic Parkinsonism: Therapy may be initiated with a single daily dose of 0.5 to 1 mg at bedtime. In some patients, this will be adequate; in others, 4 to 6 mg daily may be required.

Some patients experience optimal relief by taking the entire daily dose at bedtime; others respond more favorably to divided doses 2 to 4 times daily.

Therapy with other agents should not be terminated abruptly when therapy with benztropine is initiated, but may be reduced or discontinued gradually. Benztropine may be administered concomitantly with levodopa or a levodopa/carbidopa combination, in which case the dose of each may need adjustment.

Drug-induced Extrapyramidal Symptoms: Benztropine mesylate should not be used beyond the period necessary to counteract the extrapyramidal manifestations. In the majority of patients, the use of anticholinergic agents is not required after 3 months of antipsychotic therapy. Although therapy with the drug causing parkinsonism can frequently be continued without change of dosage when adjunctive therapy with benztropine is used, a reduction in dosage of the psychotropic drug might be indicated.

Patients must be closely observed for severe reactions and benztropine discontinued temporarily if they appear (see Precautions and Adverse Effects).

Adults: In treating extrapyramidal disorders caused by antipsychotics, the recommended dosage is 1 to 4 mg once or twice daily, orally or parenterally. Dosage must be individualized.

In acute dystonic reactions, 2 mg of benztropine given im or iv relieves the condition quickly. After that, 1 to 2 mg given orally twice daily for 2 to 3 days usually prevents recurrence.

When extrapyramidal disorders develop soon after initiation of treatment with antipsychotics, they are likely to be transient. One to 2 mg given orally 2 or 3 times daily usually provides relief within 1 or 2 days. After 1 or 2 weeks, the need for continued therapy with benztropine should be re-evaluated.

Children ≥ 3 years of age: 0.02 to 0.05 mg/kg/dose po/im/iv once or twice daily.

Benzydamine

Local Analgesic

CPhA Monograph

Date of Preparation: November 2004

Date of Revision: March 2009

This monograph has been compiled by CPhA and reviewed by experts. It may contain information different from that found in Health Canada-approved Product Monographs. The reader is referred to the *CPS* Editorial Policy for more information.

SUMMARY PRODUCT INFORMATION:

Route of Administration	Dosage Form	Product Strength
Local/Topical	Solution containing 10% ethanol	Benzydamine 0.15%

INDICATIONS AND CLINICAL USE: Benzydamine is indicated for:

- the symptomatic relief of oropharyngeal mucositis secondary to radiation therapy
- relief of pain in acute sore throat

Other Uses: The International Society for Oral Oncology and Multinational Association of Supportive Care in Cancer Society's guidelines for prevention and treatment of cancer therapy-induced oral and gastrointestinal mucositis recommend benzydamine for prevention of radiation-induced mucositis in patients with head and neck cancer receiving moderate-dose radiation therapy [*Cancer* 2007;109(5):820-31].

There is some evidence that vaginal use of benzydamine may relieve radiation-induced vaginal mucositis in women undergoing pelvic radiotherapy [*Cochrane Database Syst Rev* 2003;(1):CD003750].

Small studies of prophylactic benzydamine application prior to intubation have shown reduced incidence and severity of postoperative sore throat [*Anesth Analg* 2006;103(4):1001-3, *Anesth Analg* 2004;99(3):710-2].

CONTRAINDICATIONS:

- Patients who are hypersensitive to benzydamine or to any ingredient in the formulation or component of the container.

WARNINGS AND PRECAUTIONS: General: Benzydamine solution is meant for local use and should not be swallowed.

Ingestion of food or hot liquids while the mouth feels numb should be avoided due to risk of patients burning the mouth or biting the tongue or cheeks.

Renal: Caution is advised in patients with renal impairment as benzydamine is absorbed through the oral mucosa and eliminated unchanged by the kidneys.

Special Populations: Pregnant Women: Some benzydamine is absorbed through the oral mucosa. No information is available on the safety of benzydamine use during pregnancy or lactation.

Nursing Women: See Pregnant Women.

Pediatrics (birth to 16 years old): Safety and efficacy have not been established in children ≤5 years.

ADVERSE REACTIONS: Benzydamine can cause numbness, stinging or burning in the mouth (8–10%) and nausea/vomiting (2%). This can be attenuated by diluting benzydamine 0.15% solution with equal parts lukewarm water.

Rarely, cough, dry mouth/thirst, sedation and headache have been reported with benzydamine use.

DRUG INTERACTIONS: Drug-Drug Interactions: There are no reports of drug interactions involving benzydamine.

DOSAGE AND ADMINISTRATION: For relief of oropharyngeal mucositis in patients undergoing radiotherapy: 15 mL for each gargle or rinse, held in the mouth for at least 30 seconds then expelled, 3 to 4 times daily. Therapy should begin the day prior to radiotherapy and should be continued throughout and after radiotherapy for as long as necessary.

For acute sore throat (e.g., tonsillitis or pharyngitis): use 15 mL as a gargle then expel, every 1.5 to 3 hours.

For prevention of mucositis associated with radiation therapy for cancer of the head or neck a dose of 15 mL for 2 minutes, 4 to 8 times daily has been used [*Cancer* 2001;92(4):875-85].

In women undergoing pelvic radiotherapy, benzydamine 0.1% was administered as a vaginal douche twice daily for 2 weeks, to prevent or relieve radiation-induced vaginal mucositis [*Cochrane Database Syst Rev* 2003;(1):CD003750].

To reduce the incidence and severity of post-operative sore throat, patients gargled with 15 mL benzydamine hydrochloride 0.15% solution diluted to 30 mL with distilled water, for 30 seconds, 5 minutes prior to intubation [*Anesth Analg* 2006;103(4):1001-3].

Dosage in Renal Impairment: No dosage adjustment is necessary. However, caution is advised in patients with renal impairment. Benzydamine is absorbed through the oral mucosa and eliminated unchanged by the kidneys.

OVERDOSAGE:

For management of a suspected drug overdose, CPhA recommends that you contact your **regional Poison Control Centre**. See the *CPS* Directory section for a list of Poison Control Centres.

ACTION AND CLINICAL PHARMACOLOGY: Benzydamine is an indazole nonsteroidal anti-inflammatory medication with topical anesthetic, analgesic and antimicrobial activity. It does not interfere with arachidonic acid metabolism and is a weak inhibitor of prostaglandin synthesis. Benzydamine's anti-inflammatory effects may be due to: inhibition of production of pro-inflammatory cytokines; inhibition of generation of reactive oxygen species by neutrophils; membrane stabilization.

Pharmacokinetics: Adults: Absorption: Approximately 11% of the drug used as a mouthwash is absorbed, whereas oral ingestion results in close to 100% absorption. Topical use of benzydamine as a mouthwash produces higher tissue concentrations and lower peak plasma levels than oral administration, leading to greater efficacy and less risk of side effects. The state of the mucosa does not seem to influence absorption. Peak plasma levels after use of benzydamine mouthwash are obtained at about 2 hours, though tissue concentration peaks 15–30 minutes after application. The $t_{½}$ for benzydamine mouthwash is 10 hours.

Excretion: Benzydamine is excreted in the urine primarily as unchanged drug.

STORAGE AND STABILITY: Store at room temperature.

Berinert®

human C1 esterase inhibitor

C1 Esterase Inhibitor

CSL Behring

Date of Revision: May 28, 2010

SUMMARY PRODUCT INFORMATION:

Route of Administration	Dosage Form/ Strength	Clinically Relevant Nonmedicinal Ingredients
Intravenous injection	Lyophilised powder, 500 U/vial	Glycine, sodium chloride and sodium citrate. For a complete listing see Dosage Forms, Composition and Packaging.

DESCRIPTION: Berinert is a purified, pasteurised, lyophilised concentrate of human C1 esterase inhibitor (C1-INH) to be reconstituted for intravenous administration. It is prepared from large pools of human plasma. Each Berinert vial contains 500 U C1-INH. One standard unit of C1-INH concentrate is equal to the amount of C1-INH in 1 mL of fresh citrated human plasma, which is equivalent to 270 mg/L or 2.5 μM/L.

INDICATIONS AND CLINICAL USE: Berinert (Human C1 esterase inhibitor) is indicated for the treatment of acute abdominal or facial attacks of hereditary angioedema (HAE) of moderate and severe intensity*.

The safety and efficacy of Berinert for prophylactic therapy has not been established.

Geriatrics (>65 years of age): Safety and efficacy of Berinert in the geriatric population have not been established.

Pediatrics (3-16 years of age): The safety and efficacy of Berinert in this age group has not been systematically evaluated. The clinical study did not include a sufficient number of subjects in this age group to determine if they respond differently from older subjects included in the study.

CONTRAINDICATIONS: Berinert is contraindicated in individuals who have a known hypersensitivity or have had an anaphylactic or severe systemic reaction to C1-INH preparations or to any ingredient in the formulation or component of the container.

For a complete listing, see Dosage Forms, Composition and Packaging.

WARNINGS AND PRECAUTIONS:

Serious Warnings and Precautions

- Products made from human plasma may contain infectious agents such as viruses and, theoretically, the agent responsible for the Creutzfeldt-Jakob disease (CJD).

General: Berinert is made from human plasma and may contain pathogens such as viruses and, theoretically, the agent responsible for the Creutzfeldt-Jakob disease (CJD). The risk that such products will transmit an infectious agent has been reduced by implementing stringent measures to reduce the risk of contamination by pathogens.

The current manufacturing process includes multiple steps that reduce the risk of viral transmission. Since 22 February 2001 (Date of licensure of the product formulation as of today), no proven case of virus transmission has been attributed to Berinert.

Despite these measures, human plasma-derived products may still potentially transmit diseases. There is also the possibility that unknown infectious agents may be present in such products. All infections thought by a physician to have been possibly transmitted by this product should be reported by the latter or another healthcare provider to CSL Behring at 1-613-783-1892.

The physician or healthcare provider should discuss the risks and benefits of this product with the patient.

Cardiovascular: Up to now, the development of thrombosis has been reported in association with Berinert when used (off-label) and at higher than labeled doses (greater than 90 U/kg body weight) in newborns and young children with congenital heart anomalies during or after cardiac surgery under extracorporeal circulation.

Allergic Reactions: As with all pharmaceutical agents, allergic reactions may occur. If symptoms of allergic or early signs of hypersensitivity reactions (including hives, generalized urticaria, tightness of the chest, wheezing, hypotension, and anaphylaxis) occur, immediately discontinue the administration of Berinert and take appropriate measures as required.

Special Populations: Pregnant Women: Animal reproduction studies have not been conducted with Berinert. In a retrospective case collection study, 20 pregnant women ranging in age from 20 to 35 years who received Berinert with repeated doses, up to 3500 U per attack, reported no complications during delivery and no harmful effects on their 34 neonates. In pregnant women, the benefits of treatment should be weighed against the potential risks.

Nursing Women: Berinert has not been evaluated in nursing mothers with HAE. Berinert should be given to nursing mothers only if clearly needed.

Pediatrics: The safety and efficacy of Berinert was not systematically evaluated in children.

* An HAE attack of moderate intensity is characterized by a degree of discomfort caused by clinical HAE symptoms that results in some interference with daily activities. An HAE attack of severe intensity is characterized by a degree of discomfort caused by clinical HAE symptoms that makes it impossible to perform daily activities.

Geriatrics: Safety and efficacy of Berinert in the geriatric population have not been established. Clinical studies with Berinert included four subjects greater than 65 years old. There were an insufficient number of subjects in this age group to determine whether they respond differently from younger subjects.

ADVERSE REACTIONS: Adverse Drug Reaction Overview: The most serious adverse reaction reported in subjects in clinical studies who received Berinert is an increase in the severity of pain associated with HAE.

The most common adverse reactions that have been reported in greater than 4% of the subjects who received Berinert are HAE, headache, abdominal pain, nausea, muscle spasms, pain, diarrhea, and vomiting.

The other common adverse reactions that have been reported in 1% to 4 % of the subjects who received Berinert are back pain, dysgeusia, edema peripheral, abdominal distension and upper respiratory tract infection.

Clinical Trial Adverse Drug Reactions: Because clinical trials are conducted under very specific conditions the adverse reaction rates observed in the clinical trials may not reflect the rates observed in practice and should not be compared to the rates in the clinical trials of another drug. Adverse drug reaction information from clinical trials is useful for identifying drug-related adverse events and for approximating rates.

Pivotal Study: In a pivotal Phase III clinical study, 124 subjects experiencing an acute moderate to severe abdominal or facial HAE attack were treated with Berinert (either a 10 U per kg body weight dose, 20 U per kg body weight dose), or placebo (physiological saline solution). Table 1, Table 2 and Table 3 list the associated Adverse Events (AEs) that occurred in more than 4% of the subjects up to 4 hours, 72 hours and 9 days respectively after the end of a Berinert infusion, **irrespective of causality**.

Table 1: Berinert

Adverse Reactions[a] Occurring Up to 4 Hours After Initial Infusion in More Than 4% of Subjects, Irrespective of Causality[b]

Adverse Reactions	Number (%) of Subjects Reporting Adverse Reactions Berinert 20 units/kg (n=43)	Number (%) of Subjects Reporting Adverse Reactions Placebo Group (n=42)
Nausea[b]	3 (7%)	5 (11.9%)
Dysgeusia	2 (4.7%)	0 (0)
Abdominal pain[b]	2 (4.7%)	3 (7.1%)
Vomiting[b]	1 (2.3%)	3 (7.1%)
Diarrhea[b]	0 (0)	4 (9.5%)
Headache	0 (0)	2 (4.8%)

[a] The study protocol specified that adverse events that began within 72 hours of blinded study medication administration were to be classified as at least possibly related to study medication (ie, adverse reactions).

[b] The following abdominal symptoms were identified in the protocol as associated with HAE abdominal attacks: abdominal pain, bloating, cramps, nausea, vomiting, and diarrhea.

Table 2: Berinert

Adverse Reactions[a] Occurring in More Than 4% of Subjects Up to 72 Hours After Infusion of Initial or Rescue Medication[b] by Intent-to-Treat, Irrespective of Causality

Adverse Reactions Number (%) of Subjects	Reporting Adverse Reactions[b,c] Berinert 20 units/kg (n=43)	Number (%) of Subjects Reporting Adverse Reactions[b,c] Placebo Group (n=42)
Nausea	3 (7%)	11 (26.2%)
Headache	3 (7%)	5 (11.9%)
Abdominal pain	3 (7%)	5 (11.9%)
Dysgeusia	2 (4.7%)	1 (2.4%)
Vomiting	1 (2.3%)	7 (16.7%)
Pain	1 (2.3%)	4 (9.5%)
Muscle spasms	1 (2.3%)	4 (9.5%)
Diarrhea	0 (0)	8 (19%)
Back pain	0 (0)	2 (4.8%)
Facial pain	0 (0)	2 (4.8%)

[a] The study protocol specified that adverse events that began within 72 hours of blinded study medication administration were to be classified as at least possibly related to study medication (ie, adverse reactions).

[b] If a subject experienced no relief or insufficient relief of symptoms within 4 hours after infusion, investigators had the option to administer a blinded second infusion ("rescue" treatment) of Berinert (20 units/kg for the placebo group or 10 units/kg for the 10 units/kg group), or placebo (for the 20 units/kg group).

[c] Adverse reactions following either initial treatment and/or blinded "rescue" treatment. Because more subjects in the placebo randomization group than in the Berinert randomization group received rescue treatment, the median observation period in this analysis for subjects randomized to placebo was slightly longer than for subjects randomized to receive Berinert.

Table 3: Berinert

Incidence of Adverse Events by Descending Frequency Occurring in More Than 4% of Subjects Receiving Berinert Up to 9 Days after Infusion, Irrespective of Causality

Adverse Event	Number of Subjects Reporting AE (n=108)	Percent
Hereditary angioedema	14	13.0
Headache	13	12.0
Abdominal pain[a]	7	6.5
Nausea[a]	7	6.5
Muscle spasms	6	5.6
Pain	6	5.6

(cont'd)

Table 3: Berinert *(cont'd)*

Incidence of Adverse Events by Descending Frequency Occurring in More Than 4% of Subjects Receiving Berinert Up to 9 Days after Infusion, Irrespective of Causality

Adverse Event	Number of Subjects Reporting AE (n=108)	Percent
Diarrhea[a]	5	4.6
Vomiting[a]	5	4.6

[a] Symptoms were considered to be related to the underlying disease. Any increase in intensity or new occurrence of these symptoms after study medication administration was considered to be an AE.

Extension Study: In a supportive Phase III extension study, 56 subjects with 559 acute moderate to severe abdominal or facial attacks received a 20 U/kg body weight dose of Berinert. Table 4 lists the associated AEs that occurred in this extension study in more than 4% of subjects up to 72 hours or 9 days after the end of a Berinert infusion, **irrespective of causality**.

Table 4: Berinert

Incidence of Adverse Events by Descending Frequency Occurring in More Than 4% of Subjects Receiving Berinert Up to 72 Hours or 9 Days after Infusion, Irrespective of Causality

Adverse Event	Number (%) of Subjects Reporting Adverse Events up to 72 hours (n=56)	Number (%) of Subjects Reporting Adverse Events up to 72 hours (n=56)
Headache	3 (5.4%)	4 (7.1%)
Abdominal pain	3 (5.4%)	3 (5.4%)
Hereditary angioedema	2 (3.6%)	4 (7.1%)
Nasopharyngitis	2 (3.6%)	3 (5.4%)

Less Common Clinical Trial Adverse Drug Reactions (<1%): The following lists the associated Adverse Events (AEs) that occurred in less than 1% of the subjects up to 9 days after the end of a Berinert infusion in a Pivotal phase III clinical study CE1145_3001, **irrespective of causality** (grouped by SOC).
Ear and Labyrinth Disorders: ear pain.
Gastrointestinal Disorders: abdominal pain upper, dysphagia, eructation, lip swelling, retching, toothache, haemorrhoidal haemorrhage.
General Disorders and Administration Site Conditions: face edema, pyrexia, puncture site reaction.
Hepatobiliary Disorders: biliary colic.
Infections and Infestations: bronchitis, cystitis, influenza.
Investigations: blood pressure increase, increased body temperature.
Musculoskeletal and Connective Tissue Disorders: tendonitis, joint swelling.
Psychiatric Disorders: anxiety.
Renal and Urinary Disorders: haematuria, renal pain.
Respiratory, Thoracic and Mediastinal Disorders: cough, pharyngolaryngeal pain, rhinorrhoea, throat irritation.
Post-Market Adverse Drug Reactions: Because postmarketing reporting of adverse reactions is voluntary and from a population of uncertain size, it is not always possible to reliably estimate the frequency of these reactions or establish a causal relationship to product exposure.

Adverse reactions reported in patients receiving Berinert for treatment of HAE include allergic/anaphylactic reactions, injection-site pain, injection-site redness, chills, and fever.

The following adverse reactions, identified by system organ class, have been attributed to Berinert during post approval use.
Immune System Disorders: allergic/anaphylactic reactions.
General/Body as a Whole: pain on injection, redness at injection site, chills, fever.

DRUG INTERACTIONS: No formal drug interaction studies have been conducted with Berinert, and to date no relevant interactions are known.

DOSAGE AND ADMINISTRATION: Recommended Dose and Dosage Adjustment: The recommended dose of Berinert for the treatment of acute **abdominal and facial** HAE episodes **of moderate or severe intensity** is 20 units (U) per kg body weight administered by intravenous injection.
Administration: It is recommended that Berinert be administered by slow intravenous injection at a rate of 4 mL/minute.

Berinert should not be mixed with other medicinal products and should be administered by a separate infusion line.
Reconstitution: Use the Mix2Vial filter transfer set provided with Berinert (see Dosage Forms, Composition and Packaging).
Ensure that the diluent and product vials are at room temperature. Then, follow these steps to reconstitute Berinert:

1. Remove the caps from both vials to expose the central portions of the rubber stoppers.
2. Clean the surface of the rubber stoppers with an alcohol swab and allow them to dry.
3. Open the Mix2Vial package by peeling away the lid. To maintain sterility, leave the Mix2Vial set in its clear outer package.
4. Place the diluent vial on a level surface and hold the vial tightly. Grasp the Mix2Vial package and firmly snap the blue end of the Mix2Vial set onto the stopper of the diluent vial.
5. While holding the diluent vial, carefully remove the outer package from the Mix2Vial set. Make sure to pull off only the package, not the Mix2Vial set.
6. With the product vial firmly on a surface, invert the diluent vial with the Mix2Vial set attached and firmly snap the transparent end onto the stopper of the product vial. The diluent will transfer into the product vial automatically.
7. With the diluent and product vials still attached to the Mix2Vial set, gently swirl the product vial to ensure the product is fully dissolved. Do not shake the vial.
8. With one hand, grasp the product vial and with the other hand grasp the diluent vial; then turn the diluent vial counterclockwise to separate it from the Mix2Vial set/product vial.
9. Draw air into an empty, sterile syringe. With the product vial upright, screw the syringe to the Mix2Vial set. Press the syringe plunger to inject air into the product vial. Keeping the syringe plunger pressed, invert the product vial and draw the solution into the syringe by slowly pulling the plunger back.
10. Once the solution has been transferred into the syringe, firmly grasp the barrel of the syringe (keeping the plunger facing down) and unscrew the syringe from the Mix2Vial set. Attach the syringe to an infusion set or another suitable administration set.

Do not refrigerate after reconstitution. To ensure product sterility, reconstitute and administer Berinert using aseptic techniques. Berinert contains no preservatives, the reconstituted product should be administered immediately.

The reconstituted solution should be a colorless and clear solution. Inspect Berinert visually for particulate matter and discoloration prior to administration. Do not use if the solution is cloudy or contains particulates.

OVERDOSAGE:
Up to now, the development of thrombosis has been reported in association with Berinert when used (off-label) and at higher than labeled doses (greater than 90 U/kg body weight) in newborns and young children with congenital heart anomalies during or after cardiac surgery under extracorporeal circulation.

For management of a suspected drug overdose, contact your regional Poison Control Centre. See the *CPS* Directory section for a list of Poison Control Centres.

ACTION AND CLINICAL PHARMACOLOGY: Mechanism of Action: C1 esterase inhibitor is a normal constituent of human plasma and belongs to the group of serine protease inhibitors (serpins) that includes antithrombin III, alpha1-protease inhibitor, alpha2-antiplasmin, and heparin cofactor II. As with the other inhibitors in this group, C1 esterase inhibitor has an important inhibiting potential on several of the major cascade systems of the human body, including the complement system, the intrinsic coagulation (contact) system, the fibrinolytic system, and the coagulation cascade. Regulation of these systems is performed through the formation of complexes between the proteinase and the inhibitor, resulting in inactivation of both and consumption of the C1 esterase inhibitor.

C1 esterase inhibitor, which is usually activated during the inflammatory process, inactivates its substrate by covalently binding to the reactive site. C1 esterase inhibitor is the only known inhibitor for the subcomponent of the complement component 1 (C1r), C1s, coagulation factor XIIa, and kallikrein. Additionally, C1 esterase inhibitor is the main inhibitor for coagulation factor XIa of the intrinsic coagulation cascade.

HAE patients have low levels of endogenous or functional C1 esterase inhibitor. Although the events that induce attacks of angioedema in HAE patients are not well defined, it has been postulated that increased vascular permeability and the clinical manifestation of HAE attacks may be primarily mediated through contact system activation. Suppression of contact system activation by C1 esterase inhibitor through the inactivation of plasma kallikrein and factor XIIa is thought to modulate this vascular permeability by preventing the generation of bradykinin.

Administration of Berinert to patients with C1 esterase inhibitor deficiency replaces the missing or malfunctioning protein in patients. The plasma concentration of C1 esterase inhibitor in healthy volunteers is approximately 270 mg/L.
Pharmacodynamics: No pharmacodynamic studies in humans have been performed for Berinert, but due to the pharmacological profile of C1-INH and the pathophysiological changes observed in subjects with HAE, it is assumed that intravenously administered C1-INH has an identical pharmacodynamic profile to that of endogenous C1-INH in the plasma of healthy subjects.
Pharmacokinetics: The pharmacokinetics (PK) of Berinert were evaluated in an open-label, uncontrolled, single-center study in 40 subjects (34 adults and 6 children under 18 years of age) with either mild or severe HAE. The 25 subjects with mild HAE were treated on demand for an acute attack; the 15 subjects with severe HAE were treated on a prophylactic basis. All subjects received a single intravenous injection of Berinert ranging from 500 U to 1500 U. The median dose was 1058 U (range: 526-1010 U), the median dose per kg body weight was 14.5 U/kg (range: 9.9-22.1 U/kg). Blood was sampled to determine C1 esterase inhibitor activity at baseline and for up to 72 hours after the infusion. In addition, the in vivo recovery (IVR) was calculated for the first 4 hours after the infusion.

The median volume of distribution at steady state for Berinert in all subjects was 45.4 mL/kg body weight, which corresponds to 3.2 L for a person weighing 70 kg. The median systemic clearance was 1.0 mL/kg/hour (70 mL/h for a person weighing 70 kg), resulting in an overall median elimination half-life of 36.1 hours.

STORAGE AND STABILITY: When stored at temperatures of 2 to 25°C, Berinert is stable for the period indicated by the expiration date on the carton and vial label (up to 30 months). Keep Berinert in its original carton until ready to use. Do not freeze. Protect from light.

INFORMATION FOR THE PATIENT: Published in e-CPS, available by subscription at www.e-cps.ca.

DOSAGE FORMS, COMPOSITION AND PACKAGING: Each vial contains: lyophilized human C1 esterase inhibitor (C1-INH) 500 U. Nonmedicinal ingredients: glycine, sodium chloride and sodium citrate. Single-use vials of concentrate for reconstitution with 10 mL of Sterile Water for Injection (Diluent). Each product package consists of a carton containing the vials of Berinert and Sterile Water for Injection (Diluent) and the Mix2Vial transfer set. The components used in the packaging for Berinert are latex-free.

Besifloxacin

CPhA Monograph

see *Fluoroquinolones*

The reader is invited to consult CPhA's monograph **Fluoroquinolones.**

Besivance™

besifloxacin

Antibacterial (ophthalmic)

Bausch & Lomb

Date of Preparation: October 23, 2009

SUMMARY PRODUCT INFORMATION:

Route of Administration	Dosage Form/ Strength	Clinically Relevant Nonmedicinal Ingredients
Ophthalmic Topical	7.5 mL bottle containing 5 mL of 0.6% w/v sterile ophthalmic suspension	Contains poloxamer 407, polycarbophil, benzalkonium chloride. For a complete listing see Dosage Forms, Composition and Packaging.

INDICATIONS AND CLINICAL USE: BESIVANCE (besifloxacin ophthalmic suspension) 0.6% w/v is indicated for the treatment of patients one year of age and older with bacterial conjunctivitis caused by susceptible strains of the following organisms:
Aerobic, Gram-Positive: CDC coryneform group G: *S. aureus*, *S. epidermidis*, *S. mitis*, *S. oralis*, *S. pneumoniae*.
Aerobic, Gram-Negative: *H. influenzae*.
Geriatrics (>60 years of age): No overall differences in safety and effectiveness have been observed between elderly and younger patients.
Pediatrics (<1 year old): The safety and efficacy of BESIVANCE in patients less than one year of age have not been established.

CONTRAINDICATIONS: BESIVANCE is contraindicated in patients with known hypersensitivity to this drug, to other quinolones, or to any ingredient in the formulation or component of the container. For a complete listing, see Dosage Forms, Composition and Packaging.

WARNINGS AND PRECAUTIONS: General; Not for injection into the eye. For topical ophthalmic use only.

BESIVANCE is a sterile suspension for topical ophthalmic use only, and should not be injected subconjunctivally, nor should it be introduced directly into the anterior chamber of the eye. There are no data to support use of BESIVANCE in patients with concomitant corneal injury/damage.
Contact Lenses: Patients should be advised **not** to wear contact lenses if they have signs and symptoms of bacterial conjunctivitis or during the course of therapy with BESIVANCE.
Growth of Resistant Organisms with Prolonged Use: As with other anti-infectives, prolonged use of BESIVANCE may result in overgrowth of non-susceptible organisms, including fungi. If super-infection occurs, discontinue use and institute alternative therapy. Whenever clinical judgment dictates, the patient should be examined with the aid of magnification, such as slit-lamp biomicroscopy and, where appropriate, fluorescein staining.
Carcinogenesis and Mutagenesis: Long-term studies in animals to determine the carcinogenic potential of besifloxacin have not been performed.
Immune: Anaphylaxis and Hypersensitivity: Besifloxacin is only commercially available for topical ophthalmic administration. While anaphylaxis or other hypersensitivity reactions have not been observed with topical ophthalmic use of besifloxacin in humans, the potential for such reactions should be considered since patients with known hypersensitivity to fluoroquinolones were excluded from clinical trials.

In patients receiving systemically administered quinolones, serious and occasionally fatal hypersensitivity (anaphylactic) reactions have been reported, some following the first dose. Some reactions were accompanied by cardiovascular collapse, loss of consciousness, angioedema (including laryngeal, pharyngeal or facial edema), airway obstruction, dyspnea, urticaria, and itching.

If any allergic reaction occurs, BESIVANCE should be discontinued and appropriate therapy should be administered as clinically indicated.

Special Populations: Pregnant Women: Since there are no adequate and well-controlled studies in pregnant women, BESIVANCE should be used during pregnancy only if the potential benefit justifies the potential risk to the fetus.

In an oral embryofetal development study in rats, the No Observable Adverse Effect Level (NOAEL) for besifloxacin was 100 mg/kg/day for both parental and reproductive toxicity based on maternal mortality, decreased uterine weight, increased resorptions and post-implantation loss, and reduced fetal bodyweight together with a delay in fetal ossification at the highest dose of 1000 mg/kg/day. This NOAEL is approximately 3333 times the highest recommended total daily human ophthalmic dose (based on a three times daily dosing regimen with 50 µL eye drops in both eyes of a 60 kg patient). In a similar study in rabbits, the fetal and maternal NOAEL was 2 mg/kg/day based on abortions and early deliveries, decreased uterine weight, increased resorptions and post-implantation loss and reduced fetal bodyweight at the highest dose of 20 mg/kg/day. This NOAEL is approximately 67 times the highest recommended total daily human ophthalmic dose. In a prenatal and postnatal development study in rats, the NOAEL for parental toxicity was 10 mg/kg/day (approximately 333 times the highest recommended total daily human ophthalmic dose), based on decreased body weight and food intake at 100 mg/kg/day, and the NOAEL for reproductive performance of parental females and development of their pups was 100 mg/kg/day (approximately 3333 times the highest recommended total daily human ophthalmic dose), based on litter size reduction, decreased survival, developmental retardation, and delayed sexual maturation of the pups at 1000 mg/kg/day. The exposure-based safety factors for embryofetal and prenatal/postnatal development, calculated using the lowest NOAEL dose of 2 mg/kg in the rabbit compared to human exposure following ocular administration is greater than 150-fold.

Nursing Women: Besifloxacin has not been measured in human milk, although it can be presumed to be excreted in human milk. Caution should be exercised when BESIVANCE is administered to a nursing mother.

Pediatrics (<1 year of age): The safety and effectiveness of BESIVANCE in infants below one year of age have not been established. The efficacy of BESIVANCE in treating bacterial conjunctivitis in pediatric patients one year or older has been demonstrated in controlled clinical trials.

There is no evidence that the ophthalmic administration of quinolones has any effect on weight bearing joints, even though systemic administration of some quinolones has been shown to cause arthropathy in immature animals.

Geriatrics (>60 years of age): No overall differences in safety and effectiveness have been observed between elderly and younger patients.

ADVERSE REACTIONS: Adverse Drug Reaction Overview: A total of 2377 patients were enrolled in three safety and efficacy trials, 1187 into the BESIVANCE group, 614 into a vehicle group, and 576 into an active control group. BESIVANCE was administered three times daily for five days. The population treated with BESIVANCE was between 1 and 98 years old with clinical signs and symptoms of bacterial conjunctivitis.

No serious adverse reactions related to BESIVANCE were reported.

Overall, 75/1187 (6.3%) subjects treated with BESIVANCE had a treatment-emergent non-ocular adverse event.

Similarly, 139/1187 (11.7%) study eyes treated with BESIVANCE had a treatment-emergent ocular adverse event.

15/1187 (1.3%) of subjects treated with BESIVANCE discontinued treatment due to an AE.

The most frequently reported treatment-emergent ocular adverse events in the study eye were blurred vision (2.1%), eye pain (1.9%), and eye irritation (1.4%).

Clinical Trial Adverse Drug Reactions: Because clinical trials are conducted under very specific conditions the adverse reaction rates observed in the clinical trials may not reflect the rates observed in practice and should not be compared to the rates in the clinical trials of another drug. Adverse drug reaction information from clinical trials is useful for identifying drug-related adverse events and for approximating rates.

Bacterial Conjunctivitis Trials: The rates of the most common treatment-emergent ocular adverse events irrespective of causality observed in eyes treated with BESIVANCE during the three bacterial conjunctivitis clinical trials are displayed in Table 1.

Table 1: BESIVANCE

Incidence (%) of Treatment-Emergent Adverse Events Irrespective of Causality that Occurred in ≥1% of Study Eyes/Patients Treated with BESIVANCE or Vehicle in Bacterial Conjunctivitis Studies (Population: Safety[a])

Adverse Events	Besifloxacin n=1187 (%)	Vehicle n=614 (%)
Eye Disorders		
Vision Blurred	25 (2.1%)	24 (3.9%)
Eye Irritation	17 (1.4%)	18 (2.9%)
Eye Pain	22 (1.9%)	11 (1.8%)
Conjunctivitis	14 (1.2%)	15 (2.4%)
Eye Pruritus	13 (1.1%)	10 (1.6%)
Conjunctivitis Bacterial	7 (0.6%)	9 (1.5%)
Nervous System Disorders		
Headache	21 (1.8%)	11 (1.8%)

[a] Safety population includes subjects treated for bacterial conjunctivitis that were randomized and received at least one dose of the study drug in the three safety and efficacy studies. BESIVANCE was tested in all three studies, while the vehicle was tested in only two of the studies.

The most frequently reported treatment-related ocular adverse events (possibly, probably or definitely related) in the study eye were blurred vision (1.9%), eye irritation (1.3%), and eye pain (1.2%).

Less Common Clinical Trial Adverse Drug Reactions (<1%) : Treatment-related adverse events (possibly, probably or definitely related) reported in 0.1 to 1.0% of eyes receiving BESIVANCE included:

Eye Disorders: eye pruritus, dry eye, conjunctivitis, conjunctivitis bacterial, punctate keratitis, conjunctival oedema, eye discharge, corneal infiltrates, corneal staining, eyelid margin crusting, keratoconjunctivitis sicca, foreign body sensation in eyes, conjunctival follicles, dry skin, eye disorder, instillation site pain, photophobia, visual disturbance.

Nervous System Disorders: headache.

DRUG INTERACTIONS: Overview: No specific interaction studies have been performed. Results from in vitro and in vivo metabolism studies demonstrated that the overall extent of besifloxacin metabolism was very low. Topical ophthalmic use of besifloxacin is not expected to elicit any potential systemic PK drug interactions because systemic exposure to besifloxacin is low following topical administration to humans (see Action and Clinical Pharmacology, Pharmacokinetics).

Drug-Drug Interactions: No specific drug-drug interaction studies were conducted.

Drug-Food Interactions: Interactions of BESIVANCE with food have not been established.

Drug-Herb Interactions: Interactions of BESIVANCE with herbal products have not been established.

Drug-Laboratory Test Interactions: Interactions of BESIVANCE with laboratory tests have not been established.

DOSAGE AND ADMINISTRATION: Dosing Considerations: BESIVANCE (besifloxacin ophthalmic suspension) 0.6% is administered by instillation into the affected eye(s). It is indicated for topical ophthalmic use only, and should **not** be administered systemically, injected subconjunctivally, or introduced directly into the anterior chamber of the eye. BESIVANCE is **not for injection.**

Recommended Dose and Dosage Adjustment: The recommended dosage regimen for BESIVANCE in the treatment of patients one year of age and older with bacterial conjunctivitis is to instill one drop in the affected eye(s) 3 times a day for 7 days.

Missed Dose: If a dose of this medication has been missed, it should be taken as soon as possible. However, if it is almost time for the next dose, the missed dose should be skipped and return to the regular dosing schedule. Do not double doses.

Administration: Patients should be advised to thoroughly wash hands prior to using BESIVANCE.

Patients should be advised to avoid contaminating the applicator tip with material from the eye, fingers or other source.

Patients should be instructed to invert closed bottle (upside down) and shake once before each use. Remove cap with bottle still in the inverted position. Tilt head back, and with bottle inverted, gently squeeze bottle to instill one drop into the affected eye(s).

OVERDOSAGE:
No information is available on overdosage of BESIVANCE. A topical overdose of BESIVANCE may be flushed from the eye(s) with warm tap water.

> For management of a suspected drug overdose, contact your **regional Poison Control Centre**. See the *CPS* Directory section for a list of Poison Control Centres.

ACTION AND CLINICAL PHARMACOLOGY: Mechanism of Action: Besifloxacin is an 8-chloro fluoroquinolone with a N-1 cyclopropyl group that has activity against Gram-positive and Gram-negative bacteria.

The antibacterial action of besifloxacin results from dual inhibition of DNA gyrase and topoisomerase IV. DNA gyrase is an essential enzyme required for replication, transcription and repair of bacterial DNA. Topoisomerase IV is an essential enzyme required for partitioning of the chromosomal DNA during bacterial cell division.

Pharmacodynamics: Due to low systemic exposure of besifloxacin, QT prolongation in patients is unlikely (see Action and Clinical Pharmacology, Pharmacokinetics).

Pharmacokinetics: See Table 2.

Table 2: BESIVANCE

Summary of Besifloxacin Pharmacokinetic Parameters Following Topical Ocular Administration in Humans

Tissue	Dose Regime/Study Day	C_{max}	$t_{½}$ (h)	$AUC_{(0-t)}$
Plasma[a]	0.6% TID Day 1	0.37±0.27 ng/mL	4.3±2.2	$AUC_{(0-6)}$1.45±0.87 ng*h/mL
	0.6% TID Day 6[b]	0.43±0.30 ng/mL	6.8±2.1	$AUC_{(0-6)}$ 1.95±1.31 ng*h/mL $AUC_{(0-12)}$ 3.21±2.50 ng*h/mL
Tears[c]	0.6% Single Dose Day 1	610±540 µg/g	3.4	$AUC_{(0-24)}$ 1232 µg*h/g

[a] Data from human subjects with clinically diagnosed bilateral bacterial conjunctivitis.
[b] Subjects received 3 doses per day for 5 days and a single dose on Day 6 (16 doses total).
[c] Data from healthy human volunteers; values represent data from Full Analysis Set (FAS) population.

Absorption: Plasma concentrations of besifloxacin were measured in adult patients with suspected bacterial conjunctivitis who received BESIVANCE bilaterally three times a day (16 doses total). Following the first and last dose, variability in plasma besifloxacin concentrations between subjects was large, and the maximum plasma besifloxacin concentration in each patient was less than 1.3 ng/mL.

Distribution: The concentration of besifloxacin in tear fluid was measured in healthy adult subjects who received a single drop of BESIVANCE. Following a single administration, the mean besifloxacin concentration observed in samples collected 24 hours after a single administration was 1.6 µg/g. In vitro, besifloxacin was approximately 39-44% bound to proteins in human plasma and was approximately evenly distributed between plasma and the cellular components of human blood.

Metabolism: Results from in vitro studies with human hepatocytes and nonclinical in vivo studies demonstrate that besifloxacin is metabolically stable, with little or no chiral interconversion to the (−) enantiomer. Following in vitro incubation with hepatocytes from multiple species, a total of eight metabolites were observed; however, the relative amount of each metabolite was small and the overall extent of metabolism was very low.

Excretion: Following repeated topical ocular administration to humans, besifloxacin was eliminated from the systemic circulation with an apparent half-life of 6.8 hours. Excretion of besifloxacin has not been studied in humans.

Special Populations and Conditions: The pharmacokinetics of besifloxacin have not been studied specifically in special populations (e.g., pediatrics, geriatrics, gender, race, genetic polymorphism) or certain conditions (e.g., hepatic insufficiency, renal insufficiency).

STORAGE AND STABILITY: Store at 15-25°C. Protect from light.

SPECIAL HANDLING INSTRUCTIONS: There are no special handling instructions for BESIVANCE.

INFORMATION FOR THE PATIENT: Published in e-CPS, available by subscription at www.e-cps.ca.

DOSAGE FORMS, COMPOSITION AND PACKAGING: Each mL of sterile ophthalmic suspension contains: besifloxacin 6 mg (0.6%). Preservative: benzalkonium chloride 0.01%. Nonmedicinal ingredients: edetate disodium dihydrate, mannitol, poloxamer 407, polycarbophil, sodium chloride, sodium hydroxide and water for injection. White low density polyethylene (LDPE) bottles of 7.5 mL (containing 5 mL of suspension) with a controlled dropper tip and tan polypropylene cap. Tamper evidence is provided with a shrink band around the cap and neck area of the package.

(Shown in Product Identification Section)

Betaderm Ⓟ

betamethasone valerate

Topical Corticosteroid

Taro

SUPPLIED: Cream: 0.05%: Each g contains: betamethasone as betamethasone 17-valerate 0.05% in a water washable aqueous base of ceteareth-15, cetyl alcohol, chlorocresol, mineral oil, phosphoric acid, polyethylene glycol 1000, propylene glycol, purified water, sodium hydroxide, stearyl alcohol and white petrolatum. Jars of 454 g. Store at room temperature (15-30°C).

0.1% : Each g contains: betamethasone as betamethasone 17-valerate 0.1% in a water washable aqueous base of cetyl alcohol, chlorocresol, mineral oil, phosphoric acid, polyoxyethylene cetyl ether, propylene glycol, purified water, sodium hydroxide, sodium phosphate monobasic, stearyl alcohol and white petrolatum. Tubes of 15 g. Jars of 454 g. Store at room temperature (15-30°C).

Ointment: 0.05%: Each g contains: betamethasone as betamethasone 17-valerate 0.05% in a base consisting of fractionated coconut oil and white petrolatum and chlorocresol as a preservative. Jars of 454 g. Store at room temperature (15-30°C).

0.1%: Each g contains: betamethasone as betamethasone 17-valerate 0.1% in a base consisting of fractionated coconut oil and white petrolatum and chlorocresol as a preservative. Jars of 454 g. Store at room temperature (15-30°C).

Scalp Lotion: Each g contains: betamethasone as betamethasone 17-valerate 0.1% in a base of carbomer, isopropyl alcohol, purified water and sodium hydroxide. Plastic bottles of 75 mL. Store at room temperature (15-30°C).

Betadine® Topical Preparations

povidone-iodine

Antiseptic

Purdue Pharma

Date of Revision: November 16, 2009

INDICATIONS: Mouth-wash/Gargle: As a mouth-wash for routine use. Eliminates or reduces offensive mouth odours. As a gargle or mouth-wash, as primary or adjunctive therapy in infections of the mouth and throat such as aphthous stomatitis, Vincent's infection, pharyngitis, oral moniliasis, tonsillitis and following oral surgery and dental procedures. Because of its effectiveness as a germicide, it may be used following oral surgery and dental procedures and to help relieve the pain and irritation of minor sore throat.

Ointment: The treatment of minor skin infections. For the prevention of infection in burns, cuts, abrasions, poison ivy rash, poison oak rash and insect bites.
Solution: For the preparation of skin prior to surgery and injections. Use full strength for pre- and post-operative skin and mucus membrane antisepsis, prophylaxis and treatment of wounds, lacerations and burns, bacterial and mycotic infections of the skin, trichomonal, monilial and non-specific vaginitis, cervicitis, oral infections, and dental procedures. Film-forming, non-staining, water-soluble for the preparation of skin prior to surgery and injections. Dependable topical germicide.
Surgical Scrub: Pre- and post-operative scrubbing or washing, pre- and post-operative use on patients, general use in physician's office. Phosphate-free antiseptic sudsing skin cleanser. A microbicidal cleanser for the pre-operative and post-operative scrubbing or washing by hospital operating personnel and for general use in the physician's office.

CONTRAINDICATIONS: Not to be used in known hypersensitivity to iodine or povidone. Not to be used in hyperfunction of the thyroid (hyperthyroidism), other manifest thyroid diseases, as well as before and after radioactive iodine therapy. It should not be used prior to radioiodine scintigraphy (thyroid gland) or radioiodine treatment of thyroid carcinoma.

WARNINGS: See Precautions.

PRECAUTIONS: General: For external use only. Avoid contact with eyes. If contact occurs, flush eyes with water. In pre-operative preparation, avoid "pooling" beneath the patient. Prolonged exposure to wet solution may cause irritation or rarely, severe skin reactions. Chemical burns of skin due to "pooling" may occur (chemical burn of skin). Discontinue use and consult a physician promptly if skin irritation, contact dermatitis, hypersensitivity or allergic reaction develops. These may be signs of a serious condition. Do not heat prior to application. Keep out of the reach of children.

Patients with goiter, thyroid nodules, or other thyroid diseases (thyroid disorder) are at risk of developing thyroid hyperfunction (hyperthyroidism) from the administration of large amounts of iodine. In this patient population, povidone-iodine solution should not be applied for an extended period of time and to large areas of the skin unless strictly indicated. Even after the end of the treatment one should look for the early symptoms of possible hyperthyroidism and if necessary the thyroid function should be monitored.

Newborns and small infants are at increased risk of developing hypothyroidism from the administration of large amounts of iodine. Because of the permeable nature of their skin and the increased sensitivity to iodine, the use of povidone-iodine should be kept to the absolute minimum in newborns and small infants. A check of the child's thyroid function (e.g., T_4 levels and TSH levels) may be necessary. Any possible oral ingestion of povidone-iodine by the infant must be absolutely avoided. Betadine Mouth-wash/Gargle: Consult your physician promptly for severe or persistent sore throat, or sore throat accompanied by high fever, headache, nausea or vomiting. Betadine Ointment: In case of deep puncture or serious burns, consult a physician. If infection increases, discontinue use and consult a physician.

Drug Interactions: Drug Interactions and Other Forms of Interactions: The PVP-iodine complex is effective at pH values of between 2.0 and 7.0. It has to be expected that the complex will react with protein and other unsaturated organic compounds, leading to impairment of its effectiveness.

The concomitant use of wound-treatment preparations containing enzymatic components leads to weakening of the effects of both substances. Products containing mercury, silver, hydrogen peroxide, alkali, tannic acid and taurolidine may interact with povidone-iodine and should not be used concomitantly.

Povidone-iodine products when used concomitantly or immediately after application of octenidine containing antiseptics in the same or adjacent sites may lead to transient dark discolorations in the areas involved.

Note: Due to the oxidative effect of povidone-iodine solution various diagnostic agents can show false-positive lab results (e.g. tests with toluidine or gum guaiac for the determination of hemoglobin or glucose in the stool or the urine).

Absorption of iodine from povidone iodine solution may interfere with thyroid function tests. During the use of povidone-iodine solution the iodine uptake of the thyroid can be lowered; this can lead to interference with various investigations (thyroid scintigraphy, determination of PBI [protein-bound iodine], radioiodine diagnostics) and can make a planned treatment of the thyroid with iodine (radioiodine therapy) impossible. After the end of the treatment, an appropriate interval should be allowed before a new scintigram is carried out.

Pregnancy: During pregnancy and lactation, povidone-iodine solution should only be used if strictly indicated and its use should be kept to the absolute minimum. Because of the ability of iodine to pass through the placenta and be secreted in breast milk, and because of the increased sensitivity of the fetus and newborn to iodine, no large amounts of povidone-iodine should be administrated during pregnancy and lactation. Moreover, iodine is concentrated in the breast milk, as compared with the serum. Povidone-iodine use may induce transient hypothyroidism with elevation of TSH (thyroid stimulating hormone) in the fetus or in the newborn. A check of the child's thyroid function may be necessary. Any possible oral ingestion of the solution by the infant must be absolutely avoided.

Lactation: See Pregnancy.

ADVERSE EFFECTS: Rarely, hypersensitive skin reactions may occur (e.g. delayed contact-allergic reactions (delayed type hypersensitivity reaction), which can appear in the form of pruritus, erythema, small blisters or similar manifestations).

Very rarely, acute, generalized, allergic reactions (anaphylactic reactions) with drop in blood pressure (blood pressure decreased) and/or dyspnea as well as cases of acute skin and mucosal swelling (angioedema) have been reported.

The long-term use of povidone-iodine solution for the treatment of wounds and burns over extensive areas of the skin can lead to a notable uptake of iodine. In isolated cases, patients with a history of thyroid disease can develop hyperfunction of the thyroid (iodine induced hyperthyroidism), sometimes with symptoms such as tachycardia or restlessness.

Following uptake of large amounts of povidone-iodine (e.g., in the treatment of burns), the appearance of additional disorders of electrolyte imbalance and abnormal blood osmolarity, impairment of renal function with acute renal failure and metabolic acidosis have been described in the use of iodine-containing products.

OVERDOSE:

Symptoms: Acute iodine toxicity is manifested by abdominal symptoms, anuria, circulatory collapse, pulmonary edema and metabolic abnormalities.

Treatment: Treatment is symptomatic and supportive.

> For management of a suspected drug overdose, CPhA recommends that you contact your **regional Poison Control Centre**. See the *CPS* Directory section for a list of Poison Control Centres.

DOSAGE: Mouth-wash/Gargle: For use as needed. As a routine mouth-wash: use full strength or dilute to taste. Effective up to dilution of 1 part Betadine with 2 parts water. As a gargle or mouth-wash: use full strength for 30 seconds, hourly, or as directed by physician or dentist.
Ointment: Apply directly to affected area once or twice daily unless directed otherwise by a healthcare practitioner.
Solution: Pre-operative use on patients: Clean the affected area. Following cleansing of the operative area with Betadine Surgical Scrub, Apply apply Betadine Solution at full strength as often as needed as a paint or wet soak. Allow to dry before applying surgical drapes and avoid "pooling" beneath the patient. Prolonged exposure to the solution may cause irritation or rarely, severe skin reaction. In rare instance of local irritation or sensitivity, discontinue use promptly.
Patients with wounds, burns, skin lesions: Apply as needed once or twice daily. For wounds, burns, and skin lesions, apply directly to affected area once or twice daily unless directed otherwise by a healthcare practitioner.
Surgical Scrub: Preoperative scrubbing by operating personnel: wet hands with water. Pour 5 mL on the palm of the hand and spread over both hands. Without adding more water, rub the scrub thoroughly over all the areas for about 5 minutes. Use a soft brush, if desired. Clean thoroughly under fingernails. Add a little water to develop copious suds. Rinse thoroughly under running water. Complete the wash by scrubbing with another 5 mL if desired.
Preoperative use on patients: wet the operative area with water. Apply scrub (1 mL is sufficient to cover an area of 125 to 200 cm^2) and rub thoroughly for about 5 minutes. Then develop a lather and rinse off by aid of sterile gauze saturated with water. The area may then be painted with solution and allowed to dry.
Use in physician's office: Use for washing whenever a germicidal soap is required. For maximum degerming of the hands proceed as follows: Wet hands with water. Pour 5 mL on the palm of the hand and spread over both hands. Without adding more water, rub the scrub thoroughly over all the areas for about 5 minutes. Use a soft brush, if desired. Clean thoroughly under fingernails. Add a little water to develop copious suds. Rinse thoroughly under running water. Complete the wash by scrubbing with another 5 mL if desired. To prepare the patient's skin proceed as follows: Wet the operative area with water. Apply scrub (1 mL is sufficient to cover an area of 125 to 200 cm^2) and rub thoroughly for about 5 minutes. Then develop a lather and rinse off by aid of sterile gauze saturated with water. The area may then be painted with solution and allowed to dry.

SUPPLIED: Mouth-wash/Gargle: Each mL of solution contains: povidone-iodine USP 1% and alcohol 8%. Nonmedicinal ingredients: alcohol, eucalyptus oil, glycerine, menthol, methyl salicylate, sodium cyclamate, sodium hydroxide and water. Bottles of 250 mL. Flammable. Keep away from open flame and sources of heat. Store at 15-25 °C.

Ointment: Each g contains: povidone-iodine USP 10% (1% available iodine) in a water-soluble polyethylene glycol ointment base. Nonmedicinal ingredients: polyethylene glycol, sodium bicarbonate and water. Tubes of 20 g. Store at 15-25 °C.
Solution: Each mL of solution contains: povidone-iodine USP 10% (1% available iodine). Nonmedicinal ingredients: citric acid, disodium hydrogen phosphate, glycerine, nonoxynol-9, sodium hydroxide and water. Plastic bottles of 100 and 500 mL. Store at 15-25 °C.
Surgical Scrub: Each mL of liquid contains: povidone-iodine USP 7.5% (0.75% available iodine). Nonmedicinal ingredients: ammonium nonoxynol-4 sulfate, lauric myristic diethanolamide, potassium iodate, sodium hydroxide and water. Plastic bottles of 500 mL. Store at 15-25 °C.

Betagan® Ⓟ
levobunolol HCl
Glaucoma Therapy

Allergan

PHARMACOLOGY: Levobunolol is a noncardioselective beta-adrenoceptor antagonist, equipotent at both $beta_1$ and $beta_2$ receptors. Levobunolol is approximately 60 times more potent than the dextro isomer in its beta-blocking activity, yet equipotent in its potential for direct myocardial depression. Accordingly, the levo isomer, levobunolol, is used. Levobunolol does not have significant local anesthetic (membrane-stabilizing) effect or intrinsic sympathomimetic activity.

Beta-adrenergic receptor blockade reduces cardiac output in both healthy subjects and patients with heart disease. In patients with severe impairment of myocardial function, beta-adrenergic receptor blockade may inhibit the stimulatory effect of the sympathetic nervous system necessary to maintain adequate cardiac function.

Beta-adrenergic receptor blockade in the bronchi and bronchioles results in increased airway resistance from unopposed parasympathetic activity. Such an effect in patients with asthma or other bronchospastic conditions is potentially dangerous.

Levobunolol, when instilled into the eye, will lower elevated intraocular pressure (IOP), as well as normal IOP, whether or not accompanied by glaucoma. Elevated IOP is a major risk factor in the pathogenesis of glaucomatous visual field loss. The higher the level of intraocular pressure, the greater the likelihood of optic nerve damage and visual field loss.

The onset of action with 1 drop of levobunolol can be detected within 1 hour after treatment, with maximum effect seen between 2 and 6 hours. A significant decrease in IOP can be maintained for up to 24 hours with once daily dosing of levobunolol 0.5%.

Measurements of aqueous flow and total outflow facility suggest that levobunolol lowers IOP primarily by decreasing aqueous humor production. Levobunolol reduces IOP with little or no effect on pupil size or accommodation, in contrast to the miosis which cholinergic agents are known to produce. The blurred vision and night blindness often associated with miotics would not be expected. This is particularly important in patients with central lens opacities who would experience decreased visual acuity with pupillary constriction.

Levobunolol has been shown to be as effective as timolol in lowering intraocular pressure.

In controlled clinical studies of up to 2 years duration, IOP was well controlled in approximately 80% of subjects treated with levobunolol 0.5% b.i.d. The mean IOP decreases from baseline were between 6.87 and 7.81 mm Hg. No significant effects on pupil size, tear production or corneal sensitivity were observed. Topically applied levobunolol at concentrations of 0.5 and 1%, decreased heart rate and blood pressure in some patients. The IOP-lowering effect of levobunolol was well maintained over the course of these studies.

In a 3-month controlled clinical study, once-daily application of levobunolol 0.5% controlled the IOP of 72% of subjects, producing an overall mean decrease in IOP of 7.0 mm Hg. Once-daily application of timolol 0.5% controlled the IOP of 64% of subjects, producing a mean decrease in IOP of 4.5 mm Hg. The difference in overall mean decreases in IOP was statistically significant.

In 2 subsequent 3-month trials comparing levobunolol 0.5% with timolol 0.5% administered once daily, overall differences between the 2 drugs were not significant. A greater percentage of subjects in both the levobunolol groups and the timolol groups maintained adequately lowered intraocular pressure in the latter 2 studies, probably because subjects with severe ocular hypertension, unlikely to be controlled by therapy with a beta-blocker alone, were excluded from the study.

In one 3-month study and one 1-year study, levobunolol 0.25% twice daily controlled the IOP of approximately 63 and 70% of the subjects, respectively. The overall mean decreases from baseline were 5.4 and 5.1 mm Hg respectively.

In another 3-month clinical study, the mean decrease in IOP was significantly greater (more than 2 mm Hg) in the 0.25 and 0.5% levobunolol twice-daily treatment groups than in the levobunolol 0.5% twice-daily treatment group.

The prophylactic effect of topical 0.5% levobunolol HCl on IOP elevations after neodymium: YAG laser posterior capsulotomies was investigated in a controlled study. One drop was administered 30 to 120 minutes prior to the capsulotomy. Eight subjects (38%) in the vehicle treatment group and none in the levobunolol group experienced increases from baseline in IOP of 10 mm Hg or greater. Mean reductions in IOP from baseline ranged from 2.1 to 2.9 mm Hg in the levobunolol group, while in the vehicle treatment group, IOP increases (4.4 to 6.4 mm Hg) were observed at hours 1, 2, and 3 following capsulotomy.

In a controlled study, 0.5% levobunolol or placebo were administered immediately after a unilateral extracapsular cataract extraction and implantation of a posterior chamber intraocular lens. Treatment continued on a once-daily basis for 7 days. The incidence of IOP elevations from baseline ≥ 10 mm Hg was 8 subjects (40%) in the vehicle group and 4 subjects (19%) in the levobunolol group. Mean IOP increased from baseline up to 8.6 mm Hg at 24 hours in the vehicle group and up to 2 mm Hg at 24 hours in the levobunolol group.

In another controlled study, levobunolol 0.5% was significantly more effective than betaxolol 0.5% or placebo in preventing increased IOP after cataract extraction and posterior chamber lens placement. Two drops of the assigned medication were administered to the study eye after surgery. A significant mean increase in intraocular pressure from the preoperative to the early postoperative period was noted in the groups treated with betaxolol (6.73 mm Hg), placebo (5.35 mm Hg) and timolol (3.83 mm Hg). Levobunolol-treated eyes showed a mean decrease in pressure of 0.43 mm Hg.

An IOP of 30 mm Hg or greater was found in 3 placebo-treated eyes (15%), 4 betaxolol-treated eyes (20%), 1 timolol-treated eye (5%), and none of the levobunolol-treated eyes. Five placebo-treated eyes (25%), 6 betaxolol-treated eyes (30%), 5 timolol-treated eyes (25%), and 1 levobunolol-treated eye (5%) experienced a pressure rise of 10 mm Hg or greater.

INDICATIONS: The control of intraocular pressure in patients with chronic open-angle glaucoma or mild to moderate ocular hypertension.

CONTRAINDICATIONS: In those individuals with bronchial asthma or with a history of bronchial asthma, or severe chronic obstructive pulmonary disease; sinus bradycardia; second- and third-degree atrioventricular block; overt cardiac failure; cardiogenic shock; or hypersensitivity to any component of this product.

WARNINGS: As with other topically applied ophthalmic drugs, levobunolol may be absorbed systemically. The same adverse reactions found with systemic administration of beta-adrenergic blocking agents may occur with topical administration.

Contains sodium metabisulfite, a sulfite that may cause allergic-type reactions including anaphylactic symptoms and life-threatening or less severe asthmatic episodes in certain susceptible people. The overall prevalence of sulfite sensitivity in the general population is unknown and probably low. Sulfite sensitivity is seen more frequently in asthmatic than in nonasthmatic people.

Keep out of reach of children. For external use only. Do not touch dropper tip to any surface, since this may contaminate the solution. Protect from light and excessive heat. Discard any unused solution after end of treatment period.

PRECAUTIONS: Use with caution in patients with known contraindications to systemic use of beta-adrenoceptor blocking agents. These include abnormally low heart rate and heart block more severe than first degree. Congestive heart failure should be adequately controlled before beginning therapy with levobunolol. In patients with a history of cardiac disease, especially arrhythmia and bradycardia, pulse rates should be monitored.

Use with caution in patients with known hypersensitivity to other beta-adrenoceptor blocking agents.

Use with caution in patients with known diminished pulmonary function.

Lactation: It is not known whether this drug is excreted in human milk. Systemic beta-blockers and topical timolol maleate are known to be excreted in human milk. Caution should be exercised when levobunolol is administered to a nursing woman.
Children: Safety and effectiveness in children have not been established.

Drug Interactions: Levobunolol may have additive effects in patients taking systemic antihypertensive drugs. These possible additive effects may include hypotension, including orthostatic hypotension, bradycardia, dizziness, and/or syncope. Conversely, systemic beta-adrenoceptor blocking agents may potentiate the ocular hypotensive effect of levobunolol.

Close observation of the patient is recommended when a beta-blocker is administered to patients receiving catecholamine-depleting drugs such as reserpine, because of possible additive effects and the production of hypotension and/or marked bradycardia, which may produce vertigo, syncope, or postural hypotension.

ADVERSE EFFECTS: Transient burning, stinging or itching, blepharoconjunctivitis and decreases in heart rate and blood pressure have been reported occasionally with the use of levobunolol. Iridocyclitis, headache, transient ataxia, dizziness, lethargy, urticaria and pruritus have been reported rarely. Decreased corneal sensitivity has been noted in a small number of patients. The following additional adverse reactions have been reported with ophthalmic use of beta$_1$ and beta$_2$ (nonselective) adrenergic receptor blocking agents:
Body as a whole: headache.
Cardiovascular: arrhythmia, syncope, heart block, cerebral vascular accident, cerebral ischemia, congestive heart failure, palpitation.
Digestive: nausea.
Psychiatric: depression.
Integumentary: hypersensitivity, including localized and generalized rash.
Respiratory: bronchospasm (predominantly in patients with pre-existing bronchospastic disease), respiratory failure.
Endocrine: masked symptoms of hypoglycemia in insulin-dependent diabetics.
Special Senses: signs and symptoms of keratitis, blepharoptosis, visual disturbances including refractive changes (due to withdrawal of miotic therapy in some cases), diplopia, ptosis.

Other reactions associated with the oral use of nonselective adrenergic receptor blocking agents should be considered potential effects with ophthalmic use of these agents.

OVERDOSE:

Symptoms: Overdose has not been reported to date. Should accidental ocular overdosage occur, flush eye(s) with water or normal saline. If accidentally ingested, efforts to decrease further absorption may be appropriate (gastric lavage). The most common signs and symptoms to be expected with overdosage of a systemic beta-adrenergic blocking agent are symptomatic bradycardia, hypotension, bronchospasm, and acute cardiac failure. Should these symptoms occur, discontinue therapy and initiate appropriate supportive therapy.

Treatment: See Symptoms.

> For management of a suspected drug overdose, CPhA recommends that you contact your **regional Poison Control Centre**. See the *CPS* Directory section for a list of Poison Control Centres.

DOSAGE: The recommended starting dose is 1 drop of levobunolol 0.25% twice a day in the affected eye(s). If the clinical response is not adequate, the dosage may be changed to 1 drop of levobunolol 0.5% twice a day in the affected eye(s). Levobunolol 0.5% once a day has been found to be effective in controlling IOP in many patients with mild to moderate open-angle glaucoma and ocular hypertension. As with any new medication, careful monitoring of patients is advised.

Dosages above 1 drop of levobunolol 0.5% twice a day are not generally more effective. If the patient's IOP is not at a satisfactory level on this regimen, concomitant therapy with dipivefrin and/or epinephrine, and/or pilocarpine and other miotics, and/or systemically administered carbonic anhydrase inhibitors, such as acetazolamide, can be instituted.

SUPPLIED: Each mL of sterile ophthalmic solution contains: levobunolol HCl 5 mg (0.5%). Nonmedicinal ingredients: benzalkonium chloride 0.004% (as preservative), edetate disodium, polyvinyl alcohol (Liquifilm), potassium phosphate monobasic, sodium chloride, sodium metabisulfite, sodium phosphate dibasic, sodium hydroxide or hydrochloric acid to adjust pH. Plastic dropper bottles of 3 mL (hospitals only), 5 and 10 mL. Protect from light and excessive heat.

Betaject® Pr

betamethasone sodium phosphate—betamethasone acetate
Glucocorticoid

Sandoz

SUPPLIED: Each mL of sterile, aqueous injectable suspension contains: betamethasone acetate 3 mg and betamethasone sodium phosphate equivalent to betamethasone 3 mg. Nonmedicinal ingredients: benzalkonium chloride and disodium edetate (as preservatives), dibasic sodium phosphate, monobasic sodium phosphate, sodium hydroxide and/or hydrochloric acid (to adjust pH) and water for injection. Multidose vials of 1 and 5 mL, boxes of 10 and 1, respectively. Store between 2 and 30°C. Protect from light. Protect from freezing. Discard within 28 days of initial use.

Betaloc® Pr

metoprolol tartrate
Beta-adrenoceptor Blocking Agent

AstraZeneca

Date of Preparation: June 26, 2000
Date of Revision: September 17, 2009

PHARMACOLOGY: BETALOC (metoprolol tartrate) is a β-adrenoceptor blocking agent. In vitro and in vivo animal studies have shown that it has a preferential effect on β$_1$-adrenoreceptors, chiefly located in cardiac muscle. This preferential effect is not absolute, however, and at higher doses, BETALOC also inhibits β$_2$-adrenoreceptors, chiefly located in the bronchial and vascular musculature. It is used in the treatment of hypertension, angina pectoris and to reduce mortality in patients with myocardial infarction.

The mechanism of the **antihypertensive** effect has not been established. Among the factors that may be involved are: competitive ability to antagonize catecholamine-induced tachycardia at the beta-receptor sites in the heart, thus decreasing heart rate, cardiac contractility and cardiac output; inhibition of renin release by the kidneys; inhibition of the vasomotor centres.

By blocking catecholamine-induced increases in heart rate, in velocity and extent of myocardial contraction and in blood pressure, metoprolol reduces the oxygen requirements of the heart at any given level of effort, thus making it useful in the long-term management of **angina pectoris**. However, in patients with heart failure, β-adrenoceptor blockade may increase oxygen requirements by increasing left ventricular fibre length and end-diastolic pressure.

The mechanisms involved in **reducing mortality in patients with acute myocardial infarction** are not fully understood.

Pharmacokinetics: In man, absorption of BETALOC is rapid and complete, with oxidative metabolism occurring in the liver primarily via cytochrome P450 2D6. Plasma levels following oral administration, however, approximate 50% of levels following i.v. administration, indicating about 50% first-pass metabolism.

Intersubject plasma levels achieved are highly variable after oral administration, although they show good reproducibility within each individual. Peak plasma concentrations are attained after approximately 1.5 to 2 hours with conventional metoprolol formulations, and after approximately 4 to 5 hours with sustained-release formulations. Upon repeated oral administration, the percentage of the dose systemically available is higher than after a single dose and also increases dose-dependently. Ingestion together with food may raise the systemic availability of an oral dose by approximately 30 to 40%. Only a small fraction of the drug (about 12%) is bound to human serum albumin. Metoprolol undergoes oxidative metabolism in the liver primarily by the CYP2D6 isoenzyme. Elimination is mainly by biotransformation in the liver, and the plasma half-life averages 3.5 hours (extremes: 1 and 9 hours). The total clearance rate is approximately 1 L/min and the protein binding rate is approximately 5 to 10%. Less than 5% of an oral dose of BETALOC is recovered unchanged in the urine; the rest is excreted by the kidneys as metabolites that appear to have no clinical significance.

The systemic availability and half-life of BETALOC in patients with renal failure do not differ to a clinically significant degree from those in normal subjects. The excretion of metabolites, however, is reduced. Significant accumulation of metabolites was observed in patients with a GFR of approximately 5 mL/min, but this accumulation does not influence the β-blocking effects of metoprolol. Consequently, no reduction in dosage is usually needed in patients with chronic renal failure.

Elderly subjects show no significant changes in the plasma concentrations of metoprolol as compared with young persons. However, plasma concentrations of the major pharmacologically active metabolites were higher in the elderly.

Liver cirrhosis may increase the bioavailability of metoprolol and reduce its total clearance.

Pharmacodynamics: Significant β-blocking effect (as measured by reduction of exercise heart rate) occurs within 1 hour after oral administration, and its duration is dose-related. For example, a 50% reduction of the maximum registered effect after single oral doses of 20, 50 and 100 mg occurred at 3.3, 5.0 and 6.4 hours, respectively, in normal subjects. After repeated oral dosages of 100 mg twice daily, a significant reduction in exercise systolic blood pressure was evident at 12 hours.

Following i.v. administration of BETALOC, the half-life of the distribution phase is approximately 12 minutes; the urinary recovery of unchanged drug is approximately 10%. When the drug was infused over a 10 minute period, in normal volunteers, maximum β-blockade was achieved at approximately 20 minutes. Doses of 5 and 15 mg yielded a maximal reduction in exercise-induced heart rate of approximately 10 and 15%, respectively. The effect on exercise heart rate decreased linearly with time at the same rate for both doses, and disappeared at approximately 5 hours and 8 hours for the 5 mg and 15 mg doses, respectively.

Equivalent maximal beta-blocking effect is achieved with oral and i.v. doses in the ratio of approximately 2.5:1.

There is a linear relationship between the log of plasma levels and reduction of exercise heart rate. However, antihypertensive activity does not appear to be related to plasma levels. Because of variable plasma levels attained with a given dose and lack of a consistent relationship of antihypertensive activity to dose, selection of proper dosage requires individual titration.

In several studies of patients with acute myocardial infarction, i.v. followed by oral administration of BETALOC caused a reduction in heart rate, systolic blood pressure and cardiac output. Stroke volume, diastolic blood pressure, and pulmonary artery end diastolic pressure remained unchanged.

Studies in hypertensive and angina patients have shown plasma levels of 28 to 46 ng/mL 12 hours after regular tablets and 19 to 45 ng/mL 24 hours after BETALOC DURULES and were comparable to the peak levels after 100 mg regular tablets.

INDICATIONS: Hypertension: BETALOC (metoprolol tartrate) is indicated in patients with mild or moderate hypertension. It may be used alone or in combination with other antihypertensive agents (see Dosage).

The combination of BETALOC with a diuretic or peripheral vasodilator has been found to be compatible and generally more effective than metoprolol tartrate alone. Limited experience with other antihypertensive agents has not shown evidence of incompatibility with BETALOC.

BETALOC is not recommended for the emergency treatment of hypertensive crises.

Angina Pectoris: BETALOC is indicated for the long-term treatment of angina pectoris due to ischemic heart disease.

Myocardial Infarction: BETALOC is indicated in the treatment of hemodynamically stable patients with definite or suspected acute myocardial infarction to reduce cardiovascular mortality.

Treatment with i.v. BETALOC can be initiated as soon as the patient's clinical condition allows (see Dosage, Contraindications and Warnings). BETALOC i.v. should be administered by a qualified health professional who is experienced in the use of antihypertension i.v. agents and who has been trained in the management of patients with myocardial infarction. Alternatively, in patients with proven myocardial infarction, oral treatment can begin within 3 to 10 days of the acute event (see Dosage). Data are not available as to whether benefit would ensue if the treatment is initiated later.

Clinical trials have shown that patients in whom the myocardial infarction was unconfirmed, received no benefit from early BETALOC therapy.

The COMMIT trial has shown that allocation to the intravenous then oral BETALOC regimen in a patient population of Chinese origin with 25% of patients in Killip Class II-III resulted in an excess of cardiogenic shock, (5.0% vs. 3.9% on placebo) mainly during the first 24 hours after admission. (See Warnings.)

CONTRAINDICATIONS: BETALOC (metoprolol tartrate) should not be used in the presence of:

1. known hypersensitivity to metoprolol and related derivatives;
2. sinus bradycardia;
3. sick sinus syndrome;
4. second- and third-degree AV block;
5. right ventricular failure secondary to pulmonary hypertension;
6. overt heart failure;
7. cardiogenic shock;
8. severe peripheral arterial circulatory disorders;
9. anesthesia with agents that produce myocardial depression, e.g. ether.
10. The i.v. form is also contraindicated in the presence of asthma and other obstructive respiratory diseases (for oral treatment, see Precautions, Bronchospastic Diseases).

Myocardial Infarction Patients—Additional Contraindications: BETALOC is contraindicated in patients with a heart rate <45 beats/min; significant heart block greater than first degree (PR interval ≥0.24 s); systolic blood pressure <100 mmHg; or moderate to severe cardiac failure (see Warnings).

WARNINGS: Cardiac Failure: Special caution should be exercised when administering BETALOC (metoprolol tartrate) to patients with a history of heart failure. Sympathetic stimulation is a vital component supporting circulatory function in congestive heart failure, and inhibition with β-blockade always carries the potential hazard of further depressing myocardial contractility and precipitating cardiac failure. The positive inotropic action of digitalis may be reduced by the negative inotropic effect of metoprolol tartrate when the two drugs are used concomitantly. The effects of β-blockers and digitalis are additive in depressing A-V conduction and may induce bradycardia. This also applies to combinations with calcium antagonists of the verapamil type or some antiarrhythmics (see Precautions, Drug Interactions).

In patients without a history of cardiac failure, continued depression of the myocardium over a period of time can, in some cases, lead to cardiac failure and/or hypotension (systolic blood pressure ≤90 mmHg). Therefore, at the first sign or symptom of impending cardiac failure, patients should be fully digitalized and/or given a diuretic and the response observed closely. If cardiac failure continues, despite adequate digitalization and diuretic therapy, BETALOC therapy should be reduced or withdrawn.

Abrupt Cessation of Therapy: Patients with angina should be warned against abrupt discontinuation of BETALOC. There have been reports of severe exacerbation of angina and of myocardial infarction or ventricular arrhythmias occurring in patients with angina pectoris, following abrupt discontinuation of beta-blocker therapy. The last 2 complications may occur with or without preceding exacerbation of angina pectoris. Therefore, when discontinuation of BETALOC is planned in patients with angina pectoris or previous myocardial infarction, the dosage should be gradually reduced over a period of at least 10 to 14 days, in diminishing doses, to 25 mg once a day for the last 6 days. During this period the patient should be carefully observed. In situations of greater urgency, metoprolol tartrate therapy should be discontinued stepwise and under conditions of closer observation. If angina markedly worsens or acute coronary insufficiency develops, it is recommended that treatment with metoprolol should be reinstituted promptly, at least temporarily.

Patients should be warned against interruption or discontinuation of therapy without the physician's advice. Because coronary artery disease is common and may be unrecognized, it may be prudent not to discontinue BETALOC therapy abruptly even in patients treated only for hypertension.

Oculomucocutaneous Syndrome: Various skin rashes and conjunctival xerosis have been reported with β-blockers, including metoprolol tartrate. Oculomucocutaneous syndrome, a severe syndrome whose signs include conjunctivitis sicca and psoriasiform rashes, otitis and sclerosing serositis, has occurred with chronic use of one β-adrenergic-blocking agent (practolol). This syndrome has not been observed with BETALOC or any other such agent. However, physicians should be alert to the possibility of such reactions and should discontinue treatment in the event that they occur.

Severe Sinus Bradycardia: Severe sinus bradycardia may occur with the use of BETALOC from unopposed vagal activity remaining after blockade of β$_1$-adrenergic receptors. Very rarely a pre-existing AV conduction disorder of moderate degree may become aggravated, possibly leading to AV block. In such cases, dosage should be reduced. Atropine, isoproterenol or dobutamine should be considered in patients with acute myocardial infarction.

Thyrotoxicosis: Although metoprolol has successfully been used for the symptomatic (adjuvant) therapy of thyrotoxicosis, possible deleterious effects from long-term use of BETALOC have not been adequately appraised. β-blockade may mask the clinical signs of continuing hyperthyroidism or complications and give a false impression of improvement. Therefore, abrupt withdrawal of metoprolol tartrate may be followed by an exacerbation of the symptoms of hyperthyroidism, including thyroid storm.

Myocardial Infarction Patients—Additional Warnings: Acute Intervention: During acute intervention in myocardial infarction, i.v. metoprolol should only be used by experienced staff under circumstances where resuscitation and monitoring equipment are available.

Cardiac Failure: Depression of the myocardium with BETALOC may lead to cardiac failure (see general Warnings above). Special caution should be exercised when administering BETALOC to patients with a history of cardiac failure or those with a minimal cardiac reserve. Should failure occur, treatment should be as described in Warnings.

Severe Sinus Bradycardia: See general Warnings for severe sinus bradycardia.

AV Conduction: BETALOC slows AV conduction and may produce significant first- (PR interval ≥0.26 s), second-, or third-degree heart block. Acute myocardial infarction also produces heart block.

If heart block occurs, BETALOC should be discontinued and atropine (0.25 to 0.5 mg) should be administered i.v. If treatment with atropine is not successful, cautious administration of isoproterenol or installation of a cardiac pacemaker should be considered.

Hypotension: If hypotension (systolic blood pressure ≤90 mmHg) occurs, BETALOC should be discontinued, and the hemodynamic status of the patient and the extent of myocardial damage carefully assessed. Invasive monitoring of central venous, pulmonary capillary wedge, and arterial pressures may be required. Appropriate therapy with fluids, positive inotropic agents, balloon counterpulsation, or other treatment modalities should be instituted. If hypotension is associated with sinus bradycardia or AV block, treatment should be directed at reversing these (see above).

Patients of Chinese Origin with Acute Myocardial Infarction: It has been shown that allocation to the intravenous then oral BETALOC regimen resulted in a significant increase in the development of cardiogenic shock [5% BETALOC vs. 3.9% placebo] mainly during the first 24 hours after admission in a Chinese population with 25% of patients in Killip Class II-III.

PRECAUTIONS: Bronchospastic Diseases: **Patients with bronchospastic diseases should, in general, not receive β-blockers.** Because of its relative β_1-selectivity, however, BETALOC (metoprolol tartrate) may be used with caution in patients with bronchospastic disease who do not respond to, or cannot tolerate, other antihypertensive treatment. Since β_1-selectivity is not absolute, a β_2-stimulating agent should preferably be administered concomitantly, and the lowest possible dose of BETALOC should be used. In these circumstances it would be prudent initially to administer BETALOC in smaller doses 3 times daily, instead of larger doses 2 times daily, to avoid the higher plasma levels associated with the longer dosing interval (see Dosage).

Because it is unknown to what extent β_2-stimulating agents may exacerbate myocardial ischemia and the extent of infarction, these agents should not be used prophylactically in patients with proven or suspected acute myocardial infarction. If bronchospasm not related to congestive heart failure occurs, BETALOC should be discontinued. A theophylline derivative or a β_2-agonist may be administered cautiously, depending on the clinical condition of the patient. Both theophylline derivatives and β_2-agonists may produce serious cardiac arrhythmias.

Diabetes and Hypoglycemia: BETALOC should be administered with caution to diabetic patients subject to spontaneous hypoglycemia (most of these patients are insulin treated). β-adrenergic blockers may mask the premonitory signs and symptoms of acute hypoglycemia, but this is mainly attributed to unselective β-adrenergic blockers.

Liver Function: BETALOC should be used with caution in patients with impaired liver function. Liver function tests should be performed at regular intervals during long-term treatment. Dose adjustment is normally not needed in patients suffering from liver cirrhosis because metoprolol has low protein binding (5 to 10%). When there are signs of serious impairment of liver function (e.g., shunt-operated patients) a dose reduction should be considered.

Allergen Immunotherapy: There may be increased difficulty in treating an allergic type reaction in patients on β-blockers. In these patients, the reaction may be more severe due to pharmacologic effects of the β-blockers and problems with fluid changes. Epinephrine should be administered with caution since it may not have its usual effects in the treatment of anaphylaxis. On the one hand, larger doses of epinephrine may be needed to overcome the bronchospasm, while on the other these doses can be associated with excessive α-adrenergic stimulation with consequent hypertension, reflex bradycardia and heart-block, and possible potentiation of bronchospasm. Alternatives to the use of large doses of epinephrine include vigorous supportive care such as fluids and the use of β-agonists including parenteral salbutamol or isoproterenol to overcome bronchospasm and norepinephrine to overcome hypotension.

Patients Undergoing Surgery: It is not advisable to withdraw β-adrenoceptor blocking drugs prior to surgery in the majority of patients especially in those with risk of overt or silent coronary heart disease. However, care should be taken to avoid using anesthetic agents that may depress the myocardium. Vagal dominance, if it occurs, may be corrected with atropine (1 to 2 mg i.v.).

Some patients receiving β-blocking drugs have been subject to protracted severe hypotension during anesthesia. Difficulty in restarting and maintaining the heartbeat has also been reported.

Acute initiation of high-dose metoprolol to patients undergoing non-cardiac surgery should be avoided, since it has been associated with bradycardia, hypotension and stroke including fatal outcome in patients with cardiovascular risk factors.

Since metoprolol is a competitive inhibitor of β-adrenoceptor agonists, its effects may be reversed, if necessary, by sufficient doses of such agonists as isoproterenol or dobutamine.

Peripheral Artery Disorders: Metoprolol may aggravate the symptoms of peripheral arterial circulatory disorders, mainly due to its blood pressure lowering effect.

Pheochromocytoma: Where a β-blocker is prescribed for a patient known to be suffering from a pheochromocytoma, an α-blocker should be given concomitantly.

Occupational Hazards: Reaction Time: β-blockers may adversely affect the patient's reaction time. Patients should be advised to avoid operating automobiles and machinery or engaging in other tasks requiring alertness until the patient's response to therapy with BETALOC has been determined.

Pregnancy: Metoprolol crosses the placental barrier. Since BETALOC has not been studied in human pregnancy, it should not be given to pregnant women. The use of any drug in patients of child-bearing potential requires that the anticipated benefit be weighed against the possible hazards.

Lactation: Metoprolol is excreted in breast milk in very small quantities. Caution should be exercised when BETALOC is administered to a nursing woman.

Children: The safety and efficacy of BETALOC in children has not been established.

Geriatrics: Caution is indicated when using BETALOC in elderly patients. An excessively pronounced decrease in blood pressure or pulse rate may cause the blood supply to vital organs to fall to inadequate levels.

Drug Interactions: Antihypertensives: BETALOC dosage should be adjusted according to the individual requirements of the patient especially when used concomitantly with other antihypertensive agents (see Dosage).

MAO Inhibitors and Adrenergic Neuron Blockers: Patients receiving MAO inhibitors or catecholamine-depleting drugs (such as reserpine or guanethidine) should be closely monitored because the added β-adrenergic-blocking action of BETALOC may produce an excessive reduction of sympathetic activity. BETALOC should not be combined with other β-blockers. Similarly, patients taking Selective Serotonin Reuptake Inhibitors (SSRIs), such as paroxetine, fluoxetine, and sertraline, in combination with BETALOC, should be aware that the plasma concentration of metoprolol may be raised. This occurs as metoprolol is metabolized via cytochrome P450 2D6, which is inhibited by SSRIs.

Calcium Entry Blockers: As with other β-blockers, BETALOC should not be given to patients receiving calcium antagonists of the verapamil type. However, in exceptional cases, when in the opinion of the physician concomitant use is considered essential, such use should be instituted gradually in a hospital setting under careful supervision. Negative inotropic, dromotropic, and chronotropic effects may occur when BETALOC is given together with calcium antagonists. Verapamil and diltiazem may reduce the clearance of metoprolol.

Antiarrhythmic Agents: β-blockers may enhance the negative inotropic and negative dromotropic effect of antiarrhythmic agents such as quinidine and amiodarone. Coadministration of these and other antiarrythmics (e.g. propafenone) may raise plasma levels of metoprolol.

Digitalis Glycosides: Digitalis glycosides, in association with β-blockers, may increase atrioventricular conduction time and may induce bradycardia.

Clonidine Withdrawal Syndrome: The hypertensive crisis which may follow the withdrawal of clonidine may be accentuated in the presence of β-blockade. It has been proposed that withdrawal of the β-blocker several days before the clonidine may reduce the danger of rebound effects.

Oral Antidiabetics: The dosage of oral antidiabetics may have to be readjusted in patients receiving β-blockers (see Precautions).

Indomethacin: Concurrent treatment with indomethacin may decrease the antihypertensive effect of β-blockers.

Cytochrome P450 Inducers and Inhibitors: Metoprolol is a metabolic substrate for the cytochrome P450 isoenzyme CYP2D6. Drugs that act as enzyme-inducing and enzyme-inhibiting substances may exert an influence on the plasma level of metoprolol. Plasma levels of metoprolol may be raised by coadministration of compounds metabolised by CYP2D6, such as antihistamines, histamine-2-receptor antagonists (e.g. cimetidine, ranitidine), antidepressants, antipsychotics and COX-2-inhibitors. The plasma concentration of metoprolol is lowered by rifampin and may be raised by alcohol and hydralazine.

Lidocaine: Metoprolol may reduce the clearance of lidocaine.

Inhalation Anesthetics: In patients receiving β-blocker therapy, inhalation anesthetics enhance the cardiodepressant effect.

ADVERSE EFFECTS: The most common adverse events reported are exertional tiredness, gastrointestinal disorders and disturbances of sleep patterns. The most serious adverse events reported are congestive heart failure, bronchospasm and hypotension.

* Excess frequency of 0.4% compared with placebo in a study of 46 000 patients with acute myocardial infarction where the frequency of cardiogenic shock was 2.3% in the metoprolol group and 1.9% in the placebo group in the subset of patients with low shock risk index. The shock risk index was based on the absolute risk of shock in each individual patient derived from age, sex, time delay, Killip class, blood pressure, heart rate, ECG abnormality, and prior history of hypertension. The patient group with low shock risk index corresponds to the patients in which metoprolol is recommended for use in acute myocardial infarction.

† Extreme caution should be exercised when giving i.v. metoprolol to patients with heart rates between 45 and 60 and/or pulmonary rales less than 10 cm. Therapy should be discontinued in patients if the heart rate drops below 45 or the systolic blood pressure drops below 100 mmHg.

Reported adverse events according to organ systems are:

Cardiovascular: congestive heart failure (see Warnings); secondary effects of decreased cardiac output, which include: syncope, vertigo, lightheadedness and postural hypotension; severe bradycardia; lengthening of PR interval; second and third degree AV block; sinus arrest; cardiac arrhythmias; palpitations; chest pains; edema; cold extremities; claudication; gangrene in patients with pre-existing severe peripheral circulatory disorders; hot flushes; cardiogenic shock in patients with acute myocardial infarction*

In a placebo controlled study in patients with acute myocardial infarction, the incidences of cardiovascular reactions are found in Table 1.

Table 1: BETALOC

Cardiovascular Reactions

	Metoprolol	Placebo
Hypotension (systolic BP <90 mmHg)	27.4%	23.2%
Bradycardia (heart rate <40 beats/min)	15.9%	6.7%
Second- or third-degree heart block	4.7%	4.7%
First-degree heart block (PR ≥0.26 s)	5.3%	1.9%
Heart failure	27.5%	29.6%

CNS: headache, dizziness, mental depression, lightheadedness, concentration impaired, anxiety, weakness, fatigue, sedation, somnolence or insomnia, vivid dreams/nightmares, vertigo, paresthesia, hallucination, nervousness, impotence/sexual dysfunction, amnesia/memory impairment, confusion.

Gastrointestinal: diarrhea, constipation, flatulence, heartburn, nausea and vomiting, abdominal pain, dryness of mouth, hepatitis.

Respiratory: shortness of breath, wheezing, bronchospasm, status asthmaticus, rhinitis.

Allergic/Dermatological (see Warnings): skin rash (exanthema, urticaria, psoriasiform and dystrophic skin lesion, aggravated psoriasis); sweating; pruritus; photosensitivity.

Eye, Ear, Nose and Throat (EENT): blurred vision and non-specific visual disturbances; dry and/or itching eyes; conjunctivitis; tinnitus; hearing difficulties in doses exceeding those recommended; taste disturbances.

Miscellaneous: muscle cramps; exertional tiredness; weight gain; loss of hair; arthritis; Peyronie's disease; arthralgia.

Clinical Laboratory: The following laboratory parameters have been rarely elevated: transaminases, BUN, alkaline phosphatase and bilirubin. Isolated cases of thrombocytopenia and leukopenia have been reported.

OVERDOSE:

Symptoms: The most common signs to be expected with overdosage of a β-adrenoceptor blocking agent are hypotension, bradycardia, congestive heart failure, bronchospasm and hypoglycemia. Atrioventricular block, cardiogenic shock and cardiac arrest may develop. In addition, impairment of consciousness (or even coma), nausea, vomiting and cyanosis may occur.

Concomitant ingestion of alcohol, antihypertensives, quinidine, or barbiturates aggravate the signs and symptoms.

The first manifestations of overdosage set in 20 minutes to 2 hours after drug administration.

Treatment: If an overdose occurs, in all cases therapy with BETALOC (metoprolol tartrate) should be discontinued and the patient hospitalized and observed closely. To prevent absorption of any drug still present in the gastrointestinal tract, gastric lavage or activated charcoal should be used. In addition, if required, the following therapeutic measures are suggested:

Bradycardia and Hypotension: Initially 1 to 2 mg of atropine sulfate should be given i.v. and/or a cardiac pacemaker should be used. If a satisfactory effect is not achieved, norepinephrine or dopamine may be administered after preceding treatment with atropine (see Precautions concerning the use of epinephrine in β-blocked patients). Treatment with glucagon or administration of calcium ions may also be considered.

Congestive Heart Failure: conventional therapy.

Bronchospasm: Bronchospasm can usually be reversed by bronchodilators such as β_2-agonists.

Hypoglycemia: i.v. glucose.

It should be remembered that BETALOC is a competitive antagonist of isoproterenol and hence, large doses of isoproterenol can be expected to reverse many of the effects of excessive doses of BETALOC. However, the complications of excess isoproterenol e.g., hypotension and tachycardia, should not be overlooked.

For management of a suspected drug overdose, CPhA recommends that you contact your **regional Poison Control Centre**. See the *CPS* Directory section for a list of Poison Control Centres.

DOSAGE: Hypertension: BETALOC (metoprolol tartrate) is usually used in conjunction with other antihypertensive agents, particularly a thiazide diuretic, but may be used alone (see Indications).

The dose must always be adjusted to the individual requirements of the patient, in accordance with the following guidelines.

BETALOC treatment should be initiated with doses of 50 mg b.i.d. If an adequate response is not seen after 1 week, dosage should be increased to 100 mg b.i.d. In some cases the daily dosage may need to be increased by further 100 mg increments at intervals of not less than 2 weeks up to a maximum of 200 mg b.i.d., which should not be exceeded. The usual maintenance dose is within the range of 100 to 200 mg daily.

When BETALOC is combined with another antihypertensive agent which is already being administered, BETALOC should be added initially at a dose of 50 mg b.i.d. After 1 or 2 weeks the daily dosage may be increased if required, in increments of 100 mg, at intervals of not less than 2 weeks, until adequate blood pressure control is obtained.

Angina Pectoris: The recommended dosage range for BETALOC is 100 to 400 mg/day in divided doses.

Treatment should be initiated with 50 mg b.i.d. for the first week.

If response is not adequate, the daily dosage should be increased by 100 mg for the next week. The usual maintenance dose is 200 mg/day.

The need for further increases should be closely monitored at weekly intervals and the dosage increased in 100 mg increments to a maximum of 400 mg/day in 2 or 3 divided doses.

A BETALOC dose of 400 mg/day should not be exceeded.

Slow-release BETALOC DURULES: BETALOC DURULES (200 mg slow release tablets) are intended only for maintenance dosing in those patients requiring doses of 100 to 400 mg/day. Treatment must always be initiated and individual titration of dosage carried out using the regular tablets. Dosing with half or whole DURULES may be preferred for maintenance because of the convenience of once daily administration. One half BETALOC DURULES will provide 100 mg slow release metoprolol. The following maintenance doses may now be accommodated: 100 mg = ½ DURULES, 200 mg = 1 DURULES, 300 mg = 1+½ DURULES, 400 mg = 2 DURULES.

Whole tablets may sometimes seem to appear in the stool; these will only be the matrices which have remained intact after the active substance has been leached out.

Myocardial Infarction: In addition to the usual contraindications: **Only patients with suspected acute myocardial infarction who meet the following criteria are suitable for therapy as described:** systolic blood pressure ≥100 mmHg; heart rate† ≥45 beats/min; PR interval <0.24 s; rales† <10 cm and adequate peripheral circulation.

Early Treatment: During the early phase of definite or suspected acute myocardial infarction, treatment with BETALOC can be initiated as soon as possible after the patient's arrival in the hospital. Such treatment should be initiated in a coronary care or similar unit immediately after the patient's hemodynamic condition has stabilized.

Treatment in this early phase should begin with the i.v. administration of 3 bolus injections of 5 mg of BETALOC each. The injections should be given at approximately 2 minute intervals. During the i.v. administration of BETALOC, blood pressure, heart rate, and electrocardiogram should be carefully monitored. If any of the injections are associated with adverse cardiovascular effects, i.v. administration should be stopped immediately and the patient should be observed carefully and appropriate therapy instituted.

In patients who tolerate the full i.v. dose (15 mg), BETALOC tablets, 50 mg every 6 hours should be initiated 15 minutes after the last i.v. dose and continued for 48 hours. Thereafter, patients should receive a maintenance dosage of 100 mg twice daily (see Late Treatment below).

Patients who appear not to tolerate the full i.v. dose should be started on either 25 mg or 50 mg every 6 hours (depending on the degree of intolerance) 15 minutes after the last i.v. dose or as soon as their clinical condition allows. In patients with severe intolerance, treatment with BETALOC should be discontinued (see Warnings).

Late Treatment (for proven myocardial infarction patients only): Patients with contraindications to treatment during the early phase of myocardial infarction, patients who appear not to tolerate the full early treatment, and patients in whom the physician wishes to delay therapy for any other reason should be started on BETALOC tablets, 100 mg twice daily, as soon as their clinical condition allows. Treatment can begin within 3 to 10 days of the acute event. Therapy should be continued for at least 3 months. Although the efficacy of treatment with BETALOC beyond 6 months has not been conclusively established, data from studies with other β-blockers suggest that the treatment should be continued for 1 to 3 years.

Impaired Liver Function: Dose adjustment is normally not needed in patients suffering from liver cirrhosis because metoprolol has low protein binding (5 to 10%). When there are signs of serious impairment of liver function (e.g., shunt-operated patients) a dose reduction should be considered.

Note: Parenteral drug products should be inspected visually for particulate matter and discoloration prior to administration whenever solution and container permit.

SUPPLIED: Tablets: 50 mg: Each compressed, white, scored, biconvex, circular tablet, contains: metoprolol tartrate 50 mg (engraved A/BB). Nonmedicinal ingredients: colloidal silica, lactose, magnesium stearate, microcrystalline cellulose, polyvinyl pyrrolidone and sodium starch glycolate. Bottles of 100. Store at 15 to 30°C.

100 mg: Each compressed, white, scored, biconvex circular tablet, contains: metoprolol tartrate 100 mg (engraved A/ME). Nonmedicinal ingredients: colloidal silica, lactose, magnesium stearate, microcrystalline cellulose, polyvinyl pyrrolidone and sodium starch glycolate. Bottles of 100. Store at 15 to 30°C.

DURULES: Each white, biconvex rod-shaped film-coated tablet contains: metoprolol tartrate 200 mg (scored and engraved A/MD). Nonmedicinal ingredients: aluminum silicate, ethylcellulose, hydroxypropyl methylcellulose, magnesium stearate, paraffin, polyethylene glycol and titanium dioxide. Bottles of 100. Store at 15 to 30°C.

Injection: Each mL of aqueous injectable solution contains: metoprolol tartrate 1 mg. Also contains sodium chloride 45 mg (9 mg/mL). Glass vials of 5 mL. Store at 15 to 30°C, protected from light.

(Shown in Product Identification Section)

Betamethasone

CPhA Monograph

see Corticosteroids: Eye Ear Nose

see Corticosteroids: Systemic

see Corticosteroids: Topical

Betaseron®

interferon beta-1b

Immunomodulator

Bayer

Date of Revision: December 4, 2009

SUMMARY PRODUCT INFORMATION:

Route of Administration	Dosage Form/ Strength	Clinically Relevant Nonmedicinal Ingredients
Subcutaneous	Lyophilized powder: 0.3 mg of interferon beta-1b/single-use vial Diluent: 1.2 mL of sodium chloride 0.54% solution/single-use syringe	Albumin human, USP For a complete listing see Dosage Forms, Composition and Packaging.

DESCRIPTION: BETASERON (interferon beta-1b) is a purified, sterile, lyophilized protein product produced by recombinant DNA techniques and formulated for use by injection.

INDICATIONS AND CLINICAL USE: BETASERON (interferon beta-1b) is indicated for:

- the treatment of patients with a single demyelinating event accompanied by at least two clinically silent lesions typical of multiple sclerosis (MS) on magnetic resonance imaging, to delay progression to definite MS. Before initiating treatment with BETASERON, alternate diagnoses should first be excluded.
- the reduction of the frequency of clinical exacerbations in ambulatory patients with relapsing-remitting multiple sclerosis. Relapsing-remitting MS is characterized by recurrent attacks of neurologic dysfunction followed by complete or incomplete recovery.
- the slowing of progression in disability and the reduction of the frequency of clinical exacerbations in patients with secondary-progressive multiple sclerosis.

The safety and efficacy of BETASERON in primary progressive MS have not been evaluated.

Pediatrics (<18 years of age): Safety and efficacy in children under 18 years of age have not been established.

CONTRAINDICATIONS:

- Patients with a history of hypersensitivity to natural or recombinant interferon beta, albumin human or to any other ingredient in the formulation. For a complete listing, see Dosage Forms, Composition and Packaging.
- Pregnant women.

WARNINGS AND PRECAUTIONS: Cardiovascular: Rare cases of cardiomyopathy have been reported. If this occurs, and a relationship to BETASERON (interferon beta-1b) is suspected, treatment should be discontinued.

Symptoms of flu syndrome observed with BETASERON therapy may prove stressful to patients with severe cardiac conditions. Patients with cardiac disease such as angina, congestive heart failure, or arrhythmia should be monitored closely for worsening of their clinical conditions.

Dependence/Tolerance: No evidence or experience suggests that abuse or dependence occurs with BETASERON therapy; however, the risk of dependence has not been systematically evaluated.

Endocrine and Metabolism: Rare cases of thyroid dysfunction (hyper- as well as hypothyroidism) associated with the use of BETASERON have been reported.

Hepatic/Biliary/Pancreatic: Rare post-market cases of serious hepatic injury, including autoimmune hepatitis, hepatitis and hepatic failure, have been reported with interferon beta treatment for multiple sclerosis.

It is recommended that liver function testing occur at baseline, every month for the first 6 months of treatment and at 6-month intervals thereafter. Dose reduction or discontinuation of therapy should be considered if alanine aminotransferase (ALT) levels increase 5 times above the upper limit of normal.

Interferon beta therapy should be initiated with caution in patients with a history of significant liver disease or alcohol abuse and in patients with clinical evidence of acute liver disease.

Caution must be exercised when prescribing drugs with documented hepatotoxicity to patients on interferon beta therapy for multiple sclerosis.

In rare cases, pancreatitis has been observed with BETASERON use, often associated with hypertriglyceridemia.

Hypersensitivity: Serious hypersensitivity reactions (rare but severe acute reactions such as bronchospasm, anaphylaxis and urticaria) may occur.

Immune: The administration of cytokines to patients with pre-existing monoclonal gammopathy has been associated with the development of systemic capillary leak syndrome with shock-like symptoms and fatal outcome.

Immunogenicity: As with all therapeutic proteins, there is a potential for immunogenicity. Serum samples in controlled clinical trials were collected every 3 months for monitoring of development of antibodies to BETASERON.

In the different controlled clinical trials, between 23% and 41% of the patients developed serum interferon beta-1b neutralizing activity confirmed by at least two consecutive positive titres; of these patients, between 43% and 55% converted to a stable antibody negative status (based on two consecutive negative titres) during the subsequent observational period of the respective study.

The development of neutralizing activity is associated with a reduction in clinical efficacy only with regard to relapse activity. Some analyses suggest that this effect might be larger in patients with higher titre levels of neutralizing activity.

In the study of patients with a single clinical event suggestive of multiple sclerosis, neutralizing activity measured every 6 months was observed at least once in 32% (88) of the patients treated early with BETASERON; of these, 47% (41) returned to negative status over a 3 year period. Within this period, the development of neutralizing activity was not associated with a reduction in clinical efficacy (with regard to time to clinically definite multiple sclerosis (CDMS), and time to confirmed EDSS progression).

New adverse events have not been associated with the development of neutralizing activity.

It has been demonstrated in vitro that BETASERON cross reacts with natural interferon beta. However, this has not been investigated in vivo and its clinical significance is uncertain.

There are sparse and inconclusive data on patients who have developed neutralizing activity and have completed BETASERON therapy.

The decision to continue or discontinue treatment should be based on clinical disease activity rather than on neutralizing activity status.

Neurologic: Rare cases of seizures have been reported with interferon beta therapy. BETASERON should be administered with caution to patients with a history of seizure disorders.

This product contains human albumin and hence carries an extremely remote risk for transmission of viral diseases. A theoretical risk for transmission of Creutzfeldt-Jakob disease (CJD) is also considered extremely remote.

The effect of BETASERON on the ability to drive and use machinery has not been investigated.

Psychiatric: In the RR-MS clinical trial, one suicide and four attempted suicides were observed among 372 study patients during a 3-year period. All five patients received BETASERON (three in the 0.05 mg [1.6 MIU] group and two in the 0.25 mg [8.0 MIU] group). There were no attempted suicides in patients on study who did not receive BETASERON. In the SP-MS study there were 5 suicide attempts in the placebo group and 3 in the BETASERON group including one patient in each group who committed suicide. Depression and suicide have been reported to occur in patients receiving interferon alpha, a related compound. Patients treated with BETASERON should be informed that depression and suicidal ideation may be a side effect of the treatment and should report these symptoms immediately to the prescribing physician. Patients exhibiting depression should be monitored closely and cessation of therapy should be considered.

Sexual Function/Reproduction: Studies in female rhesus monkeys with normal menstrual cycles, at doses up to 0.33 mg (10.7 MIU)/kg/day (equivalent to 32 times the recommended human dose based on body surface area comparison) showed no apparent adverse effects on the menstrual cycle or on associated hormonal profiles (progesterone and estradiol) when administered over 3 consecutive menstrual cycles. The extrapolability of animal doses to human doses is not known. Effects of BETASERON on women with normal menstrual cycles are not known.

Special Populations: Pregnant Women: BETASERON was not teratogenic at doses up to 0.42 mg (13.3 MIU)/kg/day in rhesus monkeys, but demonstrated dose-related abortifacient activity when administered at doses ranging from 0.028 mg (0.89 MIU)/kg/day (2.8 times the recommended human dose based on body surface area comparison) to 0.42 mg (13.3 MIU)/kg/day (40 times the recommended human dose based on body surface area comparison). The extrapolability of animal doses to human doses is not known. Lower doses were not studied in monkeys. Spontaneous abortions while on treatment were reported in 4 patients who participated in the BETASERON RR-MS clinical trial, whereas there was one induced abortion in each of the placebo and BETASERON groups in the SP-MS trial. BETASERON given to rhesus monkeys on gestation days 20 to 70 did not cause teratogenic effects; however, it is not known if teratogenic effects exist in humans. There are no adequate and well-controlled studies in pregnant women.

Women of Childbearing Age: Women of childbearing potential should take reliable contraceptive measures. If the patient becomes pregnant or plans to become pregnant while taking BETASERON, the patient should discontinue therapy. It is not known if interferons alter the efficacy of oral contraceptives.

Nursing Women: It is not known whether BETASERON is excreted in human milk. Given that many drugs are excreted in human milk, there is a potential for serious adverse reactions in nursing infants, therefore a decision should be made whether to discontinue nursing or discontinue BETASERON treatment.

Pediatrics (<18 years of age): Safety and efficacy in children under 18 years of age have not been established.

Information to Be Provided to the Patient: Patients should be informed of the potential risk of liver injury with interferon beta therapy, and of the requirement for frequent laboratory testing for liver function (see Monitoring and Laboratory Tests). Patients should be informed of the symptoms suggesting liver dysfunction, such as jaundice, malaise, fatigue, nausea, vomiting, abdominal pain, dark urine and pruritus, and advised to consult their physician immediately if such symptoms arise.

Patients should be instructed in injection techniques to assure the safe self-administration of BETASERON (see below and Information for the Patient).

Instruction on Self-injection Technique and Procedures: It is recommended that the first injection be administered by, or under the direct supervision of, a physician. Appropriate instructions for reconstitution of BETASERON and self-injection, using aseptic techniques, should be given to the patient. A careful review of Information for the Patient is also recommended.

Patients should be cautioned against the re-use of needles or syringes and instructed in safe disposal procedures. Information on how to acquire a puncture-resistant container for disposal of used needles and syringes should be given to the patient along with instructions for safe disposal of full containers.

Overall, 80% of patients in the two controlled clinical trials reported injection site reactions at one or more times during therapy. Post-marketing experience has been consistent with this finding, with infrequent reports of injection site necrosis.

The onset of injection site necrosis usually appears early in therapy with most cases reported to have occurred in the first two to three months of therapy. The number of sites where necrosis has been observed was variable.

Rarely, the area of necrosis has extended to subcutaneous fat or fascia. Response to treatment of injection site necrosis with antibiotics and/or steroids has been variable. In some of these patients elective debridement and, less frequently, skin grafting took place to facilitate healing which could take from three to six months.

Some patients experienced healing of necrotic skin lesions while BETASERON therapy continued. In other cases new necrotic lesions developed even after therapy was discontinued. The nature and severity of all reported reactions should be carefully assessed.

To minimize the risk of injection site necrosis patients should be advised to use an aseptic injection technique and rotate the injection sites with each dose. Patient understanding and use of aseptic self-injection technique and procedures should be periodically re-evaluated.

The incidence of injection site reactions may be reduced by the use of an autoinjector. In the pivotal study of patients with a single clinical event suggestive of MS an autoinjector was used by the majority of patients. Injection site reactions, as well as injection site necrosis, were observed less frequently in this study than in the other pivotal studies.

Flu-like symptoms are not uncommon following initiation of therapy with BETASERON. In the controlled MS clinical trials, acetaminophen and non-steroidal anti-inflammatory drugs (NSAIDs) were permitted for relief of fever or myalgia.

Patients should be cautioned not to change the dosage or the schedule of administration without medical consultation.

Awareness of Adverse Reactions: Patients should be advised about the common adverse events associated with the use of BETASERON, particularly injection site reactions and the flu-like symptom complex (see Adverse Reactions).

Patients should be cautioned to report depression or suicidal ideation (see Warnings and Precautions, Psychiatric).

Patients should be advised about the abortifacient potential of BETASERON (see Warnings and Precautions, Special Populations, Pregnant Women).

Monitoring and Laboratory Tests: The following laboratory tests are recommended prior to initiating BETASERON therapy and at periodic intervals thereafter: thyroid function test, hemoglobin, complete and differential white blood cell counts, platelet counts and blood chemistries including liver function tests. It is recommended that liver function testing occur at baseline, every month for the first 6 months of treatment and at 6-month intervals thereafter. Dose reduction or discontinuation of therapy should be considered if alanine aminotransferase (ALT) levels increase 5 times above the upper limit of normal. A pregnancy test, chest roentgenogram and ECG should also be performed prior to initiating BETASERON therapy.

In the controlled MS trials, patients were monitored every 3 months. The study protocol stipulated that BETASERON therapy be discontinued in the event the absolute neutrophil count fell below 750/mm³. When the absolute neutrophil count had returned to a value greater than 750/mm³, therapy could be restarted at a 50% reduced dose. No patients were withdrawn or dose-reduced for neutropenia or lymphopenia. Similarly, if AST/ALT levels exceeded 10 times the upper limit of normal, or if the serum bilirubin exceeded 5 times the upper limit of normal, therapy was discontinued. In each instance, hepatic enzyme abnormalities returned to normal following discontinuation of therapy. When measurements had decreased to below these levels, therapy could be restarted at a 50% dose reduction, if clinically appropriate. Dose was reduced in two patients due to increased liver enzymes; one continued on treatment and one was ultimately withdrawn.

In the study conducted in patients with a single clinical event suggestive of MS, five BETASERON patients (1.7%) were withdrawn due to increased hepatic enzymes (AST/ALT), two of them after a dose reduction.

ADVERSE REACTIONS: Adverse Drug Reaction Overview: The most frequently observed adverse reactions are a flu-like symptom complex (fever, chills, arthralgia, malaise, sweating, headache or myalgia) and injection site reactions. Flu-like symptoms may be reduced by administration of acetaminophen or NSAIDs. Dose titration was used at the start of treatment in the clinically isolated syndrome and secondary-progressive MS studies in order to increase the tolerability of BETASERON (see Dosage and Administration).

Clinical Trial Adverse Drug Reactions: The following adverse events were observed in placebo-controlled clinical studies of BETASERON (interferon beta-1b), at the recommended dose of 0.25 mg (8 MIU), in patients with relapsing-remitting MS (n=124) and secondary-progressive MS (n=360), and in patients with a single clinical event suggestive of MS (n=292). Because clinical trials are conducted under very specific conditions the adverse reaction rates observed in the clinical trials may not reflect the rates observed in practice and should not be compared to the rates in the clinical trials of another drug. Adverse drug reaction information from clinical trials is useful for identifying drug-related adverse events and for approximating rates.

Relapsing-remitting MS: Injection site reactions (85%) and injection site necrosis (5%) occurred after administration of BETASERON. Inflammation, pain, hypersensitivity, necrosis, and non-specific reactions were significantly associated (P<0.05) with the 0.25 mg (8 MIU) BETASERON-treated group, compared to placebo. Only inflammation, pain, and necrosis were reported as severe events. The incidence rate for injection site reactions was calculated over the course of 3 years. This incidence rate decreased over time, with 79% of patients experiencing the event during the first 3 months of treatment compared to 47% during the last 6 months. The median time to the first occurrence of an injection site reaction was 7 days. Patients with injection site reactions reported these events 183.7 days per year. Three patients withdrew from the 0.25 mg (8 MIU) BETASERON-treated group for injection site pain.

Flu-like symptom complex was reported in 76% of the patients treated with 0.25 mg (8 MIU) BETASERON. A patient was defined as having a flu-like symptom complex if flu-like syndrome or at least two of the following symptoms were concurrently reported: fever, chills, myalgia, malaise or sweating. Only myalgia, fever, and chills were reported as severe in more than 5% of the patients. The incidence rate for flu-like symptom complex was also calculated over the course of 3 years. The incidence rate of these events decreased over time, with 60% of patients experiencing the event during the first 3 months of treatment compared to 10% during the last 6 months. The median time to the first occurrence of flu-like symptom complex was 3.5 days and the median duration per patient was 7.5 days per year.

Twenty-one (28%) of the 76 females of childbearing age treated at 0.25 mg (8 MIU) BETASERON and 10 (13%) of the 76 females of childbearing age treated with placebo reported menstrual disorders. All reports were of mild to moderate severity and included: intermenstrual bleeding and spotting, early or delayed menses, decreased days of menstrual flow, and clotting and spotting during menstruation.

Mental disorders such as depression, anxiety, emotional lability, depersonalization, suicide attempts and confusion were observed in this study. Two patients withdrew for confusion. One suicide and four attempted suicides were also reported. It is not known whether these symptoms may be related to the underlying neurological basis of MS, to BETASERON treatment, or to a combination of both. Some similar symptoms have been noted in patients receiving interferon alpha and both interferons are thought to act through the same receptor. Patients who experience these symptoms should be monitored closely and cessation of therapy should be considered.

Additional common clinical and laboratory adverse events associated with the use of BETASERON are listed in the following paragraphs. These events occurred at an incidence of 5% or more in the 124 MS patients treated with 0.25 mg (8 MIU) BETASERON every other day for periods of up to three years in the controlled trial, and at an incidence that was at least twice that observed in the 123 placebo patients. Common adverse clinical and laboratory adverse events associated with the use of BETASERON were: injection site reaction (85%); lymphocyte count <1500/mm^3 (82%); ALT >5 times baseline value (19%); absolute neutrophil count <1500/mm^3 (18%); menstrual disorder (17%); WBC <3000/mm^3 (16%); palpitation (8%); dyspnea (8%); cystitis (8%); hypertension (7%); breast pain (7%); tachycardia (6%); gastrointestinal disorders (6%); total bilirubin >2.5 times baseline value (6%); somnolence (6%); laryngitis (6%); pelvic pain (6%); menorrhagia (6%); injection site necrosis (5%); peripheral vascular disorders (5%).

A total of 277 MS patients have been treated with BETASERON in doses ranging from 0.025 mg (0.8 MIU) to 0.5 mg (16 MIU). During the first three years of treatment, withdrawals due to clinical adverse events or laboratory abnormalities not mentioned above included: fatigue (2%, 6 patients); cardiac arrhythmia (<1%, 1 patient); allergic urticarial skin reaction to injections (<1%, 1 patient); headache (<1%, 1 patient); unspecified adverse events (<1%, 1 patient); "felt sick" (<1%, 1 patient).

Table 1 enumerates adverse events and laboratory abnormalities that occurred at an incidence of 2% or more among the 124 MS patients treated with 0.25 mg (8 MIU) BETASERON every other day for periods of up to three years in the controlled trial and at an incidence that was at least 2% more than that observed in the 123 placebo patients. Reported adverse events have been re-classified using the standard COSTART glossary to reduce the total number of terms employed in Table 1. In Table 1, terms so general as to be uninformative, and those events where a drug cause was remote have been excluded.

Table 1: BETASERON

Incidence of Adverse Events and Laboratory Abnormalities (Regardless of Causality) ≥2% and >2% Difference (BETASERON vs. Placebo) in the Relapsing-remitting MS Study

System Organ Class Adverse Event	Placebo n=123	BETASERON 0.25 mg (8 MIU) n=124
Infections and Infestations		
Sinusitis	26%	36%
Laryngitis	2%	6%
Neoplasms, Benign, Malignant and Unspecified		
Cyst	2%	4%
Breast Neoplasm	0%	2%
Blood and Lymphatic System Disorders		
Lymphadenopathy	11%	14%
Endocrine Disorders		
Goiter	0%	2%
Metabolism and Nutrition Disorders		
Glucose <55 mg/dL	13%	15%
Weight Gain	0%	4%
Weight Loss	2%	4%
Psychiatric Disorders		
Depression	24%	25%
Anxiety	13%	15%
Nervousness	5%	8%
Suicide Attempt	0%	2%

(cont'd)

Table 1: BETASERON *(cont'd)*

Incidence of Adverse Events and Laboratory Abnormalities (Regardless of Causality) ≥2% and >2% Difference (BETASERON vs. Placebo) in the Relapsing-remitting MS Study

System Organ Class Adverse Event	Placebo n=123	BETASERON 0.25 mg (8 MIU) n=124
Nervous System Disorders		
Dizziness	28%	35%
Hypertonia	24%	26%
Myasthenia	10%	13%
Migraine	7%	12%
Somnolence	3%	6%
Confusion	2%	4%
Speech Disorder	1%	3%
Convulsion	0%	2%
Hyperkinesia	0%	2%
Amnesia	0%	2%
Eye Disorders		
Conjunctivitis	10%	12%
Abnormal Vision	4%	7%
Cardiac Disorders		
Palpitation[a]	2%	8%
Tachycardia	3%	6%
Vascular Disorders		
Hypertension	2%	7%
Peripheral Vascular Disorder	2%	5%
Hemorrhage	1%	3%
Respiratory, Thoracic and Mediastinal Disorders		
Dyspnea[a]	2%	8%
Gastrointestinal Disorders		
Diarrhea	29%	35%
Abdominal Pain	24%	32%
Constipation	18%	24%
Vomiting	19%	21%
Gastrointestinal Disorder	3%	6%
Skin and Subcutaneous Tissue Disorders		
Sweating[a]	11%	23%
Alopecia	2%	4%
Necrosis	0%	2%
Musculoskeletal and Connective Tissue Disorders		
Myalgia[a]	28%	44%
Pelvic Pain	3%	6%
Renal and Urinary Disorders		
Cystitis	4%	8%
Urinary Urgency	2%	4%
Reproductive System and Breast Disorders		
Dysmenorrhea	11%	18%
Menstrual Disorder[a]	8%	17%
Metrorrhagia	8%	15%
Breast Pain	3%	7%
Menorrhagia	3%	6%
Fibrocystic Breast	1%	3%

(cont'd)

Table 1: BETASERON *(cont'd)*

Incidence of Adverse Events and Laboratory Abnormalities (Regardless of Causality) ≥2% and >2% Difference (BETASERON vs. Placebo) in the Relapsing-remitting MS Study

System Organ Class Adverse Event	Placebo n=123	BETASERON 0.25 mg (8 MIU) n=124
General Disorders and Administration Site Conditions		
Injection Site Reaction[a]	37%	85%
Headache	77%	84%
Flu-like Symptom Complex[a]	56%	76%
Fever[a]	41%	59%
Pain	48%	52%
Asthenia[a]	35%	49%
Chills[a]	19%	46%
Malaise[a]	3%	15%
Generalized Edema	6%	8%
Injection Site Necrosis[a]	0%	5%
Investigations		
Lymphocytes <1500/mm³	67%	82%
ALT >5 Times Baseline[a]	6%	19%
ANC <1500/mm³[a]	6%	18%
WBC <3000/mm³[a]	5%	16%
Total Bilirubin >2.5 Times Baseline	2%	6%
Urine Protein >1+	3%	5%
AST >5 Times Baseline[a]	0%	4%

[a] Significantly associated with BETASERON treatment (P<0.05).

It should be noted that the figures cited in Table 1 cannot be used to predict the incidence of side effects in the course of usual medical practice where patient characteristics and other factors differ from those that prevailed in the clinical trials. The cited figures do provide the prescribing physician with some basis for estimating the relative contribution of drug and nondrug factors to the side effect incidence rate in the population studied.

Secondary-progressive MS: The incidence of adverse events that occurred in at least 2% of patients treated with 8 MIU BETASERON or placebo for up to three years, or where an adverse event was reported at a frequency at least 2% higher with BETASERON than that observed for placebo-treated patients in the secondary-progressive study, is presented in Table 2. Adverse events significantly associated with BETASERON compared to placebo (p<0.05) are also indicated in Table 2.

Table 2: BETASERON

Incidence of Adverse Events (Regardless of Causality) ≥2% or >2% Difference (BETASERON vs. Placebo) in the Secondary-progressive MS Study

System Organ Class Adverse Event	Placebo n=358	BETASERON 0.25 mg (8 MIU) n=360
Infections and Infestations		
Rhinitis	32%	28%
Urinary Tract Infection	25%	22%
Pharyngitis	20%	16%
Infection	11%	13%
Bronchitis	12%	9%
Sinusitis	6%	6%
Pneumonia	5%	5%
Abscess[a]	2%	4%
Upper Respiratory Tract Infection	2%	3%
Herpes Simplex	2%	3%
Herpes Zoster	2%	1%
Blood and Lymphatic System Disorders		
Leukopenia[a]	5%	10%
Lymphadenopathy	1%	3%
Anemia	5%	2%
Ecchymosis	2%	1%
Immune System Disorders		

(cont'd)

Table 2: BETASERON *(cont'd)*

Incidence of Adverse Events (Regardless of Causality) ≥2% or >2% Difference (BETASERON vs. Placebo) in the Secondary-progressive MS Study

System Organ Class Adverse Event	Placebo n=358	BETASERON 0.25 mg (8 MIU) n=360
Allergic Reaction	3%	2%
Metabolism and Nutrition Disorders		
Weight Loss	3%	2%
Hypercholesterolemia	2%	1%
Psychiatric Disorders		
Depression	31%	27%
Insomnia	8%	12%
Emotional Lability	11%	8%
Anxiety	5%	6%
Nervousness	3%	4%
Nervous System Disorders		
Headache	41%	47%
Hypertonia[a]	31%	41%
Myasthenia	40%	39%
Neuropathy	41%	38%
Paresthesia	39%	35%
Abnormal Gait	34%	34%
Ataxia	23%	19%
Dizziness	14%	14%
Incoordination	13%	11%
Vertigo	12%	8%
Paralysis	10%	8%
Somnolence	8%	8%
Tremor	9%	6%
Sleep Disorder	5%	6%
Hypesthesia	4%	6%
Neuralgia	7%	5%
Movement Disorder	6%	5%
Migraine	3%	4%
Spastic Paralysis	1%	3%
Speech Disorder	5%	2%
Dysarthria	4%	2%
Convulsion	2%	2%
Hyperesthesia	2%	2%
Optic Neuritis	2%	2%
Amnesia	3%	1%
Hemiplegia	2%	1%
Thinking Abnormal	2%	1%
Myoclonus	2%	0%
Eye Disorders		
Abnormal Vision	15%	11%
Amblyopia	10%	7%
Diplopia	9%	7%
Eye Pain	5%	4%
Eye Disorder	2%	3%
Conjunctivitis	3%	2%

(cont'd)

Table 2: BETASERON *(cont'd)*

Incidence of Adverse Events (Regardless of Causality) ≥2% or >2% Difference (BETASERON vs. Placebo) in the Secondary-progressive MS Study

System Organ Class Adverse Event	Placebo n=358	BETASERON 0.25 mg (8 MIU) n=360
Ear and Labyrinth Disorders		
Otitis Media	3%	2%
Deafness	3%	1%
Ear Disorder	2%	1%
Tinnitus	2%	1%
Cardiac Disorders		
Palpitation	3%	2%
Syncope	3%	2%
Tachycardia	1%	2%
Vascular Disorders		
Vasodilatation	4%	6%
Peripheral Vascular Disorder	5%	5%
Hypertension[a]	2%	4%
Hypotension	4%	2%
Hemorrhage	2%	2%
Respiratory, Thoracic and Mediastinal Disorders		
Cough Increased	10%	5%
Dyspnea	2%	3%
Sore Throat	1%	2%
Asthma	2%	1%
Thorax Pain	2%	1%
Voice Alteration	2%	1%
Gastrointestinal Disorders		
Nausea	13%	13%
Constipation	12%	12%
Abdominal Pain[a]	6%	11%
Diarrhea	10%	7%
Gastroenteritis	5%	6%
Vomiting	6%	4%
Dysphagia	5%	4%
Gastrointestinal Disorder	5%	4%
Tooth Disorder	4%	4%
Dyspepsia	4%	4%
Anorexia	2%	4%
Flatulence	1%	3%
Fecal Incontinence	3%	2%
Gastritis	2%	2%
Gastrointestinal Pain	0%	2%
Gingivitis	0%	2%
Dry Mouth	2%	1%
Colitis	2%	0%
Skin and Subcutaneous Tissue Disorders		
Rash[a]	12%	20%
Sweating Increased	6%	6%
Pruritus	6%	6%
Skin Disorder	4%	4%

(cont'd)

Table 2: BETASERON *(cont'd)*

Incidence of Adverse Events (Regardless of Causality) ≥2% or >2% Difference (BETASERON vs. Placebo) in the Secondary-progressive MS Study

System Organ Class Adverse Event	Placebo n=358	BETASERON 0.25 mg (8 MIU) n=360
Eczema	4%	2%
Alopecia	2%	2%
Acne	2%	2%
Dry Skin	3%	1%
Subcutaneous Hematoma	3%	1%
Seborrhea	2%	1%
Musculoskeletal and Connective Tissue Disorders		
Back Pain	24%	26%
Myalgia[a]	9%	23%
Arthralgia	20%	20%
Pain in Extremity	12%	14%
Neck Pain	6%	5%
Chest Pain	4%	5%
Bone Fracture (not spontaneous)	5%	3%
Muscle Cramps	3%	3%
Spontaneous Bone Fracture	3%	3%
Arthritis	1%	2%
Joint Disorder	1%	2%
Renal and Urinary Disorders		
Urinary Incontinence	15%	8%
Urinary Urgency	7%	8%
Urinary Tract Disorder	10%	7%
Cystitis	9%	7%
Increased Urinary Frequency	5%	6%
Urinary Retention	6%	4%
Dysuria	2%	2%
Nocturia	1%	2%
Pyelonephritis	0%	2%
Kidney Pain	2%	0%
Reproductive System and Breast Disorders		
Metrorrhagia	6%	12%
Menstrual Disorder	13%	9%
Impotence	4%	7%
Vaginitis	4%	3%
Amenorrhea	4%	3%
Menopause	4%	2%
Menorrhagia	4%	2%
Vaginal Moniliasis	2%	2%
Prostatic Disorder	1%	2%
Breast Pain	2%	1%
General Disorders and Administration Site Conditions		
Asthenia	58%	63%
Flu Syndrome[a]	40%	61%
Injection Site Inflammation[a]	4%	48%
Injection Site Reaction[a]	10%	46%
Fever[a]	13%	40%

(cont'd)

Table 2: BETASERON *(cont'd)*

Incidence of Adverse Events (Regardless of Causality) ≥2% or >2% Difference (BETASERON vs. Placebo) in the Secondary-progressive MS Study

System Organ Class Adverse Event	Placebo n=358	BETASERON 0.25 mg (8 MIU) n=360
Pain	25%	31%
Chills[a]	7%	23%
Injection Site Pain	5%	9%
Malaise	5%	8%
Peripheral Edema	7%	7%
Injection Site Necrosis[a]	0%	5%
Chills and Fever[a]	0%	3%
Injection Site Hemorrhage	2%	2%
Investigations		
Laboratory Test Abnormal	1%	3%
Liver Function Test Abnormal	1%	3%
ALT Increased	2%	2%
Injury, Poisoning and Procedural Complications		
Accidental Injury	17%	14%

[a] Significantly associated with BETASERON treatment (P<0.05).

Seventy-four (74) patients discontinued treatment due to adverse events (23 on placebo and 51 on BETASERON). Injection site reactions were significantly associated with early termination of treatment in the BETASERON group compared to placebo (p<0.05). The highest frequency of adverse events leading to discontinuation involved the nervous system, of which depression (7 on placebo and 11 on BETASERON) was the most common.

Single clinical event suggestive of MS: The incidence of all adverse events reported during the two-year study duration that occurred in ≥1% of patients treated with 8 MIU BETASERON and with a higher frequency versus the placebo group is presented in Table 3. The most frequent adverse events reported for BETASERON were injection site reaction (48.3%), flu syndrome (44.2%), headache (26.7%) and asthenia (21.6%).

The frequency of some adverse events decreased substantially from the first year to the second year of the study. The proportion of BETASERON-treated patients experiencing flu syndrome was reduced from 42% in the first year to 13% in the second year. Also, injection site reactions occurred less frequently during the second year (30%) than during the first year (46%).

Table 3: BETASERON

Incidence of Adverse Events (Regardless of Causality) ≥1% Occurring More Frequently in BETASERON (vs. Placebo) Patients With a Single Demyelinating Event Suggestive of MS

System Organ Class Adverse Event (Preferred Term, MedDRA Version 9.0)	Placebo (n=176)	BETASERON 0.25 mg (8 MIU) (n=292)
Infections and Infestations		
Infection	3.4%	5.8%
Herpes Simplex	1.1%	1.4%
Tooth Abscess	0.6%	1.0%
Herpes Zoster	0%	1.0%
Blood and Lymphatic System Disorders		
Leukopenia[a]	5.7%	18.2%
Lymphadenopathy	0.6%	1.4%
Thrombocytopenia	0.6%	1.4%
Immune System Disorders		
Hypersensitivity	1.7%	4.5%
Endocrine Disorders		
Hypothyroidism	1.1%	1.4%
Metabolism and Nutrition Disorders		
Hypoglycemia	0%	1.0%
Psychiatric Disorders		
Insomnia	4.0%	8.2%
Affect Lability	2.3%	4.1%
Nervousness	1.1%	1.4%
Nervous System Disorders		
Headache[a]	17.0%	26.7%
Optic Neuritis	2.3%	2.7%

(cont'd)

Table 3: BETASERON *(cont'd)*

Incidence of Adverse Events (Regardless of Causality) ≥1% Occurring More Frequently in BETASERON (vs. Placebo) Patients With a Single Demyelinating Event Suggestive of MS

System Organ Class Adverse Event (Preferred Term, MedDRA Version 9.0)	Placebo (n=176)	BETASERON 0.25 mg (8 MIU) (n=292)
Migraine	1.7%	2.4%
Hypertonia	1.1%	2.1%
Visual Field Defect	0%	1.4%
Hemiplegia	0.6%	1.0%
Myoclonus	0%	1.0%
Eye Disorders		
Visual Disturbance[a]	0.6%	3.4%
Eye Pain	2.8%	3.1%
Vision Blurred	0%	1.7%
Conjunctivitis	1.1%	1.4%
Diplopia	0.6%	1.0%
Cardiac Disorders		
Palpitations	0.6%	1.4%
Tachycardia	0%	1.4%
Vascular Disorders		
Hypertension	0%	2.1%
Hypotension	0%	1.4%
Respiratory, Thoracic and Mediastinal Disorders		
Cough	2.3%	2.4%
Epistaxis	0.6%	1.4%
Gastrointestinal Disorders		
Vomiting[a]	1.1%	5.1%
Abdominal Pain	2.8%	4.8%
Diarrhea	1.7%	4.1%
Tooth Disorder	1.7%	2.4%
Gastritis	0.6%	1.7%
Aphthous Stomatitis	0.6%	1.4%
Constipation	0.6%	1.0%
Glossodynia	0%	1.0%
Skin and Subcutaneous Tissue Disorders		
Rash[a]	2.8%	11.0%
Hyperhidrosis	1.1%	2.1%
Pruritus	1.1%	2.1%
Urticaria	0.6%	2.1%
Skin Disorder	0%	1.4%
Psoriasis	0.6%	1.0%
Eczema	0%	1.0%
Musculoskeletal and Connective Tissue Disorders		
Back Pain	6.8%	9.9%
Pain in Extremity	3.4%	6.2%
Arthralgia	5.7%	5.8%
Renal and Urinary Disorders		
Proteinuria	1.1%	2.7%
Urinary Incontinence	0.6%	1.0%
Micturition Urgency	0.6%	1.0%
Nocturia	0%	1.0%

(cont'd)

Table 3: BETASERON *(cont'd)*

Incidence of Adverse Events (Regardless of Causality) ≥1% Occurring More Frequently in BETASERON (vs. Placebo) Patients With a Single Demyelinating Event Suggestive of MS

System Organ Class Adverse Event (Preferred Term, MedDRA Version 9.0)	Placebo (n=176)	BETASERON 0.25 mg (8 MIU) (n=292)
Reproductive System and Breast Disorders		
Dysmenorrhea[b]	0%	2.4%
Ejaculation Disorder[c]	0%	2.4%
Metrorrhagia[b]	0%	1.9%
Vaginal Candidiasis[b]	0%	1.4%
Impotence[c]	0%	1.2%
General Disorders and Administration Site Conditions		
Injection Site Reaction[a]	8.5%	48.3%
Influenza-like Illness[a]	18.2%	44.2%
Asthenia	17.0%	21.6%
Pyrexia[a]	4.5%	13.0%
Injection Site Pain	2.8%	5.8%
Chills[a]	1.1%	5.5%
Pain	4.0%	4.1%
Gait Disturbance	0.6%	2.1%
Malaise	0.6%	1.0%
Chest Pain	0%	1.0%
Injection Site Inflammation	0%	1.0%
Injection Site Necrosis	0%	1.0%
Investigations		
Alanine Aminotransferase Increased[a]	4.5%	15.4%
Aspartate Aminotransferase Increased[a]	2.8%	11.0%
Liver Function Test Abnormal[a]	1.1%	5.5%
Laboratory Test Abnormal	1.7%	2.1%
Gamma-glutamyltransferase Increased	0.6%	1.0%
Injury, Poisoning and Procedural Complications		
Injury	4.0%	5.5%
Subcutaneous Hematoma	2.8%	3.4%
Post-procedural Complication	0%	1.4%

[a] Significantly associated with BETASERON treatment (P<0.05).
[b] Incidence in females only (n=207).
[c] Incidence in males only (n=85).

Serious adverse events were reported by equal proportions (6.8%) of patients in the two treatment groups. Eight BETASERON patients (2.7%) experienced adverse events which led to premature discontinuation of the study.

A 3-year integrated analysis combined safety data from the 2-year placebo-controlled study and the pre-planned follow-up study. The incidence of adverse events reported in ≥10% of overall patients is presented in Table 4.

Flu-like symptoms and injection site reactions were observed less frequently than in the other pivotal trials. To increase tolerability of BETASERON, dose titration was performed and NSAIDs were administered at start of therapy. Moreover, an autoinjector was used by the majority of patients throughout the study.

Other events observed during pre-marketing evaluation of various doses of BETASERON in 1440 patients are listed in the paragraphs that follow. Given that most of the events were observed in open and uncontrolled studies, the role of BETASERON in their causation cannot be reliably determined.

Blood and Lymphatic System Disorders: chronic lymphocytic leukemia, hemoglobin less than 9.4 g/100 mL, petechia, platelets less than 75 000/mm³ and splenomegaly.

Cardiac Disorders: angina pectoris, arrhythmia, atrial fibrillation, cardiomegaly, cardiac arrest, cerebral ischemia, endocarditis, heart failure, myocardial infarct, pericardial effusion, syncope, ventricular extrasystoles and ventricular fibrillation.

Ear and Labyrinth Disorders: deafness, ear pain, otitis externa and otitis media.

Endocrine Disorders: Cushing's syndrome, diabetes insipidus, diabetes mellitus, hypothyroidism and inappropriate ADH.

Eye Disorders: blepharitis, blindness, dry eyes, diplopia, iritis, keratoconjunctivitis, mydriasis, photophobia, retinitis and visual field defect.

Gastrointestinal Disorders: aphthous stomatitis, ascites, cardiospasm, cheilitis, cholecystitis, cholelithiasis, duodenal ulcer, dry mouth, enteritis, esophagitis, fecal impaction, fecal incontinence, flatulence, gastritis, gingivitis, glossitis, hematemesis, ileus, increased salivation, intestinal obstruction, melena, nausea, oral leukoplakia, oral moniliasis, pancreatitis, proctitis, salivary gland enlargement, stomach ulcer, taste loss, taste perversion and tenesmus.

General Disorders and Administration Site Conditions: edema, hernia, hypothermia and photosensitivity.

Hepatobiliary Disorders: alkaline phosphatase greater than 5 times baseline value, hepatitis and hepatomegaly.

Immune System Disorders: anaphylactoid reaction.

Infections and Infestations: abscess, cellulitis, infection, periodontal abscess, peritonitis and sepsis.

Metabolism and Nutrition Disorders: alcohol intolerance, calcium greater than 11.5 mg/dL, glucose greater than 160 mg/dL, glycosuria, hypoglycemic reaction, ketosis and thirst.

Musculoskeletal and Connective Tissue Disorders: arthritis, arthrosis, bursitis, dystonia, leg cramps, muscle atrophy, myopathy, myositis, ptosis and tenosynovitis.

Neoplasms, Benign, Malignant and Unspecified: adenoma, carcinoma of the lung, hepatic neoplasia, sarcoma, skin benign neoplasm, skin carcinoma, spider angioma and uterine neoplasm.

Nervous System Disorders: abnormal gait, acute brain syndrome, aphasia, ataxia, brain edema, chronic brain syndrome, coma, delirium, encephalopathy, facial paralysis, foot drop, hemiplegia, hydrocephalus, hypalgesia, hyperesthesia, incoordination, libido decreased, meningitis, neuralgia, neuropathy, nystagmus, oculogyric crisis, ophthalmoplegia, papilledema, paralysis, reflexes decreased, shock, subdural hematoma, torticollis and tremor.

Psychiatric Disorders: agitation, apathy, delusions, dementia, depersonalization, euphoria, hallucinations, manic reaction, neurosis, paranoid reaction, psychosis and stupor.

Renal and Urinary Disorders: anuria, BUN greater than 40 mg/dL, hematuria, kidney calculus, kidney failure, kidney tubular disorder, nephritis, nocturia, oliguria, polyuria, urethritis, urinary incontinence and urinary retention.

Reproductive System and Breast Disorders: balanitis, breast engorgement, cervicitis, epididymitis, gynecomastia, impotence, leukorrhea, salpingitis and uterine fibroids enlarged.

Respiratory, Thoracic and Mediastinal Disorders: apnea, asthma, atelectasis, cyanosis, hemoptysis, hiccup, hyperventilation, hypoventilation, hypoxia, interstitial pneumonia, lung edema, parosmia, pleural effusion, pneumonia and pneumothorax.

Skin and Subcutaneous Tissue Disorders: contact dermatitis, erythema nodosum, exfoliative dermatitis, furunculosis, hirsutism, leukoderma, lichenoid dermatitis, maculopapular rash, psoriasis, seborrhea, skin hypertrophy, skin necrosis, skin ulcer, urticaria and vesiculobullous rash.

Vascular Disorders: cerebral hemorrhage, gastrointestinal hemorrhage, hypotension, intracranial hypertension, postural hypotension, pulmonary embolus, rectal hemorrhage, subarachnoid hemorrhage, thrombophlebitis, thrombosis, vaginal hemorrhage, varicose vein, vasospasm and venous pressure increased.

Abnormal Hematologic and Clinical Chemistry Findings: Relapsing-remitting MS: In the relapsing-remitting MS study, the most common laboratory abnormalities included: lymphocyte count <1500/mm³ (82%); ALT >5 times baseline value (19%); absolute neutrophil count <1500/mm³ (18%) (no patients had absolute neutrophil counts <500/mm³); WBC <3000/mm³ (16%); total bilirubin >2.5 times baseline value (6%).

Three patients were withdrawn from treatment with 0.25 mg (8 MIU) BETASERON for abnormal liver enzymes including one following dose reduction (see Warnings and Precautions, Monitoring and Laboratory Tests).

Table 4: BETASERON

Incidence of Adverse Events ≥10% of Overall Patients in Integrated 3-Year Analysis

System Organ Class Adverse Event (Preferred term, MedDRA version 11.0)	Delayed Treatment (n=176)	Early Treatment (n=292)
Infections and Infestations		
Upper respiratory tract infection	29.5%	26.0%
Pharyngitis	13.6%	12.7%
Blood and Lymphatic System Disorders		
Leukopenia	12.5%	22.3%
Psychiatric Disorders		
Depression	20.5%	15.4%
Insomnia	10.2%	10.6%
Nervous System Disorders		
Multiple sclerosis relapse	43.2%	30.1%
Headache	27.8%	31.8%
Paresthesia	24.4%	25.0%
Skin and Subcutaneous Tissue Disorders		
Rash	8.5%	14.4%
Musculoskeletal and Connective Tissue Disorders		
Back pain	10.2%	13.0%
General Disorders and Administration Site Conditions		
Injection site reaction (various kinds)[a]	41.5%	57.2%
Flu-like symptom complex[b]	47.7%	51.4%
Asthenia	26.7%	25.7%
Pyrexia	9.7%	15.8%
Investigations		
ALT increased	6.8%	15.8%

[a] " Injection site reaction (various kinds)" comprises all adverse events occurring at the injection site, ie, the terms "injection site edema", "injection site hemorrhage", "injection site hypersensitivity", "injection site inflammation", "injection site mass", "injection site necrosis", "injection site pain", and "injection site reaction".
[b] "Flu-like symptom complex" denotes the terms "flu syndrome" and/or a combination of at least two adverse events from "fever", "chills", "myalgia", "malaise", or "sweating".
Abbreviations: ALT—alanine aminotransferase.

Secondary-progressive MS: Significantly more patients on active therapy (14.4% vs 4.7% on placebo) had elevated ALT values (>5 times baseline value). Elevations were also observed in AST and gamma-GT values in the BETASERON group throughout the study. In the BETASERON group, most ALT abnormalities resolved spontaneously with continued treatment whereas some resolved upon dose reduction or temporary discontinuation of treatment.

Lymphopenia (<1500/mm³) was observed in 90.9% of BETASERON patients compared to 74.3% of placebo patients and neutropenia (<1400/mm³) was noted in 18.0% BETASERON and 5.1% placebo patients.

Single clinical event suggestive of MS: The following laboratory abnormalities were reported at a significantly higher incidence in the BETASERON group: lymphocyte count <1500/mm³: BETASERON 79.1% vs placebo 45.5%; ALT >5 times baseline value: BETASERON 17.8% vs placebo 4.5%; absolute neutrophil count <1500/mm³: BETASERON 10.6% vs placebo 2.3%; WBC <3000/mm³: BETASERON 10.6% vs placebo 1.7%; AST >5 times baseline value: BETASERON 6.2% vs placebo 0.6%.

Bilirubin values of Grade 3 or 4 were reported in five BETASERON patients and in one placebo patient.

Five patients discontinued BETASERON due to elevated liver function tests (see Warnings and Precautions, Monitoring and Laboratory Tests).

There were no relevant differences between the BETASERON and placebo groups for lipid profile, thyroid function parameters, other serum chemistry parameters or urinalysis parameters.

Post-Market Adverse Drug Reactions: Rare post-marketing cases of adverse hepatic reactions have been reported, including autoimmune hepatitis, hepatitis and hepatic failure requiring liver transplantation.

DRUG INTERACTIONS: Drug-Drug Interactions: Interactions between BETASERON and other drugs have not been evaluated. Although studies designed to examine drug interactions have not been done, it was noted that BETASERON patients (n=180) have received corticosteroid or ACTH treatment of relapses for periods of up to 28 days.

BETASERON administered in three cancer patients over a dose range of 0.025 mg (0.8 MIU) to 2.2 mg (71 MIU) led to a dose-dependent inhibition of antipyrine elimination. The effect of alternate-day administration of 0.25 mg (8 MIU) BETASERON on drug metabolism in MS patients is unknown.

Interferons have been reported to reduce the activity of hepatic cytochrome P450-dependent enzymes in humans and animals. Caution should be exercised when BETASERON is administered in combination with agents that have a narrow therapeutic index and are largely dependent on the hepatic cytochrome P450 system for clearance.

Drug-Food Interactions: Interactions with food have not been established.

Drug-Herb Interactions: Interactions with herbal products have not been established.

Drug-Laboratory Test Interactions: Interactions with laboratory tests have not been established.

DOSAGE AND ADMINISTRATION: Dosing Considerations: For subcutaneous use only.

BETASERON (interferon beta-1b) should only be prescribed by (or following consultation with) clinicians who are experienced in the diagnosis and management of multiple sclerosis.

Recommended Dose and Dosage Adjustment: The recommended dose of BETASERON for both relapsing-remitting and secondary-progressive MS patients is 0.25 mg (8 MIU) injected subcutaneously every other day.

Dose titration was used at the start of treatment in the clinically isolated syndrome and secondary-progressive MS studies in order to increase the tolerability of BETASERON.

In the study in patients with a single clinical event suggestive of MS (clinically isolated syndrome), dosage was increased as shown in Table 5.

Table 5: BETASERON

Schedule for Dose Titration[a]

Treatment Day	Dose	Volume
1, 3, 5	0.0625 mg (2 MIU)	0.25 mL
7, 9, 11	0.125 mg (4 MIU)	0.5 mL
13, 15, 17	0.1875 mg (6 MIU)	0.75 mL
≥19	0.250 mg (8 MIU)	1.0 mL

[a] Titration scheme as used in the study in patients with a single clinical event suggestive of multiple sclerosis. The titration period may be adjusted if any significant adverse reaction occurs.

In the secondary-progressive MS study, patients initiated treatment with half the dose (4 MIU s.c. every other day) for a period of 2 weeks prior to escalating to the recommended dose of 8 MIU (s.c. every other day).

Efficacy of treatment for longer than 2 years has not been substantially demonstrated in relapsing-remitting multiple sclerosis. For secondary-progressive multiple sclerosis, safety and efficacy data beyond 3 years are not available.

In patients with a single clinical event suggestive of MS, efficacy has been demonstrated over a period of three years.

Missed Dose: If an injection is missed, it should be given as soon as feasible. The next injection should be given two days later.

Administration: Reconstitution: To reconstitute lyophilized BETASERON for injection, use the vial adapter to inject the entire contents of the prefilled diluent syringe containing Sodium Chloride 0.54% Solution into the BETASERON vial. Gently swirl the vial of BETASERON to dissolve the drug completely; do not shake. Inspect the reconstituted product visually and discard the product before use if it contains particulate matter or is discolored. After reconstitution with diluent, each mL of solution contains 0.25 mg (8 MIU) interferon beta-1b, 13 mg Albumin Human USP and 13 mg Mannitol USP.

Vial Content	Volume of Diluent to be Added to Vial	Approximate Available Volume	Nominal Concentration per mL
0.3 mg interferon beta-1b	1.2 mL	1.2 mL	0.25 mg/mL

Subcutaneous Injection: Withdraw 1 mL of reconstituted solution from the vial back into the syringe, fitted with a ½-inch needle, and inject the solution subcutaneously. Sites for self-injection include arms, abdomen, buttocks and thighs. All components are suitable for single use only; unused portions should be discarded (see Information for the Patient, Proper Use of this Medication section for self-injection procedure.)

ACTION AND CLINICAL PHARMACOLOGY: Mechanism of Action: Interferons are a family of naturally occurring proteins, which have molecular weights ranging from 15 000 to 21 000 daltons. Three major classes of interferons have been identified: alpha, beta and gamma. Interferon beta-1b, interferon alpha, and interferon gamma have overlapping yet distinct biologic activities. The activities of interferon beta are species-restricted and, therefore, the most pertinent pharmacological information on BETASERON (interferon beta-1b) is derived from studies of human cells in culture and in vivo.

Interferon beta-1b has been shown to possess both antiviral and immunomodulatory activities. The mechanisms by which BETASERON exerts its actions in multiple sclerosis (MS) are not clearly understood. However, it is known that the biologic response-modifying properties of interferon beta-1b are mediated through its interactions with specific cell receptors found on the surface of human cells. The binding of interferon beta-1b to these receptors induces the expression of a number of interferon-induced gene products (e.g., 2',5'-oligoadenylate synthetase, protein kinase, and indoleamine 2,3-dioxygenase) that are believed to be the mediators of the biological actions of interferon beta-1b. A number of these interferon-induced products have been readily measured in the serum and cellular fractions of blood collected from patients treated with interferon beta-1b.

Pharmacokinetics: Given that serum concentrations of interferon beta-1b are low or not detectable following subcutaneous administration of 0.25 mg (8 MIU) or less of BETASERON (interferon beta-1b), pharmacokinetic information in MS patients receiving the recommended dose of BETASERON is not available. Following single and multiple daily subcutaneous administrations of 0.5 mg (16 MIU) BETASERON to healthy volunteers (n=12), serum interferon beta-1b concentrations were generally below 100 IU/mL. Peak serum interferon beta-1b concentrations occurred between 1 to 8 hours, with a mean peak serum interferon concentration of 40 IU/mL. Bioavailability, based on a total dose of 0.5 mg (16 MIU) BETASERON given as two subcutaneous injections at different sites, was approximately 50%.

After intravenous administration of BETASERON (0.006 mg [0.2 MIU] to 2.0 mg [64 MIU]), similar pharmacokinetic profiles were obtained from healthy volunteers (n=12) and from patients with diseases other than MS (n=142). In patients receiving single intravenous doses up to 2.0 mg (64 MIU), increases in serum concentrations were dose proportional. Mean serum clearance values ranged from 9.4 mL/min kg^{-1} to 28.9 mL/min kg^{-1} and were independent of dose. Mean terminal elimination half-life values ranged from 8.0 minutes to 4.3 hours and mean steady-state volume of distribution values ranged from 0.25 L/kg to 2.88 L/kg. Three-times-a-week intravenous dosing for 2 weeks resulted in no accumulation of interferon beta-1b in the serum of patients. Pharmacokinetic parameters after single and multiple intravenous doses of BETASERON were comparable.

STORAGE AND STABILITY: Before Reconstitution: Store between 2-25°C. Excursions between 25 and 30°C are permitted as long as they do not exceed a maximum of 30 days. Do not freeze. Do not use beyond the expiration date indicated on the labels of the BETASERON vial and the prefilled diluent syringe.

After Reconstitution: The reconstituted product contains no preservative. If not used immediately, store under refrigeration between 2 and 8°C **and use within 3 hours of reconstitution**. Do not freeze.

INFORMATION FOR THE PATIENT: Published in e-CPS, available by subscription at www.e-cps.ca.

DOSAGE FORMS, COMPOSITION AND PACKAGING: Each single-use vial of lyophilized powder contains: interferon beta-1b 0.3 mg (9.6 MIU), 15 mg albumin human USP and 15 mg mannitol USP.

BETASERON is supplied in:

- A carton containing 15 single-use packs;
- A 3-month pack containing 3×15 single-use packs; and
- An Initiation Pack of 12 for initial dose titration, containing 4 differently coloured and numbered triple packs (containing a total of 12 doses).

The single-use pack is supplied in a blister pack or in a carton. Each single-use pack contains the necessary components to prepare and inject a single dose of BETASERON:

Single-use Blister Pack: 1 vial of medication, 1 prefilled diluent syringe (containing 1.2 mL of Sodium Chloride 0.54% solution), 1 vial adapter with attached 27 gauge, ½" needle and 3 alcohol wipes. **The single-use blister pack can only be used with the BETAJECT III autoinjector.**

Single-use Carton: 1 vial of medication, 1 prefilled diluent syringe (containing 1.2 mL of Sodium Chloride 0.54% solution), 1 vial adapter with attached 30 gauge, ½" needle and 2 alcohol wipes. **The single-use carton can only be used with the BETAJECT Lite or BETAJECT Comfort autoinjector.**

The Initiation Pack contains 4 differently coloured and numbered triple packs:

- Yellow with number "1" (for treatment days 1, 3, and 5; 0.25 mL syringe marking)
- Red with number "2" (for treatment days 7, 9, and 11; 0.5 mL syringe marking)
- Green with number "3" (for treatment days 13, 15, and 17; 0.75 mL syringe marking)
- Blue with number "4" (for treatment days 19, 21, and 23; 0.25, 0.5, 0.75 and 1.0 mL syringe markings)

Each **triple** pack contains 3 vials of medication, 3 prefilled diluent syringes (containing 1.2 mL of sodium chloride 0.54% solution), 3 vial adapters with attached 30 gauge, ½" needle, and 6 alcohol wipes.

The Initiation Pack can only be used with the BETAJECT Lite or BETAJECT Comfort autoinjector.

(Shown in Product Identification Section)

Betnesol® Ⓟ

betamethasone sodium phosphate

Topical Corticosteroid

Paladin

Date of Revision: May 1, 2009

INDICATIONS: Enema: For local use as a retention enema in ulcerative colitis.

CONTRAINDICATIONS: Systemic infections, live virus immunization, hypersensitivity.

PRECAUTIONS: Following administration of Betnesol (betamethasone sodium phosphate) Enema, there is some systemic absorption of the steroid, which can be a therapeutic advantage, as combined systemic and local therapy can be beneficial, certainly in some cases. However, adrenal function can be affected; thus it is necessary to take such precautions as apply during and after systemic therapy.

In patients on corticosteroid therapy subjected to unusual stress, increased dosage of rapidly acting corticosteroids before, during and after the stressful situation is indicated. Corticosteroid treatment may reduce the response of the pituitary-adrenal axis to stress and relative insufficiency may persist for up to 1 year after withdrawal or prolonged therapy.

While on corticosteroid therapy patients should not be vaccinated against smallpox because of potential complications. Conversely, patients with vaccinia should not receive corticosteroid therapy. Other immunization procedures should not be undertaken in patients who are on corticosteroids, especially on high doses, because of possible hazards of neurological complications and a lack of antibody response. Patients without a definite history of chickenpox should be advised to avoid close contact with chickenpox or herpes zoster. If exposed to chickenpox or herpes zoster, patients should seek urgent medical attention. If the patient is a child, then the parents must be aware that exposure to chickenpox must be avoided. Passive immunization with varicella/zoster immunoglobulin (VZIG) is needed by exposed nonimmune patients who are receiving systemic corticosteroids or who have used them within the previous 3 months. VZIG should be given not later than 10 days from exposure to chickenpox. If a diagnosis of chickenpox is confirmed, the illness warrants specialist care and urgent treatment. A diagnosis of chickenpox should be considered in any patient receiving corticosteroids who presents with a fever or systemic illness. Corticosteroids should not be stopped and a dose increase may be necessary.

If corticosteroids are indicated in patients with latent tuberculosis or tuberculin reactivity, close observation is necessary as reactivation of the disease may occur. During prolonged corticosteroid therapy, these patients should receive chemoprophylaxis.

Corticosteroids may mask some signs of infection and new infections may appear during their use. There may be impaired resistance to and inability to localize infection when corticosteroids are used. If corticosteroids have to be used in the presence of bacterial infections, institute appropriate vigorous anti-infective therapy.

Use corticosteroids cautiously in patients with ocular herpes simplex because of possible corneal ulceration and perforation. Corticosteroids may worsen diabetes mellitus, osteoporosis, hypertension, glaucoma and epilepsy.

Prolonged use of corticosteroids may produce posterior subcapsular cataracts, glaucoma with possible damage to the optic nerves, and may enhance the establishment of secondary ocular infections due to fungi or viruses.

Corticosteroid therapy may cause hyperacidity or peptic ulcer. Since appearance of peptic ulcer may be asymptomatic until perforation or hemorrhage occurs, take x-rays when treatment is prolonged or when there is gastric distress. An ulcer regimen including an antacid should be considered as a prophylactic measure during prolonged therapy.

Use the lowest possible dose of corticosteroid to control the condition under treatment, and when dosage reduction is possible, the reduction should be gradual.

Average and large doses of hydrocortisone or cortisone can cause elevation of blood pressure, salt, and water retention, and increased potassium excretion. These effects are less likely to occur with the synthetic derivatives except when used in large doses. Because of the possibility of fluid retention, care must be taken when corticosteroids are administered to patients with congestive heart failure. Dietary salt restriction and potassium supplementation may be necessary. All corticosteroids increase calcium excretion.

Drug induced secondary adrenocortical insufficiency may be minimized by gradual dosage reduction. This type of relative insufficiency may persist for months after discontinuation of therapy, therefore, in any stress situation occurring during that period, reinstitute hormone therapy. If the patient is receiving steroids already, the dosage may have to be increased. Since mineralocorticoid secretion may be impaired, salt and/or a mineralocorticoid should be administered concurrently.

Use steroids with caution in nonspecific ulcerative colitis if there is a probability of impending perforation, abscess or other pyogenic infection; diverticulitis, fresh intestinal anastomoses; active or latent peptic ulcer; renal insufficiency; hypertension; osteoporosis; and myasthenia gravis. Fat embolism has been reported as a possible complication of hypercortisonism.

There is an enhanced effect of corticosteroids on patients with hypothyroidism and in those with cirrhosis.

In patients with liver failure, blood levels of corticosteroid may be increased, as with other drugs which are metabolized by the liver.

Psychic derangements may appear when corticosteroids are used, ranging from euphoria, insomnia, mood swings, personality changes, and severe depression, to frank psychotic manifestations. Also, existing emotional instability or psychotic tendencies may be aggravated by corticosteroids.

Care should be taken when there is a history of severe affective disorders (especially a previous history of steroid psychosis), steroid myopathy or peptic ulceration.

Steroids may increase or decrease motility and number of spermatozoa in some patients.

Advise patients to inform subsequent physicians of the prior use of corticosteroids.

Geriatrics: The risks and benefits of corticosteroid therapy for the elderly patient should be carefully weighed, considering the more serious consequences of the common side effects in old age, especially osteoporosis, diabetes, hypertension, susceptibility to infection and thinning of the skin.

Pediatrics: Systemic corticosteroids may cause growth retardation in infancy, childhood and adolescence. Treatment should be limited to the minimum dosage for the shortest possible time.

Growth and development of infants and children on prolonged corticosteroid therapy should be carefully observed.

Pregnancy: Since adequate human reproduction studies have not been done with corticosteroids, the use of these drugs in pregnancy or women of childbearing potential requires that the possible benefits of the drug be weighed against the potential hazards to the mother and embryo or fetus. Infants born of mothers who have received substantial doses of corticosteroids during pregnancy should be carefully observed for signs of hypoadrenalism.

Administration of corticosteroids to pregnant animals can cause abnormalities of fetal development including cleft palate and intrauterine growth retardation. The relevance of these findings in humans has not been established, however, patients should avoid extensive use in pregnancy.

Lactation: Since adequate human reproduction studies have not been done with corticosteroids, the use of these drugs in nursing mothers requires that the possible benefits of the drug be weighed against the potential hazards. Corticosteroids are excreted in small amounts in breast milk and infants of mothers taking pharmacological doses of steroids should be monitored carefully for signs of adrenal suppression.

Drug Interactions: Corticosteroids may reduce the effects of anticholinesterases in myasthenia gravis, cholecystographic x-ray media, salicylates and nonsteroidal anti-inflammatory drugs (NSAIDs).

Estrogens may potentiate the effects of glucocorticoids, whereas phenytoin, phenobarbital, ephedrine and rifampin may reduce the effects of glucocorticoids. Dosage adjustments may be required in these cases.

Increase or decrease the action of concomitantly administered anticoagulants.

Increase renal clearance of acetylsalicylic acid (ASA).

Test Interactions : Corticosteroids may suppress reactions to skin tests.

ADVERSE EFFECTS: The following adverse events have been reported following the systemic (other betamethasone sodium phosphate dosage forms) and/or local (such as Betnesol Enema) use of betamethasone sodium phosphate.

Fluid and Electrolyte Disturbances: sodium retention; fluid retention; congestive heart failure in susceptible patients; potassium loss; hypokalemic alkalosis; hypertension; benign intracranial hypertension; psychic instability.

Musculoskeletal: muscle weakness; steroid myopathy; loss of muscle mass; osteoporosis; vertebral compression fractures; aseptic necrosis of femoral and humeral heads; pathologic fracture of long bones.

Gastrointestinal : peptic ulcer and possible subsequent perforation and hemorrhage; pancreatitis; abdominal distention; ulcerative esophagitis.

Dermatologic: impaired wound healing; thin fragile skin; petechiae and ecchymoses; erythema; increased sweating; may suppress reactions to skin tests.

Neurological: convulsions; increased intracranial pressure with papilledema (pseudotumor cerebri) usually after treatment; vertigo; headache.

Endocrine: menstrual irregularities, development of Cushingoid state; suppression of growth in children; secondary adrenocortical and pituitary unresponsiveness, particularly in times of stress, as in trauma, surgery or illness; decreased carbohydrate tolerance; manifestations of latent diabetes mellitus; increased requirements for insulin or oral hypoglycemic agents in diabetes.

Ophthalmic: posterior subcapsular cataracts; increased intraocular pressure; glaucoma; exophthalmos.

Metabolic: negative nitrogen balance due to protein catabolism.

Other: hypersensitivity, thromboembolism; features of hypercortisolism, aseptic osteonecrosis.

OVERDOSE:

For management of a suspected drug overdose, CPhA recommends that you contact your **regional Poison Control Centre**. See the *CPS* Directory section for a list of Poison Control Centres.

DOSAGE: Normally, one Betnesol (betamethasone sodium phosphate) Enema is used nightly, for 2 to 4 weeks. More prolonged treatment is permissible in patients showing progressive improvement. If the response is inadequate, it is undesirable to persist with medical treatment to a point where surgical measures are unduly delayed.

SUPPLIED: Each disposable plastic bag of 100 mL contains: betamethasone 5 mg (as betamethasone sodium phosphate) in buffered solution. Boxes of 7×100 mL. Store below 25°C. Protect from light.

Betoptic® S Ⓟ

betaxolol HCl

Antiglaucoma Agent

Alcon

SUPPLIED: Each mL of sterile, isotonic, aqueous suspension contains: betaxolol 0.25% (0.28% betaxolol HCl) with benzalkonium chloride (as preservative), mannitol, poly (styrenedivinyl benzene) sulfonic acid, carbomer 934P, edetate disodium, hydrochloric acid and/or sodium hydroxide (to adjust pH) and purified water. Drop-Tainer dispensers of 5 and 10 mL. Store at room temperature (15 to 30°C).

Bexxar® Therapy

tositumomab—iodine I 131 tositumomab

Antineoplastic Radioimmunotherapeutic

GlaxoSmithKline

Date of Revision: December 20, 2007

SUMMARY PRODUCT INFORMATION:

Route of Administration	Dosage Form/ Strength	Clinically Relevant Nonmedicinal Ingredients
Intravenous	Intravenous/ 35 mg/2.5 mL 225 mg/16.1 mL	Not applicable For a complete listing see Dosage Forms, Composition and Packaging.

DESCRIPTION: Physical Characteristics: Iodine-131 decays with beta and gamma emissions with a physical half life of 8.04 days. The principal beta emission has a mean energy of 191.6 keV and the principal gamma emission has an energy of 364.5 keV.

External Radiation: The specific gamma ray constant for iodine-131 is 2.2 R/millicurie hour at 1 cm. The first half-value layer is 0.24 cm lead (Pb) shielding. A range of values is shown in Table 1 for the relative attenuation of the radiation emitted by this radionuclide that results from interposition of various thicknesses of Pb. To facilitate control of the radiation exposure from this radionuclide, the use of a 2.55 cm thickness of Pb will attenuate the radiation emitted by a factor of about 1000.

Table 1: BEXXAR
Radiation Attenuation by Lead Shielding

Shield Thickness (Pb) cm	Attenuation Factor
0.24	0.5
0.89	10^{-1}
1.60	10^{-2}
2.55	10^{-3}
3.7	10^{-4}

The fraction of iodine-131 radioactivity that remains in the vial after the date of calibration is calculated as follows:
Fraction of remaining radioactivity of iodine-131 after × days = $2^{-(x/8.04)}$
Physical decay is presented in Table 2.

INDICATIONS AND CLINICAL USE: BEXXAR therapy (tositumomab and iodine I 131 tositumomab) is indicated for:

- the treatment of patients with CD20 positive relapsed or refractory, low grade, follicular, or transformed non-Hodgkin's lymphoma, including patients with rituximab-refractory non-Hodgkin's lymphoma.

This product should be administered under the supervision of a qualified health professional who is appropriately qualified in the use of radioimmunotherapy and the management of patients with non-Hodgkin's lymphoma (NHL). Appropriate management of therapy and complications is only possible when adequate diagnostic and treatment facilities are readily available.

Table 2: BEXXAR
Physical Decay Chart: Iodine-131: Half-Life 8.04 Days

Days	Fraction Remaining
0[a]	1.000
1	0.917
2	0.842
3	0.772
4	0.708
5	0.650
6	0.596
7	0.547
8	0.502
9	0.460
10	0.422
11	0.387
12	0.355
13	0.326
14	0.299

[a] (Calibration day).

CONTRAINDICATIONS: BEXXAR therapy (tositumomab and iodine I 131 tositumomab) is contraindicated in patients with known hypersensitivity to murine proteins or any component of BEXXAR.

WARNINGS AND PRECAUTIONS:

Serious Warnings and Precautions

Special Requirements: BEXXAR therapy (tositumomab and iodine I 131 tositumomab) contains a radioactive component and should be administered only by physicians and other health care professionals qualified by training in the safe use and handling of therapeutic radionuclides.

Thyroid-blocking therapy must be initiated at least 24 hour before receiving the dosimetric dose and continued for 14 days after the therapeutic dose of BEXXAR to decrease the risk of hypothyroidism (see Warnings and Precautions, Endocrine and Metabolism and Dosage and Administration).

Hypersensitivity Reactions, Including Anaphylaxis: Serious hypersensitivity reactions, including some with fatal outcome, have been reported with BEXXAR. Medications for the treatment of severe hypersensitivity reactions should be available for immediate use. Patients who develop severe hypersensitivity reactions should have infusions of BEXXAR discontinued and receive medical attention (see Warnings and Precautions, Immune).

Prolonged and Severe Cytopenias: The majority of patients who received BEXXAR experienced severe thrombocytopenia and neutropenia. BEXXAR should not be administered to patients with >25% lymphoma marrow involvement and/or impaired bone marrow reserve (see Warnings and Precautions, Hematologic and Adverse Reactions).

Pregnancy: BEXXAR can cause fetal harm when administered to a pregnant woman.

General: BEXXAR therapy (tositumomab and iodine I 131 tositumomab) is a biologic product with a radioactive component and should be administered only under the supervision of a health professional who is experienced in the use of radionuclides. Appropriate management of therapy and complications is only possible when adequate diagnostic and treatment facilities are readily available.

Radionuclide Precautions: Iodine I 131 tositumomab is radioactive. It may be received, used and administered only by authorized personnel. Its receipt, storage, use, transfer and disposal are subject to the regulations and/or appropriate licenses of local competent official organizations. As in the use of any other radioactive material, care should be taken to minimize radiation exposure to patients consistent with proper patient management, and to minimize radiation exposure to occupational workers.

Contamination: The following measures should be taken by the patient for up to 2 weeks after receiving the radiopharmaceutical.

Therapeutic Dose: Avoidance of contact with infants, young children and pregnant women. Sleeping in a separate bed (separated by a distance of at least 2 to 3 meters). Maintain an appropriate distance of 2 meters from others. Travel alone in a private automobile if possible, otherwise maintain as great a distance as possible between patient and driver. Toilet should be used instead of urinal. Male patients should sit to use the toilet. Toilet should be flushed several times after use. Separate laundry and eating utensils and wash items separately.

Carcinogenesis and Mutagenesis: No long-term animal studies have been performed to establish the carcinogenic or mutagenic potential of BEXXAR or to determine its effects on fertility in males or females. However, radiation is a potential carcinogen and mutagen. Administration of BEXXAR results in delivery of a significant radiation dose to the testes. The radiation dose to the ovaries has not been established. There have been no studies to evaluate whether administration of BEXXAR causes hypogonadism, premature menopause, azoospermia, and/or mutagenic alterations to germ cells. There is a potential risk that BEXXAR may cause toxic effects on the male and female gonads. Effective contraceptive methods should be used during treatment and for 12 months following administration of BEXXAR.

Secondary Malignancies: Although there were 995 patients in the investigator assessment, 10 patients were determined to have MDS/AML prior to BEXXAR and were then excluded from the independent, masked pathology review. Based on an independent, masked pathology review, myelodysplastic syndrome (MDS) and/or acute leukemia developed in 32/985 (3.2%) patients after receiving BEXXAR. This analysis yields an annualised incidence of 1.3% per year (95% CI: 0.9%-1.8% per year).

Most patients had extensive exposure to common alkylating agents and/or to topoisomerase II inhibiting agents, which have all been documented as risk factors for the development of MDS and leukemia. It is unknown to what extent BEXXAR plays a role in the development of MDS and/or leukemia in patients with NHL.

Endocrine and Metabolism: Hypothyroidism: Use of BEXXAR may result in hypothyroidism. Thyroid-blocking therapy must be initiated at least 24 hours before receiving the dosimetric dose and continue for 14 days after the therapeutic dose of BEXXAR to decrease the risk of hypothyroidism. TSH levels should be monitored before and after BEXXAR. After treatment, patients should be monitored for elevation of TSH and/or signs or symptoms of hypothyroidism every 6 months for the first 2 years, and annually thereafter.

Hematologic: Prolonged and Severe Cytopenias: (See Serious Warnings and Precautions and Adverse Reactions, Hematologic Events.) The most common adverse reactions associated with BEXXAR were grade 3 or grade 4 cytopenias. These consisted primarily of grade 3 or 4 thrombocytopenia (53%) and grade 3 or 4 neutropenia (63%). The time to nadir was 4 to 7 weeks and the duration of cytopenias was approximately 30 days. Thrombocytopenia, neutropenia, and anemia persisted for more than 90 days following administration of BEXXAR in 16 (7%), 15 (7%), and 12 (5%) patients respectively (this includes patients with transient recovery followed by recurrent cytopenia). Due to the variable nature in the onset of cytopenias, complete blood counts should be obtained weekly following BEXXAR and should continue until levels recover.

The safety of BEXXAR has not been established in patients with >25% lymphoma marrow involvement, platelet count $<100\times10^9$/L or neutrophil count $<1.5\times10^9$/L.

Immune: Hypersensitivity Reactions Including Anaphylaxis: (See Adverse Reactions: Immunogenicity.) Severe hypersensitivity reactions may result in fatal outcomes during and following administration of BEXXAR. Emergency supplies including medications for the treatment of hypersensitivity reactions, e.g., epinephrine, antihistamines, and corticosteroids, should be available for immediate use in the event of an allergic reaction during administration of BEXXAR. Patients who have received murine proteins should be screened for human anti-murine antibodies (HAMA). Patients who are positive for HAMA may be at increased risk of anaphylaxis and serious hypersensitivity reactions during administration of BEXXAR.

Immunization: The safety of immunization with live viral vaccines following administration of BEXXAR has not been studied. The ability of patients who have received BEXXAR to generate a primary or anamnestic humoral response to any vaccine has not been studied.

Renal Function: Iodine I 131 tositumomab and iodine-131 are excreted primarily by the kidneys. Impaired renal function may decrease the rate of excretion of the radiolabelled iodine and increase patient exposure to the radioactive component of BEXXAR. There are no data regarding the safety of administration of BEXXAR in patients with impaired renal function.

Special Populations: Pregnant Women: Ideally examinations and treatments using radiopharmaceuticals, in women of child-bearing capability should be performed during the first ten days following the onset of menses. Use of BEXXAR may cause fetal harm when administered to a pregnant woman. Iodine-131 may cause harm to the fetal thyroid gland when administered to pregnant women. Review of the literature has shown that transplacental passage of radioiodide may cause severe, and possibly irreversible, hypothyroidism in neonates. While there are no adequate and well-controlled studies of BEXXAR in pregnant animals or humans, use of BEXXAR in women of childbearing age should be deferred until the possibility of pregnancy has been ruled out. If the patient becomes pregnant while being treated with BEXXAR, the patient should be apprised of the potential hazard to the fetus.

Nursing Women: Radioiodine is excreted in breast milk and may reach concentrations equal to or greater than maternal plasma concentrations. Immunoglobulins are also known to be excreted in breast milk. The absorption potential and potential for adverse effects of the monoclonal antibody component (tositumomab) in the infant are not known. Therefore, formula feedings should be substituted for breast feedings before starting treatment. Women should be advised to discontinue nursing.

Pediatrics (<18 years of age): The safety and effectiveness of BEXXAR in pediatric patients has not been evaluated.

Geriatrics (>65 years of age): Clinical studies of BEXXAR did not include sufficient numbers of patients aged 65 and over to determine whether they respond differently from younger patients. In clinical studies, 230 patients received BEXXAR at the recommended dose. Of these, 27% (61 patients) were age 65 or older and 4% (10 patients) were age 75 or older. While the incidence of severe hematologic toxicity was lower, the duration of severe hematologic toxicity was longer in those age 65 or older as compared to patients less than 65 years of age. Due to the limited experience, greater sensitivity of some older individuals cannot be ruled out.

Monitoring and Laboratory Tests: A complete blood count (CBC) with differential and platelet count should be obtained prior to, and at least weekly following, administration of BEXXAR and should continue until levels recover. More frequent monitoring is indicated in patients with evidence of moderate or more severe cytopenias (see Warnings and Precautions). Thyroid stimulating hormone (TSH) levels should be monitored before treatment with BEXXAR, and then every 6 months for the first 2 years, and annually thereafter. Serum creatinine levels should be measured prior to administration of BEXXAR.

Administration of BEXXAR may result in the development of human anti-murine antibodies (HAMA). The presence of HAMA may affect the accuracy of the results of in vitro and in vivo diagnostic tests and may affect the toxicity profile and efficacy of therapeutic agents that rely on murine antibody technology. Patients who are HAMA positive may be at increased risk for serious allergic reactions and other side effects if they undergo in vivo diagnostic testing or treatment with murine monoclonal antibodies.

ADVERSE REACTIONS: Clinical Trial Adverse Drug Reactions: Because clinical trials are conducted under very specific conditions the adverse reaction rates observed in the clinical trials may not reflect the rates observed in practice and should not be compared to the rates in the clinical trials of another drug. Adverse drug reaction information from clinical trials is useful for identifying drug-related adverse events and for approximating rates.

The most serious adverse reactions observed in the clinical trials were prolonged and severe cytopenias, which were generally reversible, and the sequelae of cytopenias, which included infections (sepsis) and hemorrhage in thrombocytopenic patients, allergic reactions (bronchospasm and angioedema), secondary leukemia, and myelodysplasia (see Warnings and Precautions).

The most common adverse reactions occurring in the clinical trials included neutropenia, thromobocytopenia, and anemia. Less common but severe adverse reactions included pneumonia, pleural effusion, and dehydration.

Data regarding adverse events were primarily obtained in 230 patients with non-Hodgkin's lymphoma enrolled in five clinical trials using the recommended dose and schedule. Patients had a median follow-up of 39 months and 79% of the patients were followed at least 12 months for survival and selected adverse events. Patients had a median of 3 prior chemotherapy regimens, a median age of 55 years, 60% were male, 27% had transformation to a higher grade histology, 29% were intermediate grade and 2% high grade histology (IWF), and 68% had Ann Arbor stage IV disease. Patients enrolled in these studies were not permitted to have prior hematopoietic stem cell transplantation or irradiation to more than 25% of the red marrow. In the expanded access program, which included 765 patients, data regarding clinical serious adverse events and HAMA and TSH levels were used to supplement the characterization of delayed adverse events (see Adverse Reactions, Hypothyroidism, Secondary Leukemia and Myelodysplastic Syndrome (MDS), Immunogenicity).

Table 3 lists adverse events that occurred in ≥1% of patients in clinical trials.

Table 3: BEXXAR

Incidence of Adverse Experiences Regardless of Relationship to Study Drug Occurring in ≥1% of the Patients Treated with BEXXAR Therapy (N=230)

Body System Preferred Term	All Grades[a]	Grade III/IV
Total	**n=224 (97%)**	**n=180 (78%)**
Non-Hematologic AEs		
Body as a Whole	**81%**	**12%**
Asthenia	46%	2%
Fever	37%	2%
Infection[b]	21%	<1%
Pain	19%	1%
Chills	18%	1%
Headache	16%	0%
Abdominal Pain	15%	3%
Back Pain	8%	1%
Chest Pain	7%	0%
Neck Pain	6%	1%
Malaise	4%	<1%
Sepsis	4%	3%
Injection Site Reaction	3%	0%
Face Oedema	2%	0%

(cont'd)

Table 3: BEXXAR *(cont'd)*

Incidence of Adverse Experiences Regardless of Relationship to Study Drug Occurring in ≥1% of the Patients Treated with BEXXAR Therapy (N=230)

Body System Preferred Term	All Grades[a]	Grade III/IV
Total	**n=224 (97%)**	**n=180 (78%)**
Pelvic Pain	2%	0%
Cellulitis	2%	0%
Injection Site Hypersensitivity	1%	0%
Flu Syndrome	1%	0%
Cardiovascular System	**26%**	**3%**
Hypotension	7%	1%
Vasodilation	5%	0%
Tachycardia	5%	0%
Cardiovascular Disorder	3%	0%
Deep Thrombophlebitis	2%	<1%
Palpitation	2%	0%
Syncope	2%	<1%
Postural Hypotension	1%	0%
Digestive System	**56%**	**9%**
Nausea	36%	3%
Vomiting	15%	1%
Anorexia	14%	0%
Diarrhea	12%	0%
Constipation	6%	<1%
Dyspepsia	6%	<1%
Dysphagia	2%	<1%
Stomatitis	2%	<1%
Flatulence	2%	0%
Gastrointestinal Carcinoma[c]	2%	2%
Rectal Disorder	2%	0%
Gastritis	1%	0%
Melena	1%	0%
Mouth Ulceration	1%	0%
Ulcerative Stomatitis	1%	0%
Endocrine System	**7%**	**0%**
Hypothyroidism[c]	7%	0%
Hemic and Lymphatic System	**66%**	**65%**
Myeloproliferative Disorder	10%	10%
Ecchymosis	4%	<1%
Acute Myeloblastic Leukemia[c]	3%	3%
Lymphadenopathy	2%	0%
Lymphoma Like Reaction	2%	1%
Petechia	2%	0%
Metabolic and Nutritional Disorders	**21%**	**3%**
Peripheral Edema	9%	0%
Weight Loss	6%	<1%
Oedema	3%	<1%
Dehydration	3%	<1%
Hypercalcaemia	2%	<1%
Musculoskeletal System	**23%**	**3%**
Myalgia	13%	<1%

(cont'd)

Table 3: BEXXAR (cont'd)

Incidence of Adverse Experiences Regardless of Relationship to Study Drug Occurring in ≥1% of the Patients Treated with BEXXAR Therapy (N=230)

Body System Preferred Term	All Grades[a]	Grade III/IV
Total	**n=224 (97%)**	**n=180 (78%)**
Arthralgia	10%	1%
Pathological Fracture	2%	<1%
Arthritis	1%	<1%
Myasthenia	1%	0%
Nervous System	**26%**	**3%**
Dizziness	5%	0%
Somnolence	5%	0%
Insomnia	4%	0%
Anxiety	3%	0%
Confusion	2%	1%
Paresthesia	2%	0%
Peripheral Neuritis	1%	0%
Depression	1%	0%
Respiratory System	**44%**	**8%**
Cough Increased	21%	1%
Pharyngitis	12%	0%
Dyspnea	11%	3%
Rhinitis	10%	0%
Pneumonia	6%	3%
Epistaxis	4%	0%
Bronchitis	4%	<1%
Sinusitis	3%	0%
Lung Disorder	3%	<1%
Pleural Effusion	3%	2%
Asthma	2%	0%
Skin and Appendages	**44%**	**5%**
Rash	17%	<1%
Pruritus	10%	0%
Sweating	8%	<1%
Skin Carcinoma[c]	7%	3%
Urticaria	4%	0%
Herpes Zoster	4%	0%
Skin Disorder	3%	0%
Skin Ulcer	3%	1%
Herpes Simplex	2%	0%
Special Senses	**8%**	**<1%**
Conjunctivitis	2%	0%
Ear Disorder	2%	0%
Urogenital System	**14%**	**3%**
Urinary Tract Infection	4%	<1%
Urinary Frequency	2%	0%
Dysuria	1%	0%
Bladder Carcinoma[c]	1%	<1%

[a] AEs for ANC, platelets, and hemoglobin derived from laboratory data. Only Grade 3/4 hematologic AEs are reported from laboratory data.

[b] The COSTART term for infection includes a subset of infections (e.g., upper respiratory infection). Other terms are mapped to preferred terms (e.g., pneumonia and sepsis).

[c] Please refer to the Delayed Adverse Reactions for details.

Hematologic Events: Hematologic toxicity was the most frequently observed adverse event in clinical trials with BEXXAR therapy (tositumomab and iodine I 131 tositumomab) (see Table 4). Sixty-three (27%) of 230 patients received one or more hematologic supportive care measures following the therapeutic dose (see Warnings and Precautions) 12% received filgrastim, 7% received Epoetin alfa, 15% received platelet transfusions, and 16% received packed red blood cell transfusions. Twenty-eight (12%) patients experienced hemorrhagic events; the majority were mild to moderate. Table 4 provides a detailed description of the hematologic toxicity.

Table 4: BEXXAR

Hematologic Toxicity[a] (N=230)

Endpoint	Values
Platelets	
Median nadir (×10⁹/L)	43
Per patient incidence[a] platelets <50×10⁹/L	53% (n=123)
Median[b] duration of platelets <50×10⁹/L (days)	32
Grade 3/4 without recovery to Grade 2, N (%)	16 (7%)
Per patient incidence[c] platelets <25×10⁹/L	21% (n=47)
ANC	
Median nadir (×10⁹/L)	0.69
Per patient incidence[a] ANC<1×10⁹/L	63% (n=145)
Median[b] duration of ANC<1×10⁹/L (days)	31
Grade 3/4 without recovery to Grade 2, N (%)	15 (7%)
Per patient incidence[c] ANC <0.5×10⁹/L	25% (n=57)
Hemoglobin	
Median nadir (g/L)	100
Per patient incidence[a] <80 g/L	29% (n=66)
Median[b] duration of hemoglobin <80 g/L (days)	23
Grade 3/4 without recovery to Grade 2, N (%)	12 (5%)
Per patient incidence[c] hemoglobin <65 g/L	5% (n=11)

[a] Grade 3/4 toxicity was assumed if patient was missing 2 or more weeks of hematology data between Week 5 and Week 9.

[b] Duration of Grade 3/4 of 1000+ days (censored) was assumed for those patients with undocumented grade 3/4 and no hematologic data on or after Week 9.

[c] Grade 4 toxicity was assumed if patient had documented Grade 3 toxicity and was missing 2 or more weeks of hematology data between Week 5 and Week 9.

Infectious Events: One hundred and thirty of 230 (57%) patients developed one or more adverse events possibly related to infection. The majority of these were viral (rhinitis, pharyngitis, flu symptoms, or herpes) or other minor infections. Twenty of 230 (9%) patients experienced 24 infections that were considered to be serious, because the patient was hospitalized for management of the infection. Documented infections included pneumonia, bacteremia, septicemia, bronchitis and skin infections.

Hypersensitivity Reactions: Fourteen patients (6%) experienced one or more of the following adverse events: allergic reaction, face edema, injection site hypersensitivity, anaphylactoid reaction, laryngismus, and serum sickness.

Gastrointestinal Toxicity: Eighty-seven patients (38%) experienced one or more gastrointestinal adverse events, including nausea, emesis, abdominal pain, and diarrhea. These events were temporally related to the infusion of the antibody. Nausea, vomiting, and abdominal pain were often reported within days of infusion, whereas diarrhea was generally reported days to weeks after infusion.

Infusional Toxicity: A constellation of symptoms, including fever, rigors or chills, sweating, hypotension, dyspnea, bronchospasm, and nausea have been reported during or within 48 hours of infusion. Sixty-seven patients (29%) reported fever, rigors/chills, or sweating within 14 days following the dosimetric dose. Adjustment of the rate of infusion to control adverse reactions occurred in 16 patients (7%); seven patients required adjustments for only the dosimetric infusion, two required adjustments for only the therapeutic infusion, and seven required adjustments for both the dosimetric and the therapeutic infusions. Adjustments included reduction in the rate of infusion by 50%, temporary interruption of the infusion, and in 2 patients, infusion was permanently discontinued.

Less Common Clinical Trial Adverse Drug Reactions (<1%): The following list the adverse experiences regardless of relationship to study drug occurring in <1% of the patients treated with BEXXAR therapy.

Body as a Whole: abdomen enlarged, accidental injury, allergic reaction, anaphylactoid reaction, ascites, carcinoma, chest pain substernal, chills and fever, cyst, hernia, injection site edema, injection site pain, neck rigidity and serum sickness.

Cardiovascular System: aortic stenosis, arrhythmia, atrial flutter, cardiomegaly, cerebral hemorrhage, hemorrhage, migraine, peripheral vascular disorder, pulmonary embolus, shock, thrombophlebitis and thrombosis.

Digestive System: abnormal stools, carcinoma of mouth, cholecystitis, colitis, dry mouth, eructation, gastroenteritis, gastrointestinal disorder, gastrointestinal hemorrhage, gingivitis, glossitis, gum hemorrhage, hepatitis, increased appetite, intestinal obstruction, jaundice, liver function tests abnormal, nausea and vomiting, oral moniliasis, periodontal abscess, tenesmus and ulcerative colitis.

Hemic and Lymphatic System: chronic leukemia, leukemia, lymphedema.

Metabolic and Nutritional Disorders: generalized edema, hyperuricemia, hypoglycemia, hypokalemia, hyponatremia, hypovolemia and weight gain.

Musculoskeletal System: arthrosis, bone disorder, bone pain, muscle atrophy, tendon disorder and tenosynovitis.

Nervous System: abnormal gait, agitation, amnesia, ataxia, depersonalization, encephalopathy, foot drop, hypertonia, hypokinesia, nervousness, neuralgia, neuropathy, paralysis, subdural hematoma, thinking abnormal and tremor.

Respiratory System: aspiration pneumonia, atelectasis, carcinoma of lung, hemoptysis, hyperventilation, hypoxia, laryngismus, lung hemorrhage, pneumothorax and voice alteration.

Skin and Appendages: acne, erythema nodosum, fungal dermatitis, hair disorder, maculopapular rash, pustular rash, skin benign neoplasm, skin discoloration, skin melanoma, skin nodule and vesiculobullous rash.

Special Senses: abnormal vision, amblyopia, diplopia, dry eyes, ear pain, lacrimation disorder, parosmia, taste loss, taste perversion, tinnitus and vestibular disorder.

Urogenital System: breast carcinoma, breast pain, genital edema, hydronephrosis, kidney failure, kidney function abnormal, nocturia, oliguria, prostatic carcinoma, urinary incontinence, urinary retention, urinary tract disorder, urinary urgency and urination impaired.

Delayed Adverse Reactions: Delayed adverse reactions, including hypothyroidism, HAMA, and myelodysplasia/leukemia, were assessed in 230 patients included in clinical studies and 765 patients included in expanded access programs. The entry characteristics of patients included from the expanded access programs were similar to the characteristics of patients enrolled in the clinical studies, except that the median number of prior chemotherapy regimens was fewer (2 vs 3) and the proportion with low-grade histology was higher (77% vs 70%) in patients from the expanded access programs.

Hypothyroidism: Twelve percent (27/230) of the patients included from the clinical studies had an elevated TSH level (8%) or no TSH level obtained (4%) prior to treatment. Of the 203 patients documented to be euthyroid at entry, 137 (67%) patients had at least one follow-up TSH value. The overall incidence of hypothyroidism in the clinical study patients was 18% with cumulative incidences of 11% and 19% at 2 and 5 years respectively. New events have been observed up to 90 months post-treatment. Of the 765 patients in the expanded access programs, 670 patients did not have elevated TSH upon study entry. Of these, 455 patients had at least one post-treatment TSH value available and were not taking thyroid hormonal treatment upon study entry. With a median follow-up period of 33 months, the incidence of hypothyroidism based on elevated TSH or initiation of thyroid replacement therapy in these 455 patients was 13% with a median time to development of hypothyroidism of 15 months. The cumulative incidences of hypothyroidism at 2 and 5 years in these patients were 9% and 17% respectively.

Immunogenicity: Immune response to murine antibody may be masked in patients after administration of BEXXAR. Eighty of the 788 patients (10%) with a negative baseline HAMA and follow-up converted to a positive HAMA. The median time to a positive HAMA was 167 days (range: 5-3400 days). After administration of BEXXAR, the 1-, 2-, and 5-year cumulative incidences of testing positive for HAMA were 9% (95% CI: 7%-11%), 9% (95% CI: 8%-12%), and 10% (95% CI: 8%-12%), respectively. There was an apparent plateau in the cumulative incidence between 1 and 2 years.

The data reflect the percentage of patients whose test results were considered positive for HAMA in an ELISA assay that detects antibodies to the Fc portion of IgG_1 murine immunoglobulin and are highly dependent on the sensitivity and specificity of the assay. Additionally, the observed incidence of antibody positivity in an assay may be influenced by several factors including sample handling, concomitant medications, and underlying disease. For these reasons, comparison of the incidence of HAMA in patients treated with BEXXAR with the incidence of HAMA in patients treated with other products may be misleading.

Secondary Leukemia and Myelodysplastic Syndrome (MDS): There were 34 new cases of MDS/secondary leukemia reported among 995 (3.4%) patients included in clinical studies and expanded access programs, with a median follow-up of 2.4 years. The overall incidence of MDS/secondary leukemia among the 230 patients included in the clinical studies, was 10% (24/230), with a median follow-up of 39 months and a median time to development of MDS of 34 months. The cumulative incidence of MDS/secondary leukemia was 4.7% at 2 years and 15% at 5 years. Among the 765 patients included in the expanded access program, where the median duration of follow-up was shorter (27 months), the overall incidence of MDS/secondary leukemia was 3% (20/765) and the median time to development of MDS was 31 months. In the expanded access population, the cumulative incidence of MDS/secondary leukemia was 1.6% at 2 years and 6% at 5 years.

In a study of 76 previously untreated patients with low-grade non-Hodgkin's lymphoma who received BEXXAR, no patients developed MDS with a median follow-up of 5.1 years.

Secondary Malignancies: There were 65 reports of second malignancies, excluding secondary leukemia. The most common included non-melanomatous skin cancers, breast, lung, bladder, and head and neck cancers. Some of these events included recurrence of an earlier diagnosis of cancer.

DRUG INTERACTIONS: Drug-Drug Interactions: No formal drug-drug interaction studies have been performed. Due to the frequent occurrence of severe and prolonged thrombocytopenia, the potential benefits of medications that interfere with platelet function and/or anticoagulation should be weighed against the potential increased risk of bleeding and hemorrhage.

DOSAGE AND ADMINISTRATION: BEXXAR therapy (tositumomab and iodine I 131 tositumomab) is suitable for administration on an outpatient basis with appropriate license conditions as granted by the Canadian Nuclear Safety Commission (CNSC). BEXXAR is intended as a single course of treatment. The safety of multiple courses of BEXXAR therapy, or combination of this regimen with other forms of irradiation or chemotherapy, has not been evaluated.

Dosing Considerations: The safety of BEXXAR was established only in the setting of patients receiving thyroid blocking agents and premedication to ameliorate/prevent infusion reactions (see Concomitant Medications).

Concomitant Medications: The safety of BEXXAR was established in studies in which all patients received the following concurrent medications:

- Thyroid protective agents: Saturated solution of potassium iodide (SSKI) 4 drops orally three times daily; Lugol's solution 20 drops orally three times daily; or potassium iodide tablets 130 mg orally daily. Thyroid protective agents should be initiated at least 24 hours prior to administration of the iodine I 131 tositumomab dosimetric dose and continued until 2 weeks after administration of the iodine I 131 tositumomab therapeutic dose.
- **Patients should not receive the dosimetric dose of iodine I 131 tositumomab if they have not yet received at least three doses of SSKI, three doses of Lugol's solution, or one dose of 130 mg potassium iodide tablet (at least 24 hours prior to the dosimetric dose).**
- Acetaminophen 650 mg orally and diphenhydramine 50 mg orally 30 minutes prior to administration of tositumomab in the dosimetric and therapeutic steps.

Dosage: BEXXAR consists of four components administered in two discrete steps: the dosimetric step, followed 7-14 days later by a therapeutic step.

Dosimetric Step:

- Tositumomab 450 mg intravenously in 50 mL 0.9% sodium chloride over 60 minutes. Reduce the rate of infusion by 50% for mild to moderate infusional toxicity; interrupt infusion for severe infusional toxicity. After complete resolution of severe infusional toxicity, infusion may be resumed with a 50% reduction in the rate of infusion.
- Iodine I 131 tositumomab (containing 185 MBq (5.0 mCi) iodine-131 and 35 mg tositumomab) intravenously in 30 mL 0.9% Sodium Chloride over 20 minutes. Reduce the rate of infusion by 50% for mild to moderate infusional toxicity; interrupt infusion for severe infusional toxicity. After complete resolution of severe infusional toxicity, infusion may be resumed with a 50% reduction in the rate of infusion.

Therapeutic Step: Note: Do not administer the therapeutic step if biodistribution is altered (see Assessment of Biodistribution of Iodine I 131 Tositumomab).

- Tositumomab 450 mg intravenously in 50 mL 0.9% Sodium Chloride over 60 minutes. Reduce the rate of infusion by 50% for mild to moderate infusional toxicity; interrupt infusion for severe infusional toxicity. After complete resolution of severe infusional toxicity, infusion may be resumed with a 50% reduction in the rate of infusion.
- Iodine I 131 tositumomab (see Calculation of Iodine-131 Activity for Therapeutic Dose). Reduce the rate of infusion by 50% for mild to moderate infusional toxicity; interrupt infusion for severe infusional toxicity. After complete resolution of severe infusional toxicity, infusion may be resumed with a 50% reduction in the rate of infusion.
- Patients with platelet counts ≥150×10⁹/L: The recommended dose is the activity of iodine-131 calculated to deliver 75 cGy total body irradiation and 35 mg tositumomab, administered intravenously over 20 minutes.
- Patients with NCI Grade 1 thrombocytopenia (platelet counts ≥100×10⁹/L but <150×10⁹/L): The recommended dose is the activity of iodine-131 calculated to deliver 65 cGy total body irradiation and 35 mg tositumomab, administered intravenously over 20 minutes.

Figure 1 shows an overview of the dosing schedule.

Dosimetry: The following section describes the procedures for image acquisition for collection of dosimetry data, interpretation of biodistribution images, calculation of residence time, and calculation of activity hours. Please read all sections carefully.

Image Acquisition and Interpretation: Manufacturer-specific quality control procedures should be followed for the gamma camera/computer system, the collimator, and the dose calibrator. Less than 20% variance between maximum and minimum pixel count values in the useful field of view is acceptable on iodine-131 intrinsic flood fields and variability <10% is preferable. Iodine-131-specific camera uniformity corrections are strongly recommended, rather than applying lower energy correction to the Iodine-131 window. Camera extrinsic uniformity should be assessed at least monthly using ^{99m}Tc or ^{57}Co as a source with imaging at the appropriate window.

Additional (non-routine) quality control procedures are required. To assure the accuracy and precision of the patient total body counts, the gamma camera must undergo validation and daily quality control on each day it is used to collect patient images.

Each imaging day, 3 separate anterior whole body scans are acquired, one each for the source, background, and patient. The source, background and patient scans are acquired in whole body mode using the exact same scanning parameters for all 3 scans. The source and background counts are obtained first and the camera sensitivity (i.e., constant counting efficiency) is established prior to obtaining the patient count.

The total counts from each scan are separately recorded. Please note that some equipment may require drawing a Region of Interest (ROI) around the whole body field of view to obtain total counts from the whole body scan. Use whatever procedure is necessary for the type of camera used.

Gamma Camera Set-Up: The same camera, collimator, scanning speed, energy window, and setup must be used for all studies.

The gamma camera must be capable of whole body imaging and have a large or extra large field of view with a digital interface. The camera and computer must be set up for scanning as follows:

- High-energy or medium-energy parallel hole collimator
- 20-25% symmetric window centred on the 364-keV photo peak of iodine
- Matrix: appropriate whole body matrix
- Scanning speed: 30-100 cm/minute as appropriate for collimator (314-414 keV)

Counts from Calibrated Source for Quality Control: Camera sensitivity for iodine-131 must be determined each day. Determination of the gamma camera's sensitivity is obtained by scanning a calibrated activity of iodine-131 (e.g., 7400-9250 kBq (200-250 µCi) in at least 20 mL of saline within a sealed pharmaceutical vial). The radioactivity of the iodine-131 source is first determined using a NIST-traceable-calibrated clinical dose calibrator at the iodine-131 setting.

Background Counts: The background count is obtained from a scan with no radioactive source. This should be obtained following the count of the calibrated source just prior to obtaining the patient count.

Figure 1: BEXXAR

Effective Recommended Dose—Dosing Schedule

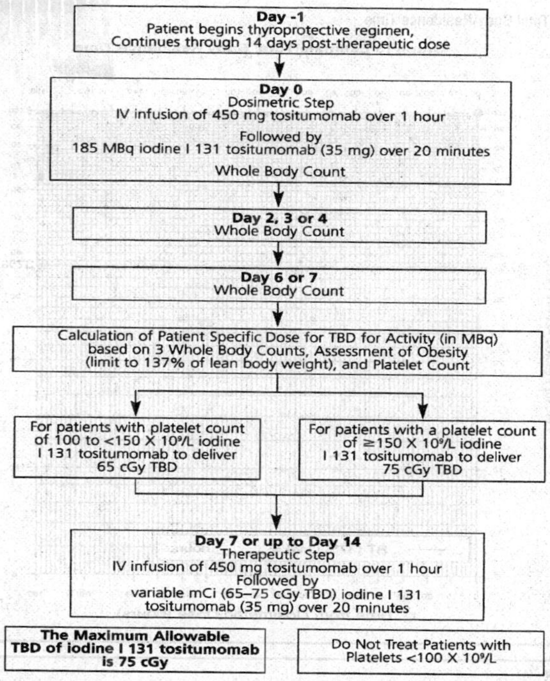

If abnormally high background counts are measured, the source should be identified and, if possible, removed. If abnormally low background counts are measured, the camera energy window setting and collimator should be verified before repeating the background counts.

The counts per kBq (µCi) are obtained by dividing the background-corrected source count by the calibrated activity for that day. For a specific camera and collimator, the counts per kBq (µCi) should be relatively constant. When values vary more than 10% from the established ratio, the reason for the discrepancy should be ascertained and corrected and the source count repeated.

Patient Total Body Counts: Acquire anterior whole body images for gamma camera counts. For any particular patient, the same gamma camera must be used for all scans. To obtain proper counts, extremities must be included in the images, and arms should not cross over the body. The scans should be centred on the midline of the patient. Record the time of the start of the radiolabelled dosimetric infusion and the time of the start of each count acquisition.

Gamma camera counts will be obtained at the three imaging time points:

Count 1: Within an hour of end of the infusion of the iodine I 131 tositumomab dosimetric dose prior to patient voiding.

Count 2: Two to 4 days after administration of the iodine I 131 tositumomab dosimetric dose and immediately following patient voiding.

Count 3: Six to 7 days after the administration of the iodine I 131 tositumomab dosimetric dose and immediately following patient voiding.

Tumour or organ imaging is not required.

Assessment of Biodistribution of Iodine I 131 Tositumomab: The biodistribution of iodine I 131 tositumomab should be assessed by either evaluation of the total body residence time or visual examination of whole body gamma camera images from the first image taken at the time of Count 1 (within an hour of the end of the infusion) and from the second image taken at the time of Count 2 (at 2 to 4 days after administration). To resolve ambiguities, an evaluation of the third image at the time of Count 3 (6 to 7 days after administration) may be necessary. Biodistribution should not be evaluated on the third image. If either of these methods indicate that the biodistribution is altered when compared to expected biodistribution as described below, the tositumomab iodine I 131 therapeutic dose should not be administered. A Nuclear Medicine Physician and/or Radiation Oncologist (as appropriate) should be consulted to determine whether the gamma scans indicate that the biodistribution is altered when compared to expected biodistribution as described below.

Anterior images obtained using a high energy or medium energy collimator used at 30-100 cm/min (as appropriate) are adequate for evaluation.

Expected Biodistribution: Total Body Residence Time: The median total body residence time is 90 hours with an expected range of 50 to 150 hours.

Whole Body Camera Imaging: On the first image, obtained shortly after the dosimetric dose injection, most of the activity is in the blood pool (heart and major blood vessels) and the uptake in normal liver and spleen is generally less than in the heart. On the second image, obtained 2-4 days after administration of the dosimetric dose, the activity in the blood pool decreases significantly and is generally moderately decreased in liver and spleen. Images may show uptake by thyroid, kidneys, stomach, and urinary bladder, and minimal uptake in the lungs. Tumour uptake in soft tissues and in normal organs may be seen as areas of increased intensity in the later images. If tumour is present in the spleen, focal or moderately intense splenic uptake is an expected pattern. Visualization of tumours is desirable, but not required for the expected biodistribution pattern.

Altered Biodistribution: Total Body Residence Time: Total body residence times outside the range of 50 to 150 hours are considered altered. (Note: If the results are outside the range, first verify the camera acquisition and the calculations of the total body residence time).

Whole Body Camera Imaging: On the first day, if the blood pool is not visualized on the first imaging study or if there is diffuse intense tracer uptake in the liver and/or spleen or uptake suggestive of urinary obstruction the biodistribution is altered. Diffuse lung uptake greater than that of blood pool on the first day would not be expected unless there was pulmonary involvement with tumour.

Calculation of Iodine-131 Activity for Therapeutic Dose: There are two options for calculation of the Iodine-131 activity for the therapeutic dose. The derived values and calculation of the therapeutic dose may be determined manually [see "The Dosimetry Workbook"] or calculated automatically using the BEXXAR Dosimetry Software.

The methods for determining the activity hours (MBq h or mCi h), residence time (h), and desired total body dose (cGy) are described below:

Residence Time (h): For each timepoint, calculate the background corrected total body count by subtracting the background count from the patient's anterior total body count. The percent of injected activity remaining at each timepoint is calculated by dividing the background-corrected total body count from that timepoint by the background-corrected total body count from Day 0 and multiplying by 100. The time from the start of the dosimetric dose of iodine I 131 tositumomab to the acquisition of each total body count should be calculated in hours. The residence time (h) is determined by plotting the time from the start of the infusion and the percent injected activity values for the last two patient count acquisition timepoints in Figure 2.

A best-fit line is then drawn from 100% (the pre-plotted day 0 value) through the two plotted points (if the line does not intersect the two points, one point must lie above the best-fit line and one point must lie the same distance below the best-fit line). The residence time (h) is read from the x axis of the graph at the point where the fitted line intersects the horizontal 37% injected activity line.

Activity Hours (MBq·h): In order to determine the activity hours (MBq·h), look up the patient's maximum effective mass derived from the patient's sex and height in Table 5. If the patient's actual weight is less than the maximum effective mass, the actual weight should be used in the activity hours table (see Table 6). If the patient's actual weight is greater than the maximum effective mass, the maximum effective mass from Table 5 should be used.

Figure 2: BEXXAR
Graph to Estimate Total Body Residence Time

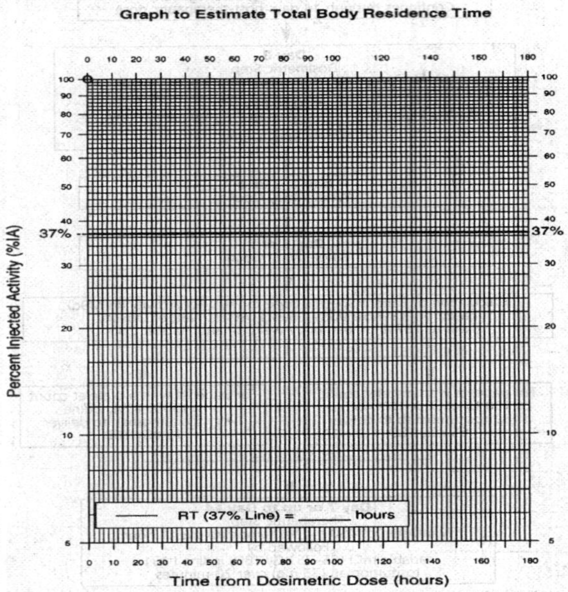

Table 5: BEXXAR
Dosimetry—Maximum Effective Mass

Men			Women		
Height (ft'-in")	Height (cm)	Maximum Effective Mass (kg)	Height (ft'-in")	Height (cm)	Maximum Effective Mass (kg)
4'-5"	134.5	40.5	4'-5"	134.5	40.7
4'-6"	137.0	44.2	4'-6"	137.0	43.8
4'-7"	140.0	47.9	4'-7"	140.0	47.0
4'-8"	142.0	51.6	4'-8"	142.0	50.2
4'-9"	145.0	55.3	4'-9"	145.0	53.3
4'-10"	147.5	59.0	4'-10"	147.5	56.5
4'-11"	150.0	62.7	4'-11"	150.0	59.7
5'-0"	152.5	66.3	5'-0"	152.5	62.8
5'-1"	155.0	70.0	5'-1"	155.0	66.0
5'-2"	157.5	73.7	5'-2"	157.5	69.2
5'-3"	160.0	77.4	5'-3"	160.0	72.3
5'-4"	162.5	81.1	5'-4"	162.5	75.5
5'-5"	165.0	84.8	5'-5"	165.0	78.7
5'-6"	167.5	88.5	5'-6"	167.5	81.8
5'-7"	170.0	92.2	5'-7"	170.0	85.0
5'-8"	172.5	95.8	5'-8"	172.5	88.2
5'-9"	175.5	99.5	5'-9"	175.5	91.3
5'-10"	178.0	103.2	5'-10"	178.0	94.5
5'-11"	180.5	106.9	5'-11"	180.5	97.7
6'-0"	183.0	110.6	6'-0"	183.0	100.8
6'-1"	185.5	114.3	6'-1"	185.5	104.0
6'-2"	188.0	118.0	6'-2"	188.0	107.2
6'-3"	190.5	121.7	6'-3"	190.5	110.3
6'-4"	193.0	125.4	6'-4"	193.0	113.5
6'-5"	195.5	129.0	6'-5"	195.5	116.7
6'-6"	198.0	132.7	6'-6"	198.0	119.8

(cont'd)

Table 5: BEXXAR *(cont'd)*
Dosimetry—Maximum Effective Mass

Men			Women		
Height (ft'-in")	Height (cm)	Maximum Effective Mass (kg)	Height (ft'-in")	Height (cm)	Maximum Effective Mass (kg)
6'-7"	200.5	136.4	6'-7"	200.5	123.0
6'-8"	203.0	140.0	6'-8"	203.0	126.2
6'-9"	205.5	143.8	6'-9"	205.5	129.3
6'-10"	208.5	147.5	6'-10"	208.5	132.5
6'-11"	211.0	151.2	6'-11"	211.0	135.7
7'-0"	213.5	154.9	7'-0"	213.5	138.8

Multiply pounds by 0.454 to obtain kilograms. To calculate the maximum effective mass for patient heights not included in above table, use the following formulas:
Males: Maximum effective mass (kg)=65.76+1.452 (height in cm −152)
Females: Maximum effective mass (kg)=62.34+1.247 (height in cm −152)
Adapted from: Zasadny KR et al.

Table 6: BEXXAR
Dosimetry: Activity Hours

Mass[a] (kg)	Activity Hours (MBq· h)
40.0	171606
40.5	173530
41.0	175491
41.5	177452
42.0	179376
42.5	181337
43.0	183261
43.5	185185
44.0	187109
44.5	189033
45.0	190920
45.5	192844
46.0	194768
46.5	196655
47.0	198542
47.5	200466
48.0	202353
48.5	204240
49.0	206127
49.5	207977
50.0	209864
50.5	211788
51.0	213675
51.5	215562
52.0	217486
52.5	219373
53.0	221260
53.5	223147
54.0	225034
54.5	226921
55.0	228808
55.5	230658
56.0	232545
56.5	234395

(cont'd)

Table 6: BEXXAR *(cont'd)*
Dosimetry: Activity Hours

Mass[a] (kg)	Activity Hours (MBq· h)
57.0	236282
57.5	238132
58.0	239982
58.5	241832
59.0	243682
59.5	245532
60.0	247382
60.5	249269
61.0	251119
61.5	253006
62.0	254856
62.5	256706
63.0	258593
63.5	260443
64.0	262293
64.5	264143
65.0	265993
65.5	267806
66.0	269656
66.5	271506
67.0	273319
67.5	275169
68.0	276982
68.5	278832
69.0	280645
69.5	282458
70.0	284271
70.5	286121
71.0	287971
71.5	298821
72.0	291671
72.5	293484
73.0	295334
73.5	297147
74.0	298997
74.5	300810
75.0	302660
75.5	304473
76.0	306286
76.5	308099
77.0	309912
77.5	311725
78.0	313538
78.5	315351
79.0	317164
79.5	318977
80.0	320790
80.5	322566

(cont'd)

Table 6: BEXXAR *(cont'd)*
Dosimetry: Activity Hours

Mass[a] (kg)	Activity Hours (MBq· h)
81.0	324379
81.5	326192
82.0	327968
82.5	329781
83.0	331557
83.5	333370
84.0	335146
84.5	336922
85.0	338698
85.5	340474
86.0	342287
86.5	344063
87.0	345839
87.5	347578
88.0	349354
88.5	351130
89.0	352906
89.5	354645
90.0	356421
90.5	358234
91.0	360010
91.5	361823
92.0	363599
92.5	365375
93.0	367188
93.5	368964
94.0	370740
94.5	372516
95.0	374329
95.5	376105
96.0	377881
96.5	379657
97.0	381433
97.5	383209
98.0	384948
98.5	386724
99.0	388500
99.5	390276
100.0	392015
100.5	393791
101.0	395530
101.5	397306
102.0	399045
102.5	400821
103.0	402560
103.5	404299
104.0	406075
104.5	407814

(cont'd)

Table 6: BEXXAR *(cont'd)*

Dosimetry: Activity Hours

Mass[a] (kg)	Activity Hours (MBq· h)
105.0	409553
105.5	411292
106.0	413031
106.5	414770
107.0	416509
107.5	418248
108.0	419987
108.5	421726
109.0	423465
109.5	425204
110.0	426906
110.5	428645
111.0	430384
111.5	432086
112.0	433825
112.5	435527
113.0	437266
113.5	438968
114.0	440670
114.5	442409
115.0	444111
115.5	445813
116.0	447515
116.5	449217
117.0	450919
117.5	452621
118.0	454323
118.5	456025
119.0	457727
119.5	459429
120.0	461131
120.5	462833
121.0	464572
121.5	466274
122.0	467976
122.5	469678
123.0	471417
123.5	473119
124.0	474821
124.5	476523
125.0	478225
125.5	479927
126.0	481629
126.5	483331
127.0	485033
127.5	486735
128.0	488400
128.5	490102

(cont'd)

Table 6: BEXXAR *(cont'd)*

Dosimetry: Activity Hours

Mass[a] (kg)	Activity Hours (MBq· h)
129.0	491804
129.5	493469
130.0	495171
130.5	496873
131.0	498538
131.5	500240
132.0	501905
132.5	503607
133.0	505272
133.5	506937
134.0	508639
134.5	510304
135.0	511969
135.5	513634
136.0	515336
136.5	517001
137.0	518666
137.5	520331
138.0	521996
138.5	523661
139.0	525326
139.5	526954

[a] The minimum of the patient's actual weight (kg) or maximum effective mass (kg) from Table 5. For values between 140 kg and 160 kg, use the following formula:
Activity Hours (MBq·h)=14287+(88.74) (Wt in kg-140).

Calculation of Iodine-131 Activity for the Iodine I 131 Tositumomab Therapeutic Dose: The following equation is used to calculate the activity of iodine-131 required for delivery of the desired total body dose of radiation.

$$\text{Iodine-131 (cGy) Activity (MBq}^{a}\text{)} = \frac{\text{Activity Hours (MBq·h)}}{\text{Residence Time (h)}} \times \frac{\text{Desired Total Body Dose (cGy)}}{75\text{ cGy}}$$

[a] 1 mCi=37 MBq.

Instructions for Preparation and Use: Preparation of BEXXAR: General: Read all directions thoroughly and assemble all materials before preparing the dose for administration.

The iodine I 131 tositumomab dosimetric and therapeutic doses should be measured by a suitable radioactivity calibration system immediately prior to administration. The dose calibrator must be operated in accordance with the manufacturer's specifications and quality control for the measurement of iodine-131.

All supplies used for preparation and administration of BEXXAR therapy should be sterile. Use appropriate aseptic technique and radiation precautions for the preparation of the components for BEXXAR.

Gloves (i.e., latex, vinyl, etc.) should be utilized in the preparation and administration of the product. Iodine I 131 tositumomab doses should be prepared, assayed, and administered by personnel who are licensed to handle and/or administer radionuclides. Appropriate shielding should be used during preparation and administration of the product.

Restrictions on patient contact with others and release from the hospital must follow all applicable regulations and/or appropriate licenses of local competent official organizations.

Preparation for the Dosimetric Step: Tositumomab Dose: Method:

1. Using an aseptic needle, withdraw and dispose of 32 mL of saline from a 50 mL bag of sterile 0.9% sodium chloride for injection, USP.
2. Withdraw the entire contents from each of the two 225 mg vials (a total of 450 mg tositumomab in 32 mL) and transfer to the infusion bag containing 18 mL of 0.9% Sodium Chloride for Injection, USP to yield a final volume of 50 mL.
3. Gently mix the solution by inverting/rotating the bag. **Do not shake.**
4. The diluted tositumomab may be stored for up to 24 hours when stored refrigerated at 2°C-8°C and for up to 8 hours at room temperature.

Note: tositumomab solution may contain particulates that are generally white in nature. The product should appear clear to opalescent, colourless to slightly yellow.

Preparation of Iodine I 131 Tositumomab Dosimetric Dose: Method:

1. Allow minimum 60 minutes (may require up to 120 minutes) for thawing (at ambient temperature) of the iodine I 131 tositumomab dosimetric vial with appropriate lead shielding.
2. Based on the activity concentration of the vial (see actual product specification sheet for the vial supplied in the dosimetric package), calculate the volume required for an iodine I 131 tositumomab activity of 185 MBq (5.0 mCi).
3. Withdraw the calculated volume from the iodine I 131 tositumomab vial.
4. Transfer this volume to the shielded preparation vial.
5. Assay the dose to ensure that the appropriate activity (MBq) has been prepared.
    a. If the assayed dose is 185 MBq (5.0 mCi) (+/−10%) proceed with step 6.
    b. If the assayed dose does not contain 185 MBq (5.0 mCi) (+/−10%) recalculate the activity concentration of the iodine I 131 tositumomab at this time, based on the volume and the activity in the preparation vial. Recalculate the volume required for an iodine I 131 tositumomab activity of 185 MBq (5.0 mCi). Using the same 30 mL syringe, add or subtract the appropriate volume from the iodine I 131 tositumomab vial so that the preparation vial contains the volume required for an iodine I 131 tositumomab activity of 185 MBq (5.0 mCi) (+/−10%). Re-assay the preparation vial and proceed with step 6.
6. Calculate the amount of tositumomab contained in the solution of iodine I 131 tositumomab in the shielded preparation vial, based on the volume and protein concentration (see actual product specification sheet supplied in the dosimetric package).

7. If the shielded preparation vial contains less than 35 mg, calculate the amount of additional tositumomab needed to yield a total of 35 mg protein. Calculate the volume needed from the 35 mg vial of tositumomab, based on the protein concentration. Withdraw the calculated volume of tositumomab from the 35 mg vial of tositumomab, and transfer this volume to the shielded preparation vial. The preparation vial should now contain a total of 35 mg of tositumomab.
8. Add a sufficient quantity of 0.9% sodium chloride for injection, USP to the shielded preparation vial to yield a final volume of 30 mL. Gently mix the solutions.
9. Withdraw the entire contents from the preparation vial into a 30 mL or larger syringe with a large bore needle (18-20 gauge).
10. Assay and record the activity.

Administration: Administration of the Dosimetric Step: BEXXAR is administered via an IV tubing set with an in-line 0.22 micron filter. **The same IV tubing set and filter must be throughout the entire dosimetric or therapeutic step. A change in filter can result in loss of drug.** If a new IV line without an in-line filter is connected to the patient's intravenous access, prime the IV line with 0.9% sodium chloride prior to the iodine I 131 tositumomab infusion.

Tositumomab Infusion: A 0.22 micron in-line filter should be attached to the primary IV infusion set and the bag of sterile 0.9% Sodium Chloride for Injection. Prime lines. Attach tositumomab bags and infuse tositumomab over 60 minutes. After completion of the tositumomab infusion, inject 50 mL saline into empty tositumomab bag and mix. Flush primary IV infusion set and the in-line IV filter set for 10 minutes. Discard the tositumomab bag.

Iodine I 131 Tositumomab Dosimetric Infusion: Set syringe pump to deliver the entire 185 MBq (5.0 mCi) (35 mg) dose of iodine I 131 tositumomab over 20 minutes. At the end of the infusion, attach a syringe with 30 mL of 0.9% sodium chloride to the 3-way stopcock and back flush (rinse) the syringe. Infuse the 30 mL rinse into the patient over 10 minutes (infusion rate of 180 mL/hour).

Determination of Dose for the Therapeutic Step (see Calculation of Iodine-131 Activity for Therapeutic Dose): The methodology for determining and calculating the patient-specific dose of iodine-131 activity (MBq or mCi) to be administered in the therapeutic step involves the following three steps:

1. Following infusion of the iodine I 131 tositumomab dosimetric dose, obtain total body gamma camera counts and whole body images:
   - Within one hour of infusion and prior to urination;
   - 2-4 days after infusion of the dosimetric dose, following urination;
   - 6-7 days after infusion of the dosimetric dose, following urination.
2. Assess biodistribution. If biodistribution is altered, the therapeutic step should not be administered.
3. Calculate iodine-131 activity for the therapeutic dose. This step can be completed manually or calculate automatically using the BEXXAR dosimetry software.

For more detail regarding image acquisition and therapeutic dose calculations see Dosimetry.

Preparation for the Therapeutic Step (7 to 14 days following dosimetric dose): Tositumomab Dose: Refer to Preparation for the Dosimetric Step. Tositumomab Dose

Preparation of Iodine I 131 Tositumomab Therapeutic Dose: Method:

1. Allow minimum 60 (may require up to 120 minutes) for thawing (at ambient temperature) of the iodine I 131 tositumomab therapeutic vial with appropriate lead shielding.
2. Calculate the dose of iodine I 131 tositumomab required (see Calculation of Iodine-131 Activity for Therapeutic Dose).
3. Based on the activity concentration of the vial (see actual product specification sheet for each vial supplied in the therapeutic package), calculate the volume required for the iodine I 131 tositumomab activity required for the therapeutic dose.
4. Using one or more 30 mL syringe withdraw the calculated volume from the iodine I 131 tositumomab vials.
5. Transfer this volume to the shielded preparation vial.
6. Assay the dose to ensure that the appropriate activity (MBq or mCi) has been prepared.
   a. If the assayed dose is the calculated dose (+/−10%) needed for the therapeutic step, proceed with step 7.
   b. If the assayed dose does not contain the desired dose (+/−10%), re-calculate the activity concentration of the iodine I 131 tositumomab at this time, based on the volume and the activity in the preparation vial. Re-calculate the volume required for an iodine I 131 tositumomab activity for the therapeutic dose. Using the same syringe, add or subtract the appropriate volume from the iodine I 131 tositumomab vial so that the preparation vial contains the volume required for the iodine I 131 tositumomab activity required for the therapeutic dose. Re-assay the preparation vial. Proceed to step 7.
7. Calculate the amount of tositumomab protein contained in the solution of iodine I 131 tositumomab in the shielded preparation vial, based on the volume and protein concentration (see product specification sheet).
8. If the shielded preparation vial contains less than 35 mg, calculate the amount of additional tositumomab needed to yield a total of 35 mg protein. Calculate the volume needed from the 35 mg vial of tositumomab, based on the protein concentration. Withdraw the calculated volume of tositumomab from the 35 mg vial of tositumomab, and transfer this volume to the shielded preparation vial. The preparation vial should now contain a total of 35 mg of tositumomab.
   Note: If the dose of iodine I 131 tositumomab requires the use of 2 vials of iodine I 131 tositumomab or the entire contents of a single vial of iodine I 131 tositumomab, there may be no need to add protein from the 35 mg vial of tositumomab.
9. Add a sufficient quantity of 0.9% sodium chloride for injection, USP to the shielded preparation vial to yield a final volume of 30 mL. Gently mix the solutions.
10. Withdraw the entire volume from the preparation vial into a sterile 30 mL or 60 mL syringe using a large bore needle.
11. Assay and record the activity.

Administration of the Therapeutic Step: Note: Release from the hospital must follow all applicable federal and institutional regulations.

BEXXAR therapy can be administered on an outpatient basis with specific instructions to minimize radiation dose to others.

Tositumomab Infusion: Refer to Administration of the Dosimetric Step, Tositumomab Infusion.

Iodine I 131 Tositumomab Therapeutic Infusion: Set syringe pump to deliver the entire therapeutic dose of iodine I 131 tositumomab over 20 minutes.

After completion of the infusion of iodine I 131 tositumomab, close the stopcock to the syringe. Flush the secondary IV infusion set and the extension set with 0.9% sodium chloride from the 50 mL bag of sterile, 0.9% sodium chloride for injection, USP.

OVERDOSAGE:

Some patients have received more than 75 cGy total body dose of radiation. The maximum dose of BEXXAR therapy (tositumomab and iodine I 131 tositumomab) that was administered in clinical trials was 88 cGy. Three patients were treated with a total body dose of 85 cGy of iodine I 131 tositumomab in a dose escalation study. Two of the 3 patients developed Grade 4 toxicity of 5 weeks duration with subsequent recovery. In addition, accidental overdose of BEXXAR occurred in one patient at a total body dose of 88 cGy. The patient developed Grade 3 hematologic toxicity of 18 days duration. Patients who receive an accidental overdose of iodine I 131 tositumomab should be monitored closely for cytopenias and radiation-related toxicity. The effectiveness of hematopoietic stem cell transplantation as a supportive care measure for marrow injury has not been studied; however, the timing of such support should take into account the pharmacokinetics of BEXXAR and decay rate of the iodine-131 in order to minimize the possibility of irradiation of infused hematopoietic stem cells.

For management of a suspected drug overdose, CPhA recommends that you contact your **regional Poison Control Centre**. See the *CPS* Directory section for a list of Poison Control Centres.

ACTION AND CLINICAL PHARMACOLOGY: BEXXAR therapy (tositumomab and iodine I 131 tositumomab) is an anti-neoplastic radioimmunotherapeutic monoclonal antibody-based regimen composed of the monoclonal antibody, tositumomab, and the radiolabeled monoclonal antibody, iodine I 131 tositumomab.

Mechanism of Action: The high-energy beta particles emitted by I-131 are cytotoxic over distances of approximately 1-2 mm (the average path length is 0.8 mm and the maximum path length is 2.4 mm), thus permitting eradication of antigen-negative tumour cells by crossfire from neighbouring antibody-coated cells. In addition to cell death associated with ionizing radiation from the radioisotope, possible mechanisms of action of BEXXAR include induction of apoptosis, complement-dependent cytotoxicity (CDC), and antibody-dependent cellular cytotoxicity (ADCC) mediated by the antibody.

Pharmacokinetics: The median blood clearance following administration of 485 mg of protein (450 mg dose of tositumomab followed by a 35 mg dose of tositumomab containing the appropriate MBq (mCi) of iodine I 131 tositumomab) in 110 patients with non-Hodgkin's lymphoma (NHL) was 68.2 mg/h (range: 30.2-260.8 mg/h). Patients with high tumour burden, splenomegaly, or bone marrow involvement were noted to have a faster clearance, shorter terminal half-life, and larger volume of distribution. The total body clearance, as measured by total body gamma camera counts, was mono-exponential and dependent on the same factors noted for blood clearance. The effective half-life was 65 hours.

Elimination of iodine-131 occurs by decay (see Table 2) and excretion in the urine. Urine was collected for 49 dosimetric doses. After 5 days, the whole body clearance was 67% of the injected dose. Ninety-eight percent of the clearance was accounted for in the urine.

Radiation Dosimetry: Estimations of radiation-absorbed doses for iodine I 131 tositumomab were performed using sequential whole body images and the MIRDOSE 3 software program. The estimated radiation-absorbed doses to organs and marrow from a course of the BEXXAR therapy (tositumomab and iodine I 131 tositumomab) are presented in Table 7. The average tumour dose was 12 times the total body dose and higher than any of the average organ doses.

Table 7: BEXXAR

Estimated Radiation-Absorbed Organ Doses

	BEXXAR mGy/MBq Median	BEXXAR mGy/MBq Range
From Organ ROIs		
Thyroid	2.71	1.4–6.2
Kidneys	1.96	1.5–2.5
ULI Wall	1.34	0.8–1.7
LLI Wall	1.30	0.8–1.6
Heart Wall	1.25	0.5–1.8
Spleen	1.14	0.7–5.4
Testes	0.83	0.3–1.3
Liver	0.82	0.6–1.3
Lungs	0.79	0.5–1.1
Red Marrow	0.65	0.5–1.1
Stomach Wall	0.40	0.2–0.8
From Whole Body ROIs		
Urine Bladder Wall	0.64	0.6–0.9
Bone Surfaces	0.41	0.4–0.6
Pancreas	0.31	0.2–0.4
Gall Bladder Wall	0.29	0.2–0.3
Adrenals	0.28	0.2–0.3
Ovaries	0.25	0.2–0.3
Small Intestine	0.23	0.2–0.3
Thymus	0.22	0.1–0.3
Uterus	0.20	0.2–0.2
Muscle	0.18	0.1–0.2
Breasts	0.16	0.1–0.2
Skin	0.13	0.1–0.2
Brain	0.13	0.1–0.2
Total Body	0.24	0.2–0.3

STORAGE AND STABILITY: Tositumomab: Vials of tositumomab (35 mg and 225 mg) should be stored refrigerated at 2-8°C prior to dilution. Do not use beyond expiration date. Protect from strong light. **Do not shake.** Do not freeze. Discard any unused portions left in the vial.

Solutions of diluted tositumomab are stable for up to 24 hours when stored refrigerated at 2-8°C and for up to 8 hours at room temperature. However, it is recommended that the diluted solution be stored refrigerated at 2-8°C prior to administration because it does not contain preservatives. Any unused portion must be discarded. Do not freeze solutions of diluted tositumomab.

Iodine I 131 Tositumomab: Store frozen in the original lead pots. Do not use beyond the expiration date on the label of the lead pot. The dosimetric dose has a 16 day shelf life and the therapeutic dose has a shelf life of 5 days when stored frozen.

Thawed dosimetric and therapeutic doses of iodine I 131 tositumomab should be stored in the upright position. Thawed doses are stable up to 8 hours at 2-8°C or at room temperature. Because solutions of iodine I 131 tositumomab diluted for infusion contain no preservatives, it is recommended that the diluted solution be stored refrigerated at 2-8°C prior to administration (do not freeze). Any unused portion must be discarded according to federal regulations.

SPECIAL HANDLING INSTRUCTIONS: As in the use of any other radioactive material, care should be taken to minimize radiation exposure to patients consistent with proper patient management, and to minimize radiation exposure to occupational workers. See Dosage and Administration.

INFORMATION FOR THE PATIENT: Published in e-CPS, available by subscription at www.e-cps.ca.

DOSAGE FORMS, COMPOSITION AND PACKAGING: Tositumomab: Tositumomab is supplied as a sterile, pyrogen-free, clear to opalescent, colourless to slightly yellow, preservative-free liquid concentrate. It is supplied at a nominal concentration of 14 mg/mL tositumomab in 35 mg and 225 mg single-use vials. The formulation contains 10% (w/v) maltose, 145 mM sodium chloride, 10 mM phosphate, 17.5 mM potassium hydroxide, and Water for Injection, USP. The pH is approximately 7.2.

Iodine I 131 Tositumomab: Iodine I 131 tositumomab is supplied as a sterile, clear, preservative-free liquid for IV administration. The formulation for the dosimetric and the therapeutic dosage forms contains 4.4%-6.6% (w/v) povidone, 1-2 mg/mL maltose (dosimetric dose) or 9-15 mg/mL maltose (therapeutic dose), 8.5-9.5 mg/mL sodium chloride, 1.22 mg/mL phosphoric acid, 1.05-6.57 mg/mL potassium hydroxide and 0.9-1.3 mg/mL ascorbic acid. The pH is approximately 7.0.

BEXXAR therapy: The components of the BEXXAR therapy (tositumomab, iodine I 131 tositumomab) for the dosimetric or therapeutic step are scheduled to arrive on the same day. These components include a tositumomab therapy kit with two single-use 225 mg vials (16.1 mL) and one single-use 35 mg vial (2.5 mL) of tositumomab supplied by GlaxoSmithKline Inc.

Iodine I 131 Tositumomab Dosimetric Dose Vial: Each lead pot for preparation of the iodine I 131 tositumomab dosimetric dose contains: one single-use vial with not less than 20 mL of iodine I 131 tositumomab at nominal protein and activity concentrations of 0.1 mg/mL and 22.57 MBq/mL (0.61 mCi/mL) (at calibration), respectively supplied by MDS Nordion.

Iodine I 131 Tositumomab Therapeutic Dose Vial: Each lead pot for preparation of the iodine I 131 tositumomab therapeutic dose contains: one single-use vial with not less than 20 mL of iodine I 131 tositumomab at nominal protein and activity concentrations of 1.1 mg/mL and 207.2 MBq/mL (5.6 mCi/mL) (at calibration), respectively, supplied by MDS Nordion.

BEXXAR Therapy: BEXXAR is supplied in two discrete steps as follows: BEXXAR Dosimetric Step: A carton containing two single-use 225 mg vials and one single-use 35 mg vial of tositumomab supplied by GlaxoSmithKline Inc. and a package containing a single-use vial of iodine I 131 tositumomab (22.57 MBq/mL (0.61 mCi/mL) at calibration), supplied by MDS Nordion.
BEXXAR Therapeutic Step: A carton containing two single-use 225 mg vials and one single-use 35 mg vial of tositumomab, supplied by GlaxoSmithKline Inc. and a package containing one or two single-use vials of iodine I 131 tositumomab (207.2 MBq/mL (5.6 mCi/mL) at calibration), supplied by MDS Nordion.

Bezalip® SR ℞

bezafibrate

Lipid Metabolism Regulator

Actavis

Date of Preparation: May 26, 2008
Date of Revision: July 26, 2010

SUMMARY PRODUCT INFORMATION:

Route of Administration	Dosage Form/ Strength	Clinically Relevant Nonmedicinal Ingredients
Oral	Sustained release tablet 400 mg	Lactose For a complete listing of nonmedicinal ingredients, see Dosage Forms, Composition and Packaging.

INDICATIONS AND CLINICAL USE: BEZALIP SR (bezafibrate) is indicated as an adjunct to diet and other therapeutic measures for:

- Treatment of patients with hypercholesterolemia Type IIa and IIb mixed hyperlipidemia, to regulate lipid and apoprotein levels (reduce serum TG, LDL cholesterol and apolipoprotein B, increase HDL cholesterol and apolipoprotein A).
- Treatment of adult patients with high to very high triglyceride levels, Fredrickson classification Type IV and V hyperlipidemias, who are at a high risk of sequelae and complications (i.e. pancreatitis) from their dyslipidemia.

BEZALIP SR may not be adequate therapy in some patients with familial combined hyperlipidemia with type IIb and type IV hyperlipoproteinemia. Initial therapy for dyslipidemia should include at least an equivalent of the American Heart Association (AHA) step 1 diet.

There is evidence from coronary angiographic studies to show that triglyceride-rich lipoproteins are an important factor in the progression of coronary artery disease. A 5-year double-blind, placebo-controlled intervention trial (bezafibrate coronary atherosclerosis intervention trial (BECAIT)) has demonstrated that bezafibrate retards or prevents the progression of atheroma in young post-infarction patients (<45 years). The results show that long-term treatment with bezafibrate, can retard the progression of focal atheroma resulting in a reduced cardiac morbidity. Analysis of treatment effect at each patient's last assessment showed that the change in minimum lumen diameter (MLD) was 0.13 mm less in the bezafibrate group than the placebo group (p=0.049). The 5-year cumulative coronary event rate (defined as sudden coronary death, fatal or non-fatal reinfarction, CABG or PTCA) was significantly lower for bezafibrate (3/47; 6.4%) versus placebo (11/45; 24.4%) treated patients (p=0.02).

CONTRAINDICATIONS:

- Hepatic impairment, including primary biliary cirrhosis.
- Renal impairment (serum creatinine levels >1.5 mg/100 mL, i.e., >135 µmol/L, or creatinine clearance <60 mL/min or in patients undergoing dialysis) (see Warnings and Precautions, Musculoskeletal and Action and Clinical Pharmacology, Pharmacokinetics, Renal Insufficiency).
- Pre-existing gallbladder disease (see Warnings and Precautions).
- Hypersensitivity to bezafibrate, to any component of the product or to other fibrates.
- Photoallergic or phototoxic reactions to fibrates.
- Pregnancy or lactation.
- BEZALIP SR (bezafibrate) is not indicated for the treatment of Type I hyperlipoproteinemia.
- Combination therapy of BEZALIP SR 400 mg with HMG-CoA reductase inhibitors in patients with predisposing factors for myopathy e.g. preexisting renal impairment, severe infection, trauma, surgery, disturbances of the hormonal or electrolyte balance (see Drug Interactions).

WARNINGS AND PRECAUTIONS: General: Bezafibrate clinically, pharmacologically and chemically shows similarities with clofibrate. Physicians prescribing BEZALIP SR (bezafibrate) should also be familiar with the risks and benefits of clofibrate.

If BEZALIP SR is chosen for treatment, the prescribing physician should discuss the proposed therapy and inform the patient of the expected benefits and potential risks associated with long-term administration (see Warnings and Precautions).

Drug Interactions: See Drug Interactions.

Hematologic: Mild hemoglobin, leucocyte and platelet decreases have occurred occasionally following initiation of BEZALIP SR therapy. However, these levels stabilize during long-term administration. Periodic blood counts are recommended during the first 12 months of BEZALIP SR administration.

Hepatic/Biliary/Pancreatic: Liver Function: Abnormal liver function tests have been observed occasionally during BEZALIP SR administration, including elevated transaminases, and decreased or, rarely, increased alkaline phosphatase. However, these abnormalities are reversible upon discontinuation of the drug. Therefore, periodic liver function tests (AST, ALT, and GGT [if originally elevated]) in addition to other baseline tests are recommended after 3 to 6 months and at least yearly thereafter. BEZALIP SR therapy should be terminated if drug related abnormalities persist.

Hepatobiliary Disease: In patients with a past history of jaundice or hepatic disorder, BEZALIP SR should be used with caution.

Cholelithiasis: BEZALIP SR may increase cholesterol excretion into the bile, and may lead to cholelithiasis. Appropriate diagnostic procedures should be performed if cholelithiasis-related signs and symptoms should occur. BEZALIP SR therapy should be discontinued if gallstones are found.

Musculoskeletal: Treatment with drugs of the fibrate class including bezafibrate has been associated on rare occasions with myositis or rhabdomyolysis, usually in patients with impaired renal function (see Contraindications). Myopathy should be considered in any patient with diffuse myalgias, muscle tenderness/weakness, or marked elevations in creatine phosphokinase levels. Patients should be advised to report unexplained muscle pain, tenderness or weakness promptly, particularly if accompanied by malaise or fever. CPK levels should be assessed in patients reporting these symptoms, and BEZALIP SR therapy should be discontinued if markedly elevated CPK levels (10 times the upper limit of normal) occur or myopathy is diagnosed.

Teratology: Standard tests for teratology, fertility and peri- and post-natal effects in animals have shown a relative absence of risk, however, embryotoxicity has occurred in animals at toxic doses.

Special Populations: Pregnant Women: Strict birth control procedures must be exercised by women of childbearing potential. If pregnancy occurs despite birth control procedures, BEZALIP SR should be discontinued. Women planning a pregnancy should discontinue BEZALIP SR several months prior to conception (see Contraindications).

Nursing Women: In the absence of data concerning the presence of bezafibrate in human breast milk, BEZALIP SR should not be used by nursing mothers (see Contraindications).

Pediatrics: Limited experience is available in children at a dose of 10-20 mg/kg/day. Therefore, in the absence of adequate information concerning the long-term safety, BEZALIP SR should be used with caution in treating children.

Geriatrics (>70 years of age): BEZALIP SR 400 mg sustained release tablets should not be used in elderly patients as the creatinine clearance after 70 years of age is normally lower than 60 mL/min (see Dosage and Administration).

Monitoring and Laboratory Tests: Adequate pretreatment laboratory studies should be performed to ensure patients have elevated serum cholesterol and/or triglycerides with or without low HDL levels. Periodic determinations of serum lipids, fasting glucose, creatinine, ALT, CGT and CPK should be considered during BEZALIP treatment, particularly during the first months of therapy.

ADVERSE REACTIONS: Clinical Trial Adverse Drug Reactions: In 2 separate double-blind placebo controlled trials, a total of 88 patients on 200 mg bezafibrate tid and 87 patients on placebo were evaluated for adverse events. Listed in Table 1 are those adverse events with a positive induced risk occurring during the first 2 months of bezafibrate treatment.

A double-blind, placebo controlled study was undertaken in young patients (<45 years) who had previously suffered a myocardial infarction. Patients were evaluated for safety during 5 years of treatment with either 200 mg tid bezafibrate (n=47) or placebo (n=45). Table 2 lists the cumulative incidence of the most common adverse events at 1, 2 and 5 years, irrespective of relationship to study drug.

Table 1: BEZALIP SR

Adverse Events

	2-Month Cumulative Incidence (%)		
Body System	**Bezafibrate 200 mg t.i.d. (n=88)**	**Placebo (n=87)**	**Induced Risk (%)**
Body as a Whole	13.6	11.4	+2.6
Allergic Reaction	1.1	—	+1.1
Migraine	1.1	—	+1.1
Pain	1.1	—	+1.1
Digestive System	17.0	11.9	+5.9
Dyspepsia	3.4	—	+3.4
Flatulence	4.5	—	+4.5
Gastritis	5.7	4.6	+1.1
Hemic and Lymphatic System	1.1	—	+1.1
Anemia	1.1	—	+1.1
Nervous System	4.6	8.2	−3.9
Dizziness	2.3	—	+2.3
Insomnia	1.1	—	+1.1
Skin and Appendages	4.5	3.6	+1.0
Eczema	1.1	—	+1.1
Pruritus	3.4	—	+3.4

Table 2: BEZALIP SR

Adverse Events

	Cumulative Incidence Rate (%) at					
	1 Year		2 Years		5 Years	
	Bezafibrate (n=47)	**Placebo (n=45)**	**Bezafibrate (n=47)**	**Placebo (n=45)**	**Bezafibrate (n=47)**	**Placebo (n=45)**
Elevated AST	24	18	37	23	49	46
Elevated ALT	21	22	33	34	57	66
Gastritis	13	13	15	16	14	24
Elevated CK	11	2	15	9	30	52
Dyspepsia	6	2	9	2	11	10
Abdominal Pain	6	13	9	13	14	13
Headache	4	2	4	2	4	2
Diarrhea	9	4	11	4	16	12
Upper Respiratory Tract Infection	4	4	9	12	14	14
Rash	4	7	9	7	14	9
Pharyngitis	4	2	4	5	12	7
Bronchitis	2	0	7	0	16	3
Tenosynovitis	0	2	5	5	12	5
Flu Syndrome	0	2	7	2	22	5

The most common adverse reactions observed in clinical trial patients treated for up to 5 years with bezafibrate and from surveillance studies in countries where bezafibrate has been marketed since as early as 1978, also include:

Dermatologic: pruritus, urticaria or erythema and isolated cases of photosensitivity.

Gastrointestinal: epigastric distress, flatulence, nausea, diarrhea, constipation.

Less common adverse reactions observed include:

CNS: headache, dizziness.

Immune System: hypersensitivity.

Musculoskeletal: muscular weakness, myalgia and muscle cramps.

Renal and Urinary Disorders: acute renal failure.

Skin and Appendages: alopecia, Stevens-Johnson syndrome, toxic epidermal necrolysis.

In isolated cases, the occurrence of gallstones, cholestasis, cholelithiasis, thrombocytopenia (i.e., purpura), pancytopenia and erectile dysfunction have been reported.

Abnormal liver function test have been observed occasionally during bezafibrate therapy including elevated transaminases and decreased or rarely increased alkaline phosphatase. However, after five years of placebo-controlled double-blind therapy, the cumulative event rates for elevations in ALT and AST were similar between the placebo and bezafibrate groups (see Table 2).

Mild decreases in hemoglobin, leukocytes and erythrocytes, and slight increase in platelets have been observed occasionally in patients receiving bezafibrate therapy. A decline of alkaline phosphatase has been shown so consistently that it could be used as an indicator of patient compliance. A parallel decrease of gamma-glutamyl transferase has also been noted.

Slight increase in serum creatinine may occur. In patients with existing renal failure, if dosage recommendations are not followed, myositis and rhabdomyolysis may develop (see Warnings and Precautions).

Bezafibrate also has the potential to provoke CPK elevations which generally subsides when the drug is discontinued (see Warnings and Precautions).

DRUG INTERACTIONS: Drug-Drug Interactions: Concomitant Anticoagulants: Caution should be exercised when oral anticoagulants are given with BEZALIP SR (bezafibrate). The dosage of anticoagulants should be reduced up to 50% to maintain the prothrombin time at the desired level to prevent bleeding complications. Careful frequent (perhaps weekly) monitoring of prothrombin time is therefore recommended until it has been definitely determined that the prothrombin level has been stabilized.

HMG-CoA Reductase Inhibitors: Interaction between fibrates and HMG-Co A reductase inhibitors (statins) may vary in nature and intensity depending on the combination of the administered drugs.

Due to the risk of rhabdomyolysis, bezafibrate should only be administered together with HMG-CoA reductase inhibitors in exceptional cases when strictly indicated. Patients receiving this combination therapy must be informed carefully of the symptoms of myopathy and monitored closely. Combination therapy must be discontinued immediately at the first signs of myopathy. This combination therapy must not be used in patients with predisposing factors for myopathy (impaired renal function, severe infection, trauma, surgery, disturbances of the hormonal or electrolyte balance and a high alcohol intake).

Cyclosporine: Severe myositis and rhabdomyolysis have occurred when a cyclosporine was administered with a fibrate. Therefore, the benefits and risks of using BEZALIP SR concomitantly with cyclosporine should be carefully considered.

Immuno-Suppressant Therapies: In isolated cases, reversible impairment of renal function (accompanied by a corresponding increase in the serum creatinine level) has been reported in organ transplant patients receiving immuno-suppressant therapy and concomitant bezafibrate. Renal function should be closely monitored in these patients and in the event of relevant significant changes in laboratory parameters, bezafibrate should be discontinued.

Insulin and Sulphonylurea: Serious hypoglycaemia may result in the combinatory use of bezafibrate and hypoglycaemic agents.

MAO-Inhibitors: MAO-inhibitors (with hepatotoxic potential) must not be administered together with BEZALIP.

Resins: When bezafibrate is used concurrently with cholestyramine or any other resin, an interval of at least 2 h should be maintained between the two drugs, since the absorption of bezafibrate is impaired by cholestyramine.

Estrogens: Since estrogens may lead to a rise in lipid levels, the prescribing of BEZALIP SR in patients taking estrogens or estrogen-containing contraceptives must be critically considered on an individual basis.

Drug-Food Interactions: The rate and degree of absorption of bezafibrate is reduced by approximately 50% in the presence of cholestyramine but is only slightly reduced in the presence of food.

DOSAGE AND ADMINISTRATION: Dosing Considerations:

- Since a reduction of total mortality has not been established, BEZALIP SR (bezafibrate) should be administered only to those patients described in Indications and Clinical Use. If a significant serum lipid response is not obtained in three months, BEZALIP SR should be discontinued.
- In patients with impaired renal function (serum creatinine >1.5 mg/100 mL, i.e. >135 µmol/L or creatinine clearance <60 mL/min), the BEZALIP SR 400 mg sustained release tablet should not be used.
- **Initial Therapy:** Before instituting BEZALIP SR therapy, attempts should be made to control serum lipids with appropriate diet, exercise and weight loss in obese patients, as well as other medical problems, such as diabetes mellitus and hypothyroidism. In patients at high risk, consideration should be given to the control of other risk factors such as smoking, excessive alcohol intake, hormonal contraceptive use, and inadequately controlled hypertension.
- **Long-Term Therapy:** Since long-term administration of BEZALIP SR is recommended, the potential risks and benefits should be carefully weighed.

Recommended Dose and Dosage Adjustment: The dosage is one BEZALIP SR 400 mg sustained release tablet once daily.

Missed Dose: Take the missed dose as soon as you remember it. However, if it is almost time for the next dose, skip the missed dose and continue your regular dosing schedule. Do not take 2 doses at the same time.

Administration: The 400 mg sustained-release tablet should be taken in the morning or evening with or after meals. The sustained release tablet should be swallowed without chewing with sufficient fluid. When BEZALIP SR 400 mg tablets are administered concurrently with resins, an interval of 2 hours should be maintained between the two drugs (see Warnings and Precautions).

OVERDOSAGE:

While there has been no reported case of overdosage, symptomatic and supportive measures should be taken. Because bezafibrate is highly bound to plasma proteins, hemodialysis should not be considered.

In patients with existing impaired renal function, if dosage recommendations are not followed, overdosage may occur and severe rhabdomyolysis may develop. Administration of BEZALIP SR (bezafibrate) must be stopped immediately and renal function must be carefully monitored (see Warnings and Precautions).

> For management of a suspected drug overdose, CPhA recommends that you contact your **regional Poison Control Centre**. See the *CPS* Directory section for a list of Poison Control Centres.

ACTION AND CLINICAL PHARMACOLOGY: Mechanism of Action: The fibrates, including BEZALIP SR (bezafibrate) , lower elevated serum lipids by decreasing the low density lipoprotein (LDL) fraction rich in cholesterol and the very low density lipoprotein (VLDL) fraction rich in triglycerides. In addition, fibrates (including BEZALIP SR) increase the high density lipoprotein (HDL) cholesterol fraction.

The mechanisms of action of the fibrates have not been definitely established. Work carried out to date, including the information derived from animal studies, suggests that the major modes of action of the fibrates likely encompass the following:

- VLDL catabolism by increased lipoprotein and hepatic triglyceride lipase activities
- attenuation of triglyceride biosynthesis by acetyl-CoA carboxylase enzyme inhibition
- attenuation of cholesterol biosynthesis by inhibition of the rate-limiting 3-hydroxy-3-methylglutaryl-coenzyme A reductase (HMG-CoA reductase).

Pharmacodynamics: Due to their major action on lipoprotein and hepatic triglyceride lipase, the fibrates appear to produce a greater reduction on the VLDL than on the LDL fraction. Therapeutic doses of BEZALIP SR (bezafibrate) produce variable elevations of HDL cholesterol, a reduction in the content of LDL cholesterol, and a substantial reduction in the triglyceride content of the VLDL fraction. In the course of the intensified degradation of triglyceride-rich lipoproteins (chylomicrons, VLDL) precursors for the formation of HDL are formed which explains an increase in HDL. Furthermore, cholesterol biosynthesis is reduced by bezafibrate, which is accompanied by a stimulation of the LDL-receptor-mediated lipoprotein catabolism. Changes by BEZALIP SR in the lipid components (VLDL-triglycerides, VLDL-cholesterol, LDL-cholesterol, HDL-cholesterol) are usually paralleled by changes in the corresponding apolipoproteins: apolipoprotein B is reduced, while apolipoprotein A1 and A2 may be increased.

Bezafibrate also exerts an effect on thrombogenic factors: in addition to an inhibition of platelet aggregation, a significant decrease in elevated plasma fibrinogen levels as well as a reduction of blood viscosity can be achieved.

Some data may indicate that a reduction in blood glucose concentration due to an increase in glucose tolerance may be observed in diabetic patients. In the same patients, the concentration of fasting and postprandial free fatty acids may be reduced by bezafibrate.

Pharmacokinetics: Absorption: A peak concentration of about 6 mg/L is reached after 3-4 h with the 400 mg sustained release tablet.

Distribution: In human serum, 94-96% of bezafibrate is bound to protein. The apparent volume of distribution is about 17 L. There is no accumulation of the drug following repeated administration for periods of 28 days to 1 year.

Metabolism: After administration of ^{14}C-labelled bezafibrate, 95% of the administered dose was excreted within 48 hours in the urine and the remainder was found in the feces. In the urine, about 50% was present as unchanged bezafibrate, about 25% as bezafibrate glucuronide and the remainder as metabolites, one of which was identified as hydroxy-bezafibrate, which does not have any lipid-lowering properties in animals. Clofibric acid was not found as a metabolite.

Excretion: The elimination is rapid, with excretion almost exclusively renal. Within 48 h, 95% of the activity of the ^{14}C-labelled drug is recovered in the urine and 3% in the feces. The rate of renal clearance ranges from 3.4 to 6.0 L/h. The elimination half-life of bezafibrate is 1-2 h. The elimination of bezafibrate is reduced in patients with renal insufficiency. BEZALIP SR 400 mg tablets are contraindicated in patients with renal impairment (see Contraindications).

Special Populations and Conditions: Pediatrics: Limited experience is available in children.

Geriatrics: Pharmacokinetic investigations in the elderly suggest that elimination may be delayed in cases of impaired liver function. Liver disease (except fatty liver) is a contraindication (see Hepatic Insufficiency below).

Hepatic Insufficiency: Liver disease (except fatty liver) is a contraindication.

Renal Insufficiency: In patients with severe renal failure, important accumulation of fibrates are observed with large increases in the half-life. There is a correlation between creatinine clearance and the elimination half-life of bezafibrate. Because bezafibrate is highly bound to plasma proteins, hemodialysis should not be considered. Bezafibrate is contraindicated in patients with renal impairment (serum creatinine levels >1.5 mg /100 mL, i.e. >135 µmol/L, or creatinine clearance <60 mL/min) including in patients undergoing dialysis (see Contraindications and Warnings and Precautions).

STORAGE AND STABILITY: BEZALIP SR (bezafibrate) tablets should be stored at room temperature (15-30°C). Protect from high humidity.

INFORMATION FOR THE PATIENT: Published in e-CPS, available by subscription at www.e-cps.ca.

DOSAGE FORMS, COMPOSITION AND PACKAGING: Each round, white, sustained-release film-coated tablet, printed on one side: "D9", contains: bezafibrate 400 mg. Nonmedicinal ingredients: colloidal silicon dioxide, hydroxypropyl methylcellulose 2208 & 2910, lactose, magnesium stearate, methyl methacrylate, polyethyl acrylate, polyethylene glycol 10 000, polysorbate 80, povidone K25, sodium citrate, sodium lauryl sulfate, talc and titanium dioxide. Blister packs of 30.

(Shown in Product Identification Section)

Biaxin®

clarithromycin

Antibiotic

Abbott

Biaxin BID®

clarithromycin

Antibiotic

Abbott

Biaxin® XL

clarithromycin

Antibiotic

Abbott

Date of Preparation: May 8, 1992
Date of Revision: August 31, 2009

Note: When used in combination with acid antisecretory drugs and other antimicrobials for the eradication of *H. pylori*, the product monograph for those agents should be consulted.

SUMMARY PRODUCT INFORMATION:

Route of Administration	Dosage Form/ Strength	Clinically Relevant Nonmedicinal Ingredients
Oral	Film-coated tablets/ 250 mg and 500 mg	Cellulosic polymers, croscarmellose sodium, D&C Yellow No. 10, magnesium stearate, povidone, pregelatinized starch (250 mg only), propylene glycol, silicon dioxide, sorbic acid, sorbitan monooleate, stearic acid, talc, titanium dioxide and vanillin
	Extended-release tablets/ 500 mg	Cellulosic polymers, Quinoline Yellow Lake E104, lactose monohydrate, magnesium stearate, propylene glycol, sorbitan monooleate, talc, titanium dioxide and vanillin
	Oral suspension/ 125 mg/5 mL and 250 mg/5 mL	Artificial and natural fruit flavour, citric acid, carbopol, castor oil, hydroxypropyl methylcellulose phthalate, maltodextrin, potassium sorbate, povidone, silicon dioxide, sucrose or sugar, titanium dioxide and xanthan gum

INDICATIONS AND CLINICAL USE: Biaxin BID (clarithromycin tablets, USP, film-coated): BIAXIN BID (clarithromycin tablets, USP, film-coated) may be indicated in the treatment of mild to moderate infections caused by susceptible strains of the designated microorganisms in the diseases listed below:

Upper Respiratory Tract: Pharyngitis/tonsillitis, caused by *S. pyogenes* (Group A beta-hemolytic streptococci).

Acute maxillary sinusitis caused by *S. pneumoniae*, *H. influenzae*, and *M. (Branhamella) catarrhalis*.

Lower Respiratory Tract: Acute bacterial exacerbation of chronic bronchitis caused by *S. pneumoniae*, *H. influenzae* (including beta-lactamase producing strains), *M. (Branhamella) catarrhalis* (including beta-lactamase producing strains).

Pneumonia caused by *S. pneumoniae* and *M. pneumoniae*.

Uncomplicated Skin and Skin Structure Infections: Uncomplicated Skin and Skin Structure Infections caused by *S. pyogenes*, *S. aureus*.

Mycobacterial Infections: BIAXIN BID (clarithromycin tablets, USP, film-coated) is indicated for the prevention of disseminated *M. avium* complex (MAC) disease in patients with advanced HIV infection, and for the treatment of disseminated mycobacterial infections due to *M. avium* and *M. intracellulare*.

Eradication of *H. pylori*: BIAXIN BID (clarithromycin tablets, USP, film-coated) in the presence of acid suppression (with omeprazole) with another antibiotic (amoxicillin) is indicated for the eradication of *H. pylori* that may result in decreased recurrence of duodenal ulcer in patients with active duodenal ulcers and who are *H. pylori* positive.

For additional information on the use of BIAXIN BID in triple therapy for the treatment of *H. pylori* infection and active duodenal ulcer recurrence, refer to the Hp-PAC Product Monograph.)

BIAXIN XL (clarithromycin extended-release tablets): BIAXIN XL (clarithromycin extended-release tablets) may be indicated in the treatment of mild to moderate infections caused by susceptible strains of the designated microorganisms in the diseases listed below:

Upper Respiratory Tract: Acute maxillary sinusitis due to *H. influenzae*, *M. catarrhalis*, or *S. pneumoniae*.

Lower Respiratory Tract: Acute bacterial exacerbation of chronic bronchitis due to *H. parainfluenzae*, *H. influenzae*, *M. catarrhalis*, *S. aureus*, or *S. pneumoniae*.

Community-acquired pneumonia due to *H. influenzae*, *H. parainfluenzae*, *M. catarrhalis*, *S. pneumoniae*, *C. pneumoniae* (TWAR), or *M. pneumoniae*.

The efficacy and safety of BIAXIN XL in treating other infections for which BIAXIN BID and BIAXIN are approved have not been established.

BIAXIN (clarithromycin for oral suspension, USP): BIAXIN (clarithromycin for oral suspension, USP) is indicated for the treatment of infections due to susceptible organisms, in the following conditions:

Upper Respiratory Tract: Pharyngitis caused by *S. pyogenes* (Group A β-hemolytic streptococci).

Acute otitis media caused by *H. influenzae*, *M. catarrhalis*, or *S. pneumoniae*.

Lower Respiratory Tract: Mild to moderate community-acquired pneumonia caused by *S. pneumoniae*, *C. pneumoniae*, or *M. pneumoniae*.

Uncomplicated Skin and Skin Structure Infections: Uncomplicated skin and skin structure infections (i.e., impetigo and cellulitis) caused by *S. aureus* or *S. pyogenes*.

Mycobacterial Infections: Disseminated mycobacterial infections due to *M. avium* and *M. intracellulare*.

Geriatrics (>65 years of age): Dosage adjustment should be considered in elderly patients with severe renal impairment. For a brief discussion please see Warnings and Precautions, Special Populations, Geriatrics (>65 years of age).

Pediatrics (6 months-12 years of age): Dosing recommendations for children are based on body weight. Please see Dosage and Administration, Table 17 for determining dosage. For a brief discussion please see Warnings and Precautions, Special Populations, Pediatrics (6 months-12 years of age).

CONTRAINDICATIONS: BIAXIN BID (clarithromycin tablets, USP, film-coated), BIAXIN XL (clarithromycin extended-release tablets) and BIAXIN (clarithromycin for oral suspension, USP) are contraindicated in patients with a known hypersensitivity to clarithromycin, erythromycin, other macrolide antibacterial agents or to any ingredient in the formulation or component of the container. (See Dosage Forms, Composition and Packaging.)

Clarithromycin is contraindicated as concurrent therapy with astemizole, terfenadine, cisapride, pimozide, ergotamine or dihydroergotamine. There have been post-marketing reports of drug interactions when clarithromycin and/or erythromycin are co-administered with cisapride, astemizole, pimozide, or terfenadine resulting in cardiac arrhythmias (QT prolongation, ventricular tachycardia, ventricular fibrillation, and torsades de pointes) most likely due to inhibition of hepatic metabolism of these drugs by erythromycin and clarithromycin. Fatalities have been reported (see Drug Interactions, Drug-Drug Interactions).

WARNINGS AND PRECAUTIONS:

Serious Warnings and Precautions

- Clarithromycin should not be used in **pregnancy** except where no alternative therapy is appropriate, particularly during the first 3 months of pregnancy. If pregnancy occurs while taking the drug, the patient should be apprised of the potential hazard to the fetus. See Warnings and Precautions, Special Populations.
- The concomitant administration of clarithromycin and drugs metabolized by CYP3A and/or transported by P-gp may result in significant safety concerns (see Drug Interactions).

General: Clarithromycin should be administered with caution to any patient who has demonstrated some form of drug allergy, particularly to structurally related-drugs. If an allergic reaction to clarithromycin occurs, administration of the drug should be discontinued. Serious hypersensitivity reactions may require epinephrine, antihistamines, or corticosteroids.

Long-term use may, as with other antibiotics, result in colonization with increased numbers of non-susceptible bacteria and fungi. If superinfections occur, appropriate therapy should be instituted.

There have been post-marketing reports of colchicine toxicity with concurrent use of clarithromycin and colchicine. In patients with impaired renal function and/or who are elderly, colchicine and clarithromycin should not be used concurrently due to the risk of colchicine toxicity. Deaths have been reported in some such patients (see Drug Interactions, Drug-Drug Interactions, Colchicine and Adverse Reactions, Post-Market Adverse Drug Reactions).

Several studies of HIV-positive patients receiving clarithromycin for treatment of MAC infection have shown poorer survival in those patients randomized to receive doses higher than 500 mg b.i.d. The explanation for the poorer survival associated with doses higher than 500 mg b.i.d. has not been determined. Treatment or prophylaxis of MAC infection with clarithromycin should not exceed the approved dose of 500 mg b.i.d.

Exacerbation of symptoms of myasthenia gravis and new onset of symptoms of myasthenic syndrome has been reported in patients receiving clarithromycin therapy.

Use of clarithromycin with other drugs may lead to drug-drug interactions. For established or potential drug-drug interactions and their mechanisms, see Contraindications and Drug Interactions, Drug-Drug Interactions.

Carcinogenesis and Mutagenesis: Long-term studies in animals have not been performed to evaluate the carcinogenic potential of clarithromycin.

The following in vitro mutagenicity tests have been conducted with clarithromycin: Salmonella/mammalian microsome test, bacterial induced mutation frequency test, in vitro chromosome aberration test, rat hepatocyte DNA synthesis assay, mouse lymphoma assay, mouse dominant lethal study, mouse micronucleus test. All tests had negative results except the in vitro chromosome aberration test which was weakly positive in one test and negative in another. In addition, a Bacterial Reverse-Mutation Test (Ames Test) has been performed on clarithromycin metabolites with negative results.

Gastrointestinal: *C. difficile*-Associated Disease: *C. difficile*-associated disease (CDAD) has been reported with use of many antibacterial agents, including clarithromycin. CDAD may range in severity from mild diarrhea to fatal colitis. It is important to consider this diagnosis in patients who present with diarrhea, or symptoms of colitis, pseudomembranous colitis, toxic megacolon, or perforation of colon subsequent to the administration of any antibacterial agent. CDAD has been reported to occur over two months after the administration of antibacterial agents.

Treatment with antibacterial agents may alter the normal flora of the colon and may permit overgrowth of *C. difficile*. *C. difficile* produces toxins A and B, which contribute to the development of CDAD. CDAD may cause significant morbidity and mortality. CDAD can be refractory to antimicrobial therapy.

If the diagnosis of CDAD is suspected or confirmed, appropriate therapeutic measures should be initiated. Mild cases of CDAD usually respond to discontinuation of antibacterial agents not directed against *C. difficile*. In moderate to severe cases, consideration should be given to management with fluids and electrolytes, protein supplementation, and treatment with an antibacterial drug clinically effective against *C. difficile*. Surgical evaluation should be instituted as clinically indicated; as surgical intervention may be required in certain severe cases (see Adverse Reactions).

Hepatic/Biliary/Pancreatic: Clarithromycin is principally excreted by the liver and kidney. In patients with both hepatic and renal impairments or in the presence of severe renal impairment, decreased dosage of clarithromycin or prolonged dosing intervals might be appropriate (see Dosage and Administration, Recommended Dose and Dosage Adjustment).

Renal: Clarithromycin is principally excreted by the liver and kidney. In patients with both hepatic and renal impairments or in the presence of severe renal impairment, decreased dosage of clarithromycin or prolonged dosing intervals might be appropriate (see Dosage and Administration, Recommended Dose and Dosage Adjustment).

For the eradication of *H. pylori*, amoxicillin and clarithromycin should not be administered to patients with renal impairment since the appropriate dosage in this patient population has not yet been established.

Sensitivity/Resistance: The development of resistance (11 out of 19 breakthrough isolates in one study) has been seen in HIV positive patients receiving clarithromycin for prophylaxis and treatment of MAC infection.

To avoid failure of the eradication treatment with a potential for developing antimicrobial resistance and a risk of failure with subsequent therapy, patients should be instructed to follow closely the prescribed regimen.

Antibiotic Resistance in Relation to *H. pylori* Eradication: Triple and Dual Therapy with Omeprazole. Among the 113 triple therapy recipients with pretreatment *H. pylori* isolates susceptible to clarithromycin, 2/102 patients (2%) developed resistance after treatment with omeprazole, clarithromycin, and amoxicillin. Among patients who received triple therapy, 6/108 (5.6%) patients had pretreatment *H. pylori* isolates resistant to clarithromycin. Of these 6 patients, 3 (50%) had *H. pylori* eradicated at follow-up, and 3 (50%) remained positive after treatment. In 5/113 (4.4%) patients, no susceptibility data for clarithromycin pretreatment were available. Twenty-six patients 26/104 (25%) with pretreatment isolates susceptible to clarithromycin developed resistance after treatment with omeprazole and clarithromycin. Development of clarithromycin resistance should be considered as a possible risk especially when less efficient treatment regimens are used.

Special Populations: Pregnant Women: There are no adequate and well-controlled studies in pregnant women. The benefits against risk, particularly during the first 3 months of pregnancy should be carefully weighed by a physician (see Warnings and Precautions, Serious Warnings and Precautions). Four teratogenicity studies in rats (three with oral doses and one with intravenous doses up to 160 mg/kg/day administered during the period of major organogenesis) and two in rabbits (at oral doses up to 125 mg/kg/day or intravenous doses of 30 mg/kg/day administered during gestation days 6 to 18) failed to demonstrate any teratogenicity from clarithromycin. Two additional oral studies in a different rat strain at similar doses and similar conditions demonstrated a low incidence of cardiovascular anomalies at doses of 150 mg/kg/day administered during gestation days 6 to 15. Plasma levels after 150 mg/kg/day were 2 times the human serum levels.

Four studies in mice revealed a variable incidence of cleft palate following oral doses of 1000 mg/kg/day during gestation days 6 to 15. Cleft palate was also seen at 500 mg/kg/day. The 1000 mg/kg/day exposure resulted in plasma levels 17 times the human serum levels. In monkeys, an oral dose of 70 mg/kg/day produced fetal growth retardation at plasma levels that were 2 times the human serum levels.

Embryonic loss has been seen in monkeys and rabbits.

Nursing Women: The safety of clarithromycin for use during breast feeding of infants has not been established. Clarithromycin is excreted in human milk.

Preweaned rats, exposed indirectly via consumption of milk from dams treated with 150 mg/kg/day for 3 weeks, were not adversely affected, despite data indicating higher drug levels in milk than in plasma.

Pediatrics (6 months-12 years of age): Use of clarithromycin tablets in children under 12 years of age has not been studied.

Use of clarithromycin for oral suspension, USP in children under 6 months has not been studied. In pneumonia, clarithromycin granules were not studied in children younger than 3 years.

The safety of clarithromycin has not been studied in MAC patients under the age of 20 months.

Neonatal and juvenile animals tolerated clarithromycin in a manner similar to adult animals. Young animals were slightly more intolerant to acute overdosage and to subtle reductions in erythrocytes, platelets and leukocytes, but were less sensitive to toxicity in the liver, kidney, thymus and genitalia.

Increased valproate and phenobarbital concentrations and extreme sedation were noted in a 3-year old patient coincident with clarithromycin therapy. Cause and effect relationship cannot be established. However, monitoring of valproate and phenobarbital concentrations may be considered.

Geriatrics (>65 years of age): Dosage adjustment should be considered in elderly patients with severe renal impairment. In a steady-state study in which healthy elderly subjects (age 65 to 81 years old) were given 500 mg every 12 hours, the maximum concentrations of clarithromycin and 14-OH clarithromycin were increased. The AUC was also increased. These changes in pharmacokinetics parallel known age-related decreases in renal function. In clinical trials, elderly patients did not have an increased incidence of adverse events when compared to younger patients.

ADVERSE REACTIONS: Adverse Drug Reaction Overview: The majority of side effects observed in clinical trials involving 3563 patients treated with BIAXIN BID were of a mild and transient nature. Fewer than 3% of adult patients without mycobacterial infections discontinued therapy because of drug-related side-effects. The most common drug-related adverse reactions in adults taking BIAXIN BID were nausea, diarrhea, abdominal pain, dyspepsia, headache, taste perversion and vomiting. In pediatric patients taking BIAXIN (oral suspension), the most frequently reported events were diarrhea, vomiting, abdominal pain, dyspepsia, taste perversion and infection. The most frequently reported events in adults taking BIAXIN XL were diarrhea, abnormal taste and nausea.

Clinical Trial Adverse Drug Reactions: General Statement: Because clinical trials are conducted under very specific conditions, the adverse reaction rates observed in the clinical trials may not reflect the rates observed in practice and should not be compared to the rates in the clinical trials of another drug. Adverse drug reaction information from clinical trials is useful for identifying drug-related adverse events and for approximating rates.

BIAXIN BID (clarithromycin tablets, USP, film-coated): Patients with Respiratory Tract or Skin Infections: Adverse Reactions: Table 1 provides a listing of adverse reactions from clinical trials or post-marketing surveillance as well as adverse events reported during post-marketing surveillance. Adverse events reported during post-marketing surveillance may include patients treated for various infections and are not limited to patients with respiratory tract or skin infections.

In studies of adults with pneumonia comparing clarithromycin to erythromycin base or erythromycin stearate, there were significantly fewer adverse events involving the digestive system in patients treated with clarithromycin.

Abnormal Laboratory Values: Changes in laboratory values with possible clinical significance reported during clinical studies or during post-marketing surveillance are displayed in Table 2.

Patients with Mycobacterial Infections: In patients with acquired immune deficiency syndrome (AIDS) and other immunocompromised patients treated with the higher doses of clarithromycin over long periods of time for prevention or treatment of mycobacterial infections, it was often difficult to distinguish adverse events possibly associated with clarithromycin administration from underlying signs of HIV disease or intercurrent illness. Other adverse reactions have been observed in different patient populations and during post-marketing surveillance. Please also refer to Adverse Reactions, Clinical Trial Adverse Drug Reactions, Patients with Respiratory Tract or Skin Infections.

Table 1: BIAXIN BID

Patients with Respiratory Tract or Skin Infections—BIAXIN BID

System Organ Class	Adverse Reaction/Adverse Event
General Disorders and Administration Site Conditions	Asthenia Pain Chest pain
Infections and Infestations	Infection Colitis pseudomembranous Candidiasis Rhinitis Pharyngitis Vaginal candidiasis Vaginal infection
Musculoskeletal and Connective Tissue Disorders	Back pain Myalgia
Investigations	Increased liver enzymes
Cardiac Disorders[a]	Electrocardiogram QT prolonged Ventricular tachycardia Torsades de pointes
Gastrointestinal Disorders	Constipation Flatulence Dry mouth Glossitis Stomatitis Gastrointestinal disorder Tongue discolouration Tooth discolouration Pancreatitis
Metabolism and Nutrition Disorders	Anorexia Hypoglycemia[b]
Hepatobiliary Disorders	Hepatomegaly Hepatic function abnormal Hepatitis Hepatitis cholestatic Jaundice (cholestatic and hepatocellular) Hepatic failure[c]
Nervous System Disorders	Dizziness Somnolence Convulsion Parosmia Dysgeusia Ageusia
Ear and Labyrinth Disorders	Vertigo Tinnitus Ear disorder Deafness[d]
Psychiatric Disorders	Nervousness Anxiety Insomnia Nightmare Depression Confusional state Disorientation Depersonalisation Hallucination Psychotic disorder

(cont'd)

Table 1: BIAXIN BID *(cont'd)*

Patients with Respiratory Tract or Skin Infections—BIAXIN BID

System Organ Class	Adverse Reaction/Adverse Event
Respiratory, Thoracic and Mediastinal Disorders	Cough Dyspnea Asthma
Skin and Subcutaneous Tissue Disorders	Pruritus Rash Hyperhidrosis Urticaria Stevens-Johnson syndrome Toxic epidermal necrosis
Immune System Disorders	Anaphylactic reaction Myasthenia gravis
Eye Disorders	Visual disturbance Conjunctivitis
Renal and Urinary Disorders	Hematuria Nephritis interstitial
Reproductive System and Breast Disorders	Dysmenorrhea
Blood and Lymphatic System Disorders	Eosinophilia Anemia Leukopenia Thrombocythemia Thrombocytopenia

[a] As with other macrolides, QT prolongation, ventricular tachycardia, and torsades de pointes have been reported with clarithromycin.
[b] There have been reports of hypoglycemia, some of which have occurred in patients on concomitant oral hypoglycemic agents or insulin.
[c] Hepatic dysfunction may be severe and is usually reversible. Hepatic failure with fatal outcome has been reported and generally has been associated with serious underlying diseases and/or concomitant medications.
[d] There have been reports of hearing loss with clarithromycin which is usually reversible upon withdrawal of therapy.

Table 2: BIAXIN BID

Abnormal Hematologic and Clinical Chemistry Findings in Patients with Respiratory Tract or Skin Infections Treated with BIAXIN BID

System Organ Class	Laboratory Values	Frequency
Investigations	Alanine aminotransferase increased Aspartate aminotransferase increased Gamma-glutamyltransferase increased Blood alkaline phosphatase increased Blood lactate dehydrogenase increased Blood bilirubin increased Blood creatinine increased White blood cell count decreased	Uncommon (Less than 1%)
	Prothrombin time prolonged Blood urea increased	1% 4%

Prophylaxis: Adverse Reactions: Discontinuation due to adverse events was required in 18% of AIDS patients receiving clarithromycin 500 mg b.i.d., compared to 17% of patients receiving placebo in a randomized, double-blind study. Primary reasons for discontinuation in the clarithromycin-treated patients include headache, nausea, vomiting, depression and taste perversion. The most frequently reported adverse events with an incidence of 2% or greater, excluding those due to the patient's concurrent condition, are listed in Table 3. Among these events, taste perversion was the only event that had significantly higher incidence in the clarithromycin-treated compared to the placebo-treated group.

Table 3: BIAXIN BID

Percentage of Adverse Events[a] in Immunocompromised Adult Patients Receiving Prophylaxis Against *M. avium* Complex

System Organ Class[b]	Adverse Reaction	Clarithromycin (n=339) %	Placebo (n=339) %
Gastrointestinal Disorders	Abdominal pain	5.0%	3.5%
	Nausea	11.2%	7.1%
	Diarrhea	7.7%	4.1%
	Vomiting	5.9%	3.2%
	Dyspepsia	3.8%	2.7%
	Flatulence	2.4%	0.9%
Nervous System Disorders	Dysgeusia	8.0%	0.3%
	Headache	2.7%	0.9%
Skin and Subcutaneous Tissue Disorders	Rash	3.2%	3.5%

[a] Includes those events possibly or probably related to study drug and excludes concurrent conditions.
[b] ≥2% Adverse Event Incidence Rates for either treatment group.

Abnormal Laboratory Values: In immunocompromised patients receiving prophylaxis against *M. avium*, those laboratory values outside the extreme high or low limit for the specified test were analyzed (see Table 4).

Treatment of Patients with Mycobacterial Infections: Adverse Reactions: Excluding those patients who discontinued therapy due to complications of their underlying non-mycobacterial diseases (including death), approximately 14% of the patients discontinued therapy due to drug-related adverse events.

In adult patients, the most frequently reported adverse events with an incidence of 3% or greater, excluding those due to the patient's concurrent condition, are listed in Table 5 by the total daily dose the patient was receiving at the time of the event. A total of 867 patients were treated with clarithromycin for mycobacterial infections. Of these, 43% reported one or more adverse events. Most of these events were described as mild to moderate in severity, although 14% were described as severe.

Incidence of adverse events was higher in patients taking 4000 mg total daily doses compared to lower doses (see Table 5).

Table 4: BIAXIN BID

Percentage of Patients[a] Exceeding Extreme Laboratory Value in Immunocompromised Patients Receiving Prophylaxis Against *M. avium* Complex

System Organ Class	Laboratory Values	Clarithromycin 500 mg b.i.d.		Placebo	
Investigations	Hemoglobin decreased <8 g/dL	4/118	3%	5/103	5%
	Platelet count decreased $<50\times10^9/L$	11/249	4%	12/250	5%
	White blood cell count decreased $<1\times10^9/L$	2/103	4%	0/95	0%
	Aspartate aminotransferase increased >5×ULN[b]	7/196	4%	5/208	2%
	Alanine aminotransferase increased >5×ULN[b]	6/217	3%	4/232	2%
	Blood alkaline phosphatase increased >5×ULN[b]	5/220	2%	5/218	2%

[a] Includes only patients with baseline values within the normal range or borderline high (hematology variables) and within the normal range or borderline low (chemistry variables).
[b] ULN—Upper Limit of Normal.

Table 5: BIAXIN BID

Percentage of Adverse Events[a] in Immunocompromised Adult Patients Treated with Clarithromycin for Mycobacterial Infections

		Presented by Total Daily Dose at Time of the Event		
System Organ Class	Adverse Reaction	1000 mg (n=463)	2000 mg (n=516)	4000 mg (n=87)
Gastrointestinal Disorders	Nausea	11%	16%	40%
	Vomiting	7%	9%	24%
	Abdominal Pain	5%	7%	20%
	Diarrhea	4%	6%	17%
	Flatulence	1%	2%	7%
	Constipation	1%	<1%	5%
	Dry Mouth	<1%	0%	5%
Nervous System Disorders	Dysgeusia	6%	7%	29%
	Headache	2%	2%	7%
Skin and Subcutaneous Tissue Disorders	Rash	4%	3%	2%
Investigations	Aspartate aminotransferase increased	2%	2%	11%
	Alanine aminotransferase increased	1%	1%	9%
Respiratory, Thoracic and Mediastinal Disorders	Dyspnea	<1%	<1%	7%
Psychiatric Disorders	Insomnia	<1%	<1%	6%
Ear and Labyrinth Disorders	Hearing impaired[b]	3%	2%	5%

[a] Related adverse events considered to be definitely, probably, possibly or remotely related to study events.
[b] Sum of patients with deafness, ear disorder, partial transitory deafness, and/or tinnitus.
Legend: n=number of adverse events.

A limited number of pediatric AIDS patients have been treated with clarithromycin suspension for mycobacterial infections. The most frequently reported adverse events, excluding those due to the patient's concurrent condition, are listed in Table 6 by the total daily dose of clarithromycin the patient received.

Abnormal Laboratory Values: In immunocompromised patients treated with clarithromycin for mycobacterial infections, evaluations of laboratory values were made by analysing those values outside the seriously abnormal level (i.e., the extreme high or low limit) for the specified test (see Table 7 and Table 8).

Patients with *H. Pylori* Infection—Triple Therapy: (clarithromycin/omeprazole/amoxicillin): Adverse Reactions: A summary of drug-related adverse event incidence rates is presented in Table 9.

(Other adverse reactions have been observed in different patient populations and during post-marketing surveillance. Please also refer to Adverse Reactions, Clinical Trial Adverse Drug Reactions, Patients with Respiratory Tract or Skin Infections.)

Patients with *H. Pylori* Infection—Dual Therapy: (clarithromycin/omeprazole): Adverse Reactions: Of 346 patients, 156 (45%) reported at least one adverse event. Adverse events associated with the Gastrointestinal disorders, Nervous system disorders, and Infections and infestations system organ class (SOC) were the most commonly reported adverse events among clarithromycin/omeprazole-treated patients. One hundred and two patients (29%) reported gastrointestinal disorder events. The most common adverse events reported in the Gastrointestinal disorder SOC were nausea (5%) diarrhea (4%), vomiting (3%), and abdominal pain (3%). Eighty-three patients (24%) reported adverse events in the Nervous system disorders SOC. Dysgeusia (15%), headache (5%), and dizziness (2%) were the most frequently reported events in the Nervous system disorders SOC. Twenty-nine patients (8%) reported adverse events in the Infections and infestations SOC. Infection (3%) was the most frequently reported adverse event in the Infections and infestations SOC. Adverse events by system organ class for all patients treated with clarithromycin and omeprazole are presented in Table 10.

(Other adverse reactions have been observed in different patient populations and during post-marketing surveillance. Please also refer to Adverse Reactions, Clinical Trial Adverse Drug Reactions, Patients with Respiratory Tract or Skin Infections.)

The most commonly reported adverse events for the 346 patients who received clarithromycin and omeprazole were: taste perversion (15%), nausea (5%), headache (5%), diarrhea (4%), vomiting (3%), abdominal pain (3%), and infection (3%).

Table 11 presents adverse events reported by 1% or more of clarithromycin/omeprazole-treated patients.

Twelve (4%) of the clarithromycin/omeprazole-treated patients prematurely discontinued from study drug therapy due to adverse events. The most frequently reported adverse events leading to withdrawal included taste perversion, nausea, and headache. Three patients treated with clarithromycin and omeprazole died during follow-up periods; none of the deaths were considered by the investigator to be related to study drug administration.

Few laboratory abnormalities were observed among clarithromycin/ omeprazole-treated patients. The incidence of possibly clinically significant hematology and serum chemistry variables was <1% for any variable evaluated.

Table 6: BIAXIN

Number of Pediatric AIDS Patients Treated with Clarithromycin for Mycobacterial Infections Who Experienced Adverse Events

System Organ Class	Adverse Event	Presented by Total Daily Dose at Time of the Event		
		<15 mg/kg/day (n=19)	15–<25 mg/kg/day (n=13)	≥25 mg/kg/day (n=12)
Ear and Labyrinth Disorders	Tinnitus	2	0	0
	Deafness	1	1	0
Gastrointestinal Disorders	Vomiting	1	0	0
	Nausea	1	0	0
	Abdominal pain	1	0	0
	Pancreatitis	1	0	0
Skin and Subcutaneous Tissue Disorders	Purpuric rash	1	0	0
Investigations	Amylase increased	0	0	1

Table 7: BIAXIN BID

Percentage of Immunocompromised Adult Patients Treated with Clarithromycin for Mycobacterial Infections who had On-Treatment Laboratory Values that Were Outside the Seriously Abnormal Level

System Organ Class	Laboratory Values	Seriously Abnormal Level	Presented by Total Daily Dose		
			1000 mg	2000 mg	4000 mg
Investigations	Aspartate aminotransferase increased	>5×ULN	3%	2%	4%
	Alanine aminotransferase increased	>5×ULN	2%	2%	7%
	Platelet count decreased	$<50\times10^9$/L	2%	2%	4%
	White blood cell count decreased	$<1\times10^9$/L	0%	2%	0%
	Blood urea increased	>50 mg/dL	<1%	<1%	4%

Legend: ULN=Upper Limit of Normal.

Table 8: BIAXIN

Number of Pediatric AIDS Patients Treated with Clarithromycin for Mycobacterial Infections who had On-Treatment Laboratory Values that Were Outside the Seriously Abnormal Level

System Organ Class	Laboratory Values	Seriously Abnormal Level	Presented by Total Daily Dose		
			<15 mg/kg/day	15–<25 mg/kg/day	≥25 mg/kg/day
Investigations	Alanine aminotransferase increased	>5×ULN	0	1	0
	Blood bilirubin increased	>12 mg/dL	1	0	0
	Platelet count decreased	$<50\times10^9$/L	0	1	0
	Blood urea increased	>50 mg/dL	0	1	0

Legend: ULN=Upper Limit of Normal.

Table 9: BIAXIN BID

Summary of Drug-Related Adverse Event Incidence Rates by System Organ Class

System Organ Class	Patients with Drug-Related Adverse Events (% of Patients Treated)[a]	
	Omeprazole + Clarithromycin + Amoxicillin (n=137)	Omeprazole + Clarithromycin (n=130)
Gastrointestinal Disorders	24 (18%)	21 (16%)
General Disorders and Administration Site Conditions	5 (4%)	0 (0%)
Nervous System Disorders	15 (11%)	30 (23%)
Cardiac Disorders	0 (0%)	1 (1%)
Investigations	9 (7%)	0 (0%)
Infections and Infestations	1 (1%)	1 (1%)

(cont'd)

Table 9: BIAXIN BID *(cont'd)*

Summary of Drug-Related Adverse Event Incidence Rates by System Organ Class

System Organ Class	Patients with Drug-Related Adverse Events (% of Patients Treated)[a]	
	Omeprazole + Clarithromycin + Amoxicillin (n=137)	Omeprazole + Clarithromycin (n=130)
Hepatobiliary Disorders	2 (1%)	0 (0%)
Psychiatric Disorders	1 (1%)	1 (1%)
Ear and Labyrinth Disorders	1 (1%)	2 (2%)
Respiratory, Thoracic and Mediastinal Disorders	1 (1%)	0 (0%)
Skin and Subcutaneous Tissue Disorders	3 (2%)	1 (1%)
Eye Disorders	0 (0%)	1 (1%)
Reproductive System and Breast Disorders	1 (1%)	0 (0%)

[a] Patients with more than one event within a system organ class are counted only once in the total for that system organ class.
Note: There is a statistical difference (Fisher's exact two-sided, p-value = 0.009) between omeprazole + clarithromycin + amoxicillin (11%) versus omeprazole + clarithromycin (23%) in regard to nervous system disorders.

Table 10: BIAXIN BID

Summary of Adverse Event Incidence by System Organ Class all Patients Treated with Clarithromycin/Omeprazole

System Organ Class[a]	Number (%) of Patients (N=346)
Infections and Infestations	29 (8%)
Neoplasma Benign, Malignant and Unspecified	2 (<1%)
Metabolism and Nutrition Disorders	1 (<1%)
Psychiatric Disorders	12 (3%)
Nervous System Disorders	83 (24%)
Eye Disorders	2 (<1%)
Ear and Labyrinth Disorders	1 (<1%)
Cardiac Disorders	6 (2%)
Vascular Disorders	1 (<1%)
Respiratory, Thoracic and Mediastinal Disorders	5 (1%)
Gastrointestinal Disorders	102 (29%)
Hepatobiliary Disorders	1 (<1%)
Skin and Subcutaneous Tissue Disorders	11 (3%)
Musculoskeletal and Connective Tissue Disorders	12 (3%)
Renal and Urinary Disorders	2 (<1%)
General Disorders and Administration Site Conditions	24 (7%)
Investigations	8 (2%)
Injury, Poisoning and Procedural Complications	3 (1%)
Total[b]	156 (45%)

[a] Patients with more than one event within a system organ class are counted only once in the total for that system organ class.
[b] Patients with event in more than one system organ class are counted only once in the total.

BIAXIN XL (clarithromycin extended-release tablets): Adverse Reactions: Fewer than 2% of adult patients taking BIAXIN XL (clarithromycin extended-release tablets) discontinued therapy because of drug-related side effects. The most frequently reported adverse events in adults taking clarithromycin extended-release tablets were diarrhea (6%), abnormal taste (7%), and nausea (3%). Most of these events were described as mild or moderate in severity. Of the reported adverse events, less than 1% were described as severe.

There have been rare reports of clarithromycin extended-release tablets in the stool, many of which have occurred in patients with anatomic (including ileostomy or colostomy) or functional gastrointestinal disorders with shortened GI transit times.

(Other adverse reactions have been observed in different patient populations and during post-marketing surveillance. Please also refer to Adverse Reactions, Clinical Trial Adverse Drug Reactions, Patients with Respiratory Tract or Skin Infections.)

BIAXIN (clarithromycin for oral suspension, USP): Adverse Reactions: The safety profile of BIAXIN (clarithromycin for oral suspension, USP) is similar to that of the 250 mg tablet in adult patients. **(Other adverse reactions have been observed in different patient populations and during post-marketing experience. Please also refer to Adverse Reactions, Clinical Trial Adverse Drug Reactions, Patients with Respiratory Tract or Skin Infections.)**

As with other macrolides, hepatic dysfunction, including increased liver enzymes, and hepatocellular and/or cholestatic hepatitis, with or without jaundice, has been infrequently reported with BIAXIN. This hepatic dysfunction may be severe and is usually reversible. In very rare instances, hepatic failure with fatal outcome has been reported and generally has been associated with serious underlying diseases and/or concomitant medications.

Allergic reactions ranging from urticaria and mild skin eruptions to anaphylaxis and Stevens-Johnson syndrome/toxic epidermal necrolysis have occurred with orally administered clarithromycin.

There have been rare reports of pancreatitis and convulsions.

Of the 1829 patients who received clarithromycin for oral suspension, 571 (31%) reported at least one adverse event. The adverse events reported are summarized in Table 12.

The majority of the patients reported adverse event in the Gastrointestinal disorders system organ class (SOC) (19%), and the Infections and infestations SOC (9%).

The events occurring most frequently in the Gastrointestinal disorder SOC were diarrhea (7%), vomiting (7%), abdominal pain (3%), dyspepsia (3%) and nausea (1%).

Other adverse events included infection (3%), rhinitis (2.2%), rash (2.2%), increased cough (2.1%), fever (2.2%), headache (1.6%), conjunctivitis (1.1%), dysgeusia(3%) and transient elevation of AST (0.9%).

The majority of adverse events were considered by the investigators to have either mild or moderate severity. 375/1829 patients (21%) had a mild adverse events, 175/1829 patients (10%) had moderate adverse events and 20/1829 patients (1%) had severe adverse events.

In the two U.S. acute otitis media studies of clarithromycin versus antimicrobial/beta-lactamase inhibitor, the incidence of adverse events in all patients treated, primarily diarrhea (15% vs. 38%) and diaper rash (3% vs.11%) in young children, was clinically or statistically lower in the clarithromycin arm versus the control arm.

In another U.S. otitis media study of clarithromycin versus cephalosporin, the incidence of adverse events in all patients treated, primarily diarrhea and vomiting, did not differ clinically or statistically for the two agents.

Table 11: BIAXIN BID

Rank-Order of Adverse Events for Patients who Received Clarithromycin and Omeprazole

System Organ Class	Adverse Event[a]	Number (%) of Patients
Nervous System Disorders	Dysgeusia	53 (15%)
	Headache	16 (5%)
	Dizziness	7 (2%)
Gastrointestinal Disorders	Nausea	18 (5%)
	Diarrhea	15 (4%)
	Vomiting	12 (3%)
	Abdominal pain	11 (3%)
	Tongue discoloration	8 (2%)
	Constipation	5 (1%)
	Dry mouth	4 (1%)
Infections and Infestations	Infection	9 (3%)
	Rhinitis	7 (2%)
	Pharyngitis	5 (1%)
General Disorders and Administration Site Conditions	Pain	6 (2%)
	Asthenia	4 (1%)
	Chills	4 (1%)
	Influenza	4 (1%)
Musculoskelatal and Connective Tissue Disorders	Back pain	5 (1%)
Skin and Subcutaneous Tissue Disorders	Rash	4 (1%)

[a] Events reported in at least 1% of the clarithromycin/omeprazole population.

Table 12: BIAXIN

Adverse Events Reported in Pediatric Clinical Trials

System Organ Class	Number (%) of Patients N=1829
Infections and Infestations	172 (9%)
Neoplasms Benign, Malignant and Unspecified (Including Cysts And Polyps)	1 (<1%)
Blood and The Lymphatic System Disorders	14 (<1%)
Metabolism and Nutrition Disorders	9 (<1%)
Psychiatric Disorders	12 (0.7%)
Nervous System Disorders	41 (2%)
Eye Disorders	22 (1%)
Ear and Labyrinth Disorders	25 (1%)
Vascular Disorders	2 (<1%)
Respiratory, Thoracic and Mediastinal Disorders	61 (3%)
Gastrointestinal Disorders	355 (19%)
Skin and Subcutaneous Disorders	66 (4%)
Musculoskeletal and Connective Tissue Disorders	2 (<1%)
Renal and Urinary Disorders	5 (<1%)
Reproductive System and Breast Disorders	2 (<1%)
General Disorders and Administration Site Conditions	56 (3%)
Investigations	29 (2%)
Injury, Poisoning and Procedural Complications	19 (1%)
Total[a]	571 (31%)

[a] Patients with more than one event within a system organ class are only counted once in the total for that system organ class. Patients with events in more than one system organ class are counted only once in the overall total.

Post-Market Adverse Drug Reactions: The following list of adverse events is a compilation of adverse reactions from Post-marketing Surveillance and Post-marketing Clinical Studies for all clarithromycin formulations. See Table 13.

Table 13: BIAXIN/BIAXIN BID/BIAXIN XL

Post-Market Adverse Drug Reactions

System Organ Class	Adverse Event
Blood and Lymphatic System Disorders	Leukopenia Thrombocytopenia
Cardiac Disorders[a]	Electrocardiogram QT prolonged Ventricular tachycardia Torsades de pointes
Gastrointestinal Disorders	Dyspepsia Vomiting Glossitis Stomatitis Tongue discoloration Tooth discoloration Pancreatitis
Infections and Infestations	Candidiasis
Hepatobiliary Disorders	Hepatic function abnormal Hepatitis Hepatitis cholestatic Hepatic failure[b] Jaundice (cholestatic and hepatocellular)
Investigations	Increased liver enzymes
Metabolism and Nutrition Disorders	Hypoglycemia[c]
Nervous System Disorders	Dizziness Vertigo Alteration of sense of smell Convulsions Ageusia Anosmia
Psychiatric Disorders	Anxiety Insomnia Bad dreams Confusion Disorientation Hallucination Psychosis Depersonalization Depression
Skin and Subcutaneous Tissue Disorders	Urticaria Mild skin eruptions Stevens-Johnson syndrome Toxic epidermal necrosis
Immune System Disorders	Anaphylaxis Myasthenia gravis
Ear and Labyrinth Disorders	Tinnitus Hearing loss[d]
Renal and Urinary Disorders	Interstitial nephritis

[a] As with other macrolides, QT prolongation, ventricular tachycardia, and torsades de pointes have been reported with clarithromycin.
[b] Hepatic dysfunction may be severe and is usually reversible. Hepatic failure with fatal outcome has been reported and generally has been associated with serious underlying diseases and/or concomitant medications.
[c] There have been reports of hypoglycemia, some of which have occurred in patients on concomitant oral hypoglycemic agents or insulin.
[d] There have been reports of hearing loss with clarithromycin which is usually reversible upon withdrawal of therapy.

Colchicine: There have been post-marketing reports of colchicine toxicity with concomitant use of clarithromycin and colchicine, especially in the elderly, some of which occurred in patients with renal insufficiency. Deaths have been reported in some such patients (see Warnings and Precautions, General and Drug Interactions, Drug-Drug Interactions).

DRUG INTERACTIONS:

Serious Drug Interactions

- Concomitant administration of clarithromycin with astemizole, cisapride, pimozide, terfenadine, ergotamine, or dihydroergotamine is contraindicated (see Contraindications and Drug Interactions, Drug-Drug Interactions).
- Clarithromycin is an inhibitor of the cytochrome P450 3A isoform subfamily (CYP3A) and the P-glycoprotein transporter (P-gp). The concomitant administration of clarithromycin and drugs metabolized by CYP3A and/or transported by P-gp may lead to an increase in the plasma concentrations of the co-administered drug which could result in clinically significant safety concerns.

Overview: Many categories of drugs are metabolized by CYP3A and/or transported by P-gp located in the liver and in the intestine. Some drugs may inhibit or induce the activities of CYP3A and/or P-gp. Administration of such inhibitors or inducers may impact upon the metabolism. In some cases serum concentrations may be increased and in others decreased. Care must therefore be exercised when co-administering such drugs.

Effects of Clarithromycin on Other Drugs: Clarithromycin is an inhibitor of CYP3A and P-gp. This inhibition may lead to increased or prolonged serum levels of those drugs also metabolized by CYP3A or transported by P-gp when co-administered with clarithromycin. For such drugs the monitoring of their serum concentrations may be necessary.

Clarithromycin should be used with caution in patients receiving treatment with other drugs known to be CYP3A and/or P-gp substrates, especially if the CYP3A/P-gp substrate has a narrow safety margin (e.g., carbamazepine) and/or the substrate is extensively metabolized by CYP3A or transported by P-gp. Dosage adjustments may be considered, and when possible, serum concentrations of these drugs should be monitored closely in patients concurrently receiving clarithromycin.

With certain drugs, co-administration of clarithromycin should be avoided, e.g. oral midazolam (see Table 14).

Effects of Other Drugs on Clarithromycin: Clarithromycin is a substrate of CYP3A. Co-administration of strong inducers of the cytochrome P450 metabolism system may accelerate the metabolism of clarithromycin and thus lower exposure to clarithromycin while increasing exposure to its metabolite 14-OH-clarithromycin which could impair the intended therapeutic effect. Co-administration of potent CYP3A inhibitors may lead to increased exposure to clarithromycin and decreased exposure to its metabolite 14-OH-clarithromycin. Clarithromycin dosage adjustment or consideration of alternative treatments may be required.

Bi-Directional Drug Interactions: Bi-directional drug interactions are complex and may occur if both of the interacting drugs are substrates and inhibitors/ inducers of CYP3A.

Additional Mechanisms: Interactions with clarithromycin have been reported with drugs metabolized by cytochrome P450 isoforms other than CYP3A system. Additional mechanisms, such as effects upon absorption, may also be responsible for interaction between drugs, including zidovudine and clarithromycin.
Drug-Drug Interactions: Some of the drug-drug interactions which have been reported between clarithromycin-macrolides and other drugs or drug categories are listed in Table 14. The drugs listed in this table are based on drug interactions case reports, clinical trials, or potential interactions due to the expected mechanism of the interaction.
Combination Therapy with Omeprazole and/or Amoxicillin: For more information on drug interactions for omeprazole and amoxicillin, refer to their respective Product Monographs, under Drug Interactions.
Drug-Food Interactions: BIAXIN BID (clarithromycin tablets, USP, film-coated) and BIAXIN (clarithromycin for oral suspension, USP) may be given with or without meals. BIAXIN XL (clarithromycin extended-release tablets) must be taken with food.
Drug-Herb Interactions: Interactions with herbal products have not been established.
Drug-Laboratory Test Interactions: Interactions with laboratory tests have not been established.

DOSAGE AND ADMINISTRATION:

Dosing Considerations: BIAXIN BID (clarithromycin tablets, USP, film-coated) and BIAXIN (clarithromycin for oral suspension, USP) may be given with or without meals. BIAXIN XL (clarithromycin extended-release tablets) must be taken with food.

In patients with both hepatic and renal impairments or in the presence of severe renal impairment, decreased dosage of clarithromycin or prolonged dosing intervals might be appropriate (see Dosage and Administration, Recommended Dose and Dosage Adjustment).

In children with renal impairment and a creatinine clearance less than 30 mL/min, the dosage of BIAXIN should be reduced by one-half, i.e., up to 250 mg once daily, or 250 mg twice daily in more severe infections. Dosage should not be continued beyond 14 days in these patients.

Recommended Dose and Dosage Adjustment: BIAXIN BID (clarithromycin tablets, USP, film-coated): Adults with Respiratory Tract or Skin Infections: The adult dosage of BIAXIN BID is 250 mg to 500 mg every 12 hours (see Table 15) for 7 to 14 days. For infections caused by less susceptible organisms, the upper dosage should be used.

In the treatment of Group A streptococcus infections, therapy should be continued for 10 days. The usual drug of choice in the treatment of streptococcal infections and the prophylaxis of rheumatic fever is penicillin administered by either the i.m or the oral route.

Clarithromycin is generally effective in the eradication of *S. pyogenes* from the nasopharynx; however, data establishing the efficacy of clarithromycin in the subsequent prevention of rheumatic fever are not presently available.

Renal Impairment: In patients with renal impairment and a creatinine clearance less than 30 mL/min., the dosage of BIAXIN BID should be reduced by one-half, i.e., 250 mg once daily, or 250 mg twice daily in more severe infections. Dosage should not be continued beyond 14 days in these patients. The safety and efficacy of 500 mg clarithromycin in patients with severe renal impairment has not been established.

Table 14: BIAXIN/BIAXIN BID/BIAXIN XL
Established or Potential Drug-Drug Interactions

Clarithromycin	Ref	Effect	Clinical Comments
Astemizole/ Terfenadine	CT	terfenadine-acid metabolite concentrations increase ↑ QT interval	Macrolides have been reported to alter the metabolism of terfenadine resulting in increased serum levels of terfenadine which has occasionally been associated with cardiac arrhythmias such as QT prolongation, ventricular tachycardia, ventricular fibrillation and torsade de pointes (see Contraindications). In a study involving 14 healthy volunteers, the concomitant administration of BIAXIN BID tablets and terfenadine resulted in a two to three-fold increase in the serum levels of the acid metabolite of terfenadine, MDL 16, 455, and in prolongation of the QT interval. Similar effects have been observed with concomitant administration of astemizole and other macrolides.
Atazanavir	CT	↑ clarithromycin levels ↑ atazanavir AUC	Both clarithromycin and atazanavir are substrates and inhibitors of CYP3A, and there is evidence of a bi-directional drug interaction. Co-administration of clarithromycin (500 mg twice daily) with atazanavir (400 mg once daily) resulted in a 2-fold increase in exposure to clarithromycin and a 70% decrease in exposure to 14-OH-clarithromycin, with a 28% increase in the AUC of atazanavir. Because of the large therapeutic window for clarithromycin, no dosage reduction should be necessary in patients with normal renal function. For patients with moderate renal function (creatinine clearance 30 to 60 mL/min), the dose of clarithromycin should be decreased by 50%. For patients with creatinine clearance <30 mL/min, the dose of clarithromycin should be decreased by 75% using an appropriate clarithromycin formulation. Doses of clarithromycin greater than 1000 mg per day should not be co-administered with protease inhibitors.
Carbamazepine	C	↑ levels of carbamazepine	Clarithromycin administration in patients receiving carbamazepine has been reported to cause increased levels of carbamazepine. Blood level monitoring of carbamazepine may be considered.
Cisapride/Pimozide	C	↑ levels of cisapride ↑ levels of pimozide	Elevated cisapride levels have been reported in patients receiving clarithromycin and cisapride concomitantly. This may result in QT prolongation and cardiac arrhythmias including ventricular tachycardia, ventricular fibrillation and torsade de pointes. Similar effects have been observed in patients taking clarithromycin and pimozide concomitantly (see Contraindications).
Colchicine	C	Potential colchicine toxicity	Colchicine is a substrate for both CYP3A and the efflux transporter, P-glycoprotein (Pgp). Clarithromycin and other macrolides are known to inhibit CYP3A and Pgp. When clarithromycin and colchicine are administered together, inhibition of Pgp and/or CYP3A by clarithromycin may lead to increased exposure to colchicine. Patients should be monitored for clinical symptoms of colchicine toxicity (see Warnings and Precautions, General and Adverse Reactions, Post-Market Adverse Drug Reactions).
Cyclosporine	C	↑ levels of cyclosporine	There have been reports of elevated cyclosporine serum concentrations when clarithromycin and cyclosporine are used concurrently. Cyclosporine levels should be monitored and the dosage should be adjusted as necessary. Patients should also be monitored for increased cyclosporine toxicity.
Didanosine	CT	No change in didanosine pharmacokinetics in HIV-infected patients (n=12)	Simultaneous administration of BIAXIN BID tablets and didanosine to 12 HIV-infected adult patients resulted in no statistically significant change in didanosine pharmacokinetics.

(cont'd)

Table 14: BIAXIN/BIAXIN BID/BIAXIN XL *(cont'd)*
Established or Potential Drug-Drug Interactions

Clarithromycin	Ref	Effect	Clinical Comments
Digoxin	C	↑ levels of digoxin	Digoxin is thought to be a substrate for the efflux transporter, P-gp. Clarithromycin is known to inhibit P-gp. When clarithromycin and digoxin are administered together, inhibition of P-gp by clarithromycin may lead to increased exposure to digoxin. Elevated digoxin serum concentrations have been reported in patients receiving BIAXIN BID tablets and digoxin concomitantly. In post-marketing surveillance some patients have shown clinical signs consistent with digoxin toxicity, including potentially fatal arrhythmias. Serum digoxin levels should be carefully monitored while patients are receiving digoxin and clarithromycin simultaneously.
Disopyramide/ Quinidine	C	↑ levels of disopyramide, resulting ventricular fibrillation and QT prolongation (rarely reported) Torsades de pointes	Increased disopyramide plasma levels, resulting in ventricular fibrillation and QT prolongation, coincident with the co-administration of disopyramide and clarithromycin have rarely been reported. There have been post-marketed reports of torsades de pointes occurring with concurrent use of clarithromycin and quinidine or disopyramide. Electrocardiograms should be monitored for QTc prolongation during co-administration of clarithromycin with these drugs. Serum levels of these medications should be monitored during clarithromycin therapy.
Ergotamine/ Dihydroergotamine	C	Potential ischemic reactions Potential ergot toxicity	Post-marketing reports indicate that co-administration of clarithromycin with ergotamine or dihydroergotamine has been associated with acute ergot toxicity characterized by severe peripheral vasospasm, dysesthesia, and ischemia of the extremities and other tissues including the central nervous system. Concomitant administration of clarithromycin and these medicinal products is contraindicated (see Contraindications).
Fluconazole	CT	↑ clarithromycin C_{min} and AUC	Concomitant administration of fluconazole 200 mg daily and clarithromycin 500 mg twice daily to 21 healthy volunteers led to increases in the mean steady-state clarithromycin C_{min} and AUC of 33% and 18%, respectively. Steady-state concentrations of 14-OH clarithromycin were not significantly affected by concomitant administration of fluconazole. No clarithromycin dose adjustment is necessary.
Itraconazole	CT, P	↑ levels of clarithromycin ↑ levels of itraconazole	Both clarithromycin and itraconazole are substrates and inhibitors of CYP3A, leading to a bidirectional drug interaction. Clarithromycin may increase the plasma levels of itraconazole, while itraconazole may increase the plasma levels of clarithromycin. Patients taking itraconazole and clarithromycin concomitantly should be monitored closely for signs or symptoms of increased or prolonged pharmacologic effect.
Lansoprazole/ Omeprazole	CT	Mild change of lansoprazole and 14-OH clarithromycin concentrations	One study demonstrated that concomitant administration of clarithromycin and lansoprazole resulted in mild changes of serum concentrations of lansoprazole and 14-OH clarithromycin. However, no dosage adjustment is considered necessary based on these data.
		↑ omeprazole C_{max} and AUC_{0-24}	Clarithromycin 500 mg three times daily was given in combination with omeprazole 40 mg once daily to healthy subjects. The steady-state plasma concentrations of omeprazole were increased (i.e., C_{max}, AUC_{0-24}, and $t_{1/2}$ increased by 30%, 89%, and 34%, respectively), by concomitant administration of clarithromycin. The mean 24-hour gastric pH value was 5.2 when omeprazole was administered alone and 5.7 when co-administered with clarithromycin.
		↑ levels of clarithromycin	To a lesser extent, omeprazole administration increases the serum concentrations of clarithromycin. Omeprazole administration also increases tissue and mucus concentrations of clarithromycin.
Lovastatin/ Simvastatin	C	Rhabdomyolysis (rarely reported)	Rhabdomyolysis coincident with the co-administration of clarithromycin and the HMG-CoA reductase inhibitors, lovastatin and simvastatin, has rarely been reported.
Atorvastatin	C		Concurrent use of atorvastatin and clarithromycin may result in increased atorvastatin exposure and an increased risk of rhabdomyolysis.
Ritonavir/Indinavir	CT	↑ clarithromycin C_{max}, C_{min}, and AUC	A pharmacokinetic study demonstrated that the concomitant administration of ritonavir 200 mg q8h and clarithromycin 500 mg q12h resulted in a marked inhibition of the metabolism of clarithromycin. The clarithromycin C_{max} increased by 31%, C_{min} increased 182% and AUC increased by 77% with concomitant administration of ritonavir. An essentially complete inhibition of the formation of 14-[R]-hydroxy-clarithromycin was noted. Because of the large therapeutic window for clarithromycin, no dosage reduction should be necessary in patients with normal renal function. However, for patients with renal impairment, the following dosage adjustments should be considered: For patients with CL_{CR} 30 to 60 mL/min the dose of clarithromycin should be reduced by 50%. For patients with CL_{CR} <30 mL/min the dose of clarithromycin should be decreased by 75%. Doses of clarithromycin greater than 1g/day should not be co-administered with ritonavir.
		↑ indinavir AUC ↑ clarithromycin AUC	One study demonstrated that the concomitant administration of clarithromycin and indinavir resulted in a metabolic interaction; the clarithromycin AUC increased by 53% and the indinavir AUC was increased by 20%, but the individual variation was large. No dose adjustment is necessary with normal renal function.

(cont'd)

Table 14: BIAXIN/BIAXIN BID/BIAXIN XL *(cont'd)*

Established or Potential Drug-Drug Interactions

Clar-ithromycin	Ref	Effect	Clinical Comments
Saquinavir	CT	↑ saquinavir AUC and C_{max} ↑ clarithromycin AUC	Both clarithromycin and saquinavir are substrates and inhibitors of CYP3A, and there is evidence of a bi-directional drug interaction. Concomitant administration of clarithromycin (500 mg bid) and saquinavir (soft gelatin capsules, 1200 mg tid) to 12 healthy volunteers resulted in steady-state AUC and C_{max} values of saquinavir which were 177% and 187% higher than those seen with saquinavir alone. Clarithromycin AUC and C_{max} values were approximately 40% higher than those seen with clarithromycin alone. No dose adjustment is required when the two drugs are co-administered for a limited time at the doses/ formulations studied. Observations from drug interaction studies using the soft gelatin capsule formulation may not be representative of the effects seen using the saquinavir hard gelatin capsule. Observations from drug interaction studies performed with saquinavir alone may not be representative of the effects seen with saquinavir/ ritonavir therapy. When saquinavir is co-administered with ritonavir, consideration should be given to the potential effects of ritonavir on clarithromycin.
Tacrolimus	P	Potential ↑ in tacrolimus concentrations	Concomitant administration of tacrolimus and clarithromycin may result in increased plasma levels of tacrolimus and increased risk of toxicity.
Theophylline	P	Potential ↑ in theophylline concentrations	Clarithromycin use in patients who are receiving theophylline may be associated with an increase of serum theophylline concentrations. Monitoring of serum theophylline concentrations should be considered for patients receiving high doses of theophylline or with baseline concentrations in the upper therapeutic range.
Tolterodine	P	↑ serum tolterodine concentrations	The primary route of metabolism for tolterodine is via the 2D6 isoform of cytochrome P450 (CYP2D6). However, in a subset of the population devoid of CYP2D6, the identified pathway of metabolism is via CYP3A. In this population subset, inhibition of CYP3A results in significantly higher serum concentrations of tolterodine. A reduction of tolterodine dosage may be necessary in the presence of CYP3A inhibitors, such as clarithromycin in the CYP2D6 poor metabolizer population.
Verapamil	C	Potential ↑ in verapamil concentrations	Hypotension, bradyarrhythmias, and lactic acidosis have been observed in patients receiving concurrent verapamil, belonging to the calcium channel blockers drug class.
Warfarin/ Aceno-coumarol	C	↑ anticoagulant effect	There have been reports of increased anticoagulant effect when clarithromycin and oral anticoagulants are used concurrently. Anticoagulant parameters should be closely monitored. Adjustment of the anticoagulant dose may be necessary. Clarithromycin has also been reported to increase the anticoagulant effect of acenocoumarol.
Zidovudine	C	Potential ↓ in zidovudine concentrations	Simultaneous oral administration of BIAXIN BID tablets and zidovudine to HIV-infected adult patients may result in decreased steady-state zidovudine concentrations. Clarithromycin appears to interfere with the absorption of simultaneously administered oral zidovudine, and therefore, this interaction can be largely avoided by staggering the doses of clarithromycin and zidovudine. This interaction does not appear to occur in pediatric HIV-infected patients taking clarithromycin suspension with zidovudine or dideoxyinosine. Similar interaction studies have not been conducted with clarithromycin extended-release (ER) and zidovudine.
Phospho-diesterase Inhibitors	P	↑ phosphodiesterase inhibitor exposure	Sildenafil, tadalafil, and vardenafil are metabolized, at least in part, by CYP3A, and CYP3A may be inhibited by concomitantly administered clarithromycin. Co-administration of clarithromycin with sildenafil, tadalafil or vardenafil would likely result in increased phosphodiesterase inhibitor exposure. Reduction of sildenafil, tadalafil and vardenafil dosages should be considered when these drugs are co-administered with clarithromycin.
Triazolobenzo-diazepines	CT, C, P	↑ midazolam AUC	When midazolam was co-administered with clarithromycin tablets (500 mg twice daily), midazolam AUC was increased 2.7-fold after intravenous administration of midazolam and 7-fold after oral administration. Concomitant administration of oral midazolam and clarithromycin should be avoided. If intravenous midazolam is co-administered with clarithromycin, the patient must be closely monitored to allow dose adjustment of midazolam. The same precautions should also apply to other benzodiazepines that are metabolized by CYP3A, including triazolam and alprazolam. For benzodiazepines which are not dependent on CYP3A for their elimination (temazepam, nitrazepam, lorazepam), a clinically important interaction with clarithromycin is unlikely. There have been post-marketing reports of drug interactions and central nervous system (CNS) effects (e.g., somnolence and confusion) with the concomitant use of clarithromycin and triazolam. Monitoring the patient for increased CNS pharmacological effects is suggested.
Others/Drugs Metabolized by CYP3A	C/P	Potential increase in serum concentration	Interactions with erythromycin and/or clarithromycin have been reported with a number of other drugs metabolized by CYP3A, such as alfentanil, bromocriptine, cilostazol, methylprednisolone, or vinblastine. Serum concentrations of drugs metabolized by CYP3A should be monitored closely in patients concurrently receiving erythromycin or clarithromycin.

(cont'd)

Table 14: BIAXIN/BIAXIN BID/BIAXIN XL *(cont'd)*

Established or Potential Drug-Drug Interactions

Clar-ithromycin	Ref	Effect	Clinical Comments
Others/Drugs Metabolized by Cytochrome P450 Isoforms other than CYP3A	C/P	Potential change in serum concentration	Interactions with erythromycin and/or clarithromycin have been reported with drugs metabolized by other cytochrome P450 isoforms (i.e., not CYP3A), such as hexobarbital, phenytoin, and valproate. Serum concentrations of these drugs should be monitored closely in patients concurrently receiving erythromycin or clarithromycin.
Others/Drug Inducers of the Cytochrome P450 System	CT, P	↓ levels of clarithromycin ↑ levels of rifabutin	Strong inducers of the cytochrome P450 metabolism system such as efavirenz, nevirapine, rifampin, rifabutin, and rifapentine[a] may accelerate the metabolism of clarithromycin and thus lower the plasma levels of clarithromycin, while increasing those of 14-OH-clarithromycin, a metabolite that is also microbiologically active. Since the microbiological activities of clarithromycin and 14-OH-clarithromycin are different for different bacteria, the intended therapeutic effect could be impaired during concomitant administration of clarithromycin and enzyme inducers. Clarithromycin has been reported to increase serum and tissue concentration of rifabutin and thus may increase the risk of toxicity.

[a] Not marketed in Canada.
Interactions with other drugs have not been established.
Legend: C=case study; CT=clinical trial; P=potential.

Table 15: BIAXIN BID

Adult Dosage Guidelines

Infection	Dosage (b.i.d.)	Duration
Upper Respiratory Tract	**250–500 mg**	
Pharyngitis/tonsillitis	250 mg	10 days
Acute maxillary sinusitis	500 mg	7–14 days
Lower Respiratory Tract	**250–500 mg**	
Acute exacerbation of chronic bronchitis and pneumonia	250–500 mg	7–14 days
Uncomplicated Skin and Skin Structure Infections	**250 mg**	7–14 days

Hepatic Impairment: In patients with both hepatic and renal impairments or in the presence of severe renal impairment, decreased dosage of clarithromycin or prolonged dosing intervals may be appropriate. Clarithromycin may be administered without dosage adjustment in the presence of hepatic impairment if there is normal renal function.

Eradication of *H. Pylori*: Triple Therapy: BIAXIN BID/omeprazole/amoxicillin: The recommended dose is clarithromycin 500 mg b.i.d. in conjunction with amoxicillin 1 g b.i.d. and omeprazole 20 mg daily for 10 days.

For more information on omeprazole or amoxicillin, refer to their respective Product Monographs, under Dosage and Administration.

(For additional information on the use of BIAXIN BID in triple therapy for the treatment of *H. pylori* infection and active duodenal ulcer recurrence, refer to the Hp-PAC Product Monograph.)

Dual Therapy: BIAXIN BID/omeprazole: In patients who are sensitive to penicillin-based therapy (e.g. amoxicillin), dual therapy with clarithromycin and omeprazole may provide a feasible alternative.

The recommended dose is clarithromycin 500 mg t.i.d plus omeprazole 40 mg q.d. for 14 days, followed by 20 mg omeprazole q.d. for 14 days.

Optimal therapeutic regimens consisting of a shorter treatment duration for the eradication of *H. pylori* are yet to be determined.

Adults with Mycobacterial Infections: Prophylaxis: The recommended dose of BIAXIN BID for the prevention of disseminated *M. avium* disease is 500 mg b.i.d.

Treatment: Clarithromycin is recommended as the primary agent for the treatment of disseminated infection due to MAC. Clarithromycin should be used in combination with other antimycobacterial drugs which have shown in vitro activity against MAC, including ethambutol and rifampin. Although no controlled clinical trial information is available for combination therapy with clarithromycin, the U.S. Public Health Service Task Force has provided recommendations for the treatment of MAC.

The recommended dose for mycobacterial infections in adults is 500 mg b.i.d.

Treatment of disseminated MAC infections in AIDS patients should continue for life if clinical and mycobacterial improvement are observed.

BIAXIN XL (clarithromycin extended-release tablets): Adults with Respiratory Tract Infection: The adult dosage is 1000 mg every 24 hours for 5, 7 or 14 days. Clarithromycin extended-release tablets must be taken with food. Clarithromycin extended-release tablets should be swallowed whole and not chewed, broken or crushed. Table 16 provides dosage guidelines.

Table 16: BIAXIN XL

Adult Dosage Guidelines

Infection	Dosage (Once daily)	Duration (days)
Acute maxillary sinusitis	1000 mg	14
Acute bacterial exacerbation of chronic bronchitis	1000 mg	5 or 7
Community-acquired pneumonia	1000 mg	7

Renal Impairment: Based on a study done with BIAXIN BID, patients with severe renal impairment (CR_{CL} <30 mL/min) have greater clarithromycin exposure than patients with normal renal function (CR_{CL} ≥80 mL/min). Clarithromycin C_{max} was about 3.3 times higher and AUC was about 4.2 times higher in the patients with severe renal impairment. The maximum daily clarithromycin dose for patients with severe renal impairment is 500 mg. The safety and efficacy of 500 mg clarithromycin in patients with severe renal impairment has not been established.

In the same study, patients with moderate renal impairment (CR_{CL} 30-79 mL/min) had greater clarithromycin exposure than patients with normal renal function, but the elevations were much less than those observed in severe renal impairment. Compared to the subjects with normal renal function, the clarithromycin C_{max} was about 52% higher and the AUC was about 74% higher in the patients with moderate renal impairment. No clarithromycin dose adjustment is required for patients with moderate renal impairment.

Hepatic Impairment: Based on studies done with BIAXIN BID, no adjustment of dosage is necessary for subjects with moderate or severe hepatic impairment but with normal renal function.

BIAXIN (clarithromycin for oral suspension, USP): The recommended daily dosage of BIAXIN (clarithromycin for oral suspension, USP) is 15 mg/kg/day, in divided doses every 12 hours, not to exceed 1000 mg/day. The usual duration of treatment is for 5 to 10 days depending on the pathogen involved and the severity of the condition. Treatment for pharyngitis caused by Streptococcal spp. should be 10 days.

In children with renal impairment and a creatinine clearance less than 30 mL/min, the dosage of BIAXIN should be reduced by one-half, i.e., up to 250 mg once daily, or 250 mg twice daily in more severe infections. Dosage should not be continued beyond 14 days in these patients.

Table 17 is a suggested guide for determining dosage.

Table 17: BIAXIN

BIAXIN Oral Suspension. Pediatric Dosage Guidelines. Based on Body Weight in kg

	125 mg/5 mL	250 mg/5 mL
Weight[a]	**Dosage (mL) given twice daily**	**Dosage (mL) given twice daily**
8–11 kg (1–2 years)[b]	2.5	1.25
12–19 kg (2–4 years)	5	2.5
20–29 kg (4–8 years)	7.5	3.75
30–40 kg (8–12 years)	10	5

[a] Children <8 kg should be dosed on a per kg basis (approximately 7.5 mg/kg b.i.d.). .
[b] Approximate ages.

Children with Mycobacterial Infections: Clarithromycin is recommended as the primary agent for the treatment of disseminated infection due to MAC. Clarithromycin should be used in combination with other antimycobacterial drugs which have shown in vitro activity against MAC, including ethambutol and rifampin. Although no controlled clinical trial information is available for combination therapy with clarithromycin, the U.S. Public Health Service Task Force has provided recommendations for the treatment of MAC.

In children, the recommended dose is 7.5 mg/kg b.i.d. up to 500 mg b.i.d. clarithromycin per day in two divided doses. Dosing recommendations for children are shown in Table 17.

Treatment of disseminated MAC infections in AIDS patients should continue for life if clinical and mycobacterial improvement are observed.

Missed Dose: If a dose of clarithromycin is missed, the patient should take the dose as soon as possible and then return to their normal scheduled dose. However, if a dose is skipped, the patient should not double the next dose.

Administration: BIAXIN BID may be taken with or without food.

BIAXIN XL (clarithromycin extended-release tablets) must be taken with food. The tablets should be swallowed whole and not chewed, broken or crushed.

BIAXIN (clarithromycin for oral suspension, USP) may be taken with or without food.

Directions for Reconstitution: 125 mg/5 mL: 150 mL size: 79 mL of water should be added to the granules in the bottle and shaken to yield 150 mL of reconstituted suspension.

105 mL size: 55 mL of water should be added to the granules in the bottle and shaken to yield 105 mL of reconstituted suspension.

55 mL size: 29 mL of water should be added to the granules in the bottle and shaken to yield 55 mL of reconstituted suspension.

Directions for Reconstitution: 250 mg/5 mL: 105 mL size: 54 mL of water should be added to the granules in the bottle and shaken to yield 105 mL of reconstituted suspension.

Shake well before use. The reconstituted suspension must not be refrigerated. Any reconstituted unused medication should be discarded after 14 days. The graduated syringe included in the package should be rinsed between uses. Do not leave syringe in bottle. Do not store reconstituted suspension in syringe.

OVERDOSAGE:

Reports indicate that the ingestion of large amounts of clarithromycin can be expected to produce gastrointestinal symptoms. Adverse reactions accompanying overdosage should be treated by the prompt elimination of unabsorbed drug and supportive measures.

Clarithromycin is protein bound (70%). No data are available on the elimination of clarithromycin by hemodialysis or peritoneal dialysis.

> For management of a suspected drug overdose, contact your **regional Poison Control Centre**. See the *CPS* Directory section for a list of Poison Control Centres.

ACTION AND CLINICAL PHARMACOLOGY: Mechanism of Action: General: Clarithromycin exerts its antibacterial action by binding to the 50S ribosomal subunit of susceptible bacteria and suppressing protein synthesis.

Pharmacodynamics: Eradication of *H. pylori*: *H. pylori* is now established as a major etiological factor in duodenal ulcer disease. The presence of *H. pylori* may damage the mucosal integrity due to the production of enzymes (catalase, lipases, phospholipases, proteases, and urease), adhesins and toxins; the generated inflammatory response contributes to mucosal damage.

The concomitant administration of an antimicrobial(s) such as clarithromycin and an antisecretory agent, improves the eradication of *H. pylori* as compared to individual drug administration. The higher pH resulting from antisecretory treatment, optimizes the environment for the pharmacologic action of the antimicrobial agent(s) against *H. pylori*.

Pharmacokinetics: Clarithromycin Tablets, USP, film-coated: A summary of clarithromycin pharmacokinetic parameters following the administration of clarithromycin film-coated tablets is provided in Table 18.

Table 18: BIAXIN BID

Clarithromycin Pharmacokinetic Parameters Following the Administration of Clarithromycin Film-coated Tablets

	C_{max} (mg/L)	t_{max} (hr)	$t_{½}$ (hr)	AUC_{0-t} (mg·hr/L)
Single Dose				
250 mg				
Mean	1	1.5	2.7	5.47
500 mg				
Mean	1.77	2.2	—	11.66
Multiple Doses				
250 mg b.i.d.				
Mean	1	—	3 to 4	6.34
500 mg b.i.d.				
Mean	3.38	2.1	5 to 7	44.19

Clarithromycin Extended-Release Tablets: A summary of clarithromycin pharmacokinetic parameters following the administration of clarithromycin extended-release tablets is provided in Table 19.

Table 19: BIAXIN XL

Clarithromycin Pharmacokinetic Parameters Following the Administration of Clarithromycin Extended-Release Tablets

	C_{max} (mg/L)	t_{max} (hr)	AUC_{0-t} (mg·hr/L)
2×500 mg once daily			
Mean (fasting conditions)	2.21	5.5	33.72
2×500 mg once daily			
Mean (fed conditions)	3.77	5.6	48.09

Clarithromycin for Oral Suspension, USP: A summary of clarithromycin pharmacokinetic parameters in adult volunteers following the administration of clarithromycin for oral suspension is provided in Table 20.

Table 20: BIAXIN

Clarithromycin Pharmacokinetic Parameters in Adult Subjects Following the Administration of Clarithromycin for Oral Suspension

250 mg/10 mL	C_{max} (mg/L)	t_{max} (hr)	$t_{½}$ (hr)	$AUC_{0-\infty}$ (mg·hr/L)
Mean (fasting conditions)	1.24	3.3	3.7	7.2
Mean (fed conditions)	0.95	5.3	3.7	6.5

A summary of clarithromycin pharmacokinetic parameters in pediatric patients following the administration of clarithromycin for oral suspension is provided in Table 21.

Table 21: BIAXIN

Clarithromycin Pharmacokinetic Parameters in Pediatric Patients Following the Administration of Clarithromycin for Oral Suspension

	C_{max} (mg/L)	t_{max} (hr)	AUC_{0-t} (mg·hr/L)
Single Dose (125 mg/5 mL)			
Mean (fasting conditions)	3.59	3.1	10
Mean (fed conditions)	4.58	2.8	14.2
Multiple Doses (7.5 mg/kg b.i.d.)			
Mean (fasting conditions)	4.6	2.8	15.7

Absorption: Clarithromycin Film-Coated Tablets: The absolute bioavailability of 250 mg and 500 mg clarithromycin tablets is approximately 50%. Food slightly delays the onset of clarithromycin absorption but does not affect the extent of bioavailability. Therefore, BIAXIN BID tablets may be given without regard to meals.

In fasting healthy human subjects, peak serum concentrations are attained within 2 hours after oral dosing. Steady-state peak serum clarithromycin concentrations, which are attained within 2 to 3 days, are approximately 1 mg/L with a 250 mg dose twice daily and 2 to 3 mg/L with a 500 mg dose twice daily. The elimination half-life of clarithromycin is about 3 to 4 hours with 250 mg twice daily dosing but increases to about 5 to 7 hours with 500 mg administered twice daily.

Clarithromycin displays non-linear pharmacokinetics at clinically relevant doses, producing greater than proportional increases in AUC with increasing dose. The degree of non-linearity is reduced on chronic clarithromycin administration (i.e., at steady state). The non-linearity of the pharmacokinetics of the principle metabolite, 14-OH clarithromycin, is slight at the recommended doses of 250 mg and 500 mg administered twice daily. With 250 mg twice daily, 14-OH clarithromycin attains a peak steady state concentration of about 0.6 mg/L and has an elimination half-life of 5 to 6 hours. With a 500 mg twice daily dose, the peak steady-state of 14-OH concentrations of clarithromycin are slightly higher (up to 1 mg/L) and its elimination half-life is about 7 hours. With either dose, the steady-state concentration of this metabolite is generally attained within 2 to 3 days.

Adult Patients with HIV. Steady-state concentrations of clarithromycin and 14-OH clarithromycin observed following administration of 500 mg doses of clarithromycin twice a day to adult patients with HIV infection were similar to those observed in healthy volunteers. However, at the higher clarithromycin doses which may be required to treat mycobacterial infections, clarithromycin concentrations can be much higher than those observed at 500 mg clarithromycin doses. In adult HIV-infected patients taking 2000 mg/day in two divided doses, steady-state clarithromycin C_{max} values ranged from 5 to10 mg/L. C_{max} values as high as 27 mg/L have been observed in HIV-infected adult patients taking 4000 mg/day in two divided doses of clarithromycin tablets.

Elimination half-lives appeared to be lengthened at these higher doses as well. The higher clarithromycin concentrations and longer elimination half-lives observed at these doses are consistent with the known non-linearity in clarithromycin pharmacokinetics.

Clarithromycin and omeprazole. Clarithromycin 500 mg t.i.d. and omeprazole 40 mg q.d. were studied in fasting healthy adult subjects. When clarithromycin was given alone as 500 mg q8h, the mean steady state C_{max} value was approximately 3.8 μg/mL and the mean C_{min} value was approximately 1.8 μg/mL. The mean AUC_{0-8} for clarithromycin was 22.9 μg·hr/mL. The T_{max} and half life were 2.1 hrs and 5.3 hrs, respectively, when clarithromycin was dosed at 500 mg t.i.d. When clarithromycin was administered with omeprazole, increases in omeprazole half-life and AUC_{0-24} were observed. For all subjects combined, the mean omeprazole AUC_{0-24} was 89% greater and the harmonic mean for omeprazole $t_{½}$ was 34% greater when omeprazole was administered with clarithromycin than when omeprazole was administered alone. When clarithromycin was administered with omeprazole, the steady state C_{max}, C_{min}, and AUC_{0-8} of clarithromycin were increased by 10%, 27%, and 15%, respectively over values achieved when clarithromycin was administered with placebo.

Clarithromycin Extended-Release Tablets: Clarithromycin extended-release tablets provided extended absorption of clarithromycin from the gastrointestinal tract after oral administration. Relative to an equal dose of immediate-release clarithromycin film-coated tablets, clarithromycin extended-release tablets provide lower and later steady-state peak plasma concentrations, but equivalent 24-hour AUCs for both clarithromycin and its microbiologically-active metabolite, 14-OH clarithromycin.

While the extent of formation of 14-OH clarithromycin following administration of clarithromycin extended-release tablets (2×500 mg once daily) under steady-state conditions is not affected by food, administration under fasting conditions is associated with approximately 30% lower clarithromycin AUC relative to administration with food. Similarly, single-dose administration of clarithromycin extended-release (500 mg once daily) is associated with a 25% lower clarithromycin AUC relative to administration of clarithromycin immediate-release film-coated tablets (250 mg b.i.d.). Therefore, it is recommended that BIAXIN XL (clarithromycin extended-release tablets be given with food.

Figure 1 illustrates the steady-state clarithromycin plasma concentration-time profile for BIAXIN XL (2×500 mg once daily) relative to BIAXIN (500 mg twice daily).

Figure 1: Biaxin XL

Steady-State Clarithromycin Plasma Concentration-Time Profile for BIAXIN XL (2×500 mg Once Daily) Relative to BIAXIN (500 mg Twice Daily)

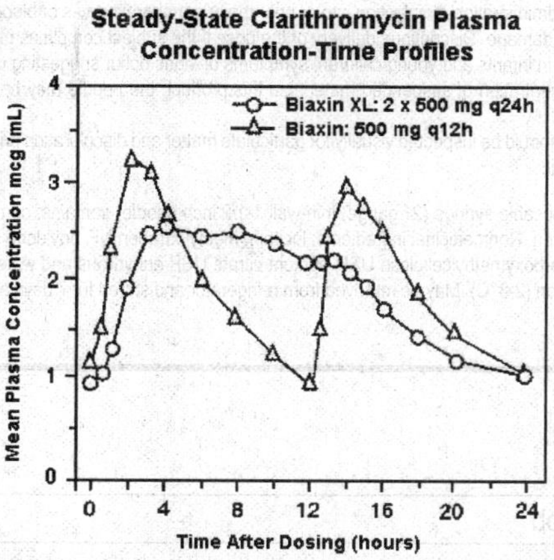

In healthy human subjects, steady-state peak plasma clarithromycin concentrations of approximately 2 to 3 mg/L were achieved about 5 to 8 hours after oral administration of 2×500 mg clarithromycin extended-release tablets once daily; for 14-OH clarithromycin, steady-state peak plasma concentrations of approximately 0.8 mg/L were attained 6 to 9 hours after dosing. Steady-state peak plasma concentrations of approximately 1 to 2 mg/L were achieved about 5 to 6 hours after oral administration of a single 500 mg clarithromycin extended-release tablet once daily; for 14-OH clarithromycin, steady-state peak plasma concentrations of approximately 0.6 mg/L were attained about 6 hours after dosing.

Clarithromycin for Oral Suspension, USP: Adult Volunteers. Single and multiple dose adult volunteer studies showed that the suspension formulation was not significantly different from the tablet formulation in terms of C_{max} of clarithromycin and AUC, although the onset and/or rate of absorption of the suspension formulation was slower than that of the tablet. As with the tablet formulation, steady state is achieved by the fifth dose of a 12 hour multiple-dose suspension regimen.

Children. In children taking 15 to 30 mg/kg/day in two divided doses, steady-state clarithromycin C_{max} values generally ranged from 8 to 20 µg/mL. C_{max} values as high as 23 µg/mL have been observed in HIV-infected pediatric patients taking 30 mg/kg/day in two divided doses. In children requiring antibiotic therapy, administration of 7.5 mg/kg q12h doses of clarithromycin as the suspension generally resulted in steady-state peak plasma concentrations of 3 to 7 µg/mL for clarithromycin, and 1 to 2 µg/mL for 14-OH clarithromycin. In HIV-infected children taking 15 mg/kg every 12 hours, steady-state clarithromycin peak concentrations generally ranged from 6 to 15 µg/mL A single and multiple dose study conducted in pediatric patients showed that food leads to a slight delay in the onset of absorption, but does not affect the overall bioavailability of clarithromycin.

Clarithromycin and its 14-OH metabolite penetrate into middle ear effusion (MEE) of patients with secretory otitis media.

For adult patients, the bioavailability of 10 mL of the 125 mg/5mL suspension is similar to a 250 mg tablet.

Single dose adult volunteer studies show that the reformulated (125 mg/5 mL and 250 mg/5 mL) and the current (125 mg/5 mL) clarithromycin for oral suspension have comparable bioavailability under fasting and non-fasting conditions.

Distribution: Clarithromycin distributes readily into body tissues and fluids, and provides tissue concentrations that are higher than serum concentrations. Examples from tissue and serum concentrations are presented in Table 22.

Table 22: BIAXIN BID

Representative Clarithromycin Tissue and Serum Concentrations Following the Administration of 250 mg b.i.d of Clarithromycin Film-Coated Tablets

	Concentrations	
Tissue Type	**Tissue (µg/g)**	**Serum (mg/L)**
Tonsil	1.6	0.8
Lung	8.8	1.7
Leukocytes[a]	9.2	1.0

[a] In vitro data.

Metabolism: Clarithromycin is principally excreted by the liver and kidney. The major metabolite found in urine is 14-OH-clarithromycin.

Excretion: At 250 mg twice daily, approximately 20% of an orally administered dose of clarithromycin film-coated tablet is excreted in the urine as the unchanged parent drug. The urinary excretion of unchanged clarithromycin is somewhat greater (approximately 30%) with 500 mg twice daily dosing. The renal clearance of clarithromycin is, however, relatively independent of the dose size and approximates the normal glomerular filtration rate. The major metabolite found in urine is 14-OH-clarithromycin which accounts for an additional 10 to 15% of the dose with twice daily dosing at either 250 mg or 500 mg. Most of the remainder of the dose is eliminated in the feces, primarily via the bile. About 5-10% of the parent drug is recovered from the feces. Fecal metabolites are largely products of N-demethylation, 14-hydroxylation or both.

Special Populations and Conditions: Pediatrics: Refer to Absorption.

Geriatrics: Dosage adjustment should be considered in elderly with severe renal impairment. In a steady-state study in which healthy elderly subjects (age 65 to 81 years old) were given 500 mg of clarithromycin every 12 hours, the maximum concentrations of clarithromycin and 14-OH clarithromycin were increased. The AUC was also increased. These changes in pharmacokinetics parallel known age-related decreases in renal function. In clinical trials, elderly patients did not have an increased incidence of adverse events when compared to younger patients.

Hepatic Insufficiency: The steady-state concentrations of clarithromycin in subjects with impaired hepatic function did not differ from those in normal subjects; however, the 14-OH clarithromycin concentrations were lower in the hepatically impaired subjects. The decreased formation of 14-OH clarithromycin was at least partially offset by an increase in renal clearance of clarithromycin in subjects with impaired hepatic function when compared to healthy subjects (see Warnings and Precautions, Hepatic/Biliary/Pancreatic and Dosage and Administration, Recommended Dose and Dosage Adjustment).

Renal Insufficiency: The elimination of clarithromycin was impaired in patients with impaired renal function. The daily dose of clarithromycin should be limited to 500 mg in patients with severe renal impairment (CR_{CL} <30 mL/min) (see Warnings and Precautions, Renal and Dosage and Administration, Recommended Dose and Dosage Adjustment).

STORAGE AND STABILITY: BIAXIN BID (clarithromycin tablets, USP, film-coated): Store film-coated tablets between 15 and 25°C in a tightly closed container. Protect from light.

BIAXIN XL (clarithromycin extended-release tablets): Store extended-release tablets between 15 and 25°C in a tightly closed container. Protect from light.

BIAXIN (clarithromycin for oral suspension, USP): Store granules for suspension between 15 and 25°C in a tightly closed bottle. Protect from light. The reconstituted suspension must not be refrigerated. Any reconstituted unused medication should be discarded after 14 days. The graduated syringe included in the package should be rinsed between uses. Do not leave syringe in bottle. Do not store reconstituted suspension in syringe.

INFORMATION FOR THE PATIENT: Published in e-CPS, available by subscription at www.e-cps.ca.

DOSAGE FORMS, COMPOSITION AND PACKAGING: BIAXIN: HDPE bottle which allows capacity for shaking consists of a: granulation of clarithromycin with carbopol and povidone (K90) which is coated with HP-55 polymer (hydroxypropylmethylcellulose phthalate). Nonmedicinal ingredients: castor oil, citric acid, flavor (artificial and natural fruit), maltodextrin, potassium sorbate, silicon dioxide, sucrose, titanium dioxide and xanthan gum. Water is added to reconstitute the suspension prior to use. When reconstituted, the concentration of clarithromycin is 125 mg/5 mL or 250 mg/5 mL. HDPE bottles of 55, 105 and 150 mL (125 mg/5 mL) and 105 mL (250 mg/5 mL). A graduated syringe is included in the package.

BIAXIN BID: 250 mg: Each oval, printed with Abbott logo on one side, yellow, film-coated tablet contains: clarithromycin 250 mg. Nonmedicinal ingredients: cellulosic polymers, croscarmellose sodium, D&C Yellow No. 10, magnesium stearate, povidone, pregelatinized starch, propylene glycol, silicon dioxide, sorbic acid, sorbitan monooleate, stearic acid, talc, titanium dioxide and vanillin. Tartrazine-free. HDPE bottles of 100.

500 mg: Each oval, printed with Abbott logo on one side, pale yellow, film-coated tablet contains: clarithromycin 500 mg. Nonmedicinal ingredients: cellulosic polymers, croscarmellose sodium, D&C Yellow No. 10, magnesium stearate, povidone, propylene glycol, silicon dioxide, sorbic acid, sorbitan monooleate, stearic acid, talc, titanium dioxide and vanillin. Tartrazine-free. HDPE bottles of 100.

BIAXIN XL: Each oval, debossed, yellow, film-coated, extended-release tablet contains: clarithromycin 500 mg. Nonmedicinal ingredients: cellulosic polymers, lactose monohydrate, magnesium stearate, propylene glycol, Quinoline Yellow Lake E104, sorbitan monooleate, talc, titanium dioxide and vanillin. Tartrazine-free. HDPE bottles of 60. Also available in 7-Day Treatment PAC (14 tablets) and 10-Day Treatment PAC (20 tablets).

(Shown in Product Identification Section)

Bicalutamide Tablets ℞

bicalutamide

Nonsteroidal Antiandrogen

Accord Healthcare

SUPPLIED: Each white to off white, round, biconvex, film-coated tablet, debossed with 'B50' on one side and plain on other side contains: bicalutamide 50 mg. Nonmedicinal ingredients: hypromellose E 5, lactose monohydrate, magnesium stearate, polyethylene glycol, povidone K-30, sodium starch glycolate and titanium dioxide. Blister strips of 15 tablets, packages of 30 tablets. Bottles of 30 and 100. Store between 15-30°C.

Bicillin® L-A ℞

penicillin G benzathine

Antibiotic

King Pharmaceuticals

Date of Preparation: October 27, 2006
Date of Revision: June 1, 2007

PHARMACOLOGY: Penicillin G exerts a bactericidal action against penicillin-susceptible microorganisms during the stage of active multiplication. It acts through the inhibition of biosynthesis of cell-wall mucopeptide. It is not active against the penicillinase-producing bacteria, which include many strains of staphylococci.

The following in vitro data are available, but their clinical significance is unknown. Penicillin G exerts high in vitro activity against staphylococci (except penicillinase-producing strains), streptococci (Groups A, C, G, H, L and M), and pneumococci. Other organisms susceptible to penicillin G are *N. gonorrhoeae*, *C. diphtheriae*, *B. anthracis*, Clostridia species, *A. bovis*, *S. moniliformis*, *L. monocytogenes* and Leptospira species. *T. palidium* is extremely susceptible to the bactericidal action of penicillin G.

Sensitivity Plate Testing: If the Kirby-Bauer method of disc sensitivity is used, a 20-unit penicillin disc should give a zone greater than 28 mm when tested against a penicillin-sensitive bacterial strain.

Pharmacokinetics: Intramuscular penicillin G benzathine is absorbed very slowly into the bloodstream from the intramuscular site and converted by hydrolysis to penicillin G. This combination of hydrolysis and slow absorption results in blood serum levels much lower but much more prolonged than other parenteral penicillins.

Intramuscular administration of 300 000 units of penicillin G benzathine in adults results in blood levels of 0.03 to 0.05 units per mL, which are maintained for 4 to 5 days. Similar blood levels may persist for 10 days following administration of 600 000 units and for 14 days following administration of 1 200 000 units. Blood concentrations of 0.003 units per mL may still be detectable 4 weeks following administration of 1 200 000 units.

Approximately 60% of penicillin G is bound to serum protein. The drug is distributed throughout the body tissues in widely varying amounts. Highest levels are found in the kidneys with lesser amounts in the liver, skin, and intestines. Penicillin G penetrates into all other tissues to a lesser degree with a very small level found in the cerebrospinal fluid. With normal kidney function the drug is excreted rapidly by tubular excretion. In neonates and young infants and in individuals with impaired kidney function, excretion is considerably delayed.

INDICATIONS: Intramuscular penicillin G benzathine is indicated in the treatment of infections due to penicillin-G-sensitive microorganisms that are susceptible to the low and very prolonged serum levels common to this particular dosage form. Therapy should be guided by bacteriological studies (including sensitivity tests) and by clinical response.

The following infections will usually respond to adequate dosage of intramuscular penicillin G benzathine.

Streptococcal Infections (Group A without bacteremia): mild-to-moderate infections of the upper respiratory tract (e.g., pharyngitis).

Venereal Infections: syphilis, yaws, bejel, and pinta.

Medical Conditions in which Penicillin G Benzathine Therapy is indicated as Prophylaxis: Rheumatic fever and/or chorea—Prophylaxis with penicillin G benzathine has proven effective in preventing recurrence of these conditions. It has also been used as follow-up prophylactic therapy for rheumatic heart disease and acute glomerulonephritis.

CONTRAINDICATIONS: A history of a previous hypersensitivity reaction to any of the penicillins is a contraindication.

WARNINGS: Not for intravenous use. Do not inject intravenously or admix with other intravenous solutions. There have been reports of inadvertent intravenous administration of penicillin G benzathine which has been associated with cardiorespiratory arrest and death. Prior to administration of this drug, carefully read Warnings, Adverse Effects and Dosage.

Penicillin G benzathine should only be prescribed for the indications listed in this monograph.

Anaphylaxis: **Serious and occasionally fatal hypersensitivity (anaphylactic) reactions have been reported in patients on penicillin therapy. These reactions are more likely to occur in individuals with a history of penicillin hypersensitivity and/or a history of hypersensitivity to multiple allergens. There have been reports of individuals with a history of penicillin hypersensitivity who have experienced severe reactions when treated with cephalosporins. Before initiating therapy with Bicillin L-A, careful inquiry should be made concerning previous hypersensitivity reactions to penicillins, cephalosporins, or other allergens. If an allergic reaction occurs, Bicillin L-A should be discontinued and appropriate therapy instituted. Serious anaphylactic reactions require immediate emergency treatment with epinephrine, oxygen, intravenous steroids and airway management, including intubation should also be administered as indicated.**

Pseudomembraneous Colitis: Pseudomembraneous colitis has been reported with nearly all antibacterial agents, including penicillin and may range in severity from mild to life-threatening. Therefore, it is important to consider this diagnosis in patients who present with diarrhea subsequent to the administration of any antibacterial agent.

Treatment with antibacterial agents alters the normal flora of the colon and may permit overgrowth of clostridia. Studies indicate that a toxin produced by *C. difficile* is one primary cause of "antibiotic-associated colitis".

After the diagnosis of pseudomembraneous colitis has been established, appropriate therapeutic measures should be initiated. Mild cases of pseudomembraneous colitis usually respond to drug discontinuation alone. In moderate to severe cases, consideration should be given to management with fluids and electrolytes, protein supplementation, and treatment with an antibacterial drug clinically effective against *C. difficile* colitis.

Do not inject into or near an artery or nerve. Injection into or near a nerve may result in permanent neurological damage.

Inadvertent intravascular administration, including inadvertent direct intra-arterial injection or injection immediately adjacent to arteries, of Bicillin L-A and other penicillin preparations has resulted in severe neurovascular damage, including transverse myelitis with permanent paralysis, gangrene requiring amputation of digits and more proximal portions of extremities, and necrosis and sloughing at and surrounding the injection site. Such severe effects have been reported following injections into the buttock, thigh, and deltoid areas.

Other serious complications of suspected intravascular administration which have been reported include immediate pallor, mottling or cyanosis of the extremity both distal and proximal to the injection site followed by bleb formation; severe edema requiring anterior and/or posterior compartment fasciotomy in the lower extremity. The above-described severe effects and complications have most often occurred in infants and small children. Prompt consultation with an appropriate specialist is indicated if any evidence of compromise of the blood supply occurs at, proximal to, or distal to the site of injection. (See Contraindications, Precautions and Dosage.)

Quadriceps femoris fibrosis and atrophy have been reported following repeated intramuscular injections of penicillin preparations into the anterolateral thigh.

PRECAUTIONS: Penicillin should be used with caution in individuals with histories of significant allergies and/or asthma.

Care should be taken to avoid intravenous or intraarterial administration, or injection into or near major peripheral nerves or blood vessels, since such injection may produce neurovascular damage. (See Contraindications, Precautions and Dosage.)

The use of antibiotics may result in overgrowth of nonsusceptible organisms. Constant observation of the patient is essential. If new infections due to bacteria or fungi appear during therapy, the drug should be discontinued and appropriate measures taken.

Whenever allergic reactions occur, penicillin should be withdrawn unless, in the opinion of the physician, the condition being treated is life-threatening and amenable only to penicillin therapy.

In streptococcal infections, therapy must be sufficient to eliminate the organism; otherwise, the sequelae of streptococcal disease may occur. Cultures should be taken following completion of treatment to determine whether streptococci have been eradicated.

Pregnancy: There are no adequate and well controlled studies in pregnant women showing conclusively that harmful effects of this drug on the fetus can be excluded.

Penicillins readily cross the placenta and the effect, if any, on the fetus is not known. Although generally considered to be safe, Bicillin L-A should be used during pregnancy only if clearly needed.

Lactation: Soluble penicillin G is excreted in breast milk. The effect on the infant, if any, is not known. Caution should be used when Bicillin L-A is administered to a nursing woman.

Drug Interactions: Tetracycline, a bacteriostatic antibiotic, may antagonize the bactericidal effect of penicillin, and concurrent use of these drugs should be avoided. The rate of excretion of the penicillins is decreased by concomitant administration of probenecid; probenecid prolongs, as well as increases, blood levels of the penicillins.

Laboratory Tests: In prolonged therapy with penicillin and particularly with high-dosage schedules, periodic evaluation of the renal and hematopoietic systems is recommended.

Laboratory Test Interactions: Penicillins can interfere with the copper sulfate reagent method of testing for glycosuria, resulting in falsely elevated or falsely decreased readings. Such interference does not occur with the glucose oxidase method.

ADVERSE EFFECTS: As with other penicillins, untoward reactions of the sensitivity phenomena are likely to occur, particularly in individuals who have previously demonstrated hypersensitivity to penicillins or in those with a history of allergy, asthma, hay fever or urticaria.

As with other treatments for syphilis, the Jarisch-Herzheimer reaction has been reported.

The following adverse reactions have been reported with penicillin G:

General: Hypersensitivity reactions including the following: skin eruptions (maculopapular to exfoliative dermatitis), erythema, cellulitis, paresthesia, urticaria, laryngeal edema, fever, eosinophilia; other serum sickness-like reactions (including chills, fever, edema, arthralgia and prostration); and anaphylaxis including shock and death.

Note: Urticaria, other skin rashes and serum sickness-like reactions may be controlled with antihistamines and, if necessary, systemic corticosteroids. Whenever such reactions occur, penicillin G should be discontinued unless, in the opinion of the physician, the condition being treated is life-threatening and amenable only to treatment with penicillin G. Serious anaphylactic reactions require immediate emergency treatment with epinephrine. Oxygen, intravenous steroids, and airway management, including intubation, should also be administered, as indicated.

Gastrointestinal: pseudomembranous colitis. Onset of pseudomembranous colitis symptoms may occur during or after antibacterial treatment.

Hematologic: hemolytic anemia, leukopenia, thrombocytopenia. There has been one report of pancytopenia in an elderly patient, who received concomitant methotrexate and flucloxacillin.

Neurologic: neuropathy.

Urogenital: nephropathy.

The following adverse events have been temporally associated with parenteral administration of penicillin G benzathine, although a causal relationship has not necessarily been established.

Body as a Whole: hypersensitivity reactions including allergic vasculitis, pruritus, fatigue, asthenia and pain; aggravation of existing disorder; headache.

Cardiovascular: cardiac arrest; hypotension; tachycardia; ventricular arrhythmia, palpitations; pulmonary hypertension; pulmonary embolism; vasodilation; vasovagal reactions; cerebrovascular accident; syncope.

Gastrointestinal: nausea, vomiting; blood in stool; intestinal necrosis.

Hemic and Lymphatic: lymphadenopathy.

Injection Site: injection site reactions including pain, inflammation, lump, abscess, cellulitis, necrosis, edema, hemorrhage, cellulites, hypersensitivity, atrophy, ecchymosis, and skin ulcer. Neurovascular reactions including warmth, vasospasm, pallor, mottling, gangrene, numbness of the extremities, cyanosis of the extremities, and neurovascular damage.

Metabolic: elevated BUN, creatinine and AST.

Musculoskeletal: joint disorder, periostitis, exacerbation of arthritis, myoglobinuria, rhabdomyolysis.

Nervous System: nervousness, tremors, dizziness, somnolence; confusion, memory impairment; anxiety; euphoria; transverse myelitis, seizures; coma.

A syndrome manifested by a variety of CNS symptoms, such as severe agitation with confusion, visual and auditory hallucinations, and a fear of impending death (Hoigne's syndrome), has been reported after administration of penicillin G procaine and less commonly, after injection of the combination of penicillin G benzathine and penicillin G procaine. Other symptoms associated with this syndrome, such as psychosis, seizures, dizziness, tinnitus, cyanosis, palpitations, tachycardia and/or abnormal perception in taste, also may occur.

Respiratory: hypoxia, apnea, dyspnea.

Skin: diaphoresis.

Special Senses: blurred vision, blindness.

Urogenital: neurogenic bladder; hematuria; proteinuria; renal failure; impotence; priapism.

OVERDOSE:

There have been no reported overdosages with Bicillin L-A. Penicillin in overdosage has the potential to cause neuromuscular hyper-irritability or convulsive seizures. Since there is no antidote, treatment should be symptomatic and supportive.

> For management of a suspected drug overdose, CPhA recommends that you contact your **regional Poison Control Centre**. See the *CPS* Directory section for a list of Poison Control Centres.

DOSAGE: Bicillin L-A is intended for intramuscular injection only. Do not inject into or near an artery or nerve, or intravenously, or admixed with other intravenous solutions (see Warnings).

The following dosages are recommended:

Streptococcal Group A: upper respiratory infections (e.g. pharyngitis):

Adults: a single dose of 1.2 million I.U.

Older Children: a single dose of 900 000 I.U.

Children and Infants Under 27 Kg: a single dose of 300 000 to 600 000 I.U.

Venereal Infections: Syphilis: Primary, Secondary, and Early Latent: 2.4 million I.U. (1 dose).

Late Latent and Tertiary (not involving the central nervous system): 2.4 million I.U. at 7-day intervals for three doses.

Congenital: under 2 years of age: 50 000 I.U./kg/body weight; ages 2-12 years: adjust dosage based on adult dosage schedule.

Persons co-infected with HIV may require a longer course of treatment, as well as closer and longer follow-up.

Yaws, Bejel and Pinta: a single dose of 1.2 million I.U.

Prophylaxis: For rheumatic fever and glomerulonephritis.

Following an acute attack, penicillin G benzathine (parenteral) may be given in doses of 1 200 000 I.U. once a month or 600 000 I.U. every 2 weeks.

Directions for Use: **BICILLIN L-A is intended for intramuscular injection only. Do not inject into or near an artery or nerve, or intravenously, or admixed with other intravenous solutions (see Warnings).**

Administer by **deep, intramuscular injection** in the upper, outer quadrant of the buttock. In infants and small children, the midlateral aspect of the thigh may be preferable. When doses are repeated, vary the injection site. Care should be taken to avoid intravenous or intraarterial administration, or injection into or near major peripheral nerves or blood vessels, since such injection may produce neurovascular damage. Discontinue delivery of the dose if the subject complains of severe immediate pain at the injection site or if, especially in infants and young children, symptoms or signs occur suggesting onset of severe pain.

Because of the high concentration of suspended material in this product, the needle may be blocked if the injection is not made at a slow, steady rate.

Parenteral drug products should be inspected visually for particulate matter and discoloration prior to administration, whenever solution and container permit.

SUPPLIED: Each 2 mL disposable syringe (21 gauge, thin-wall 1-1/2 inch needle) contains: penicillin G benzathine 1 200 000 I.U. as an aqueous suspension. Nonmedicinal ingredients: lecithin, methylparaben NF, povidone USP C200, propylparaben NF sterile pulverized, sodium carboxymethylcellulose USP, sodium citrate USP anhydrous and water for injection USP. Packages of 10. Store under refrigeration (2-8°C). May be removed from refrigerator and stored for 7 days at a temperature not exceeding 30°C. Keep from freezing.

BiCNU® Pr

carmustine

Antineoplastic

Bristol-Myers Squibb

Date of Revision: August 24, 2007

Caution: Carmustine is a potent drug and should be used only by physicians experienced with cancer chemotherapeutic drugs (see Warnings and Precautions). Blood counts as well as renal and hepatic function tests should be taken regularly. Discontinue the drug if abnormal depression of bone marrow or abnormal renal or hepatic function is seen.

PHARMACOLOGY: Carmustine alkylates DNA and RNA and has been shown to inhibit several enzymes by carbamoylation of amino acids in proteins. Carmustine is not cross-resistant with other alkylating agents.

It is thought that the antineoplastic and toxic activities of BiCNU may be due to metabolites. In a series of in vivo and in vitro experiments with formate ^{14}C, adenine-8-^{14}C and DL-leucine-4,5-^{3}H, Wheeler and Bowdon obtained results indicating that carmustine interferes with the de novo synthesis of purine nucleotides and with the conversion of purine nucleotides to components of DNA but to a much lesser extent of RNA. Inhibition of DNA synthesis occurred in the absence of inhibition of the synthesis of protein. In a more recent study, D.P. Groth et al confirmed that carmustine altered de novo purine biosynthesis. It is suggested that carmustine inhibits a reaction(s) involved with the insertion of the C-8 position of the purine ring. These biochemical effects are similar to those described by Wheeler and Alexander for the accepted biological alkylating agents like nitrogen mustards and suggest the inclusion of carmustine in this class of agents.

On the other hand, by chemical evaluation the alkylating properties of carmustine have been shown to be quite weak compared to the above mentioned alkylating agents and it is still an open question whether this activity is sufficient to account for the observed biological effects of carmustine.

Because of the high lipid solubility and the relative lack of ionization at a physiological pH, carmustine readily crosses the blood brain barrier. I.V. administered carmustine is rapidly degraded, with no intact drug detectable after 15 minutes. Approximately 60 to 70% of a total dose is excreted in the urine in 96 hours and about 10% as respiratory CO_2. The fate of the remainder is undetermined.

INDICATIONS: As adjuvant therapy to surgery and radiotherapy or in combination therapy with other chemotherapeutic agents in the following:

Primary Brain Tumors: Carmustine is a small molecule which is virtually un-ionized in aqueous solution at pH 7 and is therefore highly lipid soluble. These characteristics allow it to cross the blood brain barrier and make it attractive in the treatment of brain tumors. An overall 47% response rate with carmustine compares favorably with any other method of treating brain tumors, such as glioblastoma, brainstemglioma, medulloblastoma, astrocytoma, ependymoma, and metastatic brain tumors.

Malignant Lymphomas: Hodgkin's disease, non-Hodgkin's lymphomas either alone or in combination with other chemotherapeutic agents. Carmustine has a striking antineoplastic effect against Hodgkin's disease even when the tumor has become resistant to standard chemotherapeutic agents including radiotherapy.

Virtually all of these studies in which carmustine was used to treat patients with Hodgkin's disease resulted in a 40 to 50% response rate.

Multiple Myeloma: Carmustine is effective in the treatment of myeloma producing improvement in 30% of the patients. In combination with prednisone, it is particularly active in that it shows 70% response. Carmustine has been used as part of a 5-drug regimen (melphalan, cyclophosphamide, prednisone and vincristine) in 29 patients with a 90% response rate.

Malignant Melanoma (disseminated): In combination with vincristine sulfate, carmustine has been shown to give response rates up to 45% in malignant melanoma.

Gastrointestinal Carcinoma: A 12.5% response rate was obtained with carmustine in the therapy of gastrointestinal cancer. Such a result suggests the use of carmustine only after other more appropriate agents have failed in advanced disease.

CONTRAINDICATIONS: In individuals who have demonstrated a previous hypersensitivity to it or any component of its formulation.

WARNINGS: Pulmonary Toxicity: Early onset pulmonary toxicity usually occurs within 3 years of therapy and is characterized by pulmonary infiltrates and/or fibrosis, and cases of fatal pulmonary toxicity have occurred. Age of onset has been reported from 1 year and 10 months to 72 years of age. Risk factors include smoking, the presence of a respiratory condition, pre-existing radiographic abnormalities, sequential or concomitant thoracic irradiation, and association with other agents that cause lung damage. The incidence appears to be dose related with total cumulative doses of 1200 to 1500 mg/m² being associated with increased likelihood of lung fibrosis.

Cases of late pulmonary fibrosis, occurring up to 17 years after treatment, have also been reported. In a recent long-term follow-up of 17 patients who survived childhood brain tumors, 8 (47%) died of lung fibrosis. Of these 8 deaths, 2 occurred within 3 years of treatment, and 6 occurred 8 to 13 years after treatment. Of the patients who died, the median age at treatment was 2.5 years (ranging from 1 to 12); the median age of the long-term survivors was 10 years (5 to 16 years at treatment). All 5 patients treated below the age of 5 years have died of pulmonary fibrosis. In this series, dose of carmustine did not influence fatal outcome nor did coadministration of vincristine or spinal irradiation. Of the remaining survivors available for follow-up, evidence of lung fibrosis was detected in all patients. The risks and benefits of carmustine therapy must be carefully considered, especially in young patients, due to the extremely high risk of pulmonary toxicity.

Bone marrow suppression, notably thrombocytopenia and leukopenia, which may contribute to bleeding and overwhelming infections in an already compromised patient, is a common and severe toxic effect of carmustine.

The occurrence of acute leukemia and bone marrow dysplasias have been reported in patients following nitrosourea therapy.

Carmustine has been administered directly into the carotid artery; this procedure is investigational and has been associated with ocular toxicity.

PRECAUTIONS: Carmustine should be administered by individuals experienced with antineoplastic therapy. Since delayed bone marrow toxicity is the major toxicity, complete blood counts should be monitored frequently for at least 6 weeks after a dose. Repeat doses of carmustine should not be given more frequently than every 6 weeks. The bone marrow toxicity of carmustine is cumulative, and therefore dosage adjustment must be considered on the basis of nadir blood counts from prior dose (see Dosage, Table 1).

Liver and renal function should also be monitored.

Baseline pulmonary function studies should be conducted along with frequent pulmonary function tests during treatment. Patients with a baseline below 70% of the predicted Forced Vital Capacity (FVC) or Carbon Monoxide Diffusing Capacity (DL_{co}) are particularly at risk.

Since pulmonary toxicity has been reported to occur with a frequency ranging up to 30%, patients on carmustine therapy should be instructed to report immediately any signs of respiratory complications. In such cases, therapy should be discontinued and evaluation of respiratory gas exchange and spirometry should be performed. If necessary, patients should then be treated with corticosteroids.

Pregnancy: Safe use in pregnancy has not been established. Carmustine is embryotoxic and teratogenic in rats and embryotoxic in rabbits at dose levels equivalent to the human dose. Carmustine also affects fertility in male rats at doses somewhat higher than the human dose. Carmustine is carcinogenic in rats and mice, producing a marked increase in tumor incidence in doses approximating those employed clinically. The benefit to the mother versus the risk of toxicity to the mother and fetus must be carefully weighed.
Lactation: It is not known whether carmustine is excreted in human milk. Because of the potential for serious adverse events in nursing infants, nursing should be discontinued while taking carmustine.
Children: Carmustine should be used with extreme caution in children due to the high risk of pulmonary toxicity (see Adverse Effects).
Geriatric: No data from clinical studies of BiCNU are available for patients 65 years of age and over to determine whether they respond differently than younger patients. Other reported clinical experience has not identified differences in responses between elderly and younger patients. In general, dose selection for an elderly patient should be cautious, usually starting at the low end of the dose range, reflecting the greater frequency of decreased hepatic, renal, or cardiac function and of concomitant disease or other drug therapy.

BiCNU and its metabolites are substantially excreted by the kidney, and the risk of toxic reactions to this drug may be greater in patients with impaired renal function. Because elderly patients are more likely to have decreased renal function, care should be taken in dose selection and renal function should be monitored.
Drug Interactions: Greater myelotoxicity (e.g. leukopenia and neutropenia) has been reported when carmustine was combined with cimetidine.

ADVERSE EFFECTS: Hematopoietic: thrombocytopenia (platelets below 100 000 cells/mm^3) and leukopenia (leukocytes below 4000 cells/mm^3).

Delayed myelosuppression is a frequent and serious adverse event associated with carmustine administration. It usually occurs 4 to 6 weeks after drug administration and is dose-related. Platelet nadirs occur at 4 to 5 weeks; leukocyte nadirs occur at 5 to 6 weeks post-therapy. Myelosuppression is the major dose limiting factor with carmustine as is with so many drugs of this type. Thrombocytopenia is generally more severe than leukopenia; however, both may be dose-limiting toxicities. Anemia also occurs but it is generally less severe.

Carmustine may produce cumulative myelosuppression (see Warnings).

The occurrence of acute leukemia and bone marrow dysplasias have been reported in patients following long-term nitrosourea therapy.

Greater myelotoxicity (e.g. leukopenia and neutropenia) has been reported when carmustine was combined with cimetidine (see Precautions, Drug Interactions).
Pulmonary Toxicity: Carmustine-induced pulmonary toxicity has been reported to occur with a frequency ranging up to 30% (see Warnings).
Hepatic: Carmustine produces reversible hepatic toxicity which is manifested by increased transaminase, alkaline phosphatase and bilirubin levels when high doses are employed. It has been rarely noted at therapeutic doses. Hepatotoxicity is delayed up to 60 days after dosing.
Skin: Burning and hyperemia at the site of injection are common, but true thrombosis is rare. Accidental contact of reconstituted carmustine with the skin has caused hyperpigmentation of the affected areas. Within 2 hours after rapid i.v. administration of carmustine, intense flushing of the skin and suffusion of the conjunctiva could last for about 4 hours. Skin rash has also been reported.
Renal: Renal abnormalities consisting of decreases in kidney size, progressive azotemia and renal failure have been reported in patients who receive large cumulative doses after prolonged therapy with carmustine and related nitrosoureas. Kidney damage has also been reported occasionally in patients receiving lower total doses.
Neurological: There have been rare instances of encephalopathy reported.
Gastrointestinal: Nausea and vomiting frequently appear within 2 hours and usually last 4 to 6 hours and are dose-related. Prior administration of antiemetics and sedatives is effective in diminishing and sometimes preventing this adverse event.
Endocrine: Gynecomastia has been observed in a few rare cases.
Cardiovascular: hypotension, tachycardia.
Other: Muscular pain has been infrequently reported. Neuroretinitis, chest pain, headache, allergic reactions.

OVERDOSE:
Treatment: In the case of overdosage, the patient should be treated symptomatically.

For management of a suspected drug overdose, CPhA recommends that you contact your **regional Poison Control Centre.** See the *CPS* Directory section for a list of Poison Control Centres.

DOSAGE: The recommended dose of carmustine as a single agent in previously untreated patients is 200 mg/m^2 i.v. every 6 weeks. This may be given as a single dose or divided into daily injections such as 100 mg/m^2 on 2 successive days. When carmustine is used in combination with other myelosuppressive drugs or in patients in whom bone marrow reserve is depleted, the doses should be adjusted accordingly.

A repeat course of carmustine should not be given until circulating blood elements have returned to acceptable levels (platelets above 100 000 cells/mm^3, leukocytes above 4000 cells/mm^3) this usually occurs within 6 weeks. Blood counts should be monitored frequently and repeat courses should not be given before 6 weeks because of delayed toxicity.

Doses subsequent to the initial dose should be adjusted according to the hematologic response of the patient to the preceding dose. The schedule in Table 1 is suggested as a guide to dosage adjustment.

Table 1: BiCNU
Dosage Adjustment

Nadir After Prior Dose		
Leukocytes	**Platelets**	**Percent of Prior Dose to be Given**
>4000	>100 000	100%
>3000-3999	>75 000-99 999	100%
>2000-2999	>25 000-74 999	70%
<2000	<25 000	50%

Reconstitution: Preparation of I.V. Solutions: To facilitate reconstitution, allow the supplied sterile diluent (absolute alcohol) to come to controlled room temperature (15 to 30°C) before mixing.

Dissolve carmustine completely with 3 mL of the supplied sterile diluent and then aseptically add 27 mL of Sterile Water for Injection, USP to the alcohol solution. Each mL of the resulting solution will contain 3.3 mg of carmustine in 10% ethanol. (Solution in the ethanol must be complete before sterile water for injection is added.) Accidental contact of reconstituted carmustine with the skin has caused transient hyperpigmentation of the affected areas. If carmustine lyophilized material or solution contacts the skin, immediately wash thoroughly with soap and water. If carmustine lyophilized material or solution contacts mucosa, flush thoroughly with water.

Reconstitution as recommended results in a clear, colorless to light yellow solution which may be further diluted with Sodium Chloride for Injection, USP or 5% Dextrose for Injection, USP. The reconstituted solution should be used i.v. only and should be administered by i.v. infusion over a 1 to 2 hour period. Injection of carmustine over shorter periods of time may produce intense pain and burning at the site of injection (see Adverse Effects).
Stability of Reconstituted Solutions: The lyophilized dosage formulation contains no preservatives and is not intended as a multiple dose vial.

After reconstitution as recommended carmustine is stable for 24 hours under refrigeration (2 to 8°C).

The reconstituted solution further diluted with 500 mL of Sodium Chloride Injection, USP or 5% Dextrose Injection, USP, **in glass containers**, results in a solution which should be utilized within 8 hours and be protected from light. These solutions are also stable for 24 hours under refrigeration (2 to 8°C) and an additional 6 hours at room temperature (25°C) protected from light. Further diluted carmustine should be used immediately if not refrigerated.

Note: Reconstituted vials stored under refrigeration should be examined for crystal formation prior to use. If crystals are observed, they may be redissolved by warming the vial to room temperature and agitation.
Handling and Disposal: Preparation of carmustine should be done in a vertical laminar flow hood (Biological Safety Cabinet—Class II). Personnel preparing carmustine should wear PVC gloves, safety glasses, disposable gowns and masks. All needles, syringes, vials and other materials which have come in contact with carmustine should be segregated and incinerated at 1000°C or more. Sealed containers may explode. Intact vials should be returned to the manufacturer for destruction. Proper precautions should be taken in packaging these materials for transport. Personnel regularly involved in the preparation and handling of carmustine should have biannual blood examinations.

SUPPLIED: Each 30 mL amber glass vial contains: carmustine 100 mg with a 3 mL vial or ampoule of absolute ethanol as sterile diluent. Nonmedicinal ingredients: none. Boxes of 10.

The unopened vial may have a physical appearance ranging from lacy flakes to a congealed mass, with no evident degradation of the active ingredient, carmustine. Do not use if product has liquified.

Unopened vials of the dry powder should be shipped and stored under refrigeration (2 to 8°C). Alternatively, carmustine may be shipped on dry ice and subsequently stored under refrigeration (2 to 8°C). The recommended storage of unopened vials prevents significant decomposition until expiration date indicated on package. Normal room temperature storage (22°C) of the unopened vials will result in a slow decomposition of the drug (approximately 3%) in 36 days.
Note: Carmustine has a low melting point (approximately 30.5 to 32°C). Vials of the drug exposed to this temperature or above will cause the drug to liquify and appear as an oil film in the bottom of the vials. This is a sign of decomposition and vials should be discarded. If there is a question of adequate refrigeration upon receipt of this product, immediately inspect the larger vial in each individual carton. For inspection, hold the vial to a bright light. The carmustine will appear as a very small amount of dry flakes or dry congealed mass. If this is evident, carmustine is suitable for use and should be refrigerated immediately.

Glass containers were used for the stability data provided in this section. Only use glass containers for BiCNU administration.
Special Instructions: Handling and Disposal: Procedures for proper handling and disposal of anti-cancer drugs should be considered. Several guidelines on this subject have been published. There is no general agreement that all of the procedures recommended in the guidelines are necessary or appropriate.

Accidental contact of reconstituted BiCNU with the skin has caused burning and hyperpigmentation of the affected area.

Personnel preparing BiCNU should wear safety glasses and disposable gowns and masks. To minimize the risk of dermal exposure, always wear impervious gloves when handling vials containing BiCNU lyophilized powder for injection. This includes all handling activities in clinical settings, pharmacies, storerooms, and home healthcare settings, including during unpacking and inspection, transport within a facility, and dose preparation and administration.

Biltricide® Ⓟ
praziquantel
Antihelminthic

Bayer

Date of Preparation: March 7, 1997
Date of Revision: November 30, 2007

PHARMACOLOGY: Mechanism of Action: Praziquantel induces a rapid contraction of schistosomes by a specific effect on the permeability of the cell membrane. The drug further causes vacuolization and disintegration of the schistosome tegument. The effect is more marked on adult worms compared to young worms. An increased calcium influx may play an important role.

Secondary effects are inhibition of glucose uptake, lowering of glycogen levels and stimulation of lactate release. The action of praziquantel is limited very specifically to trematodes and cestodes; nematodes (including filariae) are not affected.
Clinical Pharmacology: After oral administration, praziquantel is rapidly absorbed (approximately 80%), subjected to a first pass effect, metabolized and eliminated by the kidneys. Maximal serum concentration is achieved 1 to 3 hours after dosing. The half-life of praziquantel in serum is 0.8 to 1.5 hours.
INDICATIONS: For the treatment of infections due to the following species of schistosoma: (*S. haematobium*, *S. japonicum*, *S. mansoni*, and *S. mekongi*), and infections due to the liver flukes *C. sinensis*/*O. viverrini*. (Approval of this indication was based on studies in which the two species were not differentiated.)
CONTRAINDICATIONS: In patients who have previously shown hypersensitivity to the drug or to any of the excipients. Since parasite destruction within the eye may cause irreversible lesions, ocular cysticercosis should not be treated with praziquantel.

The concomitant administration of praziquantel with strong inducers of cytochrome P450 such as rifampin must be avoided as therapeutically effective plasma levels of praziquantel may not be achieved.
WARNINGS: Information to Be Provided to the Patient: There may possibly be effects on vigilance. Patients should be warned not to drive a car and not to operate machinery on the day of praziquantel treatment and during the subsequent 24 hours as their ability to do so may be temporarily impaired by the use of praziquantel.
Children: Safety in children under 4 years of age has not been established.
Pregnancy: No adequate and well-controlled studies have been conducted with praziquantel in pregnant women (see Precautions).
PRECAUTIONS: General: Nephrotoxic effects of praziquantel have not been observed. Since 80% of praziquantel and its derivatives are excreted in the kidneys, excretion may be delayed in patients with impaired renal function.

Caution should be taken in patients with uncompensated liver insufficiency or with hepatosplenic schistosomiasis. Because of reduced drug metabolization in the liver, considerably higher and longer lasting concentrations of unmetabolized praziquantel can occur in the vascular system and/or collateral circulation, leading to prolonged plasma half-life. If necessary, the patient may be hospitalized for the duration of treatment. Mild increases in liver enzymes have also been reported in some patients.

Patients suffering from cardiac irregularities should be monitored during treatment.

When schistosomiasis or fluke infection is found in patients living in or coming from areas with endemic human cysticercosis, it is advisable to hospitalize the patient for the duration of treatment.

As praziquantel can exacerbate central nervous system pathology due to schistosomiasis, paragonimiasis, or *T. solium* cysticercosis, as a general rule this drug should not be administered to individuals reporting a history of epilepsy and/or other signs of potential central nervous systems involvement such as subcutaneous nodules suggestive of cysticercosis.
Pregnancy: An increase in the abortion rate was found in rats at 3 times the single human therapeutic dose. Although animal reproduction studies have not brought to light any evidence that the mother or the unborn child might be harmed, these studies are not always predictive of human response. Praziquantel should not be used in pregnancy unless the potential benefit of treating women of reproductive age and pregnant women far outweighs the risk to their health and to the health of their babies (see Warnings).
Lactation: Praziquantel appears in the milk of nursing women at a concentration of 20 to 25% that of maternal serum. Breastfeeding should be suspended for the day(s) of treatment and the following 72 hours. The physician should evaluate if the potential benefit clearly outweighs the potential risk (taking into consideration the quality of available alternative artificial nutrition).
Drug Interactions: Many categories of drugs are known to inhibit or induce the drug metabolizing family of P450 enzymes located in the liver and intestine. Coadministration of such drugs may impact upon their metabolisms. In some cases serum concentration or bioavailability may be increased and in others decreased. Care must therefore be exercised when coadministering such drugs. Praziquantel is believed to be metabolized via the P450 enzyme system. The following lists some of the drug interactions which have been reported so far with praziquantel. Other causes such as effects upon absorption among others may also exist.

Concomitant administration of praziquantel with strong inducers of cytochrome P450 such as rifampin must be avoided because therapeutically effective levels of praziquantel may not be achieved.

Coadministration with praziquantel of anticonvulsants like phenytoin, fosphenytoin, carbamazepine and phenobarbital or with chloroquine or dexamethasone have been reported to lower praziquantel bioavailability and serum levels. Similar trends have been reported with glucose and bicarbonate.

Cimetidine, miconazole and ketoconazole have been shown to inhibit P450 enzyme mediated metabolism. When coadministered with praziquantel, increased bioavailability and serum levels of praziquantel have been reported. Praziquantel on the other hand has been shown to reduce albendazole bioavailability and serum levels.
ADVERSE EFFECTS: Adverse reactions vary according to dose and duration of praziquantel medication. Furthermore, they are dependent on the parasite species, extent of parasitization, duration of infection and localization of the parasites in the body.

Adverse reactions are based on publications and on spontaneous reports sorted by CIOMS III categories of frequency and MedDRA System Organ Classes (in internationally agreed order). Frequencies of adverse reactions are mainly based on data from medical literature.

The following adverse reactions have been observed after praziquantel administration. It is often not clear whether the complaints reported by patients or the undesired effects recorded by the physician are caused by praziquantel itself (direct relation), or may be considered to be an endogenous reaction to the death of the parasites (indirect relation) or are symptomatic observations of the infestation (no relation). It may be difficult to differentiate between the possible variations.

Table 1: Biltricide

Adverse Drug Reactions

Very Common ≥10%	Common ≥1 to <10%	Uncommon ≥0.1 to <1%	Rare ≥0.01 to <0.1%	Very Rare <0.01%
Immune System Disorders				
				Allergic reaction Polyserositis Eosinophilia
Nervous System Disorders				
Headache Dizziness	Vertigo Somnolence (including drowsiness)			Seizures
Cardiac Disorders				
				Unspecific arrhythmias
Gastrointestinal Disorders				
Gastrointestinal and abdominal pains Nausea Vomiting	Anorexia Diarrhea (very rarely bloody diarrhea)			
Skin and Subcutaneous Tissue Disorders				
	Urticaria			Puritus
Musculoskeletal, Connective Tissue and Bone				
	Myalgia			
General Disorders and Administration Site Conditions				
	Feeling unwell Fever			

Mild increases in liver enzymes have been reported in some patients.

OVERDOSE:

Symptoms: No data are available regarding overdosage in humans.

Treatment: In the event of an overdose, a fast-acting laxative is recommended. In rats and mice the acute oral LD_{50} was approximately 2500 mg/kg and in dogs the oral LD_{50} was less than 200 mg/kg.

> For management of a suspected drug overdose, CPhA recommends that you contact your **regional Poison Control Centre**. See the *CPS* Directory section for a list of Poison Control Centres.

DOSAGE: Doses should be individualized depending on the diagnosis. Based on clinical experience, the following dosages are recommended.

Schistosomiasis: 3×20 mg/kg body weight as a 1-day treatment. Using Table 2, the number of tablets to be taken 3 times on the same day can be determined.

Table 2: Biltricide

Dosing in Schistosomiasis

Body Weight in kg	20–25	26–33	34–41	42–48	49–56	57–63	64–70	71–78	79–86
Dose (mg)	450	600	750	900	1050	1200	1350	1500	1650
Number of Tablets Corresponding to 1×20 mg/kg[a]	3/4	1	1¼	1½	1¾	2	2¼	2½	2¾

[a] Each 600 mg oblong tablet has 3 scores. When broken, each of the 4 segments contains 150 mg of active ingredient.

The recommended dose for clonorchiasis and opisthorchiasis is 3×25 mg/kg body weight as a 1-day treatment. See Table 3.

Table 3: Biltricide

Dosing in Clonorchiasis and Opisthorchiasis

Body Weight in kg	22–26	27–33	34–38	39–44	45–50	51–56	57–62	63–68	69–75
Dose (mg)	600	750	900	1050	1200	1350	1500	1650	1800
Number of Tablets Corresponding to 25 mg/kg[a]	1	1¼	1½	1¾	2	2¼	2½	2¾	3

[a] Each 600 mg oblong tablet has 3 scores. When broken, each of the 4 segments contains 150 mg of active ingredient.

Administration: The tablets should be swallowed whole with a little liquid, preferably during or after meals. Keeping the tablets (or segments thereof) in the mouth may reveal a bitter taste which can cause gagging or vomiting.

The interval between administration should be at least 4 hours and not more than 6 hours. When broken, each of the 4 segments contains 150 mg of active ingredient so that the dosage can be easily adjusted to the patient's body weight.

Children: Safety and efficacy in children under 4 years of age have not been established (see Warnings).

INFORMATION FOR THE PATIENT: Published in e-CPS, available by subscription at www.e-cps.ca.

SUPPLIED: Each white, film-coated, oblong tablet, with 3 scores on both sides and engraved BAYER on one side and LG on the other, contains: praziquantel 600 mg. Nonmedicinal ingredients: cornstarch, magnesium stearate, microcrystalline cellulose, polyvidone 25, sodium lauryl sulfate, polyethylene glycol 4000, methylhydroxypropylcellulose and titanium dioxide. When broken, each of the four segments contains 150 mg of the active ingredient so that the dosage can be easily adjusted to the patient's body weight. Segments are broken off by pressing the score (notch) with thumbnails. If one quarter of a tablet is required, this is best achieved by breaking the segment from the outer end. Bottles of 6. Store at room temperature below 30°C. Protect from light and excessive humidity.

(Shown in Product Identification Section)

Biobase™

ethyl alcohol

Antiseptic Vehicle for Topical Preparations

Odan

Biobase-G™

glycolic acid—ethyl alcohol

Antiseptic Vehicle for Topical Preparations

Odan

SUPPLIED: Biobase: Each mL of unscented solution contains: ethyl alcohol 70% v/v. Nonmedicinal ingredients: ceteareth-20, citric acid and purified water. Plastic bottles of 50 and 100 mL with a brushed nylon applicator to prevent clogging and control flow.

Biobase-G: 6%: Each mL of unscented solution contains: glycolic acid 6% w/v and ethyl alcohol 20% w/v. Nonmedicinal ingredients: citric acid, ethyl alcohol, laureth-4, purified water and sodium hydroxide. pH 3.5. Plastic bottles of 50 and 100 mL with a brushed nylon applicator to prevent clogging and control flow.

8%: Each mL of unscented solution contains: glycolic acid 8% w/v and ethyl alcohol 20% w/v. Nonmedicinal ingredients: citric acid, ethyl alcohol, laureth-4, purified water and sodium hydroxide. pH 3.5. Plastic bottles of 50 and 100 mL with a brushed nylon applicator to prevent clogging and control flow.

10%: Each mL of unscented solution contains: glycolic acid 10% w/v and ethyl alcohol 20% w/v. Nonmedicinal ingredients: citric acid, ethyl alcohol, laureth-4, purified water and sodium hydroxide. pH 3.5. Plastic bottles of 50 and 100 mL with a brushed nylon applicator to prevent clogging and control flow.

BioGaia Chewable Tablets

lactobacillus reuteri protectis

Natural Health Product—Probiotic

Ferring

INDICATIONS: Provides live microorganisms to benefit health and/or to confer a health benefit.

CONTRAINDICATIONS: Do not use if you are experiencing nausea, fever, vomiting, bloody diarrhea or severe abdominal pain. Do not use if you have an immune-compromised condition e.g. AIDS, lymphoma, patients undergoing long-term corticosteroid treatment.

WARNINGS AND PRECAUTIONS: Discontinue use and consult a health care practitioner if symptoms of digestive upset (e.g. diarrhea) occur, worsen, or persist beyond 3 days.

OVERDOSE:

> For management of a suspected drug overdose, CPhA recommends that you contact your **regional Poison Control Centre**. See the *CPS* Directory section for a list of Poison Control Centres.

DOSAGE: Children: Chew at least one tablet a day for good digestive health until your symptoms subside.
Adults: Chew at least one tablet a day for good digestive health until your symptoms subside.

SUPPLIED: Each chewable tablet contains: lactobacillus reuteri 100 million cfu. Nonmedicinal ingredients: citric acid, anhydrous, isomalt, lemon-lime flavour and xylitol. Store at room temperature.

BioGaia Drops

lactobacillus reuteri protectis

Natural Health Product—Probiotic

Ferring

INDICATIONS: Provides live microorganisms to benefit health and/or to confer a health benefit.

CONTRAINDICATIONS: Do not use if you are experiencing nausea, fever, bloody diarrhea or severe abdominal pain. Do not use if you have an immune compromised condition (e.g. AIDS, lymphoma, patients undergoing long-term corticosteroid treatment).

WARNINGS AND PRECAUTIONS: Discontinue use and consult a health care practitioner if symptoms of digestive upset (e.g. diarrhea) occur, worsen, or persist beyond 3 days.

OVERDOSE:

> For management of a suspected drug overdose, CPhA recommends that you contact your **regional Poison Control Centre**. See the *CPS* Directory section for a list of Poison Control Centres.

DOSAGE: Children: Shake well before use. Take 5 drops per day (equivalent to 100 million active lactobacillus reuteri).
Adults: Shake well before use. Take 5 drops per day (equivalent to 100 million active lactobacillus reuteri).

SUPPLIED: Five drops contain: lactobacillus reuteri 100 million cfu. Nonmedicinal ingredients: medium chain triglycerides, silicone dioxide and sunflower oil. Keep refrigerated.

Biomega

fish oil—vitamin D3

Herbal Product

USANA Health Sciences

SUPPLIED: Each capsule contains: fish oil 1000 mg and vitamin D_3 2.5 µg. Nonmedicinal ingredients: gelatin, glycerin, lemon oil, maize oil, purified water and tocopherols excipient NF.

(Shown in Product Identification Section)

Bionet®

benzocaine—cetylkonium chloride

Local Anti-infective—Analgesic

Church & Dwight

INDICATIONS: The symptomatic treatment of mild infection and relief of pain in gum, pharyngeal, tonsillar and other oral disorders such as aphthous ulcers, stomatitis and gingivitis. May also be used postoperatively in tonsillectomy, dental surgery and tooth extraction.

CONTRAINDICATIONS: Benzocaine sensitivity.

WARNINGS: No data supplied by the manufacturer.

PRECAUTIONS: Severe or persistent sore throat accompanied by high fever, headache, nausea and vomiting may be serious, consult a physician promptly. Do not use for more than 2 days or administer to children under 2 years of age unless directed by a physician.

If benzocaine sensitization develops, discontinue Bionet administration.

ADVERSE EFFECTS: No data supplied by the manufacturer.

OVERDOSE:

Benzocaine has a low toxicity while the probable human lethal dose for cetylkonium is estimated to lie in the range of 50 to 500 mg/kg.

Symptoms: Overdosage of benzocaine will produce giddiness, motor unrest, cardiac palpitations, respiratory difficulties, tremors, clonic convulsions, arterial hypotension, dilated pupils and pallor. Quaternary ammonium salts ingested in large quantities evince the following symptomatology: burning of mouth and throat, apprehension, restlessness, confusion, weakness, CNS depression, muscular weakness with asphyxia.

Treatment: If respiration fails, start artificial respiration. 0.5 mL of 1:1 000 epinephrine given i.v. may be needed to improve circulation, or large quantities of milk or gastric lavage, if it can be performed promptly. In children, induce emesis and if there is no immediate response, use gastric lavage. Avoid alcohol.

> For management of a suspected drug overdose, CPhA recommends that you contact your **regional Poison Control Centre**. See the *CPS* Directory section for a list of Poison Control Centres.

DOSAGE: Allow lozenge to dissolve slowly in the mouth. Repeat every 2 hours or as required, until infection subsides.

SUPPLIED: Each white, round, even, biconvex, uncoated, peppermint flavored lozenge, contains: cetylkonium chloride 5 mg (cetyldimethyl benzyl ammonium chloride) and benzocaine 7.5 mg. Nonmedicinal ingredients: flavor, magnesium stearate, povidone, sucrose and tragacanth. Energy: 22 kJ (5.2 kcal). Alcohol-, gluten-, sodium- and tartrazine-free. Push-through packages of 16.

(Shown in Product Identification Section)

Bi-PegLyte™

PEG 3350—electrolytes—bisacodyl

Gastrointestinal Lavage

PendoPharm

Date of Preparation: May 6, 2009

SUMMARY PRODUCT INFORMATION:

Route of Administration	Dosage Form/ Strength	Clinically Relevant Nonmedicinal Ingredients
Oral	PEG 3350 and Electrolytes For Oral Solution: Per sachet: polyethylene glycol 59.5 g, sodium sulphate 5.74 g, sodium bicarbonate 1.69 g, sodium chloride 1.46 g, potassium chloride 0.76 g. Bisacodyl delayed release tablet USP 5 mg	Flavours, sodium saccharine (sachets), lactose (tablets). For a complete listing see Dosage Forms, Composition and Packaging.

INDICATIONS AND CLINICAL USE: Bi-PegLyte Bowel Prep Kit (PEG 3350 and Electrolytes for Oral Solution USP and Bisacodyl Delayed Release Tablets USP) is indicated for cleansing of the colon as a preparation for colonoscopy in adults.

Pediatrics: Safety and effectiveness of Bi-PEGLYTE Bowel Prep Kit (PEG 3350 and Electrolytes for Oral Solution USP and Bisacodyl Delayed Release Tablets USP) in pediatric patients has not been established.

CONTRAINDICATIONS: Patients who are hypersensitive to this drug or to any ingredient in the formulation or component of the container. For a complete listing, see Dosage Forms, Composition and Packaging.

Patients with:

- Ileus
- Gastric retention
- Gastrointestinal (GI) obstruction
- Bowel perforation
- Toxic colitis
- Toxic megacolon
- Acute surgical abdomen
- Appendicitis
- Rectal bleeding
- Gastroenteritis
- Diverticulitis

WARNINGS AND PRECAUTIONS: General: Use of Bi-PegLyte is not recommended when abdominal pain, nausea, or vomiting are present.

No additional flavorings or ingredients may be added to the solution.

Carcinogenesis and Mutagenesis: Long-term carcinogenic and reproductive studies with animals have not been performed.

Gastrointestinal: Bi-PegLyte Bowel Prep Kit should be used with caution in patients with severe ulcerative colitis Patients with impaired gag reflex and patients prone to regurgitation or aspiration during administration of PEG/Electrolyte solution should be closely observed. If GI obstruction or perforation is suspected, appropriate studies should be performed to rule out these conditions before administration. If a patient experiences severe bloating, distension or abdominal pain, administration of the solution should be slowed or temporarily discontinued until the symptoms abate. Patients suffering from an acute exacerbation of inflammatory bowel disease have not been studied.

Ischemic colitis has been reported with use of a sodium sulphate-free PEG electrolyte solution and bisacodyl 20 mg bowel prep kit for colon preparation prior to colonoscopy (see Adverse Reactions). If patients develop severe abdominal pain or rectal bleeding, patients should be evaluated as soon as possible.

Immune: Cases of urticaria, rhinorrhea, dermatitis and anaphylactic reactions have been reported with PEG-based products which may represent allergic reactions.

Neurologic: Use of large volume (4 L) PEG-based colon preparation products have resulted in reports of generalized tonic-clonic seizures in patients with no prior history of seizures. Electrolyte abnormalities, such as hyponatremia and hypokalemia, as well as severe vomiting and excessive beverage consumption have been associated with these cases. A correction of fluid and electrolyte abnormalities resolved the neurologic irregularity. Therefore, in patients with known or suspected hyponatremia, or in patients using concomitant medications that increase the risk of electrolyte abnormalities (such as diuretics), Bi-PegLyte Bowel Prep Kit should be used with caution. In these patients, baseline and post-colonoscopy laboratory tests (sodium, potassium, calcium, creatinine, and BUN) should be monitored.

Renal: The close monitoring of patients with impaired water handling who experience severe vomiting should be performed, including measurement of electrolytes (sodium, potassium, calcium, BUN and creatinine).

Special Populations: Pregnant Women: Reproduction studies of oral doses of bisacodyl tablets have been performed in rats administered up to 70 times the human dose, and have revealed no evidence of impaired fertility damage to the fetus. At the dose which equated to 70 times the human dose, there was some evidence of lower litter survival at weaning. There are, however, no adequate and well-controlled studies in pregnant women, hence bisacodyl tablets should be used during pregnancy only at the discretion of the physician.

Animal reproduction studies have not been conducted with PEG/Electrolyte powder, and it is also not known whether PEG/Electrolyte powder can affect reproductive capacity or harm the fetus when administered to a pregnant patient. Bi-PegLyte Bowel Prep Kit should be given to a pregnant patient only if clearly needed.

Nursing Women: It is not known whether this drug is excreted in human milk. Because many drugs are excreted in human milk, caution should be exercised when Bi-PegLyte Bowel Prep Kit is administered to a nursing woman.

Pediatrics: Safety and effectiveness of Bi-PegLyte Bowel Prep Kit in pediatric patients has not been established.

Geriatrics (>60 years of age): There are isolated reports of serious post-marketing events following the administration of PEG-based products in patients over 60 years of age (acute pulmonary edema after vomiting and aspirating the PEG-based solution, asystole, esophageal perforation, and upper GI bleeding from a Mallory-Weiss tear). Caution is required in patients with renal and cardiac dysfunction in whom fluid and electrolyte shifts are of extra risk.

ADVERSE REACTIONS: Adverse Drug Reaction Overview: Nausea, abdominal fullness and bloating are the most frequent adverse reactions occurring in up to 50% of patients taking 4 L PEG/Electrolyte preparations. Less frequent adverse reactions to the 4 L preparation are abdominal cramps, vomiting and anal irritation. These adverse effects are transient.

A number of clinical studies in the literature have demonstrated that administration of 2 L PEG-ELS products similar to the PEG/Electrolyte product found in Bi-PegLyte, in conjunction with bisacodyl tablets (15 or 20 mg), result in significantly less nausea and vomiting (approximately 43% and 50% respectively) than administration of a 4 L product. In addition, the 2 L + bisacodyl regimen also resulted in less pain, bloating, fullness, anal irritation and overall feeling of discomfort, resulting in better patient compliance.

Cramping and abdominal discomfort has occurred in some patients after bisacodyl administration; no systemic effects have been reported.

Post-Market Adverse Drug Reactions: The following rare adverse events have been reported following administration of 4 L of the PEG/Electrolyte product found in this kit (Peglyte):

Cardiovascular: bradycardia, acute pulmonary edema, hypotension.
Eye: sensitivity to light, painful irritated eyes.
Gastrointestinal: rectal bleeding (occult blood in stool), sores in mouth.
General and Administration Site Conditions: chills, loss of appetite.
Hematologic: anemia.
Metabolism and Nutrition: fluid imbalance, hypoglycaemia.
Musculoskeletal and Connective Tissue: muscle pain.
Nervous System: headaches, unconscious, coma, seizures, shakes.
Psychiatric: confused feeling, disorientation.
Respiratory, Thoracic and Mediastinal: aspiration.
Skin and Subcutaneous Tissue: oily hair and skin, facial swelling, leg swelling.

Isolated cases of urticaria, rhinorrhea and dermatitis have been reported which may represent allergic reactions.

There have been rare reported cases of PEG-ELS-induced colitis, arrhythmia, pancreatitis and cardiac arrest, although these may occur less frequently with regimens that use a lower volume of PEG-ELS (2 L vs 4 L).

The following adverse reactions have been identified during post approval use of a sodium sulphate-free PEG electrolyte solution and bisacodyl 20 mg bowel prep kit for colon preparation:

Gastrointestinal: In patients over 60 years of age, there are isolated reports of serious post-marketing events following the administration of PEG-based products. These adverse reactions include acute pulmonary edema after vomiting and aspirating the PEG-based solution, asystole, esophageal perforation, and upper GI bleeding from a Mallory-Weiss tear. In addition, the following serious adverse reactions were seen during administration of 4 L of PEG-3350 colon cleansing preparation: two deaths in end stage renal failure patients who developed diarrhea, vomiting and dysnatremia.

Ischemic colitis has been reported with use of a sodium sulphate-free 2 L PEG electrolyte solution and bisacodyl 20 mg bowel prep kit for colon prior to colonoscopy. However, the use of the sodium sulphate-free PEG electrolyte solution and bisacodyl 20 mg bowel prep kit for colon preparation has not been causally associated with these cases of ischemic colitis (see Warnings and Precautions).

Neurologic: The use of large volume (4 L) PEG-based colon preparation has resulted in reports of generalized tonic-clonic seizures (see Warnings and Precautions).

DRUG INTERACTIONS: Oral medications administered within 1 hour of the start of administration of the PEG/Electrolyte solution may be flushed from the gastrointestinal tract and not absorbed.

DOSAGE AND ADMINISTRATION: Recommended Dose and Dosage Adjustment: The recommended Bi-PegLyte Bowel Prep Kit oral dosage regimen for adults on the day prior to colonoscopy is the entire contents of one kit.

Administration: No solid food or milk (clear liquids only) should be taken on the day of the preparation. No antacids should be taken within one hour of taking the bisacodyl tablets.

Step 1: The 3 bisacodyl tablets (15 mg) should be taken with water. Do not chew or crush.

Step 2: Prepare the PEG/Electrolyte solution as follows:

1. Dissolve the entire contents of one sachet in 1 L (32 ounces) of water and mix rapidly. No additional ingredients, e.g. flavouring, should be added to the solution.
2. Refrigerate the solution as chilling improves the taste.
3. Use the solution within 48 hours of mixing and discard unused portion.

Step 3: Wait for a bowel movement (or maximum of 6 hours).

After a bowel movement, or if there is no bowel movement within 6 hours of taking the bisacodyl tablets, rapidly drink a glassful (240 mL) of PEG/Electrolyte solution every 10 minutes until the entire 1 litre solution is finished. Repeat Step 2 with the other PEG/Electrolyte powder sachet, drinking 240 mL of solution every 10 minutes or as directed by a physician. The patients should be instructed to drink all of the solution.

Watery bowel movements should begin within 1 hour and continue for 1 to 2 hours after finishing. Lavage is complete when fecal discharge is clear.

Reconstitution: Oral Solutions: Each pouch of PEG/Electrolyte powder is to be added to one (1) litre of water (32 ounces) and mixed rapidly.

Reconstituted solution should be used within 48 hours after mixing if stored at room temperature. Discard unused portion.

OVERDOSAGE:

There are no specific antidotes that are required to be administered in the event of overdose; however, supportive care may be required in order to prevent dehydration and/or electrolyte imbalance.

> For management of a suspected drug overdose, contact your regional Poison Control Centre. See the *CPS* Directory section for a list of Poison Control Centres.

ACTION AND CLINICAL PHARMACOLOGY: Mechanism of Action: PEG/Electrolyte solution cleanses the bowel by induction of diarrhea. The osmotic activity of polyethylene glycol 3350, in combination with the electrolyte concentration, results in virtually no net absorption or secretion of ions or water. Accordingly, large volumes may be administered without significant changes in fluid and electrolyte balance.

pms-Bisacodyl is a contact stimulant laxative, administered either orally or rectally, which acts directly on the colonic mucosa to produce normal peristalsis throughout the large intestine.

On contact with the mucosa or submucosal plexi of the large intestine, pms-Bisacodyl stimulates sensory nerve endings to produce parasympathetic reflexes resulting in increased peristaltic contractions of the colon. It has also been shown to promote fluid and ion accumulation in the colon, which increases the laxative effect.

pms-Bisacodyl is very poorly absorbed, if at all, in the small intestine following oral administration, or in the large intestine following rectal administration.

STORAGE AND STABILITY: The Bi-PegLyte Bowel Prep Kit carton should be stored at room temperature (15-30°C). The reconstituted PEG/Electrolyte solution should be used within 48 hours after mixing if stored at room temperature. Discard unused portion.

INFORMATION FOR THE PATIENT: Published in e-CPS, available by subscription at www.e-cps.ca.

DOSAGE FORMS, COMPOSITION AND PACKAGING: Bi-PegLyte Bowel Prep Kit (PEG 3350 and Electrolytes for Oral Solution USP and Bisacodyl Delayed Release Tablets USP) contains two sachets of PEG/Electrolyte powder (PEG 3350 and Electrolytes for Oral Solution USP, 70 g each) and one blisterpack containing three (3) tablets of pms-Bisacodyl Enteric Coated Tablets (Bisacodyl delayed release tablets USP).

Each 70 g sachet of PEG/Electrolyte powder fruit flavored, to be dissolved in 1 L of water, contains: polyethylene glycol 3350 59.55 g, sodium sulphate 5.74 g, sodium bicarbonate 1.69 g, sodium chloride 1.46 g, potassium chloride 0.76 g, flavours 0.64 g, sodium saccharine 0.14 g.

The mmol/L equivalents of the PEG/Electrolyte ingredient concentrations are as follows: polyethylene glycol 18 mmol/L, sodium 126 mmol/L, potassium 10 mmol/L, chloride 35 mmol/L, sulphate 40 mmol/L. The osmolarity of a prepared solution of PEG/Electrolytes ranges from 235-305 mOsmol.

Each yellow, enteric coated tablet contains: bisacodyl USP 5 mg. Nonmedicinal ingredredients: colloidal silicon dioxide, FD&C Yellow No. 6, glycerol triacetate, hydroxypropyl methylcellulose, lactose monohydrate, magnesium stearate, methylated silica methylcellulose, microcrystalline cellulose, PEG 8000, polydextrose, polydimethylsiloxane, polyethylene glycol, polyvinyl acetate phthalate, purified water, sodium alginate, sodium bicarbonate, sodium carboxymethylcellulose, sorbitan tristearate, stearic acid, talc, titanium dioxide and triethyl citrate. Blisterpacks of 3.

Biphentin®

methylphenidate HCl

Central Nervous System Stimulant

Purdue Pharma

Date of Preparation: March 8, 2006
Date of Revision: June 19, 2009

PHARMACOLOGY: Methylphenidate is a central nervous system (CNS) stimulant. The mode of action of stimulants in Attention-Deficit Hyperactivity Disorder (ADHD) is not completely understood, but they are thought to act primarily through indirect mechanisms, such as release of dopamine and norepinephrine from neuronal pools, and inhibition of neurotransmitter reuptake.

There is some evidence suggesting that the mechanism whereby methylphenidate produces its mental and behavioural effects in children is related to a dose-dependent blockade of the dopamine transporter and an increase in extracellular dopamine. While the evidence regarding how these effects relate to the condition of the CNS is not conclusive, it is likely that an increase in dopamine transporter activity is part of the underlying mechanistic basis of ADHD.

Pharmacokinetics: Pharmacokinetics of Methylphenidate: Methylphenidate is rapidly and extensively absorbed following oral administration—with peak blood levels obtained in 1 to 3 hours.

Methylphenidate is excreted almost entirely in the urine. The primary route of metabolism for methylphenidate is desterification to the inactive metabolite ritalinic acid (α-phenyl-2-piperidine acetic acid), which represents 60-81% of the administered dose, and 6-oxy-α-phenyl-2-piperidine acetic acid (9-12% of the administered dose). Unchanged drug accounts for less than 1% of the administered dose. First pass metabolism results in an absolute bioavailability of 30% with large inter-individual differences (11-52%).

Methylphenidate is eliminated from plasma with a mean half-life of 2.4 hours in children and 2.1 hours in adults. The apparent systemic clearance, for a 0.3 mg/kg dose, is 10.2 and 10.5 L/h/kg in children and adults, respectively. These data indicate that the pharmacokinetic behavior of methylphenidate in hyperactive children is similar to that in normal adults. The apparent distribution volume of methylphenidate in children is approximately 20 L/kg, with substantial variability (11 to 33 L/kg).

In blood, methylphenidate and its metabolites are distributed between plasma (57%) and erythrocytes (43%). Methylphenidate and its metabolites exhibit low plasma protein binding (approximately 15%).

Pharmacokinetics and Pharmacodynamics of Biphentin: In a single dose study in healthy adult volunteer subjects, Biphentin (methylphenidate hydrochloride controlled release capsules, 20 mg) was fully bioavailable, relative to two separate 10 mg doses of an immediate-release reference formulation (Ritalin), under both fasted and fed conditions (relative AUC, 96% and 107%, respectively). In a single dose study in young children (6-12 years) with ADHD, Biphentin, when given at a dose equal to the patient's pre-study methylphenidate dose (mean dose 38.6 mg), following a child's typical breakfast, was fully bioavailable relative to the same daily dose of immediate-release methylphenidate (Ritalin) given as two separate doses (relative AUC, 101%).

Biphentin was designed to be an alternative to separate doses of immediate release methylphenidate by providing a biphasic plasma concentration time profile when given as a single dose. The rate of increase in plasma methylphenidate concentration with the controlled release formulation was similar to that with the immediate-release formulation. In adults the initial peak concentration occurred at 1.7 hours post-dose for Biphentin and at 1.8 hours post-dose for the immediate-release formulation, when given under fasting conditions, and at 2.0 hours post-dose and 2.5 hours post-dose, respectively, when given with food. The initial maximum concentration (C_{max}) achieved with the controlled release formulation was 76% (fasted) and 84% (fed) of that of immediate-release methylphenidate. In young children, being treated for ADHD with methylphenidate, the initial peak concentration occurred at 2.6 hours post-dose for Biphentin and at 2.1 hours post-dose for the immediate-release formulation, when given at doses equal to the children's pre-study maintenance doses. The initial maximum concentration achieved with the controlled release formulation was 79% of that of immediate-release methylphenidate.

A double-blind, placebo-controlled, crossover comparison of the pharmacodynamics of Biphentin and immediate-release methylphenidate in children (age 6 to 17 years) with ADHD demonstrated equivalent improvements on the same daily dose, with a similar time-course, on both behavioural and cognitive parameters, relative to placebo. Biphentin was given as a single morning dose while immediate-release methylphenidate was given at the same daily dose, in equally divided doses in the morning and at lunchtime. Improvements relative to placebo were noted within 1 hour on Biphentin and persisted into the early evening.

INDICATIONS: Biphentin (methylphenidate hydrochloride controlled release capsules) is indicated for treatment of Attention-Deficit Hyperactivity Disorder (ADHD) in: **children (6-11 years of age), adolescents (12-18 years of age), adults (>18 years of age).**

Children (<6 years of age): Biphentin should not be used in children under 6 years, since safety and efficacy in this age group have not been established.

Geriatrics (>65 years of age): No data available.

A diagnosis of ADHD (DSM-IV) implies the presence of hyperactive-impulsive or inattentive symptoms that caused impairment and that were present before age 7 years. The symptoms must be persistent, must be more severe than is typically observed in individuals at a comparable level of development, must cause clinically significant impairment, e.g. in social, academic, or occupational functioning, and must be present in two or more settings, e.g. school (or work) and at home. The symptoms must not be better accounted for by another mental disorder. For the Inattentive Type, at least 6 of the following symptoms must have persisted for at least 6 months: lack of attention to details/careless mistakes, lack of sustained attention, poor listener, failure to follow through on tasks, poor organization, avoids tasks requiring sustained mental effort, loses things, easily distracted, forgetful. For the Hyperactive-Impulsive Type, at least 6 of the following symptoms must have persisted for at least 6 months: fidgeting/squirming, leaving seat, inappropriate running/climbing, difficulty with quiet activities, "on the go," excessive talking, blurting answers, can't wait turn, intrusive. For a Combined Type diagnosis, both inattentive and hyperactive-impulsive criteria must be met.

Special Diagnostic Considerations: The specific etiology of ADHD is unknown, and there is no single diagnostic test. Adequate diagnosis requires the use not only of medical but of special psychological, educational, and social resources. Learning may or may not be impaired. The diagnosis must be based upon a complete history and evaluation of the patient and not solely on the presence of the required number of DSM-IV characteristics.

Need for Comprehensive Treatment Program: Biphentin is indicated as an integral part of a total treatment program for ADHD that may include other measures (psychological, educational, social) for patients with this syndrome. Drug treatment may not be indicated for all patients with this syndrome. Drug treatment is not intended for use in the patient who exhibits symptoms secondary to environmental factors and/or other primary psychiatric disorders, including psychosis. Appropriate educational placement is essential in children and adolescents with this diagnosis and psychosocial intervention is often helpful. When remedial measures alone are insufficient, the decision to prescribe drug treatment will depend upon the physician's assessment of the chronicity and severity of the patient's symptoms.

Long-Term Use: The effectiveness of Biphentin for long-term use, i.e. for more than 4 weeks, has not been systematically evaluated in placebo-controlled trials. Therefore, the physician who elects to use Biphentin for extended periods should periodically re-evaluate the long-term usefulness of the drug for the individual patient (see Dosage).

CONTRAINDICATIONS: Anxiety, tension, agitation, thyrotoxicosis, advanced arteriosclerosis, symptomatic cardiovascular disease, moderate to severe hypertension or glaucoma.

Patients who are hypersensitive to methylphenidate hydrochloride or to any other ingredient in the formulation or component of the container. For a complete listing of excipients, see Supplied.

Patients with motor tics or with a family history or diagnosis of Tourette's syndrome (verbal tics) (see Adverse Effects).

During treatment with monoamine oxidase inhibitors, and also within a minimum of 14 days following discontinuation of a monoamine oxidase inhibitor (hypertensive crises may result) (see Precautions, Drug Interactions).

WARNINGS:

Serious Warnings and Precautions
- **Drug Dependence** (see Drug Dependence/Tolerance)

General: Biphentin (methylphenidate hydrochloride controlled release capsules) has not been compared to other controlled release methylphenidate preparations on the Canadian market, and therefore is not interchangeable.

Children: Theoretically there exists a pharmacological potential for all ADHD drugs to increase the risk of sudden/cardiac death. Although confirmation of an incremental risk for adverse cardiac events arising from treatment with ADHD medications is lacking, prescribers should consider this potential risk.

All drugs with sympathomimetic effects prescribed in the management of ADHD should be used with caution in patients who: a) are involved in strenuous exercise or activities, b) use other stimulants, or c) have a family history of sudden/cardiac death.

Prior to the initiation of treatment, a personal and family history (including assessment for a family history sudden death or ventricular arrhythmia) and physical exam should be obtained to assess for the presence of cardiac disease. In patients with relevant risk factors and based on the clinician's judgement, further cardiovascular evaluation may be considered (e.g. electrocardiogram and echocardiogram). Patients who develop symptoms such as exertional chest pain, unexplained syncope, or other symptoms suggestive of cardiac disease during ADHD treatment should undergo a prompt cardiac evaluation.

Cardiovascular: Sudden Death and Pre-existing Structural Cardiac Abnormalities or Other Serious Heart Problems: Children and Adolescents: Sudden death has been reported in association with stimulant drugs used for ADHD treatment at usual doses in children and adolescents with structural cardiac abnormalities or other serious cardiac problems. Although some serious heart problems alone carry an increased risk of sudden death, Biphentin generally should not be used in children or adolescents with known serious structural cardiac abnormalities, cardiomyopathy, serious heart rhythm abnormalities, or other serious cardiac problems that may place them at increased vulnerability to the sympathomimetic effects of a stimulant drug.

Adults: Sudden death, stroke, and myocardial infarction have been reported in adults taking stimulant drugs at usual doses for ADHD. Although the role of stimulants in these adult cases is also unknown, adults have a greater likelihood than children of having serious structural cardiac abnormalities, cardiomyopathy, serious heart rhythm abnormalities, coronary artery disease, or other serious cardiac problems. Adults with such abnormalities should also generally not be treated with stimulant drugs.

Pre-existing Cardiovascular and Cerebral Vascular Conditions: CNS stimulants should be used with caution in patients with a condition of the cardiovascular or cerebrovascular system, taking into account risk predictors for these conditions. Patients should be screened for pre-existing or underlying cardiovascular or cerebrovascular conditions before initiation of treatment with stimulants and monitored for new conditions of the heart or brain during the course of treatment.

Hypertension: Hypertension may occur during methylphenidate treatment in some patients. Caution is particularly indicated in treating patients whose underlying medical conditions might be compromised by increases in blood pressure or heart rate, e.g., those with pre-existing hypertension, heart failure, recent myocardial infarction or hyperthyroidism.

Blood pressure should be monitored at appropriate intervals in patients receiving stimulants, especially in patients with pre-existing conditions that may result in hypertension.

Drug Dependence/Tolerance: Biphentin should be given cautiously to emotionally unstable patients, such as those with a history of drug dependence or alcoholism, because such patients may increase dosage on their own initiative.

Chronic abuse can lead to marked tolerance and psychological dependence with varying degrees of abnormal behaviour. Frank psychotic episodes can occur, especially with parenteral abuse.

Careful supervision is required during drug withdrawal, since severe depression and underlying hyperactivity can be unmasked. Long-term follow-up may be required because of the patient's basic personality disturbances.

Endocrine and Metabolism: Long-Term Suppression of Growth: Sufficient data on the safety of long-term use of methylphenidate in children are not yet available. Although a causal relationship has not been established, suppression of growth (i.e., weight gain, and/or height) has been reported with the long-term use of stimulants in children. Therefore, patients requiring long-term therapy should be carefully monitored. Patients who are not growing or gaining weight as expected should have their treatment interrupted.

Psychiatric: Depression and Psychotic Disorders: Biphentin should not be used to treat severe exogenous or endogenous depression. Clinical experience suggests that in psychotic children, administration of methylphenidate may exacerbate symptoms of behavioural disturbance and thought disorder.

Bipolar Illness: Particular care should be taken in using stimulants to treat ADHD in patients with comorbid bipolar disorder because of concern for possible induction of a mixed/manic episode in such patients. Prior to initiating treatment with a stimulant, patients with comorbid depressive symptoms should be adequately screened to determine if they are at risk for bipolar disorder; such screening should include a detailed psychiatric history, including a family history of suicide, bipolar disorder and depression.

Emergence of New Psychotic or Manic Symptoms: Treatment emergent psychotic or manic symptoms e.g., hallucinations, delusional thinking, or mania in children and adolescents without a prior history of psychotic illness or mania can be caused by stimulants at usual doses. If such symptoms occur, consideration should be given to a possible causal role of the stimulant, and discontinuation of treatment may be appropriate. In a pooled analysis of multiple short-term, placebo-controlled studies, such symptoms occurred in about 0.1% (4 patients with events out of 3482 exposed to methylphenidate or amphetamine for several weeks at usual doses) of stimulant-treated patients compared to 0 in placebo-treated patients.

Aggression: Aggressive behaviour or hostility is often observed in children and adolescents with ADHD, and has been reported in clinical trials and the postmarketing experience of some medications indicated for the treatment of ADHD. Although there is no systematic evidence that stimulants cause aggressive behaviour or hostility, patients beginning treatment for ADHD should be monitored for the appearance of or worsening of aggressive behaviour or hostility.

Fatigue: Biphentin should not be used for the prevention or treatment of normal fatigue states.

Neurologic: Seizures: There is some clinical evidence that methylphenidate may lower the convulsive threshold in patients with prior history of seizures, with prior EEG abnormalities in the absence of seizures and, very rarely, in patients with no prior EEG evidence or history of seizures. Clinical experience has shown that a small number of patients may experience an increase in seizure frequency when treated with methylphenidate. If seizure frequency rises, the drug should be discontinued.

Ophthalmologic: Visual Disturbance: Symptoms of visual disturbances have been encountered in rare cases. Difficulties with accommodation and blurring of vision have been reported.

Pregnancy: Studies to establish safe use of methylphenidate in pregnant women have not been conducted. Therefore, Biphentin should not be given to pregnant women unless the potential benefit outweighs the risk to the fetus.

Lactation: It is not known whether methylphenidate and/or its metabolites pass into breast milk. For safety reasons, the physician should assess the patient's medical condition and advise on the following options: refrain from breast-feeding infants while taking Biphentin, or discontinue the drug while nursing.

Pediatrics (<6 years of age): Biphentin should not be used in children under six years, since safety and efficacy in this age group have not been established. Long-term effects of methylphenidate in children have not been well established (see Warnings, Endocrine and Metabolism).

PRECAUTIONS: Drug treatment is not indicated in all cases of Attention Deficit Hyperactivity Disorder and should be considered only in light of the complete history and evaluation. The decision to prescribe Biphentin (methylphenidate hydrochloride controlled release capsules) should depend on the physician's assessment of the chronicity and severity of the patient's symptoms and their appropriateness for his/her age. Treatment should not depend solely on the presence of one or more abnormal behavioural characteristics. Where these symptoms are associated with acute stress reactions, treatment with methylphenidate is usually not indicated.

Patients with an element of agitation may react adversely; discontinue therapy if necessary.

Patients with motor tics or with a family history or diagnosis of Tourette's syndrome may be at risk for exacerbation of these conditions, although available evidence does not support a direct association with stimulant therapy.

Periodic laboratory tests are advised during prolonged therapy. The tests should include, but not be limited to, haematological parameters, including complete blood count, differential and platelet counts, and liver enzymes.

Long-term effects of methylphenidate have not been well established.

Because methylphenidate may affect performance, patients should be cautious when driving or operating machinery.

Drug Interactions: Alcohol may exacerbate the CNS adverse effect of psychoactive drugs. Therefore, patients undergoing Biphentin therapy should be advised to avoid alcohol during treatment.

Because of possible increases in blood pressure and heart rate, Biphentin should be used cautiously with drugs with similar pharmacological actions.

Inhibition of Drug Metabolism by Methylphenidate: Human pharmacologic studies have shown that methylphenidate may inhibit the metabolism of coumarin anticoagulants (e.g., warfarin), anticonvulsants (e.g., phenobarbital, phenytoin, primidone) and some antidepressants (tricyclics and selective serotonin reuptake inhibitors). Downward dose adjustment of these drugs may be required when given concomitantly with methylphenidate. It may be necessary to adjust the dosage and monitor plasma drug concentrations (or, in the case of coumarin, coagulation times) when initiating or discontinuing concomitant methylphenidate.

Monoamine Oxidase Inhibitors: Methylphenidate is contraindicated during treatment with monoamine oxidase inhibitors, and also within a minimum of 14 days following discontinuation of a monoamine oxidase inhibitor (hypertensive crises may result). The same precautions apply to Biphentin (see Contraindications).

Clonidine: Serious adverse events have been reported in concomitant use with clonidine, although no causality for the combination has been established. The safety of using methylphenidate in combination with clonidine or other centrally acting alpha-2 agonists has not been systematically evaluated.

ADVERSE EFFECTS: Adverse events in children (6-11 years of age) and adolescents (12-18 years of age) with ADHD were evaluated in two Canadian randomized controlled clinical trials of Biphentin (methylphenidate hydrochloride controlled release capsules) in comparison with placebo and immediate release methylphenidate. Table 1 and Table 2 list all adverse events occurring at an incidence of 1% or more, from both studies, in children (6-11 years of age) and adolescents (12-18 years of age), whether considered by the clinical investigator to be related to the study drug or not.

Adverse events in adults with ADHD were evaluated in a Canadian randomized controlled trial in comparison with placebo. A summary of adverse events occurring at an incidence of 1% or more is given in Table 3, which includes all events, whether considered by the clinical investigator to be related to the study drug or not.

Table 1: Biphentin

Adverse Events[a] Reported in Biphentin Clinical Trials in Children 6-11 Years of Age (≥1%)

	Biphentin % (n=68)	IR Methylphenidate % (n=68)
Body as a Whole		
Headache	11.8	8.8
Abdominal Pain	8.8	8.8
Flu Syndrome	5.9	7.4
Pain	2.9	1.5
Infection	2.9	2.9
Asthenia	1.5	2.9
Malaise	1.5	0.0
Photosensitivity Reaction	1.5	0.0
Chills	1.5	4.4
Fever	1.5	1.5
Allergic Reaction	1.5	0.0
Neoplasm (benign nasal polyp)	0.0	1.5
Cardiovascular		
Hypertension	1.5	0.0
Vasodilatation	1.5	0.0
Central Nervous System		
Insomnia	22.1	14.7
Somnolence	11.8	4.4
Nervousness	8.8	8.8
Depression	7.4	4.4
Apathy	7.4	4.4
Emotional Lability	2.9	8.8
Obsessive Behaviour	2.9	2.9
Vocal Tics	2.9	0.0
Speech Disorder	2.9	1.5
Motor Tics	2.9	1.5

(cont'd)

Table 1: Biphentin *(cont'd)*

Adverse Events[a] Reported in Biphentin Clinical Trials in Children 6-11 Years of Age (≥1%)

	Biphentin % (n=68)	IR Methylphenidate % (n=68)
Rebound	4.4	1.5
Sleep Disorder	1.5	2.9
Dizziness	1.5	0.0
Anxiety	1.5	0.0
Euphoria	1.5	1.5
Stereotypies	1.5	0.0
Depersonalization	0.0	1.5
Agitation	0.0	1.5
Hallucinations	0.0	1.5
Hyperkinesia	0.0	1.5
Tremor	0.0	1.5
Digestive		
Anorexia	22.1	19.1
Nausea	5.9	2.9
Increased Appetite	2.9	0.0
Vomiting	2.9	1.5
Diarrhea	0.0	2.9
Respiratory		
Pharyngitis	2.9	2.9
Asthma	1.5	1.5
Cough Increased	1.5	5.9
Rhinitis	0.0	1.5
Bronchitis	0.0	1.5
Skin and Appendages		
Rash	5.9	2.9
Eczema	1.5	0.0
Skin Discolouration	1.5	0.0
Special Senses		
Abnormal Vision	1.5	0.0
Conjunctivitis	1.5	0.0
Corneal Lesion	1.5	0.0
Otitis Media	1.5	0.0

[a] Events are listed regardless of the causality assessment by the clinical investigator.

Table 2: Biphentin

Adverse Events[a] Reported in Biphentin Clinical Trials in Adolescents 12-18 Years of Age (≥1%)

	Biphentin % (n=40)	IR Methylphenidate % (n=40)
Body as a Whole		
Headache	25.0	22.5

(cont'd)

Table 2: Biphentin *(cont'd)*

Adverse Events[a] Reported in Biphentin Clinical Trials in Adolescents 12-18 Years of Age (≥1%)

	Biphentin % (n=40)	IR Methylphenidate % (n=40)
Flu Syndrome	7.5	7.5
Abdominal Pain	5.0	10.0
Asthenia	2.5	2.5
Infection	0.0	2.5
Pain	0.0	2.5
Cardiovascular		
Palpitation	2.5	0.0
Tachycardia	0.0	2.5
Syncope	0.0	2.5
Central Nervous System		
Nervousness	27.5	25.0
Somnolence	15.0	7.5
Dizziness	7.5	10.0
Insomnia	7.5	12.5
Depersonalization	7.5	0.0
Depression	2.5	5.0
Emotional Lability	5.0	5.0
Sleep Disorder	2.5	2.5
Vocal Tics	2.5	2.5
Apathy	2.5	0.0
Obsessive Behaviour	2.5	0.0
Vertigo	2.5	2.5
Anxiety	0.0	2.5
Rebound	0.0	2.5
Neurosis	0.0	2.5
Digestive		
Anorexia	7.5	27.5
Nausea	5.0	5.0
Increased Appetite	5.0	12.5
Vomiting	2.5	2.5
Diarrhea	2.5	0.0
Metabolic and Nutrition		
Thirst	0.0	2.5
Musculoskeletal		
Arthralgia	2.5	2.5
Respiratory		
Pharyngitis	5.0	2.5

(cont'd)

Table 2: Biphentin *(cont'd)*

Adverse Events[a] Reported in Biphentin Clinical Trials in Adolescents 12-18 Years of Age (≥1%)

	Biphentin % (n=40)	IR Methylphenidate % (n=40)
Cough Increased	0.0	5.0
Asthma	0.0	2.5
Sinusitis	0.0	2.5
Skin and Appendages		
Pruritus	0.0	2.5
Urogenital		
Dysmenorrhea	0.0	2.5

[a] Events are listed regardless of the causality assessment by the clinical investigator.

Table 3: Biphentin

Adverse Events[a] Reported in Biphentin Clinical Trials in Adults (≥1%)

	Biphentin % (n=50)	Placebo % (n=50)
Body as a Whole		
Headache	28.0	24.0
Asthenia	8.0	10.0
Abdominal Pain	4.0	6.0
Fever	4.0	0.0
Pain	2.0	6.0
Chest Pain	2.0	2.0
Accidental Injury	2.0	0.0
Body Odour	2.0	0.0
Allergic Reaction	2.0	0.0
Chills	0.0	2.0
Hernia	0.0	2.0
Flu Syndrome	0.0	2.0
Infection	0.0	4.0
Cardiovascular		
Tachycardia	6.0	4.0
Palpitation	2.0	2.0
Peripheral Vascular Disease	2.0	0.0
Central Nervous System		
Nervousness	24.0	4.0
Insomnia	22.0	10.0
Anxiety	18.0	0.0
Dry Mouth	12.0	2.0
Emotional Lability	10.0	2.0
Depression	8.0	2.0
Agitation	6.0	4.0
Akathisia	6.0	0.0

(cont'd)

Table 3: Biphentin *(cont'd)*

Adverse Events[a] Reported in Biphentin Clinical Trials in Adults (≥1%)

	Biphentin % (n=50)	Placebo % (n=50)
Dizziness	4.0	2.0
Hypertension	4.0	2.0
Abnormal Thinking	4.0	0.0
Somnolence	2.0	4.0
Depersonalization	2.0	2.0
Twitching	2.0	2.0
Confusion	2.0	0.0
Neurosis	2.0	0.0
Paresthesia	2.0	0.0
Vasodilatation	2.0	0.0
Personality Disorder	0.0	2.0
Rebound	0.0	2.0
Digestive		
Anorexia	26.0	6.0
Nausea	20.0	8.0
Dyspepsia	4.0	4.0
Nausea and Vomiting	2.0	0.0
Constipation	2.0	0.0
Vomiting	2.0	0.0
Diarrhea	0.0	6.0
Haemic and Lymphatic		
Ecchymosis	0.0	2.0
Metabolic and Nutrition		
Weight Loss	2.0	0.0
Musculoskeletal		
Arthralgia	2.0	2.0
Myalgia	0.0	2.0
Respiratory		
Rhinitis	4.0	0.0
Cough Increased	2.0	0.0
Pharyngitis	2.0	0.0
Epistaxis	0.0	2.0
Hiccough	0.0	2.0
Skin and Appendages		
Sweating	6.0	0.0
Special Senses		
Abnormal Vision	2.0	0.0
Ear Disorder	2.0	0.0

[a] Events are listed regardless of the causality assessment by the clinical investigator.

The prescriber should be aware that these figures cannot be used to predict the incidence of adverse events in the course of usual medical practice where patient characteristics and other factors differ from those which prevailed in the clinical trials. Similarly, the cited frequencies cannot be compared with figures obtained from other clinical investigations involving different treatments, uses, and investigators. The cited figures, however, do provide the prescribing physician with some basis for estimating the relative contribution of drug and non-drug factors to the adverse event incidence rate in the population studied.

There were no adverse events reported to have occurred in <1% of the children in the Biphentin clinical trials.

There were no adverse events reported to have occurred in <1% of the adolescents in the Biphentin clinical trials.

There were no adverse events reported to have occurred in <1% of the adults in the Biphentin clinical trial.

Abnormal Hematologic and Clinical Chemistry Findings: None.

Adverse Events Reported with Other Methylphenidate Hydrochloride Products: Nervousness and insomnia are the most common adverse reactions reported with other methylphenidate products. Other reactions include hypersensitivity (including skin rash, urticaria, fever, arthralgia, exfoliative dermatitis, erythema multiforme with histopathological findings of necrotizing vasculitis, and thrombocytopenic purpura); anorexia; nausea; dizziness; headache; dyskinesia; drowsiness; blood pressure and pulse changes, both up and down; tachycardia; sudden cardiac death; angina; abdominal pain; weight loss during prolonged therapy. There have been rare reports of Tourette's syndrome. Toxic psychosis has been reported. Although a definite causal relationship has not been established, the following have been reported in patients taking other methylphenidate products: instances of abnormal liver function, e.g., hepatic coma; isolated cases of cerebral arteritis and/or occlusion; leukopenia and/or anaemia; transient depressed mood; a few instances of scalp hair loss. Very rare reports of neuroleptic malignant syndrome (NMS) have been received, and in most of these, patients were concurrently receiving therapies associated with NMS. In a single report, a ten-year-old boy who had been taking methylphenidate for approximately 18 months experienced an NMS-like event within 45 minutes of ingesting his first dose of venlafaxine. It is uncertain whether this case represented a drug-drug interaction, a response to either drug alone, or some other cause.

OVERDOSE:

Symptoms: Signs and symptoms of acute overdose, resulting principally from overstimulation of the central nervous system and from excessive sympathomimetic effects, may include the following: agitation, cardiac arrhythmias, confusion, convulsions (may be followed by coma), delirium, euphoria, flushing, hallucinations, headache, hyperpyrexia, hyperreflexia, hypertension, muscle twitching, mydriasis and dryness of mucus membranes, palpitations, sweating, tachycardia, tremors and vomiting.

Treatment: Management consists of providing supportive measures. The patient must be protected against self-injury and against external stimuli that would exacerbate overstimulation already present. If signs and symptoms are not too severe and the patient is conscious, gastric contents may be evacuated by induction of emesis or gastric lavage. In the presence of severe intoxication, use a carefully titrated dosage of short-acting barbiturate before performing gastric lavage.

Intensive care must be provided to maintain adequate circulation and respiratory exchange. External cooling procedures may be required to reduce hyperpyrexia.

Efficacy of peritoneal dialysis or extracorporeal hemodialysis for methylphenidate overdosage has not been established.

For management of a suspected drug overdose, CPhA recommends that you contact your **regional Poison Control Centre**. See the *CPS* Directory section for a list of Poison Control Centres.

DOSAGE: Dosing Considerations: Biphentin (methylphenidate hydrochloride controlled release capsules) has not been compared to other controlled release methylphenidate preparations on the Canadian market, and therefore is not interchangeable.

Biphentin should be administered starting at the lowest possible dose. Dosage should then be individually and slowly adjusted, to the lowest effective dosage, since individual patient response to Biphentin varies widely.

Biphentin should not be used in patients with symptomatic cardiovascular disease and should generally not be used in patients with known structural cardiac abnormalities (see Contraindications and Warnings).

Children: Theoretically there exists a pharmacological potential for all ADHD drugs to increase the risk of sudden/cardiac death. Although confirmation of an incremental risk for adverse cardiac events arising from treatment with ADHD medications is lacking, prescribers should consider this potential risk.

All drugs with sympathomimetic effects prescribed in the management of ADHD should be used with caution in patients who: a) are involved in strenuous exercise or activities, b) use other stimulants, or c) have a family history of sudden/cardiac death. Prior to the initiation of treatment, a personal and family history (including assessment for a family history of sudden death or ventricular arrhythmia) and physical exam should be obtained to assess for the presence of cardiac disease. In patients with relevant risk factors and based on the clinician's judgement, further cardiovascular evaluation may be considered (e.g. electrocardiogram and echocardiogram). Patients who develop symptoms such as exertional chest pain, unexplained syncope, or other symptoms suggestive of cardiac disease during ADHD treatment should undergo a prompt cardiac evaluation.

Particular care should be taken in patients with symptoms of a psychiatric illness as there is a increased risk of comorbid disorder symptoms during stimulant treatment for ADHD (see Warnings).

Patients who are considered to need extended treatment with Biphentin should undergo periodic evaluation of their cardiovascular status (see Warnings).

Caution should be exercised in prescribing concomitant drugs.

Dosage of Biphentin should be individualized according to the needs and responses of the patient.

Biphentin capsules should be swallowed whole and must never be crushed or chewed. The contents may be sprinkled on these soft foods: apple sauce, ice cream or yogurt.

If paradoxical aggravation of symptoms or other adverse effects occur, reduce dosage, or if necessary, discontinue the drug.

Biphentin should be periodically discontinued to assess the patient's condition. Improvement may be sustained when the drug is either temporarily or permanently discontinued.

Children (6 Years and Over): In patients not currently treated with methylphenidate, Biphentin should be initiated in low doses, as a single daily dose in the morning. Dosage should be individualized on the basis of factors such as age, body weight and individual response.

The usual initial dose should be 10-20 mg/day orally.

Patients currently receiving immediate-release formulations of methylphenidate may be converted to the same daily dose of Biphentin, as a single daily dose in the morning.

The total daily dose may be adjusted in weekly increments of 10 mg/day up to a maximum of 60 mg/day. In some children, higher doses (maximum 1 mg/kg/day) may be necessary and in such cases, careful monitoring for adverse events should be implemented.

If adverse events occur, the dosage should be reduced or, if necessary, the drug should be discontinued.

If improvement is not observed after appropriate dosage adjustment the drug should be discontinued.

Adults: Biphentin is to be administered as a single daily dose in the morning. The usual initial dose should be 10-20 mg/day orally. The daily dose should be titrated weekly, in increments of 10 mg, according to individual response, up to a maximum dose of 80 mg/day.

INFORMATION FOR THE PATIENT: Published in e-CPS, available by subscription at www.e-cps.ca.

SUPPLIED: 10 mg: Each controlled release capsule with white body and light turquoise blue cap, imprinted with Biphentin and 10 mg, contains: methylphenidate HCl 10 mg. Nonmedicinal ingredients: gelatin, hydroxypropyl methylcellulose, methyl acrylic acid copolymer, polyethylene glycol, sugar beads, talc and triethyl citrate; capsule shell: FD&C Blue No. 1 and titanium dioxide. Store in a cool, dry place between 15 and 30°C. Protect from moisture. Opaque plastic bottles of 100.

15 mg: Each controlled release capsule with white body and orange cap, imprinted with Biphentin and 15 mg, contains: methylphenidate HCl 15 mg. Nonmedicinal ingredients: gelatin, hydroxypropyl methylcellulose, methyl acrylic acid copolymer, polyethylene glycol, sugar beads, talc and triethyl citrate; capsule shell: D&C Red No. 28, D&C Yellow No. 10, FD&C Red No. 40 and titanium dioxide. Opaque plastic bottles of 100. Store in a cool, dry place between 15 and 30°C. Protect from moisture.

20 mg: Each controlled release capsule with white body and yellow cap, imprinted with Biphentin and 20 mg, contains: methylphenidate HCl 20 mg. Nonmedicinal ingredients: gelatin, hydroxypropyl methylcellulose, methyl acrylic acid copolymer, polyethylene glycol, sugar beads, talc and triethyl citrate; capsule shell: D&C Red No. 33, D&C Yellow No. 10 and titanium dioxide. Opaque plastic bottles of 100. Store in a cool, dry place between 15 and 30°C. Protect from moisture.

30 mg: Each controlled release capsule with white body and blue violet cap, imprinted with Biphentin and 30 mg, contains: methylphenidate HCl 30 mg. Nonmedicinal ingredients: gelatin, hydroxypropyl methylcellulose, methyl acrylic acid copolymer, polyethylene glycol, sugar beads, talc and triethyl citrate; capsule shell: FD&C Blue No. 1, FD&C Red No. 3 and titanium dioxide. Opaque plastic bottles of 100. Store in a cool, dry place between 15 and 30°C. Protect from moisture.

40 mg: Each controlled release capsule with white body and pink cap, imprinted with Biphentin and 40 mg, contains: methylphenidate HCl 40 mg. Nonmedicinal ingredients: gelatin, hydroxypropyl methylcellulose, methyl acrylic acid copolymer, polyethylene glycol, sugar beads, talc and triethyl citrate; capsule shell: D&C Red No. 28, FD&C Blue No. 1, FD&C Red No. 40 and titanium dioxide. Opaque plastic bottles of 100. Store in a cool, dry place between 15 and 30°C. Protect from moisture.

50 mg: Each controlled release capsule with white body and light green cap, imprinted with Biphentin and 50 mg, contains: methylphenidate HCl 50 mg. Nonmedicinal ingredients: gelatin, hydroxypropyl methylcellulose, methyl acrylic acid copolymer, polyethylene glycol, sugar beads, talc and triethyl citrate; capsule shell: D&C Yellow No. 10, FD&C Green No. 3 and titanium dioxide. Opaque plastic bottles of 50. Store in a cool, dry place between 15 and 30°C. Protect from moisture.
60 mg: Each controlled release capsule with white body and iron grey cap, imprinted with Biphentin and 60 mg, contains: methylphenidate HCl 60 mg. Nonmedicinal ingredients: gelatin, hydroxypropyl methylcellulose, methyl acrylic acid copolymer, polyethylene glycol, sugar beads, talc and triethyl citrate; capsule shell: Black Iron oxide and titanium dioxide. Opaque plastic bottles of 50. Store in a cool, dry place between 15 and 30°C. Protect from moisture.
80 mg: Each controlled release capsule with white body and reddish orange cap, imprinted with Biphentin and 80 mg, contains: methylphenidate HCl 80 mg. Nonmedicinal ingredients: gelatin, hydroxypropyl methylcellulose, methyl acrylic acid copolymer, polyethylene glycol, sugar beads, talc and triethyl citrate; capsule shell: FD&C Red No. 40, FD&C Yellow No. 6, D&C Yellow No. 10 and titanium dioxide. Opaque plastic bottles of 50. Store in a cool, dry place between 15 and 30°C. Protect from moisture.

(Shown in Product Identification Section)

Bismutal

bismuth camphocarbonate—guaifenesin

Sore Throat Treatment

Rougier Pharma

SUPPLIED: Each white to creamy white opaque rectal suppository contains: bismuth camphocarbonate 150 mg and guaifenesin 250 mg. Nonmedicinal ingredients: semisynthetic glycerides. Boxes of 2.

Bisoprolol Ⓟ

Beta-adrenergic Blocking Agent, Selective

CPhA Monograph

Date of Preparation: August 2010

> This monograph has been compiled by CPhA and reviewed by experts. It may contain information different from that found in Health Canada-approved Product Monographs. The reader is referred to the *CPS* Editorial Policy for more information.

SUMMARY PRODUCT INFORMATION:

Route of Administration	Dosage Form	Strength
Oral	Tablet	5 mg, 10 mg

INDICATIONS AND CLINICAL USE: Health Canada-approved Indication:
- management of patients with mild to moderate hypertension. It may be used alone or in combination with other antihypertensive agents, particularly thiazide diuretics.

Uses Without Health Canada Approval:
- treatment of heart failure.
- prophylaxis of chronic angina pectoris.

CONTRAINDICATIONS: Bisoprolol is contraindicated in patients with:
- hypersensitivity to bisoprolol or to any ingredient in the formulation or component of the container.
- sinus bradycardia
- cardiogenic shock or decompensated heart failure
- right ventricular failure secondary to pulmonary hypertension
- second or third degree A-V block

WARNINGS AND PRECAUTIONS:

> **Serious Warnings and Precautions**
> Abrupt discontinuation of bisoprolol therapy can lead to severe exacerbation of angina and myocardial infarction. If bisoprolol is to be discontinued, gradually reduce the dose over a period of 2 weeks and closely observe the patient.

Cardiovascular: Beta-blockers, including bisoprolol, can precipitate worsening heart failure. It is important to follow the recommended dose titration schedule to minimize the likelihood of worsening heart failure (see Dosage and Administration). In patients with no history of heart failure, continued use of beta-blockers can, in rare instances, lead to cardiac failure. If heart failure develops discontinue bisoprolol and monitor the patient for resolution of symptoms.

Beta-blockade may aggravate symptoms of arterial insufficiency in patients with peripheral vascular disease.

Beta-blocking effects of bisoprolol may result in severe sinus bradycardia.

Bisoprolol may cause severe hypotension and myocardial depression in patients undergoing anesthesia.

Endocrine and Metabolism: Bisoprolol may mask the signs of hyperthyroidism (e.g., tachycardia). Abrupt discontinuation of bisoprolol in patients with thyrotoxicosis may precipitate the symptoms of hyperthyroidism, including thyroid storm.

Use beta-blockers with caution in diabetic patients, especially those with labile diabetes or those prone to hypoglycemia. Bisoprolol may mask the symptoms of hypoglycemia, such as tachycardia.

Immune: It has been reported that patients with a history of anaphylactic reactions have a more severe response to the allergen if they are receiving beta-blockers. The response to epinephrine used to treat the allergic reaction may be attenuated and larger doses of epinephrine may be needed.

Respiratory: Bisoprolol is relatively cardioselective, though in general, patients with bronchospastic disease should not use bisoprolol, except when other antihypertensive treatments have failed. When used in this situation, the lowest possible dose should be used, a bronchodilator (beta$_2$-adrenergic agonist) should be available and the patient's respiratory status monitored.

Special Populations: Pregnant Women: The safety of bisoprolol in pregnancy has not been established. Interuterine growth retardation has been reported with some beta-blockers. Greatest weight reductions occur with drug exposure during the 2nd trimester. Bisoprolol should be used during pregnancy only when the possible benefits outweigh the potential risks.

Nursing Women: Bisoprolol is excreted in breast milk. If bisoprolol therapy in the mother is necessary, the nursing infant should be monitored for signs of beta-blockade such as bradycardia, hypotension and hypoglycemia.

Pediatrics: Appropriate dosing of bisoprolol in children has not been established.

Geriatrics: When used in elderly patients with essential hypertension the response rates and mean decreases in diastolic blood pressure were similar to that in younger patients, but there was a tendency for older patients to require higher doses of bisoprolol. Observed reductions in heart rate were slightly greater in the elderly than in the young and the degree of heart rate reduction was dose-related.

ADVERSE REACTIONS: Adverse Drug Reactions Overview: Adverse reactions that appear to be dose-related are: bradycardia, diarrhea, asthenia, fatigue and sinusitis. Most frequent adverse reactions are: arthralgia, dizziness, headache, insomnia, diarrhea, nausea, coughing, rhinitis, upper respiratory tract infection, fatigue and peripheral edema.

More Common Adverse Drug Reactions (≥1%): Table 1 lists the more common adverse effects of bisoprolol.

Less Common Adverse Drug Reactions (<1%): Cardiovascular: palpitation, embolism, extrasystoles, myocardial infarction, Raynaud-like disorder, hypertension (rebound), heart failure, AV block, tachycardia, arrhythmia.

Central Nervous System: decreased concentration/memory, involuntary muscle contraction, syncope, coma, encephalopathy, speech disorder, hallucination, confusion.

Allergic/Dermatologic: rash, pruritus, alopecia, exfoliative dermatitis, skin photosensitivity, epidermal necrolysis, erythema multiforme, scleroderma, skin discolouration, urticaria, diaphoresis.

Ear/Nose/Throat: anosmia.

Endocrine and Metabolism: abnormal lacrimation, hypoglycemia, weight gain.

Gastrointestinal: taste abnormalities, ageusia.

Genitourinary: Peyronie's disease, galactorrhea, mastalgia, still-birth.

Hematologic: purpura, vasculitis, peripheral ischemia.

Immune: increased reactivity and sensitivity to allergens (see Warnings and Precautions).

Musculoskeletal: twitching, tremor.

Ophthalmologic: ocular pain/pressure, conjunctivitis, visual disturbances.

Respiratory: asthma/bronchospasm, shortness of breath, pulmonary edema.

Table 1: Bisoprolol

More Common Adverse Drug Reactions (≥1%)

Body System	Effect
Cardiovascular	Generalized edema, peripheral edema, chest pain, bradycardia, hypotension
CNS	Headache, fatigue, dizziness, hypoaesthesia, paraesthesia, fever
Ear/Nose/Throat	Earache, dry mouth
Gastrointestinal	Diarrhea, nausea, abdominal pain, vomiting, dyspepsia
Musculoskeletal	Arthralgia, myalgia, muscle cramps
Psychiatric	Insomnia, somnolence
Respiratory	Upper respiratory tract infection, rhinitis, wheezing, coughing, dyspnea
Sexual Function	Decreased libido, impotence

DRUG INTERACTIONS: Drug-Drug Interactions: See Table 2.

Table 2: Bisoprolol

Drug-Drug Interactions

Interacting Drug	Effect	Clinical Comment
Alpha agonists (e.g., phenylephrine)	Exaggerated hypertensive response of alpha agonist.	Monitor blood pressure.
Amiodarone	Increased bradycardic effect of bisoprolol.	Monitor for signs of bradycardia.
Calcium channel blockers (e.g., nifedipine)	Increased hypotensive effects of bisoprolol; can lead to bradycardia and heart failure.	Monitor for signs of hypotension and decreased heart rate.
Catecholamine-depleting drugs (e.g., guanethidine)	Excessive reduction of sympathetic activity.	Monitor for signs of bradycardia and/or hypotension.
Clonidine	Exacerbated rebound hypertension.	Discontinue bisoprolol 3 to 5 days before stopping clonidine. If replacing clonidine with bisoprolol, initiate bisoprolol 5 to 7 days after stopping clonidine.
Insulin	Increased hypoglycemic effect of insulin.	Monitor for signs of hypoglycemia.
Methacholine	Increased effects of methacholine.	Avoid combination or use with caution.
NSAIDs	Decreased antihypertensive effect of bisoprolol.	Monitor blood pressure and adjust bisoprolol dose as necessary when either starting or stopping an NSAID.
Propafenone	Increased serum concentration of bisoprolol.	Monitor patient and adjust dose of bisoprolol if necessary.
Rifampin	Decreased bisoprolol levels.	Monitor clinical response to bisoprolol and adjust dose if necessary.

DOSAGE AND ADMINISTRATION: Recommended Dose and Dosage Adjustment: Adults: See Table 3.

Geriatrics: Dosage adjustment is not necessary in otherwise healthy elderly patients.

Renal Impairment: See Table 4.

Dosage in Dialysis: Bisoprolol is not dialyzable. Dose replacement or adjustment is not necessary in patients undergoing dialysis.

Hepatic Impairment: Half-life of bisoprolol may increase in patients with severe hepatic impairment. Initial dose should be 2.5 mg once daily. Dose should be carefully titrated to a maximum of 10 mg daily with frequent monitoring.

OVERDOSAGE:

> For management of a suspected drug overdose, CPhA recommends that you contact your **regional Poison Control Centre**. See the *CPS* Directory section for a list of Poison Control Centres.

ACTION AND CLINICAL PHARMACOLOGY: Mechanism of Action: Bisoprolol is a selective and competitive inhibitor of beta1-adrenoceptors. It has no significant membrane stabilizing activity or intrinsic sympathomimetic activity. At higher doses, bisoprolol loses its cardioselectivity and also inhibits beta$_2$-adrenoceptors located in bronchial and vascular smooth muscles. Antihypertensive effect of bisoprolol may involve decrease of cardiac output by beta-blockade, inhibition of renin release by the kidneys, and decrease in sympathetic outflow from the vasomotor centres in the brain. Bisoprolol significantly reduces heart rate, increases sinus node recovery time, and prolongs AV node refractory periods and conduction.

Pharmacokinetics: Adults: Absorption: Bisoprolol is well absorbed after oral administration. Bioavailability is greater than 80%. Peak plasma concentration occurs within about 2 to 4 hours after administration. Absorption is unaffected by food.

Distribution: Bisoprolol has a large volume of distribution (2.93 L/kg). Serum protein binding of bisoprolol is about 30%.

Metabolism: Extensively hepatic (50%). Bisoprolol undergoes N-dealkylation and O-dealkylation, with subsequent oxidation to inactive carboxylic acids.

Excretion: The plasma half-life of bisoprolol is about 9-12 hours. Plasma half-life increases to 27-36 hours in patients with ClCr <40 mL/min, and increases up to two-fold in patients with serious liver disorder. Bisoprolol is eliminated renally (50% unchanged, remainder as inactive metabolites). Less than 2% of the oral dose of bisoprolol is excreted in the feces.

Table 3: Bisoprolol

Dose in Adult Patients

Indication	Route	Initial Dose	Dose Titration	Usual Dose	Maximum Dose	Clinical Comment
Hypertension[a]	Oral	2.5–5 mg once daily	Increase to 10 mg, then 20 mg once daily	10–20 mg once daily	20 mg once daily	Individualize dosage according to the response to patient's blood pressure and tolerance. Doses >20 mg provide minimal added benefit.
Heart failure[b] (Not an approved use in Canada)	Oral	1.25 mg once daily	If required, double the dose every 2–4 weeks	10 mg once daily	10 mg once daily	Increase dose gradually. Monitor for signs and symptoms of heart failure.
Chronic angina pectoris (Not an approved use in Canada)	Oral			5–10 mg once daily	20 mg once daily	If bisoprolol is to be discontinued, taper slowly over 2 weeks with minimal physical exercise (see Warnings and Precautions).

[a] Canadian guidelines on the management of hypertension [*Can J Cardiol* 2008;24(6):465-75] available from www.hypertension.ca.
[b] The Canadian Cardiovascular Society guidelines on the management of heart failure [*Can J Cardiol* 2006;22(1):23-45] available from www.hfcc.ca.

Table 4: Bisoprolol

Dose in Adult Patients with Renal Impairment

Route	Creatinine Clearance	Dosage Adjustment	Clinical Comment
Oral	<40 mL/min	Initial: 2.5 mg once daily Maximum: 10 mg once daily	Increase dose with caution.

Special Populations: Race: African-Americans on bisoprolol monotherapy may experience smaller reductions in blood pressure than patients of other races [*Rev Cardiovasc Med* 2008;9(2):84-95].

Bisphosphonates: Oral

alendronate sodium
clodronate disodium
etidronate disodium
risedronate sodium hemi-pentahydrate

Bone Metabolism Regulator

CPhA Monograph

Date of Revision: November 2007

This monograph has been compiled by CPhA and reviewed by experts. It may contain information different from that found in Health Canada-approved Product Monographs. The reader is referred to the *CPS* Editorial Policy for more information.

SUMMARY PRODUCT INFORMATION:

Drug[a]	Dosage Form	Strength
Alendronate	Liquid	70 mg/75 mL
	Tablet	5 mg, 10 mg, 40 mg, 70 mg
Clodronate	Capsule	400 mg
Etidronate	Tablet	200 mg, 400 mg
Risedronate	Tablet	5 mg, 30 mg, 35 mg, 75 mg

[a] Table contains single-entity oral bisphosphonates only.

PHARMACOLOGY: Bisphosphonates (previously called diphosphonates) are stable analogues of pyrophosphate. After binding to bone surfaces, they slow the formation of hydroxyapatite crystals and delay their aggregation into large clusters. They also interfere with the resorptive action and promote apoptosis (programmed cell death) of osteoclasts, resulting in decreased depth and rate of formation of new bone remodeling units. Lifelong accumulation of remodeling deficits begins shortly after bone growth stops and is thought to be the underlying mechanism of age-related bone loss. By inhibiting this process, bisphosphonates increase bone mass and decrease susceptibility to fracture. An additional proposed mechanism of action is inhibition of osteocyte and osteoblast apoptosis, thereby increasing the life span of osteocytes and decreasing bone fragility. This monograph focuses on the use of oral bisphosphonates.

The bisphosphonates have been classified as 1st, 2nd or 3rd generation agents, based on the type of side chain on the carbon atom, their relative antiresorptive potencies and when they were developed. Of the oral agents available in Canada, etidronate and clodronate, with short alkyl or halide side chains, are considered 1st generation. Alendronate, with its amino terminal group, is considered a 2nd generation agent and is sometimes referred to as an aminobisphosphonate. Risedronate possesses a cyclic side chain and is a 3rd generation bisphosphonate.

The antiresorptive properties of bisphosphonates have widespread clinical applications. In the treatment of Paget's disease of bone, bisphosphonate therapy results in reduction of elevated alkaline phosphatase levels and relief of bone pain. Bisphosphonates have been shown to maintain and increase bone mass and decrease the incidence of vertebral and non-vertebral fractures in the prevention and treatment of primary and secondary osteoporosis. They are also used in the management of hypercalcemia of malignancy, metastatic and osteolytic bone disease and in bone imaging.

Pharmacokinetics: Bisphosphonates are poorly absorbed from the gastrointestinal tract. Typically, absorption ranges from 0.6 to 3% of an oral dose and is significantly reduced in the presence of calcium, other divalent cations or food or beverages other than plain water. Bisphosphonates are not metabolized. After binding to bone surfaces and exerting their effects on osteoclasts, they are retained in the bone for months or years and are slowly released with the process of bone turnover. The portion of absorbed drug that is not bound to bone is excreted by the kidney unchanged.

INDICATIONS: Bisphosphonates have many clinical uses including prevention and treatment of primary and secondary osteoporosis, Paget's disease of bone, hypercalcemia, primary hyperparathyroidism (when surgery is not possible), multiple myeloma and osteolysis associated with bone metastases of malignant tumors.

Table 1 lists the labeled indications for the oral bisphosphonates.

CONTRAINDICATIONS: All bisphosphonates are contraindicated in patients with hypersensitivity to any bisphosphonate. Alendronate is contraindicated in patients with abnormalities of the esophagus that delay emptying, such as stricture or achalasia, in patients who cannot stand or sit upright for at least 30 minutes, in patients with hypocalcemia and in patients with creatinine clearance <0.58 mL/s. Alendronate oral solution should not be given to patients at increased risk of aspiration. Clodronate is contraindicated in patients with serum creatinine >440 μmol/L, severe inflammation of the gastrointestinal tract and concomitant treatment with other bisphosphonates. It is also contraindicated in patients who are pregnant or breastfeeding. Etidronate is contraindicated in patients with clinically overt osteomalacia, until appropriate treatment has been initiated for it. Risedronate is contraindicated in patients with hypocalcemia.

WARNINGS: Bisphosphonates may cause upper gastrointestinal disorders such as dysphagia, esophagitis, esophageal ulcer and gastric ulcer. Esophageal injury has been more commonly associated with aminobisphosphonates such as alendronate. There appears to be a higher risk of esophageal injury if the patient does not remain upright following the dose. It is recommended that patients take bisphosphonates on an empty stomach with a full glass of water and remain in an upright position for at least 30 minutes after a dose.

Because bisphosphonates are excreted renally, caution and appropriate monitoring are advised for patients with renal failure (see Contraindications).

In the treatment of Paget's disease with etidronate, it can take months to realize the maximum benefit of therapy. Caution is advised regarding treatment beyond the recommended duration of therapy, because of the potential for impaired mineralization of new bone. A drug-free interval is recommended between courses of treatment for Paget's disease (see Dosage).

PRECAUTIONS: Gastrointestinal: To minimize the risk of upper gastrointestinal irritation or injury, bisphosphonates should be taken on an empty stomach with a full glass of plain water. They should not be taken with food, calcium, other medications, or any beverage other than water. Patients should remain in an upright position (sitting or standing) for 30 minutes after a dose. Manufacturers' recommendations vary for the different agents with respect to the time of day and how long before a meal they should be taken (see Dosage).

Dosing instructions should be clearly explained and reinforced. Advise patients to stop taking the bisphosphonate and consult their physician if symptoms of esophageal injury develop, such as difficulty swallowing, retrosternal pain or new or worsening heartburn.

Caution is advised for patients with a history of gastrointestinal disorders, especially delayed esophageal transit time. Alendronate is contraindicated in patients with delayed esophageal emptying.

Bone Metabolism: Hypocalcemia and other disturbances of bone and mineral metabolism should be effectively treated prior to bisphosphonate therapy. Because mild decreases in serum calcium and phosphorus have been observed with some bisphosphonates, maintaining adequate intake of calcium and vitamin D is recommended. Calcium interferes with the absorption of the bisphosphonate and should be taken at a different time of the day. In the case of cyclic etidronate therapy, some experts advise that calcium and vitamin D supplements not be taken during the 14-day etidronate phase; however, they can be taken 2 hours before or after etidronate in situations where the physician deems it appropriate. For information on recommended intake of calcium and vitamin D, see the CPhA monographs, *Calcium Salts: Oral* and *Vitamin D*.

Dose and time-dependent impairment of new bone mineralization can occur with continuous etidronate dosing regimens. This can lead to accumulation of unmineralized osteoid with bone pain and fractures, similar to the clinical manifestations of osteomalacia. Extended periods of continuous use should be approached cautiously.

General: Although osteonecrosis of the jaw is more commonly seen in cancer patients receiving intravenous bisphosphonates, cases have been reported in patients taking oral therapy. Some experts advise that patients have a dental exam and any dental procedures before starting therapy or within three months if possible, especially those with risk factors (e.g., cancer, chemotherapy, corticosteroids, head and neck radiotherapy or poor oral hygiene). Patients should also make their dentist aware they are taking a bisphosphonate. Some clinicians also recommend a regular dental exam as well as good oral hygiene in patients taking a bisphosphonate.

Pregnancy: No published data are available on the use of oral bisphosphonates in pregnancy. Based on animal studies, bisphosphonates are thought to cross the placenta. With very little human data, risks versus benefits must be weighed carefully.

Lactation: It is not known whether bisphosphonates are excreted in breast milk. Bisphosphonates have poor oral bioavailability. Because plasma concentrations are low it is unlikely that it would be excreted into milk in clinically relevant concentrations.

Drug Interactions: Because bisphosphonates are highly bound to bone, are not metabolized, are not highly protein bound and do not induce or inhibit microsomal enzyme systems, they do not possess an obvious potential for interacting with other drugs. Their absorption can, however, be greatly decreased in the presence of food, calcium and other cations or beverages other than plain water.

A possible association with an increased incidence of gastric ulceration has been reported with concomitant use of NSAIDs and alendronate. When used with NSAIDs, clodronate has been reported to be associated with renal dysfunction but synergistic action has not been established.

Drug-Laboratory Test Interactions: Bisphosphonates could potentially interfere with the binding of bone-imaging diagnostic agents to bone.

ADVERSE EFFECTS: Oral bisphosphonates are generally well tolerated, especially when taken as recommended by appropriately selected patients (see Dosage and Contraindications). Gastrointestinal effects such as dyspepsia and nausea are the most frequently reported side effects. Esophageal injury is thought to be more common with the use of aminobisphosphonates such as alendronate (see Warnings and Precautions). Nausea and diarrhea occur in a significant percentage of patients treated with etidronate in doses greater than 5 mg/kg/day, but are less common at doses used for osteoporosis.

Localized osteonecrosis of the jaw has been reported rarely with oral bisphosphonate treatment. It is generally associated with local infections or tooth extraction (see Precautions).

Rarely, the following adverse effects have been reported with the use of bisphosphonates, although a causal relationship has not always been established: acute-phase reactions involving fever and lymphopenia, bone, joint or muscle pain, leukemia, skin reactions, arthralgias and ocular effects (e.g., inflammation, pain, iritis).

OVERDOSE:

Symptoms: Clinical experience with oral bisphosphonate overdose is extremely limited. Expected signs and symptoms might include gastrointestinal upset, esophageal symptoms, diarrhea and hypocalcemia.

Treatment: Suggested measures for management of bisphosphonate overdose include giving milk or antacids orally to bind unabsorbed drug, correcting electrolyte imbalances such as hypocalcemia, keeping the patient upright and monitoring of renal function. It has been suggested that vomiting should not be induced because of the possible risk of esophageal irritation.

For management of a suspected drug overdose, CPhA recommends that you contact your **regional Poison Control Centre**. See the *CPS* Directory section for a list of Poison Control Centres.

DOSAGE: Table 2 lists the oral bisphosphonate dosage for each indication. Bisphosphonates should be taken on an empty stomach with a full glass of plain water. They should not be taken with other medications, calcium or other divalent cations, or any beverage other than plain water. Some additional specific recommendations from the manufacturers regarding administration are footnoted in Table 2.

Tablets and capsules should be swallowed whole, not sucked or chewed. Adequate intake of calcium and vitamin D should be maintained during bisphosphonate therapy (see Precautions).

Table 1: Bisphosphonates: Oral

Labeled Indications

Bisphosphonate	Paget's Disease of Bone	Hypercalcemia of Malignancy	Osteolysis Secondary to Bone Metastases	Prevention of Postmenopausal Osteoporosis	Treatment of Postmenopausal Osteoporosis	Treatment and Prevention of Corticosteroid-Induced Osteoporosis in Men and Women	Treatment of Primary Osteoporosis in Men
Alendronate	Yes	—	—	Yes	Yes	Yes	Yes
Clodronate	—	Yes[a]	Yes[a]	—	—	—	—
Etidronate	Yes	Yes[a]	—	Yes	Yes	Yes[b]	—
Risedronate	Yes	—	—	Yes	Yes	Yes	Yes[c]

[a] Oral maintenance therapy is used following iv therapy.
[b] Prevention only.
[c] To improve bone mineral density.

Table 2: Bisphosphonates: Oral[a]

Dosage

Indication	Alendronate[b]	Clodronate[c]	Etidronate[d]	Risedronate[e]
Paget's Disease of Bone	40 mg daily for 6 months. Retreatment may be considered after a 6-month post-treatment evaluation period.	—	5 mg/kg/day for up to 6 months. Doses >10 mg/kg/day should be used with caution and not for longer than 3 months. Doses >20 mg/kg/day are not recommended. Retreatment may be considered after a 90-day etidronate-free period.	30 mg daily for 2 months. Retreatment may be considered following a post-treatment evaluation of at least 2 months.
Hypercalcemia of Malignancy (following a course of iv therapy)	—	1600 to 2400 mg daily. May be divided into 2 daily doses if necessary to improve gastrointestinal tolerance. Maximum daily dose: 3200 mg.	20 mg/kg/day for 30 days or longer, depending on serum calcium levels. Treatment for longer than 90 days is not recommended.	—
Osteolysis Secondary to Bone Metastases (following a course of iv therapy)	—	As for hypercalcemia of malignancy.	—	—
Prevention of Post-menopausal Osteoporosis	5 mg daily	—	90-day cycle: etidronate 400 mg daily for 14 days, then calcium carbonate 1250 mg daily for 76 days.	5 mg daily OR 35 mg once weekly
Treatment of Post-menopausal Osteoporosis	10 mg daily OR 70 mg once weekly OR one bottle of 70 mg oral solution once weekly	—	As for prevention of postmenopausal osteoporosis, above	5 mg daily OR 35 mg once weekly OR 75 mg on two consecutive days per month, on the same calendar days each month
Treatment of Primary Osteoporosis in Men	10 mg daily OR 70 mg once weekly OR one bottle of 70 mg oral solution once weekly	—	—	35 mg once weekly
Prevention and Treatment of Corticosteroid-induced Osteoporosis in Men and Women	5 mg daily. Postmenopausal women not taking estrogen: 10 mg daily.	—	For prevention only. Dose as for prevention of postmenopausal osteoporosis.	5 mg daily

[a] Bisphosphonates should be taken on an empty stomach with a full glass of plain water. They should not be taken with food, other medications, calcium or other divalent cations, or any beverage other than plain water.
[b] After administration, patients must not lie down for at least 30 minutes and until after their first food of the day; should not be taken at bedtime or before rising for the day.
[c] See individual product monographs for administration directions.
[d] Nothing but plain water by mouth for 2 hours before and after each dose.
[e] Take at least 30 minutes before the first food or drink (other than plain water) and/or any other medication of the day.

Blenoxane™ ℞

bleomycin sulfate

Antineoplastic—Antibiotic

Bristol

Date of Preparation: March 20, 1981
Date of Revision: May 28, 1999

Caution: Bleomycin should be administered under the supervision of a qualified physician experienced in the use of cancer chemotherapeutic agents. Adequate diagnostic and treatment facilities should be available to allow appropriate management of therapy and possible complications.

Patients receiving bleomycin must be observed carefully and frequently during and after therapy. It should be used with extreme caution in patients with significant impairment of renal function or compromised pulmonary function.

PHARMACOLOGY: Although the exact mechanism of action of bleomycin is unknown, available evidence indicates that the main mode of action is inhibition of DNA synthesis with some evidence of inhibition of RNA and protein synthesis

The major route of excretion of bleomycin is the kidney, with 60 to 70% of an administered dose recovered in the urine as active bleomycin. Renal dysfunction can significantly prolong excretion.

In patients with a creatinine clearance of >35 mL/min, the serum or plasma terminal elimination half-life of bleomycin is approximately 115 minutes. In patients with a creatinine clearance of <35 mL/min, the plasma or serum terminal elimination half-life increases exponentially as the creatinine clearance decreases.

When administered intrapleurally in the treatment of malignant pleural effusion, bleomycin acts as a sclerosing agent. Following intrapleural administration, resultant bleomycin plasma concentrations suggest a systemic absorption rate of approximately 45% (see Precautions).

INDICATIONS: Bleomycin should be considered an adjuvant to surgery and radiation therapy. It has been shown to be useful in the management of the following neoplasms:

Squamous Cell Carcinoma: head and neck including mouth, tongue, tonsil, nasopharynx, oropharynx, sinus, palate, lip, buccal mucosa, gingiva and epiglottis; skin; larynx and paralarynx.

Bleomycin is also indicated in squamous cell carcinomas of the penis, cervix, and vulva.

The response to bleomycin is poorer in patients with head and neck cancer who have received previous irradiation.

Lymphomas: Hodgkin's disease and non-Hodgkin's lymphoma.

Testicular Carcinoma: embryonal cell carcinoma, choriocarcinoma and teratocarcinoma. Studies to date have revealed that the use of vinblastine sulfate with bleomycin increases the response rate of testicular tumors.

Malignant Pleural Effusion: When administered by intrapleural injection, bleomycin has been shown to be useful in the treatment of malignant pleural effusion and in the prevention of recurrence.

Other Malignancies: Bleomycin has been shown to produce responses in some renal carcinomas and soft tissue sarcomas.

CONTRAINDICATIONS: In patients who have demonstrated hypersensitivity to the drug.

WARNINGS: Bleomycin should be administered under the supervision of a qualified physician experienced in the use of cancer chemotherapeutic agents. Adequate diagnostic and treatment facilities should be available to allow appropriate management of therapy and possible complications.

Patients receiving bleomycin must be observed carefully and frequently during and after therapy. It should be used with extreme caution in patients with significant impairment of renal function or compromised pulmonary function.

Pulmonary toxicities occur in 10% of treated patients. In approximately 1% of treated patients, nonspecific pneumonitis induced by bleomycin progresses to pulmonary fibrosis, and death. Pulmonary toxicity is more frequent in patients over 70 years of age and in those receiving total doses greater than 400 units. Although pulmonary toxicity is age and dose related, the toxicity is unpredictable. Renal impairment is a risk factor in the development of pulmonary toxicity. Frequent monitoring is essential (see Adverse Effects).

Idiosyncratic reactions similar to anaphylaxis have been reported in 1% of patients with lymphoma who were treated with bleomycin. Since these reactions usually occur after the first or second dose, careful monitoring is essential after these doses (see Adverse Effects).

Renal and hepatic toxicity, beginning as a deterioration in renal or liver function tests, have been reported infrequently. These toxicities may occur, however, at any time after initiation of therapy.

Pregnancy: Bleomycin may cause fetal harm when administered to a pregnant woman. Women of childbearing potential should be advised to avoid becoming pregnant during therapy with bleomycin. If bleomycin is used during pregnancy or if the patient becomes pregnant while receiving this drug, the patient should be apprised of the potential hazard.

Lactation: It is not known if bleomycin is excreted in human milk. Because many drugs are excreted in human milk and because of the potential for serious adverse reactions in nursing infants from bleomycin, a decision should be made to discontinue nursing or to discontinue the drug, taking into account the importance of the drug to the mother. The benefits and risks of nursing against discontinuing the drug must be weighed carefully.

PRECAUTIONS: Bleomycin should be used as indicated. The physician must carefully weigh the therapeutic benefit versus risk of toxicity.

Bleomycin should be administered preferably to patients who are hospitalized and who can be observed carefully and frequently during and after therapy. It should be used with extreme caution in patients with significant impairment of renal function or compromised pulmonary function due to disease other than malignancy, and in patients over 70 years of age because of the apparent increased danger of pulmonary toxicity.

To monitor the onset of pulmonary toxicity, x-rays of the chest should be taken every 1 to 2 weeks. If pulmonary changes are noted, treatment should be discontinued until it can be determined whether the cause is drug related. Pneumonitis due to bleomycin should be treated with corticosteroids in an effort to prevent progression to pulmonary fibrosis. Infectious pneumonitis should receive appropriate antibiotic therapy.

Following intrapleural administration, resultant bleomycin plasma concentrations suggest a systemic absorption of approximately 45%. Thus, in the determination of cumulative exposure to bleomycin, systemic exposure following intrapleural administration of bleomycin for injection needs to be taken into account.

Since bleomycin is eliminated predominantly through renal excretion, the administration of nephrotoxic drugs with bleomycin may reduce its renal clearance, potentially leading to bleomycin-related toxicity (see Pharmacology, Warnings, Dosage and Adverse Effects).

An association between decreased renal function and enhanced bleomycin-related toxicities has been reported. Pharmacokinetic/pharmacodynamic relationships suggest that enhancement of toxicity is a consequence of reduced renal clearance of bleomycin resulting in prolonged elimination half-life and increased area-under-the plasma-concentration vs time-curve compared to patients with normal renal function. Dosage reductions of 40 to 75% have been recommended for patients with creatinine clearance values ≤40 mL/min.

ADVERSE EFFECTS: Pulmonary: Pulmonary toxicity is potentially the most serious side effect of bleomycin (see Warnings).

The identification of patients with pulmonary toxicity due to bleomycin has been extremely difficult. The reason for this is the lack of specificity of the clinical syndrome, the x-ray changes and even the tissue changes seen on examination of biopsy and autopsy specimens.

Bleomycin-induced pneumonitis apparently produces dyspnea and fine rales that are in no way different from those produced by infectious pneumonias, or the signs and symptoms produced by primary or metastatic lung disease in some patients.

On x-ray, bleomycin-induced pneumonitis produces patchy opacities, usually of the lower lung fields, that look the same as infectious bronchopneumonia or even lung metastases in some patients.

The microscopic tissue changes due to bleomycin toxicity are frequently present as bronchiolar squamous metaplasia, reactive macrophages, atypical alveolar epithelial cells, fibrinous edema and interstitial fibrosis. The acute stage may involve capillary changes and subsequent fibrinous exudation into alveoli producing a change similar to hyaline membrane formation and progressing to a diffuse interstitial fibrosis resembling the Hamman-Rich syndrome. These microscopic findings are non specific and are similar to the changes produced in radiation pneumonitis, pneumocystis pneumonitis, and at times reaction to long-standing malignant pulmonary disease.

Serial pulmonary function tests in 156 patients receiving bleomycin therapy revealed some demonstrable alteration in approximately 20%. The most common changes were a decrease in total lung volume and a decrease in vital capacity. However, no predictive correlation between these changes and the development of pulmonary fibrosis could be ascertained.

To monitor the onset of pulmonary toxicity, x-rays of the chest should be taken every 1 to 2 weeks. If pulmonary changes are noted, treatment should be discontinued until it can be determined if they are drug related. Studies have suggested that sequential measurement of the pulmonary diffusion capacity for carbon monoxide (DL_{co}) during treatment with bleomycin may be an indicator to subclinical pulmonary toxicity. It is recommended that the DL_{co} be monitored monthly if it is to be employed to detect pulmonary toxicities, and thus the drug should be discontinued when the DL_{co} falls below 30 to 35% of the pretreatment value.

Patients who have received bleomycin are at greater risk of developing pulmonary toxicity when oxygen is administered at surgery. While long exposure to very high oxygen concentrations is a known cause of lung damage, after bleomycin administration, lung damage can occur at lower concentrations than usually would be considered safe. Suggestive preventive measures are: maintain $FI\ O_2$ at concentrations approximately that of room air (25%) during surgery and the postoperative period; carefully monitor fluid replacement, focusing more on colloid administration than crystalloid administration.

Sudden onset of an acute chest pain syndrome suggestive of pleuropericarditis has been rarely reported during bleomycin infusion. Although each patient must be individually evaluated, further courses of bleomycin do not appear to be contraindicated.

Pulmonary adverse events have been reported rarely following the intrapleural administration of bleomycin.

Skin and Mucous Membranes: Cutaneous effects are the most frequent side effects occurring in approximately 50% of treated patients. Skin and mucous membrane reactions include stomatitis, alopecia, hyperpigmentation, thickening, ulceration, erythema, hyperkeratosis, nail changes, rash, vesiculation, tenderness, pruritus, hyperesthesia, peeling, striae and bleeding. In 2% of treated patients it was necessary to discontinue bleomycin therapy because of these toxicities. Cutaneous toxicity is a relatively late manifestation developing usually in the 2nd and 3rd week of treatment after 150 to 200 units of bleomycin had been administered and, in general, was related to total cumulative dose. Scleroderma-like skin changes have also been reported as part of postmarketing surveillance.

Idiosyncratic Reactions: In approximately 1% of patients with lymphoma who were treated with bleomycin, an idiosyncratic reaction, similar clinically to anaphylaxis, has been reported. The reaction may be immediate or delayed for several hours and occurs usually after the first or second dose. It consists of hypotension, fever, chills, mental confusion and wheezing. Treatment is symptomatic, including volume expanders, pressor agents, antihistamines, and corticosteroids.

Other: Fever, chills and vomiting were frequently reported side effects. Anorexia and weight loss are common and may persist long after termination of bleomycin. Pain at the tumor site, phlebitis, and other local reactions were reported infrequently. Malaise has also been reported as part of postmarketing surveillance.

Vascular toxicities coincident with the use of bleomycin in combination with other antineoplastic agents have been reported rarely. The events are clinically heterogeneous and may include myocardial infarction, cerebrovascular accident, thrombotic microangiopathy (hemolytic-uremic syndrome) or cerebrovascular arteritis.

There are also reports of Raynaud's phenomenon occurring in patients treated with bleomycin in combination with vinblastine with or without cisplatin or, in few cases, with bleomycin as a single agent. It is currently unknown if the cause of Raynaud's phenomenon in these cases is the disease, underlying vascular compromise, bleomycin, vinblastine, hypomagnesemia, or a combination of any of these factors.

Bleomycin occasionally has been associated with local pain following intrapleural administration. Hypotension requiring symptomatic treatment has been reported infrequently. Very rarely death has been reported in association with bleomycin pleurodesis in very seriously ill patients.

Toxicity to the renal, hepatic and central nervous systems are rare, but as with any potent drug, these symptoms should be monitored. It is noteworthy that there has been no evidence of bone marrow or immunological depression. This is contrary to the currently available antineoplastic drugs.

OVERDOSE:
No data supplied by the manufacturer.

> For management of a suspected drug overdose, CPhA recommends that you contact your **regional Poison Control Centre**. See the *CPS* Directory section for a list of Poison Control Centres.

DOSAGE: The following dosage schedule is recommended:

Squamous Cell Carcinoma, Non-Hodgkin's Lymphoma, Testicular Carcinoma: 0.25 to 0.50 units/kg (10 to 20 units/m²) given i.v. or i.m. weekly or twice weekly.

Hodgkin's Disease: 0.25 to 0.50 units/kg (10 to 20 units/m²) i.v., i.m. or s.c. weekly or twice weekly. After a 50% response, the maintenance dose of 1 unit daily or 5 units weekly i.v. or i.m. should be given.

Malignant Pleural Effusion: 60 units administered as a single intrapleural injection (see Reconstitution).

Because of the possibility of an anaphylactoid reaction, patients with lymphoma should be started with 2 units or less for the first 2 doses. If no acute reaction occurs, then the regular dose schedule may be followed.

Pulmonary toxicity from bleomycin appears to be dose related with a striking increase when the total dose is over 400 units. Total doses over 400 units should be given with great caution.

Improvement or responses in testicular carcinoma and Hodgkin's lymphoma are usually prompt and noted within 2 weeks. When responses are not seen within this period of time, continued therapy with bleomycin should be re-evaluated.

Responses in patients with squamous cell cancers are slow, requiring up to 3 weeks before onset of response is noted.

Note: When bleomycin is used in combination with other antineoplastic agents, pulmonary toxicities may occur at lower doses. Bleomycin-related toxicities also may be more frequent in patients with impaired renal function and dose modification has been suggested. Dosage reductions of 40 to 75% have been recommended for patients with creatinine clearance values ≤40 mL/min.

Bleomycin may be given by i.m., i.v., intra-arterial, s.c. or intrapleural routes.

Reconstitution: I.M. or S.C.: Dissolve the contents of a bleomycin vial in 1 to 5 mL of Sterile Water for Injection, Sodium Chloride for Injection or Bacteriostatic Water for Injection.

I.V. or Intra-arterial: Dissolve the contents of the vial in 5 to 20 mL of Sodium Chloride Injection 0.9% and administer slowly over a period of 10 minutes.

Intrapleural Infusion: Dissolve 60 units of bleomycin in 50 to 100 mL of Sodium Chloride Injection 0.9%, and administer as a rapid push through a thoracostomy tube following drainage of excess pleural fluid and the confirmation of complete lung expansion. The thoracostomy tube is then clamped and the patient is moved from the supine to the left and right lateral positions during the next 4 hours. The clamp is then removed and suction re-established. The amount of time the thoracostomy tube remains in place following sclerosis is based on individual patient requirements.

In general, intrapleural injection of local anesthetics or systemic narcotic analgesia is not required.

Stability of Reconstituted Solutions: Reconstituted bleomycin solution may be stored in refrigerator above freezing point for up to 48 hours.

Diluted bleomycin is stable at 25°C for 24 hours in 0.9% Sodium Chloride Injection and for up to 8 hours in 20% w/v Mannitol in Water. Discard the solution if precipitate forms in Mannitol.

Special Instructions for Handling and Disposal:

1. Preparation of bleomycin should be done in a vertical laminar flow hood (Biological Safety Cabinet-Class II).
2. Personnel preparing bleomycin should wear PVC gloves, safety glasses, disposable gowns and masks.
3. All needles, syringes, vials and other materials which have come in contact with bleomycin should be segregated and incinerated at 1000°C or more. Sealed containers may explode. Intact vials should be returned to the Manufacturer for destruction. Proper precautions should be taken in packaging these materials for transport.
4. Personnel regularly involved in the preparation and handling of bleomycin should have biannual blood examinations.

SUPPLIED: Each vial contains: sterile bleomycin sulfate equivalent to bleomycin 15 units. Nonmedicinal ingredients: none. Note: A unit of bleomycin is equal to the formerly used milligram activity. The term milligram activity is a misnomer and was changed to units to be more precise. Store the dry powder at 2 to 8°C.

Bleomycin Sulphate for Injection USP Ⓟ

bleomycin sulfate

Antineoplastic

Hospira

SUPPLIED: Each vial of sterile lyophilised powder contains: bleomycin sulphate equivalent to 15 units of bleomycin. Sodium hydroxide or sulfuric acid may be used as pH adjusters. Contains no preservatives. Single use vials, cartons of 1. Store between 2 and 8°C. Protect from light. Discard unused portion.

Blephamide® Ⓟ

sulfacetamide sodium—prednisolone acetate

Antibacterial—Anti-inflammatory

Allergan

SUPPLIED: Each mL of sterile ophthalmic suspension contains: sulfacetamide sodium 10% and prednisolone acetate 0.2%. Nonmedicinal ingredients: benzalkonium chloride 0.0044% (as preservative), edetate disodium, polysorbate 80, polyvinyl alcohol (Liquifilm), potassium phosphate monobasic, sodium phosphate dibasic and sodium thiosulfate. Plastic dropper bottles of 5 and 10 mL.

BLES® Ⓟ

bovine lipid extract surfactant

Lung Surfactant (Bovine)

BLES

Date of Revision: August 13, 2010

SUMMARY PRODUCT INFORMATION:

Route of Administration	Dosage Form/ Strength	Clinically Relevant Nonmedicinal Ingredients
Intratracheal instillation	Suspension/27 mg phospholipid/mL	For a complete listing of nonmedicinal ingredients, see Dosage Forms, Composition and Packaging.

DESCRIPTION: BLES (bovine lipid extract surfactant) is extracted from bovine lung surfactant. The manufacturing process removes hydrophilic proteins, the majority of which would be surfactant-associated protein SP-A, and selects for hydrophobic phospholipids and surfactant-associated proteins SP-B and SP-C.

INDICATIONS AND CLINICAL USE:

- BLES (bovine lipid extract surfactant) is indicated for rescue treatment of Neonatal Respiratory Distress Syndrome (NRDS/Hyaline Membrane Disease).

For infants with NRDS confirmed by x-ray and who require mechanical ventilation, with arterial to alveolar oxygen ratio (Pa_{O2}/PA_{O2}) <0.22, BLES is to be given as soon as possible after the oxygenation criteria are met.

The use of BLES in infants less than 380 g or greater than 4460 g birth weight has not been evaluated in controlled trials.

CONTRAINDICATIONS: Use of BLES (bovine lipid extract surfactant) is contraindicated in infants with active pulmonary haemorrhage.

WARNINGS AND PRECAUTIONS:

> **Serious Warnings and Precautions**
> - **Administer in a highly supervised clinical setting.**
> - **BLES can affect oxygenation and lung compliance rapidly. In some infants, hyperoxia may occur within minutes of administration.**
> - **Transient episodes of bradycardia and decreased oxygen saturation may occur during dosing.**

General: BLES (bovine lipid extract surfactant) is intended for intratracheal use only (see Dosage and Administration).

Use of BLES should be restricted to a highly supervised clinical setting with immediate availability of experienced neonatologists and other clinicians experienced with intubation, ventilator management, and general care of premature infants.

A higher rate of sepsis has been described in those infants treated with BLES than those in the control arm. Health professionals caring for these infants should be aware of this increased risk, take appropriate precautionary measures and be vigilant for any signs and symptoms of sepsis.

Carcinogenesis and Mutagenesis: No studies have been performed to investigate the carcinogenesis or mutagenesis of BLES.

Immunogenicity: Long-term studies comparing BLES to placebo (sham air) treatment demonstrated no significant differences in development of allergic manifestations.

Ophthalmologic: Hyperoxia may occur within minutes of administration of BLES. If hyperoxia develops and oxygen saturation is in excess of 95%, Fi_{O2} should be reduced until saturation is 90 to 95%, to decrease the risk of retinopathy of prematurity.

Respiratory: Vigilant clinical attention should be given to all infants prior to, during and after administration of BLES. Infants receiving BLES should be monitored for oxygenation with a transcutaneous oxygen probe or oxygen saturation monitor as well as occasional blood gas measurements. In addition, carbon dioxide (CO_2) levels should be monitored with transcutaneous CO_2 probe correlated with blood gas readings.

BLES can rapidly affect oxygenation and lung compliance. If the improvement in chest expansion seems excessive, peak ventilator inspiratory pressures should be reduced immediately, to avoid overdistension and pulmonary air leaks. Monitor tidal volume after dosing, as sudden lung compliance may occur without much chest movement.

During the dosing procedure, transient episodes of bradycardia and decreased oxygen saturation have been reported (see Adverse Reactions). If these occur, the dosing procedure should be stopped and appropriate measures to alleviate the condition initiated. After stabilization, the dosing procedure can be resumed.

Administration techniques used with other surfactant products, such as slow administration or the use of small test aliquots, are not recommended with BLES. Unlike other products that require a slow drip to prevent reflux, BLES has a much lower viscosity and a higher protein content that promote a more rapid distribution. Slow administration may lead to uneven distribution, resulting in uneven lung compliance.

If the dose fails to subside in the ETT with additional pressures recommended in the Dosage and Administration section, consider the possibility of a mucous plug.

Mucous Plugs: Infants whose ventilation becomes markedly impaired during or shortly after dosing may have mucous plugging of the endotracheal tube, particularly if pulmonary secretions were prominent prior to drug administration. Suctioning of all infants prior to dosing may lessen the chance of mucous plugs obstructing the endotracheal tube. After dosing, exogenous surfactant may encourage the transport of resident mucus. If endotracheal tube obstruction from such plugs is suspected, and suctioning is unsuccessful in removing the obstruction, the blocked endotracheal tube should be replaced immediately.

Monitoring and Laboratory Tests: Correction of acidosis, hypotension, hypoglycemia and hypothermia is recommended prior to administration.

ADVERSE REACTIONS: Adverse Drug Reaction Overview: Very common adverse events occurring in ≥10% of infants who received BLES (bovine lipid extract surfactant), in descending order of frequency, were patent ductus arteriosus, decreased post-dose pulmonary function values, intraventricular haemorrhage of all grades, sepsis, retinopathy of prematurity, bradycardia and severe intraventricular haemorrhage.

Common adverse events occurring in ≥1% and <10% of infants who received BLES, in descending order of frequency, were pulmonary interstitial emphysema, periventricular leukomalacia, pneumothorax, pulmonary haemorrhage, endotracheal tube complications, necrotizing enterocolitis, respiratory acidosis, convulsions, hypotension, apnoea, hydrocephalus and pneumonia.

Due to the rapid effect of BLES on lung compliance and oxygenation, infants should be monitored for respiratory parameters and any of the common adverse events.

Clinical Trial Adverse Drug Reactions: Because clinical trials are conducted under very specific conditions, the adverse drug reaction rates observed in the clinical trials may not reflect the rates observed in practice and should not be compared to the rates in the clinical trials of another drug. Adverse drug reaction information from clinical trials is useful for identifying drug-related adverse events and for approximating rates.

In a double-blinded, comparative, multicentre clinical trial comparing the safety and efficacy of BLES and Exosurf Neonatal (colfosceril palmitate; Glaxo Wellcome), 568 infants received BLES and 565 received Exosurf for rescue treatment of NRDS.

Adverse events occurring in ≥1% of infants treated with BLES are summarized by body system and in order of decreasing frequency in Table 1. The incidence of these events in Exosurf-treated infants is provided for comparison.

Table 1: BLES

Adverse Events in ≥1% of Infants Treated with BLES Compared with Infants Treated with Exosurf

Body System/Event	BLES N=568 %	Exosurf N=565 %	Statistically Significant p-value
Infections			
Sepsis	28	23	<0.05
Nervous System Disorders			
Intraventricular haemorrhage, total	29	29	—
Intraventricular haemorrhage, Grades III and IV	12	11	—
Periventricular leukomalacia	8	7	—
Convulsion	2	1	—
Hydrocephalus	1	<1	—
Eye Disorders			
Retinopathy of prematurity	19	20	—
Cardiac Disorders			
Patent ductus arteriosus	44	44	—
Bradycardia	13	15	—
Vascular Disorders			
Hypotension	2	2	—
Respiratory Disorders			
Pulmonary interstitial emphysema	9	17	<0.0005
Pneumothorax	8	12	<0.05
Pulmonary haemorrhage	8	7	—
Endotracheal tube complication	6	6	—
Respiratory acidosis[a]	4	2	<0.05
Apnoea	2	4	—
Pneumonia	1	<1	<0.05
Gastrointestinal Disorders			
Necrotizing enterocolitis	6	7	—
Investigations			
Decreased pulmonary function[b]	39	41	—

[a] Almost all incidences of respiratory acidosis occurred at one study site.
[b] The term "decreased pulmonary function" covered incidences of a fall in saturation or oxygenation, or an increase in CO_2 values after dosing.

The most frequent events reported to occur in either treatment group were patent ductus arteriosus in almost half of the infants, and decreased pulmonary function (defined as incidences of a fall in saturation or oxygenation, or an increase in CO_2 values after dosing) in approximately one third of infants. These events occurred with similar frequency in either treatment group, and are anticipated complications when infants in distress are handled.

Sepsis and pneumonia occurred significantly more frequently in BLES-treated infants than in those who received Exosurf. Notwithstanding this higher incidence of sepsis, death due to infections was comparable between the two arms of the study.

Although the incidence of pulmonary haemorrhage was low (<1%) within the first two hours after dosing, it was observed to increase to 8% before discharge from intensive care. This was not significantly different from the incidence of pulmonary haemorrhage with Exosurf. For the 750-1250 gram birth weight group receiving BLES, 7 of 32 deaths (22%) were attributed to pulmonary haemorrhage.

There was a significantly greater incidence of respiratory acidosis following treatment with BLES. All incidences of respiratory acidosis occurred within two hours of dosing, and almost all incidences following either surfactant occurred at one study centre, perhaps due to too rapid weaning of the ventilatory pressure and rate with decreased minute ventilation.

Significantly fewer infants who received BLES developed pulmonary interstitial emphysema or pneumothorax than did those who were treated with Exosurf. This may reflect the increased ventilatory requirements of infants who received Exosurf. Thus, a reduction in ventilatory pressure following treatment with BLES may protect infants from pulmonary air leaks.

Table 2 summarizes the adverse events that were reported to occur within two hours post-dose, in ≥1% of infants treated with BLES. The incidence of these events in Exosurf-treated infants is provided for comparison.

Table 2: BLES

Adverse Events within Two Hours of Dosing in ≥1% of Infants Treated with BLES or Exosurf

Body System/Event	BLES N=568 %	Exosurf N=565 %	Statistically Significant p-value
Cardiac Disorders			
Bradycardia	11	14	—
Respiratory System Disorders			
Endotracheal tube complications	6	6	—
Respiratory acidosis[a]	4	2	<0.05
Pulmonary haemorrhage	<1	1	—
Investigations			
Decreased pulmonary function[b]	39	41	—

[a] Almost all incidences of respiratory acidosis occurred at one study site.
[b] The term "decreased pulmonary function" covered incidences of a fall in saturation or oxygenation, or an increase in CO_2 values.

Decreased pulmonary function (reported incidences of a fall in saturation or oxygenation, or an increase in CO_2 values), bradycardia and endotracheal tube complications occurred with the same frequency in each treatment group, and are commonly associated with handling and treatment of premature infants. As discussed above, respiratory acidosis occurred, for the most part, at one site and may have been due to inadequate monitoring of lung compliance at that site.

Other adverse events that were reported to occur within two hours after administration of BLES, but at a frequency of <1% were: acidosis; hypertension; hypotension; hypoxia; patent ductus arteriosus; pneumonia; pneumothorax; and pulmonary haemorrhage.

Less Common Clinical Trial Adverse Drug Reactions: Uncommon adverse events that were reported to occur in <1% of infants treated with BLES were:

Infections and Infestations: miscellaneous infections other than pneumonia.
Blood and Lymphatic Systems: neonatal coagulation disorder, neonatal jaundice; thrombocytopenia.
Endocrine Disorders: hypercalcaemia; hypoglycaemia.
Metabolism and Nutritional: acidosis; hyperkalemia.
Nervous System Disorders: abnormal electroencephalogram; cerebral infarction; encephalopathy; ependymitis; meningitis.
Cardiac Disorders: cardiac arrest; cardiomegaly; cor pulmonale; hypertrophic cardiomyopathy; pneumopericardium; pulmonary oedema; pulmonary valve stenosis; supraventricular tachycardia.
Vascular Disorders: haemorrhage; hypertension.
Respiratory Disorders: asphyxia; bronchopulmonary dysplasia; hypoxia; pulmonary hypertension.
Gastrointestinal Disorders: enteritis; gastrointestinal haemorrhage; gastrointestinal reflux; ileus; intestinal perforation; pneumoperitoneum.
Hepato-biliary Disorders: hepatomegaly.
Skin Disorders: cellulitis.
Renal and Urinary Disorders: anuria; hydronephrosis; hydroureter; nephrocalcinosis.
General Disorders: growth retardation; neonatal hypothermia.

Abnormal Hematologic and Clinical Chemistry Findings: Laboratory values were not collected in clinical trials. However, respiratory acidosis was reported as an adverse event in 4% of infants receiving BLES and 2% of those receiving Exosurf (p<0.05). Respiratory acidosis occurred primarily at one study centre. Lung compliance and oxygenation should be monitored closely, as ventilation parameters may change rapidly after dosing (see Warnings and Precautions).

Post-Market Adverse Drug Reactions: No new adverse reactions have been reported, nor has there been an increase in the incidence of known adverse reactions identified in the clinical trials.

Three infants at one site, who were administered very small aliquots of 1 mL at a time without rotation of the infant, developed pulmonary haemorrhage, intraventricular haemorrhage and/or periventricular leukomalacia, and died. The very small doses given without rotation may have led to uneven surfactant distribution and uneven lung compliance.

DRUG INTERACTIONS: There are no known drug interactions between BLES and other substances. BLES is not known to interfere with laboratory results.

Clinical experience with BLES has shown it to be safe and effective when used with nitric oxide therapy, high frequency oscillation and extracorporeal membranous oxygenation.

DOSAGE AND ADMINISTRATION: Dosing Considerations: BLES (bovine lipid extract surfactant) is intended for **intratracheal** instillation only after an endotracheal airway has been established.

BLES does not require reconstitution or filtering before use. Vials are for single use only, to ensure sterility. Once at room temperature, gently swirl or invert the vial to suspend the lipid and disperse any agglomerates. Inspect the vial for homogeneity. It is normal for warmed vials to have an even dispersion of fine but visible flecks of lipid. Contents should appear as an off-white to light yellow suspension. If contents are a darker colour or will not disperse evenly, discard the vial. Report this and the lot number to the manufacturer.

BLES should be warmed to at least room temperature, but no higher than body temperature before being administered. Warming can be accomplished in the following ways (times are approximate):

Method of Warming	Refrigerated Vials	Frozen Vials
In the hand	5 min.	10 to 15 min.
On the counter	20 min.	60 min.
In a 37°C water bath	2 min.	5 min.

Recommended Dose and Dosage Adjustment: The recommended dosage of BLES is 5 mL/kg at 27 mg of phospholipids/mL, which equals 135 mg phospholipid/kg. As many as 3 subsequent doses of BLES can be given within the first 5 days of life. See Repeat Doses for details. Table 3 suggests the total dosage for a range of birth weights.

Table 3: BLES

Dosing Chart

Weight (g)	Total Dose (mL)	Weight (g)	Total Dose (mL)
600–650	3.2	1301–1350	6.8
651–700	3.5	1351–1400	7.0

(cont'd)

Table 3: BLES *(cont'd)*

Dosing Chart

Weight (g)	Total Dose (mL)	Weight (g)	Total Dose (mL)
701–750	3.8	1401–1450	7.2
751–800	4.0	1451–1500	7.5
801–850	4.2	1501–1550	7.8
851–900	4.5	1551–1600	8.0
901–950	4.8	1601–1650	8.2
951–1000	5.0	1651–1700	8.5
1001–1050	5.2	1701–1750	8.8
1051–1100	5.5	1751–1800	9.0
1101–1150	5.8	1801–1850	9.2
1151–1200	6.0	1851–1900	9.5
1201–1250	6.2	1901–1950	9.8
1251–1300	6.5	1951–2000	10.0

Administration: Dosing Procedures: The infant should be suctioned and allowed to recover before commencing the procedure. Ensure proper placement of the endotracheal tube (ETT) via chest auscultation and radiograph, if available (1-2 cm below the vocal cords, 1-2 cm above the carina). **Do not instill BLES down the right mainstem bronchus.**

Draw the full dose into a syringe with a large gauge needle, and fit the needle with a sterile #5 Fr feeding tube which has been cut to an appropriate length so that it will reach the distal tip of the ETT. Discharge the syringe to fill the feeding tube with surfactant. Briefly disconnect the infant from the ventilator so that the feeding tube may be threaded into the ETT. Alternately, to allow simultaneous mechanical ventilation or hand bagging, pass the feeding tube through the suction valve of a closed suctioning adaptor attached to the ETT.

Instill as a single bolus dose or up to three aliquots, as tolerated, with the infant supine for the first aliquot, then rotated to the left and right for subsequent aliquots. Instill each aliquot or dose over 2 to 3 seconds. After each aliquot is instilled, the infant should be ventilated manually for 30 seconds, using pressures sufficient to achieve good chest expansion before returning the infant to the ventilator. If the infant remains on mechanical ventilation during dosing, raise the pressure by 1 to 2 cm H_2O, if necessary, to assist with emptying the ETT. Allow approximately 1-2 minutes recovery time after each aliquot. Ensure oxygen saturation readings are about 95% before commencing the next aliquot.

The volume of surfactant will rise in the ETT during administration. If the surfactant is slow to subside, interrupt administration and hand ventilate until the ETT is clear before continuing. If the surfactant fails to subside, investigate the possibility of a mucous plug. Small aliquots or a slow drip are not recommended, as this may lead to poor surfactant distribution and uneven lung compliance.

Monitoring After Administration: Once instillation is complete, new mechanical ventilatory parameters need to be established according to the Tcp_{O2}/Tcp_{CO2} readings, the oxygen saturation monitor and chest expansion. Tcp_{O2}/Tcp_{CO2} readings are preferred in infants of lower gestation (less than 32 weeks), and oxygen saturation readings preferred with older infants. Monitor tidal volume closely, as sudden lung compliance may occur without much chest movement. Start at pre-instillation settings and wean the pressures (PIP/PEEP), Fi_{O2} and the ventilator rate, as indicated by the infant's status. Follow-up blood gases one hour after dosing is a standard procedure for any infant who has received BLES (Pa_{O2} should be between 60-70 torr, Pa_{CO2} should be kept between 35-45 torr, and pH between 7.35-7.45). Avoid suctioning for 2 hours post-BLES, unless absolutely necessary. Due to the immediate effect of BLES on lung compliance and oxygenation (usually within 5 to 30 minutes), Fi_{O2} should be decreased accordingly, to prevent hyperoxia. Chest expansion should be observed closely and ventilatory pressures (PIP/PEEP) decreased accordingly. High oxygen saturation levels (>95%) or high Tcp_{O2}/Tcp_{CO2} readings (as confirmed by comparison to blood gas measurements) indicate the infant should be weaned off Fi_{O2}, ventilator rates and pressures. Blood gas readings should be 60-70 torr for Pa_{O2} and 35-45 torr for Pa_{CO2}. Failure to wean appropriately may result in a pneumothorax.

Infants whose ventilation becomes markedly impaired during or shortly after dosing may have mucous plugging of the ETT, particularly if pulmonary secretions were prominent prior to drug administration. In addition, surfactant may promote the movement of resident mucus. If suctioning is unsuccessful in removing the obstruction, the blocked ETT should be replaced immediately.

Repeat Doses: Neonates can receive up to 3 additional doses of BLES within the first 5 days of life. The criteria for an additional dose are a positive response to the previous dose, and an increase in respiratory support as signalled by a gradual increase in Fi_{O2}. This increase must be at least 10% greater than the Fi_{O2} required after the initial response to the previous dose of BLES.

All infants exhibiting respiratory deterioration should be evaluated for a patent ductus arteriosus (PDA), pneumothorax and pulmonary haemorrhage before retreatment with BLES. The regimen for repeat doses is the same as for the initial dose. See Dosing Procedures for details.

OVERDOSAGE:
No evidence of human overdose with BLES (bovine lipid extract surfactant) has been documented. Based on animal data, overdosage may result in acute airway obstruction.

> For management of a suspected drug overdose, CPhA recommends that you contact your **regional Poison Control Centre**. See the *CPS* Directory section for a list of Poison Control Centres.

ACTION AND CLINICAL PHARMACOLOGY: Mechanism of Action: BLES (bovine lipid extract surfactant) restores surfactant activity in neonates with respiratory distress syndrome (NRDS), thereby improving gaseous exchange by decreasing alveolar surface tension and promoting lung compliance in the infant with NRDS.

BLES is an extract of natural bovine surfactant which contains numerous phospholipids, with dipalmitoylphosphatidylcholine (DPPC) being the most abundant. It also includes hydrophobic surfactant-associated proteins SP-B and SP-C, which facilitate their dispersion. When administered intratracheally, BLES is rapidly adsorbed, forming an active phospholipid monolayer at the air-fluid interface.

The metabolic fate of BLES has not been investigated.

BLES can have an immediate effect on lung compliance, usually within 5 to 30 minutes after treatment with a single dose. Clinical experience with BLES has shown that BLES significantly improved gas exchange and lung compliance by the 4-hour time-point. Fraction of inspired oxygen (Fi_{O2}) and ventilatory requirements were significantly decreased, and there was a reduction in the severity of NRDS and its associated complications.

STORAGE AND STABILITY: BLES (bovine lipid extract surfactant) has a shelf life of 36 months when stored frozen below −10°C. Do not use past expiry date on label. Store vials in cartons until ready for use.

Alternately, BLES may be stored refrigerated (2-8°C) for up to 10 months within the labelled expiry date. In the space provided on the vial labelling, record the new expiry date of up to 10 months from the day it is removed from the freezer. Refrigerated vials should not be returned to the freezer.

If a vial has been warmed for use but not opened, it may be returned to its previous storage condition a maximum of 2 times. In the space provided on the vial labelling, record the number of times the vial has been warmed and returned to storage.

SPECIAL HANDLING INSTRUCTIONS: There are no special handling instructions.

INFORMATION FOR THE PATIENT: Published in e-CPS, available by subscription at www.e-cps.ca.

DOSAGE FORMS, COMPOSITION AND PACKAGING: Each mL of suspension for intratracheal instillation contains: phospholipids 27 mg and surfactant-associated proteins SP-B and SP-C 176 to 500 µg, with sodium chloride and calcium chloride. Preservative-free. Sterile, single use clear glass vials of 3, 4, and 5 mL, packaged individually or in cartons of 10.

(Shown in Product Identification Section)

B-natal Lozenge
pyridoxine HCl
Natural Health Product

Ferring

INDICATIONS: To help in the maintenance of good health. Helps to prevent vitamin B_6 deficiency.

WARNINGS AND PRECAUTIONS: Vitamin B_6 is contraindicated in those hypersensitive to any component of vitamin B_6. Individuals who are being treated with levodopa without concurrently taking carbidopa should avoid taking B-natal.

OVERDOSE:

> For management of a suspected drug overdose, CPhA recommends that you contact your **regional Poison Control Centre**. See the *CPS* Directory section for a list of Poison Control Centres.

DOSAGE: Adults: Take one B-natal as needed. Do not exceed 3 B-Natals in a 24 hour period. The recommended dosage is safe for use in pregnant women as stated in Health Canada guidelines.

SUPPLIED: Each lozenge contains: vitamin B_6 25 mg (as pyridoxine hydrochloride). Nonmedicinal ingredients: blue food colouring, green apple flavour (artificial), malic acid, simple sugar, sugar and yellow food colouring. Storage: 15 to 25°C. Protect from excess light and moisture.

B-natal Therapop
pyridoxine HCl
Natural Health Product

Ferring

INDICATIONS: To help the maintenance of good health. Helps to prevent vitamin B_6 deficiency.

WARNINGS AND PRECAUTIONS: Vitamin B_6 is contraindicated in those hypersensitive to any component of vitamin B_6. Individuals who are being treated with levodopa without concurrently taking carbidopa should avoid taking B-Natal.

OVERDOSE:

> For management of a suspected drug overdose, CPhA recommends that you contact your **regional Poison Control Centre**. See the *CPS* Directory section for a list of Poison Control Centres.

DOSAGE: Adults: Take one B-natal as needed. Do not exceed 3 B-Natals in a 24 hour period. The recommended dosage is safe for use in pregnant women as stated in Health Canada guidelines.

SUPPLIED: Each Therapop contains: vitamin B_6 25 mg (as pyridoxine hydrochloride). Nonmedicinal ingredients: blue food colouring, cherry flavour, red food colouring, simple sugar and sugar. Storage: 15 to 25°C. Protect from excess light and moisture.

The reader is invited to consult CPhA's monograph **Bisphosphonates: Oral**.

Bonefos®
clodronate disodium
Bone Metabolism Regulator—Antihypercalcemic Agent

Bayer

Date of Revision: January 18, 2010

SUMMARY PRODUCT INFORMATION:

Route of Administration	Dosage Form/ Strength	Clinically Relevant Nonmedicinal Ingredients
Intravenous (IV) For slow infusion	Solution/60 mg/mL	No clinically relevant nonmedicinal ingredients For a complete listing see Dosage Forms, Composition and Packaging.
Oral	Capsule/400 mg	Lactose For a complete listing see Dosage Forms, Composition and Packaging.

INDICATIONS AND CLINICAL USE: BONEFOS (clodronate disodium) is indicated:
- for the management of hypercalcemia of malignancy;
- as an adjunct in the management of osteolysis resulting from bone metastases of malignant tumors.

Prior to treatment with BONEFOS, renal excretion of excess calcium should be promoted by restoration and maintenance of adequate fluid balance and urine output.

In responsive patients, intravenous infusion of BONEFOS decreases the flux of calcium from the bones by inhibiting the osteoclastic activity and bone resorption, thus reducing the calcium level in the blood.

Treatment with oral clodronate following intravenous infusion has been found to prolong the duration of action (see Dosage and Administration).

Geriatrics: No data is available. As older patients may have decreased renal function, please refer to Warnings and Precautions, Renal.

Pediatrics: The safety and efficacy of BONEFOS in children have not been established.

CONTRAINDICATIONS:
- Renal functional impairment when serum creatinine exceeds 440 µmol/L (5.0 mg/dL) (see Warnings and Precautions).
- Severe inflammation of the gastrointestinal tract.
- Pregnancy and lactation.
- Concomitant treatment with other bisphosphonates
- Hypersensitivity to bisphosphonates, clodronate disodium or to any ingredient in the formulation or component of the container. For a complete listing, see Summary Product Information and Dosage Forms, Composition and Packaging.

WARNINGS AND PRECAUTIONS: General: The recommended daily dose of **iv BONEFOS must be diluted in 500 mL of 0.9% sodium chloride injection USP or 5% dextrose injection USP and administered as a slow intravenous infusion lasting at least two hours. BONEFOS should not be mixed with other intravenous infusions.** No other drugs or nutrients should be added to the diluted infusion solution (see Dosage and Administration). BONEFOS (clodronate disodium) should **not** be given as a bolus injection **since rapid bolus injection may precipitate acute renal failure, severe local reactions, and thrombophlebitis.** Extravasation should be avoided. Local reactions may occur (see Adverse Reactions).

Patients must be adequately hydrated before and during the treatment period. This is particularly important when administering clodronate as an intravenous infusion and in patients with hypercalcemia and/or impaired renal function (see Adverse Reactions). Excess calcium impairs the renal concentrating mechanisms resulting in polyuria and excessive fluid loss. Nausea and lethargy caused by hypercalcemia can also reduce oral fluid intake leading to a profound negative fluid balance. Isotonic saline should be administered at a rate determined by the severity of hypercalcemia, the degree of dehydration and the cardiovascular status of the patient (see Warnings and Precautions, Renal).

Administration of Oral Dosage Form: The drug should be taken on an empty stomach, with a glass of plain water, at least two hours before or after food or any other oral drugs, because food or other drugs may decrease the amount of clodronate disodium absorbed by the body.

Osteonecrosis of the Jaw: Osteonecrosis of the jaw (ONJ) has been reported in patients with cancer receiving treatment regimens including bisphosphonates. Many of these patients were also receiving chemotherapy and corticosteroids. The majority of reported cases have been associated with dental procedures such as tooth extraction. Many had signs of local infection, including osteomyelitis.

A dental examination with appropriate preventative dentistry should be considered prior to treatment with bisphosphonates in patients with concomitant risk factors (e.g., cancer, chemotherapy, radiotherapy, corticosteroids, poor oral hygiene).

While on treatment, these patients should avoid invasive dental procedures if possible. For patients who develop ONJ while on bisphosphonate therapy, dental surgery may exacerbate the condition. For patients requiring dental procedures, there are no data available to suggest whether discontinuation of bisphosphonate treatment reduces the risk of ONJ. Clinical judgement of the treating physician should guide the management plan of each patient based on individual benefit/risk assessment.

Endocrine and Metabolism: Hypocalcemia: Intravenous or oral administration of clodronate may present a risk of hypocalcemia. When given intravenously, the drug tends to chelate blood calcium during therapy which may contribute to hypocalcemia. Asymptomatic hypocalcemia is a common adverse reaction which occurs in approximately 3% of treated patients. Symptomatic hypocalcemia is rare. Symptomatic hypocalcemia can be reversed by the administration of calcium gluconate.

Serum Phosphate: Hyperphosphatemia has not been reported during clodronate therapy. However, transient hypophosphatemia can occur following therapy with clodronate.

Hyperparathyroidism: Increased serum parathyroid hormone levels have been observed in patients receiving clodronate and are attributed to a homeostatic response to the fall in serum calcium. The clinical importance has not been established.

Neurologic: The effect of BONEFOS on the ability to drive and use machinery is not known.

Renal: Administration of clodronate may aggravate renal function in some patients. Intravenous administration of doses notably higher than those recommended may cause severe renal damage, especially if the infusion rate is too high. Appropriate monitoring of the renal function during and after intravenous infusion is required. Since the drug is excreted by the kidneys, it is essential to establish that the excretion of the fluid load and of the drug would not present an excessive medical risk. Adequate fluid intake must be maintained during clodronate treatment. If during therapy there is deterioration of renal function, the intravenous infusion must be stopped.

Clodronate should be used with caution in patients with renal impairment. When the benefits of the use of clodronate in renal impairment outweigh the risks, dose adjustment should be considered, otherwise, the drug should be withheld. Data for dose adjustment in relation to renal function have been derived from a study involving 24 subjects with chronic renal impairment of varying severity and 24 healthy volunteers with normal renal function. Based on the results of this study, dose reductions are recommended depending on the degree of renal insufficiency (see Dosage and Administration). Serum creatinine and blood urea nitrogen should be monitored when the drug is administered intravenously in patients with impaired renal function.

Note: Caution should be exercised in determining dosage adjustment for patients with malignancy and severe skeletal disease, given the potential for wide variation in nonrenal clearance in such patients.

Special Populations: Pregnant Women: The safety and efficacy of BONEFOS in pregnant women has not been established (see Contraindications).

Nursing Women: There is no clinical experience with BONEFOS in lactating women and it is not known whether BONEFOS passes into breast milk (see Contraindications).

Pediatrics: The safety and efficacy of BONEFOS in children have not been established.

Geriatrics: No data is available. As older patients may have decreased renal function, please refer to Warnings and Precautions, Renal.

Impaired Renal Function: Clodronate is eliminated mainly via the kidneys. A study examining the pharmacokinetics of clodronate in renally impaired subjects that enrolled a total of 60 subjects in 4 groups (18 subjects with mild, 12 with moderate, and 16 with severe renal insufficiency, and 14 healthy volunteers) demonstrates a clear increase in the mean clodronate serum $AUC_{(0-24h)}$ with decreasing renal function after daily oral clodronate administration. There was no increase in adverse events with worsening renal function. No dose adjustment is considered necessary for subjects with mild renal impairment. Dosage adjustment in patients with moderate and severe renal impairment is recommended (see Dosage and Administration).

Monitoring and Laboratory Tests: As many patients with hypercalcemia have other electrolyte abnormalities at presentation, appropriate attention must be given to maintaining electrolyte balance. Serum electrolytes should be monitored at least daily and supplementation provided as needed during treatment of hypercalcemia (see Adverse Reactions).

Calcium levels should be monitored throughout the treatment. Corrected (adjusted) serum calcium values may be calculated using established algorithms, such as:

$Ca_{adj}=Ca_t-0.71\ (A-A_m)$

Ca_{adj}=adjusted calcium concentration (mg/100 mL)

Ca_t=total calcium concentration (mg/100 mL)

A=albumin concentration (g/100 mL)

A_m=mean normal albumin concentration of the given laboratory (g/100 mL)

Serum creatinine and blood urea nitrogen should be monitored when the drug is administered intravenously in patients with impaired renal function.

ADVERSE REACTIONS: Adverse Drug Reaction Overview: Bisphosphonates are generally well tolerated, especially when taken properly by appropriately selected patients (see Dosage and Administration and Contraindications).

Adverse Drug Reactions: The following adverse reactions have been observed with both oral and intravenous treatment with clodronate, although the frequency of reactions may differ.

Gastrointestinal: Gastrointestinal disturbances including nausea, vomiting, gastric pain and diarrhea were the most frequently reported adverse events with oral clodronate and occurred in approximately 10% of patients. These reactions were usually mild. In rare cases, treatment had to be discontinued. Difficulty in swallowing the capsule, irritation of the mouth and ulcerative pharyngitis were rarely reported.

Renal: Severe renal damage has occurred, especially after bolus injection or rapid intravenous infusion of high doses of clodronate. Fatal renal failure, which may have been related to the underlying hypercalcemia and dehydration, has occurred in patients receiving intravenous clodronate.

Respiratory: Very rare instances of bronchoconstriction have been observed in patients with acetylsalicylic acid-sensitive asthma.

Skin and Subcutaneous Tissue Disorders: Some cases of skin disorders, usually manifesting as erythematous or maculopapular lesions, have been reported. Immediate hypersensitivity reactions seem to be rare. Local reaction may occur following extravasation.

Abnormal Hematologic and Clinical Chemistry Findings: Renal: Occasional mild to moderate abnormalities in renal function (increase in mean serum creatinine concentrations, transient proteinuria) occurred after iv clodronate therapy.

Biochemical Changes: Asymptomatic hypocalcemia is a common adverse reaction which occurs in approximately 3% of treated patients. Symptomatic hypocalcemia is rare. Although not yet reported during BONEFOS (clodronate disodium) therapy, hyperphosphatemia has been known to occur with other bisphosphonates.

Endocrine: Secondary hyperparathyroidism may develop as a result of BONEFOS therapy. This is a homeostatic response to the fall in serum calcium and will reverse upon discontinuation of therapy.

Hepato-biliary: During a 12-month study of 610 postmenopausal osteopenic women randomized to receive placebo or clodronate, elevations of aminotransferases were common, exceeding the normal range in up to 18% of clodronate-treated subjects versus up to 7% of placebo-treated subjects. Aminotransferases were elevated to more than twice the normal range in 1.8% (9/491) of clodronate-treated subjects. No serious adverse events due to liver disease were reported during the 12 months of follow-up. Changes in serum concentrations of alkaline phosphatase have been observed. In patients with metastatic diseases, alkaline phosphatase may also be elevated due to liver and bone metastases.

Post-Market Adverse Drug Reactions: Musculoskeletal and Connective Tissue Disorders: Isolated cases of osteonecrosis of the jaw have been reported, primarily in patients who were previously treated with amino-bisphosphonates such as zoledronate and pamidronate. Osteonecrosis of the jaw has other well-documented multiple risk factors. It is not possible to determine if these events are related to bisphosphonates, to concomitant drugs or other therapies (e.g., chemotherapy, radiotherapy, corticosteroids), to the patient's underlying disease or to other co-morbid risk factors (e.g., anemia, infection, pre-existing oral disease).

Severe bone, joint, and/or muscle pain has been reported in patients taking BONEFOS; however, such reports have been infrequent. The onset of symptoms varied from days to several months after starting BONEFOS.

Renal and Urinary Disorders: Impairment of renal function (elevation of serum creatinine and proteinuria) and severe renal damage have been reported, especially after rapid intravenous infusion of high doses of clodronate (see Dosage and Administration, Dosing Considerations, Renal Impairment).

Single cases of renal failure, in rare cases with fatal outcome, have been reported, especially with concomitant use of nonsteroidal anti-inflammatory drugs (NSAIDs), most often diclofenac.

Respiratory, Thoracic and Mediastinal Disorders: Impairment of respiratory function in patients with acetylsalicylic acid-sensitive asthma and hypersensitivity reactions manifesting as respiratory disorder have been reported.

DRUG INTERACTIONS: Drug-Drug Interactions: See Table 1.

Table 1: BONEFOS

Drug-Drug Interactions with Clodronate

Drug	Effect	Management
NSAIDs, especially diclofenac	Increased potential of renal dysfunction	Caution. Closely monitor serum creatinine levels.
Aminoglycosides, corticosteroids, phosphate, calcitonin, mithramycin, loop diuretics	Increased incidence of hypocalcemia	Caution or avoid. Closely monitor serum calcium levels.
Estramustine phosphate	Increased toxicity due to increased serum levels of estramustine. Estramustine levels can increase by up to 80%.	Caution. Therapeutic monitoring of serum estramustine levels recommended.
Calcium-containing iv solutions, e.g., Ringer's solution	Chelates to clodronate	Avoid mixing with clodronate iv infusion.
Antacid or drug containing calcium, iron, magnesium or aluminum	Chelates to clodronate, significantly reducing bioavailability	Avoid. Take oral clodronate two hours before or after meals and other drugs.

- Clodronate has been reported to be associated with renal dysfunction when used simultaneously with NSAIDs, most often diclofenac.
- The use of clodronate with other agents indicated for the reduction of calcium, such as corticosteroids, phosphate, calcitonin, mithramycin or loop diuretics, may result in increased hypocalcemic effect depending on tumor type and pathophysiological situation.
- Due to increased risk of hypocalcemia, caution should be exercised when using clodronate together with aminoglycosides.
- Bisphosphonates are not known to affect the antineoplastic activity of most anticancer agents, including carmustine, cyclophosphamide, doxorubicin and fluorouracil. However, concomitant use of estramustine phosphate with clodronate has been reported to increase the serum concentration of estramustine by up to 80%.
- Clodronate iv solutions must not be mixed with calcium-containing solutions, such as Ringer's solution, since clodronate forms poorly soluble complexes with divalent cations.
- For oral administration, simultaneous administration with food, liquids or drugs containing divalent cations (i.e., calcium, magnesium, aluminum or iron), such as antacids or iron preparations, leads to significantly reduced bioavailability of clodronate.
- Clodronate is compatible with 0.9% saline and 5% dextrose injections.

Drug-Food Interactions: The drug should be taken on an empty stomach, with a glass of plain water, at least two hours before or after food or any other oral drugs, because food or other drugs may decrease the amount of clodronate disodium absorbed by the body.

Clodronate should in no case be taken with milk or food containing calcium or other divalent cations because they impair the absorption of clodronate.

Drug-Herb Interactions: Interactions with herbal products have not been established.

Drug-Laboratory Test Interactions: Interactions with laboratory tests have not been established.

DOSAGE AND ADMINISTRATION: Dosing Considerations: Renal Impairment: Since clodronate is eliminated mainly via the kidneys, it should be used with caution in patients with renal impairment. Dosage should be reduced in patients with renal impairment, and daily doses exceeding 1600 mg should not be used continuously (see Contraindications and Warnings and Precautions).

Limited data suggest that clodronate can be effectively removed from plasma by standard hemodialysis immediately following clodronate infusion but is poorly removed by peritoneal dialysis. No formal study has been conducted for a regimen recommendation of clodronate use in subjects undergoing hemodialysis or peritoneal dialysis.

Intravenous Infusion: The following dose reductions are recommended depending on the degree of renal insufficiency: See Table 2.

Table 2: BONEFOS

Intravenous Dose Reductions for Renal Impairment

Degree of Renal Failure: Creatinine Clearance (mL/min)	Percent of Normal Dose
50–80	75–100%
12–50	50–75%
<12	50%

Oral Administration: The following dose reductions are recommended depending on the degree of renal impairment: See Table 3.

Caution should be exercised in determining dosage adjustment for patients with malignancy and severe skeletal disease, given the potential for wide variation in nonrenal clearance in such patients.

Recommended Dose and Dosage Adjustment: Intravenous Infusion: The recommended adult dose is 300 mg per day (one 5 mL ampoule).

Table 3: BONEFOS

Oral Dose Reductions for Renal Impairment

Degree of Renal Insufficiency	Creatinine Clearance (mL/min)	Dose
Mild	50–80	No dose reduction recommended
Moderate	30–50	25% reduction
Severe	<30	50% reduction

Oral Administration: Hypercalcemia Due to Malignancy: The oral recommended daily maintenance dose following intravenous therapy is in the range of 1600 mg (four capsules) to 2400 mg (six capsules) given preferably as a single dose or in two divided doses. The maximal recommended daily dose is 3200 mg (eight capsules).
Osteolytic Bone Metastases Due to Malignancy: In patients with increased bone resorption, but no hypercalcemia, the recommended starting dose is 1600 mg/day. The dose may be increased if this is deemed clinically appropriate. However, the daily dose should not exceed 3200 mg.
Retreatment: Controlled studies have not been undertaken for retreatment with clodronate. Limited clinical experience has suggested that patients developing hypercalcemia following termination of therapy with clodronate or during oral administration may be retreated either with a higher oral dosage (up to 3200 mg/day) or with the iv infusion preparation (300 mg/day).
Administration: Intravenous Infusion: The contents of the ampoule must be diluted in 500 mL of 0.9% sodium chloride injection or 5% dextrose injection and administered by infusion lasting at least two hours. The compatibility of BONEFOS with other admixed drugs or injection solutions has not been studied. Treatment should be continued until plasma calcium levels return to normal, which is generally achieved after two to five days of treatment. Treatment should not be prolonged beyond seven days. Adequate hydration should be ensured, and renal function and serum calcium levels should be monitored before and during treatment. The length of time that a clinically acceptable serum calcium level is maintained after infusion of clodronate varies considerably from patient to patient.
Oral Administration: BONEFOS capsules should be swallowed whole, and should not be taken with food (see Warnings and Precautions). The drug should be taken on an empty stomach, with a glass of plain water, at least two hours before or after food or any other oral drugs.

When twice daily dosing is used, the first dose should be taken as recommended above. The second dose should be taken between meals, more than two hours after and one hour before eating, drinking (other than plain water), or taking any other oral drugs.

Reconstitution: Parenteral Products:

Ampoule Size	Volume of Diluent to Be Used	Approximate Available Volume	Nominal Concentration per mL
300 mg/5 mL	500 mL of 0.9% saline injection or 500 mL of 5% dextrose injection	505 mL	0.6 mg/mL

One 5 mL ampoule should be diluted in 500 mL of 0.9% (9 mg/mL) saline injection or 5% (50 mg/mL) dextrose injection and administered as an infusion over at least two hours.

The diluted product may be stored for up to 24 hours at room temperature.

OVERDOSAGE:
There is a lack of documented experience on acute overdosing with clodronate. An overdose of the intravenous preparation can result in renal damage. Renal function should be monitored. Overdosage may result in hypocalcemia. Careful monitoring for several days for signs and symptoms of hypocalcemia, in addition to monitoring of serum calcium levels, is recommended in cases where the dose given was too high in relation to initial serum calcium levels (see Warnings and Precautions).

Treatment of overdose should be symptomatic. Adequate hydration should be ensured, and oral or parenteral calcium supplementation may be required to restore plasma calcium levels. Milk or antacids may be given to bind the unabsorbed clodronate following acute oral overdosage.

> For management of a suspected drug overdose, CPhA recommends that you contact your **regional Poison Control Centre**. See the *CPS* Directory section for a list of Poison Control Centres.

ACTION AND CLINICAL PHARMACOLOGY: Mechanism of Action: Clodronate belongs to the class of bisphosphonates which bind to hydroxyapatite and inhibit formation and dissolution of calcium crystals in vitro.

Bisphosphonates, including clodronate, act on the bony skeleton causing reduction of normal and abnormal bone resorption. The most likely mechanism of action of clodronate appears to be suppression of osteoclast activity, resulting in reduction of bone resorption. However, clodronate may also have indirect inhibitory effects through osteoblastic cells, which control the recruitment and activity of osteoclasts.
Pharmacodynamics: In responsive patients, inhibition of increased bone resorption by clodronate leads to reduction of hypercalcemia of malignancy presenting with or without demonstrable skeletal metastases.

During and also after intravenous administration of clodronate the elevated serum calcium decreases, in some instances to hypocalcemic levels. The decrease in serum calcium concentration is rapid with significant reductions usually attained within two days after starting intravenous therapy and continuing for five to six days after discontinuing therapy.

Clodronate is not metabolized, and absorbed drug is excreted unchanged by the kidneys. The kidneys have a prominent role in calcium homeostasis. In addition to skeletal osteolysis, renal dysfunction becomes a contributor to the pathogenesis of hypercalcemia. At the time of diagnosis most hypercalcemic patients are significantly dehydrated. The antagonistic effects of calcium on the action of antidiuretic hormone impair the renal concentration mechanisms resulting in polyuria and excessive fluid loss. Hydration status is further compromised by reduction of oral fluid intake due to nausea, vomiting and mental status. Prior to initiation of therapy with BONEFOS (clodronate disodium) for treatment of hypercalcemia, the state of the negative fluid balance requires vigorous and adequate hydration with isotonic saline (0.9%). Normalization of blood calcium levels by clodronate in adequately hydrated patients may also normalize plasma parathyroid hormone (PTH) levels without resulting impairment of desired clodronate effects (decrease in urinary calcium, hydroxyproline and phosphate excretion).
Pharmacokinetics: Intravenous Administration: After an iv dose, clodronate exhibits a plasma concentration profile which fits a two-compartment model with $t_{½α}$ approximately 0.3 h and $t_{½β}$ approximately 2 h. The $t_{½}$ of the terminal elimination phase is approximately 13 h, and accounts for 10-15% of renal excretion. Total clearance is about 110 mL/min and renal clearance is approximately 90 mL/min.
Distribution: Volume of distribution is approximately 20 L. The substance which is bound to bone is about 20% of the absorbed amount. The binding of clodronate to serum proteins is variable, between 2%-36%.
Metabolism: Clodronate is not metabolized.
Excretion: Clodronate is eliminated mainly via the kidneys and 60-80% of the absorbed dose will be found in urine within 48 hours. The substance which is bound to bone (about 20% of the absorbed amount) will be excreted more slowly, at a rate depending on the turnover of the bone.
Oral Administration: Absorption: Following a single oral dose, the absorption of clodronate is rapid and the peak serum concentration is reached within 30 minutes. Absorption is estimated at 1-3% of the ingested dose.
Metabolism: Clodronate is not metabolized.
Excretion: Unabsorbed drug is excreted unchanged in the feces.
STORAGE AND STABILITY: BONEFOS (clodronate disodium) capsules and intravenous infusion should be stored between 15 and 30°C.

The diluted intravenous solution may be stored for up to 24 hours at room temperature.
INFORMATION FOR THE PATIENT: Published in e-CPS, available by subscription at www.e-cps.ca.
DOSAGE FORMS, COMPOSITION AND PACKAGING: Capsules: Each yellow, hard gelatin capsule contains: anhydrous clodronate (as the tetrahydrate) 400 mg. Nonmedicinal ingredients: calcium stearate, colloidal anhydrous silica, gelatin, iron oxide (red and yellow), lactose, talc and titanium dioxide. High density polyethylene bottles of 120.
IV Infusion: Each mL of iv infusion contains: clodronate tetrahydrate corresponding to anhydrous clodronate, 60 mg. Nonmedicinal ingredients: sodium hydroxide (to adjust the pH) and water for injection. Ampuls of 5 mL, packages of 5.

Boostrix®

combined diphtheria, tetanus, acellular pertussis (adsorbed) vaccine

Active Immunizing Agent Against Infection by Diphtheria, Tetanus and Whooping Cough

GlaxoSmithKline

Date of Revision: October 21, 2009

SUMMARY PRODUCT INFORMATION:

Route of Administration	Dosage Form/ Strength	Clinically Relevant Nonmedicinal Ingredients
Intramuscular	Suspension for injection/not less than 2.5 limit of flocculation ('Lf'), or 2 IU ('International Units') of diphtheria toxoid; not less than 5 Lf (20 IU) of tetanus toxoid; 8 µg of pertussis toxoid, 8 µg of filamentous hemagglutinin and 2.5 µg of pertactin (69 kDa outer membrane protein)	Aluminum adjuvant (as aluminum hydroxide and aluminum phosphate), sodium chloride and water for injection

DESCRIPTION: BOOSTRIX (combined diphtheria, tetanus, acellular pertussis (adsorbed) vaccine) is presented as a turbid white suspension in a single dose vial or prefilled syringe. Upon storage, a white deposit and clear supernatant can be observed.
INDICATIONS AND CLINICAL USE: BOOSTRIX (combined diphtheria, tetanus, acellular pertussis (adsorbed) vaccine) is indicated for:

- Booster vaccination against diphtheria, tetanus and pertussis of individuals from the age of four years onwards.
  BOOSTRIX is not intended for primary immunization.

CONTRAINDICATIONS:

- BOOSTRIX (combined diphtheria, tetanus, acellular pertussis (adsorbed) vaccine) is contraindicated in patients who are hypersensitive to any component of the vaccine or subjects having shown signs of hypersensitivity after previous administration of diphtheria, tetanus, or pertussis vaccines. For a complete listing, see Dosage Forms, Composition and Packaging.
- BOOSTRIX is contraindicated if the subject has experienced an encephalopathy of unknown etiology, occurring within 7 days following previous vaccination with pertussis containing vaccine. In these circumstances, adult-type combined diphtheria tetanus vaccine should be used.
- BOOSTRIX should not be administered to subjects who have experienced transient thrombocytopenia or neurological complications following an earlier immunization against diphtheria and/or tetanus.

WARNINGS AND PRECAUTIONS: General: It is good clinical practice that immunization should be preceded by a review of the medical history (especially with regard to previous immunization and possible occurrence of undesirable events) and a clinical examination.

As with any other vaccine, BOOSTRIX (combined diphtheria, tetanus, acellular pertussis (adsorbed) vaccine) may not protect 100% of individuals receiving the vaccine.

BOOSTRIX should under no circumstances be administered intravenously.

As with other vaccines, the administration of BOOSTRIX should be postponed in subjects suffering from acute severe febrile illness. The presence of a minor infection is not a contraindication.

If any of the following events occur in temporal relation to administration of whole-cell DTP or acellular DTP vaccine, the decision to give subsequent doses of vaccine containing the pertussis component should be carefully considered. There may be circumstances, such as high incidence of pertussis, in which the potential benefits outweigh possible risks, particularly since these events have not been proven to cause permanent sequelae: temperature of ≥40.5°C within 48 hours of vaccination, not due to another identifiable cause; collapse or shock like state (hypotonic hyporesponsive episode) within 48 hours of vaccination; persistent, inconsolable crying lasting ≥3 hours, occurring within 48 hours of vaccination; convulsions with or without fever, occurring within 3 days of vaccination.
Neurologic: In children with progressive neurological disorders, including infantile spasms, uncontrolled epilepsy or progressive encephalopathy, it is better to defer pertussis (Pa or Pw) immunization until the condition is corrected or stable. However, the decision to give pertussis vaccine must be made on an individual basis after careful consideration of the risks and benefits.

A history or a family history of convulsions and a family history of an adverse event following DTP vaccination do not constitute contraindications.
Hematologic: BOOSTRIX should be administered with caution to subjects with thrombocytopenia or a bleeding disorder since bleeding may occur following an intramuscular administration to these subjects. Firm pressure should be applied to the injection site (without rubbing) for at least 2 minutes.
Immune: HIV infection is not considered as a contraindication for diphtheria, tetanus and pertussis vaccination. The expected immunological response may not be obtained after vaccination.
Sensitivity: As with other injectable vaccines, appropriate medication (eg. Epinephrine 1:1000) should be readily available for immediate use in case of anaphylaxis or anaphylactoid reactions following administration of the vaccine. For this reason, the vaccinee should remain under medical supervision for 30 minutes after immunization.
Special Populations: Pregnant Women: Adequate human data on the use of BOOSTRIX during pregnancy are not available.

As with other inactivated vaccines, one does not expect vaccination with BOOSTRIX to be harmful to the fetus. However, the vaccine should be used during pregnancy only when clearly needed, and when the possible advantages outweigh the possible risks for the fetus.
Nursing Women: Adequate human data on the use during lactation and adequate animal reproductive studies are not available.
ADVERSE REACTIONS: Clinical Trial Adverse Drug Reactions: Because clinical trials are conducted under very specific conditions the adverse reaction rates observed in the clinical trials may not reflect the rates observed in practice and should not be compared to the rates in the clinical trials of another drug. Adverse drug reaction information from clinical trials is useful for identifying drug-related adverse events and for approximating rates.

A total of 1243 vaccinees have received a dose of BOOSTRIX (combined diphtheria, tetanus, acellular pertussis (adsorbed) vaccine) in clinical studies of which 1032 were over 10 years of age.

During controlled clinical studies, diary cards were used to monitor signs and symptoms in all vaccinees following administration of a dose of BOOSTRIX. Table 1 summarizes data from two pivotal studies for solicited local and general symptoms reported during a 15 day follow up period after vaccination. Onset of the majority of local and general symptoms occurred within 48 hours of vaccination. All symptoms resolved without sequelae. A causal relationship between these events and vaccination has not necessarily been established.
Clinical Studies in Children, Adolescents and Adults : In controlled clinical studies, the most commonly reported solicited reactions were those at the site of injection. They included pain, redness and swelling. In a study which involved children, in which parents who spontaneously contacted the investigator to report swelling were asked to bring in their child for examination, notable swellings (as judged by the investigator) were observed with a frequency of 0.5% following dTpa vaccination. None of these cases were considered to correspond to the phenomenon of whole limb swelling as previously reported following DT and DTP vaccination. All local symptoms resolved without any sequelae.

Systemic adverse events, considered to be probably or suspected to be related to vaccination, very commonly reported in adolescents and adults were malaise, fatigue and headache. Commonly reported symptoms in children included diarrhea. Irritability, loss of appetite and vomiting were reported only for 4-6 year old children.

Fever >39.0°C, considered as probably or suspected to be related to vaccination, was infrequently reported in adolescents and adults and commonly reported in children 4-6 years of age.

All unsolicited symptoms were very rarely reported. These included increased sweating, hypertonia, arthrosis, myalgia, pruritus and lymphadenopathy.

Very rare allergic reactions including anaphylactoid reactions, have been reported following vaccination with DTPa-containing vaccines.

Extremely rare cases of collapse or shock-like state (hypotonic hyporesponsive episode) and convulsions within 2 to 3 days of vaccination have been reported in DTPa and DTPa combination vaccines. All of the subjects recovered totally and spontaneously without sequelae. At the present time, there have been no collapse or shock-like episodes reported following administration of BOOSTRIX.

DRUG INTERACTIONS: Drug-Drug Interactions: Concomitant use with other inactivated vaccines or with immunoglobulin has not been studied. It is unlikely the coadministration will result in interference with the immune responses. When considered necessary, BOOSTRIX (combined diphtheria, tetanus, acellular pertussis (adsorbed) vaccine) can be administered simultaneously with other vaccines or immunoglobulin, at a different injection site.

As with other vaccines, patients receiving immunosuppressive therapy or patients with immunodeficiency may not achieve an adequate response.
Drug-Lifestyle Interactions: The vaccine is unlikely to produce an effect on the ability to drive and use machines.

Table 1: BOOSTRIX

Summary Data From 2 Pivotal Studies for Solicited Local and General Symptoms Reported During a 15 Day Follow up Period Vaccination

	Incidence (%)					
	BOOSTRIX administered to adolescent subjects aged 10-17 years	Adolescent comparator group who received separate Td and aP (ap) vaccines		BOOSTRIX administered to adult subjects aged 18 years	Adult comparator group who received separate Td and aP (ap) vaccines	
Solicited Symptoms	BOOSTRIX N=448	Td N=60	aP N=59	BOOSTRIX N=438	Td[a] N=54	aP[a] N=55
Local reactions						
Pain (All)	**79.0**	83.3	67.8	**72.6**	85.2	56.4
(Grade 3)	**3.8**	10.0	8.5	**0.7**	0	3.65
Redness (All)	**33.0**	53.3	15.3	**32**	38.9	20.0
(≥50 mm)	**5.8**	16.7	0	**2.5**	7.4	0
Swelling (All)	**35.0**	46.7	15.3	**20.8**	29.6	10.9
(≥50 mm)	**7.8**	10.0	1.7	**2.5**	5.6	0
General Symptoms						
Fever (≥37.5°C)	**8.9**	8.3	5.1	**18.5**	33.3	12.7
Fever (≥39.1°C)	**0.4**	0	0	**0.2**	0	0
Malaise	**27.7**	26.7	20.3	**19.2**	20.4	14.5
Fatigue	**56.2**	50.0	40.7	**27.2**	25.9	23.6
Vomiting	**4.0**	5.0	3.4	**3.4**	3.7	5.5
Headache	**51.3**	51.7	35.6	**37.0**	44.4	47.3
Dizziness	**20.5**	26.7	13.6	**10.0**	3.7	9.1

a These data are from the first vaccination of either of these comparator vaccine.
Legend: Td=Tetanus + diphtheria toxoid; aP=acellular pertussis.

DOSAGE AND ADMINISTRATION: Recommended Dose: A single 0.5 mL dose of the vaccine is recommended.
Tetanus Prophylaxis in Wound Management: Table 2 summarizes the recommended use of immunizing agents in wound management. It is important to ascertain the number of doses of toxoid previously given and the interval since the last dose. When a tetanus booster dose is required, the combined preparation of tetanus and diphtheria toxoid formulated for adults (Td) is preferred. Appropriate cleansing and debridement of wounds is imperative, and use of antibiotics may be considered.

Some individuals with humoral immune deficiency, including those with HIV infection, may not respond adequately to tetanus toxoid. Therefore, tetanus immune globulin (TIG) should be used in addition to tetanus toxoid if a wound occurs that is not clean, regardless of the time elapsed since the last booster.

Table 2: BOOSTRIX

Guide to Tetanus Prophylaxis in Wound Management

	Clean, Minor Wounds		All Other Wounds	
History of Tetanus Immunization	**Td or Tdap[a]**	**Tig[b]**	**Td or Tdap[a]**	**Tig**
Uncertain of <3 doses of an immunization series[c]	Yes	No	Yes	Yes
≥3 doses received in an immunization series[c]	No[d]	No	No[e]	No[f]

a Adult type combined tetanus and diphtheria toxoids or a combined preparation of diphtheria, tetanus and acellular pertussis. If the patient is <7 years old a tetanus toxoid-containing vaccine is given as part of the routine childhood immunization.
b Tetanus immune globulin, given at a separate site from Td (or Tdap).
c The immunization series for tetanus is described in the text (Schedule and Dosage).
d Yes, if >10 years since last booster.
e Yes, if >5 years since last booster. More frequent boosters not required and can be associated with increased adverse events. The bivalent toxoid, Td, is not considered to be significantly more reactogenic than T alone and is recommended for use in this circumstance. The patient should be informed that Td (or Tdap) has never been given.
f Yes, if individuals are known to have a significant humoral immune deficiency state (e.g. HIV, agammaglobulinemia) since immune response to tetanus toxoid may be suboptimal.

Administration: Do not remove the white back-stop from the syringe. Prior to administration, ensure that the plunger rod is firmly attached to the rubber stopper by turning the plunger clockwise until slight resistance is felt. **Do not** over tighten. Remove syringe LUER Tip-cap and needle cap. Attach needle by pressing and twisting in a clockwise rotation until secured to the syringe.

Prior to vaccination, the vaccine should be well shaken in order to obtain a homogeneous turbid white suspension and visually inspected for any foreign particulate matter and/or variation of physical aspect prior to administration. In the event of either being observed, discard the vaccine.

BOOSTRIX (combined diphtheria, tetanus, acellular pertussis (adsorbed) vaccine) should not be mixed with other vaccines in the same syringe.

BOOSTRIX is for deep muscular injection.

Repeat vaccination against diphtheria and tetanus should be performed at intervals as per official recommendations (generally 10 years). It is not necessary to recommence primary vaccination, should the officially recommended interbooster interval be exceeded.

OVERDOSAGE:
No case of overdose has been reported.

For management of a suspected drug overdose, CPhA recommends that you contact your **regional Poison Control Centre**. See the *CPS* Directory section for a list of Poison Control Centres.

ACTION AND CLINICAL PHARMACOLOGY: Diphtheria: Diphtheria is a serious communicable disease, primarily a localized and generalized intoxication caused by diphtheria toxin, an extracellular protein metabolite of toxigenic strains of *C. diphtheriae*. The disease occurs most frequently in unimmunized or partially immunized individuals. The incidence of diphtheria in Canada has decreased from 9000 cases reported in 1924 to extremely low levels. Only one or two cases have been reported annually in recent years. The case fatality rate remains 5 to 10%, with the highest death rates in the very young and elderly. If immunization levels are allowed to fall and adults do not receive booster doses, disease re-emergence may appear as demonstrated in the Commonwealth of Independent States (former Soviet Union), where tens of thousands of cases with substantial mortality have been reported. Protection against disease is due to the development of neutralizing antibodies to the diphtheria toxin. Following adequate immunization with diphtheria toxoid, it is generally accepted that protection persists for at least 10 years. Serum antitoxin levels of at least 0.01 antitoxin units per mL are generally regarded as protective. This significantly reduces both the risk of developing diphtheria and the severity of clinical illness. Immunization with diphtheria toxoid does not, however, eliminate carriage of *C. diphtheriae* in the pharynx or nose or on the skin.
Tetanus: Tetanus is an intoxication manifested primarily by neuromuscular dysfunction caused by a potent exotoxin released by *C. tetani*. Immunization is highly effective, provides long lasting protection and is recommended for the entire population. Only 1 to 7 with an average of 5 cases of tetanus are reported annually in Canada while no deaths have been recorded since 1995. The disease continues to occur almost exclusively among persons who are unvaccinated or inadequately vaccinated or whose vaccination histories are unknown or uncertain.

Spores of *C. tetani* are ubiquitous. Naturally acquired immunity to tetanus toxin does not occur. Thus, universal primary immunization and timed booster doses to maintain adequate tetanus antitoxin levels are necessary to protect all age groups. Protection against disease is due to the development of neutralizing antibodies to the tetanus toxin. Tetanus toxoid is a highly effective antigen and a completed primary series generally induces serum antitoxin levels of at least 0.01 antitoxin units per mL, a level which has been reported to be protective. It is generally accepted that protection persists for at least 10 years. To maintain immunity to tetanus following completion of primary immunization, booster doses administered as Td are recommended at 10 yearly intervals.
Pertussis: Pertussis (whooping cough) is a disease of the respiratory tract caused by *B. pertussis*. Pertussis is highly communicable (attack rates in unimmunized household contacts of up to 90% have been reported) and can affect individuals of any age; however, severity is greatest among young infants. Precise epidemiologic data do not exist, since bacteriological confirmation of pertussis can be obtained in less than half of the suspected cases. Most reported illness from *B. pertussis* occurs in infants and young children in whom complications can be severe. Older children, adolescents and adults, in whom classic signs of pertussis infection are often absent, may go undiagnosed, and may serve as reservoirs of disease and may act as the primary source of transmission of the bacillus to infants.

Pertussis epidemics are cyclic, occur every 3 to 4 years and outbreaks continue to occur due to 1) the decline in immunity in individuals who received the whole cell vaccine during childhood; 2) a decline in the population that may have acquired natural infection with longer lasting immunity; 3) improvements in diagnosis and surveillance; and 4) possible genetic changes in current strains compared with the strains of *B. pertussis* from which the original whole cell vaccine was prepared. With the licensure of acellular pertussis vaccines, which have better safety and efficacy profiles, the use of whole cell pertussis vaccines is no longer recommended in Canada.

During the 1980s pertussis incidence was low, but has increased since 1990 in spite of high vaccine coverage. Over the past 10 years, the annual number of reported cases of pertussis in Canada has ranged from 2400 to 10 000 although these figures likely under represent the true incidence because of incomplete reporting.

Active surveillance for pertussis has found that 1 to 25% of patients with prolonged cough had *B. pertussis* infection. Using a combination of laboratory methods, the Sentinel Health Unit Surveillance System has documented pertussis infection in 9 to 20% of non improving cough illness of 7 days or more in adolescents and adults.

Canadian studies have estimated that the secondary attack rate of pertussis in adolescents and adults by household contact ranged between 12 and 14% in contacts aged 12 to 17 years, 11 to 18% for those 18 to 29 years of age and 8 to 33% in those 30 years of age or older. It can be concluded that between 10 to 25% of adolescents and adults are susceptible to pertussis and thus play a role in its transmission.

Antigenic components of *B. pertussis* believed to contribute to protective immunity include: pertussis toxin; filamentous hemagglutinin; and pertactin (69 kDa). Although the role of these antigens in providing protective immunity in humans is not well understood, clinical trials which evaluated candidate acellular DTP vaccines manufactured by GlaxoSmithKline supported the efficacy of three component INFANRIX (DTPa). Recently published data suggests a higher importance of the PT and pertactin (69 kDa) components in providing protection against pertussis.
Protective Efficacy of Pertussis: There is currently no correlate of protection defined for pertussis; however, the protective efficacy of GlaxoSmithKline DTPa (INFANRIX) vaccine against WHO defined typical pertussis (≥21 days of paroxysmal cough with laboratory confirmation) was demonstrated in the following 3 dose primary studies:
A Prospective Blinded Household Contact Study Performed in Germany (3, 4, 5 months schedule): Based on data collected from secondary contacts in households where there was an index case with typical pertussis, the protective efficacy of the vaccine was 88.7%. Protection against laboratory confirmed mild disease, defined as 14 days or more of cough of any type was 73 and 67% when defined as 7 days or more of cough of any type
An NIH Sponsored Efficacy Study Performed in Italy (2, 4, 6 months schedule): The vaccine efficacy was found to be 84%. When the definition of pertussis was expanded to include clinically milder cases with respect to type and duration of cough, the efficacy of INFANRIX was calculated to be 71% against >7 days of any cough and 73% against >14 days of any cough. In a follow up of the same cohort, the efficacy was confirmed up to 5 years after completion of primary vaccination without administration of a booster dose of pertussis.

As infants cannot begin their pertussis vaccination course until they are at least 6 weeks old and three doses of vaccine need to be given, vaccination does not confer complete protection until infants have received all 3 doses. Several studies have shown that adults are a significant source of pertussis in the first week of life. It could be expected that immunization of immediate close contacts of newborn infants, such as parents, grandparents and healthcare workers, would reduce exposure of pertussis to infants not yet adequately protected through immunization. Booster immunization with BOOSTRIX, an acellular pertussis vaccine with reduced antigen content of diphtheria toxoids and pertussis, has demonstrated that the vaccine was immunogenic and well tolerated in clinical studies in which adolescents and adults have received BOOSTRIX.

STORAGE AND STABILITY: BOOSTRIX (combined diphtheria, tetanus, acellular pertussis (adsorbed) vaccine) must be stored at 2 to 8°C. Do not use beyond the expiry date printed on the label and packaging.

Upon removal from the refrigerator, the vaccine is stable for 8 hours at 21°C.

Do not freeze; discard if vaccine has been frozen.

INFORMATION FOR THE PATIENT: Published in e-CPS, available by subscription at www.e-cps.ca.

DOSAGE FORMS, COMPOSITION AND PACKAGING: BOOSTRIX (combined diphtheria, tetanus, acellular pertussis (adsorbed) vaccine) contains diphtheria toxoid, tetanus toxoid, three purified pertussis antigens [pertussis toxoid (PT), filamentous haemagglutinin (FHA) and pertactin (69 kDalton outer membrane protein)] adsorbed onto aluminum salts. The final vaccine is formulated in saline. Prefilled syringes, packages of 1 and 10.

BOOSTRIX meets the World Health Organization requirements for manufacture of biological substances and for diphtheria and tetanus vaccines.

Botox® Ⓟ

botulinum toxin type A

Neuromuscular Paralytic Agent

Allergan

Date of Revision: September 26, 2008

SUMMARY PRODUCT INFORMATION:

Route of Administration	Dosage Form/ Strength	Clinically Relevant Nonmedicinal Ingredients
• Intramuscular use for all indication except hyperhidrosis • Intradermal use for hyperhidrosis only	Sterile vacuum-dried concentrate; powder for solution for injection; 100 Allergan units per vial	Albumin (human) For a complete listing see Dosage Forms, Composition and Packaging.

INDICATIONS AND CLINICAL USE: BOTOX (Botulinum toxin type A for injection) is indicated:
- for the treatment of blepharospasm associated with dystonia, including benign essential blepharospasm or VII nerve disorders in patients 12 years of age or older,
- for the treatment of strabismus in patients 12 years of age or older. BOTOX is ineffective in chronic paralytic strabismus except to reduce antagonist contracture in conjunction with surgical repair,
- to reduce the subjective symptoms and objective signs of cervical dystonia (spasmodic torticollis) in adults,
- in the management of focal spasticity, including the treatment of upper limb spasticity associated with stroke in adults,
- in the treatment of dynamic equinus foot deformity due to spasticity in pediatric cerebral palsy patients, two years of age or older, and
- for the treatment of hyperhidrosis of the axilla in patients 18 years of age or older.

Geriatrics (>65 years of age): Studies specifically designed to determine the dose in elderly patients have not been performed. Dosages for the elderly are as for other adults. Initial dosing should begin at the lowest recommended dose for the specific indication.

Pediatrics (<18 years of age): The safety and effectiveness of BOTOX in the treatment of blepharospasm or strabismus have not been investigated in children under 12 years of age.

The safety and effectiveness of BOTOX in the treatment of cervical dystonia has not been investigated in children under 16 years of age.

The safety and effectiveness of BOTOX in the management of focal spasticity, including the treatment of upper limb spasticity associated with stroke has not been investigated in children and adolescents under 18 years of age.

The safety and effectiveness of BOTOX in the treatment of dynamic equinus foot deformity due to spasticity in pediatric cerebral palsy patients has not been investigated in children under two years of age.

CONTRAINDICATIONS: BOTOX is contraindicated in:
- patients who are hypersensitive to botulinum toxin type A or to any ingredient in the formulation or component of the container. For a complete listing, see Dosage Forms, Composition and Packaging.
- the presence of infection at the proposed injection site(s).

WARNINGS AND PRECAUTIONS:

Serious Warnings and Precautions
- The term "Allergan unit" upon which dosing is based, is a specific measurement of toxin activity that is unique to Allergan's formulation of botulinum toxin type A. Therefore, the "Allergan units" used to describe BOTOX activity are different from those used to describe that of other botulinum toxin preparations and the units representing BOTOX activity are not interchangeable with other products.
- BOTOX should only be given by physicians with the appropriate qualifications and experience in the treatment and the use of required equipment.
- Follow the recommended dosage and frequency of administration for BOTOX (see Warnings and Precautions, General and Dosage and Administration).

General: Use BOTOX only as directed.

Do not use dosage recommendations and potency Units applied to other botulinum toxin products when using BOTOX.

The safe and effective use of BOTOX (Botulinum toxin type A for injection) depends upon proper storage of the product, selection of the correct dose, and proper reconstitution and administration techniques.

Physicians administering BOTOX should be familiar with the relevant anatomy of the area involved and any alterations to the anatomy due to prior surgical procedures. An understanding of standard electromyographic techniques is also required for treatment of strabismus, and may be useful for the treatment of cervical dystonia, and focal spasticity associated with pediatric cerebral palsy and upper limb spasticity in adults.

Caution should be used when BOTOX is used in the presence of inflammation at the proposed injection site(s) or when excessive weakness or atrophy is present in the target muscle.

Muscle weakness remote to the site of injection and other serious adverse effects (e.g. dysphagia, aspiration pneumonia) have been rarely reported in both pediatric and adult patients, in some cases associated with a fatal outcome.

Patients or caregivers should be advised to seek immediate medical care if swallowing, speech or respiratory disorders arise.

Patients with a history of underlying neurological disorders, dysphagia and/or aspiration should be treated with extreme caution. The botulinum toxin product should be used under specialist supervision in these patients and should only be used if the benefit of treatment is considered to outweigh the risk.

Injection specific dosage and administration recommendations should be followed. In treating adult patients, including when combining indications, the maximum cumulative dose should generally not exceed 360 Units, up to a maximum of 6 U/kg, in a 3 month interval. In treating pediatric patients, the maximum cumulative dose should generally not exceed 6 Units/kg, up to a maximum of 200 Units, in a 3 month interval.

One unit (U) of BOTOX corresponds to the calculated median intraperitoneal lethal dose (LD_{50}) in mice. The method utilized for performing the assay is specific to Allergan's product, BOTOX. Due to specific details of this assay such as the vehicle, dilution scheme and laboratory protocols for the various mouse LD_{50} assays, Units of biological activity of BOTOX cannot be compared to nor converted into Units of any other botulinum toxin or any toxin assessed with any other specific assay method. Therefore, differences in species sensitivities to different botulinum neurotoxin serotypes precludes extrapolation of animal-dose activity relationships to human dose estimates. The specific activity of BOTOX is approximately 20 units/nanogram of neurotoxin protein complex.

This product contains human serum albumin, a derivative of human blood. Based on effective donor screening and product manufacturing processes, it carries an extremely remote risk for transmission of viral diseases. A theoretical risk for transmission of Creutzfeldt-Jakob disease (CJD) also is considered extremely remote. No cases of transmission of viral diseases or CJD have ever been identified for albumin.

Dynamic Equinus Foot Deformity Due to Spasticity in Pediatric Cerebral Palsy: BOTOX is a treatment of spasticity that has only been studied in association with usual standard of care regimens, and is not intended as a replacement for these treatment modalities. BOTOX is not likely to be effective in improving range of motion at a joint affected by a fixed contracture.

Carcinogenesis and Mutagenesis: Studies in animals have not been performed to evaluate the carcinogenic potential of BOTOX. BOTOX was not mutagenic in in vitro and in vivo mutagenicity studies.

Cardiovascular: There have been rare reports following administration of botulinum toxin of adverse events involving the cardiovascular system, including arrhythmia and myocardial infarction, some with fatal outcomes. Some of these patients had risk factors including preexisting cardiovascular disease. The exact relationship of these events to BOTOX/BOTOX COSMETIC is unknown.

Ear/Nose/Throat: Cervical Dystonia: Dysphagia is a commonly reported adverse event following treatment of cervical dystonia patients with all types of botulinum toxins. Patients with cervical dystonia should be informed of the possibility of experiencing dysphagia which may be mild, but could be severe. Consequent to the dysphagia there is the potential for aspiration, dyspnea and occasionally the need for tube feeding. In rare cases, dysphagia followed by aspiration pneumonia and death has been reported.

Injections into the levator scapulae may be associated with an increased risk of upper respiratory infection and dysphagia.

Dysphagia has contributed to decreased food and water intake resulting in weight loss and dehydration. Patients with subclinical dysphagia may be at increased risk of experiencing more severe dysphagia following a BOTOX injection.

Limiting the dose injected into both sternocleidomastoid muscles to less than 100 units may decrease the occurrence of dysphagia. Patients with smaller neck muscle mass, or patients who receive bilateral injections into the sternocleidomastoid muscle, have been reported to be at greater risk of dysphagia. Dysphagia is attributable to the localized diffusion of the toxin to the oesophageal musculature.

Patients or caregivers should be advised to seek immediate medical care if swallowing, speech or respiratory disorders arise.

Immune: Formation of neutralizing antibodies to botulinum toxin type A may reduce the effectiveness of BOTOX treatment by inactivating the biological activity of the toxin. The critical factors for neutralizing antibody formation have not been well characterized. The results from some studies suggest that BOTOX injections at more frequent intervals or at higher doses may lead to greater incidence of antibody formation. When appropriate, the potential for antibody formation may be minimized by injecting with the lowest effective dose given at the longest feasible intervals between injections.

As with all biologic products, an anaphylactic reaction may occur. Necessary precautions should be taken and epinephrine should be available.

Serious and/or immediate hypersensitivity reactions such as anaphylaxis and serum sickness have been rarely reported, as well as other manifestations of hypersensitivity including urticaria, soft tissue edema, and dyspnea. Some of these reactions have been reported following the use of BOTOX either alone or in conjunction with other products associated with similar reactions. One fatal case of anaphylaxis has been reported in which lidocaine was used as the diluent for BOTOX and consequently the causal agent cannot be reliably determined. If such a reaction occurs, further injection should be discontinued and appropriate medical therapy immediately.

Neurologic: Extreme caution should be exercised when administering BOTOX to individuals with peripheral motor neuropathic diseases (e.g. amyotrophic lateral sclerosis, or motor neuropathy) or neuromuscular junction disorders (e.g. myasthenia gravis or Lambert-Eaton syndrome). Patients with neuromuscular junction disorders may be at increased risk of clinically significant systemic effects including severe dysphagia and respiratory compromise from typical doses of BOTOX. There have been rare cases of administration of botulinum toxin to patients with known or unrecognized neuromuscular junction disorders where the patients have shown extreme sensitivity to the systemic effects of typical clinical doses. In some of these cases, dysphagia has lasted several months and required placement of a gastric feeding tube. **When exposed to very high doses, patients with neurologic disorders, e.g. pediatric cerebral palsy or adult spasticity, may also be at increased risk of clinically significant systemic effects.**

New onset or recurrent seizures have been reported, typically in patients who are predisposed to experiencing these events. The reports in children were reports predominantly from cerebral palsy patients treated for spasticity. The exact relationship of these events to the botulinum toxin injection has not been established.

Ophthalmologic: Blepharospasm: Reduced blinking following BOTOX injection into the orbicularis oculi muscle can lead to corneal exposure, persistent epithelial defect, and corneal ulceration, especially in patients with VII nerve disorders. One case of corneal perforation in an aphakic eye requiring corneal grafting has occurred because of this effect. Careful testing of corneal sensation in eyes previously operated upon, avoidance of injection into the lower lid area to avoid ectropion, and vigorous treatment of any epithelial defect should be employed. This may require protective drops, ointment, therapeutic soft contact lenses, or closure of the eye by patching or other means.

Because of the anticholinergic activity of botulinum toxin, caution should be exercised when treating patients at risk for angle closure glaucoma, including patients with anatomically narrow angles. Acute angle closure glaucoma has been reported very rarely following periorbital injections of botulinum toxin.

Strabismus: BOTOX is ineffective in chronic paralytic strabismus except to reduce antagonist contracture in conjunction with surgical repair. The efficacy of BOTOX in deviations over 50 prism diopters, in restrictive strabismus, in Duane's syndrome with lateral rectus weakness, and in secondary strabismus caused by prior surgical over-recession of the antagonist is doubtful. In order to enhance efficacy, multiple injections over time may be required.

During the administration of BOTOX for the treatment of strabismus, retrobulbar hemorrhages sufficient to compromise retinal circulation have occurred from needle penetrations into the orbit. It is recommended that appropriate instruments to decompress the orbit be accessible. Ocular (globe) penetrations by needles have also occurred. An ophthalmoscope to diagnose this condition should be available.

Inducing paralysis in one or more extraocular muscles may produce spatial disorientation, double vision, or past-pointing. Covering the affected eye may alleviate these symptoms.

Skin: As is expected for any injection procedure, localized pain, inflammation, paresthesia, hypoaesthesia, tenderness, swelling/edema, erythema, localized infection, bleeding and/or bruising have been associated with the injection. Needle-related pain and/or anxiety have resulted in vasovagal responses, including transient symptomatic hypotension and syncope. Care should be taken when injecting near vulnerable anatomic structures.

Primary Hyperhidrosis of the Axillae: Medical history and physical examination, along with specific additional investigations as required, should be performed to exclude potential causes of secondary hyperhidrosis (e.g. hyperthyroidism or phaeochromocytoma). This will avoid symptomatic treatment of hyperhidrosis without the diagnosis and/or treatment of underlying disease.

Special Populations: Pregnant Women: There are no adequate and well-controlled studies of BOTOX administration in pregnant women. Studies in animals have shown reproductive toxicity. The potential risk for humans is unknown. BOTOX should not be used during pregnancy unless clearly necessary. If this drug is used during pregnancy, or if the patient becomes pregnant while taking this drug, the patient should be apprised of the potential risks, including abortion or fetal malformations, which have been observed in rabbits.

Nursing Women: It is not known whether this drug is excreted in human milk. Because many drugs are excreted in human milk, caution should be exercised when BOTOX is administered to a nursing woman.

Pediatrics (2-18 years of age): There have been very rare spontaneous reports of death sometimes associated with aspiration pneumonia in children with severe cerebral palsy after treatment with botulinum toxin. A causal association to BOTOX has not been established in these cases. Post-marketing reports of possible distant spread of toxin have been very rarely reported in pediatric patients with co-morbidities, predominantly with cerebral palsy, who received >8 U/kg. Extreme caution should be exercised when treating pediatric patients who have significant neurologic debility, dysphagia, or have a recent history of aspiration pneumonia or lung disease.

The safety and effectiveness of BOTOX in the treatment of blepharospasm or strabismus have not been investigated in children under 12 years of age.

The safety and effectiveness of BOTOX in the treatment of cervical dystonia has not been investigated in children under 16 years of age.

The safety and effectiveness of BOTOX in the management of focal spasticity, including upper limb spasticity associated with stroke and primary hyperhidrosis of the axillae, has not been investigated in children and adolescents under 18 years of age.

The safety and effectiveness of BOTOX in the treatment of dynamic equinus foot deformity due to spasticity in pediatric cerebral palsy patients has not been investigated in children under two years of age.

Geriatrics (>65 years of age): Studies specifically designed to determine dose in elderly patients have not been performed. Dosages for the elderly are as for other adults. Initial dosing should begin at the lowest recommended dose for the specific indication.

Monitoring and Laboratory Tests: There are no specific requirements for laboratory test monitoring when patients are treated with BOTOX.

ADVERSE REACTIONS: Adverse Drug Reaction Overview: In general, adverse reactions occur within the first few days following injection and while generally transient may have duration of several months or, in rare cases, longer.

Local muscle weakness represents the expected pharmacological action of botulinum toxin in muscle tissue. However, weakness of adjacent muscles associated with local diffusion and/or injection technique has been reported. Muscle weakness remote to the site of injection and other serious adverse effects (e.g. dysphagia, aspiration pneumonia) have been rarely reported in both pediatric and adult patients, some associated with a fatal outcome.

As is expected for any injection procedure, localized pain, inflammation, paresthesia, hypoaesthesia, tenderness, swelling/oedema, erythema, localized infection, bleeding and/or bruising have been associated with the injection. Needle-related pain and/or anxiety have resulted in vasovagal responses, including transient symptomatic hypotension and syncope.

Clinical Trial Adverse Drug Reactions: Because clinical trials are conducted under very specific conditions the adverse reaction rates observed in the clinical trials may not reflect the rates observed in practice and should not be compared to the rates in the clinical trials of another drug. Adverse drug reaction information from clinical trials is useful for identifying drug-related adverse events and for approximating rates.

For each indication the frequency of adverse reactions documented during clinical trials is given. The following lists events that occurred in ≥1% of subjects. The frequency is defined as follows: very common (≥1/10); common (≥1/100, <1/10).

Blepharospasm: Safety data compiled from controlled clinical trials and open label studies involving 1732 patients treated with BOTOX, the following adverse reactions were reported.

Eye Disorders: Very common: eyelid ptosis. Common: punctate keratitis, lagophthalmos, dry eye, photophobia, eye irritation, lacrimation increase.

Skin and Subcutaneous Tissue Disorder: Common: ecchymosis.

Strabismus: Safety data compiled from clinical trials involving approximately 2058 patients treated with BOTOX, the following adverse reactions were reported.

Eye Disorders: Very common: eyelid ptosis, eye movement disorder.

Cervical Dystonia: Safety data compiled from placebo controlled, double-blind trial involving 231 patients treated with BOTOX, the following adverse reactions were reported.

Infections and Infestations: Common: rhinitis, upper respiratory tract infection.
Nervous System Disorders: Common: dizziness, hypertonia, hypoaesthesia, somnolence, headache.
Gastrointestinal Disorders: Very common: dysphagia. Common: dry mouth, nausea.
Musculoskeletal and Connective Tissue Disorders: Very common: muscular weakness. Common: musculoskeletal stiffness.
General Disorders and Administration Site Conditions: Very common: pain. Common: asthenia, malaise, influenza like illness.
Pediatric Cerebral Palsy: Safety data compiled from two double-blind, randomized, placebo controlled and an open-label extension studies involving approximately 304 patients treated with BOTOX. The following adverse reactions were reported.
Infections and Infestations : Very common: viral infection, ear infection.
Nervous System Disorders: Common: somnolence, gait disturbance, paraesthesia.
Skin and Subcutaneous Tissue Disorders: Common: rash.
Musculoskeletal and Connective Tissue Disorders: Common: myalgia, muscular weakness, pain in extremity.
Renal and Urinary Disorders: Common: urinary incontinence.
Injury, Poisoning and Procedural Complications: Common: fall.
General Disorders and Administration Site Conditions: Common: malaise, injection site pain, asthenia.
Focal Spasticity, Including the Treatment of Upper Limb Spasticity Associated with Stroke in Adult: Safety data compiled from double-blind and open label studies involving 339 patients treated with BOTOX. The following adverse reactions were reported.
Nervous System Disorders: Common: hypertonia.
Skin and Subcutaneous Tissue Disorders: Common: ecchymosis.
Musculoskeletal and Connective Tissue Disorders: Common: muscular weakness, pain in extremity.
General Disorders and Administration Site Conditions: Common: injection site pain, pyrexia, influenza like illness.
Primary Hyperhidrosis of the Axillae: Safety data compiled from double-blind and open-label studies involving 397 patients treated with BOTOX. The following adverse reactions were reported.
Nervous System Disorders: Common: headache, paresthesia.
Vascular Disorders: Common: hot flush.
Gastrointestinal Disorders: Common: nausea.
Skin and Subcutaneous Tissue Disorders: Common: hyperhidrosis, skin odor abnormal, pruritus, subcutaneous nodule, alopecia.
Musculoskeletal and Connective Tissue Disorders: Common: pain in extremity.
General Disorders and Administration Site Conditions: Very common: injection site pain. Common: pain, injection site edema, injection site hemorrhage, injection site hypersensitivity, injection site irritation, asthenia.
Note: increase in non-axillary sweating was reported in 4.5% of patients within one month after injection and showed no pattern with respect to anatomical sites affected. Resolution was seen in approximately 30% of the patients within four months.
Less Common Clinical Trial Adverse Drug Reactions (<1%): For each indication the frequency of adverse reactions documented during clinical trials is given. The frequency is defined as follows: Uncommon (≥1/1000, <1/100); rare (≥1/10 000, <1/1000); very rare (<1/10 000).
Blepharospasm: Nervous System Disorders: Uncommon: dizziness, facial palsy.
Eye Disorders: Uncommon: keratitis, ectropion, diplopia, entropion, vision blurred. Rare: eyelid oedema. Very rare: ulcerative keratitis, corneal epithelium defect, corneal perforation.
Skin and Subcutaneous Tissue Disorder: Uncommon: rash.
General Disorders and Administration Site Conditions: Uncommon: fatigue.
Strabismus: Eye Disorders: Uncommon: ocular retrobulbar hemorrhages, eye penetration, Holmes-Adie pupil. Rare: vitreous hemorrhage.
Cervical Dystonia: Eye Disorders: Uncommon: diplopia, eyelid ptosis.
General Disorders and Administration Site Conditions: Uncommon: pyrexia.
Focal Spasticity, Including the Treatment of Upper Limb Spasticity Associated with Stroke in Adults: Nervous System Disorders: Uncommon: hypoaesthesia, headache, paraesthesia.
Vascular Disorders: Uncommon: orthostatic hypotension.
Gastrointestinal Disorders: Uncommon: nausea.
Skin and Subcutaneous Tissue Disorders: Uncommon: dermatitis, pruritus, rash.
Musculoskeletal and Connective Tissue Disorders: Uncommon: arthralgia, bursitis.
General Disorders and Administration Site Conditions: Uncommon: asthenia, pain, injection site hypersensitivity, malaise.
Abnormal Hematologic and Clinical Chemistry Findings: No specific trends in abnormal hematologic or clinical chemistry findings have been reported.
Post-Market Adverse Drug Reactions: BOTOX and BOTOX COSMETIC contain the same active ingredient in the same formulation. Therefore, adverse events observed with the use of BOTOX COSMETIC also have the potential to be associated with the use of BOTOX.

Adverse events after treatment with botulinum toxin include rare spontaneous reports of death, sometimes associated with anaphylaxis, dysphagia, respiratory compromise, pneumonia, and/or other significant debility. There have also been rare reports of adverse events involving the cardiovascular system, including arrhythmia and myocardial infarction, some with fatal outcomes. Some of these patients had risk factors including pre-existing cardiovascular disease. New onset or recurrent seizures have also been reported, typically in patients who are predisposed to experiencing these events. The exact relationship of these events to the botulinum toxin injection has not been established.

The following other adverse events have been reported since the drug has been marketed: abdominal pain; diarrhea; vomiting; pyrexia; anorexia; vision blurred; visual disturbance, hypoacusis; tinnitus; vertigo; facial palsy, facial paresis; brachial plexopathy; radiculopathy; syncope; hypoaesthesia; malaise; myalgia; myasthenia gravis; paraesthesia; allergic reaction, skin rash (including erythema multiforme, urticaria and psoriasiforme eruption); pruritus; hyperhidrosis; alopecia, including madarosis.

Angle closure glaucoma has been reported very rarely following BOTOX treatment for blepharospasm.

These reactions are reported voluntarily from a population of uncertain size. The exact relationship of these events to botulinum toxin is unknown.

DRUG INTERACTIONS: Overview: No specific interactions have been reported.
Drug-Drug Interactions: See Table 1.
Drug-Food Interactions: Interactions with food have not been established.
Drug-Herb Interactions: Interactions with herbal products have not been established.
Drug-Laboratory Test Interactions: Interactions with laboratory tests have not been established.

DOSAGE AND ADMINISTRATION: Dosing Considerations:

- **Intramuscular Use for All Indications except Hyperhidrosis**
- **Intradermal Use for Hyperhidrosis only**
- BOTOX (Botulinum toxin type A for injection) should only be given by physicians with the appropriate qualifications and experience in the treatment and the use of required equipment.
- The term "Allergan unit" upon which dosing is based, is a specific measurement of toxin activity that is unique to Allergan's formulation of botulinum toxin type A. Therefore, the "Allergan units" used to describe BOTOX activity are different from those used to describe that of other botulinum toxin preparations and the units representing BOTOX activity are not interchangeable with other products.
- The use of one vial for more than one patient is not recommended because the product and diluent do not contain a preservative.
- Follow the recommended dosage and frequency of administration for each indication.
- Generally, optimum dose levels and the number of injection sites per muscle have not been established for all indications. Treatment should be initiated at the lowest effective dose. This dose can be gradually increased in subsequent treatments to the maximum recommended dose, if needed.
- Injection intervals of BOTOX should be according the specific indication. In treating adult patients, when combining indications, the maximum cumulative dose should generally not exceed 6 units/kg, up to a maximum of 360 units, in a 3 month interval. In treating pediatric patients, the maximum cumulative dose should generally not exceed 6 units/kg, up to a maximum of 200 units, in a 3 month interval.

Recommended Dose and Dosage Adjustment: Blepharospasm: For blepharospasm, diluted BOTOX (see Table 4) is injected using a sterile, 27-30 gauge needle with or without electromyographic guidance. The initial recommended dose is 1.25 U to 2.5 U (0.05 mL to 0.1 mL volume at each site) injected into the medial and lateral pretarsal orbicularis oculi of the upper lid and into the lateral pre-tarsal orbicularis oculi of the lower lid.

In general, the initial effect of the injections is seen within three days and reaches a peak at one to two weeks post-treatment. Treatment effects last approximately three months, following which the procedure can be repeated indefinitely.

At repeat treatment sessions, the dose may be increased up to two-fold if the response from the initial treatment is considered insufficient (i.e., defined as an effect that lasts no longer than two months). However the re appears to be little benefit obtainable from injecting more than 5 U per site. Some tolerance may be found when BOTOX is used in treating blepharospasm if treatments are given more frequently than every three months, and it is rare to have the effect be permanent.

The cumulative dose of BOTOX for treatment of blepharospasm in a two month period should not exceed 200 U.

Avoiding injection near the levator palpebrae superioris may reduce the complication of ptosis. Avoiding medial lower lid injections, and thereby reducing diffusion into the inferior oblique, may reduce the complication of diplopia.

Table 1: BOTOX

Established or Potential Drug-Drug Interactions

Proper Name of Drug	Ref	Effect	Clinical Comment
Aminoglycoside antibiotics or spectinomycin, or other medicinal products that interfere with neuromuscular transmission (e.g. neuromuscular blocking agents, both depolarizing (succinylcholine) and non-depolarizing (tubocurarine derivatives), lincosamides, polymyxins, quinidine, magnesium sulfate, and anticholinesterases).	T	Theoretically, the effect of botulinum toxin type A may be potentiated.	The effect of botulinum toxin may be potentiated by aminoglycoside antibiotics or spectinomycin, or other drugs that interfere with neuromuscular transmission (e.g. tubocuraine-type muscle relaxants). Caution should be exercised when BOTOX is used with aminoglycosides (e.g. streptomycin, tobramycin, neomycin, gentamycin, netilmicin, kanamycin, amikacin), spectinomycin, polymyxins, tetracyclines, lincomycin or any other drugs that interfere with neuromuscular transmission.
Different botulinum neurotoxin serotypes	T	Unknown	The effect of administering different botulinum neurotoxin serotypes at the same time or within several months of each other is unknown. Excessive weakness may be exacerbated by administration of another botulinum toxin prior to the resolution of the effects of a previously administered botulinum toxin.

Legend: C=case study; CT=clinical trial; T=theoretical.

Strabismus: BOTOX is intended for injection into extraocular muscles utilizing the electrical activity recorded from the tip of the injection needle as a guide to placement within the target muscle. Injection without surgical exposure or electromyographic guidance should not be attempted. Physicians should be familiar with electromyographic techniques.

To prepare the eye for BOTOX injection, it is recommended that several drops of a local anesthetic and an ocular decongestant be given several minutes prior to injection.

Note: The recommended volume of BOTOX injected for treatment of strabismus is 0.05 mL to 0.15 mL per muscle.

The initial listed doses of the diluted BOTOX (see Table 4) typically create paralysis of injected muscles beginning one to two days after injection and increasing in intensity during the first week. The paralysis lasts for 2-6 weeks and gradually resolves over a similar time period. Overcorrections lasting over six months have been rare.

About one-half of patients will require subsequent doses because of inadequate paralytic response of the muscle to the initial dose, or because of mechanical factors such as large deviations or restrictions, or because of the lack of binocular motor fusion to stabilize the alignment.

I. Initial doses in units (abbreviated as U). Use the lower listed doses for treatment of small deviations. Use the larger doses only for large deviations.
   A. For vertical muscles, and for horizontal strabismus of less than 20 prism diopters: 1.25 U to 2.5 U in any one muscle.
   B. For horizontal strabismus of 20 prism diopters to 50 prism diopters: 2.5 U to 5 U in any one muscle.
   C. For persistent VI nerve palsy of one month or longer duration: 1.25 U to 2.5 U in the medial rectus muscle.
II. Subsequent doses for residual or recurrent strabismus.
   A. It is recommended that patients be reexamined 7-14 days after each injection to assess the effect of that dose.
   B. Patients experiencing adequate paralysis of the target muscle that require subsequent injections should receive a dose comparable to the initial dose.
   C. Subsequent doses for patients experiencing incomplete paralysis of the target muscle may be increased up to two-fold compared to the previously administered dose.
   D. Subsequent injections should not be administered until the effects of the previous dose have dissipated as evidenced by substantial function in the injected and adjacent muscles.
   E. The maximum recommended dose as a single injection for any one muscle is 25 U.
   F. The recommended volume of BOTOX injected for treatment of strabismus is 0.05 mL to 0.15 mL per muscle.

Cervical Dystonia (spasmodic torticollis): Several dosing regimens have been used in clinical trials for treatment of cervical dystonia with BOTOX. Dosing must be tailored to the individual patient based on the patient's head and neck position, localization of pain and muscle hypertrophy, patient's bodyweight, and patient response. In initial controlled clinical trials to establish safety and efficacy for cervical dystonia, doses of diluted BOTOX ranged from 140 U to 280 U. However, in clinical practice, a range of 200 U to 360 U have been used effectively.

A 25, 27 or 30 gauge needle may be used for superficial muscles, and a 22 gauge needle may be used for deeper musculature. For cervical dystonia, localization of the involved muscles with electromyographic guidance may be useful.

Multiple injection sites allow BOTOX to have more uniform contact with the innervation areas of the dystonic muscle, and are especially useful in larger muscles. The optimal number of injection sites is dependent upon the size of the muscle to be chemically denervated.

Clinical improvement generally occurs within the first two weeks after injection. The maximum clinical benefit generally occurs approximately six weeks post-injection. Repeat doses should be administered when the clinical effect of a previous injection diminishes, but not more frequently than every two months. The interval between injections reported in the clinical trials showed substantial variation (from 2 to 32 weeks), with a typical duration of approximately 12 to 16 weeks, depending on patient's individual symptoms and responses.

Table 2 is intended to give dosing guidelines for injection of BOTOX in the treatment of cervical dystonia.

This information is provided as guidance for the initial injection. The extent of muscle hypertrophy and the muscle groups involved in the dystonic posture may change with time necessitating alterations in the dose of toxin and muscles to be injected. The exact dosage and sites injected must be individualized for each patient.

Focal Spasticity: The exact dosage and number of injection sites should be tailored to the individual based on the size, number and location of muscles involved, the severity of spasticity, presence of local muscle weakness, and the patient response to previous treatment. In clinical trials, the doses did not exceed 360 U divided among selected muscles (typically in the flexor muscles of the elbow, wrist and fingers) at any treatment session. Clinical improvement in mus cle tone generally occurs within two weeks following treatment with the peak effect seen four to six weeks following treatment. In clinical studies, patients were reinjected at 12 to 16 week intervals. The degree of muscle spasticity at the time of reinjection may necessitate alterations in the dose of BOTOX and muscles to be injected.

Table 3 is intended to give dosing guidelines for injection of BOTOX in the treatment of upper limb spasticity associated with stroke.

In controlled and open non-controlled clinical trials doses usually between 200 and 240 units, and up to 360 units divided among selected muscles have been used at a given treatment session.

In controlled clinical trials patients were followed for 12 weeks after single treatment. Improvement in muscle tone occurred within two weeks with the peak effect generally seen within four to six weeks. In an open, non-controlled continuation study, most of the patients were re-injected after an interval of 12 to 16 weeks, when the effect on muscle tone had diminished.

These patients received up to four injections with a maximal cumulative dose of 960 units over 54 weeks. If it is deemed appropriate by the treating physician, repeat doses may be administered, when the effect of a previous injection has diminished. Re-injections should not occur before 12 weeks. The degree and pattern of muscle spasticity at the time of reinjection may necessitate alterations in the dose of BOTOX and muscles to be injected. The lowest effective dose should be used.

A 25, 27 or 30 gauge needle may be used for superficial muscles, and a 22-gauge needle may be used for deeper musculature. For focal spasticity, localization of the involved muscles with electromyographic guidance or nerve stimulation techniques may be useful.

Multiple injection sites allow BOTOX to have more uniform contact with the innervation areas of the muscle and are especially useful in larger muscles.

Table 2: BOTOX

Dosage Guide for Cervical Dystonia

Classification	Muscle Groupings	Total Dosage; Number of Sites
Type I Head rotated toward side of shoulder elevations	Sternocleidomastoid Levator scapulae Scalene Splenius capitis Trapezius	50–100 U; at least 2 sites 50 U; 1–2 sites 25–50 U; 1–2 sites 25–75 U; 1–3 sites 25–100 U; 1–8 sites
Type II Head rotation only	Sternocleidomastoid	25–100 U; at least 2 sites if >25 U given
Type III Head tilted toward side of shoulder elevation	Sternocleidomastoid Levator scapulae Scalene Trapezius	25–100 U; at posterior border; at least 2 sites if >25 U given 25–100 U; at least 2 sites 25–75 U; at least 2 sites 25–100 U; 1–8 sites
Type IV Bilateral posterior cervical muscle spasm with elevation of the face	Splenius capitis and cervicis	50–200 U; 2–8 sites, treat bilaterally

Table 3: BOTOX

Dosing Guidelines in Upper Limb Spasticity Associated with Stroke

Muscle	Total Dosage; Number of Sites
Biceps brachii	100–200 U; up to 4 sites
Flexor digitorum profundus	15–50 U; 1–2 sites
Flexor digitorum sublimis	15–50 U; 1–2 sites
Flexor carpi radialis	15–60 U; 1–2 sites
Flexor carpi ulnaris	10–50 U; 1–2 sites
Adductor Pollicis	20 U; 1–2 sites
Flexor Pollicis Longus	20 U; 1–2 sites

Dynamic Equinus Foot Deformity Due to Spasticity in Pediatric Cerebral Palsy Patients, Two Years of Age or Older: For the treatment of equinus foot deformity due to spasticity in pediatric cerebral palsy, diluted BOTOX is injected using a sterile 23-26 gauge needle. In clinical trials, the total dose of 4 U/kg was administered by injecting BOTOX into each of two sites in the medial and lateral heads of the gastrocnemius muscle of the affected lower limb(s). In diplegia, the initial recommended total dose is 6 units/kg body weight divided between the affected limbs.

Clinical improvement generally occurs within the first two weeks after injection. Repeat doses should be administered when the clinical effect of a previous injection diminishes but not more frequently than every two months. The average duration of the therapeutic effect reported in an open-label clinical trial of 207 patients was 3.1 to 3.6 months. In this study, although the dose was 4 U/kg, the number of Units injected did not exceed 200 U.

Hyperhidrosis of the Axilla: BOTOX is reconstituted with 0.9% non-preserved sterile saline (100 U/4 mL). Using a 30 gauge needle, 50 U of BOTOX (2 mL) is injected intradermally, evenly distributed in multiple sites approximately 1-2 cm apart within the hyperhidrotic area of the axilla. The hyperhidrotic area may be defined using standard staining techniques, for example Minor's iodine-starch test.

Lack of Response: There are several potential explanations for a lack or diminished response to an individual treatment with BOTOX. These may include inadequate dose selection, selection of inappropriate muscles for injection, muscles inaccessible to injection, underlying structural abnormalities such as muscle contractures or bone disorders, change in pattern of muscle involvement, patient perception of benefit compared with initial results, inappropriate storage or reconstitution, as well as neutralizing antibodies to botulinum toxin. A neutralizing antibody is defined as an antibody that inactivates the biological activity of the toxin. However, there have been patients who continued to respond to therapy and demonstrated presence of neutralizing antibodies; the proportion of patients which lose their response to botulinum toxin therapy and have demonstrable levels of neutralizing antibodies is small.

The critical factors for neutralizing antibody production are the frequency and dose of injection. Some cervical dystonia patients acquired immunity to botulinum toxin when injected at two to three week intervals with doses exceeding 300 units in a 30 day period. Some tolerance may be observed when BOTOX is used in treating blepharospasm if treatments are given more frequently than every three months. To reduce the potential for neutralizing antibody formation, it is recommended that injection intervals should be no more frequent than two months. In general, the dose should not exceed 360 U in any two month period. For the treatment of blepharospasm, the cumulative dose of BOTOX in a two month period should not exceed 200 U.

A suggested course of action when patients do not respond to BOTOX injections is:

1. wait the usual treatment interval;
2. consider reasons for lack of response listed above;
3. more than one treatment course should be considered before classification of a patient as a non-responder;
4. test patient serum for neutralizing antibody presence.

Missed Dose: Missed doses may be administered as soon as is practical.

Table 4: BOTOX

Dilution

Quantity of Diluent Added (0.9% Sodium Chloride Injection)	Resulting Dose Units/0.1 mL 100 U Vials
1.0 mL	10.0 U
2.0 mL	5.0 U
4.0 mL	2.5 U
8.0 mL	1.25 U

Administration: An injection of BOTOX is prepared by drawing into a sterile 1 mL tuberculin syringe an amount of the properly diluted toxin (see Table 4) slightly greater than the intended dose. Air bubbles in the syringe barrel are expelled and the syringe may be attached to the electromyographic injection needle, preferably a 1.5 inch, 27 gauge needle. Injection volume in excess of the intended dose is expelled through the needle into an appropriate waste container to assure patency of the needle and to confirm that there is no syringe-needle leakage. A new sterile needle and syringe should be used to enter the vial on each occasion for dilution or removal of BOTOX.

Reconstitution: Parenteral Products: To reconstitute vacuum-dried BOTOX, use sterile normal saline without a preservative; 0.9% Sodium Chloride Injection is the only recommended diluent. Draw up the proper amount of diluent in the appropriate size syringe. Since BOTOX is denatured by bubbling or similar violent agitation, inject the diluent into the vial gently. Discard the vial if a vacuum does not pull the diluent into the vial. Record the date and time of reconstitution on the space on the label. BOTOX should be administered within twenty-four hours after reconstitution. During this time period, reconstituted BOTOX should be stored in a refrigerator (2 to 8°C). Reconstituted BOTOX should be clear, colorless and free of particulate matter. Parenteral drug products should be inspected visually for particulate matter and discoloration prior to administration and whenever the solution and the container permit.

Note: These dilutions are calculated for an injection volume of 0.1 mL. A decrease or increase in the BOTOX dose is also possible by administering a smaller or larger injection volume (i.e., 0.05 mL (50% decrease in dose) to 0.15 mL (50% increase in dose)).

OVERDOSAGE:

In the event of overdosage or injection error, additional information may be obtained by contacting Allergan, Inc. at (800) 433-8871.

Overdose of BOTOX is a relative term and depends upon dose, site of injection, and underlying tissue properties. Signs and symptoms of overdose are not apparent immediately post-injection. Should accidental injection or oral ingestion occur, or overdose be suspected, the person should be medically monitored for up to several weeks for progressive signs or symptoms of muscular weakness distant from the site of injection that may include ptosis, diplopia, swallowing and speech disorders, generalized weakness or respiratory failure. These patients should be considered for further medical evaluation and appropriate medical therapy immediately instituted, which may include hospitalization.

For management of a suspected drug overdose, CPhA recommends that you contact your **regional Poison Control Centre**. See the *CPS* Directory section for a list of Poison Control Centres.

ACTION AND CLINICAL PHARMACOLOGY: Mechanism of Action: BOTOX (Botulinum toxin type A for injection) is a sterile, vacuum-dried form of purified botulinum neurotoxin type A complex, produced from a culture of the Hall strain of *C. botulinum* grown in a medium containing N-Z amine, glucose and yeast extract. It is purified to a crystalline complex consisting of the neurotoxin, a non-toxic protein and four major hemagglutinin proteins.

BOTOX blocks neuromuscular conduction by binding to receptor sites on motor nerve terminals, entering the nerve terminals, and inhibiting the release of acetylcholine. When injected intramuscularly at therapeutic doses, BOTOX produces partial chemical denervation of the muscle resulting in localized muscle paralysis. When chemically denervated, the muscle may atrophy, axonal sprouting may occur, and extrajunctional acetylcholine receptors may develop. There is evidence that reinnervation of the muscle may occur, thus reversing muscle weakness produced by localized injection of BOTOX.

One Allergan unit of BOTOX corresponds to the calculated median intraperitoneal lethal dose (LD_{50}) in mice, performed in a mouse potency assay. This assay method is specific to Allergan's product, BOTOX. Due to specific method details such as the vehicle, dilution scheme and laboratory protocols for the various mouse LD_{50} assays, units of biological activity of BOTOX can not be compared to or converted into units of any other botulinum toxin activity. The specific activity of BOTOX is approximately 20 units/nanogram of neurotoxin protein complex.

Pharmacodynamics: When injected into neck muscles, BOTOX reduces both objective signs and subjective symptoms of cervical dystonia (spasmodic torticollis). These improvements include reduced angle of head turning, reduced shoulder elevation, decreased size and strength of hypertrophic muscles, and decreased pain. Based on the results of well-controlled studies, 40-58% of patients with cervical dystonia would be expected to have a significant improvement in their symptoms.

The paralytic effect on muscles injected with BOTOX reduces the excessive, abnormal contractions of blepharospasm associated with dystonia.

When used for the treatment of strabismus, it has been postulated that the administration of BOTOX affects muscle pairs by inducing an atrophic lengthening of the injected muscle and a corresponding shortening of the antagonist muscle.

Following injection of BOTOX some distant muscles have shown increased electrophysiologic neuromuscular jitter. This effect is not associated with other types of electrophysiologic abnormalities, or with clinical signs of weakness or symptoms regarding either safety or efficacy.

In the treatment of pediatric cerebral palsy patients with dynamic equinus foot deformity due to spasticity, BOTOX injections into the gastrocnemius produce an improvement in ankle position (reduction in equinus) and an improvement in gait pattern due to increased heel-to-floor contact.

In the treatment of hyperhidrosis of the axilla (N=320), BOTOX-treated patients demonstrated a responder rate based on gravimetric assessment of 95% at week 1 and 82% at week 16. The mean percentage reduction in sweat production in the BOTOX-treated patients ranged from 83% at week 1 to 69% at week 16. Treatment response has been reported to persist for 4 to 7 months (average of 5.2 months) in patients (N=12) treated with 50 U per axilla. Repeat injections should be administered when effects from previous injections subside.

When used for the treatment of focal spasticity BOTOX injected into upper limb muscles reduces the objective signs and subjective symptoms of spasticity. Improvements include reduction of muscle tone, increase in range of motion, and in some patients reduction of spasticity-related disability.

Pharmacokinetics: It is believed that little systemic distribution of therapeutic doses of BOTOX occurs. BOTOX is not expected to be presented in the peripheral blood at measurable levels following IM or intradermal injection at the recommended doses. The recommended quantities of neurotoxin administered at each treatment session are not expected to result in systemic, overt distant clinical effects, i.e. muscle weakness, in patients without other neuromuscular dys function. However, clinical studies using single fiber electromyographic techniques have shown subtle electrophysiologic findings consistent with neuromuscular inhibition (i.e. "jitter") in muscles distant to the injection site, but these were unaccompanied by any clinical signs or symptoms of neuromuscular inhibition from the effects of botulinum toxin.

STORAGE AND STABILITY:

- Store the vacuum-dried product either in a refrigerator at 2-8°C, or in a freezer at or below −5°C.
- Administer BOTOX within 24 hours after the vial is removed from the freezer and reconstituted.
- During these 24 hours, reconstituted BOTOX should be stored in a refrigerator (2 to 8°C).
- Reconstituted BOTOX should be clear, colorless and free of particulate matter.
- Do not freeze reconstituted BOTOX.
- At the time of use, product acceptability should be confirmed relative to the expiration date indicated on the product vial and outer box.

SPECIAL HANDLING INSTRUCTIONS: All vials, including expired vials, or equipment used with the drug should be disposed of carefully as is done with all medical waste.

INFORMATION FOR THE PATIENT: Published in e-CPS, available by subscription at www.e-cps.ca.

DOSAGE FORMS, COMPOSITION AND PACKAGING: Each sterile vial contains: *Clostridium botulinum* toxin type A 100 units (U), human serum albumin 0.5 mg and sodium chloride 0.9 mg in a vacuum-dried form without a preservative. One Allergan unit (U) corresponds to the calculated median lethal dose (LD_{50}) in mice using reconstituted BOTOX and injected intraperitoneally.

Botox Cosmetic® ℞

botulinum toxin type A (purified neurotoxin complex)

Neuromuscular Paralytic Agent

Allergan

Date of Revision: September 26, 2008

SUMMARY PRODUCT INFORMATION:

Route of Administration	Dosage Form/ Strength	Clinically Relevant Nonmedicinal Ingredients
Intramuscular	Sterile vacuum-dried concentrate; powder for solution for injection; 100 Allergan units per vial	Albumin (human) For a complete listing see Dosage Forms, Composition and Packaging.

INDICATIONS AND CLINICAL USE: BOTOX COSMETIC (Botulinum toxin type A for injection) is indicated:

- for the treatment of upper facial rhytides, including forehead, lateral canthus, and glabellar lines.

Geriatrics (>65 years of age): Studies specifically designed to determine the dose in elderly patients have not been performed. Dosages for the elderly are as for other adults. Initial dosing should begin at the lowest recommended dose for the specific indication.

Pediatrics (<18 years of age): Use of BOTOX COSMETIC is not recommended in children.

CONTRAINDICATIONS: BOTOX COSMETIC is contraindicated in:

- patients who are hypersensitive to botulinum toxin type A or to any ingredient in the formulation or component of the container. For a complete listing, see Dosage Forms, Composition and Packaging.
- the presence of infection at the proposed injection site(s).

WARNINGS AND PRECAUTIONS:

Serious Warnings and Precautions

- The term "Allergan unit" upon which dosing is based, is a specific measurement of toxin activity that is unique to Allergan's formulation of botulinum toxin type A. Therefore, the "Allergan units" used to describe BOTOX COSMETIC activity are different from those used to describe that of other botulinum toxin preparations and the units representing BOTOX COSMETIC activity are not interchangeable with other products.
- BOTOX COSMETIC should only be given by physicians with the appropriate qualifications and experience in the treatment and the use of required equipment.
- Follow the recommended dosage and frequency of administration for BOTOX COSMETIC (see Warnings and Precautions, General and Dosage and Administration).

General: BOTOX and BOTOX COSMETIC contain the same active ingredient in the same formulation. Therefore adverse events observed with the use of BOTOX also have the potential to be associated with the use of BOTOX COSMETIC.

Use BOTOX COSMETIC only as directed.

Do not use dosage recommendations and potency Units applied to other botulinum toxin products when using BOTOX COSMETIC.

The safe and effective use of BOTOX COSMETIC (Botulinum toxin type A for injection) depends upon proper storage of the product, selection of the correct dose, and proper reconstitution and administration techniques.

Caution should be used when BOTOX COSMETIC is used in the presence of inflammation at the proposed injection site(s) or when excessive weakness or atrophy is present in the target muscle.

Muscle weakness remote to the site of injection and other serious adverse effects (e.g. dysphagia when injected into the neck region) have been very rarely reported in the cosmetic application.

Patients or caregivers should be advised to seek immediate medical care if swallowing, speech or respiratory disorders arise.

Patients with a history of underlying neurologic disorders, dysphagia and/or aspiration should be treated with extreme caution. The botulinum toxin product should be used under specialist supervision in these patients and should only be used if the benefit of treatment is considered to outweigh the risk.

Injection intervals of BOTOX COSMETIC should be no more frequent than every two months. Indication specific dosage and administration recommendations should be followed. If combined with non-cosmetic indications, the maximum cumulative dose should generally not exceed 6 units/kg, up to a maximum of 360 Units, in a 3 month interval.

One unit (U) of BOTOX COSMETIC corresponds to the calculated median intraperitoneal lethal dose (LD_{50}) in mice. The method utilized for performing the assay is specific to Allergan's product, BOTOX COSMETIC. Due to specific details of this assay such as the vehicle, dilution scheme and laboratory protocols for the various mouse LD_{50} assays, Units of biological activity of BOTOX COSMETIC cannot be compared to nor converted into Units of any other botulinum toxin or any toxin assessed with any other specific assay method. Therefore, differences in species sensitivities to different botulinum neurotoxin serotypes precludes extrapolation of animal-dose activity relationships to human dose estimates. The specific activity of BOTOX COSMETIC is approximately 20 units/nanogram of neurotoxin protein complex.

This product contains human serum albumin, a derivative of human blood. Based on effective donor screening and product manufacturing processes, it carries an extremely remote risk for transmission of viral diseases. A theoretical risk for transmission of Creutzfeldt-Jakob disease (CJD) also is considered extremely remote. No cases of transmission of viral diseases or CJD have ever been identified for albumin.

Carcinogenesis and Mutagenesis: Studies in animals have not been performed to evaluate the carcinogenic potential of BOTOX COSMETIC. BOTOX COSMETIC was not mutagenic in in vitro and in vivo mutagenicity studies.

Cardiovascular: There have been rare reports following administration of botulinum toxin of adverse events involving the cardiovascular system, including arrhythmia and myocardial infarction, some with fatal outcomes. Some of these patients had risk factors including preexist ing cardiovascular disease. The exact relationship of these events to BOTOX COSMETIC/BOTOX is unknown.

Immune: Formation of neutralizing antibodies to botulinum toxin type A may reduce the effectiveness of BOTOX COSMETIC treatment by inactivating the biological activity of the toxin. The critical factors for neutralizing antibody formation have not been well characterized. The results from some studies suggest that BOTOX injections at more frequent intervals or at higher doses may lead to greater incidence of antibody formation. When appropriate, the potential for antibody formation may be minimized by injecting with the lowest effective dose given at the longest feasible intervals between injections.

As with all biologic products, an anaphylactic reaction may occur. Necessary precautions should be taken and epinephrine should be available.

Serious and/or immediate hypersensitivity reactions such as anaphylaxis and serum sickness have been rarely reported, as well as other manifestations of hypersensitivity including urticaria, soft tissue edema, and dyspnea. Some of these reactions have been reported following the use of BOTOX COSMETIC either alone or in conjunction with other products associated with similar reactions. If such a reaction occurs, further injection should be discontinued and appropriate medical therapy immediately instituted. One fatal case of anaphylaxis has been reported in which the patient died after being injected with BOTOX COSMETIC diluted with 5 mL of 1% lidocaine. The causal role of BOTOX COSMETIC, lidocaine, or both cannot be reliably determined.

Neurologic: Extreme caution should be exercised when administering BOTOX COSMETIC to individuals with peripheral motor neuropathic diseases (e.g., amyotrophic lateral sclerosis, or motor neuropathy) or neuromuscular junction disorders (e.g., myasthenia gravis or Lambert-Eaton syndrome). Patients with neuromuscular junction disorders may be at increased risk of clinically significant systemic effects including severe dysphagia and respiratory compromise from typical doses of BOTOX COSMETIC. There have been rare cases of administration of a botulinum toxin to patients with known or unrecognized neuromuscular junction disorders where the patients have shown extreme sensitivity to the systemic effects of typical clinical doses. In some of these cases, dysphagia has lasted several months and required placement of a gastric feeding tube. **When exposed to very high doses, patients with neurologic disorders, e.g., pediatric cerebral palsy or adult spasticity, may also be at increased risk of clinically significant systemic effects.**

Ophthalmologic: In order to reduce the complications of ptosis, avoid injection near the levator palpebrae superioris, particularly in patients with larger brow-depressor complexes. Medial corrugator injections should be placed at least 1 cm above the bony supraorbital ridge. To reduce the occurrence of diplopia, injections of the lateral canthal lines should be outside the bony orbit, not medial to the vertical line through the lateral canthus. To reduce the occurrence of lip ptosis, injections should be above the insertion of the zygomaticus muscles.

Skin: As is expected for any injection procedure, localized pain, inflammation, paresthesia, hypoaesthesia, tenderness, swelling/edema, erythema, localized infection, bleeding and/or bruising have been associated with the injection. Needle-related pain and/or anxiety have resulted in vasovagal responses, including transient symptomatic hypotension and syncope. Care should be taken when injecting near vulnerable anatomic structures.

Special Populations: Pregnant Women: There are no adequate and well-controlled studies of BOTOX COSMETIC administration in pregnant women. Studies in animals have shown reproductive toxicity. The potential risk for humans is unknown. **BOTOX COSMETIC should not be used during pregnancy.** If this drug is used during pregnancy, or if the patient becomes pregnant while taking this drug, the patient should be apprised of the potential risks, including abortion or fetal malformations, which have been observed in rabbits.

Nursing Women: It is not known whether this drug is excreted in human milk. Because many drugs are excreted in human milk, caution should be exercised when BOTOX COSMETIC is administered to a nursing woman.

Pediatrics (2-18 years of age): Use of BOTOX COSMETIC is not recommended in children.

Geriatrics (>65 years of age): Studies specifically designed to determine the dose in elderly patients have not been performed. Dosages for the elderly are as for other adults. Initial dosing should begin at the lowest recommended dose for the specific indication.

Monitoring and Laboratory Tests: There are no specific requirements for laboratory test monitoring when patients are treated with BOTOX COSMETIC.

ADVERSE REACTIONS: Adverse Drug Reaction Overview: In general, adverse reactions occur within the first few days following injection and while generally transient may have duration of several months or, in rare cases, longer.

Local muscle weakness represents the expected pharmacological action of botulinum toxin in muscle tissue. However, weakness of adjacent muscles associated with local diffusion and/or injection technique has been reported. Muscle weakness remote to the site of injection and other serious adverse effects (e.g. dysphagia when injected into the neck region) have been very rarely reported in the cosmetic application.

As is expected for any injection procedure, localized pain, inflammation, paresthesia, hypoaesthesia, tenderness, swelling/oedema, erythema, localized infection, bleeding and/or bruising have been associated with the injection. Needle-related pain and/or anxiety have resulted in vasovagal responses, including transient symptomatic hypotension and syncope.

Clinical Trial Adverse Drug Reactions: Because clinical trials are conducted under very specific conditions the adverse reaction rates observed in the clinical trials may not reflect the rates observed in practice and should not be compared to the rates in the clinical trials of another drug. Adverse drug reaction information from clinical trials is useful for identifying drug-related adverse events and for approximating rates.

Safety was evaluated in two multicenter, double-blind, placebo-controlled, parallel group studies of identical design for the treatment of glabellar lines (N=535; 405 in the BOTOX COSMETIC-treated group and 130 in the placebo-treated group). The most frequently reported treatment-related adverse events were headache (9.4% in the BOTOX COSMETIC-treated group and 15.4% in the placebo-treated group) and blepharoptosis (3.2% in the BOTOX COSMETIC-treated group and 0% in the placebo-treated group). Blepharoptosis is consistent with the pharmacologic action of BOTOX COSMETIC, and may be technique related.

Adverse events that were reported as treatment-related and were reported in 1-3% of BOTOX COSMETIC-treated patients are listed in decreasing order of incidence: injection site pain/burning/stinging (2.5%), face pain (2.2%), erythema (1.7%), local muscle weakness (1.7%), injection site edema (1.5%), ecchymosis (1.0%), skin tightness (1.0%), paresthesia (1.0%) and nausea (1.0%). Most adverse events reported were of mild-to-moderate severity and all were transient. In a multicenter, open-label, repeat injection study, 318 patients who had participated in one of the two double-blind studies and who had glabellar line severity of at least mild severity at maximum frown received 2 additional treatments of BOTOX COSMETIC. In this study, adverse events were comparable in type, incidence, severity, and causality to those reported in the two placebo-controlled, double-blind studies.

In clinical studies where BOTOX COSMETIC was administered for the treatment of forehead or periorbital wrinkles, treatment-related adverse events have been consistent with those for glabellar lines. Adverse events that were reported as treatment-related after treatment of horizontal forehead lines with 16 U of BOTOX COSMETIC include: headache (20%), bruising (10%), eyelid swelling (15%), and aching or itching forehead (10%). Injecting well above the brow reduces the risk of ptosis.

Treatment-related adverse events associated with treatment of periorbital wrinkles include mild bruising (4-25%) and headache (5.6%); these events occurred at a similar rate on the placebo-treated side. In addition, eyelid droop or shape change, and pain have been reported. Rare cases of diplopia and an asymmetric smile due to injection of zygomaticus major have been reported. These complications can be avoided with adherence to the recommended injection location (see Warnings and Precautions and Dosage and Administration).

Abnormal Hematologic and Clinical Chemistry Findings: No specific trends in abnormal hematologic or clinical chemistry findings have been reported.

Post-Market Adverse Drug Reactions: BOTOX and BOTOX COSMETIC contain the same active ingredient in the same formulation. Therefore, adverse events observed with the use of BOTOX COSMETIC also have the potential to be associated with the use of BOTOX.

Adverse events after treatment with botulinum toxin include rare spontaneous reports of death, sometimes associated with anaphylaxis, dysphagia, respiratory compromise, pneumonia, and/or other significant debility. There have also been rare reports of adverse events involving the cardiovascular system, including arrhythmia and myocardial infarction, some with fatal outcomes. Some of these patients had risk factors including pre-existing cardiovascular disease. New onset or recurrent seizures have also been reported, typically in patients who are predisposed to experiencing these events. The exact relationship of these events to the botulinum toxin injection has not been established.

The following other adverse events have been reported since the drug has been marketed: abdominal pain; diarrhea; vomiting; pyrexia; anorexia; vision blurred; visual disturbance, hypoacusis; tinnitus; vertigo; facial palsy, facial paresis; brachial plexopathy; radiculopathy; syncope; hypoaesthesia; malaise; myalgia; myasthenia gravis; paraesthesia; allergic reaction, skin rash (including erythema multiforme, urticaria and psoriasiform eruption); pruritus; hyperhidrosis; alopecia, including madarosis.

These reactions are reported voluntarily from a population of uncertain size. The exact relationship of these events to botulinum toxin is unknown.

DRUG INTERACTIONS: Overview: No specific interactions have been reported.

Drug-Drug Interactions: See Table 1.

Table 1: BOTOX COSMETIC

Established or Potential Drug-Drug Interactions

Proper Name of Drug	Ref	Effect	Clinical Comment
Aminoglycoside antibiotics or spectinomycin, or other medicinal products that interfere with neuromuscular transmission (e.g. neuromuscular blocking agents, both depolarizing (succinylcholine) and non-depolarizing (tubocurarine derivatives), lincosamides, polymyxins, quinidine, magnesium sulfate, and anticholinesterases).	T	Theoretically, the effect of botulinum toxin type A may be potentiated	The effect of botulinum toxin may be potentiated by aminoglycoside antibiotics or spectinomycin, or other drugs that interfere with neuromuscular transmission (e.g. tubocuraine-type muscle relaxants). Caution should be exercised when BOTOX COSMETIC is used with aminoglycosides (e.g. streptomycin, tobramycin, neomycin, gentamycin, netilmicin, kanamycin, amikacin), spectinomycin, polymyxins, tetracyclines, lincomycin or any other drugs that interfere with neuromuscular transmission.
Different botulinum neurotoxin serotypes	T	Unknown	The effect of administering different botulinum neurotoxin serotypes at the same time or within several months of each other is unknown. Excessive weakness may be exacerbated by administration of another botulinum toxin prior to the resolution of the effects of a previously administered botulinum toxin.

Legend: C=case study; CT=clinical trial; T=theoretical.

Drug-Food Interactions: Interactions with food have not been established.

Drug-Herb Interactions: Interactions with herbal products have not been established.

Drug-Laboratory Test Interactions: Interactions with laboratory tests have not been established.

DOSAGE AND ADMINISTRATION: Dosing Considerations:

- **For Intramuscular Use Only**
- BOTOX COSMETIC (Botulinum toxin type A for injection) should only be given by physicians with the appropriate qualifications and experience in the treatment and the use of required equipment.
- The term "Allergan unit" upon which dosing is based, is a specific measurement of toxin activity that is unique to Allergan's formulation of botulinum toxin type A. Therefore, the "Allergan units" used to describe BOTOX COSMETIC activity are different from those used to describe that of other botulinum toxin preparations and the units representing BOTOX COSMETIC activity are not interchangeable with other products.
- The use of one vial for more than one patient is not recommended because the product and diluent do not contain a preservative.
- Treatment should be initiated at the lowest recommended dose. This dose can be gradually increased in subsequent treatments to the maximum recommended dose, if needed.
- Injection intervals of BOTOX COSMETIC should be no more frequent than every two months. Indication specific dosage and administration recommendations should be followed. In treating adult patients, if combined with non-cosmetic indications, the maximum cumulative dose should generally not exceed 6 Units/kg, up to a maximum of 360 units, in a 3 month interval.

Recommended Dose and Dosage Adjustment: BOTOX COSMETIC is reconstituted only with 0.9% sterile non-preserved saline. Dilutions resulting in 4.0 U-7.0 U per 0.1 mL are generally recommended.

Glabellar lines: 4 U should be administered intramuscularly using a 30 gauge needle in each of 5 sites, 2 in each corrugator muscle and 1 in the procerus muscle for a total dose of 20 U. In order to reduce the complication of ptosis, injection near the levator palpebrae superioris should be avoided, particularly in patients with larger brow-depressor complexes. Medial corrugator injections should be placed at least 1 cm above the bony supraorbital ridge.

Forehead lines: 2-6 U should be injected intramuscularly at each of 4 injection sites in the frontalis muscle, every 1-2 cm along either side of a deep forehead crease, 2-3 cm above the eyebrows, for a total dose of up to 24 U.

Lateral canthus lines: Generally, 2-6 U should be injected bilaterally at each of 1-3 injection sites at a 2-3 mm depth, lateral to the lateral orbital rim, where most lines are seen when a smile is forced. Injection should be at least 1 cm outside the bony orbit, not medial to the vertical line through the lateral canthus, and not close to the inferior margin of the zygoma.

An injection of BOTOX COSMETIC is prepared by drawing into a sterile 1.0 mL tuberculin syringe an amount of the properly diluted toxin (see Table 2) slightly greater than the intended dose. Air bubbles in the syringe barrel are expelled and the syringe may be attached to the electromyographic injection needle, preferably a 1.5 inch, 27 gauge needle. Injection volume in excess of the intended dose is expelled through the needle into an appropriate waste container to assure patency of the needle and to confirm that there is no syringe-needle leakage. A new sterile needle and syringe should be used to enter the vial on each occasion for dilution or removal of BOTOX COSMETIC.

Lack of Response: There are several potential explanations for a lack or diminished response to an individual treatment with BOTOX COSMETIC. These may include inadequate dose selection, selection of inappropriate muscles for injection, muscles inaccessible to injection, underlying structural abnormalities such as muscle contractures or bone disorders, change in pattern of muscle involvement, patient perception of benefit compared with initial results, inappropriate storage or reconstitution, as well as neutralizing antibodies to botulinum toxin. A neutralizing antibody is defined as an antibody that inactivates the biological activity of the toxin. However, there have been patients who continued to respond to therapy and demonstrated presence of neutralizing antibodies; the proportion of patients which lose their response to botulinum to xin therapy and have demonstrable levels of neutralizing antibodies is small.

The critical factors for neutralizing antibody production are the frequency and dose of injection. To reduce the potential for neutralizing antibody formation, it is recommended that injection intervals of BOTOX COSMETIC should be no more frequent than two months. More frequent injections should not be required, as BOTOX COSMETIC treatment reduces the severity of the facial lines for up to 120 days.

A suggested course of action when patients do not respond to BOTOX COSMETIC injections is:

1. wait the usual treatment interval;
2. consider reasons for lack of response listed above;
3. more than one treatment course should be considered before classification of a patient as a non-responder;
4. test patient serum for neutralizing antibody presence.

Missed Dose: Missed doses may be administered as soon as is practical.

Administration: An injection of BOTOX COSMETIC is prepared by drawing into a sterile 1.0 mL tuberculin syringe an amount of the properly diluted toxin (see Table 2) slightly greater than the intended dose. Air bubbles in the syringe barrel are expelled and the syringe may be attached to the electromyographic injection needle, preferably a 1.5 inch, 27 gauge needle. Injection volume in excess of the intended dose is expelled through the needle into an appropriate waste container to assure patency of the needle and to confirm that there is no syringe-needle leakage. A new sterile needle and syringe should be used to enter the vial on each occasion for dilution or removal of BOTOX COSMETIC.

Reconstitution: Parenteral Products: To reconstitute vacuum-dried BOTOX COSMETIC, use sterile normal saline without a preservative; 0.9% Sodium Chloride Injection is the only recommended diluent. Draw up the proper amount of diluent in the appropriate size syringe. Since BOTOX COSMETIC is denatured by bubbling or similar violent agitation, inject the diluent into the vial gently. Discard the vial if a vacuum does not pull the diluent into the vial. Record the date and time of reconstitution on the space on the label. BOTOX COSMETIC should be administered within twenty-four hours after reconstitution.

During this time period, reconstituted BOTOX COSMETIC should be stored in a refrigerator (2 to 8°C). Reconstituted BOTOX COSMETIC should be clear, colorless and free of particulate matter. Parenteral drug products should be inspected visually for particulate matter and discoloration prior to administration and whenever the solution and the container permit.

Table 2: BOTOX COSMETIC Dilution

Resulting Dose: Units per 0.1 mL	Quantity of Diluent Added (0.9% Sodium Chloride for Injection) 100 U Vial
7.5 U	1.3 mL
5.0 U	2.0 mL
2.5 U	4.0 mL

OVERDOSAGE:

In the event of overdosage or injection error, additional information may be obtained by contacting Allergan, Inc. at (800) 433-8871.

Overdose of BOTOX COSMETIC is a relative term and depends upon dose, site of injection, and underlying tissue properties. Signs and symptoms of overdose are not apparent immediately post-injection. Should accidental injection or oral ingestion occur, or overdose be suspected, the person should be medically monitored for up to several weeks for progressive signs or symptoms of muscular weakness distant from the site of injection that may include ptosis, diplopia, swallowing and speech disorders, generalized weakness or respiratory failure. These patients should be considered for further medical evaluation and appropriate medical therapy immediately instituted, which may include hospitalization.

> For management of a suspected drug overdose, CPhA recommends that you contact your **regional Poison Control Centre**. See the *CPS* Directory section for a list of Poison Control Centres.

ACTION AND CLINICAL PHARMACOLOGY: Mechanism of Action: BOTOX COSMETIC (Botulinum toxin type A for injection) is a sterile, vacuum-dried form of purified botulinum neurotoxin type A complex, produced from a culture of the Hall strain of *C. botulinum* grown in a medium containing N-Z amine, glucose and yeast extract. It is purified to a crystalline complex consisting of the neurotoxin, a non-toxic protein and four major hemagglutinin proteins.

BOTOX COSMETIC blocks neuromuscular conduction by binding to receptor sites on motor nerve terminals, entering the nerve terminals, and inhibiting the release of acetylcholine. When injected intramuscularly at therapeutic doses, BOTOX COSMETIC produces partial chemical denervation of the muscle resulting in localized muscle paralysis. When chemically denervated, the muscle may atrophy, axonal sprouting may occur, and extrajunctional acetylcholine receptors may develop. There is evidence that reinnervation of the muscle may occur, thus reversing muscle weakness produced by localized injection of BOTOX COSMETIC.

One Allergan unit of BOTOX COSMETIC corresponds to the calculated median intraperitoneal lethal dose (LD_{50}) in mice, performed in a mouse potency assay. This assay method is specific to Allergan's product, BOTOX COSMETIC. Due to specific method details such as the vehicle, dilution scheme and laboratory protocols for the various mouse LD_{50} assays, units of biological activity of BOTOX COSMETIC can not be compared to or converted into units of any other botulinum toxin activity. The specific activity of BOTOX COSMETIC is approximately 20 units/nanogram of neurotoxin protein complex.

Pharmacodynamics: When injected into neck muscles, BOTOX COSMETIC reduces both objective signs and subjective symptoms of cervical dystonia (spasmodic torticollis). These improvements include reduced angle of head turning, reduced shoulder elevation, decreased size and strength of hypertrophic muscles, and decreased pain. Based on the results of well-controlled studies, 40-58% of patients with cervical dystonia would be expected to have a significant improvement in their symptoms.

The paralytic effect on muscles injected with BOTOX COSMETIC reduces the excessive, abnormal contractions of blepharospasm associated with dystonia.

When used for the treatment of strabismus, it has been postulated that the administration of BOTOX COSMETIC affects muscle pairs by inducing an atrophic lengthening of the injected muscle and a corresponding shortening of the antagonist muscle.

Following injection of BOTOX COSMETIC some distant muscles have shown increased electrophysiologic neuromuscular jitter. This effect is not associated with other types of electrophysiologic abnormalities, or with clinical signs of weakness or symptoms regarding either safety or efficacy.

In the treatment of pediatric cerebral palsy patients with dynamic equinus foot deformity due to spasticity, BOTOX COSMETIC injections into the gastrocnemius produce an improvement in ankle position (reduction in equinus) and an improvement in gait pattern due to increased heel-to-floor contact.

In the treatment of hyperhidrosis of the axilla (N=320), BOTOX COSMETIC-treated patients demonstrated a responder rate based on gravimetric assessment of 95% at week 1 and 82% at week 16. The mean percentage reduction in sweat production in the BOTOX COSMETIC-treated patients ranged from 83% at week 1 to 69% at week 16. Treatment response has been reported to persist for 4 to 7 months (average of 5.2 months) in patients (N=12) treated with 50 U per axilla. Repeat injections should be administered when effects from previous injections subside.

When used for the treatment of focal spasticity BOTOX COSMETIC injected into upper limb muscles reduces the objective signs and subjective symptoms of spasticity. Improvements include reduction of muscle tone, increase in range of motion, and in some patients reduction of spasticity-related disability.

Pharmacokinetics: It is believed that little systemic distribution of therapeutic doses of BOTOX COSMETIC occurs. BOTOX COSMETIC is not expected to be presented in the peripheral blood at measurable levels following IM or intradermal injection at the recommended doses. The recommended quantities of neurotoxin administered at each treatment session are not expected to result in systemic, overt distant clinical effects, i.e. muscle weakness, in patients without other neuromuscular dysfunction. However, clinical studies using single fiber electromyographic techniques have shown subtle electrophysiologic findings consistent with neuromuscular inhibition (i.e. "jitter") in muscles distant to the injection site, but these were unaccompanied by any clinical signs or symptoms of neuromuscular inhibition from the effects of botulinum toxin.

STORAGE AND STABILITY:

- Store the vacuum-dried product either in a refrigerator at 2-8°C, or in a freezer at or below −5°C.
- Administer BOTOX COSMETIC within 24 hours after the vial is removed from the freezer and reconstituted.
- During these 24 hours, reconstituted BOTOX COSMETIC should be stored in a refrigerator (2 to 8°C).
- Reconstituted BOTOX COSMETIC should be clear, colorless and free of particulate matter.
- Do not freeze reconstituted BOTOX COSMETIC.
- At the time of use, product acceptability should be confirmed relative to the expiration date indicated on the product vial and outer box.

SPECIAL HANDLING INSTRUCTIONS: All vials, including expired vials, or equipment used with the drug should be disposed of carefully as is done with all medical waste.

INFORMATION FOR THE PATIENT: Published in e-CPS, available by subscription at www.e-cps.ca.

DOSAGE FORMS, COMPOSITION AND PACKAGING: Each sterile vial contains: *Clostridium botulinum* toxin type A neurotoxin complex (900kD) 100 units (U), human serum albumin 0.5 mg and sodium chloride 0.9 mg in a vacuum-dried form without a preservative. One Allergan unit (U) corresponds to the calculated median lethal dose (LD_{50}) in mice using reconstituted BOTOX COSMETIC and injected intraperitoneally.

Bravelle™ P

urofollitropin

Gonadotropin

Ferring

Date of Preparation: June 3, 2005
Date of Revision: November 28, 2007

SUMMARY PRODUCT INFORMATION:

Route of Administration	Dosage Form/ Strength	Clinically Relevant Nonmedicinal Ingredients
Subcutaneous or Intramuscular Injection	75 IU FSH activity per vial	Lactose monohydrate, Polysorbate 20 (Tween 20), Phosphate buffer (sodium phosphate dibasic, heptahydrate and phosphoric acid)

INDICATIONS AND CLINICAL USE: BRAVELLE (Urofollitropin for injection, purified) in conjunction with hCG is indicated for:

- Multiple follicular development (controlled ovarian stimulation)
- Ovulation induction in patients who have previously received pituitary suppression. This includes patients participating in Assisted Reproductive Technology (ART) program.

Selection of Patients: General: Careful attention should be given to the diagnosis of infertility in the selection of candidates for BRAVELLE (Urofollitropin for Injection, Purified) therapy.

1. Before treatment with BRAVELLE is instituted, a thorough gynecologic and endocrinologic evaluation must be performed, except for those patients enrolled in an In Vitro Fertilization (IVF) program. The evaluation may include a hysterosalpingography (to rule out uterine and tubal pathology). Anovulation should be confirmed by menstrual history, observation of basal body temperature pattern, serial vaginal smears, examination of cervical mucus, and determination of serum (or urine) progesterone, urinary pregnanediol and endometrial biopsy. Patients with tubal pathology should receive urofollitropins only if enrolled in an in vitro fertilization program.
2. Primary ovarian failure should be excluded by the determination of gonadotropin levels.
3. Careful examination should be made to rule out the presence of an early pregnancy.
4. Patients in late reproductive life have a greater predilection to endometrial carcinoma as well as a higher incidence of anovulatory disorders. Cervical dilation and curettage should always be done for diagnosis before starting BRAVELLE therapy in such patients who demonstrate abnormal uterine bleeding or other signs of endometrial abnormalities.
5. Evaluation of the husband's fertility potential should be included in the workup.

Prior to therapy with BRAVELLE patients should be informed of the duration of treatment and monitoring of their condition that will be required. Possible adverse reactions (see Adverse Reactions) and the risk of multiple births should be discussed.

Pregnant Women: BRAVELLE (Urofollitropin for Injection, Purified) is contraindicated in pregnant women.

Pediatric and Geriatric Populations: BRAVELLE (Urofollitropin for Injection, Purified) is not used in pediatric or geriatric populations.

CONTRAINDICATIONS: BRAVELLE (Urofollitropin for Injection, Purified) is contraindicated in women who exhibit:

1. A high circulating FSH level indicating primary ovarian failure.
2. Uncontrolled thyroid and adrenal dysfunction.
3. An organic intracranial lesion such as pituitary tumor.
4. The presence of any causes of infertility other than anovulation unless they are candidates for assisted reproductive procedures.
5. Abnormal bleeding of undetermined origin.
6. Ovarian cysts or enlargement not due to polycystic ovary syndrome.
7. Prior hypersensitivity to urofollitropins.
8. BRAVELLE is not indicated in women who are pregnant or lactating. There are limited human data on the effects of BRAVELLE when administered during pregnancy.

WARNINGS AND PRECAUTIONS: General: BRAVELLE (Urofollitropin for Injection, Purified) is a drug that should only be used by physicians who are experienced in the management of fertility disorders and only when facilities for appropriate clinical and endocrinologic evaluations are available. It is a potent gonadotropic substance capable of causing mild to severe adverse reactions in women. Urofollitropin therapy requires a certain time commitment by physicians and supportive health professionals, and its use requires the availability of appropriate monitoring facilities (see Laboratory Tests). In female patients it must be used with a great deal of care.

The drug substance of this drug product is manufactured from human urine. Although the risk is theoretical, and no case of transmission of an infectious agent linked to the use of urine-derived gonadotropins has ever been identified, the risk of transmitting infectious agents cannot be completely excluded.

Overstimulation of the Ovary During BRAVELLE Therapy: Ovarian Enlargement: Mild to moderate uncomplicated ovarian enlargement which may be accompanied by abdominal distension and/or abdominal pain, occurs in approximately 20% of those treated with follitropin and hCG, and generally regresses without treatment within two or three weeks.

In order to minimize the hazard associated with the occasional abnormal ovarian enlargement which may occur with FSH-hCG therapy, the lowest dose consistent with expectation of good results should be used. Careful monitoring of ovarian response can further minimize the risk of overstimulation.

If the ovaries are abnormally enlarged on the last day of BRAVELLE therapy, hCG should not be administered in the course of therapy; this will reduce the chance of developing the Ovarian Hyperstimulation Syndrome.

Ovarian Hyperstimulation Syndrome (OHSS): OHSS is a medical event distinct from uncomplicated ovarian enlargement. OHSS may progress rapidly to become a serious medical event. It is characterized by an apparent dramatic increase in vascular permeability, which can result in a rapid accumulation of fluid in the peritoneal cavity, thorax, and potentially, the pericardium. The early warning signs of development of OHSS are severe pelvic pain, nausea, vomiting, and weight gain. The following symptomatology has been seen with cases of OHSS: abdominal pain, abdominal distension, gastrointestinal symptoms including nausea, vomiting and diarrhea, severe ovarian enlargement, weight gain, dyspnea, and oliguria. Clinical evaluation may reveal hypovolemia, hemoconcentration, electrolyte imbalances, ascites, hemoperitoneum, pleural effusions, hydrothorax, acute pulmonary distress, and thromboembolic events (see Pulmonary and Vascular Complications). Transient liver function test abnormalities suggestive of hepatic dysfunction, which may be accompanied by morphologic changes on liver biopsy, have been reported in association with the Ovarian Hyperstimulation Syndrome (OHSS).

In the clinical study of ovulation induction, 6 of 72 (8.33 %) BRAVELLE treated women developed OHSS and two were classified as severe. Cases of OHSS are more common, more severe and more protracted if pregnancy occurs. OHSS develops rapidly; therefore patients should be followed for at least two weeks after hCG administration. Most often, OHSS occurs after treatment has been discontinued and reaches its maximum at about 7 to 10 days after treatment. Usually, in cases where OHSS may be developing prior to hCG administration (see Laboratory Tests), the hCG should be withheld.

If severe OHSS occurs, treatment **must** be stopped and the patient should be hospitalized.

A physician experienced in the management of the syndrome, or who is experienced in the management of fluid and electrolyte imbalances should be consulted.

Pulmonary and Vascular Complications: Serious pulmonary conditions (e.g. atelectasis, acute respiratory distress syndrome) have been reported. In addition, thromboembolic events both in association with, and separate from, the Ovarian Hyperstimulation Syndrome have been reported following urofollitropin therapy. Intravascular thrombosis and embolism, which may originate in venous or arterial vessels, can result in reduced blood flow to critical organs or the extremities. Sequelae of such events have included venous thrombophlebitis, pulmonary embolism, pulmonary infarction, cerebral vascular occlusion (stroke), and arterial occlusion resulting in loss of limb. In rare cases, pulmonary complications and/or thromboembolic events have resulted in death.

Other Reproductive Complications: Multiple ovulations with resulting multiple births occur frequently following treatment with gonadotropins and hCG. Prior to gonadotropin and hCG therapy, the patient and her partner should be informed of the possibility and risks associated with multiple births.

Multiple pregnancies have occurred following treatment with BRAVELLE SC and IM in a clinical trial for ovulation induction in which BRAVELLE SC, BRAVELLE IM and a recombinant FSH product were directly compared. The rates of multiple pregnancies appear in Table 1.

The multiple pregnancy rates for the In Vitro Fertilization (IVF) studies appear in Table 2.

Hypersensitivity/Anaphylactic Reactions: Hypersensitivity anaphylactic reactions associated with urofollitropins administered have been reported in some patients. These reactions presented as generalized urticaria, facial edema, angioneurotic edema, and/or dyspnea suggestive of laryngeal edema. The relationship of these symptoms to uncharacterized urinary proteins is uncertain.

Renal and Hepatic: The safety and efficacy of BRAVELLE (Urofollitropin for Injection, Purified) in renal and hepatic insufficiency have not been studied.

Special Populations: Nursing Women: It is not known whether this drug is excreted in human milk. Because many drugs are excreted in human milk and because of the potential for serious adverse reactions in the nursing infant from BRAVELLE (Urofollitropin for Injection, Purified), a decision should be made whether to discontinue nursing or to discontinue the drug, taking into account the importance of the drug to the mother.

Table 1: BRAVELLE

Multiple Pregnancies-Primary Efficacy Responders in Ovulation Induction Study

Parameter (%)	BRAVELLE SC N=26	BRAVELLE IM N=28	Recombinant FSH SC N=35	p-value
Total number of continuing pregnancies	9 (34.6)	7 (25.0)	10 (28.6)	
Total number of multiple pregnancies	6 (23.1)	2 (7.1)	4 (11.4)	
Singlets	3 (11.5)	5 (17.9)	6 (17.1)	0.261
Twins	4 (15.4)	0	2 (5.7)	
Triplets	2 (7.7)	0	0	
Quadruplets	0	1 (4.8)	2 (5.7)	
Quintuplets	0	0	0	
Sextuplets	0	1 (4.8)	0	

Monitoring and Laboratory Tests: Laboratory Tests: The combination of both estradiol levels and ultrasonography are useful for monitoring the growth and development of follicles, timing of hCG administration, as well as minimizing the risk of the Ovarian Hyperstimulation Syndrome and multiple gestations.

The clinical confirmation of ovulation is determined by:

a. A rise in basal body temperature;
b. Increase in serum progesterone, and
c. Menstruation following the shift in basal body temperature.

When used in conjunction with indices of progesterone production, sonographic visualization of the ovaries will assist in determining if ovulation has occurred. Sonographic evidence of ovulation may include the following:

a. Fluid in the cul-de-sac;
b. Ovarian stigmata; and
c. Collapsed follicle.

Because of the subjectivity of the various tests for the determination of follicular maturation and ovulation, it cannot be overemphasized that the physician should choose tests with which he/she is thoroughly familiar.

ADVERSE REACTIONS: Clinical Trial Adverse Drug Reactions: Because clinical trials are conducted under very specific conditions the adverse reaction rates observed in the clinical trials may not reflect the rates observed in practice and should not be compared to the rates in the clinical trials of another drug. Adverse drug reaction information from clinical trials is useful for identifying drug-related adverse events and for approximating rates.

The safety of BRAVELLE (Urofollitropin for Injection, Purified) was examined in three clinical studies that enrolled a total of 251 patients receiving BRAVELLE including 72 for ovulation induction and 179 for IVF (In Vitro Fertilization).

Adverse events occurring with ≥1% incidence in the clinical study patients receiving BRAVELLE are listed in Table 3.

The following other adverse events occurred in BRAVELLE treated patients with a frequency <1%:

Body as a Whole: allergic reaction, chest pain, fever, flu syndrome, infection, itchy throat, malaise, shingles.
Cardiovascular: thrombosis.
Digestive: abnormal stools, melena, upset stomach.
Endocrine: endocrine disorder.
Metabolic/Nutritional: weight gain.
Musculoskeletal: leg cramps.
Nervous System: dizziness, dystonia.
Respiratory: bronchitis, rhinitis.
Skin/Appendages: acne, herpes simplex, pruritus.
Special Senses: conjunctivitis, sty.
Urogenital: abortion, dysmenorrhea, kidney calculus, urinary frequency, urinary incontinence, vaginitis.

The following medical events have been reported subsequent to pregnancies resulting from gonadotropin therapy in published clinical studies:

1. Spontaneous abortion.
2. Ectopic pregnancy.
3. Premature labor.
4. Postpartum fever.
5. Congenital abnormalities.

The following adverse reactions have been previously reported during urofollitropin for injection, purified therapy:

1. Pulmonary and vascular complications (see Warnings and Precautions).
2. Adnexal torsion (as a complication of ovarian enlargement).
3. Mild to moderate ovarian enlargement.
4. Hemoperitoneum.
5. There have been infrequent reports of ovarian neoplasms, both benign and malignant, in women who have undergone multiple drug regimens for ovulation induction; however, a causal relationship has not been established.

No local injection site reactions were observed following administration of BRAVELLE; however, pain and irritation at the injection site were statistically significantly less frequent with BRAVELLE than with comparator, recombinant hFSH.

DRUG INTERACTIONS: Drug-Drug Interactions: No drug/drug interaction studies have been conducted for BRAVELLE (Urofollitropin for Injection, Purified) in humans.

DOSAGE AND ADMINISTRATION: Dosing Considerations: Infertile Patients with Oligo-Anovulation: The dose of BRAVELLE (Urofollitropin for Injection, Purified) to stimulate development of ovarian follicles must be individualized for each patient. The lowest dose consistent with achieving good results based on clinical experience and reported clinical data should be used.

Recommended Dose and Dosage Adjustment: Infertile Patients with Oligo-Anovulation/Ovulation Induction: The recommended initial dose of BRAVELLE for patients who have received GnRH agonist or antagonist pituitary suppression is 150 IU daily for the first 5 days of treatment. Based on clinical monitoring (including serum estradiol levels and vaginal ultrasound results), subsequent dosing should be adjusted according to individual patient response.

Adjustments in dose should not be made more frequently than once every 2 days and should not exceed more than 75 to 150 IU per adjustment. The maximum daily dose of BRAVELLE should not exceed 450 IU and in most cases dosing beyond 12 days is not recommended.

If patient response to BRAVELLE is appropriate, hCG (5000 to 10 000 USP units) should be given one day following the last dose of BRAVELLE. The hCG should be withheld if the serum estradiol is greater than 2000 pg/mL, if the ovaries are abnormally enlarged or if abdominal pain occurs, and the patient should be advised to refrain from intercourse. These precautions may reduce the risk of Ovarian Hyperstimulation Syndrome and multiple gestations. Patients should be followed closely for at least 2 weeks after hCG administration. If there is inadequate follicle development or ovulation without subsequent pregnancy, the course of treatment with BRAVELLE may be repeated. The couple should be encouraged to have intercourse daily, beginning on the day prior to the administration of hCG until ovulation becomes apparent from the indices employed for the determination of progestational activity. In the light of the foregoing indices and parameters mentioned, it should become obvious that, unless a physician is willing to devote considerable time to these patients and be familiar with and conduct the necessary laboratory studies, he/she should not use BRAVELLE.

Assisted Reproductive Technologies (ART)/In Vitro Fertilization (IVF): The recommended initial dose of BRAVELLE (Urofollitropin for Injection, Purified) for patients who have received GnRH agonist or antagonist pituitary suppression is 225 IU for the first 5 days of treatment. Based on clinical monitoring (including serum estradiol levels and vaginal ultrasound results), subsequent dosing should be adjusted according to individual patient response. Adjustments in dose should not be made more frequently than once every 2 days and should not exceed more than 75 to 150 IU per adjustment. The maximum daily dose of BRAVELLE given should not exceed 450 IU and in most cases dosing beyond 12 days is not recommended.

Once adequate follicular development is evident, hCG (5000-10 000 USP units) should be administered to induce final follicular maturation in preparation for oocyte retrieval. The administration of hCG must be withheld in cases where the ovaries are abnormally enlarged on the last day of therapy. This should reduce the chance of developing OHSS.

Administration: Dissolve the contents of one or more vials of BRAVELLE (Urofollitropin for Injection, Purified) in one mL sterile saline for injection, USP and **administer subcutaneously or intramuscularly** immediately. Any unused reconstituted material should be discarded. Parenteral drug products should be inspected visually for particulate matter and discoloration prior to administration, whenever solution and container permit.

Table 2: BRAVELLE

Multiple Pregnancies—Primary Efficacy Responders in In Vitro Fertilization Studies

	Study 1				Study 2		
Parameter (%)	BRAVELLE SC N=56	BRAVELLE IM N=55	Recombinant FSH SC N=56	p-value	BRAVELLE SC N=57	Recombinant FSH SC N=59	p-value
Total number of continuing pregnancies	25 (44.6)	19 (32.2)	17 (29.3)		23 (40.3)	27 (45.8)	
Total number of multiple pregnancies	7 (12.5)	9 (16.4)	9 (16.1)		8 (14.0)	11 (18.6)	
Singlets	18 (32.1)	10 (18.2)	8 (13.2)		15 (26.3)	16 (27.1)	
Twins	5 (8.9)	7 (12.7)	7 (12.5)	0.816	5 (8.8)	10 (16.9)	0.6179
Triplets	1 (1.8)	1 (1.8)	2 (3.6)		3 (5.3)	1 (1.7)	
Quadruplets	1 (1.8)	1 (1.8)	0		0	0	

For patients requiring a single injection from multiple vials of BRAVELLE, up to 6 vials can be reconstituted with 1 mL of Sterile Saline for Injection, USP. This can be accomplished by reconstituting a single vial. Then draw the entire contents of the first vial into a syringe, and inject the contents into a second vial of lyophilized BRAVELLE. Gently swirl the second vial and check to make sure that the solution is clear and free of particles. This step can be repeated with 4 additional vials for a total of up to 6 vials of lyophilized BRAVELLE into 1 mL of diluent.

The injection site should be swabbed with a disinfectant to remove any surface bacteria. Clean about two inches around the point where the needle will go in and let the disinfectant dry at least one minute before proceeding.

Subcutaneous Administration: The recommended sites for subcutaneous injection are either side of the lower abdomen (around the navel) in alternating fashion with the actual injection site varied a little with each injection. Pinch up a large area of skin between the finger and thumb. The needle should be inserted at the base of the pinched-up skin at a 45° angle. Subcutaneous injection of BRAVELLE into the thigh is not recommended unless the lower abdomen is not usable because of scarring, surgical deformity or other medical conditions. Subcutaneous injection of BRAVELLE may be carried out by patients or their partners, provided proper instructions are given by the physician. Self-administration of BRAVELLE should only be performed by patients who are well motivated, adequately trained and with access to expert advice.

Intramuscular Administration: The best site for intramuscular administration is the upper outer quadrant of the buttock muscle near the hip. The area contains few blood vessels and major nerves. Stretching the skin helps the needle to go in more easily and pushes the tissue beneath the skin out of the way. This helps the solution to disperse correctly. The needle should be inserted right up to the hilt at an angle of 90° to the skin surface. Pushing in with a quick thrust causes the least discomfort.

Drug Abuse and Dependence: There have been no reports of abuse or dependence with follitropins.

Table 3: BRAVELLE

Incidence of Adverse Events ≥1% Reported in the Clinical Trial

Adverse Events Body System/Preferred Term	BRAVELLE SC N=155	BRAVELLE IM N=96	Recombinant SC N=157
Body as a Whole			
Abdomen Enlarged	2 (1.3%)	1 (1.0%)	4 (2.5%)
Abdominal Cramps	11 (7.1%)	5 (5.2%)	13 (8.3%)
Abdominal Fullness	7 (4.5%)	0 (0.0%)	3 (1.9%)
Abdominal Pain	7 (4.5%)	4 (4.2%)	10 (6.4%)
Accidental Injury	0 (0.0%)	1 (1.0%)	0 (0.0%)
Allergic Reaction	2 (1.3%)	1 (1.0%)	0 (0.0%)
Back Pain	2 (1.3%)	0 (0.0%)	3 (1.9%)
Fever	0 (0.0%)	1 (1.0%)	0 (0.0%)
Flu Syndrome	0 (0.0%)	1 (1.0%)	0 (0.0%)
Headache	22 (14.2%)	13 (13.5%)	18 (11.5%)
Injection Site Hemorrhage	2 (1.3%)	1 (1.0%)	0 (0.0%)
Injection Site Pain	0 (0.0%)	0 (0.0%)	2 (1.3%)
Injection Site Reaction	6 (3.9%)	1 (1.0%)	5 (3.2%)
Knee Edema	0 (0.0%)	1 (1.0%)	0 (0.0%)
Malaise	0 (0.0%)	1 (1.0%)	3 (1.9%)
Neck Pain	0 (0.0%)	2 (2.1%)	0 (0.0%)
Pain	10 (6.5%)	7 (7.3%)	3 (1.9%)
Pelvic Pain	4 (2.6%)	4 (4.2%)	5 (3.2%)
Cardiovascular			
Tachycardia	0 (0.0%)	1 (1.0%)	0 (0.0%)
Digestive			
Constipation	2 (1.3%)	3 (3.1%)	4 (2.5%)
Diarrhea	2 (1.3%)	2 (2.1%)	2 (1.3%)
Nausea	14 (9.0%)	9 (9.4%)	17 (10.8%)
Vomiting	2 (1.3%)	5 (5.2%)	7 (4.5%)
Metabolic/Nutritional			
Dehydration	0 (0.0%)	1 (1.0%)	0 (0.0%)
Musculoskeletal			
Joint Disorder	0 (0.0%)	1 (1.0%)	0 (0.0%)
Nervous			
Anxiety	2 (1.3%)	0 (0.0%)	0 (0.0%)
Depression	0 (0.0%)	1 (1.0%)	0 (0.0%)
Emotional Lability	2 (1.3%)	3 (3.1%)	2 (1.3%)
Hypertension	0 (0.0%)	1 (1.0%)	0 (0.0%)
Insomnia	0 (0.0%)	0 (0.0%)	2 (1.3%)
Respiratory			

(cont'd)

Table 3: BRAVELLE *(cont'd)*

Incidence of Adverse Events ≥1% Reported in the Clinical Trial

Adverse Events Body System/Preferred Term	BRAVELLE SC N=155	BRAVELLE IM N=96	Recombinant SC N=157
Cough Increased	2 (1.3%)	0 (0.0%)	0 (0.0%)
Nasal Congestion	2 (1.3%)	0 (0.0%)	0 (0.0%)
Respiratory Disorder	8 (5.2%)	1 (1.0%)	6 (3.8%)
Sinusitis	3 (1.9%)	0 (0.0%)	4 (2.5%)
Skin/Appendages			
Exfoliative Dermatitis	0 (0.0%)	1 (1.0%)	0 (0.0%)
Pruritus	0 (0.0%)	2 (2.1%)	2 (1.3%)
Rash	3 (1.9%)	4 (4.2%)	5 (3.2%)
Skin Disorder	0 (0.0%)	1 (1.0%)	0 (0.0%)
Sweating	0 (0.0%)	1 (1.0%)	0 (0.0%)
Urogenital			
Abdominal Cramps	6 (3.9%)	5 (5.2%)	9 (5.7%)
Breast Tenderness	3 (1.9%)	1 (1.0%)	0 (0.0%)
Cervix Disorder	2 (1.3%)	0 (0.0%)	0 (0.0%)
Cystitis	0 (0.0%)	1 (1.0%)	0 (0.0%)
Hot Flash	7 (4.5%)	1 (1.0%)	0 (0.0%)
Infection Fungal	2 (1.3%)	1 (1.0%)	2 (1.3%)
OHSS	10 (6.5%)	5 (5.2%)	7 (4.5%)
Ovarian Disorder	3 (1.9%)	3 (3.1%)	2 (1.3%)
Pelvic Cramps	4 (2.6%)	0 (0.0%)	0 (0.0%)
Post-Retrieval Pain	12 (7.7%)	0 (0.0%)	12 (7.6%)
Pregnancy Disorder	2 (1.3%)	0 (0.0%)	0 (0.0%)
Urinary Tract Infection	5 (3.2%)	1 (1.0%)	3 (1.9%)
Uterine Disorder	0 (0.0%)	1 (1.0%)	0 (0.0%)
Uterine Spasm	4 (2.6%)	4 (4.2%)	6 (3.8%)
Vaginal Discharge	4 (2.6%)	0 (0.0%)	0 (0.0%)
Vaginal Hemorrhage	10 (6.5%)	6 (6.3%)	13 (8.3%)
Vaginal Pruritus	0 (0.0%)	2 (2.1%)	0 (0.0%)
Vaginal Spotting	4 (2.6%)	0 (0.0%)	4 (2.5%)
Vaginitis	0 (0.0%)	0 (0.0%)	3 (1.9%)

OVERDOSAGE:
Aside from possible ovarian hyperstimulation and multiple gestations (see Warnings and Precautions), little is known concerning the consequences of acute overdosage with BRAVELLE (Urofollitropin for Injection, Purified).

For management of a suspected drug overdose, CPhA recommends that you contact your **regional Poison Control Centre**. See the *CPS* Directory section for a list of Poison Control Centres.

ACTION AND CLINICAL PHARMACOLOGY: Mechanism of Action: BRAVELLE (Urofollitropin for Injection, Purified) is a highly purified preparation of human follicle stimulating hormone (hFSH) extracted from the urine of postmenopausal women. Human FSH consists of two non-covalently linked glycoproteins designated as the α and β subunits. The alpha subunit has 92 amino acids of which two are modified by attachment of carbohydrates. The β subunit has 111 amino acids of which two are modified by attachment of carbohydrates. BRAVELLE is biologically standardized for FSH activity in terms of the Second International Reference Preparation for Human Menopausal Gonadotropins established in September 1964 by the Expert Committee on Biological Standards of the World Health Organization.

Follicle Stimulating Hormone (FSH) is essential for normal female and male gamete growth and maturation, and gonadal steroid production. Deficiencies in the endogenous production of FSH may lead to infertility. FSH is critical at the onset and duration of follicular development, and consequently for the timing and number of follicles reaching maturity in females. The primary action of follitropin in women with gonadal dysfunction is the stimulation of follicular development and steroid production. Follitropin may also be used to promote multiple follicular development in medically assisted reproduction programs. In order to induce ovulation, in the absence of an endogenous luteinizing hormone (LH) surge, human chorionic gonadotropin (hCG) must be given after follitropin administration once follicular maturation has occurred.

Pharmacokinetics: Single doses of 225 IU and multiple daily doses (7 days) of 150 IU of FSH were administered to healthy volunteer female subjects while their endogenous FSH was suppressed. Serum FSH concentrations were determined in sixteen subjects who received FSH subcutaneously (SC) and 13 who received the drug intramuscularly (IM). Based on the steady state ratio of FSH C_{max} and AUC, SC and IM administration of FSH were not bioequivalent. Multiple doses of FSH IM resulted in C_{max} and AUC of 77.7% and 81.8% compared to multiple doses of FSH SC which may result in higher dosage used in IM.

The FSH pharmacokinetic parameters for single and multiple dose BRAVELLE, administered SC and IM are in Table 4.

Absorption: The maximum plasma concentration of FSH was attained at 20.5 and 17.4 hours following SC and IM single dose administration, respectively. However, following multiple dosing, it was attained at approximately 10 hours following both routes of administration.

Distribution: Human tissue or organ distribution of FSH has not been studied for BRAVELLE.

Metabolism: Metabolism of FSH has not been studied for BRAVELLE in humans.

Excretion: The mean elimination half-lives of FSH for SC and IM single dosing are 31.8 and 37 hours, respectively. However, following multiple dosing (×7 days) they are 20.6 and 15.2 hours for SC and IM, respectively.

Table 4: BRAVELLE

FSH Pharmacokinetic Parameters Following BRAVELLE Administration

Pharmacokinetic Parameters	Single Dose (225 IU)		Multiple Dose×7 (150 IU)	
	SC	IM	SC	IM
C_{max} (mIU/mL)	6.0 (1.7)	8.8 (4.5)	14.8 (2.9)	11.5 (2.9)
T_{max} (hrs)	20.5 (7.7)	17.4 (12.2)	9.6 (2.1)	11.3 (8.4)
AUC_{abs} (mIU·hr/mL)	379 (111)	331 (179)	234.7 (77.0)	192.1 (52.3)
$T_{1/2}$ (hrs)	31.8	37	20.6	15.2
K_{el} (L/min)	0.0218	0.0209	0.0336	0.0457
V (mL)	16 835.6 (74.9)	29 936.7 (15 353.7)	21 168.8 (3151.1)	16 601.9 (4296.7)
K_a(hr-1)	0.0500 (0.0231)	0.1408 (0.1227)	0.0905 (0.0383)	0.0358 (0.0108)

STORAGE AND STABILITY: Store at 15-25°C. Protect from light.
Reconstituted Solutions: Use immediately after reconstitution. Discard unused material.

SPECIAL HANDLING INSTRUCTIONS: No special handling instructions.

INFORMATION FOR THE PATIENT: Published in e-CPS, available by subscription at www.e-cps.ca.

DOSAGE FORMS, COMPOSITION AND PACKAGING: Each vial of sterile, lyophilized, white to off-white powder or pellet, contains 75 IU of follicle stimulating hormone (FSH) activity, plus 20 mg of lactose as the monohydrate and 0.005 mg tween in a sterile, lyophilized form, for subcutaneous or intramuscular injection. The final product contains sodium phosphate buffer (sodium phosphate dibasic and phosphoric acid). BRAVELLE contains 1-2% luteinizing hormone (LH) activity based on bioassay. Human Chorionic Gonadotropin (hCG) is not detected in BRAVELLE. Each vial is available with an accompanying vial of sterile diluent containing 2 mL of 0.9% Sodium Chloride Injection, USP. Box of 5 vials + 5 vials diluent. Box of 100 vials + 100 vials diluent.

Bretylium Tosylate Injection USP Ⓟ

bretylium tosylate

Antiarrhythmic

Sandoz

SUPPLIED: Each mL of solution contains: bretylium tosylate 50 mg. Nonmedicinal ingredients: sodium hydroxide and/or hydrochloric acid to adjust pH and water for injection. Single use amber vials of 10 mL, boxes of 5. Store between 15 and 30°C. Protect from light.

Brevibloc® Ⓟ

esmolol HCl

Beta-adrenergic Receptor Blocking Agent

Baxter

Brevibloc Premixed® Ⓟ

esmolol HCl

Beta-adrenergic Receptor Blocking Agent

Baxter

Date of Preparation: October 25, 1995
Date of Revision: June 10, 2008

SUMMARY PRODUCT INFORMATION:

Route of Administration	Dosage Form/ Strength	Clinically Relevant Nonmedicinal Ingredients
Injection	10 mL (10 mg/mL) Vials	Sodium acetate trihydrate, glacial acetic acid, sodium chloride, hydrochloric acid, sodium hydroxide, water for injection
Injection	250 mL (10 mg/mL) Premixed Bags	

INDICATIONS AND CLINICAL USE: BREVIBLOC Injection/BREVIBLOC PREMIXED Injection (esmolol hydrochloride) is indicated for:

- the perioperative management of tachycardia and hypertension in patients in whom there is a concern for compromised myocardial oxygen balance and who, in the judgement of the physician, are clearly at risk of developing haemodynamically-induced myocardial ischemia.
- the rapid control of ventricular rate in patients with atrial fibrillation or atrial flutter in acute situations when the use of a short-acting agent is desirable.

BREVIBLOC Injection/BREVIBLOC PREMIXED Injection is not indicated for use in chronic settings.

Geriatrics: The safety and effectiveness of BREVIBLOC (esmolol hydrochloride) in elders have not been established.
Pediatrics: The safety and effectiveness of BREVIBLOC (esmolol hydrochloride) in children have not been established.

CONTRAINDICATIONS: BREVIBLOC Injection/BREVIBLOC PREMIXED Injection (esmolol hydrochloride) is contraindicated in patients who require inotropic agents and/or vasopressors to maintain systemic blood pressure and cardiac output.

BREVIBLOC Injection/BREVIBLOC PREMIXED Injection is also contraindicated in patients with hypotension, sinus bradycardia, second and third degree A-V block, right ventricular failure secondary to pulmonary hypertension, overt cardiac failure, or cardiogenic shock (see Warnings and Precautions).

WARNINGS AND PRECAUTIONS:

> **Serious Warnings and Precautions**
> **During the administration of BREVIBLOC Injection/BREVIBLOC PREMIXED Injection (esmolol hydrochloride) patients should be carefully monitored, with particular attention to heart rate and blood pressure.**

General: Abrupt Cessation of Therapy with BREVIBLOC (esmolol hydrochloride): Abrupt cessation of BREVIBLOC Injection/BREVIBLOC PREMIXED Injection in patients has not been reported to produce the withdrawal effects which may occur with abrupt withdrawal of beta-blockers following chronic use in coronary artery disease patients. However, caution should be used in discontinuing BREVIBLOC (esmolol hydrochloride) infusions abruptly in these patients.

The use of intravenous verapamil with a beta-blocker may cause severe depression of ventricular function. Accordingly, patients with atrial fibrillation or atrial flutter who have received verapamil should only be administered BREVIBLOC Injection/BREVIBLOC PREMIXED Injection if the benefits outweigh the risk.

Cardiovascular: Hypotension: The administration of BREVIBLOC Injection/BREVIBLOC PREMIXED Injection has been associated with excessive hypotension. The hypotensive effect of BREVIBLOC Injection/BREVIBLOC PREMIXED Injection is dose related and may increase in the presence of both narcotic analgesics and inhalational anaesthetics. In patients with low pretreatment blood pressure or with a propensity to develop hypotension (e.g., hypovolemic patients) BREVIBLOC (esmolol hydrochloride) should be used with special caution, and only when in the physician's judgement the potential benefits outweigh the risk. In the event of hypotension, the dosage of BREVIBLOC Injection/BREVIBLOC PREMIXED Injection should be reduced or the drug should be discontinued.

Sinus Bradycardia: Severe bradycardia and cardiac arrest may occur with the use of BREVIBLOC (esmolol hydrochloride). Therefore, in patients with low pretreatment heart rates BREVIBLOC (esmolol hydrochloride) should be used with special caution, and only when in the physician's judgement the potential benefits outweigh the risk. In the event of bradycardia, the dosage of BREVIBLOC Injection/BREVIBLOC PREMIXED Injection should be reduced or the drug should be discontinued.

Cardiac Failure: Sympathetic stimulation is a vital component supporting circulatory function in patients with congestive heart failure. Inhibition with beta-blockade always carries the potential hazard of further depressing myocardial contractility. Therefore, special caution should be exercised when administering BREVIBLOC Injection/BREVIBLOC PREMIXED Injection to patients with a history of heart failure. Beta-blockers act selectively without abolishing the inotropic action of digitalis on the heart muscle. The effects of beta-blockers and digitalis are additive in depressing A-V nodal conduction. Even in patients with no history of cardiac failure, continued depression of the myocardium over a period of time can, in some cases, lead to cardiac failure. Therefore, at the first sign or symptom of impending cardiac failure, the dosage of BREVIBLOC (esmolol hydrochloride) should be reduced or the drug should be withdrawn. Because of the short elimination half-life of BREVIBLOC (esmolol hydrochloride), these measures may be sufficient but specific treatment may also be considered.

Endocrine and Metabolism: Diabetes Mellitus/Hypoglycaemia: BREVIBLOC Injection/BREVIBLOC PREMIXED Injection should be administered with caution to patients subject to spontaneous hypoglycaemia, or to diabetic patients (especially those with labile diabetes) who are receiving insulin or oral hypoglycaemic agents. Beta-adrenergic blockers may mask the premonitory signs and symptoms of acute hypoglycaemia.

Renal: Renal Impairment: The pharmacokinetics of BREVIBLOC Injection/BREVIBLOC PREMIXED Injection (esmolol hydrochloride) are unchanged in kidney-impaired patients except that the volume of distribution is increased. However, the acid metabolite of BREVIBLOC (esmolol hydrochloride) is primarily excreted unchanged by the kidney, thus BREVIBLOC Injection/BREVIBLOC PREMIXED Injection should be administered with caution to patients with impaired renal function. The elimination half-life of the acid metabolite was prolonged ten-fold and the plasma level was considerably elevated in patients with end-stage renal disease.

Respiratory: Bronchospastic Diseases: Patients with bronchospastic diseases should not, in general, receive beta-blockers. Because of its relative beta-1 selectivity and titratability, BREVIBLOC Injection/BREVIBLOC PREMIXED Injection may be used with caution in patients with bronchospastic diseases. Since beta-1 selectivity is not absolute, BREVIBLOC (esmolol hydrochloride) should be carefully titrated to obtain the lowest possible effective dose. In the event of bronchospasm, the infusion should be terminated immediately and a beta-2 stimulating agent may be administered if conditions warrant.

Special Populations: Pregnant Women: There are no studies in pregnant women. BREVIBLOC (esmolol hydrochloride) should be used during pregnancy only if the potential benefit justifies the potential risk to the fetus.

Nursing Women: It is not known whether BREVIBLOC (esmolol hydrochloride) is excreted in human milk. Caution, however, should be exercised when BREVIBLOC Injection/BREVIBLOC PREMIXED Injection is administered to a nursing mother.

Pediatrics: The safety and effectiveness of BREVIBLOC (esmolol hydrochloride) in children have not been established.

Geriatrics: The safety and effectiveness of BREVIBLOC (esmolol hydrochloride) in elders have not been established.

Monitoring and Laboratory Tests: During the administration of BREVIBLOC (esmolol hydrochloride) patients should be carefully monitored, with particular attention to heart rate and blood pressure.

ADVERSE REACTIONS: Clinical Trial Adverse Drug Reactions: During Management of Perioperative Tachycardia and Associated Hypertension: In clinical trials 763 patients were treated with BREVIBLOC Injection (esmolol hydrochloride) in operative settings.

BREVIBLOC Injection as a bolus of 100 mg and 200 mg was given in a total of 367 patients during clinical studies. Hypotension was reported in 16% among esmolol treated patients compared to 8% in the placebo group (187 patients). Bradycardia occurred in 4% of patients, in both the esmolol and placebo groups.

Other adverse effects with a frequency of less than 1% occurred as frequently in the esmolol as it did with the placebo group. They were: bronchospasm, pain at injection and wheezing.

When BREVIBLOC (esmolol hydrochloride) was infused in 396 patients, hypotension was the most commonly observed side effect in 5% of patients. The other reported adverse effect was bradycardia (heart rate less than 50 beats per minute), observed in 1% of patients. Other adverse effects occurring with a less than 1% incidence were the following: S-T segment depression, ECG changes, myocardial ischemia, junctional rhythm, hypertension, atrial fibrillation, bronchospasm, agitation, nausea, vomiting, urticaria and itching.

None of these side effects were judged to be severe, and all resolved after the discontinuation of BREVIBLOC (esmolol hydrochloride).

During Management of Atrial Fibrillation and Atrial Flutter: Most adverse effects reported in clinical trials with BREVIBLOC Injection in 390 patients with atrial fibrillation and atrial flutter have been mild and transient. The most serious adverse reaction observed was symptomatic hypotension (12%). BREVIBLOC (esmolol hydrochloride) was discontinued in about 11% of the patients. Other adverse reactions, grouped by system, are:

Cardiovascular: symptomatic hypotension (diaphoresis, dizziness) (12%), asymptomatic hypotension (25%), diaphoresis (9%), premature ventricular contraction and dyspnea (1%).
Central Nervous System: dizziness (3%), somnolence (3%), headache (3%), confusion, agitation (2%), fatigue (1%).
Gastrointestinal: nausea (6%), vomiting (1%).
Local Dermatological Reactions: inflammation (2%), induration (2%), I.V. infiltration (2%).

Less Common Clinical Trial Adverse Drug Reactions (<1%): Cardiovascular: pallor, flushing, bradycardia (<50 beats per minute), chest pain, syncope, pulmonary edema, junctional rhythm, heart block, increased PAP, abnormal ECG, narrowed pulse pressure, recurrence of SVT, angina, ventricular ectopy, peripheral ischemia (<1%).
Central Nervous System: paraesthesia, asthenia, depression, abnormal thinking, anxiety, anorexia, one brief episode of grand mal seizure (30 seconds), lightheadedness, weakness, irritability, drowsiness (<1%).
Gastrointestinal: dyspepsia, constipation, dry mouth, abdominal discomfort (<1%).
Local Dermatological Reactions: clamminess, edema, erythema, skin discolouration, ecchymosis, burning, enlarged macular area (<1%).
Respiratory: bronchospasm, wheezing, dyspnea, nasal congestion, rhonchi, pharyngitis, rales, pleural effusion, atelectasis and common cold, pleural pain (<1%).
Miscellaneous: urinary retention, dysuria, oliguria, speech disorder, abnormal vision, midscapular pain, rigors, fever (<1%).

Post-Market Adverse Drug Reactions: In addition, the following adverse events have occurred under conditions where a causal association is uncertain:
Cardiovascular: arteriospasm coronary, cardiac failure congestive, electromechanical dissociation, myocardial infarction, supraventricular extrasystoles, ventricular extrasystoles, ventricular fibrillation, hypertensive crisis, atrioventricular block.
Dermatological Reactions: blister, skin exfoliation.
Respiratory: respiratory failure.
Urogenital: renal tubular necrosis.
Neurological: neuropathy.

DRUG INTERACTIONS: Drug-Drug Interactions: Catecholamine-depleting drugs, (e.g., reserpine) may have an additive effect when given with beta-blocking agents. Patients treated concurrently with BREVIBLOC (esmolol hydrochloride) and a catecholamine depletor should, therefore, be closely observed for evidence of hypotension or marked bradycardia.

When digoxin and BREVIBLOC (esmolol hydrochloride) were concomitantly administered intravenously to normal volunteers, a 10-20% increase in digoxin blood level was observed at some time points. Digoxin did not affect BREVIBLOC (esmolol hydrochloride) pharmacokinetics.

When the interaction of intravenous morphine and BREVIBLOC (esmolol hydrochloride) was studied in normal subjects, no effect on morphine blood level was seen. However the steady-state blood levels of BREVIBLOC Injection/BREVIBLOC PREMIXED Injection were increased by 46% in the presence of morphine, but no other pharmacokinetic parameters were changed.

The effect of BREVIBLOC (esmolol hydrochloride) on the duration of succinylcholine-induced neuromuscular blockade was studied in patients undergoing surgery. The onset of neuromuscular blockade by succinylcholine was unaffected by BREVIBLOC Injection/BREVIBLOC PREMIXED Injection, but the duration of neuromuscular blockade was prolonged from five to eight minutes.

A study of interaction between BREVIBLOC (esmolol hydrochloride) and warfarin showed that concomitant administration of BREVIBLOC Injection and warfarin does not alter warfarin plasma levels. BREVIBLOC (esmolol hydrochloride) concentrations were equivocally higher when given with warfarin, but this is not likely to be clinically important.

Please see Warnings and Precautions for the use of intravenous verapamil with BREVIBLOC.
Drug-Food Interactions: Interactions with food have not been established.
Drug-Herb Interactions: Interactions with herbal products have not been established.
Drug-Laboratory Test Interactions: Interactions with laboratory tests have not been established.

DOSAGE AND ADMINISTRATION: Recommended Dose and Dosage Adjustment: Management of Perioperative Tachycardia and Hypertension: Intubation: For the management of postintubation tachycardia and hypertension, give 1.5 mg/kg (up to a maximum of 100 mg) as a bolus injection (over 30 seconds) 1 to 2 minutes before intubation.
For Intra- and Postoperative Tachycardia and Hypertension: For intraoperative and postoperative treatment of tachycardia and/or hypertension give 1.5 mg/kg as a bolus injection (over 30 seconds) followed by 0.15 mg/kg/min infusion. Adjust infusion rate as required up to 0.3 mg/kg/min to maintain desired heart rate and/or blood pressure.
Management of Atrial Fibrillation and Atrial Flutter: Responses to BREVIBLOC Injection/BREVIBLOC PREMIXED Injection (esmolol hydrochloride) usually (over 95%) occur within the range of 0.05 to 0.2 mg/kg/min. The average effective dosage is approximately 0.1 mg/kg/min (7 mg/70 kg/min) although dosages as low as 0.025 mg/kg/min have been sufficient in some patients. Dosages as high as 0.3 mg/kg/min have been used but provided little added effect with an increased rate of adverse effects, and are not recommended. Dosage of BREVIBLOC (esmolol hydrochloride) must be individualized by titration in which each step consists of a loading dose followed by a maintenance infusion.

To initiate treatment, administer a loading dose infusion of 0.5 mg/kg/min of BREVIBLOC Injection/BREVIBLOC PREMIXED Injection for one minute followed by a four-minute maintenance infusion of 0.05 mg/kg/min. If the therapeutic response is inadequate at this point, repeat the same loading dose and increase the maintenance infusion to 0.1 mg/kg/min.

Continue the titration procedure as above, repeating the loading dose (0.5 mg/kg/min for one minute), and increasing the maintenance infusion by increments of 0.05 mg/kg/min (for four minutes). As the desired heart rate or a safety end point (e.g., lowered blood pressure) is approached, omit the loading dose and reduce the incremental dose of the maintenance infusion from 0.05 mg/kg/min to 0.025 mg/kg/min or lower. Also if desired, increase the interval between titration steps from five to ten minutes.

Maintenance dosages above 0.2 mg/kg/min have not been shown to have significantly increased benefits. The effectiveness of dosages above 0.3 mg/kg/min has not been studied.

If a safety end point is exceeded, discontinue the infusion of BREVIBLOC (esmolol hydrochloride) and re-start at a lower dose. In the event of an adverse reaction, the dosage infusion of BREVIBLOC (esmolol hydrochloride) should be discontinued. If a reaction occurs at the site of the local infusion, an alternate infusion site should be used. Avoid the use of butterfly needles. The use of BREVIBLOC (esmolol hydrochloride) infusions up to 24 hours has been well documented.

BREVIBLOC Injection/BREVIBLOC PREMIXED Injection (esmolol hydrochloride) 10 mg/mL (100 mg/10 mL vial and 2500 mg/250 mL premixed bag) do not require dilution.
Directions for Use: Parenteral drug products should be inspected visually for particulate matter and discoloration prior to administration, whenever solution and container permit. Samples containing visible particles should be discarded.
BREVIBLOC Injection (10 mg/mL) Ready-to-use Vial: This dosage form is prediluted to provide ready-to-use, iso-osmotic solution of 10 mg/mL esmolol hydrochloride in sodium chloride recommended for BREVIBLOC intravenous administration. It may be used to administer the appropriate BREVIBLOC (esmolol hydrochloride) loading dosage infusions by hand-held syringe while the maintenance infusion is being prepared.
BREVIBLOC PREMIXED Injection (10 mg/mL) INTRAVIA Bag: This dosage form is prediluted to 250 mL to provide a ready-to-use, iso-osmotic solution of 10 mg/mL esmolol hydrochloride in sodium chloride. BREVIBLOC PREMIXED Injection (10 mg/mL) is provided in ready-to-use bags with two ports, a medication port and a delivery port. **The medication port is to be used solely for withdrawing an initial bolus from the bag; the medication withdrawal port is not intended for repeat bolus administration. The sterility of the premixed bag cannot be assured after repeat withdrawals from the bag. The use of aseptic technique is required when withdrawing the bolus dose. Do not add any additional medications to BREVIBLOC PREMIXED Injection.** Each bag is for single-patient use only and contains no preservative. It is advised that once drug has been withdrawn from BREVIBLOC PREMIXED Injection, the bag should be used within 24 hours, with any unused portion discarded.

The BREVIBLOC PREMIXED Injection contains esmolol hydrochloride at a concentration of 10 mg/mL. The initial loading dose can be removed from the medication port of the premixed bag.

Please refer to Special Handling Instructions for Preparation for Intravenous Administration.
Missed Dose: This section is not applicable as BREVIBLOC Injection/BREVIBLOC PREMIXED Injection is an IV drug titrated by a physician.

OVERDOSAGE:
Overdosage with BREVIBLOC (esmolol hydrochloride) can produce bradycardia, congestive heart failure, hypotension, bronchospasm, electromechanical dissociation, drowsiness, loss of consciousness, hypoglycaemia and cardiac arrest.

Cases of massive accidental overdoses of BREVIBLOC (esmolol hydrochloride) have occurred due to dilution errors. Some of these overdoses have been fatal while others resulted in permanent disability. Bolus doses in the range of 625 mg to 3500 mg (12.5-70 mg/kg) have been fatal. Patients have recovered completely from overdoses as high as 1750 mg given over one minute or doses of 7500 mg given over one hour for cardiovascular surgery. The patients who survived appear to be those whose cardiovascular circulation could be supported until the effects of BREVIBLOC Injection/BREVIBLOC PREMIXED Injection resolved.

The first step in the management of toxicity should be to discontinue the BREVIBLOC (esmolol hydrochloride) infusion. Then, because of its approximately 9-minute elimination half-life and based on the observed clinical effects, the following measures should also be considered:

1. **General:** BREVIBLOC Injection/BREVIBLOC PREMIXED Injection (esmolol hydrochloride) is a competitive antagonist of isoproterenol and hence larger doses of isoproterenol may be needed to reverse many of the effects of excessive dosage of BREVIBLOC. However, the complications of excessive isoproterenol should not be overlooked.
2. **Bradycardia:** Atropine or another anticholinergic drug.
3. **Heart block (second or third degree):** Isoproterenol or transvenous cardiac pacemaker.
4. **Congestive heart failure:** Conventional therapy such as diuretic and/or digitalis glycoside. In shock due to inadequate cardiac contractility: dopamine, dobutamine, isoproterenol.
5. **Hypotension (depending on associated factors):** Epinephrine, rather than isoproterenol, or norepinephrine may be useful in addition to atropine and digitalis.
6. **Bronchospasm:** Aminophylline or isoproterenol or other beta-2 agonists.
7. **Hypoglycaemia:** Intravenous glucose.

For management of a suspected drug overdose, CPhA recommends that you contact your **regional Poison Control Centre**. See the *CPS* Directory section for a list of Poison Control Centres.

ACTION AND CLINICAL PHARMACOLOGY: Mechanism of Action: BREVIBLOC Injection/BREVIBLOC PREMIXED Injection (esmolol hydrochloride) is a beta-adrenergic receptor blocking agent with predominant blocking effect on beta-1 receptors. It does not possess significant intrinsic sympathomimetic or membrane stabilizing activity. BREVIBLOC Injection/BREVIBLOC PREMIXED Injection, which is administered only intravenously, has a rapid onset and a short duration of action.
Pharmacodynamics: In human electrophysiology studies, BREVIBLOC (esmolol hydrochloride) produced effects typical of a beta-blocker: a decrease in the heart rate, increase in sinus cycle length, prolongation of the sinus node recovery time, prolongation of the AH interval during normal sinus rhythm and during atrial pacing, and an increase in antegrade Wenckebach cycle length.

Studies in normal volunteers have confirmed the beta-blocking activity of BREVIBLOC (esmolol hydrochloride), showing reduction in heart rate at rest and during exercise, and attenuation of isoproterenol-induced increases in heart rate. Blood levels of BREVIBLOC (esmolol hydrochloride) have been shown to correlate with extent of beta-blockade.

Bolus injections of 50 and 100 mg BREVIBLOC (esmolol hydrochloride), given intraoperatively during general anaesthesia, decreased heart rate by more than 20% within two minutes. Systolic blood pressure fell by 17% within five minutes. The effects lasted for up to ten minutes.

When given 1.5 to 2 minutes before intubation, 100 and 200 mg bolus injections of BREVIBLOC (esmolol hydrochloride) attenuated the heart rate and blood pressure response to endotracheal intubation. No effects were detectable five minutes after the administration of BREVIBLOC Injection.

The haemodynamics were studied during continuous intravenous infusions in patients with elevated heart rate and acute ischemic heart disease (e.g., unstable angina pectoris or acute myocardial infarction). Titrated infusions of BREVIBLOC (esmolol hydrochloride), from 0.05 to 0.3 mg/kg/min, lowered heart rate and blood pressure. There were small increases in the left ventricular end diastolic pressure and pulmonary capillary wedge pressure, but were not considered to be clinically significant. Cardiac index, however, decreased. Cardiac index returned to pretreatment levels within 30 minutes after discontinuation of the infusion.

The relative cardioselectivity of BREVIBLOC Injection was demonstrated in mildly asthmatic patients. BREVIBLOC (esmolol hydrochloride) infusions (0.1, 0.2 and 0.3 mg/kg/min) produced no significant increases in specific airway resistance when compared to placebo. At 0.3 mg/kg/min, BREVIBLOC Injection (esmolol hydrochloride) produced slightly enhanced bronchomotor sensitivity to dry-air stimulus but was not considered clinically significant.
Pharmacokinetics: Absorption: Following bolus injections of BREVIBLOC (esmolol hydrochloride) to healthy volunteers, the distribution and elimination half-lives averaged 1.4 and 10.9 minutes respectively. The blood concentrations of BREVIBLOC (esmolol hydrochloride) were below quantifiable limits within 10 minutes.
Distribution: Following a loading infusion of 0.5 mg/kg/min over one minute, BREVIBLOC (esmolol hydrochloride) infusions of 0.050 to 0.3 mg/kg/min reach steady-state blood levels within five minutes with corresponding blood levels from $1.56\times10_{-4}$ to 9.93×10^{-4} mg/mL. Steady-state blood levels increase linearly with dose over the dose range of 0.05-0.3 mg/kg/min. If a loading dose is not used, approximately 30 minutes are required to reach steady-state blood levels. Fifty-five percent of the amount in blood is bound to plasma proteins while the acid metabolite is only 10% bound. After cessation of the infusion, the blood levels of BREVIBLOC (esmolol hydrochloride) decrease rapidly with an elimination half-life of nine minutes.
Metabolism: The total body clearance of BREVIBLOC (esmolol hydrochloride) is about 20 L/hr/kg. Since this is greater than cardiac output, the metabolism of BREVIBLOC (esmolol hydrochloride) is not limited by the rate of blood flow to metabolizing tissues such as the liver. The central and total volume of distribution were found to be 1.9 L/kg and 3.3 L/kg, respectively.
Excretion: Esterases in the red blood cell cytosol hydrolyse the ester link of BREVIBLOC (esmolol hydrochloride) resulting in the formation of the corresponding free acid and methanol. This acid metabolite, which shows approximately 1/1500th the beta-blocking activity of esmolol in animal studies, has an elimination half-life of about 3.7 hours and is excreted in the urine with a clearance approximately equivalent to the glomerular filtration rate. Excretion of the acid metabolite is significantly decreased in patients with renal disease, with elimination half-life increased to about ten-fold that of patients with normal renal function, and plasma level was considerably elevated.

After several hours of infusion, at rates up to 0.3 mg/kg/min, methanol blood levels approximated endogenous levels (<10 µg/mL) and were less than 2% of levels usually associated with methanol toxicity.

Less than two percent of BREVIBLOC (esmolol hydrochloride) is excreted unchanged in urine. After 24 hours, approximately 73-88% of the dose is recovered in the urine as the acid metabolite.
Special Populations and Conditions: Pediatrics: The safety and effectiveness of BREVIBLOC (esmolol hydrochloride) in children have not been established.
Geriatrics: The safety and effectiveness of BREVIBLOC (esmolol hydrochloride) in elders have not been established.
Gender: No data is available.
Race: No data is available.
Hepatic Insufficiency: The pharmacokinetics of BREVIBLOC Injection/BREVIBLOC PREMIXED Injection and of its major metabolite are unaltered in patients with hepatic cirrhosis.
Renal Insufficiency: In patients with end-stage renal disease, on haemo- or peritoneal dialysis, the pharmacokinetics of BREVIBLOC (esmolol hydrochloride) were unchanged except for an increase in the volume of distribution in patients on peritoneal dialysis. The elimination half-life of the acid metabolite is increased about ten times in patients with renal disease.
Genetic Polymorphism: No data is available.

STORAGE AND STABILITY: Vial: Store at 15 to 25°C.
Premixed Bag: Store at 15 to 25°C. Protect from freezing. Avoid excessive heat.

SPECIAL HANDLING INSTRUCTIONS: Caution: When using BREVIBLOC PREMIXED Injection (10 mg/mL), do not use plastic containers in series connections. Such use could result in an embolism due to residual air being drawn from the primary container before administration of the fluid from the secondary container is completed.

Do not introduce additives to BREVIBLOC Injection/BREVIBLOC PREMIXED Injection.
To Open BREVIBLOC PREMIXED Bag: Do not remove unit from overwrap until ready to use. Do not use if overwrap has been previously opened or damaged. The overwrap is a moisture barrier. The inner bag maintains sterility of the solution.

Tear overwrap at notch and remove premixed bag. Some opacity of the plastic due to moisture absorption during the sterilization process may be observed. This is normal and does not affect the solution quality or safety. The opacity will diminish gradually.

Check for minute leaks by squeezing inner bag firmly. If leaks are found, discard solution as sterility may be impaired.

Do not use unless the solution is clear, colourless to light yellow, and the plastic protector on the delivery port is intact. Do not use if the solution is cloudy or a precipitate is present.
Preparation for Intravenous Administration: (use aseptic technique)

1. Suspend premixed bag from eyelet support.
2. Remove plastic protector from delivery port at bottom of bag.
3. Attach administration set. Refer to complete directions accompanying set.

INFORMATION FOR THE PATIENT: Published in e-CPS, available by subscription at www.e-cps.ca.

DOSAGE FORMS, COMPOSITION AND PACKAGING: BREVIBLOC: Each mL of clear, colourless to light yellow, sterile, nonpyrogenic, iso-osmotic solution contains: esmolol HCl 10 mg. Nonmedicinal ingredients: glacial acetic acid, USP, hydrochloric acid, NF, as needed to adjust pH, sodium acetate trihydrate, USP, sodium chloride, USP, sodium hydroxide, as needed to adjust pH and water for injection, USP. Osmolarity: 312 mOsmol/L. Amber glass single dose vials of 10 mL, boxes of 25.
BREVIBLOC PREMIXED: Each mL of clear, colourless to light yellow, sterile, nonpyrogenic, iso-osmotic solution contains: esmolol HCl 10 mg. Nonmedicinal ingredients: glacial acetic acid, USP, hydrochloric acid, NF, as needed to adjust pH, sodium acetate trihydrate, USP, sodium chloride, USP, sodium hydroxide, as needed to adjust pH and water for injection, USP. Osmolarity: 312 mOsmol/L. Non-latex, non-PVC INTRAVIA bags premixed bags of 250 mL with two PVC ports. The INTRAVIA bag is manufactured from a specially designed multilayer plastic (PL 2408). Solutions in contact with the plastic container leach out certain chemical compounds from the plastic in very small amounts; however, biological testing was supportive of the safety of the plastic container materials. Boxes of 10.

Brevicon® 0.5/35 Ⓟ
norethindrone—ethinyl estradiol
Oral Contraceptive

Pfizer

Brevicon® 1/35 Ⓟ
norethindrone—ethinyl estradiol
Oral Contraceptive

Pfizer

PHARMACOLOGY: Estrogen-progestogen combinations act primarily through the mechanism of gonadotropin suppression due to the estrogenic and progestational activity of their components. Although the primary mechanism of action is inhibition of ovulation, alterations in the cervical mucus and the endometrium may also contribute to effectiveness.

INDICATIONS: Prevention of pregnancy.

CONTRAINDICATIONS: History of or actual thrombophlebitis or thromboembolic disorders; history of or actual cerebrovascular disorders; history of or actual myocardial infarction or coronary arterial disease; active liver disease or history of or actual benign or malignant liver tumors; history of or known or suspected carcinoma of the breast; history of or known or suspected estrogen-dependent neoplasia; undiagnosed abnormal vaginal bleeding; any ocular lesion arising from ophthalmic vascular disease, such as partial or complete loss of vision or defect in visual fields; when pregnancy is suspected or diagnosed.

WARNINGS: Predisposing Factors for Coronary Artery Disease: Cigarette smoking increases the risk of serious cardiovascular side effects and mortality. Birth control pills increase this risk, especially with increasing age. Convincing data are available to support an upper age limit of 35 years for oral contraceptive use by women who smoke.

Other women who are independently at high risk for cardiovascular disease include those with diabetes, hypertension, abnormal lipid profile, or a family history of these. Whether oral contraceptives accentuate this risk is unclear.

In low risk, nonsmoking women of any age, the benefits of oral contraceptive use outweigh the possible cardiovascular risks associated with low-dose formulations. Consequently, oral contraceptives may be prescribed for these women up to the age of menopause.

Cigarette smoking increases the risk of serious adverse effects on the heart and blood vessels. This risk increases with age and becomes significant in oral contraceptive users over 35 years of age. Women should be counselled not to smoke.

Discontinue Medication at the Earliest Manifestation of the Following:

A. Thromboembolic and cardiovascular disorders such as: thrombophlebitis, pulmonary embolism, cerebrovascular disorders, myocardial ischemia, mesenteric thrombosis, and retinal thrombosis.
B. Conditions that predispose to venous stasis and to vascular thrombosis, e.g., immobilization after accidents or confinement to bed during long-term illness. Other nonhormonal methods of contraception should be used until regular activities are resumed. For use of oral contraceptives when surgery is contemplated, see Precautions.
C. Visual defects—partial or complete.
D. Papilledema or ophthalmic vascular lesions.
E. Severe headache of unknown etiology or worsening of pre-existing migraine headache.

PRECAUTIONS: Physical Examination and Follow-up: Before oral contraceptives are used, a thorough history and physical examination should be performed, including a blood pressure determination. Breasts, liver, extremities and pelvic organs should be examined and a Papanicolaou smear should be taken if the patient has been sexually active.

The first follow-up visit should be done 3 months after oral contraceptives are prescribed. Thereafter, examinations should be performed at least once a year or more frequently if indicated. At each annual visit, examination should include those procedures that were done at the initial visit as outlined above or per recommendations of the Canadian Workshop on Screening for Cancer of the Cervix. Their suggestion was that, for women who had 2 consecutive negative Pap smears, screening could be continued every 3 years up to the age of 69.

Pregnancy: Fetal abnormalities have been reported to occur in the offspring of women who have taken estrogen-progestogen combinations in early pregnancy. Rule out pregnancy as soon as it is suspected.

Lactation: The use of oral contraceptives during the period a mother is breast-feeding her infant may not be advisable. The hormonal components are excreted in breast milk and may reduce its quantity and quality. The long-term effects on the developing child are not known.

Hepatic Function: Patients who have had jaundice including a history of cholestatic jaundice during pregnancy should be given oral contraceptives with great care and under close observation.

The development of severe generalized pruritus or icterus requires that the medication be withdrawn until the problem is resolved.

If a patient develops jaundice that proves to be cholestatic in type, the use of oral contraceptives should not be resumed. In patients taking oral contraceptives, changes in the composition of the bile may occur and an increased incidence of gallstones has been reported.

Hepatic nodules have been reported to be associated with use of oral contraceptives, particularly in long-term users of oral contraceptives. These nodules include benign hepatic adenomas, focal nodular hyperplasia and other hepatic lesions. In addition, hepatocellular carcinoma has been reported. Although these lesions are extremely rare, they have caused fatal intra-abdominal hemorrhage and should be considered in women presenting with an abdominal mass, acute abdominal pain, or evidence of intra-abdominal bleeding.

Hypertension: Patients with essential hypertension whose blood pressure is well-controlled may be given oral contraceptives but only under close supervision. If a significant elevation of blood pressure in previously normotensive or hypertensive subjects occurs at any time during the administration of the drug, cessation of medication is necessary.

Migraine and Headache: The onset or exacerbation of migraine or the development of headache of a new pattern which is recurrent, persistent or severe, requires discontinuation of oral contraceptives and evaluation of the cause.

Diabetes: Current low dose oral contraceptives exert minimal impact on glucose metabolism. Diabetic patients, or those with a family history of diabetes, should be observed closely to detect any worsening of carbohydrate metabolism. Patients predisposed to diabetes who can be kept under close supervision may be given oral contraceptives. Young diabetic patients whose disease is of recent origin, well-controlled, and not associated with hypertension or other signs of vascular disease such as ocular fundal changes should be monitored more frequently while using oral contraceptives.

Ocular Disease: Patients who are pregnant or are taking oral contraceptives may experience corneal edema that may cause visual disturbances and changes in tolerance to contact lenses, especially of the rigid type. Soft contact lenses usually do not cause disturbances. If visual changes or alterations in tolerance to contact lenses occur, temporary or permanent cessation of wear may be advised.

Breasts: Increasing age and a strong family history are the most significant risk factors for the development of breast cancer. Other established risk factors include obesity, nulliparity and late age at first full-term pregnancy. The identified groups of women that may be at increased risk of developing breast cancer before menopause are long-term users of oral contraceptives (more than 8 years) and starters at early age. In a few women, the use of oral contraceptives may accelerate the growth of an existing but undiagnosed breast cancer. Since any potential increased risk related to oral contraceptive use is small, there is no reason to change prescribing habits at present.

Women receiving oral contraceptives should be instructed in self-examination of their breasts. Their physicians should be notified whenever any masses are detected. A yearly clinical breast examination is also recommended because, if a breast cancer should develop, drugs that contain estrogen may cause a rapid progression.

Vaginal Bleeding: Persistent irregular vaginal bleeding requires assessment to exclude underlying pathology.

Fibroids: Patients with fibroids (leiomyomata) should be carefully observed. Sudden enlargement, pain, or tenderness requires discontinuation of the use of oral contraceptives.

Emotional Disorders: Patients with a history of emotional disturbances, especially the depressive type, may be more prone to have a recurrence of depression while taking oral contraceptives. In cases of a serious recurrence, a trial of an alternate method of contraception should be made which may help to clarify the possible relationship. Women with premenstrual syndrome (PMS) may have a varied response to oral contraceptives, ranging from symptomatic improvement to worsening of the condition.

Metabolic and Endocrine Diseases: In metabolic or endocrine diseases and when metabolism of calcium and phosphorus is abnormal, careful clinical evaluation should precede medication and a regular follow-up is recommended.

Connective Tissue Disease: The use of oral contraceptives in some women has been associated with positive lupus erythematous cell tests and with clinical lupus erythematous. In some instances, exacerbation of rheumatoid arthritis and synovitis have been observed.

Laboratory Tests: Results of laboratory tests should be interpreted in light of the fact that the patient is on oral contraceptives. The laboratory tests listed below are modified.

A. Liver function tests: Aspartate serum transaminase (AST): variously reported elevations. Alkaline phosphatase and gamma glutamine transaminase (GGT): slightly elevated.

B. Coagulation tests: Minimal elevation of test values reported for such parameters as Factors VII, VIII, IX and X. Increased platelet aggregation. Decreased antithrombin III.

C. Thyroid function tests: Protein binding of thyroxine is increased as indicated by increased total serum thyroxine concentrations and decreased T_3 resin uptake.

D. Lipoproteins: Small changes of unproven clinical significance may occur in lipoprotein cholesterol fractions.

E. Gonadotropins: LH and FSH levels are suppressed by the use of oral contraceptives. Wait 2 weeks after discontinuing the use of oral contraceptives before measurements are made.

Tissue Specimens: Pathologists should be advised of oral contraceptive therapy when specimens obtained from surgical procedures and Pap smears are submitted for examination.

Return to Fertility: After discontinuing oral contraceptive therapy, the patient should delay pregnancy until at least 1 normal spontaneous cycle has occurred in order to date the pregnancy. An alternative contraceptive method should be used during this time.

Amenorrhea: Women having a history of oligomenorrhea, secondary amenorrhea, or irregular cycles may remain anovulatory or become amenorrheic following discontinuation of estrogen-progestin combination therapy.

Amenorrhea, especially if associated with breast secretion, that continues for 6 months or more after withdrawal, warrants a careful assessment of hypothalamic-pituitary function.

Thromboembolic Complications—Postsurgery: There is an increased risk of postsurgery thromboembolic complications in oral contraceptive users, after major surgery. If feasible, oral contraceptives should be discontinued and an alternative method substituted at least 1 month prior to **major** elective surgery. Oral contraceptives should not be resumed until the first menstrual period after hospital discharge following surgery.

Drug Interactions: The concurrent administration of oral contraceptives with other drugs may result in an altered response to either agent. Reduced effectiveness of the oral contraceptive, should it occur, is more likely with the low dose formulations. It is important to ascertain all drugs that a patient is taking, both prescription and nonprescription, before oral contraceptives are prescribed.

Refer to the revised 1994 Report on Oral Contraceptives, Health Canada, for possible drug interactions with oral contraceptives.

Noncontraceptive Benefits of Oral Contraceptives: Several health advantages other than contraception have been reported.
Effects on menses: Increased menstrual cycle regularity; decreased menstrual blood loss; decreased incidence of iron deficiency anemia secondary to reduced menstrual blood loss; decreased incidence of dysmenorrhea.
Effects related to ovulation inhibition: Decreased incidence of functional ovarian cysts; decreased incidence of ectopic pregnancy.
Effects on other organs of the reproductive tract: Decreased incidence of acute salpingitis; decreased incidence of endometrial cancer (50%); decreased incidence of ovarian cancer (40%); potential beneficial effects on endometriosis; improvement of acne vulgaris, hirsutism, and other androgen-mediated disorders.
Effects on breasts: Decreased incidence of benign breast disease (fibroadenomas and fibrocystic breast disease); decreased incidence of breast biopsies.

The noncontraceptive benefits of oral contraceptives should be considered in addition to the efficacy of these preparations when counselling patients regarding contraceptive method selection.

Oral contraceptives **do not protect** against sexually transmitted diseases (STDs) including HIV/AIDS. For protection against STDs, it is advisable to use latex condoms **in combination with** oral contraceptives.

ADVERSE EFFECTS: An increased risk of the following serious adverse reactions has been associated with the use of oral contraceptives: thrombophlebitis; pulmonary embolism; mesenteric thrombosis; neuro-ocular lesions, e.g., retinal thrombosis; myocardial infarction; cerebral thrombosis; cerebral hemorrhage; hypertension; benign hepatic tumors; gallbladder disease.

The following adverse reactions also have been reported in patients receiving oral contraceptives: Nausea and vomiting, usually the most common adverse reactions, occur in approximately 10% or less of patients during the first cycle. Other reactions, as a general rule, are seen less frequently or only occasionally.

Other Adverse Reactions: gastrointestinal symptoms (such as abdominal cramps and bloating); breakthrough bleeding; spotting; change in menstrual flow; dysmenorrhea; amenorrhea during and after treatment; infertility after discontinuance of treatment; edema; chloasma or melasma which may persist; breast changes: tenderness, enlargement, and secretion; change in weight (increase or decrease); endocervical hyperplasias; possible diminution in lactation when given immediately post-partum; cholestatic jaundice; migraine; increase in size of uterine leiomyomata; rash (allergic); mental depression; reduced tolerance to carbohydrates; vaginal candidiasis; premenstrual-like syndrome; intolerance to contact lenses; change in corneal curvature (steepening); cataracts; optic neuritis; retinal thrombosis; changes in libido; chorea; changes in appetite; cystitis-like syndrome; rhinitis; headache; nervousness; dizziness; hirsutism; loss of scalp hair; erythema multiforme; erythema nodosum; hemorrhagic eruption; vaginitis; porphyria; impaired renal function; Raynaud's phenomenon; auditory disturbances; hemolytic uremic syndrome; pancreatitis; arterial thromboembolism.

OVERDOSE:

Symptoms: Numerous cases of the ingestion by children of estrogen-progestogen combinations have been reported. Although mild nausea may occur, there appears to be no other reaction.

Treatment: Treatment should be limited to a laxative such as citrate of magnesia with the aim of removing unabsorbed material as rapidly as possible.

For management of a suspected drug overdose, CPhA recommends that you contact your **regional Poison Control Centre**. See the *CPS* Directory section for a list of Poison Control Centres.

DOSAGE: Information for the Patient on How to Take the Birth Control Pill:

1. **Read these directions:**
   - before you start taking your pills, and
   - any time you are not sure what to do.
2. **Look at your pill pack** to see if it has 21 or 28 pills:
   - 21-Pill Pack: 21 active pills (with hormones) taken daily for 3 weeks, and then take no pills for 1 week

     or
   - 28-Pill Pack: 21 active pills (with hormones) taken daily for 3 weeks, and then 7 "reminder" pills (no hormones) taken daily for 1 week.

   Also check the pill pack for instructions on (1) where to start and (2) directions to take pills (see package insert for illustrations).
3. It is recommended that you use a second method of birth control (e.g., latex condoms and spermicidal foam or gel) for the first 7 days of the first cycle of pill use. This will provide a back-up in case pills are forgotten while you are getting used to taking them.
4. **When receiving any medical treatment, be sure to tell your doctor that you are using birth control pills.**
5. **Many women have spotting or light bleeding or may feel sick to their stomach during the first 3 months on the pill.** If you do feel sick, do not stop taking the pill. The problem will usually go away. If it does not go away, check with your doctor or clinic.
6. **Missing pills also can cause some spotting or light bleeding**, even if you make up the missed pills. You also could feel a little sick to your stomach on the days you take 2 pills to make up for missed pills.
7. **If you miss pills at any time, you could get pregnant. The greatest risks for pregnancy are:**
   - when you start a pack late, or
   - when you miss pills at the beginning or at the very end of the pack.
8. **Always be sure you have ready:**
   - **another kind of birth control** (such as latex condoms and spermicidal foam or gel) to use as a backup in case you miss pills, and
   - **an extra, full pack of pills.**
9. **If you experience vomiting or diarrhea, or if you take certain medicines**, such as antibiotics, your pills may not work as well. Use a backup method, such as latex condoms and spermicidal foam or gel, until you can check with your doctor or clinic.
10. **If you forget more than 1 pill 2 months in a row**, talk to your doctor or clinic about how to make pill-taking easier or about using another method of birth control.
11. **If your questions are not answered here, call your doctor or clinic.**

When to start the first pack of pills: Be sure to read these instructions:

- before you start taking your pills, and
- any time you are not sure what to do.

Decide with your doctor or clinic what is the best day for you to start taking your first pack of pills. Your pills may be either a 21-day or a 28-day type.

A. 21-Day Combination: With this type of birth control pill, you are on pills for 21 days and off pills for 7 days. You must not be off the pills for more than 7 days in a row.

1. **The first day of your menstrual period (bleeding) is Day 1 of your cycle.** Your doctor may advise you to start taking the pills on Day 1, on Day 5, or on the first Sunday after your period begins. If your period starts on Sunday, start that same day.
2. Take 1 pill at approximately the same time every day for 21 days; **then take no pills for 7 days**. Start a new pack on the 8th day. You will probably have a period during the 7 days off the pill. (This bleeding may be lighter and shorter than your usual period.)

B. 28-Day Combination: With this type of birth control pill, you take 21 pills that contain hormones and 7 pills that contain no hormones.

1. **The first day of your menstrual period (bleeding) is Day 1 of your cycle.** Your doctor may advise you to start taking the pills on Day 1, on Day 5, or on the first Sunday after your period begins. If your period starts on Sunday, start that same day.
2. Take 1 pill at approximately the same time every day for 28 days. Begin a new pack the next day, **not missing any days**. Your period should occur during the last 7 days of using that pill pack.

What to do during the month:

1. **Take a pill at approximately the same time every day until the pack is empty.**
   - Try to associate taking your pill with some regular activity such as eating a meal or going to bed.
   - Do not skip pills even if you have bleeding between monthly periods or feel sick to your stomach (nausea).
   - Do not skip pills even if you do not have sex very often.
2. When you finish a pack:
   - **21 pills: Wait 7 days** to start the next pack. You will have your period during that week.
   - **28 pills:** Start the next pack **on the next day**. Take 1 pill every day. Do not wait any days between packs.

What to do if you miss pills: Table 1 outlines the actions you should take if you miss 1 or more of your birth control pills. Match the number of pills missed with the appropriate starting time for your type of pill pack.

Table 1: Brevicon 0.5/35/1/35
What to Do if You Miss Pills

Sunday Start	Other Than Sunday Start
Miss 1 pill	**Miss 1 pill**
Take it as soon as you remember, and take the next pill at the usual time. This means that you might take 2 pills in one day.	Take it as soon as you remember, and take the next pill at the usual time. This means that you might take 2 pills in one day.
Miss 2 pills in a row	**Miss 2 pills in a row**
First 2 Weeks: 1. Take 2 pills the day you remember and 2 pills the next day. 2. Then take 1 pill a day until you finish the pack. 3. Use a backup method of birth control if you have sex in the 7 days after you miss the pills. **Third Week:** 1. Keep taking 1 pill a day until Sunday. 2. On Sunday, safely discard the rest of the pack and start a new pack that day. 3. Use a backup method of birth control if you have sex in the 7 days after you miss the pills. 4. You may not have a period this month. **If you miss 2 periods in a row, call your doctor or clinic.**	**First 2 Weeks:** 1. Take 2 pills the day you remember and 2 pills the next day. 2. Then take 1 pill a day until you finish the pack. 3. Use a backup method of birth control if you have sex in the 7 days after you miss the pills. **Third Week:** 1. Safely dispose of the rest of the pill pack and start a new pack that same day. 2. Use a backup method of birth control if you have sex in the 7 days after you miss the pills. 3. You may not have a period this month. **If you miss 2 periods in a row, call your doctor or clinic.**
Miss 3 or more pills in a row	**Miss 3 or more pills in a row**
Anytime in the Cycle: 1. Keep taking 1 pill a day until Sunday. 2. On Sunday, safely discard the rest of the pack and start a new pack that day. 3. Use a backup method of birth control if you have sex in the 7 days after you miss the pills. 4. You may not have a period this month. **If you miss 2 periods in a row, call your doctor or clinic.**	**Anytime in the Cycle:** 1. Safely dispose of the rest of the pill pack and start a new pack that same day. 2. Use a backup method of birth control if you have sex in the 7 days after you miss the pills. 3. You may not have a period this month. **If you miss 2 periods in a row, call your doctor or clinic.**

Note: 28-Day Pack: If you forget any of the 7 "reminder" pills (without hormones) in Week 4, just safely dispose of the pills you missed. Then keep taking 1 pill each day until the pack is empty. You do not need to use a backup method.

Always be sure you have on hand:

- a backup method of birth control (such as latex condoms and spermicidal foam or gel) in case you miss pills, and
- an extra, full pack of pills.

If you forget more than 1 pill 2 months in a row, talk to your doctor or clinic about ways to make pill-taking easier or about using another method of birth control.

Dosage: **A. 21-Day Pack:** With this type of birth control pill, the patient is 21 days on pills with 7 days off pills. The patient must not be off the pills for more than 7 days in a row.

1. **The first day of the patient's menstrual period (bleeding) is day 1 of a cycle.** The doctor may advise the patient to start taking the pills on Day 1, on Day 5, or on the first Sunday after a period begins. If a period starts on Sunday, the patient starts that same day.
2. The pack must be labelled correctly before starting. The pack is pre-printed with a Sunday starting day. If the patient is starting on a day other than a Sunday, she should use the Flexi-start sticker labels provided. The patient peels off the label with the chosen starting day and applies it over the pre-printed days on top of the card.
3. The patient takes 1 pill at approximately the same time every day for 21 days; **then she takes no pills for 7 days**. She starts a new pack on the 8th day. She will probably have a period during the 7 days off the pill. (This bleeding may be lighter and shorter than a usual period.)

B. 28-Day Pack: With this type of birth control pill, the patient takes 21 pills which contain hormones and 7 pills which contain no hormones.

1. **The first day of the patient's menstrual period (bleeding) is day 1 of a cycle.** The doctor may advise the patient to start taking the pills on Day 1, on Day 5, or on the first Sunday after a period begins. If a period starts on Sunday, the patient starts that same day.
2. The pack must be labelled correctly before starting. The pack is pre-printed with a Sunday starting day. If the patient is starting on a day other than a Sunday, she should use the Flexi-start sticker labels provided. The patient peels off the label with the chosen starting day and applies it over the pre-printed days on top of the card.
3. The patient takes 1 pill at approximately the same time every day for 28 days. She begins a new pack the next day, **not missing any days on the pills.** The patient's period should occur during the last 7 days of using that pill pack.

What to do during the month:

1. **The patient takes a pill at approximately the same time every day until the pack is empty.**
   - The patient should try to associate taking the pill with some regular activity like eating a meal or going to bed.
   - The patient must not skip pills even if she has bleeding between monthly periods or feels sick to her stomach (nausea).
   - The patient must not skip pills even if she does not have sex very often.
2. **When a pack is finished:**
   - **21 Pills: The patient must wait 7 days** to start the next pack. A period will begin during that week.
   - **28 Pills:** The patient starts the next pack **on the next day**. She takes 1 pill every day. She does not wait any days between packs.

INFORMATION FOR THE PATIENT: Published in e-CPS, available by subscription at www.e-cps.ca.

SUPPLIED: Brevicon 0.5/35: Each blue circular tablet, impressed "SEARLE" on one side and "BX" on the other, contains: norethindrone 0.5 mg and ethinyl estradiol 0.035 mg. Inert orange-colored tablets, impressed "SEARLE" on one side and "P" on the other. Nonmedicinal ingredients: active tablets: cornstarch, FD&C Blue No. 2, lactose, magnesium stearate and povidone; placebo tablets: FD&C Yellow No. 6 Lake, lactose hydrous, magnesium stearate and microcrystalline cellulose. Dispensers of 21 (21 active tablets) and 28 (21 active and 7 inert tablets) days. Store below 25°C.

Brevicon 1/35: Each white circular tablet, impressed "SEARLE" on one side and "BX" on the other, contains: norethindrone 1 mg and ethinyl estradiol 0.035 mg. Inert orange-colored tablets are impressed "SEARLE" on one side and "P" on the other. Nonmedicinal ingredients: Active tablets: cornstarch, lactose, magnesium stearate and povidone. Placebo tablets: FD&C Yellow No. 6 Lake, lactose hydrous, magnesium stearate and microcrystalline cellulose. Dispensers of 21 (21 active tablets) and 28 (21 active and 7 inert tablets) days.

(Shown in Product Identification Section)

Bricanyl® Turbuhaler® ℞

terbutaline sulfate

Bronchodilator

AstraZeneca

Date of Preparation: April 18, 2000
Date of Revision: December 20, 2005

PHARMACOLOGY: Terbutaline sulfate produces bronchodilation by stimulation of the β_2-adrenergic receptors in bronchial smooth muscle, thereby causing relaxation of muscle fibres. This action is manifested by an increase in pulmonary function as demonstrated by FEV_1 measurements. Terbutaline also produces a decrease in airway and pulmonary resistance.

Following inhalation of terbutaline Turbuhaler, a significant improvement in pulmonary function measurements is well established after 5 minutes. Twenty to 30% of the metered dose is deposited in the lungs with an inspiration flow rate of about 60 L/min.

The maximal response is usually attained between 15 and 60 minutes following administration. Significant bronchodilator activity has been observed to persist for 4 to 7 hours.

INDICATIONS: As a bronchodilator for the symptomatic relief of bronchial asthma and for relief of reversible bronchospasm which may occur in association with bronchitis and emphysema.

CONTRAINDICATIONS: Known hypersensitivity to sympathomimetic amines and, like other sympathomimetic amines, should not be used in patients with tachyarrhythmias.

WARNINGS: Like other β_2-agonist inhalers, terbutaline should not be used on a regular daily basis without appropriate concomitant anti-inflammatory therapy (see Dosage).

Terbutaline should be used with caution in patients with diabetes, hypertension, hyperthyroidism and a history of seizures. As with other sympathomimetic bronchodilator agents, terbutaline should be administered cautiously to cardiac patients, especially those with associated arrhythmias, and coronary insufficiency, to elderly or to patients who are unusually responsive to sympathomimetic amines. Due to the hyperglycemic effects of β_2-agonists, additional blood glucose controls are recommended initially in diabetic patients.

Occasionally, patients have been reported to have developed severe paradoxical bronchospasm with repeated use of sympathomimetic inhalant preparations. In such instances, the preparation should be discontinued immediately and alternate therapy instituted. Fatalities, the exact cause of which are unknown, have been reported following excessive use of inhaled preparations containing sympathomimetic amines. Cardiac arrest was noted in several instances.

Beta-receptor blocking agents (including eye-drops), especially those which are noncardioselective, may partially or totally inhibit the effect of beta-receptor stimulants. Severe resistant bronchospasm may be produced with the use of beta-blockers in asthmatic patients.

Potentially serious hypokalemia may result from β_2-agonist therapy, mainly from parenteral or nebulized administration. Particular caution is advised in acute severe asthma as this may be potentiated by hypoxia and concomitant treatment with xanthine derivatives, steroids and diuretics; it is recommended that serum potassium levels be monitored in such situations.

Pregnancy: The safe use of terbutaline has not been established in human pregnancy. The use of this drug in pregnancy, lactation, or women of childbearing potential requires that the expected therapeutic benefit of the drug be weighed against its possible hazards to the mother or child. Animal reproductive studies have shown no adverse effects on fetal development.

Transient hypoglycemia has been reported in newborn preterm infants after maternal β_2-agonist treatment.

Systemic β_2-agonists should be used with caution before childbirth in view of their inhibiting effect on uterine contractions.

Lactation: Terbutaline is excreted in breast milk. Caution should be exercised when terbutaline is administered to nursing women.

Children: Terbutaline is not presently recommended for children below 6 years of age due to limited clinical data in this pediatric group.

PRECAUTIONS: If therapy does not produce a significant improvement or if the patient's condition gets worse, medical advice must be sought in order to determine a new plan of treatment. In the case of acute or rapidly worsening dyspnea, a doctor should be consulted immediately.

Increasing use of β_2-agonists to control symptoms of bronchial obstruction, especially administration on a regular basis or in high amounts, indicates deterioration of asthma control. Under these conditions, the patient's therapy plan has to be revised. It is inadequate simply to increase the use of bronchodilators under these circumstances, in particular over extended periods of time (see Dosage). The revised treatment regimen should include concomitant use of other antiasthma drugs, such as anti-inflammatory agents.

To ensure optimal delivery of terbutaline to the bronchial tree, the patient should be properly instructed in the use of Turbuhaler.

In patients in whom the administration of terbutaline induces cardiac irregularities, the administration of the drug should be stopped. If a reduced response to terbutaline becomes apparent, the patient should seek medical advice.

In patients requiring concomitant treatment with terbutaline and a beta-blocker, it is recommended that a beta-blocker (e.g., metoprolol) with less predominant β_2-blocking effects be considered. If concomitant treatment is necessary, patients should be monitored carefully for possible deterioration in pulmonary function and the need to adjust the dosage of either drug (see Drug Interactions).

Immediate hypersensitivity reactions and exacerbation of bronchospasm have been reported after terbutaline administration.

Drug Interactions: Sympathomimetic Bronchodilators and Epinephrine: The concomitant use of terbutaline with other sympathomimetic bronchodilators or epinephrine is not generally recommended since their combined effect on the cardiovascular system may be deleterious to the patient. If additional adrenergic drugs are to be administered by any route to the patient using terbutaline, the adrenergic drugs must be used with caution. Such concomitant use, however, should be individualized and not given on a routine basis. If regular coadministration is required, alternative therapy should be considered.

MAO Inhibitors and Tricyclic Antidepressants: Terbutaline should be administered with caution in patients being treated with MAO inhibitors or tricyclic antidepressants, since the action of terbutaline on the vascular system may be potentiated.

Beta-Adrenergic Receptor Blockers: Beta-adrenergic receptor blocking agents not only block the pulmonary effect of terbutaline but may produce severe asthmatic attacks in asthmatic patients. Therefore, patients requiring treatment for both bronchospastic disease and hypertension should be treated with medication other than beta-adrenergic blocking agents for their hypertension.

Bricanyl Turbuhaler contains terbutaline sulfate which is sensitive to moisture. Patients should be instructed to avoid exhaling into the device and to replace the cover after using Turbuhaler.

ADVERSE EFFECTS: When treatment with terbutaline is started, the following adverse reactions can be classified as frequent (i.e. >1/100): tremor, palpitations, restlessness, headache, muscle cramps, nervousness. Other reported reactions include increased heart rate, tachycardia, ectopic beats, drowsiness, nausea, vomiting, sweating and dizziness. As for all β_2-agonists, cardiac arrhythmias, e.g., atrial fibrillation, supraventricular tachycardia and extrasystoles have been rarely reported.

These adverse reactions are all characteristic of sympathomimetic amines and initial dose titrations will often reduce these reactions. With the possible exception of muscle cramps, all have been spontaneously reversible within the first 2 weeks of treatment. Urticaria and exanthema may also occur.

Sleep disturbances and behavioral disturbances, such as agitation, hyperactivity and restlessness, have been observed.

As with other inhalation therapy, the potential for paradoxical bronchospasm should be kept in mind with terbutaline. If it occurs, the preparation should be discontinued immediately and alternative therapy instituted.

Potentially serious hypokalemia may result from β_2-agonist therapy.

OVERDOSE:

Symptoms: The symptoms of overdosage are similar to those described under Adverse Effects, and are attributable to excessive β-adrenergic stimulation.

Treatment: To antagonize the effect of excessive stimulation, the judicious use of a β-adrenergic blocking agent such as propranolol may be considered, bearing in mind the danger of inducing an asthmatic attack.

For management of a suspected drug overdose, CPhA recommends that you contact your **regional Poison Control Centre**. See the *CPS* Directory section for a list of Poison Control Centres.

DOSAGE: Dosage should be individualized, and patient response should be monitored by the prescribing physician on an ongoing basis.

Adults and Children ≥6 Years: The generally recommended dose of terbutaline is 1 inhalation (0.5 mg) taken as required. This will usually be adequate to relieve bronchospasm in the majority of patients, however, if required, a second dose may be taken, preferably after waiting 5 minutes for the effect of the first dose to be obtained. If a more severe attack has not been relieved by the second administration, higher doses may be required. In these cases, patients should immediately consult their doctor or the nearest hospital.

More than 6 doses (6 inhalations of terbutaline) should not be necessary in any 24-hour period.

If a previously effective dosage regimen fails to provide the usual relief, or the effects of a dose last for less than 3 hours, medical advice should be sought immediately; this is a sign of seriously worsening asthma that requires reassessment of therapy.

Treatment with β_2-agonists in bronchial asthma should be on demand, e.g., symptoms oriented. **Patients must not use them on a daily basis for control of bronchospasm without using other concomitant antiasthma medication(s) according to the present practice for asthma treatment to control airway inflammation.**

The daily dose of terbutaline should not be increased without adequate reassessment of the therapy plan.

As with other β_2-agonists, increasing demand for terbutaline in bronchial asthma is a sign of poor asthma control and indicates that the treatment plan should be revised.

When prescribing terbutaline to children, it is necessary to ascertain that they can follow the instructions for use. Terbutaline is not recommended for use in children below the age of 6 years.

Note: The medication from terbutaline Turbuhaler is delivered to the lungs as the patient inhales and, therefore, it is important to instruct the patient to breathe in forcefully and deeply through the mouthpiece. The patient may not taste or feel any medication when using terbutaline Turbuhaler due to the small amount of drug dispensed.

INFORMATION FOR THE PATIENT: Published in e-CPS, available by subscription at www.e-cps.ca.

SUPPLIED: Each Turbuhaler contains: 50 or 200 doses of micronized terbutaline sulfate. Each inhalation from the multiple-dose powder inhaler contains: terbutaline sulfate 0.5 mg; no additives or carrier substances are included in the inhalation. Turbuhaler cannot be refilled and should be discarded when empty. Store with the cover tightened, at room temperature between 15 and 30°C, in a dry place, away from moisture.

(Shown in Product Identification Section)

Bromazepam ☒

CPhA Monograph

see *Benzodiazepines*

Bromocriptine ℞

Dopamine Agonist

CPhA Monograph

Date of Preparation: November 2008

This monograph has been compiled by CPhA and reviewed by experts. It may contain information different from that found in Health Canada-approved Product Monographs. The reader is referred to the *CPS* Editorial Policy for more information.

SUMMARY PRODUCT INFORMATION:

Route of Administration	Dosage Form	Strength
Oral	Tablet	2.5 mg
	Capsule	5 mg

INDICATIONS AND CLINICAL USE: Bromocriptine is indicated for:

- treatment of galactorrhea, with or without amenorrhea, due to hyperprolactinemia
- treatment of prolactin-dependent menstrual disorders and infertility, e.g., secondary to amenorrhea, ovulatory insufficiency or short luteal phase
- treatment of prolactin-secreting adenomas: as a treatment for inoperable macroadenomas, as an adjunct to surgery to facilitate adenoma removal, or as an alternative to surgery in patients with microadenomas
- treatment of prolactin-dependent male hypogonadism
- as an adjunct to surgery or radiotherapy for acromegaly, or as monotherapy in special cases
- monotherapy of early Parkinson's disease or as an adjunct to levodopa in advanced cases with motor complications

Unapproved uses of bromocriptine include management of neuroleptic malignant syndrome and restless legs syndrome.

Because of the risk of serious adverse effects including seizures and severe hypotension or hypertension, bromocriptine is no longer recommended for suppression of lactation following childbirth.

CONTRAINDICATIONS:

- Patients who are hypersensitive to bromocriptine or other ergot derivatives or any ingredient in the formulation or component of the container
- Uncontrolled hypertension
- Pregnancy-related hypertensive disorders
- Severe ischemic heart disease or peripheral vascular disease

WARNINGS AND PRECAUTIONS:

Serious Warnings and Precautions

- Rarely, bromocriptine has been associated with pleuropulmonary and/or retroperitoneal fibrosis; see Adverse Reactions.
- Sudden onset of sleep or somnolence has been reported with dopamine agonist therapy in patients with Parkinson's disease; patients must be warned of the possible impairment of their ability to perform hazardous tasks such as driving a vehicle or operating machinery.
- Symptomatic hypotension commonly occurs, especially in the early days of therapy; conversely, hypertension has occurred rarely.

Cardiovascular: Dose-related hypotension, including first-dose syncope, postural hypotension and severe prolonged hypotension, can occur in patients taking bromocriptine. Blood pressure should be monitored periodically, especially when therapy is initiated and in patients taking other hypotensive drugs.

Rarely, hypertension has also occurred.

Gastrointestinal: Based on older case reports of peptic ulceration and bleeding in patients taking bromocriptine for acromegaly, it is recommended that bromocriptine be used with caution or alternate therapy be considered in patients with a history of peptic ulcer disease.

Hepatic/Biliary/Pancreatic: Bromocriptine is metabolized in the liver. Although no specific guidelines are available, caution is advised in patients with significant hepatic impairment, and dosage adjustment may be indicated.

Ophthalmologic: During treatment of macroprolactinoma, visual field examinations are recommended to monitor effects on the optic chiasm caused by changes in the dimensions of the prolactinoma. Rapid visual field loss requires evaluation by a neurosurgeon.

Perioperative Considerations: Bromocriptine therapy can be continued in the perioperative period when appropriate.

Psychiatric: Because psychotic symptoms such as hallucinations have occurred in association with bromocriptine therapy, the drug should be used cautiously in patients with a history of psychotic disorders.

Renal: Although bromocriptine is not renally eliminated, caution is advised in patients with renal failure as there is little experience with its use in this population. Dosage adjustment is not routinely recommended based on renal function.

Respiratory: See Boxed Serious Warnings and Precautions.

Sexual Function/Reproduction: Women being treated for galactorrhea and/or prolactin-induced amenorrhea need to be aware that fertility may be restored during bromocriptine therapy. Women who are sexually active during this treatment period are advised to use a barrier (nonhormonal) contraceptive method until such time as fertility is established and pregnancy is desired.

Special Populations: Pregnant Women: Bromocriptine has not been associated with an increased risk of congenital birth defects and is sometimes used during pregnancy to suppress the growth of macroprolactinomas. Visual field examinations are indicated during pregnancy to monitor effects of changing tumor size on the optic chiasm.

Women who receive bromocriptine during the postpartum period should be closely monitored for cardiovascular effects such as hypotension or hypertension. It is because of serious cardiovascular effects and seizures in the postpartum population that bromocriptine is no longer indicated for suppression of lactation following childbirth.

Nursing Women: Because it suppresses lactation, bromocriptine is not compatible with breastfeeding.

Pediatrics: Bromocriptine is sometimes used in children ≥11 years in the management of hyperprolactinemic conditions. The usual adult precautions apply when bromocriptine is used in this setting.

Monitoring and Laboratory Tests: To assess effectiveness of therapy, serum prolactin is measured in patients treated for hyperprolactinemia; for acromegaly, growth hormone levels are monitored. To monitor for adverse effects, blood pressure should be periodically measured, and visual field examinations are performed in patients with macroprolactinomas.

Occupational Hazards: Patients should be warned that bromocriptine-induced somnolence or sudden onset of sleep can impair their ability to perform hazardous tasks such as operating machinery or driving a motor vehicle.

ADVERSE REACTIONS: More Common Adverse Drug Reactions: See Table 1.

Table 1: Bromocriptine
More Common Adverse Drug Reactions (≥1%)

Body System	Effect	Clinical Comment
Central Nervous System	Headache (19%), vertigo (17%), fatigue (7%), lightheadedness (5%)	May respond to temporary dosage reduction and/or gradual re-titration. Patients should be warned about the possibility of vertigo or lightheadedness and how these adverse effects may affect their ability to perform hazardous tasks such as driving.
Cardiovascular	Hypotension	Monitor for symptomatic hypotension, especially for the first three days after initiating therapy.
Gastrointestinal	Nausea (20–50%), abdominal cramps (4%), constipation (3–14%) or diarrhea (3%)	May be attenuated by administration with food or temporary dosage reduction
Respiratory	Nasal congestion (4–5%)	

Less Common Adverse Drug Reactions (<1%): Cardiovascular: Bromocriptine has been associated with cold-induced vasoconstriction in the fingers. This usually responds to dosage reduction and can also be avoided by keeping the fingers warm.

While hypotension occurs more frequently especially during initial therapy (see Table 1), hypertension has also been reported, rarely.

Central Nervous System: Rarely, cerebrospinal fluid rhinorrhea has occurred in patients taking bromocriptine for the treatment of large prolactinomas.

Seizures and stroke have occurred rarely in women who took bromocriptine postpartum to suppress lactation; bromocriptine is no longer recommended for this indication.

Exacerbation or precipitation of manic episodes, hallucinations and other psychotic symptoms have occurred in patients taking bromocriptine. Concomitant therapy with levodopa may increase the risk of these effects.

Respiratory: Pleuropulmonary changes including pleural effusion, pleural thickening and pulmonary infiltrates have occurred rarely. Previous asbestos exposure may be a predisposing factor. Patients taking bromocriptine who experience unexplained pleuropulmonary symptoms should be investigated thoroughly to rule out serious lung changes necessitating immediate withdrawal of the drug. Retroperitoneal fibrosis has also occurred rarely. Pleuropulmonary changes and retroperitoneal fibrosis are usually associated with long-term use and may be dose-related.

DRUG INTERACTIONS: Overview: Concomitant therapy with other ergot alkaloids (e.g., cabergoline, ergotamine derivatives, ergonovine, methysergide) should be avoided due to the theoretical risk of additive vasoconstrictive effects.

Drug-Drug Interactions: See Table 2.

Table 2: Bromocriptine
Drug-Drug Interactions

Interacting Drug	Effect	Clinical Comment
Antihypertensive Drugs	Possible additive hypotensive effects	Monitor blood pressure as appropriate; therapy may need to be altered or adjusted.
Antipsychotic Drugs	The dopamine antagonistic effects of antipsychotics oppose the therapeutic effects of bromocriptine.	The combination should be avoided when possible; it may be less pronounced with quetiapine or clozapine compared to first-generation antipsychotics or to other "atypical" agents.
Cyclosporine	Bromocriptine therapy may result in decreased cyclosporine clearance.	Monitor cyclosporine serum concentrations and decrease dose if required.
Nitroglycerin	Ergot derivatives such as bromocriptine may antagonize the vasodilatory effects of nitroglycerin	Avoid combination when possible.
Inhibitors of CYP3A4 (e.g., erythromycin, clarithromycin, grapefruit juice, ketoconazole, ritonavir)	Possible increased bromocriptine serum concentrations	Avoid one of the interacting drugs if a reasonable alternative exists. If concomitant therapy is used, monitor for increased effects of bromocriptine when the CYP3A4 inhibitor is initiated, or decreased effects when it is discontinued; adjust bromocriptine dose as necessary.
Inducers of CYP3A4 (e.g., carbamazepine, dexamethasone, phenobarbital, phenytoin, primidone, rifampin)	Possible decreased bromocriptine serum concentrations	Monitor for decreased therapeutic effect of bromocriptine if CYP3A4 inducer initiated, converse if discontinued; adjust bromocriptine dose as necessary.

Table 3: Bromocriptine

Dose in Adult Patients

Indication	Route	Initial Dose	Dose Titration	Usual Dose	Maximum Dose	Duration of Therapy	Clinical Comment
Hyperprolactinemic Disorders (e.g., amenorrhea, galactorrhea, male hypogonadism, infertility, prolactin-secreting adenomas)	Oral	1.25–2.5 mg daily	Increase by 2.5 mg daily every 3–7 days	2.5–15 mg daily in 2–3 divided doses	Up to 30 mg daily has been used for amenorrhea and/or galactorrhea; for male hypogonadism up to 40 mg daily has been used	Continue until optimal therapeutic response achieved	Because bromocriptine therapy often results in the return of fertility, a barrier contraceptive method should be used until the desired time to conceive.
Acromegaly	Oral	1.25–2.5 mg at bedtime	May increase by 1.25–2.5 mg daily every 3–7 days	20–30 mg daily in 4 divided doses	Usual maximum 30 mg per day	Continue until optimal therapeutic response achieved	Growth hormone level should be measured monthly to assess response to therapy. In patients receiving radiotherapy of the pituitary, bromocriptine therapy should be discontinued on a trial basis for approximately 4–8 weeks annually to assess ongoing need for the drug. If signs/symptoms of acromegaly recur or growth hormone levels rise, resumption of bromocriptine therapy may be considered.
Parkinson's Disease	Oral	1.25 mg twice daily	Increase by 2.5 mg/day every 2–4 weeks as required	15–30 mg/day in 3 divided doses	Usual maximum 30 mg per day		
Restless Legs Syndrome	Oral	7.5 mg at bedtime	N/A	7.5 mg at bedtime	7.5 mg at bedtime		Non-approved use.
Neuroleptic Malignant Syndrome	Oral; nasogastric tube	2.5 mg every 6–8 hours	May increase to 2.5–5 mg 2–6 times per day	2.5–5 mg 2–6 times/day	40 mg/day	Continue for 10 days, then taper slowly	Non-approved use.

Table 4: Bromocriptine

Dose in Pediatric Patients

Indication	Route	Age	Initial Dose	Dose Titration	Usual Dose	Maximum Dose	Duration of Therapy	Clinical Comment
Hyperprolactinemic Disorders	Oral	11–15 y	1.25–2.5 mg daily	Increase by 2.5 mg daily every 3–7 days	2.5–10 mg daily in 2–3 divided doses	Usual maximum 10 mg daily	Continue until optimal therapeutic response achieved	Doses should be taken with food.
	Oral	≥16 y	Refer to adult dosing (see Table 3)					

Drug-Herb Interactions: Though kava should no longer be available in Canada, it should be noted that kava may antagonize the dopaminergic effects of bromocriptine; concomitant administration should be avoided.

DOSAGE AND ADMINISTRATION: Recommended Dose and Dosage Adjustment: Bromocriptine should be taken with food. See Table 3 and Table 4.

Hepatic Impairment: Although no specific guidelines are established, dosage adjustment may be necessary in patients with significant hepatic impairment as the drug is almost completely metabolized in the liver.

Renal Impairment: Dosage adjustment is not routinely recommended in patients with renal impairment.

OVERDOSAGE:

> For management of a suspected drug overdose, CPhA recommends that you contact your regional Poison Control Centre. See the *CPS* Directory section for a list of Poison Control Centres.

ACTION AND CLINICAL PHARMACOLOGY: Bromocriptine is a semisynthetic ergot alkaloid with dopaminergic properties, exhibiting strong agonist activity at dopamine D2 receptors and a partial agonist effect on dopamine D1 receptors. Bromocriptine's dopaminergic activity is utilized in many clinical settings such as Parkinson's disease, restless legs syndrome and neuroleptic malignant syndrome. Bromocriptine also suppresses growth hormone production and decreases prolactin secretion and is used in the management of many conditions related to hyperprolactinemia in both males and females (see Indications and Clinical Use).

Pharmacokinetics: Bromocriptine is well absorbed following oral administration, and is subject to a high hepatic extraction ratio and first-pass metabolism which results in approximately 6-7% of the original dose reaching the systemic circulation unchanged. Peak plasma concentrations are reached in 1 to 1.5 hours.

Bromocriptine is approximately 90-96% bound to serum albumin. As a substrate of CYP3A4, bromocriptine is almost completely metabolized in the liver to inactive metabolites that are subsequently eliminated through biliary excretion in the feces. The elimination half-life of bromocriptine is approximately 2-8 h.

STORAGE AND STABILITY: Bromocriptine tablets and capsules should be stored in airtight, light-resistant containers at a temperature <25°C.

Budesonide

CPhA Monograph

see *Corticosteroids: Eye Ear Nose*

see *Corticosteroids: Inhaled*

Bugs Bunny™ and friends

multiple vitamins and minerals

Vitamin—Mineral Supplement

Bayer Consumer Care

SUPPLIED: Multiple Vitamins Complete: Each flavored, chewable, shaped tablet contains: vitamin A (as acetate) 480 µg (1600 IU), thiamine (vitamin B_1) (thiamine mononitrate) 1.5 mg, riboflavin (vitamin B_2) (riboflavin) 1.5 mg, vitamin B_6 (pyridoxine hydrochloride) 1 mg, vitamin B_{12} (cyanocobalamin) 3 µg, biotin (biotin) 30 µg, vitamin C (sodium ascorbate) 50 mg, vitamin D (cholecalciferol) 10 µg (400 IU), vitamin E (dl-alpha-tocopheryl acetate) 4.5 mg (10 IU), folate (folic acid) 0.1 mg, niacinamide (niacinamide) 8 mg, pantothenic acid (calcium d-pantothenate) 10 mg, calcium (calcium phosphate dibasic) 160 mg, copper (cupric oxide) 1 mg, iron (ferrous fumarate) 4 mg and phosphorus (calcium phosphate dibasic) 125 mg. Nonmedicinal ingredients: aspartame, butylated hydroxytoluene, carrageenan, citric acid, FD&C Blue # 2, FD&C Red # 3, FD&C Red # 40, FD&C Yellow # 6, flavors (cherry, grape, lemon, orange, raspberry and tutti-frutti), gelatin, glycerides of stearic and palmytic acids, hydrogenated vegetable oil, magnesium stearate, malic acid, monoammonium glycyrrhizinate, pectin, silica gel, sodium aluminosilicate, sodium benzoate, sodium citrate, sorbic acid, sorbitol, soybean oil, starch, stearic acid, sucrose and triglycerides. Bottles of 60.

Buminate

albumin (human), USP

Blood Product—Human Plasma Derivative

Baxter

Date of Preparation: June 18, 2009

SUMMARY PRODUCT INFORMATION:

Route of Administration	Dosage Form/ Strength	Clinically Relevant Nonmedicinal Ingredients
Intravenous	Solution for infusion: 5% and 25%	None of the nonmedicinal ingredients are clinically relevant. The sodium content is 145±15 mEq/L. For a complete listing see Dosage Forms, Composition and Packaging.

DESCRIPTION: BUMINATE 5%, Albumin (Human), 5% Solution and BUMINATE 25%, Albumin (Human), 25% Solution are sterile, nonpyrogenic preparations of albumin in a single dosage form for intravenous administration prepared from human venous plasma using the Cohn-Oncley cold ethanol fractionation process.

Each 100 mL of BUMINATE 5% contains 5 g of albumin.

Each 100 mL of BUMINATE 25% contains 25 g of albumin.

This product is prepared from large pools of human plasma, which may contain the causative agents of hepatitis and other viral diseases (see Warnings and Precautions). The likelihood of the presence of viable hepatitis viruses has been minimized by testing the plasma at three stages for the presence of hepatitis viruses, by fractionation steps with demonstrated virus removal capacity and by heating the product for 10-11 hours at 60°C. This procedure has been shown to be an effective method of inactivating hepatitis virus in albumin solutions even when those solutions were prepared from plasma known to be infective.

BUMINATE 5% and BUMINATE 25% contain no blood group isoagglutinins thereby permitting administration without regard to the recipient's blood group.

INDICATIONS AND CLINICAL USE:

1. Hypovolemia

   Hypovolemia is a possible indication for BUMINATE 5% and BUMINATE 25%. Its effectiveness in reversing hypovolemia depends largely upon its ability to draw interstitial fluid into the circulation. It is most effective with patients who are well hydrated.

   When hypovolemia is long-standing and hypoalbuminemia exists accompanied by adequate hydration or edema, 25% albumin is preferable to 5% protein solutions. However, in the absence of adequate or excessive hydration, 5% protein solutions should be used or 25% Albumin should be diluted with crystalloid.

   Although crystalloid solutions and colloid-containing plasma substitutes can be used in emergency treatment of shock and in other similar conditions where the restoration of blood volume is urgent, Albumin (Human) has a prolonged intravascular half-life. When blood volume deficit is the result of hemorrhage, compatible red blood cells or whole blood should be administered as quickly as possible.

   Recent studies have provided additional information suggesting that the use of albumin neither increases nor decreases mortality, compared to normal saline, when used for treatment of hypovolemic patients.

2. Hypoalbuminemia

   A. General

   Hypoalbuminemia is another possible indication for use of BUMINATE 5% or BUMINATE 25%. Hypoalbuminemia can result from one or more of the following:

   (1) Inadequate production (malnutrition, burns, major injury, infections, etc.)

   (2) Excessive catabolism (burns, major injury, pancreatitis, etc.)

   (3) Loss from the body (hemorrhage, excessive renal excretion, burn exudates, etc.)

   (4) Redistribution within the body (major surgery, various inflammatory conditions, etc.)

   When albumin deficit is the result of excessive protein loss, the effect of administration of albumin will be temporary unless the underlying disorder is reversed. In most cases, increased nutritional replacement of amino acids and/or protein with concurrent treatment of the underlying disorder will restore normal plasma albumin levels more effectively than albumin solutions. Occasionally hypoalbuminemia accompanying severe injuries, infections or pancreatitis cannot be quickly reversed and nutritional supplements may fail to restore serum albumin levels. In these cases, BUMINATE 5% or BUMINATE 25% might be a useful therapeutic adjunct.

B. Burns

An optimum regimen for the use of albumin, electrolytes and fluid in the early treatment of burns has not been established, however, in conjunction with appropriate crystalloid therapy, BUMINATE 5% or BUMINATE 25% may be indicated for treatment of oncotic deficits after the initial 24 hour period following extensive burns and to replace the protein loss which accompanies any severe burn. In severe burns immediate therapy in the first 24 hours must include large volumes of crystalloid solutions.

C. Adult Respiratory Distress Syndrome (ARDS)—BUMINATE 25%—A characteristic of ARDS is a hypoproteinemic state, which may be causally related to the interstitial pulmonary edema. Although uncertainty exists concerning the precise indication of albumin infusion in these patients, if there is a pulmonary overload accompanied by hypoalbuminemia, 25% albumin solution may have a therapeutic effect when used with a diuretic.

D. Nephrosis—BUMINATE 25% may be a useful aid in treating edema in patients with severe nephrosis who are receiving steroids and/or diuretics.

3. Cardiopulmonary Bypass Surgery—BUMINATE 5% or BUMINATE 25% have been recommended prior to or during cardiopulmonary bypass surgery, although no clear data exist indicating its advantage over crystalloid solutions.

There is no valid reason for use of Albumin as an intravenous nutrient.

CONTRAINDICATIONS:

- Albumin administration must not be diluted with water for injections as this may cause hemolysis in recipients. There exists a risk of potentially fatal hemolysis and acute renal failure from inappropriate use of Sterile Water for Injection as a diluent for BUMINATE 5% and BUMINATE 25%.
- Patients with a history of allergic reactions to albumin or to any of the excipients or components of the container (see Dosage Forms, Composition and Packaging).
- Patients with a history of an incompatibility reaction to such preparations (see Adverse Reactions).
- Patients with cardiac failure, pulmonary edema or severe and chronic anemia because of the risk of acute circulatory overload.
- Patients with chronic renal insufficiencies due to the potential for accumulations of aluminum; BUMINATE 5% and BUMINATE 25% have been reported to contain trace amounts of aluminum and accumulations of aluminum in patients with chronic renal insufficiencies have led to toxic manifestations such as hypercalcemia, vitamin D-refractory osteodystrophy, anemia, and severe progressive encephalopathy. Therefore, when large volumes of BUMINATE 5%, Albumin (Human), 5% Solution or BUMINATE 25%, Albumin (Human), 25% Solution are contemplated for administration to such patients, serious consideration of these potential risks relative to the anticipated benefits should be given.

WARNINGS AND PRECAUTIONS:

Serious Warnings and Precautions
- Risk of transmitting infectious agents (see General)
- Must **not** be diluted with water for injection (see General; see also Contraindications and Dosage and Administration)

The physician should discuss the risks and benefits of this product with the patient, before administering to the patient (see General).

General: Because this product is made from human plasma, it may carry a risk of transmitting infectious agents, e.g., viruses and, theoretically, the variant Creutzfeldt-Jakob disease (vCJD) agent. This also applies to unknown or emerging viruses and other pathogens.

The risk of transmitting an infectious agent has been reduced by screening plasma donors for prior exposure to certain viruses, by testing for the presence of certain current virus infections, and by inactivating and/or removing certain viruses. The measures taken are considered effective for enveloped viruses such as HIV, HBV, and HCV, and for the non-enveloped viruses HAV and Parvovirus B19.

Despite these measures, such products could still transmit disease. Based on effective donor screening and product manufacturing processes, the risk for disease transmission is considered extremely remote. No cases of transmission of viral diseases or vCJD have ever been identified for albumin.

All infections thought by a physician to have been possibly transmitted by this product, should be reported by the physician, or other healthcare provider to Baxter Healthcare Corporation at 1-800-423-2862. It is strongly recommended that every time that Albumin (Human) is administered to a patient, the name and batch number of the product are recorded in order to maintain a link between the patient and the batch of the product.

Albumin (Human) solutions must not be diluted with water for injection. There exists a risk of potentially fatal hemolysis and acute renal failure from the inappropriate use of Sterile Water for Injection as a diluent for Albumin (Human). Acceptable diluents include 0.9% sodium chloride or 5% dextrose in water (see Dosage and Administration).

Certain components used in the packaging of this product contain natural latex.

Cardiovascular: Hemodynamics: Do not administer without very close monitoring of hemodynamics; look for evidence of cardiac or respiratory failure, renal failure, or increasing intra-cranial pressure.

Hypervolemia/Hemodilution: Albumin (Human) should be used with caution in conditions where hypervolemia and its consequences or hemodilution could represent a special risk for the patient. Examples of such conditions are:

- Decompensated cardiac insufficiency
- Hypertension
- Esophageal varices
- Pulmonary edema
- Hemorrhagic diathesis
- Compensated severe chronic anemia
- Severe anemia
- Renal and post-renal failure
- Brain edema

The rate of administration should be adjusted according to the solution concentration and the patient's hemodynamic measurements (see Dosage and Administration). Rapid administration might cause circulatory overload and pulmonary edema. At the first clinical signs of cardiovascular overload (increased respiratory rate, laboured breathing, tachycardia, rales on auscultation of the lungs, headache, dyspnea, jugular vein congestion), or increased blood pressure, raised central venous pressure and pulmonary edema, the infusion is to be stopped immediately and patient's hemodynamic parameters carefully monitored.

When BUMINATE 5% is used following injuries or surgery, the quick rise in blood pressure which follows administration makes it necessary to monitor the patient to detect and treat severed blood vessels that may not have bled at a lower blood pressure. Patients should always be carefully monitored to guard against circulatory overload.

A rise in blood pressure after BUMINATE 25% infusion necessitates careful observation of the injured or post-operative patient in order to detect and treat severed blood vessels that may not have bled at a lower blood pressure.

Immune: Suspicion of allergic or anaphylactic type reactions requires immediate discontinuation of the injection. In case of shock, standard medical treatment for shock should be implemented.

Renal: Not recommended for administration to dialysis patients.

Use with caution in patients with renal and post-renal failure (see Cardiovascular, Hypervolemia/Hemodilution).

Special Populations: Pregnant Women: There are no adequate data from the use of BUMINATE 5% and BUMINATE 25% in pregnant women. Physicians should carefully consider the potential risks and benefits for each specific patient before prescribing Albumin (Human).

Nursing Women: There are no adequate data from the use of BUMINATE 5% or BUMINATE 25% in lactating women. BUMINATE 5% or BUMINATE 25% should only be administered to lactating women if the benefit clearly outweighs any potential risk to the nursing infant.

Pediatrics: The safety and effectiveness of BUMINATE 5% or BUMINATE 25% solution has not been established in pediatric patients, but no risks additional to those seen in adults have been identified when BUMINATE 5% or BUMINATE 25% solution has been administered to these patients.

Buminate Albumin (Human) solutions are not recommended for administration to infants.

Geriatrics: No studies have been conducted to evaluate the safety and effectiveness in the geriatric population.

Monitoring and Laboratory Tests: Large Volumes: If comparatively large volumes are to be replaced, controls of coagulation and hematocrit are necessary. Care must be taken to ensure adequate substitution of other blood constituents (coagulation factors, electrolytes, platelets, and erythrocytes). Appropriate hemodynamic monitoring should be undertaken.

Electrolyte Status: When Albumin (Human) is given, the electrolyte status of the patient should be monitored and appropriate steps taken to restore or maintain the electrolyte balance.

Blood Pressure: A rise in blood pressure after Albumin (Human) infusion necessitates careful observation of the injured or post-operative patient in order to detect and treat severed blood vessels that may not have bled at a lower blood pressure.

ADVERSE REACTIONS: Adverse Drug Reaction Overview: There are no data available on adverse reactions from controlled clinical trials conducted with BUMINATE 5% or BUMINATE 25%.

Post-Market Adverse Drug Reactions: The following adverse reactions have been reported in the post-marketing experience. These reactions are listed by MedDRA System Organ Class (SOC), then by Preferred Term in order of severity.

Immune System Disorders: anaphylactic shock, anaphylactic reactions, hypersensitivity/allergic reactions.

Nervous System Disorders: headache.

Cardiac Disorders: tachycardia.

Vascular Disorders: hypotension, flushing.

Respiratory, Thoracic, and Mediastinal Disorders: dyspnea.

Gastrointestinal Disorders: vomiting, nausea, dysguesia.

Skin and Subcutaneous Tissue Disorders: urticaria, rash, pruritus.

General Disorders and Administration Site Conditions: pyrexia, chills.

DRUG INTERACTIONS: No interaction studies have been performed with Albumin (Human).*

DOSAGE AND ADMINISTRATION: Dosing Considerations:

- Dosage must be individualized.
- Solution must be administered intravenously.
- Albumin (Human) solutions should not be mixed with other medicinal products including blood and blood components, but can be used concomitantly with other parenterals such as whole blood, plasma, saline, dextrose or sodium lactate when deemed medically necessary.
- Albumin (Human) solutions should not be mixed with protein hydrolysates or solutions containing alcohol since these combinations may cause the proteins to precipitate.
- Do not add supplementary medication.
- Patient should receive adequate hydration.
- Monitor the patient and adjust the dosage and rate of infusion to the patient's circulatory situation to guard against circulatory overload and hypervolemia.
- Ensure adequate substitution of other blood constituents (coagulation factors, electrolytes, platelets and erythrocytes), if large volumes are to be replaced.
- Monitor hemodynamic performance regularly; this may include:
  - arterial blood pressure and pulse rate
  - central venous pressure
  - pulmonary artery wedge pressure
  - urine output
  - electrolyte
  - hematocrit/hemoglobin
- BUMINATE 5% may be administered rapidly to individuals with reduced plasma volume except if patient has a history of cardiac or circulatory disease (should be administered slowly at 5 to 10 mL per minute to avoid too rapid a rise in the blood pressure).
- BUMINATE 25% must be administered intravenously at a rate not to exceed 1 mL/min to patients with normal blood volume. More rapid administration might cause circulatory overload and pulmonary edema.
- BUMINATE 5% and BUMINATE 25% solutions must not be diluted with water for injection as this may cause hemolysis in recipients. (See Contraindications.)

Recommended Dose and Dosage Adjustment: The concentration of the albumin preparation, dosage and the infusion-rate should be adjusted to the patient's individual requirements. The dose required depends on the size of the patient, the severity of trauma or illness and on continuing fluid and protein losses.

Measures of adequacy of circulating volume and not plasma albumin levels should be used to determine the dose required.

The quantity of BUMINATE 5% given may be increased to a total of 1.0 g albumin per kilogram of body weight (i.e. 20 mL per kilogram), but administration should be monitored by careful observation of the patient.

The addition of four volumes of normal saline or 5% dextrose to 1 volume of BUMINATE 25% gives a solution, which is approximately isotonic and isosmotic with citrated plasma.

In the absence of active hemorrhage, the total dose of BUMINATE 25% should not exceed the normal circulating albumin mass, i.e. 2 grams per kg body weight.

1. **Hypovolemia/Hypovolemic Shock**

For patients with significant plasma volume deficits, albumin replacement is best administered in the form of BUMINATE 5%.

The initial dose of BUMINATE 5% administered should be 250 to 500 mL for older children and adults and 12 to 20 mL per kilogram of body weight for young children. It may be repeated after 30 minutes intervals if the response is not adequate.

For BUMINATE 25%, as a guideline, the initial treatment should be in the range of 100 to 200 mL for adults and 2.5 to 5 mL per kilogram body weight for children. This may be repeated after 15 to 30 minutes, if the response is not adequate.

Upon administration of additional albumin or if hemorrhage has occurred, hemodilution and a relative anemia will follow. This condition should be controlled by the supplemental administration of compatible red blood cells or compatible whole blood.

2. **Burns**

The optimal therapeutic regimen for administration of crystalloid and colloid solutions after extensive burns has not been established.

When BUMINATE 5% is administered after the first 24 hours following burns, an initial dose of 500 mL is recommended.

When BUMINATE 25% is administered after the first 24 hours following burns, the dose should be determined according to the patient's condition and response to treatment.

3. **Hypoalbuminemia**

Hypoalbuminemia is usually accompanied by a hidden extravascular albumin deficiency of equal magnitude. This total body albumin deficit must be considered when determining the amount of albumin necessary to reverse the hypoalbuminemia.

Administration: Do not use unless solution is clear of particulate matter and seal is intact. BUMINATE 5% and BUMINATE 25% are a transparent or slightly opalescent solutions that may have a greenish tint or may vary from a pale straw to an amber color. Parenteral drug products should be inspected visually for particulate matter and discoloration prior to administration, whenever solution and container permit.

This product must not be used after the expiry date given on the label.

Do not use if turbid.

1. Remove cap from bottle to expose center portion of rubber stopper.
2. Clean stopper with germicidal solution.

Follow directions for use printed on the administration set container. Make certain that the administration set contains an adequate filter (15-micron or smaller).

Do not begin administration more than 4 hours after the container has been entered.

Discard unused portion.

OVERDOSAGE:

Hypervolemia may occur if the dosage and rate of infusion are too high. (See Warnings and Precautions, Cardiovascular.)

For management of a suspected drug overdose, CPhA recommends that you contact your **regional Poison Control Centre**. See the *CPS* Directory section for a list of Poison Control Centres.

ACTION AND CLINICAL PHARMACOLOGY: Mechanism of Action: Albumin is responsible for 70-80% of the colloid osmotic pressure of normal plasma, thus making it useful in regulating the volume of circulating blood. Albumin is also a transport protein and binds naturally occurring, therapeutic and toxic materials in the circulation.

Pharmacodynamics: BUMINATE 5% is osmotically equivalent to an equal volume of normal human plasma and will increase circulating plasma volume by an amount approximately equal to the volume infused.

* None known based upon the absence of data from clinical trials, literature searches, and safety reports.

BUMINATE 25% is osmotically equivalent to approximately five times its volume of human plasma. When injected intravenously, 25% albumin will draw about 3.5 times its volume of additional fluid into the circulation within 15 minutes, except when the patient is markedly dehydrated. This extra fluid reduces hemoconcentration and blood viscosity.

Pharmacokinetics: Total body albumin is estimated to be 350 g for a 70 kg man and is distributed throughout the extracellular compartments; more than 60% is located in the extravascular fluid compartment. The half-life of albumin is 15 to 20 days with a turnover of approximately 15 g per day.

The minimum plasma albumin level necessary to prevent or reverse peripheral edema is unknown. Some investigators recommend that plasma albumin levels be maintained at approximately 2.5 g/dL. This concentration provides a plasma oncotic value of 20 mm Hg.

Duration of Effect: The degree and duration of volume expansion depends upon the initial blood volume. With patients treated for diminished blood volume, the effect of infused albumin may persist for many hours; however, in patients with normal volume, the duration will be shorter.

STORAGE AND STABILITY: Store at room temperature, not to exceed 30°C. Avoid freezing to prevent damage to the bottle.

Stability testing for BUMINATE 25% showed that aluminum concentration increased over time reaching levels that could exceed 1000 ppb over the shelf life of the product. (See Contraindications.)

INFORMATION FOR THE PATIENT: Published in e-CPS, available by subscription at www.e-cps.ca.

DOSAGE FORMS, COMPOSITION AND PACKAGING: 5%: BUMINATE 5% is a transparent or slightly opalescent solution, which may have a greenish tint or may vary from a pale straw to an amber colour. The solution has been adjusted to physiological pH with sodium bicarbonate and/or sodium hydroxide. BUMINATE 5% is stabilized with N-acetyltryptophan (0.004 M) and sodium caprylate (0.004 M). The sodium content is 145±15 mEq/L. The solution contains no preservative and none of the coagulation factors found in fresh whole blood or plasma. Bottles of 250 and 500 mL containing 12.5 or 25.0 g of albumin respectively.

25%: BUMINATE 25% is a transparent or slightly opalescent solution, which may have a greenish tint or may vary from a pale straw to an amber colour. The solution has been adjusted to physiological pH with sodium bicarbonate and/or sodium hydroxide. BUMINATE 25% is stabilized with N-acetyltryptophan (0.02 M) and sodium caprylate (0.02 M). The sodium content is 145±15 mEq/L. The solution contains no preservative and none of the coagulation factors found in fresh whole blood or plasma. Bottles of 20, 50, and 100 mL containing 5.0, 12.5 or 25.0 g of albumin, respectively.

Buprenorphine Ⓝ

CPhA Monograph

see *Opioids*

Burinex® Ⓟ

bumetanide

Diuretic

LEO Pharma

PHARMACOLOGY: Bumetanide is a loop diuretic. The diuretic effect of bumetanide results largely from the inhibition of sodium reabsorption in the ascending limb of the loop of Henle. This is shown by a marked reduction in freewater clearance during hydration and tubular solute-free water reabsorption during hydropenia.

Bumetanide may have an additional action in the proximal tubule, since phosphaturia has been observed during bumetanide induced diuresis and the renal clearance of bumetanide is decreased by probenecid. The proximal tubular activity does not seem to be related to an inhibition of carbonic anhydrase. Potassium excretion is increased by bumetanide in a dose-related fashion.

Following oral administration to normal subjects, bumetanide is rapidly and almost completely (>80%) absorbed from the gastrointestinal tract. The time to reach peak blood levels is 0.5 to 2 hours. Plasma protein binding of bumetanide is approximately 95%.

Bumetanide is rapidly eliminated, the plasma half-life being 1.5 hours. The majority (approx. 80%) of an oral dose of bumetanide is recovered in the urine (about 60% of this as unchanged bumetanide, the remainder as metabolites).

After oral administration of 1 mg of bumetanide diuresis begins within 30 minutes with a peak effect between 1 and 2 hours. Diuresis is nearly completed after 3 to 4 hours.

Pharmacological and clinical studies have shown that 1 mg bumetanide produces a diuretic response similar to that of approximately 40 mg furosemide.

INDICATIONS: For the treatment of edema associated with congestive heart failure, cirrhosis of the liver and renal disease including the nephrotic syndrome.

CONTRAINDICATIONS: In patients who are anuric, in hepatic coma and in states of severe electrolyte depletion until the condition is improved or corrected. Bumetanide is contraindicated in patients hypersensitive to bumetanide and other sulfonamide derivatives.

WARNINGS:

> Bumetanide is a potent diuretic which, if given in excessive amounts, can lead to profound diuresis with water and electrolyte depletion. Therefore, careful medical supervision is required and dose and dosage schedule have to be adjusted to the individual patient's needs (see Dosage).

The dose of bumetanide should be adjusted to patient's need. Excessive doses or too frequent administration can lead to profound water loss, electrolyte depletion, dehydration, reduction in blood volume and circulatory collapse with a possibility of vascular thrombosis and embolism, particularly in elderly patients.

Hypokalemia can occur as a consequence of bumetanide administration. Prevention of hypokalemia requires particular attention in the following conditions: patients receiving digitalis and diuretics for congestive heart failure, hepatic cirrhosis and ascites, states of aldosterone excess with normal renal function, potassium-losing nephropathy, certain diarrheal states, or other states where hypokalemia is thought to represent particular added risks to the patient, (i.e., history of ventricular arrhythmias).

In patients with hepatic cirrhosis and ascites, sudden alterations of electrolyte balance may precipitate hepatic encephalopathy and coma.

Serum electrolyte determination should be performed frequently.

Ototoxicity: In cats, dogs and guinea pigs, bumetanide has been shown to produce ototoxicity. In these test animals bumetanide was 5 to 6 times more potent than furosemide and, since the diuretic potency of bumetanide is about 40 to 60 times greater, it is anticipated that blood levels necessary to produce ototoxicity will rarely be achieved. The potential exists, however, and must be considered a risk particularly with therapy at high doses, repeated frequently in the face of renal excretory function impairment. Potentiation of aminoglycoside ototoxicity has not been tested for bumetanide. Like other members of this class of diuretics, bumetanide probably shares this risk.

Patients allergic to sulfonamides may show hypersensitivity to bumetanide.

PRECAUTIONS: Serum potassium should be measured periodically and potassium supplements or potassium sparing diuretics may be required especially when high doses are used for prolonged periods. Particular caution with potassium concentration is necessary in patients receiving digitalis glycosides or potassium depleting steroids. Periodic determination of other electrolytes are also advised, particularly in patients on low salt diets.

It may be advisable to hospitalize patients with hepatic cirrhosis and ascites prior to initiating therapy. Sudden alterations of fluid and electrolyte balance in patients with cirrhosis may precipitate hepatic encephalopathy and coma; therefore, strict observation is necessary during the period of diuresis. Supplemental potassium chloride and, if required, an aldosterone antagonist are helpful in preventing hypokalemia and metabolic alkalosis.

It is essential to replace electrolyte losses and to maintain fluid balance so as to avoid any risk of electrolyte depletion, hypovolemia or hypotension.

Since rigid sodium restriction is conducive to both hyponatremia and hypokalemia, such restriction is not advisable in patients on bumetanide therapy.

Bumetanide may increase urinary calcium excretion with resultant hypocalcemia.

Reversible elevation of BUN and creatinine may occur, especially in association with dehydration and in patients with renal insufficiency. Marked increases in BUN and creatinine or the development of oliguria during treatment of patients with progressive renal disease is an indication for discontinuation.

Hyperuricemia may occur; it has been asymptomatic in cases reported to date.

Studies in normal subjects receiving bumetanide revealed no adverse effects on glucose tolerance, plasma insulin, glucagon and growth hormone levels but the possibility of an effect on glucose metabolism exists. Periodic determinations of blood sugar should be done, particularly in patients with diabetes or suspected of latent diabetes.

Patients under treatment should be observed regularly for possible occurrence of blood dyscrasias, liver damage, or idiosyncratic reactions which have been reported rarely in foreign marketing experience.

Drug Interactions: Drugs with Ototoxic Potential: Bumetanide may, in view of its ototoxic potential, enhance the ototoxic effect of aminoglycosides and simultaneous administration should generally be avoided especially in patients with impaired renal function.

Drugs with Nephrotoxic Potential: There has been no experience on the concurrent use of bumetanide with drugs known to have nephrotoxic potential. Simultaneous administration of these drugs should be avoided.

Cardiac Glycosides: Low serum potassium levels can occur as a consequence of bumetanide administration. Hypokalemia may increase the sensitivity of the myocardium to the toxic effects of digitalis. Thus correction of the hypokalemic state is required and the dose may need adjustment.

Lithium: Lithium should generally not be given with diuretics such as bumetanide. Concurrent administration of diuretics such as bumetanide and lithium may reduce lithium clearance. Adjustment of lithium dosage may be necessary. To minimize potential lithium toxicity close clinical observation and more frequent determination of serum lithium are required.

Probenecid: Pretreatment with probenecid reduces both the natriuresis and hyperreninemia produced by bumetanide. This antagonistic effect of probenecid on bumetanide natriuresis is not due to a direct action on sodium excretion but is probably secondary to its inhibitory effect on renal tubular secretion of bumetanide. Thus, probenecid should not be administered concurrently with bumetanide.

Indomethacin: Indomethacin blunts the increases in urine volume and sodium excretion seen during bumetanide treatment and inhibits the bumetanide-induced increase in plasma renin activity. Concurrent therapy with bumetanide is thus not recommended.

Antihypertensives: Bumetanide may potentiate the effect of antihypertensive drugs. Therefore, the dose of the latter may need adjustment when bumetanide is used to treat edema in hypertensive patients.

Pregnancy: Bumetanide is neither teratogenic nor embryotoxic in mice when given in doses up to 3 400 times the maximum human therapeutic dose.

Bumetanide has been shown to be nonteratogenic, but it has a slight embryotoxic effect in rats when given in oral doses of 100 mg/kg/day and in rabbits at doses of 0.1 mg/kg/day. In one study, moderate growth retardation and increased incidence of delayed ossification of sternebrae were observed in rats at oral doses of 100 mg/kg/day. These effects were associated with maternal weight reduction during dosing. No such adverse effects were observed at 30 mg/kg/day.

In rabbits, a dose-related decrease in litter size and an increase in resorption rate were noted at oral doses of 0.1 and 0.3 mg/kg/day. A slightly increased incidence of delayed ossification of sternebrae occurred at 0.3 mg/kg/day; however, no effects were seen at 0.03 mg/kg/day. The sensitivity of the rabbit to bumetanide parallels the marked pharmacologic and toxicologic effects of the drug in this species.

Bumetanide was not teratogenic in the hamster at an oral dose of 0.5 mg/kg/day.

There are no studies in pregnant women. Bumetanide should be given to a pregnant woman only if the potential benefit justifies the potential risk to the fetus.

Lactation: Since bumetanide passes into the breast milk, the drug should not be given to nursing mothers.

Children: The safety and effectiveness of bumetanide in the pediatric age group below the age of 18 have not been established.

ADVERSE EFFECTS: The most frequent clinical adverse reactions observed with bumetanide are muscle cramps (1.1%), dizziness (1.1%), hypotension (0.8%), headache (0.6%), nausea (0.6%), and encephalopathy (in patients with preexisting liver disease) (0.6%). One or more of these adverse reactions have been reported in approximately 4.1% of bumetanide-treated patients.

Less frequent clinical adverse reactions to bumetanide are impaired hearing (0.5%), pruritus (0.4%), ECG changes (0.4%), weakness (0.2%), hives (0.2%), abdominal pain (0.2%), arthritic pain (0.2%), musculoskeletal pain (0.2%), rash (0.2%), and vomiting (0.2%). One or more of these adverse reactions have been reported in approximately 2.9% of bumetanide-treated patients.

Other clinical adverse reactions, which have each occurred in approximately 0.1% of patients, are vertigo, chest pain, ear discomfort, fatigue, dehydration, sweating, hyperventilation, dry mouth, upset stomach, renal failure, asterixis, itching, nipple tenderness, diarrhea, premature ejaculation and difficulty maintaining an erection.

Laboratory abnormalities reported have included hyperuricemia (18.4%), hypochloremia (14.9%), hypokalemia (14.7%), azotemia (10.6%), hyponatremia (9.2%), increased serum creatinine (7.4%), hyperglycemia (6.6%), and variations in phosphorus (4.5%), CO_2 content (4.3%), bicarbonate (3.1%) and calcium (2.4%). Although manifestations of the pharmacologic action of bumetanide, these conditions may become more pronounced by intensive therapy.

Diuresis induced by bumetanide may also rarely be accompanied by changes in LDH (1.0%), total serum bilirubin (0.8%), serum proteins (0.7%), AST (0.6%), ALT (0.5%), alkaline phosphatase (0.4%), cholesterol (0.4%) and creatinine clearance (0.3%). Also reported have been thrombocytopenia (0.2%), deviations in hemoglobin (0.8%), prothrombin time (0.8%), hematocrit (0.6%), WBC (0.3%), platelet counts (0.2%) and differential counts (0.1%). Increases in urinary glucose (0.7%) and urinary protein (0.3%) have also been seen.

OVERDOSE:

Symptoms: Profound water loss and electrolyte depletion, dehydration, reduction of blood volume and circulatory collapse with a possibility of vascular thrombosis and embolism. Electrolyte depletion may be manifested by weakness, dizziness, mental confusion, anorexia, lethargy, vomiting and cramps.

Treatment: Discontinue the drug. Institute water and electrolyte replacement with careful monitoring of urine and electrolyte output and serum electrolyte levels.

> For management of a suspected drug overdose, CPhA recommends that you contact your **regional Poison Control Centre**. See the *CPS* Directory section for a list of Poison Control Centres.

DOSAGE: Dosage should be individualized with careful monitoring of patient response.

The usual total oral daily dosage is 0.5 to 2.0 mg and in most patients may be given as a single dose.

If the diuretic response to an initial 1 mg dose is not adequate, a second or third dose may be given at 4 to 5 hour intervals. The maximum recommended daily dose is 10 mg.

An intermittent dose schedule, whereby bumetanide is given on alternate days or for 3 to 4 days with rest periods of 1 to 2 days in between is recommended as the safest and most effective method for the continued control of edema.

In patients with hepatic failure the dosage should be kept to a minimum, and if necessary, dosage increased very carefully. A maintenance dose as low as 0.5 mg daily should be considered and the daily dose should not exceed 5 mg (see Warnings).

SUPPLIED: 1 mg: Each 8 mm, white, circular, scored tablet, marked 133 and with an Assyrian lion on the other side, contains: bumetanide 1 mg. Nonmedicinal ingredients: agar, colloidal anhydrous silica, lactose, magnesium stearate, maize starch, polysorbate 80, polyvidone and talc. Blister packs of 30 (3 packs of 10 tablets each). Store at room temperature (15-25°C) protected from light and high humidity.

5 mg: Each 10 mm, white, circular, tablet, marked with a score line and 5 mg on one face, contains: bumetanide 5 mg. Nonmedicinal ingredients: agar, colloidal anhydrous silica, lactose, magnesium stearate, maize starch, polysorbate 80, polyvidone and talc. Blister packs of 30 (3 packs of 10 tablets each). Store at room temperature (15-25°C) protected from light and high humidity.

(Shown in Product Identification Section)

Buro-Sol® Otic Solution

aluminum acetate—benzethonium chloride

Antipruritic—Astringent

Stiefel, a GSK company

SUPPLIED: Each bottle contains: aluminum acetate 0.5% and benzethonium chloride 0.03% in a dilute acetic acid solution. Plastic bottles with ear dropper of 15 and 60 mL.

Buro-Sol® Powder

aluminum acetate—benzethonium chloride

Antipruritic—Astringent

Stiefel, a GSK company

SUPPLIED: Each 2.36 g powder packet dissolved in 450 mL water produces: a clear aluminum acetate solution 0.35% USP (1:15 Burow's Solution) with benzethonium chloride 0.023% stable for 90 days at room temperature kept in a glass or rigid plastic container. Boxes of 10.

Buscopan®

hyoscine butylbromide

Antispasmodic

Boehringer Ingelheim

Date of Revision: April 30, 2008

SUMMARY PRODUCT INFORMATION:

Route of Administration	Dosage Form/ Strength	Clinically Relevant Nonmedicinal Ingredients
Oral	Tablets, 10 mg	acacia, carnauba wax, castor oil, lactose, magnesium stearate, maize starch, sucrose, polyethylene glycol, shellac, talc, tartaric acid, titanium dioxide, and white wax
Parenteral	Ampoules, 20 mg/mL	sodium chloride and water for injection

INDICATIONS AND CLINICAL USE: BUSCOPAN (hyoscine butylbromide) tablets are indicated for:

- The relief of smooth muscle spasm of the gastrointestinal and genitourinary systems.

BUSCOPAN ampoules are indicated for:

- The relief of acute genitourinary or gastrointestinal spasm (e.g., renal or biliary colic), or to produce smooth muscle relaxation prior to radiological procedures such as pyelography or other diagnostic procedures where spasm may be a problem (e.g., gastro-duodenal endoscopy).

Geriatrics: No data is available.
Pediatrics: No data is available.

CONTRAINDICATIONS:

- Hypersensitivity to hyoscine butylbromide, or atropinics (see Warnings and Precautions) or to any of the product excipients (see Dosage Forms, Composition and Packaging).
- BUSCOPAN (hyoscine butylbromide) tablets are contraindicated in patients with myasthenia gravis, megacolon, glaucoma or obstructive prostatic hypertrophy.
- Parenteral administration is contraindicated in patients with myasthenia gravis, untreated narrow angle glaucoma, prostatic hypertrophy with urinary retention, stenotic lesions of the gastrointestinal tract, tachycardia, angina, cardiac failure and megacolon.
- BUSCOPAN ampoules should not be given by intramuscular injection to patients being treated with anticoagulant drugs since intramuscular haematoma may occur. In these patients, the subcutaneous or intravenous routes may be used.

WARNINGS AND PRECAUTIONS: General: Therapy should be discontinued if the patient reports any unusual visual disturbances or pressure pain within the eye.

Patients intolerant of one belladonna alkaloid or derivative may also be intolerant of other belladonna alkaloids or derivatives such as hyoscine butylbromide.

After parenteral administration of BUSCOPAN, cases of anaphylaxis, including episodes of shock have been observed. As with all drugs causing such reactions, patients receiving BUSCOPAN by injection should be kept under observation.

BUSCOPAN (hyoscine butylbromide) tablets and ampoules should be used with caution in patients with prostatic enlargement. BUSCOPAN may precipitate or aggravate urinary retention in patients with the following conditions: nonobstructive prostatic hypertrophy, urinary retention (or the predisposition to) or obstructive uropathy such as a bladder neck obstruction due to prostatic hypertrophy (see Contraindications). In addition, exercise caution in patients inclined to tachyarrhythmia.

One sugar-coated tablet of 10 mg contains 41.2 mg sucrose, resulting in 411.8 mg sucrose per maximum recommended daily dose. Patients with the rare hereditary condition of fructose intolerance should not take this medicine.

Cardiovascular: As large doses of anticholinergics/systemic antispasmodics may cause an increase in heart rate, due care is necessary in patients with cardiac disease, especially cardiac arrhythmias, congestive heart failure, coronary artery disease and mitral stenosis. The increase in heart rate may also be undesirable in patients with unstable cardiovascular status in an acute hemorrhage situation.

Gastrointestinal: Exercise caution in patients with reflux esophagitis or gastrointestinal tract obstructive disease (i.e., achalasia and pyloroduodenal stenosis) due to the ability of anticholinergics/systemic antispasmodics to decrease smooth muscle motility and tone resulting in gastric retention.

Anticholinergics may aggravate hiatal hernia associated with reflux esophagitis, myasthenia gravis or pyloric obstruction.

In patients with ulcerative colitis, large anticholinergic doses may suppress intestinal motility, possibly causing paralytic ileus or resulting in obstruction; also, use may precipitate or aggravate toxic megacolon.

Ophthalmologic: The parenteral administration of hyoscine butylbromide, particularly of higher doses, has been reported to cause transient disturbances of accommodation which recede spontaneously. Therefore, patients should be cautioned about potential visual problems and the need to exercise care while driving or operating machinery after receiving BUSCOPAN ampoules.

The mydriatic effect of anticholinergics/systemic antispasmodics may result in increased intraocular pressure. BUSCOPAN should be used with caution in patients with angle-closure glaucoma or with this predisposition, as anticholinergics/systemic antispasmodics may precipitate an acute angle-closure glaucoma attack (see Contraindications).

Patients should seek urgent ophthalmological advice in case they should develop a painful eye with loss of vision after injection of BUSCOPAN.

Special Populations: Pregnant Women: Safety during pregnancy has not yet been established. Limited preclinical data has not indicated a hazard; nevertheless, the usual precautions regarding the use of drugs during pregnancy, especially during the first trimester, should be observed.

Nursing Women: Safety during lactation has not been established. No specific studies have been conducted on the excretion of this drug in breast milk. The benefits of hyoscine butylbromide use during lactation should therefore be weighed against possible effects on the infant.

Pediatrics: BUSCOPAN is not currently recommended for use in children.

Geriatrics: Geriatric patients are especially susceptible to the anticholinergic side effects of constipation, dryness of mouth and urinary retention (especially in males). If these side effects continue or are severe, discontinuation of medication should be considered.

Due care is necessary when anticholinergics are administered to geriatric patients due to the danger of precipitating undiagnosed glaucoma.

Administration of anticholinergics/systemic antispasmodics to elderly patients with intestinal atony or in debilitated patients may result in obstruction.

ADVERSE REACTIONS: Adverse Drug Reaction Overview: Many of the listed undesirable effects can be assigned to the anticholinergic properties of BUSCOPAN. Anticholinergic side effects of BUSCOPAN are generally mild and self-limited.

Accumulated clinical and postmarketing experience indicates that the following adverse reactions can be expected with the use of BUSCOPAN Ampoules and Tablets: xerostomia (dry mouth), dyshidrosis, visual accomodation disorders, tachycardia, dyspnea, and urinary retention.

There have been rare reports of dizziness, blood pressure decreased and flushing.

Skin reactions and other hypersensitivity, angioedema and fixed drug eruptions have been reported rarely.

There have been very rare reports of anaphylactic reactions and anaphylactic shock including fatal outcome.

Adverse events reported during therapy with BUSCOPAN include increased pulse rate, diarrhea, nausea, retinal pigmentation, and glaucoma.

DRUG INTERACTIONS: Overview: As hyoscine butylbromide can reduce the motility and secretory activity of the gastrointestinal system, the systemic absorption and pharmacologic effects of other oral medications may be delayed.

Drug-Drug Interactions:

Table 1: BUSCOPAN

Established or Potential Drug-Drug Interactions

Hyoscine Butylbromide	Effect	Clinical comment
Tricyclic antidepressants	Can potentiate the anticholinergic effect of parenterally administered hyoscine butylbromide.	
Antihistamines	Can potentiate the anticholinergic effect of parenterally administered hyoscine butylbromide.	
Quinidine	Can potentiate the anticholinergic effect of parenterally administered hyoscine butylbromide.	
Disopyramide	Can potentiate the anticholinergic effect of parenterally administered hyoscine butylbromide.	
Amantadine	Can potentiate the anticholinergic effect of parenterally administered hyoscine butylbromide.	
MAO inhibitors	May result in intensified anticholinergic side effects of hyoscine butylbromide. Also, may block detoxification of anticholinergics thus potentiating their action.	
Anticholinergics	May intensify anticholinergic effects. May increase the severity of potassium chloride induced gastrointestinal lesions.	
Dopamine antagonists such as metoclopramide.	May result in diminution of the effects of both drugs on the gastrointestinal tract.	
Beta-adrenergic agents	May enhanced tachycardic effects.	
Antacids or adsorbent antidiarrheals	May reduce the absorption of anticholinergics, resulting in decreased therapeutic effectiveness.	Anticholinergics such as hyoscine butylbromide should be given at least one hour before these medications.

Drug-Food Interactions: Interactions with food have not been established.
Drug-Herb Interactions: Interactions with herbs have not been established.
Drug-Laboratory Test Interactions: Interactions with laboratory tests have not been established.

DOSAGE AND ADMINISTRATION: Dosing Considerations: Individual response to BUSCOPAN (hyoscine butylbromide) may vary and doses should be adjusted accordingly.

Recommended Dose and Dosage Adjustment: Tablets: One to two 10 mg tablets per day up to a maximum of 6 tablets per day. In prolonged illness which requires repeated dosing, 1 tablet 3 to 5 times a day is recommended.

Ampoules: One half (10 mg/0.5 mL) to one ampoule (20 mg/1 mL) administered parenterally by intramuscular, subcutaneous, or intravenous routes, at an injection rate of 1 mL/min. No dilution of the ampoule is necessary prior to administration. The maximum dose should not exceed 100 mg/day (5 ampoules).

Missed Dose: In case a dose has been missed, take the next dose as scheduled. Do not double the dose.

Administration: Tablets should be swallowed whole with a glass of water.

The rapid action of injected BUSCOPAN is advantageous in acutely ill patients and in those situations where prompt spasmolytic activity facilitates diagnostic procedures such as radiological examinations. BUSCOPAN ampoules may also be used intramuscularly 10-15 minutes before radiological examinations of the stomach to slow peristaltic movements.

Dilution and Stability of Parenteral BUSCOPAN: Although dilution prior to administration is not required, BUSCOPAN solution is compatible with the following solutions, should dilution be desirable: Ringers Solution, Ringers Lactate, NaCl 0.9%, Laevulose 5%, Glucose 10%.

Solutions must be mixed under sterile conditions and are stable for 8 hours.

OVERDOSAGE:

Symptoms: Single oral doses of up to 590 mg and quantities of active drug up to 1090 mg within 5 hours have produced dry mouth, tachycardia, slight drowsiness and transient visual disorders. Other symptoms include urinary retention, reddening of the skin, and inhibition of gastrointestinal motility.

Other symptoms which occurred in animals and which may be encountered in humans include: shock, Cheyne-Stokes respiration, respiratory paralysis, clonic spasms, paresis of the striated muscle, coma, paralytic ileus and cystoparalysis.

Treatment: In the case of an oral overdose, perform gastric lavage with activated charcoal followed by magnesium sulfate (15%). BUSCOPAN overdose symptoms respond to parasympathomimetics.

For patients with glaucoma, administer pilocarpine locally. If necessary, parasympathomimetics should be administered, e.g. neostigmine 0.5-2.5 mg i.m. or i.v. Cardiovascular complications should be treated according to usual therapeutic principles. In case of respiratory paralysis: intubation, artificial respiration.

Catheterisation may be required for urinary retention.

Other overdosage symptoms should be treated with standard supportive therapy.

For management of a suspected drug overdose, CPhA recommends that you contact your **regional Poison Control Centre**. See the *CPS* Directory section for a list of Poison Control Centres.

ACTION AND CLINICAL PHARMACOLOGY: Mechanism of Action: BUSCOPAN (hyoscine butylbromide) is an antispasmodic agent which relaxes the smooth muscle of the gastrointestinal, biliary and urinary tracts. It is believed to act predominantly at the parasympathetic ganglia in the walls of the viscera of these organs. Structurally, BUSCOPAN exists as a quaternary ammonium compound and as a single positively charged cation throughout the entire pH range.

Pharmacokinetics: Absorption: BUSCOPAN undergoes rapid tissue absorption after oral administration. In the rat, it concentrates in the gastrointestinal tract, liver and kidney tissues.

Distribution: The high tissue affinity of the substance is further reflected in the extremely short distribution half-life ($t_{1/2\alpha}$) in the plasma of approximately 2-3 minutes. Despite low systemic bioavailability, hyoscine butylbromide remains available in high concentrations at the site of action. Plasma levels of radioactivity in man peak within 3 hours of enteral administration.

Metabolism: Protein binding in the human plasma occurs at 8-13% and in a 4.4% human serum albumin solution at 3-11%. Hyoscine butylbromide does not readily cross the blood brain barrier.

Excretion: A high portion of the absorbed hyoscine butylbromide (^{14}C) undergoes elimination in an unchanged form within the first few hours of administration in man and animals. Later in elimination, the metabolized portion predominates. In man, following the administration of intravenous ^{14}C-labelled substance, the elimination followed a three-phase course: $t_{1/2\alpha}$=3.5 min., $t_{1/2\beta}$=0.8 hours; $t_{1/2}$=14.0 hours. Following oral administration, the terminal elimination half-life is 4.8 hours. Metabolites from rat urine detected in quantities ranging from 4 to 44% include three main metabolites (phenyl acetic acid-scopine ester-butochloride, 4-hydroxytropic acid-scopine ester-butochloride, scopine butobromide) and four minor metabolites (including AD 12 and Ba 790).

STORAGE AND STABILITY: BUSCOPAN tablets and ampoules should be protected from light and heat. BUSCOPAN ampoules should be protected from freezing. Products should be stored at room temperature and are stable up to the expiration date indicated on the label.

INFORMATION FOR THE PATIENT: Published in e-CPS, available by subscription at www.e-cps.ca.

DOSAGE FORMS, COMPOSITION AND PACKAGING: Ampuls: Each mL contains: hyoscine butylbromide 20 mg. Nonmedicinal ingredients: sodium chloride and water for injection. Sodium: <1 mmol (<10 mg)/dose. Ampuls of 1 mL. Packages of 10. **Tablets:** Each round, white, sugar-coated tablet contains: hyoscine butylbromide 10 mg. Nonmedicinal ingredients: acacia, carnauba wax, castor oil, lactose, magnesium stearate, maize starch, polyethylene glycol, shellac, sucrose, talc, tartaric acid, titanium dioxide, and white wax. Bottles of 100 and 500.

(Shown in Product Identification Section)

Butalbital Ⓒ

CPhA Monograph

see *Barbiturates*

Butorphanol Ⓝ

CPhA Monograph

see *Opioids*

BuTrans® 5 Ⓝ

buprenorphine

Opioid Analgesic

Purdue Pharma

BuTrans® 10 Ⓝ

buprenorphine

Opioid Analgesic

Purdue Pharma

BuTrans® 20 Ⓝ

buprenorphine

Opioid Analgesic

Purdue Pharma

Date of Preparation: February 5, 2010
Date of Revision: July 19, 2010

SUMMARY PRODUCT INFORMATION:

Route of Administration	Dosage Form/Strength	Nonmedicinal Ingredients
Transdermal	Patch Three strengths with 5, 10 and 20 mg buprenorphine per patch, delivering 5, 10 and 20 µg/h buprenorphine respectively for 7 days	Aluminum acetylacetonate, levulinic acid, oleyl oleate, polyacrylate, polyethylene terephthalate, povidone.

INDICATIONS AND CLINICAL USE: Adults: BuTrans (buprenorphine transdermal patch) is indicated for:

- the management of persistent pain of moderate intensity in adults requiring continuous opioid analgesia for an extended period of time.

Geriatrics (>65 years of age): In elderly patients, BuTrans may have altered pharmacokinetics due to poor fat stores, muscle wasting or altered clearance (see Dosage and Administration). Therefore, it may be appropriate, according to clinical judgment, to initiate these patients on the lowest available BuTrans strength with dose titration to achieve satisfactory pain relief with acceptable side effects.

Pediatrics (<18 years of age): The safety and efficacy of BuTrans has not been studied in the pediatric population. Therefore, use of BuTrans is not indicated in patients under 18 years of age.

CONTRAINDICATIONS: BuTrans (buprenorphine transdermal patch) is contraindicated in:

- Patients who are hypersensitive to this drug or to any ingredient in the formulation or component of the container. For a complete listing of excipients, see Dosage Forms, Composition and Packaging;
- Patients who have ileus of any type;
- Patients with suspected surgical abdomen (e.g., acute appendicitis or pancreatitis);
- Patients with mild, intermittent or short duration pain that can otherwise be managed;
- The management of acute pain, including use in out-patient or day surgeries;
- The management of peri-operative pain (see Warnings and Precautions, Peri-Operative Considerations);
- Patients with acute asthma or other obstructive airway, and status asthmaticus;
- Patients with acute respiratory depression, elevated carbon dioxide levels in the blood, and cor pulmonale;
- Patients with acute alcoholism or alcohol dependence, delirium tremens, and convulsive disorders;
- Patients with severe CNS depression, increased cerebrospinal or intracranial pressure, and head injury;
- Patients taking monoamine oxidase (MAO) inhibitors (or within 14 days of such therapy);
- Women during pregnancy, labour and delivery or breast-feeding;
- Opioid dependent patients and for narcotic withdrawal treatment;
- Patients suffering from myasthenia gravis;
- Patients who have severe hepatic insufficiency.

WARNINGS AND PRECAUTIONS: General: BuTrans (buprenorphine transdermal patch) should ONLY be prescribed to patients who require continuous opioids for pain management. Initiation doses higher than the 5 mg patch should not be used in opioid naïve patients (see Dosage and Administration, Patients Not Already Taking Opioids (Opioid-Naïve)).

BuTrans is not indicated for use in children under 18 years of age, as dosage requirements for the safe and efficacious use of BuTrans have not been established for this patient population.

BuTrans should only be prescribed by persons knowledgeable in the continuous administration of potent opioids, in the management of patients receiving potent opioids for treatment of pain, and in the detection and management of respiratory depression including the use of opioid antagonists.

Since serum buprenorphine concentrations decline gradually after patch removal (approximately 50% in 12 hours [range 10-24 h]), patients who have experienced serious adverse events should be monitored for at least 24 hours after BuTrans removal or until the adverse reaction has subsided.

Due to the formation of a subcutaneous depot of buprenorphine, not only does continued exposure occur after patch removal but, in the case of removal prior to attainment of peak buprenorphine exposure, buprenorphine plasma levels may continue to increase after removal of BuTrans patches.

As with other CNS depressants, patients who have received BuTrans should be monitored especially for signs of respiratory depression until a stable maintenance dose is reached.

BuTrans patches are intended for transdermal use on intact skin only; use on compromised skin can lead to increased exposure to buprenorphine.

Placing BuTrans in the mouth, chewing it, swallowing it, or using it in any way other than indicated may cause choking or overdose that could result in death.

Patients should be cautioned not to consume alcohol while using BuTrans as it may increase the chance of experiencing dangerous side effects.

Risk of Unintentional Increase of Drug Exposure: Patients with Fever: A pharmacokinetic study showed no alteration of buprenorphine plasma concentrations in subjects with mild fever induced by endotoxin administration. However, because increased blood flow to the skin may enhance absorption, patients with severe febrile illness should be monitored for side effects and may require dose adjustment.

Application of External Heat: While wearing the BuTrans transdermal patch, patients should be advised to avoid exposing the BuTrans site to external heat sources, such as heating pads, electric blankets, heated water beds, heat or tanning lamps, hot water bottles, hot baths, saunas, hot whirlpool spa baths and sunbathing, as an increase in absorption of buprenorphine may occur and result in serious medical consequences.

Accidental Exposure to BuTrans: Serious medical consequences, including death, may occur if people are accidentally exposed to buprenorphine transdermal patch. Examples of accidental exposure include transfer of a buprenorphine transdermal patch while hugging, sharing a bed, or moving a patient.

Acute Abdominal Conditions: As with other µ-opioid receptor agonists, the administration of BuTrans may obscure the diagnosis or clinical course in patients with acute abdominal conditions.

Cardiovascular: Hypotensive Effects: BuTrans should be administered with caution to patients at risk for hypotension. Buprenorphine, like other opioids, may cause severe hypotension in patients with depleted blood volume or after agents acting on vasomotor tone such as phenothiazines or general anesthetics. Patients receiving BuTrans as their first around-the-clock opioid may be at increased risk of hypotension or orthostatic syncope, similar to that seen with other opioids.

Concomitant Use of CYP3A4 Inhibitors: The concomitant use of BuTrans with cytochrome P450 3A4 inhibitors such as ritonavir, ketoconazole, itraconazole, troleandomycin, clarithromycin, nelfinavir, nefazodone, verapamil, diltiazem, amiodarone, amprenavir, fosamprenavir, aprepitant, fluconazole, erythromycin and grapefruit juice may result in an increase in buprenorphine plasma concentrations, which could increase dose related toxicity, including potential fatal respiratory depression. In this situation, special patient care and observation is appropriate (see Drug Interactions).

Concomitant Use of CYP3A4 Inducers: The interaction between buprenorphine and CYP3A4 enzyme inducers has not been studied. Co-administration of BuTrans and enzyme inducers (e.g., phenobarbital, carbamazepine, phenytoin, and rifampin) could lead to increased clearance which might result in reduced efficacy.

Dependence/Tolerance: BuTrans can produce drug dependence of the opiate type. Diversion of buprenorphine has been reported.

Buprenorphine is a partial µ-opioid agonist. Chronic use of buprenorphine can result in the development of a limited degree of physical dependence. Withdrawal (abstinence syndrome), is generally mild, begins after two days and may last up to two weeks. Reports of physical dependence and withdrawal syndrome with BuTrans treatment are uncommon.

BuTrans should not be prescribed for patients with known physical dependence on other opioids. Due to its antagonist component BuTrans may not substitute for other opioids in such patients. Caution should be exercised when prescribing BuTrans to patients known to have, or suspected of having, problems with other drug or alcohol abuse or serious mental illness.

BuTrans has no approved use in the management of addictive disorders.

All buprenorphine products have some potential for opioid abuse and dependence. However, reports of abuse with BuTrans are uncommon. The development of addiction to opioid analgesics in properly managed patients with pain has been reported to be uncommon, which is consistent with the clinical trial results and post-marketing experience for BuTrans.

Careful record-keeping of prescribing information, including quantity, frequency, and renewal requests is strongly advised. Patients should be advised to properly store and dispose of the product.

Disposal of BuTrans: BuTrans should be kept out of sight and reach of children before and after use.

Upon removal, the used patch should be folded so that the adhesive side of the patch adheres to itself, and then flushed down the toilet immediately or consult with a pharmacist about other disposal options. If the adhesive from the drug accidentally contacts the skin other than the intended application site, the area should be washed with clear water. Patients should dispose of any remaining patches from a prescription as soon as they are no longer needed. Unused patches should be removed from their pouch. The protective liner should be removed and the patch should be folded in half and flushed down the toilet, or consult with a pharmacist about other disposal options (see Dosage and Administration, Safety and Handling).

Hepatic/Biliary/Pancreatic: Because buprenorphine is extensively metabolized by the liver, the activity of BuTrans may be increased and/or extended in those individuals with impaired hepatic function or those receiving other agents known to decrease hepatic clearance. Patients with severe hepatic impairment may accumulate buprenorphine during BuTrans treatment. Consideration of alternate therapy should be given, and BuTrans should not be used in such patients (see Special Populations, Hepatic Impairment).

Buprenorphine has been shown to increase intracholedochal pressure, as do other opioids, and cause spasm of the Sphincter of Oddi and should be used with caution in patients with biliary tract disease, including acute pancreatitis. Opioids may also cause an increase in serum amylase concentration.

Immune: Allergic Reactions: Cases of acute and chronic hypersensitivity to buprenorphine have been reported in clinical trials in other buprenorphine marketed products. The most common signs and symptoms include rashes, hives and pruritus. Cases of bronchospasm, angioneurotic edema and anaphylactic shock have been reported. A history of hypersensitivity to buprenorphine or any component of the formulation is a contraindication to BuTrans use.

Neurologic: Interaction with Other Central Nervous System Depressants: Buprenorphine, like all opioid analgesics, should be dosed with caution in patients who are concurrently taking other CNS depressants that may cause respiratory depression, hypotension, profound sedation, or may potentially result in coma or death. Such agents include alcohol, antihistamines, antipsychotics, benzodiazepines, centrally acting anti-emetics, general anaesthetics, other opioid analgesics, phenothiazines and sedatives or hypnotics. When such combined therapy is contemplated, a substantial reduction in the dose of one or both agents should be considered and patients carefully monitored (see Drug Interactions).

Head Injury and Increased Intracranial Pressure: BuTrans should not be used in patients who may be particularly susceptible to the intracranial effects of CO_2 retention such as those with evidence of increased intracranial pressure, impaired consciousness, shock, or coma. Respiratory depression may be exacerbated in the presence of head injury, intracranial lesions (e.g., space occupying tumours) or increased intracranial pressure. Pupillary responses and effects on consciousness resulting from buprenorphine may mask neurologic signs of increasing intracranial pressure. Opioids may obscure the clinical course of patients with head injury.

Opiate Withdrawal Effects: Buprenorphine is a partial agonist at the µ-opioid receptor and chronic administration produces dependence of the opiate type, characterized by withdrawal upon abrupt discontinuation or rapid taper. The withdrawal syndrome is generally milder than seen with full agonists and may be delayed in onset.

Neonatal Withdrawal: BuTrans is contraindicated in opioid dependent patients, for narcotic withdrawal treatment or in pregnant women (see Contraindications). In France, neonatal withdrawal has been reported in infants of women treated with sublingual buprenorphine for drug-addiction during pregnancy. Time to onset of withdrawal symptoms ranged from Day 1 to Day 8 of life with most occurring on Day 1 (69%). The most commonly-reported manifestations include abnormal crying, agitation, hypertonia, tremor and convulsions. Respiratory depression has occurred in neonates whose mothers had taken high doses, even for a short duration of time in the third trimester.

Peri-Operative Considerations: BuTrans is contraindicated for peri-operative pain relief. In the case of planned chordotomy or other pain-relieving operations, patients should not be treated with BuTrans for at least 48 hours before the operation and BuTrans should not be used in the immediate post-operative period. Thereafter if BuTrans is to be continued after the patient recovers from the post-operative period, a new dosage should be administered in accordance with the changed need for pain relief. The risk of withdrawal in opioid-tolerant patients should be addressed as clinically indicated (see Opiate Withdrawal Effects).

The administration of analgesics in the peri-operative period should be managed by healthcare providers with adequate training and experience (e.g., by an anesthesiologist) (see Contraindications).

Potential for Abuse and Diversion: BuTrans patches contain a large amount of a potent opioid, buprenorphine, which along with other opioids has potential for abuse and associated risk of fatal overdose due to respiratory depression. The high buprenorphine content in BuTrans patches may be a target for abuse and diversion, with alternative routes of administration potentially resulting in overdose due to uncontrolled delivery of the opioid. This risk should be considered when prescribing or dispensing BuTrans in situations where the healthcare professional is concerned about increased risk of misuse, abuse or diversion.

Concerns about abuse, addiction and diversion should not prevent the proper management of pain. Patients should be assessed for their clinical risks for opioid abuse or addiction prior to being prescribed opioids. All patients receiving opioids should be routinely monitored for signs of misuse and abuse.

Since BuTrans may be diverted for non-medical use, careful record keeping of prescribing information, including quantity, frequency, and renewal requests is strongly advised. Proper assessment of the patient, proper prescribing practices, periodic re-evaluation of therapy, and proper dispensing and storage are appropriate measures that help to limit abuse of opioid drugs (see Dependence/Tolerance).

Psychomotor Impairment: Opioid analgesics, including buprenorphine, can have a depressant effect on mental and/or physical responses. Caution must be exercised in activities requiring mental alertness such as driving a car or operating heavy machinery, especially when doses are being adjusted or when other CNS active drugs are being added to the treatment regimen. This impairment may be potentiated by concomitant depressant medications such as other opioids, phenothiazines, alcohol, sedatives, hypnotics, or other CNS depressants. Patients using BuTrans should not drive or operate dangerous machinery unless they are tolerant to the effects of the drug.

Respiratory Depression: As with other potent opioids, clinically significant respiratory depression may occur in patients receiving buprenorphine. Some cases of death due to respiratory depression have been reported, particularly when addicts have intravenously abused buprenorphine, usually in combination with benzodiazepines, or with concomitant administration of buprenorphine with other depressants such as alcohol or other opioids. Opioids, including buprenorphine, should be used with caution in patients with compromised respiratory function (e.g., chronic obstructive pulmonary disease, cor pulmonale, decreased respiratory reserve, hypoxia, hypercapnia or pre-existing respiratory depression), in the elderly and in debilitated patients. Particular caution is advised if BuTrans is to be administered to patients taking, or recently receiving, drugs with CNS/respiratory depressant effects.

IN THE CASE OF OVERDOSE, THE PRIMARY MANAGEMENT SHOULD BE THE REESTABLISHMENT OF ADEQUATE VENTILATION WITH MECHANICAL ASSISTANCE OF RESPIRATION, IF REQUIRED. NALOXONE MAY NOT BE EFFECTIVE IN REVERSING ANY RESPIRATORY DEPRESSION PRODUCED BY BUPRENORPHINE (SEE Overdosage).

Respiratory depression is a risk of starting opioid agonist medications, especially in elderly, debilitated patients. Respiratory depression usually follows large initial doses in non-tolerant patients, or when opioids are given in conjunction with other agents that depress respiration.

Although BuTrans is a partial opioid agonist, buprenorphine may cause hypoventilation at analgesic doses, especially in patients who have an underlying pulmonary condition or who receive usual doses of opioids or other CNS drugs associated with hypoventilation in addition to BuTrans (see Drug Interactions regarding the use of concomitant CNS active drugs).

Comparative effects of BuTrans have not been evaluated, but in clinical trials (up to doses of BuTrans 40 µg/hr), respiratory failure was reported as a rare adverse event (i.e., <0.1%, but at least in more than 1 patient [see Adverse Reactions]).

If respiratory depression from BuTrans occurs, it may persist beyond the removal of the patch. Patients with hypoventilation should be observed for at least several hours and until their respiratory rate has recovered.

In patients with respiratory depression, symptomatic treatment following standard intensive care measures should be instituted (see Overdosage).

Use in Patients with Chronic Pulmonary Disease: Buprenorphine should be used with caution in patients with chronic pulmonary disease, patients with decreased respiratory reserve and others with potentially compromised respiration. Normal analgesic doses of opioids may further decrease respiratory drive in these patients to the point of respiratory failure.

Patient Counselling Information: A patient information sheet is included in the package of BuTrans patches dispensed to the patient.

Patients receiving BuTrans patches should be given the following instructions by the physician:

1. Patients should be informed that accidental ingestion or use by individuals (including children) other than the patient for whom it was originally prescribed, may lead to severe, even fatal, consequences.
2. Patients should be advised that BuTrans patches contain buprenorphine, an opioid pain medicine.
3. Patients should be advised that each BuTrans patch may be worn continuously for 7 days, and that each patch should be applied to a different skin site after removal of the previous transdermal patch.
4. Patients should be advised that the application sites should be rotated whenever a patch is replaced. After the patch is removed, a 3-week interval is required before the same site can be re-used as a strategy to prevent skin irritation and/or reduce the potential for increased drug absorption.
5. Patients should be advised that BuTrans patches should be applied to intact, non-irritated and non-irradiated skin on a flat surface such as the upper chest, upper back, side of chest, or upper outer arm. Additionally, patients should be advised of the following:
   - If BuTrans is part of an overall strategy to suitably manage pain in patients with cognitive impairment, the potential of each patient to remove the patch(es) and place them in the mouth or on others should be considered when recommending rotation sites;
   - Hair at the application site should be clipped (not shaved) prior to patch application;
   - If the site of BuTrans application must be cleansed prior to application of the patch, do so with clear water;
   - Allow the skin to dry completely prior to patch application;
   - Do not use soaps, oils, lotions, alcohol, or any other agents that may irritate the skin or alter its characteristics.
6. Patients should be advised that BuTrans should be applied immediately upon removal from the sealed package and after removal of the protective liner.

   Additionally, patients should be advised of the following:
   - The BuTrans patch should not be used if the seal is broken, or if it is altered, cut, or damaged in any way prior to application. The transdermal patch should be pressed firmly in place with the palm of the hand for 30 seconds, making sure the contact is complete, especially around the edges;
   - The patch should **not** be folded.
7. Patients should be advised that while wearing the patch, they should avoid exposing the BuTrans application site to direct external heat sources, such as:
   - heating pads;
   - electric blankets;
   - heat lamps;
   - saunas;
   - hot tubs;
   - heated water beds.
8. Patients should be advised that there is a potential for temperature-dependent increase in buprenorphine release from the patch that could result in an overdose of buprenorphine. If patients develop a high fever while wearing the patch they should contact their physician.
9. Patients should be advised that if they experience problems with adhesion of the BuTrans patch, they may tape the edges of the patch with first aid tape.
10. Patients should be advised that if the patch falls off before 7 days a new patch may be applied to a different skin site.
11. When BuTrans is no longer needed (used or unused), patients should be advised to fold the patch (so that the adhesive side adheres to itself) and immediately flush it down the toilet, or consult with a pharmacist about other disposal options.
12. Patients should be instructed that, if the drug adhesive layer accidentally contacts the skin other than the intended application site, the area should be washed clean with clear water and not soap, alcohol, or other chemicals, because these products may increase the ability of buprenorphine to go through the skin.
13. Patients should be advised that the dose of BuTrans should **never** be adjusted without the prescribing health care professional's instruction.
14. Patients should be advised that BuTrans may impair mental and/or physical ability required for the performance of potentially hazardous tasks (e.g., driving, operating machinery).
15. Patients should be advised to refrain from any potentially dangerous activity when initially starting on BuTrans or when their dose is being adjusted, until it is established that they have not been adversely affected.
16. Patients should be advised that BuTrans should not be combined with alcohol or other centrally acting agents, such as: sleep medications, tranquilizers, sedatives and hypnotics because dangerous additive effects may occur, resulting in serious injury or death.
17. Patients should be advised to consult their physician or pharmacist if other medications are being, or will be, used with BuTrans.
18. Patients should be advised of the potential for severe constipation.
19. Patients should be advised that if they have been receiving treatment with BuTrans and cessation of therapy is indicated, it may be appropriate to taper the BuTrans dose, rather than abruptly discontinue it, due to the risk of precipitating withdrawal symptoms. Withdrawal symptoms are generally milder than seen with full agonists, and begin after two days and may last up to two weeks.
20. Patients should be advised that BuTrans contains buprenorphine, a drug with a potential for abuse.
21. Patients, family members and caregivers should be advised to protect BuTrans from theft or misuse in the work or home environment.
22. Patients should be advised that BuTrans should never be given to anyone other than the individual for whom it was prescribed because of the risk of death or other serious medical problems to that person, for whom it was not intended.
23. Patients should be instructed to keep BuTrans in a secure place out of sight and reach of children due to the risk of **fatal respiratory depression**.
24. Women of childbearing potential who become or are planning to become pregnant should be advised to consult a physician prior to initiating or continuing therapy with BuTrans.
25. Patients should be informed that, if the patch dislodges and accidentally sticks to the skin of another person, they should immediately take the patch off, wash the exposed area with water (and not soap, alcohol, or other chemicals, because these products may increase the ability of buprenorphine to go through the skin) and seek immediate medical attention for the accidentally exposed individual.

Special Populations: Special Risk Groups: Use of BuTrans, like all opioid analgesics, is associated with increased potential risks and should be used only with caution in the following conditions: adrenocortical insufficiency (e.g., Addison's disease); CNS depression or coma; high-risk debilitated patients; myxedema or hypothyroidism; prostatic hypertrophy or urethral stricture and toxic psychosis.

The administration of buprenorphine, like other opioid analgesics, may obscure the diagnosis or clinical course in patients with acute abdominal conditions. Buprenorphine may aggravate convulsions in patients with convulsive disorders and may induce or aggravate seizures in some clinical settings.

Pregnant Women: There are no data from the use of BuTrans in pregnant women. Rodent studies with some opioids, including buprenorphine, have indicated the possibility of embryotoxic effects. In humans, it is not known whether buprenorphine can cause fetal harm when administered during pregnancy or can affect reproductive capacity. Towards the end of pregnancy high oral doses of buprenorphine may induce respiratory depression in the neonate even after a short period of administration. Long-term administration of buprenorphine during the last three months of pregnancy may cause a withdrawal syndrome in the neonate. Buprenorphine crosses the placental barrier. BuTrans should not be used during pregnancy or in women of childbearing potential who are not using effective contraception.

Labour and Delivery: The safety of BuTrans given during labour and delivery has not been established.

Nursing Women: Buprenorphine has been detected in low concentrations in human milk, thus nursing mothers treated with BuTrans should not breast-feed or the use of BuTrans during lactation should be avoided.

Gender: No differences in plasma buprenorphine concentrations were detected between males and females treated with BuTrans.

Geriatrics (>65 years of age): The pharmacokinetic profile of BuTrans is similar in healthy elderly and younger adult subjects. Elderly subjects trended toward higher plasma concentrations of buprenorphine immediately after removal of BuTrans. In a pharmacokinetic study in healthy volunteers, mean plasma concentrations changed from 88.11 pg/mL at the time of patch removal at steady state to a peak of 90.77 pg/mL one hour after patch removal in younger adults (n=12). By three hours after patch removal, mean plasma levels had declined to less than 88.11 pg/mL (i.e., 73.76 pg/mL). Mean plasma concentrations in healthy elderly adults (n=12) changed from 90.68 pg/mL at patch removal to a peak of 99.56 pg/mL 12 hours after patch removal. By 18 hours after patch removal, mean plasma concentrations had declined to less than 90.68 pg/mL (i.e., 84.18 pg/mL) in healthy elderly adults. Both groups subsequently eliminated buprenorphine at similar rates.

In a safety study evaluating the recommended dose-escalation schedule, the pharmacokinetics in healthy elderly were similar to healthy younger adults.

Pediatrics (<18 years of age): BuTrans has not been studied in children and is not indicated for patients less than 18 years of age. The safety and efficacy of BuTrans in children have not been established.

Renal Impairment: A pharmacokinetic study showed that pharmacokinetic parameters for buprenorphine were similar in patients with severe renal impairment compared with normal adults. This study confirmed with multiple-dose use, that the accumulation of buprenorphine metabolites did not decrease the clearance of the parent molecule in chronic use. Therefore, no special dose adjustment of buprenorphine is necessary in patients with renal impairment.

Hepatic Impairment: In a pharmacokinetic study utilizing intravenous buprenorphine, there were no differences in clearance of buprenorphine between mild to moderate hepatically impaired subjects relative to healthy adult subjects. These data show no need for dosage adjustment when using BuTrans in patients with mild to moderate hepatic impairment.

Patients with severe hepatic impairment may accumulate buprenorphine during BuTrans treatment. Consideration of alternate therapy should be given, and BuTrans should not be used in such patients.

ADVERSE REACTIONS: Adverse Drug Reaction Overview: Serious adverse drug reactions which may be associated with BuTrans (buprenorphine transdermal patch) therapy in clinical use are those observed with other opioid analgesics, including respiratory depression (especially when used with other CNS depressants) and hypotension. Care must be exercised when using BuTrans in patients who are using benzodiazepines or other agents with CNS activity.

The adverse drug reactions seen on initiation of therapy with BuTrans in clinical studies are those often observed with other opioid analgesics (nausea, vomiting, dizziness, somnolence, constipation, pruritus and dry mouth). The frequency of these events depends on the dose, the clinical setting, the patient's level of opioid tolerance, and factors specific to the individual. They should be expected and managed as part of opioid analgesic therapy.

The most common adverse effects in six randomized titration-to-effect placebo-controlled clinical trials with BuTrans were anorexia, application site erythema, application site pruritus, asthenia, constipation, dizziness, dry mouth, headache, hyperhidrosis, insomnia, nausea, somnolence and vomiting. Opioid-agonist related adverse events tend to reduce over time, except for constipation.

A summary of adverse events for the randomized parallel-design titration-to-effect placebo controlled clinical trials occurring at an incidence of ≥1% is provided in Table 1. A summary of adverse events for the randomized crossover-design titration-to-effect placebo controlled clinical trials occurring at an incidence of ≥1% is provided in Table 2. A summary of adverse events, occurring at an incidence of ≥1% in a clinical trial in patients shown to be tolerant and responsive to a BuTrans (5-20 µg/h) patch during a run-in period of 3 weeks maximum, prior to randomization is provided in Table 3. Table 1, Table 2 and Table 3 include all events which occurred more frequently with active treatment than with placebo, whether considered by the clinical investigator to be related to the study drug or not. A summary of the less common clinical trial adverse events follows these Tables.

Clinical Trial Adverse Drug Reactions: Because clinical trials are conducted under very specific conditions the adverse reaction rates observed in the clinical trials may not reflect the rates observed in practice and should not be compared to the rates in the clinical trials of another drug. Adverse drug reaction information from clinical trials is useful for identifying drug-related adverse events and for approximating rates.

The stated frequencies of adverse events represent the proportion of individuals who experienced at least once, a treatment-emergent adverse event regardless of causality. An event was considered treatment emergent if it occurred for the first time or worsened while receiving therapy following baseline evaluation.

Table 1: BuTrans

Adverse Events ≥1% for Parallel-Design Titration-to-Effect Clinical Trials (BP96-0604, BP99-0203, BP98-1201, BUP3002)

SOC MedDRA Preferred Term	BuTrans (N=392)	Placebo (N=261)
Ear and Labyrinth Disorders		
Tinnitus	1.3	0.4
Eye Disorders		
Vision blurred	1.5	0.4
Gastrointestinal Disorders		
Constipation	13.5	5.4
Diarrhea	3.1	1.9
Dry mouth	7.1	1.5

(cont'd)

Table 1: BuTrans *(cont'd)*

Adverse Events ≥1% for Parallel-Design Titration-to-Effect Clinical Trials (BP96-0604, BP99-0203, BP98-1201, BUP3002)

SOC MedDRA Preferred Term	BuTrans (N=392)	Placebo (N=261)
Nausea	22.7	7.7
Stomach discomfort	2.0	1.1
Vomiting	11.2	1.5
General Disorders and Administration Site Conditions		
Application site erythema	7.1	1.5
Application site pain	1.5	0.8
Application site pruritus	15.1	11.9
Application site vesicles	1.0	0.0
Asthenia	1.3	1.1
Fatigue	5.1	1.1
Pain	1.5	1.5
Peripheral edema	7.4	3.4
Pyrexia	1.5	0.4
Infections and Infestations		
Influenza	1.3	0.4
Sinusitis	1.0	0.4
Urinary tract infection	2.6	2.3
Injury, Poisoning and Procedural Complications		
Fall	3.8	1.5
Skin Laceration	1.3	1.1
Investigations		
Blood pressure increased	1.0	0.4
Metabolism and Nutrition Disorders		
Anorexia	2.0	0.8
Musculoskeletal and Connective Tissue Disorders		
Arthralgia	2.0	1.9
Back pain	2.6	1.5
Joint swelling	2.6	0.8
Muscle spasms	1.3	0.8
Muscular weakness	1.0	0.4
Pain in extremity	2.8	2.3
Nervous System Disorders		
Dizziness	16.3	7.7
Headache	16.1	11.5
Hypoesthesia	2.3	0.8
Migraine	1.0	0.8
Paraesthesia	2.0	0.8
Tremor	2.0	0.4
Somnolence	13.5	4.6
Psychiatric Disorders		
Agitation	1.0	0.0
Anxiety	1.8	0.8
Depression	1.3	0.8
Disorientation	1.0	0.4
Insomnia	2.8	1.9
Nervousness	1.0	0.4
Respiratory, Thoracic and Mediastinal Disorders		

(cont'd)

Table 1: BuTrans *(cont'd)*

Adverse Events ≥1% for Parallel-Design Titration-to-Effect Clinical Trials (BP96-0604, BP99-0203, BP98-1201, BUP3002)

SOC MedDRA Preferred Term	BuTrans (N=392)	Placebo (N=261)
Cough	1.3	0.4
Dyspnea	2.8	1.1
Skin and Subcutaneous Tissue Disorders		
Hyperhidrosis	4.3	1.1
Pruritus	4.1	0.8
Pruritus generalized	1.5	0.8
Rash	2.0	1.1

Table 2: BuTrans

Adverse Events ≥1% for Crossover-Design Titration-to-Effect Clinical Trials (020-006 and 020-007)

SOC MedDRA Preferred Term	BuTrans (N=146)	Placebo (N=133)
Cardiac Disorders		
Palpitations	3.4	0.8
Ear and Labyrinth Disorders		
Tinnitus	1.4	0.0
Vertigo	1.4	0.0
Gastrointestinal Disorders		
Abdominal pain upper	3.4	2.3
Constipation	21.9	13.5
Dry mouth	10.3	1.5
Gastroesophageal reflux disease	1.4	0.0
Nausea	45.9	18.0
Vomiting	18.5	4.5
General Disorders and Administration Site Conditions		
Application site bruising	1.4	0.0
Application site pain	2.1	1.5
Application site pruritus	25.3	24.8
Application site rash	3.4	3.0
Asthenia	12.3	8.3
Fatigue	9.6	3.0
Influenza-like illness	2.1	0.0
Peripheral edema	8.9	0.8
Immune System Disorders		
Urticaria	1.4	0.0
Infections and Infestations		
Influenza	2.1	1.5
Urinary tract infection	2.1	0.8
Metabolism and Nutrition Disorders		
Anorexia	13.0	11.3
Musculoskeletal and Connective Tissue Disorders		
Musculoskeletal stiffness	1.4	0.8
Myalgia	2.1	0.0
Nervous System Disorders		
Dizziness	27.4	6.0
Headache	11.6	6.0
Migraine	2.7	1.5
Paraesthesia	1.4	0.8

(cont'd)

Table 2: BuTrans *(cont'd)*

Adverse Events ≥1% for Crossover-Design Titration-to-Effect Clinical Trials (020-006 and 020-007)

SOC MedDRA Preferred Term	BuTrans (N=146)	Placebo (N=133)
Somnolence	24.0	6.0
Tremor	4.1	2.3
Psychiatric Disorders		
Agitation	2.7	1.5
Anxiety	2.1	0.8
Nightmare	1.4	0.8
Skin and Subcutaneous Tissue Disorders		
Erythema	1.4	0.0
Hyperhidrosis	16.4	9.0
Pruritus	1.4	0.8
Surgical and Medical Procedures		
Endodontic procedure	1.4	0.0
Vascular Disorders		
Hot flush	4.1	1.5

In clinical trials in which BuTrans was compared to active controls, expected opioid effects (nausea, vomiting, dry mouth, pruritus, dizziness, somnolence), on initiation of therapy in non-tolerant individuals, reached their maximum 1-2 days after BuTrans application and usually decreased with continued use.

Less Common Clinical Trial Adverse Drug Reactions: Untoward events associated with the exposure were recorded by clinical investigators using terminology of their own choosing. Consequently, it is not possible to provide a meaningful estimate of the proportion of individuals experiencing adverse events without first grouping similar types of untoward events into a smaller number of standardized event categories.

Reported adverse events were classified using the Medical Dictionary for Regulatory Activities, version 10.0.

The events listed below present treatment emergent adverse events reported during the clinical development program of buprenorphine in a total of 5561 patients in the Phase 3 controlled and open-label clinical trials. Excluded from this list are those events already listed in Table 1, Table 2 and Table 3.

Table 3: BuTrans

Adverse Events ≥1% for Patients shown to be Tolerant and Responsive to a BuTrans (5-20 µg/h) Patch during a Run-in Period of 3 Weeks Maximum, Prior to Randomization (Study BUP3012)

SOC MedDRA Preferred Term	BuTrans (N=164)	Placebo (N=162)
Gastrointestinal Disorders		
Abdominal pain	1.2	0.0
Constipation	7.1	5.2
Diarrhea	1.5	1.5
Dry mouth	2.8	2.1
Nausea	8.9	8.9
Vomiting	2.1	0.9
General Disorders and Administration Site Conditions		
Application site erythema	3.1	1.5
Application site pruritus	4.6	3.4
Application site rash	2.1	0.6
Fatigue	2.5	1.5
Peripheral edema	3.4	0.6
Infections and Infestations		
Urinary tract infection	1.2	0.3
Musculoskeletal and Connective Tissue Disorders		
Back pain	2.5	2.1
Pain in extremity	1.2	1.2
Nervous System Disorders		
Dizziness	6.1	3.7
Psychiatric Disorders		
Anxiety	1.2	0.3

It is important to emphasize that, although the events reported occurred during treatment with buprenorphine, they were not necessarily caused by it. The events are categorized by body system and listed according to the following criteria: frequent: adverse events that occurred on one or more occasions in at least 1/100 patients; infrequent: adverse events that occurred in less than 1/100 patients but at least in 1/1000 patients; and rare: adverse events that occurred in less than 1/1000, but in at least more than 1 patient.

Blood and Lymphatic System Disorders: Infrequent: anemia, lymphadenopathy. Rare: leukocytosis.

Cardiac Disorders: Infrequent: angina pectoris, atrial fibrillation, bradycardia, cardiac failure congestive, myocardial infarction, tachycardia. Rare: acute coronary syndrome, acute myocardial infarction, angina unstable, arrhythmia, atrioventricular block first degree, bundle branch block left, cardiac flutter, cardiomegaly, coronary artery disease, extrasystoles, sinus bradycardia, supraventricular extrasystoles, ventricular extrasystoles.

Ear and Labyrinth Disorders: Infrequent: cerumen impaction, ear pain. Rare: ear discomfort, ear haemorrhage, inner ear disorder, middle ear effusion, otorrhoea, tympanic membrane hyperaemia.

Endocrine Disorders: Rare: hyperthyroidism, hypothyroidism.

Eye Disorders: Infrequent: cataract, conjunctivitis, dry eye, eye pruritus, eye swelling, vision blurred. Rare: asthenopia, blepharospasm, conjunctival haemorrhage, diplopia, eye disorder, eye irritation, eye pain, eyelid irritation, lacrimation increased, lenticular opacities, miosis, myopia, ocular hyperaemia, photopsia, visual acuity reduced, visual disturbance.

Gastrointestinal Disorders: Frequent: dyspepsia. Infrequent: abdominal discomfort, abdominal distension, abdominal pain lower, colonic polyp, dental caries, dysphagia, flatulence, food poisoning, gastric ulcer, gastritis, haemorrhoids, lip swelling, oral pain, rectal haemorrhage, toothache. Rare: abdominal haematoma, abdominal hernia, abdominal mass, abdominal tenderness, colitis, Crohn's disease, diverticulum, eructation, faeces discoloured, faeces hard, frequent bowel movements, gastrointestinal haemorrhage, gastrointestinal pain, gingival pain, haematochezia, haemorrhoidal haemorrhage, hiatus hernia, hypoaesthesia oral, inguinal hernia, intestinal obstruction, irritable bowel syndrome, mouth ulceration, oesophageal spasm, oral discomfort, oral mucosal blistering, pancreatitis, paraesthesia oral, peptic ulcer, retching, stomatitis, swollen tongue, tooth disorder, umbilical hernia.

General Disorders and Administration Site Conditions: Frequent: application site irritation, chest pain. Infrequent: application site dermatitis, application site discharge, application site discolouration, application site dryness, application site excoriation, application site exfoliation, application site inflammation, application site oedema, application site papules, application site paraesthesia, application site reaction, application site scab, application site swelling, chest discomfort, chills, drug withdrawal syndrome, energy increased, feeling abnormal, feeling hot, feeling jittery, gait disturbance, irritability, malaise, oedema, thirst. Rare: application site anaesthesia, application site bleeding, application site hypersensitivity, application site induration, application site odour, application site perspiration, application site urticaria, application site warmth, axillary pain, cyst, discomfort, face oedema, facial pain, feeling cold, feeling hot and cold, feeling of relaxation, generalised oedema, hernia, hunger, inadequate analgesia, inflammation, inflammatory pain, local swelling, lower extremity mass, pitting oedema, pre-existing condition improved, sensation of pressure, sluggishness, swelling, temperature intolerance, therapeutic response unexpected.

Hepatobiliary Disorders: Rare: cholecystitis, cholecystitis acute, cholelithiasis, gallbladder disorder.

Immune System Disorders: Infrequent: hypersensitivity, seasonal allergy. Rare: drug hypersensitivity, urticaria.

Infections and Infestations: Frequent: bronchitis, nasopharyngitis, upper respiratory tract infection. Infrequent: application site pustules, cellulitis, cystitis, diverticulitis, ear infection, eye infection, folliculitis, fungal infection, gastroenteritis, gastroenteritis viral, herpes zoster, kidney infection, laryngitis, localised infection, lower respiratory tract infection, oral herpes, otitis media, pharyngitis, pharyngitis streptococcal, pneumonia, tooth abscess, tooth infection, viral infection. Rare: abscess, application site cellulitis, application site infection, body tinea, fungal skin infection, furuncle, gingival infection, Helicobacter infection, Herpes simplex, infected sebaceous cyst, labyrinthitis, lobar pneumonia, mastoiditis, onychomycosis, oral candidiasis, oral fungal infection, osteomyelitis, otitis externa, respiratory tract infection, rhinitis, sepsis, skin candida, Staphylococcal infection, tinea pedis, tonsillitis, vaginal candidiasis, vaginal infection, viral upper respiratory tract infection, vulvovaginal mycotic infection, vulvovaginitis, wound infection.

Injury, Poisoning and Procedural Complications: Infrequent: arthropod bite, back injury, contusion, excoriation, foot fracture, injury, joint dislocation, joint injury, joint sprain, limb injury, muscle strain, procedural pain, road traffic accident, thermal burn. Rare: accident, animal bite, arthropod sting, bite, concussion, corneal abrasion, epicondylitis, eye injury, facial bones fracture, foreign body in eye, hand fracture, head injury, hip fracture, laceration, ligament rupture, lower limb fracture, medical device site reaction, meniscus lesion, mouth injury, neck injury, rib fracture, scratch, skeletal injury, sunburn, tooth fracture, upper limb fracture, whiplash injury, wrist fracture.

Investigations: Infrequent: alanine aminotransferase increased, aspartate aminotransferase increased, blood creatinine increased, blood glucose increased, blood potassium decreased, blood potassium increased, blood sodium decreased, blood triglycerides increased, blood urea increased, blood uric acid increased, blood urine present, body temperature increased, cardiac murmur, glucose urine present, haematocrit decreased, haemoglobin decreased, heart rate increased, liver function test abnormal, weight decreased, weight increased, white blood cell count increased. Rare: blood alkaline phosphatase increased, blood bilirubin increased, blood chloride decreased, blood cholesterol increased, blood glucose decreased, blood lactate dehydrogenase increased, blood pressure decreased, blood pressure diastolic increased, blood thyroid stimulating hormone, body temperature fluctuation, breath sounds abnormal, carbon dioxide decreased, electrocardiogram QT corrected interval, electrocardiogram T wave abnormal, eosinophil count decreased, gamma-glutamyltransferase increased, gastric pH decreased, haemoglobin increased, heart rate irregular, *H. pylori* identification, hepatic enzyme increased, lymphocyte count increased, neutrophil count decreased, platelet count decreased, platelet count increased, prostate examination abnormal, protein urine present, red blood cell count decreased, respiratory rate decreased, urine analysis abnormal, urine ketone body present, urine output decreased, white blood cells urine positive.

Metabolism and Nutrition Disorders: Infrequent: decreased appetite, dehydration, diabetes mellitus, fluid retention, gout, hypercholesterolaemia, hyperglycaemia, hyperlipidaemia, hypokalaemia. Rare: diabetes mellitus inadequate control, diabetes mellitus non insulin-dependent, electrolyte imbalance, hyperkalaemia, hyperphagia, hypertriglyceridaemia, hyperuricaemia, hypoglycaemia, hyponatraemia, hypovolaemia, increased appetite, lactose intolerance, malnutrition.

Musculoskeletal and Connective Tissue Disorders: Frequent: musculoskeletal pain, neck pain. Infrequent: arthritis, bone pain, bursitis, costochondritis, exostosis, flank pain, groin pain, intervertebral disc protrusion, joint crepitation, joint range of motion decreased, joint stiffness, muscle twitching, musculoskeletal chest pain, osteoarthritis, pain in jaw, rotator cuff syndrome, tendonitis. Rare: arthropathy, bunion, coccydynia, fibromyalgia, joint effusion, lumbar spinal stenosis, muscle tightness, musculoskeletal discomfort, musculoskeletal disorder, osteoporosis, periarthritis, plantar fasciitis, rheumatoid arthritis, sensation of heaviness, synovial cyst, trigger finger.

Neoplasms Benign, Malignant and Unspecified (including cysts and polyps): Rare: basal cell carcinoma, benign breast neoplasm, lipoma seborrheic keratosis, skin cancer.

Nervous System Disorders: Infrequent: amnesia, balance disorder, burning sensation, carpal tunnel syndrome, coordination abnormal, disturbance in attention, dysarthria, dysgeusia, lethargy, memory impairment, mental impairment, neuropathy peripheral, sciatica, sedation, sinus headache, syncope, tension headache, transient ischaemic attack. Rare: ageusia, carotid artery stenosis, cerebrovascular accident, convulsion, depressed level of consciousness, dizziness postural, facial palsy, formication, hyperaesthesia, hypersomnia hyporeflexia nerve compression, neuralgia, neuropathy, poor quality sleep, presyncope, restless legs syndrome, subarachnoid haemorrhage.

Psychiatric Disorders: Infrequent: abnormal dreams, confusional state, depressed mood, euphoric mood, hallucination, libido decreased, mood swings, panic attack. Rare: affect lability, anorgasmia, anxiety disorder, crying, delirium, initial insomnia, listless, loss of libido, major depression, mood altered, nicotine dependence, paranoia, restlessness, sleep disorder, stress, tension, thinking abnormal, tic.

Renal and Urinary Disorders: Infrequent: dysuria, haematuria, micturition urgency, nephrolithiasis, pollakiuria, urinary hesitation, urinary retention. Rare: acute prerenal failure, bladder spasm, chromaturia, incontinence, micturition frequency decreased, nocturia, polyuria, proteinuria, renal cyst, renal failure, renal failure acute, renal pain, urinary incontinence.

Reproductive System and Breast Disorders: Infrequent: breast mass, dysmenorrhoea, erectile dysfunction. Rare: benign prostatic hyperplasia, breast discharge, breast pain, breast tenderness, ejaculation delayed, ejaculation disorder, ejaculation failure, genital rash, menstruation irregular, metrorrhagia, pelvic pain, priapism, prostatic disorder, prostatitis, sexual dysfunction, vaginal discharge, vaginal haemorrhage.

Respiratory, Thoracic and Mediastinal Disorders: Frequent: pharyngolaryngeal pain. Infrequent: asthma, chronic obstructive pulmonary disease, epistaxis, hiccups, nasal congestion, respiratory disorder, respiratory tract congestion, rhinitis allergic, rhinorrhea, sinus congestion, sneezing, upper respiratory tract congestion, wheezing, yawning. Rare: allergic sinusitis, bronchospasm, dry throat, dysphonia, dyspnoea exertional, emphysema, nasal discomfort, nasal dryness, paranasal sinus hypersecretion, pharyngeal erythema, pleural effusion, postnasal drip, productive cough, pulmonary embolism, pulmonary hypertension, pulmonary oedema, rales, respiratory failure, rhonchi, sinus disorder, throat irritation, throat tightness.

Skin and Subcutaneous Tissue Disorders: Infrequent: acne, alopecia, blister, cold sweat, dermatitis, dermatitis allergic, dermatitis contact, dry skin, eczema, night sweats, psoriasis, rash erythematous, rash generalised, rash papular, rash pruritic, skin irritation, skin lesion, swelling face. Rare: angioedema, decubitus ulcer, dermal cyst, ecchymosis, heat rash, hyperkeratosis, hypoaesthesia facial, ingrowing nail, petechiae, piloerection, rash macular, skin burning sensation, skin discolouration, skin exfoliation, skin ulcer.
Social Circumstances: Infrequent: drug abuser. Rare: menopause.
Surgical and Medical Procedures: Rare: knee arthroplasty, tooth extraction, tooth repair.
Vascular Disorders: Frequent: hypertension. Infrequent: flushing, haematoma, hypotension. Rare: aortic aneurysm, deep vein thrombosis, hypertensive crisis, orthostatic hypotension, pallor, varicose vein.
Post-Market Adverse Drug Reactions: Other adverse reactions (≥1% frequency) not observed in clinical trials, that have been reported in post-marketing data include vasodilation.

DRUG INTERACTIONS: Overview: Additive Effects of Other CNS Depressants: BuTrans (buprenorphine transdermal patch) should be dosed with caution in patients who are currently taking other CNS depressants or other drugs that may cause respiratory depression, hypotension, profound sedation, or may potentially result in coma. Such agents include alcohol, antihistamines, antipsychotics, anxiolytics, barbiturates, benzodiazepines, centrally acting antiemetics, clonidine and related substances, general anaesthetics, neuroleptics, other opioid derivatives (analgesic and antitussive), phenothiazines and sedatives or hypnotics. When such combined therapy is contemplated, a substantial reduction in the dose of one or both agents should be considered and patients carefully monitored (see Warnings and Precautions, Neurologic, Interaction with Other Central Nervous System Depressants). Patients should also be warned that these combinations increase central nervous system depression and can make driving vehicles and operating machinery hazardous (see Warnings and Precautions, Psychomotor Impairment).
Drug-Drug Interactions: CYP 3A4 Inhibitors: Buprenorphine is primarily metabolized by glucuronidation and to a lesser extent (about 30%) by CYP3A4. Concomitant treatment with CYP3A4 inhibitors (ritonavir, ketoconazole, itraconazole, troleandomycin, clarithromycin, nelfinavir, nefazodone, verapamil, diltiazem, and amiodarone, amprenavir, fosamprenavir, aprepitant, fluconazole, erythromycin and grapefruit juice) may lead to elevated plasma concentrations with an increase in dose related toxicity of buprenorphine including potentially fatal respiratory depression (see Warnings and Precautions, Concomitant Use of CYP3A4 Inhibitors). The interaction between buprenorphine and CYP3A4 enzyme inducers has not been studied. Co-administration of BuTrans and enzyme inducers (e.g., phenobarbital, carbamazepine, phenytoin, and rifampin) could lead to increased clearance which might result in reduced efficacy.
MAO Inhibitors: MAO inhibitors intensify the effects of opioid drugs which can cause anxiety, confusion and decreased respiration. Buprenorphine is contraindicated in patients receiving MAO inhibitors or who have used them within the previous 14 days (see Contraindications and Warnings and Precautions).
Warfarin: The potential exists for INR elevation in patients who are concomitantly taking warfarin.
Anesthetics: Reductions in hepatic blood flow induced by some general anesthetics (halothane) and other drugs may result in a decreased rate of hepatic elimination of buprenorphine.
Flunitrazepam: Deaths have been reported in the addict population when buprenorphine was coadministered with flunitrazepam. This adverse drug interaction cannot be explained by a pharmacokinetic drug-drug interaction. Caution must be exercised with the combined use of buprenorphine and flunitrazepam and a dosage reduction in one or both drugs should be considered.
Drug-Herb Interactions: Interactions with herbal products have not been established.
Drug-Laboratory Test Interactions: Interactions with laboratory tests have not been established.

DOSAGE AND ADMINISTRATION: General: BuTrans (buprenorphine transdermal patch) should only be prescribed by persons knowledgeable in the continuous administration of potent opioids, in the management of patients receiving potent opioids for treatment of pain, and in the detection and management of respiratory depression including the use of opioid antagonists.
Dosing Considerations: BuTrans is intended to be used for the continual release of buprenorphine transdermally over a 7-day period per patch, for the management of persistent pain of moderate intensity. BuTrans can be used in either opioid naïve patients or patients previously treated with PRN (as needed) analgesics when the analgesic requirement has progressed to a need for continuous opioid analgesia.

BuTrans doses must be individualized based upon the status of each patient and should be assessed at regular intervals after application. Proper optimization of doses scaled to the relief of the individual's pain should aim at the regular administration of the lowest dose of BuTrans which provides pain relief with acceptable side effects. The dosage of the drug must be individualized according to the response and tolerance of the patient. An important factor to be considered in determining the appropriate dose is the extent of pre-existing opioid tolerance (see Conversion from Opioid or Fixed-Ratio Opioid/Non-Opioid Combination Drugs). Initiation on the lowest available strength of BuTrans with appropriate dose titration is suggested for the elderly and other groups discussed in Warnings and Precautions.

The patch should be worn for 7 days before changing to a new patch at the same dose. A new skin site should be selected when changing to a new patch. After the patch is removed, a 3-week interval is required before the same site can be re-used.

BuTrans should not be used in individuals less than 40 kg in weight. BuTrans may have altered pharmacokinetics due to poor fat stores, muscle wasting or altered clearance.

Opioid analgesics may be only partially effective in relieving dysesthetic pain, postherpetic neuralgia, stabbing pains, activity-related pain and some forms of headache. That is not to say that patients with these types of pain should not be given an adequate trial of opioid analgesics, but it may be necessary to refer such patients at an early time to other forms of pain therapy.

BuTrans has potential for abuse and diversion (see Warnings and Precautions).
Initial BuTrans Dose Selection: BuTrans is designed to allow for once weekly dosing, i.e., dosing every 7 days. Treatment with BuTrans should generally be initiated at the lowest available dose (BuTrans 5).
Patients Not Already Taking Opioids (Opioid-Naïve): In situations when it is clinically indicated to initiate opioid therapy with a maintenance (around-the-clock) opioid in an opioid naïve patient, clinical trials have shown that such patients may successfully initiate opioid therapy with BuTrans. **The lowest dose available (BuTrans 5) should always be used as the initial dose and titrated as required. If the patient requires rescue medication, see Management of Patients Requiring Rescue Medication.**
Conversion from Opioid or Fixed-Ratio Opioid/Non-Opioid Combination Drugs: BuTrans has been studied as an alternative opioid analgesic in patients taking up to 80 mg of oral morphine-equivalents a day. **Such patients should be started on BuTrans 5 or BuTrans 10 and be provided with adequate rescue medication and titrated as required (see Management of Patients Requiring Rescue Medication).**
Patch Application: BuTrans should be applied to non-irritated, intact skin of the upper outer arm, upper chest, upper back or the side of the chest. BuTrans should be applied to a relatively hairless or nearly hairless skin site. If none are available, the hair at the site should be clipped, not shaven. Application site should be rotated whenever a patch is replaced or added. **Application sites should be re-used at no less than 3-week intervals.**

If the application site must be cleaned, it should be done with clear water only. Soaps, alcohol, oils, lotions or abrasive devices must not be used. The skin site must be dry before the patch is applied. BuTrans should be immediately applied after removal from the sealed pouch. Following removal of the protective layer, the transdermal patch should be pressed firmly in place with the palm of the hand for approximately 30 seconds, making sure the contact is complete, especially around the edges. If the edges of the patch begin to peel off, the edge may be taped down with suitable skin tape. Bathing, showering or swimming should not affect the patch. While wearing BuTrans, patients should be advised to avoid exposing the patch site to direct external heat sources (see Warnings and Precautions).
Dose Titration: Proper optimization of doses scaled to the relief of the individual's pain should aim at regular administration of the lowest dose of controlled release buprenorphine (BuTrans) which will achieve the overall treatment goal of satisfactory pain relief with acceptable side effects. On average, steady-state blood levels are achieved after 3 days. **It is recommended that doses of BuTrans be slowly titrated—with dosage adjustment generally separated by 7 days. The dose of BuTrans should not be increased before 3 days as the plasma concentrations continue to increase following application. Subsequent increases of BuTrans dosage must be individualized according to the pain relief and tolerance of the patient with adequate rescue pain medication, as required (see Management of Patients Requiring Rescue Medication).** If pain repeatedly occurs at the end of the dosing interval it is generally an indication for a dosage increase rather than more frequent administration of controlled release buprenorphine (BuTrans). **The maximum recommended patch dose is 20 µg/h every 7 days.**

To increase the dose, the patch that is currently being worn should be removed, disposed of properly, and the next higher strength of BuTrans should be used. Application sites should be rotated whenever a patch is replaced or added. Application sites should be re-used at no less than 3-week intervals. It is recommended that no more than two patches be applied at the same time.

No change in dose titration is required in patients with renal impairment or mild to moderate hepatic impairment. Patients with severe hepatic impairment may accumulate buprenorphine and BuTrans should not be used in such patients.

Management of Patients Requiring Rescue Medication: In clinical trials with BuTrans, acetaminophen and acetaminophen with codeine combinations were used as rescue medications. If episodes of pain are encountered with appropriate adjustments of the BuTrans dose, fentanyl products should not be used as rescue medication in patients taking BuTrans. Selection of rescue medication should be based on individual patient conditions. For patients whose dose has been titrated to the recommended maintenance dose, without attainment of adequate analgesia, the total daily dose may be increased, unless precluded by side effects.

If dose limiting adverse events occur before the therapeutic goal of mild or no pain is achieved, the events should be treated with appropriate medications such as laxatives or anti-nauseants. Once adverse events are under control, upward titration should continue to an acceptable level of pain control.

If adequate pain control cannot be achieved with the maximum patch dose of BuTrans 20 µg/h every 7 days, the patient should be converted to an alternative around-the-clock µ-opioid agonist, and the dose of the alternative analgesic further titrated, as appropriate.
Managing Expected Opioid Adverse Experiences: Many patients receiving opioids, especially those who are opioid naïve, will experience side effects. Clinical trials have shown that these effects are most bothersome during the initial application and can be minimized by starting at BuTrans 5 and gradually increasing the dose as needed. Although the side effects from BuTrans are often transient, some may require treatment. Adverse events such as constipation should be anticipated and treated with a stimulant laxative and/or stool softener. Patients do not usually become tolerant to the constipating effects of opioids.

Other opioid related side effects such as sedation and nausea are usually self-limited and often do not persist beyond the first few days. If nausea persists and is unacceptable to the patient, treatment with antiemetics or other modalities may relieve these symptoms and should be considered.
Discontinuation of BuTrans Therapy: After removal of BuTrans, plasma concentrations decrease gradually, and the analgesic effect is maintained for a certain amount of time. This needs to be considered when use of BuTrans is to be followed by other opioids. As a general rule, a subsequent opioid should not be administered within 24 hours of removal of a BuTrans patch. As part of an overall strategy to suitably manage pain in this period, the use of appropriate rescue medication and/or careful monitoring during this time should be considered. Buprenorphine concentrations decline, decreasing approximately 50% in 12 hours (range 10-24 h). (See Action and Clinical Pharmacology, Pharmacokinetics.)
Safety and Handling: The buprenorphine contained in BuTrans is supplied in sealed transdermal patches. If the adhesive from the drug accidentally contacts the skin other than intended application site, the area should be washed with water. Do not use soap, alcohol or other solvents to remove the adhesive because they may enhance the absorption of the drug. When changing the patch, remove the used BuTrans patch, fold it over itself, and discard it (flush down the toilet or consult with a pharmacist about other disposal options).

OVERDOSAGE:
Symptoms: The manifestations of BuTrans (buprenorphine transdermal patch) overdose are an extension of its pharmacologic actions, but in overdose the antagonist properties may predominate. Symptoms include respiratory depression, sedation, drowsiness, nausea, vomiting and marked miosis. Respiratory depression has been absent in some cases of buprenorphine overdose. However, respiratory depression, including apnea, has occurred in other overdose situations.
Treatment: Support: Establish and maintain a patent airway, assist or control respiration as indicated, and maintain adequate body temperature and fluid balance. Oxygen, intravenous fluids, vasopressors, and other supportive measures should be employed as indicated.
Topical Exposure: Remove any patch in contact with the patient and dispose of it properly.
Ingestion of BuTrans: Administer activated charcoal (either 1 g/kg or 50 g) with an accompanying cathartic (e.g., 70% sorbitol, 1 mL/kg) to reduce buprenorphine absorption.
Opioid Antagonist: A specific opioid antagonist such as naloxone may reverse the effects of buprenorphine. The dose of naloxone required to antagonize the respiratory depressant effects of BuTrans may be in the range of 5 to 12 mg intravenously which is significantly higher than that used for a narcotic such as morphine. The onset of naloxone effect may also be delayed by 30 minutes or more. Maintenance of adequate ventilation is essential when managing a BuTrans overdose and more important than specific antidote treatment with a narcotic antagonist, such as naloxone.

For management of a suspected drug overdose, contact your regional Poison Control Centre. See the *CPS* Directory section for a list of Poison Control Centres.

ACTION AND CLINICAL PHARMACOLOGY: Mechanism of Action: Buprenorphine is a lipophilic, partial agonist with potent activity at the µ-opioid receptor. Buprenorphine produces dose related analgesia up to doses of 1.0 mg subcutaneously. The exact mechanism of analgesia is not known, but it involves the binding to µ-opioid receptors in the central nervous system (CNS) and peripheral tissues. The drug may also alter the pain threshold (threshold of afferent nerve endings to noxious stimuli). Buprenorphine is highly lipophilic and binds with high affinity to µ-, κ-, and δ-opioid receptors. Buprenorphine binds and dissociates from the µ-receptor slowly, which may account for the prolonged duration of analgesia and, in part, for the limited physical dependence potential of the drug as well as explain why the administration of a narcotic antagonist (e.g., naloxone) does not readily reverse the respiratory depression, if it occurs.

Buprenorphine is also a kappa-receptor antagonist, but the clinical relevance of this finding has not been established. Like other opioid agonists, buprenorphine may produce increases in cerebrospinal fluid pressure, cause altered mentation, mental clouding or amnesia following intravenous administration.

Buprenorphine acts to reduce blood pressure in a manner similar to other opioids.

Opioids have been associated with effects on the neuraxis, resulting in alterations in plasma cortisol, growth hormone, and the immune system. The clinical significance of these opioid-induced changes in humans is unknown.

Like other opioids, buprenorphine may cause nausea, vomiting and constipation. Use of opioids may also result in an increase in biliary tract pressure as a result of spasm of the Sphincter of Oddi.

Buprenorphine causes dose-related miosis and produces urinary retention in some patients.
Pharmacokinetics: The composition of the three strengths of BuTrans (5, 10, 20) is identical except for size. The amount of buprenorphine released from each patch per hour is proportional to the surface area of the patch. The skin is the limiting barrier to diffusion from the patch into the bloodstream. Flux rate through the skin was determined in two studies by three methods of analysis each yielding similar results. Buprenorphine flux for the 7 day application period was established to be 5, 10 and 20 µg/h for the 7 day application period for the BuTrans 5, 10 and 20, respectively.

Each BuTrans transdermal patch provides a steady delivery of buprenorphine for up to 7 days (see Figure 1). Steady state concentrations were achieved during the first application after day 3.

Figure 1: BuTrans

Buprenorphine Plasma Concentrations (pg/mL). Mean (±1.5 SEM), BuTrans 10 Application for 7 days (N=23 healthy subjects)

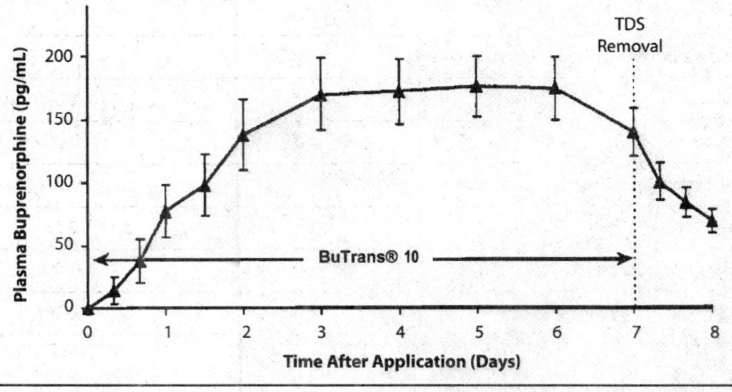

BuTrans 5, 10 and 20 provide dose-proportional increases in total exposure (AUC) over a 7 day application period (see Table 4). Dose-proportional increases in steady state plasma concentrations were maintained with BuTrans application for up to 60 days and accumulation of plasma buprenorphine did not occur (see Figure 2). After removal of BuTrans, buprenorphine concentrations decline, decreasing approximately 50% in 12 hours (range 10-24 h).

Table 4: BuTrans

Pharmacokinetic Metrics of BuTrans in Healthy Subjects (Single 7 day Application) Mean±Standard Deviation

Dose	N	AUC (pg.h/mL)	Average Concentration (pg/mL)	C_{max} (pg/mL)
BuTrans 5	12	12 647±2015	75.3±12.0	176±34
BuTrans 10	12	24 311±2355	145±14.0	191±19
BuTrans 20	9	51 106±6156	304±36.6	471±77

Figure 2: BuTrans

Buprenorphine Plasma Concentrations (pg/mL). Mean (±1.5 SEM), 7 day wear of BuTrans 5, 10 or 20 for 60 days

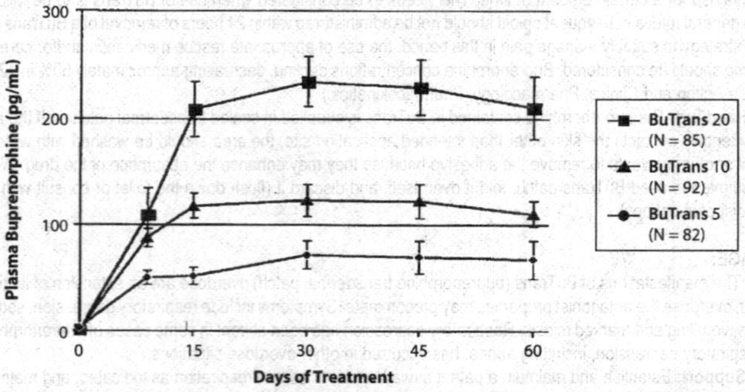

Application Site: A study in healthy subjects demonstrated that the pharmacokinetic profile of buprenorphine delivered by BuTrans is similar when applied to the upper outer arm, upper chest, upper back or the side of the chest (midaxillary line, 5th intercostal space).

In a study of healthy subjects receiving BuTrans repeatedly to the same site, immediate reapplication caused increased absorption. For this reason, rotation of application sites is recommended.

In a study of healthy subjects, application of a heating pad directly on the BuTrans patch caused a transient, 26-55% increase in blood concentrations of buprenorphine. Concentrations returned to normal within 5 hours after the heat was removed. For this reason, applying an external heat source directly, such as a heating pad, to the BuTrans patch during wear is not recommended. A heating pad applied to a BuTrans site, immediately after patch removal, did not alter absorption from the skin depot.

Absorption: Following BuTrans application, buprenorphine diffuses from the patch through the skin. In clinical pharmacology studies, the median time for BuTrans 10 to deliver detectable buprenorphine concentrations (25 pg/mL) was approximately 17 hours. The absolute bioavailability of BuTrans relative to IV, following a 7 day application is approximately 15% for all treatments (BuTrans 5, 10, 20). Plasma levels following sublingual buprenorphine doses of 4 mg to 16 mg have been reported to be in the range of 2000-4420 pg/mL. Plasma levels of oral sublingual buprenorphine are much higher in comparison to the plasma levels obtained in BuTrans 20 patch administration (471 pg/mL).

Distribution: Buprenorphine is approximately 96% bound to plasma proteins. Studies of IV buprenorphine have shown a large volume of distribution, implying extensive distribution of buprenorphine. In a study of IV buprenorphine in healthy subjects, the volume of distribution at steady state was 430 L, reflecting the large volume of distribution and lipophilicity of the drug.

Following IV administration, buprenorphine and its metabolites are secreted into bile, and within several minutes, distribute into the cerebrospinal fluid (CSF). CSF buprenorphine concentrations appear to be approximately 15 to 25% of concurrent plasma concentrations.

Metabolism and Excretion: Buprenorphine metabolism in the skin following BuTrans application is negligible. Following transdermal application, buprenorphine is eliminated via hepatic metabolism, with subsequent biliary excretion and renal excretion of soluble metabolites. Hepatic metabolism, through CYP3A4 and UGT1A1/1A3 enzymes, results in two primary metabolites—norbuprenorphine and buprenorphine 3-O-glucuronide, respectively. Norbuprenorphine is also glucuronidated prior to elimination. Buprenorphine is also eliminated in the feces. Following intramuscular administration of 2 µg/kg, approximately 70% of the dose was excreted in feces within 7 days. The total clearance of buprenorphine is approximately 55 L/h in postoperative patients.

Norbuprenorphine is the only known active metabolite of buprenorphine. It has been shown to be a respiratory depressant in rats, but only at concentrations at least 50 fold greater than observed following application of BuTrans 20.

Reductions in hepatic blood flow induced by some general anaesthetics (e.g., halothane) and other drugs may result in a decreased rate of hepatic elimination of the drug. Since buprenorphine elimination and metabolism is not solely dependent on the CYP450 enzyme system, inhibition of the CYP3A4 enzyme would not decrease buprenorphine clearance by non-CYP450 pathways, such as direct glucuronidation. BuTrans metabolism is not expected to be affected by the usual doses of drugs inhibiting CYP450 pathways. Based on in vitro studies in human microsomes and hepatocytes, buprenorphine does not appear to have the potential to inhibit metabolism by CYP450 isoenzymes at concentrations obtained with BuTrans use.

Endotoxin Challenge: In a crossover study of healthy subjects receiving endotoxin or placebo challenge during BuTrans wear, the AUC and C_{max} were similar despite a physiologic response to endotoxin. Therefore, BuTrans' performance is unlikely to be significantly affected during intercurrent mild febrile illness.

Special Populations and Conditions: Pediatrics: BuTrans has not been studied in children and is not indicated for patients less than 18 years of age.

Geriatrics: The pharmacokinetic profile of BuTrans is similar in healthy elderly and young adult subjects, although elderly subjects trended toward higher plasma concentrations of buprenorphine immediately after removal of BuTrans, than young adult subjects. Both groups eliminated buprenorphine at similar rates after patch removal.

Gender: No differences in plasma buprenorphine concentrations were detected between males and females treated with BuTrans.

Race: No data available.

Hepatic Insufficiency: In a pharmacokinetic study utilizing intravenous buprenorphine, there were no differences in clearance of buprenorphine between mild to moderate hepatically impaired subjects relative to healthy adult subjects. These data show no need for dosage adjustment when using BuTrans in patients with mild to moderate hepatic impairment.

Renal Insufficiency: Buprenorphine pharmacokinetics were similar in patients with severe renal impairment compared to normal adults (see Warnings and Precautions, Special Populations).

Genetic Polymorphism: No data available.

Cardiovascular: In a thorough QTc study, the effects of BuTrans on the QT interval were assessed in healthy volunteers. BuTrans 10 µg/h was not different from placebo. BuTrans 20 µg/h was not studied. BuTrans 40 µg/h (not a recommended dose) was associated with a mean prolongation of the QT interval of 5.9 msec compared to placebo.

STORAGE AND STABILITY: Store at 15-30°C. Do not freeze.

SPECIAL HANDLING INSTRUCTIONS: BuTrans (buprenorphine transdermal patch) should be kept in a safe place out of the sight and reach of children before and after use. Do not give to others. BuTrans patches should not be divided, cut or damaged in any other way.

The buprenorphine contained in BuTrans is supplied in sealed transdermal patches. If the adhesive from the drug accidentally contacts the skin other than the intended application site, the area should be washed with water. Do not use soap, alcohol or other solvents to remove the adhesive because they may enhance the absorption of the drug. When changing the patch, remove the used BuTrans, fold it over itself, and discard it (flush down the toilet) immediately upon removal, or consult with a pharmacist about other disposal options.

INFORMATION FOR THE PATIENT: Published in e-CPS, available by subscription at www.e-cps.ca.

DOSAGE FORMS, COMPOSITION AND PACKAGING: BuTrans (buprenorphine transdermal patch) is a rectangular or square, beige coloured patch consisting of a protective liner and functional layers. Proceeding from the outer surface toward the surface adhering to the skin, the layers are (1) a beige coloured web backing layer of polyester material; (2) an adhesive matrix rim without buprenorphine; (3) a separating foil over the adhesive matrix; (4) the buprenorphine containing adhesive matrix with inactive ingredients including aluminum acetylacetonate, levulinic acid, oleyl oleate, polyacrylate (dry solids), povidone; and (5) a release liner (see Figure 3). Before use, the release liner covering the adhesive layer is removed and discarded.

Figure 3: BuTrans

Cross Section Diagram of BuTrans

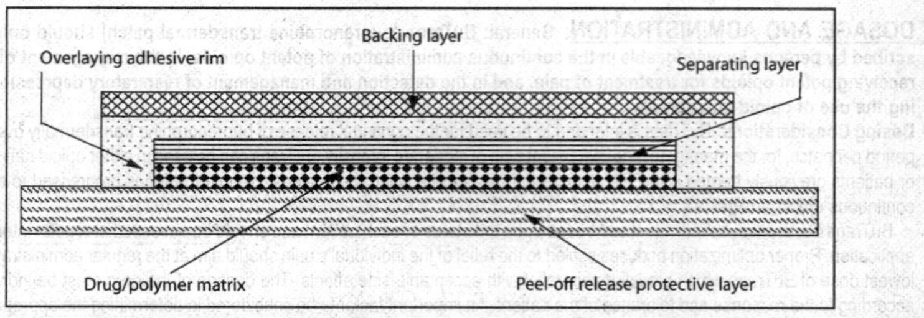

Three different strengths of BuTrans (buprenorphine transdermal patch) are available: BuTrans 5, BuTrans 10 and BuTrans 20 (see Table 5). The composition of all three strengths is identical except for size. The active component of the patch is buprenorphine. The remaining components are pharmacologically inactive. The amount of buprenorphine base mixed in the adhesive matrix is the same for each of the strengths (10% by weight). The amount of buprenorphine released from each patch per hour is proportional to the surface area of the patch.

Table 5: BuTrans

Strengths

Total Buprenorphine Content (mg)	Delivery Rate (µg/h)	Active Surface Area (cm²)
BuTrans 5	5	6.25
BuTrans 10	10	12.5
BuTrans 20	20	25.0

BuTrans 5, 10 and 20 Transdermal Patches are available in cartons of 4 patches.

(Shown in Product Identification Section)

Choose

PrCaduet®

amlodipine besylate/atorvastatin calcium

The unique combination of PrNORVASC® and PrLIPITOR® with[1]:

Improved Patient Retention

- Patient retention was **35% higher** after 6 months with CADUET vs. separate NORVASC and LIPITOR (67.7% vs. 49.9%, $p<0.0001$)[2†]

Covered by most provincial formularies*

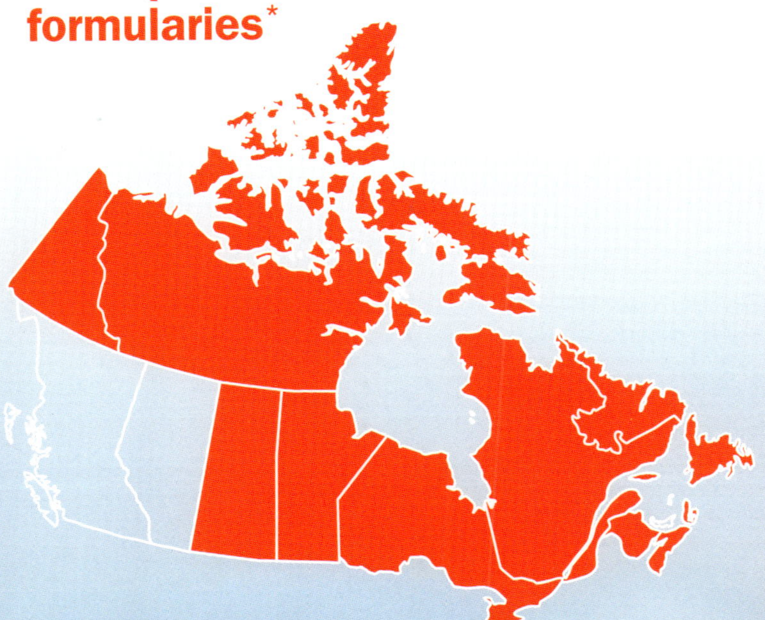

*See respective Formularies for details (not covered in BC, AB, PEI).

Pfizer Working together for a healthier world™

CADUET (amlodipine besylate/atorvastatin calcium) is indicated in patients for whom treatment with both amlodipine besylate and atorvastatin calcium is appropriate, specifically, patients at cardiovascular risk. Please refer to the Product Monographs of NORVASC (amlodipine besylate) and LIPITOR (atorvastatin calcium).

CADUET is not for initial therapy. The dose of CADUET should be determined by the titration of individual components. For information on contraindications and adverse events, please see the Product Monograph.

CADUET is contraindicated in patients with hypersensitivity to any component of this medication, the atorvastatin calcium, amlodipine besylate or other dihydropyridines. CADUET is contraindicated in patients with severe hypotension (less than 90 mmHg systolic) and in patients with active liver disease or unexplained persistent elevations of serum transaminases exceeding 3 times the upper limit of normal.

CADUET is also contraindicated in pregnancy and for nursing women: Cholesterol and other products of cholesterol biosynthesis are essential components for fetal development (including synthesis of steroids and cell membranes). CADUET should be administered to women of childbearing age only when such patients are highly unlikely to conceive and have been informed of the possible harm. If the patient becomes pregnant while taking CADUET, the drug should be discontinued immediately and the patient apprised of the potential harm to the fetus. Atherosclerosis being a chronic process, discontinuation of lipid metabolism regulating drugs during pregnancy should have little impact on the outcome of long-term therapy of primary hypercholesterolemia.

Very rare cases of rhabdomyolysis with acute renal failure secondary to myoglobinuria, have been reported with the atorvastatin calcium component of CADUET and with other HMG-CoA reductase inhibitors.

Caution should be exercised in such patients who are also severely renally impaired, elderly, or are concomitantly being administered digoxin or CYP 3A4 inhibitors.

If increases in alanine aminotransferase (ALT) or aspartate aminotransferase (AST) show evidence of progression, particularly if they rise to greater than 3 times the upper limit of normal and are persistent, the dosage of the atorvastatin calcium component of CADUET should be reduced or the drug discontinued.

In a double-blind, controlled clinical trial of all available CADUET doses (5/10 mg to 10/80 mg amlodipine besylate/atorvastatin calcium respectively), the most frequently reported adverse events among patients who took concurrent amlodipine besylate and atorvastatin calcium were peripheral edema (9.9%), headache (5.3%), respiratory tract infection (4.9%), dizziness (2.4%), abdominal pain (2.3%), asthenia (2.1%), and vasodilatation (2.0%).

Product Monograph available at: www.pfizer.ca

† Retention defined as proportion of days covered ≥80%. Retrospective, longitudinal, cohort study based on United States pharmacy claims. Patients newly initiated on CADUET or separate NORVASC and LIPITOR were followed for 180 days from the index date to calculate study outcomes. In an additional analysis, patient adherence at 1 year was evaluated for a subset of patients from the primary analysis who had at least 1 full year of follow-up data (n=3561). The main outcome measure was proportion of days covered (PDC), meaning the proportion of days in the study period that the treatment regimen is available to the patient, as observed from pharmacy claims data. Patients must have access to both medications on a given day during the observation period in order for this day to be considered "covered".

References: 1. CADUET Product Monograph. Pfizer Canada Inc., August 2009.
2. Patel BV *et al.* Adherence with single-pill amlopidine/atorvastatin versus a two-pill regimen. *Vascular Health and Risk Management* 2008;4(3):673-81.

C

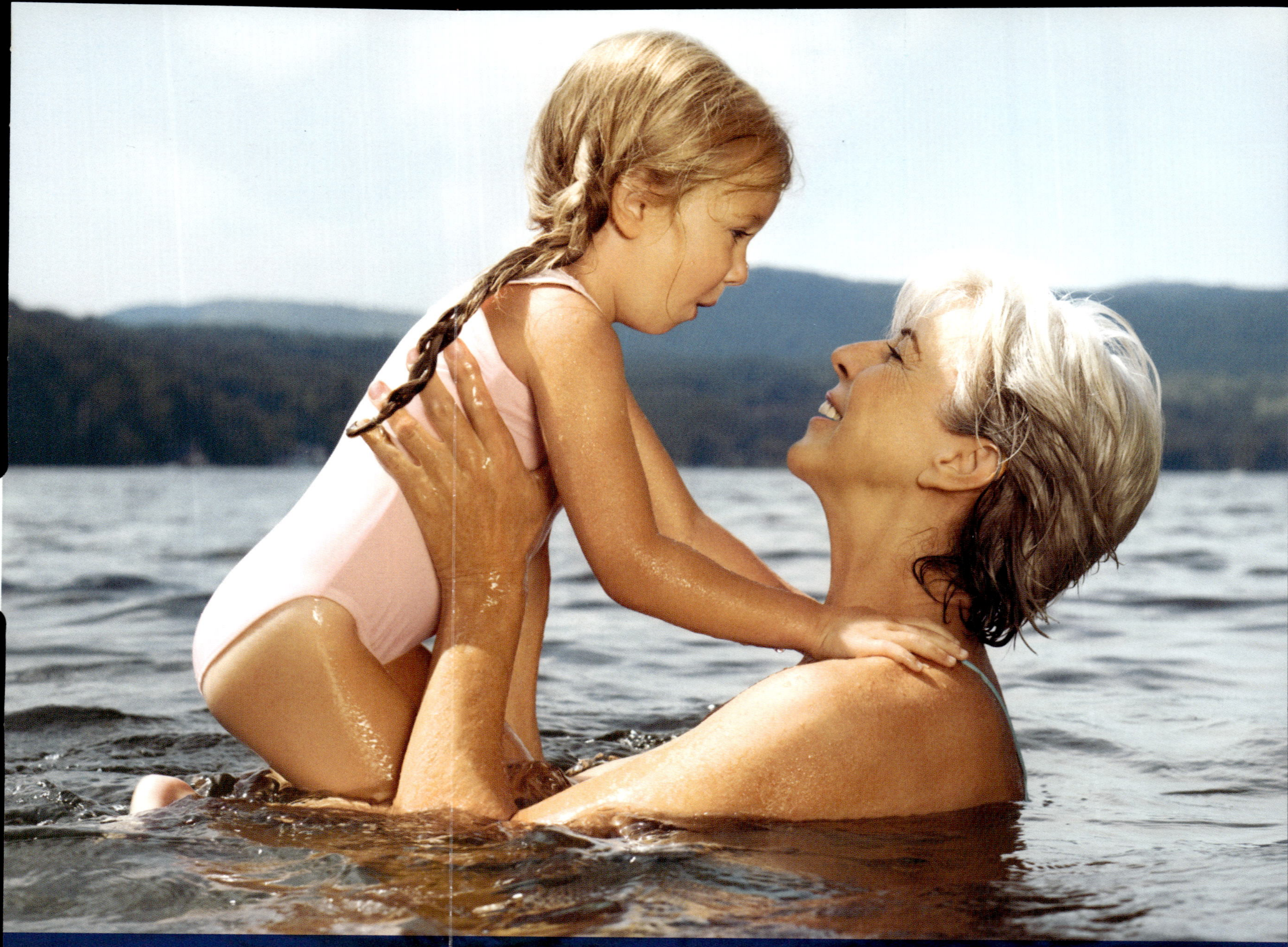

BE CELECTIVE

CELEBREX is indicated for relief of symptoms associated with Osteoarthritis, adult Rheumatoid Arthritis, and Ankylosing Spondylitis. CELEBREX is also indicated for the short-term (≤7 days) management of moderate to severe acute pain in adults in conditions such as the following: musculoskeletal and/or soft tissue trauma including sprains; postoperative orthopaedic; pain following dental extraction.[3]

For patients with an increased risk of developing CV and/or GI adverse events, other management strategies that do NOT include the use of NSAIDs should be considered first (see CONTRAINDICATIONS and WARNINGS AND PRECAUTIONS).[3]

Use of CELEBREX should be limited to the lowest effective dose for the shortest possible duration of treatment in order to minimize the potential risk for cardiovascular or gastrointestinal adverse events (see CONTRAINDICATIONS and WARNINGS AND PRECAUTIONS).[3]

CELEBREX, as a NSAID, does NOT treat clinical disease or prevent its progression. CELEBREX, as a NSAID, only relieves symptoms and decreases inflammation for as long as the patient continues to take it.[3]

CELEBREX is contraindicated in: the peri-operative setting of coronary artery bypass graft (CABG) surgery; in patients during the third trimester of pregnancy, because of risk of premature closure of the ductus arteriosus and prolonged parturition; in women who are breastfeeding, because of the potential for serious adverse reactions in nursing infants; in patients with severe uncontrolled heart failure; known hypersensitivity to celecoxib or to any of the components/excipients; demonstrated allergic-type reactions to sulfonamides; and patients with a history of asthma, urticaria, or allergic-type reactions after taking ASA or other NSAIDs; in patients with active gastric/duodenal/peptic ulcer, active GI bleeding; cerebrovascular bleedings; inflammatory bowel disease; severe liver impairment or active liver disease; severe renal impairment (creatinine clearance <30 mL/min or 0.5 mL/sec) or deteriorating renal disease. CELEBREX is contraindicated in the paediatric population under 18 years of age. Safety and efficacy of CELEBREX have not been established in this population.[3]

Serious Warnings and Precautions[3]

Risk of Cardiovascular (CV) Adverse Events: Ischemic Heart Disease, Cerebrovascular Disease, Congestive Heart Failure (NYHA II-IV).

CELEBREX is a nonsteroidal anti-inflammatory drug (NSAID). Use of some NSAIDs is associated with an increased incidence of cardiovascular adverse events (such as myocardial infarction, stroke or thrombotic events) which can be fatal. The risk may increase with duration of use. Patients with cardiovascular disease or risk factors for cardiovascular disease may be at greater risk.

Caution should be exercised in prescribing CELEBREX to any patient with ischemic heart disease (including but NOT limited to acute myocardial infarction, history of myocardial infarction and/or angina), cerebrovascular disease (including but NOT limited to stroke, cerebrovascular accident, transient ischemic attacks and/or amaurosis fugax) and/or congestive heart failure (NYHA II-IV).

Use of NSAIDs, such as CELEBREX, can promote sodium retention in a dose-dependent manner, through a renal mechanism, which can result in increased blood pressure and/or exacerbation of congestive heart failure.

Randomized clinical trials with CELEBREX have not been designed to detect differences in cardiovascular events in a chronic setting. Therefore, caution should be exercised when prescribing CELEBREX.

When managing pain and inflammation

SELECT CELEBREX®

The #1 dispensed NSAID in Canada among:[1]

- GPs
- Rheumatologists
- Gastroenterologists
- Cardiologists

CELEBREX demonstrated:

- **Superior pain relief** in OA vs. naproxen[2]
  - Reduction in pain from baseline of -29.5% with CELEBREX 200 mg/day vs. -21.8% with naproxen 1000 mg/day on WOMAC* pain subscale at week 12 ($p<0.001$)
- **Lower GI ulceration rate** vs. naproxen[3]
  - 7.5% for CELEBREX 200 mg BID vs. 34.6% for naproxen 500 mg BID during 12 weeks of treatment ($p<0.05$)
- **Onset of action within 35 minutes** in post-orthopaedic surgery (vs. >8 hours with placebo, $p<0.05$)[4]

Risk of Gastrointestinal (GI) Adverse Events.

Use of NSAIDs, such as CELEBREX, is associated with an increased incidence of gastrointestinal adverse events (such as peptic/duodenal ulceration, perforation, obstruction and gastrointestinal bleeding).

Risk in Pregnancy: Caution should be exercised in prescribing CELEBREX during the first and second trimesters of pregnancy. CELEBREX is CONTRAINDICATED for use during the third trimester because of risk of premature closure of the ductus arteriosus and uterine inertia (prolonged parturition).

The most common adverse events were headaches (15.8% vs. 20.2% placebo), upper respiratory tract infections (8.1% vs. 6.7% placebo), dyspepsia (8.8% vs. 6.2% placebo), diarrhea (5.6% vs. 3.8% placebo) and abdominal pain (4.1% vs. 2.8% placebo). See the Product Monograph for complete details.[3]

No clinically significant drug-drug interactions with phenytoin, tolbutamide, glyburide and ketoconazole. Potential interactions do exist with warfarin, lithium and fluconazole. See Product Monograph. NSAIDs may diminish the antihypertensive effects of ACE inhibitors. This interaction should be given consideration. With the exception of the use of low-dose ASA for cardiovascular protection, the use of CELEBREX in addition to any other NSAID is NOT recommended because of the absence of any evidence demonstrating synergistic benefits and the potential for additive adverse reactions. General warnings for NSAIDs should be borne in mind.[3]

For complete information regarding CELEBREX, please refer to the approved Product Monograph.

OA = osteoarthritis
* WOMAC (Western Ontario and McMaster Universities Osteoarthritis Index), consisting of 3 subscales: pain, stiffness, and physical function.

Pfizer Working together for a healthier world™

CELECOXIB CELEBREX®

CA0109CE000E

C

The reader is invited to consult CPhA's monograph **Calcium Channel Blockers** and **HMG-CoA Reductase Inhibitors.**

Caduet®

amlodipine besylate—atorvastatin calcium

Antihypertensive—Antianginal—Lipid Metabolism Regulator

Pfizer

Date of Preparation: December 5, 2003
Date of Revision: August 21, 2009

SUMMARY PRODUCT INFORMATION:

Route of Administration	Dosage Form/ Strength	Clinically Relevant Nonmedicinal Ingredients
Oral	Tablet (amlodipine/atorvastatin): 5/10 mg, 5/20 mg, 5/40 mg, 5/80 mg and 10/10 mg, 10/20 mg, 10/40 mg, 10/80 mg	Calcium carbonate, croscarmellose sodium, microcrystalline cellulose, pregelatinized starch, polysorbate 80, hydroxypropyl cellulose, purified water, colloidal silicon dioxide (anhydrous), magnesium stearate, Opadry II White 85F28751 or Opadry II Blue 85F10919

INDICATIONS AND CLINICAL USE: CADUET (amlodipine besylate/atorvastatin calcium) is indicated in patients for whom treatment with both amlodipine and atorvastatin is appropriate, specifically, patients at cardiovascular risk.

Please refer to the Product Monographs of LIPITOR (atorvastatin calcium) and NORVASC (amlodipine besylate).

CADUET is not for initial therapy. The dose of CADUET should be determined by the titration of individual components (see Dosage and Administration section of the Product Monographs of LIPITOR and NORVASC).

CONTRAINDICATIONS: CADUET is contraindicated in patients with hypersensitivity to any component of this medication, the atorvastatin, amlodipine or other dihydropyridines. CADUET is contraindicated in patients with severe hypotension (less than 90 mmHg systolic) and in patients with active liver disease or unexplained persistent elevations of serum transaminases exceeding 3 times the upper limit of normal.

CADUET is also contraindicated in pregnancy and for nursing women: Cholesterol and other products of cholesterol biosynthesis are essential components for fetal development (including synthesis of steroids and cell membranes). CADUET should be administered to women of childbearing age only when such patients are highly unlikely to conceive and have been informed of the possible harm. If the patient becomes pregnant while taking CADUET, the drug should be discontinued immediately and the patient apprised of the potential harm to the fetus. Atherosclerosis being a chronic process, discontinuation of lipid metabolism regulating drugs during pregnancy should have little impact on the outcome of long-term therapy of primary hypercholesterolemia (see Warnings and Precautions).

WARNINGS AND PRECAUTIONS: General: Before instituting therapy with CADUET, an attempt should be made to control elevated serum lipoprotein levels with appropriate diet, exercise, and weight reduction in overweight patients, and to treat other underlying medical problems (see Indications and Clinical Use). Patients should be advised to inform subsequent physicians of the prior use of atorvastatin or any other lipid-lowering agents.

Pharmacokinetic Interactions: The use of HMG CoA reductase inhibitors like some other lipid-lowering therapies has been associated with severe myopathy, including rhabdomyolysis, which may be more frequent when they are coadministered with drugs that inhibit the cytochrome P450 enzyme system. The atorvastatin component of CADUET is metabolized by cytochrome P450 isoform 3A4 and, as such, may interact with agents that inhibit this enzyme. (See Muscle Effects and Drug Interactions, Cytochrome P-450 Mediated Interactions.)

Muscle Effects: Effects on skeletal muscle such as myalgia, myopathy and very rarely, rhabdomyolysis have been reported in patients treated with the atorvastatin component of CADUET.

Very rare cases of rhabdomyolysis with acute renal failure secondary to myoglobinuria, have been reported with the atorvastatin component of CADUET and with other HMG-CoA reductase inhibitors.

Myopathy, defined as muscle aching or muscle weakness in conjunction with increases in creatine kinase (CK) values to greater than 10 times the upper limit of normal, should be considered in any patient with diffuse myalgia, muscle tenderness or weakness, and/or marked elevation of CPK. Patients should be advised to report promptly unexplained muscle pain, tenderness or weakness, particularly if accompanied by malaise or fever. Patients who develop any signs or symptoms suggestive of myopathy should have their CK levels measured. CADUET therapy should be discontinued if markedly elevated CPK levels occur or myopathy is diagnosed or suspected.

Pre-disposing Factors for Myopathy/Rhabdomyolysis: The atorvastatin component of CADUET, as with other HMG-CoA reductase inhibitors, should be prescribed with caution in patients with pre-disposing factors for myopathy/rhabdomyolysis. Such factors include: personal or family history of hereditary muscular disorders; previous history of muscle toxicity with another HMG-CoA reductase inhibitor; concomitant use of a fibrate, or niacin; hypothyroidism; alcohol abuse; excessive physical exercise; age >70 years; renal impairment; hepatic impairment; diabetes with hepatic fatty change; surgery and trauma; frailty; situations where an increase in plasma levels of active ingredient may occur.

CADUET therapy should be temporarily withheld or discontinued in any patient with an acute serious condition suggestive of a myopathy or having a risk factor predisposing to the development of renal failure secondary to rhabdomyolysis (such as sepsis, severe acute infection, hypotension, major surgery, trauma, severe metabolic, endocrine and electrolyte disorders, and uncontrolled seizures).

The risk of myopathy and rhabdomyolysis during treatment with HMG-CoA reductase inhibitors is increased with concurrent administration of cyclosporine, fibric acid derivatives, erythromycin, clarithromycin, niacin (nicotinic acid), azole antifungals or nefazodone. As there is no experience to date with the use of atorvastatin given concurrently with these drugs, with the exception of pharmacokinetic studies conducted in healthy subjects with erythromycin and clarithromycin, the benefits and risks of such combined therapy should be carefully considered (see Pharmacokinetic Interactions and Drug Interactions).

Drug/Laboratory Test Interactions: The atorvastatin component of CADUET may elevate serum transaminase and CPK levels (from skeletal muscle). In the differential diagnosis of chest pain in a patient on therapy with CADUET, cardiac and noncardiac fractions of these enzymes should be determined.

Beta-blocker Withdrawal: The amlodipine component of CADUET gives no protection against the dangers of abrupt beta-blocker withdrawal and such withdrawal should be done by the gradual reduction of the dose of beta-blocker.

Peripheral Edema: Mild to moderate peripheral edema was the most common adverse event in clinical trials with the amlodipine component of CADUET (see Adverse Reactions). The incidence of peripheral edema was dose-dependent and ranged in frequency from 3.0 to 10.8% in 5 to 10 mg dose range. Care should be taken to differentiate this peripheral edema from the effects of increasing left ventricular dysfunction.

Cardiovascular: Increased Angina and/or Myocardial Infarction: Rarely, patients, particularly those with severe obstructive coronary artery disease, have developed documented increased frequency, duration and/or severity of angina or acute myocardial infarction on starting calcium channel blocker therapy or at the time of dosage increase. The mechanism of this effect has not been elucidated.

Outflow Obstruction (Aortic Stenosis): CADUET should be used with caution in the presence of fixed left ventricular outflow obstruction (aortic stenosis).

Use in Patients with Congestive Heart Failure: Although generally calcium channel blockers should only be used with caution in patients with heart failure, it has been observed that the amlodipine component of CADUET had no overall deleterious effect on survival and cardiovascular morbidity in both short-term and long-term clinical trials in these patients. While a significant proportion of the patients in these studies had a history of ischemic heart disease, angina or hypertension, the studies were not designed to evaluate the treatment of angina or hypertension in patients with concomitant heart failure.

Hypotension: The amlodipine component of CADUET may occasionally precipitate symptomatic hypotension. Careful monitoring of blood pressure is recommended, especially in patients with a history of cerebrovascular insufficiency, and those taking medications known to lower blood pressure.

Effect on Ubiquinone (CoQ_{10}) Levels: Significant decreases in circulating ubiquinone levels in patients treated with atorvastatin and other statins have been observed. The clinical significance of a potential long-term statin-induced deficiency of ubiquinone has not been established. It has been reported that a decrease in myocardial ubiquinone levels could lead to impaired cardiac function in patients with borderline congestive heart failure.

Effect on Lipoprotein (a): In some patients, the beneficial effect of lowered total cholesterol and LDL-C levels may be partly blunted by a concomitant increase in Lp(a) lipoprotein concentrations. Present knowledge suggests the importance of high Lp(a) levels as an emerging risk factor for coronary heart disease. It is thus desirable to maintain and reinforce lifestyle changes in high risk patients placed on atorvastatin therapy.

Patients with Severe Hypercholesterolemia: Higher drug dosages (80 mg/day) required for some patients with severe hypercholesterolemia (including familial hypercholesterolemia) are associated with increased plasma levels of the atorvastatin component of CADUET. **Caution should be exercised in such patients who are also severely renally impaired, elderly, or are concomitantly being administered digoxin or CYP 3A4 inhibitors** (see Pharmacokinetic Interactions; Muscle Effects; Drug Interactions and Dosage and Administration).

Endocrine and Metabolism: Endocrine Function: HMG-CoA reductase inhibitors interfere with cholesterol synthesis and, as such, might theoretically blunt adrenal and/or gonadal steroid production. Clinical studies with the atorvastatin component of CADUET and other HMG-CoA reductase inhibitors have suggested that these agents do not reduce plasma cortisol concentration or impair adrenal reserve, and do not reduce basal plasma testosterone concentration. However, the effects of HMG-CoA reductase inhibitors on male fertility have not been studied in adequate numbers of patients. The effects, if any, on the pituitary-gonadal axis in premenopausal women are unknown.

Patients treated with the atorvastatin component of CADUET who develop clinical evidence of endocrine dysfunction should be evaluated appropriately. Caution should be exercised if an HMG-CoA reductase inhibitor or other agent used to lower cholesterol levels is administered to patients receiving other drugs (e.g. ketoconazole, spironolactone or cimetidine) that may decrease the levels of endogenous steroid hormones.

Hepatic/Biliary/Pancreatic: Hepatic Effects: In clinical trials with the atorvastatin component of CADUET, persistent increases in serum transaminases greater than 3 times the upper limit of normal occurred in <1% of patients who received atorvastatin. When the dosage of atorvastatin was reduced, or when drug treatment was interrupted or discontinued, serum transaminase levels returned to pretreatment levels. The increases were generally not associated with jaundice or other clinical signs or symptoms. Most patients continued treatment with a reduced dose of atorvastatin without clinical sequelae.

Liver function tests should be performed before the initiation of treatment, and periodically thereafter: Special attention should be paid to patients who develop elevated serum transaminase levels, and in these patients measurements should be repeated promptly and then performed more frequently.

If increases in alanine aminotransferase (ALT) or aspartate aminotransferase (AST) show evidence of progression, particularly if they rise to greater than 3 times the upper limit of normal and are persistent, the dosage of the atorvastatin component of CADUET should be reduced or the drug discontinued.

CADUET, as well as other products containing HMG-CoA reductase inhibitors, should be used with caution in patients who consume substantial quantities of alcohol and/or have a past history of liver disease. Active liver disease or unexplained transaminase elevations are contraindications to the use of the atorvastatin component of CADUET; if such a condition should develop during therapy, CADUET should be discontinued.

There are no adequate studies in patients with liver dysfunction and dosage recommendations have not been established. In a small number of patients with mild to moderate hepatic impairment in which a single dose of 5 mg of the amlodipine component of CADUET was given, half-life has been prolonged (see Action and Clinical Pharmacology, Pharmacokinetics and Metabolism). CADUET should therefore be administered with caution in these patients and careful monitoring should be performed. A lower starting dose of the amlodipine component of CADUET may be required (see Dosage and Administration).

Ophthalmologic: Effect on the Lens: Current long-term data from clinical trials do not indicate an adverse effect of the atorvastatin component of CADUET on the human lens.

Renal: Renal Insufficiency: Plasma concentrations and LDL-C lowering efficacy of the atorvastatin component of CADUET were shown to be similar in patients with moderate renal insufficiency compared with patients with normal renal function. However, since several cases of rhabdomyolysis have been reported in patients with a history of renal insufficiency of unknown severity, as a precautionary measure and pending further experience in renal disease, the lowest dose (10 mg/day) of atorvastatin should be used in these patients. Similar precautions apply in patients with severe renal insufficiency (creatinine clearance <30 mL/min [<0.5 mL/sec]); the lowest dosage should be used and implemented cautiously (see Muscle Effects; Drug Interactions and Dosage and Administration).

Sensitivity/Resistance: Hypersensitivity: An apparent hypersensitivity syndrome has been reported with other HMG-CoA reductase inhibitors which has included 1 or more of the following features: anaphylaxis, angioedema, lupus erythematous-like syndrome, polymyalgia rheumatica, vasculitis, purpura, thrombocytopenia, leukopenia, hemolytic anemia, positive ANA, ESR increase, eosinophilia, arthritis, arthralgia, urticaria, asthenia, photosensitivity, fever, chills, flushing, malaise, dyspnea, toxic epidermal necrolysis, erythema multiforme, including Stevens-Johnson syndrome. Although to date hypersensitivity syndrome has not been described as such, the atorvastatin component of CADUET should be discontinued if hypersensitivity is suspected.

Special Populations: Pregnant Women: The atorvastatin component of CADUET is contraindicated during pregnancy (see Contraindications).

There are no data on the use of atorvastatin during pregnancy. CADUET should be administered to women of childbearing age only when such patients are highly unlikely to conceive and have been informed of the potential hazards. If the patient becomes pregnant while taking CADUET, the drug should be discontinued and the patient apprised of the potential risk to the fetus.

In Studies with Amlodipine: Although amlodipine was not teratogenic in the rat and rabbit, some dihydropyridine compounds have been found to be teratogenic in animals. In rats, amlodipine has been shown to prolong both the gestation period and the duration of labor. There is no clinical experience with amlodipine in pregnant women.

Nursing Women: It is not known whether the amlodipine component of CADUET is excreted in human milk. In rats, milk concentrations of atorvastatin are similar to those in plasma. It is not known whether the atorvastatin component of CADUET is excreted in human milk. Because of the potential for adverse reactions in nursing infants, women taking CADUET should not breast-feed (see Contraindications).

Pediatrics: There have been no studies conducted to determine the safety or effectiveness of amlodipine/atorvastatin (combination product) in pediatric populations. However, there have been studies with pediatrics with amlodipine alone and atorvastatin alone (see below).

Amlodipine: The effect of amlodipine on blood pressure in patients less than 6 years of age is not known. Pediatric safety and efficacy studies beyond 8 weeks of duration have not been conducted. (Please refer to the Product Monograph for NORVASC (amlodipine besylate).)

Atorvastatin: Severe Dyslipidemias in Pediatric Patients: Safety and effectiveness of atorvastatin in patients 10-17 years of age (N=140) with heterozygous familial hypercholesterolemia have been evaluated in a controlled clinical trial of 6 months duration in adolescent boys and postmenarchal girls. Patients treated with atorvastatin had a safety and tolerability profile generally similar to that of placebo. Doses greater than 20 mg have not been studied in this patient population. (Please refer to the Product Monograph for LIPITOR (atorvastatin calcium).)

Safety and effectiveness of atorvastatin in pediatric patients has not been determined in the prevention of myocardial infarction. (Please refer to the Product Monograph for LIPITOR (atorvastatin calcium).)

Geriatrics: Amlodipine: In elderly patients (>65 years), clearance of amlodipine is decreased with a resulting increase in AUC of approximately 40-60%. In general, dose selection of the amlodipine component of CADUET for an elderly patient should be cautious, usually starting at the low end of the dosing range, reflecting the greater frequency of decreased hepatic, renal, or cardiac function, and of concomitant disease or other drug therapy (see Action and Clinical Pharmacology, Pharmacokinetics and Metabolism). In clinical trials, the incidence of adverse reactions in elderly patients was approximately 6% higher than that of younger population (<65 years). Adverse reactions include edema, muscle cramps and dizziness. The amlodipine component of CADUET should be used cautiously in elderly patients. Dosage adjustment is advisable (see Dosage and Administration).

Atorvastatin: Treatment experience in adults 70 years or older (N=221) with doses of atorvastatin up to 80 mg/day has demonstrated that the safety and effectiveness of atorvastatin in this population was similar to that of patients <70 years of age. Pharmacokinetic evaluation of atorvastatin in subjects over the age of 65 years indicates an increased AUC. As a precautionary measure, the lowest dose of the atorvastatin component of CADUET should be administered initially.

Elderly patients may be more susceptible to myopathy (see Muscle Effects, Pre-disposing Factors for Myopathy/Rhabdomyolysis).

ADVERSE REACTIONS: Clinical Trial Adverse Drug Reactions: CADUET—Hypertension and Dyslipidemia: CADUET (amlodipine besylate/atorvastatin calcium) has been evaluated for safety in 1092 patients in 2 double-blind, placebo-controlled studies treated for co-morbid hypertension and dyslipidemia. In these studies, no unexpected adverse experiences particular to this combination have been observed. Adverse experiences have been limited to those that were reported previously with amlodipine and/or atorvastatin.

In general, treatment with CADUET was well tolerated. For the most part, adverse experiences have been mild or moderate in severity. In these controlled clinical trials, adverse events or laboratory abnormalities leading to discontinuation occurred in 5.1% of patients treated with both amlodipine and atorvastatin compared to 4.0% of patients given placebo. The most common safety-related reasons for discontinuation from these studies in the combination treatment groups were headache and peripheral edema.

In a double-blind, controlled clinical trial of all available CADUET doses (5/10 mg to 10/80 mg amlodipine/atorvastatin respectively), the incidences of treatment-emergent adverse events (all causalities) that occurred in at least 1% of all combination treatment groups, pooled across all the combination doses, are summarized in Table 1.

Table 1: CADUET

Adverse Events (All Causality) >1% of Patients taking Concurrent Amlodipine and Atorvastatin

Body System COSTART Preferred Term	Placebo N=111 (%)	AML Only N=221 (%)	ATO Only N=443 (%)	AML+ATO N=885 (%)
Body as a Whole	**16 (14.4)**	**28 (12.7)**	**69 (15.6)**	**137 (15.5)**
Abdominal pain	0 (0.0)	2 (0.9)	10 (2.3)	20 (2.3)
Asthenia	3 (2.7)	4 (1.8)	8 (1.8)	19 (2.1)
Back pain	1 (0.9)	4 (1.8)	5 (1.1)	15 (1.7)
Flu syndrome	1 (0.9)	0 (0.0)	8 (1.8)	9 (1.0)
Headache	11 (9.9)	11 (5.0)	34 (7.7)	47 (5.3)
Cardiovascular	**8 (7.2)**	**16 (7.2)**	**26 (5.9)**	**67 (7.6)**
Palpitation	2 (1.8)	4 (1.8)	4 (0.9)	17 (1.9)
Vasodilatation	3 (2.7)	2 (0.9)	3 (0.7)	18 (2.0)
Digestive	**10 (9.0)**	**16 (7.2)**	**39 (8.8)**	**77 (8.7)**
Constipation	1 (0.9)	3 (1.4)	2 (0.5)	15 (1.7)
Diarrhea	2 (1.8)	2 (0.9)	5 (1.1)	17 (1.9)
GGT increased	0 (0.0)	1 (0.5)	6 (1.4)	16 (1.8)
Nausea	3 (2.7)	3 (1.4)	7 (1.6)	9 (1.0)
Metabolic and Nutritional	**6 (5.4)**	**32 (14.5)**	**21 (4.7)**	**133 (15.0)**
Alkaline phosphatase increased	0 (0.0)	0 (0.0)	2 (0.5)	10 (1.1)
Hyperglycemia	0 (0.0)	1 (0.5)	4 (0.9)	10 (1.1)
Peripheral edema	3 (2.7)	27 (12.2)	5 (1.1)	88 (9.9)
AST increased	1 (0.9)	1 (0.5)	3 (0.7)	13 (1.5)
ALT increased	0 (0.0)	1 (0.5)	5 (1.1)	15 (1.7)
Musculoskeletal	**7 (6.3)**	**12 (5.4)**	**25 (5.6)**	**35 (4.0)**
Arthralgia	4 (3.6)	3 (1.4)	4 (0.9)	10 (1.1)
Myalgia	2 (1.8)	3 (1.4)	8 (1.8)	14 (1.6)
Nervous	**9 (8.1)**	**12 (5.4)**	**25 (5.6)**	**47 (5.3)**
Dizziness	3 (2.7)	7 (3.2)	5 (1.1)	21 (2.4)
Respiratory	**9 (8.1)**	**12 (5.4)**	**28 (6.3)**	**69 (7.8)**
Pharyngitis	1 (0.9)	1 (0.5)	3 (0.7)	9 (1.0)
Respiratory tract infection	5 (4.5)	7 (3.2)	17 (3.8)	43 (4.9)
Skin and Appendages	**4 (3.6)**	**4 (1.8)**	**6 (1.4)**	**32 (3.6)**
Rash	1 (0.9)	1 (0.5)	3 (0.7)	15 (1.7)

Legend: AML=amlodipine; ATO=atorvastatin.

The incidence (%) of dose-related adverse events was consistent with those seen for amlodipine and/or atorvastatin.

In this clinical trial, the most frequently reported adverse events among patients who took concurrent amlodipine and atorvastatin were peripheral edema (9.9%), headache (5.3%), respiratory tract infection (4.9%), dizziness (2.4%), abdominal pain (2.3%), asthenia (2.1%), and vasodilatation (2.0%).

In this controlled clinical trial, similar percentages of patients who took concurrent amlodipine and atorvastatin (5.6%) versus patients who took placebo (4.5%), amlodipine only (5.4%), or atorvastatin only (4.1%) discontinued due to adverse safety experiences. Only 1 subject discontinued due to laboratory abnormalities. The most common safety-related reasons for discontinuation from the study in the combination treatment groups were peripheral edema (1.5%) and headache (1.4%), but these events led to the discontinuation of subjects in the combination treatment groups no more frequently than they did among subjects treated with either amlodipine alone or atorvastatin alone within this study.

The following information is based on the clinical experience with the parent compounds, NORVASC and LIPITOR.

Amlodipine Component of CADUET: General: Amlodipine besylate has been administered to 1714 patients (805 hypertensive and 909 angina patients) in controlled clinical trials (vs placebo alone and with active comparative agents). Most adverse reactions reported during therapy were of mild to moderate severity.

Hypertension: In the 805 hypertensive patients treated with amlodipine in controlled clinical trials, adverse effects were reported in 29.9% of patients and required discontinuation of therapy due to side effects in 1.9% of patients. The most common adverse reactions in controlled clinical trials were: edema (8.9%), and headache (8.3%).

The following adverse reactions were reported with an incidence of >0.5% in the controlled clinical trials program (n=805):

Cardiovascular: edema (8.9%), palpitations (2.0%), tachycardia (0.7%), postural dizziness (0.5%).

Skin and Appendages: pruritus (0.7%).

Musculoskeletal: muscle cramps (0.5%).

Central and Peripheral Nervous Systems: headache (8.3%), dizziness (3.0%), paresthesia (0.5%).

Autonomic Nervous System: flushing (3.1%), increased sweating (0.9%), dry mouth (0.7%).

Psychiatric: somnolence (1.4%).

Gastrointestinal: nausea (2.4%), abdominal pain (1.1%), dyspepsia (0.6%), constipation (0.5%).

General: fatigue (4.1%), pain (0.5%).

Angina: In the controlled clinical trials in 909 angina patients treated with amlodipine, adverse effects were reported in 30.5% of patients and required discontinuation of therapy due to side effects in 0.6% of patients. The most common adverse reactions reported in controlled clinical trials were: edema (9.9%) and headache (7.8%).

The following adverse reactions occurred at an incidence of >0.5% in the controlled clinical trials program (n=909):

Cardiovascular: edema (9.9%), palpitations (2.0%), postural dizziness (0.6%).

Skin and Appendages: rash (1.0%), pruritus (0.8%).

Musculoskeletal: muscle cramps (1.0%).

Central and Peripheral Nervous Systems: headache (7.8%), dizziness (4.5%), paresthesia (1.0%), hypoesthesia (0.9%).

Autonomic Nervous System: flushing (1.9%).

Psychiatric: somnolence (1.2%), insomnia (0.9%), nervousness (0.7%).

Gastrointestinal: nausea (4.2%), abdominal pain (2.2%), dyspepsia (1.4%), diarrhea (1.1%), flatulence (1.0%), constipation (0.9%).

Respiratory System: dyspnea (1.1%).

Special Senses: vision abnormal (1.3%), tinnitus (0.6%).

General: fatigue (4.8%), pain (1.0%), asthenia (1.0%).

Atorvastatin component of CADUET: Dyslipidemia: Atorvastatin is generally well-tolerated. Adverse reactions have usually been mild and transient. In controlled clinical studies (placebo-controlled and active-controlled comparative studies with other lipid lowering agents) involving 2502 patients, <2% of patients were discontinued due to adverse experiences attributable to atorvastatin. Of these 2502 patients, 1721 were treated for at least 6 months and 1253 for 1 year or more.

Adverse experiences occurring at an incidence >1% in patients participating in placebo-controlled clinical studies of atorvastatin and reported to be possibly, probably or definitely drug related are shown in Table 2.

Table 2: CADUET

Associated Adverse Events Reported in >1% of Patients in Placebo-Controlled Clinical Trials

	Placebo % (n=270)	Atorvastatin % (n=1122)
Gastrointestinal		
Constipation	1	1
Diarrhea	1	1
Dyspepsia	2	1
Flatulence	2	1
Nausea	0	1
Nervous System		
Headache	2	1
Miscellaneous		
Pain	<1	1
Myalgia	1	1
Asthenia	<1	1

The following additional adverse events were reported in clinical trials; not all events listed below have been associated with a causal relationship to atorvastatin therapy: Muscle cramps, myositis, myopathy, paresthesia, peripheral neuropathy, pancreatitis, hepatitis, cholestatic jaundice, anorexia, vomiting, alopecia, pruritus, rash, impotence, hyperglycemia, and hypoglycemia.

Less Common Clinical Trial Adverse Drug Reactions: Amlodipine—Angina: Amlodipine has been evaluated for safety in about 11 000 patients with hypertension and angina. The following events occurred in <1% but >0.1% of patients in comparative clinical trials (double-blind comparative vs placebo or active agents; n=2615) or under conditions of open trials or marketing experience where a causal relationship is uncertain.

Cardiovascular: arrhythmia (including ventricular tachycardia and atrial fibrillation), bradycardia, hypotension, peripheral ischemia, syncope, tachycardia, postural dizziness, postural hypotension, vasculitis.

Central and Peripheral Nervous Systems: hypoesthesia, peripheral neuropathy, tremor, vertigo.

Gastrointestinal: anorexia, constipation, dysphagia, vomiting, gingival hyperplasia.

General: allergic reaction, asthenia*, back pain, hot flushes, malaise, rigors, weight gain.

Musculoskeletal System: arthralgia, arthrosis, myalgia.

Psychiatric: sexual dysfunction (male* and female), insomnia, nervousness, depression, abnormal dreams, anxiety, depersonalization.

Respiratory System: epistaxis.

Skin and Appendages: pruritus*, rash erythematous, rash maculopapular, erythema multiforme.

Special Senses: conjunctivitis, diplopia, eye pain, tinnitus.

Urinary System: micturition frequency, micturition disorder, nocturia.

Autonomic Nervous System: dry mouth, sweating increased.

Metabolic and Nutritional: hyperglycemia, thirst.

Hemopoietic: leucopenia, purpura, thrombocytopenia.

The following events occurred in <0.1% of patients: cardiac failure, skin discoloration, urticaria, skin dryness, Stevens-Johnson syndrome, alopecia, twitching, ataxia, hypertonia, migraine, apathy, amnesia, gastritis, pancreatitis, increased appetite, coughing, rhinitis, parosmia, taste perversion, and xerophthalmia.

Isolated cases of angioedema have been reported. Angioedema may be accompanied by breathing difficulty.

Abnormal Hematologic and Clinical Chemistry Findings: Atorvastatin: Laboratory Tests: Increases in serum transaminase levels have been noted in clinical trials (see Warnings and Precautions).

* These events occurred in less than 1% in placebo-controlled trials, but the incidence of these side effects was between 1% and 2% in all multiple dose studies.

Post-Market Adverse Drug Reactions: Amlodipine: In post-marketing experience, jaundice and hepatic enzyme elevations (mostly consistent with cholestasis or hepatitis), in some cases severe enough to require hospitalization, have been reported in association with the use of amlodipine.

Atorvastatin: The following adverse events have also been reported during post-marketing experience with the atorvastatin component of CADUET, regardless of causality assessment: Very rare reports: severe myopathy with or without rhabdomyolysis (see Warnings and Precautions, Muscle Effects, Renal Insufficiency and Drug Interactions). Isolated reports: Gynecomastia, thrombocytopenia, arthralgia and allergic reactions including urticaria, angioneurotic edema, anaphylaxis and bullous rashes (including erytheme multiforme, Stevens-Johnson syndrome and toxic epidermal necrolysis) and fatigue, back pain, chest pain, malaise, dizziness, amnesia, peripheral edema, weight gain, abdominal pain, insomnia, hypoesthesia, tinnitus, tendon rupture, and dysgeusia. These may have no causal relationship to atorvastatin.

Ophthalmologic Observations: See Warnings and Precautions, Ophthalmologic.

DRUG INTERACTIONS: Overview: Pharmacokinetic interaction studies conducted with drugs in healthy subjects may not detect the possibility of a potential drug interaction in some patients due to differences in underlying diseases and use of concomitant medications (see also Warnings and Precautions, Geriatrics, Renal Insufficiency and Patients with Severe Hypercholesterolemia).

Data from a drug-drug interaction study involving 10 mg of amlodipine and 80 mg of atorvastatin in healthy subjects indicate that the pharmacokinetics of amlodipine are not altered when the drugs are coadministered. The effect of amlodipine on the pharmacokinetics of atorvastatin showed no effect on the C_{max} but the AUC of atorvastatin increased by 18% (90% confidence interval: 109 to 127%) in the presence of amlodipine.

No drug interaction studies have been conducted with CADUET and other drugs, although studies have been conducted in the individual amlodipine and atorvastatin components, as described below:

Cytochrome P-450 Mediated Interactions: Drugs known to be inhibitors of the cytochrome P450 system include: azole antifungals, cimetidine, cyclosporine, erythromycin, quinidine, warfarin.

Drugs known to be inducers of the cytochrome P450 system include: phenobarbital, phenytoin, rifampin.

Drugs known to be biotransformed via the cytochrome P450 system include: benzodiazepines, flecainide, imipramine, propafenone, and theophylline.

Amlodipine: As with all drugs, care should be exercised when treating patients with multiple medications. Dihydropyridine calcium channel blockers undergo biotransformation by the cytochrome P450 system, mainly via CYP 3A4 isoenzyme. Coadministration of the amlodipine component of CADUET with other drugs which follow the same route of biotransformation may result in altered bioavailability of amlodipine or these drugs. Dosages of similarly metabolized drugs, particularly those of low therapeutic ratio, and especially in patients with renal and/or hepatic impairment, may require adjustment when starting or stopping concomitantly administered amlodipine to maintain optimum therapeutic blood levels.

The amlodipine component of CADUET has a low (rate of first-pass) hepatic clearance and consequent high bioavailability, and thus, may be expected to have a low potential for clinically relevant effects associated with elevation of amlodipine plasma levels when used concomitantly with drugs that compete for or inhibit the cytochrome P450 system.

In clinical trials, the amlodipine component of CADUET has been safely administered with thiazide diuretics, beta blockers, angiotensin converting enzyme inhibitors, long acting nitrates, sublingual nitroglycerin, digoxin, warfarin, non steroidal anti-inflammatory drugs, antibiotics, and oral hypoglycemic drugs.

Atorvastatin: The atorvastatin component of CADUET is metabolized by the cytochrome P450 isoenzyme, CYP 3A4. Erythromycin, a CYP 3A4 inhibitor, increased atorvastatin plasma levels by 40%. Coadministration of CYP 3A4 inhibitors, such as grapefruit juice, some macrolide antibiotics (i.e. erythromycin, clarithromycin), immunosuppressants (cyclosporine), azole antifungal agents (i.e. itraconazole, ketoconazole), protease inhibitors, or the antidepressant, nefazodone, may have the potential to increase plasma concentrations of HMG CoA reductase inhibitors, including atorvastatin. Caution should thus be exercised with concomitant use of these agents (see Warnings and Precautions, Pharmacokinetic Interactions, Muscle Effects, Renal Insufficiency and Endocrine Function; Dosage and Administration).

Concomitant Therapy with Other Lipid Metabolism Regulators: Based on post-marketing surveillance, gemfibrozil, fenofibrate, other fibrates, and lipid lowering doses of niacin (nicotinic acid) may increase the risk of myopathy when given concomitantly with HMG-CoA reductase inhibitors, probably because they can produce myopathy when given alone (see Warnings and Precautions, Muscle Effects). Therefore, combined drug therapy should be approached with caution.

Inducers of cytochrome P450 3A: Concomitant administration of atorvastatin with inducers of cytochrome P450 3A4 (eg efavirenz, rifampin) can lead to variable reductions in plasma concentrations of atorvastatin. Due to the dual interaction mechanism of rifampin, (cytochrome P450 3A4 induction and inhibition of hepatocyte uptake transporter OATP1B1), simultaneous coadministration of atorvastatin with rifampin resulted in a mean increase in Cmax and AUC of atorvastatin of 12 and 190%, respectively. In contrast, a delayed administration of atorvastatin after administration of rifampin has been associated with a significant reduction (approximately 80%) in atorvastatin plasma concentrations.

Drug-Drug Interactions: The drugs listed in Table 3 are based on either drug interaction case reports or studies, or predicted interactions due to the expected magnitude and seriousness of the interaction (ie. those identified as contraindicated).

Table 3: CADUET

Established or Predicted Drug-Drug Interactions[a]

	Effect		
	Amlodipine	**Atorvastatin**	**Clinical comment**
Amlodipine		↔ in the AUC, C_{max} or T_{max} of atorvastatin ↔ in blood pressure or heart rate	
Antacids (aluminum- and magnesium-based)	↔ on the disposition of amlodipine	↓ in plasma concentrations of atorvastatin by ~35% ↔ in LDL-C reduction triglyceride-lowering effect may be affected	
Antipyrine		↔ in the PK of antipyrine	Antipyrine was used as a non-specific model for drugs metabolized by the microsomal hepatic enzyme system (cytochrome P450 system). Interactions with other drugs metabolized via the same cytochrome isozymes are not expected.
Beta-blockers	blood pressure lowering effect of beta-blockers may be ↑ by amlodipine		Patients should be carefully monitored.
Bile Acid Sequestrants		↓ in plasma concentration of atorvastatin by ~26%	See Action and Clinical Pharmacology. When atorvastatin is used concurrently with colestipol or any other resin, an interval of at least 2 hours should be maintained between the two drugs, since the absorption of atorvastatin may be impaired by the resin.

(cont'd)

Table 3: CADUET *(cont'd)*

Established or Predicted Drug-Drug Interactions[a]

	Effect		
	Amlodipine	**Atorvastatin**	**Clinical comment**
Cimetidine	↔ in the PK of amlodipine	↔ in plasma concentration of atorvastatin ↔ in LDL-C reduction ↓ triglyceride lowering effect from 34% to 26%	
Cyclosporine	↔ in the PK of cyclosporine		
Diltiazem Hydrochloride		Steady-state diltiazem increases the exposure, based on AUC_{LASTs}, of a single dose of atorvastatin by approximately 50%.	
Digoxin	↔ in serum digoxin levels or digoxin renal clearance	↔ in digoxin PK by coadministration with atorvastatin 10 mg daily ↑ in digoxin concentrations ~20% following coadministration with atorvastatin 80 mg daily	Patients taking digoxin should be monitored appropriately.
Fibric Acid Derivatives (Gemfibrozil, Fenofibrate, Bezafibrate) and Niacin (Nicotinic Acid)		↑ in the risk of myopathy during treatment with other drugs in this class, including atorvastatin	Although there is limited experience with the use of atorvastatin given concurrently with fibric acid derivatives and niacin, the benefits and risks of such combined therapy should be carefully considered. See Warnings and Precautions, Muscle Effects.
Macrolide antibiotics		↑ in atorvastatin plasma levels by ~40% with erythromycin and ~80% with clarithromycin ↔ in atorvastatin plasma levels with azithromycin	See Warnings and Precautions, Muscle Effects.
Oral Contraceptives and Hormone Replacement Therapy		↑ in AUC of norethindrone by ~30% and ethinyl estradiol by ~20%	These increases should be considered when selecting an oral contraceptive. In clinical studies, atorvastatin was used concomitantly with estrogen replacement therapy without evidence to date of clinically significant adverse interactions.
Protease Inhibitor (nelfinavir mesylate)		↑ in AUC by 74% and C_{max} by 122% of atorvastatin by nelfinavir mesylate	Nelfinavir is a known CYP3A4 inhibitor.
Quinapril		↔ in PK profile of atorvastatin	
Sildenafil	↔ in AUC or C_{max} of amlodipine mean additional ↓ of supine systolic and diastolic blood pressure was 8 mmHg and 7 mmHg, respectively		
Warfarin	↔ in warfarin-induced prothrombin response time	↔ in warfarin-induced prothrombin response time	

[a] For more detailed drug interaction information please refer to individual Product Monographs for NORVASC and LIPITOR.

Legend: ↔ = no change; ↑ = increase; ↓ = decrease; ~ = approximately; AUC = area under the curve; C_{max} = maximal concentrations; LDL-C = low density lipoprotein cholesterol; PK = pharmacokinetics; T_{max} = time to maximal concentrations.

Drug-Food Interactions: Grapefruit Juice: Amlodipine: Published data indicate that through inhibition of the cytochrome P450 system, grapefruit juice can increase plasma levels and augment pharmacodynamic effects of some dihydropyridine calcium channel blockers. Following oral administration of 10 mg amlodipine to 20 male volunteers, pharmacokinetics of amlodipine were similar when amlodipine was administered with and without grapefruit juice.

Atorvastatin: Coadministration of grapefruit juice has the potential to increase plasma concentrations of HMG-CoA reductase inhibitors including LIPITOR. The equivalent of 1.2 L per day resulted in a 2.5 fold increase in AUC of atorvastatin.

DOSAGE AND ADMINISTRATION: CADUET is a combination product containing amlodipine besylate and atorvastatin calcium. CADUET is not intended for initial therapy.

General Considerations: The dosage of CADUET must be individualized on the basis of both effectiveness and tolerance for each component which should be determined by titration as described below.

CADUET can be administered once daily, at any time of the day, with or without food.

Amlodipine (essential hypertension and chronic stable angina): Use in Adults: For both hypertension and angina, the recommended initial dose of amlodipine besylate is 5 mg once daily. If necessary, dose can be increased after 1-2 weeks to a maximum dose of 10 mg once daily.

Use in the Elderly or in Patients with Impaired Renal Function: The recommended initial dose in patients over 65 years of age or patients with impaired renal function is 5 mg once daily. If required, increasing in the dose should be done gradually and with caution (see Warnings and Precautions, Renal, Renal Insufficiency; Special Populations, Geriatrics).

Use in Patients with Impaired Hepatic Function: Dosage requirements have not been established in patients with impaired hepatic function. When amlodipine is used in these patients, the dosage should be carefully and gradually adjusted depending on patients tolerance and response. A lower starting dose of 2.5 mg once daily should be considered (see Warnings and Precautions, Hepatic/Biliary/Pancreatic, Hepatic Effects).

Use in Children: There have been no studies conducted to determine the safety or effectiveness of CADUET in pediatric populations.

The effective antihypertensive oral dose in pediatric patients ages 6 17 years is 2.5 mg to 5 mg once daily. Doses in excess of 5 mg daily have not been studied; dose should be determined based upon the medical need of the patients (see Warnings and Precautions Special Populations, Pediatrics).

Atorvastatin (hyperlipidemia): Patients should be placed on a standard cholesterol-lowering diet before receiving atorvastatin, and should continue on this diet during treatment with atorvastatin. If appropriate, a program of weight control and physical exercise should be implemented.

Prior to initiating therapy with atorvastatin, secondary causes for elevations in plasma lipid levels should be excluded. A lipid profile should also be performed.

Primary Hypercholesterolemia and Combined (Mixed) Dyslipidemia, Including Familial Combined Hyperlipidemia: The recommended starting dose of atorvastatin is 10 or 20 mg once daily, depending on patient's LDL-C reduction required. Patients who require a large reduction in LDL-C (more than 45%) may be started at 40 mg once daily. The dosage range of atorvastatin is 10 to 80 mg once daily. Doses can be given at any time of the day with or without food, and should preferably be given in the evening. A significant therapeutic response is evident within 2 weeks, and the maximum response is usually achieved within 2-4 weeks. The response is maintained during chronic therapy. Adjustments of dosage, if necessary, should be made at intervals of 2 to 4 weeks. The maximum dose is 80 mg/day.

The dosage of atorvastatin should be individualized according the baseline LDL-C, total-C/HDL-C ratio and/or TG levels to achieve the recommended desired lipid values at the lowest dose needed to achieve LDL-C desired level. Lipid levels should be monitored periodically and, if necessary, the dose of atorvastatin adjusted based on desired lipid levels recommended by guidelines.

Severe Dyslipidemias: In patients with severe dyslipidemias, including homozygous and heterozygous familial hypercholesterolemia and dysbetalipoproteinemia (Type III), higher dosages (up to 80 mg/day) may be required (see Warnings and Precautions, Pharmacokinetic Interactions, Muscle Effects; Drug Interactions).

Heterozygous Familial Hypercholesterolemia in Pediatric Patients (10-17 years of age): There have been no studies conducted to determine the safety or effectiveness of CADUET in pediatric populations.

In this population, the recommended starting dose of LIPITOR is 10 mg/day; the maximum recommended dose is 20 mg/day (doses greater than 20 mg/day have not been studied in this patient population). Doses should be individualized according to the recommended goal of therapy (see Warnings and Precautions, Special Populations, Pediatrics). Adjustments should be made at intervals of 4 weeks or more.

Prevention of Cardiovascular Disease: Clinical trials conducted that evaluated atorvastatin in the primary prevention of myocardial infarction used a dose of 10 mg atorvastatin once daily.

For secondary prevention of myocardial infarction, optimal dosing may range from 10 mg to 80 mg atorvastatin once daily, to be given at the discretion of the prescriber, taking into account the expected benefit and safety considerations relevant to the patient to be treated.

Concomitant Therapy: See Drug Interactions, Overview, Cytochrome P-450 Mediated Interactions; Drug-Drug Interactions; Drug-Food Interactions.

Dosage in Patients with Renal Insufficiency: See Warnings and Precautions, Renal.

OVERDOSAGE:

There is no information on overdosage with CADUET in humans.

Amlodipine: Symptoms: Overdosage can cause excessive peripheral vasodilation with marked and probably prolonged hypotension and possibly a reflex tachycardia. In humans, experience with overdosage of the amlodipine component of CADUET is limited. When amlodipine was ingested at doses of 105-250 mg some patients remained normotensive with or without gastric lavage while another patient experienced hypotension (90/50 mmHg) which normalized following plasma expansion. A patient who took 70 mg of amlodipine with benzodiazepine developed shock which was refractory to treatment and died. In a 19-month old child who ingested 30 mg of amlodipine (about 2 mg/kg) there was no evidence of hypotension but tachycardia (180 bpm) was observed. Ipecac was administered 3.5 hrs after ingestion and on subsequent observation (overnight) no sequelae were noted.

Treatment: Clinically significant hypotension due to overdosage requires active cardiovascular support, including frequent monitoring of cardiac and respiratory function, elevation of extremities, and attention to circulating fluid volume and urine output. A vasoconstrictor (such as norepinephrine) may be helpful in restoring vascular tone and blood pressure, provided that there is no contraindication to its use. As amlodipine is highly protein bound, hemodialysis is not likely to be of benefit. Intravenous calcium gluconate may be beneficial in reversing the effects of calcium channel blockade. Clearance of amlodipine is prolonged in elderly patients and in patients with impaired liver function. Since amlodipine absorption is slow, gastric lavage may be worthwhile in some cases.

Atorvastatin: There is no specific treatment for the atorvastatin component of CADUET overdosage. Should an overdose occur, the patient should be treated symptomatically and supportive measures instituted as required. Due to extensive drug binding to plasma proteins, hemodialysis is not expected to significantly enhance atorvastatin clearance.

> For management of a suspected drug overdose, CPhA recommends that you contact your **regional Poison Control Centre**. See the *CPS* Directory section for a list of Poison Control Centres.

ACTION AND CLINICAL PHARMACOLOGY: Mechanism of Action: CADUET (amlodipine besylate/atorvastatin calcium), is a combination tablet which combines 2 mechanisms of action: the dihydropyridine calcium antagonist (calcium entry blocker or calcium ion antagonist) action of amlodipine and the HMG-CoA reductase inhibition of atorvastatin. The amlodipine component of CADUET inhibits the transmembrane influx of calcium ions into vascular smooth muscle and cardiac muscle. The atorvastatin component of CADUET is a selective, competitive inhibitor of HMG-CoA reductase, the rate-limiting enzyme that converts 3-hydroxy-3-methylglutaryl-coenzyme A to mevalonate, a precursor of sterols, including cholesterol.

The Antihypertensive/Antianginal Action of CADUET: Experimental data suggest that amlodipine binds to both dihydropyridine and nondihydropyridine binding sites. The contractile processes of cardiac and vascular smooth muscle tissues are dependent upon the movement of extracellular calcium ions into these cells through specific ion channels. Amlodipine inhibits calcium ion influx across cell membranes selectively, with a greater effect on vascular smooth muscle cells than on cardiac muscle cells. Serum calcium concentration is not affected by amlodipine. Within the physiologic pH range, amlodipine is an ionized compound and its kinetic interaction with the calcium channel receptor is characterized by the gradual association and dissociation with the receptor binding site.

- Hypertension: The mechanism by which amlodipine reduces arterial blood pressure involves direct peripheral arterial vasodilation and reduction in peripheral vascular resistance.
- Angina: The precise mechanism by which amlodipine relieves angina has not been fully delineated. Amlodipine is a dilator of peripheral arteries and arterioles which reduces the total peripheral resistance and, therefore, reduces the workload of the heart (afterload). The unloading of the heart is thought to decrease ischemia and relieve effort angina by reducing myocardial energy oxygen consumption and oxygen requirements.

The Antidyslipidemic Action of CADUET: Atorvastatin lowers plasma cholesterol and lipoprotein levels by inhibiting HMG-CoA reductase and cholesterol synthesis in the liver and by increasing the number of hepatic LDL receptors on the cell-surface for enhanced uptake and catabolism of LDL.

Atorvastatin reduces LDL-C and the number of LDL particles. Atorvastatin also reduces VLDL-C, serum TG and IDL, as well as the number of apo B containing particles, but increases HDL-C. Elevated serum cholesterol due to elevated LDL-C is a major risk factor for the development of cardiovascular disease. Low serum concentration of HDL-C is an independent risk factor. Elevated plasma TG is also a risk factor for cardiovascular disease, particularly if due to increased IDL, or associated with decreased HDL-C or increased LDL-C.

Epidemiologic, clinical and experimental studies have established that high LDL-C, low HDL-C and high plasma TG promote human atherosclerosis, and are risk factors for developing cardiovascular disease. Some studies have also shown that the total (TC):HDL-C ratio (TC:HDL-C) is the best predictor of coronary artery disease. In contrast, increased levels of HDL-C are associated with decreased cardiovascular risk. Drug therapies that reduce levels of LDL-C or decrease TG while simultaneously increasing HDL-C have demonstrated reductions in rates of cardiovascular mortality and morbidity.

Pharmacodynamics: CADUET: Studies have been conducted in which placebo, amlodipine alone, atorvastatin alone, and the 8 dose combinations of amlodipine and atorvastatin have been administered once daily, in patients with co-morbid dyslipidemia and hypertension. Analyses of changes in systolic blood pressure demonstrated that there was no overall modification of amlodipine's effect on systolic blood pressure when the drug was taken in combination with atorvastatin compared to amlodipine alone. Analyses of changes in LDL-C demonstrated that there was no overall modification of atorvastatin's effect on LDL-C when the drug was taken in combination with amlodipine compared with atorvastatin alone.

Amlodipine: Hemodynamics: Following administration of recommended doses to patients with hypertension, amlodipine produces vasodilation resulting in a reduction of supine and standing blood pressures. These decreases in blood pressure are not accompanied by any significant change in heart rate or plasma catecholamine levels with chronic dosing. With chronic once daily oral administration (5 and 10 mg once daily), antihypertensive effectiveness is maintained throughout the 24-hour dose interval with minimal peak to trough differences in blood pressure reduction. Since the vasodilation induced by amlodipine is gradual in onset, acute hypotension has rarely been reported after oral administration of amlodipine. In normotensive patients with angina, amlodipine has not been associated with any clinically significant reductions in blood pressure or changes in heart rate.

Negative inotropic effects have not been observed when amlodipine was administered at the recommended doses to man, but has been demonstrated in animal models. Hemodynamic measurements of cardiac function at rest and during exercise (or pacing) in angina patients with normal ventricular function have generally demonstrated a small increase in cardiac index without significant influence on dP/dt or on left ventricular end diastolic pressure or volume.

In hypertensive patients with normal renal function, therapeutic doses of amlodipine resulted in a decrease in renal vascular resistance and an increase in glomerular filtration rate and effective renal plasma flow without change in filtration fraction.

Electrophysiologic Effects: Amlodipine does not change sinoatrial nodal function or atrioventricular conduction in intact animals, or man. In patients with chronic stable angina, intravenous administration of 10 mg of amlodipine and a further 10 mg of amlodipine after a 30-minute interval produced peripheral vasodilation and afterload reduction, but did not significantly alter A-H and H-V conduction and sinus node recovery time after pacing. Similar results were obtained in patients receiving amlodipine and concomitant beta-blockers. In clinical studies in which amlodipine was administered in combination with beta-blockers to patients with either hypertension or angina, no adverse effects on electrocardiographic parameters were observed. In clinical trials with angina patients, amlodipine as monotherapy did not alter electrocardiographic intervals.

Atorvastatin: Human Pharmacology: The lowering of total cholesterol, LDL-C and apo B have been shown to reduce the risk of cardiovascular events and mortality.

Atorvastatin is a selective, competitive inhibitor of HMG-CoA reductase. In both subjects and in patients with homozygous and heterozygous familial hypercholesterolemia, nonfamilial forms of hypercholesterolemia, mixed dyslipidemia, hypertriglyceridemia, and dysbetalipoproteinemia, atorvastatin has been shown to reduce levels of total-C, LDL-C, apo B and total TG, and raises HDL-C levels.

Epidemiologic and clinical studies have associated the risk of coronary artery disease (CAD) with elevated levels of total-C, LDL-C and decreased levels of HDL-C. These abnormalities of lipoprotein metabolism are considered as major contributors to the development of the disease. Like LDL, cholesterol-enriched lipoproteins, including VLDL, IDL and remnants can also promote atherosclerosis. Elevated plasma triglycerides are frequently found in a triad with low HDL-C levels and small LDL particles, as well as in association with non-lipid metabolic risk factors for coronary heart disease (metabolic syndrome). Clinical studies have also shown that serum triglycerides can be an independent risk factor for CAD. CAD risk is especially increased if the hypertriglyceridemia is due to increased intermediate density lipoproteins (IDL) or associated with decreased HDL or increased LDL-C. In addition, high TG levels are associated with an increased risk of pancreatitis. Although epidemiological and preliminary clinical evidence link low HDL-C levels and high triglyceride levels with coronary artery disease and atherosclerosis, the independent effect of raising HDL or lowering TG on the risk of coronary and cerebrovascular morbidity and mortality has not been demonstrated in prospective, well-controlled outcome studies. Other factors, e.g. interactions between lipids/lipoproteins and endothelium, platelets and macrophages, have also been incriminated in the development of human atherosclerosis and of its complications. Regardless of the intervention used (low-fat/low-cholesterol diet, partial ileal bypass surgery or pharmacologic therapy), effective treatment of hypercholesterolemia/dyslipidemia has consistently been shown to reduce the risk of CAD.

Atorvastatin reduces LDL-C and the number of LDL particles, lowersVLDL-C and serum TG, reduces the number of apo B containing particles, and also increases HDL-C. Atorvastatin is effective in reducing LDL-C in patients with homozygous familial hypercholesterolemia, a condition that rarely responds to any other lipid-lowering medication. In addition to the above effects, atorvastatin reduces IDL-C and apolipoprotein E (apo E) in patients with dysbetalipoproteinemia (Type III).

In patients with Type II dyslipidemia, atorvastatin improved endothelial dysfunction. Atorvastatin significantly improved flow-mediated endothelium-dependent dilatation induced by reactive hyperemia, as assessed by brachial ultrasound ($p<0.01$).

Pharmacokinetics: Absorption: CADUET: Following oral administration of therapeutic doses of CADUET tablets, 2 distinct peak plasma concentrations are observed. The first peak is attributable to atorvastatin and occurs within 1 to 2 hours after dosing. The second peak is attributable to amlodipine and occurs between 6 and 12 hours after dosing. The rate and extent of absorption (bioavailability) of both amlodipine and atorvastatin from CADUET combination tablet are not significantly different from those observed during coadministration of separate amlodipine and atorvastatin tablets, as assessed by C_{max}: 101% (90% CI: 98, 104) and AUC: 100% (90% CI: 97, 103) for the amlodipine component and C_{max}: 94% (90% CI: 85, 104) and AUC: 105% (90% CI: 99, 111) for the atorvastatin component, respectively.

The bioavailability of amlodipine from the CADUET tablet was not affected under the fed state as assessed by C_{max} and AUC. Food decreases the rate and extent of absorption of atorvastatin from the CADUET tablets by approximately 32% and 11%, respectively. Similar reductions in plasma concentrations were observed with atorvastatin in the fed state without a reduction in LDL-C effect.

Amlodipine: After oral administration of therapeutic doses of amlodipine, absorption occurs gradually with peak plasma concentration reached between 6 and 12 hours. Absolute bioavailability has been estimated to be between 64 and 90%. The bioavailability of amlodipine is not altered by the presence of food.

Atorvastatin: Atorvastatin is rapidly absorbed after oral administration; maximal plasma concentrations occur within 1 to 2 hours. Extent of absorption and plasma atorvastatin concentrations increase in proportion to atorvastatin dose. The absolute bioavailability (parent drug) of atorvastatin is approximately 12% and the systemic availability of HMG-CoA reductase inhibitory activity is approximately 30%. The low systemic availability is attributed to presystemic clearance in gastrointestinal mucosa and/or first-pass metabolism in the liver. Although food decreases the rate and extent of drug absorption by approximately 25% and 9%, as assessed by C_{max} and AUC respectively, LDL-C reduction and HDL-C elevation are similar when atorvastatin is given with and without food. Plasma atorvastatin concentrations are lower (approximately 30% for C_{max} and AUC) following drug administration in the evening compared with morning dosing. However, LDL-C reduction and HDL-C elevation are the same regardless of the time of drug administration.

Distribution: Amlodipine: Ex vivo studies have shown that approximately 93% of the circulating drug is bound to plasma proteins in hypertensive patients. Steady state plasma levels of amlodipine are reached after 7 to 8 days of consecutive daily dosing.

Atorvastatin: Mean volume of distribution of atorvastatin is approximately 381 L. Atorvastatin is ≥98% bound to plasma proteins. A blood/plasma ratio of approximately 0.25 indicates poor drug penetration into red blood cells. Based on observations in rats, atorvastatin is likely to be secreted in human milk (see Contraindications, Warnings and Precautions).

Metabolism: Amlodipine: Amlodipine is metabolized through the cytochrome P450 system, mainly via CYP 3A4 isoenzyme. Amlodipine is extensively (about 90%) converted to inactive metabolites (via hepatic metabolism).

Atorvastatin: Atorvastatin is extensively metabolized to ortho- and para-hydroxylated derivatives by cytochrome P450 system via the CYP 3A4 isoenzyme and to various beta-oxidation products. In vitro, inhibition of HMG-CoA reductase by ortho- and para-hydroxylated metabolites is equivalent to that of atorvastatin. Approximately 70% of circulating inhibitory activity for HMG-CoA reductase is attributed to active metabolites. In animals, the ortho-hydroxy metabolite undergoes further glucuronidation. Atorvastatin and its metabolites are eliminated by biliary excretion.

Excretion: Amlodipine: Elimination from the plasma is biphasic with a terminal elimination half-life of about 35-50 hours. Ten percent (10%) of the parent compound and 60% of the metabolites are excreted in the urine.

Atorvastatin: Atorvastatin is eliminated primarily in bile following hepatic and/or extrahepatic metabolism; however, the drug does not appear to undergo significant enterohepatic recirculation. Mean plasma elimination half-life of atorvastatin in humans is approximately 14 hours, but the half-life for inhibitory activity for HMG-CoA reductase is 20 to 30 hours due to the contribution of longer-lived active metabolites. Less than 2% of a dose of atorvastatin is recovered in urine following oral administration.

Special Populations and Conditions: Pediatrics: Pharmacokinetic data in the pediatric population are not available.

Geriatrics: Amlodipine: In elderly hypertensive patients (mean age 69 years) there was a decrease in clearance of amlodipine from plasma as compared to young volunteers (mean age 36 years) with a resulting increase in the area under the curve (AUC) of about 60%.

Atorvastatin: Plasma concentrations of atorvastatin are higher (approximately 40% for C_{max} and 30% for AUC) in healthy elderly subjects (age 65 years or older) compared with younger individuals. LDL-C reduction, however, is comparable to that seen in younger patient populations.

Gender: Atorvastatin: Plasma concentrations of atorvastatin in women differ (approximately 20% higher for C_{max} and 10% lower for AUC) from those in men; however, there is no clinically significant difference in LDL-C reduction between men and women.

Race: Atorvastatin: Plasma concentrations of atorvastatin are similar in black and white subjects.

Hepatic Insufficiency: Amlodipine: Following single oral administration of 5 mg of amlodipine, patients with chronic mild-moderate hepatic insufficiency showed about 40% increase in AUC of amlodipine as compared to normal volunteers. This was presumably due to a reduction in clearance of amlodipine as the terminal elimination half-life was prolonged from 34 hrs in young normal subjects to 56 hrs in the elderly patients with hepatic insufficiency.

Atorvastatin: Plasma concentrations of atorvastatin are markedly increased (approximately 16-fold in C_{max} and 11-fold in AUC) in patients with chronic alcoholic liver disease (Childs-Pugh B).

Renal Insufficiency: Amlodipine: The pharmacokinetics of amlodipine are not significantly influenced by renal impairment. Plasma concentrations in the patients with moderate to severe renal failure were higher than in the normal subjects. Accumulation and mean elimination half-life in all patients were within the range of those observed in other pharmacokinetic studies with amlodipine in normal subjects.

Atorvastatin: Plasma concentrations and LDL-C lowering efficacy of atorvastatin are similar in patients with moderate renal insufficiency compared with patients with normal renal function. However, since several cases of rhabdomyolysis have been reported in patients with a history of renal insufficiency of unknown severity, as a precautionary measure and pending further experience in renal disease, the lowest dose (10 mg/day) of atorvastatin should be used in these patients. Similar precautions apply in patients with severe renal insufficiency (creatinine clearance <30 mL/min [<0.5 mL/sec]); the lowest dosage should be used and implemented cautiously (see Warnings and Precautions, Muscle Effects; Drug Interactions and Dosage and Administration).

STORAGE AND STABILITY: Store at 25°C; excursions permitted to 15-30°C.

SPECIAL HANDLING INSTRUCTIONS: Not applicable.

INFORMATION FOR THE PATIENT: Published in e-CPS, available by subscription at www.e-cps.ca.

DOSAGE FORMS, COMPOSITION AND PACKAGING: 5 mg/10 mg: Each white tablet, engraved with "Pfizer" on one side and CDT 051 on the other side, contains: amlodipine besylate 5 mg and atorvastatin calcium 10 mg. Nonmedicinal ingredients: calcium carbonate, colloidal silicon dioxide (anhydrous), croscarmellose sodium, hydroxypropyl cellulose, magnesium stearate, microcrystalline cellulose, Opadry II White 85F28751, polysorbate 80, pregelatinized starch and purified water. High-density polyethylene (HDPE) bottles of 90, containing desiccant, with child-resistant closure.

5 mg/20 mg: Each white tablet, engraved with "Pfizer" on one side and CDT 052 on the other side, contains: amlodipine besylate 5 mg and atorvastatin calcium 20 mg. Nonmedicinal ingredients: calcium carbonate, colloidal silicon dioxide (anhydrous), croscarmellose sodium, hydroxypropyl cellulose, magnesium stearate, microcrystalline cellulose, Opadry II White 85F28751, polysorbate 80, pregelatinized starch and purified water. High-density polyethylene (HDPE) bottles of 90, containing desiccant, with child-resistant closure.

5 mg/40 mg: Each white tablet, engraved with "Pfizer" on one side and CDT 054 on the other side, contains: amlodipine besylate 5 mg and atorvastatin calcium 40 mg. Nonmedicinal ingredients: calcium carbonate, colloidal silicon dioxide (anhydrous), croscarmellose sodium, hydroxypropyl cellulose, magnesium stearate, microcrystalline cellulose, Opadry II White 85F28751, polysorbate 80, pregelatinized starch and purified water. High-density polyethylene (HDPE) bottles of 90, containing desiccant, with child-resistant closure.

5 mg/80 mg: Each white tablet, engraved with "Pfizer" on one side and CDT 058 on the other side, contains: amlodipine besylate 5 mg and atorvastatin calcium 80 mg. Nonmedicinal ingredients: calcium carbonate, colloidal silicon dioxide (anhydrous), croscarmellose sodium, hydroxypropyl cellulose, magnesium stearate, microcrystalline cellulose, Opadry II White 85F28751, polysorbate 80, pregelatinized starch and purified water. High-density polyethylene (HDPE) bottles of 90, containing desiccant, with child-resistant closure.

10 mg/10 mg: Each blue tablet, engraved with "Pfizer" on one side and CDT 101 on the other side, contains: amlodipine besylate 10 mg and atorvastatin calcium 10 mg. Nonmedicinal ingredients: calcium carbonate, colloidal silicon dioxide (anhydrous), croscarmellose sodium, hydroxypropyl cellulose, magnesium stearate, microcrystalline cellulose, Opadry II Blue 85F10919, polysorbate 80, pregelatinized starch and purified water. High-density polyethylene (HDPE) bottles of 90, containing desiccant, with child-resistant closure.

10 mg/20 mg: Each blue tablet, engraved with "Pfizer" on one side and CDT 102 on the other side, contains: amlodipine besylate 10 mg and atorvastatin calcium 20 mg. Nonmedicinal ingredients: calcium carbonate, colloidal silicon dioxide (anhydrous), croscarmellose sodium, hydroxypropyl cellulose, magnesium stearate, microcrystalline cellulose, Opadry II Blue 85F10919, polysorbate 80, pregelatinized starch and purified water. High-density polyethylene (HDPE) bottles of 90, containing desiccant, with child-resistant closure.

10 mg/40 mg: Each blue tablet, engraved with "Pfizer" on one side and CDT 104 on the other side, contains: amlodipine besylate 10 mg and atorvastatin calcium 40 mg. Nonmedicinal ingredients: calcium carbonate, colloidal silicon dioxide (anhydrous), croscarmellose sodium, hydroxypropyl cellulose, magnesium stearate, microcrystalline cellulose, Opadry II Blue 85F10919, polysorbate 80, pregelatinized starch and purified water. High-density polyethylene (HDPE) bottles of 90, containing desiccant, with child-resistant closure.

10 mg/80 mg: Each blue tablet, engraved with "Pfizer" on one side and CDT 108 on the other side, contains: amlodipine besylate 10 mg and atorvastatin calcium 80 mg. Nonmedicinal ingredients: calcium carbonate, colloidal silicon dioxide (anhydrous), croscarmellose sodium, hydroxypropyl cellulose, magnesium stearate, microcrystalline cellulose, Opadry II Blue 85F10919, polysorbate 80, pregelatinized starch and purified water. High-density polyethylene (HDPE) bottles of 90, containing desiccant, with child-resistant closure.

(Shown in Product Identification Section)

Caelyx® Ⓟ

doxorubicin HCl, pegylated liposomal

Antineoplastic

Schering-Plough

Date of Revision: March 26, 2007

SUMMARY PRODUCT INFORMATION:

Route of Administration	Dosage Form/ Strength	Clinically Relevant Nonmedicinal Ingredients
Intravenous Injection	2 mg/mL	For a complete listing see Dosage Forms, Composition and Packaging.

INDICATIONS AND CLINICAL USE: CAELYX (Pegylated Liposomal Doxorubicin Hydrochloride for Injection) is indicated for:

- monotherapy for patients with metastatic breast cancer, where there is an increased cardiac risk associated with conventional doxorubicin.
- advanced ovarian carcinoma in women who have failed standard first-line therapy. Platinum-and paclitaxel- based chemotherapy is the current standard first-line treatment regimen.
- AIDS-related Kaposi's sarcoma (KS) in patients with low CD4 counts (<200 CD4 lymphocytes/mm³) and extensive mucocutaneous or visceral disease whose disease has progressed despite therapy or who are intolerant to prior systemic combination chemotherapy comprising of at least two of the following agents: a vinca alkaloid, bleomycin and doxorubicin (or another anthracycline).

CONTRAINDICATIONS:

- CAELYX (Pegylated Liposomal Doxorubicin Hydrochloride for Injection) is contraindicated in patients who have a history of hypersensitivity reactions to a conventional formulation of doxorubicin or the components of CAELYX.
- Should not be administered while breast-feeding.

WARNINGS AND PRECAUTIONS:

Serious Warnings and Precautions

- **Cardiotoxicity including congestive heart failure and cardiomyopathy may occur (see Warnings and Precautions, Cardiovascular);**
- **Acute infusion reactions (see General, Infusion Reactions);**
- **Myelosuppression (see Warnings and Precautions, Hematologic, Myelosuppression);**
- **CAELYX should only be administered by physicians experienced with cancer chemotherapeutic drugs.**

General: CAELYX is a unique formulation of doxorubicin hydrochloride and must not be used interchangeably with other formulations of doxorubicin hydrochloride.

Infusion Reactions: Serious and sometimes life-threatening infusion reactions may occur within minutes of starting the infusion of CAELYX. These reactions have been described as allergic-like or anaphylactoid-like and are defined by the following COSTART terms: allergic reaction, anaphylactoid reaction, asthma, face edema, hypotension, vasodilatation, urticaria, back pain, chest pain, chills, fever, hypertension, tachycardia, dyspepsia, nausea, dizziness, dyspnea, pharyngitis, rash, pruritus, sweating, injection site reaction and drug interaction. Very rarely, convulsions have been observed in relation to infusion reactions.

Temporarily stopping the infusion usually resolves these symptoms without further therapy. However, medication to treat these symptoms (e.g. antihistamines, corticosteroids, adrenaline, and anticonvulsants), as well as emergency equipment should be available for immediate use. In most patients, treatment can be resumed after all symptoms have resolved without recurrence. Infusion-associated reactions rarely recur after the first treatment cycle. To minimize the risk of infusion reactions, the initial dose should be administered at a rate no greater than 1 mg/minute (see Dosage and Administration).

In patients with solid tumors, 100 out of 929 patients (10.8%) were described as having an infusion-associated reaction during treatment with CAELYX. Permanent treatment discontinuation rates were infrequently reported at 2%.

In the pivotal breast cancer trials, a similar incidence of infusion reactions (32/254-13%) was observed. The rate of permanent treatment discontinuation was 2% (4/254).

In the ovarian cancer population (subset of the solid tumor cohort), 51/510 (10%) patients reported treatment-related infusion reaction adverse events. Five patients (<1%) (reporting nine events) discontinued due to treatment-related infusion reactions.

In patients with AIDS-KS, infusion-associated reactions were characterized by flushing, shortness of breath, facial edema, headache, chills, back pain, tightness in the chest and throat and/or hypotension and can be expected at the rate of 5% to 10%. Very rarely, convulsions have been observed in relation to infusion reactions. Many patients were able to tolerate further infusions without complications, however, eight patients discontinued CAELYX therapy because of an infusion reaction.

Injection Site Effects: CAELYX (Pegylated Liposomal Doxorubicin Hydrochloride for Injection) should be considered an irritant and precautions should be taken to avoid extravasation (see Dosage and Administration).

In studies with rabbits, lesions that were induced by subcutaneous injection of CAELYX were minor and reversible compared to more severe and irreversible lesions and tissue necrosis that were induced after subcutaneous injection of conventional doxorubicin hydrochloride.

Toxicity Potentiation: The doxorubicin in CAELYX may potentiate the toxicity of other anticancer therapies. Exacerbation of cyclophosphamide-induced hemorrhagic cystitis and enhancement of the hepatotoxicity of 6-mercaptopurine have been reported with the conventional formulation of doxorubicin hydrochloride. Radiation-induced toxicity to the myocardium, mucosae, skin and liver have been reported to be increased by the administration of doxorubicin hydrochloride.

Cardiovascular: Special attention must be given to the cardiac toxicity exhibited by doxorubicin hydrochloride. Although uncommon, acute left ventricular failure has occurred, particularly in patients who have received total dosage of doxorubicin exceeding the currently recommended limit of 550 mg/m² body surface. This limit appears to be lower (400 mg/m² body surface) in patients who have received radiotherapy to the mediastinal area or concomitant therapy with other potentially cardiotoxic agents such as cyclophosphamide. The incidence of CAELYX associated cardiotoxicity was significantly lower than that with conventional doxorubicin hydrochloride.

Caution should be observed in patients who have received other anthracyclines or anthracenediones. The total dose of doxorubicin HCl administered to the individual patient should also take into account any previous or concomitant therapy with related compounds such as daunorubicin. Congestive heart failure and/or cardiomyopathy may be encountered after discontinuation of therapy.

Patients with a history of cardiovascular disease should be administered CAELYX only when the potential benefit of treatment outweighs the risk.

Cardiac function particularly left ventricular ejection fraction (LVEF) at baseline and periodically should be monitored by MUGA scan or echography. The evaluation of left ventricular function is considered to be mandatory before each additional administration of CAELYX that exceeds a lifetime cumulative anthracycline dose of 450 mg/m² body surface.

Congestive heart failure and/or cardiomyopathy may occur suddenly, without prior ECG changes and may also be encountered several weeks after discontinuation of therapy.

Hematologic: Myelosuppression: In AIDS-KS and other patient populations treated with CAELYX, many patients presented with baseline myelosuppression due to such factors as their HIV disease, numerous concomitant medications, or tumors involving bone marrow. In the AIDS-KS population, myelosuppression appears to be the dose-limiting adverse event. Leukopenia is the most common adverse event (about 60%) experienced in this population; anemia (about 20%) and thrombocytopenia (about 10%) can also be expected.

In patients with ovarian cancer treated at a dose of 50 mg/m² body surface, myelosuppression was generally mild to moderate, reversible, and was not associated with episodes of neutropenic infection or sepsis. A similar low incidence of myelosuppression was seen in patients with metastatic breast cancer receiving CAELYX in a first-line clinical trial, although febrile neutropenia was seen in 3/254 (1.2 %) patients receiving CAELYX 50 mg/m² body surface, every 4 weeks.

Leukopenia (33.2%) was the most frequently reported hematological adverse event, followed by, anemia (32.2%), neutropenia (31.6%) and thrombocytopenia (10.7%). Life-threatening (Grade IV) hematological effects were extremely rare (1.6%, 0.4%, 2.9%, 0.2% respectively). Growth factor support was required infrequently (<5%) and transfusion support was required in approximately 15% of patients.

Because of this potential for bone marrow suppression, careful hematologic monitoring is required during use of CAELYX. Complete blood counts, including platelet counts, should be obtained frequently and at a minimum prior to each dose of CAELYX. With the recommended dosage schedule, leukopenia is usually transient. Hematologic toxicity may require dose reduction or suspension or delay of CAELYX therapy.

Persistent severe myelosuppression, although not seen in patients with breast or ovarian cancer, may result in superinfection or hemorrhage.

CAELYX may potentiate the toxicity of other anticancer therapies. In particular, hematologic toxicity may be more severe when CAELYX is administered in combination with other agents that cause bone marrow suppression. Patients treated with CAELYX may require growth factors to support their blood counts.

As with other DNA-damaging antineoplastic agents, secondary acute myeloid leukemias and myelodysplasias have been reported in patients having received combined treatment with doxorubicin. Therefore, any patient treated with doxorubicin or CAELYX should be kept under hematologic supervision.

Hepatic/Biliary/Pancreatic: The pharmacokinetics of CAELYX have not been studied in patients with hepatic impairment. Doxorubicin is known to be eliminated in large part by the liver. Thus CAELYX dosage should be reduced in patients with impaired hepatic function (see Action and Clinical Pharmacology and Dosage and Administration). Prior to CAELYX administration, evaluation of hepatic function is recommended using conventional clinical laboratory tests such as AST, ALT, alkaline phosphatase and bilirubin.

Diabetics: Precautions should be taken when using CAELYX in diabetics, since CAELYX is diluted in a (5%) Dextrose Injection USP solution.

Skin: Palmar-Plantar Erythrodysesthesia (PPE): In 254 breast cancer patients treated with CAELYX at a dose of 50 mg/m² body surface, every 4 weeks, 42 patients (17%) reported Grade III PPE, and no cases of Grade IV PPE were reported. Discontinuations due to PPE were infrequent (17 patients, 7%).

In 512 ovarian cancer patients treated with CAELYX at a dose of 50 mg/m² body surface, 100 patients (19.5%) reported Grade III treatment-related PPE and 3 patients (0.6%) reported Grade IV treatment-related PPE, with 19 patients (3.7%) discontinuing.

In 705 patients with AIDS-related Kaposi's sarcoma treated with CAELYX at 20 mg/m² body surface, 24 patients (3.4%) developed PPE with 3 patients (0.9%) discontinuing.

Palmar-plantar erythrodysesthesia is characterized by painful, macular reddening skin eruptions characterized by swelling, pain, and, for some patients, desquamation of the skin on the hands and the feet.

PPE was generally seen after 2 or 3 cycles of treatment but may occur earlier. In most patients the reaction is mild and resolves in one to two weeks with or without treatment with corticosteroids so that prolonged delay of therapy need not occur. However, dose modification may be required to manage PPE. (See Dosage and Administration, Dose Modifications Guidelines.) The reaction can be severe and debilitating in some patients and may require discontinuation of treatment.

Strategies to prevent and treat PPE, which may be initiated for 4 to 7 days after treatment with CAELYX include keeping hands and feet cool, by exposing them to cool water (soaks, baths, or swimming), avoiding excessive heat/hot water and keeping them unrestricted (no socks, gloves, or shoes that are tight fitting). PPE appears to be primarily related to the dose schedule and can be reduced by extending the dose interval 1-2 weeks or reducing the dose. In some settings, pyridoxine has been tried to ameliorate the symptoms of PPE.

Radiation Therapy: Skin recall reaction due to prior radiotherapy has occurred with CAELYX administration.

Special Populations: Pregnant Women: CAELYX should not be administered to pregnant women. Women of childbearing potential should be advised to avoid pregnancy while they or their male partner are receiving CAELYX and in the six months following discontinuation of CAELYX therapy.

CAELYX can cause fetal harm when administered to pregnant women. CAELYX is embryotoxic in rat and embryotoxic and abortifacient in rabbits. Teratogenicity cannot be ruled out.

Nursing Women: It is not known whether this drug is excreted in human milk. Due to the potential for serious adverse reactions in nursing infants from CAELYX, mothers should discontinue nursing prior to taking this drug.

Pediatrics: The safety and effectiveness of CAELYX in pediatric patients have not been established.

Geriatrics (>60 years of age): Experience with CAELYX in patients over 60 years of age is limited. (See Action and Clinical Pharmacology.)

ADVERSE REACTIONS: Clinical Trial Adverse Drug Reactions: Breast Cancer: Breast Cancer Patients: 254 patients with advanced breast cancer who had not received prior chemotherapy for metastatic disease were treated with CAELYX at a dose of 50 mg/m² body surface, every 4 weeks in a phase III clinical trial. The most frequently reported treatment related adverse effects included palmar-plantar erythrodysesthesia (PPE) (48.0%) and nausea (37.0%) (Table 1). These effects were mostly mild and reversible, with severe (Grade III) cases reported in 17.0% and 3.0% respectively, and no reported incidences of life-threatening (Grade IV) cases for either PPE or nausea. Infrequently, these effects resulted in permanent treatment discontinuation (7.0% and 0% respectively). Pronounced alopecia (or total hair loss) was seen in only 7.0% of CAELYX-treated patients as compared with 54.0% of patients treated with doxorubicin.

Hematologic adverse effects were infrequently reported, were mostly mild or moderate in severity, and manageable. Anemia, neutropenia, leukopenia and thrombocytopenia were infrequently reported at incidences of 5.0%, 4.0%, 2.0%, and 1.0%, respectively. Life-threatening (Grade IV) hematologic effects were reported at incidences of <1.0 %. The need for either growth factor support or transfusion support was minimal (5.1% and 5.5% of patients, respectively). Febrile neutropenia was reported in 3/254 (1.2%) patients treated with CAELYX and 8/255 (3.1%) patients treated with doxorubicin.

Abnormal Hematologic and Clinical Chemistry Findings: Clinically significant laboratory abnormalities (Grades III and IV) in this breast cancer group included increases in total bilirubin (2.4%) and AST (1.6%). Increases in ALT were less frequent (<1%). No clinically significant increases in serum creatinine were reported. Clinically significant hematologic measurements were infrequent and low as measured by leukopenia (4.3%), anemia (3.9%), neutropenia (1.6%) and thrombocytopenia (1.2%). Sepsis was reported at an incidence of 1%.

Table 1: CAELYX

Treatment Related Undesirable Effects Reported in ≥5% of CAELYX-treated Patients by Severity and Body System in Breast Cancer Clinical Trial (I97–328)

AE Body System	I97–328 All Severities %	I97–328 Grades 3/4 %
Body as a Whole		
Asthenia	10	1
Erythema	7	<1
Fatigue	12	<1
Fever	8	0
Weakness	6	<1
Gastrointestinal System		
Abdominal Pain	8	1
Anorexia	11	1
Constipation	8	<1
Diarrhea	7	1
Mouth Ulceration	5	<1
Mucositis Nose	23	4
Nausea	37	3
Stomatitis	22	5
Vomiting	19	<1
Red Blood Cell Disorders		
Anemia	5	1
Skin and Appendages		
Alopecia	20	0
PPE[a]	48	17
Pigmentation Abnormal	8	<1
Rash	10	2

[a] Palmar-Plantar Erythrodysesthesia (hand-foot syndrome). No cases of Grade IV (life-threatening) PPE were reported.

Undesirable effects reported between ≥1% and <5% in 254 CAELYX-treated breast cancer patients, not previously reported in CAELYX clinical trials were breast pain, leg cramps, edema, leg edema, peripheral neuropathy, oral pain, ventricular arrhythmia, folliculitis, bone pain, musculo-skeletal pain, thrombocythemia, cold sores (non-herpetic), fungal infection, epistaxis, upper respiratory tract infection, bullous eruption, dermatitis, erythematous rash, dry skin, pruritus, skin discoloration, scaly skin, nail disorder, lacrimation, blurred vision, flushing, weight decrease, dyspepsia and dyspnea.

Ovarian Cancer: Ovarian Cancer Trials (Phase II and III): Information on the adverse reactions is based on the experience in 512 patients with ovarian cancer treated at a dose of 50 mg/m² body surface. The median cumulative dose in the ovarian cancer trials was 150.6 mg/m², median cycle length was 30.0 days, and median days on drug was 65.5 days.

Of these 512 patients, a total of 509 patients (99.4%) in the ovarian cancer trials, reported a total of 5026 adverse events, and 484 (94.5%) patients reported treatment-related adverse events. Treatment-related fatal adverse events were reported in 4 (0.8%) patients, while Grade IV (life-threatening) treatment-related adverse events were reported by 38 (7.4%) patients.

Myelosuppression was mostly mild or moderate and manageable. Leukopenia (33.2%) was the most frequently reported hematological adverse event, followed by anemia (32.2%), neutropenia (31.6%) and thrombocytopenia (10.7%). Life-threatening (Grade IV) haematological effects were extremely rare (1.6%, 0.4%, 2.9%, 0.2% respectively). Growth factor support was required infrequently (<5%) and transfusion support was required in approximately 15% of patients.

Frequently reported treatment related adverse effects included palmar-plantar erythrodysesthesia (PPE) (46.1%) and stomatitis (38.9%). These effects were mainly mild, with severe (Grade III) cases reported in 19.5% and 8.0% respectively, and life threatening (Grade IV) cases reported in 0.6% and 0.8% respectively. These resulted infrequently in permanent treatment discontinuation (<5% and <1% respectively).

Other frequently reported drug related effects (≥5%) included nausea (38.1%), asthenia (34.0%), rash (25.0%), vomiting (24.4%), alopecia (17.4%), constipation (12.9%), anorexia (12.1%), mucous membrane disorder (14.5%), diarrhea (11.7%), abdominal pain (8.2%), fever (9.4%), paresthesia (7.6%), pain (7.4%), skin discoloration (6.1%), pharyngitis (6.4%), dry skin (5.9%), dyspepsia (5.5%) and somnolence (5.1%).

Less frequently (1 to <5%) reported undesirable effects included peripheral edema, oral moniliasis, vasodilatation, mouth ulceration, pruritus, allergic reaction, dehydration, dyspnea, vesiculobullous rash, chills, infection, weight loss, esophagitis, skin disorder, exfoliative dermatitis, cardiovascular disorder, chest pain, dizziness, maculopapular rash, gastritis, myalgia, back pain, depression, insomnia, dysphagia, increased cough, sweating, nausea and vomiting, malaise, taste perversion, urinary tract infection, conjunctivitis, acne, gingivitis, herpes zoster, hypochromic anemia, anxiety, vaginitis, headache, flatulence, dry mouth, cachexia, neuropathy, hypertonia, skin ulcer and dysuria.

Summary of Frequently Reported (≥1%) Related Adverse Events by Severity (Grade 3,4), Body System and COSTART Preferred Term Reported in Ovarian Cancer Patients: See Table 2.

Table 2: CAELYX

Summary of Frequently Reported (≥1%) Related Adverse Events by Severity (Grade 3,4), Body System and COSTART Preferred Term Reported in Ovarian Cancer Patients

Adverse Event	Ovarian Cancer Patients treated with CAELYX n=512		
No. (%) of Patients Reporting Treatment-related Adverse Events	n=484 (94.5%)		
	Grade 3	Grade 4	All Severities
Body as a Whole			
Asthenia	34 (6.6)	0	174 (34.0)
Mucous Membrane Disorder	16 (3.1)	0	74 (14.5)
Digestive System			
Stomatitis	41 (8.0)	5 (0.8)	199 (38.9)
Nausea	21 (4.1)	1 (0.2)	195 (38.1)
Vomiting	22 (4.3)	3 (0.6)	125 (24.4)
Hemic and Lymphatic System			
Leukopenia	36 (7.0)	8 (1.6)	170 (33.2)
Anemia	28 (5.5)	2 (0.4)	165 (32.2)
Neutropenia	46 (9.0)	15 (2.9)	162 (31.6)
Thrombocytopenia	6 (1.2)	1 (0.2)	55 (10.7)
Skin and Appendages			
Hand-foot Syndrome[a]	100 (19.5)	3 (0.6)	236 (46.1)
Rash	17 (3.3)	1 (0.2)	128 (25.0)
Alopecia	6 (1.2)	0	89 (17.4)

[a] Palmar-Plantar Erythrodysesthesia (PPE).

Abnormal Hematologic and Clinical Chemistry Findings: In the subset of patients with ovarian cancer, clinically significant laboratory abnormalities occurring in clinical trials with CAELYX included increases in total bilirubin (usually in patients with liver metastases) (5%) and serum creatinine levels (5%). Clinically significant measurements, measured by Grades III and IV neutropenia (11.4%), anemia (5.7%), and thrombocytopenia (1.2%) were low. Increases in AST were less frequently (<1%) reported. Sepsis related to leukopenia was observed infrequently (<1%).

Pivotal Phase III Trial—Ovarian Cancer: In the pivotal phase III ovarian cancer trial, the toxicity profiles of the two agents: CAELYX and topotecan were very different.

Hematologic toxicity was more frequent and usually grade 3, 4 in the topotecan-treated patients in comparison with CAELYX (neutropenia 77% vs 12%, thrombocytopenia 34% vs 1%, and anemia 28% vs 5% respectively). Grade 3, 4 hematologic adverse events were observed in 90% of topotecan-treated patients compared with 55% of CAELYX-treated patients.

Most drug-related adverse events associated with CAELYX were mild to moderate in severity with the exceptions of palmar-plantar erythrodysesthesia (PPE) and stomatitis. However, PPE and stomatitis were managed successfully with dose modifications and rarely resulted in study discontinuation (4% for PPE and 1% for stomatitis).

There was no evidence of a relationship between cumulative CAELYX dose and change from baseline for LVEF (Left Ventricular Ejection Fraction).

Topotecan-associated toxicities more often resulted in morbidity and life-threatening sequelae than the primary CAELYX-related adverse events.

In the pivotal phase III ovarian cancer study, comparing CAELYX vs topotecan, three deaths in the topotecan group due to neutropenic sepsis were considered treatment-related. There were no treatment-related deaths in the CAELYX group. There were no cases of treatment-related sepsis or neutropenic fever in the CAELYX group (see Table 3).

Table 3: CAELYX

Treatment Related Adverse Events Reported by >10% of Patients in Either Ovarian Cancer Treatment Group (Pivotal Phase III Study)

	CAELYX (n=239)			Topotecan (n=235)		
Any Adverse Event	All Grades 222 (93%)	Grade III 132 (55%)	Grade IV 20 (8%)	All Grades 232 (99%)	Grade III 176 (75%)	Grade IV 158 (67%)
Body as a Whole						
Asthenia	75 (31%)	13 (5%)	0	104 (44%)	17 (7%)	0
Mucous Membrane Disorder	33 (14%)	8 (3%)	0	7 (3%)	0	0
Fever	28 (12%)	0	0	49 (21%)	6 (3%)	5 (2%)
Abdominal Pain	20 (8%)	3 (1%)	0	29 (12%)	3 (1%)	1 (<1%)
Digestive System						
Stomatitis	95 (40%)	19 (8%)	1 (<1%)	35 (15%)	1 (<1%)	0

(cont'd)

Table 3: CAELYX *(cont'd)*

Treatment Related Adverse Events Reported by >10% of Patients in Either Ovarian Cancer Treatment Group (Pivotal Phase III Study)

	CAELYX (n=239)			Topotecan (n=235)		
Any Adverse Event	**All Grades 222 (93%)**	**Grade III 132 (55%)**	**Grade IV 20 (8%)**	**All Grades 232 (99%)**	**Grade III 176 (75%)**	**Grade IV 158 (67%)**
Nausea	85 (36%)	6 (3%)	1 (<1%)	127 (54%)	12 (5%)	2 (1%)
Vomiting	58 (24%)	11 (5%)	2 (1%)	81 (35%)	14 (6%)	2 (1%)
Constipation	33 (14%)	0	0	58 (25%)	3 (1%)	1 (<1%)
Diarrhea	28 (12%)	4 (2%)	0	49 (21%)	5 (2%)	1 (<1%)
Anorexia	26 (11%)	1 (<1%)	0	32 (14%)	1 (<1%)	0
Hematopoietic and Lymphatic System						
Leukopenia	87 (36%)	21 (9%)	3 (1%)	149 (63%)	82 (35%)	35 (15%)
Anemia	85 (36%)	12 (5%)	1 (<1%)	169 (72%)	58 (25%)	8 (3%)
Neutropenia	84 (35%)	19 (8%)	10 (4%)	191 (81%)	33 (14%)	145 (62%)
Thrombocytopenia	31 (13%)	3 (1%)	0	152 (65%)	40 (17%)	40 (17%)
Skin and Appendages						
PPE[a]	117 (49%)	53 (22%)	2 (1%)	2 (1%)	0	0
Rash	58 (24%)	10 (4%)	0	18 (8%)	1 (<1%)	0
Alopecia	38 (16%)	3 (1%)	0	115 (49%)	14 (6%)	0

[a] Palmar-Plantar Erythrodysesthesia.

AIDS-KS: Information on adverse events is based on the experience reported in 711 patients with AIDS-KS enrolled in four open-label studies, as well as 254 patients enrolled in two controlled trials. The majority of patients were treated with 20 mg/m² (body surface) of CAELYX every two to three weeks.

Open-Label Trials: In the open-label trials, the median cumulative dose of CAELYX (Pegylated Liposomal Doxorubicin Hydrochloride for Injection) was 120 mg/m² body surface. Overall, the immune status was poor in 90.1% of the patients enrolled in these studies, with a median CD4 count of 20 cells/mm³.

As expected, patients were receiving many concomitant medications. Over half (58.1%) of the patients were taking one of the four available antiretroviral medications; zidovudine (AZT) was the most frequently employed in 34.3% of patients, with didanosine (ddI), zalcitabine (ddC) and stavudine (d4T) also used in decreasing order of frequency. Use and frequency of other antivirals was frequent: 55.7% received acyclovir at sometime during the trial, 28.9% received ganciclovir and 16.4% received foscarnet. Systemic antifungals were frequently employed with fluconazole being used by 75.7% of patients. Prophylactic therapy of opportunistic infections was used; sulfamethoxazole/trimethoprim being used the most, in 54.9% of patients.

In many instances, it was difficult to determine whether adverse events resulted from CAELYX, from concomitant therapy, or from the patients' underlying disease(s). Of the 711 patients for whom adverse events data are recorded, 84.6% reported one or more adverse events that were considered by the investigators to be possibly related, probably related or related to treatment with CAELYX. For patients who discontinued therapy, death was the most common reason (32.3% of patients). Adverse reactions only infrequently (5.3%) led to discontinuation of treatment.

Controlled Trials: In the two controlled studies, the median dose of CAELYX administered per cycle was 20mg/m² body surface, and the mean duration of therapy with CAELYX was 81.1 days. The majority of patients were classified as poor risk. In all three groups, subcutaneous KS lesions were present in more than 98.4% of patients, 21.7% of patients had evidence of pulmonary KS, and 15.7% of gastrointestinal involvement. In all of the three groups, the majority of patients had CD4 cell counts of less than 50 cells/mm³.

Fewer CAELYX-treated patients died during the course of the controlled trials (16.9%). Early termination due to adverse events was observed in 10.6% of CAELYX-treated patients. In general, the safety profile of the patients treated in the controlled studies was consistent with the one of the patients that were treated with CAELYX in the open-label trials. Table 4 shows all events occurring at ≥5% in the open-label and controlled trials, that were considered by investigators, at least possibly related to the study drug.

Table 4: CAELYX

Possibly or Probably Drug-related Adverse Events by Body System and COSTART Preferred Term—Including Open-label Studies—Reported in ≥5% of AIDS-KS Patients

	CAELYX (Open-label)[a]	CAELYX (Comparator)[b]	ABV[c]	BV[d]
Number of Patients	711	254	125	120
Number of Patients Reporting Adverse Events	566 (79.6%)	192 (75.6%)	114 (91.2%)	92 (76.7%)
	Number of Patients by Body System and Preferred COSTART Term Incidence			
Body as a Whole	**165 (23.2%)**	**55 (21.7%)**	**72 (57.6%)**	**43 (35.8%)**
Asthenia	67 (9.4%)	29 (11.4%)	37 (29.6%)	10 (8.3%)
Fever	62 (8.7%)	13 (5.1%)	38 (30.4%)	22 (18.3%)
Headache	30 (4.2%)	7 (2.8%)	9 (7.2%)	4 (3.3%)
Abdominal Pain	16 (2.3%)	3 (1.2%)	7 (5.6%)	1 (0.8%)
Chills	8 (1.1%)	2 (0.8%)	8 (6.4%)	6 (5.0%)
Pain	10 (1.4%)	3 (1.2%)	7 (5.6%)	2 (1.7%)
Laboratory Test Abnormal	3 (0.4%)	8 (3.1%)	0	7 (5.8%)
Chills and Fever	2 (0.3%)	2 (0.8%)	6 (4.8%)	6 (5.0%)

(cont'd)

Table 4: CAELYX *(cont'd)*

Possibly or Probably Drug-related Adverse Events by Body System and COSTART Preferred Term—Including Open-label Studies—Reported in ≥5% of AIDS-KS Patients

	CAELYX (Open-label)[a]	CAELYX (Comparator)[b]	ABV[c]	BV[d]
Malaise	3 (0.4%)	2 (0.8%)	6 (4.8%)	1 (0.8%)
Cardiovascular System	**2 (0.3%)**	**1 (0.4%)**	**6 (4.8%)**	**1 (0.8%)**
Phlebitis	2 (0.3%)	1 (0.4%)	6 (4.8%)	1 (0.8%)
Digestive System	**207 (29.1%)**	**57 (22.4%)**	**77 (61.6%)**	**37 (30.8%)**
Nausea	91 (12.8%)	36 (14.2%)	54 (43.2%)	14 (11.7%)
Diarrhea	53 (7.5%)	10 (3.9%)	11 (8.8%)	3 (2.5%)
Stomatitis	45 (6.3%)	12 (4.7%)	4 (3.2%)	2 (1.7%)
Nausea and Vomiting	29 (4.1%)	2 (0.8%)	15 (12.0%)	10 (8.3%)
Vomiting	25 (3.5%)	8 (3.1%)	17 (13.6%)	3 (2.5%)
Oral Moniliasis	40 (5.6%)	2 (0.8%)	2 (1.6%)	4 (3.3%)
Anorexia	8 (1.1%)	6 (2.4%)	17 (13.6%)	3 (2.5%)
Constipation	12 (1.7%)	2 (0.8%)	8 (6.4%)	9 (7.5%)
Hemic and Lymphatic System	**471 (66.2%)**	**144 (56.7%)**	**63 (50.4%)**	**49 (40.8%)**
Leukopenia	435 (61.2%)	138 (54.3%)	56 (44.8%)	46 (38.3%)
Anemia	145 (20.4%)	19 (7.5%)	14 (11.2%)	9 (7.5%)
Thrombocytopenia	66 (9.3%)	15 (5.9%)	6 (4.8%)	12 (10.0%)
Hypochromic Anemia	68 (9.6%)	9 (3.5%)	6 (4.8%)	6 (5.0%)
Nervous System	**15 (2.1%)**	**10 (3.9%)**	**30 (24.0%)**	**28 (23.3%)**
Paresthesia	6 (0.8%)	6 (2.4%)	14 (11.2%)	14 (11.7%)
Neuropathy	4 (0.6%)	3 (1.2%)	9 (7.2%)	11 (9.2%)
Peripheral Neuritis	6 (0.8%)	2 (0.8%)	10 (8.0%)	5 (4.2%)
Skin and Appendages	**81 (11.4%)**	**30 (11.8%)**	**55 (44.0%)**	**12 (10.0%)**
Alopecia	63 (8.9%)	18 (7.1%)	53 (42.4%)	10 (8.3%)
Rash	19 (2.7%)	12 (4.7%)	5 (4.0%)	2 (1.7%)

[a] Patients treated with CAELYX in the open-label studies.
[b] Patients treated with CAELYX in the controlled studies (vs ABV or BV).
[c] ABV (Adriamycin, bleomycin, vincristine).
[d] BV (bleomycin, vincristine).

Incidence 1% to 5% (Possibly or Probably Related) in CAELYX-treated AIDS-KS Patients: Body as a Whole: allergic reaction, anaphylactoid reaction, back pain, chest pain, flu syndrome, infection, mucous membrane disorder, pain.
Cardiovascular: hypotension, tachycardia, vasodilatation.
Digestive System: aphthous stomatitis, dyspepsia, dysphagia, glossitis, liver function tests abnormal, mouth ulceration.
Hemic and Lymphatic System: hemolysis, pancytopenia, prothrombin increased.
Metabolic/Nutritional: bilirubinemia, AST increased, ALT increased, weight loss.
Nervous System: dizziness, emotional lability, somnolence.
Respiratory System: dyspnea, pneumonia.
Skin and Appendages: dry skin, herpes simplex, pruritus.
Others: retinitis, albuminuria.
Incidence Less Than 1% (Possibly or Probably Related) in CAELYX-Treated AIDS-KS Patients: Body as a Whole: abscess, cellulitis, substernal chest pain, cryptococcosis, facial edema, hypothermia, immune system disorder, injection site hemorrhage, injection site pain, injection site reaction, moniliasis, neoplasm, radiation injury, sepsis.
Cardiovascular System: arrhythmia, bradycardia, bundle branch block, cardiomegaly, cardiovascular disorder, congestive heart failure, deep thrombophlebitis, heart failure, hemorrhage, migraine, palpitation, pericardial effusion, peripheral vascular disorder, supraventricular extrasystoles, syncope, thrombophlebitis, thrombosis, ventricular arrhythmia, ventricular extrasystoles.
Digestive System: bloody diarrhea, cholestatic jaundice, colitis, dry mouth, eructation, esophageal ulcer, esophagitis, fecal impaction, gastritis, GI hemorrhage, gingivitis, hematemesis, hepatic failure, hepatitis, hepatosplenomegaly, increased appetite, jaundice, leukoplakia of mouth, liver damage, melena, pancreatitis, rectal disorder, sclerosing cholangitis, tenesmus, ulcerative proctitis, ulcerative stomatitis.
Endocrine System: diabetes mellitus.
Hemic and Lymphatic System: eosinophilia, erythrocytes abnormal, lymphadenopathy, lymphangitis, lymphedema, lymphoma like reaction, marrow depression, petechia, purpura, thromboplastin decreased.
Metabolic/Nutritional: BUN increased, cachexia, creatinine increased, dehydration, edema, hypercalcemia, hyperkalemia, hyperlipemia, hypernatremia, hyperphosphatemia, hyperuricemia, hypoglycemia, hypokalemia, hypomagnesemia, hypophosphatemia, hypoproteinemia, ketosis, LDH increased, peripheral edema, weight gain.
Musculoskeletal System: arthralgia, bone disorder, bone pain, joint disorder, myalgia, myasthenia, myositis.
Nervous System: abnormal dreams, abnormal gait, acute brain syndrome, anxiety, cerebrovascular accident, confusion, convulsion, depression, dysarthria, dyskinesia, hypertonia, hypokinesia, hypotonia, insomnia, nervousness, nystagmus, paralysis, reflexes decreased, thinking abnormal, vertigo.
Respiratory System: asthma, bronchitis, cough increased, hiccup, hyperventilation, lung disorder, pharyngitis, pleural effusion, pneumothorax, rhinitis, sinusitis.
Skin and Appendages: acne, cutaneous moniliasis, eczema, erythema nodosum, exfoliative dermatitis, furunculosis, herpes zoster, leukoderma, maculopapular rash, psoriasis, pustular rash, seborrhea, skin discoloration, skin necrosis, skin ulcer.
Special Senses: abnormal vision, blindness, conjunctivitis, diplopia, eye disorder, eye pain, optic neuritis, otitis media, taste perversion, tinnitus.
Urogenital System: balanitis, cystitis, dysuria, genital edema, glycosuria, hematuria, kidney failure, kidney function abnormal, prostatic disorder, testis disorder, urine abnormality.
Post-Market Adverse Drug Reactions: Very rarely, convulsions have been observed in relation to infusion reactions. (Please see Warnings and Precautions, General, Infusion Reactions.)

As reported in clinical trials and post-marketing, myelosuppression associated with anemia, thrombocytopenia, leukopenia, and rarely (>1/10 000 <1/1000) febrile neutropenia, has been reported in CAELYX-treated patients.

Following the marketing of CAELYX, serious skin conditions including erythema multiforme, Stevens Johnson syndrome and toxic epidermal necrolysis have been reported very rarely (<1/10 000).

Patients with cancer are at increased risk for thromboembolic disease. In patients treated with CAELYX, cases of thrombophlebitis, venous thrombosis, and pulmonary embolism are seen uncommonly (≥1/1000 <1/100).

DRUG INTERACTIONS: Overview: No formal drug interaction studies have been conducted with CAELYX. CAELYX may interact with drugs known to interact with the conventional formulation of doxorubicin hydrochloride.

In patients who have received concomitant cyclophosphamide or taxanes, no new additive toxicities were noted.

Drug-Food Interactions: CAELYX interactions with food have not been established.

Drug-Herb Interactions: CAELYX interactions with herbal products have not been established.

Drug-Laboratory Interactions: CAELYX interactions with laboratory tests have not been established.

DOSAGE AND ADMINISTRATION: Recommended Dose and Dosage Adjustment: CAELYX (Pegylated Liposomal Doxorubicin Hydrochloride for Injection) exhibits unique pharmacokinetic properties and must not be used interchangeably with other formulations of doxorubicin hydrochloride.

Breast Cancer/Ovarian Cancer Patients: CAELYX is administered intravenously at a dose of 50 mg/m² body surface, once every 4 weeks for as long as the disease does not progress, and the patient shows no evidence of clinical cardiotoxicity and continues to tolerate treatment.

For doses <90 mg: dilute CAELYX in 250 mL (50 mg/mL) (5%) Dextrose USP solution for infusion.

For doses ≥90 mg: dilute CAELYX in 500 mL (50 mg/mL) (5%) Dextrose USP solution for infusion.

The use of any diluent other than Dextrose 5% in water for infusion, or the presence of any bacteriostatic agent such as benzyl alcohol may cause precipitation of CAELYX.

To minimize the risk of infusion reactions, the initial dose is administered at a rate no greater than 1 mg/minute. If no infusion reaction is observed, subsequent CAELYX infusions may be administered over a 60-minute period.

In the breast cancer trial program, modification of the infusion was permitted for those patients experiencing an infusion reaction as follows:

5 % of the total dose was infused slowly over the first 15 minutes. If tolerated without reaction, the infusion rate was doubled for the next 15 minutes. If tolerated, the infusion was completed over the next hour for a total infusion time of 90 minutes.

Subsequent CAELYX infusions may be administered over a 60 minute period.

Serious and sometimes life-threatening infusion reactions, which are characterized by allergic-like or anaphylactoid-like reactions, with symptoms including asthma, flushing, urticarial rash, chest pain, fever, hypertension, tachycardia, pruritus, sweating, shortness of breath, facial oedema, chills, back pain, tightness in the chest and throat and/or hypotension may occur within minutes of starting the infusion of CAELYX (see Warnings and Precautions). Temporarily stopping the infusion usually resolves these symptoms without further therapy. However, medications to treat these symptoms (e.g., antihistamines, corticosteroids, and adrenaline), as well as emergency equipment should be available for immediate use. In most patients treatment can be resumed after all symptoms have resolved, without recurrence. Infusion reactions rarely recur after the first treatment cycle. To minimize the risk of infusion reactions, the initial dose should be administered at a rate no greater than 1 mg/minute (see Recommended Dose and Dosage Adjustment).

AIDS-KS Patients: CAELYX should be administered intravenously at a dose of 20 mg/m² body surface (equivalent to doxorubicin HCl) once every two-to-three weeks. Intervals shorter than 10 days should be avoided as drug accumulation and increased toxicity cannot be ruled out. Patients should be treated for as long as they respond satisfactorily and tolerate treatment.

The appropriate dose of CAELYX is diluted in 250 mL of (5%) Dextrose Injection USP and administered by intravenous infusion over 30 minutes. CAELYX should not exceed 90 mg per infusion. Rapid infusion may increase the risk of infusion-related reactions (see Warnings and Precautions, General, Infusion Reactions). It is recommended that the CAELYX infusion line be connected through the side port of an intravenous infusion of (5%) Dextrose USP Intravenous Infusion to achieve further dilution and minimize the risk of thrombosis and extravasation.

CAELYX should be considered an irritant and precautions should be taken to avoid extravasation. On intravenous administration of CAELYX, extravasation may occur with or without an accompanying stinging or burning sensation and even if blood returns well on aspiration of the infusion needle. If any signs or symptoms of extravasation have occurred, the infusion should be immediately terminated and restarted in another vein. The application of ice over the site of extravasation for approximately 30 minutes may be helpful in alleviating the local reaction.

Do not administer as a bolus injection or undiluted solution. CAELYX must not be given by the intramuscular or subcutaneous route.

Caution should be exercised in handling CAELYX solution. The use of gloves is required. If CAELYX comes into contact with skin or mucosa, wash immediately and thoroughly with soap and water.

Partially used vials should be discarded. CAELYX should be handled and disposed of in a manner consistent with that of other anti-cancer drugs. There are several guidelines on this subject.

Incompatibilities: Until specific compatibility data are available, it is not recommended that CAELYX be mixed with other drugs.

Dose Modifications: Dose adjustment is required in patients with history of prior anthracyclines use, prior mediastinal irradiation, concurrent cyclophosphamide therapy, pre-existing cardiovascular disease.

To manage adverse events such as palmar-plantar erythrodysesthesia (PPE), stomatitis or hematologic toxicity, the dose may be reduced or delayed. Guidelines for CAELYX dose modification secondary to these adverse effects are provided in the following tables. The toxicity grading in these tables is based on the National Cancer Institute Common Toxicity Criteria (NCI-CTC).

The tables for PPE and stomatitis (Table 5, Table 6) provide the schedule followed for dose modification in clinical trials in the treatment of breast cancer or ovarian cancer (modification of the recommended 4 week treatment cycle). If these toxicities occur in patients with AIDS related KS, the recommended 2 to 3 week treatment cycle can be modified in a similar manner.

The table for hematologic toxicity (Table 7) provides the schedule followed for dose modification in clinical trials in the treatment of patients with breast or ovarian cancer only. Dose modification in patients with AIDS-KS is addressed in Table 8, Table 9 and Table 10.

Guidelines For CAELYX Dose Modification in Breast or Ovarian Cancer Patients: See Table 5, Table 6 and Table 7.

Table 5: CAELYX

Palmar-Plantar Erythrodysesthesia

Toxicity Grade at Current Assessment	Week After Prior CAELYX Dose: Weeks 4 & 5	Week After Prior CAELYX Dose: Week 6
Grade-1- (mild erythema, swelling, or desquamation not interfering with daily activities)	Redose unless patient has experienced a previous Grade 3 or 4 skin toxicity, in which case wait an additional week	Decrease dose by 25%; return to 4-week interval
Grade-2- (erythema, desquamation, or swelling interfering with, but not precluding normal physical activities; small blisters or ulcerations less than 2 cm in diameter)	Wait an additional week	Decrease dose by 25%; return to 4-week interval
Grade-3- (blistering, ulceration, or swelling interfering with walking or normal daily activities; cannot wear regular clothing)	Wait an additional week	Withdraw patient
Grade-4- (diffuse or local process causing infectious complications, or a bedridden state or hospitalization)	Wait an additional week	Withdraw patient

Table 6: CAELYX

Stomatitis

Toxicity Grade at Current Assessment	Week after Prior CAELYX Dose: Weeks 4 & 5	Week after Prior CAELYX Dose: Week 6
Grade-1- (painless ulcers, erythema, or mild soreness)	Redose unless patient has experienced a previous Grade 3 or 4 stomatitis in which case wait an additional week	Decrease dose by 25%; return to 4-week interval or withdraw patient per physician's assessment
Grade-2- (painful erythema, edema, or ulcers, but can eat)	Wait an additional week	Decrease dose by 25%; return to 4-week interval or withdraw patient per physician's assessment
Grade-3- (painful erythema, edema, or ulcers, but cannot eat)	Wait an additional week	Withdraw patient
Grade-4- (requires parenteral or enteral support)	Wait an additional week	Withdraw patient

Table 7: CAELYX

Hematological Toxicity (ANC or Platelets)—Management of Patients with Breast or Ovarian Cancer

Grade	ANC	Platelets	Modification
1	1500–1900	75 000–150 000	Resume treatment with no dose reduction
2	1000–<1500	50 000–<75 000	Wait until ANC ≥1500 and platelets ≥75 000; redose with no dose reduction
3	500–<1000	25 000–<50 000	Wait until ANC ≥1500 and platelets ≥75 000; redose with no dose reduction
4	<500	<25 000	Wait until ANC ≥1500 and platelets ≥75 000; decrease dose by 25% or continue full dose with growth factor support

The dose modifications shown in Table 8, Table 9 and Table 10 are recommended for managing possible adverse events in AIDS-KS patients.

Guidelines For CAELYX Dose Modification in AIDS-KS Patients: See Table 8, Table 9 and Table 10.

Table 8: CAELYX

Palmar-Plantar Erythrodysesthesia

Toxicity Grade	Symptoms	Weeks Since Last Dose: 3	Weeks Since Last Dose: 4
0	No symptoms	Redose at 2- to 3-week interval	Redose at 2- to 3-week interval
1	Mild erythema, swelling, or desquamation not interfering with daily activities	Redose unless patient has experienced a previous grade 3 or 4 skin toxicity in which case wait an additional week	Redose at 25% dose reduction; return to 3-week interval
2	Erythema, desquamation, or swelling interfering with, but not precluding normal physical activities; small blisters or ulcerations less than 2 cm in diameter	Wait an additional week	Redose at 50% dose reduction; return to 3-week interval
3	Blistering, ulceration, or swelling interfering with walking or normal daily activities; cannot wear regular clothing	Wait an additional week	Discontinue CAELYX
4	Diffuse or local process causing infectious complications, or a bedridden state or hospitalization	Wait an additional week	Discontinue CAELYX

Table 9: CAELYX

Hematological Toxicity

Grade	ANC (10^9 cells/L)	Platelets (10^9 cells/L)	Modification
1	1.5–1.9	75–150	None
2	1.0–<1.5	50–<75	None
3	0.5–0.999	25–<50	Wait until ANC ≥1 and/or platelets ≥50 then redose at 25% dose reduction
4	<0.5	<25	Wait until ANC ≥1 and/or platelets ≥50 then redose at 50% dose reduction

Patients with impaired hepatic function: AIDS-KS Patients: Experience with CAELYX in treating AIDS-KS patients with hepatic impairment is limited. Therefore, based on experience with doxorubicin HCl, it is recommended that CAELYX dosage be reduced if the bilirubin is elevated as follows: Serum bilirubin 21 to 51 µmol/L (1.2-3.0 mg/dL), give 50% of normal dose; >51 µmol/L, give 25% of normal dose.

Table 10: CAELYX

Stomatitis

Grade	Symptoms	Modification
1	Painless ulcers, erythema, or mild soreness	None
2	Painful erythema, edema, or ulcers, but can eat	Wait 1 week and if symptoms improve redose at 100% dose
3	Painful erythema, edema, or ulcers, and cannot eat	Wait 1 week and if symptoms improve redose at 25% dose reduction
4	Requires parenteral or enteral support	Wait 1 week and if symptoms improve redose at 50% dose reduction

Breast Cancer/Ovarian Cancer Patients: CAELYX pharmacokinetics determined in a small number of ovarian cancer patients with elevated total bilirubin levels do not differ from patients with normal total bilirubin; however, until further experience is gained, the CAELYX dosage in patients with impaired hepatic function should be reduced based on the experience from the breast and ovarian clinical trial program as follows:

- At initiation of therapy, if the bilirubin is between 21 to 51 µmol/L (1.2-3.0 mg/dL), the first dose is reduced by 25%.
- If the bilirubin is >51 µmol/L (3.0 mg/dL), the first dose is reduced by 50%.
- If the patient tolerates the first dose without an increase in serum bilirubin or liver enzymes, the dose for cycle 2 can be increased to the next dose level, i.e. if reduced by 25% for the first dose, increase to full dose for cycle 2; if reduced by 50% for the first dose, increase to 75% of full dose for cycle 2.
- The dosage can be increased to full dose for subsequent cycles if tolerated.

Prior to CAELYX administration, evaluate hepatic function using conventional clinical laboratory tests such as ALT/AST, alkaline phosphatase, and bilirubin.

Patients with Impaired Renal Function: As doxorubicin is metabolized by the liver and excreted in the bile, dose modification is not required with CAELYX. Population-based analysis confirms that changes in renal function over the range tested (estimated creatinine clearance 30-156 mL/min) do not alter the pharmacokinetics of CAELYX. No pharmacokinetic data are available in patients with creatinine clearance of less than 30 mL/min.

AIDS-KS Patients with Splenectomy: As there is no experience with CAELYX in patients who have had splenectomy, treatment with CAELYX is not recommended.

Reconstitution: Parenteral Products: Caution must be exercised in handling CAELYX solution. The use of gloves is required. If CAELYX comes into contact with skin or mucosa, wash immediately and thoroughly with soap and water. CAELYX must be handled and disposed of in a manner consistent with that of other anticancer medicinal products.

The appropriate dose of CAELYX, up to a maximum of 90 mg, must be diluted in 250 mL of (5%) Dextrose Injection USP, prior to administration. For doses ≥90 mg, dilute CAELYX in 500 mL of (5%) Dextrose USP Injection, prior to administration. Aseptic technique must be strictly observed since no preservative or bacteriostatic agent is present in CAELYX.

- Do not use with In-Line Filters.
- Do not mix with other drugs.
- Do not use with any diluent other than (5%) Dextrose Injection USP.
- Do not use any bacteriostatic agent, such as benzyl alcohol.

It is recommended that the CAELYX infusion line be connected through the side port of an intravenous infusion of (50 mg/mL) (5%) Dextrose USP. Infusion may be given through a peripheral vein.

CAELYX is not a clear solution but a translucent, red liposomal dispersion. Parenteral drug products should be inspected visually for particulate matter and discoloration prior to administration.

Do not use material that shows evidence of precipitation or any other particulate matter. Discard unused portion.

If the patient experiences early symptoms or signs of infusion reaction, immediately discontinue the infusion, give appropriate premedications (antihistamine and/or short acting corticosteroid) and restart at a slower rate.

OVERDOSAGE:

Acute overdosage with doxorubicin HCl causes increases in mucositis, leukopenia and thrombocytopenia.

Treatment of acute overdosage consists of treatment of the severely myelosuppressed patient with hospitalization, antibiotics, platelet and granulocyte transfusions and symptomatic treatment of mucositis.

Chronic overdosage with cumulative doses of doxorubicin HCl exceeding 550 mg/m² body surface, increases the risk of cardiomyopathy and resultant congestive heart failure. Doxorubicin HCl cardiomyopathy has been reported to be associated with a persistent reduction in the voltage of QRS wave, a prolongation of the systolic time interval and a reduction of the left ventricular ejection fraction (LVEF). Treatment consists of vigorous management of congestive heart failure with digitalis preparations and diuretics. Reduction of afterload with vasodilating agents has been recommended.

For management of a suspected drug overdose, CPhA recommends that you contact your **regional Poison Control Centre**. See the *CPS* Directory section for a list of Poison Control Centres.

ACTION AND CLINICAL PHARMACOLOGY: Mechanism of Action: The active ingredient of CAELYX (Pegylated Liposomal Doxorubicin Hydrochloride for Injection) is doxorubicin HCl. The mechanism of action of doxorubicin HCl is thought to be related to its ability to bind DNA and inhibit nucleic acid synthesis. Cell structure studies have demonstrated rapid cell penetration and perinuclear chromatin binding, rapid inhibition of mitotic activity and nucleic acid synthesis, and induction of mutagenesis and chromosomal aberrations.

CAELYX is doxorubicin HCl encapsulated in long-circulating STEALTH liposomes. Liposomes are microscopic vesicles composed of a phospholipid bilayer that are capable of encapsulating active drugs. The STEALTH liposomes of CAELYX are formulated with surface-bound methoxypolyethylene glycol (MPEG), a process often referred to as pegylation, to protect liposomes from detection by the mononuclear phagocyte system (MPS) and to increase blood circulation time.

STEALTH liposomes have a half-life of approximately 73.9 hours in humans. They are stable in blood, and direct measurement of liposomal doxorubicin shows that at least 90% of the drug (the assay used cannot quantify less than 5-10% free doxorubicin) remains liposome-encapsulated during circulation.

It is hypothesized that because of their small size (ca. 100 nm) and persistence in the circulation, the pegylated CAELYX liposomes are able to penetrate the altered and often compromised vasculature of tumors. This hypothesis is supported by studies using colloidal gold-containing STEALTH liposomes, which can be visualized microscopically. Evidence of penetration of STEALTH liposomes from blood vessels and their entry and accumulation in tumors has been seen in mice with C-26 colon carcinoma tumors. Once the STEALTH liposomes distribute to the tissue compartment, the encapsulated doxorubicin HCl becomes available. The exact mechanism of release is not understood.

Pharmacokinetics: Population Pharmacokinetics: The pharmacokinetics of CAELYX was evaluated in 120 patients from 10 different clinical trials using the population pharmacokinetic approach. The pharmacokinetics of CAELYX over the dose range of 10 mg/m² to 60 mg/m² body surface, was best described by a two compartment non-linear model with zero order input and Michaelis-Menten elimination. The mean intrinsic clearance of CAELYX was 0.030 L/h/m² (range 0.008 to 0.152 L/h/m²) and the mean central volume of distribution was 1.93 L/m² (range 0.96-3.85 L/m²) approximating the plasma volume. The apparent half-life ranged from 24-231 hours, with a mean of 73.9 hours. The apparent non-linearity suggests that the clearance of CAELYX is saturable, and that greater than dose-proportional increases in exposure occur as the dose is increased.

Breast Cancer: The pharmacokinetics of CAELYX determined in 18 patients with breast carcinoma were similar to the pharmacokinetics determined in the larger population of 120 patients with various cancers. The mean intrinsic clearance was 0.0160 L/h/m² (range 0.0080-0.027 L/h/m²), the mean central volume of distribution was 1.46 L/m² (range 1.10-1.64 L/m²). The mean apparent half-life was 71.5 hours (range 45.2-98.5 hours).

Ovarian Cancer: The pharmacokinetics of CAELYX determined in 11 patients with ovarian carcinoma were similar to the pharmacokinetics determined in the larger population of 120 patients with various cancers. The mean intrinsic clearance was 0.021 L/h/m² (range 0.009-0.041 L/h/m²), the mean central volume of distribution was 1.95 L/m² (range 1.67-2.40 L/m²). The mean apparent half-life was 75.0 hours (range 36.1-125 hours).

AIDS-KS: The plasma pharmacokinetics, and tumor localization of CAELYX were studied in 42 patients with AIDS- related Kaposi's sarcoma (KS) who received single doses of 10 or 20 mg/m² body surface, administered by a 30-minute infusion. Twenty-three of these patients received single doses of both 10 and 20 mg/m² body surface, with 3-week wash-out period between doses. The pharmacokinetic parameter values of CAELYX are presented in Table 11.

Table 11: CAELYX

Pharmacokinetic Parameters in CAELYX-treated Patients (Mean±SD)

	Dose	
Parameter (units)	**10 mg/m² body surface (n=23)**	**20 mg/m² body surface (n=23)**
Peak Plasma Concentration (µg/mL)	4.12±0.215	8.34±0.49
Plasma Clearance (L/h/m²)	0.0556±0.01	0.041±0.004
Steady-state Volume of Distribution (L/m²)	2.83±0.145	2.72±0.120
AUC (µg/mL·h)	277±32.9	590±58.7
First Phase (λ_1) Half-life (h)	4.7±1.1	5.2±1.4
Second Phase (λ_2) Half-life (h)	52.3±5.6	55.0±4.8

Across this dosage range, CAELYX displayed linear pharmacokinetics. Disposition occurred in two phases after CAELYX administration, with a relatively short first phase (~5 hours) and a prolonged second phase (~55 hours) that accounted for the majority of the area under the curve (AUC).

In contrast to the pharmacokinetics of doxorubicin, which display a large volume of distribution, the steady state volume of distribution of CAELYX indicated that CAELYX was confined mostly to the vascular fluid volume. Plasma protein binding of CAELYX has not been determined; however, the plasma protein binding of doxorubicin is approximately 70%.

Doxorubicinol, the major metabolite of doxorubicin, was detected at very low levels (range: 0.8 to 26.2 ng/mL) in the plasma of patients who received 10 or 20 mg/m² (body surface) of CAELYX. The plasma clearance of CAELYX was slow, with a mean clearance value of 0.042 L/h/m² at a dose of 20 mg/m² body surface.

Kaposi's sarcoma lesions and normal skin biopsies were obtained at 48 and 96 hours post infusion of 10 or 20 mg/m² (body surface) of CAELYX in 22 patients. Significantly higher doxorubicin concentrations were found in KS lesions than in normal skin biopsies at both sampling times and dose levels. The median doxorubicin concentrations ranged from 2-fold to 20-fold higher in KS lesions than in normal skin.

Tissue Distribution: The concentration of CAELYX in AIDS-KS lesions was a median of 21 times higher than in normal skin at 48 hours post-treatment. Population pharmacokinetic analyses suggested that there were small differences in the volume of distribution between tumor types, with the largest volume of distribution in patients with AIDS-KS (2.24 L/m²), and the smallest volume of distribution in patients with breast carcinoma (1.12 L/m²). The volume of distribution in the ovarian carcinoma population is 1.56 L/m².

Pharmacokinetics of CAELYX in Elderly Patients: The population based pharmacokinetic analysis included patients from 21 to 73 years of age. The results of this analysis suggested that age did not influence the pharmacokinetic profile of CAELYX.

Pharmacokinetics of CAELYX in Patients with Impaired Renal Function: As doxorubicin is metabolized by the liver and excreted in the bile, dose modification should not be required with CAELYX. Population-based analysis confirms that changes in renal function over the range tested (estimated creatinine clearance 30-156 mL/min) do not alter the pharmacokinetics of CAELYX. No pharmacokinetic data are available in patients with creatinine clearance of less than 30 mL/min.

Pharmacokinetics of CAELYX in Patients with Hepatic Insufficiency: Based upon population pharmacokinetics, bilirubin concentrations did not affect the pharmacokinetics of CAELYX. It should be noted however, that few patients with elevated bilirubin were included in the analysis and that the highest bilirubin in the study was 4.0 mg/dL. Until more data are available demonstrating the safety of CAELYX in this patient population, suggested dosing reductions mentioned under Dosage and Administration should be followed.

STORAGE AND STABILITY:

- CAELYX should not be used after the expiry date stated on the label and carton.
- Unopened vials of CAELYX should be stored at 2-8°C. Avoid freezing.
- After dilution:
  - Chemical and physical in-use stability has been demonstrated for 24 hours at 2 to 8°C.
  - From a microbiological point of view, the product should be used immediately. If not used immediately, in-use storage times and conditions prior to use are the responsibility of the user and should not be longer than 24 hours at 2 to 8°C.
  - Partially used vials must be discarded.
- CAELYX should not be used if it shows evidence of precipitation or any other particulate matter.
- CAELYX should not be used if it shows a discoloration of the solution.
- Keep out of reach and sight of children.

INFORMATION FOR THE PATIENT: Published in e-CPS, available by subscription at www.e-cps.ca.

DOSAGE FORMS, COMPOSITION AND PACKAGING: Each mL of a sterile, translucent, red liposomal dispersion, contains: doxorubicin HCl 2 mg in a pegylated liposomal formulation in water for injection and a pH of 6.0 to 7.0.

The STEALTH liposome carriers are composed of N-(carbamoyl-methoxypolyethylene glycol 2000)-1,2-distearoyl-sn-glycero-3-phosphoethanolamine sodium salt (MPEG-DSPE), 3.19 mg/mL; fully hydrogenated soy phosphatidylcholine (HSPC), 9.58 mg/mL; and cholesterol, 3.19 mg/mL. Each mL also contains 2 mg of ammonium sulfate, 1.55 mg of histidine as a buffer, hydrochloric acid and/or sodium hydroxide for pH control and 94 mg of sucrose to maintain isotonicity. Greater than 90% of the drug is encapsulated in the STEALTH liposomes.

Single use, glass vials of 10 mL (20 mg) and 25 mL (50 mg).

Cafergot® ℞

ergotamine tartrate—caffeine

Migraine Therapy

Novartis Pharmaceuticals

Date of Revision: March 18, 2009

PHARMACOLOGY: The mechanism of action of CAFERGOT in relieving migraine is not completely understood. Ergotamine is a ligand at serotoninergic 5-HT$_1$ receptors (5-HT$_{1A}$, 5-HT$_{1B}$, 5-HT$_{1D}$, and 5-HT$_{1F}$), 5-HT$_2$ receptors, adrenergic receptors (α_1 and α_2), and dopaminergic receptors (D_1 and D_2). The addition of caffeine to ergotamine tartrate facilitates the absorption of ergotamine and may increase migraine pain relief effects.

Ergotamine is rapidly and incompletely (approximately 62% of the oral dose) absorbed by the gastrointestinal tract. Peak plasma levels are reached about 2 hours after ingestion. Ergotamine is extensively metabolized in the liver. The bioavailability of unchanged drug is about 2% when the drug is administered orally. It has been suggested that the therapeutic effects of the drug are partially due to active metabolites. Protein binding amounts to 98%. Parent drug and metabolites are mainly excreted with the bile. Their elimination from plasma is biphasic with a half-life of 2.7 hours and 21 hours, respectively.

Caffeine is rapidly and almost completely absorbed; it is to a large extent metabolized. The metabolites are mainly excreted in the urine. Plasma elimination half-life is about 3.5 hours, protein binding 35%.

Pharmacokinetics: Interactions: Ergotamine has been shown to be both an inhibitor and substrate of cytochrome P450 3A4 catalyzed reactions. Pharmacokinetic interactions (increased blood levels of ergotamine) have been reported in patients treated with ergotamine and macrolide antibiotics (e.g., troleandomycin, clarithromycin, erythromycin), and in patients treated with ergotamine and protease inhibitors (e.g., ritonavir) presumably due to inhibition of cytochrome P450 3A4 metabolism of ergotamine (see Contraindications). No pharmacokinetic interactions involving other cytochrome P450 isoenzymes are known.

INDICATIONS: CAFERGOT (ergotamine tartrate and caffeine) is indicated in acute attacks of migraine with or without aura.

CAFERGOT Tablets are not intended for the prophylactic therapy of migraine or for use in the management of hemiplegic, basilar, or ophthalmoplegic migraine (see Contraindications).

CONTRAINDICATIONS:

CAFERGOT is contraindicated in:

- Any known hypersensitivity to ergot alkaloids, caffeine, or any other components of the formulation.
- Concomitant treatment of any potent CYP 3A4 inhibitors, including macrolide antibiotics (e.g., clarithromycin, erythromycin, troleandomycin), HIV protease or reverse transcriptase inhibitors (e.g., delavirdine, indinavir, nelfinavir, and ritonavir), and azole antifungals (e.g., ketoconazole, itraconazole, voriconazole).

  Coadministration of ergotamine with potent CYP 3A4 inhibitors has been associated with acute ergot toxicity (ergotism) characterized by vasospasm and vascular ischemia of the extremities, with some cases resulting in amputation. Ergotism can also involve signs and symptoms of vascular ischemia of other tissues such as renal, cardiac, cerebral or gastrointestinal vasospasm. There have been rare reports of cerebral ischemia in patients on protease or reverse transcriptase inhibitor therapy when CAFERGOT (ergotamine tartrate and caffeine) was coadministered, at least one resulting in death. Because of the increased risk for ergotism and other serious vasospastic adverse events, ergotamine use is contraindicated with these drugs and other potent inhibitors of CYP 3A4 (see Warnings, CYP 3A4 Inhibitors and also Precautions, Drug Interactions).
- Concomitant treatment with vasoconstrictive agents (including ergot alkaloids, triptans and other 5-HT_1 receptor agonists) (see Precautions, Drug Interactions).
- Confirmed or suspected central or peripheral ischemic diseases, such as coronary vascular disease, stroke, transient ischemic attack, peripheral vascular disorders; obliterative vascular disease, because of the vasoconstrictor action of ergotamine.
- Complicated migraine, migraine with prolonged aura, temporal arteritis; hemiplegic or basilar migraine.
- Heart disease, inadequately controlled hypertension.
- Septic conditions, shock.
- Severe renal or hepatic impairment.
- Women who are or may be pregnant because ergotamine has oxytocic and vasoconstrictor effects on the placenta and umbilical cord.
- Nursing mothers. Ergotamine is excreted in breast milk and may cause symptoms of vomiting, diarrhea, weak pulse and unstable blood pressure in infants.

WARNINGS:

> **Warning:** Serious and/or life threatening ischemia has been associated with the coadministration of CAFERGOT with potent CYP 3A4 inhibitors including protease inhibitors and macrolide antibiotics. Because CYP 3A4 inhibition elevates the serum levels of CAFERGOT, the risk for vasospasm leading to cerebral ischemia, cardiac ischemia and/or ischemia of the extremities is increased. Hence, concomitant use of these medications is contraindicated. (See also Contraindications.)

CYP 3A4 Inhibitors: Coadministration of ergotamine with potent CYP 3A4 inhibitors such as HIV protease or reverse transcriptase inhibitors or macrolide antibiotics has been associated with serious adverse events; for this reason, these drugs should not be given concomitantly with ergotamine (see Contraindications). While these reactions have not been reported with less potent CYP 3A4 inhibitors, there is a potential risk for serious toxicity including vasospasm when these drugs are used with ergotamine. Examples of less potent CYP 3A4 inhibitors include: saquinavir, nefazodone, fluconazole, fluoxetine, grapefruit juice, fluvoxamine, zileuton, metronidazole, and clotrimazole. These lists are not exhaustive, and the prescriber should consider the effects on CYP 3A4 of other agents being considered for concomitant use with ergotamine.

Fibrotic Complications: There have been reports of patients on CAFERGOT therapy developing retroperitoneal and/or pleuropulmonary fibrosis. There have also been rare reports of fibrotic thickening of the aortic, mitral, tricuspid, and/or pulmonary valves with long term continuous use of CAFERGOT. CAFERGOT should not be used for chronic daily administration (see Dosage).

PRECAUTIONS: Although signs and symptoms of ergotism rarely develop, care should be exercised to remain within the limits of recommended dosage. Excessive or prolonged dosage is not recommended since vasospasms may occur. Such symptoms as tingling in the fingers or toes should be reported to the physician immediately and the drug should be discontinued at once.

Owing to its vasoconstrictor properties, ergotamine may cause myocardial ischemia or, in rare cases, infarction, even in patients with no known history of coronary heart disease.

Patients who are being treated with CAFERGOT should be informed of the maximum doses allowed and of the first symptoms of overdosage: hypoesthesia, paresthesia (e.g., numbness, tingling) in the fingers and toes, non-migraine-related nausea and vomiting, symptoms of myocardial ischemia (e.g., precordial pain) and symptoms of ergotism including cerebral ischemia (e.g., limb weakness, blurred vision and slurred speech).

CAFERGOT is only indicated for the treatment of acute migraine attacks and not for prevention.

Like all drugs, CAFERGOT must be kept out of the reach of children.

If contrary to recommendations ergotamine-containing drugs including CAFERGOT are used excessively over years, they may induce fibrotic changes, in particular of the pleura and the retroperitoneum. There have also been rare reports of fibrotic changes of the cardiac valves (see Warnings).

Patients with mild to moderate hepatic impairment, especially cholestatic patients should be appropriately monitored.

The occurrence of drug-induced headaches has been reported during prolonged and uninterrupted treatment with CAFERGOT.

Drug Interactions: Ergot alkaloids have been shown to be both inhibitors and substrates of CYP 3A4. The concomitant use of cytochrome P450 3A4 (CYP 3A4) inhibitors such as macrolide antibiotics (e.g., troleandomycin, erythromycin, clarithromycin), HIV protease or reverse transcriptase inhibitors (e.g., ritonavir, indinavir, nelfinavir, or delavirdine) or azole antifungals (e.g., ketoconazole, itraconazole, voriconazole) and CAFERGOT must be avoided (see Contraindications), since this can result in an elevated exposure to ergotamine and ergot toxicity (vasospasm and ischemia of the extremities and other tissues). No pharmacokinetic interactions involving other cytochrome P450 isoenzymes are known.

Among patients treated concomitantly with ergotamine-containing preparations and propranolol a few cases of vasospastic reactions have been reported. Concurrent use of vasoconstrictor agents including preparations containing ergot alkaloids, and 5-HT_1 receptor agonists (triptans), and nicotine (e.g., heavy smoking) must be avoided since this may result in enhanced vasoconstriction (see Contraindications).

Selective Serotonin Reuptake Inhibitors/Serotonin Norepinephrine Reuptake Inhibitors and Serotonin Syndrome: There have been very few case reports of serotonin syndrome after i.v. administration of a related compound (dihydroergotamine) concomitantly with SSRI/SNRI. No such interactions have been reported to date with CAFERGOT (ergotamine and caffeine). However, cases of life-threatening serotonin syndrome have been reported during combined use of selective serotonin reuptake inhibitors (SSRIs)/serotonin norepinephrine reuptake inhibitors (SNRIs) and triptans. Therefore, if concomitant treatment with CAFERGOT and SSRIs (e.g., fluoxetine, fluvoxamine, paroxetine, sertraline) or SNRIs (e.g., venlafaxine) is clinically warranted, careful observation of the patient is advised, particularly during treatment initiation and dose increases. Serotonin syndrome symptoms may include mental status changes (e.g., agitation, hallucinations, coma), autonomic instability (e.g., tachycardia, labile blood pressure, hyperthermia), neuromuscular aberrations (e.g., hyperreflexia, incoordination) and/or gastrointestinal symptoms (e.g., nausea, vomiting, diarrhea).

CAFERGOT should not be used in patients on estrogen-based contraceptives or those who are smoking. Estrogen-based contraceptives and cigarette are independent risk factors of thrombosis. The interactions of ergotamine, estrogen-based contraceptives, and smoking are complex; the combination of these conditions may significantly increase the risk of thrombosis.

ADVERSE EFFECTS: Postmarketing Experience: The most common of all side effects are nausea and vomiting. Depending on the dose of ergotamine, signs and symptoms of vasoconstriction may occur.

Adverse reactions are ranked under heading of frequency, the most frequent first, using the following convention: very common (≥1/10); common (≥1/100, <1/10); uncommon (≥1/1000, <1/100); rare (≥1/10 000, <1/1000) very rare (<1/10 000), including isolated reports.

Immune System: Rare: hypersensitivity reactions (such as skin rash, face edema, urticaria and dyspnea).

Nervous System: Common: dizziness. Uncommon: paresthesia (e.g., tingling), hypoesthesia (e.g., numbness).

Ear and Labyrinth: Rare: vertigo.

Cardiac: Uncommon: cyanosis. Rare: bradycardia, tachycardia. Very rare: myocardial ischemia, myocardial infarction.

Vascular: Uncommon: peripheral vasoconstriction. Rare: increase in blood pressure. Very rare: gangrene.

Respiratory, Thoracic and Mediastinal: Rare: dyspnea.

Gastrointestinal: Common: nausea and vomiting (not migraine related), abdominal pain. Uncommon: diarrhea.

Skin and Subcutaneous Tissue: Rare: rash, face edema, urticaria.

Musculoskeletal and Connective Tissue: Uncommon: pain in extremities. Rare: myalgia.

General Disorders and Administration Site Conditions: Uncommon: weakness in extremities.

Investigations: Rare: absence of pulse.

Injury, Poisoning and Procedural Complications: Rare: ergotism (intense arterial vasoconstriction, producing signs and symptoms of vascular ischemia of the extremities and other tissues [such as renal, cardiac, cerebral, or gastrointestinal vasospasm]).

If ergotamine containing drugs are used excessively over years, they may induce fibrotic changes, in particular of the pleura and the retroperitoneum. There have also been rare reports of fibrotic changes of the cardiac valves.

The occurrence of drug-induced headaches has been reported during prolonged and uninterrupted treatment with CAFERGOT (see Precautions).

OVERDOSE:

Symptoms: In humans, the minimum lethal dose of ergotamine ranges from 15 to 20 mg. The following cases of ergotamine tartrate overdosage are cited to provide broad guidelines only:

1) An overdosage of 44 mg ergotamine tartrate taken by an adult female, presumably all absorbed, was followed by recovery on supportive therapy only.

2) A 14-month-old child died following the ingestion of 12 mg ergotamine tartrate. Although vomiting was induced shortly after ingestion, the child was not exposed to expert treatment for some 13 hours after ingestion.

Ergotamine poisoning results in nausea, vomiting, diarrhea, thirst, muscle pain, cold and pale skin, itching, a rapid and weak pulse, bradycardia or tachycardia, pain suggestive of angina, rise and/or fall of blood pressure (usually in that order), mental confusion, dizziness, headache, depression, drowsiness, hypotension, convulsion, shock, possible unconsciousness, coma, symptoms and complications of ergotism. Ergotism may present with an intense arterial vasoconstriction, producing signs and symptoms of vascular ischemia of the extremities such as numbness, tingling and pain in the extremities, cyanosis, and absence of pulse. If the condition is allowed to progress untreated, gangrene may result. Ergotism can also involve signs and symptoms of vascular ischemia of other tissues such as renal, cardiac, cerebral, or gastrointestinal vasospasm. Most cases of ergotism are associated with chronic intoxication and/or overdose. Neurological changes can rarely include convulsions and hemiplegia. Respiratory depression can occur.

Treatment: In the case of orally ingested drug, administration of activated charcoal is recommended. In the case of very recent oral intake gastric lavage may be considered.

Treatment should be symptomatic and supportive. In the event of severe vasospastic reactions, i.v. administration of a peripheral vasodilator such as nitroprusside, phentolamine or dihydralazine, local application of warmth to the affected area, and nursing care to prevent tissue damage are recommended. In the event of coronary constriction, appropriate treatment such as nitroglycerine should be initiated.

> For management of a suspected drug overdose, contact your **regional Poison Control Centre**. See the *CPS* Directory section for a list of Poison Control Centres.

DOSAGE: CAFERGOT (ergotamine tartrate and caffeine) should be given **at the first symptoms of an attack. CAFERGOT should not be administered prophylactically.**

Adults: CAFERGOT Tablets: The first time CAFERGOT is taken, an initial dose of 2 tablets of CAFERGOT is recommended. If relief is not obtained within half an hour, a further tablet should be taken; this may be repeated at half-hourly intervals (see Maximum Daily Dosage).

For **subsequent attacks** the initial dose may be increased up to 3 tablets, depending on the dose required in previous attacks. If necessary, additional doses may be taken at half-hourly intervals up to the maximum dosage indicated below.

Children (6 to 12 years): The initial dose is one tablet of CAFERGOT; additional doses of one tablet may be given twice only, if required, in the course of an attack.

If supplemental antimigraine medication is required, a minimum of 6 to 8 hours should elapse before the use of any ergotamine or dihydroergotamine-containing preparations; and at least 24 hours should elapse before the use of a triptan. Conversely, CAFERGOT should not be taken until at least 6 hours have elapsed following the use of a triptan or ergotamine or dihydroergotamine-containing preparations.

Maximum Dose per Attack per Day: Adults: 6 mg ergotamine tartrate = 6 tablets.

Children: 3 mg ergotamine tartrate = 3 tablets.

Maximum Weekly Dose: Adults: 10 mg ergotamine tartrate = 10 tablets.

Children: 5 mg ergotamine tartrate = 5 tablets.

INFORMATION FOR THE PATIENT: Published in e-CPS, available by subscription at www.e-cps.ca.

SUPPLIED: Each circular, flat, speckled yellowish-white with isolated dots of pigment, compressed tablet, flat-faced, bevelled edge, 9 mm in diameter, with "XL" and a score on one side, contains: ergotamine tartrate USP 1 mg and caffeine USP 100 mg. Nonmedicinal ingredients: cellulose microcrystalline, iron oxide pigment yellow, magnesium stearate, maize starch, talc and tartaric acid. Cartons of 10 blisters of 10 tablets each. Store tablets below 25°C, protect from light.

(Shown in Product Identification Section)

Calcijex® Ⓟ

calcitriol

Vitamin D3 Metabolite

Abbott

SUPPLIED: Each mL of sterile, isotonic, clear, aqueous solution contains: calcitriol 1 µg or 2 µg, edetate disodium (stabilizer) 1 mg, polysorbate 20 4 mg, sodium chloride 1.5 mg, sodium ascorbate (stabilizer) 10 mg. Dibasic sodium phosphate, anhydrous and monobasic sodium phosphate, monohydrate as buffers. The pH of the solution is approximately 7. Preservative-free. Ampuls of 1mL.

Store at room temperature; however, brief exposure up to 40°C does not adversely affect the product. Protect from light, excessive heat.

Parenteral drug products should be inspected visually for particulate matter and discoloration prior to administration, whenever solution and container permit. Discard unused portion.

Calcimar® Ⓟ

calcitonin salmon

Calcium Regulator

sanofi-aventis

SUPPLIED: Each mL of sterile solution contains: calcitonin salmon 200 IU per mL with 0.5% phenol USP as a conservation agent. Sodium chloride, sodium acetate, acetic acid and sodium hydroxide have been added to regulate tonicity. Multidose vials of 2 mL. Store refrigerated (2 to 8°C). Stable for 2 weeks at room temperature (15-30°C).

Note: 1 International Unit is equivalent to 1 MRC unit.

Calcite 500 + D 400
calcium carbonate—vitamin D
Calcium Supplement—Vitamin D Supplement

Riva

Calcite 500 + D 800
calcium carbonate—vitamin D
Calcium Supplement—Vitamin D Supplement

Riva

Calcite D 500
calcium carbonate—vitamin D
Calcium Supplement—Vitamin D Supplement

Riva

SUPPLIED: Calcite 500 + D 400: Each blue, film-coated, oblong, biconvex tablet plain both sides contains: calcium carbonate 1250 mg from oyster shell which provides 500 mg (25 mEq) elemental calcium and 400 IU of vitamin D_3 (cholecalciferol). Nonmedicinal ingredients: carnauba wax, croscarmellose sodium, brilliant blue FCF (FDC Blue No. 1) aluminium lake, magnesium stearate, microcrystalline cellulose, polyethylene glycol, polyvinyl alcohol, talc and titanium dioxide. HDPE bottles of 60, 100 and 500. Store between 15 and 30°C in tight and light resistant containers.
Calcite 500 + D 800: Each film-coated, oblong, biconvex tablet plain on both sides contains: calcium carbonate 1250 mg from oyster shell which provides 500 mg (25 mEq) elemental calcium and 800 IU of vitamin D_3 (cholecalciferol). Nonmedicinal ingredients: carnauba wax, croscarmellose sodium, magnesium stearate, microcrystalline cellulose, polyethylene glycol, polyvinyl alcohol, talc and titanium dioxide. HDPE bottles of 60, 100 and 500. Store between 15 and 30°C in tight and light resistant containers.
Calcite D 500: Each green, film-coated, oblong, biconvex tablet engraved "RIVA" on one side and plain on the other contains: calcium carbonate 1250 mg from oyster shell which provides 500 mg (25 mEq) elemental calcium and 125 IU of vitamin D_3 (cholecalciferol). Nonmedicinal ingredients: brilliant blue FCF (FDC Blue no. 1) aluminum lake, carnauba wax, croscarmellose sodium, hypromellose, magnesium stearate, microcrystalline cellulose, polydextrose, polyethylene glycol, quinoleine yellow WS (D&C Yellow #10) aluminum lake, titanium dioxide and triacetin. HDPE bottles of 100. Store between 15 and 30°C in tight and light resistant containers.

Calcitriol ℞
CPhA Monograph

see *Vitamin D*

Calcium 500
calcium carbonate
Mineral Supplement

Trianon

Calcium D 500
calcium carbonate—vitamin D
Vitamin—Mineral Supplement

Trianon

SUPPLIED: Calcium 500: Each green, film-coated, biconvex, oblong-shaped tablet contains: calcium carbonate 1250 mg which provides calcium 500 mg (25 mEq) obtained from oyster shell. Nonmedicinal ingredients: carnauba wax, cellulose, colloidal silicon dioxide, magnesium stearate, Opadry green dye (D&C yellow 10 aluminum lake, FD&C blue 1 aluminum lake, hydroxypropyl methylcellulose, polydextrose, polyethylene glycol, titanium dioxide and triacetin). Alcohol, gluten-, sulfite- and tartrazine-free. Bottles of 100 and 500.
Calcium D 500: Each gray, film-coated, biconvex, oblong-shaped tablet contains: calcium carbonate 1250 mg which provides calcium 500 mg (25 mEq) obtained from oyster shell and vitamin D 125 IU. Nonmedicinal ingredients: carnauba wax, cellulose, colloidal silicon dioxide, magnesium stearate, Opadry gray dye (FD&C blue 2 aluminum lake, FD&C red 40 aluminum lake, FD&C yellow 6 aluminum lake, hydroxypropyl methylcellulose, polyethylene glycol, polysorbate 80 and titanium dioxide). Alcohol, gluten-, sulfite- and tartrazine-free. Bottles of 100.

Calcium Channel Blockers ℞
amlodipine besylate
diltiazem HCl
felodipine
flunarizine HCl
nifedipine
nimodipine
verapamil HCl

Antianginal—Antiarrhythmic—Antihypertensive—Adjunct in the Management of Subarachnoid Hemorrhage—Migraine Prophylaxis

CPhA Monograph

Date of Revision: October 2006

This monograph has been compiled by CPhA and reviewed by experts. It may contain information different from that found in Health Canada-approved Product Monographs. The reader is referred to the *CPS* Editorial Policy for more information.

PHARMACOLOGY: Many drugs affect calcium ion movement in smooth and cardiac muscle. This general monograph focuses on the calcium channel blockers (CCBs) affecting the cardiovascular system.

CCBs (also referred to as slow channel blockers, calcium entry blockers or calcium antagonists) are a chemically and pharmacologically heterogeneous group of drugs, but physiologically they all share the ability to selectively antagonize the calcium ion movements that are responsible for the excitation-contraction coupling in the cardiovascular system.

There are two main classes of CCBs: dihydropyridines (nifedipine, amlodipine, felodipine and nimodipine) and nondihydropyridines which include diltiazem (a benzothiazepine) and verapamil (a phenylalkylamine). Flunarizine is an antihistamine with calcium channel blocking activity.

CCBs exert their effect at the voltage-gated (or slow) calcium channels of the plasma membrane. CCBs block transmembrane influx of calcium through the slow channel into the cardiac muscle and vascular smooth muscle, without significantly affecting the transmembrane influx of sodium through the fast channel. This results in a reduction of free calcium ions in the muscle tissue and no change in serum calcium concentrations. The effects on the cardiovascular system include depression of mechanical contraction of myocardial and smooth muscle and depression of both impulse formation (automaticity) and conduction velocity.

The different pharmacologic profiles for these agents are in part based on their ability to bind to different receptor sites at the calcium channel. Dihydropyridines are strong vasodilators, acting via relaxation of vascular smooth muscle cells. They have little direct effect on myocardial contractility or SA/AV nodal conduction. However, they cause tachycardia and increased cardiac output via reflex sympathetic activity. These drugs also cause peripheral edema, presumably through precapillary vasodilation. The nondihydropyridines (diltiazem and verapamil) have an increased effect on AV nodal conduction compared to that of the dihydropyridines; while they also cause vasodilation via relaxation of vascular smooth muscle, their vasodilatory effects are only one-tenth the magnitude of nifedipine's. All CCBs interfere somewhat with blood coagulation by inhibiting platelet aggregation.

Angina: The precise mechanism by which CCBs relieve angina has not been fully determined but it is believed to be brought about largely by vasodilatory effects on the coronary and peripheral vasculature. This increases blood flow to the ischemic area of the myocardium and reduces oxygen demand by decreasing the afterload.

Arrhythmia: Verapamil and diltiazem depress AV nodal conduction and prolong functional refractory periods, which is the basis for their use in supraventricular arrhythmias.

Hypertension: The mechanism by which CCBs reduce arterial blood pressure involves direct peripheral arterial vasodilation and reduction in peripheral vascular resistance.

Other Uses: Nimodipine, which has a more marked effect on the cerebral circulation than on the peripheral circulation, is used in the management of subarachnoid hemorrhage. Although the mechanism of action is not fully understood, current evidence suggests that nimodipine increases collateral circulation due to dilation of the small cerebral resistance vessels and/or prevention of calcium overload in the neurons. Flunarizine may relieve or prevent reactive vasodilation of migraine sufferers by inhibiting the vasoconstriction during the prodromal phase.

Pharmacokinetics: All CCBs are well absorbed from the gastrointestinal tract following oral administration. They undergo considerable first-pass metabolism by the liver resulting in reduced bioavailability; amlodipine has a lower rate of first-pass hepatic clearance.

CCBs are metabolized by the cytochrome P450 system, as substrates of CYP3A4, and excreted renally or fecally to varying degrees. Verapamil is also a substrate of CYP1A2, CYP2C9 and CYP2C19. Most metabolites of CCBs are inactive; however, verapamil and diltiazem have metabolites with pharmacologic activity.

The potential exists for interactions with other drugs metabolized by the same pathway, or in particular, those that induce or inhibit this enzymatic system (see Drug Interactions). Plasma concentrations of CCBs are increased in elderly patients and patients with hepatic impairment, e.g., cirrhosis or impaired hepatic blood flow.

Renal impairment has little effect on the pharmacokinetic profile of most CCBs since renal elimination of unchanged drug or active metabolites is minimal. In the case of verapamil, however, the extent of renal elimination of its metabolites is 70%. Although the principal metabolite, norverapamil, is reported to possess only 20% of the cardiovascular activity of verapamil, caution is advised when verapamil is used in patients with renal impairment.

Table 1 presents the pharmacokinetic parameters of the available CCBs.

Table 1: Calcium Channel Blockers
Pharmacokinetic Parameters (Oral Administration)

Calcium Channel Blocker	Absorption (%)	Bioavailability (%)	Time to Peak Concentration (hours)	Protein Binding (%)	Elimination Half-life (hours)	Main Route of Elimination
Dihydropyridines						
Amlodipine	NA[a]	60 to 65	6 to 12	95	35 to 50	Hepatic
Felodipine, extended-release	≈100	20	2.5 to 5	99	11 to 16	Hepatic
Nifedipine, immediate-release	90	45 to 75	0.5 to 2	92 to 98	2 to 5	Hepatic
Nifedipine, prolonged action (PA)	NA[a]	50 to 70	4	98	NA[a]	Hepatic
Nifedipine, extended-release (XL)	78%	86 (relative to immediate-release)	6	92 to 98	10	Hepatic
Nimodipine	>90	13	1.5	99	1 (early) 8 to 9 (terminal)	Hepatic
Nondihydropyridines						
Diltiazem, immediate-release	80 to 90	40 to 67	2 to 4	70 to 80	3.5 to 6 (5 to 8 with high and repetitive dosage)	Hepatic

(cont'd)

Table 1: Calcium Channel Blockers *(cont'd)*

Pharmacokinetic Parameters (Oral Administration)

Calcium Channel Blocker	Absorption (%)	Bioavailability (%)	Time to Peak Concentration (hours)	Protein Binding (%)	Elimination Half-life (hours)	Main Route of Elimination
Diltiazem, sustained-release (SR)	80	40%	7 to 11	70 to 80	5 to 7	Hepatic
Diltiazem, controlled-delivery (CD)	80	40%	10 to 14	70 to 80	5 to 8	Hepatic
Verapamil, immediate-release	> 90	20 to 35	1 to 2	90	2.8 to 7.4 (4.5 to 12 with repetitive dosage)	Hepatic
Verapamil, sustained-release: Isoptin SR		20 to 35[b]	4 to 8		6 to 9	Hepatic
Verapamil, sustained-release: Chronovera			11			Hepatic
Other						
Flunarizine	well absorbed	NA[a]	2 to 4	99	19 days	Hepatic

[a] Data not available.
[b] When administered under fasting conditions.

INDICATIONS: CCBs are used mainly to treat hypertension, angina and cardiac arrhythmias. Clinical applications of the specific agents may reflect differences in their pharmacokinetic/pharmacodynamic profiles, the availability of data from clinical trials, or the labeled indications for a particular agent. Many of the CCBs available in Canada are marketed as second-line antihypertensive agents for the treatment of mild to moderate hypertension, either alone or in combination with other drugs, particularly thiazide diuretics; however, the current Canadian Recommendations for the Management of Hypertension include long-acting dihydropyridine CCBs as acceptable first-line agents in uncomplicated hypertension. Immediate-release (short-acting) formulations, particularly nifedipine, should not be used for the treatment of hypertension (see Warnings).

Amlodipine, diltiazem, nifedipine extended-release and verapamil immediate-release and sustained-release are indicated for second-line management of effort-associated chronic stable angina pectoris without evidence of vasospasm.

Immediate-release formulations of diltiazem, nifedipine and verapamil may be useful in unstable angina when spasm of the coronary vessels is known to be a contributing factor; generally, patients should be hospitalized for treatment.

Oral verapamil is used as adjunctive therapy in the management of obstructive hypertrophic cardiomyopathy where surgery is not otherwise indicated.

Other uses: Although not approved for Raynaud's phenomenon, nifedipine has been effective and is considered the drug of choice for the management of this condition. The extended-release form of nifedipine should be used. Other CCBs may be considered, although they are probably less effective.

The iv formulations of diltiazem and verapamil are indicated for temporary control of rapid ventricular rate in atrial fibrillation or atrial flutter. They should not be used in patients with atrial fibrillation or atrial flutter associated with an accessory bypass tract such as Wolff-Parkinson-White syndrome or Lown-Ganong-Levine syndrome. They are also used for the rapid conversion of paroxysmal supraventricular tachycardia to sinus rhythm. When clinically advisable, appropriate vagal maneuvers (e.g., the Valsalva maneuver) should be attempted prior to iv administration of diltiazem or verapamil.

Nimodipine is the only CCB indicated as adjunctive therapy in the management of a recent subarachnoid hemorrhage from a ruptured intracranial aneurysm. Nimodipine has been shown to decrease the severity and incidence of delayed ischemic neurologic deficits.

Flunarizine, a selective calcium entry blocker is the only agent in this group indicated for the prophylaxis of migraine with or without aura. There is limited evidence on the use of other CCBs in the prophylaxis of migraine.

Table 2 lists the current labelled indications of the various CCBs available in Canada.

CONTRAINDICATIONS: In patients with known hypersensitivity to a particular calcium channel blocker, the specific agent in question is contraindicated. All CCBs are contraindicated in patients who have or are prone to severe hypotension or cardiogenic shock; in patients with extreme bradycardia; patients with severe congestive heart failure and/or severe left ventricular dysfunction (i.e., ejection fraction <40%) unless secondary to a supraventricular tachycardia that is amenable to oral CCB therapy; in patients receiving drugs that are known to affect cardiac conduction; in patients with second- or third-degree AV block, sick sinus syndrome or patients with atrial flutter or atrial fibrillation and an accessory bypass tract (e.g., Wolff-Parkinson-White, Lown-Ganong-Levine syndrome) except in the presence of a functioning ventricular pacemaker.

CCBs should not be used routinely in patients who survive a myocardial infarction and in particular, a dihydropyridine should be used only when a compelling indication exists. Diltiazem and verapamil are contraindicated in postmyocardial infarction patients with moderate or severe left ventricular dysfunction.

Concomitant use of iv CCBs with beta-blockers (especially iv) or cardiac depressant drugs that can produce a reduction in myocardial contractility and AV conduction is contraindicated.

Use of iv verapamil and diltiazem in patients with wide complex ventricular tachycardia (QRS >0.12 s) can result in marked hemodynamic deterioration and ventricular fibrillation. It is important to accurately diagnose wide complex QRS tachycardia of supraventricular origin prior to administration of iv verapamil or diltiazem.

Dihydropyridines should be avoided in patients with advanced valvular aortic stenosis. Reduction of diastolic pressure in these patients may worsen rather than improve myocardial oxygen delivery.

Flunarizine is contraindicated in patients with depression, Parkinson's syndrome, or other extrapyramidal disorders.

WARNINGS: Cardiovascular: There is an increased risk of cardiovascular events in patients with chronic stable angina who are treated with immediate-release nifedipine as monotherapy. The increased risk is due primarily to a greater frequency of episodes of angina. Sustained-release preparations and concurrent use of beta-blockers do not appear to be associated with an increased risk.

Nifedipine can cause deterioration in some heart failure patients. Felodipine and amlodipine exert less negative inotropic effect than nifedipine and may improve some hemodynamic parameters but not exercise tolerance. Long-term therapy with these agents has been associated with fluid retention and clinical deterioration. Diltiazem may improve outcomes in heart failure caused by specific etiologies such as cardiomyopathy.

CCBs should be used with care in patients prone to excessive hypotension; in patients with acute cerebral infarction, hemorrhage, edema, severely raised intracranial pressure or cerebrovascular insufficiency; in patients with outflow obstruction of the left ventricle (aortic stenosis).

Table 2: Calcium Channel Blockers

Labelled Indications

Calcium Channel Blocker	Hypertension	Stable Angina	Atrial Fibrillation	Supraventricular Tachycardia	Coronary Spasm	Obstructive Hypertrophic Cardiomyopathy	Subarachnoid Hemorrhage	Migraine Prophylaxis
Dihydropyridines								
Amlodipine	Yes	Yes	—	—	—	—	—	—
Felodipine, extended-release	Yes	—	—	—	—	—	—	—
Nifedipine, immediate-release	—	Yes[a]	—	—	Yes	—	—	—
Nifedipine, prolonged-action (PA)	Yes	—	—	—	—	—	—	—
Nifedipine, extended-release (XL)	Yes	Yes	—	—	—	—	—	—
Nimodipine	—	—	—	—	—	—	Yes	—
Nondihydropyridines								
Diltiazem, immediate-release	—	Yes[a]	Yes	—	Yes	—	—	—
Diltiazem, injectable	—	—	Yes	Yes	—	—	—	—
Diltiazem, sustained-release (SR)	Yes	Yes	—	—	—	—	—	—
Diltiazem, controlled-delivery (CD)	Yes	Yes	—	—	—	—	—	—
Verapamil, immediate-release	Yes	Yes[a]	Yes	Yes	Yes	Yes	—	—
Verapamil, injectable	—	—	Yes	Yes	—	—	—	—
Verapamil, sustained-release[b]	Yes[b]	Yes[b]	—	—	—	—	—	—
Other								
Flunarizine	—	—	—	—	—	—	—	Yes

[a] Immediate release preparations are not recommended as monotherapy for stable angina.
[b] Labeled indications vary by brand. Please see individual product monographs.

In patients with angina or arrhythmias using antihypertensive drugs, especially beta-blockers, the additional hypotensive effect of CCBs should be taken into consideration. Greater incidence of adverse effects may occur (i.e., headaches, flushing) because of excessive vasodilation.

Dihydropyridines should not be used for acute reduction of blood pressure. Strokes have occurred when immediate-release formulations were used.

Acute Hepatic Injury: Rarely, symptoms consistent with acute hepatic injury as well as significant elevations in liver enzymes have occurred. These were reversible on drug discontinuation.

Beta-blocker Withdrawal: Dihydropyridines give no protection against the dangers of abrupt beta-blocker withdrawal (increased angina) and such withdrawal should be done by the gradual reduction of the dose of beta-blocker.

Duchenne's Muscular Dystrophy: Verapamil, especially iv, may decrease neuromuscular transmission in these patients and can precipitate respiratory muscle failure. It should be used with caution in these patients.

Hypertrophic Cardiomyopathy: Serious adverse effects may occur in patients with hypertrophic cardiomyopathy who are treated with verapamil. These effects include pulmonary edema, sinus bradycardia, 2nd degree AV block and sinus arrest.

PRECAUTIONS: Cardiovascular: CCBs produce arterial and arteriolar vasodilation; hypotension and a compensatory increase in heart rate may occur, especially with dihydropyridines. Blood pressure and heart rate should be monitored during initial therapy or increases in doses, especially in patients prone to hypotension, those with a history of cerebrovascular insufficiency, and those who are taking medications known to lower blood pressure.

Discontinuation: Abrupt withdrawal of CCBs may cause increased frequency and duration of chest pain. Dosages should be gradually tapered off.

Gingival Hyperplasia: Nifedipine, diltiazem, felodipine, amlodipine and verapamil have been implicated in drug-induced gingival hyperplasia. The reported prevalence of clinically significant hyperplasia varies widely but is generally felt to be from 3 to 10%. Males are 3 times as likely as females to develop clinically significant gingival hyperplasia (a link to androgen metabolism has been suggested). Good dental hygiene is crucial in minimizing this adverse effect.

Peripheral Edema: Mild to moderate peripheral edema associated with arterial vasodilation occurs primarily in the lower extremities; care should be taken to distinguish peripheral edema alone from heart failure and chronic venous insufficiency.

Pregnancy: A study on the pregnancy outcome of 78 women who had been exposed to CCBs in the first trimester did not find higher rates of major malformations or perinatal complications compared with controls. Maternal hypertension was the most important factor responsible for low birth weight babies in the group taking CCBs. Nifedipine and possibly other CCBs may delay labour.

Lactation: All CCBs are excreted in maternal milk in significant concentrations. The importance of the drug to the mother should be taken into account when deciding whether or not to discontinue nursing or discontinue the drug.

Children: Limited experience in pediatric patients indicates that results of treatment are similar to those in adults. Patients less than 6 months of age may not respond to iv verapamil; this resistance may be related to a developmental difference in AV node responsiveness.

Elderly: Administer cautiously to elderly patients, especially those with a history of hypotension or cerebrovascular insufficiency since the incidence of adverse reactions is higher. Elderly patients are also more likely to have sick sinus syndrome, which is a contraindication to CCB use. Nifedipine, diltiazem and verapamil have been associated with an increased risk of gastrointestinal hemorrhage in the elderly as compared with beta-blockers, and may present an increased risk of cancer.

Diabetic patients may require adjustment of their control dosages. Close monitoring of blood glucose level is recommended.

Impaired Liver Function: Use with caution in the patients with impaired liver function. A dose reduction may be necessary. Close monitoring for excessive pharmacological response (pulse, blood pressure and abnormal prolongation of the PR interval) is recommended.

Occupational Hazard: Sedation and/or drowsiness occurs in some patients treated with flunarizine and some other calcium channel blockers.

Drug Interactions: CCBs are metabolized by the hepatic microsomal cytochrome P450 isoenzyme, CYP3A4. Verapamil is also a substrate for CYP1A2, CYP2C9 and CYP2C19. Coadministration of CCBs with other drugs which follow the same route of biotransformation may result in altered bioavailability. Dosages of similarly metabolized drugs may require adjustment when starting or stopping concomitantly administered CCBs, to maintain optimum therapeutic serum levels. Amlodipine has a low rate of first-pass hepatic clearance and may have a lower potential for interacting with drugs that are metabolized by cytochrome P450.

Amlodipine, diltiazem, nifedipine and verapamil can also inhibit CYP3A4, which can significantly affect the pharmacokinetics of drugs metabolized by this enzyme such as carbamazepine and cyclosporine.

Table 3 lists some of the documented interactions involving CCBs.

Table 3: Calcium Channel Blockers

Drug and Food Interactions

Drug or Food Interacting with Calcium Channel Blockers	Potential Effect
ASA	Diltiazem or verapamil may enhance the antiplatelet activity of ASA. Patients should be monitored for prolonged bleeding time.
Beta-blockers	Hypotension, additive depressant effects on myocardial contractility, heart rate and AV conduction.
Carbamazepine	Diltiazem has caused carbamazepine toxicity when initiated in patients stabilized on carbamazepine, by inhibiting CYP3A4. If this combination is used, patients should be monitored for signs of carbamazepine toxicity. In addition, carbamazepine, as an inducer of CYP3A4, could increase the clearance and decrease the effectiveness of CCBs.
Cyclosporine	Decreased clearance of cyclosporine, probably due to inhibition of CYP3A4, leads to increased cyclosporine levels with possible renal toxicity. Known to occur with diltiazem and verapamil. With appropriate cyclosporine dosage adjustment, CCBs may have a renoprotective effect vs. cyclosporine nephrotoxicity.
Digoxin	Diltiazem and verapamil can reduce digoxin clearance causing increased serum digoxin concentrations with additive effects on AV node conduction. Digoxin level should be monitored and adjusted appropriately.
Grapefruit juice	Decreased clearance of felodipine, nifedipine, nimodipine and verapamil, due to inhibition of intestinal CYP3A4. Grapefruit juice should be avoided in patients taking these drugs.
Rifampin	Through induction of CYP3A4, rifampin has decreased the effectiveness of diltiazem by increasing its metabolism. Diltiazem dose may need to be increased if this combination is used.

Drug-Food Interactions: see Table 3, grapefruit juice.

ADVERSE EFFECTS: This list is not exhaustive; individual product monographs should be consulted for any specific adverse effect.

In therapeutic dosages, CCBs are generally well tolerated and have a relatively low incidence of adverse effects. Most are transient and mild in severity, occur within the first few weeks of therapy, do not require drug discontinuation and occasionally may be minimized with dosage adjustment. Side effects tend to be dose-related and occur most frequently during periods of dose titration. Adverse effects may be exaggerated in older patients (over 65).

The most common adverse effects and those that most frequently result in discontinuation are cardiovascular and nervous system effects related to the vasodilatory action of CCBs, e.g., pedal edema, flushing, palpitations, headache. Serious side effects include angina, congestive heart failure (due to negative inotropic and chronotropic effects) or pulmonary edema, tachycardia, bradycardia, excessive hypotension, skin rashes; arthritis and transient blindness (for nifedipine); extrapyramidal effects, galactorrhea and mental depression (for flunarizine).

Cardiovascular: pedal edema (caused by precapillary vasodilation and not by salt and water retention), peripheral or facial edema, swelling, hypotension, syncope, bradycardia, tachycardia (caused by reflex activation of the sympathetic system and also peripheral vasodilation), angina (occurs when titrating the dose up or down).

Central Nervous System: The most common are headache and dizziness or lightheadedness (rapid blood pressure fall). Others include asthenia, paresthesia, somnolence, fatigue, nervousness, giddiness and insomnia.

Dermatological: rash, increased sweating, chills, photosensitivity reaction, urticaria, pruritus, hair loss.

Gastrointestinal: Nausea is the most common. Others include constipation (caused by interaction of the calcium channel blocker, e.g., verapamil, with calcium channels in smooth muscle of the gut), diarrhea, vomiting, gastrointestinal distress or bleeding and heartburn. One study reported that in an elderly population, CCBs were associated with an increased risk of gastrointestinal hemorrhage compared with beta-blockers. The risks for verapamil, diltiazem and nifedipine did not differ significantly. Vasodilation and mild platelet inhibition were postulated by the authors to be the reason for the finding.

Gingival Hyperplasia: The prevalence of clinically significant gingival hyperplasia with chronic use of CCBs is low (see Precautions).

Musculoskeletal: joint stiffness, muscle pain and cramps.

Respiratory: nasal or chest congestion, shortness of breath, dyspnea, wheezing, cough, respiratory infections.

Others: micturition disorder; weight gain and/or increased appetite with flunarizine.

OVERDOSE:

Symptoms: CCB overdose is increasingly common and mortality is high. Consultation with a regional poison centre is strongly advised in all patients with CCB overdose.

Hypotension is the most common manifestation of CCB overdose. Impaired myocardial contractility and bradycardia are other important features. Verapamil and diltiazem have more pronounced negative inotropic and chronotropic effects than the dihydropyridines (e.g. amlodipine, felodipine and nifedipine). Dihydropyridines are primarily vasodilators, and reflex tachycardia may occur following overdose. Extreme hypotension can lead to lethargy, dizziness, syncope, altered mental status, metabolic acidosis and renal failure. Profound calcium channel blockade inhibits insulin release and can result in hyperglycemia. Seizures have been reported.

The onset of symptoms will generally be evident within 2 to 3 hours of ingestion of an immediate release formulation. The onset of symptoms may be delayed for 6 to 8 hours after ingestion of a sustained release formulation. Many reports describe patients with major hemodynamic deterioration long after ingestion (> 24 hours), particularly with sustained-release products.

Treatment: Ensure adequate oxygenation and airway protection. Establish intravenous access, obtain a 12–lead ECG and begin continuous cardiac monitoring. Patients with signs or symptoms of CCB toxicity should be admitted to an intensive care unit.

Although it should not be routinely performed, gastric lavage may be considered on the advice of a Poison Control Centre in the unusual case where a patient presents within one hour of a large ingestion and vomiting has not occurred. However, lavage may increase vagal tone and exacerbate bradydysrhythmias. This may be prevented by atropine. Administration of activated charcoal is recommended within 2 hours of overdose (multidose activated charcoal has no role in this setting). Whole bowel irrigation with polyethylene glycol solution may be considered for patients without ileus who have minimal systemic toxicity and who have ingested a sustained-release formulation. Give 1-2 L/h by nasogastric tube (up to 500 mL/h in children) and continue until the rectal effluent is clear.

Intravascular volume expansion with rapid infusion of saline is the initial treatment for hypotension and maintenance of the patient's hemodynamic status. Atropine may be given for symptomatic bradycardia: 1.0 mg i.v. (0.02 mg/kg in children), but it often produces no meaningful increase in heart rate,

IV calcium is used to reverse negative inotropy and impaired conduction. Reasonable recommendations for poisoned adults include an initial iv bolus of 13 to 25 mEq of calcium: 10 to 20 mL of a 10% calcium chloride solution or 30 to 60 mL of a 10% calcium gluconate solution (if 10 mL vials are available, this amounts to 1 to 2 vials of 10% calcium chloride or 3 to 6 vials of 10% calcium gluconate, Table 4). This is then followed by either repeat boluses every 15 to 20 minutes for 3 or 4 doses, or a continuous infusion of 0.5 mEq/kg/h (0.2 to 0.4 mL/kg/h of 10% calcium chloride or 0.6 to 1.2 mL/kg/h of 10% calcium gluconate). Further doses depend on the response. There is no difference in the efficacy of calcium chloride or calcium gluconate, but calcium chloride dihydrate contains 13.6 mEq of elemental calcium per gram and calcium gluconate contains 4.3 mEq of elemental calcium per gram. Thus, if calcium gluconate is used rather than calcium chloride, three times the volume must be used to administer the same dose of elemental calcium. If there is any suspicion that digoxin was ingested in the overdose, calcium should not be given until after specific therapy for digoxin toxicity has been completed.

Table 4: Calcium Channel Blockers

Administration of Intravenous Calcium for Calcium Channel Blocker Overdose

	Calcium chloride (dihydrate)	Calcium gluconate
10% Solution	1 g $CaCl_2 \cdot H_2O$/10 mL 1.36 mEq elemental Ca^{++}/mL	1 g Ca^{++} gluconate/10 mL 0.45 mEq elemental Ca^{++}/mL
Adults	10–20 mL (1–2 10 mL vials) by slow iv push. Repeat every 15 to 20 minutes as necessary.	30–60 mL (3–6 10 mL vials) by slow iv push. Repeat every 15 to 20 minutes as necessary.
Children	0.2 mL/kg by slow iv push. Repeat every 15 to 20 minutes as necessary.	0.6 mL/kg by slow iv push. Repeat every 15 to 20 minutes as necessary.

Vasopressors are often given for calcium channel blocker overdose. However, there is some evidence that vasopressors lessen myocardial efficiency. The choice of agent depends on many factors; no single agent has been consistently effective. Norepinephrine is a reasonable initial agent, but in any patient requiring vasopressors, consideration should be given to high-dose insulin therapy (below).

Many authorities recommend early and aggressive treatment with insulin in combination with continuous dextrose infusion to maintain euglycemia. This should be done in conjunction with a regional poison centre. Treatment generally consists of a bolus dose (0.25 to 0.5 units regular insulin per kilogram), followed by infusion of 0.25 to 1.0 units per kilogram per hour. Exceptional patients may require even higher doses. Improvement in cardiac function and blood pressure are thought to result from improved myocardial utilization of carbohydrates.

Glucagon can be considered for patients with refractory hypotension following calcium channel blocker overdose, or in patients with concomitant beta-adrenergic antagonist overdose. Phosphodiesterase inhibitors such as milrinone have been used as second-line inotropic agents in combination with another inotrope and invasive hemodynamic monitoring.

As CCBs are highly protein bound, hemodialysis is not likely to be of benefit. Seizures can be treated with iv diazepam.

For management of a suspected drug overdose, CPhA recommends that you contact your **regional Poison Control Centre**. See the *CPS* Directory section for a list of Poison Control Centres.

DOSAGE: Oral: Although the absorption of some CCBs is slowed by the presence of food, bioavailability is not considered to be significantly affected. Grapefruit juice, however, does have a marked effect on bioavailability (see Table 3). Consistency in the timing of doses relative to meals is advised.

Hypertension: The initial dosage of a CCB must be individualized mainly due to the risk of hypotension, taking into consideration factors such as the age of the patient, renal and/or hepatic failure, or diuretic therapy. Patients at increased risk should receive lower initial doses.

Optimal doses are usually lower in patients also receiving diuretics since additive antihypertensive effects can be expected. Careful titration of the CCB is advised with attention to the possibility of excessive blood pressure reduction.

Once therapy has been initiated, the dosage of the CCB should be gradually titrated to achieve the desired effect. At a given dosage regimen, the full reduction in blood pressure may take at least 3 weeks. Therefore, in order to assess adequately the response to a particular dose level, there should be an interval of at least 3 weeks between increases in dose.

Angina: In general, there should be an interval of at least 3 days between increases in dose in order to adequately assess the response to a particular dose level. In hospitalized patients under close supervision, the titration phase may proceed more rapidly. In patients with vasospastic angina, the last dose of the day may be given at bedtime to help minimize angina pain which, in such patients, frequently occurs in early morning. After anginal symptoms are controlled, dosage should be gradually reduced to the lowest level that will maintain relief of symptoms.

Switching from Regular to Prolonged- or Extended-release Formulations: Patients can be changed to prolonged- or extended-release formulations at the same total daily dose as the regular formulation. In some patients, the dosage of the sustained-release formulation may require adjustment.

Discontinuation: Abrupt withdrawal of CCBs may cause increased frequency and duration of chest pain. It is generally recommended that the dose be gradually decreased.

Table 5 lists dosage recommendations for CCBs in the treatment of hypertension and angina, including initial, maintenance and maximum dosages. More detailed information may be found within individual product monographs including specific dosage recommendations for different indications, titration guidelines and dosage adjustments in renal or hepatic failure.

Migraine Prophylaxis: The dose of flunarizine is 10 mg/day, administered in the evening. Maximum benefits may not be seen before the patient has completed several weeks of continuous treatment. Therapy should be continued for at least 6 to 8 weeks before assessing response.

Obstructive Hypertrophic Cardiomyopathy: The usual starting dose of verapamil is 80 to 120 mg TID or QID. Higher doses (up to 600 to 720 mg/day) may be required. In some patients, therapy should be started in hospital as significant clinical deterioration can occur.

Raynaud's Phenomenon: The dose of nifedipine is 20 mg (prolonged-action) or 30 mg (extended-release) taken 30 to 60 minutes before cold exposure. Other CCBs have been used but are considered less effective than nifedipine.

Subarachnoid Hemorrhage: The usual recommended dose of nimodipine is 60 mg administered orally every 4 hours for 21 days after diagnosis of subarachnoid hemorrhage. Patients with hepatic insufficiency should receive 30 mg orally every 4 hours for 21 days. Treatment should begin as soon as possible or within 4 days of subarachnoid hemorrhage.

If the patient is unable to swallow, the capsule contents may be aspirated into a syringe, emptied into the patient's nasogastric tube and washed down with 30 mL of normal saline.

Nimodipine may be continued perioperatively.

IV: Atrial Fibrillation/Atrial Flutter: Continuous ECG and blood pressure monitoring are recommended during the administration period. Diltiazem may be administered direct iv or by continuous iv infusion, at a dose of 0.25 mg/kg initially, then 10 mg/h (up to 15 mg/h) for 24 hours. Verapamil should be given as a slow iv injection over at least 2 minutes (over at least 3 minutes in elderly patients). The initial iv dose of verapamil is 5 to 10 mg (0.075 to 0.15 mg/kg). A dose of 10 mg (0.15 mg/kg) may be given 30 minutes after the first dose if the initial response is not adequate. A single dose of 10 mg should not be exceeded. Oral therapy should replace iv therapy as soon as possible. The usual oral dosage of verapamil for prevention of recurrent paroxysmal supraventricular tachycardia is 240 to 480 mg daily, in 3 or 4 divided doses.

Special Patient Populations: Elderly: Patients over 65 years of age may develop elevated plasma concentrations of the CCB with standard doses; lower dosages may be warranted in these patients. CCBs should be administered cautiously to elderly patients and the dosage should be carefully and gradually adjusted depending on patient tolerance and response. The risk of peripheral edema and gastrointestinal hemorrhage is increased in these patients (see Adverse Effects).

Impaired Hepatic Function: Dosage requirements have not been established. CCBs should be administered cautiously. A lower starting dose should be considered. Patients on verapamil should be monitored carefully for abnormal prolongation of the PR interval or other signs of overdosage. CCBs should not be used in patients with severe hepatic dysfunction.

Impaired Renal Function: There are few available data concerning dosage requirements in patients with renal insufficiency. If CCBs must be used in these patients, dosage should be carefully and gradually adjusted.

Table 5: Calcium Channel Blockers

Oral Dosage in Hypertension or Angina

Calcium Channel Blocker	Usual Initial Dose	Usual Maintenance Dose	Recommended Maximum Dosage
Calcium channel blockers indicated for hypertension or angina			
Amlodipine	Hypertension or angina: 5 mg daily	Hypertension or angina: 5 to 10 mg daily	10 mg daily
Diltiazem, controlled-delivery (CD)	Hypertension: 120 to 240 mg once daily Angina: 120 to 180 mg daily	Hypertension or angina: 240 to 360 mg once daily	360 mg daily
Diltiazem, sustained-release (SR)	Hypertension: 120 to 240 mg/day in 2 to 3 divided doses Angina: For initiation of therapy, immediate-release tablets are recommended.	Hypertension or angina: 120 to 360 mg daily (in 2 to 3 divided doses) Optimum: 240 to 360 mg daily	360 mg/day
Nifedipine, extended-release (XL)	Hypertension or angina: 30 mg once daily	Hypertension or angina: 30 to 60 mg once daily	90 mg daily
Verapamil, immediate-release	Hypertension: 80 mg TID Angina: up to 80 mg QID	Hypertension: 160 mg TID; Angina: 120 mg TID to QID	480 mg/day
Verapamil, sustained-release (Chronovera)	180 mg at bedtime	Hypertension: 180 to 480 mg at bedtime Angina: 180 to 360 mg at bedtime	480 mg at bedtime
Calcium channel blockers indicated for hypertension only			
Felodipine, extended-release	5 mg daily	2.5 to 10 mg daily	10 mg daily
Nifedipine, prolonged-action (PA)	10 to 20 mg BID	20 mg BID	80 mg/day
Verapamil, sustained-release (Isoptin SR)	180 to 240 mg/day	180 to 240 mg BID	480 mg/day
Calcium channel blockers indicated for angina only (in combination therapy)			
Diltiazem, immediate-release	30 mg QID	240 mg/day in 3 to 4 divided doses	360 mg/day
Nifedipine, immediate-release	10 mg TID	10 to 20 mg TID	120 mg/day

The reader is referred to individual product monographs for more detailed information on dosage recommendations for specific indications or special patient groups such as children, elderly or debilitated patients or those with hepatic or renal failure.

Calcium Chloride

calcium chloride

Calcium Replenisher

Hospira

SUPPLIED: Each mL contains: calcium chloride dihydrate 100 mg in Water for Injection. May contain hydrochloric acid and/or sodium hydroxide. Hypertonic solution to be used with caution. Must not be given by i.m. or s.c. injection. Abboject syringes of 10 mL, boxes of 10. Lifeshield syringes of 10 mL, boxes of 10. Protect from freezing. Avoid excessive heat.

Calcium Salts: Oral

calcium acetate
calcium carbonate
calcium citrate
calcium glucoheptonate
calcium gluconate
calcium lactate
calcium phosphate

Calcium Therapy

CPhA Monograph

Date of Revision: October 2010

This monograph has been compiled by CPhA and reviewed by experts. It may contain information different from that found in Health Canada-approved Product Monographs. The reader is referred to the *CPS* Editorial Policy for more information.

PHARMACOLOGY: Calcium is the most abundant mineral in the human body and is essential for maintaining the functional integrity of nervous and musculoskeletal systems as well as cell membrane and capillary permeability. The majority (99%) of body calcium is contained in bone with the remainder equally distributed between intra- and extracellular fluids. Calcium is an activator in many enzymatic reactions and is necessary for nerve impulse transmission, renal function, respiration and blood coagulation.

Pharmacokinetics: Calcium is actively absorbed, mainly in the duodenum and proximal jejunum. Calcium must be in a soluble, ionized form to be absorbed. Factors such as an acidic intestinal pH, the presence of vitamin D, and pregnancy and lactation tend to favour calcium absorption. However, absorption may be impeded in the elderly, or by a deficiency of parathyroid hormone, calcitonin or vitamin D, the presence of anions or fatty acids which may precipitate or complex with calcium, or in certain disease states such as achlorhydria, renal osteodystrophy, steatorrhea or uremia. Calcium from supplements is absorbed to a greater extent when doses of 500 mg or less are given.

Once absorbed, most calcium is rapidly incorporated into skeletal muscle; the remainder is equally distributed between intra- and extracellular fluids. Normal total serum calcium concentrations range from 2.2 to 2.6 mmol/L, although only the ionized fraction is physiologically active. Of the total serum calcium, 50% is ionized, 5% is complexed with anions such as phosphates or citrates and 45% is protein bound. Hyperproteinemia is associated with an increase in total serum calcium; hypoproteinemia has the opposite effect. Acidosis favours an increase in ionic calcium concentration, while alkalosis leads to a decrease in the ionized fraction.

CSF calcium concentrations tend to be similar to the serum concentration of ionized calcium, i.e., approximately 50% of total serum calcium.

Calcium crosses the placenta, reaching higher levels in fetal blood than in maternal blood. Calcium is excreted in breast milk.

Calcium is excreted mainly in the feces, either by passing through the gut unabsorbed or through biliary or pancreatic secretion into the gut lumen. Very small amounts of calcium are excreted in the urine as most renally filtered calcium is reabsorbed. Urinary excretion of calcium is promoted by growth hormone, calcitonin and nonthiazide diuretics, whereas parathyroid hormone, vitamin D, thiazide diuretics or a decrease in ionized calcium concentration tend to decrease the amount of calcium excreted in the urine. Calcium is also excreted in sweat.

INDICATIONS: Oral calcium salts are classified by Health Canada as a natural health product (NHP).

Calcium is used orally as a dietary supplement in patients whose intake is inadequate or should be increased, e.g., children, adolescents, postmenopausal women, the elderly. Oral calcium is also used in the treatment of osteoporosis, osteomalacia, hypoparathyroidism, tetany, pseudohypoparathyroidism or hypocalcemia secondary to anticonvulsant therapy.

Although caution is advised when calcium salts are used in patients with renal failure because of the possibility of hypercalcemia, calcium acetate and calcium carbonate are used to control hyperphosphatemia in patients with chronic renal failure, by forming insoluble phosphates in the gut that are excreted fecally.

Calcium carbonate is used in the symptomatic management of dyspepsia and mild gastroesophageal reflux disease.

CONTRAINDICATIONS: Hypercalcemia and hypercalciuria (e.g., in hyperparathyroidism, vitamin D overdosage, decalcifying tumors such as plasmacytoma, bone metastases); severe cardiac disease; ventricular fibrillation; calcium loss due to immobilization.

WARNINGS: See Precautions.

PRECAUTIONS: Calcium salts should be used with caution in patients with cardiac or renal disease, sarcoidosis, or in patients receiving digoxin (particularly if calcium is given parenterally). When calcium carbonate is used to bind phosphates in patients with chronic renal failure, appropriate monitoring for the potential development of hypercalcemia is recommended.

A meta-analysis showed an association between calcium supplements (taken without supplemental vitamin D) and an increased risk of myocardial infarction [*BMJ* 2010;341:c3691]. High doses of calcium supplements should not be used by postmenopausal women who do not need extra calcium or who need only a modest amount to reach a total daily intake of 1200 mg. Health Canada recommends that patients not exceed 1500 mg/day from supplements alone.

High dietary intake of calcium is thought to decrease the risk of symptomatic renal calculi, presumably by decreasing the absorption and promoting the urinary excretion of oxalate. However, calcium from oral supplements may predispose some individuals to the risk of symptomatic stones. Proposed explanations for this incongruity include the possible importance of the timing of calcium ingestion relative to oxalate consumption, and the possibility that other factors present in dietary sources of calcium may affect oxalate absorption or excretion.

Studies done in recent years have shown that many calcium supplements contain varying amounts of lead. Supplements derived from bone meal, fossil or oyster shells, or dolomite contain the highest amounts. Certain patients may be at higher risk such as children or patients who rely on supplementation to meet their daily calcium requirements. Patients on chronic calcium therapy, especially children, infants, pregnant or breastfeeding women and chronic renal failure or dialysis patients, may be advised to avoid products derived from dolomite, fossil or oyster shells or bone meal, in favor of sources with lower lead content such as refined calcium carbonate or chelated calcium (gluconate and lactate salts).

Drug Interactions: See Table 1.

In addition to the specific medications mentioned in this monograph, the rate and/or extent of absorption of other oral medications may vary when taken concurrently with calcium supplements, especially the carbonate salt. Patients should generally be advised to separate calcium administration from administration of other drugs by several hours.

ADVERSE EFFECTS: Calcium salts can cause gastric irritation or constipation.

Hypercalcemia is unlikely to develop in patients with normal renal function who are taking oral calcium salts; however, it could occur if large doses are given to patients with chronic renal failure. Symptoms of mild hypercalcemia may be absent, or could include anorexia, nausea and vomiting; if hypercalcemia becomes more severe, CNS effects such as confusion, delirium and coma may occur.

The milk-alkali syndrome, characterized by metabolic alkalosis, hypercalcemia, renal calcinosis and possible renal failure, has occurred in patients ingesting excessive amounts of calcium used in association with absorbable antacid (e.g., calcium carbonate). Factors that may increase the risk of milk-alkali syndrome include dehydration and renal impairment.

Table 1: Calcium Salts: Oral

Drug Interactions

Interacting Drug	Effect	Clinical Comment
Bisphosphonates, oral (alendronate, clodronate, etidronate, risedronate)	Calcium decreases absorption.	Give alendronate or risedronate 30 minutes before calcium; separate administration of clodronate or etidronate and calcium by 2 hours.
Digoxin	Concomitant administration may enhance inotropic effects of digoxin, leading to cardiac arrhythmias.	Particularly a concern with i.v. calcium.
Iron supplements	Calcium decreases absorption of iron.	Separate administration times by several hours.
Levothyroxine	May form an insoluble chelate with calcium, reducing levothyroxine absorption.	Separate administration by at least 4 hours.
Phenytoin	May form a nonabsorbable complex with calcium.	Separate administration times by several hours.
Quinolones, oral	Calcium salts decrease absorption.	Administer oral quinolone at least 2 hours before or 6 hours after calcium.
Tetracyclines	Calcium decreases absorption of tetracyclines.	Administration times should be separated by 3–4 hours.

OVERDOSAGE:

Symptoms: Acute ingestion of calcium salts may cause mild gastric symptoms but has not caused hypercalcemia or other toxicity. Chronic ingestion of calcium salts may produce more significant toxicity (see Adverse Effects).

Treatment: Acute ingestion of calcium salts seldom requires treatment. Symptomatic hypercalcemia following chronic ingestion may require fluid resuscitation to correct extracellular volume depletion and the establishment of a diuresis and occasionally, if the serum calcium is extremely high, hemodialysis or peritoneal dialysis.

> For management of a suspected drug overdose, CPhA recommends that you contact your **regional Poison Control Centre**. See the *CPS* Directory section for a list of Poison Control Centres.

DOSAGE: Dietary Intake: Increased dietary intake of calcium is preferred over supplementation whenever possible. Food sources include dairy products (e.g., cheese, milk, yogurt), canned salmon or sardines (with bones), fortified beverages (e.g., soy, fruit juices), dried figs, legumes (e.g., beans) and almonds.

Supplementation: Requirements for supplemental calcium vary according to life stage group, actual dietary intake of calcium, serum calcium levels and clinical indication. Based on these considerations, the dosage of supplemental calcium can be calculated to meet the potential shortfall between the recommended and actual intake. Health Canada's recommendations for calcium intake are presented in Table 2.

Table 2: Calcium Salts: Oral

Recommended Adequate Intake (AI) of Calcium From All Sources (Diet and Supplements)

Life Stage Group	Age	Elemental Ca^{++} (mg/day)
Infants[a] and Children	Birth to 6 months	210
	7 to 12 months	270
	1 to 3 years	500
	4 to 8 years	800
	9 to 18 years	1300
Adults	19 to 50 years	1000
	>50 years	1200[b]
Pregnancy or Breastfeeding	No change from AI for appropriate age	

[a] For all healthy infants, Adequate Intake (AI) is based on estimated mean intakes of human milk.
[b] Along with calcium, supplemental vitamin D 400 IU/day is recommended for patients >50 y.

Calcium supplements contain varying amounts of lead, depending on the source (see Precautions). Lead content should be among the many factors considered when recommending a calcium supplement to a patient.

Oral calcium supplement doses >500 mg/day should be administered in divided doses for optimal absorption. Other than calcium citrate, calcium salts should be taken with food. Doses of syrup may be diluted in water, fruit juice or formula for children or infants.

With advancing age or in the presence of achlorhydria, calcium absorption from the gastrointestinal tract is reduced; calcium dosage may need to be adjusted accordingly. Vitamin D supplementation can increase the absorption of oral calcium.

Table 3 lists the various calcium salts and their elemental calcium content.

Table 3: Calcium Salts: Oral

Elemental Calcium Content

Calcium Salt	Percentage Elemental Ca^{++}	Elemental Ca^{++} (mmol/g)[a]
Calcium acetate	25.3	6.3
Calcium carbonate	40	10
Calcium citrate	21	5.3
Calcium glucoheptonate	8	2.1
Calcium gluconate	9	2.3
Calcium lactate	13	3.3
Calcium phosphate dibasic anhydrous	29	7.3
Calcium phosphate dibasic dihydrate	23	5.8
Calcium phosphate tribasic	40	10

[a] Conversion: 1 g elemental calcium = 25 mmol = 50 mEq.

Prevention of Hyperphosphatemia: In patients with chronic renal failure, the dosage of calcium acetate or carbonate used to prevent hyperphosphatemia is titrated to maintain the desired phosphate level while preventing hypercalcemia. The usual dosage is 500 to 700 mg elemental calcium with each meal (see Table 3).

Calcium Salts: Parenteral

calcium chloride

calcium gluconate

Calcium Therapy

CPhA Monograph

Date of Revision: November 2007

> This monograph has been compiled by CPhA and reviewed by experts. It may contain information different from that found in Health Canada-approved Product Monographs. The reader is referred to the *CPS* Editorial Policy for more information.

SUMMARY PRODUCT INFORMATION:

Drug[a]	Dosage Form	Strength
Calcium chloride	Injectable solution	10% (0.68 mmol/mL)
Calcium gluconate	Injectable solution	10% (0.23 mmol/mL)

[a] Table includes single-entity parenteral calcium products only. For specific product information consult Health Canada's Drug Product Database http://www.hc-sc.gc.ca/dhp-mps/prodpharma/databasdon/index_e.html.

PHARMACOLOGY: Calcium is the most abundant mineral in the human body and is essential for maintaining the functional integrity of nervous and musculoskeletal systems as well as cell membrane and capillary permeability. The majority (99%) of body calcium is contained in bone with the remainder equally distributed between intra- and extracellular fluids. Calcium is an activator in many enzymatic reactions and is necessary for nerve impulse transmission, renal function, respiration and blood coagulation.

Pharmacokinetics: Once absorbed into the bloodstream, most calcium is rapidly incorporated into skeletal muscle; the remainder is equally distributed between intra- and extracellular fluids. Normal total serum calcium concentrations range from 2.2 to 2.6 mmol/L, although only the ionized fraction is physiologically active. Of the total serum calcium, 50% is ionized, 5% is complexed with anions such as phosphates or citrates and 45% is protein bound. Hyperproteinemia is associated with an increase in total calcium; hypoproteinemia has the opposite effect. Acidosis favors an increase in ionic calcium concentration, while alkalosis leads to a decrease in the ionized fraction.

CSF calcium concentrations tend to be similar to the serum concentration of ionized calcium, i.e., approximately 50% of total serum calcium.

Calcium crosses the placenta, reaching higher levels in fetal blood than in maternal blood, and is excreted in breast milk.

Calcium is excreted mainly in the feces, either as a result of passing through the gut unabsorbed or through biliary or pancreatic secretion into the gut lumen. Very small amounts of calcium are excreted in the urine as most renally filtered calcium is reabsorbed. Urinary excretion of calcium is promoted by growth hormone, calcitonin and nonthiazide diuretics, whereas parathyroid hormone, vitamin D, thiazide diuretics or a decrease in ionized calcium concentration tend to decrease the amount of calcium excreted in the urine. Calcium is also excreted in sweat.

INDICATIONS: The treatment of hypocalcemia for those conditions requiring a prompt increase in serum calcium concentrations, such as neonatal tetany and tetany due to parathyroid deficiency, vitamin D deficiency and alkalosis; the prevention of hypocalcemia during exchange transfusions of citrated blood; the treatment of hyperkalemia when there is ECG evidence of secondary cardiac toxicity.

Calcium salts have also been administered as adjunctive therapy in a number of conditions, including the following: insect bites or stings (e.g., black widow spider), sensitivity reactions characterized by urticaria or angioedema, magnesium sulfate overdosage, or lead colic.

The use of calcium is not recommended in cardiac arrest except in cases of calcium channel blocker overdose, hyperkalemia or severe hypocalcemia.

CONTRAINDICATIONS: Hypercalcemia and hypercalciuria (e.g., in hyperparathyroidism, vitamin D overdosage, decalcifying tumors such as plasmocytoma, bone metastases); severe renal disease; calcium loss due to immobilization.

WARNINGS: See Precautions.

PRECAUTIONS: Parenteral calcium must be used cautiously in patients with cardiac disease.

Because concurrent use of iv calcium with digitalis glycosides may increase the risk of cardiac arrhythmias, the use of iv calcium in digitalized patients should be avoided. If absolutely necessary, iv calcium should be given slowly and in small amounts, with ECG monitoring.

When severe hypocalcemia co-exists with hyperphosphatemia (>6 mmol/L), patients should be treated for hyperphosphatemia prior to the administration of iv calcium; the aim is to achieve a proper calcium/phosphate ratio in order to prevent extraskeletal deposition of calcium. Correction of hyperphosphatemia may require measures such as discontinuing exogenous phosphate, administration of oral aluminum hydroxide, or dialysis.

High dose calcium therapy by any of the parenteral routes should always be accompanied by very careful monitoring of serum concentration and urinary calcium excretion, particularly in children. Serum calcium concentrations should generally be maintained between 2.2 and 2.6 mmol/L. Cardiac monitoring is also recommended.

Drug Interactions: Digitalis glycosides (see Precautions). Parenteral calcium is precipitated by carbonates, bicarbonates, phosphates, sulfates and tartrates in addition to iv solutions containing various drugs. Specialized references should be consulted for compatability information.

ADVERSE EFFECTS: Cardiovascular: Hypotension, bradycardia, cardiac arrhythmias, syncope and cardiac arrest may occur with too rapid iv administration.

Local: **Tissue irritation and necrosis may occur with im or sc injection, or if extravasation occurs during iv administration, particularly with the chloride salt.**

OVERDOSE:

Symptoms: Markedly elevated plasma calcium level, weakness, lethargy, intractable nausea and vomiting, coma and sudden death.

Treatment: To rapidly lower serum calcium to safe levels, administer sodium chloride by iv infusion plus a potent natriuretic agent, e.g., furosemide, to increase renal clearance of calcium.

> For management of a suspected drug overdose, CPhA recommends that you contact your **regional Poison Control Centre**. See the *CPS* Directory section for a list of Poison Control Centres.

DOSAGE: Table 1 lists the elemental calcium content of the available parenteral calcium salts.

Table 1: Calcium Salts: Parenteral
Elemental Calcium Content

Calcium Salt	% elemental Ca++	Elemental Ca++/g (mmol)[a]
Calcium chloride	27	6.8
Calcium gluconate	9	2.3

[a] 1 g elemental calcium = 25 mmol = 50 mEq.

IV: Calcium injections must be administered slowly, through a small needle into a large vein, to minimize venous irritation. The rate of administration should not exceed 0.35 to 0.9 mmol/minute. Injection should be stopped if patient complains of discomfort. Patients should remain recumbent for a short period following injection.

Table 2 lists dosages of iv calcium for various indications as well as corresponding volumes of available calcium injection solutions.

Table 2: Calcium Salts: Parenteral
Dosage

Indication	Dose of Elemental Calcium (mmol)	Volume (mL) of Calcium Chloride[a] 10% Injection, 0.68 mmol Ca++/mL	Volume (mL) of Calcium Gluconate[b] 10% Injection, 0.23 mmol Ca++/mL	Comments
Emergency treatment of hypocalcemia	Adults: 3.5 to 7	—[b]	15 to 30	May be repeated every 1 to 3 days depending on response.
	Children: 0.5 to 3.5	—[b]	2 to 15	
	Infants: < 0.5	—[b]	< 2	
Hyperkalemia-induced cardiac arrhythmias	Adults: 1.125 to 7	1.7 to 10.3	4.8 to 30	Monitor ECG. May repeat in 1 to 2 minutes if necessary.
Hypermagnesemia	Adults: 2.5 to 5	3.7 to 7.4	10.7 to 21.5	Repeat according to response.
Hypocalcemic tetany	Adults: 2.25 to 8	3.3 to 11.8	9.7 to 34.3	Once daily until tetany controlled.
	Children: 0.25 to 0.7/kg	0.4 to 1/kg	1.1 to 3/kg	Give 3 to 4 times daily until tetany controlled.
	Neonates: 1.2/kg/day	1.8/kg	5.5/kg	Give in divided doses.
Prevention of hypocalcemia during exchange transfusions	Adults: 0.68	1	—[a]	Concurrently with each 100 mL citrated blood.
	Neonates: 0.23	0.34	—[a]	After each 100 mL citrated blood.
Cardiopulmonary resuscitation[c]	Adults: 3.5 to 7	5.1 to 10.3	—[a]	Repeat at 10-minute intervals as necessary.
	Children: 0.135/kg	0.2/kg	—[a]	Repeat at 10-minute intervals as necessary.

[a] Calcium chloride is often recommended as the preferred salt when calcium is used in cardiopulmonary resuscitation or to prevent hypocalcemia during transfusions.
[b] Most clinicians consider calcium gluconate the preferred salt for the treatment of hypocalcemia, especially if acidosis is also present.
[c] Calcium should not be used in cardiopulmonary resuscitation except in the presence of hypocalcemia, hyperkalemia or overdose involving calcium channel blockers or beta-blockers.

IM: Calcium chloride should never be injected im as it may cause severe necrosis and sloughing when injected into tissue. Other calcium salts should only be administered im when iv access cannot be established.

Calmylin Original with Codeine Ⓝ

codeine phosphate—ammonium chloride—diphenhydramine HCl

Antihistamine—Antitussive—Expectorant

Rougier Pharma

Calmylin PSE with Codeine Ⓝ

codeine phosphate—guaifenesin—pseudoephedrine HCl

Decongestant—Antitussive—Expectorant

Rougier Pharma

SUPPLIED: Calmylin Original with Codeine: Each 5 mL of clear red syrup with a raspberry odor contains: codeine phosphate 3.33 mg, ammonium chloride 125 mg and diphenhydramine HCl 12.5 mg. Nonmedicinal ingredients: alcohol, artificial coloring and flavoring, FD&C Yellow #6, glycerin, menthol, methylparaben, propylparaben, purified water, simethicone, sorbitol and sucrose. Bottles of 100, 250 and 350 mL.

Calmylin PSE with Codeine: Each 5 mL of red, clear syrup with a raspberry odor syrup contains: codeine phosphate 3.33 mg, guaifenesin 100 mg and pseudoephedrine HCl 30 mg. Nonmedicinal ingredients: alcohol, artificial coloring and flavoring, citric acid, FD&C Yellow #6, glycerin, maltitol, menthol, methylparaben, propylene glycol, propylparaben, purified water, sodium chloride, sodium citrate, sodium cyclamate and sorbitol. Bottles of 100 and 250 mL.

Store between 15 and 30°C.

Caltine® Ⓟ

calcitonin salmon

Paget's Disease Therapy—Hypercalcemia Treatment

Ferring

PHARMACOLOGY: Salmon calcitonin participates in the regulation of the homeostasis of calcium by acting primarily on bone, in Paget's disease, presumably by an initial blocking effect on accelerated bone resorption. The rate of bone turnover appears to be decreased.

The pharmacologic activity of salmon calcitonin is the same as that of the endogenously produced hormone, but salmon calcitonin is substantially more potent on a weight basis and has a longer duration of action. Calcitonin acts predominantly on bone to depress bone resorption, but also has direct effects on the kidneys and the gastrointestinal tract. As a result of the inhibition of release of calcium from bone, and the stimulation of urinary calcium excretion, calcitonin tends to lower blood calcium.

Following parenteral administration, the hypocalcemic effect of calcitonin is apparent in about 15 minutes, peaks at approximately 4 hours, and lasts for 8 to 24 hours.

The lowering of serum calcium with calcitonin can, under certain conditions, be as much as 3 to 4 mg%. Chronic administration of calcitonin results in a parallel diminution of 2 parameters of bone turnover, namely, serum alkaline phosphatase levels, and total hydroxyproline excretion in the urine. The extent to which calcitonin can inhibit bone resorption depends on the existing rate of bone resorption (the higher the rate of bone resorption, the more evident the inhibition of bone resorption following calcitonin administration). Thus, these biochemical effects are more prominent in patients with generalized Paget's disease, or hypercalcemia, than in healthy adults, who have a relatively low rate of bone resorption.

Paget's disease is characterized by a mixed picture of bone resorption, increased vascularity, high bone turnover and irregular bone formation. One or more bones may be affected, and an increased alkaline phosphatase is often found on a routine laboratory screen. Clinical features can include bone pain, deformities, nerve and blood vessel compression, increased cardiac output, spontaneous fractures and osteogenic sarcoma. Immobilization of patients with Paget's disease may lead to hypercalcemia, hypercalciuria, and renal calculus formation.

Salmon calcitonin has been shown to be effective in relieving bone pain in 60 to 80% of patients with Paget's disease. A similar proportion show a parallel diminution of alkaline phosphatase levels in the serum (reflecting increased bone formation), and of total hydroxyproline excretion in the urine (reflecting breakdown of collagen-containing bone matrix) in the same proportions (average 50%). Significant pain relief is usually evident within 2 months after initiation of therapy, with the maximum relief being obtained within 6 to 12 months.

The biochemical changes produced by calcitonin have been shown to correlate with changes toward more normal bone, as evidenced by radiologic assessments showing slowing or even regression of resorption fronts in pagetic lesions, the observation of rapid healing of pathological fractures during treatment, with the prevention of immobilization hypercalcemia, and the decreased fracture rate during therapy.

In Paget's disease, orthopedic surgery is associated with complications due to softness of bone and/or excessive bleeding in about 50% of cases. In patients pretreated with calcitonin prior to surgery, no complications were found.

Other symptoms of Paget's disease that may show a beneficial effect with calcitonin treatment are high output cardiac failure, and symptoms due to, or mimicking neurologic compression.

In most patients with hypercalcemia treated with calcitonin, the hypocalcemic response was partial, with the serum calcium decreasing from a dangerously high level to a more tolerable or mildly hypercalcemic range. Often, there was an accompanying clinical improvement, allowing resumption of eating and further improvement, and, where applicable, the institution of definitive treatment for the underlying disease. In patients with multiple myeloma, a stable normocalcemia was achieved in all those with mild hypercalcemia, and about half of those with severe hypercalcemia. Prolonged normocalcemia after cessation of calcitonin therapy has been reported.

INDICATIONS: Paget's Disease of Bone: For the management of symptomatic Paget's disease of bone (osteitis deformans).
Hypercalcemia: For the early treatment of hypercalcemic emergencies (eg. hypercalcemic patients with carcinoma—with or without metastases, multiple myeloma or primary hyperparathyroidism), along with other appropriate agents, in cases where a rapid reduction in serum calcium concentration is required, until more specific treatment of the underlying disorder is instituted. The drug may also be added to the existing therapeutic regimens for the treatment of hypercalcemia, such as i.v. fluids and furosemide, oral phosphates, corticosteroids or other agents.

Salmon calcitonin may be used in patients with azotemia and those with limited cardiac reserve in whom i.v. fluids may be contraindicated.

CONTRAINDICATIONS: Hypersensitivity to salmon calcitonin.

WARNINGS: Administration of salmon calcitonin has been associated with serious allergic type reactions, such as bronchospasm, swelling of the tongue or throat, tachycardia, hypotension, collapse and anaphylactic shock and in 1 case death due to anaphylaxis (see Precautions).
Children: There are no adequate safety and efficacy data supporting the use of calcitonin in children. The relationship between juvenile Paget's disease to Paget's disease in adults has not been established and salmon calcitonin has been used only rarely in children.
Pregnancy: Salmon calcitonin has been shown to decrease fetal birth weights in rabbits when given in doses 14 to 56 times the human therapeutic doses. It is not known whether salmon calcitonin can cause fetal harm when administered to pregnant women. Therefore the drug should be used during pregnancy only when the potential benefits justify the possible risks to the fetus.
Lactation: Salmon calcitonin inhibits lactation in animals, and the drug should therefore not be administered to nursing mothers.

PRECAUTIONS: The possibility of a systemic allergic reaction should be borne in mind, and appropriate measures of treatment of a hypersensitivity reaction should be readily available. Skin testing should be considered prior to initiating salmon calcitonin therapy and the drug should not be given to patients with a positive skin test. The following procedure is suggested for the skin test:

Prepare a dilution of 10 IU/mL by withdrawing 1/10 mL (0.1 mL) in a tuberculin syringe and filling it to 1 mL with Dextrose injection 5% USP (or Saline Injection, USP). Mix well, discard 0.9 mL and inject intracutaneously 0.1 mL (approximately 1 IU) on the inner aspect of the forearm. Observe the injection site 15 minutes after injection. The appearance of more than a mild erythema or wheal constitutes a positive response.

The possibility of hypocalcemic tetany following salmon calcitonin administration should be considered, and calcium injection should be readily available, particularly during administration of the first several doses of salmon calcitonin.

Patients receiving salmon calcitonin for long periods should have periodic examinations of urine sediment as coarse granular casts and casts containing renal tubular epithelial cells were reported in some volunteers in a study of the effect of calcitonin salmon on immobilization osteoporosis.

Radiographic evidence of marked progressive pagetic lesions, possibly with some loss of definition of periosteal margins, must be evaluated carefully to rule out the possibility of osteogenic sarcoma since the frequency of this tumor is increased in patients with Paget's disease of bone.

Careful instructions in sterile injection technique should be given to the patient, and to other persons who may administer salmon calcitonin.

ADVERSE EFFECTS: Adverse effects with salmon calcitonin are usually mild, although in about 10% of patients, adverse effects may be severe enough to require discontinuance of the drug.

Adverse effects of salmon calcitonin most frequently involve the gastrointestinal tract. Nausea, with or without vomiting, is the most common adverse effect (incidence of about 20 to 40%), but it usually disappears with continued use. Other less common adverse effects on the gastrointestinal tract include: anorexia, diarrhea, epigastric pain, abdominal pain and an unusual taste.

Three cases of hypertension have been reported following the use of salmon calcitonin.

Flushing of face, ears, hands, and feet may occur (incidence of 10 to 35%), usually within minutes after salmon calcitonin injection, but this effect is usually well tolerated. Tenderness and/or tingling of the palms and soles has also been reported.

A local inflammatory reaction may occur at the site of injection: swelling, pain, erythema, urticaria have been occasionally reported (incidence of about 10%). A few cases of generalized urticaria have been reported with both salmon and human forms of calcitonin.

During the first few days of the drug administration, some patients may experience diuresis and increased urinary sodium excretion but this usually returns to the baseline levels within 5 to 7 days. Urinary frequency may occur during this time.

Antibodies to salmon calcitonin have been reported in 30 to 50% of patients after 2 to 18 months of therapy, but in no instance have these elevated antibody titers been associated with any systemic allergic or anaphylactic effect, and only rarely have antibodies been associated with the development of clinical resistance to calcitonin.

One case of symptoms of hypocalcemic tetany accompanying administration of human calcitonin has been reported (paresthesia, increased irritability). These symptoms disappeared on administration of calcium salts.

Administration of salmon calcitonin has been associated with serious allergic type reactions, such as bronchospasm, swelling of the tongue or throat, tachycardia, hypotension, collapse and anaphylactic shock and in 1 case death due to anaphylaxis.

OVERDOSE:

Treatment: In general, no corrective action needs to be taken, other than to discontinue treatment temporarily and maintain the patient under observation. Supportive treatment may be indicated. Provisions for parenteral calcium administration should be available during the first several administrations of calcitonin in case of hypocalcemic tetany.

> For management of a suspected drug overdose, CPhA recommends that you contact your **regional Poison Control Centre**. See the *CPS* Directory section for a list of Poison Control Centres.

DOSAGE: Dosage is expressed in terms of IU (International Units). An International Unit for salmon calcitonin is defined as the activity contained in 0.02525 mg of the International Reference Preparation of Calcitonin, Salmon for Bioassay.

Paget's Disease: The recommended adult dosage in Paget's disease of bone is 100 IU (1 mL) daily administered s.c. or i.m. The effect of the drug should be monitored by determinations of serum alkaline phosphatase and urinary hydroxyproline excretion before initiating salmon calcitonin therapy and every 3 to 6 months during chronic therapy. Decreases in these parameters are usually seen within the first few months of therapy, as is relief of bone pain.

Adjustments in dosage should be guided by clinical and radiologic response and by changes in biochemical parameters. When clinical or biochemical improvement occurs, the patient can often be maintained at a dose of 50 IU/day or at 50 to 100 IU 3 times/week. A dose of 100 IU/day should be continued in more severe cases. Benefits of long-term calcitonin therapy generally persist for weeks or months after drug withdrawal, usually followed by return to the pretreatment status.

The possibility of substantial antibody formation should be investigated. Although specialized tests for antibody titer are not widely available, the following test will detect titers that interfere with the action of calcitonin.

After overnight fasting, a sample of the patient's blood is taken for determination of serum calcium and 100 IU of salmon calcitonin are injected i.m. The patient is then permitted to eat his usual breakfast. At 3 and 6 hours post-injection, additional blood samples are drawn. The serum calcium values are then compared. A decrease of 0.5 mg% or more from the fasting level at 3 and 6 hours is usually seen in the responsive patient. Decreases of 0.3 mg% or less constitute an inadequate response to calcitonin in the patient with active Paget's disease. If the hypocalcemic action of calcitonin is lost, further therapy with salmon calcitonin will not be effective. In these cases, patient compliance should also be assessed in the event of relapse.

Hypercalcemia: For the management of hypercalcemia, the recommended initial dosage is 4 IU/kg every 12 hours by s.c. or i.m. injection. If the response to this dosage is not satisfactory after 1 to 2 days, dosage may be increased up to 8 IU/kg every 12 hours. If there is no satisfactory improvement after another 2 days, dosage may be increased to a maximum of 8 IU/kg every 6 hours.

Administration: Calcitonin salmon may be administered s.c. or i.m. Prior to initiation of salmon calcitonin therapy, a skin test using calcitonin salmon should be performed (see Precautions). When the injection volume exceeds 2 mL, the i.m. route is preferable and multiple sites of injection should be used. The s.c. route of administration is preferred for self-administration. Patients and/or other individuals who are administering calcitonin salmon should be carefully instructed about proper techniques including aseptic precautions. Because treatment with salmon calcitonin is usually prolonged, injection sites should be alternated.

INFORMATION FOR THE PATIENT: Published in e-CPS, available by subscription at www.e-cps.ca.

SUPPLIED: Each mL contains: synthetic salcatonin (BP) 100 IU, sodium acetate 0.489 mg, sodium chloride 0.067 mg, acetic acid and sodium hydroxide to adjust toxicity and pH. pH: 3.9 to 4.5. Prescored glass ampuls of 100 IU (1 mL). Store at refrigerator temperature (2 to 8°C).

Caltrate®
calcium carbonate
Calcium Supplement

Pfizer Consumer Healthcare

Caltrate® with Vitamin D
calcium carbonate—vitamin D
Calcium Supplement

Pfizer Consumer Healthcare

Caltrate® Plus
calcium carbonate—vitamin D—magnesium—zinc—copper—manganese
Calcium Supplement

Pfizer Consumer Healthcare

Caltrate® Select
calcium carbonate—vitamin D
Calcium Supplement

Pfizer Consumer Healthcare

INDICATIONS: As a dietary supplement where calcium intake may be inadequate: during childhood, adolescence, pregnancy, lactation, and in postmenopausal women and the aged.

In the treatment of calcium deficiency states which may occur in diseases such as hypoparathyroidism (acute and chronic); pseudohypoparathyroidism, postmenopausal and senile osteoporosis, rickets and osteomalacia.

CONTRAINDICATIONS: Hypercalcemia and hypercalciuria (e.g., hyperparathyroidism, vitamin D overdosage, decalcifying tumors such as plasmocytoma; bone metastases); severe renal disease; and in calcium loss due to immobilization.

PRECAUTIONS: In mild hypercalciuria (exceeding 300 mg/24 hours) as well as in chronic renal failure, or where there is evidence of stone formation in the urinary tract, adequate checks must be kept on urinary calcium excretion. If necessary, dosage should be reduced or calcium therapy discontinued.

High vitamin D intake should be avoided during calcium therapy unless especially indicated.

Certain dietary substances interfere with the absorption of calcium. These include oxalic acid (found in large quantities in rhubarb and spinach), phytic acid (bran and whole cereals) and phosphorus.

Administration of corticosteroids may interfere with calcium absorption.

Calcium compounds reduce blood concentrations of oral tetracyclines. Concomitant use should be avoided or doses of the drugs should not be taken within 3 hours of each other.

Caltrate Plus contains 20 µg of vitamin K. The Adequate Intake (AI) for vitamin K is 90 µg and 120 µg for women and men, respectively. Higher levels than the AI have the potential to interact with anticoagulant therapy.

Do not exceed the recommended daily dose.

Keep out of reach of children.

ADVERSE EFFECTS: Occasional constipation may occur with high calcium carbonate intake.

Abdominal distension, abdominal pain, diarrhea and vomiting may occur when taking calcium carbonate supplements.

OVERDOSE:

In case of accidental overdose, contact a physician or poison control centre immediately, even if there are no symptoms.

> For management of a suspected drug overdose, CPhA recommends that you contact your **regional Poison Control Centre**. See the *CPS* Directory section for a list of Poison Control Centres.

DOSAGE: 1 or 2 tablets a day at mealtime or as recommended by a physician.

Caltrate with Vitamin D Soft Chews: Children (6 to under 12 years) one chew daily at mealtime. Adults (12 years and over) one or two chews daily at mealtime or as recommended by a physician.

Take a few hours before or after taking other medications.

SUPPLIED: Caltrate: Each white, oval, scored, film-coated tablet, engraved "600 g" and "Caltrate", contains: calcium carbonate USP 1500 mg providing 600 mg (30 mEq) elemental calcium. Nonmedicinal ingredients: cornstarch, croscarmellose sodium, hypromellose, magnesium stearate, polysorbate 80, titanium dioxide and triacetin. Energy: <4.2 kJ (1 kcal). Gelatin- and sugar-free. Bottles of 60. All Caltrate products are bisulfite-, gluten-, lactose-, potassium-, preservative- and tartrazine-free. Suitable for sodium restricted diets. Store at controlled room temperature 15 to 30°C.

Caltrate with Vitamin D: Tablets: Each light tan, oval, scored, film-coated tablet, engraved "Caltrate" and "D600", contains: calcium carbonate USP 1500 mg providing 600 mg (30 mEq) elemental calcium and vitamin D_3 (cholecalciferol) 5 µg/200 IU. Nonmedicinal ingredients: acacia, alpha tocopherol, cornstarch, croscarmellose sodium, FD&C yellow No. 6, hypromellose, magnesium stearate, medium chain triglycerides, polysorbate 80, sucrose, titanium dioxide, triacetin and tricalcium phosphate. Energy: <4.2 kJ (1 kcal). Gelatin-free. Bottles of 60 and 120. All Caltrate products are bisulfite-, gluten-, lactose-, potassium-, preservative- and tartrazine-free. Suitable for sodium restricted diets. Store at controlled room temperature 15 to 30°C.

Vanilla Soft Chews: Each vanilla flavoured (cream colour) square chew contains: calcium carbonate 1500 mg providing 600 mg (30 mEq) elemental calcium and vitamin D_3 (cholecalciferol) 10 µg/400 IU. Nonmedicinal ingredients: acacia gum, gelatin, liquid glucose, palm oil, sucrose and vanilla flavour. Energy: <37.7 kJ (9 kcal). Packages of 60. All Caltrate products are bisulfite-, gluten-, lactose-, potassium-, preservative- and tartrazine-free. Suitable for sodium restricted diets. Store at controlled room temperature 15 to 30°C.

Chocolate Soft Chews: Each chocolate flavoured (mocha colour) square chew contains: calcium carbonate 1500 mg providing 600 mg (30 mEq) elemental calcium and vitamin D_3 (cholecalciferol) 10 µg/400 IU. Nonmedicinal ingredients: acacia gum, chocolate flavour, cocoa, gelatin, liquid glucose, palm oil and sucrose. Energy: <37.7 kJ (9 kcal). Packages of 60. All Caltrate products are bisulfite-, gluten-, lactose-, potassium-, preservative- and tartrazine-free. Suitable for sodium restricted diets. Store at controlled room temperature 15 to 30°C.

Strawberry Soft Chews: Each strawberry flavoured (pink colour) square chew contains: calcium carbonate 1500 mg providing 600 mg (30 mEq) elemental calcium and vitamin D_3 (cholecalciferol) 10 µg/400 IU. Nonmedicinal ingredients: acacia gum, FD&C red No. 40, gelatin, liquid glucose, palm oil, strawberry and vanilla flavours and sucrose. Energy: <37.7 kJ (9 kcal). Packages of 60. All Caltrate products are bisulfite-, gluten-, lactose-, potassium-, preservative- and tartrazine-free. Suitable for sodium restricted diets. Store at controlled room temperature 15 to 30°C.

Caltrate Plus: Chewables: Each pale, purple, scored, flat/round chewable tablet, engraved "Caltrate" and "U 3", contains: calcium carbonate USP 1500 mg providing 600 mg (30 mEq) elemental calcium, vitamin D_3 (cholecalciferol) 10 µg/400 IU, vitamin K_1 20 µg, magnesium (as oxide) 50 mg, zinc (as oxide) 7.5 mg, copper (as oxide) 1 mg and manganese (as sulfate) 1.8 mg. Nonmedicinal ingredients: acacia gum, aspartame (phenylalanine), cornstarch, crospovidone, FD&C blue No. 2 and red No. 40, flavours, gelatin, magnesium stearate, mannitol, medium chain triglycerides, modified food starch, natural and artificial flavour, palm oil, silicon dioxide, sodium ascorbate, sorbitol, stearic acid, sucrose and vitamin E. Energy: <4.2 kJ (1 kcal). Bottles of 50. All Caltrate products are bisulfite-, gluten-, lactose-, potassium-, preservative- and tartrazine-free. Suitable for sodium restricted diets. Store at controlled room temperature 15 to 30°C.

Tablets: Each light tan, oval, scored, film-coated tablet, engraved "Caltrate" and "+400", contains: calcium carbonate USP 1500 mg providing 600 mg (30 mEq) elemental calcium, vitamin D_3 (cholecalciferol) 10 µg/400 IU, vitamin K_1 20 µg, magnesium (as oxide) 50 mg, zinc (as oxide) 7.5 mg, copper (as oxide) 1 mg and manganese (as sulfate) 1.8 mg. Nonmedicinal ingredients: acacia gum, cornstarch, croscarmellose sodium, FD&C blue No. 1, FD&C red No. 40, FD&C yellow No. 6, glucose, hypromellose, magnesium stearate, mannitol, medium chain triglycerides, microcrystalline cellulose, modified food starch, polysorbate 80, sucrose, titanium dioxide, triacetin, tricalcium phosphate and vitamin E. Energy: <4.2 kJ (1 kcal). Gelatin-free. Bottles of 60 and 120. All Caltrate products are bisulfite-, gluten-, lactose-, potassium-, preservative- and tartrazine-free. Suitable for sodium restricted diets. Store at controlled room temperature 15 to 30°C.

Caltrate Select: Each beige, oval, scored, film-coated tablet, engraved "Caltrate" and "S400" contains: calcium carbonate USP 1500 mg providing 600 mg (30 mEq) elemental calcium and vitamin D_3 (cholecalciferol) 10 µg/400 IU. Nonmedicinal ingredients: acacia, alpha tocopherol, cornstarch, croscarmellose sodium, FD&C yellow No. 6, magnesium stearate, medium chain triglycerides, polyethylene glycol, polyvinyl alcohol, sucrose, talc, titanium dioxide and tricalcium phosphate. Energy: <4.2 kJ (1 kcal). Gelatin-free. Bottles of 50. All Caltrate products are bisulfite-, gluten-, lactose-, potassium-, preservative- and tartrazine-free. Suitable for sodium restricted diets. Store at controlled room temperature 15 to 30°C.

Campral® Ⓟ
acamprosate calcium
Alcohol Abstinence Aid

Mylan

Date of Preparation: March 14, 2007

SUMMARY PRODUCT INFORMATION:

Route of Administration	Dosage Form/ Strength	Clinically Relevant Nonmedicinal Ingredients
Oral	Tablet/333 mg	No known clinically relevant nonmedicinal ingredients. For a complete listing see Dosage Forms, Composition and Packaging.

INDICATIONS AND CLINICAL USE: Adults: CAMPRAL (acamprosate calcium) is indicated for the maintenance of abstinence from alcohol in patients with alcohol dependence who are abstinent at treatment initiation. Treatment with CAMPRAL should be part of a comprehensive management program that includes counselling.

The efficacy of CAMPRAL in promoting abstinence has not been demonstrated in subjects who have not undergone detoxification and not achieved alcohol abstinence prior to beginning CAMPRAL treatment. The efficacy of CAMPRAL in promoting abstinence from alcohol in polysubstance abusers has not been adequately assessed.

Geriatrics (>65 years of age): Forty-one of the 4234 patients in double-blind, placebo-controlled, clinical trials of CAMPRAL were 65 years of age or older. There were too few patients in this age group to evaluate any differences in safety or efficacy in geriatric patients compared to younger patients. However, since renal function diminishes in elderly patients and acamprosate is excreted unchanged in urine, acamprosate plasma concentrations are likely to be higher in the elderly population compared to younger adults. (See Warnings and Precautions, Special Populations, Geriatrics (>65 years of age).)

Pediatrics (<18 years of age): The safety and efficacy of CAMPRAL have not been established in the pediatric population.

CONTRAINDICATIONS:

- Patients who are hypersensitive to this drug or to any ingredient in the formulation or component of the container. For a complete listing, see Dosage Forms, Composition and Packaging.
- Patients with severe renal impairment (creatinine clearance ≤30 mL/min).
- In nursing women.

WARNINGS AND PRECAUTIONS: General: CAMPRAL treatment should only be initiated after detoxification or weaning therapy, once the patient is abstinent from alcohol.

CAMPRAL does not constitute treatment for the withdrawal period.

CAMPRAL does not prevent the harmful effects of continuous alcohol abuse.

Renal: No dose adjustment is recommended in patients with mild renal impairment (creatinine clearance of 80-50 mL/min). Treatment with CAMPRAL in patients with moderate renal impairment (creatinine clearance of 30-50 mL/min) requires a reduction of the dose (see Dosage and Administration). Patients with severe renal impairment (creatinine clearance of ≤30 mL/min) should not be given CAMPRAL (see Contraindications).

Dependence/Tolerance: CAMPRAL did not produce any evidence of withdrawal symptoms in patients in clinical trials at therapeutic doses. Post marketing data, retrospectively collected, provided no evidence of drug abuse or dependence.

Driving and Operating Machinery: Although in controlled studies CAMPRAL has not been shown to impair psychomotor coordination, any psychoactive drug may impair judgment, thinking, or motor skills. Patients should be cautioned about operating hazardous machinery, including automobiles, until they are reasonably certain that CAMPRAL therapy does not affect their ability to engage in such activities.

Psychiatric: Suicidality: In controlled clinical trials of acamprosate, adverse events of a suicidal nature (suicidal ideation, suicide attempts, completed suicides) were infrequent overall, but were more common in acamprosate-treated patients than in patients treated with placebo (1.4% vs. 0.5% in studies of 6 months or less; 2.4% vs. 0.8% in year-long studies). Completed suicides occurred in 3 of 2272 (0.13%) patients in the pooled acamprosate group from all controlled studies and 2 of 1962 patients (0.10%) in the placebo group. Adverse events coded as "depression" were reported at similar rates in acamprosate-treated and placebo-treated patients. Because the interrelationship between alcohol dependence, depression and suicidality is well-recognized and complex, rigorous clinical monitoring is recommended in alcohol-dependent patients, including those treated with acamprosate.

Special Populations: Pregnant Women and Women of Child-bearing Potential: The safety of this product for use in human pregnancy has not been established. Acamprosate may be used during pregnancy only after a careful benefit/risk assessment, when the patient cannot abstain from drinking alcohol without being treated with acamprosate and when there is consequently a risk of foetotoxicity or teratogenicity due to alcohol.

Acamprosate calcium has been shown to be teratogenic in rats when given in doses that are approximately equal to the human dose (on a mg/m² basis) and in Burgundy Tawny rabbits when given in doses that were approximately 3 times the human dose (on a mg/m² basis). No developmental effects were observed in New Zealand white rabbits at doses up to approximately 8 times the human dose (on a mg/m² basis).

The findings in animals should be considered in relation to known adverse developmental effects of ethyl alcohol, which include the characteristics of foetal alcohol syndrome (craniofacial dysmorphism, intrauterine and postnatal growth retardation, retarded psychomotor and intellectual development) and milder forms of neurological and behavioural disorders in humans).

Nursing Women: In animal studies, acamprosate calcium was excreted in the milk of lactating rats dosed orally with acamprosate calcium. It is not known whether acamprosate calcium is excreted in human milk, therefore, CAMPRAL is contraindicated for use in nursing mothers (see Contraindications).

Pediatrics (18 years of age): The safety and efficacy of CAMPRAL have not been established in the pediatric population, therefore, acamprosate is not recommended for use in patients under 18 years of age.

Geriatrics (>65 years of age): The safety and efficacy of acamprosate have not been established in patients older than 65 years of age. CAMPRAL is excreted unchanged in the urine, and the elderly are more likely to have decreased renal function. Therefore, care should be taken in dose selection. (See Dosage and Administration.)

Hepatic: No dose adjustment is needed in patients with mild to moderate liver impairment (Child-Pugh A and B). No pharmacokinetic study has been done in the severely liver impaired patients (Child-Pugh C), however, physicians should carefully consider the potential risks and benefits of using acamprosate, when the patient cannot abstain from drinking alcohol without being treated with acamprosate.

ADVERSE REACTIONS: Adverse Drug Reaction Overview: Adverse events associated with CAMPRAL tend to be mild and transient in nature. They are predominantly gastrointestinal or dermatological in nature.

Diarrhoea, and less frequently, vomiting and abdominal pain are the gastrointestinal adverse reaction. Pruritus is the predominant dermatological adverse reaction. An occasional maculopapular rash and rare cases of bullous skin reactions have been reported.

Clinical Trial Adverse Drug Reactions: Adverse Events Leading to Discontinuation: For studies where adverse events were reported either by worksheet or spontaneously, among the 1749 alcohol dependent patients who received CAMPRAL 1998/2000 mg/day in placebo-controlled trials, 8% discontinued treatment due to an adverse event, as compared to 6% of 1962 patients receiving placebo. Among patients receiving CAMPRAL 1998/2000 mg/day in studies collecting spontaneous adverse events, only diarrhea was associated with the discontinuation of more than 1% of patients. Diarrhea occurred at a higher rate among patients taking CAMPRAL (2%) versus patients taking placebo (<1%).

Common Adverse Events Reported in Controlled Trials: Common, non-serious adverse events were collected spontaneously in some controlled studies and using a checklist in other studies. The overall profile of adverse events was similar using either method. Table 1 shows those events that occurred in any CAMPRAL treatment group at a rate of 3% or greater and greater than the placebo group in controlled clinical trials with spontaneously reported adverse events. The reported frequencies of adverse events represent the proportion of individuals who experienced, at least once, a treatment-emergent adverse event of the type listed, without regard to the causal relationship of the events to the drug.

Table 1: CAMPRAL

Events Occurring at a Rate of at Least 3% and Greater than Placebo in any CAMPRAL Treatment Group in Controlled Clinical Trials with Spontaneously Reported Adverse Events

Body System/Preferred Term	Number of Patients (%) with Events			
	CAMPRAL[a] 1332 mg/day	CAMPRAL[a] 1998 mg/day[c]	CAMPRAL[a] Pooled[d]	Placebo
Number of Patients in Treatment Group	397	1539	2019	1706
Number (%) of patients with an AE	248 (62%)	910 (59%)	1231 (61%)	955 (56%)
Body as a Whole	**121 (30%)**	**513 (33%)**	**685 (34%)**	**517 (30%)**
Accidental Injury[a]	17 (4%)	44 (3%)	70 (3%)	52 (3%)
Asthenia	29 (7%)	79 (5%)	114 (6%)	93 (5%)
Pain	6 (2%)	56 (4%)	65 (3%)	55 (3%)
Digestive System	**85 (21%)**	**440 (29%)**	**574 (28%)**	**344 (20%)**
Anorexia	20 (5%)	35 (2%)	57 (3%)	44 (3%)
Diarrhea	39 (10%)	257 (17%)	329 (16%)	166 (10%)
Flatulence	4 (1%)	55 (4%)	63 (3%)	28 (2%)
Nausea	11 (3%)	69 (4%)	87 (4%)	58 (3%)
Nervous System	**150 (38%)**	**417 (27%)**	**598 (30%)**	**500 (29%)**
Anxiety[b]	32 (8%)	80 (5%)	118 (6%)	98 (6%)
Depression	33 (8%)	63 (4%)	102 (5%)	87 (5%)
Dizziness	15 (4%)	49 (3%)	67 (3%)	44 (3%)
Dry Mouth	13 (3%)	23 (1%)	36 (2%)	28 (2%)
Insomnia	34 (9%)	94 (6%)	137 (7%)	121 (7%)
Paresthesia	11 (3%)	29 (2%)	40 (2%)	34 (2%)
Skin and Appendages	**26 (7%)**	**150 (10%)**	**187 (9%)**	**169 (10%)**
Pruritus	12 (3%)	68 (4%)	82 (4%)	58 (3%)

(cont'd)

Table 1: CAMPRAL *(cont'd)*

Events Occurring at a Rate of at Least 3% and Greater than Placebo in any CAMPRAL Treatment Group in Controlled Clinical Trials with Spontaneously Reported Adverse Events

Body System/Preferred Term	Number of Patients (%) with Events			
	CAMPRAL[a] 1332 mg/day	CAMPRAL[a] 1998 mg/day[c]	CAMPRAL[a] Pooled[d]	Placebo
Sweating	11 (3%)	27 (2%)	40 (2%)	39 (2%)

[a] Includes events coded as "fracture" by sponsor.
[b] Includes events coded as "nervousness" by sponsor.
[c] Includes 258 patients treated with acamprosate calcium 2000 mg/day, using a different dosage strength and regimen.
[d] Includes all patients in the first two columns as well as 83 patients treated with acamprosate calcium 3000 mg/day, using a different dosage strength and regimen.

Other Events Observed During the Pre-marketing Evaluation of CAMPRAL: Following is a list of terms that reflect treatment-emergent adverse events reported by patients treated with CAMPRAL in 20 clinical trials (4461 patients treated with CAMPRAL, 3526 of whom received the maximum recommended dose of 1998 mg/day for up to one year in duration). This listing does not include those events already listed above; events for which a drug cause was considered remote; event terms which were so general as to be uninformative; and events reported only once which were not likely to be acutely life-threatening.

Events are further categorized by body system and listed in order of decreasing frequency according to the following definitions: frequent adverse events are those occurring in at least 1/100 patients (only those not already listed in the summary of adverse events in controlled trials appear in this listing); infrequent adverse events are those occurring in 1/100 to 1/1000 patients; rare events are those occurring in fewer than 1/1000 patients.

Body as a Whole: Frequent: headache, abdominal pain, back pain, infection, flu syndrome, chest pain, chills, suicide attempt; Infrequent: fever, intentional overdose, malaise, allergic reaction, abscess, neck pain, hernia, intentional injury; Rare: ascites, face edema, photosensitivity reaction, abdomen enlarged, sudden death.

Cardiovascular System : Frequent: palpitation, syncope; Infrequent: hypotension, tachycardia, hemorrhage, angina pectoris, migraine, varicose vein, myocardial infarct, phlebitis, postural hypotension; Rare: heart failure, mesenteric arterial occlusion, cardiomyopathy, deep thrombophlebitis, shock.

Digestive System : Frequent: vomiting, dyspepsia, constipation, increased appetite; Infrequent: liver function tests abnormal, gastroenteritis, gastritis, dysphagia, eructation, gastrointestinal hemorrhage, pancreatitis, rectal hemorrhage, liver cirrhosis, esophagitis, hematemesis, nausea and vomiting, hepatitis; Rare: melena, stomach ulcer, cholecystitis, colitis, duodenal ulcer, mouth ulceration, carcinoma of liver.

Endocrine System: Rare: goiter, hypothyroidism.

Hemic and Lymphatic System: Infrequent: anemia, ecchymosis, eosinophilia, lymphocytosis, thrombocytopenia; Rare: leukopenia, lymphadenopathy, monocytosis.

Metabolic and Nutritional Disorders: Frequent: peripheral edema, weight gain; Infrequent: weight loss, hyperglycemia, AST increased, ALT increased, gout, thirst, hyperuricemia, diabetes mellitus, avitaminosis, bilirubinemia; Rare: alkaline phosphatase increased, creatinine increased, hyponatremia, lactic dehydrogenase increased.

Musculoskeletal System: Frequent: myalgia, arthralgia; Infrequent: leg cramps; Rare: rheumatoid arthritis, myopathy.

Nervous System: Frequent: somnolence, libido decreased, amnesia, thinking abnormal, tremor, vasodilatation, hypertension; Infrequent: convulsion, confusion, libido increased, vertigo, withdrawal syndrome, apathy, suicidal ideation, neuralgia, hostility, agitation, neurosis, abnormal dreams, hallucinations, hypesthesia; Rare: alcohol craving, psychosis, hyperkinesia, twitching, depersonalization, increased salivation, paranoid reaction, torticollis, encephalopathy, manic reaction.

Respiratory System: Frequent: rhinitis, cough increased, dyspnea, pharyngitis, bronchitis; Infrequent: asthma, epistaxis, pneumonia; Rare: laryngismus, pulmonary embolus.

Skin and Appendages: Frequent: rash; Infrequent: acne, eczema, alopecia, maculopapular rash, dry skin, urticaria, exfoliative dermatitis, vesiculobullous rash; Rare: psoriasis.

Special Senses: Frequent: abnormal vision, taste perversion; Infrequent: tinnitus, amblyopia, deafness; Rare: ophthalmitis, diplopia, photophobia.

Urogenital System: Frequent: impotence; Infrequent: metrorrhagia, urinary frequency, urinary tract infection, sexual function abnormal, urinary incontinence, vaginitis; Rare: kidney calculus, abnormal ejaculation, hematuria, menorrhagia, nocturia, polyuria, urinary urgency.

Abnormal Hematologic and Clinical Chemistry Findings: Overall, there was no evidence of any negative effect of acamprosate calcium on hematologic or clinical chemistry parameters during the course of clinical trials in alcohol-dependent patients of up to one year in duration.

Post-Market Adverse Drug Reactions: It is estimated that more than 1.6 million alcohol-dependent patients have been treated with CAMPRAL since market introduction. Although no causal relationship to CAMPRAL has been found, the following serious adverse events have been reported to be temporally associated with CAMPRAL treatment in at least 3 patients and are not described elsewhere in the monograph: acute kidney failure.

DRUG INTERACTIONS: Overview: Acamprosate calcium had no inducing potential on the cytochrome CYP1A2 and 3A4 systems, and in vitro enzyme inhibition studies suggest that acamprosate calcium does not inhibit in vivo metabolism mediated by cytochrome CYP1A2, 2C9, 2C19, 2D6, 2E1, or 3A4.

Drug-Drug Interactions: The pharmacokinetics of acamprosate calcium were unaffected when co-administered with alcohol, disulfiram or diazepam. Similarly, the pharmacokinetics of ethanol, diazepam and nordiazepam, imipramine and desipramine, naltrexone and 6-beta naltrexol were unaffected following co-administration with acamprosate calcium. However, co-administration of CAMPRAL with naltrexone led to a 33% increase in the C_{max} and a 25% increase in the AUC of acamprosate calcium. No adjustment of dosage is recommended in such patients.

An open-label study in patients receiving febarbamate, difebarbamate, phenobarbital, meprobamate, or oxazepam, showed that acamprosate calcium could be initiated safely during the acute detoxification phase with these medications.

Other concomitant therapies: In clinical trials, CAMPRAL has been safely administered in combination with antidepressants, anxiolytics, hypnotics and sedatives, and non-opioid analgesics.

Drug-Food Interactions: Administration of CAMPRAL with food diminishes its bioavailability compared with administration of the drug in the fasting state. Although dosing may be done without regard to a meal, dosing with meals was employed during clinical trials and is suggested as an aid to compliance in those patients who regularly eat three meals daily.

Drug-Herb Interactions: Interactions with herbal products have not been established.

Drug-Laboratory Test Interactions: In clinical studies, CAMPRAL had no detrimental effects on standard laboratory tests, including tests that evaluated hepatic and renal function.

Drug-Lifestyle Interactions: The concomitant intake of alcohol and CAMPRAL does not affect the pharmacokinetics of either alcohol or CAMPRAL.

DOSAGE AND ADMINISTRATION: Dosing Considerations: Placebo controlled studies demonstrated the efficacy of CAMPRAL as an adjunct to counselling. Treatment with CAMPRAL should be part of a comprehensive management program that includes counselling.

Renal impairment (see Recommended Dose and Dosage Adjustment).

In some patients, daily dose could be lowered temporarily for tolerability reasons.

The recommended treatment duration is 1 year.

Adults: Recommended Dose and Dosage Adjustment: The recommended dose of CAMPRAL is two 333 mg tablets taken three times daily. Treatment with CAMPRAL should be initiated as soon as possible after detoxification and should be maintained if the patient relapses. Re-detoxification may be required according to clinical judgement.

Dosage in Renal Impairment: No dose adjustment is recommended in patients with mild renal impairment (creatinine clearance of 80-50 mL/min). For patients with moderate renal impairment (creatinine clearance of 30-50 mL/min), a dose of one 333 mg tablet taken three times daily is recommended. Patients with severe renal impairment (creatinine clearance of ≤30 mL/min) should not be given CAMPRAL (see Contraindications).

Missed Dose: Double doses of CAMPRAL tablets should not be taken. If a dose is missed or the patient does not remember whether the dose was taken, he/she should be instructed to take the next dose at the scheduled time.

Administration: CAMPRAL tablets are enteric coated and should be swallowed whole, not split or crushed or chewed. Although dosing may be done without regard to a meal, dosing with meals was employed during clinical trials and is suggested as an aid to compliance in those patients who regularly eat three meals daily.

OVERDOSAGE:
In all reported cases of acute overdosage with CAMPRAL (total reported doses of up to 56 g of acamprosate calcium), the main symptom was diarrhea. No case of hypercalcaemia has ever been reported. A risk of hypercalcemia may be considered in chronic overdosage. Treatment of overdose should be symptomatic and supportive.

For management of a suspected drug overdose, CPhA recommends that you contact your **regional Poison Control Centre**. See the *CPS* Directory section for a list of Poison Control Centres.

ACTION AND CLINICAL PHARMACOLOGY: Mechanism of Action: Acamprosate calcium is a synthetic compound which dissociates into two molecules of acetylhomotaurine and one calcium ion. Acetylhomotaurine has a chemical structure similar to that of the endogenous amino acid homotaurine, which is a structural analogue of the amino acid neurotransmitter γ-aminobutyric acid and the amino acid neuromodulator taurine. Acetylation of its amine function facilitates passage of acetylhomotaurine through the blood brain barrier. Acamprosate calcium modulates glutamatergic and GABAergic neurotransmission and modifies neuronal excitability.

The mechanism of action of acamprosate calcium in maintenance of alcohol abstinence is not completely understood. In animal studies, acamprosate calcium acts centrally and appears to restore the normal balance between neuronal excitation and inhibition that becomes altered as a result of chronic alcohol exposure.

Pharmacodynamics: Acamprosate calcium has negligible CNS activity outside of its effects on alcohol dependence, exhibiting no anticonvulsant, antidepressant, or anxiolytic activity in animals or effects on psychometric tests in healthy volunteers.

The administration of CAMPRAL is not associated with the development of tolerance or dependence in animal studies, nor would it be expected to precipitate withdrawal symptoms in patients physically dependent on opioids, by virtue of its mechanism of action.

CAMPRAL is not alcohol aversive therapy and does not cause a disulfiram-like reaction as a result of ethanol ingestion.

Pharmacokinetics: Pharmacokinetic studies of acamprosate were based on acetylhomotaurine determination in urine and plasma.

Absorption: The absolute bioavailability of CAMPRAL after oral administration is about 11%. Steady-state plasma concentrations of acamprosate calcium are reached within 5 days of dosing. Steady-state peak plasma concentrations after CAMPRAL doses of 2×333 mg tablets TID average 350 ng/mL and occur at 3-8 hours post-dose. Coadministration of CAMPRAL with food decreases bioavailability by 20% compared with its administration in the fasting state. This decrease is not clinically significant and no adjustment of dose is necessary.

Distribution: The volume of distribution for acamprosate calcium following intravenous administration of acamprosate is estimated to be 72-109 liters (approximately 1 L/kg), and the volume of distribution at steady-state is estimated to be 24 liters. The binding of acamprosate to plasma proteins is negligible.

Metabolism: Acamprosate calcium does not undergo metabolism following oral and intravenous administration.

Excretion: After oral dosing of 2×333 mg of CAMPRAL, the terminal half-life of acamprosate was about 20-33 hours. Following oral administration of ^{14}C-acamprosate calcium, urinary excretion accounted for 11% of the administered dose, i.e. 100% of the absorbed drug, while fecal excretion accounted for the remainder.

Special Populations and Conditions: Pediatrics: The pharmacokinetics of CAMPRAL have not been evaluated in a pediatric population.

Geriatrics: The pharmacokinetics of CAMPRAL have not been evaluated in a geriatric population. However, since renal function diminishes in elderly patients and acamprosate is excreted unchanged in urine, its plasma concentrations are likely to be higher in the elderly population compared with younger adults.

Gender: CAMPRAL does not exhibit any significant pharmacokinetic differences between male and female subjects.

Race: No specific study of CAMPRAL pharmacokinetics in various racial groups has been performed.

Hepatic Insufficiency: Acamprosate calcium is not metabolized by the liver and the pharmacokinetics of acamprosate calcium are not altered in patients with mild to moderate hepatic impairment (groups A and B of the Child-Pugh classification). No adjustment of dosage is recommended in such patients.

No pharmacokinetic study has been done in the severely liver impaired patients (Child-Pugh C), however, physician should carefully consider the potential risks and benefits of using acamprosate, when the patient cannot abstain from drinking alcohol without being treated with acamprosate.

Renal Insufficiency: Peak plasma concentrations of acamprosate after administration of a single dose of 2×333 mg CAMPRAL tablets to patients with moderate or severe renal impairment were about 2-fold and 4-fold higher, respectively, compared to healthy subjects. Similarly, elimination half-life of acamprosate was about 1.8-fold and 2.6-fold longer, respectively, compared to healthy subjects. There is a linear relationship between creatinine clearance values and total apparent plasma clearance, renal clearance and plasma half-life of acamprosate calcium.

No dose adjustment is recommended in patients with mild renal impairment (creatinine clearance of 80-50 mL/min).

A dose of 1×333 mg TID is recommended in patients with moderate renal impairment (creatinine clearance of 30-50 mL/min, see Warnings and Precautions, Renal).

Patients with severe renal impairment (creatinine clearance ≤30 mL/min) must not be given CAMPRAL (see Contraindications).

Alcohol-Dependent Subjects: Cross-study comparison of CAMPRAL at doses of 2×333 mg TID indicated similar pharmacokinetics between alcohol-dependent subjects and healthy subjects.

STORAGE AND STABILITY: Store at controlled room temperature (15-30°C).

Others: Keep in a safe place out of the reach of children.

INFORMATION FOR THE PATIENT: Published in e-CPS, available by subscription at www.e-cps.ca.

DOSAGE FORMS, COMPOSITION AND PACKAGING: Each delayed-release, enteric-coated, white, round-shaped tablet with "333" on one side, contains: acamprosate calcium 333 mg. Nonmedicinal ingredients: anionic copolymer of methacrylic acid and acrylic acid ethyl ester, colloidal anhydrous silica, crospovidone, magnesium silicate, magnesium stearate, microcrystalline cellulose, propylene glycol, sodium starch glycolate and talc. Boxes of 84 (12×7 blisters).

(Shown in Product Identification Section)

Camptosar® Ⓟ
irinotecan HCl trihydrate
Antineoplastic

Pfizer

Date of Revision: June 29, 2009

SUMMARY PRODUCT INFORMATION:

Route of Administration	Dosage Form/ Strength	Clinically Relevant Nonmedicinal Ingredients
Intravenous	Solution/20 mg/mL	Sorbitol For a complete listing see Dosage Forms, Composition and Packaging.

INDICATIONS AND CLINICAL USE: CAMPTOSAR (irinotecan hydrochloride trihydrate) is indicated as a component of first-line therapy for patients with metastatic carcinoma of the colon or rectum.

CAMPTOSAR is also indicated as a single agent for the treatment of patients with metastatic carcinoma of the colon or rectum whose disease has recurred or progressed following 5-fluorouracil-based therapy.

CAMPTOSAR should be administered only under the supervision of a physician who is experienced in the use of cancer chemotherapeutic agents. Appropriate management of complications is possible only when adequate diagnostic and treatment facilities are readily available.

Geriatrics: Evidence from clinical and pharmacokinetic studies suggests that patients 65 years of age or older should be closely monitored because of a greater risk of late diarrhea in this population. Specific dosing recommendations may apply to this population depending upon the regimen used (see Warnings and Precautions, General, Geriatrics and Dosage and Administration).

Pediatrics: The safety and effectiveness of CAMPTOSAR in the pediatric population have not been established (see Warnings and Precautions).

CONTRAINDICATIONS: CAMPTOSAR (irinotecan hydrochloride trihydrate) is contraindicated in patients who are hypersensitive to this drug or to any ingredient in the formulation or component of the container. For a complete listing, see Dosage Forms, Composition and Packaging.

Co-administration of CAMPTOSAR with azole antifungals (ketoconazole, fluconazole, itraconazole), known CYP3A4 inhibitors, is contraindicated because this can lead to an increase in the relative exposure to the active metabolite SN-38 and can therefore possibly lead to increased toxicity.

In patients receiving concomitant CAMPTOSAR and ketoconazole, exposure to SN-38 was increased by approximately 110%. Patients should discontinue ketoconazole at least 1 week prior to starting irinotecan therapy. See Warnings and Precautions regarding potential drug-drug interactions with other CYP3A4 inhibitors and inducers.

Patients with hereditary fructose intolerance should not be given CAMPTOSAR, as this product contains sorbitol.

WARNINGS AND PRECAUTIONS:

Serious Warnings and Precautions
- CAMPTOSAR (irinotecan hydrochloride trihydrate) should be administered only under the supervision of a physician who is experienced in the use of cancer chemotherapeutic agents.
- Severe early and late forms of diarrhea leading to dehydration and electrolyte imbalance (see Warnings and Precautions and Adverse Reactions, Adverse Drug Reaction Overview).
- Typhlitis, ulcerative and ischemic colitis, ileus and intestinal perforation (see Warnings and Precautions and Adverse Reactions, Post-Market Adverse Drug Reactions).
- Severe myelosuppression with grade 3-4 neutropenia (see Warnings and Precautions and Adverse Reactions, Adverse Drug Reaction Overview).

General: Patients at Particular Risk: Physicians should exercise particular caution in monitoring the effects of CAMPTOSAR in patients with poor performance status. Patients with performance status of 3 or 4 should not receive CAMPTOSAR. In patients receiving either CAMPTOSAR /5-FU/LV or 5-FU/LV in clinical trials comparing these agents, higher rates of hospitalisation, neutropenic fever, thromboembolism, first-cycle treatment discontinuation, and early deaths were observed in patients with a baseline performance status of 2, than in patients with a baseline performance status of 0 or 1. Close monitoring is recommended in patients who have previously received pelvic/abdominal irradiation and in the elderly as these patients may be less tolerant of the toxic effects of the drug. The use of CAMPTOSAR has not been established in patients with significant hepatic dysfunction (see Warnings and Precautions, Hepatic/Biliary/Pancreatic). There are known and suspected drug-drug interactions (see Contraindications, Drug Interactions below, and Drug Interactions).

Drug Interactions: CYP3A4 Inhibitors:
- Co-administration of CAMPTOSAR with azole antifungals (ketoconazole, fluconazole, itraconazole) is contraindicated (see Contraindications).
- Co-administration of CAMPTOSAR with other CYP3A4 inhibitors (e.g., cimetidine, fluoroquinolone antibiotics [ciprofloxacin and norfloxacin in patients with compromised renal function], macrolide antibiotics (azithromycin, clarithromycin, erythromycin), atazanavir sulfate, grapefruit juice, and CYP3A4-inhibitory calcium channel blockers (verapamil, diltiazem, and nifedipine) could lead to an increase in the relative exposure to the active metabolite SN-38 and therefore possibly increased toxicity (see Drug Interactions and Dosage and Administration).

The appropriate starting dose of CAMPTOSAR when co-administered with CYP3A4 inhibitors has not been determined.

CYP3A4 Inducers:
- The co-administration of CAMPTOSAR with CYP3A4 inducers (e.g., St. John's Wort, phenytoin, phenobarbital, carbamazepine, glucocorticoids, rifampin) leads to a reduction in the plasma concentration of the active metabolite SN-38, which could potentially lead to a reduction of efficacy (see Drug Interactions).

The appropriate starting dose of CAMPTOSAR when co-administered with CYP3A4 inducers has not been determined.

Irradiation Therapy: The concurrent administration of CAMPTOSAR with irradiation is not recommended.

Extravasation: CAMPTOSAR is administered by intravenous infusion. Care should be taken to avoid extravasation. The infusion site should be monitored for signs of inflammation or other adverse effects. If extravasation occurs, flushing the site with sterile water and/or applying ice to the area are recommended.

Carcinogenesis and Mutagenesis: Carcinogenicity studies have not been conducted. Rats administered 2 mg/kg or 25 mg/kg irinotecan IV once weekly for 13 weeks and allowed to recover for 91 weeks had a significant linear trend with dose for the incidence of combined uterine horn endometrial stromal polyps and endometrial stromal sarcomas. Irinotecan and SN-38 were not mutagenic in bacterial in vitro assays (Ames assay). Irinotecan was clastogenic both in vitro (chromosome aberrations in Chinese hamster ovary cells) and in vivo (micronucleus test in mice). Therefore, irinotecan may be able to induce chromosomal damage in human spermatozoa. For this reason, males undergoing CAMPTOSAR treatment should discuss effective contraceptive methods with their doctors.

Cardiovascular: All thromboembolic events (includes angina pectoris, arterial thrombosis, cerebral infarct, cerebrovascular accident, deep thrombophlebitis, embolus lower extremity, heart arrest, myocardial infarct, myocardial ischemia, peripheral vascular disorder, pulmonary embolus, sudden death, thrombophlebitis, thrombosis and vascular disorder) when considered together, have been commonly observed in patients receiving CAMPTOSAR. The specific cause of these events has not been determined. See also Adverse Reactions, Clinical Trial Adverse Drug Reactions.

Myocardial ischemic events have been uncommonly observed in patients receiving CAMPTOSAR. In some cases, a causal association with administration of CAMPTOSAR could not be excluded. See Adverse Reactions, Post-Market Adverse Drug Reactions.

Endocrine and Metabolism: Hyperglycemia has been reported in patients receiving CAMPTOSAR. This has usually been observed in patients with a history of diabetes or evidence of glucose intolerance prior to administration of CAMPTOSAR (see also Drug Interactions, Drug-Drug Interactions, Dexamethasone).

Gastrointestinal: Diarrhea: CAMPTOSAR can induce both an early (occurring during or shortly after infusion of CAMPTOSAR) and a late (generally occurring more than 24 hours after CAMPTOSAR administration) form of diarrhea that appear to be mediated by different mechanisms.

Early onset diarrhea is cholinergic in nature. It is usually transient and only infrequently is severe. It may be accompanied by symptoms of rhinitis, increased salivation, miosis, lacrimation, diaphoresis, flushing, and intestinal hyperperistalsis that can cause abdominal cramping. Early diarrhea may be alleviated by the use of atropine. Prophylactic or therapeutic administration of 0.25 to 1 mg of intravenous or subcutaneous atropine should be considered (unless contraindicated) (see Dosage and Administration).

Late onset diarrhea can be prolonged, may lead to dehydration, electrolyte imbalance, or infection, and can be life-threatening. The mechanism of action of late onset diarrhea is unknown. All grade late onset diarrhea occurred in 80% of patients and **late diarrhea should be treated promptly with loperamide**. Patients with diarrhea should be carefully monitored, and given fluid and electrolyte replacement if they become dehydrated. Patients should be given antibiotic support (see Drug Interactions) if they develop ileus, fever, or severe neutropenia. After the first treatment, subsequent chemotherapy should be delayed until patients return to pre-treatment bowel function for at least 24 hours without need for antidiarrhea medication. Patients experiencing clinically significant (grade ≥2) late diarrhea, should have subsequent doses of CAMPTOSAR decreased (see Dosage and Administration).

Management of Late Onset Diarrhea: At the initiation of chemotherapy, patients should be given a sufficient supply of loperamide and instructed on its appropriate use. The prompt use of oral loperamide for controlling and treating the diarrhea is recommended and is higher than the usual dosage recommendation. Pre-treatment with loperamide before the onset of late diarrhea is not recommended. Instead, at the first episode of late-onset diarrhea (ie. poorly formed stools or more frequent bowel movement), patients are to take 4 mg loperamide, followed by 2 mg loperamide every two hours until they are free of diarrhea for at least 12 hours. During the night, the dose of loperamide may be 4 mg administered every 4 hours. Loperamide is not recommended to be used for more than 48 consecutive hours at these doses, because of the risk of paralytic ileus.

Inflammatory Bowel Disease and/or Bowel Obstruction: Cases of colitis complicated by ulceration, bleeding, ileus, and infection have been observed. Cases of ileus without preceding colitis have also been reported. Patients experiencing ileus should receive prompt antibiotic support (see Drug Interactions) and must not be treated with irinotecan until resolution of the bowel obstruction.

Nausea and Vomiting: CAMPTOSAR is emetogenic (see Adverse Reactions). Pre-medication with anti-emetic agents is recommended for patients receiving CAMPTOSAR. In clinical studies with the weekly dosage schedule, this pre-medication has mostly consisted of 10 mg dexamethasone given in conjunction with another type of anti-emetic agent. Anti-emetic agents should be given on the day of treatment, starting at least 30 minutes before administration of CAMPTOSAR. Physicians should also consider providing patients with an anti-emetic regimen for subsequent use as needed.

Hematologic: CAMPTOSAR commonly causes neutropenia, leukopenia, and anemia, any of which may be severe and therefore should not be used in patients with severe bone marrow failure. Therapy with CAMPTOSAR should be temporarily omitted if neutropenic fever occurs or if the absolute neutrophil count drops below $1.5 \times 10^9/L$. After the patient recovers to an absolute neutrophil count ≥1.5×10⁹/L, subsequent doses of CAMPTOSAR should be reduced depending upon the level of neutropenia observed (see Dosage and Administration). Severe neutropenia resulting in deaths due to sepsis have been reported in patients treated with CAMPTOSAR. Neutropenic complications should be managed promptly with antibiotic support (see Drug Interactions). Routine administration of colony stimulating factor is not necessary; however, physicians should consider the use of colony-stimulating factors in patients experiencing clinically significant neutropenia (≥grade 2).

In one study an increased risk of neutropenia was observed in patients homozygous for the UGT1A1*28 allele, who received single-agent CAMPTOSAR at a dose of 350 mg/m². Individuals with certain genetic polymorphisms in the UGT1A1 gene (eg. UGT1A1 *28/*28 genotype) have reduced UGT1A1 activity, which in turn increases the concentration of SN-38, the active metabolite of irinotecan (see Action and Clinical Pharmacology, Pharmacokinetics).

Patients with the UGT1A1*28 allele, treated with combination regimens that deliver doses of CAMPTOSAR in the range of 100-180 mg/m², in combination with 5-FU/LV, the risk of grade 4 neutropenia was lower than in studies where CAMPTOSAR was administered at doses of 300-350 mg/m² as a single agent (see Adverse Reactions, Hematology).

As in the case with all patients, dose modification should be considered based on individual patient tolerance to treatment (see Dosage and Administration).

Hepatic/Biliary/Pancreatic: Increases in serum levels of liver enzymes and bilirubin have been reported in clinical trials and in the post-market period (see Adverse Reactions, Adverse Drug Reaction Overview).

The use of CAMPTOSAR in patients with significant hepatic dysfunction has not been established. CAMPTOSAR was not administered to patients with serum bilirubin >35 µmol/L, or transaminase >3 times the upper limit of normal if no liver metastases, or transaminase >5 times the upper limit of normal with liver metastases (see Dosage and Administration).

In clinical trials of weekly dosage schedule, patients with modestly elevated baseline serum total bilirubin levels (17-35 µmol/L) had a significantly greater likelihood of experiencing first-cycle grade 3 or 4 hematologic toxicities including neutropenia than those with bilirubin levels that were less than 17 µmol/L. Patients with deficient glucuronidation of bilirubin, such as those with Gilbert's syndrome, may also be at greater risk of myelosuppression when receiving therapy with CAMPTOSAR. An association between baseline bilirubin elevations and an increased risk of late diarrhea has not been observed in studies of the weekly dosage schedule (see Dosage and Administration).

Immune: Hypersensitivity reactions including severe anaphylactic or anaphylactoid reactions have been reported (see Adverse Reactions).

Administration of live or live attenuated vaccines in patients immunocompromised by chemotherapeutic agents including irinotecan, may result in serious or fatal infections. Vaccination with a live vaccine should be avoided in patients receiving irinotecan. Killed or inactivated vaccines may be administered; however, the response to such vaccines may be diminished.

Neurologic: Speech Disorders: There have been post-market reports of speech disorders (e.g., dysarthria, stuttering, change in voice, garbled or slurred speech, difficulty speaking) in patients treated with irinotecan. In some cases, the speech disorder occurred in the context of other symptoms such as numbness or tingling of the tongue or mouth or symptoms attributed to cholinergic syndrome, hypersensitivity/allergy, cerebrovascular events, or intracranial neoplasia. In some cases, however, the speech disorder occurred in the absence of other symptoms and recurred with subsequent infusions of irinotecan. In most of these cases, the speech disorders occurred during or shortly after infusion of irinotecan and resolved spontaneously within minutes to hours following discontinuation of the irinotecan infusion. The cause of speech disorders in patients treated with irinotecan has not been determined.

Driving and Operating Machinery: Patients should be warned about the potential for fatigue, dizziness or visual disturbances which may occur following the administration of irinotecan, and advised not to drive or operate machinery if these symptoms occur.

Renal: Increases in serum creatinine or blood urea nitrogen have been observed. Rare cases of renal impairment and acute renal failure have been identified. These events have generally been attributed to complications of infection or to dehydration related to nausea, vomiting and/or diarrhea, which are common and sometimes severe adverse events following CAMPTOSAR treatment. Rare instances of renal dysfunction due to tumour lysis syndrome have also been reported.

The influence of renal insufficiency on the pharmacokinetics of CAMPTOSAR has not been evaluated.

Respiratory: Interstitial pulmonary disease presenting as pulmonary infiltrates is uncommon during CAMPTOSAR therapy (see Adverse Reactions). Interstitial pulmonary disease can be fatal. Risk factors possibly associated with the development of interstitial pulmonary disease include pre-existing lung disease, use of pneumotoxic drugs, radiation therapy, and colony stimulating factors. Patients with risk factors should be closely monitored for respiratory symptoms before and during irinotecan therapy.

Special Populations: Pregnant Women: CAMPTOSAR has been shown to be embryotoxic in rats and rabbits at a dose of 6 mg/kg/day. It is teratogenic in rats at doses greater than 1.2 mg/kg/day, and in rabbits at 6 mg/kg/day. Treatment-related changes in the fetuses included external and visceral abnormalities, skeletal variations and abnormalities. CAMPTOSAR may cause fetal harm when administered to a pregnant woman. If the drug is used during pregnancy, or if the patient becomes pregnant while receiving this drug, the patient should be informed of the potential hazard to the fetus. Women of childbearing potential should be advised to avoid becoming pregnant while receiving CAMPTOSAR.

Nursing Women: In rats, radioactivity appeared in the milk within 5 minutes of intravenous administration of radiolabeled irinotecan and was concentrated up to 65-fold at 4 hours after administration relative to plasma concentrations. It is not known whether irinotecan is excreted in human milk. Because many drugs are excreted in human milk and because of the potential for serious adverse reactions in nursing infants, it is recommended that nursing be discontinued when receiving therapy with CAMPTOSAR.

Pediatrics: The safety and effectiveness of CAMPTOSAR in the pediatric population have not been established.

Geriatrics: Patients greater than 65 years of age should be closely monitored because of a greater risk of late diarrhea in this population (see Adverse Reactions). The starting dose of CAMPTOSAR in patients 70 years and older for the once-every-3-week-dosage schedule should be 300 mg/m² (see Dosage and Administration).

Monitoring and Laboratory Tests: Careful monitoring of white blood cell count with differential, hemoglobin and platelet count is recommended before each dose of CAMPTOSAR. Liver function should be monitored before initiation of treatment and monthly, or as clinically indicated. (See Adverse Reactions, Adverse Drug Reaction Overview.)

ADVERSE REACTIONS: Adverse Drug Reaction Overview: Gastrointestinal: Nausea, vomiting and diarrhea are common adverse events following treatment with CAMPTOSAR (irinotecan hydrochloride trihydrate) and can be severe. When observed, nausea and vomiting usually occur during or shortly after infusion of CAMPTOSAR. In the clinical studies testing the every 3-week-dosage schedule, the median time to the onset of late diarrhea was 5 days after CAMPTOSAR infusion. In the clinical studies evaluating the weekly dosage schedule, the median time to onset of late diarrhea was 11 days following administration of CAMPTOSAR. All grade late diarrhea occurred in approximately 80% in this patient population. For patients on the 125 mg/m² weekly dose, the median duration of any grade late diarrhea was 3 days. The median duration was 7 days for those patients reporting grades 3 or 4 late diarrhea on this same weekly dose.

Results from a retrospective analysis have shown that the frequency of grade 3 and 4 late diarrhea by age was significantly greater in patients ≥65 years than in patients <65 years of age. However, results from a prospective study treating patients with metastatic colorectal cancer refractory to one 5-FU-based chemotherapeutic regimen, on a 125 mg/m² weekly dosage schedule (4 weeks on, 2 weeks off) did not demonstrate any statistically significant difference in the rate of treatment-emergent grade 3-4 late diarrhea in patients ≥65 years of age versus patients <65 years of age. It should be noted however, that a statistically significant increase in the incidence of treatment-emergent early diarrhea in patients ≥65 years of age versus patients <65 years of age was found. Furthermore, a 10% reduction in median relative weekly dose intensity was required in patients ≥65 years versus patients <65 years in order to achieve tolerability. In the early Japanese trials, there is some information that patients with considerable ascites or pleural effusions were at increased risk for neutropenia or diarrhea.

Hematology: Typical adverse hematologic events of CAMPTOSAR included neutropenia, leukopenia (including lymphocytopenia), and anemia. Serious thrombocytopenia is uncommon. When evaluated in the trials of weekly administration, the frequency of grade 3 or 4 neutropenia was significantly increased in patients who had prior pelvic or abdominal irradiation. In the clinical studies evaluating the weekly dosage schedule, neutropenic fever (concurrent NCI grade 4 neutropenia and fever of grade 2 or greater) occurred in 3.0% of the patients. Only 5.6% of patients received G-CSF for the treatment of neutropenia. NCI grade 3 or 4 anemia was noted in 6.9% of the patients. Blood transfusions were given to 9.9% of the patients. There were no significant differences in the frequency of grade 3 and 4 neutropenia by age or gender (see Warnings and Precautions and Dosage and Administration, Single-agent and Combination Dosage Schedules). In the early Japanese trials, there is some information that patients with considerable ascites or pleural effusions were at increased risk for neutropenia or diarrhea.

Individuals with certain polymorphs of UGT1A1, such as UGT1A1*28, may have reduced activity of this enzyme. Approximately 10% of the North American population is homozygous for the UGT1A1*28 allele (also referred to as UGT1A1 7/7 genotype).

In a single arm study of 66 patients with solid tumors or lymphomas who received CAMPTOSAR as a single-agent at a dose of 350 mg/m² on a once every 3 weeks schedule, 3 out of 6 patients with UGT1A1 *28/*28 genotype had grade 4 neutropenia versus 3 out of 24 patients with the UGT1A1 *1/*28 genotype, and 0 out of 29 patients with the UGT1A1 *1/*1 genotype (see Warnings and Precautions).

In a study which compared CAMPTOSAR (100-125 mg/m²) in combination with bolus 5-FU/LV (IFL regimen), oxaliplatin (85 mg/m²) in combination with infusional 5-FU/LV (FOLFOX4 regimen) and a combination of oxaliplatin (85 mg/m²) plus CAMPTOSAR (200 mg/m²) (IROX regimen), the incidence of grade 4 neutropenia is shown in Table 1.

Table 1: CAMPTOSAR

Rates of Grade 4 Neutropenia for UGT1A1*28 Genotype by Treatment

UGT1A1 Genotype	IFL[a] n=109	FOLFOX4[b] n=285	IROX[c] n=103
6/6	6.8% (3/44)	19.4% (26/134)	9.6% (5/52)
6/7	11.1% (6/54)	22.2% (28/126)	15.0% (6/40)
7/7	18.2% (2/11)	36.0% (9/25)	54.5% (6/11)

[a] IFL: irinotecan 100-125 mg/m² followed by leucovorin 20 mg/m² and 5-FU 400 mg/m² given as a bolus on days 1, 8, 15, and 22 followed by a 2-week rest in repeated 6-week cycles.

[b] FOLFOX4: oxaliplatin 85 mg/m² on day 1, leucovorin 200 mg/m² on days 1 and 2, and 5-FU 400 mg/m² given as a bolus followed by 600 mg/m² given as a 22 hr continuous infusion on days 1 and 2 administered in repeated 2-week cycles.

[c] Oxaliplatin 85 mg/m² followed by irinotecan 200 mg/m² administered on day 1 of repeated 3-week cycles.

In a study to investigate the role of UGT1A1*28 polymorphism in the development of toxicity in patients treated with CAMPTOSAR and infusional 5-FU/LV at doses of 180 mg/m², 1 out of 22 patients with the UGT1A1 *28/*28 genotype had grade 4 neutropenia, versus 6 out of 114 patients with the UGT1A1 *1/*28 and 2 out of 114 for patients with the UGT1A1 *1/*1 genotype.

Whole Body: Asthenia, fever, and abdominal pain are generally the most common events of this type.

Cholinergic Symptoms: Patients may have cholinergic symptoms of rhinitis, increased salivation, miosis, lacrimation, diaphoresis, flushing, and intestinal hyperperistalsis that can cause abdominal cramping and early diarrhea. If these symptoms occur, they manifest during or shortly after drug infusion. They are thought to be related to the anticholinesterase activity of the irinotecan parent compound and are more likely to occur at higher irinotecan dose levels. The timing of the symptoms is most consistent with the occurrence of peak irinotecan serum levels during parental administration.

Hepatic: In the clinical studies evaluating the weekly dosage schedule, NCI grade 3 or 4 liver enzyme abnormalities were observed in less than 10% of patients. These events typically occur in patients with known hepatic metastases.

Dermatologic: Alopecia has been reported during treatment with CAMPTOSAR. Rashes have also been reported but did not result in discontinuation of treatment.

Respiratory: Severe pulmonary events are infrequent. Early effects such as dyspnea have been reported (see Warnings and Precautions). In the clinical studies evaluating the weekly dosage schedule, over half the patients with dyspnea had lung metastases. The extent to which malignant pulmonary involvement or other pre-existing lung disease may have contributed to dyspnea in these patients is unknown.

Potentially life threatening interstitial disease presenting with dyspnea, fever and pulmonary infiltrates (reticulonodular pattern on chest x-ray) is uncommon during CAMPTOSAR therapy. Usually seen in Japanese studies the contribution of CAMPTOSAR to these events was difficult to assess because these patients also had lung tumours and some had pre-existing non-malignant pulmonary disease.

Neurologic: Insomnia and dizziness can occur, but are not usually considered to be directly related to the administration of CAMPTOSAR. Dizziness may sometimes represent symptomatic evidence of orthostatic hypotension in patients with dehydration (see Warnings and Precautions).

Cardiovascular: Vasodilation (flushing) may occur during administration of CAMPTOSAR. Bradycardia may also occur, but has not required intervention. These effects have been attributed to the cholinergic syndrome sometimes observed during or shortly after infusion of CAMPTOSAR. All thromboembolic events, when considered together, have commonly been observed in patients receiving CAMPTOSAR (see Warnings and Precautions, Cardiovascular). The specific cause of these events has not been determined.

Hypersensitivity: Hypersensitivity reactions including severe anaphylactic or anaphylactoid reactions have been observed (see Warnings and Precautions).

Clinical Trial Adverse Drug Reactions: Combination-Agent (Irinotecan/5-FU/LV) Therapy: A total of 955 patients with metastatic colorectal cancer received regimens of CAMPTOSAR in combination with 5-FU/LV, 5-FU/LV alone, or CAMPTOSAR alone. In the two phase 3 studies, 370 patients received CAMPTOSAR in combination with 5-FU/LV, 362 patients received 5-FU/LV alone, and 223 patients received CAMPTOSAR alone (see Table 7 in Dosage and Administration for recommended combination regimens).

In Study 1, 49 (7.3%) patients died within 30 days of last study treatment: 21 (9.3%) received CAMPTOSAR in combination with 5-FU/LV, 15 (6.8%) received 5-FU/LV alone, and 13 (5.8%) received CAMPTOSAR alone. Deaths potentially related to treatment occurred in 2 (0.9%) patients who received CAMPTOSAR in combination with 5-FU/LV (2 neutropenic fever/sepsis), 3 (1.4%) patients who received 5-FU/LV alone (1 neutropenic fever/sepsis, 1 CNS bleeding during thrombocytopenia, 1 unknown) and 2 (0.9%) patients who received CAMPTOSAR alone (2 neutropenic fever). Deaths from any cause within 60 days of first study treatment were reported for 15 (6.7%) patients who received CAMPTOSAR in combination with 5FU/LV, 16 (7.3%) patients who received 5FU/LV alone and 15 (6.7%) patients who received CAMPTOSAR alone. Discontinuations due to adverse events were reported for 17 (7.6%) patients who received CAMPTOSAR in combination with 5-FU/LV, 14 (6.4%) patients who received 5-FU/LV alone, and 26 (11.7%) patients who received CAMPTOSAR alone.

In Study 1, data on hospitalization included hospitalization required as a consequence of chemotherapy-induced adverse events and hospitalizations that may have resulted from complications due to cancer or intercurrent illnesses. One hundred and thirteen (50.2%) patients of 225 who received CAMPTOSAR in combination with 5FU/LV were hospitalized. Sixty-eight (30.2%) patients were hospitalized once, 28 (12.4%) patients were hospitalized twice and 17 (7.6%) patients were hospitalized more than two times. Ninety-nine (44.4%) patients of 223 treated with CAMPTOSAR alone were hospitalized. Seventy-one (31.8%) patients were hospitalized once, 21 (9.4%) were hospitalized twice and 7 (3.1%) were hospitalized more than two times. Eighty-six (39.3%) patients of 219 treated with 5 FU/LV were hospitalized. Sixty (27.4%) patients were hospitalized once, 20 (9.1%) patients were hospitalized twice and 6 (2.7%) were hospitalized more than two times.

In Study 2, 10 (3.5%) patients died within 30 days of last study treatment: 6 (4.1%) received CAMPTOSAR in combination with 5-FU/LV and 4 (2.8%) received 5-FU/LV alone. There was one potentially treatment related death, which occurred in a patient who received CAMPTOSAR in combination with 5-FU/LV (0.7%, neutropenic sepsis). Deaths from any cause within 60 days of first study treatment were reported for 3 (2.1%) patients who received CAMPTOSAR in combination with 5FU/LV and 2 (1.4%) patients who received 5FU/LV alone. Discontinuations due to adverse events were reported for 9 (6.2%) patients who received CAMPTOSAR in combination with 5-FU/LV and 1 (0.7%) patients who received 5-FU/LV alone.

In Study 2, data on hospitalization included hospitalization required as a consequence of chemotherapy-induced adverse events. Fifty (34.5%) patients of 145 who received CAMPTOSAR in combination with 5FU/LV were hospitalized. Thirty-five (24.1%) patients were hospitalized once, 8 (5.5%) patients were hospitalized twice and 7 (4.8%) patients were hospitalized more than two times. Twenty-nine (20.3%) patients of 143 treated with 5FU/LV were hospitalized. Twenty-one (14.7%) patients were hospitalized once, 6 (4.2%) patients were hospitalized twice and 2 (1.4%) patients were hospitalized more than two times.

The most clinically significant adverse events (all grades 1-4) for patients receiving CAMPTOSAR-based therapy were diarrhea, nausea, vomiting, neutropenia, and alopecia. The most clinically significant adverse events for patients receiving 5-FU/LV therapy were diarrhea, neutropenia, neutropenic fever, and mucositis. In Study 1, grade 4 neutropenia, neutropenic fever (defined as grade 2 fever and grade 4 neutropenia), and mucositis were observed less often with weekly CAMPTOSAR /5-FU/LV than with monthly administration of 5-FU/LV.

Table 2 and Table 3 list the clinically relevant adverse events reported in Studies 1 and 2, respectively.

Single-Agent Therapy: Weekly Dosage Schedule: In three clinical studies evaluating the weekly dosage schedule, 304 patients with metastatic carcinoma of the colon or rectum that had recurred or progressed following 5-FU-based therapy were treated with CAMPTOSAR.

Seventeen of the patients died within 30 days of the administration of CAMPTOSAR. In five cases (1.6%, 5/304), the deaths were potentially drug-related. These five patients experienced a constellation of medical events that included known effects of CAMPTOSAR. One of these patients died of neutropenic sepsis without fever. Neutropenic fever, defined as NCI grade 4 neutropenia and grade 2 or greater fever, occurred in nine (3.0%) other patients. These patients recovered with supportive care. Thirteen (4.3%) patients discontinued CAMPTOSAR treatment because of medical events.

One hundred and nineteen (39.1%) of the 304 patients were hospitalized a total of 156 times because of adverse events; 81 (26.6%) patients were hospitalized for events judged to be related to administration of CAMPTOSAR. The primary reasons for drug-related hospitalization were diarrhea, with or without nausea and/or vomiting (18.4%); neutropenia/leukopenia, with or without diarrhea and/or fever (8.2%); and nausea and/or vomiting (4.9%).

Adjustments in the dose of CAMPTOSAR were made during the cycle of treatment and for subsequent cycles based on individual patient tolerance. The first dose of at least one cycle of CAMPTOSAR was reduced for 67% of patients who began the studies at the 125 mg/m² starting dose. Within-cycle dose reductions were required for 32% of the cycles initiated at the 125 mg/m² dose level. The most common reasons for dose reduction were late diarrhea, neutropenia, and leukopenia.

Table 2: CAMPTOSAR

Study 1: Percent (%) of Patients Experiencing Clinically Relevant Adverse Events in Combination Therapies[a]

	Study 1					
	CAMPTOSAR + Bolus 5-FU/LV Weekly×4 q 6 Weeks N=225		Bolus 5-FU/LV Daily×5 q 4 Weeks N=219		CAMPTOSAR Weekly×4 q 6 Weeks N=223	
Adverse Event	Grade 1-4	Grade 3 and 4	Grade 1-4	Grade 3 and 4	Grade 1-4	Grade 3 and 4
Total Adverse Events	100	53.3	100	45.7	99.6	45.7
Gastrointestinal						
Diarrhea						
late	84.9	22.7	69.4	13.2	83.0	31.0
grade 3	—	15.1	—	5.9	—	18.4
grade 4	—	7.6	—	7.3	—	12.6
early	45.8	4.9	31.5	1.4	43.0	6.7
Nausea	79.1	15.6	67.6	8.2	81.6	16.1
Abdominal Pain	63.1	14.6	50.2	11.5	67.7	13.0
Vomiting	60.4	9.7	46.1	4.1	62.8	12.1
Anorexia	34.2	5.8	42.0	3.7	43.9	7.2
Constipation	41.3	3.1	31.5	1.8	32.3	0.4
Mucositis	32.4	2.2	76.3	16.9	29.6	2.2
Hematologic						
Neutropenia	96.9	53.8	98.6	66.7	96.4	31.4
grade 3	—	29.8	—	23.7	—	19.3
grade 4	—	24.0	—	42.5	—	12.1
Leukopenia	96.9	37.8	98.6	23.3	96.4	21.5
Anemia	96.9	8.4	98.6	5.5	96.9	4.5
Neutropenic Fever	—	7.1	—	14.6	—	5.8
Thrombocytopenia	96.0	2.6	98.6	2.7	96.0	1.7
Neutropenic Infection	—	1.8	—	0	—	2.2
Body as a Whole						
Asthenia	70.2	19.5	64.4	11.9	69.1	13.9
Pain	30.7	3.1	26.9	3.6	22.9	2.2
Fever	42.2	1.7	32.4	3.6	43.5	0.4
Infection	22.2	0	16.0	1.4	13.9	0.4
Metabolic and Nutritional						
↑Bilirubin	87.6	7.1	92.2	8.2	83.9	7.2
Dermatologic						
Exfoliative Dermatitis	0.9	0	3.2	0.5	0	0
Rash	19.1	0	26.5	0.9	14.3	0.4
Alopecia[b]	43.1	—	26.5	—	46.1	—
Respiratory						
Dyspnea	27.6	6.3	16.0	0.5	22.0	2.2
Cough	26.7	1.3	18.3	0	20.2	0.4
Pneumonia	6.2	2.7	1.4	1.0	3.6	1.3
Neurologic						
Dizziness	23.1	1.3	16.4	0	21.1	1.8
Somnolence	12.4	1.8	4.6	1.8	9.4	1.3
Confusion	7.1	1.8	4.1	0	2.7	0

(cont'd)

Table 2: CAMPTOSAR *(cont'd)*

Study 1: Percent (%) of Patients Experiencing Clinically Relevant Adverse Events in Combination Therapies[a]

	Study 1					
	CAMPTOSAR + Bolus 5-FU/LV Weekly×4 q 6 Weeks N=225		Bolus 5-FU/LV Daily×5 q 4 Weeks N=219		CAMPTOSAR Weekly×4 q 6 Weeks N=223	
Adverse Event	Grade 1-4	Grade 3 and 4	Grade 1-4	Grade 3 and 4	Grade 1-4	Grade 3 and 4
Cardiovascular						
Vasodilatation	9.3	0.9	5.0	0	9.0	0
Hypotension	5.8	1.3	2.3	0.5	5.8	1.7
Thromboembolic Events[c]	9.3	—	11.4	—	5.4	—

[a] Severity of adverse events based on NCI CTC (version 1.0).
[b] Complete hair loss=Grade 2.
[c] Includes angina pectoris, arterial thrombosis, cerebral infarct, cerebrovascular accident, deep thrombophlebitis, embolus lower extremity, heart arrest, myocardial infarct, myocardial ischemia, peripheral vascular disorder, pulmonary embolus, sudden death, thrombophlebitis, thrombosis, vascular disorder.

Note: Combination toxicities (gastrointestinal and cardiovascular syndromes) may occur simultaneously and both contribute to the toxicity profile.

Table 3: CAMPTOSAR

Study 2: Percent (%) of Patients Experiencing Clinically Relevant Adverse Events in Combination Therapies[a]

	Study 2			
	CAMPTOSAR +5-FU/LV Infusional D 1 and 2 q 2 Weeks N=145		5-FU/LV Infusional D 1 and 2 q 2 Weeks N=143	
Adverse Event	Grade 1-4	Grade 3 and 4	Grade 1-4	Grade 3 and 4
Total Adverse Events	100	72.4	100	39.2
Gastrointestinal				
Diarrhea				
late	72.4	14.4	44.8	6.3
grade 3	—	10.3	—	4.2
grade 4	—	4.1	—	2.1
Cholinergic Syndrome[b]	28.3	1.4	0.7	0
Nausea	66.9	2.1	55.2	3.5
Abdominal Pain	17.2	2.1	16.8	0.7
Vomiting	44.8	3.5	32.2	2.8
Anorexia	35.2	2.1	18.9	0.7
Constipation	30.3	0.7	25.2	1.4
Mucositis	40	4.1	28.7	2.8
Hematologic				
Neutropenia	82.5	46.2	47.9	13.4
grade 3	—	36.4	—	12.7
grade 4	—	9.8	—	0.7
Leukopenia	81.3	17.4	42	3.5
Anemia	97.2	2.1	90.9	2.1
Neutropenic Fever	—	3.4	—	0.7
Thrombocytopenia	32.6	0	32.2	0
Neutropenic Infection	—	2.1	—	0
Body as a Whole				
Asthenia	57.9	9	48.3	4.2
Pain	64.1	9.7	61.5	8.4
Fever	22.1	0.7	25.9	0.7
Infection	35.9	7.6	33.6	3.5
Metabolic and Nutritional				
↑Bilirubin	19.1	3.5	35.9	10.6
Dermatologic				

(cont'd)

Table 3: CAMPTOSAR *(cont'd)*

Study 2: Percent (%) of Patients Experiencing Clinically Relevant Adverse Events in Combination Therapies[a]

	Study 2			
	CAMPTOSAR +5-FU/LV Infusional D 1 and 2 q 2 Weeks N=145		5-FU/LV Infusional D 1 and 2 q 2 Weeks N=143	
Adverse Event	**Grade 1-4**	**Grade 3 and 4**	**Grade 1-4**	**Grade 3 and 4**
Hand and Foot Syndrome	10.3	0.7	12.6	0.7
Cutaneous Signs	17.2	0.7	20.3	0
Alopecia[c]	56.6	—	16.8	—
Respiratory				
Dyspnea	9.7	1.4	4.9	0
Cardiovascular				
Hypotension	3.4	1.4	0.7	0
Thromboembolic Events[d]	11.7	—	5.6	—

[a] Severity of adverse events based on NCI CTC (version 1.0).
[b] Includes rhinitis, increased salivation, miosis, lacrimation, diaphoresis, flushing, abdominal cramping or diarrhea (occurring during or shortly after infusion of irinotecan).
[c] Complete hair loss=Grade 2.
[d] Includes angina pectoris, arterial thrombosis, cerebral infarct, cerebrovascular accident, deep thrombophlebitis, embolus lower extremity, heart arrest, myocardial infarct, myocardial ischemia, peripheral vascular disorder, pulmonary embolus, sudden death, thrombophlebitis, thrombosis, vascular disorder.
Note: Combination toxicities (gastrointestinal and cardiovascular syndromes) may occur simultaneously and both contribute to the toxicity profile.

The adverse events in Table 4 are based on the experience of the 304 patients enrolled in the three studies.

Table 4: CAMPTOSAR

Adverse Events Occurring in >10% of 304 Patients with Previously Treated Metastatic Carcinoma of the Colon or Rectum[a]

	% of Patients Reporting	
Body System and Event	**NCI Grades 1-4**	**NCI Grades 3 and 4**
Gastrointestinal		
Diarrhea (late)[b]	87.8	30.6
7–9 stools/day (grade 3)	—	(16.4)
≥10 stools/day (grade 4)	—	(14.1)
Nausea	86.2	16.8
Vomiting	66.8	12.5
Anorexia	54.9	5.9
Diarrhea (early)[c]	50.7	7.9
Constipation	29.9	2.0
Flatulence	12.2	0
Stomatitis	11.8	0.7
Dyspepsia	10.5	0
Hematologic		
Leucopenia	63.2	28.0
Anemia	60.5	6.9
Neutropenia	53.9	26.3
0.5 to <1.0×10⁹/L (grade 3)	—	(14.8)
<0.5×10⁹/L (grade 4)	—	(11.5)
Body as a Whole		
Asthenia	75.7	12.2
Abdominal Cramping/Pain	56.9	16.4
Fever	45.4	0.7
Pain	23.7	2.3
Headache	16.8	0.7
Back Pain	14.5	1.6
Chills	13.8	0.3
Minor Infection[d]	14.5	0

(cont'd)

Table 4: CAMPTOSAR *(cont'd)*

Adverse Events Occurring in >10% of 304 Patients with Previously Treated Metastatic Carcinoma of the Colon or Rectum[a]

	% of Patients Reporting	
Body System and Event	**NCI Grades 1-4**	**NCI Grades 3 and 4**
Edema	10.2	1.3
Abdominal Enlargement	10.2	0.3
Metabolic and Nutritional		
↓ Body Weight	30.3	0.7
Dehydration	14.8	4.3
↑ Alkaline Phosphatase	13.2	3.9
↑ AST	10.5	1.3
Dermatologic		
Alopecia	60.5	NA[e]
Sweating	16.4	0
Rash	12.8	0.7
Respiratory		
Dyspnea	22.0	3.6
↑ Coughing	17.4	0.3
Rhinitis	15.5	0
Neurologic		
Insomnia	19.4	0
Dizziness	14.8	0
Cardiovascular		
Vasodilation (Flushing)	11.2	0

[a] Severity of adverse events based on NCI CTC (version 1.0).
[b] Occurring >24 hours after administration of CAMPTOSAR.
[c] Occurring ≤24 hours after administration of CAMPTOSAR.
[d] Primarily upper respiratory infections.
[e] Not applicable; complete hair loss=NCI grade 2.

Once-Every-3-Week Dosage Schedule: A total of 535 patients with metastatic colorectal cancer whose disease had progressed following prior 5-FU therapy participated in the two phase 3 studies: 316 received CAMPTOSAR, 129 received 5-FU, and 90 received best supportive care.

Eleven (3.5%) patients treated with CAMPTOSAR died within 30 days of treatment. In three cases (1%, 3/316), the deaths were potentially related to CAMPTOSAR treatment and were attributed to neutropenic infection, grade 4 diarrhea and asthenia, respectively. One (0.8%, 1/129) patient treated with 5-FU died within 30 days of treatment; this death was attributed to grade 4 diarrhea.

Fifty-five percent (295/535) of patients were hospitalized at least once due to serious adverse events: 60% (188/316) of patients received CAMPTOSAR, 63% (57/90) received best supportive care, and 39% (50/129) received 5-FU- based therapy. Eight percent (25/316) of patients treated with CAMPTOSAR and 7% (9/129) treated with 5-FU-based therapy discontinued treatment due to adverse events.

Table 5 lists the grade 3 and 4 adverse events reported in the 535 patients enrolled in the two studies (V301 and V302) evaluating the once-every-3-week dosage schedule.

Table 5: CAMPTOSAR

Percent of Patients Experiencing Grade 3 and 4 Adverse Events in Comparative Studies of Once-Every-3-Week CAMPTOSAR Therapy[a]

	Study V301		Study V302	
Adverse Event	**CAMPTOSAR n=189**	**BSC[b] n=90**	**CAMPTOSAR n=127**	**5-FU[c] n=129**
Total Grade 3/4 Adverse Events	79.4	66.7	69.3	54.3
Gastrointestinal				
Diarrhea	21.7	5.6	22.0	10.9
Vomiting	13.8	7.8	14.2	4.7
Nausea	13.8	3.3	11.0	3.9
Abdominal Pain	13.8	15.6	8.7	7.8
Constipation	9.5	7.8	7.9	6.2
Anorexia	5.3	6.7	5.5	3.9
Mucositis	1.6	1.1	2.4	5.4
Hematologic				
Leukopenia/Neutropenia	22.2	0	14.2	2.3
Anemia	7.4	6.7	6.3	3.1

(cont'd)

Table 5: CAMPTOSAR *(cont'd)*

Percent of Patients Experiencing Grade 3 and 4 Adverse Events in Comparative Studies of Once-Every-3-Week CAMPTOSAR Therapy[a]

Adverse Event	Study V301		Study V302	
	CAMPTOSAR n=189	BSC[b] n=90	CAMPTOSAR n=127	5-FU[c] n=129
Hemorrhage	5.3	3.3	0.8	3.1
Thrombocytopenia	1.1	0	3.9	1.6
Infection				
without grade 3/4 neutropenia	8.5	3.3	0.8	3.9
with grade 3/4 neutropenia	1.1	0	1.6	0
Fever				
without grade 3/4 neutropenia	2.1	1.1	1.6	0
with grade 3/4 neutropenia	2.1	0	3.9	1.6
Body as a Whole				
Pain	18.5	22.2	16.5	13.2
Asthenia	14.8	18.9	13.4	11.6
Cholinergic Syndrome	12.2	0	1.6	0
Metabolic and Nutritional				
Hepatic[d]	8.5	6.7	8.7	6.2
Dermatologic				
Hand and Foot Syndrome	1.6	0	0.8	4.7
Cutaneous Signs[e]				3.1
Respiratory[f]	10.1	7.8	4.7	7
Neurologic[g]	12.2	13.3	8.7	3.9
Cardiovascular[h]	8.5	3.3	3.9	1.6
Other[i]	31.7	27.8	11.8	14

a Severity of adverse events based on NCI CTC (version 1.0).
b BSC=best supportive care.
c One of the following 5-FU regimens were used: (1) Leucovorin, 200 mg/m² iv over 2 hr; followed by 5-FU, 400 mg/m² iv bolus; followed by 5-FU, 600 mg/m² continuous iv infusion over 22 hr on days 1 and 2 every 2 wk. (2) 5-FU, 250 to 300 mg/m²/day protracted continuous iv infusion until toxicity. (3) 5-FU, 2 to 3 g/m²/day iv over 24 hr every wk for 6 wk with or without leucovorin, 20 to 500 mg/m²/day every wk iv for 6 wk with 2-wk rest between cycles.
d Hepatic includes events such as ascites and jaundice.
e Cutaneous signs include events such as rash.
f Respiratory includes events such as dyspnea and cough.
g Neurologic includes events such as somnolence.
h Cardiovascular includes events such as dysrhythmias, ischemia, and mechanical cardiac dysfunction.
i Other includes events such as accidental injury, hepatomegaly, syncope, vertigo, and weight loss.

Post-Market Adverse Drug Reactions: The following events have been identified during postmarketing use of CAMPTOSAR in clinical practice.

Infrequent cases of colitis, including typhlitis, ulcerative and ischemic colitis, have been observed. This can be complicated by ileus or what was described as toxic megacolon, ulceration, bleeding, obstruction, and infection. Rare cases of intestinal perforation have been reported. Cases of ileus without preceding colitis have also been observed. Patients experiencing ileus should receive prompt antibiotic support (see Warnings and Precautions). Hiccups have also been reported.

Rare cases of hyponatremia mostly related to diarrhea and vomiting have been reported.

Increases in serum levels of transaminases (i.e., AST and ALT), GGT and bilirubin in the absence of progressive liver metastasis have been observed; rare cases of symptomatic pancreatitis or asymptomatic elevated pancreatic enzymes have been observed.

Infrequent cases of renal insufficiency, hypotension or circulatory failure have been observed in patients who experienced episodes of dehydration associated with diarrhea and/or vomiting, or sepsis (see Warnings and Precautions).

Early effects such as muscular contraction or cramps and paresthesia have been reported.

Severe pulmonary events are infrequent. Interstitial pulmonary disease presenting as pulmonary infiltrates is uncommon during irinotecan therapy. Early effects such as dyspnea have been reported (see Warnings and Precautions).

Myocardial ischemic events, with some cases resulting in fatality, have been observed in patients treated with CAMPTOSAR, the majority of whom had underlying cardiac disease, other known risk factors for cardiac disease and/or were treated with other concomitant cytotoxic chemotherapy (see Warnings and Precautions).

Speech disorders have been reported in patients treated with irinotecan. See Warnings and Precautions, Neurologic.

DRUG INTERACTIONS: Overview: CAMPTOSAR (irinotecan hydrochloride trihydrate) is metabolized by carboxyl esterase to an active metabolite, SN-38, and oxidized by CYP3A4 to two relatively inactive metabolites (APC and NPC). SN-38 is glucuronidated to an inactive conjugate (see Action and Clinical Pharmacology, Pharmacokinetics). Pharmacokinetic drug-drug and drug-herbal interactions have been shown in (Table 6). These have most often been attributed to inhibition or induction of CYP3A4, though multiple mechanisms have been suggested to contribute to the interactions (induction/inhibition of carboxyl esterase, UDP-glucuronyl transferase 1A1, and drug transporters).

In vitro drug interaction studies reveal that the metabolism of irinotecan to its active metabolite SN-38 by carboxylesterase enzymes is not inhibited by 5-fluorouracil (5-FU). Data from a phase 1 clinical study involving CAMPTOSAR, 5-FU, and leucovorin (LV) in 26 patients with solid tumours indicate that the disposition of irinotecan and its active metabolite SN-38 are not substantially altered when the drugs are co-administered. In vivo or in vitro drug interaction studies to evaluate the influence of irinotecan on the disposition of 5-FU and LV have not been conducted.

Co-administration with CYP3A4 inhibitors (e.g., cimetidine, macrolide antibiotics [azithromycin, clarithromycin, erythromycin], azole antifungals [fluconazole, ketoconazole, itraconazole], grapefruit juice, CYP3A4-inhibitory calcium channel blockers such as verapamil, diltiazem, and nifedipine) can potentially lead to significantly increased formation of SN-38 and potential toxicity. This interaction has been documented in cancer patients with the co-administration of CAMPTOSAR and ketoconazole, a potent enzyme inhibitor, where the relative exposure to the CYP3A4-mediated metabolite APC was reduced by 87%, whereas the relative exposure to the active metabolite SN-38 increased by 100%.

Exposure to fluoroquinolones such as ciprofloxacin or norfloxacin may be increased in patients with compromised renal function due to dehydration or colorectal cancer complications. In these circumstances co-administration of CAMPTOSAR and CYP3A4-inhibitory fluoroquinolone antibiotics could potentially lead to increased SN-38 exposure and enhanced toxicity.

Similarly, co-administration of CAMPTOSAR with CYP3A4 inducers (e.g., carbamazepine, phenobarbital, phenytoin, glucocorticoids, St. John's Wort) leads to reduction in plasma levels of the active metabolite SN-38, which may have a deleterious impact on treatment outcome. This interaction has been documented in cancer patients with the co-administration of CAMPTOSAR with St. John's Wort and with the co-administration of CAMPTOSAR with phenytoin.

The prescribing information of concomitant medications should also be consulted to identify potential interactions.

Drug-Drug Interactions: See Table 6.

Table 6: CAMPTOSAR

Pharmacokinetic Interactions

	Ref[a]	Effect	Clinical Comment
CYP3A4 Inhibitors			**Potential for Increased Toxicity**
Azole Antifungals			See Contraindications.
Ketoconazole	CT	SN-38 ~110% increased, APC ~90% decreased	
Fluconazole, itraconazole	T		
Cimetidine	T		See Warnings and Precautions.
Fluoroquinolone Antibiotics			
Ciprofloxacin, norfloxacin	T		
Macrolide Antibiotics			
Azithromycin, clarithromycin, erythromycin	T		
Calcium Channel Blockers			
Diltiazem, verapamil, nifedipine	T		
Grapefruit juice	T		
Atazanavir sulfate	T	See Atazanavir Product Monograph and below	
CYP3A4 Inducers			**Potential for Decreased Efficacy**
Anticonvulsants			See Warnings and Precautions and Drug-Herb Interactions.
Carbamazepine, phenobarbital, phenytoin	CT, C	Irinotecan decreased ~60%, SN-38 decreased ~75%	
St. John's wort	C	SN-38 decreased ~40%	
Glucocorticoids			
Dexamethasone	T		
Rifampin	T		

a Level of Evidence; C=Case Study, CT=Clinical Trial, T=Theoretical.

Appropriate starting dose for patients taking drugs shown or anticipated to alter the kinetics of CAMPTOSAR has not been formally defined. Co-administration of azole antifungals and irinotecan is contraindicated and patients should discontinue ketoconazole at least 1 week prior to starting CAMPTOSAR therapy (see Contraindications). Patients should not drink grapefruit juice during treatment. Consideration should be given to starting or substituting to non-enzyme-inducing anticonvulsants at least one week prior to initiation of CAMPTOSAR therapy in patients requiring anticonvulsant treatment. Co-administration of atazanavir sulfate, a CYP3A4 and UGT1A1 inhibitor has the potential to increase systemic exposure to SN-38, the active metabolite of irinotecan. Physicians should take this into consideration when co-administering these drugs (see Warnings and Precautions).

Pharmacodynamic Interactions: Antineoplastic Agents: Adverse events due to CAMPTOSAR, such as myelosuppression and diarrhea, would be expected to be enhanced by combination with other anti-neoplastic agents having similar adverse effects.

Laxatives: It would be expected that laxative use during CAMPTOSAR therapy may worsen the incidence or severity of diarrhea.

Diuretics: The use of diuretics should be carefully monitored because of the potential risk of dehydration secondary to vomiting and/or diarrhea induced by CAMPTOSAR. The physician may wish to withhold diuretics during CAMPTOSAR dosing, and certainly during periods of active vomiting or diarrhea.

Dexamethasone: Lymphocytopenia has been reported in patients receiving CAMPTOSAR. It is possible that the administration of dexamethasone as an anti-emetic prophylaxis may have enhanced the likelihood of this effect. However, in these reports, serious opportunistic infections were not observed and no complications were specifically attributed to lymphocytopenia.

Hyperglycemia has been reported in patients receiving CAMPTOSAR. This has usually been observed in patients with a history of diabetes mellitus or evidence of glucose intolerance prior to administration of CAMPTOSAR. It is probable that dexamethasone, given as anti-emetic prophylaxis, contributed to hyperglycemia in some patients.

Prochlorperazine: The incidence of akathisia in clinical trials of the weekly dosage schedule was greater (8.5%, 4 of 47 patients) when prochlorperazine was administered on the same day as CAMPTOSAR than when these drugs were given on separate days (1.3%, 1 of 80 patients). However, the 8.5% incidence of akathisia is within the range reported for use of prochlorperazine when given as premedication for other chemotherapies.

Neuromuscular Blocking Agents: Interaction between CAMPTOSAR and neuromuscular blocking agents cannot be ruled out since irinotecan has anticholinesterase activity. Drugs with anticholinesterase activity may prolong the neuromuscular blocking effects of suxamethonium and the neuromuscular blockade of non-depolarizing drugs may be antagonized.

Drug-Herb Interactions: St. John's Wort: Exposure to the active metabolite SN-38 is reduced by approximately 40% in patients taking concomitant St. John's wort and CAMPTOSAR. St. John's wort should be discontinued at least 1 week prior to the first cycle of CAMPTOSAR (see Warnings and Precautions).

Drug-Laboratory Test Interactions: There are no known interactions between CAMPTOSAR and laboratory tests.

DOSAGE AND ADMINISTRATION: Recommendations Common to Combination and Single Agent CAMPTOSAR (irinotecan hydrochloride trihydrate for injection) Schedules:

- Dosing of patients is not recommended with (see Warnings and Precautions):
  - serum bilirubin >35 µmol/L, transaminase >3 times ULN if no liver metastases, or transaminase >5 times ULN with liver metastases
  - ECOG performance status 3 or 4
- Recommended laboratory tests (see Warnings and Precautions) before/during therapy:
  - white blood cell count with differential, hemoglobin and platelet count before each dose
  - liver function before initiation of treatment and monthly or as clinically indicated
- Dose reduction may be considered for patients (see Warnings and Precautions):
  - aged ≥70 years
  - with prior pelvic/abdominal radiotherapy

- with performance status of 2
- with moderately elevated bilirubin levels (17-35 µmol/L)
- with Gilbert's syndrome
- Dose schedules, dose modifications and dose delay:
  - patients should be carefully monitored for toxicity and assessed prior to each treatment
  - dosage schedule and dose modifications for combination therapy are summarized in Table 7 and Table 8 and for single agent therapy in Table 9 and Table 10.
  - dose modifications should be based on the worst preceding toxicity. Patients should return to pre-treatment bowel function without requiring antidiarrhea medications for at least 24 hours before the next chemotherapy administration. Patients experiencing clinically significant (defined as grade ≥2) diarrhea, abdominal cramping, or neutropenia on the day of treatment administration should have treatment delayed until they recover and subsequent doses should be decreased.
  - a new cycle of therapy should not begin until the toxicity has recovered to NCI grade 1 or less. Treatment may be delayed 1 to 2 weeks to allow for recovery from treatment-related toxicity. If the patient has not recovered, consideration should be given to discontinuing therapy.
  - provided intolerable toxicity does not develop, treatment with additional cycles may be continued indefinitely as long as patients continue to experience clinical benefit.

It is recommended that patients receive premedication with antiemetic agents. Prophylactic or therapeutic administration of atropine should be considered in patients experiencing cholinergic symptoms. Besides the dosage modification, prompt use of oral loperamide is recommended in order to control and treat the diarrhea (see Warnings and Precautions, Gastrointestinal).

Recommended Dose and Dosage Adjustment: CAMPTOSAR Combination-Agent Therapy—Dosage Schedules: CAMPTOSAR should be administered as an intravenous infusion over 90 minutes. For all regimens, the dose of Leucovorin (LV) should be administered immediately after CAMPTOSAR, with the administration of 5-Fluorouracil (5-FU) to occur immediately after receipt of LV. The recommended regimens are shown in Table 7.

Table 7: CAMPTOSAR

Combination-Agent Dosage Schedules and Dose Modifications[a]

Regimen 1 6-wk cycle	CAMPTOSAR	125 mg/m² IV over 90 min once-weekly (days 1, 8, 15, 22) then 2-week rest		
	LV Bolus	20 mg/m² IV bolus once-weekly (days 1, 8, 15, 22) then 2-week rest		
	5-FU Bolus	500 mg/m² IV bolus once-weekly (days 1, 8, 15, 22) then 2-week rest		
		Starting Dose and Modified Dose Levels (mg/m²)		
		Starting Dose	Dose Level-1	Dose Level-2
	CAMPTOSAR	125	100	75
	LV Bolus	20	20	20
	5-FU Bolus	500	400	300
Regimen 2 6-wk cycle	CAMPTOSAR	180 mg/m² IV over 90 min once every 2 weeks (days 1, 15, 29) then 1-week rest		
	LV Infusion	200 mg/m² IV over 2 h on days 1, 2 every 2 weeks (days 1, 2, 15, 16, 29, 30) then 1-week rest		
	5-FU Bolus	400 mg/m² IV bolus immediately followed by		
	5-FU Infusion[b]	600 mg/m² IV over 22 h on days 1, 2 every 2 weeks (days 1, 2, 15, 16, 29, 30) 1-week rest		
		Starting Dose and Modified Dose Levels (mg/m²)		
		Starting Dose	Dose Level-1	Dose Level-2
	CAMPTOSAR	180	150	120
	LV Infusion	200	200	200
	5-FU Bolus	400	320	240
	5-FU Infusion[b]	600	480	360

[a] Dose reductions beyond dose level −2 by decrements of ~20% may be warranted for patients continuing to experience toxicity.
[b] Infusion follows bolus administration.

CAMPTOSAR Combination-Agent Therapy—Dose Modifications: Patients should be carefully monitored for toxicity and assessed prior to each treatment, especially during the first cycle of therapy. Doses of CAMPTOSAR and 5-FU should be modified as necessary to accommodate individual patient tolerance to treatment. Based on the recommended dose-levels described in Table 7, Combination-Agent Dosage Regimens & Dose Modifications, subsequent doses should be adjusted as suggested in Table 8, Recommended Dose Modifications for Combination Schedules.

Table 8: CAMPTOSAR

Recommended Dose Modifications for CAMPTOSAR/5-Fluorouracil(5-FU)/Leucovorin (LV) Combination Schedule

Patients should return to pre-treatment bowel function without requiring antidiarrhea medications for at least 24 hours before the next chemotherapy administration. A new cycle of therapy should not begin until the granulocyte count has recovered to ≥1.5×10⁹/L, and the platelet count has recovered to ≥100×10⁹/L, and treatment-related diarrhea is fully resolved. Treatment should be delayed 1 to 2 weeks to allow for recovery from treatment-related toxicities. If the patient has not recovered after a 2-week delay, consideration should be given to discontinuing therapy.

Toxicity NCI CTC grade[a] (Value)	During a Cycle of Therapy	At the Start of Subsequent Cycles of Therapy[b]
No Toxicity	Maintain dose level	Maintain dose level
Neutropenia		
1 (1500 to 1999/mm³)	Maintain dose level	Maintain dose level
2 (1000 to 1499/mm³)	↓1 dose level	Maintain dose level
3 (500 to 999/mm³)	Omit dose until resolved to ≤grade 2 then ↓1 dose level	↓1 dose level
4 (<500/mm³)	Omit dose until resolved to ≤grade 2 then ↓2 dose levels	↓2 dose levels

(cont'd)

Table 8: CAMPTOSAR *(cont'd)*

Recommended Dose Modifications for CAMPTOSAR/5-Fluorouracil(5-FU)/Leucovorin (LV) Combination Schedule

Patients should return to pre-treatment bowel function without requiring antidiarrhea medications for at least 24 hours before the next chemotherapy administration. A new cycle of therapy should not begin until the granulocyte count has recovered to ≥1.5×10⁹/L, and the platelet count has recovered to ≥100×10⁹/L, and treatment-related diarrhea is fully resolved. Treatment should be delayed 1 to 2 weeks to allow for recovery from treatment-related toxicities. If the patient has not recovered after a 2-week delay, consideration should be given to discontinuing therapy.

Toxicity NCI CTC grade[a] (Value)	During a Cycle of Therapy	At the Start of Subsequent Cycles of Therapy[b]
Neutropenic fever (grade 4 neutropenia & ≥grade 2 fever)	Omit dose until resolved then ↓2 dose levels	↓2 dose levels
Other Hematologic Toxicities	Dose modifications for leukopenia or thrombocytopenia during a cycle of therapy and at the start of subsequent cycles of therapy are also based on NCI toxicity criteria and are the same as recommended for neutropenia above.	
Diarrhea		
1 (2–3 stools/day >pretx[c])	Delay dose until resolved to baseline then give same dose	Maintain dose level
2 (4–6 stools/day >pretx[c])	Omit dose until resolved to baseline then ↓1 dose level	Maintain dose level
3 (7–9 stools/day >pretx[c])	Omit dose until resolved to baseline then ↓1 dose level	↓1 dose level
4 (≥10 stools/day >pretx[c])	Omit dose until resolved to baseline then ↓2 dose levels	↓2 dose levels
Other Non-Hematologic Toxicities[d]		
1	Maintain dose level	Maintain dose level
2	Omit dose, then ↓1 dose level when resolved to ≤grade 1	Maintain dose level
3	Omit dose, then ↓1 dose level when resolved to ≤grade 2	↓1 dose level
4	Omit dose, then ↓2 dose levels when resolved to ≤grade 2	↓2 dose levels
	For mucositis/stomatitis decrease only 5-FU, not CAMPTOSAR	**For mucositis/stomatitis decrease only 5-FU, not CAMPTOSAR**

[a] National Cancer Institute Common Toxicity Criteria.
[b] Relative to the starting dose used in the previous cycle.
[c] Pretreatment.
[d] Excludes alopecia, anorexia, asthenia.

CAMPTOSAR Single-Agent Therapy—Dosage Schedules: CAMPTOSAR should be administered as an intravenous infusion over 90 minutes for both the weekly and once-every-3-week dosage schedules. Single-agent dosage regimens are shown in Table 9.

Table 9: CAMPTOSAR

Single-Agent Regimens of CAMPTOSAR and Dose Modifications

Weekly Regimen[a]	125 mg/m² IV over 90 min once-weekly (days 1, 8, 15, 22) followed by a 2-week rest		
	Starting Dose and Modified Dose Levels (mg/m²)		
	Starting Dose	Dose Level-1	Dose Level-2
	125	100	75
Once-Every-3-Week Regimen[b]	350 mg/m² IV over 90 min, once weekly every 3 weeks		
	Starting Dose and Modified Dose Levels (mg/m²)		
	Starting Dose	Dose Level-1	Dose Level-2
	350	300	250

[a] Subsequent doses may be adjusted as high as 150 mg/m² or to as low as 50 mg/m² in 25 to 50 mg/m² decrements depending upon individual patient tolerance.
[b] Subsequent doses may be adjusted as low as 200 mg/m² in 50 mg/m² decrements depending upon individual patient tolerance.

CAMPTOSAR Single-Agent Therapy—Dose Modifications: Patients should be carefully monitored for toxicity and doses of CAMPTOSAR should be modified as necessary to accommodate individual patient tolerance to treatment. Based on recommended dose-levels described in Table 9, Single-Agent Regimens of CAMPTOSAR and Dose-Modifications, subsequent doses should be adjusted as suggested in Table 10, Recommended Dose Modifications for Single-Agent Schedules. The 350 mg/m² dose has not been evaluated in patients who are 70 years and older and the recommended starting dose is therefore 300 mg/m².

Administration: Parenteral Products: The CAMPTOSAR vial is for single use only. Unused portions must be discarded. CAMPTOSAR must be diluted prior to infusion, using 5% Dextrose Injection (preferred) or 0.9% Sodium Chloride Injection to a final concentration range of 0.12 to 3.0 mg/mL. Other drugs should not be added to the infusion solution.

The infusion solutions, when packaged in low-density polyethylene (LDPE) or polyvinyl chloride (PVC) containers, are physically and chemically stable for up to 28 days at controlled room temperature (15 to 30°C) or at refrigerated temperatures (2 to 8°C), if protected from light. If stored at room temperature (15 to 30°C) but exposed to light, the infusion solutions are physically and chemically stable for 72 hours (3 days). **Freezing CAMPTOSAR and admixtures of CAMPTOSAR may result in precipitation of the drug and should be avoided.**

Because of possible microbial contamination during dilution, it is recommended that the admixture be prepared immediately prior to use and infusion commenced as soon as practicable after preparation. If not used immediately, in-use storage times and conditions prior to use are the responsibility of the user and would normally not be longer than 24 hours at 2 to 8°C, or 6 hours at 15 to 30°C, unless reconstitution/dilution has taken place in controlled and validated aseptic conditions.

Parenteral drug products should be inspected visually for particulate matter and discolouration prior to administration whenever solution and container permit.

Table 10: CAMPTOSAR

Recommended Dose Modifications for Single-Agent Schedules[a]

Patients should return to pre-treatment bowel function without requiring antidiarrhea medications for at least 24 hours before the next chemotherapy administration. A new cycle of therapy should not begin until the granulocyte count has recovered to ≥1.5×10⁹/L, and the platelet count has recovered to ≥100×10⁹/L, and treatment-related diarrhea is fully resolved. Treatment should be delayed 1 to 2 weeks to allow for recovery from treatment-related toxicities. If the patient has not recovered after a 2-week delay, consideration should be given to discontinuing therapy.

Toxicity NCI Grade[b] (value)	During a Cycle of Therapy	At the Start of Subsequent Cycles of Therapy (After Adequate Recovery), Compared with the Starting Dose in the Previous Cycle[c]	
	Weekly	Weekly	Once Every 3 Weeks
No Toxicity	Maintain dose level	↑25 mg/m² up to a maximum dose of 150 mg/m²	Maintain dose level
Neutropenia			
1 (1500 to 1999/mm³)	Maintain dose level	Maintain dose level	Maintain dose level
2 (1000 to 1499/mm³)	↓25 mg/m²	Maintain dose level	Maintain dose level
3 (500 to 999/mm³)	Omit dose, then ↓25 mg/m² when resolved to ≤grade 2	↓25 mg/m²	↓50 mg/m²
4 (<500/mm³)	Omit dose, then ↓50 mg/m² when resolved to ≤grade 2	↓50 mg/m²	↓50 mg/m²
Neutropenic Fever (grade 4 neutropenia & ≥grade 2 fever)	Omit dose, then ↓50 mg/m² when resolved	↓50 mg/m²	↓50 mg/m²
Other Hematologic Toxicities	Dose modifications for leukopenia, thrombocytopenia and anemia during a cycle of therapy and at the start of subsequent cycles of therapy are also based on NCI toxicity criteria and are the same as recommended for neutropenia above.		
Diarrhea			
1 (2–3 stools/day >pretx[c])	Maintain dose level	Maintain dose level	Maintain dose level
2 (4–6 stools/day >pretx[c])	↓25 mg/m²	Maintain, if the only grade 2 toxicity	Maintain dose level
3 (7–9 stools/day >pretx[c])	Omit dose, then ↓25 mg/m² when resolved to ≤grade 2	↓25 mg/m², if the only grade 3 toxicity	↓50 mg/m²
4 (≥10 stools/day >pretx[c])	Omit dose, then ↓50 mg/m² when resolved to ≤grade 2	↓50 mg/m²	↓50 mg/m²
Other Non-Hematologic Toxicities[d]			
Grade 1	Maintain dose level	Maintain dose level	Maintain dose level
Grade 2	↓25 mg/m²	↓25 mg/m²	↓50 mg/m²
Grade 3	Omit dose, then ↓25 mg/m² when resolved to ≤grade 2	↓25 mg/m²	↓50 mg/m²
Grade 4	Omit dose, then ↓50 mg/m² when resolved to ≤grade 2	↓50 mg/m²	↓50 mg/m²

a National Cancer Institute Common Toxicity Criteria.
b All dose modifications should be based on the worst preceding toxicity.
c Pretreatment.
d Excludes alopecia, anorexia, asthenia.

OVERDOSAGE:
Single doses of up to 750 mg/m² of CAMPTOSAR (irinotecan hydrochloride trihydrate) have been given in some trials and there have been reports of overdosage at doses up to approximately twice the recommended therapeutic dose, which may be fatal. The most significant adverse reactions reported were severe neutropenia and severe diarrhea. There is no known antidote for overdosage of CAMPTOSAR. Maximum supportive care should be instituted to prevent dehydration due to diarrhea and to treat any infectious complications. Complete blood count (CBC), platelets, electrolytes, liver and renal function should be monitored in cases of overdosage and patients should be monitored for signs and symptoms of respiratory distress.

For management of a suspected drug overdose, contact your **regional Poison Control Centre**. See the *CPS* Directory section for a list of Poison Control Centres.

ACTION AND CLINICAL PHARMACOLOGY: Mechanism of Action: CAMPTOSAR (irinotecan hydrochloride trihydrate) is an antineoplastic agent of the topoisomerase I inhibitor class. Irinotecan is a semi-synthetic derivative of camptothecin, an alkaloid extract from plants such as Camptotheca acuminata. Camptothecins interact specifically with the enzyme topoisomerase I, which relieves torsional strain in DNA by inducing reversible single-strand breaks. Irinotecan and its active metabolite SN-38 bind to the topoisomerase I-DNA complex and prevent religation of these single-strand breaks.

Irinotecan serves as a water-soluble precursor of the lipophilic metabolite SN-38, which is formed from irinotecan primarily by liver carboxylesterase enzymes. The SN-38 metabolite is approximately 1000 times more potent than irinotecan as an inhibitor of topoisomerase I purified from human and rodent tumour cell lines. The precise contribution of SN-38 to the activity of CAMPTOSAR in humans has not been completely defined. Both irinotecan and SN-38 exist in an active lactone form and an inactive hydroxy acid anion form. An acidic pH promotes the formation of the lactone whereas a basic pH favours the hydroxy acid anion form.

Pharmacokinetics: After intravenous infusion of CAMPTOSAR in humans, irinotecan plasma levels decline in a multiexponential manner. A summary of mean irinotecan and SN-38 pharmacokinetic parameters in patients with metastatic carcinoma of the colon and rectum (dosed at 125 or 340 mg/m²) is tabulated in Table 11.

Table 11: CAMPTOSAR

Summary of Mean (±Standard Deviation) Irinotecan and SN-38 Pharmacokinetic Parameters in Patients with Solid Tumors

	125 mg/m² (n=64)		340 mg/m² (n=6)	
	Irinotecan	SN-38	Irinotecan	SN-38
C_{max} (ng/mL)	1660±797	26.3±11.9	3392±874	56.0±28.2
AUC_{0-24} (ng·h/mL)	10 200±3270	229±108	20 604±6027	474±245
$t_{1/2}$ (h)	5.8[a]±0.7	10.4[a]±3.1	11.7[b]±1.0	21.0[b]±4.3
V_{area} (L/m²)	110±48.5	—	234±69.6	—
CL (L/h/m²)	13.3±6.01	—	13.9±4.0	—

a Plasma specimens collected for 24 hours following the end of the 90-minute infusion.
b Plasma specimens collected for 48 hours following the end of the 90-minute infusion. Because of the longer collection period, these values provide a more accurate reflection of the terminal elimination half-lives of irinotecan and SN-38.

Legend: C_{max}=maximum plasma concentration; AUC_{0-24}=area under plasma concentration-time curve from 0 to 24 hours after end of infusion; $t_{1/2}$=terminal elimination half-life; V_{area}=volume of distribution of terminal elimination phase; CL=total systemic clearance.

Over the recommended dose range of 50 to 350 mg/m², the AUC of irinotecan increases linearly with dose. The AUC of SN-38 increases less than proportionally with dose. Irinotecan exhibits moderate plasma protein binding (30 to 68% bound). SN-38 is approximately 95% bound to human plasma proteins, mainly albumin.

The complete disposition of irinotecan in humans has not been fully elucidated. The metabolic conversion of irinotecan to SN-38 is mediated by carboxylesterase enzymes primarily in the liver. SN-38 subsequently undergoes conjugation by UDP-glucuronyl transferase 1A1 (UGT1A1) to form a glucuronide metabolite (SN-38 glucuronide). UGT1A1 enzyme activity is reduced in individuals with certain genetic polymorphisms, such as UGT1A1*28. Approximately 10% of the North American population is homozygous for the UGT1A1*28 allele (also known as UGT1A1 7/7).

In a prospective study, in which irinotecan was administered as a single-agent (350 mg/m²) on a once every 3 week schedule, patients homozygous for the UGT1A1*28 allele (UGT1A1 7/7) had higher systemic exposures to SN-38 than those who were homozygous for the wild-type UGT1A1 allele (UGT1A1 *1/*1) (see Warnings and Precautions, Hematologic and Adverse Reactions, Hematology). The urinary excretion of irinotecan (11 to 20%), SN-38 (<1%), and SN-38 glucuronide (3%) is low.

Irinotecan is oxidized by cytochrome P450 isozyme 3A4 (CYP3A4) to yield two relatively inactive metabolites, APC (7-ethyl-l0-[4-N-(5-aminopentanoic acid)-l-piperidino]-carbonyloxycamptothecin) and the minor metabolite, NPC (7-ethyl-l0-(4 amino-1-piperidino)carbonyloxycamptothecin). See Figure 1.

Figure 1: CAMPTOSAR

Metabolism

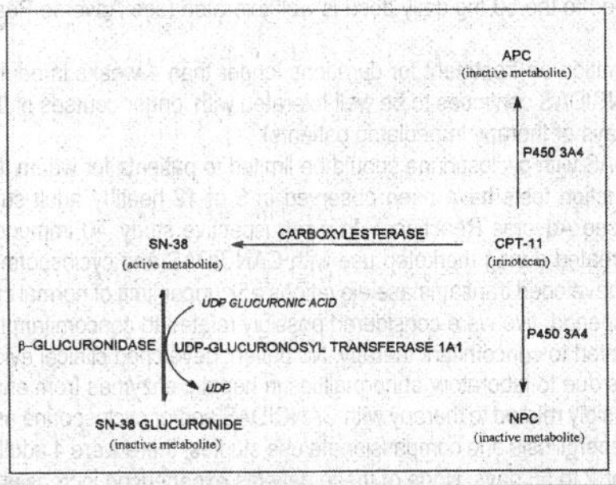

In one pharmacokinetic study of patients administered a starting dose of irinotecan 125 mg/m², the terminal half-life of irinotecan was statistically significantly longer in patients who were 65 years or older compared to patients younger than 65 years (6.0 hours versus 5.5 hours, respectively). Dose-normalized AUC_{0-24} was 14.8% higher, C_{max} was 11.3% higher and clearance was 17.5% lower in patients 65 years and older compared with patients younger than 65 years. Also, dose normalized AUC_{0-24} of SN-38 was 11.2% higher in subjects age 65 years and over compared to subjects less than 65 years, but this result was not statistically significant.

In a different pharmacokinetic study that was prospectively designed to investigate the effect of age on irinotecan toxicity, no statistically significant differences in irinotecan pharmacokinetics were seen in patients ≥65 years compared to those <65 years administered a single 125 mg/m² irinotecan dose. Irinotecan C_{max} and AUC_{0-24} were, respectively, 0.7% and 0.3% lower in patients ≥65 years compared to patients who were <65 years. Values for SN-38 C_{max} and AUC_{0-24} were, respectively, 1.8% lower and 0.8% higher in patients ≥65 years compared to patients <65 years and values for SN-38 glucuronide C_{max} and AUC_{0-24} were, respectively, 1.0% and 3.1% lower in patients ≥65 years compared to patients who were <65 years.

The reason for the conflicting results between the two pharmacokinetic studies is not known. Clinically, however, particular caution should be exercised when administering irinotecan to elderly patients as these patients may be less tolerant of the toxic effects of the drug. See Warnings and Precautions and Adverse Reactions, Adverse Drug Reaction Overview.

Special Populations and Conditions: Renal Insufficiency: The influence of renal insufficiency on the pharmacokinetics of irinotecan has not been formally studied.

Hepatic Insufficiency: Irinotecan clearance is diminished in patients with hepatic dysfunction while relative exposure to the active metabolite SN-38 is increased. The magnitude of these effects is proportional to the degree of liver impairment as measured by elevations in serum total bilirubin and transaminase concentrations (see Dosage and Administration and Warnings and Precautions).

Gender: There is no clinically important gender influence on the pharmacokinetics of irinotecan; the influence of race has not been studied.

STORAGE AND STABILITY: Store at controlled room temperature (15 to 30°C). Protect from light. CAMPTOSAR (irinotecan hydrochloride trihydrate) is available in an amber-coloured polypropylene vial or in an amber glass vial that is packaged in plastic blister to protect from breakage. It is recommended that the vial remain in the carton until time of use. The CAMPTOSAR glass vial should be inspected for damage and visible signs of leaks before removing the plastic blister. If there are signs of breakage or leakage from the vial, do not open the plastic blister. Incinerate the unopened package.

SPECIAL HANDLING INSTRUCTIONS: As with other potentially toxic anti-cancer agents, care should be exercised in the handling and preparation of infusion solutions containing CAMPTOSAR (irinotecan hydrochloride trihydrate). Preparation of CAMPTOSAR should be done in a vertical laminar flow hood. The use of gloves, safety glasses and protective clothing is recommended. If CAMPTOSAR solution contacts the skin, wash the skin immediately and thoroughly with soap and water. If CAMPTOSAR contacts the mucous membranes, flush thoroughly with water. All waste material that has come in contact with CAMPTOSAR should be properly segregated, sealed and incinerated.

INFORMATION FOR THE PATIENT: Published in e-CPS, available by subscription at www.e-cps.ca.

DOSAGE FORMS, COMPOSITION AND PACKAGING: Each mL of sterile, clear, light yellow aqueous solution contains: irinotecan HCl trihydrate 20 mg. Nonmedicinal ingredients: lactic acid, sorbitol and water for injection. Sodium hydroxide and/or hydrochloric acid may be used to adjust the pH to 3.0 to 3.8. Single use vials of 2, 5 and 15 mL.

Cancidas® 🄿
caspofungin acetate
Antifungal

Merck Frosst

Date of Revision: April 15, 2010

SUMMARY PRODUCT INFORMATION:

Route of Administration	Dosage Form/ Strength	Clinically Relevant Nonmedicinal Ingredients
Intravenous infusion	50 mg vial, 70 mg vial	For a complete listing see Dosage Forms, Composition and Packaging.

DESCRIPTION: CANCIDAS (caspofungin acetate) is a sterile, lyophilized product for intravenous (IV) infusion that contains a semisynthetic lipopeptide (echinocandin) compound synthesized from a fermentation product of Glarea lozoyensis. CANCIDAS is a member of a class of antifungal drugs (echinocandins) that inhibits the synthesis of β (1, 3)-D-glucan, an integral component of the fungal cell wall.

INDICATIONS AND CLINICAL USE: CANCIDAS is indicated for use in adults and children 12 months and older for:

- Empirical therapy for presumed fungal infections in febrile, neutropenic patients.
- Treatment of Invasive Candidiasis including candidemia, intra-abdominal abscesses, peritonitis and pleural space infections. CANCIDAS has not been studied in candida endocarditis, osteomyelitis or meningitis.
- Treatment of Esophageal Candidiasis.
- Treatment of Invasive Aspergillosis in patients who are refractory to or intolerant of other therapies. The indication is based on results from an open-label, non-comparative study that enrolled 69 adult patients with documented invasive aspergillosis refractory to or intolerant of other therapies. CANCIDAS has not been studied as initial therapy for invasive aspergillosis.

Geriatrics (≥65 years of age): In a limited number of patients ≥65 years of age, no overall differences in safety or efficacy have been observed between elderly and younger patients.

Pediatrics (≤17 years of age): The safety and effectiveness of CANCIDAS in pediatric patients aged 12 months to 17 years of age are supported by evidence from adequate and well-controlled studies in adults, pharmacokinetic data in pediatric patients and additional data from prospective studies in pediatric patients 12 months to 17 years of age.

CANCIDAS has not been studied in pediatric patients with Candida endocarditis, osteomyelitis, and meningitis. CANCIDAS has also not been studied as initial therapy for invasive aspergillosis in pediatric patients.

The safety and efficacy of CANCIDAS has not been adequately studied in neonates and infants under 3 months of age and children aged 3 to 11 months.

CONTRAINDICATIONS: CANCIDAS is contraindicated in patients with hypersensitivity to any component of this product.

WARNINGS AND PRECAUTIONS: General: The efficacy of a 70 mg dose regimen in adult patients who are not clinically responding to the 50 mg daily dose is not known. Limited safety data suggest that an increase in dose to 70 mg daily in patients who have not clinically responded to the 50 mg daily dose is well tolerated (see Adverse Reactions and Dosage and Administration).

There is limited safety information on treatment for durations longer than 4 weeks in adult and pediatric patients; however, available data suggest that CANCIDAS continues to be well tolerated with longer courses of therapy (up to 162 days of therapy in adult patients and up to 87 days of therapy in pediatric patients).

Concomitant use of CANCIDAS with cyclosporine should be limited to patients for whom the potential benefit outweighs the potential risk. Elevated liver function tests have been observed in 5 of 12 healthy adult subjects who received concomitant CANCIDAS and cyclosporine (see Adverse Reactions). In a retrospective study, 40 immunocompromised patients, including 37 transplant recipients, were treated during marketed use with CANCIDAS and cyclosporine for 1 to 290 days (median 17.5 days). Fourteen patients (35%) developed transaminase elevations >5× upper limit of normal or >3× baseline during concomitant therapy or the 14-day follow-up period; five were considered possibly related to concomitant therapy. One patient had elevated bilirubin considered possibly related to concomitant therapy. No patient developed clinical evidence of hepatotoxicity or serious hepatic events. Discontinuations due to laboratory abnormalities in hepatic enzymes from any cause occurred in four patients. Of these, 2 were considered possibly related to therapy with CANCIDAS and/or cyclosporine as well as to other possible causes.

In the prospective invasive aspergillosis and compassionate use studies, there were 4 adult patients treated with CANCIDAS (50 mg/day) and cyclosporine for 2 to 56 days. None of these patients experienced increases in hepatic enzymes.

Given the limitations of these data, CANCIDAS and cyclosporine should only be used concomitantly in those patients for whom the potential benefit outweighs the potential risk. Patients who develop abnormal liver function tests during concomitant therapy should be monitored and the risk/benefit of continuing therapy should be evaluated.

Hepatic/Biliary/Pancreatic: Laboratory abnormalities in liver function tests have been seen in healthy volunteers and adult and pediatric patients treated with CANCIDAS. In some adult and pediatric patients with serious underlying conditions who were receiving multiple concomitant medications with CANCIDAS, cases of clinically significant hepatic dysfunction, hepatitis and hepatic failure have been reported; a causal relationship to CANCIDAS has not been established. Patients who develop abnormal liver function tests during CANCIDAS therapy should be monitored for evidence of worsening hepatic function and the risk/benefit of continuing CANCIDAS therapy should be re-evaluated.

Special Populations: Pregnant Women: There are no adequate and well controlled studies in pregnant women. CANCIDAS should be used in pregnancy only if the potential benefit justifies the potential risk to the fetus.

Caspofungin was shown to be embryotoxic in rats and rabbits. Findings included incomplete ossification of the skull and torso and an increased incidence of cervical rib in rats. An increased incidence of incomplete ossifications of the talus/calcaneus was seen in rabbits. Caspofungin also produced increases in resorptions in rats and rabbits and periimplantation losses in rats. These findings were observed at doses which produced exposures similar to those seen in patients treated with a 70 mg dose. Caspofungin crossed the placental barrier in rats and rabbits and was detected in the plasma of fetuses of pregnant animals dosed with CANCIDAS.

Nursing Women: It is not known whether caspofungin is excreted in human milk. Caspofungin has been found in the milk of lactating laboratory animals. Women receiving CANCIDAS should not breast-feed.

Pediatrics (≤17 years of age): The safety and effectiveness of CANCIDAS in pediatric patients aged 12 months to 17 years of age are supported by evidence from adequate and well-controlled studies in adults, pharmacokinetic data in pediatric patients and additional data from prospective studies in pediatric patients 12 months to 17 years of age.

The safety and efficacy of CANCIDAS has not been adequately studied in neonates and infants under 3 months of age and children aged 3 to 11 months.

Postmarketing hepatobiliary adverse reactions have been reported in pediatric patients with serious underlying medical conditions (see Warnings and Precautions, Hepatic/Biliary/Pancreatic).

Geriatrics (≥65 years of age): Clinical studies of CANCIDAS did not include sufficient numbers of patients aged 65 and over to determine whether they respond differently from younger patients. In a limited number of patients ≥65 years of age, no overall differences in safety or efficacy have been observed between elderly and younger patients. Plasma concentrations of caspofungin in healthy older men and women (≥65 years of age) were increased slightly (approximately 28% in area under the curve [AUC]) compared to young healthy men. In patients who were treated empirically or who had invasive candidiasis, a similar modest effect of age was seen in older patients relative to younger patients. No dose adjustment is recommended for the elderly; however, greater sensitivity of some older individuals cannot be ruled out.

Patients with Special Diseases or Conditions : Hepatic Insufficiency: Adult patients with mild hepatic insufficiency (Child-Pugh score 5 to 6) do not need a dosage adjustment. For adult patients with moderate hepatic insufficiency (Child-Pugh score 7 to 9), CANCIDAS 35 mg daily is recommended based upon pharmacokinetic data. However, where recommended, a 70 mg loading dose should still be administered on Day 1. There is no clinical experience in adult patients with severe hepatic insufficiency (Child-Pugh score >9) and in pediatric patients with any degree of hepatic insufficiency (see Dosage and Administration).

Renal Insufficiency: Mild to advanced renal insufficiency does not alter significantly caspofungin plasma concentrations and does not require a change in dosing. Caspofungin is not dialyzable, thus supplementary dosing is not required following hemodialysis.

ADVERSE REACTIONS: Adverse Drug Reaction Overview: Possible histamine-mediated symptoms have been reported including reports of rash, facial swelling, pruritus, or sensation of warmth or bronchospasm. Anaphylaxis has been reported during administration of CANCIDAS.

Adverse Drug Reaction Overview from Clinical Trials in Adult Patients: In clinical studies, 1865 adult individuals received single or multiple doses of CANCIDAS: 564 febrile, neutropenic patients (empirical therapy study), 382 patients with invasive candidiasis, 297 patients with esophageal and/or oropharyngeal candidiasis, 228 patients with invasive aspergillosis, and 394 individuals in phase I studies. In the empirical therapy study patients had received chemotherapy for malignancy or had undergone hematopoietic stem-cell transplantation. In the studies involving patients with documented Candida infections, the majority of the patients had serious underlying medical conditions (e.g., hematologic or other malignancy, recent major surgery, HIV [with CD4 counts less than 50/mm³]) requiring multiple concomitant medications. Patients in the noncomparative Aspergillus study often had serious predisposing medical conditions (e.g., bone marrow or peripheral stem cell transplants, hematologic malignancy, solid tumors or organ transplants) requiring multiple concomitant medications.

Reported drug related clinical and laboratory abnormalities among all adults treated with CANCIDAS (total 1780) were typically mild and rarely led to discontinuation.

Common (>1/100)	General	Fever, headache, chills, abdominal pain, pain
	GI	Nausea, diarrhea, vomiting
	Liver	Elevated liver enzyme levels (AST, ALT, alkaline phosphatase, direct and total bilirubin)
	Kidney	Increased serum creatinine
	Blood	Anemia (decreased hemoglobin and hematocrit)
	Cardiac	Tachycardia
	Metabolism	Hypokalaemia (blood potassium decreased)
	Peripheral Vascular	Phlebitis/thrombophlebitis, infusion-site pruritus, infused-vein complication, flushing
	Bone	Arthralgia
	Respiratory	Dyspnea
	Skin	Rash, pruritus, sweating, erythema

Adverse Drug Reaction Overview from Clinical Trials in Pediatric Patients: In clinical studies, 171 pediatric patients received single or multiple doses of CANCIDAS: 104 febrile, neutropenic patients; 56 patients with invasive candidiasis; 1 patient with esophageal candidiasis; and 10 patients with invasive aspergillosis. The overall clinical safety profile of CANCIDAS in pediatric patients is comparable to that in adult patients.

Reported drug-related clinical and laboratory abnormalities among all pediatric patients treated with CANCIDAS (total 171) were typically mild and rarely led to discontinuation.

Common (>1/100)	General	Fever, headache, chills
	Liver	Elevated liver enzyme levels (AST, ALT)
	Cardiac	Tachycardia
	Peripheral Vascular	Catheter site pain, flushing, hypotension
	Skin	Rash, pruritus

Clinical Trial Adverse Drug Reactions: Because clinical trials are conducted under very specific conditions the adverse reaction rates observed in the clinical trials may not reflect the rates observed in practice and should not be compared to the rates in the clinical trials of another drug. Adverse drug reaction information from clinical trials is useful for identifying drug-related adverse events and for approximating rates.

Clinical Trial Experience in Adult Patients: Empirical Therapy: In the randomized, double-blinded empirical therapy study, patients received either CANCIDAS 50 mg/day (following a 70 mg loading dose) or AmBisome (amphotericin B liposome for injection) (3.0 mg/kg/day). Drug-related clinical adverse experiences occurring in ≥2% of the patients in either treatment group are presented in Table 1.

Table 1: CANCIDAS

Drug-Related[a] Clinical Adverse Experiences Among Patients with Persistent Fever and Neutropenia. Incidence ≥2% for at Least One Treatment Group by Body System

	CANCIDAS 50 mg[b] N=564 % (n)	AmBisome 3 mg/kg[c] N=547 % (n)
Clinical Adverse Experiences	47.0 (265)	59.6 (326)
Body as a Whole		
Fever	17.0 (96)	19.4 (106)
Chills	13.8 (78)	24.7 (135)
Perspiration/Diaphoresis	2.8 (16)	2.2 (12)
Flushing	1.8 (10)	4.2 (23)
Abdominal Pain	1.4 (8)	2.4 (13)
Cardiovascular System		
Tachycardia	1.4 (8)	2.4 (13)
Hypertension	1.1 (6)	2.0 (11)
Digestive System		
Nausea	3.5 (20)	11.3 (62)
Vomiting	3.5 (20)	8.6 (47)
Diarrhea	2.7 (15)	2.4 (13)
Metabolism and Nutrition		

(cont'd)

Table 1: CANCIDAS *(cont'd)*

Drug-Related[a] Clinical Adverse Experiences Among Patients with Persistent Fever and Neutropenia. Incidence ≥2% for at Least One Treatment Group by Body System

	CANCIDAS 50 mg[b] N=564 % (n)	AmBisome 3 mg/kg[c] N=547 % (n)
Hypokalemia	3.7 (21)	4.2 (23)
Musculoskeletal System		
Back Pain	0.7 (4)	2.7 (15)
Nervous System & Psychiatric		
Headache	4.3 (24)	5.7 (31)
Respiratory System		
Dyspnea	2.0 (11)	4.2 (23)
Tachypnea	0.4 (2)	2.0 (11)
Skin & Skin Appendage		
Rash	6.2 (35)	5.3 (29)

[a] Determined by the investigator to be possibly, probably, or definitely drug-related.
[b] 70 mg on Day 1, then 50 mg daily for the remainder of treatment; daily dose was increased to 70 mg for 73 patients.
[c] 3.0 mg/kg/day; daily dose was increased to 5.0 mg/kg for 74 patients.

The proportion of patients with drug-related clinical adverse experiences was higher in the AmBisome group (59.6%) than in the CANCIDAS group (47.0%). Only rash, perspiration, and diarrhea were numerically higher in the CANCIDAS group with the remaining adverse experiences being numerically higher in the AmBisome group. Numerically higher frequencies of clinical adverse experiences were observed in the CANCIDAS group compared with the AmBisome group for serious rash (4 vs 0), discontinuations due to drug-related adverse experiences in the skin/skin appendages (10 vs 3), discontinuations due to drug-related hepatobiliary adverse events (4 vs 0).

Also reported was an isolated, serious adverse experience of hyperbilirubinemia considered possibly related to CANCIDAS.

Infusion-related Reactions: The proportion of patients who experienced an infusion-related adverse event was significantly lower ($p<0.001$) in the group treated with CANCIDAS (35.1%) than in the group treated with AmBisome (51.6%).

The frequency of severe infusion-related fever was higher in the CANCIDAS group compared with the AmBisome group (12 vs 6). However, the frequency of moderate or severe infusion-related fever was lower in the CANCIDAS group than in the AmBisome group (61 vs 76).

Invasive Candidiasis: In an initial randomized, double-blinded invasive candidiasis study, patients received either CANCIDAS 50 mg/day (following a 70 mg loading dose) or amphotericin B 0.6 to 1.0 mg/kg/day. Drug-related clinical adverse experiences occurring in ≥2% of the patients in either treatment group are presented in Table 2.

Table 2: CANCIDAS

Drug-Related Clinical Adverse Experiences Among Patients with Invasive Candidiasis[a]. Incidence ≥2% for at Least One Treatment Group by Body System

	CANCIDAS 50 mg[b] (n=114) % (n)	Amphotericin B 0.6–1.0 mg/kg (n=125) % (n)
Body as a Whole		
Fever	7.0 (8)	23.2 (29)
Chills	5.3 (6)	26.4 (33)
Cardiovascular System		
Hypertension	1.8 (2)	6.4 (8)
Tachycardia	1.8 (2)	10.4 (13)
Hypotension	0.9 (1)	2.4 (3)
Peripheral Vascular System		
Phlebitis/Thrombophlebitis	3.5 (4)	4.8 (6)
Digestive System		
Vomiting	3.5 (4)	8.0 (10)
Diarrhea	2.6 (3)	0.8 (1)
Nausea	1.8 (2)	5.6 (7)
Jaundice	0.9 (1)	3.2 (4)
Metabolic/Nutritional/Immune		
Hypokalemia	0.9 (1)	5.6 (7)
Nervous System & Psychiatric		
Tremor	1.8 (2)	2.4 (3)
Respiratory System		
Tachypnea	0	10.4 (13)
Skin & Skin Appendage		

(cont'd)

Table 2: CANCIDAS *(cont'd)*

Drug-Related Clinical Adverse Experiences Among Patients with Invasive Candidiasis[a]. Incidence ≥2% for at Least One Treatment Group by Body System

	CANCIDAS 50 mg[b] (n=114) % (n)	Amphotericin B 0.6–1.0 mg/kg (n=125) % (n)
Rash	0.9 (1)	3.2 (4)
Sweating	0.9 (1)	3.2 (4)
Erythema	0	2.4 (3)
Urogenital System		
Renal Insufficiency	0.9 (1)	5.6 (7)
Renal Insufficiency, acute	0	5.6 (7)

[a] Determined by the investigator to be possibly, probably, or definitely drug related.
[b] Patients received CANCIDAS 70 mg on Day 1, then 50 mg daily for the remainder of their treatment.

The incidence of drug-related clinical adverse experiences was significantly lower among patients treated with CANCIDAS (28.9%) than among patients treated with amphotericin B (58.4%). Also, the proportion of patients who experienced an infusion-related adverse event was significantly lower in the CANCIDAS group (20.2%) than in the amphotericin B group (48.8%).

In a second randomized, double-blinded invasive candidiasis study, patients received either CANCIDAS 50 mg/day (following a 70 mg loading dose) or CANCIDAS 150 mg/day. Drug-related clinical adverse experiences occurring in ≥2.0% of the patients in either treatment group are presented in Table 3. In addition, the proportion of patients who experienced any adverse reaction was similar in the 2 treatment groups; however, this study was not large enough to detect differences in rare or unexpected adverse events. In this study, three (3.0%) patients in the 150 mg group and none in the 70/50 mg group had at least one serious drug-related adverse experience (toxic hepatitis, leukopenia, and hyperbilirubinemia).

Table 3: CANCIDAS

Drug-Related[a] Clinical Adverse Experiences Among Patients with Invasive Candidiasis Incidence ≥2.0% for at Least One Treatment Group by System Organ Class or Preferred Term

Adverse Experience (MedDRA v11.0 System Organ Class and Preferred Term)	CANCIDAS 50 mg[b] N=104 (percent)	CANCIDAS 150 mg N=100 (percent)
All Systems, Any Adverse Experience	**13.5**	**14.0**
General Disorders and Administration Site Conditions	**6.7**	**7.0**
Injection site erythema	0.0	2.0
Injection site phlebitis	3.8	2.0
Injection site swelling	1.0	2.0
Metabolism and Nutrition Disorders	**1.9**	**2.0**
Hypokalemia	1.0	2.0
Nervous System Disorders	**0.0**	**2.0**
Headache	0.0	2.0

[a] Determined by the investigator to be possibly, probably, or definitely drug-related. Within any system organ class, individuals may experience more than 1 adverse experience.
[b] Patients received CANCIDAS 70 mg on Day 1, then 50 mg daily for the remainder of their treatment.

Esophageal and/or Oropharyngeal Candidiasis: Drug-related clinical adverse experiences occurring in ≥2% of patients with esophageal and/or oropharyngeal candidiasis are presented in Table 4.

Table 4: CANCIDAS

Drug-Related Clinical Adverse Experiences Among Patients with Esophageal and/or Oropharyngeal Candidiasis[a]. Incidence ≥2% for at Least One Treatment Dose (Per Comparison) by Body System

	CANCIDAS 50 mg[b] (N=83) % (n)	Fluconazole 200 mg[b] (N=94) % (n)	CANCIDAS 50 mg[c] (N=80) % (n)	CANCIDAS 70 mg[c] (N=65) % (n)	Amphotericin B 0.5 mg/kg[c] (N=89) % (n)
Body as a Whole					
Fever	3.6 (3)	1.1 (1)	21.3 (17)	26.2 (17)	69.7 (62)
Pain, abdominal	3.6 (3)	2.1 (2)	2.5 (2)	†	9.0 (8)
Chills	†	†	2.5 (2)	1.5 (1)	75.3 (67)
Pain	†	†	1.3 (1)	4.6 (3)	5.6 (5)
Edema, facial	†	†	†	3.1 (2)	†
Flu-like Illness	†	†	†	3.1 (2)	†
Warm Sensation	†	†	†	1.5 (1)	4.5 (4)
Asthenia/Fatigue	†	†	†	†	6.7 (6)
Malaise	†	†	†	†	5.6 (5)
Edema/Swelling	†	†	†	†	5.6 (5)
Cardiovascular System					

(cont'd)

Table 4: CANCIDAS *(cont'd)*

Drug-Related Clinical Adverse Experiences Among Patients with Esophageal and/or Oropharyngeal Candidiasis[a], Incidence ≥2% for at Least One Treatment Dose (Per Comparison) by Body System

	CANCIDAS 50 mg[b] (N=83) % (n)	Fluconazole 200 mg[b] (N=94) % (n)	CANCIDAS 50 mg[c] (N=80) % (n)	CANCIDAS 70 mg[c] (N=65) % (n)	Amphotericin B 0.5 mg/kg[c] (N=89) % (n)
Tachycardia	†	†	1.3 (1)	†	4.5 (4)
Vasculitis	†	†	†	†	3.4 (3)
Peripheral Vascular					
Infused Vein Complication	12.0 (10)	8.5 (8)	2.5 (2)	1.5 (1)	†
Phlebitis/ Thrombophlebitis	15.7 (13)	8.5 (8)	11.3 (9)	13.8 (9)	22.5 (20)
Digestive System					
Nausea	6.0 (5)	6.4 (6)	2.5 (2)	3.1 (2)	21.3 (19)
Diarrhea	3.6 (3)	2.1 (2)	1.3 (1)	3.1 (2)	11.2 (10)
Vomiting	1.2 (1)	3.2 (3)	1.3 (1)	3.1 (2)	13.5 (12)
Anorexia	†	†	1.3 (1)	†	3.4 (3)
Gastritis	†	2.1 (2)	†	†	†
Musculoskeletal System					
Myalgia	1.2 (1)	†	†	3.1 (2)	2.2 (2)
Pain, back	†	†	†	†	2.2 (2)
Pain, musculoskeletal	†	†	1.3 (1)	†	4.5 (4)
Hemic & Lymphatic System					
Anemia	†	†	3.8 (3)	†	9.0 (8)
Metabolic/Nutritional/Immune					
Anaphylaxis	†	†	†	†	2.2 (2)
Nervous System & Psychiatric					
Headache	6.0 (5)	1.1 (1)	11.3 (9)	7.7 (5)	19.1 (17)
Insomnia	1.2 (1)	†	†	†	2.2 (2)
Paresthesia	†	†	1.3 (1)	3.1 (2)	1.1 (1)
Dizziness	†	2.1 (2)	†	1.5 (1)	1.1 (1)
Tremor	†	†	†	†	7.9 (7)
Respiratory System					
Tachypnea	†	†	1.3 (1)	†	4.5 (4)
Skin & Skin Appendage					
Pruritus	1.2 (1)	†	2.5 (2)	1.5 (1)	†
Erythema	1.2 (1)	†	1.3 (1)	1.5 (1)	7.9 (7)
Rash	†	†	1.3 (1)	4.6 (3)	3.4 (3)
Sweating	†	†	1.3 (1)	†	3.4 (3)
Induration	†	†	†	3.1 (2)	6.7 (6)

[a] Relationship to drug was determined by the investigator to be possibly, probably, or definitely drug related. Patients who received CANCIDAS 35 mg daily in these studies are not included in this table.
[b] Derived from a Phase III comparator-controlled clinical study.
[c] Derived from Phase II comparator-controlled clinical studies.
Legend: †=incidence 0.0%.

Invasive Aspergillosis: In the open-label, noncomparative aspergillosis study, in which patients received CANCIDAS (70 mg loading dose on Day 1 followed by 50 mg daily), the following drug-related clinical adverse experiences were observed with an incidence of ≥2%: fever (2.9%), infused-vein complications (2.9%), nausea (2.9%), vomiting (2.9%) and flushing (2.9%).

Also reported in this patient population were pulmonary edema, adult respiratory distress syndrome (ARDS), and radiographic infiltrates.

Clinical Trial Experience in Pediatric Patients: The overall safety of caspofungin was assessed in 171 pediatric patients who received single or multiple doses of CANCIDAS: 104 febrile, neutropenic patients; 56 patients with invasive candidiasis; 1 patient with esophageal candidiasis; and 10 patients with invasive aspergillosis. Table 5 shows the incidence of drug-related clinical adverse experiences reported in ≥2.0% of pediatric patients in clinical studies. The most common drug-related clinical adverse experiences in pediatric patients treated with CANCIDAS were fever (11.7%), rash (4.7%), and headache (2.9%).

One patient (0.6%) receiving CANCIDAS, and three patients (11.5%) receiving AmBisome developed a serious drug-related clinical adverse experience. Two patients (1.2%) were discontinued from CANCIDAS and three patients (11.5%) were discontinued from AmBisome due to a drug-related clinical adverse experience. The proportion of patients who experienced an infusion-related adverse event was 21.6% in the group treated with CANCIDAS and 34.6% in the group treated with AmBisome.

Table 5: CANCIDAS

Drug-Related Clinical Adverse Experiences Among Pediatric Patients[a], Incidence ≥2% for at Least One Treatment Dose by Body System

	CANCIDAS Any dose[b] N=171 (%)	CANCIDAS 50 mg/m2[c] N=56 (%)	AmBisome 3 mg/kg[c] N=26 (%)
Cardiac Disorders			
Tachycardia	1.2	1.8	11.5
Gastrointestinal Disorders			
Nausea	0.0	0.0	3.8
Vomiting	0.6	1.8	7.7
General Disorders & Administration Site Conditions			
Adverse Drug Reaction	0.0	0.0	3.8
Catheter Site Pain	1.2	3.6	0.0
Chills	1.8	1.8	7.7
Fever	11.7	28.6	23.1
Hepatobiliary Disorders			
Hepatitis, toxic	0.0	0.0	3.8
Hyperbilirubinemia	0.0	0.0	3.8
Jaundice	0.0	0.0	3.8
Metabolism & Nutrition Disorders			
Hypokaliemia	0.6	0.0	3.8
Nervous System Disorders			
Headache	2.9	8.9	0.0
Respiratory, Thoracic, & Mediastinal Disorders			
Dyspnea	0.0	0.0	3.8
Laryngospasm	0.0	0.0	3.8
Skin & Subcutaneous Tissue Disorders			
Angioneurotic Edema	0.0	0.0	3.8
Circumoral Edema	0.0	0.0	3.8
Pruritus	1.8	3.6	0.0
Rash	4.7	8.9	0.0
Vascular Disorders			
Flushing	1.8	3.6	0.0
Hypotension	1.8	3.6	3.8

[a] Relationship to drug was determined by the investigator to be possibly, probably or definitely drug-related.
[b] Derived from all pediatric clinical studies.
[c] Derived from Phase II comparator-controlled clinical study of empirical therapy.

Abnormal Hematologic and Clinical Chemistry Findings: Laboratory Abnormalities in Adult Patients: Empirical Therapy: Drug-related laboratory adverse experiences occurring in ≥2% of the patients in either treatment group are presented in Table 6.

Table 6: CANCIDAS

Drug-Related[a] Laboratory Adverse Experiences Among Patients with Persistent Fever and Neutropenia. Incidence ≥2% for at Least One Treatment Group by Laboratory Test Category

	CANCIDAS 50 mg[b] N=564 % (n)†	AmBisome 3.0 mg/kg[c] N=547 % (n)†
Drug Related Laboratory Abnormalities	22.5 (127)	32.0 (175)
Blood Chemistry		
Alanine aminotransferase increased	8.7 (49)	8.9 (48)
Alkaline phosphatase increased	7.0 (39)	12.0 (65)
Aspartate aminotransferase increased	7.0 (39)	7.6 (41)
Direct serum bilirubin increased	2.6 (10)	5.2 (20)
Total serum bilirubin increased	3.0 (17)	5.2 (28)

(cont'd)

Table 6: CANCIDAS *(cont'd)*

Drug-Related[a] Laboratory Adverse Experiences Among Patients with Persistent Fever and Neutropenia. Incidence ≥2% for at Least One Treatment Group by Laboratory Test Category

	CANCIDAS 50 mg[b] N=564 % (n)†	AmBisome 3.0 mg/kg[c] N=547 % (n)†
Hypokalemia	7.3 (41)	11.8 (64)
Hypomagnesemia	2.3 (12)	2.6 (13)
Serum creatinine increased	1.2 (7)	5.5 (30)

a Determined by the investigator to be possibly, probably, or definitely drug-related.
b 70 mg on Day 1, then 50 mg daily for the remainder of treatment; daily dose was increased to 70 mg for 73 patients.
c 3.0 mg/kg/day; daily dose was increased to 5.0 mg/kg for 74 patients.
Legend: †=Not all tests were conducted for some patients.

The proportion of patients with drug-related laboratory adverse experiences was higher in the AmBisome group (32.0%) than in the CANCIDAS group (22.5%). Each drug-related laboratory adverse experience with a frequency of ≥2% in at least one treatment group was numerically higher in the AmBisome group than in the CANCIDAS group.

Numerically higher frequencies of clinically significant laboratory abnormalities were observed in the CANCIDAS group compared with the AmBisome group for increased AST >2.5×ULN (9.7% vs 5.1%), increased AST >2.5×baseline (30.0% vs 27.9%); and increased ALT >2.5×baseline (30.4% vs 27.6%). Numerically lower frequencies of clinically significant laboratory abnormalities were observed in the CANCIDAS group than the AmBisome group for increased alkaline phosphatase >2.5×ULN (6.5% vs 10.6%), increased alkaline phosphatase >2.5×baseline (10.6% vs 20.4%), and increased total bilirubin >2.5×ULN (7.1% vs 9.7%). The frequencies of other clinically significant laboratory abnormalities were similar in the two groups.

Nephrotoxicity: To evaluate the effect of CANCIDAS and AmBisome on renal function, nephrotoxicity was defined as doubling of serum creatinine relative to baseline or an increase of ≥1 mg/dL in serum creatinine if baseline serum creatinine was above the upper limit of the normal range. Among patients whose baseline creatinine clearance was >30 mL/min, the incidence of nephrotoxicity was significantly lower in the group treated with CANCIDAS (2.6%) than in the group treated with AmBisome (11.5%).

Invasive Candidiasis: The incidence of drug-related laboratory adverse experiences in patients with invasive candidiasis was significantly lower among patients receiving CANCIDAS (24.3%) than among patients receiving amphotericin B (54.0%).

Drug-related laboratory adverse experiences occurring in ≥2% of the patients in an initial invasive candidiasis study are presented in Table 7.

Table 7: CANCIDAS

Drug-Related Laboratory Adverse Experiences Among Patients with Invasive Candidiasis[a]. Incidence ≥2% for at Least One Treatment Group by Laboratory Test Category

	CANCIDAS 50 mg[b] (n=114) % (n)†	Amphotericin B 0.6–1.0 mg/kg (n=125) % (n)†
Blood Chemistry		
ALT increased	3.7 (4)	8.1 (10)
AST increased	1.9 (2)	9.0 (11)
Blood urea increased	1.9 (2)	15.8 (19)
Direct serum bilirubin increased	3.8 (3)	8.4 (8)
Serum alkaline phosphatase increased	8.3 (9)	15.6 (19)
Serum bicarbonate decreased	0	3.6 (4)
Serum creatinine increased	3.7 (4)	22.6 (28)
Serum phosphate increased	0	2.7 (3)
Serum potassium decreased	9.9 (11)	23.4 (29)
Serum potassium increased	0.9 (1)	2.4 (3)
Total serum bilirubin increased	2.8 (3)	8.9 (11)
Hematology		
Hematocrit decreased	0.9 (1)	7.3 (9)
Hemoglobin decreased	0.9 (1)	10.5 (13)
Urinalysis		
Urine protein increased	0	3.7 (4)

a Determined by the investigator to be possibly, probably, or definitely drug related.
b Patients received CANCIDAS 70 mg on Day 1, then 50 mg daily for the remainder of their treatment.
Legend: †=Not all tests were conducted for some patients.

The percentage of patients with either a drug-related clinical adverse experience or a drug-related laboratory adverse experience was significantly lower among patients receiving CANCIDAS (42.1%) than among patients receiving amphotericin B (75.2%). Furthermore, a significant difference between the two treatment groups was observed with regard to incidence of discontinuation due to drug-related clinical or laboratory adverse experience; incidences were 3/114 (2.6%) in the CANCIDAS group and 29/125 (23.2%) in the amphotericin B group.

To evaluate the effect of CANCIDAS and amphotericin B on renal function, nephrotoxicity was defined as doubling of serum creatinine relative to baseline or an increase of ≥1 mg/dL in serum creatinine if baseline serum creatinine was above the upper limit of the normal range. In a subgroup of patients whose baseline creatinine clearance was >30 mL/min, the incidence of nephrotoxicity was significantly lower in the CANCIDAS group than in the amphotericin B group.

In a second randomized, double-blinded invasive candidiasis study, patients received either CANCIDAS 50 mg/day (following a 70 mg loading dose) or CANCIDAS 150 mg/day. Drug-related laboratory adverse experiences occurring in ≥2.0% of the patients in either treatment group are presented in Table 8.

Table 8: CANCIDAS

Drug-Related[a] Laboratory Adverse Experiences Among Patients with Invasive Candidiasis Incidence ≥2.0% for at Least One Treatment Group by System Organ Class or Preferred Term

Adverse Experience (MedDRA v11.0 System Organ Class and Preferred Term)	CANCIDAS 50 mg[b] N=104 (percent)	CANCIDAS 150 mg N=100 (percent)
All Systems, Any Adverse Experience	**7.8**	**7.1**
Alanine Aminotransferase increased	2.0	2.0
Alkaline Phosphatase increased	6.9	2.0
Aspartate Aminotransferase increased	4.0	2.0

a Determined by the investigator to be possibly, probably, or definitely drug-related. Within any system organ class, individuals may experience more than 1 adverse experience.
b Patients received CANCIDAS 70 mg on Day 1, then 50 mg daily for the remainder of their treatment.

Esophageal and/or Oropharyngeal Candidiasis: Drug-related laboratory abnormalities occurring in ≥2% of patients with esophageal and/or oropharyngeal candidiasis are presented in Table 9.

Table 9: CANCIDAS

Drug-Related Laboratory Abnormalities Reported Among Patients with Esophageal and/or Oropharyngeal Candidiasis[a]. Incidence ≥2% (for at Least One Treatment Dose) by Laboratory Test Category

	CANCIDAS 50 mg[b] (N=163) % (n)††	CANCIDAS 70 mg[c] (N=65) % (n)††	Fluconazole 200 mg[b] (N=94) % (n)††	Amphotericin B 0.5 mg/kg[c] (N=89) % (n)††
Blood Chemistry				
ALT increased	10.6 (17)	10.8 (7)	11.8 (11)	22.7 (20)
AST increased	10.5 (17)	10.8 (7)	12.9 (12)	22.7 (20)
Blood urea increased	†	†	1.2 (1)	10.3 (9)
Direct serum bilirubin increased	0.6 (1)	†	3.3 (3)	2.5 (2)
Serum albumin decreased	8.6 (14)	4.6 (3)	5.4 (5)	14.9 (13)
Serum alkaline phosphatase increased	10.5 (17)	7.7 (5)	11.8 (11)	19.3 (17)
Serum bicarbonate decreased	0.9 (1)	†	†	6.6 (4)
Serum calcium decreased	1.9 (3)	†	3.2 (3)	1.1 (1)
Serum creatinine increased	†	1.5 (1)	2.2 (2)	28.1 (25)
Serum potassium decreased	3.7 (6)	10.8 (7)	4.3 (4)	31.5 (28)
Serum potassium increased	0.6 (1)	†	2.2 (2)	1.1 (1)
Serum sodium decreased	1.9 (3)	1.5 (1)	3.2 (3)	1.1 (1)
Serum uric acid increased	0.6 (1)	†	†	3.4 (3)
Total serum bilirubin increased	†	†	3.2 (3)	4.5 (4)
Total serum protein decreased	3.1 (5)	†	3.2 (3)	3.4 (3)
Hematology				
Eosinophils increased	3.1 (5)	3.1 (2)	1.1 (1)	1.1 (1)
Hematocrit decreased	11.1 (18)	1.5 (1)	5.4 (5)	32.6 (29)
Hemoglobin decreased	12.3 (20)	3.1 (2)	5.4 (5)	37.1 (33)
Lymphocytes increased	†	1.6 (1)	2.2 (2)	†
Neutrophils decreased	1.9 (3)	3.1 (2)	3.2 (3)	1.1 (1)
Platelet count decreased	3.1 (5)	1.5 (1)	2.2 (2)	3.4 (3)
Prothrombin time increased	1.3 (2)	1.5 (1)	†	2.3 (2)
WBC count decreased	6.2 (10)	4.6 (3)	8.6 (8)	7.9 (7)
Urinalysis				
Urine blood increased	†	†	†	4.0 (2)
Urine casts increased	†	†	†	8.0 (4)
Urine pH increased	0.8 (1)	†	†	3.6 (2)
Urine protein increased	1.2 (2)	†	3.3 (3)	4.5 (4)
Urine RBC's increased	1.1 (1)	3.8 (1)	5.1 (4)	12.0 (6)
Urine WBC's increased	†	7.7 (2)	†	24.0 (12)

a Relationship to drug was determined by the investigator to be possibly, probably, or definintely drug-related. Patients who received CANCIDAS 35 mg daily in these studies are not included in this table.
b Derived from Phase II and Phase III comparator-controlled clinical studies.
c Derived from Phase II comparator-controlled studies.
Legend: †=Incidence 0.0%; ††=Not all tests were conducted for some patients.

Invasive Aspergillosis: Drug-related laboratory abnormalities reported with an incidence ≥2% in patients treated with CANCIDAS in the noncomparative aspergillosis study were: serum alkaline phosphatase increased (2.9%), serum potassium decreased (2.9%), eosinophils increased (3.2%), urine protein increased (4.9%), and urine RBCs increased (2.2%).
Concomitant Therapy with Cyclosporine: In one clinical study, 3 of 4 subjects who received CANCIDAS 70 mg daily on Days 1 through 10, and also received two 3 mg/kg doses of cyclosporine 12 hours apart on Day 10, developed transient elevations of ALT on Day 11 that were 2 to 3 times the upper limit of normal (ULN). In a separate panel of subjects in the same study, 2 of 8 subjects who received CANCIDAS 35 mg daily for 3 days and cyclosporine (two 3 mg/kg doses administered 12 hours apart) on Day 1 had small increases in ALT (slightly above the ULN) on Day 2. In another clinical study, 2 of 8 healthy men developed transient ALT elevations of less than 2×ULN. In this study, cyclosporine (4 mg/kg) was administered on Days 1 and 12, and CANCIDAS was administered (70 mg) daily on Days 3 through 13. In one subject, the ALT elevation occurred on Days 7 and 9 and, in the other subject, the ALT elevation occurred on Day 19. These elevations returned to normal by Day 27. In all groups, elevations in AST paralleled ALT elevations but were of lesser magnitude. In these clinical studies, cyclosporine (one 4 mg/kg dose or two 3 mg/kg doses) increased the AUC of caspofungin by approximately 35% (see Warnings and Precautions).
Laboratory Abnormalities in Pediatric Patients: Table 10 shows the incidence of drug-related laboratory adverse experiences reported in ≥2.0% of pediatric patients in clinical studies. The overall laboratory safety profile in pediatric patients is comparable to that in adult patients. The most common drug-related laboratory adverse experiences in pediatric patients treated with CANCIDAS were increased ALT (6.5%) and increased AST (7.6%).

Table 10: CANCIDAS

Drug-Related Laboratory Adverse Experiences Among Pediatric Patients[a], Incidence ≥2% for at Least One Treatment Dose by Body System

	CANCIDAS Any dose[b] N=171 (%)	CANCIDAS 50 mg/m²[c] N=56 (%)	AmBisome 3 mg/kg[c] N=26 (%)
Blood Chemistry Test			
ALT increased	6.5	3.6	0.0
AST increased	7.6	1.8	0.0
Blood bilirubin increased	0.6	1.8	4.0
Blood phosphorus decreased	2.0	1.8	0.0
Blood potassium decreased	3.5	3.6	11.5
Blood sodium decreased	0.0	0.0	3.8
Direct bilirubin increased	0.0	0.0	6.3

[a] Relationship to drug was determined by the investigator to be possibly, probably or definitely drug-related.
[b] Derived from all pediatric clinical studies.
[c] Derived from Phase II comparator-controlled clinical study of empirical therapy.

None of the patients receiving CANCIDAS or AmBisome developed a serious drug-related adverse event or were discontinued from therapy due to a drug-related laboratory adverse experience.
Overall Safety Experience of CANCIDAS in Clinical Trials: The overall safety of CANCIDAS was assessed in 2036 individuals (including 1642 adult or pediatric patients and 394 volunteers) from 34 clinical studies. These individuals received single or multiple (once daily) doses of CANCIDAS, ranging from 5 mg to 210 mg. Full safety data is available from 1951 individuals, as the safety data from 85 patients enrolled in 2 compassionate use studies was limited solely to serious adverse reactions. Treatment emergent adverse reactions, regardless of causality, which occurred in ≥5% of all individuals who received CANCIDAS in these trials, are shown in Table 11.
Overall, 1665 of the 1951 (85.3%) patients/volunteers who received CANCIDAS experienced an adverse reaction.

Table 11: CANCIDAS

Treatment-Emergent[a] Adverse Reactions in Patients Who Received CANCIDAS in Clinical Trials[b]—Incidence ≥5% for at Least One Treatment Group by System Organ Class or Preferred Term

Adverse Reaction[c] (MedDRA v10 System Organ Class and Preferred Term)	CANCIDAS (N=1951) N	(%)
All Systems, Any Adverse Reaction	**1665**	**(85.3)**
Investigations	**901**	**(46.2)**
Alanine Aminotransferase Increased	258	(13.2)
Aspartate Aminotransferase Increased	233	(11.9)
Blood Alkaline Phosphatase Increased	232	(11.9)
Blood Potassium Decreased	220	(11.3)
Blood Bilirubin Increased	117	(6.0)
General Disorders and Administration Site Conditions	**843**	**(43.2)**
Pyrexia	381	(19.5)
Chills	192	(9.8)
Edema Peripheral	110	(5.6)
Gastrointestinal Disorders	**754**	**(38.6)**
Diarrhea	273	(14.0)
Nausea	166	(8.5)
Vomiting	146	(7.5)
Abdominal Pain	112	(5.7)
Infections and Infestations	**730**	**(37.4)**
Pneumonia	115	(5.9)
Respiratory, Thoracic, and Mediastinal Disorders	**613**	**(31.4)**
Cough	111	(5.7)
Skin and Subcutaneous Tissue Disorders	**520**	**(26.7)**
Rash	159	(8.1)
Erythema	98	(5.0)
Nervous System Disorders	**412**	**(21.1)**
Headache	193	(9.9)
Vascular Disorders	**344**	**(17.6)**
Hypotension	118	(6.0)

(cont'd)

[a] Defined as an adverse reaction, regardless of causality, while on CANCIDAS or during the 14-day post-CANCIDAS follow-up period.
[b] Incidence for each preferred term is ≥5% among individuals who received at least 1 dose of CANCIDAS.
[c] Within any system organ class, individuals may experience more than 1 adverse event.

Clinical Trial Adverse Drug Reactions (<5%): Clinically significant adverse reactions, regardless of causality or incidence which occurred in these trials, are listed below.
Blood and Lymphatic System Disorders: anaemia, coagulopathy, febrile neutropenia, neutropenia, thrombocytopenia.
Cardiac Disorders: arrhythmia, atrial fibrillation, bradycardia, cardiac arrest, myocardial infarction, tachycardia.
Gastrointestinal Disorders: abdominal distension, abdominal pain upper, constipation, dyspepsia.
General Disorders and Administration Site Conditions: asthenia, fatigue, infusion site pain/pruritus/swelling, mucosal inflammation, edema.
Hepatobiliary Disorders: hepatic failure, hepatomegaly, hepatotoxicity, hyperbilirubinemia, jaundice.
Immune System Disorders: bacteremia, sepsis, urinary tract infection.
Metabolism and Nutrition Disorders: anorexia, decreased appetite, fluid overload, hypomagnesemia, hypercalcemia, hyperglycemia, hypokalemia.
Musculoskeletal and Connective Tissue Disorders: arthralgia, back pain, pain in extremity.
Nervous System Disorders: convulsion, dizziness, somnolence, tremor.
Psychiatric Disorders: anxiety, confusional state, depression, insomnia.
Renal and Urinary Disorders: hematuria, renal failure.
Respiratory, Thoracic and Mediastinal Disorders: dyspnea, epistaxis, hypoxia, tachypnea.
Skin and Subcutaneous Tissue Disorders: erythema, petechiae, skin lesion, urticaria.
Vascular Disorders: flushing, hypertension, phlebitis.
Post-Market Adverse Drug Reactions: In addition to adverse events identified in clinical trials, the following events have been identified since market introduction of CANCIDAS. Because they are reported spontaneously from a population of unknown size, estimates of frequency cannot be made. The following events have been chosen for inclusion due to their seriousness, frequency of reporting, potential causal connection to CANCIDAS, or a combination of these factors.
The following post-marketing adverse events have been reported:
Gastrointestinal Disorders: pancreatitis.
Hepatobiliary Disorders: hepatic necrosis, rare cases of hepatic dysfunction.
Metabolism and Nutrition Disorders: hypercalcemia.
Renal and Urinary Disorders: clinically significant renal dysfunction.
Skin and Subcutaneous Tissue Disorders: erythema multiforme, Stevens-Johnson, skin exfoliation, toxic epidermal necrolysis.
General Disorders and Administration Site Conditions: swelling and peripheral edema.
Postmarketing hepatobiliary adverse reactions have been reported in pediatric patients with serious underlying medical conditions (see Warnings and Precautions, Hepatic/Biliary/Pancreatic).
DRUG INTERACTIONS: Overview: Studies in vitro show that caspofungin acetate is not an inhibitor of any enzyme in the cytochrome P450 (CYP) system at or up to 5 times the concentration expected in human use. In clinical studies, caspofungin did not induce the CYP3A4 metabolism of other drugs. Caspofungin is not a substrate for P-glycoprotein and is a poor substrate for cytochrome P450 enzymes.
Studies in healthy adult volunteers show that the pharmacokinetics of caspofungin are not significantly altered by itraconazole, amphotericin B, mycophenolate, nelfinavir or tacrolimus. Caspofungin has no significant effect on the pharmacokinetics of itraconazole, amphotericin B, rifampin or the active metabolite of mycophenolate.
Drug-Drug Interactions: Tacrolimus: For adult patients receiving both caspofungin and tacrolimus, standard monitoring of tacrolimus blood concentrations and appropriate tacrolimus dosage adjustments are recommended. Caspofungin reduced the blood AUC of tacrolimus by approximately 20%, maximal blood concentration (C_{max}) by 16%, and 12-hour blood concentration (C_{12hr}) by 26% in healthy adult subjects when tacrolimus (2 doses of 0.1 mg/kg 12 hours apart) was administered on the 10th day of CANCIDAS 70 mg daily, as compared to results from a control period in which tacrolimus was administered alone.
Cyclosporine: In two adult clinical studies, cyclosporine (one 4 mg/kg dose or two 3 mg/kg doses) increased the AUC of caspofungin by approximately 35%. CANCIDAS did not increase the plasma levels of cyclosporine. There were transient increases in liver ALT and AST when CANCIDAS and cyclosporine were co-administered. (see Warnings and Precautions and Adverse Reactions).
Rifampin: Results from two clinical drug interaction studies in healthy adult volunteers indicate that rifampin both induces and inhibits caspofungin disposition with net induction at steady state. In one study, rifampin and caspofungin were co-administered for 14 days with both therapies initiated on the same day. In the second study, rifampin was administered alone for 14 days to allow the induction effect to reach steady state, and then rifampin and caspofungin were co-administered for an additional 14 days. When the induction effect of rifampin was at steady state, there was little change in caspofungin AUC or end-of-infusion concentration, but caspofungin trough concentrations were reduced by approximately 30%. The inhibitory effect of rifampin was demonstrated when rifampin and caspofungin treatments were initiated on the same day, and a transient elevation in caspofungin plasma concentrations occurred on Day 1 (approximately 60% increase in AUC). This inhibitory effect was not seen when caspofungin was added to preexisting rifampin therapy, and no elevation in caspofungin concentrations occurred. When CANCIDAS is co-administered to adult patients with rifampin (or other inducers of drug clearance, see Other Medications), use of a daily dose of 70 mg of CANCIDAS may be considered (see Dosage and Administration).
Other Medications: Results from population pharmacokinetic screening in adults suggest that co-administration of inducers of drug clearance (efavirenz, nevirapine, phenytoin, dexamethasone or carbamazepine) with CANCIDAS may result in clinically meaningful reductions in caspofungin concentrations. Available data suggest that the inducible drug clearance mechanism involved in caspofungin disposition is likely an uptake transport process, rather than metabolism. Therefore, when CANCIDAS is co-administered to adult patients with inducers of drug clearance, such as efavirenz, nevirapine, rifampin, dexamethasone, phenytoin, or carbamazepine, use of a daily dose of 70 mg of CANCIDAS may be considered (see Dosage and Administration).

In pediatric patients, results from regression analyses of pharmacokinetic data suggest that co-administration of dexamethasone with CANCIDAS may result in clinically meaningful reductions in caspofungin trough concentrations. This finding may indicate that pediatric patients will have similar reductions with inducers as seen in adults. When CANCIDAS is coadministered to pediatric patients with inducers of drug clearance, such as rifampin, efavirenz, nevirapine, phenytoin, dexamethasone, or carbamazepine, a CANCIDAS dose of 70 mg/m² daily (not to exceed an actual daily dose of 70 mg) should be considered.

Drug-Food Interactions: Interactions with food have not been established.

Drug-Herb Interactions: Interactions with herbs have not been established.

Drug-Laboratory Test Interactions: Interactions with laboratory tests have not been established.

DOSAGE AND ADMINISTRATION: **Dosing Considerations: Do not mix or co-infuse CANCIDAS with other medications.** There are no data available on the compatibility of CANCIDAS with other intravenous substances, additives, or medications. Do not use diluents containing dextrose (α-D-glucose), as CANCIDAS is not stable in diluents containing dextrose.

CANCIDAS should be administered by slow intravenous infusion over approximately 1 hour.

Recommended Dose and Dosage Adjustment in Adult Patients: Empirical Therapy for presumed fungal infections in febrile, neutropenic patients: A single 70 mg loading dose should be administered on Day 1, followed by 50 mg daily thereafter. CANCIDAS should be administered by slow intravenous infusion over approximately 1 hour. Duration of treatment should be based on the patient's clinical response. Empirical therapy should be continued until resolution of neutropenia. Patients found to have a fungal infection should be treated for a minimum of 14 days; treatment should continue for at least 7 days after both neutropenia and clinical symptoms are resolved. If the 50 mg dose is well tolerated but does not provide an adequate clinical response, the daily dose can be increased to 70 mg. Although an increase in efficacy with 70 mg daily has not been demonstrated, limited safety data suggest that an increase in dose to 70 mg daily is well tolerated.

Invasive Candidiasis: A single 70 mg loading dose should be administered on Day 1, followed by 50 mg daily thereafter. CANCIDAS should be administered by slow intravenous infusion over approximately 1 hour. Duration of treatment of invasive candidiasis should be dictated by the patient's clinical and microbiological response. In general, antifungal therapy should continue for at least 14 days after the last positive culture. Patients who remain persistently neutropenic may warrant a longer course of therapy pending resolution of the neutropenia.

Esophageal Candidiasis: Fifty (50) mg should be administered daily by slow intravenous infusion over approximately 1 hour. Duration of treatment should be dictated by the patient's clinical response. Because of the risk of relapse of oropharyngeal candidiasis in HIV-infected patients with esophageal and/or oropharyngeal candidiasis at baseline, suppressive oral therapy could be considered. A 70 mg loading dose has not been studied with this indication.

Invasive Aspergillosis: A single 70 mg loading dose should be administered on Day 1, followed by 50 mg daily thereafter. CANCIDAS should be administered by slow intravenous infusion over approximately 1 hour. Duration of treatment should be based upon the severity of the patient's underlying disease, recovery from immunosuppression, and clinical response. The efficacy of a 70 mg dose regimen in patients who are not clinically responding to the 50 mg daily dose is not known. Limited safety data suggest that an increase in dose to 70 mg daily is well tolerated. The efficacy of doses above 70 mg has not been adequately studied in patients with invasive aspergillosis.

Adult Patients Receiving Concomitant Inducers of Drug Clearance: When CANCIDAS is co-administered with inducers of drug clearance, such as efavirenz, nevirapine, rifampin, dexamethasone, phenytoin, or carbamazepine, use of a daily dose of 70 mg of CANCIDAS may be considered (see Drug Interactions).

No dosage adjustment is necessary for elderly patients (65 years of age or older).

No dosage adjustment is necessary based on gender, race, or renal impairment.

Patients with Hepatic Insufficiency: Adult patients with mild hepatic insufficiency (Child-Pugh score 5 to 6) do not need a dosage adjustment. For adult patients with moderate hepatic insufficiency (Child-Pugh score 7 to 9), CANCIDAS 35 mg daily is recommended based upon pharmacokinetic data. However, where recommended, a 70 mg loading dose should still be administered on Day 1. There is no clinical experience in adult patients with severe hepatic insufficiency (Child-Pugh score >9) and in pediatric patients with any degree of hepatic insufficiency.

Recommended Dose and Dosage Adjustment in Pediatric Patients (≤17 years of age): CANCIDAS should be administered in pediatric patients by slow IV infusion over approximately 1 hour.

Dosing in pediatric patients (12 months to 17 years of age) should be based on the patient's body surface area (see Dosage and Administration, Preparation of CANCIDAS for Infusion in Pediatric Patients (≤17 years of age)). For all indications, a single 70 mg/m² loading dose (not to exceed an actual dose of 70 mg) should be administered on Day 1, followed by 50 mg/m² daily thereafter (not to exceed an actual dose of 70 mg daily). Duration of treatment should be individualized to the indication, as described for each indication in adults (see Dosage and Administration, Recommended Dose and Dosage Adjustment in Adult Patients).

If the 50 mg/m² daily dose is well tolerated but does not provide an adequate clinical response, the daily dose can be increased to 70 mg/m² daily (not to exceed an actual daily dose of 70 mg). Although an increase in efficacy with 70 mg/m² daily has not been demonstrated, limited safety data suggest that an increase in dose to 70 mg/m² daily is well tolerated.

When CANCIDAS is co-administered to pediatric patients with inducers of drug clearance, such as rifampin, efavirenz, nevirapine, phenytoin, dexamethasone, or carbamazepine, use of a CANCIDAS dose of 70 mg/m² daily (not to exceed an actual daily dose of 70 mg) should be considered (see Drug Interactions).

The efficacy and safety of CANCIDAS have not been adequately studied in neonates and infants under 3 months of age and children aged 3 to 11 months.

Missed Dose: The injection schedule will be set by the physician, who will monitor the response and condition to determine what treatment is needed.

Administration: Directions for Reconstitution and Dilution: Preparation of CANCIDAS for Infusion in Adults: Preparation of the 70 mg Day 1 loading-dose infusion for adults:

1. Equilibrate the refrigerated vial of CANCIDAS to room temperature.
2. Aseptically add 10.5 mL of either 0.9% Sodium Chloride Injection, Sterile Water for Injection, Bacteriostatic Water for Injection with methylparaben and propylparaben, or Bacteriostatic Water for Injection with 0.9% benzyl alcohol to the vial*. Do not mix with diluents containing dextrose (α-D-glucose) as CANCIDAS is not stable in diluents containing dextrose. This reconstituted solution may be stored for up to 1 hour at 15 to 25°C.†
3. Aseptically transfer 10 mL‡ of reconstituted CANCIDAS to an IV bag (or bottle) containing 250 mL 0.9%, 0.45%, or 0.225% Sterile Saline for Injection, or Lactated Ringer's Injection. Do not mix with diluents containing dextrose (α-D-glucose) as CANCIDAS is not stable in diluents containing dextrose. This infusion solution should be used without delay. It can, however, be stored for up to 24 hours at 15 to 25°C or for 48 hours refrigerated at 2 to 8°C. (If a 70 mg vial is unavailable, see Alternative Infusion Preparation Methods, Preparation of 70 mg Day 1 loading dose from two 50 mg vials.)

Preparation of the daily 50 mg infusion for adults:

1. Equilibrate the refrigerated vial of CANCIDAS to room temperature.
2. Aseptically add 10.5 mL of either 0.9% Sodium Chloride Injection, Sterile Water for Injection, Bacteriostatic Water for Injection with methylparaben and propylparaben, or Bacteriostatic Water for Injection with 0.9% benzyl alcohol to the vial*. Do not mix with diluents containing dextrose (α-D-glucose) as CANCIDAS is not stable in diluents containing dextrose. This reconstituted solution may be stored for up to 1 hour at 15 to 25°C.†
3. Aseptically transfer 10 mL‡ of reconstituted CANCIDAS to an IV bag (or bottle) containing 250 mL 0.9%, 0.45%, or 0.225% Sterile Saline for Injection, or Lactated Ringer's Injection. Do not mix with diluents containing dextrose (α-D-glucose) as CANCIDAS is not stable in diluents containing dextrose. This infusion solution should be used without delay. It can, however, be stored for up to 24 hours at 15 to 25°C or 48 hours refrigerated at 2 to 8°C. (If a reduced infusion volume is medically necessary, see Alternative Infusion Preparation Methods, Preparation of 50 mg daily doses at reduced volume for adults.)

Alternative Infusion Preparation Methods for adults: Preparation of 70 mg Day 1 loading dose from two 50 mg vials: Reconstitute two 50 mg vials with 10.5 mL of diluent each (see Preparation of the daily 50 mg infusion for adults). Aseptically transfer a total of 14 mL of the reconstituted CANCIDAS from the two vials to 250 mL 0.9%, 0.45%, or 0.225% Sterile Saline for Injection, or Lactated Ringer's Injection. Do not mix with diluents containing dextrose (α-D-glucose) as CANCIDAS is not stable in diluents containing dextrose. This infusion solution should be used without delay. It can, however, be stored for up to 24 hours at 15 to 25°C or 48 hours refrigerated at 2 to 8°C.

* The white to off-white compact powder will dissolve completely. Mix gently until a clear solution is obtained.

† As with all parenteral drug products, intravenous admixtures should be inspected visually for clarity, particulate matter, precipitate, discolouration and leakage prior to administration whenever solution and container permit. Solutions showing haziness, particulate matter, precipitate, discolouration or leakage should not be used.

‡ CANCIDAS is formulated to provide the full labeled vial dose (70 mg or 50 mg) when 10 mL is withdrawn from the vial.

Preparation of 50 mg daily doses at reduced volume for adults: When medically necessary, the 50 mg daily doses can be prepared by adding 10 mL of reconstituted CANCIDAS to 100 mL of 0.9%, 0.45%, or 0.225% Sterile Saline for Injection, or Lactated Ringer's Injection. Do not mix with diluents containing dextrose (α-D-glucose) as CANCIDAS is not stable in diluents containing dextrose. This infusion solution should be used without delay. It can, however, be stored for up to 24 hours at 15 to 25°C or 48 hours refrigerated at 2 to 8°C (see Preparation of the daily 50 mg infusion for adults).

Preparation of a 35 mg daily dose from a 70 mg vial for adult patients with moderate hepatic insufficiency: Reconstitute one 70 mg vial (see Preparation of the 70 mg Day 1 loading-dose infusion for adults). Aseptically transfer 5 mL of the reconstituted CANCIDAS from the vial to 250 mL or, if medically necessary, to 100 mL of 0.9%, 0.45%, or 0.225% Sterile Saline for Injection, or Lactated Ringer's Injection. Do not mix with diluents containing dextrose (α-D-glucose) as CANCIDAS is not stable in diluents containing dextrose. This infusion solution should be used without delay. It can however, be stored for up to 24 hours at 15 to 25°C or 48 hours refrigerated at 2 to 8°C.

Preparation of a 35 mg daily dose from a 50 mg vial for adult patients with moderate hepatic insufficiency: Reconstitute one 50 mg vial (see Preparation of the daily 50 mg infusion for adults). Aseptically transfer 7 mL of the reconstituted CANCIDAS from the vial to 250 mL of 0.9%, 0.45%, or 0.225% Sterile Saline for Injection, or Lactated Ringer's Injection or, if medically necessary, to 100 mL of 0.9%, 0.45%, or 0.225% Sterile Saline for Injection, or Lactated Ringer's Injection. Do not mix with diluents containing dextrose (α-D-glucose) as CANCIDAS is not stable in diluents containing dextrose. This infusion solution should be used without delay. It can, however, be stored for up to 24 hours at 15 to 25°C or 48 hours refrigerated at 2 to 8°C.

Table 12: CANCIDAS

Preparation of the Patient Infusion Solutions in Adults

Dose[a]	Volume of Reconstituted CANCIDAS for Transfer to I.V. Bag or Bottle	Typical Preparation (Reconstituted CANCIDAS Added to 250 mL)		Reduced Volume Infusion (Reconstituted CANCIDAS Added to 100 mL)	
		Infusion Volume (mL)	Final Concentration (mg/mL)	Infusion Volume (mL)	Final Concentration (mg/mL)
70 mg	10 mL	260	0.28	not recommended	
70 mg (from two 50 mg vials)[b]	14 mL	264	0.28	not recommended	
50 mg	10 mL	260	0.20	110	0.47
35 mg for moderate hepatic insufficiency (from one 70 mg vial)	5 mL	255	0.14	105	0.34
35 mg for moderate hepatic insufficiency (from one 50 mg vial)	7 mL	257	0.14	107	0.34

[a] 10.5 mL should be used for reconstitution of all vials.

[b] If a 70 mg vial is not available, the 70 mg dose can be prepared from two 50 mg vials.

Preparation of CANCIDAS for Infusion in Pediatric Patients (≤17 years of age): Calculation of Body Surface Area (BSA) for pediatric dosing: Before preparation of infusion, calculate the body surface area (BSA) of the patient using the following formula (Mosteller Formula):

$$\text{BSA (m}^2\text{)} = \sqrt{\frac{\text{Height (cm)} \times \text{Weight (kg)}}{3600}}$$

Preparation of the 70 mg/m² infusion for pediatric patients ≥12 months of age (using a 70 mg vial):

1. Determine the actual loading dose to be used in the pediatric patient by using the patient's BSA (as calculated above) and the following equation:
   BSA (m²) × 70 mg/m² = Loading Dose
   The maximum loading dose on Day 1 should not exceed 70 mg regardless of the patient's calculated dose.
2. Equilibrate the refrigerated vial of CANCIDAS to room temperature.
3. Aseptically add 10.5 mL of 0.9% Sodium Chloride Injection, Sterile Water for Injection or Bacteriostatic Water for Injection with methylparaben and propylparaben.* This reconstituted solution may be stored for up to 1 hour at 15 to 25°C.† This will give a final caspofungin concentration in the vial of 7.2 mg/mL.
4. Remove the volume of drug equal to the calculated loading dose (Step 1) from the vial. Aseptically transfer this volume (mL)‡ of reconstituted CANCIDAS to an IV bag (or bottle) containing 250 mL of 0.9%, 0.45%, or 0.225% Sodium Chloride Injection, or Lactated Ringer's Injection. Alternatively, the volume (mL)‡ of reconstituted CANCIDAS can be added to a reduced volume of 0.9%, 0.45%, or 0.225% Sodium Chloride Injection or Lactated Ringer's Injection, not to exceed a final concentration of 0.5 mg/mL. This infusion solution should be used without delay. It can, however, be stored for up to 24 hours at 15 to 25°C or 48 hours refrigerated at 2 to 8°C.
5. If the calculated loading dose is <50 mg, then the dose may be prepared from the 50 mg vial [follow Steps 2-4 from Preparation of the 50 mg/m² infusion for pediatric patients ≥12 months of age (using a 50 mg vial)]. The final caspofungin concentration in the 50 mg vial after reconstitution is 5.2 mg/mL.

Preparation of the 50 mg/m² infusion for pediatric patients ≥12 months of age (using a 50 mg vial):

1. Determine the daily maintenance dose to be used in the pediatric patient by using the patient's BSA (as calculated above) and the following equation:
   BSA (m²) × 50 mg/m² = Daily Maintenance Dose
   The daily maintenance dose should not exceed 70 mg regardless of the patient's calculated dose.
2. Equilibrate the refrigerated vial of CANCIDAS to room temperature.
3. Aseptically add 10.5 mL of 0.9% Sodium Chloride Injection, Sterile Water for Injection or Bacteriostatic Water for Injection with methylparaben and propylparaben.* This reconstituted solution may be stored for up to 1 hour at 15 to 25°C.† This will give a final caspofungin concentration in the vial of 5.2 mg/mL.
4. Remove the volume of drug equal to the calculated loading dose (Step 1) from the vial. Aseptically transfer this volume (mL)‡ of reconstituted CANCIDAS to an IV bag (or bottle) containing 250 mL of 0.9%, 0.45%, or 0.225% Sodium Chloride Injection, or Lactated Ringer's Injection. Alternatively, the volume (mL)‡ of reconstituted CANCIDAS can be added to a reduced volume of 0.9%, 0.45%, or 0.225% Sodium Chloride Injection or Lactated Ringer's Injection, not to exceed a final concentration of 0.5 mg/mL. This infusion solution should be used without delay. It can, however, be stored for up to 24 hours at 15 to 25°C or 48 hours refrigerated at 2 to 8°C.
5. If the actual daily maintenance dose is >50 mg, then the dose may be prepared from the 70 mg vial [follow Steps 2-4 from Preparation of the 70 mg/m² infusion for pediatric patients ≥12 months of age (using a 70 mg vial)]. The final caspofungin concentration in the 70 mg vial after reconstitution is 7.2 mg/mL.

OVERDOSAGE:

In clinical studies, the highest dose was 210 mg, which was administered as a single dose to 6 healthy adult subjects, and was generally well tolerated.

Caspofungin is not dialyzable.

In clinical trials, one pediatric patient (16 years of age) received a single dose of caspofungin of 113 mg (on Day 1) followed by 80 mg daily for an additional 7 days. These dosages were generally well tolerated.

For management of a suspected drug overdose, contact your regional Poison Control Centre. See the *CPS* Directory section for a list of Poison Control Centres.

ACTION AND CLINICAL PHARMACOLOGY: Mechanism of Action: CANCIDAS is a sterile, lyophilized product for intravenous (IV) infusion that contains a semisynthetic lipopeptide (echinocandin) compound synthesized from a fermentation product of Glarea lozoyensis. CANCIDAS is a member of a class of antifungal drugs (echinocandins) that inhibits the synthesis of β (1, 3)-D-glucan, an integral component of the fungal cell wall.

Pharmacodynamics: Caspofungin acetate, inhibits the synthesis of β (1, 3)-D-glucan, an essential component of the cell wall of many filamentous fungi and yeast. β (1, 3)-D-glucan is not present in mammalian cells. Caspofungin has shown activity in regions of active cell growth of the hyphae of *A. fumigatus*.

Caspofungin has in vitro activity against various pathogenic fungi of the Aspergillus and Candida species.

Interpretive standards (or breakpoints) for caspofungin against Candida species are applicable only to tests performed using CLSI microbroth dilution reference method M27-A3 for minimum inhibitory concentrations (MIC) read as a partial inhibition endpoint at 24 hours. The MIC values for caspofungin using CLSI microbroth dilution reference method M27-A3 should be interpreted according to the criteria provided in Table 13.

Table 13: CANCIDAS

Susceptibility Interpretive Criteria for Caspofungin Against Candida Species

	Broth Microdilution MIC[a] (μg/mL) at 24 hours		
Pathogen	**Susceptible**	**Indeterminate**	**Resistant**
Candida species	≤2	(b)	(b)

[a] A report of "Susceptible" indicates that the pathogen is likely to be inhibited if the antimicrobial compound in the blood reaches the concentrations usually achievable.

[b] The current absence of data on caspofungin-resistant isolates precludes defining any categories other than "Susceptible." Isolates yielding test results suggestive of a "Non-Susceptible" category should be retested, and if the result is confirmed, the isolate should be submitted to a reference laboratory for further testing.

There are no established breakpoints for caspofungin against Candida species using the European Committee for Antimicrobial Susceptibility Testing (EUCAST) method.

No standardized techniques for susceptibility testing or interpretive breakpoints have been established for Aspergillus species and other filamentous fungi using either the CLSI or EUCAST method.

Pharmacokinetics: Plasma concentrations of caspofungin decline in a polyphasic manner following single 1-hour intravenous infusions. A short α-phase occurs for 1 to 2 hours immediately post-infusion, followed by a β-phase with a half-life of 9 to 11 hours. An additional γ-phase also occurs with a half-life of 27 hours. Distribution, rather than excretion or biotransformation, is the dominant mechanism influencing plasma clearance. Approximately 75% of a radioactive dose was recovered: 41% in urine and 34% in feces. Caspofungin is slowly metabolized by hydrolysis and N-acetylation. Caspofungin also undergoes spontaneous chemical degradation to an open-ring peptide compound. At later time points (≥5 days post-dose), there is a low level (≤7 pmol/mg protein, or ≤1.3% of administered dose) of covalent binding of radiolabel in plasma following single-dose administration of [^{3}H] caspofungin acetate, which may be due to two reactive intermediates formed during the chemical degradation of caspofungin. There is little excretion or biotransformation of caspofungin during the first 30 hours after administration. Caspofungin is extensively bound to albumin (approximately 97%), and it is slowly metabolized by hydrolysis and N-acetylation. A small amount of caspofungin is excreted unchanged in urine (approximately 1.4% of dose). Renal clearance of parent drug is low.

STORAGE AND STABILITY: Vials: The lyophilized single-dose vials should be stored at 2 to 8°C. Discard unused portion.

Reconstituted Concentrate: Reconstituted CANCIDAS may be stored at 15 to 25°C for up to 1 hour prior to the preparation of the patient infusion solution.

Patient Infusion Solution: The final patient infusion solution in the IV bag or bottle should be used without delay. It can, however, be stored for up to 24 hours at 15 to 25°C or up to 48 hours refrigerated at 2 to 8°C.

INFORMATION FOR THE PATIENT: Published in e-CPS, available by subscription at www.e-cps.ca.

DOSAGE FORMS, COMPOSITION AND PACKAGING: 50 mg: Each single-use vial of a white to off-white compact powder for infusion contains: caspofungin 50 mg as caspofungin acetate. Nonmedicinal ingredients: acetic acid and/or sodium hydroxide to adjust pH, glacial acetic acid, mannitol and sucrose. Preservative-free. Single-dose vials with a red aluminum seal and a plastic flip-off cap.

70 mg: Each single-use vial of a white to off-white compact powder for infusion contains: caspofungin 70 mg as caspofungin acetate. Nonmedicinal ingredients: acetic acid and/or sodium hydroxide to adjust pH, glacial acetic acid, mannitol and sucrose. Preservative-free. Single-dose vials with a yellow-orange aluminum seal and a plastic flip-off cap.

CanesOral®

fluconazole

Antifungal

Bayer Consumer Care

CanesOral® Combi-Pak

fluconazole—clotrimazole

Antifungal

Bayer Consumer Care

Date of Preparation: February 23, 2010

SUMMARY PRODUCT INFORMATION:

Product	Route of Administration	Dosage Form/ Strength	Clinically Relevant Nonmedicinal Ingredients
CANESORAL	Oral	Capsule, 150 mg	Lactose. For a complete listing of nonmedicinal ingredients see Dosage Forms, Composition and Packaging.
CANESTEN External Cream	Vaginal	Cream, 10 mg/g	For a complete listing of nonmedicinal ingredients see Dosage Forms, Composition and Packaging.

INDICATIONS AND CLINICAL USE: CANESORAL (fluconazole) is indicated for the single-dose treatment of vaginal candidiasis (yeast infections due to Candida) and is clinically proven to cure most vaginal yeast infections.

CANESORAL COMBI-PAK contains CANESORAL (fluconazole) and CANESTEN External Cream (clotrimazole) which is indicated for the topical treatment of external irritation caused by vulvovaginal candidiasis.

CONTRAINDICATIONS: CANESORAL (fluconazole) and CANESTEN External Cream (clotrimazole) are contraindicated in patients who have shown hypersensitivity to clotrimazole, fluconazole or to any of the excipients used. See Dosage Forms, Composition and Packaging for a complete listing of excipients. There is no information regarding cross hypersensitivity between fluconazole and other azole antifungal agents. Caution should be used in prescribing fluconazole to patients with hypersensitivity to other azoles.

Co-administration of terfenadine* is contraindicated in patients receiving fluconazole at multiple doses of 400 mg or higher based upon results of a multiple dose interaction study (see Warnings and Precautions).

Co-administration of cisapride* is contraindicated in patients receiving fluconazole (see Warnings and Precautions).

WARNINGS AND PRECAUTIONS: CANESORAL (fluconazole) is indicated for single dose only. Some (not all) adverse experiences have been reported in patients following exposure to multiple doses of fluconazole.

Clinically significant warnings and precautions for CANESORAL (fluconazole) and CANESTEN External Cream (clotrimazole) are listed below.

* Not marketed.

CANESORAL (fluconazole): General: The convenience of the single oral dose fluconazole regimen for the treatment of vaginal yeast infections **should be weighed against the acceptability of a higher incidence of drug related adverse events** with fluconazole (26%) versus intravaginal agents (16%) in comparative clinical studies where no difference in efficacy was demonstrated (see Adverse Reactions).

Fluconazole administered in combination with ethinyl estradiol- and levonorgestrel-containing oral contraceptives produced an overall mean increase in ethinyl estradiol and levonorgestrel levels; however, in some patients there were decreases up to 47% and 33% of ethinyl estradiol and levonorgestrel levels, respectively (see Drug Interactions). The data presently available indicate that the decreases in some individual ethinyl estradiol and levonorgestrel AUC values with fluconazole treatment may be the result of random variation. While there is evidence that fluconazole can inhibit the metabolism of ethinyl estradiol and levonorgestrel, there is no evidence that fluconazole is a net inducer of ethinyl estradiol or levonorgestrel metabolism. The clinical significance of these effects is presently unknown.

Cardiovascular: QT Prolongation: Some azoles, including fluconazole, have been associated with prolongation of the QT interval on the electrocardiogram. During post-marketing surveillance, there have been very rare cases of QT prolongation and torsade de pointes in patients taking fluconazole. These reports included seriously ill patients with multiple confounding risk factors, such as structural heart disease, electrolyte abnormalities and concomitant medications that may have been contributory. Fluconazole should be administered with caution to patients with these potentially proarrhythmic conditions (see Warnings and Precautions, Drug Interactions and Adverse Reactions).

Dermatologic: In very rare cases, during the treatment of systemic and vaginal infections, patients have developed exfoliative skin disorders (Stevens-Johnson Syndrome, Toxic Epidermal Necrolysis) during treatment with fluconazole.

Hepatic/Biliary/Pancreatic: In the treatment of systemic infections, multiple doses of fluconazole have been associated with rare cases of serious hepatic toxicity, including fatalities primarily in patients with serious underlying medical conditions. In cases of fluconazole-associated hepatotoxicity, no obvious relationship to total daily dose, duration of therapy, sex or age of the patient has been observed. Fluconazole hepatotoxicity has usually, but not always, been reversible on discontinuation of therapy.

Immune: In rare cases, anaphylaxis and angioedema has been reported in patients using fluconazole.

CANESTEN External Cream (clotrimazole): CANESTEN External Cream is not for ophthalmic use.

As with all topical agents, skin sensitization may result. Use of CANESTEN topical preparations should be discontinued should such reactions occur, and appropriate therapy instituted.

Special Populations: CANESORAL (fluconazole): Pregnant Women: Single-dose oral fluconazole 150 mg does not appear to increase the risk of congenital anomalies. There have been reports of multiple congenital abnormalities in infants whose mothers were treated with high dose (400-800 mg/day) fluconazole therapy for coccidioidomycosis (an unapproved indication). Exposure to fluconazole began during the first trimester in all cases and continued for three months or longer. Fluconazole should not be used in pregnant women unless the potential benefit outweighs the potential risk to the fetus. Women of child-bearing potential taking fluconazole for vaginal candidiasis should consider using adequate contraception.

Fluconazole was administered orally to pregnant rabbits during organogenesis in two studies, at 5, 10 and 20 mg/kg and at 5, 25 and 75 mg/kg respectively. Maternal weight gain was impaired at all dose levels, and abortions occurred at 75 mg/kg (approximately 9.4× the maximum recommended human dose); no adverse fetal effects were detected. In several studies in which pregnant rats were treated orally with fluconazole during organogenesis, maternal weight gain was impaired and placental weights were increased at the 25 mg/kg dose. There were no fetal effects at 5 or 10 mg/kg; increases in fetal anatomical variants (supernumerary ribs, renal pelvis dilation) and delays in ossification were observed at 25 and 50 mg/kg and higher doses. At doses ranging from 80 mg/kg to 320 mg/kg (approximately 10-40× the maximum recommended human dose) embryolethality in rats was increased and fetal abnormalities included wavy ribs, cleft palate and abnormal cranio-facial ossification. These effects are consistent with the inhibition of estrogen synthesis in rats and may be a result of known effects of lowered estrogen on pregnancy, organogenesis and parturition.

Nursing Women: CANESORAL is secreted in human breast milk at concentrations similar to plasma, hence its use in nursing mothers is not recommended.

Pediatrics: CANESORAL should not be used by girls less than 12 years of age unless advised by a physician.

CANESTEN External Cream (clotrimazole): Pregnant Women: Although intravaginal application of clotrimazole has shown negligible absorption from both normal and inflamed human vaginal mucosa, CANESTEN External Cream should not be used in the first trimester of pregnancy unless the physician considers it essential to the welfare of the patient.

Nursing Women: CANESTEN EXTERNAL CREAM (clotrimazole): It is not known if clotrimazole is secreted in breast milk.

Pediatrics: CANESTEN EXTERNAL CREAM (clotrimazole) should not be used by girls less than 12 years of age unless advised by a physician.

ADVERSE REACTIONS: Clinical Trial Adverse Drug Reactions: CANESORAL (fluconazole): In patients with vaginal candidiasis treated with fluconazole (150 mg) as a single oral dose, the adverse events documented in two controlled North American trials were as follows: see Table 1.

Table 1: CANESORAL

Adverse Events

	Percent of Patients with Side Effects	
	Fluconazole (n=448)	**Intravaginal Products (n=422)**
Drug Related Side Effects	26.1	15.9
Nausea	6.7	0.7
Abdominal Pain	5.6	1.7
Diarrhea	2.7	0.5
Dyspepsia	1.3	0.2
Headache	12.9	6.6
Application Site Reactions	0.0	4.5
Dizziness	1.3	0.0
Taste Perversion	1.3	0.0
Most of the reported side effects were mild to moderate in severity.		

Less Common Clinical Trial Adverse Drug Reactions: Occasional allergic reactions including pruritus and urticaria were reported.

Post-Market Adverse Drug Reactions: In marketing experience of single dose fluconazole, rare cases of anaphylactic reaction and angioedema have been reported.

In addition, the following adverse experiences have been reported in patients under conditions (e.g. open trials, marketing experience fluconazole) where a causal relationship is uncertain or in patients treated with multiple doses of fluconazole:

Cardiovascular: QT prolongation, torsade de pointes (see Warnings and Precautions, Cardiovascular, QT Prolongation).

Central and Peripheral Nervous System: seizures.

Dermatologic: alopecia, exfoliative skin disorders including Stevens-Johnson syndrome and toxic epidermal necrolysis (see Warnings and Precautions).

Gastrointestinal: vomiting.

Hematopoietic and Lymphatic: leukopenia including neutropenia and agranulocytosis, thrombocytopenia.

Immunologic: face edema.

Body as a Whole: face edema, urticaria.

Liver/Biliary: hepatic failure, hepatitis, hepatocellular necrosis, jaundice.

Metabolic/Nutritional: hypercholesterolemia, hypertriglyceridemia, hypokalemia.

CANESTEN EXTERNAL CREAM (clotrimazole): Experimental, therapeutic, and large scale clinical studies have shown CANESTEN EXTERNAL CREAM to be well tolerated after topical application.

Erythema, stinging, blistering, peeling, edema, pruritus, urticaria, and general irritation of the skin have been reported infrequently.

Two of 419 (0.5%) patients treated with the 1% vaginal cream experienced adverse reactions judged to be possibly drug related. These were intercurrent cystitis and vaginal burning. Neither necessitated discontinuation of treatment. None were of serious consequence and no complications occurred.

DRUG INTERACTIONS: Drug-Drug Interactions: CANESORAL (fluconazole): Clinically or potentially significant drug interactions between fluconazole and the following agents/classes have been observed.

Benzodiazepines (Short Acting): Following oral or intravenous administration of midazolam, fluconazole resulted in substantial increases in midazolam concentrations and psychomotor effects. This effect on midazolam appears to be more pronounced following oral administration of fluconazole than with fluconazole administered intravenously. If concomitant benzodiazepine therapy, such as midazolam or triazolam, is necessary in patients being treated with fluconazole, consideration should be given to decreasing the benzodiazepine dosage.

Cimetidine: Absorption of orally administered fluconazole does not appear to be affected by gastric pH. Fluconazole 100 mg was administered as a single oral dose alone and two hours after a single dose of cimetidine 400 mg to six healthy male volunteers. After the administration of cimetidine, there was a significant decrease in fluconazole AUC (area under the plasma concentration-time curve) and C_{max}. There was a mean ± SD decrease in fluconazole AUC of 13%±11% (range: -3.4 to -31%) and C_{max} decreased 19%±14% (range: -5 to -40%). However, the administration of cimetidine 600 mg to 900 mg intravenously over a 4-hour period (from 1 hour before to 3 hours after a single oral dose of fluconazole 200 mg) did not affect the bioavailability or pharmacokinetics of fluconazole in 24 healthy male volunteers.

Coumarin-Type Anticoagulants: In a clinical trial, there was a significant increase in prothrombin time response (area under the prothrombin time-time curve) following a single dose of warfarin (15 mg) administered to 13 normal male volunteers following oral fluconazole 200 mg administered daily for 14 days as compared to the administration of warfarin alone. There was a mean ± SD increase in the prothrombin time response (area under the prothrombin time-time curve) of 7%±4% (range: -2 to 13%). Mean is based on data from 12 subjects as one of 13 subjects experienced a 2-fold increase in his prothrombin time response.

During the post-marketing experience, as with some azole antifungals, bleeding events (bruising, epistaxis, gastrointestinal bleeding, hematuria, and melena) have been reported, in association with increases in prothrombin time in patients receiving fluconazole concurrently with warfarin.

Prothrombin time may be increased in patients receiving concomitant fluconazole and coumarin-type anticoagulants.

Cyclosporine: Cyclosporine AUC and C_{max} were determined before and after the administration of fluconazole 200 mg daily for 14 days in eight renal transplant patients who had been on cyclosporine therapy for at least 6 months and on a stable cyclosporine dose for at least 6 weeks. There was a significant increase in cyclosporine AUC, C_{max}, C_{min} (24-hour concentration), and a significant reduction in apparent oral clearance following the administration of fluconazole. The mean ± SD increase in AUC was 92%±43% (range: 18 to 147%). The C_{max} increased 60%±48% range (range: -5 to 133%). The C_{min} increased 157%±96% (range: 33 to 360%). The apparent oral clearance decreased 45%±15% (range: -15 to -60%). Fluconazole administered at 100 mg daily dose does not affect cyclosporine pharmacokinetic levels in patients with bone marrow transplants. Fluconazole may significantly increase cyclosporine levels in renal transplant patients with or without renal impairment.

Drugs Prolonging the QTc Interval: The use of fluconazole in patients concurrently taking drugs metabolized by the Cytochrome P-450 system may be associated with elevations in the serum levels of these drugs.

Astemizole†: Definitive interaction studies with fluconazole have not been conducted. The use of fluconazole may be associated with elevations in serum levels of astemizole. Caution should be used when coadministering fluconazole with astemizole. Patients should be carefully monitored.

Cisapride†: There have been reports of cardiac events including torsade de pointes in patients to whom fluconazole and cisapride were coadministered. Co-administration of cisapride is contraindicated in patients receiving fluconazole. (see Contraindications).

Terfenadine†: Because of the occurrence of serious cardiac dysrhythmias secondary to prolongation of the QTc interval in patients receiving azole antifungals in conjunction with terfenadine, interaction studies have been performed. In one study, 6 healthy volunteers received terfenadine 60 mg BID for 15 days. Fluconazole 200 mg was administered daily from days 9 through 15. Fluconazole did not affect terfenadine plasma concentrations. Terfenadine acid metabolite AUC increased 36%± 36% (range: 7 to 102%) from day 8 to day 15 with the concomitant administration of fluconazole. There was no change in cardiac repolarization as measured by Holter QTc intervals. However, another study at a 400 mg and 800 mg daily dose of fluconazole demonstrated that fluconazole taken in doses of 400 mg per day or greater significantly increases plasma levels of terfenadine when taken concomitantly. Therefore the combined use of fluconazole at doses of 400 mg or higher with terfenadine is contraindicated (see Contraindications). Patients should be carefully monitored if they are being concurrently prescribed fluconazole at multiple doses lower than 400 mg/day with terfenadine.

Hydrochlorothiazide: Concomitant oral administration of 100 mg fluconazole and 50 mg hydrochlorothiazide for 10 days in 13 normal volunteers resulted in a significant increase in fluconazole AUC and C_{max} compared to fluconazole given alone. There was a mean ± SD increase in fluconazole AUC and C_{max} of 45%±31% (range: 19 to 114%) and 43%±31% (range: 19 to 122%), respectively. These changes are attributed to a mean ± SD reduction in renal clearance of 30%±12% (range -10 to -50%).

Oral Contraceptives: Oral contraceptives were administered as a single dose both before and after the oral administration of fluconazole 50 mg once daily for 10 days in 10 healthy women. There was no significant difference in ethinyl estradiol or levonorgestrel AUC after the administration of fluconazole. The mean increase in ethinyl estradiol AUC was 6% (range: -47 to 108%) and levonorgestrel AUC increased 17% (range: -33 to 141%).

Twenty-five normal females received daily doses of both 200 mg fluconazole or placebo for two, ten-day periods. The treatment cycles were one month apart with all subjects receiving fluconazole during one cycle and placebo during the other. The order of study treatment was random. Single doses of an oral contraceptive tablet containing levonorgestrel and ethinyl estradiol were administered on the final treatment day (day 10) of both cycles. Following administration of 200 mg of fluconazole, the mean percentage increase of AUC for levonorgestrel compared to placebo was 25% (range: -12 to 82%) and the mean percentage increase for ethinyl estradiol compared to placebo was 38% (range: -11 to 101%). Both of these increases were statistically significantly different from placebo.

Oral Hypoglycemics: The effects of fluconazole on the pharmacokinetics of the sulfonylurea oral hypoglycemic agents tolbutamide, glipizide, and glyburide were evaluated in three placebo-controlled studies in normal volunteers. All subjects received the sulfonylurea alone as a single dose and again as a single dose following the administration of fluconazole 100 mg daily for 7 days. In these three studies, 22/46 (47.8%) of fluconazole-treated patients and 9/22 (40.1%) of placebo-treated patients experienced symptoms consistent with hypoglycemia.

Tolbutamide: In 13 normal male volunteers, there was a significant increase in tolbutamide (500 mg single dose) AUC and C_{max} following the administration of fluconazole. There was a mean ± SD increase in tolbutamide AUC of 26%±9% (range: 12 to 39%). Tolbutamide C_{max} increased 11%±9% (range: 6 to 27%).

Glipizide: The AUC and C_{max} of glipizide (2.5 mg single dose) were significantly increased following the administration of fluconazole in 13 normal male volunteers. There was a mean ± SD increase in AUC of 49%±13% (range: 27 to 73%) and an increase in C_{max} of 19%±23% (range: -11 to 79%).

Glyburide: The AUC and C_{max} of glyburide (5 mg single dose) were significantly increased following the administration of fluconazole in 20 normal male volunteers. There was a mean ± SD increase in AUC of 44%±29% (range: -13 to 115%) and C_{max} increased 19%±19% (range: -23 to 62%). Five subjects required oral glucose following the ingestion of glyburide after 7 days of fluconazole administration.

Clinically significant hypoglycemia may be precipitated by the use of fluconazole with oral hypoglycemic agents; one fatality has been reported from hypoglycemia in association with combined fluconazole and glyburide use. Fluconazole reduces the metabolism of tolbutamide, glyburide, and glipizide and increases the plasma concentration of these agents.

Phenytoin: Fluconazole increases the plasma concentrations of phenytoin. Phenytoin AUC was determined after 4 days of phenytoin dosing (200 mg daily, orally for 3 days, followed by 250 mg intravenously for one dose) both with and without the administration of fluconazole (oral fluconazole 200 mg daily for 16 days) in 10 normal male volunteers. There was a significant increase in phenytoin AUC. The mean ± SD increase in phenytoin AUC was 88%±68% (range: 16 to 247%). The absolute magnitude of this interaction is unknown because of the intrinsically non-linear disposition of phenytoin.

Rifabutin: There have been reports that an interaction exists when fluconazole is administered concomitantly with rifabutin, leading to increased serum levels of rifabutin. There have been reports of uveitis in patients to whom fluconazole and rifabutin were coadministered.

† Not marketed in Canada.

Rifampin: Administration of a single oral 200 mg dose of fluconazole after 15 days of rifampin administered as 600 mg daily in 8 healthy male volunteers resulted in a significant decrease in fluconazole AUC and a significant increase in apparent oral clearance of fluconazole. There was a mean ± SD reduction in fluconazole AUC of 23%±9% (range: -13 to -42%). Apparent oral clearance of fluconazole increased 32%±17% (range: 16 to 72%). Fluconazole half-life decreased from 33.4±4.4 hours to 26.8±3.9 hours.

Rifampin enhances the metabolism of concurrently administered fluconazole.

Tacrolimus: There have been reports that an interaction exists when fluconazole is administered concomitantly with tacrolimus, leading to increased serum levels of tacrolimus. There have been reports of nephrotoxicity in patients to whom fluconazole and tacrolimus were coadministered.

Theophylline: The pharmacokinetics of theophylline were determined from a single intravenous dose of aminophylline (6 mg/kg) before and after the oral administration of fluconazole 200 mg daily for 14 days in 16 normal male volunteers. There were significant increases in theophylline AUC, C_{max} and half-life with a corresponding decrease in clearance. The mean ± SD theophylline AUC increased 21%±16% (range: -5 to 48%). The C_{max} increased 13%±17% (range: -13 to 40%). Theophylline clearance decreased 16%±11% (range: -32 to 5%). The half-life of theophylline increased from 6.6±1.7 hours to 7.9±1.5 hours.

Zidovudine: Plasma zidovudine concentrations were determined on two occasions (before and following fluconazole 200 mg daily for 15 days) in 13 volunteers with AIDS or ARC who were on a stable zidovudine dose for at least two weeks. There was a significant increase in zidovudine AUC following the administration of fluconazole. The mean ± SD increase in AUC was 20%±32% (range: -27 to 104%). The metabolite, GZDV, to parent drug ratio significantly decreased after the administration of fluconazole, from 7.6±3.6 to 5.7±2.2.

Drugs exhibiting no significant pharmacokinetic interactions with fluconazole:

Antacids: Administration of Maalox (20 mL) to 14 normal male volunteers immediately prior to a single dose of fluconazole 100 mg had no effect on the absorption or elimination of fluconazole.

Interaction studies with other medications have not been conducted, but such interactions may occur.

Drug-Food Interactions: Interactions with foods have not been established.

Drug-Herb Interactions: Interactions with herbal products have not been established.

CANESTEN External Cream (clotrimazole): There are no known drug interactions with topical clotrimazole.

DOSAGE AND ADMINISTRATION: Dosing Considerations: CANESORAL (fluconazole): The recommended dosage of CANESORAL for vaginal candidiasis is 150 mg as a single oral dose.

Recommended Dose and Dosage Adjustment: There is no need to adjust single dose therapy for vaginal candidiasis because of impaired renal function.

CANESTEN External Cream (clotrimazole): Use only in conjunction with CANESORAL Capsules. The cream should be spread onto the irritated area once or twice daily as needed, for up to seven consecutive days.

Vaginal Candidiasis may be accompanied by irritation in the vaginal area. Therefore, concomitant local treatment with CANESTEN External Cream applied to the irritated vaginal area and as far as the anal region twice a day is advisable. CANESTEN External Cream applied on the glans penis may prevent re-infection by the partner.

OVERDOSAGE:

CANESORAL (fluconazole): Symptoms: There have been reports of overdosage with fluconazole and in one reported case, a 42-year-old patient infected with human immunodeficiency virus developed hallucinations and exhibited paranoid behaviour after reportedly ingesting 8200 mg of fluconazole. The patient was admitted to the hospital, and his condition resolved within 48 hours.

Treatment: In the event of overdose, symptomatic treatment (with supportive measures and gastric lavage if necessary) may be adequate. Fluconazole is largely excreted in urine. A three hour hemodialysis session decreases plasma levels by approximately 50%.

Mice and rats receiving very high doses of fluconazole, whether orally or intravenously, displayed a variety of nonspecific, agonal signs such as decreased activity, ataxia, shallow respiration, ptosis, lacrimation, salivation, urinary incontinence and cyanosis. Death was sometimes preceded by clonic convulsions.

CANESTEN External Cream (clotrimazole): Acute overdosage with topical application of CANESTEN External Cream is unlikely and would not be expected to lead to a life-threatening situation.

For management of a suspected drug overdose, CPhA recommends that you contact your **regional Poison Control Centre**. See the *CPS* Directory section for a list of Poison Control Centres.

ACTION AND CLINICAL PHARMACOLOGY: CANESORAL (fluconazole): Mechanism of Action: Fluconazole is a highly selective inhibitor of fungal cytochrome P-450 sterol C-14-α-demethylation. Mammalian cell demethylation is much less sensitive to fluconazole inhibition. The subsequent loss of normal sterols correlates with the accumulation of 14-α-methyl sterols in fungi and may be responsible for the fungistatic activity of fluconazole.

Pharmacodynamics: The effects of fluconazole on the metabolism of carbohydrates, lipids, adrenal and gonadal hormones were assessed. In normal volunteers, fluconazole administration at doses ranging from 200 to 400 mg once daily for up to 14 days was associated with small and inconsistent effects on testosterone concentrations, endogenous corticosteroid concentrations, and the ACTH-stimulated cortisol response. In addition, fluconazole appears to have no clinically significant effects on carbohydrate or lipid metabolism in man.

Pharmacokinetics: Fluconazole is a polar bis-triazole antifungal drug. Studies have shown that fluconazole exhibits specificity as an inhibitor of the fungal as opposed to mammalian cytochrome P-450 mediated reactions, including those involved in steroid biosynthesis and drug metabolism. Many of the clinical advantages of fluconazole are a result of its unique pharmacokinetic properties.

Absorption: The pharmacokinetic properties of fluconazole are similar following administration by the intravenous or oral routes and do not appear to be affected by gastric pH. In normal volunteers, the bioavailability of orally administered fluconazole is over 90% compared with intravenous administration. Essentially all of the administered drug reaches systemic circulation; thus, there is no evidence of first-pass metabolism of the drug. In addition, no adjustment in dosage is necessary when changing from p.o. to i.v. or vice versa.

Peak plasma concentrations (C_{max}) in fasted normal volunteers occur rapidly following oral administration, usually between 1 and 2 hours of dosing with a terminal plasma elimination half-life of approximately 30 hours (range 20-50 hours) after oral administration. The long plasma elimination half-life provides the basis for once daily dosing with fluconazole in the treatment of fungal infections.

In fasted normal volunteers, administration of a single oral 150 mg dose of fluconazole produced a mean C_{max} of 2.70 μg/mL (range: 1.91 to 3.70 μg/mL).

In normal volunteers, oral bioavailability as measured by C_{max} and AUC was not affected by food when fluconazole was administered as a single 50 mg capsule; however, T_{max} was doubled.

Distribution: The apparent volume of distribution of fluconazole approximates that of total body water. Plasma protein binding is low (11-12%) and is constant over the concentration range tested (0.1 mg/L to 10 mg/L). This degree of protein binding is not clinically meaningful.

A single oral 150 mg dose of fluconazole administered to 27 patients penetrated into vaginal tissue, resulting in tissue: plasma ratios ranging from 0.94 to 1.14 over the first 48 hours following dosing.

A single oral 150 mg dose of fluconazole administered to 14 patients penetrated into vaginal fluid, resulting in fluid: plasma ratios ranging from 0.36 to 0.71 over the first 72 hours following dosing.

Metabolism and Excretion: Fluconazole is cleared primarily by renal excretion, with approximately 80% of the administered dose appearing in the urine as unchanged drug. Following administration of radiolabeled fluconazole, greater than 90% of the radioactivity is excreted in the urine. Approximately 11% of the radioactivity in urine is due to metabolites. An additional 2% of the total radioactivity is excreted in feces.

The pharmacokinetics of fluconazole do not appear to be affected by age alone but are markedly affected by reduction in renal function. There is an inverse relationship between the elimination half-life and creatinine clearance. There is no need to adjust single dose therapy for vaginal candidiasis because of impaired renal function.

CANESTEN EXTERNAL CREAM (clotrimazole): Mechanism of Action: CANESTEN EXTERNAL CREAM (clotrimazole) acts primarily by damaging the permeability barrier in the cell membrane of fungi. CANESTEN EXTERNAL CREAM (Clotrimazole) brings about inhibition of ergosterol biosynthesis, an essential constituent of fungal cell membranes. If ergosterol synthesis is completely or partially inhibited, the cell is no longer able to construct an intact cell membrane. This leads to death of the fungus.

Exposure of *C. albicans* to clotrimazole causes leakage of intracellular phosphorus compounds into the ambient medium with a concomitant breakdown of cellular nucleic acids and potassium efflux. The onset of these events is rapid and extensive after exposure of the organism to the drug, and causes a time-dependent and concentration-dependent inhibition of fungal growth.

Pharmacokinetics: The pharmacokinetics of topically applied clotrimazole in human subjects have been evaluated by Duhm et al. who reported on the penetration of radioactive clotrimazole 1% cream and 1% solution into intact and acutely inflamed skin. Six hours after application of the drug, the concentration of clotrimazole found in skin layers varied from 100 µg/cm³ in the stratum corneum to 0.5 to 1.0 µg/cm³ in the stratum reticulare and <0.1 µg/cm³ in the subcutis. No measurable amount of radioactivity (0.001 µg/mL) was found in the serum within 48 hours after application of 0.5 mL of the solution or 0.8 g of the cream.

STORAGE AND STABILITY: CANESORAL (fluconazole) should be stored at room temperature, between 15-30°C.

CANESTEN External Cream (clotrimazole) should be stored between 2-30°C.

INFORMATION FOR THE PATIENT: Published in e-CPS, available by subscription at www.e-cps.ca.

DOSAGE FORMS, COMPOSITION AND PACKAGING: Capsules: Each hard white gelatin capsule, marked with "CanesOral" in pink colour on the body of the capsule contains: fluconazole 150 mg. Nonmedicinal ingredients: colloidal silicon dioxide, D&C Red #7, gelatin, lactose monohydrate, magnesium stearate, pregelatinized starch, propylene glycol, sodium laurel sulphate and titanium dioxide. Unit dose blister pack of 1 capsule.

External Cream: Each g of external cream contains: clotrimazole 10 mg in a vanishing cream base. Nonmedicinal ingredients: benzyl alcohol, cetostearyl alcohol, cetyl esters wax, octyldodecanol, polysorbate 60, sorbitan monostearate and water. Tube of 10 g.

CANESORAL COMBI-PAK is supplied in a box which contains CANESORAL and CANESTEN External Cream.

Canesten® Topical
clotrimazole
Antifungal

Bayer Consumer Care

PHARMACOLOGY: Clotrimazole acts primarily by damaging the permeability barrier in the cell membrane of fungi. Clotrimazole brings about inhibition of ergosterol biosynthesis, an essential constituent of fungal cell membranes. If ergosterol synthesis is completely or partially inhibited, the cell is no longer able to construct an intact cell membrane. This leads to death of the fungus.

Exposure of *C. albicans* to clotrimazole causes leakage of intracellular phosphorus compounds into the ambient medium with a concomitant breakdown of cellular nucleic acids and potassium efflux. The onset of these events is rapid and extensive after exposure of the organism to the drug, and causes a time-dependent and concentration-dependent inhibition of fungal growth.

Pharmacokinetics: Metabolism studies performed after oral or i.v. administration have shown that in most species studied, levels of clotrimazole in tissue and serum are low. The majority of the drug is excreted as metabolites in the feces, with small amounts excreted in the urine. Human studies indicate slow excretion following oral administration of ^{14}C-labeled clotrimazole (greater than 6 days). After intraperitoneal and s.c. administration, very low levels have been observed in the urine. The absorption and organ distribution of the drug is very poor when administered parenterally.

The pharmacokinetics of topically applied clotrimazole in human subjects have been evaluated by Duhm et al. who reported on the penetration of radioactive clotrimazole 1% cream and 1% solution into intact and acutely inflamed skin. Six hours after application of the drug, the concentration of clotrimazole found in skin layers varied from 100 µg/cm³ in the stratum corneum to 0.5 to 1 µg/cm³ in the stratum reticulare and <0.1 µg/cm³ in the subcutis. No measurable amount of radioactivity (0.001 µg/mL) was found in the serum within 48 hours after application of 0.5 mL of the solution or 0.8 g of the cream.

In animal experiments, clotrimazole exerts an in vitro and in vivo, dose-dependent stimulating effect on certain microsomal enzyme systems which is approximately equal to that of phenobarbital in its inductive potential. However, this stimulating effect subsides rapidly when treatment is discontinued. The enzyme-inductive effect of clotrimazole has been found to be intact in adrenalectomized animals.

Results of 22 mycologically controlled double-blind, 1 mycologically controlled single-blind, and 4 mycologically controlled open studies show that 1% solution and cream are effective in the treatment of tinea cruris, tinea corporis, tinea pedis, tinea versicolor and cutaneous candidiasis. For the cream, mycological cure rates were 80% for tinea cruris/tinea corporis, 67% for tinea pedis, 88% for tinea versicolor and 92% for cutaneous candidiasis as compared to 4.7%, 0%, 37.5% and 0%, respectively, for the vehicle control (total of 238 patients). The corresponding values for the solution are 92% for tinea cruris/tinea corporis, 64% for tinea pedis, 83% for tinea versicolor, 83% for cutaneous candidiasis, 100% for *C. paronychia* and 93% for mixed dermatophytoses as compared to 30%, 31%, 64%, 28% and 0%, respectively, (there is no corresponding value for mixed dermatophytoses) for the vehicle control (total of 874 patients).

INDICATIONS: For the topical treatment of the following dermal infections: tinea pedis, tinea cruris and tinea corporis due to *T. rubrum*, *T. mentagrophytes* and *E. floccosum*; candidiasis due to *C. albicans*; tinea versicolor due to *M. furfur*; diaper rash infected by *C. albicans*.

CONTRAINDICATIONS: Hypersensitivity to clotrimazole.

PRECAUTIONS: As with all topical agents, skin sensitization may result. Use of clotrimazole topical preparations should be discontinued should such reactions occur, and appropriate therapy instituted.

Pregnancy: Although the topical application of clotrimazole has resulted in very low serum and tissue levels, the use of clotrimazole topical preparations by pregnant or lactating women is not recommended unless it is on the advice of a physician.

Lactation: See Pregnancy.

Clotrimazole topical preparations are not suitable for treating fungal infections of the nail or scalp.

Occlusive dressings should not be applied over clotrimazole topical preparations unless directed by a physician. **It is noted that diapers would not be considered occlusive dressings because of frequent changes and airings, normal hygiene practices and the use of newer more breathable and absorbent diapers.**

The topical preparations are not for ophthalmic use.

ADVERSE EFFECTS: Experimental, therapeutic, and large scale clinical studies have shown clotrimazole to be well tolerated after topical application.

Erythema, stinging, blistering, peeling, edema, pruritus, urticaria and general irritation of the skin have been reported infrequently.

Out of a total of 184 patients treated with the 1% cream, irritation was reported in 12 and soreness in 1 patient; therapy was discontinued in 3 patients. In comparison, 1 case of increased inflammation and pruritus and 1 case of folliculitis was reported in the 54 patients treated with the vehicle control.

OVERDOSE:

For management of a suspected drug overdose, CPhA recommends that you contact your **regional Poison Control Centre**. See the *CPS* Directory section for a list of Poison Control Centres.

DOSAGE: Children: (For the treatment of diaper rash): Thinly apply and gently massage sufficient topical cream onto the affected and surrounding skin areas twice daily at a diaper change (in the morning and evening). Do not use for more than 14 days. If symptoms worsen or there is no improvement after 2 weeks, consult a physician.

Adults: (For the treatment of jock itch, athletes foot and ringworm): Thinly apply and gently massage sufficient topical cream into the affected and surrounding skin areas twice daily, in the morning and evening. For the treatment to be completely successful the topical cream should be applied regularly and in sufficient quantities.

Clinical improvement with relief of pruritus, usually occurs within the first week of treatment. The symptoms of jock itch and ringworm usually resolve within 2 to 4 weeks. Athlete's foot may require at least 4 weeks. In mycoses of the foot, treatment should be continued—even when it has led to rapid subjective improvement—for about 2 weeks after all symptoms have disappeared so that relapses may be prevented. If the signs and symptoms of the infection have not been resolved after 4 weeks of treatment with clotrimazole, a physician should be consulted.

If a cure is not mycologically confirmed, treatment should, as a rule, be continued for 2 weeks after all clinical symptoms have disappeared. Candida infections are generally treated for only 2 weeks.

Added hygienic measures are of special importance in the management of the often refractory fungal diseases of the foot. After washing, the feet—particularly between the toes—should be dried thoroughly to avoid trapped moisture. Well-fitting, ventilated shoes and cotton or wool socks are recommended to ensure a successful treatment outcome and to help prevent a recurrence.

INFORMATION FOR THE PATIENT: Published in e-CPS, available by subscription at www.e-cps.ca.

SUPPLIED: Each g of topical cream contains: clotrimazole 10 mg in a vanishing cream base. Nonmedicinal ingredients: benzyl alcohol, cetostearyl alcohol, cetyl esters wax, octyl dodecanol, polysorbate 60, sorbitan monostearate and water. Tubes of 15 and 30 g. Plastic tubs of 500 g. Store below 30°C. Avoid freezing.

Canesten® Vaginal
clotrimazole
Antifungal

Bayer Consumer Care

PHARMACOLOGY: Clotrimazole acts primarily by damaging the permeability barrier in the cell membrane of fungi. Clotrimazole brings about inhibition of ergosterol biosynthesis, an essential constituent of fungal cell membranes. If ergosterol synthesis is completely or partially inhibited, the cell is no longer able to construct an intact cell membrane. This leads to death of the fungus.

Exposure of *C. albicans* to clotrimazole causes leakage of intracellular phosphorus compounds into the ambient medium with a concomitant breakdown of cellular nucleic acids and potassium efflux. The onset of these events is rapid and extensive after exposure of the organism to the drug, and causes a time-dependent and concentration-dependent inhibition of fungal growth.

Pharmacokinetics: Metabolism studies performed after oral or i.v. administration have shown that in most species studied, levels of clotrimazole in tissue and serum are low. The majority of the drug is excreted as metabolites in the feces, with small amounts excreted in the urine. Human studies indicate slow excretion following oral administration of ^{14}C-labeled clotrimazole (greater than 6 days). After intraperitoneal and s.c. administration, very low levels have been observed in the urine. The absorption and organ distribution of the drug is very poor when administered parenterally.

The pharmacokinetics of topically applied clotrimazole in human subjects have been evaluated by Duhm et al. who reported on the penetration of radioactive clotrimazole 1% cream and 1% solution into intact and acutely inflamed skin. Six hours after application of the drug, the concentration of clotrimazole found in skin layers varied from 100 µg/cm³ in the stratum corneum to 0.5 to 1 µg/cm³ in the stratum reticulare and <0.1 µg/cm³ in the subcutis. No measurable amount of radioactivity (0.001 µg/mL) was found in the serum within 48 hours after application of 0.5 mL of the solution or 0.8 g of the cream.

Intravaginal application of ^{14}C-labeled clotrimazole inserts containing 100 mg of active substance in human subjects has shown that the amount absorbed is less than 1/200 of that absorbed after the oral administration of 1.5 g of clotrimazole. The maximum serum concentration values were between 0.016 and 0.05 µg/mL from 1 to 3 days after intravaginal application. Intravaginal application in human subjects of 5 mL ^{14}C-labeled clotrimazole vaginal cream containing 50 mg of active substance has shown that the systemic absorption of clotrimazole from the vaginal cream is quantitatively proportional to that from the vaginal inserts.

In animal experiments, clotrimazole exerts an in vitro and in vivo, dose-dependent, stimulating effect on certain microsomal enzyme systems which is approximately equal to that of phenobarbital in its inductive potential. However, this stimulating effect subsides rapidly when treatment is discontinued. The enzyme-inductive effect of clotrimazole has been found to be intact in adrenalectomized animals.

In 11 double-blind and 1 large multicentre open study, treatment of 814 patients with the 100 mg insert for 6 to 7 days resulted in an average mycological cure rate of 79% (range of 67 to 91%). In studies comparing the 3- and 7-day regimen, 168 patients were treated with one clotrimazole vaginal insert (100 mg) daily for 7 days. Overall and mycological cure rates were 67 and 70%, respectively.

In 8 double-blind studies and 1 single-blind study involving 432 patients using the 1% cream for 7 days, the average mycological cure rate was 72% with a range of 55 to 90%.

Oral contraceptives did not significantly alter mycological cure rates and overall success. In a limited number of pregnant women, both the 1% cream and the 100 mg insert appeared to be effective, although the cure rates seemed to be somewhat lower.

In clinical trials involving 200 mg clotrimazole vaginal inserts, 498/611 patients (82%) had a negative culture for Candida sp. 4 weeks following treatment.

In clinical trials with clotrimazole 2% vaginal cream, 266/303 patients (88%) had a negative culture for Candida sp. 4 weeks following treatment.

In clinical trials with clotrimazole 500 mg vaginal inserts, 158/231 patients (68%) had a negative culture for Candida sp. 4 weeks following treatment.

In clinical trials with clotrimazole 10% vaginal cream, 592/726 patients (82%) had a negative culture for Candida sp. 4 weeks following treatment.

INDICATIONS: Canesten Combi-Pak ComforTAB 1: For the 1-day treatment of vaginal candidiasis.
Canesten Combi-Pak Cream 1: For the 1-day treatment of vaginal candidiasis.
Canesten Cream 1: For the 1-day treatment of vaginal candidiasis.
Canesten Combi-Pak ComforTAB 3: For the 3-day treatment of vaginal candidiasis.
Canesten Cream 3: For the 3-day treatment of vaginal candidiasis.
Canesten Cream 6: For the 6-day treatment of vaginal candidiasis.
Canesten External Cream Refill: For the topical treatment of external irritation associated with vulvovaginal candidiasis.

CONTRAINDICATIONS: Hypersensitivity to clotrimazole.

PRECAUTIONS: Clotrimazole vaginal inserts are not for oral use.

Not for ophthalmic use.

As with all topical agents, skin sensitization may result. Use of clotrimazole preparations should be discontinued should such reactions occur, and appropriate therapy instituted.

Pregnancy: Although intravaginal application of clotrimazole has shown negligible absorption from both normal and inflamed human vaginal mucosa, clotrimazole vaginal preparations should not be used in the first trimester of pregnancy unless the physician considers it essential to the welfare of the patient.

The use of applicators may be undesirable in some pregnant patients and digital insertion of the inserts may be considered.

ADVERSE EFFECTS: Experimental, therapeutic, and large scale clinical studies have shown clotrimazole to be well tolerated after topical application.

Erythema, stinging, blistering, peeling, edema, pruritus, urticaria and general irritation of the skin have been reported infrequently.

Two of 419 (0.5%) patients treated with the 1% vaginal cream experienced adverse reactions judged to be possibly drug related. These were intercurrent cystitis and vaginal burning. Neither necessitated discontinuation of treatment. None were of serious consequence and no complications occurred.

The 100 mg inserts were also well tolerated. Only a few cases consisting primarily of burning sensation and mild skin reactions were reported. In studies comparing the 3- and 7-day regimen, 4 of 212 patients (1.9%) in the 7-day group reported adverse reactions possibly related to treatment. These included: irritation, burning, cramping, itching, redness, abdominal bloating, bleeding and rash. In an additional 9 double-blind comparative studies, 5 out of 219 patients on the 7-day regimen with the 100 mg insert experienced similar types of adverse reactions, none of which necessitated discontinuation of treatment. In a large open multicentre and 2 double-blind studies employing the 100 mg insert in a 6-day regimen, 11 out of 595 (1.8%) patients complained of possible drug-related side effects. Mild burning occurred in 4 patients while other reactions such as skin rash, lower abdominal cramps, slight urinary frequency and burning or irritation in the sexual partner occurred rarely. In no case was it necessary to discontinue treatment.

In clinical trials involving 200 mg clotrimazole vaginal inserts, 24/832 patients (2.9%) experienced an adverse reaction. 2/217 patients (0.9%) who received 2% clotrimazole vaginal cream in clinical trials experienced an adverse reaction. In clinical trials involving 500 mg clotrimazole vaginal inserts, 12/515 patients (2.3%) experienced an adverse reaction. 26/796 (3.3%) of patients in clinical trials involving 10% clotrimazole vaginal cream experienced an adverse reaction. Most adverse reactions involved local itching and burning. Only rarely was it necessary to discontinue treatment.

OVERDOSE:

For management of a suspected drug overdose, CPhA recommends that you contact your **regional Poison Control Centre**. See the *CPS* Directory section for a list of Poison Control Centres.

DOSAGE: Canesten Combi-Pak ComforTAB 1: The recommended dose is 1 vaginal tablet intravaginally for 1 day, preferably at bedtime. The External Cream should be spread onto irritated area once or twice a day as needed, for up to 7 consecutive days.

Canesten Combi-Pak Cream 1: The recommended dose is 1 full applicator intravaginally (as a single-dose therapy), preferably at bedtime. The External Cream should be spread onto the irritated area once or twice a day as needed, for up to 7 consecutive days.

Canesten Cream 1: The recommended dose is 1 full applicator intravaginally (as a single-dose therapy) preferably at bedtime.

Canesten Combi-Pak ComforTAB 3: The recommended daily dose is 1 vaginal tablet intravaginally for 3 consecutive days, preferably at bedtime. The External Cream should be spread onto the irritated area once or twice a day as needed, for up to 7 consecutive days.
Canesten Cream 3: The recommended daily dose is 1 full applicator intravaginally for 3 consecutive days, preferably at bedtime.
Canesten Cream 6: The recommended daily dose is 1 full applicator intravaginally for 6 consecutive days, preferably at bedtime.
External Cream Refill: Use only in conjunction with Canesten Vaginal Tablets or Vaginal Creams. The cream should be spread onto the irritated area once or twice daily as needed, for up to 7 consecutive days.

Vaginal candidiasis may be accompanied by irritation in the vaginal area. Therefore, concomitant local treatment with vaginal cream (or External Cream) applied to the irritated vaginal area and as far as the anal region twice a day is advisable. External cream (or vaginal cream) applied on the glans penis may prevent re-infection by the partner.
Note: The cream or insert should be inserted deep intravaginally by means of the applicator (see Precautions). The plunger should then be depressed slowly.

General hygienic measures such as twice daily tub baths and avoidance of tight underclothing are important in vaginal infections.

INFORMATION FOR THE PATIENT: Published in e-CPS, available by subscription at www.e-cps.ca.

SUPPLIED: Canesten Combi-Pak ComforTAB 1: Each insert contains: clotrimazole 500 mg and each g of External Cream contains: clotrimazole 10 mg. Nonmedicinal ingredients: benzyl alcohol, calcium lactate, cetostearyl alcohol, cetyl esters wax, cornstarch, crospovidone, hypromellose, lactic acid, lactose, magnesium stearate, microcrystalline cellulose, octyldodecanol, polysorbate 60, silicon dioxide, sorbitan monostearate and water. Boxes of 1 strip of 1 Canesten 500 mg Vaginal Insert with one plastic applicator, one 10 g tube of Canesten 1% External Cream and patient instructions. Store below 30°C. Avoid freezing.
Canesten Combi-Pak Cream 1: Each g of vaginal cream contains: clotrimazole 100 mg and each g of External Cream contains: clotrimazole 10 mg. Nonmedicinal ingredients: benzyl alcohol, cetostearyl alcohol, cetyl esters wax, isopropyl myristate, octyldodecanol, polysorbate 60, sorbitan monostearate and water. Boxes containing one 5 g pre-filled applicator with plunger of Canesten 10% Vaginal Cream, one 10 g tube of Canesten 1% External Cream and patient instructions. Store below 30°C. Avoid freezing.
Canesten Cream 1 (10% clotrimazole): Each g contains: clotrimazole 100 mg in a vanishing cream base. Nonmedicinal ingredients: benzyl alcohol, cetostearyl alcohol, cetyl esters wax, isopropyl myristate, polysorbate 60, sorbitan monostearate and water. Boxes containing one 5 g pre-filled applicator with a plunger in a blister pack and patient instructions. Store below 30°C. Avoid freezing.
Canesten Combi-Pak ComforTAB 3: Each insert contains: clotrimazole 200 mg and each g of External Cream contains: clotrimazole 10 mg. Nonmedicinal ingredients: adipic acid, benzyl alcohol, cetostearyl alcohol, cetyl esters wax, cornstarch, lactose, magnesium stearate, octyldodecanol, polysorbate 60, polysorbate 80, silicon dioxide, sodium bicarbonate, sorbitan monostearate, stearic acid and water. Boxes of 1 strip of 3 Canesten 200 mg Vaginal Inserts with one plastic applicator, one 10 g tube of Canesten 1% External Cream and patient instructions. Store below 30°C. Avoid freezing.
Canesten Cream 3 (2% clotrimazole): Each g contains: clotrimazole 20 mg in a vanishing cream base. Nonmedicinal ingredients: benzyl alcohol, cetostearyl alcohol, cetyl esters wax, octyldodecanol, polysorbate 60, sorbitan monostearate and water. Tubes of 25 g in a carton with 3 disposable plastic applicators and patient instructions. 25 g of vaginal cream is sufficient for 3 intravaginal applications with additional cream for extravaginal use if required. Store below 30°C. Avoid freezing.
Canesten Cream 6 (1% clotrimazole): Each g contains: clotrimazole 10 mg in a vanishing cream base. Nonmedicinal ingredients: benzyl alcohol, cetostearyl alcohol, cetyl esters wax, octyldodecanol, polysorbate 60, sorbitan monostearate and water. Tubes of 50 g in a carton with 6 disposable plastic applicators and patient instructions. 50 g of vaginal cream is sufficient for 6 intravaginal applications with additional cream for extravaginal use if required. Store below 30°C. Avoid freezing.
Canesten External Cream Refill (1% clotrimazole): Each g contains: clotrimazole 10 mg: Nonmedicinal ingredients: benzyl alcohol, cetostearyl alcohol, cetyl esters wax, octyldodecanol, polysorbate 60, sorbitan monostearate and water. Tubes of 15 g. Store below 30°C. Avoid freezing.

Canthacur®
cantharidin
Vesicant—Wart Remover

Paladin

SUPPLIED: Each mL contains: cantharidin 0.7% in an adherent film-forming vehicle. Bottles of 7.5 mL. Flammable. Keep away from heat, fire and flame. Close tightly immediately after use. Store at room temperature.

Canthacur®-PS ℞
cantharidin—podophyllin—salicylic acid
Vesicant—Wart Remover

Paladin

SUPPLIED: Each mL contains: cantharidin 1%, podophyllin 5% and salicylic acid 30% in an adherent film-forming vehicle. Bottles of 7.5 mL. Flammable. Keep away from heat, fire and flame. Close tightly immediately after use. Store at room temperature.

Cantharone®
cantharidin
Vesicant—Wart Remover

Dormer

SUPPLIED: Each bottle of 7.5 mL contains: cantharidin 0.7% in a film-forming vehicle of acetone, ethocol and flexible collodion, ether 35% and alcohol 11%. Close tightly immediately after use. Keep away from heat.

Cantharone Plus® ℞
cantharidin—salicylic acid—podophyllin
Vesicant—Wart Remover

Dormer

SUPPLIED: Each bottle of 7.5 mL contains: salicylic acid 30%, podophyllin 2%, cantharidin 1% in a film-forming vehicle of octylphenylpolyethylene glycol, cellosolve, ethocel, collodion, castor oil and acetone. Close tightly. Highly flammable.

Capex™ ℞
fluocinolone acetonide
Synthetic Corticosteroid

Galderma

PHARMACOLOGY: Pharmacodynamics: Like other topical corticosteroids, fluocinolone acetonide has anti-inflammatory, antipruritic, and vasoconstrictive properties. The mechanism of the anti-inflammatory activity of the topical steroids in general is unclear. Various laboratory methods, including skin blanching assays, are used to compare and predict potencies and/or clinical efficacies of the topical corticosteroids. There is evidence of recognizable correlation between vasoconstrictor potency and therapeutic efficacy in man. Generally, fluocinolone acetonide is considered to be in the low range of corticosteroid potency.
Pharmacokinetics: The extent of percutaneous absorption of topical corticosteroids is determined by many factors including the vehicle, the integrity of the epidermal barrier, and the use of occlusive dressings. Topical corticosteroids can be absorbed from normal intact skin. Inflammation and/or other disease processes in the skin increase percutaneous absorption.

Once absorbed through the skin, topical corticosteroids are handled through the same metabolic and elimination pathways as after systemic administration.
Additional Information: Local Treatment—Topical Application: Topical efficacy depends on the inherent glucocorticoid activity (or potency) of the steroid, the concentration in the preparation, permeability coefficient, the vehicle and excipients and local metabolic processes. Except for serious conditions, low-potency glucocorticoids are preferred by many authorities because adverse effects on the skin appear to be less severe than with high potency agents, even if the latter are used at appropriately lower concentrations. Only hydrocortisone and its acetate are available for nonprescription topical use.

Drugs with a high lipid-water distribution coefficient penetrate well from absorbable or non-oleaginous vehicles and tend to remain longer in the skin than water-soluble agents, exerting a more extended local action but lesser systemic side effects, especially if the drug is metabolized rapidly systemically. However, it is desirable that the agents be metabolized in the skin so that less is delivered to the systemic circulation.

Steroids that have the 17-OH group substituted and/or which are fluorinated are metabolized poorly locally and hence may have a significant potential for systemic effects; for this reason, special caution is urged when such compounds are used in children.

Occlusive dressings may be used, especially for low-potency, poorly penetrant steroids. The stratum corneum under the dressing becomes macerated and more permeable. However, such dressings increase absorption into the bloodstream and hence favor systemic effects.
Anti-inflammatory Properties: Cortisol and the synthetic analogs of cortisol have the capacity to prevent or suppress the development of the local heat, redness, swelling, and tenderness by which inflammation is recognized. At the microscopic level, they inhibit not only the early phenomena of the inflammatory process (edema, fibrin deposition, capillary dilation, migration of leukocytes into the inflamed area, and phagocytic activity) but also the later manifestations (capillary proliferation, fibroblast proliferation, deposition of collagen, and, still later, cicatrization).

Although understanding of these effects is unsatisfactory, many observations have been made that have therapeutic relevance and that must be taken into account in explanatory formulations. Perhaps the most important of these for the physician is that corticosteroids inhibit the inflammatory response whether the inciting agent is radiant, mechanical, chemical, infectious, or immunological. In clinical terms, the administration of corticosteroids for their anti-inflammatory effects is palliative therapy; the underlying cause of the disease remains; the inflammatory manifestations are merely suppressed.

It is this suppression of inflammation and its consequences that has made the corticosteroids such valuable therapeutic agents-indeed, at times lifesaving. It is also this property that gives them a nearly unique potential for therapeutic disaster. The signs and symptoms of inflammation are expressions of the disease process that are often used by the physician in diagnosis and in evaluating the effectiveness of treatment. These may be missing in patients treated with corticosteroids.

Anti-inflammatory effects depend upon the direct local action of the steroids. Topical or systemic glucocorticoids often markedly improve certain skin diseases, such as pruritus, psoriasis, dermatitis herpetiformis and eczema; pemphigus; erythema multiforme, exfoliative dermatitis and mycosis fungoides usually require systemic treatment, which may be life-saving.

INDICATIONS: Treatment of seborrheic dermatitis of the scalp. Fluocinolone shampoo has not been proven, by clinical trials, to be effective in other corticosteroid-responsive dermatoses.

CONTRAINDICATIONS: In those patients with a history of hypersensitivity to any of the components of the preparation. Topical application to the eye is absolutely contraindicated, especially in the presence of ophthalmological infections.

WARNINGS: Fluocinolone shampoo is considered an eye irritant. If the product is accidentally introduced into the eyes, liberal rinsing with water should be immediately performed.

PRECAUTIONS: General: Systemic absorption of topical corticosteroids can produce reversible hypothalamic-pituitary-adrenal (HPA) axis suppression with the potential for glucocorticosteroid insufficiency after withdrawal of treatment. Manifestations of Cushing's syndrome, hyperglycemia, and glucosuria can also be produced in some patients by systemic absorption of topical corticosteroids while on treatment.

Patients receiving a large dose of a higher potency topical steroid applied to a large surface area or under occlusion should be evaluated periodically for evidence of HPA axis suppression. This may be done by using the ACTH stimulation, A.M. plasma cortisol, and urinary free cortisol tests.

Patients receiving superpotent corticosteroids should not be treated for more than 2 weeks at a time, and only small areas should be treated at any one time due to the increased risk of HPA suppression.

If HPA axis suppression is noted, an attempt should be made to withdraw the drug, to reduce the frequency of application, or to substitute a less potent corticosteroid. Recovery of HPA axis function is generally prompt and complete upon discontinuation of topical corticosteroids. Infrequently, signs and symptoms of glucocorticosteroid insufficiency may occur requiring supplemental systemic corticosteroids.

Children may be more susceptible to systemic toxicity from equivalent doses due to their larger skin surface to body mass ratios.

If irritation develops, fluocinolone shampoo should be discontinued and appropriate therapy instituted. Allergic contact dermatitis with corticosteroids is usually diagnosed by observing failure to heal rather than noting a clinical exacerbation as with most topical products not containing corticosteroids. Such an observation should be corroborated with appropriate diagnostic patch test.

If concomitant skin infections are present or develop, an appropriate antifungal or antibacterial agent should be used. If a favorable response does not occur promptly, use of fluocinolone shampoo should be discontinued until the infection has been adequately controlled.
Children: Safety and effectiveness in children and infants have not been established. Because of a higher ratio of skin surface area to body mass, children are at a greater risk than adults of HPA-axis-suppression when they are treated with topical corticosteroids. They are therefore also at greater risk of glucocorticosteroid insufficiency after withdrawal of treatment, and of Cushing's syndrome while on treatment. Adverse effects including striae have been reported with inappropriate use of topical corticosteroids in infants and children.

HPA axis suppression, Cushing's syndrome, and intracranial hypertension have been reported in children receiving topical corticosteroids. Manifestations of adrenal suppression in children include linear growth retardation, delayed weight gain, low plasma cortisol levels, and absence of response to ACTH stimulation. Manifestations of intracranial hypertension include bulging fontanelle, headaches, and bilateral papilledema.
Pregnancy: Teratogenic Effects: Pregnancy Category C: Corticosteroids have been shown to be teratogenic in laboratory animals when administered systemically at relatively low dosage levels. Some corticosteroids have been shown to be teratogenic after dermal application in laboratory animals. No studies have been done on fluocinolone shampoo to show teratologic effects on animals.
Lactation: Systemically administered corticosteroids appear in human milk and could suppress growth, interfere with endogenous corticosteroid production, or cause other untoward effects. It is not known whether topical administration of corticosteroids could result in sufficient systemic absorption to produce detectable quantities in human milk. Because many drugs are excreted in human milk, caution should be exercised when fluocinolone shampoo is administered to a nursing woman.
Carcinogenesis, Mutagenesis, Impairment of Fertility: Long-term animal studies have not been performed to evaluate the carcinogenic potential or the effect on fertility of fluocinolone shampoo.
Information to Be Provided to the Patient: Patients using topical corticosteroids should receive the following information and instructions: This medication is to be used as directed by the physician. It is for external use only. Avoid contact with the eyes. In case of contact, wash eyes liberally with water.

This medication should not be used for any disorder other than that for which it was prescribed.

The treated area should not be bandaged or otherwise covered or wrapped so as to be occlusive unless directed by the physician.

Patients should report to their physician any signs of local adverse reaction.

Fluocinolone shampoo mixture is to be discarded after 3 months.
Laboratory Tests: The following tests may be helpful in evaluating patients for HPA axis suppression: ACTH stimulation test, A.M plasma cortisol test, and urinary free cortisol test.
Drug Interactions: No studies have been done on fluocinolone shampoo to show any drug interaction. Generally, there are known drug interactions caused by glucocorticoids, not necessarily from topical application.

Glucocorticoids decrease the hypoglycemic activity of insulin and oral hypoglycemics, so that a change in dose of the antidiabetic drugs may be necessitated. The usual doses of mineralocorticoids and large doses of some glucocorticoids cause hypokalemia and may exaggerate the hypokalemic effects of thiazides and high-ceiling diuretics.

In combination with amphotericin-B, they also may cause hypokalemia. Glucocorticoids appear to enhance the ulcerogenic effects of NSAIDs. They decrease the plasma levels of salicylates, and salicylism may occur on discontinuing steroids. Glucocorticoids may increase or decrease the effects of prothrombopenic anticoagulants. Estrogens, phenobarbital, phenytoin and rifampin increase the metabolic clearance of adrenal steroids and hence necessitate dose adjustments.

ADVERSE EFFECTS: In controlled clinical trials, the total incidence of adverse reactions associate with the use of fluocinolone shampoo was less than 1%. There was no evidence of skin atrophy or increased irritation in patients treated in the controlled clinical trials.

The following additional local adverse reactions have been reported infrequently with other topical corticosteroids, and they may occur more frequently with the use of occlusive dressings, especially with higher potency corticosteroids. These reactions are listed in an approximate decreasing order of occurrence: dryness, folliculitis, allergic contact dermatitis, secondary infection, skin atrophy, striae, miliaria, burning, itching, irritation, and hypopigmentation.

OVERDOSE:

Topically applied fluocinolone shampoo can be absorbed in sufficient amounts to produce systemic effects (see Precautions).

For management of a suspected drug overdose, CPhA recommends that you contact your **regional Poison Control Centre**. See the *CPS* Directory section for a list of Poison Control Centres.

DOSAGE: The pharmacist must empty the contents of the fluocinolone capsule into the shampoo base prior to dispensing to the patient. This product should be shaken well prior to use. **No more than approximately 30 mL of the medicated shampoo should be applied to the scalp area once daily, worked into a lather and allowed to remain on the scalp for about 5 minutes.** The hair and scalp should then be rinsed completely twice. It has been found, through patient responses, that the shampoo lathers better if the hair is fully wet before applying the shampoo.

Capex shampoo is supplied as a 2-component package: a capsule containing the active ingredient, fluocinolone; and 118 mL of the shampoo base in a 180 mL bottle. The pharmacist must mix the capsule contents into the shampoo base at the time of dispensing; hence, is supplied to patients as mixed Capex shampoo.

Directions for Mixing: **The contents of the capsule is mixed into the shampoo base prior to dispensing to the patients. The mixed form, when dispensed to the patient, should be disposed of after 3 months.**

INFORMATION FOR THE PATIENT: Published in e-CPS, available by subscription at www.e-cps.ca.

SUPPLIED: Capex shampoo is marketed as a 2-component product: Capsule and Shampoo base. Capsule: Each capsule contains: fluocinolone acetonide 12 mg. Nonmedicinal ingredients: dibasic calcium phosphate dihydrate and talc. Shampoo Base: 118.28 mL is packaged in a 180 mL bottle. Nonmedicinal ingredients: aluminum acetate basic, benzalkonium chloride, boric acid powder, citric acid anhydrous, cocamido-ether-sulfate complex, cocoamine oxide, D&C Yellow #10, FD&C Blue #1, herbal fragrance #10396, lauramide DEA, magnesium aluminum silicate, methylparaben, oat flour, propylene glycol, propylparaben and purified water.

Capex shampoo is dispensed to the patient as the mixture form in 180 mL bottles (capsule mixed into the shampoo base by the pharmacist). Keep the (mixed) dispensed dosage form at room temperature, approximately 15 to 30°C and shaken well before each use. Keep unmixed dosage form at controlled room temperature of 15 to 30°C.

The reader is invited to consult CPhA's monograph **ACE Inhibitors**.

Capoten™

captopril

Angiotensin Converting Enzyme Inhibitor

Bristol-Myers Squibb

Date of Preparation: August 28, 1981
Date of Revision: November 8, 2006

PHARMACOLOGY: Captopril is an angiotensin converting enzyme inhibitor which is used in the treatment of hypertension and heart failure.

The mechanism of action of captopril has not yet been fully elucidated. It appears to lower blood pressure and be an adjunct in the therapy of congestive heart failure primarily through suppression of the renin-angiotensin-aldosterone system; however, there is no consistent correlation between renin levels and response to the drug. Renin, an enzyme synthesized by the kidneys, is released into the circulation where it acts on a plasma globulin substrate to produce angiotensin I, a relatively inactive decapeptide. Angiotensin I is then converted by angiotensin converting enzyme (ACE) to angiotensin II, a potent endogenous vasoconstrictor substance. Angiotensin II also stimulates aldosterone secretion from the adrenal cortex, thereby contributing to sodium and fluid retention.

Captopril prevents the conversion of angiotensin I to angiotensin II by inhibition of ACE, a peptidyldipeptide carboxy hydrolase.

ACE is identical to "bradykininase", and captopril may also interfere with the degradation of the vasopressor peptide, bradykinin. However, the effectiveness of captopril in therapeutic doses appears to be unrelated to potentiation of the actions of bradykinin. Increased concentrations of bradykinin or prostaglandin E_2 may also have a role in the therapeutic effect of captopril, especially in low-renin hypertension.

Inhibition of ACE results in decreased plasma angiotensin II and increased plasma renin activity (PRA), the latter resulting from loss of negative feedback on renin release caused by reduction in angiotensin II. The reduction of angiotensin II leads to decreased aldosterone secretion, and, as a result, small increases in serum potassium may occur along with sodium and fluid loss.

The antihypertensive effects persist for a longer period of time than does demonstrable inhibition of circulating ACE. It is not known whether the ACE present in vascular endothelium is inhibited longer than the ACE in circulating blood.

Administration of captopril results in a reduction of peripheral arterial resistance in hypertensive patients with either no change, or an increase, in cardiac output. There is an increase in renal blood flow following administration of captopril and glomerular filtration rate is usually unchanged. In instances of rapid reduction of long-standing or severely elevated blood pressure, the glomerular filtration rate may decrease transiently.

Peak reductions of blood pressure usually occur within 60 to 90 minutes after oral administration of a single dose of captopril. The duration of effect appears to be dose related. The reduction in blood pressure may be progressive, so to achieve maximal therapeutic effects, several weeks of therapy may be required. The blood pressure lowering effects of captopril and thiazide-type diuretics appear to be additive. In contrast, captopril and beta-blockers have a less than additive effect.

Blood pressure is lowered to about the same extent in both standing and supine positions. Orthostatic effects and tachycardia are infrequent but may occur in volume-depleted patients. Abrupt withdrawal of captopril has not been associated with a rapid increase in blood pressure.

The antihypertensive effect of angiotensin converting enzyme inhibitors is generally lower in black patients than in non-blacks.

In patients with heart failure, captopril significantly decreased systemic vascular resistance (afterload), reduced pulmonary capillary wedge pressure (preload) and pulmonary vascular resistance, increased cardiac output (stroke index), and increased exercise tolerance time (ETT). Clinical improvement has been observed in some patients where acute hemodynamic effects were minimal.

Captopril has been studied in patients with diabetic nephropathy, most of whom had hypertension, with type I insulin-dependent diabetes mellitus, retinopathy and proteinuria ≥500 mg/day, in a multicenter, double-blind, placebo controlled trial. In this study, captopril has shown to decrease the rate of progression of renal insufficiency and to reduce associated clinical sequelae for the combined end-point of end-stage renal disease (dialysis or renal transplantation) or death (from all causes). The effect on reduction of all-cause mortality alone was not statistically significant. No dosage adjustment was made according to creatinine clearance. Patients who had already progressed to severe renal failure were not included in the clinical trial.

Studies in rats and cats indicate that captopril does not cross the blood-brain barrier to any significant extent.

Pharmacokinetics: Following oral administration of therapeutic doses of captopril, rapid absorption occurs with peak blood levels at about 1 hour. The presence of food in the gastrointestinal tract reduces absorption by about 30 to 40%. Based on C-14 labeling, average minimal absorption is approximately 70 to 75%. In a 24-hour period, over 95% of the absorbed dose is eliminated in the urine; 40 to 50% is unchanged drug although it appears this percentage may be smaller in patients with congestive heart failure; most of the remainder is the disulfide dimer of captopril and captopril-cysteine disulfide.

Approximately 25 to 30% of the circulating drug is bound to plasma proteins. The apparent elimination half-life for total radioactivity in blood is about 4 hours. The half-life of unchanged captopril is approximately 2 hours.

In patients with normal renal function, absorption and disposition of a labeled dose are not altered after 7 days of captopril administration. In patients with renal impairment, however, retention of captopril occurs (see Dosage).

INDICATIONS: Hypertension: Captopril is indicated for the treatment of essential or renovascular hypertension. It is usually administered in association with other drugs, particularly thiazide diuretics. The blood pressure lowering effects of captopril and thiazides are approximately additive.

In using captopril, consideration should be given to the risk of neutropenia/agranulocytosis (see Warnings).

Patients with Normal Renal Function: Captopril should normally be used in those patients in whom treatment with diuretics or beta-blockers was found ineffective or has been associated with unacceptable adverse effects.

Captopril can be tried as an initial agent in those patients with severe hypertension or in those in whom the use of diuretics and/or beta-blockers is contraindicated or in patients with medical conditions in which those drugs frequently cause serious adverse effects.

Patients with Impaired Renal Function: In these patients, particularly those with collagen vascular disease, captopril should be reserved for hypertensives who have either developed unacceptable side effects on other drugs, or have failed to respond satisfactorily to drug combinations (see Precautions).

Congestive Heart Failure: Captopril is indicated in the treatment of congestive heart failure as concomitant therapy with a diuretic in patients who have not responded adequately to digitalis and diuretics or in whom the administration of digitalis is contraindicated or has been associated with unacceptable side effects. captopril therapy must be initiated under close medical supervision.

Myocardial Infarction: Captopril is indicated to improve survival, delay the onset of symptomatic heart failure and reduce hospitalizations for heart failure following myocardial infarction in clinically stable patients with left ventricular dysfunction manifested as an ejection fraction of ≤40%.

Diabetic Nephropathy: Captopril is indicated for the treatment of diabetic nephropathy (proteinuria ≥500 mg/day) in patients with type I insulin-dependent diabetes mellitus and retinopathy.

CONTRAINDICATIONS: Captopril is contraindicated in patients with a history of hypersensitivity to the drug and in patients with a history of angioedema related to previous treatment with an ACE inhibitor.

WARNINGS:

Serious Warning
When used in pregnancy, angiotensin converting enzyme (ACE) inhibitors can cause injury or even death of the developing fetus. When pregnancy is detected, captopril should be discontinued as soon as possible.

Angioedema: Angioedema has been reported in patients treated with ACE inhibitors, including captopril. Angioedema associated with laryngeal involvement may be fatal. If laryngeal stridor or angioedema of the face, tongue, or glottis occurs, captopril should be discontinued immediately, the patient treated appropriately in accordance with accepted medical care, and carefully observed until the swelling disappears. In instances where swelling is confined to the face and lips, the condition generally resolves without treatment, although antihistamines may be useful in relieving symptoms. Where there is involvement of the tongue, glottis or larynx, likely to cause airway obstruction, appropriate therapy (including but not limited to 0.3 to 0.5 mL of s.c. epinephrine solution 1:1000) should be administered promptly (see Adverse Effects).

The incidence of angioedema during ACE inhibitor therapy has been reported to be higher in black than in non-black patients.

Patients with a history of angioedema unrelated to ACE inhibitor therapy may be at increased risk of angioedema while receiving an ACE inhibitor (see Contraindications).

Proteinuria: Total urinary proteins greater than 1 g/day were seen in less than 1% of patients receiving captopril (captopril). These have been predominantly in those who had prior renal disease, or in those receiving relatively high doses (in excess of 150 mg/day), or both. In patients without prior evidence of renal disease, the incidence of proteinuria was 0.5%. In those patients without prior evidence of renal disease receiving 150 mg or less per day, the incidence was 0.2%. Parameters of renal function, such as BUN and serum creatinine, were seldom altered in the patients with proteinuria. In most cases, proteinuria subsided or cleared within 6 months whether or not captopril was continued, but some patients had persistent proteinuria. Nephrotic syndrome occurred in about one-fifth of the proteinuria patients.

Membranous glomerulopathy was found in biopsies taken from proteinuric patients. A causal relationship to captopril has not been established since pretreatment biopsies were not taken and membranous glomerulopathy has been shown to occur in hypertensive patients not receiving captopril.

Since most cases of proteinuria occurred by the eighth month of therapy, patients with prior renal disease or those receiving captopril at doses greater than 150 mg/day should have urinary protein estimations (dipstick on first morning urine, or quantitative 24-hour urine) prior to therapy, at approximately monthly intervals for the first 9 months of treatment, and periodically thereafter. When proteinuria is persistent, 24-hour quantitative determinations provide greater precision. For patients who develop proteinuria exceeding 1 g/day, or proteinuria that is increasing, the benefits and risks of continuing captopril should be evaluated.

Neutropenia/Agranulocytosis: Neutropenia (<1000/mm³) with myeloid hypoplasia has resulted from use of captopril. About half of the neutropenic patients developed systemic or oral cavity infections or other features of the syndrome of agranulocytosis.

The risk of neutropenia is dependent on the clinical status of the patient: In clinical trials in patients with hypertension who have normal renal function (serum creatinine less than 1.6 mg/dL and no collagen disease), neutropenia has been seen in 1 patient out of over 8600 exposed.

In patients with some degree of renal failure (serum creatinine at least 1.6 mg/dL) but no collagen vascular disease, the risk of neutropenia in clinical trials was about 1 per 500, a frequency over 15 times that for uncomplicated hypertension. Daily doses of captopril were relatively high in these patients, particularly in view of their diminished renal function. In patients with renal failure, use of allopurinol concomitantly with captopril has been associated with neutropenia.

In patients with collagen vascular disease (e.g., systemic lupus erythematosus, scleroderma) and impaired renal function, neutropenia occurred in 3.7% of patients in clinical trials.

While none of the over 750 patients in formal clinical trials of heart failure developed neutropenia, it has occurred during the subsequent clinical experience. About half of the reported cases had serum creatinine >1.6 mg/dL and more than 75% were in patients also receiving procainamide. In heart failure, it appears that the same risk factors for neutropenia are present.

Neutropenia has been detected within 3 months after captopril was started. Bone marrow examinations in patients with neutropenia consistently showed myeloid hypoplasia, frequently accompanied by erythroid hypoplasia and decreased numbers of megakaryocytes (e.g., hypoplastic bone marrow and pancytopenia); anemia and thrombocytopenia were sometimes seen.

In general, neutrophils returned to normal in about 2 weeks after captopril was discontinued, and serious infections were limited to clinically complex patients. About 13% of the cases of neutropenia have ended fatally, but almost all fatalities were in patients with serious illness, having collagen vascular disease, renal failure, heart failure or immunosuppressant therapy, or a combination of these complicating factors.

Evaluation of the hypertensive or heart failure patient should always include assessment of renal function.

If captopril is used in patients with impaired renal function, white blood cell and differential counts should be evaluated prior to starting treatment and at approximately 2-week intervals for about 3 months, then periodically.

In patients with collagen vascular disease or who are exposed to other drugs known to affect the white cells or immune response, particularly when there is impaired renal function, captopril should be used only after an assessment of benefit and risk, and then with caution.

All patients treated with captopril should be told to report any signs of infection (e.g., sore throat, fever). If infection is suspected, white cell counts should be performed without delay.

Since discontinuation of captopril and other drugs has generally led to prompt return of the white count to normal, upon confirmation of neutropenia (neutrophil count <1000/mm³) the physician should withdraw captopril and closely follow the patient's course.

Since captopril decreases aldosterone production, elevation of serum potassium may occur rarely, especially in patients with renal failure (see Precautions, Drug Interactions).

Hypotension: Excessive hypotension was seen in hypertensive patients but is a possible consequence of captopril use in severely salt/volume-depleted persons such as those treated vigorously with diuretics, for example patients with severe congestive heart failure (see Precautions, Drug Interactions).

In heart failure, where the blood pressure was either normal or low, decreases in mean blood pressure greater than 20% were recorded in about half of the patients. This transient hypotension may occur after any of the first several doses and produces either no symptoms or brief mild lightheadedness, although in rare instances, it has been associated with arrhythmia or conduction defects. Hypotension was the reason for discontinuation of drug in 3.6% of patients with heart failure.

Because of the potential fall in blood pressure in these patients, therapy should be started under close medical supervision. A low starting dose may minimize the hypotensive effect (see Dosage). Patients should be followed closely for the first 2 weeks of treatment and whenever the dose of captopril, or diuretic, is increased. Similar considerations may apply to patients with ischemic heart or cerebrovascular disease in whom an excessive fall in blood pressure could result in myocardial infarction or cerebrovascular accident. Hypotension in itself is not a reason to discontinue captopril. If associated symptoms are troublesome or persist, they are usually relieved by a reduction in the dose of either captopril or diuretic.

Pregnancy: ACE inhibitors can cause fetal and neonatal morbidity and mortality when administered to pregnant women. When pregnancy is detected, captopril should be discontinued as soon as possible.

The use of ACE inhibitors during the second and third trimesters of pregnancy has been associated with fetal and neonatal injury including hypotension, neonatal skull hypoplasia, anuria, reversible or irreversible renal failure, and death. Oligohydramnios has also been reported, presumably resulting from decreased fetal renal function, associated with fetal limb contractures, craniofacial deformation, and hypoplastic lung development.

Prematurity, patent ductus arteriosus, and other structural cardiac malformations, as well as neurologic malformations, have also been reported following exposure in the first trimester of pregnancy.

Infants with a history of in utero exposure to ACE inhibitors should be closely observed for hypotension, oliguria, and hyperkalemia. If oliguria occurs, attention should be directed toward support of blood pressure and renal perfusion. Exchange transfusion or dialysis may be required as a means of reversing hypotension and/or substituting for impaired renal function, however, limited experience with those procedures has not been associated with significant clinical benefit.

Captopril may be removed from the general circulation by hemodialysis.

Animal Data: Captopril was embryocidal in rabbits when given in doses 2 to 70 times (on a mg/kg basis) the maximum recommended human dose, and low incidences of craniofacial malformations were seen. These effects in rabbits were most probably due to the particularly marked decrease in blood pressure caused by the drug in this species. Captopril was also embryocidal in sheep when given in doses similar to those given in humans. Captopril given to pregnant rats at 400 times the recommended human dose continuously during gestation and lactation caused a reduction in neonatal survival.

No teratogenic effects have been observed after large doses of captopril were administered to hamsters and rats.

Lactation: The presence of concentrations of ACE inhibitor have been reported in human milk. Use of ACE inhibitors is not recommended during breat-feeding.

PRECAUTIONS: Renal Impairment: As a consequence of inhibiting the renin-angiotensin-aldosterone system, changes in renal function have been seen in susceptible individuals. In patients whose renal function may depend on the activity of the renin-angiotensin-aldosterone system, such as patients with bilateral renal artery stenosis, unilateral renal artery stenosis to a solitary kidney, or severe congestive heart failure, treatment with agents that inhibit this system has been associated with oliguria, progressive azotemia, and rarely, acute renal failure and/or death. In susceptible patients, concomitant diuretic use may further increase risk.

Use of captopril should include appropriate assessment of renal function.

Hyperkalemia: Elevations in serum potassium have been observed in some patients treated with ACE inhibitors, including captopril. When treated with ACE inhibitors, patients at risk for the development of hyperkalemia include those with: renal insufficiency; diabetes mellitus; and those using concomitant potassium-sparing diuretics, potassium supplements or potassium-containing salt substitutes; or other drugs associated with increases in serum potassium (e.g., heparin). The incidence of hyperkalemia related or possibly related to therapy in the diabetic patients studied with nephropathy and proteinuria was 3.6% and was a reason for discontinuation of the drug in 1% of the patients. Hyperkalemia was defined as persistent elevation of serum potassium to 6.0 mg/dL or more in the absence of a remediable cause, such as other drugs, volume depletion, exogenous potassium supplements, etc.

Impaired Liver Function: Elevations of liver enzymes and/or serum bilirubin, cases of cholestatic jaundice, and of hepatocellular injury with or without secondary cholestasis, have occurred during therapy with captopril in patients without pre-existing liver abnormalities. In most cases the changes were reversible on discontinuation of the drug. Should the patient receiving captopril experience any unexplained symptoms (see Information to Be Provided to the Patient), particularly during the first weeks or months of treatment, it is recommended that a full set of liver enzyme tests and other necessary investigations be carried out. Discontinuation of captopril should be considered when appropriate.

There are no adequate studies in patients with cirrhosis and/or liver dysfunction. captopril should be used with particular caution in patients with pre-existent liver abnormalities. Such patients should have their baseline liver function tests obtained before administration of the drug. Close monitoring of response and metabolic effects should apply to these patients.

Cough: Cough has been reported with the use of captopril. Characteristically, ACE inhibitor-induced cough is nonproductive, persistent and resolves after discontinuation of therapy or lowering of the dose. captopril-induced cough should be considered as part of the differential diagnosis of the cough.

Valvular Stenosis: There is concern, on theoretical grounds, that patients with aortic stenosis might be at particular risk of decreased coronary perfusion when treated with vasodilators because they do not develop as much afterload reduction.

Surgery/Anesthesia: In patients undergoing major surgery or during anesthesia with agents that produce hypotension, captopril will block angiotensin II formation secondary to compensatory renin release. This may lead to hypotension which can be corrected by volume expansion.

Anaphylactoid Reactions During Membrane Exposure: Anaphylactoid reactions have been reported in patients dialyzed with high-flux membranes (e.g., polyacrylonitrile [PAN]) and treated concomitantly with an ACE inhibitor. Dialysis should be stopped immediately if symptoms such as nausea, abdominal cramps, burning, angioedema, shortness of breath and severe hypotension occur. Symptoms are not relieved by antihistamines. In these patients consideration should be given to using a different type of dialysis membrane or a different class of antihypertensive agents.

Anaphylactoid Reactions During Desensitization: There have been isolated reports of patients experiencing sustained life-threatening anaphylactoid reactions while receiving ACE inhibitors during desensitizing treatment with hymenoptera (bees, wasps) venom. In the same patients, these reactions have been avoided when ACE inhibitors were temporarily withheld for at least 24 hours, but they have reappeared upon inadvertent rechallenge.

Children: Safety and effectiveness in children have not been established although there is limited experience with the use of captopril in children from 2 months to 15 years of age with secondary hypertension and varying degrees of renal insufficiency. Dosage, on a weight basis, was comparable to that used in adults. Captopril should be used in children only if other measures for controlling blood pressure have not been effective.

Information to Be Provided to the Patient: **Patients should be told that taking captopril during pregnancy can cause injury and even death to the developing fetus. Patients should be advised to stop taking the medication and to contact their physician as soon as possible if they become pregnant while taking captopril.**

Patients should be advised that captopril may pass into breast milk and that they should not breast-feed while taking captopril.

Patients should be told to report promptly any indication of infection (e.g., sore throat, fever), which may be a sign of neutropenia, or of progressive edema, which might be related to proteinuria and nephrotic syndrome.

All patients should be cautioned that excessive perspiration and dehydration may lead to an excessive fall in blood pressure because of reduction in fluid volume. Other causes of volume depletion such as vomiting or diarrhea may also lead to a fall in blood pressure; patients should be advised to consult with the physician.

Patients should be advised to return to the physician if he/she experiences any symptoms possibly related to liver dysfunction. This would include viral like symptoms in the first weeks to months of therapy (such as fever, malaise, muscle pain, rash or adenopathy which are possible indicators of hypersensitivity reactions), or if abdominal pain, nausea or vomiting, loss of appetite, jaundice, itching or any other unexplained symptoms occur during therapy.

Patients should be warned against interruption or discontinuation of antihypertensive medications without the physician's advice.

Patients treated for severe congestive heart failure should be cautioned to increase their physical activity slowly.

Drug Interactions: Diuretic Therapy: Patients on diuretics and especially those in whom diuretic therapy was recently instituted, as well as those on severe dietary salt restriction or dialysis, may occasionally experience a precipitous reduction of blood pressure usually within the first hour after receiving the initial dose of captopril (see Warnings).

When feasible the hypotensive effects may be minimized by either discontinuing the diuretic or increasing the salt intake approximately 1 week prior to initiation of treatment with captopril. Alternatively, provide medical supervision for at least 1 hour after the initial dose. If hypotension occurs, the patient should be placed in a supine position and, if necessary, receive an intravenous infusion of normal saline. This transient hypotensive response is not a contraindication to further doses which can be given without difficulty once the blood pressure has increased after volume expansion.

Agents Having Vasodilator Activity: Data on the effect of concomitant use of other vasodilators in patients receiving captopril for heart failure are not available; therefore, nitroglycerin or other nitrates (as used for management of angina) or other drugs having vasodilator activity should, if possible, be discontinued before starting captopril. If resumed during captopril therapy, such agents should be administered cautiously, and perhaps at lower dosage.

Agents Causing Renin Release: Captopril's effect will be augmented by antihypertensive agents that cause renin release. For example, diuretics (e.g., thiazides) may activate the renin-angiotensin-aldosterone system.

Agents Affecting Sympathetic Activity: The sympathetic nervous system may be especially important in supporting blood pressure in patients receiving captopril alone or with diuretics. Therefore, agents affecting sympathetic activity (e.g., ganglionic blocking agents or adrenergic neuron blocking agents) should be used with caution. Beta-adrenergic blocking drugs add some further antihypertensive effect to captopril, but the overall response is less than additive.

In heart failure, special caution is necessary since sympathetic stimulation is a vital component supporting circulatory function and inhibition with beta-blockade always carries a potential hazard of further depressing myocardial contractility.

Agents Increasing Serum Potassium: Since captopril decreases aldosterone production, elevation of serum potassium may occur. Potassium-sparing diuretics such as spironolactone, triamterene, or amiloride or potassium supplements should be given only for documented hypokalemia, and then with caution, since they may lead to a significant increase of serum potassium. Salt substitutes which contain potassium should also be used with caution.

Inhibitors of Endogenous Prostaglandin Synthesis: It has been reported that indomethacin may reduce the antihypertensive effect of captopril, especially in cases of low renin hypertension. Other nonsteroidal anti-inflammatory agents (e.g., ASA) may also have this effect.

The blood pressure lowering effects of captopril and beta-blockers are less than additive.

In patients with renal failure, the use of allopurinol concomitantly with captopril has been associated with neutropenia.

In patients with heart failure, the use of procainamide concomitantly with captopril has been associated with neutropenia.

Drug/Laboratory Test Interaction: Captopril may cause false-positive reactions for urinary acetone and for dipstick tests for urinary ketones.

ADVERSE EFFECTS: Hypertension and Congestive Heart Failure: Reported incidences are based on clinical trials involving approximately 7000 patients treated with captopril.

Renal: Approximately 1 of every 100 patients developed proteinuria (see Warnings).

Each of the following has been reported in approximately 1 to 2 of 1000 patients and are of uncertain relationship to drug use: renal insufficiency, renal failure, polyuria, oliguria and urinary frequency.

Hematologic: Neutropenia/agranulocytosis has occurred (see Warnings). Cases of anemia, thrombocytopenia and pancytopenia have been reported.

Dermatologic: A rash occurred in 8.5% of patients with normal renal function and 13% of patients with evidence of prior renal functional impairment. It was dose related, having occurred in 7% of patients at doses of 150 mg or less per day. The rash is usually maculopapular, but rarely urticarial, and generally occurs during the first 4 weeks of therapy. The rash is usually mild and disappears within a few days of dosage reduction, short-term treatment with an antihistaminic agent, and/or discontinuing therapy; remission may occur even if captopril is continued. Pruritus, without rash, occurs in about 2 of 100 patients. Between 7 and 10% of patients with skin rash have shown an eosinophilia and/or positive ANA titers. A reversible associated pemphigoid-like lesion, and photosensitivity, have also been reported.

Allergic: Angioedema of the face, mucous membranes of the mouth, or of the extremities has been observed in approximately 1 of 1000 patients and is reversible on discontinuance of captopril therapy. Serum sickness and bronchospasm have been reported. One case of laryngeal edema has been reported.

Cardiovascular: Hypotension may occur; see Warnings and Precautions, Drug Interactions for discussion of hypotension on initiation of captopril therapy.

Tachycardia, chest pain, and palpitations have each been observed in approximately 1 of 100 patients.

Angina pectoris, myocardial infarction, Raynaud's syndrome and congestive heart failure have each occurred in 2 to 3 of 1000 patients.

Flushing or pallor has been reported in 2 to 5 of 1000 patients.

Alterations in Taste: 2% of patients receiving 150 mg or less per day of captopril developed a diminution or loss of taste perception. At doses in excess of 150 mg/day, 7% of patients experienced this effect. Taste impairment is reversible and usually self-limited (2 to 3 months) even with continued drug administration. Weight loss may be associated with the loss of taste.

The following have been reported in about 0.5 to 2% of patients:

Gastrointestinal: gastric irritation, abdominal pain, nausea, vomiting, diarrhea, anorexia, constipation, aphthous ulcers and peptic ulcer.

Central Nervous System: dizziness, headache, malaise, fatigue, insomnia and paresthesia.

Others: dry mouth, dyspnea, cough, alopecia, impotence, loss of libido, disturbed vision, and itching and/or dry eyes.

Other clinical adverse effects reported since the drug was marketed are listed below by body system. In many cases, an incidence or causal relationship cannot be accurately determined.

General: asthenia, gynecomastia.

Cardiovascular: cardiac arrest, cerebrovascular accident, syncope.

Dermatologic: bullous pemphigus, Stevens-Johnson syndrome.

Gastrointestinal: pancreatitis, glossitis.

Hematologic: anemia, including aplastic and hemolytic.

Hepatobiliary: hepatitis, including rare cases of necrosis, cholestasis (see Precautions).

Metabolic: symptomatic hyponatremia.

Musculoskeletal: myalgia, myasthenia.

Nervous/Psychiatric: ataxia, confusion, depression, nervousness, somnolence.

Respiratory: bronchospasm, eosinophilic pneumonitis, rhinitis.

Special Senses: blurred vision.

As with other ACE inhibitors, a syndrome has been reported which includes: fever, myalgia, arthralgia, rash or other dermatologic manifestations, eosinophilia and an elevated ESR. Findings have usually resolved with discontinuation of treatment.

Altered Laboratory Findings: Elevations of liver enzymes and/or serum bilirubin have occurred (see Precautions).

Rare cases of cholestatic jaundice and hepatocellular injury with or without secondary cholestasis, have been reported in association with captopril administration.

Elevation of BUN and serum creatinine may occur, especially in patients who are volume-depleted or who have renovascular hypertension. In instances of rapid reduction of long-standing or severely elevated blood pressure, the glomerular filtration rate may decrease transiently, also resulting in transient rises in serum creatinine and BUN.

Small increases in the serum potassium concentration frequently occur, especially in patients with renal impairment (see Precautions).

Diabetic Nephropathy: In 400 patients treated with captopril, the overall adverse reactions profile appeared to be similar to the above. However, the following adverse reactions have occurred more frequently in women than in men: dizziness (31% vs 20%), cough (23% vs 17%) and pharyngitis (20% vs 14%). In 395 patients treated with placebo, the incidences were: dizziness (22%), cough (15%) and pharyngitis (11%) in women and men combined.

The incidence of hypotension or orthostatic hypotension was 5.3% and was a reason for discontinuation of the drug in 1.8% of the patients.

The incidence of hyperkalemia related or possibly related to therapy in the diabetic patients studied with nephropathy and proteinuria was 3.6% and was a reason of discontinuation of the drug in 1% of the patients. Hyperkalemia was defined as persistent elevation of serum potassium to 6.0 mg/dL or more in the absence of a remediable cause, such as other drugs, volume depletion, exogenous potassium supplements, etc.

In patients with serum creatinine ≥1.5 mg/dL, the incidence of a marked abnormality in hemoglobin (a drop >3 g/dL) was 6% in patients treated with captopril versus 0% in those on placebo.

OVERDOSE:

Treatment: In the event of overdosage, correction of hypotension would be of primary concern. Volume expansion with an i.v. infusion of normal saline is the treatment of choice for restoration of blood pressure.

Captopril may be removed from the general circulation by hemodialysis.

For management of a suspected drug overdose, CPhA recommends that you contact your **regional Poison Control Centre**. See the *CPS* Directory section for a list of Poison Control Centres.

DOSAGE: Captopril tablets should be taken 1 hour before meals. **Dosage must be individualized.**

Adults: Hypertension: Initiation of therapy requires consideration of recent antihypertensive drug treatment, the extent of blood pressure elevation, salt restriction, and other clinical circumstances. If possible, discontinue the patient's previous antihypertensive drug regimen for 1 week before starting captopril. If this is impossible, especially in severe hypertension, the diuretic should be continued.

Initial Dose: 25 mg 2 or 3 times a day. If a satisfactory reduction of blood pressure has not been achieved after 1 or 2 weeks, the dose may be increased to 50 mg 2 or 3 times a day. The dose of captopril in hypertension usually does not exceed 150 mg daily. Therefore, if the blood pressure has not been satisfactorily controlled after 1 to 2 weeks at this dose (and the patient is not already receiving a diuretic), a modest dose of thiazide-type diuretic (e.g., hydrochlorothiazide 25 mg daily) should be added. The diuretic dose may be increased at 1 to 2 week intervals until its highest usual antihypertensive dose is reached.

If captopril is being started in a patient already receiving a diuretic, therapy should be initiated under close medical supervision (see Warnings and Precautions, Drug Interactions regarding hypotension), with dosage and titration of captopril as noted above.

In severe hypertension, if further blood pressure reduction is required, the dose of captopril may be increased to 100 mg 2 or 3 times a day, and then, if necessary, to 150 mg 2 or 3 times a day, while continuing the diuretic. The usual dose range is 25 to 150 mg 2 or 3 times a day. A maximum daily dose of 450 mg given in 3 equally divided doses should not be exceeded.

For patients with accelerated or malignant hypertension, when temporary discontinuation of current antihypertensive therapy is not practical or desirable, or when prompt titration to more normotensive blood pressure levels is indicated, the diuretic should be continued but other concurrent antihypertensive medication stopped and captopril dosage promptly initiated at 25 mg 3 times a day, under close medical supervision. When necessitated by the patient's clinical condition, the daily dose of captopril may be increased every 24 hours under continuous medical supervision until a satisfactory blood pressure response is obtained or the maximum dose of captopril is reached. In this regimen, addition of a more potent diuretic, e.g., furosemide, may also be indicated.

Beta-blockers may also be used in conjunction with captopril therapy (see Precautions, Drug Interactions), but the effects of the 2 drugs are less than additive.

Heart Failure: Initiation of therapy requires consideration of recent diuretic therapy and the possibility of severe salt/volume depletion. In patients with either normal or low blood pressure, who have been vigorously treated with diuretics and who may be hyponatremic and/or hypovolemic, a starting dose of 6.25 or 12.5 mg 3 times a day may minimize the magnitude or duration of the hypotensive effect (see Warnings, Hypotension). For these patients, titration to the usual daily dosage can then occur within the next several days.

For most patients the usual initial daily dosage is 25 mg 3 times daily. After a dose of 50 mg 3 times daily is reached, further increases in dosage should be delayed, where possible, for at least 2 weeks to determine if a satisfactory response occurs. Most patients studied have had a satisfactory clinical improvement at 50 or 100 mg 3 times daily. A maximum daily dose of 450 mg of captopril should not be exceeded.

Captopril is to be used in conjunction with a diuretic. Captopril therapy must be initiated under very close medical supervision.

Left Ventricular Dysfunction after Myocardial Infarction: The recommended dose for long-term use in patients following a myocardial infarction is a target maintenance dose of 50 mg 3 times daily.

Therapy may be initiated as early as 3 days following a myocardial infarction. After a single dose of 6.25 mg, captopril therapy should be initiated at 12.5 mg 3 times daily. captopril should then be increased to 25 mg 3 times daily during the next several days and to a target dose of 50 mg 3 times daily over the next several weeks as tolerated (see Pharmacology).

Captopril may be used in patients treated with other post-myocardial infarction therapies, e.g., thrombolytics, ASA, beta-blockers.

Diabetic Nephropathy: The recommended daily dose of captopril for long-term use to treat diabetic nephropathy is 25 mg 3 times daily.

If further blood pressure reduction is required, other antihypertensive agents such as diuretics, beta-adrenoceptor-blockers, centrally-acting agents or vasodilators may be used in conjunction with captopril.

Dosage Adjustment in Renal Impairment: Because captopril is excreted primarily by the kidneys, excretion rates are reduced in patients with impaired renal function. These patients will take longer to reach steady-state levels of captopril and will reach higher steady-state levels for a given daily dose than patients with normal renal function. Therefore, these patients may respond to smaller or less frequent doses.

Captopril is removed by hemodialysis.

Renal Impairment Due to Diabetic Nephropathy (With or Without Hypertension): Captopril at doses of 25 mg 3 times daily was well-tolerated in patients with diabetic nephropathy and mild to moderate renal impairment (see Precautions, Hyperkalemia). Accordingly, no dose adjustment based on creatinine clearance is recommended for these patients.

Captopril has not been studied in patients with diabetic nephropathy and severe renal impairment (creatinine clearance ≤30 mL/min/1.73m²). These patients can be expected to have a higher steady-state concentration for a given daily dose than those with normal or mild-moderate renal impairment, and therefore may respond to smaller or less frequent doses. Doses may be adjusted based on clinical observation.

Renal Impairment Not Due to Diabetic Nephropathy: For patients with significant renal impairment not due to diabetic nephropathy, initial daily dosage of captopril should be reduced, and smaller increments utilized for titration, which should be quite slow (1- to 2-week intervals). After the desired therapeutic effect has been achieved, the dose should be slowly back-titrated to determine the minimal effective dose. When concomitant diuretic therapy is required, a loop diuretic (e.g., furosemide), rather than a thiazide diuretic, is preferred in these patients with impaired renal function (see Precautions, Anaphylactoid Reactions During Membrane Exposure).

Table 1 is based on theoretical considerations and may be useful as a guide to minimize drug accumulation.

Table 1: Capoten

Recommended Dosage Interval in Patients with Renal Impairment Not Due to Diabetic Nephropathy

Creatinine Clearance (mL/min/1.73 m²)	Dosage Interval (Hours)
>75	8
75 to 35	12 to 24
34 to 20	24 to 48
19 to 8	48 to 72
7 to 5	72 to 108 (3 to 4.5 days)

SUPPLIED: 25 mg: Each white, square tablet, quadrisect scored on one side and imprinted CAPOTEN 25 on the other, contains: captopril 25 mg. Nonmedicinal ingredients: cornstarch, lactose, microcrystalline cellulose and stearic acid. Bottles of 100. Store at room temperature (15 to 30°C). Protect from moisture. Keep bottles tightly closed.

50 mg: Each white, oval tablet, biconvex with a full bisecting score on one side and imprinted CAPOTEN 50 on the other, contains: captopril 50 mg. Nonmedicinal ingredients: cornstarch, lactose, microcrystalline cellulose and stearic acid. Bottles of 100. Store at room temperature (15 to 30°C). Protect from moisture. Keep bottles tightly closed.

(Shown in Product Identification Section)

Capsaicin
Topical Analgesic

CPhA Monograph

Date of Preparation: July 2006

This monograph has been compiled by CPhA and reviewed by experts. It may contain information different from that found in Health Canada-approved Product Monographs. The reader is referred to the *CPS* Editorial Policy for more information.

SUMMARY PRODUCT INFORMATION:

Route of Administration	Dosage Form	Strength
Topical	cream	0.025%
	cream	0.05%
	cream	0.075%
	cream	0.025% plus menthol 4%
	cream	0.025% plus menthol 4%, camphor 3% and eucalyptus oil 0.5%
	gel	0.025% plus menthol 3%
	gel	0.035% plus menthol 3%
	liquid	0.025% plus camphor 3.5% and methyl salicylate 18%
	ointment	0.025% plus menthol 4%
	ointment	0.05% plus menthol 4%
	patch	0.004% plus camphor 1%, dementholized mint oil 0.6%, eucalyptus oil 0.5% and menthol 0.3%

INDICATIONS AND CLINICAL USE: Capsaicin is indicated for:

- topical treatment of pain syndromes

Capsaicin has been used topically for the treatment of pain due to diabetic neuropathy, post-herpetic neuralgia, osteoarthritis and rheumatoid arthritis.

Capsaicin cream has been reported to be statistically significantly more effective than vehicle alone in large randomized double-blind, vehicle controlled trials in patients with osteoarthritis, chronic neuropathic pain, including painful diabetic neuropathy, and post-herpetic neuralgia. Capsaicin has been shown to be as effective as orally administered amitriptyline in patients with painful diabetic neuropathy, and as effective as topical doxepin cream in patients with chronic neuropathic pain.

Capsaicin has also been found to be effective for the treatment of pruritic psoriasis and for idiopathic intractable pruritus ani.

The onset of action occurs after 14 to 28 days, while peak effect is achieved after 4 to 6 weeks of continuous therapy with capsaicin. Following application, the action of capsaicin has been noted to last several hours.

CONTRAINDICATIONS:

- Patients who are hypersensitive to capsaicin or to the fruits of Capsicum plants or to any ingredient in the formulation or component of the container.
- Capsaicin should not be used on broken or irritated skin.

WARNINGS AND PRECAUTIONS: Ophthalmologic: Avoid contact with eyes. After application, wash hands thoroughly to prevent spreading capsaicin to eyes and mucous membranes. Flush eyes with water if contact does occur.

Special Populations: The effects of capsaicin according to age or other factors in special populations have not been studied.

Pregnant Women: Safety in pregnancy has not been established, however, there are no documented problems in humans.

Nursing Women: It has not been determined if capsaicin is excreted into breast milk. In the unlikely case that capsaicin is applied to the nipple or areola, remove completely before breastfeeding.

Pediatrics: Use of capsaicin in children under the age of 2 years is not recommended.

ADVERSE REACTIONS: Adverse Drug Reactions Overview: See Table 1.

Table 1: Capsaicin

More Common Adverse Drug Reactions (≥1%)

Body System	Effect	Incidence	Clinical Comment
Dermatologic	Local burning, stinging or erythema	44–81%	This is a transient effect most prominent in the first week of treatment, which diminishes or disappears with continued use at the recommended dose. If capsaicin is applied less frequently than recommended or used intermittently, the burning effect may persist.
Respiratory	Coughing	5–12%	Likely due to inhalation of dried capsaicin residue. Can be prevented by washing the treated skin 30 to 40 minutes after application.

DRUG INTERACTIONS: Overview: No interactions with capsaicin have been identified.

DOSAGE AND ADMINISTRATION: Recommended Dose and Dosage Adjustment: Adults: See Table 2.

Table 2: Capsaicin

Dose in Adult Patients

Indication	Route	Dose	Clinical Comment
Pain syndromes	Topical	Apply cream or ointment sparingly 3 or 4 times daily to the affected area.	Therapeutic response may not be apparent for 1 to 2 weeks in arthritic disorders or 2 to 4 weeks in neuralgias.

Pediatrics: For children older than 2 years of age, refer to adult dosing (see Table 2).

Administration: Rub in well until little residue remains on the skin. If capsaicin is used on hands, refrain from washing hands for a minimum of 30 minutes. Heating pads should not be used and hot baths or showers should be avoided immediately prior to or following application of capsaicin since warm water or excessive sweating may intensify the localized burning sensation caused by capsaicin.

OVERDOSAGE:

For management of a suspected drug overdose, CPhA recommends that you contact your **regional Poison Control Centre**. See the *CPS* Directory section for a list of Poison Control Centres.

ACTION AND CLINICAL PHARMACOLOGY: Mechanism of Action: Capsaicin is a natural product derived from the fruit of plants in the genus Capsicum. Capsaicin depletes substance P from peripheral sensory C-type neurons, which, after repeat application, is presumed to reduce transmission of pain impulses to the CNS. Capsaicin also interacts with vanilloid (V1) receptors on sensory efferent neurons. Prolonged exposure to capsaicin stimulates and desensitizes V1 receptors, which are gated cation channels that are modulated by noxious stimuli.

Pharmacokinetics: Adults: Summary of Pharmacokinetic Parameters: Absorption: Percutaneous absorption of capsaicin is concentration and vehicle dependent, while the stratum corneum is believed to be the rate-limiting barrier. The effect of the vehicle correlates with alcohol content since this reflects greater capsaicin solubility and thus greater concentration can be achieved in the stratum corneum. Volatile alcohol-based vehicles facilitate capsaicin uptake into the skin better than nonvolatile glycols or oil-based vehicles.

Metabolism: In animal studies following intravenous administration, capsaicin was metabolized in the liver by the cytochrome P450 enzyme system mostly to dihydrocapsaicin, an active capsaicinoid.

Excretion: Elimination of capsaicin from the stratum corneum is vehicle independent and the half-life is estimated to be 24 hours following application. Intravenously administered capsaicin and its metabolites are excreted in the urine.

STORAGE AND STABILITY: Store in a cool place, protect from light and freezing.

Captopril

CPhA Monograph

see *ACE Inhibitors*

Carbachol

Parasympathomimetic Agent—Miotic

CPhA Monograph

Date of Revision: November 2003

> This monograph has been compiled by CPhA and reviewed by experts. It may contain information different from that found in Health Canada-approved Product Monographs. The reader is referred to the *CPS* Editorial Policy for more information.

PHARMACOLOGY: Carbachol is a parasympathomimetic agent that directly stimulates cholinergic receptors. Unlike acetylcholine, carbachol is resistant to inactivation by cholinesterase, resulting in a more prolonged action.

Carbachol is used primarily for its ocular hypotensive effect. Following ocular application, carbachol causes contraction of the ciliary muscle which pulls open the pores of the trabecular meshwork, facilitating aqueous humor outflow. Contraction of the ciliary muscle also causes accommodative spasm. Miosis is caused by the cholinergic stimulation of the papillary sphincter by the drug. Carbachol does not penetrate the cornea readily; benzalkonium chloride is used to enhance corneal penetration.

Pharmacokinetics: Following topical application of carbachol to the conjunctival sac, miosis occurs within 10 to 20 minutes, lasting 4 to 8 hours. Maximal reduction in intraocular pressure occurs in 4 hours and lasts for 8 hours.

Following intraocular administration, miosis occurs within 2 to 5 minutes and persists for about 24 hours. Reduction in intraocular pressure also lasts for approximately 24 hours.

INDICATIONS: Ophthalmic: 0.01% solutions have been used in ocular surgery to produce miosis following delivery of the lens in round pupil cataract extraction as well as in penetrating keratoplasty, iridectomy and anterior segment surgery where miosis is desired.

1.5 and 3% solutions are used for the reduction of intraocular pressure in chronic, primary, open-angle glaucoma.

CONTRAINDICATIONS: Hypersensitivity to carbachol, or to any ingredient in its commercial formulation; iritis, or other conditions in which pupillary constriction is undesirable.

WARNINGS: Carbachol should be used with extreme caution in the presence of the following conditions: asthma, acute heart failure, corneal abrasion, hyperthyroidism, urinary tract obstruction, Parkinson's disease, active peptic ulcer, or gastrointestinal spasm.

PRECAUTIONS: Patients requiring topical ophthalmic treatment should be advised about the transient ocular and frontal headache which usually accompanies the initial few days of therapy.

ADVERSE EFFECTS: The most frequent adverse effect following ophthalmic application is a burning or stinging sensation. Conjunctival hyperemia, blurred vision, twitching of eyelids, eye pain and headache frequently occur. Rarely, retinal detachment has occurred.

Ophthalmic administration has rarely been associated with systemic cholinergic side effects.

Systemic side effects may include bradycardia, sweating, asthma, nausea, faintness, vomiting, diarrhea, salivation and abdominal cramps. Atropine may be required for serious toxicity.

OVERDOSE:

> For management of a suspected drug overdose, CPhA recommends that you contact your **regional Poison Control Centre**. See the *CPS* Directory section for a list of Poison Control Centres.

DOSAGE: Ophthalmic: Topical: Instil 1 or 2 drops of carbachol 1.5% or 3% topical ophthalmic solution into the conjunctival sac 2 or 3 times daily, or as directed.

To minimize systemic absorption and drainage into the nose and throat, finger pressure may be applied to the lacrimal sac for 1 to 2 minutes following administration. Alternatively, simple lid closure for 2 to 5 minutes suspends the pumping action of fluid down the nasolacrimal system that occurs with blinking.

Following topical administration, excess solution should be removed from the hands and eye area.

Intraocular: 0.1 to 0.5 mL carbachol 0.01% ophthalmic injection solution is introduced into the anterior chamber to produce miosis during ocular surgery.

Carbocaine®

mepivacaine HCl

Local Anesthetic

Hospira

PHARMACOLOGY: Mepivacaine stabilizes the neuronal membrane and prevents the initiation and transmission of nerve impulses, thereby effecting local anesthesia. Its pharmacological properties are somewhat similar to those of lidocaine, which it resembles chemically. Its action is more rapid in onset and somewhat more prolonged than that of lidocaine. It has been employed for all types of infiltration and regional nerve block anesthesia.

Onset of anesthesia is rapid, the time of onset for sensory block ranging from about 3 to 20 minutes depending upon such factors as the anesthetic technique, the type of block, the concentration of the solution and the individual patient. The degree of motor blockade produced is dependent on the concentration of the solution. The 1% concentration will block sensory and sympathetic conduction without loss of motor function and will be effective in small superficial nerve blocks. The 2% concentration of mepivacaine will produce complete sensory and motor block of any nerve group.

The duration of anesthesia also varies depending upon the technique and type of block, the concentration and the individual. Mepivacaine will normally provide anesthesia which is adequate for 2 to 2½ hours of surgery. It has been reported that vasoconstrictors do not significantly prolong anesthesia with mepivacaine, but epinephrine (1:200 000) may be added to the mepivacaine solution to promote local hemostasis and to delay systemic absorption of the anesthetic.

The drowsiness and lassitude seen with lidocaine have not been commonly noted with mepivacaine. Mepivacaine has shown excellent tissue compatibility; irritation or tissue damage has not been observed.

INDICATIONS: For production of local or regional anesthesia by local infiltration, peripheral nerve block techniques, and central neural techniques including epidural and caudal blocks.

CONTRAINDICATIONS: Hypersensitivity to mepivacaine or amide-type local anesthetics or to other components of mepivacaine solutions.

WARNINGS: Local anesthetics should only be employed by clinicians who are well versed in diagnosis and management of dose-related toxicity and other acute emergencies which might arise from the block to be employed, and then only after insuring the immediate availability of oxygen, other resuscitative drugs, cardiopulmonary resuscitative equipment, and the personnel resources needed for proper management of toxic reactions and related emergencies (see also Adverse Effects and Precautions). Delay in proper management of dose-related toxicity, underventilation from any cause, and/or altered sensitivity may lead to acidosis, cardiac arrest and, possibly death.

Local anesthetic solutions containing antimicrobial preservatives (i.e., those supplied in multiple-dose vials) should not be used for epidural or caudal anesthesia because safety has **not** been established with regard to intrathecal injection, either intentionally or inadvertently, of such preservatives.

It is essential that aspiration for blood or cerebrospinal fluid (where applicable) be done prior to injecting any local anesthetic, both the original dose and all subsequent doses, to avoid intravascular or subarachnoid injection. However, a negative aspiration does not ensure against an intravascular or subarachnoid injection.

Mepivacaine with epinephrine or other vasopressors should not be used concomitantly with ergot-type oxytocic drugs, because a severe persistent hypertension may occur. Likewise, solutions of mepivacaine containing a vasoconstrictor, such as epinephrine, should be used with extreme caution in patients receiving monoamine oxidase inhibitors (MAOI) or antidepressants of the triptyline or imipramine types, because severe prolonged hypertension may result.

Local anesthetic procedures should be used with caution when there is inflammation and/or sepsis in the region of the proposed injection.

Mixing or the prior or intercurrent use of any local anesthetic with mepivacaine cannot be recommended because of insufficient data on the clinical use of such mixtures.

These solutions are not intended for spinal anesthesia or dental use.

PRECAUTIONS: General: During major regional nerve block, the patient should have i.v. fluids running via an indwelling catheter to assure a functioning i.v. pathway. Injections should be made slowly, with frequent aspirations before and during the injection to avoid intravascular injection. Current opinion favors fractional administration with constant attention to the patient, rather than rapid bolus injection. Syringe aspirations should also be performed before and during each supplemental injection in continuous (intermittent) catheter techniques. An intravascular injection is still possible even if aspirations for blood are negative.

During the administration of epidural anesthesia, it is recommended that a test dose be administered initially and the effects monitored before the full dose is given. When using a continuous catheter technique, test doses should be given prior to both the original and all reinforcing doses, because plastic tubing in the epidural space can migrate into a blood vessel or through the dura. When clinical conditions permit, an effective test dose should contain epinephrine (10 to 15 μg have been suggested) to serve as a warning of unintended intravascular injection. If injected into a blood vessel, this amount of epinephrine is likely to produce an epinephrine response within 45 seconds, consisting of an increase of pulse and blood pressure, circumoral pallor, palpitations, and nervousness in the unsedated patient. The sedated patient may exhibit only a pulse rate increase of 20 or more beats/minute for 15 or more seconds. Therefore, following the test dose, the heart rate should be monitored for a heart rate increase. The test dose should also contain an amide anesthetic to detect an unintended intrathecal administration. This will be evidenced within a few minutes by signs of spinal block. A negative outcome from the test dose does not guarantee that the epidural needle is accurately placed.

Injection of repeated doses of local anesthetics may cause significant increases in plasma levels with each repeated dose due to slow accumulation of the drug or its metabolites or to slow metabolic degradation. Tolerance to elevated blood levels varies with the status of the patient. Debilitated elderly patients, and acutely ill patients should be given reduced doses commensurate with their age and physical status. Local anesthetics should also be used with caution in patients with severe disturbances of cardiac rhythm, shock, heart block or hypotension.

Local anesthetic solutions containing a vasoconstrictor should be used cautiously and in carefully restricted quantities in areas of the body supplied by end arteries or having otherwise compromised blood supply such as digits, nose, external ear, penis. Patients with hypertensive vascular disease may exhibit exaggerated vasoconstrictor response. Ischemic injury or necrosis may result.

Mepivacaine should be used with caution in patients with known allergies and sensitivities.

Use mepivacaine cautiously in patients with hepatic and renal disease, and in patients with impaired cardiovascular function.

Serious dose-related cardiac arrhythmias may occur if preparations containing a vasoconstrictor such as epinephrine are employed in patients during or following the administration of potent inhalation anesthetics. In deciding whether to use these products concurrently in the same patient, the combined action of both agents upon the myocardium, the concentration and volume of vasoconstrictor used, and the time since injection, when applicable, should be taken into account. If epinephrine is used, a 1:200 000 concentration is preferred.

Many drugs used during the conduct of anesthesia are considered potential triggering agents for familial malignant hyperthermia. Because it is not known whether amide-type local anesthetics may trigger this reaction and because the need for supplemental general anesthesia cannot be predicted in advance, it is suggested that a standard protocol for management should be available.

Head and Neck Area: Small doses of local anesthetics injected into the head and neck area may produce adverse reactions similar to systemic toxicity seen with unintentional intravascular injections of larger doses. The injection procedures require the utmost care.

Pregnancy: Obstetrical anesthesia: Animal reproduction studies have not been conducted with mepivacaine. There are no adequate well-controlled studies in pregnant women of the effect of mepivacaine on the developing fetus. Mepivacaine should be used during pregnancy only if the potential benefit justifies the potential risk to the fetus. This does not preclude the use of mepivacaine at term for obstetrical anesthesia or analgesia.

Maternal hypotension has resulted from regional anesthesia. Local anesthetics produce vasodilation by blocking sympathetic nerves.

Epidural, paracervical, caudal, or pudendal anesthesia may alter the forces of parturition through changes in uterine contractility or maternal expulsive efforts. In one study, paracervical block anesthesia was associated with a decrease in the mean duration of first stage labor and facilitation of cervical dilation. Epidural anesthesia has been reported to prolong the second stage of labor by removing the parturient's reflex urge to bear down or by interfering with motor function. The use of obstetrical anesthesia may increase the need for forceps assistance.

The use of some local anesthetic drug products during labor and delivery may be followed by diminished muscle strength and tone for the first day or two of life. The long-term significance of these observations is unknown.

Fetal bradycardia may occur in 20 to 30% of patients receiving paracervical block anesthesia with the amide-type local anesthetics and may be associated with fetal acidosis. Fetal heart rate should always be monitored during paracervical anesthesia. Added risk appears to be present in prematurity, postmaturity, toxemia of pregnancy, and fetal distress. The physician should weigh the possible advantages against dangers when considering paracervical block in these conditions. Careful adherence to recommended dosage is of the utmost importance in obstetrical paracervical block. Failure to achieve adequate analgesia with recommended doses should arouse suspicion of intravascular or fetal intracranial injection.

Cases compatible with unintended fetal intracranial injection of local anesthetic solution have been reported following intended paracervical or pudendal block or both.

Case reports of maternal convulsions and cardiovascular collapse following use of some local anesthetics for paracervical block in early pregnancy (as anesthesia for elective abortion) suggest that systemic absorption under these circumstances may be rapid. Injection should be made slowly and with frequent aspiration. Allow a 5-minute interval between sides.

It is extremely important to avoid aortocaval compression by the gravid uterus during administration of regional block to parturients and the patient must be maintained in the left lateral decubitus position.

Lactation: It is not known whether local anesthetic drugs are excreted in human milk.

ADVERSE EFFECTS: Reactions to mepivacaine are characteristic of those associated with other amide-type local anesthetics: A major cause of adverse reactions to this group of drugs is excessive plasma levels, which may be due to overdosage, inadvertent intravascular injection or slow metabolic degradation. Transient slight stinging on injection has been noted occasionally.

CNS reactions are characterized by excitation and/or depression. Disorientation, restlessness, anxiety, dizziness, tinnitus, blurred vision or tremors may occur, possibly proceeding to convulsions. However, excitement may be transient or absent, with depression being the first manifestation of an adverse reaction. This may quickly be followed by drowsiness merging into unconsciousness and respiratory arrest. Other CNS effects may be nausea, vomiting, chills and constriction of the pupils.

High doses or inadvertent intravascular injection may lead to high plasma levels and related depression of the myocardium, decreased cardiac output, heart block, hypotension (or sometimes hypertension) bradycardia, ventricular arrhythmias and possibly cardiac arrest.

Allergic-type reactions are rare and may occur as a result of sensitivity to the local anesthetic or to other formulation ingredients, such as the antimicrobial preservative methylparaben, contained in multiple-dose vials. Cross-sensitivity among members of amide-type local anesthetic group has been reported. The usefulness of screening for sensitivity has not been definitely established.

Neurologic effects following epidural or caudal anesthesia may include spinal block of varying magnitude (including high or total spinal block); hypotension secondary to spinal block; urinary retention; fecal and urinary incontinence; loss of perineal sensation and sexual function; persistent anesthesia, paresthesia, weakness, paralysis of the lower extremities and loss of sphincter control, all of which may have slow, incomplete or no recovery; headache; backache; septic meningitis; meningismus, slowing of labor; increased incidence of forceps delivery; cranial nerve palsies due to traction on nerves from loss of cerebrospinal fluid; neuritis; numbness.

OVERDOSE:

Treatment: Toxic effects of local anesthetics require symptomatic treatment; there is no specific cure. The physician should be prepared to maintain an airway and to support ventilation with oxygen and assisted or controlled respiration as required. Supportive treatment of the cardiovascular system includes i.v. fluids and, when appropriate, vasopressors (preferably those that stimulate the myocardium).

Convulsions may be controlled with oxygen and i.v. administration, in small increments, of a barbiturate or muscle relaxant, as follows: preferably, an ultra short-acting barbiturate such as thiopental or thiamylal; if this is not available, a short-acting barbiturate (e.g. secobarbital or pentobarbital) or a short-acting muscle relaxant (succinylcholine). I.V. muscle relaxants and barbiturates should only be administered by those familiar with their use.

For management of a suspected drug overdose, CPhA recommends that you contact your **regional Poison Control Centre**. See the *CPS* Directory section for a list of Poison Control Centres.

DOSAGE: The dose of any local anesthetic administered varies with the anesthetic procedure, the area to be anesthetized, the vascularity of the tissues, the number of neuronal segments to be blocked, the depth of anesthesia and degree of muscle relaxation required, the duration of anesthesia desired, individual tolerance and the physical condition of the patient. The recommended single adult dose for unsedated, healthy, normal-sized individuals should not usually exceed 400 mg. The following dosages have generally proved satisfactory and are therefore suggested as a guide. The smallest dose and concentration required to produce the desired result should be administered. The recommended dosage is based on requirements for the average adult and should be reduced for elderly or debilitated patients.

Nerve Block (e.g., cervical, brachial, intercostal, pudendal): From 5 to 40 mL of a 1% solution, or 5 to 20 mL of a 2% solution, depending on the area and extent of block. Pudendal block: one half of total dose injected each side.

Paracervical Block: Maximum of up to 20 mL of a 1% solution (half-dose injected slowly each side, 5 minutes between sides) per 90-minute period.

Transvaginal Block: Up to 30 mL of a 1% solution (half-dose injected each side).

Caudal and Epidural Block: From 15 to 30 mL of a 1% solution, from 10 to 20 mL of a 2% solution containing no preservative.

Infiltration: Up to 40 mL of a 1% solution (or an equivalent amount in a more dilute solution, depending on the area of the operative field).

Therapeutic Block (in management of pain): From 1 to 5 mL of a 1 or 2% solution.

Pediatric doses should be measured as a percentage of total adult dose based on body weight (not exceeding 5 to 6 mg/kg). In children under 3 years of age or weighing less than 14 kg, 1% solutions should be employed.

Mepivacaine solution may be diluted with an equal part of sodium chloride injection USP. Dosages in excess of the aforementioned amounts have been administered without serious side effects. Due caution should be exercised in the use of larger dosages and in general a total dosage of 7 mg/kg should not be exceeded. Under no circumstances should administration be repeated at intervals less than 1.5 hours. The total dose for 24 hours should not exceed 1000 mg.

SUPPLIED: Infiltration and Nerve Block: Each mL of solution contains: mepivacaine HCl 10 mg in water for injection. Nonmedicinal ingredients: sodium chloride and methylparaben. May also contain sodium hydroxide and/or hydrochloric acid (for pH adjustment). Gluten-, lactose- and sulfite-free. Multiple dose vials of 50 mL (1%), boxes of 5.

Caudal and Epidural Block: Each mL of solution contains: mepivacaine HCl 10 mg in water for injection. Nonmedicinal ingredients: calcium chloride (dihydrate), potassium chloride and sodium chloride. May also contain sodium hydroxide and/or hydrochloric acid (for pH adjustment). Gluten-, lactose-, preservative- and sulfite-free. Single dose vials of 30 mL (1%), boxes of 10.

Caudal and Epidural Block: Each mL of solution contains: mepivacaine HCl 20 mg in water for injection. Nonmedicinal ingredients: calcium chloride (dihydrate), potassium chloride and sodium chloride. May also contain sodium hydroxide and/or hydrochloric acid (for pH adjustment). Gluten-, lactose-, preservative- and sulfite-free. Single dose vials of 20 mL (2%), boxes of 10.

Carbolith® Ⓟ

lithium carbonate

Antimanic

Valeant

PHARMACOLOGY: Preclinical studies have shown that lithium alters sodium transport in nerve and muscle cells and effects a shift toward intraneuronal metabolism of catecholamines, but the specific biochemical mechanism of lithium action in mania is unknown.

Pharmacokinetics: Lithium ions are rapidly absorbed from the gastrointestinal tract and plasma lithium peaks are reached 2 to 4 hours after lithium administration. The distribution of lithium in the body approximates that of total body water, but its passage across the blood-brain barrier is slow and at equilibration the CSF lithium level reaches only approximately half the plasma concentration.

Lithium undergoes a biphasic elimination pathway with an alpha half-life of 5 hours and beta half-life of 18 hours.

Lithium is excreted primarily in urine with less than 1% being eliminated with the feces. Lithium is filtered by the glomeruli and 80% of the filtered lithium is reabsorbed in the tubules, probably by the same mechanism responsible for sodium reabsorption.

The renal clearance of lithium is proportional to its plasma concentration. About 50% of a single dose of lithium is excreted in 24 hours. A low salt intake resulting in low tubular concentration of sodium will increase lithium reabsorption and might result in retention or intoxication.

Renal lithium clearance tends to be remarkably constant in the same individual but decreases with age and when sodium intake is lowered. The dose necessary to maintain a given concentration of serum lithium depends on the ability of the kidney to excrete lithium. However, renal lithium excretion may vary greatly between individuals and lithium dosage must, therefore, be adjusted individually. In clinical reports, it has been noted that serum lithium may rise an average of 0.2 to 0.4 mEq or mmol/L after intake of 300 mg and 0.3 to 0.6 mEq or mmol/L after intake of 600 mg of lithium carbonate. It has been suggested that manic patients retain larger amounts of lithium during the active manic phase, but recent studies have been unable to confirm a clear difference in excretion patterns. However, patients in a manic state seem to have an increased tolerance to lithium.

Once Daily Administration: Clinical trials comparing once daily at bedtime dosing versus 2 to 4 times-a-day dosing have shown that urinary volume is significantly decreased with single daily dosing.

Total daily doses of lithium required to reach therapeutic levels were lower with the once-daily dosage schedule than with the divided dosage schedule.

In addition, administration of a single bedtime dose of lithium may result in initial post-absorptive symptoms—which are believed to be associated with rapid rise in serum lithium levels—to occur at night while the patient is sleeping.

In one study, significantly less sclerotic glomeruli, atrophic tubules and interstitial fibrosis were observed in patients on a single daily dosage regimen, as compared to patients on a multiple daily dosage regimen.

INDICATIONS: In the lithium treatment of manic episodes of manic-depressive illness. Maintenance therapy has been found to be useful in preventing or diminishing the frequency of subsequent relapses in bipolar manic-depressive patients (with a history of mania). Typical symptoms of mania, as an affective disorder, include pressure of speech, motor hyperactivity, reduced need for sleep, flight of ideas, grandiosity, or poor judgment, aggressiveness, and possibly hostility. When given to a patient experiencing a manic episode, lithium may produce a normalization of symptomatology within 1 to 3 weeks.

CONTRAINDICATIONS: Lithium should generally not be given to patients with significant renal or cardiovascular disease, severe debilitation or dehydration, or sodium depletion, and to patients receiving diuretics, since the risk of lithium toxicity is very high in such patients. If the psychiatric indication is life-threatening, and if such a patient fails to respond to other measures, lithium treatment may be undertaken with extreme caution, including daily serum lithium determinations and adjustments to the usually low doses ordinarily tolerated by these individuals. In such instances, hospitalization is necessary.

WARNINGS: Lithium toxicity is closely related to serum lithium levels, and can occur at doses close to the therapeutic levels. Facilities for prompt and accurate serum lithium determinations should be available before initiating therapy.

The ability to tolerate lithium is greater during the acute manic phase and decreases when manic symptoms subside (see Dosage).

Impaired Renal Function: Chronic lithium therapy is frequently associated with a decrease in renal concentrating capacity with development of thirst, polyuria, micturia, weight gain and altered kidney function tests, occasionally presenting as nephrogenic diabetes insipidus. Such patients should be carefully managed to avoid dehydration with resulting lithium retention and toxicity. The evidence suggests that impaired renal function during chronic therapy may be in most instances, only partially reversible when lithium is discontinued.

Prevention of renal toxicity and other toxic effects of long-term therapy requires a firm diagnosis of bipolar manic depressive illness; careful screening for pre-existing renal and other diseases; establishment of standardized 12-hour serum lithium levels which are as low as possible yet clinically effective; maintaining control of treatment by monitoring serum lithium levels and exercising clinical and laboratory surveillance over possible side effects or signs of lithium intoxication; exercising maximum control of at-risk patients; insuring that long-term lithium therapy is maintained only when clinical response has been clearly established; and adjusting the dosage schedule and preparation used so as to obtain temporarily periods of lithium concentrations as low as possible in the kidney.

Glomerular sclerosis and interstitial fibrosis as well as tubular lesions have been reported in patients on chronic lithium therapy. When kidney function is assessed for baseline data prior to starting lithium therapy or thereafter, routine urinalysis and other tests may be used to evaluate tubular function (e.g., urine specific gravity or osmolality or 24-hour urine volume) and glomerular function (e.g., serum creatinine or creatinine clearance).

During lithium therapy, progressive or sudden changes in renal function, even within the normal range indicate the need for re-evaluation of treatment including dosage and frequency of lithium administration, and a reassessment of the risk-benefit of long-term lithium therapy.

Pregnancy: Data from lithium birth registries suggest an increase in cardiac and other anomalies, especially Ebstein's anomaly; nephrogenic diabetes insipidus, euthyroid goiter and hypoglycemia have occurred in infants born to women who took lithium during pregnancy. Therefore, lithium should not be used during pregnancy or in women of childbearing potential unless it cannot be substituted by other appropriate therapy and in the opinion of the physician the expected benefits outweigh the possible hazards to the fetus.

Lactation: Lithium is excreted in human milk. Nursing should not be undertaken during lithium therapy except in rare and unusual circumstances where, in the view of the physician, the potential benefits to the mother outweigh possible hazards to the child.

Children: Since information regarding the safety and effectiveness of lithium in children under 12 years of age is not available, the use of lithium carbonate in such patients is not recommended at this time.

PRECAUTIONS: To maximize benefits, minimize the risks, and reduce as much as possible the adverse effects of lithium therapy, it is essential to provide proper information to patients and relatives about the treatment regimen and control procedures required during treatment, as well as an explanation of the expected benefits and the most commonly experienced immediate and long-term side effects. In most cases, appropriate written material should be provided to supplement verbal information.

Outpatients and their families should be warned that the patient must discontinue therapy and contact the physician if such clinical signs of lithium toxicity as diarrhea, vomiting, tremor, mild ataxia, drowsiness, or muscular weakness occur.

Occupational Hazards: Further, since lithium may impair mental and/or physical abilities, patients should be cautioned about undertaking activities requiring alertness (e.g., operating vehicles or machinery).

Previously existing underlying thyroid disorders do not necessarily constitute a contraindication to lithium therapy; where hypothyroidism exists, careful monitoring of the thyroid function during lithium stabilization and maintenance allows for correction of changing thyroid parameters, if any. Where hypothyroidism occurs during lithium stabilization and maintenance, supplemental thyroid treatment may be used.

Lithium decreases sodium re-absorption by the renal tubules which would lead to sodium depletion. Therefore, it is essential for the patient to maintain a normal diet, including salt, and an adequate fluid intake (2 500 to 3 000 mL), at least during the initial stabilization period. Decreased tolerance to lithium has been reported to ensue from protracted sweating or diarrhea and, if such occurs, supplemental fluid and salt should be administered. In addition to sweating and diarrhea, concomitant infection with elevated temperatures may also necessitate a temporary reduction or cessation of medication.

Drug Interactions: Combined Use of Haloperidol and Lithium: An encephalopathy resembling the malignant neuroleptic syndrome (characterized by weakness, lethargy, fever, tremulousness and confusion, extrapyramidal symptoms, leukocytosis, elevated serum enzymes, BUN and FBS) followed by irreversible brain damage has occurred in a few patients treated with lithium plus haloperidol. A causal relationship between these events and concomitant administration of lithium and haloperidol has not been clearly established; however, patients receiving such combined therapy should be monitored closely for early evidence of neurological toxicity such as rigidity and/or hyperpyrexia and treatment discontinued promptly if such signs appear.

Combined Use of Phenothiazines and Lithium: Both pharmacokinetic interactions and clinical toxicity with the combined use of these agents have been described. Lithium-induced reductions in plasma chlorpromazine levels, phenothiazine-induced increases in red cell uptake of lithium and chlorpromazine-induced increases in renal lithium excretion have been reported. Clinically, occasional cases of neurotoxicity have been reported and may be more likely to occur with thioridazine than other phenothiazines, when combined with lithium. Therefore, the clinician should be alert for altered response to either drug when used in combination and when either drug is withdrawn.

The action of neuromuscular blocking agents may be prolonged in patients receiving lithium. Therefore, caution should be exercised when the combination is required. A temporary omission of a few doses of lithium can reduce the risks of this interaction.

Indomethacin has been reported to increase steady-state plasma lithium levels by 30 to 59%. There is also evidence that other nonsteroidal anti-inflammatory agents may have a similar effect. When such combinations are used, increased frequency of monitoring plasma lithium levels is recommended.

There are reports that concurrent use of methyldopa or tetracycline may increase the risk of lithium toxicity.

Concurrent use of lithium and carbamazepine or phenytoin might result in an increased risk of CNS toxicity. The administration of aminophylline or theophylline to patients on lithium therapy may require increased lithium doses to maintain the psychotropic effect. Patients stabilized on lithium therapy who receive a thiazide diuretic may require a reduction of lithium dosage to avoid accumulation and toxicity, since there is often a 20 to 40% reduction of renal lithium clearance. Furosemide appears to be less likely to affect lithium clearance.

ADVERSE EFFECTS: Mild side effects may be encountered even when serum lithium levels remain below 1 mEq/L. The most frequent side effects are the initial postabsorptive symptoms, believed to be associated with a rapid rise in serum lithium levels. They include nausea, abdominal pain, vomiting, diarrhea, vertigo, muscle weakness, sleepiness and a dazed feeling, and frequently disappear after stabilization of therapy. The more common and persistent adverse reactions are: fine tremor of the hands which is not responsive to antiparkinson drugs, and at times, fatigue, thirst and polyuria (renal toxicity). These side effects may subside with continued treatment or a temporary reduction or cessation of dosage. If persistent, a lowering or cessation of dosage and reassessment of lithium therapy is indicated.

Mild to moderate toxic reactions may occur at lithium levels from 1.5 to 2 mEq/L, and moderate to severe reactions at levels above 2 mEq/L. Permanent neurological damage has been reported after exposure to toxic levels of lithium.

A number of patients may experience lithium accumulation during initial therapy, increasing to toxic levels and requiring immediate discontinuation of the drug. Some elderly patients with lower renal clearances for lithium may also experience different degrees of lithium toxicity, requiring reduction or temporary withdrawal of medication. However, in patients with normal renal clearance the toxic manifestations appear to occur in a fairly regular sequence related to serum lithium levels. The usually transient gastrointestinal symptoms are the earliest side effects to occur. A mild degree of fine tremor of the hands may persist throughout therapy. Thirst and polyuria may be followed by increased drowsiness, ataxia, tinnitus and blurred vision, indicating early intoxication. As intoxication progresses the following manifestations may be encountered: confusion, increasing disorientation, muscle twitching, hyperreflexia, nystagmus, seizures, diarrhea, vomiting, and eventually coma and death.

The following toxic reactions have been reported and appear to be related to serum lithium levels, including levels within the therapeutic range.

Neuromuscular: tremor, muscle hyperirritability (fasciculations, twitching, clonic movements of whole limbs), ataxia, choreoathetotic movements, hyperactive deep tendon reflexes.

Central Nervous System: blackout spells, epileptiform seizures, slurred speech, dizziness, vertigo, incontinence of urine or feces, somnolence, psychomotor retardation, restlessness, confusion, stupor, coma.

Cardiovascular: cardiac arrhythmia, hypotension, peripheral circulatory collapse.

Gastrointestinal: anorexia, nausea, vomiting, diarrhea.
Genitourinary: albuminuria, oliguria, polyuria, glycosuria.
Dermatologic: drying and thinning of hair, anesthesia of skin, acne, chronic folliculitis, xerosis cutis, alopecia and exacerbation of psoriasis.
Autonomic Nervous System: blurred vision, dry mouth.
Thyroid Abnormalities: euthyroid goiter and/or hypothyroidism (including myxedema) accompanied by lower T_3 and T_4 levels and elevated TSH. Iodine^{131} uptake may be elevated. On the average 5 to 15% of patients on long-term lithium therapy manifest clinical signs or have altered serum hormone levels (see Precautions). Paradoxically, rare cases of hyperthyroidism have been reported.
EEG Changes: diffuse slowing, widening of frequency spectrum, potentiation and disorganization of background rhythm.
ECG Changes: reversible flattening, isoelectricity or inversion of T waves.
Miscellaneous: fatigue, lethargy, transient scotomata, dehydration, weight loss, tendency to sleep.

Miscellaneous reactions frequently unrelated to dosage include: transient EEG and ECG changes, leukocytosis, headache, diffuse non-toxic goiter with or without hypothyroidism, transient hyperglycemia, generalized pruritus with or without rash, cutaneous ulcers, albuminuria, worsening of organic brain syndrome, excessive weight gain, edematous swelling of ankles or wrists, and thirst or polyuria, sometimes resembling diabetes insipidus, and metallic taste.

A single instance has been reported of the development of painful discoloration of fingers and toes and coldness of the extremities within one day of starting treatment with lithium. The mechanism through which these symptoms (resembling Raynaud's syndrome) developed is not known. Recovery followed discontinuance.

Serious reactions to long-term therapy: In addition to other possible adverse reactions, the main concern during chronic lithium therapy centers on the kidney function, the thyroid, parathyroid, the bones and skin.

OVERDOSE:

Symptoms: Lithium toxicity is closely related to the concentration of lithium in the blood and is usually associated with serum concentrations in excess of 1.5 mEq/L or mmol/L. Early signs of toxicity which may occur at lower serum concentrations were described under Adverse Effects and usually respond to reduction of dosage. Lithium intoxication has been preceded by the appearance or aggravation of the following symptoms: sluggishness, drowsiness, lethargy, coarse tremors or muscle twitchings, loss of appetite, vomiting, and diarrhea. Occurrence of these symptoms requires immediate cessation of medication and careful clinical reassessment and management. Signs and symptoms of lithium intoxication have already been described under Adverse Effects.

Treatment: No specific antidote for lithium poisoning is known. Early symptoms of lithium toxicity can usually be treated by reduction or cessation of dosage of the drug and resumption of the treatment at a lower dose after 24 to 48 hours. In severe cases of lithium poisoning, the first and foremost goal of treatment consists of elimination of this ion from the patient and supportive care.

Recommended treatment consists of: gastric lavage, correction of fluid and electrolyte imbalance and regulation of kidney function. Urea, mannitol and aminophylline all produce significant increases in lithium excretion. Hemodialysis is an effective and rapid means of removing the ion from the severely toxic patient. Infection prophylaxis, regular chest x-ray, and preservation of adequate respiration are essential.

> For management of a suspected drug overdose, CPhA recommends that you contact your **regional Poison Control Centre**. See the *CPS* Directory section for a list of Poison Control Centres.

DOSAGE: Selection of patients and approach to lithium therapy: The results of lithium therapy depend largely on the nature and course of the illness itself, rather than on the symptoms. The selection of patients for long-term treatment requires a clearcut diagnosis of primary affective disorder, the condition for which the stabilizing effects of lithium have been found useful. The variables that have been more consistently associated with response to lithium therapy in patients with a primary affective disorder are: the good quality of remissions with good function and no significant symptomatology during the free intervals between previous episodes of illness; low frequency of episodes, typically 1 or 2 (and not more than 3 or 4) per year; and symptomatology during the acute episodes that meet strict criteria for a primary affective disorder (DSM-III; Research Diagnosis Criteria).

Screening for lithium candidates should include at least, a medical history and physical examination with emphasis on the CNS, urinary, cardiovascular, gastrointestinal and endocrine systems and the skin. It should also include: routine 24-hour urine volume, serum creatinine, record of weight, and ECG, possibly electrolytes and TSH, and for long-term treatment, creatinine clearance and a urine concentration test. Other examinations and tests should be used when indicated. Monitoring lithium treatment should include, for each visit, mental status, physical examination, weight, 12-hour serum lithium and a check for lithium side effects and compliance. It should also include serum creatinine every 2 months, plasma thyroid hormone and TSH every 6 to 12 months, particularly in female patients, and attention to renal and thyroid function should be maintained throughout, with tests used for baseline screening repeated as required.

The first objective of treatment is to establish an effective and safe daily dosage of lithium with the aid of standardized 12-hour serum lithium levels maintained within the therapeutic range, as high as necessary for efficacy, and with the patient as much as possible free of significant side effects. Three daily doses should be used initially, at least until the daily dosage is established. The next aim is to move to an optimal dose, which should be as low as possible, consistent with protection against relapse. During follow-up, an adjustment to lower dosages may be required to minimize adverse effects, and a change in the lithium preparation used and/or the frequency of dosing, either towards multiple doses or towards a single dose, may be necessary to handle absorption-related adverse effects or concern over possible renal toxicity. Intermittent lithium treatment in carefully selected patients has been recommended by some lithium experts, but should not be undertaken without careful planning and great caution. The cooperation of patients and relatives is required throughout. Before deciding on the institution of long-term treatment, it is essential to establish that the patient has clearly responded to a course of stabilizing lithium therapy and that the risk of such therapy is acceptable. Maintaining a patient with a lithium non-responsive condition on long-term therapy poses an unacceptable risk. A decision with regards to long-term therapy can be made during a time-limited trial of lithium therapy with frequent reassessment of outcome. The following are among the factors to be reassessed before a decision is made; careful reconfirmation of the diagnosis of primary affective disorder; the health status of the patient; the side effects of lithium therapy experienced by the patient, and the response to treatment. Assessment of response to treatment is based strictly on firm evidence of relapse prevention during a reasonable trial period, but can be assisted by consideration of the predictors of response outlined above. Great pains should be taken to exclude false responders and false non-responders. It should also be borne in mind that non-responders are more susceptible to the adverse effects of lithium.

Acute Mania: The therapeutic dose for the treatment of acute mania should be based primarily on the patient's clinical condition. It must be individualized for each patient according to blood concentrations and clinical response. The dosage should be adjusted to obtain serum concentrations between 0.8 and 1.2 mEq or mmol/L (in blood samples drawn before the patient has had his first lithium dose of the day).

In properly screened adult patients, with good renal function, the suggested initial daily dosage for acute mania is 900 to 1800 mg (15 to 20 mg/kg), divided into 3 doses. In view of the large variability of renal lithium excretion between individuals, it is suggested that lithium treatment be started at a dose between 600 and 900 mg/day, reaching gradually a level of 1 200 to 1 800 mg in 3 divided doses. Depending on the patient's clinical condition, the initial dosage should be adjusted to produce the desired serum lithium concentration. The weight of the patient should also influence the choice of the initial dose.

Geriatrics: Lithium should be used cautiously and in reduced doses in the elderly patient, usually in the range of 600 to 1 200 mg/day. Serum lithium concentrations should be monitored frequently and kept below 1.0 mEq/L or mmol/L.

Maintenance Therapy: After the acute manic episode subsides, the dosage should be rapidly reduced to achieve serum concentrations between 0.6 and 1.0 mEq or mmol/L, since there is evidence at this time of a decreased tolerance to lithium. The average suggested dosage at this stage is 900 mg/day (approximately 25 mEq), divided into 3 doses, with a range usually between 500 and 1 200 mg/day. If a satisfactory response to antimanic lithium is not obtained in 14 days, consider discontinuing lithium therapy. When the manic attack is controlled, maintain lithium administration during the expected duration of the manic phase, since early withdrawal might lead to relapse. It is essential to maintain clinical supervision of the patient and monitor lithium concentrations as required during treatment (see Precautions).

Once patients are stabilized on a maintenance dose with a multiple dosing schedule, and once stable therapeutic blood levels are reached, the dosage schedule may be changed to a once daily dosage administration.

The total daily dose, when administered as a single daily dose, may be approximately 5 to 30% lower than when given in divided doses over the day.

It is essential to maintain clinical supervision of the patient and to monitor serum lithium levels both when using the divided daily dosage regimen and when transferring to the once daily administration dosage regimen.

In uncomplicated cases receiving maintenance therapy during remission, serum lithium levels should be monitored at least every 2 months.

Patients abnormally sensitive to lithium may exhibit toxic signs at serum levels of 1 to 1.4 mEq/L.

Elderly patients often respond to reduced dosage and may exhibit signs of toxicity at serum levels ordinarily tolerated by other patients.

Note: Blood samples for serum lithium determination should be drawn immediately prior to the next dose when lithium concentrations are relatively stable (i.e., 12±1 hours after the previous dose of lithium). Total reliance must not be placed on serum levels alone. Adequate patient evaluation requires both clinical assessment and laboratory analysis.

Children: Lithium is not recommended for routine use in children under 12 years of age since information in this age group is not yet available.

SUPPLIED: 150 mg (Lactose-free): Each orange and white capsule printed ICN C11 contains: lithium carbonate USP 150 mg. Nonmedicinal ingredients: talc; shell: FD&C Red #3, FD&C Yellow #6, gelatin and titanium dioxide. Lactose-free. Bottles of 100 and 1 000.

300 mg (Lactose-free): Each flesh-colored capsule printed ICN C12 contains: lithium carbonate USP 300 mg. Nonmedicinal ingredients: talc; shell: FD&C Red #2, FD&C Yellow #6, gelatin and titanium dioxide. Lactose-free. Bottles of 100 and 1 000.

600 mg: Each aqua-blue opaque-colored capsule printed ICN C13 contains: lithium carbonate USP 600 mg. Nonmedicinal ingredients: lactose and talc; shell: FD&C Blue #1, gelatin and titanium dioxide. Bottles of 100.

Carbonic Anhydrase Inhibitors: Systemic ℞

acetazolamide
methazolamide

Carbonic Anhydrase Inhibitors

CPhA Monograph

Date of Revision: November 2005

> This monograph has been compiled by CPhA and reviewed by experts. It may contain information different from that found in Health Canada-approved Product Monographs. The reader is referred to the *CPS* Editorial Policy for more information.

PHARMACOLOGY: Carbonic anhydrase inhibitors (CAIs) are nonbacteriostatic sulfonamides that reduce the formation of hydrogen and bicarbonate ions from carbon dioxide and water. In the kidneys, this causes a decrease in hydrogen ion secretion and an increase in sodium, potassium, bicarbonate and water excretion at the proximal tubules resulting in an alkaline diuresis. Inhibition of carbonic anhydrase in the ciliary process of the eye results in a decrease in production of bicarbonate and aqueous humor, thus reducing intraocular pressure in patients with glaucoma. It is suggested that the anticonvulsant effects of CAIs are due to carbonic anhydrase inhibition in the CNS which retards abnormal, paroxysmal and excessive discharge from neurons.

Pharmacokinetics: After oral administration, CAIs are absorbed from the GI tract, and distributed primarily into erythrocytes, the eyes, the plasma and the CNS. Acetazolamide is excreted unchanged by the kidneys. Methazolamide is partially metabolized by the liver and 15 to 30% is excreted unchanged.

INDICATIONS: CAIs are used in the adjunctive treatment of chronic simple (open-angle) glaucoma, secondary glaucoma, and preoperatively in acute angle-closure glaucoma where delay of surgery is desired in order to lower intraocular pressure. Acetazolamide is also used to prevent symptoms of high-altitude sickness, as an adjunct in the treatment of absence seizures and in the treatment of edema, hydrocephalus and periodic paralysis.

Currently, oral CAIs are rarely used in the treatment of glaucoma because of their serious adverse effects. Therapy has shifted toward the use of topical CAIs which are better tolerated and have fewer side effects. The role of acetazolamide as a diuretic or an anticonvulsant is also limited because tolerance to CAIs develop quickly. Intermittent use is more effective than long-term use.

CONTRAINDICATIONS: CAIs are contraindicated in patients with liver disease or dysfunction. Administration of CAIs to patients with cirrhosis can cause hepatic encephalopathy. Acetazolamide should be avoided in patients with creatinine clearance of less than 10 mL/min. Methazolamide is contraindicated in patients with renal insufficiency. CAIs should not be given to patients with low serum potassium or sodium levels, suprarenal gland failure or hyperchloremic acidosis. Long-term use of CAIs for the treatment of noncongestive angle-closure glaucoma is contraindicated since decreased intraocular pressure may mask worsening glaucoma.

WARNINGS: See Precautions.

PRECAUTIONS: It is recommended that a complete blood count be performed at baseline and at regular intervals (at least once every 6 months) during CAI therapy. If there are any significant changes, the drug should be discontinued. Regular monitoring of electrolytes is also recommended. The dose of acetazolamide should be adjusted in patients with renal impairment. Patients with previous sulfonamide sensitivity should take CAIs with caution since cross-sensitivity between antibacterial and other diuretic sulfonamides have been reported. CAIs should be used with caution in patients with respiratory acidosis or those with severe loss of respiratory capacity since they can precipitate or aggravate acidosis. Diabetics should be advised that blood or urine glucose levels may increase. Patients taking CAIs should avoid tasks that require mental alertness or physical coordination until they know how the drug will affect them.

Pregnancy: Teratogenicity has been demonstrated in animal studies. There are no well-controlled studies in pregnant women. CAIs should not be used in pregnancy, especially the first trimester, unless the benefits outweigh the risks.

Lactation: Safety for use in nursing mothers has not been established because the extent of CAI excretion into breast milk is uncertain. The American Academy of Pediatrics considers acetazolamide to be compatible with breast-feeding. There are no data available for methazolamide.

Children: No randomized controlled studies exist; however, acetazolamide has been used in children to treat glaucoma, seizures and hydrocephalus.

Drug Interactions: Anticonvulsants: CAIs may increase the risk of osteomalacia caused by anticonvulsants such as phenytoin, phenobarbital or primidone.
Cisapride: Hypokalemia caused by acetazolamide increases the risk for cardiac arrhythmias.
Cyclosporine: Acetazolamide may increase cyclosporine trough levels with possible nephrotoxicity and neurotoxicity.
Drugs Excreted Renally: Urinary alkalinization caused by CAIs may lead to a decrease in effect of phenobarbital and salicylates, and an increased effect of amphetamines, memantine, procainamide, quinidine and possibly tricyclic antidepressants.
Potassium-related: Low potassium caused by CAIs may increase the risk of digoxin toxicity, and hypokalemia secondary to other drugs (e.g., diuretics, amphotericin) may worsen.
Primidone serum and urine concentration may be decreased with concomitant CAI use.
Salicylates: CAI-induced acidosis increases the CNS penetration of salicylates. Salicylates also increase the accumulation and thus the toxicity of CAIs.
Topiramate: When topiramate (a weak CAI) is used in combination with other CAIs, the risk of developing renal stones may be increased.

ADVERSE EFFECTS: Adverse reactions that occur most often (> 10%) with CAIs are malaise, diarrhea, anorexia, metallic taste and polyuria. Drowsiness, dizziness and depression are also common, occurring at a rate of 1 to 10%. The following have also been reported at a rate of < 1%.
Central Nervous System: tinnitus, paresthesia (a numbness and tingling feeling in the extremities), convulsions, weakness, fatigue, nervousness, disorientation, confusion, ataxia, tremor, headache, lassitude and flaccid paralysis.
Dermatologic: Photosensitivity, urticaria and rash including Stevens-Johnson syndrome, erythema multiforme and toxic epidermal necrolysis have been reported.
Gastrointestinal: Abdominal cramping, dyspepsia and nausea have commonly occurred. Melena, constipation and dryness of the mouth have occasionally occurred.
Hematologic: More serious adverse reactions include bone marrow depression, thrombocytopenia, thrombocytopenia purpura, leukopenia, pancytopenia, agranulocytosis, aplastic and hemolytic anemia.
Renal and Metabolic: metabolic acidosis (incidence increases to 50% for acetazolamide in the elderly), hypokalemia, hyperglycemia, renal calculi.
Miscellaneous: hepatic failure, myopia, impotence.

OVERDOSE:

Symptoms: Drowsiness, anorexia, hypoglycemia, nausea, vomiting, dizziness, paresthesia, ataxia, tremor and tinnitus.

Treatment: Treatment is symptomatic and supportive. Hypoglycemia can be corrected with i.v. dextrose. Monitor electrolytes and blood pH. Acidosis may respond to bicarbonate administration and potassium supplementation may be necessary.

> For management of a suspected drug overdose, CPhA recommends that you contact your **regional Poison Control Centre**. See the *CPS* Directory section for a list of Poison Control Centres.

DOSAGE: Acetazolamide can be given p.o. or i.v. Acetazolamide for injection is available through the Special Access Programme, Health Canada (see Appendix). The extended-release capsule is indicated only for use in glaucoma and high altitude sickness. I.M. administration is not recommended because the alkaline pH can cause pain. Methazolamide is given only orally. Orally administered CAIs should be taken with food to decrease GI side effects.

Geriatrics: Initial starting dose of acetazolamide is 250 mg once or twice daily. The lowest effective dose should be used.

Glaucoma (see Indications): CAIs should be used as adjunct to other glaucoma therapy. The adult dose of methazolamide for glaucoma is 50 to 100 mg 2 or 3 times a day. The adult dose of acetazolamide for chronic simple (open angle) glaucoma is 250 mg to 1 g p.o. daily in divided doses. Doses greater than 1 g/day have no additional effects. The usual dose of acetazolamide for secondary glaucoma and preoperative treatment of acute angle-closure glaucoma is 250 mg p.o. every 4 hours. For rapid lowering of intraocular pressure or for patients unable to take the oral tablet, 500 mg of acetazolamide can be given i.v. and repeated 2 to 4 hours later if necessary. In children the usual oral dose of acetazolamide for glaucoma is 8 to 30 mg/kg/day in 3 divided doses. For acute glaucoma, acetazolamide 20 to 40 mg/kg/day i.v. in 4 divided doses may be given. Do not exceed 1 g/day for both the oral and i.v. dose, regardless of weight.

Epilepsy (see Indications): Acetazolamide should be used as adjunctive therapy in the prophylactic management of seizures. The oral dose for both adults and children is 8 to 30 mg/kg daily in 1 to 4 divided doses. In adults, acetazolamide should be started at 250 mg p.o. daily and increased to a maximum of 1 g/day. Doses above 1 g have no added benefit. The usual dose range is 375 mg to 1 g daily. The extended-release capsule is not recommended for the treatment of epilepsy.

Edema (see Indications): For the treatment of edema secondary to drugs or congestive heart failure, the usual adult dose of acetazolamide is 250 to 375 mg daily. The dose in children is 5 mg/kg p.o. or i.v. given daily in the morning. For best results, acetazolamide should be given on alternate days. Increasing the dose does not increase diuresis and will only increase the side effects of acetazolamide. Failure of therapy is usually due to overdosage or too frequent dosage.

High Altitude Sickness: Usual adult dose of acetazolamide is 0.5 to 1 g daily in 2 to 3 divided doses given 48 hours before the ascent and continued as needed. For rapid ascent, the 1 g dose is recommended.

Carboplatin Injection ℞

carboplatin

Antineoplastic

Hospira

SUPPLIED: Each mL of sterile aqueous solution contains: carboplatin 10 mg. Nonmedicinal ingredients: none. Preservative-free. Single use vials of 5, 15, 45 and 60 mL, cartons of 1. Store between 15 and 25°C. Protect from light. Discard unused portion.

> The reader is invited to consult CPhA's monograph **Calcium Channel Blockers**.

Cardizem® CD ℞

diltiazem HCl

Antihypertensive—Antianginal

Biovail Pharmaceuticals

Date of Preparation: August 13, 2008

PHARMACOLOGY: CARDIZEM CD capsules are formulations of diltiazem HCl, which is a calcium ion influx inhibitor (calcium entry blocker or calcium ion antagonist).

Mechanism of Action: The therapeutic effect of this group of drugs is believed to be related to their specific cellular action of selectively inhibiting transmembrane influx of calcium ions into cardiac muscle and vascular smooth muscle. The contractile processes of these tissues are dependent upon the movement of extracellular calcium into the cells through specific ion channels. Diltiazem blocks transmembrane influx of calcium through the slow channel without affecting to any significant degree the transmembrane influx of sodium through the fast channel. This results in a reduction of free calcium ions available within cells of the above tissues. Diltiazem does not alter total serum calcium.

Angina: The precise mechanism by which diltiazem relieves angina has not been fully determined, but it is believed to be brought about largely by its vasodilator action.

In angina due to coronary spasm, diltiazem increases myocardial oxygen delivery by dilating both large and small coronary arteries and by inhibiting coronary spasm at drug levels which cause little negative inotropic effect. The resultant increases in coronary blood flow are accompanied by dose-dependent decreases in systemic blood pressure and decreases in peripheral resistance.

In angina of effort it appears that the action of diltiazem is related to the reduction of myocardial oxygen demand. This is probably caused by a decrease in blood pressure brought about by the reduction of peripheral resistance and of heart rate.

Hypertension: The antihypertensive effect of diltiazem is believed to be brought about largely by its vasodilatory action on peripheral blood vessels with resultant decrease in peripheral vascular resistance.

Hemodynamic and Electrophysiologic Effects: Diltiazem produces antihypertensive effects both in the supine and standing positions. Resting heart rate is usually slightly reduced. During dynamic exercise, increases in diastolic pressure are inhibited while maximum achievable systolic pressure is usually unaffected. Heart rate at maximum exercise is reduced.

Studies to date, primarily in patients with normal ventricular function, have shown that cardiac output, ejection fraction, and left ventricular end-diastolic pressure have not been affected.

Chronic therapy with diltiazem produces no change, or a decrease, in circulating plasma catecholamines. However, no increased activity of the renin-angiotensin-aldosterone axis has been observed. Diltiazem inhibits the renal and peripheral effects of angiotensin II.

In man i.v. diltiazem in doses of 20 mg prolongs AH conduction time and AV node functional and effective refractory periods by approximately 20%. Chronic oral administration of diltiazem in doses up to 540 mg/day has resulted in small increases in PR interval. Second-degree and third-degree AV block have been observed (see Warnings). In patients with sick sinus syndrome, diltiazem significantly prolongs sinus cycle length (up to 50% in some cases).

Pharmacokinetics: Diltiazem is well absorbed from the gastrointestinal tract and is subject to an extensive first-pass effect giving absolute bioavailability (compared to i.v. dosing) of about 40%. Therapeutic blood levels appear to be in the 50 to 200 ng/mL range and the plasma elimination half-life (beta-phase) following single or multiple drug administration is approximately 3.5 to 6.0 hours. In vitro human serum binding studies revealed that 70 to 80% of diltiazem is bound to plasma proteins.

Diltiazem undergoes extensive hepatic metabolism in which only 2 to 4% of the drug appears unchanged in the urine and 6 to 7% appears as metabolites. The metabolic pathways of diltiazem include N- and O-demethylation (via cytochrome P450), deacetylation (via plasma and tissue esterases), in addition to conjugation (via sulfation and glucuronidation). In vitro studies have demonstrated that CYP 3A4 is the principal CYP isoenzyme involved in N-demethylation. The major metabolite, desacetyl diltiazem, is present in the plasma at levels 10 to 20% of the parent drug and is 25 to 50% as potent as diltiazem in terms of coronary vasodilation.

Single oral doses of 30 to 120 mg of Cardizem immediate release tablets result in detectable plasma levels within 30 to 60 minutes and peak plasma levels 2 to 4 hours after drug administration. There is a departure from linearity of accumulation of diltiazem when Cardizem tablets are administered to steady-state in normal subjects. A 240 mg daily dose (60 mg q.i.d.) gave plasma levels 2.3 times higher than a 120 mg daily dose (30 mg q.i.d.) and a 360 mg daily dose (90 mg q.i.d.) had levels 1.7 times higher than the 240 mg daily dose.

CARDIZEM CD (Once-a-day) Capsules: More than 95% of drug is absorbed from the CARDIZEM CD formulation. A single 360 mg dose of the capsule results in detectable plasma levels within 2 hours and peak plasma levels between 10 and 14 hours. When CARDIZEM CD was taken with a high fat content breakfast, the extent of diltiazem absorption was not affected but was delayed. Dose-dumping does not occur. The apparent elimination half-life after single or multiple dosing is 5 to 8 hours. A departure from linearity similar to that seen with Cardizem tablets is observed. As the dose of CARDIZEM CD capsules is increased from a daily dose of 120 to 240 mg, there is an increase in the area under the curve (AUC) of 2.7 times. When the dose is increased from 240 to 360 mg there is an increase in AUC of 1.6 times.

A study which compared patients with normal hepatic function to liver cirrhosis patients noted an increase in half-life and a 69% increase in bioavailability in the hepatically impaired patients. A single dose study in patients with severely impaired renal function showed no difference in the half-life of diltiazem as compared to patients with normal renal function (see Precautions and Dosage).

INDICATIONS: Angina: CARDIZEM CD is indicated for the management of chronic stable angina (effort-associated angina) without evidence of vasospasm in patients who remain symptomatic despite adequate doses of beta-blockers and/or organic nitrates or who cannot tolerate those agents.

CARDIZEM CD may be tried in combination with beta-blockers in chronic stable angina patients with normal ventricular function. When such concomitant therapy is introduced, patients must be monitored closely (see Warnings).

Since the safety and efficacy of CARDIZEM CD capsules in the management of unstable or vasospastic angina have not been substantiated, use of this formulation for these indications is not recommended.

Hypertension: For the treatment of mild to moderate essential hypertension. CARDIZEM CD should normally be used in those patients in whom treatment with diuretics or beta-blockers has been ineffective, or has been associated with unacceptable adverse effects.

CARDIZEM CD can be tried as an initial agent in those patients in whom the use of diuretics and/or beta-blockers is contraindicated, or in patients with medical conditions in which these drugs frequently cause serious adverse effects.

Safety of concurrent use of CARDIZEM CD with other antihypertensive agents has not been established.

CONTRAINDICATIONS: Diltiazem HCl is contraindicated: In patients with sick sinus syndrome except in the presence of a functioning ventricular pacemaker; in patients with second or third degree AV block; in patients with known hypersensitivity to diltiazem; in patients with hypotension (less than 90 mmHg systolic); and, in myocardial infarction patients who have left ventricular failure manifested by pulmonary congestion; in pregnancy and in women of childbearing potential. Fetal malformations and adverse effects on pregnancy have been reported in animals. In repeated dose studies a high incidence of vertebral column malformations were present in the offspring of mice receiving more than 50 mg/kg of diltiazem orally. Nursing Mothers: (See Precautions).

In the offspring of mice receiving a single oral dose of 50 or 100 mg/kg on day 12 of gestation, the incidence of cleft palate and malformed extremities was significantly higher. Vertebral malformations were most prevalent when they received the drug on day 9. In rats, a significantly higher fetal death rate was present when 200 and 400 mg/kg were given orally on days 9 to 14 of gestation. Single oral dose studies in rats resulted in a significant incidence of skeletal malformations in the offspring of the group receiving 400 mg/kg on day 11. In rabbits, all pregnant dams receiving 70 mg/kg orally from day 6 to 18 of gestation aborted; at 35 mg/kg, a significant increase in skeletal malformations was recorded in the offspring.

WARNINGS: Cardiac Conduction: Diltiazem prolongs AV node refractory periods without significantly prolonging sinus node recovery time, except in patients with sick sinus syndrome. This effect may rarely result in abnormally slow heart rates (particularly in patients with sick sinus syndrome) or second- or third-degree AV block (6 of 1208 patients or 0.5%).

First degree AV block was observed in 5.8% of patients receiving CARDIZEM CD (see Adverse Effects).

Concomitant use of diltiazem with agents known to affect cardiac conduction (such as beta-blockers, digitalis or amiodarone) may result in additive effects on cardiac conduction (see Precautions, Drug Interactions).

Congestive Heart Failure: Because diltiazem has a negative inotropic effect in vitro and it affects cardiac conduction, the drug should only be used with caution and under careful medical supervision in patients with congestive cardiac failure (see also Contraindications).

Use with Beta-blockers: The combination of diltiazem and beta-blockers warrants caution since in some patients additive effects on heart rate, AV conduction, blood pressure or left ventricular function have been observed. Close medical supervision is recommended.

Generally, diltiazem should not be given to patients with impaired left ventricular function while they receive beta-blockers. However, in exceptional cases when, in the opinion of the physician, concomitant use is considered essential, such use should be instituted gradually in a hospital setting.

Diltiazem gives no protection against the dangers of abrupt beta-blocker withdrawal and such withdrawal should be done by the gradual reduction of the dose of beta-blocker.

Hypotension: Since diltiazem lowers peripheral vascular resistance, decreases in blood pressure may occasionally result in symptomatic hypotension. In patients with angina or arrhythmias using antihypertensive drugs, the additional hypotensive effect of diltiazem should be taken into consideration.

Patients with Myocardial Infarction: Use of immediate release diltiazem at 240 mg/day started 3 to 15 days after a myocardial infarction was associated with an increase in cardiac events in patients with pulmonary congestion, and no overall effect on mortality. Although there has not been a study of CARDIZEM CD in acute myocardial infarction reported, their use may have effects similar to those of immediate release diltiazem in acute myocardial infarction.

Acute Hepatic Injury: In rare instances, significant elevations in alkaline phosphatase, CPK, LDH, AST, ALT and symptoms consistent with acute hepatic injury have been observed. These reactions have been reversible upon discontinuation of drug therapy. Although a causal relationship to diltiazem has not been established in all cases a drug induced hypersensitivity reaction is suspected (see Adverse Effects). As with any drug given over prolonged periods, laboratory parameters should be monitored at regular intervals.

PRECAUTIONS: Dermatological Events: Dermatological events (see Adverse Effects) may be transient and may disappear despite continued use of diltiazem. However, skin eruptions progressing to erythema multiforme and/or exfoliative dermatitis have also been infrequently reported. Should a dermatological reaction persist, the drug should be discontinued.

Impaired Hepatic or Renal Function: Diltiazem should be used with caution in patients with renal or hepatic impairment. Because diltiazem is extensively metabolized by the liver and excreted by the kidney and in bile, monitoring of laboratory parameters of renal or hepatic function is recommended and cautious dosage titration are recommended in patients with impaired hepatic or renal function (see Adverse Effects).

Children: The safety and effectiveness of diltiazem in children has not yet been established.

Lactation: Diltiazem has been reported to be excreted in human milk. One report of oral diltiazem usage suggests that concentrations in breast milk may approximate serum levels. Since diltiazem safety in newborns has not been established, it should not be given to nursing mothers.

Geriatrics: Administration of diltiazem to elderly patients (over or equal to 65 years of age) requires caution. The incidence of adverse reactions is approximately 13% higher in this group. Those adverse reactions which occur more frequently include: peripheral edema, bradycardia, palpitation, dizziness, rash and polyuria. Therefore, particular care in titration is advisable (see Dosage).

Drug Interactions: Due to the potential for additive effects, caution and careful titration are warranted in patients receiving CARDIZEM CD concomitantly with other agents know to affect cardiac contractility and/or conduction.

Cytochrome P450 System: As with all drugs, care should be exercised when treating patients with multiple medications. Calcium channel blockers undergo biotransformation by the cytochrome P450 system. Coadministration of diltiazem with other drugs which follow the same route of biotransformation may result in altered bioavailability. Dosages of similarly metabolized drugs, particularly those of low therapeutic ratio, and especially in patients with renal and/or hepatic impairment, may require adjustment when starting or stopping concomitantly administered diltiazem to maintain optimum therapeutic blood levels.

Drugs known to be inhibitors of the cytochrome P450 system include: azole antifungals, cimetidine, cyclosporine, erythromycin, quinidine, warfarin.

Drugs known to be inducers of the cytochrome P450 system include: phenobarbital, phenytoin, rifampin.

Drugs known to be biotransformed via P450 include: benzodiazepines, flecainide, imipramine, propafenone, terfenadine, theophylline.

Amiodarone: Severe conduction system abnormalities including heart block of varying degree, sinus arrest and a low cardiac output state of life-threatening severity have been reported following concomitant use of diltiazem and amiodarone. These drugs may also have additive effects on cardiac conduction and contractility.

Anesthetics: The depression of cardiac contractility, conductivity, and automaticity as well as the vascular dilation associated with anesthetics may be potentiated by calcium channel blockers. When used concomitantly, anesthetics and calcium channel blockers should be titrated carefully.

Benzodiazepines: Diltiazem significantly increases peak plasma levels and the elimination half-life of triazolam and midazolam.

Beta-blockers: The concomitant administration of diltiazem with beta adrenergic blocking drugs warrants caution and careful monitoring. Such an association may have an additive effect on heart rate, on AV conduction or on blood pressure (see Warnings). Appropriate dosage adjustments may be necessary. A study in 5 normal subjects showed that diltiazem increased propranolol bioavailability by approximately 50%.
Calcium Antagonists: Limited clinical experience suggests that in certain severe conditions not responding adequately to verapamil or to nifedipine, using diltiazem in conjunction with either of these drugs may be beneficial.
Carbamazepine: Concomitant administration of diltiazem with carbamazepine has been reported to result in elevated serum levels of carbamazepine (40 to 72% increase) resulting in toxicity in some cases. Patients receiving these drugs concurrently should be monitored for a potential drug interaction.
Cimetidine: A study in 6 healthy volunteers has shown a significant increase in peak diltiazem plasma levels (58%) and area under the curve (53%) after a 1-week course of cimetidine at 1200 mg/day and a single dose of oral diltiazem 60 mg. Ranitidine produced smaller, nonsignificant increases. Patients currently receiving diltiazem therapy should be carefully monitored for a change in pharmacological effect when initiating and discontinuing therapy with cimetidine. An adjustment in the diltiazem dose may be warranted.
Cyclosporine: Concomitant administration of diltiazem and cyclosporine has resulted in an increase in cyclosporine concentrations. A pharmacokinetic interaction between diltiazem and cyclosporine has been observed during studies involving renal and cardiac transplant patients. In renal and cardiac transplant recipients, a reduction of cyclosporine dose ranging from 15 to 48% was necessary to maintain cyclosporine trough concentrations similar to those seen prior to the addition of diltiazem. If these agents are to be administered concurrently, cyclosporine concentrations should be monitored, especially when diltiazem therapy is initiated, adjusted or discontinued. Downward titration of the cyclosporine dose may be necessary. The effect of cyclosporine on diltiazem plasma concentrations has not been evaluated.
Digitalis: Diltiazem and digitalis glycosides may have an additive effect in prolonging AV conduction. In clinical trials, concurrent administration of diltiazem and digoxin have resulted in increases in serum digoxin levels with prolongation of AV conduction. This increase may result from a decrease in renal clearance of digoxin. Patients on concomitant therapy, especially those with renal impairment, should be carefully monitored. The dose of digoxin may need downward adjustment.
Lovastatin: In a 10-subject study, coadministration of diltiazem with lovastatin resulted in a 3 to 4 times increase in mean lovastatin AUC and C_{max} versus lovastatin alone; no change in pravastatin AUC and C_{max} was observed during diltiazem coadministration. Diltiazem plasma levels were not significantly affected by lovastatin or pravastatin.
Rifampin: Administration of diltiazem with rifampin markedly reduced plasma diltiazem concentrations and the therapeutic effect of diltiazem.
Short- and Long-Acting Nitrates: Diltiazem may be safely coadministered with nitrates, but there have been few controlled studies to evaluate the antianginal effectiveness of this combination.

ADVERSE EFFECTS: See also Overall Cardizem Safety Profile.

Angina: The safety of CARDIZEM CD, administered at doses up to 360 mg a day, was evaluated in 365 patients with chronic stable angina treated in controlled and open-label clinical trials. Adverse events were reported in 21.1% of patients, and required discontinuation in 2.2% of patients.

The most common adverse effects reported were: first degree AV block (5.8%), dizziness (3.0%), headache (3.0%), asthenia (2.7%), bradycardia (2.5%), and angina pectoris (1.6%).

The following percentage of adverse effects, divided by system, was reported:
Cardiovascular: first degree AV block (5.8%), bradycardia (2.5%), angina pectoris (1.6%), peripheral edema (1.4%), palpitations (1.1%), and ventricular extrasystoles (0.8%).
Central Nervous System: dizziness (3.0%), headache (3.0%), asthenia (2.7%), insomnia (1.1%), nervousness (0.8%).
Dermatological: rash (0.8%).
Gastrointestinal: nausea (1.4%), diarrhea (0.5%).
Other: amblyopia (0.5%).

The following additional adverse effects have occurred with an incidence of less than 0.5% in clinical trials: bundle branch block, ventricular tachycardia, ECG abnormality, supraventricular extrasystoles, chest pain, syncope, postural hypotension, paresthesia, tremor, depression, mental confusion, impotence, abdominal pain, constipation, gastrointestinal disorder, epistaxis, nuchal rigidity, myalgia.

Hypertension: A safety evaluation was carried out in controlled studies in 378 hypertensive patients treated with CARDIZEM CD at doses up to 360 mg a day. Adverse effects were reported in 30.7% of patients and required discontinuation of therapy in 2.1%.

The most common adverse effects were: headache (8.7%), edema (4.0%), bradycardia (3.7%), dizziness (3.4%), ECG abnormality (2.9%), asthenia (2.6%) and first degree AV block (2.1%).

The following percentage of adverse effects, divided by system, was reported:
Cardiovascular: edema peripheral (4.0%), bradycardia (3.7%), ECG abnormalities (2.9%), first degree AV block (2.1%), arrhythmia (1.6%), vasodilation (flushing) (1.6%), bundle branch block (0.8%), cardiomegaly (0.5%), hypotension (0.5%).
Central Nervous System: headache (8.7%), dizziness (3.4%), asthenia (2.6%), somnolence (1.3%), nervousness (1.1%).
Gastrointestinal: constipation (1.3%), dyspepsia (1.3%), diarrhea (0.6%).
Laboratory Tests: ALT increase (0.8%).
Other: leukopenia (1.1%), nocturia (0.5%).

The following additional adverse effects have occurred with an incidence of less than 0.5% in clinical trials: systolic murmur, supraventricular extrasystoles, migraine, tachycardia, increased appetite, increase in weight, albuminuria, bilirubinemia, hyperuricemia, thirst, insomnia, vertigo, nausea, pruritus, rash, increased perspiration, polyuria, amblyopia, tinnitus, and elevations in creatine kinase, alkaline phosphatase, and AST.

Overall Cardizem Safety Profile: In clinical trials of diltiazem involving over 3300 patients, the most common adverse reactions were headache (4.6%), edema (4.6%), dizziness (3.5%), asthenia (2.7%), first degree AV block (2.4%), bradycardia (1.7%), flushing (1.5%), nausea (1.4%), rash (1.2%), and dyspepsia (1.0%).

In addition, the following events were reported with a frequency of less than 1.0%.
Cardiovascular: angina, arrhythmia, bundle branch block, tachycardia, ventricular extrasystoles, congestive heart failure, syncope, palpitations, AV block (second or third degree), hypotension, ECG abnormalities.
Dermatological: petechiae, pruritus, photosensitivity, urticaria.
Gastrointestinal: anorexia, diarrhea, dysgeusia, mild elevations of AST, ALT, LDH, and alkaline phosphatase (see Warnings), vomiting, weight increase, thirst, constipation.
Nervous System: amnesia, depression, gait abnormality, nervousness, somnolence, hallucinations, paresthesia, personality change, tinnitus, tremor, abnormal dreams, insomnia.
Other: amblyopia, CPK increase, dyspnea, epistaxis, eye irritation, hyperglycemia, sexual difficulties, nasal congestion, nocturia, osteo-articular pain, impotence, dry mouth, polyuria, hyperuricemia.
Postmarketing Surveillance: The following postmarketing events have been reported infrequently in patients receiving Cardizem: acute generalized exanthematous pustulosis, allergic reactions, alopecia, asystole, erythema multiforme (including Stevens-Johnson syndrome, toxic epidermal necrolysis), exfoliative dermatitis (see Precautions), extrapyramidal symptoms, gingival hyperplasia, hemolytic anemia, detached retina, increased bleeding time, leukopenia, myopathy, purpura, retinopathy, and thrombocytopenia. Isolated cases of angioedema have been reported. Angioedema may be accompanied by breathing difficulty. In addition, events such as myocardial infarction have been observed which are not readily distinguishable from the natural history of the disease in these patients. A number of well-documented cases of generalized rash, some characterized as leukocytoclastic vasculitis, have been reported. However, a definitive cause and effect relationship between these events and Cardizem therapy is yet to be established.

OVERDOSE:

Symptoms: There have been reports of diltiazem overdose in amounts ranging from <1 to 18 g. In cases with a fatal outcome, the majority involved multiple drug ingestion.

Events observed following diltiazem overdose included bradycardia, hypotension, heart block and cardiac failure.

Treatment: The effectiveness of i.v. calcium administration to reverse the pharmacological effects of diltiazem overdose has been inconsistent. In a few reported cases, overdose with calcium channel blockers associated with hypotension and bradycardia that was initially refractory to atropine became more responsive to atropine after the patients received i.v. calcium. In some cases i.v. calcium has been administered (1 g calcium chloride or 3 g calcium gluconate) over 5 minutes, and repeated every 10 to 20 minutes as necessary. Calcium gluconate has also been administrated as a continuous infusion at a rate of 2 g/hour for 10 hours. Infusions of calcium for 24 hours or more may be required. Patients should be monitored for signs of hypercalcemia.

In the event of overdosage or exaggerated response, appropriate supportive measures should be employed in addition to gastric lavage. Limited data suggest that plasmapheresis or charcoal hemoperfusion may hasten diltiazem elimination. The following measures may be considered:
Bradycardia: Administer atropine. If there is no response to vagal blockade, administer isoproterenol cautiously.
High Degree AV Block: Treat as for bradycardia above. Fixed high degree AV block should be treated with cardiac pacing.
Cardiac Failure: Administer inotropic agents (isoproterenol, dopamine or dobutamine) and diuretics.
Hypotension: Administer fluids and vasopressors (e.g., dopamine or norepinephrine).

Actual treatment and dosage should depend on the severity of the clinical situation.

For management of a suspected drug overdose, CPhA recommends that you contact your **regional Poison Control Centre**. See the *CPS* Directory section for a list of Poison Control Centres.

DOSAGE: Angina: Dosages for the treatment of angina should be adjusted to each patient's needs, starting with a dose of 120 mg to 180 mg once daily. Individual patients may respond to higher doses of up to 360 mg once daily. When necessary, titration should be carried out over a 7 to 14 day period.

Patients controlled on diltiazem alone or in combination with other medications may be safely switched to CARDIZEM CD capsules at the nearest equivalent total daily dose. Subsequent titration to higher or lower doses may be necessary and should be initiated as clinically warranted.

There is limited experience with doses above 360 mg, however, the incidence of adverse reactions increases as the dose increases with first degree AV block, dizziness, and sinus bradycardia bearing the strongest relationship to dose. Therefore, doses greater than 360 mg are not recommended.

Hypertension: Dosage should be individualized depending on patient's tolerance and responsiveness to CARDIZEM CD capsules. When used as monotherapy, usual starting doses are 180 to 240 mg once daily, although some patients may respond to 120 mg once daily. Maximum antihypertensive effect is usually observed after approximately 2 to 4 weeks of therapy; therefore, dosage adjustments should be scheduled accordingly. The usual dosage range studied in clinical trials was 240 to 360 mg once daily.

A maximum daily dose of 360 mg once daily should not be exceeded.

The dosage of CARDIZEM CD or concomitant antihypertensive agents may need to be adjusted when adding one to the other. See Warnings and Precautions regarding use with beta-blockers.

Geriatrics: Pharmacokinetics of diltiazem in elderly patients has not been fully elucidated. Preliminary results in elderly patients (over 65 years old) suggest that a lower dosage might be required in this age group (see Precautions).

There are few available data concerning dosage requirements in patients with impaired renal or hepatic function. If diltiazem must be used in these patients, the dosage should be carefully and gradually adjusted depending on patient tolerance and response (see Precautions).

CARDIZEM CD capsules should not be chewed or crushed.

INFORMATION FOR THE PATIENT: Published in e-CPS, available by subscription at www.e-cps.ca.

SUPPLIED: 120 mg: Each light turquoise blue, controlled delivery capsule, comprised of an opaque cap and body printed in blue with cardizem CD 120 mg on the body and containing white to off-white beads, contains: diltiazem HCl 120 mg. Nonmedicinal ingredients: acetyltributyl citrate, beeswax, Blue FD&C No. 1, castor oil, cornstarch, ethylcellulose, fumaric acid, gelatin, polymethyl methacrylate, silica, simethicone, stearic acid, sucrose, talc and titanium dioxide. Bisulfites-, gluten- and tartrazine-free. Bottles of 100.

180 mg: Each controlled delivery capsule, comprised of a blue opaque cap and a light turquoise opaque body printed in blue with cardizem CD 180 mg on the body and containing white to off-white beads, contains: diltiazem HCl 180 mg. Nonmedicinal ingredients: acetyltributyl citrate, beeswax, Blue FD&C No. 1, castor oil, cornstarch, ethylcellulose, fumaric acid, gelatin, polymethyl methacrylate, silica, simethicone, stearic acid, sucrose, talc and titanium dioxide. Bisulfites-, gluten- and tartrazine-free. Bottles of 100.

240 mg: Each controlled delivery capsule, comprised of a blue opaque cap and body printed with cardizem CD 240 mg on the body and containing white to off-white beads, contains: diltiazem HCl 240 mg. Nonmedicinal ingredients: acetyltributyl citrate, beeswax, Blue FD&C No. 1, castor oil, cornstarch, ethylcellulose, fumaric acid, gelatin, polymethyl methacrylate, silica, simethicone, stearic acid, sucrose, talc and titanium dioxide. Bisulfites-, gluten- and tartrazine-free. Bottles of 100.

300 mg: Each controlled delivery capsule, comprised of a blue opaque cap and grey opaque body printed with cardizem CD 300 mg on the body and containing white to off-white beads, contains: diltiazem HCl 300 mg. Nonmedicinal ingredients: acetyltributyl citrate, beeswax, Blue FD&C No. 1, castor oil, cornstarch, ethylcellulose, fumaric acid, gelatin, iron oxide, polymethyl methacrylate, silica, simethicone, stearic acid, sucrose, talc and titanium dioxide. Bisulfites-, gluten- and tartrazine-free. Bottles of 100.

Keep between 15 and 30°C. Protect from light.

(Shown in Product Identification Section)

Cardura-1™ Ⓟ
doxazosin mesylate
Antihypertensive—Symptomatic Treatment of Benign Prostatic Hyperplasia (BPH)

Pfizer

Cardura-2™ Ⓟ
doxazosin mesylate
Antihypertensive—Symptomatic Treatment of Benign Prostatic Hyperplasia (BPH)

Pfizer

Cardura-4™ Ⓟ
doxazosin mesylate
Antihypertensive—Symptomatic Treatment of Benign Prostatic Hyperplasia (BPH)

Pfizer

Date of Preparation: December 13, 1991
Date of Revision: November 23, 2009

PHARMACOLOGY: The mechanism of action of doxazosin is selective blockade of alpha$_1$ subtype of postsynaptic, postjunctional alpha-adrenergic receptors.
Pharmacodynamics: Hypertension: Administration of doxazosin results in a reduction in systemic vascular resistance. In patients with hypertension there is little change in cardiac output. Maximum reductions in blood pressure usually occur 2 to 6 hours after dosing and are associated with a small increase in standing heart rate. Doxazosin has a greater effect on blood pressure and heart rate in the standing position. Tolerance has not been observed in long-term therapy.

Systolic and diastolic blood pressure is lowered in both the supine and standing positions. In clinical trials, blood pressure responses were measured at the end of the dosing interval (24 hours), with the usual supine response 6 to 11 mmHg systolic and 5 to 9 mmHg diastolic. The response in the standing position tended to be larger by 3 to 5 mmHg. Peak blood pressure effects (1 to 6 hours) were larger by about 50 to 75% (i.e., trough values were about 55 to 70% of peak effect), with the larger peak-trough differences seen in systolic pressures. There was no apparent difference in the blood pressure response of Caucasians and Blacks or of patients above and below age 65.

During controlled clinical studies, predominantly normocholesterolemic patients receiving doxazosin had small but statistically significant reductions in total serum cholesterol (2.7%) and LDL cholesterol (4.3%), and increase in the HDL/total cholesterol ratio (4.3%) relative to placebo. No significant changes were observed in high-density lipoprotein fraction and triglycerides compared to placebo.
Benign Prostatic Hyperplasia (BPH): Benign Prostatic Hyperplasia (BPH) is a common cause of urinary outflow obstruction in aging males. Severe BPH may lead to urinary retention and renal damage. A static and a dynamic component contribute to the symptoms and reduced urinary flow rate associated with BPH. The static component is related to an increase in prostate size caused, in part, by a proliferation of smooth muscle cells in the prostatic stroma.

However, the severity of BPH symptoms and the degree of urethral obstruction do not correlate well with the size of the prostate. The dynamic component of BPH is associated with an increase in smooth muscle tone in the prostate and bladder neck. The degree of tone in this area is mediated by α_1-adrenoceptors which are present in high density in the prostatic stroma, prostatic capsule and bladder neck. Blockage of the α_1-receptor decreases urethral resistance and may relieve the obstruction and BPH symptoms. In 30 to 70% of patients with symptomatic BPH, placebo has also shown a remarkable and sometimes dramatic effect in controlled short-term studies.

The symptoms may subside or fade away without treatment in approximately 20% of patients.

Doxazosin antagonizes phenylephrine-induced contractions, in vitro, in the human prostate. Doxazosin is bound with high affinity to the α_{1A}-adrenoceptor subtype, thought to be the predominant functional type in the prostate.

The effect of doxazosin in BPH is thought to result from selective blockade of the α_{1A}-adrenoceptors located in the prostatic muscular stroma, capsule and bladder neck. This action results in relief of the urinary outlet obstruction and symptomatology associated with BPH.

In controlled clinical trials in over 900 patients, the efficacy of doxazosin was evaluated. In 2 studies doxazosin 4 to 8 mg once daily significantly improved maximum urinary flow rate (MFR) 2.3 to 3.3 mL/s (placebo 0.1 to 0.7 mL/s). Significant improvements were usually noticed within 2 weeks of commencing doxazosin treatment and a significantly larger proportion of patients (32 to 42%) responded with MFR improvements ≥3 mL/s (placebo 13 to 17%). Average flow rate also improved with doxazosin treatment, (1.3 to 2.1 mL/s vs placebo 0.2 to 0.3 mL/s). Doxazosin also resulted in a significant relief of the obstructive and irritative symptoms associated with BPH.

Using invasive urodynamics in a controlled clinical trial in 43 BPH patients, doxazosin 2 mg improved MFR 3.4 mL/s, and reduced urethral resistance 7.5 to 13.5 cmH_2O (placebo, MFR-0.6 mL/s and resistance of 3.3 cmH_2O).

In a 29-week controlled BPH trial in 100 patients, doxazosin was significantly more effective than placebo in improving urinary flow rates and reducing BPH symptoms; the effect was sustained over the entire treatment period. No tolerance to the effect of doxazosin on urodynamics or BPH symptomatology was observed in patients treated for up to 4 years in open-label studies.

Both hypertensive and normotensive BPH patients treated with doxazosin demonstrate statistically significant improvements in urodynamics and symptomatology compared to placebo.

Pharmacokinetics: After oral administration of therapeutic doses of doxazosin, absorption occurs with peak blood levels at about 2 hours. Bioavailability is approximately 65%. Food has little or no effect on the bioavailability.

Approximately 98% of the circulating drug is bound to plasma proteins. Plasma elimination is biphasic with a terminal elimination half-life of about 22 hours. There is an accumulation of plasma doxazosin levels following steady state dosing, consistent with the terminal elimination half-life.

In a study of elderly hypertensive patients the pharmacokinetic parameters of doxazosin at steady state were similar to those observed in a previous study of young and elderly healthy subjects who received a single oral dose of doxazosin.

In a cross-over study in 24 normotensive subjects, the pharmacokinetics and safety of doxazosin were shown to be similar with morning and evening dosing regimens. Doxazosin may, therefore, be administered as a single daily morning or evening dose (see Dosage).

Doxazosin is extensively metabolized, mainly by O-demethylation of the quinazoline nucleus or hydroxylation of the benzodioxan moiety. Excretion is mainly via the feces with 9% of the dose excreted in urine as doxazosin (<0.5%) or metabolites. Less than 5% is excreted as the unchanged drug, mainly in the feces.

The disposition of doxazosin in patients with normal renal insufficiency is similar to that in patients with normal renal function. Only limited data are available in patients with liver impairment and on the effects of drugs known to influence hepatic metabolism (e.g., cimetidine) (see Precautions, Patients with Impaired Liver Function).

INDICATIONS: Hypertension: In the treatment of mild to moderate essential hypertension. It is employed in a general treatment program in association with a thiazide diuretic and/or other antihypertensive agents, as needed, for proper patient response.

Doxazosin may be tried as a sole therapy in those patients in whom treatment with other agents caused adverse effects or is inappropriate.

Benign Prostatic Hyperplasia (BPH): Doxazosin is also indicated for the treatment of symptoms of benign prostatic hyperplasia (BPH). The onset of effect is rapid, with improvement in peak flow and symptoms observed within 1 to 2 weeks. The effect on these variables was maintained over the entire study duration (up to 4 years). Doxazosin may be used in BPH patients who are either hypertensive or normotensive. While the reduction in blood pressure in normotensive patients with BPH is clinically insignificant, patients with hypertension and BPH have both conditions effectively treated with doxazosin monotherapy (see Dosage for dosage regimens).

A number of clinical conditions can mimic symptomatic BPH (i.e., stricture of urethra, stricture of bladder neck, urinary bladder stones, neurogenic bladder dysfunction secondary to diabetes, Parkinsonism, etc.). These conditions should therefore be ruled out before doxazosin therapy is initiated.

CONTRAINDICATIONS: Patients with a known sensitivity to doxazosin or quinazolines.

WARNINGS: Syncope and "First Dose" Effect: Doxazosin can cause marked hypotension, especially postural hypotension and syncope in association with the first dose or first few doses of therapy. A similar effect can occur if therapy is reinstated following interruption for more than a few doses. Postural effects are most likely to occur between 2 and 6 hours after dose.

In controlled studies of doxazosin the incidence of syncopal episodes was 0.7%. An initial dose of 1 mg/day resulted in a 4% incidence of postural side effects with no cases of syncope. In controlled clinical trials for BPH in normotensive patients, there was a 0.2% occurrence of syncope with doxazosin. In controlled trials in patients with both BPH and hypertension receiving doxazosin, the incidence of syncope was 0.8%.

The likelihood of syncopal episodes or excessive hypotension can be minimized by limiting the initial dose of doxazosin to 1 mg, by increasing the dosage slowly and by introducing any additional antihypertensive drugs into the patient's regimen with caution (see Dosage).

Patients should be advised of the possibility of syncopal and orthostatic symptoms, and to avoid driving or hazardous tasks for 24 hours: after the initial dose of doxazosin, after the dose is increased, and after interruption of therapy when treatment is resumed. They should be cautioned to avoid situations where injury could result should syncope occur.

If syncope occurs, the patient should be placed in the supine position. If this measure is inadequate, volume expansion with i.v. fluids or vasopressor therapy may be used. A transient hypotensive response is not a contraindication to further doses of doxazosin.

Orthostatic Hypotension: While syncope is the most severe orthostatic effect of doxazosin, other symptoms of lowered blood pressure such as dizziness, lightheadedness or vertigo can occur. These were common in clinical trials in hypertension, occurring in up to 23% of all patients treated and causing discontinuation of therapy in about 2%. In placebo-controlled titration trials, there was an increased frequency of orthostatic effects in patients given 8 mg or more (10%) compared to patients given 1 to 4 mg (5%) or placebo (3%).

In placebo-controlled trials in BPH, the incidence of orthostatic hypotension with doxazosin was ≤1%. With maintenance doses of up to 8 mg/day in normotensive patients with BPH, the average decreases in both sitting and standing blood pressure were small: 5/2 mmHg with doxazosin and 1/1 mmHg with placebo.

Patients with occupations in which such events represent potential problems should be treated with particular caution.

Concomitant administration of doxazosin with a PDE-5 inhibitor such as sildenafil, tadalafil or vardenafil, should be used with caution as it may lead to symptomatic hypotension.

Patients should be advised of the need to lie down when symptoms of lowered blood pressure occur, and to be careful when arising from a lying position. If dizziness, lightheadedness or palpitations are bothersome, they should be reported to the physician so that dose adjustment can be considered. Patients should also be told that drowsiness or somnolence can occur with doxazosin, requiring caution in people who must drive or operate heavy machinery.

If hypotension occurs, place the patient in the recumbent position and institute supportive measures as necessary.

Priapism: Rarely (probably less frequently than once in every several thousand patients), α_1-antagonists such as doxazosin have been associated with priapism. Because this condition can lead to permanent impotence if not promptly treated, patients should be advised about the seriousness of the condition.

Hematological Events: Analysis of hematologic data from patients receiving doxazosin in controlled clinical trials showed that the mean white blood cell (WBC) (n=474) and mean neutrophil counts (n=419) were decreased by 2.4% and 1.0% respectively, compared to placebo. A search through a data base of 2400 patients revealed 4 cases in which drug-related neutropenia could not be ruled out. Two had a single low value on the last day of treatment. Two had stable, nonprogressive neutrophil counts in the 1000/mm^3 range over periods of 20 and 40 weeks. No patients became symptomatic as a result of the low WBC or neutrophil counts.

In BPH patients treated with doxazosin, the incidence of clinically significant WBC abnormalities was 0.4%.

In postmarketing experience, rare cases of hematopoietic events such as leukopenia and thrombocytopenia have been reported.

Hepatic Events: In postmarketing experience, rare cases of abnormal liver function tests, cholestasis, jaundice and hepatitis have been reported.

Peripheral Edema: Fluid retention resulting in weight gain may occur during doxazosin therapy. In placebo-controlled monotherapy trials, patients receiving doxazosin gained a mean of 0.6 kg compared to a mean loss of 0.1 kg for placebo-treated patients. The overall incidence of body weight gain reported as a side effect in controlled clinical trials was 0.8%.

PRECAUTIONS: General: Doxazosin therapy does not modify the natural history of benign prostatic hyperplasia (BPH). It does not retard or stop the progression of BPH, nor does it improve urine flow sufficiently to significantly reduce the residual urine volume. However, significant reduction of the mean residual volume has been shown in patients with baseline residual volumes of >50 mL. The patient may continue to be at risk of developing urinary retention and other BPH complications during doxazosin therapy.

Long-term Safety and Efficacy: The long-term safety and efficacy (i.e., >4 years) have not yet been established for the use of doxazosin in the treatment of benign prostatic hyperplasia.

Prostatic Cancer: Carcinoma of the prostate and BPH cause many of the same symptoms. These two diseases frequently coexist. Therefore, patients thought to have BPH should be examined prior to starting doxazosin therapy to rule out the presence of carcinoma of the prostate.

Doxazosin should not be used in patients with PSA >10 ng/mL unless cancer of the prostate has been ruled out.

Patients with Impaired Liver Function: As with any drug wholly metabolized by the liver, doxazosin should be administered with caution to patients with evidence of impaired hepatic function or to patients receiving drugs known to influence hepatic metabolism.

Patients with Impaired Renal Function: The use of doxazosin in patients with impaired renal function requires careful monitoring. Clinical studies indicate that the disposition of doxazosin in patients with renal insufficiency is similar to that in patients with normal renal function, however, accumulation of the drug with chronic dosing may occur. Less than 10% of the dose of doxazosin is excreted in the urine as unchanged drug and metabolites.

Concomitant Conditions: Doxazosin should not be prescribed to patients with symptomatic BPH who have the following concomitant conditions:

Chronic urinary retention, high residual urine (over 200 mL), peak urine flow of 5 mL/s or less, history of prior prostatic surgery, chronic fibrous or granulomatous prostatitis, urethral stricture, history of pelvic irradiation, presence of prostatic calculi, presence of large median lobe of prostate, presence of calculi in urinary bladder, recent history of epididymitis, gross hematuria, presence of neurogenic bladder dysfunction (diabetes mellitus, parkinsonism, uninhibited neurogenic bladder, etc.), hydronephrosis, presence of carcinoma of the prostate. Nor should doxazosin be prescribed to patients having experienced a myocardial infarction, transient ischemic attacks, or cerebrovascular accident within the past 6 months.

Pregnancy: There are no studies in pregnant women. Doxazosin is not recommended in pregnant women unless the potential benefit outweighs the potential risk to mother and fetus.

Doxazosin crosses the placental barrier.

Studies in pregnant rabbits and rats at daily oral doses of up to 40 and 20 mg/kg, respectively, have revealed no evidence of teratogenic effect. A dosage regimen of 82 mg/kg/day in the rabbit was associated with reduced fetal survival, an increase in embryomortality as well as increases in fetal and placental weights.

In peri- and postnatal studies in rats, postnatal development at maternal doses of 40 or 50 mg/kg/day of doxazosin was delayed as evidenced by slower body weight gain and a slightly later appearance of anatomical features and reflexes.

Lactation: Studies in lactating rats indicate that doxazosin accumulates in rat breast milk. It is not known whether this drug is excreted in human milk. Caution should be exercised when doxazosin is administered to a nursing mother and, in general, nursing should be interrupted.

Children: The use of doxazosin is not recommended in children since safety and efficacy have not been established.

Geriatrics: Doxazosin should be used cautiously in elderly patients because of the possibility of postural hypotension. There was an age-related trend towards an increased incidence of postural hypotension and postural dizziness in elderly hypertensive patients treated with this drug.

Cardiac Toxicity in Animals: An increased incidence of myocardial necrosis or fibrosis was displayed by Sprague-Dawley rats after 6 months of dietary administration at concentrations calculated to provide 80 mg doxazosin/kg/day and after 12 months of dietary administration at concentrations calculated to provide 40 mg doxazosin/kg/day.

Myocardial fibrosis was observed in both rats and mice treated in the same manner with 40 mg doxazosin/kg/day for 18 months. No cardiotoxicity was observed at lower doses (up to 10 or 20 mg/kg/day, depending on the study) in either species.

These lesions were not observed after 12 months of oral dosing in dogs and Wistar rats at maximum doses of 20 and 100 mg/kg/day respectively. There is no evidence that similar lesions occur in humans.

Drug Interactions: Doxazosin is highly (98%) bound to plasma protein. In vitro data in human plasma indicate that doxazosin has no effect on protein binding of digoxin, warfarin, phenytoin or indomethacin.

Doxazosin has been administered to patients receiving thiazide diuretics, beta-adrenergic blocking agents and nonsteroidal anti-inflammatory drugs. No unexpected interactions were reported. An additive hypotensive effect was observed when doxazosin was coadministered with thiazide diuretics and beta-adrenergic blocking agents. There is limited experience with doxazosin in combination with ACE inhibitors or calcium channel blockers.

Digoxin: Serum digoxin concentrations were not affected by treatment with doxazosin.

Cimetidine: In a randomized, open-label, cross-over study in 22 male subjects, the single co-administration of 1 mg doxazosin with 400 mg b.i.d. cimetidine resulted in a 10% increase in mean AUC of doxazosin (p=0.006), and a slight but not statistically significant increase in mean C_{max} and mean half-life of doxazosin. The effect of further administration of cimetidine has not been studied.

PDE-5 Inhibitors: Symptomatic hypotension has been reported during the concomitant use of PDE-5 inhibitors (e.g. sildenafil, tadalafil, vardenafil) and doxazosin (see Warnings).

ADVERSE EFFECTS: Hypertension: Doxazosin has been administered to approximately 4 000 patients in clinical trials of whom 1 679 patients were included in controlled trials. The most serious adverse event occurring in the controlled clinical trials was syncope occurring in 0.7% of patients and resulting in a discontinuation rate of 0.2%.

The most frequent adverse events in controlled clinical trials were: headache (16.5%), fatigue/malaise (14.8%), dizziness (14.6%), postural dizziness (8.7%) and edema (6.6%). Discontinuation of doxazosin due to adverse events was required in 7% of patients.

Adverse events which occurred with an incidence of ≥1% in the controlled clinical trials in patients with mild to moderate essential hypertension were as shown in Table 1.

Table 1: Cardura

Adverse Events

Adverse Event	Incidence (n=1679) (%)
All Adverse Events	49.0
Headache	16.5
Fatigue	14.8
Dizziness	14.6
Postural Dizziness	8.7
Edema	6.6
Somnolence	4.9
Nausea	3.9
Dyspnea	3.9
Decrease in Platelets	3.9
Palpitation	3.6
Sexual Dysfunction	3.5

(cont'd)

Table 1: Cardura *(cont'd)*
Adverse Events

Adverse Event	Incidence (n=1679) (%)
Dry Mouth	3.4
Vertigo	3.0
Rhinitis	3.0
Diarrhea	2.9
Chest Pain	2.7
Asthenia	2.7
Vision/Accommodation Abnormalities	2.4
Decrease in White Blood Cells	2.4
Anxiety/Nervousness	2.3
Insomnia	2.2
Dyspepsia	2.1
Rash	1.7
Paresthesia	1.7
Muscle Cramps	1.7
Tachycardia	1.6
Depression/Apathy	1.6
Hypoesthesia	1.6
Abdominal Pain	1.6
Decrease in Hematocrit	1.6
Increased Sweating	1.4
Flatulence	1.4
Decrease in Hemoglobin	1.4
Pain (general body)	1.3
Myalgia	1.3
Constipation	1.3
Conjunctivitis/Eye Pain	1.2
Micturition Frequency	1.2
Polyuria	1.0
Decrease in Neutrophil Count	1.0

The following other adverse events occurred in hypertensive patients with an incidence of <1% in controlled clinical trials (n=1679): postural hypotension, arrhythmia, syncope, pruritus, arthralgia, agitation, flushing, tremor, paroniria, tinnitus, vomiting, epistaxis, sinusitis, bronchospasm/bronchitis, urinary incontinence, urinary disorder, face edema, weight increase, general edema, angina pectoris, peripheral ischemia, hypotension, paresis, twitching, migraine, amnesia, movement disorders, emotional lability, abnormal thinking, depersonalization, pallor, hypertonia, ataxia, thirst, gout, hypokalemia, lymphadenopathy, purpura, breast pain, alopecia, dry skin, eczema, taste perversion, photophobia, abnormal lacrimation, increased appetite, anorexia, fecal incontinence, coughing, pharyngitis, hot flushes, back pain, infection, fever/rigors and muscle weakness.

Benign Prostatic Hyperplasia: Doxazosin has been administered once daily to 665 both hypertensive and normotensive patients with BPH in controlled clinical trials. The most serious adverse event occurring in the controlled trials was syncope (0.5%).

The most frequent adverse events in controlled trials were dizziness (15.6%), headache (9.8%) and fatigue (8%).

Discontinuation rate of doxazosin due to adverse events was 9%.

Adverse events which occurred with an incidence of ≥1% in the controlled clinical trials in normotensive or hypertensive patients with BPH were as shown in Table 2.

Table 2: Cardura
Adverse Events

Adverse Event	Incidence	
	Short Term[a] (n=665) %	Long Term[b] (n=450) %
All Adverse Events	45.0	66.0
Dizziness	15.6	20.7
Headache	9.8	12.2
Fatigue	8.0	11.6
Somnolence	3.0	4.9
Edema	2.7	4.9
Dyspnea	2.6	<1
Diarrhea	2.3	3.8
Abdominal Pain	2.3	1.8
Pain	2.0	5.1
Back Pain	1.8	2.9
Dyspepsia	1.8	2.4
Hypotension	1.7	2.5
Nausea	1.5	3.1
Dry Mouth	1.4	<1
Abnormal Vision	1.4	2.2
Palpitation	1.2	1.8
Chest Pain	1.2	3.8
Insomnia	1.2	1.3
Urinary Tract Infection	1.2	1.1
Anxiety	1.1	<1
Respiratory Disorder	1.1	2.5
Impotence	1.1	4.9
Increased Sweating	1.1	<1
Leg Cramps	<1	1.6
Hypertonia	<1	1.1
Paresthesia	<1	1.1
Tremor	—	1.1
Asthenia	<1	1.1
Depression	<1	3.1
Decreased Libido	<1	2.7
Constipation	<1	1.3
Prostatic Disorder	<1	1.8
Ejaculation Failure	<1	1.1
Urinary Retention	<1	1.6
Dermatitis	—	1.3
Rash	<1	1.3
Arthralgia	<1	1.3
Arrhythmia	—	1.1
Myocardial Infarction	<1	1.3
Hematuria	<1	1.8
Tinnitus	<1	1.3

[a] Placebo-controlled clinical trials; treated with doxazosin from 1 to 203 days.
[b] Open label extension of 3 placebo-controlled clinical trials; treated for up to 50 months.

The following other adverse events occurred in normotensive or hypertensive patients with BPH with an incidence of <1% in short-term controlled clinical trials (n=665): tachycardia, angina, syncope, postural hypotension, pruritus, rash, myalgia, paresthesia, flushing, conjunctivitis, tinnitus, decreased libido, depression, nervousness, flatulence, rhinitis, epistaxis, carcinoma, dysuria, asthenia, influenza-like symptoms, viral infection, fever, weight increase, malaise, myocardial infarction, bradycardia, sudden death, pallor, hyperglycemia, gout, lymphadenopathy, prostatic disorder, ejaculation failure, epididymitis, dry skin, genital pruritus, urticaria, maculopapular rash, erythematous rash, aggravated psoriasis, eczema, hypoesthesia, hypertonia, leg cramps, confusion, speech disorder, ataxia, abnormal thinking, depersonalization, paroniria, emotional lability, impaired concentration, amnesia, earache, taste perversion, eye pain, visual field defect, cataract, melena, constipation, vomiting, gingivitis, increased appetite, coughing, bronchospasm, bronchitis, upper respiratory tract infection, sinusitis, pneumonia, urinary retention, micturition disorder, abnormal urine, renal pain, urinary incontinence, cystitis, arthritis, tendon disorder, arthralgia, hernia, rigors, hot flushes, allergy, sepsis, fungal infection, hematuria and subarachnoid hemorrhage.

The following other adverse events occurred in normotensive or hypertensive patients with BPH with an incidence of <1% in long-term controlled clinical trials (n=450): convulsions, encephalopathy, hypokinesia, migraine, fever, malaise, rigor, enlarged abdomen, allergic reaction/allergy, weight increase, nervousness, amnesia, anxiety, depersonalization, impaired concentration, abnormal thinking, flatulence, melena, vomiting, rectal hemorrhage, abnormal semen, tooth disorder, increased appetite, diverticulitis, esophagitis, gastric ulcer, tenesmus, tongue disorder, tooth hypoplasia, syncope, aneurysm, cardiac failure, abnormal ECG, hypertension, epistaxis, pharyngitis, rhinitis, bronchitis, pulmonary carcinoma, epididymitis, perineal pain, cystitis, dysuria, polyuria, urinary incontinence, oliguria, abnormal urine, increased sweating, seborrhea, maculopapular rash, skin disorder, nail disorder, photosensitivity reaction, pruritus, skin hypertrophy, urticaria, conjunctivitis, diplopia, eye abnormality, eye pain, myopia, visual field defect, myalgia, arthritis, polymyalgia rheumatica, atrial fibrillation, tachycardia, extra systoles, angina pectoris, myocardial ischemia, flushing, dry mouth, aggravated hypertension, sexual dysfunction, purpura, deafness, earache, cerebrovascular disorder/accident, intermittent claudication, carcinoma, herpes simplex, herpes zoster, fungal infection, otitis media, dehydration, hyperglycemia, hyperuricemia, cholelithiasis, AST increase, ALT increase and breast neoplasm.

Data from long-term (up to 50 months), open BPH studies (n=450) indicate higher rates of dizziness in younger hypertensive (27%) and normotensive (22%) patients, impotence in younger hypertensive (8%) patients, and discontinuation rates in patients due to adverse events (16.7%) compared to data from short-term placebo-controlled BPH studies (n=665).

Uncontrolled Trials and Postmarketing Experience: The following additional adverse events have also been reported in patients with essential hypertension and in normotensive or hypertensive patients with BPH: parosmia, renal calculus, priapism, ejaculation disorders such as retrograde ejaculation, jaundice, cholestasis and hepatitis.

Laboratory Abnormalities: No clinically relevant adverse effects were noted on serum potassium, serum glucose, uric acid, blood urea nitrogen or creatinine. Decreases in white blood cells, neutrophils, platelets (see Warnings), hemoglobin and hematocrit have been reported. Abnormal liver function tests have occurred.

OVERDOSE:

No data are available regarding overdosage with doxazosin in humans.

Treatment: Should administration of doxazosin lead to hypotension, support of the cardiovascular system is of first importance. Restoration of blood pressure and normalization of heart rate may be accomplished by keeping the patient in the supine position. If this measure is inadequate, shock should first be treated with volume expanders. If necessary, vasopressors should be used. Renal function should be monitored and supported as needed. As doxazosin is highly protein bound, dialysis may not be of benefit.

> For management of a suspected drug overdose, CPhA recommends that you contact your **regional Poison Control Centre**. See the *CPS* Directory section for a list of Poison Control Centres.

DOSAGE: Dosage must be individualized. Doxazosin may be administered either in the morning or in the evening.

The absorption of doxazosin is not affected by food.

When doxazosin is being added to the existing antihypertensive therapy, the patient should be carefully monitored for the occurrence of hypotension (see Warnings, Syncope and "First Dose" Effect). If a diuretic or other antihypertensive agent is being added to a doxazosin regimen, reducing the dose of doxazosin and retitration, with careful monitoring, may be necessary.

If doxazosin administration is discontinued for several days, or longer, therapy should be reinstituted using the initial dosing regimen.

Hypertension: 1 to 16 mg Once Daily: The initial dose of doxazosin in patients with hypertension is 1 mg given once daily and this dose should not be exceeded. This starting dose is intended to minimize postural hypotensive effects. The maximum reduction in blood pressure normally occurs between 2 and 6 hours after a dose.

The dose may be slowly increased to achieve the desired blood pressure response. The usual dose range is 1 to 8 mg once daily. The maximum recommended daily dose is 16 mg once daily.

Increases in dose beyond 4 mg increased the likelihood of excessive postural effects including syncope, postural dizziness/vertigo and postural hypotension. At a titrated dose of 16 mg once daily, the frequency of postural effects is about 12% compared to 3% for placebo.

Benign Prostatic Hyperplasia: 1 to 8 mg Once Daily: The initial dosage of doxazosin is 1 mg given once daily (see Warnings, Syncope and "First Dose" Effect). Depending on the individual patient's urodynamics and BPH symptomatology, dosage may then be increased to 2 mg and thereafter to 4 mg and 8 mg once daily, the maximum recommended dose. The recommended titration interval is 1 to 2 weeks. Blood pressure should be evaluated routinely in these patients.

Doxazosin should be discontinued if the drug has been increased to the maximum tolerated dose and improvement in urinary flowmetry is less than 25% or if doxazosin side effects are more bothersome than BPH symptoms, or if the patient develops a urinary complication secondary to BPH while on doxazosin therapy.

INFORMATION FOR THE PATIENT: Published in e-CPS, available by subscription at www.e-cps.ca.

SUPPLIED: 1 mg: Each capsular scored white tablet, engraved ASTRA on one side and CARDURA with 1 on the other side, contains: doxazosin mesylate equivalent to doxazosin 1 mg. Nonmedicinal ingredients: lactose, magnesium stearate, microcrystalline cellulose, sodium lauryl sulfate and sodium starch glycolate. Opaque plastic (high density polyethylene) bottles of 100. Store at room temperature, 15 to 30°C.

2 mg: Each capsular scored white tablet, engraved ASTRA on one side and CARDURA with 2 on the other side, contains: doxazosin mesylate equivalent to doxazosin 2 mg. Nonmedicinal ingredients: lactose, magnesium stearate, microcrystalline cellulose, sodium lauryl sulfate and sodium starch glycolate. Opaque plastic (high density polyethylene) bottles of 100. Store at room temperature, 15 to 30°C.

4 mg: Each capsular shaped yellow to orange scored tablet, with upper engraved "Cardura", lower bisected and engraved "4 mg", contains: doxazosin mesylate equivalent to doxazosin 4 mg. Nonmedicinal ingredients: FD&C Yellow #6 Aluminum Lake, lactose, magnesium stearate, microcrystalline cellulose, sodium lauryl sulfate and sodium starch glycolate. Opaque plastic (high density polyethylene) bottles of 100. Store at room temperature, 15 to 30°C.

(Shown in Product Identification Section)

Carnitor® ℞

levocarnitine

Carnitine Replenisher

Sigma-Tau

PHARMACOLOGY: Levocarnitine is a naturally occurring substance required in mammalian energy metabolism. It has been shown to facilitate long-chain fatty acid entry into cellular mitochondria, thereby delivering substrate for oxidation and subsequent energy production. Fatty acids are utilized as an energy substrate in all tissues except the brain. In skeletal and cardiac muscle, fatty acids are the main substrate for energy production.

Primary systemic carnitine deficiency is characterized by low concentrations of levocarnitine in plasma, RBC, and/or tissues. It has not been possible to determine which symptoms are due to carnitine deficiency and which are due to an underlying organic acidemia, as symptoms of both abnormalities may be expected to improve with levocarnitine. The literature reports that carnitine can promote the excretion of excess organic or fatty acids in patients with defects in fatty acid metabolism and/or specific organic acidopathies that bioaccumulate acylCoA esters.

Secondary carnitine deficiency can be a consequence of inborn errors of metabolism or iatrogenic factors such as hemodialysis. Levocarnitine may alleviate the metabolic abnormalities of patients with inborn errors that result in accumulation of toxic organic acids. Conditions for which this effect has been demonstrated are: glutaric aciduria II, methyl malonic aciduria, propionic acidemia, and medium chain fatty acylCoA dehydrogenase deficiency. Autointoxication occurs in these patients due to the accumulations of acylCoA compounds that disrupt intermediary metabolism. The subsequent hydrolysis of the acylCoA compound to its free acid results in acidosis which can be life-threatening. Levocarnitine clears the acylCoA compound by formation of acylcarnitine, which is quickly excreted. Carnitine deficiency is defined biochemically as abnormally low plasma concentrations of free carnitine, less than 20 µmol/L at one week post term and may be associated with low tissue and/or urine concentrations. Further, this condition may be associated with a plasma concentration ratio of acylcarnitine/levocarnitine greater than 0.4 or abnormally elevated concentrations of acylcarnitine in the urine. In premature infants and newborns, secondary deficiency is defined as plasma levocarnitine concentrations below age-related normal concentrations.

End Stage Renal Disease (ESRD) patients on maintenance hemodialysis may have low plasma carnitine concentrations and an increased ratio of acylcarnitine/carnitine because of reduced intake of meat and dairy products, reduced renal synthesis and dialytic losses. Certain clinical conditions common in hemodialysis patients such as malaise, muscle weakness, cardiomyopathy and cardiac arrhythmias may be related to abnormal carnitine metabolism.

Pharmacokinetic and clinical studies with levocarnitine have shown that administration of levocarnitine to ESRD patients on hemodialysis results in increased plasma levocarnitine concentrations. In one study, BUN, creatinine, and phosphorus blood levels decreased with levocarnitine administration. In another study, increases in hematocrit, decreases in hypotensive episodes, and improvement in well-being have been observed, although not statistically significant.

INDICATIONS: Oral Solution, Tablets and Injection: In the treatment of primary systemic carnitine deficiency. In the reported cases, the clinical presentation consisted of recurrent episodes of Reye-like encephalopathy, hypoketotic hypoglycemia, and/or cardiomyopathy. Associated symptoms included hypotonia, muscle weakness and failure to thrive. A diagnosis of primary carnitine deficiency requires that serum, red cell and/or tissue carnitine levels be low and that the patient does not have a primary defect in fatty acid or organic acid oxidation (see Pharmacology). In some patients, particularly those presenting with cardiomyopathy, carnitine supplementation rapidly alleviated signs and symptoms. Treatment should include, in addition to carnitine, supportive and other therapy as indicated by the condition of the patient.

Levocarnitine is also indicated for acute and chronic treatments of patients with an inborn error of metabolism which results in a secondary carnitine deficiency.

Injection: Levocarnitine injection is also indicated for the prevention and treatment of carnitine deficiency in patients with end stage renal disease who are undergoing dialysis.

CONTRAINDICATIONS: None known.

WARNINGS: None.

PRECAUTIONS: General: The safety and efficacy of oral levocarnitine has not been evaluated in patients with renal insufficiency. Chronic administration of high doses of oral levocarnitine in patients with severely compromised renal function or in ESRD patients on dialysis may result in accumulation of the potentially toxic metabolites, trimethylamine (TMA) and trimethylamine-N-oxide (TMAO), since these metabolites are normally excreted in the urine.

Oral Solution: For oral/internal use only. Gastrointestinal reactions may result from a too rapid consumption of carnitine. The oral solution may be consumed alone, or dissolved in drinks or other liquid foods to reduce taste fatigue. It should be consumed slowly and doses should be spaced evenly throughout the day to maximize tolerance.

Injection: The injection is for i.v. use only.

Oral Solution, Tablets and Injection:

Pregnancy: Category B: Reproductive studies have been performed in rats and rabbits at doses up to 3.8 times the human dose on the basis of surface area and have revealed no evidence of impaired fertility or harm to the fetus due to levocarnitine. There are, however, no adequate and well controlled studies in pregnant women. Because animal reproduction studies are not always predictive of human response, this drug should be used during pregnancy only if clearly needed.

Lactation: Levocarnitine supplementation in nursing mothers has not been specifically studied.

Studies in dairy cows indicate that the concentration of levocarnitine in milk is increased following exogenous administration of levocarnitine. In nursing mothers receiving levocarnitine, any risks to the child of excess carnitine intake need to be weighed against the benefits of levocarnitine supplementation to the mother. Consideration may be given to discontinuation of nursing or of levocarnitine treatment.

ADVERSE EFFECTS: Oral Solution and Tablets: Various mild gastrointestinal complaints have been reported during the long-term administration of oral L- or D,L-carnitine; these include transient nausea and vomiting, abdominal cramps, and diarrhea. Mild myasthenia has been described only in uremic patients receiving D,L-carnitine. Gastrointestinal adverse reactions with levocarnitine oral solution dissolved in liquids might be avoided by a slow consumption of the solution or by a greater dilution. Decreasing the dosage often diminishes or eliminates drug-related patient body odor or gastrointestinal symptoms when present. Tolerance should be monitored very closely during the first week of administration, and after any dosage increases.

Seizures have been reported to occur in patients with or without pre-existing seizure activity, receiving either oral or i.v. levocarnitine. In patients with pre-existing seizure activity, an increase in seizure frequency and/or severity has been reported.

Injection: Transient nausea and vomiting have been observed. Less frequent adverse reactions are body odor, nausea, and gastritis. An incidence for these reactions is difficult to estimate due to the confounding effects of the underlying pathology.

Seizures have been reported to occur in patients with or without pre-existing seizure activity, receiving either oral or i.v. levocarnitine. In patients with pre-existing seizure activity, an increase in seizure frequency and/or severity has been reported.

Table 1 lists the adverse events that have been reported in two double-blind, placebo-controlled trials in patients on chronic hemodialysis. Events occurring at ≥5% are reported without regard to causality.

Table 1: Carnitor

Adverse Events with a Frequency ≥5% Regardless of Causality by Body System

	Placebo (n=63)	Levocarnitine 10 mg (n=34)	Levocarnitine 20 mg (n=62)	Levocarnitine 40 mg (n=34)	Levocarnitine 10, 20 and 40 mg (n=130)
Body as a Whole					
Abdominal Pain	17	21	5	6	9
Accidental Injury	10	12	8	12	10
Allergic Reaction	5	6			2
Asthenia	8	9	8	12	9
Back Pain	10	9	8	6	8
Chest Pain	14	6	15	12	12
Fever	5	6	5	12	7
Flu Syndrome	40	15	27	29	25
Headache	16	12	37	3	22
Infection	17	15	10	24	15
Injection Site Reaction	59	38	27	38	33
Pain	49	21	32	35	30
Cardiovascular					
Arrhythmia	5	3		3	2
Atrial Fibrillation			2	6	2
Cardiovascular Disorder	6	3	5	6	5
Electrocardiogram Abnormal		3		6	2
Hemorrhage	6	9	2	3	4
Hypertension	14	18	21	21	20
Hypotension	19	15	19	3	14

(cont'd)

Table 1: Carnitor *(cont'd)*

Adverse Events with a Frequency ≥5% Regardless of Causality by Body System

	Placebo (n=63)	Levocarnitine 10 mg (n=34)	Levocarnitine 20 mg (n=62)	Levocarnitine 40 mg (n=34)	Levocarnitine 10, 20 and 40 mg (n=130)
Palpitations		3	8		5
Tachycardia	5	6	5	9	6
Vascular Disorder	2		2	6	2
Digestive					
Anorexia	3	3	5	6	5
Constipation	6	3	3	3	3
Diarrhea	19	9	10	35	16
Dyspepsia	10	9	6		5
Gastrointestinal Disorder	2	3		6	2
Melena	3	6			2
Nausea	10	9	5	12	8
Stomach Atony	5				
Vomiting	16	9	16	21	15
Endocrine System					
Parathyroid Disorder	2	6	2	6	4
Hemic/Lymphatic					
Anemia	3	3	5	12	6
Metabolic/Nutritional					
Hypercalcemia	3	15	8	6	9
Hyperkalemia	6	6	6	6	6
Hypervolemia	17	3	3	12	5
Peripheral Edema	3	6	5	3	5
Weight Decrease	3	3	8	3	5
Weight Increase	2	3		6	2
Musculoskeletal					
Leg Cramps	13		8		4
Myalgia	6				
Nervous					
Anxiety	5		2		1
Depression	3	6	5	6	5
Dizziness	11	18	10	15	13
Drug Dependence	2	6			2
Hypertonia	5	3			1
Insomnia	6	3	6		4
Paresthesia	3	3	3	12	5
Vertigo		6			2
Respiratory					
Bronchitis			5	3	3
Cough Increase	16		10	18	9
Dyspnea	19	3	11	3	7
Pharyngitis	33	24	27	15	23
Respiratory Disorder	5				
Rhinitis	10	6	11	6	9
Sinusitis	5		2	3	2
Skin And Appendages					

(cont'd)

Table 1: Carnitor *(cont'd)*

Adverse Events with a Frequency ≥5% Regardless of Causality by Body System

	Placebo (n=63)	Levocarnitine 10 mg (n=34)	Levocarnitine 20 mg (n=62)	Levocarnitine 40 mg (n=34)	Levocarnitine 10, 20 and 40 mg (n=130)
Pruritus	13		8	3	5
Rash	3		5	3	3
Special Senses					
Amblyopia	2		6		3
Eye Disorder	3	6	3		3
Taste Perversion			2	9	3
Urogenital					
Urinary Tract Infection	6	3	3		2
Kidney Failure	5	6	6	6	6

OVERDOSE:

Symptoms: There have been no reports of toxicity from levocarnitine overdosage. Levocarnitine is easily removed from plasma by dialysis. The i.v. LD_{50} of levocarnitine in rats is 5.4 g/kg and the oral LD_{50} of levocarnitine in mice is 19.2 g/kg. Carnitine may cause diarrhea.

Treatment: Overdosage should be treated with supportive care.

For management of a suspected drug overdose, CPhA recommends that you contact your **regional Poison Control Centre**. See the *CPS Directory* section for a list of Poison Control Centres.

DOSAGE: Oral Solution: For oral use only. **Not for parenteral use.**

Adults: The recommended dosage is 1 to 3 g/day for a 50 kg subject which is equivalent to 10 to 30 mL/day oral solution. Higher doses should be administered only with caution and only where clinical and biochemical considerations make it seem likely that higher doses will be of benefit. Dosage should start at 1 g/day (10 mL/day), and be increased slowly while assessing tolerance and therapeutic response. Monitoring should include periodic blood chemistries, vital signs, plasma carnitine concentrations, and overall clinical condition.

Infants and Children: The recommended dosage is 50 to 100 mg/kg/day which is equivalent to 0.5 mL/kg/day oral solution. Higher doses should be administered only with caution and only where clinical and biochemical considerations make it seem likely that higher doses will be of benefit. Dosage should start at 50 mg/kg/day, and be increased slowly to a maximum of 3 g/day (30 mL/day) while assessing tolerance and therapeutic response. Monitoring should include periodic blood chemistries, vital signs, plasma carnitine concentrations, and overall clinical condition.

Oral solution may be consumed alone or dissolved in drinks or other liquid food. Doses should be spaced evenly throughout the day (every 3 or 4 hours) preferably during or following meals and should be consumed slowly in order to maximize tolerance.

Tablets: For oral administration only.

Adults: The recommended oral dosage is 990 mg; 2 or 3 times a day using the 330 mg tablets, depending on clinical response.

Infants and Children: The recommended oral dosage is between 50 and 100 mg/kg/day in divided doses, with a maximum of 3 g/day. Dosage should begin at 50 mg/kg/day. The exact dosage will depend on clinical response.

Monitoring should include periodic blood chemistries, vital signs, plasma carnitine concentrations and overall clinical condition.

Injection: Metabolic Disorders: Levocarnitine injection is administered i.v. The recommended dose is 50 mg/kg given as a slow 2 to 3 minute bolus injection or by infusion. Often a loading dose is given in patients with severe metabolic crisis, followed by an equivalent dose over the following 24 hours. It should be administered q3h or q4h, and never less than q6h either by infusion or by i.v. injection. All subsequent daily doses are recommended to be in the range of 50 mg/kg or as therapy may require. The highest dose administered has been 300 mg/kg.

It is recommended that a plasma carnitine concentration be obtained prior to beginning this parenteral therapy. Weekly and monthly monitoring is recommended as well. This monitoring should include blood chemistries, vital signs, plasma carnitine concentrations (the plasma free carnitine concentration should be between 35 and 60 μmol/L at baseline) and overall clinical condition.

ESRD Patients on Hemodialysis: The recommended dose is 20 mg/kg dry body weight as a slow 2 to 3 minute bolus injection into the venous return line after each dialysis session. It is recommended that therapy begin after being on hemodialysis for a period of 6 months. Postdialysis levocarnitine plasma levels approach physiological levels after approximately 2 months of therapy at 20 mg/kg. After 2 months of therapy and based on clinical assessment, the dose may be adjusted to 5 mg/kg after each dialysis session.

Compatibility and Stability: Carnitor injection is compatible and stable when mixed in parenteral solutions of sodium chloride 0.9% or lactated Ringers' in concentrations ranging from 250 mg/500 mL (0.5 mg/mL) to 4200 mg/500 mL (8 mg/mL) and stored at room temperature (25°C) for up to 24 hours in PVC plastic bags.

Parenteral drug products should be inspected visually for particulate matter and discoloration prior to administration, whenever solution and container permit.

Pediatric Dosage: See Dosage.

SUPPLIED: Injection: Each mL of sterile, aqueous solution, **for i.v. use only**, contains: levocarnitine 200 mg. pH adjusted to 6.0 to 6.5 with hydrochloric acid and/or sodium hydroxide. Preservative-free (levocarnitine will support microbial growth). Single dose vials of 5 mL, cartons of 5. Store at room temperature (15 to 30°C). Avoid excessive heat. Protect from freezing. Discard unused portion after opening.

Oral Solution: Each 10 mL of clear, cherry flavored solution, **for oral use only**, contains: levocarnitine 1 g. Nonmedicinal ingredients: artificial cherry flavor, D,L-malic acid, methyl- and propylparaben (as preservatives), purified water and sucrose syrup. pH is approximately 5. Multiple-unit plastic containers of 118 mL, cases of 24. Store at room temperature (15 to 30°C). Avoid excessive heat. Protect from freezing. Store upright.

Tablets: Each white, biconvex tablet, embossed with "CARNITOR ST", **for oral use only**, contains: levocarnitine 330 mg. Nonmedicinal ingredients: magnesium stearate, microcrystalline cellulose and povidone. Single unit blisters of laminated aluminum foil in cards of 10, cartons of 90 (9 cards/carton). Store at room temperature (15 to 30°C). Avoid excessive heat. Protect from freezing. Do not store after removal from foil packaging: contents hygroscopic.

Carters Little Pills

bisacodyl

Laxative

Church & Dwight

INDICATIONS: Short-term treatment for occasional acute or chronic constipation, and irregularity. Use as part of a bowel-cleansing regimen in preparing the patient for surgery, or for preparing the colon for x-ray endoscopic examination. (This drug does not replace colonic irrigation prior to surgery.)

May also be used in postoperative restoration of normal bowel hygiene.

CONTRAINDICATIONS: Stimulant laxatives are contraindicated for patients with acute surgical abdomen, appendicitis, rectal bleeding, gastroenteritis or intestinal obstruction.

WARNINGS: The frequent or prolonged use of this drug may lead to laxative dependence.

Keep out of the reach of children.

PRECAUTIONS: A physician's consultation is strongly advised when treating constipation associated with colitis, carcinoma of the colon, or diverticulitis.

Pregnancy: Caution and/or a physician's advice is warranted when treating constipation during pregnancy and lactation.

Lactation: See Pregnancy.

This drug should not be used in the presence of nausea/vomiting, fever, abdominal pain, or symptoms of appendicitis.

Rectal bleeding or failure to produce a bowel movement after taking this drug may indicate a serious problem; in such case, the drug should be discontinued and a physician consulted.

ADVERSE EFFECTS: No systemic side effects have been reported. Occasional mild abdominal cramps occurred in some patients.

OVERDOSE:

Treatment: No specific antidotes are required in cases of overdosage; however, supportive care may be required to prevent dehydration and/or electrolyte imbalance.

> For management of a suspected drug overdose, CPhA recommends that you contact your **regional Poison Control Centre**. See the *CPS* Directory section for a list of Poison Control Centres.

DOSAGE: Adults and children 12 years of age and older: single daily dose of 2 (10 mg) or, exceptionally, 3 (15 mg) tablets. Children 6 to under 12 years of age: single daily dose of 1 (5 mg) tablet. Children under 6 years of age: use only as directed by a physician.

Desired effects are to be expected within 8 to 12 hours if taken at bedtime, or within 6 hours if taken before breakfast.

Tablets must be swallowed whole, not crushed or chewed.

Tablets should not be swallowed within 2 hours prior to or after taking other medications, to prevent having the desired effect of these drugs reduced or delayed.

SUPPLIED: Each tablet contains: bisacodyl USP 5 mg. Nonmedicinal ingredients: calcium phosphate, calcium sulfate, carnauba wax, cellulose, gelatin, kaolin, magnesium stearate, methacrylic acid copolymer, polyethylene glycol pregelatinized starch, silicon dioxide, sucrose, talc, titanium dioxide, white wax. Blister packs, cartons of 25 and 75.

Carvedilol

Beta-adrenergic Blocking Agent

CPhA Monograph

Date of Preparation: April 2008

> This monograph has been compiled by CPhA and reviewed by experts. It may contain information different from that found in Health Canada-approved Product Monographs. The reader is referred to the *CPS* Editorial Policy for more information.

SUMMARY PRODUCT INFORMATION:

Route of Administration	Dosage Form	Strength
Oral	Tablet	3.125 mg, 6.25 mg, 12.5 mg, 25 mg

INDICATIONS AND CLINICAL USE: Carvedilol is indicated for treatment of mild, moderate or severe heart failure of ischemic or nonischemic origin.

The Canadian Cardiovascular Society Consensus Conference on Heart Failure 2006 made the following general recommendations with respect to the use of beta blockers in patients with heart failure, all of which apply to carvedilol: all patients with a left ventricular ejection fraction ≤40% should receive a beta blocker shown to be beneficial in large-scale clinical trials; patients with New York Heart Association (NYHA) class IV symptoms should be stable before the introduction of a beta blocker; beta blockers should generally not be introduced in patients with acute heart failure, heart failure with symptomatic hypotension (after adjusting other therapies), significant bradycardia, significant atrioventricular (AV) block (without a pacemaker) and/or severe reactive airways disease. Stable chronic obstructive pulmonary disease is not a contraindication to the use of beta blockers in this setting; the initial dose of a beta blocker should be low and titrated slowly to the target dose used in large-scale clinical trials or the maximum tolerated dose if the target dose cannot be achieved [Canadian Cardiovascular Society consensus conference recommendations on heart failure 2006: diagnosis and management. *Can J Cardiol* 2006;22(1):23-45].

In large-scale clinical trials carvedilol was added to ongoing therapy for heart failure, which comprised diuretics, angiotensin converting enzyme (ACE) inhibitors and digoxin. Beta blockers have also been used as a background therapy in large-scale clinical trials of angiotensin II receptor blockers (candesartan, valsartan), aldosterone antagonists (eplerenone, spironolactone) and the combination of isosorbide dinitrate plus hydralazine.

Carvedilol has been shown to significantly reduce mortality when compared with placebo (3.2% vs 7.8%, p=0.001), and to decrease the risk of sudden death (1.7% vs 3.8%), death from progressive pump failure (0.7 vs 3.3%) and the risk of cardiovascular hospitalizations (14.1% vs 19.6%, p=0.036) in a large randomized multicentre clinical trial [The effect of carvedilol on morbidity and mortality in patients with chronic heart failure. U.S. Carvedilol Heart Failure Study Group. *N Engl J Med* 1996;334(21):1349-55].

Carvedilol is also used for the management of clinically stable patients with left ventricular dysfunction (left ventricular ejection fraction ≤40%) after myocardial infarction [Effect of carvedilol on outcome after myocardial infarction in patients with left-ventricular dysfunction: the CAPRICORN randomised trial. *Lancet* 2001;357(9266):1385-90], treatment of hypertension [Comparison of a new vasodilating beta-blocker, carvedilol, with atenolol in the treatment of mild to moderate essential hypertension. *Am J Hypertens* 1994;7(2):129-36; [Comparison of acebutolol with and without hydrochlorothiazide versus carvedilol with and without hydrochlorothiazide in black patients with mild to moderate systemic hypertension. *Am J Cardiol* 1999;84(1):70-5], stable angina pectoris [Effectiveness of three different doses of carvedilol for exertional angina. Carvedilol-Angina Study Group. *Am J Cardiol* 1998;82(8):927-31; [Comparison of safety and efficacy of carvedilol and metoprolol in stable angina pectoris. *Am J Cardiol* 1999;83(5):643-9] and portal hypertension in patients with cirrhosis [Randomized comparison of long-term carvedilol and propranolol administration in the treatment of portal hypertension in cirrhosis. *Hepatology* 2002;36(6):1367-73], although it is not approved for these indications in Canada.

Geriatrics: The pattern and frequency of adverse events in elderly patients with heart failure was similar to that reported in younger patients with heart failure enrolled in clinical trials. However, because plasma levels of carvedilol are generally higher in elderly individuals the maximum tolerated dose may be lower in elderly patients than in younger patients.

Pediatrics: In pediatric patients with heart failure there was no difference in the percentage of patients who experienced improvement, worsening or no change in clinical status after 8 months of treatment with carvedilol or placebo in a randomized, double-blind, multicentre trial [Carvedilol for children and adolescents with heart failure: a randomized controlled trial. *JAMA* 2007;298(10):1171-9]. There was a possible beneficial trend in children with a systemic left ventricle (i.e., those with congenital heart defects resulting in an absent or poorly functioning left ventricle), but not in those without a systemic left ventricle.

CONTRAINDICATIONS:

- Hypersensitivity to carvedilol
- Decompensated cardiac failure
- Asthma or other bronchospastic condition
- Second or third degree atrioventricular block or sick sinus syndrome unless a permanent pacemaker has been inserted
- Cardiogenic shock
- Severe hypotension
- Severe bradycardia
- Clinically apparent hepatic dysfunction as evidenced by the presence of ascites, esophageal varices, jaundice or spider angiomata.

WARNINGS AND PRECAUTIONS:

> **Serious Warnings and Precautions**
> - Abrupt cessation of therapy: severe exacerbations of angina, myocardial infarction and ventricular arrhythmias have occurred after abrupt withdrawal of beta blockers.
> - Beta blockers including carvedilol can precipitate worsening heart failure. Worsening of heart failure is most likely to occur after initiating or increasing the dosage of carvedilol. It is important to follow the recommended dose titration schedule to minimize the likelihood of worsening heart failure.

Allergic Reactions: Carvedilol may antagonize the action of epinephrine when the latter is used to treat allergic reactions. Larger than usual doses of epinephrine may be required to treat anaphylaxis.

Cardiovascular: Hypotension: Hypotension including postural hypotension may be precipitated by carvedilol. Hypotension is more likely to occur during initiation of treatment; thus, it is important to follow the dosage recommendations (see Dosage and Administration).

Bradycardia: Severe bradycardia may occur after initiating treatment with carvedilol. The dosage should be reduced or the drug withdrawn in such cases.

Endocrine and Metabolism: Diabetes mellitus: Beta blockers may mask some of the signs of hypoglycemia, particularly autonomic signs such as tachycardia, in patients with diabetes. Beta blockers may lead to worsening hyperglycemia.

Thyrotoxicosis: Beta blockers may mask the clinical signs of hyperthyroidism, particularly tachycardia. Abrupt withdrawal of a beta blocker may result in an exacerbation of hyperthyroidism and may precipitate thyroid storm.

Hepatic/Biliary/Pancreatic: Carvedilol undergoes extensive hepatic metabolism including significant first-pass metabolism. Thus, the bioavailability of carvedilol may be increased in patients with hepatic dysfunction.

Perioperative Considerations: Caution with anesthetic agents that depress myocardial function.

Renal Function: Worsening of renal function may occur upon initiation of carvedilol in patients with heart failure. Patients with pre-existing renal insufficiency, hypotension (systolic blood pressure <100 mm Hg), ischemic heart disease and/or diffuse vascular disease are at increased risk of worsening renal function. Renal function should be monitored before and after initiating treatment with carvedilol and after increasing the dose. If clinically significant worsening of renal function occurs during treatment with carvedilol the dose should be reduced or treatment withdrawn.

Special Populations: Pregnant or Nursing Women: Pregnancy category C. Post-implantation loss of pregnancy has been observed in animals treated with carvedilol. Use of beta blockers during pregnancy has been associated with persistent bradycardia, hypotension and intrauterine growth retardation. Neonatal hypoglycemia has been reported in infants after maternal use of beta blockers at parturition or during breast-feeding.

Pediatrics: Carvedilol is not approved for use in children, although the drug has been evaluated in children with heart failure aged 3 months to 18 years in clinical trials. The safety and efficacy of carvedilol in this setting is not well established.

Geriatrics: Plasma levels are approximately 50% higher in elderly than in younger patients.

Monitoring and Laboratory Tests: Blood pressure, heart rate electrocardiogram, serum creatinine and liver function tests in all patients, and blood sugar in patients with diabetes or those at risk of developing diabetes.

Occupational Hazards: Patients may experience dizziness and syncope after the initiation of carvedilol. Patients should be counseled to avoid driving or operating potentially dangerous machinery if they experience dizziness upon initiation of carvedilol or after dosage adjustments.

ADVERSE REACTIONS: Adverse Drug Reactions Overview: In patients with mild to moderate heart failure, hypotension or postural hypotension occurred in 9.7% of patients randomized to carvedilol and in 3.6% of those randomized to placebo. In patients with severe heart failure, hypotension or postural hypotension occurred in 15.1% of patients randomized to carvedilol and in 8.7% of those randomized to placebo. Among patients treated with carvedilol in these trials, syncope was reported in 3.4% of patients with mild-to-moderate heart failure (vs 2.5% with placebo), and in 2.9% of those with severe heart failure (vs 2.3% with placebo). In patients with left ventricular dysfunction after myocardial infarction the incidence of hypotension or postural hypotension was 20.2% among those treated with carvedilol (vs 12.6% with placebo). Syncope was reported by 3.9% of carvedilol recipients and 1.9% of placebo recipients in this trial. Bradycardia occurs more often in patients receiving carvedilol for heart failure (9%) or after myocardial infarction (6.5%) than for hypertension (2%). Hypotension occurs most often during the first 30 days of treatment. Patients should be advised to take carvedilol with food to minimize the risk of postural hypotension.

More Common Adverse Drug Reactions: Adverse reactions that occurred more frequently in recipients of carvedilol than placebo in large, randomized, multicentre trials conducted exclusively in patients with heart failure are shown in Table 1. Only events that occurred in >3% of carvedilol recipients are shown.

Table 1: Carvedilol

More Common Adverse Drug Reactions

	Mild-to-Moderate Heart Failure[a]		Severe Heart Failure[b]	
Event	**Carvedilol, % (n=765)**	**Placebo, % (n=437)**	**Carvedilol, % (n=1156)**	**Placebo, % (n=1133)**
Dizziness	32	19	24	17
Fatigue	24	22	—	—
Hypotension	9	3	14	8
Hyperglycemia	12	8	5	3
Diarrhea	12	6	5	3
Increased body weight	10	7	12	11
Asthenia	7	7	11	9
Bradycardia	9	1	10	3
Increased cough	8	9	5	4
Nausea	9	5	4	3
Headache	8	7	5	3
Syncope	3	3	8	5
Peripheral edema	2	1	7	6
Generalized edema	5	3	6	5
Arthralgia	6	5	1	1
Increased blood urea nitrogen	6	5	—	—

(cont'd)

Table 1: Carvedilol *(cont'd)*

More Common Adverse Drug Reactions

Event	Mild-to-Moderate Heart Failure[a]		Severe Heart Failure[b]	
	Carvedilol, % (n=765)	Placebo, % (n=437)	Carvedilol, % (n=1156)	Placebo, % (n=1133)
Increased non-protein nitrogen	6	5	—	—
Angina pectoris	2	3	6	4
Vomiting	6	4	1	2
Increased digoxin level	5	4	2	1
Abnormal vision	5	2	—	—
Rales	4	4	4	2
Hypercholesterolemia	4	3	1	1
Dependent edema	4	2	—	—

[a] Most of these patients were enrolled in the US Carvedilol Heart Failure studies [The effect of carvedilol on morbidity and mortality in patients with chronic heart failure. U.S. Carvedilol Heart Failure Study Group. *N Engl J Med* 1996;334(21):1349-55].
[b] Data from the COPERNICUS trial [Effect of carvedilol on survival in severe chronic heart failure. *N Engl J Med* 2001;344(22):1651-8].

Less Common Adverse Drug Reactions (≤3%): Cardiovascular: aggravated angina pectoris, AV block, bundle branch block, complete AV block, fluid overload, myocardial ischemia, postural hypotension, palpitation, hypertension, peripheral ischemia.
Central and Peripheral Nervous System: convulsions (rare), hypesthesia, hypokinesia, migraine, paresthesia, vertigo.
Allergic/Dermatologic: alopecia, pruritus, erythematous rash, exfoliative dermatitis, maculopapular rash, psoriaform rash, photosensitivity.
Endocrine and Metabolism: diabetes mellitus, hyperuricemia, hypoglycemia, hyponatremia, glycosuria, hypervolemia, hypokalemia, weight loss, hyperkalemia.
Gastrointestinal: melena, periodontitis.
Hematologic: anemia, decreased prothrombin, leucopenia, purpura, thrombocytopenia.
Hepatic/Biliary/Pancreatic: elevated serum ALT, AST, bilirubin, alkaline phosphatase and/or GGT levels.
Musculoskeletal: muscle cramps.
Psychiatric: aggravated depression, emotional lability, impaired concentration, nervousness, paroniria (morbid dreams), somnolence.
Pulmonary: bronchospasm.
Renal and Urinary: albuminuria, hematuria, increased frequency of micturition, increased serum creatinine, renal insufficiency, urinary incontinence.
Sexual Function/Reproduction: decreased libido, male impotence.
Special Senses: blurred vision, tinnitus.
Abnormal Hematologic and Clinical Chemistry Findings: See Table 2.

Table 2: Carvedilol

Abnormal Hematologic and Clinical Chemistry Findings

Test	Effect	Clinical Comment
Blood glucose	Increase	Monitor blood glucose at baseline and during treatment with carvedilol. Adjust doses of antihyperglycemic medications if necessary. Counsel patients accordingly.
Serum creatinine	Increase	Patients at risk are those with pre-existing renal insufficiency, hypotension (SBP <100 mm Hg), ischemic heart disease and/or diffuse vascular disease. Monitor serum creatinine before and after initiating treatment with carvedilol and after increasing the dose. If renal function worsens, reduce the dose or withdraw treatment.

DRUG INTERACTIONS: Overview: The combination of carvedilol and other drugs with antihypertensive effects may result in an additive or exaggerated hypotensive effect. Concomitant use of carvedilol and drugs that affect cardiac conduction (e.g., diltiazem, verapamil, antiarrhythmic agents) may result in cardiac conduction abnormalities and hemodynamic compromise.

Carvedilol undergoes oxidative metabolism mediated by hepatic cytochrome P450 isozymes, the most important of which is CYP2D6. Thus the pharmacokinetics of the drug may be altered when coadministered with strong inhibitors of CYP2D6.

No pharmacokinetic drug-drug interaction was detected in studies designed to evaluate the potential for drug interactions between carvedilol and glyburide, hydrochlorothiazide, torsemide or warfarin.

Drug-Drug Interactions: See Table 3.

Table 3: Carvedilol

Drug-Drug Interactions

Interacting Drug	Effect	Clinical Comment
Amiodarone	Amiodarone inhibited the metabolism of carvedilol in heart failure patients [Stereoselective effect of amiodarone on the pharmacokinetics of racemic carvedilol. *Drug Metab Pharmacokinet* 2005;20(6):423-7]. The S(−) enantiomer of carvedilol was affected to a greater extent than the R(+) enantiomer.	Monitor patients for signs of carvedilol excess if amiodarone is initiated in patients stabilized on carvedilol. Adjust the dose of carvedilol as needed.
Cimetidine	The steady-state area under the plasma concentration versus time curve (AUC) of carvedilol increased by 30% when coadministered with cimetidine.	Use an alternative H_2-receptor antagonist.
Cyclosporine	The trough concentration of cyclosporine increased when carvedilol therapy was initiated in renal transplant recipients.	Monitor patients for signs of cyclosporine excess if carvedilol is initiated in patients stabilized on cyclosporine. Monitor serum concentrations of cyclosporine and adjust the dose of cyclosporine as needed.

(cont'd)

Table 3: Carvedilol *(cont'd)*

Drug-Drug Interactions

Interacting Drug	Effect	Clinical Comment
Digoxin	Carvedilol increases serum digoxin concentrations.	Monitor patients for signs of digoxin excess and measure serum digoxin concentrations if carvedilol is initiated in patients stabilized on digoxin. Adjust the dose of digoxin as needed.
Fluoxetine	Fluoxetine selectively inhibited CYP2D6-mediated metabolism and decreased the clearance of carvedilol in heart failure patients who were extensive metabolizers of CYP2D6 substrates [Effect of fluoxetine on carvedilol pharmacokinetics, CYP2D6 activity, and autonomic balance in heart failure patients. *J Clin Pharmacol* 2001;41(1):97-106]. The R(+) enantiomer was affected to a greater extent than the S(−) enantiomer.	Despite the significant effects of fluoxetine on carvedilol metabolism there was no significant difference in adverse events, blood pressure or heart rate over 4 weeks.
Rifampin	The AUC of carvedilol decreased by 70% when coadministered with rifampin.	If a patient on carvedilol must be treated with rifampin, increased dosages of carvedilol may be required. Monitor patients and adjust the dose when introducing and withdrawing rifampin.

DOSAGE AND ADMINISTRATION: Dosing Considerations: Patients with heart failure should be clinically stable for at least 4 weeks before initiating treatment with carvedilol. This includes being on stable doses of ACE inhibitors (if tolerated) and diuretics with or without digoxin.

In patients with heart failure the initial dose of carvedilol must be low (i.e., 3.125 mg BID) and the dose should be increased slowly to the target dose or the maximum tolerated dose. Abrupt withdrawal or major reductions in the dose of carvedilol should be avoided. If a patient becomes hypotensive, consideration may be given to reducing the dosage of other medications or changing the timing of administration of other medications (i.e., an ACE inhibitor) before reducing the dose of carvedilol.

Objective improvement in cardiac function may not be apparent for 6 to 12 months after initiating treatment with a beta blocker in a patient with heart failure.

If fluid retention and/or worsening heart failure occur after initiation of carvedilol, consider increasing the dose of diuretic and delaying titration of the dose of carvedilol. It may be necessary to reduce the dose of carvedilol or temporarily discontinue the drug in some patients. If the dosage of carvedilol is decreased because of worsening heart failure, the dosage should not be increased until the symptoms have been stabilized for at least 2 weeks.

The dosage of carvedilol should be reduced if the pulse falls below 55 beats per minute. Caution patients who experience dizziness or fatigue to avoid driving or hazardous activities when initiating treatment or increasing the dose. These events are most likely to occur within 2 hours after administration.

Recommended Dose and Dosage Adjustment: Adults: See Table 4.

Table 4: Carvedilol

Oral Dose in Adult Patients

Indication	Initial Dose	Dose Titration	Target Dose	Clinical Comment
Heart failure	3.125 mg BID	Double the dose at 2- to 4-week intervals (i.e., 6.25 mg BID, then 12.5 mg BID, then 25 mg BID)	25 mg BID	Titrate to the maximum tolerated dose if the target dose cannot be achieved
Hypertension	6.25 mg BID	As needed to achieve target systolic/diastolic blood pressure	Maximum dose is 25 mg BID	Not an approved indication in Canada

Dialysis: Carvedilol is not removed by hemodialysis or peritoneal dialysis. Administration of supplemental doses is not recommended after dialysis sessions.
Hepatic Impairment: Carvedilol is contraindicated in patients with severe liver dysfunction, but patients with mild liver disease may receive carvedilol. The starting dose does not need to be altered in these patients, but because of the potential for higher plasma levels and an increased likelihood of vasodilation the dosage should be increased more cautiously than in patients without liver dysfunction. The maximum tolerated dose at the end of the dosage titration period may be lower in such patients than in similar individuals without liver dysfunction.
Genetic Polymorphism: Carvedilol undergoes stereoselective hepatic metabolism mediated by CYP2D6 (see Pharmacokinetics: Adults).
Missed Dose: If the patient misses a dose they should be advised to take it as soon as they remember, unless it is time for the next dose. They should be advised to resume their normal schedule without taking 2 doses at the same time.
Administration: Carvedilol should be taken with food to minimize the risk of orthostatic hypotension.

OVERDOSAGE:

For management of a suspected drug overdose, CPhA recommends that you contact your **regional Poison Control Centre**. See the *CPS* Directory section for a list of Poison Control Centres.

ACTION AND CLINICAL PHARMACOLOGY: Mechanism of Action: Carvedilol is a nonselective beta-adrenergic receptor antagonist with $alpha_1$-antagonist activity. The potency of the drug is 10-fold greater at beta-adrenergic than alpha-adrenergic receptors. Carvedilol produces bradycardia through its $beta_1$-antagonist activity, and hypotension primarily through its $alpha_1$-adrenergic antagonist activity. $Beta_1$-blockade prevents reflex tachycardia in response to the decrease in systemic vascular resistance. The drug also inhibits release of renin mediated via beta-adrenergic receptors.

The $beta_1$-receptor antagonist activity of carvedilol is attributable primarily to the S(−) enantiomer and the $alpha_1$-receptor antagonist activity of the drug is primarily associated with the R(+) enantiomer.

In patients with heart failure, carvedilol has been shown to significantly reduce heart rate, blood pressure, pulmonary artery pressure and pulmonary capillary wedge pressure. After 3 months of administration there were significant reductions in heart rate, pulmonary artery pressure, right atrial pressure, systemic vascular resistance, and a significant increase in stroke volume index.

Pharmacokinetics: Adults: Absorption: Peak plasma concentrations of carvedilol occur approximately 1 hour after oral administration to fasting individuals. The absolute bioavailability of the drug ranges from 25% to 35% because of extensive first-pass metabolism. When administered with food the rate of absorption is reduced, but the extent of absorption is unchanged.
Distribution: The volume of distribution of carvedilol is estimated to be 115 L indicating extensive extravascular distribution. Plasma concentrations of carvedilol are dose proportional after oral administration. At therapeutic doses carvedilol is highly bound (>98%) to plasma proteins (primarily albumin) in a concentration independent manner. Plasma levels of R(+) carvedilol are generally 2 to 3 times higher than those of S(−) carvedilol after oral administration.
Metabolism and Excretion: Carvedilol undergoes extensive hepatic metabolism mediated predominantly by CYP2D6 and CYP2C9 and to a lesser extent by CYP1A2, CYP2E1 and CYP3A4. Carvedilol has three major and one minor pharmacologically active metabolites all of which exist as 2 enantiomers. The metabolites are produced at differing rates by the same CYP isozymes. S(−) carvedilol is metabolized more rapidly than R(+) carvedilol in vitro and in vivo. The metabolites are present in concentrations that are 10 to 50 times lower than the parent enantiomers.

Carvedilol undergoes stereoselective hepatic metabolism mediated by CYP2D6. Poor metabolizers of debrisoquin (i.e., those with low CYP2D6 activity) have plasma levels of R(+) carvedilol that are 2 to 3 times higher than those in extensive metabolizers of debrisoquin.

Biliary-fecal excretion is the major elimination pathway for the metabolites of carvedilol. Less than 2% of an administered oral dose of carvedilol is excreted unchanged in the urine. The mean elimination half-life ($t_{1/2}$) of R(+) carvedilol is 5 to 9 hours and that of S(−) carvedilol is 7 to 11 hours.

Special Populations: Geriatrics: The area under the plasma concentration vs time curve (AUC) is higher in elderly subjects aged 65 to 76 years compared with younger subjects aged 18 to 43 years. In elderly individuals the mean AUC of S(−) carvedilol was 50% higher and that of R(+) carvedilol 23% higher than that in younger individuals.

Cirrhotic Liver Disease: In patients with hepatic cirrhosis the absolute bioavailability of carvedilol is 4 times higher than in healthy volunteers and the median C_{max} and AUC values are increased by 4-fold to 7-fold.

Casodex® Ⓟ

bicalutamide

Nonsteroidal Antiandrogen

AstraZeneca

Date of Revision: May 10, 2010

SUMMARY PRODUCT INFORMATION:

Route of Administration	Dosage Form/ Strength	Clinically Relevant Nonmedicinal Ingredients
Oral	Tablet/50 mg	Lactose monohydrate For a complete listing see Dosage Forms, Composition and Packaging.

INDICATIONS AND CLINICAL USE: CASODEX (bicalutamide) 50 mg is indicated for use in combination therapy with either an LHRH analogue or surgical castration in the treatment of metastatic (Stage D2) prostate cancer.

Pediatrics: The safety and effectiveness of CASODEX in children has not been established.

CONTRAINDICATIONS: CASODEX (bicalutamide) is contraindicated in the following:

- Patients who are hypersensitive to the drug or any of its components. For a complete listing, see Dosage Forms, Composition and Packaging.
- Patients with localized prostate cancer otherwise undergoing watchful waiting (see Warnings and Precautions).
- Women: The safety and effectiveness of CASODEX in women has not been studied.
- Children: The safety and effectiveness of CASODEX in children has not been studied.

WARNINGS AND PRECAUTIONS:

CASODEX (bicalutamide) should only be prescribed by a qualified healthcare professional who is experienced with the treatment of prostate cancer and the use of anti-androgens.

- CASODEX 150 mg/day dose should not be used (see Warnings and Precautions, General).
- Rare hepatic failure, including fatal outcomes (see Warnings and Precautions, Hepatic/Biliary/Pancreatic).
- Uncommon interstitial lung disease, including fatal outcomes (see Warnings and Precautions, Respiratory).

General: During treatment with CASODEX, somnolence has been reported and those patients who experience this symptom should observe caution when driving or using machines.

Localized Prostate Cancer patients: CASODEX (bicalutamide) 150 mg is **not** to be administered.

Evidence from a large on-going clinical study demonstrates that at 5.4 year median follow-up, the use of CASODEX 150 mg as immediate therapy for the treatment of localized prostate cancer in patients otherwise undergoing watchful waiting is associated with increased mortality. Health Canada previously assessed CASODEX 150 mg versus castration in the locally advanced patient population and found level 1 scientific evidence (one of the 2 randomized clinical trials) of increased mortality in CASODEX 150 mg treated patients.

Patients taking CASODEX 50 mg per day for the treatment of metastatic prostate cancer are not affected by this new information.

Anti-Androgen Withdrawal Syndrome: In some patients with metastatic prostate cancer, anti-androgens (steroidal and non-steroidal), may promote, rather than inhibit, the growth of prostate cancer. A decrease in PSA and/or clinical improvement following discontinuation of antiandrogens has been reported. It is recommended that patients prescribed an antiandrogen, who have PSA progression, should have the antiandrogen discontinued immediately and be monitored for 6-8 weeks for a withdrawal response prior to any decision to proceed with other prostate cancer therapy.

Gynaecomastia, Breast Pain: Gynaecomastia has been reported in patients receiving CASODEX. For metastatic (M1) patients receiving CASODEX 50 mg, concomitant surgical or medical castration may reduce the effects of gynaecomastia.

Hepatic/Biliary/Pancreatic: CASODEX is extensively metabolized in the liver. Data suggests that the elimination of CASODEX may be slower in subjects with severe hepatic impairment and this could lead to increased accumulation of CASODEX. Therefore, CASODEX should be used with caution in patients with moderate to severe hepatic impairment.

Hepatotoxicity including rare hepatic failure has been observed with CASODEX, and fatal outcomes have been reported. CASODEX therapy should be discontinued if changes are severe (also see Adverse Reactions, Post-Market Adverse Drug Reactions).

Respiratory: Uncommon cases of interstitial lung disease (some cases have been fatal) have been reported with CASODEX (also see Adverse Reactions, Post-Market Adverse Drug Reactions). Interstitial lung disease has been reported most often at doses greater than 50 mg. CASODEX (bicalutamide) 150 mg is **not** to be administered.

If patients present with worsening of respiratory symptoms such as dyspnoea, cough and fever, CASODEX should be interrupted and prompt investigation initiated. If Interstitial Lung Disease is confirmed, CASODEX should be discontinued and the patient treated appropriately.

Special Populations: Pregnant Women: CASODEX is contraindicated in females. CASODEX may cause fetal harm when administered to pregnant women. The male offspring of rats (but not rabbits) receiving doses of 10 mg/kg/day and above, were observed to have reduced anogenital distance and hypospadias in reproductive toxicology studies. These pharmacological effects have been observed with other antiandrogens. No other teratogenic effects were observed in rabbits (receiving doses up to 200 mg/kg/day) or rats (receiving doses up to 250 mg/kg/day).

Nursing Women: See Pregnant Women.

Pediatrics: The safety and effectiveness of CASODEX (non-steroidal antiandrogen) in children has not been established.

Monitoring and Laboratory Tests: Regular assessments of serum Prostate Specific Antigen (PSA) may be helpful in monitoring patients' response.

Anemia has been observed in patients with androgen deprivation therapy. Hemoglobin levels should be monitored.

Since transaminase abnormalities and jaundice, rarely severe, have been reported with the use of CASODEX, periodic liver function tests should be considered. If clinically indicated, discontinuation of therapy should be considered. Abnormalities are usually reversible upon discontinuation.

Since CASODEX may elevate plasma testosterone and estradiol levels, fluid retention could occur. Accordingly, CASODEX should be used with caution in those patients with cardiac disease.

A reduction in glucose tolerance has been observed in males receiving CASODEX in combination with LHRH agonists. This may manifest as diabetes or loss of glycaemic control in those with pre-existing diabetes. Consideration should therefore be given to monitoring blood glucose in patients receiving CASODEX in combination with LHRH agonists.

ADVERSE REACTIONS: Adverse Drug Reaction Overview: CASODEX in Metastatic Patients: In patients with advanced prostate cancer, treated in the multicentre, double-blind controlled clinical trial comparing CASODEX 50 mg once daily with flutamide 250 mg three times a day, each in combination with an LHRH analogue, the most frequent adverse experiences included hot flushes (53%), asthenia (22%), constipation (22%), nausea (14%), peripheral edema (13%), anemia (13%), haematuria (12%), abdominal pain (11%), dizziness (10%), gynecomastia (9%), rash (9%), chest pain (8%), erectile dysfunction (7%), flatulence (7%), dyspepsia (7%), decreased appetite (6%), breast tenderness (6%), weight increase (5%), depression (4%), dry skin (4%), alopecia (4%), pruritus (3%), somnolence (3%), decreased libido (2%), hirsutism (2%), hypersensitivity reactions (1%) including angioedema and urticaria, and a serious infrequent adverse experience includes cardiac failure (0.8%).

Adverse event reports of abnormal liver function test results occurred in 7% of patients. These changes were frequently transient and rarely severe, resolving or improving with continued therapy or following cessation of therapy.

Hepatic failure and interstitial lung disease (see Warnings and Precautions) have been observed in post-marketed data and fatal outcomes have been reported for both.

CASODEX (bicalutamide), in general has been well tolerated with few withdrawals due to adverse events. The most common adverse events leading to withdrawal of study medication were abnormal liver function tests (1.5%), hot flushes (1.0%), and nausea and vomiting (0.7%).

After a 160 week follow-up, there were 213/401 deaths in the CASODEX-LHRH arm and 235/407 deaths in the flutamide-LHRH arm of the trial. There were 30 vs. 18 deaths due to adverse events in the two arms respectively and in both arms, the most common causes of death due to adverse events were attributed to the cardiovascular system (see Cardiovascular under the Clinical Trial Adverse Drug Reactions sub-section below).

Cardiac failure was observed in a pharmaco-epidemiology study of LHRH agonists and anti-androgens used in the treatment of prostate cancer. The risk appears to be increased when CASODEX was used in combination with LHRH agonists.

Clinical Trial Adverse Drug Reactions: The following adverse experiences were reported within the same clinical trial with an incidence of ≥5%, regardless of causality (see Table 1).

Table 1: CASODEX

Incidence of Adverse Events (≥ 5% in Either Treatment Group) Regardless of Causality

Adverse Event	Treatment Group Number of Patients (%)	
	CASODEX Plus LHRH Analogue (n=401)	**Flutamide Plus LHRH Analogue (n=407)**
Hot Flushes	211 (53)	217 (53)
Pain (General)	142 (35)	127 (31)
Back Pain	102 (25)	105 (26)
Asthenia	89 (22)	87 (21)
Constipation	87 (22)	69 (17)
Pelvic Pain	85 (21)	70 (17)
Infection	71 (18)	57 (14)
Nausea	56 (14)	54 (13)
Peripheral Edema	53 (13)	42 (10)
Anemia[a]	51 (13)	60 (15)
Dyspnea	51 (13)	32 (8)
Diarrhea	49 (12)	107 (26)
Nocturia	49 (12)	55 (14)
Hematuria	48 (12)	26 (6)
Abdominal Pain	46 (11)	46 (11)
Dizziness	41 (10)	35 (9)
Bone Pain	37 (9)	43 (11)
Gynecomastia	36 (9)	30 (8)
Rash	35 (9)	30 (7)
Urinary Tract Infection	35 (9)	36 (9)
Chest Pain	34 (8)	34 (8)
Hypertension	34 (8)	29 (7)
Cough Increased	33 (8)	24 (6)
Pharyngitis	32 (8)	23 (6)
Paresthesia	31 (8)	40 (10)
Increased Liver Enzyme Test[b]	30 (7)	46 (11)
Weight Loss	30 (7)	39 (10)
Headache	29 (7)	27 (7)
Flu Syndrome	28 (7)	20 (5)
Myasthenia	27 (7)	19 (5)
Insomnia	27 (7)	39 (10)
Erectile Dysfunction	27 (7)	35 (9)
Flatulence	26 (7)	22 (5)
Hyperglycemia	26 (7)	27 (7)
Dyspepsia	26 (7)	23 (6)
Decreased Appetite	25 (6)	29 (7)
Sweating	25 (6)	20 (5)
Bronchitis	24 (6)	11 (3)

(cont'd)

Table 1: CASODEX *(cont'd)*

Incidence of Adverse Events (≥ 5% in Either Treatment Group) Regardless of Causality

Adverse Event	Treatment Group Number of Patients (%)	
	CASODEX Plus LHRH Analogue (n=401)	**Flutamide Plus LHRH Analogue (n=407)**
Breast Pain (tenderness)	23 (6)	15 (4)
Urinary Frequency	23 (6)	29 (7)
Alkaline Phosphatase Increased	22 (5)	24 (6)
Weight Increased	22 (5)	18 (4)
Arthritis	21 (5)	29 (7)
Anxiety	20 (5)	9 (2)
Urinary Retention	20 (5)	14 (3)
Urinary Impaired	19 (5)	15 (4)
Pneumonia	18 (4)	19 (5)
Pathological Fracture	17 (4)	32 (8)
Depression	16 (4)	33 (8)
Vomiting	16 (4)	28 (7)
Rhinitis	15 (4)	22 (5)
Urinary Incontinence	15 (4)	32 (8)

[a] Anemia includes hypochromic anemia and iron deficiency anemia.
[b] Abnormal liver function tests reported as adverse events.

In addition, the following adverse experiences were reported by investigators within the same clinical trials (as possible adverse drug reactions in the opinion of investigating clinicians) with a frequency of less than 5%, during treatment with CASODEX 50 mg plus an LHRH analogue. No causal relationship of these experiences to drug treatment has been made.

Cardiovascular: In the pivotal trial of 813 patients comparing CASODEX 50 mg once daily with Flutamide 250 mg three times a day, each in combination with an LHRH analogue, an imbalance of deaths related to cardiovascular adverse events was noted (CASODEX-LHRH therapy: 18 deaths; Flutamide-LHRH therapy: 9 deaths) however, there is difficulty in interpreting this imbalance as the exposure was longer on the CASODEX-LHRH arm by a mean of 13 weeks. Other cardiovascular-related experiences reported include angina pectoris, congestive heart failure, myocardial infarction, heart arrest, coronary artery disorder, syncope, atrial fibrillation, cerebrovascular accident, deep thrombophlebitis, arrhythmia, bradycardia, cerebral ischemia, hemorrhage.
Central Nervous System: hypertonia, confusion, somnolence, decreased libido, neuropathy, nervousness.
Endocrine System: diabetes mellitus.
Gastrointestinal: melena, rectal hemorrhage, dry mouth, dysphagia, gastrointestinal disorder, periodontal abscess, gastrointestinal carcinoma, rectal disorder, intestinal obstruction, gastritis.
Hematological: ecchymosis, thrombocytopenia.
Immune System Disorders: hypersensitivity, angioedema and urticaria.
Metabolic and Nutritional: edema, BUN increased, creatinine increased, dehydration, gout, hypercholesteremia, hypoglycemia, hypercalcemia.
Musculoskeletal: leg cramps, bone disorders, myalgia.
Respiratory System: lung disorder, asthma, epistaxis, sinusitis, pleural effusion, voice alteration.
Skin and Appendages: dry skin, alopecia, pruritus, herpes zoster, skin carcinoma, skin disorder, skin hypertrophy, hirsutism, skin ulcer.
Special Senses: cataract, abnormal vision, conjunctivitis.
Urogenital: dysuria, urinary urgency, hydronephrosis, urinary tract disorder, bladder stenosis, kidney calculus, prostatic disorder, balanitis.
Whole Body: neoplasm, neck pain, fever, chills, sepsis, hernia, cyst, injection site reaction, allergic reaction, neck rigidity, face edema.
Abnormal Hematologic and Clinical Chemistry Findings: Laboratory abnormalities including elevated AST, ALT, bilirubin, BUN, creatinine and decreased haemoglobin and white cell count have been reported in both CASODEX-LHRH analogue treated and flutamide-LHRH analogue treated patients. Increased liver enzyme tests and decreases in haemoglobin were reported less frequently with CASODEX-LHRH analogue therapy. Other changes were reported with similar incidence in both treatment groups.
Post-Market Adverse Drug Reactions: The following adverse reactions have been identified during post-approval use of CASODEX:
Hepato-Biliary Disorders: hepatic failure (fatal outcomes have been reported).
Respiratory: interstitial lung disease (fatal outcomes have been reported).
Hematologic: anaemia.

DRUG INTERACTIONS: Drug-Drug Interactions: Clinical studies with CASODEX (bicalutamide) have not demonstrated any drug/drug interactions with LHRH analogues.

In vitro studies have shown that the R-enantiomer is an inhibitor of CYP 3A4, with lesser inhibitory effects on CYP 2C9, 2C19 and 2D6 activity. Although in vitro studies have suggested the potential for CASODEX to inhibit cytochrome 3A4, a number of clinical studies show the magnitude of any inhibition is unlikely to be of clinical significance for the majority of substances which are metabolised by cytochrome P450. Nevertheless, such an increase in AUC could be of clinical relevance for drugs with a narrow therapeutic index (e.g. cyclosporin).

In vitro studies have shown that CASODEX can displace the coumarin anticoagulant, warfarin, from its protein binding sites. It is recommended that if CASODEX is started in patients who are already receiving coumarin anticoagulants prothrombin time should be closely monitored and adjustment of the anticoagulant dose may be necessary.
Drug-Food Interactions: Interactions with food have not been established.
Drug-Herb Interactions: Interactions with herbal products have not been established.
Drug-Laboratory Test Interactions: Interactions with laboratory tests have not been established.

DOSAGE AND ADMINISTRATION: Recommended Dose and Dosage Adjustment: CASODEX 50 mg in metastatic disease: The recommended dose for CASODEX (bicalutamide) therapy in combination with an LHRH analogue or surgical castration is one 50 mg tablet once daily with or without food. CASODEX treatment should be started at the same time as treatment with an LHRH analogue or after surgical castration.
Dosing Considerations in Special Populations: Renal or Hepatic Impairment: No dosage adjustment is necessary for patients with renal or mild hepatic impairment. Increased accumulation may occur in patients with moderate to severe hepatic impairment (see Warnings and Precautions).

OVERDOSAGE:
A single dose of CASODEX (bicalutamide) that results in symptoms of an overdose considered to be life-threatening has not been established. In animal studies, CASODEX demonstrated a low potential acute toxicity. The LD_{50} in mice and rats was greater than 2000 mg/kg. Long-term clinical trials have been conducted with doses up to 200 mg of CASODEX daily and these doses have been well tolerated.

There is no specific antidote; treatment of an overdose should be symptomatic. In the management of an overdose with CASODEX, vomiting may be induced if the patient is alert. It should be remembered that in this patient population multiple drugs may have been taken. Dialysis is not likely to be helpful since CASODEX is highly protein bound and is extensively metabolized. General supportive care, including frequent monitoring of vital signs and close observation of the patient, is indicated.

> For management of a suspected drug overdose, contact your regional Poison Control Centre. See the *CPS* Directory section for a list of Poison Control Centres.

ACTION AND CLINICAL PHARMACOLOGY: Pharmacodynamics: CASODEX (bicalutamide) is a non-steroidal antiandrogen, devoid of other endocrine activity. Bicalutamide competitively inhibits the action of androgens by binding to cytosol androgen receptors in target tissue. This inhibition results in regression of prostatic tumours. CASODEX is a racemate and the (R)-enantiomer is primarily responsible for the antiandrogenic activity of CASODEX.
Pharmacokinetics: The absorption, distribution, metabolism and excretion of bicalutamide has been investigated after administration of a single 50 mg oral dose to volunteers. The results indicated that the dose was extensively absorbed and was excreted almost equally in urine (36%) and faeces (43%) over a 9 day collection period. There is no evidence of any clinically significant effect of food on bioavailability. Steady state plasma concentrations of the (R)-enantiomer of approximately 9 µg/mL are observed during daily administration of 50 mg doses of CASODEX. At steady state, the active (R)-enantiomer accounts for 99% of the circulating plasma bicalutamide concentration. Bicalutamide is highly protein bound (racemate 96%, (R)-enantiomer 99.6%). On daily administration, the (R)-enantiomer accumulates about 10-fold in plasma, consistent with an elimination half-life of approximately one week. The (S)-enantiomer is very rapidly cleared relative to the (R)-enantiomer. Bicalutamide is extensively metabolized via both oxidation and glucuronidation with approximately equal renal and biliary elimination of the metabolites.
Special Populations and Conditions: Pediatrics: The pharmacokinetics of the (R)-enantiomer are unaffected by age.
Geriatrics: The pharmacokinetics of the (R)-enantiomer are unaffected by age.
Hepatic Insufficiency: The pharmacokinetics of the (R)-enantiomer are unaffected by mild to moderate hepatic impairment. Patients with severe hepatic impairment eliminate the (R)-enantiomer from plasma more slowly.
Renal Insufficiency: The pharmacokinetics of the (R)-enantiomer are unaffected by renal impairment.

STORAGE AND STABILITY: Store between 15-30°C.

INFORMATION FOR THE PATIENT: Published in e-CPS, available by subscription at www.e-cps.ca.

DOSAGE FORMS, COMPOSITION AND PACKAGING: Each white, film-coated tablet, intagliated with CDX50 on one side and a logo (an arrow attached to the arc of a circle) on the other side, contains: bicalutamide 50 mg. Nonmedicinal ingredients: lactose monohydrate, magnesium stearate, methylhydroxypropylcellulose, polyethylene glycol, polyvidone, sodium starch glycolate and titanium dioxide. Blister strips of 15 tablets, 30 tablets per package.

(Shown in Product Identification Section)

Catapres® 🅿
clonidine HCl
Antihypertensive

Boehringer Ingelheim

Date of Revision: April 24, 2009

SUMMARY PRODUCT INFORMATION:

Route of Administration	Dosage Form/ Strength	All Nonmedicinal Ingredients
Oral	Tablets 0.1 mg, 0.2 mg	CATAPRES tablets 0.1 mg and 0.2 mg contain: colloidal silica, dibasic calcium phosphate, lactose, maize starch, polyvinylpyrrolidone, soluble starch and stearic acid. 0.2 mg also contains FD&C Yellow #6. See Dosage Forms, Composition and Packaging.

INDICATIONS AND CLINICAL USE: CATAPRES (clonidine hydrochloride) is indicated for the treatment of hypertension. It may be used alone or in combination with thiazide diuretics. Clonidine should normally be used in those patients in whom treatment with diuretic or beta-blocker was found ineffective or has been associated with unacceptable adverse effects.

CATAPRES can also be tried as an initial agent in those patients in whom use of diuretics and/or beta blockers is contraindicated or in patients with medical conditions in which these drugs frequently cause serious adverse effects.
Pediatrics (<18 years of age): Safety and effectiveness in children have not been established.

CONTRAINDICATIONS: CATAPRES is contraindicated in patients with severe bradyarrhythmia resulting from either sick sinus syndrome or atrioventricular (AV) block of 2nd or 3rd degree; patients with sinus node function impairment.

Patients who are hypersensitive to this drug or to any ingredients in the formulation or component of the container. For a complete listing, see Dosage Forms, Composition and Packaging.

In case of rare hereditary conditions that may be incompatible with the excipient, lactose, (see Warnings and Precautions) the use of the product is contraindicated.

WARNINGS AND PRECAUTIONS: General: Patients should be instructed not to discontinue therapy without consulting their physician. A pronounced withdrawal reaction with symptoms suggesting sympathetic over-activity may develop within 12 to 48 hours when clonidine is discontinued. High serum levels of catecholamines have been found during such episodes (see Drug Interactions). When discontinuing CATAPRES (clonidine hydrochloride) therapy, the physician should reduce the dose gradually over 2 to 4 days to avoid a possible rapid rise in blood pressure and associated subjective symptoms such as nervousness, agitation, restlessness, palpitations, tremor, nausea and headache. Rare instances of hypertensive encephalopathy and death have been recorded after abrupt cessation of CATAPRES therapy. A withdrawal reaction is most likely to occur in patients who have been receiving large doses (greater than 1.2 mg/day) or in those who are continuing to receive a concomitant beta-blocker. If therapy is to be discontinued in patients receiving clonidine and a β adrenergic blocking agent concomitantly, the β blocker should be first phased out gradually before clonidine therapy is discontinued.

It has been demonstrated that an excessive rise in blood pressure, should it occur, can be reversed by resumption of CATAPRES therapy or by intravenous phentolamine.

Clonidine is not indicated in pheochromocytoma. However, **in contrast to guanethidine and reserpine the drug has no crisis-inducing properties**, in this condition.

Clonidine does not affect the urinary vanilmandelic acid (VMA) and catecholamine excretion significantly in patients with pheochromocytoma, so that no false positive or false negative results will occur during the administration of the drug.

CATAPRES tablets contain up to 216.1 mg of lactose per maximum recommended daily dose (0.6 mg). Patients with the rare hereditary conditions of galactose intolerance e.g. galactosaemia should not take this medicine.
Pediatrics (<18 years of age): Safety and effectiveness in children have not been established.
Cardiovascular: Because it lowers blood pressure, CATAPRES (clonidine hydrochloride) should be used with caution in patients with severe coronary insufficiency, recent myocardial infarction, cerebrovascular disease or chronic renal failure.

CATAPRES should be used with caution in patients with mild to moderate bradyarrhythmia such as low sinus rhythm, with disorders of cerebral or peripheral perfusion, polyneuropathy, and constipation, and in patients with heart failure or severe coronary heart disease.

The dosage of clonidine hydrochloride should be increased gradually to minimize the sedative effect of the drug. This is of particular importance in those patients who operate automobiles and potentially dangerous machinery.

Depending on the dose given, CATAPRES can lower the heart rate and pulse rate. In patients with diseases affecting the rhythmic and atrioventricular (AV) conduction system of the heart, arrhythmias have been observed after high doses.

CATAPRES should be monitored particularly carefully in patients with heart failure or severe coronary heart disease.

A few instances of a condition resembling Raynaud's phenomenon have been reported. Caution should therefore be observed if patients with Raynaud's disease or thromboangiitis obliterans are to be treated with clonidine.
Dependence/Tolerance: Tolerance may develop in some patients, necessitating a re-evaluation of therapy. This usually consists of an increase in dosage or concomitant administration of a diuretic to enhance the hypotensive response to the drug.

Ophthalmologic: In several studies clonidine hydrochloride produced a dose-dependent increase in the incidence and severity of spontaneously occurring retinal degeneration in albino rats treated for six months or longer. In view of this retinal degeneration, eye examinations were performed in 908 patients prior to the start of clonidine hydrochloride therapy, who were then examined periodically thereafter. In 353 of these 908 patients, examinations were performed for periods of 24 months or longer. Except for the dryness of the eyes, no drug-related abnormal ophthalmologic findings were recorded and clonidine hydrochloride did not alter retinal function as shown by specialized tests such as the electroretinogram and macular dazzle. It is recommended that as an integral part of their overall long-term care, patients treated with CATAPRES should receive periodic eye examinations.

Patients who wear contact lenses should be warned that treatment with CATAPRES may cause decreased lacrimation (see Adverse Reactions).

Peri-Operative Considerations: Administration of CATAPRES should be continued to within four hours of surgery and resumed as soon as possible thereafter. The blood pressure should be carefully monitored and appropriate measures instituted to control it as necessary.

Psychiatric: Patients with a known history of depression should be carefully supervised while under treatment with clonidine, as there have been occasional reports of further depressive episodes occurring in such patients.

Renal: Clonidine and its metabolites are extensively excreted with the urine. Renal insufficiency requires particularly careful adjustment of dosage.

As with any drug excreted primarily in the urine, smaller doses of the drug are often effective in treating patients with a degree of renal failure. In patients exhibiting renal failure or insufficiency, periodic determination of the BUN is indicated. If, in the physician's opinion, a rising BUN is significant, the drug should be stopped.

Special Populations: Pregnant Women: Reproduction studies performed in rabbits at doses up to approximately 3 times the maximum recommended daily human dose (MRDHD) of clonidine hydrochloride has revealed no evidence of teratogenic or embryotoxic potential in rabbits. When rats were given clonidine hydrochloride alone in doses as low as one-third the MRDHD, some embryotoxicity was evident.

There are, however, no adequate and well controlled studies in pregnant women. Because animal reproduction studies are not always predictive of human response, this drug should be used during pregnancy only if clearly needed.

Careful monitoring of the mother and child is recommended. Clonidine hydrochloride passes the placenta barrier and may lower the heart rate of the fetus. A postpartum transient rise in blood pressure in the newborn cannot be excluded. There is no adequate experience regarding the long-term effect of prenatal exposure.

Nursing Women: The use of CATAPRES during lactation is not recommended due to a lack of supporting information.

Pediatrics (<18 years of age): Safety and effectiveness in children have not been established.

ADVERSE REACTIONS: Adverse Drug Reaction Overview: Most adverse effects are mild and generally tend to diminish with continuation of therapy. The most common (which appear to be dose-related) are dry mouth (about 40%), drowsiness (about 33%), dizziness (about 16%), constipation and sedation (each in about 10%).

The most serious reactions have been reported upon abrupt discontinuation of the drug (see Warnings and Precautions).

Clinical Trial Adverse Drug Reactions: Because clinical trials are conducted under very specific conditions the adverse reaction rates observed in the clinical trials may not reflect the rates observed in practice and should not be compared to the rates in the clinical trials of another drug. Adverse drug reaction information from clinical trials is useful for identifying drug-related adverse events and for approximating rates.

The following less frequent adverse reactions have been reported in patients receiving clonidine hydrochloride.

Cardiac Disorders: bradyarrhythmia, about 0.5%. Rare cases of sinus bradycardia and atrioventricular block have been reported, both with and without the use of concomitant digitalis.

Endocrine: gynecomastia, about 0.1%.

Eye Disorder: accommodation disorder, lacrimation decreased (caution: contact lens wearers).

Gastrointestinal Disorders: nausea and vomiting, about 5% of patients; colonic pseudo-obstruction, constipation, dry mouth, salivary gland pain.

General Disorders and Administration Site Conditions: fatigue, about 4%, malaise, about 1%.

Investigations: blood glucose increased rarely.

Nervous System Disorders: headache, about 1%, dizziness, paresthesia, sedation.

Psychiatric Disorders: confusional state, delusional perception, depression, about 1%; hallucinations, libido decreased, nightmares, sleep disorder.

Reproductive System and Breast Disorders: decreased sexual activity, erectile dysfunction about 3% of patients.

Respiratory, Thoracic and Mediastinal Disorders: nasal dryness.

Skin and Subcutaneous Disorders: rash, about 1 % of patients; pruritus, about 0.7%; urticaria, about 0.5%; and alopecia, about 0.2%.

Vascular Disorders: orthostatic hypotension, about 3% of patients, Raynaud's phenomenon has been reported rarely.

Other: weakness, about 10% of patients; dryness, burning of the eyes.

The following adverse events have been reported during therapy with Catapres: anorexia (about 1%); mild transient abnormalities in liver function tests (about 1%); weight gain (about 1%); nervousness and agitation (each about 3%); insomnia (about 0.5%); palpitations and tachycardia (each about 0.5%); angioneurotic edema (about 0.5%); nocturia (about 1%); difficulty in micturition (about 0.2%); urinary retention (about 0.1%); discontinuation syndrome (about 1%); muscle or joint pain (about 0.6%) and cramps of the lower limbs (about 0.3%).

Behavioural changes; restlessness; anxiety; delirium; blurred vision; pallor; weakly positive Coombs' test; increased sensitivity to alcohol and fever have also been reported.

Rarely: hepatitis, parotitis; transient elevation of serum creatine phosphokinase; congestive heart failure and electro cardiographic abnormalities i.e. conduction disturbances and arrhythmias have been reported.

Also, there have been isolated reports of continual dry mouth leading to an accelerated rate of dental caries, in patients receiving clonidine hydrochloride.

DRUG INTERACTIONS: Overview: The reduction in blood pressure induced by clonidine can be further potentiated by concurrent administration of other anti-hypertensive agents such as diuretics, vasodilators, β blockers, calcium antagonists and ACE-inhibitors, but not α_1-blocking agents.

Concomitant use of β-blockers and/or cardiac glycosides can further lower heart rate (bradycardia) or cause dysrhythmia (atrioventricular block) in isolated cases.

It cannot be ruled out that concomitant administration of a beta-receptor blocker will cause or potentiate peripheral vascular disorders.

The antihypertensive effect of clonidine may be reduced or abolished and orthostatic regulation disturbances may be provoked or aggravated by concomitant administration of tricyclic antidepressants or neuroleptics with alpha-receptor blocking properties.

If clonidine hydrochloride and tricyclic antidepressants are administered as concurrent therapy, an increase in the dosage of CATAPRES may be necessary. Amitriptyline in combination with clonidine hydrochloride enhances the manifestation of corneal lesions in rats.

Substances with $alpha_2$ receptor blocking properties such as phenolamine or tolazoline may abolish the $alpha_2$-receptor mediated effects of clonidine in a dose-dependent manner. Therefore, depending upon the dose administered, tolazoline is suitable as an antidote.

Concurrent use of appetite suppressants (with the exception of fenfluramine) and clonidine hydrochloride may decrease the hypotensive effects of clonidine hydrochloride. Concurrent use of fenfluramine and clonidine hydrochloride may increase the hypotensive effects of clonidine hydrochloride.

Sympathomimetic amines, indomethacin and possibly other non-steroidal anti-inflammatory agents may reduce the antihypertensive effects of clonidine hydrochloride. Substances which raise blood pressure or induce a Na^+ and water retaining effect such as non steroidal anti- inflammatory agents can reduce the therapeutic effect of clonidine. The patient should be carefully monitored to confirm that the desired effect is being obtained.

Clonidine hydrochloride may enhance the CNS-depressive effects of alcohol, barbiturates or other sedatives.

Withdrawal of clonidine hydrochloride may result in an excess of circulating catecholamines (see Warnings and Precautions). Therefore, caution should be exercised in concomitant use of drugs which affect the metabolism, tissue uptake or pressor effects of these amines (monoamine oxidase (MAO) inhibitors, tricyclic antidepressants and beta blocking agents, respectively).

The concomitant use of clonidine with methylphenidate has resulted in serious adverse reactions, including death, in children with attention-deficit/hyperactivity (ADHD).

DOSAGE AND ADMINISTRATION: Dosing Considerations: Treatment of hypertension requires regular medical supervision.

The dose of CATAPRES (clonidine hydrochloride) must be adjusted according to the patient's individual blood pressure response.

Recommended Dose and Dosage Adjustment: Initial Dose: 0.1 mg tablet twice daily (morning and bedtime).

Maintenance Dose: After a period of 2-4 weeks, further increments of 0.1 mg per day may be necessary until the desired response is achieved. In those instances where it is not possible to have equal amounts of drug at each of the dosing intervals, taking the larger portion of the total daily dose at bedtime may minimize transient adjustment effect of dry mouth and drowsiness.

The therapeutic doses most commonly employed have ranged from 0.2 mg to 0.6 mg per day given in divided doses. Usually doses above 0.6 mg per day do not result in a further marked reduction in blood pressure.

Discontinuation of Treatment: If CATAPRES (clonidine hydrochloride) is to be discontinued, reduce dosage gradually (see Warnings and Precautions).

Missed Dose: If a dose of CATAPRES is missed, patients should take the dose as soon as possible and then return to their normal schedule.

Administration: The tablets should be swallowed whole with water.

Use in Elderly: Elderly patients may benefit from a lower initial dose.

Use in Impaired Renal Function: Doses must be adjusted according to the degree of impairment and patients should be carefully monitored. Since only a minimal amount of clonidine is removed during routine hemodialysis, there is no need to give supplemental clonidine during dialysis.

Use in Impaired Hepatic Function: Dosage instructions for patients with impaired hepatic function have not been established.

Use in Children: The safety and efficacy of clonidine have not been established in children.

OVERDOSAGE:

The signs and symptoms of clonidine hydrochloride overdosage include generalised sympathetic depression and include pupillary constriction, hypotension, hypothermia, bradycardia, lethargy, irritability, weakness, somnolence including coma, diminished or absent reflexes, vomiting and hypoventilation. With large overdoses, reversible cardiac induction defects or arrhythmias, coma, respiratory depression including apnoea, seizures and transient hypertension have been reported.

In a patient who ingested 100 mg clonidine hydrochloride, plasma clonidine levels were 60 ng/mL (one hour), 190 ng/mL (1.5 hours), 370 ng/mL (two hours) and 120 ng/mL (5.5 and 6.5 hours). This patient developed hypertension followed by hypotension, bradycardia, apnoea, hallucinations, semicoma, and premature ventricular contractions. The patient fully recovered after intensive treatment.

Clonidine overdosage usually responds to symptomatic treatment, volume expansion for hypotension and careful cardiovascular monitoring. Gastric lavage, followed by administration of activated charcoal if a large dose has been taken, can be initiated within two hours of ingestions if the airway can be protected. Routine hemodialysis is of limited benefit since a maximum of 5% of circulating clonidine is removed.

Intravenous naloxone has been used as antidotes to clonidine poisoning, with inconsistent results. If other efforts fail, these agents may provide some benefit in reversing the effects of clonidine.

> For management of a suspected drug overdose, CPhA recommends that you contact your **regional Poison Control Centre**. See the *CPS* Directory section for a list of Poison Control Centres.

ACTION AND CLINICAL PHARMACOLOGY: Mechanism of Action: Clonidine hydrochloride is an α adrenergic agonist which also has some α adrenergic antagonist effects. The antihypertensive effect of clonidine hydrochloride is thought to be due to central α_2 adrenergic stimulation, which results in a decreased sympathetic outflow to the heart, kidneys, and peripheral vasculature and thus decreased peripheral vascular resistance, decreased systolic and diastolic blood pressure and decreased heart rate. Renal blood flow and glomerular filtration rate remain essentially unchanged. Normal postural reflexes are intact and therefore orthostatic symptoms are mild and infrequent. Acute studies with clonidine hydrochloride in humans have demonstrated a moderate reduction (15% to 20%) of cardiac output in the supine position with no change in the peripheral resistance; at a 45° tilt there is a smaller reduction in cardiac output and a decrease of peripheral resistance. During long-term therapy, cardiac output tends to return to control values, while peripheral resistance remains decreased. Slowing of the pulse rate has been observed in most patients given clonidine, but the drug does not alter normal hemodynamic response to exercise.

Other studies in patients have provided evidence of a reduction in plasma renin activity and in the excretion of aldosterone and catecholamines, but the exact relationship of these pharmacologic actions to the antihypertensive effect has not been fully elucidated.

Prolonged treatment with clonidine hydrochloride in animals causes a decrease in the responsiveness of the vascular smooth muscle to catecholamines and angiotensin. The change in vascular response may be of importance in explaining the chronic hypotensive effect in man.

Acute administration of clonidine stimulates the release of growth hormone in children and adults, but the drug does not produce sustained elevation of growth hormone during chronic administration.

Pharmacodynamics: CATAPRES (clonidine hydrochloride) acts relatively rapidly. The patient's blood pressure declines within 30 to 60 minutes after an oral dose, the maximum decrease occurring within 2 to 4 hours.

In man, the blood pressure reduction due to clonidine does not cause significant alterations in renal blood flow in the supine position. In the erect position, a consistent decrease in renal vascular resistance is seen.

Pharmacokinetics: Absorption: The plasma level of CATAPRES peaks in approximately 3 to 5 hours. In humans, a significant plasma level (0.20 μg% of clonidine) can be detected one hour after oral administration of a single dose of 390 mg.

Distribution: Clonidine is 50% bound to plasma proteins.

Metabolism: About 50% of the absorbed dose is metabolized in the liver. Four different metabolites have been detected in humans.

Excretion: Following oral administration about 40-60% of the absorbed dose is recovered in the urine as unchanged drug in 24 hours.

The plasma half-life ranges from 12 to 16 hours, but the half-life increases up to 41 hours in patients with severe impairment of renal function. In humans, 65% of the orally administered drug is excreted in the urine, and an estimated 22% in the faeces.

Special Populations and Conditions: Renal Insufficiency: Doses must be adjusted according to the degree of impairment and patients should be carefully monitored. Since only a minimal amount of clonidine is removed during routine hemodialysis, there is no need to give supplemental clonidine during dialysis.

STORAGE AND STABILITY: CATAPRES should be stored at room temperature (15-30°C).

INFORMATION FOR THE PATIENT: Published in e-CPS, available by subscription at www.e-cps.ca.

DOSAGE FORMS, COMPOSITION AND PACKAGING: 0.1 mg: Each round, white, flat tablet with bevelled edges, one side scored with each half bearing the imprint O1C, the reverse side bearing the Ingelheim Tower, contains: clonidine HCl 0.1 mg. Nonmedicinal ingredients: colloidal silica, dibasic calcium phosphate, lactose, maize starch (dried), polyvinylpyrrolidone, soluble starch and stearic acid. Bottles of 100.

0.2 mg: Each round, orange, flat tablet with bevelled edges, one side scored with each half bearing the imprint O2C, the reverse side bearing the Ingelheim Tower, contains: clonidine HCl 0.2 mg. Nonmedicinal ingredients: colloidal silica, dibasic calcium phosphate, FD&C Yellow #6, lactose, maize starch, polyvinylpyrrolidone, soluble starch and stearic acid. Bottles of 100.

Cathflo® Pr

alteplase, recombinant

Fibrinolytic Agent

Roche

Date of Revision: September 6, 2003

PHARMACOLOGY: Alteplase is an enzyme (serine protease) that has the property of fibrin-enhanced conversion of plasminogen to plasmin. It produces limited conversion of plasminogen in the absence of fibrin. Alteplase binds to fibrin in a thrombus and converts the entrapped plasminogen to plasmin, thereby initiating local fibrinolysis.

In patients with acute myocardial infarction, studies have shown that alteplase is rapidly cleared from the plasma, with an initial half life of less than 5 minutes. Clearance is mediated primarily by the liver.

When recombinant alteplase is administered according to the instructions in Dosage, circulating plasma levels of alteplase will not reach pharmacologic concentrations. If a 2 mg dose of alteplase were administered by bolus injection directly into the systemic circulation (rather than instilled into the catheter), the concentration of circulating alteplase would return to endogenous circulating levels of 5 to 10 ng/mL within 30 minutes.

INDICATIONS: For the restoration of function to central venous access devices.

CONTRAINDICATIONS: Should not be administered to patients with known hypersensitivity to alteplase or any component of the formulation (i.e., l-arginine, phosphoric acid and polysorbate 80).

WARNINGS: Catheter dysfunction may be caused by a variety of conditions other than thrombus formation, such as catheter malposition, mechanical failure, constriction caused by a suture, and lipid deposits or drug precipitates within the lumen of the catheter.

During attempts to determine catheter occlusion, vigorous suction should not be applied because of the risk of damage to the vascular wall or collapse of soft walled catheters. Excessive pressure should be avoided when any medication, including recombinant alteplase, is instilled into the catheter. Such force could cause rupture of the catheter or expulsion of the clot into the circulation.

PRECAUTIONS: General: The most frequent adverse reaction associated with all thrombolytics in all approved indications is bleeding. Known conditions have been associated with an increased risk of bleeding with the use of thrombolytics. Patients with known conditions associated with bleeding events were excluded from the pivotal trials; thus recombinant alteplase has not been studied in this patient population. Caution should be exercised with patients who have active internal bleeding or who have had any of the following within 48 hours: coronary artery bypass graft surgery, obstetrical delivery, organ biopsy, or puncture of noncompressible vessels. In addition, caution should be exercised with patients who have hemostatic defects (including those secondary to severe hepatic or renal disease) or any condition in which bleeding constitutes a significant hazard or would be particularly difficult to manage because of its location, or who are at high risk for embolic complications (e.g., recent pulmonary embolism, deep vein thrombosis, endarterectomy). Death and permanent disability have been reported in patients who have experienced stroke and other serious bleeding episodes when receiving pharmacologic doses of a thrombolytic.

Should serious bleeding in a critical location (e.g., intracranial, gastrointestinal, retroperitoneal, pericardial) occur, treatment with recombinant alteplase should be stopped and the drug should be withdrawn from the catheter.

When treating infected catheters, risks for systemic infection include surgical replacement of the catheter and successful thrombolysis; both may release localized infection into systemic circulation. In the pivotal safety trial, 4 patients developed sepsis from 16 minutes to 3 days following alteplase treatment. All 4 patients responded to antibiotic therapy. Recombinant alteplase should be used with caution in the presence of known or suspected infection in the catheter. As with all catheterization procedures, care should be used to maintain aseptic technique.

Drug Interactions: The interaction of recombinant alteplase with other drugs has not been formally studied. Concomitant use of drugs affecting coagulation and/or platelet function has not been studied.

Laboratory Tests: Potential interactions between recombinant alteplase and laboratory tests have not been studied.

Geriatrics: No incidents of ICH, embolic events, or major bleeding events were observed in geriatric patients. The effect of alteplase on common age-related comorbidities has not been studied. In general, caution should be used in geriatric patients with conditions known to increase the risk of bleeding (see Precautions, General).

Children: Alteplase has been studied in patients from 2 to 16 years of age. No study drug related adverse events were observed in these pediatric patients. Patients with low body weights ≥10 kg and <30 kg received up to 2 doses of alteplase, with each dose equal to 110% of the internal lumen volume of the dysfunctional CVAD (to a maximum dose of 2 mg). The treatment efficacy in these subsets of patients was similar to that observed in adult patients. Alteplase has not been studied in patients who are younger than 2 years of age or who weigh less than 10 kg.

Pregnancy: The use of recombinant alteplase in pregnant women has not been studied. Animal toxicity studies have indicated no maternal or fetal toxicity at 33 times the human dose for restoration of function to occluded CVADs. Recombinant alteplase should be used during pregnancy only if the potential benefit justifies the potential risk to the fetus.

Lactation: It is not known whether recombinant alteplase is excreted in human milk. Because many drugs are excreted in human milk, caution should be exercised when recombinant alteplase is administered to a nursing woman.

Readministration: In clinical trials for restoration of function to CVADs, patients received a single treatment of up to 2 doses of 2 mg/2 mL (4 mg total of alteplase). The readministration of recombinant alteplase on subsequent occasions has not been studied. Antibody formation was not studied in clinical trial. However, in acute myocardial infarction (AMI) trials, transient antibody formation was observed in less than 0.5% of AMI patients administered a single i.v. dose of 100 mg Activase rt-PA (alteplase recombinant).

In the event that an anaphylactoid reaction were to occur upon the administration of recombinant alteplase, appropriate therapy should be initiated.

ADVERSE EFFECTS: Because clinical trials are conducted under widely varying conditions, adverse reaction rates observed in the clinical trials of a drug cannot be directly compared to rates in the clinical trials of another drug and may not reflect the rates observed in practice. The adverse reaction information from clinical trials does, however, provide a basis for identifying the adverse events that appear to be related to drug use and for approximating rates.

In the pivotal trials, patients were excluded if they were at high risk for bleeding or embolic stroke, had a known condition for which bleeding constituted a significant hazard, had received a fibrinolytic agent within 24 hours, or had known right to left shunt, a patent foramen ovale, or an atrial or ventricular septal defect.

In the pivotal trials during the 30-day post-treatment period, no incidents of ICH, major hemorrhages, embolic events or death were reported as related to alteplase administration. Patients had indwelling catheters to treat underlying disease. Complications observed after alteplase instillation were attributed to underlying illness, concomitant medications, or disease progression.

The most serious adverse events occurring in <0.5% of patients in the pivotal trials were sepsis, gastrointestinal bleeding and venous thrombosis. The cases of gastrointestinal bleeding and venous thrombosis were deemed unrelated to alteplase.

Treatment of infected dysfunctional catheters, whether using thrombolysis or surgically replacing the CVAD, may release localized infected clot or fluid into the systemic circulation. In the pivotal trials, sepsis was reported in 4 of 1135 treated patients. These events occurred from 16 minutes to 3 days following alteplase instillation. All 4 patients had positive catheter cultures within 24 hours before or after symptom onset. Two of the 4 patients had positive peripheral blood cultures within 24 hours before or after symptom onset. Two of the 4 patients had pre-existing fever.

In the pivotal trials, there were no observed differences in the adverse reaction profile in the following subpopulations: age, sex, low body weight or catheter type. Adverse reaction profiles associated with specific comorbidities or concomitant medications have not been documented.

Recombinant alteplase was studied in one randomized, double-blind, placebo-controlled trial and one open label trial. The data described in Table 1 reflects the experience with alteplase in 1144 patients.

Table 1: Cathflo

Demographic Characteristics and Dose Information for the Pivotal Trials

Demographic Group		Efficacy Trial (N=149)	Safety Trial (N=995)
Age Range		2–87 years	2–92 years
Geriatric (65 years and over)		30	282
Pediatric (2–16 years)		12	114
Low Body Weight (10 to <30 kg)		5	65
Sex Distribution	Female:	82 (35.0%)	562 (56.5%)
	Male:	67 (45.0%)	433 (43.5%)
Number of Doses of Active Drug Recorded:	0	23 (15.4%)	0 (0%)
	1	94 (63.1%)	786 (78.0%)
	2	32 (21.5%)	209 (21.0%)

Allergic Reactions: No allergic-type reactions were observed in the pivotal trials in patients treated with up to two 2 mg/2 mL (4 mg) doses of recombinant alteplase instilled into the catheter lumen for 30 minutes to 4 hours (see Precautions, Readministration).

OVERDOSE:
No data supplied by the manufacturer.

For management of a suspected drug overdose, CPhA recommends that you contact your **regional Poison Control Centre**. See the *CPS* Directory section for a list of Poison Control Centres.

DOSAGE: Usual Dose: Recombinant alteplase is for intracatheter administration (instillation into the dysfunctional catheter). For patients weighing 30 kg and over, the dose of recombinant alteplase is 2 mg, with a dose volume of 2 mL. The recommended dose for patients weighing less than 30 kg is 110% of the internal lumen volume of their CVAD, not to exceed 2 mL. There is no efficacy and safety information on dosing in excess of 2 mg per dose. Studies have not been performed with total doses greater than 4 mg (two 2 mg doses).

Preparation and Administration: Preparation of Solution:

1. Reconstitute recombinant alteplase to a final concentration of 1 mg/mL:
2. Aseptically withdraw 2.2 mL of Sterile Water for Injection, USP (diluent is not provided). Do not use Bacteriostatic Water for Injection, USP, for reconstitution as it has not been studied clinically.
3. Inject the 2.2 mL of Sterile Water for Injection, USP, into the recombinant alteplase vial, directing the diluent stream into the powder. Slight foaming is not unusual; let the vial stand undisturbed to allow large bubbles to dissipate.
4. Mix by gently swirling until the contents are completely dissolved. **Do not shake.** The reconstituted preparation results in a colorless to pale yellow transparent solution containing 1 mg/mL recombinant alteplase at a pH of approximately 7.3.
5. Recombinant alteplase contains no antibacterial preservatives and should be reconstituted immediately before use. The solution may be used within 8 hours following reconstitution when stored at 2 to 30°C.
6. Withdraw 2 mL (2 mg) of solution from the reconstituted vial.

No other medication should be added to solutions containing recombinant alteplase.

Administration:

1. Inspect the product prior to administration for foreign matter and discolouration.
2. Instill the appropriate dose of recombinant alteplase (see Usual Dose) into the occluded catheter.
3. After 30 minutes of dwell time, assess catheter function by attempting to aspirate blood. If the catheter is functional, go to Step 6. If the catheter is not functional, go to Step 4.
4. After 120 minutes of dwell time, assess catheter function by attempting to aspirate blood and catheter contents. If the catheter is functional, go to Step 6. If the catheter is not functional, go to Step 5.
5. If catheter function is not restored after one dose of recombinant alteplase, a second dose may be instilled. Repeat the procedure beginning with Step 2.
6. If catheter function has been restored, aspirate 4 to 5 mL of blood to remove recombinant alteplase and residual clot, discard aspirate and gently irrigate the catheter with 0.9% Sodium Chloride.

Any unused solution should be discarded.

SUPPLIED: Each vial of sterile, white to pale yellow, lyophilized powder contains: recombinant alteplase 2 mg. Nonmedicinal ingredients: l-arginine, phosphoric acid and polysorbate 80. Cartons of 10. Store lyophilized recombinant alteplase at refrigerated temperature 2 to 8°C. Do not use beyond the expiration date on the vial. Protect the lyophilized material during extended storage from excessive exposure to light.

Caverject®

alprostadil

Prostaglandin

Pfizer

PHARMACOLOGY: Alprostadil is a prostaglandin with various pharmacological actions that include vasodilation and inhibition of platelet aggregation, inhibition of gastric secretion, stimulation of intestinal smooth muscle and stimulation of uterine smooth muscle.

Alprostadil, when given to impotent men by intracavernous injection, induces erections within 5 to 20 minutes after administration. The duration of erection is dose-dependent. The mechanism of penile erection involves a complex series of neurovascular events. Alprostadil injected intracavernosally causes tumescence by increasing cavernous blood flow through relaxation of trabecular smooth muscle and dilation of cavernosal arteries.

With regards to the action of alprostadil on penile structures, in most animal species tested, alprostadil had relaxant effects on retractor penis and corpus cavernosum urethra in vitro. Alprostadil also relaxed isolated preparations of human corpus cavernosum and spongiosum, as well as cavernous arterial segments previously contracted by either noradrenaline or $PGF_{2\alpha}$. In pigtail monkeys (Macaca nemestrina), alprostadil increased cavernous arterial blood flow in vivo. The degree and duration of cavernous smooth muscle relaxation in this animal model was dose-dependent.

Other actions of PGE_1 involve the cardiovascular system, CNS, autonomic nervous system, respiratory system, gastrointestinal system and hematopoietic system.

Pharmacokinetics: Absorption: The absolute bioavailability of alprostadil following intracavernosal injection has not been determined.

Distribution: Following a 20 µg intracavernosal injection of alprostadil, mean peripheral plasma concentrations of alprostadil were 89 pg/mL and 102 pg/mL at 30 and 60 minutes post-injection respectively, which were not significantly greater than baseline levels of endogenous alprostadil at 96 pg/mL. Alprostadil is bound primarily to plasma albumin (81%) and to a lesser degree to α-globulin IV-4 fraction (55%). No significant binding could be demonstrated with erythrocytes or white cells.

Metabolism: Alprostadil is rapidly converted to compounds which are further metabolized prior to excretion. In man, a single pass through the lung effectively metabolizes approximately 80% of the available PGE_1 primarily by beta- and omega-oxidation. Therefore, any alprostadil which may enter the systemic circulation following intracavernosal injection is rapidly metabolized. However, pulmonary clearance of PGE_1 can be affected by disease states such as acute respiratory distress syndrome (ARDS), with a resultant reduction in the pulmonary extraction ratio.

After intracavernosal administration of 20 µg of alprostadil, peripheral levels of the primary metabolite 15-oxo-13,14-dihydro-PGE_1 increased, reaching a peak at 30 minutes and falling to pre-dose levels by 60 minutes post-injection.

Excretion: The major route of elimination of the metabolites of alprostadil is through the kidney. Urinary excretion of an i.v. dose is essentially complete (90%) within 24 hours of administration. The remainder of the dose is excreted in the feces. There is no evidence to suggest any tissue retention of PGE_1 or its metabolites after an i.v. administration.

Pharmacokinetics in Special Populations: Geriatrics: The potential effect of age on the pharmacokinetics of alprostadil has not been formally evaluated. In patients with ARDS, the mean (±SD) pulmonary extraction of alprostadil was 72%±15% in 11 elderly patients aged 65 years or older (mean 71±6 years) and 65%±20% in 6 young patients aged 35 years or younger (mean 28±5 years).

Children: Plasma alprostadil concentrations were evaluated in 10 neonates (gestational age 34 weeks in 2 infants and 38 to 40 weeks in 8 infants) receiving steady-state i.v. infusions of alprostadil to treat underlying cardiac malformations. Alprostadil infusion rates ranged from 5 to 50 ng/kg/min (median 45 ng/kg/min), with resultant plasma concentrations in the range of 22 to 530 pg/mL (median 56 pg/mL). The individual clearance of alprostadil in neonates is highly variable as reflected by the wide range of plasma concentrations observed.

Gender: The influence of gender on the pharmacokinetics of alprostadil has not been formally studied. Two studies evaluated pulmonary extraction in 23 patients with ARDS following i.v. administration of alprostadil. The 17 males had a pulmonary extraction of 66% compared to 69% in the 6 female patients, suggesting no gender influence.

Race: The influence of race on the pharmacokinetics of alprostadil has not been formally studied.

Renal and Hepatic Insufficiency: The effects of renal and hepatic insufficiency on the pharmacokinetics of alprostadil have not been formally studied. Since systemic clearance of alprostadil is primarily by first-pass metabolism through the lungs, it is not expected that altered renal or hepatic function will have a major influence on the pharmacokinetics of alprostadil.

Pulmonary Disease: In one study, pulmonary extraction of alprostadil given i.v. was found to be reduced by 15% in patients with ARDS (66%) compared to patients with normal respiratory function (78%). In a second study of 14 patients with ARDS or at risk of developing ARDS, the mean extraction efficiency of alprostadil was 67% ranging from subnormal (11%) to normal (90%).

INDICATIONS: For the intracavernosal treatment of erectile dysfunction due to neurogenic, vasculogenic, psychogenic, or mixed etiology. Intracavernosal alprostadil may also be useful as an adjunct to diagnostic tests in the diagnosis of erectile dysfunction.

CONTRAINDICATIONS: Patients with a known hypersensitivity to the drug. Patients who have any condition that may predispose them to priapism such as sickle cell anemia or trait, multiple myeloma or leukemia. Patients with anatomical deformations of the penis, such as angulation, cavernosal fibrosis, Peyronie's disease. Patients with penile implants.

Caverject should not be used in women or children and is **not for use in newborns.**

Alprostadil should not be used in men for whom sexual activity is inadvisable or contraindicated.

WARNINGS: Prolonged erection (4 to 6 hours) and/or priapism (>6 hours) are known to occur following intracavernosal administration of vasoactive substances, including alprostadil. In clinical studies, prolonged erection occurred in 4% of patients and 0.4% experienced priapism.

The patient should be instructed to immediately report to his physician, or if unavailable, to seek immediate medical assistance for an erection persisting more than 3 hours. Treatment of prolonged erection/priapism should be according to established medical practice (see Overdose, Symptoms and Treatment). If priapism is not treated immediately, penile tissue damage and permanent loss of potency may result.

In the majority of cases, spontaneous detumescence occurred. To minimize the chances of prolonged erection or priapism, alprostadil should be titrated slowly to the lowest effective dose (see Dosage).

PRECAUTIONS: General: Underlying treatable medical causes of erectile dysfunction must be diagnosed and treated prior to initiating therapy with alprostadil.

The results of clinical studies with alprostadil indicate an overall incidence of penile fibrosis, including Peyronie's disease, of 3% (55/1 861). In one long-term (up to 18 months duration) self-injection study, the incidence of fibrosis reported was 7.8% (53/683). Regular follow-up of patients, with careful examination of the penis, is strongly recommended to detect signs of penile fibrosis. Treatment with alprostadil should be discontinued in patients who develop penile angulation, cavernosal fibrosis or Peyronie's disease.

Patients on anticoagulants such as warfarin or heparin may have an increased propensity for bleeding after intracavernosal injection.

An injection of alprostadil can induce a small amount of bleeding at the injection site (see Adverse Effects—hematoma, ecchymosis, hemorrhage). In patients infected with blood-borne diseases, this may increase the transmission of blood-borne diseases between partners.

The safety and efficacy of combinations of alprostadil and other vasoactive agents have not been systematically studied. Therefore, the use of such combinations is not recommended.

Drug Interactions: The potential for pharmacokinetic drug-drug interactions between alprostadil and other agents has not been formally studied.

Information to Be Provided to the Patient: Patients using a self-injection program of therapy should receive proper instruction in both intracavernosal injection and aseptic technique (see Information for the Patient). Physicians should ensure that patients are able to demonstrate competence and skill with the injection procedure prior to initiating self-injection.

The initial treatment dose is established in the physicians office. The lowest effective dose sufficient to induce an erection lasting up to 1 hour should be used. The patient may expect an erection to occur within 5 to 20 minutes. Patients who require dosage adjustments and are self-injecting alprostadil, should not increase or decrease their dose without the advice of their physician. Generally, patients should not use alprostadil more than once a day and not more than 3 times a week, with at least 24 hours between each use.

Alprostadil is labelled for "single use only". Patients should discard any unused solution after withdrawing the proper volume for their dose. The vial should not be shaken once reconstituted.

Reconstituted vials of alprostadil which on visual inspection appear cloudy, colored or contain particulate matter, should be discarded.

Patients who experience an erection lasting longer than 2 hours should attempt to detumesce using methods prescribed by their physician.

Patients should be advised on the possible adverse effects associated with the use of alprostadil; the most frequent being mild to moderate penile pain after injection. A patient should report to his physician if he complains of: any penile pain not previously present, an increased intensity of pain, nodules or hard tissue appearing in the penis, or curvature of the erect penis. There is the potential for infection with any type of injection, therefore patients should also report any occurrences of penile redness, swelling, or tenderness. The importance of regular physician visits to assess the continued safety and efficacy of alprostadil treatment should be stressed to the patient.

A potentially serious adverse reaction with intracavernosal therapy is priapism. Accordingly, the patient should be instructed to contact the physician's office immediately or, if unavailable, to seek immediate medical assistance if an erection persists for longer than 3 hours.

In clinical trials, the use of concomitant medicines such as antihypertensives, diuretics, antidiabetic agents (including insulin) or NSAIDs, did not affect the safety or efficacy of alprostadil.

The use of alprostadil intracavernosally does not offer any protection from the spread of sexually transmitted diseases. Individuals using alprostadil should be properly counselled with regards to protective measures to safeguard against the spread of sexually transmitted diseases, including human immunodeficiency virus (HIV) infection.

Patients should be instructed not to reuse or share needles or syringes. The patient should not allow anyone else to use this medicine. Patients should dispose of used needles, syringes, and vials, safely and properly (see Information for the Patient).

A patient administration guide, found in every package, provides a step-by-step method for the proper preparation and administration of alprostadil. Patients should be instructed to carefully follow this guide for self-injection.

Carcinogenesis, Mutagenesis and Impairment of Fertility: Long-term carcinogenicity studies have not been conducted. Reproductive studies in the rat with alprostadil at doses of up to 0.2 mg/kg/day did not adversely affect or alter spermatogenesis, conferring a 200-fold margin of safety at usual human doses. A battery of mutagenicity assays including, bacterial mutation (Ames), alkaline elution, rat micronucleus, sister chromatid exchange, CHO/HGPRT mammalian cell forward gene mutation and unscheduled DNA synthesis (UDS), revealed no potential for mutagenesis.

A one-year irritancy study was conducted in male Cynomolgus monkeys. Three groups of 5 animals received twice weekly intracavernosal injections of either 3 or 8.25 µg alprostadil or vehicle. A further 2 groups of 6 animals were given 8.25 µg alprostadil or vehicle twice weekly, as above, and in addition, multiple doses during weeks 44, 48 and 52. Three monkeys receiving vehicle and 3 monkeys receiving 8.25 µg alprostadil were held for evaluation following a 4-week recovery period. No evidence of alprostadil-related penile or systemic tissue lesions were found. Local irritation noted in control and treated monkeys was considered to be related to the injection procedure itself and any penile lesions found were reversible. After the 4-week recovery period, a regression in histological changes in the penis was observed.

ADVERSE EFFECTS: Local Adverse Events: The following local adverse events (see Table 1) were reported from controlled and uncontrolled clinical trials, including an uncontrolled 18-month safety study.

Table 1: Caverject

Local Adverse Events

Local Event (Reported in ≥1% of Patients)	No. (%) of Patients (n=1861)	
Penile pain	696	(37)
Pain after injection	580	(31)
Pain at the injection site	370	(20)
Prolonged erection (4-6 h)	82	(4)
Penile fibrosis[a]	55	(3)
Injection site hematoma	63	(3)
Penis disorder[b]	46	(3)
Injection site ecchymosis	32	(2)
Penile rash	21	(1)
Penile edema	18	(1)

[a] Includes generalized or deep fibrosis, penile curvature/deviation, and Peyronie's disease.
[b] Includes numbness, yeast infection, irritation, sensitivity, phimosis, pruritus, erythema, venous leak, penile skin tear, strange feeling in penis, burning sensation in penis and itch at tip of penis.

Penile Pain: Penile pain after intracavernosal administration of alprostadil was reported at least once by 37% of patients in clinical studies of up to 18 months in duration. The intensity of pain was rated mild or moderate in the majority of cases. Three percent of patients discontinued treatment because of penile pain. The frequency of penile pain was 2% in 294 patients who received 1 to 3 injections of placebo.

Prolonged Erection/Priapism: In clinical trials, prolonged erection was defined as an erection that lasted for 4 to 6 hours; priapism was defined as an erection that lasted 6 hours or longer (see Warnings).

Hematoma/Ecchymosis: The frequency of hematoma and ecchymosis was 3 and 2%, respectively. In most cases, hematoma/ecchymosis was judged to be a complication of a faulty injection technique. Accordingly, proper instruction of the patient in self-injection is of importance to minimize the potential of hematoma/ecchymosis (see Dosage).

Local events observed in <1% of the patients include: balanitis, lack of efficacy, injection site hemorrhage, injection site inflammation, injection site itching, injection site reaction, injection site swelling, injection site edema, trauma, urethral bleeding, urethral disorder, penile hematoma, penile warmth, priapism (>6 h), numbness, yeast infection, irritation, sensitivity, phimosis, pruritus, erythema, venous leak, painful erection and abnormal ejaculation.

Systemic Adverse Events: The following systemic adverse event information (see Table 2) was derived from controlled and uncontrolled studies, including an uncontrolled 18-month safety study.

Table 2: Caverject

Systemic Adverse Events

Systemic Event[a] by Body System[b] (Reported in ≥1% of Patients)[c]	No. (%) of Patients (n=1861)	
Body as a Whole	245	(13)
Upper respiratory infection	76	(4)
Flu syndrome	42	(2)
Headache	37	(2)
Trauma[d]	33	(2)
Localized pain[e]	32	(2)
Back pain	22	(1)
Localized abdominal pain	10	(<1)
Respiratory	123	(7)
Sinusitis	43	(2)
Nasal congestion	25	(1)
Cough	21	(1)
Bronchitis	18	(1)
Pharyngitis	16	(<1)
Urogenital	121	(7)
Prostatic disorder[f]	28	(2)
Urinary tract infection	16	(<1)
Testicular pain	16	(<1)
Hematuria	10	(<1)
Cardiovascular	80	(4)
Hypertension	39	(2)
CNS	66	(4)
Dizziness	22	(1)
Digestive	86	(5)
Nausea	14	(<1)
Tooth abscess	12	(<1)
Diarrhea	11	(<1)
Dyspepsia	11	(<1)
Skin and Appendages	49	(3)
Rash	11	(<1)

[a] Number (%) patients reporting the event, with patients reporting the same event more than once counted only once.
[b] Number (%) patients reporting a drug-related event within body system, with patients reporting more than one event within the body system counted only once.
[c] No significant adverse events were reported by 294 patients who received 1 to 3 injections of placebo.
[d] Includes injuries, fractures, abrasions, lacerations, dislocations.
[e] Includes pain in various anatomical structures other than injection site.
[f] Includes prostatitis, pain, hypertrophy, enlargement.

Systemic events reported in 1% of patients and judged by investigators to be possibly related to the use of alprostadil include: testicular pain, scrotal disorder, scrotal edema, hematuria, testicular disorder, impaired urination, urinary frequency, pelvic pain, hypotension, vasodilation, peripheral vascular disorder, supraventricular extrasystole, vasovagal reactions, hypesthesia, non-generalized weakness, diaphoresis, rash, non-application site pruritus, skin neoplasm, nausea, dry mouth, increased serum creatinine, leg cramps and mydriasis.

Hemodynamic changes, manifested as decreases in blood pressure and increases in pulse rate, were observed during clinical studies, principally at doses above 20 µg and above 30 µg of alprostadil respectively, and appeared to be dose-dependent. However, these changes were clinically unimportant; only 3 patients discontinued the treatment because of symptomatic hypotension.

Alprostadil had no clinically important effect on serum or urine laboratory tests.

OVERDOSE:

Symptoms: The pharmacotoxic signs of alprostadil are similar in all animal species and include depression, soft stool or diarrhea and rapid breathing. In mice, the lowest acute LD_{50} was 12 mg/kg which is 12 000 times greater than the maximum recommended human dose of 60 µg.

In man, prolonged erection and/or priapism are known to occur following intracavernosal administration of vasoactive substances. Given the dose-response relationship of alprostadil with erection duration, the therapeutic dose range should be determined individually for each patient by his physician during the initial office instruction. Inadvertent or intentional overdosing is the most common cause of prolonged pharmacological erection. In clinical trials with alprostadil, overdosage was not observed. If intracavernous overdose of alprostadil occurs, the patient should be under medical supervision until any systemic effects have resolved and/or until penile detumescence has occurred. Symptomatic treatment of any systemic symptoms would be appropriate.

Patients should be instructed to report any erections persisting for more than 3 hours to a physician. The treatment of priapism/prolonged erection should be according to established medical practice. Physicians may refer to 2 suggested protocols for detumescence presented below.

Detumescence Protocols: 1. Aspirate 40 to 60 mL from either right or left corpora using vacutainer and holder as for drawing blood. Use landmarks as for intracavernosal injection. Patient will often detumesce while aspirating. Apply ice for 20 minutes post-aspiration if erection remains. If 1) unsuccessful then, 2. Have patient lie in supine position. Dilute 10 mg phenylephrine into 20 mL water for injection (0.05%). With an insulin syringe, inject 0.1 to 0.2 mL (50 to 100 µg) into the corpora every 2 to 5 minutes, until detumescence occurs. The occasional patient may experience very transient bradycardia and hypertension when given phenylephrine injections, therefore monitor patient's blood pressure and pulse every 10 minutes. Patients at risk include those with cardiac arrhythmias and diabetics. Refer to the prescribing information for phenylephrine before use. **Do not** give to patients on MAOIs. When phenylephrine is used within the first 12 hours of erection, the majority of patients will respond. 3. If the above measures fail to detumesce the patient, a urologist should be consulted as soon as possible, especially if the erection has been present for many hours. If priapism is not treated immediately, penile tissue damage and/or permanent loss of potency may result.

Treatment: See Symptoms.

> For management of a suspected drug overdose, CPhA recommends that you contact your **regional Poison Control Centre**. See the *CPS* Directory section for a list of Poison Control Centres.

DOSAGE: Administration: Alprostadil is administered by direct intracavernosal injection. A 0.5 inch 27- to 30-gauge needle is generally recommended. Alprostadil is injected into either of two corpora cavernosum along the dorso-lateral aspects of the proximal third of the penis. Avoid any area where there are visible veins. The injection site should be changed for each injection (i.e., alternate sides of penis). Within either area, the point of injection should also be changed each time and the injection site must be cleansed with an alcohol swab.

Therapeutic/Effective Dose: Appropriate initial doses and maintenance doses are recommended based on the etiology of the erectile dysfunction. In all cases, the dose should be titrated on an individual basis by the physician, and the lowest effective dose always employed as the therapeutic dose. An effective dose is defined as one which produces an erection sufficient for intercourse with an erection duration not exceeding 1 hour. The following guidelines for dose titration are recommended.

Initial Titration in Physician's Office: Erectile Dysfunction of Vasculogenic, Psychogenic or Mixed Etiology: Dosage titration should be initiated at 2.5 µg of alprostadil. If there is a partial response, the dose may be increased by 2.5 µg to a dose of 5 µg and then in increments of 5 to 10 µg, depending upon erectile response, until the effective dose is reached (see Therapeutic/Effective Dose). If there is no response to the initial 2.5 µg dose, the second dose may be increased to 7.5 µg, followed by increments of 5 to 10 µg. The patient must remain in the physician's office until complete detumescence is achieved. If there is no response, then the next higher dose may be given within 1 hour. If there is a response, then there should be at least a 24-hour interval before the next dose is given.

Erectile Dysfunction of Pure Neurogenic Etiology: Dosage titration should be initiated at 1.25 µg of alprostadil. The dose may be increased by 1.25 µg to a dose of 2.5 µg, followed by an increment of 2.5 µg to a dose of 5 µg and then in 5 µg increments until the effective dose is reached (see Therapeutic/Effective Dose). The patient must remain in the physician's office until complete detumescence is achieved. If there is no response, then the next higher dose may be given within 1 hour. If there is a response, then there should be at least a 24-hour interval before the next dose is given.

In one clinical study involving 579 patients, the majority of patients (56%) were titrated to doses of >5 µg but ≤ 20 µg. The mean dose at the end of the titration phase was 17.8 µg of alprostadil.

Maintenance Therapy: The initial injection of alprostadil must be delivered by a medically trained health care professional. Before beginning a self-injection program of therapy, the physician must ensure that the patient (or his partner) aptly demonstrates skill and competence with the injection procedure, and uses appropriate sterile technique. A patient package insert is available to patients for referral (see Information for the Patient).

The dose selected for self-injection therapy is established during dose titration in the physician's office. The correct dose is the lowest effective dose. The dose should be reduced if the erection persists for longer than 1 hour; however, the physician should take into consideration the patient's preferences when defining the dose for self-injection. An erection lasting >3 hours is to be treated as a medical emergency. A physician should be consulted for any dose adjustments, if required. The dose should be adjusted in accordance with the titration guidelines described above. Regular follow-up visits, at least every 3 months, are recommended in order to assess the safety and efficacy of the therapy.

Maximum Recommended Dose Limits: Daily dose should not exceed **60 µg**. **Not** more than once daily and **not** more than 3 times weekly, with at least 24 hours between each dose. Do not inject alprostadil into an erect penis.

There is no evidence that tolerance to the effects of alprostadil develops with continued use. The long-term use of alprostadil has been documented for up to 6 months in an uncontrolled self-injection study. The mean dose after 6 months was 20.7 µg.

A vial of Caverject delivers 1 dose only. Instructions for proper disposal of the syringe, needle and vial should be followed (see Information for the Patient).

Diagnostic Dose: Pharmacologic Testing: An initial dose of 2.5 µg is employed with subsequent upward titration in 2.5 µg increments. Patients are monitored for the occurrence of an erection following an intracavernosal injection of alprostadil.

Adjunct to Laboratory Investigations: A single dose of alprostadil sufficient to induce a rigid erection is used. For use with Doppler imaging/Duplex Ultrasonography, ^{133}Xenon washout tests, Radionuclide Phallography and Penile Arteriography for the visualization and assessment of the penile vasculature.

Reconstituted Solutions: See Table 3. Alprostadil is reconstituted with the addition of 1 mL bacteriostatic water for injection (BWFI). Vial content after reconstitution is approximately 1.13 mL which allows 1.0 mL to be delivered to the patient. An excess of alprostadil is added to compensate for loss due to adsorption to the vial and syringe. The resultant solution contains 20 µg/mL of alprostadil, 172 mg/mL lactose, 47 µg/mL sodium citrate, and 8.4 mg/mL benzyl alcohol. Once reconstituted, no additional substances should be injected into the vial.

Once reconstituted, the alprostadil solution must be used immediately. Do not freeze the reconstituted solution. A solution which appears cloudy, colored or contains particles should be discarded.

Table 3: Caverject

Parenteral Products Reconstitution

Vial Amount	Volume of Diluent Added	Nominal Concentration
23.2 µg	1 mL BWFI	20 µg/mL

Legend:
BWFI=bacteriostatic water for injection.

INFORMATION FOR THE PATIENT: Published in e-CPS, available by subscription at www.e-cps.ca.

SUPPLIED: 20 µg: Each case contains: a single dose vial of alprostadil 20 µg sterile powder, 1 mL prefilled syringe of BWFI diluent, a 27-gauge 0.5 inch needle, 2 alcohol swabs and Patient Administration Leaflet. These cases are fitted with a lock designed for safe and convenient disposal of the contents after use. Once reconstituted, each mL contains: alprostadil 20 µg, lactose monohydrate 172 mg, sodium citrate dihydrate 47 µg, benzyl alcohol 8.4 mg, and sterile water for injection q.s. Cartons of 5.

20 µg, Diagnostic Vials: Each single-dose vial contains: alprostadil 20 µg sterile powder. Packs of 5.

The unreconstituted lyophilized sterile powder (20 µg vials) should be stored between 2 to 30°C.

CaVit D

calcium carbonate—vitamin D

Calcium Supplement with Vitamin D

Rougier Pharma

SUPPLIED: Each pale salmon FC, oblong biconvex tablet, engraved 'CaVit D' on one side and scored on the other side contains: calcium 500 mg (as calcium carbonate) and vitamin D 400 IU (as cholecalciferol). Nonmedicinal ingredients: acacia gum, croscarmellose sodium, FD&C Yellow #6 aluminum lake, glyceryl behenate, maltodextrin, microcrystalline cellulose, polyethylene glycol, polyvinyl alcohol, talc and titanium dioxide. Bottles of 120. Store between 15 and 30°C.

Cayston™ Ⓟ

aztreonam

Antibiotic

Gilead Sciences

Date of Preparation: September 9, 2009

CAYSTON, indicated for the management of cystic fibrosis patients with chronic pulmonary *P. aeruginosa* infections, has been issued marketing authorization with conditions, pending the results of studies to verify its clinical benefit. Patients should be advised of the nature of the authorization.

SUMMARY PRODUCT INFORMATION:

Route of Administration	Dosage Form/Strength	Nonmedicinal Ingredients
Inhalation	Sterile lyophilized powder for reconstitution 75 mg aztreonam/vial	Lysine Diluent (0.17% sodium chloride)

INDICATIONS AND CLINICAL USE: CAYSTON (aztreonam for inhalation solution) is indicated for the management of cystic fibrosis (CF) patients with chronic pulmonary *P. aeruginosa* infections.

Demonstration of longer-term safety and efficacy of CAYSTON is limited to uncontrolled, open-label clinical trial data obtained over nine cycles of therapy.

Safety and efficacy have not been demonstrated in patients with FEV_1 <25% or >75% predicted or in patients colonized with *B. cepacia* complex.

Sputum culture and susceptibility testing performed periodically will provide information on changing microbial flora and the possible emergence of bacterial resistance.

Geriatrics (>65 years of age): Clinical studies with CAYSTON did not include sufficient numbers of patients aged 65 years old and over to determine whether they responded differently from younger patients.

Pediatrics (<18 years of age): Safety and efficacy have not been studied in patients under the age of 6 years.

CONTRAINDICATIONS: CAYSTON (aztreonam for inhalation solution) is contraindicated in patients with a known allergy to aztreonam or to any ingredient in the formulation or any components of the container. For a complete listing see Dosage Forms, Composition and Packaging.

WARNINGS AND PRECAUTIONS: General: CAYSTON should only be used with the Altera Nebulizer System manufactured by PARI Respiratory Equipment, Inc. CAYSTON is not for oral, intravenous, subcutaneous, intramuscular, or intrathecal administration.

CAYSTON has been specifically formulated with the amino acid lysine. Do not use other formulations of aztreonam (e.g., aztreonam for injection) in the Altera Nebulizer System. Aztreonam for injection has not been formulated for inhalation, and contains arginine, a substance known to cause pulmonary inflammation.

Certain antibiotics (eg. cefoxitin, imipenem) may induce high levels of beta-lactamase in vitro in some gram-negative aerobes such as Enterobacter and Pseudomonas sp., resulting in antagonism to many beta-lactam antibiotics including aztreonam. These in vitro findings suggest that such beta-lactamase inducing antibiotics should not be used concurrently with aztreonam lysine.

Carcinogenesis and Mutagenesis: A 104-week rat inhalation toxicology study of aztreonam lysine using dose levels 7 to 27 times the maximum human recommended dose demonstrated no drug-related increase in malignant tumors. Both aztreonam for injection (aztreonam arginine) and aztreonam lysine demonstrated no evidence of mutagenic potential in in vitro and in vivo laboratory models.

Immune: Allergic Reactions: Severe allergic reactions have been reported following administration of aztreonam for injection (aztreonam arginine) to patients with no known history of exposure to aztreonam. CAYSTON is contraindicated in patients with a known history of aztreonam allergy. If an allergic reaction to CAYSTON does occur, stop administration of the drug and initiate treatment as appropriate. The occurrence of rash may be indicative of an allergic reaction to CAYSTON.

A history of allergy to beta-lactam antibiotics, such as penicillins, cephalosporins, and/or carbapenems, may be a risk factor for an allergic reaction to CAYSTON, since cross-reactivity may occur. Caution is advised when administering CAYSTON to patients if they have a history of beta-lactam allergy.

Respiratory: Bronchospasm: Bronchospasm is a potential complication associated with nebulized therapies. Reduction of ≥15% in forced expiratory volume in 1 second (FEV_1) immediately following administration of study medication after pretreatment with a bronchodilator was observed in 3% of patients treated with CAYSTON and 4% of patients receiving placebo.

Special Populations: Pregnant Women: No adequate and well-controlled studies of CAYSTON or aztreonam for injection (aztreonam arginine) have been conducted in pregnant women. Because animal reproduction studies are not always predictive of human response, CAYSTON should be used during pregnancy only if the potential benefit outweighs the risk.

Aztreonam for injection (aztreonam arginine) has been shown to cross the placenta and enter fetal circulation. No evidence of embryo- or fetotoxicity or teratogenicity has been shown in studies with pregnant rats and rabbits treated with daily doses up to 15 and 5 times, respectively, the human dose of aztreonam for injection (aztreonam arginine). The systemic concentration of aztreonam following inhaled administration of 75 mg CAYSTON (3 times a day) is approximately 1% of the concentration resulting from a 500 mg dose of aztreonam for injection (aztreonam arginine).

Nursing Women: The safety of CAYSTON in breast-fed infants of mothers who received CAYSTON has not been established.

Following administration of aztreonam for injection (aztreonam arginine), aztreonam is excreted in human milk at concentrations that are less than one percent of those determined in simultaneously obtained maternal serum. Systemic concentration of aztreonam following inhaled administration of CAYSTON is approximately 1% of the concentration resulting from a standard dose of aztreonam for injection (aztreonam arginine). Therefore, aztreonam exposure in breast-fed infants due to mothers receiving CAYSTON is likely to be extremely low.

Pediatrics (<18 years of age): Safety and efficacy have not been studied in patients under the age of 6 years.

Geriatrics (>65 years of age): Clinical studies with CAYSTON did not include sufficient numbers of patients aged 65 years old and over to determine whether they responded differently from younger patients.

Renal Impairment: Aztreonam is known to be excreted renally and therefore administration of CAYSTON in patients with renal impairment should be undertaken with caution.

Hepatic Impairment: There are no data on the use of CAYSTON in patients with severe hepatic impairment (ALT or AST greater than 5 times the upper limit of normal). No drug-related worsening of hepatic function was observed in patients in clinical trials with baseline ALT or AST less than 5 times the upper limit of normal.

ADVERSE REACTIONS: Adverse Drug Reaction Overview: In clinical studies, CAYSTON was generally well-tolerated with an adverse event profile consistent with the signs and symptoms of cystic fibrosis. In the placebo-controlled studies AIR-CF1 and AIR-CF2, the most common adverse drug reaction (based on adverse events assessed by the Investigator to be possibly or probably related to study medication) was cough, occurring in 15% of patients treated with CAYSTON versus 10% of patients treated with placebo (Table 1). The majority of adverse reactions in CAYSTON-treated patients in the placebo-controlled Phase 3 studies were mild (21%) to moderate (8%) in severity, as judged by the Investigator. Adverse reactions of severe intensity were reported with the same incidence in both the placebo and CAYSTON treatment groups, 2%. Patient discontinuations due to adverse events occurred at a higher rate in placebo-treated patients (16%) vs. CAYSTON-treated patients (7%). Most study discontinuations were associated with signs and symptoms of pulmonary exacerbations. The most common adverse event resulting in study drug discontinuation in both treatment groups was cough.

Patients 6 years and older were included in clinical studies with CAYSTON. Fifty-five patients under 18 years of age received CAYSTON in the placebo-controlled studies. In CAYSTON clinical studies no dose adjustments were made for pediatric patients. Pyrexia was more commonly reported in pediatric than adult patients in the placebo-controlled studies.

Clinical Trial Adverse Drug Reactions: Because clinical studies are conducted under very specific conditions the adverse reaction rates observed in the clinical studies may not reflect the rates observed in practice and should not be compared to the rates in the clinical studies of another drug. Adverse drug reaction information from clinical studies is useful for identifying drug related adverse events and for approximating rates.

The safety of CAYSTON was evaluated in 344 patients from two Phase 3 placebo controlled studies (AIR-CF1 and AIR-CF2) and one Phase 3 uncontrolled open label follow-on study (AIR-CF3). In these studies patients with *P. aeruginosa* initiated treatment with doses of 75 mg of CAYSTON 2 or 3 times a day for 28 days. Seventy-nine patients were 6-17 years of age and 265 patients were 18 years of age and older. In the uncontrolled open label study, 171 patients initiated the ninth 28-day course of CAYSTON.

In studies AIR-CF1 and AIR-CF2, 215 CF patients received CAYSTON 75 mg 2 times or 3 times a day for 28 days. Table 1 displays adverse reactions, assessed as at least possibly related to treatment by the investigator, reported in ≥1% of patients treated with CAYSTON in Phase 3 placebo-controlled studies (AIR-CF1 and AIR-CF2), compared with the incidence observed following multiple courses of therapy in the uncontrolled, open-label follow-on study (AIR-CF3).

Table 1: CAYSTON

Adverse Reactions[a] Occurring in ≥1% of CAYSTON Treated Patients over Multiple Courses of Therapy from the Placebo-controlled Phase 3 Studies (AIR-CF1 and AIR-CF2) and the Uncontrolled, Open-label Follow-on Study (AIR-CF3)[b]

	Integrated AIR-CF1 and AIR-CF2		AIR-CF3[c]			
System Organ Class Preferred Term	Placebo Pooled (N=160) n (%)	CAYSTON Pooled (N=215) n (%)	CAYSTON Pooled Course 1 (N=274) n (%)	CAYSTON Pooled Course 3 (N=246) n (%)	CAYSTON Pooled Course 6 (N=188) n (%)	CAYSTON Pooled Course 9 (N=171) n (%)
Respiratory, Thoracic and Mediastinal Disorders						
Cough	16 (10.0)	33 (15.3)	31 (11.3)	10 (4.1)	7 (3.7)	2 (1.2)
Wheezing	5 (3.1)	6 (2.8)	2 (0.7)	1 (0.4)	1 (0.5)	0 (0.0)
Chest discomfort	2 (1.3)	5 (2.3)	7 (2.6)	1 (0.4)	1 (0.5)	0 (0.0)
Pharyngolaryngeal pain	4 (2.5)	4 (1.9)	6 (2.2)	0 (0.0)	1 (0.5)	0 (0.0)
Crackles lung	2 (1.3)	3 (1.4)	0 (0.0)	0 (0.0)	0 (0.0)	0 (0.0)
Dysphonia	3 (1.9)	3 (1.4)	1 (0.4)	2 (0.8)	0 (0.0)	0 (0.0)
Dyspnea	3 (1.9)	3 (1.4)	6 (2.2)	2 (0.8)	1 (0.5)	1 (0.6)
Productive cough	11 (6.9)	3 (1.4)	7 (2.6)	0 (0.0)	0 (0.0)	0 (0.0)
Throat irritation	2 (1.3)	3 (1.4)	2 (0.7)	0 (0.0)	0 (0.0)	0 (0.0)
Hemoptysis	4 (2.5)	2 (0.9)	7 (2.6)	3 (1.2)	1 (0.5)	0 (0.0)
Nasal congestion	1 (0.6)	2 (0.9)	3 (1.1)	0 (0.0)	1 (0.5)	0 (0.0)
Respiratory tract congestion	5 (3.1)	1 (0.5)	1 (0.4)	3 (1.2)	0 (0.0)	0 (0.0)
Musculoskeletal and Connective Tissue Disorders						
Arthralgia	0 (0.0)	0 (0.0)	2 (0.7)	4 (1.6)	1 (0.5)	1 (0.6)
Nervous System Disorders						
Headache	1 (0.6)	3 (1.4)	4 (1.5)	1 (0.4)	1 (0.5)	0 (0.0)

[a] Adverse reactions are those AEs judged by the investigator to have a causality of possible or probable. This does not include all AEs reported.
[b] Planned study durations in days (treatment + follow-up): AIR-CF2 (28+56), AIR-CF1 (28+14).
Planned study duration for AIR-CF3: up to nine 28-day courses, each course followed by 28 days off treatment.
[c] In addition to the events listed for courses 1, 3, 6, 9 for study AIR-CF3, dyspnea exertional (1.0%) and pleuritic pain (1.0%) were observed during course 4.

Less Common Clinical Trial Adverse Drug Reactions (>0.5% to <1%): In addition to the events listed in Table 1, the following uncommon adverse reactions, assessed as at least possibly related to treatment by the Investigator, were reported in >0.5% to <1% of patients treated with CAYSTON in the Phase 3 placebo-controlled studies:

Respiratory, Thoracic and Mediastinal: non-cardiac chest pain, sneezing, sputum discolored, dyspnea exacerbated, dyspnea exertional.

Gastrointestinal: diarrhea, vomiting.

Investigations: pulmonary function test decreased.

In addition to the events listed above, other adverse events reasonably associated with treatment in placebo-controlled studies include: pyrexia (12%), rhinorrhea (8%), bronchospasm (3%) (see Warnings and Precautions) and rash (2%).

Abnormal Hematologic and Clinical Chemistry Findings: No abnormal hematologic and chemistry findings were observed. However, reduction in elevated white blood cell and elevated neutrophil counts were observed in the CAYSTON treatment group relative to placebo, consistent with antibiotic therapy.

DRUG INTERACTIONS: Drug-Drug Interactions: No formal clinical studies of drug interactions with CAYSTON have been conducted. In clinical studies of CAYSTON, many patients used commonly prescribed CF therapies such as TOBI (tobramycin inhalation solution), Pulmozyme (dornase alfa), pancreatic enzymes, oral/inhaled steroids, and/or azithromycin concomitantly with CAYSTON.

Drug-Food Interactions: Interactions of CAYSTON with food have not been established.

Drug-Herb Interactions: Interactions of CAYSTON with herbs have not been established.

Drug-Laboratory Test Interactions: Interactions of CAYSTON with laboratory tests have not been established.

DOSAGE AND ADMINISTRATION: General: CAYSTON is administered by inhalation over a 2 to 3 minute period, using the Altera Nebulizer System. CAYSTON should only be used with an Altera Nebulizer System. CAYSTON should not be used with any other nebulizer. CAYSTON should not be mixed with any other drugs in the Altera Nebulizer Handset. Do not put other drugs in the Altera Nebulizer Handset. Patients should use a bronchodilator before each dose of CAYSTON. Short acting bronchodilators can be taken between 15 minutes and 4 hours and long acting bronchodilators can be taken between 30 minutes and 12 hours prior to each dose of CAYSTON. For patients receiving several respiratory therapies, the recommended order is: 1) bronchodilator 2) chest physiotherapy, 3) other inhaled medications, and 4) CAYSTON.

CAYSTON is for inhalation administration only.

Like all other nebulized treatments, the amount of CAYSTON delivered to the lungs will depend upon patient factors as well as the nebulization system used and its performance. Using the Altera Nebulizer System under in vitro conditions, the mean emitted dose (% nominal) was approximately 60 mg (80% of label dose) with a fine particle fraction of approximately 90% as measured by cascade impaction.

Recommended Dose and Dosage Adjustment: The recommended dosage for both adults and pediatric patients 6 years of age and older is one single-use vial (75 mg) of CAYSTON administered 3 times a day for a 28-day course (followed by 28 days without CAYSTON therapy). Dosage is not based on weight or adjusted for age. All patients should be administered a 75 mg dose 3 times a day. Each dose should be taken at least 4 hours apart.

Missed Dose: In case of a missed dose, the dose can still be taken provided there is a period of at least 4 hours between each dose.

CAYSTON Reconstitution: CAYSTON must be administered immediately after reconstitution. Do not reconstitute CAYSTON until ready to administer a dose.

Take one amber glass vial containing CAYSTON and one diluent ampule from the carton. To open the glass vial, carefully remove the metal ring by pulling the tab and remove the gray rubber stopper. Twist the tip off the diluent ampule and squeeze the liquid into the glass vial. Replace the rubber stopper, then gently swirl the vial until contents have completely dissolved.

CAYSTON Administration: Remove the rubber stopper, then pour the reconstituted CAYSTON into the Altera Nebulizer Handset. Turn the unit on. Place the mouthpiece of the handset in your mouth and breathe normally only through your mouth. Administration typically takes between 2 and 3 minutes. Further instruction for patients on how to administer drug is provided in Information for the Patient. Instructions for testing nebulizer functionality and cleaning the handset are provided in the Instructions for Use included with the Altera Nebulizer System.

OVERDOSAGE:
Adverse reactions specifically associated with overdose of CAYSTON have not been identified.

> For management of a suspected drug overdose, contact your regional Poison Control Centre. See the *CPS* Directory section for a list of Poison Control Centres.

ACTION AND CLINICAL PHARMACOLOGY: Mechanism of Action: Aztreonam exhibits activity in vitro against a broad spectrum of gram-negative aerobic pathogens including *P. aeruginosa*. Aztreonam binds to penicillin-binding proteins of susceptible bacteria, which leads to inhibition of bacterial cell wall synthesis, followed by filamentation and cell lysis.

Aztreonam activity is not significantly inhibited by sputum in the CF lung.

Pharmacokinetics: Absorption: Sputum Concentrations: Individual patients' sputum aztreonam concentrations exhibited considerable variability. Ten minutes following a single dose of 75 mg CAYSTON, the mean (range) sputum level in 195 patients with CF was 726 (0-6010) µg/g, which is approximately 10 times that of the aztreonam MIC_{90} for all isolates of *P. aeruginosa* observed at baseline for patients treated with CAYSTON in the Phase 3 placebo-controlled studies (64 µg/mL). Mean (range) sputum levels of aztreonam at Days 0, 14, and 28 of 75 mg 3 times a day CAYSTON dosing were 984 (8-6010) µg/g, 793 (2-2780) µg/g, and 715 (1-2800) µg/g, respectively, indicating no increased accumulation of aztreonam following 3 times a day dosing.

Plasma Concentrations: Individual patients' plasma aztreonam concentrations exhibited considerable variability. One hour following a single dose of 75 mg CAYSTON (at approximately peak plasma concentration), the mean (range) plasma level in patients with CF was 0.59 (0-2.92) µg/mL. Mean (range) peak plasma levels at Days 0, 14, and 28 of 75 mg 3 times a day CAYSTON dosing were 0.55 (0-1.62) µg/mL, 0.67 (0.01-1.66) µg/mL, and 0.65 (0-1.74) µg/mL, respectively, indicating no systemic accumulation of aztreonam following 3 times a day dosing. In contrast, the serum concentration of aztreonam following administration of a 500 mg dose of aztreonam for injection (aztreonam arginine) is approximately 54 µg/mL.

Distribution: Local and systemic tissue distribution following inhalation exposure has not been clinically characterized.

Metabolism: The in vitro metabolic stability and metabolism of aztreonam was demonstrated in pulmonary S9 fractions from healthy human donors as well as rats, dogs, and cynomolgus monkeys and pulmonary microsomes from human donors. Incubations were conducted at 3 and 50 µM to examine the metabolic stability of aztreonam by monitoring the rate of disappearance and also the formation of metabolites. Hepatocyte incubations were conducted in suspension for 6 hours at 37°C. Aztreonam is stable in pulmonary subcellular fractions in all species examined with little metabolism of the parent compound. As predicted by the high metabolic stability, no significant metabolites were observed by UV absorbance or high sensitivity linear ion trap LC/MS/MS. No oxidative metabolites were observed in hepatocyte or pulmonary incubations and no glucuronide and sulfate conjugates or esterase hydrolysis products were detected.

Excretion: The elimination half-life of aztreonam from serum is approximately 2.1 hours for inhalation administration, similar to what has been reported for aztreonam for injection (aztreonam arginine). Systemically absorbed aztreonam is eliminated about equally by active tubular secretion and glomerular filtration.

Special Populations and Conditions: Age: There was no clinically relevant effect of age on the pharmacokinetics of CAYSTON.

Gender: There was no clinically relevant effect of gender on the pharmacokinetics of CAYSTON.

Hepatic Insufficiency: Pharmacokinetic studies have not been performed with CAYSTON in patients with hepatic impairment

Renal Insufficiency: Pharmacokinetic studies have not been performed with CAYSTON in patients with renal impairment.

STORAGE AND STABILITY: Prior to Reconstitution: CAYSTON vials should be stored in a refrigerator at 2 to 8°C and may be stored by patients at room temperature (up to 25°C) for up to 28 days. Diluent ampules may be refrigerated or stored at room temperature (15 to 30°C).

Do not use CAYSTON if it has been stored at room temperature for more than 28 days. Unused vials of CAYSTON stored at room temperature for more than 28 days should be discarded. Do not store back in the refrigerator. Do not use CAYSTON beyond the expiration date stamped on the vial. Do not use diluent beyond the expiration date embossed on the ampule.

Following Reconstitution: CAYSTON should be used immediately upon reconstitution. Do not reconstitute more than one dose at a time.

Do not use diluent or reconstituted CAYSTON if it is cloudy or if there are particles in the solution.

SPECIAL HANDLING INSTRUCTIONS: The reconstituted solution should be used immediately and should not be stored. Do not reconstitute CAYSTON until ready to administer a dose (seeInformation for the Patient, for detailed instructions for administration).

INFORMATION FOR THE PATIENT: Published in e-CPS, available by subscription at www.e-cps.ca.

DOSAGE FORMS, COMPOSITION AND PACKAGING: A dose of CAYSTON consists of a single-use 2 mL vial of sterile, lyophilized powder (75 mg aztreonam and the nonmedicinal ingredient lysine) and a low-density polyethylene ampule containing 1 mL of sterile diluent (0.17% sodium chloride). The formulations contain no preservatives. CAYSTON is reconstituted and administered by inhalation using the Altera Nebulizer System. Each kit of CAYSTON contains 84 sterile vials of CAYSTON and 88 sterile diluent ampules packed in two cartons each with a 14-day supply (42 vials of CAYSTON packaged in two trays and one tray of 44 diluent ampules). The four additional diluent ampules are provided in case of spillage.

CeeNU® Ⓟ

lomustine

Antineoplastic

Bristol-Myers Squibb

Date of Preparation: July 4,1974
Date of Revision: February 24, 2009

Caution: CeeNU (lomustine-CCNU) is a potent drug and should be used only by physicians experienced with cancer chemotherapeutic drugs (see Warnings and Precautions). Blood counts as well as renal and hepatic function tests should be taken regularly. Discontinue the drug if abnormal depression of bone marrow is seen.

PHARMACOLOGY: It is generally agreed that lomustine acts as an alkylating agent but, as with other nitrosoureas, it may also inhibit several key enzymatic processes.

Lomustine may be given orally. Following oral administration of radioactive lomustine at doses ranging from 30 mg/m^2 to 100 mg/m^2, about half of the radioactivity given was excreted within 24 hours. The serum half-life of the drug and/or metabolites ranges from 16 hours to 2 days. Tissue levels are comparable to plasma levels at 15 minutes after i.v. administration.

Because of the high lipid solubility and the relative lack of ionization at physiological pH, lomustine crosses the blood-brain barrier quite effectively. Levels of radioactivity in the CSF are 50% or greater than those measured concurrently in plasma.

INDICATIONS: Adjuvant therapy to surgery and radiotherapy or in combination therapy with other chemotherapeutic agents in the following:

1. Brain tumors: both primary and metastatic, in patients who have already received appropriate surgical and/or radiotherapeutic procedures.
2. Lung cancer: squamous cell, anaplastic large cell, and adenocarcinoma. Lomustine has been used alone and in combination with other appropriate antineoplastic drugs, such as cyclophosphamide.
3. Malignant melanoma: alone or in combination with other active drugs, such as vincristine.
4. Hodgkin's disease: alone or in combination with other active drugs.
5. Breast carcinoma: in advanced disease after conventional therapy has failed.

Lomustine has been used in renal cell carcinoma although the response rate is low in this resistant cancer. Responses have also been observed with non-Hodgkin's lymphoma, ovarian and pancreatic carcinoma but data are insufficient to make a definite recommendation.

CONTRAINDICATIONS: Known hypersensitivity to lomustine. Severe leukopenia and/or thrombocytopenia.

WARNINGS: Lomustine should be administered by individuals experienced in the use of antineoplastic therapy.

Delayed bone marrow suppression, notably thrombocytopenia and leukopenia, which may contribute to bleeding and overwhelming infections in an already compromised patient, is the most common and severe of the toxic effects of lomustine.

Blood counts should be monitored weekly for at least 6 weeks after a dose (see Adverse Effects). At the recommended dosage, courses of lomustine should not be given more frequently than every 6 weeks.

The bone marrow toxicity of lomustine is cumulative and therefore dosage adjustment must be considered on the basis of nadir blood counts from prior dose (see Dosage, Table 1).

Caution should be used in administering lomustine to patients with decreased circulating platelets, leukocytes or erythrocytes (see Dosage).

Pulmonary toxicity from lomustine appears to be dose related (see Adverse Effects).

Long-term use of nitrosoureas has been reported to be possibly associated with the development of secondary malignancies.

Liver and renal function tests should be monitored periodically (see Adverse Effects).

Pregnancy: Safe use in pregnancy has not been established. Lomustine is embryotoxic and teratogenic in rats and embryotoxic in rabbits at dose levels equivalent to the human dose. If this drug is used during pregnancy, or if the patient becomes pregnant while taking (receiving) this drug, the patient should be apprised of the potential hazard to the fetus. Women of childbearing potential should be advised to avoid becoming pregnant.

Carcinogenesis, Mutagenesis, Impairment of Fertility: Lomustine is carcinogenic in rats and mice, producing a marked increase in tumor incidence in doses approximating those employed clinically.

Nitrosourea therapy does have carcinogenic potential. The occurrence of acute leukemia and bone marrow dysplasias has been reported in patients following nitrosourea therapy.

Lomustine also affects fertility in male rats at doses somewhat higher than the human dose.

Lactation: It is not known whether this drug is excreted in human milk. Because many drugs are excreted in human milk and because of the potential for serious adverse reactions in nursing infants from lomustine, a decision should be made whether to discontinue nursing or to discontinue the drug, taking into account the importance of the drug to the mother.

PRECAUTIONS: Due to delayed bone marrow suppression, blood counts should be monitored weekly for at least 6 weeks after a dose.

Baseline pulmonary function studies should be conducted along with frequent pulmonary function tests during treatment. Patients with a baseline below 70% of the predicted Forced Vital Capacity (FVC) or Carbon Monoxide Diffusing Capacity (DL_{CO}) are particularly at risk.

Since lomustine may cause liver dysfunction, it is recommended that liver function tests be monitored periodically.

Renal function tests should also be monitored periodically.

ADVERSE EFFECTS: Gastrointestinal: Nausea and vomiting may occur 3 to 6 hours after an oral dose and usually lasts less than 24 hours. The frequency and duration may be reduced by the use of antiemetics prior to dosing and by the administration of lomustine to fasting patients.

Hematologic Toxicity: The most frequent and most serious toxicity of lomustine is delayed myelosuppression. It usually occurs 4 to 6 weeks after drug administration and is dose related. Thrombocytopenia occurs at about 4 weeks post-administration and persists for 1 to 2 weeks. Leukopenia occurs at 5 to 6 weeks after a dose of lomustine and persists for 1 to 2 weeks.

Approximately 65% of patients receiving 130 mg/m^2 develop white blood cell counts below 5000/mm^3. Thirty-six percent developed white blood cell counts below 3000/mm^3. Thrombocytopenia is generally more severe than leukopenia. However, both may be dose-limiting toxicities.

Lomustine may produce cumulative myelosuppression, manifested by more depressed indices or longer duration of suppression after repeated doses.

The occurrence of acute leukemia and bone marrow dysplasias have been reported in patients following long-term nitrosourea therapy. Anemia also occurs, but is less frequent and less severe than thrombocytopenia or leukopenia.

Pulmonary Toxicity: Pulmonary toxicity characterized by pulmonary infiltrates and/or fibrosis has been reported rarely with lomustine. Onset of toxicity has occurred after an interval of 6 months or longer from the start of therapy with cumulative dose of lomustine usually greater than 1100 mg/m^2. There is one report of pulmonary toxicity at a cumulative dose of only 600 mg.

Delayed onset pulmonary fibrosis occurring up to 15 years after treatment has been reported in patients with intracranial tumors who received related nitrosoureas during their childhood and early adolescence.

Other Toxicities: Stomatitis, alopecia, anemia have been reported infrequently.

Neurological reactions such as disorientation, lethargy, ataxia and dysarthria have been noted in some patients receiving lomustine. However, the relationship to medication in these patients is unclear.

Nephrotoxicity: Renal abnormalities consisting of decrease in kidney size, progressive azotemia and renal failure have been reported in patients who receive large cumulative doses after prolonged therapy with lomustine and related nitrosoureas. Kidney damage has also been reported occasionally in patients receiving lower total doses.

Hepatotoxicity: A reversible type of hepatic toxicity, manifested by increased transaminase, alkaline phosphatase and bilirubin levels, has been reported in a small percentage of patients receiving lomustine.

OVERDOSE:

Treatment: In case of overdosage, treat the patient symptomatically.

For management of a suspected drug overdose, CPhA recommends that you contact your **regional Poison Control Centre**. See the *CPS* Directory section for a list of Poison Control Centres.

DOSAGE: The recommended dose of lomustine in adults and children is 130 mg/m^2 as a single dose by mouth every 6 weeks. In individuals with compromised bone marrow function, reduce the dose to 100 mg/m^2 every 6 weeks.

A repeat course of lomustine should not be given until circulating blood elements have returned to acceptable levels (platelets above 100 000/mm^3; leukocytes above 4000/mm^3). Monitor blood counts weekly and do not give repeat courses before 6 weeks because the hematologic toxicity is delayed and cumulative.

Doses subsequent to the initial dose should be adjusted according to the hematologic response of the patient to the preceding dose. The schedule in Table 1 is suggested as a guide to dosage adjustments.

Table 1: CeeNU

Dosage Adjustment Guide

Nadir After Prior Dose		
Leukocytes	**Platelets**	**Percentage of Prior Dose to be Given**
>4000	>100 000	100%
3000–3999	75 000–99 999	100%
2000–2999	25 000–74 999	70%
<2000	<25 000	50%

When lomustine is used in combination with myelosuppressive drugs, the doses should be adjusted accordingly.

Handing and Disposal: Preparation of lomustine should be done in a vertical laminar flow hood (Biological Safety Cabinet-class II). Lomustine capsules should not be placed in automated counting machines. The counting and pouring of lomustine should be done carefully and the equipment used should be rinsed with water and then thoroughly cleaned with detergent and water. Personnel handing lomustine should wear gloves, safety glasses, a mask and disposable protective clothing. Vials and other materials which have come in contact with lomustine should be segregated and incinerated at 1000°C or more. Sealed containers may explode. Intact vials should be returned to the manufacturer for destruction. Proper precautions should be taken in packaging these materials for transport. Personnel regularly involved in the preparation and handling of lomustine should have bi-anual blood examinations.

SUPPLIED: 10 mg: Each capsule with a white cap and body, imprinted with "BRISTOL" over "3030" on the cap and with "10 MG" on the body, contains: lomustine 10 mg. Nonmedicinal ingredients: mannitol and magnesium stearate; capsule shell: gelatin, printing ink and titanium dioxide. A desiccant packet is enclosed in each bottle of capsules. Bottles of 20.

40 mg: Each capsule with a white cap and moss green body, imprinted with "BRISTOL" over "3031" on the cap and with "40 MG" on the body, contains: lomustine 40 mg. Nonmedicinal ingredients: mannitol and magnesium stearate; capsule shell: FD&C blue No. 2, gelatin, printing ink, titanium dioxide and yellow iron oxide. A desiccant packet is enclosed in each bottle of capsules. Bottles of 20.

100 mg: Each capsule with a moss green cap and body, imprinted with "BRISTOL" over "3032" on the cap and with "100 MG" on the body, contains: lomustine 100 mg. Nonmedicinal ingredients: mannitol and magnesium stearate; capsule shell: FD&C blue No. 2, gelatin, printing ink, titanium dioxide and yellow iron oxide. A desiccant packet is enclosed in each bottle of capsules. Bottles of 20.

Unopened bottles of lomustine capsules are stable for 36 months at room temperature. **Protect from light.** Avoid excessive heat (over 40°C).

(Shown in Product Identification Section)

Cefaclor ℞
Antibiotic

CPhA Monograph

Date of Preparation: November 2004
Date of Revision: September 2009

This monograph has been compiled by CPhA and reviewed by experts. It may contain information different from that found in Health Canada-approved Product Monographs. The reader is referred to the *CPS* Editorial Policy for more information.

SUMMARY PRODUCT INFORMATION:

Route of Administration	Dosage Form	Product Strength
Oral	Capsule	250 mg, 500 mg
	Suspension	125 mg/5 mL, 250 mg/5 mL, 375 mg/5 mL

INDICATIONS AND CLINICAL USE:

- Cefaclor is no longer routinely recommended for the treatment of acute otitis media in childhood because it lacks activity against penicillin-resistant *S. pneumoniae* and has marginal activity against *H. influenzae*.
- The use of cefaclor is limited in the treatment of lower respiratory tract infections including pneumonia, bronchitis and pulmonary complications resulting from cystic fibrosis because it lacks activity against penicillin-resistant *S. pneumoniae* and has no activity against atypical pathogens.
- Cefaclor is no longer recommended for the treatment of upper respiratory tract infections such as pharyngitis. Penicillin is the drug of choice for the treatment of group A streptococcal pharyngitis [Practice guidelines for the diagnosis and management of group A streptococcal pharyngitis. *Clin Infect Dis* 2002;35(2):113-25].
- Cefaclor is not recommended for the treatment of skin and soft-tissue infections; however, second-generation cephalosporins such as cefuroxime may be used as empirical therapy for the treatment of skin and soft tissues infections. First-generation cephalosporins such as cephalexin are recommended for uncomplicated skin and soft-tissue bacterial infections caused by gram-positive organisms unless resistance is present. Re-evaluate patients 24 to 48 hours after receipt of antibiotics [Practice guidelines for the diagnosis and management of skin and soft-tissue infections. *Clin Infect Dis* 2005;41(10):1373-406].
- Cefaclor is no longer recommended for the treatment of urinary tract infections including cystitis and mild pyelonephritis (patient is hemodynamically stable and not vomiting). Some clinicians may recommend cefaclor as continuous prophylaxis in patients with recurrent urinary tract infections [Antibiotics for preventing recurrent urinary tract infection in non-pregnant women. *Cochrane Database Syst Rev* 2004;(3):CD001209].

CONTRAINDICATIONS:

- Patients who are hypersensitive to cefaclor or to any ingredient in the formulation.
- Patients who are hypersensitive to cephalosporins or to other beta-lactam antibiotics.

WARNINGS AND PRECAUTIONS:

Serious Warnings and Precautions

- Cefaclor has been associated with severe allergic reactions including anaphylactic reactions. For this reason a history of allergic reactions, including the type and severity of the reaction, should be obtained before prescribing and administering cefaclor.
- Cross-sensitivity between penicillins and cephalosporins is estimated to be very low. Current opinion on the true incidence of cross-sensitivity is about 1%. The beta-lactam subunit is not considered the primary allergenic determinant; rather, the side chain predicts cross-reactivity. After thorough investigation into the nature of the allergy, a cephalosporin can be considered in a penicillin allergic patient provided there is no history of an immediate-sensitivity reaction. Although the risk of cross-reaction is predicted to be low the patient should be monitored for signs of a sensitivity reaction.
- Patients with a history of immediate-sensitivity reaction to penicillin (e.g., anaphylaxis, bronchospasm and/or hypotension) are considered to be at increased risk of similar reactions to cephalosporins, including cefaclor. For this reason, administration of cefaclor should be avoided in patients with a history of severe allergic reactions to penicillin antibiotics unless skin testing is performed to rule out cross-sensitivity.
- Cephalosporin antibiotics including cefaclor have been associated with *C. difficile*-associated diarrhea and colitis.

Hepatic: Transient elevation of liver enzymes and cholestatic jaundice have occurred rarely during cephalosporin therapy (<1%).
Immune: Cefaclor is associated with more reports of serum sickness-like reactions consisting of pruritic and urticarial rash, painful and swollen joints (arthralgia or arthritis) and fever than any other cephalosporin. It may result from inherited defects in the metabolism of reactive metabolites. Serum sickness-like reactions with cefaclor are reported more frequently in children. The incidence is highest in young children (less than 6 years of age) and those with a history of allergy. They are more likely to occur during or following a second or subsequent course of cefaclor [*Ann Pharmacother* 1992;26(7-8):910-4]. This reaction occurs in approximately 0.5% of patients taking cefaclor, usually 2 to 21 days after initiation of cefaclor therapy. Patients improve within a few days upon discontinuation of cefaclor. Symptoms may resolve sooner with corticosteroid and antihistamine therapy. A history of serum sickness-like reaction to cefaclor is not a contraindication to the use of other β-lactam antibiotics.
Renal: Nephrotoxicity has been reported rarely with cephalosporins, and is more likely in older individuals, or in patients who are taking other nephrotoxic drugs concomitantly or have pre-existing renal impairment. Since cefaclor is cleared renally, dosage adjustment is recommended in patients with impaired renal function (see Table 5).
Special Populations: Pregnant Women: Pregnancy Category B_M. Although it has not been unequivocally established that there is not an increased risk of birth defects with the use of cefaclor, it is generally accepted that cephalosporins are safe to use during pregnancy.
Nursing Women: Cefaclor is excreted in breast milk in low concentrations. Potential risks to the infant include altered bowel flora, diarrhea, obscured diagnosis of fever and hypersensitivity reactions. Cephalosporins are generally considered to be compatible with breast-feeding.
Pediatrics (birth to 16 years old): Safety and efficacy of cefaclor in infants less than one month of age has not been established. Serum sickness-like reactions occur more frequently in young children, especially those under 6 years of age (see Warnings and Precautions).

ADVERSE REACTIONS:

Table 1: Cefaclor
Common Adverse Drug Reactions

Body System	Incidence (%)
Gastrointestinal	
Diarrhea	≤1.5
Hematologic	
Eosinophilia	2
Immune	
Urticaria	1
Morbilliform Eruptions	1

Less Common Adverse Drug Reactions (<1%): CNS: reversible hyperactivity, nervousness, insomnia, confusion, hypertonia, headache, dizziness, somnolence.
Gastrointestinal: nausea, vomiting, dyspepsia, pseudomembranous colitis.
Genitourinary: genital pruritus, vaginal moniliasis, vaginitis.
Hematologic: thrombocytopenia, transient lymphocytosis and leukopenia, hemolytic anemia, aplastic anemia, agranulocytosis, reversible neutropenia.
Hepatic: transient elevation of AST, ALT and alkaline phosphatase, cholestatic jaundice.
Immune: Stevens-Johnson syndrome, toxic epidermal necrolysis, angioedema, anaphylaxis, serum sickness-like reactions.
Renal: interstitial nephritis, transient elevation of BUN or serum creatinine, abnormal urinalysis.
Skin: pruritus, rash.

DRUG INTERACTIONS: Drug-Drug Interactions:

Table 2: Cefaclor
Drug-Drug Interactions

Interacting Drug	Effect	Clinical Comment
Aminoglycosides	The combination of aminoglycosides and cephalosporins may increase the incidence of nephrotoxicity.	Monitor aminoglycoside levels and kidney function.
Probenecid	Probenecid inhibits renal tubular excretion of cefaclor, thereby ↓ elimination of cefaclor.	This interaction has been exploited to increase serum levels of penicillins.
Tetracyclines (doxycycline, minocycline, tetracycline)	Bacteriostatic action of tetracyclines may inhibit the bactericidal activity of penicillins.	The combination of penicillins and tetracycline is avoided in pneumococcal meningitis and scarlet fever because tetracycline reduces the effectiveness of penicillin. The clinical significance of the interaction in other infections is unknown.

Drug-Food Interactions: Food does not affect the extent of absorption of cefaclor.
Drug-Laboratory Interactions: Cefaclor may cause a false-positive test for glucose in the urine and may cause a positive direct Coombs' test.

DOSAGE AND ADMINISTRATION: Recommended Dose and Dosage Adjustment: In general, the dose of cefaclor in treating an infection in adults is 250 to 500 mg po every 8 hours.

Table 3: Cefaclor
Dose in Adult Patients

Indication	Usual Dose	Duration of Treatment	Detailed Information
Recurrent urinary tract infection, continuous prophylaxis	250 mg po daily at bedtime	6 to 12 months	There are no published guidelines. Recommendation is based on a Cochrane systematic review [Antibiotics for preventing recurrent urinary tract infection in non-pregnant women. *Cochrane Database Syst Rev* 2004;(3):CD001209].

Geriatric Patients: No dosage adjustment needed in geriatric patients.

Table 4: Cefaclor
Dose in Pediatric Patients Other Than Neonates

Indication	Usual Dose	Maximum Dose	Duration of Treatment	Detailed Information
Otitis Media, acute	40 mg/kg daily divided Q8H or Q12H	2 g daily	10 days	Cefaclor is no longer routinely recommended in the treatment of acute otitis media in children.

Table 5: Cefaclor
Dose in Pediatric Patients with Renal Impairment

Creatinine Clearance	Dose Adjustment
30–50 mL/min	Usual dose
10–29 mL/min	Usual dose
<10 mL/min	50% of usual dose

Renal Impairment in Adults: No dose adjustment is required.
Dosage in Dialysis: 250 mg to 500 mg after hemodialysis. For peritoneal dialysis, give 250 mg to 500 mg every 8 hours.
Hepatic Impairment: No dose adjustment is required in patients with hepatic impairment.
Administration: Administer orally, with or without food.

OVERDOSAGE:

For management of a suspected drug overdose, CPhA recommends that you contact your **regional Poison Control Centre**. See the *CPS* Directory section for a list of Poison Control Centres.

ACTION AND CLINICAL PHARMACOLOGY: Cefaclor is a second-generation cephalosporin which is bactericidal against sensitive organisms. It inhibits peptidoglycan synthesis in the bacterial cell wall leading to the formation of a defective cell wall with eventual lysis and cell death. The spectrum of activity of cefaclor includes penicillin-sensitive gram-positive *S. pneumoniae* and gram-negative susceptible bacteria such as *H. influenzae*, *M. catarrhalis*, *E. coli* and Klebsiella species. Cefaclor possesses little or no activity against methicillin-resistant *S. aureus*, Enterococcus species, Enterobacteriaceae producing inducible β-lactamases and extended spectrum β-lactamases, Chlamydia, Mycoplasma and Listeria species. Cefuroxime axetil, cefixime or amoxicillin-clavulanate are more stable against β-lactamase producing *H. influenzae* than cefaclor. Penicillin-resistant *S. pneumoniae* are considered resistant to all first- and second-generation cephalosporins. They often remain susceptible to amoxicillin (high-dose) and third-generation cephalosporins.
Pharmacokinetics: Cefaclor is rapidly absorbed after oral administration with a bioavailability of about 90-95%. Peak serum concentration occurs within 1 hour under fasting conditions. Cefaclor distributes into tissues and fluids including bone, pleural and synovial fluid. Its volume of distribution ranges from 0.24 to 0.35 L/kg. Cefaclor is not highly protein bound (22 to 25%). The elimination half-life of cefaclor ranges from 0.5 to 1 hour in patients with normal renal function. In end-stage renal disease, the half-life is prolonged (about 3 hours). Cefaclor is excreted unchanged in the urine.
STORAGE AND STABILITY: After reconstitution, cefaclor oral solutions have an expiry of 14 days in the refrigerator.

Cefazolin

Antibacterial—Anti-infective

CPhA Monograph

Date of Preparation: November 2005
Date of Revision: September 2009

This monograph has been compiled by CPhA and reviewed by experts. It may contain information different from that found in Health Canada-approved Product Monographs. The reader is referred to the *CPS* Editorial Policy for more information.

SUMMARY PRODUCT INFORMATION:

Route of Administration	Dosage Form	Strength
Injectable (IM, IV)	Powder for injection	0.5, 1, 10, 20 g vial

INDICATIONS AND CLINICAL USE: Cefazolin is a first-generation cephalosporin with a spectrum of activity including gram-negative bacteria such as *P. mirabilis*, *E. coli*, Klebsiella and Moraxella species, and gram-positive bacteria such as methicillin-sensitive *S. aureus* (MSSA), penicillin-sensitive *S. pneumoniae* and β-haemolytic Streptococci.

Cefazolin possesses little or no activity against methicillin-resistant *S. aureus*, penicillin-resistant *S. pneumoniae*, Enterococcus species, Listeria species, Haemophilus species, Enterobacteriaceae producing inducible β-lactamases and extended spectrum β-lactamases, Pseudomonas species, anaerobic gram-negative bacilli, Pasteurella species, Eikenella species and atypical species such as Chlamydia and Mycoplasma.

Cefazolin is used in the following clinical settings to treat or prevent infections caused by susceptible organisms:

- Treatment of impetigo, cellulitis and erysipelas caused by MSSA. Cephalosporins are generally safe in possibly penicillin-allergic patients who are judged not to be at risk for immediate hypersensitivity reactions.
  Cloxacillin iv may be preferred as it has a narrower spectrum, aimed at gram positives; however, cefazolin is often preferred because of fewer doses per day, better stability when reconstituted, less irritation to the veins and it is less viscous when used in pumps (especially for home iv use).
  Also used in treatment of necrotizing infections of the skin, fascia and muscle [*Clin Infect Dis* 2005;41:1373-1406].
- Treatment of hematogenous osteomyelitis due to MSSA when culture and in vitro susceptibility results are known.
- Treatment of pyomyositis due to MSSA.
- Alternative treatment for MSSA community-acquired pneumonia [*Clin Infect Dis* 2007;44 (Suppl 2):S27-S72].
- Empiric treatment of acute, uncomplicated urinary tract infections when oral therapy is not feasible.
- Treatment of pyelonephritis. Because of increased resistance to first generation cephalosporins in the community, cefazolin should only be used when culture and in vitro susceptibility results are known. Fluroquinolones and trimethoprim-sulfamethoxazole are primary regimens for empiric treatment of acute pyelonephritis. Cefazolin is an option for treating pyelonephritis in pregnancy when the organism is susceptible and iv therapy is required.
- Peri-operative prophylaxis of surgical site infections.
- Prevention of intrapartum streptococcus group B infection of the infant in penicillin-allergic women not considered to be at risk of immediate hypersensitivity reactions [*MMWR* 2002;51(RR11):1-25].
- Treatment of infective endocarditis of native valves caused by cloxacillin-susceptible staphylococci strains. Given in combination with gentamicin, as treatment for penicillin-allergic patients who are not considered to be at risk of immediate hypersensitivity reactions. Treatment of infective endocarditis caused by *S. pyogenes* and highly penicillin susceptible *S. pneumoniae* in combination with gentamicin [*Circulation* 2005;111:3167-3184].
- Prevention of infective endocarditis in susceptible patients. Oral amoxicillin is preferred; however, parenteral cefazolin is recommended by the American Heart Association guidelines as an alternative in patients who are unable to take oral medications including patients who are allergic to penicillins and ampicillin [*Circulation* 2007;116:1736-1754].

Patients with any of the following conditions may benefit from cefazolin iv for prevention of infective endocarditis while undergoing certain dental or surgical procedures: prosthetic heart valves or prosthetic material used for the cardiac valve region, previous infective endocarditis, heart transplantation recipients who develop cardiac valvulopathy, congenital heart disease (unrepaired cyanotic congenital heart disease, including palliative shunts and conduits); repaired congenital heart disease with residual defects at the site or adjacent to the site of a prosthetic patch or prosthetic device which inhibits endothelialization; completely repaired congenital heart defect with prosthetic material or device, whether placed by surgery or by catheter intervention, during the first six months after the procedure [*Circulation* 2007;116: 1736-1754]. These are dental procedures that involve manipulation of gingival tissue or the periapical region of teeth or perforation of the oral mucosa, procedures on respiratory tract involving incision or biopsy of respiratory mucosa and procedures in patients with infected skin, skin structures or musculoskeletal tissue.

Antibiotic prophylaxis against infective endocarditis is not recommended for genitourinary or gastrointestinal tract procedures.

Cefazolin is no longer recommended for treatment of animal bites because of poor in vitro activity against *P. multocida*. Cefazolin is no longer recommended for treatment of human bites because of resistance of *E. corrodens*, a prominent aerobic pathogen, to first-generation cephalosporins [*Clin Infect Dis* 2005;41:1373-1406].

Cefazolin is an alternative to penicillins for the treatment of staphylococcal and nonenterococcal streptococcal infections.

Cefazolin does not penetrate the cerebrospinal fluid sufficiently to be used in the treatment of bacterial meningitis. Among cephalosporins, only the third-generation agents should be used in this clinical setting.

Cephalosporins, including cefazolin, have a long history of use for the treatment of infections in pregnancy and breast-feeding.

Orally administered probenecid inhibits urinary excretion of cefazolin, allowing once daily administration in home-based intravenous therapy programs or for the outpatient treatment of mild-to-moderate community-acquired skin and soft tissue infections.

Cefazolin has poor activity against Bacteroides species and is not suitable as monotherapy for the treatment of infections or the prophylaxis of surgical procedures involving the bowel. However, the combination of cefazolin plus intravenous metronidazole, which is active against anaerobes, is an inexpensive regimen that may be used for the treatment of community-acquired intra-abdominal infections.

CONTRAINDICATIONS:

- Patients who are hypersensitive to cefazolin or to any ingredient in the formulation.
- Patients who are hypersensitive to other cephalosporin antibiotics.

WARNINGS AND PRECAUTIONS:

Serious Warnings and Precautions

- Cefazolin has been associated with severe allergic reactions including anaphylactic reactions. For this reason a history of allergic reactions, including the type and severity of the reaction, should be obtained before prescribing and administering cefazolin.
- Cross-sensitivity between penicillins and cephalosporins is estimated to be very low. Current opinion on the true incidence of cross-sensitivity is about 1%. The beta-lactam subunit is not considered the primary allergenic determinant; rather, the side chain predicts cross-reactivity. After thorough investigation into the nature of the allergy, a cephalosporin can be considered in a penicillin allergic patient provided there is no history of an immediate-sensitivity reaction. Although the risk of cross-reaction is predicted to be low the patient should be monitored for signs of a sensitivity reaction.
- Patients with a history of immediate-sensitivity reaction to penicillin (e.g., anaphylaxis, bronchospasm and/or hypotension) are considered to be at increased risk of similar reactions to cephalosporins, including cefazolin. For this reason, administration of cefazolin should be avoided in patients with a history of severe allergic reactions to penicillin antibiotics unless skin testing is performed to rule out cross-sensitivity.
- Cephalosporin antibiotics including cefazolin have been associated with *C. difficile*-associated diarrhea and colitis.
- Cefazolin should not be administered into lateral ventricles of the brain as this causes seizures.

Special Populations: Pregnant Women: Pregnancy Category B_M. Cefazolin crosses the placenta. It is generally accepted that cephalosporins are safe to use during pregnancy.

Nursing Women: Cefazolin is distributed into breast milk in low concentrations. Potential effects on the nursing infant include disruption of the gut microbial flora or interference with accurate fever work-up. The American Academy of Pediatrics considers cefazolin to be compatible with breastfeeding.

ADVERSE REACTIONS: More Common Adverse Drug Reactions: See Table 1.

Table 1: Cefazolin

More Common Adverse Drug Reactions (≥1%)

Body System	Effect	Clinical Comment
Dermatologic	Rash, urticaria, pruritus	Manifestation of allergic reactions, which may be severe; hypersensitivity reactions can also include fever and chills, joint pain and/or inflammation
Gastrointestinal	Diarrhea	Generally mild. Resolves upon withdrawal of treatment
Neurologic	Headache	Generally mild

Less Common Adverse Drug Reactions (<1%): Gastrointestinal: *C. difficile*-associated diarrhea and colitis.
Hematologic: transient neutropenia, thrombocytopenia, hemolytic anemia (case report).
Hepatic/Biliary/Pancreatic: elevated serum liver transaminase levels.
Immune: hypersensitivity reactions (e.g., Stevens-Johnson syndrome, toxic epidermal necrolysis, erythema multiforme).
Neurologic: seizures in patients undergoing hemodialysis (case report).
Renal: interstitial nephritis (in combination with methenamine: case report).
Miscellaneous: serum sickness-like reaction (case report).

DRUG INTERACTIONS: Drug-Drug Interactions: See Table 2.

Table 2: Cefazolin

Drug-Drug Interactions

Interacting Drug	Effect	Clinical Comment
Probenecid	Inhibits renal tubular secretion of cefazolin, resulting in higher and more prolonged serum concentrations of cefazolin.	Co-administration of oral probenecid with cefazolin has been used therapeutically to reduce the frequency of administration of cefazolin.

Drug-Laboratory Interactions: Cefazolin may cause a positive direct and indirect Coombs' test. Reported in 3% or more of patients receiving a cephalosporin. Mechanism is usually nonimmunogenic (a cephalosporin-globulin complex binds to the erythrocyte and reacts nonspecifically with Coomb's serum). Actual immune-mediated hemolytic reactions have been reported rarely with first-generation agents such as cefazolin.

DOSAGE AND ADMINISTRATION: Recommended Dose and Dosage Adjustment: Adults: See Table 3.

Table 3: Cefazolin

Dose in Adult Patients

Indication	Route	Dose	Duration of Therapy	Clinical Comment
Treatment of community-acquired skin and soft tissue infections caused by MSSA (i.e., impetigo, cellulitis, erysipelas)	IV	1 g Q8H, maximum 12 g/day	10 days depending on response to therapy. Switch to a suitable oral antibiotic as soon as feasible.	As an alternative to parenteral cloxacillin. Recommended in penicillin-allergic patients not at high risk of immediate hypersensitivity reaction. Also used in the treatment of necrotizing infections of the skin, fascia and muscle. Cefazolin has been administered at a dose of 2 g Q12H for home-based treatment of skin and soft tissue infections.
Treatment of hematogenous osteomyelitis	IV	2 g Q8H, maximum 12 g/day	4–6 weeks	Treatment of hematogenous osteomyelitis due to MSSA when culture and in vitro susceptibility tests are known. Switch to a suitable oral antibiotic as soon as feasible.
Treatment of pyomyositis due to MSSA	IV	2 g Q8H, maximum 12 g/day	Average duration: 3–4 weeks. Duration of therapy may be prolonged if multiple muscle groups are involved or there has been delay in initiating therapy.	
Alternative treatment for methicillin-sensitive *S. aureus* community-acquired pneumonia	IV	1–2 g Q8H	10 days depending on response to therapy.	
Treatment of acute, uncomplicated urinary tract infections	IV	1 g Q8-12H		Empiric treatment for when oral therapy is not feasible.
Treatment of pyelonephritis	IV	1 g Q8H		Because of increased resistance to first generation cephalosporins in the community, cefazolin should only be used when culture and in vitro susceptibility results are known. Cefazolin is an option for treating pyelonephritis in pregnancy when the organism is susceptible and iv therapy is required.
Surgical prophylaxis for: high-risk biliary tract[a] or gastroduodenal[b] surgery, vaginal or abdominal hysterectomy, high-risk cesarean section[c], therapeutic abortion, craniotomy, CSF shunt surgery	IV	1–2 g starting 30 minutes to 1 hour prior to procedure	Single dose	2 g dose may be used for patients weighing >80 kg
Surgical prophylaxis for vascular surgery (e.g., abdominal aorta reconstruction, procedures involving a groin incision, brachial artery repair)	IV	1–2 g starting 30 minutes to 1 hour prior to procedure	Single dose	2 g dose may be used for patients weighing >80 kg
Surgical prophylaxis for colorectal surgery including appendectomy	IV	1 g starting 30 minutes to 1 hour prior to procedure	In combination with metronidazole iv 500 mg; single dose	
Surgical prophylaxis for head and neck surgery	IV	1 g starting 30 minutes to 1 hour prior to procedure	Single dose	
Surgical prophylaxis for urologic surgery and/or procedures	IV	1 g starting 30 minutes to 1 hour prior to procedure	Single dose	
Surgical prophylaxis for total prosthetic joint replacement	IV	1 g starting 30 minutes to 1 hour prior to procedure	May continue post-operatively Q8H for 24 hours	

(cont'd)

Table 3: Cefazolin *(cont'd)*

Dose in Adult Patients

Indication	Route	Dose	Duration of Therapy	Clinical Comment
Surgical prophylaxis for open heart surgery procedures (e.g., prosthetic valve, coronary artery bypass)	IV	1 g starting 30 minutes to 1 hour prior to procedure	Continue post-operatively Q8H for 24 to 48 hours	2 g dose may be used for patients weighing >80 kg
Surgical prophylaxis for pulmonary resection	IV	1 g starting 30 minutes to 1 hour prior to procedure	Continue post-operatively Q8H until chest tubes are removed for a maximum of 48 hours	
Prevention of group B streptococcal infection in neonates	IV	Starting at onset of labor or rupture of membranes: 2 g initially, then 1 g Q8H	Until delivery (or labor is stopped)	As an alternative to penicillin G in women who are allergic to penicillin but are not considered to be at risk of immediate hypersensitivity reactions. Consult local guidelines or those of the Society of Obstetricians and Gynaecologists of Canada for selection of patients for prophylaxis [*JOGC* 2004;26(9):826–832].
Treatment of native-valve endocarditis caused by cloxacillin-susceptible strains of Staphylococci	IV	cefazolin 2 g q8h (6 g/24 hours) ± gentamicin 3 mg/kg per 24 hours iv/im divided in 2 to 3 doses	Cefazolin: 6 weeks Gentamicin: 3–5 days	As an alternative to cloxacillin in patients who are allergic to penicillin but are not considered to be at risk of immediate hypersensitivity reactions [*Circulation* 2005;111: e394–e434].
Treatment of native-valve endocarditis in patients with highly susceptible *S. pneumoniae*, *S. pyogenes*, *S. gallolyticus subsp. gallolyticus* (formerly *S. bovis*) with penicillin G MIC >0.1 µg/mL to <0.5 µg/mL (intermediate sensitivity)	IV	cefazolin 2 g Q8H (6 g/24 hours) ± gentamicin 3 mg/kg per 24 hours iv/im divided in 2 to 3 doses	Cefazolin: 4 weeks Gentamicin: 2 weeks	Cefazolin is an alternative to penicillin G in patients who are allergic to penicillin but are not considered to be at risk of immediate hypersensitivity reactions. For penicillin-susceptible *S. pneumoniae* (MIC ≤1 µg/mL), treat with penicillin, cefazolin or ceftriaxone [*Circulation* 2005;111: e394–e434]; note that ceftriaxone is not indicated for intermediate sensitivity (MIC >0.1 µg/mL to <0.5 µg/mL).
Prevention of infective endocarditis prior to dental procedures	IM/IV	1 g 30–60 minutes before the procedure	Single dose	As an alternative to oral amoxicillin in patients who are allergic to penicillin, not considered to be at risk of immediate hypersensitivity reaction and unable to take oral medications.

[a] High-risk patients are aged >60 years, with obstructive jaundice, previous biliary surgery, acute cholecystitis, common duct stone, or non-functioning gall bladder. Not recommended in low-risk patients.
[b] High-risk patients are those with gastrointestinal bleeding, gastrointestinal obstruction, gastric ulcer or malignancy, decreased gastric motility, decreased gastric acidity or morbid obesity. Not recommended in low-risk patients.
[c] High-risk patients are those with premature rupture of membranes and/or onset of labor [*Clin Infect Dis* 2004;38:1706-1715]. Not recommended in low-risk patients.
Abbreviations: MSSA = methicillin-sensitive *S. aureus*

Pediatrics: See Table 4.

Table 4: Cefazolin

Dose in Pediatric Patients

Indication	Route	Dose	Duration of Treatment	Clinical Comment
Treatment of mild to moderately severe infections	IM/IV	25–50 mg/kg/day in divided doses Q6–8H	Depends on susceptibility of organisms and response to therapy.	Switch to a suitable oral antibiotic as soon as feasible.
Treatment of severe infections	IM/IV	100 mg/kg/day in divided doses Q6–8H	Depends on susceptibility of organisms and response to therapy.	Switch to a suitable oral antibiotic as soon as feasible.
Treatment of impetigo and for skin and soft-tissue infections	IV	50 mg/kg daily divided Q8H	Depends on susceptibility of organisms and response to therapy.	For penicillin-allergic patients except those with immediate hypersensitivity reactions.
Treatment of native-valve infective endocarditis who are culture positive for MSSA	IV	100 mg/kg per 24 hours divided Q8H plus gentamicin 3 mg/kg per 24 hours divided Q8H	Cefazolin: 6 weeks Gentamicin: 3–5 days	As an alternative to cloxacillin in patients who are allergic to penicillin but are not considered to be at risk of immediate hypersensitivity reactions.

(cont'd)

Table 4: Cefazolin *(cont'd)*

Dose in Pediatric Patients

Indication	Route	Dose	Duration of Treatment	Clinical Comment
Prevention of infective endocarditis prior to dental procedures	IM/IV	50 mg/kg 30 to 60 minutes before the procedure	Single dose	As an alternative to oral amoxicillin in patients who are allergic to penicillin, not considered at risk of immediate hypersensitivity reactions and unable to take oral medications.
Surgical prophylaxis for prosthetic valve or pacemaker insertion, high risk[a] esophageal and gastroduodenal surgery, neurosurgery (craniotomy), orthopedic surgery (internal fixation of fractures or prosthetic joints), thoracic surgery (noncardiac)	IV	25 mg/kg at least 30 minutes prior to surgical incision	Single dose	Single dose of cefazolin should be sufficient. Redosing may be needed for surgeries which take longer than 4 hours or if there is major blood loss.
Surgical prophylaxis for head and neck surgery (incision through oral or pharyngeal mucosa)	IV	25 mg/kg given at least 30 minutes before surgical incision	Single dose in combination with gentamicin 2 mg/kg	Single dose of cefazolin should be sufficient. Redosing may be needed for surgeries which take longer than 4 hours or if there is major blood loss.

[a] High risk if esophageal obstruction, decreased gastric acidity or gastrointestinal motility is present or patient is morbidly obese.
Abbreviations: MSSA = methicillin-sensitive *S. aureus*

Renal Impairment, Adults: See Table 5.

Table 5: Cefazolin

Dose in Adult Patients with Renal Impairment

Route	Creatinine Clearance (mL/minute)	Recommended Dose and Dosing Interval
IM/IV	>50	100% of dose, Q8H
IM/IV	10 to 50	100% of dose, Q12H
IM/IV	<10	50% of dose, Q24–48H

Renal Impairment, Pediatrics: See Table 6.

Table 6: Cefazolin

Dose in Pediatric Patients with Renal Impairment

Route	Creatinine Clearance (mL/minute)	Recommended Dose and Dosing Interval
IM/IV	30–50	100% of dose, Q8H
IM/IV	10–29	25 mg/kg dose Q12H
IM/IV	<10	25 mg/kg dose Q24H

Dosage in Dialysis: In patients receiving hemodialysis, cefazolin should be administered at a dose of 15-20 mg/kg after each dialysis session. In patients receiving continuous ambulatory peritoneal dialysis, cefazolin should be administered at a dose of 500 mg Q12H.

OVERDOSAGE:

For management of a suspected drug overdose, CPhA recommends that you contact your **regional Poison Control Centre**. See the *CPS* Directory section for a list of Poison Control Centres.

ACTION AND CLINICAL PHARMACOLOGY: Mechanism of Action: Cefazolin and other cephalosporin antibiotics interfere with peptidoglycan synthesis in bacterial cell walls by interacting with penicillin binding proteins. Cephalosporins, including cefazolin, are considered to be bactericidal and the effectiveness of the drug in killing bacteria is not considered to be concentration-dependent. Maximal bactericidal activity of cephalosporins is achieved at concentrations that are four times the minimal inhibitory concentration. Cephalosporins produce persistent suppression of bacterial growth (post-antibiotic effect) that lasts for several hours in the case of gram-positive bacteria, but not in the case of gram-negative bacteria.
Pharmacokinetics: Adults: See Table 7.

Table 7: Cefazolin

Pharmacokinetics Following IV Administration to Adults

Peak serum concentration after 1 g dose	193 mg/L
Plasma protein binding (%)	74 to 86%
Primary route of elimination	Excreted unchanged in the urine
Terminal elimination half-life	1.9 h
Terminal elimination half-life in end-stage renal disease	10 h

STORAGE AND STABILITY: Reconstituted powder for injection is stable at room temperature for 24 hours and for 10 days when stored at 5°C.

Cefazolin for Injection Pr

cefazolin sodium

Antibiotic

Apotex

Date of Preparation: July 5, 2007
Date of Revision: February 4, 2008

SUMMARY PRODUCT INFORMATION:

Route of Administration	Dosage Form/ Strength	Clinically Relevant Nonmedicinal Ingredients
Parenteral (I.V/I.M)	Powder for injection 1 g and 10 g cefazolin per vial	The formulation does not contain any nonmedicinal ingredients

INDICATIONS AND CLINICAL USE: Cefazolin for Injection is indicated in the treatment of the following serious infections due to susceptible strains of the listed organisms:

Respiratory Tract Infections caused by *S. pneumoniae*, *K. pneumoniae*, *H. influenzae*, *S. aureus* (penicillin-sensitive and penicillin-resistant) and group A beta-hemolytic streptococci.

Urinary Tract Infections caused by *E. coli*, *P. mirabilis*, *K. pneumoniae* and some strains of enterobacter and enterococci. See Note below.

Skin and Soft Tissue Infections caused by *S. aureus* (penicillin-sensitive and penicillin-resistant), group A beta-hemolytic streptococci and other strains of streptococci.

Bone and Joint Infections caused by *S. aureus*.

Septicemia caused by *S. pneumoniae*, *S. aureus* (penicillin-sensitive and penicillin-resistant), *P. mirabilis*, *E. coli* and *K. pneumoniae*. See Note below.

Endocarditis caused by *S. aureus* (penicillin-sensitive and penicillin-resistant) and group A beta-hemolytic streptococci.

Determine susceptibility of the causative organism to cefazolin sodium by performing appropriate culture and susceptibility studies.

Note: Most strains of Enterococci, indole positive proteus (*P. vulgaris*), *E. cloacae*, *M. morganii*, *P. rettgeri* and methicillin-resistant staphylococci are resistant. Serratia, Pseudomonas, and *A. calcoaceticus* (formerly Mima and Herellea species) are almost uniformly resistant to cefazolin.

Perioperative Prophylaxis: In patients undergoing potentially contaminated surgical procedures, and in patients in whom infection would pose a serious risk (e.g., during open-heart surgery and prosthetic arthroplasty), the preoperative, intraoperative and postoperative administration of Cefazolin for Injection may reduce the incidence of certain postoperative infections. Identification of the causative organisms should be made by culture should signs of infection occur, so that appropriate therapy may be instituted.

CONTRAINDICATIONS: Cefazolin sodium is contraindicated in patients with known allergy to the cephalosporin group of antibiotics.

WARNINGS AND PRECAUTIONS: Warnings: Cefazolin sodium should be used with caution in penicillin—allergic patients. There is clinical evidence of partial cross—allergenicity of the penicillins and the cephalosporins. There are instances of patients who have had reactions to both penicillins and cephalosporins (including fatal anaphylaxis after parenteral use). Clinical and laboratory evidence of partial cross—allerginicity of the two drug classes exists.

Cefazolin sodium should be administered cautiously and then only when absolutely necessary to any patient who has demonstrated some form of allergy particularly to drugs. Immediate emergency treatment with epinephrine is indicated for serious anaphylactoid reactions. As indicated, oxygen, intravenous steroids, and airway management, including intubation, should also be employed.

There have been reports of pseudomembranous colitis with the use of cephalosporins. It is, therefore, important to consider its diagnosis in patients who develop diarrhea in association with antibiotic use.

Precautions: General: The overgrowth of non-susceptible organisms may result from the prolonged use of cefazolin sodium. It is essential that the patient be carefully observed. In patients with a history of lower gastrointestinal disease, particularly colitis, cefazolin sodium should be prescribed with caution.

Clinitest tablets, but not enzyme—based tests such as Clinistix and Tes-Tape, may falsely indicate glucose in the urine of patients on cefazolin.

Positive direct and indirect Coombs' tests have been reported during treatment with cefazolin. These may also occur in neonates whose mothers received cephalosporins before delivery. The clinical significance of this effect has not been established.

Renal: Caution should be exercised in treating patients with pre-existing renal damage although cefazolin has not shown evidence of nephrotoxicity.

Patients with low urinary output due to impaired renal function should be administered reduced daily dosages of cefazolin. (See Dosage in Patients with Reduced Renal Function.) Blood levels of cefazolin in dialysis patients remain fairly high and should be monitored.

In beta-hemolytic streptococcal infections, treatment should be continued at least 10 days, to minimize possible complications associated with the disease.

Special Populations: Pregnant Women: The safe use of cefazolin sodium during pregnancy has not been established.

Nursing Women: Very low concentrations of cefazolin sodium are found in the milk of nursing mothers. Cefazolin sodium should be administered with caution to nursing women.

Pediatrics: The safe use of cefazolin sodium in premature infants and infants under one month of age have not been established.

ADVERSE REACTIONS: During clinical trials and post-marketing experience with cefazolin sodium the following adverse reactions have been observed.

Clinical Trial/Post-Market Adverse Drug Reactions: Because clinical trials are conducted under very specific conditions the adverse reaction rates observed in the clinical trials may not reflect the rates observed in practice and should not be compared to the rates in the clinical trials of another drug. Adverse drug reaction information from clinical trials is useful for identifying drug-related adverse events and for approximating rates.

Gastrointestinal: diarrhea, oral candidiasis (oral thrush), vomiting, nausea, stomach cramps, anorexia. During antibiotic treatment symptoms of pseudomembranous colitis can appear. There have been rare reports of nausea and vomiting.

Allergic: Allergic reactions occur infrequently and include: anaphylaxis, eosinophilia, itching, drug fever, skin rash.

Hematologic: neutropenia, anemia, leukopenia, thromocythemia, positive direct and indirect antiglobulin (Coombs') tests.

Hepatic and Renal: Without clinical evidence of renal or hepatic impairment transient increases in AST, ALT, BUN and alkaline phosphates levels have been observed. Transient hepatitis and cholestatic jaundice have been reported rarely, as with some penicillins and some other cephalosporins.

Local Reactions: Phlebitis at the site of injection occurred rarely. Infrequently there is pain at the site of injection following intramuscular injection. Some induration has been reported.

Other Reactions: vulvar pruritus, genital moniliasis, vaginitis and anal pruritus.

DRUG INTERACTIONS: The renal tubular secretion of cefazolin sodium may be decreased when probenecid is used concurrently, resulting in increased and prolonged cefazolin blood levels.

DOSAGE AND ADMINISTRATION: Dosing Considerations: After reconstitution cefazolin sodium may be administered either intramuscularly or intravenously. In both cases total daily dosages are the same.

Recommended Dose and Dosage Adjustment: Adults: See Table 1.

Cefazolin sodium has been administered in dosages of 6 g per day in serious infections such as endocarditis.

Treatment should be continued for at least 10 days in beta-haemolytic streptococcal infections to minimize possible complications associated with the disease.

Dosage in Patients with Reduced Renal Function: After an initial loading dose appropriate to the severity of the infection, the following reduced dosage schedule is recommended: See Table 2.

Table 1: Cefazolin for Injection
Recommended Dose

Type of Infection	Dose	Frequency
Mild infections caused by susceptible Gram-positive cocci	250 to 500 mg	Every 8 hours
Acute, uncomplicated urinary tract infections[a]	1 g	Every 12 hours
Moderate to severe infections	500 mg to 1 g	Every 6 to 8 hours

[a] This dosage recommendation applies to intramuscular use. The efficacy of cefazolin sodium when administered intravenously at 12-hour intervals has not been established.

Table 2: Cefazolin for Injection
Dosage in Patients with Reduced Renal Function

Creatinine Clearance (mL/s)	Serum Creatinine (µmol /L)	Dosage
≥0.91	≤140	250 mg to 1 g every 6–12 hours
0.58–0.90	141–273	250 mg to 1 g every 8–12 hours
0.18–0.57	274–406	125 mg to 500 mg every 12 hours
≤0.17	≥407	125 mg to 500 mg every 18 hours

Perioperative Prophylactic Use: The recommended dosage regimen to prevent postoperative infection in contaminated or potentially contaminated surgery is:

a. 1 gram intravenously (i.v.) or intramuscularly (i.m.) administered 1/2 hour to 1 hour prior to the start of surgery so that at the time of the initial surgical incision adequate antibiotic levels are present in the serum and tissues.
b. For lengthy operative procedures (e.g., 2 hours or more) 0.5 to 1 gram administered i.v. or i.m. during surgery. (Administration should be modified according to the duration of the operative procedure and the time of greatest exposure to infective organisms).
c. Postoperatively, 0.5 to 1 gram intravenously or intramuscularly every 6 to 8 hours postoperatively. The prophylactic administration of cefazolin sodium may be continued for 3 to 5 days following the completion of surgery where the occurrence of infection may be particularly devastating (e.g., open-heart surgery and prosthetic arthroplasty).

Children: A total daily dosage of 25 to 50 mg per kg of body weight, divided into three or four equal doses, is effective for most mild to moderately severe infections in children.

For severe infections total daily dosage may be increased to 100 mg per kg of body weight. The use of cefazolin in premature infants and in infants under one month is not recommended since safety for use in these patients has not been established. See Table 3 and Table 4.

Table 3: Cefazolin for Injection
Pediatric Dosage Guide (25 mg/kg/day)

Weight	25 mg/kg/day Divided into 3 Doses		25 mg/kg/day Divided into 4 Doses	
kg	Approximate Single Dose mg/q8h	Volume Needed of 125 mg/mL[a] Solution	Approximate Single Dose mg/q6h	Volume Needed of 125 mg/mL[a] Solution
4.5	40 mg	0.35 mL	30 mg	0.25 mL
9.0	75 mg	0.60 mL	55 mg	0.45 mL
13.6	115 mg	0.90 mL	85 mg	0.70 mL
18.1	150 mg	1.20 mL	115 mg	0.90 mL
22.7	190 mg	1.50 mL	140 mg	1.10 mL

[a] 125 mg/mL concentration may be obtained by reconstituting the 500 mg vial with 3.8 mL of diluent.

Table 4: Cefazolin for Injection
Pediatric Dosage Guide (50 mg/kg/day)

Weight	50 mg/kg/day Divided into 3 Doses		50 mg/kg/day Divided into 4 Doses	
kg	Approximate Single Dose mg/q8h	Volume Needed of 225 mg/mL[a] Solution	Approximate Single Dose mg/q6h	Volume Needed of 225 mg/mL[a] Solution
4.5	75 mg	0.35 mL	55 mg	0.25 mL
9.0	150 mg	0.70 mL	110 mg	0.50 mL
13.6	225 mg	1.00 mL	170 mg	0.75 mL
18.1	300 mg	1.35 mL	225 mg	1.00 mL
22.7	375 mg	1.70 mL	285 mg	1.25 mL

[a] 225 mg/mL concentration may be obtained by reconstituting the 500 mg vial with 2 mL of diluent.

Treatment with 60% of normal daily dose may be administered in divided doses every 12 hours to children with mild to moderate renal impairment (Clcr 0.67-1.17 mL/s). Children with moderate renal impairment (Clcr 0.33-0.67 mL/s) should be given 25 percent of the normal daily dose in equally divided doses every 12 hours, and children with severe renal impairment (Clcr 0.08-0.33 mL/s) should receive 10 percent of the normal daily dose every 24 hours.

All dosage recommendations apply after an initial loading dose.

Administration: Cefazolin sodium may be administered intravenously or intramuscularly after reconstitution.

Intramuscular: Inject the reconstituted solution into a large muscle mass. Pain on injection of cefazolin sodium occurs infrequently.

Intravenous: Direct i.v. (bolus) injection: Inject the appropriately diluted reconstituted solution slowly over 3 to 5 minutes directly into a vein or through tubing for patients receiving parenteral fluids.

Intermittent or Continuous Infusion: The reconstituted solution can be administered along with primary intravenous fluid management programs in a volume control set or in a separate secondary i.v. container.

Reconstitution: Parenteral Products: Parenteral drug products should be **shaken well** when reconstituted, and inspected visually for particulate matter prior to administration. The reconstituted solutions should be discarded, if particulate matter is evident.

Reconstituted solutions may range in colour from pale yellow to yellow without a change in potency. For intramuscular and direct intravenous injection, the reconstituted solutions should be stored in original containers (Type I USP glass vial and grey bromobutyl rubber stopper).

For Intramuscular Injection: Single Dose Vials: Reconstitute according to Table 5. **Shake well.**

Table 5: Cefazolin for Injection
Single Dose Vial Reconstitution Table

Strength	Diluent	Volume to be Added to Vial (mL)	Approximate Available Volume (mL)	Nominal Concentration (mg/mL)
500 mg	Sterile Water for Injection or	3.8	4.0	125
	Sodium Chloride 0.9% Injection	2.0	2.2	225
1 g	Sterile water for Injection	2.5	3.0	334

For Direct Intravenous (bolus) Injection: Single Dose Vials: Reconstitute as directed in Table 5. **Shake well.** A minimum of 10 mL of Sterile Water for Injection should be used to dilute the reconstituted solution. The reconstituted solutions should be stored in glass containers.

Pharmacy Bulk Vial: The Pharmacy Bulk Vial is intended for use in hospitals with recognized IV admixture programs and is restricted to **the preparation of admixtures for infusion. It is not for direct infusion.**

The Pharmacy Bulk Vial is intended for multiple dispensing of doses for intravenous use only, employing a single puncture. Reconstitute according to Table 6. **Shake well.** Visually inspect for particulate matter and discard the solution if present. Further dilute aliquot doses in one of the solutions listed below. Any unused reconstituted solution should be discarded after 8 hours.

Table 6: Cefazolin for Injection
Pharmacy Bulk Vial Reconstitution Table

Strength	Volume of Diluent to Add	Approximate Available Volume	Approximate Concentration
10 g	45 mL	50 mL	200 mg/mL
	96 mL	100 mL	100 mg/mL

For intermittent or continuous intravenous infusion, reconstituted cefazolin sodium may be further diluted as follows and stored in Large Volume Parenterals.

Single Dose Vials: Reconstitute according to Table 5. **Shake well.** Further dilute in 50 to 100 mL of one of the following solutions: Sodium Chloride 0.9%; Dextrose 5% or 10% in water; Dextrose 5% in Lactated Ringer's Injection; Dextrose 5% and Sodium Chloride Injection 0.9% (also maybe used with Dextrose 5% and Sodium Chloride Injection 0.45% or 0.2%); Lactated Ringer's Injection; Ringer's Injection; Sodium Bicarbonate 5% in Sterile Water for Injection.

Pharmacy Bulk Vial: Reconstitute according to Table 6. **Shake well.** Further dilute aliquots in 50 to 100 mL of Sterile Water for Injection or one of the solutions listed above.

The further diluted solutions should be used within 24 hours, at room temperature or 72 hours if stored under refrigeration from the time of initial puncture.

OVERDOSAGE:
There is a lack of experience with acute cefazolin sodium overdosage. Supportive therapy should be instituted according to symptoms in cases of suspected overdosage.

> For management of a suspected drug overdose, CPhA recommends that you contact your **regional Poison Control Centre**. See the *CPS* Directory section for a list of Poison Control Centres.

ACTION AND CLINICAL PHARMACOLOGY: Mechanism of Action: Cefazolin sodium is a cephalosporin antibiotic for parenteral administration. Cefazolin exerts its bactericidal effect by inhibiting bacterial cell wall synthesis. Cefazolin is about 85% bound to serum protein. The peak level in serum is approximately 32-42 mg/mL after an intramuscular (i.m.) injection of 500 mg. Over 80% of injected cefazolin is excreted in the urine during first 24 hours after i.m. injection; most is excreted during the first 4-6 hours.

Clinical Pharmacology: The blood levels of cefazolin listed in Table 7 and Table 8 were determined following intramuscular and intravenous administration.

Table 7: Cefazolin for Injection
Serum Concentration (mg/mL) Following Administration

	Time after Intravenous Injection in Minutes					
Cefazolin	**5**	**15**	**30**	**60**	**120**	**240**
1 g	188.4	135.8	106.8	73.7	45.6	16.5

Table 8: Cefazolin for Injection
Serum Concentration (mg/mL) Following Administration

	Time after Intramuscular Injection in Hours					
Cefazolin	**½**	**1**	**2**	**4**	**6**	**8**
1 g	65.8	68.3	60.6	29.3	11.2	6.5
500 mg	36.2	36.8	37.9	15.5	6.3	3.0
250 mg	15.5	17.0	13.0	5.1	2.5	<1.5

The serum half-life is approximately 1.8 hours following intravenous administration and 2.0 hours after intramuscular administration.

The mean peak serum levels of cefazolin in hospitalized patients are approximately equivalent to those seen in normal volunteers.

Healthy volunteers received a continuous intravenous infusion 3.5 mg/kg for 1 hour (approximately 250 mg) and 1.5 mg/kg hourly for the next two hours (approximately 100 mg). A steady serum level of 28 mg/mL was attained at the third hour.

Cefazolin levels in synovial fluid and serum are similar four hours after drug administration. Levels in cord blood are equivalent to 40% of those found in maternal blood.

In patients without obstructive biliary disease, serum levels of cefazolin can be up to five times lower than bile levels of cefazolin. However, bile levels of cefazolin are considerably lower than serum levels in patients with obstructive biliary disease.

Cefazolin is excreted unchanged in the urine. Approximately 60% of the drug is excreted in the first six hours, and this increases to 70%-80% within 24 hours. Peak urine concentrations of approximately 2400 μg/mL and 4000 μg/mL are achieved following intramuscular doses of 500 mg and 1 gram, respectively.

STORAGE AND STABILITY: Cefazolin for Injection should be stored between 15 and 25°C, protected from light.

Reconstituted vials of cefazolin sodium may be stored for 24 hours at controlled room temperature not exceeding 25°C, or for 72 hours under refrigeration (2 to 8°C), protected from light.

SPECIAL HANDLING INSTRUCTIONS: Not applicable.

INFORMATION FOR THE PATIENT: Published in e-CPS, available by subscription at www.e-cps.ca.

DOSAGE FORMS, COMPOSITION AND PACKAGING: Each clear glass vial of sterile powder contains: cefazolin sodium equivalent to 1 g of cefazolin. Each Pharmacy Bulk Vial of sterile powder contains: cefazolin sodium equivalent to 10 g of cefazolin.

Cefazolin for Injection USP Pr
cefazolin sodium
Antibiotic

Sandoz

SUPPLIED: 500 mg: Each vial of sterile powder contains: cefazolin 500 mg (as cefazolin sodium). Nonmedicinal ingredients: none. Glass vials of 15 mL, boxes of 10. Store between 15 and 25°C. Protect from light.

1 g: Each vial of sterile powder contains: cefazolin 1 g (as cefazolin sodium). Nonmedicinal ingredients: none. Glass vials of 15 mL, boxes of 10. Store between 15 and 25°C. Protect from light.

10 g: Each vial of sterile powder contains: cefazolin 10 g (as cefazolin sodium). Nonmedicinal ingredients: none. Pharmacy bulk glass bottles of 100 mL, boxes of 1. Store between 15 and 25°C. Protect from light.

Cefotaxime Sodium for Injection, BP Pr
cefotaxime sodium
Antibiotic

Hospira

Date of Preparation: April 4, 2008

PHARMACOLOGY: Cefotaxime Sodium is a semi-synthetic, 2-aminothiazolyl cephalosporin antibiotic for parenteral use. In vitro studies indicate that the antibacterial action of Cefotaxime Sodium results from inhibition of cell wall synthesis. It is stable against the action of most β-lactamases.

INDICATIONS: Treatment: Cefotaxime Sodium for Injection, BP may be indicated for the treatment of infections caused by susceptible strains of the designated micro-organisms in the diseases listed below.

Lower Respiratory Tract Infections: Pneumonia and lung abscess caused by *S. pneumoniae* (formerly *D. pneumoniae*), other streptococci (excluding enterococci, e.g. *S. faecalis*), *S. aureus* (penicillinase and non-penicillinase producing), *E. coli*, *H. influenzae*, (including ampicillin resistant strains) and unspecified Klebsiella species.

Urinary Tract Infections: Caused by *E. coli*, unspecified Klebsiella species (including *K. pneumoniae*), *P. mirabilis*, indole positive Proteus, *S. marcescens* and *S. epidermidis*. Also, uncomplicated gonorrhea caused by *N. gonorrhoeae*, including penicillin resistant strains.

Bacteremia/Septicemia: Caused by *E. coli*, unspecified Klebsiella strains and *S. marcescens*.

Skin Infections: Caused by *S. aureus* (penicillinase and non-penicillinase producing), *S. epidermidis*, group A streptococci, *E. coli*, *P. mirabilis* and indole positive Proteus.

Intra-Abdominal Infections: Caused by *E. coli*, and unspecified Klebsiella species.

Gynecological Infections: Including pelvic inflammatory disease, endometritis and pelvic cellulitis caused by *E. coli*, Group A streptococci and *S. epidermidis*; anaerobic bacteria including unspecified Peptococcus and Peptostreptococcus strains and some strains of *B. fragilis*. In several cases, although clinical cures were achieved, bacteriological follow-up was not available.

Cefotaxime Sodium, like other cephalosporins, has no activity against *C. trachomatis*. Therefore, when cephalosporins are used in the treatment of patients with pelvic inflammatory disease and *C. trachomatis* is one of the suspected pathogens, appropriate anti-chlamydial coverage should be added.

Central Nervous System Infections: Meningitis and ventriculitis caused by *H. influenzae*, *N. meningitidis*, *S. pneumoniae*, *K. pneumoniae* and *E. coli*. Cefotaxime Sodium is not active against *L. monocytogenes*.

Clinical experience with Cefotaxime Sodium in anaerobic infections is limited. Cefotaxime Sodium has been used with some success in wound and intra-abdominal infections against some strains of unidentified Bacteroides and anaerobic cocci.

Cefotaxime Sodium has been shown to be active against some strains of Pseudomonas.

In the treatment of infections encountered in immunosuppressed and granulocytopenic patients, results of therapy with Cefotaxime Sodium have not been impressive.

Cefotaxime Sodium should not be considered in the treatment of enterococcal infections, i.e. *S. faecalis*.

Specimens for bacteriologic culture should be obtained prior to therapy in order to isolate and identify the causative organisms and to determine their susceptibilities to Cefotaxime Sodium. Therapy may be instituted before results of susceptibility studies are known; antibiotic treatment should be re-evaluated once these results become available.

Prophylactic Use: The administration of Cefotaxime Sodium for Injection, BP perioperatively (preoperatively, intraoperatively and postoperatively) may reduce the incidence of certain infections in patients undergoing elective surgical procedures (e.g. abdominal or vaginal hysterectomy, gastrointestinal and genitourinary tract surgery) that may be classified as contaminated or potentially contaminated.

In patients undergoing caesarian section who are considered to be at increased risk of infection, intraoperative (after clamping the umbilical cord) and postoperative use of Cefotaxime Sodium for Injection, BP may also reduce the incidence of certain postoperative infections.

Effective use for elective surgery depends on the time of administration (see Dosage).

For patients undergoing gastrointestinal surgery, preoperative bowel preparation by mechanical cleansing as well as with a non-absorbable antibiotic (e.g. neomycin) is recommended.

If there are signs of infection, specimens for culture should be obtained for identification of the causative organism so that appropriate therapy may be instituted.

CONTRAINDICATIONS: Cefotaxime Sodium for Injection, BP is contraindicated in patients who have shown hypersensitivity to cefotaxime sodium, the cephalosporin or the penicillin groups of antibiotics.

WARNINGS: Anaphylactic Reactions: **Before therapy with Cefotaxime Sodium for Injection, BP is instituted, it must be carefully determined whether the patient has had previous hypersensitivity reactions to cefotaxime, cephalosporins, penicillins or other drugs. Since cross allergy exists between penicillins and cephalosporins in 5 to 10% of cases, Cefotaxime Sodium for Injection, BP should be given with extreme caution to patients with type 1 hypersensitivity reactions to penicillin. Antibiotics, including Cefotaxime Sodium for Injection, BP should be administered with caution to any patient who has demonstrated some form of allergy, particularly to drugs. If an allergic reaction to Cefotaxime Sodium for Injection, BP occurs, the drug should be discontinued and the patient treated with the usual agents (e.g. epinephrine, antihistamines, pressor amines or corticosteroids).**

Speed of I.V. Injection: During post-marketing surveillance, a potentially life-threatening arrhythmia was reported in very few patients who received a rapid bolus injection of cefotaxime through a central venous catheter. Therefore, cefotaxime should only be administered as instructed in Dosage.

C. difficile Associated Disease (e.g. pseudomembranous colitis): Treatment with broad spectrum antibiotics, such as Cefotaxime Sodium for Injection, BP, alters the normal flora of the colon and may permit overgrowth of *C. difficile* or other Clostridia. It has been established that a toxin produced by *C. difficile* is one primary cause of antibiotic-associated colitis.

Pseudomembranous colitis has been reported with the use of cephalosporins (and other broad spectrum antibiotics); therefore, it is important to consider its diagnosis in patients who develop diarrhea during the administration of Cefotaxime Sodium for Injection, BP. This colitis can range from mild to life-threatening in severity. The diagnosis of this rare but possibly fatal condition is confirmed by endoscopy and/or histology. Screening of feces for this pathogen and above all its cytotoxin, is the best way to diagnose *C. difficile* associated disease.

C. difficile **associated disease can be favoured by fecal stasis.**

Mild cases of colitis may respond to discontinuation of Cefotaxime Sodium for Injection, BP and replacement with a suitable specific antibiotic. Moderate to severe cases should be managed with fluid, electrolyte and protein supplementation as indicated. When the colitis is not relieved by discontinuance of Cefotaxime Sodium for Injection, BP administration or when it is severe, an antibiotic specifically effective in antibiotic-associated pseudomembranous colitis (e.g. vancomycin) or other suitable therapy may be indicated. Other possible causes of colitis should also be considered (see Adverse Effects).

PRECAUTIONS: Cefotaxime Sodium for Injection, BP should be prescribed with caution in individuals with a history of lower gastrointestinal disease, particularly colitis.

General: Prolonged use of Cefotaxime Sodium for Injection, BP may result in the overgrowth of nonsusceptible organisms. Constant evaluation of the patient's condition is essential. If superinfection occurs, therapy should be discontinued and appropriate measures taken.

As with other beta-lactam antibiotics, granulocytopenia and, more rarely, agranulocytosis may develop during treatment with Cefotaxime Sodium for Injection, BP particularly if given over long periods. For courses of treatment lasting longer than 10 days, blood counts should therefore be monitored and treatment stopped in the event of neutropenia.

Cefotaxime Sodium for Injection BP, like other parenteral anti-infective drugs, may be locally irritating to tissues. In most cases, perivascular extravasation of Cefotaxime Sodium for Injection, BP responds to changing of the infusion site. In rare instances, extensive perivascular extravasation of Cefotaxime Sodium for Injection, BP may result in tissue damage and require surgical treatment. To minimize the potential for tissue inflammation, infusion sites should be monitored regularly and changed when appropriate.

Pregnancy: Cefotaxime crosses the placental barrier. However, the safety of Cefotaxime Sodium for Injection, BP in pregnancy has not been established and it should not be used during pregnancy.

Use of Cefotaxime Sodium for Injection, BP in women of child-bearing potential requires that the anticipated benefits be weighed against the possible risks.

Lactation: Since cefotaxime is excreted in human milk in low concentrations, either breast feeding or treatment of the mother should be discontinued as necessary.

Patients with Special Diseases and Conditions: Although Cefotaxime Sodium rarely produces alterations in kidney function, evaluation of renal status is recommended, especially in severely ill patients receiving high doses.

Patients with markedly impaired renal function should be placed on the special dosage schedule recommended under Dosage, because normal dosage in these individuals is likely to produce excessive and prolonged serum antibiotic concentrations. If Cefotaxime Sodium for Injection, BP and aminoglycosides are to be administered to the same patient, these antibiotics should be administered separately and not as a mixed injection (see Dosage, Reconstitution, Incompatibilities). Renal function must be monitored in all such cases.

The sodium content of cefotaxime (48.2 mg/g) should be taken into account in patients necessitating sodium restriction.

Drug Interactions: Probenecid interferes with the renal tubular transfer of cephalosporins, thereby delaying their excretion and increasing their plasma concentrations.

As with other cephalosporins, cefotaxime sodium may potentiate the nephrotoxic effects of nephrotoxic drugs.

Laboratory Tests: Positive direct Coombs' test is known to develop in individuals during treatment with the cephalosporin group of antibiotics, including cefotaxime sodium.

In laboratory tests a false positive reaction to glucose may occur with reducing substances but not with the use of specific glucose oxidase methods.

ADVERSE EFFECTS: Clinical Trials: The most frequent adverse reactions with their frequency of occurrence are:

Central Nervous System (0.2%): headache.

Gastrointestinal (1.7%): colitis, diarrhea, nausea and vomiting. Symptoms of pseudomembranous colitis can appear during or after Cefotaxime Sodium treatment.

Genitourinary System (<1%): moniliasis, vaginitis.

Hematologic System (<1%): As with other β-lactam antibiotics, neutropenia and, more rarely, agranulocytosis may develop during treatment with Cefotaxime Sodium, particularly if given over long periods. Furthermore, transient leukopenia, eosinophilia and thrombocytopenia have also been reported.

Some individuals have developed positive direct Coombs' test during treatment with Cefotaxime Sodium and other cephalosporin antibiotics (see Precautions, Laboratory Tests). Rare cases of hemolytic anemia have been reported.

Hypersensitivity (1.8%): rash, pruritus, fever.

Kidney (<1%): Increased BUN has occasionally been observed.

Liver (<1%): Transient elevations in AST, ALT, serum LDH, and serum alkaline phosphatase levels have been reported.

Local (5%): injection site inflammation with intravenous administration. Pain, induration and tenderness after intramuscular injection.

Other Adverse Events Including Post-Marketing Surveillance Data: Anaphylactic Reactions: Angioedema, bronchospasm, malaise possibly culminating in shock, may rarely occur.

Cardiovascular: Potentially life-threatening arrythmia following rapid bolus infusion has been reported in very few patients who received rapid intravenous administration of Cefotaxime Sodium through a central venous catheter (see Warnings, Speed of I.V. Injection).

Central Nervous System: Administration of high doses of β-lactam antibiotics, including Cefotaxime Sodium, particularly in patients with renal insufficiency may result in encephalopathy (e.g. impairment of consciousness, abnormal movements and convulsions).

Cutaneous: rash, pruritus and less frequently urticaria. As with other cephalosporins, isolated cases of bullous eruptions (erythema multiforme, Stevens-Johnson syndrome, toxic epidermal necrolysis) have been reported.

Gastrointestinal: During treatment with Cefotaxime Sodium, abdominal pain may occur. As with all other broad spectrum antibiotics diarrhea may sometimes be a symptom of enterocolitis, which may, in some cases, be accompanied by blood in stools. A particular form of enterocolitis that can occur with antibiotics is pseudomembranous colitis which is in most cases due to *C. difficile* (see Warnings, *C. difficile* Associated Disease (e.g. pseudomembranous colitis)).

Kidney: Decreases in renal function (increase of creatinine) have been observed with cephalosporins, including Cefotaxime Sodium, particularly when co-prescribed with aminoglycosides.

As with some other cephalosporins, rare cases of interstitial nephritis have been reported in patients treated with Cefotaxime Sodium.

Liver: Transient elevations in gamma-GT and bilirubin levels have been reported.

Other: Superinfection: as with other antibiotics, the use of Cefotaxime Sodium, especially if prolonged, may result in overgrowth of nonsusceptible organisms. Repeated evaluation of the patient's condition is essential. If superinfection occurs during therapy, appropriate measures should be taken.

As reported with other antibiotics for the treatment of borreliosis, a Jarisch-Herxheimer reaction may develop during the first days of treatment.

The occurrence of one or more of the following symptoms has been reported after several week's treatment of borreliosis: skin rash, itching, fever, leucopenia, increase in liver enzymes, difficulty of breathing, joint discomfort. To some extent, these manifestations are consistent with the symptoms of the underlying disease for which the patient is being treated.

OVERDOSE:

Symptoms: There is a risk of reversible encephalopathy in cases of administration of high doses of β-lactam antibiotics including Cefotaxime Sodium for Injection, BP.

Treatment: No specific antidote exists.

For management of a suspected drug overdose, contact your regional Poison Control Centre. See the *CPS* Directory section for a list of Poison Control Centres.

DOSAGE: Cefotaxime Sodium for Injection, BP may be administered intramuscularly or intravenously after reconstitution (see Table 3 and Table 4 with recommended mode of reconstitution according to route of administration).

Dosage: Treatment for adults and children with body weight of 50 kg or more: The dosage of Cefotaxime Sodium for Injection, BP should be determined by susceptibility of the causative organisms, severity of the infection and condition of the patient.

The maximum daily dosage should not exceed 12 g.

Treatment for Neonates, Infants and Children: The following dosage schedule is recommended:

Neonates (birth to 1 month): 0-1 week of age: 50 mg/kg per dose IV every 12 hours.

1-4 weeks of age: 50 mg/kg per dose IV every 8 hours.

Infants and Children (1 month to 12 years): For body weights less than 50 kg, the recommended daily dose is 50 to 100 mg/kg IM or IV of body weight divided into 4 to 6 equal doses, or up to 180 mg/kg/day for severe infections (including central nervous system infections).

For body weights 50 kg or more, the usual adult dosage should be used. **The maximum daily dosage should not exceed 12 g.**

Table 1: Cefotaxime Sodium for Injection, BP

Guidelines for Dosage of Cefotaxime Sodium for Injection, BP for Adults and Children with Body Weight of 50 Kg or More

Type of Infection	Daily Dose (g)	Frequency and Route
Uncomplicated gonorrhea	1	1 g IM single dose
Uncomplicated infections	2	1 g every 12 hours IM or IV
Moderately severe to severe infections	3-6	1-2 g every 8 hours IM or IV
Very severe infections (e.g., septicemia, CNS)	6-8	2 g every 6-8 hours IV
Life-threatening infections	up to 12	2 g every 4 hours IV

Table 2: Cefotaxime Sodium for Injection, BP

Guidelines for Dosage of Cefotaxime Sodium for Injection, BP for Neonates, Infants and Children

Patients	Age or Weight	Dose	Route	Dose Interval
Neonates	0 to 1 week	50 mg/kg/**dose**	IV	Every 12 hours
Neonates	1 to 4 weeks	50 mg/kg/**dose**	IV	Every 8 hours
Infants and Children	<50 kg	50 to 100 mg/kg/**day** (up to 180 mg/kg/day for severe infections, including meningitis)	IV or IM	Divided into 4 to 6 equal doses
Children	≥50 kg	adult dosage		

Duration of Treatment: Administration of Cefotaxime Sodium for Injection, BP should be continued for a minimum of 48 to 72 hours after the patient defervesces or after evidence of bacterial eradication has been obtained; a minimum of 10 days of treatment is recommended for infections caused by Group A beta-hemolytic streptococci in order to guard against the risk of rheumatic fever or glomerulonephritis; frequent bacteriologic and clinical appraisal is necessary during therapy of chronic urinary tract infections and may be required for several months after therapy has been completed; persistent infections may require prolonged treatment. Doses less than those recommended should not be employed.

Prophylactic use: Surgery Patients: To prevent postoperative infection in contaminated or potentially contaminated surgery, recommended doses are as follows:

- 1 g IM or IV administered ½ to 1½ hours prior to the initial surgical incision to ensure that adequate antibiotic levels are present in the serum and tissues at the start of surgery.
- 1 g IM or IV administered 1½ to 2 hours following the first dose; for lengthy operative procedures, additional intraoperative doses may be administered, if necessary, at appropriate intervals (1½ to 2 hours) during surgery.
- 1 g IM or IV administered within 2 hours following completion of surgery

The total cumulative prophylactic dose should not exceed 6 g in a 12 hour period.

Caesarian Section Patients: The first dose of 1 g is administered IV as soon as the umbilical cord is clamped. The second and third doses should be given as 1 g IM or IV at 6 and 12 hours after the first dose.

Dosage for Patients with Impaired Renal Function: In patients with estimated creatinine clearance of less than 20 mL/min/1.73m², the dose of Cefotaxime Sodium for Injection, BP should be halved (see Precautions, Patients with Special Diseases and Conditions).

If serum creatinine values alone are available, the following formula (based on sex, weight and age of the patient) may be used to convert these values into creatinine clearance.

$$\text{Males: } \frac{\text{Weight (kg)} \times (140 - \text{age in years})}{72 \times \text{serum creatinine (mg/dL)}}$$

Females: 0.85×above value.

In Hemodialyzed Patients: 1 to 2 g daily, depending on the severity of the infection; on the day of hemodialysis, Cefotaxime Sodium for Injection, BP must be administered after the dialysis session.

Administration: Intramuscular: Cefotaxime Sodium for Injection, BP should be injected well within the body of a relatively large muscle such as the upper outer quadrant of the buttock (i.e. gluteus maximus); aspiration is necessary to avoid inadvertent injection into a blood vessel.

Intravenous: The intravenous route is preferable for patients with bacteremia, bacterial septicemia, or other severe or life-threatening infections, or for patients who may be poor risks because of lowered resistance resulting from such debilitating conditions as malnutrition, trauma, surgery, diabetes, heart failure, or malignancy, particularly if shock is present or impending.

For bolus administration, the solution containing Cefotaxime Sodium for Injection, BP must be injected over a period of 3 to 5 minutes (see Warnings, Speed of I.V. Injection).

Using an infusion system, it may also be given over a longer period of time through the tubing system by which the patient may be receiving other intravenous solutions. Butterfly or scalp vein type needles are preferred for this type of infusion. However, during infusion of the solution containing Cefotaxime Sodium for Injection, BP, it is advisable to discontinue temporarily the administration of other solutions at the same site (see Reconstitution, Incompatibilities).

Reconstitution: For Intramuscular Use: Cefotaxime Sodium for Injection, BP should be reconstituted with Sterile Water for Injection in accordance with the volumes recommended in Table 3.

Table 3: Cefotaxime Sodium for Injection, BP

Reconstitution Table for Intramuscular Use

	Volume to Be Added to Vial (mL)[a]	Approximate Available Volume (mL)	Approx. Average Concentration (mg/mL)
500 mg vial	2	2.2	230
1 g vial	3	3.4	300
2 g vial	5	6.0	330

[a] Shake to dissolve.

For Intravenous Use: For Intravenous Bolus Use: The 500 mg, 1 and 2 g vials should be reconstituted with at least 10 mL of Sterile Water for Injection.

For Intravenous Infusion Use: Reconstituted solution may be further diluted with 50 to 1000 mL of the fluids recommended for IV infusion.

Table 4: Cefotaxime Sodium for Injection, BP

Reconstitution Table for Intravenous Use

	Volume to Be Added to Vial (mL)[a]	Approximate Available Volume (mL)	Approx. Average Concentration (mg/mL)
500 mg vial	10	10.2	50
1 g vial	10	10.4	95
2 g vial	10	11.0	180

[a] Shake to dissolve.

Solutions for IV Infusion: Further dilution may be undertaken only in glass bottles.

Cefotaxime Sodium for Injection, BP is compatible with the following infusion fluids: Water for Injection, 0.9% NaCl Injection, 5% Dextrose Injection, 0.9% NaCl and 5% Dextrose Injection.

Incompatibilities: Solutions of Cefotaxime Sodium for Injection, BP must not be admixed with aminoglycoside solutions. If Cefotaxime Sodium for Injection, BP and aminoglycosides are to be administered to the same patient, they must be administered separately and not as a mixed injection.

Solutions of Cefotaxime Sodium for Injection, BP should not be prepared with diluents having a pH above 7.5 such as Sodium Bicarbonate Injection.

Stability and Storage: Solutions of Cefotaxime Sodium for Injection, BP range from light yellow to amber, depending on concentration and the diluent used. Store at controlled room temperature (15-30°C) protected from light. Single dose vials. Discard unused portion.

Cefotaxime Sodium for Injection, BP reconstituted in the original vial as described under Reconstitution maintains satisfactory potency for 12 hours at room temperature (25°C) and for 24 hours under refrigeration (2-8°C). Only freshly prepared reconstituted solutions may be further diluted with 50 to 1000 mL of the recommended infusion fluids in glass bottles. Such solutions maintain satisfactory potency for 12 hours at room temperature (25°C) and for 24 hours under refrigeration (2-8°C). Any unused solutions should be discarded.

Cefotaxime Sodium for Injection, BP solutions exhibit maximum stability in the pH 5 to 7 range.

Special Instructions: Parenteral drug products should be inspected visually for particulate matter and discoloration prior to administration. Solutions of Cefotaxime Sodium for Injection, BP range from light yellow to amber, depending on concentration and diluent used. The dry powder as well as solutions tend to darken, depending on storage conditions.

As with all parenteral drug products, intravenous admixtures should be inspected visually for clarity, particulate matter, precipitate, discoloration and leakage prior to administration, whenever solution and container permit. Solutions showing haziness, particulate matter, precipitate, discoloration or leakage should not be used. Discard unused portion.

SUPPLIED: Each vial of sterile, creamy white powder contains: cefotaxime sodium 500 mg, 1 g and 2 g. Single dose vials, boxes of 10.

Cefoxitin Pr

Antibacterial—Anti-infective

CPhA Monograph

Date of Preparation: October 2006
Date of Revision: August 2009

This monograph has been compiled by CPhA and reviewed by experts. It may contain information different from that found in Health Canada-approved Product Monographs. The reader is referred to the *CPS* Editorial Policy for more information.

SUMMARY PRODUCT INFORMATION:

Route of Administration	Dosage Form	Strength
Injectable (IM, IV)	Powder for injection	1 g, 2 g, 10 g vials

INDICATIONS AND CLINICAL USE: Cefoxitin is a parenteral cephamycin antibacterial agent that is grouped with the second-generation cephalosporins. The following gram-positive organisms are generally considered to be susceptible to cefoxitin: methicillin-susceptible *S. aureus* (although activity is reduced in comparison to first-generation cephalosporins), penicillin-susceptible *S. pneumoniae*, *S. pyogenes*, group B streptococci and viridans streptococci. The following gram-negative organisms are generally considered to be susceptible to cefoxitin: community-acquired strains of *E. coli*, *H. influenzae*, *K. pneumoniae*, *M. catarrhalis* and *P. mirabilis*. Cefoxitin has activity against *N. gonorrhoeae*, including penicillinase-producing strains although resistance is increasingly reported. Cefoxitin is active against anaerobic species including most, but not all, strains of *B. fragilis* and *Eikenella corrodens*.

Cefoxitin is indicated for the parenteral treatment of bacterial infections caused by susceptible organisms. These generally include the following clinical situations:

- treatment of hospital inpatients with pelvic inflammatory disease. Intravenous cefoxitin plus oral or iv doxycycline is considered to be a suitable primary regimen.
- treatment of mild-to-moderate community-acquired intra-abdominal infections attributable to mixed gastrointestinal flora. Such infections include diverticulitis, appendix rupture and bowel perforation.
- treatment of mild-to-moderate mixed aerobic/anaerobic soft tissue infections, including diabetic foot infections and animal or human bites.

Cefoxitin is also used to prevent surgical site infections primarily for gastrointestinal surgery but is also considered an alternative agent for gynecological surgery prophylaxis.

Cephalosporins, including cefoxitin, have a long history of use for the treatment of infections in pregnancy and breastfeeding.

It is recommended that cefoxitin not be used as monotherapy for blood stream infections attributed to *B. fragilis* in severely ill patients, because up to 15% of strains of this organism may not be susceptible to the drug.

Among the cephalosporin antibacterial agents, cefoxitin, cefotetan, ceftazidime and cefixime have the least activity against methicillin-susceptible *S. aureus*. For this reason cefoxitin is not an agent of choice for empirical or definitive treatment of infections caused by this organism.

The following organisms are generally resistant to cefoxitin: methicillin-resistant *S. aureus*, penicillin-resistant *S. pneumoniae*, enterococci and hospital-acquired gram-negative organisms, notably Pseudomonas spp. and *E. cloacae*. The causative organisms of "atypical" pneumonia (Legionella, Mycoplasma and Chlamydia spp.), *L. monocytogenes* and intracellular pathogens are resistant to all cephalosporins, including cefoxitin.

Resistance to cefoxitin appears to be due to the production of AmpC-type beta-lactamases and reduced outer membrane porin production. Cefoxitin remains susceptible to extended-spectrum beta-lactamases in vitro. The clinical significance of this is unknown, in particular because concurrent resistance determinants, such as ampC and loss of porin expression, may be present and testing of such is not readily available.

Cefoxitin does not penetrate the cerebrospinal fluid sufficiently to be used in the treatment of bacterial meningitis. Among cephalosporins, only the third-generation agents should be used in this clinical setting.

CONTRAINDICATIONS:

- Patients who are hypersensitive to cefoxitin or to any ingredient in the formulation.
- Patients who are hypersensitive to other cephalosporin antibiotics.

WARNINGS AND PRECAUTIONS:

Serious Warnings and Precautions

- Cefoxitin has been associated with severe allergic reactions including anaphylactic reactions. For this reason a history of allergic reactions, including the type and severity of the reaction, should be obtained before prescribing and administering cefoxitin.
- Cross-sensitivity between penicillins and cephalosporins is estimated to be very low. Current opinion on the true incidence of cross-sensitivity is about 1%. The beta-lactam subunit is not considered the primary allergenic determinant; rather, the side chain predicts cross-reactivity. After thorough investigation into the nature of the allergy, a cephalosporin can be considered in a penicillin allergic patient provided there is no history of an immediate-sensitivity reaction. Although the risk of cross-reaction is predicted to be low the patient should be monitored for signs of a sensitivity reaction.
- Patients with a history of immediate-sensitivity reaction to penicillin (e.g., anaphylaxis, bronchospasm and/or hypotension) are considered to be at increased risk of similar reactions to cephalosporins, including cefoxitin. For this reason, administration of cefoxitin should be avoided in patients with a history of severe allergic reactions to penicillin antibiotics unless skin testing is performed to rule out cross-sensitivity.
- Cephalosporin antibiotics including cefoxitin have been associated with *C. difficile*-associated diarrhea and colitis.

ADVERSE REACTIONS: More Common Adverse Drug Reactions: See Table 1.

Table 1: Cefoxitin

More Common Adverse Drug Reactions (≥1%)

Body System	Effect	Clinical Comment
Dermatologic	Rash, urticaria, pruritus	Manifestations of allergic reactions.
Gastrointestinal	Diarrhea	Generally mild; resolves upon withdrawal of treatment.
Local Reactions	Pain and tenderness after im injection using water	May be reconstituted with lidocaine 0.5 or 1% solution (without epinephrine) to reduce discomfort.

Less Common Adverse Drug Reactions (<1%): Cardiovascular: hypotension.
Gastrointestinal: nausea and vomiting. *C. difficile*-associated diarrhea and colitis. Severe persistent diarrhea including cases that arise after withdrawal of treatment may be attributable to *C. difficile* and should be evaluated accordingly.
Hematologic: transient neutropenia, thrombocytopenia and anemia. Aplastic anemia, pancytopenia and hemolytic anemia have been reported in association with cephalosporin antibiotics.
Hepatic/Biliary/Pancreatic: elevated serum transaminase levels.
Immune: hypersensitivity reactions; angioedema, eosinophilia, serum sickness-like reactions, anaphylaxis.
Renal: elevated BUN, elevated serum creatinine, interstitial nephritis, renal toxicity (rare).

DRUG INTERACTIONS: Drug-Drug Interactions: See Table 2.

Table 2: Cefoxitin

Drug-Drug Interactions

Interacting Drug	Effect	Clinical Comment
Aminoglycosides	The combination of aminoglycosides and cephalosporins may increase the incidence of nephrotoxicity.	Monitor kidney function.
Anticoagulants	Increased anticoagulant effect.	An 8% bleeding rate has been reported in patients receiving the combination of an anticoagulant and cefoxitin. The mechanism may involve interference with vitamin K production. Monitor INR in patients receiving concurrent anticoagulants and adjust the dose accordingly. Vitamin K may be administered in the event that bleeding occurs.
Probenecid	Inhibits renal tubular secretion of cefoxitin, resulting in higher and prolonged serum concentrations of cefoxitin.	Coadministration of oral probenecid with cefoxitin has been used therapeutically in the outpatient treatment of pelvic inflammatory disease.

Drug-Laboratory Interactions: A false-positive reaction for glucose may be produced by cefoxitin in urine when copper reduction tests such as Benedict's, Fehling's solution or Clinitest tablets are used; this is, however, not seen with enzyme-based tests.

Cefoxitin may cause a positive direct Coombs' test.

Falsely elevated serum or urine creatinine measurements may occur during cefoxitin treatment when using tests that employ the Jaffé reaction.

DOSAGE AND ADMINISTRATION: Recommended Dose and Dosage Adjustment: Geriatric patients should receive the usual adult doses of cefoxitin, although adjustments for renal dysfunction may be required more frequently in this population. See Table 3.

Table 3: Cefoxitin

Dose in Adult Patients

Indication	Route	Usual Dose	Maximum Dose	Duration of Therapy	Clinical Comment
Treatment of Infection					
Inpatient treatment of pelvic inflammatory disease	IV	2 g Q6H in combination with oral or iv doxycycline 100 mg Q12H	12 g/day	Parenteral and oral therapy should be administered for a total of 14 days.	Switch to oral antibiotics as soon as feasible.
Outpatient treatment of pelvic inflammatory disease	IM	2 g single dose in combination with a single oral dose of probenecid 1 g, plus doxycycline 100 mg twice daily for 14 days	2 g	Single dose	Other more convenient regimens are recommended as first choice for the treatment of this condition.

(cont'd)

Table 3: Cefoxitin *(cont'd)*

Dose in Adult Patients

Indication	Route	Usual Dose	Maximum Dose	Duration of Therapy	Clinical Comment
Intra-abdominal infections (peritonitis, diverticulitis, acute cholecystitis)	IV	1–2 g Q6–8H	12 g/day	Dependent upon susceptibility of organisms and response to therapy. Generally 7 to 10 days of parenteral and oral therapy is administered.	Switch to a suitable oral antibiotic as soon as feasible.
Urinary tract infection	IV	1–2 g Q6–8H	12 g/day	Dependent upon susceptibility of organisms and response to therapy. A total of 14 days of parenteral and oral therapy is generally recommended for pyelonephritis.	Many other agents available and preferred as first line therapy. Switch to a suitable oral antibiotic as soon as feasible.
Skin and soft tissue infection	IV	1–2 g Q6–8H	12 g/day	Dependent upon susceptibility of organisms and response to therapy.	Switch to a suitable oral antibiotic as soon as feasible.
Prophylaxis of Infection					
Gastrointestinal surgery, including appendectomy	IV	1–2 g 30 to 60 minutes prior to surgery	12 g/day	Pre-op plus intraoperatively Q2–3H for surgeries >4 hours.	Some clinicians continue Q6H after surgery for up to 24 hours. This practice is generally not necessary and may promote resistant organisms.

Pediatrics: See Table 4.

Table 4: Cefoxitin

Dose in Pediatric Patients

Indication	Route	Age	Usual Dose	Maximum Dose	Duration of Therapy	Clinical Comment
As indicated for adults (see Table 3)	IM/IV	≥3 months of age	80–160 mg/kg/day divided Q4–6H	12 g/day	Dependent upon susceptibility of organisms and response to therapy.	Switch to a suitable oral antibiotic as soon as feasible.
Surgical prophylaxis	IV	≥3 months of age	20–40 mg/kg 30 to 60 minutes prior to surgery	12 g/day	Pre-op plus Q2–3H for surgeries >4 hours' duration or significant blood loss.	

Renal Impairment: See Table 5.

Table 5: Cefoxitin

Dose in Adult Patients with Renal Impairment

Route	Creatinine Clearance (mL/min)	Dosage Adjustment
IM/IV	30–50	1–2 g Q8–12H
IM/IV	10–29	1–2 g Q12–24H
IM/IV	5–9	0.5–1 g Q12–24H
IM/IV	<5	0.5–1 g Q24–48H

Dialysis: A 1-2 g dose should be administered after each dialysis session.
Hepatic Impairment: No dosage adjustments are required in patients with hepatic impairment.
Administration: Cefoxitin may be administered by iv or im injection. For im injection, the dose may be prepared with 2 mL of either sterile water for injection or lidocaine HCl 0.5 or 1% solution (without epinephrine), for each 1 g of cefoxitin powder.

OVERDOSAGE:

For management of a suspected drug overdose, CPhA recommends that you contact your **regional Poison Control Centre**. See the *CPS* Directory section for a list of Poison Control Centres.

ACTION AND CLINICAL PHARMACOLOGY: Mechanism of Action: Similar to the mode of action of cephalosporin antibiotics, cefoxitin and other cephamycins interfere with peptidoglycan synthesis in bacterial cell walls by covalently binding to penicillin-binding proteins. Cefoxitin is bactericidal and its effectiveness in killing bacteria is not considered to be concentration-dependent. Maximal bactericidal activity of cephalosporins and cephamycins is achieved at concentrations that are four times the minimal inhibitory concentration. Cephalosporins and cephamycins produce persistent suppression of bacterial growth (i.e., the post-antibiotic effect) that lasts for several hours in the case of gram-positive bacteria, but not in the case of gram-negative bacteria.
Pharmacokinetics: Adults: See Table 6.

Table 6: Cefoxitin

Summary of the Pharmacokinetic Properties of Cefoxitin After a 1 g Injection in Adults

Peak serum concentration after 1 g iv dose	110 µg/mL
Plasma protein binding	41–79%
Primary route of elimination	Renal excretion (90%)
Terminal elimination half-life	0.8–1.0 h
Terminal elimination half-life in end-stage renal disease	10–22 h
CSF concentration after 1 g iv dose	1.2–22 µg/mL

STORAGE AND STABILITY: Reconstituted powder for injection is stable at room temperature for 24 hours.

Cefprozil Pr
Antibiotic

CPhA Monograph

Date of Preparation: July 2008
Date of Revision: September 2009

This monograph has been compiled by CPhA and reviewed by experts. It may contain information different from that found in Health Canada-approved Product Monographs. The reader is referred to the *CPS* Editorial Policy for more information.

SUMMARY PRODUCT INFORMATION:

Route of Administration	Dosage Form	Strength
Oral	Tablet	250 mg, 500 mg
	Powder for solution	125 mg/5 mL, 250 mg/5 mL

INDICATIONS AND CLINICAL USE: Cefprozil is used predominantly for certain respiratory conditions because of its activity against sensitive *S. pneumoniae*, *H. influenza* and *M. catarrhalis*. It is used in the following clinical settings to treat infections caused by susceptible organisms:

- Alternative treatment to penicillin G or amoxicillin in adults with community-acquired pneumonia with penicillin-sensitive *S. pneumoniae* (MIC <2 µg/mL).
- Treatment of acute otitis media in children who have failed high-dose amoxicillin treatment or who do not like the taste of cefuroxime axetil suspension. Also, second-line therapy in adults with acute otitis media.
- Treatment of pharyngitis due to Group A β-hemolytic *S. pyogenes* in children and adults who are allergic to penicillin but who do not have an immediate hypersensitivity type reaction to β-lactam antibiotics. Penicillin is the treatment of choice for Group A streptococcal pharyngitis.
- Alternative therapy for the treatment of acute bacterial sinusitis in children and adults who have failed first-line agents or who cannot tolerate cefuroxime axetil.
- Treatment of acute exacerbations of chronic obstructive pulmonary disease (COPD) in patients with 2 of the 3 symptoms of increased sputum purulence, increased sputum volume and increased dyspnea, and who have no other risk factors that may increase the likelihood of treatment failure or association of more virulent and/or resistant bacteria.
- Second-line therapy for the treatment of uncomplicated urinary tract infections in children between the ages of 2 months and 12 years.

Though cefprozil is indicated for treating skin and soft tissue infections, current guidelines recommend cefazolin iv and cephalexin po, as alternatives to cloxacillin iv/po, for the treatment of skin and soft tissue infections due to methicillin-sensitive *S. aureus*.

CONTRAINDICATIONS:

- Patients who are hypersensitive to cefprozil or to any ingredient in the formulation.
- Patients who are hypersensitive to cephalosporins or to other β-lactam antibiotics.

WARNINGS AND PRECAUTIONS:

Serious Warnings and Precautions

- Cefprozil has been associated with severe allergic reactions including anaphylactic reactions. For this reason a history of allergic reactions, including the type and severity of the reaction, should be obtained before prescribing and administering cefprozil.
- Cross-sensitivity between penicillins and cephalosporins is estimated to be very low. Current opinion on the true incidence of cross-sensitivity is about 1%. The beta-lactam subunit is not considered the primary allergenic determinant; rather, the side chain predicts cross-reactivity. After thorough investigation into the nature of the allergy, a cephalosporin can be considered in a penicillin allergic patient provided there is no history of an immediate-sensitivity reaction. Although the risk of cross-reaction is predicted to be low the patient should be monitored for signs of a sensitivity reaction.
- Patients with a history of immediate-sensitivity reaction to penicillin (e.g., anaphylaxis, bronchospasm and/or hypotension) are considered to be at increased risk of similar reactions to cephalosporins, including cefprozil. For this reason, administration of cefprozil should be avoided in patients with a history of severe allergic reactions to penicillin antibiotics unless skin testing is performed to rule out cross-sensitivity.
- Cephalosporin antibiotics including cefprozil have been associated with *C. difficile*-associated diarrhea and colitis.

Dermatologic: Cefprozil should be used with caution if infectious mononucleosis is suspected, due to an increased incidence of maculopapular rash when it is used in this setting.
Renal: Nephrotoxicity has been reported rarely with cephalosporins, and is more likely in older individuals, or in patients who are taking other nephrotoxic drugs concomitantly or have pre-existing renal impairment. Since cefprozil is renally cleared, dosage adjustment is recommended in patients with impaired renal function (see Table 5 and Table 6).
Special Populations: Pregnant Women: Pregnancy Category B_M. Although it has not been unequivocally established that there is not an increased risk of birth defects with the use of cefprozil, it is generally accepted that cephalosporins are safe to use during pregnancy.
Nursing Women: Cefprozil is excreted in breast milk in low concentrations. Potential risks to the infant include altered bowel flora, diarrhea, obscured diagnosis of fever and hypersensitivity reactions. According to the American Academy of Pediatrics, cefprozil is compatible with breastfeeding.
Pediatrics: Safety and efficacy of cefprozil in infants less than 6 months of age has not been established. In newborn infants, there have been reports of accumulation of other cephalosporins possibly because of prolonged half-life of cephalosporins in this age group.
Geriatrics: Clearance of cefprozil may be reduced in this population. Monitor renal function and adjust dose accordingly (see Table 5).
ADVERSE REACTIONS: Adverse Drug Reactions Overview: More Common Adverse Drug Reactions: See Table 1.

Table 1: Cefprozil

More Common Adverse Drug Reactions (≥1%)

Body System	Effect	Clinical Comment
Gastrointestinal	Diarrhea, nausea, vomiting	
Dermatologic	Rash (hypersensitivity)	Commonly seen in children more than in adults.

Less Common Adverse Drug Reactions (<1%): Central Nervous System: dizziness, confusion, fever, headache, insomnia, somnolence, hyperactivity.
Allergic/Dermatologic: generalized maculopapular rash, Stevens-Johnson syndrome, exfoliative dermatitis.
Gastrointestinal: abdominal pain.
Genitourinary: vaginal yeast infections, genital pruritus.
Hematologic: leukopenia, transient decreases in leukocyte count and eosinophilia, thrombocytopenia.
Hepatic/Biliary/Pancreatic: hepatitis, cholestatic jaundice, transient elevations of aspartate aminotransferase, alanine transaminase, alkaline phosphatase and bilirubin.
Renal: elevated BUN and serum creatinine.
Miscellaneous: serum sickness-like reactions.

DRUG INTERACTIONS: Drug-Drug Interactions: See Table 2.

Table 2: Cefprozil

Drug-Drug Interactions

Interacting Drug	Effect	Clinical Comment
Probenecid	Probenecid inhibits renal tubular excretion of cefprozil, thereby ↓ elimination of cefprozil.	This interaction has been exploited to increase serum levels of penicillins. The area under the curve for cefprozil is doubled with concomitant administration of probenecid.

Drug-Food Interactions: Cefprozil can be taken with or without food; the pharmacokinetics of cefprozil are not altered when taking it with food.
Drug-Laboratory Interactions: A false-positive reaction for glucose may be produced by cefprozil in urine when copper reduction tests such as Benedict's, Fehling's solution or Clinitest tablets, are used; this is, however, not seen with enzyme-based tests. A false-negative reaction for glucose may be produced by cefprozil in the blood when using the ferricyanide test.

DOSAGE AND ADMINISTRATION: Dosing Considerations:

- To promote less variation in peak and trough serum levels of cefprozil, administer around-the-clock, e.g., Q12H not BID.
- The reconstituted oral suspension is stable under refrigeration, between 2 to 8°C, for up to 14 days; discard unused portion afterwards.

Recommended Dose and Dosage Adjustment: Adults: See Table 3.

Table 3: Cefprozil

Dose in Adult Patients

Indication	Usual Dose	Duration of Therapy	Clinical Comment
Pneumonia	500 mg po Q12H	Optimal duration is unknown. Historically, duration ranged from 10 to 14 days depending on whether the patient is to be hospitalized, virulence of etiologic agent, and presence of comorbidities and rate of response.	Alternative therapy to penicillin G or amoxicillin for penicillin-sensitive *S. pneumoniae* (MIC <2 μg/mL). Cefprozil has no activity against atypical pathogens.
Sinusitis	250–500 mg po Q12H	10 to 14 days	
Pharyngitis	500 mg po daily	10 days	
Acute Otitis Media	250–500 mg po Q12H	10 days	
Acute exacerbations of COPD	500 mg po Q12H	10 days	Second-generation oral cephalosporins are considered first-line therapy in patients with COPD with no risk factors[a] and who have 2 of 3 symptoms: increased sputum purulence, increased sputum volume and dyspnea.

[a] Risk factors include one of the following: FEV_1 <50% predicted, ≥4 exacerbations per year, ischemic heart disease, use of home oxygen, chronic oral steroid use.

Pediatrics: See Table 4.

Table 4: Cefprozil

Dose in Pediatric Patients

Indication	Usual Dose	Duration of Therapy	Clinical Comment
Acute otitis media	>6 months to 12 years: 30 mg/kg po daily divided Q12H, maximum 1 g daily	<2 y: 10 days ≥2 y: 5–7 days	Consider cefprozil if the patient has failed high-dose amoxicillin therapy or cannot tolerate cefuroxime axetil suspension.
Sinusitis	>6 months to 12 years: 30 mg/kg po daily divided Q12H, maximum 1 g daily	10 to 14 days	Compared to cefuroxime axetil, cefprozil has inferior coverage of Haemophilus species and penicillin-intermediate *S. pneumoniae*.

(cont'd)

Table 4: Cefprozil *(cont'd)*

Dose in Pediatric Patients

Indication	Usual Dose	Duration of Therapy	Clinical Comment
Pharyngitis	2 to 12 years: 15 mg/kg po daily divided Q12H, maximum 1 g daily	10 days	A meta-analysis of cephalosporin versus penicillin treatment of group A streptococcal tonsillopharyngitis, concluded that cephalosporins had a better bacteriologic and clinical cure rate than penicillins, but may increase selection pressure.
Uncomplicated urinary tract infection	2 months to 12 years: 30 mg/kg po daily divided Q12H	7 to 10 days	

Renal Impairment: See Table 5 and Table 6.

Table 5: Cefprozil

Dose in Adult Patients with Renal Impairment

Creatinine Clearance	Dose and Interval Adjustment
>50 mL/min	100% of dose at usual interval
10–50 mL/min	50% of dose at usual interval
<10 mL/min	50% of dose at usual interval

Table 6: Cefprozil

Dose in Pediatrics with Renal Impairment

Creatinine Clearance	Dose and Interval Adjustment
30–50 mL/min	100% of dose at usual interval
10–29 mL/min	7.5 mg/kg at usual interval
<10 mL/min	7.5 mg/kg at usual interval

Dialysis: Cefprozil is removed by hemodialysis. In adults, administer an additional dose of 250 mg after hemodialysis. In children on hemodialysis, the dose of cefprozil to be administered is 7.5 mg/kg Q12H. A supplemental dose of 5 mg/kg should be given post-dialysis to children.
Hepatic Impairment: No dose adjustment is necessary when administering cefprozil in patients with hepatic impairment.

OVERDOSAGE:

For management of a suspected drug overdose, CPhA recommends that you contact your **regional Poison Control Centre**. See the *CPS* Directory section for a list of Poison Control Centres.

ACTION AND CLINICAL PHARMACOLOGY: Mechanism of Action: Cefprozil is a bactericidal second-generation cephalosporin. It inhibits peptidoglycan synthesis in the bacterial cell wall leading to the formation of a defective cell wall with eventual lysis and cell death.

The spectrum of activity of cefprozil includes methicillin-susceptible *S. aureus* (MSSA), penicillin-sensitive *S. pneumoniae*, β-haemolytic Streptococci, Moraxella and Pasteurella species. Cefprozil possesses little or no activity against methicillin-resistant *S. aureus*, penicillin-resistant *S. pneumoniae*, Enterococcus species, *S. saprophyticus*, Enterobacteriaceae-producing inducible β-lactamases and extended spectrum β-lactamases, anaerobic gram-negative bacilli, and Chlamydia, Pseudomonas, Bordetella and Mycoplasma species.

Pharmacokinetics: Adults: Absorption: Cefprozil is well absorbed after oral administration in fasting and nonfasting subjects, with a bioavailability of about 90%. Peak plasma concentration occurs within 1.5 hours under fasting conditions. Mean peak serum concentrations of 6.1, 10.5 and 18.3 μg/mL were achieved in 12 young and healthy, fasting male volunteers who received single doses of 250 mg, 500 mg or 1 g of cefprozil, respectively.
Distribution: The plasma half-life of cefprozil is 1.3 hours and is prolonged in patients with renal insufficiency (5.2-6 hours). Cefprozil is not highly protein-bound (35-45%); binding is independent of drug concentrations in the range of 2 to 20 μg/mL. In healthy adults with normal renal function, the volume of distribution of cefprozil is estimated to be 0.23 L/kg. Cefprozil distributes into tissues and fluids including tonsillar and adenoidal tissues, and middle ear fluid.
Excretion: Cefprozil is excreted unchanged in the urine by glomerular filtration and tubular secretion. Average cefprozil concentrations in the urine following single doses of 250 mg, 500 mg and 1 g over the first 4 hours in 12 young and healthy, fasting male volunteers, were 700, 1000 and 2900 μg/mL, respectively. Renal clearance of cefprozil is between 1.78 and 2.53 mL/minute/kg.

Ceftin® Ⓟ

cefuroxime axetil

Antibiotic

GlaxoSmithKline

Date of Revision: November 19, 2008

PHARMACOLOGY: Cefuroxime axetil is an orally active prodrug of cefuroxime. After oral administration, cefuroxime axetil, as CEFTIN, is absorbed from the gastrointestinal tract and rapidly hydrolyzed by nonspecific esterases in the intestinal mucosa and blood to release cefuroxime into the blood stream. Conversion to cefuroxime, the microbiologically active form, occurs rapidly. The inherent properties of cefuroxime are unaltered after its administration as cefuroxime axetil. Cefuroxime exerts its bactericidal effect by binding to an enzyme or enzymes referred to as penicillin-binding proteins (PBPs) involved in bacterial cell wall synthesis.

This binding results in inhibition of bacterial cell wall synthesis and subsequent cell death. Specifically, cefuroxime shows high affinity for PBP 3, a primary target for cefuroxime in gram-negative organisms such as *E. coli*.

INDICATIONS: CEFTIN (cefuroxime axetil) is indicated for the treatment of patients with mild to moderately severe infections caused by susceptible strains of the designated organisms in the following diseases:

Upper Respiratory Tract Infections: Pharyngitis and tonsillitis caused by *S. pyogenes*. Otitis Media caused by *S. pneumoniae*, *S. pyogenes* (group A beta-hemolytic streptococci), *H. influenzae* (beta-lactamase negative and beta-lactamase positive strains) or *M. catarrhalis*. Sinusitis caused by *M. catarrhalis*, *S. pneumoniae* or *H. influenzae* (including ampicillin-resistant strains).
Lower Respiratory Tract Infections: Pneumonia or bronchitis caused by *S. pneumoniae*, *H. influenzae* (including ampicillin-resistant strains), *H. parainfluenzae*, *K. pneumoniae* or *M. catarrhalis*.
Skin Structure Infections: Skin structure infections caused by *S. aureus*, *S. pyogenes* or *S. agalactiae*.
Gonorrhea: Acute uncomplicated urethritis and cervicitis caused by *N. gonorrheae*.

Bacteriologic studies to determine the causative organism and its susceptibility to cefuroxime should be performed. Once these results become available, antibiotic treatment should be adjusted if required.

CONTRAINDICATIONS: CEFTIN (cefuroxime axetil) is contraindicated for patients who have shown Type 1 hypersensitivity to cefuroxime, to any of its components, or to any of the cephalosporin group of antibiotics.

WARNINGS: Before therapy with CEFTIN (cefuroxime axetil) is instituted, careful inquiry should be made to determine whether the patient has had previous hypersensitivity reactions to cefuroxime, cephalosporins, penicillin, or other drugs. CEFTIN should be administered with caution to any patient who has demonstrated some form of allergy, particularly to drugs. There is some clinical and laboratory evidence of partial cross-allergenicity of the cephalosporins and penicillin. Special care is indicated in patients who have experienced anaphylactic reaction to penicillins or other beta-lactams. If an allergic reaction to CEFTIN occurs, treatment should be discontinued and standard agents (e.g. epinephrine, antihistamines, corticosteroids) administered as necessary.

Pseudomembranous colitis has been reported to be associated with the use of CEFTIN and other broad-spectrum antibiotics. Therefore, it is important to consider its diagnosis in patients administered CEFTIN who develop diarrhea. Treatment with broad spectrum antibiotics, including CEFTIN, alters the normal flora of the colon and may permit overgrowth of Clostridia. Studies indicate that a toxin produced by *C. difficile* is one primary cause of antibiotic associated colitis. Mild cases of colitis may respond to drug discontinuance alone. Moderate to severe cases should be managed with fluid, electrolyte, and protein supplementation as indicated. When the colitis is severe or not relieved by discontinuance of CEFTIN administration, consideration should be given to the administration of oral vancomycin or other suitable therapy. Other possible causes of colitis should also be considered.

CEFTIN suspension contains aspartame, which is a source of phenylalanine and so should be avoided in patients with phenylketonuria.

PRECAUTIONS: General: Broad-spectrum antibiotics including CEFTIN (cefuroxime axetil) should be administered with caution to individuals with a history of gastrointestinal disease, particularly colitis.

The concomitant administration of aminoglycosides and some cephalosporins has caused nephrotoxicity. There is no evidence that CEFTIN, when administered alone, is nephrotoxic, although transient elevations of BUN and serum creatinine have been observed in clinical studies. However, the effect of administering CEFTIN concomitantly with aminoglycosides is not known.

Studies suggest that the concomitant use of potent diuretics, such as furosemide and ethacrynic acid, may increase the risk of renal toxicity with cephalosporins.

As with other antibiotics, use of CEFTIN may result in the overgrowth of Candida. Prolonged use may also result in the overgrowth of other non-susceptible organisms (e.g. enterococci and *C. difficile*), which may require interruption of treatment. Repeated evaluation of the patient's condition is essential. If superinfection occurs during therapy, appropriate measures should be taken. Should an organism become resistant during antibiotic therapy, CEFTIN should be discontinued and another appropriate antibiotic should be substituted.

The sucrose content of CEFTIN suspension (see Supplied) should be taken into account when treating diabetic patients.

Pregnancy: The safety of CEFTIN in pregnancy has not been established. The use of CEFTIN in pregnant women requires that the likely benefit from the drug be weighed against the possible risk to the mother and fetus. Animal studies following parenteral administration have shown cefuroxime to affect bone calcification in the fetus and to cause maternal toxicity in the rabbit. Reproduction studies that have been performed in mice and rats at oral doses of up to 50 to 160 times the human dose have revealed no evidence of impaired fertility or harm to the fetus due to cefuroxime axetil. There are, however, no adequate and well-controlled studies in pregnant women. Because animal reproduction studies are not always predictive of human response, this drug should be used during pregnancy only if clearly needed.

Lactation: Since cefuroxime is excreted in human milk, consideration should be given to discontinuing nursing temporarily during treatment with CEFTIN.

Drug Interactions: Drugs which reduce gastric acidity may result in a lower bioavailability of CEFTIN compared with that of the fasting state and tend to cancel the effect of post-prandial absorption.

In common with other antibiotics, cefuroxime axetil may affect the gut flora, leading to lower estrogen reabsorption and reduced efficacy of combined oral contraceptives.

Drug-Laboratory Test Interactions: A false-positive reaction for glucose in the urine may occur with copper reduction tests (Benedict's or Fehling's solution or with Clinitest Tablets) but not with enzyme-based tests for glycosuria (e.g., Clinistix, Tes-Tape). As a false-negative result may occur in the ferricyanide test, it is recommended that either the glucose oxidase or hexokinase method be used to determine blood plasma glucose levels in patients receiving CEFTIN.

Cefuroxime does not interfere with the assay of serum and urine creatinine by the alkaline picrate method.

Cephalosporins as a class tend to be absorbed onto the surface of red cell membranes and react with antibodies directed against the drug to produce a positive Coombs' test (which can interfere with cross-matching of blood) and, very rarely, hemolytic anemia.

Occupational Hazards: Ability to Perform Tasks That Require Judgement, Motor or Cognitive Skills: As this medicine may cause dizziness, patients should be warned to be cautious when driving or operating machinery.

ADVERSE EFFECTS: The following adverse reactions have been reported:

Gastrointestinal (approximately 8% of patients): diarrhea (5.6%), nausea (2.4%), vomiting (2%), loose stools (1.3%). Reports of abdominal pain have occurred.

Hepatic (3% of patients): transient increases of hepatic enzyme levels (ALT, AST, LDH).

CNS (2.2% of patients): headache and dizziness.

Hypersensitivity (1.3% of patients): rashes (0.6%), pruritus (0.3%), urticaria (0.2%), shortness of breath and rare reports of bronchospasm. Hypersensitivity reactions to CEFTIN may occur in patients who report delayed hypersensitivity to penicillins (see Warnings). As with other cephalosporins, there have been rare reports of drug fever.

Hematologic: increased erythrocyte sedimentation rate, eosinophilia, decreased hemoglobin and, very rarely, hemolytic anemia.

Miscellaneous: The following adverse reactions have been observed to occur, although infrequently, in association with parenteral cefuroxime sodium and may be potential adverse effects of oral cefuroxime axetil: drowsiness, vaginitis, positive direct Coombs test, and transient increases in serum bilirubin, creatinine, alkaline phosphatase and urea nitrogen (BUN). In addition, the incidence of diaper rash (1.4%) has been associated with CEFTIN suspension in children.

Postmarketing Experience with CEFTIN Products: In addition to adverse events reported during clinical trials, the following events have been identified during clinical practice in patients treated with CEFTIN Tablets or with CEFTIN for Oral Suspension and were reported spontaneously. Data are generally insufficient to allow an estimate of incidence or to establish causation.

General: The following hypersensitivity reactions have been reported: anaphylaxis, angioedema, pruritus, rash, serum sickness-like reaction, urticaria.

Gastrointestinal: pseudomembranous colitis (see Warnings).

Hematologic: thrombocytopenia, and leucopenia (sometimes profound).

Hepatic: Jaundice (predominantly cholestatic) and hepatitis have been reported very rarely.

Infections and Infestations: Candida overgrowth.

Neurologic: seizure.

Skin: erythema multiforme, Stevens-Johnson syndrome, toxic epidermal necrolysis.

Urologic: renal dysfunction.

OVERDOSE:

Treatment: Other than general supportive treatment, no specific antidote is known. Excessive serum levels of cefuroxime can be reduced by dialysis. For treatment of hypersensitivity reactions, see Warnings.

For management of a suspected drug overdose, CPhA recommends that you contact your **regional Poison Control Centre**. See the *CPS* Directory section for a list of Poison Control Centres.

DOSAGE: CEFTIN (cefuroxime axetil) may be given orally without regard to meals. Absorption is enhanced when CEFTIN is administered with food. In comparative bioavailability studies in healthy adults, CEFTIN suspension was not bioequivalent to CEFTIN tablets. The area under the curve for the suspension averaged 91% of that for the tablet, while the C_{max} for the suspension averaged 71% of the C_{max} of the tablets.

CEFTIN suspension contains aspartame, which is a source of phenylalanine and so should be avoided in patients with phenylketonuria. (See Warnings.)

Tablets: Adults and Children (12 Years of Age and Older): The usual recommended dosage is 250 mg twice a day. However, dosage may be modified according to the type of infection present, as indicated in Table 1.

Table 1: CEFTIN Tablets

Dosage According to the Type of Infection

Type of Infection	Dosage
Pharyngitis, tonsillitis, sinusitis, bronchitis, skin structure infections	250 mg twice daily
More severe infections e.g., pneumonia	500 mg twice daily
Uncomplicated gonorrhea	1000 mg single dose

There are presently no data available on the effects of CEFTIN in patients with renal impairment. However, in patients where there is significant impairment, a reduction in CEFTIN dosage may be required.

Infants and Children Less Than 12 Years of Age: CEFTIN tablets are not recommended for children less than 12 years of age.

Oral Suspension: Infants and Children 3 Months to 12 Years of Age: There is no experience in infants under the age of 3 months.

There is no clinical trial experience with the use of CEFTIN suspension in the treatment of lower respiratory tract infections.

The recommended dosage of CEFTIN suspension for various types of infections is indicated in Table 2, Table 3 and Table 4.

Table 2: CEFTIN Suspension

Recommended Dosage for Various Infections

Type of Infection	Dosage
Otitis media, skin structure infections	15 mg/kg twice daily Maximum dose 1 g/day
Pharyngitis, tonsillitis	10 mg/kg twice daily Maximum dose 500 mg/day

Table 3: CEFTIN Suspension

Recommended Dosage for Pharyngitis and Tonsillitis Infections

Weight (kg)	Dosage mg/day	Doses/day	Multidose Bottle mL/dose
6	125	2	2.5
13	250	2	5.0
19	375	2	7.5
25	500	2	10.0
>25	500	2	10.0

Table 4: CEFTIN Suspension

Recommended Dosage for Otitis Media and Skin Structure Infections

Weight (kg)	Dosage mg/day	Doses/day	Multidose Bottle mL/dose
4	125	2	2.5
8	250	2	5.0
13	375	2	7.5
17	500	2	10.0
21	625	2	12.5
25	750	2	15.0
29	875	2	17.5
33	1000	2	20.0
>33	1000	2	20.0

The usual duration of treatment for CEFTIN tablets and CEFTIN for oral suspension is 7 to 10 days. For β-hemolytic streptococcal infections, therapy should be continued for at least 10 days.

Directions for Reconstituting Suspension in Bottles: Prepare a suspension at time of dispensing, as follows: 1) Shake the bottle to loosen the granules, and remove the cap. 2) Add the total amount of water for reconstitution all at once (see Table 5) and replace cap. 3)**Invert the bottle and rock the bottle vigorously until the sound of the granules against the container disappears.** 4) Turn the bottle into an upright position and shake vigorously. Each 5 mL provides 125 mg cefuroxime. 5) Refrigerate immediately at between 2 and 8°C.

Note: Shake the bottle vigorously until the suspension can be heard moving in the bottle before each use. Replace cap securely after each opening. If desired, the dose of the reconstituted suspension may be added to one of the following cold beverages immediately prior to administration: milk (i.e. skim, 2% or homogenized), fruit juice (i.e. apple, orange, or grape) or lemonade.

Note: CEFTIN granules should **not** be reconstituted in **hot beverages.**

Table 5: CEFTIN Suspension

Reconstitution Instructions

Labelled Volume (mL)	Amount of Water for Reconstitution (mL)
70	27
100	37

INFORMATION FOR THE PATIENT: Published in e-CPS, available by subscription at www.e-cps.ca.

SUPPLIED: Suspension: Dry, white to pale yellow, tutti-frutti-flavored granules. After reconstitution, each 5 mL contains: cefuroxime 125 mg (as cefuroxime axetil). Nonmedicinal ingredients: acesulfame potassium, aspartame, polyvinyl pyrrolidone, stearic acid, sucrose (about 3 g/5 mL), tutti frutti flavoring and xanthan gum. Bottles of 70 and 100 mL, containing 1.75 g and 2.5 g cefuroxime (as cefuroxime axetil), respectively. Store granules between 2 and 30°C. The reconstituted suspension must be stored immediately between 2 and 8°C in a refrigerator, and discarded after 10 days.

Tablets: 250 mg: Each white to off-white, film-coated, capsule-shaped, biconvex tablet, engraved with "GXES7" on one side, contains: cefuroxime 250 mg (as cefuroxime axetil). Nonmedicinal ingredients: colloidal silicon dioxide, croscarmellose sodium, hydrogenated vegetable oil, hydroxypropyl methylcellulose, methylparaben, microcrystalline cellulose, propylene glycol, propylparaben, sodium benzoate, sodium lauryl sulfate and titanium dioxide. Bottles of 60. Store between 15 and 30°C.

500 mg: Each white to off-white, film-coated, capsule-shaped, biconvex tablet, engraved with "GXEG2" on one side, contains: cefuroxime 500 mg (as cefuroxime axetil). Nonmedicinal ingredients: colloidal silicon dioxide, croscarmellose sodium, hydrogenated vegetable oil, hydroxypropyl methylcellulose, methylparaben, microcrystalline cellulose, propylene glycol, propylparaben, sodium benzoate, sodium lauryl sulfate and titanium dioxide. Bottles of 60. Store between 15 and 30°C.

(Shown in Product Identification Section)

Ceftriaxone

Antibacterial

CPhA Monograph

Date of Preparation: November 2007
Date of Revision: September 2009

This monograph has been compiled by CPhA and reviewed by experts. It may contain information different from that found in Health Canada-approved Product Monographs. The reader is referred to the *CPS* Editorial Policy for more information.

SUMMARY PRODUCT INFORMATION:

Route of Administration	Dosage Form	Strength
IM, IV	Dry powder vial for reconstitution	0.25 g, 1 g, 2 g; 10 g bulk vials available to hospitals with iv admixture programs

INDICATIONS AND CLINICAL USE: Ceftriaxone is a third-generation cephalosporin antibacterial agent. Compared to first- and second-generation cephalosporins, ceftriaxone has enhanced activity against aerobic gram-negative organisms such as Enterobacteriaceae; while retaining good activity against streptococci (except enterococci), it is less active against staphylococci. Ceftriaxone is used in the following clinical settings to treat or prevent infections caused by susceptible organisms:

- Treatment of lower respiratory tract infections such as nosocomial or community-acquired pneumonia.
- Treatment of complicated or uncomplicated urinary tract infections.
- Treatment of septicemia.
- Treatment of skin and skin structure infections.
- Treatment of bone and joint infections including osteomyelitis and septic arthritis.
- Treatment of intra-abdominal infections (not as monotherapy if *B. fragilis* may be involved).
- Treatment of meningitis.
- Post-exposure prophylaxis for contacts of patients with invasive meningococcal disease.
- Treatment of brain abscesses and other CNS infections such as subdural empyema, in conjunction with other antimicrobials.
- Treatment of uncomplicated or disseminated gonorrhea.
- Treatment of native valve or prosthetic valve endocarditis.
- Treatment of Lyme disease.
- Empiric anti-infective treatment of victims of sexual assault, in conjunction with other antimicrobial agents.

Ceftriaxone has been effective in treating Shigella infections caused by *S. sonnei* or *S. flexneri*, and is preferred over ampicillin when the susceptibility of the organism is unknown or in areas where ampicillin-resistant strains have been reported.

Ceftriaxone has been used in the empiric management of febrile neutropenia, in combination with an aminoglycoside.

While it has some activity against *T. pallidum*, ceftriaxone is not considered a first-line agent in the treatment of syphilis.

Ceftriaxone has been used to treat chancroid (genital ulcers caused by *H. ducreyi*) but is not a first-line agent; treatment failures have occurred in patients who are HIV positive.

Ceftriaxone is effective in the prevention of many postsurgical infections but is generally not recommended for this purpose when less expensive agents with a narrower spectrum of activity would be equally effective.

CONTRAINDICATIONS:

- Patients who are hypersensitive to ceftriaxone or to any ingredient in the formulation.
- Patients who are hypersensitive to other cephalosporin antibiotics.

WARNINGS AND PRECAUTIONS:

Serious Warnings and Precautions

- Ceftriaxone has been associated with severe allergic reactions including anaphylactic reactions. For this reason a history of allergic reactions, including the type and severity of the reaction, should be obtained before prescribing and administering ceftriaxone.
- Cross-sensitivity between penicillins and cephalosporins is estimated to be very low. Current opinion on the true incidence of cross-sensitivity is about 1%. The beta-lactam subunit is not considered the primary allergenic determinant; rather, the side chain predicts cross-reactivity. After thorough investigation into the nature of the allergy, a cephalosporin can be considered in a penicillin allergic patient provided there is no history of an immediate-sensitivity reaction. Although the risk of cross-reaction is predicted to be low the patient should be monitored for signs of a sensitivity reaction.
- Patients with a history of immediate-sensitivity reaction to penicillin (e.g., anaphylaxis, bronchospasm, and/or hypotension) are considered to be at increased risk of similar reactions to cephalosporins, including ceftriaxone. For this reason, administration of ceftriaxone should be avoided in patients with a history of severe allergic reactions to penicillin antibiotics unless skin testing is performed to rule out cross-sensitivity.
- Cephalosporin antibiotics including ceftriaxone have been associated with *C. difficile*-associated diarrhea and colitis.

General: Prolonged therapy with ceftriaxone may result in the overgrowth of organisms not susceptible (or initially susceptible) to ceftriaxone, particularly *C. albicans*, enterococci, *B. fragilis* or *P. aeruginosa*, Citrobacter or Enterbacter species.

Special Populations: Pregnant Women: Ceftriaxone crosses the placenta and is usually considered safe to use in pregnancy when clearly necessary.

Nursing Women: Ceftriaxone is distributed into breast milk in low concentrations. Potential effects on the nursing infant include disruption of the gut microbial flora or interference with accurate fever work-up. The American Academy of Pediatrics considers ceftriaxone to be compatible with breast-feeding.

Pediatrics: Because it can displace bilirubin from serum albumin, ceftriaxone should be avoided in hyperbilirubinemic neonates, particularly those born prematurely. Cefotaxime is a reasonable alternative in this setting.

Ceftriaxone that has been reconstituted with sterile water preserved with benzyl alcohol should not be administered to neonates.

Fatal reactions involving ceftriaxone-calcium precipitates in the lungs and kidneys have been reported following administration of calcium-containing iv solutions to neonates also receiving ceftriaxone.

ADVERSE REACTIONS: More Common Adverse Drug Reactions: See Table 1.

Table 1: Ceftriaxone

More Common Adverse Drug Reactions (≥ 1%)

Body System	Effect	Estimated Frequency	Clinical Comment
Hematologic	Eosinophilia Thrombocytosis Leukopenia	6% 5% 2%	Generally reversible upon discontinuation
Hepatic	Elevated AST, ALT	4–5%	Monitor and consider discontinuing ceftriaxone if elevations are marked
Dermatologic	Rash	2%	Manifestations of allergic reactions, which may be severe
Gastrointestinal	Transient diarrhea	5–10%	Generally mild; resolves upon withdrawal of treatment
General	Pain, induration, tenderness at im injection site	1–2%	Pain on im injection may be mitigated by reconstituting ceftriaxone with lidocaine 1% solution (**without** epinephrine)

Less Common Adverse Drug Reactions (< 1%): Cardiovascular: phlebitis with iv administration.

Gastrointestinal: *C. difficile*-associated diarrhea and colitis. Severe persistent diarrhea including cases that arise after withdrawal of treatment may be attributable to *C. difficile* and should be evaluated accordingly.

Hematologic: aplastic anemia, pancytopenia and hemolytic anemia have been reported in association with cephalosporin antibiotics.

Hepatic/Biliary/Pancreatic: elevated alkaline phosphatase, bilirubin; jaundice.

Immune: hypersensitivity reactions.

Neurologic: dizziness, headache.

Abnormal Hematologic and Clinical Chemistry Findings: See Table 2.

Table 2: Ceftriaxone

Abnormal Hematologic and Clinical Chemistry Findings

Test	Effect	Clinical Comment
Coombs' test	Positive direct and indirect test result	Positive test is indicative of immune-mediated hemolysis. The direct test detects antibodies bound to erythrocytes; the indirect test detects antibodies in serum. The condition usually resolves upon withdrawal of drug treatment. The reaction may interfere with hematologic studies or transfusion cross-matching procedures. A false-positive Coomb's test result may be detected in neonates whose mothers received a cephalosporin antibiotic before delivery.

DRUG INTERACTIONS: Drug-Drug Interactions: See Table 3.

Table 3: Ceftriaxone

Drug-Drug Interactions

Interacting Drug	Effect	Clinical Comment
Calcium-containing intravenous solutions, including TPN or Ringer's solution	Ceftriaxone-calcium precipitate	Cases of fatal reactions involving precipitates in the lungs and kidneys of neonates have been reported.
Coumarin anticoagulants, e.g., wafarin, nicoumalone (acenocoumarol)	Possible increased anticoagulant effect when coadministered with cephalosporins	The mechanism may involve interference with vitamin K production. Monitor INR and adjust the anticoagulant dose accordingly. Vitamin K may be administered if bleeding occurs.

DOSAGE AND ADMINISTRATION: Recommended Dose and Dosage Adjustment: Ceftriaxone can be administered im or iv. For severe or life-threatening infections the iv route is preferred.

Adults: See Table 4.

Table 4: Ceftriaxone

Dose in Adult Patients

Indication	Route	Usual Dose	Maximum Dose	Duration of Therapy	Clinical Comment
Lower respiratory tract infections	IV	1–2 g/day in 1 or 2 divided doses	4 g/day	4–14 days[a]	
Urinary tract infections, complicated or uncomplicated	IM[b]/IV	1–2 g/day in 1 or 2 divided doses	4 g/day	4–14 days[a]	Generally reserved as second-line therapy in patients with severe cases of complicated UTI or pyelonephritis
Septicemia	IV	1–2 g/day in 1 or 2 divided doses	4 g/day	4–14 days[a]	Depending on the suspected source of infection, empiric therapy may require additional antimicrobial agents

(cont'd)

Table 4: Ceftriaxone *(cont'd)*
Dose in Adult Patients

Indication	Route	Usual Dose	Maximum Dose	Duration of Therapy	Clinical Comment
Skin and skin structure infections	IM[b]/IV	1–2 g/day in 1 or 2 divided doses	4 g/day	4–14 days[a]	
Bone and joint infections (e.g., osteomyelitis, septic arthritis)	IV	1–2 g/day in 1 or 2 divided doses	4 g/day	4–6 weeks	
Intra-abdominal infections	IV	1–2 g/day in 1 or 2 divided doses	4 g/day	4–14 days[a]	Not to be used as monotherapy when *B. fragilis* may be involved
Meningitis	IV	2 g Q12–24H	4 g/day	7 days for susceptible strains of *H. influenzae* 10–14 days for *S. pneumoniae* 21 days for Enterobacteriaceae such as *E. coli*, Klebsiella spp	
Post-exposure prophylaxis for close contacts[c] (> 12 y) of patients with invasive meningococcal disease	IM[b]	250 mg (single dose)	N/A	One dose	Close contacts defined in footnote [c]
Brain abscess	IV	2 g Q12H	4 g/day	Duration of therapy is unclear; assessment of clinical response is guided by neuroimaging.	
Gonorrhea, uncomplicated	IM[b]	125–250 mg (single dose)	NA	One dose	Give in conjunction with presumptive treatment for concomitant chlamydial infection (e.g., azithromycin 1 g po single dose or doxycycline 100 mg po BID×7 days)
Gonococcal conjunctivitis	IM[b]	1 g (single dose)	NA	One dose	
Gonorrhea, disseminated	IM[b]/IV	1 g Q24H	Usual maximum 1 g/day	Switch to appropriate oral therapy (e.g., cefixime, fluoroquinolone) 24–48 h after infection begins to resolve, to complete a minimum 7-day course	
Prophylaxis in sexual assault victims	IM[b]	125 mg (single dose)	N/A	One dose	Give in conjunction with a single dose of either metronidazole 2 g po or azithromycin 1 g po or a 7-day course of doxycycline 100 mg po BID.
Lyme disease	IV	2 g Q24H	2 g daily	10–28 days (average 14 days)	
Endocarditis	IM[b]/IV	2 g Q24H	2 g daily	4 weeks	

[a] Continue therapy for at least 48 to 72 hours after signs and symptoms of the infection have resolved.
[b] To minimize discomfort, the preferred diluent for im ceftriaxone is lidocaine 1% **without** epinephrine.
[c] Close contacts are persons who may have had direct contact with the infected person's oral or nasal secretions, including those who live in the same home or share a bed, children and staff in a day care centre, those who share any object that has been in the mouth (e.g., beverages, lipstick, musical instrument mouthpieces) or airline passengers sitting on either side of an infected patient (not across the aisle) for flights of at least 8 hours. Classmates or colleagues are not close contacts unless any of the above conditions are met.
Abbreviations: N/A = not applicable

Pediatrics: Children over the age of 12 years may receive the appropriate adult dose, depending on the type and severity of the infection. For children 12 years of age or younger, the dose of ceftriaxone for most serious infections (other than meningitis) is 50–75 mg/kg/day, maximum 2 g/day, either as one daily dose or 2 divided doses given every 12 hours. Table 5 lists some specific dosage recommendations for pediatric patients.

Renal Impairment: Ceftriaxone dosage adjustment is generally not needed for patients with renal failure, provided hepatic function is intact.

Dialysis: Because ceftriaxone is not removed by hemodialysis, supplemental dosing is not required following dialysis sessions. A supplemental dose of 1g Q12H is recommended for patients receiving peritoneal dialysis.

Hepatic Impairment: No dosage adjustments are required in patients with hepatic impairment, provided renal function is intact.

Administration: Ceftriaxone may be administered by iv or im injection.

For iv injection, reconstitute vials with sterile water to a concentration of 100 mg/mL. Reconstituted solution may be administered over 5 minutes or diluted further in normal saline or dextrose 5% solution for intermittent infusion.

Table 5: Ceftriaxone
Dose in Pediatric Patients

Indication	Route	Age	Usual Dose	Maximum Dose	Duration of Therapy	Clinical Comment
Otitis media	IM[a]	≤ 12 y	50 mg/kg (single dose)	1 g	One dose	
Meningitis	IV	≤ 12 y	100 mg/kg Q12H × 3 doses then 100 mg/kg q24H	4 g/day	Duration of therapy is unclear; assessment of clinical response is guided by neuroimaging.	
Post-exposure prophylaxis for close contacts[b] of patients with invasive meningococcal disease	IM[a]	≤ 12 y	125 mg (single dose)	N/A	One dose	Close contacts defined in footnote [b]
Endocarditis	IM[a]/IV	≤ 12 y	100 mg/kg Q24H	2 g/day	4 weeks	
Gonorrhea, uncomplicated	IM[a]	≤ 12 y	Weight ≤ 45 kg: 125 mg (single dose) Weight > 45 kg: 250 mg (single dose)	N/A	One dose	Give in conjunction with presumptive treatment for concomitant chlamydial infection (single dose of azithromycin 12–15 mg/kg po, max 1 g, for children ≤ 9 years; doxycycline 5 mg/kg/day po in divided doses, max 100 mg BID, for children > 9 years)
Gonorrhea, disseminated	IM[a]/IV	≤ 12 y	Weight ≤ 45 kg: 50 mg/kg Q24H	1 g/day	7 days	
Prevention of gonococcal infections in neonates born to mothers with documented gonococcal infection, or treatment of gonoccocal ophthalmia neonatorum	IM[a]/IV	Newborn	25–50 mg/kg (single dose at birth)	125 mg	One dose	Give in conjunction with presumptive treatment for chlamydial infection, unless it is documented that the mother is negative (≤ 7 days and ≤ 2 kg—erythromycin[c] 20 mg/kg/day po in divided doses; ≤ 7 days and > 2 kg—erythromycin[c] 30 mg/kg/day po in divided doses; > 7 days—erythromycin[c] 40 mg/kg/day po in divided doses)
Treatment of gonoccocal ophthalmia neonatorum	IM[a]/IV	Newborn	25–50 mg/kg (single dose at birth)	125 mg	One dose	
Lyme disease	IV	≤ 12 y	50–75 mg/kg Q24H	2 g/day	10–28 days (average 14 days)	

[a] To minimize discomfort, the preferred diluent for im ceftriaxone is lidocaine 1% **without** epinephrine.
[b] Close contacts are children who may have had direct contact with the infected person's oral or nasal secretions, including those who live in the same home or share a bed, children and staff in the same day care centre, those who share any object that has been in the mouth (e.g., beverages, lipstick, musical instrument mouthpieces) or airline passengers sitting on either side of an infected patient (not across the aisle) for flights of at least 8 hours. Classmates are **not** close contacts unless any of the above conditions are met.
[c] The use of erythromycin in infants under 6 weeks of age has been associated with infantile hypertrophic pyloric stenosis (IHPS). The risks and benefits of using erythromycin in this setting should be explained to parents.
Abbreviations:
N/A = not applicable.

For im injection, vials may be reconstituted with sterile water, normal saline, dextrose 5% solution, bacteriostatic water for injection or lidocaine 1% solution **without** epinephrine, to a final concentration of 250-350 mg/mL. Reconstituted solution should be administered by deep intragluteal injection, with no more than 1 g injected at a single site. To minimize discomfort on im injection, lidocaine 1% solution **without** epinephrine is the preferred diluent. Vials reconstituted with lidocaine 1% solution should **never** be administered iv.

OVERDOSAGE:

For management of a suspected drug overdose, CPhA recommends that you contact your **regional Poison Control Centre**. See the *CPS* Directory section for a list of Poison Control Centres.

ACTION AND CLINICAL PHARMACOLOGY: Mechanism of Action: The proposed mechanism of action of cephalosporins, including ceftriaxone, is interference with mucopeptide synthesis in bacterial cell walls through covalent binding with penicillin-binding proteins. This results in defective cell walls that eventually lyse, culminating in cell death. Maximal bacterial killing occurs with cephalosporin concentrations four times the minimal inhibitory concentration (MIC). Cephalosporins exhibit a post-antibiotic effect with gram-positive organisms but not gram-negative bacilli. The major determinant of the bactericidal effect of cephalosporins is the length of time the serum drug concentration exceeds the MIC.

Pharmacokinetics: Adults:

Summary of the Pharmacokinetic Properties of Ceftriaxone in Adults

Peak serum concentration after an iv dose	1 g: 123–151 µg/mL
	2 g: 223–276 µg/mL
Time to peak concentration	IV: 30 min
	IM: 1–3 h
Plasma protein binding (%)	83–96% (50% lower in infants and children)
Route of elimination	Renal: 33–67%, unchanged
	Biliary: 35–45% (subsequent intestinal metabolism occurs)
Terminal elimination half-life	6–9 h
CSF concentration after 100 mg/kg iv dose	20 µg/mL at 2 hours

STORAGE AND STABILITY: Sterile dry powder vials should be stored at room temperature (between 15 and 30°C).

Ceftriaxone for Injection BP ℞
ceftriaxone sodium
Antibiotic

Sandoz

SUPPLIED: 0.25 g: Each vial of white or yellowish, crystalline, slightly hygroscopic sterile powder contains: ceftriaxone 0.25 g in the form of the sodium salt. Nonmedicinal ingredients: none. Boxes of 10×0.25 g vials. Store between 15 and 30°C and protect from light.
1 g: Each vial of white or yellowish, crystalline, slightly hygroscopic sterile powder contains: ceftriaxone 1 g in the form of the sodium salt. Nonmedicinal ingredients: none. Boxes of 10×1 g vials. Store between 15 and 30°C and protect from light.
2 g: Each vial of white or yellowish, crystalline, slightly hygroscopic sterile powder contains: ceftriaxone 2 g in the form of the sodium salt. Nonmedicinal ingredients: none. Boxes of 10×2 g vials. Store between 15 and 30°C and protect from light.
10 g: Each vial of white or yellowish, crystalline, slightly hygroscopic sterile powder contains: ceftriaxone 10 g in the form of the sodium salt. Nonmedicinal ingredients: none. Boxes of 1×10 g vial. Store between 15 and 30°C and protect from light.

Ceftriaxone for Injection USP ℞
ceftriaxone sodium
Antibiotic

Apotex

Date of Revision: July 18, 2008

PHARMACOLOGY: In vitro studies indicate that the bactericidal action of ceftriaxone results from the inhibition of cell-wall synthesis. In *E. coli*, ceftriaxone showed a high affinity for penicillin binding proteins (PBP) 1a and 3 and a moderate affinity for 1b and 2. In *H. influenzae*, the highest affinity was shown for PBP 4 and PBP 5. The binding affinity to PBP 4 was 35-fold that of PBP 3, 10-fold that of PBP 2 and approximately 100-fold that of PBP 1. The morphological changes resulting from the PBP binding include filament formation or cell wall and septal thickening, and then cell lysis.

INDICATIONS: The treatment of the following infections when caused by susceptible strains of the designated micro-organisms:

Lower respiratory tract infections caused by *E. coli, H. influenzae, K. pneumoniae* and species, *S. aureus, S. pneumoniae* and species (excluding enterococci).

Urinary tract infections (complicated and uncomplicated) caused by *E. coli*, Klebsiella species, *P. mirabilis* and *P. vulgaris*.

Bacterial septicemia caused by *E. coli, H. influenzae, K. pneumoniae, S. aureus* and *S. pneumoniae*, (excluding enterococci).

Skin and skin structure infections caused by *K. pneumoniae* and species, *P. mirabilis, S. aureus, S. epidermidis* and Streptococcus species (excluding enterococci).

Bone and joint infections caused by *S. aureus, S. pneumoniae* and Streptococcus species (excluding enterococci).

Intra-abdominal infections caused by *E. coli* and *K. pneumoniae*.

Meningitis caused by *H. influenzae, N. meningitidis*, and *S. pneumoniae*. Ceftriaxone for injection should not be used for the treatment of meningitis caused by *L. monocytogenes*.

Uncomplicated gonorrhea (cervical/urethral, pharyngeal and rectal) caused by *N. gonorrhoeae* (penicillinase and nonpenicillinase producing strains).

Susceptibility Testing: Specimens for bacteriologic culture should be obtained prior to therapy in order to identify the causative organisms and to determine their susceptibilities to ceftriaxone. Therapy may be instituted before results of susceptibility testing are known. However, modification of the treatment may be required once these results become available.

Prophylaxis: The preoperative administration of a single 1 g dose of ceftriaxone sodium may reduce the incidence of postoperative infections in patients undergoing vaginal or abdominal hysterectomy, coronary artery bypass surgery, or in patients at risk of infection undergoing biliary tract surgery. If signs of post surgical infection should appear, specimens for culture should be obtained for identification of the causative organism(s) so that the appropriate therapy may be instituted.

CONTRAINDICATIONS: Ceftriaxone for Injection USP is contraindicated in patients with known allergy to ceftriaxone, other cephalosporins or penicillins.

Hyperbilirubinemic neonates and preterm neonates should not be treated with ceftriaxone. In vitro studies have shown that ceftriaxone can displace bilirubin from its binding to serum albumin and bilirubin encephalopathy can possibly develop in these patients (see Precautions).

In neonates Ceftriaxone for Injection must not be administered concurrently with calcium-containing intravenous solutions, including continuous calcium-containing infusions such as parenteral nutrition because of the risk of precipitation of ceftriaxone-calcium salt (see Warnings and Adverse Effects). Cases of fatal reactions with calcium-ceftriaxone precipitates in lung and kidneys have been described in neonates. In some cases the infusion lines and the times of administration of ceftriaxone and calcium-containing solutions differed. As a theoretical consideration and based on 5 half-lives of ceftriaxone (at which point negligible amounts of the original ceftriaxone dose would be present), ceftriaxone for injections and IV calcium-containing solutions should not be administered within 5 days of each other in neonates and in infants up to 10 weeks of age (by ten weeks of age the ceftriaxone half-life is generally less than 10 hours).

For information regarding all other patients, see Warnings.

WARNINGS: Before therapy with ceftriaxone sodium is instituted, careful inquiry should be made concerning previous hypersensitivity reactions to ceftriaxone, other cephalosporins, penicillins or other allergens. Ceftriaxone for injection should only be administered with caution to any patient who has demonstrated any form of allergy particularly to drugs. Serious and occasionally fatal hypersensitivity (anaphylactoid) reactions have been reported in patients receiving cephalosporins. The reactions are more likely to occur in persons with a history of sensitivity to multiple allergens. Ceftriaxone for injection should be administered with caution to patients with type I hypersensitivity reaction to penicillin. If an allergic reaction occurs, the administration of ceftriaxone for injection should be discontinued and appropriate therapy instituted.

Pseudomembranous colitis has been reported with the use of ceftriaxone sodium, (and with broad-spectrum and other antibiotics). Therefore, it is important to consider its diagnosis in patients administered ceftriaxone for injection who develop diarrhea. Treatment with broad-spectrum antibiotics, including ceftriaxone for injection, alters the normal flora of the colon and may permit overgrowth of Clostridia. Studies indicate that a toxin produced by *C. difficile* is one primary cause of antibiotic-associated colitis. Mild cases of colitis may respond to drug discontinuation alone. Moderate to severe cases should be managed with fluid, electrolyte, and protein supplementation as indicated. When the colitis is not relieved by discontinuation of ceftriaxone for injection administration or when it is severe, consideration should be given to the administration of vancomycin or other suitable therapy. Other possible causes of the colitis should also be considered.

Interaction with Calcium-Containing Products: In the available scientific literature there are no reports of intravascular calcium-ceftriaxone precipitates in patients other than neonates treated with ceftriaxone and calcium-containing intravenous solutions or any other calcium-containing products. However, the theoretical possibility exists for an interaction between ceftriaxone and calcium-containing intravenous solutions in all patients. Therefore ceftriaxone should not be mixed with or administered to any patient simultaneously with calcium-containing intravenous solutions or products, even via different infusion lines. As a further theoretical consideration and based on 5 half-lives of ceftriaxone for almost complete clearance of the drug, ceftriaxone and calcium-containing intravenous solutions should not be administered within 48 hours of each other in any patient (see Contraindications for information regarding neonates).

There have been reports of sonographic abnormalities in the gallbladder of patients treated with ceftriaxone sodium; some of these patients also had symptoms of gallbladder disease. These abnormalities appear on sonography as an echo without acoustical shadowing suggesting sludge or as an echo with acoustical shadowing which may be misinterpreted as gallstones. The chemical nature of the sonographically-detected material has been determined to be predominantly a ceftriaxone-calcium salt. The condition appears to be transient and reversible upon discontinuation of ceftriaxone sodium and institution of conservative management. Therefore, Ceftriaxone for Injection should be discontinued in patients who develop signs and symptoms suggestive of gallbladder disease and/or the sonographic findings described above. The effect of pre-existing gallbladder disease is not known.

Cases of pancreatitis, possibly of biliary obstruction etiology, have been rarely reported in patients treated with ceftriaxone sodium. Most patients presented with risk factors for biliary stasis and biliary sludge, e.g. preceding major therapy, severe illness and total parenteral nutrition. A trigger or cofactor role of ceftriaxone sodium related biliary precipitation can not be ruled out. Ceftriaxone sodium may cause renal lithiasis through precipitation of calcium ceftriaxonate. When using this product in subjects with hypercalciuria or a history of renal lithiasis, benefit must be weighed against risk. Very rare cases of nephrolithiasis (renal precipitation) have been reported, mostly in children older than 3 years and who have been treated with either high daily doses (e.g. ≥80 mg/kg/day) or total doses exceeding 10 grams and presenting other risk factors (e.g. fluid restrictions, confinement to bed, etc.). This event may be symptomatic, may lead to renal insufficiency, and appears to be reversible upon discontinuation of ceftriaxone sodium.

Sonography for biliary sludge or renal lithiasis is recommended in cases of right hypochondrial and/or abdominal pain. Ceftriaxone for injections treatment should be withdrawn to allow signs and symptoms to resolve.

PRECAUTIONS: General: Alterations in prothrombin time (see Adverse Effects) and hypoprothrombinemia have occurred rarely in patients treated with ceftriaxone sodium. Patients with impaired vitamin K synthesis or low vitamin K stores (e.g., chronic hepatic disease and malnutrition) may require monitoring of hematology and coagulation parameters during ceftriaxone for injection treatment. Vitamin K administration (10 mg weekly) may be necessary if the prothrombin time is prolonged before or during treatment.

Prolonged treatment with ceftriaxone sodium may result in overgrowth of non-susceptible organisms and organisms initially sensitive to the drug. Development of resistant organisms during the administration of ceftriaxone for injection in clinical trials has been observed in 6% of the 94 patients infected with *P. aeruginosa*, in 33% of 3 patients infected with Citrobacter species and in 10% of the 10 patients infected with Enterobacter species. If superinfection occurs, appropriate measures should be taken.

Ceftriaxone for Injection should be administered with caution to individuals with a history of gastrointestinal disease, particularly colitis.

Renal and Hepatic Impairment: Although transient elevations of BUN and serum creatinine have been observed in clinical studies, there is no other evidence that ceftriaxone sodium, when administered alone, is nephrotoxic.

In severe renal impairment (creatinine clearance of less than 10 mL/min), periodic monitoring of serum ceftriaxone concentrations is recommended. The maximum daily dose should not exceed 2 g. In severe renal impairment associated with clinically significant hepatic impairment, close monitoring of serum ceftriaxone concentrations, at regular intervals, is recommended. If there is evidence of accumulation, dosage should be decreased accordingly.

Drug Interactions: Interactions between ceftriaxone sodium and other drugs have not been fully evaluated.

Pregnancy: The safety of ceftriaxone sodium in the treatment of infections during pregnancy has not been established. Ceftriaxone sodium should only be used during pregnancy if the likely benefit outweighs the potential risk to the fetus and/or the mother. Ceftriaxone has been detected in the umbilical cord blood, amniotic fluid and placenta. At parturition, 1 hour after a 2 g I.V. dose of ceftriaxone for injection, average ceftriaxone concentrations in maternal serum, umbilical cord serum, amniotic fluid, and placenta were 106±40 µg/mL, 19.5±11.5 µg/mL, 3.8±3.2 µg/mL and 20.9±4.4 µg/g.

Lactation: Ceftriaxone is excreted in human milk at low concentrations, (e.g., the peak concentration of total drug in milk ranged between 0.45 to 0.65 µg/mL, approximately five hours after the administration of 1 g I.V. or I.M.). The clinical significance of this is unknown; therefore, caution should be exercised when ceftriaxone for injection is administered to a nursing mother.

Neonates: The safety of ceftriaxone sodium in neonates (birth to one month of age) has not been established. In vitro studies have shown that ceftriaxone can displace bilirubin from serum albumin. Ceftriaxone for Injection should not be used in neonates (especially premature), at risk of developing bilirubin encephalopathy (see Contraindications).

Elderly Patients: The elimination of ceftriaxone may be reduced in elderly patients possibly due to impairment of both renal and hepatic function.

Drug-Laboratory Test Interactions: Ceftriaxone may interfere with urine glucose determinations utilizing the copper-reduction test (Clinitest), but not utilizing the glucose-oxidase test (Diastix or Tes Tape). In patients treated with ceftriaxone for injection the Coombs' test may rarely become false-positive; and ceftriaxone, like other antibiotics, may result in false-positive tests for galactosemia.

ADVERSE EFFECTS: During clinical trials and post-marketing experience with ceftriaxone sodium the following adverse reactions have been observed:

Clinical Adverse Experiences: Dermatological: rash (1.3%); exanthema, allergic dermatitis and pruritus (0.1-1.0%); urticaria (post-marketing reports). Isolated cases of severe cutaneous adverse reactions (erythema multiforme, Stevens-Johnson Syndrome, or Lyell's Syndrome/toxic epidermal necrolysis) have also been reported.

Hematological: anemia (0.1-1.0%); auto-immune hemolytic anemia and serum sickness (<0.1%); granulocytopenia (post-marketing reports). Isolated cases of agranulocytosis (<500/mm^3) have been reported, most of them after 10 days of treatment and following total doses of 20 g or more.

Hepatic: jaundice, reports (in asymptomatic and symptomatic patients) of ultrasonographic shadows suggesting precipitations in the gallbladder and reports of gallbladder sludge (<0.1%).

Urogenital: moniliasis and vaginitis (0.1-1.0%); oliguria and nephrolithiasis (post-marketing reports).

Gastrointestinal: diarrhea (3.3%); nausea, vomiting, dysgeusia and gastric pain (0.1-1.0%); abdominal pain, colitis, flatulence, dyspepsia, pseudomembranous colitis and stomatitis (<0.1%); glossitis (post-marketing reports).

Neurological: dizziness and headache (0.1-1.0%); ataxia and paresthesia (<0.1%).

Miscellaneous: fever, chills, diaphoresis, malaise, burning tongue, flushing, edema and anaphylactic shock (0.1-1.0%); bronchospasm, palpitations and epistaxis (<0.1%); glottic/laryngeal edema (post-marketing reports).

Other: Ceftriaxone must not be mixed with or administered simultaneously with calcium-containing intravenous solutions or products, even via different infusion lines. Cases of fatal reactions with calcium-ceftriaxone precipitates in lung and kidneys have been described in neonates. In some cases the infusion lines and times of administration of ceftriaxone and calcium-containing intravenous solutions differed.

Local Reactions at Injection Site: pain (9.4%)*, induration and tenderness (1-2%); phlebitic reactions (0.1-1.0%); thrombophlebitis (<0.1%).
Laboratory Abnormalities: Hematologic: eosinophilia (4.6%), thrombocytosis (5.1%), leukopenia (2.0%); neutropenia, lymphopenia, thrombocytopenia, increase or decrease in hematocrit, prolongation of prothrombin time and decrease in hemoglobin (0.1-1.0%); leucocytosis, lymphocytosis, monocytosis, basophilia and decrease in prothrombin time (<0.1%). (See Precautions for information on alterations in prothrombin time.)
Hepatic: increase in AST (4.0%)†, ALT (4.8%)†, increase in alkaline phosphatase (1.0%); increase in bilirubin (0.1-1.0%).
Urinary: increase in BUN (1.1%)‡; increase in creatinine, erythrocyturia, proteinuria and presence of casts in urine (0.1-1.0%); glycosuria (<0.1%).

OVERDOSE:
Ultrasonographic shadows suggesting precipitations in the kidneys accompanied by calcium ceftriaxone precipitate in the urine was observed in one patient dosed with ceftriaxone sodium at 10 g/day (2.5 times the maximum recommended dose). No other case of overdosage has been reported to date with ceftriaxone for injection. No specific information on symptoms or treatment is available. Excessive serum concentration of ceftriaxone cannot be reduced by hemodialysis or peritoneal dialysis. Treatment should be symptomatic.

For management of a suspected drug overdose, contact your **regional Poison Control Centre**. See the *CPS* Directory section for a list of Poison Control Centres.

DOSAGE: Ceftriaxone for Injection may be administered intravenously or intramuscularly after reconstitution.
Dosage and route of administration should be determined by the severity of infection, susceptibility of the causative organisms, and condition of the patient. The intravenous route is preferable for patients with septicemia or other severe or life-threatening infections.
Adults: See Table 1.

Table 1: Ceftriaxone for Injection
Dose in Adult Patients

Type of Infection	Route	Dose	Frequency	Total Daily Dose
Moderate and Severe Infections	I.V. or I.M.	1 or 2 g[a]	q 24 h	1 or 2 g
		0.5 or 1 g	q 12 h	1 or 2 g
There is limited experience with daily doses of 3-4 g administered as a single dose or two equally divided doses. The total daily dose should not exceed 4 g.				
Uncomplicated Gonorrhea	I.M.	250 mg	Single Dose	—

Infants and Children (one month to 12 years of age) : See Table 2.

Table 2: Ceftriaxone for Injection
Dose in Infants and Children (one month to 12 years of age)

Type of Infection	Route	Dose	Frequency	Total Daily Dose
Serious Miscellaneous Infections	I.V. or I.M.	25 or 37.5 mg/kg	q 12 h	50 or 75 mg/kg
The total daily dose should not exceed 2 g. If body weight is 50 kg or more the adult dose should be used.				
Meningitis	I.V. or I.M.	50 mg/ kg[a]	q 12 h	100 mg/kg

[a] With or without a loading dose of 75 mg/kg. The total daily dose should not exceed 4 g.

With the exception of gonorrhea, which is treated with a single dose, the administration of Ceftriaxone for Injection should be continued for a minimum of 48 to 72 hours after the patient defervesces or after evidence of bacterial eradication has been obtained, usually 4 to 14 days. In bone and joint infections the average duration of treatment during clinical trials was 6 weeks, with a range of 1 to 13 weeks, depending on the severity of the infection.
When treating infections caused by beta hemolytic streptococcus, it is recommended that therapy be continued for at least 10 days. The average duration of therapy for infections associated with beta hemolytic streptococcus during clinical trials was 2 weeks, with a range of 1 to 5 weeks, depending on the site and severity of the infection.
Prophylaxis (Vaginal or Abdominal Hysterectomy, Coronary Artery Bypass Surgery, Biliary Tract Surgery): For preoperative use as prophylaxis before vaginal or abdominal hysterectomy or coronary artery bypass surgery or biliary tract surgery in patients at risk of infection, a single dose of 1 g administered 1/2 to 2 hours before surgery is recommended.
Impairment of Renal and/or Hepatic Function: In patients with mild to moderate renal impairment, changes in the dosage regimen are not required, **provided liver function is intact**. In cases of preterminal renal failure (creatinine clearance less than 10 mL/min), periodic monitoring of serum ceftriaxone concentrations is recommended. The daily dosage should be limited to 2 g or less. In patients with liver damage, there is no need for the dosage to be reduced **provided renal function is intact**. In cases of coexistent renal and clinically significant hepatic insufficiency, close monitoring of serum ceftriaxone concentrations, at regular intervals, is recommended. If there is evidence of accumulation, dosage should be decreased accordingly.
Administration: Intramuscular: The reconstituted solution of Ceftriaxone for Injection should be administered by deep intragluteal injection. It is recommended that not more than 1 g be injected at a single site. Pain on intramuscular injection is usually mild and less frequent when Ceftriaxone for Injection is administered in sterile 1% Lidocaine solution.
Intravenous (bolus) Injection: The reconstituted solution should be administered over approximately 5 minutes. If the distal port of an intravenous administration set is used, stop the primary flow, inject the reconstituted Ceftriaxone for Injection solution and then restart the primary flow. This will prevent mixing with the primary fluid and possible incompatibilities.
Short Intravenous Infusion: The further diluted intravenous solution should be given over a period of 10 to 15 minutes in infants and children and 20 to 30 minutes in adults.
Note: Ceftriaxone for Injection solution should not be physically mixed with aminoglycoside antibiotics nor administered at the same site because of possible chemical incompatibility. There have also been literature reports of physical incompatibilities between ceftriaxone and vancomycin, amsacrine, or fluconazole.
Ceftriaxone must not be mixed with or administered simultaneously with calcium-containing intravenous solutions or products, even via different infusion lines. Cases of fatal reactions with calcium-ceftriaxone precipitates in lung and kidneys have been described in neonates. In some cases the infusion lines and times of administration of ceftriaxone and calcium-containing solutions differed.
Reconstitution: For Intramuscular Use: Reconstitute ceftriaxone for injection with the appropriate diluent: Sterile Water for Injection; 0.9% Sodium Chloride Injection; 5% Dextrose Injection; Bacteriostatic Water for Injection; 1% Lidocaine Solution.
Reconstitute as follows: See Table 3 and Table 4.

* Pain on intramuscular injection is usually mild and less frequent when the drug is administered in sterile 1% Lidocaine solution.
† Incidence is more frequent in patients less than one year old.
‡ Incidence is more frequent in patients less than one year old and over 50 years old.

Table 3: Ceftriaxone for Injection
Regular Volume Reconstitution Table (I.M.)

Vial Size	Volume to be Added to Vial mL	Approximate Available Volume mL	Approximate Average Concentration g/mL
0.25 g	0.9	1	0.25
1 g	3.3	4	0.25
2 g	6.6	8	0.25

Shake well until dissolved

Table 4: Ceftriaxone for Injection
Low Volume Reconstitution Table (I.M.)

Vial Size	Volume to be Added to Vial mL	Approximate Available Volume mL	Approximate Average Concentration g/mL
0.25 g	Not recommended for this vial size		
1 g	2.2	2.8	0.35
2 g	4.4	5.6	0.35

Shake well until dissolved.
Note: Solutions prepared for intramuscular use or any solution containing lidocaine or bacteriostatic water for injection should never be administered intravenously.
For Intravenous Use: Reconstitute only with Sterile Water for Injection.
Reconstitute as follows: See Table 5.

Table 5: Ceftriaxone for Injection
Reconstitution Table (I.V.)

Vial Size	Volume to be Added to Vial mL	Approximate Available Volume mL	Approximate Average Concentration g/mL
0.25 g	2.4	2.5	0.1
1 g	9.6	10.1	0.1
2 g	19.2	20.5	0.1

Shake well until dissolved. The prepared solution may be further diluted to the desired volume with any of the Solutions for I.V. Infusion listed below.
Solutions for I.V. Infusion: 0.9% Sodium Chloride Injection; 5% Dextrose Injection; Dextrose and Sodium Chloride Injection.
Pharmacy Bulk Vial Reconstitution for Preparation of Intravenous Infusion Solutions: The closure of the pharmacy bulk vial shall be penetrated only one time after reconstitution, using a suitable sterile transfer device or dispensing set which allows measured dispensing for the contents.

Table 6: Ceftriaxone for Injection
Reconstitution Table for Bulk Pharmacy Vial

Vial Size	Volume to be Added to Vial mL	Approximate Available Volume mL	Approximate Average Concentration g/mL
10 g	95	101	0.1

Shake well until dissolved. Withdraw the required amount and dilute with one of the Solutions for I.V. Infusion. Any unused solution remaining within a period of 8 hours should be discarded.
Stability and Storage Recommendations: Ceftriaxone for injection should be stored at a controlled room temperature (between 15 and 30°C) and protected from light.
Reconstituted Solutions—Stability and Storage Recommendations:

1. For Intramuscular Use: Solutions should be reconstituted immediately before use. If storage is required, these solutions may be stored under refrigeration and should be used within 48 hours.
2. For I.V. Bolus Injection (without further dilution): Reconstituted solutions should be administered within 24 hours when stored at room temperature and within 72 hours when refrigerated (2-8°C).
3. For I.V. Infusion: Further diluted reconstituted solutions should be administered within 24 hours when stored at room temperature.
   a) Solutions further diluted with 0.9% Sodium Chloride Injection, or with 5% Dextrose Injection should be administered within 72 hours when stored under refrigeration (2-8°C).
   b) Solutions further diluted with Dextrose and Sodium Chloride Injection as diluent should not be refrigerated. These solutions are not physically compatible when refrigerated.
4. Extended Use of Intravenous Admixtures: Although intravenous admixtures may often be physically and chemically stable for longer periods, **due to microbiological considerations, they are usually recommended for use within a maximum of 24 hours at room temperature or 72 hours when refrigerated (2-8°C)**. Hospitals and institutions that have recognized admixture programs and use validated aseptic techniques for preparation of intravenous solutions may extend the storage times for ceftriaxone for injection admixtures with 0.9% Sodium Chloride Injection or 5% Dextrose Injection in glass or polyvinyl chloride infusion containers, in concentrations of 3-40 mg/mL, to seven days when stored under refrigeration (2-8°C).
   Warning: As with all parenteral drug products, intravenous admixtures should be visually inspected prior to administration, whenever solution and container permit. Solutions showing any evidence of haziness or cloudiness, particulate matter, precipitation, discolouration or leakage should not be used.
5. Frozen I.V. Infusion Solutions: Hospitals and institutions that have recognized admixture programes and use validated aseptic techniques for preparation of intravenous solutions may freeze and store ceftriaxone for injection I.V. infusion solutions when prepared in accordance with the following instructions.
   I.V. infusion solutions prepared from reconstituted ceftriaxone for injection (ceftriaxone sodium) further diluted with 5% Dextrose Injection or 0.9% Sodium Chloride Injection, in flexible polyvinyl chloride infusion containers, in concentrations up to 40 mg ceftriaxone per mL, may be stored at −10 to −20°C for periods up to three months.
   The frozen solutions should be thawed in a refrigerator (2-8°C) overnight and should subsequently be used within 24 hours when stored at room temperature or seven days when stored under refrigeration (2-8°C).
   After thawing, check for leaks by squeezing the bag firmly. If leaks are found, discard the container as sterility may be impaired. Do not use unless the solution is clear and seals/outlet ports are intact. Ceftriaxone solutions range from light yellow to amber in colour. Parenteral drug products should be inspected visually for particulate matter and discolouration prior to administration whenever the solution and container permit.
   Do not refreeze the previously frozen ceftriaxone I.V. infusion solutions.

Incompatibility: **Ceftriaxone for Injection should not be added to solutions containing calcium such as Hartmann's solution and Ringer's solution (see Contraindications and Warnings).**

Ceftriaxone for Injection should not be physically mixed with other antimicrobial agents, vancomycin, amsacrine, or fluconazole.

Ceftriaxone for Injection should not be added to blood products, protein hydrolysates or amino acids.

SUPPLIED: Each vial of sterile white to pale yellow crystalline powder contains: ceftriaxone sodium (expressed in terms of anhydrous free acid) equivalent to 0.25 g, 1 g or 2 g; and as a Pharmacy Bulk vial containing the equivalent of ceftriaxone 10 g (not for direct administration). The availability of the pharmacy bulk vial is restricted to hospitals with a recognized intravenous admixture programme. Nonmedicinal ingredients: none. Sodium content of each g of ceftriaxone is approximately 83 mg (3.6 mEq sodium ion). The pH of freshly reconstituted solutions usually ranges from 6 to 8. Solutions are yellowish in colour.

Ceftriaxone Sodium for Injection, BP Ⓟ

ceftriaxone sodium

Antibiotic

Hospira

SUPPLIED: Each vial contains sterile powder equivalent to 250 mg, 500 mg and 1 g in 10 mL vial sizes, and 2 g in 50 mL vial size of ceftriaxone, cartons of 10. Each Pharmacy Bulk Vial contains sterile powder equivalent to 10 g in 100 mL vial size of ceftriaxone (not for direct administration), single cartons. **The availability of the pharmacy bulk vial is restricted to hospitals with a recognized intravenous admixture program.** Nonmedicinal ingredients: None. Sodium content of each g of Ceftriaxone Sodium for Injection, BP is approximately 83 mg (3.6 mEq sodium ion). Solutions are yellowish in colour.

Cefuroxime Ⓟ

Antibiotic

CPhA Monograph

Date of Preparation: October 2009

This monograph has been compiled by CPhA and reviewed by experts. It may contain information different from that found in Health Canada-approved Product Monographs. The reader is referred to the *CPS* Editorial Policy for more information.

SUMMARY PRODUCT INFORMATION:

Route of Administration	Dosage Form	Strength
Injectable (iv, im)	Dry powder for reconstitution	750 mg, 1.5 g; 7.5 g bulk vials available to hospitals with iv admixture program

INDICATIONS AND CLINICAL USE: Cefuroxime is a second-generation cephalosporin with enhanced activity against gram-negative bacteria compared to first-generation cephalosporins but less activity against gram-positive bacteria (see Action and Clinical Pharmacology). Generally, first-generation cephalosporins or penicillins are preferred for gram-positive infections when susceptible to these agents. In addition, third-generation cephalosporins are preferred agents over cefuroxime for serious infections caused by gram-negative organisms.

Cefuroxime sodium is indicated in the following clinical settings to treat or prevent infections caused by susceptible organisms:

- Lower respiratory tract infections
- Urinary tract infections (alternative agent)
- Skin and soft tissue infections
- Bone and joint infections (alternative agent)
- Preoperative prophylaxis
  - Open heart surgery
  - Noncardiac surgical procedures (e.g., vaginal hysterectomy)
- Gonorrhea: Cefuroxime has been used for uncomplicated gonorrhea; however, the 2006 Canadian Sexually Transmitted Infections guidelines do not list cefuroxime as an alternative for gonococcal infections [www.phac-aspc.gc.ca/std-mts/sti-its/pdf/sti-its-eng.pdf]. Eradication rates are not generally as high as other accepted regimens [*MMWR Recomm Rep* 2006;55(RR-11):1-94].
- Meningitis: Cefuroxime has been used in the treatment of meningitis but is not considered a drug of choice. Third-generation cephalosporins have been found to be clinically superior to cefuroxime in the treatment of meningitis [*Clin Infect Dis* 2004;39(9):1267-84].

CONTRAINDICATIONS:

- Patients who are hypersensitive to cefuroxime or to any ingredient in the formulation

WARNINGS AND PRECAUTIONS:

Serious Warnings and Precautions

- Cefuroxime has been associated with severe allergic reactions including anaphylactic reactions. For this reason a history of allergic reactions, including the type and severity of the reaction, should be obtained before prescribing and administering cefuroxime.
- Cross-sensitivity between penicillins and cephalosporins is estimated to be very low. Current opinion on the true incidence of cross-sensitivity is about 1%. The beta-lactam subunit is not considered the primary allergenic determinant; rather, the side chain predicts cross-reactivity. After thorough investigation into the nature of the allergy, a cephalosporin can be considered in a penicillin-allergic patient provided there is no history of an immediate-sensitivity reaction. Although the risk of cross-reaction is predicted to be low the patient should be monitored for signs of a sensitivity reaction.
- Patients with a history of immediate-sensitivity reaction to penicillin (e.g., anaphylaxis, bronchospasm and/or hypotension) are considered to be at increased risk of similar reactions to cephalosporins, including cefuroxime. For this reason, administration of cefuroxime should be avoided in patients with a history of severe allergic reactions to penicillin antibiotics unless skin testing is performed to rule out cross-sensitivity.
- Cephalosporin antibiotics including cefuroxime have been associated with *C. difficile*-associated diarrhea and colitis.

General: Cefuroxime may be associated with increased PT/INR, particularly in patients with poor nutritional status, hepatic or renal disease.

Renal: Nephrotoxicity has been reported rarely with cephalosporins, and is more likely in older individuals, or in patients who are taking other nephrotoxic drugs concomitantly or have pre-existing renal impairment. Since cefuroxime is cleared renally, dosage adjustment is recommended in patients with impaired renal function (see Dosage and Administration).

Sensitivity/Resistance: Prolonged use of cefuroxime may result in overgrowth of non-susceptible organisms.

Special Populations: Pregnant Women: Pregnancy Category B_M. Cefuroxime sodium crosses the placenta. It is generally accepted that cephalosporins are safe to use during pregnancy.

Nursing Women: Cefuroxime sodium is excreted in breast milk in low concentrations. Potential risks to the infant include altered bowel flora, diarrhea, obscured diagnosis of fever and hypersensitivity reactions. Cephalosporins are generally considered to be compatible with breast-feeding.

Pediatrics: Mild to severe hearing loss has been reported in a few pediatric patients receiving cefuroxime for the treatment for meningitis, although meningitis itself is associated with hearing loss. This may be due to the reduced efficacy in CSF sterilization compared to 3rd generation cephalosporins. Safety and effectiveness in pediatric patients below 3 months of age have not been established.

ADVERSE REACTIONS: Adverse Drug Reactions Overview: Adverse reactions to cefuroxime are similar to those of other cephalosporins.

More Common Adverse Drug Reactions (≥1%): Table 1 lists the more common adverse effects of cefuroxime.

Table 1: Cefuroxime

More Common Adverse Drug Reactions (≥1%)

Body System	Effect	% Incidence
Hematologic	Decreased hemoglobin and hematocrit	10
	Eosinophilia	7
Hepatic/Biliary/Pancreatic	Elevated liver function tests	4
Local Reactions	Mild to moderate pain at injection site	Up to 95% when given im
	Thrombophlebitis	2

Less Common Adverse Drug Reactions (<1%): Central Nervous System: headache, dizziness, somnolence, hyperactivity, psychotic reaction including disorientation, fluctuating consciousness, and episodes of restlessness, agitation and anxiety (case report), seizure.

Dermatologic: rash, erythema multiforme, Stevens-Johnson syndrome, toxic epidermal necrolysis, serum sickness-like reactions, anaphylaxis.

Ear/Nose/Throat: hearing loss reported in children receiving cefuroxime for meningitis.

Gastrointestinal: nausea, vomiting, *C. difficile*-associated diarrhea, colitis.

Hematologic: transient neutropenia and leukopenia, thrombocytopenia, hemolytic anemia, increased prothrombin time, increased erythrocyte sedimentation rate, agranulocytosis.

Hepatic/Biliary/Pancreatic: transient elevation in AST, ALT, alkaline phosphatase, LDH, and bilirubin concentrations, jaundice.

Immune: anaphylaxis and hypersensitivity reactions, angioedema.

Renal: acute interstitial nephritis, increased BUN, increased serum creatinine.

Other: stiffness at injection site.

DRUG INTERACTIONS: Drug-Drug Interactions: Drug-drug interactions involving cefuroxime are listed in Table 2.

Table 2: Cefuroxime

Drug-Drug Interactions

Interacting Drug	Effect	Clinical Comment
Aminoglycosides (e.g., amikacin, gentamicin, tobramycin)	Increased risk of nephrotoxicity; increased bactericidal activity against certain pathogens	Monitor aminoglycoside levels and renal function; discontinue one or both drugs, and use alternative therapy if renal dysfunction develops; may also be used therapeutically for synergistic effect.
Coumarin anticoagulants, e.g., warfarin, nicoumalone (acenocoumarol)	Possible increased anticoagulant effect when coadministered with cephalosporins	The mechanism may involve interference with vitamin K production. Monitor INR and adjust the anticoagulant dose accordingly. Vitamin K may be administered if bleeding occurs.
Probenecid	Probenecid inhibits the renal tubular excretion of cefuroxime thereby decreasing elimination of cefuroxime; may result in increased and prolonged serum concentrations of cefuroxime	This interaction has been exploited to increase serum levels of penicillins.

Drug-Laboratory Interactions: A false-positive reaction for glucose may be produced by cefuroxime in urine when copper reduction tests such as Benedict's, Fehling's solution or Clinitest tablets are used; this is, however, not seen with enzyme-based tests.

Cefuroxime may cause a positive direct Coombs' test.

DOSAGE AND ADMINISTRATION: Dosing Considerations: For severe life-threatening infections cefuroxime sodium should be given by the iv route.

Recommended Dose and Dosage Adjustment: Adults: See Table 3.

Table 3: Cefuroxime

Dose in Adult Patients

Indication	Route	Usual Dose	Maximum Dose
Mild to moderate infections	IV/IM	750 mg iv Q8H	6 g/day
Severe infections including bone and joint infections	IV	1.5 g iv Q8H	6 g/day or 9 g/day if used for meningitis (although cefuroxime not recommended for this indication)
Surgical prophylaxis — noncardiac	IV/IM	1.5 g iv 30–60 minutes before initial incision	May continue 750 mg iv/im Q8H for prolonged procedure to a maximum of 24 hours (i.e., 3 doses including induction)
Surgical prophylaxis — cardiac	IV	1.5 g iv at induction of anesthesia and Q12H for 24 to 48 hours	6 g (4 doses); there is no evidence that continuing beyond 48 hours is any more effective.

Pediatrics: See Table 4.

Table 4: Cefuroxime

Dose in Pediatric Patients (1 month to 12 years)

Indication	Route	Usual Dose	Maximum Dose
Mild to moderate infections	IV/IM	50–100 mg/kg/day divided Q6–8H	2 g/dose; 6 g/day
Severe infections including bone and joint infections	IV/IM	150 mg/kg/day divided Q8H	2 g/dose; 6 g/day
Surgical prophylaxis — noncardiac	IV/IM	50 mg/kg iv 30–60 minutes before initial incision	May continue iv/im Q8H for prolonged procedure to a maximum of 24 hours (i.e., 3 doses including induction)

(cont'd)

Table 4: Cefuroxime *(cont'd)*

Dose in Pediatric Patients (1 month to 12 years)

Indication	Route	Usual Dose	Maximum Dose
Surgical prophylaxis — cardiac	IV	50 mg/kg iv at induction of anesthesia and Q12H for 24 to 48 hours	1.5 g/dose; 4 doses; there is no evidence that continuing beyond 48 hours is any more effective.

Renal Impairment: See Table 5.

Table 5: Cefuroxime

Dose in Adult Patients with Renal Impairment

Route	Creatinine Clearance (mL/min)	Dosage Adjustment
IV/IM	>50	Q8H
IV/IM	10–50	Q8–12H
IV/IM	<10	Q24H

Dosage in Dialysis: A supplemental dose should be given after dialysis.
Hepatic Impairment: No dosage adjustments are required in patients with hepatic impairment.
Administration: Cefuroxime sodium may be given by iv or im injection after reconstitution. When administering im inject deep into a large muscle mass. For iv bolus injection slowly inject over a period of 3 to 5 minutes. For intermittent iv infusion administer over 30 minutes.

OVERDOSAGE:

For management of a suspected drug overdose, CPhA recommends that you contact your **regional Poison Control Centre**. See the *CPS* Directory section for a list of Poison Control Centres.

ACTION AND CLINICAL PHARMACOLOGY: Mechanism of Action: Cefuroxime is a second generation cephalosporin that exerts its bactericidal activity through inhibition of peptidoglycan synthesis in the bacterial cell wall, leading to the formation of a defective cell wall with eventual lysis and cell death.

The in vitro activity of cefuroxime includes gram-positive aerobic bacteria such as penicillinase-producing and non-penicillinase-producing strains of *S. aureus*, most strains of *S. epidermidis*, α-hemolytic and β-hemolytic streptococci, and *S. pneumoniae*. Gram-negative aerobic bacteria include some Enterobacteriaceae (e.g., *C. freundii*, *E. aerogenes*, *E. coli*, *K. pneumoniae*, *P. multocida*, *P. mirabilis*, Salmonella and Shigella), *H. influenzae* (including ampicillin-resistant strains) and *H. parainfluenzae*, *N. gonorrhoeae* and *N. meningitidis*. Cefuroxime is also active against some anaerobic bacteria including Actinomyces, Clostridium (not difficile), Fusobacterium, Peptostreptococcus, Propionibacterium and Veillonella.

Cefuroxime has little or no activity against staphylococci resistant to penicillinase-resistant penicillins, Enterococcus species, *L. monocytogenes*, *P. aeruginosa*, *A. calcoaceticus*, *P. vulgaris*, Legionella, Campylobacter species, Providencia species, Serratia species, *C. difficile*, and *B. fragilis*.

Pharmacokinetics: Adults: Absorption: Cefuroxime 750 mg im results in peak plasma levels of 35 to 40 µg/mL after 30 to 40 minutes compared to 73 µg/mL 5 minutes after the same dose given iv.
Distribution: Cefuroxime is widely distributed into body tissues and fluids and passes readily across the placenta, will pass into breast milk and uninflamed meninges. The extent of plasma protein binding is approximately 33-50%.
Excretion: Cefuroxime is primarily renally excreted with approximately 89% excreted unchanged in urine in 8 hours; 90-100% within 24 hours. The serum half-life ranges from 1 to 2 hours after im or iv administration and is increased by 30% when administered with probenecid, which is sometimes used to prolong its therapeutic effect. The half-life increases as renal function declines and can reach 20 hours when creatinine clearance falls below 10 mL/min.

STORAGE AND STABILITY: According to the manufacturer reconstituted solution should be used within 4 hours if kept between 15 and 25°C or 48 hours if stored under refrigeration.

Cefzil™ Pr
cefprozil
Antibiotic

Bristol-Myers Squibb

Date of Preparation: March 29, 1995
Date of Revision: October 21, 2008

PHARMACOLOGY: CEFZIL (cefprozil) is a semisynthetic broad spectrum cephalosporin antibiotic intended for oral administration. It has in vitro activity against a broad range of gram positive and gram negative bacteria. The bactericidal action of cefprozil results from inhibition of cell-wall synthesis.
Pharmacokinetics: Cefprozil is well absorbed following oral administration in both fasting and nonfasting subjects. The oral bioavailability of cefprozil is about 90%. The pharmacokinetics of cefprozil are not altered when administered with meals, or when coadministered with antacid. Average plasma concentrations after administration of cefprozil to fasting subjects are shown in Table 1. Urinary recovery accounts for 60% of the administered dose.

Table 1: CEFZIL

Mean Plasma Concentrations

Dosage	Mean Plasma Cefprozil[a] Concentrations (µg/mL) Peak ~1.5 h	4 h	8 h	8-hour Urinary Excretion
250 mg	6.1	1.7	0.2	60%
500 mg	10.5	3.2	0.4	62%
1 g	18.3	8.4	1.0	54%

[a] Data represent mean values from 12 healthy, young male volunteers.

During the first 4-hour period after drug administration, the average urine concentrations following the 250 mg, 500 mg, and 1 g doses were approximately 170 µg/mL, 450 µg/mL and 600 µg/mL, respectively.

The average plasma half-life in normal subjects is 1.3 hours. Plasma protein binding is approximately 36% and is independent of concentration in the range of 2 to 20 µg/mL. There is no evidence of accumulation of cefprozil in the plasma in individuals with normal renal function following multiple oral doses of up to 1 g every 8 hours for 10 days.
Renal Insufficiency: In patients with reduced renal function, the plasma half-life prolongation is related to the degree of the renal dysfunction and may be prolonged up to 5.2 hours. In patients with complete absence of renal function, the plasma half-life of cefprozil averaged 5.9 hours. The half-life is shortened during hemodialysis to 2.1 hours. Excretion pathways in patients with markedly impaired renal function have not been determined (see Precautions and Dosage).
Hepatic Insufficiency: In patients with impaired hepatic function, no differences in pharmacokinetic parameters were observed, when compared to normal control subjects.
Geriatrics: Following administration of a single 1 g dose of cefprozil, the average AUC observed in healthy elderly subjects (≥65 years of age) was approximately 35 to 60% higher than that of healthy young adults and the average AUC in females was approximately 15 to 20% higher than in males. The magnitude of these age and gender-related variations in the pharmacokinetics of cefprozil are not sufficient to necessitate dosage adjustments.
Children: Comparable pharmacokinetic parameters of cefprozil are observed between pediatric patients (6 months to 12 years) and adults following oral administration. The maximum plasma concentrations are achieved at 1 to 2 hours after dosing. The plasma elimination half-life is approximately 1.5 hours. The AUC of cefprozil to pediatric patients after 7.5, 15 and 30 mg/kg doses is similar to that observed in normal adult subjects after 250, 500 and 1000 mg doses, respectively.

INDICATIONS: CEFZIL (cefprozil) is indicated for the treatment of the following infections caused by susceptible strains of the designated microorganisms:
Upper Respiratory Tract: **Pharyngitis/tonsillitis** caused by group A β-hemolytic (GABHS) *S. pyogenes*.

Substantial data establishing the efficacy of cefprozil in the subsequent prevention of rheumatic fever are not available at present, although no case was reported during its evaluation in over 978 pediatric and 831 adult patients in controlled clinical trials.

Otitis media caused by *S. pneumoniae*, *H. influenzae*. *M. (Branhamella) catarrhalis*.

Acute sinusitis caused by *S. pneumoniae*, *H. influenzae*, (beta-lactamase positive and negative strains), and *M. (Branhamella) catarrhalis*.
Skin and Skin Structure: **Uncomplicated skin and skin-structure infections** caused by *S. aureus* (including penicillinase-producing strains) and *S. pyogenes*.
Urinary Tract: **Uncomplicated urinary tract infections** (including acute cystitis) caused by *E. coli*, *K. pneumoniae*, *P. mirabilis*.

Cultures and susceptibility studies should be performed when appropriate.

CONTRAINDICATIONS: CEFZIL (cefprozil) is contraindicated in patients with known allergy to the cephalosporin class of antibiotics or to any component of the preparations (see Supplied).

WARNINGS: Before therapy with CEFZIL (cefprozil) is instituted, careful inquiry should be made to determine whether the patient has had previous hypersensitivity reactions to CEFZIL (cefprozil), cephalosporins, penicillins, or other drugs. If this product is to be given to penicillin-sensitive patients, caution should be exercised because cross-sensitivity among beta-lactam antibiotics has been clearly documented and may occur in up to 10% of patients with a history of penicillin allergy.

If an allergic reaction to Cefzil occurs, discontinue the drug. Serious acute hypersensitivity reactions may require treatment with epinephrine and other emergency measures, including oxygen, i.v. fluids, i.v. antihistamines, corticosteroids, pressor amines, and airway management, as clinically indicated.
Gastrointestinal: *C. difficile*-associated disease: *C. difficile*-associated disease (CDAD) has been reported with use of many antibacterial agents, including CEFZIL (cefprozil). CDAD may range in severity from mild diarrhea to fatal colitis. It is important to consider this diagnosis in patients who present with diarrhea, or symptoms of colitis, pseudomembranous colitis, toxic megacolon, or perforation of colon subsequent to the administration of any antibacterial agent. CDAD has been reported to occur over 2 months after the administration of antibacterial agents.

Treatment with antibacterial agents may alter the normal flora of the colon and may permit overgrowth of *C. difficile*. *C. difficile* produces toxins A and B, which contribute to the development of CDAD. CDAD may cause significant morbidity and mortality. CDAD can be refractory to antimicrobial therapy.

If the diagnosis of CDAD is suspected or confirmed, appropriate therapeutic measures should be initiated. Mild cases of CDAD usually respond to discontinuation of antibacterial agents not directed against *C. difficile*. In moderate to severe cases, consideration should be given to management with fluids and electrolytes, protein supplementation, and treatment with an antibacterial agent clinically effective against *C. difficile*. Surgical evaluation should be instituted as clinically indicated, as surgical intervention may be required in certain severe cases (see Adverse Effects).

PRECAUTIONS: General: Evaluation of renal status before and during therapy is recommended, especially in seriously ill patients. In patients with known or suspected renal impairment (see Dosage), careful clinical observation and appropriate laboratory studies should be done prior to and during therapy. The total daily dose of CEFZIL (cefprozil) should be reduced in patients with creatinine clearance values ≤30 mL/min because high and/or prolonged plasma antibiotic concentrations can occur from usual doses in such individuals. Cephalosporins, including CEFZIL, should be given with caution to patients receiving concurrent treatment with potent diuretics since these agents are suspected of adversely affecting renal function.

Prolonged use of CEFZIL may result in the overgrowth of nonsusceptible organisms. Careful observation of the patient is essential. If superinfection occurs during therapy, appropriate measures should be taken.

Positive direct Coombs' tests have been reported during treatment with cephalosporin antibiotics.

Cefprozil should be prescribed with caution in individuals with a history of gastrointestinal disease particularly colitis.
Drug Interactions: Nephrotoxicity has been reported following concomitant administration of aminoglycoside antibiotics and cephalosporin antibiotics. Concomitant administration of probenecid doubled the area under the curve for cefprozil.

If an aminoglycoside is used concurrently with cefprozil, especially if high dosages of the former are used or if therapy is prolonged, renal function should be monitored because of the potential nephrotoxicity and ototoxicity of aminoglycoside antibiotics.
Drug/Laboratory Test Interactions: Cephalosporin antibiotics may produce a false positive reaction for glucose in the urine with copper reduction tests (Benedict's or Fehling's solution or with Clinitest tablets), but not with enzyme-based tests (glucose oxidase) for glycosuria. A false negative reaction may occur in the ferricyanide test for blood glucose. The presence of cefprozil in the blood does not interfere with the assay of plasma or urine creatinine by the alkaline picrate method.
Pregnancy: Reproduction studies have been performed in mice, rats, and rabbits at doses 14, 7 and 0.7 times the maximum human daily dose (1000 mg) based upon mg/m², and have revealed no evidence of harm to the fetus due to cefprozil. There are, however, no adequate and well-controlled studies in pregnant women. Because animal reproduction studies are not always predictive of human response, this drug should be used during pregnancy only if the potential benefit justifies the potential risk.
Lactation: Less than 1% of a maternal dose is excreted in human milk. Caution should be exercised when CEFZIL is administered to a nursing mother. Consideration should be given to temporary discontinuation of nursing and use of formula feeding.
Children: The use of CEFZIL in the treatment of acute sinusitis in these age groups is supported by evidence from adequate and well-controlled studies of cefprozil in adults and from pediatric pharmacokinetic studies.

Safety and effectiveness in children below the age of 6 months have not been established. Accumulation of other cephalosporin antibiotics in newborn infants (resulting from prolonged drug half-life in this age group) has been reported.
Geriatrics: Cefprozil has not been studied in the chronically ill or institutionalized elderly subjects. In these subjects, drug clearance by the kidney may be reduced even with normal serum creatinine clearance. Reduction of dose or of frequency of administration may be indicated.

ADVERSE EFFECTS: The adverse reactions to CEFZIL (cefprozil) are similar to those observed with other orally administered cephalosporins. Cefprozil was usually well tolerated in controlled clinical trials. Approximately 2% of patients discontinued cefprozil therapy due to adverse events.

The most common adverse events (of probable or unknown relationship to study drug) observed in 4227 patients treated with cefprozil in clinical efficacy trials are:
Gastrointestinal: diarrhea (2.7%), nausea (2.3%), vomiting (1.4%) and abdominal pain (0.9%).
Hepatobiliary: As with some penicillins and some other cephalosporin antibiotics, cholestatic jaundice has been reported rarely.
Hypersensitivity: rash (1.2%), erythema (0.1%), pruritus (0.3%) and urticaria (0.07%). Such reactions have been reported more frequently in children than in adults. Signs and symptoms usually occur a few days after initiation of therapy and subside within a few days after cessation of therapy.
Central Nervous System: Dizziness, hyperactivity, headache, nervousness, insomnia, confusion, and drowsiness have been reported rarely (<1%) and causal relationship is uncertain. All were reversible.
Other: genital pruritus (0.8%) and vaginitis (0.7%).
Laboratory Abnormalities: Transitory abnormalities in clinical laboratory test results of uncertain etiology have been reported during clinical trials as follows:
Hepatobiliary: elevations of AST, ALT, alkaline phosphatase, and bilirubin.
Hematopoietic: transiently decreased leukocyte count and eosinophilia.
Renal: slight elevations in BUN and serum creatinine.

Adverse reactions reported from post-marketing experience and which were not seen in the clinical trials include anaphylaxis, angioedema, serum sickness, colitis including pseudomembraneous colitis, erythema multiforme, fever, Stevens-Johnson syndrome, thrombocytopenia and exfoliative dermatitis. Tooth discoloration has been reported during post-marketing surveillance. The association between these events and Cefzil administration is unknown.

In addition to the adverse reactions listed above which have been observed in patients treated with cefprozil, the following adverse reactions and altered laboratory tests have been reported for cephalosporin-class antibiotics. Toxic epidermal necrolysis, renal dysfunction, toxic nephropathy, aplastic anemia, hemolytic anemia, hemorrhage, prolonged prothrombin time, positive Coombs' tests, elevated LDH, pancytopenia, neutropenia, agranulocytosis.

Several cephalosporins have been implicated in triggering seizures, particularly in patients with renal impairment, when the dosage was not reduced (see Dosage and Overdose). If seizures associated with drug therapy occur, the drug should be discontinued. Anticonvulsant therapy can be given if clinically indicated.

OVERDOSE:

Symptoms: Since no case of overdosage has been reported to date, no specific information on symptoms or treatment of overdosage is available. In animal toxicology studies, single doses as high as 5000 mg/kg were without serious or lethal consequences.

Treatment: Cefprozil is eliminated primarily by the kidneys. In case of severe overdosage, especially in patients with compromised renal function, hemodialysis will aid in the removal of cefprozil from the body.

For management of a suspected drug overdose, contact your **regional Poison Control Centre**. See the *CPS* Directory section for a list of Poison Control Centres.

DOSAGE: CEFZIL (cefprozil) is administered orally (with or without food), in the treatment of infections due to susceptible bacteria in the following doses:

Adults (13 years and older): Upper respiratory tract (pharyngitis/tonsillitis): 500 mg q24h. Acute sinusitis: 250 mg or 500 mg q12h. Skin and skin structure: 250 mg q12h or 500 mg q24h. Uncomplicated urinary tract: 500 mg q24h.

Children (2 to 12 years): Skin and skin structure: 20 mg/kg q24h. See Table 2.

Table 2: CEFZIL

Dosage in Children (2-12 years): Skin and Skin Structure (20 mg/kg q24h)

		Multi-dose bottle			
		125 mg/5 mL		250 mg/5 mL	
Age[a] (years)	Weight (kg)	tsp/dose	mL/dose	tsp/dose	mL/dose
2–3	11–14	2.0	10.0	1.0	5.0
4–6	15–21	3.0	15.0	1.5	7.5
7–8	22–26	—	—	2.0	10.0
9–10	28–31	—	—	2.5	12.5
11	35	—	—	3.0	15.0

[a] Ages given are a useful guide only. Correct dosage should be determined by weight.

Infants and Children (6 months to 12 years): Otitis media: 15 mg/kg q12h. See Table 3.

Table 3: CEFZIL

Dosage in Infants and Children (6 months-12 years): Otitis Media (15 mg/kg q12h)

		Multi-dose bottle			
		125 mg/5 mL		250 mg/5 mL	
Age[a] (years)	Weight (kg)	tsp/dose	mL/dose	tsp/dose	mL/dose
6 months–1 year	7–9	1.0	5.0	0.5	2.5
2	11–12	1.5	7.5	0.75	3.75
3–4	14–15	—	—	1.0	5.0
5–6	17–21	—	—	1.25	6.25
7–8	22–26	—	—	1.5	7.5
9–10	28–31	—	—	1.75	8.75
11–12	35–39	—	—	2.0	10.0

[a] Ages given are a useful guide only. Correct dosage should be determined by weight.

Upper respiratory tract (pharyngitis/tonsillitis): 7.5 mg/kg q12h. See Table 4.

Table 4: CEFZIL

Dosage in Infants and Children (6 months-12 years): Upper Respiratory Tract (Pharyngitis/Tonsillitis) (7.5 mg/kg q12h)

		Multi-dose bottle			
		125 mg/5 mL		250 mg/5 mL	
Age[a] (years)	Weight (kg)	tsp/dose	mL/dose	tsp/dose	mL/dose
6 months–1 year	7–9	0.5	2.5	—	—
2–6	11–21	1.0	5.0	0.5	2.5
7–9	22–28	—	—	0.75	3.75
10–11	31–35	—	—	1.0	5.0
12	41	—	—	1.25	6.25

[a] Ages given are a useful guide only. Correct dosage should be determined by weight.

Acute Sinusitis: 7.5 mg/kg q12h or 15 mg/kg q12h. Follow dosing instructions as for otitis media and upper respiratory tract presented in Table 3 and Table 4.

The maximum pediatric daily dose should not exceed the maximum daily dose recommended for adults (e.g., 1 g/day).

Duration of Therapy: Duration of therapy in the majority of clinical trials was 10 to 15 days. The duration of treatment should be guided by the patient's clinical and bacteriological response. In the treatment of acute uncomplicated cystitis, a 7-day oral therapy is usually sufficient. In the treatment of infections due to *S. pyogenes*, a therapeutic dosage of cefprozil should be administered for at least 10 days.

Renal Impairment: Cefprozil may be administered to patients with impaired renal function. No dosage adjustment is necessary for patients with creatinine clearance values >30 mL/min. For those with creatinine clearance values ≤ 30 mL/min, 50% of the standard dose should be given at the standard dosing interval. Cefprozil is in part removed by hemodialysis; therefore, cefprozil should be administered after the completion of hemodialysis.

Reconstitution: Prior to dispensing, the pharmacist must constitute the dry powder with water as described in Table 5.

Table 5: CEFZIL

Reconstitution Table

Cefzil Powder for Oral Suspension	Bottle Size (mL)	Diluent (water) Added to Bottle (mL)	Approximate Available Volume (mL)	Final Concentration
125 mg/5 mL	75	54	75	125 mg/5 mL
	100	72	100	125 mg/5 mL
250 mg/5 mL	75	54	75	250 mg/5 mL
	100	72	100	250 mg/5 mL

For ease in preparation, the water can be added in 2 portions. Shake well after each addition and prior to use.

Storage of Reconstituted Suspension: The constituted CEFZIL oral suspension must be stored in the refrigerator (2 to 8°C) for up to 14 days. Keep container tightly closed. Discard unused portion after 14 days.

SUPPLIED: Powder for Oral Suspension: 125 mg/5 mL: Each 5 mL of constituted, bubble-gum flavored solution contains: anhydrous cefprozil 125 mg. Nonmedicinal ingredients: aspartame, citric acid, colloidal silicone dioxide, FD&C yellow No. 6, flavors (natural and artificial), glycine, microcrystalline cellulose, polysorbate 80, simethicone, sodium benzoate, sodium carboxymethylcellulose, sodium chloride and sucrose. Bottles of 75 and 100 mL.

250 mg/5 mL: Each 5 mL of constituted, bubble-gum flavored solution contains: anhydrous cefprozil 250 mg. Nonmedicinal ingredients: aspartame, citric acid, colloidal silicone dioxide, FD&C yellow No. 6, flavors (natural and artificial), glycine, microcrystalline cellulose, polysorbate 80, simethicone, sodium benzoate, sodium carboxymethylcellulose, sodium chloride and sucrose. Bottles of 75 and 100 mL.

Tablets: 250 mg: Each light orange, caplet-shaped, film-coated tablet engraved with 7720 on one side and with 250 on the other side, contains: anhydrous cefprozil 250 mg. Nonmedicinal ingredients: FD&C yellow No. 6, hydroxypropylmethylcellulose, magnesium stearate, microcrystalline cellulose, polyethylene glycol, polysorbate 80, simethicone, sodium starch glycolate and titanium dioxide. Bottles of 100.

500 mg: Each white, caplet-shaped, film-coated tablet, engraved with 7721 on one side and with 500 on the other side, contains: anhydrous cefprozil 500 mg. Nonmedicinal ingredients: hydroxypropylmethylcellulose, magnesium stearate, microcrystalline cellulose, polyethylene glycol, polysorbate 80, simethicone, sodium starch glycolate and titanium dioxide. Bottles of 100.

Store the tablets and powder for oral suspension at room temperature (15 to 30°C) and protect from light and excessive humidity.

(Shown in Product Identification Section)

Celebrex® ℞

celecoxib

Nonsteroidal Anti-inflammatory Drug (NSAID)

Pfizer

Date of Revision: April 9, 2010

SUMMARY PRODUCT INFORMATION:

Route of Administration	Dosage Form/ Strength	Clinically Relevant Nonmedicinal Ingredients
Oral	Capsules, 100 mg and 200 mg	Lactose monohydrate For a complete listing see the Dosage Forms, Composition and Packaging.

INDICATIONS AND CLINICAL USE: CELEBREX (celecoxib) is indicated for relief of symptoms associated with:

- Osteoarthritis,
- Adult Rheumatoid Arthritis, and
- Ankylosing Spondylitis.

CELEBREX (celecoxib) is also indicated for the short-term (≤7 days) management of moderate to severe acute pain in adults in conditions such as the following:

- musculoskeletal and/or soft tissue trauma including sprains,
- postoperative orthopaedic, and
- pain following dental extraction.

For patients with an increased risk of developing CV and/or GI adverse events, other management strategies that do not include the use of NSAIDs should be considered first. (See Contraindications and Warnings and Precautions.)

Use of CELEBREX should be limited to the lowest effective dose for the shortest possible duration of treatment in order to minimize the potential risk for cardiovascular or gastrointestinal adverse events. (See Contraindications and Warnings and Precautions.)

CELEBREX, as a NSAID, does **not** treat clinical disease or prevent its progression.

CELEBREX, as a NSAID, only relieves symptoms and decreases inflammation for as long as the patient continues to take it.

Geriatrics (>65 years of age): Evidence from clinical studies and postmarket experience suggests that use in geriatric population is associated with differences in safety (see Warnings and Precautions, Special Populations, Geriatrics (>65 years of age)).

Pediatrics (<18 years of age): Safety and Efficacy have not been established in the paediatric population (see Contraindications).

CONTRAINDICATIONS: CELEBREX is contraindicated in:

- the peri-operative setting of coronary artery bypass graft surgery (CABG). Although CELEBREX has **not** been studied in this patient population, a selective COX-2 inhibitor NSAID studied in such a setting has led to an increased incidence of cardiovascular/thromboembolic events, deep surgical infections and sternal wound complications.
- the third trimester of pregnancy, because of risk of premature closure of the ductus arteriosus and prolonged parturition
- women who are breastfeeding, because of the potential for serious adverse reactions in nursing infants
- severe uncontrolled heart failure
- known hypersensitivity to celecoxib or to any of the components/excipients
- demonstrated allergic-type reactions to sulfonamides
- history of asthma, urticaria, or allergic-type reactions after taking ASA or other NSAIDs (i.e. complete or partial syndrome of ASA-intolerance—rhinosinusitis, urticaria/angioedema, nasal polyps, asthma). Fatal anaphylactoid reactions have occurred in such individuals. Individuals with the above medical problems are at risk of a severe reaction even if they have taken NSAIDs in the past without any adverse reaction. The potential for cross-reactivity between different NSAIDs must be kept in mind (see Warnings and Precautions, Hypersensitivity Reactions, Anaphylactoid Reactions).
- active gastric/duodenal/peptic ulcer, active gastrointestinal bleeding
- cerebrovascular bleedings
- inflammatory bowel disease
- severe liver impairment or active liver disease
- severe renal impairment (creatinine clearance <30 mL/min or 0.5 mL/sec) or deteriorating renal disease (individuals with lesser degrees of renal impairment are at risk of deterioration of their renal function when prescribed NSAIDs and must be monitored) (see Warnings and Precautions, Renal)
- known hyperkalemia (see Warnings and Precautions, Renal, Fluid and Electrolyte Balance).
- Safety and Efficacy of CELEBREX have not been established in the paediatric population under 18 years of age.

WARNINGS AND PRECAUTIONS:

Serious Warnings and Precautions
Risk of Cardiovascular (CV) Adverse Events: Ischemic Heart Disease, Cerebrovascular Disease, Congestive Heart Failure (NYHA II-IV) (see Warnings and Precautions, Cardiovascular).

CELEBREX is a non-steroidal anti-inflammatory drug (NSAID). Use of some NSAIDs is associated with an increased incidence of cardiovascular adverse events (such as myocardial infarction, stroke or thrombotic events) which can be fatal. The risk may increase with duration of use. Patients with cardiovascular disease or risk factors for cardiovascular disease may be at greater risk.

Caution should be exercised in prescribing CELEBREX to any patient with ischemic heart disease (including but not limited to acute myocardial infarction, history of myocardial infarction and/or angina), cerebrovascular disease (including but not limited to stroke, cerebrovascular accident, transient ischemic attacks and/or amaurosis fugax) and/or congestive heart failure (NYHA II-IV).

Use of NSAIDs, such as CELEBREX, can promote sodium retention in a dose-dependent manner, through a renal mechanism, which can result in increased blood pressure and/or exacerbation of congestive heart failure. (See also Warnings and Precautions, Renal, Fluid and Electrolyte Balance.)

Randomized clinical trials with CELEBREX have not been designed to detect differences in cardiovascular events in a chronic setting. Therefore, caution should be exercised when prescribing CELEBREX.

Risk of Gastrointestinal (GI) Adverse Events (see Warnings and Precautions, Gastrointestinal (GI)).

Use of NSAIDs, such as CELEBREX, is associated with an increased incidence of gastrointestinal adverse events (such as peptic/duodenal ulceration, perforation, obstruction and gastrointestinal bleeding).

Risk in Pregnancy: Caution should be exercised in prescribing CELEBREX during the first and second trimesters of pregnancy. CELEBREX is contraindicated for use during the third trimester because of risk of premature closure of the ductus arteriosus and uterine inertia (prolong parturition). (See Contraindications.)

General: Frail or debilitated patients may tolerate side effects less well and therefore special care should be taken in treating this population. **To minimize the potential risk for an adverse event, the lowest effective dose should be used for the shortest possible duration.** As with other NSAIDs, caution should be used in the treatment of elderly patients who are more likely to be suffering from impaired renal, hepatic or cardiac function. For high risk patients, alternate therapies that do not involve NSAIDs should be considered.

CELEBREX is **not** recommended for use with other NSAIDs , with the exception of low-dose ASA for cardiovascular prophylaxis, because of the absence of any evidence demonstrating synergistic benefits and the potential for additive adverse reactions (see Drug Interactions, Drug-Drug Interactions, Acetylsalicylic Acid (ASA) or Other NSAIDs).

Cardiovascular: CELEBREX is a non-steroidal anti-inflammatory drug (NSAID). Use of some NSAIDs is associated with an increased incidence of cardiovascular adverse events (such as myocardial infarction, stroke or thrombotic events) which can be fatal (see Adverse Reactions). The risk may increase with dose and duration of use. Patients with cardiovascular disease or risk factors for cardiovascular disease may be at greater risk.

Caution should be exercised in prescribing CELEBREX to patients with risk factors for cardiovascular disease, cerebrovascular disease or renal disease, such as any of the following (NOT an exhaustive list):

- **Hypertension**
- **Dyslipidemia/Hyperlipidemia**
- **Diabetes Mellitus**
- **Congestive Heart Failure (NYHA I)**
- **Coronary Artery Disease (Atherosclerosis)**
- **Peripheral Arterial Disease**
- **Smoking**
- **Creatinine Clearance <60 mL/min or 1 mL/sec**

Use of NSAIDs, such as CELEBREX, can lead to new hypertension or can worsen pre-existing hypertension, either of which may increase the risk of cardiovascular events as described above. Thus blood pressure should be monitored regularly. Consideration should be given to discontinuing CELEBREX should hypertension either develop or worsen with its use.

Use of NSAIDs, such as CELEBREX, can induce fluid retention and edema, and may exacerbate congestive heart failure, through a renal-mediated mechanism. (See Warnings and Precautions, Renal, Fluid and Electrolyte Balance.)

For patients with a high risk of developing an adverse CV event, other management strategies that do **not** include the use of NSAIDs should be considered first. **To minimize the potential risk for an adverse CV event, the lowest effective dose should be used for the shortest possible duration.**

One of three randomized clinical trials of about 3 years duration showed a dose-related increase in serious cardiovascular events (mainly myocardial infarction), detectable at doses of CELEBREX 200 mg twice daily or more, compared to placebo.

Endocrine and Metabolism: Corticosteroids: CELEBREX (celecoxib) is not a substitute for corticosteroids. It does **not** treat corticosteroid insufficiency. Abrupt discontinuation of corticosteroids may lead to exacerbation of corticosteroid-responsive illness. Patients on prolonged corticosteroid therapy should have their therapy tapered slowly if a decision is made to discontinue corticosteroids (see Drug Interactions, Drug-Drug Interactions, Glucocorticoids).

Gastrointestinal (GI): Serious GI toxicity (sometimes fatal), such as peptic/duodenal ulceration, inflammation, perforation, obstruction and gastrointestinal bleeding, can occur at any time, with or without warning symptoms, in patients treated with NSAIDs, such as CELEBREX. Minor upper GI problems, such as dyspepsia, commonly occur at any time. Health care providers should remain alert for ulceration and bleeding in patients treated with CELEBREX, even in the absence of previous GI tract symptoms. Most spontaneous reports of fatal GI events are in elderly or debilitated patients and therefore special care should be taken in treating this population. **To minimize the potential risk for an adverse GI event, the lowest effective dose should be used for the shortest possible duration.** For high risk patients, alternate therapies that do not involve NSAIDs should be considered (see Warnings and Precautions, Special Populations, Geriatrics (>65 years of age)).

Patients should be informed about the signs and/or symptoms of serious GI toxicity and instructed to discontinue using CELEBREX and seek emergency medical attention if they experience any such symptoms. The utility of periodic laboratory monitoring has **not** been demonstrated, nor has it been adequately assessed. Most patients who develop a serious upper GI adverse event on NSAID therapy have no symptoms. Upper GI ulcers, gross bleeding, or perforation caused by NSAIDs, appear to occur in approximately 1% of patients treated for 3 to 6 months, and in about 2% to 4% of patients treated for one year. These trends continue, thus increasing the likelihood of developing a serious GI event at some time during the course of therapy. Even short-term therapy has its risks.

Caution should be taken if prescribing CELEBREX to patients with a prior history of peptic/duodenal ulcer disease and/or gastrointestinal bleeding as these individuals have a greater than 10-fold higher risk for developing a GI bleed when taking NSAID than patients with neither of these risk factors. Other risk factors for GI ulceration and bleeding include the following: *H. pylori* infection, increased age, prolonged use of NSAID therapy, excess alcohol intake, smoking, poor general health status or concomitant therapy with any of the following:

- Anticoagulants (e.g. warfarin)
- Antiplatelet agents (e.g. ASA, clopidogrel)
- Oral corticosteroids (e.g. prednisone)
- Selective Serotonin Reuptake Inhibitors (SSRIs) (e.g. citalopram, paroxetine, fluoxetine, sertraline)

There is no definitive evidence that the concomitant administration of histamine H2-receptor antagonists and/or antacids will either prevent the occurrence of gastrointestinal side effects or allow the continuation of CELEBREX when and if these adverse reactions appear.

CELEBREX (celecoxib) exhibited a low incidence of gastroduodenal ulceration and serious clinically significant GI events within clinical trials (see Adverse Reactions, Clinical Trial Adverse Drug Reactions—New Drug Submission (NDS) Arthritis Trials). In a prospective long-term outcome study (CLASS), there were no significant differences in the incidence of complicated ulcers between patients who received a higher-than-therapeutic dose of CELEBREX (400 mg BID) for OA and RA, in the presence of concomitant ASA (N=882 patients), compared to ibuprofen 800 mg TID and diclofenac 75 mg BID. The incidence of complicated and symptomatic ulcers was lower for CELEBREX than for Ibuprofen in patients not taking ASA. In active-controlled studies, the endoscopic gastroduodenal ulceration rate observed with all doses of CELEBREX was less than what was seen with the NSAID comparator and, in placebo-controlled studies, was similar to that seen with placebo.

Genitourinary: Some NSAIDs are associated with persistent urinary symptoms (bladder pain, dysuria, urinary frequency), hematuria or cystitis. The onset of these symptoms may occur at any time after the initiation of therapy with a NSAID. Should urinary symptoms occur, in the absence of alternate explanation, treatment with CELEBREX should be stopped to ascertain if symptoms disappear. This should be done before urological investigations or treatments are carried out.

Hematologic: NSAIDs inhibiting prostaglandin biosynthesis interfere with platelet function to varying degrees; patients who may be adversely affected by such an action, such as those on anticoagulants or suffering from hemophilia or platelet disorders should be carefully observed when CELEBREX is administered.

CELEBREX does not generally affect platelet counts, prothrombin time (PT), or partial thromboplastin time (PTT), and does not appear to inhibit platelet aggregation at indicated dosages.

Anticoagulants: Numerous studies have shown that the concomitant use of NSAIDs and anticoagulants increases the risk of bleeding. Concurrent therapy of CELEBREX with warfarin requires close monitoring of the international normalized ratio (INR).

Even with therapeutic INR monitoring, increased bleeding may occur.

Antiplatelet Effects: NSAIDs inhibit platelet aggregation and have been shown to prolong bleeding time in some patients. Unlike acetylsalicylic acid (ASA), their effect on platelet function is quantitatively less, or of shorter duration, and is reversible. CELEBREX does not appear to inhibit platelet aggregation at indicated dosages.

CELEBREX and other NSAIDs have no proven efficacy as antiplatelet agents and should **not** be used as a substitute for Acetylsalicylic Acid (ASA) or other antiplatelet agents for prophylaxis of cardiovascular thromboembolic diseases. Antiplatelet therapies (e.g. ASA) should **not** be discontinued. There is some evidence that use of NSAIDs with ASA can markedly attenuate the cardioprotective effects of ASA (see Drug Interactions, Drug-Drug Interactions, Acetylsalicylic Acid (ASA) or Other NSAIDs).

Concomitant administration of CELEBREX with low dose ASA increases the risk of GI ulceration and associated complications.

Blood Dyscrasias: Blood dyscrasias (such as neutropenia, leukopenia, thrombocytopenia, aplastic anemia and agranulocytosis) associated with the use of non-steroidal anti-inflammatory drugs (NSAIDs) are rare, but could occur with severe consequences.

Anemia is sometimes seen in patients receiving NSAIDs, including CELEBREX. This may be due to fluid retention, GI blood loss, or an incompletely described effect upon erythropoiesis. Patients on long-term treatment with NSAIDs, including CELEBREX, should have their hemoglobin or hematocrit checked if they exhibit any signs or symptoms of anemia or blood loss.

In controlled clinical trials the incidence of anemia was 0.6% with CELEBREX and 0.4% with placebo. Serious potentially fatal bleeding events have been reported, predominantly in the elderly, in patients receiving CELEBREX concurrently with warfarin or similar agents (see Drug Interactions, Drug-Drug Interactions and Adverse Reactions, Post-Market Adverse Drug Reactions).

Hepatic/Biliary/Pancreatic: As with other NSAIDs, borderline elevations of one or more liver enzyme tests (AST, ALT, alkaline phosphatase) may occur in up to 15% of patients. These laboratory abnormalities may progress, may remain essentially unchanged, or may be transient with continuing therapy.

In controlled clinical trials of CELEBREX, the incidence of borderline elevations of liver tests was 6% for CELEBREX and 5% for placebo, and approximately 0.2% of patients taking CELEBREX and 0.3% of patients taking placebo had notable elevations of ALT and AST.

A patient with symptoms and/or signs suggesting liver dysfunction, or in whom an abnormal liver test has occurred, should be evaluated for evidence of the development of a more severe hepatic reaction while on therapy with CELEBREX. Severe hepatic reactions, including liver necrosis and hepatic failure (with fatal outcome or requiring liver transplant), fulminant hepatitis (with fatal outcome), and jaundice have been reported with CELEBREX.

Although such reactions are rare, if abnormal liver tests persist or worsen, if clinical signs and symptoms consistent with liver disease develop (e.g. jaundice), or if systemic manifestations occur (e.g., eosinophilia, associated with rash, etc.), CELEBREX should be discontinued (see Contraindications).

If there is a need to prescribe this drug in the presence of impaired liver function, it must be done under strict observation.

Hypersensitivity Reactions: Allergies to Sulfonamides: (See Contraindications.)

Anaphylactoid Reactions: As with NSAIDs in general, anaphylactoid reactions have occured in patients without known prior exposure to CELEBREX. In post-marketing experience, very rare cases of anaphylactic/anaphylactoid reactions and angioedema have been reported in patients receiving CELEBREX. CELEBREX should **not** be given to patients with the ASA-triad. This symptom complex typically occurs in asthmatic patients who experience rhinitis with or without nasal polyps, or who exhibit severe, potentially fatal bronchospasm after taking ASA or other NSAIDs (see Contraindications).

ASA-Intolerance: CELEBREX should not be given to patients with the complete or partial syndrome of ASA-intolerance (rhinosinusitis, urticaria/angioedema, nasal polyps, asthma) in whom asthma, anaphylaxis, urticaria/angioedema, rhinitis or other allergic manifestations are precipitated by ASA or other NSAIDs. Fatal anaphylactoid reactions have occurred in such individuals. As well, individuals with the above medical problems are at risk of a severe reaction even if they have taken NSAIDs in the past without any adverse reaction (see Contraindications).

Cross-Sensitivity: Patients sensitive to one NSAID may be sensitive to any of the other NSAID as well.

Serious Skin Reactions: See Warnings and Precautions, Skin.

Immune: See Warnings and Precautions, Infection, Aseptic Meningitis.

Infection: CELEBREX in common with other NSAIDs, may mask signs and symptoms of an underlying infectious disease.

Aseptic Meningitis: Rarely, with some NSAIDs, the symptoms of aseptic meningitis (stiff neck, severe headaches, nausea and vomiting, fever or clouding of consciousness) have been observed. Patients with autoimmune disorders (systemic lupus erythematosus, mixed connective tissues diseases, etc.) seem to be pre-disposed. Therefore, in such patients, the physician must be vigilant to the development of this complication.

Neurologic: Some patients may experience drowsiness, dizziness, blurred vision, vertigo, tinnitus, hearing loss, insomnia or depression with the use of NSAIDs, such as CELEBREX. If patients experience such adverse reaction(s), they should exercise caution in carrying out activities that require alertness.

Ophthalmologic: Blurred and/or diminished vision has been reported with the use of NSAIDs. If such symptoms develop CELEBREX should be discontinued and an ophthalmologic examination performed. Ophthalmic examination should be carried out at periodic intervals in any patient receiving CELEBREX for an extended period of time.

Peri-Operative Considerations: Coronary Artery Bypass Graft Surgery: See Contraindications.

Psychiatric: See Warnings and Precautions, Neurologic.

Renal: Long-term administration of NSAIDs to animals has resulted in renal papillary necrosis and other abnormal renal pathology. In humans, there have been reports of acute interstitial nephritis, hematuria, low grade proteinuria and occasionally nephrotic syndrome.

Renal insufficiency due to NSAID use is seen in patients with pre-renal conditions leading to reduction in renal blood flow or blood volume. Under these circumstances, renal prostaglandins help maintain renal perfusion and glomerular filtration rate (GFR). In these patients, administration of a NSAID may cause a reduction in prostaglandin synthesis leading to impaired renal function. Patients at greatest risk of this reaction are those with pre-existing renal insufficiency (GFR <60 mL/min or 1 mL/s), dehydrated patients, patients on salt restricted diets, those with congestive heart failure, cirrhosis, liver dysfunction, taking angiotensin-converting enzyme inhibitors, angiotensin-II receptor blockers, cyclosporin, diuretics, and those who are elderly. In such patients, renal function should be monitored. Serious or life-threatening renal failure has been reported in patients with normal or impaired renal function after short term therapy with NSAIDs. Even patients at risk who demonstrate the ability to tolerate a NSAID under stable conditions may decompensate during periods of added stress (e.g. dehydration due to gastroenteritis). Discontinuation of NSAIDs is usually followed by recovery to the pre-treatment state.

Clinical trials with CELEBREX have shown renal effects similar to those observed with comparator NSAIDs (see Contraindications).

Caution should be used when initiating treatment with NSAIDS, such as CELEBREX, in patients with considerable dehydration. Such patients should be rehydrated prior to initiation of therapy. Caution is also recommended in patients with pre-existing kidney disease.

Advanced Renal Disease: No information is available from controlled clinical studies regarding the use of CELEBREX in patients with advanced kidney disease. In post-marketing experience, serious renal failure, including the need for dialysis, and fatalities have been reported in patients with impaired renal function. Therefore, treatment with CELEBREX, as with NSAIDs, is not recommended in these patients with advanced renal disease. Kidney function should be monitored, especially in high-risk populations, such as the elderly, patients with cardiovascular disease and diabetes mellitus, as well as in the setting of concomitant use of diuretics and ACE inhibitors (see Contraindications).

Fluid and Electrolyte Balance: Use of NSAIDs, such as CELEBREX, can promote sodium retention in a dose-dependent manner, which can lead to fluid retention and edema, and consequences of increased blood pressure and exacerbation of congestive heart failure. Thus, caution should be exercised in prescribing CELEBREX in patients with a history of congestive heart failure, compromised cardiac function, hypertension, increased age or other conditions predisposing to fluid retention (see Warnings and Precautions, Cardiovascular).

Use of NSAIDs, such as CELEBREX, can increase the risk of hyperkalemia, especially in patients with diabetes mellitus, renal failure, increased age, or those receiving concomitant therapy with adrenergic blockers, angiotensin-converting enzyme inhibitors, angiotensin-II receptor antagonists, cyclosporin, or some diuretics.

Electrolytes should be monitored periodically (see Contraindications).

Fluid retention has been observed in 2.1% of patients taking CELEBREX in clinical trials (see Adverse Reactions, Clinical Trial Adverse Drug Reactions—New Drug Submission (NDS) Arthritis Trials). In a prospective long-term outcome study (CLASS), hypertension was observed in 2.0%, 3,1% and 2.0% of patients receiving 400 mg BID CELEBREX (N=3987), 800 mg TID ibuprofen (N=1985) and 75 mg BID diclofenac (N=1996), respectively. The corresponding rates for edema were: 3.7%, 5.2% and 3.5%, respectively (see Adverse Reactions, Clinical Trial Adverse Drug Reactions—New Drug Submission (NDS) Arthritis Trials).

Respiratory: ASA-induced asthma is an uncommon but very important indication of ASA and NSAID sensitivity. It occurs more frequently in patients with asthma who have nasal polyps.

Sexual Function/Reproduction: The use of CELEBREX, as with any drug known to inhibit cyclooxygenase/prostaglandin synthesis, may impair fertility and is not recommended in women attempting to conceive. Therefore, in women who have difficulties conceiving, or who are undergoing investigation of infertility, withdrawal of CELEBREX should be considered.

Skin: In rare cases, serious skin reactions such as Stevens-Johnson syndrome, toxic epidermal necrolysis, exfoliative dermatitis and erythema multiforme have been associated with the use of some NSAIDs. Because the rate of these reactions is low, they have usually been noted during post-marketing surveillance in patients taking other medications also associated with the potential development of these serious skin reactions. Thus, causality is **not** clear. These reactions are potentially life threatening but may be reversible if the causative agent is discontinued and appropriate treatment instituted. Patients should be advised that if they experience a skin rash they should discontinue their NSAID and contact their physician for assessment and advice, including which additional therapies to discontinue.

Serious skin reactions, some of them fatal, including exfoliative dermatitis, Stevens-Johnson syndrome, and toxic epidermal necrolysis, have been reported very rarely in association with the use of CELEBREX (see Adverse Reactions, Post-Market Adverse Drug Reactions). Patients appear to be at higher risk for these events early in the course of therapy: the onset of the event occurring in the majority of cases within the first month of treatment. CELEBREX should be discontinued at the first appearance of skin rash, mucosal lesions, or any other sign of hypersensitivity.

Special Populations: Pregnant Women: CELEBREX is contraindicated for use during the third trimester of pregnancy because of risk of premature closure of the ductus arteriosus and the potential to prolong parturition.

Caution should be exercised in prescribing CELEBREX during the first and second trimesters of pregnancy.

Inhibition of prostaglandin synthesis may adversely affect pregnancy and/or the embryo-fetal development. Data from epidemiological studies suggest an increased risk of miscarriage and of cardiac malformation after use of a prostaglandin synthesis inhibitor in early pregnancy.

In animals, administration of a prostaglandin synthesis inhibitor has been shown to result in increased pre- and post-implantation loss and embryo-fetal lethality. In addition, increased incidences of various malformations, including cardiovascular, have been reported in animals given a prostaglandin synthesis inhibitor during the organogenetic period.

Nursing Women: (See Contraindications.)

Pediatrics (<18 years of age): (See Contraindications.)

Geriatrics (>65 years of age): Patients older than 65 years (referred to in this document as older or elderly) and frail or debilitated patients are more susceptible to a variety of adverse reactions from NSAIDs. The incidence of these adverse reactions increases with dose and duration of treatment. In addition, these patients are less tolerant to ulceration and bleeding. Most reports of fatal GI events are in this population. Older patients are also at risk of lower esophageal injury including ulceration and bleeding. For such patients, consideration should be given a starting dose lower than the one usually recommended, with individual adjustment when necessary and under close supervision.

CELEBREX has been studied in elderly patients. Of the total number of patients who received CELEBREX in clinical trials, more than 3300 patients (25 %) were 65-74 years of age, while approximately 1300 additional patients (10 %) were 75 years and over (see Adverse Reactions). While the incidence of adverse experiences tended to be higher in elderly patients, no substantial differences in safety and effectiveness were observed between these subjects and younger patients (see Warnings and Precautions, Gastrointestinal (GI) and Adverse Reactions, Adverse Drug Reaction Overview).

CYP2C9 Poor Metabolizers: Patients who are known, or suspected to be CYP2C9 poor metabolizers based on previous history/experience with other CYP2C9 substrates should be administered celecoxib with caution. The maximum recommended dose in CYP2C9 poor metabolizers is 100 mg daily. (See Drug Interactions and Dosage and Administration.)

Monitoring and Laboratory Tests: Cardiovascular: (Hypertension): Blood pressure should be monitored regularly during therapy with CELEBREX.

Hematologic: Patients on long-term treatment with NSAIDs, including CELEBREX, should have their hemoglobin, hematocrit, and blood cell count checked if they exhibit any signs or symptoms of anemia or blood loss.

Concurrent therapy of CELEBREX with warfarin requires close monitoring of the international normalized ratio (INR).

Hepatic: Patient with symptoms and/or signs of liver dysfunction, or in whom an abnormal liver function test has occurred, should be monitored carefully for evidence of the development of a more severe hepatic reaction while on therapy with CELEBREX. If abnormal liver tests persist or worsen, CELEBREX should be discontinued.

Renal: Renal function (serum creatinine and serum urea etc.) should be monitored in high-risk populations, such as the elderly, patients with advanced renal disease, patients with cardiovascular disease and diabetes mellitus, as well as in the setting of concomitant use of diuretics and ACE inhibitors (see Contraindications). If abnormal renal tests persist or worsen, CELEBREX should be discontinued.

Patients on long-term treatment with NSAIDs, including CELEBREX, should have their electrolytes such as serum potassium checked regularly if they exhibit any signs or symptoms of renal disease.

ADVERSE REACTIONS: Adverse Drug Reaction Overview: Of the CELEBREX (celecoxib) treated patients in controlled trials, approximately 4250 were patients with OA, approximately 2100 were patients with RA, and approximately 1050 were patients with post-surgical pain. More than 8500 patients have received a total daily dose of CELEBREX of 200 mg (100 mg BID or 200 mg QD) or more, including more than 400 treated at 800 mg (400 mg BID). Approximately 3900 patients have received CELEBREX at these doses for 6 months or more; approximately 2300 of these have received it for 1 year or more and 124 of these have received it for 2 years or more.

CELEBREX has been studied in elderly patients. Of the total number of patients who received CELEBREX in clinical trials, more than 3300 patients were 65-74 years of age, while approximately 1300 additional patients were 75 years and over. While the incidence of adverse experiences tended to be higher in elderly patients, no substantial differences in safety and effectiveness were observed between these subjects and younger patients. In GI endoscopy studies involving over 800 elderly patients, the rate of gastroduodenal ulceration was not different in elderly patients compared to the young. Other reported clinical experience has not identified differences in response between the elderly and younger patients, but greater sensitivity of some older individuals cannot be ruled out.

In clinical studies comparing renal function as measured by the GFR, urea and creatinine, and platelet function as measured by bleeding time and platelet aggregation, the results were not different between elderly and young volunteers.

Clinical Trial Adverse Drug Reactions—New Drug Submission (NDS) Arthritis Trials: Table 1 lists all adverse events, regardless of causality, occurring in ≥2% of patients receiving CELEBREX from 12 controlled studies conducted in patients with osteoarthritis and rheumatoid arthritis that included a placebo and/or a positive control group.

Table 1: CELEBREX

Events Occurring in ≥2% of Celebrex Patients From Original NDS Arthritis Trials

	CELEBREX 100–200 mg BID and 200 mg QD (n=4146) (%)	Placebo (n=1864) (%)	Naproxen 500 mg BID (n=1366) (%)	Ibuprofen 800 mg TID (n=387) (%)	Diclofenac 75 mg BID (n=345) (%)
Gastrointestinal					
Abdominal pain	4.1	2.8	7.7	9.0	9.0
Diarrhea	5.6	3.8	5.3	9.3	5.8
Dyspepsia	8.8	6.2	12.2	10.9	12.8
Flatulence	2.2	1.0	3.6	4.1	3.5

(cont'd)

Table 1: CELEBREX *(cont'd)*

Events Occurring in ≥2% of Celebrex Patients From Original NDS Arthritis Trials

	CELEBREX 100–200 mg BID and 200 mg QD (n=4146) (%)	Placebo (n=1864) (%)	Naproxen 500 mg BID (n=1366) (%)	Ibuprofen 800 mg TID (n=387) (%)	Diclofenac 75 mg BID (n=345) (%)
Nausea	3.5	4.2	6.0	3.4	6.7
Body as a Whole					
Back pain	2.8	3.6	2.2	2.6	0.9
Peripheral edema	2.1	1.1	2.1	1.0	3.5
Injury-accidental	2.9	2.3	3.0	2.6	3.2
Central and Peripheral Nervous Systems					
Dizziness	2.0	1.7	2.6	1.3	2.3
Headache	15.8	20.2	14.5	15.5	15.4
Psychiatric					
Insomnia	2.3	2.3	2.9	1.3	1.4
Respiratory					
Pharyngitis	2.3	1.1	1.7	1.6	2.6
Rhinitis	2.0	1.3	2.4	2.3	0.6
Sinusitis	5.0	4.3	4.0	5.4	5.8
Upper respiratory tract infection	8.1	6.7	9.9	9.8	9.9
Skin					
Rash	2.2	2.1	2.1	1.3	1.2

In placebo- or active-controlled clinical trials, the discontinuation rate due to adverse events was 7.1% for patients receiving CELEBREX and 6.1% for patients receiving placebo. Among the most common reasons for discontinuation due to adverse events in the CELEBREX treatment groups were dyspepsia and abdominal pain (cited as reasons for discontinuation in 0.8% and 0.7% of CELEBREX patients, respectively). Among patients receiving placebo, 0.6% discontinued due to dyspepsia and 0.6% withdrew due to abdominal pain.

The adverse event profile from the long-term outcomes trial (at 4- and 2-fold the recommended doses for OA and RA respectively) is similar to those reported in the arthritis-controlled trials. In the arthritis-controlled trials, the CELEBREX endoscopic gastroduodenal ulceration rate was consistently less than what was seen with the NSAID comparators. In the long-term outcome study however, there was no statistically significant difference for the incidence of complicated ulcers (perforation, obstruction, or bleeding) among the CELEBREX 400 mg BID and NSAID comparators. The major differences in study design and patient populations preclude direct comparison between the GI endpoint results in the arthritis controlled and the long-term outcome trials.

The incidences of withdrawals due to adverse events and the incidences of selected serious adverse events (i.e., those causing hospitalization or felt to be life-threatening or otherwise medically significant) observed in this trial are shown in Table 2. No significant differences were seen across treatment groups in the incidences of serious adverse events (see Table 2).

Table 2: CELEBREX

Summary of Withdrawal and Serious Cardiovascular Adverse Event Data from the CLASS Trial. Incidence Rates (%) in all OA and RA Patients and in Patients without ASA

	Celecoxib 400 mg BID	Diclofenac 75 mg BID	Ibuprofen 800 mg TID
All Patients	(n=3987)	(n=1996)	(n=1985)
All withdrawals	22.4	26.5[a]	23.0
Withdrawals for GI symptoms	12.2	16.6[a]	13.4
Serious adverse events	6.8	5.6	6.0
Myocardial infarction (fatal and nonfatal)	0.5	0.2	0.5
Deep vein thrombosis	0.2	0.3	0.0
Cardiac failure	0.2	0.1	0.5
Unstable angina	0.2	0.2	0.0
Cerebrovascular disorder	0.1	0.3	0.3
Patients Without ASA	(n=3105)	(n=1551)	(n=1573)
All withdrawals	21.2	25.4[a]	22.5
Withdrawals for GI symptoms	11.5	15.4[a]	13.2
Serious adverse events	5.0	4.2	4.3
Myocardial infarction (fatal and nonfatal)	0.2	0.1	0.1
Deep vein thrombosis	0.2	0.2	0.0

(cont'd)

Table 2: CELEBREX *(cont'd)*

Summary of Withdrawal and Serious Cardiovascular Adverse Event Data from the CLASS Trial. Incidence Rates (%) in all OA and RA Patients and in Patients without ASA

	Celecoxib 400 mg BID	Diclofenac 75 mg BID	Ibuprofen 800 mg TID
Cardiac failure	0.1	<0.1	0.3
Unstable angina	<0.1	0.0	0.0
Cerebrovascular disorder	<0.1	0.3	0.1

[a] p<0.05 vs celecoxib.

The following adverse events occurred in 0.1-1.9% of patients regardless of causality: CELEBREX (100-200 mg BID or 200 mg QD).

Gastrointestinal: constipation, diverticulitis, dry mouth, dysphagia, eructation, esophagitis, gastritis, gastroenteritis, gastroesophageal reflux, hemorrhoids, hiatal hernia, melena, stomatitis, tenesmus, tooth disorder, vomiting.
Cardiovascular: aggravated hypertension, angina pectoris, coronary artery disorder, myocardial infarction.
General: allergy aggravated, allergic reaction, asthenia, chest pain, cyst NOS, edema generalized, face edema, fatigue, fever, hot flushes, influenza-like symptoms, pain, peripheral pain.
Resistance Mechanism Disorders: herpes simplex, herpes zoster, infection bacterial, infection fungal, infection soft tissue, infection viral, moniliasis, moniliasis genital, otitis media.
Central, Peripheral Nervous Systems: leg cramps, hypertonia, hypoesthesia, migraine, neuralgia, neuropathy, paresthesia, vertigo.
Female Reproductive: breast fibroadenosis, breast neoplasm, breast pain, dysmenorrhea, menstrual disorder, vaginal hemorrhage, vaginitis.
Male Reproductive: prostatic disorder.
Hearing and Vestibular: deafness, ear abnormality, earache, tinnitus.
Heart Rate and Rhythm: palpitation, tachycardia.
Liver and Biliary System: ALT increased, AST increased, hepatic function abnormal.
Metabolic and Nutritional: urea increased, CPK increased, diabetes mellitus, hypercholesterolemia, hyperglycemia, hypokalemia, NPN increase, creatinine increased, alkaline phosphatase increased, weight increase.
Musculoskeletal: arthralgia, arthrosis, bone disorder, fracture accidental, myalgia, neck stiffness, synovitis, tendinitis.
Platelets (bleeding or clotting): ecchymosis, epistaxis, thrombocythemia.
Psychiatric: anorexia, anxiety, appetite increased, depression, nervousness, somnolence.
Hemic: anemia.
Respiratory: bronchitis, bronchospasm, bronchospasm aggravated, coughing, dyspnea, laryngitis, pneumonia.
Skin and Appendages: alopecia, dermatitis, nail disorder, photosensitivity reaction, pruritus, rash erythematous, rash maculopapular, skin disorder, skin dry, sweating increased, urticaria.
Application Site Disorders: cellulitis, dermatitis contact, injection site reaction, skin nodule.
Special Senses: taste perversion.
Urinary System: albuminuria, cystitis, dysuria, hematuria, micturition frequency, renal calculus, urinary incontinence, urinary tract infection.
Vision: blurred vision, cataract, conjunctivitis, eye pain, glaucoma.

Adverse Events From Ankylosing Spondylitis Studies: A total of 896 patients were treated with CELEBREX in placebo- and active-controlled ankylosing spondylitis studies for a maximum duration of 12 weeks. CELEBREX was also studied in one long-term open label extension study up to 2 years in 215 patients with ankylosing spondylitis. The average daily dose was 200 mg. The types of adverse events reported in the ankylosing spondylitis studies were generally similar to those reported in the arthritis studies. The percentage of patients with hypertension (6.1%) and serious GI adverse events (3.7%) in the 2-year, openlabel extension study, were greater than those reported in the 12week studies, respectively of 0.7% and 0.0 %. The most common Gastro-Intestinal disorders reported in the 2-year extension study compared to those reported in the 12week studies include Diarrhea (15.0% vs. 4.5%), Abdominal Pain upper (13.6 % vs. 3.8%), Dyspepsia (9.8% vs. 3.7%), Nausea (5.6% vs. 2.8%) and Abdominal Pain (5.6% vs. 1.5%). The percentage of patients with cardio-vascular events (1.4%) in the 2-year open-label extension study was similar to that observed in the CLASS trials.

Adverse Events From Analgesia and Dysmenorrhea Studies: Approximately 1700 patients were treated with CELEBREX in analgesia and dysmenorrhea studies. All patients in post-oral surgery pain studies received a single dose (up to 400 mg) of study medication. Doses up to 600 mg/day of CELEBREX were studied in primary dysmenorrhea and post-orthopaedic surgery pain studies. The types of adverse experiences in the analgesia and dysmenorrhea studies were similar to those reported in arthritis studies. The only new adverse event reported was alveolar osteitis (dry socket) in the post-oral surgery pain studies.

In approximately 700 patients treated with CELEBREX in the post-general and orthopaedic surgery pain studies, the most commonly reported adverse experiences were nausea, vomiting, headache, dizziness and fever.

Other serious adverse reactions which occur rarely (estimated <0.1%) regardless of causality: the following adverse events have occurred rarely in patients taking CELEBREX.

Cardiovascular: syncope, congestive heart failure, ventricular fibrillation, pulmonary embolism, cerebrovascular accident, peripheral gangrene, thrombophlebitis.
Gastrointestinal: intestinal obstruction, intestinal perforation, gastrointestinal bleeding, colitis with bleeding, esophageal perforation, pancreatitis, cholelithiasis, ileus.
Hemic and Lymphatic: thrombocytopenia.
Liver and Biliary System: cholelithiasis, hepatitis, jaundice, liver failure.
Metabolic: hypoglycemia.
Nervous System: ataxia.
Renal: acute renal failure.
General: sepsis, sudden death.

Serious Cardiovascular Adverse Events: Long-term Studies Involving Patients with Sporadic Adenomatous Polyps: Two studies involving patients with sporadic adenomatous polyps were conducted with celecoxib: the APC trial (Adenoma Prevention with Celecoxib) and the PreSAP trial (Prevention of Colorectal Sporadic Adenomatous Polyps). In the APC trial, there was a dose-related increase in the composite endpoint of cardiovascular death, myocardial infarction, or stroke (adjudicated) with celecoxib compared to placebo over 3 years of treatment. The PreSAP trial did not demonstrate a statistically significant increased risk for the same composite endpoint, as shown in Table 3.

Serious Cardiovascular Adverse Events in the APC and PreSAP Trials:

Table 3: CELEBREX

Number (%) of Subjects [Hazards Ratio[a] (95% Confidence Interval) Compared to Placebo]

	APC Trial			PreSAP Trial	
	Placebo	Celecoxib 200 mg BID	Celecoxib 400 mg BID	Placebo	Celecoxib 400 mg QD
Adjudicated Endpoint[b]	N=679	N=685	N=671	N=628	N=933
CV death	1 (0.1)	5 (0.7) [4.9 (0.6, 42.2)]	6 (0.9) [6.2 (0.7, 51.4)]	4 (0.6)	4 (0.4) [0.7 (0.2, 2.7)]
CV death or MI	4 (0.6)	14 (2.0) [3.5 (1.1, 10.6)]	15 (2.2) [3.9 (1.3, 11.7)]	7 (1.1)	13 (1.4) [1.3 (0.5, 3.2)]

(cont'd)

Table 3: CELEBREX *(cont'd)*

Number (%) of Subjects [Hazards Ratio[a] (95% Confidence Interval) Compared to Placebo]

	APC Trial			PreSAP Trial	
	Placebo	Celecoxib 200 mg BID	Celecoxib 400 mg BID	Placebo	Celecoxib 400 mg QD
Adjudicated Endpoint[b]	N=679	N=685	N=671	N=628	N=933
CV death, MI, or stroke (APTC endpoint)	6 (0.9)	17 (2.5) [2.8 (1.1, 7.2)]	20 (3.0) [3.4 (1.4, 8.5)]	12 (1.9)	21 (2.3) [1.2 (0.6, 2.4)]

[a] Hazards ratios are based on event rates per subject-year of exposure to study medication.
[b] Includes only serious adverse events, for all randomized subjects, adjudicated and categorized according to a pre-specified scheme by an independent Cardiovascular Safety Committee blinded to randomized treatment assignments.

Legend: BID=twice daily; QD=once daily; N=number of subjects treated; CV=cardiovascular; MI=myocardial infarction; APTC=Antiplatelet Trialists' Collaboration; HF=heart failure.

Investigator Reports of Adverse Reaction From Long-term, Placebo-controlled Polyp Prevention Studies: Indications and dosages of the PreSAP and APC trials are not approved in Canada. Exposure to CELEBREX in the APC and PreSAP trials was 400 to 800 mg daily for up to 3 years; Among adverse reactions that occurred in higher percentages of patients than in the arthritis pre- marketing trials (treatment durations up to 12 weeks; (see Adverse Reactions, Clinical Trial Adverse Drug Reactions—New Drug Submission (NDS) Arthritis Trials), hypertension was reported at an incidence of 12.5 % in the celecoxib group (400-800 mg daily dose) compared to 9.8% in the placebo group.

Abnormal Hematologic and Clinical Chemistry Findings: During the controlled clinical trials, there was an increased incidence of hyperchloremia in patients receiving celecoxib compared with patients on placebo. Other laboratory abnormalities that occurred more frequently in the patients receiving celecoxib included hypophosphatemia, and elevated urea. These laboratory abnormalities were also seen in patients who received comparator NSAIDs in these studies. The clinical significance of these abnormalities has not been established.

Post-Market Adverse Drug Reactions: Additional reports of serious adverse events temporally associated with CELEBREX during worldwide post-marketing experience are included below. Because these events are reported voluntarily from a population of uncertain size, it is not always possible to reliably estimate their frequency or clearly establish a causal relationship to CELEBREX exposure.

Blood and Lymphatic System Disorders: pancytopenia, agranulocytosis, aplastic anemia, leukopenia.
Immune System Disorders: serious allergic reactions, anaphylactic shock.
Psychiatric Disorders: confusion, hallucinations.
Nervous System Disorders: aggravated epilepsy, aseptic meningitis, ageusia, anosmia.
Ear and Labyrinth Disorders: decreased hearing.
Eye Disorders: conjunctivitis.
Cardiac Disorders: congestive heart failure, heart failure, myocardial infarction.
Vascular Disorders: vasculitis, cerebral hemorrhage, pulmonary embolism (some with fatal outcome).
Respiratory, Thoracic and Mediastinal Disorders: bronchospasm.
Gastrointestinal Disorders: gastrointestinal hemorrhage, acute pancreatitis.
Hepatobiliary Disorders: liver failure (with fatal outcome), fulminant hepatitis (with fatal outcome), liver necrosis, hepatitis, jaundice.
Skin and Subcutaneous Tissue Disorders: angioedema, isolated reports of skin exfoliation including: Stevens-Johnson syndrome, epidermal necrolysis, erythema multiforme.
Reproductive System and Breast Disorders: menstrual disorder.
Musculoskeletal and Connective Tissue Disorders: myositis.
Renal and Urinary Disorders: acute renal failure, interstitial nephritis, hyponatremia.
General Disorders and Administration Site Conditions: chest pain.

Serious bleeding (some of them fatal) have been reported, predominantly in the elderly, in association with increases in prothrombin time in patients receiving CELEBREX concurrently with warfarin or similar agents (see Drug Interactions).

DRUG INTERACTIONS: Overview: General: Celecoxib metabolism is predominantly mediated via cytochrome P450 2C9 in the liver (commonly used drugs which are also substrates and/or inhibitors for cytochrome P450 2C9 include warfarin, fluoxetine, fluconazole, phenytoin, and tolbutemide). Co-administration of celecoxib with drugs that are known to inhibit 2C9 should be done with caution. Furthermore, patients who are known or suspected to be poor CYP2C9 metabolizers based on previous history/experience with other CYP2C9 substrates should be administered celecoxib with caution as they may have abnormally high plasma levels due to reduced metabolic clearance. Consider starting treatment at half the lowest recommended dose.

In vitro studies indicate that celecoxib, although not a substrate, is a relatively weak inhibitor of cytochrome P450 2D6. Therefore, there is a potential for an in vivo drug interaction with drugs that are metabolized by P450 2D6.

In vitro studies indicate that celecoxib is not an inhibitor of cytochrome P450 2C9, 2C19 or 3A4.

Drug-Drug Interactions: Acetylsalicylic Acid (ASA) or Other NSAIDs: The use of CELEBREX in addition to any other NSAID, including over-the-counter ones (such as ASA and ibuprofen) for analgesic and/or anti-inflammatory effects is **not** recommended because of the absence of any evidence demonstrating synergistic benefits and the potential for additive adverse reactions.

The exception is the use of low dose ASA for cardiovascular protection, when another NSAID is being used for its analgesic/anti-inflammatory effect, keeping in mind that combination NSAID therapy is associated with additive adverse reactions.

Some NSAIDs (e.g. ibuprofen) may interfere with the antiplatelet effects of low dose ASA, possibly by competing with ASA for access to the active site of cyclooxygenase-1.

As with all other NSAIDs the concomitant administration of ASA with CELEBREX results in an increased rate of GI ulceration or other complications, compared to use of CELEBREX alone. In the long-term outcomes study (at 4- and 2-fold the recommended doses for OA and RA respectively), there was no statistically significant difference for the incidence of complicated ulcers between CELEBREX and comparator groups in patients taking ASA. Concomitant low dose ASA use increased the rate of complicated ulcers to four times that of patients not taking ASA. Resulting incidence rate for complicated ulcers in patients taking CELEBREX and ASA was 1.02%.

Antacids: Co-administration of CELEBREX with an aluminum- and magnesium-containing antacid resulted in a reduction in plasma celecoxib concentrations with a decrease of 37% in C_{max} and 10% in AUC.

Anticoagulants: Anticoagulant activity should be monitored, particularly in the first few days, after initiating or changing CELEBREX therapy in patients receiving warfarin or similar agents, since these patients are at an increased risk of bleeding complications. The effect of celecoxib on the anticoagulant effect of warfarin was studied in a group of healthy subjects receiving daily doses of 2-5 mg of warfarin (dose sufficient to prolong prothrombin times to 1.2 to 1.7 times their baseline values). In these subjects, celecoxib did not alter the anticoagulant effect of warfarin as determined by prothrombin time. However, in post-marketing experience, serious bleeding events (some of them fatal) have been reported, predominantly in the elderly, in association with increases in prothrombin time, in patients receiving CELEBREX concurrently with warfarin or similar agents. (See Adverse Reactions, Post-Market Adverse Drug Reactions.)

Antihypertensives: NSAIDs may diminish the antihypertensive effects of Angiotensin Converting Enzyme (ACE) inhibitors. This interaction should be given consideration. Combinations of ACE inhibitors, angiotensin-II antagonists, or diuretics with NSAIDs might have an increased risk for acute renal failure and hyperkalemia. Blood pressure and renal function (including electrolytes) should be monitored more closely in this situation, as occasionally there can be a substantial increase in blood pressure

Although prospective studies of CELEBREX with ACE inhibitors have not been conducted, no adverse reactions indicative of elevations in blood pressure were seen in clinical trials in which arthritis patients were taking CELEBREX concurrently with ACE inhibitors (n=305).

Antiplatelet Agents: There is an increased risk of bleeding, via inhibition of platelet function, where antiplatelet agents are combined with NSAIDs. CELEBREX does not generally affect platelet counts, prothrombin time (PT), or partial thromboplastin time (PTT), and does not appear to inhibit platelet aggregation at indicated dosages (see Warnings and Precautions, Hematologic, Antiplatelet Effects).

Cyclosporin and Tacrolimus: Although this interaction has not been studied with celecoxib, co-administration of cyclosporin or tacrolimus and any NSAID may increase the nephrotoxic effect of cyclosporin or tacrolimus due to the NSAID's effect on renal prostaglandins. Renal function should be monitored when celecoxib and either of these drugs is used in combination.

Digoxin: No interaction data is available for the co-administration of celecoxib and digoxin. However an increase in serum digoxin level has been noted with some NSAIDS.

Diuretics: Clinical studies, as well as post marketing observations, have shown that NSAIDs can reduce the effects of diuretics. This response has been attributed to inhibition of renal prostaglandin synthesis. Although prospective studies of CELEBREX with diuretics have not been conducted, no adverse reactions indicative of elevations in blood pressure were seen in clinical trials in which arthritis patients were taking CELEBREX concurrently with diuretics (n=485). No adverse reactions indicative of sodium retention or renal impairment were seen in clinical trials in patients taking CELEBREX concurrently with diuretics.

Fluconazole: Concomitant administration of fluconazole at 200 mg QD resulted in a two-fold increase in celecoxib plasma concentration. This increase is due to the inhibition of celecoxib metabolism via P450 2C9 by fluconazole (see Action and Clinical Pharmacology, Pharmacokinetics, Metabolism). CELEBREX should be introduced at the lowest recommended dose in patients receiving fluconazole.

Glucocorticoids: Some studies have shown that the concomitant use of NSAIDs and oral glucocorticoids increase the risk of GI side effects such as ulceration and bleeding. This is especially the case in older (>65 years of age) individuals.

Ketoconazole: CELEBREX did not have a significant effect on the pharmacokinetics of ketoconazole.

Lithium: In a study conducted in healthy subjects, mean steady-state lithium plasma levels increased approximately 17% in subjects receiving lithium 450 mg BID with CELEBREX 200 mg BID as compared to subjects receiving lithium alone. Patients on lithium treatment should be closely monitored when CELEBREX is introduced or withdrawn.

Methotrexate: CELEBREX did not have a significant effect on the pharmacokinetics of methotrexate.

Oral Hypoglycemics: The effect of celecoxib on the pharmacokinetics and/or pharmacodynamics of glyburide and tolbutemide has been studied and clinically important interactions have not been found.

Phenytoin: CELEBREX did not have a significant effect on the pharmacokinetics of phenytoin.

Other Drug Interactions: No drug interaction data are available for CELEBREX and the co-administration of the following products: acetaminophen, alcohol, aminoglycosides, bone marrow depressants, butemide, cholestyramine, colchicine, corticosteroids, gold compounds, indapamide, insulin, nephrotoxic agents, non-steroidal anti-inflammatory agents, oral contraceptives, potassium supplements, probenecid, valproic acid, zidovudine.

Drug-Food Interactions: When CELEBREX capsules were taken with a high fat meal, peak plasma levels were delayed for about 1 to 2 hours with an increase in total absorption (AUC) of 10% to 20%. Under fasting conditions, at doses above 200 mg, there is less than a proportional increase in C_{max} and AUC, which is thought to be due to the low solubility of the drug in aqueous media.

Drug-Herb Interactions: The interaction of CELEBREX with herbal medications or supplements has not been studied.

Drug-Laboratory Test Interactions: Interactions with laboratory tests have not been established.

DOSAGE AND ADMINISTRATION:

Dosing Considerations : Hepatic Impairment: CELEBREX capsule should be introduced at the lowest dose in patients with mild hepatic impairment (Child-Pugh 5-6). The daily recommended dose of CELEBREX capsules in patients with moderate hepatic impairment (Child-Pugh 7-9) should be reduced by 50% and should be given at the lowest dose of 100 mg once daily (see Action and Clinical Pharmacology, Pharmacokinetics, Special Populations and Conditions). CELEBREX is contraindicated in patients with severe hepatic impairment (Child-Pugh >9) (see Contraindications).

Renal Insufficiency: No dosage adjustment is necessary for patients with creatinine clearance >30 mL/min (see Action and Clinical Pharmacology, Pharmacokinetics, Special Populations and Conditions). CELEBREX is contraindicated in patients with severe renal impairment (estimated creatinine clearance <30 mL/min) (see Contraindications).

Elderly (>65 years of age): In the elderly, frail and debilitated, the dosage should be reduced to the lowest level providing control of symptoms, and adjusted when necessary (see Warnings and Precautions, Special Populations, Geriatrics (>65 years of age)).

CYP2C9 Poor Metabolizers: Patients who are known, or suspected to be CYP2C9 poor metabolizers based on previous history/experience with other CYP2C9 substrates should be administered celecoxib with caution. The maximum recommended dose in CYP2C9 poor metabolizers is 100 mg daily (see Drug Interactions and Warnings and Precautions, Special Populations).

Recommended Dose and Dosage Adjustment—18 Years of Age and Older: Use of CELEBREX should be limited to the lowest effective dose for the shortest possible duration of treatment (see Contraindications and Warnings and Precautions).

Osteoarthritis: The recommended daily dose of CELEBREX (celecoxib) is 200 mg administered as a single dose or as two divided doses (100 mg twice per day). Maximum dose=200 mg a day.

Rheumatoid Arthritis: The recommended starting dose of CELEBREX is 100 mg twice per day, which may be increased to 200 mg twice per day if necessary. Maximum dose=200 mg twice a day.

Ankylosing Spondylitis: The recommended daily dose of CELEBREX (celecoxib) is 200 mg administered as a single dose or as two divided doses (100 mg twice a day). Maximum dose=200 mg a day.

Management of Acute Pain: The recommended dose of CELEBREX is 400 mg as a single dose on the first day followed by 200 mg once daily on subsequent days up to a maximum of 7 days. Patients may be instructed to take an additional dose of 200 mg on any given day, if needed. Maximum dose=400 mg a day for up to 7 days.

Administration: CELEBREX can be taken with or without food.

Missed Dose: Patients who miss one or more doses of CELEBREX (celecoxib) should not increase the dose of CELEBREX to compensate for the missed dose or doses, but should continue therapy as soon as possible, then take the next dose at the scheduled time.

OVERDOSAGE:

No overdoses of CELEBREX were reported during clinical trials. Doses up to 2400 mg/day for up to 10 days in 12 patients did not result in serious toxicity.

Symptoms following acute NSAID overdoses are usually limited to lethargy, drowsiness, nausea, vomiting, and epigastric pain, which are generally reversible with supportive care. Gastrointestinal bleeding can occur. Hypertension, acute renal failure, respiratory depression and coma may occur, but are rare. Anaphylactoid reactions have been reported with therapeutic ingestion of NSAIDs, and may occur following an overdose.

Patients should be managed by symptomatic and supportive care following an NSAID overdose. There are no specific antidotes. No information is available regarding the removal of celecoxib by hemodialysis, but based on its high degree of plasma protein binding (>97%) dialysis is unlikely to be useful in overdose. Emesis and/or activated charcoal (60 to 100 g in adults, 1 to 2 g/kg in children) and/or osmotic cathartic may be indicated in patients seen within 4 hours of ingestion with symptoms or following a large overdose. Forced diuresis, alkalinization of urine, hemodialysis, or hemoperfusion may not be useful due to high protein binding.

> For management of a suspected drug overdose, contact your regional Poison Control Centre. See the *CPS Directory* section for a list of Poison Control Centres.

ACTION AND CLINICAL PHARMACOLOGY: Mechanism of Action: CELEBREX (celecoxib) is a non-steroidal anti-inflammatory drug that exhibits anti-inflammatory, analgesic, and anti-pyretic activities in animals. The mechanism of action of CELEBREX is believed to be related to inhibition of cyclooxygenase-2 (COX-2). COX-2 is expressed at high levels in inflamed tissues where it is induced by mediators of inflammation. COX-2 also plays physiological roles in a limited number of tissues, including those of the female reproductive tract, the kidney and possibly the vascular endothelium. COX-2 has the same catalytic activity as COX-1. COX-1 is expressed constitutively in most tissues including the gastrointestinal tract, kidney, lungs, brain, and platelets. The prostaglandins produced by COX-1 play key roles in the maintenance of physiological functions such as platelet aggregation and are among the factors that maintain the GI mucosal barrier. At therapeutic concentrations (see Dosage and Administration) celecoxib inhibits COX-2 and does not inhibit COX-1.

Pharmacokinetics: The pharmacokinetics of celecoxib have been evaluated in approximately 1500 individuals. In addition to healthy, young and elderly volunteers (male and female), pharmacokinetic measurements have been done in patients and also in special populations including individuals with hepatic or renal impairment.

Absorption: Peak plasma levels of celecoxib occur approximately 3 hours after an oral dose. Both peak plasma levels (C_{max}) and area under the curve (AUC) are roughly dose proportional across the clinical dose range of 100-200 mg studied. Under fasting conditions, at higher doses, there is a less than proportional increase in C_{max} and AUC which is thought to be due to the low solubility of the drug in aqueous media. Because of the low solubility, absolute bioavailability studies have not been conducted. With multiple dosing, steady state conditions are reached on or before day 5.

The pharmacokinetic parameters of celecoxib in a group of healthy subjects are shown in Table 4.

Food Effects: When CELEBREX (celecoxib) capsules were taken with a high fat meal, peak plasma levels were delayed for about 1 to 2 hours with an increase in total absorption (AUC) of 10% to 20%. Co-administration of CELEBREX with an aluminum- and magnesium-containing antacid resulted in a reduction in plasma celecoxib concentrations with a decrease of 37% in C_{max} and 10% in AUC. CELEBREX capsules can be administered without regard to the timing of meals.

Table 4: CELEBREX

Summary of Single Dose (200 mg) Disposition Kinetics of Celecoxib in Healthy Subjects[a]

Mean (% CV) Pharmacokinetic (PK) Parameter Values (95% Confidence Interval)				
C_{max} (ng/mL)	T_{max} (h)	Effective $t_{1/2}$ (h)	V_{ss}/F (L)	CL/F (L/h)
705 (38) (484.2–925.0)	2.8 (37) (1.95–3.71)	11.2 (31) (8.3–14.0)	429 (34) (307.2–551.5)	27.7 (28) (21.3–34.1)

[a] Subjects under fasting conditions (n=36, 19-52 years).

Distribution: In healthy subjects, celecoxib is highly protein bound (~97%) within the clinical dose range. In vitro studies indicate that celecoxib binds primarily to albumin and, to a lesser extent, α_1-acid glycoprotein. The apparent volume of distribution at steady state (V_{ss}/F) is approximately 400 L, suggesting extensive distribution into the tissues. Celecoxib is not preferentially bound to red blood cells.

Metabolism: Celecoxib metabolism is primarily mediated via cytochrome P450 2C9. Three metabolites, a primary alcohol, the corresponding carboxylic acid and its glucuronide conjugate, have been identified in human plasma. These metabolites are inactive as COX-1 or COX-2 inhibitors. Cytochrome P450 2C9 activity is reduced in individuals with genetic polymorphisms that lead to reduced enzyme activity, such as those homozygous for the CYP2C9*3 polymorphism. Patients who are known or suspected to be P450 2C9 poor metabolizers based on a previous history should be administered celecoxib with caution as they may have abnormally high plasma levels due to reduced metabolic clearance. The maximum recommended dose in CYP2C9 poor metabolizers is 100 mg daily. (See Warnings and Precautions, Special Populations, CYP2C9 Poor Metabolizers and Drug Interactions.)

In a pharmacokinetic study of celecoxib 200 mg administered once daily in healthy volunteers, genotyped as either CYP2C9*1/*1, CYP2C9*1/*3, or CYP2C9*3/*3, the median C_{max} and AUC_{0-24} of celecoxib on Day 7 were approximately 4-fold and 7-fold, respectively, in subjects genotyped as CYP2C9*3/*3 compared to other genotypes. In three separate single dose studies, involving a total of 5 subjects genotyped as CYP2C9*3/*3, single-dose AUC_{0-24} increased by approximately 3-fold compared to normal metabolizers. It is estimated that the frequency of the homozygous *3/*3 genotype is 0.3-1.0% among different ethnic groups.

Excretion: Celecoxib is eliminated predominantly by hepatic metabolism with little (<3%) unchanged drug recovered in the urine and feces. Following a single oral dose of radiolabelled drug, approximately 57% of the dose was excreted in the feces and 27% was excreted into the urine. The primary metabolite in both urine and feces was the carboxylic acid metabolite (73% of dose) with low amounts of the glucuronide also appearing in the urine. It appears that the low solubility of the drug prolongs the absorption process making terminal half-life ($t_{1/2}$) determinations more variable. The effective half-life is approximately 11 hours under fasted conditions. The apparent plasma clearance (CL/F) is about 500 mL/min.

Special Populations and Conditions: Geriatrics: At steady state, elderly subjects (over 65 years old) had a 40% higher C_{max} and a 50% higher AUC compared to the young subjects. In elderly females, celecoxib C_{max} and AUC are higher than those for elderly males, but these increases are predominantly due to lower body weight in elderly females. Dose adjustment in the elderly is not generally necessary. However, for elderly patients of less than 50 kg in body weight, initiate therapy at the lowest recommended dose, and as with all other NSAIDs, exercise caution in the use of higher doses.

Race: Meta-analysis of pharmacokinetic studies has suggested an approximately 40% higher AUC of celecoxib in black patients compared to Caucasians. The cause and clinical significance of this finding is unknown.

Hepatic Insufficiency: A pharmacokinetic study in subjects with mild (Child-Pugh 5-6) and moderate (Child-Pugh 7-9) hepatic impairment has shown that steady-state celecoxib AUC is increased about 40% and 180%, respectively, above that seen in healthy control subjects. Therefore, CELEBREX capsules should be introduced at a reduced dose in patients with moderate hepatic impairment. Patients with severe hepatic impairment have not been studied. The use of CELEBREX in patients with severe hepatic impairment is not recommended (see Contraindications).

Renal Insufficiency: In a cross-study comparison, celecoxib AUC was approximately 40% lower in patients with chronic renal insufficiency (GFR 35-60 mL/min) than that seen in subjects with normal renal function. No significant relationship was found between GFR and celecoxib clearance. Patients with severe renal insufficiency have not been studied (see Contraindications).

STORAGE AND STABILITY: Store at room temperature (15-30°C).

Keep in a safe place out of reach of children and pets.

INFORMATION FOR THE PATIENT: Published in e-CPS, available by subscription at www.e-cps.ca.

DOSAGE FORMS, COMPOSITION AND PACKAGING: 100 mg: Each white to off-white hard gelatin capsule, with blue ink band on body marked in white with "100" and with blue ink band on cap marked in white with "7767", contains: celecoxib 100 mg. Nonmedicinal ingredients: croscarmellose sodium, lactose monohydrate, magnesium stearate, povidone and sodium lauryl sulfate; shell: edible ink (indigotine [E132]), gelatin and titanium dioxide (E171). Bottles of 100 and 500.

200 mg: Each white to off-white hard gelatin capsule, with gold ink band on body marked in white with "200" and with gold ink band on cap marked in white with "7767", contains: celecoxib 200 mg. Nonmedicinal ingredients: croscarmellose sodium, lactose monohydrate, magnesium stearate, povidone and sodium lauryl sulfate; shell: edible ink (ferric oxide [E172]), gelatin and titanium dioxide (E171). Bottles of 100 and 500.

(Shown in Product Identification Section)

Celestone® Soluspan® ℞

betamethasone sodium phosphate—betamethasone acetate

Injectable Glucocorticoid

Schering-Plough

PHARMACOLOGY: Celestone Soluspan is a combination of soluble and slightly soluble betamethasone esters that provides potent anti-inflammatory, antirheumatic and antiallergic effects in the treatment of corticosteroid-responsive disorders. Prompt therapeutic activity is achieved by betamethasone sodium phosphate, which is absorbed quickly after injection. Sustained activity is provided by betamethasone acetate, which is only slightly soluble and becomes a repository for slow absorption, thereby controlling symptoms over a prolonged period.

INDICATIONS: I.M. injection in allergic, dermatologic, rheumatic, and other conditions responsive to systemic corticosteroids, including bursitis; **injection directly into the affected tissues** in bursitis and associated inflammatory disorders of tendons such as tenosynovitis, and inflammatory disorders of muscle such as fibrositis and myositis; **intra-articular and periarticular injection** in rheumatoid arthritis and osteoarthritis; **intralesional injection** in various dermatologic conditions; and **local injection** in certain inflammatory and cystic disorders of the foot.

CONTRAINDICATIONS: Herpes simplex of the eye and systemic fungal infections. Regional corticosteroid therapy is contraindicated in areas that are locally infected, although infection elsewhere in the body is not a contraindication to the use of corticosteroids regionally.

WARNINGS: No data supplied by the manufacturer.

PRECAUTIONS: Strict aseptic technique is mandatory in the use of Celestone Soluspan injection. Celestone Soluspan is not intended for intravenous or subcutaneous use.

Following intra-articular injection, a portion of the administered dose of Celestone Soluspan is absorbed systemically. In patients being treated concomitantly with peroral and parenteral corticosteroids, especially those receiving large doses, the systemic absorption of the drug should be considered in determining intra-articular dosage.

In patients on corticosteroid therapy subjected to unusual stress, increased dosage of rapidly acting corticosteroids before, during and after the stressful situation is indicated.

While on corticosteroid therapy, patients should not be vaccinated against smallpox because of potential complications. Conversely, patients with vaccinia should not receive corticosteroid therapy. Other immunization procedures should not be undertaken in patients receiving corticosteroids, especially high doses, because of possible hazards of neurological complications and a lack of antibody response. However, immunization procedures may be undertaken in patients who are receiving corticosteroids as replacement therapy, e.g., for Addison disease.

Patients who are on immunosuppressant doses of corticosteroids should be warned to avoid exposure to chickenpox or measles and, if exposed, to obtain medical advice. This is of particular importance to children.

The use of corticosteroids in active tuberculosis should be restricted to those cases of fulminating or disseminated tuberculosis in which the corticosteroid is used for management in conjunction with an appropriate antituberculous regimen. If corticosteroids are indicated in patients with latent tuberculosis or tuberculin reactivity, close observation is necessary since reactivation of the disease may occur. During prolonged corticosteroid therapy, patients should receive chemoprophylaxis. If rifampin is used in a chemoprophylactic program, its enhancing effect on metabolic hepatic clearance of corticosteroids should be considered; adjustment in corticosteroid dosage may be required.

Corticosteroids may mask some signs of infection, and new infections may appear during use. There may be decreased resistance and inability to localize infection when corticosteroids are used. If corticosteroids have to be used in the presence of bacterial infections, institute appropriate vigorous anti-infective therapy.

Prolonged corticosteroid use may produce posterior subcapsular cataracts (especially in children), glaucoma with possible damage to the optic nerves, and may enhance secondary ocular infections due to fungi or viruses. Ophthalmologic examination should be done periodically, especially in patients on long-term therapy (more than six weeks).

Average and large doses of corticosteroids can cause elevation of blood pressure, salt and water retention, and increased excretion of potassium. These effects are less likely to occur with the synthetic derivatives except when used in large doses. Dietary salt restriction and potassium supplementation may be considered. All corticosteroids increase calcium excretion.

The lowest possible dose of corticosteroid should be used to control the condition under treatment; when dosage reduction is possible, the reduction should be gradual.

Drug-induced secondary adrenocortical insufficiency may be minimized by gradual dosage reduction. Such relative insufficiency may persist for months after discontinuation of therapy; therefore, if stress occurs during that period, corticotherapy should be reinstituted. If the patient is receiving corticosteroids already, dosage may have to be increased. Since mineralocorticoid secretion may be impaired, salt and/or a mineralocorticosteroid should be administered concurrently.

Because rare instances of anaphylactoid reactions have occurred in patients receiving parenteral corticosteroid therapy, appropriate precautionary measures should be taken prior to administration, especially when the patient has a history of allergy to any drug.

Use acetylsalicylic acid (ASA) cautiously in conjunction with corticosteroids in hypoprothrombinemia.

Celestone Soluspan injection should be administered intramuscularly with caution to patients with idiopathic thrombocytopenic purpura.

Intramuscular injections of corticosteroids should be given deep into large muscle masses to avoid local tissue atrophy.

Corticosteroids should be used with caution in: nonspecific ulcerative colitis, if there is a probability of impending perforation, abscess, or other pyogenic infection; diverticulitis; fresh intestinal anastomoses; active or latent peptic ulcer; renal insufficiency; hypertension; osteoporosis; and myasthenia gravis. Fat embolism has been reported as a possible complication of hypercorticism.

There is an enhanced effect of corticosteroids on patients with hypothyroidism and in those with cirrhosis.

Psychic derangement may appear when corticosteroids are used, ranging from euphoria, insomnia, mood swings, personality changes, and severe depression to frank psychotic manifestations. Also, existing emotional instability or psychotic tendencies may be aggravated by corticosteroids.

Growth and development in infants and children on prolonged corticosteroid therapy should be carefully observed.

Steroids may increase or decrease motility and number of spermatozoa in some patients.

Advise patients to inform subsequent physicians of the prior use of corticosteroids.

Corticosteroids may suppress reactions to skin tests.

Corticosteroids should not be injected into unstable joints, infected areas or intervertebral spaces. Repeated injections into joints of osteoarthritis may increase joint destruction. Avoid injecting corticosteroids directly into the substance of tendons because delayed appearance of tendon rupture has resulted.

Following intra-articular corticosteroid therapy, care should be taken by the patient to avoid overuse of the joint in which symptomatic benefit has been obtained.

Examination of any joint fluid present is necessary to exclude a septic process. Local injection into a previously infected joint is to be avoided. A marked increase in pain and local swelling, further restriction of joint motion, fever and malaise are suggestive of septic arthritis. If the diagnosis of sepsis is confirmed, appropriate antimicrobial therapy should be instituted.

Since complications of glucocorticosteroid treatment are dependent on dose, size and duration of treatment, a risk/benefit decision must be made with each patient.

With long-term corticosteroid therapy, transfer from parenteral to oral administration should be considered after weighing the potential benefits and risks.

Dosage adjustments may be required with remission or exacerbation of the disease process, the patient's individual response to therapy and exposure of the patient to emotional or physical stress such as serious infection, surgery or injury. Monitoring may be necessary for up to one year following cessation of long-term or high-dose corticosteroid therapy.

Pregnancy: Since adequate human reproduction studies have not been done with corticosteroids, the use of these drugs in pregnancy, nursing mothers or women of childbearing potential requires that the possible benefits of the drug be weighed against the hazards to the mother and embryo, fetus or infant. Infants born to mothers who have received substantial doses of corticosteroids during pregnancy should be carefully observed for signs of hypoadrenalism.

When mothers were given betamethasone injections prenatally, the infants had transient suppression of fetal growth hormone and presumably of those pituitary hormones which regulate corticosteroid production by both the definitive and fetal zones of the fetal adrenal glands. However, the suppression of fetal hydrocortisone did not interfere with the pituitary-adrenocortical responses to stress after birth.

Women who have been on corticosteroids during pregnancy should be monitored during and after labor and delivery for any indication of adrenal insufficiency because of the stresses associated with childbirth.

Corticosteroids cross the placental barrier and appear in breast milk of nursing mothers. Because transplacental passage of corticosteroids occurs, newborn and young infants born of mothers who were dosed with corticosteroids throughout most or some portion of their pregnancy should be examined carefully for signs of adrenal insufficiency and the possible very rare occurrence of congenital cataracts.

Because of the potential for unwanted adverse effects from Celestone Soluspan in nursing infants, a decision should be made whether to discontinue nursing or to discontinue the drug, taking into account the importance of the drug to the mother.

Since use of corticosteroids prophylactically beyond the 32nd week of gestation is still controversial, the risk/benefit ratio should be considered for mother and fetus when using corticosteroids beyond this gestational period.

Corticosteroids are **not** indicated in the management of hyaline membrane disease after birth and should not be administered to pregnant women with pre-eclampsia, eclampsia, or evidence of placental damage.

Lactation: See Pregnancy.

Drug Interactions: Concurrent use of phenobarbital, phenytoin, rifampin or ephedrine may enhance the metabolism and clearance of corticosteroids, reducing their therapeutic effects.

Patients receiving both a corticosteroid and an estrogen should be observed for excessive corticosteroid effects.

Concurrent use of corticosteroids with potassium-depleting diuretics may enhance hypokalemia. Concurrent use of corticosteroids with cardiac glycosides may enhance the possibility of arrhythmias or digitalis toxicity associated with hypokalemia. Corticosteroids may enhance the potassium depletion caused by amphotericin B. In all patients taking any of these drug therapy combinations, serum electrolyte determinations, particularly potassium levels, should be monitored closely.

Concurrent use of corticosteroids with coumarin-type anticoagulants may increase or decrease the anticoagulant effects, possibly requiring adjustment in dosage.

Combined effects of nonsteroidal anti-inflammatory drugs or alcohol with glucocorticosteroids may result in an increased occurrence or increased severity of gastrointestinal ulceration.

Corticosteroids may decrease blood salicylate concentrations. ASA should be used cautiously in conjunction with corticosteroids in hypoprothrombinemia.

Dosage adjustments of an antidiabetic drug may be necessary when corticosteroids are given to diabetics.

Concomitant glucocorticosteroid therapy may inhibit the response to somatotropin.

Laboratory Test Interactions: Corticosteroids may affect the nitroblue tetrazolium test for bacterial infection and produce false negative results.

ADVERSE EFFECTS: There have been a few cases of crystal deposition but no reports of dimpling of the skin after intradermal injection. Nevertheless, because dimpling of the skin is attributable to atrophy of subcutaneous fat and is seen with other injectable corticosteroids, s.c. injection should be avoided. Pain has not been reported.

Fluid and Electrolyte Disturbances: sodium retention, potassium loss, hypokalemic alkalosis; fluid retention; congestive heart failure in susceptible patients; hypertension.

Musculoskeletal: muscle weakness; corticosteroid myopathy; loss of muscle mass; aggravation of myasthenic symptoms in myasthenia gravis; osteoporosis; vertebral compression fractures; aseptic necrosis of femoral and humeral heads; pathologic fracture of long bones; tendon rupture; joint instability (from repeated intra-articular injections).

Gastrointestinal: hiccups; peptic ulcer with possible perforation and hemorrhage; pancreatitis; abdominal distention; ulcerative esophagitis.

Dermatologic: impaired wound healing; skin atrophy; thin fragile skin; petechiae and ecchymoses; facial erythema; increased sweating; suppressed reactions to skin tests; reactions such as allergic dermatitis, urticaria, angioneurotic edema.

Neurological: convulsions; increased intracranial pressure with papilledema (pseudotumor cerebri) usually after treatment; vertigo; headache.

Endocrine: menstrual irregularities; development of Cushingoid state; suppression of growth in children; secondary adrenocortical and pituitary unresponsiveness, particularly in times of stress, as in trauma, surgery or illness; decreased carbohydrate tolerance; manifestations of latent diabetes mellitus; increased requirements of insulin or oral hypoglycemic agents in diabetics.

Ophthalmic: posterior subcapsular cataracts; increased intraocular pressure; glaucoma; exophthalmos.

Metabolic: negative nitrogen balance due to protein catabolism.

Psychiatric: euphoria, mood swings; severe depression to frank psychotic manifestations; personality changes; hyperirritability; insomnia.

Other: hypersensitivity, thromboembolism, anaphylactoid and hypotensive or shock-like reactions.

Additional adverse reactions related to parenteral corticosteroid therapy include rare instances of blindness associated with intralesional therapy around the face and head, hyperpigmentation or hypopigmentation, subcutaneous and cutaneous atrophy, sterile abscess, postinjection flare (following intra-articular use) and charcot-like arthropathy.

OVERDOSE:

Symptoms: Acute overdosage with glucocorticosteroids, including betamethasone, is not expected to lead to a life-threatening situation. Except at the most extreme dosages, a few days of excessive glucocorticosteroid dosing is unlikely to produce harmful results in the absence of specific contraindications, such as in patients with diabetes mellitus, glaucoma, or active peptic ulcer, or in patients on medications such as digitalis, coumarin-type anticoagulants or potassium-depleting diuretics.

Treatment: Complications resulting from the metabolic effects of the corticosteroid or from deleterious effects of the basic or concomitant illnesses or resulting from drug interactions should be handled as appropriate. Maintain adequate fluid intake and monitor electrolytes in serum and urine, with particular attention to sodium and potassium balance. Treat electrolyte imbalance if necessary.

> For management of a suspected drug overdose, CPhA recommends that you contact your **regional Poison Control Centre**. See the *CPS* Directory section for a list of Poison Control Centres.

DOSAGE: Shake well before using. Dosage must be adjusted according to the severity of the condition, the response obtained, and the patient's tolerance to the corticosteroid. For systemic effect, treatment is initiated with 1 mL i.m. in most conditions and repeated weekly, or more often, if necessary. In severe illnesses such as status asthmaticus or disseminated lupus erythematosus, 2 mL might be required initially. In dermatologic disorders, including neurodermatitis, psoriasis, hypertrophic lichen planus, lichen simplex, eczema, contact dermatitis, and dermatitis medicamentosa, i.m. dosage is usually 1 mL at intervals of 3 days to a week. In respiratory tract disorders, including bronchial asthma, hay fever, allergic bronchitis, and perennial allergic rhinitis, i.m. dosage is usually 1 to 2 mL at weekly intervals. Bursitis may be treated with i.m. injections of 1 mL repeated weekly if necessary.

The initial dose should be maintained or adjusted until a satisfactory response is observed. If a satisfactory clinical response does not occur after a reasonable period of time, treatment with Celestone Soluspan should be discontinued and other appropriate therapy initiated.

For local effect, in acute bursitis (subdeltoid, subacromial and prepatellar), 1 intrabursal injection of 1 mL relieves pain and restores full range of movement in a few hours. Several intrabursal injections at intervals of 1 to 2 weeks are usually required in recurrent acute bursitis and in acute exacerbations of chronic bursitis. Partial relief of pain and some increase in mobility may be expected in both conditions after 1 or 2 injections. In tendonitis, myositis, fibrositis, tenosynovitis, peritendonitis, and periarticular inflammatory conditions, 3 or 4 local injections of 1 mL each at intervals of 1 to 2 weeks between injections are given in most cases. Injection should be made into the affected tendon sheaths rather than into the tendons themselves. In periarticular inflammatory conditions, the painful area should be infiltrated. In ganglions of joint capsules, 0.5 mL is injected directly into the ganglion cysts. In rheumatoid arthritis and osteoarthritis, relief of pain, soreness and stiffness may be experienced in 2 to 4 hours after intra-articular injection. Using sterile technique, a 20 to 24 gauge needle on an empty syringe for aspiration is inserted into the synovial cavity and a few drops of synovial fluid are withdrawn to confirm that the needle is in the joint. The aspirating syringe is replaced by the syringe containing Celestone Soluspan and the injection is then made into the joint (see Table 1).

Table 1: Celestone Soluspan

Intra-articular Injection

Size of Joint	Location	Dose (mL)
Very Large	Hip	1.0 to 2.0
Large	Knee Ankle Shoulder	1.0
Medium	Elbow Wrist	0.5 to 1.0
Small (Metacarpophalangeal, interphalangeal) (Sternoclavicular)	Hand Chest	0.25 to 0.5

Pain with intra-articular injection of Celestone Soluspan has not been a problem. However, should the physician want to administer it with a local anesthetic, it can be mixed in the syringe with an equal volume of 1% or 2% lidocaine hydrochloride, procaine hydrochloride, or similar local anesthetics using formulations which do not contain parabens. Anesthetics containing methylparaben, propylparaben, phenol, etc. should be avoided. The required dose of Celestone Soluspan is first withdrawn from the vial into the syringe. The local anesthetic is then drawn in, and the syringe is shaken briefly. Do not inject local anaesthetic into the vial of Celestone Soluspan.

Dermatologic conditions that have responded to intralesional treatment with Celestone Soluspan include: localized neurodermatitis, psoriasis, nummular eczema, alopecia areata, hypertrophic lichen planus, circumscribed lichen simplex, keloids, and chronic discoid lupus erythematosus. In intralesional treatment, 0.2 mL of Celestone Soluspan is injected intradermally (not s.c.) per square centimeter of lesion using a tuberculin syringe with a 25 gauge, 13 mm needle. Care should be taken to deposit a uniform depot of medication intradermally. A total of no more than 1 mL at weekly intervals is recommended.

Disorders of the foot responsive to corticosteroids injected locally: For most injections into the foot, a tuberculin syringe with a 25 gauge, 2 cm needle is used. Treatment is given at intervals of 3 days to a week. In bursitis under heloma durum (hard corn), bursitis under heloma molle (soft corn), synovial cysts, and Morton's neuralgia (metatarsalgia) 0.25 to 0.5 mL are recommended. For bursitis under calcaneal spurs, bursitis over hallux rigidus (flexion deformity of the great toe), bursitis over digiti quinti varus (inward deviation of the fifth toe), tenosynovitis, and periostitis of the cuboid, 0.5 mL is recommended; in acute gouty arthritis, 0.5 to 1 mL are recommended.

SUPPLIED: Each mL of sterile aqueous suspension contains: betamethasone acetate USP 3 mg and betamethasone sodium phosphate USP equivalent to 3 mg betamethasone USP. Nonmedicinal ingredients: benzalkonium chloride, disodium edetate, sodium phosphate dibasic, sodium phosphate monobasic and water. Vials of 1 mL. Boxes of 10 and multiple dose vials of 5 mL. Store between 2 and 30°C. Protect from light.

The reader is invited to consult CPhA's monograph **Selective Serotonin Reuptake Inhibitors**.

Celexa®

citalopram HBr

Antidepressant

Lundbeck

Date of Preparation: January 28, 1999
Date of Revision: November 17, 2006

PHARMACOLOGY: Citalopram is a highly selective and potent serotonin (5-hydroxytryptamine, 5-HT) reuptake inhibitor with minimal effects on the neuronal reuptake of norepinephrine (NE) and dopamine (DA). The ability of citalopram to potentiate serotonergic activity in the CNS via inhibition of the neuronal reuptake of serotonin is thought to be responsible for its antidepressant action. Tolerance to the inhibition of serotonin reuptake is not induced by long-term (14 days) treatment of rats with citalopram.

Citalopram has no or very low affinity for a series of receptors including serotonin 5-HT_{1A}, 5-HT_2, dopamine D_1 and D_2, α_1-, α_2-, β-adrenergic, histamine H_1, muscarinic cholinergic, benzodiazepine, gamma aminobutyric acid (GABA) and opioid receptors.

Pharmacokinetics: Absorption: Following the administration of a single oral dose of citalopram (40 mg) to healthy male volunteers, peak blood levels occurred at about 4 hours (range 1 to 6 hours). The absolute bioavailability of citalopram was about 80% (range 52 to 93%) relative to an i.v. dose. Absorption was not affected by food.

Distribution: After i.v. infusion in healthy male volunteers, the apparent volume of distribution $(V_d)\beta$ was about 12 L/kg (range 9 to 17 L/kg), indicating a pronounced tissue distribution; $(V_d)\beta$ oral was about 17 L/kg (range 14 to 21 L/kg). The binding of citalopram and its demethylated metabolites to human plasma proteins is about 80%.

Steady-state: The single- and multiple-dose pharmacokinetics of citalopram are linear and dose-proportional in a dose range of 10 to 60 mg/day. Steady-state plasma levels are achieved in patients in 1 to 2 weeks. At a daily dose of 40 mg, the average plasma concentration is about 83 ng/mL (n=114) with a range from 30 to 200 ng/mL. Citalopram does not accumulate during long-term treatment. A clear relationship between citalopram plasma levels and therapeutic response or side effects has not been established.

Metabolism: Citalopram is metabolized in the liver to demethylcitalopram (DCT), didemethylcitalopram (DDCT), citalopram-N-oxide, and a deaminated propionic acid derivative. In vitro studies show that DCT, DDCT and citalopram-N-oxide also inhibit the neuronal reuptake of serotonin but are less selective and less potent than the parent compound and are of minor clinical importance. Unchanged citalopram is the predominant compound in plasma. In vitro studies indicated that the biotransformation of citalopram to its demethyl metabolites depends on both CYP 2C19 and CYP 3A4, with a small contribution from CYP 2D6.

Elimination: The elimination half-life of citalopram ($t_{1/2}$) is approximately 37 hours (range: 30 to 42 hours) which allows recommendation of once-daily dosing. The systemic citalopram plasma clearance (Cl_S) is 0.33 L/min. Citalopram is eliminated primarily via the liver (85%) and the remainder via the kidneys; approximately 12% (range 6 to 21%) of the daily dose is excreted in urine as unchanged citalopram.

Special Populations: Geriatrics: Elderly patients (4 males and 7 females aged 73 to 90 years), received a 20 mg/day dose of citalopram for 3 to 4 weeks. In the elderly, steady-state plasma levels were elevated (106 ng/mL), half-life prolonged (1.5 to 3.75 days) and clearance decreased (0.08 to 0.3 L/min). Elevation of citalopram plasma levels occurred at an earlier age in females than in males. In this population, lower doses and a lower maximum dose of citalopram are recommended (see Precautions and Dosage).

Reduced Hepatic Function: The pharmacokinetics of citalopram were compared in patients with reduced hepatic function (3 female and 6 male patients aged 41 to 60 years) to those seen in 12 healthy male volunteers (aged 21 to 43 years). In patients with reduced hepatic function the half-life of citalopram was approximately doubled (83 hours vs 37 hours), steady-state citalopram concentrations increased by 61% and oral clearance decreased by 37%. Consequently the use of citalopram in patients with reduced hepatic function should be approached with caution and lower maximal doses should be prescribed (see Precautions and Dosage).

Reduced Renal Function: In patients with mild to moderate reduction of the renal function (4 female and 3 male patients aged 30 to 55 years), citalopram was being eliminated more slowly than in 12 healthy male volunteers (aged 21 to 43 years); half-lives being 49 hours vs 37 hours. However, mild to moderate renal impairment had no major influence on the kinetics of citalopram. At present, no information is available for chronic treatment of patients with severely reduced renal function (creatinine clearance <20 mL/min) (see Precautions).

Clinical Trials: The efficacy of citalopram in the treatment of depression was established in 5 placebo-controlled studies in patients who met the DSM-III or DSM-III-R criteria for major depression. Response to treatment was evaluated by the Hamilton Depression Rating Scale (HAMD) and/or the Montgomery Asberg Depression Rating Scale (MADRS), as well as the Clinical Global Impression (CGI) Severity Scale. On the HAMD and MADRS, total scores, selected single items, and percentage of responders (defined as patients whose HAMD/MADRS total score decreased by at least 50% vs baseline) were assessed.

In a 6-week fixed-dose, dose-response study, patients received citalopram, at doses of 10, 20, 40, or 60 mg/day or placebo (n=129 to 131 per group). The 40 and 60 mg/day doses were titrated, with patients reaching these designated doses within 4 and 8 days, respectively. The study showed that the 40 and 60 mg/day doses were significantly more effective than placebo, although the 60 mg/day dose was not more effective than the 40 mg/day dose. The lower doses did not show statistically significant superiority over placebo, except on the MADRS; on this scale the percent of responders was significantly higher in all the citalopram-treated groups than in the placebo-treated group.

The second study was a 4-week flexible-dose study in which 85% of the depressed patients met the criteria for melancholia. At entry, 89 and 91 patients were randomized to the citalopram and placebo groups, respectively. This was the only study in which more male than female patients participated (64 vs 36%). The initial dose of citalopram, 20 mg/day, could be titrated to the maximal tolerated dose or a maximum dose of 80 mg/day. Patients treated with citalopram showed significantly greater improvement than patients treated with placebo. At week 4, the average daily dose was 63 mg, with 52% of patients receiving the 80 mg/day dose.

In a 6-week fixed-dose study, patients received citalopram, 20 or 40 mg/day, or placebo (n=64 to 70 per group). Patients treated with citalopram, 40 mg/day, showed significantly greater improvement than placebo-treated patients. The difference between the lower dose of citalopram and placebo was not significant.

In another 6-week fixed-dose study, patients received citalopram, 20 or 40 mg/day or placebo (n=88 to 97 per group). Although citalopram-treated patients improved to a somewhat greater degree than the placebo-treated patients, the differences between drug and control groups did not reach statistical significance due to a high placebo response, i.e., substantial improvement in the placebo group.

A 6-week, flexible-dose study was conducted in elderly, depressed patients (the mean age of male and female patients was 75 and 77 years, respectively) to determine the antidepressant effect and safety of citalopram in this subpopulation. The number of patients who received citalopram and placebo was 98 and 51, respectively. The study allowed patients to enter with lower baseline HAMD scores than are usually acceptable (≥18 in clinical trials). However, only a small percentage of patients had HAMD scores of less than 18 at entry. The dose of citalopram was titrated from a starting dose of 10 mg/day to a maximum dose of 30 mg/day. Patients treated with citalopram showed significantly greater improvement than patients treated with placebo. The final dose of citalopram was 10, 20 and 30 mg/day in 5%, 51% and 44% of patients, respectively.

The effectiveness of citalopram in preventing relapse was assessed in 2 long-term studies. Depressed patients who responded to citalopram during an initial 6 or 8 weeks of acute treatment (fixed doses of 20 or 40 mg/day in one study and flexible doses of 20 to 60 mg/day in the second study) were randomized to continue on citalopram or receive placebo. The number of patients who received citalopram and placebo was 257 and 116, respectively. In both studies, patients who continued on citalopram experienced significantly lower relapse rates over the subsequent 6 months compared to those receiving placebo. In the fixed-dose study, the relapse rates were similar at the 20 and 40 mg/day doses, namely 10% and 12%, respectively. Of the placebo-treated patients, 31% experienced relapse. In the flexible-dose study, the relapse rates were 14% and 24% in the citalopram- and placebo-treated patients, respectively. While the majority of patients (76%) were maintained on 20 or 40 mg/day of citalopram during most of the study, some patients received 60 mg/day, while a few patients were maintained on less than 20 mg/day.

INDICATIONS: For the symptomatic relief of depressive illness.

The relapse rate was significantly lower in citalopram-treated patients than in placebo-treated patients in 2 placebo-controlled studies, that were conducted over a 24-week period in patients who responded to 6 or 8 weeks of acute treatment with citalopram (see Pharmacology, Clinical Trials). Nevertheless, the physician who elects to use citalopram for extended periods should periodically reevaluate the long-term usefulness of the drug for the individual patient.

CONTRAINDICATIONS: In patients with known hypersensitivity to citalopram hydrobromide or the excipients of the drug product.

Monoamine oxidase inhibitors (MAOIs): In patients, receiving selective serotonin reuptake inhibitors (SSRIs) in combination with a MAOI, there have been reports of serious, sometimes fatal, reactions including hyperthermia, rigidity, myoclonus, autonomic instability with possible rapid fluctuations of vital signs, and mental status changes, including extreme agitation progressing to delirium and coma. These reactions have also been reported in patients who have recently discontinued SSRI treatment and have been started on a MAOI. Some cases presented with features resembling serotonin syndrome. Therefore, citalopram should not be used in combination with a MAOI or within 14 days of discontinuing treatment with a MAOI. Similarly, at least 14 days should elapse after discontinuing citalopram treatment before starting a MAOI.

Pimozide: Citalopram should not be used in combination with the anti-psychotic drug pimozide, as results from a controlled study with racemic citalopram indicate that concomitant use is associated with an increased risk of QTc prolongation compared to pimozide alone. This apparent pharmacodynamic interaction occured in the absence of a clinically significant pharmacokinetic interaction; the mechanism is unknown (see Precautions, Drug Interactions).

WARNINGS: Potential Association with Behavioral and Emotional Changes, Including Self-Harm: Pediatrics: Placebo-Controlled Clinical Trial Data: Recent analyses of placebo-controlled clinical trial safety databases from SSRIs and other newer antidepressants suggest that use of these drugs in patients under the age of 18 may be associated with behavioral and emotional changes, including an increased risk of suicidal ideation and behavior over that of placebo.

The small denominators in the clinical trial database, as well as the variability in placebo rates, preclude reliable conclusions on the relative safety profiles among these drugs.

Adults and Pediatrics: Additional data: There are clinical trial and post-marketing reports with SSRIs and other newer antidepressants, in both pediatrics and adults, of severe agitation-type adverse events coupled with self-harm and harm to others. The agitation-type events include: akathisia, agitation, disinhibition, emotional lability, hostility, aggression, depersonalization. In some cases, the events occurred within several weeks of starting treatment.

Rigorous clinical monitoring for suicidal ideation or other indicators of potential for suicidal behavior is advised in patients of all ages. This includes monitoring for agitation-type emotional and behavioral changes.

Discontinuation Symptoms: Patients currently taking citalopram should not be discontinued abruptly, due to risk of discontinuation symptoms. At the time that a medical decision is made to discontinue an SSRI or other newer antidepressant drug, a gradual reduction in the dose rather than an abrupt cessation is recommended.

PRECAUTIONS: Suicide: The possibility of a suicide attempt is inherent in depression and may persist until remission occurs. Therefore, high risk patients should be closely supervised throughout therapy with citalopram and consideration should be given to the possible need for hospitalization. In order to minimize the opportunity for overdosage, prescription for citalopram should be written for the smallest quantity of drug consistent with good patient management (see Potential Association with Behavioral and Emotional Changes, Including Self-Harm under Warnings).

Activation of Mania/Hypomania: In placebo-controlled trials with citalopram, some of which included patients with bipolar disorder, mania/hypomania was reported in 0.1% of 1027 patients treated with citalopram vs none of the 426 patients treated with placebo. Activation of mania/hypomania has also been reported in a small proportion of patients with major affective disorders treated with other marketed antidepressants. If a patient enters a manic phase, citalopram should be discontinued.

Seizures: Citalopram has not been systematically evaluated in patients with a seizure disorder. These patients were excluded from clinical studies during the premarketing testing of citalopram. In clinical trials, seizures occurred in 0.25% of patients treated with citalopram and in 0.23% of patients treated with placebo. Like other antidepressants, citalopram should be used with caution in patients with a history of seizure disorder. The drug should be discontinued in any patient who develop seizures.

Discontinuation of Treatment with citalopram: When discontinuing treatment, patients should be monitored for symptoms which may be associated with discontinuation (e.g. dizziness, abnormal dreams, sensory disturbances [including paresthesias and electric shock sensations], agitation, anxiety, emotional indifference, impaired concentration, headache, migraine, tremor, nausea, vomiting and sweating) or other symptoms which may be of clinical significance (see Adverse Effects). A gradual reduction in the dosage over several weeks, rather than abrupt cessation is recommended whenever possible. If intolerable symptoms occur following a decrease in the dose or upon discontinuation of treatment, dose titration should be managed on the basis of the patient's clinical response. (See Adverse Effects and Dosage).

Serotonin Syndrome: Rarely, the occurrence of serotonin syndrome has been reported in patients receiving SSRIs. A combination of symptoms, possibly including agitation, confusion, tremor, myoclonus and hyperthermia, may indicate the development of this condition.

Serotonergic Drugs: There have been rare postmarketing reports describing patients with weakness, hyperreflexia and incoordination, following the concomitant use of a SSRI and the antimigraine drug sumatriptan, a 5-HT_1 agonist. Such interaction should be considered if citalopram is to be used in combination with a 5-HT_1 agonist. St-John's Wort: In common with other SSRI's, pharmacodynamic interactions between citalopram and the herbal remedy St-John's Wort may occur and may result in undesirable effects.

Hyponatremia: Hyponatremia and SIADH (syndrome of inappropriate antidiuretic hormone secretion) have been reported as a rare adverse event with use of citalopram as with other SSRIs. Elderly female patients in particular seem to be a group at risk.

Pregnancy: The safety of citalopram during pregnancy and lactation has not been established. Therefore, citalopram should not be used during pregnancy, unless, in the opinion of the physician, the expected benefits to the patient markedly outweigh the possible hazards to the fetus.

Post-marketing reports indicate that some neonates exposed to SSRIs such as citalopram and other antidepressants late in the third trimester have developed complications requiring prolonged hospitalization, respiratory support, and tube feeding. Such complications can arise immediately upon delivery. Reported clinical findings have included respiratory distress, cyanosis, apnea, seizures, temperature instability, feeding difficulty, vomiting, hypoglycemia, hypotonia, hypertonia, hyperreflexia, tremor, jitteriness, irritability and constant crying. These features are consistent with either a direct toxic effect of SSRIs and other newer antidepressants, or, possibly, a drug discontinuation syndrome. It should be noted that, in some cases, the clinical picture is consistent with serotonin syndrome (see Precautions, Serotonin Syndrome). When treating a pregnant woman with citalopram during the third trimester, the physician should carefully consider the potential risks and benefits of treatment (see Dosage).

Lactation: See Pregnancy. Citalopram is excreted in human milk. Citalopram should not be administered to nursing mothers unless, in the opinion of the treating physician, the expected benefits to the patient markedly outweigh the possible hazards to the child.

Children: Safety and effectiveness in patients below the age of 18 have not been established.

Geriatrics: In premarketing clinical trials, 800 elderly patients (≥65 years of age) have been treated with citalopram. Of these patients 298 were ≥75 years old. In a pharmacokinetic study (n=11, age 73 to 90 years), clearance was substantially decreased and half-life prolonged (see Pharmacology, Pharmacokinetics). In a 6-week placebo-controlled study, approximately equal numbers of patients received citalopram at 20 or 30 mg/day, as the final dose. In about 5% of patients, the final dose was 10 mg/day (see Pharmacology, Clinical Trials). Consequently, elderly patients should be administered lower doses and a lower maximum dose (see Dosage).

Hepatic Impairment: In subjects with hepatic impairment, citalopram clearance was significantly decreased and plasma concentrations, as well as elimination half-life significantly increased (see Pharmacology, Pharmacokinetics). Consequently, the use of citalopram in hepatically impaired patients should be approached with caution and a lower maximum dosage is recommended (see Dosage).

Renal Impairment: No dosage adjustment is needed in patients with mild to moderate renal impairment. Since, no information is available on the pharmacokinetic or pharmacodynamic effects of citalopram in patients with severely reduced renal function (creatinine clearance <20 mL/min), citalopram should be used with caution in these patients.

Patients with Cardiac Disease: Citalopram has not been systematically evaluated in patients with a recent history of myocardial infarction or unstable heart disease. Patients with these diagnoses were generally excluded from clinical trials during the drug's premarketing assessment. However, the electrocardiograms of patients, who received citalopram in clinical trials, indicate that citalopram was not associated with the development of clinically significant ECG abnormalities.

In clinical trials, citalopram caused small but statistically significant decreases in heart rate (see Adverse Effects, ECG). Consequently, caution should be observed when citalopram is initiated in patients with pre-existing slow heart rate.

Diabetic Patients: Citalopram has not been systematically evaluated in diabetic patients since diabetes constituted an exclusion criterion. Although 13 patients did receive insulin during the studies, this number is too small to determine whether citalopram affects the response to insulin. Rare events of hypoglycemia were reported. Citalopram should be used with caution in diabetic patients on insulin or other antidiabetic drugs.

Occupational Hazards: Interference with Cognitive and Motor Performance: In studies in normal volunteers, citalopram in doses of 40 mg/day did not impair cognitive function or psychomotor performance. However, psychotropic medications may impair judgement, thinking or motor skills. Consequently, patients should be cautioned against driving a car or operating hazardous machinery until they are reasonably certain that citalopram does not affect them adversely.

Electroconvulsive Therapy (ECT): The safety and efficacy of the concurrent use of citalopram and ECT have not been studied.

Bleeding Disorders: There have been reports of cutaneous bleeding abnormalities such as ecchymosis and purpura with SSRIs. Caution is advised in patients taking SSRIs, particularly in concomitant use with drugs known to affect platelet function (e.g., atypical antipsychotics and phenothiazines, most tricyclic antidepressants, ASA, and NSAIDs) as well as in patients with a history of bleeding disorders.

Drug Interactions: MAOIs: For interactions between citalopram and MAOIs, see Contraindications.

General: The studies described in this section were carried out in young, healthy, mostly male volunteers. In addition, some of the studies, namely interactions with metoprolol, warfarin, digoxin, imipramine, and levomepromazine, utilized only single doses of these drugs, although citalopram was given repeatedly to attain steady state. Thus, data are not available in patients who would be receiving these drugs on an ongoing basis at therapeutic doses.

Metoprolol: Coadministration of citalopram (40 mg/day for 22 days) and the β-adrenergic blocking agent metoprolol (single dose of 150 mg), resulted in a 2-fold increase in the plasma levels of metoprolol. However, the effect of metoprolol on blood pressure and heart rate was not affected.

Warfarin: Administration of citalopram (40 mg/day for 21 days), did not affect either the pharmacokinetics or the pharmacodynamics (prothrombin time) of a single, 25 mg dose of warfarin.

Digoxin: Administration of citalopram (40 mg/day for 21 days) did not affect the pharmacokinetics of digoxin (single dose of 1 mg), although the serum levels of citalopram were slightly lower in the presence of digoxin.

Imipramine: Coadministration of citalopram (40 mg/day for 10 days) and the tricyclic antidepressant, imipramine (single dose of 100 mg), did not affect the pharmacokinetics of either drug. However, in the presence of citalopram, the concentration of desipramine, the metabolite of imipramine, increased by approximately 50% and its half-life was prolonged. The results indicate that citalopram does not interfere with the demethylation of imipramine to desipramine but does inhibit the metabolism of desipramine to its 2-hydroxy metabolite. Consequently, concomitant treatment with citalopram and imipramine/desipramine should be undertaken with caution.

Levomepromazine: Coadministration of citalopram (40 mg/day for 10 days) and levomepromazine (single dose of 50 mg), did not affect the pharmacokinetics of either drug.

Lithium: Coadministration of citalopram (40 mg/day for 10 days) and lithium (30 mmol/day for 5 days), did not affect the pharmacokinetics of either drug. However, since lithium may increase serotonergic neurotransmission, concomitant treatment with these 2 drugs should be undertaken with caution.

Cimetidine: Citalopram 40 mg/day was administered for 29 days. During the last 8 days of treatment, cimetidine (400 mg b.i.d.) was added to the treatment regimen. In the presence of cimetidine, a potent inhibitor of hepatic cytochrome P450 enzymes, the C_{max} and AUC of citalopram was increased by 39% and 41%, respectively. Thus, caution should be exercised at the upper end of the dose range of citalopram when it is used concomitantly with high doses of cimetidine.

Carbamazepine: Carbamazepine, titrated to 400 mg/day, was given for 21 days alone and then in combination with citalopram (40 mg/day) for an additional 14 days. Citalopram did not affect the plasma levels of either carbamazepine, a CYP 3A4 substrate, or its metabolite, carbamazepine-epoxide. However, since carbamazepine is a microsomal enzyme inducer, the possibility that carbamazepine may increase the clearance of citalopram should be considered if the two drugs are given concomitantly.

Pimozide: In a double-blind crossover study in healthy young adults, a single dose of pimozide 2 mg co-administered with racemic citalopram 40 mg given once daily for 11 days was associated with a mean increase in QTc values at Tmax of approximately 12 ms compared to pimozide when given with placebo. The mechanism of this apparent pharmacodynamic interaction is not known.

Cytochrome P450 Isozymes: Using in vitro models of human liver microsomes, the biotransformation of citalopram to its demethyl metabolites was shown to depend on both CYP 2C19 and CYP 3A4, with a small contribution from CYP 2D6. Studies have also indicated that citalopram is a weak inhibitor of CYP 2D6 and CYP 2C19 and a weak or negligible inhibitor of CYP 3A4 and CYP 1A2. One in vitro study using human liver microsomes has shown that ketoconazole and omeprazole reduced the rate of formation of the demethylcitalopram metabolite of citalopram to 45-60% and 75-85% of control, respectively. As data are not available from multi-dose pharmacokinetic studies, the possibility that the clearance of citalopram will be decreased when citalopram is administered with a potent inhibitor of CYP 3A4 (e.g., ketoconazole, itraconazole, fluconazole or erythromycin), or a potent inhibitor of CYP 2C19 (e.g., omeprazole), should be considered.

Various scientific publications have acknowledged that the main components in grapefruit juice may act as a CYP3A4 inhibitor. Citalopram is also metabolized by other isoenzymes not affected by grapefruit juice, namely CYP2C19 and CYP2D6. Although there is a theoretical possibility of pharmacokinetic drug interactions resulting from co-administration of citalopram with grapefruit juice, the onset of an interaction is considered unlikely.

Alcohol: Although citalopram did not potentiate the cognitive and psychomotor effects of alcohol in volunteers, the concomitant use of alcohol and citalopram should be avoided.

Other Drugs: No pharmacodynamic interactions have been noted in clinical trials where citalopram has been given concomitantly with benzodiazepines (anxiolytics/hypnotics), analgesics (NSAIDs, non-NSAIDs), antihistamines, antihypertensives or other cardiovascular drugs. Pharmacokinetic interactions between citalopram and these drugs were not specifically studied.

ADVERSE EFFECTS: During the premarketing clinical development, 3652 patients received citalopram for the treatment of depression. Of these patients, 66% were females and 34% were males. The mean age of the patients was 50 years, with 70% being <60 years old (30% <40 years old, 40% 40 to 59 years old) and 30% being ≥60 years old. Adverse events observed with citalopram are in general mild and transient. They usually attenuate during the first one or two weeks of treatment.

Adverse Findings Observed in Short-term, Placebo-controlled Trials: Adverse Reactions Leading to Discontinuation of Treatment: From the short-term (4 to 6 weeks) placebo-controlled, Phase III clinical trials, 15.9% (163/1 027) of the citalopram-treated patients discontinued treatment due to an adverse event. The discontinuation rate in the placebo-treated patients was 7.7% (33/426).

The events associated with discontinuation of citalopram in 1% or more of patients at a rate of at least twice that of placebo, were as follows: nausea (4.1% vs 0.0%), insomnia (2.4% vs 1.2%), somnolence (2.4% vs 1.2%), dizziness (2.3% vs 0.7%), vomiting (1.3% vs 0.0%), agitation (1.2% vs 0.0%), asthenia (1.1% vs 0.5%), and dry mouth (1.1% vs 0.2%).

Incidence of Adverse Events in Placebo-controlled Studies: Table 1 enumerates the incidence of treatment emergent adverse events that occurred in 1 027 depressed patients who received citalopram at doses ranging from 10 to 80 mg/day in placebo-controlled trials of up to 6 weeks in duration. Events included are those occurring in 2% or more of patients treated with citalopram, and for which the incidence in patients treated with citalopram was greater than the incidence in placebo-treated patients. Reported adverse events were classified using the standard World Health Organization (WHO)-based dictionary terminology.

The prescriber should be aware that these figures cannot be used to predict the incidence of adverse events in the course of usual medical practice where patient characteristics and other factors differ from those which prevailed in the clinical trials. Similarly, the cited frequencies cannot be compared with figures obtained from other clinical investigations involving different treatments, uses, and investigators. The cited figures, however, do provide the prescribing physician with some basis for estimating the relative contribution of drug and non-drug factors to the adverse event incidence rate in the population studied.

Table 1: Celexa

Treatment-emergent Adverse Events[a]—Incidence in Placebo-controlled Clinical Trials

	Percentage of Patients Reporting	
Body System/Adverse Event	**Citalopram (n=1027)**	**Placebo (n=426)**
Body as a Whole		
Fatigue	5.2	3.1
Fever[b]	2.4	0.2
Autonomic Nervous System		
Dry mouth[b]	19.4	12.2
Sweating increased	10.5	8.0
Central and Peripheral Nervous Systems		
Tremor	8.4	6.3

(cont'd)

Table 1: Celexa *(cont'd)*

Treatment-emergent Adverse Events[a]—Incidence in Placebo-controlled Clinical Trials

	Percentage of Patients Reporting	
Body System/Adverse Event	**Citalopram (n=1027)**	**Placebo (n=426)**
Gastrointestinal System		
Nausea[b]	20.6	13.4
Diarrhea	8.1	5.4
Dyspepsia	4.3	3.5
Vomiting	3.9	2.6
Abdominal pain	3.1	2.1
Psychiatric		
Somnolence[b]	17.3	9.9
Anorexia[b]	4.2	1.6
Nervousness	3.6	3.5
Anxiety	3.3	2.1
Agitation[b]	2.4	0.7
Libido decreased[b]	2.2	0.2
Yawning[b]	2.1	0
Reproductive, Female[c]		
Dysmenorrhea (<50 years)	2.7	1.6
Reproductive, Male[d]		
Ejaculation disorder[b]	6.2	1.1
Impotence[d]	3.2	0.6
Respiratory System		
Upper respiratory tract infection	5.1	4.7
Rhinitis	4.9	3.3
Pharyngitis	3.4	2.8
Sinusitis[b]	2.4	0.2
Urinary System		
Micturition disorder	2.3	2.1

[a] Events included are those occurring in 2% or more of patients treated with Celexa, and for which the incidence in patients treated with Celexa was greater than the incidence in placebo-treated patients.
[b] Statistically significantly higher incidence in the citalopram group (p<0.05).
[c] Denominator used was for females only (n=623 for Celexa; n=245 for Placebo).
[d] Denominator used was for males only (n=404 for Celexa; n=181 for Placebo).

The following events had an incidence on placebo ≥ citalopram: asthenia, back pain, headache, dizziness, constipation, palpitation, insomnia, abnormal vision.

Most Frequent Adverse Events: Adverse events that occurred in citalopram-treated patients in the course of the short-term, placebo-controlled trials with an incidence greater than, or equal to, 10% were: nausea, dry mouth, somnolence, and increased sweating (Table 1).

Dose Dependency of Adverse Events: The potential relationship between the dose of citalopram and the incidence of an adverse event was examined in a fixed dose short-term, placebo-controlled study in which patients received citalopram at doses of 10, 20, 40 or 60 mg/day. The incidence of diarrhea, dry mouth, fatigue, insomnia, increased sweating, nausea and somnolence was dose-related.

Male and Female Sexual Dysfunction with SSRIs: While sexual dysfunction is often part of depression and other psychiatric disorders, there is increasing evidence that treatment with selective serotonin reuptake inhibitors (SSRIs) may induce sexual side effects. This is a difficult area to study because patients may not spontaneously report symptoms of this nature, and therefore, it is thought that sexual side effects with SSRIs may be underestimated.

In placebo-controlled, short-term clinical trials, the reported incidence of decreased libido, ejaculation disorders (primarily ejaculation delay and ejaculation failure), and impotence in male depressed patients receiving citalopram (n=404) was 3.7%, 6.2%, and 3.2%, respectively. In female depressed patients receiving citalopram (n=623), the reported incidence of decreased libido and anorgasmia was 1.3% and 1.1%, respectively. The reported incidence of each of these adverse events was ≤1% among male and female depressed patients receiving placebo.

Weight Changes: Patients treated with citalopram in controlled trials experienced a weight loss of about 0.5 kg compared to no change for placebo patients.

ECG: Retrospective analyses of ECG in citalopram-treated (n=779 <60 years and n=313 ≥60 years) and placebo-treated (n=74 <60 years and n=43 ≥60 years) patients indicated that citalopram decreases heart rate. In patients <60 years old, the mean decrease was approximately 5 bpm, while in patients ≥60 years old, mean decreases ranged between 5 to 10 bpm. Following the initial drop, heart rate remained decreased but stable over prolonged periods of time (up to one year in over 100 younger and over 50 elderly patients). The effect was reversible within approximately a week after stopping treatment.

In the 6-week, fixed dose, dose-response study, the mean decreases in heart rate ranged between 2 to 6 bpm in the 20 to 60 mg/day dose range, but the effect did not seem to be dose-related and was independent of gender. In placebo-treated patients heart rates remained unaffected. The differences in heart rates between citalopram- and placebo-treated patients were statistically significant. ECG parameters, including QT interval, remained unaffected.

Adverse Reactions following Discontinuation of Treatment (or Dose Reduction): There have been reports of adverse reactions upon the discontinuation of citalopram (particularly when abrupt), including but not limited to the following: dizziness, abnormal dreams, sensory disturbances (including paresthesias and electric shock sensations), agitation, anxiety, emotional indifference, impaired concentration, headache, migraine, tremor, nausea, vomiting and sweating or other symptoms which may be of clinical significance (see Precautions and Dosage).

Patients should be monitored for these or any other symptoms. A gradual reduction in the dosage over several weeks, rather than abrupt cessation is recommended whenever possible. If intolerable symptoms occur following a decrease in the dose or upon discontinuation of treatment, dose titration should be managed on the basis of the patient's clinical response. These events are generally self-limiting. Symptoms associated with discontinuation have been reported for other selective serotonin reuptake inhibitors (see Precautions and Dosage).

Additional Adverse Events Observed During the Premarketing Evaluation of Citalopram: The events listed below include all adverse events that were reported in the overall development program of citalopram (n=3652). All reported events are included except those already listed in Table 1 and those events which occurred in only one patient. It is important to emphasize that, although the events reported occurred during treatment with citalopram, they were not necessarily caused by it. The events are enumerated using the following criteria: frequent: adverse events that occurred on one or more occasions in at least 1/100 patients; infrequent: adverse events that occurred in less than 1/100 patients but at least in 1/1000 patients; rare: adverse events that occurred in fewer than 1/1000 patients.

Body as a Whole: General Disorders: Frequent: Influenza-like symptoms, non-pathological trauma, pain. Infrequent: alcohol intolerance, allergic reaction, allergy, chest pain, edema, hot flushes, leg pain, malaise, rigors, syncope. Rare: peripheral edema, sudden death, traumatic injury.

Cardiovascular Disorders: Frequent: postural hypotension, tachycardia. Infrequent: angina pectoris, arrhythmia, bradycardia, cardiac failure, cerebrovascular disorders, edema dependent, extrasystoles, flushing, hypertension, hypotension, myocardial infarction, myocardial ischemia, peripheral ischemia. Rare: aggravated hypertension, bundle branch block, cardiac arrest, coronary artery disorder, ECG abnormal, heart disorder, phlebitis, supraventricular extrasystoles.

Central and Peripheral Nervous System Disorders: Frequent: migraine, paraesthesia. Infrequent: abnormal gait, ataxia, convulsions, dysphonia, dystonia, extrapyramidal disorder, hyperkinesia, hypertonia, hypoesthesia, hypokinesia, involuntary muscle contractions, leg cramps, neuralgia, speech disorder, vertigo. Rare: abnormal coordination, convulsions grand mal, hyperesthesia, ptosis, sensory disturbance, stupor.

Collagen Disorders: Rare: rheumatoid arthritis.

Endocrine Disorders: Rare: goiter, gynecomastia, hypothyroidism.

Gastrointestinal System Disorders: Frequent: flatulence. Infrequent: colitis, dental abscess, dysphagia, eructation, gastritis, gastroenteritis, gastrointestinal disorder (not specified), hemorrhoids, increased saliva, teeth-grinding, toothache. Rare: appendicitis, esophagitis, gastric ulcer, gastroesophageal reflux, gingivitis, stomatitis, tooth disorder, ulcerative stomatitis.

Hematopoietic and Lymphatic Disorders: Infrequent: anemia, epistaxis, leukocytosis, purpura. Rare: coagulation disorder, gingival bleeding, granulocytopenia, hematoma, leukopenia, lymphadenopathy, lymphocytosis, pulmonary embolism.

Liver and Biliary System Disorders: Infrequent: cholecystitis, cholelithiasis, increased gamma-GT, increased ALT. Rare: bilirubinemia, increased AST, jaundice.

Metabolic and Nutritional Disorders: Frequent: appetite decreased, weight decrease, weight increase. Infrequent: leg edema, xerophthalmia. Rare: dehydration, edema, hypoglycemia, hypokalemia, increased alkaline phosphatase, obesity, thirst.

Musculoskeletal System Disorders: Infrequent: arthralgia, arthritis, arthrosis, dystonia, muscle weakness, myalgia. Rare: bone disorder, bursitis, osteoporosis, tendon disorder.

Neoplasm: Rare: breast neoplasm malignant female.

Psychiatric Disorders: Frequent: abnormal dreaming, aggravated depression, amnesia, apathy, confusion, depression, impaired concentration, increased appetite, sleep disorder, suicide attempt. Infrequent: abnormal thinking, aggressive reaction, delusion, depersonalization, drug abuse, drug dependence, emotional lability, euphoria, hallucination, increased libido, manic reaction, neurosis, paranoid reaction, paroniria, psychosis, psychotic depression. Rare: catatonic reaction, hysteria, personality disorder.

Reproductive Disorders, Female: Frequent: abnormal orgasm. Infrequent: amenorrhea, breast pain, lactation nonpuerperal, menorrhagia, menstrual disorder, premenstrual syndrome, salpingitis, unintended pregnancy, vaginal dryness, vaginitis. Rare: breast enlargement, vaginal hemorrhage.

Reproductive Disorders, Male: Infrequent: penis disorder, prostatic disorder, testis disorder.

Resistance Mechanism Disorders: Infrequent: abscess, fungal infection, herpes simplex infection, otitis media, viral infection. Rare: bacterial infection, moniliasis, sepsis.

Respiratory System Disorders: Infrequent: bronchitis, coughing, dyspnea, pneumonia. Rare: asthma, bronchospasm, increased sputum, laryngitis, pneumonitis, respiratory disorder.

Skin and Appendage Disorders: Frequent: pruritus, rash. Infrequent: acne, alopecia, dermatitis, dry skin, eczema, photosensitivity reaction, psoriasis, rash erythematous, rash maculo-papular, skin discoloration, urticaria. Rare: cellulitis, decreased sweating, hypertrichosis, melanosis, pruritus ani.

Special Senses, Vision, Hearing and Vestibular Disorders: Frequent: abnormal accommodation. Infrequent: conjunctivitis, earache, eye pain, mydriasis, taste perversion, tinnitus. Rare: eye abnormality, keratitis, photophobia.

Urinary System Disorders: Frequent: polyuria. Infrequent: abnormal urine, cystitis, hematuria, micturition frequency, urinary incontinence, urinary retention, urinary tract infection. Rare: dysuria, facial edema, oliguria, renal calculus, renal pain.

Events Observed During the Postmarketing Evaluation of Citalopram: Adverse events which have been reported to be temporally (but not necessarily causally) associated with citalopram treatment in at least 3 patients since its market introduction include: abnormal hepatic function, acute renal failure, aggravated condition, aggravated migraine, akathisia, anaphylaxis, angioedema, asthma, choreoathetosis, convulsions NOS, decreased drug level, decreased prothrombin time, delirium, dyskinesia, ecchymosis, eosinophilia, epidermal necrolysis, erythema multiforme, gastrointestinal hemorrhage, gynecological problems, hemolytic anemia, hepatitis, hypersensitivity NOS, hyperprolactinemia, hypomania, hyponatremia, increased drug level, increased prothrombin time, menometrorrhagia, myoclonic jerks, neuroleptic malignant syndrome, neuropathy, nystagmus, pancreatitis, pancytopenia, purpura NOS, rhabdomyolysis, serotonin syndrome, SIADH, spontaneous abortion/fetal death, suicide ideation, thrombocytopenia, vasodilatation, ventricular arrhythmia, torsades de pointes, withdrawal syndrome.

OVERDOSE:

Symptoms: Citalopram has a wide margin of safety in overdose. Cases of overdoses involved the ingestion of citalopram either alone or in combination with other drugs and/or alcohol. Cases of overdoses of citalopram ranging from 180 mg to 2000 mg have been reported during the premarketing clinical development. All patients recovered. One patient, ingesting over 1500 mg citalopram, had reversible ECG abnormalities, the most important of which was prolongation of QTc.

Citalopram is given to patients at potential risk of suicide and reports of attempted suicide have been received after its market introduction. Post-marketing reports of drug overdoses involving citalopram have included fatalities with citalopram alone as well as non-fatal overdoses of up to 5200 mg. In many cases, details regarding the precise dose of citalopram or combination with other drugs and/or alcohol are often lacking. Although most patients recovered without sequelae, fatalities have been reported at doses of citalopram up to 3920 mg.

Fatal cases of serotonin syndrome have been reported in patients who took overdoses of moclobemide (Manerix) and citalopram. The plasma concentrations of moclobemide were between 16 and 90 mg/L (therapeutic range: 1 to 3 mg/L) and those of citalopram between 0.3 and 1.7 mg (therapeutic concentration: 0.3 mg/L). This indicates that a relatively low dose of citalopram, given with an overdose of moclobemide represents a serious risk for the patient.

Symptoms most often accompanying citalopram overdose included dizziness, sweating, nausea, vomiting, tremor, and somnolence. In more rare cases, observed symptoms included confusion, loss of consciousness, convulsions, coma, sinus tachycardia, cyanosis, hyperventilation and rhabdomyolysis.

Treatment: Establish and maintain an airway to ensure adequate ventilation and oxygenation. Gastric lavage and use of activated charcoal should be considered. Cardiac and vital sign monitoring are recommended, along with general symptomatic and supportive measures. There are no specific antidotes for citalopram.

Due to the large volume of distribution of citalopram, forced diuresis, dialysis, hemoperfusion and exchange transfusion are unlikely to be of benefit. In managing overdosage, the possibility of multiple drug involvement must be considered.

> For management of a suspected drug overdose, CPhA recommends that you contact your **regional Poison Control Centre**. See the *CPS* Directory section for a list of Poison Control Centres.

DOSAGE: **Citalopram is not indicated for use in children under 18 years of age** (see Warnings, Potential Association with Behavioral and Emotional Changes, Including Self-Harm).

General: Citalopram should be administered once daily, in the morning or evening, with or without food.

Adults: Citalopram should be administered as a single oral dose of 20 mg/day. In patients who do not respond adequately, an increase of dosage to 40 mg/day should be considered. Certain patients may require 60 mg/day. However, in a dose-response study, the 60 mg/day dose did not demonstrate an advantage regarding effectiveness over the 40 mg/day dose. Dose increases should usually occur in increments of 20 mg, at intervals of no less than 1 week.

Treatment of Pregnant Women During The Third Trimester: Post-marketing reports indicate that some neonates exposed to SSRIs such as citalopram and other newer antidepressants late in the third trimester have developed complications requiring prolonged hospitalization, respiratory support, and tube feeding (see Precautions). When treating pregnant women with citalopram during the third trimester, the physician should carefully consider the potential risks and benefits of treatment. The physician may consider tapering citalopram in the third trimester.

Geriatrics: A single oral dose of 20 mg/day is the recommended dose for most elderly patients. Some patients may respond to a 10 mg/day dose (see Pharmacology, Clinical Trials). The dose may be titrated to a maximum of 40 mg/day if needed and tolerated. As with other SSRIs, caution should be exercised in treating elderly female patients who may be more susceptible to adverse events such as hyponatremia and SIADH (syndrome of inappropriate antidiuretic hormone secretion) (see Precautions).

Hepatic Impairment: Patients with reduced hepatic function should receive dosages of no more than 30 mg/day.

Renal Impairment: No dosage adjustment is necessary for patients with mild to moderate renal impairment. Since there is no information available on the pharmacokinetic or pharmacodynamic effects of citalopram in patients with severe renal impairment, citalopram should be used with caution in these patients.

Maintenance Treatment: Evaluation of citalopram in 2 placebo- controlled studies has shown that its antidepressant efficacy was maintained for periods of up to 24 weeks, following 6 or 8 weeks of initial treatment (total of 32 weeks) (see Pharmacology, Clinical Trials). In the flexible dose study, the great majority of patients were receiving 20 or 40 mg/day doses both at 12 and 24 weeks. During maintenance therapy, the dosage should be kept at the lowest effective level and patients should be periodically reassessed to determine the need for continued treatment.

Switching Patients To or From a Monoamine Oxidase Inhibitor (MAOI): At least 14 days should elapse between discontinuation of a MAOI and initiation of therapy with citalopram. Similarly, at least 14 days should be allowed after stopping citalopram before starting a MAOI (see Contraindications).

Discontinuation of Citalopram Treatment: Symptoms associated with the discontinuation or dosage reduction of citalopram have been reported. Patients should be monitored for these and other symptoms when discontinuing treatment or during dosage reduction (see Precautions and Adverse Effects).

A gradual reduction in the dose over several weeks rather than abrupt cessation is recommended whenever possible. If intolerable symptoms occur following a decrease in the dose or upon discontinuation of treatment, dose titration should be managed on the basis of the patient's clinical response (see Precautions and Adverse Effects).

Children: See Warnings, Potential Association with Behavioral and Emotional Changes, Including Self-Harm.

INFORMATION FOR THE PATIENT: Published in e-CPS, available by subscription at www.e-cps.ca.

SUPPLIED: 20 mg: Each film-coated, white, oval, scored tablet, marked "C" and "N" symmetrically around the score, contains: citalopram 20 mg (as citalopram HBr). Nonmedicinal ingredients: copolyvidone, cornstarch, croscarmellose sodium, glycerin, lactose monohydrate, magnesium stearate, methylhydroxypropyl cellulose, microcrystalline cellulose, polyethylene glycol 400 and titanium dioxide. Blister packages of 30. Bottles of 100 and 250.

40 mg: Each film-coated, white, oval, scored tablet, marked "C" and "R" symmetrically around the score, contains: citalopram 40 mg (as citalopram HBr). Nonmedicinal ingredients: copolyvidone, cornstarch, croscarmellose sodium, glycerin, lactose monohydrate, magnesium stearate, methylhydroxypropyl cellulose, microcrystalline cellulose, polyethylene glycol 400 and titanium dioxide. Blister packages of 30.

Store in a dry place at room temperature between 15 and 30°C.

(Shown in Product Identification Section)

CellCept® Ⓟ

mycophenolate mofetil
Immunosuppressant

Roche

CellCept® i.v. Ⓟ

mycophenolate mofetil HCl
Immunosuppressant

Roche

Date of Preparation: November 2, 1995
Date of Revision: February 23, 2010

SUMMARY PRODUCT INFORMATION:

Route of Administration	Dosage Form/ Strength	Clinically Relevant Nonmedicinal Ingredients
Oral	Capsules/250 mg	None
	Tablets/500 mg	None
	Powder/200 mg/mL (reconstituted)	Aspartame (see Warnings and Precautions, Endocrine and Metabolism, Phenylketonurics.)
Intravenous	Lyophilized powder/500 mg/vial (as hydrochloride)	Polysorbate 80 (TWEEN) (see Contraindications.)
For a complete listing of nonmedicinal ingredients see Dosage Forms, Composition and Packaging.		

INDICATIONS AND CLINICAL USE: CellCept (mycophenolate mofetil) is indicated for:

Adults:

- The prophylaxis of organ rejection in patients receiving allogeneic renal, cardiac or hepatic transplants. CellCept should be used concomitantly with cyclosporine and corticosteroids.
- CellCept i.v. (mycophenolate mofetil hydrochloride for intravenous infusion) is an alternative dosage form to CellCept capsules, tablets and oral suspension. CellCept i.v. should be administered within 24 hours following transplantation. CellCept i.v. can be administered for up to 14 days; patients should be switched to oral CellCept as soon as they can tolerate oral medication.

Pediatrics (2-18 years of age):

- CellCept is indicated for the prophylaxis of organ rejection in pediatric patients (2 to 18 years) receiving allogeneic renal transplants. CellCept should be used concomitantly with cyclosporine and corticosteroids.

CONTRAINDICATIONS:

- CellCept (mycophenolate mofetil) is contraindicated in patients with a hypersensitivity to mycophenolate mofetil, mycophenolic acid or any component of the drug product (see Dosage Forms, Composition and Packaging).
- CellCept i.v. (mycophenolate mofetil hydrochloride for injection) is contraindicated in patients who are allergic to Polysorbate 80 (TWEEN) (see Dosage Forms, Composition and Packaging).

WARNINGS AND PRECAUTIONS:

> **Serious Warnings and Precautions**
> **Increased susceptibility to infection and the possible development of lymphoma may result from immunosuppression. Only physicians experienced in immunosuppressive therapy and management of solid organ transplant patients should use CellCept (mycophenolate mofetil). Patients receiving the drug should be managed in facilities equipped and staffed with adequate laboratory and supportive medical resources. The physician responsible for maintenance therapy should have complete information requisite for the follow-up of the patient.**

Carcinogenesis and Mutagenesis: Patients receiving immunosuppressive regimes involving combinations of drugs, including CellCept, as part of an immunosuppressive regimen are at increased risk of developing lymphomas and other malignancies, particularly of the skin. The risk appears to be related to the intensity and duration of immunosuppression rather than to the use of any specific agent. As with all patients at an increased risk for skin cancer, exposure to sunlight and UV light should be limited by wearing protective clothing and using a sunscreen with a high protection factor.

Lymphoproliferative disease or lymphoma developed in 0.4%-1% of patients receiving CellCept (2 g or 3 g) with other immunosuppressive agents in controlled clinical trials of renal, cardiac and hepatic transplant patients (see Adverse Reactions).

Endocrine and Metabolism: Because CellCept is an inosine monophosphate dehydrogenase (IMPDH) inhibitor, on theoretical grounds it should be avoided in patients with rare hereditary deficiency of hypoxanthine-guanine phosphoribosyl-transferase (HGPRT) such as Lesch-Nyhan and Kelley-Seegmiller syndrome.

Phenylketonurics: CellCept Oral Suspension contains aspartame, a source of phenylalanine (0.56 mg phenylalanine per mL suspension).

Gastrointestinal: CellCept should be administered with caution in patients with active serious digestive system disease. Gastrointestinal bleeding (requiring hospitalization) has been observed in approximately 3% of renal, in 1.7% of cardiac and in 5.4% of hepatic transplant patients treated with CellCept 3 g daily. CellCept has been associated with an increased incidence of digestive system adverse events, including infrequent cases of gastrointestinal tract ulceration, and rarely perforation (colon, gall bladder). Most patients receiving CellCept were also receiving other drugs that are known to be associated with these complications. Patients with active peptic ulcer disease were excluded from enrollment in studies with mycophenolate mofetil.

Immune: Oversuppression of the immune system can also increase susceptibility to infection, including opportunistic infections, fatal infections and sepsis. CellCept has been administered in combination with the following agents in clinical trials: anti-thymocyte globulin [equine] (Atgam) induction, muromonab-CD3 (Orthoclone OKT3), cyclosporine (Sandimmune, Neoral), and corticosteroids. The efficacy and safety of the use of CellCept in combination with other immunosuppressive agents has not been determined.

Such infections include latent viral reactivation, such as by polyomaviruses. Cases of progressive multifocal leukoencephalopathy (PML) associated with the JC virus, sometimes fatal, have been reported in CellCept treated patients. The reported cases had risk factors for PML, including immunosuppressant therapies and impairment of immune function. In immunosuppressed patients, physicians should consider PML in the differential diagnosis in patients reporting neurological symptoms and consultation with a neurologist should be considered as clinically indicated.

BK virus-associated nephropathy has been observed during the use of CellCept in patients post renal transplant. This infection can be associated with serious outcomes, sometimes leading to renal graft loss. Patient monitoring may help detect patients at risk for BK virus-associated nephropathy. Reduction in immunosuppression should be considered for patients who develop evidence of BK virus-associated nephropathy.

Cases of pure red cell aplasia (PRCA) have been reported in patients treated with CellCept in combination with other immunosuppressive agents. The mechanism for mycophenolate mofetil induced PRCA is unknown. In some cases PRCA was found to be reversible with dose reduction or cessation of CellCept therapy. In transplant patients however reduced immunosuppression may place the graft at risk.

In patients receiving CellCept (2 g or 3 g) in controlled studies for prevention of renal, cardiac or hepatic rejection, fatal infection/sepsis occurred in approximately 2% of renal and cardiac patients and in 5% of hepatic patients (see Adverse Reactions).

Severe neutropenia (absolute neutrophil count [ANC] $<0.5\times10^3/\mu L$) developed in up to 2.0% of renal, up to 2.8% of cardiac and up to 3.6% hepatic transplant patients receiving CellCept 3 g daily (see Adverse Reactions).

Patients receiving CellCept should be monitored for neutropenia (see Warnings and Precautions, Monitoring and Laboratory Tests and Dosage and Administration, Dosage Adjustment). The development of neutropenia may be related to CellCept itself, concomitant medications, viral infections, or some combination of these causes. If neutropenia develops (ANC $<1.3\times10^3/\mu L$), dosing with CellCept should be interrupted or the dose reduced, appropriate diagnostic tests performed, and the patient managed appropriately. Neutropenia has been observed most frequently in the period from 31 to 180 days post-transplant for patients treated for prevention of renal, cardiac and hepatic rejection.

Patients receiving CellCept should be instructed to report immediately any evidence of infection, unexpected bruising, bleeding or any other manifestation of bone marrow depression.

Renal: Administration of doses of CellCept greater than 1 g administered twice a day to renal transplant patients with severe chronic renal impairment (GFR <25 mL/min/1.73 m^2) should be avoided and patients should be carefully observed (see Action and Clinical Pharmacology, Pharmacokinetics, Special Populations and Conditions, Renal Insufficiency and Dosage and Administration, Dosage Adjustment, Renal Impairment).

No data are available for cardiac or hepatic transplant patients with severe chronic, renal impairment. CellCept should be used for cardiac or hepatic transplant patients with severe, chronic, renal impairment if the potential benefits outweigh the potential risks.

Special Populations: Pregnant Women: There are no adequate and well-controlled studies in pregnant women. However, an increased risk of first trimester pregnancy loss and congenital malformations of heart, ear, face, hand, eye, vertebrae, oesophagus, and multiple congenital abnormalities have been reported in offspring of patients exposed to mycophenolate mofetil in combination with other immunosuppressants during pregnancy. CellCept has been shown to have teratogenic effects in animals, it may cause fetal harm when administered to a pregnant woman. Therefore, CellCept should not be used in pregnant women unless the potential benefit justifies the potential risk to the fetus.

Women of childbearing potential should be instructed of the potential risks during pregnancy. Effective contraception must be used before beginning CellCept therapy, during therapy, and for 6 weeks following discontinuation of therapy, even where there has been a history of infertility, unless due to hysterectomy. Two reliable forms of contraception must be used simultaneously unless abstinence is the chosen method (see Drug Interactions). If pregnancy does occur during treatment, the physician and patient should discuss the desirability of continuing the pregnancy (see Information for the Patient).

Women of childbearing potential should have a negative serum or urine pregnancy test with a sensitivity of at least 50 mIU/mL within 1 week prior to beginning therapy. It is recommended that CellCept therapy should not be initiated by the physician until a report of a negative pregnancy test has been obtained.

Nursing Women: Studies in rats have shown mycophenolate mofetil is excreted in milk. It is not known whether this drug is excreted in human milk. Because many drugs are excreted in human milk and because of the potential for serious adverse reactions in nursing infants from mycophenolate mofetil, a decision should be made whether to discontinue nursing or to discontinue the drug, taking into account the importance of the drug to the mother (see Information for the Patient).

Pediatrics (2 years to 18 years): Safety and efficacy in children receiving allogeneic cardiac or hepatic transplants have not been established.

For pediatric patients receiving renal transplants also see Action and Clinical Pharmacology, Pharmacokinetics, Special Populations and Conditions, Pediatrics, Adverse Reactions, Pediatrics and Dosage and Administration, Pediatrics (2 to 18 years).

Geriatrics: Elderly patients may be at an increased risk of adverse events compared with younger individuals.

Monitoring and Laboratory Tests: Complete blood counts should be performed weekly during the first month, twice monthly for the second and third months of treatment, then monthly through the first year (see Warnings and Precautions, Immune and Dosage and Administration).

Information to Be Provided to the Patient: Patients should be informed of the need for repeated appropriate laboratory tests while they are receiving CellCept (see Warnings and Precautions, Immune). Patients should be given complete dosage instructions and informed of the increased risk of lymphoproliferative disease and certain other malignancies.

ADVERSE REACTIONS: Clinical Trial Adverse Drug Reactions: Because clinical trials are conducted under very specific conditions the adverse reaction rates observed in the clinical trials may not reflect the rates observed in practice and should not be compared to the rates in the clinical trials of another drug. Adverse drug reaction information from clinical trials is useful for identifying drug-related adverse events and for approximating rates.

Adverse Drug Reaction Overview: The adverse event profile associated with the use of immunosuppressive drugs is often difficult to establish owing to the presence of underlying disease and the concurrent use of many other medications. The principal adverse reactions associated with the administration of CellCept (mycophenolate mofetil) include diarrhea, leukopenia, sepsis and vomiting, and there is evidence of a higher frequency of certain types of infections.

The adverse event profile associated with the administration of CellCept i.v. (mycophenolate mofetil hydrochloride for injection) has been shown to be similar to that observed after administration of oral dosage forms of CellCept.

CellCept (oral): The incidence of adverse events for CellCept was determined in randomized comparative double-blind trials in prevention of rejection in renal (2 active, 1 placebo controlled trials), cardiac (1 active controlled trial) and hepatic (1 active controlled trial) transplant patients.

Safety data are summarized in Table 1 for all active controlled trials in renal (2 trials), cardiac (1 trial) and hepatic (1 trial) transplant patients. Approximately 53% of renal patients, 65% of the cardiac patients and 45% of the hepatic patients have been treated for more than one year.

Adverse events, whether or not deemed to be causally associated with the study medication, reported in ≥10% of patients in treatment groups are presented in Table 1.

Table 1: CellCept

Adverse Events in Controlled Studies in Prevention of Renal, Cardiac or Hepatic Allograft Rejection (Reported in ≥10% of Adult Patients Randomized to CellCept)

	Renal Studies			Cardiac Study		Hepatic Study	
	CellCept 2 g/day (n=336) %	CellCept 3 g/day (n=330) %	Azathioprine 1–2 mg/kg/day or 100–150 mg/day (n=326) %	CellCept 3 g/day (n=289) %	Azathioprine 1.5–3 mg/kg/day (n=289) %	CellCept 3 g/day (n=277) %	Azathioprine 1–2 mg/kg/day (n=287) %
Body as a Whole							
Pain	33.0	31.2	32.2	75.8	74.7	74.0	77.7
Abdominal pain	24.7	27.6	23.0	33.9	33.2	62.5	51.2
Fever	21.4	23.3	23.3	47.4	46.4	52.3	56.1
Headache	21.1	16.1	21.2	54.3	51.9	53.8	49.1
Infection	18.2	20.9	19.9	25.6	19.4	27.1	25.1
Sepsis	17.6	19.7	15.6	18.7	18.7	27.4	26.5
Asthenia	13.7	16.1	19.9	43.3	36.3	35.4	33.8
Chest pain	13.4	13.3	14.7	26.3	26.0	15.9	13.2
Back pain	11.6	12.1	14.1	34.6	28.4	46.6	47.4
Accidental injury	—	—	—	19.0	14.9	11.2	15.0
Chills	—	—	—	11.4	11.4	10.8	10.1
Ascites	—	—	—	—	—	24.2	22.6
Abdomen enlarged	—	—	—	—	—	18.8	17.8
Hernia	—	—	—	—	—	11.6	8.7
Peritonitis	—	—	—	—	—	10.1	12.5
Cardiovascular							
Hypertension	32.4	28.2	32.2	77.5	72.3	62.1	59.6

(cont'd)

Table 1: CellCept *(cont'd)*

Adverse Events in Controlled Studies in Prevention of Renal, Cardiac or Hepatic Allograft Rejection (Reported in ≥10% of Adult Patients Randomized to CellCept)

	Renal Studies			Cardiac Study		Hepatic Study	
	CellCept 2 g/day (n=336) %	CellCept 3 g/day (n=330) %	Azathioprine 1–2 mg/kg/day or 100–150 mg/day (n=326) %	CellCept 3 g/day (n=289) %	Azathioprine 1.5–3 mg/kg/day (n=289) %	CellCept 3 g/day (n=277) %	Azathioprine 1–2 mg/kg/day (n=287) %
Hypotension	—	—	—	32.5	36.0	18.4	20.9
Cardiovascular disorder	—	—	—	25.6	24.2	—	—
Tachycardia	—	—	—	20.1	18.0	22.0	15.7
Arrhythmia	—	—	—	19.0	18.7	—	—
Bradycardia	—	—	—	17.3	17.3	—	—
Pericardial effusion	—	—	—	15.9	13.5	—	—
Heart failure	—	—	—	11.8	8.7	—	—
Digestive							
Diarrhea	31.0	36.1	20.9	45.3	34.3	51.3	49.8
Constipation	22.9	18.5	22.4	41.2	37.7	37.9	38.3
Nausea	19.9	23.6	24.5	54.0	54.3	54.5	51.2
Dyspepsia	17.6	13.6	13.8	18.7	19.4	22.4	20.9
Vomiting	12.5	13.6	9.2	33.9	28.4	32.9	33.4
Nausea and vomiting	10.4	9.7	10.7	11.1	7.6	—	—
Oral moniliasis	10.1	12.1	11.3	11.4	11.8	10.1	10.1
Flatulence	—	—	—	13.8	15.6	12.6	9.8
Anorexia	—	—	—	—	—	25.3	17.1
Liver function tests abnormal	—	—	—	—	—	24.9	19.2
Cholangitis	—	—	—	—	—	14.1	13.6
Hepatitis	—	—	—	—	—	13.0	16.0
Cholestatic jaundice	—	—	—	—	—	11.9	10.8
Hemic and Lymphatic							
Anemia	25.6	25.8	23.6	42.9	43.9	43.0	53.0
Leukopenia	23.2	34.5	24.8	30.4	39.1	45.8	39.0
Thrombocytopenia	10.1	8.2	13.2	23.5	27.0	38.3	42.2
Hypochromic anemia	7.4	11.5	9.2	24.6	23.5	13.7	10.8
Leukocytosis	7.1	10.9	7.4	40.5	35.6	22.4	21.3
Ecchymosis	—	—	—	16.6	8.0	—	—
Metabolic and Nutritional							
Peripheral edema	28.6	27.0	28.2	64.0	53.3	48.4	47.7
Hypercholesteremia	12.8	8.5	11.3	41.2	38.4	—	—
Hypophosphatemia	12.5	15.8	11.7	—	—	14.4	9.1
Edema	12.2	11.8	13.5	26.6	25.6	28.2	28.2
Hypokalemia	10.1	10.0	8.3	31.8	25.6	37.2	41.1
Hyperkalemia	8.9	10.3	16.9	14.5	19.7	22.0	23.7
Hyperglycemia	8.6	12.4	15.0	46.7	52.6	43.7	48.8
Creatinine increased	—	—	—	39.4	36.0	19.9	21.6
BUN increased	—	—	—	34.6	32.5	10.1	12.9
Lactic dehydrogenase increased	—	—	—	23.2	17.0	—	—
Bilirubinemia	—	—	—	18.0	21.8	14.4	18.8
Hypervolemia	—	—	—	16.6	22.8	—	—
Generalized edema	—	—	—	18.0	20.1	14.8	16.0
Hyperuricemia	—	—	—	16.3	17.6	—	—
AST increased	—	—	—	17.3	15.6	—	—
Hypomagnesemia	—	—	—	18.3	12.8	39.0	37.6

(cont'd)

Table 1: CellCept *(cont'd)*

Adverse Events in Controlled Studies in Prevention of Renal, Cardiac or Hepatic Allograft Rejection (Reported in ≥10% of Adult Patients Randomized to CellCept)

	Renal Studies			Cardiac Study		Hepatic Study	
	CellCept 2 g/day (n=336) %	**CellCept 3 g/day (n=330) %**	**Azathioprine 1–2 mg/kg/day or 100–150 mg/day (n=326) %**	**CellCept 3 g/day (n=289) %**	**Azathioprine 1.5–3 mg/kg/day (n=289) %**	**CellCept 3 g/day (n=277) %**	**Azathioprine 1–2 mg/kg/day (n=287) %**
Acidosis	—	—	—	14.2	16.6	—	—
Weight gain	—	—	—	15.6	15.2	—	—
ALT increased	—	—	—	15.6	12.5	—	—
Hyponatremia	—	—	—	11.4	11.8	—	—
Hyperlipemia	—	—	—	10.7	9.3	—	—
Hypocalcemia	—	—	—	—	—	30.0	30.0
Hypoproteinemia	—	—	—	—	—	13.4	13.9
Hypoglycemia	—	—	—	—	—	10.5	9.1
Healing abnormal	—	—	—	—	—	10.5	8.7
Musculoskeletal System							
Leg cramps	—	—	—	16.6	15.6	—	—
Myasthenia	—	—	—	12.5	9.7	—	—
Myalgia	—	—	—	12.5	9.3	—	—
Nervous System							
Tremor	11.0	11.8	12.3	24.2	23.9	33.9	35.5
Insomnia	8.9	11.8	10.4	40.8	37.7	52.3	47.0
Dizziness	5.7	11.2	11.0	28.7	27.7	16.2	14.3
Anxiety	—	—	—	28.4	23.9	19.5	17.8
Paresthesia	—	—	—	20.8	18.0	15.2	15.3
Hypertonia	—	—	—	15.6	14.5	—	—
Depression	—	—	—	15.6	12.5	17.3	16.7
Agitation	—	—	—	13.1	12.8	—	—
Somnolence	—	—	—	11.1	10.4	—	—
Confusion	—	—	—	13.5	7.6	17.3	18.8
Nervousness	—	—	—	11.4	9.0	10.1	10.5
Respiratory							
Infection	22.0	23.9	19.6	37.0	35.3	15.9	19.9
Dyspnea	15.5	17.3	16.6	36.7	36.3	31.0	30.3
Cough increased	15.5	13.3	15.0	31.1	25.6	15.9	12.5
Pharyngitis	9.5	11.2	8.0	18.3	13.5	14.1	12.5
Lung disorder	—	—	—	30.1	29.1	22.0	18.8
Sinusitis	—	—	—	26.0	19.0	11.2	9.8
Rhinitis	—	—	—	19.0	15.6	—	—
Pleural effusion	—	—	—	17.0	13.8	34.3	35.9
Asthma	—	—	—	11.1	11.4		—
Pneumonia	—	—	—	10.7	10.4	13.7	11.5
Atelectasis	—	—	—	—	—	13.0	12.9
Skin and Appendages							
Acne	10.1	9.7	6.4	12.1	9.3	—	—
Rash	—	—	—	22.1	18.0	17.7	18.5
Skin disorder	—	—	—	12.5	8.7	—	—
Pruritus	—	—	—	—	—	14.1	10.5
Sweating	—	—	—	—	—	10.8	10.1
Special Senses							
Amblyopia	—	—	—	14.9	6.6	—	—

(cont'd)

Table 1: CellCept *(cont'd)*

Adverse Events in Controlled Studies in Prevention of Renal, Cardiac or Hepatic Allograft Rejection (Reported in ≥10% of Adult Patients Randomized to CellCept)

	Renal Studies			Cardiac Study		Hepatic Study	
	CellCept 2 g/day (n=336) %	CellCept 3 g/day (n=330) %	Azathioprine 1–2 mg/kg/day or 100–150 mg/day (n=326) %	CellCept 3 g/day (n=289) %	Azathioprine 1.5–3 mg/kg/day (n=289) %	CellCept 3 g/day (n=277) %	Azathioprine 1–2 mg/kg/day (n=287) %
Urogenital							
Urinary tract infection	37.2	37.0	33.7	13.1	11.8	18.1	17.8
Hematuria	14.0	12.1	11.3	—	—	—	—
Kidney tubular necrosis	6.3	10.0	5.8	—	—	—	—
Kidney function abnormal	—	—	—	21.8	26.3	25.6	28.9
Oliguria	—	—	—	14.2	12.8	17.0	20.6

The placebo-controlled renal transplant study generally showed fewer adverse events occurring in ≥10% of patients. In addition, those that occurred were not only qualitatively similar to the azathioprine-controlled renal transplant studies, but also occurred at lower rates, particularly for infection, leukopenia, hypertension, diarrhea and respiratory infection. However, the following adverse events were reported in the placebo-controlled renal transplant study but not reported in the azathioprine-controlled renal transplant studies with an incidence of ≥10%: urinary tract disorder, bronchitis and pneumonia.

The above data demonstrate that in three pivotal trials for prevention of renal rejection, patients receiving 2 g per day of CellCept had an overall better safety profile than did patients receiving 3 g per day of CellCept.

The above data demonstrate that the types of adverse events observed in multicentre controlled trials in renal, cardiac and hepatic transplant patients are qualitatively similar except for those that are unique to the specific organ involved.

Sepsis, which was generally CMV viremia, was slightly more common in renal transplant patients treated with CellCept compared to patients treated with azathioprine. The incidence of sepsis was comparable in patients treated with CellCept or azathioprine in cardiac and hepatic studies.

In the digestive system, diarrhea was increased in renal and cardiac transplant patients receiving CellCept compared to patients receiving azathioprine, but was comparable in hepatic transplant patients treated with CellCept or azathioprine.

The incidence of malignancies among the 1483 patients treated in controlled trials for the prevention of renal allograft rejection who were followed for ≥1 year was similar to the incidence reported in the literature for renal allograft recipients.

Lymphoproliferative disease or lymphoma developed in 0.4%-1% of patients receiving CellCept (2 g or 3 g daily) with other immunosuppressive agents in controlled clinical trials of renal, cardiac and hepatic transplant patients followed for at least 1 year (see Warnings and Precautions, Carcinogenesis and Mutagenesis). Non-melanoma skin carcinomas occurred in 1.6%-4.2% of patients, other types of malignancy in 0.7%-2.1% of patients. Three-year safety data in renal and cardiac transplant patients did not reveal any unexpected changes in incidence of malignancy compared to the 1-year data.

Severe neutropenia (ANC <0.5×10³/µL) developed in up to 2.0% of renal transplant patients, up to 2.8% of cardiac transplant patients and up to 3.6% of hepatic transplant patients receiving CellCept 3 g daily (see Warnings and Precautions, Immune and Monitoring and Laboratory Tests and Dosage Administration, Dosage Adjustment).

Table 2 shows the incidence of opportunistic infections that occurred in the renal, cardiac and hepatic transplant populations in the azathioprine-controlled prevention trials.

The following other opportunistic infections occurred with an incidence of less than 4% in patients treated with CellCept in the above azathioprine-controlled studies: Herpes zoster, visceral disease; Candida, urinary tract infection, fungemia/disseminated disease, tissue invasive disease; Cryptococcosis; Aspergillus/Mucor; *P. carinii*.

In the placebo-controlled renal transplant study, the same pattern of opportunistic infection was observed compared to the azathioprine-controlled renal studies, with a notably lower incidence of the following: Herpes simplex and CMV tissue-invasive disease.

In patients receiving CellCept (2 g or 3 g) in controlled studies for prevention of renal, cardiac or hepatic rejection, fatal infection/sepsis occurred in approximately 2% of renal and cardiac patients and in 5% of hepatic patients (see Warnings and Precautions, Immune).

In cardiac transplant patients, the overall incidence of opportunistic infections was approximately 10% higher in patients treated with CellCept than in those receiving azathioprine, but this difference was not associated with excess mortality due to infection/sepsis among patients treated with CellCept.

The following adverse events were reported with ≥3%-<10% incidence in renal, cardiac and hepatic transplant patients treated with CellCept, in combination with cyclosporine and corticosteroids (see Table 3).

Table 2: CellCept

Viral and Fungal Infections in Controlled Studies in Prevention of Renal, Cardiac or Hepatic Transplant Rejection

	Renal Studies			Cardiac Study		Hepatic Study	
	CellCept 2 g/day %	CellCept 3 g/day %	Azathioprine 1–2 mg/kg/day or 100–150 mg/day %	CellCept 3 g/day %	Azathioprine 1.5–3 mg/kg/day %	CellCept 3 g/day %	Azathioprine 1–2 mg/kg/day %
Herpes simplex	16.7	20.0	19.0	20.8	14.5	10.1	5.9
CMV							
–Viremia/syndrome	13.4	12.4	13.8	12.1	10.0	14.1	12.2
–Tissue invasive disease	8.3	11.5	6.1	11.4	8.7	5.8	8.0
Herpes zoster	6.0	7.6	5.8	10.7	5.9	4.3	4.9
–Cutaneous disease	6.0	7.3	5.5	10.0	5.5	4.3	4.9
Candida	17.0	17.3	18.1	18.7	17.6	22.4	24.4
–Muco-cutaneous	15.5	16.4	15.3	18.0	17.3	18.4	17.4

Table 3: CellCept

Adverse Events Reported in ≥3%-<10% of Adult Patients Treated with CellCept in Combination with Cyclosporine and Corticosteroids

Body System	Renal	Cardiac	Hepatic
Body as a Whole	abdomen enlarged, accidental injury, chills occurring with fever, cyst, face edema, flu syndrome, hemorrhage, hernia, malaise, pelvic pain	abdomen enlarged, cellulitis, chills occurring with fever, cyst, face edema, flu syndrome, hemorrhage, hernia, malaise, neck pain, pelvic pain	abscess, cellulitis, chills occurring with fever, cyst, flu syndrome, hemorrhage, lab test abnormal, malaise, neck pain
Cardiovascular	angina pectoris, atrial fibrillation, cardiovascular disorder, hypotension, palpitation, peripheral vascular disorder, postural hypotension, tachycardia, thrombosis, vasodilatation	angina pectoris, atrial fibrillation, atrial flutter, congestive heart failure, extrasystole, heart arrest, palpitation, pallor, peripheral vascular disorder, postural hypotension, pulmonary hypertension, supraventricular tachycardia, supraventricular extrasystoles, syncope, vasospasm, ventricular extrasystole, ventricular tachycardia, venous pressure increased	arrhythmia, arterial thrombosis, atrial fibrillation, bradycardia, palpitation, syncope, vasodilatation
Digestive	anorexia, esophagitis, flatulence, gastritis, gastroenteritis, gastrointestinal hemorrhage, gastrointestinal moniliasis, gingivitis, gum hyperplasia, hepatitis, ileus, infection, liver function tests abnormal, mouth ulceration, rectal disorder	anorexia, dysphagia, esophagitis, gastritis, gastroenteritis, gastrointestinal disorder, gingivitis, gum hyperplasia, infection, jaundice, liver damage, liver function tests abnormal, melena, rectal disorder, stomatitis	dysphagia, esophagitis, gastritis, gastrointestinal disorder, gastrointestinal hemorrhage, ileus, infection, jaundice, melena, mouth ulceration, nausea and vomiting, rectal disorder, stomach ulcer
Endocrine	diabetes mellitus, parathyroid disorder	Cushing's syndrome, diabetes mellitus, hypothyroidism	diabetes mellitus
Hemic and Lymphatic	ecchymosis, polycythemia	petechia, prothrombin time increased, thromboplastin time increased	coagulation disorder, ecchymosis, pancytopenia, prothrombin time increased

(cont'd)

Table 3: CellCept *(cont'd)*

Adverse Events Reported in ≥3%-<10% of Adult Patients Treated with CellCept in Combination with Cyclosporine and Corticosteroids

Body System	Renal	Cardiac	Hepatic
Metabolic and Nutritional	acidosis, alkaline phosphatase increased, creatinine increased, dehydration, gamma glutamyl transpeptidase increased, hypercalcemia, hyperlipemia, hyperuricemia, hypervolemia, hypocalcemia, hypoglycemia, hypoproteinemia, lactic dehydrogenase increased, AST increased, ALT increased, weight gain	abnormal healing, alkaline phosphatase increased, alkalosis, dehydration, gout, hypocalcemia, hypochloremia, hypoglycemia, hypoproteinemia, hypophosphatemia, hypovolemia, hypoxia, respiratory acidosis, thirst, weight loss	acidosis, alkaline phosphatase increased, dehydration, hypercholesteremia, hyperlipemia, hyperphosphatemia, hypervolemia, hyponatremia, hypoxia, hypovolemia, AST increased, ALT increased, weight gain, weight loss
Musculoskeletal	arthralgia, joint disorder, leg cramps, myalgia, myasthenia	arthralgia, joint disorder	arthralgia, leg cramps, myalgia, myasthenia, osteoporosis
Nervous	anxiety, depression, hypertonia, paresthesia, somnolence	convulsion, emotional lability, hallucinations, neuropathy, thinking abnormal, vertigo	agitation, convulsion, delirium, dry mouth, hypertonia, hypesthesia, neuropathy, psychosis, thinking abnormal, somnolence
Respiratory	asthma, bronchitis, lung edema, lung disorder, pleural effusion, pneumonia, rhinitis, sinusitis	apnea, atelectasis, bronchitis, epistaxis, hemoptysis, hiccup, lung edema, neoplasm, pain, pneumothorax, respiratory disorder, sputum increased, voice alteration	asthma, bronchitis, epistaxis, hyperventilation, lung edema, pneumothorax, respiratory disorder, respiratory moniliasis, rhinitis
Skin and Appendages	alopecia, fungal dermatitis, hirsutism, pruritus, rash, skin benign neoplasm, skin carcinoma, skin disorder, skin hypertrophy, skin ulcer, sweating	fungal dermatitis, hemorrhage, pruritus, skin benign neoplasm, skin carcinoma, skin hypertrophy, skin ulcer, sweating	acne, fungal dermatitis, hemorrhage, hirsutism, skin benign neoplasm, skin disorder, skin ulcer, vesiculobullous rash
Special Senses	amblyopia, cataract (not specified), conjunctivitis	abnormal vision, conjunctivitis, deafness, ear disorder, ear pain, eye hemorrhage, tinnitus, lacrimation disorder	abnormal vision, amblyopia, conjunctivitis, deafness
Urogenital	albuminuria, dysuria, hydronephrosis, impotence, pain, pyelonephritis, urinary frequency, urinary tract disorder	dysuria, hematuria, impotence, kidney failure, nocturia, prostatic disorder, urine abnormality, urinary frequency, urinary incontinence, urinary retention	acute kidney failure, dysuria, hematuria, kidney failure, scrotal edema, urinary frequency, urinary incontinence

Pediatrics: The type and frequency of adverse events in a clinical study in 100 pediatric patients 3 months to 18 years of age dosed with CellCept oral suspension 600 mg/m² twice daily (up to 1 g twice daily) were generally similar to those observed in adult patients dosed with CellCept capsules at a dose of 1 g twice daily. However, the following treatment-related adverse events occurred with a frequency of ≥10% in children and were more frequent in the pediatric population, particularly in children under 6 years of age, when the frequency of treatment-related adverse events were compared to adults: diarrhea, anemia, leucopenia, sepsis and infection.

CellCept i.v.: The adverse event profile of CellCept i.v. was determined from a single, double-blind, controlled comparative study of the safety of 2 g/day of intravenous and oral CellCept in renal transplant patients in the immediate post-transplant period (administered for the first 5 days). The potential venous irritation of CellCept i.v. was evaluated by comparing the adverse events attributable to peripheral venous infusion of CellCept i.v. with those observed in the IV placebo group; patients in this group received active medication by the oral route.

Adverse events attributable to peripheral venous infusion were phlebitis and thrombosis, both observed at 4% in patients treated with CellCept i.v.

In the active controlled study in hepatic transplant patients, 2 g/day of CellCept i.v. was administered in the immediate post-transplant period (up to 14 days). The safety profile of intravenous CellCept was similar to that of intravenous azathioprine.

Post-Market Adverse Drug Reactions: The following adverse events, not mentioned above, were reported in clinical trials and in postmarketing experience in patients treated with CellCept:

Congenital Disorders: An increased risk of first trimester pregnancy loss and congenital malformations of heart, ear, face, hand, eye, vertebrae, oesophagus, and multiple congenital abnormalities have been reported in offspring of patients exposed to mycophenolate mofetil in combination with other immunosuppressants during pregnancy.

Digestive: colitis (sometimes caused by cytomegalovirus), pancreatitis, isolated cases of intestinal villous atrophy.

Hemic and Lymphatic: Cases of pure red cell aplasia (PRCA) have been reported in patients treated with CellCept in combination with other immunosuppressive agents.

Resistance Mechanism Disorders: Serious life-threatening infections such as meningitis and infectious endocarditis have been reported occasionally and there is evidence of a higher frequency of certain types of infection such as tuberculosis and atypical mycobacterial infection.

Cases of progressive multifocal leukoencephalopathy (PML), sometimes fatal, have been reported in CellCept treated patients. The reported cases had risk factors for PML, including immunosuppressant therapies and impairment of immune function.

BK virus-associated nephropathy has been observed in patients treated with CellCept. This infection can be associated with serious outcomes, sometimes leading to renal graft loss.

DRUG INTERACTIONS: Drug-Drug Interactions: It is recommended that CellCept (mycophenolate mofetil) should not be administered concomitantly with azathioprine because both have the potential to cause bone marrow suppression and such concomitant administration has not been studied clinically.

In view of the significant reduction in the AUC of mycophenolic acid (MPA) by cholestyramine, caution should be used in the concomitant administration of CellCept with drugs that interfere with enterohepatic recirculation because of the potential to reduce the efficacy of CellCept.

Patients should be advised that during treatment with CellCept vaccinations may be less effective and the use of live attenuated vaccines should be avoided. Prescribers should refer to the Canadian Immunization Guideline for further guidance.

Drug interaction studies with mycophenolate mofetil have been conducted with acyclovir, antacids, cholestyramine, cyclosporine A, ganciclovir, tacrolimus, oral contraceptives, and trimethoprim/sulfamethoxazole. Drug interaction studies have not been conducted with other drugs that may be commonly administered to renal, cardiac or hepatic transplant patients. CellCept has not been administered concomitantly with azathioprine.

Acyclovir: Coadministration of mycophenolate mofetil (1 g) and acyclovir (800 mg) to twelve healthy volunteers resulted in no significant change in MPA AUC and C_{max}. However, the phenolic glucuronide of MPA (MPAG) and acyclovir plasma AUCs were increased 10.6% and 21.9%, respectively. Because MPAG plasma concentrations are increased in the presence of renal impairment, as are acyclovir concentrations, the potential exists for mycophenolate and acyclovir or its prodrug e.g., valacyclovir to compete for tubular secretion, further increasing the concentrations of both drugs.

Antacids with Magnesium and Aluminum Hydroxides: Absorption of a single dose of mycophenolate mofetil (2 g) was decreased when administered to rheumatoid arthritis patients also taking Maalox TC (10 mL four times daily). The C_{max} and AUC values for MPA were 38% and 17% lower, respectively, than when mycophenolate mofetil was administered alone under fasting conditions. CellCept may be administered to patients who are also taking antacids containing magnesium and aluminum hydroxides; however, it is recommended that CellCept and the antacid not be administered simultaneously.

Cholestyramine: Following single dose administration of 1.5 g mycophenolate mofetil to normal healthy subjects pretreated with 4 g three times daily of cholestyramine for 4 days, there was a mean 40% reduction in the AUC of MPA. This decrease is consistent with interruption of enterohepatic recirculation by irreversible binding, in the intestine, of recirculating MPAG with cholestyramine. Some degree of enterohepatic recirculation is also anticipated following IV administration of CellCept. Therefore, CellCept is not recommended to be given with cholestyramine or other agents that may interfere with enterohepatic recirculation.

Cyclosporine: CellCept has been investigated with Sandimmune but not with the Neoral formulation. Cyclosporine (Sandimmune) pharmacokinetics (at doses of 275 mg/day to 415 mg/day) were unaffected by single and multiple doses of 1.5 g twice daily of mycophenolate mofetil in ten stable renal transplant patients. The mean (±SD) AUC_{0-12} and C_{max} of cyclosporine after 14 days of multiple doses of mycophenolate mofetil were 3290 (±822) ng·h/mL and 753 (±161) ng/mL, respectively, compared to 3245 (±1088) ng·h/mL and 700 (±246) ng/mL, respectively, 1 week before administration of mycophenolate mofetil. The effect of cyclosporine on mycophenolate mofetil pharmacokinetics could not be evaluated in this study; however, plasma concentrations of MPA were similar to that for healthy volunteers. In renal transplant patients concomitant administration of CellCept and cyclosporine resulted in reduced MPA exposures by 30-50% compared with patients receiving the combination of sirolimus and similar doses of CellCept.

Ganciclovir: Following single-dose administration to twelve stable renal transplant patients, no pharmacokinetic interaction was observed between mycophenolate mofetil (1.5 g) and IV ganciclovir (5 mg/kg). Mean (±SD) ganciclovir AUC and C_{max} (n=10) were 54.3 (±19.0) µg·h/mL and 11.5 (±1.8) µg/mL, respectively after coadministration of the two drugs, compared to 51.0 (±17.0) µg·h/mL and 10.6 (±2.0) µg/mL, respectively after administration of IV ganciclovir alone. The mean (±SD) AUC and C_{max} of MPA (n=12) after coadministration were 80.9 (±21.6) µg·h/mL and 27.8 (±13.9) µg/mL, respectively compared to values of 80.3 (±16.4) µg·h/mL and 30.9 (±11.2) µg/mL, respectively after administration of mycophenolate mofetil alone. Therefore, no substantial alteration of MPA pharmacokinetics is anticipated and mycophenolate mofetil dose adjustment is not required. However, because MPAG plasma concentrations are increased in the presence of renal impairment, as are ganciclovir concentrations, the potential exists for the two drugs to compete for tubular secretion and thus further increases in concentrations of both drugs may occur. In patients with renal impairment in which mycophenolate mofetil and ganciclovir or its prodrug e.g., valganciclovir are coadministrated, the dose recommendations for ganciclovir, or its prodrug e.g., valganciclovir should be observed and patients monitored carefully.

Rifampicin: After correction for dose a 70% decrease in MPA exposure (AUC_{0-12h}) has been observed with concomitant rifampicin administration in a single heart-lung transplant patient. It is therefore recommended to monitor MPA exposure levels and to adjust CellCept doses accordingly to maintain clinical efficacy when the drugs are administered concomitantly.

Tacrolimus: Exposure to tacrolimus concomitantly administered with CellCept had no effect on the AUC or C_{max} of MPA in hepatic transplant recipients. A similar finding was observed in a recent study in kidney transplant recipients.

In renal transplant patients it was shown that the tacrolimus concentration did not appear to be altered by CellCept.

However, in hepatic transplant patients, there was a 20% increase in tacrolimus AUC when multiple doses of CellCept (1.5 g twice daily) were administered to patients on tacrolimus.

Oral Contraceptives: Following single dose administration to healthy women, no pharmacokinetic interaction was observed between mycophenolate mofetil (1 g) and two tablets of Ortho-Novum 7/7/7 (1 mg norethindrone [NET] and 35 µg ethinyl estradiol [EE]).

Similarly, a study of coadministration of CellCept (1 g twice daily) and combined oral contraceptives containing ethinylestradiol (0.02 mg-0.04 mg) and levonorgestrel (0.05 mg-0.20 mg), desogestrel (0.15 mg) or gestodene (0.05 mg-0.10 mg), showed that the pharmacokinetics of oral contraceptives were unaffected by coadministration of CellCept. This study was conducted in 18 women with psoriasis over 3 menstrual cycles and showed no clinically relevant influence of CellCept on serum levels of progesterone, LH and FSH, thus indicating no influence of CellCept on the ovulation-suppressing action of the oral contraceptives.

Although these studies demonstrate the lack of a gross pharmacokinetic interaction, one cannot exclude the possibility of changes in the pharmacokinetics of the oral contraceptive under long term dosing conditions with CellCept which might adversely affect the efficacy of the oral contraceptive.

Trimethoprim/Sulfamethoxazole, Norfloxacin and Metronidazole: Following single dose administration of mycophenolate mofetil (1.5 g) to twelve healthy male volunteers on day 8 of a 10 day course of Bactrim DS (trimethoprim 160 mg/sulfamethoxazole 800 mg) administered twice daily, no effect on the bioavailability of MPA was observed. The mean (±SD) AUC and C_{max} of MPA after concomitant administration were 75.2 (±19.8) µg·h/mL and 34.0 (±6.6) µg/mL, respectively compared to 79.2 (±27.9) µg·h/mL and 34.2 (±10.7) µg/mL, respectively after administration of mycophenolate mofetil alone.

No effect on the systemic exposure of MPA was observed when CellCept was concomitantly administered with any antibiotic separately. In contrast, the systemic exposure (AUC) of MPA was reduced by 10%, 19%, and 33% when CellCept was concomitantly administered with norfloxacin, metronidazole, and norfloxacin plus metronidazole, respectively, following a single dose of CellCept (statistically significant only for the differences seen in norfloxacin plus metronidazole when compared to baseline (P=.01)).

Ciprofloxacin and Amoxicillin Plus Clavulanic Acid: Reductions in pre-dose (trough) MPA concentrations of 54% have been reported in renal transplant recipients in the days immediately following commencement of oral ciprofloxacin or amoxicillin plus clavulanic acid. Effects tended to diminish with continued antibiotic use and cease after discontinuation. The change in pre-dose level may not accurately represent changes in overall MPA exposure therefore clinical relevance of these observations is unclear.

Live Vaccines: Live vaccines should not be given to patients with an impaired immune response. The antibody response to other vaccines may be diminished (see Warnings and Precautions, Immune).

Other Interactions: The measured value for renal clearance of MPAG indicates removal occurs by renal tubular secretion as well as glomerular filtration. Consistent with this, coadministration of probenecid, a known inhibitor of tubular secretion, with mycophenolate mofetil in monkeys raises plasma AUC of MPAG by 3-fold. Thus, other drugs known to undergo renal tubular secretion may compete with MPAG and thereby raise plasma concentrations of MPAG or the other drug undergoing tubular secretion.

Drugs that alter the gastrointestinal flora may interact with mycophenolate mofetil by disrupting enterohepatic recirculation. Interference of MPAG hydrolysis may lead to less MPA available for absorption.

Concomitant administration of sevelamer and CellCept in adults and pediatric patients decreased the MPA C_{max} and AUC_{0-12} by 30% and 25 %, respectively. This data suggests that sevelamer or other calcium free phosphate binders should not be administered simultaneously with CellCept to minimize the impact on the absorption of MPA.

DOSAGE AND ADMINISTRATION: Dosing Considerations:

- CellCept (mycophenolate mofetil) should be used concomitantly with standard cyclosporine and corticosteroid therapy.

CellCept Capsules, Tablets and Powder for Oral Suspension:

- The initial oral dose of CellCept should be given as soon as possible following renal, cardiac or hepatic transplantation. Food had no effect on MPA AUC, but has been shown to decrease MPA C_{max} by 40%. It is recommended that CellCept be administered on an empty stomach.

Note: If required CellCept Oral Suspension can be administered via a nasogastric tube with a minimum size of 8 French.

CellCept i.v.:

- CellCept i.v. is an alternative dosage form to CellCept capsules and tablets recommended for patients unable to take CellCept capsules or tablets. CellCept i.v. should be administered within 24 hours following transplantation. CellCept i.v. can be administered for up to 14 days; patients should be switched to oral CellCept as soon as they can tolerate oral medication.

Caution: CellCept i.v. solution should never be administered by rapid or bolus intravenous injection.

Recommended Dose: Adults: Renal Transplantation: A dose of 1 g administered orally or intravenously (over 2 hours) twice a day (daily dose of 2 g) is recommended for use in renal transplant patients. Although a dose of 1.5 g administered twice daily (daily dose of 3 g) was used in clinical trials and was shown to be safe and effective, no efficacy advantage could be established for renal transplant patients. Patients receiving 2 g per day of CellCept in these trials demonstrated an overall better safety profile than did patients receiving 3 g per day of CellCept.

Cardiac Transplantation: A dose of 1.5 g twice daily administered intravenously (over **no less than 2 hours**) or 1.5 g twice daily oral (daily dose of 3 g) is recommended for use in adult cardiac transplant patients.

Hepatic Transplantation: A dose of 1 g twice daily administered intravenously (over **no less than 2 hours** or 1.5 g twice daily oral (daily dose of 3 g) is recommended for use in adult hepatic transplant patients.

Pediatrics (2 to 18 years): The recommended dose of CellCept oral suspension for renal transplant patients is 600 mg/m² body surface area twice daily (up to a maximum of 2 g daily).

Patients with a body surface area of 1.25 to 1.5 m² may be dosed with CellCept capsules at a dose of 750 mg twice daily (1.5 g daily dose). Patients with a body surface area >1.5 m² may be dosed with CellCept capsules or tablets at a dose of 1 g twice daily (2 g daily dose).

Dosage Adjustment: Renal Impairment: In renal transplant patients with severe chronic renal impairment (GFR <25 mL/min/1.73 m²) outside the immediate post-transplant period, doses of CellCept greater than 1 g administered twice a day should be avoided. These patients should also be carefully observed (see Action and Clinical Pharmacology, Pharmacokinetics, Special Populations and Conditions, Renal Insufficiency).

No data are available for cardiac or hepatic transplant patients with severe chronic renal impairment. CellCept should be used for cardiac or hepatic transplant patients with severe chronic renal impairment if the potential benefits outweigh the potential risks.

If neutropenia develops (ANC <1.3×10³/µL), dosing with CellCept should be interrupted or the dose reduced, appropriate diagnostic tests performed, and the patient managed appropriately (see Warnings and Precautions, Immune, Monitoring and Laboratory Tests and Adverse Reactions).

Delayed Renal Graft Function Post Transplant: No dose adjustment is recommended for these patients, however, they should be carefully observed (see Action and Clinical Pharmacology, Pharmacokinetics, Special Populations and Conditions, Renal Insufficiency).

Administration: CellCept (tablets, capsules) should be administered orally, and should be taken on an empty stomach (see Actions and Clinical Pharmacology, Absorption).

It is recommended that CellCept Powder for Oral Suspension be reconstituted by the pharmacist prior to dispensing to the patient (see Dosage and Administration, Reconstitution, Preparation of Oral Suspension).

CellCept i.v. must be reconstituted and diluted to a concentration of 6 mg/mL using 5% Dextrose Injection USP (see Dosage and Administration, Reconstitution, Preparation of Infusion Solution (6 mg/mL)). CellCept i.v. is incompatible with other intravenous infusion solutions. **Following reconstitution, CellCept i.v. must be administered by slow intravenous infusion over a period of no less than 2 hours by either peripheral or central vein.**

Reconstitution: Preparation of Oral Suspension:

1. Tap the closed bottle several times to loosen the powder.
2. Measure 94 mL of purified water in a graduated cylinder.
3. Add approximately half of the total amount of the purified water for reconstitution to the bottle and shake the closed bottle well for about 1 minute.
4. Add the remainder of water and shake the closed bottle well for about 1 minute.
5. Remove the child-resistant cap and push bottle adapter into neck of bottle.
6. Close bottle with child-resistant cap tightly. This will assure the proper seating of the bottle adapter in the bottle and child-resistant status of the cap.

Dispense with patient information leaflet and oral dispensers. Oral dispensers are for use with CellCept oral suspension only. It is recommended to write the date of expiration of the reconstituted suspension on the bottle label in the space provided. (The shelf life of the reconstituted suspension is 60 days.)

Net contents after reconstitution of the oral suspension is 175 mL, containing 200 mg/mL mycophenolate mofetil. Store reconstituted suspension at 15 to 30°C. Do not freeze. Discard any unused portion 60 days after reconstitution.

Preparation of Infusion Solution (6 mg/mL): CellCept i.v. does not contain an antibacterial preservative; therefore reconstitution and dilution of the product must be performed under aseptic conditions.

CellCept i.v. infusion solution must be prepared in two steps: the first step is a reconstitution step with 5% Dextrose Injection, USP and the second step is a dilution step with 5% Dextrose Injection, USP. A detailed description of the preparation is given below:

Step 1:

a. Two (2) vials of CellCept i.v. are used for preparing each 1 g dose, whereas three (3) vials are needed for each 1.5 g dose. Reconstitute the contents of each vial by injecting 14 mL of 5% Dextrose Injection, USP.
b. Gently shake the vial to dissolve the drug.
c. Inspect the resulting slightly yellow solution for particulate matter and discoloration prior to further dilution. Discard the vial if particulate matter or discoloration is observed.

Step 2:

a. To prepare a 1 g dose, further dilute the contents of the two reconstituted vials (approx. 2×15 mL) into 140 mL of 5% Dextrose Injection USP. To prepare a 1.5 g dose, further dilute the contents of the three reconstituted vials (approx. 3×15 mL) into 210 mL of 5% Dextrose Injection USP. The final concentration of both solutions is 6 mg mycophenolate mofetil per mL.
b. As with all parenteral drug products, diluted solution should be inspected visually for clarity, particulate matter, precipitate, discoloration and leakage prior to administration whenever solution and container permit. Solutions showing haziness, particulate matter, precipitate, discoloration or leakage should not be used. Discard unused portion.

If the infusion solution is not prepared immediately prior to administration, the commencement of administration of the infusion solution should be within 4 hours from reconstitution and dilution of the drug product. Keep solutions at 15 to 30°C.

CellCept i.v. should not be mixed or administered concurrently via the same infusion catheter with other intravenous drugs or infusion admixtures.

OVERDOSAGE:

Reports of overdoses with mycophenolate mofetil have been received from clinical trials and during post-marketing experience. In many of these cases no adverse events were reported. In those overdose cases in which adverse events were reported, the events fall within the known safety profile of the drug.

It is expected that an overdose of mycophenolate mofetil could possibly result in oversuppression of the immune system and increase susceptibility to infections and bone marrow suppression (see Warnings and Precautions, Immune). If neutropenia develops, dosing with CellCept should be interrupted or the dose reduced (see Warnings and Precautions, Immune).

The highest dose administered to renal transplant patients in clinical trials has been 4 g per day. In limited experience with cardiac and hepatic transplant patients in clinical trials, the highest doses used were 4 g or 5 g per day. At doses of 4 g or 5 g per day, there appears to be a higher rate, compared to the use of 3 g per day or less, of gastrointestinal intolerance (nausea, vomiting, and/or diarrhea), and occasional hematologic abnormalities, principally neutropenia, leading to a need to reduce or discontinue dosing.

At clinically encountered concentrations, MPA and MPAG are not removed by hemodialysis. However, at high MPAG plasma concentrations (>100 µg/mL), small amounts of MPAG are removed. By interfering with enterohepatic recirculation of the drug, bile acid sequestrants, such as cholestyramine reduce the MPA AUC.

For management of a suspected drug overdose, contact your regional Poison Control Centre. See the *CPS Directory* section for a list of Poison Control Centres.

ACTION AND CLINICAL PHARMACOLOGY: Mechanism of Action: Mycophenolate mofetil (MMF) has been demonstrated in experimental animal models to prolong the survival of allogeneic transplants (kidney, heart, liver, intestine, limb, small bowel, pancreatic islets, and bone marrow). MMF has also been shown to reverse ongoing acute rejection in the canine renal and rat cardiac allograft models. MMF also inhibited proliferative arteriopathy in experimental models of aortic and heart allografts in rats, as well as in primate cardiac xenografts. MMF was used alone or in combination with other immunosuppressive agents in these studies. MMF has been demonstrated to inhibit immunologically-mediated inflammatory responses in animal models and to inhibit tumor development and prolong survival in murine tumor transplant models.

MMF is rapidly absorbed following oral administration and hydrolyzed to form MPA, which is the active metabolite. MPA is a potent, selective, uncompetitive and reversible inhibitor of inosine monophosphate dehydrogenase (IMPDH), and therefore inhibits the de novo pathway of guanosine nucleotide synthesis without incorporation into DNA. Because T- and B-lymphocytes are critically dependent for their proliferation on de novo synthesis of purines whereas other cell types can utilize salvage pathways, MPA has potent cytostatic effects on lymphocytes. MPA inhibits proliferative responses of T- and B-lymphocytes to both mitogenic and allospecific stimulation. Addition of guanosine or deoxyguanosine reverses the cytostatic effects of MPA on lymphocytes. MPA also suppresses antibody formation by B-lymphocytes. MPA prevents the glycosylation of lymphocyte and monocyte glycoproteins that are involved in intercellular adhesion to endothelial cells and may inhibit recruitment of leukocytes into sites of inflammation and graft rejection. MMF did not inhibit early events in the activation of human peripheral blood mononuclear cells, such as the production of interleukin-1 (IL-1) and interleukin-2 (IL-2), but did block the coupling of these events to DNA synthesis and proliferation.

Pharmacokinetics: Following oral and IV administration, MMF undergoes rapid and complete metabolism to MPA, the active metabolite. Oral absorption of the drug is rapid and essentially complete. The parent drug MMF can be measured systemically during the intravenous infusion; however, shortly (about 5 minutes) after the infusion is stopped or after oral administration, MMF concentration is below the limit of quantitation (0.4 µg/mL).

Absorption: In 12 healthy volunteers, the mean absolute bioavailability of oral MMF relative to IV MMF (based on MPA AUC) was 94%. The area under the plasma-concentration time curve (AUC) for MPA appears to increase in a dose-proportional fashion in renal transplant patients receiving multiple doses of MMF up to a daily dose of 3 g (see Table 4 for pharmacokinetic parameters). Effect of Food: Food (27 g fat, 650 calories) had no effect on the extent of absorption (MPA AUC) of MMF when administered at doses of 1.5 g twice daily to renal transplant patients. However, MPA C_{max} was decreased by 40% in the presence of food (see Dosage and Administration).

Distribution: The mean (±SD) apparent volume of distribution of MPA in twelve healthy volunteers is approximately 3.6 (±1.5) and 4.0 (±1.2) L/kg following IV and oral administration, respectively. MPA, at clinically relevant concentrations, is 97% bound to plasma albumin. MPAG is 82% bound to plasma albumin at MPAG concentration ranges that are normally seen in stable renal transplant patients; however, at higher MPAG concentrations (observed in patients with renal impairment or delayed graft function), the binding of MPA may be reduced as a result of competition between MPAG and MPA for protein binding. Mean blood to plasma ratio of radioactivity concentrations was approximately 0.6 indicating that MPA and MPAG do not extensively distribute into the cellular fractions of blood.

In vitro studies to evaluate the effect of other agents on the binding of MPA to human serum albumin (HSA) or plasma proteins showed that salicylate (at 25 mg/dL with HSA) and MPAG (at ≥460 µg/mL with plasma proteins) increased the free fraction of MPA. At concentrations exceeding those encountered clinically, cyclosporine, digoxin, naproxen, prednisone, propranolol, tacrolimus, theophylline, tolbutamide, and warfarin did not increase the free fraction of MPA. MPA at concentrations as high as 100 µg/mL had little effect on the binding of warfarin, digoxin or propranolol, but decreased the binding of theophylline from 53% to 45% and phenytoin from 90% to 87%.

Metabolism: Following oral and intravenous dosing, MMF undergoes complete metabolism to MPA, the active metabolite. Metabolism to MPA occurs presystemically after oral dosing. MPA is metabolized principally by glucuronyl transferase to form the phenolic glucuronide of MPA (MPAG) which is not pharmacologically active.

In vivo, MPAG is converted to free MPA via enterohepatic recirculation. The following metabolites of the 2-hydroxyethyl-morpholino moiety are also recovered in the urine following oral administration of MMF to healthy subjects: N-(2-carboxymethyl)-morpholine, N-(2-hydroxyethyl)-morpholine, and the N-oxide of N-(2-hydroxyethyl)-morpholine.

Secondary peaks in the plasma MPA concentration-time profile are usually observed 6-12 hours post-dose. The coadministration of cholestyramine (4 g three times daily) resulted in approximately a 40% decrease in the MPA AUC (largely as a consequence of lower concentrations in the terminal portion of the profile). These observations suggest that enterohepatic recirculation contributes to MPA plasma concentrations.

Renal insufficiency has no consistent effect on MPA pharmacokinetics. Mean MPA AUC was increased by 50% in severe renal impairment (GFR <25 mL/min/1.73 m²), however, there was considerable variation about the mean. For MPAG, there is an increase (3-6 fold) in mean AUC (see Actions and Clinical Pharmacology, Special Populations and Conditions, Renal Insufficiency).

Excretion: Negligible amount of drug is excreted as MPA (<1% of dose) in the urine. Orally administered radiolabeled MMF resulted in complete recovery of the administered dose; with 93% of the administered dose recovered in the urine and 6% recovered in feces. Most (about 87%) of the administered dose is excreted in the urine as MPAG. At clinically encountered concentrations MPA is not removed by hemodialysis. Similarly, MPAG concentrations normally encountered are unaffected by hemodialysis, however, at high MPAG plasma concentrations (>100 µg/mL), small amounts of this metabolite are removed. Mean (±SD) apparent half-life and plasma clearance of MPA are 17.9 (±6.5) hours and 193 (±48) mL/min following oral administration and 16.6 (±5.8) hours and 177 (±31) mL/min following IV administration, respectively.

Special Populations and Conditions: Pharmacokinetics in Healthy Volunteers, Renal, Cardiac and Hepatic Transplant Patients: Shown in Table 4 are the mean (±SD) pharmacokinetic parameters for MPA following the administration of oral MMF given as single doses to healthy volunteers and multiple doses to renal, cardiac and hepatic transplant patients. In the early post-transplant period (<40 days post-transplant), renal, cardiac and hepatic transplant patients had mean MPA AUCs approximately 30% lower and C_{max} approximately 40% lower compared to the late transplant period (3-6 months post-transplant).

MPA AUC values obtained following administration of 1 g twice daily intravenous CellCept to renal transplant patients in the early post-transplant phase are comparable to those observed following 1 g twice daily oral CellCept. In hepatic transplant patients, administration of 1 g twice daily intravenous CellCept followed by 1.5 g twice daily oral CellCept resulted in MPA AUC values similar to those found in renal transplant patients administered 1 g CellCept twice daily.

Table 4: CellCept

Pharmacokinetic Parameters for MPA [mean (±SD)] Following Administration of MMF to Healthy Volunteers (Single Dose), Renal, Cardiac and Hepatic Transplant Patients (Multiple Doses)

	Dose/ Route	T_{max} (h)	C_{max} (µg/mL)	Total AUC (µg·h/mL)
Healthy Volunteer (single dose)	1 g/oral	0.80 (±0.36) (n=129)	24.5 (±9.5) (n=129)	63.9 (±16.2) (n=117)
Renal Transplant Patients (twice daily dosing) Time After Transplantation	**Dose/ Route**	**T_{max} (h)**	**C_{max} (µg/mL)**	**Interdosing Interval AUC_{0-12} (µg·h/mL)**
5 days	1 g/i.v.	1.58 (±0.46) (n=31)	12.0 (±3.82) (n=31)	40.8 (±11.4) (n=31)
6 days	1 g/oral	1.33 (±1.05) (n=31)	10.7 (±4.83) (n=31)	32.9 (±15.0) (N=31)
Early (<40 days)	1 g/oral	1.31 (±0.76) (n=25)	8.16 (±4.50) (n=25)	27.3 (±10.9) (n=25)
Early (<40 days)	1.5 g/oral	1.21 (±0.81) (n=27)	13.5 (±8.18) (n=27)	38.4 (±15.4) (n=27)
Late (>3 months)	1.5 g/oral	0.90 (±0.24) (n=23)	24.1 (±12.1) (n=23)	65.3 (±35.4) (n=23)
Cardiac Transplant Patients (twice daily dosing) Time After Transplantation	**Dose/ Route**	**T_{max} (h)**	**C_{max} (µg/mL)**	**Interdosing Interval AUC_{0-12} (µg·h/mL)**

(cont'd)

Table 4: CellCept *(cont'd)*

Pharmacokinetic Parameters for MPA [mean (±SD)] Following Administration of MMF to Healthy Volunteers (Single Dose), Renal, Cardiac and Hepatic Transplant Patients (Multiple Doses)

Early (day before discharge)	1.5 g/oral	1.8 (±1.3) (n=11)	11.5 (±6.8) (n=11)	43.3 (±20.8) (n=9)
Late (>6 months)	1.5 g/oral	1.1 (±0.7) (n=52)	20.0 (±9.4) (n=52)	54.1[a] (±20.4) (n=49)
Hepatic Transplant Patients (twice daily dosing) Time After Transplantation	**Dose/ Route**	**T_{max} (h)**	**C_{max} (µg/mL)**	**Interdosing Interval AUC_{0-12} (µg·h/mL)**
4–9 days	1.0 g/i.v.	1.50 (±0.517) (n=22)	17.0 (±12.7) (n=22)	34.0 (±17.4) (n=22)
Early (5–8 days)	1.5 g/oral	1.15 (±0.432) (n=20)	13.1 (±6.76) (n=20)	29.2 (±11.9) (n=20)
Late (3 months)	1.5 g/oral	1.44 (±1.03) (n=9)	16.3 (±11.9) (n=9)	38.6 (±10.8) (n=9)
Late (>6 months)	1.5 g/oral	1.37 (±0.477) (n=9)	19.6 (±9.86) (n=9)	52.5 (±14.4) (n=9)

[a] AUC_{0-12} values quoted are extrapolated from data from samples collected over 4 hours.

Renal and Hepatic Insufficiency: Shown in Table 5 are the mean (±SD) pharmacokinetic parameters for MPA following the administration of oral MMF given as single doses to non-transplant subjects with renal and hepatic impairment.

Table 5: CellCept

Pharmacokinetic Parameters for MPA [mean (±SD)] Following Single Doses of MMF Capsules in Chronic Renal and Hepatic Impairment

Renal Impairment (no. of patients)	**Dose**	**T_{max} (h)**	**C_{max} (µg/mL)**	**AUC_{0-96} (µg·h/mL)**
Healthy Volunteers GFR >80 mL/min/1.73 m² (n=6)	1 g	0.75 (±0.27)	25.3 (±7.99)	45.0 (±22.6)
Mild Renal Impairment GFR 50–80 mL/min/1.73 m² (n=6)	1 g	0.75 (±0.27)	26.0 (±3.82)	59.9 (±12.9)
Moderate Renal Impairment GFR 25–49 mL/min/1.73 m² (n=6)	1 g	0.75 (±0.27)	19.0 (±13.2)	52.9 (±25.5)
Severe Renal Impairment GFR <25 mL/min/1.73 m² (n=7)	1 g	1.00 (±0.41)	16.3 (±10.8)	78.6 (±46.4)
Hepatic Impairment (no. of patients)	**Dose**	**T_{max} (h)**	**C_{max} (µg/mL)**	**AUC_{0-48} (µg·h/mL)**
Healthy Volunteers (n=6)	1 g	0.63 (±0.14)	24.3 (±5.73)	29.0 (±5.78)
Alcoholic Cirrhosis (n=18)	1 g	0.85 (±0.58)	22.4 (±10.1)	29.8 (±10.7)

Renal Insufficiency: In a single-dose study, MMF was administered as capsule or intravenous infusion over 40 minutes. The mean plasma MPA AUC observed after oral dosing to volunteers with severe chronic renal impairment (glomerular filtration rate [GFR] <25 mL/min/1.73 m²) was about 75% higher relative to the mean observed in healthy volunteers (GFR >80 L/min/1.73 m²). However, the mean single dose plasma MPAG AUC was 3-6 fold higher in volunteers with severe renal impairment than in volunteers with mild renal impairment or healthy volunteers, consistent with the known renal elimination of MPAG. No data are available on the safety of long-term exposure to this level of MPAG.

Plasma MPA AUC observed after single dose (1 g) intravenous dosing to volunteers (n=4) with severe chronic renal impairment (GFR <25 mL/min/1.73 m²) was 62.4 µg·h/mL (±19.3). Multiple dosing of MMF in patients with severe chronic renal impairment has not been studied (see Dosage and Administration, Recommended Dose and Dosage Adjustment, Renal Impairment).

Subjects with severe chronic renal impairment who have received single doses of MMF showed higher mean plasma MPA and MPAG AUCs relative to subjects with lesser degrees of renal impairment or normal healthy subjects. No data are available on the safety of long-term exposure to these levels of MPAG.

Delayed Renal Graft Function Post-Transplant: In patients with delayed renal graft function post-transplant, mean MPA AUC_{0-12} was comparable, but MPAG AUC_{0-12} was 2-3 fold higher, compared to that seen in post-transplant patients without delayed renal graft function. In the three pivotal studies of prevention of rejection, 298 of 1483 patients (20%) experienced delayed graft function. Although patients with delayed graft function have a higher incidence of certain adverse events (anemia, thrombocytopenia, hyperkalemia) than patients without delayed graft function, these events were not more frequent in patients receiving CellCept than azathioprine or placebo. No dose adjustment is recommended for these patients, however, they should be carefully observed. See Dosage and Administration, Dosage Adjustment, Delayed Renal Graft Function Post Transplant).

Hemodialysis: At clinically encountered concentrations, MPA is not removed by hemodialysis. Similarly, MPAG concentrations normally encountered are unaffected by hemodialysis, however, at high MPAG concentrations (>100 µg/mL), hemodialysis removes only small amounts of MPAG.

Hepatic Insufficiency: In a single dose (1 g, oral) study of 18 volunteers with alcoholic cirrhosis and 6 healthy volunteers, hepatic MPA glucuronidation processes appeared to be relatively unaffected by hepatic parenchymal disease when pharmacokinetic parameters of healthy volunteers and alcoholic cirrhosis patients within this study were compared. However, it should be noted that for unexplained reasons, the healthy volunteers in this study had about a 50% lower AUC as compared to healthy volunteers in other studies, thus making comparisons between volunteers with alcoholic cirrhosis and healthy volunteers difficult. Effects of hepatic disease on this process probably depend on the particular disease. Hepatic disease with other etiologies may show a different effect. In a single-dose (1 g) intravenous study of 6 volunteers with alcoholic cirrhosis, MPA AUC was 44.1 µg·h/mL (±15.5).

Pediatrics: The pharmacokinetic parameters of MPA and MPAG have been evaluated in 55 pediatric patients (ranging from 1 year to 18 years of age) receiving CellCept oral suspension at a dose of 600 mg/m² twice daily (up to a maximum of 1 g twice daily) after allogeneic renal transplantation. This dose achieved MPA AUC values in pediatric patients similar to those seen in adult renal transplant patients receiving CellCept capsules at a dose of 1g twice daily in the early post-transplant period. As observed in adults, early post-transplant MPA AUC values were approximately 45%-53% lower than those observed in the later post-transplant period (>3 months). MPA AUC values were similar in the early and late post-transplant period across the 1-18 year age range.

Geriatrics: Pharmacokinetics in the elderly has not been formally evaluated.

Gender: Data obtained from several studies were pooled to examine any gender-related differences in the pharmacokinetics of MPA (data were adjusted to 1 g oral dose). Mean (±SD) MPA AUC_{0-12} for males (n=79) was 32.0 (±14.5) and for females (n=41) was 36.5 (±18.8) µg·h/mL while mean (±SD) MPA C_{max} was 9.96 (±6.19) in the males and 10.6 (±5.64) µg/mL in the females. These differences are not of clinical significance.

STORAGE AND STABILITY: CellCept Capsules 250 mg: Store at 15 to 30°C. Store in original package.
CellCept Tablets 500 mg: Store at 15 to 30°C. Protect from light. Store in original package.
CellCept Oral Suspension: Store dry powder at 15 to 30°C.
CellCept Intravenous: Store powder at 15 to 30°C. Reconstituted/Infusion Solutions: Store at 15 to 30°C.

SPECIAL HANDLING INSTRUCTIONS: Because MMF has demonstrated teratogenic effects in rats and rabbits, CellCept (mycophenolate mofetil) tablets should not be crushed and CellCept capsules should not be opened or crushed. Avoid inhalation or direct contact with skin or mucous membranes of the powder contained in CellCept capsules and CellCept Powder for Oral Suspension (before or after reconstitution). Caution should be exercised in the handling and preparation of solutions of CellCept i.v. Avoid skin contact of the solution. If such contact occurs, wash thoroughly with soap and water; rinse eyes with plain water. Should a spill occur, wipe up using paper towels wetted with water to remove spilled powder or suspension.

INFORMATION FOR THE PATIENT: Published in e-CPS, available by subscription at www.e-cps.ca.

DOSAGE FORMS, COMPOSITION AND PACKAGING: CellCept: Capsules: Each oblong, blue/brown, two-piece hard gelatin capsule, printed in black with "CellCept 250" on the blue cap and "Roche" on the brown body, contains: mycophenolate mofetil 250 mg. Nonmedicinal ingredients: croscarmellose sodium, magnesium stearate, povidone (K-90) and pregelatinized starch; capsule shell: black iron oxide, gelatin, indigotine (FD&C blue #2) aluminum lake, potassium hydroxide, red iron oxide, shellac, titanium dioxide and yellow iron oxide. Blister packs of 10, boxes of 10.

Powder for Oral Suspension: Available as a white to off-white powder blend for reconstitution to a white to off-white fruit flavor suspension containing 200 mg/mL of mycophenolate mofetil. Each bottle of CellCept powder for oral suspension contains 35 g of MMF in a 110 g powder for oral suspension. Nonmedicinal ingredients: aspartame, citric acid, colloidal silicon dioxide, fruit flavor, methylparaben, sodium citrate, sorbitol, soybean lecithin and xanthan gum. Bottle of 225 mL with bottle adapter and 2 oral dispensers*. The deliverable volume after reconstitution is 165 mL.

Tablets: Each lavender-colored, caplet-shaped, film coated tablet, engraved with "CellCept 500" on one side and "Roche" on the other, contains: mycophenolate mofetil 500 mg. Nonmedicinal ingredients: croscarmellose sodium, hydroxypropyl cellulose, hydroxypropyl methylcellulose, indigotine (FD&C blue #2) aluminum lake, iron oxide, magnesium stearate, microcrystalline cellulose, polyethylene glycol 400, povidone (K-90) and titanium dioxide. Blister packs of 10, boxes of 5.

CellCept i.v.: Each vial of sterile, white to off-white lyophilized powder **for i.v. infusion** contains: the equivalent of mycophenolate mofetil 500 mg as the hydrochloride salt. Nonmedicinal ingredients: citric acid, polysorbate 80 and sodium hydroxide and/or hydrochloric acid to adjust pH. Sterile vials of 20 mL, cartons of 4. Each vial is intended for single use only.

(Shown in Product Identification Section)

Celsentri® Ⓟ

maraviroc

CCR5 Antagonist

ViiV Healthcare ULC

Date of Revision: May 17, 2010

SUMMARY PRODUCT INFORMATION:

Route of Administration	**Dosage Form/ Strength**	**Clinically Relevant Nonmedicinal Ingredients**
Oral	Film-coated tablets; 150, 300 mg maraviroc	Not applicable For a complete listing see Dosage Forms, Composition and Packaging.

INDICATIONS AND CLINICAL USE: CELSENTRI (maraviroc), in combination with other antiretroviral agents, is indicated for adult patients infected with CCR5-tropic HIV-1.

This indication is based on safety and efficacy data from 2 double-blind, placebo-controlled trials in treatment-experienced patients and one double-blind, comparative study in treatment-naïve patients.

The following points should be considered when initiating therapy with CELSENTRI:

- Adult patients infected with only CCR5-tropic HIV-1 should use CELSENTRI.
- CCR5 tropism should be confirmed using a highly sensitive tropism assay prior to initiation of CELSENTRI therapy. Outgrowth of pre-existing low-level CXCR4- or dual/mixed-tropic HIV-1 not detected by tropism testing at screening has been associated with virologic failure on CELSENTRI.
- CELSENTRI is not recommended in patients infected with dual/mixed or CXCR4-tropic HIV-1; efficacy in this patient population was not demonstrated in a Phase 2 Study.
- In treatment-naïve subjects, more subjects treated with CELSENTRI experienced virologic failure and developed lamivudine resistance compared to efavirenz.

Pediatrics (<16 years of age): The safety and efficacy of CELSENTRI have not been established in pediatric patients.

Geriatrics (>65 years of age): In general, caution should be exercised when administering CELSENTRI in elderly patients (see Warnings and Precautions, Special Populations).

CONTRAINDICATIONS: CELSENTRI (maraviroc) is contraindicated in patients with hypersensitivity to maraviroc or any component of this medication. For a complete listing, see Dosage Forms, Composition and Packaging.

WARNINGS AND PRECAUTIONS:

> **Serious Warnings and Precautions**
> **Hepatotoxicity has been reported with CELSENTRI use. A systemic allergic reaction, including pruritic rash, eosinophilia or elevated IgE may occur prior to the development of hepatotoxicity. Patients with signs or symptoms of acute hepatitis or allergic reaction should be evaluated immediately and, if required discontinuation of CELSENTRI treatment should be considered (see Warnings and Precautions, Hepatic/Biliary/Pancreatic).**

General: CELSENTRI (maraviroc) should be taken as part of an antiretroviral combination regimen. As with other antiretrovirals, CELSENTRI should be optimally combined with other antiretrovirals to which the patient's virus is sensitive. Physicians should ensure that appropriate dose adjustment of CELSENTRI is made when CELSENTRI is coadministered with CYP3A4 inhibitors and/or inducers since maraviroc concentrations and its therapeutic effects may be affected (see Drug Interactions).

Tropism testing should be performed prior to initiation of therapy using a highly sensitive tropism assay; however tropism assays may not detect low levels of dual/mixed or CXCR4-tropic variants. CELSENTRI did not demonstrate efficacy in a Phase 2 study of patients infected with dual/mixed or CXCR4-using virus.

The long-term impact of CELSENTRI-mediated inhibition of the CCR5 coreceptor is the subject of ongoing studies.

* Oral dosing dispenser manufactured by F. Hoffmann-La Roche Ltd., 4070 Basel, Switzerland.

Cardiovascular: CELSENTRI should be used with caution in patients with a history of cardiovascular disease or who are at risk for cardiovascular events. Cases of myocardial ischemia and myocardial infarction were reported in 11 subjects (1.3%) receiving CELSENTRI in Phase 3 studies in treatment-experienced studies [total exposure 609 patient-years (300 on once daily + 309 on twice daily CELSENTRI)]. These events mostly occurred in subjects with pre-existing cardiac disease or cardiac risk factors, which confounded the assessment of CELSENTRI causality.

In the Phase 2b/3 study in treatment-naïve patients, 3 subjects (0.8%) who received CELSENTRI had events related to ischemic heart diseases and 5 subjects (1.4%) who received efavirenz had such events (total exposure 506 and 508 patient-years for CELSENTRI and efavirenz, respectively).

Postural Hypotension and Syncope: CELSENTRI-related cases of postural hypotension and syncope were reported during Phase 3 studies in HIV-infected patients (treatment-naïve and treatment-experienced) who received the drug at the recommended dose (see Adverse Drug Reaction Overview). At dosing higher than the recommended dose, CELSENTRI-related cases of postural hypotension and syncope were observed during Phase 1 studies in healthy volunteers.

Caution should be used when administering CELSENTRI in patients who have a history of postural hypotension or who are on concomitant medications known to lower blood pressure.

Immune: Immune Reconstitution Syndrome: During the initial phase of treatment, patients responding to antiretroviral therapy may develop an inflammatory response to indolent or residual opportunistic infections (such as MAC, CMV, PCP and TB), which may necessitate further evaluation and treatment.

Potential Risk of Infection and Malignancy: The antagonistic action of CELSENTRI on the CCR5 coreceptor may impair immune function and potentially increase the risk of developing infections and/or malignancy.

The rates of certain infections (upper respiratory tract and Herpes virus) were higher in subjects receiving CELSENTRI, while others (pneumonia) were lower as compared to those in patients on placebo in Phase 3 treatment-experienced studies (see Adverse Reactions). The overall incidence and severity of infection and AIDS-defining category C infections were similar in the CELSENTRI and placebo treatment arms.

In the Phase 2b/3 study in treatment-naïve patients, the incidence of AIDS-defining Category C events when adjusted for exposure was 1.8 for CELSENTRI compared to 2.4 for efavirenz per 100 patient-years of exposure.

Patients on CELSENTRI treatment should be carefully monitored for symptoms of infection.

There were no increased reports of malignancies in subjects treated with CELSENTRI during Phase 3 studies. Long-term follow-up is required to assess whether CELSENTRI increases the risk of malignancy. The exposure-adjusted rate for malignancies per 100 patient-years of exposure in treatment-experienced studies was 4.6 for CELSENTRI compared to 9.3 on placebo. In treatment-naïve patients, the rates were 1.0 and 2.4 per 100 patient-years of exposure for CELSENTRI and efavirenz, respectively.

Hepatic/Biliary/Pancreatic: A case of possible CELSENTRI-induced hepatotoxicity with allergic features has been reported in a study of healthy volunteers. In addition, an increase in hepatic adverse reactions with CELSENTRI was observed during studies of treatment-experienced subjects with HIV infection, although there was no overall increase in ACTG Grade 3/4 liver function test abnormalities. There were fewer cases of hepatobiliary disorders reported in treatment-naïve patients on CELSENTRI but the overall incidence of hepatic adverse events and ACTG Grade 3/4 liver function test abnormalities in treatment-naïve patients was similar between CELSENTRI and efavirenz (see Adverse Reactions).

Discontinuation of CELSENTRI should be considered in any patient with signs or symptoms of acute hepatitis, in particular if drug-related hypersensitivity is suspected or with increased liver transaminases combined with rash or other systemic symptoms of potential hypersensitivity (e.g. pruritic rash, eosinophila or elevated IgE).

Caution should also be used when administering CELSENTRI to patients with pre-existing liver dysfunction or who are co-infected with viral hepatitis B or C. If there is evidence of worsening of liver disease in such patients, interruption or discontinuation of treatment must be considered.

The safety and efficacy of CELSENTRI have not been specifically studied in patients with significant underlying liver disorders. However drug levels were increased in patients with moderate hepatic impairment (see Action and Clinical Pharmacology, Special Populations and Conditions, Hepatic Impairment).

In Phase 3 studies, approximately 6% of subjects were co-infected with Hepatitis B virus and approximately 6% were co-infected with Hepatitis C virus. Thus, the number of co-infected subjects was too small to assess the risk for hepatic adverse events with CELSENTRI administration in this patient population (see Action and Clinical Pharmacology, Special Populations and Conditions, Hepatic Impairment).

Renal: Renal Impairment: The safety and efficacy of maraviroc have not been specifically studied in patients with renal impairment, therefore maraviroc should be used with caution in this population. In the absence of metabolic inhibitors, renal clearance accounts for less than 25% of total clearance of maraviroc. However, in the presence of metabolic inhibitors, renal clearance may account for up to 70% of total clearance of maraviroc, hence renal impairment may result in increased maraviroc exposures in this case. Therefore, maraviroc should be used with caution in patients with renal impairment (CL_{cr} <80 mL/min) who are also taking potent CYP3A4 inhibitors (see Dosage and Administration).

Special Populations: Pregnancy, Fertility and Reproduction: Embryofetal development studies in rats and rabbits revealed no evidence of harm to the fetus from maraviroc. Pre- and post-natal developmental studies showed a slight increase in motor activity in male offspring at both weaning and as adults at the high dose, while no effects were seen in female offspring. The subsequent development of these offspring, including fertility and reproductive performance, was not affected by the maternal administration of maraviroc.

No meaningful clinical data on exposure during pregnancy are available. Because animal reproduction studies are not always predictive of human response, maraviroc should be used during pregnancy only if the potential benefit justifies the potential risk to the fetus.

Antiretroviral Pregnancy Registry: To monitor maternal-fetal outcomes of pregnant women exposed to CELSENTRI and other antiretroviral agents, an Antiretroviral Pregnancy Registry has been established. Physicians are encouraged to register patients by calling ViiV Healthcare ULC's Drug Safety Department (1-877-393-8448).

Nursing Women: It is recommended that HIV-infected women not breast-feed their infants under any circumstances to avoid the transmission of HIV infection. Studies in lactating rats indicate that maraviroc is extensively secreted into rat milk. It is not known whether maraviroc is secreted into human milk. Mothers should be instructed not to breast-feed if they are receiving CELSENTRI because of both the potential for HIV transmission and any possible undesirable effects in nursing infants.

Pediatrics (<16 years of age): The pharmacokinetics, safety and efficacy of maraviroc in pediatric patients have not been established. Therefore, maraviroc should not be used in this patient population.

Geriatrics (>65 years of age): There were insufficient numbers of subjects aged 65 and over in the clinical studies to determine whether they respond differently from younger subjects. In general, caution should be exercised when administering CELSENTRI in elderly patients, also reflecting the greater frequency of decreased hepatic and renal function, of concomitant disease and other drug therapy.

Gender and Race: Population pharmacokinetic analysis of pooled phase 1/2a data indicated that while gender did not affect pharmacokinetics, a typical Asian subject showed a 26.5% higher exposure than a typical Caucasian. However a study designed to evaluate pharmacokinetic differences between Caucasians and Singaporeans showed no differences.

Population pharmacokinetic modeling of data from the treatment-naïve patients study (MERIT) showed a 17.5% higher average concentration in the typical Black subject compared with the typical Caucasian subject. The typical female subject had a 13.7% higher average concentration compared with the typical male.

The maraviroc exposure differences are small and therefore unlikely to pose efficacy, safety or tolerability risks. Dosage adjustment is not necessary based on gender or race.

Patients Co-infected with Hepatitis B and/or Hepatitis C Virus: The safety and efficacy of CELSENTRI have not been studied specifically in patients co-infected with Hepatitis B or Hepatitis C virus. CELSENTRI should be used in caution with this population.

Dose Adjustment: Physicians should ensure that appropriate dose adjustment of CELSENTRI is made when CELSENTRI is co-administered with potent CYP3A4 inhibitors and/or inducers since CELSENTRI concentrations and its therapeutic effects may be affected (see Drug Interactions or Dosage and Administration). Please also refer to the respective product monographs of the other antiretroviral medicinal products used in the combination.

ADVERSE REACTIONS: Adverse Drug Reaction Overview: The overall safety profile of CELSENTRI (maraviroc) is based on over 2000 patients and healthy volunteers who received at least 1 dose of maraviroc during various clinical studies. Specifically, the adverse event profile of CELSENTRI is based on 1374 HIV-1 infected patients who received at least one dose of CELSENTRI during clinical studies. This includes 426 treatment-experienced patients and 360 treatment-naïve patients who received the recommended dose 300 mg twice daily and a further 588 treatment-experienced and treatment-naïve patients who received 300 mg once daily. Assessment of treatment related adverse reactions is based on pooled data at the recommended dose from two Phase 2b/3 studies in treatment-experienced adults patients (MOTIVATE 1 and MOTIVATE 2) and one study in treatment-naïve adult patients (MERIT) in CCR5-tropic HIV-1 infected patients.

Assessment of adverse drug reactions is based on data at the recommended dose from two Phase 3 studies in treatment-experienced adult patients (MOTIVATE 1 and MOTIVATE 2 pooled data) and one study in treatment-naïve adult patients (MERIT) in CCR5-tropic HIV-1 infected. The median duration of maraviroc therapy for subjects in these studies was 48 weeks, with the total exposure on CELSENTRI twice daily at 309 patient-years versus 111 patient-years on placebo.

During these 2 studies, approximately 50.5% of maraviroc patients reported at least 1 treatment-related AE with the most frequently reported adverse reactions at the recommended dose regardless of the incidence compared to OBT alone were diarrhoea, nausea and headache. Most of the adverse events reported were judged to be mild to moderate in severity. The most commonly reported grade 3 or 4 adverse events in subjects receiving 300 mg of CELSENTRI twice daily in these two studies were liver function analyses (5.16%) and febrile disorders (2.58%). All other grade 3 or 4 adverse events were reported in less than 2% of the subjects.

Eighty-eight subjects (20.7%) receiving 300 mg twice daily reported at least 1 SAE with 13 (3.1%) subjects with an SAE considered at least possibly treatment-related: elevated transaminases, generalised rash, mucormycosis, myositis, increased nausea and vomiting, syncope and pancytopaenia, diarrhoea, syncope and orthostatic hypotension, increased hepatic enzymes, pneumonia, esophageal carcinoma, loss of consciousness, hepatic failure, bile duct cancer, and metastases to liver, bone and peritoneum.

In the two treatment-experienced studies, the rates of discontinuation due to adverse events were 4.5% in subjects receiving CELSENTRI twice daily + optimized background therapy (OBT) compared to 5.3% in those receiving placebo + OBT. Adverse events that led to discontinuations in 2 or more patients are: LFTs increased/abnormal (3 on maraviroc BID), abdominal pain upper (1 on maraviroc BID), rash (1 on maraviroc BID), and pyrexia (1 on maraviroc BID). In the treatment-naïve study the rates of permanent discontinuation were lower in patients receiving maraviroc 300 mg twice daily compared to those receiving efavirenz.

Dizziness or postural dizziness occurred in 8.4% and 8.2% on CELSENTRI and placebo, respectively, with 2 subjects (0.5%) on CELSENTRI permanently discontinuing therapy (1 due to syncope, 1 due to orthostatic hypotension) versus 1 subject on placebo (0.5%) permanently discontinuing therapy due to dizziness.

Clinical Trial Adverse Drug Reactions: Because clinical trials are conducted under widely varying conditions, adverse reaction rates observed in the clinical trials of a drug cannot be directly compared to rates in the clinical trials of another drug and may not reflect the rates observed in practice.

Studies in Treatment-Experienced Patients (MOTIVATE 1 and MOTIVATE 2): Assessment of treatment-emergent adverse events is based on the pooled data from 2 studies in treatment-experienced patients with CCR5-tropic HIV-1. The median duration of therapy was 48 weeks for patients receiving maraviroc and 21 weeks for patients receiving placebo. The population was 89% male and 84% white, with mean age of 46 years (range 17-75 years). Patients received dose equivalents of 300 mg maraviroc once or twice daily.

The most common adverse events reported with CELSENTRI twice daily therapy with frequency rates higher than placebo, regardless of causality, were cough, pyrexia, upper respiratory tract infections, rash and dizziness. In these 2 studies, the rates of discontinuation due to adverse events were 4.5% in patients receiving CELSENTRI twice daily + optimized background therapy (OBT) compared to 5.3% in those receiving placebo + OBT. Most of the adverse events reported were judged to be mild to moderate in severity. The data described in Table 1 occurred with CELSENTRI twice daily dosing.

The total number of subjects reporting infections were 233 (54.7%) and 84 (40.2%) in the CELSENTRI twice daily and placebo groups, respectively. The differences between the CELSENTRI and placebo groups may be explained by the longer treatment duration in the CELSENTRI arm. The exposure-adjusted frequency (rate per 100 patient-years) of these events was similar: 133 for both CELSENTRI and placebo, respectively. Dizziness or postural dizziness occurred in 8.4% and 8.2% on CELSENTRI and placebo, respectively, with 2 patients (0.5%) on CELSENTRI permanently discontinuing therapy (1 due to syncope, 1 due to orthostatic hypotension) versus 1 patient on placebo (0.5%) permanently discontinuing therapy due to dizziness.

Treatment-emergent adverse events, regardless of causality, from Studies in treatment-experienced patients are summarized in Table 1. Events occurring at ≥2% of subjects and at a numerically higher rate in subjects treated with CELSENTRI + OBT are included; events that occurred at the same or a higher rate on placebo + OBT after rounding are not displayed.

Table 1: CELSENTRI

Percentage of Patients at Twice Daily Dosing with Treatment-Emergent Adverse Events (All Causality) (≥2% on CELSENTRI +OBT[b] and at Higher Rate Compared to Placebo + OBT) Pooled Studies Week 48 in Treatment-Experienced Patients (MOTIVATE 1 and MOTIVATE 2)

	CELSENTRI + OBT Twice Daily[a] N=426 (%)	Placebo + OBT N=209 (%)
Eye Disorders		
Conjunctival infections, irritations and inflammations	2.3	1.4
Ocular infections, inflammations and associated manifestations	2.1	1.0
Gastrointestinal Disorders		
Constipation	5.9	2.9
Stomatitis, ulceration	2.3	1.9
Gastrointestinal signs and symptoms	2.3	1.9
General Disorders and Administration Site Conditions		
Pyrexia	12.9	8.6
Pain and discomfort	3.8	2.9
Edema	3.3	2.9
General signs and symptoms	3.1	2.4
Body temperature perception	2.1	1.9
Infections and Infestations[c]		
Upper respiratory tract infection	22.8	12.9
Herpes infection	7.7	4.3
Sinusitis	6.8	3.3
Bronchitis	6.6	4.8
Folliculitis	3.8	1.9
Pneumonia	2.3	5.3
Anogenital warts	2.1	1.4
Influenza	2.1	0.5

(cont'd)

Table 1: CELSENTRI *(cont'd)*

Percentage of Patients at Twice Daily Dosing with Treatment-Emergent Adverse Events (All Causality) (≥2% on CELSENTRI +OBT[b] and at Higher Rate Compared to Placebo + OBT) Pooled Studies Week 48 in Treatment-Experienced Patients (MOTIVATE 1 and MOTIVATE 2)

	CELSENTRI + OBT Twice Daily[a] N=426 (%)	Placebo + OBT N=209 (%)
Otitis media	2.1	0.5
Metabolism and Nutrition Disorders		
Appetite disorders	7.5	6.7
Musculoskeletal and Connective Tissue Disorders		
Joint related signs and symptoms	6.8	2.9
Muscle pains	3.1	0.5
Neoplasms Benign, Malignant and Unspecified		
Skin neoplasms benign	3.1	1.4
Nervous System Disorders		
Dizziness/postural dizziness	8.7	8.1
Paresthesias and dysesthesias	4.9	2.9
Sensory abnormalities	4.0	1.4
Disturbances in consciousness	3.8	2.9
Peripheral neuropathies	3.8	2.9
Psychiatric Disorders		
Disturbances in initiating and maintaining sleep	7.7	5.3
Depressive disorders	4.2	2.9
Anxiety disorders	3.5	3.3
Renal and Urinary Disorders		
Bladder and urethral symptoms	4.9	1.4
Urinary tract signs and symptoms	2.8	1.4
Respiratory, Thoracic and Mediastinal Disorders		
Coughing and associated symptoms	13.8	5.3
Upper respiratory tract signs and symptoms	6.1	3.3
Nasal congestion and inflammations	4.2	2.9
Breathing abnormalities	3.5	2.4
Bronchospasm and obstruction	2.1	1.9
Paranasal sinus disorders	2.8	0.5
Skin and Subcutaneous Tissue Disorders		
Rash	10.8	5.3
Apocrine and eccrine gland disorders	4.9	3.8
Dermal and epidermal conditions	4.5	4.3
Pruritus	3.8	1.9
Lipodystrophies	3.3	0.5
Erythemas	2.3	1.0
Vascular Disorders		
Vascular hypertensive disorders	3.1	1.9

[a] 300 mg dose equivalent.
[b] OBT: optimized background therapy.
[c] **MedDRA High Level Terms are shown in order to group related terms for all disorders except Infections and Infestations, which shows MedDRA Preferred Terms with the following related terms grouped:**
Bronchitis: bronchitis, acute bronchitis, bacterial bronchitis.
Herpes Simplex Infection: genital Herpes, Herpes simplex, Herpes virus, Herpes ophthalmic, oral Herpes, proctitis Herpes.
Influenza: influenza, influenza-like illness.
Pneumonia: pneumonia, lobar pneumonia, pneumonia bacterial, bronchopneumonia.
Sinusitis: sinusitis, acute sinusitis, chronic sinusitis, sinobronchitis.
Upper Respiratory Tract Infection: upper respiratory tract infection, laryngitis, laryngopharyngitis, nasopharyngitis, pharyngitis, respiratory tract infection, rhinitis, viral respiratory tract infection.

Less Common Clinical Trial Adverse Drug Reactions: The following adverse events occurred in <2% of CELSENTRI-treated patients. These events have been included because of their seriousness but a causal relationship to CELSENTRI has not been established. Events attributed to the patient's underlying HIV infection are not listed.
Blood and Lymphatic System Disorders: bone marrow failure, marrow depression, coagulopathy, hemolytic anemia, hypoplastic anemia, leukopenia, lymphadenopathy, neutropenia, pancytopenia.
Cardiac Disorders: unstable angina, acute cardiac failure, coronary artery disease, coronary artery occlusion, myocardial infarction, myocardial ischemia.
Ear and Labyrinth Disorders: deafness.
Eye Disorders: cataract, eyelid ptosis, glaucoma, retinal tear.
Gastrointestinal Disorders: hemorrhagic diarrhea, pancreatitis, rectal hemorrhage, small intestinal obstruction, esophageal varices.
Hepatobiliary Disorders: hepatic cirrhosis, hepatic failure, cholestatic jaundice, portal vein thrombosis.
Infections and Infestations: endocarditis, infective myositis, viral meningitis, pneumonia, treponema infections, septic shock.
Metabolism and Nutrition Disorders: diabetes mellitus, tetany.
Musculoskeletal and Connective Tissue Disorders: myositis, osteonecrosis, rhabdomyolysis, blood creatine kinase (CK) increased.
Neoplasms Benign and Malignant: abdominal neoplasm, anal cancer, anaplastic large cell lymphomas T- and null-cell types, bile duct neoplasms malignant, endocrine neoplasms malignant and unspecified, basal cell carcinoma, Bowen's disease, lipoma, lymphoma, metastases to liver, cholangiocarcinoma, esophageal carcinoma, seborrheic keratosis, squamous cell carcinoma, sweat gland tumor, tongue neoplasm (malignant stage unspecified).
Nervous System Disorders: areflexia, cerebrovascular accident, convulsion, epilepsy, facial palsy, loss of consciousness, nervous system disorder, neuritis, Parkinsonism, petit mal epilepsy, polyneuropathy, tremor (excluding congenital).
Psychiatric Disorders: hallucination, auditory hallucination, suicidal ideation.
Renal and Urinary Disorders: oliguria, polyuria, renal failure, acute renal failure.
Respiratory, Thoracic and Mediastinal Disorders: bronchospasm, hemoptysis, respiratory distress, respiratory failure.
Skin and Subcutaneous Tissue Disorders: exfoliative dermatitis, purpura.
Vascular Disorders: aortic arteriosclerosis, peripheral embolism, vasculitis, venous thrombosis.
Laboratory Abnormalities: Table 2 shows the treatment-emergent Grade 3-4 laboratory abnormalities that occurred in ≥2% of patients receiving CELSENTRI.

Table 2: CELSENTRI

Maximum Shift in Laboratory Test Values (Without Regard to Baseline) Incidence ≥2% of Grade 3-4 Abnormalities (ACTG Criteria) Studies in Treatment-Experienced Patients (MOTIVATE 1 and MOTIVATE 2) Pooled Analysis, 48 Weeks

Laboratory Parameter Preferred Term	Limit	CELSENTRI Twice Daily + OBT N=421[a] %	Placebo + OBT N=207[a] %
Aspartate aminotransferase	>5.0×ULN	4.8	2.9
Alanine aminotransferase	>5.0×ULN	2.6	3.4
Total bilirubin	>5.0× ULN	5.5	5.3
Amylase	>2.0× ULN	5.7	5.8
Lipase	>2.0× ULN	4.9	6.3
Absolute neutrophil count	<750/mm³	4.3	2.4

[a] Percentages based on total patients evaluated for each laboratory parameter.

Study in Treatment-naïve Patients (MERIT): Treatment-emergent Adverse Events: The most common adverse events of at least moderate severity (incidence >5%) in a double-blind comparative controlled study in which 721 treatment-naïve patients received CELSENTRI 300 mg BID (N=360) or efavirenz (N=361) in combination with zidovudine/lamivudine for 48 weeks were gastrointestinal events, upper respiratory tract infections, asthenia, and headaches.

Treatment-emergent adverse events that occurred in ≥2% of patients in either the CELSENTRI or efavirenz treatment groups and with at least moderate severity (Grades 2-4) are summarized in Table 3.

Table 3: CELSENTRI

Percentage of Subjects with Selected Treatment-Emergent Adverse Events (All Causality, ≥2% in Either Treatment Group and of At Least Moderate Severity) 96 Weeks Data in Treatment-naïve Patients (MERIT)

	CELSENTRI + ZDV/LMV 300 mg BID N=360 (%)	EFAVIRENZ + ZDV/LMV 600 mg QD N=361 (%)
Blood and Lymphatic System Disorders		
Anemias	4.0	2.0
Neutropenias	3.0	3.0
Ear and Labyrinth Disorders		
Inner ear signs and symptoms	0.6	2.0
Gastrointestinal Disorders		
Nausea and vomiting symptoms	13.0	10.0
Diarrhea	5.0	7.0
Gastrointestinal and abdominal pains	6.0	7.0
Flatulence, bloating and distention	3.0	2.0
General Disorders and Administration Site Conditions		
Asthenic conditions	10.0	8.0
Febrile disorders	3.0	2.0
Infections and Infestations[a]		
Upper respiratory tract infection	11.0	7.0
Bronchitis	8.0	4.0
Influenza	4.0	3.0
Herpes simplex infection	2.0	1.0
Bacterial infections	2.0	0.3

(cont'd)

Table 3: CELSENTRI *(cont'd)*

Percentage of Subjects with Selected Treatment-Emergent Adverse Events (All Causality, ≥2% in Either Treatment Group and of At Least Moderate Severity) 96 Weeks Data in Treatment-naïve Patients (MERIT)

	CELSENTRI + ZDV/LMV 300 mg BID N=360 (%)	EFAVIRENZ + ZDV/LMV 600 mg QD N=361 (%)
Sinusitis	3.0	2.0
Abdominal and GI infections	3.0	4.0
Herpes zoster/varicella	3.0	3.0
Pneumonia	3.0	2.0
Skin structures and soft tissue infections	1.0	3.0
Treponema infections	0.8	2.0
Injury, Poisoning and Procedural Complications		
Non-site specific injuries	0.6	2.0
Metabolism and Nutrition Disorders		
Appetite disorders	2.0	3.0
Musculoskeletal and Connective Tissue Disorders		
Musculoskeletal and connective tissue signs and symptoms	4.0	6.0
Joint related signs and symptoms	2.0	1.0
Nervous System Disorders		
Headaches	8.0	9.0
Neurological signs/symptoms	3.0	10.0
Disturbances in consciousness	3.0	3.0
Mental impairment (excl dementia and memory loss)	0.3	2.0
Psychiatric Disorders		
Disturbances in initiating and maintaining sleep	4.0	5.0
Parasomnias	2.0	5.0
Depressive disorders	3.0	4.0
Anxiety symptoms	2.0	2.0
Respiratory, Thoracic and Mediastinal Disorders		
Coughing and associated symptoms	2.0	2.0
Skin and Subcutaneous Tissue Disorders		
Rash	2.0	6.0
Dermatitis and eczema	0.6	2.0
Pruritus	0.6	2.0
Vascular Disorders		
Vascular hypertensive disorders	2.0	2.0

[a] **MedDRA High Level Terms are shown in order to group related terms for all disorders except Infections and Infestations, which shows MedDRA Preferred Terms with the following related terms grouped:**
Bronchitis: bronchitis, acute bronchitis, bacterial bronchitis.
Herpes Simplex Infection: genital Herpes, Herpes simplex, Herpes virus, Herpes ophthalmic, oral Herpes, proctitis Herpes.
Influenza: influenza, influenza-like illness.
Pneumonia: pneumonia, lobar pneumonia, pneumonia bacterial, bronchopneumonia.
Sinusitis: sinusitis, acute sinusitis, chronic sinusitis, sinobronchitis.
Upper Respiratory Tract Infection: upper respiratory tract infection, laryngitis, laryngopharyngitis, nasopharyngitis, pharyngitis, respiratory tract infection, rhinitis, viral respiratory tract infection.

Laboratory Abnormalities:

Table 4: CELSENTRI

Maximum Shift in Laboratory Test Values (Without Regard to Baseline) Incidence ≥2% of Grade 3-4 Abnormalities (ACTG Criteria) 96 Weeks Data in Treatment-Naïve Patients (MERIT Study)

Laboratory Parameter Preferred Term	Limit	CELSENTRI 300 mg BID + ZDV/LMV N=353[a] %	Efavirenz 600 mg QD + ZDV/LMV N=350[a] %
Aspartate aminotransferase	>5.0×ULN	4.0	4.0
Alanine aminotransferase	>5.0×ULN	3.9	4.0
Creatine kinase		3.9	4.8

(cont'd)

Table 4: CELSENTRI *(cont'd)*

Maximum Shift in Laboratory Test Values (Without Regard to Baseline) Incidence ≥2% of Grade 3-4 Abnormalities (ACTG Criteria) 96 Weeks Data in Treatment-Naïve Patients (MERIT Study)

Laboratory Parameter Preferred Term	Limit	CELSENTRI 300 mg BID + ZDV/LMV N=353[a] %	Efavirenz 600 mg QD + ZDV/LMV N=350[a] %
Amylase	>2.0×ULN	4.3	6.0
Absolute neutrophil count	<750/mm^3	5.7	4.9
Hemoglobin	<7.0 g/dL	2.9	2.3

[a] N=total number of subjects evaluable for laboratory abnormalities.
Percentages based on total patients evaluated for each laboratory parameter. If the same subject in a given treatment group had >1 occurrence of the same abnormality, only the most severe is counted.

Less Common Adverse Events: The following adverse events occurred in <2% of CELSENTRI-treated patients. These events have been included because of their seriousness and either increased frequency on CELSENTRI or are potential risks due to the mechanism of action. Events attributed to the patient's underlying HIV infection are not listed.
Cardiac Disorders: unstable angina, acute cardiac failure, coronary artery disease, coronary artery occlusion, myocardial infarction, myocardial ischemia.
Hepatobiliary Disorders: hepatic cirrhosis, hepatic failure, cholestatic jaundice, hypertransaminasemia, jaundice.
Infections and Infestations: *C. difficile* colitis, meningitis, pneumonia, septic shock.
Musculoskeletal and Connective Tissue Disorders: myositis, osteonecrosis, rhabdomyolysis, blood CK increased.
Neoplasms benign, Malignant and Unspecified (including Cysts and Polyps): abdominal neoplasm, anal cancer, basal cell carcinoma, Bowen's disease, cholangiocarcinoma, diffuse large B-cell lymphoma, lymphoma, metastases to liver, esophageal carcinoma, nasopharyngeal carcinoma, squamous cell carcinoma, squamous cell carcinoma of skin, tongue neoplasm (malignant stage unspecified).
Nervous System Disorders: cerebrovascular accident, convulsions, facial palsy, hemianopia, loss of consciousness, visual field defect.
Post-Market Adverse Drug Reactions: The following events have been identified during post-approval use of CELSENTRI:
Gastrointestinal Disorders: dysphagia, swollen tongue.
Neoplasms Benign, Malignant, and Unspecified (incl cysts and polyps): myelodysplastic syndrome.
Pregnancy, Puerperium and Perinatal Conditions: abortion spontaneous.
Skin and Subcutaneous Tissue Disorders: Stevens-Johnson syndrome, lipodystrophy acquired.

Because they are reported voluntarily from a population of unknown size, estimates of frequency or causal relationship with Celsentri cannot be established.

DRUG INTERACTIONS: Overview: Maraviroc is a substrate of cytochrome P450 CYP3A4. Coadministration of CELSENTRI (maraviroc) with medicinal products that induce CYP3A4 may decrease maraviroc concentrations and reduce its therapeutic effects. Coadministration of CELSENTRI with medicinal products that inhibit CYP3A4 may increase maraviroc plasma concentrations. Dose adjustment of CELSENTRI is recommended when CELSENTRI is coadministered with potent CYP34A inhibitors and/or inducers (see Table 7).

Drug-Drug Interactions: Effect of Maraviroc on the Pharmacokinetics of Concomitant Drugs: Maraviroc is unlikely to inhibit the metabolism of coadministered drugs that are metabolized by cytochrome P450 enzymes because it does not inhibit the seven major cytochrome P450 isoenzymes (CYP1A2, CYP2B6, CYP2C8, CYP2C9, CYP2C19, CYP2D6 and CYP3A4) at clinically relevant concentrations in vitro (IC_{50} >30 μM).

Drug interaction studies were performed with maraviroc and other drugs likely to be coadministered or commonly used as probes for pharmacokinetic interactions (see Table 5 and Table 6). Maraviroc had no effect on the pharmacokinetics of zidovudine or lamivudine, suggesting no interactions with renal clearance or non-P450 metabolism. Maraviroc had no clinically relevant effect on the pharmacokinetics of midazolam, the oral contraceptives ethinyloestradiol and levonorgestrel, no effect on the urinary 6β-hydroxycortisol/cortisol ratio, suggesting no induction of CYP3A4 in vivo. Despite lack of in vitro inhibition of CYP2D6, maraviroc caused an increase in debrisoquine metabolic ratio at 600 mg QD although not at 300 mg BID.

Maraviroc inhibits P-glycoprotein in vitro (IC_{50} is 183 μM). Systemic effects of P-glycoprotein are unlikely to be of relevance. Maraviroc could inhibit P-glycoprotein in the gut and may thus affect bioavailability of certain drugs.

Effect of Concomitant Drugs on the Pharmacokinetics of Maraviroc: Maraviroc is a substrate of CYP3A4 and Pgp and hence its pharmacokinetics are likely to be modulated by inhibitors and inducers of these enzymes/transporters. The CYP3A4/Pgp inhibitors ketoconazole, lopinavir/ritonavir, ritonavir, darunavir/ritonavir, saquinavir/ritonavir and atazanavir±ritonavir all increased the C_{max} and AUC of maraviroc (see Table 7). The CYP3A4 inducers rifampin, efavirenz and etravirine decreased the C_{max} and AUC of maraviroc (see Table 7).

Tipranavir/ritonavir (net CYP3A4 inhibitor/Pgp inducer) did not affect the steady state pharmacokinetics of maraviroc. Substrates and inhibitors of renal clearance (cotrimoxazole and tenofovir) did not affect the pharmacokinetics of maraviroc (see Table 7).

Table 5: CELSENTRI

Established and Other Potentially Significant Drug Interactions: Alterations in Dose or Regimen May be Recommended Based on Drug Interaction Studies or Predicted Interaction (see Table 6 and Table 7)

Drug Class: Drug Name	Clinical Comment
HIV Antiviral Agents: Non-Nucleoside Reverse Transcriptase Inhibitors (NNRTIs):	
Efavirenz	An interaction trial between maraviroc (100 mg twice daily [BID]) and efavirenz (600 mg once daily [QD]) has been performed. In the presence of efavirenz, a decrease of 45% for maraviroc exposure (AUC) was observed. Lower exposure could potentially lead to treatment failure, and therefore the dose of CELSENTRI should be increased to 600 mg BID with efavirenz in the absence of a PI (except tipranavir/ritonavir) or other potent CYP3A4 inhibitor.
Nevirapine	An interaction trial conducted in HIV-infected subjects taking a single dose of maraviroc (300 mg) with nevirapine (200 mg BID), lamivudine (150 mg BID.) and tenofovir (300 mg QD) demonstrated that maraviroc exposure was not significantly affected. The combination of CELSENTRI and nevirapine, lamivudine and tenofovir can be used without dose adjustments.
Delavirdine (not studied)	No interaction trial in healthy volunteers between maraviroc and delavirdine was conducted. Population pharmacokinetics in HIV-infected patients (n=10) determined that delavirdine behaved as a CYP3A4 inhibitor, and increased maraviroc concentrations. Therefore, the CELSENTRI dose should be decreased to 150 mg BID if used with delavirdine.
Etravirine	An interaction trial between maraviroc (300 mg BID) and etravirine (200 mg BID) has been performed. In the presence of these agents, a decrease in the exposure (AUC) of maraviroc was observed (AUC ratio 0.47). Maraviroc did not affect the exposures of etravirine. The CELSENTRI dose should therefore be increased to 600 mg BID with etravirine in the absence of a PI (except tipranavir/ritonavir) or other potent CYP3A4 inhibitor.

(cont'd)

Table 5: CELSENTRI *(cont'd)*

Established and Other Potentially Significant Drug Interactions: Alterations in Dose or Regimen May be Recommended Based on Drug Interaction Studies or Predicted Interaction (see Table 6 and Table 7)

Drug Class: Drug Name	Clinical Comment
Nucleoside Reverse Transcriptase Inhibitors (NRTIs):	
Tenofovir	An interaction trial between maraviroc (300 mg BID) and tenofovir (300 mg BID) has been performed. In the presence of these agents, there was no clinically relevant change in the exposure (AUC) of maraviroc. The effect of maraviroc on tenofovir was not studied and no effect is expected. Therefore the 300 mg BID CELSENTRI dose can be used.
Lamivudine	An interaction trial between maraviroc (300 mg BID) and lamivudine (150 mg BID) has been performed. In the presence of these agents, there was no clinically relevant change in the exposure (AUC) of lamivudine. The effect of lamivudine on maraviroc levels was not assessed and no change is expected. Therefore the 300 mg BID CELSENTRI dose can be used.
Zidovudine	An interaction trial between maraviroc (300 mg BID) and zidovudine (300 mg BID) has been performed. In the presence of these agents, there was no clinically relevant change in the exposure (AUC) of zidovudine. The effect of zidovudine on maraviroc levels was not assessed and no change is expected. Therefore the 300 mg BID CELSENTRI dose can be used.
Raltegravir	An interaction trial between maraviroc (300 mg BID) and raltegravir (400 mg BID) has been performed. No clinically significant interaction was observed between maraviroc and raltegravir. CELSENTRI 300 mg BID and raltegravir can be co-administered without dose adjustment.
Protease Inhibitors (PIs):	
Atazanavir	An interaction trial between maraviroc (300 mg BID) and atazanavir (400 mg QD) has been performed. In the presence of atazanavir, an increase in maraviroc exposure (AUC) was observed (ratio 3.57). The effect of maraviroc on atazanavir was not studied and no effect is expected. The CELSENTRI dose should therefore be decreased to 150 mg BID in the presence of atazanavir.
Atazanavir/ritonavir	An interaction trial between maraviroc (300 mg BID) and atazanavir/ritonavir (300 mg/100 mg QD) has been performed. In the presence of atazanavir/ritonavir, an increase in maraviroc exposure (AUC) was observed (ratio 4.88). The effect of maraviroc on atazanavir/ritonavir was not studied and no effect is expected. The CELSENTRI dose should therefore be decreased to 150 mg BID in the presence of atazanavir/ritonavir.
Lopinavir/ritonavir	Two interaction trials between maraviroc (300 mg BID) and lopinavir/ritonavir (400 mg/100 mg BID) have been performed. In the presence of lopinavir/ritonavir, an increase in maraviroc exposure (AUC) was observed (ratios 3.95 and 3.83). The effect of maraviroc on lopinavir/ritonavir was not studied and no effect is expected. The CELSENTRI dose should therefore be decreased to 150 mg BID in the presence of lopinavir/ritonavir.
Saquinavir/ritonavir	Two interaction trials between maraviroc (100 mg BID) and saquinavir/ritonavir (1000 mg/100 mg BID) have been performed. In the presence of saquinavir/ritonavir, an increase in maraviroc exposure (AUC) was observed (ratios 8.32 and 9.77). The effect of maraviroc on saquinavir/ritonavir was not studied and no effect is expected. The CELSENTRI dose should therefore be decreased to 150 mg BID in the presence of saquinavir/ritonavir.
Darunavir/ritonavir	An interaction trial between maraviroc (150 mg BID) and darunavir/ritonavir (600 mg/100 mg BID) has been performed. In the presence of darunavir/ritonavir, an increase in maraviroc exposure (AUC) was observed (ratio 4.05). Darunavir and ritonavir levels were consistent with historical data. Dose should therefore be decreased to 150 mg BID in the presence of darunavir/ritonavir.
Tipranavir/ritonavir	An interaction trial between maraviroc (150 mg BID) and tipranavir/ritonavir (500 mg/200 mg BID) has been performed. In the presence of these agents, there was no clinically relevant change in the exposure (AUC) of maraviroc. Tipranavir levels were consistent with historical data. Therefore the 300 mg BID CELSENTRI dose can be used.
Saquinavir	An interaction trial between maraviroc (100 mg BID) and saquinavir (1200 mg TID) has been performed. In the presence of saquinavir, an increase in maraviroc exposure (AUC) was observed (ratio 4.25). The effect of maraviroc on saquinavir was not studied and no effect is expected. The CELSENTRI dose should therefore be decreased to 150 mg BID in the presence of saquinavir.
Ritonavir	An interaction trial between maraviroc (100 mg BID) and ritonavir (100 mg BID) has been performed. In the presence of ritonavir, an increase in maraviroc exposure (AUC) was observed (ratio 2.61). The effect of maraviroc on ritonavir was not studied and no effect is expected. The CELSENTRI dose should therefore be decreased to 150 mg BID in the presence of ritonavir.
Nelfinavir (not studied)	No interaction trial in healthy volunteers between maraviroc and nelfinavir was conducted. However, nelfinavir is considered to be a potent CYP3A4 inhibitor and would be expected to increase maraviroc concentration. The CELSENTRI dose should therefore be decreased to 150 mg BID in the presence of nelfinavir.
Indinavir (not studied)	No interaction trial in healthy volunteers between maraviroc and indinavir was conducted. Population pharmacokinetics in HIV-infected patients (n=10) determined that indinavir behaved as a potent CYP3A4 inhibitor. The CELSENTRI dose should therefore be decreased to 150 mg BID in the presence of indinavir.
NNRTI + PI:	
Efavirenz + Lopinavir/ritonavir	An interaction trial between maraviroc (300 mg BID) and lopinavir/ritonavir (400 mg/100 mg BID) + efavirenz (600 mg QD) has been performed. In the presence of these agents, an increase in the exposure (AUC) of maraviroc was observed (AUC ratio 2.53). The effect of maraviroc on lopinavir/ritonavir + efavirenz was not studied and no effect is expected. The CELSENTRI dose should therefore be decreased to 150 mg BID in the presence of lopinavir/ritonavir + efavirenz.

(cont'd)

Table 5: CELSENTRI *(cont'd)*

Established and Other Potentially Significant Drug Interactions: Alterations in Dose or Regimen May be Recommended Based on Drug Interaction Studies or Predicted Interaction (see Table 6 and Table 7)

Drug Class: Drug Name	Clinical Comment
Efavirenz + Saquinavir/ritonavir	An interaction trial between maraviroc (100 mg BID) and saquinavir/ritonavir (1000 mg/100 mg BID) + efavirenz (600 mg QD) has been performed. In the presence of these agents, an increase in the exposure (AUC) of maraviroc was observed (AUC ratio 5.00). The effect of maraviroc on saquinavir/ritonavir + efavirenz was not studied and no effect is expected. The CELSENTRI dose should therefore be decreased to 150 mg BID in the presence of saquinavir/ritonavir + efavirenz.
Etravirine + Darunavir/ritonavir	An interaction trial between maraviroc (150 mg BID) and etravirine (200 mg BID) + darunavir/ritonavir (600 mg/100 mg BID) has been performed. In the presence of these agents, an increase in the exposure (AUC) of maraviroc was observed (AUC ratio 3.10). The effect of maraviroc on etravirine + darunavir/ritonavir is not clinically significant. The CELSENTRI dose should therefore be decreased to 150 mg BID in the presence of etravirine + darunavir/ritonavir.
Efavirenz + Didanosine EC + Tenofovir	An interaction trial conducted in HIV-infected subjects taking a single dose of maraviroc (300 mg) and efavirenz (600 mg QD) + didanosine EC (250 mg QD) + tenofovir (300 mg QD) has been performed. In the presence of efavirenz + didanosine + tenofovir, a decrease of 52% for maraviroc exposure (AUC) was observed. The effect of maraviroc on efavirenz, didanosine and tenofovir was not studied and no effect is expected. Lower maraviroc exposure could potentially lead to treatment failure, and therefore the combination of CELSENTRI and efavirenz + didanosine + tenofovir should not be used without a dosage increase to 600 mg BID for CELSENTRI.
Other HIV Combinations:	
Efavirenz + Lamivudine/zidovudine	An interaction trial conducted in HIV-infected subjects taking a single dose of maraviroc (300 mg) and efavirenz (600 mg QD) + lamivudine/zidovudine (150 mg/ 300 mg BID) has been performed. In the presence of efavirenz + lamivudine/zidovudine, a decrease of 53% for maraviroc exposure (AUC) was observed. The effect of maraviroc on efavirenz, lamivudine and zidovudine was not studied and no effect is expected. Lower maraviroc exposure could potentially lead to treatment failure, and therefore in the presence of efavirenz + lamivudine/zidovudine. The CELSENTRI dose should therefore be increased to 600 mg BID.
Nevirapine + Lamivudine + Tenofovir	An interaction trial conducted in HIV-infected subjects taking a single dose of maraviroc (300 mg) nevirapine (200 mg BID) + lamivudine (150 mg BID) + tenofovir (300 mg QD) has been performed. In the presence of these agents, there was no clinically relevant change in the exposure (AUC) of maraviroc. The effect of maraviroc on nevirapine, lamivudine and tenofovir was not studied and no effect is expected. This indicates that the 300 mg BID CELSENTRI dose can be used.
Lopinavir/ritonavir + Lamivudine + Stavudine	An interaction trial conducted in HIV-infected subjects taking a single dose of maraviroc (300 mg) and lopinavir/ritonavir (400 mg/100 mg BID) + lamivudine (150 mg BID) + stavudine (40 mg BID) has been performed. In the presence of lopinavir/ritonavir + lamivudine + stavudine, an increase in maraviroc exposure (AUC) was observed (ratio 2.65). The effect of maraviroc on lopinavir/ritonavir + lamivudine + stavudine was not studied and no effect is expected. The CELSENTRI dose should therefore be decreased to 150 mg BID in the presence of lopinavir/ritonavir + lamivudine + stavudine.
Antifungals/Antibacterials:	
Ketoconazole	An interaction trial between maraviroc (100 mg BID) and ketoconazole (400 mg QD) has been performed. In the presence of ketoconazole, an increase in maraviroc exposure (AUC) was observed (ratio 5.01). The effect of maraviroc on ketoconazole was not studied and no effect is expected. The CELSENTRI dose should therefore be decreased to 150 mg BID in the presence of ketoconazole.
Itraconazole (not studied)	No interaction trial in healthy volunteers between maraviroc and itraconazole was conducted. However, like ketoconazole (see Table 8) itraconazole is a potent CYP3A4 inhibitor and would be expected to increase the exposure of CELSENTRI. The CELSENTRI dose should therefore be decreased to 150 mg BID in the presence of itraconazole.
Voriconazole (not studied)	No interaction trial in healthy volunteers between maraviroc and voriconazole was conducted. However, voriconazole is considered to be a moderate CYP3A4 inhibitor and the CELSENTRI dose of 300 mg BID should be administered with caution.
Fluconazole (not studied)	No interaction trial in healthy volunteers between maraviroc and fluconazole was conducted. However, fluconazole is considered to be a moderate CYP3A4 inhibitor and the CELSENTRI dose of 300 mg BID should be administered with caution.
Rifampin	An interaction trial between maraviroc (100 mg BID) and rifampin (600 mg QD) has been performed. In the presence of rifampin, a decrease of 63% for maraviroc exposure (AUC) was observed. Lower exposure could potentially lead to treatment failure, and therefore in the presence of rifampin the CELSENTRI dose should be increased to 600 mg BID.
Sulfamethoxazole/ trimethoprim	An interaction trial between maraviroc (300 mg BID) and sulfamethoxazole/trimethoprim (800 mg/160 mg BID) has been performed. In the presence of these agents, there was no clinically relevant change in the exposure (AUC) of maraviroc indicating that the 300 mg BID CELSENTRI dose can be used.
Telithromycin and Clarithromycin (not studied)	No interaction trials in healthy volunteers between maraviroc and telithromycin or clarithromycin were conducted. However, like ketoconazole (see Table 8) telithromycin and clarithromycin are potent CYP3A4 inhibitors and would be expected to increase the exposure of CELSENTRI. The CELSENTRI dose should therefore be decreased to 150 mg BID in the presence of either telithromycin or clarithromycin.
Analgesics:	
Midazolam	An interaction trial between maraviroc (300 mg BID) and midazolam (7.5 mg QD) has been performed. In the presence of maraviroc, an increase of 18% for midazolam exposure (AUC) was observed, indicating that maraviroc is not an inhibitor of the CYP3A4 enzyme.

(cont'd)

Table 5: CELSENTRI *(cont'd)*

Established and Other Potentially Significant Drug Interactions: Alterations in Dose or Regimen May be Recommended Based on Drug Interaction Studies or Predicted Interaction (see Table 6 and Table 7)

Drug Class: Drug Name	Clinical Comment
Methadone (not studied)	No interaction trial in healthy volunteers between maraviroc and methadone was conducted. No interaction is expected.
Buprenorphine (not studied)	No interaction trial in healthy volunteers between maraviroc and buprenorphine was conducted. No interaction is expected.
Phosphodiesterase-5 Inhibitors:	
Sildenafil (not studied)	No interaction trial in healthy volunteers between maraviroc and sildenafil was conducted. Though no pharmacokinetic interaction is expected, both CELSENTRI and the PDE-5 inhibitors have reported hypotension adverse effects, as such the CELSENTRI dose of 300 mg BID should be administered with caution.
Oral Contraceptives:	
Ethinylestradiol and Levonorgestrel	An interaction trial between maraviroc (100 mg BID) and ethinylestradiol (30 µg QD) and levonorgestrel (150 µg QD) has been performed. In the presence of maraviroc, there was no observed change in the exposure (AUC) of either ethinylestradiol or levonorgestrel, suggesting no potential for an interaction with these oral contraceptives.
Antivirals:	
HCV Agents (not studied)	No interaction trial in healthy volunteers between maraviroc and pegylated interferon and ribavirin was conducted. No interaction is expected.
Lipid Lowering Medicinal Products:	
Statins (not studied)	No interaction trial in healthy volunteers between maraviroc and a statin was conducted. No interaction is expected.

Table 6: CELSENTRI

Drug Interactions: Effect of Maraviroc on the Pharmacokinetics of Co-administered Drugs

Coadministered Drug	Dose of Coadministered Drug	Dose of Maraviroc	N	Ratio (90% CI) of Coadministered Drug Pharmacokinetic Parameters with/without Maraviroc (no effect=1.00)		
				C_{max}	AUC_t	C_{min}
Midazolam	7.5 mg QD	300 mg BID	12	↑1.21 (0,92, 1,60)	1.18 (1,04, 1,34)	ND
Ethinylestradiol	30 µg QD	100 mg BID	15	↑0.98 (0.91, 1.06)	1.00 (0.95, 1.05)	1.16 (1.08, 1.26)
Levonorgestrel	150 µg QD	100 mg BID	15	↑1.00 (0.93, 1.08)	0.99 (0.92, 1.04)	0.99 (0.93, 1.06)
Etravirine	200 mg BID	300 mg BID	14	↑1.05 (0.95, 1.17)	1.06 (0.99, 1.14)	1.08 (0.98, 1.19)
Darunavi/Ritonavir + Etravirine	600 mg BID/100 mg BID + 200 mg BID	150 mg BID	10	↑0.96 (0.84, 1.10) 1.02 (0.80, 1.30) 1.08 (0.98, 1.20)	0.86 (0.76, 0.96) 0.93 (0.75, 1.16) 1.00 (0.86, 1.15)	0.77 (0.69, 0.85) 0.74 (0.63, 0.86) 0.81 (0.65, 1.01)
Raltegravir	400 mg BID	300 mg BID	17	↑0.67 (0.41, 1.08)	0.63 (0.44, 0.90)	0.72 (0.58, 0.90)
Zidovudine/ Lamivudine	300 mg BID/150 mg BID	300 mg BID	12	↑0.92 (0.68, 1.24) 1.16 (0.88, 1.54)	0.98 (0.79, 1.22) 1.14 (0.98, 1.32)	1.22 (0.99, 1.49) 1.35 (1.14, 1.61)

ND: not determined.

Table 7: CELSENTRI

Drug Interactions: Effect of Co-administered Drugs on the Pharmacokinetics of Maraviroc

Coadministered Drug	Dose of Coadministered Drug	Dose of Maraviroc	N	PK Change	Ratio (90% CI) of Maraviroc Pharmacokinetic Parameters with/without Coadministered Drug (no effect=1.00)		
					C_{max}	AUC	C_{min}
CYP3A4 and/or P-gp Inhibitors							
Ketoconazole	400 mg QD	100 mg BID	12	↑	3.38 (2.38, 4.78)	5.01 (3.98, 6.29)	3.75 (3.01, 4.69)
Saquinavir	1200 mg TID	100 mg BID	12	↑	3.32 (2.45, 4.49)	4.25 (3.47, 5.19)	ND
Lopinavir/ ritonavir	400 mg/ 100 mg BID	100 mg BID	8	↑	1.61 (0.99, 2.63)	3.83 (2.81, 5.21)	ND

(cont'd)

Table 7: CELSENTRI *(cont'd)*

Drug Interactions: Effect of Co-administered Drugs on the Pharmacokinetics of Maraviroc

Coadministered Drug	Dose of Coadministered Drug	Dose of Maraviroc	N	PK Change	Ratio (90% CI) of Maraviroc Pharmacokinetic Parameters with/without Coadministered Drug (no effect=1.00)		
					C_{max}	AUC	C_{min}
Lopinavir/ ritonavir	400 mg/ 100 mg BID	300 mg BID	11	↑	1.97 (1.66, 2.34)	3.95 (3.43, 4.56)	9.24 (7.98, 10.7)
Ritonavir	100 mg BID	100 mg BID	8	↑	1.28 (0.79, 2.09)	2.61 (1.92, 3.56)	4.55 (3.37, 6.13)
Saquinavir/ ritonavir	1000 mg/ 100 mg BID	100 mg BID	8	↑	4.23 (2.60, 6.88)	8.32 (6.11, 11.30)	ND
Saquinavir/ ritonavir	1000 mg/ 100 mg BID	100 mg BID	11	↑	4.78 (3.41, 6.71)	9.77 (7.87, 12.10)	11.3 (8.96, 14.1)
Atazanavir	400 mg QD	300 mg BID	12	↑	2.09 (1.72, 2.55)	3.57 (3.30, 3.87)	4.19 (3.65, 4.80
Atazanavir/ ritonavir	300 mg/ 100 mg QD	300 mg BID	12	↑	2.67 (2.32, 3.08)	4.88 (4.40, 5.41)	6.67 (5.78, 7.70
Lopinavir/ ritonavir + Lamivudine + Stavudine	400/100 mg BID + 150 mg BID + 40 mg BID	300 mg single dose	5	↑	1.80[a] (1.03, 3.14)	2.65[a] (1.61, 4.35)	ND
Darunavir/ ritonavir	600 mg/ 100 mg BID	150 mg BID	15	↑	2.29 (1.46, 3.59)	4.05 (2.95, 5.59)	8.00 (6.35, 10.1)
CYP3A4 and/or P-gp Inducers							
Efavirenz	600 mg QD	100 mg BID	12	↓	0.49 (0.38, 0.63)	0.55 (0.49, 0.62)	0.55 (0.43, 0.72)
Efavirenz + Lamivudine/ zidovudine	600 mg QD + 150 mg BID/ 300 mg BID	300 mg single dose	8	↓	0.67[a] (0.41, 1.09)	0.46[a] (0.30, 0.72)	ND
Efavirenz + Didanosine EC + Tenofovir DF	600 mg QD + 250 mg QD + 300 mg QD	300 mg single dose	8	↓	0.76[a] (0.47, 1.25)	0.48[a] (0.31, 0.75)	ND
Rifampin	600 mg QD	100 mg BID	12	↓	0.34 (0.26, 0.43)	0.37 (0.33, 0.41)	0.22 (0.17, 0.28)
Etravirine	200 mg BID	300 mg BID	14	↓	0.40 (0.28, 0.57)	0.47 (0.38, 0.58)	0.47 (0.38, 0.58)
Nevirapine + Lamivudine + Tenofovir DF	200 mg BID + 300 mg QD + 300 mg QD	300 mg single dose	8	↔	1.54[a] (0.94, 2.51)	1.01[a] (0.65, 1.55)	ND
CYP3A4 and/or P-gp Inhibitors + Inducers							
Lopinavir/ ritonavir + Efavirenz	400 mg/ 100 mg BID + 600 mg QD	300 mg BID	11	↑	1.25 (1.01, 1.55)	2.53 (2.24, 2.87)	6.29 (4.72, 8.39)
Saquinavir/ ritonavir + Efavirenz	1000 mg/ 100 mg BID + 600 mg QD	100 mg BID	11	↑	2.26 (1.64, 3.11)	5.00 (4.26, 5.87)	8.42 (6.46, 10.97)
Darunavir/ Ritonavir + Etravirine	600 mg/100 mg BID + 200 mg BID	150 mg BID	10	↑	1.77 (1.20, 2.60)	3.1 (2.57, 3.74)	5.27 (4.51, 6.15)
Tipranavir/ ritonavir	500 mg/ 200 mg BID	150 mg BID	12	↔	0.86 (0.61, 1.21)	1.02 (0.85, 1.23)	1.80 (0.85, 1.23)
Raltegravir	400 mg BID	300 mg BID	17	↔	0.79 (0.67, 0.94)	0.86 (0.80, 0.92)	0.90 (0.85, 0.96)
Renal Substrates/Inhibitors							
Sulfamethoxazole/ trimethoprim	800 mg/ 160 mg BID	300 mg BID	15	↔	1.19 (1.04, 1.37)	1.11 (1.01, 1.21)	0.90 (0.80, 1.00)
Tenofovir DF	300 mg QD	300 mg BID	12	↔	1.04 (0.90, 1.19)	1.03 (0.98, 1.09)	ND

[a] In HIV patients, compared to historical controls.
ND: not determined.

Drug-Food Interactions: Coadministration of a 300 mg tablet with a high fat breakfast reduced maraviroc C_{max} and AUC by 33% in healthy volunteers. There were no food restrictions in the studies that demonstrated the efficacy and safety of maraviroc. Therefore, maraviroc can be taken with or without food at the recommended dose (see Dosage and Administration).

Drug-Herb Interactions: Concomitant use of maraviroc and St. John's wort (Hypericum perforatum) or products containing St. John's wort is not recommended. Coadministration of maraviroc with St. John's wort is expected to substantially decrease maraviroc concentrations and may result in suboptimal levels of maraviroc and lead to loss of virologic response and possible resistance to maraviroc.

Drug-Laboratory Test Interactions: Interactions with laboratory tests have not been established.

DOSAGE AND ADMINISTRATION:

Dosing Considerations: CELSENTRI (maraviroc) must be taken every day in combination with other antiretroviral agents. The recommended dose is 300 mg twice daily but adjustments are recommended based on the patient's concomitant medications. CELSENTRI can be taken with or without food.

Recommended Dose and Dosage Adjustment: Adults: The recommended dose of CELSENTRI is 300 mg twice daily. A dose adjustment may be needed due to the potential for drug interactions (see Table 8 and Drug Interactions, Drug-Drug Interactions, Table 5).

Table 8: CELSENTRI

Recommended Dosing Regimen

Concomitant Medications	CELSENTRI Dose
Potent CYP3A4 inhibitors (with or without a CYP3A4 inducer) including: • protease inhibitors (except tipranavir/ritonavir) • delavirdine • ketoconazole, itraconazole, clarithromycin, telithromycin	150 mg twice daily
Potent CYP3A4 inducers (without a potent CYP3A4 inhibitor) including: • efavirenz • rifampin • etravirine • carbamazepine, phenobarbital and phenytoin	600 mg twice daily
Other concomitant medications, including all other antiretrovirals including tipranavir/ritonavir, raltegravir, all NRTIs and enfuvirtide	300 mg twice daily

Pediatrics (<16 years of age): The pharmacokinetics, safety and efficacy of maraviroc in pediatric patients have not been established. Therefore, maraviroc should not be used in this patient population.

Geriatrics (>65 years of age): There were insufficient numbers of subjects aged 65 and over in the clinical studies to determine whether they respond differently from younger subjects. In general, caution should be exercised when administering CELSENTRI in elderly patients, also reflecting the greater frequency of decreased hepatic and renal function, of concomitant disease and other drug therapy.

Renal Impairment: The safety and efficacy of maraviroc have not been specifically studied in patients with renal impairment, therefore maraviroc should be used with caution in this population. In the absence of metabolic inhibitors, renal clearance accounts for less than 25% of total clearance of maraviroc. However, in the presence of metabolic inhibitors, renal clearance may account for up to 70% of total clearance of maraviroc, hence renal impairment may result in increased maraviroc exposures in this case. Therefore, maraviroc should be used with caution in patients with renal impairment (CL_{cr} <80 mL/min) who are also taking potent CYP3A4 inhibitors.

Table 9 provides dose interval adjustment guidelines based on simulations of increasing renal impairment in patients being coadministered potent CYP3A4 inhibitors. The safety and efficacy of these dose interval adjustments have not been clinically evaluated. Therefore, clinical response to treatment and renal function should be closely monitored in these patients.

Table 9: CELSENTRI

Dose Interval Adjustments Based on Simulations of Increasing Renal Impairment in Patients Being Coadministered Potent CYP3A4 Inhibitors

	Creatinine Clearance (CLcr) (mL/min)		
Recommended CELSENTRI Dose Interval	**50–80 mL/min**	**30–50 mL/min**	**<30 mL/min**
If coadministered without potent CYP3A4 inhibitors or coadministered with tipranavir/ritonavir	Every 12 hours	Every 12 hours	Every 12 hours
If coadministered with potent CYP3A4 inhibitors (e.g. PIs including lopinavir/ritonavir, darunavir/ritonavir, atazanavir/ritonavir (except tipranavir/ritonavir), saquinavir/ritonavir), ketoconazole, itraconazole, clarithromycin, telithromycin)	Every 24 hours	Every 24 hours	Every 24 hours
If coadministered with saquinavir/ritonavir	Every 24 hours	Every 48 hours	Every 72 hours

Missed Dose: If a dose is missed, patients should take the next dose as soon as possible. A dose should not be doubled.

OVERDOSAGE:

There is no specific antidote for overdose with maraviroc. Treatment of overdose should consist of general supportive measures including keeping the patient in a supine position, careful assessment of patient vital signs, blood pressure and ECG. Administration of activated charcoal may be used to aid in removal of unabsorbed drug. Since maraviroc is moderately protein bound, dialysis may be beneficial in removal of this medicine.

The highest dose administered in clinical studies was 1200 mg. The dose limiting adverse event was postural hypotension.

Prolongation of the QT interval was seen in dogs and monkeys at plasma concentrations 6 and 12 times, respectively, those expected in humans at the maximum recommended dose of 300 mg twice daily. However, no significant QT prolongation was seen in the Phase 3 clinical studies using the recommended doses of maraviroc or in a specific pharmacokinetic study to evaluate the potential of maraviroc to prolong the QT interval (see Action and Clinical Pharmacology, Pharmacokinetics, Effects on Electrocardiogram).

For management of a suspected drug overdose, contact your regional Poison Control Centre. See the *CPS* Directory section for a list of Poison Control Centres.

ACTION AND CLINICAL PHARMACOLOGY: Mechanism of Action: Maraviroc is a member of a therapeutic class called CCR5 antagonists. Maraviroc selectively binds to the human chemokine CCR5 coreceptor and inhibits the interaction of the envelope glycoprotein (gp120) from CCR5-tropic HIV-1 strains with CCR5 coreceptor. Binding of gp120 to CCR5 coreceptor is an essential step in the HIV-1 entry process for CCR5-tropic viruses (i.e. viruses that use only CCR5 coreceptor for entry). Maraviroc has no activity against viruses that can use CXCR4 as their coreceptor. These CXCR4-using viruses include dual-tropic viruses (which can use either CCR5 or CXCR4 coreceptors), mixed-tropic viruses (which consist of a mixture of CCR5-tropic and CXCR4-tropic viruses) or CXCR4-tropic viruses (which can use only CXCR4 coreceptor for entry).

Pharmacodynamics: Maraviroc inhibits the replication of CCR5-tropic laboratory strains and clinical isolates of HIV-1 in models of acute T-cell infection.

Exposure Response Relationship in Treatment-Experienced Subjects: The relationship between maraviroc modeled plasma trough concentration (C_{min}) (1-9 samples per patient taken on up to 7 visits) and virologic response (<400 copies/mL viral RNA at 24 weeks, discontinuation=failure) was evaluated in 594 treatment-experienced HIV-1-infected subjects with varied optimized background antiretroviral regimens in treatment-experienced patients studies (MOTIVATE 1 and MOTIVATE 2). Table 10 illustrates the proportion of subjects with virologic success (%) at 24 weeks within each C_{min} quartile for maraviroc 150 mg twice daily and 300 mg twice daily compared with equivalent placebo plus optimized background therapy.

The C_{min} exposure response relationships shown in Table 10 above are specific to 300 mg twice daily dosing given in the absence of potent CYP3A4/Pgp inhibitors and 150 mg twice daily in the presence of potent CYP3A4/Pgp inhibitors. Near maximal response is achieved between C_{min} Quartiles 2 and 4.

Exposure Response Relationship in Treatment-Naïve Subjects: The relationship between maraviroc modeled plasma trough concentration (C_{min}) (1-12 samples per patient taken on up to 8 visits) and virologic response (<50 copies/mL viral RNA at 48 weeks, discontinuation=failure) was evaluated in 294 treatment-naïve HIV-1-infected subjects receiving maraviroc 300 mg twice daily in combination with zidovudine/lamivudine in treatment-naïve patients study (MERIT). Table 11 illustrates the proportion of subjects with virologic success (%) within each C_{min} quartile.

Table 10: CELSENTRI

Treatment-Experienced Subjects with Virologic Success by C_{min} Quartile (Q1-Q4)

	150 mg BID (with CYP3A inhibitors)			300 mg BID (without CYP3A inhibitors)		
	n	**Median C_{min}**	**% Subjects with Virologic Success**	**n**	**Median C_{min}**	**% Subjects with Virologic Success**
Placebo	160	—	30.6	35	—	28.6
Q1	78	33	52.6	22	13	50.0
Q2	77	87	63.6	22	29	68.2
Q3	78	166	78.2	22	46	63.6
Q4	78	279	74.4	22	97	68.2

Table 11: CELSENTRI

Treatment-Naïve Subjects with Virologic Success by C_{min} Quartile (Q1-Q4)

	300 mg BID		
	n	**Median C_{min}**	**% Subjects with Virologic Success**
Q1	75	23	57.3
Q2	72	39	72.2
Q3	73	56	74.0
Q4	74	81	83.8

The relationship between low C_{min} and lack of virologic success shown in Q1 in Table 11 is explained by poor adherence to antiretroviral treatment. Fifteen of 32 subjects (47%) in Q1 who were classed as failures (discontinuation=failure) at 48 weeks had no measurable maraviroc concentration on one or more visits indicating poor adherence to treatment.

Pharmacokinetics: Healthy volunteer (phase 1) and phase 2a asymptomatic patient exposures are derived from non-compartmental analysis using full pharmacokinetic profiles while the phase 2b/3 patient exposures are derived from population modeling of sparse samples after outpatient dosing. See Table 12.

Table 12: CELSENTRI

Mean Maraviroc Pharmacokinetic Parameters

	Maraviroc Dose	N	AUC_{12} (ng·h/mL)	C_{max} (ng/mL)	C_{min} (ng/mL)
Healthy volunteers (phase 1)	300 mg twice daily	64	2908	888	43.1
Asymptomatic HIV patients (phase 2a)	300 mg twice daily	8	2550	618	33.6
Treatment-experienced HIV patients (phase 3)[a]	300 mg twice daily	94	1513	266	37.2
	150 mg twice daily (+ CYP3A inhibitor)	375	2463	332	101
Treatment-naïve HIV patients (phase 2b/3)[a]	300 mg twice daily	344	1865	287	60

[a] Estimated exposures from modeling phase 3 data may differ from noncompartmental analysis of phase 1/2a study data due to methodology, sparse sampling, food effects, compliance and concomitant medications.

Absorption: Peak maraviroc plasma concentrations are attained 0.5-4 h following single oral doses of 1-1200 mg administered to uninfected volunteers. The pharmacokinetics of oral maraviroc are not dose proportional over the dose range.

The absolute bioavailability of a 100 mg dose is 23% and is predicted to be 33% at 300 mg. Maraviroc is a substrate for the efflux transporter P-glycoprotein.

Effect of Food on Oral Absorption: Coadministration of a 300 mg tablet with a high fat breakfast reduced maraviroc C_{max} and AUC by 33% in healthy volunteers. There were no food restrictions in the studies that demonstrated the efficacy and safety of maraviroc. Therefore, maraviroc can be taken with or without food at the recommended dose (see Dosage and Administration).

Distribution: Maraviroc is bound (approximately 76%) to human plasma proteins, and shows moderate affinity for albumin and alpha-1 acid glycoprotein. The volume of distribution of maraviroc is approximately 194 L.

Preclinical data in the rat indicate CSF exposure with concentrations ~10% of free plasma concentrations.

Metabolism: Studies in humans and in vitro studies using human liver microsomes and expressed enzymes have demonstrated that maraviroc is principally metabolized by the cytochrome P450 system to metabolites that are essentially inactive against HIV-1. In vitro studies indicate that CYP3A4 is the major enzyme responsible for maraviroc metabolism. In vitro studies also indicate that polymorphic enzymes CYP2C9, CYP2D6 and CYP2C19 do not contribute significantly to the metabolism of maraviroc.

Maraviroc is the major circulating component (~42% drug related radioactivity) following a single oral dose of 300 mg [^{14}C]-maraviroc to healthy male volunteers. The most significant circulating metabolite in humans is a secondary amine (~22% radioactivity) formed by N-dealkylation. This polar metabolite has no significant pharmacological activity. Other metabolites are products of mono-oxidation and are only minor components of plasma drug related radioactivity.

Excretion: The terminal half-life of maraviroc following oral dosing to steady-state in healthy subjects was 14-18 hours. A mass balance/excretion study was conducted using a single 300 mg dose of ^{14}C labeled maraviroc. Approximately 20% of the radiolabel was recovered in the urine and 76% was recovered in the feces over 168 hours. Maraviroc was the major component present in urine (mean of 8% dose) and feces (mean of 25% dose). The remainder was excreted as metabolites.

Effects on Electrocardiogram: A placebo-controlled, randomized, crossover study to evaluate the effect on the QT interval of healthy male and female volunteers was conducted with 3 single oral doses of maraviroc and moxifloxacin. The placebo-adjusted mean maximum increases in QTc from baseline after 100, 300 and 900 mg of maraviroc were −2.3, −0.6, and 1.0 msec, respectively, and 12.9 msec for moxifloxacin 400 mg. No subject in any group had an increase in QTc of ≥60 msec from baseline. No subject experienced an interval exceeding the potentially clinically relevant threshold of 500 msec. No clinically significant QT prolongation was seen in the studies in treatment-experienced and treatment-naïve subjects with HIV using the recommended doses of maraviroc.

Special Populations and Conditions: Hepatic Impairment: Maraviroc is primarily metabolized and eliminated by the liver. A study compared the pharmacokinetics of a single 300 mg dose of CELSENTRI in patients with mild (Child-Pugh Class A, n=8), and moderate (Child-Pugh Class B, n=8) hepatic impairment compared to healthy subjects (n=8). Geometric mean ratios for C_{max} and AUC_{last} were 11% and 25% higher respectively for subjects with mild hepatic impairment, and 32% and 46% higher respectively for subjects with moderate hepatic impairment compared to subjects with normal hepatic function. The pharmacokinetics of maraviroc have not been studied in subjects with severe hepatic impairment (see Warnings and Precautions).

Renal Insufficiency: The safety and efficacy of maraviroc have not been specifically studied in patients with renal impairment, therefore maraviroc should be used with caution in this population. In the absence of metabolic inhibitors, renal clearance accounts for less than 25% of total clearance of maraviroc. However, in the presence of metabolic inhibitors, renal clearance may account for up to 70% of total clearance of maraviroc, hence renal impairment may result in increased maraviroc exposures in this case (see Dosage and Administration).

STORAGE AND STABILITY: CELSENTRI (maraviroc) film-coated tablets should be stored at 15 to 30°C in a USP tight container.

INFORMATION FOR THE PATIENT: Published in e-CPS, available by subscription at www.e-cps.ca.

DOSAGE FORMS, COMPOSITION AND PACKAGING: 150 mg: Each blue, biconvex, oval, film-coated tablet, debossed with "Pfizer" on one side and "MVC 150" on the other, contains: maraviroc 150 mg. Nonmedicinal ingredients: dibasic calcium phosphate (anhydrous), magnesium stearate, microcrystalline cellulose and sodium starch glycolate; film-coating [Opadry II Blue (85G20583)]: FD&C blue #2 aluminum lake, polyethylene glycol (macrogol 3350), polyvinyl alcohol, soya lecithin, talc and titanium dioxide. High density polyethylene bottles (HDPE) with polypropylene child resistant (CR) closures and an aluminium foil/polyethylene heat induction seal of 30, 60, 120 and 180. Polyvinyl chloride (PVC) blisters with aluminium foil backing, cartons of 30, 60, 90 and 180 (2×90).

300 mg: Each blue, biconvex, oval, film-coated tablet, debossed with "Pfizer" on one side and "MVC 300" on the other, contains: maraviroc 300 mg. Nonmedicinal ingredients: dibasic calcium phosphate (anhydrous), magnesium stearate, microcrystalline cellulose and sodium starch glycolate; film-coating [Opadry II Blue (85G20583)]: FD&C blue #2 aluminum lake, polyethylene glycol (macrogol 3350), polyvinyl alcohol, soya lecithin, talc and titanium dioxide. High density polyethylene bottles (HDPE) with polypropylene child resistant (CR) closures and an aluminium foil/polyethylene heat induction seal of 30, 60, 120 and 180. Polyvinyl chloride (PVC) blisters with aluminium foil backing, cartons of 30, 60, 90 and 180 (2×90).

(Shown in product Identification Section)

Centrum®
multiple vitamins and minerals
Vitamin-Mineral Supplement

Pfizer Consumer Healthcare

Centrum Advantage®
multiple vitamins and minerals
Vitamin-Mineral Supplement

Pfizer Consumer Healthcare

Centrum Cardio®
multiple vitamins and minerals
Vitamin-Mineral Supplement

Pfizer Consumer Healthcare

Centrum Forte®
multiple vitamins and minerals
Vitamin-Mineral Supplement

Pfizer Consumer Healthcare

Centrum Performance®
multiple vitamins and minerals
Vitamin-Mineral Supplement

Pfizer Consumer Healthcare

Centrum Protegra®
multiple vitamins and minerals
Vitamin-Mineral Supplement

Pfizer Consumer Healthcare

Centrum Select®
multiple vitamins and minerals
Vitamin-Mineral Supplement

Pfizer Consumer Healthcare

Centrum Select® Chewables
multiple vitamins and minerals
Vitamin-Mineral Supplement

Pfizer Consumer Healthcare

INDICATIONS: For use as a nutritional supplement.

Helps maintain good health, helps metabolize carbohydrates, fats or proteins, helps maintain immune function, helps maintain eyesight and helps in development of bones.

Centrum Cardio: Helps promote healthy cholesterol levels for cardiovascular health.

CONTRAINDICATIONS: In the presence of hemochromatosis, hemosiderosis, hemolytic anemia.

PRECAUTIONS: There is enough iron in this product to seriously harm a child.

Keep out of reach of children.

As with any drug, if you are pregnant or nursing, contact a healthcare professional before taking.

If taking other supplements, read label, since supplements may contain the same ingredient.

Do not exceed recommended daily dose/amount.

Do not use if you have a copper storage or metabolism disorder such as Wilsons' disease.

Oral iron preparations may aggravate existing peptic ulcer, regional enteritis and ulcerative colitis. Oral iron preparations can impair the absorption of tetracycline antibiotics. Antacids given concomitantly with iron compounds decrease iron absorption.

Centrum Forte, Centrum Select and Centrum Select Chewables: Contain <25 µg of vitamin K. The Adequate Intake (AI) for vitamin K is 90 µg and 120 µg for women and men, respectively. Higher levels than the AI have the potential to interact with anticoagulant therapy.

Centrum Cardio: Sitosterolemics: Contains phytosterols (sitosterols).

ADVERSE EFFECTS: Rarely, in iron sensitive patients, mild gastrointestinal upset may occur.

OVERDOSE:

In case of accidental overdose, contact a physician or poison control centre immediately, even if there are no symptoms.

> For management of a suspected drug overdose, CPhA recommends that you contact your **regional Poison Control Centre**. See the *CPS* Directory section for a list of Poison Control Centres.

DOSAGE: Centrum, Centrum Forte, Centrum Performance, Centrum Select: 1 tablet daily with food. Take a few hours before or a few hours after taking other medications.

Centrum Advantage, Centrum Protegra and Centrum Cardio: 2 tablets daily with food. Take a few hours before or a few hours after taking other medications.

SUPPLIED: Centrum: Each light peach, scored, oval, film-coated tablet, engraved "C" and "U1" contains: vitamins: beta-carotene (a source of vitamin A) 1800 µg/3000 IU, vitamin A (vitamin A acetate) 300 µg/1000 IU, vitamin E (dl-α-tocopheryl acetate) 11 mg/25 IU, vitamin C (ascorbic acid) 90 mg, folic acid (folate) 0.4 mg, vitamin B_1 (thiamine mononitrate) 2.25 mg, vitamin B_2 (riboflavin) 3.2 mg, niacin (niacinamide) 15 mg, vitamin B_6 (pyridoxine HCl) 3 mg, vitamin B_{12} (cyanocobalamin) 14 µg, vitamin D_3 (cholecalciferol) 10 µg/400 IU, biotin 45 µg, pantothenic acid (calcium pantothenate) 10 mg; minerals: calcium (calcium carbonate and phosphate) 175 mg, phosphorus (calcium phosphate) 125 mg, iodine (potassium iodide) 0.15 mg, iron (ferrous fumarate) 10 mg, magnesium (magnesium oxide) 50 mg, copper (cupric oxide) 2 mg; other ingredients: lutein 250 µg. Nonmedicinal ingredients: ascorbyl palmitate, BHT, citric acid, corn starch, crospovidone, FD&C Yellow No. 6, gelatin, hydrogenated soybean oil, hypromellose, lactose, magnesium stearate, methyl cellulose, microcrystalline cellulose, mineral oil, modified food starch, polysorbate, silicon dioxide, sodium alumino-silicate, sodium ascorbate, sodium benzoate, sodium citrate, sodium lauryl sulfate, sorbic acid, stearic acid, sucrose, titanium dioxide and triethyl citrate. Energy: <4.2 kJ (1 kcal). Sodium: <0.22 mmol (5 mg). Gluten-, parabens-, peanut oil- and tartrazine (FD&C Yellow No. 5)-free. Bottles of 60 and 100.

Centrum Advantage: Each dark green, scored, oval, film-coated tablet, engraved "C" and "U4" contains: vitamins: beta-carotene (a source of vitamin A) 900 µg/1500 IU, vitamin A (vitamin A acetate) 150 µg/500 IU, vitamin E (dl-α-tocopheryl acetate) 45 mg/100 IU, vitamin C (ascorbic acid) 125 mg, folic acid (folate) 0.3 mg, vitamin B_1 (thiamine mononitrate) 1.25 mg, vitamin B_2 (riboflavin) 2.5 mg, niacin (niacinamide) 7.5 mg, vitamin B_6 (pyridoxine HCl) 2.5 mg, vitamin B_{12} (cyanocobalamin) 50 µg, vitamin D_3 (cholecalciferol) 10 µg/400 IU, biotin 22.5 µg, pantothenic acid (calcium pantothenate) 5 mg; minerals: calcium (calcium carbonate) 200 mg, iodine (potassium iodide) 0.075 mg, iron (ferrous fumarate) 2 mg, magnesium (magnesium oxide) 50 mg, copper (copper sulfate) 0.5 mg, manganese (manganese sulfate) 2.5 mg, potassium (potassium chloride) 20 mg, chromium (chromium chloride) 50 µg, molybdenum (sodium molybdate) 22.5 µg, selenium (sodium selenate) 35 µg, zinc (zinc oxide) 3.75 mg; other ingredients: lutein 1 mg and lycopene 1 mg. Nonmedicinal ingredients: ascorbyl palmitate, citric acid, corn starch, croscarmellose sodium, crospovidone, D&C Yellow No. 10, dibasic calcium phosphate, FD&C Blue No. 1, FD&C Yellow No. 6, gelatin, hydrogenated soybean oil, hypromellose, lactose monohydrate, magnesium stearate, methyl cellulose, microcrystalline cellulose, mineral oil light, polysorbate 80, silicon dioxide, sodium benzoate, sodium citrate, sodium lauryl sulfate, sorbic acid, stearic acid, sucrose, titanium dioxide and triethyl citrate. Energy: <4.2 kJ (1 kcal). Sodium: <0.22 mmol (5 mg). Gluten-, parabens-, peanut oil- and tartrazine (FD&C Yellow No. 5)-free. Bottles of 60 and 100.

Centrum Cardio: Each white, scored, oval, film-coated tablet, engraved "C" and "C" contains: vitamins: beta-carotene (a source of vitamin A) 600 µg/1000 IU, vitamin A (vitamin A acetate) 300 µg/1000 IU, vitamin E (dl-α-tocopheryl acetate) 5.3 mg/11.75 IU, vitamin C (ascorbic acid) 60 mg, folic acid (folate) 0.2 mg, vitamin B_1 (thiamine mononitrate) 0.7 mg, vitamin B_2 (riboflavin) 0.875 mg, niacin (niacinamide) 10 mg, vitamin B_6 (pyridoxine HCl) 2 mg, vitamin B_{12} (cyanocobalamin) 1.5 µg, vitamin D_3 (cholecalciferol) 2.5 µg/100 IU, biotin 31.25 µg, pantothenic acid (calcium pantothenate) 3.75 mg, vitamin K_1 15 mg; minerals: calcium (calcium carbonate and phosphate) 81 mg, phosphorus (calcium phosphate) 62.5 mg, iodine (potassium iodide) 0.05 mg, iron (ferrous fumarate) 2.5 mg, magnesium (magnesium oxide) 50 mg, copper (cupric oxide) 0.5 mg, manganese (manganese sulfate) 1 mg, potassium (potassium chloride) 20 mg, chromium (chromium chloride) 20 µg, selenium (sodium selenate) 15 µg, zinc (zinc oxide) 2.5 mg; other ingredients: phytosterols 500 mg. Nonmedicinal ingredients: acacia gum, ascorbyl palmitate, BHT, calcium stearate, citric acid, corn starch, croscarmellose sodium, dibasic calcium phosphate, gelatin, glucose, hypromellose, magnesium stearate, maltodextrin, medium chain triglycerides, microcrystalline cellulose, modified food starch, silicon dioxide, sodium ascorbate, sodium benzoate, sodium citrate, sorbic acid, sucrose and titanium dioxide. Energy: <4.2 kJ (1 kcal). Sodium: <0.22 mmol (5 mg). Gluten-, parabens-, peanut oil- and tartrazine (FD&C Yellow No. 5)-free. Bottles of 14, 50 and 90.

Centrum Forte: Each orange, scored, oval, film-coated tablet, engraved "C" and "C3" contains: vitamins: beta-carotene (a source of vitamin A) 1800 µg/3000 IU, vitamin A (vitamin A acetate) 300 µg/1000 IU, vitamin E (dl-α-tocopheryl acetate) 34 mg/75 IU, vitamin C (ascorbic acid) 90 mg, folic acid (folate) 0.6 mg, vitamin B_1 (thiamine mononitrate) 2.25 mg, vitamin B_2 (riboflavin) 3.2 mg, niacin (niacinamide) 15 mg, vitamin B_6 (pyridoxine HCl) 5 mg, vitamin B_{12} (cyanocobalamin) 20 µg, vitamin D_3 (cholecalciferol) 15 µg/600 IU, biotin 45 µg, pantothenic acid (calcium pantothenate) 10 mg, vitamin K_1 25 µg; minerals: calcium (calcium carbonate) 200 mg, iodine (potassium iodide) 0.15 mg, iron (ferrous fumarate) 10 mg, magnesium (magnesium oxide) 50 mg, copper (copper sulfate) 1 mg, manganese (manganese sulfate) 5 mg, potassium (potassium chloride) 80 mg, chromium (chromium chloride) 35 µg, molybdenum (sodium molybdate) 45 µg, selenium (sodium selenate) 55 µg, zinc (zinc oxide) 7.5 mg; other ingredients: lutein 500 µg and lycopene 600 µg. Nonmedicinal ingredients: acacia gum, ascorbyl palmitate, BHT, citric acid, corn starch, croscarmellose sodium, crospovidone, dibasic calcium phosphate, FD&C Yellow No. 6, food starch modified, gelatin, hydrogenated soybean oil, hypromellose, lactose monohydrate, magnesium stearate, methyl cellulose, microcrystalline cellulose, mineral oil light, modified food starch, polysorbate 80, silicon dioxide, sodium ascorbate, sodium benzoate, sodium citrate, sodium lauryl sulfate, sorbic acid, stearic acid, sucrose, titanium dioxide and triethyl citrate. Energy: <4.2 kJ (1 kcal). Sodium: <0.22 mmol (5 mg). Gluten-, parabens-, peanut oil- and tartrazine (FD&C Yellow No. 5)-free. Bottles of 60, 100 and 250.

Centrum Performance: Each orange, oval, scored, film-coated tablet, engraved "C" and "G 1" contains: vitamins: beta-carotene (a source of vitamin A)) 1200 µg/2000 IU, vitamin A (vitamin A acetate) 300 µg/1000 IU, vitamin E (dl-α-tocopheryl acetate) 27 mg/60 IU, vitamin C (ascorbic acid) 120 mg, folic acid (folate) 0.6 mg, vitamin B_1 (thiamine mononitrate) 4.5 mg, vitamin B_2 (riboflavin) 5.1 mg, niacin (niacinamide) 15 mg, vitamin B_6 (pyridoxine HCl) 6 mg, vitamin B_{12} (cyanocobalamin) 20 µg, vitamin D_3 (cholecalciferol) 10 µg/400 IU, biotin 40 µg, pantothenic acid (calcium pantothenate) 10 mg; minerals: calcium (calcium phosphate) 162 mg, phosphorous (calcium phosphate) 125 mg, iodine (potassium iodide) 0.15 mg, iron (ferrous fumarate) 8 mg, magnesium (magnesium oxide) 50 mg, copper (copper sulfate) 1 mg, manganese (manganese sulfate) 4 mg, potassium (potassium chloride) 80 mg, chromium (chromium chloride) 25 µg, molybdenum (sodium molybdate) 50 µg, selenium (sodium selenate) 55 µg, zinc (zinc oxide) 7.5 mg, nickel (nickel sulfate) 5 µg, tin (stannous chloride) 10 µg, vanadium (sodium metavanadate) 10 µg, silicon (sodium metasilicate) 10 µg. Herbal ingredients: ginseng root (Panax Ginseng) standardized extract 50 mg. Nonmedicinal ingredients: ascorbyl palmitate, citric acid, corn starch, crospovidone, FD&C Red No. 40, FD&C Yellow No. 6, gelatin, hypromellose, lactose momohydrate, magnesium stearate, methyl cellulose, microcrystalline cellulose, mineral oil light, polysorbate 80, silicon dioxide, sodium ascorbate, sodium benzoate, sodium citrate, sodium lauryl sulfate, sorbic acid, stearic acid, sucrose, titanium dioxide and triethyl citrate. Energy: <4.2 kJ (1 kcal). Sodium: <0.22 mmol (5 mg). Gluten-, parabens-, peanut oil- and tartrazine (FD&C Yellow No. 5)-free. Bottles of 75.

Centrum Protegra: Each light peach, scored, oval, film-coated tablet, engraved "C" and "U14" contains: vitamins: beta-carotene (a source of vitamin A) 3000 µg/5000 IU, vitamin A (vitamin A acetate) 150 µg/500 IU, vitamin E (dl-α-tocopheryl acetate) 45 µg/100 IU, vitamin C (ascorbic acid) 125 mg, folic acid (folate) 0.35 mg, vitamin B_1 (thiamine mononitrate) 1.15 mg, vitamin B_2 (riboflavin) 1.6 mg, niacin (niacinamide) 7.5 mg, vitamin B_6 (pyridoxine HCl) 5 mg, vitamin B_{12} (cyanocobalamin) 12.5 µg, vitamin D_3 (cholecalciferol) 5 µg/200 IU, biotin 22.5 µg, pantothenic acid (calcium pantothenate) 5 mg; minerals: calcium (calcium carbonate and phosphate) 87.5 mg, phosphorus (calcium phosphate) 62.5 mg, iodine (potassium iodide) 0.075 mg, iron (ferrous fumarate) 5 mg, magnesium (magnesium oxide) 50 mg, copper (cupric oxide) 1 mg, manganese (manganese sulfate) 2.5 mg, potassium (potassium chloride) 20 mg, chromium (chromium chloride) 12.5 µg, molybdenum (sodium molybdate) 12.5 µg, selenium (sodium selenate) 12.5 µg, zinc (zinc oxide) 7.5 mg, nickel (nickel sulfate) 2.5 µg, tin (stannous chloride) 5 µg, vanadium (sodium metavanadate) 5 µg, silicon (sodium metasilicate) 5 µg; other ingredients: lutein 250 µg. Nonmedicinal ingredients: ascorbyl palmitate, BHT, citric acid, corn starch, crospovidone, FD&C Yellow No. 6, gelatin, hydrogenated soybean oil, hypromellose, lactose, magnesium stearate, methyl cellulose, microcrystalline cellulose, mineral oil, modified food starch, polysorbate, silicon dioxide, sodium alumino-silicate, sodium ascorbate, sodium benzoate, sodium citrate, sodium lauryl sulfate, sorbic acid, soybean oil, stearic acid, sucrose, titanium dioxide and triethyl citrate. Energy: <4.2 kJ (1 kcal). Sodium: <0.22 mmol (5 mg). Gluten-, parabens-, peanut oil- and tartrazine (FD&C Yellow No. 5)-free. Bottles of 80 and 120.

Centrum Select: Each orange, scored, oval, film-coated tablet, engraved "C" and "C1" contains: vitamins: beta-carotene (a source of vitamin A) 1800 µg/3000 IU, vitamin A (vitamin A acetate) 300 µg/1000 IU, vitamin E (dl-α-tocopheryl acetate) 34 mg/75 IU, vitamin C (ascorbic acid) 90 mg, folic acid (folate) 0.6 mg, vitamin B_1 (thiamine mononitrate) 2.25 mg, vitamin B_2 (riboflavin) 3.2 mg, niacin (niacinamide) 15 mg, vitamin B_6 (pyridoxine HCl) 8 mg, vitamin B_{12} (cyanocobalamin) 25 µg, vitamin D_3 (cholecalciferol) 15 µg/600 IU, biotin 45 µg, pantothenic acid (calcium pantothenate) 10 mg, vitamin K_1 25 µg; minerals: calcium (calcium carbonate) 200 mg, iodine (potassium iodide) 0.15 mg, iron (ferrous fumarate) 4 mg, magnesium (magnesium oxide) 50 mg, copper (copper sulfate) 1 mg, manganese (manganese sulfate) 5 mg, potassium (potassium chloride) 80 mg, chromium (chromium chloride) 100 µg, molybdenum (sodium molybdate) 45 µg, selenium (sodium selenate) 55 µg, zinc (zinc oxide) 7.5 mg; other ingredients: lutein 500 µg and lycopene 600 µg. Nonmedicinal ingredients: acacia gum, ascorbyl palmitate, BHT, citric acid, corn starch, croscarmellose sodium, crospovidone, dibasic calcium phosphate, FD&C Yellow No. 6, gelatin, hydrogenated soybean oil, hypromellose, lactose monohydrate, magnesium stearate, methylcellulose, microcrystalline cellulose, mineral oil light, modified food starch, polysorbate 80, silicon dioxide, sodium ascorbate, sodium benzoate, sodium citrate, sodium lauryl sulfate, sorbic acid, stearic acid, sucrose, titanium dioxide and triethyl citrate. Energy: <4.2 kJ (1 kcal). Sodium: <0.22 mmol (5 mg). Gluten-, parabens-, peanut oil- and tartrazine (FD&C Yellow No. 5)-free. Bottles of 60, 100 and 250.

Centrum Select Chewables: Each pale pink, scored, flat/round chewable tablet, engraved "Select" and "L50", contains: vitamins: beta-carotene (a source of vitamin A) 1800 µg/3000 IU, vitamin A (vitamin A acetate) 300 µg/1000 IU, vitamin E (dl-α-tocopheryl acetate) 34 mg/75 IU, vitamin C (ascorbic acid) 90 mg, folic acid (folate) 0.6 mg, vitamin B_1 (thiamine mononitrate) 2.25 mg, vitamin B_2 (riboflavin) 3.2 mg, niacin (niacinamide) 15 mg, vitamin B_6 (pyridoxine HCl) 8 mg, vitamin B_{12} (cyanocobalamin) 25 µg, vitamin D_3 (cholecalciferol) 10 µg/400 IU, biotin 45 µg, vitamin K_1 25 µg, pantothenic acid (calcium pantothenate) 10 mg; minerals: calcium (calcium carbonate and phosphate) 200 mg, phosphorus (calcium phosphate) 125 mg, iodine (potassium iodide) 0.15 mg, iron (ferrous fumarate) 4 mg, magnesium (magnesium oxide) 50 mg, copper (cupric oxide) 2 mg, manganese (manganese sulfate) 5 mg, chromium (chromium chloride) 100 µg, molybdenum (sodium molybdate) 45 µg, selenium (sodium selenate) 55 µg, zinc (zinc oxide) 3 mg, nickel (nickel sulfate) 5 µg, tin (stannous chloride) 0.010 mg, vanadium (sodium metavanadate) 10 µg, silicon (sodium metasilicate) 0.010 mg; other ingredients: lutein 500 µg, lycopene 600 µg. Nonmedicinal ingredients: acacia gum, ascorbyl palmitate, aspartame (phenylalanine), BHT, citric acid, corn starch, crospovidone, dibasic calcium phosphate, flavor, gelatin, glycerides, hydrogenated soybean oil, lactose monohydrate, magnesium stearate, maltodextrin, mannitol, microcrystalline cellulose, modified food starch, mono and diglycerides, ponceau 4R, silicon dioxide, sodium alumino silicate, sodium ascorbate, sodium benzoate, sodium citrate, sorbic acid, sorbitol, stearic acid and sucrose. Phenylketonurics: contains phenylalanine. Energy: <0.71 kJ (0.17 kcal). Sodium: <0.22 mmol (5 mg). Gluten-, parabens-, peanut oil- and tartrazine (FD&C Yellow No. 5)-free. Bottles of 60.

Centrum Junior® Complete

multiple vitamins and minerals

Vitamin-Mineral Supplement

Pfizer Consumer Healthcare

INDICATIONS: For use as a nutritional supplement for children.

CONTRAINDICATIONS: Centrum Junior Complete: In the presence of hemochromatosis, hemosiderosis, hemolytic anemia.

PRECAUTIONS: Product contains iron, which can be harmful to children if taken in large doses.

There is enough iron in this package to seriously harm a child.

Keep out of reach of children.

If taking other supplements, read label, since supplements may contain the same ingredient.

Do not exceed recommended daily dose/amount.

Centrum Junior Complete contains iron. Oral iron preparations may aggravate existing peptic ulcer, regional enteritis and ulcerative colitis. Oral iron preparations can impair the absorption of tetracycline antibiotics. Antacids given concomitantly with iron compounds decrease iron absorption.

OVERDOSE:

In case of accidental overdose, contact a physician or poison control centre immediately, even if there are no symptoms.

> For management of a suspected drug overdose, CPhA recommends that you contact your **regional Poison Control Centre**. See the *CPS* Directory section for a list of Poison Control Centres.

DOSAGE: Children 4-12 years: Chew 1 tablet daily with food. Take a few hours before or a few hours after taking other medications.

SUPPLIED: Each round tablet, engraved "animal imprint" on both sides, contains: vitamins: beta-carotene (a source of vitamin A) 1200 µg/2000 IU, vitamin A (as acetate) 300 µg/1000 IU, vitamin E (dl-α-tocopheryl acetate) 4.5 mg/10 IU, vitamin C (37.5 mg from ascorbic acid; 37.5 mg from sodium ascorbate) 75 mg, folic acid (folate) 0.1 mg, vitamin B_1 (thiamine mononitrate) 1 mg, vitamin B_2 (riboflavin) 1 mg, niacinamide 10 mg, vitamin B_6 (pyridoxine HCl) 1 mg, vitamin B_{12} (cyanocobalamin) 2 µg, vitamin D_3 10 µg/400 IU, biotin 30 µg, pantothenic acid (calcium d-pantothenate) 5 mg; minerals: calcium (calcium carbonate) 250 mg, iodine (potassium iodide) 0.15 mg, iron (carbonyl iron) 5 mg, magnesium 50 mg, copper (cupric sulfate) 0.5 mg and zinc (zinc oxide) 3 mg. Nonmedicinal ingredients: ascorbyl palmitate, carboxymethylcellulose sodium, citric acid, cornstarch, dibasic calcium phosphate, flavours, gelatin, hydrogenated palm oil, lactose monohydrate, magnesium stearate, maltodextrin, microcrystalline cellulose, modified food starch, mono and diglycerides, polydextrose, silicon dioxide, sodium ascorbate, sodium benzoate, sodium citrate, sorbic acid, stearic acid, sucrose and xylitol. Energy: 9.8 kJ (2.4 kcal). Gluten-, parabens-, peanut oil- and tartrazine (FD&C Yellow No. 5)-free. Bottles of 60, assorted flavours and colours.

Centrum® Materna®

multiple vitamins and minerals

Prenatal/Postpartum Supplement

Pfizer Consumer Healthcare

INDICATIONS: Prenatal/postpartum vitamin and mineral supplement. Helps prevent neural tube defects when taken daily prior to becoming pregnant and during early pregnancy.

CONTRAINDICATIONS: Iron therapy is contraindicated in the presence of hemochromatosis, hemosiderosis, hemolytic anemia.

Do not use if you have a copper storage or metabolism disorder, such as Wilson's disease.

PRECAUTIONS: Product contains iron, which can be harmful to children if taken in large doses.

There is enough iron in this package to seriously harm a child.

Keep out of reach of children.

If taking other supplements, read label, since supplements may contain the same ingredient.

Do not exceed recommended daily dose/amount.

Folic acid may obscure pernicious anemia in that the peripheral blood picture may revert to normal while neurological manifestations remain progressive. Oral iron preparation may aggravate existing peptic ulcer, regional enteritis and ulcerative colitis. Antacids given concomitantly with iron compounds decrease iron absorption.

Take a few hours before or a few hours after taking other medications.

ADVERSE EFFECTS: Rarely, in iron-sensitive patients, mild gastrointestinal upsets may occur.

OVERDOSE:

In case of accidental overdose, contact a physician or poison control centre immediately, even if there are no symptoms.

> For management of a suspected drug overdose, CPhA recommends that you contact your **regional Poison Control Centre**. See the *CPS* Directory section for a list of Poison Control Centres.

DOSAGE: Women 19 years of age or older: 1 tablet daily with food prior to conception, during pregnancy and when breast-feeding.

SUPPLIED: Each light pink, oval, scored, film-coated tablet, engraved "MATERNA" and "M4", contains: vitamins: beta-carotene (source of vitamin A) 1500 µg/2500 IU, vitamin A (vitamin A acetate) 300 µg/1000 IU, vitamin E (dl-a tocopheryl acetate) 13.5 mg/30 IU, vitamin C (ascorbic acid) 85 mg, folic acid (folate) 1 mg, vitamin B_1 (thiamine mononitrate) 1.4 mg, vitamin B_2 (riboflavin) 1.4 mg, niacin (niacinamide) 18 mg, vitamin B_6 (pyridoxine hydrochloride) 1.9 mg, vitamin B_{12} (cyanocobalamin) 2.6 µg, vitamin D_3 (cholecalciferol) 10 µg/400 IU, biotin 30 µg, pantothenic acid (calcium pantothenate) 6 mg; minerals: calcium (calcium carbonate) 250 mg, iodine (potassium iodide) 220 µg, iron (ferrous fumarate) 27 mg, magnesium (magnesium oxide) 50 mg, copper (cupric sulfate) 1 mg, manganese (manganese sulfate) 2 mg, chromium (chromium chloride) 30 µg, molybdenum (sodium molybdate) 50 µg, selenium (sodium selenate) 30 µg and zinc (zinc oxide) 7.5 mg. Nonmedicinal ingredients: ascorbyl palmitate, BHT, calcium phosphate, celluloses, citric acid, corn starch, crospovidone, FD&C Red No. 40, gelatin, hypromellose, lactose, magnesium stearate, mineral oil, polysorbate 80, silicon dioxide, sodium benzoate, sodium citrate, sodium lauryl sulfate, sorbic acid, soybean oil, stearic acid, sucrose, titanium dioxide and triethyl citrate. Gluten-, parabens-, peanut oil- and tartrazine (FD&C Yellow No. 5)-free. Bottles of 100. Protect from moisture. Store at room temperature (15-30°C).

Cephalexin ℞

Antibiotic

CPhA Monograph

Date of Preparation: November 2005

Date of Revision: September 2009

> This monograph has been compiled by CPhA and reviewed by experts. It may contain information different from that found in Health Canada-approved Product Monographs. The reader is referred to the *CPS* Editorial Policy for more information.

SUMMARY PRODUCT INFORMATION:

Route of Administration	Dosage Form	Product Strength
Oral	Tablet	250 mg, 500 mg
	Suspension	125 mg/5 mL, 250 mg/5 mL

PHARMACOLOGY: Cephalexin is a semisynthetic first-generation cephalosporin with bactericidal activity against sensitive organisms. It inhibits peptidoglycan synthesis in the bacterial cell wall leading to the formation of a defective cell wall with eventual lysis and cell death. The spectrum of activity of cephalexin includes methicillin-susceptible *S. aureus* (MSSA) and β-haemolytic Streptococci, Enterobacteriaceae, *E. coli* and Klebsiella. Cephalexin possesses little or no activity against methicillin-resistant *S. aureus* (MRSA), penicillin-intermediate and penicillin-resistant *S. pneumoniae*, Enterococcus species, Enterobacteriaceae producing inducible and extended β-lactamases, Haemophilus, Pseudomonas, Pasteurella, Eikenella, Capnocytophaga, Bordetella, Chlamydia and Mycoplasma species and anaerobic gram-negative bacilli. Penicillin-resistant *S. pneumoniae* is considered resistant to all first- and second-generation cephalosporins but often remains susceptible to high-dose amoxicillin and third-generation cephalosporins. Although active in vitro against Salmonella, cephalexin is not recommended due to poor intracellular penetration. For antibiotic susceptibility, many laboratories do not test specifically for cephalexin but for cephalothin; the results of the latter are considered valid for the former.

Pharmacokinetics: Cephalexin is completely absorbed after oral administration. Following single doses of 250 mg, 500 mg or 1 g, in healthy, fasting adults, peak serum concentrations of 9 µg/mL, 18 µg/mL or 32 µg/mL occur within 1 hour, respectively. Less than 10% of absorbed drug is bound to serum protein. The half-life of cephalexin in adults with normal renal function ranges from 0.5 to 1.2 hours. In adults with end-stage renal disease, the half-life is prolonged (~16 hours). More than 80% is excreted as cephalexin in the urine, through glomerular filtration and tubular secretion.

Cephalexin is acid-stable. Food in the stomach causes a delay in onset and a lower peak concentration but does not decrease the total amount of cephalexin absorbed. Concomitant probenecid prolongs the half-life of cephalexin.

INDICATIONS: Cephalexin is used in the following clinical settings to treat or prevent infections caused by susceptible organisms:

- Treatment of uncomplicated skin and soft-tissue bacterial infections, including impetigo, carbuncles and cellulitis, caused by gram-positive organisms. Re-evaluate patients 24 to 48 hours after receiving the cephalexin [*Clin Infect Dis* 2005;41(10):1373-406].
- Treatment of postpartum breast abscess or mastitis.
- Treatment of septic bursitis.
- Treatment of group A streptococcal pharyngitis. Penicillin V is the recommended drug of choice for the treatment of group A streptococcal pharyngitis. Cephalexin is used as an alternative in penicillin-allergic patients who are not considered to be at risk of immediate hypersensitivity reactions [*Clin Infect Dis* 2002;35(2):113-25].
- Treatment of asymptomatic bacteriuria in pregnancy. Also used in traumatic pre-operative genitourinary procedures involving mucosal bleeding [*Clin Infect Dis* 2005;40(5):643-54].
- Treatment of acute cystitis in pregnant women [Anti-infective Review Panel. *Anti-infective guidelines for community-acquired infections.* Toronto (ON): MUMS Guideline Clearinghouse; 2005].
- Oral step-down treatment of acute osteomyelitis after initial iv therapy for MSSA once the patient's condition has stabilized.
- Prevention of infective endocarditis in susceptible patients. Oral amoxicillin is preferred; however, oral cephalexin is recommended as an oral alternative in penicillin-allergic patients who are not considered to be at risk of immediate hypersensitivity reactions [*Circulation* 2007;116(15):1736-54].

Patients with any of the following conditions may benefit from cephalexin for prevention of infective endocarditis while undergoing certain dental or surgical procedures so as to prevent severe outcomes: prosthetic heart valves or prosthetic material used for the cardiac valve region, previous infective endocarditis, heart transplantation recipients who develop cardiac valvulopathy, congenital heart disease, i.e., unrepaired cyanotic congenital heart disease, including palliative shunts and conduits; repaired congenital heart disease with residual effects at the site or adjacent to the site of a prosthetic patch or prosthetic device which inhibits endothelialization; completely repaired congenital heart defect with prosthetic material or device, whether placed by surgery or by catheter intervention, during the first six months after the procedure [*Circulation* 2007;116(15):1736-54]. Antibiotic prophylaxis against infective endocarditis is recommended in the aforementioned patients for dental procedures that involve manipulation of gingival tissue or the periapical region of teeth or perforation of the oral mucosa, procedures on respiratory tract involving incision or biopsy of respiratory mucosa and procedures in patients with infected skin, skin structures or musculoskeletal tissue; however, antibiotic prophylaxis against infective endocarditis is not recommended for genitourinary or gastrointestinal tract procedures [*Circulation* 2007;116(15):1736-54].

Cephalexin is no longer recommended for the treatment of animal bites because of poor in vitro activity against *P. multocida*. Cephalexin is no longer recommended for the treatment of human bites because of resistance of *E. corrodens*, a prominent aerobic pathogen, to first-generation cephalosporins [*Clin Infect Dis* 2005;41(10):1373-406].

CONTRAINDICATIONS:

- Patients who are hypersensitive to cephalexin or to any ingredient in the formulation.
- Patients who are hypersensitive to cephalosporins or to other β-lactam antibiotics.

WARNINGS AND PRECAUTIONS:

Serious Warnings and Precautions
- Cephalexin has been associated with severe allergic reactions including anaphylactic reactions. For this reason a history of allergic reactions, including the type and severity of the reaction, should be obtained before prescribing and administering cephalexin.
- Cross-sensitivity between penicillins and cephalosporins is estimated to be very low. Current opinion on the true incidence of cross-sensitivity is about 1%. The beta-lactam subunit is not considered the primary allergenic determinant; rather, the side chain predicts cross-reactivity. After thorough investigation into the nature of the allergy, a cephalosporin can be considered in a penicillin allergic patient provided there is no history of an immediate-sensitivity reaction. Although the risk of cross-reaction is predicted to be low the patient should be monitored for signs of a sensitivity reaction.
- Patients with a history of immediate-sensitivity reaction to penicillin (e.g., anaphylaxis, bronchospasm and/or hypotension) are considered to be at increased risk of similar reactions to cephalosporins, including cephalexin. For this reason, administration of cephalexin should be avoided in patients with a history of severe allergic reactions to penicillin antibiotics unless skin testing is performed to rule out cross-sensitivity.
- Cephalosporin antibiotics including cephalexin have been associated with *C. difficile*-associated diarrhea and colitis.

Hematologic: Rarely, mild, transient neutropenia and other blood dyscrasias have occurred with cephalosporins.
Renal: Nephrotoxicity has been reported rarely with cephalosporins, and is more likely in older individuals, or in patients who are taking other nephrotoxic drugs concomitantly or have pre-existing renal impairment. Since cephalexin is renally cleared, dose adjustment is recommended in patients with impaired renal function (see Table 4).
Hepatic: Transient elevation of liver enzymes (AST and ALT) has occurred rarely during cephalosporin therapy.
Special Populations: *Pregnant Women:* Pregnancy Category B_M. Although it has not been unequivocally established that there is not an increased risk of birth defects with the use of cephalexin, it is generally accepted that cephalosporins are safe to use during pregnancy.
Nursing Women: Cephalexin is excreted in breast milk in low concentrations. Potential risks to the infant include altered bowel flora, diarrhea, obscured diagnosis of fever and hypersensitivity reactions. Cephalosporins are generally considered to be compatible with breast-feeding.
Drug Interactions: See Table 1.

Table 1: Cephalexin
Drug Interactions

Interacting Drug	Effect	Clinical Comment
Probenecid	Probenecid inhibits renal tubular excretion of cephalexin, which may result in decreased elimination of cephalexin.	This interaction has been exploited to increase serum levels of penicillins and most cephalosporins.

Drug/Laboratory Test Interactions: Cephalexin may produce a false positive reaction for glucose in the urine with Benedict or Fehling's solution or with Clinitest tablets, but not with Tes-Tape (Glucose Enzymatic Test Strip, USP).
Positive direct Coombs' tests have been reported during treatment with the cephalosporins. This can interfere with cross-matching for transfusion, hematologic studies or Coombs' testing of neonates whose mothers received a cephalosporin prior to delivery.

PRECAUTIONS: See Warnings and Precautions.

ADVERSE EFFECTS: Side effects include nausea, vomiting and diarrhea. These are usually mild and transient and rarely require discontinuation of the drug.
Hematologic: eosinophilia, hemolytic anemia, neutropenia, thrombocytopenia.
Hepatic: cholestatic jaundice (rare), transient hepatitis (rare).
Immune: serum sickness-like reaction.
Renal: interstitial nephritis, acute tubular necrosis.

OVERDOSE:

For management of a suspected drug overdose, CPhA recommends that you contact your **regional Poison Control Centre**. See the *CPS* Directory section for a list of Poison Control Centres.

DOSAGE: Cephalexin is given orally. The usual adult dose is 1 g/day in divided doses every 6 hours. If a total daily dose of greater than 4 g is required, consider parenteral cephalosporin or the addition of probenecid. In children >1 year, the usual dose is 25 to 100 mg/kg administered in divided doses every 6 hours with a daily maximum of 4 g. The usual duration of therapy is 7 to 10 days. For most indications, QID dosing is most often prescribed and conventionally considered sufficient. See Table 2 and Table 3.

Table 2: Cephalexin
Dose in Adult Patients

Indication	Usual Dose	Duration of Treatment	Clinical Comment
Impetigo	250–500 mg po Q6H	7 to 10 days	For Streptococci and MSSA. Duration of treatment dependent on clinical response. Consider if widespread infection, patient is immunocompromised, has valvular disease or if not improved with topical therapy within 24–48 hours.
Skin and soft tissue infections	500 mg po Q6H	7 to 10 days	Cloxacillin is the drug of choice for MSSA skin and soft tissue infections due to its narrower spectrum of activity, although cephalexin is better absorbed.
Group A Streptococcal pharyngitis	500 mg po Q12H	10 days	Not for patients with immediate hypersensitivity reactions to β-lactam antibiotics.
Postpartum mastitis with or without breast abscess	500 mg po Q6H	7 to 10 days	Not for MRSA infection.
Septic bursitis	500 mg po Q6H	2 to 3 weeks	
Asymptomatic bacteriuria in pregnancy	250 mg po Q6H	7 to 14 days	Also for patients who are not pregnant and undergoing traumatic pre-operative genitourinary procedures involving mucosal bleeding (e.g., transurethral resection of the prostate) to minimize postprocedure bacteremia and sepsis [*Clin Infect Dis* 2005; 40(5):643-54].

(cont'd)

Table 2: Cephalexin *(cont'd)*
Dose in Adult Patients

Indication	Usual Dose	Duration of Treatment	Clinical Comment
Acute cystitis in pregnancy	250 mg po QID	7 days	Follow-up with urine cultures 1 to 2 weeks after treatment completion; monthly urine cultures recommended thereafter until delivery.
Endocarditis prevention	2 g po per dose	Single dose	Give 30 to 60 minutes prior to procedure.
Osteomyelitis, acute	500 mg to 1000 mg po Q6H	4 to 6 weeks	The dose stated is step-down following an initial course of iv antimicrobial therapy. The total course should be 4 to 6 weeks including the initial iv antimicrobial.

Table 3: Cephalexin
Dose in Infants (>28 days) and Older Children

Indication	Usual Dose	Duration of Treatment	Clinical Comment
Impetigo	25–50 mg/kg po daily divided Q6H	7 to 10 days	For Streptococci and Staphylococci species. Duration of treatment dependent on clinical response.
Skin and soft tissue infections	25 mg/kg po daily divided Q6H	7 to 10 days	Cloxacillin is the drug of choice for MSSA skin and soft tissue infections. Do not use cephalexin in patients with a history of immediate hypersensitivity reactions to β-lactam antibiotics.
Group A Streptococcal pharyngitis	25–50 mg/kg po daily divided Q12H	10 days	Not for patients with a history of immediate hypersensitivity reactions to β-lactam antibiotics.
Osteomyelitis (following iv therapy)	100–150 mg/kg po daily divided Q6H	4 to 6 weeks	Consider oral step-down therapy from iv antimicrobial therapy once patient has stabilized.
Endocarditis prevention	50 mg/kg po per dose; maximum: 2 g	Single dose	Give 30 to 60 minutes prior to procedure.

Renal Impairment: See Table 4.

Table 4: Cephalexin
Dose in Adult Patients with Renal Impairment

Creatinine Clearance	Recommended Dosing Interval
>50 mL/min	Q6–8H
10–50 mL/min	Q8–12H
<10 mL/min	Q12–24H

Cerezyme® Pr
imiglucerase
Enzyme Replacement Therapy
Genzyme

Date of Preparation: March 31, 2006

SUMMARY PRODUCT INFORMATION:

Route of Administration	Dosage Form/Strength	Clinically Relevant Nonmedicinal Ingredients
Intravenous infusion	Lyophilized powder for reconstitution and intravenous infusion 200 Units 400 Units	There are no clinically relevant nonmedicinal ingredients. For a complete listing, see Dosage Forms, Composition and Packaging.

DESCRIPTION: CEREZYME (imiglucerase for injection) is an analogue of β-glucocerebrosidase produced by recombinant DNA technology. The lysosomal enzyme catalyses the hydrolysis of glucocerebroside to glucose and ceramide.

INDICATIONS AND CLINICAL USE: CEREZYME (imiglucerase for injection) is indicated for long-term enzyme replacement therapy in patients with a confirmed diagnosis of non-neuronopathic (Type 1) or chronic neuronopathic (Type 3) Gaucher disease who exhibit non-neurological manifestations of the disease.
The non-neurological manifestations of Gaucher disease include one or more of the following conditions:
- anaemia after exclusion of other causes, such as iron deficiency
- thrombocytopenia
- bone disease after exclusion of other causes such as Vitamin D deficiency
- hepatomegaly or splenomegaly

Pediatrics (2-16 years of age): The safety and effectiveness of CEREZYME have been established in children and adolescents (from 2 up to 16 years of age). Use of CEREZYME in these age groups is supported by evidence from well-controlled studies of CEREZYME and CEREDASE (alglucerase injection) in adults and pediatric patients, with additional data obtained from the literature and from long term follow-up information.

CONTRAINDICATIONS:
- Patients who are severely hypersensitive to this drug or to any ingredient in the formulation or component of the container (see Warnings and Precautions). For a complete listing, see Dosage Forms, Composition and Packaging.

WARNINGS AND PRECAUTIONS: General: Therapy with CEREZYME (imiglucerase for injection) should be directed by physicians knowledgeable in the management of patients with Gaucher disease.
Treatment with CEREZYME should be approached with caution in patients who have exhibited symptoms of hypersensitivity to the product (see Immune and Adverse Reactions).

Caution is advisable in administration of CEREZYME to patients previously treated with placental-derived β-glucocerebrosidase (CEREDASE, alglucerase injection) and who have developed antibody or who have exhibited symptoms of hypersensitivity to placental-derived β-glucocerebrosidase (CEREDASE, alglucerase injection).

Carcinogenesis and Mutagenesis: Studies have not been conducted in either animals or humans to assess the potential effects of CEREZYME on carcinogenesis or mutagenesis.

Immune: Hypersensitivity reactions to CEREZYME may occur (see Adverse Reactions). Treatment should be carefully evaluated if there is significant clinical evidence of hypersensitivity to the product. The decision to continue treatment should be based on an evaluation of the benefits relative to the potential risks.

Anaphylactoid reaction has been reported in less than 1% of the patient population. Further treatment with CEREZYME should be conducted with caution. Most patients have successfully continued therapy after a reduction in rate of infusion and pretreatment with antihistamines and/or corticosteroids.

Approximately 15% of patients treated and tested to date have developed IgG antibody to CEREZYME during the first year of therapy. Patients who developed IgG antibody largely did so within 6 months of treatment and rarely developed antibodies to CEREZYME after 12 months of therapy. Approximately 46% of patients with detectable IgG antibodies experienced symptoms of hypersensitivity, however the presence of IgG antibodies did not prohibit the continuance of treatment.

Respiratory: In less than 1% of the patient population, pulmonary hypertension has also been observed during treatment with CEREZYME. Pulmonary hypertension is a known complication of Gaucher disease, and has been observed both in patients receiving and not receiving CEREZYME. No causal relationship with CEREZYME has been established. Patients with respiratory symptoms should be evaluated for the presence of pulmonary hypertension.

Special Populations: A comprehensive set of response parameters and treatment guidelines have been established and should be followed for the evaluation of Gaucher patients' response to therapy. An ongoing database, known as the International Collaborative Gaucher Group (ICGG) Registry, has been established for the world-wide collection of uniform data to improve the understanding of the disease and the clinical response to enzyme replacement therapy. The Registry may be contacted at 1-800-745-4447. The Gaucher Registry should be used by Canadian physicians as a monitoring vehicle for all Gaucher patients in Canada. Enrollment of patients is the responsibility of the treating physician. The Registry will be used to monitor the long term effectiveness of enzyme replacement therapy when used in the community. All references to specific patients should be made by initials or Registry identification (ID) number, not by name.

The parameters monitored by the Registry include haemoglobin, platelet count, spleen and liver volume, and location and degree of skeletal involvement. Recommended primary assessments and assessment schedules for various evaluations for untreated patients and those on ERT are presented in Table 1 and Table 2.

Table 1: CEREZYME

Initial Assessment

A complete history of patient and family, preferably including a pedigree
A comprehensive physical examination (annual)
Quality of life (annual): Patient-reported functional health and well-being (SF-36 Health Survey)
Blood tests Primary tests: • Hemoglobin • Platelet count Biochemical markers (one or more of these biochemical markers should be consistently monitored in conjunction with other clinical assessments of disease activity; chitotriosidase, when available as a validated procedure, may be the most sensitive indicator of changing disease activity, and is therefore preferred, although approximately 5% of the general population do not express any chitotriosidase activity due to genetic variability in enzyme expression): • Chitotriosidase • ACE • TRAP Additional blood tests (to be evaluated selectively based on each patient's age and clinical status): • WBC, PT, and PTT • Iron, iron binding capacity, ferritin, vitamin B_{12} • AST and/or ALT; alkaline phosphatase; calcium, phosphorous, albumin, total protein, total and direct bilirubin • Serum immunoelectrophoresis • Hepatitis profile
β-glucosidase and mutation analysis
Antibody sample[a]
Visceral (contiguous transaxial 10-mm thick sections for sum of region of interest) Spleen volume (volumetric MRI or CT) Liver volume (volumetric MRI or CT)
Skeletal MRI (coronal; T1- and T2-weighted) of the entire femora X-ray (AP view of the entire femora)[b] and lateral view of the spine DXA lumbar spine and femoral neck
Pulmonary (recommended every 12–24 months for patients with borderline or above normal pulmonary pressures at baseline) ECG, chest x-ray, and Doppler echocardiogram (right ventricular systolic pressure) for patients >18 years old

[a] A baseline sample to be stored at Genzyme Corporation; an optional subsequent sample at 6 months after starting enzyme replacement therapy (ERT). The samples will be tested only if clinically indicated such as for a suspected immune-mediated adverse event, or for suspected loss of ERT effectiveness.

[b] Optimally from hips to below knees.

Legend: ACE: angiotension-converting enzyme; TRAP: tartrate-resistant acid phosphatase; AP: anterior-posterior; ALT: alanine transaminase; AST: aspartate transaminase; CT: computed tomography; DXA: dual energy x-ray absorptiometry; MRI: magnetic resonance imaging; PT: prothrombin time; PTT: partial thromboplastin time; WBC: white blood cells.

Medical or health care professionals are encouraged to register Gaucher patients, including those with chronic neuronopathic manifestations of the disease, in the "ICGG Gaucher Registry".

For more information please consult the Registry website: www.gaucherregistry.com.

Pregnant Women: It is not known whether CEREZYME can cause fetal harm when administered to pregnant women or if it can affect reproductive capacity. CEREZYME should not be administered during pregnancy except when the indication and need are clear and the potential benefit is judged by the physician to substantially justify the risk.

Nursing Women: There is no clinical experience with lactating women and it is not known whether CEREZYME is excreted in human milk. Because many drugs are excreted in human milk, caution should be exercised when CEREZYME is administered to nursing women.

Pediatrics (<2 years of age): There is limited data for pediatric patients under the age of two. The safety and effectiveness of CEREZYME have been established in children and adolescents (from 2 to 16 years of age).

Monitoring and Laboratory Tests: Patients with antibodies to CEREZYME have a higher risk of hypersensitivity reactions, although not all patients with symptoms of hypersensitivity have detectable IgG antibodies. It is suggested that patients be monitored periodically during the first year of therapy (approximately every 3 months) and at approximately 18 months for IgG antibody formation.

Table 2: CEREZYME

Ongoing Monitoring[a]

Parameters	Patients Not on Enzyme Therapy		Patients on Enzyme Therapy: Not Achieved Therapeutic Goals		Patients on Enzyme Therapy: Achieved Therapeutic Goals	Patients on Enzyme Therapy: At Time of Dose Change or Significant Clinical Complication
	Every 12 months	Every 12–24 months	Every 3 months	Every 12 months	Every 12–24 months	
A comprehensive physical examination	X			X	X (annual)	
SF-36 (QOL) survey	X			X	X (annual)	X
Blood Tests						
Hemoglobin	X		X		X	X
Platelet Count	X		X		X	X
Biochemical Markers[b] Chitotriosidase ACE TRAP	X		X		X	X
Additional blood tests	To be followed appropriately if abnormal based on each patient's age and clinical status.					
Visceral (contiguous transaxial 10 mm thick sections for sum of region of interest)						
Spleen volume (volumetric MRI or CT)		X		X	X	X
Liver volume (volumetric MRI or CT)		X		X	X	X
Skeletal[c]						
MRI of entire femora (coronal; T1- & T2-weighted)[d]		X			X	X
X-ray[d,e]		X				
DXA		X				
Pulmonary	Recommended every 12–24 months for patients with borderline or above normal pulmonary pressures at baseline.					

[a] A comprehensive physical examination should be performed at least annually.

[b] One or more of these biochemical markers should be consistently monitored every 12 months and in conjunction with other clinical assessments of disease activity and response to treatment; chitotriosidase, when available as a validated procedure, may be the most sensitive indicator of changing disease activity, and is therefore preferred.

[c] Anatomical sites not included here should be evaluated if symptoms develop in such locations.

[d] AP view of the entire femora (optimally from hips to below knees), and lateral view of the spine.

[e] Optional in absence of new symptoms or evidence of disease progression.

ADVERSE REACTIONS: Clinical Trial Adverse Drug Reactions: Clinical studies are conducted under very specific conditions and the adverse event rates observed in clinical studies may not reflect the rates observed in general practice.

The following safety information is based on the 3 pre-marketing clinical studies completed prior to registration of CEREZYME (imiglucerase for injection): the Pivotal study (RC91-0110), the Extension study (RC92-0501) and the Israeli study (RC92-0301). All patients were Type 1 Gaucher patients. CEREZYME naïve patients refer to those patients who were randomized to receive CEREZYME for 6 months at a dose of 60 U/kg every 2 weeks during the Pivotal study and continued on CEREZYME during the Extension study. CEREZYME cross-over patients refer to those patients who were randomized to receive Ceredase during the Pivotal study then were switched to CEREZYME during the Extension study. Some dose reductions based on maintenance of efficacy occurred during the Extension study. The 10 patients in the Israeli study received CEREZYME for 18 to 24 months at doses of either 15 U/kg every other week or 2.5 U/kg three times weekly. See Table 3.

Table 3: CEREZYME

All Related Adverse Events (≥1%) in CEREZYME Treated Patients During the Pivotal, Extension and Israeli Studies (by COSTART Body System)

	CEREZYME naïve (N=15) No. (%)	CEREZYME cross-over (N=15) No. (%)	CEREZYME Israeli Study (N=10) No. (%)
Body as a Whole			
Headache	4 (27)	0 (0)	0 (0)
Abdominal Pain	0 (0)	0 (0)	1 (10)
Fever	0 (0)	1 (6.7)	0 (0)
Chest Pain	0 (0)	1 (6.7)	0 (0)

(cont'd)

Table 3: CEREZYME *(cont'd)*

All Related Adverse Events (≥1%) in CEREZYME Treated Patients During the Pivotal, Extension and Israeli Studies (by COSTART Body System)

	CEREZYME naïve (N=15) No. (%)	CEREZYME cross-over (N=15) No. (%)	CEREZYME Israeli Study (N=10) No. (%)
Cardiovascular System			
Hypotension	1 (6.7)	0 (0)	0 (0)
Vasodilation	0 (0)	1 (6.7)	1 (10)
Digestive System			
Nausea	1 (6.7)	0 (0)	1 (10)
Diarrhea	0 (0)	1 (6.7)	0 (0)
Nervous System			
Dizziness	1 (6.7)	0 (0)	0 (0)
Emotional Lability	0 (0)	1 (6.7)	0 (0)
Paresthesia	0 (0)	1 (6.7)	0 (0)
Hyperesthesia	0 (0)	0 (0)	1 (10)
Nervousness	0 (0)	0 (0)	1 (10)
Skin and Appendages			
Pruritus	1 (6.7)	1 (6.7)	0 (0)
Rash	1 (6.7)	0 (0)	0 (0)
Rash Macular-papular	0 (0)	1 (6.7)	0 (0)
Urogenital System			
Oliguria	1 (6.7)	0 (0)	0 (0)

During the 3 pre-marketing clinical studies, no additional adverse events were reported as potentially related to CEREZYME treatment. No serious adverse events were reported in any of the 3 studies.

A completed post-marketing clinical study conducted in Japan (protocol 8-98) investigated the use of CEREZYME in patients with neuronopathic Gaucher disease. During this study, one Type 3 Gaucher patient experienced an adverse event of nail disorder which was considered potentially related to CEREZYME therapy. No additional adverse events were reported that were related to CEREZYME.

Post-Market Adverse Drug Reactions: Additional adverse events have been identified during post-marketing use of CEREZYME. Due to the voluntary nature of post-marketing reporting and the continuous accrual and loss of patients over time, actual patient exposure and event frequencies are difficult to obtain and are therefore estimates. Post-marketing reports in patients treated with CEREZYME revealed that approximately 13.8% of patients experienced adverse drug reactions. Some of the adverse events were related to the route of administration. These include discomfort, pruritus, burning, swelling or sterile abscess at the site of venipuncture. Each of these events were found to occur in <1% of the total patient population.

Symptoms suggestive of hypersensitivity have been noted in approximately 6.6% of patients. Onset of such symptoms has occurred during or shortly after infusions; these symptoms include pruritis, flushing, rash, urticaria, angioedema, chest discomfort, dyspnea, coughing, cyanosis, and hypotension. Anaphylactoid reaction has also been reported (see Warnings and Precautions, Immune). Each of these events were found to occur in <1.5% of the total patient population. Pre-treatment with antihistamines and/or corticosteroids and reduction in the rate of infusion has allowed continued use of CEREZYME in most patients.

Additional adverse reactions that have been reported in approximately 6.5% of patients treated with CEREZYME include nausea, abdominal pain, vomiting, diarrhea, rash, fatigue, headache, fever, dizziness, chills, backache, and tachycardia. Each of these events were found to occur in <1.5% of the total patient population.

In addition to the adverse reactions that have been observed in patients treated with CEREZYME, transient peripheral edema has been reported for this therapeutic class of drug.

Antibody Formation: A voluntary immunosurveillance program was initiated in 1991 to better determine the extent of antibody formation in patients receiving alglucerase, which was then extended to patients receiving imiglucerase treatment. Genzyme offers this service to the Gaucher-treating physicians world-wide. As part of the immunosurveillance program, patients are monitored for the development of IgG antibodies to the enzyme using an ELISA test. The resultant absorbance values are compared to a cut-off established from a normal human serum distribution study. Confirmation by the radioimmunoprecipitation (RIP) test of the "above normal range" ELISA indicates that the patient developed antibodies to glucocerebrosidase.

During post-marketing safety surveillance of imiglucerase, the seroconversion rate in patients treated with imiglucerase only has remained at approximately 15%. This overall seroconversion rate is consistent with the rate of antibody formation in patients treated with imiglucerase only reported in the US Pivotal/Extended (3/15, 20%) and Israeli (1/10, 10%) Studies. Patients who develop IgG antibody largely do so within 6 months of treatment and rarely develop antibodies to imiglucerase after 12 months of therapy. Infusion-associated reactions have been reported in approximately half of patients with detectable IgG antibodies to imiglucerase. The most commonly reported symptoms, which are mostly mild to moderate in nature, include pruritus, rash, urticaria, headache, dyspnea and chills. Reactions in most cases are managed by a slower infusion rate and/or pretreatment with anti-pyretics or antihistamines. Patients with antibodies to imiglucerase have a higher risk of infusion-associated reactions; however, not all patients experiencing infusion-associated reactions have detectable IgG antibodies. It is suggested that patients be monitored periodically for IgG antibody formation.

DRUG INTERACTIONS: Drug-Drug Interactions: Interactions with other drugs have not been established.

Drug-Food Interactions: Interactions with food have not been established.

Drug-Herb Interactions: Interactions with herbal products have not been established.

Drug-Laboratory Test Interactions: Interactions with laboratory tests have not been established.

DOSAGE AND ADMINISTRATION: Dosing Considerations:

- Disease severity may dictate that treatment be initiated at a relatively high dose or relatively frequent administration. Dosage adjustments should be made on an individual basis, and may increase or decrease, based on achievement of therapeutic goals as assessed by routine comprehensive evaluations of the patient's clinical non-neurological manifestations.
- The efficacy of CEREZYME (imiglucerase for injection) on neurological symptoms of chronic neuronopathic Gaucher patients has not been established and no special dosage regimen can be recommended for these manifestations.
- In situations where CEREZYME will be administered in a home care environment, it is suggested that the health care professional be trained and prepared for the possibility of an allergic-type reaction.

Recommended Dose and Dosage Adjustment: CEREZYME is administered by intravenous infusion over 1-2 hours. The maximum recommended infusion rate is 1 unit/kg/minute.

Dosage should be individualized to each patient. Treatment may be initiated from 2.5 units/kg of body weight 3 times a week up to 60 U/kg administered as frequently as once every two weeks. Initial dosage may vary, however, 60 units/kg every 2 weeks is the dosage for which most data are available.

Higher doses (up to 120 U/kg every 2 weeks) have been given safely to Type 3 patients.

The vials are single use only. All unused portions must be discarded. To avoid discarding partially used vials, the dose administered at each infusion may be slightly adjusted. Relatively low toxicity, combined with the extended time course of the response, permits small dosage adjustments, but the total dose administered each month should remain substantially unchanged.

Administration: Preparation of Solution for Intravenous Infusion:

1. Using aseptic technique, reconstitute each 200 U vial of CEREZYME with 5.1 mL or each 400 U vial of CEREZYME with 10.2 mL of Sterile Water for Injection, USP, without preservatives. (Reconstitution yields a total volume of 5.3 mL for the 200 U vial and 10.6 mL for the 400 U vial). This results in a final concentration of 40 U/mL for each 200 U vial or each 400 U vial.
2. Gently swirl each vial to mix the solution. **Important: Avoid excessive agitation during the reconstitution.**
3. Bubbles may be present in the solution following reconstitution. Let the solution sit for several minutes to allow any bubbles to dissipate and the lyophilized product to be thoroughly dissolved.
4. The reconstituted preparation results in a clear solution. Inspect vials visually for particulate matter or discolouration before further dilution. Vials exhibiting particulate matter or discolouration should not be used.

Dilution:

1. The total volume following dilution may vary from 100-200 mL. The amount of Normal Saline within the range used for dilution does not affect the amount of CEREZYME administered to the patient.
2. Using aseptic technique, withdraw the contents of each vial and dilute it with 0.9% Sodium Chloride Injection, USP (Normal Saline) to a total volume of 100-200 mL.
3. When more than 20 vials of CEREZYME are required, the drug itself prior to dilution yields a volume of 100 mL. The upper range (200 mL) for total volume offers the flexibility for ensuring dilution of the drug in these instances.

Since CEREZYME does not contain any antibacterial preservatives, it must be reconstituted and diluted **immediately prior to administration**.

OVERDOSAGE:

Experience with doses up to 240 U/kg every two weeks has been reported. At that dose, there have been no reports of obvious toxicity.

> For management of a suspected drug overdose, CPhA recommends that you contact your **regional Poison Control Centre**. See the *CPS* Directory section for a list of Poison Control Centres.

ACTION AND CLINICAL PHARMACOLOGY: Mechanism of Action: CEREZYME (imiglucerase for injection) is an analogue of β-glucocerebrosidase produced by recombinant DNA technology. The lysosomal enzyme catalyses the hydrolysis of glucocerebroside to glucose and ceramide. Gaucher disease is an autosomal genetic disorder characterized by a deficiency of β-glucocerebrosidase activity, resulting in accumulation of glucocerebroside in the lysosomes of tissue macrophages in the liver, spleen, bone marrow and occasionally in lung and kidney. Secondary hematologic sequelae include severe anaemia and thrombocytopenia in addition to the characteristic progressive hepatosplenomegaly, skeletal complications, including osteonecrosis and osteopenia with secondary pathological fractures.

In clinical trials, CEREZYME improved the symptoms associated with Gaucher disease. CEREZYME improved anaemia and thrombocytopenia, reduced spleen and liver size, decreased cachexia and improved Gaucher disease related skeletal involvement and quality of life. Patients reported beneficial results in their general health, energy levels, mobility and reduction of bone pain while on therapy.

Patients have been shown to consistently respond to therapy regardless of the heterogeneity or severity of Gaucher disease. Pediatric patients generally respond to enzyme replacement therapy more quickly than adults. The skeletal response in both pediatric and adult patients to enzyme replacement therapy is generally slower than the hematologic and organ response. The initial primary uptake sites of CEREZYME are the spleen and liver.

Pharmacokinetics: During one hour intravenous infusions of four doses (7.5, 15, 30, 60 U/Kg) of CEREZYME steady-state enzymatic activity was achieved by 30 minutes. Following infusion, plasma enzymatic activity declined rapidly with a half-life ranging from 3.6 to 10.4 minutes. Plasma clearance ranged from 9.8 to 20.3 mL/min/Kg, (mean±S.D, 14.5±4.0 mL/min/Kg). The volume of distribution corrected for weight ranged from 0.09 to 0.15 L/Kg (0.12±0.02 L/kg). These variables appear to be independent of dose or duration of infusion.

Within the dose range of 7.5 to 60 U/kg, elimination half-life, plasma clearance, and volume of distribution values appear to be independent of the infused dose, suggesting that macrophage uptake was not saturated.

The pharmacokinetics of CEREZYME do not appear to be different from placental-derived β-glucocerebrosidase (CEREDASE, alglucerase injection).

STORAGE AND STABILITY: See Table 4.

Table 4: CEREZYME

Lyophilized Vial

CEREZYME (imiglucerase for injection)	Temperature	Recommended Maximum Storage Time
Lyophilized vial	2–8°C	Do not use past expiry date on label.
Lyophilized Vial	23–27°C	Do not exceed 48 hours.

Reconstituted Solutions: Stability of reconstituted and diluted solutions are noted in Table 5.

Table 5: CEREZYME

Reconstituted Solutions

CEREZYME Condition	Temperature	Recommended Maximum Storage Time
Reconstituted Vial (WFI)	2–8°C	Up to 12 hours
Reconstituted Vial (WFI)	28–32°C	Up to 12 hours
Diluted with 0.9% NaCl	2–8°C	Up to 24 hours
Diluted with 0.9% NaCl	20–25°C	Up to 24 hours

Note: Reconstituted vials of CEREZYME are single use only. Use the vials immediately upon reconstitution. Although not recommended, CEREZYME, after reconstitution with Sterile Water for Injection has been shown to be stable for up to 12 hours when stored at room temperature (25°C) and at 2-8°C. Additionally, CEREZYME when diluted with saline, has been shown to be stable for up to 24 hours when stored at room temperature and at 2-8°C.

INFORMATION FOR THE PATIENT: Published in e-CPS, available by subscription at www.e-cps.ca.

DOSAGE FORMS, COMPOSITION AND PACKAGING: 200 Units/Vial: Each vial (blue label) of sterile, non-pyrogenic, white to off-white lyophilized powder for intravenous infusion contains: imiglucerase 212 units (which allows for a withdrawal dose of 200 units), mannitol 170 mg, sodium citrates 70 mg, polysorbate 80 NF 0.53 mg. Preservative-free. Type I glass vials of 20 mL capped with a 20 mm plastic cap and a flip-off aluminum crimp seal. Individual cartons are available in shrink-wrapped bundles of 100, 108 and 120 vials.

400 Units/Vial: Each vial (red label) of sterile, non-pyrogenic, white to off-white lyophilized powder for intravenous infusion contains: imiglucerase 424 units (which allows for a withdrawal dose of 400 units), mannitol 340 mg, sodium citrates 140 mg, polysorbate 80 NF 1.06 mg. Preservative-free. Type I glass vials of 20 mL capped with a 20 mm plastic cap and a flip-off aluminum crimp seal. Individual cartons are available in shrink-wrapped bundles of 100, 108 and 120 vials.

The total sodium citrate composition is made up of trisodium citrate and disodium hydrogen citrate in a ratio of 26:9. Citric acid and/or sodium hydroxide may be present to adjust the pH to approximately 6.3.

Vial Size	Volume of Diluent to be Added to Vial	Approximate Available Volume	Nominal concentration per mL
200 units	5.1 mL Sterile Water for Injection, USP	5.0 mL	40 U/mL
400 units	10.2 mL Sterile Water for Injection, USP	10.0 mL	40 U/mL

Cerumol®

paradichlorobenzene—chlorbutol—oil of turpentine

Cerumenolytic

Paladin

SUPPLIED: Each mL of clear oily preparation contains: paradichlorobenzene PCB (1949) 2%, chlorbutol BP 5% and oil of turpentine BP 10%. Nonmedicinal ingredients: peanut oil. Bottles of 11 mL, packaged in sealed boxes and supplied with a dropper. The product must be used within six months following the insertion of the dropper. Store at room temperature (between 15 and 30°C).

Cervarix™

human papillomavirus vaccine types 16 and 18 (recombinant, AS04 adjuvanted)

Active Immunizing Agent

GlaxoSmithKline

Date of Revision: July 12, 2010

SUMMARY PRODUCT INFORMATION:

Route of Administration	Dosage Form/ Strength per 0.5 mL dose	Clinically Relevant Nonmedicinal Ingredients
Intramuscular injection	Suspension for injection/20 µg Human Papillomavirus (HPV) type 16 L1 protein, 20 µg Human Papillomavirus (HPV) type 18 L1 protein	3-0-desacyl-4'-monophosphoryl lipid A (MPL), aluminum hydroxide, hydrated sodium chloride, sodium dihydrogen phosphate dihydrate, water for injection

DESCRIPTION: CERVARIX (Human Papillomavirus vaccine Types 16 and 18 [Recombinant, AS04 adjuvanted]) is a non-infectious recombinant, AS04-adjuvanted vaccine.

This vaccine contains recombinant C-terminally truncated L1 proteins from HPV type-16 and type-18 each assembled as virus-like particles (VLPs). The HPV-16 and HPV-18 L1 antigens are prepared by recombinant DNA technology using a Baculovirus expression system in Trichoplusia ni cells.

HPV-16 and HPV-18 L1 antigens in CERVARIX are adjuvanted with AS04. The adjuvant system, AS04, is composed of 3-O-desacyl-4'-monophosphoryl lipid A (MPL) adsorbed onto aluminum (as hydroxide salt).

INDICATIONS AND CLINICAL USE: CERVARIX is a vaccine indicated in females from 10 to 25 years of age for the prevention of cervical cancer (squamous cell cancer and adenocarcinoma) by protecting against the following precancerous or dysplastic lesions caused by oncogenic Human Papillomavirus (HPV), types 16 and 18:

- Cervical intraepithelial neoplasia (CIN) grade 2 and grade 3
- Cervical adenocarcinoma in situ (AIS)
- Cervical intraepithelial neoplasia (CIN) grade 1

CONTRAINDICATIONS: CERVARIX should not be administered in:

- females with a known hypersensitivity to any component in the vaccine. For a complete listing, see Dosage Forms, Composition and Packaging.

WARNINGS AND PRECAUTIONS: General: CERVARIX is a prophylactic vaccine. It does not prevent progression of HPV-related lesions present at the time of vaccination.

CERVARIX does not provide protection against all oncogenic HPV types and may not prevent infection with HPV-16/18 or subsequent progression to Cervical Carcinoma, in all vaccine recipients.

CERVARIX is not a treatment for current HPV infection, precancerous lesions, or cervical cancer.

It is good clinical practice that the vaccination should be preceded by a review of the medical history (especially with regard to previous vaccination and possible occurrence of undesirable events) and a clinical examination if indicated.

Vaccination is for primary prevention and is not a substitute for regular cervical screening (secondary prevention) or for precautions against exposure to HPV and other sexually transmitted diseases. All women should continue to follow recommended cervical cancer screening procedures.

Prior to administration, the healthcare provider should review the immunization history for possible vaccine hypersensitivity and previous vaccination-related adverse reactions to allow an assessment of benefits and risks. As with any injectable vaccine, appropriate medical treatment and supervision should always be readily available in case of a rare anaphylactic event following the administration of the vaccine.

Precautions should be taken to avoid intravascular administration.

Febrile Illness: As with other vaccines, administration of CERVARIX should be postponed in individuals suffering from acute severe febrile illness. However, the presence of a minor infection, such as a cold, should not result in the deferral of vaccination.

Hematologic: As with all vaccines administered intramuscularly, CERVARIX should be given with caution to individuals with thrombocytopenia or any coagulation disorder since bleeding may occur following an intramuscular administration to these individuals.

Immune: As with any vaccine, a protective immune response may not be elicited in all vaccine recipients.

There are no data on the use of CERVARIX in individuals with impaired immune responsiveness such as HIV infected patients or patients receiving immunosuppressive treatment. For those individuals an adequate immune response may not be elicited. The duration of protection has not been established.

Syncope: Because vaccinees may develop syncope, sometimes resulting in falling with injury, observation for 15 minutes after administration is recommended. Syncope, sometimes associated with tonic-clonic movements and other seizure-like activity, has been reported following vaccination with CERVARIX. When syncope is associated with tonic-clonic movements, the activity is usually transient and typically responds to restoring cerebral perfusion by maintaining a supine or Trendelenburg position.

Special Populations: Pregnant Women: Vaccination should not be undertaken in women who are pregnant and vaccinees should be advised to take adequate precautions to avoid pregnancy for 2 months following vaccination.

Patients and healthcare providers are encouraged to report any exposure to CERVARIX vaccine during Pregnancy by calling 1-800-387-7374.

Spontaneous Abortions: Outcomes Around Time of Vaccination: In 761 women who had their last menstrual period within 30 days prior to, or 45 days after a vaccine dose and for whom pregnancy outcome was known, spontaneous abortion occurred in a higher proportion of women who received CERVARIX (13.6%) compared to those receiving a control substance (9.6%). It is not known if this is due to a vaccine related effect.

Nursing Women: The effect on breastfed infants of the administration of CERVARIX to their mothers has not been evaluated in clinical studies. CERVARIX should only be used during breast-feeding when the possible advantages outweigh the possible risks.

Serological data suggest a transfer of anti-HPV-16 and anti-HPV-18 antibodies via the milk during the lactation period in rats. However, it is unknown whether vaccine-induced antibodies are excreted in human breast milk.

Pediatrics: CERVARIX is not indicated for children younger than 10 years of age (see Adverse Reactions). Safety and effectiveness in pediatric patients younger than 10 years of age have not been established.

ADVERSE REACTIONS: Clinical Trial Adverse Drug Reactions: Because clinical trials are conducted under very specific conditions, the adverse reaction rates observed in the clinical trials may not reflect the rates observed in practice and should not be compared to the rates in the clinical trials of another drug. Adverse drug reactions information from clinical trials is useful for identifying drug-related adverse events for approximating rates.

Studies in Females 10 Through 25 Years of Age: The safety of CERVARIX was evaluated by pooling data from controlled and uncontrolled clinical trials involving 23 713 females 10 through 25 years of age in the pre-licensure clinical development program. In these studies, 12 785 females (10 through 25 years of age [of these; 1193 of the female children were 10 through 14 years of age and 6316 were 15 through 17 years of age]) received at least one dose of CERVARIX and 10 298 females received at least one dose of a control [Hepatitis A Vaccine containing 360 EL.U. (10 through 14 years of age), Hepatitis A Vaccine containing 720 EL.U. (15 through 25 years of age), or $Al(OH)_3$ (500 µg, 15 through 25 years of age)].

Compliance with the full vaccination course was equally high in both the HPV vaccine and control groups.

Data on solicited local and general adverse events were collected by subjects or parents using standardized diary cards for 7 consecutive days following each vaccine dose (i.e., day of vaccination and the next 6 days). Unsolicited adverse events were recorded with diary cards for 30 days following each vaccination (day of vaccination and 29 subsequent days). Parents and/or subjects were also asked at each study visit about the occurrence of any adverse events and instructed to immediately report serious adverse events throughout the study period. These studies were conducted in North America, Latin America, Europe, Asia, and Australia.

Solicited Adverse Events: The reported frequencies of solicited local injection site reactions (pain, redness, and swelling) and general adverse events (fatigue, fever, gastrointestinal symptoms, headache, arthralgia, myalgia, and urticaria) within 7 days after vaccination in females 10 through 25 years of age are presented in Table 1. An analysis of solicited local injection site reactions by dose is presented in Table 2. Local reactions were reported more frequently with CERVARIX when compared with the control groups; in ≥84% of recipients of CERVARIX, these local reactions were mild to moderate in intensity. Compared with dose 1, pain was reported less frequently after doses 2 and 3 of CERVARIX, in contrast to redness and swelling where there was a small increased incidence. There was no increase in the frequency of general adverse events with successive doses.

Table 1: CERVARIX

Rates of Solicited Local Adverse Reactions and General Adverse Events in Females 10 Through 25 Years of Age Within 7 Days of Vaccination (Total Vaccinated Cohort[a])

Adverse Reaction/Event	CERVARIX[g] (10–25 yrs) %	HAV 720[b] (15–25 yrs) %	HAV 360[c] (10–14 yrs) %	$Al(OH)_3$ Control[d] (15–25 yrs) %
Local Adverse Reaction	N=6431	N=3079	N=1027	N=549
Pain	91.8	78.0	64.2	87.2
Redness	48.0	27.6	25.2	24.4
Swelling	44.1	19.8	17.3	21.3
General Adverse Event	N=6432	N=3079	N=1027	N=549
Fatigue	55.0	53.7	42.3	53.6
Headache	53.4	51.3	45.2	61.4
GI[e]	27.8	27.3	24.6	32.8
Fever (≥99.5°F)	12.8	10.9	16.0	13.5
Rash	9.6	8.4	6.7	10.0
	N=5881	N=3079	N=1027	—
Myalgia[f]	49.1	44.9	33.1	—
Arthralgia[f]	20.8	17.9	19.9	—
Urticaria[f]	7.4	7.9	5.4	—

[a] Total vaccinated cohort included subjects with at least one documented dose (N).
[b] HAV 720=Hepatitis A Vaccine control group [720 EL.U. of antigen and 500 µg $Al(OH)_3$].
[c] HAV 360=Hepatitis A Vaccine control group [360 EL.U. of antigen and 250 µg of $Al(OH)_3$].
[d] $Al(OH)_3$ Control=control containing 500 µg $Al(OH)_3$.
[e] GI=Gastrointestinal symptoms, including nausea, vomiting, diarrhea, and/or abdominal pain.
[f] Adverse events solicited in a subset of subjects.
[g] The number of subjects in the CERVARIX group for Local Adverse Reactions and General Adverse Events varies (6431 and 6432 respectively). The number of subjects included in the analysis is the number of subjects with a documented dose (for Local Adverse Reactions, there was one less subject with a documented dose).
Studies: HPV-001, 008 diary card subset, 012, 013, 014, 016.

The pattern of solicited local adverse reactions and general adverse events following administration of CERVARIX was similar between the age cohorts (10 through 14 years and 15 through 25 years).

Unsolicited Adverse Events by Subject: The frequency of unsolicited adverse events that occurred within 30 days of vaccination (≥1% for CERVARIX and greater than any of the control groups) in females 10 through 25 years of age are presented in Table 3.

Serious Adverse Events (SAEs): In the pooled safety database, inclusive of controlled and uncontrolled studies, which enrolled females 10 through 72 years of age, 5.3% (862/16 142) of subjects who received CERVARIX and 5.9% (814/13 811) of subjects who received control reported at least one serious adverse event, without regard to causality, during the entire follow-up period (up to 7.4 years). Among females 10 through 25 years of age enrolled in these clinical studies, 6.4% of subjects who received CERVARIX and 7.2% of subjects who received the control reported at least one serious adverse event during the entire follow-up period (up to 7.4 years).

Deaths: In completed and ongoing studies which enrolled 57 323 females 9 through 72 years of age, 37 deaths were reported during the 7.4 years of follow-up: 20 in subjects who received CERVARIX (0.06%, 20/33 623) and 17 in subjects who received control (0.07%, 17/23 700). Causes of death among subjects were consistent with those reported in adolescent and adult female populations. The most common causes of death were motor vehicle accident (5 subjects who received CERVARIX; 5 subjects who received control) and suicide (2 subjects who received CERVARIX; 5 subjects who received control), followed by neoplasm (3 subjects who received CERVARIX; 2 subjects who received control), autoimmune disease (3 subjects who received CERVARIX; 1 subject who received control), infectious disease (3 subjects who received CERVARIX; 1 subject who received control), homicide (2 subjects who received CERVARIX; 1 subject who received control), cardiovascular disorders (2 subjects who received CERVARIX), and death of unknown cause (2 subjects who received control). Among females 10 through 25 years of age, 31 deaths were reported (0.05%, 16/29 467 of subjects who received CERVARIX and 0.07%, 15/20 192 of subjects who received control).

New Onset Autoimmune Diseases (NOADs): The pooled safety database, which included controlled and uncontrolled trials which enrolled females 10 through 25 years of age, was searched for new medical conditions indicative of potential new onset autoimmune diseases. Overall, the incidence of potential NOADs, as well as NOADs in the group receiving CERVARIX was 0.8% (95/12 533) and comparable to the pooled control group (0.8%, 87/10 730) during the 4.3 years of follow-up (mean 3.0 years) (Table 4). In the largest randomized, controlled trial (Study HPV-008) which enrolled females 15 through 25 years of age

Table 2: CERVARIX

Rates of Solicited Local Adverse Reactions in Females 10 Through 25 Years of Age by Dose Within 7 Days of Vaccination (Total Vaccinated Cohort[a])

	CERVARIX (10–25 yrs) %			HAV 720[b] (15–25 yrs) %			HAV 360[c] (10–14 yrs) %			Al(OH)3 Control[d] (15–25 yrs) %		
	Post-Dose			Post-Dose			Post-Dose			Post-Dose		
Adverse Reaction	**1**	**2**	**3**	**1**	**2**	**3**	**1**	**2**	**3**	**1**	**2**	**3**
N	**6415**	**6197**	**5936**	**3070**	**2919**	**2758**	**1027**	**1021**	**1011**	**546**	**521**	**500**
Pain	86.9	76.2	78.7	65.6	54.4	56.1	48.5	38.5	36.9	79.1	66.8	72.4
Pain, Grade 3[e]	7.5	5.7	7.7	2.0	1.4	2.0	0.8	0.2	1.6	9.0	6.0	8.6
Redness	27.8	29.6	35.6	16.6	15.2	16.1	15.6	13.3	12.1	11.5	11.5	15.6
Redness, >50 mm	0.2	0.5	1.0	0.1	0.1	0.0	0.1	0.2	0.1	0.2	0.0	0.0
Swelling	22.7	25.2	32.7	10.5	9.4	10.5	9.4	8.6	7.6	10.3	10.4	12.0
Swelling, >50 mm	1.2	1.0	1.3	0.2	0.2	0.2	0.4	0.3	0.0	0.0	0.0	0.0

[a] Total vaccinated cohort included subjects with at least one documented dose (N).
[b] HAV 720=Hepatitis A Vaccine control group [720 EL.U. of antigen and 500 µg $Al(OH)_3$].
[c] HAV 360=Hepatitis A Vaccine control group [360 EL.U. of antigen and 250 µg of $Al(OH)_3$].
[d] $Al(OH)_3$ Control=control containing 500 µg $Al(OH)_3$.
[e] Defined as spontaneously painful or pain that prevented normal daily activities.

and which included active surveillance for potential NOADs, the incidence of potential NOADs and NOADs was 0.8% among subjects who received CERVARIX (78/9319) and 0.8% among subjects who received Hepatitis A Vaccine [720 EL.U. of antigen and 500 µg $Al(OH)_3$] control (77/9235).

Less Common Clinical Trial Adverse Drug Reactions (<1%): Blood and Lymphatic System Disorders: Uncommon: lymphadenopathy.

Table 3: CERVARIX

Rates of Unsolicited Adverse Events in Females 10 Through 25 Years of Age Within 30 Days of Vaccination (≥1% For CERVARIX and Greater Than HAV 720, HAV 360, or $Al(OH)_3$ Control) (Total Vaccinated Cohort[a])

Adverse Event	CERVARIX[e] % N=6654	HAV 720[b] % N=3186	HAV 360[c] % N=1032	$Al(OH)_3$ Control[d] % N=581
Headache	5.3	7.6	3.3	9.3
Nasopharyngitis	3.6	3.4	5.9	3.3
Influenza	3.2	5.6	1.3	1.9
Pharyngolaryngeal pain	2.9	2.7	2.2	2.2
Dizziness	2.2	2.6	1.5	3.1
Upper respiratory tract infection	2.0	1.3	6.7	1.5
Chlamydia infection	2.0	4.4	0.0	0.0
Dysmenorrhea	2.0	2.3	1.9	4.0
Pharyngitis	1.5	1.8	2.2	0.5
Injection site bruising	1.4	1.8	0.7	1.5
Vaginal infection	1.4	2.2	0.1	0.9
Injection site pruritus	1.3	0.5	0.6	0.2
Back pain	1.1	1.3	0.7	3.1
Urinary tract infection	1.0	1.4	0.3	1.2

[a] Total vaccinated cohort included subjects with at least one documented dose (N).
[b] HAV 720=Hepatitis A Vaccine control group [720 EL.U. of antigen and 500 µg $Al(OH)_3$].
[c] HAV 360=Hepatitis A Vaccine control group [360 EL.U. of antigen and 250 µg of $Al(OH)_3$].
[d] $Al(OH)_3$ Control=control containing 500 µg $Al(OH)_3$.
[e] The number of subjects in the CERVARIX group varies between Table 1 and Table 3 because Table 3 included subjects from studies HPV-001, 003, 004, 005, 008 diary card subset, 012, 013, 014, 016.

Table 4: CERVARIX

Incidence of New Medical Conditions Indicative of Potential New Onset Autoimmune Disease and New Onset Autoimmune Disease Throughout the Follow-up Period Regardless of Causality in Females 10 Through 25 Years of Age (Total Vaccinated Cohort[a])

	CERVARIX (N=12 533) n (%)[c]	Pooled Control Group[b] (N=10 730) n (%)[c]
Total Number of Subjects With at Least One Medical Condition	**95 (0.8)**	**87 (0.8)**
Arthritis[d]	9 (0.1)	4 (0.0)
Celiac disease	2 (0.0)	5 (0.0)
Dermatomyositis	0 (0.0)	1 (0.0)
Diabetes mellitus insulin-dependent (Type 1 or unspecified)	5 (0.0)	5 (0.0)
Erythema nodosum	3 (0.0)	0 (0.0)
Hyperthyroidism[e]	14 (0.1)	15 (0.1)
Hypothyroidism[f]	30 (0.2)	28 (0.3)
Inflammatory bowel disease[g]	8 (0.1)	4 (0.0)
Multiple sclerosis	4 (0.0)	1 (0.0)
Myelitis transverse	1 (0.0)	0 (0.0)
Optic neuritis/Optic neuritis retrobulbar	3 (0.0)	1 (0.0)
Psoriasis[h]	8 (0.1)	11 (0.1)
Raynaud's phenomenon	0 (0.0)	1 (0.0)
Rheumatoid arthritis	4 (0.0)	3 (0.0)
Systemic lupus erythematosus[i]	2 (0.0)	3 (0.0)
Thrombocytopenia[j]	1 (0.0)	1 (0.0)
Vasculitis[k]	1 (0.0)	3 (0.0)
Vitiligo	2 (0.0)	2 (0.0)

[a] Total vaccinated cohort included subjects with at least one documented dose (N).
[b] Pooled Control Group=Hepatitis A Vaccine control group [720 EL.U. of antigen and 500 µg $Al(OH)_3$], Hepatitis A Vaccine control group [360 EL.U. of antigen and 250 µg of $Al(OH)_3$], and a control containing 500 µg $Al(OH)_3$.
[c] n (%): number and percentage of subjects with medical condition.
[d] Term includes reactive arthritis and arthritis.
[e] Term includes Basedow's disease, goiter, and hyperthyroidism.
[f] Term includes thyroiditis, autoimmune thyroiditis, and hypothyroidism.
[g] Term includes colitis ulcerative, Crohn's disease, proctitis ulcerative, and inflammatory bowel disease.
[h] Term includes psoriatic arthropathy, nail psoriasis, guttate psoriasis, and psoriasis.
[i] Term includes systemic lupus erythematosus and cutaneous lupus erythematosus.
[j] Term includes idiopathic thrombocytopenic purpura and thrombocytopenia.
[k] Term includes leukocytoclastic vasculitis and vasculitis.

General Disorders and Administration Site Conditions: Uncommon: other injection site reactions such as induration and local paresthesia.

Post-Market Adverse Drug Reactions: The following events have been spontaneously reported during post-approval use of CERVARIX. This list includes serious events or events which have suspected causal association to CERVARIX. Because these events are reported voluntarily from a population of uncertain size, it is not always possible to reliably estimate their frequency or establish a causal relationship to vaccination.

Immune System Disorders: Allergic reactions (including anaphylactic and anaphylactoid reactions), angioedema and erythema multiforme have been rarely reported (≥1/10 000 to <1/1000).

Nervous System Disorders: Syncope or vasovagal responses to injection (sometimes accompanied by tonic-clonic movements) have been rarely reported (≥1/10 000 to <1/1000).

DRUG INTERACTIONS: Drug-Drug Interactions: Use with other vaccines: Studies to evaluate the concomitant administration of CERVARIX and other vaccines (conjugate meningococcal vaccine, Hepatitis B vaccine, Hepatitis A and B vaccine and adult/adolescent formulations of tetanus, diphtheria, acellular pertussis (dTpa)) are currently on-going.

Data have not been generated on the concomitant administration of CERVARIX and other vaccines. If CERVARIX is to be given at the same time as another injectable vaccine, the vaccines should always be administered at different injection sites. CERVARIX should not be mixed with any other vaccine in the same syringe or vial.

Use with Hormonal Contraceptives: In clinical efficacy studies, approximately 60% of females who received CERVARIX used hormonal contraceptives. There is no evidence that the use of hormonal contraceptives has an impact on the efficacy of CERVARIX.

Use with Systemic Immunosuppressive Medications: As with other vaccines it may be expected that, in patients receiving immunosuppressive therapy, an adequate response may not be achieved.

Drug-Food Interactions: Interactions with food have not been established.

Drug-Herb Interactions: Interactions with herbal products have not been established.

Drug-Laboratory Test Interactions: Interactions with laboratory tests have not been established

Drug-Lifestyle Interactions: Effects on the ability to drive and use machines: No studies on the effects on the ability to drive or use machines have been performed.

DOSAGE AND ADMINISTRATION: Recommended Dose and Dosage Adjustment: The primary vaccination course consists of three doses.

The recommended vaccination schedule is 0, 1, 6 months. If flexibility in the vaccination schedule is necessary, the second dose can be administered between 1 month and 2.5 months after the first dose and the third dose can be administered between 5 months and 9 months after the first dose. The necessity for a booster has not been established.

Administration: CERVARIX is for intramuscular injection in the deltoid region. Do not administer this product intradermally, or subcutaneously and precautions should be taken to avoid intravascular administration.

A fine white deposit with a clear, colourless supernatant may be observed upon storage of the syringe/vial. This does not constitute a sign of deterioration.

The content of the syringe/vial should be inspected visually both before and after shaking for any foreign particulate matter and/or abnormal physical appearance prior to administration. In the event of either being observed, discard the vaccine.

Shake well before use.

Any unused product or waste material should be disposed of in accordance with local requirements.

Preparation for Administration: The syringe comes fully assembled. **Do not remove the white back-stop from the syringe.** Prior to administration, ensure that the plunger rod is firmly attached to the rubber stopper by turning the plunger clockwise until slight resistance is felt. **Do not** over tighten. Holding the syringe barrel in one hand (avoid holding the syringe plunger), remove the syringe LUER Tip-cap and needle cap by twisting anticlockwise. Attach needle by pressing and twisting in a clockwise rotation until secured to the syringe. Remove the needle protector, which on occasion can be a little stiff. Administer the vaccine. See Figure 1.

Figure 1: CERVARIX Syringe

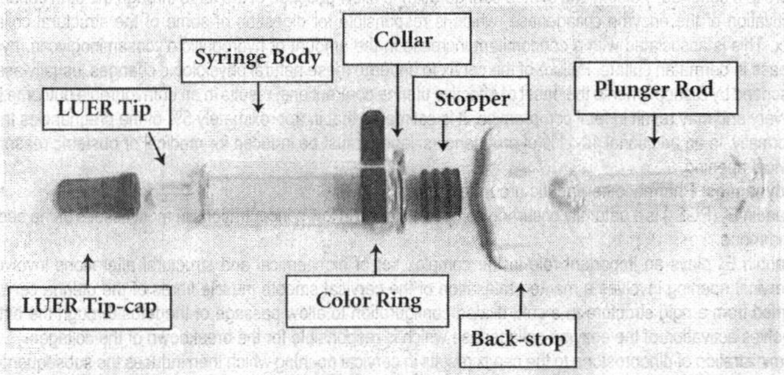

OVERDOSAGE:
Insufficient data are available.

> For management of a suspected drug overdose, contact your regional Poison Control Centre. See the *CPS* Directory section for a list of Poison Control Centres.

ACTION AND CLINICAL PHARMACOLOGY: Disease Burden: Worldwide, oncogenic Human Papillomavirus (HPV) types are the necessary cause of cervical cancer. Compelling epidemiological evidence confirms that persistent infection with oncogenic HPV types is responsible for virtually all cases of invasive cervical cancer. Based on a large consensus among experts, the most common HPV types identified in invasive cervical cancer worldwide were, in decreasing order of frequency, HPV-16, -18, -45, -31, -33, -52, -58, -35, -59, -56, -39, -51, -73, -68 and -66. HPV types -16 and -18 are responsible for more than 70% of invasive cervical cancers. Together, HPV types -16, -18, -31 and -45 account for up to 80.3% of cases. In the United States, the most common HPV genotypes detected in invasive cancers are HPV type −16 (HPV-16, 53.2%), HPV-18 (13.1%), and HPV-45 (6.1%) and those in in situ cancers were HPV-16 (56.3%), HPV-31 (12.6%), and HPV-33 (8.0%). HPV is a highly prevalent family of viruses. Up to 80% of females who have ever been sexually active will acquire an HPV infection in their lifetime, which in some cases may cause cervical cancer. Oncogenic HPV types have been found in up to 75% of HPV infections.

Cervical cancers begin as asymptomatic precancerous lesions and usually develop gradually over many years. Cervical lesions are described according to the degree of cytopathology found on the Pap* smear, with progression in degree of dysplasia.

HPV is generally transmitted via skin-to-skin contact during sexual activity. Papillomavirus entry into cells may take as little as 2 to 4 hours. Condoms reduce the risk of HPV infection, but are not fully effective. The period between exposure to the infection and the development of a specific lesion is extremely variable, making it virtually impossible for most individuals to determine exactly when, and from whom, they were exposed to the virus.

Studies have shown that prior infection with HPV does not provide females with reliable immunity against subsequent infections or reduce the risk of an HPV infection becoming persistent. Approximately 50% of females generate antibodies against initial HPV infections. In females that do generate anti-HPV antibodies, levels are typically low and slow to develop and are not reliably protective. Since antibody levels in women that have cleared an HPV infection are either low or not-existent, women may be susceptible to the same or different HPV type in the future. In the absence of detectable anti-HPV antibodies, generating immune memory in response to HPV infection in previously exposed women has not been demonstrated to provide protection against future infection or disease.

In Canada, cervical cancer affects females of all ages and among females aged 20 to 44, cervical cancer ranks as second most common to breast cancer. The proportion of HPV-16 and HPV-18 related cervical cancer cases in North America is 76% and increases to 84% when HPV-16, -18, -45, and -31 are included. The annual rate of new diagnoses of cervical cancer in Canada is 8.9/100 000 and the annual mortality rate is 2.5/100 000. The annual rate of new diagnoses of adenocarcinoma of the cervix may be as high as 1.83/100 000 in Canada. Despite the significant reduction in the burden of disease from cervical cancer since the introduction of cervical cancer screening, new cases and deaths from cervical cancer continue, with approximately 1300 new cases and 380 deaths from cervical cancer estimated in 2008.

Infections with multiple oncogenic HPV types are common in sexually active females with cytologic abnormalities; however, almost all cervical cancer is attributable to a single HPV type. Natural history studies of HPV infection support that the risk of progression to cervical precancers and cervical cancers increases with persistent infection. In fact, HPV persistent infections tend to occur at a higher percentage with HPV-16 than with other oncogenic HPV types and that the risk of progression to cervical cancer is higher for HPV-16, -18 and -45 than other HPV types.

Worldwide, the proportion of cervical intraepithelial neoplasia (CIN) grades 2 and 3, and invasive cervical cases associated with HPV-16 and HPV-18 are 52.3% and 70.3% respectively. HPV-16 predominates in squamous cell carcinomas (55.2%) as well as in cervical adenocarcinomas (48.4%), whereas HPV-18 has been detected more than twice as frequently in adenocarcinoma (36.3%) as compared to squamous cervical carcinomas (12.8%).

Overall, incidence and mortality rates due to cervical cancer have shown a steady decline in the past 30 years due to the introduction of Pap screening programs. The reduction has been driven primarily by decreases in the rates of cervical squamous cell carcinomas, the predominant histological type. Rates of adenocarcinoma and adenosquamous carcinomas have increased over this period, particularly in females 20 to 34 years of age. Rates have plateaued in the last 5 years, suggesting that further prevention strategies beyond Pap screening may be necessary. Given that adenocarcinomas occur further in the endocervical canal, they are often more difficult to detect through normal cytological screening.

Until recently, cervical cancer screening programs have allowed for detection and removal of precancerous lesions (secondary prevention). Primary prevention of these lesions via vaccination can provide an additional opportunity to prevent cervical cancer by prevention of the infection which initiates the disease process.

Mechanism of Action: CERVARIX is a non-infectious recombinant vaccine prepared from the highly purified virus-like particles (VLPs) of the major capsid L1 protein of oncogenic HPV types 16 and 18. Since the VLPs contain no viral DNA, they cannot infect cells, reproduce or cause disease.

High and sustained antibodies against HPV are associated with protection against HPV-related infection and/or disease. Animal studies suggest that the efficacy of L1 VLP vaccines is predominantly mediated by the development of neutralizing antibody (humoral) immune responses. Vaccination with HPV L1 capsid proteins predominately induces serum neutralizing IgG antibodies; however, transudation of anti-HPV IgG neutralizing antibodies from the serum to the cervical mucosa is thought to provide a mechanism to prevent HPV entry into cervical epithelial cells which might otherwise lead to infection and cervical cancer. CERVARIX studies have demonstrated that there is a correlation between levels of anti-HPV antibodies in serum samples relative to anti-HPV antibodies in cervicovaginal secretion samples. While the minimum level of antibodies required to prevent HPV infection are not yet known, anti-papillomavirus antibodies have been shown to be sufficient to prevent infection and/or disease. These data suggest that the mechanism of action of L1 VLP vaccines is primarily mediated through a vaccine-induced antibody-mediated immune response.

The adjuvant in CERVARIX is AS04 which has been shown in clinical trials to induce a stronger and sustained immune response compared to the same antigens adjuvanted with aluminum salt [$Al(OH)_3$] alone.

STORAGE AND STABILITY: Store in a refrigerator at 2 to 8°C. Do not freeze. Store in the original package in order to protect from light.

The expiry date of the vaccine is indicated on the label and packaging. Do not use after the expiry date shown on the label.

CERVARIX should be administered as soon as possible after being removed from the refrigerator. However, stability data generated indicated that CERVARIX remains stable and can be administered in case the vaccine has been stored outside the refrigerator up to three days at temperatures between 8 and 25°C or up to one day at temperatures between 25 and 37°C. If exposed to temperatures >37°C, discard vaccine.

INFORMATION FOR THE PATIENT: Published in e-CPS, available by subscription at www.e-cps.ca.

DOSAGE FORMS, COMPOSITION AND PACKAGING: Each 0.5 mL dose of suspension for injection contains: Human Papillomavirus type 16 L1 protein† 20 µg and Human Papillomavirus type 18 L1 protein† 20 µg. Nonmedicinal ingredients: aluminum hydroxide, hydrated ($Al(OH)_3$)†, sodium chloride, sodium dihydrogen phosphate dihydrate, 3-0-desacyl-4'- monophosphoryl lipid A (MPL)‡ and water for injection. Pre-filled syringes (type I glass) with a plunger stopper (rubber butyl) with or without needles in pack sizes of 1 and 10. Note: Multiple safety needle tips are compatible with this system. Vials (type I glass) with a stopper (rubber butyl) in pack sizes of 1, 10 and 100. Pre-filled syringe components contain latex and vial components are latex-free.

Cervidil™ Pr

dinoprostone

Prostaglandin

Ferring

Date of Preparation: April 1, 1997
Date of Revision: July 20, 2006

SUMMARY PRODUCT INFORMATION:

Route of Administration	Dosage Form/ Strength	Clinically Relevant Nonmedicinal Ingredients
Vaginal	10 mg	Hydrogel polymer Prepared with: macrogol 8000, dicyclohexylmethane-4,4'diisocyanate, 1,2,6-hexanetriol, polyester retrieval system

DESCRIPTION: CERVIDIL is a thin, flat, semi-transparent polymeric slab which is rectangular in shape with rounded corners contained within a knitted polyester retrieval system.

Each insert contains 10 mg dinoprostone (prostaglandin E_2) dispersed throughout its matrix, and releases approximately 0.3 mg/hour PGE_2 over a 12 hour period. The reservoir of 10 mg dinoprostone serves to maintain constant release.

The retrieval system consists of a one-piece knitted polyester pouch and withdrawal tape. This ensures easy and reliable removal of the insert when the patient's requirement for PGE_2 has been fulfilled or an obstetric event makes it necessary to stop further drug administration.

INDICATIONS AND CLINICAL USE: CERVIDIL (dinoprostone) is indicated for:

- Initiation and/or continuation of cervical ripening in patients at or near term in whom there is a medical or obstetrical indication for the induction of labour.

Geriatrics (>65 years of age): CERVIDIL has not been studied in this patient population and is not recommended for use.

Pediatrics (<18 years of age): CERVIDIL has not been studied in this patient population and is not recommended for use.

CONTRAINDICATIONS: CERVIDIL is contraindicated in:

- Patients who are hypersensitive to this drug or to any ingredient in the formulation or component of the container. For a complete listing, see Dosage Forms, Composition and Packaging.
- Patients in whom there is clinical suspicion or definite evidence of fetal distress where delivery is not imminent;
- Patients with placenta previa or unexplained vaginal bleeding during this pregnancy;
- Patients in whom there is evidence or strong suspicion of marked cephalopelvic disproportion;
- Patients in whom oxytocic drugs are contraindicated or when prolonged contraction of the uterus may be detrimental to fetal safety or uterine integrity (previous cesarean section or major uterine surgery);
- Multipara with 6 or more previous term pregnancies;
- Patients with a history of difficult labour and/or traumatic delivery;
- Patients with overdistension of uterus (multiple pregnancy, polyhydramnios);
- Patients with fetal malpresentation;
- Patients with a history of epilepsy whose seizures are poorly controlled;
- CERVIDIL should not be used simultaneously with other oxytocics (see Warnings and Precautions);
- CERVIDIL should not be used when there is a history of, or current pelvic inflammatory disease, unless adequate prior treatment has been instituted.

WARNINGS AND PRECAUTIONS:

> **Serious Warnings and Precautions**
> **For Hospital Use Only:** CERVIDIL should be administered only by trained obstetrical personnel in a hospital setting with appropriate obstetrical care facilities.

General: Since prostaglandins potentiate the effect of oxytocin, CERVIDIL must be removed before oxytocin administration is initiated and the patient's uterine activity carefully monitored for uterine hyperstimulation.

If uterine hyperstimulation is encountered or if labour commences, the vaginal insert should be removed. CERVIDIL should also be removed prior to amniotomy. The vaginal insert should be removed if there is evidence of maternal systemic adverse PGE_2 effects such as nausea, vomiting, hypotension or tachycardia.

* Pap (Papanicolaou test detects abnormal cervical cells).

† L1 protein in the form of non-infectious virus-like particles (VLPs) produced by recombinant DNA technology using a Baculovirus expression system.

‡ The GlaxoSmithKline proprietary AS04 adjuvant system is composed of aluminum hydroxide and 3-0-desacyl-4'- monophosphoryl lipid A (MPL).

The experience of CERVIDIL in patients with ruptured membranes is limited. Therefore, CERVIDIL should be used with caution in those patients. Since the release of dinoprostone from the insert can be affected in the presence of amniotic fluid, special attention should be given to uterine activity and fetal condition.

Caution should be exercised in the administration of CERVIDIL for cervical ripening in patients with a history of previous uterine hypertonicity, glaucoma, or a history of childhood asthma, even though there have been no asthma attacks in adulthood or unexplained genital bleeding during the current pregnancy.

Women aged 35 and over (occasionally also younger women), women with complications during pregnancy and women at gestational age above 40 weeks, have a higher risk for developing disseminated intravascular coagulation (DIC). These factors may enhance the risk of disseminated intravascular coagulation in women with pharmacologically induced labour. Therefore, dinoprostone should be used with caution in these women. In the immediate post-partum phase the physician should look carefully for early signs of developing DIC (e.g. fibrinolysis).

Uterine activity, fetal status and the progression of cervical dilatation and effacement should be carefully monitored whenever the dinoprostone vaginal insert is in place. Any evidence of uterine hyperstimulation, sustained uterine contractions, fetal distress, or other fetal or maternal adverse reactions, should be a cause for consideration of removal of the insert. The possibility of uterine rupture and/or cervical laceration should be born in mind where hypertonic myometrial contractions are sustained.

Cephalopelvic relationships should be carefully evaluated before the use of CERVIDIL.

Prolonged treatment of newborn infants with prostaglandin E_1 can induce proliferation of bone. There is no evidence that short term administration of prostaglandin E_2 can cause similar bone effects.

Patients with severe renal disease and/or severe hepatic disease accompanied by metabolic aberrations should be dosed with caution.

Carcinogenesis and Mutagenesis: Long-term carcinogenicity and fertility studies have not been conducted with CERVIDIL (dinoprostone vaginal insert). No evidence of mutagenicity has been observed with prostaglandin E_2 in the Unscheduled DNA Synthesis Assay, the Micronucleus Test, or Ames Assay.

Special Populations: Pregnant Women: Animal studies indicate that the prostaglandins may be teratogenic. No effect would be expected clinically, when used as indicated, since CERVIDIL (dinoprostone vaginal insert) is administered after the period of organogenesis. Any dose of the drug that produces sustained increased uterine tone could put the embryo or fetus at risk.

Nursing Women: CERVIDIL is not indicated for use during early or other phases of pregnancy or during lactation.

Monitoring and Laboratory Tests: After insertion, the patient should remain supine and monitored for 2 hours for any evidence of uterine hyperstimulation, change in fetal heart rate or maternal blood pressure or heart rate.

If any of these changes occur, removal of CERVIDIL should be considered.

ADVERSE REACTIONS: Clinical Trial Adverse Drug Reactions: Because clinical trials are conducted under very specific conditions the adverse reaction rates observed in the clinical trials may not reflect the rates observed in practice and should not be compared to the rates in the clinical trials of another drug. Adverse drug reaction information from clinical trials is useful for identifying drug-related adverse events and for approximating rates.

CERVIDIL is well tolerated. In placebo-controlled trials in which 658 women were entered and 320 received active therapy (218 without retrieval system, 102 with retrieval system), the following events were reported.

Table 1: CERVIDIL

Total Drug Related Adverse Events

	Controlled Studies[a]		Study 101-801[b]	
	Active (%)	Placebo (%)	Active (%)	Placebo (%)
Uterine hyperstimulation with fetal distress	2.8	0.3	2.9	0
Uterine hyperstimulation without fetal distress	4.7	0	2.0	0
Fetal distress without uterine hyperstimulation	3.8	1.2	2.9	1.0
N	320	338	102	104

[a] Controlled studies (with and without retrieval system).
[b] Controlled study (with retrieval system).

Drug related fever, nausea, vomiting, diarrhea, and abdominal pain were noted in less than 1% of patients who received CERVIDIL.

Table 2 outlines the frequency of reported adverse events.

Table 2: CERVIDIL

Frequency of Reported Adverse Events

Frequency	MedDRA System Organ Class	Adverse Events (MedDRA Preferred Term)
Common (>1/100, <1/10)	Pregnancy, puerperium and perinatal conditions	Abnormal labour affecting fetus Fetal heart rate disorder Fetal distress syndrome Uterine hypertonus
Uncommon (>1/1000, <1/100)	Gastro-intestinal disorders	Nausea, vomiting, diarrhea
Rare (>1/10 000, <1/1000)	Blood and lymphatic system disorders Reproductive system and breast disorders Pregnancy, puerperium and perinatal conditions	Disseminated intravascular coagulation Uterine rupture

An increased risk of post-partum disseminated intravascular coagulation has been reported in patients whose labour was induced by pharmacological means, either with dinoprostone or oxytocin. The frequency of this adverse event, however, appears to be rare (<1 per 1000 pregnancies).

Very rare cases of anaphylactic reactions have been reported with the use of dinoprostone.

In Study 101-801 (with the retrieval system) all cases of hyperstimulation reversed within 2 to 13 minutes of removal of the product. Tocolytics were required in one of the five cases.

In cases of fetal distress, when product removal was thought advisable, there was a return to normal rhythm and no neonatal sequelae.

Five minute Apgar scores were 7 or above in 98.2% (646/658) of studied neonates whose mothers participated in placebo-controlled studies with CERVIDIL. A 3 year pediatric follow-up study in 121 infants whose mothers received PGE_2, found no significant differences from a control group on physical examination or psychomotor evaluation.

Post-Market Adverse Drug Reactions: In post marketing experience reports, uterine rupture has been reported rarely in association with the use of CERVIDIL (see Warnings and Precautions and Contraindications).

DRUG INTERACTIONS: Overview: CERVIDIL may augment the activity of oxytocic agents and their concomitant use is not recommended. A dosing interval of at least 30 minutes is recommended for the sequential use of oxytocin following the removal of the dinoprostone vaginal insert. No other drug interactions have been identified.

DOSAGE AND ADMINISTRATION: To remove CERVIDIL from the packaging, first tear the foil along the top of the sachet. Do not use scissors or sharp implements to cut the foil as this may damage the product. Use the retrieval system to gently pull the product out of the sachet. After removal from the patient, ensure that the entire product (vaginal delivery system and retrieval system) has been removed from the vagina.

Recommended Dose and Dosage Adjustment: The dosage of dinoprostone in the vaginal insert is 10 mg designed to be released at approximately 0.3 mg/hour over a 12 hour period. CERVIDIL should be removed upon onset of active labour or 12 hours after insertion.

One CERVIDIL is placed transversely in the posterior fornix of the vagina immediately after removal from its foil package. The insertion of the vaginal insert does not require sterile conditions. The vaginal insert must not be used without its retrieval system. There is no need for previous warming of the product. A minimal amount of K-Y jelly (or other water-miscible lubricant) may be used to assist in insertion of CERVIDIL. Care should be taken not to permit excess contact or coating with the lubricant and thus prevent optimal swelling and release of dinoprostone from the vaginal insert. Patients should remain in the supine position for 2 hours following insertion, but thereafter may be ambulatory.

OVERDOSAGE:

CERVIDIL is used as a single dosage in a single application. Overdosage is usually manifested by uterine hyperstimulation which may be accompanied by fetal distress and is responsive to removal of the insert. Other treatment must be symptomatic, since to date, clinical experience with prostaglandin antagonists is insufficient.

The use of beta-adrenergic agents should be considered in the event of undesirable increased uterine activity.

For management of a suspected drug overdose, CPhA recommends that you contact your **regional Poison Control Centre**. See the *CPS* Directory section for a list of Poison Control Centres.

ACTION AND CLINICAL PHARMACOLOGY: Mechanism of Action: Dinoprostone (PGE_2) is a naturally-occurring biomolecule. It is found in low concentrations in most tissues of the body and functions as a local hormone. As with any local hormone, it is very rapidly metabolized in the tissues of synthesis. The rate limiting step for inactivation is regulated by the enzyme 15-hydroxyprostaglandin dehydrogenase (PGDH). Any PGE_2 that escapes local inactivation is rapidly cleared to the extent of 95% on the first pass through the pulmonary circulation.

In pregnancy, PGE_2 is secreted continuously by the fetal membranes and placenta and plays an important role in the final events leading to the initiation of labour. It is known that PGE_2 stimulates the production of $PGF_{2\alpha}$ which in turn sensitizes the myometrium to endogenous or exogenously administrated oxytocin. Although PGE_2 is capable of initiating uterine contractions and may interact with oxytocin to increase uterine contractility, the available evidence indicates, that in the concentrations found during the early part of labour, PGE_2 plays an important role in cervical ripening without affecting uterine contractions. This distinction serves as the basis for considering cervical ripening and induction of labour, usually by the use of oxytocin, as two separate processes.

PGE_2 plays an important role in the complex set of biochemical and structural alterations involved in cervical ripening. Cervical ripening involves a marked relaxation of the cervical smooth muscle fibers of the uterine cervix which must be transformed from a rigid structure to a softened, yielding and dilated configuration to allow passage of the fetus through the birth canal. This process involves activation of the enzyme collagenase, which is responsible for digestion of some of the structural collagen network of the cervix. This is associated with a concomitant increase in the amount of hydrophilic glycosaminoglycan, hyaluronic acid, and a decrease in dermatan sulfate. Failure of the cervix to undergo these natural physiologic changes, usually assessed by the method described by Bishop, prior to the onset of effective uterine contractions, results in an unfavourable outcome for successful vaginal delivery and may result in fetal compromise. It is estimated that in approximately 5% of the pregnancies the cervix does not ripen normally. In an additional 10-11% of pregnancies, labour must be induced for medical or obstetric reasons prior to the time of cervical ripening.

Pharmacodynamics: Pharmacotherapeutic group: oxytocics.

Prostaglandin E_2 (PGE_2) is a naturally occurring compound found in low concentrations in most tissues of the body. It functions as a local hormone.

Prostaglandin E_2 plays an important role in the complex set of biochemical and structural alterations involved in cervical ripening. Cervical ripening involves a marked relaxation of the cervical smooth muscle fibres of the uterine cervix which must be transformed from a rigid structure to a soft, dilated configuration to allow passage of the fetus through the birth canal. This process involves activation of the enzyme collagenase which is responsible for the breakdown of the collagen.

Local administration of dinoprostone to the cervix results in cervical ripening which then induces the subsequent events which complete labour.

Pharmacokinetics: PGE_2 is rapidly metabolised primarily in the tissue of synthesis.

No correlation could be established between PGE_2 release and plasma concentrations of its metabolite, PGE_m. The relative contributions of endogenously and exogenously released PGE_2 to the plasma levels of the metabolite PGE_m could not be determined.

The reservoir of 10 mg dinoprostone serves to maintain a controlled and constant release. The release rate is approximately 0.3 mg per hour over 12 hours in women with intact membranes whereas release is higher and more variable in women with premature rupture of membranes. CERVIDIL releases dinoprostone to the cervical tissue continuously at a rate which allows cervical ripening to progress until complete, and with the facility to remove the dinoprostone source when the clinician decides that cervical ripening is complete or labour has started, at which point no further dinoprostone is required.

STORAGE AND STABILITY: Store in a freezer between −20 and −10°C

INFORMATION FOR THE PATIENT: Published in e-CPS, available by subscription at www.e-cps.ca.

DOSAGE FORMS, COMPOSITION AND PACKAGING: Each vaginal insert contains: dinoprostone 10 mg (prostaglandin E_2) dispersed throughout its matrix described as 236 mg of a cross-linked polyethylene oxide/urethane polymer which is a semi-transparent, beige colored, flat, 0.8 mm thick rectangular slab with rounded corners measuring 29 mm by 9.5 mm. The insert and its retrieval system, made of polyester yarn, are nontoxic and when placed in a moist environment, absorb water, swell, and release dinoprostone. Cartons of 1 containing 1 insert within a retrieval system, enclosed in a foil (aluminum/polyethylene) pack.

C.E.S.® Ⓟ

conjugated estrogens

Estrogens

Valeant

Date of Preparation: June 3, 2009

SUMMARY PRODUCT INFORMATION:

Route of Administration	Dosage Form/ Strength	Clinically Relevant Nonmedicinal Ingredients
Oral	Tablets/0.3 mg, 0.625 mg, 0.9 mg, and 1.25 mg	Lactose (see Warnings and Precautions, Endocrine and Metabolism, Other Conditions) For a complete listing see Dosage Forms, Composition and Packaging.

INDICATIONS AND CLINICAL USE: C.E.S. (conjugated estrogens tablets, CSD) is indicated for:

In female patients:

- Relief of menopausal and postmenopausal symptoms occurring in naturally or surgically induced estrogen deficiency states including vaginal and vulvar atrophy (with or without pruritus). **When prescribing solely for the treatment of symptoms of vulvar and vaginal atrophy, topical vaginal products should be considered.**
- Prevention and treatment of osteoporosis in naturally occurring or surgically induced estrogen-deficiency states. This is in addition to other important therapeutic measures such as adequate diet, calcium and vitamin D intake, cessation of smoking, as well as regular physical weight bearing exercise. C.E.S. for prevention and treatment of osteoporosis is to be considered in light of other available therapies (see Warnings and Precautions, Boxed Warnings).
- Hypoestrogenism due to hypogonadism, castration, or primary ovarian failure.
- Atrophic vaginitis.

In patients with intact uteri, C.E.S. should always be supplemented by administration of a progestin whose role is to prevent endometrial hyperplasia/carcinoma.

In male patients:

- Inoperable progressing prostatic cancer (for palliation only when castration is not feasible, or when castration failed or delayed escape following a response to castration occurred).

Geriatrics (>65 years of age): See above indications.
Pediatrics (<16 years of age): C.E.S. is not indicated for use in children.

CONTRAINDICATIONS: Treatment with C.E.S. (conjugated estrogens) is contraindicated in patients with any of the following conditions:
- Patients who are hypersensitive to this drug or to any ingredient in the formulation or component of the container. For a complete listing, see Dosage Forms, Composition and Packaging.
- Liver dysfunction or disease as long as liver function tests have failed to return to normal.
- Known or suspected estrogen-dependent malignant neoplasia (e.g. endometrial cancer).
- Endometrial hyperplasia.
- Known, suspected, or past history of breast cancer.
- Undiagnosed abnormal genital bleeding.
- Known or suspected pregnancy (see Warnings and Precautions, Special Populations, Pregnant Women).
- Active or past history of arterial thromboembolic disease (e.g., stroke, myocardial infarction, coronary heart disease).
- Active or past history of confirmed venous thromboembolism (such as deep vein thrombosis or pulmonary embolism) or active thrombophlebitis.
- Partial or complete loss of vision due to ophthalmic vascular disease.
- During breastfeeding since estrogens pass into breast milk.
- Classical migraine.

WARNINGS AND PRECAUTIONS:

Serious Warnings and Precautions
The Women's Health Initiative (WHI) trial examined the health benefits and risks of oral combined estrogen plus progestin therapy (n=16 608) and oral estrogen-alone therapy (n=10 739) in postmenopausal women aged 50 to 79 years.
The estrogen plus progestin arm of the WHI trial (mean age 63.3 years) indicated an increased risk of myocardial infarction (MI), stroke, invasive breast cancer, pulmonary emboli and deep vein thrombosis in postmenopausal women receiving treatment with combined conjugated equine estrogens (CEE, 0.625 mg/day) and medroxyprogesterone acetate (MPA, 2.5 mg/day) for 5.2 years compared to those receiving placebo.
The estrogen-alone arm of the WHI trial (mean age 63.6 years) indicated an increased risk of stroke and deep vein thrombosis in hysterectomized women treated with CEE-alone (0.625 mg/day) for 6.8 years compared to those receiving placebo.
Therefore, the following should be given serious consideration at the time of prescribing:
- Estrogens with or without progestins **should not** be prescribed for primary or secondary prevention of cardiovascular diseases.
- Estrogens with or without progestins should be prescribed at the **lowest effective dose** for the approved indication.
- Estrogens with or without progestins should be prescribed for the **shortest period** possible for the approved indication.
- The use of C.E.S. for the prevention or treatment of osteoporosis should be considered in light of other available therapies.

Carcinogenesis and Mutagenesis: Breast Cancer: Available epidemiological data indicate that the use of combined estrogen plus progestin by postmenopausal women is associated with an increased risk of invasive breast cancer.
In the estrogen plus progestin arm of the WHI trial, among 10 000 women over a one-year period, there were:
- 8 more cases of invasive breast cancer (38 on combined HRT versus 30 on placebo).

The WHI study also reported that the invasive breast cancers diagnosed in the estrogen plus progestin group were similar in histology but were larger (mean [SD], 1.7 cm [1.1] vs 1.5 cm [0.9], respectively; P=0.04) and were at a more advanced stage compared with those diagnosed in the placebo group. The percentage of women with abnormal mammograms (recommendations for short-interval follow-up, a suspicious abnormality, or highly suggestive of malignancy) was significantly higher in the estrogen plus progestin group versus the placebo group. This difference appeared at year one and persisted in each year thereafter.
In the estrogen-alone arm of the WHI trial, there was no statistically significant difference in the rate of invasive breast cancer in hysterectomized women treated with conjugated equine estrogens versus women treated with placebo.
It is recommended that estrogens not be given to women with existing breast cancer or those with a previous history of the disease (see Contraindications).
There is a need for caution in prescribing estrogens for women with known risk factors associated with the development of breast cancer, such as strong family history of breast cancer (first degree relative) or who present a breast condition with an increased risk (abnormal mammograms and/or atypical hyperplasia at breast biopsy).
Other known risk factors for the development of breast cancer such as nulliparity, obesity, early menarche, late age at first full term pregnancy and at menopause should also be evaluated.
It is recommended that women undergo mammography prior to the start of HRT treatment and at regular intervals during treatment, as deemed appropriate by the treating physician and according to the perceived risks for each patient.
The overall benefits and possible risks of hormone replacement therapy should be fully considered and discussed with patients. It is important that the modest increased risk of being diagnosed with breast cancer after 4 years of treatment with combined estrogen plus progestin HRT (as reported in the results of the WHI trial) be discussed with the patient and weighed against its known benefits.
Instructions for regular self-examination of the breasts should be included in this counselling.
Endometrial Hyperplasia and Endometrial Carcinoma: Estrogen-only HRT increases the risk of endometrial hyperplasia/carcinoma if taken by women with intact uteri. Estrogen should be prescribed with an appropriate dosage of a progestin for women with intact uteri in order to prevent endometrial hyperplasia/carcinoma.
Ovarian Cancer: Some recent epidemiologic studies have found that the use of hormone replacement therapy (estrogen-alone and estrogen plus progestin therapies), in particular for five or more years, has been associated with an increased risk of ovarian cancer.
Cardiovascular: The results of the Heart and Estrogen/progestin Replacement Studies (HERS and HERS II) and the Women's Health Initiative (WHI) trial indicate that the use of estrogen plus progestin is associated with an increased risk of coronary heart disease (CHD) in postmenopausal women. The results of the WHI trial indicate that the use of estrogen-alone and estrogen plus progestin is associated with an increased risk of stroke in postmenopausal women.
WHI Trial Findings: In the combined estrogen plus progestin arm of the WHI trial, among 10 000 women over a one-year period, there were:
- 8 more cases of stroke (29 on combined HRT versus 21 on placebo)
- 7 more cases of CHD (37 on combined HRT versus 30 on placebo).

In the estrogen-alone arm of the WHI trial of women with prior hysterectomy, among 10 000 women over a one-year period, there were/was:
- 12 more cases of stroke (44 on estrogen-alone therapy versus 32 on placebo)
- no statistically significant difference in the rate of CHD.

HERS and HERS II Findings: In the Heart and Estrogen/progestin Replacement Study (HERS) of postmenopausal women with documented heart disease (n=2763, average age 66.7 years), a randomized placebo-controlled clinical trial of secondary prevention of coronary heart disease (CHD), treatment with 0.625 mg/day oral conjugated equine estrogen (CEE) plus 2.5 mg oral medroxyprogesterone acetate (MPA) demonstrated no cardiovascular benefit. Specifically, during an average follow-up of 4.1 years, treatment with CEE plus MPA did not reduce the overall rate of CHD events in postmenopausal women with established coronary heart disease. There were more CHD events in the hormone-treated group than in the placebo group in year 1, but not during the subsequent years.
From the original HERS trial, 2321 women consented to participate in an open label extension of HERS known as HERS II. Average follow-up in HERS II was an additional 2.7 years, for a total of 6.8 years overall. After 6.8 years, hormone therapy did not reduce the risk of cardiovascular events in women with CHD.
Blood Pressure: Women using hormone replacement therapy sometimes experience increased blood pressure. Blood pressure should be monitored with HRT use. Elevation of blood pressure in previously normotensive or hypertensive patients should be investigated and HRT may have to be discontinued.
Ear/Nose/Throat: Otosclerosis: Estrogens should be used with caution in patients with otosclerosis.
Endocrine and Metabolism: Glucose and Lipid Metabolism: A worsening of glucose tolerance and lipid metabolism has been observed in a significant percentage of peri- and post-menopausal patients. Therefore, diabetic patients or those with a predisposition to diabetes should be observed closely to detect any alterations in carbohydrate or lipid metabolism, especially in triglyceride blood levels.
Women with familial hyperlipidemias need special surveillance. Lipid lowering measures are recommended additionally, before treatment is started.
Heme Metabolism: Women with porphyria need special surveillance.
Calcium and Phosphorus Metabolism: Because the prolonged use of estrogens influences the metabolism of calcium and phosphorus, estrogens should be used with caution in patients with metabolic and malignant bone diseases associated with hypercalcemia and in patients with renal insufficiency.
Hypothyroidism: Patients who require thyroid hormone replacement therapy and who are also taking estrogen should have their thyroid function monitored regularly to assure that thyroid hormone levels remain in an acceptable range (see Drug Interactions, Drug-Laboratory Test Interactions).
Other Conditions: C.E.S. contains lactose. In patients with rare hereditary galactose intolerance, lactase deficiency or glucose-galactose malabsorption, the severity of the condition should be taken into careful consideration before prescribing C.E.S.. The patients should be closely monitored.
Genitourinary: Vaginal Bleeding: Abnormal vaginal bleeding, due to its prolongation, irregularity or heaviness, occurring during therapy should prompt appropriate diagnostic measures to rule out the possibility of uterine malignancy and the treatment should be re-evaluated.
Uterine Leiomyomata: Pre-existing uterine leiomyomata may increase in size during estrogen use. Growth, pain or tenderness of uterine leiomyomata requires discontinuation of medication and appropriate investigation.
Endometriosis: Symptoms and physical findings associated with a previous diagnosis of endometriosis may reappear or become aggravated with estrogen use.
Hematologic: Venous Thromboembolism: Available epidemiological data indicate that use of estrogen with or without progestin by postmenopausal women is associated with an increased risk of developing venous thromboembolism (VTE).
In the estrogen plus progestin arm of the WHI trial, among 10 000 women on combined HRT over a one-year period, there were 18 more cases of venous thromboembolism, including 8 more cases of pulmonary embolism.
In the estrogen-alone arm of the WHI trial, among 10 000 women on estrogen therapy over a one-year period, there were 7 more cases of venous thromboembolism, although there was no statistically significant difference in the rate of pulmonary embolism.
Generally recognized risk factors for VTE include a personal history, a family history (the occurrence of VTE in a direct relative at a relatively early age may indicate genetic predisposition), severe obesity (body mass index >30 kg/m²) and systemic lupus erythematosus. The risk of VTE also increases with age and smoking.
The risk of VTE may be temporarily increased with prolonged immobilization, major surgery or trauma. In women on HRT, attention should be given to prophylactic measures to prevent VTE following surgery. Also, patients with varicose veins should be closely supervised. The physician should be alert to the earliest manifestations of thrombotic disorders (thrombophlebitis, retinal thrombosis, cerebral embolism and pulmonary embolism). If these occur or are suspected, hormone therapy should be discontinued immediately, given the risks of long-term disability or fatality.
If feasible, estrogens should be discontinued at least 4 weeks before major surgery which may be associated with an increased risk of thromboembolism, or during periods of prolonged immobilization.
Hepatic/Biliary/Pancreatic: Gallbladder Diseases: A two-to four-fold increase in the risk of gallbladder disease requiring surgery in women receiving postmenopausal estrogens has been reported.
Hepatic Hemangioma: Particular caution is indicated in women with hepatic hemangiomas as estrogens may cause an exacerbation of this condition.
Jaundice: Caution is advised in patients with a history of liver and/or biliary disorders. If cholestatic jaundice develops during treatment, the treatment should be discontinued and appropriate investigations carried out.
Liver Function Tests: Liver function tests should be done periodically in subjects who are suspected of having hepatic disease. For information on endocrine and liver function tests, see Monitoring and Laboratory Tests.
Immune: Angioedema: Estrogens may induce or exacerbate symptoms of angioedema, in particular in women with hereditary angioedema.
Systemic Lupus Erythematosus: Particular caution is indicated in women with systemic lupus erythematosus.
Neurologic: Cerebrovascular Insufficiency: Patients who develop visual disturbances, classical migraine, transient aphasia, paralysis or loss of consciousness should discontinue medication.
Dementia: Available epidemiological data indicate that the use of combined estrogen plus progestin in women age 65 and over may increase the risk of developing probable dementia.
The Women's Health Initiative Memory Study (WHIMS), a clinical substudy of the WHI, was designed to assess whether postmenopausal hormone replacement therapy (oral estrogen plus progestin or oral estrogen-alone) reduces the risk of dementia in women aged 65 and over (age range 65-79 years) and free of dementia at baseline.
In the estrogen plus progestin arm of the WHIMS (n=4532), women with intact uteri were treated with daily 0.625 mg conjugated equine estrogens (CEE) plus 2.5 mg medroxyprogesterone acetate (MPA) or placebo for an average of 4.05 years. The results, when extrapolated to 10 000 women treated over a one-year period showed:
- 23 more cases of probable dementia (45 on combined HRT versus 22 on placebo).

In the estrogen-alone arm of the WHIMS (n=2947), women with prior hysterectomy were treated with daily 0.625 mg CEE or placebo for an average of 5.21 years. The results, when extrapolated to 10 000 women treated over a one-year period showed:
- 12 more cases of probable dementia (37 on estrogen-alone versus 25 on placebo), although this difference did not reach statistical significance.

When data from the estrogen plus progestin arm of the WHIMS and the estrogen-alone arm of the WHIMS were combined, as per the original WHIMS protocol, in 10 000 women over a one-year period, there were:
- 18 more cases of probable dementia (41 on estrogen plus progestin or estrogen-alone versus 23 on placebo).

Epilepsy: Particular caution is indicated in women with epilepsy, as estrogens with or without progestins may cause an exacerbation of this condition.
Peri-Operative Considerations: If feasible, estrogens should be discontinued at least 4 weeks before major surgery which may be associated with an increased risk of thromboembolism, or during periods of prolonged immobilization.
Renal: Fluid Retention: Estrogens may cause fluid retention. Therefore, particular caution is indicated in cardiac or renal dysfunction, or asthma. If, in any of the above-mentioned conditions, a worsening of the underlying disease is diagnosed or suspected during treatment, the benefits and risks of treatment should be reassessed based on the individual case.
Special Populations: Pregnant Women: Estrogen therapy during pregnancy is associated with an increased risk of fetal congenital reproductive-tract disorders. In females there is an increased risk of vaginal adenosis, squamous cell dysplasia of the cervix, and cancer later in life; in the male, of urogenital abnormalities. Although some of these changes are benign, it is not known whether they are precursors of malignancy (see Contraindications).
Nursing Women: Estrogens should not be used during breastfeeding since they pass into breast milk (see Contraindications).
Monitoring and Laboratory Tests: Before C.E.S (conjugated estrogens) is administered, the patient should have a complete physical examination including blood pressure determination. Breasts and pelvic organs should be appropriately examined and a Papanicolaou smear should be performed. Endometrial biopsy should be done only when indicated. Baseline tests should include mammography, measurements of blood glucose, calcium, triglycerides and cholesterol, and liver function tests.
The first follow-up examination should be done within 3-6 months after initiation of treatment to assess response to treatment. Thereafter, examinations should be made at intervals at least once a year. Appropriate investigations should be arranged at regular intervals as determined by the physician.
The importance of regular self-examination of the breasts should be discussed with the patient.

ADVERSE REACTIONS: Adverse Drug Reaction Overview: See Warnings and Precautions regarding potential induction of malignant neoplasms and adverse effects similar to those of oral contraceptives.
The following adverse reactions have been reported with estrogen/progestin combination in general:
Blood and Lymphatic System Disorders: altered coagulation tests (see Warnings and Precautions, Drug-Laboratory Test Interactions).
Cardiac Disorders: palpitations; increase in blood pressure (see Warnings and Precautions); coronary thrombosis.
Endocrine Disorders: increased blood sugar levels; decreased glucose tolerance.
Eye Disorders: neuro-ocular lesions (e.g., retinal thrombosis, optic neuritis); visual disturbances; steepening of the corneal curvature; intolerance to contact lenses.
Gastrointestinal Disorders: nausea; vomiting; abdominal discomfort (cramps, pressure, pain, bloating).
General Disorders and Administration Site Conditions: fatigue; changes in appetite; changes in body weight; changes in libido.
Hepatobiliary Disorders: gallbladder disorder; asymptomatic impaired liver function; cholestatic jaundice.
Musculoskeletal and Connective Tissue Disorders: Musculoskeletal pain including leg pain not related to thromboembolic disease (usually transient, lasting 3-6 weeks) may occur.
Nervous System Disorders: aggravation of migraine episodes; headaches; dizziness; neuritis.
Psychiatric Disorders: mental depression; nervousness; irritability.
Renal and Urinary Disorders: cystitis; dysuria; sodium retention; edema.

Reproductive System and Breast Disorders: breakthrough bleeding; spotting; change in menstrual flow; dysmenorrhea; vaginal itching/discharge; dyspareunia; endometrial hyperplasia; pre-menstrual-like syndrome; reactivation of endometriosis; changes in cervical erosion and amount of cervical secretion; breast swelling and tenderness.
Skin and Subcutaneous Tissue Disorders: chloasma or melasma, which may persist when drug is discontinued; erythema multiforme; erythema nodosum; haemorrhagic eruption; loss of scalp hair; hirsutism and acne.
Vascular Disorders: isolated cases of: thrombophlebitis; thromboembolic disorders.
Clinical Trial Adverse Drug Reactions: Data are not available.
Less Common Clinical Trial Adverse Drug Reactions: Data are not available.
Abnormal Hematologic and Clinical Chemistry Findings: Data are not available.
Post-Market Adverse Drug Reactions: The following post-marketing adverse drug reactions have been reported for C.E.S.:
Cardiovascular Disorders: myocardial infarction, increase blood pressure, palpitation.
Gastrointestinal Disorders: abdominal pain, bloating, dyspepsia, nausea, vomiting, diarrhoea, gallbladder disorder.
General Disorders and Administration Site Conditions: allergic reaction, headache, hot flushes, lack of drug effect, sweating, weight increase, chills, fatigue, dizziness, feeling strange, pain.
Eye Disorders: dry eyes.
Musculoskeletal and Connective Tissue Disorders: arthralgia, muscle cramp, pain legs, bursitis, arthritis aggravated.
Neoplasm Benign, Malignant and Unspecified (incl cysts and polyps): breast cancer.
Nervous System Disorders: cerebral infarction, stroke, muscle weakness, swallowing difficult, facial palsy, abnormal coordination, memory impairment.
Psychiatric Disorders: anger, anxiety, insomnia, depression, irritability, thinking abnormal, impaired concentration.
Reproductive System and Breast Disorders: postmenopausal bleeding, uterine hemorrhage, breast tenderness, menstrual disorders, atrophic vaginitis, menorrhagia.
Skin and Subcutaneous Tissue Disorders: chloasma, skin hyperpigmentation, papular rash, rash, urticaria, pruritus, dermatitis.
Vascular Disorders: venous deep thrombosis.
Others: antinuclear factor test positive.

If adverse symptoms persist, the prescription of HRT should be re-considered.

DRUG INTERACTIONS: Overview: Estrogens may diminish the effectiveness of anticoagulants, antidiabetic and antihypertensive agents.

Preparations inducing liver enzymes (e.g., barbiturates, hydantoins, carbamazepine, meprobamates, phenylbutazone or rifampicin) may interfere with the activity of orally administered estrogens.

Drug-Drug Interactions: The following section contains information on drug interactions with ethinyl estradiol-containing products (specifically, oral contraceptives) that have been reported in the public literature. It is unknown whether such interactions occur with drug products containing other types of estrogens. Therapeutic monitoring is recommended.

1. The metabolism of ethinyl estradiol is increased by rifampin and anticonvulsants such as phenobarbital, phenytoin and carbamazepine. Coadministration of troglitazone and certain ethinyl estradiol containing drug products (e.g., oral contraceptives containing ethinyl estradiol) reduce the plasma concentrations of ethinyl estradiol by 30%.

   Ascorbic acid and acetaminophen may increase AUC and/or plasma concentrations of ethinyl estradiol. Coadministration of atorvastatin and certain ethinyl estradiol containing drug products (e.g., oral contraceptives containing ethinyl estradiol) increase AUC values for ethinyl estradiol by 20%.

   Clinical pharmacokinetic studies have not demonstrated any consistent effect of antibiotics (other than rifampin) on plasma concentrations of synthetic steroids.
2. Drug products containing ethinyl estradiol may inhibit the metabolism of other compounds. Increased plasma concentrations of cyclosporin, prednisolone, and theophylline have been reported with concomitant administration of certain drugs containing ethinyl estradiol (e.g., oral contraceptives containing ethinyl estradiol). In addition, these drugs containing ethinyl estradiol may induce the conjugation of other compounds.

   Decreased plasma concentrations of acetaminophen and increased clearance of temazepam, salicylic acid, morphine and clofibric acid have been noted when these drugs were administered with certain ethinyl estradiol containing drug products (e.g., oral contraceptives containing ethinyl estradiol).

Drug-Food Interactions: As other inhibitors of CYP3A4, grapefruit juice may increase plasma concentration of 17 β-estradiol, possibly resulting in side effects.

Drug-Herb Interactions: It was found that some herbal products (e.g., St. John's wort) which are available as over-the-counter (OTC) products might interfere with steroid metabolism and therefore, alter the efficacy and safety of estrogen/progestin products.

Physicians and other health care providers should be made aware of other non-prescription products concomitantly used by the patient, including herbal and natural products obtained from widely spread health stores.

Drug-Laboratory Test Interactions: The results of certain endocrine and liver function tests may be affected by estrogen-containing products:

- increased prothrombin time and partial thromboplastin time; increased levels of fibrinogen and fibrinogen activity; increased coagulation factors VII, VIII, IX, X; increased norepinephrine-induced platelet aggregability; decreased antithrombin III;
- increased thyroxine-binding globulin (TBG), leading to increased circulating total thyroid hormone (T_4) as measured by column or radioimmunoassay; T_3 resin uptake is decreased, reflecting the elevated TBG; free T_4 concentration is unaltered;
- other binding proteins may be elevated in serum i.e., corticosteroid binding globulin (CBG), sex-hormone binding globulin (SHBG), leading to increased circulating corticosteroids and sex steroids respectively; free or biologically active hormone concentrations are unchanged;
- impaired glucose tolerance;
- increased serum triglycerides and phospholipids concentration;

The results of the above laboratory tests should not be considered reliable unless therapy has been discontinued for two to four weeks.

The pathologist should be informed that the patient is receiving hormone replacement therapy (HRT) when relevant specimens are submitted.

Drug-Lifestyle Interactions: Acute alcohol ingestion during HRT may lead to elevations in circulating estradiol levels.

DOSAGE AND ADMINISTRATION:

Dosing Considerations: Conjugated estrogens therapy may be given continuously with no interruption in therapy, or in cyclical regimens (regimens such as 25 days on drug followed by 5 days off drug) as is medically appropriate on an individualized basis.

Continuous, noncyclic therapy may be indicated in hysterectomized women or in cases where the signs and symptoms of estrogen deficiency become problematic during the treatment-free interval. In women with an intact uterus, a progestin should be coadministered for a **minimum** of 10 days, but preferably at least 12 to 14 days per cycle to avoid overstimulation of the endometrium. In addition, progestin should be administered to minimize the occurrence of endometrial hyperplasia. Unexpected or abnormal vaginal bleeding in such patients requires institution of prompt diagnostic measures to rule out the possibility of uterine malignancy. Since progestins are administered to reduce the risk of hyperplastic changes of the endometrium, patients without a uterus do not require a progestin for this purpose.

Recommended Dose and Dosage Adjustment: Usual Dosage Range: Menopausal Symptoms: 0.625 to 1.25 mg daily, cyclically or continuously as is medically required. Adjust dosage upward or downward according to severity of symptoms and response of the patient. For maintenance, adjust dosage to lowest level providing effective control.

Osteoporosis (loss of bone mass): 0.625 mg daily.

Hypoestrogenism Due to: 1) Female hypogonadism: 0.3 mg to 0.625 mg daily, administered cyclically (e.g., 3 weeks on and 1 week off) or continuously as required. Doses are adjusted depending on the severity of symptoms and responsiveness of the endometrium.

2) Female castration or primary ovarian failure: 1.25 mg daily, cyclically or continuously as required. Adjust dosage upward or downward according to severity of symptoms and lowest level that will provide effective control.

Atrophic Vaginitis: 0.3 mg to 1.25 mg daily depending upon the tissue response of the individual patient. Administer cyclically or continuously as required.

Vulvar Atrophy: 0.3 mg to 1.25 mg daily depending upon the tissue response of the individual patient. Administer cyclically or continuously as required.

Missed Dose: If a patient misses a dose, it should be taken as soon as possible. If it is close to the patient's next scheduled dose, the missed dose should be skipped, and the patient should continue with her normal schedule. The patient should not take two doses at the same time.

Administration: Oral.

C.E.S. should be prescribed with an appropriate dosage of a progestin for women with intact uteri in order to prevent endometrial hyperplasia/carcinoma. Progestin therapy is not required as part of hormone replacement therapy in women who have had a previous hysterectomy.

OVERDOSAGE:
Symptoms: Numerous reports of ingestion of large doses of estrogen products and estrogen-containing oral contraceptives by young children have not revealed acute serious ill effects. Over dosage with estrogen may cause nausea, breast discomfort, fluid retention, bloating or vaginal bleeding in women.
Treatment: Symptomatic treatment should be given.

> For management of a suspected drug overdose, contact your regional Poison Control Centre. See the *CPS* Directory section for a list of Poison Control Centres.

ACTION AND CLINICAL PHARMACOLOGY: Mechanism of Action: Conjugated estrogens are a mixture of estrogens derived from plant sterols and contain the sodium salts of water-soluble estrogen sulfates. C.E.S. (conjugated estrogens) is derived from plant sterols only. Conjugated estrogens contain estrone, equilin, 17-α-dihydroequilin, 17-α-estradiol, equilenin and 17-α-dihydroequilenin as salts of their sulfate esters.

Estrogen drug products act by regulating the transcription of a limited number of genes. They may act directly at the cell's surface via non-"estrogen receptor" mechanism or directly with the estrogen receptor inside the cell. Estrogens diffuse through cell membranes, distribute themselves throughout the cell, bind to and activate the nuclear estrogen receptor, a DNA-binding protein found in estrogen-responsive tissues. The activated estrogen receptor binds to specific DNA sequences, or hormone-response elements, which enhance the transcription of adjacent genes and in turn lead to the observed effects. Estrogen receptors have been identified in the wall of blood vessels, in tissues of the reproductive tract, breast, pituitary, hypothalamus, liver, and bone of women.

Estrogens are important in the development and maintenance of the female reproductive system and secondary sex characteristics. By a direct action, they cause growth and development of the uterus, Fallopian tubes, and vagina. Together with other hormones, such as pituitary hormones and progesterone, they cause enlargement of the breasts through promotion of ductal growth, stromal development, and the accretion of fat. Estrogens are involved together with other hormones, especially progesterone, in the processes of the ovulatory menstrual cycle and pregnancy, and affect the release of pituitary gonadotropins. They also contribute to the shaping of the skeleton, maintenance of tone and elasticity of urogenital structures, changes in the epiphyses of the long bones that allow for the pubertal growth spurt and its termination, and pigmentation of the nipples and genitals.

Pharmacodynamics: Conjugated estrogens used in therapeutic preparations are soluble in water and are well absorbed from the gastrointestinal tract after release from the drug formulation.

Estrogen Deficiency and Vasomotor Symptoms: As a result of the decrease in ovarian hormones, about 75% of menopausal women experience vasomotor symptoms such as hot flushes and sweating, and these symptoms are seen whether menopause is surgically induced or spontaneous. Vasomotor symptoms may begin before the cessation of menses.

Estrogen Deficiency and Osteoporosis: The rate of bone mass decline is accelerated for several years following natural or induced menopause. Conjugated estrogens reduce postmenopausal bone loss. Up to 60% reduction in hip and wrist fractures in women given estrogen within a few years of menopause has been documented in case-control studies. Other studies suggest that estrogen reduces the rate of vertebral fractures.

In postmenopausal women already diagnosed as having osteoporosis and vertebral fractures, treatment with conjugated estrogens may prevent further loss of bone mass. Even when started as late as six years after menopause, estrogen prevents further loss of bone mass for as long as the treatment is continued. When estrogen therapy is discontinued, bone mass declines at a rate comparable to that of the immediate postmenopausal period.

Effects on the Endometrium: An increased risk of endometrial hyperplasia, a possible precursor of endometrial adenocarcinoma, has been associated with the use of unopposed estrogen therapy. The results of clinical studies indicate that the addition of a progestin to an estrogen replacement regimen reduces the incidence of endometrial hyperplasia and the attendant risk of adenocarcinoma in women with intact uteri without interfering with the efficacy of estrogen replacement therapy for its approved indications.

Effect on Bleeding Patterns: With a continuous therapy, bleeding patterns such as absence of bleeding to irregular bleeding, may occur. However, it is frequently light spotting or moderate bleeding.

Pharmacokinetics: Absorption: Conjugated estrogens used in therapeutic preparations are soluble in water and are well absorbed from the gastrointestinal tract after release from the drug formulation.

Distribution: Administered estrogens and their esters are handled within the body essentially the same way as the endogenous hormones. Metabolic conversion of estrogen occurs primarily in the liver (first pass effect), but also at local target tissue sites. Complex metabolic processes result in a dynamic equilibrium of circulating conjugated and unconjugated estrogenic forms which are continually interconverted, especially between estrone and estradiol and between esterified and nonesterified forms. Although naturally occurring estrogens circulate in the blood largely bound to sex hormone-binding globulin (SHBG) and albumin, only unbound estrogens enter target tissue cells. A significant proportion of the circulating estrogen exists as sulfate conjugates, especially estrone sulfate, which serves as a circulating reservoir for the formation of more active estrogenic species.

Metabolism: When given orally, naturally occurring estrogens and their esters are extensively metabolized (first pass effect) and circulate primarily as estrone sulfate, with smaller amounts of other conjugated and unconjugated estrogenic species. This results in limited oral potency. By contrast, synthetic estrogens, such as ethinyl estradiol and the nonsteroidal estrogens, are degraded very slowly in the liver and other tissues, which results in their high intrinsic potency.

Excretion: A certain proportion of the estrogen is excreted into the bile, then reabsorbed from the intestine and returned to the liver through the portal venous system. During this enterohepatic recirculation, estrogens are desulfated and resulfated and undergo degradation through conversion to less active estrogens (estriol and other estrogens), oxidation to nonestrogenic substances (catecholestrogens, which interact with catecholamine metabolism, especially in the CNS), and conjugation with glucuronic acids (which are then rapidly excreted in the urine).

Special Populations and Conditions: No pharmacokinetic studies were conducted in special populations, including patients with renal or hepatic impairment.

Estrogen Pharmacology: Estrogens occur naturally in several forms. The primary source of estrogen in normally cycling women is the ovarian follicle, which secretes 70 to 500 µg of estradiol daily, depending on the phase of the menstrual cycle. Estradiol is converted primarily to estrone, which circulates in roughly equal proportion to estradiol, and to small amounts of estriol. After menopause, most endogenous estrogen stems from the conversion of androstenedione, which is secreted by the adrenal cortex, to estrone in peripheral tissues.

Thus, estrone, especially in its sulfate ester form, is the most abundant circulating estrogen in postmenopausal women. Although circulating estrogens exist in a dynamic equilibrium of metabolic interconversions, estradiol is the principal intracellular human estrogen and is substantially more potent than estrone or estriol at the receptor site.

An increased risk of endometrial hyperplasia, a possible precursor of endometrial adenocarcinoma, has been associated with the use of unopposed estrogen therapy. The results of clinical studies indicate that the addition of a progestin to an estrogen replacement regimen reduces the incidence of endometrial hyperplasia and the attendant risk of adenocarcinoma in women with intact uteri without interfering with the efficacy of estrogen replacement therapy for its approved indications.

STORAGE AND STABILITY: Store at room temperature (15-30°C).

Keep out of reach of children.

SPECIAL HANDLING INSTRUCTIONS: None required.

INFORMATION FOR THE PATIENT: Published in e-CPS, available by subscription at www.e-cps.ca.

DOSAGE FORMS, COMPOSITION AND PACKAGING: 0.3 mg: Each oval, green, sugar-coated tablet contains: conjugated estrogens CSD 0.3 mg. Nonmedicinal ingredients: calcium carbonate, calcium sulphate, carnauba wax, D&C Yellow No. 10, FD&C Blue No. 1, FD&C Blue No. 2, FD&C Yellow No. 6, hydroxypropyl cellulose, hydroxypropyl methylcellulose, magnesium stearate, methylparaben, microcrystalline cellulose, povidone, sodium benzoate, sucrose, talc, titanium dioxide and white wax. Bottles of 100.

0.625 mg: Each oval, maroon, sugar-coated tablet contains: conjugated estrogens CSD 0.625 mg. Nonmedicinal ingredients: calcium carbonate, calcium phosphate, calcium sulphate, carnauba wax, colloidal silicon dioxide, lactose, magnesium carbonate, FD&C Blue No. 2, FD&C Red No. 40, methylparaben, microcrystalline cellulose, povidone, sodium benzoate, starch, sucrose, talc, titanium dioxide, stearic acid and white wax. Bottles of 100 and 1000.

0.9 mg: Each oval, pink, sugar-coated tablet contains: conjugated estrogens CSD 0.9 mg. Nonmedicinal ingredients: calcium carbonate, calcium sulphate, carnauba wax, erythrosine aluminum lake, hydroxypropyl methyl cellulose, magnesium stearate, methylparaben, microcrystalline cellulose, povidone, sodium benzoate, sucrose, talc, titanium dioxide and white wax. Bottles of 100.

1.25 mg: Each oval, yellow, sugar-coated tablet contains: conjugated estrogens CSD 1.25 mg. Nonmedicinal ingredients: acacia, calcium carbonate, calcium phosphate, calcium sulphate, carnauba wax, colloidal silicon dioxide, lactose, magnesium carbonate, D&C Yellow No. 10, FD&C Yellow No. 6, methylparaben, microcrystalline cellulose, pharmaceutical glaze, starch, sucrose, talc, titanium dioxide, stearic acid and white wax. Bottles of 100.

Cesamet® Ⓝ

nabilone

Antiemetic

Valeant

Date of Preparation: June 3, 2008
Date of Revision: March 17, 2009

PHARMACOLOGY: CESAMET (nabilone) is a synthetic cannabinoid with antiemetic properties which have been found to be of value in the management of some patients with nausea and vomiting associated with cancer chemotherapy. It also has sedative and psychotropic effects.

After oral administration, comparable peak plasma levels of nabilone and of its carbinol metabolite were attained within 2 hours. The combined plasma concentrations of nabilone and of its carbinol metabolite accounted for, at most, 10 to 20% of the total radiocarbon concentration in plasma. The plasma half-life of nabilone was approximately 2 hours, while that of the total radiocarbon was of the order of 35 hours.

Of the 2 major possible metabolic pathways, stereo-specific enzymatic reduction and direct enzymatic oxidation, the latter appears to be the more important in man.

The drug and its metabolites are eliminated mainly in the feces (approximately 65%) and to a lesser extent in the urine (approximately 20%). The major excretory pathway is the biliary system.

INDICATIONS: Adults: >18 years: CESAMET (nabilone) is indicated for the management of severe nausea and vomiting associated with cancer chemotherapy.

Children: <18 years: The safety and efficacy of CESAMET in the pediatric population have not been established and its use is not recommended in this patient population.

Geriatrics: >65 years: CESAMET should be used with caution in the elderly. (See Precautions.)

CONTRAINDICATIONS: CESAMET (nabilone) is contraindicated in patients with known sensitivity to marijuana or other cannabinoid agents, and in those with a history of psychotic reactions.

WARNINGS: CESAMET (nabilone) should be used with extreme caution in patients with severe liver dysfunction and in those with a history of non-psychotic emotional disorders.

CESAMET should not be taken with alcohol, sedatives, hypnotics, or other psychotomimetic substances.

CESAMET should not be used during pregnancy, in nursing mothers or in pediatric patients, since its safety under these conditions has not been established.

PRECAUTIONS: Occupational Hazards: Since CESAMET (nabilone) will often impair the mental and/or physical abilities required for the performance of potentially hazardous tasks, such as driving a car and operating machinery, the patient should be warned accordingly and should not be permitted to drive or engage in dangerous tasks until the effects of nabilone are no longer present.

Adverse psychotropic reactions can persist for 48 to 72 hours following cessation of treatment.

Since CESAMET elevates supine and standing heart rates and causes postural hypotension, it should be used with caution in the elderly and in patients with hypertension or heart disease.

Drug Interactions: Potential interactions between CESAMET, and diazepam; sodium secobarbital; alcohol; or codeine, were evaluated. The depressant effects of the combinations were additive. Psychomotor function was particularly impaired with concurrent use of diazepam.

Pediatrics: The safety and efficacy in children under the age of 18 has not been established. Therefore the use of CESAMET in this patient population is not recommended.

ADVERSE EFFECTS: The most frequently observed adverse reactions to nabilone and their incidences reported in the course of clinical trials were as follows: drowsiness (66.0%), vertigo (58.8%), psychological high (38.8%), dry mouth (21.6%), depression (14.0%), ataxia (12.8%), blurred vision (12.8%), sensation disturbance (12.4%), anorexia (7.6%), asthenia (7.6%), headache (7.2%), orthostatic hypotension (5.2%), euphoria (4.0%) and hallucinations (2.0%).

The following adverse reactions were observed in less than 1% of the patients who were administered nabilone in the course of the clinical trials: tachycardia, tremors, syncope, nightmares, distortion in the perception of time, confusion, dissociation, dysphoria, psychotic reactions and seizures.

Spontaneously Reported Adverse Events: The following adverse reactions listed in order of decreasing frequency by body system have been reported since CESAMET has been marketed. All events are listed regardless of causality assessment.

Blood and Hematopoietic: leukopenia.

Cardiovascular: hypotension and tachycardia.

Eye and Ear: visual disturbances.

Gastrointestinal: dry mouth, nausea, vomiting and constipation.

Nervous System: hallucinations, CNS depression, CNS stimulation, ataxia, stupor, vertigo, convulsion and circumoral paresthesia.

Psychiatric: somnolence, confusion, euphoria, depression, dysphoria, depersonalization, anxiety, psychosis and emotional lability.

Miscellaneous and Ill-defined Conditions: dizziness, headache, insomnia, abnormal thinking, chest pain, lack of effect, and face edema.

OVERDOSE:

Symptoms: Signs and symptoms which might be expected to occur are psychotic episodes including hallucinations, anxiety reactions, respiratory depression and coma (experience with cases of overdosage of more than 10 mg/day has not yet been reported).

Treatment: Overdose may be considered to have occurred, even at prescribed dosages, if disturbing psychiatric symptoms are present. In these cases, the patient should be observed in a quiet environment and supportive measures, including reassurance, should be used. Subsequent doses should be withheld until patients have returned to their baseline mental status; routine dosing may then be resumed if clinically indicated. In such instances, a lower initiating dose is suggested.

If psychotic episodes occur, the patient should be managed conservatively, if possible. For moderate psychotic episodes and anxiety reactions, verbal support and comforting may be sufficient. In more severe cases, antipsychotic drugs may be useful; however, the utility of antipsychotic drugs in cannabinoid psychosis has not been systematically evaluated. Support for their use is drawn from limited experience using anti-psychotic agents to manage cannabis overdoses. Because of the potential for drug-drug interactions (e.g., additive CNS depressant effects due to nabilone and chlorpromazine), such patients should be closely monitored.

Protect the patient's airway and support ventilation and perfusion. Meticulously monitor and maintain, within acceptable limits, the patient's vital signs, blood gases, serum electrolytes, etc. Absorption of drugs from the gastrointestinal tract may be decreased by giving activated charcoal, which, in many cases, is more effective than emesis or lavage; consider charcoal instead of or in addition to gastric emptying. Repeated doses of charcoal over time may hasten elimination of some drugs that have been absorbed. Safeguard the patient's airway when employing gastric emptying or charcoal.

The use of forced diuresis, peritoneal dialysis, hemodialysis, charcoal hemoperfusion or cholestyramine has not been reported. In the presence of normal renal function, most of a dose of nabilone is eliminated through the biliary system.

Treatment for respiratory depression and comatose state consists of symptomatic and supportive therapy. Particular attention should be paid to the occurrence of hypothermia. If the patient becomes hypotensive, consider fluids, inotropes and/or vasopressors.

For management of a suspected drug overdose, CPhA recommends that you contact your **regional Poison Control Centre**. See the *CPS* Directory section for a list of Poison Control Centres.

DOSAGE: Adults: The usual dosage of CESAMET is 1 mg or 2 mg twice a day. The first dose should be given the night before initiating administration of chemotherapeutic medication. The second dose is usually administered 1 to 3 hours before chemotherapy. If required, administration of CESAMET can be continued up to 24 hours after the chemotherapeutic agent is given. The maximum recommended daily dose is 6 mg in divided doses.

CESAMET is available in 0.25 mg and 0.5 mg strengths for dose adjustment within the therapeutic range. Dose adjustment may be required for the purposes of response and tolerance in individual patients. Overdosage may occur even at prescribed dosages, if disturbing psychiatric symptoms are present. In these cases, the patient should be observed in a quiet environment and supportive measures, including reassurance, should be used. Subsequent doses should be withheld until patients have returned to their baseline mental status; routine dosing may then be resumed if clinically indicated. In such instances, a lower initiating dose is suggested.

CESAMET contains nabilone in a capsule dosage form and is intended only for oral administration.

INFORMATION FOR THE PATIENT: Published in e-CPS, available by subscription at www.e-cps.ca.

SUPPLIED: 0.25 mg: Each No. 4 hard gelatin capsule, opaque green cap and white body, imprinted ICN logo on the cap and 3103 on the body, contains: nabilone 0.25 mg. Nonmedicinal ingredients: D&C Yellow #10, FD&C Blue #1, FD&C Red #40, gelatin, starch, povidone and titanium dioxide. Bottles of 50. Store at controlled room temperature at 15-30°C.

0.5 mg: Each No. 4 hard gelatin capsule, opaque red cap and white body, imprinted ICN logo on the cap and 3102 on the body, contains: nabilone 0.5 mg. Nonmedicinal ingredients: D&C Red #33, D&C Yellow #10, FD&C Red #40, gelatin, povidone, starch and titanium dioxyde. Bottles of 50. Store at controlled room temperature at 15-30°C.

1 mg: Each No. 2 hard gelatin capsule, opaque blue cap and white body, imprinted ICN logo on the cap and 3101 on the body, contains: nabilone 1 mg. Nonmedicinal ingredients: FD&C Blue #2 (indigo carmine), gelatin, povidone, red iron oxide, starch and titanium dioxide. Bottles of 50. Store at controlled room temperature at 15-30°C.

Cetrotide™ Ⓟ

cetrorelix acetate

GnRH Antagonist

EMD Canada

PHARMACOLOGY: Cetrotide (cetrorelix acetate for injection) is a synthetic decapeptide with gonadotropin-releasing hormone (GnRH) antagonistic activity. Cetrorelix acetate is an analog of native GnRH with substitutions of amino acids at positions 1, 2, 3, 6, and 10. The molecular formula is Acetyl-D-3-(2'-naphtyl)-alanine-D-4-chlorophenylalanine-D-3-(3'-pyridyl)-alanine-L-serine-L-tyrosine-D-citruline-L-leucine-L-arginine-L-proline-D-alanine-amide, and the molecular weight is 1431.06, calculated as the anhydrous free base.

GnRH induces the production and release of luteinizing hormone (LH) and follicle stimulating hormone (FSH) from the gonadotrophic cells of the anterior pituitary. Due to a positive estradiol (E_2) feedback at midcycle, GnRH liberation is enhanced resulting in an LH-surge. This LH-surge induces the ovulation of the dominant follicle, resumption of oocyte meiosis and subsequently luteinization as indicated by rising progesterone levels.

Cetrotide competes with natural GnRH for binding to membrane receptors on pituitary cells and thus controls the release of LH and FSH in a dose-dependent manner. The onset of LH suppression is approximately one hour with the 3 mg dose and two hours with the 0.25 mg dose. This suppression is maintained by continuous treatment and there is a more pronounced effect on LH than on FSH. An initial release of endogenous gonadotropins has not been detected with Cetrotide, which is consistent with an antagonist effect.

The effects of Cetrotide on LH and FSH are reversible after discontinuation of treatment. In women, Cetrotide delays the LH-surge, and consequently ovulation, in a dose-dependent fashion. FSH levels are not affected at the doses used during controlled ovarian stimulation. Following a single 3 mg dose of Cetrotide, duration of action of at least 4 days has been established. A dose of Cetrotide 0.25 mg every 24 hours has been shown to maintain the effect.

Clinical Studies: Seven hundred and thirty two (732) patients were treated with Cetrotide in five (two Phase 2 dose-finding and three Phase 3) clinical trials. The clinical trial population consisted of Caucasians (95.5%) and Black, Asian, Arabian and Others (4.5%). Women were between 19 and 40 years of age (mean: 32 years). The studies excluded subjects with polycystic ovary syndrome (PCOS), subjects with low or no ovarian reserve, and subjects with stage III-IV endometriosis.

Two dose regimens were investigated in these clinical trials, either a single dose per treatment cycle or multiple dosing. In the Phase 2 studies, a single dose of 3 mg was established as the minimal effective dose for the inhibition of premature LH surges with a protection period of at least 4 days. When Cetrotide is administered in a multidose regimen, 0.25 mg was established as the minimal effective dose. The extent and duration of LH-suppression is dose dependent.

In the Phase 3 program, efficacy of the single 3 mg dose regimen of Cetrotide and the multiple 0.25 mg dose regimen of Cetrotide was established separately in two adequate and well controlled clinical studies utilizing active comparators. A third non-comparative clinical study evaluated only the multiple 0.25 mg dose regimen of Cetrotide. The ovarian stimulation treatment with recombinant FSH or human menopausal gonadotropin (hMG) was initiated on day 2 or 3 of a normal menstrual cycle. The dose of gonadotropins was administered according to the individual patient's disposition and response.

In the single dose regimen study, Cetrotide 3 mg was administered on the day of controlled ovarian stimulation (COS) when adequate estradiol levels (400 pg/mL) were obtained, usually on day 7 (range day 5-12). If human chorionic gonadotropin (hCG) was not given within 4 days of the 3 mg dose of Cetrotide, then 0.25 mg of Cetrotide was administered daily beginning 96 hours after the 3 mg injection until and including the day of hCG administration.

In the two multiple dose regimen studies, Cetrotide 0.25 mg was started on day 5 or 6 of COS. Both gonadotropins and Cetrotide were continued daily (multiple dose regimen) until the injection of hCG.

In the two active comparative studies, results showed that on stimulation day 6/7 there were more small follicles in the Cetrotide patient group than in the comparator patient groups. This was reversed on the day of hCG administration, when the number of small (11-14 mm) follicles was generally lower in the Cetrotide than in the comparator groups. There was no or only a small difference with regard to the medium-size or large follicles (20 mm and over) on the day of hCG administration.

Levels of E_2 increased continuously and a pronounced increase in E_2 levels was seen the day before hCG administration in both groups (Cetrotide and comparator). On the day of hCG administration, E_2 levels were clearly higher and the increase was faster in the comparator groups than in the Cetrotide group. These higher E_2 levels in the comparator groups correlate with a higher number of **small follicles** in this group.

The fertilization rate of Cetrotide treatment versus the comparator patient groups was also similar.

Oocyte pick-up (OPU) followed by in vitro fertilization (IVF) or intracytoplasmic sperm injection (ICSI) as well as embryo transfer (ET) were subsequently performed. The results for Cetrotide are summarized in Table 1.

Table 1: Cetrotide

Results of Phase 3 Clinical Studies with Cetrotide 3 mg in a Single Dose (sd) Regimen and 0.25 mg in a Multiple Dose (md) Regimen

Parameter	Cetrotide 3 mg (sd, Active Comparative Study)	Cetrotide 0.25 mg (md, Active Comparative Study)	Cetrotide 0.25 mg (md, Non-Comparative Study)
No. of subjects	115	159	303
hCG administered [%]	98.3	96.2	96.0
Oocyte pick-up [%]	98.3	94.3	93.1
LH-surge [%] (LH≥10 U/L and P[a] ≥ 1 ng/mL)[b]	0.0	1.9	1.0
Serum E_2 [pg/mL] at day hCG[c,d]	1125 (470–2952)	1064 (341–2531)	1185 (311–3676)

(cont'd)

Table 1: Cetrotide *(cont'd)*

Results of Phase 3 Clinical Studies with Cetrotide 3 mg in a Single Dose (sd) Regimen and 0.25 mg in a Multiple Dose (md) Regimen

Parameter	Cetrotide 3 mg (sd, Active Comparative Study)	Cetrotide 0.25 mg (md, Active Comparative Study)	Cetrotide 0.25 mg (md, Non-Comparative Study)
Serum LH [U/L] at day hCG[c,d]	1.0 (0.5–2.5)	1.5 (0.5–7.6)	1.1 (0.5–3.5)
No. of follicles ≥11 mm at day hCG[e]	11.2±5.5	10.8±5.2	10.4±4.5
No. of oocytes:			
IVF[e]	9.2±5.2	7.6±4.3	8.5±5.1
ICSI[e]	10.0±4.2	10.1±5.6	9.3±5.9
Fertilization rate:			
IVF[e]	0.48±0.33	0.62±0.26	0.60±0.26
ICSI[e]	0.66±0.29	0.63±0.29	0.61±0.25
No. of embryos transferred[e]	2.6±0.9	2.1±0.6	2.7±1.0
Clinical pregnancy rate [%]			
per attempt	22.6	20.8	19.8
per subject with ET	26.3	24.1	23.3

[a] Progesterone.
[b] Following initiation of Cetrotide therapy.
[c] Morning values.
[d] Median with 5th–95th percentiles.
[e] Mean standard deviation.

In addition to IVF and ICSI, one pregnancy was obtained after intrauterine insemination. In the five Phase 2 and Phase 3 clinical trials, 184 pregnancies have been reported out of a total of 732 patients (including 21 pregnancies following the replacement of frozen-thawed embryos).

In the 3 mg regimen, 9 patients received an additional dose of 0.25 mg of Cetrotide and two other patients received two additional doses of 0.25 mg Cetrotide. The median number of days of Cetrotide multiple dose treatment was 5 (range 1-15) in both studies.

Limited data are available in repeated administration of Cetrotide in the same patient (for multiple cycles). Accordingly, it is unknown (up until now) whether the efficacy remains unchanged, or whether immunogenicity and/or sensitization has been developed with the use of Cetrotide in the same patient for more than one cycle.

INDICATIONS: Cetrotide (cetrorelix acetate for injection) is indicated for the prevention of premature ovulation in patients undergoing controlled ovarian stimulation.

CONTRAINDICATIONS: Cetrotide (cetrorelix acetate for injection) is contraindicated under the following conditions:
1. hypersensitivity to cetrorelix acetate, extrinsic peptide hormones or mannitol;
2. known hypersensitivity to GnRH or any other GnRH analogs;
3. known or suspected pregnancy, and lactation (see Precautions);
4. moderate or severe impairment of hepatic or renal function.

WARNINGS: Cetrotide (cetrorelix acetate for injection) should be prescribed by physicians who are experienced in fertility treatment. Before starting treatment with Cetrotide, pregnancy must be excluded (see Contraindications and Precautions).

PRECAUTIONS: General: Caution is advised in patients with hypersensitivity to GnRH analogs. These patients should be carefully monitored after the first injection. Therefore, it is recommended that a physician supervises the first administration. Special care should be taken in women with signs and symptoms of active allergic conditions or known history of allergic predisposition. Treatment with Cetrotide (cetrorelix acetate for injection), is not advised in women with severe allergic conditions.

Efficacy and safety (immunogenicity and/or sensitization) have not been extensively evaluated in women undergoing multiple treatment cycles with Cetrotide. However, hypersensitivity, antibody formation, and acute anaphylactic reaction have been reported with GnRH analogs. Therefore, special care should be taken upon using the drug in the same patient for more than one cycle.

Information to Be Provided to the Patient: Prior to therapy with Cetrotide, patients should be informed of the duration of treatment and monitoring procedures that will be required. The risk of possible adverse reactions should be discussed (see Adverse Effects). Cetrotide should not be prescribed if a patient is pregnant. If Cetrotide is prescribed to patients for self-administration, information for proper use is given in the Patient Insert (see Information for the Patient).

Drug Interactions: No formal drug interaction studies have been performed with Cetrotide. In clinical studies, no interaction between exogenous gonadotropins and Cetrotide was observed.

Carcinogenesis, Mutagenesis, Impairment of Fertility: Long-term carcinogenicity studies in animals have not been performed with cetrorelix acetate. Cetrorelix acetate was not genotoxic in vitro (Ames test, HPRT test, chromosome aberration test) or in vivo (chromosome aberration test, mouse micronucleus test). Cetrorelix acetate induced polyploidy in CHL-Chinese hamster lung fibroblasts, but not in V79-Chinese hamster lung fibroblasts, cultured peripheral human lymphocytes or in an in vitro micronucleus test in the CHL-cell line. Treatment with 0.46 mg/kg cetrorelix acetate for 4 weeks resulted in complete infertility in female rats which was reversed 8 weeks after cessation of treatment.

Pregnancy: Cetrotide is contraindicated in pregnant women.

When administered to rats for the first seven days of pregnancy, cetrorelix acetate did not affect the development of the implanted conceptus at doses up to 38 µg/kg (approximately 1 times the recommended human therapeutic dose based on body surface area). However, a dose of 139 µg/kg (approximately 4 times the human dose) resulted in a resorption rate and a post-implantation loss of 100%.

When administered from day 6 to near term to pregnant rats and rabbits, very early resorptions and total implantation losses were seen in rats at doses from 4.6 µg/kg (0.2 times the human dose) and in rabbits at doses from 6.8 µg/kg (0.4 times the human dose). In animals that maintained their pregnancy, there was no increase in the incidence of fetal abnormalities.

The fetal resorption observed in animals is a logical consequence of the alteration in hormonal levels effected by the antigonadotrophic properties of Cetrotide, which could result in fetal loss in humans as well. Therefore, this drug should not be used in pregnant women.

Lactation: It is not known whether Cetrotide is excreted in human milk. Because many drugs are excreted in human milk, and because the effects of Cetrotide on lactation and/or the breast-fed child have not been determined, Cetrotide should not be used by nursing mothers.

ADVERSE EFFECTS: The safety of Cetrotide (cetrorelix acetate for injection) in 949 patients undergoing controlled ovarian stimulation in clinical studies was evaluated. Women were between 19 and 40 years of age (mean: 32). 94.0% of them were Caucasian. Cetrotide was given in doses ranging from 0.1 mg to 5 mg as either a single or multiple dose.

Table 2 shows systemic adverse events from the beginning of Cetrotide treatment until confirmation of pregnancy by ultrasound at an incidence ≥1% in Cetrotide treated subjects undergoing COS.

Table 2: Cetrotide

Adverse Events

Adverse Events in ≥1% (WHO preferred term)	Cetrotide N=949 % (n)
Ovarian Hyperstimulation Syndrome[a]	3.5 (33)
Nausea	1.3 (12)
Headache	1.1 (10)

[a] Intensity moderate or severe, or WHO Grade II or III, respectively.

Local site reactions (e.g. redness, swelling and pruritus) have been reported. Usually, they were of a transient nature and mild intensity. Rare cases of hypersensitivity reactions including anaphylactoid reactions have been observed.

Two stillbirths were reported in Phase 3 studies of Cetrotide.

Ovarian Hyperstimulation Syndrome (OHSS): During or following controlled ovarian stimulation an ovarian hyperstimulation syndrome can occur. This event must be considered as an intrinsic risk of the stimulation procedure with gonadotropins (refer to the relevant gonadotropin Product Monograph for warning symptoms etc.).

In this potentially serious medical event, the ovaries are massively enlarged, and intravascular fluid volume shifts into the peritoneal space, resulting in hypovolemia, oliguria, hemoconcentration, and massive ascites. The syndrome can usually be avoided by closely monitoring the patient and withholding the hCG if ovarian response becomes excessive.

Congenital Anomalies: Clinical follow-up studies of 316 newborns of women administered Cetrotide were reviewed. One infant of a set of twin neonates was found to have anencephaly at birth and died after four days. The other twin was normal. Developmental findings from ongoing baby follow-up included a child with a ventricular septal defect and another child with bilateral congenital glaucoma.

Four pregnancies that resulted in therapeutic abortion in Phase 2 and Phase 3 controlled ovarian stimulation studies had major anomalies (diaphragmatic hernia, trisomy 21, Klinefelter syndrome, polymalformation, and trisomy 18). In three of these four cases, intracytoplasmic sperm injection (ICSI) was the fertilization method employed; in the fourth case, in vitro fertilization (IVF) was the method employed.

The minor congenital anomalies reported include: supernumerary nipple, bilateral strabismus, imperforate hymen, congenital nevi, hemangiomata, and QT syndrome.

The causal relationship between the reported anomalies and Cetrotide is unknown. Multiple factors, genetic and others (including, but not limited to ICSI, IVF, gonadotropins, and progesterone) make causal attribution difficult to study.

OVERDOSE:
There have been no reports of overdosage with Cetrotide (cetrorelix acetate for injection) 0.25 mg or 3 mg in humans. Single doses up to 120 mg Cetrotide have been well tolerated in patients treated for other indications without signs of overdosage.

For management of a suspected drug overdose, CPhA recommends that you contact your **regional Poison Control Centre**. See the *CPS* Directory section for a list of Poison Control Centres.

DOSAGE: Ovarian stimulation therapy with gonadotropins (FSH, hMG) is started on cycle Day 2 or 3. The dose of gonadotropins should be adjusted according to individual response. The response should be primarily based on the number and size of the developing follicles as evidenced by ultrasound. This may be more reliable than by the amount of circulating estradiol. Cetrotide (cetrorelix acetate for injection) may be administered subcutaneously either once daily (0.25 mg dose) or once (3 mg dose) during the early- to mid-follicular phase.

In the single dose regimen, 3 mg of Cetrotide is administered when the serum estradiol level is indicative of an appropriate stimulation response, usually on stimulation day 7 (range day 5-9). If hCG has not been administered within four days after injection of Cetrotide 3 mg, Cetrotide 0.25 mg should be administered once daily until the day of hCG administration.

In the multiple dose regimen, 0.25 mg of Cetrotide is administered on either stimulation day 5 (morning or evening) or day 6 (morning) and continued daily until the day of hCG administration.

When assessment by ultrasound shows a sufficient number of follicles of adequate size (≥17 mm in diameter), hCG is administered to induce ovulation and final maturation of the oocytes. No hCG should be administered if the ovaries show an excessive response to the treatment with gonadotropins to reduce the chance of developing ovarian hyperstimulation syndrome (OHSS).

Administration: Cetrotide 0.25 mg and 3 mg can be administered by the patient herself after appropriate instructions by her doctor.

Reconstituted Solutions: Parenteral Products: The reconstituted product is to be administered subcutaneously. Use immediately after reconstitution.

As with all parenteral drug products, reconstituted solutions should be inspected visually for clarity, particulate matter, precipitate, discolouration and leakage prior to administration. Solution showing haziness, particulate matter, precipitate, discolouration or leakage should not be used. Discard unused portions.

INFORMATION FOR THE PATIENT: Published in e-CPS, available by subscription at www.e-cps.ca.

SUPPLIED: 0.25 mg: Each single dose vial (multiple dose regimen) of sterile lyophilized powder contains: 0.25 mg of cetrorelix as cetrorelix acetate and 54.80 mg of mannitol. Cartons of one packaged tray. Each packaged tray contains: one glass vial containing 0.25 mg of cetrorelix acetate, one prefilled glass syringe with 1 mL of Sterile Water for Injection, Ph.Eur., one 20 gauge needle (yellow), one 27 gauge needle (grey), and two alcohol swabs. Store between 2 and 25°C. **Do not freeze.** Keep the container in the outer carton to protect it from light. Do not use the product after the expiry date indicated on the label.

3 mg: Each single dose vial (single dose regimen) of sterile lyophilized powder contains: 3 mg of cetrorelix as cetrorelix acetate and 164.40 mg of mannitol. Cartons of one packaged tray. Each packaged tray contains: one glass vial containing 3 mg of cetrorelix acetate, one prefilled glass syringe with 3 mL of Sterile Water for Injection, Ph.Eur, one 20 gauge needle (yellow), one 27 gauge needle (grey), and two alcohol swabs. Store between 2 and 25°C. **Do not freeze.** Keep the container in the outer carton to protect it from light. Do not use the product after the expiry date indicated on the label.

Champix® Ⓟ

varenicline tartrate

Smoking-Cessation Aid

Pfizer

Date of Revision: May 28, 2010

SUMMARY PRODUCT INFORMATION:

Route of Administration	Dosage Form/Strength	All Nonmedicinal Ingredients
Oral	Tablet: 0.5 mg and 1 mg	Anhydrous dibasic calcium phosphate, colloidal silicon dioxide, croscarmellose sodium, magnesium stearate, and microcrystalline cellulose. The film-coating contains hypromellose, polyethylene glycol, titanium dioxide and triacetin. The 1 mg tablet also contains FD&C Blue #2/Indigo Carmine Aluminum Lake as a colouring agent.

INDICATIONS AND CLINICAL USE: Adults: CHAMPIX (varenicline tartrate) is indicated for: smoking-cessation treatment in adults in conjunction with smoking-cessation counselling.

See Serious Warnings and Precautions, Psychiatric Symptoms.

Geriatrics (>65 years of age): No dosage adjustment is necessary for healthy elderly patients. However, varenicline is known to be substantially excreted by the kidney, and the risk of toxic reactions to this drug may be greater in patients with impaired renal function. Because elderly patients are more likely to have decreased renal function, care should be taken in dose selection, and it may be useful to monitor renal function (see Warnings and Precautions, Special Populations, Geriatrics (>65 years of age)).

Pediatrics (<18 years of age): The safety and efficacy of varenicline in pediatric patients have not been established, therefore its use in this patient population is not recommended (see Warnings and Precautions, Special Populations, Pediatrics (<18 years of age)).

CONTRAINDICATIONS: Patients who are hypersensitive to varenicline or to any ingredient in the formulation or component of the container.

WARNINGS AND PRECAUTIONS:

Serious Warnings and Precautions

Psychiatric Symptoms:

There have been post-marketing reports of serious neuropsychiatric symptoms in patients being treated with CHAMPIX (varenicline tartrate), including depressed mood, agitation, aggression, hostility, changes in behavior, suicide related events, including ideation, behavior, attempted suicide and suicide, as well as worsening of pre-existing psychiatric disorder. **These events have occurred in patients with and without pre-existing psychiatric disorders (see also Warnings and Precautions, Psychiatric Symptoms).**

Some reported cases may have been complicated by the symptoms of nicotine withdrawal in patients who stopped smoking. Depressed mood may be a symptom of nicotine withdrawal. Depression, rarely including suicidal ideation, has been reported in smokers undergoing a smoking cessation attempt without medication. However, some of these symptoms have occurred in patients taking CHAMPIX who continued to smoke. All patients being treated with CHAMPIX should be observed for neuropsychiatric symptoms.

Important Recommendations Regarding Psychiatric Symptoms:

- The benefits and risks of all options for quitting smoking should be discussed with the patient before initiating treatment.
- All patients attempting to quit smoking with CHAMPIX, as well as their families and caregivers, should be alerted about the need to monitor for depressed mood, agitation, aggression, hostility, suicidal ideation or behavior, or changes in behavior or thinking that are not typical for the patient.
- Patients should be instructed to stop taking CHAMPIX immediately and contact their doctor if they experience, or if others observe, these symptoms. In many post-marketing cases, resolution of symptoms after discontinuation of CHAMPIX was reported, although in some cases the symptoms persisted; therefore, ongoing monitoring and supportive care should be provided until symptoms resolve.
- **Regarding alcohol intake:** Patients should be advised that alcohol intake may increase the risk of experiencing psychiatric adverse events during treatment with CHAMPIX.
- **Regarding patients with psychiatric history:** Patients with concomitant psychiatric conditions, even if well controlled, or with a history of psychiatric symptoms, should be diligently monitored by a healthcare professional for new or worsened psychiatric events.

Psychiatric Symptoms: (See also Adverse Reactions, Post-Market Adverse Events.)

There have been post-marketing reports of serious neuropsychiatric symptoms in patients being treated with CHAMPIX, including anxiety, psychosis, mood swings, depressed mood, agitation, hostility, changes in behaviour or thinking, suicidal ideation, suicide behavior and suicide, as well as worsening of pre-existing psychiatric illness (previously diagnosed or not) (see Serious Warnings and Precautions).

There are a number of confounding factors which may have contributed, including effects of nicotine withdrawal due to partial or complete smoking discontinuation; concomitant, or history of psychiatric conditions, and the concomitant use of other CNS drugs and/or alcohol. However, there are cases for which these confounding factors did not appear to be present, including cases where symptoms occurred within the first week of initiating CHAMPIX, and prior to initiating smoking cessation. There have been other cases where symptoms developed following cessation of CHAMPIX therapy.

It is not known whether these events are occurring at a rate and severity which is different from the background rate for smoking cessation in the general population, or in the psychiatric population (treated or untreated), or different from the rates for other drugs in the class of smoking cessation (see Adverse Reactions, Neuropsychiatric Adverse Events in Randomized, Double-Blind, Placebo-Controlled Clinical Studies of Varenicline).

Pre-Existing Psychiatric Disorders or Symptoms: Patients with serious psychiatric disorders such as schizophrenia, bipolar disorder, and major depressive disorder did not participate in the pre-marketing studies of CHAMPIX and the safety and efficacy of CHAMPIX in such patients has not been studied (see also Special Populations, Use of CHAMPIX in Patients with Concomitant Conditions, Psychiatric Patients).

Patients with concomitant psychiatric conditions, even if well controlled, or with a history of psychiatric symptoms, should be diligently monitored by a health care professional for new or worsened psychiatric events.

Concomitant Illness: The full consequences of using this product in patients with concomitant illness have not been studied, and caution should be exercised (see Special Populations, Use of CHAMPIX in Patients with Concomitant Conditions).

Angioedema and Hypersensitivity Reactions: There have been post-marketing reports of hypersensitivity reactions, including angioedema, in patients treated with CHAMPIX (see Adverse Reactions, Post-Market Adverse Events). Clinical signs included swelling of the face, mouth (tongue, lips and gums), neck (pharynx and larynx) and extremities. There were rare reports of life-threatening angioedema requiring urgent medical attention due to respiratory compromise. Patients experiencing these symptoms should be instructed to discontinue treatment with CHAMPIX and contact a healthcare provider immediately.

Serious Skin Reactions: There have also been post-marketing reports of rare but severe cutaneous reactions, including Stevens-Johnson syndrome and erythema multiforme, in patients using CHAMPIX (see Adverse Reactions, Post-Market Adverse Events). As these skin reactions can be life-threatening, patients should be instructed to discontinue treatment at the first sign of rash or skin reaction and contact a healthcare provider immediately.

Nicotine Replacement Therapy (NRT): The concomitant use of NRT with CHAMPIX (varenicline tartrate) may result in an increase in adverse reactions. In a clinical drug interaction study (N=24), the incidences of nausea, headache, vomiting, dizziness, dyspepsia and fatigue were greater for the combination of NRT and varenicline than for NRT alone (see Drug Interactions). The safety and efficacy of the combination treatment with CHAMPIX and NRT have not been studied. Due to the proposed mechanism of action of varenicline, it is not anticipated that co-administration with NRT would confer additional benefit compared with CHAMPIX alone.

Effect of Smoking-Cessation: Physiological changes resulting from smoking-cessation, with or without treatment with CHAMPIX, may alter the pharmacokinetics or pharmacodynamics of some drugs for which dosage adjustment may be necessary (examples include theophylline, warfarin and insulin). As smoking induces cytochrome P450 (CYP) isoenzyme 1A2, smoking-cessation may result in an increase of plasma levels of CYP1A2 substrates.

Nausea: Nausea was the most common adverse event associated with CHAMPIX treatment. Nausea was generally described as mild or moderate and often transient; however, for some subjects, it was persistent over several months. The incidence of nausea was dose-dependent. Initial dose-titration was beneficial in reducing the occurrence of nausea. Nausea was reported by approximately 30% of patients treated with CHAMPIX 1 mg BID after an initial week of dose titration. In patients taking CHAMPIX 0.5 mg BID, the incidence of nausea was 16% following initial titration. Approximately 3% of subjects treated with CHAMPIX 1 mg BID in studies involving 12 weeks of treatment discontinued treatment prematurely because of nausea. For patients with intolerable nausea, dose reduction should be considered (see Dosage and Administration, Recommended Dose and Dosage Adjustment).

Accidental Injury, Including While Driving, Operating Machinery: There have been post-marketing reports of traffic accidents, near-miss incidents in traffic, and other accidental injuries in patients taking CHAMPIX. In some cases, the patients reported somnolence, dizziness, loss of consciousness (blackouts), seizures or difficulty concentrating.

Therefore, patients should be advised not to engage in potentially hazardous activities, such as driving a car or operating dangerous machines, until they know how CHAMPIX may affect them.

Carcinogenesis and Mutagenesis: Carcinogenesis: Lifetime carcinogenicity studies were performed in CD-1 mice and Sprague Dawley rats. There was no evidence of a carcinogenic effect in mice administered varenicline by oral gavage for 2 years at doses up to 20 mg/kg/day (47 times the maximum recommended human daily exposure based on the area under the curve (AUC). Rats were administered varenicline (1, 5, and 15 mg/kg/day) by oral gavage for 2 years. In male rats (n=65 per sex per dose group), incidences of hibernoma (tumor of the brown fat) was increased at the mid dose (1 tumor, 5 mg/kg/day, 23 times the maximum recommended human daily exposure based on AUC) and at the maximum dose (2 tumors, 15 mg/kg/day, 67 times the maximum recommended human daily exposure based on AUC). The clinical relevance of this finding to humans has not been established. There was no evidence of carcinogenicity in female rats.

Mutagenesis: Varenicline was not genotoxic, with or without metabolic activation, in the following assays: Ames bacterial mutation assay; mammalian CHO/HGPRT assay; and tests for cytogenetic aberrations in vivo in rat bone marrow and in vitro in human lymphocytes.

Dependence/Tolerance: Animal Studies: The subjective nicotine-like effects of varenicline were investigated in drug discrimination studies. At 1 mg/kg, there was complete substitution of varenicline for nicotine in a paradigm of nicotine-associated lever pressing for food reward. In an efficacy model, varenicline pretreatment dose-dependently reduced nicotine self administration under a fixed-ratio schedule. Under a progressive ratio schedule rats worked harder for nicotine than for varenicline.

Human Studies : The rewarding potential of varenicline (1 mg and 3 mg doses) was compared with that of amphetamines in subjects experienced with psychomotor stimulants. The pattern for both smokers and non-smokers was consistent with a profile of a drug that, while having some pharmacological activity, did not produce amphetamine-like subjective effects.

Sexual Function/Reproduction: Impairment of Fertility: There was no evidence of impairment of fertility in either male or female Sprague-Dawley rats administered varenicline succinate up to 15 mg/kg/day (67 and 36 times, respectively, the maximum recommended human daily exposure based on AUC at 1 mg BID). However, a decrease in fertility was noted in the offspring of pregnant rats who were administered varenicline succinate at an oral dose of 15 mg/kg/day (36 times the maximum recommended human daily exposure based on AUC at 1 mg BID). This decrease in fertility in the offspring of treated female rats was not evident at an oral dose of 3 mg/kg/day (9 times the maximum recommended human daily exposure based on AUC at 1 mg BID).

Information to Be Provided to the Patient: Consumer Information is included in the package of CHAMPIX dispensed to the patient.

Prior to prescribing CHAMPIX, physicians should:

- Discuss with the patient the expected benefits and risks of CHAMPIX, as well as those of all smoking-cessation options.
- Inform the patients that quitting smoking, with or without CHAMPIX, may be associated with nicotine withdrawal symptoms (including depression or agitation) or exacerbation of pre-existing psychiatric disorder.
- Patients should be advised not to engage in potentially hazardous tasks, such as driving a car or operating dangerous machines, until they know how CHAMPIX may affect them. In some cases, patients have reported somnolence, dizziness, loss of consciousness, seizures or difficulty concentrating while driving.
- Inform the patient that there have been post-marketing reports of serious neuropsychiatric symptoms in patients being treated with CHAMPIX, including anxiety, psychosis, mood swings, aggression, depressed mood, agitation, hallucinations, hostility, changes in behavior or thinking, suicidal ideation, suicidal behavior and suicide, as well as worsening of pre-existing psychiatric disorder.
- Inform the patient that these events have occurred in people with previous psychiatric disorder, as well as those with no previous history.
- Encourage the patient to reveal any history of psychiatric disorder prior to initiating treatment.
- Patients with a history of serious psychiatric disorder should be informed that this patient population did not participate in the pre-marketing studies of CHAMPIX, and therefore the safety and efficacy of CHAMPIX in such patients have not been studied.
- Patients with concomitant psychiatric conditions, even if well controlled, or with a history of psychiatric symptoms, should be informed that if they are prescribed CHAMPIX, they will be diligently monitored by their physician for new or worsened psychiatric events.

Patients receiving CHAMPIX should be given the following instructions by the physician:

- Patients should be instructed to read the patient information leaflet supplied with every CHAMPIX prescription before starting their CHAMPIX pills. This leaflet is approved by Health Canada and is Part III of the CHAMPIX Product Monograph.
- Patients should also be provided with educational materials and necessary counseling to support an attempt at quitting smoking, including a review of the overall smoking cessation plan with the physician.
- Patients should call 1-800-CHAMPIX for a list of provincial Smoking Cessation resources (toll-free quit line) which can be used to support a quit attempt.
- Patients should be informed that there are two choices of CHAMPIX doses, based on physician judgment and patient preference: after one week titration, the dose can go up to 1.0 mg twice daily, or remain at 0.5 mg twice daily. Based on the limited data available, the two doses do not appear different in terms of either quit rates, or rates of serious psychiatric side effects (see Dosage and Administration, Dosing Considerations).
- Patients should be instructed on how to titrate CHAMPIX, beginning at a dose of 0.5 mg per day. Prescribers should explain that one 0.5 mg tablet should be taken daily for the first three days, and that for the next four days, two 0.5 mg tablets should be taken daily: one in the morning and one in the evening.
- Following one week of titration, there are two dosing options, the dose can remain at 0.5 mg twice daily or can go up to 1.0 mg twice daily, depending on the dosing regimen chosen.
- Patients should be informed that the maximum dose of CHAMPIX is 1.0 mg twice a day.
- If needed, the dose can be changed depending on how well the patient tolerates CHAMPIX and how effective the doctor and patient consider it is in helping the patient quit smoking.
- Patients should be encouraged to continue in their quit attempt if they have early lapses after their quit date.
- Patients should be encouraged to inform friends and family members/caregivers of their quit attempt which includes treatment with CHAMPIX and ask for their support and help in monitoring for any changes in behavior or thinking that are not typical for the patient.
- Patients should be informed that if they develop agitation, hostility, depressed mood or changes in behavior or thinking that are not typical for them, or develop suicidal ideation or suicidal behavior, CHAMPIX should be discontinued immediately, and symptoms reported to their healthcare provider.
- Patients should be advised that drinking alcohol may increase the risk of experiencing psychiatric adverse events during treatment with CHAMPIX.
- Patients should be informed that they may experience vivid, unusual or strange dreams during treatment with CHAMPIX.
- Patients should be informed that nausea is the most common adverse event associated with CHAMPIX and is usually transient. CHAMPIX should be taken after eating and with a full glass of water. Patients should be advised that if they are persistently troubled by this symptom, a dose reduction may be considered.
- Patients should be informed that there have been reports of **angioedema**, with swelling of the face, mouth (tongue, lips and gums) and neck (pharynx and larynx) that can lead to life-threatening respiratory compromise. Patients should be instructed to discontinue CHAMPIX and seek immediate emergency medical attention if they experience these symptoms.
- Patients should be informed that **serious skin reactions**, such as Stevens-Johnson syndrome and erythema multiforme, were reported by some patients taking CHAMPIX. Patients should be advised to stop taking CHAMPIX at the first sign of rash with mucosal lesions or skin reaction and seek immediate emergency medical attention.

Special Populations: Use of CHAMPIX in Patients with Concomitant Conditions: Psychiatric Patients: Patients with serious psychiatric disorders such as schizophrenia, bipolar disorder, and major depressive disorder did not participate in the pre-marketing clinical trials. Smoking-cessation with or without pharmacotherapy, has been associated with the exacerbation of underlying psychiatric illness; the impact on this population of a smoking-cessation product with nicotinic partial agonist properties is unknown. Care should be taken with patients with a history of psychiatric illness and patients should be advised accordingly. **Patients with concomitant psychiatric conditions, even if well controlled, or with a history of psychiatric symptoms, should be diligently monitored by a healthcare professional for new or worsened psychiatric events** (see Warnings and Precautions, Serious Warnings and Precautions, and also Pre-Existing Psychiatric Disorders or Symptoms).

Patients with Epilepsy: The use of CHAMPIX has not been studied in patients with epilepsy. There have been post-marketing reports of seizures in patients using varenicline. It is not known for how many of these there is a prior history or risk of a seizure disorder.

Patients with Irritable Bowel or Other Gastrointestinal (GI) Problems: The use of CHAMPIX has not been studied in patients with irritable bowel syndrome or other GI problems.

Patients Exposed to Chemotherapy : The use of CHAMPIX has not been studied in patients exposed to emetogenic chemotherapy.

Pregnant Women: There are no adequate data from the use of CHAMPIX in pregnant women. Studies in animals have shown reproductive toxicity. The potential risk for humans is unknown. CHAMPIX should not be used during pregnancy.

Nonteratogenic Effects: Varenicline succinate has been shown to have an adverse effect on the fetus in animal reproduction studies. Administration of varenicline succinate to pregnant rabbits resulted in reduced fetal weights at an oral dose of 30 mg/kg/day (50 times the human AUC at 1 mg BID); this reduction was not evident following treatment with 10 mg/kg/day (23 times the maximum recommended daily human exposure based on AUC). In addition, in the offspring of pregnant rats treated with varenicline succinate there were decreases in fertility and increases in auditory startle response at an oral dose of 15 mg/kg/day (36 times the maximum recommended human daily exposure based on AUC at 1 mg BID).

Nursing Women: Animal studies have shown that varenicline can be transferred to nursing pups. It is not known whether varenicline is excreted in human milk. Because many drugs are excreted in human milk and because the potential for adverse reactions in nursing infants from CHAMPIX is unknown, a decision should be made whether to discontinue nursing or to discontinue the drug.

Pediatrics (<18 years of age): Safety and efficacy of CHAMPIX in pediatric patients have not been established; therefore, CHAMPIX is not recommended for use in patients under 18 years of age.

Geriatrics (>65 years of age): A combined single and multiple-dose pharmacokinetic study demonstrated that the pharmacokinetics of 1 mg varenicline given once daily (QD) or BID to 16 healthy elderly male and female smokers (aged 65-75 years) for 7 consecutive days was similar to that of younger subjects. No overall differences in safety or effectiveness were observed between these subjects and younger subjects, and other reported clinical experience has not identified differences in responses between the elderly and younger patients, but greater sensitivity of some older individuals cannot be ruled out.

Varenicline is known to be substantially excreted by the kidney, and the risk of toxic reactions to this drug may be greater in patients with impaired renal function. Because elderly patients are more likely to have decreased renal function, care should be taken in dose selection, and it may be useful to monitor renal function (see Dosage and Administration, Special Populations, Geriatrics (>65 years of age)).

Renal Impairment: A multiple dose pharmacokinetic study was conducted in patients with normal renal function, with mild, moderate, or severe renal impairment (estimated creatinine clearance: >80 mL/min, >50 and ≤80 mL/min, ≥30 and ≤50 mL/min, and <30 mL/min, respectively) or end-stage renal disease (ESRD). Varenicline pharmacokinetics was unchanged in subjects with mild renal impairment. Relative to subjects with normal renal function, varenicline exposure increased 1.5-fold in patients with moderate renal impairment and 2.1-fold in patients with severe renal impairment. In subjects with ESRD, varenicline was efficiently removed by hemodialysis. The recommended dose of CHAMPIX is reduced in patients with severe renal impairment. CHAMPIX is not recommended in patients with ESRD. (See Action and Clinical Pharmacology, Special Populations and Conditions, Renal Impairment, and Dosage and Administration, Special Populations, Patients with Impaired Renal Function.)

ADVERSE REACTIONS: Clinical Trial Adverse Drug Reactions: Smoking-cessation with or without treatment is associated with various symptoms. For example, dysphoric or depressed mood, insomnia, irritability, frustration or anger, anxiety, difficulty concentrating, restlessness, decreased heart rate, increased appetite or weight gain have been reported in patients attempting to stop smoking.

Overview: Pre-marketing clinical trials included approximately 2300 patients treated for at least 12 weeks, approximately 700 for 6 months, and approximately 100 for one year. In general, onset of adverse events was in the first few weeks of therapy and severity was generally mild to moderate. No differences were observed by age, race or gender with regard to the incidence of adverse reactions, although patient numbers in elderly, and in non-caucasian races were too limited to allow conclusions.

Commonly Observed Adverse Events: The most commonly observed adverse events associated with CHAMPIX (>5% and twice the rate seen in placebo-treated patients) were nausea, abnormal dreams, constipation, flatulence, and vomiting.

For patients exposed to the maximum recommended dose of 1 mg BID following initial dosage titration, the incidence of nausea was 30%, compared with 16% in 0.5 mg BID and approximately 10% in placebo-treated patients. Nausea was generally described as mild to moderate and often transient; however, for some subjects, it was persistent throughout the treatment period.

Adverse Events Leading to Discontinuation: In Phase 2 and 3 placebo-controlled studies, the treatment discontinuation rate due to adverse events in patients randomized to 12 weeks treatment with the recommended maximum dose of 1 mg BID was 12% for CHAMPIX compared to 10% for placebo. In this group, the adverse events most frequently resulting in treatment discontinuation in CHAMPIX treated patients were as follows: nausea (2.7% vs 0.6% for placebo), insomnia (1.3% vs 1.2% for placebo), fatigue/malaise/asthenia (1.0% vs 0.5% for placebo), and dizziness (0.7% vs 0.4% for placebo).

Table 1 shows the adverse events for CHAMPIX and placebo in the 12-week fixed dose studies with titration in the first week (Studies 1 (titrated arm only), 3, and 4). MedDRA High Level Group Terms (HLGT) reported in ≥5% of patients in the CHAMPIX 1 mg BID dose group, and more commonly than in the placebo group, are listed, along with subordinate Preferred Terms (PT) reported in ≥1% of CHAMPIX patients (and at least 0.5% more frequently than placebo). Closely related Preferred Terms such as 'Insomnia', 'Initial insomnia', 'Middle insomnia', 'Early morning awakening' were grouped, but individual patients reporting two or more grouped events were only counted once.

Table 1: CHAMPIX

Common Treatment-Emergent Adverse Events (%) in the Fixed-Dose, Placebo-Controlled Studies (≥1% in the 1 mg BID CHAMPIX group, and 1 mg BID CHAMPIX at least 0.5% more than placebo)

System Organ Class High Level Group Term Preferred Term	CHAMPIX 0.5 mg BID N=129	CHAMPIX 1 mg BID N=821	Placebo N=805
Gastrointestinal			
GI Signs and Symptoms			
Nausea	16	30	10
Abdominal Pain[a]	5	7	5
Flatulence	9	6	3
Dyspepsia	5	5	3
Vomiting	1	5	2
GI Motility/Defecation Conditions			
Constipation	5	8	3
Gastroesophageal Reflux Disease	1	1	0
Salivary Gland Conditions			
Dry Mouth	4	6	4
Psychiatric Disorders			
Sleep Disorder/Disturbances			
Insomnia[b]	19	18	13
Abnormal Dreams	9	13	5
Sleep Disorder	2	5	3
Nightmare	2	1	0
Nervous System			
Headaches			
Headache	19	15	13
Neurological Disorders NEC			
Dysgeusia	8	5	4
Somnolence	3	3	2
Lethargy	2	1	0
General Disorders			
General Disorders NEC			
Fatigue/Malaise/Asthenia	4	7	6
Respir/Thoracic/Mediast			
Respiratory Disorders NEC			
Rhinorrhea	0	1	0
Dyspnea	2	1	1
Upper Respiratory Tract Disorder	7	5	4
Skin/Subcutaneous Tissue			
Epidermal and Dermal Conditions			
Rash	1	3	2
Pruritus	0	1	1
Metabolism and Nutrition			
Appetite/General Nutrition. Disorders			
Increased Appetite	4	3	2
Decreased Appetite/Anorexia	1	2	1

(cont'd) Table 1: CHAMPIX (cont'd)

[a] Includes PTs Abdominal (pain, pain upper, pain lower, discomfort, tenderness, distension) and Stomach discomfort.
[b] Includes PTs Insomnia/Initial insomnia/Middle insomnia/Early morning awakening.
Legend: NEC: not elsewhere classified.

Initial dose titration was beneficial in reducing the occurrence of nausea.

An additional 12 weeks of CHAMPIX 1 mg BID was well-tolerated in patients who had completed 12 weeks of treatment and had stopped smoking. Adverse events resulted in treatment discontinuation in 1.7% of patients who received CHAMPIX compared with 1.3% of placebo patients.

Safety Study: One Year Double-Blind Drug-Treatment: The overall pattern and the frequency of adverse events during a 52-week trial with CHAMPIX 1 mg BID (n=251 subjects randomized to CHAMPIX arm, and n=126 to placebo arm) were similar to those described in Table 1, except for the following events which were seen to be increased relative to placebo, as compared to the profile for 12 week drug exposure: nausea (40% vs 8% placebo); and the pooled terms of: abdominal pain (17% vs 3% placebo), and increased blood pressure (11% vs 6% placebo). Few of these events were recorded as severe.

Neuropsychiatric Adverse Events in Randomized, Double-Blind, Placebo-Controlled Clinical Studies of Varenicline: Pooled Data Including Ten Smoking Cessation Trials: Table 2 provides the incidence of all causality, treatment-emergent neuropsychiatric adverse events with varenicline as compared to placebo (≥0.2% more than placebo) in adult smokers, adverse event summarized from all randomized, placebo-controlled, double-blind varenicline studies (10 studies) completed by 31 December 2008, regardless of Study Dose or Duration. Four of these are described in the Clinical Trials section. There were no suicidal and self injurious behaviors reported (suicide ideation and suicide attempt) in the varenicline group versus 2 events (0.1%) in the placebo group.

Table 2: CHAMPIX

All-Causality Treatment-Emergent Neuropsychiatric Adverse Events (%) in Ten Completed Phase 2/4 Placebo-Controlled Studies (≥0.2% more than placebo)

Neuropsychiatric Adverse Events	Varenicline (N=3091) % (n)	Placebo (N=2005) % (n)
Psychiatric Disorders[a]		
Depressed Mood Disorders and Disturbances	**2.8 (88)**	**1.9 (38)**
Depression	1.6 (51)	1.2 (24)
Depressed Mood	1.0 (32)	0.6 (12)
Disturbances in Thinking and Perception	**0.4 (13)**	**0.1 (2)**
Thinking Abnormal	0.2 (7)	– (1)
Mood Disorders and Disturbances NEC	**2.4 (73)**	**1.5 (30)**
Affect Lability	0.6 (20)	0.3 (6)
Mood Swings	0.3 (10)	0.1 (2)
Apathy	0.2 (5)	– (1)
Psychiatric Disorders NEC	**0.5 (16)**	**0.3 (6)**
Sleep Disorders and Disturbances	**25.1 (776)**	**14.5 (291)**
Insomnia	13.9 (431)	9.5 (191)

(cont'd)

Table 2: CHAMPIX *(cont'd)*

All-Causality Treatment-Emergent Neuropsychiatric Adverse Events (%) in Ten Completed Phase 2/4 Placebo-Controlled Studies (≥0.2% more than placebo)

Neuropsychiatric Adverse Events	Varenicline (N=3091) % (n)	Placebo (N=2005) % (n)
Abnormal Dreams	9.9 (305)	3.6 (73)
Sleep Disorder	3.1 (97)	1.7 (35)
Middle Insomnia	1.1 (35)	0.3 (7)
Initial Insomnia	1.0 (30)	0.6 (12)
Nightmare	0.5 (17)	0.3 (7)
Early Morning Awakening	0.4 (13)	0.1 (3)
Nervous System Disorders[b]		
Mental Impairment Disorders	**4.0 (124)**	**3.6 (73)**
Disturbance in Attention	3.4(104)	3.1 (63)
Amnesia	0.3 (9)	0.1 (2)
Neurological Disorders NEC	**16.4 (507)**	**13.0 (260)**
Dysgeusia	6.2 (193)	3.2 (64)
Somnolence	3.4 (105)	2.4 (49)
Lethargy	0.8 (25)	0.4 (8)

[a] Number (%) of subjects with adverse events by: **Psychiatric Disorders System Organ Class: All High Level Group Terms (HLGT)** and Preferred Terms (PTs) reported in each HLGT that are ≥0.2 % greater than placebo.
[b] Number (%) of subjects with adverse events by: **Nervous System Disorders System Organ Class Selected HLGTs** and PTs reported in each HLGT that are ≥0.2 % greater than placebo.
MedDRA version 11; included data up to 30 days after last dose of drug.
Legend: NEC: not elsewhere classified.

Data from One Phase 2 Trial with Two Varenicline Doses: Data are shown from the Phase 2 trial (12 weeks duration) that included both efficacious doses, 0.5 mg BID and 1.0 mg BID.

Table 3: CHAMPIX

All-Causality Treatment-Emergent Neuropsychiatric Adverse Events (%) in One Phase 2 Dose Response Study that Included Both, 0.5 mg BID and 1.0 mg BID Doses, (≥1% greater than placebo for any varenicline dose regimen)

Neuropsychiatric Adverse Events[a]	0.5 mg BID (N=253) % (n)	1.0 mg BID (N=253) % (n)	Placebo (N=121) % (n)
Total Psychiatric Disorders			
Depressed Mood Disorders and Disturbances	**4.3 (11)**	**3.2 (8)**	**3.3 (4)**
Depressed Mood	1.2 (3)	0.8 (2)	– (0)
Disturbances in Thinking and Perception	**1.2 (3)**	**0.8 (2)**	**– (0)**
Thinking Abnormal	1.2 (3)	– (0)	– (0)
Mood Disorders and Disturbances NEC	**2.8 (7)**	**3.6 (9)**	**3.3 (4)**
Affect Lability	0.8 (2)	2.0 (5)	0.8 (1)
Sexual Dysfunction, Disturbances and Gender Identity Disorders	**0.4 (1)**	**1.6 (4)**	**– (0)**
Libido Decreased	– (0)	1.6 (4)	– (0)
Sleep Disorders and Disturbances	**34.4 (87)**	**36.4 (92)**	**15.7 (19)**
Insomnia	20.6 (52)	22.9 (58)	9.9 (12)
Abnormal Dreams	12.6 (32)	18.2 (46)	4.1(5)
Sleep Disorder	2.4 (6)	4.0 (10)	0.8 (1)
Initial Insomnia	3.2 (8)	1.2 (3)	1.7 (2)
Early Morning Awakening	1.2 (3)	0.8 (2)	– (0)
Nervous System Disorders[b]			
Mental Impairment Disorders	**6.3 (16)**	**9.9 (25)**	**4.1 (5)**
Disturbance in Attention	5.9 (15)	7.9 (20)	4.1 (5)
Amnesia	– (0)	1.2 (3)	– (0)
Neurological Disorders NEC	**22.9 (58)**	**24.9 (63)**	**14.0 (17)**
Dysgeusia	11.9 (30)	12.6 (32)	4.1 (5)
Somnolence	3.6 (9)	7.1 (18)	1.7 (2)
Lethargy	1.2 (3)	2.8 (7)	– (0)

(cont'd)

Table 3: CHAMPIX *(cont'd)*

All-Causality Treatment-Emergent Neuropsychiatric Adverse Events (%) in One Phase 2 Dose Response Study that Included Both, 0.5 mg BID and 1.0 mg BID Doses, (≥1% greater than placebo for any varenicline dose regimen)

Neuropsychiatric Adverse Events[a]	0.5 mg BID (N=253) % (n)	1.0 mg BID (N=253) % (n)	Placebo (N=121) % (n)
Hypoaesthesia	0.4 (1)	1.2 (3)	– (0)

[a] Number (%) of subjects with adverse events by: **Psychiatric Disorders System Organ Class: High Level Group Terms (HLGT)** and Preferred Terms (PTs) reported in each HLGT >1 % greater than placebo.
[b] Number (%) of subjects with adverse events by: **Nervous System Disorders System Organ Class:** Selected HLGTs and PTs reported in each HLGT that are >1 % greater than placebo.
MedDRA version 11; included data up to 30 days after last dose of drug.
Legend: NEC: not elsewhere classified.

Less Common Clinical Trial Adverse Drug Reactions: In the paragraphs that follow, the frequency of less commonly reported adverse events from clinical trials is presented. The variability associated with adverse event reporting and the terminology used to describe adverse events limit the value of the quantitative frequency estimates provided. It is important to emphasize that although the events reported occurred during treatment with CHAMPIX, they were not necessarily caused by it. All reported events are included except those already listed in Table 1, those too general to be informative, and those not reasonably associated with the use of the drug. In some cases, separate event terms have been consolidated to facilitate meaningful presentation. Events are further classified within system organ class categories and enumerated in order of decreasing frequency using the following definitions: frequent (occurring in at least 1/100 patients), infrequent (occurring in <1/100 to 1/1000 patients) and rare (occurring in fewer than 1/1000 patients).

Blood and Lymphatic System Disorders: Infrequent: anemia, lymphadenopathy. Rare: leukocytosis, thrombocytopenia, splenomegaly.

Cardiac Disorders: Infrequent: angina pectoris, arrhythmia, atrial fibrillation, bradycardia, ventricular extrasystoles, myocardial infarction, palpitations, tachycardia. Rare: cardiac flutter, coronary artery disease, cor pulmonale, acute coronary syndrome.

Ear and Labyrinth Disorders: Infrequent: tinnitus, vertigo. Rare: deafness, Meniere's disease.

Endocrine Disorders: Infrequent: thyroid gland disorders.

Eye Disorders: Infrequent: conjunctivitis, dry eye, eye irritation, scotoma, scleral discolouration, vision blurred, visual disturbance, eye pain, mydriasis, myopia, lacrimation increased, photophobia. Rare: acquired night blindness, blindness transient, cataract subcapsular, ocular vascular disorder, vitreous floaters.

Gastrointestinal Disorders: Frequent: diarrhea, gingivitis. Infrequent: change of bowel habit, abnormal feces, aphthous stomatitis, gingival pain, tongue coated, dysphagia, enterocolitis, eructation, gastritis, gastrointestinal hemorrhage, hematemesis, hematochezia, mouth ulceration, esophagitis. Rare: gastric ulcer, intestinal obstruction, pancreatitis acute.

General Disorders and Administration Site Conditions: Frequent: chest pain, influenza like illness, edema, thirst. Infrequent: chest discomfort, chills, circadian rhythm sleep disorder, feeling cold, cyst, pyrexia.

Hepatobiliary Disorders: Infrequent: gall bladder disorder.

Immune System Disorders: Infrequent: hypersensitivity. Rare: drug hypersensitivity.

Infections and Infestations: Infrequent: bronchitis, nasopharyngitis, sinusitis, fungal infection, viral infection.

Investigations: Frequent: liver function test abnormal, weight increased. Infrequent: blood pressure increased, electrocardiogram abnormal, electrocardiogram T wave amplitude decreased, electrocardiogram ST segment depression, heart rate increased, platelet count decreased, semen abnormal, C-reactive protein increased, blood calcium decreased, muscle enzyme increased, urine analysis abnormal.

Metabolism and Nutrition Disorders: Infrequent: polydipsia, diabetes mellitus, hyperlipidemia, hypokalemia. Rare: hyperkalemia, hypoglycemia.

Musculoskeletal and Connective Tissue Disorders: Frequent: arthralgia, back pain, muscle cramp, musculoskeletal pain, myalgia. Infrequent: arthritis, chest wall pain, costochondritis, joint stiffness, muscle spasms, osteoporosis. Rare: myositis.

Nervous System Disorders: Frequent: disturbance in attention, dizziness, sensory disturbance, somnolence. Infrequent: amnesia, coordination abnormal, dysarthria, dysphoria, hypertonia, hypoesthesia, hypogeusia, libido increased, libido decreased, migraine, parosmia, psychomotor hyperactivity, restlessness, restless legs syndrome, syncope, tremor. Rare: balance disorder, cerebrovascular accident, convulsion, facial palsy, mental impairment, multiple sclerosis, nystagmus, psychomotor skills impaired, transient ischemic attack, visual field defect.

Psychiatric Disorders: Frequent: anxiety, depression, emotional disorder, irritability, restlessness. Infrequent: aggression, agitation, disorientation, dissociation, mood swings, panic reaction, bradyphrenia, thinking abnormal. Rare: euphoric mood, hallucination, psychotic disorder, suicidal ideation, suicide.

Renal and Urinary Disorders: Frequent: polyuria. Infrequent: glycosuria, nephrolithiasis, nocturia, urine abnormality, urethral syndrome. Rare: renal failure acute, urinary retention.

Reproductive System and Breast Disorders: Frequent: menstrual disorder. Infrequent: erectile dysfunction, menorrhagia, vaginal discharge, sexual dysfunction.

Respiratory, Thoracic and Mediastinal Disorders: Frequent: epistaxis, respiratory disorders. Infrequent: asthma, cough, hoarseness, pharyngolaryngeal pain, throat irritation, respiratory tract congestion, sinus congestion, post nasal drip, rhinorrhea, snoring. Rare: pleurisy, pulmonary embolism.

Skin and Subcutaneous Tissue Disorders: Frequent: hyperhydrosis, rash generalized. Infrequent: acne, dermatitis, dry skin, eczema, erythema, psoriasis, night sweats, urticaria. Rare: photosensitivity reaction.

Vascular Disorders: Frequent: hot flush, hypertension. Infrequent: hypotension, peripheral ischemia, thrombosis.

Post-Market Adverse Events: The following adverse events have been reported during post-approval use of CHAMPIX. Because these events are reported voluntarily from a population of uncertain size, it is not always possible to reliably estimate their frequency or establish a causal relationship to drug exposure.

Psychiatric Symptoms: There have been reports of depressed mood, agitation, aggression, hostility, anxiety, changes in behavior or thinking, mania, psychosis, hallucinations, paranoia, delusion, homicidal ideation, mood swings, suicidal ideation and completed suicide in patients attempting to quit smoking while taking CHAMPIX (see Warnings and Precautions, Psychiatric Symptoms). Of the cases with information provided, the majority reported possible contributing factors, including primarily prior psychiatric history and/or concurrent psychiatric medications. Smoking status at the time of event onset was not reported in most cases.

Smoking cessation with or without treatment is associated with nicotine withdrawal symptoms and the exacerbation of underlying psychiatric illness. The role of CHAMPIX in these reports is not known (see also Warnings and Precautions, Psychiatric Symptoms).

Hypersensitivity and Serious Skin Reactions: There have also been reports of hypersensitivity reactions, including angioedema and of rare but severe cutaneous reactions including Stevens-Johnson syndrome and erythema multiforme in patients taking CHAMPIX (see Warnings and Precautions, Angioedema and Hypersensitivity Reactions and Serious Skin Reactions).

DRUG INTERACTIONS: Overview: Based on varenicline pharmacokinetic characteristics, and clinical experience to date, it appears unlikely that CHAMPIX would produce or be subject to clinically meaningful drug interactions.

Drug interaction studies were performed with varenicline and: cimetidine, metformin, digoxin, warfarin, transdermal nicotine and bupropion.

No clinically meaningful pharmacokinetic drug interactions have been identified, other than potential for interaction with cimetidine in patients with severe renal impairment (see Cimetidine).

Drugs Cleared by, or Which Affect, Cytochrome P450 Enzymes: In vitro studies demonstrated that varenicline does not inhibit cytochrome P450 enzymes (IC50 >6400 ng/mL). The P450 enzymes tested for inhibition were: 1A2, 2A6, 2B6, 2C8, 2C9, 2C19, 2D6, 2E1, and 3A4/5. Also, in human hepatocytes in vitro, varenicline did not induce the activity of cytochrome P450 enzymes 1A2 and 3A4.

Therefore, varenicline is unlikely to alter the pharmacokinetics of compounds that are primarily metabolised by cytochrome P450 enzymes.

Furthermore, since metabolism of varenicline represents less than 10% of its clearance, drugs known to affect the cytochrome P450 system are unlikely to alter the pharmacokinetics of CHAMPIX (see Action and Clinical Pharmacology, Pharmacokinetics) and therefore a dose adjustment of CHAMPIX should not be required for these types of drugs.

Drugs Cleared by, or Which Affect, Renal Secretion: In vitro studies demonstrated that varenicline does not inhibit human renal transport proteins at therapeutic concentrations. Therefore, drugs that are cleared by renal secretion (e.g., Metformin) are unlikely to be affected by varenicline.

In vitro studies demonstrated the active renal secretion of varenicline is mediated by the human organic cation transporter, hOCT2. In patients with normal renal function coadministration with inhibitors of hOCT2 does not require a dose adjustment of CHAMPIX as the increase in systemic exposure to CHAMPIX is not expected to be clinically meaningful except in cases of severe renal impairment, (see Cimetidine, and Other Inhibitors of hOCT2).

Drug-Drug Interactions: Drug-drug interaction studies were limited to approximately two week studies in healthy young adult volunteers who smoked.

Single Dosing for One of the Two Drugs: Cimetidine: Co-administration of varenicline (2 mg single dose) with an hOCT2 inhibitor, cimetidine (300 mg four times daily (QID) at steady-state) to 12 smokers increased the systemic exposure of varenicline by 29% (90% CI: 21.5%, 36.9%) due to a reduction in varenicline renal clearance. No dosage adjustment is recommended based on concomitant cimetidine administration in subjects with normal renal function or in patients with mild to moderate renal impairment. In patients with severe renal impairment, the concomitant use of cimetidine and varenicline should be avoided. (See Dosage and Administration, Recommended Dose and Dosage Adjustment, Special Populations, Patients with Impaired Renal Function.)

Other Inhibitors of hOCT2: Other inhibitors of hOCT2 have not been directly studied. Cimetidine causes greater in vivo drug interactions with renally cleared compounds than other inhibitors of hOCT2. Consequently, co-administration of other inhibitors of hOCT2 with varenicline would not require dosage adjustment in patients with normal renal function or moderate renal impairment. In patients with severe renal impairment, the concomitant use of varenicline and other inhibitors of hOCT2, such as trimethoprim, ranitidine or levofloxacin should be avoided. (See Dosage and Administration, Recommended Dose and Dosage Adjustment, Special Populations, Patients with Impaired Renal Function.)

Co-Administration with Other Drugs Eliminated via hOCT2: Based on the lack of interaction between varenicline and metformin, interactions between varenicline and other cationic drugs eliminated via hOCT2 are unlikely.

Warfarin: Varenicline (1 mg BID steady-state) did not alter the pharmacokinetics of a single 25 mg dose of (R, S)-warfarin in 24 smokers. Prothrombin time (INR) was not affected by CHAMPIX. Smoking-cessation itself may result in changes to warfarin pharmacokinetics (see Warnings and Precautions).

Multiple Dosing for Both Drugs: Metformin: When co-administered to 30 smokers, varenicline (1 mg BID) did not alter the steady-state pharmacokinetics of metformin (500 mg BID), which is a substrate of hOCT2. Metformin had no effect on varenicline steady-state pharmacokinetics.

Digoxin: Varenicline (1 mg BID) did not alter the steady-state pharmacokinetics of digoxin administered as a 0.25 mg daily dose in 18 smokers. Steady-state pharmacokinetics of varenicline remained unchanged by digoxin co-administration.

Use with Other Therapies for Smoking-Cessation: Safety and efficacy of varenicline in combination with other smoking-cessation therapies, such as bupropion or nicotine replacement therapy, have not been studied.

Bupropion: Varenicline (1 mg BID) did not alter the steady-state pharmacokinetics of bupropion (150 mg BID) in 46 smokers. Steady-state pharmacokinetics of varenicline remained unchanged by bupropion co-administration.

Nicotine Replacement Therapy (NRT): When varenicline (1 mg BID) and NRT (transdermal, 21 mg/day) were co-administered to 24 smokers for 12 days, there was a statistically significant decrease in average systolic blood pressure (mean 2.6 mmHg) measured on the final day of the study. In this study, the incidence of nausea, headache, vomiting, dizziness, dyspepsia and fatigue were greater for the combination of varenicline and NRT than for NRT alone. Due to the partial agonist nicotinic activity of varenicline, it is not anticipated that co-administration with NRT would confer additional benefits compared with CHAMPIX alone, and may result in increased side effects (see Warnings and Precautions).

Drug-Food Interactions: Oral bioavailability of CHAMPIX is unaffected by food.

Drug-Herb Interactions: CHAMPIX has no known drug-herb interactions.

Drug-Laboratory Test Interactions: CHAMPIX has no known drug-laboratory test interactions.

DOSAGE AND ADMINISTRATION:

Dosing Considerations: Smoking-cessation therapies are more likely to succeed for patients who are motivated to stop smoking and who are provided additional counselling and/or support services. In the clinical trials on which approval was based, CHAMPIX was used with supportive counseling. Physicians should review the patient's overall smoking-cessation plan that includes treatment with CHAMPIX.

The majority of clinical evidence in efficacy and safety was based on a 1.0 mg BID dose. There is little clinical experience with doses above the maximum recommended dose of 1 mg BID.

There is limited data available for dose comparison. In the one randomized clinical trial that included both 1.0 mg BID and 0.5 mg BID arms and that was designed to compare each of the two doses to placebo, and not to each other, the quit rates for 1.0 mg BID (n=253), 0.5 mg BID (n=253) and placebo (n=121) were:

- for Weeks 9 to 12: 51%, 45%, and 12% respectively, and
- for Weeks 9 to 52: 23%, 19% and 4% respectively.

Based on the limited data available, it cannot be concluded that there is a difference between the two doses in the rate of serious neuropsychiatric events (see Adverse Reactions, Neuropsychiatric Adverse Events in Randomized, Double-Blind, Placebo-Controlled Clinical Studies of Varenicline).

CHAMPIX should be taken after eating and with a full glass of water.

Patients with Impaired Renal Function: For patients with severe renal impairment, daily dosage should be adjusted accordingly (see Recommended Dose and Dosage Adjustment, Special Populations, Patients with Impaired Renal Function).

Recommended Dose and Dosage Adjustment: Adults: The patient should set a date to stop smoking. CHAMPIX dosing should start 1-2 weeks before this date.

Following one week of titration, there is a choice of two doses for CHAMPIX: 0.5 mg BID or 1.0 mg BID.

As shown in the table below, the two titration schedules are identical from Day 1 to Day 7, separating at Day 8 when the patient either remains on 0.5 mg BID or moves up to 1.0 mg BID.

	Dosing Regimen	
Day	**0.5 mg BID**	**1.0 mg BID**
Days 1–3:	0.5 mg once daily	0.5 mg once daily
Days 4–7:	0.5 mg twice daily	0.5 mg twice daily
Days 8–onward	0.5 mg twice daily	1.0 mg twice daily

The choice of dosing regimen should be based on physician judgment and patient preference, following discussion with the patient (see also Dosing Considerations).

Once CHAMPIX treatment is initiated, the dose may be changed, temporarily or permanently, according to patient and physician judgments on tolerability and efficacy.

Patients should be treated with CHAMPIX for 12 weeks. For patients who have successfully stopped smoking at the end of 12 weeks, an additional course of 12 weeks treatment with CHAMPIX may be considered.

No data are available on the efficacy of an additional 12 week course of treatment for patients who do not succeed in stopping smoking or who relapse after treatment.

Dose tapering may be considered. Regardless of whether the treatment course is 12 or 24 weeks, risk of smoking-cessation relapse is elevated in the period immediately following the end of drug treatment. In addition, dose tapering may help minimize discontinuation symptoms (e.g., increase in irritability, urge to smoke, depression, and/or insomnia), observed in up to 3% of patients at the end of treatment.

Special Populations: Patients with Impaired Renal Function: No dosage adjustment is necessary for patients with mild (estimated creatinine clearance >50 mL/min and ≤80 mL/min) to moderate (estimated creatinine clearance ≥30 mL/min and ≤50 mL/min) renal impairment. For patients who experience intolerable adverse events, dosing may be reduced.

For patients with severe renal impairment, the recommended dose of CHAMPIX is 0.5 mg twice daily. Dosing should begin at 0.5 mg once daily for the first 3 days then increased to 0.5 mg twice daily. Based on insufficient clinical experience with CHAMPIX in patients with end-stage renal disease, treatment is not recommended in this patient population (see also Warnings and Precautions, Special Populations, Renal Impairment).

Patients with Hepatic Impairment: No dosage adjustment is necessary for patients with hepatic impairment.

Psychiatric Patients, Patients with Epilepsy, Patients Undergoing Chemotherapy, Patients with GI Disturbances such as Irritable Bowel, and in General, Patients with Heart Disease or COPD: The use of CHAMPIX has not been studied in these patient populations (see Warnings and Precautions, Special Populations).

Dosing in Elderly Patients: No dosage adjustment is necessary for elderly patients with normal renal function. However, varenicline is known to be substantially excreted by the kidney, and the risk of toxic reactions to this drug may be greater in patients with impaired renal function. Because elderly patients are more likely to have decreased renal function, care should be taken in dose selection, and it may be useful to monitor renal function (see Warnings and Precautions, Special Populations, Geriatrics (>65 years of age)).

Use in Children: Safety and effectiveness of CHAMPIX in pediatric patients have not been established; therefore, CHAMPIX is not recommended for use in patients under 18 years of age.

OVERDOSAGE:

Symptoms: Consistent with its pharmacological profile, CHAMPIX resulted in increased incidences of nausea and vomiting when given at doses greater than the recommended dose of 1 mg BID.

Treatment: Varenicline has been shown to be dialyzed in patients with end-stage renal disease (see Action and Clinical Pharmacology, Special Populations and Conditions, Renal Insufficiency), however, there is no experience with dialysis following overdose.

> For management of a suspected drug overdose, contact your regional Poison Control Centre. See the *CPS Directory* section for a list of Poison Control Centres.

ACTION AND CLINICAL PHARMACOLOGY:

Mechanism of Action: The efficacy of CHAMPIX in smoking-cessation is believed to be a result of varenicline's partial agonist activity at the α4β2 nicotinic acetylcholine receptor (ie agonist activity to a lesser degree than nicotine), while simultaneously preventing nicotine binding (ie antagonist activity).

In vitro, varenicline binds with higher affinity to the α4β2 receptor subtype than to other common nicotinic receptors (>500-fold α3β4; >3500-fold α7; >20,000-fold α1βγδ), or to non-nicotinic receptors and transporters (>2000-fold).

Electrophysiology studies in vitro and neurochemical studies in vivo have shown that varenicline acts as a partial agonist at α4β2 nicotinic acetylcholine receptors. In the absence of nicotine, varenicline's agonist activity is at a significantly lower level than nicotine, but sufficient to activate the central nervous mesolimbic dopamine system, believed to be the neuronal mechanism underlying reinforcement and reward experienced upon smoking. In the presence of nicotine, which competes for the same human α4β2 nicotinic acetylcholine receptor (nAChR) binding site, varenicline prevented nicotine from activating the α4β2 receptor, since it has higher affinity for this site and this prevented full stimulation of the central nervous mesolimbic dopamine system.

Varenicline is also a partial agonist at α3β4 receptors, but a full agonist at α7 receptors and a full agonist at 5-HT3 receptors.

Varenicline has moderate affinity for the 5-HT3 serotonergic receptor (Ki=350 nM), at which it acts as a weak, full agonist (EC_{50}=0.96 μM). Varenicline-induced nausea shortly after dosing, when gastrointestinal levels are predicted to be temporarily high, may be due to activation of this peripheral receptor, in addition to a possible role for peripheral α3β4 and/or central α4β2 nAChRs.

Pharmacokinetics: See Table 4.

Table 4: CHAMPIX

Summary of Mean with Standard Deviation Varenicline Pharmacokinetic Parameters in Adult Male and Female Smokers

	C_{max} (ng/mL)	T_{max}[a] (hr)	$AUC_{0\text{-}24}$ (ng·h/mL)	$t_{½}$ (hr)	Clearance[b] (L/hr)	Volume of distribution[b] (L)
1 mg[c] BID	9.22 (2.05)	3.00 [1.00–8.00]	194[d] (42.7)	33.0[e] (14.4)	10.4 (25%CV)	337 (50%CV)

a T_{max} presented as median [range].
b Apparent clearance and central volume of distribution estimated from a population PK analysis conducted on pooled data from 1878 subjects (49.2% females); presented as typical value (interindividual coefficient of variation).
c Derived from three multiple-dose studies (N=103).
d N=64.
e N=46.

Absorption: Maximum plasma concentrations of varenicline occur typically within 3-4 hours after oral administration. Following administration of multiple oral doses of varenicline to healthy volunteers, steady-state conditions were reached within 4 days. Varenicline exhibits linear kinetics when given as single (0.1 to 3 mg) or repeated (1 to 3 mg/day) doses. In a mass balance study, absorption of varenicline is virtually complete after oral administration and systemic availability is high. Oral bioavailability of varenicline is unaffected by food or time-of-day dosing.

Distribution: Plasma protein binding of varenicline is low (≤20%) and independent of both age and renal function.

Metabolism: Varenicline tartrate undergoes minimal metabolism, with approximately 92% of recovered drug-related entity in urine being unchanged varenicline. Metabolite profiles (for circulation and urine) were similar for smokers and non-smokers, and are from the following minor routes of metabolism: N-carbomyl glucuronidation, N-formylation and conjugation with a hexose sugar.

Excretion: The elimination half-life of varenicline tartrate is approximately 24 hours. Renal elimination of varenicline is the major elimination route, primarily through glomerular filtration along with active tubular secretion via the organic cationic transporter, OCT2.

Special Populations and Conditions: There were no clinically meaningful differences seen in varenicline tartrate pharmacokinetics due to being elderly, race, gender, smoking status, or use of concomitant medications, as demonstrated in specific pharmacokinetic studies and in population pharmacokinetic analyses.

Pediatrics: When 22 adolescent smokers aged 12 to 17 years (inclusive) received a single 0.5 mg and 1 mg dose of varenicline the pharmacokinetics of varenicline was approximately dose proportional between the 0.5 mg and 1 mg doses. Systemic exposure, as assessed by $AUC_{0-\infty}$, and renal clearance of varenicline tartrate were comparable to those of an adult population. An increase of 30% in C_{max} and a shorter elimination half-life (10.9 h) were observed in adolescents compared with adults.

Because the safety and effectiveness of varenicline in pediatric patients have not been established, varenicline is not recommended for use in patients under 18 years of age.

Geriatrics: A combined single and multiple-dose pharmacokinetic study demonstrated that the pharmacokinetics of 1 mg varenicline given once or twice daily to 16 healthy elderly male and female smokers (aged 65-75 years) for 7 consecutive days was similar to that of younger subjects.

Because elderly patients are more likely to have decreased renal function, care should be taken in dose selection, and it may be useful to monitor renal function (see Dosage and Administration, Special Populations, Geriatrics).

Hepatic Insufficiency: Due to the absence of significant hepatic metabolism, varenicline tartrate pharmacokinetics should be unaffected in patients with hepatic insufficiency, except in the case that there is accompanying renal compromise (see Dosage and Administration). The potential for clinically meaningful drug interactions between varenicline and metabolic inhibitors/inducers is low.

Renal Insufficiency: Varenicline tartrate pharmacokinetics were studied in subjects with normal, mild, moderate, severe renal impairment and end-stage renal disease (n=6 per arm), following 0.5 mg once daily administration for 12 days.

Varenicline pharmacokinetics were essentially unchanged in subjects with mild renal impairment (estimated creatinine clearance >50 mL/min and ≤80 mL/min).

In patients with moderate renal impairment (estimated creatinine clearance ≥30 mL/min and ≤50 mL/min), varenicline exposure [AUCτ] increased 1.5-fold compared with subjects with normal renal function (estimated creatinine clearance >80 mL/min).

In subjects with severe renal impairment (estimated creatinine clearance <30 mL/min), varenicline exposure [AUCτ] was increased 2.1-fold.

In subjects with end-stage renal disease (ESRD), undergoing a three hour session of hemodialysis for three days a week, varenicline exposure [AUCτ] was increased 2.7-fold; varenicline was efficiently removed by hemodialysis (see Dosage and Administration, Recommended Dose and Dosage Adjustment, Special Populations, Patients with Impaired Renal Function).

STORAGE AND STABILITY: Store at room temperature (15-30°C).

INFORMATION FOR THE PATIENT: Published in e-CPS, available by subscription at www.e-cps.ca.

DOSAGE FORMS, COMPOSITION AND PACKAGING: 0.5 mg: Each capsular, biconvex, white to off-white film-coated tablet, debossed with "*Pfizer*" on one side and "CHX 0.5" on the other side contains: varenicline 0.5 mg (as tartrate). Nonmedicinal ingredients: anhydrous dibasic calcium phosphate, colloidal silicon dioxide, croscarmellose sodium, magnesium stearate and microcrystalline cellulose; film-coating: hypromellose, polyethylene glycol, titanium dioxide and triacetin. High-density polyethylene (HDPE) bottles of 56.

1 mg: Each capsular, biconvex, light blue film-coated tablet ,debossed with "*Pfizer*" on one side and "CHX 1.0" on the other side contains: varenicline 1 mg (as tartrate). Nonmedicinal ingredients: anhydrous dibasic calcium phosphate, colloidal silicon dioxide, croscarmellose sodium, magnesium stearate and microcrystalline cellulose; film-coating: hypromellose, polyethylene glycol, titanium dioxide and triacetin. Also contains FD&C Blue #2/Indigo Carmine Aluminum Lake as a colouring agent. Continuation pack: Includes blister strips of 28 tablets (combination of 2 strips of 14 tablets).
Initial dosing pack: Includes 0.5 mg tablets in blister strips of 11 tablets and 1 mg tablets in blister strips of 14 tablets.

(Shown in Product Identification Section)

Charcoal, Activated
Poison Antidote

CPhA Monograph

Date of Revision: October 2006

This monograph has been compiled by CPhA and reviewed by experts. It may contain information different from that found in Health Canada-approved Product Monographs. The reader is referred to the *CPS* Editorial Policy for more information.

PHARMACOLOGY: Activated charcoal is a fine, black, odorless and tasteless powder. It is formed in a two-step process beginning with the heat-induced chemical decomposition of organic materials such as wood, coconut or peat followed by "activation" at high temperatures by a variety of agents such as steam or carbon dioxide. This last step increases the adsorptive (binding) capacity of the charcoal by forming an internal network of pores with a huge surface area.

Activated charcoal adsorbs many organic and inorganic substances, including drugs, thereby decreasing the extent of their absorption from the gastrointestinal tract. In order for this process to occur, the activated charcoal must come into direct contact with the substance ingested.

In vitro studies indicate that binding begins within about 1 minute of charcoal coming into contact with the agent to be adsorbed, but that equilibrium may not be reached for 10 to 25 minutes. Based on volunteer studies, the effectiveness of activated charcoal in preventing the absorption of ingested substances decreases with time; the greatest benefit is seen when it is administered within 1 hour of the toxic ingestion.

Multiple doses of activated charcoal may be used in an attempt to increase the elimination rate of a small number of ingested toxins by interrupting enteroenteric, enterohepatic or enterogastric circulation. This is sometimes termed "gut dialysis".

Some commercial preparations of activated charcoal also contain sorbitol. Sorbitol acts as a sweetener and cathartic.

Pharmacokinetics: Activated charcoal is not absorbed or metabolized and is eliminated unchanged in the feces along with any bound drug.

INDICATIONS: Activated charcoal is used to prevent absorption of ingested substances from the GI tract in the treatment of poisoning by many drugs and chemicals. However, activated charcoal is ineffective in adsorbing caustic or corrosive alkalies and acids, ethanol, methanol, sodium chloride, lead, lithium, iron salts, boric acid and other mineral acids. The current position statement of the American Academy of Clinical Toxicology and the European Association of Poison Centres and Clinical Toxicologists (AACT/EAPCCT) recommends that the administration of activated charcoal may be considered if a patient has ingested a potentially toxic amount of a poison (known to be adsorbed to charcoal) up to one hour previously. However, benefit after one hour cannot be excluded. They also advise that single-dose activated charcoal should not be used routinely in the management of most poisoned patients.

Multiple-dose activated charcoal (MDAC) may be used to enhance elimination of selected drugs already absorbed into the body (see Pharmacology). This use is controversial. The 1999 position statement of the AACT/EAPCCT recommends MDAC be considered only if a patient has ingested a life-threatening amount of carbamazepine, dapsone, phenobarbital, quinine or theophylline. This position statement has been endorsed by the Canadian Association of Poison Control Centres. However, some experts advocate a broader role for MDAC. These clinicians suggest MDAC be considered in circumstances when a significant amount of the toxic agent is likely to remain in the gastrointestinal tract after a single dose of activated charcoal (e.g., massive ingestions, sustained-release formulations, concretions, slowed gastrointestinal motility).

CONTRAINDICATIONS: Activated charcoal is contraindicated if a patient has an unprotected airway (e.g., decreased level of consciousness without endotracheal intubation). It is relatively contraindicated for use in a caustic ingestion because it does not adsorb these agents and may obscure the view during endoscopy. However, it may be administered if necessary for co-ingested agents that are systemic toxins. Because activated charcoal can cause vomiting, it is also contraindicated for use in ingestions of pure petroleum distillates that are not well adsorbed and carry a high risk of aspiration.

Multiple doses of activated charcoal are contraindicated if an intestinal obstruction or signs of decreased peristalsis (e.g., decreased bowel sounds, abdominal distension, and ileus) are present.

WARNINGS: See Precautions.

PRECAUTIONS: *Drug Interactions:* Activated charcoal may decrease the effectiveness of other orally administered drugs (i.e., drugs administered with therapeutic intent). If activated charcoal interrupts the enterohepatic circulation of the drug in question, this effect may not be completely abolished by separating administration of the drug from that of charcoal.

Pregnancy: Because activated charcoal is not absorbed, it would not be expected to harm the fetus or appear in breast milk.

Lactation: See Pregnancy.

Children: Commercially available products combining charcoal and sorbitol should be used cautiously, if at all, in children. Children are especially vulnerable to fluid and electrolyte abnormalities that may be caused by cathartics such as sorbitol. **If these preparations are used, fluid and electrolyte status should be monitored carefully, and only one dose of a sorbitol-containing preparation administered. If further doses of charcoal are required, preparations that do NOT contain sorbitol should be used.**

ADVERSE EFFECTS: Activated charcoal is generally well tolerated. The most common adverse effects are nausea, vomiting (15%) and constipation. Constipation may be more common in patients who are not ambulatory due to a depressed level of consciousness. Vomiting may be more common when activated charcoal is administered with sorbitol. Bowel obstruction or pseudo-obstruction has been described rarely after MDAC. Pulmonary aspiration has occurred. However, complications following aspiration of activated charcoal are consistent with those following aspiration of gastric contents. Transient corneal abrasions have been reported after accidental ocular spillage of activated charcoal.

OVERDOSE:

For management of a suspected poisoning, CPhA recommends that you contact your **regional Poison Control Centre**. See the *CPS* Directory section for a list of Poison Control Centres.

DOSAGE: The optimal dose of activated charcoal for poisoned patients is unknown. When indicated, it should be administered as soon as possible after ingestion of the poison. It may be administered orally or via nasogastric or orogastric tube. All formulations should be shaken well for at least 1 minute prior to administration. Only activated charcoal formulated as a suspension should be used in the management of poisoning; tablets and capsules should not be used for this indication.

Initial Dose: Adults and children: 1 g/kg body weight when the amount of ingested toxin is unknown or when known in a 10:1 ratio of activated charcoal to toxin, up to an amount that is safely administered and tolerated. For massive ingestions, an initial dose of 2 g/kg body weight may be indicated. Sorbitol-containing preparations should only be given once, and the dose of these preparations should never exceed 1g/kg body weight.

Multiple Dose Activated Charcoal (MDAC): Initial dose as above, then 0.25 to 0.5 g/kg body weight given every 1 to 6 hours. Alternatively, some experts recommend that after an initial adult dose of 50 to 100 g, activated charcoal should be given at a minimum rate of 12.5 g/h or equivalent (e.g., 25 g every 2 hours).

Criteria for stopping MDAC are not well defined. In general, no more than 3 or 4 doses in total should be administered unless recommended by a Poison Specialist.

In 2004, the ACCT/EAPCCT suggested that the routine use of a cathartic in combination with activated charcoal is not recommended. If a cathartic is used, it should be limited to a single dose to minimize adverse effects.

If vomiting interferes with administration, an antiemetic may be administered intravenously. In addition, the administration of smaller doses of charcoal more frequently may decrease the likelihood of vomiting.

Chloral Hydrate
Sedative—Hypnotic

CPhA Monograph

Date of Revision: July 2009

This monograph has been compiled by CPhA and reviewed by experts. It may contain information different from that found in Health Canada-approved Product Monographs. The reader is referred to the *CPS* Editorial Policy for more information.

SUMMARY PRODUCT INFORMATION:

Route of Administration	Dosage Form	Strength
Oral	Syrup	100 mg/mL

PHARMACOLOGY: The mechanism of action of chloral hydrate is not well understood. The CNS depressant effect of the drug may be due to its active metabolite, trichloroethanol. Tolerance to the sedative effects may develop over a 5- to 14-day period of continued use.

Pharmacokinetics: Chloral hydrate is rapidly absorbed following oral or rectal administration. Following a hypnotic dose, onset of sleep is approximately 30–60 minutes, with a duration of action of 4–8 hours.

Chloral hydrate is rapidly and extensively metabolized in the liver and erythrocytes by alcohol dehydrogenase to its major active metabolite, trichloroethanol. A small amount of chloral hydrate and a larger portion of trichloroethanol are oxidized to a minor, less active metabolite, trichloroacetic acid, in the liver and kidneys. This metabolite is excreted in the urine and bile, together with trichloroethanol in free or conjugated form.

The average half-life of trichloroethanol in adults is 8 hours, ranging from 4–12 hours. The half-life is prolonged in children (10 hours), preterm neonates (37 hours) and term neonates (28 hours). Trichloroethanol is 70–80% bound to plasma proteins and is widely distributed to all body tissues including CSF, breast milk and placenta.

The half-life of trichloroacetic acid is longer, up to 100 hours. It is highly protein bound (94%), primarily to albumin, and may be responsible for interactions with other drugs with significant protein binding. On multiple dosing, trichloracetic acid can displace bilirubin or warfarin from binding sites, potentially resulting in hyperbilirubinemia or hypoprothrombinemia.

INDICATIONS: For short-term use as a sedative or hypnotic. Tolerance to these effects often develops after a 2-week period. Chloral hydrate has also been used prior to surgery or other procedures to reduce anxiety or to produce sedation or sleep, without depressing respiration or cough reflex.

CONTRAINDICATIONS: Patients with severe impairment of renal or hepatic function, a history of idiosyncratic reaction to chloral hydrate, or hypersensitivity to chloral hydrate or any component of the formulation.

WARNINGS: Abuse and Dependence: Chloral hydrate should be used as a hypnotic only for short-term use (<2 weeks). Prolonged use of chloral hydrate may produce tolerance and physical and/or psychological dependence. Sudden withdrawal after prolonged use may result in hallucinations and symptoms similar to delirium tremens (sometimes fatal), therefore chloral hydrate should be tapered gradually. Chloral hydrate should be avoided in patients with a history of drug abuse or dependence.

Self-harm: Due to the risk of toxicity associated with overdose, chloral hydrate should be given in limited quantities to patients with clinical depression/suicidality.

Cardiac Disorders: In patients with severe cardiac disease, chloral hydrate should be avoided due to the possibility of cardiac arrhythmias and hypotension associated with larger doses.

Gastrointestinal: Because of its irritant properties, oral use of chloral hydrate should be avoided in patients with gastritis, esophagitis or gastric or duodenal ulcer. Rectal use should be avoided in patients with proctitis or colitis.

Children: Chloral hydrate should not be administered to children by nonmedical personnel or in an unsupervised medical setting. Patients should be monitored for CNS and respiratory depressive effects, particularly with concurrent use of other sedatives or opioids. Deaths associated with the use of chloral hydrate for sedation prior to diagnostic or therapeutic procedures have been reported, particularly in pediatric patients. In addition, particular care must be taken in calculating and administering the proper dose.

Sedation with chloral hydrate in children with adenoidal hypertrophy and obstructive sleep apnea has been reported to cause episodes of life-threatening respiratory obstruction. Children with obstructive sleep apnea from other causes may be at risk as well. Laryngeal edema resulting in severe respiratory difficulty in a child has also been reported.

PRECAUTIONS: Occupational Hazards: Due to chloral hydrate's sedative effects, patients should be warned against driving, operating dangerous machinery or engaging in other activities requiring mental alertness and physical coordination after taking the drug.

Drug Interactions: Anticoagulants, Oral: Chloral hydrate may transiently enhance the hypoprothrombinemic response to warfarin, especially within the first 2 weeks of therapy, by displacing warfarin from plasma protein binding sites. When chloral hydrate is added or removed from the therapeutic regimen, or when dosage changes are made, frequent prothrombin time determinations are recommended.

CNS depressants (including alcohol): Additive CNS effects may occur when chloral hydrate is given concurrently with other CNS depressants, e.g., alcohol, barbiturates, benzodiazepines.

Drug-Laboratory Test Interactions: Chloral hydrate may interfere with fluorometric determinations of urine catecholamines. Chloral hydrate should not be administered within 48 hours prior to the test.

Pregnancy: Chloral hydrate crosses the placenta. Safety has not been established. Chronic use during pregnancy may cause withdrawal symptoms in the neonate.

Lactation: Small amounts of chloral hydrate are excreted in breast milk and may cause drowsiness in the infant.

Children: Gastric irritation and vomiting may occur following administration of the oral liquid. To minimize unpleasant taste and reduce gastric irritation, each dose of oral liquid should be well diluted with water or other liquid such as fruit juice or ginger ale.

Due to the prolonged half-lives of chloral hydrate's metabolites, excessive CNS depression may occur due to accumulation following repeated dosing. The degree of sedation should be monitored and caregivers cautioned against exceeding prescribed dosage.

Neonates should be monitored for increased bilirubin concentrations as hyperbilirubinemia may occur due to competition of chloral hydrate metabolites with bilirubin for hepatic glucuronidation.

Geriatrics: In elderly patients likely to have age-related hepatic/renal function impairment, and in debilitated patients or those patients prone to CNS depression, reduction of dose may be necessary to avoid oversedation or other adverse effects.

Respiratory: Careful monitoring is required in patients with respiratory insufficiency.

ADVERSE EFFECTS: Gastrointestinal: The most frequent adverse effect of chloral hydrate is gastrointestinal irritation, manifested by nausea, vomiting, diarrhea and stomach pain. Unpleasant taste and flatulence may also occur. These effects can be minimized by taking chloral hydrate with a full glass of fluid. Ileus in an infant has been reported.

Central Nervous System: Adverse effects of chloral hydrate due to CNS depressant effects include: lightheadedness, ataxia, nightmares, drowsiness, vertigo, headache, confusion and malaise. Most CNS effects occur infrequently. Hangover effect can occur, although it is less commonly observed than with barbiturates and some benzodiazepines. Rarely, paradoxical and idiosyncratic reactions (hallucinations, delirium, unusual excitement, disorientation, incoherence, paranoia) have occurred.

Cardiovascular: Large doses of chloral hydrate have been reported to produce hypotension, ventricular and atrial arrhythmias, torsades de pointes, depression of myocardial contractility and shortening of refractory period.

Respiratory: Life-threatening respiratory obstruction episodes have been reported in young children (see Warnings).

Dermatologic: Dermatologic reactions are not common, but include: erythematous rash, urticaria, angioedema, eczematoid dermatitis, scarlatiniform exanthema, bullous lesions, non-thrombocytopenic purpura and erythema multiforme. Some cutaneous reactions are accompanied by fever. Chloral hydrate is an irritant when applied to the skin and mucous membranes.

Metabolic: Chloral hydrate has been reported to precipitate attacks of acute intermittent porphyria. Rarely, ketonuria has been reported.

Hematologic: Leukopenia and eosinophilia have been reported.

Ophthalmologic: Chloral hydrate has produced oculotoxicities manifesting as ptosis, allergic conjunctivitis or keratoconjunctivitis.

Other: Increases in middle ear pressure in infants and children have been reported.

OVERDOSE:

Symptoms: Acute poisoning resembles barbiturate intoxication, producing symptoms of CNS depression and deep coma, respiratory depression, hypotension and cardiac arrhythmias. The main cause of death appears to be arrhythmias, which can include ventricular fibrillation, ventricular tachycardia and torsades de pointes. Individuals with known cardiac dysfunction are highly susceptible to toxicity.

Gastritis, nausea and vomiting are common. Gastric necrosis, perforation, gastrointestinal hemorrhage and esophageal stricture have also been reported. Other signs may include pinpoint pupils, cyanosis, hypothermia, muscle flaccidity and pulmonary edema. Renal damage (albuminuria) and hepatic damage (jaundice) may occur.

The usual lethal dose is 10 g; however, fatalities have occurred with as little as 4 g and survival has been documented after the ingestion of 30 g of chloral hydrate.

Chronic poisoning may manifest with symptoms of gastritis, skin rash, peripheral vasodilation, hypotension, renal damage and myocardial depression.

Treatment: Patients who have ingested chloral hydrate in overdose occasionally require respiratory and hemodynamic support. This may include intubation, ventilation, boluses of isotonic iv fluids and inotropic agents. Chloral hydrate-induced arrhythmias are often resistant to conventional antiarrhythmics; iv β-blockers are considered the treatment of choice. Hemodialysis significantly increases clearance of both parent drug and trichloroethanol. Once the patient's airway is secured, activated charcoal should be administered.

> For management of a suspected drug overdose, CPhA recommends that you contact your **regional Poison Control Centre**. See the *CPS* Directory section for a list of Poison Control Centres.

DOSAGE: Dosage must be individualized. Doses for oral and rectal routes are equivalent. Chloral hydrate can be administered rectally as a retention enema by dissolving liquid in cottonseed or olive oil or in a hydrophillic polyethylene glycol base.

Doses of chloral hydrate liquid should be diluted with water or other liquid (such as fruit juice or ginger ale) to reduce gastric irritation and improve taste.

Chloral hydrate should be avoided in patients with moderate to severe renal failure (creatinine clearance <0.8 mL/s), or in patients with severe hepatic dysfunction. No dosage adjustment is necessary for patients with mild renal failure.

Hypnotic: Adults: 500–1000 mg, 15–30 minutes before bedtime.

Geriatrics: Initial 250 mg, 15–30 minutes before bedtime.

Children: 50 mg/kg at bedtime, maximum 1000 mg per single dose. See Warnings, Children

Sedative: Adults: 250 mg 3 times daily after meals, maximum 2000 mg/day.

Premedicant: Adults: 500–1000 mg, 30 minutes prior to procedure.

Children: 25–50 mg/kg, 30 minutes prior to procedure. May repeat in 30 minutes if necessary, using half the dose. Maximum 1000 mg per single dose. See Warnings, Children.

Chloral Hydrate-Odan™ ℞

chloral hydrate

Sedative—Hypnotic

Odan

SUPPLIED: Each 5 mL of the clear red-orange flavored syrup contains: 500 mg of chloral hydrate USP. Nonmedicinal ingredients: citric acid, D&C Yellow #10, FD&C Red #40, glycerin, methylparaben, orange flavor, propylene glycol, purified water, sodium benzoate, sodium citrate, sodium hydroxide and sucrose. Plastic white opaque bottles of 500 mL. Store in a tight, light-resistant container preferably between 15 and 30°C. Protect from freezing.

Chloramphenicol ℞

Antibiotic

CPhA Monograph

Date of Revision: May 2009

> This monograph has been compiled by CPhA and reviewed by experts. It may contain information different from that found in Health Canada-approved Product Monographs. The reader is referred to the *CPS* Editorial Policy for more information.

SUMMARY PRODUCT INFORMATION:

Drug	Route of Administration	Dosage Form	Strength
Chloramphenicol Sodium Succinate	Injectable	Powder	1 g/vial
Chloramphenicol	Topical	Ophthalmic Solution	0.25%, 0.5%
		Ophthalmic Ointment	1%
Chloramphenicol/ Hydrocortisone Acetate	Topical	Ophthalmic/Otic Solution	chloramphenicol 0.2% plus hydrocortisone acetate 1%
		Ophthalmic/Otic Ointment	chloramphenicol 1% plus hydrocortisone acetate 1%

PHARMACOLOGY: Chloramphenicol, which was originally isolated from *Streptomyces venezuelae* and is now synthetically produced, exerts mainly a bacteriostatic effect on a wide range of gram-positive and gram-negative organisms and is active against Rickettsia, Chlamydia and Mycoplasma. It is bactericidal against *H. influenzae*, *S. pneumoniae* and *N. meningitidis* and is also very active against *S. typhi*. The sodium succinate ester is inactive until hydrolyzed to free chloramphenicol which occurs rapidly in vivo. The mechanism of action of chloramphenicol is through inhibition of protein synthesis by binding to the 50S ribosomal subunit. There is some evidence that chloramphenicol inhibits protein synthesis in rapidly proliferating mammalian cells. This may be the cause of reversible bone marrow depression but does not seem related to the development of idiopathic aplastic anemia (see Adverse Effects). Both natural and acquired resistance to chloramphenicol has been seen in strains of *P. aeruginosa*, Staphylococcus and Enterobacteriaceae, particularly Shigella, Salmonella and Escherichia. Bacteria may become resistant by becoming impermeable to chloramphenicol, or by producing an enzyme that inactivates it by adding an acetyl group. The latter mechanism is plasmid-mediated, and may be associated with resistance to other antibiotics.

Pharmacokinetics: Chloramphenicol sodium succinate is hydrolyzed to free chloramphenicol following iv administration, presumably by esterases in the liver, kidneys and lungs. The rate and extent of hydrolysis and renal elimination of the succinate ester are subject to a high degree of interindividual variation; however, an average of 30% is eliminated by the kidney as unchanged ester.

Chloramphenicol is approximately 60% bound to serum proteins and is widely distributed in the body, including the CSF. Plasma protein binding is significantly lower in premature infants and patients with severe liver dysfunction, resulting in a higher proportion of free drug in serum. These individuals may therefore have a lower therapeutic range than the general population.

CSF concentrations range from 21 to 50% of serum concentrations with uninflamed meninges and 45 to 89% of serum concentrations with inflamed meninges. Chloramphenicol crosses the placenta and is distributed into breast milk.

Chloramphenicol is metabolized in the liver, mainly by conjugation with glucuronic acid; only about 5 to 15% of an oral dose is excreted unchanged in the urine. The half-life of chloramphenicol is 1.5 to 4 hours in adults with normal renal and hepatic function. The plasma half-life is increased in patients with markedly reduced hepatic function. In patients with impaired renal function, the half-life of chloramphenicol itself is not significantly altered although the half-life of the inactive metabolites may be prolonged. Following iv administration, patients with renal impairment may achieve higher chloramphenicol concentrations due to decreased renal excretion of the succinate ester.

Since the processes for glucuronide conjugation and renal excretion in neonates may be immature, the half-life of the drug in neonates less than 3 days old may be in excess of 24 hours and about 10 hours for infants 10 to 16 days old. The dosage and administration interval should be adjusted using measured serum concentrations.

Plasma concentrations of chloramphenicol are not affected by peritoneal dialysis and only small amounts of the drug are removed by hemodialysis.

INDICATIONS: The use of chloramphenicol should be reserved for the treatment of serious infections caused by susceptible organisms when less toxic antimicrobials are ineffective or contraindicated.

Chloramphenicol is used as an alternative to first-line agents in the acute treatment of typhoid fever caused by *S. typhi*, as well as invasive salmonellosis. It should not be used to eliminate the carrier state.

Chloramphenicol has been used for the treatment of bacterial meningitis caused by susceptible strains of *H. influenzae*, *S. pneumoniae* and *N. meningitidis* when standard therapy is ineffective or contraindicated. Chloramphenicol should **not** be used to treat meningitis caused by *S. pneumoniae* unless the causative strain is known to have a chloramphenicol minimum bactericidal concentration of 4 μg/mL or less. Chloramphenicol is also used to treat brain abscesses caused by *B. fragilis* or other susceptible organisms.

Chloramphenicol is used as an alternative agent in the treatment of rickettsial infections, such as typhus or Rocky Mountain spotted fever, when tetracyclines cannot be given. It can also be used to treat severe *H. influenzae* infections other than meningitis, e.g., epiglottitis.

Chloramphenicol can be used as an alternative agent in the treatment of infections caused by Actinomyces, Bacteroides, Brucella and Burkholderia spp. In vitro testing suggests vancomycin-resistant enterococci may be susceptible to chloramphenicol but in vivo efficacy has not been established.

Chloramphenicol can be used as an alternative agent in the treatment of the following agents of bioterrorism: anthrax, plague and tularemia.

Chloramphenicol may be used locally in the treatment of superficial infections of the eye or external ear, caused by susceptible organisms, when less potentially toxic topical agents are not appropriate.

CONTRAINDICATIONS: Chloramphenicol is contraindicated in individuals with a history of previous hypersensitivity or toxic reaction to it.

WARNINGS: Serious and sometimes fatal reactions have occurred in patients taking chloramphenicol, even during short-term systemic therapy and possibly after long-term local application. These include blood dyscrasias such as aplastic anemia, hypoplastic anemia, thrombocytopenia and granulocytopenia. Two forms of bone marrow suppression are known to occur; a rare idiosyncratic, non-dose-related, irreversible reaction (aplastic anemia) with a high mortality rate (>50%) and a common, dose-related, reversible type. While hematologic studies may detect early peripheral blood changes, they are not useful in predicting irreversible bone marrow depression which precedes the development of aplastic anemia. Most cases of aplastic anemia have occurred weeks or months after completion of therapy. This reaction has limited its usefulness as an antimicrobial agent in current therapies.

A severe and potentially fatal reaction known as the gray baby syndrome has occurred in premature and newborn infants receiving large doses of chloramphenicol. Most commonly, chloramphenicol therapy had been initiated in the first 48 hours after birth; however, it has occurred in children as old as 2 years and in infants born to mothers who received chloramphenicol in the final stages of labor. Symptoms include failure to feed, abdominal distention, vomiting, blue-gray skin color, hypothermia, irregular breathing and cardiovascular collapse. Death can occur within hours. The syndrome has been attributed to excessive serum concentrations of chloramphenicol due to immature hepatic and renal elimination processes. If the syndrome is detected early and chloramphenicol is stopped, the infant may recover completely.

Chloramphenicol must not be used when less toxic agents can be expected to be effective.

PRECAUTIONS: It is essential that hematologic studies be conducted prior to and every 2 days during therapy with chloramphenicol. The drug should be discontinued if reticulocytopenia, leukopenia, thrombocytopenia, anemia or other hematologic abnormalities occur (see Warnings).

Chloramphenicol has a narrow therapeutic index and ideally plasma concentrations should be monitored. Although this test is no longer readily available in most laboratories efforts should be made to procure this service. For most infections peak concentrations should be between 10 and 20 μg/mL and trough concentrations between 5 and 10 μg/mL (see Dosage). Toxicity is generally associated with levels above 40 μg/mL.

Ocular symptoms such as a bilateral decrease in visual acuity or central scotomas may herald the onset of chloramphenicol-induced optic neuritis which rarely may result in blindness. Chloramphenicol must be discontinued immediately if optic or peripheral neuritis occurs.

Natural or plasmid-mediated resistance to chloramphenicol is known to occur in strains of staphylococci, Salmonella, Shigella, *E. coli* and rarely, *H. influenzae*.

As with other antibiotics, therapy with chloramphenicol may result in the overgrowth of nonsusceptible organisms including bacteria, viruses or fungi.

Repeated courses of chloramphenicol should be avoided whenever possible.

Otic preparations should not be used in patients with a perforated tympanic membrane.

When chloramphenicol is used topically in combination with corticosteroids, the signs of suprainfection may be masked.

Concomitant therapy with other drugs that may cause bone marrow suppression should be avoided (see Precautions, Drug Interactions).

Chloramphenicol should be used with caution in patients with acute intermittent porphyria or the Mediterranean form of G-6-PD deficiency. Chloramphenicol use may precipitate hemolysis in patients with a severe deficit of G-6-PD.

Pregnant Women: Chloramphenicol readily crosses the placenta. Birth defects in humans have not been documented; however, it should be used with caution in pregnancy at term or during labour because of potential toxicity in premature or full-term infants, including gray baby syndrome (see Warnings).

Nursing Women: Chloramphenicol is excreted in human breast milk and should not be used in nursing mothers because of the possibility of adverse effects (e.g., bone marrow suppression) in the infant.

Neonates: Caution should be used in therapy of premature and full-term infants to avoid toxicity including gray baby syndrome (see Warnings). Serum drug levels should be monitored.

Drug Interactions: See Table 1 for important drug interactions. Chloramphenicol inhibits hepatic microsomal enzymes, including CYP2C9, and may interfere with the metabolism of chlorpropamide, phenobarbital, phenytoin, tacrolimus, tolbutamide, warfarin or other drugs metabolized by the microsomal system. Dosages of these drugs may need to be adjusted accordingly. Conversely, drugs such as rifampin or phenobarbital which induce microsomal enzymes may increase the metabolism and reduce serum concentrations of chloramphenicol.

Table 1: Chloramphenicol

Drug-Drug Interactions

Interacting Drug	Effect	Clinical Comment
Anemia therapy (folic acid, iron salts, vitamin B_{12})	Delayed or reduced response to these agents due to impairment of hematopoiesis. May result in increased levels of serum iron by inhibition of heme synthesis.	If avoidance of chloramphenicol is not possible monitor response to anemia therapy and iron levels.
Antibacterials (aminoglycosides, cephalosporins, penicillins)	Possible antagonism of these agents by chloramphenicol.	Reports are conflicting and combinations of these agents have been used successfully. It would be prudent to avoid when possible, particularly for infections requiring bactericidal activity such as meningitis.

(cont'd)

Table 1: Chloramphenicol *(cont'd)*

Drug-Drug Interactions

Interacting Drug	Effect	Clinical Comment
Anticoagulants	↑ anticoagulant effect by inhibiting the hepatic metabolism of the anticoagulant or by interfering with vitamin K production by intestinal bacteria.	Monitor INR.
Barbiturates	↑ barbiturate levels ↓ chloramphenicol levels	Monitor for toxicity of barbiturate and serum levels of chloramphenicol.
Hydantoins	↑ hydantoin levels ↓ chloramphenicol serum levels	Monitor serum levels of both drugs.
Rifampin	↓ chloramphenicol serum levels	Monitor chloramphenicol serum levels and adjust dosage accordingly.
Sulfonylureas	↓ metabolism of sulfonylureas resulting in ↑ serum levels and potential hypoglycemia.	Monitor blood glucose levels.
Myelosuppressive drugs and radiation	Additive bone marrow suppression.	Avoid combination.

ADVERSE EFFECTS: Central Nervous System: Headache, mild depression, mental confusion and delirium have been described in patients receiving chloramphenicol.

Optic and peripheral neuritis have been reported, usually following long-term therapy. If this occurs, the drug should be promptly discontinued.

Gastrointestinal: nausea, vomiting and diarrhea. Following oral administration, disturbances of the oral and intestinal flora may cause stomatitis, glossitis and enterocolitis. An unpleasant taste has been reported following rapid iv administration. Jaundice has been reported rarely.

Gray Baby Syndrome: A toxic reaction which can occur in premature and newborn infants receiving large doses of chloramphenicol. It is characterized by abdominal distention, vomiting, blue-gray skin color, hypothermia, irregular breathing and cardiovascular collapse, followed by death in a few hours or days. If chloramphenicol is stopped early after the onset of symptoms, the infant may recover completely (see Warnings and Precautions).

Hematologic: Serious and sometimes fatal blood dyscrasias including aplastic anemia, hypoplastic anemia, thrombocytopenia and granulocytopenia have occurred during systemic or topical therapy with chloramphenicol. Two types of bone marrow suppression may occur. One is dose-related and generally reversible, tending to occur when serum levels exceed 25 µg/mL or with an adult dose above 4 g daily. Aplastic anemia, however, is an irreversible, idiosyncratic reaction occurring in approximately 1 in 25 000 to 40 000 patients treated and is not related to dose or duration of therapy. The onset of aplastic anemia may not occur until weeks or months following the discontinuation of chloramphenicol. See Warnings and Precautions.

Hypersensitivity: Fever, macular and vesicular rashes, angioedema and urticaria may occur, especially after topical use. Jarisch-Herxheimer reactions (JHR) have been reported in patients taking chloramphenicol. The reaction starts 2 to 6 hours after exposure to antimicrobial therapy and generally resolves within 16 to 24 hours. Patients may initially experience fever (≥38°C) with chills. Diaphoresis may occur. Other common symptoms include myalgias, increased heart rate and respiratory rate, headache, malaise and hypotension. Treatment of JHR is supportive and includes fluid resuscitation and administration of antipyretics. JHR should not be mistaken for an allergic reaction to chloramphenicol.

Local: Transient burning or stinging may occur upon instillation of ophthalmic preparations. Hypersensitivity or inflammatory reactions have been reported rarely. Bone marrow hypoplasia has also occurred rarely following local use of chloramphenicol.

OVERDOSE:

Symptoms: Nausea and vomiting may occur, particularly after oral ingestion. Metabolic acidosis may occur after acute or chronic ingestion and may precede the onset of hypotension, hypothermia and abdominal distention. Infrequently, acute overdose may lead to sudden cardiovascular collapse. Sustained high serum levels may be associated with many other adverse effects (see Warnings, Precautions and Adverse Effects).

Treatment: In cases of recent oral ingestion, induction of emesis or administration of activated charcoal with or without a cathartic may be indicated in certain cases. Charcoal hemoperfusion may be helpful in removing chloramphenicol from circulation.

For management of a suspected drug overdose, CPhA recommends that you contact your **regional Poison Control Centre.** See the *CPS* Directory section for a list of Poison Control Centres.

DOSAGE: When given iv direct, chloramphenicol should be administered as a 10 g/100 mL solution over at least 1 minute. Alternatively, it may be given as an iv infusion at a concentration of ≤20 mg/mL over 10–30 minutes. Oral preparations of chloramphenicol are no longer available. The iv solution chloramphenicol sodium succinate can be given orally. The bitter taste can be masked by first dissolving the iv solution in water, then diluting in milk.

Chloramphenicol has a narrow therapeutic index and ideally plasma concentrations should be monitored. For most infections peak concentrations should be between 10 and 20 µg/mL and trough concentrations between 5 and 10 µg/mL. For meningitis, peak and trough concentrations should be maintained between 15 and 25 µg/mL and 5 and 15 µg/mL, respectively. Serum samples should be drawn 0.5 to 1.5 hours after completion of iv administration for peak serum levels.

Oral and IV: Adults: 50 mg/kg/day in divided doses at 6-hour intervals. Patients with infections due to moderately resistant organisms or CNS infections may require higher doses of up to 100 mg/kg/day to achieve therapeutic serum or CSF levels, but the dose should be decreased as soon as possible to 50 mg/kg daily. Maximum daily dose is 4 g. Adults with impairment of hepatic or renal function may have reduced ability to metabolize and excrete the drug. In instances of impaired metabolic processes, dosages should be adjusted appropriately (see Precautions).

Children and infants over 4 weeks of age: Dosage of 50 mg/kg/day divided at 6-hour intervals is effective against most susceptible organisms. Severe infections (e.g., septicemia or meningitis): up to 100 mg/kg/day divided at 6-hour intervals. Dose should be decreased as soon as possible to 50 mg/kg daily. Maximum daily dose is 4 g.

Children with impaired hepatic or renal function require dosage adjustment based on serum chloramphenicol levels when possible (see Precautions).

Dose in Neonates: See Table 2.

Table 2: Chloramphenicol

Dose in Neonates

Indication	Age, Weight	Dose	Clinical Comment
Serious infections when less toxic antimicrobials are ineffective or contraindicated	≤7 days	25 mg/kg daily Q24H	**Appropriate dosing is extremely important in neonates with immature metabolic processes as severe toxicity such as gray baby syndrome may occur. Serum concentration monitoring is particularly important in this age group and should be performed whenever possible (see Warnings and Precautions)**
	>7 days, ≤2 kg	25 mg/kg daily Q24H	
	>7 days, >2 kg	50 mg/kg daily Q12H	

IM administration is controversial and generally should not be used, because studies have reported varying serum levels.

Local: Ophthalmic: Preparations (e.g., a thin strip of ointment approximately 1 cm long or 1 drop of solution) may be applied in the conjunctival sac every 3 hours for the first 48 hours, at which time the dosing interval may be increased.

Otic: Instil 2 or 3 drops into the ear canal every 6 to 8 hours.

Chlordiazepoxide

CPhA Monograph

see *Benzodiazepines*

Chloroquine

Antimalarial—Antiparasitic

CPhA Monograph

Date of Preparation: November 2003

Date of Revision: October 2006

This monograph has been compiled by CPhA and reviewed by experts. It may contain information different from that found in Health Canada-approved Product Monographs. The reader is referred to the *CPS* Editorial Policy for more information.

SUMMARY PRODUCT INFORMATION:

Route of Administration	Dosage Form	Product Strength
Oral	Tablet	250 mg (150 mg base)

INDICATIONS AND CLINICAL USE: Chloroquine is indicated for the prevention and treatment of malaria caused by susceptible strains of *P. malariae*, *P. ovale*, *P. falciparum* or *P. vivax*. Chloroquine must be combined with primaquine for the treatment of malaria caused by *P. vivax* or *P. ovale*.

Chloroquine is also used in the treatment of extraintestinal amebiasis. Unapproved uses include treatment of rheumatoid arthritis and lupus erythematosus

Pediatrics: Chloroquine has been used in children to treat and prevent malaria and to treat extraintestinal amebiasis.

CONTRAINDICATIONS: Patients who are hypersensitive to chloroquine or to other 4-aminoquinoline compounds or to any ingredient in the formulation or component of the container. Retinal or visual field changes attributable to 4-aminoquinoline compounds or to any other etiology. Chloroquine may be used in these patients for the treatment of acute attacks of malaria caused by susceptible strains of plasmodia if the benefits outweigh the risks.

WARNINGS AND PRECAUTIONS: General: Patients on long-term chloroquine therapy should be examined periodically for muscle weakness (including knee and ankle reflex tests). If there is evidence of muscle weakness, chloroquine should be discontinued. Chloroquine may exacerbate porphyria in patients with the condition.

Hematologic: A complete blood count should be checked periodically while on long-term chloroquine therapy. If any adverse hematologic effects are detected, chloroquine should be discontinued. Chloroquine should be used with caution in patients with glucose-6-phosphate dehydrogenase (G-6-PD) deficiency since hemolysis and acute renal failure have occurred in these patients receiving chloroquine.

Hepatic/Biliary/Pancreatic: Since chloroquine may concentrate in the liver, it should be used with caution in conjunction with other hepatotoxic drugs or in patients with hepatic disease or alcoholism

Ophthalmologic: Dose-related, irreversible retinal damage has been associated with long-term or high-dose chloroquine therapy. If chloroquine is to be used long term, ophthalmologic examinations (including visual acuity, expert slit lamp, funduscopic and visual field tests) should be performed at baseline and periodically during therapy. If there are any abnormalities, discontinue chloroquine immediately and observe the patient for possible progression.

Skin: Chloroquine may exacerbate psoriasis in patients with the disease.

Special Populations: Pregnant Women: Birth defects have not been associated with the use of chloroquine in pregnancy. Therapeutic use is not known to convey a significant risk of ocular toxicity to the infant. Chloroquine should only be used in pregnancy when the benefit outweighs the risk.

Nursing Women: Chloroquine is excreted in breast milk, however the amount is not considered to be harmful to a nursing infant. The American Academy of Pediatrics considers chloroquine to be compatible with breastfeeding. Chloroquine should be used with caution in infants with G-6-PD deficiency.

Pediatrics: Since chloroquine overdoses are often fatal, extreme care should be taken when administrating doses to children. Chloroquine should be kept out of reach of children.

DRUG INTERACTIONS: See Table 1.

Table 1: Chloroquine

Drug-Drug Interactions

Interacting Drug	Reference	Effect	Clinical Comment
Aluminum and Magnesium Salts	CT	↓ absorption of chloroquine	Separate doses of antacids and chloroquine by 4 hours
Chlorpromazine	CT	chloroquine may ↑ chlorpromazine concentrations	Monitor patient for increased neuroleptic effects
Cimetidine	CT	cimetidine may ↓ metabolism of chloroquine	May need to lower chloroquine dose when administered with cimetidine
Cyclosporine	C	chloroquine may ↑ cyclosporine concentrations	Monitor cyclosporine levels
Hepatotoxic Agents		See Warnings and Precautions	
Methotrexate	CT	chloroquine may ↓ the efficacy of methotrexate	Monitor patient for loss of efficacy
Penicillamine	CT	chloroquine may ↑ the effect of penicillamine	No special precautions appear necessary

Legend:
C=case study.
CT=clinical trial.
T=theoretical.

ACTION AND CLINICAL PHARMACOLOGY: The precise mechanism of action of chloroquine is unknown. The antimalarial effect may involve chloroquine binding to DNA, interfering with protein synthesis or inhibition of DNA and RNA polymerase. Chloroquine is active against the erythrocytic stages of plasmodium strains. The mechanism of action of chloroquine in the treatment of extraintestinal amebiasis, rheumatoid arthritis and lupus erythematosus is unknown.

Pharmacokinetics: See Table 2.

Table 2: Chloroquine

Summary of Pharmacokinetic Parameters in Adults

	$t_{1/2}$ (h)	Clearance	Volume of Distribution
Single Dose Mean	72–120	0.35 L/kg/h	116–285 L/kg

Absorption: Chloroquine tablets are absorbed rapidly and almost completely with a bioavailability of 89%. The time to peak concentration is 1-2 hours.
Distribution: Chloroquine is extensively distributed into body tissues (i.e., eyes, heart, kidneys, liver, lungs) with an apparent volume of distribution of 116-285 L/kg. Chloroquine is moderately bound to protein (50-65%).
Metabolism: Chloroquine is partially metabolized by the liver. The major metabolite is desethylchloroquine which is active. Chloroquine inhibits CYP2D6.
Excretion: 70% of chloroquine is excreted unchanged in the urine.

ADVERSE REACTIONS: Adverse Drug Reaction Overview: See Table 3.

Table 3: Chloroquine

Common Adverse Drug Reactions

Body System	Incidence
Gastrointestinal	
Nausea	>1%
Diarrhea	>1%

Less Common Adverse Drug Reactions: Cardiovascular: EKG changes, hypotension.
Gastrointestinal: anorexia, vomiting.
Hematologic: blood dyscrasias.
Ophthalmologic: blurred vision, retinopathy.
Miscellaneous: fatigue, personality changes, hair bleaching, stomatitis.

DOSAGE AND ADMINISTRATION: Adults: See Table 4.

Table 4: Chloroquine

Dose in Adult Patients

Indication	Initial Dose	Usual Dose	Duration of Treatment	Detailed Information
Malaria Prophylaxis	500 mg (300 mg base) weekly	500 mg (300 mg base) weekly	1–2 weeks prior to exposure and continued for 4 weeks after leaving the endemic area	Use a loading dose of 1000 mg if chloroquine is not initiated 2 weeks prior to exposure.
Malaria Treatment	1000 mg followed by 500 mg after 6–8 hours (day 1)	500 mg daily (day 2 and 3)	3 days	1000 mg followed by an additional 500 mg dose given 6, 24 and 48 hours after.
Extraintestinal Amebiasis	1000 mg daily for 2 days	500 mg daily	2–3 weeks	Administer in conjunction with an intestinal amebicide.
Rheumatoid Arthritis	250 mg daily	250 mg daily		Use the lowest effective dose. A response to chloroquine therapy may not occur for 4–6 weeks.
Lupus Erythematosus	250 mg daily	250 mg daily		Use in conjunction with topical steroids. When systemic and local manifestations subside, gradually taper chloroquine and discontinue.

Pediatrics: See Table 5.

Table 5: Chlroroquine

Dose in Pediatric Patients

Indication	Initial Dose	Usual Dose	Maximum Dose	Duration of Treatment	Detailed Information
Malaria Prophylaxis	8.3 mg/kg (5 mg/kg base) weekly	8.3 mg/kg (5 mg/kg base) weekly	Do not exceed adult dose	1–2 weeks prior to exposure and continued for 4 weeks after leaving the endemic area	Give 16.7 mg/kg (10 mg/kg base) in 2 divided doses 6 hours apart prior to initiating usual dose if chloroquine is not initiated 2 weeks prior to exposure.
Malaria Treatment	16.7 mg/kg (10 mg/kg base)	8.3 mg/kg (5 mg/kg base)	Do not exceed adult dose	2 days	16.7 mg/kg (10 mg/kg base) initially followed by 8.3 mg/kg (5 mg/kg base) given 6, 24 and 48 hours after.
Extraintestinal Amebiasis	16.7 mg/kg (10 mg/kg base) daily	16.7 mg/kg (10 mg/kg base) daily	Do not exceed adult dose	2–3 weeks	Administer in conjuction with an intestinal amebicide.

Renal Impairment: See Table 6.

Table 6: Chloroquine

Dose in Adult Patients with Renal Impairment

Indication	Route	Creatinine Clearance	Dose Adjustment
Malaria Treatment	Oral	>10 mL/min	no adjustment
		<10 mL/min	decrease dose by 50%

Hepatic Impairment: Since chloroquine may concentrate in the liver, it should be used with caution in patients with hepatic disease.
Missed Dose: If chloroquine is taken weekly, the missed dose should be taken as soon as the patient remembers. Wait 7 days before taking the next dose. If chloroquine is taken daily, the missed dose should be take as soon as the patient remembers. If it is almost time for the next dose, the missed dose should not be taken and the patient should return to the regular dosage schedule.
Administration: Oral: Chloroquine can be given with food to minimize GI adverse effects. Take at the same time and day every week. Tablets may be crushed and mixed with a flavoured vehicle.

OVERDOSE:
Signs and Symptoms: Chloroquine overdose is extremely toxic and symptoms often develop within minutes. Apnea, hypotension, respiratory and cardiovascular compromise can be precipitous. CNS involvement includes decreased level of consciousness, seizures and coma.
Recommended Management: It is recommended that a Poison Control Centre be contacted to obtain expert advice on the management of chloroquine overdose.

Early and aggressive management of chloroquine overdose substantially reduces mortality rates. Closely observe ECG, serum potassium, arterial blood gases and vital signs, especially for hypotension. For hypotension unresponsive to iv fluids, epinephrine iv infusion should be started at a dose of 0.25 µg/kg/min and titrated until a systolic blood pressure over 100 mm Hg is achieved. Diazepam, 2 mg/kg iv infused over 30 minutes, may be used to decrease the cardiotoxicity of chloroquine and to control seizures. A single dose of activated charcoal should be considered at a dose of 1 g/kg for patients who present within 2 hours of ingestion. Chloroquine is not removed by hemodialysis, peritoneal dialysis or charcoal hemoperfusion.

For management of a suspected drug overdose, CPhA recommends that you contact your **regional Poison Control Centre**. See the *CPS* Directory section for a list of Poison Control Centres.

Chlorpheniramine
Antihistamine

CPhA Monograph

Date of Preparation: October 2007
Date of Revision: November 2008

This monograph has been compiled by CPhA and reviewed by experts. It may contain information different from that found in Health Canada-approved Product Monographs. The reader is referred to the *CPS* Editorial Policy for more information.

SUMMARY PRODUCT INFORMATION:

Route of Administration	Dosage Form	Strength
Oral[a]	Tablet, immediate release	4 mg
	Tablet, long-acting[a]	12 mg

[a] Also available in combination products.

INDICATIONS AND CLINICAL USE: Chlorpheniramine is used in adults and children ≥6 years for the symptomatic relief of allergic states such as allergic rhinitis, acute and chronic urticaria and atopic and contact dermatitis. Patients with pruritus from insect bites, neurodermatitis, pruritus ani or vulvae, or patients with generalized pruritus may derive benefit from chlorpheniramine therapy. It can also be used in the management of exanthematous eruptions seen in measles and chickenpox.

Chlorpheniramine has also been used in the management of chronic upper airway cough syndrome (previously referred to as postnasal drip syndrome).
Geriatrics: Chlorpheniramine use should be avoided in elderly patients because of their increased susceptibility to anticholinergic adverse effects such as drowsiness, dry mouth and urinary retention (see Adverse Reactions).
Pediatrics: Caution is advised in young children as paradoxical excitement has been reported. Safety and effectiveness of chlorpheniramine in children <6 years has not been established. A Centers for Disease Control report attributed the cause of death in 3 infants to overdose of cough and cold medications [*MMWR Morb Mortal Wkly Rep* 2007;56(1):1-4]. A Cochrane systematic review concluded that over-the-counter cough and cold medications were not more effective than placebo in reducing acute cough due to upper respiratory tract infection in children [*Cochrane Database Syst Rev* 2008;(1):CD001831]. A critical review of clinical trials between 1950 and 1991 concluded that over-the-counter cough and cold medications did not improve symptoms of upper respiratory tract infection [*JAMA* 1993;269(17):2258-63].

CONTRAINDICATIONS:
- Patients who are hypersensitive to chlorpheniramine or to any ingredient in the formulation or component of the container.
- Newborn or premature infants.
- Patients receiving monamine oxidase inhibitor therapy.

WARNINGS AND PRECAUTIONS: Cardiovascular: Use with caution in patients with a history of cardiovascular disease due to chlorpheniramine's ability to cause tachycardia and hypotension.
Gastrointestinal: Chlorpheniramine can reduce gastrointestinal motility. Use caution in patients with GI obstruction such as stenosing peptic ulcer and pyloroduodenal obstruction.
Genitourinary: Urinary retention is an adverse effect of chlorpheniramine. Use caution in patients with urinary obstruction due to prostatic hyperplasia or bladder neck obstruction.
Neurologic: Reports of convulsions have been documented in patients with seizure disorders who used chlorpheniramine.
Ophthalmologic: Patients with angle-closure glaucoma should avoid using drugs with anticholinergic effects, including chlorpheniramine, due to its ability to increase intraocular pressure.
Respiratory: Patients with chronic lung disease including asthma or COPD should use chlorpheniramine under the supervision of a physician.
Special Populations: Pregnant Women: Pregnancy Category B: There is no evidence that exposure to chlorpheniramine during 1st trimester of pregnancy increases the risk of congenital defects above the baseline risk. Although there are reports of association between in utero exposure to first-generation antihistamines during the last 2 weeks of pregnancy and retrolental fibroplasias in premature infants, chlorpheniramine is recommended as a drug of choice in the management of allergic disease in pregnancy. If used during pregnancy, the lowest effective dose should be used for the shortest duration.
Nursing Women: Chlorpheniramine is distributed in breast milk but does not appear to have any serious and harmful effects to children during breast-feeding. The lowest effective dose should be used for the shortest duration. Larger doses or prolonged duration of treatment may cause irritability and drowsiness in the infants. Use chlorpheniramine at bedtime after the last feeding of the day as this may minimize symptoms in the infant, or offer a nonsedating antihistamine that is compatible with breast-feeding as an alternative.
Pediatrics: Avoid chlorpheniramine in premature and newborn infants (see Contraindications). Evidence to support the use of first-generation antihistamines in cough and cold products in children younger than 6 years of age is lacking. There are rare reports of serious adverse events associated with the misuse of these products in this age group.
Geriatrics: The elderly may be more susceptible to adverse effects of chlorpheniramine such as dizziness, sedation, anticholinergic effects and hypotension. Chlorpheniramine and other first-generation antihistamines should be avoided in elderly patients.

ADVERSE REACTIONS: Adverse Drug Reactions Overview: Up to 50% of patients taking chlorpheniramine may experience dose-related adverse effects of which CNS and anticholinergic effects (drowsiness, dizziness, dry mouth, blurred vision, vaginal dryness and difficulty urinating) are the most prominent. Elderly patients are more susceptible to these effects. Serious toxicity has been reported with chlorpheniramine but appears to be rare.

More Common Adverse Drug Reactions (≥1%): See Table 1.

Table 1: Chlorpheniramine
More Common Adverse Drug Reactions

Body System	Effect	Clinical Comment
Cardiovascular/ CNS	Common: sedation, dizziness, fatigue Rare: CNS stimulation (insomnia, irritability, restlessness, tremor, nightmares, hallucination, convulsions)	Patients with focal cerebral cortical lesions are at increased risk of CNS stimulation. Sedation may be minimized with gradual dosing; avoid driving, piloting airplanes or boats or operating heavy machinery. To avoid daytime drowsiness, can take chlorpheniramine before bed and not in the middle of the night.
Ear/Nose/Throat	Dry mouth	
Gastrointestinal	Loss of appetite, nausea, vomiting, epigastric distress, constipation or diarrhea	
Genitourinary	Urinary retention, urinary frequency, dysuria, impotence	
Neurologic	Lack of coordination	
Ophthalmologic	↑ intraocular pressure	See Warnings and Precautions.

Less Common Adverse Drug Reactions (<1%): Cardiovascular: extrasystole.
Central Nervous System: confusion, dyskinesias, headaches, nervousness.
Allergic/Dermatologic: allergic dermatitis, photosensitization.
Ear/Nose/Throat: tinnitus.
Endocrine and Metabolism: increased appetite, weight gain.
Hematologic: thrombocytopenia, leucopenia, agranulocytosis and hemolytic anemia have been reported rarely.

DRUG INTERACTIONS: Overview: Any drugs that cause CNS depression or anticholinergic side effects should be used with caution with chlorpheniramine.

Drug-Drug Interactions: See Table 2.

Table 2: Chlorpheniramine
Drug-Drug Interactions

Interacting Drug	Effect	Clinical Comment
Alcohol and other CNS depressants, e.g., tricyclic antidepressants	Additive CNS depressive effects	Avoid combination. If used concomitantly, monitor for additive CNS depressive effects, e.g., confusion, drowsiness, respiratory depression and weakness.
CYP3A4 inhibitors, e.g., clarithromycin, erythromycin, ketoconazole	May ↑ chlorpheniramine levels	If used concomitantly, monitor for signs of ↑ chlorpheniramine levels such as sedation. Monitor for ↑ side effects with chlorpheniramine when a CYP3A4 inhibitor is added and for ↓ clinical effects when the CYP3A4 inhibitor is discontinued.
Phenytoin	↑ serum phenytoin through inhibition of phenytoin metabolism shown in one case report; additive CNS depressant effects	If used concomitantly, monitor phenytoin serum levels. Observe for signs and symptoms of phenytoin toxicity such as ataxia, nystagmus, diplopia, vomiting and tinnitus. Upon initiation or discontinuation of chlorpheniramine, monitor phenytoin serum levels. If used concomitantly, monitor for additive CNS depressant effects, e.g., confusion, drowsiness, respiratory depression and weakness.

Drug-Laboratory Interactions: Chlorpheniramine may interfere with allergy skin test antigens by masking the response via histamine antagonism. Discontinue chlorpheniramine at least two to four days prior to the skin test.

DOSAGE AND ADMINISTRATION: Dosing Considerations: Patients receiving other CNS depressants or anticholinergic drugs are more susceptible to the adverse effects of chlorpheniramine. Initiating treatment at a lower dose may reduce the likelihood of adverse effects. Chlorpheniramine should be avoided in elderly patients or used with extreme caution at the lowest effective dose. Pediatric patients under the age of 6 years may experience paradoxical excitement rather than sedation. Avoid if possible, or use with caution at the lowest effective dose.

Recommended Dose and Dosage Adjustment: Adults: See Table 3.

Table 3: Chlorpheniramine
Dose in Adult Patients

Indication	Dose	Clinical Comment
Allergic Rhinitis	Tablets, immediate-release: 4 mg po Q4–6H, max 24 mg/24 h Tablets, long-acting: 12 mg po Q12H, max 24 mg/24 h	For prevention of seasonal allergic rhinitis, can use 4 mg po QHS, then increase to 8 mg TID PRN over a 2-week period; start prior to allergy season. For the elderly, consider lower doses due to higher susceptibility to adverse reactions.
Chronic Upper Airway Cough Syndrome	4–8 mg po HS	Use in combination with a decongestant (e.g., pseudoephedrine) for cough associated with nonallergic rhinitis.

Pediatrics: See Table 4.

Table 4: Chlorpheniramine
Dose in Pediatric Patients

Indication	Dose	Clinical Comment
Allergic Rhinitis	Tablets, regular: ≥12 y: 4 mg po Q4–6H, max 24 mg/24 h; 6–11 y: 2 mg po Q4–6H, max 12 mg/24 h; 2–5 y: 1 mg po Q4–6H, max 6 mg/24 h Tablets, long-acting: ≥12 y: 12 mg po Q12H, max 24 mg/24 h	Can use 0.35 mg/kg/day in divided doses every 4–6 hours

Renal Impairment: No dose adjustment is necessary.
Hepatic Impairment: Chlorpheniramine is cleared via the liver; therefore, a dose adjustment may be necessary in patients with compromised hepatic function.

OVERDOSAGE:

> For management of a suspected drug overdose, CPhA recommends that you contact your **regional Poison Control Centre**. See the *CPS* Directory section for a list of Poison Control Centres.

ACTION AND CLINICAL PHARMACOLOGY: Mechanism of Action: Chlorpheniramine, a first-generation antihistamine, is a propylamine that belongs to the alkylamine class of antihistamines. It blocks the H_1 receptor, thereby inhibiting the action of histamine on smooth muscle cells, such as the gastrointestinal and respiratory tracts. By blocking vasodilation and reducing capilliary permeability, chlorpheniramine reduces edema and wheal formation associated with histamine release.

Pharmacokinetics: Adults: Absorption: Chlorpheniramine is rapidly absorbed from the gastrointestinal tract after oral administration. Peak concentrations of 16-71 ng/mL occurs within 2-3 hours following oral administration of the immediate-release chlorpheniramine tablets. For the extended-release formulation, peak concentrations of 16-71 ng/mL are reached within 5.7-8.1 hours (peak concentration: 17-76 ng/mL). Administration with food may delay absorption but oral bioavailability is not affected.
Distribution: In vitro, 69-72% of chlorpheniramine is bound to plasma proteins. Apparent steady-state volume of distribution in adults is 2.5-3.2 L/kg following iv administration of chlorpheniramine and 3.8 L/kg in children.
Metabolism: Chlorpheniramine undergoes extensive metabolism in the gastrointestinal mucosa as well as first-pass hepatic metabolism. Metabolites are inactive.
Excretion: Following a single oral dose of chlorpheniramine maleate, about 20% of the chlorpheniramine is eliminated via renal excretion in healthy individuals with normal renal and hepatic function. In adults with normal renal and hepatic function, the terminal elimination half-life is 24 h (range 12-43 h). In children with normal renal and hepatic function, the terminal elimination half-life averages 9.6-13.1 h.

Chlorpromazine

Antipsychotic—Antiemetic

CPhA Monograph

Date of Revision: October 2010

> This monograph has been compiled by CPhA and reviewed by experts. It may contain information different from that found in Health Canada-approved Product Monographs. The reader is referred to the *CPS* Editorial Policy for more information.

SUMMARY PRODUCT INFORMATION:

Route of Administration	Dosage Form	Strength
Oral	Tablet	25 mg, 50 mg, 100 mg
IM, IV	Injectable solution	25 mg/mL

PHARMACOLOGY: Chlorpromazine is a low-potency aliphatic phenothiazine antipsychotic. The ability of phenothiazines to ameliorate the positive symptoms of psychotic disorders (hallucinations, delusions) is believed to be mediated by antagonism of postsynaptic dopamine D_2 receptors in the mesolimbic tract. Relief of nausea may involve antagonism of D_2, histamine H_1 and muscarine M_1 receptors. Extrapyramidal side effects and hyperprolactinemia have been attributed to antagonism of postsynaptic D_2 receptors in the nigrostriatal and tuberoinfundibular dopaminergic tracts, respectively.

Chlorpromazine also demonstrates moderate to high affinity for H_1 receptors (may result in sedation, weight gain), alpha$_1$ adrenergic receptors (orthostatic hypotension, reflex tachycardia) and M_1 receptors (anticholinergic side effects).

Pharmacokinetics: Chlorpromazine is readily absorbed from the gastrointestinal tract; however, its bioavailability is variable due to considerable first-pass metabolism by the liver. Liquid concentrates may have greater bioavailability than tablets. Food does not appear to affect bioavailability consistently. IM administration bypasses much of the first-pass effect and higher plasma concentrations are achieved. The onset of action after im administration is usually 15 to 30 minutes and after oral administration 30 to 60 minutes.

Chlorpromazine is highly bound to plasma proteins (>90%), principally albumin. It is not dialyzable. It is distributed widely throughout the body; it crosses the blood brain barrier and the placenta and is distributed into breast milk. Volume of distribution is approximately 20 L/kg.

Chlorpromazine is metabolized extensively by the cytochrome P450 isoenzymes CYP2D6 (major pathway), CYP1A2 and CYP3A4; at least 12 different metabolites are known. Less than 1% is excreted unchanged. Most metabolites are excreted in the urine as unconjugated or conjugated compounds. The half-life of chlorpromazine is approximately 30 hours.

INDICATIONS: Health Canada-approved indications include:
- management of mania and psychotic disorders such as schizophrenia
- prevention and treatment of nausea and vomiting

Uses without Health Canada approval: Chlorpromazine has been used in the management of symptoms associated with attacks of acute intermittent porphyria such as nausea, vomiting and restlessness/anxiety, as an adjunct in the management of tetanus, and in the management of intractable hiccups.

CONTRAINDICATIONS:
- Patients who are hypersensitive to chlorpromazine or to any ingredient in the formulation or component of the container.
- Patients with:
  - severe CNS depression or coma
  - bone marrow suppression
  - blood dyscrasias
  - severe hepatic disease

WARNINGS:

> **Serious Warnings and Precautions**
> - The use of phenothiazines such as chlorpromazine has been associated with acute and chronic extrapyramidal reactions including dystonias, akathisia, parkinsonian symptoms, neuroleptic malignant syndrome (NMS) and tardive dyskinesia (TD). NMS can be life-threatening, especially when not recognized and addressed early, and TD may not resolve after drug discontinuation. See Adverse Effects.
> - The use of antipsychotic agents in elderly patients has been associated with a dose-related increase in all-cause mortality, with an inverse relationship to duration of use. The risk may be higher with first-generation or "conventional" antipsychotics compared to second-generation or "atypical" agents [*N Engl J Med* 2005;353:2335-41; *CMAJ* 2007;176(5):627-32. doi:10.1503/cmaj.061250]. The use of antipsychotics in older patients should be carefully considered, and first-generation agents should be avoided whenever possible.

PRECAUTIONS: Abrupt Withdrawal: Sudden discontinuation of antipsychotics can result in symptoms such as nausea, vomiting, diarrhea, sweating, insomnia and confusion. Psychosis and movement disorders can also be precipitated. Antipsychotics should be discontinued gradually when possible.

Anticholinergic Effects: Paralytic ileus resulting from the anticholinergic action of chlorpromazine may occur, especially in the elderly. Administer with caution in patients with angle closure glaucoma, urinary retention or prostatic hyperplasia.

Cardiovascular: Chlorpromazine may cause hypotension, particularly following parenteral use. Patients should be supine when receiving im injections and remain supine or sitting for 30 minutes afterward. Blood pressure should be measured before and after injections.

Nonspecific, usually reversible ECG changes have been reported with chlorpromazine. A small number of reports have associated chlorpromazine with QTc interval prolongation and torsades de pointes. Use chlorpromazine with caution in patients with cardiovascular disease.

CNS: See also Warnings and Adverse Effects. Chlorpromazine may lower the seizure threshold. Use the drug cautiously in patients with a history of seizures or additional risk factors such as acute alcohol withdrawal.

Dermatologic: Photosensitivity may occur. Patients should apply a broad-spectrum sunscreen prior to sunlight exposure.

Endocrine: Patients with hypocalcemia may be more susceptible to dystonic reactions (see Adverse Effects). Chlorpromazine can elevate prolactin levels and can lead to galactorrhea, amenorrhea, gynecomastia and sexual dysfunction (men and women). The correlation between prolactin levels and these adverse effects is low.

Phenothiazines affect thermoregulation. Use chlorpromazine with caution in patients who may be exposed to extreme heat or cold.

Hematologic: Blood dyscrasias including agranulocytosis have occurred in patients taking antipsychotics. These reactions are rare with phenothiazines, and most have occurred between the fourth and tenth week of treatment. Monitor patients during that time for the appearance of sore throat, fever and weakness. If these symptoms occur, discontinue the drug if STAT white blood cell and differential counts confirm a suspected hematologic reaction.

Hepatic: Chlorpromazine should be used with caution in patients who have impaired liver function or alcoholic liver disease. CNS depression may be potentiated. If bilirubinemia or icterus occurs, discontinue the drug and perform liver function tests.

Respiratory: Use cautiously in patients with respiratory difficulties as CNS depression may cause respiratory failure in these patients.

Ocular: Chlorpromazine has been associated with retinopathy, pigmentary lens deposits and cataract formation. Discontinue chlorpromazine if retinal changes are observed (see also Adverse Effects).

Occupational Hazards: Warn patients that chlorpromazine may impair their ability to safely perform activities requiring full mental alertness, such as driving or operating machinery. Potentiation of the effects of alcohol may also occur.

Drug Interactions: For drug-drug interactions, see Table 1.

Table 1: Chlorpromazine

Drug-Drug Interactions

Interacting Drug	Effect	Comment
Anticholinergic agents (e.g., antihistamines, antiparkinsonian drugs, atropine, tricyclic antidepressants)	Additive anticholinergic side effects (e.g., constipation, urinary retention, blurred vision, dry eyes, dry mouth, cognitive impairment).	Monitor for increased anticholinergic effects.
Anticonvulsants	Chlorpromazine may lower the seizure threshold. Chlorpromazine may also inhibit the metabolism of some anticonvulsants, and its metabolism may be induced by some agents such phenytoin.	Anticonvulsant therapy should be monitored closely and may require dosage adjustment.
CNS depressants	Chlorpromazine may enhance the CNS depressant effects of drugs including alcohol, anticonvulsants, antihistamines, barbiturates, benzodiazepines, MAO inhibitors, opioid analgesics and tricyclic antidepressants.	Monitor therapy to prevent or manage excessive sedation or respiratory depression.
CYP2D6 substrates (e.g., amitriptyline, atomoxetine, duloxetine, metoprolol, propranolol, tamoxifen, tamsulosin) or strong inhibitors (e.g., bupropion, fluoxetine, paroxetine, quinidine, ritonavir)	Substrates: decreased clearance of substrates due to inhibition of CYP2D6 by chlorpromazine. Strong inhibitors: decreased chlorpromazine clearance.	Avoid combination or monitor for increased effects of chlorpromazine or interacting drug and adjust dose as required.
Dopaminergic agents (e.g., bromocriptine, cabergoline, levodopa, pramipexole, ropinirole)	Chlorpromazine may antagonize the dopaminergic effects of these drugs resulting in decreased efficacy.	Avoid combination.
Drugs that prolong the QTc interval (e.g., amiodarone, clarithromycin, disopyramide, domperidone, erythromycin, indapamide, lithium, moxifloxacin, pimozide, procainamide, quetiapine, quinidine, quinine, tricyclic antidepressants, ziprasidone)	Potential additive QTc prolongation.	Avoid combination.
Lithium	Lithium may enhance the neurotoxic effects of chlorpromazine. Rare cases of severe neurotoxicity have been reported.	If lithium and chlorpromazine are used concurrently, monitor closely for signs of adverse neurologic effects, especially if serum concentrations of lithium are in the upper range.

Cigarette Smoking: Hepatic metabolism may be induced by smoking, leading to decreased plasma concentrations of chlorpromazine. Conversely, levels may increase if smoking is discontinued during chlorpromazine therapy.

Drug-Herb Interactions: Avoid concurrent use of phenothiazines with kava kava, gotu kola, valerian and St. John's wort because these herbs may increase CNS depression. Kava kava may also provide additive dopamine antagonism. Avoid dong quai because of a possible increased risk of photosensitization.

Pregnancy: Most studies have found chlorpromazine to be nonteratogenic and otherwise relatively safe for use during pregnancy, when used occasionally in low doses. Avoid using chlorpromazine near term because of the danger of maternal hypotension and possible adverse effects in the neonate (e.g., lethargy, jaundice, extrapyramidal effects).

Lactation: Phenothiazines are distributed into breast milk in small amounts. If the decision is made to use chlorpromazine during lactation, use the lowest effective dose for the shortest possible time to minimize the risk of adverse effects such as sedative and anticholinergic effects in the infant.

Geriatrics: See Warnings, Serious Warnings and Precautions. If chlorpromazine is used in elderly patients, use reduced dosages; elderly patients are more susceptible to the therapeutic and adverse effects of phenothiazines, particularly postural hypotension, cognitive impairment, extrapyramidal effects and anticholinergic effects such as constipation, urinary retention and blurred vision.

Children: Children with acute illnesses such as viral infections, CNS infections or dehydration may be more susceptible to dystonic reactions to phenothiazines.

ADVERSE EFFECTS: Adverse effects with different phenothiazines vary in type, frequency and mechanism; some are dose related, while others involve individual patient sensitivity.

In general, members of the aliphatic group of phenothiazines have strong sedative, hypotensive and anticholinergic properties and mild to moderate extrapyramidal effects. More common adverse effects (incidence ≥2 %) are described in Table 2.

Table 2: Chlorpromazine

More Common Adverse Effects (≥2%)

Body System	Effect	Comment
Autonomic Nervous System	Anticholinergic effects such as dry mouth, dry eyes, blurred vision, constipation, urinary retention (particularly problematic for men with benign prostatic hyperplasia)	Anticholinergic effects may improve spontaneously with continued therapy. Treatment options include reducing dose of chlorpromazine or switching to an antipsychotic with less propensity to cause anticholinergic effects.
	Syncope, impaired temperature regulation	
Central Nervous System	Sedation, memory impairment, confusion, delirium	Dose-related; elderly patients more susceptible.
	Acute onset extrapyramidal effects such as parkinsonism, akathisia, dystonic reactions	Less common with low-potency antipsychotics such as chlorpromazine; use lowest effective dose for shortest possible time and regularly re-evaluate need for continued therapy. Management options include dosage reduction, switching to a 2nd generation antipsychotic, medications such as benzodiazepines (akathisia), anticholinergic agents (dystonia, parkinsonism) or beta-blockers (akathisia).
	Late onset movement disorders such as tardive dyskinesia (TD), characterized by rhythmical involuntary movements of the tongue, face, mouth or jaw (e.g., protrusion of the tongue, puffing of the cheeks, puckering of the mouth and chewing movements)	There is no evidence-based drug treatment for this syndrome. Management includes discontinuing the antipsychotic, switching to a 2nd generation agent. Fine vermicular movements of the tongue may be an early sign of TD and discontinuing the drug when this occurs might prevent full onset of the syndrome.
Cardiovascular	Hypotension, tachycardia, ECG changes (e.g., QTc prolongation)	Hypotension more common with low-potency agents; older patients more susceptible.
Dermatologic	Photosensitivity, photoallergic reactions	Recommend use of sunscreen.
Endocrine	Weight gain, dysglycemia, hyperlipidemia, hyperprolactinemia (manifestations can include galactorrhea, gynecomastia, amenorrhea, sexual dysfunction)	Encourage healthy diet and lifestyle to minimize cardiovascular risk factors; hyperprolactinemic symptoms may respond to dosage reduction.
Ocular	Lenticular pigmentation	May manifest as glare or halo around lights; associated with long-term therapy.
	Retinitis pigmentosa, cataracts	Reduced vision and blindness can occur; periodic eye examination recommended.
	Pigmentation of cornea, conjunctiva, sclera, eyelids (slate-blue color)	Associated with long-term therapy; may be irreversible.
Genitourinary	Sexual dysfunction including anorgasmia, ejaculatory dysfunction, erectile dysfunction	May remit with continued therapy; dosage reduction may be helpful.

Less Common Adverse Effects (<2%): Central Nervous System: Neuroleptic Malignant Syndrome (NMS): This rare but potentially fatal syndrome characterized by muscle rigidity, fever/hyperthermia, labile blood pressure and fluctuating levels of consciousness, can occur in patients taking chlorpromazine and other antipsychotics. NMS appears to occur more commonly in young males. Dehydration is an additional risk factor. Patients need to be aware of the importance of adequate hydration, particularly in situations involving environmental exposure to extreme heat.

Hematologic: agranulocytosis, leukopenia, granulocytopenia, eosinophilia, thrombocytopenia, anemia, aplastic anemia, pancytopenia. Agranulocytosis occurs in fewer than 0.01% of patients receiving chlorpromazine. See also Precautions.

Hepatic: cholestatic jaundice; symptoms generally subside following discontinuation of the drug but cholestasis may be prolonged.

OVERDOSAGE:

Symptoms: Symptoms of chlorpromazine overdose are an extension of its pharmacologic actions. The primary symptoms observed are extrapyramidal reactions, hypotension and sedation. Mild or early intoxication may appear as restlessness and confusion, which may progress to coma. Altered temperature regulation can occur; both hypothermia and hyperthermia have been reported. Neuroleptic malignant syndrome can occur in overdose, though it most often occurs with therapeutic doses (see Adverse Effects). Other symptoms may include anticholinergic manifestations (mydriasis, dry mouth, agitation, urinary retention, decreased bowel sounds), tachycardia, cardiac arrhythmias, seizures, miosis and respiratory and/or vasomotor collapse.

Treatment: Patients who have ingested chlorpromazine in overdose occasionally require respiratory and hemodynamic support. This may include intubation, ventilation, boluses of isotonic iv fluids, and inotropic support. Once the patient's airway is adequately protected, 1 dose of activated charcoal (1 g/kg body weight) can be administered up to 120 minutes after oral overdose, to minimize absorption of chlorpromazine. The utility of this intervention decreases with time, and it may not influence clinical outcome. Patients with seizures should be treated with benzodiazepines, or, if necessary, barbiturates. Ventricular arrhythmias are uncommon, and may be treated with boluses of sodium bicarbonate (typically 1–2 mEq/kg) as well as antiarrhythmics such as lidocaine. In the rare patient with torsades de pointes, iv magnesium sulfate and/or an overdrive pacemaker should be used. Acute dystonic reactions may be treated with iv benztropine or diphenhydramine.

For management of a suspected drug overdose, CPhA recommends that you contact your **regional Poison Control Centre**. See the *CPS* Directory section for a list of Poison Control Centres.

DOSAGE: Dosage should be initiated at a low level and increased gradually, carefully noting the clinical response. Patients on long-term therapy should be evaluated periodically to determine the need for continued therapy. Avoid using first-generation antipsychotic agents in elderly patients when possible (see Warnings, Serious Warnings and Precautions). In general, lower doses are recommended for children, elderly or debilitated patients, and in patients with first-episode psychosis. See Precautions and Adverse Effects.

Oral: Psychotic Disorders: Adults: 25 to 75 mg daily in 2 to 4 divided doses. The daily dose may be increased twice weekly by 20 to 50 mg until symptoms are controlled. Optimum therapeutic response may not occur for weeks or months. The usual maximum recommended daily dose is 1 g. After optimal control of symptoms is achieved, the dose should be reduced to the lowest amount that will maintain relief of symptoms. During maintenance therapy the drug can be administered once or twice daily with the largest dose at bedtime.

Children ≥6 Months: 0.5 to 1 mg/kg/dose every 4 to 6 hours. Maximum dose if child's weight <22.7 kg is 40 mg daily; if 22.7 to 45.5 kg, 75 mg daily.

Acute Intermittent Porphyria (not an approved use in Canada): Adults: 25 to 50 mg 3 to 4 times daily.

Intractable Hiccups (not an approved use in Canada): Adults: 25 to 50 mg 3 to 4 times daily. If not controlled in 2 to 3 days, 25 to 50 mg may be given im.

Relief of Nausea and Vomiting (not an approved use in Canada): Adults: 10 to 25 mg every 4 hours. Increase dose as needed and tolerated.

Children: 0.5 to 1 mg/kg/dose every 4 to 6 hours. Maximum dose if child's weight <22.7 kg is 40 mg daily; if 22.7 to 45.5 kg, 75 mg daily.

Parenteral: The im route is used primarily when rapid action is required to control acute severe symptomatology. The iv route is sometimes used. IM injections should be administered slowly, deep into the upper quadrant of the buttock. Oral administration should be substituted as soon as possible. To minimize the risk of hypotension, have the patient lie down for at least 30 minutes following injection.

Chlorpromazine ampoules should be protected from light. Pink or discolored solutions should be discarded.

Psychotic Disorders: Adults: 25 mg im followed by doses of 25 to 50 mg im in 1 hour if required. Doses can be increased over several days to a maximum of 400 mg every 4 to 6 hours.

Children ≥6 Months: 0.5 to 1 mg/kg/dose every 6 to 8 hours. Maximum dose if child's weight <22.7 kg is 40 mg/day; if 22.7 to 45.5 kg, 75 mg/day.

Acute Intermittent Porphyria (not an approved use in Canada): Adults: 25 mg im 3 or 4 times daily.

Adjunctive Treatment of Tetanus (not an approved use in Canada): Adults: 25 to 50 mg im 3 to 4 times daily; may be given direct iv. Children: 0.55 mg/kg im or iv. Maximum dose if child's weight <22.7 kg is 40 mg/day; if 22.7 to 45.5 kg, 75 mg/day.

Intractable Hiccups (not an approved use in Canada): Adults: If oral therapy not effective, 25 to 50 mg im. If still not effective, 25 to 50 mg may be diluted in 500 to 1000 mL normal saline and infused slowly iv.

Relief of Nausea and Vomiting (not an approved use in Canada): Adults: 25 to 50 mg every 3 to 4 hours.

Children: 0.5 to 1 mg/kg/dose every 6 to 8 hours as necessary. Maximum dose if child's weight <22.7 kg is 40 mg daily; if 22.7 to 45.5 kg, 75 mg daily.

Chlorpropamide

CPhA Monograph

see *Sulfonylureas*

Chlorthalidone

CPhA Monograph

see *Thiazide Diuretics*

Cholecalciferol

CPhA Monograph

see *Vitamin D*

Cholestyramine

Antidiarrheal—Antihypercholesterolemic—Bile Acid Sequestrant

CPhA Monograph

Date of Preparation: August 2006
Date of Revision: April 2010

This monograph has been compiled by CPhA and reviewed by experts. It may contain information different from that found in Health Canada-approved Product Monographs. The reader is referred to the *CPS* Editorial Policy for more information.

SUMMARY PRODUCT INFORMATION:

Route of Administration	Dosage Form	Strength
Oral	Powder for Suspension	4 g/9 g
	Powder for Suspension (Light)[a]	4 g/5 g

[a] This product contains aspartame. Please consult product monograph for details.

INDICATIONS AND CLINICAL USE: Health Canada-approved indications include:

- treatment of elevated serum cholesterol as an adjunct to diet and exercise in patients with primary hypercholesterolemia (elevated LDL-cholesterol)
- treatment of pruritus associated with partial biliary obstruction
- treatment of diarrhea associated with excess fecal bile acids due to short bowel syndrome

Uses Without Health Canada Approval: Cholestyramine has been used in the treatment of pruritus associated with partial biliary cirrhosis and in the treatment of diarrhea associated with pseudomembranous colitis, erythroprotoporphyria and hyperoxaluria. It has also been used in the removal of drugs (e.g., cardiac glycosides, leflunomide) or toxins (heptachlor, a pesticide) from the gastrointestinal tract, including removal of drugs that undergo enterohepatic recycling.

Bile acid sequestrants are alternatives to HMG-CoA reductase inhibitors (statins) for the treatment of hypercholesterolemia. At a daily dose of 8 to 10 g/day, cholestyramine reduces LDL-cholesterol concentrations by 10-20%. It has been demonstrated to reduce the rate of coronary heart disease related death and nonfatal myocardial infarction. The LDL-lowering properties of bile acid sequestrants, including cholestyramine, are additive to those of other cholesterol-lowering drugs. The addition of a bile acid sequestrant to a statin can produce a 12% to 16% reduction in LDL cholesterol beyond that achieved with a statin alone. The LDL-cholesterol-lowering activity of 4 g of cholestyramine is estimated to be equivalent to 5 g of colestipol, another bile acid sequestrant.

Treatment with bile acid sequestrants may increase plasma HDL-cholesterol and triglyceride concentrations.

CONTRAINDICATIONS:

- Patients who are hypersensitive to cholestyramine or to any ingredient in the formulation.
- Complete biliary obstruction. Cholestyramine is unlikely to be effective in these patients as no bile products reach the intestine.

WARNINGS AND PRECAUTIONS:

Serious Warnings and Precautions

- Cholestyramine should never be administered in its dry powder form. Always prepare a suspension with water or other fluid (see Dosage and Administration) before ingestion.
- Cholestyramine can cause hyperchloremic acidosis because it is a chloride ion exchange resin. Children may be more susceptible to this effect.
- Cholestyramine may worsen pre-existing constipation.
- Bile acid sequestrants, including cholestyramine, can bind to and impair absorption of fat-soluble vitamins. With long-term use this may lead to hypoprothrombinemia secondary to vitamin K deficiency and an increased bleeding tendency. Patients receiving long-term therapy may require supplements of vitamins A, D and K.
- Bile acid sequestrants, including cholestyramine have the capacity to bind drugs. Many interactions are possible (see Drug Interactions)
- Cholestyramine may reduce serum or red cell levels of folate.
- Some formulations of cholestyramine may contain aspartame, which when metabolized in the gastrointestinal tract produces substantial quantities of phenylalanine. Patients with phenylketonuria and others who must restrict intake of phenylalanine should be cautioned accordingly.

Special Populations: Pregnant Women: Cholestyramine is unlikely to cause direct harm to the fetus because it is not absorbed from the gastrointestinal tract. The interference with absorption of fat soluble vitamins, especially vitamins A and K, may be detrimental. In general, pregnancy-related dyslipidemia does not require treatment.

Nursing Women: The interference with absorption of fat soluble vitamins may be detrimental to the mother or the fetus as long-term use could result in deficiencies. Dyslipidemia in nursing women does generally not require treatment.

Pediatrics: Cholestyramine has been evaluated for the treatment of familial hypercholesterolemia in children aged 6 to 18 years, and for the management of diarrhea in infants.

Monitoring and Laboratory Tests: Serum lipids should be monitored before initiating treatment and periodically during treatment with cholestyramine. Periodic measurement of serum electrolytes and INR is also advised.

ADVERSE REACTIONS: More Common Adverse Drug Reactions: See Table 1.

Table 1: Cholestyramine
More Common Adverse Drug Reactions

Body System	Effect	Clinical Comment
Gastrointestinal	Constipation (dose-related in approximately 20% of patients), bloating and flatulence (abates with continued therapy), nausea, gas, upper abdominal pain.	Constipation is more common with high doses (>24 g/day) and in the elderly. If constipation occurs, decrease the dose or interrupt therapy temporarily. Consider increasing fluid and fibre in the diet.

Less Common Adverse Drug Reactions: Allergic/Dermatologic: pruritus, rash.
Gastrointestinal: abdominal pain, anorexia, biliary colic, bloating, diarrhea, distention, dyspepsia, heartburn, indigestion, irritation of the skin, tongue and perianal area, nausea, vomiting, fecal impaction.
Hematologic: anemia, ecchymosis.
Metabolic: raises triglyceride levels.
Abnormal Hematologic and Clinical Chemistry Findings: See Table 2.

Table 2: Cholestyramine
Abnormal Hematologic and Clinical Chemistry Findings

Test	Effect	Clinical Comment
Serum electrolytes	Hyperchloremic acidosis	Large quantities of chloride are released from cholestyramine in the gastrointestinal tract and may be absorbed into the systemic circulation in place of intestinal bicarbonate. This effect is more prevalent at high doses and in children. May be offset by reducing dietary chloride intake. Monitor electrolytes periodically during treatment.
INR	Increased	Hypoprothrombinemia due to impaired vitamin K absorption may develop. Monitor INR periodically during prolonged use.

DRUG INTERACTIONS: Overview: Cholestyramine is a chloride-containing anion-exchange resin with a high affinity for anionic substances; thus it has the capacity to bind to many drugs. This results in impaired absorption of the drug from the gastrointestinal tract. Cholestyramine can also increase the rate of clearance of drugs that are enterohepatically recycled. It should be assumed that a drug has the potential to interact with cholestyramine unless clinical studies have suggested otherwise. Advise patients to take other drugs at least 1 hour before or 4 to 6 hours after taking cholestyramine (or as great an interval as possible) to minimize the potential effect of cholestyramine on the absorption of the drug. In the case of drugs that are enterohepatically recycled, modifying the time of administration may not mitigate against the effects of cholestyramine.

Of note, cholestyramine does not interfere with the absorption of ASA, carbamazepine, or phenytoin.

Although cholestyramine has been shown to reduce the absorption of HMG Co-A reductase inhibitors, the cholesterol lowering effects are additive when they are administered together.

Drug-Drug Interactions: See Table 3.
Drug-Food Interactions: Impaired absorption of fat soluble vitamins.

DOSAGE AND ADMINISTRATION: Dosing Considerations: Cholestyramine should not be taken in its dry powder form. The powder should be mixed with 60 to 180 mL of water, milk, fruit juice or other noncarbonated beverage. The powder may also be incorporated into soups or pulpy fruits such as apple sauce or crushed pineapple because of their high moisture content.

Treatment should be started with one daily dose so that the patient can build up tolerance to the anticipated gastrointestinal effects of the drug. The dose can then be increased every 5 to 7 days until the desired frequency is reached.

Patients should be advised to take other drugs at least 1 hour before or 4 to 6 hours after taking cholestyramine (or as great an interval as possible) to minimize the potential effect of cholestyramine on the absorption of the drug.

Cholestyramine should not be used in patients with bloody diarrhea.

Recommended Dose and Dosage Adjustment: Adults: See Table 4.
Pediatrics: See Table 5.

In children a dosage of 8 to 16 g/day administered in 2 or 3 divided doses has been used. The drug may be initiated at a dose of 2 to 4 g twice daily and then increased to achieve the desired effect.

OVERDOSAGE:

For management of a suspected drug overdose, CPhA recommends that you contact your **regional Poison Control Centre**. See the *CPS* Directory section for a list of Poison Control Centres.

ACTION AND CLINICAL PHARMACOLOGY: Mechanism of Action: Cholestyramine is a nonabsorbable chloride-containing anion-exchange resin. The drug acts by releasing chloride ions and binding to bile acids in the gastrointestinal tract. Excretion of this complex in the feces interrupts enterohepatic recycling of bile acids. This results in a compensatory increase in LDL-receptor activity of liver cells which hastens the breakdown of LDL-cholesterol in plasma. Plasma triglyceride levels may increase during treatment with cholestyramine possibly due to increased VLDL concentrations.

Cholestyramine may bind other acids or negatively charged substances which have a greater affinity for the resin than chloride ions. This is an important mechanism contributing to numerous potential drug interactions.

Table 3: Cholestyramine

Drug-Drug Interactions

Interacting Drug	Effect	Clinical Comment
Acetaminophen	Absorption of acetaminophen is reduced by 60% when given together with cholestyramine.	Administer acetaminophen ≥1 hour prior to or 4–6 hours after administration of cholestyramine.
Amiodarone	Cholestyramine reduces absorption of amiodarone from the gut and may interfere with enterohepatic recycling of the drug. Thus serum levels of amiodarone decrease when it is co-administered with cholestyramine.	Consider an alternate agent for dyslipidemia. As cholestyramine may interfere with enterohepatic recycling of amiodarone, spacing administration of the two drugs is unlikely to mitigate the effects of cholestyramine on amiodarone blood levels. Higher doses of amiodarone may be necessary in patients receiving ongoing treatment with cholestyramine. Upon discontinuation of cholestyramine, adjust amiodarone dose and monitor for amiodarone toxicity, e.g., arrhythmia, pneumonitis, thyroid abnormalities.
Hydrocortisone	Cholestyramine impairs absorption of hydrocortisone from the gastrointestinal tract resulting in lower exposure to hydrocortisone.	Higher doses of hydrocortisone may be required in patients receiving ongoing treatment with cholestyramine. Prednisone is an alternative corticosteroid, the pharmacokinetics of which do not appear to be affected by cholestyramine.
Digoxin	Cholestyramine reduces absorption of digoxin and may interfere with enterohepatic recirculation of the drug.	Consider an alternate agent for dyslipidemia. Monitor serum levels and for signs of ineffectiveness of digoxin after cholestyramine introduction. Monitor for altered response to digoxin when initiating, discontinuing or changing the dose of cholestyramine. Also, when the interval between the doses of cholestyramine and digoxin is changed, adjust dose of digoxin accordingly.
Ezetimibe	Cholestyramine reduces systemic exposure to ezetimibe (↓ mean AUC by 55%).	Administer ezetimibe ≥1 hour prior or 4–6 hours after administration of cholestyramine.
Furosemide	The diuretic response to furosemide is markedly reduced in patients receiving concurrent cholestyramine.	Administer furosemide ≥1 hour prior to or 4–6 hours after administration of cholestyramine. Monitor for altered response to furosemide when initiating, discontinuing or changing the dose of cholestyramine and when the interval between the doses of cholestyramine and furosemide is changed. Adjust dose of furosemide accordingly.
Glipizide	Cholestyramine binds to glipizide and impairs gastrointestinal absorption of the drug.	Administer glipizide ≥1 hour prior to or 4–6 hours after administration of cholestyramine. Monitor blood sugar levels and adjust the dose of glipizide accordingly if used together with cholestyramine.
Hydrochlorothiazide	Cholestyramine binds to hydrochlorothiazide and impairs gastrointestinal absorption of the drug.	Higher dosages of hydrochlorothiazide may be required to control blood pressure in patients receiving cholestyramine. Administer hydrochlorothiazide ≥1 hour prior to or 4–6 hours after administration of cholestyramine to partially overcome this effect.
Leflunomide	Cholestyramine binds the active metabolite of leflunomide which undergoes enterohepatic recycling. This significantly reduces serum levels and hastens elimination of the drug.	Avoid concurrent use. This interaction is potentially useful in the event of leflunomide overdose and in patients who experience serious leflunomide-related toxicity which mandates withdrawal of the drug.

(cont'd)

Table 3: Cholestyramine *(cont'd)*

Drug-Drug Interactions

Interacting Drug	Effect	Clinical Comment
Lorazepam	Cholestyramine interferes with enterohepatic recirculation of lorazepam, thereby reducing the elimination half-life and increasing the rate of clearance of the drug.	Adjust the dose of lorazepam if necessary.
Methotrexate	Cholestyramine interferes with enterohepatic recirculation of methotrexate, thereby reducing the elimination half-life and increasing the rate of clearance of the drug.	Consider an alternate agent for dyslipidemia. Adjust dose of methotrexate to compensate for reduced exposure during treatment with cholestyramine. Monitor for altered response to methotrexate when initiating, discontinuing or changing the dose of cholestyramine. Also, when the interval between the doses of cholestyramine and methotrexate is changed, adjust dose of methotrexate accordingly.
Metronidazole	Cholestyramine interferes with absorption of metronidazole from the gastrointestinal tract.	Administer metronidazole ≥1 hour prior to or 4–6 hours after cholestyramine. Monitor for reduced therapeutic effect of metronidazole and adjust dose accordingly.
Mycophenolate	Cholestyramine interferes with absorption of mycophenolate from the gastrointestinal tract.	Administer mycophenolate ≥1 hour prior to or 4–6 hours after cholestyramine. Monitor serum levels of mycophenolate during concomitant administration and adjust the dose of mycophenolate accordingly.
NSAIDs—diclofenac	Cholestyramine significantly reduces absorption of diclofenac from the gastrointestinal tract.	Consider use of an alternative NSAID. Administer diclofenac ≥1 hour prior to or 4–6 hours after administration of cholestyramine.
NSAIDs—ibuprofen	Cholestyramine may bind ibuprofen and impair gastrointestinal absorption of the drug.	Administer ibuprofen ≥1 hour prior to or 4–6 hours after administration of cholestyramine.
NSAIDs— meloxicam, piroxicam, tenoxicam	Cholestyramine interferes with enterohepatic recirculation of meloxicam, piroxicam and tenoxicam, thereby reducing the elimination half-life and increasing the rate of clearance of these drugs.	Consider using alternative NSAIDs.
Propranolol	Cholestyramine interferes with absorption of propranolol from the gastrointestinal tract.	Administer propranolol ≥1 hour prior to or 4–6 hours after cholestyramine. Adjust the dose of propranolol to achieve the desired outcome.
Raloxifene	Cholestyramine interferes with enterohepatic recirculation of raloxifene, thereby reducing exposure to the drug.	Avoid concurrent use.
Thyroid hormone (levothyroxine, liothyronine)	Cholestyramine impairs absorption of thyroid hormone from the gastrointestinal tract.	The magnitude of the interaction can be minimized by administering the two agents 4 to 6 hours apart. Monitor thyroid function during treatment with cholestyramine and adjust dose of thyroid hormone accordingly.
Warfarin	Cholestyramine impairs absorption of warfarin from the gastrointestinal tract.	Warfarin undergoes enterohepatic recycling. Separating the time of administration will only partially mitigate this interaction. Cholestyramine also impairs absorption of vitamin K from the large intestine; thus, the ultimate effect of cholestyramine on the INR in a patient receiving warfarin is difficult to predict. Monitor INR closely and adjust the dose of warfarin accordingly in patients receiving both drugs concurrently or when withdrawing cholestyramine.

Table 4: Cholestyramine

Dose in Adult Patients

Indication	Initial Dose	Dose Titration	Usual Dose	Maximum Dose	Duration of Therapy	Clinical Comment
Hypercholesterolemia	4 g po once daily	Increase frequency at 5- to 7-day intervals.	4 g po 3 to 4 times daily	24 g po daily	Duration of treatment is indeterminate.	Cholestyramine may be given twice daily if desired (morning and bedtime).
Pruritus associated with partial biliary obstruction	4 g po once daily	Titrate to desired effect.	4 g po 1 to 3 times daily	16 g po daily	Relief usually occurs within 1 to 3 weeks of initiation of treatment. Symptom returns within 1 to 2 weeks of stopping therapy.	See Hypercholesterolemia.
Diarrhea associated with excess fecal bile acids	4 g po once daily	Titrate to desired effect.			Relief should occur within 3 days of initiation of therapy. If no relief occurs, alternative therapy should be initiated.	See Hypercholesterolemia.

Table 5: Cholestyramine
Dose in Pediatric Patients

Indication	Initial Dose	Dose Titration	Usual Dose	Duration of Therapy	Clinical Comment
Hyper-cholesterolemia	≤10 y: 2 g po daily; range: 1–4 g >10 y: 2 g po daily; maximum daily dose 8 g	Titrate to desired effect.	8–16 g po daily divided 2–3 times	Indeterminate	Not an approved use in Canada.

Pharmacokinetics: Adults: Absorption: Cholestyramine is not absorbed from the gastrointestinal tract.

Cialis® Ⓟ

tadalafil

Treatment of Erectile Dysfunction

Lilly

Date of Preparation: September 8, 2003
Date of Revision: March 5, 2009

SUMMARY PRODUCT INFORMATION:

Route of Administration	Dosage Form/ Strength	Clinically Relevant Nonmedicinal Ingredients
Oral	Tablet—2.5 mg, 5 mg, 10 mg and 20 mg	Lactose monohydrate For a complete listing see Dosage Forms, Composition and Packaging.

INDICATIONS AND CLINICAL USE: CIALIS (tadalafil) is indicated for the treatment of erectile dysfunction in men.

Geriatrics (>65 years of age): No dosage adjustment is required in male elderly patients (see Warnings and Precautions, Geriatrics).

Pediatrics (<18 years of age): CIALIS has not been evaluated in individuals less than 18 years old.

CONTRAINDICATIONS: CIALIS (tadalafil) has been shown to potentiate the hypotensive effects of nitrates. This is thought to result from the combined effects of nitrates and tadalafil on the nitric oxide/cGMP pathway. **Therefore, administration of CIALIS to patients who are using any form of organic nitrate (e.g., oral, sublingual, transdermal, by inhalation), either regularly and/or intermittently, is contraindicated, due to the risk of developing potentially life-threatening hypotension.**

CIALIS should not be prescribed to patients for whom nitrates are prescribed, even though the patient may not have actually used the nitrate therapy.

In a patient prescribed CIALIS, where nitrate administration is deemed medically necessary in a life-threatening situation, at least 48 hours should have elapsed after the last dose of CIALIS before nitrate administration is considered. In such circumstances, nitrates should only be administered under close medical supervision with appropriate hemodynamic monitoring.

CIALIS should not be used in patients with a known hypersensitivity to tadalafil or any component of the tablet (see Dosage Forms, Composition and Packaging).

WARNINGS AND PRECAUTIONS: Sexual activity carries a potential cardiac risk for patients with pre-existing cardiovascular disease. Therefore, treatments for erectile dysfunction, including CIALIS (tadalafil), should not be used in men with cardiac disease for whom sexual activity is inadvisable. The following groups of patients with cardiovascular disease were not included in clinical trials:

- patients with a myocardial infarction within the last 90 days
- patients with unstable angina or angina occurring during sexual intercourse
- patients with New York Heart Association Class 2 or greater heart failure in the last 6 months
- patients with uncontrolled arrhythmias, hypotension (<90/50 mm Hg), or uncontrolled hypertension (>170/100)
- patients with a stroke within the last 6 months.

Additionally, there is no controlled clinical data on the safety or efficacy of CIALIS in the following groups; if prescribed, this should be done with caution:

- patients with severe renal insufficiency (creatinine clearance <30 mL/min)
- patients with severe hepatic insufficiency (Child-Pugh Class C).

Patients with left ventricular outflow obstruction, (e.g., aortic stenosis and idiopathic hypertrophic subaortic stenosis) can be sensitive to the action of vasodilators, including PDE5 inhibitors.

Priapism was not reported in clinical trials with CIALIS. However, priapism has been reported rarely in post-marketing surveillance with PDE5 inhibitors, including tadalafil. The incidence of priapism may increase when PDE5 inhibitors are used in combination with intrapenile injections containing vasoactive agents. Patients who experience erections lasting 4 hours or more should be instructed to seek immediate medical assistance. If priapism is not treated immediately, penile tissue damage and permanent loss of potency may result.

The safety and efficacy of CIALIS in conjunction with other medications used for the treatment of ED have not been studied. Thus the use of such combinations is not recommended.

General Precautions: The evaluation of erectile dysfunction should include a determination of potential underlying causes and the identification of appropriate treatment following an appropriate medical assessment.

CIALIS should be used with caution in patients who have conditions that might predispose them to priapism (such as sickle cell anemia, multiple myeloma, or leukemia).

Agents for the treatment of erectile dysfunction should be used with caution in patients with anatomical deformation of the penis (such as angulation, cavernosal fibrosis or Peyronie's disease).

Post-marketing reports of sudden loss of vision have occurred rarely, in temporal association with the use of PDE5 inhibitors. It is not clear whether these are related directly to the use of PDE5 inhibitors or to other factors. There may be an increased risk to patients who have already experienced Non-Arteritic Ischemic Optic Neuropathy (NAION).

In humans, CIALIS has no effect on bleeding time when taken alone or with acetylsalicylic acid (ASA).

There is no safety information on the administration of CIALIS to patients with bleeding disorders or active peptic ulceration. Therefore, CIALIS should be administered with caution to these patients.

Caution is advised when PDE5 inhibitors are coadministered with alpha blockers. PDE5 inhibitors, including CIALIS, and alpha adrenergic blocking agents are both vasodilators with blood-pressure-lowering effects. When vasodilators are used in combination, an additive effect on blood pressure may be anticipated. In some patients, concomitant use of these two drug classes can lower blood pressure significantly (see Drug Interactions, Action and Clinical Pharmacology), which may lead to symptomatic hypotension (e.g., fainting). Consideration should be given to the following:

Patients should be stable on alpha-blocker therapy prior to initiating a PDE5 inhibitor. Patients who demonstrate hemodynamic instability on alpha-blocker therapy alone are at increased risk of symptomatic hypotension with concomitant use of PDE5 inhibitors.

In those patients already taking an optimized dose of PDE5 inhibitor, alpha-blocker therapy should be initiated at the lowest dose. Stepwise increase in alpha-blocker dose may be associated with further lowering of blood pressure when taking a PDE5 inhibitor.

Safety of combined use of PDE5 inhibitors and alpha blockers may be affected by other variables, including intravascular volume depletion and other antihypertensive drugs.

Otologic: Sudden decrease or loss of hearing has been reported in a few number of postmarketing and clinical trials with the use of PDE5 inhibitors, including CIALIS. These events, which may be accompanied by tinnitus and dizziness, have been reported in temporal association to the intake of PDE5 inhibitors, including CIALIS. It is not possible to determine whether these events are related directly to the use of PDE5 inhibitors or other factors (see Adverse Reactions, Post-Market Adverse Drug Reactions, and Information for the Patient). Physicians should advise patients to stop taking CIALIS and seek prompt medical attention in case of sudden decrease or loss of hearing.

Special Populations: Geriatrics: Of the total number of patients in the primary efficacy and safety studies of CIALIS, 27% were ages 65 and over. No differences in safety or effectiveness were observed between these patients and younger patients. No dose adjustment is required in elderly patients.

Use in Patients with Renal Impairment: In a clinical pharmacology study, administration of CIALIS 10 mg to patients with moderate renal failure (creatinine clearance=31 to 50 mL/min) was less well tolerated, with more back pain experienced, than in patients with mild renal failure (creatinine clearance=51 to 80 mL/min) and healthy subjects. However, when CIALIS 20 mg was administered to patients undergoing hemodialysis there were no complaints of back pain. Hemodialysis contributed negligibly to tadalafil elimination. Daily use of CIALIS 10 or 20 mg should be avoided in patients with renal impairment. A starting dose of 10 mg prior to anticipated sexual activity should be considered for these patients, but no more frequently than on alternate days, and not exceeding 3 times a week. If the 10 mg dose is tolerated but insufficiently effective, the dose may be increased to 20 mg. If the 10 mg dose is not tolerated, CIALIS On-Demand dosing should be discontinued (see Dosage and Administration).

CIALIS 5 mg for Once-a-Day use may be considered for patients with mild to moderate renal impairment. The dosage may be decreased to 2.5 mg Once-a-Day, based on individual tolerability.

Use in Patients with Hepatic Impairment: In a clinical pharmacology study, administration of CIALIS 10 mg to patients with mild and moderate hepatic impairment (Child-Pugh Class A and B) did not result in increased exposure (AUC) to tadalafil, in comparison to healthy subjects. Daily use of CIALIS 10 or 20 mg should be avoided in patients with hepatic impairment. A starting dose of 10 mg prior to anticipated sexual activity should be considered for these patients, but no more frequently than on alternate days, and not exceeding 3 times a week. If the 10 mg dose is tolerated but insufficiently effective, the dose may be increased to 20 mg. If the 10 mg dose is not tolerated, CIALIS On-Demand dosing should be discontinued (see Dosage and Administration).

CIALIS 5 mg for Once-a-Day use may be considered for patients with hepatic impairment. The dosage may be decreased to 2.5 mg Once-a-Day, based on individual tolerability.

Pregnant Women: CIALIS is not indicated for use in newborns, children or women.

There are no studies of tadalafil in pregnant women.

Nursing Women: See Pregnant Women.

Pediatrics: See Pregnant Women.

Information to Be Provided to the Patient: Physicians should discuss with patients the contraindication of CIALIS with regular and/or intermittent use of organic nitrates.

Physicians should also discuss with patients the potential for CIALIS to augment the blood pressure lowering effect of alpha blockers and antihypertensive medications (see Drug Interactions, Action and Clinical Pharmacology).

Physicians should consider the potential cardiac risk of sexual activity in patients with pre-existing cardiovascular disease. Patients who experience symptoms upon initiation of sexual activity should be advised to refrain from further sexual activity and should report the episode to their physician.

Daily use of CIALIS 10 or 20 mg should be avoided in patients with renal or hepatic impairment and those taking protease inhibitors (e.g., ritonavir) or other potent CYP3A4 inhibitors (e.g., ketoconazole). A starting dose of 10 mg prior to anticipated sexual activity should be considered for these patients, but no more frequently than on alternate days, and not exceeding 3 times a week. If the 10 mg dose is tolerated but insufficiently effective, the dose may be increased to 20 mg. If the 10 mg dose is not tolerated, CIALIS On-Demand dosing should be discontinued (see Dosage and Administration).

CIALIS 5 mg for Once-a-Day use may be considered for these patients. The dosage may be decreased to 2.5 mg Once-a-Day, based on individual tolerability.

Priapism was not reported in clinical trials with CIALIS. However, priapism has been reported rarely in post-marketing surveillance with PDE5 inhibitors, including tadalafil. The incidence of priapism may increase when PDE5 inhibitors are used in combination with intrapenile injections containing vasoactive agents (e.g., Caverject). Patients who experience erections lasting 4 hours or more should be instructed to seek immediate medical assistance. If priapism is not treated immediately, penile tissue damage and permanent loss of potency may result.

Tadalafil should be used with caution in patients who have conditions that might predispose them to priapism (such as sickle cell anemia, multiple myeloma, or leukemia), or in patients with anatomical deformation of the penis (such as angulation, cavernosal fibrosis or Peyronie's disease).

Physicians should discuss with patients the increased risk of Non-Arteritic Anterior Ischemic Optic Neuropathy (NAION) in individuals who have already experienced NAION in one eye, including whether such individuals could be adversely affected by use of vasodilators, such as PDE5 inhibitors. Patients should stop taking CIALIS and consult their physician if they experience changes in, or loss of vision in one or both eyes.

Physicians should advise patients to stop taking PDE5 inhibitors, including CIALIS, and seek prompt medical attention in the event of sudden decrease or loss of hearing. These events, which may be accompanied by tinnitus and dizziness, have been reported in temporal association to the intake of PDE5 inhibitors, including CIALIS. It is not possible to determine whether these events are related directly to the use of PDE5 inhibitors or to other factors (see Adverse Reactions, Post-Market Adverse Drug Reactions, and Information for the Patient).

Long-term human studies with subjects 45 years or older have shown that CIALIS therapy may decrease sperm concentration in some patients, but the clinical relevance of this to human fertility is unknown.

CIALIS works only in the presence of sexual stimulation.

The use of CIALIS offers no protection against sexually transmitted diseases. Counselling of patients about the protective measures necessary to guard against sexually transmitted diseases, including Human Immunodeficiency Virus (HIV), should be considered.

ADVERSE REACTIONS: CIALIS (tadalafil) was administered to over 4000 subjects (aged 19 to 86 years) during clinical trials worldwide. Over 230 patients were treated for longer than one year and over 720 patients were treated for over 6 months.

In controlled Phase 2/3 clinical trials for On-Demand dosing, the discontinuation rate due to adverse events in CIALIS-treated patients (1.7%) was not significantly different from that in placebo-treated patients (1.1%). The discontinuation rate due to adverse events in clinical trials with CIALIS for Once-a-Day use was also not significantly different between CIALIS- and placebo-treated patients (3.2% versus 2.8%). In these studies, the adverse events reported with CIALIS were generally mild or moderate, transient, and decreased with continued dosing.

In controlled Phase 2/3 clinical trials, the following adverse events were reported: (see Table 1):

Additional reported adverse events where a causal relationship is uncertain (but plausible) and which occurred in <2% of patients receiving CIALIS included dizziness (1.7%), swelling of eyelids (0.3%), sensations described as eye pain (0.3%), and conjunctival hyperemia (0.3%). Across all clinical studies, reports of changes in colour vision were rare (<0.1%). Sudden decrease or loss of hearing was reported rarely (<0.1%) in clinical trials.

Post-Market Adverse Drug Reactions: In post-marketing surveillance, adverse events that have been reported very rarely in temporal association in patients taking tadalafil include:

Body as a Whole: hypersensitivity reactions including rash, urticaria, facial edema, Stevens-Johnson syndrome, and exfoliative dermatitis.

Cardiovascular and Cerebrovascular: Serious cardiovascular events, including myocardial infarction, sudden cardiac death, unstable angina pectoris, ventricular arrhythmia, stroke, transient ischemic attacks, chest pain, palpitations, and tachycardia, have been reported either post marketing and/or in clinical trials. Most of the patients in whom these events have been reported had pre-existing cardiovascular risk factors. However, it is not possible to definitively determine whether these events are related directly to these risk factors, to CIALIS, to sexual activity, or to a combination of these or other factors.

Hypotension (more commonly reported when tadalafil is given to patients who are already taking antihypertensive agents), hypertension, and syncope.

Skin and Subcutaneous Tissues: hyperhidrosis (sweating).

Gastrointestinal: abdominal pain and gastroesophageal reflux.

Nervous System: migraine, transient global amnesia.

Respiratory System: epistaxis (nose bleed).

Special Senses: blurred vision, nonarteritic anterior ischemic optic neuropathy, retinal vein occlusion, visual field defect.

Otologic: Cases of sudden decrease or loss of hearing have been reported post-marketing in temporal association with the use of PDE5 inhibitors, including CIALIS. In some of the cases, medical conditions and other factors were reported that may have also played a role in the otologic adverse events. In many cases, medical follow-up information was limited. It is not possible to determine whether these reported events are related directly to the use of CIALIS, to the patient's underlying risk factors for hearing loss, a combination of these factors, or to other factors (see Warnings and Precautions and Information for the Patient).

Urogenital: priapism, prolonged erection, spontaneous penile erection.

Table 1: CIALIS

Adverse Events Reported by ≥2% of Patients Treated with CIALIS, and More Frequent on Drug than Placebo, in Phase 2/3 Clinical Trials

	CIALIS Dosing Regimen:			
	On-Demand (10, 20 mg) % Patients		Once-a-Day (2.5, 5 mg) % Patients	
Event	CIALIS (N=1561)	Placebo (N=758)	CIALIS (N=500)	Placebo (N=248)
Headache	11	4	4	5
Dyspepsia	7	1	4	2
Back Pain	4	3	3	1
Myalgia	4	1	2	1
Nasal Congestion	4	2	2	0
Flushing	4	1	2	1

DRUG INTERACTIONS: CIALIS is not expected to cause clinically significant inhibition or induction of the clearance of drugs metabolized by CYP450 isoforms. Studies have confirmed that tadalafil does not inhibit or induce CYP450 isoforms, including CYP1A2, CYP3A4, CYP2C9, CYP2C19, CYP2D6, and CYP2E1.

CYP1A2 Substrate: CIALIS 10 mg had no clinically significant effect on the pharmacokinetics of theophylline. When CIALIS 10 mg was administered to subjects taking theophylline, a small augmentation (3 beats per minute) of the increase in heart rate associated with theophylline was observed.

CYP3A4 Substrates: CIALIS 10 or 20 mg had no clinically significant effect on exposure (AUC) to midazolam or lovastatin.

CYP2C9 Substrate: CIALIS 10 and 20 mg doses had no clinically significant effect on exposure (AUC) to S-warfarin or R-warfarin, nor did CIALIS affect changes in prothrombin time induced by warfarin.

CIALIS is a substrate of and principally metabolized by CYP3A4. Studies have shown that drugs that inhibit or induce CYP3A4 can alter tadalafil exposure.

CYP3A4 Inhibitor: Ketoconazole (400 mg daily), a selective and potent inhibitor of CYP3A4, increased tadalafil AUC by 312% and C_{max} by 22% following a CIALIS 20 mg dose. Ketoconazole (200 mg daily) increased tadalafil AUC by 107% and C_{max} by 15% following a CIALIS 10 mg dose.

HIV Protease Inhibitor: Ritonavir (200 mg twice daily), an inhibitor of CYP3A4, CYP2C9, CYP2C19, and CYP2D6, increased tadalafil AUC by 124%, with no change in C_{max}, following a CIALIS 20 mg dose.

Daily use of CIALIS 10 or 20 mg should be avoided in patients taking protease inhibitors (e.g., ritonavir) or other potent CYP3A4 inhibitors (e.g., ketoconazole). A starting dose of 10 mg prior to anticipated sexual activity should be considered for these patients, but no more frequently than on alternate days, and not exceeding 3 times a week. If the 10 mg dose is tolerated but insufficiently effective, the dose may be increased to 20 mg. If the 10 mg dose is not tolerated, CIALIS On-Demand dosing should be discontinued (see Dosage and Administration).

CIALIS 5 mg for Once-a-Day use may be considered for these patients. The dosage may be decreased to 2.5 mg Once-a-Day, based on individual tolerability.

Grapefruit juice being a weak inhibitor of CYP3A4 gut wall metabolism, may give rise to modest increases in plasma levels of tadalafil.

CYP3A4 Inducer: Rifampin (600 mg daily), a selective CYP3A4 inducer, reduced tadalafil AUC by 88% and C_{max} by 46%, following a CIALIS 10 mg dose.

Antihypertensive Agents: In clinical pharmacology studies, the potential for CIALIS 10 or 20 mg to augment the hypotensive effects of antihypertensive agents was examined. Major classes of antihypertensive agents were studied, including calcium channel blockers (amlodipine), angiotensin converting enzyme (ACE) inhibitors (enalapril), beta-adrenergic receptor blockers (metoprolol), thiazide diuretics (bendrofluazide), and angiotensin II receptor blockers (various types and doses, alone or in combination with thiazides, calcium channel blockers, beta-blockers, and/or alpha-blockers). CIALIS had no clinically significant interaction with any of these classes. Analysis of Phase 3 clinical trial data also showed no difference in adverse events in patients taking CIALIS with or without antihypertensive medications.

Alpha-adrenergic Receptor-blocking Agents: Consistent with the vasodilatory effects of alpha-blockers and PDE5 inhibitors, the concomitant use of CIALIS with non-selective alpha-blockers may lead to symptomatic hypotension in some patients. Patients should be stable on alpha-blocker therapy prior to initiating a PDE5 inhibitor (see Warnings and Precautions, Action and Clinical Pharmacology).

No significant decreases in blood pressure were observed when CIALIS 10 or 20 mg doses were administered to subjects taking the selective alpha[1]-adrenergic blocker, alfuzosin, or the selective alpha[1A]-adrenergic blocker, tamsulosin. CIALIS may be administered with selective alpha[1 or 1A] blockers such as alfuzosin or tamsulosin.

When CIALIS 20 mg was administered to healthy subjects taking the maximum recommended dose (4 mg or 8 mg daily) of the alpha[1]-adrenergic blocker, doxazosin, there was an augmentation of the blood-pressure-lowering effect of doxazosin. Caution should be exercised when prescribing CIALIS to patients who are taking alpha[1] blockers, such as doxazosin, as simultaneous administration may lead to symptomatic hypotension in some patients.

Prior to prescribing CIALIS, physicians should carefully consider whether their patients with certain underlying conditions could be adversely affected by vasodilatory effects, especially in combination with sexual activity. Patients with increased susceptibility to vasodilators include those with left ventricular outflow obstruction (e.g., aortic stenosis, hypertrophic obstructive cardiomyopathy), or those with the rare syndrome of multiple system atrophy, manifesting as severely impaired autonomic control of blood pressure.

Alcohol: CIALIS did not affect alcohol concentrations, and alcohol did not affect tadalafil concentrations. At high doses of alcohol (0.7 g/kg, mean maximum blood concentration 0.08%), the addition of CIALIS 10 or 20 mg did not induce statistically significant mean blood pressure decreases. In some subjects, postural dizziness and orthostatic hypotension were observed. When CIALIS was administered with lower doses of alcohol (0.6 g/kg), hypotension was not observed and dizziness occurred with similar frequency to alcohol alone.

Alcohol consumption may decrease the ability to attain an erection and may also temporarily decrease blood pressure. PDE5 inhibitors, including tadalafil, are vasodilators and may augment the blood-pressure-lowering effect of alcohol.

H_2 Antagonists: An increase in gastric pH resulting from administration of H_2 antagonists, e.g., nizatidine, had no significant effect on the pharmacokinetics of CIALIS 10 mg dose.

Antacids (magnesium hydroxide/aluminum hydroxide): Simultaneous administration of an antacid (magnesium hydroxide/aluminum hydroxide) and CIALIS 10 mg reduced the apparent rate of absorption of tadalafil without altering exposure (AUC) to tadalafil.

Acetylsalicylic Acid (ASA): CIALIS 20 mg did not potentiate the increase in bleeding time caused by ASA.

DOSAGE AND ADMINISTRATION: **Dosage Consideration:** The management of erectile dysfunction should be individualized. Dosage and regimen should be discussed between the physician and the patient based on effectiveness and tolerability.

CIALIS On-Demand Dosing: The recommended dose of CIALIS is 20 mg taken prior to anticipated sexual activity, without regard to food. The dose may be adjusted based on individual tolerability and effectiveness. The maximum recommended dosing frequency is once per day. CIALIS doses of 10 mg and 20 mg are intended for use prior to anticipated sexual activity and are not recommended for continuous daily use.

CIALIS has been shown to be effective within 30 minutes of taking the tablet, and up to 36 hours later. Patients may initiate sexual activity at varying time points relative to dosing, in order to determine their own optimal window of responsiveness.

For On-Demand dosing, CIALIS may be administered with selective alpha-[1 or 1A] blockers such as alfuzosin or tamsulosin, and no dosage adjustment of CIALIS is required. However, when prescribing CIALIS to patients who are taking non-selective alpha-blockers such as doxazosin, the recommended starting dose is 10 mg.

Daily use of CIALIS 10 or 20 mg should be avoided in patients with renal or hepatic impairment and those taking protease inhibitors (e.g., ritonavir) or other potent CYP3A4 inhibitors (e.g., ketoconazole). A starting dose of 10 mg prior to anticipated sexual activity should be considered for these patients, but no more frequently than on alternate days, and not exceeding 3 times a week. If the 10 mg dose is tolerated but insufficiently effective, the dose may be increased to 20 mg. If the 10 mg dose is not tolerated, CIALIS On-Demand dosing should be discontinued (see Action and Clinical Pharmacology, Pharmacokinetics in Special Populations and Conditions and Warnings and Precautions, Drug Interactions).

CIALIS for Once-a-Day Use: The recommended dose of CIALIS is 5 mg per day, taken at approximately the same time each day, and without regard to food.

The dosage may be decreased to 2.5 mg once a day, based on individual tolerability.

No dose adjustment is required when CIALIS Once-a-Day is used in combination with alpha-blockers.

No dose adjustment is required in patients with mild to moderate renal or hepatic impairment, and those taking protease inhibitors (e.g., ritonavir) or other potent CYP3A4 inhibitors (e.g., ketoconazole). CIALIS for Once-a-Day use is not recommended for patients with severe renal impairment.

OVERDOSAGE:
Symptoms and Treatment of Overdosage: Single doses of up to 500 mg tadalafil have been given to healthy subjects, and multiple doses of 100 mg/day for 21 days have been given to patients. Adverse events (e.g., headache, dyspepsia) were similar to those seen at lower doses.

In cases of overdose, standard supportive measures should be adopted as required. Renal dialysis is not expected to accelerate clearance, as tadalafil is highly bound to plasma proteins.

Treatment of Priapism: All patients should be counselled to contact a physician if they experience any erection persisting for more than 4 hours. Priapism should be treated according to established medical practice. One algorithm aimed primarily at treating priapism secondary to pharmacological agents is presented below:

Procedure 1—External Perineal Compression: Although frequently unsuccessful, the use of prolonged external perineal compression, including ice, may be applied as a temporizing measure. If procedure 1 is unsuccessful, proceed to procedure 2.

Procedure 2—Penile Aspiration: Place the patient in the supine position and assure local anesthesia of the penis. The penile shaft should be punctured at either the 2 o'clock or the 10 o'clock position, and 20-30 mL of blood aspirated from the corpus cavernosum. If detumescence has occurred, the penis should be dressed with an elasticized bandage to ensure continued emptying of the corpora and to compress the puncture site(s). If procedure 2 is unsuccessful, proceed to procedure 3.

Procedure 3—Intracavernous Injection of an Alpha-Adrenergic Agonist: If aspiration alone fails to achieve detumescence, the corpus cavernosum can be injected with a solution of phenylephrine (10 mg in 19 mL of 0.9% saline=500 µg/mL, and inject 0.1-0.2 mL every 2-5 minutes, for up to 10 doses). Clinicians should refer to the prescribing information for phenylephrine prior to its use.

If the above algorithm fails to detumesce the patient, a urologist should be consulted immediately. Penile tissue damage and/or permanent loss of potency may result if priapism is not treated immediately.

For management of a suspected drug overdose, contact your regional Poison Control Centre. See the *CPS* Directory section for a list of Poison Control Centres.

ACTION AND CLINICAL PHARMACOLOGY: CIALIS (tadalafil), an oral treatment for erectile dysfunction, is a potent, selective, reversible inhibitor of cyclic guanosine monophosphate (cGMP)-specific phosphodiesterase type 5 (PDE5).

Mechanism of Action: When sexual stimulation causes the local release of nitric oxide in the corpus cavernosum, nitric oxide then activates the enzyme guanylyl cyclase, which results in increased levels of cGMP. The increased levels of cGMP in the corpus cavernosum produce smooth muscle relaxation and inflow of blood into the penile tissues, thereby producing an erection. PDE5 degrades cGMP in the corpus cavernosum, and the inhibition of PDE5 by CIALIS maintains increased levels of cGMP in the corpus cavernosum. CIALIS has no effect on penile blood flow in the absence of sexual stimulation.

Studies in vitro have shown that tadalafil is a potent inhibitor of PDE5. PDE5 is an enzyme found in corpus cavernosum smooth muscle, vascular and visceral smooth muscle, skeletal muscle, platelets, kidney, lung, and cerebellum. The effect of tadalafil is more selective on PDE5 than on other phosphodiesterases. Tadalafil is >10 000-fold more selective for PDE5 than for PDE1, PDE2, PDE4, and PDE7 enzymes, which are found in the heart, brain, blood vessels, liver, and other organs. Tadalafil is >10 000-fold more selective for PDE5 than for PDE3, an enzyme found in the heart and blood vessels. This selectivity for PDE5 over PDE3 is important because PDE3 is an enzyme involved in cardiac contractility. Additionally, tadalafil is approximately 700-fold more potent for PDE5 than for PDE6, an enzyme which is found in the retina and is responsible for phototransduction. Tadalafil is also >9000-fold more potent for PDE5 than for PDE8 through PDE10. Tadalafil is 14-fold more potent for PDE5 than for PDE11A1 and 40-fold more potent for PDE5 than for PDE11A4, two of the four known forms of PDE11. PDE11 is an enzyme found in human prostate, testes, skeletal muscle and in other tissues. In vitro, tadalafil inhibits human recombinant PDE11A1 and, to a lesser degree, PDE11A4 activities at concentrations within the therapeutic range. The physiological role and clinical consequence of PDE11 inhibition in humans have not been defined.

Pharmacodynamics: Studies of CIALIS on Blood Pressure and Heart Rate: CIALIS 10 or 20 mg doses administered to healthy subjects produced no significant difference compared to placebo in supine systolic and diastolic blood pressure (difference in the mean maximal decrease of 1.6/0.8 mm Hg, respectively), and in standing systolic and diastolic blood pressure (difference in the mean maximal decrease of 0.2/4.6 mm Hg, respectively). In addition, there was no significant effect on heart rate.

When CIALIS and certain oral antihypertensive medications (amlodipine, enalapril, metoprolol, bendrofluazide, angiotensin II receptor blockers) were assessed in drug interaction studies, CIALIS 10 or 20 mg doses did not result in clinically significant augmentation of the antihypertensive effects of those medications (see Drug Interactions). Analysis of Phase 3 clinical trial data also showed no difference in adverse events in patients taking CIALIS with or without antihypertensive medications.

Larger effects were recorded among subjects receiving concomitant nitrates (see Contraindications).

The potential hemodynamic interactions of CIALIS with a non-selective alpha blocker (doxazosin 4, 8 mg), a selective [1A] alpha blocker (tamsulosin 0.4 mg) and a selective [1] alpha blocker (alfuzosin 10 mg) were investigated in randomized, double-blind, crossover design studies. Blood pressure (BP) and heart rate were recorded before dosing and for 24 hours after dosing.

CIALIS 20 mg augmented the hypotensive effect of 8 mg doxazosin by producing a mean maximal decrease in standing systolic BP (SBP) that was significantly greater than placebo (a mean difference of 9.8 mm Hg). Analysis of BP outliers showed that the number of subjects with a standing SBP of less than 85 mm Hg was greater after doxazosin plus tadalafil (28%) versus doxazosin plus placebo (6%). A further clinical pharmacology study was performed in order to investigate the lower dose of 4 mg doxazosin. The changes produced in that study were comparable to those observed in the earlier study.

In subjects on tamsulosin, CIALIS 10 and 20 mg produced mean maximal decreases in standing SBP that were similar to placebo (mean difference of 1.7 and 2.3 mm Hg, respectively). No subject taking tamsulosin had a decrease in standing SBP less than 85 mm Hg. In subjects receiving alfuzosin, CIALIS 20 mg also produced a maximal decrease in SBP that was not significantly different from that after placebo (mean difference of 4.35 mm Hg). One subject taking alfuzosin had an asymptomatic SBP of less than 85 mm Hg.

No vasodilatory adverse events were observed when tadalafil was administered with tamsulosin or alfuzosin. Two such events (dizziness, vertigo) were reported following administration of CIALIS with doxazosin. No syncope was reported in these studies.

Studies of CIALIS on Other Cardiac/Hemodynamic Parameters: In patients with stable coronary artery disease (CAD) and demonstrable ischemia with exercise, CIALIS 10 mg was non-inferior to placebo with respect to effect on time to ischemia. In a separate double-blind, placebo-controlled study to evaluate the effects of CIALIS on myocardial perfusion in patients with CAD, CIALIS 20 mg had no significant effect on myocardial blood flow, both at rest and during pharmacological stress with dobutamine.

Tadalafil at doses up to 500 mg did not significantly change cardiac output and did not significantly impact patients' hemodynamic response to exercise. The effect of CIALIS has not been evaluated in cardiac catheterization studies.

No tadalafil-related changes in electrocardiographic measures, including QTc interval, were observed following administration of CIALIS single doses up to 500 mg and multiple doses of up to 100 mg once-daily for 21 days, to healthy subjects or patients. ECGs were obtained pre- and post-dose, spanning the period from the expected T_{max} of tadalafil (2 hours) to the expected T_{max} of the primary metabolite (methylcatechol glucuronide, 24 hours).

In clinical pharmacology studies, CIALIS 10 and 20 mg had no clinically significant effect on acetylsalicylic acid-induced prolongation of bleeding time or warfarin-induced changes in prothrombin time (see Drug Interactions). Also, in clinical studies there was no evidence of bleeding-related adverse events associated with CIALIS treatment.

Studies of CIALIS on Vision: In a study to assess the effects of a single dose of tadalafil 40 mg on vision, no impairment of colour discrimination (blue/green) was detected using the Farnsworth-Munsell 100-hue test. This finding is consistent with the low affinity of tadalafil for PDE6 compared to PDE5 (see Action and Clinical Pharmacology, Mechanism of Action). In addition, no effects were observed on visual acuity, electroretinograms, intraocular pressure, or pupillometry. Across all clinical studies with CIALIS 10 or 20 mg, reports of changes in colour vision were rare (<0.1% of patients).

Studies of CIALIS on Sperm Characteristics: Three studies were conducted in men, ages 45-70 years, to assess the potential effect on spermatogenesis of CIALIS 10 mg (one 6-month study) and 20 mg (one 6-month and one 9-month study) administered once daily. In all 3 studies, there were no adverse effects on sperm morphology or sperm motility. There were also no significant changes in mean concentrations of the reproductive hormones, testosterone, luteinizing hormone or follicle-stimulating hormone with either 10 or 20 mg of CIALIS compared to placebo. No decrease in sperm concentration was observed in the study of 20 mg CIALIS taken for 6 months. In the study of 10 mg CIALIS for 6 months and the study of 20 mg CIALIS for 9 months, results showed a statistically significant decrease in mean sperm concentration relative to placebo. The clinical relevance of this to human fertility is unknown. In the 9-month study (n=125 [CIALIS 20 mg], n=128 [placebo]), decreases in sperm concentration were in a few patients (but not all) associated with higher ejaculatory frequency, which may have resulted from CIALIS-related improvement in sexual function.

The amount of tadalafil found in the ejaculate of most subjects on repeated CIALIS dosing was negligible; however, a few subjects showed unexplained higher levels of tadalafil in their ejaculate.

Studies of CIALIS on Erectile Function: The efficacy and safety of tadalafil at doses of 2 to 100 mg have been evaluated in clinical trials up to 24 weeks duration, involving over 4000 patients. CIALIS 10 mg or 20 mg On Demand or CIALIS 2.5 mg or 5 mg for Once-a-Day use, is effective in improving erectile function in men with ED. Erectile function effects of CIALIS were dose-related. In clinical studies assessing patients' ability to engage in successful and satisfying sexual intercourse, CIALIS demonstrated highly statistically significant improvement compared with placebo. Additionally, partners of patients on CIALIS had statistically significant greater satisfaction with sexual intercourse compared with partners of patients on placebo.

Overall, CIALIS consistently showed efficacy in a broad and representative population that included patients with ED of various severities (Mild, Moderate, Severe), etiologies (including patients with diabetes), ages (21 to 86 years), and ethnicities. Patients on CIALIS therapy demonstrated consistent and statistically significant improvement in erectile function, compared to patients on placebo. The period of responsiveness to CIALIS was evaluated in an "at-home" setting and by office-based RIGISCAN. These studies demonstrated that CIALIS 20 mg significantly improved patients' ability to have successful sexual intercourse as early as 16 minutes after dose administration and up to 36 hours after dose administration. The treatment effect did not diminish over time.

Pharmacokinetics: Absorption: Tadalafil is rapidly absorbed after oral administration and the mean maximum observed plasma concentration (C_{max} of 189 µg/L at 10 mg and 378 µg/L at 20 mg) is achieved at a median time of 2 hours after dosing. The absolute bioavailability of tadalafil has not been determined.

The rate and extent of absorption of tadalafil are not influenced by food, thus CIALIS may be taken with or without food. The time of dosing (morning versus evening) had no clinically relevant effects on the rate and extent of absorption.

Distribution: The mean volume of distribution is approximately 64 L at steady-state, indicating that tadalafil is distributed into tissues. At therapeutic concentrations, 94% of tadalafil in plasma is bound to proteins. Protein binding is not affected by impaired renal function.

Less than 0.0005% of the administered dose appeared in the semen of healthy subjects.

Metabolism: Tadalafil is predominantly metabolized by the cytochrome P450 (CYP) 3A4 isoform. The major circulating metabolite is the methylcatechol glucuronide. This metabolite is at least 13 000-fold less potent than tadalafil for PDE5. Consequently, it is not expected to be clinically active at observed metabolite concentrations.

Excretion: The mean oral clearance for tadalafil is 2.5 L/h, and the mean half-life is 17.5 hours in healthy subjects. Tadalafil is excreted predominantly as inactive metabolites, mainly in the feces (approximately 61% of the dose) and to a lesser extent in the urine (approximately 36% of the dose).

Tadalafil pharmacokinetics in healthy subjects are linear with respect to time and dose. Over a dose range of 2.5 to 20 mg, exposure (AUC) increases proportionally with dose. Steady-state plasma concentrations are attained within 5 days of once-daily dosing.

Pharmacokinetics determined with a population approach in patients with erectile dysfunction are similar to pharmacokinetics in subjects without erectile dysfunction.

Special Populations and Conditions: Geriatrics: The mean AUC value (4881 µg·h/L for 10 mg dose) in male subjects aged 65 to 78 years was approximately 25% higher than AUC (3896 µg·h/L) for subjects aged 19 to 45 years, while age had negligible effect on C_{max} values. This effect of age is not clinically significant and does not require a dose adjustment (see Warnings and Precautions, Geriatrics).

Pediatrics: Tadalafil has not been evaluated in individuals less than 18 years old.

Hepatic Insufficiency: In a clinical pharmacology study using CIALIS 10 mg, tadalafil exposure (AUC) in subjects with mild and moderate hepatic impairment (Child-Pugh Class A and B) was comparable to exposure in healthy subjects. Daily use of CIALIS 10 or 20 mg should be avoided in patients with hepatic impairment. A starting dose of 10 mg prior to anticipated sexual activity should be considered for these patients, but no more frequently than on alternate days, and not exceeding 3 times a week. If the 10 mg dose is tolerated but insufficiently effective, the dose may be increased to 20 mg. If the 10 mg dose is not tolerated, CIALIS On-Demand dosing should be discontinued (see Warnings and Precautions, Use in Patients with Hepatic Impairment and Dosage and Administration).

CIALIS 5 mg for Once-a-Day use may be considered for patients with hepatic impairment. The dosage may be decreased to 2.5 mg once a day, based on individual tolerability.

Renal Insufficiency: In clinical pharmacology studies using single-dose CIALIS 5 to 20 mg, tadalafil exposure (AUC) approximately doubled in subjects with mild (creatinine clearance 51 to 80 mL/min) or moderate (creatinine clearance 31 to 50 mL/min) renal insufficiency, and in subjects with end-stage renal disease on dialysis. In dialysis patients, C_{max} was 41% higher than that observed in healthy subjects. Hemodialysis contributed negligibly to tadalafil elimination. Daily use of CIALIS 10 or 20 mg should be avoided in patients with renal impairment. A starting dose of 10 mg prior to anticipated sexual activity should be considered for these patients, but no more frequently than on alternate days, and not exceeding 3 times a week. If the 10 mg dose is tolerated but insufficiently effective, the dose may be increased to 20 mg. If the 10 mg dose is not tolerated, CIALIS On-Demand dosing should be discontinued (see Warnings and Precautions, Use in Patients with Renal Impairment and Dosage and Administration).

Patients with Diabetes: Tadalafil exposure (AUC 3454 µg·h/L for a 10 mg dose) in patients with diabetes was 19% lower, and the mean maximum plasma concentration (C_{max} of 184 µg/L) was 5% lower than that observed in healthy subjects. This difference in exposure does not require a dose adjustment.

STORAGE AND STABILITY: Store at controlled room temperature, 15-30°C.

SPECIAL HANDLING INSTRUCTIONS: None.

INFORMATION FOR THE PATIENT: Published in e-CPS, available by subscription at www.e-cps.ca.

DOSAGE FORMS, COMPOSITION AND PACKAGING: 2.5 mg (for Once-a-Day use): Each yellow-orange, almond-shaped, film-coated tablet, debossed on one side with "C2½", contains: tadalafil 2.5 mg. Nonmedicinal ingredients: croscarmellose sodium, hydroxypropylcellulose, hydroxypropylmethylcellulose, iron oxide, lactose monohydrate, magnesium stearate, microcrystalline cellulose, sodium lauryl sulfate, talc, titanium dioxide and triacetin. Blister packages of 14 and 28.

5 mg (for Once-a-Day use): Each yellow, almond-shaped, film-coated tablet, debossed on one side with "C5", contains: tadalafil 5 mg. Nonmedicinal ingredients: croscarmellose sodium, hydroxypropylcellulose, hydroxypropylmethylcellulose, iron oxide, lactose monohydrate, magnesium stearate, microcrystalline cellulose, sodium lauryl sulfate, talc, titanium dioxide and triacetin. Blister packages of 14 and 28.

10 mg (for "On-Demand" dosing): Each yellow, almond-shaped, film-coated tablet, debossed on one side with "C10", contains: tadalafil 10 mg. Nonmedicinal ingredients: croscarmellose sodium, hydroxypropylcellulose, hydroxypropylmethylcellulose, iron oxide, lactose monohydrate, magnesium stearate, microcrystalline cellulose, sodium lauryl sulfate, talc, titanium dioxide and triacetin. Blister packages of 2,4 and 8.

20 mg (for "On-Demand" dosing): Each yellow, almond-shaped, film-coated tablet, debossed on one side with "C20", contains: tadalafil 20 mg. Nonmedicinal ingredients: croscarmellose sodium, hydroxypropylcellulose, hydroxypropylmethylcellulose, iron oxide, lactose monohydrate, magnesium stearate, microcrystalline cellulose, sodium lauryl sulfate, talc, titanium dioxide and triacetin. Blister packages of 2,4 and 8.

(Shown in Product Identification Section)

Ciclesonide

CPhA Monograph

see *Corticosteroids: Inhaled*

Cilazapril

CPhA Monograph

see *ACE Inhibitors*

Ciloxan®

ciprofloxacin HCl

Antibacterial

Alcon

SUPPLIED: Ointment: Each g of ophthalmic ointment contains: ciprofloxacin HCl 3.5 mg equivalent to 3 mg base. Nonmedicinal ingredients: mineral oil and white petrolatum. Metal ophthalmic ointment tubes of 3.5 g.

Solution: Each mL of ophthalmic solution contains: ciprofloxacin HCl 3.5 mg equivalent to ciprofloxacin base 3 mg. Also contains benzalkonium chloride 0.006% as preservative. Nonmedicinal ingredients: acetic acid, edetate disodium, hydrochloric acid and/or sodium hydroxide, mannitol, purified water, and sodium acetate. Plastic Drop-Tainer dispensers of 5 mL.

Store in the carton at room temperature (2 to 30°C).

Cimetidine

Histamine H2-Receptor Antagonist

CPhA Monograph

Date of Preparation: May 2009

This monograph has been compiled by CPhA and reviewed by experts. It may contain information different from that found in Health Canada-approved Product Monographs. The reader is referred to the *CPS* Editorial Policy for more information.

SUMMARY PRODUCT INFORMATION:

Route of Administration	Dosage Form	Product Strength
Oral	Tablet	200 mg, 300 mg, 400 mg, 600 mg, 800 mg

INDICATIONS AND CLINICAL USE: Cimetidine is indicated for:

- Treatment of active duodenal ulcers and prevention of recurrence.
- Treatment of active gastric ulcers and prevention of recurrence.
- Management of gastroesophageal reflux disease (GERD).

  After a successful course of initial therapy of four to eight weeks with a histamine H_2-receptor antagonist (H_2RA), approximately 20% of the patients with uninvestigated GERD will remain asymptomatic for up to 6 months after the therapy [*COMPUS* 2007;1(2):1-178. http://www.cadth.ca/media/pdf/compus_Scientific_Report_final.pdf]. In uninvestigated GERD, proton pump inhibitors (PPIs) have better efficacy than H_2RAs as initial therapy for up to four weeks with respect to reflux symptoms [*COMPUS* 2007;1(2):1-178. http://www.cadth.ca/media/pdf/compus_Scientific_Report_final.pdf].
- Treatment of nonsteroidal anti-inflammatory agent (NSAID)-induced erosions and lesions and prevention of recurrence.

  Routine concomitant anti-ulcer prophylaxis is not warranted for all patients taking NSAIDs. It is important to assess patient risk factors such as history of complicated ulcers, low-dose ASA use, concomitant anticoagulation and/or corticosteroid use, and age ≥60 years [*Am J Gastroenterol* 2009;104(3):728-38; *Circulation* 2008;118(18):1894-909]. Standard doses of H_2RAs equivalent to ranitidine 150 mg twice daily or cimetidine 400 mg twice daily have been shown to be ineffective at reducing the risk of NSAID-induced endoscopic gastric ulcers. Double doses of H_2RAs equivalent to ranitidine 300 mg twice daily have been shown to be effective at reducing the risk of NSAID-induced gastric and duodenal endoscopic ulcers [*Health Technol Assess* 2007;11(51):iii-iv, 1-164; *Cochrane Database Syst Rev* 2002;(4):CD002296; *Technology Overview* 2004;12:1-20. http://www.cadth.ca/media/pdf/261_gastro_ov_e.pdf].
- Treatment of pathological hypersecretion associated with Zollinger-Ellison syndrome, systemic mastocytosis and multiple endocrine adenomas.

  High dose PPIs may be more effective in suppressing acid than H_2RAs in patients with Zollinger-Ellison syndrome [*Gastroenterology* 1989;97(4):827-36]. H_2RAs may be used in systemic mastocytosis to lessen abdominal pain, heartburn, cramping and/or diarrhea [*Hematol Oncol Clin North Am* 2000;14(3):659-87, vii].
- Adjunctive treatment in the management of cystic fibrosis in children.

  Children ≥5 years with cystic fibrosis may be more likely to experience regurgitation and heartburn relative to their siblings [*J Pediatr* 1985;106(2):223-7]. Transient relaxation of the lower esophageal sphincter appears to be the main mechanism, which is also common in children without cystic fibrosis. There is a paucity of evidence with respect to dosing of antisecretory agents in this population.

Other Clinical Uses:

According to the American College of Gastroenterology guideline on the management of *Helicobacter pylori* infection, quadruple therapy consisting of a PPI or H_2RA, bismuth, metronidazole and tetracycline for 10 to 14 days, may be considered in patients with hypersensitivity to penicillin or in those who have previously been treated with a macrolide [*Am J Gastroenterol* 2007;102(8):1808-25]. H_2RAs may be preferred in patients who cannot tolerate PPIs. The Canadian Helicobacter Study Group Consensus prefers PPIs over H_2RAs in treatment regimens for *H. pylori* [*Can J Gastroenterol* 2004;18(9):547-54].

A Cochrane review showed benefit in dyspepsia symptoms and quality of life scores with H_2RAs and PPIs compared to placebo in patients with non-ulcer dyspepsia (NUD) [*Cochrane Database Syst Rev* 2006;(4):CD001960]. NUD is a heterogeneous condition where patients may present symptoms such as abdominal pain or discomfort, postprandial fullness, bloating, early satiety, nausea or vomiting.

Because of its side effect and drug-drug interaction profiles, and the availability of effective alternatives such as other H_2RAs and PPIs, cimetidine, an H_2RA, has fallen out of favor for various gastroenterology conditions.

Geriatrics: Monitor for drug interactions if cimetidine is initiated as this population may be on multiple medications. May increase risk of neurologic adverse effects (see Warnings and Precautions).

Pediatrics: Since data in children younger than 16 years old are limited, the manufacturers do not recommend the use of cimetidine unless the benefits outweigh the risks. Limited clinical experience with pediatric cimetidine dosing is available (see Dosage and Administration).

CONTRAINDICATIONS:

- Patients who are hypersensitive to cimetidine or to any ingredient in the formulation.

WARNINGS AND PRECAUTIONS: Cardiovascular: Cimetidine has been associated with sinus bradycardia.

Gastrointestinal: Cimetidine may mask symptoms of gastric malignancy.

Neurologic: Confusion, agitation, psychosis, paranoia, depression, anxiety, hallucinations, hostility, delirium and disorientation may occur, especially in the elderly (≥50 years) and in those with hepatic or renal insufficiency. The condition is more likely at higher doses and develops 2 to 3 days after starting cimetidine. It is reversible and resolves within 3 to 4 days of stopping cimetidine.

Peri-Operative Considerations: H_2RAs may be administered 2 hours preoperatively to decrease gastric acidity.

Renal: Since cimetidine is excreted by the kidneys, dose adjustment is needed in patients with renal failure. Increase in serum creatinine early in cimetidine therapy is frequent and possibly due to competitive renal tubular secretion. This does not signify deteriorating renal function. Interstitial nephritis has also been reported, which subsides with withdrawal of cimetidine.

Respiratory: Cimetidine and other agents which decrease gastric acid may increase the risk of community-acquired pneumonia.

Special Populations: Pregnant Women: Pregnancy Category B_M. Cimetidine crosses the placental barrier. To date, there have been no reports of increased congenital malformations ascribed to cimetidine in humans. No evidence of impaired fertility or harm to the fetus was observed in reproduction studies using rats, rabbits and mice, with cimetidine doses of up to 40 times the usual human dose. Because of its antiandrogenic properties, cimetidine has been reported to reduce sperm counts in males, and prostate and seminal vesicles in animals. The use of cimetidine in pregnancy requires that the potential benefit of the drug be weighed against the possible risk to the fetus.
Nursing Women: Cimetidine distributes into breast milk. Limited evidence suggests that the infant doses resulting from maternal cimetidine breast milk levels are much less than neonatal doses of 5 to 10 mg/kg daily. The clinical significance of an infant ingesting cimetidine from the milk, however, is currently unknown. Adverse effects to the fetus have not been reported. The American Academy of Pediatrics lists cimetidine as compatible with breastfeeding. Because of the potential of cimetidine to affect the metabolism of other drugs given concomitantly, nizatidine and famotidine may be preferred as they concentrate to a lesser degree in the breast milk [*Clin Pharm* 1991;10(8):594-624].
Pediatrics (≤16 years): Since data in children younger than 16 years old are limited, the manufacturers do not recommend the use of cimetidine unless the benefits outweigh the risks. Limited clinical experience with pediatric cimetidine dosing is available where 20 to 40 mg/kg daily has been used (see Dosage and Administration).
Geriatrics: Decreased cimetidine clearance may increase the possibility of CNS adverse effects in the elderly.
ADVERSE REACTIONS: More Common Adverse Drug Reactions (≥1%): See Table 1.

Table 1: Cimetidine
More Common Adverse Drug Reactions (≥1%)

Body System	Effect
Central Nervous System	headache
Endocrine	gynecomastia
Gastrointestinal	nausea, vomiting

Less Common Adverse Drug Reactions (<1%): Cardiovascular: arrhythmia, bradycardia, hypotension, tachycardia, heart block.
Central Nervous System: agitation, disorientation, dizziness, hallucination, mental confusion, somnolence, delirium and depression (several cases).
Dermatologic: erythema multiforme (1 case), Stevens-Johnson syndrome (1 case), toxic epidermal necrolysis (1 case), exfoliative dermatitis, generalized exfoliative erythroderma, baboon-like syndrome, reversible alopecia.
Gastrointestinal: collagenous colitis.
Hematologic: agranulocytosis, granulocytopenia (several cases), neutropenia, thrombocytopenia, pancytopenia (several cases), aplastic anemia, hemolytic anemia.
Hepatic/Biliary/Pancreatic: increased AST/ALT, pancreatitis.
Immune: delayed hypersensitivity.
Ophthalmologic: optic neuropathy.
Renal: elevated creatinine, urinary retention, acute tubulointerstitial nephritis associated with antineutrophil cytoplasmic antibody where the patient was reactive with myeloperoxidase.
Sexual Function/Reproduction: impotence, galactorrhea. Climacteric symptoms specifically hot flushes. Profuse sweating, anxiety and dizziness in young man on maintenance hemodialysis.
Miscellaneous: arthralgia, myalgia, edema of the breast, fever.
DRUG INTERACTIONS: Overview: Cimetidine inhibits cytochrome P450 enzymes specifically CYP1A2, 2C9, 2D6 and 3A4. Drugs that are metabolized by these isoenzymes may be affected when used concurrently with cimetidine. By altering the gastric pH, cimetidine may affect the absorption of certain drugs such as ketoconazole or itraconazole.
Drug-Drug Interactions: See Table 2.

Table 2: Cimetidine
Drug-Drug Interactions

Interacting Drug	Effect	Clinical Comment
Antacids	Simultaneous administration of antacids with cimetidine reduces cimetidine serum levels possibly by adsorbing to the cimetidine in the gastrointestinal tract. Data is conflicting regarding this interaction depending on single dose versus multiple dose studies.	Clinical significance unknown. If cimetidine is taken with food, take antacids 1 hour after, to avoid this potential interaction. Space antacids 1 hour before or after cimetidine administration if cimetidine is taken on an empty stomach.
Amiodarone	Cimetidine may increase amiodarone serum levels by inhibiting hepatic metabolism of amiodarone or uptake of amiodarone by hepatocytes.	Monitor amiodarone levels when cimetidine is initiated, discontinued or if there is a change in the dose. Consider using an alternate H_2-receptor antagonist.
Atazanavir	Cimetidine may decrease atazanavir levels by reducing its absorption.	Avoid combination. Separating the doses may not prevent this interaction.
Azole Antifungals, i.e., itraconazole, ketoconazole, posaconazole	By suppressing gastric acid, cimetidine may decrease absorption of azole antifungals, decreasing bioavailability and resulting in a loss of antifungal efficacy.	Avoid combination. Consider using a non-interacting antifungal such as fluconazole, voriconazole or terbinafine, if an H_2-receptor antagonist is needed. Consider giving glutamic acid hydrochloride 680 mg, 15 minutes before administration of ketoconazole, on an empty stomach, to enhance its absorption.
Benzodiazepines, i.e., alprazolam, chlordiazepoxide, clonazepam, clorazepate, diazepam, flurazepam, midazolam, triazolam	Increased serum levels of benzodiazepines undergoing oxidative metabolism in the liver or their active metabolites.	Upon initiation of cimetidine, observe for signs and symptoms of increased plasma levels of benzodiazepines such as prolonged sedation. Warn patients of possible impairment of judgment and reflexes. Consider switching to lorazepam, oxazepam or temazepam as they undergo glucuronide conjugation or consider using an alternate H_2-receptor antagonist.
Beta Blockers, i.e., carvedilol, labetalol, metoprolol, propranolol, timolol	Increased plasma levels of beta blockers that undergo significant hepatic metabolism.	Use beta blockers that are not hepatically metabolized, such as atenolol or nadolol, or use an alternate H_2-receptor antagonist such as ranitidine or famotidine.

(cont'd)

Table 2: Cimetidine *(cont'd)*
Drug-Drug Interactions

Interacting Drug	Effect	Clinical Comment
Carbamazepine	Cimetidine may transiently increase plasma levels of carbamazepine by inhibiting its metabolism. Decreased carbamazepine clearance has been shown when steady states have not been reached. Transient decrease in carbamazepine clearances were observed in trials where cimetidine was withheld until steady state carbamazepine concentrations were attained.	Upon initiation of cimetidine, observe for signs and symptoms of carbamazepine toxicity such as somnolence, dizziness, nystagmus and twitching, especially during the first few weeks of therapy. Monitor for carbamazepine levels when cimetidine is discontinued or if there is a change in dose. Consider using an alternate H_2-receptor antagonist such as ranitidine.
Carmustine	Cimetidine may increase bone marrow suppression of carmustine by an unknown mechanism.	Monitor for excessive bone marrow suppression, such as leukopenia, thrombocytopenia, neutropenia, with concomitant use of cimetidine and carmustine. An alternate H_2-receptor antagonist such as ranitidine may be theoretically less likely to interact.
Clozapine	Cimetidine may increase serum clozapine levels by decreasing its hepatic metabolism.	Avoid combination. Monitor for signs and symptoms of clozapine toxicity such as diaphoresis, dizziness, vomiting, generalized weakness and lightheadedness on standing, if cimetidine is initiated and decreased therapeutic effects when cimetidine is discontinued. Consider using an alternate H_2-receptor antagonist such as ranitidine.
Cyclosporine	Concomitant use may increase serum creatinine levels as it may compete with creatinine for renal tubular secretion; blood cyclosporine levels seem not affected by cimetidine.	Monitor serum creatinine levels if used concomitantly. Consider using an alternate H_2-receptor antagonist such as ranitidine.
Diltiazem	Cimetidine may increase serum levels of diltiazem by inhibiting hepatic metabolism of diltiazem.	Monitor patients for bradycardia or hypotension when initiating, discontinuing or changing the dose of cimetidine. Adjust diltiazem dose, if needed. Consider using an alternate H_2-receptor antagonist.
Dofetilide[a]	Cimetidine may increase plasma dofetilide levels by reducing renal and hepatic metabolism of dofetilide.	Avoid combination because it may result in QT_c interval prolongation with cimetidine co-administration. Consider using an alternate H_2-receptor antagonist such as ranitidine at doses ≤150 mg twice daily if necessary. May consider proton pump inhibitors and antacids.
Erlotinib	By suppressing gastric acid, cimetidine may decrease absorption resulting in decreased serum levels of erlotinib.	Avoid combination. Separating the doses may not prevent this interaction.
Ethanol	Cimetidine may increase ethanol peak levels by increasing its absorption and decreasing its metabolism.	Avoid combination. Combination can lead to increased risk of intoxication and worsening of symptoms related to peptic ulcer or gastroesophageal reflux disease.
Lidocaine	Cimetidine may increase lidocaine serum levels by inhibiting its metabolism, decrease its protein binding and/or decrease its volume of distribution.	Clinical significance unknown. If used concomitantly, monitor for adverse effects of lidocaine toxicity such as lightheadedness and paresthesias. Measure lidocaine plasma levels. Adjust lidocaine dose, if needed. Consider using an alternate H_2-receptor antagonist such as ranitidine, famotidine or nizatidine.
Metformin	Cimetidine may increase metformin serum levels by inhibiting its tubular secretion resulting in reduced renal clearance.	Consider using an alternate H_2-receptor antagonist such as famotidine. Monitor for signs and symptoms of lactic acidosis such as hyperventilation, tachycardia or nausea, if used concomitantly, especially in patients with reduced renal function. Adjust metformin dose, if needed.
Mirtazapine	Remeron RD product monograph lists cimetidine as an agent that increases the AUC of mirtazapine by about 60%.	Consider monitoring for somnolence and arrhythmia with concomitant use. Adjust mirtazapine dose when initiating, discontinuing or changing the dose of cimetidine.
Nifedipine	Cimetidine may increase nifedipine serum levels by inhibiting its metabolism and/or increasing its bioavailability due to increased pH.	Monitor patients for altered effects of nifedipine when initiating, discontinuing or changing the dose of cimetidine. Adjust nifedipine dose if needed.

(cont'd)

Table 2: Cimetidine *(cont'd)*

Drug-Drug Interactions

Interacting Drug	Effect	Clinical Comment
Phenytoin	Cimetidine may increase serum phenytoin levels by inhibiting its hepatic metabolism.	Avoid combination. Monitor for signs and symptoms of phenytoin toxicity such as nystagmus, ataxia or confusion with concomitant use. Monitor phenytoin levels upon initiation, discontinuation or change in dose of cimetidine.
Procainamide	Cimetidine may increase procainamide and its metabolite, N-acetylprocainamide serum levels by decreasing its clearance.	Avoid combination. Monitor serum procainamide and NAPA levels. Adjust procainamide dose, if needed.
Quinidine	Cimetidine may increase serum quinidine levels by inhibiting its hepatic metabolism and/or decreasing its renal clearance and/or increased absorption.	Avoid combination. Monitor for signs and symptoms of quinidine toxicity such as ECG abnormalities with concomitant use. Monitor quinidine serum levels upon initiation, discontinuation or change in dose of cimetidine. Consider using an alternate H_2-receptor antagonist such as ranitidine, famotidine and nizatidine.
Selective Serotonin Reuptake Inhibitors (SSRIs), i.e., citalopram, escitalopram, paroxetine	Cimetidine may increase serum levels of SSRIs by inhibiting CYP2C19.	Monitor for altered SSRI effect when cimetidine is initiated, discontinued or changed in dose. Adjust SSRI dose as needed. Consider using an alternate H_2-receptor antagonist such as ranitidine.
Sirolimus	The Rapamune product monograph lists cimetidine as an agent that may increase sirolimus blood levels.	Monitor blood sirolimus trough levels when cimetidine is initiated, discontinued or if there is a change in the dose.
Tacrolimus	Advagraf and Prograf product monographs lists cimetidine as an agent that may increase tacrolimus blood levels.	Monitor for signs and symptoms of tacrolimus toxicity such as hypomagnesemia, mild elevations of renal function makers such as creatinine, hyperreflexia, oliguria, tremor and elevations in liver enzymes with concomitant use.
Theophyllines, e.g. aminophylline, theophylline	Cimetidine may increase serum theophylline levels by inhibiting its hepatic metabolism.	Monitor for signs and symptoms of theophylline toxicity such as seizures, arrhythmias, metabolic abnormalities (e.g., hypokalemia, hypomagnesemia, hypophosphatemia) with concomitant use. Monitor theophylline levels upon initiation, discontinuation or change in dose of cimetidine. If cimetidine is initiated, a decrease in the theophylline dose may be necessary. Consider using an alternate H_2-receptor antagonist such as ranitidine, famotidine and nizatidine.
Tricyclic Antidepressants, i.e., amitriptyline, desipramine, doxepin, imipramine, nortriptyline	Cimetidine may increase serum levels of tricyclic antidepressants by inhibiting its hepatic metabolism and/or increasing its bioavailability.	Consider using an alternate H_2-receptor antagonist such as ranitidine, famotidine and nizatidine. Adjust dose of the tricyclic antidepressant as necessary, if used concomitantly. Monitor for anticholinergic symptoms such as severe dry mouth, urinary retention, dizziness and blurred vision with concomitant use.
Warfarin	Cimetidine may inhibit hepatic metabolism of warfarin therefore increasing its effects.	Avoid combination. If used concomitantly, monitor INR and signs and symptoms of bleeding when cimetidine is initiated, discontinued or if there is a change in the dose. Adjust warfarin dose as necessary. Consider using an alternate H_2-receptor antagonist such as ranitidine, famotidine and nizatidine.

[a] Available through the Special Access Programme, Health Canada.

Drug-Food Interactions: Take cimetidine with meals and at bedtime. See Action and Clinical Pharmacology, Pharmacokinetics, Absorption.

Drug-Laboratory Interactions: Patients should be off cimetidine for at least one week prior to the urea breath test for *H. pylori*, to prevent false negative results.

Cimetidine may increase levels of the following tests: alanine aminotransferase, serum alkaline phosphatase, serum amylase, serum aspartate aminotransaminase, serum bilirubin, blood urea nitrogen, serum C3 complement, serum creatinine, plasma follicle stimulating hormone, serum gamma-glutamyltransferase, serum high-density lipoprotein cholesterol, serum lactate dehydrogenase, serum lipase, serum prolactin, serum testosterone, serum uric acid.

Cimetidine may decrease levels of the following tests: blood erythrocytes, plasma insulin, plasma parathyroid hormone assay, blood platelet, urine porphobilinogen, serum testosterone, serum triiodothyronine (T_3).

DOSAGE AND ADMINISTRATION: Recommended Dose and Dosage Adjustment: Adults: See Table 3.

Table 3: Cimetidine

Dose in Adult Patients

Indication	Dose	Duration of Therapy	Clinical Comment
Duodenal ulcer, active	800 mg po once daily or 600 mg po BID or 300 mg po QID	4 weeks minimum	
Duodenal ulcer, prevention of recurrence	400 mg po daily or 300 mg po BID	At least 6 to 12 months	
Gastric ulcer, active	800 mg po once daily or 400 mg po BID or 600 mg po BID or 300 mg po QID	6 to 8 weeks minimum	
Gastric ulcer, prevention of recurrence	400 mg po once daily or 300 mg po BID	At least 6 to 12 months	
Gastroesophageal reflux disease (GERD)	800 mg po once daily or 600 mg po BID or 300 mg po QID	8 to 12 weeks	
NSAID-induced lesions, treatment	800 mg po once daily or 400 mg po BID	If duodenal ulcer: 4 weeks minimum If gastric ulcer: 6 to 8 weeks	Discontinue NSAID, if possible. Test and treat if positive for *H. pylori*. Double dose of H_2RAs effectively reduce the risk of NSAID-induced gastric and duodenal endoscopic ulcers. Standard doses are not effective.
NSAID-induced lesions, prevention of recurrence	400 mg po once daily	At least 6 to 12 months if NSAID is discontinued	If ongoing NSAID treatment required, recurrence of lesions may be prevented by continuous concomitant treatment with cimetidine. However, PPIs are more effective than H_2RAs.
Pathologic hypersecretory conditions (e.g., Zollinger-Ellison syndrome)	300 mg po QID. Maximum 2400 mg po daily	Indefinite	PPIs may be more effective in suppressing acid secretion in patients with Zollinger-Ellison syndrome. Cimetidine 400 mg po BID has been used in systemic mastocytosis.
Helicobacter pylori eradication	Cimetidine 400 mg po BID Bismuth subsalicylate 525 mg po QID (available as 262 mg tablets) Metronidazole 250 mg po QID Tetracycline 500 mg po QID	10 to 14 days	Quadruple therapy requires complex dosing frequency and high pill count. Predictors of treatment failure include poor compliance and antibiotic resistance. Consider in patients with penicillin hypersensitivity or in those previously treated with macrolides. PPIs are considered first line. H_2RA can be substituted in the quadruple therapy, if patient cannot tolerate PPIs.
Non-ulcer dyspepsia (NUD)	400 mg po BID		Relative to placebo and antacids, cimetidine showed benefit in relieving pain and nausea, but not bloating, when given for 6 weeks. Patients with NUD may benefit from cimetidine therapy as it may relieve epigastric discomfort.

Pediatrics: See Table 4.

Table 4: Cimetidine

Dose in Pediatric Patients

Age	Dose	Maximum dose	Clinical Comment
0 to 4 weeks	5 to 10 mg/kg/day in divided doses every 8 to 12 hours	The maximum dose in pediatric patients should not exceed the maximum adult dose for the same clinical use Table 3).	Data is limited.
1 month to 1 year	10 to 20 mg/kg/day in divided doses every 6 to 12 hours		
1 year to 12 years	20 to 40 mg/kg/day in divided doses every 6 hours		

Renal Impairment: See Table 5.

Table 5: Cimetidine

Dose in Adult Patients with Renal Impairment

Creatinine Clearance	Dose Adjustment
>50 mL/min	No adjustment
10–50 mL/min	Decrease dose by 50%
<10 mL/min	Decrease dose by 75%

Dosage in Dialysis: In patients with renal insufficiency, cimetidine may cause mental confusion possibly because of high plasma concentrations. Patients undergoing hemodialysis may experience gastric hypersecretion. Cimetidine should be given after hemodialysis because 5 to 20% is dialyzable. Peritoneal dialysis does not remove cimetidine and no adjustment is necessary.

Hepatic Impairment: Reduce cimetidine dose in severe liver disease. Cimetidine may cause confusion in patients with hepatic insufficiency possibly because of high plasma concentrations.

Administration: Usually taken with food and at bedtime.

OVERDOSAGE:

For management of a suspected drug overdose, CPhA recommends that you contact your **regional Poison Control Centre**. See the *CPS* Directory section for a list of Poison Control Centres.

ACTION AND CLINICAL PHARMACOLOGY: Mechanism of Action: By competitively inhibiting histamine at the H_2-receptor, cimetidine reduces gastric acid secretion under basal conditions and when stimulated with food or caffeine. In patients with peptic ulcer disease or Zollinger-Ellison syndrome, the basal gastric acid secretions are inhibited to a greater extent than meal-stimulated acid secretion at a given blood concentration of cimetidine.

Pharmacokinetics: Adults: Absorption: Cimetidine is rapidly and well absorbed following oral administration. Oral bioavailability is between 60 and 70%. When cimetidine is taken with meals, its absorption is delayed and slightly decreased; however, cimetidine is administered with food because peak concentrations and therefore maximal antisecretory effects of cimetidine are achieved when the stomach is no longer protected by the buffering capacity of food. The onset of action of cimetidine ranges from 15 to 60 minutes. Duration of action ranges from 4 to 8 hours.

Distribution: Cimetidine is 15 to 20% bound to plasma proteins. Cimetidine crosses the placenta. It also distributes into breast milk. Volume of distribution ranges from 0.8 to 1.3 L/kg which is also age-dependent, decreasing with increasing age.

Metabolism: Cimetidine is metabolized in the liver to sulfoxide and 5-hydroxymethyl derivatives and may represent 25 to 40% of the total elimination of cimetidine.

Excretion: Cimetidine is primarily excreted in the urine as unchanged drug. In patients with normal renal function, the elimination half-life of cimetidine is 2 hours. In patients with creatinine clearance of 20 to 50 mL/min, the half-life is 2.9 hours. In patients with creatinine clearance of less than 20 mL/min, the half-life is 3.7 hours. In patients who are anephric, the half-life of cimetidine is 5 hours.

Cimzia™ Ⓟ

certolizumab pegol

Biological Response Modifier

UCB

Date of Preparation: August 12, 2009
Date of Revision: May 26, 2010

CIMZIA (certolizumab pegol) should be prescribed by physicians who have sufficient knowledge of rheumatoid arthritis and who have fully familiarized themselves with the efficacy/safety profile of CIMZIA.

SUMMARY PRODUCT INFORMATION:

Route of Administration	Dosage Form/ Strength	Clinically Relevant Nonmedicinal Ingredients
Subcutaneous (SC) Injection	Solution for injection in a single-use prefilled glass syringe/200 mg/mL	None For a complete listing see Dosage Forms, Composition and Packaging.

DESCRIPTION: CIMZIA (certolizumab pegol) is a recombinant, humanized antibody Fab' fragment, with specificity for human tumor necrosis factor alpha (TNFα). The Fab' fragment is manufactured in *E. coli* and is subsequently purified and conjugated to polyethylene glycol (PEG).

INDICATIONS AND CLINICAL USE: CIMZIA (certolizumab pegol) in combination with methotrexate (MTX) is indicated for:

- reducing signs and symptoms, inducing major clinical response, and reducing the progression of joint damage as assessed by X-ray, in adult patients with moderately to severely active rheumatoid arthritis (RA).

CIMZIA may be used alone for reducing signs and symptoms in adult patients with moderately to severely active rheumatoid arthritis (RA) who do not tolerate MTX.

Geriatrics (≥65 years of age): Specific clinical studies have not been performed in elderly subjects (see Warnings and Precautions, Special Populations, Geriatrics (≥65 years of age)).

Pediatrics (<18 years of age): Safety and efficacy of CIMZIA in pediatric patients have not been established.

CONTRAINDICATIONS:

- Patients with known hypersensitivity to CIMZIA (certolizumab pegol) or any of its components. For a complete listing, see Dosage Forms, Composition and Packaging.
- Patients with active tuberculosis or other severe infections such as sepsis, abscesses and opportunistic infections.

WARNINGS AND PRECAUTIONS:

Serious Warnings and Precautions
SERIOUS INFECTIONS
SERIOUS INFECTIONS, SEPSIS, TUBERCULOSIS (INCLUDING MILIARY, DISSEMINATED AND EXTRAPULMONARY DISEASE), INVASIVE FUNGAL INFECTIONS (SUCH AS HISTOPLASMOSIS) AND OTHER OPPORTUNISTIC INFECTIONS, SOME OF WHICH HAVE BEEN FATAL, HAVE BEEN REPORTED IN PATIENTS RECEIVING TNF BLOCKING AGENTS INCLUDING CIMZIA (CERTOLIZUMAB PEGOL). MANY OF THE SERIOUS INFECTIONS REPORTED HAVE OCCURRED IN PATIENTS ON CONCOMITANT IMMUNOSUPPRESSIVE THERAPY THAT, IN ADDITION TO THEIR RHEUMATOID ARTHRITIS, COULD PREDISPOSE THEM TO INFECTIONS. CIMZIA SHOULD NOT BE GIVEN TO PATIENTS WITH A CLINICALLY IMPORTANT INFECTION, INCLUDING CHRONIC OR LOCALIZED INFECTIONS. PHYSICIANS SHOULD EXERCISE CAUTION WHEN CONSIDERING THE USE OF CIMZIA IN PATIENTS WITH A HISTORY OF RECURRING INFECTION. PATIENTS SHOULD BE MONITORED FOR SIGNS AND SYMPTOMS OF INFECTION WHILE ON AND AFTER TREATMENT WITH CIMZIA.
ANY NEW INFECTION THAT DEVELOPS WHILE ON CIMZIA, OR AFTER RECENT TREATMENT, SHOULD BE CLOSELY MONITORED. CIMZIA SHOULD BE DISCONTINUED IF A PATIENT DEVELOPS A SERIOUS INFECTION (see Warnings and Precautions, Serious Infections).
MALIGNANCY
LYMPHOMA AND OTHER MALIGNANCIES, SOME FATAL, HAVE BEEN REPORTED IN CHILDREN AND ADOLESCENT PATIENTS TREATED WITH TNF BLOCKERS, OF WHICH CIMZIA IS A MEMBER (see Warnings and Precautions, Malignancies). CIMZIA IS NOT INDICATED FOR USE IN PEDIATRIC PATIENTS.

Serious Infections: Serious and sometimes fatal infection due to bacterial, mycobacterial, invasive fungal, viral, or other opportunistic pathogens has been reported in patients receiving TNF blocking agents. Among opportunistic infections, tuberculosis (TB), histoplasmosis, aspergillosis, candidiasis, coccidioidomycosis, listeriosis, and pneumocystosis were the most common. Patients have frequently presented with disseminated rather than localized disease and are often taking concomitant immunosuppressants that, in addition to their underlying disease, could predispose them to infections.

Treatment with CIMZIA should not be initiated in patients with an active infection, including clinically important localized infections. The risks and benefits of treatment should be considered prior to initiating therapy in patients:

- with chronic or recurrent infection
- who have been exposed to tuberculosis
- who have resided or traveled in areas of endemic tuberculosis or endemic mycoses, such as histoplasmosis, coccidioidomycosis, or blastomycosis
- with underlying conditions that may predispose them to infection

CIMZIA should be discontinued if a patient develops a serious infection or sepsis. A patient who develops a new infection during treatment with CIMZIA should be closely monitored, undergo a prompt and complete diagnostic workup appropriate for an immunocompromised patient, and appropriate antimicrobial therapy should be initiated.

For patients who reside or travel in regions where mycoses are endemic, invasive fungal infection should be suspected if they develop a serious systemic illness. Appropriate empiric antifungal therapy should be considered while a diagnostic workup is being performed. Antigen and antibody testing for histoplasmosis may be negative in some patients with active infection. When feasible, the decision to administer empiric antifungal therapy in these patients should be made in consultation with a physician with expertise in the diagnosis and treatment of invasive fungal infections and should take into account both the risk for severe fungal infection and risks of antifungal therapy.

Tuberculosis: Cases of reactivation of tuberculosis or new tuberculosis infections have been observed in patients receiving CIMZIA, including patients who have previously received treatment for latent or active tuberculosis. Before initiation of therapy with CIMZIA, all patients must be evaluated for both active and inactive (latent) tuberculosis infection. This evaluation should include a detailed medical history of tuberculosis or possible previous exposure to patients with active tuberculosis and previous and/or current immunosuppressive therapy. Appropriate screening tests, e.g. tuberculin skin test and chest X-ray, should be performed in all patients and interpreted in accordance with the current Canadian Tuberculosis Standards guidelines. Prescribers are reminded of the risk of false negative tuberculin skin test results, especially in patients who are severely ill or immunocompromised.

If active tuberculosis is diagnosed, CIMZIA therapy must not be initiated. If latent tuberculosis is diagnosed or suspected, appropriate anti-tuberculosis prophylaxis should be instituted in accordance with the current Canadian Tuberculosis Standards guidelines before starting treatment with CIMZIA. In this situation, the benefit/risk balance of therapy with CIMZIA should be very carefully considered. Patients should be instructed to seek medical advice if signs/symptoms (e.g., persistent cough, wasting/weight loss, low grade fever) suggestive of a tuberculosis infection occur during or after initiation of therapy with CIMZIA (see Adverse Reactions, Adverse Drug Reaction Overview, Infections, Tuberculosis and Opportunistic Infections).

Malignancies: In clinical studies with CIMZIA and other TNF blocking agents, more cases of malignancies have been observed among patients receiving active drug than in placebo patients.

In rheumatoid arthritis placebo-controlled and open-label studies combined, most observed malignancies included lung, breast and ovarian cancers, basal cell carcinoma, and lymphoma. Three cases of lymphoma were reported in patients treated with CIMZIA (1 case in the placebo-controlled studies and 2 in the open-label studies), corresponding to a rate of 0.09 (0.02-0.27)/100 patient-years among 2367 patients. This is approximately 2-fold higher than expected in the general population. Patients with RA, particularly those with highly active disease, are at a higher risk for the development of lymphoma. Malignancies other than lymphomas and non-melanoma skin cancers were observed at a rate (95% confidence interval) of 0.61 (0.37-0.94)/100 patient-years among 2367 CIMZIA-treated patients and 0.41 (0.01-2.27)/100 patient-years among 647 placebo-treated patients.

The size of the control groups and limited duration of the controlled portions of the studies preclude the ability to draw firm conclusions but the possible risk for the development of lymphomas or other malignancies in patients treated with a TNF blocker cannot be excluded. The potential role of TNF blocking therapy in the development of malignancies is not known.

Rates in clinical trials for CIMZIA cannot be compared to rates for other TNF blockers and may not predict the rates observed in a broader patient population. Patients with rheumatoid arthritis, particularly those with highly active disease, are at a higher risk for development of lymphoma (see Adverse Reactions, Adverse Drug Reaction Overview, Malignancies).

Malignancies, some fatal, have been reported among children, adolescents, and young adults who received treatment with TNF blocking agents (initiation of therapy ≤18 years of age), of which CIMZIA is a member. Approximately half the cases were lymphomas, including Hodgkin's and non-Hodgkin's lymphomas. The other cases represented a variety of different malignancies and included rare malignancies usually associated with immunosuppression and malignancies that are not usually observed in children and adolescents. The malignancies occurred after a median of 30 months of therapy (range 1 to 84 months). Most of the patients were receiving concomitant immunosuppressants. These cases were reported post-marketing and are derived from a variety of sources including registries and spontaneous post-marketing reports.

Leukemia: Cases of acute and chronic leukemia have been reported in association with post-marketing TNF blocker use in RA and other indications. Even in the absence of TNF blocker therapy, patients with RA may be at higher risk (approximately 2-fold) than the general population for the development of leukemia.

Heart Failure: Cases of worsening congestive heart failure (CHF) and new onset CHF have been reported with TNF blockers, including CIMZIA. CIMZIA has not been formally studied in patients with CHF; however, in clinical studies in patients with CHF with another TNF blocker, worsening CHF and increased mortality due to CHF were observed. Exercise caution in patients with heart failure and monitor them carefully (see Adverse Reactions, Adverse Drug Reaction Overview, Heart Failure).

Hepatitis B Virus Reactivation: Use of TNF blockers, including CIMZIA, may increase the risk of reactivation of hepatitis B virus (HBV) in patients who are chronic carriers of this virus. In some instances, HBV reactivation occurring in conjunction with TNF blocker therapy has been fatal. The majority of these reports have occurred in patients concomitantly receiving other medications that suppress the immune system, which may also contribute to HBV reactivation. Patients at risk for HBV infection should be evaluated for prior evidence of HBV infection before initiating CIMZIA therapy. Prescribers should exercise caution in prescribing TNF blockers for patients identified as carriers of HBV. Adequate data are not available on the safety or efficacy of treating patients who are carriers of HBV with TNF blocker therapy, in conjunction with anti-viral therapy, to prevent HBV reactivation. Patients who are carriers of HBV and require treatment with TNF blockers should be closely monitored for clinical and laboratory signs of active HBV infection throughout therapy and for several months following termination of therapy. In patients who develop HBV reactivation, CIMZIA should be stopped and effective anti-viral therapy with appropriate supportive treatment should be initiated. The safety of resuming TNF blocker therapy after HBV reactivation is not known. In this situation, prescribers should exercise caution when considering resumption of CIMZIA therapy and monitor patients closely.

Hematological Reactions: Rare reports of pancytopenia, including aplastic anemia, have been reported with TNF blocking agents. Adverse events of the hematologic system, including medically significant cytopenia (e.g., leukopenia, pancytopenia, thrombocytopenia) have been infrequently reported with CIMZIA. The causal relationship of these reports to CIMZIA remains unclear. Prescribers should exercise caution in considering the use of CIMZIA in patients who have or have had significant hematologic abnormalities. All patients should be advised to seek immediate medical attention if they develop signs and symptoms suggestive of blood dyscrasias or infection (e.g., persistent fever, bruising, bleeding, pallor) while on CIMZIA. Discontinuation of CIMZIA therapy should be considered in patients with confirmed significant hematologic abnormalities.

Neurologic Reactions: Use of TNF blocking agents has been associated with rare cases of new onset or exacerbation of clinical symptoms and/or radiographic evidence of demyelinating disease. Prescribers should exercise caution in considering the use of CIMZIA in patients with pre-existing or recent-onset central nervous system demyelinating disorders. Neurological disorders, including seizure disorder, optic neuritis, and peripheral neuropathy have been reported in patients treated with CIMZIA. Causal relationship to CIMZIA remains unclear.

Use with Other Biologic Medicines: The use of CIMZIA in combination with other biologic medicines has not been studied. An increased risk of serious infections has been seen in clinical studies of other TNF blocking agents used in combination with anakinra or abatacept, with no added benefit. Because of the nature of the adverse events seen with this combination therapy, similar toxicities may also result from the combination of CIMZIA and other biologic disease modifying anti-rheumatic drugs (DMARDs). Therefore, the use of CIMZIA in combination with other biologic DMARDs is not recommended (see Drug Interactions).

Switching Between Biologic DMARDs: When switching from one biologic DMARD to another, patients should continue to be monitored for signs of infection.

Hypersensitivity: The following symptoms that could be compatible with hypersensitivity reactions have been reported rarely following CIMZIA administration to patients: angioedema, dyspnea, hypotension, rash, serum sickness, and urticaria. If such reactions occur, discontinue further administration of CIMZIA and institute appropriate therapy. There are no data on the risks of using CIMZIA in patients who have experienced a severe hypersensitivity reaction towards another TNF blocker; in these patients caution is needed.

Autoimmunity: Treatment with CIMZIA may result in the formation of autoantibodies. If a patient develops symptoms suggestive of a lupus-like syndrome following treatment with CIMZIA, treatment should be discontinued (see Adverse Reactions, Adverse Drug Reaction Overview, Autoantibodies).

Immunizations: No data are available on the response to vaccinations or the secondary transmission of infection by live vaccines in patients receiving CIMZIA. Live vaccines should not be administered concurrently with CIMZIA. The efficacy of vaccination in patients receiving CIMZIA is not known. Based on its mechanism of action, CIMZIA may blunt the effectiveness of some immunizations (see Drug Interactions).

Immunosuppression: Since TNF mediates inflammation and modulates cellular immune responses, the possibility exists for TNF blocking agents, including CIMZIA, to affect host defenses against infections and malignancies. The impact of treatment with CIMZIA on the development and course of malignancies, as well as active and/or chronic infections, is not fully understood. The use of CIMZIA in patients with severe immunosuppression has not been formally evaluated (see Adverse Reactions, Adverse Drug Reaction Overview, Infections; Tuberculosis and Opportunistic Infections; Malignancies).

Laboratory Tests: Interference with certain coagulation assays has been detected in patients treated with CIMZIA. Certolizumab pegol may cause erroneously elevated activated partial thromboplastin time (aPTT) assay results in patients without coagulation abnormalities. There is no evidence that CIMZIA therapy has an effect on in vivo coagulation. After patients receive CIMZIA, careful attention should be used in selecting the type of method used to measure coagulation (see Drug Interactions, Drug-Laboratory Test Interactions).

Carcinogenesis and Mutagenesis: Long-term animal studies of CIMZIA have not been conducted to assess its carcinogenic potential. Certolizumab pegol was not genotoxic in the Ames test, the human peripheral blood lymphocytes chromosomal aberration assay, or the mouse bone marrow micronucleus assay.

Special Populations: Pregnant Women: There are no adequate and well-controlled studies of CIMZIA in pregnant women. Since certolizumab pegol does not cross-react with mouse or rat TNFα, reproductive studies were performed in rats using a rodent anti-murine TNFα PEGylated Fab' fragment (cTN3 PF) similar to certolizumab pegol. Doses up to and including 100 mg/kg revealed no evidence of impaired fertility or harm to the fetus due to cTN3 PF. Because animal reproduction and developmental studies are not always predictive of human response, CIMZIA should be used during pregnancy only if clearly needed.

Nursing Women: It is not known whether CIMZIA is excreted in human milk or absorbed systemically. Rodent studies have shown limited excretion of cTN3 PF (a rodent anti-murine TNFa PEGylated Fab' fragment similar to certolizumab pegol) in milk. Because many drugs and immunoglobulins are excreted in human milk and because of the potential for serious adverse reactions in nursing infants from CIMZIA, a decision should be made whether to discontinue nursing or discontinue the drug, taking into account the importance of the drug to the mother.

Pediatrics (<18 years of age): Safety and efficacy of CIMZIA in pediatric patients have not been established.

Geriatrics (≥65 years of age): Specific clinical studies have not been performed in elderly subjects. Because there is a higher incidence of infections in the elderly population in general, caution should be used when treating the elderly.

ADVERSE REACTIONS: Adverse Drug Reaction Overview: The most serious adverse reactions were (see Warnings and Precautions):

- serious infections
- malignancies
- heart failure

The data described below reflect the exposure to CIMZIA (certolizumab pegol) in 2367 RA patients, including 2030 exposed for at least 6 months, 1663 exposed for at least one year and 282 for at least 2 years and 1774 in adequate and well-controlled studies. CIMZIA was studied primarily in placebo-controlled trials and in long-term follow-up studies. In placebo-controlled studies, the population had a median age of 53 years at entry; approximately 80% were female, 93% were Caucasian and all patients were suffering from active RA, with a median disease duration of 6.2 years. Most patients received the recommended dose of CIMZIA or higher.

The most commonly occurring adverse reactions, reported in a greater percentage of CIMZIA-treated patients in all placebo-controlled trials (difference ≥2%) were upper respiratory tract infections (17.6% for CIMZIA, 9.4% for placebo), lower respiratory tract and lung infections 5.6% for CIMZIA, 3.4% for placebo), musculoskeletal and connective tissue signs and symptoms (6.7% for CIMZIA, 4.2% for placebo), herpes viral infections (3.6% for CIMZIA, 1.2% for placebo), rashes, eruptions and exanthems (4.0% for CIMZIA, 1.3% for placebo), and vascular hypertensive disorders (5.1% for CIMZIA, 1.2% for placebo).

The percentage of patients who discontinued treatment due to adverse reactions during the phase III RA placebo-controlled studies were 5% for CIMZIA-treated patients and 2.5% for placebo-treated patients. The most common adverse reactions leading to discontinuation of CIMZIA were tuberculosis infections (0.5%); and pyrexia, urticaria, pneumonia, and rash (0.3%).

Deaths: In the placebo-controlled studies, 9 of 1774 patients (0.51%) who received CIMZIA at any dose, compared with 1 of 647 patients (0.15%) who received placebo, died. The most common causes leading to death in patients who received CIMZIA were cardiovascular events and/or infections. All cardiovascular deaths were in patients with pre-existing history of cardiovascular conditions.

In the combined placebo-controlled and open-label studies in patients with RA, 28 deaths occurred in patients who received CIMZIA over 3218.0 patient-years of exposure (1 death per 115 patient-years) and 1 death occurred in a placebo-treated patient over 224.9 patient-years of exposure (1 death per 225 patient-years). Cardiovascular (primarily in predisposed patients) and/or infectious events were the most common causes leading to death in patients who received CIMZIA.

Infections: The incidence of new cases of infections in placebo-controlled clinical studies in rheumatoid arthritis was 0.91 per patient-year for all CIMZIA-treated patients and 0.72 per patient-year for placebo-treated patients. The infections consisted primarily of upper respiratory tract infections, herpes infections, urinary tract infections, and lower respiratory tract infections.

In the placebo-controlled studies, there were more new cases of serious infection adverse reactions in the CIMZIA treatment groups, compared to the placebo groups (0.06 per patient-year for all CIMZIA doses vs 0.02 per patient-year for placebo). Rates of serious infections in the 200 mg every other week dose group were 0.06 per patient-year and 0.04 in the 400 mg every 4 weeks dose group. Serious infections included tuberculosis, pneumonia, cellulitis, pyelonephritis, and erysipelas. In the placebo group, no serious infection occurred in more than one subject. There is no evidence of increased risk of infections with continued exposure over time (see Warnings and Precautions, Serious Warnings and Precautions).

Tuberculosis and Opportunistic Infections: In placebo-controlled and open-label rheumatoid arthritis studies, there were 36 cases of TB reported which occurred with CIMZIA treatment and none on placebo. The majority of cases occurred in countries with high endemic rates of TB. No cases of TB have been reported in the US or Canada. Reports include cases of miliary, lymphatic, peritoneal, as well as pulmonary TB. In rare cases, tuberculosis has been fatal. Rare cases of opportunistic infections have also been reported in these clinical trials (see Warnings and Precautions, Serious Warnings and Precautions, and Serious Infections).

Malignancies: A total of 12 malignancies were identified during the placebo-controlled studies. Eleven patients (0.6%) among 1774 patients receiving CIMZIA and 1 patient (0.2%) among 647 patients receiving placebo experienced malignancies. In the controlled and uncontrolled studies, there were 30 malignancies among 2367 CIMZIA-treated patients.

Lymphoma: In rheumatoid arthritis placebo-controlled and open-label studies combined, 3 cases of lymphoma were reported in patients treated with CIMZIA (1 case in the placebo-controlled studies and 2 in the open-label studies), corresponding to a rate of 0.09 (0.02-0.27)/100 patient-years among 2367 patients. No lymphoma was reported among 647 placebo-treated patients.

Non-Lymphoma Malignancies: In the rheumatoid arthritis placebo-controlled studies, 8 patients (0.045%) treated with CIMZIA and 1 patient (0.2%) in the placebo group experienced malignancies other than lymphomas and non-melanoma skin cancers (NMSC).

In rheumatoid arthritis placebo-controlled and open-label studies combined, 20 malignancies other than lymphomas and non-melanoma skin cancers were observed at a rate (95% confidence interval) of 0.61 (0.37-0.94)/100 patient-years among 2367 CIMZIA-treated patients and 1 malignancy (bladder cancer) at a rate of 0.41 (0.01-2.27)/100 patient-years among 647 placebo-treated patients. Observed malignancies included 1 endocrine, 5 gastrointestinal, 2 breast, 1 hepatobiliary, 7 reproductive, 2 renal and urinary tract, 1 respiratory tract and 1 metastases malignancies.

Non-Melanoma Skin Cancers: In the rheumatoid arthritis placebo-controlled studies, non-melanoma skin cancers occurred in 2 patients (0.1%) receiving CIMZIA and no patient in the placebo group. In the controlled and uncontrolled studies, there were a total of 5 (6 events) non-melanoma skin cancers reported (see Warnings and Precautions, Malignancies).

Cardiovascular Disorders: In the placebo-controlled studies, the percentage of patients with any event in the cardiac disorders System Organ Class (SOC) was 3.4% in the CIMZIA-treated group (1.60 events per 100 patient-years) and 2.0% in the placebo group (1.23 events per 100 patient-years). Sixteen patients in the CIMZIA-treated group (0.9%; 1.63 per 100 patient-years) versus 3 patients in the placebo group (0.5%; 1.69 per 100 patient-years) reported a serious event in the cardiac disorders SOC.

In the CIMZIA-treated group, the most common cardiovascular events at the high level term across SOCs, compared with placebo, were vascular hypertensive disorders (5.1% vs 1.2%), rate and rhythm disorders (1.0% vs 0.2%), ischaemic coronary artery disorders (0.7% vs 0.3%), peripheral embolism and thrombosis (0.6% vs 0), and supraventricular arrhythmias (0.6% vs 0.5%). Four patients (0.2%) experienced cerebrovascular accidents (CVAs) and 4 patients (0.2%) experienced transient ischaemic attacks (TIAs) in the CIMZIA-treated group, compared with 1 patient (0.2%) who experienced a CVA in the placebo group. One patient, each, in the CIMZIA-treated and placebo groups experienced a pulmonary embolism. Three patients in the CIMZIA-treated group experienced hypertension events, including 2 vascular hypertension and 1 malignant hypertension events, compared with no patient in the placebo group.

Heart Failure: In placebo-controlled studies, 1 patient (0.1%) reported cardiac failure (0.11 per 100 patient-years) in the CIMZIA-treated patient group, compared to no patient in the placebo group. In the open-label rheumatoid arthritis studies, an additional 6 patients (0.3%) reported cardiac failure (where cardiac failure was the primary event), and of these, 3 died. All patients with cardiac failure events had other risk factors for cardiac disease.

The incidence rate per 100 patient-years of cardiac failure in both placebo-controlled and open-label studies was 0.18 (see Warnings and Precautions, Heart Failure).

Hepatic: In placebo-controlled rheumatoid arthritis studies, the adverse events of ALT elevated occurred in 2.6% of CIMZIA-treated and 2.3% of placebo-treated patients, and AST elevated occurred in 1.9% of CIMZIA and placebo-treated patients. Hepatic adverse events occurred in 1.7% of CIMZIA-treated patients and 1.1% of placebo-treated patients. In placebo-controlled and open-label rheumatoid arthritis studies combined, the incidence of hepatic adverse events in CIMZIA-treated patients was 2.07 per 100 patient-years, as compared to 2.87 per 100 patient-years during the placebo-controlled rheumatoid arthritis studies.

Autoantibodies: In placebo-controlled rheumatoid arthritis studies, there was no clinically meaningful increase in ANA or double-stranded DNA conversion noted for CIMZIA-treated patients at any dose. For subjects who were ANA negative at baseline, 16.7% of those treated with CIMZIA developed positive ANA titers, compared with 12.0% of subjects in the placebo group. Taking into account the difference in exposure between the 2 groups, there is no increased risk of developing a positive ANA with CIMZIA treatment. In both placebo-controlled and long-term follow-up studies for rheumatoid arthritis there were 3 cases of lupus-like syndrome, including one patient who had manifestations of lupus prior to treatment with CIMZIA. There have been rare reports of other immune-mediated conditions; the causal relationship to CIMZIA is not known. The impact of long-term treatment with CIMZIA on the development of autoimmune diseases is unknown.

Immunogenicity: The overall percentage of patients with antibodies to CIMZIA detectable on at least one occasion was 7% in the phase III RA placebo-controlled trials. Approximately one third (3%) of these patients had antibodies with neutralizing activity in vitro. Patients treated with concomitant immunosuppressants (methotrexate) had a lower rate of antibody development than patients not taking immunosuppressants at baseline. Antibody formation was associated with lowered drug plasma concentration and reduced efficacy. No association was seen between antibody development and the development of adverse events.

The data reflect the percentage of patients whose test results were considered positive for antibodies to certolizumab pegol in an ELISA assay, and are highly dependent on the sensitivity and specificity of the assay. Additionally, the observed incidence of antibodies in an assay may be influenced by several factors including sample handling, timing of sample collection, concomitant medications, and underlying disease. For these reasons, comparison of the incidence of antibodies to certolizumab pegol with the incidence of antibodies to other TNF blocking agents is not appropriate.

Clinical Trial Adverse Drug Reactions: Because clinical trials are conducted under very specific conditions the adverse reaction rates observed in the clinical trials may not reflect the rates observed in practice and should not be compared to the rates in the clinical trials of another drug. Adverse drug reaction information from clinical trials is useful for identifying drug-related adverse events and for approximating rates.

Table 1 summarizes the adverse reactions reported at a rate of at least 1% in patients treated with CIMZIA 200 mg every other week compared to placebo, given concomitantly with methotrexate in the phase III RA placebo-controlled studies. Table 2 summarizes the adverse reactions reported at a rate of at least 1% in patients treated with CIMZIA 400 mg every 4 weeks, compared to placebo, given without concomitant methotrexate in the phase III RA placebo-controlled study.

Table 1: CIMZIA

Adverse Reactions Reported by ≥1% of Patients Treated with CIMZIA 200 mg Dosed Every Other Week During Phase III Rheumatoid Arthritis Placebo-Controlled Studies, with Concomitant Methotrexate

Primary System Organ Class Adverse Event (Preferred Term)	Placebo + MTX (N=324) n (%)	CIMZIA 200 mg EOW + MTX (N=640) n (%)
Blood and Lymphatic System Disorders		
Eosinophilia	3 (0.9)	17 (2.7)
Leukopenia	4 (1.2)	8 (1.3)
Eye Disorders		
Conjunctivitis	1 (0.3)	8 (1.3)
Gastrointestinal Disorders		
Abdominal pain	1 (0.3)	8 (1.3)
Abdominal pain upper	1 (0.3)	11 (1.7)
Diarrhoea	5 (1.5)	10 (1.6)
Dyspepsia	7 (2.2)	15 (2.3)
Gastritis	0 (0.0)	9 (1.4)
Toothache	3 (0.9)	10 (1.6)
Vomiting	3 (0.9)	11 (1.7)
General Disorders and Administration Site Conditions		
Fatigue	7 (2.2)	19 (3.0)
Injection site discolouration	0 (0.0)	7 (1.1)
Injection site erythema	0 (0.0)	7 (1.1)
Injection site haematoma	0 (0.0)	8 (1.3)
Injection site pain	0 (0.0)	8 (1.3)
Injection site reaction	0 (0.0)	9 (1.4)
Pyrexia	6 (1.9)	21 (3.3)
Infections and Infestations		
Bronchitis	4 (1.2)	9 (1.4)
Bronchitis acute	4 (1.2)	19 (3.0)
Herpes simplex	1 (0.3)	16 (2.5)
Influenza	7 (2.2)	18 (2.8)
Nasopharyngitis	4 (1.2)	29 (4.5)
Pharyngitis	3 (0.9)	20 (3.1)
Respiratory tract infection	0 (0.0)	15 (2.3)
Respiratory tract infection viral	2 (0.6)	10 (1.6)
Rhinitis	2 (0.6)	13 (2.0)
Sinusitis	3 (0.9)	14 (2.2)
Tonsillitis	1 (0.3)	7 (1.1)
Upper respiratory tract infection	7 (2.2)	35 (5.5)
Viral infection	0 (0.0)	9 (1.4)

(cont'd)

Table 1: CIMZIA *(cont'd)*

Adverse Reactions Reported by ≥1% of Patients Treated with CIMZIA 200 mg Dosed Every Other Week During Phase III Rheumatoid Arthritis Placebo-Controlled Studies, with Concomitant Methotrexate

Primary System Organ Class Adverse Event (Preferred Term)	Placebo + MTX (N=324) n (%)	CIMZIA 200 mg EOW + MTX (N=640) n (%)
Investigations		
Activated partial thromboplastin time prolonged	2 (0.6)	12 (1.9)
Blood alkaline phosphatase increased	0 (0.0)	7 (1.1)
Gamma-glutamyltransferase increased	3 (0.9)	10 (1.6)
Hepatic enzyme increased	6 (1.9)	14 (2.2)
Musculoskeletal and Connective Tissue Disorders		
Arthralgia	6 (1.9)	16 (2.5)
Back pain	3 (0.9)	23 (3.6)
Pain in extremity	2 (0.6)	8 (1.3)
Nervous System Disorders		
Headache	12 (3.7)	31 (4.8)
Psychiatric Disorders		
Anxiety	2 (0.6)	10 (1.6)
Respiratory, Thoracic and Mediastinal Disorders		
Cough	2 (0.6)	12 (1.9)
Pharyngolaryngeal pain	0 (0.0)	9 (1.4)
Skin and Subcutaneous Tissue Disorders		
Rash	2 (0.6)	20 (3.1)
Vascular Disorders		
Hypertension	4 (1.2)	31 (4.8)

Legend: EOW=Every Other Week; MTX=Methotrexate.

Table 2: CIMZIA

Adverse Reactions Reported by ≥1% of Patients Treated with CIMZIA 400 mg Dosed Every 4 Weeks During the Phase III Rheumatoid Arthritis Placebo-Controlled Study, without Concomitant Methotrexate

Primary System Organ Class Adverse Event (Preferred Term)	Placebo (N=109) n (%)	CIMZIA 400 mg E4W (N=111) n (%)
Gastrointestinal Disorders		
Diarrhoea	3 (2.8)	8 (7.2)
Dry mouth	0 (0.0)	2 (1.8)
Gastritis	0 (0.0)	2 (1.8)
General Disorders and Administration Site Conditions		
Chest pain	1 (0.9)	3 (2.7)
Injection site rash	0 (0.0)	2 (1.8)
Injection site reaction	2 (1.8)	3 (2.7)
Infections and Infestations		
Influenza	0 (0.0)	5 (4.5)
Sinusitis	4 (3.7)	6 (5.4)
Upper respiratory tract infection	6 (5.5)	10 (9.0)
Injury, Poisoning and Procedural Complications		
Arthropod bite	0 (0.0)	2 (1.8)
Investigations		
Blood creatine phosphokinase increased	0 (0.0)	4 (3.6)
Gamma-glutamyltransferase increased	2 (1.8)	3 (2.7)
Haemoglobin decreased	1 (0.9)	2 (1.8)
Musculoskeletal and Connective Tissue Disorders		
Muscle cramp	0 (0.0)	3 (2.7)
Myalgia	0 (0.0)	2 (1.8)

(cont'd)

Table 2: CIMZIA *(cont'd)*

Adverse Reactions Reported by ≥1% of Patients Treated with CIMZIA 400 mg Dosed Every 4 Weeks During the Phase III Rheumatoid Arthritis Placebo-Controlled Study, without Concomitant Methotrexate

Primary System Organ Class Adverse Event (Preferred Term)	Placebo (N=109) n (%)	CIMZIA 400 mg E4W (N=111) n (%)
Osteoporosis	0 (0.0)	2 (1.8)
Rheumatoid arthritis aggravated	0 (0.0)	2 (1.8)
Nervous System Disorders		
Dizziness	1 (0.9)	2 (1.8)
Headache	9 (8.3)	13 (11.7)
Psychiatric Disorders		
Depression	0 (0.0)	3 (2.7)
Reproductive System and Breast Disorders		
Menometrorrhagia	0 (0.0)	2 (1.8)
Respiratory, Thoracic and Mediastinal Disorders		
Nasal congestion	1 (0.9)	2 (1.8)
Nasopharyngitis	4 (3.7)	6 (5.4)
Pharyngitis	1 (0.9)	3 (2.7)
Respiratory tract congestion	0 (0.0)	2 (1.8)
Sinus congestion	1 (0.9)	4 (3.6)
Skin and Subcutaneous Tissue Disorders		
Hypotrichosis	0 (0.0)	2 (1.8)
Pruritus	0 (0.0)	3 (2.7)

Legend: E4W=Every 4 Weeks.

Less Common Clinical Trial Adverse Drug Reactions (<1%): Other infrequent serious adverse drug reactions occurring at an incidence of less than 1% in rheumatoid arthritis patients treated with CIMZIA in placebo-controlled and open label trials were:
Blood and Lymphatic System Disorders: anaemia, thrombocytopenia.
Cardiac Disorders: cardiomyopathies (includes heart failure), ischemic coronary artery disorders (includes myocardial infarction, angina pectoris), arrhythmias (includes atrial fibrillation), palpitations, pericarditis.
Ear and Labyrinth Disorders: vertigo.
Eye Disorders: eye and eyelid inflammation.
Gastrointestinal Disorders: ascites, gastrointestinal ulceration and perforation, gastrointestinal tract inflammation (any site), stomatitis.
General Disorders and Administration Site Conditions: chills.
Hepatobiliary Disorders: hepatopathy (includes cirrhosis).
Immune System Disorders: vasculitides, lupus erythematosus, allergic disorders, sarcoidosis, serum sickness, angioneurotic edema.
Infections and Infestations: fungal infection (includes opportunistic), sepsis (includes multiorgan failure).
Metabolism and Nutrition Disorders: weight change, blood glucose changes, electrolyte imbalance.
Neoplasms Benign, Malignant and Unspecified (including cysts and polyps): solid organ tumor, benign tumor and cysts (includes skin papilloma), non-melanoma skin cancers, blood and lymphatic system malignancies, gastrointestinal tumor, melanoma.
Nervous System Disorders: peripheral neuropathies.
Psychiatric Disorders: suicide attempt.
Renal and Urinary Disorders: renal impairment, nephropathy (including nephritis).
Respiratory, Thoracic and Mediastinal Disorders: pleural effusion (and related symptoms), interstitial lung disease, pneumonitis.
Vascular Disorders: hemorrhage or bleeding (any site), hypercoagulation (includes pulmonary embolism, thrombophlebitis), cerebrovascular accident.

Post-Market Adverse Drug Reactions: Additional adverse events have been identified during post-marketing use of CIMZIA. Because these events are reported voluntarily from a population of uncertain size, it is not always possible to reliably estimate their frequency or establish a causal relationship to CIMZIA exposure. These adverse events include, but are not limited to, the following (listed by system organ class):
Gastrointestinal Disorders: intestinal obstruction.
General Disorders and Administration Site Conditions: asthenia, fistula (any site).
Nervous System Disorders: sensory abnormalities.
Pregnancy, Puerperium and Perinatal Conditions: spontaneous miscarriage.
Vascular Disorders: hypotension.

DRUG INTERACTIONS: Overview: CIMZIA (certolizumab pegol) may be used alone or in combination with methotrexate (MTX). Co-administration of certolizumab pegol with methotrexate had no significant effect on the pharmacokinetics of methotrexate.
Drug-Drug Interactions: Use with Other Biologic Medicines: An increased risk of serious infections has been seen in clinical studies of other TNF blocking agents used in combination with anakinra or abatacept, with no added benefit. Because of the nature of the adverse events seen with this combination therapy, similar toxicities may also result from the combination of CIMZIA and other biologic DMARDs. Therefore, the use of CIMZIA in combination with other biologic DMARDs is not recommended (see Warnings and Precautions, Use with Other Biologic Medicines).
Live Vaccines: Live vaccines should not be given concurrently with CIMZIA (see Warnings and Precautions, Immunizations).
Drug-Food Interactions: CIMZIA is administered as a subcutaneous injection. Interactions with food are therefore not applicable.
Drug-Herb Interactions: Interactions with herbal products have not been established.
Drug-Laboratory Test Interactions: Interference with certain coagulation assays has been detected in patients treated with CIMZIA. Certolizumab pegol may cause erroneously elevated activated partial thromboplastin time (aPTT) assay results in patients without coagulation abnormalities. This effect has been observed with the PTT-Lupus Anticoagulant (LA) and Standard Target Activated Partial Thromboplastin time (STA-PTT) tests manufactured by Diagnostica Stago, and the HemosIL APTT-SP liquid and HemosIL lyophilized silica tests manufactured by Instrumentation Laboratory. Other aPTT assays may be affected as well. Interference with thrombin time (TT) and prothrombin time (PT) assays has not been observed. There is no evidence that CIMZIA therapy has an effect on in vivo coagulation (see Warnings and Precautions, Laboratory Tests).

DOSAGE AND ADMINISTRATION: Dosing Considerations: CIMZIA (certolizumab pegol) is intended for use under the guidance and supervision of a healthcare professional. A patient may self-inject CIMZIA if a physician determines that it is appropriate, and with medical follow-up, as necessary, after proper training in subcutaneous injection technique.

CIMZIA may be used alone or in combination with methotrexate (MTX). CIMZIA should not be used in combination with other biologic disease modifying anti-rheumatic drugs (DMARDs) or other TNF blocking agents.

Recommended Dose and Dosage Adjustment: The recommended dose of CIMZIA for adult patients with rheumatoid arthritis is 400 mg (given as two subcutaneous injections of 200 mg) at Weeks 0, 2 and 4, followed by 200 mg every other week. For maintenance dosing, CIMZIA 400 mg every 4 weeks may be considered.

Missed Dose: Patients who miss a dose of CIMZIA should be advised as follows: if the next scheduled dose is within 1 week, patients should wait until the next scheduled dose. If the next scheduled dose is 1 week or longer away, patients should inject the missed dose as soon as they become aware of it, then follow with their next scheduled dose.

Administration: CIMZIA is administered by subcutaneous injection.

The solution in the pre-filled syringe should be carefully inspected visually for particulate matter and discoloration prior to administration. The solution should be a clear colorless to yellow liquid, essentially free from particulates and should not be used if cloudy or if foreign particulate matter is present. CIMZIA does not contain preservatives; therefore, unused portions of drug remaining from or in the syringe should be discarded.

Patients using CIMZIA should be instructed to inject the full amount in the syringe (1 mL), which provides 200 mg of CIMZIA, according to the directions provided in the Consumer Information Leaflet.

Injection sites should be rotated and injections should not be given into areas where the skin is tender, bruised, red or hard. When a 400 mg dose is needed, each 200 mg injection should occur at separate sites in the thigh or abdomen.

OVERDOSAGE:

Doses of up to 800 mg SC and 20 mg/kg intravenous (IV) have been administered to patients in clinical studies without evidence of dose-limiting toxicities. In cases of overdosage, it is recommended that patients are monitored closely for any signs and symptoms of adverse reactions or effects, and appropriate symptomatic treatment instituted immediately.

For management of a suspected drug overdose, CPhA recommends that you contact your **regional Poison Control Centre**. See the *CPS* Directory section for a list of Poison Control Centres.

ACTION AND CLINICAL PHARMACOLOGY: Mechanism of Action: Certolizumab pegol has a high affinity for human TNFα and binds with a K_D of 90pM. TNFα is a key pro-inflammatory cytokine with a central role in inflammatory processes. Certolizumab pegol selectively neutralizes TNFα (90% inhibitory concentration [IC_{90}] of 4 ng/mL for inhibition of human TNFα in the in vitro L929 murine fibrosarcoma cytotoxicity assay) but does not neutralize lymphotoxin α (TNFβ).

Certolizumab pegol was shown to neutralize membrane associated and soluble human TNFα in a dose-dependent manner. Incubation of monocytes with certolizumab pegol resulted in a dose-dependent inhibition of lipopolysaccharide-induced TNFα and interleukin-1β production in human monocytes.

Certolizumab pegol does not contain a fragment crystallizable (Fc) region, which is normally present in a complete antibody, and therefore does not fix complement or cause antibody-dependent cell-mediated cytotoxicity. It does not induce apoptosis in vitro in human peripheral blood-derived monocytes or lymphocytes, or neutrophil degranulation.

Pharmacodynamics: Biological activities ascribed to TNFα include the upregulation of cellular adhesion molecules and chemokines, upregulation of major histocompatibility complex (MHC) class I and class II molecules, and direct leukocyte activation. TNFα stimulates the production of downstream inflammatory mediators, including interleukin-1, prostaglandins, platelet activating factor, and nitric oxide. Elevated levels of TNFα have been implicated in the pathology of rheumatoid arthritis. CIMZIA (certolizumab pegol) binds to TNFα, inhibiting its role as a key mediator of the inflammation and joint destruction associated with rheumatoid arthritis.

Pharmacokinetics: A total of 126 healthy subjects received doses of up to 800 mg certolizumab pegol subcutaneously (SC) and up to 10 mg/kg intravenously (IV) in four pharmacokinetic studies. Data from these studies demonstrate that single IV and SC doses of certolizumab pegol have predictable dose-related plasma concentrations with a linear relationship between the dose administered and the maximum plasma concentration (C_{max}), and the Area Under the certolizumab pegol plasma concentration versus time Curve (AUC). A mean C_{max} of approximately 43 to 49 μg/mL occurred at Week 5 during the initial starting dose period using the recommended dose regimen for the treatment of patients with rheumatoid arthritis (400 mg SC at Weeks 0, 2 and 4 followed by 200 mg every other week).

Certolizumab pegol plasma concentrations were broadly dose-proportional and pharmacokinetics observed in patients with rheumatoid arthritis were consistent with those seen in healthy subjects.

Absorption: Following subcutaneous administration, peak plasma concentrations of certolizumab pegol were attained between 54 and 171 hours post-injection. Certolizumab pegol has a bioavailability (F) of approximately 80% (ranging from 76% to 88%) following SC administration compared to IV administration.

Distribution: The apparent volume of distribution (V/F) was estimated at 8.01 L in the RA population pharmacokinetic analysis.

Metabolism: PEGylation, the covalent attachment of PEG polymers to peptides, delays the metabolism and elimination of these entities from the circulation by a variety of mechanisms, including decreased renal clearance, proteolysis, and immunogenicity. Accordingly, certolizumab pegol is an antibody Fab' fragment conjugated with PEG in order to extend the terminal plasma elimination half-life ($t_{½}$) of the Fab'. The metabolism of certolizumab pegol has not been studied in human subjects. Data from animals indicate that once cleaved from the Fab' fragment the PEG moiety is mainly excreted in urine without further metabolism.

Excretion: The terminal elimination phase half-life ($t_{½}$) was approximately 14 days for all doses tested. The clearance following IV administration to healthy subjects ranged from 9.21 mL/h to 14.38 mL/h. The clearance following SC dosing was estimated as 21.0 mL/h in the RA population PK analysis, with an inter-subject variability of 30.8% (%CV) and inter-occasion variability 22.0%. The route of elimination of certolizumab pegol has not been studied in human subjects. Studies in animals indicate that the major route of elimination of the PEG component is via urinary excretion.

Special Populations and Conditions: Pediatrics (<18 years of age): Certolizumab pegol has not been studied in pediatric patients.

Geriatrics (≥65 years of age): Specific clinical studies have not been performed in elderly subjects.

Gender: Specific clinical studies have not been performed to assess the effect of gender on the pharmacokinetics of certolizumab pegol.

Race: Pharmacokinetic parameters in Japanese subjects were similar to those in Caucasian subjects following SC dosing at three dose levels in a biocomparability study.

Hepatic Impairment: Specific clinical studies have not been performed to assess the effect of hepatic impairment on the pharmacokinetics of certolizumab pegol.

Renal Impairment: Specific clinical studies have not been performed to assess the effect of renal impairment on the pharmacokinetics of certolizumab pegol. There are insufficient data to provide a dosing recommendation in moderate and severe renal impairment. The pharmacokinetics of the PEG (polyethylene glycol) fraction of certolizumab pegol is expected to be dependent on renal function but has not been assessed in renal impairment.

STORAGE AND STABILITY: Store CIMZIA (certolizumab pegol) at 2-8°C. Do not freeze. Protect from light. Do not use beyond the expiration date. Keep out of reach of children.

SPECIAL HANDLING INSTRUCTIONS: See Information for the Patient.

INFORMATION FOR THE PATIENT: Published in e-CPS, available by subscription at www.e-cps.ca.

DOSAGE FORMS, COMPOSITION AND PACKAGING: Each mL of sterile, preservative-free, clear and colourless to pale yellow, essentially free from particulates solution for subcutaneous administration, contains: certolizumab pegol 200 mg, sodium acetate 1.36 mg, sodium chloride 7.31 mg and Water for Injection, USP. pH approximately 4.7. Single-use pre-filled glass syringes of 1 mL with a fixed 25 gauge ½ inch needle, cartons containing two alcohol preps and two single use pre-filled glass syringes. The syringe components do not contain any latex or dry natural rubber.

Cipralex® Ⓟ

escitalopram oxalate

Antidepressant—Anxiolytic—Antiobsessional

Lundbeck

Date of Revision: February 1, 2010

SUMMARY PRODUCT INFORMATION:

Route of Administration	Dosage Form/ Strength	Nonmedicinal Ingredients
Oral	Tablets 10 and 20 mg	Colloidal silicon dioxide, croscarmellose sodium, hydroxypropyl methyl cellulose, magnesium stearate, microcrystalline cellulose, polyethylene glycol 400, talc, titanium dioxide (white E-171)

INDICATIONS AND CLINICAL USE: Adults:

- Cipralex (escitalopram oxalate) is indicated for the symptomatic relief of Major Depressive Disorder (MDD).
- The efficacy of Cipralex in maintaining an antidepressant response, in patients with major depressive disorder who responded during an 8-week, acute-treatment phase while taking Cipralex and were then observed for relapse during a period of up to 36 weeks, was demonstrated in a placebo-controlled trial.
- Cipralex is indicated for the symptomatic relief of anxiety causing clinically significant distress in patients with Generalized Anxiety Disorder (GAD).
- The efficacy of Cipralex in maintaining anxiolytic response for at least 6 months in patients with GAD was demonstrated in a long-term placebo-controlled trial (in patients who had initially responded to Cipralex during a 12-week open-label phase).
- Cipralex is indicated for the symptomatic relief of obsessive-compulsive disorder (OCD). The obsessions and compulsions must be experienced as intrusive, markedly distressing, time consuming or interfering significantly with the person's social or occupational functioning.
- The efficacy of Cipralex in maintaining an anti-obsessive response for up to 6 months, in patients with obsessive-compulsive disorder, was demonstrated in a long-term placebo-controlled trial in patients who initially responded to 16 weeks of Cipralex open-label treatment.
- Physicians who elect to use Cipralex for extended periods should periodically re-evaluate the usefulness of the drug for individual patients.

Geriatrics: Although there was no evidence from clinical studies suggesting that use in geriatric population is associated with differences in safety and effectiveness, a greater sensitivity of some older individuals to effects of escitalopram cannot be ruled out. A brief discussion can be found in the appropriate sections (Action and Clinical Pharmacology, Pharmacokinetics; Warnings and Precautions and Dosage and Administration).

Pediatrics: Escitalopram is not indicated for use in patients below the age of 18 (see Warnings and Precautions, General, Potential Association with Behavioural and Emotional Changes, Including Self-harm).

CONTRAINDICATIONS:

- Cipralex (escitalopram oxalate) is contraindicated in patients with known hypersensitivity to escitalopram or any of the excipients of the drug product.
- **Monoamine Oxidase Inhibitors:** Cases of serious reactions have been reported in patients receiving selective serotonin reuptake inhibitors (SSRIs) in combination with a monoamine oxidase inhibitor (MAOI) or the reversible MAOI (RIMA), moclobemide, and in patients who have recently discontinued an SSRI and have been started on a MAOI (see Drug Interactions). With the co-administration of an SSRI with MAOI, there have been reports of serious, sometimes fatal reactions including hyperthermia, rigidity, myoclonus, autonomic instability with possible fluctuations of vital signs, and mental status changes, including extreme agitation progressing to delirium and coma. Some cases presented with features resembling serotonin syndrome.

  Therefore, escitalopram should not be used in combination with a MAOI or within 14 days of discontinuing treatment with a MAOI. Similarly, at least 14 days should elapse after discontinuing escitalopram treatment before starting a MAOI.
- **Pimozide:** Escitalopram should not be used in combination with the antipsychotic drug pimozide, as results from a controlled study with racemic citalopram indicate that concomitant use is associated with an increased risk of QTc prolongation compared to pimozide alone. This apparent pharmacodynamic interaction occurred in the absence of a clinically significant pharmacokinetic interaction; the mechanism is unknown (see Drug Interactions).

WARNINGS AND PRECAUTIONS: General: Potential Association with Behavioural and Emotional Changes, Including Self-harm: Pediatrics: Placebo-Controlled Clinical Trial Data:

- **Recent analyses of placebo-controlled clinical trial safety databases from SSRIs and other newer antidepressants suggest that use of these drugs in patients under the age of 18 may be associated with behavioural and emotional changes, including an increased risk of suicidal ideation and behaviour over that of placebo.**
- **The small denominators in the clinical trial database, as well as the variability in placebo rates, preclude reliable conclusions on the relative safety profiles among these drugs.**

Adults and Pediatrics: Additional data:

- **There are clinical trials and post-marketing reports with SSRIs and other newer antidepressants, in both pediatrics and adults, of severe agitation-type adverse events coupled with self-harm and harm to others. The agitation-type events include: akathisia, agitation, emotional lability, hostility, aggression, depersonalization. In some cases, the events occurred within several weeks of starting treatment.**

Rigorous clinical monitoring for suicidal ideation or other indicators of potential for suicidal behaviour is advised in patients of all ages. This includes monitoring for agitation-type emotional and behavioural changes.

Discontinuation Symptoms: Patients currently taking escitalopram should NOT be discontinued abruptly, due to risk of discontinuation symptoms. At the time that a medical decision is made to discontinue an SSRI or other newer antidepressant drug, a gradual reduction in the dose rather than an abrupt cessation is recommended.

Discontinuation of Treatment with Escitalopram: When discontinuing treatment, patients should be monitored for symptoms that may be associated with discontinuation (e.g. dizziness, abnormal dreams, sensory disturbances [including paraesthesias and electric shock sensations], agitation, anxiety, emotional indifference, impaired concentration, headache, migraine, tremor, nausea, vomiting and sweating) or other symptoms that may be of clinical significance (see Adverse Reactions). A gradual reduction in the dosage over several weeks, rather than abrupt cessation is recommended whenever possible. If intolerable symptoms occur following a decrease in the dose or upon discontinuation of treatment, dose titration should be managed on the basis of the patient's clinical response (see Adverse Reactions and Dosage and Administration).

Escitalopram Treatment During Pregnancy—Effects on Newborns: Post-marketing reports indicate that some neonates exposed to SSRIs such as escitalopram and other antidepressants late in the third trimester have developed complications requiring prolonged hospitalization, respiratory support, and tube feeding. Such complications can arise immediately upon delivery. When treating a pregnant woman with escitalopram during the third trimester, the physician should carefully consider the potential risks and benefits of treatment (see Warnings and Precautions, Special Populations, Pregnant Women and Nursing Women and Dosage and Administration).

Interference with Cognitive and Motor Performance: In a study with healthy volunteers, racemic citalopram did not impair cognitive function or psychomotor performance. However, psychotropic medications may impair judgement, thinking or motor skills. Consequently, patients should be cautioned against driving a car or operating hazardous machinery until they are reasonably certain that escitalopram does not affect them adversely.

The following additional Precautions are listed alphabetically.

Cardiovascular: Patients with Cardiac Disease: Neither escitalopram nor racemic citalopram has been systematically evaluated in patients with a recent history of myocardial infarction or unstable heart disease. Patients with these diagnoses were generally excluded from clinical trials during the drug's premarketing assessment. However, the electrocardiograms (ECG) of patients participating in clinical trials with escitalopram and racemic citalopram indicate that the medications were not associated with the development of clinically significant ECG abnormalities. In line with other SSRIs, including racemic citalopram, escitalopram causes statistically significant, but clinically unimportant decrease in heart rate. In patients <60 years old, the mean decrease with escitalopram was approximately 2.3 bpm, while in patients ≥60 years old, the mean decrease was approximately 0.6 bpm.

Endocrine and Metabolism: Diabetic Patients: Neither escitalopram nor racemic citalopram has been systematically evaluated in diabetic patients; in the case of racemic citalopram, diabetes constituted an exclusion criterion. Rare events of hypoglycaemia were reported for racemic citalopram. Treatment with an SSRI in patients with diabetes may alter glycaemic control (hypoglycaemia and hyperglycaemia). Escitalopram should be used with caution in diabetic patients on insulin or oral hypoglycaemic drugs.

Hematologic: Bleeding Disorders: SSRIs and serotonin/norepinephrine reuptake inhibitors (SNRIs), including Cipralex, may increase the risk of bleeding events. Concomitant use of aspirin, nonsteroidal anti-inflammatory drugs (NSAIDs), warfarin, and other anticoagulants may add to this risk. Case reports and epidemiological studies (case-control and cohort design) have demonstrated an association between use of drugs that interfere with serotonin reuptake and the occurrence of gastrointestinal bleeding. There have been reports of bleeding events ranging from ecchymoses, hematomas, epistaxis, and petechiae to life-threatening haemorrhages, associated with treatment with SSRIs and SNRIs.

Caution is advised in patients taking SSRIs and SNRIs, particularly in concomitant use with drugs known to affect platelet function (e.g. atypical antipsychotics and phenothiazines, most tricyclic antidepressants, anticoagulants, platelet aggregation inhibitors, acetylsalicylic acid and NSAIDs), as well as in patients with a history of bleeding disorders or predisposing conditions (e.g., thrombocytopenia).

Hepatic/Biliary/Pancreatic: Hepatic Impairment: Based on a study conducted with escitalopram in patients with mild to moderate hepatic impairment, the half-life was approximately doubled and the exposure was increased by approximately two third, compared to subjects with normal liver function. Consequently, the use of escitalopram in hepatically impaired patients should be approached with caution and a lower dosage is recommended (see Dosage and Administration). No information is available about the pharmacokinetics of escitalopram in patients with severe hepatic impairment (Child-Pugh Criteria C). Escitalopram should be used with additional caution in patients with severe hepatic impairment.

Neurologic: Seizures: Escitalopram has not been systematically evaluated in patients with a seizure disorder. These patients were excluded from the clinical studies. In clinical trials with escitalopram, convulsions have been reported very rarely (2 out of 3981 patients) in association with treatment with escitalopram. From post-marketing data, the reporting of seizures with escitalopram is comparable to that of other antidepressants. Like other antidepressants, escitalopram should be used with caution in patients with a history of seizure disorder.

Serotonin Syndrome/Neuroleptic Malignant Syndrome (NMS)-Like Events: On rare occasions serotonin syndrome or neuroleptic malignant syndrome-like events have occurred in association with treatment with SSRIs, including escitalopram, particularly when given in combination with other serotonergic and/or neuroleptic drugs. As these syndromes may result in potentially life-threatening conditions, treatment with Cipralex should be discontinued if such events (characterized by clusters of symptoms such as hyperthermia, rigidity, myoclonus, autonomic instability with possible rapid fluctuations of vital signs, mental status changes including confusion, irritability, extreme agitation progressing to delirium and coma) occur and supportive symptomatic treatment should be initiated. Cipralex should not be used in combination with MAO inhibitors or serotonin-precursors (such as L-tryptophan, oxitriptan) and should be used with caution in combination with other serotonergic drugs (triptans, certain tricyclic antidepressants, lithium, tramadol, St. John's Wort) due to the risk of serotonergic syndrome (see Contraindications and Drug Interactions, Serotonergic Drugs, Triptans ($5HT_1$ agonists)).

Psychiatric: Suicide: The possibility of a suicide attempt is inherent in depression and may persist until remission occurs. Therefore, high-risk patients should be closely supervised throughout therapy with consideration to the possible need for hospitalization. In order to minimize the opportunity for overdosage, prescription for escitalopram should be written for the smallest quantity of drug consistent with good patient management.

Because of the well established comorbidity between depression and other psychiatric disorders, the same precautions observed when treating patients with depression should be observed when treating patients with other psychiatric disorders (see Warnings and Precautions, General, Potential Association with Behavioural and Emotional Changes, Including Self-harm).

Activation of Mania/Hypomania: In placebo-controlled trials of Cipralex (escitalopram oxalate) activation of mania/hypomania was reported in one patient of the n=715 treated with escitalopram and in none of the n=592 patients treated with placebo. Activation of mania/hypomania has also been reported in a small proportion of patients treated with racemic citalopram, and with other marketed antidepressants. As with other antidepressants, escitalopram should be used with caution in patients with a history of mania/hypomania.

Electroconvulsive Therapy (ECT): The safety and efficacy of the concurrent use of either escitalopram or racemic citalopram and ECT have not been studied.

Renal: Hyponatremia: As with other antidepressants, cases of hyponatraemia and SIADH (syndrome of inappropriate antidiuretic hormone secretion) have been reported with escitalopram and racemic citalopram as a rare adverse event. The majority of these occurrences have been in elderly individuals, some in patients taking diuretics or who were otherwise volume-depleted. Elderly female patients in particular seem to be a group at risk.

Renal Impairment: No information is available on the pharmacokinetic or pharmacodynamic effects of escitalopram on patients with renal impairment. Based on the information available for racemic citalopram, no dosage adjustment is needed in patients with mild to moderate renal impairment. Since no information is available on the pharmacokinetic or pharmacodynamic effects of either escitalopram or racemic citalopram in patients with severely reduced renal function (creatinine clearance <30 mL/min), escitalopram should be used with caution in these patients (see Dosage and Administration).

Special Populations: Pregnant Women and Nursing Women: The safety of escitalopram during human pregnancy and lactation has not been established. Therefore, escitalopram should not be used during pregnancy, unless the potential benefit to the patient outweighs the possible risk to the foetus.

Studies with escitalopram have not been performed in nursing mothers, but it is known that racemic citalopram is excreted in human milk and it is expected that escitalopram is also excreted into breast milk. Escitalopram should not be administered to nursing mothers unless the expected benefits to the patient outweigh the possible risk to the child.

Complications Following Late Third Trimester Exposure to SSRIs: Post-marketing reports indicate that some neonates exposed to SSRIs such as Cipralex and other antidepressants late in the third trimester have developed complications requiring prolonged hospitalization, respiratory support, and tube feeding. Such complications can arise immediately upon delivery. Reported clinical findings have included respiratory distress, cyanosis, apnoea, seizures, temperature instability, feeding difficulty, vomiting, hypoglycaemia, hypotonia, hypertonia, hyperreflexia, tremor, jitteriness, irritability, and constant crying. These features are consistent with either a direct toxic effect of SSRIs and other newer antidepressants, or, possibly, a drug discontinuation syndrome. It should be noted that, in some cases, the clinical picture is consistent with serotonin syndrome (see Warnings and Precautions, Serotonin Syndrome/Neuroleptic Malignant Syndrome (NMS)-Like Events). When treating a pregnant woman with Cipralex during the third trimester, the physician should carefully consider the potential risks and benefits of treatment (see Dosage and Administration).

Risk of PPHN and Exposure to SSRIs: In one epidemiological case-control study on persistent pulmonary hypertension (PPHN) with n=377 infants with PPHN and n=836 matched control infants, PPHN was six times more common in babies whose mothers took an SSRI antidepressant after the 20th week of pregnancy compared to babies whose mothers did not take an antidepressant. The study was too small to determine relative risks among the specific SSRIs. This information is considered to be preliminary at this time. The absolute risk of PPHN in the general population is reported to be 1-2 per 1000.

Pediatrics: Escitalopram is not indicated for use in patients below the age of 18 (see **Warnings and Precautions, General, Potential Association with Behavioural and Emotional Changes, Including Self-harm**).

Geriatrics: Approximately 5% of the 715 patients treated with escitalopram in clinical trials of depressive disorder were 60 years of age or over; elderly patients in these trials received daily doses between 10 and 20 mg. No overall significant differences in safety or effectiveness were observed between the elderly and younger subjects, but the number of elderly patients treated was insufficient to adequately assess for differential responses. Greater sensitivity of some older individuals to effects of escitalopram cannot be ruled out. In a multiple-dose pharmacokinetic study, the area under the curve (AUC) and half-life of escitalopram were increased by approximately 50% at steady-state in elderly subjects as compared to young subjects. Consequently, elderly patients should be administered lower doses and a lower maximum dose (see Action and Clinical Pharmacology, Pharmacokinetics and Dosage and Administration).

ADVERSE REACTIONS: Adverse Drug Reaction Overview: Adverse events information for Cipralex (escitalopram oxalate) was collected from 715 patients with major depressive disorder (MDD) who were exposed to escitalopram and from 592 patients who were exposed to placebo in double-blind, placebo-controlled trials. During clinical trials, all treatment groups were comparable with respect to gender, age and race. The mean age of patients was 41 years (18 to 76 years). Of these patients, approximately 66% were females and 34% were males.

The adverse event information for Cipralex in patients with generalized anxiety disorder (GAD) was collected from 832 patients exposed to escitalopram and from 566 patients exposed to placebo in 8-12 week double-blind, placebo-controlled trials. A total of 187 patients exposed to escitalopram and 188 patients exposed to placebo in a 24 to 76 week double-blind phase of a placebo-controlled long-term trial were also included. The demographics of the clinical trial population in GAD were similar to the population of patients included in MDD clinical trials.

The adverse event information for Cipralex in patients with obsessive-compulsive disorder (OCD) was collected from two studies with double-blind, placebo-controlled treatment periods of up to 24 weeks. In the first study, a total of 227 patients were exposed to escitalopram and 114 patients were exposed to placebo in a 24-week double-blind, placebo-controlled, fixed-dose trial with assessments at weeks 12 and 24. In the second study, 322 patients who initially responded to 16 weeks of open-label escitalopram treatment were subsequently randomized to double-blind treatment with escitalopram (n=164) or placebo (n=158) for up to 24 weeks. In total, 391 patients were exposed to escitalopram and 272 patients were exposed to placebo in these two long-term studies. The mean age of patients with OCD included in the trials was approximately 36 to 38 years (ranging from 18 to 67 years). One trial included similar proportions of males and females and the other trial had a slightly higher proportion of females than males (57% females and 43% males).

Adverse Events Observed in Controlled Trials: Adverse Events Associated with Discontinuation of Treatment: From the short-term (8-week) placebo-controlled, phase III studies in patients suffering from MDD, the incidence of discontinuation was: 17.3% (124/715) on escitalopram, 15.7% (64/408) on citalopram and 16.4% (97/592) on placebo. Discontinuation due to adverse events was more common in the active treatment groups (5.9% in escitalopram and 5.4% in citalopram) than in the placebo group (2.2%).

The events that were associated with discontinuation of escitalopram in 1% or more of patients at a rate of at least twice that of placebo were: nausea (1.5% vs 0.2%) and ejaculation failure (1.8% vs 0.0% of male patients).

Among the 832 GAD patients who received escitalopram 10-20 mg/day in placebo-controlled trials, 7.8% discontinued treatment due to an adverse event, as compared to 3.2 % of 566 patients receiving placebo. Adverse events that were associated with the discontinuation of at least 1% of patients treated with escitalopram, and for which the rate was higher than the placebo rate, were: dizziness (1.2% vs. 0.2%), fatigue (1.1% vs. 0.2%) and nausea (1.8% vs. 0.2%).

During the first 12 weeks of treatment in the 24-week placebo controlled trial, discontinuation of treatment due to adverse events was reported for 9% and 11% of the 227 OCD patients who were treated with 10 mg/day or 20 mg/day escitalopram, respectively, compared to 5% of the 114 patients receiving placebo. All patients who discontinued treatment due to adverse events in the escitalopram groups did so in the first 12 weeks. Eight percent of patients receiving placebo discontinued treatment due to an adverse event during the 24-week period. Adverse events that were associated with discontinuation of at least 1% of patients treated with escitalopram, and for which the rate was higher than the placebo rate, were: nausea (1.8% vs. 0.0%), insomnia (1.8% vs. 0.9%), and erectile dysfunction (1.1% vs. 0.0%).

Most Frequent Adverse Events: Adverse events that occurred in escitalopram-treated patients in the course of the short-term, placebo-controlled trials with an incidence greater than, or equal to, 10% were: headache and nausea. The incidence of headache was higher in the placebo group, which suggests that this is a non-specific symptom related to the underlying condition or treatment administration. The point prevalence of nausea increased during the first week (as expected with an SSRI) and then decreased to approach placebo levels by the end of the studies.

Clinical Trial Adverse Drug Reactions: Because clinical trials are conducted under very specific conditions the adverse reaction rates observed in the clinical trials may not reflect the rates observed in practice and should not be compared to the rates in the clinical trials of another drug. Adverse drug reaction information from clinical trials is useful for identifying drug-related adverse events and for approximating rates.

Major Depressive Disorder: Table 1 enumerates the incidence of treatment emergent adverse events that occurred in 715 depressed patients who received escitalopram at doses ranging from 10 to 20 mg/day in placebo-controlled trials of up to 8 weeks in duration. Events included are those occurring in 2% or more of patients treated with escitalopram, and for which the incidence in patients treated with escitalopram was greater than the incidence in placebo-treated patients. Reported adverse events were classified using the Medical Dictionary for Regulatory Activities (MedDRA), version 9.1.

Table 1: Cipralex

Treatment-Emergent Adverse Events[a]. Incidence in Placebo-Controlled Clinical Trials for Major Depressive Disorder

Body System/Adverse Event	Percentage of Patients Reporting: Escitalopram (n=715)	Placebo (n=592)
Cardiac Disorders		
Palpitations	1.4	1.2
Ear and Labyrinth Disorders		
Vertigo	1.4	0.8
Gastrointestinal Disorders		
Nausea	15.2	8.1
Diarrhoea	8.4	5.2
Dry mouth	6.6	4.6
Constipation	3.5	1.2
Dyspepsia	3.1	2.9
Abdominal pain upper	1.5	0.8
Stomach discomfort	1.1	0.3
General Disorders and Administration Site Conditions		
Fatigue	4.9	2.7
Pyrexia	1.1	0.0
Infections and Infestations		
Nasopharyngitis	4.6	3.4
Influenza	4.3	4.1
Sinusitis	2.1	1.9
Gastroenteritis	1.8	0.7
Herpes simplex	1.3	0.3
Investigations		
Weight increased	1.8	1.5
Metabolism and Nutrition Disorders		
Decreased appetite	2.4	0.7
Increased appetite	1.7	1.4
Musculoskeletal and Connective Tissue Disorders		
Arthralgia	1.4	0.5
Pain in extremity	1.4	0.8
Nervous System		

(cont'd)

Table 1: Cipralex *(cont'd)*

Treatment-Emergent Adverse Events[a]. Incidence in Placebo-Controlled Clinical Trials for Major Depressive Disorder

	Percentage of Patients Reporting	
Body System/Adverse Event	**Escitalopram (n=715)**	**Placebo (n=592)**
Dizziness	6.3	3.6
Somnolence	4.1	1.2
Sedation	2.4	0.7
Migraine	1.5	1.5
Tremor	1.5	0.7
Lethargy	1.0	0.2
Paraesthesia	1.0	0.7
Sinus headache	1.0	0.3
Psychiatric Disorders		
Insomnia	8.2	3.6
Anxiety	2.2	2.0
Libido decreased	2.1	0.3
Anorgasmy	1.8	0.2
Abnormal dreams	1.3	0.8
Respiratory, Thoracic and Mediastinal Disorders		
Pharyngolaryngeal pain	2.1	1.0
Yawning	1.5	0.2
Skin and Subcutaneous Tissue Disorders		
Hyperhidrosis	3.4	1.4
Night sweats	1.7	0.3
Rash	1.0	0.8
Vascular Disorders		
Hot flush[c]	2.2	0.0
Hot flush[b]	1.0	0.7
Reproductive System and Breast Disorders		
Ejaculation delayed[c]	3.6	0.0
Ejaculation failure[c]	2.7	0.0
Erectile dysfunction[c]	2.7	0.0
Ejaculation disorder[c]	1.3	0.0

[a] Events included are those occurring in 1% or more of patients treated with escitalopram, and for which the incidence in patients treated with escitalopram was greater than the incidence in placebo-treated patients.
[b] Denominator used was for females only (n=490 for escitalopram; n=404 for placebo).
[c] Denominator used was for males only (n=225 for escitalopram; n=188 for placebo).

The following events had a higher incidence in the placebo group compared to the escitalopram group: vomiting, abdominal pain, flatulence, upper respiratory tract infection, bronchitis, back pain, neck pain, headache.

Adverse reactions observed with escitalopram are in general mild and transient. They are most frequent during the first and/or second week of treatment and usually decrease in intensity and frequency with continued treatment and do not generally lead to a cessation of therapy.

In a clinical trial involving patients with Major Depressive Disorder that compared fixed doses of escitalopram (10 mg/day and 20 mg/day) with placebo, the most common adverse events that occurred in patients treated with escitalopram are shown in Table 2.

Table 2: Cipralex

Incidence of Common Adverse Events[a] for Major Depressive Disorder, Study MD-01

	Percentage of Patients Reporting		
Adverse Event	**Placebo (n=122)**	**Escitalopram 10 mg/day (n=119)**	**Escitalopram 20 mg/day (n=125)**
Diarrhoea	7.4	10.1	14.4
Nausea	6.6	22.7	13.6
Insomnia	1.6	10.9	11.2
Mouth dry	7.4	10.9	9.6
Dizziness	3.3	10.1	9.6
Ejaculation failure	0.0	0.0	7.3

(cont'd)

Table 2: Cipralex *(cont'd)*

Incidence of Common Adverse Events[a] for Major Depressive Disorder, Study MD-01

	Percentage of Patients Reporting		
Adverse Event	**Placebo (n=122)**	**Escitalopram 10 mg/day (n=119)**	**Escitalopram 20 mg/day (n=125)**
Nasopharyngitis	1.6	5.0	7.2
Constipation	1.6	2.5	5.6
Dyspepsia	1.6	5.9	4.0
Pharyngolaryngeal pain	0.0	5.9	1.6

[a] Events included are those occurring in 5% or more of patients treated with escitalopram (10 mg/day or 20 mg/day), and for which the incidence was greater than the incidence in placebo-treated patients.

Male and Female Sexual Dysfunction with SSRIs: While sexual dysfunction is often part of depression and other psychiatric disorders, there is increasing evidence that treatment with selective serotonin reuptake inhibitors (SSRIs) may induce sexual side effects. This is a difficult area to study because patients may not spontaneously report symptoms of this nature, and therefore, it is thought that sexual side effects with SSRIs may be underestimated.

Table 3 shows the incidence rates of sexual side effects in patients with major depressive disorder in placebo-controlled short-term trials.

Table 3: Cipralex

Incidence of Sexual Side Effects in Placebo-Controlled Clinical Trials for Major Depressive Disorder

	Percentage of Patients Reporting	
Adverse Event	**Escitalopram (n=715)**	**Placebo (n=592)**
Libido decreased	2.1	0.3
Anorgasmy	1.8	0.2
In Males Only		
Ejaculation delayed	3.6	0.0
Ejaculation failure	2.7	0.0
Erectile dysfunction	2.7	0.0
Ejaculation disorder	1.3	0.0

Generalized Anxiety Disorder: Table 4 enumerates the incidence of treatment emergent adverse events that occurred among 832 patients who received escitalopram in placebo-controlled trials for up to 8-12 weeks in duration. Events included are those occurring in 1% or more of patients treated with escitalopram, and for which the incidence in patients treated with escitalopram was greater than the incidence in placebo-treated patients. Reported adverse events were classified using the Medical Dictionary for Regulatory Activities (MedDRA), version 9.1.

The most frequent adverse events that occurred in escitalopram-treated patients in the course of the short-term, placebo-controlled trials with an incidence greater than, or equal to, 10% were: nausea, headache and insomnia.

Table 4: Cipralex

Treatment-Emergent Adverse Events[a]. Incidence in Placebo-Controlled Clinical Trials for Generalized Anxiety Disorder (8–12 weeks)

	Percentage of Patients Reporting	
Body System/Adverse Event	**Escitalopram (n=832)**	**Placebo (n=566)**
Cardiac Disorders		
Palpitations	1.3	0.4
Tachycardia	1.3	0.7
Ear and Labyrinth Disorders		
Tinnitus	1.1	0.7
Vertigo	1.0	0.2
Gastrointestinal Disorders		
Nausea	19.4	9.0
Diarrhoea	9.6	5.8
Dry mouth	7.3	4.6
Constipation	3.7	3.5
Vomiting	2.8	1.4
Abdominal pain upper	2.2	1.2
Flatulence	1.6	0.9
Toothache	1.3	0.0
General Disorders and Administration Site Conditions		
Fatigue	9.9	2.7

(cont'd)

Table 4: Cipralex *(cont'd)*

Treatment-Emergent Adverse Events[a]. Incidence in Placebo-Controlled Clinical Trials for Generalized Anxiety Disorder (8–12 weeks)

Body System/Adverse Event	Percentage of Patients Reporting: Escitalopram (n=832)	Percentage of Patients Reporting: Placebo (n=566)
Irritability	1.9	0.9
Chills	1.2	0.0
Infections and Infestations		
Nasopharyngitis	5.3	5.0
Sinusitis	1.8	1.8
Gastroenteritis	1.3	1.2
Investigations		
Weight increased	1.1	0.9
Metabolism and Nutrition Disorders		
Decreased appetite	2.5	0.7
Anorexia	1.2	0.2
Increased appetite	1.0	0.9
Musculoskeletal and Connective Tissue Disorders		
Back pain	3.0	2.5
Myalgia	1.9	0.7
Pain in extremity	1.3	0.7
Neck pain	1.2	0.9
Shoulder pain	1.0	0.7
Nervous System Disorders		
Headache	23.7	18.6
Dizziness	7.9	5.6
Somnolence	7.6	5.5
Paraesthesia	2.2	1.1
Sedation	2.2	0.2
Lethargy	1.6	0.4
Psychiatric Disorders		
Insomnia	10.1	3.7
Libido decreased	3.6	2.1
Anorgasmy	2.8	0.4
Abnormal dreams	1.8	0.9
Loss of libido	1.6	0.0
Orgasm abnormal	1.6	0.0
Nightmare	1.3	0.7
Restlessness	1.3	0.0
Depression	1.2	1.2
Sleep disorder	1.0	0.5
Renal and Urinary Disorders		
Pollakiuria	1.2	0.4
Reproductive System and Breast Disorders		
Ejaculation delayed[b]	5.6	0.8
Erectile dysfunction[b]	1.9	0.4
Respiratory, Thoracic and Mediastinal Disorders		
Yawning	2.3	0.4
Skin and Subcutaneous Tissue Disorders		
Hyperhidrosis	4.7	1.2
Night sweats	1.1	0.2
Pruritus	1.0	0.9

(cont'd)

Table 4: Cipralex *(cont'd)*

Treatment-Emergent Adverse Events[a]. Incidence in Placebo-Controlled Clinical Trials for Generalized Anxiety Disorder (8–12 weeks)

[a] Events included are those occurring in 1% or more of patients treated with escitalopram, and for which the incidence in patients treated with escitalopram was greater than the incidence in placebo-treated patients.
[b] Denominator used was for males only (n=324 for escitalopram; n=241 for placebo).

The following events had a higher incidence in the placebo group compared to the escitalopram group: dyspepsia, abdominal pain, upper respiratory tract infection, influenza, anxiety, dysmenorrhoea, pharyngolaryngeal pain, sinus congestion.

In general, the safety profile was similar in the long-term (24-76 weeks) placebo-controlled study when compared to short-term (8-12 week) trials.

In a clinical trial of patients with generalized anxiety disorder that compared 10 mg/day and 20 mg/day escitalopram with placebo, the most common adverse events that occurred in patients treated with escitalopram are shown in Table 5.

Table 5: Cipralex

Incidence of Common Adverse Events[a] for Generalized Anxiety Disorder, Study 99815

Adverse Event	Percentage of Patients Reporting: Placebo (n=139)	Escitalopram 10 mg/day (n=136)	Escitalopram 20 mg/day (n=133)
Nausea	12.9	22.1	23.3
Fatigue	4.3	11.0	17.3
Dizziness	5.8	13.2	13.5
Diarrhoea	4.3	11.8	10.5
Insomnia	2.9	12.5	10.5
Hyperhidrosis	2.9	9.6	9.0
Ejaculation delayed	0.0	6.7	7.3
Dry mouth	2.2	6.6	6.8
Somnolence	2.9	3.7	6.8
Yawning	0.0	0.7	5.3

[a] Events included are those occurring in 5% or more of patients treated with escitalopram (10 mg/day or 20 mg/day), and for which the incidence was greater than the incidence in placebo-treated patients.

Obsessive Compulsive Disorder: Table 6 enumerates the incidence of treatment emergent adverse events that occurred among 227 patients who received escitalopram in the first 12 weeks of a 24-week placebo-controlled trial. Events included are those occurring in 1% or more of patients treated with escitalopram, and for which the incidence in patients treated with escitalopram was greater than the incidence in placebo-treated patients. Reported adverse events were classified using the Medical Dictionary for Regulatory Activities (MedDRA), version 9.1.

The most frequent adverse events that occurred in escitalopram-treated patients in the course of the short-term, placebo-controlled trials with an incidence greater than, or equal to, 10% were: headache, nausea and fatigue.

Table 6: Cipralex

Treatment-Emergent Adverse Events[a]. Incidence in a Placebo-Controlled Clinical Trial for Obsessive Compulsive Disorder (first 12 weeks of a 24-week trial)

Body System/Adverse Event	Percentage of Patients Reporting: Escitalopram (n=227)	Percentage of Patients Reporting: Placebo (n=114)
Eye Disorder		
Visual disturbance	1.3	0.0
Gastrointestinal Disorders		
Nausea	23.3	12.3
Diarrhoea	6.6	4.4
Dry mouth	6.2	4.4
Constipation	2.6	2.6
Vomiting	2.6	0.9
General Disorders and Administration Site Conditions		
Fatigue	14.1	5.3
Asthenia	1.3	0.9
Infections and Infestations		
Nasopharyngitis	6.6	3.5
Sinusitis	2.2	0.9
Rhinitis	1.3	0.0

(cont'd)

Table 6: Cipralex *(cont'd)*

Treatment-Emergent Adverse Events[a]. Incidence in a Placebo-Controlled Clinical Trial for Obsessive Compulsive Disorder (first 12 weeks of a 24-week trial)

Body System/Adverse Event	Percentage of Patients Reporting	
	Escitalopram (n=227)	Placebo (n=114)
Investigations		
Weight increased	1.3	0.0
Metabolism and Nutrition Disorders		
Decreased appetite	2.2	0.9
Musculoskeletal and Connective Tissue Disorders		
Neck pain	1.8	1.8
Back pain	1.3	0.9
Nervous System		
Headache	19.4	16.7
Dizziness	7.9	5.3
Somnolence	8.4	5.3
Tremor	3.5	1.8
Migraine	1.3	0.0
Psychiatric Disorders		
Libido decreased	4.8	0.9
Restlessness	2.2	0.9
Sleep disorder	1.8	0.9
Abnormal dreams	1.3	0.0
Reproductive System and Breast Disorders		
Ejaculation delayed[c]	7.6	0.0
Menorrhagia[b]	1.5	0.0
Respiratory, Thoracic and Mediastinal Disorders		
Yawning	1.8	0.0
Skin and Subcutaneous Tissue Disorders		
Hyperhidrosis	5.7	1.8
Vascular Disorders		
Hot flush[b]	1.5	0.0

[a] Events included are those occurring in 1% or more of patients treated with escitalopram, and for which the incidence in patients treated with escitalopram was greater than the incidence in placebo-treated patients.
[b] Denominator used was for females only (n=135 for escitalopram; n=63 for placebo).
[c] Denominator used was for males only (n=92 for escitalopram; n=51 for placebo).

The following events had a higher incidence in the placebo group compared to the escitalopram group: abdominal pain upper, irritability, influenza, anorexia, increased appetite, insomnia, anxiety, erectile dysfunction.

In general, the safety profile of the placebo-controlled study at 24 weeks was similar to the one observed in the first 12 weeks of the trial.

In both phases of the long-term study of patients who were randomized to receive 24 weeks of double-blind treatment with escitalopram or placebo, following response to an initial 16 weeks of open-label escitalopram treatment, the safety profile of escitalopram was similar to the safety profile in the above mentioned placebo controlled trial. Adverse events reported by at least 2% of patients after the open-label period and during the first 2 weeks after randomization were: dizziness (15.8% placebo vs 0.6% escitalopram); nausea (5.7% placebo vs 0.6% escitalopram); headache (4.4% placebo vs 1.8% escitalopram); and insomnia (3.2% placebo vs 0.6% escitalopram).

The most common AEs that occurred during treatment with 10 mg/day and 20 mg/day escitalopram in this clinical trial are shown in Table 7.

Table 7: Cipralex

Incidence of Common Adverse Events[a] for Obsessive Compulsive Disorder (first 12 weeks of 24-week trial, Study 10205)

Adverse Event	Percentage of Patients Reporting		
	Placebo (n=114)	Escitalopram 10 mg/day (n=113)	Escitalopram 20 mg /day (n=114)
Nausea	12.3	19.5	27.2
Fatigue	5.3	11.5	16.7
Somnolence	5.3	6.2	10.5
Ejaculation delayed	0.0	4.5	10.4
Diarrhoea	4.4	4.4	7.0
Dizziness	5.3	8.8	7.0
Nasopharyngitis	3.5	7.1	6.1
Libido decreased	0.9	2.7	7.0
Dry mouth	3.5	4.4	5.3
Hyperhidrosis	1.8	6.2	5.3

[a] Events included are those occurring in 5% or more of patients treated with escitalopram (10 mg/day or 20 mg/day), and for which the incidence was greater than the incidence in placebo-treated patients.

In general, the adverse event profile that occurred among the patients who received escitalopram during the 24 weeks of the trial was similar to the profile observed in the first 12 weeks of the trial.

Weight Changes: Patients treated with escitalopram in short-term controlled trials did not differ from placebo-treated patients with regards to clinically important change in body weight. In one 24-week randomized clinical trial in patients with Social Anxiety Disorder, 8.0% of patients treated with escitalopram and 3.2% of patients treated with placebo experienced weight gain of 7% or more.

Cardiovascular Parameters: Escitalopram and placebo groups in MDD and GAD patients were compared with respect to mean change from baseline in vital signs (pulse, systolic blood pressure, and diastolic blood pressure) and the incidence of patients meeting criteria for potentially clinically significant changes from baseline in these variables. The analyses did not reveal any clinically important changes in blood pressure associated with escitalopram treatment. In line with other SSRIs, including racemic citalopram, escitalopram causes statistically significant, but clinically unimportant decrease in heart rate. In MDD patients <60 years old, the mean decrease with escitalopram was approximately 2.3 bpm, while in patients ≥60 years old, the mean decrease was approximately 0.6 bpm.

Electrocardiograms from escitalopram and placebo groups in MDD and GAD patients were compared with respect to mean change from baseline in various ECG parameters and the incidence of patients meeting criteria for potentially clinically significant changes from baseline in these variables. Escitalopram was not associated with the development of clinically significant ECG abnormalities.

Adverse Reactions Following Discontinuation of Treatment (or Dose Reduction): There have been reports of adverse reactions upon the discontinuation of SSRIs such as escitalopram (particularly when abrupt), including but not limited to the following: dizziness, abnormal dreams, sensory disturbances (including paraesthesias and electric shock sensations), agitation, anxiety, emotional indifference, impaired concentration, headache, migraine, tremor, nausea, vomiting and sweating or other symptoms which may be of clinical significance (see Warnings and Precautions and Dosage and Administration).

Patients should be monitored for these or any other symptoms. A gradual reduction in the dosage over several weeks, rather than abrupt cessation is recommended whenever possible. If intolerable symptoms occur following a decrease in the dosage or upon discontinuation of treatment, dose titration should be managed on the basis of the patient's clinical response. These events are generally self-limiting. Symptoms associated with discontinuation have been reported for other selective serotonin reuptake inhibitors (see Warnings and Precautions and Dosage and Administration).

Adverse Reactions During Treatment for Up to 44 Weeks: The treatment-emergent adverse event incidence profile of escitalopram in a longer term study in patients with major depressive disorder (MDD) consisting of a 36-week placebo-controlled relapse observation phase in responders of a preceding 8-week acute treatment phase was similar to that observed in short-term studies.

Less Common Clinical Trial Adverse Drug Reactions: Untoward events associated with the exposure were recorded by clinical investigators using terminology of their own choosing. Consequently, it is not possible to provide a meaningful estimate of the proportion of individuals experiencing adverse events without first grouping similar types of untoward events into a smaller number of standardized event categories. Reported adverse events were classified using the Medical Dictionary for Regulatory Activities, version 9.1.

The events listed below present treatment emergent adverse events reported during the clinical development program of escitalopram in depressed patients (n=896), which includes a long-term clinical trial, in GAD patients included in short-term (8-12 weeks) trials (n=832) and in one GAD long-term (24-76 weeks) trial (n=187); and in OCD patients included in a long-term (24 weeks with assessments at 12 weeks and 24 weeks) trial (n=227). Excluded from this list are those already listed in Table 1 (MDD), Table 4 (GAD) or Table 6 (OCD first 12 weeks of a 24 week trial).

It is important to emphasise that, although the events reported occurred during treatment with escitalopram, they were not necessarily caused by it. The events are categorized by body system and listed according to the following criteria: frequent: adverse events that occurred on one or more occasions in at least 1/100 patients; infrequent: adverse events that occurred in less than 1/100 patients but at least in 1/1000 patients; rare: adverse events that occurred in less than 1/1000 but at least in 1/10 000 patients.

Blood and Lymphatic System Disorders: Infrequent: anaemia, lymphadenopathy. Rare: lymphadenitis.

Cardiac Disorders: Rare: atrial fibrillation, atrial ventricular block first degree, bradycardia, extrasystoles, myocarditis, nodal rhythm, sinus bradycardia.

Congenital, Familial and Genetic Disorders: Rare: epidermal naevus, Gilbert's syndrome.

Ear and Labyrinth Disorders: Infrequent: ear disorder, ear pain, tinnitus. Rare: cerumen impaction, deafness, Meniere's disease, motion sickness, tympanic membrane perforation.

Endocrine Disorders: Rare: goiter, hyperthyroidism, thyroiditis.

Eye Disorders: Infrequent: accommodation disorder, blepharospasm, conjunctivitis, dry eye, eye pain, eye pruritus, mydriasis, photopsia, vision blurred. Rare: asthenopia, chromatopsia, eye haemorrhage, eye irritation, eye swelling, eyelid oedema, iritis, keratoconus, myopia, night blindness, retinal detachment, scotoma, vitreous detachment.

Gastrointestinal Disorders: Infrequent: abdominal discomfort, abdominal distension, Crohn's disease, dysphagia, enteritis, epigastric discomfort, food poisoning, frequent bowel movements, gastrointestinal pain, gastroesophageal reflux disease, gastritis, haemorrhoids, lip dry, rectal haemorrhage. Rare: anal fissure, colitis ulcerative, colonic polyp, eructation, gingival pain, haematemesis, haematochezia, ileitis, oral pain, pruritus ani, reflux gastritis, stomatitis, tongue black hairy, tongue disorder, tooth disorder, tooth erosion.

General Disorders and Administration Site Conditions: Infrequent: chest discomfort, chest pain, feeling abnormal, feeling jittery, influenza like illness, malaise, oedema, oedema peripheral, pain, respiratory sighs, sluggishness, thirst. Rare: early satiety, face oedema, feeling hot, hunger, local swelling, performance status decreased, sensation of blood flow.

Immune System Disorders: Infrequent: anaphylactic reaction, house dust allergy, hypersensitivity, seasonal allergy. Rare: allergic oedema.

Infections and Infestations: Infrequent: acute sinusitis, bronchitis acute, cystitis, ear infection, eye infection, folliculitis, fungal infection, gastrointestinal infection, laryngitis, lung infection, pelvic inflammatory disease (gs=Gender Specific), otitis media, pharyngitis, pharyngitis streptococcal, pneumonia, respiratory tract infection, skin infection, tooth abscess, tonsillitis, tooth infection, urinary tract infection, vaginal candidiasis (gs), viral infection, viral upper respiratory tract infection, vulvovaginal mycotic infection (gs). Rare: appendicitis, bronchitis viral, carbuncle, cellulitis, dental caries, erysipelas, furuncle, genitourinary chlamydia infection, gingival infection, impetigo, infection parasitic, mastitis, onychomycosis, otitis externa, peritonsillar abcess, pyelonephritis acute, rash pustular, salmonellosis, staphylococcal infection, streptococcal infection, tracheitis, vaginal infection, varicella, wound infection.

Injury, Poisoning and Procedural Complications: Infrequent: animal bite, ankle fracture, arthropod bite, contusion, excoriation, fall, injury, intentional overdose, joint dislocation, joint injury, joint sprain, limb injury, mouth injury, procedural pain, road traffic accident, skin laceration, sunburn, thermal burn. Rare: arthropod sting, back injury, concussion, electric shock, eye injury, facial bones fracture, foot fracture, ligament injury, muscle rupture, neck injury, post-traumatic pain, radius fracture, rib fracture, sports injury, tooth injury, ulna fracture, whiplash injury.

Investigations: Infrequent: blood glucose increased, blood pressure increased, body temperature increased, heart rate increased, weight decreased. Rare: arthroscopy, blood bilirubin increased, blood cholesterol increased, blood uric acid increased, blood urine present, electrocardiogram PR shortened, haemoglobin decreased, hepatic enzyme increased, pregnancy test positive (gs).
Metabolism and Nutrition Disorders: Infrequent: food craving. Rare: dehydration, gout, hypercholesterolaemia, hypermagnesaemia, hyperphagia, latent tetany.
Musculoskeletal and Connective Tissue Disorders: Infrequent: arthritis, joint stiffness, muscle contracture, muscle spasms, muscle tightness, muscle twitching, muscular weakness, musculoskeletal chest pain, musculoskeletal discomfort, musculoskeletal stiffness, osteoarthritis, pain in jaw. Rare: chest wall pain, costochondritis, exostosis, fibromyalgia, finger deformity, ganglion, intervertebral disc protrusion, musculoskeletal pain, plantar fasciitis, rheumatoid arthritis, sacroiliitis, sensation of heaviness, tendon disorder.
Neoplasms Benign, Malignant and Unspecified (incl. cysts and polyps): Infrequent: breast neoplasm. Rare: benign breast neoplasm, lipoma, marrow hyperplasia, skin papilloma, uterine leiomyoma (gs).
Nervous System: Infrequent: amnesia, balance disorder, burning sensation, carpal tunnel syndrome, coordination abnormal, dizziness postural, disturbance in attention, dysgeusia, hyperreflexia, hypersomnia, hypertonia, hypoaesthesia, memory impairment, muscle contractions involuntary, restless legs syndrome, sciatica, syncope, tension headache. Rare: dysaesthesia, dysphasia, facial paresis, facial spasm, head discomfort, hypogeusia, myoclonus, paralysis, psychomotor hyperactivity, sensory disturbance, sleep talking, syncope vasovagal.
Pregnancy, Puerperium and Perinatal Conditions: Infrequent: pregnancy (gs).
Psychiatric Disorders: Infrequent: agitation, apathy, bruxism, confusional state, crying, depersonalization, depressed mood, derealisation, disorientation, early morning awakening, emotional disorder, hallucination auditory, initial insomnia, libido increased, mental disorder, middle insomnia, mood swings, nervousness, obsessive-compulsive disorder, panic attack, suicidal ideation, suicide attempt, tension, thinking abnormal. Rare: aggression, emotional distress, euphoric mood, flat affect, generalized anxiety disorder, hallucination, hypomania, indifference, major depression, paranoia, psychomotor retardation, tic.
Renal and Urinary Disorders: Infrequent: dysuria, haematuria, micturition urgency, urinary hesitation. Rare: bladder dilatation, bladder discomfort, chromaturia, nocturia, renal pain, urinary incontinence.
Reproductive System and Breast Disorders: Infrequent: amenorrhoea (gs), epididymitis (gs), menstrual disorder (gs), menstruation irregular (gs), metrorrhagia (gs), orchitis noninfective (gs), painful erection (gs), pelvic pain, premenstrual syndrome (gs), postmenopausal haemorrhage (gs), sexual dysfunction, testicular pain (gs). Rare: breast discharge, breast pain, breast tenderness, genital pain, menopausal symptoms (gs), uterine spasm (gs), vaginal discharge (gs), vaginal haemorrhage (gs).
Respiratory, Thoracic and Mediastinal Disorders: Infrequent: asthma, cough, dyspnoea, epistaxis, nasal congestion, postnasal drip, rhinitis allergic, rhinorrhoea, throat irritation, wheezing. Rare: allergic sinusitis, choking, dysphonia, nasal polyps, rhinitis perennial, throat tightness, tracheal disorder.
Skin and Subcutaneous Tissue Disorders: Infrequent: acne, alopecia, dermatitis allergic, dermatitis contact, dry skin, eczema, increased tendency to bruise, rash, urticaria. Rare: cold sweat, dermal cyst, dermatitis, dermatitis acneiform, dermatitis atopic, hand dermatitis, ingrowing nail, photosensitivity reaction, rash maculo-papular, skin irritation, skin nodule, skin odor abnormal, skin warm.
Social Circumstances: Infrequent: drug abuser. Rare: family stress, stress at work.
Surgical and Medical Procedures: Infrequent: tooth extraction. Rare: colon polypectomy, gingival operation, scar excision.
Vascular Disorders: Infrequent: flushing, haematoma, hypertension, hypotension, orthostatic hypotension, peripheral coldness, varicose vein. Rare: circulatory collapse, pallor, vein disorder.
Long-Term Trial (GAD): In general, the safety profile was similar in the long-term placebo-controlled study (24-76 weeks). The following events (single or duplicate cases), which are not listed in Table 4 and Table 5 or reported above in the short-term trials, have been reported: aneurysm, arteriosclerosis, dermatitis bullous, hypercholesterolaemia, hypocalcaemia, hypokalaemia, joint dislocation, migraine, nasal septum deviation, psoriasis, scoliosis, torticollis.
Long-Term Placebo-Controlled Trial in Escitalopram Responders (OCD): In general, the safety profile was similar in the long-term (24-week) placebo-controlled phase of the trial in which patients who initially responded to 16 weeks of open label escitalopram treatment were randomized to treatment with escitalopram or placebo for up to 24 weeks. The following events (single or duplicate cases), which are not reported elsewhere, have been reported: abdominal pain lower, acute tonsillitis, blood pressure decreased, dental operation, depressive symptoms, dysarthria, dyspareunia, epicondylitis, facial pain, haematochezia, hordeolum, infrequent bowel movements, laceration, lacrimation increased, limb operation, negative thoughts, neuralgia, pain inflammation activated, subcutaneous abscess, tendon injury, wisdom teeth removal.
Post-Market Adverse Drug Reactions: Adverse events not listed above that have been reported to be temporally (but not necessarily causally) associated with escitalopram treatment since its market introduction include: aggression, alanine aminotransferase increased, amblyopia, amenorrhoea not otherwise specified (NOS), angioedema, anxiety aggravated, appetite decreased NOS, aspartate aminotransferase increased, atrial fibrillation, blood alkaline phosphatase NOS increased, blood cholesterol increased, blood glucose increased, blood pressure increased, burning sensation NOS, cardiac arrest, cerebrovascular accident, clonic convulsion, coma, completed suicide, confusional state, contusion, convulsions NOS, death NOS, delirium, diplopia, disorientation, drug level NOS increased, dysarthria, dysgeusia, dyskinesia, dysphasia, ecchymosis, electrocardiogram QT prolonged, emotional distress, epidermal necrolysis, epistaxis, erectile dysfunction NOS, extrapyramidal disorder, facial palsy, feeling abnormal, fluid retention, gait abnormal NOS, galactorrhoea, gastrointestinal haemorrhage, gingival bleeding, grand mal convulsion, haematemesis, hallucination visual, hepatitis NOS, hyperventilation, hypoglycaemia NOS, injury NOS, INR increased, irritability, leukocytosis, leukopenia NOS, liver function tests NOS abnormal, loss of consciousness, memory impairment, menometrorrhagia, muscle cramps, myocardial infarction, myocardial ischaemia, neuroleptic malignant syndrome, neurotransmitter level altered, night sweats, nightmare, orthostatic hypotension, pancreatitis NOS, panic attack, panic reaction, petit mal epilepsy, platelet count decreased, priapism, pulmonary embolism, pyrexia, renal failure acute, restlessness, rhabdomyolysis, rhinorrhoea, serotonin syndrome, SIADH, speech disorder, stomatitis, tardive dyskinesia, thrombocytopenia, torsades de pointes, trismus, urinary incontinence, vasovagal attack, ventricular tachycardia, vision blurred, visual disturbance NOS, weakness.

DRUG INTERACTIONS:

> **Serious Drug Interactions**
> - **Monoamine Oxidase Inhibitors: See Contraindications.**
> - **Pimozide: See Contraindications.**

Overview: Escitalopram is the active enantiomer of racemic citalopram. The pharmacokinetic studies described in the following sections, whether using escitalopram or racemic citalopram, were carried out in young healthy, mostly male volunteers. In addition, many of the studies utilized single doses of the specific concomitant medication, with multiple dosing of escitalopram or citalopram. Thus, data are not available in patients who would be receiving the concomitant drugs on an ongoing basis at therapeutic doses.
Drug-Drug Interactions: Monoamine Oxidase Inhibitors (MAOIs): Combined use of escitalopram and MAO inhibitors is contraindicated due to the potential for serious reactions with features resembling serotonin syndrome or neuroleptic malignant syndrome (see Contraindications and Warnings and Precautions, Serotonin Syndrome/Neuroleptic Malignant Syndrome (NMS)-Like Events).
Cytochrome P450 Isozymes: Citalopram: Based on the results of broad in vitro and in vivo testing, racemic citalopram is neither the source nor the cause of any clinically important pharmacokinetic drug-drug interactions. In vitro enzyme inhibition data did not reveal an inhibitory effect of citalopram on CYP3A4, -1A2, -2D6, -2C9, -2C19 and -2E1. Accordingly, escitalopram would be expected to have little inhibitory effect on in vivo drug metabolism mediated by the cytochrome P-450 isozymes. In addition, pharmacokinetic interaction studies with racemic citalopram have also demonstrated no clinical important interactions with carbamazepine (CYP3A4 substrate), triazolam (CYP3A4 substrate), theophylline (CYP1A2 substrate), warfarin (CYP2C9 substrate), levomepromazine (CYP2D6 inhibitor).
Escitalopram: Using in vitro models of human liver microsomes, the biotransformation of escitalopram to its demethylated metabolites was shown to depend on three parallel pathways (CYP2C19, CYP3A4 with a smaller contribution from CYP2D6) (see Dosage and Administration, CYP2C19 Poor Metabolizers).

Studies also indicate that escitalopram is a very weak or negligible inhibitor of human hepatic isoenzyme CYP1A2, 2C9, 2C19, 2E1, and 3A4, and a weak inhibitor of 2D6. Although escitalopram has a low potential for clinically significant drug interactions, caution is recommended, when escitalopram is co-administered with drugs that are mainly metabolized by CYP2D6, and that have a narrow therapeutic index.

The possibility that the clearance of escitalopram will be decreased when administered with the following drugs in a multiple-dose regimen should be considered:
- potent inhibitors of CYP3A4 (eg. fluconazole, ketoconazole, itraconazole, erythromycin), or
- potent inhibitors of CYP2C19 (eg. omeprazole, esomeprazole, fluvoxamine, lansoprazole, ticlopidine). Caution should be exercised at the upper end of the dosage range of escitalopram when it is co-administered with CYP2C19 inhibitors.

In addition, a single-dose study of escitalopram co-administered with a multiple-dose regimen of cimetidine, a non-specific CYP inhibitor, led to significant changes in most of the pharmacokinetic parameters of escitalopram.

The overall metabolic pathways for escitalopram and citalopram are qualitatively similar and the interaction potential for escitalopram is expected to closely resemble that of citalopram. Thus, this allows for extrapolation to previous studies with citalopram.
CNS Drugs: Drug interactions have not been specifically studied between either escitalopram or racemic citalopram and other centrally acting drugs. Given the primary CNS effects of escitalopram, caution should be used as with other SSRIs when escitalopram is taken in combination with other centrally acting drugs.
Serotonergic Drugs: Based on the mechanism of action of escitalopram and the potential for serotonin syndrome, caution is advised when Cipralex is co-administered with other drugs or agents that may affect the serotonergic neurotransmitter systems, such as tryptophan, triptans, serotonin reuptake inhibitors, lithium, tramadol, or St. John's Wort (see Warnings and Precautions, Serotonin Syndrome/Neuroleptic Malignant Syndrome (NMS)-Like Events). Concomitant use of Cipralex and MAO inhibitors (including linezolid, an antibiotic which is a reversible nonselective MAO inhibitor) is contraindicated (see Contraindications).
Triptans ($5HT_1$ agonists): Cases of life-threatening serotonin syndrome have been reported during combined use of selective serotonin reuptake inhibitors (SSRIs)/serotonin norepinephrine reuptake inhibitors (SNRIs) and triptans. If concomitant treatment with Cipralex and a triptan is clinically warranted, careful observation of the patient is advised, particularly during treatment initiation and dose increases (see Warnings and Precautions, Serotonin Syndrome/Neuroleptic Malignant Syndrome (NMS)-Like Events).
Racemic Citalopram: As escitalopram (Cipralex), is the active isomer of racemic citalopram (Celexa), the two drugs should not be taken together.
Alcohol Use: The interaction between escitalopram and alcohol has not been studied. Although racemic citalopram did not potentiate the cognitive and psychomotor effects of alcohol in volunteers, the concomitant use of alcohol in depressed patients taking escitalopram is not recommended.
Polymorphism: It has been observed that poor metabolizers with respect to CYP2C19 have twice as high a plasma concentration of escitalopram as extensive metabolizers. (See Dosage and Administration, CYP2C19 Poor Metabolizers.) Although no significant change in exposure was observed in poor metabolizers with respect to CYP2D6, caution is recommended when escitalopram is co-administered with medicinal products that are mainly metabolized by this enzyme, and that have a narrow therapeutic index.
Interaction Data Which Include Studies Conducted with Escitalopram: See Table 8.

Table 8: Cipralex

Established or Predicted Drug-Drug Interactions with Escitalopram

Escitalopram	Reference	Effect	Clinical Comment
Cimetidine	CT	Co-administration of cimetidine (400 mg twice daily for 5 days), a moderately potent CYP2D6, 3A4 and 1A2 inhibitor, with escitalopram (single dose of 20 mg on day 4) resulted in an increase in escitalopram AUC and C_{max} of approximately 70% and 20%, respectively.	Caution should be exercised when used concomitantly with cimetidine. A reduction in the dose of escitalopram may be necessary based on clinical judgement.
Imipramine/Desipramine: substrate for CYP2D6	CT	Co-administration of escitalopram (20 mg/day for 21 days) with the tricyclic antidepressant desipramine (single dose of 50 mg), a substrate for CYP2D6, resulted in a 50% increase in desipramine concentrations.	The clinical significance of this finding is unknown. Consequently, concomitant treatment with escitalopram and imipramine/desipramine should be undertaken with caution.
Metoprolol: substrate for CYP2D6	CT	Co-administration of 20 mg/day of escitalopram for 21 days with metoprolol (a CYP2D6 substrate) resulted in a 50% increase in the peak plasma levels of the β-adrenergic blocker with no clinically significant effects on blood pressure or heart rate.	
Omeprazole: CYP2C19 inhibitor	CT	Co-administration of omeprazole (30 mg once daily for 6 days), a CYP2C19 inhibitor, with escitalopram (single dose of 20 mg on day 5) resulted in an increase in escitalopram AUC and C_{max} of approximately 50% and 10%, respectively.	Caution should be exercised when used concomitantly with CYP2C19 inhibitors (e.g. omeprazole). A reduction in the dose of escitalopram may be necessary based on clinical judgement.
Ritonavir: substrate for CYP3A4	CT	Combined administration of a single dose of ritonavir (600 mg), a CYP3A4 substrate and a potent inhibitor of CYP3A4, and escitalopram (20 mg) did not affect the pharmacokinetics of either ritonavir or escitalopram.	

Legend: CT=Clinical Trial.

Interaction Studies Conducted with Racemic Citalopram: See Table 9.

Table 9: Cipralex

Established or Predicted Drug-Drug Interactions with Racemic Citalopram

Racemic citalopram	Reference	Effect	Clinical Comment
Carbamazepine	CT	Carbamazepine, titrated to 400 mg/day, was given for 21 days alone and then in combination with racemic citalopram (40 mg/day) for an additional 14 days. Citalopram did not affect the plasma levels of carbamazepine, a CYP3A4 substrate, or its metabolite, carbamazepine-epoxide.	Since carbamazepine is a microsomal enzyme inducer, the possibility that carbamazepine may increase the clearance of escitalopram should be considered if the two drugs are given concomitantly.
Digoxin	CT	Administration of racemic citalopram (40 mg/day for 21 days) did not affect the pharmacokinetics of digoxin (single dose of 1 mg). The serum levels of citalopram were slightly lower in the presence of digoxin but with no clinical relevance.	

(cont'd)

Table 9: Cipralex *(cont'd)*

Established or Predicted Drug-Drug Interactions with Racemic Citalopram

Racemic citalopram	Reference	Effect	Clinical Comment
Ketoconazole	CT	Combined administration of racemic citalopram (40 mg single dose) and the potent CYP3A4 inhibitor ketoconazole (200 mg single dose) decreased the C_{max} of ketoconazole by 21% and did not affect the pharmacokinetics of racemic citalopram.	
Levomepromazine	CT	Co-administration of racemic citalopram (40 mg/day for 10 days) and a CYP2D6 inhibitor, levomepromazine (single dose of 50 mg) did not affect the pharmacokinetics of either drug.	
Lithium	CT	Co-administration of racemic citalopram (40 mg/day for 10 days) and lithium (30 mmol/day for 5 days) did not affect the pharmacokinetics of either drug.	Since lithium may increase serotonergic neurotransmission, concomitant treatment with escitalopram should be undertaken with caution.
Pimozide	CT	In a double-blind crossover study in healthy young adults, a single dose of pimozide 2 mg co-administered with racemic citalopram 40 mg given once daily for 11 days was associated with a mean increase in QTc values at T_{max} of approximately 12 msec compared to pimozide when given with placebo.	The mechanism of this apparent pharmacodynamic interaction is not known. Concomitant use of citalopram or escitalopram and pimozide is contraindicated.
Theophylline	CT	Co-administration of racemic citalopram (40 mg/day for 21 days) with the CYP1A2 substrate theophylline (single dose of 300 mg) did not affect the pharmacokinetics of theophylline.	
Triazolam	CT	Combined administration of racemic citalopram (titrated to 40 mg/day for 28 days) and the CYP3A4 substrate triazolam (single dose of 0.25 mg) did not significantly affect the pharmacokinetics of either drug.	
Warfarin	CT	Administration of racemic citalopram (40 mg/day for 21 days) did not affect either the pharmacokinetics or the pharmacodynamics (prothrombin time) of a single 25 mg dose of warfarin, a CYP3A4 and CYP2C9 substrate.	

Legend: CT=Clinical Trial.

Drug-Food Interactions: Various scientific publications have acknowledged that the main components in grapefruit juice may act as CYP3A4 inhibitors. Escitalopram is also metabolized by other isoenzymes not affected by grapefruit juice, namely CYP2C19 and CYP2D6. Although there is a theoretical possibility of pharmacokinetic drug interactions resulting from co-administration of escitalopram with grapefruit juice, the onset of an interaction is considered unlikely.

Drug-Herb Interactions: St-John's Wort: In common with other SSRIs and newer antidepressants, pharmacodynamic interactions between escitalopram and the herbal remedy St-John's Wort may occur and may result in undesirable side effects.

Drug-Laboratory Test Interactions: Interactions with laboratory test have not been established.

DOSAGE AND ADMINISTRATION: Dosing Considerations:

- **Cipralex (escitalopram oxalate) is not indicated for use in children under 18 years of age (see Warnings and Precautions, Potential Association with Behavioural and Emotional Changes, Including Self-harm).**
- **General:** Escitalopram should be administered as a single daily dose, with or without food.

Recommended Dose and Dosage Adjustment: Adults: Major Depressive Disorder: Escitalopram should be administered as a single oral dose of 10 mg daily. Depending on individual patient response, an increase in the dose to a maximum of 20 mg daily should be considered. Where initial sensitivity to adverse events may be a concern, escitalopram could be started at 5 mg daily and titrated upwards as tolerated.

Generalized Anxiety Disorder: Escitalopram should be administered as a single oral dose of 10 mg daily. Depending on individual patient response, an increase in the dose to a maximum of 20 mg daily should be considered. Where initial sensitivity to adverse events may be a concern, escitalopram could be started at 5 mg daily and titrated upwards as tolerated. During long-term therapy, the dosage should be maintained at the lowest effective level and patients should be periodically reassessed to determine the need to continue treatment.

Obsessive Compulsive Disorder: Escitalopram should be administered as a single oral dose of 10 mg daily. Depending on individual patient response, an increase in the dose to a maximum of 20 mg daily should be considered. Where initial sensitivity to adverse events may be a concern, escitalopram could be started at 5 mg daily and titrated upwards as tolerated. During long-term therapy, the dosage should be maintained at the lowest effective level and patients should be periodically reassessed to determine the need to continue treatment.

Treatment of Pregnant Women During the Third Trimester: Post-marketing reports indicate that some neonates exposed to SSRIs such as Cipralex and other newer antidepressants late in the third trimester have developed complications requiring prolonged hospitalization, respiratory support, and tube feeding (see Warnings and Precautions). When treating pregnant women with Cipralex during the third trimester, the physician should carefully consider the potential risks and benefits of treatment. The physician may consider tapering Cipralex in the third trimester.

Elderly Patients: A longer half-life and decreased clearance have been demonstrated in the elderly, therefore lower doses and a lower maximum dose should be considered. It may be desirable to start at 5 mg daily and titrate upwards as needed and tolerated.

Renal Impairment: No dosage adjustment is necessary for patients with mild or moderate renal impairment. Since no information is available on the pharmacokinetic or pharmacodynamic effects of either escitalopram or racemic citalopram in patients with severely reduced renal function (creatinine clearance <30 mL/min), escitalopram should be used with caution in these patients.

Hepatic Impairment: Dosages should be restricted to the lower end of the dose range in patients with mild to moderate hepatic insufficiency. Accordingly, an initial single oral dose of 5 mg daily is recommended. Subsequently, the dose may be increased based on the patient's response and clinical judgement. A daily dose of 10 mg is the recommended maximum dose for most patients with hepatic impairment. No information is available about the pharmacokinetics of escitalopram in patients with severe hepatic impairment (Child-Pugh Criteria C). Escitalopram should be used with additional caution in patients with severe hepatic impairment.

CYP2C19 Poor Metabolizers: The metabolism of escitalopram is mainly mediated by CYP2C19. For patients who are known to be poor metabolizers with respect to CYP2C19, an initial dose of 5 mg daily is recommended. The dose may be increased based on the patient's response and clinical judgement.

Long-term Treatment: During long-term therapy, the dosage should be maintained at the lowest effective level and patients should be periodically reassessed to determine the need to continue treatment.

Switching Patients to or From a Monoamine Oxidase Inhibitor (MAOI): At least 14 days should elapse between discontinuation of a MAOI and initiation of therapy with escitalopram. Similarly, at least 14 days should be allowed after stopping escitalopram before starting a MAOI (see Contraindications).

Discontinuation of Escitalopram Treatment: Symptoms associated with the discontinuation or dosage reduction of escitalopram have been reported. Patients should be monitored for these and other symptoms when discontinuing treatment or during dosage reduction (see Warnings and Precautions and Adverse Reactions).

A gradual reduction in the dose over several weeks rather than abrupt cessation is recommended whenever possible. If intolerable symptoms occur following a decrease in the dose or upon discontinuation of treatment, dose titration should be managed on the basis of the patient's clinical response (see Warnings and Precautions and Adverse Reactions).

Children: See Potential Association with Behavioural and Emotional Changes, Including Self-harm under Warnings and Precautions.

Missed Dose: In the event that a dose is missed, the patient should take the next dose when it is due.

OVERDOSAGE:

Clinical data on escitalopram overdose are limited and many cases involve concomitant overdoses of other drugs. In the majority of cases mild or no symptoms have been reported. Fatal cases of escitalopram overdose have rarely been reported with escitalopram alone (doses unknown); the majority of cases have involved multiple drug overdose. Doses up to 800 mg of escitalopram alone have been taken without any severe symptoms.

In clinical trials with racemic citalopram, there were no reports of fatal citalopram overdoses of up to 2000 mg. Post-marketing reports of drug overdoses involving racemic citalopram have included fatalities with citalopram alone. In many cases, details regarding the precise dose of racemic citalopram or combination with other drugs and/or alcohol are often lacking. However, three fatalities with known overdoses of racemic citalopram alone have been reported in the literature (doses of 2800 mg, 2880 mg, and 3920 mg), although survival has also been reported with overdoses of up to 5200 mg.

In comparing the data from racemic citalopram with that of escitalopram, it is important to be aware that the latter product is expected to have similar pharmacodynamic effects at a lower dose of the racemic product.

Fatal cases of serotonin syndrome have been reported in patients who took overdoses of moclobemide (Manerix) and racemic citalopram. The plasma concentrations of moclobemide were between 16 and 90 mg/L (therapeutic range: 1 to 3 mg/L) and those of racemic citalopram between 0.3 and 1.7 mg/mL (therapeutic concentration: 0.3 mg/L). This indicates that a relatively low dose of citalopram, given with an overdose of moclobemide represents a serious risk for the patient.

Symptoms most often accompanying overdose of racemic citalopram included dizziness, sweating, nausea, vomiting, tremor, and somnolence. In more rare cases, observed symptoms included confusion, loss of consciousness, convulsions, coma, sinus tachycardia, cyanosis, hyperventilation and rhabdomyolysis and ECG changes (including QTc prolongation, nodal rhythm, ventricular arrhythmia, and one possible case of Torsades de pointes).

Management of Overdose: As with racemic citalopram, there is no specific antidote to escitalopram. Treatment is symptomatic and supportive. Establish and maintain an airway to ensure adequate ventilation and oxygenation. Gastric lavage and use of activated charcoal should be considered as soon as possible after oral ingestion. Cardiac and vital sign monitoring are recommended, along with general symptomatic and supportive measures.

Due to the large volume of distribution of escitalopram, forced diuresis, dialysis, haemoperfusion and exchange transfusion are unlikely to be of benefit.

In managing overdosage, the possibility of multiple drug involvement must be considered.

> For management of a suspected drug overdose, contact your regional Poison Control Centre. See the *CPS* Directory section for a list of Poison Control Centres.

ACTION AND CLINICAL PHARMACOLOGY: Escitalopram (S-citalopram) is the active enantiomer of the racemic drug citalopram. In vitro and in vivo studies have suggested that escitalopram is a highly potent and selective serotonin reuptake inhibitor (SSRI), which acts by specific competitive inhibition of the membrane transporter of serotonin (5-hydroxytryptophan, 5-HT). In addition to its high affinity to the primary binding site, escitalopram also binds with a 1000 fold lower affinity to a secondary binding site on the serotonin transporter. The clinical significance of this binding has not been established.

Escitalopram has no or very low affinity for a series of receptors including 5-HT_{1A}, 5-HT_2, dopamine D_1 and D_2 receptors, α_1, α_2, β-adrenoreceptors, histamine H_1, muscarinic cholinergic, benzodiazepine, gamma aminobutyric acid (GABA) and opioid receptors. Escitalopram does not bind to, or has low affinity for various ion channels including Na^+, Cl^-, K^+ and Ca^{++} channels.

Pharmacokinetics: The single and multiple-dose pharmacokinetics of escitalopram are linear and dose-proportional in a dose range of 10 to 30 mg/day. Biotransformation of escitalopram is mainly hepatic with a mean terminal half-life of about 27-32 hours. With once daily dosing, steady-state plasma levels are achieved within approximately 1 week. At steady state, the plasma concentration of escitalopram in young healthy subjects was approximately 2.6 times that observed after a single dose.

Absorption and Distribution: Following the administration of an oral dose (10 mg or 20 mg) of escitalopram to healthy volunteers, peak plasma levels occur at about 4 hours after dosing. Absorption of escitalopram is expected to be almost complete after oral administration and is not affected by food. After a single oral administration of escitalopram 10 mg, the apparent volume of distribution of ($Vd,\beta/F$) is about 12 L/kg to 26 L/kg. The binding of escitalopram to human plasma proteins is independent of drug plasma levels and average 55 %.

Metabolism and Excretion: The plasma clearance following oral administration is about 0,6 L/min with approximately 7% due to renal clearance. Escitalopram is metabolized in the liver to S-demethylcitalopram (S-DCT) and to S-didemethylcitalopram (S-DDCT). In humans, unchanged escitalopram is the predominant compound in plasma. After multiple-dose administration of escitalopram, the mean plasma concentrations of the metabolites S-DCT and S-DDCT are usually 28-31% and <5% of the parent compound concentration, respectively. Results from in vitro studies suggest that the metabolites (S-DCT and S-DDCT) do not contribute significantly to the clinical actions of escitalopram.

In vitro studies using human liver microsomes indicated that the biotransformation of escitalopram to its demethylated metabolites depends primarily on CYP2C19 and CYP3A4 with a smaller contribution from CYP2D6. The apparent hepatic clearance of drug amounts to approximately 90% of the administered dose. Following oral administration of escitalopram, the fraction of drug recovered as escitalopram and the metabolite S-DCT is about 8% and 10% respectively.

Special Populations and Conditions: Geriatrics: Escitalopram pharmacokinetics in subjects older than 65 years of age was compared to younger subjects in a single/multiple-dose study (n=18 subjects ≥65). After a single dose, plasma escitalopram levels were similar in young and elderly subjects. At steady state in elderly subjects, escitalopram C_{max}, AUC and half-life values were increased by approximately 35, 50 and 50%, respectively, while the clearance values were decreased. In this population, lower doses and a lower maximum dose of escitalopram are recommended (see Warnings and Precautions and Dosage and Administration).

Gender: In a multiple dose study of escitalopram (10 mg/day for 3 weeks) in 18 male (9 elderly and 9 young) and 18 female (9 elderly and 9 young) subjects, there were no differences in the weight-adjusted values of the area under the curve (AUC), C_{max}, and half-life between the male and the female subjects. No adjustment in dosage is recommended on the basis of gender difference.

Hepatic Insufficiency: In patients with mild to moderate hepatic impairment (Child-Pugh Criteria A and B), the half-life of escitalopram was approximately doubled (66 hours vs. 36 hours), and the exposure was about two-third higher than in subjects with normal liver function. Consequently, the doses in the lower end of the recommended range of escitalopram should be used for patients with hepatic dysfunction. No information is available about the pharmacokinetics of escitalopram in patients with severe hepatic impairment (Child-Pugh Criteria C). Escitalopram should be used with additional caution in patients with severe hepatic impairment (see Warnings and Precautions and Dosage and Administration).

Renal Insufficiency: No information is available about the pharmacokinetics of escitalopram in patients with reduced renal function. In n=7 patients with mild to moderate renal function impairment, oral clearance of racemic citalopram was reduced by 17% compared to normal subjects, with no clinically significant effect on the kinetics. No adjustment of dosage is recommended for such patients. At present no information is available about the pharmacokinetics of either escitalopram or racemic citalopram for the chronic treatment of patients with severely reduced renal function (creatinine clearance <30 mL/min) (see Warnings and Precautions and Dosage and Administration).

STORAGE AND STABILITY: Escitalopram tablets should be stored in a dry place at room temperature (15 and 30°C).

INFORMATION FOR THE PATIENT: Published in e-CPS, available by subscription at www.e-cps.ca.

DOSAGE FORMS, COMPOSITION AND PACKAGING: 10 mg: Each film-coated, white, oval, scored tablet, marked with "EL" on one side, contains: escitalopram 10 mg (as escitalopram oxalate). Nonmedicinal ingredients: colloidal silicon dioxide, croscarmellose sodium, hydroxypropyl methylcellulose, magnesium stearate, microcrystalline cellulose, polyethylene glycol 400, talc and titanium dioxide (white E-171). Blister packages of 30. Bottles of 100.

20 mg: Each film-coated, white, oval, scored tablet, marked with "EN" on one side, contains: escitalopram 20 mg (as escitalopram oxalate). Nonmedicinal ingredients: colloidal silicon dioxide, croscarmellose sodium, hydroxypropyl methylcellulose, magnesium stearate, microcrystalline cellulose, polyethylene glycol 400, talc and titanium dioxide (white E-171). Blister packages of 30.

(Shown in Product Identification Section)

The reader is invited to consult CPhA's monograph **Fluoroquinolones**.

Ciprodex ℞

ciprofloxacin HCl—dexamethasone

Antibacterial—Corticosteroid (Otic)

Alcon

Date of Preparation: May 6, 2004

PHARMACOLOGY: Ciprofloxacin, a fluoroquinolone antibiotic, has in vitro activity against a wide range of gram-positive and gram-negative microorganisms. The bactericidal action of ciprofloxacin results from inhibition of the enzyme, DNA gyrase, which is required for the synthesis of bacterial DNA.

Dexamethasone, a potent corticosteroid, has been shown to aid in the resolution of inflammation.

Clinical Pharmacology: Following a single bilateral 4-drop topical otic dose of CIPRODEX (Ciprofloxacin Hydrochloride & Dexamethasone) Otic Suspension to pediatric patients following tympanostomy tube insertion, measurable plasma concentrations of ciprofloxacin and dexamethasone were observed up to 6 hours. In 25 patients, the mean (±SD) peak plasma concentrations of ciprofloxacin and dexamethasone were 1.14±0.98 ng/mL and 0.86±1.19 ng/mL, respectively, and were observed typically within 15 minutes to 2 hours post-dose. For ciprofloxacin, these levels were approximately 650-fold lower than levels achieved with an oral dose of 250 to 1000 mg. This bilateral exposure resulted in a peak dexamethasone concentration approximately 9-fold lower than reported by following an oral 0.5 mg dose. Estimates of half-life averaged 3.1 hours for ciprofloxacin and 4.5 hours for dexamethasone. Both values are similar to those reported after oral doses in adults. While systemic exposure was assessed with bilateral administration, most AOMT patients in the clinical trials for this product had unilateral infections (77%).

INDICATIONS: CIPRODEX (Ciprofloxacin Hydrochloride & Dexamethasone) Otic Suspension is indicated for the treatment of infections caused by most strains of the designated microorganisms in the specific conditions listed below:

Acute Otitis Media with Otorrhea through tympanostomy tubes in pediatric patients, age 6 months and older, due to: Aerobic, Gram-Positive: *S. pneumoniae*, *S. aureus*. Aerobic, Gram-Negative: *H. influenzae*, *M. catarrhalis*, *P. aeruginosa*.

Acute Otitis Externa in pediatric, adult and elderly patients, age 1 year and older, due to: Aerobic, Gram-Positive: *S. aureus*. Aerobic, Gram-Negative: *P. aeruginosa*.

CONTRAINDICATIONS: A history of hypersensitivity to ciprofloxacin, to other quinolones including nalidixic acid, or to any of the components in this medication. Use of this product is contraindicated in viral infections of the external canal including herpes simplex infections.

WARNINGS: For topical otic use only. (This product is not approved for ophthalmic use.)

Not for injection.

CIPRODEX (Ciprofloxacin Hydrochloride & Dexamethasone) Otic Suspension should be discontinued at the first appearance of a skin rash or any other sign of hypersensitivity. Serious and occasionally fatal hypersensitivity (anaphylactic) reactions, some following the first dose, have been reported in patients receiving systemic quinolones. Serious acute hypersensitivity reactions may require immediate emergency treatment.

PRECAUTIONS: General: As with other antibacterial preparations, use of this product may result in overgrowth of nonsusceptible organisms, including yeast and fungi. If the infection is not improved after one week of treatment, alternate therapy should be considered.

If otorrhea persists after a full course of therapy, or if 2 or more episodes of otorrhea occur within 6 months, further evaluation is recommended to exclude an underlying condition such as cholesteatoma, foreign body, or a tumor.

The systemic administration of quinolones, including ciprofloxacin at doses much higher than given or absorbed by the otic route, has led to lesions or erosions of the cartilage in weight-bearing joints and other signs of arthropathy in immature animals of various species.

Spontaneous extrusion of tympanostomy tubes is not unexpected and occurred at an incidence of 1.8% in the CIPRODEX treatment group in the clinical trials.

Drug Interactions: Specific drug interaction studies have not been conducted with CIPRODEX (Ciprofloxacin Hydrochloride & Dexamethasone) Otic Suspension administered in the ear.

Pregnancy: Reproduction studies have been performed in rats and mice using oral doses of up to 100 mg/kg and IV doses up to 30 mg/kg and have revealed no evidence of harm to the fetus as a result of ciprofloxacin. In rabbits, ciprofloxacin (30 and 100 mg/kg orally) produced gastrointestinal disturbances resulting in maternal weight loss and an increased incidence of abortion, but no teratogenicity was observed at either dose. After intravenous administration of doses up to 20 mg/kg, no maternal toxicity was produced in the rabbit, and no embryotoxicity or teratogenicity was observed.

Corticosteroids are generally teratogenic in laboratory animals when administered systemically at relatively low dosage levels. The more potent corticosteroids have been shown to be teratogenic after dermal application in laboratory animals. The teratogenic potential of Dexamethasone after topical (ophthalmic) treatment has been investigated in New Zealand white rabbits. Treatment with a 0.1% suspension of Dexamethasone into the conjunctival sac on days 6 through 18 of gestation resulted in a 15.6% and 32.3% incidence of fetal anomalies in two groups of rabbits.

Animal reproduction studies have not been conducted with CIPRODEX. No adequate and well controlled studies have been performed in pregnant women. Caution should be exercised when CIPRODEX is used by a pregnant woman.

Lactation: Ciprofloxacin and corticosteroids, as a class, appear in milk following oral administration. Dexamethasone in breast milk could suppress growth, interfere with endogenous corticosteroid production, or cause other untoward effects. It is not known whether topical otic administration of ciprofloxacin or dexamethasone could result in sufficient systemic absorption to produce detectable quantities in human milk. Because of the potential for unwanted effects in nursing infants, a decision should be made whether to discontinue nursing or to discontinue the drug, taking into account the importance of the drug to the mother and the low dose used in topical otic therapy.

Children: The safety and efficacy of CIPRODEX have been established in pediatric patients 6 months and older (937 patients) in clinical trials. In pediatric patients below the age of 6 months no data on safety and efficacy are available.

No clinically relevant changes in hearing function were observed in 69 pediatric patients (age 4 to 12 years) treated with CIPRODEX and tested for audiometric parameters.

Although ciprofloxacin and other quinolones cause arthropathy in immature animals after oral administration, topical ocular administration of ciprofloxacin to immature dogs did not cause any arthropathy and there is no evidence that the otic dosage form has any effect on the weight bearing joints.

ADVERSE EFFECTS: In Phases II and III clinical trials, a total of 937 patients were treated with CIPRODEX (Ciprofloxacin Hydrochloride & Dexamethasone) Otic Suspension. This included 400 patients with acute otitis media with otorrhea and 537 patients with acute otitis externa. The reported treatment-related adverse events are listed below:

Acute Otitis Media in pediatric patients with tympanostomy tubes: The following treatment-related adverse events occurred in 0.5% or more of the patients with non-intact tympanic membranes (see Table 1).

Table 1: CIPRODEX

Treatment-related Adverse Events

Adverse Event	Incidence (N=400)
Ear discomfort	3.0%
Ear pain	2.3%
Ear precipitate (residue)	0.5%
Irritability	0.5%
Taste perversion	0.5%

The following treatment-related adverse events were each reported in a single patient: tympanostomy tube blockage; ear pruritus; tinnitus; oral moniliasis; crying; dizziness; and erythema.

Acute Otitis Externa: The following treatment-related adverse events occurred in 0.4% or more of the patients with intact tympanic membranes (see Table 2).

Table 2: CIPRODEX

Treatment-related Adverse Events

Adverse Event	Incidence (N=537)
Ear pruritus	1.5%
Ear debris	0.6%
Superimposed ear infection	0.6%
Ear congestion	0.4%
Ear pain	0.4%
Erythema	0.4%

The following treatment-related adverse events were each reported in a single patient: ear discomfort; decreased hearing; and ear disorder (tingling).

OVERDOSE:

Treatment: There is no known treatment of overdosage since overdosage in the use of topical otic preparations is a remote possibility. Discontinue medication when heavy or protracted use is suspected.

For management of a suspected drug overdose, CPhA recommends that you contact your **regional Poison Control Centre**. See the *CPS* Directory section for a list of Poison Control Centres.

DOSAGE: Shake well immediately before using.

CIPRODEX (Ciprofloxacin Hydrochloride & Dexamethasone) Otic Suspension contains 3 mg/mL (3000 µg/mL) ciprofloxacin and 1 mg/mL dexamethasone.

Acute Otitis Media in pediatric patients with tympanostomy tubes: The recommended dosage regimen for the treatment of acute otitis media in pediatric patients (6 months and up) through tympanostomy tubes is:

Four drops (0.14 mL, 0.42 mg ciprofloxacin, 0.14 mg dexamethasone) instilled into the affected ear twice daily for seven days. The suspension should be warmed by holding the bottle in the hand for one or two minutes to avoid dizziness, which may result from the instillation of a cold suspension. The patient should lie with the affected ear upward, and then the drops should be instilled. The tragus should then be pumped 5 times by pushing inward to facilitate penetration of the drops into the middle ear. This position should be maintained for 60 seconds. Repeat, if necessary, for the opposite ear. Discard unused portion after therapy is completed.

Acute Otitis Externa: The recommended dosage regimen for the treatment of acute otitis externa is:

For patients (1 year and up): Four drops (0.14 mL, 0.42 mg ciprofloxacin, 0.14 mg dexamethasone) instilled into the affected ear twice daily for seven days. The suspension should be warmed by holding the bottle in the hand for one or two minutes to avoid dizziness, which may result from the instillation of a cold suspension. The patient should lie with the affected ear upward, and then the drops should be instilled. This position should be maintained for 60 seconds to facilitate penetration of the drops into the ear canal. Repeat, if necessary, for the opposite ear. Discard unused portion after therapy is completed.

INFORMATION FOR THE PATIENT: Published in e-CPS, available by subscription at www.e-cps.ca.

SUPPLIED: Each mL of otic suspension contains: ciprofloxacin HCl (equivalent to ciprofloxacin base 3 mg) and dexamethasone 1 mg. Nonmedicinal ingredients: acetic acid, benzalkonium chloride 0.1 mg as preservative, boric acid, edetate disodium, hydroxyethyl cellulose, purified water, sodium acetate, sodium chloride and tyloxapol. Sodium hydroxide and/or hydrochloric acid may be added for adjustment of pH. The solution has a pH of approximately 5 and an osmolality of approximately 300 mOsm/kg. DROP-TAINER system of 7.5 mL, that consists of a natural polyethylene bottle and natural plug, with a white polypropylene closure. Tamper evidence is provided with a shrink band around the closure and neck area of the package. Store at room temperature, 15 to 30°C. Avoid freezing. Protect from light.

Ciprofloxacin ℞

CPhA Monograph

see *Fluoroquinolones*

The reader is invited to consult CPhA's monograph **Fluoroquinolones**.

Ciprofloxacin Injection USP ℞

ciprofloxacin

Antibacterial

Hospira

SUPPLIED: Each mL contains: ciprofloxacin 2 mg in 5% dextrose injection. Nonmedicinal ingredients: dextrose, hydrochloric acid, lactic acid, nitrogen and water for injection. pH 3.5 to 4.6. Ready-to-use PVC flexible plastic containers with laminated foil overwrap of 100 mL and 200 mL. Should be administered "as is". Protect from light, excessive heat and freezing. Store at controlled room temperature (20 to 25°C). Use promptly when container is opened. Single use, discard unused portion. As with all parenteral drug products, intravenous admixtures should be inspected visually for clarity, particulate matter, precipitate, discoloration and leakage prior to administration, whenever solution and container permit.

The reader is invited to consult CPhA's monograph **Fluoroquinolones.**

Ciprofloxacin Intravenous Infusion BP ℞

ciprofloxacin

Antibacterial

Sandoz

SUPPLIED: 200 mg: Each mL of sterile solution contains: ciprofloxacin 2 mg. Nonmedicinal ingredients: dextrose monohydrate (5.5%), lactic acid solution, 1 N hydrochloric acid and water for injection. PVC minibags of 100 mL. Store between 15 and 25°C. Protect from light, excessive heat and freezing. Use promptly when pouch is opened.

400 mg: Each mL of sterile solution contains: ciprofloxacin 2 mg. Nonmedicinal ingredients: dextrose monohydrate (5.5%), lactic acid solution, 1 N hydrochloric acid and water for injection. PVC minibags of 200 mL. Store between 15 and 25°C. Protect from light, excessive heat and freezing. Use promptly when pouch is opened.

The reader is invited to consult CPhA's monograph **Fluoroquinolones.**

Cipro® I.V. ℞

ciprofloxacin

Antibacterial

Bayer

Cipro® Oral Suspension ℞

ciprofloxacin

Antibacterial

Bayer

Cipro® Tablets ℞

ciprofloxacin HCl

Antibacterial

Bayer

Date of Preparation: February 27, 1995
Date of Revision: June 5, 2008

PHARMACOLOGY: Action: Ciprofloxacin, a synthetic fluoroquinolone, has in vitro activity against a wide range of gram-negative and gram-positive microorganisms. Its bactericidal action is achieved through inhibition of topoisomerase II (DNA gyrase) and topoisomerase IV (both Type II topoisomerases), which are required for bacterial DNA replication, transcription, repair, and recombination.

Ciprofloxacin retained some of its bactericidal activity after inhibition of RNA and protein synthesis by rifampin and chloramphenicol, respectively. These observations suggest ciprofloxacin may possess two bactericidal mechanisms, one mechanism resulting from the inhibition of DNA gyrase and a second mechanism which may be independent of RNA and protein synthesis.

The mechanism of action of fluoroquinolones, including ciprofloxacin, is different from that of penicillins, cephalosporins, aminoglycosides, macrolides, and tetracyclines. Therefore, microorganisms resistant to these classes of drugs may be susceptible to ciprofloxacin. Conversely, microorganisms resistant to fluoroquinolones may be susceptible to these other classes of antimicrobial agents. There is no cross-resistance between ciprofloxacin and the mentioned classes of antibiotics.

Clinical Pharmacology: Absorption: Following oral administration of single doses of 250 mg, 500 mg, and 750 mg of ciprofloxacin tablets ciprofloxacin is absorbed rapidly and extensively mainly from the small intestine, reaching maximum serum concentrations 1-2 hours later.

The absolute bioavailability is approximately 70-80%. Maximum serum concentrations (C_{max}) and total areas under serum concentration vs. time curves (AUC) increased in proportion to dose.

The pharmacokinetics of ciprofloxacin oral suspension 10% are virtually identical to those of tablets.

Following an intravenous infusion of ciprofloxacin the mean maximum serum concentrations were achieved at the end of infusion. Pharmacokinetics of ciprofloxacin were linear over the dose range up to 400 mg administered intravenously.

Comparison of the pharmacokinetic parameters for a bid and tid i.v. dose regimen indicated no evidence of drug accumulation for ciprofloxacin and its metabolites.

A 60-minute i.v. infusion of 200 mg ciprofloxacin or the oral administration of 250 mg ciprofloxacin both given every 12 hours produced an equivalent area under the serum concentration time curve (AUC).

A 60-minute infusion of 400 mg ciprofloxacin every 12 hours was bioequivalent to a 500 mg oral dose every 12 hours with regard to AUC.

The 400 mg i.v. dose administered over 60 minutes every 12 hours resulted in a C_{max} similar to that observed with a 750 mg oral dose.

A 60-minute infusion of 400 mg ciprofloxacin every 8 hours is equivalent with respect to AUC to 750 mg oral regimen given every 12 hours.

Distribution: The protein binding of ciprofloxacin is low (20-30%), and the substance is present in plasma largely in a non-ionized form. Ciprofloxacin can diffuse freely into the extravascular space. The large steady-state volume of distribution of 2-3 L/kg body weight shows that ciprofloxacin penetrates in tissues resulting in concentrations which clearly exceed the corresponding serum levels.

Metabolism: Small concentrations of four metabolites have been reported. They were identified as desethyleneciprofloxacin (M1), sulphociprofloxacin (M2), oxociprofloxacin (M3) and formylciprofloxacin (M4). M1 to M3 display antibacterial activity comparable to or inferior to that of nalidixic acid. M4, with the smallest quantity, is largely equivalent to norfloxacin in its antimicrobial activity.

Elimination: Ciprofloxacin is largely excreted unchanged both renally and to a smaller extent non-renally. Renal clearance is between 0.18-0.3 L/h/kg and the total body clearance between 0.48-0.60 L/h/kg. Ciprofloxacin undergoes both glomerular filtration and tubular secretion.

Non-renal clearance of ciprofloxacin is mainly due to active transintestinal secretion as well as metabolization. 1% of the dose is excreted via the biliary route. Ciprofloxacin is present in the bile in high concentrations.

General: Ciprofloxacin and metronidazole have been studied in combination and serum levels of ciprofloxacin are not significantly altered by metronidazole at the doses studied. Serum levels of metronidazole when administered orally at a dose of 500 mg q6h in combination with ciprofloxacin 500 mg PO q12h are: $AUC_{0\rightarrow6}$ 156.3 mg.h/L, C_{max} 31.3 mg/L and t_{max} 1.71 hours. Serum levels of metronidazole when administered intravenously at a dose of 500 mg IV q6h in combination with ciprofloxacin 400 mg IV q12h are: $AUC_{0\rightarrow6}$ 153.0 mg·h/L, C_{max} 33.6 mg/L and t_{max} 1.0 hours. (See Dosage.)

Following infusion of 400 mg IV Ciprofloxacin every eight hours in combination with 50 mg/kg IV piperacillin sodium every 4 hours, mean serum ciprofloxacin concentrations were 3.02 µg/mL at 30 minutes and 1.18 µg/mL between 6-8 hours after the end of infusion. The mean serum ciprofloxacin concentration given alone at 400 mg IV every eight hours was 3.67 µg/mL at 30 minutes and 1.16 µg/mL at 6 hours after the end of infusion.

INDICATIONS: Oral: CIPRO (ciprofloxacin hydrochloride tablets) and CIPRO Oral Suspension (ciprofloxacin oral suspension) may be indicated for the treatment of patients with the following infections caused by susceptible strains of the indicated microorganisms:

Respiratory Tract Infections: Acute exacerbation of chronic bronchitis caused by: *H. influenzae, M. catarrhalis, S. pneumoniae.* Acute pneumonia caused by: *E. cloacae, E. coli, H. influenzae, K. pneumoniae, P. mirabilis, P. aeruginosa, S. aureus, S. pneumoniae.*

Acute sinusitis caused by: *H. influenzae, M. catarrhalis, S. pneumoniae.*

Due to the nature of the underlying conditions which usually predispose patients to pseudomonas infections of the respiratory tract, bacterial eradications may not be achieved in patients who display clinical improvement despite evidence of in vitro sensitivity. In patients requiring subsequent courses of therapy, CIPRO should be used alternately with other antipseudomonal agents. Some strains of *P. aeruginosa* may develop resistance during treatment. Therefore, susceptibility testing should be performed periodically during therapy to detect the emergence of bacterial resistance.

Urinary Tract Infections: Upper and lower urinary tract infections, such as complicated and uncomplicated cystitis, pyelonephritis, and pyelitis, caused by: *C. diversus, C. freundii, E. cloacae, E. coli, K. pneumoniae, K. oxytoca, M. morganii, P. mirabilis, P. aeruginosa, S. marcescens, S. aureus, S. epidermidis, S. saprophyticus, S. faecalis.*

Acute Uncomplicated Cystitis: caused by: *E. coli* in females.

Chronic Bacterial Prostatitis: caused by: *E. coli.*

Skin and Soft Tissue Infections: caused by: *E. cloacae, E. coli, K. pneumoniae, P. mirabilis, P. vulgaris, P. aeruginosa, S. aureus, S. epidermidis, S. pyogenes.*

Bone and Joint Infections: caused by: *E. cloacae, P. aeruginosa, S. marcescens, S. aureus.*

Infectious Diarrhea (when antibacterial therapy is indicated): caused by: *C. jejuni, E. coli* (enterotoxigenic strains), *S. dysenteriae, S. flexneri, S. sonnei.*

Meningococcal Carriers: Treatment of asymptomatic carriers of *N. meningitidis* to eliminate meningococci from the nasopharynx. An MIC determination on the isolate from the index case should be performed as soon as possible. **Ciprofloxacin is not indicated for the treatment of meningococcal meningitis.**

Typhoid Fever (enteric fever): caused by: *S. paratyphi, S. typhi.*

Uncomplicated Gonorrhea: Cervical/urethral/rectal/pharyngeal infections caused by *N. gonorrhoea.* Because co-infection with *C. trachomatis* is common, consideration should be given to treating presumptively with an additional regimen that is effective against *C. trachomatis.*

I.V.: CIPRO I.V. (ciprofloxacin injection) may be indicated for the treatment of patients with the following infections caused by susceptible strains of the indicated microorganisms:

Respiratory Tract Infections: Acute pneumonia caused by: *E. cloacae, E. coli, H. influenzae, H. parainfluenzae, K. pneumoniae, P. mirabilis, P. aeruginosa, S. aureus, S. pneumoniae.*

Due to the nature of the underlying conditions which usually predispose patients to Pseudomonas infections of the respiratory tract, bacterial eradications may not be achieved in patients who display clinical improvement despite evidence of in vitro sensitivity. In patients requiring subsequent courses of therapy, CIPRO should be used alternately with other antipseudomonal agents. Some strains of *P. aeruginosa* may develop resistance during treatment. Therefore, susceptibility testing should be performed periodically during therapy to detect the emergence of bacterial resistance.

Urinary Tract Infections: Upper and lower complicated urinary tract infections including pyelonephritis caused by: *C. diversus, E. coli, K. pneumoniae, P. mirabilis, P. aeruginosa.*

Skin or Skin Structure Infections: caused by: *E. cloacae, E. coli, K. pneumoniae, M. morganii, P. mirabilis, P. vulgaris, P. aeruginosa, S. aureus, S. pyogenes.*

Septicemia: caused by: *E. coli, S. typhi.*

Bone: caused by: *E. cloacae, P. aeruginosa.*

Complicated Intra-abdominal infections only when used in combination with metronidazole (see Dosage): caused by: *E. coli, P. aeruginosa, K. pneumoniae, B. fragilis.*

Note: Most anaerobic bacteria, including *B. fragilis,* are resistant to ciprofloxacin. Therefore, ciprofloxacin should not be used as single agent therapy for complicated intra-abdominal infections. Efficacy against Enterococcus sp. in clinical trials has been shown to be only 75%.

Empiric Therapy in Febrile Neutropenic Patients (in combination with piperacillin sodium): (see Dosage).

Appropriate culture and susceptibility tests should be performed prior to initiating treatment in order to isolate and identify organisms causing the infection and to determine their susceptibilities to ciprofloxacin. Therapy with CIPRO, CIPRO I.V. and CIPRO Oral Suspension may be initiated before results of these tests are known. However, modification of this treatment may be required once results become available or if there is no clinical improvement. Culture and susceptibility testing performed periodically during therapy will provide information on the possible emergence of bacterial resistance. If anaerobic organisms are suspected to be contributing to the infection, appropriate therapy should be administered.

CONTRAINDICATIONS: CIPRO (ciprofloxacin hydrochloride tablets), CIPRO I.V. (ciprofloxacin injection) and CIPRO Oral Suspension (ciprofloxacin oral suspension) are contraindicated in patients who have shown hypersensitivity to ciprofloxacin or other quinolone antibacterial agents or any of the excipients.

Concurrent administration of ciprofloxacin and tizanidine is contraindicated since it may result in an undesirable increase in serum tizanidine concentrations. This can be associated with clinically relevant tizanidine-induced side effects (hypotension, somnolence, drowsiness).

WARNINGS: The safety of CIPRO (ciprofloxacin hydrochloride tablets), CIPRO I.V. (ciprofloxacin injection) and CIPRO Oral Suspension (ciprofloxacin oral suspension) in pediatric patients and adolescents (under the age of 18 years), pregnant women and nursing women has not yet been established. (See Precautions, Children, Pregnancy, and Lactation.) Damage to juvenile weight-bearing joints and lameness were observed both in rat and dog studies but not in weaned piglets. Histopathological examination of the weight-bearing joints in immature dogs revealed permanent lesions of the cartilage.

CNS and Psychiatric Effects: Convulsions, increased intracranial pressure, and toxic psychosis have been reported in patients receiving quinolones, including ciprofloxacin. Ciprofloxacin may also cause central nervous system (CNS) stimulation which may lead to tremors, restlessness, lightheadedness, confusion, hallucinations, depression, nervousness, agitation, insomnia, anxiety, paranoia, nightmares and rarely, suicidal thoughts or acts. In rare cases, depression or psychosis can progress to self-endangering behavior. These reactions may occur following the first dose. If these reactions occur in patients receiving ciprofloxacin, the drug should be discontinued and appropriate measures instituted. As with all quinolones, ciprofloxacin should be used with caution in patients with known or suspected CNS disorders, such as severe cerebral arteriosclerosis, epilepsy, and other factors that predispose to seizures or lower the seizure threshold. (See Adverse Effects.)

Cytochrome P450: Ciprofloxacin is known to be a moderate inhibitor of the CYP450 1A2 enzymes. Care should be taken when other drugs are administered concomitantly which are metabolized via the same enzymatic pathway (e.g., theophylline, methylxanthines, caffeine, duloxetine, clozapine). Increased plasma concentrations associated with drug specific side effects may be observed due to inhibition of their metabolic clearance by ciprofloxacin. (See Contraindications and Precautions, Drug Interactions.)

Hypersensitivity: Serious hypersensitivity and/or anaphylactic reactions have been reported in patients receiving quinolone therapy, including ciprofloxacin. These reactions may occur within the first 30 minutes following the first dose and may require epinephrine and other emergency measures. Some reactions have been accompanied by cardiovascular collapse, hypotension/shock, seizure, loss of consciousness, tingling, angioedema (including tongue, laryngeal, throat or facial edema/swelling), airway obstruction (including bronchospasm, shortness of breath and acute respiratory distress), dyspnea, urticaria, itching and other serious skin reactions.

Ciprofloxacin should be discontinued at the first appearance of a skin rash or any other sign of hypersensitivity. Serious acute hypersensitivity reactions may require treatment with epinephrine and other resuscitative measures, including oxygen, intravenous fluids, antihistamines, corticosteroids, pressor amines and airway management, as clinically indicated.

Serious and sometimes fatal events, some due to hypersensitivity and some due to uncertain etiology, have been reported in patients receiving therapy with all antibiotics. These events may be severe and generally occur following the administration of multiple doses. Clinical manifestations may include one or more of the following: fever, rash or severe dermatologic reactions (e.g., toxic epidermal necrolysis, Stevens-Johnson syndrome), vasculitis, arthralgia, myalgia, serum sickness, allergic pneumonitis, interstitial nephritis, acute renal insufficiency or failure, hepatitis, jaundice, acute hepatic necrosis or failure, hepatic necrosis with fatal outcome, anemia including hemolytic and aplastic, thrombocytopenia including thrombotic thrombocytopenic purpura, leukopenia, agranulocytosis, pancytopenia, and/or other hematologic abnormalities.

Gastrointestinal: *C. difficile*-associated disease: *C. difficile*-associated disease (CDAD) has been reported with the use of many antibacterial agents, including ciprofloxacin. CDAD may range in severity from mild diarrhea to fatal colitis. It is important to consider this diagnosis in patients who present with diarrhea or symptoms of colitis, pseudomembranous colitis, toxic megacolon, or perforation of the colon subsequent to the administration of any antibacterial agent. CDAD has been reported to occur over 2 months after the administration of antibacterial agents.

Treatment with antibacterial agents may alter the normal flora of the colon and many permit overgrowth of *C. difficile. C. difficile* produces toxins A and B, which contribute to the development of CDAD. CDAD may cause significant morbidity and mortality. CDAD can be refractory to antimicrobial therapy.

If the diagnosis of CDAD is suspected or confirmed, appropriate therapeutic measures should be initiated. Mild cases of CDAD usually respond to discontinuation of antibacterial agents not directed against *C. difficile*. In moderate to severe cases, consideration should be given to management with fluids and electrolytes, protein supplementation, and treatment with an antibacterial agent clinically effective against *C. difficile*. Drugs that inhibit peristalsis may delay clearance of *C. difficile* and its toxins, and therefore should not be used in the treatment of CDAD. Surgical evaluation should be instituted as clinically indicated since surgical intervention may be required in certain severe cases. (See Adverse Effects.)

PRECAUTIONS: Serious and fatal reactions have been reported in patients receiving concurrent administration of CIPRO I.V. and theophylline. These reactions include cardiac arrest, seizure, status epilepticus and respiratory failure. Similar serious adverse events have been noted with administration of theophylline alone, however, the possibility that ciprofloxacin may potentiate these reactions cannot be eliminated. If concomitant use cannot be avoided, the plasma levels of theophylline should be monitored and appropriate dosage adjustments should be made.

Tendon rupture (generally Achilles tendon) has been reported predominantly in the elderly on prior systemic treatment with glucocorticoids. At any sign of tendonitis (ie, painful swelling, inflammation), a physician should be consulted and the antibiotic treatment should be discontinued. Care should be taken to keep the affected extremity at rest and avoid any inappropriate exercise (as the risk for tendon rupture might increase otherwise). Ciprofloxacin should not be used in patients with a clear history of tendon disorders related to quinolone treatment because they may be at risk of developing tendon disorders again when re-exposed to a fluoroquinolone.

Crystalluria related to ciprofloxacin has been reported only rarely in man because human urine is usually acidic. Crystals have been observed in the urine of laboratory animals, usually from alkaline urine. Patients receiving ciprofloxacin should be well hydrated and alkalinity of the urine should be avoided. The recommended daily dose should not be exceeded.

Ciprofloxacin has been shown to produce photosensitivity reactions. Patients taking ciprofloxacin should avoid direct exposure to excessive sunlight or UV light. Therapy should be discontinued if photosensitization (i.e., sunburn-like skin reactions) occurs.

I.V. infusion should be administered by slow infusion over a period of 60 minutes. Local i.v. reactions have been reported with the i.v. administration of ciprofloxacin. These reactions are more frequent if infusion time is 30 minutes or less, or if small veins of the hand are used.

Prolonged use of ciprofloxacin may result in the overgrowth of nonsusceptible organisms. Careful observation of the patient is therefore essential, and if superinfection should occur during therapy, appropriate measures should be taken.

Pregnancy: The safety of CIPRO, CIPRO I.V. and CIPRO Oral Suspension in pregnancy have not yet been established. CIPRO, CIPRO I.V. and CIPRO Oral Suspension should not be used in pregnant women unless the likely benefits outweigh the possible risk to the fetus (see Warnings). CIPRO, CIPRO I.V. and CIPRO Oral Suspension have been shown to be nonembryotoxic and nonteratogenic in animal studies.

Lactation: Ciprofloxacin is excreted in human milk. Because of the potential for serious adverse reactions in infants nursing from women taking ciprofloxacin, a decision should be made to discontinue nursing or to discontinue the administration of CIPRO, CIPRO I.V. and CIPRO Oral Suspension, taking into account the importance of the drug to the mother and the possible risk to the infant (see Warnings).

Children: The safety and efficacy of ciprofloxacin in the pediatric population less than 18 years of age have not been established. Quinolones, including ciprofloxacin, cause arthropathy and osteochondrosis in juvenile animals of several species (see Warnings).

Geriatrics: Ciprofloxacin is substantially excreted by the kidney, and the risk of adverse reactions may be greater in patients with impaired renal function.

Renal Impairment: Since ciprofloxacin is eliminated primarily by the kidney, CIPRO, CIPRO I.V. and CIPRO Oral Suspension should be used with caution and at a reduced dosage in patients with impaired renal function. (See Dosage.)

Hepatic Impairment: In preliminary studies in patients with stable chronic liver cirrhosis (with mild to moderate hepatic impairment), no significant changes in ciprofloxacin pharmacokinetics were observed. The kinetics of ciprofloxacin in patients with acute hepatic insufficiency and stable chronic cirrhosis (with severe hepatic impairment), however, have not been fully elucidated. An increased incidence of nausea, vomiting, headache and diarrhea were observed in this patient population.

Occupational Hazards: Ability to Drive and Operate Machinery: Even when ciprofloxacin is taken exactly as prescribed, it can affect the speed of reaction to such an extent that the ability to drive or to operate machinery is impaired. This applies particularly in combination with alcohol.

Sucrose Load for Oral Suspension Formulation: As the oral suspension contains sucrose, it is unsuitable for patients with rare hereditary problems of fructose intolerance, glucose-galactose malabsorption or sucrase-isomaltase insufficiency. (See Supplied.)

Dextrose Load for Intravenous Solution Formulation: Ciprofloxacin infusion solution (bags) contain glucose. This should be taken into account in patients with diabetes mellitus. Glucose content is 5 g for the 100 mL bag and 10 g for the 200 mL bag. (See Supplied.)

Drug Interactions: Caffeine: Caffeine has been shown to interfere with the metabolism and pharmacokinetics of ciprofloxacin. Excessive caffeine intake should be avoided.

Clozapine: Following concomitant administration of 250 mg ciprofloxacin for 7 days, serum concentrations of clozapine and n-desmethylclozapine were increased by 29% and 31%, respectively (see Warnings).

Cyclosporine: Some quinolones, including ciprofloxacin, have been associated with transient increases in serum creatinine levels in patients who are concomitantly receiving cyclosporine.

Duloxetine: In clinical studies it was demonstrated that concomitant use of duloxetine with strong inhibitors of the CYP450 1A2 isozyme such as fluvoxamine, may result in an increase of AUC and C_{max} of duloxetine. Although no clinical data are available on a possible interaction with ciprofloxacin, similar effects can be expected upon concomitant administration.

Ferrous Sulfate: Oral ferrous sulfate at therapeutic doses decreases the bioavailability of oral ciprofloxacin, therefore concomitant therapy is not advised.

Food and Dairy Products: Although, ciprofloxacin may be taken with meals that include milk, simultaneous administration with dairy products alone, or with calcium-fortified products should be avoided, since decreased absorption is possible. It is recommended that ciprofloxacin be administered at least 2 hours before or 2 hours after substantial calcium intake (>800 mg) (see Dosage).

Glyburide: In particular cases, concurrent administration of ciprofloxacin and glyburide can intensify the action of glyburide (hypoglycemia).

Histamine H_2-receptor Antagonists: Histamine H_2-receptor antagonists appear to have no significant effect on the bioavailability of ciprofloxacin.

Lidocaine: It was demonstrated in healthy subjects that concomitant use of lidocaine with ciprofloxacin, a moderate inhibitor of CYP450 1A2 isozyme, reduces clearance of intravenous lidocaine by 22%. Ciprofloxacin may increase the systemic toxicity of lidocaine.

Methotrexate: Renal tubular transport of methotrexate may be inhibited by concomitant administration of ciprofloxacin, potentially leading to increased plasma levels of methotrexate. This might increase the risk of methotrexate associated toxic reactions. Therefore, patients under methotrexate therapy should be carefully monitored when concomitant ciprofloxacin therapy is indicated.

Metoclopramide: Metoclopramide accelerates the absorption of ciprofloxacin (oral), resulting in a shorter time to reach maximum plasma concentrations. No effect was seen on the bioavailability of ciprofloxacin.

Multivalent Cations: Concurrent administration of a quinolone, including ciprofloxacin, with multivalent cation-containing products such as magnesium/aluminum antacids, polymeric phosphate binders such as sevelamer, sucralfate, Videx (didanosine) chewable/buffered tablets or pediatric powder, mineral supplements or products containing calcium, iron, or zinc may substantially interfere with the absorption of the quinolone, resulting in serum and urine levels considerably lower than desired. Ciprofloxacin should be administered at least 2 hours before or 6 hours after these preparations.

NSAID: Concomitant administration of a nonsteroidal anti-inflammatory drug (fenbufen) with a quinolone (enoxacin) has been reported to increase the risk of CNS stimulation and convulsive seizures.

Probenecid: Probenecid blocks renal tubular secretion of ciprofloxacin and has been shown to produce an increase in the level of ciprofloxacin in the serum.

Ropinirole: In a clinical study it was shown that concomitant use of ropinirole with ciprofloxacin, a medium inhibitor of the CYP450 1A2 isozyme, resulted in increases in the C_{max} and AUC of ropinirole of 60 and 84%, respectively. Ciprofloxacin may increase the systemic toxicity of ropinirole.

Theophylline: Concurrent administration of ciprofloxacin with theophylline may lead to elevated serum concentrations of theophylline and prolongation of its elimination half-life. This may result in increased risk of theophylline-related adverse reactions (see Adverse Effects). If concomitant use cannot be avoided, serum levels of theophylline should be monitored and dosage adjustments made as appropriate.

Tizanidine: In a clinical study in healthy subjects there was an increase in tizanidine serum concentrations (C_{max} increase: 7-fold, range: 4 to 21-fold; AUC increase: 10-fold, range: 6 to 24-fold) when given concomitantly with ciprofloxacin. Associated with the increased serum concentrations was a potentiated hypotensive and sedative effect. Tizanidine must not be administered together with ciprofloxacin. (See Contraindications, Warnings.)

Warfarin: Quinolones have been reported to increase the effects of the oral anticoagulant warfarin and its derivatives. During concomitant administration of these drugs, the prothrombin time or other appropriate coagulation tests should be closely monitored.

ADVERSE EFFECTS: CIPRO (ciprofloxacin hydrochloride tablets), CIPRO I.V. (ciprofloxacin injection) and CIPRO Oral Suspension (ciprofloxacin oral suspension) are generally well tolerated. During worldwide clinical investigation, 16 580 courses of ciprofloxacin treatment were evaluated for drug safety.

Adverse events, possibly, probably or highly probably related to ciprofloxacin occurred in 1395 (8.8%) of patients. The adverse reactions according to treatment (oral, i.v. and sequential therapy) show that the incidence of adverse reactions was 8% for the group treated orally, 17% for the group treated with ciprofloxacin i.v. and 15.3% for the group treated sequentially. The difference between the oral and i.v. group relates to adverse vascular reactions which are known to be associated with i.v. administration.

In orally treated patients enrolled in clinical trials, the most frequently reported events, possibly, probably drug-related were: nausea (1.3%) and diarrhea (1%).

In patients treated with CIPRO I.V., the most frequently reported events, possibly, probably drug-related were: rash (1.8%), diarrhea (1%) and injection site pain (1%).

Local i.v. site reactions have been reported. These reactions are more frequent if the infusion time is 30 minutes or less. These may appear as local skin reactions which resolve rapidly upon completion of the infusion. Subsequent i.v. administration is not contraindicated unless the reactions recur or worsen.

Events possibly, probably drug-related occurring at a frequency of less than 1% with ciprofloxacin oral and i.v. treatment during clinical trials and subsequent postmarketing surveillance are as follows:

Body as a Whole: back pain, chest pain, pain, pain in extremities, moniliasis.

Cardiovascular: palpitation, phlebitis, (thrombo)-phlebitis (at infusion site), tachycardia. The following has been reported rarely ≥0.01% <0.1%): hypotension. The following have been reported very rarely (<0.01%): angina pectoris, atrial fibrillation, cardiac arrest, cerebrovascular disorder, electrocardiogram abnormality, hot flashes, hypertension, kidney vasculitis, myocardial infarct, pericarditis, pulmonary embolus, substernal chest pain, syncope (fainting), vasodilation (hot flashes).

Digestive: abdominal pain, anorexia, dry mouth, dyspepsia, dysphagia, enlarged abdomen, flatulence, gastrointestinal moniliasis, jaundice, stomatitis, vomiting, abnormal liver function test. The following have been reported rarely: moniliasis (oral), cholestatic jaundice, and pseudomembranous colitis. The following have been reported very rarely: constipation, esophagitis, gastrointestinal hemorrhage, glossitis, hepatomegaly, ileus, increased appetite, intestinal perforation, life-threatening pseudomembranous colitis with possible fatal outcome, liver damage, melena, pancreatitis, tenesmus, tooth discoloration, toxic megacolon, ulcerative stomatitis.

Hemic and Lymphatic: agranulocytosis, anaemia, eosinophilia, granulocytopenia, leukocytopenia, leukocytosis, pancytopenia. The following have been reported very rarely: altered prothrombin levels, haemolytic anaemia, marrow depression (life threatening), pancytopenia (life threatening), thrombocytopenia, thrombocytosis.

Hypersensitivity: rash. The following have been reported rarely: allergic reaction, anaphylactic/anaphylactoid reactions including facial, vascular and laryngeal edema, drug fever, hemorrhagic bullae and small nodules (papules) with crust formation showing vascular involvement (vasculitis), hepatitis, interstitial nephritis, petechiae (punctuate skin hemorrhages), pruritus, serum sickness-like reaction, Stevens-Johnson syndrome. The following have been reported very rarely: shock (anaphylactic; life-threatening), pruritic rash, erythema multiforme (minor), erythema nodosum, major liver disorders including hepatic necrosis, (very rarely progressing to life threatening hepatic failures), epidermal necrolysis (Lyell syndrome, potentially life-threatening).

I.V. Infusion Site: thrombophlebitis, injection site reaction (e.g. edema, hypersensitivity, inflammation, pain). The following have been reported very rarely: burning, erythema, pain, paresthesia, and swelling.

Metabolic and Nutritional Disorder: creatinine increased. The following have been reported rarely: edema (face) and hyperglycemia.

Musculoskeletal: The following have been reported rarely: achiness, arthralgia (joint pain), joint disorder (joint swelling), pain in the extremities, partial or complete tendon rupture (predominantly achilles tendon), tendonitis (predominantly achillotendonitis), myalgia (muscular pain). The following have been reported very rarely: myasthenia (exacerbation of symptoms of myasthenia gravis).

There have been 54 reports of arthropathies with CIPRO. Ten of these reports involved children. Arthralgia was usually the first symptom which led to rapid assessment and withdrawal of the drug. No irreversible arthropathies have been observed.

Nervous System: agitation, confusion, convulsion, dizziness, hallucinations, headache, hypesthesia, increased sweating, insomnia, somnolence, tremor (trembling). The following has been reported rarely: paresthesia (peripheral paralgesia). The following have been reported very rarely: abnormal dreams (nightmares), anxiety, apathy, ataxia, depersonalization, depression, diplopia, hemiplegia, hyperesthesia, hypertonia, increase of intracranial pressure, meningism, migraine, nervousness, neuritis, paresthesia, polyneuritis, sleep disorder, twitching, grand mal convulsions, abnormal (unsteady) gait, psychosis, intracranial hypertension. In some instances these reactions occurred after the first administration of CIPRO. In these instances, CIPRO has to be discontinued and the doctor should be informed immediately.

Other: The following have been reported rarely: asthenia (general feeling of weakness, tiredness), death.

Respiratory: dyspnea. The following have been reported very rarely: hiccup, hyperventilation, increased cough, larynx edema, lung edema, lung hemorrhage, pharyngitis, stridor, voice alteration.

Skin and Appendages: pruritus, rash, maculopapular rash. The following has been reported rarely: photosensitivity reaction. The following have been reported very rarely: alopecia, angioedema, fixed eruption, photosensitive dermatitis, petechia, urticaria.

Special Senses: abnormal vision (visual disturbances), taste perversion, tinnitus. The following have been reported rarely: transitory deafness (especially at higher frequencies), taste loss (impaired taste). The following have been reported very rarely: chromatopsia, colour blindness, conjunctivitis, corneal opacity, diplopia, ear pain, eye pain, parosmia (impaired smell), anosmia (usually reversible on discontinuation).

Urogenital: albuminuria, hematuria. The following have been reported rarely: abnormal kidney function, acute kidney failure, dysuria, leukorrhea, nephritis interstitial, urinary retention, vaginitis, vaginal moniliasis.

Laboratory Values: increased alkaline phosphatase, ALT increased, AST increased, BUN (urea) increased, cholestatic parameters increased, Gamma-GT increased, lactic dehydrogenase increased, NPN increased, transaminases increased; decreased albuminuria, bilirubinemia, creatinine clearance decreased, hypercholesteremia, hyperuricemia, increased sedimentation rate. The following have been reported rarely: acidosis, amylase increased, crystalluria, electrolyte abnormality, hematuria, hypercalcemia, hypocalcemia and lipase increased.

Most of the adverse events reported were described as only mild or moderate in severity.

Adverse reactions noted during therapy with ciprofloxacin and metronidazole in clinical trials were similar to those already noted during therapy with ciprofloxacin alone with the following additions:

Cardiovascular: peripheral edema.

Digestive: colitis, gastritis, tongue discoloration.

Hemic and Lymphatic: coagulation disorder, thrombocythemia.

Skin: fungal dermatitis, pustular rash, sweating.

Metabolic: healing abnormal, hypernatremia.

Nervous: dementia.

Urinary: kidney tumour necrosis, urinary incontinence.

The following additional adverse events, in alphabetical order, regardless of incidence or relationship to drug, have been reported during clinical trials and from worldwide post-marketing experience in patients given ciprofloxacin (includes all formulations, all dosages, all drug-therapy durations, and in all indications): arrhythmia, atrial flutter, bleeding diathesis, bronchospasm, *C. difficile* associated diarrhea, candiduria, cardiac murmur, cardiopulmonary arrest, cardiovascular collapse, cerebral thrombosis, chills, delirium, drowsiness, dysphasia, edema (conjunctivae, hands, lips, lower extremities, neck), epistaxis, exfoliative dermatitis, fever, gastrointestinal bleeding, gout (flare up), gynecomastia, hearing loss, hemoptysis, hemorrhagic cystitis, hyperpigmentation, joint stiffness, lightheadedness, lymphadenopathy, manic reaction, myoclonus, nystagmus, pain (arm, breast, epigastric, foot, jaw, neck, oral mucosa), paranoia, phobia, pleural effusion, polyuria, postural hypotension, pulmonary embolism, purpura, QT prolongation (frequency <1 per million), renal calculi, respiratory arrest, respiratory distress, restlessness, rhabdomyolysis, torsades de pointes (frequency <1 per million), toxic psychosis, unresponsiveness, urethral bleeding, urination (frequent), ventricular ectopy, ventricular fibrillation (frequency <1 per million), ventricular tachycardia (frequency <1 per million), vesicles, visual acuity (decreased) and visual disturbances (flashing lights, change in color perception, overbrightness of lights).

OVERDOSE:

Symptoms: In the event of acute, excessive oral overdosage, reversible renal toxicity, arthralgia, myalgia and CNS symptoms have been reported.

Treatment: Therefore, apart from routine emergency measures, it is recommended to monitor renal function and to administer magnesium- or calcium-containing antacids which reduce the absorption of ciprofloxacin and to maintain adequate hydration. Based on information obtained from subjects with chronic renal failure, only a small amount of ciprofloxacin (<10%) is removed from the body after hemodialysis or peritoneal dialysis.

The administration of activated charcoal as soon as possible after oral overdose may prevent excessive increase of systemic ciprofloxacin exposure.

For management of a suspected drug overdose, contact your **regional Poison Control Centre**. See the *CPS* Directory section for a list of Poison Control Centres.

DOSAGE: The determination of dosage for any particular patient must take into consideration the severity and nature of the infection, the susceptibility of the causative organism, the integrity of the patient's host-defence mechanisms and the status of renal function.

Oral: CIPRO (ciprofloxacin hydrochloride tablets) or CIPRO Oral Suspension (ciprofloxacin oral suspension) may be taken before or after meals. Absorption is faster on an empty stomach. Patients should be advised to drink fluids liberally and avoid taking dairy products or antacids containing magnesium or aluminum.

Ciprofloxacin should be administered at least 2 hours before or 6 hours after antacids and mineral supplements containing magnesium or aluminum, as well as sucralfate, Videx (didanosine) chewable/buffered tablets or pediatric powder, metal cations such as iron, and multivitamin preparations with zinc (see Precautions, Drug Interactions).

Although ciprofloxacin may be taken with meals that include milk, simultaneous administration with dairy products alone, or with calcium-fortified products should be avoided, since decreased absorption is possible. It is recommended that ciprofloxacin be administered at least 2 hours before or 2 hours after substantial calcium intake (>800 mg) (see Precautions, Drug Interactions).

Adults: The recommended dosages of oral CIPRO are shown in Table 1.

Table 1: CIPRO Tablets/Cipro Oral Suspension

Recommended Dosages for Oral CIPRO

Location of Infection	Type/Severity	Unit Dose[b]	Frequency	Daily Dose
Urinary Tract	mild/moderate	250 mg	q12h	500 mg
	severe/complicated	500 mg	q12h	1000 mg
Chronic Bacterial Prostatitis	asymptomatic/mild/moderate	500 mg	q12h	1000 mg
Respiratory Tract Bone and Joint Skin and Soft Tissue	mild/moderate	500 mg	q12h	1000 mg
	severe/complicated[a]	750 mg	q12h	1500 mg
Infectious Diarrhea	mild/moderate/severe	500 mg	q12h	1000 mg
Urogenital and Extragenital Gonorrhea	uncomplicated	500 mg	once	500 mg
Typhoid Fever	mild/moderate	500 mg	q12h	1000 mg
N. Meningitidis Nasopharyngeal Colonization	carrier state	750 mg	once	750 mg
Acute Sinusitis	moderate	500 mg	q12h	1000 mg

[a] e.g., hospital-acquired pneumonia, osteomyelitis.
[b] One teaspoon (5 mL) of 10% oral ciprofloxacin suspension = 500 mg of ciprofloxacin.

Oral Suspension: See Table 2.

See Instructions below for Use/Handling.

Table 2: CIPRO Oral Suspension

Use/Handling of Ciprofloxacin Suspension

Dosage	Volume (mL) of Oral Suspension 10%
250 mg	2.5 mL
500 mg	5 mL
750 mg	7.5 mL

Depending on the severity of the infections, as well as the clinical and bacteriological responses, the average treatment period should be approximately 7 to 14 days. Generally, treatment should last 3 days beyond the disappearance of clinical symptoms or until cultures are sterile. Patients with osteomyelitis may require treatment for a minimum of 6 to 8 weeks and up to 3 months. With acute cystitis in females, a 3- to 5-day treatment may be sufficient. With infectious diarrhea, a 5-day treatment may be sufficient. Typhoid fever should be treated for 14 days. Acute sinusitis should be treated for 10 days with 500 mg q12h. Chronic bacterial prostatitis should be treated for 28 days with 500 mg every 12 hours.

Instructions to the Pharmacist for Use/Handling of CIPRO Oral Suspension: Preparation of the suspension:

1. The small bottle contains the ciprofloxacin microcapsules; the large bottle contains the diluent.
2. Open both bottles. Child-proof cap: Press down according to the instructions on the cap while turning to the left.
3. Pour the microcapsules completely into the large bottle of diluent. **Do not add water to the suspension.**
4. Close the large bottle completely according to the instructions on the cap and shake vigorously for about 15 seconds. The suspension is ready for use.

Instructions to the Patient for Taking CIPRO Oral Suspension: **Shake vigorously each time before use for approximately 15 seconds.** Swallow the prescribed amount of suspension. Do not chew the microcapsules. Reclose the bottle completely after use according to instruction on the cap. The suspension is stable for 14 days when stored in a refrigerator or at room temperature (5 to 25°C). Store in an upright position. After treatment has been completed, any remaining suspension should not be reused.

I.V. Administration: Ciprofloxacin should be administered by i.v. infusion over a period of 60 minutes. Slow infusion into a large vein will minimize patient discomfort and reduce the risk of venous irritation.

Adults: The recommended adult dosages of CIPRO I.V. (ciprofloxacin injection) are shown in Table 3.

Definitive clinical studies have not been completed for severe infections other than in the respiratory tract.

The duration of treatment depends upon the severity of infection. Generally ciprofloxacin should be continued for at least 3 days after the signs and symptoms of infection have disappeared. The usual duration is 7 to 14 days. However, for severe and complicated infections more prolonged therapy may be required. Bone and joint infections may require treatment for 4 to 6 weeks or longer.

Sequential I.V./Oral Therapy: In patients receiving i.v. ciprofloxacin, oral ciprofloxacin may be considered when clinically indicated at the discretion of the physician. Clinical studies evaluating the use of sequential i.v./oral therapy in septicemia, however, have not been completed.

Impaired Renal Function: Ciprofloxacin is eliminated primarily by renal excretion. However, the drug is also metabolized and partially cleared through the biliary system of the liver and through the intestine (see Pharmacology). This alternate pathway of drug elimination appears to compensate for the reduced renal excretion of patients with renal impairment. Nonetheless, some modification of dosage is recommended, particularly for patients with severe renal dysfunction. Table 4 provides a guideline for dosage adjustment. However, monitoring of serum drug levels provides the most reliable basis for dosage adjustments.

Table 3: CIPRO I.V.

Recommended Adult Dosages of CIPRO I.V. (Ciprofloxacin Injection)

Location of Infection	Type/Severity	Unit Dose	Frequency	Daily Dose
Urinary Tract	moderate/severe/ complicated	200 to 400 mg	q12h	400 to 800 mg
Respiratory Tract	moderate/severe	400 mg	q8h to q12h	800 to 1200 mg
Skin or Skin Structure Blood Bone	moderate	400 mg	q12h	800 mg
Intra-abdominal	complicated	400 mg	q12h	400 mg q12h only when used in combination with metronidazole 500 mg i.v. q6h[a]
Empiric Therapy in Febrile Neutropenic Patients	severe ciprofloxacin + piperacillin sodium	400 mg 50 mg/kg	q8h q4h	1200 mg Not to exceed 24 g/day

[a] (1) Clinical success was demonstrated with a limited number of patients switched to oral therapy: (CIPRO 500 mg orally q12h plus metronidazole 500 mg orally q6h) during day 3, 4 or 5 of therapy when able to take oral medication and having shown an initial clinical response to the i.v. therapy.
(2) See Metronidazole product monograph for Prescribing Information including cautionary statements.
(3) For information on CIPRO plus metronidazole combination therapy, see Pharmacology and Adverse Effects.

Table 4: CIPRO/CIPRO I.V./CIPRO Oral Suspension

Maximum Daily Dose with Stated Creatinine Clearance or Serum Creatinine

Creatinine Clearance mL/min/1.73 m²	Maximum Daily Dose		Serum Creatinine Concentration mg/100 mL
	Oral	I.V.	
31–60	1000 mg	800 mg	1.4–1.9
≤30	500 mg	400 mg	≥2.0

Maximum daily dose, not to be exceeded when either creatinine clearance or serum creatinine are in the ranges stated.

Hemodialysis: Only a small amount of ciprofloxacin (< l0%) is removed from the body after hemodialysis or peritoneal dialysis. For hemodialysis patients, please follow dosing recommendations as described in Table 4. On dialysis days, the dose should be administered after dialysis.

When only the serum creatinine concentration is available, the following formulas (based on sex, weight and age of the patient) may be used to convert this value into creatinine clearance. The serum creatinine should represent a steady state of renal function:

Creatinine Clearance mL/s =

Males: $\dfrac{\text{Weight (kg)}\times(140-\text{age})}{49\times\text{serum creatinine }(\mu\text{mol/L})}$.

Females: 0.85×the above value.

In traditional units mL/min =

Males: $\dfrac{\text{Weight (kg)}\times(140-\text{age})}{72\times\text{serum creatinine (mg/100 mL)}}$

Females: 0.85×the above value.

Impaired Hepatic Function: No dosage adjustment is required.

Pediatric Use: The safety and efficacy of CIPRO, CIPRO I.V. and CIPRO Oral Suspension in individuals less than 18 years of age has not been established. CIPRO, CIPRO I.V. and CIPRO Oral Suspension should not be used in pediatric patients and adolescents (see Warnings).

Parenteral Products: **Intermittent I.V. Infusion:** CIPRO I.V. (ciprofloxacin injection) should be administered only by i.v. infusion over a period of 60 minutes. The drug should not be given by rapid injection. Slow infusion of a dilute solution into a large vein will minimize patient discomfort and reduce the risk of venous irritation.

If CIPRO I.V. is to be given concomitantly with another drug, each drug should be given separately in accordance with the recommended dosage and route of administration for each drug. Only CIPRO I.V. (ciprofloxacin injection) in the 10 mg/mL vials should be diluted to 1.0-2.0 mg/mL with the following recommended intravenous solutions: Sterile Water for Injection, USP; 0.9% Sodium Chloride Injection, USP; 5% Dextrose Injection, USP; 5% Dextrose in 0.225% Sodium Chloride Injection, USP; 5% Dextrose in 0.45% Sodium Chloride Injection, USP; 5% Dextrose in Electrolyte #75 Injection; l0% Dextrose Injection; l0% Fructose Injection; Ringer's Injection; Lactated Ringer's Injection, USP.

CIPRO I.V. Minibags contain ciprofloxacin at 2 mg/mL and should be administered "as is".

Ciprofloxacin Injection when diluted with the recommended intravenous solutions should be used within 24 hours at room temperature or 72 hours when refrigerated. Since ciprofloxacin is slightly light sensitive, the solutions should be protected from light during storage.

Vials: See Table 5. The intravenous dose should be prepared by aseptically withdrawing the appropriate volume of concentrate from the vials of CIPRO I.V. This should be diluted with the desired volume (80-260 mL) of a suitable intravenous solution (see recommended intravenous solutions, above). The resulting solution should be infused over a period of 60 minutes by direct infusion or through a Y-type intravenous infusion set which may already be in place. If this method or the "piggyback" method of administration is used, it is advisable to discontinue temporarily the administration of any other solutions during the infusion of CIPRO I.V.

Table 5: CIPRO I.V.
Dilution for Vials

Vial Size	Vial Strength	Volume of Diluent To Be Used Per Vial	Volume of Diluent To Be Used Per Vial
20 mL	200 mg, 1%	80–180 mL	1.0 mg/mL–2.0 mg/mL
40 mL	400 mg, 1%	160–260 mL	1.3 mg/mL–2.0 mg/mL

As with all parenteral drug products, intravenous admixtures should be inspected visually for clarity, particulate matter, precipitate, discoloration and leakage prior to administration, whenever solution and container permit.

SUPPLIED: CIPRO I.V.: Minibags: Each mL contains: ciprofloxacin 2 mg. In ready-to-use minibags of 100 and 200 mL. Protect from light. Store at controlled room temperature (15 to 25°C).
CIPRO Oral Suspension: Each 100 mL of oral suspension contains: ciprofloxacin 10 g (10%). The drug product is composed of 2 components (microcapsules and diluent) which are mixed prior to dispensing (see Dosage, Instructions to the Pharmacist for Use/Handling).
Reconstitution: See Table 6.

Table 6: CIPRO Oral Suspension
CIPRO Oral Suspension

Total Volume After Reconstitution	Ciprofloxacin Contents After Reconstitution	Ciprofloxacin Contents/Bottle
100 mL	500 mg/5 mL	10 000 mg

Store at room temperature (15 to 25°C) in an upright position. Protect from freezing. **Reconstituted product may be stored in a refrigerator or at room temperature (5 to 25°C) for 14 days.** Store in an upright position. A teaspoon is provided for the patient.
Tablets: 250 mg: Each tablet, engraved CIPRO on one side and 250 on the other, contains: ciprofloxacin HCl equivalent to ciprofloxacin 250 mg. Nonmedicinal ingredients: colloidal silicon dioxide, crospovidone, hydroxypropyl methylcellulose 2910-15, magnesium stearate, maize starch, microcrystalline cellulose, polyethylene glycol, purified water, titanium dioxide. Lactose- and tartrazine-free. Bottles of 100. Store below 30°C.
500 mg: Each tablet, engraved CIPRO on one side and 500 on the other, contains: ciprofloxacin HCl equivalent to ciprofloxacin 500 mg. Nonmedicinal ingredients: colloidal silicon dioxide, crospovidone, hydroxypropyl methylcellulose 2910-15, magnesium stearate, maize starch, microcrystalline cellulose, polyethylene glycol, purified water, titanium dioxide. Lactose- and tartrazine-free. Bottles of 100. Unit dose packages of 100. Store below 30°C.
750 mg: Each tablet, engraved CIPRO on one side and 750 on the other, contains: ciprofloxacin HCl equivalent to ciprofloxacin 750 mg. Nonmedicinal ingredients: colloidal silicon dioxide, crospovidone, hydroxypropyl methylcellulose 2910-15, magnesium stearate, maize starch, microcrystalline cellulose, polyethylene glycol, purified water, titanium dioxide. Lactose- and tartrazine-free. Bottles of 50. Unit dose packages of 100. Store below 30°C.

(Shown in Product Identification Section)

The reader is invited to consult CPhA's monograph **Fluoroquinolones**.

Cipro® XL™

ciprofloxacin

Antibacterial

Bayer

Date of Preparation: April 2, 2004
Date of Revision: June 5, 2008

PHARMACOLOGY: CIPRO XL (ciprofloxacin) extended release tablets contain ciprofloxacin, a synthetic broad-spectrum antimicrobial agent for oral administration. CIPRO XL tablets are coated, bi-layer tablets consisting of an immediate release layer and an erosion-matrix type controlled-release layer. The tablets contain a combination of two types of ciprofloxacin drug substance, ciprofloxacin hydrochloride and ciprofloxacin (base).

Ciprofloxacin, a synthetic fluoroquinolone, has in vitro activity against a wide range of gram-negative and gram-positive microorganisms. Its bactericidal action is achieved through inhibition of topoisomerase II (DNA gyrase) and topoisomerase IV (both Type II topoisomerases), which are required for bacterial DNA replication, transcription, repair, and recombination.

Ciprofloxacin retained some of its bactericidal activity after inhibition of RNA and protein synthesis by rifampin and chloramphenicol, respectively. These observations suggest ciprofloxacin may possess two bactericidal mechanisms, one mechanism resulting from the inhibition of DNA gyrase and a second mechanism which may be independent of RNA and protein synthesis.

The mechanism of action of fluoroquinolones, including ciprofloxacin, is different from that of penicillins, cephalosporins, aminoglycosides, macrolides, and tetracyclines. Therefore, microorganisms resistant to these classes of drugs may be susceptible to ciprofloxacin. Conversely, microorganisms resistant to fluoroquinolones may be susceptible to these other classes of antimicrobial agents. There is no cross-resistance between ciprofloxacin and the mentioned classes of antibiotics.

Pharmacokinetics: Clinical pharmacology studies have compared the pharmacokinetics of CIPRO XL to CIPRO (ciprofloxacin) (immediate release formulation) (CIPRO XL 500 mg vs. CIPRO 250 mg BID and CIPRO XL 1000 mg vs. CIPRO 500 mg BID, respectively), examined the effects of various meals on the pharmacokinetics of CIPRO XL, and investigated possible drug interactions.

Since the mean peak plasma concentration (C_{max}) of CIPRO XL 500 mg tablets (1.59 mg/L) does not exceed that of CIPRO 500 mg tablets (2.36 mg/L), the effect of CIPRO XL 500 mg with respect to special populations (elderly, renal impairment, hepatic impairment) (see Special Populations) and drug-drug interactions is expected to be similar to that of CIPRO 500 mg tablets, which has been extensively studied.

Since the CIPRO XL formulation entails only a slight modification of drug release, the overall performance of the CIPRO XL 1000 mg formulation with respect to special populations and drug-drug and drug-disease interactions is expected to be similar to that of CIPRO, which has been extensively studied.

Absorption: CIPRO XL tablets are formulated to release drug at a slower rate compared to CIPRO tablets, which are immediate release. Approximately 35% of the ciprofloxacin dose in the CIPRO XL tablet is contained within an immediate release component, while the remaining 65% is contained in a slow-release matrix.

CIPRO XL 500 mg: The C_{max} of once daily treatment with 500 mg CIPRO XL is 1.59 mg/L, which is 40% higher than the C_{max} of CIPRO (ciprofloxacin) 250 mg tablets (immediate release formulation) (1.14 mg/L). The mean area under the plasma-concentration time curve (AUC) over 24 hours at steady state following CIPRO XL 500 mg once daily is 7.97 mg·h/L, which is equivalent to the AUC of CIPRO 250 mg tablets BID (8.25 mg·h/L). Maximum plasma concentrations are attained between 1 and 2.5 hours after dosing of CIPRO XL 500 mg (median T_{max}=1.5 h).

Table 1 compares the pharmacokinetic parameters obtained at steady state for CIPRO XL 500 mg tablets and CIPRO 250 mg tablets BID.

Table 1: CIPRO XL
Ciprofloxacin Pharmacokinetics (Mean±SD) Following CIPRO (Ciprofloxacin) 250 mg Tablets (Immediate Release Formulation) BID and CIPRO XL (Ciprofloxacin) Modified Release 500 mg Tablets Administration

	C_{max} (mg/L)	AUC_{0-24h} (mg·h/L)	$T_{1/2}$ (h)	T_{max} (h)[a]
CIPRO XL (ciprofloxacin) extended release 500 mg tablets	1.59±0.43	7.97±1.87	6.6±1.4	1.5 (1.0–2.5)
CIPRO (ciprofloxacin) 250 mg tablets (immediate release formulation) BID	1.14±0.23	8.25±2.15	4.8±0.6	1.0 (0.5–2.5)

[a] Median (range).

CIPRO XL 1000 mg: The C_{max} of once daily treatment with 1000 mg CIPRO XL is 3.11 mg/L, which is 51% higher than the C_{max} of CIPRO (ciprofloxacin) 500 mg tablets (immediate release formulation) (2.06±0.41 mg/L). The mean area under the plasma-concentration time curve (AUC) over 24 hours at steady state following CIPRO XL 1000 mg once daily is 16.83 mg·h/L, which is equivalent to the AUC of CIPRO 500 mg tablets BID (17.04 mg·h/L). Maximum plasma concentrations are attained between 1 and 4 hours after dosing (median T_{max}=2.0 h).

Table 2 compares the pharmacokinetic parameters obtained at steady state for CIPRO XL 1000 mg and CIPRO 500 mg BID.

Table 2: CIPRO XL
Ciprofloxacin Pharmacokinetics (Mean±SD) Following CIPRO (Ciprofloxacin) 500 mg Tablets (Immediate Release Formulation) BID and CIPRO XL (Ciprofloxacin) Extended Release 1000 mg Tablets Administration

	C_{max} (mg/L)	AUC_{0-24h} (mg· h/L)	$T_{1/2}$ (h)	T_{max} (h)[a]
CIPRO XL (ciprofloxacin) extended release 1000 mg tablets	3.11±1.08	16.83±5.65	6.31±0.72	2.0 (1–4)
CIPRO (ciprofloxacin) 500 mg (immediate release formulation) BID	2.06±0.41	17.04±4.79	5.66±0.89	2.0 (0.5–3.5)

[a] Median (range).

The relative bioavailability of CIPRO XL 1000 mg compared to CIPRO 500 mg tablet BID was examined in a crossover study of 20 healthy male volunteers under fasted conditions. Mean concentrations for Day 1 are shown in Figure 1.

Figure 1: CIPRO XL
Relative Bioavailability of CIPRO XL1000 mg versus CIPRO 500 mg BID

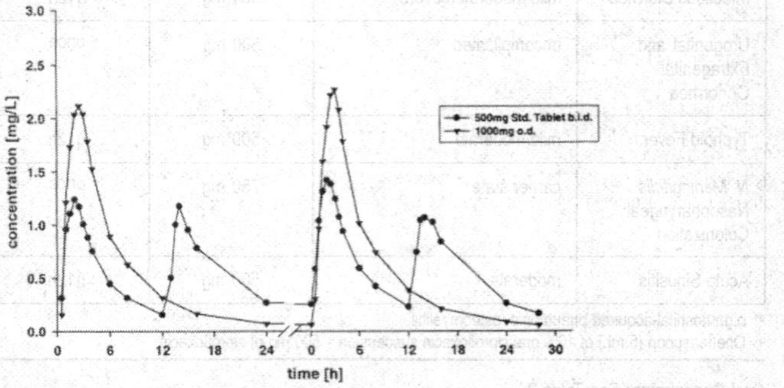

The pharmacokinetics of CIPRO XL are not altered by coadministration with food. AUC values were comparable following administration of CIPRO XL with a high-fat meal, a low-fat meal, or under fasted conditions. See Table 3.

Table 3: CIPRO XL
Pharmacokinetics of CIPRO XL (Ciprofloxacin) Extended Release 500 mg Tablets Under Fed and Fasted Conditions

Parameter	Fed	Fasted	Ratio (fed/fasted)	90% CI
AUC (mg·h/L)[a]	7.12 (21%)	7.05 (36%)	1.01	0.89–1.15
C_{max} (mg/L)[a]	1.30 (26%)	1.34 (42%)	0.97	0.79–1.18
T_{max} (h)[b]	3.5 (1.5–4.0)	1.5 (0.5–3.5)	not evaluated	

[a] Geometric mean (%CV).
[b] Median (range).

Distribution: In one study, the apparent volume of distribution (Vd_{area}) of CIPRO was estimated from kinetic data recorded after oral doses and found to be approximately 3.5 L/kg. Studies with the oral and intravenous forms of ciprofloxacin have demonstrated penetration of ciprofloxacin into a variety of tissues. A single dose study in healthy subjects has demonstrated penetration of ciprofloxacin into prostate tissue following administration of CIPRO XL 1000 mg. One and three hours after dosing, mean ciprofloxacin concentrations were greater than 4 µg/g. The binding of ciprofloxacin to serum proteins is 20% to 40%, which is not likely to be high enough to cause significant protein binding interactions with other drugs. Following administration of a single dose of CIPRO XL (500 mg or 1000 mg), ciprofloxacin concentrations in urine, collected up to 4 hours after dosing, averaged over 300 mg/L and over 500 mg/L, respectively; in urine excreted from 12 to 24 hours after dosing, ciprofloxacin concentration averaged 27 mg/L for CIPRO XL 500 mg and 58 mg/L for CIPRO XL 1000 mg.

Metabolism: Four metabolites of ciprofloxacin were identified in human urine. The primary metabolites are oxociprofloxacin (M3) and sulfociprofloxacin (M2), each accounting for roughly 3% to 8% of the total dose. Other minor metabolites are desethylene ciprofloxacin (M1) and formylciprofloxacin (M4). The relative proportion of drug and metabolite in serum corresponds to the composition found in urine. Excretion of these metabolites was essentially complete by 24 hours after dosing.

Elimination: The elimination kinetics of ciprofloxacin are similar for CIPRO XL and CIPRO (immediate release formulation). The mean serum elimination half-life ($t_{1/2}$) of CIPRO XL (ciprofloxacin) extended release is 6.6 (± 1.4) hours and 6.3 (± 0.7) hours, for the 500 mg and 1000 mg tablets, respectively. The major route of elimination of ciprofloxacin in humans is as unchanged drug in urine.

Special Populations: Renal Impairment: In patients with reduced renal function, the half-life of ciprofloxacin is slightly prolonged. Since the total drug exposure attained with CIPRO XL 500 mg does not exceed that achieved with CIPRO 500 mg tablets (immediate release formulation), which is approved as a total daily dose for use in renally impaired patients, no dosage adjustment for renal disease is required with CIPRO XL 500 mg.

For complicated urinary tract infections or acute uncomplicated pyelonephritis, where 1000 mg is the appropriate dose, the dosage of CIPRO XL should be reduced to 500 mg CIPRO XL once daily in patients with creatinine clearance below 30 mL/min (see Dosage, Impaired Renal Function).

Hepatic Impairment: In preliminary studies in patients with stable chronic liver cirrhosis (with mild to moderate hepatic impairment), no significant changes in ciprofloxacin pharmacokinetics were observed. The kinetics of ciprofloxacin in patients with acute hepatic insufficiency and stable chronic cirrhosis (with severe hepatic impairment), however, have not been elucidated.

In a study of 7 cirrhotic patients and healthy volunteers given CIPRO 750 mg every 12 hours for a total of nine doses followed by a 1 week washout and then a 30 minute infusion of CIPRO I.V. 200 mg, there was no difference in pharmacokinetics between patients with stable chronic cirrhosis (with mild to moderate hepatic impairment) and healthy volunteers.

Geriatrics: No dosage adjustment based on age alone is necessary for elderly patients. Pharmacokinetic studies of the immediate-release oral tablet (single dose) and intravenous (single and multiple dose) forms of ciprofloxacin indicate that plasma concentrations of ciprofloxacin are higher in elderly subjects (>65 years) as compared to young adults. C_{max} is increased 16% to 40%, and mean AUC is increased approximately 30%, which can be at least partially attributed to decreased renal clearance in the elderly. Elimination half-life is only slightly (~20%) prolonged in the elderly.

Since ciprofloxacin is substantially excreted by the kidney, the risk of adverse reactions may be greater in patients with impaired renal function. No significant accumulation of ciprofloxacin is anticipated in elderly subjects with renal impairment who take CIPRO XL 500 mg, therefore, no reductions in dosage are required.

However, in patients with renal impairment where CIPRO XL 1000 mg once daily is the appropriate dose, dosage may need to be reduced to CIPRO XL 500 mg once daily (see Dosage, Impaired Renal Function).

INDICATIONS: CIPRO XL (ciprofloxacin) extended release is indicated solely for the treatment of urinary tract infections, caused by susceptible strains of the designated microorganisms as listed below. **CIPRO XL and CIPRO (Ciprofloxacin) tablets (Immediate Release Formulation) are not interchangeable** (see Dosage for specific recommendations).

Uncomplicated Urinary Tract Infections (Acute Cystitis) in Females Caused by: *E. coli*, *E. faecalis*, *P. mirabilis*, *S. saprophyticus*.

Complicated Urinary Tract Infections caused by: *E. coli*, *K. pneumoniae*, *E. faecalis*, *P.mirabilis*, *P. aeruginosa*.

Acute Uncomplicated Pyelonephritis caused by: *E. coli*.

The safety and efficacy of CIPRO XL in treating infections other than uncomplicated urinary tract infection has not been demonstrated.

Appropriate culture and susceptibility tests should be performed before treatment in order to isolate and identify organisms causing infection and to determine their susceptibility to ciprofloxacin. Therapy with CIPRO XL may be initiated before results of these tests are known; once results become available, appropriate therapy should be continued.

CONTRAINDICATIONS: CIPRO XL (ciprofloxacin) extended release tablets are contraindicated in persons with a history of hypersensitivity to ciprofloxacin or any member of the quinolone class of antibacterial agents or any of the excipients.

Concurrent administration of ciprofloxacin and tizanidine is contraindicated since it may result in an undesirable increase in serum tizanidine concentrations. This can be associated with clinically relevant tizanidine-induced side effects (hypotension, somnolence, drowsiness).

WARNINGS: Children: The safety of CIPRO XL (ciprofloxacin) extended release tablets in pediatric patients and adolescents (under the age of 18 years), pregnant women and nursing women has not yet been established (see Precautions, Children,Pregnancy and Lactation). Damage to juvenile weight-bearing joints and lameness were observed both in rat and dog studies but not in weaned piglets. Histopathological examination of the weight-bearing joints in immature dogs revealed permanent lesions of the cartilage.

CNS and Psychiatric Effects: Convulsions, increased intracranial pressure, and toxic psychosis have been reported in patients receiving quinolones, including ciprofloxacin. Ciprofloxacin may also cause central nervous system (CNS) events including tremors, restlessness, lightheadedness, confusion and hallucinations, depression, nervousness, agitation, insomnia, anxiety, paranoia, nightmares and, rarely, suicidal thoughts or acts. In rare cases, depression or psychosis can progress to self-endangering behavior. These reactions may occur following the first dose. If these reactions occur in patients receiving ciprofloxacin, the drug should be discontinued and appropriate measures instituted. As with all quinolones, ciprofloxacin should be used with caution in patients with known or suspected CNS disorders, such as severe cerebral arteriosclerosis, epilepsy, and other factors that predispose to seizures or lower the seizure threshold (see Adverse Effects).

Cytochrome P450: Ciprofloxacin is known to be a moderate inhibitor of the CYP450 1A2 enzymes. Care should be taken when other drugs are administered concomitantly which are metabolized via the same enzymatic pathway (e.g., theophylline, methylxanthines, caffeine, duloxetine, clozapine). Increased plasma concentrations associated with drug specific side effects may be observed due to inhibition of their metabolic clearance by ciprofloxacin (see Contraindications and Precautions, Drug Interactions).

Hypersensitivity: Serious hypersensitivity and/or anaphylactic reactions have been reported in patients receiving quinolone therapy, including ciprofloxacin. These reactions may occur following the first dose. Some reactions have been accompanied by cardiovascular collapse, hypotension/shock, seizure, loss of consciousness, tingling, angioedema (including tongue, laryngeal, throat or facial edema/swelling), airway obstruction (including bronchospasm, shortness of breath and acute respiratory distress), dyspnea, urticaria, itching and other serious skin reactions.

Ciprofloxacin should be discontinued at the first appearance of a skin rash or any other sign of hypersensitivity. Serious acute hypersensitivity reactions may require treatment with epinephrine and other resuscitative measures, including oxygen, intravenous fluids, antihistamines, corticosteroids, pressor amines and airway management, as clinically indicated.

Serious and sometimes fatal events, some due to hypersensitivity and some due to uncertain etiology, have been reported in patients receiving therapy with all antibiotics. These events may be severe and generally occur following the administration of multiple doses. Clinical manifestations may include one or more of the following: fever, rash or severe dermatologic reactions (e.g., toxic epidermal necrolysis, Stevens-Johnson syndrome), vasculitis, arthralgia, myalgia, serum sickness, allergic pneumonitis, interstitial nephritis, acute renal insufficiency or failure, hepatitis, jaundice, acute hepatic necrosis or failure, hepatic necrosis with fatal outcome, anemia including hemolytic and aplastic, thrombocytopenia including thrombotic thrombocytopenic purpura, leukopenia, agranulocytosis, pancytopenia, and/or other hematologic abnormalities (see Contraindications and Precautions, Drug Interactions).

Gastrointestinal: *C. difficile*-associated disease: *C. difficile*-associated disease (CDAD) has been reported with the use of many antibacterial agents, including ciprofloxacin. CDAD may range in severity from mild diarrhea to fatal colitis. It is important to consider this diagnosis in patients who present with diarrhea or symptoms of colitis, pseudomembranous colitis, toxic megacolon, or perforation of the colon subsequent to the administration of any antibacterial agent. CDAD has been reported to occur over 2 months after the administration of antibacterial agents.

Treatment with antibacterial agents may alter the normal flora of the colon and may permit overgrowth of *C. difficile*. *C. difficile* produces toxins A and B, which contribute to the development of CDAD. CDAD may cause significant morbidity and mortality. CDAD can be refractory to antimicrobial therapy.

If the diagnosis of CDAD is suspected or confirmed, appropriate therapeutic measures should be initiated. Mild cases of CDAD usually respond to discontinuation of antibacterial agents not directed against *C. difficile*. In moderate to severe cases, consideration should be given to management with fluids and electrolytes, protein supplementation, and treatment with an antibacterial agent clinically effective against *C. difficile*. Drugs that inhibit peristalsis may delay clearance of *C. difficile* and its toxins, and therefore should not be used in the treatment of CDAD. Surgical evaluation should be instituted as clinically indicated since surgical intervention may be required in certain severe cases. (See Adverse Effects.)

PRECAUTIONS: Serious and fatal reactions have been reported in patients receiving concurrent administration of ciprofloxacin and theophylline. These reactions have included cardiac arrest, seizure, status epilepticus, and respiratory failure. Although similar serious adverse effects have been reported in patients receiving theophylline alone, the possibility that these reactions may be potentiated by ciprofloxacin cannot be eliminated. If concomitant use cannot be avoided, serum levels of theophylline should be monitored and dosage adjustments made as appropriate.

Tendon rupture (mainly Achilles tendon) has been reported predominantly in the elderly on prior systemic treatment with glucocorticoids. At any sign of tendonitis (eg, painful swelling, inflammation), a physician should be consulted and the antibiotic treatment should be discontinued. Care should be taken to keep the affected extremity at rest and avoid any inappropriate physical exercise (as the risk for tendon rupture might increase otherwise). Ciprofloxacin should not be used in patients with a clear history of tendon disorders related to quinolone treatment because they may be at risk of developing tendon disorders again when reexposed to a fluoroquinolone.

Crystalluria related to ciprofloxacin has been reported only rarely in man because human urine is usually acidic. Crystals have been observed in the urine of laboratory animals, usually from alkaline urine. Patients receiving ciprofloxacin should be well hydrated and alkalinity of the urine should be avoided. The recommended daily dose should not be exceeded.

Ciprofloxacin has been shown to produce photosensitivity reactions. Patients taking ciprofloxacin should avoid direct exposure to excessive sunlight or UV-light. Therapy should be discontinued if photosensitization (i.e., sunburn-like skin reactions) occurs.

Prolonged use of ciprofloxacin may result in the overgrowth of nonsusceptible organisms. Careful observation of the patient is therefore essential, and if superinfection should occur during therapy, appropriate measures should be taken.

Pregnancy: Adequate and well-controlled studies have not been performed in pregnant women. Ciprofloxacin should not be used in pregnant women unless the potential benefits outweigh the potential risk to the fetus (see Warnings).

Lactation: Ciprofloxacin is excreted in human milk. Because of the potential for serious adverse reactions in infants nursing from women taking ciprofloxacin, a decision should be made whether to discontinue the drug, taking into account the importance of the drug to the woman and possible risk to the infant (see Warnings).

Children: The safety and efficacy of ciprofloxacin in the pediatric population less than 18 years of age have not been established. Quinolones, including ciprofloxacin, cause arthropathy and osteochondrosis in juvenile animals of several species (see Warnings).

Renal Impairment: In patients with reduced renal function, the half-life of ciprofloxacin is slightly prolonged. Since the total drug exposure attained with CIPRO XL (ciprofloxacin) extended release 500 mg tablets does not exceed that achieved with CIPRO (ciprofloxacin) 500 mg tablets (immediate release formulation), which is approved as a total daily dose for use in renally impaired patients, no dosage adjustment for renal disease is required with CIPRO XL 500 mg.

For complicated urinary tract infections or acute uncomplicated pyelonephritis, where 1000 mg is the appropriate dose, the dosage of CIPRO XL should be reduced to 500 mg CIPRO XL once daily in patients with creatinine clearance below 30 mL/min (see Dosage).

Hepatic Impairment: In preliminary studies in patients with stable chronic liver cirrhosis (with mild to moderate hepatic impairment), no significant changes in CIPRO pharmacokinetics were observed. The kinetics of ciprofloxacin in patients with acute hepatic insufficiency and stable chronic cirrhosis (with severe hepatic impairment), however, have not been elucidated. An increased incidence of nausea, vomiting, headache and diarrhea were observed with the use of CIPRO in this patient population. No dosage adjustment is required with CIPRO XL in patients with stable chronic cirrhosis (with mild to moderate hepatic impairment).

Occupational Hazards: Ability to Drive and Operate Machinery: Even when ciprofloxacin is taken exactly as prescribed, it can affect the speed of reaction to such an extent that the ability to drive or to operate machinery is impaired. This applies particularly in combination with alcohol.

Geriatrics: No dosage adjustment based on age alone is necessary for elderly patients. Since ciprofloxacin is substantially excreted by the kidney, the risk of adverse reactions may be greater in patients with impaired renal function. No significant accumulation of ciprofloxacin is anticipated in elderly subjects with renal impairment who take CIPRO XL 500 mg, therefore, no reductions in dosage are required.

However, in patients with renal impairment, where CIPRO XL 1000 mg once daily is the appropriate dose, dosage may need to be reduced to CIPRO XL 500 mg once daily (see Dosage, Impaired Renal Function).

Drug Interactions: Caffeine: Ciprofloxacin has also been shown to interfere with the metabolism of caffeine. This may lead to reduced clearance of caffeine and a prolongation of its serum half-life.

Clozapine: Following concomitant administration of 250 mg ciprofloxacin for 7 days, serum concentrations of clozapine and n-desmethylclozapine were increased by 29% and 31%, respectively (see Warnings).

Cyclosporine: Some quinolones, including ciprofloxacin, have been associated with transient elevations in serum creatinine levels in patients who are concomitantly receiving cyclosporine.

Ferrous Sulfate: Oral ferrous sulfate at therapeutic doses decreases the bioavailability of oral ciprofloxacin, therefore concomitant therapy is not advised.

Food and Dairy Products: Although CIPRO XL may be taken with meals that include milk, simultaneous administration with dairy products alone, or with calcium-fortified products should be avoided, since decreased absorption is possible. It is recommended that CIPRO XL be administered at least 2 hours before or 2 hours after substantial calcium intake (>800 mg) (see Dosage).

Glyburide: In particular cases, concurrent administration of ciprofloxacin and glyburide can intensify the action of glyburide (hypoglycemia).

Histamine H_2-receptor Antagonists: Histamine H_2-receptor antagonists appear to have no significant effect on the bioavailability of ciprofloxacin.

Lidocaine: It was demonstrated in healthy subjects that concomitant use of lidocaine with ciprofloxacin, a moderate inhibitor of CYP450 1A2 isozyme, reduces clearance of intravenous lidocaine by 22%. Ciprofloxacin may increase the systemic toxicity of lidocaine.

Methotrexate: Renal tubular transport of methotrexate may be inhibited by concomitant administration of ciprofloxacin, potentially leading to increased plasma levels of methotrexate. This might increase the risk of methotrexate-associated toxic reactions. Therefore, patients under methotrexate therapy should be carefully monitored when concomitant therapy is indicated.

Metoclopramide: Metoclopramide accelerates the absorption of ciprofloxacin (oral) resulting in a shorter time to reach maximum plasma concentrations. No effect was seen on the bioavailability of ciprofloxacin.

Multivalent Cations: Concurrent administration of a quinolone, including ciprofloxacin, with multivalent cation-containing products such as magnesium/aluminum antacids, polymeric phosphate binders such as sevelamer, sucralfate, Videx (didanosine) chewable/buffered tablets or pediatric powder, mineral supplements or products containing calcium, iron, or zinc may substantially interfere with the absorption of the quinolone, resulting in serum and urine levels considerably lower than desired. CIPRO XL should be administered at least 2 hours before or 6 hours after these preparations. When CIPRO XL, given as a single 1000 mg dose, was administered 2 hours before or 4 hours after a magnesium/aluminum-containing antacid (900 mg aluminum hydroxide and 600 mg magnesium hydroxide as a single oral dose) to 18 healthy volunteers, there was a 4% and 19% reduction, respectively, in the mean C_{max} of ciprofloxacin. The reduction in the mean AUC was 24% and 26%, respectively (see Dosage).

NSAID: Concomitant administration of a nonsteroidal anti-inflammatory drug (fenbufen) with a quinolone (enoxacin) has been reported to increase the risk of CNS stimulation and convulsive seizures.

Omeprazole: Absorption of the CIPRO XL tablet was slightly diminished (20%) when given concomitantly with omeprazole.

Probenecid: Probenecid interferes with renal tubular secretion of ciprofloxacin and produces an increase in the level of ciprofloxacin in the serum. This should be considered if patients are receiving both drugs concomitantly.

Ropinirole: In a clinical study it was shown that concomitant use of ropinirole with ciprofloxacin, a medium inhibitor of the CYP450 1A2 isozyme, resulted in increases in the C_{max} and AUC of ropinirole of 60 and 84%, respectively. Ciprofloxacin may increase the systemic toxicity of ropinirole.

Theophylline: Concurrent administration of ciprofloxacin with theophylline may lead to elevated serum concentrations of theophylline and prolongation of its elimination half-life. This may result in increased risk of theophylline-related adverse reactions (see Adverse Effects). If concomitant use cannot be avoided, serum levels of theophylline should be monitored and dosage adjustments made as appropriate.

Tizanidine: In a clinical study in healthy subjects there was an increase in tizanidine serum concentrations (C_{max} increase: 7-fold, range: 4 to 21-fold; AUC increase: 10-fold, range: 6 to 24-fold) when given concomitantly with ciprofloxacin. Associated with the increased serum concentrations was a potentiated hypotensive and sedative effect. Tizanidine must not be administered together with ciprofloxacin (see Contraindications, Warnings).

Warfarin: Quinolones have been reported to enhance the effects of the oral anticoagulant warfarin and its derivatives. During concomitant administration of these drugs, the prothrombin time/INR, or other appropriate coagulation tests, should be closely monitored.

ADVERSE EFFECTS: CIPRO XL 500 mg: In a Phase III clinical trial involving 444 patients, the incidence of adverse drug reactions in patients treated with CIPRO XL (ciprofloxacin) extended release 500 mg tablets was 10%. Most adverse events reported in the trial were described as mild to moderate in severity and required no treatment. CIPRO XL 500 mg was discontinued due to adverse reactions thought to be drug-related in 0.2% of patients.

Adverse reactions, judged by investigators to be at least possibly drug-related, occurring in greater than or equal to 1% of CIPRO XL 500 mg treated patients were nausea (3%) and headache (2%).

Additional uncommon adverse reactions, judged by investigators to be at least possibly drug-related, that occurred in less than 1% of CIPRO XL 500 mg treated patients were:

Body as a Whole: abdominal pain, photosensitivity reaction.

Cardiovascular: migraine.

Digestive: anorexia, constipation, diarrhea, dyspepsia, flatulence, thirst, vomiting.

Skin/Appendages: maculopapular rash, pruritus, rash, skin disorder, vesiculobullous rash.

Special Senses: taste perversion.

Genitourinary: dysmenorrhea, vaginal candidiasis, vaginitis.

CIPRO XL 1000 mg: In a Phase III clinical trial involving 517 patients, the incidence of adverse drug reactions in patients treated with CIPRO XL (ciprofloxacin) extended release 1000 mg tablets was 13.2%. Most adverse events reported in the trial were described as mild to moderate in severity and required no treatment. CIPRO XL 1000 mg was discontinued due to adverse reactions thought to be drug-related in 3.1% of patients.

Adverse reactions, judged by investigators to be at least possibly drug-related, occurring in greater than or equal to 1% of CIPRO XL 1000 mg treated patients, were nausea (3%), diarrhea (2%), headache (1%), dizziness (1%), dyspepsia (1%) and vaginal moniliasis (1%).

Additional uncommon adverse reactions, judged by investigators to be at least possibly drug-related, that occurred in less than 1% of CIPRO XL 1000 mg treated patients were:

Body as a Whole: abdominal pain, asthenia, malaise, moniliasis, photosensitivity reaction.

Cardiovascular: bradycardia, migraine, syncope.

Digestive: anorexia, constipation, dry mouth, flatulence, liver function tests abnormal, thirst, vomiting.
Hemic/Lymphatic: prothrombin/INR decreased.
Nervous: abnormal dreams, depersonalization, depression, hypertonia, incoordination, insomnia, somnolence, tremor, vertigo.
Metabolic: hyperglycemia.
Skin/Appendages: dry skin, maculopapular rash, pruritus, rash, skin disorder, urticaria, vesiculobullous rash.
Special Senses: diplopia, taste perversion.
Urogenital: dysmenorrhea, hematuria, kidney function abnormal, vaginitis.
Ciprofloxacin: Other Formulations: The following adverse drug reactions have been reported during clinical trials and subsequent post-marketing surveillance with other formulations of ciprofloxacin.

In patients treated orally with CIPRO (tablet and suspension), the most frequently reported events, possibly, probably drug-related were: nausea (1.3%), and diarrhea (1.0%).

In patients treated with CIPRO I.V., the most frequently reported events, possibly, probably drug-related were: rash (1.8%), diarrhea (1.0%), and injection site pain (1.0%).

Events possibly or probably drug-related occurring at a frequency of less than 1% with CIPRO (ciprofloxacin) tablets (immediate release formulation) oral and CIPRO I.V. treatment during clinical trials and subsequent post-marketing surveillance are as follows:
Body as a Whole: back pain, chest pain, pain, pain in extremities, moniliasis.
Cardiovascular: palpitation, phlebitis, (thrombo)-phlebitis, tachycardia. The following have been reported very rarely (<0.01%): angina pectoris, atrial fibrillation, cardiac arrest, cerebrovascular disorder, electrocardiogram abnormality, hot flashes, hypertension, hypotension, kidney vasculitis, myocardial infarct, pericarditis, pulmonary embolus, substernal chest pain, syncope (fainting), vasodilation (hot flushes).
Digestive: abdominal pain, anorexia, dry mouth, dyspepsia, dysphagia, enlarged abdomen, flatulence, gastrointestinal moniliasis, jaundice, stomatitis, vomiting, abnormal liver function test. The following have been reported rarely (>0.01%-<0.1%): moniliasis (oral), cholestatic jaundice, pseudomembranous colitis. The following have been reported very rarely: constipation, esophagitis, gastrointestinal hemorrhage, glossitis, hepatomegaly, ileus, increased appetite, intestinal perforation, life-threatening pseudomembranous colitis with possible fatal outcome, liver damage, melena, pancreatitis, tenesmus, tooth discoloration, toxic megacolon, ulcerative stomatitis.
Hemic and Lymphatic: agranulocytosis, anaemia, eosinophilia, leukopenia (granulocytopenia), leukocytopenia, leukocytosis, pancytopenia. The following have been reported very rarely: altered prothrombin levels/INR, hemolytic anaemia, marrow depression (life threatening), pancytopenia (life threatening), thrombocytemia (thrombocytosis).
Hypersensitivity: rash. The following have been reported rarely: allergic reaction, anaphylactic/anaphylactoid reactions including facial, vascular and laryngeal edema, drug fever, vasculitis (petechia, haemorrhagic bullae, papules, crust formation), hepatitis, interstitial nephritis, petechia (punctuate skin hemorrhages), pruritus, serum sickness-like reaction, Stevens-Johnson syndrome (potentially life-threatening). The following have been reported very rarely: shock (anaphylactic; life-threatening), pruritic rash, erythema multiforme (minor), erythema nodosum, major liver disorders including hepatic necrosis (very rarely progressing to life threatening hepatic failure), epidermal necrolysis (Lyell syndrome, potentially life-threatening).
I.V. Infusion Site: thrombophlebitis, injection site reaction. The following have been reported very rarely: burning, erythema, pain, paresthesia, and swelling.
Metabolic and Nutritional Disorder: creatinine increased. The following have been reported rarely: edema (face), hyperglycemia.
Musculoskeletal: The following have been reported rarely: achiness, arthralgia (joint pain), joint disorder (joint swelling), pain in the extremities, partial or complete tendon rupture (predominantly achilles tendon), tendonitis (predominantly achillotendonitis), myalgia (muscular pain), and very rarely myasthenia (exacerbation of symptoms of myasthenia gravis).

There have been 54 reports of arthropathies with CIPRO. Ten of these reports involved children. Arthralgia was usually the first symptom which led to rapid assessment and withdrawal of the drug. No irreversible arthropathies have been observed.
Nervous System: agitation, confusion, convulsion, dizziness, hallucinations, headache, hypesthesia, increased sweating, insomnia, somnolence, tremor (trembling). The following have been reported rarely: paresthesia (peripheral paralgesia). The following have been reported very rarely: abnormal dreams (nightmares), anxiety, apathy, ataxia, depersonalization, depression, diplopia, hemiplegia, hyperesthesia, hypertonia, increase of intracranial pressure, meningism, migraine, nervousness, neuritis, polyneuritis, sleep disorder, twitching, grand mal convulsion, abnormal (unsteady) gait, psychosis, intracranial hypertension. In some instances, these reactions occurred after the first administration of CIPRO. In these instances, CIPRO is to be discontinued and the doctor should be informed immediately.
Other: The following have been reported rarely, asthenia (general feeling of weakness, tiredness), death.
Respiratory: dyspnea. The following have been reported very rarely: hiccup, hyperventilation, increased cough, larynx edema, lung edema, lung hemorrhage, pharyngitis, stridor, voice alteration.
Skin and Appendages: pruritus, rash, maculopapular rash. The following have been reported rarely: photosensitivity reaction. The following have been reported very rarely: alopecia, angioedema, fixed eruption, photosensitive dermatitis, petechia, urticaria.
Special Senses: abnormal vision (visual disturbances), taste perversion, tinnitus. The following have been reported rarely: transitory deafness (especially at higher frequencies), taste loss (impaired taste). The following have been reported very rarely: chromatopsia, colour blindness, conjunctivitis, corneal opacity, diplopia, ear pain, eye pain, parosmia (impaired smell), anosmia (usually reversible on discontinuation).
Genitourinary: albuminuria, hematuria. The following have been reported rarely: abnormal kidney function, acute kidney failure, dysuria, leukorrhea, nephritis interstitial, urinary retention, vaginitis, vaginal moniliasis.
Laboratory Values: albuminuria, alkaline phosphatase increased, ALT increased, AST increased, bilirubinemia, BUN (urea) increased, cholestatic parameters increased, decreased creatinine clearance, gamma-GT increased, hypercholesteremia, hyperuricemia, increased sedimentation rate, lactic dehydrogenase increased, NPN increased, transaminases increased. The following have been reported rarely: acidosis, amylase increased, crystalluria, electrolyte abnormality, haematuria, hypercalcemia, hypocalcemia and lipase increased.

The following additional adverse events, in alphabetical order, regardless of incidence or relationship to drug, have been reported during clinical trials and from worldwide post-marketing experience in patients given ciprofloxacin (includes all formulations, all dosages, all drug-therapy durations, and in all indications): arrhythmia, atrial flutter, bleeding diathesis, bronchospasm, *C. difficile* associated diarrhea, candiduria, cardiac murmur, cardiopulmonary arrest, cardiovascular collapse, cerebral thrombosis, chills, delirium, drowsiness, dysphasia, edema (conjunctivae, hands, lips, lower extremities, neck), epistaxis, exfoliative dermatitis, fever, gastrointestinal bleeding, gout (flare up), gynecomastia, hearing loss, hemoptysis, hemorrhagic cystitis, hyperpigmentation, joint stiffness, lightheadedness, lymphadenopathy, manic reaction, myoclonus, nystagmus, pain (arm, breast, epigastric, foot, jaw, neck, oral mucosa), paranoia, phobia, pleural effusion, polyuria, postural hypotension, pulmonary embolism, purpura, QT prolongation (frequency <1 per million), renal calculi, respiratory arrest, respiratory distress, restlessness, rhabdomyolysis, torsades de pointes (frequency <1 per million), toxic psychosis, unresponsiveness, urethral bleeding, urination (frequent), ventricular ectopy, ventricular fibrillation (frequency <1 per million), ventricular tachycardia (frequency <1 per million), vesicles, visual acuity (decreased) and visual disturbances (flashing lights, change in color perception, overbrightness of lights).

OVERDOSE:

Symptoms: In the event of acute excessive oral overdosage, reversible renal toxicity, arthralgia, myalgia and CNS symptoms have been reported.

Treatment: Therefore, apart from routine emergency measures, it is recommended to monitor renal function and to administer magnesium- or calcium-containing antacids which reduce the absorption of ciprofloxacin and to maintain adequate hydration. Based on information obtained from subjects with chronic renal failure, only a small amount of ciprofloxacin (<10%) is removed from the body after hemodialysis or peritoneal dialysis.

The administration of activated charcoal as soon as possible after oral overdose may prevent excessive increase of systemic ciprofloxacin exposure.

For management of a suspected drug overdose, contact your **regional Poison Control Centre**. See the *CPS* Directory section for a list of Poison Control Centres.

DOSAGE: CIPRO XL AND CIPRO (ciprofloxacin) tablets (immediate release formulation) are not interchangeable.
CIPRO XL should be administered once daily as described in Table 4.

Table 4: CIPRO XL
Recommended Dosage

Indication	Unit Dose CIPRO XL	Frequency	Recommended Duration
Uncomplicated Urinary Tract Infection (Acute Cystitis) in Females	500 mg	q 24h	3 days
Complicated Urinary Tract Infection	1000 mg[a]	q 24h	7–14 days
Acute Uncomplicated Pyelonephritis	1000 mg	q 24h	7–14 days

[a] For severely renally impaired patients see Impaired Renal Function below.

CIPRO XL should be administered at least 2 hours before or 6 hours after antacids and mineral supplements containing magnesium or aluminum, as well as sucralfate, Videx (didanosine) chewable/buffered tablets or pediatric powder, metal cations such as iron, and multivitamin preparations with zinc (see Precautions, Drug Interactions).

Although CIPRO XL may be taken with meals that include milk, simultaneous administration with dairy products alone, or with calcium-fortified products should be avoided, since decreased absorption is possible. It is recommended that CIPRO XL be administered at least 2 hours before or 2 hours after substantial calcium intake (>800 mg). CIPRO XL should be swallowed whole. Tablets should not be split, crushed or chewed (see Precautions, Drug Interactions).
Impaired Renal Function: CIPRO XL 500 mg: Based on pharmacokinetic data, no dosage adjustment is required with CIPRO XL 500 mg.
CIPRO XL 1000 mg: For complicated urinary tract infections or acute uncomplicated pyelonephritis, where 1000 mg is the appropriate dose, the dosage of CIPRO XL should be reduced to 500 mg CIPRO XL once daily in patients with creatinine clearance below 30 mL/min. This recommendation is based on pharmacokinetic modeling. Clinical studies with CIPRO XL have not been performed in patients with impaired renal function. For patients on hemodialysis or peritoneal dialysis, administer CIPRO XL after the dialysis procedure is completed.
Impaired Hepatic Function: Based on pharmacokinetic data, no dosage adjustment is required with CIPRO XL in patients with stable chronic cirrhosis (with mild to moderate hepatic impairment). The kinetics of ciprofloxacin in patients with acute hepatic insufficiency and stable chronic cirrhosis (with severe hepatic impairment), however, have not been elucidated.
Geriatrics: No dosage adjustment based on age alone is necessary in elderly patients. Since ciprofloxacin is substantially excreted by the kidney, the risk of adverse reactions may be greater in patients with impaired renal function. No significant accumulation of ciprofloxacin is anticipated in elderly subjects with renal impairment who take CIPRO XL 500 mg, therefore, no reductions in dosage are required.

However, in patients with renal impairment, where CIPRO XL 1000 mg once daily is the appropriate dose, dosage may need to be reduced to CIPRO XL 500 mg once daily (see Dosage, Impaired Renal Function).

INFORMATION FOR THE PATIENT: Published in e-CPS, available by subscription at www.e-cps.ca.
SUPPLIED: 500 mg: Each nearly white to slightly yellowish, film-coated, oblong-shaped, extended release tablet, coded with the word "BAYER" on one side and "C500 QD" on the reverse side, contains: ciprofloxacin 500 mg as ciprofloxacin HCl (287.5 mg, calculated as ciprofloxacin on the dried basis) and ciprofloxacin (212.6 mg, calculated on the dried basis). Nonmedicinal ingredients: crospovidone, hypromellose, magnesium stearate, polyethylene glycol, silical colloidal anhydrous, succinic acid and titanium dioxide. Bottles of 50. Store at 15 to 30°C.
1000 mg: Each nearly white to slightly yellowish, film-coated, oblong-shaped, extended release tablet, coded with the word "BAYER" on one side and "C1000 QD" on the reverse side, contains: ciprofloxacin 1000 mg as ciprofloxacin HCl (574.9 mg, calculated as ciprofloxacin on the dried basis) and ciprofloxacin (425.2 mg, calculated on the dried basis). Nonmedicinal ingredients: crospovidone, hypromellose, magnesium stearate, polyethylene glycol, silical colloidal anhydrous, succinic acid and titanium dioxide. Bottles of 50. Store at 15 to 30°C.

(Shown in Product Identification Section)

Cisplatin
Antineoplastic

CPhA Monograph

Date of Revision: November 2007

This monograph has been compiled by CPhA and reviewed by experts. It may contain information different from that found in Health Canada-approved Product Monographs. The reader is referred to the *CPS* Editorial Policy for more information.

SUMMARY PRODUCT INFORMATION:

Route of Administration	Dosage Form	Strength
Parenteral	Injectable solution	1 mg/mL

PHARMACOLOGY: Cisplatin, also known as cis-Platinum II, DDP or CDDP, is an antineoplastic agent containing platinum. The exact mechanism of action of cisplatin is not known but it is biochemically similar to bifunctional alkylating agents as it binds to DNA, producing interstrand and intrastrand crosslinks. This causes apoptosis (programmed cell death) through inhibition of DNA replication.
Pharmacokinetics: Because of the complexity of cisplatin pharmacokinetics, fate of the drug has generally been studied using assays for elemental platinum. After iv administration, peak plasma concentrations are immediate and the volume of distribution is 20 to 80 L (average 41 L/m^2). Concentrations of platinum are highest in kidney, liver and prostate, decreasing slightly in the bladder, muscle, testicle, and pancreas and are lowest in the bowel, heart, lung, cerebrum, and cerebellum. After the final administration, platinum is present in tissues as long as 180 days.

Plasma cisplatin half-life is approximately 30 minutes based on a bolus injection or iv infusion over 2 to 7 hours of doses in the range of 50 to 100 mg/m^2. Although cisplatin does not undergo normal drug-protein binding, the platinum from the drug is 90% covalently bound to plasma proteins. The half-life of the complexes is 5 days or longer.

Renal excretion accounts for 90% of the drug's elimination while less than 10% undergoes biliary excretion. The renal clearance of cisplatin and platinum compounds exceed creatinine clearance, evidence that the drug undergoes renal secretion. Approximately 10 to 40% of the administered platinum can be found in the urine in 24 hours.
INDICATIONS: Testicular cancer: In patients who have received surgical/radiotherapeutic/chemotherapeutic interventions as appropriate for the stage of testicular cancer. Cisplatin has been used as a component of therapy for metastatic testicular tumors, including nonseminomatous testicular carcinoma, seminoma testis and extragonadal germ-cell tumors.
Ovarian cancer: In patients who have received appropriate surgical or radiotherapeutic interventions, cisplatin is used in combination therapy for metastatic ovarian tumors. Cisplatin alone or in combination may also be used as second-line therapy in recurrent or refractory ovarian carcinoma in patients who have not previously been treated with the drug or in platinum-sensitive disease after an appropriate platinum-free interval.
Bladder cancer: For patients with advanced bladder cancer that is no longer controlled with local treatments such as surgery or radiotherapy, cisplatin can be administered as a single agent. The drug can also be used as neoadjuvant or adjuvant therapy with surgery and/or radiotherapeutic procedures.

Cisplatin is also used in the management of head and neck cancer, esophageal cancer, cervical cancer, non-small cell lung cancer, and small cell lung cancer, as well as other malignancies.

In pediatrics, the drug has shown activity against osteosarcoma, neuroblastoma, Wilms' tumor, some germ cell tumors, and brain tumors.

CONTRAINDICATIONS: Cisplatin should not be used in patients with demonstrated hypersensitivity to cisplatin or other platinum-containing compounds. It is also contraindicated in patients with pre-existing renal impairment or hearing impairment unless the physician and patient agree that possible risks are outweighed by potential benefits. Cisplatin should not be used in myelosuppressed patients.

WARNINGS: Cisplatin is a toxic chemotherapeutic agent that is used with risk of significant adverse effects.

The major dose-limiting toxic effect of cisplatin is cumulative nephrotoxicity which usually becomes apparent in the second week after a dose. With high-dose therapy the nephrotoxicity may occur after several days. Although the nephrotoxicity is usually reversible, high or repeated doses may lead to more severe impairment of longer duration. Irreversible (and fatal) cases have been reported. Generally, recovery from nephrotoxicity occurs within 2 to 4 weeks after cisplatin administration.

When usual doses are administered accompanied by hydration and diuresis, reports suggest that clinically important chronic renal failure does not occur when cisplatin is discontinued (see Dosage).

Serum electrolyte disturbances such as hypomagnesemia, hypocalcemia, hyponatremia, hypokalemia and hypophosphatemia have all been reported in patients receiving cisplatin therapy. These effects are likely related to renal tubular damage. Hypomagnesemia usually occurs within 3 to 4 weeks after starting therapy and becomes more severe as treatment continues. Children appear to be especially prone to hypomagnesemia associated with cisplatin. Symptoms which may accompany hypomagnesemia and/or hypocalcemia include muscle cramps, tremor and even tetany. Discontinuing cisplatin treatment and providing electrolyte supplementation usually restores normal serum electrolyte concentrations.

Cumulative ototoxicity with tinnitus and hearing loss in the high frequency range can be a significant toxicity related to cisplatin therapy. This unilateral or bilateral hearing loss may affect the ability to perceive conversational tones and the drug should be discontinued at this point or earlier. Ototoxicity may be more pronounced in children. While ototoxic effects may be related to peak cisplatin plasma concentration, it is not known whether this ototoxicity is reversible, but audiogram abnormalities appear irreversible. Cranial irradiation or concomitant use of other ototoxic medications may increase the risk of ototoxicity.

Neurotoxicity, which generally manifests as peripheral neuropathy, has occurred after single doses but usually presents after prolonged therapy (e.g., 4 to 7 months). Neuropathies may be severe with high dose or increased frequency of cisplatin. Although the usual symptoms of paresthesia in a stocking-glove distribution, areflexia and loss of proprioception and vibratory sensation are often seen during treatment, they may rarely present 3 to 8 weeks or longer after the last cisplatin dose. Since neuropathies may continue to progress after stopping treatment, cisplatin should be discontinued as soon as symptoms are reported. This neuropathy is usually reversible, but recovery is often slow.

Although cisplatin can cause leukopenia, thrombocytopenia and anemia, the hematologic toxicity is usually considered moderate and reversible. Nadirs in circulating platelets and leukocytes occur between days 18 and 23 (range 7.5 to 45) with average time to recovery of 39 days (range 13 to 62). Leukopenia and thrombocytopenia appear dose-related since they are more pronounced at doses greater than 50 mg/m².

Anemia, presenting with a decrease of 20 g hemoglobin/L from pretreatment values, occurs at approximately the same time as the other types of myelosuppression. Direct Coombs' positive hemolytic anemia has occurred, probably as a result of cisplatin sensitizing red blood cells. The anemia appears reversible when the drug is discontinued.

Cisplatin administration has been associated with anaphylactoid reactions that are characterized by facial edema, hypotension, tachycardia, flushing, wheezing and dyspnea. These reactions may occur within a few minutes of starting iv administration of cisplatin in patients who have received previous doses of cisplatin, although they have also been reported in patients who have not been previously treated with cisplatin. Reactions can be controlled with supportive measures and medications such as epinephrine, corticosteroids and antihistamines.

Infrequently, optic neuritis, papilledema and cerebral blindness have been seen in cisplatin-treated patients. These effects usually reverse upon discontinuation of the drug. With high dose or increased frequency of administration, blurred vision and altered color perception have been reported. This altered perception presents as loss of color discrimination especially in the blue-yellow axis. Funduscopic exam shows an irregularly pigmented macular area. Steroids with or without mannitol have been administered as treatment, however the efficacy of these interventions is not well documented.

PRECAUTIONS: Serum creatinine, BUN and creatinine clearance should be measured prior to starting therapy and subsequently, prior to each cycle. However, it has been suggested that serum creatinine is not a reliable guide to the measurement of glomerular filtration rate due to permanent glomerular or tubular damage. Cisplatin should generally not be given more often than every 3 to 4 weeks. Cisplatin should be administered over 6 to 8 hours. The use of hydration and mannitol may reduce nephrotoxicity. Amifostine has also been administered to patients with advanced ovarian cancer in an effort to reduce cumulative nephrotoxicity. Renal function must return to normal before administration of another cisplatin dose.

Serum magnesium, sodium, potassium and calcium should be measured before starting cisplatin therapy and before each treatment cycle. Some clinicians suggest prophylactic administration of magnesium supplementation, although it has been suggested that hypomagnesemia may occur despite these measures.

Cisplatin-associated gastrointestinal adverse effects are seen in virtually all patients treated with the drug as it is among the most emetogenic antineoplastic agents. Nausea and vomiting generally begin within 1 to 4 hours of treatment and continue up to 24 hours or even as long as a week with varing degrees of severity. Delayed and anticipatory nausea/emesis have also been reported. Factors that appear to increase the incidence of nausea and vomiting are female sex, high doses, rapid infusion and combination therapy with other emetogenic agents.

Some protocols recommend a neurokinin-1 receptor antagonist (e.g., aprepitant) in combination with a 5–HT_3 receptor antagonist (e.g., ondansetron) and an appropriate dose of dexamethasone in the prevention of emesis due to high-dose cisplatin. Selective 5-HT_3 receptor antagonists such as ondansetron (often combined with corticosteroids) are more effective than traditional agents (e.g., metoclopramide) in the management of cisplatin-induced nausea and vomiting.

Especially in children, audiometric testing should be performed prior to starting therapy and prior to all subsequent cisplatin doses. Neurologic exams should be performed regularly. Weekly peripheral blood counts and periodic liver function tests should be performed.

The literature provides inconclusive evidence of long-term effects of occupational exposure to cytotoxic agents. Caution should be exercised during the preparation and handling of cisplatin to minimize any potential hazards. Procedures for the safe handling of cytotoxic and hazardous materials should be used when handling cisplatin.

Drug Interactions: Aminoglycosides: Cisplatin causes cumulative nephrotoxicity that is potentiated by aminoglycosides. Therefore, aminoglycosides should not be used, or used with extreme caution, during or in the period shortly after cisplatin therapy. It has been suggested by some clinicians that administration of an aminoglycoside should be delayed until at least two weeks after cisplatin administration to reduce the occurrence of increased nephrotoxicity.

Loop diuretics: When given with cisplatin, loop diuretics (e.g., furosemide) may increase the risk of ototoxicity. Patients should be carefully monitored.

Phenytoin: Plasma phenytoin levels may be reduced when this drug is used with concomitant antineoplastic therapy including cisplatin. This interaction may be a result of decreased absorption and/or increased metabolism of phenytoin. Serum phenytoin concentration should be monitored in patients receiving cisplatin.

Combination use of cisplatin with agents excreted primarily by the kidneys might delay excretion of these agents (e.g., amphotericin B, bleomycin, ifosfamide, methotrexate.)

Pregnancy: As an antineoplastic agent, cisplatin may cause fetal harm when administered to pregnant women. Although risks to the fetus are possible, the drug has been used during pregnancy, but should only be considered in life-threatening situations or in severe disease where other medications are ineffective or contraindicated. Evidence suggests that cisplatin (or its platinum-containing products) appears to cross the placenta. Pregnant patients or those who become pregnant during cisplatin therapy should be informed of the potential fetal risks. Patients should be counseled to avoid becoming pregnant while receiving cisplatin treatment.

Lactation: Cisplatin has been found in breast milk. Because of the potential for serious adverse reactions in infants, nursing should not be undertaken by women being treated with cisplatin.

ADVERSE EFFECTS: Central Nervous System: Peripheral and autonomic neuropathies, dorsal column myelopathy, seizures and muscle cramps have all been reported in cisplatin-treated patients.

Gastrointestinal : Nausea, vomiting, anorexia (see Precautions) and diarrhea have been associated with cisplatin use.

Hematologic: Myelosuppression presents as leukopenia, thrombocytopenia and anemia and occurs in about 25 to 30% of patients receiving cisplatin. Acute leukemia and hemolytic anemia have also been reported. This acute leukemia has generally been seen in patients receiving treatment with other leukemogenic therapies.

Hepatic: Transient increases in bilirubin and hepatic enzymes have been reported with recommended doses. Pancreatitis has been reported.

Metabolic: Hypomagnesemia, hypocalcemia, hyponatremia, hypokalemia, hypophosphatemia, SIADH and increased plasma iron levels have all been reported.

Ophthalmic: Optic neuritis, papilledema, blurred vision, altered color perception and, infrequently, cerebral blindness have all been reported.

Renal: Dose-related renal insufficiency has been seen in 28 to 36% of patients receiving a single dose of 50 mg/m². Renal tubular damage may occur with cisplatin therapy (see Warnings and Precautions). Hyperuricemia presents with the same frequency as increases in BUN and serum creatinine and is more severe when doses greater than 50 mg/m² are administered. Uric acid peak levels occur 3 to 5 days after cisplatin dosing. Therapy with allopurinol reduces uric acid levels.

Special Senses: Of patients treated with a single dose of cisplatin 50 mg/m², approximately 31% experienced ototoxicity manifested by tinnitus or high frequency hearing loss (see Warnings and Precautions). Vestibular toxicity which presents as vertigo and vestibular dysfunction is also possible.

Miscellaneous: Cardiac abnormalities (e.g., bradycardia, left bundle-branch block, arrhythmias), hypertension, vascular toxicities (e.g., CVA, cerebral arteritis, thrombotic microangiopathy), alopecia, taste loss, rash, and hiccups have all been reported in patients receiving cisplatin therapy.

OVERDOSE:

Overdosage of cisplatin may cause death. Cisplatin overdosage has occurred because of inadvertent substitution of cisplatin for carboplatin. Carboplatin is generally administered at higher doses than cisplatin.

Acute overdosage may give rise to severe manifestations of cisplatin adverse effects including acute renal failure, deafness, ocular toxicity, myelosuppression, intractable nausea/vomiting, deafness and/or neuritis. Hepatic failure, dysarthria, paresthesias and impaired taste perception may also occur.

Treatment: Renal protection and increased platinum elimination are the principal goals of managing cisplatin overdose. Patients should be made to achieve high urine output by administration of normal saline and an osmotic diuretic such as mannitol for 6 to 24 hours after cisplatin exposure. Careful hydration is recommended with nonoliguric renal failure. Amifostine and sodium thiosulfate can be administered for nephrotoxicity.

> For management of a suspected drug overdose, CPhA recommends that you contact your **regional Poison Control Centre**. See the *CPS* Directory section for a list of Poison Control Centres.

DOSAGE: Individual institutions adopt protocols which supply the dosage of cisplatin specific to each indication as well as its method and sequence of administration with other antineoplastic agents. Check any dose > 100 mg/m² per course with the prescriber. To avoid confusion, prescriptions for cisplatin should clearly indicate a daily dosage rather than total cisplatin dosage used in one course of therapy. See Table 1 for suggested dosing of cisplatin as a single agent or in combination therapy for selected malignancies.

Table 1: Cisplatin

Dosage/Frequency of Cisplatin for Selected Malignancies[a,b]

Malignancy	Dosage/Frequency of Administration
Metastatic testicular tumors	20 mg/m² iv daily for 5 consecutive days every 3 weeks for 3-4 courses of treatment as combination therapy (e.g., etoposide with or without bleomycin depending on patient stratification).
Advanced ovarian carcinoma	75 mg/m² iv once every 3 weeks with paclitaxel; 50–100 mg/m² iv once every 3–4 weeks with cyclophosphamide; 100 mg/m² iv once every 4 weeks as a single agent
Advanced bladder cancer	50–70 mg/m² iv once every 3–4 weeks or 50 mg/m² iv once every 4 weeks, depending on extent of pretreatment

[a] Current protocols should be consulted in individual institutions for dosing recommendations.
[b] Dosing may be lowered depending on previous chemotherapy and radiation treatment as well as renal, hematologic and otic function.

Doses should not be repeated until serum creatinine is below approximately 130 µmol/L and/or BUN is below 8.9 mmol/L. Hematologic testing should be performed and no repeat courses given until blood counts reach an acceptable level (platelets ≥100 000 cells/mm³, WBC ≥4000 cells/mm³). Audiometric testing should also demonstrate that auditory acuity is within normal limits before subsequent cisplatin doses are administered.

Patients should be well-hydrated with 1 or 2 L of fluid infused over 8 to 12 hours prior to cisplatin dosing. Some experts administer lower hydration volumes over shorter intervals in ambulatory patients e.g., 500 mL of normal saline over 2 hours. Cisplatin can also be administered with saline containing mannitol. Patients should be monitored for adequate hydration and urine output (i.e., 150 to 400 mL/hr) during and for at least 4 to 6 hours after cisplatin dosing, then at least 100 to 200 mL per hour until 24 hours after cisplatin dosing.

Dosage in Renal Impairment: Cisplatin elimination in renally impaired patients has not been well studied. Use is generally avoided when creatinine clearance is less than 50 mL/minute. It has been suggested that 75% of the usual dose be administered to patients with creatinine clearance 10 to 50 mL/minute and 50% of the usual dose be given to those with creatinine clearance less than 10 mL/minute.

Pediatric dosage: Pediatric dosing of cisplatin has not been clearly established. Osteogenic sarcoma and neuroblastoma have been treated with 90 mg/m² iv once every 3 weeks or 30 mg/m² iv once weekly. Recurrent brain tumors have been treated with a dose of 60 mg/m² iv once daily for 2 consecutive days every 3 to 4 weeks.

Administration: Intravenous needles, syringes or sets containing aluminum components should not be used in preparation or administration of cisplatin solutions. A black precipitate, as well as a loss of potency, can occur because of an interaction between aluminum and platinum.

Cisplatin solution can be further diluted in 0.9% sodium chloride, 5% dextrose and 0.9% sodium chloride, 5% dextrose and 0.45% sodium chloride, 5% dextrose and 0.9% sodium chloride with mannitol, 5% dextrose and 0.45% sodium chloride with mannitol; 5% dextrose and 0.3% sodium chloride with mannitol.

All preparation should take place in a vertical laminar flow hood. Those preparing cisplatin should wear PVC gloves, safety glasses, disposable gowns and masks. Needles, syringes, vials or any other materials in contact with cisplatin should be segregated and incinerated at 1000°C or more. If cisplatin solution contacts the skin, wash immediately with soap and water. If the contact is with mucous membranes, flush thoroughly with water.

Cisplatin Injection ℞

cisplatin

Antineoplastic

Hospira

SUPPLIED: Each mL of sterile aqueous solution contains: cisplatin 1 mg. Nonmedicinal ingredients: mannitol in Water for Injection and sodium chloride. May contain hydrochloric acid as pH adjusters. Preservative-free. Single use vials of 50 and 100 mL, cartons of 1. Store between 15 and 25°C. Protect from light. Do not refrigerate or freeze cisplatin solutions since a precipitate may form. Discard unused portion.

Citalopram ℞

CPhA Monograph

see *Selective Serotonin Reuptake Inhibitors*

☞ The reader is invited to consult CPhA's monograph **Selective Serotonin Reuptake Inhibitors**.

Citalopram-Odan ℞

citalopram HBr

Antidepressant

Odan

SUPPLIED: 20 mg: Each white to off white, oval shaped, scored, film coated tablet, imprinted on the non-scored side with "O-20", contains: citalopram 20 mg (as citalopram hydrobromide). Nonmedicinal ingredients: croscarmellose sodium, crospovidone, glycerol, hypromellose, lactose monohydrate, macrogol 4000, magnesium stearate, maize starch, microcrystalline cellulose and titanium dioxide. Plastic bottles of 100 and 500. Store in a dry place and at room temperature (15 to 30°C).
40 mg: Each white to off white, oval shaped, scored, film coated tablet, imprinted on the non-scored side with "O-40", contains: citalopram 40 mg (as citalopram hydrobromide). Nonmedicinal ingredients: croscarmellose sodium, crospovidone, glycerol, hypromellose, lactose monohydrate, macrogol 4000, magnesium stearate, maize starch, microcrystalline cellulose and titanium dioxide. Plastic bottles of 100. Store in a dry place and at room temperature (15 to 30°C).

Citrodan™

magnesium citrate, anhydrous

Laxative

Odan

SUPPLIED: Each bottle of lemon-flavored, colorless solution contains: anhydrous magnesium citrate 15 g. Nonmedicinal ingredients: citrus flavor, phosphoric acid, sodium benzoate, sodium saccharin and water. Energy: <21 kJ (<5 kcal)/bottle. Sodium: <1 mmol (3.2 mg)/5 mL. Plastic bottles of 300 mL. Store at room temperature (15 to 30°C).

Citro-Mag

magnesium citrate, anhydrous

Laxative—Purgative

Rougier Pharma

SUPPLIED: Each bottle of lemon-flavored, effervescent, colorless solution, contains: anhydrous magnesium citrate 15 g. Nonmedicinal ingredients: natural and artificial flavoring, carbonic gas, purified water, sodium benzoate, sodium bicarbonate and sorbitol. Energy: 22.05 kJ (5.25 kcal)/5 mL. Sodium: <1 mmol (7.56 mg)/5 mL. Bottles of 300 mL.

Claforan® ℞

cefotaxime sodium

β-lactam Antibiotic

sanofi-aventis

Date of Revision: May 30, 2008

PHARMACOLOGY: Cefotaxime is a semi-synthetic, 2-aminothiazolyl cephalosporin antibiotic for parenteral use. In vitro studies indicate that the antibacterial action of cefotaxime results from inhibition of cell wall synthesis. It is stable against the action of most β-lactamases.

INDICATIONS: Treatment: Cefotaxime may be indicated for the treatment of infections caused by susceptible strains of the designated microorganisms in the diseases listed below:
Lower Respiratory Tract Infections: pneumonia and lung abscess caused by *S. pneumoniae*, other streptococci (excluding enterococci, e.g., *S. faecalis*), *S. aureus* (penicillinase and nonpenicillinase producing), *E. coli*, *H. influenzae*, (including ampicillin resistant strains) and unspecified Klebsiella species.
Urinary Tract Infections: caused by *E. coli*, unspecified Klebsiella species (including *K. pneumoniae*), *P. mirabilis*, indole positive Proteus, *S. marcescens* and *S. epidermidis*. Also, uncomplicated gonorrhea caused by *N. gonorrhoeae* including penicillin resistant strains.
Bacteremia/Septicemia: caused by *E. coli*, unspecified Klebsiella strains and *S. marcescens*.
Skin Infections: caused by *S. aureus* (penicillinase and non-penicillinase producing), *S. epidermidis*, Group A streptococci, *E. coli*, *P. mirabilis* and indole positive Proteus.
Intra-abdominal Infections: caused by *E. coli*, and unspecified Klebsiella species.
Gynecological Infections: including pelvic inflammatory disease, endometritis and pelvic cellulitis caused by *E. coli*, Group A streptococci and *S. epidermidis*; anaerobic bacteria including unspecified Peptococcus and Peptostreptococcus strains and some strains of *B. fragilis*. In several cases, although clinical cures were achieved, bacteriological follow-up was not available.
Cefotaxime, like other cephalosporins, has no activity against *C. trachomatis*. Therefore, when cephalosporins are used in the treatment of patients with pelvic inflammatory disease and *C. trachomatis* is one of the suspected pathogens, appropriate anti-chlamydial coverage should be added.
CNS Infections: meningitis and ventriculitis caused by *H. influenzae*, *N. meningitidis*, *S. pneumoniae*, *K. pneumoniae* and *E. coli*. Cefotaxime is not active against *L. monocytogenes*.
Clinical experience with cefotaxime in anaerobic infections is limited. It has been used with some success in wound and intra-abdominal infections against some strains of unidentified Bacteroides and anaerobic cocci.
Cefotaxime has been shown to be active against some strains of Pseudomonas.
In the treatment of infections encountered in immunosuppressed and granulocytopenic patients, results of therapy with cefotaxime have not been impressive.
Cefotaxime should not be considered in the treatment of enterococcal infections, i.e., *S. faecalis*.
Specimens for bacteriologic culture should be obtained prior to therapy in order to isolate and identify the causative organisms and to determine their susceptibilities to cefotaxime. Therapy may be instituted before results of susceptibility studies are known; antibiotic treatment should be re-evaluated once these results become available.
Prophylactic Use: The administration of cefotaxime perioperatively (preoperatively, intraoperatively and postoperatively) may reduce the incidence of certain infections in patients undergoing elective surgical procedures (e.g., abdominal or vaginal hysterectomy, gastrointestinal and genitourinary tract surgery) that may be classified as contaminated or potentially contaminated.
In patients undergoing caesarian section who are considered to be at increased risk of infection, intraoperative (after clamping the umbilical cord) and postoperative use of cefotaxime may also reduce the incidence of certain postoperative infections.
Effective use for elective surgery depends on the time of administration (see Dosage).
For patients undergoing gastrointestinal surgery, preoperative bowel preparation by mechanical cleansing as well as with a nonabsorbable antibiotic (e.g., neomycin) is recommended.
If there are signs of infection, specimens for culture should be obtained for identification of the causative organism so that appropriate therapy may be instituted.

CONTRAINDICATIONS: In patients who have shown hypersensitivity to cefotaxime sodium, the cephalosporin or the penicillin groups of antibiotics.

WARNINGS: Anaphylactic Reactions: **Before therapy with cefotaxime is instituted, it must be carefully determined whether the patient has had previous hypersensitivity reactions to cefotaxime, cephalosporins, penicillins or other drugs. Since cross allergy exists between penicillins and cephalosporins in 5 to 10 % of cases, cefotaxime should be given with extreme caution to patients with Type 1 hypersensitivity reactions to penicillin. Antibiotics, including cefotaxime should be administered with caution to any patient who has demonstrated some form of allergy, particularly to drugs. If an allergic reaction to cefotaxime occurs, the drug should be discontinued and the patient treated with the usual agents (e.g., epinephrine, antihistamine, pressor amines or corticosteroids).**
Speed of I.V. Injection: During post-marketing surveillance, a potentially life-threatening arrhythmia was reported in very few patients who received a rapid bolus injection of cefotaxime through a central venous catheter. Therefore, cefotaxime should only be administered as instructed in Dosage.
Gastrointestinal: *C. difficile*-associated disease: *C. difficile*-associated disease (CDAD) has been reported with use of many antibacterial agents, including cefotaxime. CDAD may range in severity from mild diarrhea to fatal colitis. It is important to consider this diagnosis in patients who present with diarrhea, or symptoms of colitis, pseudomembranous colitis, toxic megacolon, or perforation of colon subsequent to the administration of any antibacterial agent. CDAD has been reported to occur over 2 months after the administration of antibacterial agents.
Treatment with antibacterial agents may alter the normal flora of the colon and may permit overgrowth of *C. difficile*. *C. difficile* produces toxins A and B, which contribute to the development of CDAD. CDAD may cause significant morbidity and mortality. CDAD can be refractory to antimicrobial therapy.
If the diagnosis of CDAD is suspected or confirmed, appropriate therapeutic measures should be initiated. Mild cases of CDAD usually respond to discontinuation of antibacterial agents not directed against *C. difficile*. In moderate to severe cases, consideration should be given to management with fluids and electrolytes, protein supplementation, and treatment with an antibacterial agent clinically effective against *C. difficile*. Surgical evaluation should be instituted as clinically indicated, as surgical intervention may be required in certain severe cases (see Adverse Effects).

PRECAUTIONS: Cefotaxime should be prescribed with caution in individuals with a history of lower gastrointestinal disease, particularly colitis.
General: Prolonged use of cefotaxime may result in the overgrowth of nonsusceptible organisms. Constant evaluation of the patient's condition is essential. If superinfection occurs, therapy should be discontinued and appropriate measures taken.
As with other β-lactam antibiotics, granulocytopenia and, more rarely, agranulocytosis may develop during treatment with cefotaxime, particularly if given over long periods. For courses of treatment lasting longer than 10 days, blood counts should therefore be monitored and treatment stopped in the event of neutropenia.
Cefotaxime, like other parenteral anti-infective drugs, may be locally irritating to tissues. In most cases, perivascular extravasation of cefotaxime responds to changing of the infusion site. In rare instances, extensive perivascular extravasation of cefotaxime may result in tissue damage and require surgical treatment. To minimize the potential for tissue inflammation, infusion sites should be monitored regularly and changed when appropriate.
Pregnancy: Cefotaxime crosses the placental barrier. However, the safety of cefotaxime in pregnancy has not been established and it should not be used during pregnancy.
Use of cefotaxime in women of childbearing potential requires that the anticipated benefits be weighed against the possible risks.
Lactation: Since cefotaxime is excreted in human milk in low concentrations, either breast-feeding or treatment of the mother should be discontinued as necessary.
Patients with Special Diseases and Conditions: Although cefotaxime rarely produces alterations in kidney function, evaluation of renal status is recommended, especially in severely ill patients receiving high doses.
Patients with markedly impaired renal function should be placed on the special dosage schedule recommended under Dosage, because normal dosage in these individuals is likely to produce excessive and prolonged serum antibiotic concentrations. If CLAFORAN and aminoglycosides are to be administered to the same patient, these antibiotics should be administered separately and not as a mixed injection (see Reconstitution, Incompatibilities). Renal function must be monitored in all such cases.
The sodium content of cefotaxime sodium (48.2 mg/g) should be taken into account in patients necessitating sodium restriction.
Drug Interactions: Probenecid interferes with the renal tubular transfer of cephalosporins, thereby delaying their excretion and increasing their plasma concentrations.
As with other cephalosporins, cefotaxime may potentiate the nephrotoxic effects of nephrotoxic drugs.
Laboratory Tests: Positive direct Coombs' test is known to develop in individuals during treatment with the cephalosporin group of antibiotics, including cefotaxime sodium.
In laboratory tests a false positive reaction to glucose may occur with reducing substances but not with the use of specific glucose oxidase methods.

ADVERSE EFFECTS: Clinical Trials: The most frequent adverse reactions with their frequency of occurrence are:
CNS (0.2%): headache.
Gastrointestinal (1.7%): colitis, diarrhea, nausea and vomiting. Symptoms of pseudomembranous colitis can appear during or after cefotaxime treatment.
Genitourinary System (<1%): moniliasis, vaginitis.
Hematologic System (<1%): As with other β-lactam antibiotics, neutropenia and, more rarely, agranulocytosis may develop during treatment with cefotaxime, particularly if given over long periods. Furthermore, transient leukopenia, eosinophilia and thrombocytopenia have also been reported.
Some individuals have developed positive direct Coombs' test during treatment with cefotaxime and other cephalosporin antibiotics (see Precautions, Laboratory Tests). Rare cases of hemolytic anemia have been reported.
Hypersensitivity (1.8%): rash, pruritus, fever.
Kidney (<1%): Increased BUN has occasionally been observed.
Liver (<1%): Transient elevations in AST, ALT, serum LDH, and serum alkaline phosphatase levels have been reported.
Local (5%): Injection site inflammation with i.v. administration. Pain, induration and tenderness after i.m. injection.
Other Adverse Events including Post-marketing Surveillance Data:
Anaphylactic Reactions: angioedema, bronchospasm, malaise possibly culminating in shock, may rarely occur (see Warnings, Anaphylactic Reactions).
Cardiovascular: Potentially life-threatening arrythmia following rapid bolus infusion has been reported in very few patients who received rapid i.v. administration of cefotaxime through a central venous catheter (see Warnings, Speed of I.V. Injection).
Central Nervous System: Administration of high doses of β-lactam antibiotics, including cefotaxime, particularly in patients with renal insufficiency may result in encephalopathy (e.g., impairment of consciousness, abnormal movements and convulsions).
Cutaneous: rash, pruritus and less frequently urticaria.
As with other cephalosporins, isolated cases of bullous eruptions (erythema multiforme, Stevens-Johnson syndrome, toxic epidermal necrolysis) have been reported.
Gastrointestinal: During treatment with cefotaxime, abdominal pain may occur. As with all other broad spectrum antibiotics diarrhea may sometimes be a symptom of enterocolitis, which may, in some cases, be accompanied by blood in stools. A particular form of enterocolitis that can occur with antibiotics, including cefotaxime, is *C. difficile*-associated disease (see Warnings, Gastrointestinal, *C. difficile*-associated disease).
Kidney: Decreases in renal function (increase of creatinine) have been observed with cephalosporins including cefotaxime, particularly when coprescribed with aminoglycosides.
As with some other cephalosporins, rare cases of interstitial nephritis have been reported in patients treated with cefotaxime.
Liver: Increase in liver enzymes (ALT, AST, LDH, gamma-GT and/or alkaline phosphatase) and/or bilirubin have been reported. These laboratory abnormalities, which may also be explained by the infection, may rarely exceed twice the upper limit of the normal range and elicit a pattern of liver injury, usually cholestatic and most often asymptomatic. Hepatitis (sometimes with jaundice) has been reported.
Other: Superinfection: As with other antibiotics, the use of cefotaxime, especially if prolonged, may result in overgrowth of nonsusceptible organisms. Repeated evaluation of the patient's condition is essential. If superinfection occurs during therapy, appropriate measures should be taken.
As reported with other antibiotics for the treatment of borreliosis a Jarisch-Herxheimer reaction may develop during the first days of treatment.
The occurrence of one or more of the following symptoms has been reported after several weeks of treatment of borreliosis: skin rash, itching, fever, leukopenia, increase in liver enzymes, difficulty of breathing, joint discomfort. To some extent, these manifestations are consistent with the symptoms of the underlying disease for which the patient is being treated.

OVERDOSE:

Symptoms: There is a risk of reversible encephalopathy in cases of administration of high doses of β-lactam antibiotics including cefotaxime.

Treatment: No specific antidote exists.

For management of a suspected drug overdose, contact your regional Poison Control Centre. See the *CPS* Directory section for a list of Poison Control Centres.

DOSAGE: Cefotaxime may be administered i.m. or i.v. after reconstitution (see Table 3 and Table 4 with recommended mode of reconstitution according to route of administration).
Dosage: Treatment for Adults and Children with Body Weight of 50 kg or More: The dosage of cefotaxime should be determined by susceptibility of the causative organisms, severity of the infection and condition of the patient.

Table 1: CLAFORAN
Guidelines for Dosage of CLAFORAN (cefotaxime sodium) for Adults and Children with Body Weight of 50 kg or More

Type of Infection	Daily Dose (g)	Frequency and Route
Uncomplicated Gonorrhea	1	1 g i.m. (single dose)
Uncomplicated infections	2	1 g every 12 hours i.m. or i.v.
Moderately severe to severe infections	3 to 6	1 to 2 g every 8 hours i.m. or i.v
Very severe infections (e.g., septicemia, CNS)	6 to 8	2 g every 6 to 8 hours i.v.
Life-threatening infections	up to 12	2 g every 4 hours i.v.

The maximum daily dosage should not exceed 12 g.
Treatment for Neonates, Infants, and Children: The following dosage schedule is recommended:
Neonates (birth to 1 month): 0-1 week of age: 50 mg/kg per dose i.v. every 12 hours; 1-4 weeks of age: 50 mg/kg per dose i.v. every 8 hours.
Infants and Children (1 month to 12 years): For body weights less than 50 kg, the recommended daily dose is 50 to 100 mg/kg i.m. or i.v. divided into 4 to 6 equal doses, or up to 180 mg/kg/day for severe infections (including CNS infections).
For body weights of 50 kg or more, the usual adult dosage should be used; **the maximum daily dosage should not exceed 12 g.**
See Table 2.

Table 2: CLAFORAN
Guidelines for Dosage of CLAFORAN (cefotaxime sodium) for Neonates, Infants and Children

Patients	Age or Weight	Daily Dose	Route	Dose Interval
Neonates	0 to 1 week	50 mg/kg/**dose**	i.v.	Every 12 h
Neonates	1 to 4 weeks	50 mg/kg/**dose**	i.v.	Every 8 h
Infants and Children	<50 kg	50 to 100 mg/kg/**day** (up to 180 mg/kg/day for severe infections, including meningitis)	i.v. or i.m.	Divided into 4 to 6 equal doses
Children	≥50 kg	adult dosage		

Duration of Treatment: Administration of cefotaxime should be continued for a minimum of 48 to 72 hours after the patient defervesces or after evidence of bacterial eradication has been obtained; a minimum of 10 days of treatment is recommended for infections caused by Group A beta-hemolytic streptococci in order to guard against the risk of rheumatic fever or glomerulonephritis; frequent bacteriologic and clinical appraisal is necessary during therapy of chronic urinary tract infections and may be required for several months after therapy has been completed; persistent infections may require prolonged treatment. Doses less than those recommended should not be employed.
Prophylactic Use: Surgery Patients: To prevent postoperative infection in contaminated or potentially contaminated surgery, recommended doses are as follows: 1 g i.m. or i.v. administered 1/2 to 1½ hours prior to the initial surgical incision to ensure that adequate antibiotic levels are present in the serum and tissues at the start of surgery; 1 g i.m. or i.v. administered 1½ to 2 hours following the first dose; for lengthy operative procedures, additional intraoperative doses may be administered, if necessary, at appropriate intervals (1½ to 2 hours) during surgery; 1 g i.m. or i.v. administered within 2 hours following completion of surgery.
The total cumulative prophylactic dose should not exceed 6 g in a 12-hour period.
Caesarian Section Patients: The first dose of 1 g is administered i.v. as soon as the umbilical cord is clamped. The second and third doses should be given as 1 g i.m. or i.v. at 6 and 12 hours after the first dose.
Dosage for Patients with Impaired Renal Function: In patients with estimated creatinine clearance of less than 20 mL/min/1.73 m², the dose should be halved (see Precautions, Patients with Special Diseases and Conditions).
If serum creatinine values alone are available, the following formulas (based on sex, weight, and age of the patient) may be used to convert these values into creatinine clearance.

$$\text{Males: } Cl_{Cr}\ (\text{mL/min}) = \frac{\text{Weight (kg)} \times (140 - \text{age})}{72 \times \text{serum creatinine (mg/dL)}}$$

Females: Cl_{Cr} (mL/min) = 0.85×above value.

In Hemodialyzed Patients: 1 to 2 g daily, depending on the severity of the infection; on the day of hemodialysis, cefotaxime must be administered after the dialysis session.
Administration: I.M.: Cefotaxime should be injected well within the body of a relatively large muscle such as the upper outer quadrant of the buttock (i.e., gluteus maximus); aspiration is necessary to avoid inadvertent injection into a blood vessel.
I.V.: The i.v. route is preferable for patients with bacteremia, bacterial septicemia, or other severe or life-threatening infections, or for patients who may be poor risks because of lowered resistance resulting from such debilitating conditions as malnutrition, trauma, surgery, diabetes, heart failure, or malignancy, particularly if shock is present or impending.
For bolus administration, the solution containing cefotaxime must be injected over a period of 3 to 5 minutes (see Warnings, Speed of I.V. Injection).
Using an infusion system, it may also be given over a longer period of time through the tubing system by which the patient may be receiving other i.v. solutions. Butterfly or scalp vein type needles are preferred for this type of infusion. However, during infusion of the solution containing cefotaxime, it is advisable to discontinue temporarily the administration of other solutions at the same site (see Reconstitution, Incompatibilities).
Reconstitution: I.M.: Cefotaxime should be reconstituted with Sterile Water for Injection or Bacteriostatic Water for Injection in accordance with the volumes recommended in Table 3.
For Intravenous Use: For intravenous bolus use: 500 mg, 1 g and 2 g vials should be reconstituted with at least 10 mL of Sterile Water for Injection.
For Intravenous Infusion Use: Reconstituted solution may be further diluted with 50 to 1000 mL of the fluids recommended for i.v. infusion.
A solution of 1 g of cefotaxime in 14 mL of Sterile Water for Injection is isotonic.
Solutions for I.V. Infusion: Cefotaxime is compatible with the following infusion fluids: 0.9% NaCl injection; 5% dextrose injection; 0.9% NaCl and 5% dextrose injection; 0.45% NaCl and 5% dextrose injection; 0.2% NaCl and 5% dextrose injection; Sodium Lactate injection; 5% dextrose and 0.15% KCl injection; Plasma-Lyte 56 Electrolyte Solution in 5% dextrose injection; Ringer's injection; Lactated Ringer's solution; Lactated Ringer's with 5% dextrose injection.

Table 3: CLAFORAN
Reconstitution Table for Intramuscular Use

	Volume To Be Added To Vial (mL)[a]	Approximate Available Volume (mL)	Approximate Average Concentration (mg/mL)
500 mg vial	2	2.2	230
1 g vial	3	3.4	300
2 g vial	5	6.0	330

[a] Shake to dissolve.

Table 4: CLAFORAN
Reconstitution Table for Intravenous Use

	Volume To Be Added To Vial (mL)[a]	Approximate Available Volume (mL)	Approximate Average Concentration (mg/mL)
500 mg vial	10	10.2	50
1 g vial	10	10.4	95
2 g vial	10	11.0	180

[a] Shake to dissolve.

Incompatibilities: Solutions of CLAFORAN must not be admixed aminoglycoside solutions. If CLAFORAN and aminoglycosides are to be administered to the same patient, they must be administered separately and not as a mixed injection.
Solutions of CLAFORAN should not be prepared with diluents having a pH above 7.5 such as Sodium Bicarbonate Injection.
Stability and Storage: Solutions of CLAFORAN range from light yellow to amber, depending on concentration and the diluent used. The solutions tend to darken depending on storage conditions and should be protected from elevated temperatures and excessive light.
CLAFORAN reconstituted in the original vial as described under Reconstitution maintains satisfactory potency for 24 hours at room temperature (15-25°C) and for 48 hours under refrigeration (2-8°C). Only freshly prepared reconstituted solutions may be further diluted with 50 to 1000 mL of the recommended infusion fluids in Viaflex i.v. bags. Such solutions maintain satisfactory potency for 24 hours at room temperature (15-25°C) and for 72 hours under refrigeration (2-8°C). Any unused solutions should be discarded.
CLAFORAN solutions exhibit maximum stability in the pH 5-7 range.
Special Instructions: Parenteral drug products should be inspected visually for particulate matter and discoloration prior to administration. Solutions of CLAFORAN range from light yellow to amber, depending on concentration and diluent used. The dry powder as well as solutions tend to darken, depending on storage conditions.

SUPPLIED: A sterile, creamy white powder, in vials containing cefotaxime sodium 500 mg, 1 and 2 g. In the dry state store at room temperature. Protect from light and heat.

Claritin®
loratadine
Histamine H1-Receptor Antagonist

Schering-Plough

Claritin Kids®
loratadine
Histamine H1-Receptor Antagonist

Schering-Plough

Date of Preparation: March 30, 1998
Date of Revision: July 6, 2006

SUMMARY PRODUCT INFORMATION:

Route of Administration	Dosage Form/ Strength	Clinically Relevant Nonmedicinal Ingredients
Oral	Tablet/10 mg Rapid Dissolve Tongue Tablet/10 mg Syrup/1 mg/mL	For a complete listing see Dosage Forms, Composition and Packaging.

INDICATIONS AND CLINICAL USE: CLARITIN (loratadine) Tablets and CLARITIN (loratadine) Rapid Dissolve Tongue Tablets are indicated for:
- the relief of symptoms associated with seasonal and perennial allergic rhinitis, such as sneezing, nasal discharge and itching, and ocular itching and burning.
- the relief of symptoms and signs of chronic urticaria and other allergic dermatologic disorders.

Clinical studies to date support treatment for up to six months, thus medical recommendation is advised for longer-term use. CLARITIN Rapid Dissolve Tongue Tablets should be taken on an empty stomach.
CLARITIN KIDS (loratadine) Syrup is indicated for:
- the relief of symptoms associated with seasonal allergic rhinitis, such as sneezing, nasal discharge and itching, and ocular itching and burning.
- the relief of symptoms and signs of chronic urticaria and other allergic dermatologic disorders.

All dosage forms of CLARITIN and CLARITIN KIDS are not recommended for pregnant or lactating women.
Geriatrics: The pharmacokinetic parameters of loratadine and its major metabolite are comparable in healthy adult volunteers and healthy geriatric volunteers.
Pediatrics (2-12 years of age): In children, it is intended for short-term use only unless taken under medical supervision.

CONTRAINDICATIONS:
- Patients who are hypersensitive to this drug or to any ingredient in the formulation or component of the container. For a complete listing, see Dosage Forms, Composition and Packaging.

WARNINGS AND PRECAUTIONS: Hepatic/Biliary/Pancreatic: Patients with severe liver impairment should be administered a lower initial dose because they may have reduced clearance of loratadine; an initial dose of 5 mg once daily or 10 mg every other day is recommended.
Special Populations: Pregnant Women: The safe use of loratadine during pregnancy has not been established and is therefore not recommended.
Nursing Women: The safe use of loratadine during lactation has not been established and is therefore not recommended.
Pediatrics (2-12 years of age): The safety and efficacy of loratadine in children younger than 2 years of age have not been established. Long-term safety and efficacy of loratadine in children between the ages of 2 and 12 has not been demonstrated. Therefore, it is desirable that loratadine not be administered to children between the ages of 2 and 12 for longer than 14 days, unless recommended by a physician.

ADVERSE REACTIONS: Adverse Drug Reaction Overview: Adverse experiences reported with CLARITIN in adults during clinical trials were mild and consisted of fatigue, headache, dry mouth, sedation, gastrointestinal disorders such as nausea, gastritis, and also allergic symptoms like rash.

Nervousness and hyperkinesia were among the reported adverse experiences in pediatric patients. Gastrointestinal adverse reactions reported during pediatric trials may have been slightly more frequent in the younger patients (less than or equal to 30 kg).

During the marketing of loratadine, alopecia, anaphylaxis, abnormal hepatic function, palpitations and tachycardia have been reported rarely.

Clinical Trial Adverse Drug Reactions: Because clinical trials are conducted under very specific conditions the adverse reaction rates observed in the clinical trials may not reflect the rates observed in practice and should not be compared to the rates in the clinical trials of another drug. Adverse drug reaction information from clinical trials is useful for identifying drug-related adverse events and for approximating rates.

Table 1: CLARITIN Tablets

CLARITIN Tablets, 10 mg Once Daily vs. Placebo and Comparatives. Number (%) of Adult Patients Reporting Frequently Occurring (≥2% of loratadine treated patients) Adverse Experiences in Adults Possibly or Probably Related to Treatment: Patients Treated with CLARITIN (loratadine), Placebo and Comparatives

Adverse Experience	Loratadine 10 mg QD n=1241	Placebo n=1652	Clemastine 1 mg BID n=687	Terfenadine 60 mg BID n=506	Astemizole 10 mg OD n=342
Fatigue	54 (4)	62 (4)	62 (9)	17 (3)	22 (6)
Headache	97 (8)	104 (6)	32 (5)	40 (8)	26 (7)
Dry Mouth	49 (4)	32 (2)	22 (3)	15 (3)	2 (1)
Dryness in Nose	9 (<1)	—	6 (<1)	3 (<1)	—
Sedation[a]	99 (8)	101 (6)	151 (22)	41 (8)	50 (15)

[a] Reported as somnolence, sleepiness, drowsiness, lethargy, slow or "drugged feeling".

Adverse experiences reported with CLARITIN conventional tablets in adults during the clinical trials were mild and consisted of fatigue, headache, dry mouth, sedation, gastrointestinal disorders such as nausea, gastritis, and also allergic symptoms like rash. The incidence of sedation was similar to that of the comparative agents terfenadine, astemizole and placebo, but statistically different (p<0.01) from clemastine. See Table 1.

Table 2: CLARITIN Rapid Dissolve Tablets

CLARITIN Rapid Dissolve Tongue Tablets vs. CLARITIN Tablets vs. Placebo. Number (%) of Patients Reporting Frequently Occurring (≥2% of Loratadine Rapid Dissolve Tongue Tablet-Treated patients) Adverse Experiences Possibly or Probably Related to Treatment in Seasonal Allergic Rhinitis Studies

	Number (%) of Patients		
Adverse Experience	Loratadine 10 mg Rapid Dissolve Tongue Tablet (N=495)	Loratadine 10 mg Tablet (N=328)	Placebo (N=497)
Dry Mouth	8 (2)	8 (2)	5 (1)
Fatigue	13 (3)	12 (4)	16 (3)
Headache	40 (8)	23 (7)	55 (11)
Somnolence	22 (4)	13 (4)	13 (3)

CLARITIN Rapid Dissolve Tongue Tablets were well tolerated and did not cause local irritation or taste abnormalities. The most frequently reported adverse experience was headache. Overall, the incidence of adverse reactions was comparable to that of CLARITIN conventional tablets and to that of placebo. See Table 2.

Table 3: CLARITIN KIDS Syrup—Pediatrics

CLARITIN KIDS Syrup, 1 mg/mL, 5-10 mg Once Daily. Number (%) of Patients Reporting Frequently Occurring (≥2% of LoratadineTreatedPatients) Treatment-Related Adverse Experiences: Placebo-Controlled Clinical Trials in Pediatric Studies in Seasonal Allergic Rhinitis and Allergic Skin Disorders Studies

	Loratadine		Chlorpheniramine		
Adverse Experience	5 mg N=46	10 mg N=119	2 mg N=48	4 mg N=122	Placebo N=168
Nervousness	2 (4)	5 (4)	1 (2)	2 (2)	2 (1)
Hyperkinesia	0 (0)	4 (3)	0 (0)	1 (1)	1 (0.6)
Sedation	2 (4)	6 (5)	4 (8)	13 (11)	9 (5)
Headache	3 (6)	4 (3)	4 (8)	5 (4)	13 (8)

Table 4: CLARITIN KIDS Syrup

CLARITIN KIDS Syrup, 1 mg/mL, 5-10 mg Once Daily. Number of Patients Reporting GI Adverse Experiences in Placebo-Controlled Clinical Trials Possibly or Probably Related to Study Medication, Grouped According to Treatment, Dose, Weight, in Pediatric Studies

Adverse Experience	5 mg Dose Wt ≤30 kg (N=46)	10 mg Dose Wt >30 kg (N=119)	Placebo Wt >30 kg (N=168)
Diarrhea	1	0	0
Nausea	2	2	5
Dyspepsia	2	3	3

(cont'd)

Table 4: CLARITIN KIDS Syrup *(cont'd)*

CLARITIN KIDS Syrup, 1 mg/mL, 5-10 mg Once Daily. Number of Patients Reporting GI Adverse Experiences in Placebo-Controlled Clinical Trials Possibly or Probably Related to Study Medication, Grouped According to Treatment, Dose, Weight, in Pediatric Studies

Adverse Experience	5 mg Dose Wt ≤30 kg (N=46)	10 mg Dose Wt >30 kg (N=119)	Placebo Wt >30 kg (N=168)
Vomiting	2	0	0
Abdominal Pain	0	2	0
Total	7 (15%)	7 (5.9%)	8 (4.8%)

Adverse experiences reported in pediatric patients are shown in Table 3 and Table 4. Nervousness and hyperkinesia were among the reported adverse experiences. One case of hyperkinesia was graded as severe and was judged by the physician to be possibly related to loratadine treatment. Gastrointestinal adverse reactions reported during pediatric trials may have been slightly more frequent in the younger patients (less than or equal to 30 kg), but in older children (greater than 30 kg) are similar to placebo.

Less Common Clinical Trial Adverse Drug Reactions (<1%): In addition to those listed in Table 1, the following were reported less frequently (less than 1%): appetite increased, coughing, dizziness and palpitations.

Abnormal Hematologic and Clinical Chemistry Findings: Not applicable.

Post-Market Adverse Drug Reactions: During the marketing of loratadine, in addition to the adverse events reported during clinical trials, alopecia, anaphylaxis, abnormal hepatic function, palpitations and tachycardia have been reported rarely.

DRUG INTERACTIONS:

> **Serious Drug Interactions**
> None to report.

Overview: When administered concomitantly with alcohol, loratadine has no potentiating effects as measured by psychomotor performance studies.

Drug-Drug Interactions: Increases in plasma concentrations of loratadine have been reported after concomitant use with ketoconazole, erythromycin or cimetidine in controlled clinical trials, but without clinically significant changes (including electrocardiographic). Other drugs known to inhibit hepatic metabolism should be coadministered with caution until definitive interaction studies can be completed.

Drug-Food Interactions: See Action and Clinical Pharmacology, Pharmacokinetics, Absorption.

Drug-Herb Interactions: Interactions with herbs have not been established.

Drug-Laboratory Test Interactions: Loratadine should be discontinued approximately 48 hours prior to skin testing procedures since antihistamines may prevent or diminish otherwise positive reactions to dermal reactivity indicators.

Drug-Lifestyle Interactions: Interactions with lifestyle have not been established.

DOSAGE AND ADMINISTRATION: Dosing Considerations: Patients with severe liver impairment: an initial dose of 5 mg once daily or 10 mg every other day is recommended.

Recommended Dose and Dosage Adjustment: CLARITIN or CLARITIN KIDS should not be administered to children between 2 and 12 years of age for longer than 14 days, unless recommended by a physician.

Tablets: Adults and Children 12 Years of Age and Over: one CLARITIN tablet, 10 mg, once daily.

Rapid Dissolve Tongue Tablets: Adults and Children 12 Years of Age and Over: one CLARITIN Rapid Dissolve Tongue Tablet, 10 mg, placed in the mouth once daily.

Can be taken without water.

Should be taken on an empty stomach.

Syrup: Adults, Children Over 10 Years of Age (body weight greater than 30 kg): 10 mL (two teaspoonfuls) of CLARITIN KIDS Syrup once daily.

Children 2 Through 9 Years of Age (body weight less than or equal to 30 kg): 5 mL (one teaspoonful) of CLARITIN KIDS Syrup once daily.

OVERDOSAGE:

Somnolence, tachycardia and headache have been reported with overdoses of the conventional loratadine formulation. A single acute ingestion of 160 mg produced no adverse effects.

In the event of overdosage, treatment, which should be started immediately, is symptomatic and supportive.

Consider standard measures to remove any unabsorbed drug in the stomach, such as adsorption by activated charcoal administered as a slurry with water. The administration of gastric lavage should be considered. Physiologic saline solution is the lavage solution of choice, particularly in children. In adults, tap water can be used; however, as much as possible of the amount administered should be removed before the next instillation. Saline cathartics draw water into the bowel by osmosis, and therefore, may be valuable for their action in rapid dilution of bowel content.

Loratadine is not cleared by hemodialysis to any appreciable extent. It is not known if loratadine is removed by peritoneal dialysis.

> For management of a suspected drug overdose, CPhA recommends that you contact your **regional Poison Control Centre**. See the *CPS* Directory section for a list of Poison Control Centres.

ACTION AND CLINICAL PHARMACOLOGY: Mechanism of Action: Loratadine is a long-acting tricyclic antihistamine with selective peripheral H_1 receptor antagonistic activity. It exhibits a dose-related inhibition of the histamine-induced skin wheal and flare response in humans which is rapid in onset, is apparent at two hours and persists throughout the 24 hour observation period. Single oral doses up to 160 mg and repeat daily doses of 40 mg for up to 13 weeks were well tolerated with the incidence of sedation and dry mouth being no different from placebo.

Loratadine is well absorbed by all species studied and is almost totally metabolized.

Pharmacodynamics: Loratadine has a lower affinity for central receptors than for peripheral receptors, and it does not readily penetrate into the brain tissue.

Wheal and Flare: The antihistaminic activity and dose-response profile of loratadine were evaluated in three clinical pharmacologic studies using a histamine-induced skin wheal suppression model in healthy male volunteers. All doses were significantly more effective than placebo in suppressing the formation of histamine-induced skin wheals.

Alcohol: The ability of healthy male volunteers to concentrate was not impaired by loratadine in combination with alcohol. Loratadine did not potentiate the effects of alcohol on driving performance.

Pharmacokinetics: Absorption: ^{14}C-loratadine is rapidly absorbed reaching C_{max} values (4.7, 10.8 and 26.1 ng/mL) at 1.5, 1.0 and 1.3 hours for the 10, 20 and 40 mg dose, respectively. The loratadine elimination half-life ($T_{½}$) ranged from 7.8-11.0 hours. Descarboethoxyloratadine, the major active metabolite, reached C_{max} values (4.0, 9.9 and 16.0 ng/mL) at 3.7, 1.5 and 2.0 hours after a dose of 10, 20 and 40 mg, respectively. Its $T_{½}$ ranged from 17 to 24 hours. The accumulation indices, calculated by C_{max} and the area under the curve (AUC) ratios did not change after the 5th day, indicating little or no accumulation of either loratadine or its metabolite after a multiple once per day dosage regimen. The $T_{½}$ at steady state levels for loratadine and its metabolite were 14.4 and 18.7 hours, respectively, similar to that reported following a single oral dose.

The confidence intervals for C_{max} and AUC(I)* are within the 80-125% range indicating that the CLARITIN Rapid Dissolve Tongue Tablets were bioequivalent with respect to the active metabolite Descarboethoxyloratadine.

* AUC(I)=The area under the plasma concentration-time curve from time zero extrapolated to infinity.

Table 5: CLARITIN

Rapid Dissolve Tongue 10 mg Tablet vs. CLARITIN 10 mg Tablet (Conventional). Mean (n=18) Pharmacokinetic Parameters for Loratadine and Descarboethoxyloratadine

	Mean (%CV)			
	CLARITIN Rapid Dissolve Tongue Tablet, 10 mg		CLARITIN 10 mg Tablet	
Parameter	Loratadine	DCL[a]	Loratadine	DCL[a]
C_{max} (ng/mL)	2.56 (83)	3.72 (53)	2.11 (90)	3.66 (45)
T_{max} (h)	1.14 (72)	1.97 (129)	1.00 (34)	1.97 (98)
AUC (I) (ng·h/mL)	6.14 (100)	49.1 (50)	4.64 (106)	48.4 (44)

[a] DCL: Descarboethoxyloratadine.

Table 6: CLARITIN

CLARITIN Rapid Dissolve Tongue 10 mg Tablet vs. Loratadine Syrup 1 mg/mL. Mean (n=18) Pharmacokinetic Parameters for Loratadine and Descarboethoxyloratadine

	Mean (%CV)			
	CLARITIN Rapid Dissolve Tongue Tablet, 10 mg		Loratadine Syrup (1 mg/mL)	
Parameter	Loratadine	DCL[a]	Loratadine	DCL[a]
C_{max} (ng/mL)	2.65 (193)	3.46 (44)	3.62 (150)	3.65 (35)
T_{max} (h)	1.00 (30)	1.42 (39)	0.86 (44)	0.94 (17)
AUC (I) (ng·h/mL)	6.33 (201)	40.8 (29)	10.1 (147)	38.8 (27)

[a] DCL: Descarboethoxyloratadine.

After administration of a single 10 mg dose of loratadine as either the Rapid Dissolve Tongue Tablet, a conventional tablet, or the syrup formulation (1 mg/mL), peak plasma concentrations of loratadine and its metabolite were achieved at approximately 1 and 2 hours, respectively; mean elimination half-life of the active metabolite ranged between 19 and 21 hours. See Table 5 and Table 6.

Since loratadine is extensively metabolized there was a high inter-subject variability in the plasma drug concentrations. Hence, the percent CV of the pharmacokinetic parameters was large.

Table 7: CLARITIN

Loratadine, Administered as Either CLARITIN Rapid Dissolve Tongue 10 mg Tablet or CLARITIN 10 mg Tablet (Conventional Tablet) to Healthy Subjects (n=24) Once Daily for 10 Days

	Mean (%CV)					
	Loratadine			DCL[a]		
Parameter	Day 5	Day 7	Day 10	Day 5	Day 7	Day 10
CLARITIN Rapid Dissolve Tongue 10 mg Tablet						
C_{max} (ng/mL)	3.79 (83)	3.35 (73)	4.04 (80)	4.65 (58)	4.69 (68)	4.69 (73)
AUC(r)[b] (ng·h/mL)	12.0 (76)	11.2 (75)	12.2 (71)	71.9 (88)	82.1 (93)	72.9 (103)
CLARITIN 10 mg Tablet (Conventional Tablet)						
C_{max} (ng/mL)	3.12 (77)	3.43 (64)	3.81 (67)	4.56 (63)	5.12 (68)	4.60 (81)
AUC(r)[b] (ng·h/mL)	10.6 (67)	11.6 (61)	11.3 (64)	75.4 (94)	85.0 (99)	73.5 (114)

[a] DCL: Descarboethoxyloratadine.
[b] Area under the plasma concentration-time curve from time 0 to 24 h (for day 10, using concentration time points matching those on day 5 and 7).

Following administration of 10 mg of loratadine once daily for 10 days as either a Rapid Dissolve Tongue or a conventional tablet, plasma concentrations of loratadine and its active metabolite were at steady state by day 5 with both formulations. Mean peak plasma concentrations (T_{max}) of loratadine and its metabolite in both formulations were attained at 1.3 hours; peak to trough fluctuations observed for the Rapid Dissolve Tongue Tablet and the conventional Tablet were similar with respect to loratadine and its metabolite. Mean elimination half-life of the active metabolite was 20 hours for both formulations. See Table 7.

Effects of Food: In a single-dose, two-way crossover study with CLARITIN Rapid Dissolve Tongue Tablets, in 24 subjects, food increased the AUC of loratadine and descarboethoxyloratadine by 90% and 6% respectively. Food decreased the mean C_{max} of loratadine and descarboethoxyloratadine by 9% and 15% respectively. The time to peak plasma concentration (T_{max}) of loratadine and descarboethoxyloratadine were delayed by approximately 2.4 and 3.7 hours, respectively, when food was consumed prior to administration of CLARITIN Rapid Dissolve Tongue Tablets.

In a single-dose, randomized, two-way cross-over study with 10 mg CLARITIN Rapid Dissolve Tongue Tablets in twenty-four subjects, under fasting conditions, the mean AUC(tf)† and C_{max} values were increased by 84% and 30%, respectively, when administered without water compared to administration with water, demonstrating that bioavailability was not attenuated when CLARITIN Rapid Dissolve Tongue Tablet was dissolved on the tongue and subsequently swallowed without concomitant consumption of a liquid. The bioavailability of descarboethoxyloratadine was not different when administered without water.

Excretion: Approximately 82% of the ^{14}C-loratadine dose is excreted in the urine (40%) and faeces (42%) over a 10-day period. Approximately 27% of the dose, eliminated during the first 24 hours is present only in trace quantities in the urine. The active metabolite, descarboethoxyloratadine, represents only 0.4 to 0.6% of the administered loratadine dose.

Special Populations and Conditions: Geriatrics: The pharmacokinetic parameters of loratadine and its major metabolite are comparable in healthy adult volunteers and healthy geriatric volunteers.

STORAGE AND STABILITY: Temperature and Moisture: Tablets: Store between 15 and 30°C. Protect from exposure to excessive moisture.

Rapid Dissolve Tongue Tablets: Store between 20 and 25°C. Use immediately upon opening tablet blister. Protect from exposure to excessive moisture.

Syrup: Store between 15 and 30°C.

Others: Keep in a safe place out of reach of children.

SPECIAL HANDLING INSTRUCTIONS: None.

† AUC(tf)=The area under the plasma concentration-time curve form time zero to the final measurable sample.

INFORMATION FOR THE PATIENT: Published in e-CPS, available by subscription at www.e-cps.ca.

DOSAGE FORMS, COMPOSITION AND PACKAGING: Rapid Dissolve Tongue Tablets: Each white, round, tablet-shaped unit contains: micronized loratadine 10 mg (as base). Nonmedicinal ingredients: citric acid, gelatin, mannitol and mint flavor. Blister packages of 10 and 30.

KIDS Syrup: Each mL of clear, colorless to light yellow, fruit (peach) flavored syrup contains: loratadine 1 mg (as base). Nonmedicinal ingredients: fruit (artificial peach flavor, citric acid anhydrous, edetate disodium, glycerin, propylene glycol, purified water, sodium benzoate and sucrose). Plastic bottles of 120 mL.

Tablets: Each white, oval, shallow, deep-scored tablet, with the flask and dish logo above the score and the number 10 below, contains: loratadine 10 mg (as base). Nonmedicinal ingredients: cornstarch, lactose and magnesium stearate. Blister packages 1, 2, 10, 20, 30 and 48. Bottles of 60 and 100.

(Shown in Product Identification Section)

Claritin® Allergic Congestion Relief

oxymetazoline HCl

Nasal Decongestant

Schering-Plough

Date of Preparation: July 18, 2001
Date of Revision: July 3, 2003

PHARMACOLOGY: The sympathomimetic action of oxymetazoline hydrochloride constricts the arteriolar network within the nasal mucosa producing a prolonged decongestant effect.

INDICATIONS: The symptomatic relief of congestion of the nasopharyngeal mucous membranes in a variety of allergic disorders of the upper respiratory tract, including acute rhinitis and nasopharyngitis; acute and chronic sinusitis; acute and chronic vasomotor rhinitis; perennial allergic rhinitis and seasonal allergic rhinitis (hay fever).

CONTRAINDICATIONS: Narrow angle glaucoma, rhinitis sicca. Concurrent therapy with MAOIs. Hypersensitivity to any component. Sensitivity to even small doses of adrenergic substances as manifested by sleeplessness, dizziness, lightheadedness, weakness, tremulousness, or cardiac arrhythmias. Do not use for irrigation or displacement after sinus operations in which the dura may have been entered.

PRECAUTIONS: Do not exceed the recommended dosage. This product may cause rebound congestion if used for longer than 3 days. This product should not be used by patients who have heart disease, high blood pressure, advanced arteriosclerotic conditions, thyroid disease, diabetes, difficulty in urination due to enlargement of the prostate gland or receiving tricyclic antidepressants without careful clinical consideration. Use of the product by more than one person may spread infection. This product is not recommended for use in children under 6 years of age. This product must be kept out of the reach of children.

Systemic effects from the use of topical decongestants can occur due to rapid absorption from the nasal mucous membrane, especially when it is inflamed, and from gastrointestinal absorption if given in excess so that the nasally applied solution is swallowed. Such reactions are most likely to occur in infants, young children and the elderly.

If accidentally ingested, standard methods to remove unabsorbed drug, should be considered. There is no specific antidote for oxymetazoline. In children, oxymetazoline may produce profound CNS depression. Consultation with a Poison Control Centre should be considered and treatment will be supportive.

Pregnancy: Since no clinical data on exposed pregnancies are available with oxymetazoline, the safe use of oxymetazoline during pregnancy has not been established. Oxymetazoline is not to be used during pregnancy unless the potential benefits outweigh the risks.

To help prevent contamination from nasal secretions, rinse spray tips in hot water after each use. No more than one person should use the same nasal spray or pump.

Drug Interactions: If significant systemic absorption of oxymetazoline occurs, concomitant use of tricyclic antidepressants, maprotiline, or MAOIs, may potentiate the pressor effects of oxymetazoline.

ADVERSE EFFECTS: CLARITIN Allergic Congestion Relief is generally well tolerated; side effects are usually mild and transient and include burning, stinging or increased nasal discharge. The following adverse effects may occur with topical nasal decongestants: dryness of the nasal mucosa, sneezing, palpitations, headache, lightheadedness, insomnia. Prolonged or excessive use may cause rebound congestion.

OVERDOSE:

For management of a suspected drug overdose, CPhA recommends that you contact your **regional Poison Control Centre**. See the *CPS* Directory section for a list of Poison Control Centres.

DOSAGE: Adults and children over 12 years of age: Spray 2 or 3 times into each nostril twice a day every 12 hours. With the head upright, place the spray nozzle in the nostril without completely occluding the nostril. During each administration, the patient should bend his head slightly forward and squeeze the bottle quickly and firmly to spray the recommended number of sprays in each nostril. If symptoms persist after 3 days, consult a physician. Prolonged or excessive use may cause an increase in nasal congestion.

SUPPLIED: Each pump bottle contains: oxymetazoline HCl USP 0.05% in aqueous solution. Nonmedicinal ingredients: benzalkonium chloride, edetate disodium, monopropylene glycol, purified water, sodium phosphate monobasic monohydrate and pH adjusted with hydrochloric acid or sodium hydroxide. Conventional metered pump sprays of 25 mL. Store between 15 and 30°C.

Claritin® Allergy+Sinus

loratadine—pseudoephedrine sulfate

Histamine H1-Receptor Antagonist—Sympathomimetic Amine

Schering-Plough

Date of Preparation: May 31, 1991
Date of Revision: December 10, 2004

PHARMACOLOGY: Loratadine is a long-acting tricyclic antihistamine with selective peripheral H_1 receptor antagonistic activity. It exhibits a dose-related inhibition of the histamine-induced skin wheal and flare response in humans which is rapid in onset, is apparent at 2 hours and persists throughout the 24 hour observation period. Single oral doses up to 160 mg and repeat daily doses of 40 mg for up to 13 weeks were well tolerated with the incidence of sedation and dry mouth being no different from placebo.

^{14}C-loratadine is rapidly absorbed reaching C_{max} values (4.7, 10.8 and 26.1 ng/mL) at 1.5, 1.0 and 1.3 hours for the 10, 20 and 40 mg dose, respectively. The loratadine elimination half-life ($T_{1/2}\beta$) ranged from 7.8 to 11 hours.

Descarboethoxy-loratadine, the major active metabolite, reached C_{max} values (4.0, 9.9 and 16.0 ng/mL) at 3.7, 1.5 and 2.0 hours after a dose of 10, 20 and 40 mg, respectively. Its $T_{1/2}\beta$ ranged from 17 to 24 hours. The accumulation indices, calculated by C_{max} and the area under the curve (AUC) ratios did not change after the 5th day, indicating little or no accumulation of either loratadine or its metabolite after a multiple once per day dosage regimen. The $T_{1/2}\beta$ at steady state levels for loratadine and its active metabolite were 14.4 and 18.7 hours, respectively, similar to that reported following a single oral dose.

Approximately 82% of the ^{14}C-loratadine dose is excreted in the urine (40%) and feces (42%) over a 10-day period. Approximately 27% of the dose is eliminated in the urine during the first 24 hours largely in the conjugated form. Unchanged drug is present only in trace quantities in the urine and the active metabolite descarboethoxy-loratadine represents only 0.4 to 0.6% of the administered loratadine dose.

Pseudoephedrine sulfate, one of the naturally occurring alkaloids of Ephedra and an orally administered vasoconstrictor, produces a gradual but sustained decongestant effect facilitating shrinkage of congested mucosa in upper respiratory areas. The mucous membrane of the respiratory tract is decongested through the action of the sympathetic nerves.

INDICATIONS: For the relief of nasal and ocular symptoms of upper respiratory mucosal congestion, such as in allergic rhinitis. For short-term use only unless taken under medical supervision.

CONTRAINDICATIONS: In those patients who have shown sensitivity or idiosyncrasy to the components, to adrenergic agents or to other drugs of similar chemical structures. Also contraindicated in patients receiving MAO inhibitor therapy or within 14 days of discontinuing such treatment and in patients with narrow-angle glaucoma, urinary retention, hypertension, severe coronary artery disease and hyperthyroidism.

PRECAUTIONS: General: Sympathomimetics should be used with caution in patients with stenosing peptic ulcer, pyloroduodenal obstruction, prostatic hypertrophy or bladder neck obstruction, cardiovascular disease, increased intraocular pressure or diabetes mellitus.

Sympathomimetics should be used with caution in patients receiving digitalis.

Sympathomimetics may cause central nervous system (CNS) stimulation, excitability and convulsions or cardiovascular collapse with accompanying hypotension.

Patients with severe liver impairment should be administered a lower initial dose because they may have reduced clearance of loratadine; an initial dose of 1 tablet daily is recommended.

Geriatrics: In patients 60 years of age or older, sympathomimetics are also more likely to cause adverse reactions such as confusion, hallucination, convulsions, CNS depression and death. Consequently, caution should be exercised when administering a repeat-action formulation to this patient group.

Dependence Liability: There are no data available to indicate that abuse or dependency occurs with loratadine.

Pseudoephedrine sulfate, like other CNS stimulants, has been abused. At high doses, subjects commonly experience mood elevation, decreased appetite and a sense of increased energy, physical strength, mental capacity and alertness. Anxiety, irritability and loquacity also have been reported. With continued use, tolerance develops; the user increases the dose and ultimately toxicity occurs. Depression may follow rapid withdrawal.

Pediatrics: Safety and efficacy in children younger than 12 years of age have not yet been established.

Pregnancy: The safe use of CLARITIN ALLERGY+SINUS during pregnancy or lactation has not been established. The use of CLARITIN ALLERGY+SINUS during pregnancy is therefore not recommended.

Lactation: Loratadine and its active metabolite are eliminated in the breast milk of lactating women with milk concentrations being similar to plasma concentrations. Through 48 hours after dosing, only 0.029% of the loratadine dose is eliminated in the milk as unchanged loratadine and its active metabolite, descarboethoxy-loratadine. Pseudoephedrine has been reported to be excreted into breast milk of lactating women. The use of CLARITIN ALLERGY+SINUS (loratadine/pseudoephedrine sulfate) tablets in nursing mothers is therefore not recommended.

Other: Because of the lack of experience with long-term use of this drug, its use should be limited to 3 months unless recommended by a physician.

Drug Interactions: When administered concomitantly with alcohol, loratadine has no potentiating effect as measured by psychomotor performance studies.

When sympathomimetic drugs are given to patients receiving MAO inhibitors, hypertensive reactions, including hypertensive crises, may occur. The antihypertensive effects of methyldopa, mecamylamine, reserpine and veratrum alkaloids may be reduced by sympathomimetics. Beta-adrenergic blocking agents may also interact with sympathomimetics. Increased ectopic pacemaker activity can occur when pseudoephedrine sulfate is used concomitantly with digitalis. Antacids increase the rate of pseudoephedrine sulfate absorption; kaolin decreases it. The antibacterial agent, furazolidone, is known to cause a dose-related inhibition of MAO. Although there are no reports of a hypertensive crisis caused by the concurrent administration of pseudoephedrine and furazolidone, they should not be taken together. Care should be taken in the administration of CLARITIN ALLERGY+SINUS concomitantly with other sympathomimetic amines because the combined effects on the cardiovascular system may be harmful to the patient.

Increases in plasma concentrations of loratadine have been reported after concomitant use with ketoconazole, erythromycin or cimetidine in controlled clinical trials, but without clinically significant changes (including electrocardiographic). Other drugs known to inhibit hepatic metabolism should be coadministered with caution until definitive interaction studies can be completed.

Drug/Laboratory Test Interactions: Loratadine should be discontinued approximately 48 hours prior to skin testing procedures since antihistamines may prevent or diminish otherwise positive reactions to dermal reactivity indicators.

The in vitro addition of pseudoephedrine sulfate to sera containing the cardiac isoenzyme MB of serum creatine phosphokinase progressively inhibits the activity of the enzyme. The inhibition becomes complete over 6 hours.

ADVERSE EFFECTS: During controlled clinical studies with the recommended dosage, the incidence of adverse effects associated with CLARITIN ALLERGY+SINUS was comparable to that of placebo, with the exception of insomnia and dry mouth both of which were commonly reported. Other most frequently reported [≥5%] adverse reactions associated with CLARITIN ALLERGY+SINUS, the components and placebo are listed in Table 1.

Rare adverse reactions in decreasing order of frequency included, nausea, abdominal distress, anorexia, thirst, tachycardia, pharyngitis, rhinitis, acne, pruritus, rash, urticaria, arthralgia, confusion, dysphonia, hyperkinesia, hypoesthesia, decreased libido, paresthesia, tremor, vertigo, flushing, postural hypotension, increased sweating, eye disorders, earache, tinnitus, taste abnormality, agitation, apathy, depression, euphoria, paroniria, increased appetite, change in bowel habits, dyspepsia, eructation, hemorrhoids, tongue discoloration, tongue disorder, vomiting, transient abnormal hepatic function, dehydration, increased weight, hypertension, palpitation, migraine, bronchospasm, coughing, dyspnea, epistaxis, nasal congestion, sneezing, nasal irritation, dysuria, micturition disorder, nocturia, polyuria, urinary retention, asthenia, back pain, leg cramps, malaise and rigors.

As with other sympathomimetic amines, CNS stimulation, muscular weakness, tightness in the chest and syncope may also be encountered.

During the marketing of loratadine, alopecia, anaphylaxis and abnormal hepatic function have been reported rarely.

Table 1: CLARITIN ALLERGY+SINUS

Number (%) of Patients Reporting Adverse Experiences (Probably or Possibly Related to Treatment) ≥5% Incidence During Treatment with CLARITIN ALLERGY+SINUS, Either Component Alone (Loratadine or Pseudoephedrine) or Placebo in Clinical Studies

	A	B	C	D
Adverse Experience	**CLARITIN ALLERGY+SINUS (N=632)**	**Loratadine (N=396)**	**Pseudoephedrine (N=395)**	**Placebo (N=532)**
Dizziness	27 (4)	4 (1)	10 (5)	8 (2)
Dry mouth	93 (15)	17 (4)	41 (10)	21 (4)
Fatigue	26 (4)	22 (6)	14 (4)	13 (2)
Headache	64 (10)	48 (12)	34 (9)	52 (10)
Insomnia	113 (18)	16 (4)	66 (17)	20 (4)
Nervousness	33 (5)	11 (3)	30 (8)	5 (1)
Sedation	41 (6)	29 (7)	18 (5)	23 (4)

OVERDOSE:

In the event of overdosage, treatment, which should be started immediately, is symptomatic and supportive. Discontinuation of use, gastric lavage and support of vital functions are advised.

Symptoms: They may vary from CNS depression (sedation, apnea, diminished mental alertness, cyanosis, coma, cardiovascular collapse) to stimulation (insomnia, hallucination, tremors or convulsions) to death. Other signs and symptoms may be euphoria, excitement, tachycardia, palpitations, thirst, perspiration, nausea, dizziness, tinnitus, ataxia, blurred vision and hypertension or hypotension. Stimulation is particularly likely in children, as are atropine-like signs and symptoms (dry mouth; fixed, dilated pupils; flushing; hyperthermia; and gastrointestinal symptoms).

In large doses sympathomimetics may give rise to giddiness, headache, nausea, vomiting, sweating, thirst, tachycardia, precordial pain, palpitations, difficulty in micturition, muscular weakness and tenseness, anxiety, restlessness and insomnia. Many patients can present a toxic psychosis with delusions and hallucinations. Some may develop cardiac arrhythmias, circulatory collapse, convulsions, coma and respiratory failure.

Treatment: Emergency treatment should be started immediately. There is no specific antidote. Consider standard measures to remove any unabsorbed drug in the stomach, such as adsorption by activated charcoal administered as a slurry with water. The administration of gastric lavage should be considered. Physiologic saline solution is the lavage solution of choice, particularly in children. In adults, tap water can be used; however, as much as possible of the amount administered should be removed before the next instillation. Saline cathartics draw water into the bowel by osmosis and therefore may be valuable for their action in rapid dilution of bowel content.

Loratadine is not cleared by hemodialysis to any appreciable extent. It is not known if loratadine is removed by peritoneal dialysis.

After emergency treatment, the patient should continue to be medically monitored.

Treatment of the signs and symptoms of overdosage is symptomatic and supportive. Stimulants (analeptic agents) should not be used. Vasopressors may be used to treat hypotension. Short-acting barbiturates, diazepam or paraldehyde may be administered to control seizures. Hyperpyrexia, especially in children, may require treatment with tepid water sponge baths or hypothermic blanket. Apnea is treated with ventilatory support.

For management of a suspected drug overdose, CPhA recommends that you contact your **regional Poison Control Centre**. See the *CPS* Directory section for a list of Poison Control Centres.

DOSAGE: Adults and children 12 years of age and over: 1 tablet twice a day.

Storage and Stability: Temperature and Moisture: Store between 15 and 30°C. Protect from exposure to excessive moisture.

Others: Keep in a safe place out of reach of children.

SUPPLIED: Each white to off-white, round, biconvex, coated tablet contains: loratadine 5 mg in the tablet coating and pseudoephedrine sulfate 120 mg equally distributed between the tablet coating and the barrier-coated core. The two active components in the coating are quickly liberated; release of the decongestant in the core is delayed for several hours. Nonmedicinal ingredients: acacia, calcium sulfate, carnauba wax, cornstarch, gum rosin, lactose, magnesium stearate, microcrystalline cellulose, oleic acid, povidone, soap powder, sucrose, talc, titanium dioxide, white wax and zein. Blister packages of 10, 20 and 30.

(Shown in Product Identification Section)

Claritin® Allergy+Sinus Extra Strength

loratadine—pseudoephedrine sulfate

Histamine H1-Receptor Antagonist—Sympathomimetic Amine

Schering-Plough

Date of Preparation: October 6, 1999

Date of Revision: December 13, 2004

PHARMACOLOGY: Loratadine is a long-acting tricyclic antihistamine with selective peripheral H_1 receptor antagonistic activity. It exhibits a dose-related inhibition of the histamine-induced skin wheal and flare response in humans which is rapid in onset, is apparent at two hours and persists throughout the 24 hour observation period (Roman et al. 1986). Single oral doses up to 160 mg and repeat daily doses of 40 mg for up to 13 weeks were well tolerated with the incidence of sedation and dry mouth being no different from placebo.

^{14}C-loratadine is rapidly absorbed reaching C_{max} values (4.7, 10.8 and 26.1 ng/mL) at 1.5, 1.0 and 1.3 hours for the 10, 20 and 40 mg dose, respectively. The loratadine elimination half-life ($T_{1/2\beta}$) ranged from 7.8-11.0 hours.

Descarboethoxy-loratadine, the major active metabolite, reached C_{max} values (4.0, 9.9 and 16.0 ng/mL) at 3.7, 1.5 and 2.0 hours after a dose of 10, 20 and 40 mg, respectively. Its $T_{1/2\beta}$ ranged from 17 to 24 hours. The accumulation indices, calculated by C_{max} and the area under the curve (AUC) ratios did not change after the 5th day, indicating little or no accumulation of either loratadine or its metabolite after a multiple once per day dosage regimen. The $T_{1/2\beta}$ at steady state levels for loratadine and its active metabolite were 14.4 and 18.7 hours, respectively, similar to that reported following a single oral dose (Hilbert et al. 1987).

Approximately 82% of the ^{14}C-loratadine dose is excreted in the urine (40%) and feces (42%) over a 10-day period. Approximately 27% of the dose is eliminated in the urine during the first 24 hours largely in the conjugated form. Unchanged drug is present only in trace quantities in the urine and the active metabolite descarboethoxyloratadine represents only 0.4 to 0.6% of the administered loratadine dose.

Pseudoephedrine, one of the naturally occurring alkaloids of Ephedra and an orally administered vasoconstrictor, produces a gradual but sustained decongestant effect facilitating shrinkage of congested mucosa in upper respiratory areas. The mucous membrane of the respiratory tract is decongested through the action of the sympathetic nerves.

A drug interaction cross-over study was performed to compare CLARITIN ALLERGY+SINUS EXTRA STRENGTH extended release caplets to the individual components (loratadine 10 mg and pseudoephedrine sulfate 240 mg). Coadministration of loratadine did not affect the bioavailability of pseudoephedrine. Similarly, coadministration of pseudoephedrine did not affect the pharmacokinetics of descarboethoxyloratadine although it resulted in the slightly higher (8%) bioavailability of loratadine: C_{max}=2.79 ng/mL when administered in combination versus C_{max}=2.55 ng/mL when administered alone. This is not considered to be of clinical significance.

Another study was conducted to characterize and compare the pharmacokinetic profile of loratadine, descarboethoxyloratadine and pseudoephedrine following oral administration of CLARITIN ALLERGY+SINUS EXTRA STRENGTH given once daily and CLARITIN ALLERGY+SINUS (loratadine 5 mg/pseudoephedrine sulfate 120 mg) given every 12 hours. The results of this study show that after multiple doses to steady state, CLARITIN ALLERGY+SINUS EXTRA STRENGTH and the CLARITIN ALLERGY+SINUS comparator were equivalent with respect to the bioavailability of loratadine and descarboethoxyloratadine (based on AUC), and bioequivalent for pseudoephedrine.

INDICATIONS: CLARITIN ALLERGY+SINUS EXTRA STRENGTH (loratadine 10 mg/pseudoephedrine sulfate 240 mg) extended release caplets are indicated for the relief of symptoms associated with allergic rhinitis, including nasal and sinus congestion, sneezing, postnasal discharge and tearing and redness of the eyes. They are intended for short-term use only unless taken under medical supervision.

CONTRAINDICATIONS: CLARITIN ALLERGY+SINUS EXTRA STRENGTH (loratadine 10 mg/pseudoephedrine sulfate 240 mg) extended release caplets are contraindicated in those patients who have shown sensitivity or idiosyncrasy to their components, to adrenergic agents or to other drugs of similar chemical structures. They are also contraindicated in patients receiving MAO inhibitor therapy or within 14 days of discontinuing such treatment and in patients with narrow-angle glaucoma, urinary retention, hypertension, severe coronary artery disease and hyperthyroidism.

PRECAUTIONS: General: Sympathomimetics should be used with caution in patients with stenosing peptic ulcer, pyloroduodenal obstruction, prostatic hypertrophy or bladder neck obstruction, cardiovascular disease, increased intraocular pressure or diabetes mellitus.

Sympathomimetics should be used with caution in patients receiving digitalis.

Sympathomimetics may cause central nervous system (CNS) stimulation and convulsions or cardiovascular collapse with accompanying hypotension.

Patients with severe liver impairment should be administered a lower initial dose because they may have reduced clearance of loratadine. For CLARITIN ALLERGY+SINUS EXTRA STRENGTH, an initial dose of one caplet every other day is recommended.

Patients who have a history of difficulty in swallowing tablets or who have upper gastrointestinal narrowing or abnormal esophageal peristalsis should not use this product.

Geriatrics: In patients 60 years of age or older, sympathomimetics are also more likely to cause adverse reactions such as confusion, hallucination, convulsions, CNS depression and death. Consequently, caution should be exercised when administering a long-acting formulation to this patient group.

Dependence Liability: There are no data available to indicate that abuse or dependency occurs with loratadine.

Pseudoephedrine sulfate, like other CNS stimulants, has been abused. At high doses, subjects commonly experience mood elevation, decreased appetite and a sense of increased energy, physical strength, mental capacity and alertness. Anxiety, irritability and loquacity also have been reported. With continued use, tolerance develops; the user increases the dose and ultimately toxicity occurs. Depression may follow rapid withdrawal.

Pediatrics: Safety and efficacy of CLARITIN ALLERGY+SINUS EXTRA STRENGTH extended release caplets in children younger than 12 years of age have not yet been established.

Pregnancy: The safe use of CLARITIN ALLERGY+SINUS EXTRA STRENGTH extended release caplets during pregnancy or lactation has not been established and is therefore not recommended for use in pregnant or nursing mothers.

Lactation: Loratadine and its active metabolite are eliminated in the breast milk of lactating women with milk concentrations being similar to plasma concentrations. Through 48 hours after dosing, only 0.029% of the loratadine dose is eliminated in the milk as unchanged loratadine and its active metabolite, descarboethoxyloratadine.

Pseudoephedrine has been reported to be excreted into breast milk of lactating women. The use of CLARITIN ALLERGY+SINUS EXTRA STRENGTH extended release caplets in nursing mothers is therefore not recommended.

Long-Term Use: Because of the lack of experience with long-term use of this drug, its use should be limited to three months unless recommended by a physician.

Drug Interactions: When administered concomitantly with alcohol, loratadine has no potentiating effect as measured by psychomotor performance studies.

When sympathomimetic drugs are given to patients receiving monoamine oxidase inhibitors (MAO), hypertensive reactions, including hypertensive crises, may occur. The antihypertensive effects of methyldopa, mecamylamine, reserpine and veratrum alkaloids may be reduced by sympathomimetics. Beta-adrenergic blocking agents may also interact with sympathomimetics. Increased ectopic pacemaker activity can occur when pseudoephedrine sulfate is used concomitantly with digitalis. Antacids increase the rate of pseudoephedrine sulfate absorption; kaolin decreases it. The antibacterial agent, furazolidone, is known to cause a dose-related inhibition of MAO. Although there are no reports of a hypertensive crisis caused by the concurrent administration of pseudoephedrine and furazolidone, they should not be taken together. Care should be taken in the administration of CLARITIN ALLERGY+SINUS EXTRA STRENGTH concomitantly with other sympathomimetic amines because the combined effects on the cardiovascular system may be harmful to the patient.

Increase in plasma concentrations of loratadine have been reported after concomitant use with ketoconazole, erythromycin or cimetidine in controlled clinical trials, but without clinically significant changes (including electrocardiographic). Other drugs known to inhibit hepatic metabolism should be coadministered with caution until definitive interaction studies can be completed.

Drug/Laboratory Test Interactions: Loratadine should be discontinued approximately 48 hours prior to skin testing procedures since antihistamines may prevent or diminish otherwise positive reactions to dermal reactivity indicators.

ADVERSE EFFECTS: Adverse experiences reported during the study with CLARITIN ALLERGY+SINUS EXTRA STRENGTH (loratadine 10 mg/pseudoephedrine sulfate 240 mg) extended release caplets, administered once daily, were similar to those previously encountered during treatment with CLARITIN ALLERGY+SINUS tablets (loratadine 5 mg/pseudoephedrine sulfate 120 mg), administered twice daily. No unusual or unexpected adverse events were reported.

In clinical studies, the most frequently reported adverse events associated with CLARITIN ALLERGY+SINUS EXTRA STRENGTH extended release caplets were headache, dry mouth, insomnia and somnolence. See Table 1.

Table 1: CLARITIN ALLERGY+SINUS EXTRA STRENGTH

Number (%) of Patients Reporting Adverse Experiences (probably or possibly related to treatment) ≥5% incidence during treatment with CLARITIN ALLERGY+SINUS EXTRA STRENGTH extended release caplets, Loratadine, Pseudoephedrine sulfate or placebo in clinical studies

Adverse Experience	CLARITIN ALLERGY+ SINUS EXTRA STRENGTH (N=583)	Loratadine (N=217)	Pseudoephedrine Sulfate (N=220)	Placebo (N=370)
Dry Mouth	55 (9)	7 (3)	16 (7)	11 (3)
Headache	53 (9)	21 (10)	21 (10)	39 (11)
Insomnia	38 (7)	2 (1)	17 (8)	4 (1)
Somnolence	47 (8)	9 (4)	9 (4)	14 (4)

Rarely reported events in decreasing order of frequency included dizziness, fatigue, anorexia, nervousness, nausea, epistaxis, rhinitis, lacrimal gland disorder, asthenia, hyperkinesia, constipation, dyspepsia, palpitation, tachycardia, thirst, agitation, irritability, coughing, dyspnea, nasal irritation, and pharyngitis.

With exception of headache, which was occasionally severe, most of the adverse events associated with CLARITIN ALLERGY+SINUS EXTRA STRENGTH extended release caplets were mild to moderate in severity.

During the marketing of loratadine, alopecia, anaphylaxis, and abnormal hepatic function have been reported rarely.

There were rare postmarketing reports of mechanical upper gastrointestinal tract obstruction in patients taking the original round tablet formulation of CLARITIN ALLERGY+SINUS EXTRA STRENGTH. In many of these cases, patients have had a history of difficulty in swallowing tablets, or had known upper gastrointestinal narrowing or abnormal esophageal peristalsis.

OVERDOSE:

In the event of overdosage, treatment, which should be started immediately, is symptomatic and supportive. Discontinuation of use, gastric lavage and support vital functions are advised.

Symptoms: Somnolence, tachycardia and headache have been reported with overdoses of loratadine.

Symptoms associated with overdoses of sympathomimetics may vary from CNS depression (sedation, apnea, diminished mental alertness, cyanosis, coma, cardiovascular collapse) to stimulation (insomnia, hallucination, tremors or convulsions) to death. Other signs and symptoms may be euphoria, excitement, tachycardia, palpitations, thirst, perspiration, nausea, dizziness, tinnitus, ataxia, blurred vision and hypertension or hypotension. Stimulation is particularly likely in children, as are atropine-like signs and symptoms (dry mouth; fixed, dilated pupils; flushing; hyperthermia; and gastrointestinal symptoms).

In large doses sympathomimetics may give rise to giddiness, headache, nausea, vomiting, sweating, thirst, tachycardia, precordial pain, palpitations, difficulty in micturition, muscular weakness and tenseness, anxiety, restlessness and insomnia. Many patients can present a toxic psychosis with delusions and hallucinations. Some may develop cardiac arrhythmias, circulatory collapse, convulsions, coma and respiratory failure.

Treatment: Adsorption of any drug in the stomach may be attempted by the administration of activated charcoal as a slurry with water. Gastric lavage should be considered. Physiologic saline solution is the lavage solution of choice, particularly in children. In adults, tap water can be used; however, as much as possible of the amount administered should be removed before the next instillation. Saline cathartics draw water into the bowel by osmosis and therefore may be valuable for their action in rapid dilution of bowel content. Loratadine is not removed by hemodialysis, it is not known if loratadine is removed by peritoneal dialysis. After emergency treatment, the patient should continue to be medically monitored.

Treatment of the signs and symptoms of overdosage is symptomatic and supportive. Stimulants (analeptic agents) should not be used. Vasopressors may be used to treat hypotension. Short-acting barbiturates, diazepam or paraldehyde may be administered to control seizures. Hyperpyrexia, especially in children, may require treatment with tepid water sponge baths or hypothermic blanket. Apnea is treated with ventilatory support.

> For management of a suspected drug overdose, CPhA recommends that you contact your **regional Poison Control Centre**. See the *CPS* Directory section for a list of Poison Control Centres.

DOSAGE: Adults and children 12 years of age and over: One CLARITIN ALLERGY+SINUS EXTRA STRENGTH (loratadine 10 mg/pseudoephedrine sulfate 240 mg) extended-release caplet once daily taken whole with a glass of water, preferably upon waking. CLARITIN ALLERGY+SINUS EXTRA STRENGTH may be taken without regard to mealtime.

Patients who have a history of difficulty in swallowing tablets or who have upper gastrointestinal narrowing or abnormal esophageal peristalsis should not use this product (see Precautions and Adverse Effects).

Storage and Stability: Temperature and Moisture: Store between 15 and 30°C. Protect from exposure to excessive moisture.

Others: Keep in a safe place out of reach of children.

SUPPLIED: Each white, oval, biconvex, coated extended release caplet contains: loratadine 10 mg in the caplet coating and pseudoephedrine sulfate 240 mg in the extended-release core. The loratadine component is released immediately, whereas the pseudoephedrine sulfate component is released slowly from the core allowing for once daily administration. Nonmedicinal ingredients in caplet coating: carnauba wax, hydroxypropyl methylcellulose 2910, Opaspray White, polyethylene glycol 3350, polyethylene glycol 400, sucrose and white wax. Nonmedicinal ingredients in caplet core: dibasic calcium phosphate dihydrate, ethylcellulose, hydroxypropyl methylcellulose 2208, magnesium stearate, povidone and silicon dioxide. Blister packages of 5 and 15.

(Shown in Product Identification Section)

Claritin® Skin Itch Relief

hydrocortisone

Topical Corticosteroid

Schering-Plough

Date of Preparation: July 18, 2001
Date of Revision: July 3, 2003

INDICATIONS: For temporary relief of minor skin irritations, itching and rashes due to eczema, dermatitis, insect bites, poison ivy, poison oak, poison sumac, soaps, detergents, cosmetics and jewelry.

WARNINGS: For external use only. Do not use in or around the eyes. Do not apply to large areas of the body. Do not use to treat vulvar itching associated with vaginal discharge. Use only for 7 days maximum. If symptoms persist beyond 7 days or return after discontinuing use of the product, consult a physician.

Children: Do not use in children 2 years of age or younger, unless directed by a physician.

OVERDOSE:

> For management of a suspected drug overdose, CPhA recommends that you contact your **regional Poison Control Centre**. See the *CPS* Directory section for a list of Poison Control Centres.

DOSAGE: Apply to the affected area not more than 3 or 4 times daily.

SUPPLIED: Each g of cream contains: hydrocortisone USP 5 mg (0.5%) in a water miscible emollient base. Nonmedicinal ingredients: cetostearyl alcohol, chlorocresol, mineral oil, phosporic acid, polyethylene glycol 1000 monocetyl ether, propylene glycol, purified water, sodium hydroxide, sodium phosphate monobasic monohydrate and white petrolatum. Tubes of 20 g. Store between 15 and 30°C.

Clarus® Pr

isotretinoin

Nodular/Inflammatory and Conglobate Acne Therapy

Mylan

Date of Preparation: March 31, 2005
Date of Revision: June 10, 2009

SUMMARY PRODUCT INFORMATION:

Route of Administration	Dosage Form/ Strength	Clinically Relevant Nonmedicinal Ingredients
Oral	Capsules/10 mg	None
Oral	Capsules/40 mg	None
For a complete listing of nonmedicinal ingredients see Dosage Forms, Composition and Packaging.		

INDICATIONS AND CLINICAL USE: CLARUS (isotretinoin) is indicated for the treatment of:

- Severe Nodular and/or Inflammatory Acne
- Acne Conglobata
- Recalcitrant Acne

Because of significant side effects associated with its use, isotretinoin should be reserved for patients where the conditions listed above are unresponsive to conventional first line therapies.

CLARUS should only be prescribed by physicians knowledgeable in the use of retinoids systemically, who understand the risk of teratogenicity in females of child bearing age and who are experienced in counselling young adults for whom isotretinoin is generally indicated (see Contraindications and Warnings and Precautions, Serious Warnings and Precautions and Special Populations, Pregnant Women).

A careful assessment of the patient's mental state should be made, including whether or not they have a history of previous psychiatric illness (see Warnings and Precautions, Serious Warnings and Precautions, Psychiatric).

It is strongly recommended that each CLARUS prescription be limited to a one-month supply in order to encourage patients to return for follow-up to monitor side-effects.

Geriatrics: Clinical studies of isotretinoin did not include sufficient numbers of subjects aged 65 years and over to determine whether they respond differently from younger subjects. Although reported clinical experience has not identified differences in responses between elderly and younger patients, effects of aging might be expected to increase some risks associated with isotretinoin therapy.

Pediatrics: The use of CLARUS in pediatric patients less than 12 years of age is not recommended. The use of CLARUS for the treatment of severe recalcitrant nodular acne in pediatric patients ages 12 to 17 years should be given careful consideration, especially for those patients where a known metabolic or structural bone disease exists (see Warnings and Precautions, Special Populations, Pediatrics).

CONTRAINDICATIONS:

> - **Isotretinoin is contraindicated in pregnancy.**
>   - Females must not become pregnant while taking CLARUS or for at least one month after its discontinuation. Isotretinoin causes severe birth defects in a very high percentage of infants born to women who became pregnant during treatment with isotretinoin in any amount, even for a short period of time. Potentially any exposed fetus can be affected. There are no accurate means of determining whether an exposed fetus has been affected (see Warnings and Precautions, Special populations, Pregnant Women).
>   - If pregnancy does occur during treatment with CLARUS or for one month after its discontinuation, CLARUS treatment must be immediately stopped and the physician and patient should discuss the desirability of continuing the pregnancy.
> - CLARUS should only be prescribed by physicians knowledgeable in the use of retinoids systemically (see Indications and Clinical Use).

CLARUS is also contraindicated in the following conditions:

- breastfeeding women,
- hepatic and renal insufficiency,
- hypervitaminosis A,
- patients with excessively elevated blood lipid values,
- patients taking tetracyclines (see Warnings and Precautions, Serious Warnings and Precautions, Neurologic and Drug Interactions, Drug-Drug Interactions).
- patients who are sensitive to isotretinoin, or to any of the excipients. CLARUS capsules contain Ammonium hydroxide, beeswax yellow, gelatin, glycerin, hydrogenated vegetable oil, polyethylene glycol, polyvinyl acetate phthalate, propylene glycol, red iron oxide, yellow iron oxide, soybean oil, synthetic black iron oxide and titanium dioxide (see Dosage Forms, Composition and Packaging). CLARUS does not contain peanut oil.

WARNINGS AND PRECAUTIONS:

Serious Warnings and Precautions

- **Pregnancy Prevention:** Isotretinoin is a known teratogen contraindicated in pregnancy (see boxed Contraindications). Physicians should **only** prescribe CLARUS to females of childbearing potential if **ALL** the conditions described below under "Conditions of Use" are met.

  In addition, when prescribing this drug to female patients of childbearing potential, physicians must use Mylan Pharmaceuticals ULC Clinical Education and Awareness Resource (CLEAR), which includes comprehensive information about the potential risks of this drug, a checklist for criteria which must be met prior to prescribing this drug to female patients of childbearing potential, detailed information on birth control options, a patient informed consent for review and signature, and monthly pregnancy reminders for physicians to use at each patient visit during the treatment period.
- **Psychiatric:** Some patients treated with isotretinoin have become depressed and some attempted or committed suicide. Although a causal relationship has not been established, all patients should be screened and monitored for signs of depression during therapy (see Warnings and Precautions, Monitoring and Laboratory Tests). Before starting therapy with CLARUS physicians should determine whether the patient may be depressed or has a history of depression including a family history of major depression before starting therapy with CLARUS. If symptoms of depression develop or worsen during treatment with CLARUS, the drug should be discontinued promptly and the patient referred for appropriate psychiatric treatment as necessary. However, discontinuation of CLARUS may not alleviate symptoms and therefore further psychiatric or psychological evaluation may be necessary.
- **Neurologic:** Isotretinoin use has been associated with a number of cases of pseudotumor cerebri (benign intracranial hypertension), some of which involved concomitant use of tetracyclines (see Contraindications and Drug Interactions, Drug-Drug Interactions). Early symptoms of pseudotumor cerebri include headache, nausea and vomiting, and visual disturbances. Patients with these symptoms should be screened for papilledema and, if present, the drug should be discontinued immediately and the patient referred to a neurologist for diagnosis and care. Concomitant treatment with tetracyclines should be avoided (see Contraindications and Drug Interactions, Drug-Drug Interactions).

Conditions of Use: CLARUS is contraindicated in females of childbearing potential unless **ALL** of the following conditions apply:

1. The patient has severe disfiguring nodular and/or inflammatory acne, acne conglobata or recalcitrant acne that has not responded to standard therapy, including systemic antibiotics.
2. The patient is reliable in understanding and carrying out instructions.
3. The patient is able and willing to comply with the mandatory effective contraceptive measures.
4. The patient has received, and acknowledged understanding of, a careful oral and printed explanation of the hazards of fetal exposure to isotretinoin and the risk of possible contraception failure. This explanation may include showing a line drawing to the patient of an infant with the characteristic external deformities resulting from isotretinoin exposure during pregnancy.
5. The patient has been informed and understands the need to rapidly consult her physician if there is a risk of pregnancy.
6. The patient understands the need for rigorous follow-up on a monthly basis.
7. The patient uses effective contraception without any interruption for one month before beginning CLARUS therapy, during CLARUS therapy and for one month following discontinuation of CLARUS therapy. It is recommended that two reliable forms of contraception be used simultaneously (see Warnings and Precautions, Special Populations, Pregnant Women).
8. The patient has had two negative pregnancy tests before starting CLARUS therapy with the first pregnancy test conducted at initial assessment when the patient is qualified for CLARUS therapy by the physician. The patient has had a second serum or urine pregnancy test with a sensitivity of at least 25 mIU/mL with a negative result, performed in a licensed laboratory, within 11 days prior to initiating therapy. The patient has had two or three days of the next normal menstrual period before CLARUS therapy is initiated.
9. In the event of relapse treatment, the patient must also use the same uninterrupted and effective contraceptive measures one month prior to, during and for one month after CLARUS.

(Re items 2 to 9 see Warnings and Precautions, Special Populations, Pregnant Women).

Even female patients who normally do not employ contraception due to a history of infertility, or claim absence of sexual activity should be advised to employ contraception while taking CLARUS following the above guidelines. Even female patients who have amenorrhea must follow all the advice on effective contraception.

Information concerning the CLEAR program (see boxed Serious Warnings and Precautions) has also been provided directly to patients via the CLARUS compliance packaging. This "Patient Information" asks female patients of childbearing potential, who have not been counseled using Mylan Pharmaceuticals ULC's CLEAR program, to contact their physician for further information.

Patients should also be informed that confidential contraception counseling (provided by a health care professional) is available from Mylan Pharmaceuticals ULC.

Blood Donation: It is recommended that blood donation for transfusion purposes be deferred during therapy with isotretinoin and for one month after discontinuation of treatment. Theoretically, blood from such donors could present a small risk to the fetus if transfused to a pregnant mother during the first trimester of pregnancy.

Cardiovascular: Approximately 25% of patients receiving isotretinoin experienced an elevation in plasma triglycerides. Approximately 15% developed a decrease in high density lipoproteins and about 7% showed an increase in cholesterol levels. These effects on triglycerides, HDL and cholesterol were reversible upon reduction of the dose or cessation of isotretinoin therapy (see Adverse Reactions, Clinical Trial and Post-Market Adverse Drug Reactions, Laboratory Abnormalities).

Patients with increased tendency to develop hypertriglyceridemia include those with diabetes mellitus, obesity, increased alcohol intake and familial history.

The cardiovascular consequences of hypertriglyceridemia are not well understood, but may increase the patient's risk status. Therefore, every attempt should be made to control significant triglyceride elevation (see Warnings and Precautions, Monitoring and Laboratory Tests). Some patients have been able to reverse triglyceride elevation by reduction in weight, restriction of dietary fat and alcohol, and reduction in dose while continuing isotretinoin. An obese male patient with Darier's disease developed elevated triglycerides and subsequent eruptive xanthomas.

Ear/Nose/Throat: Impaired hearing at certain frequencies has been reported in some patients treated with isotretinoin. Patients who experience tinnitus or hearing impairment should discontinue CLARUS treatment and be referred for specialized care for further evaluation.

Endocrine and Metabolism: Patients with diabetes or a family history of diabetes may experience problems with the control of their blood sugar during isotretinoin therapy. Therefore, known or suspected diabetics should have periodic blood sugar determinations. Although no causal relationship has been established, elevated fasting blood sugars have been reported, and new cases of diabetes have been diagnosed during isotretinoin therapy (see Adverse Reactions, Clinical Trial and Post-Market Adverse Drug Reactions, Laboratory Abnormalities).

Gastrointestinal: Isotretinoin has been temporally associated with inflammatory bowel disease (including regional ileitis, colitis and hemorrhage) in patients without a prior history of intestinal disorders. Patients experiencing abdominal pain, rectal bleeding or severe diarrhea should discontinue isotretinoin immediately.

Hepatic/Biliary/Pancreatic: Liver function tests should be monitored before treatment and at regular intervals during treatment (one month after the start of treatment and at least three month intervals thereafter) unless more frequent monitoring is clinically indicated. Several cases of clinical hepatitis have been noted which are considered to be possibly or probably related to isotretinoin therapy. Additionally, mild to moderate elevations of liver enzymes have been observed in approximately 15% of individuals treated during clinical trials, some of which normalized with dosage reduction or continued administration of the drug. If normalization does not readily occur, or if hepatitis is suspected during treatment with CLARUS, the drug should be discontinued and the etiology further investigated (see Warnings and Precautions, Monitoring and Laboratory Tests).

There have been some reports of **acute pancreatitis**, which is known to be potentially fatal. This is sometimes associated with elevation of serum triglycerides in excess of 800 mg/dL or 9 mmol/L (see Adverse Reactions, Clinical Trial and Post-Market Adverse Drug Reactions, Laboratory Abnormalities). Therefore, every attempt should be made to control significant triglyceride elevation (see Warnings and Precautions, Cardiovascular). Isotretinoin should be discontinued if uncontrolled hypertriglyceridemia or symptoms of pancreatitis occur.

Immune: Anaphylactic reactions have been reported. These reactions were more serious after prior exposure to topical retinoids. Allergic cutaneous reactions and serious cases of allergic vasculitis, often with purpura (bruises and red patches) of the extremities and extracutaneous involvement have been reported. Severe allergic reactions necessitate interruption of therapy and careful monitoring.

Musculoskeletal: Effects of multiple courses of isotretinoin on the developing musculoskeletal system are unknown. There is some evidence that long-term, high-dose, or multiple courses of therapy with isotretinoin have more of an effect than a single course of therapy on the musculoskeletal system (see also Warnings And Precautions, Special Populations, Pediatrics).

In an open-label clinical trial (N=217) of a single course of therapy with isotretinoin for severe recalcitrant nodular acne in pediatric patients 12 to 17 years, bone density measurements at several skeletal sites were not significantly decreased (lumbar spine change>−4% and total hip change>−5%) or were increased in the majority of patients. One patient had a decrease in lumbar spine bone mineral density >4% based on unadjusted data. Sixteen (7.9%) patients had decreases in lumbar spine bone mineral density >4%, and all the other patients (92%) did not have significant decreases or had increases (adjusted for body mass index). Nine patients (4.5%) had a decrease in total hip bone mineral density >5% based on unadjusted data. Twenty-one (10.6%) patients had decreases in total hip bone mineral density >5%, and all the other patients (89%) did not have significant decreases or had increases (adjusted for body mass index). Follow-up studies performed in 8 of the patients with decreased bone mineral density for up to 11 months thereafter demonstrated increasing bone density in 5 patients at the lumbar spine, while the other 3 patients had lumbar spine bone density measurements below baseline values. Total hip bone mineral densities remained below baseline (range −1.6% to −7.6%) in 5 of 8 patients (62.5%).

In this clinical trial transient elevations in CPK were observed in 12% of patients, including those undergoing strenuous physical activity in association with reported musculoskeletal adverse events such as back pain, arthralgia, limb injury, or muscle sprain. In these patients, approximately half of the CPK elevations returned to normal within 2 weeks and half returned to normal within 4 weeks. No cases of rhabdomyolysis were reported in this trial.

In a separate open-label extension study of 10 patients, ages 13-18 years, who started a second course of isotretinoin 4 months after the first course, two patients showed a decrease in mean lumbar spine bone mineral density up to 3.25%.

Spontaneous reports of osteoporosis, osteopenia, bone fractures, and delayed healing of bone fractures have been seen in the isotretinoin population. While causality to isotretinoin has not been established, an effect cannot be ruled out. Longer term effects have not been studied. It is important that isotretinoin be given at the recommended doses for no longer than the recommended duration.

Although an effect of isotretinoin on bone loss is not established, physicians should use caution when prescribing isotretinoin to patients with a genetic predisposition for age-related osteoporosis, a history of childhood osteoporosis conditions, osteomalacia, or other disorders of bone metabolism. This would include patients diagnosed with anorexia nervosa and those who are on chronic drug therapy that causes drug-induced osteoporosis/osteomalacia and/or affects vitamin D metabolism, such as systemic corticosteroids and any anticonvulsant. Patients may be at increased risk when participating in sports with repetitive impact where the risks of spondylolisthesis with and without pars fractures and hip growth plate injuries in early and late adolescence are known. There are spontaneous reports of fractures and/or delayed healing in patients while on treatment with isotretinoin or following cessation of treatment with isotretinoin while involved in these activities. While causality to isotretinoin has not been established, an effect cannot be ruled out.

Hyperostosis: Due to possible occurrence of bone changes, a careful evaluation of the risk/benefit ratio should be carried out in every patient and CLARUS administration should be restricted to severe cases of acne. Bone changes including, premature epiphyseal closure, hyperostosis and calcification of tendons and ligaments have occurred after several years of administration at high doses for treating disorders of keratinization. The dose levels, duration of treatment and total cumulative dose in these patients generally far exceeded those recommended for the treatment of acne.

In clinical trials of disorders of keratinization, with a mean dose of 2.24 mg/kg/day, a high prevalence of skeletal hyperostosis was noted. Two children showed x-ray findings suggestive of premature closure of the epiphysis. Additionally, skeletal hyperostosis was noted in six of eight patients in a prospective study of disorders of keratinization.

Minimal skeletal hyperostosis and calcification of tendons have also been observed by x-rays in prospective studies of cystic acne patients treated with a single course of therapy at recommended doses. There are spontaneous reports of premature epiphyseal closure in acne patients receiving recommended doses of isotretinoin. The effect of multiple courses of isotretinoin on epiphyseal closure is unknown.

In a clinical study of 217 pediatric patients (12 to 17 years) with severe recalcitrant nodular acne, hyperostosis was not observed after 16 to 20 weeks of treatment with approximately 1 mg/kg/day of isotretinoin given in two divided doses. Hyperostosis may require a longer time frame to appear. The clinical course and significance remain unknown.

Myalgia and arthralgia (mild to moderate) may occur and may be associated with reduced tolerance to vigorous exercise (see Adverse Reactions, Clinical Trial and Post-Market Adverse Drug Reactions, Musculoskeletal). Instances of raised serum creatine phosphokinase (CPK) values have been reported in patients receiving isotretinoin, particularly those undertaking vigorous physical activity. Discontinuation of isotretinoin may be required.

Ophthalmologic: Corneal opacities have occurred in patients receiving isotretinoin for acne and more frequently when higher drug dosages were used in patients with disorders of keratinization. Dry eyes, corneal opacities, decreased night vision, keratitis, blepharitis and conjunctivitis usually resolve after discontinuation of therapy. Due to the possible occurrence of keratitis, patients with dry eyes should be monitored. All CLARUS patients experiencing visual difficulties should discontinue the drug and have an ophthalmological examination (see Adverse Reactions, Clinical Trial and Post-Market Adverse Drug Reactions, Ophthalmologic). Dry eyes, can be helped by the application of a lubricating eye ointment or by the application of tear replacement therapy. Intolerance to contact lenses may occur which may necessitate the patient to wear glasses during treatment.

A number of cases of decreased night vision have occurred during isotretinoin therapy and in rare instances have persisted after therapy (see Adverse Reactions, Clinical Trial and Post-Market Adverse Drug Reactions, Ophthalmologic). Because the onset in some patients was sudden, patients should be advised of this potential problem and warned to be cautious when driving or operating any vehicle at night. CLARUS patients experiencing visual impairment should discontinue treatment and have an ophthalmological examination. Visual problems should be carefully monitored.

Skin: Acute exacerbation of acne is occasionally seen during the initial period but this subsides with continued treatment, usually 7-10 days, and usually does not require dose adjustment.

Exposure to intense sunlight or to UV rays should be avoided. When necessary a sun-protection product with a high protection factor of a least SPF 15 should be used.

It is recommended that aggressive chemical dermabrasion and cutaneous laser treatment be avoided in patients on CLARUS and for a period of 5-6 months after the end of treatment because of the risk of hypertrophic scarring in atypical areas, and more rarely hyper- or hypo-pigmentation in treated areas.

It is recommended that wax epilation be avoided in patients on CLARUS therapy and for a period of 5-6 months after treatment because of the risk of epidermal stripping, scarring or dermatitis.

Concurrent administration of CLARUS with keratolytic or exfoliative anti-acne agents should be avoided as local irritation may increase.

Patients should be advised to use a skin-moisturizing ointment or cream and a lip balm from the start of treatment as isotretinoin is likely to cause dryness of the skin and lips.

Special Populations: Pregnant Women: There is an extremely high risk (25% or greater) that major human fetal abnormalities will occur if pregnancy occurs during treatment with isotretinoin or up to one month following its discontinuation. Potentially any exposed fetus can be affected. These abnormalities, associated with isotretinoin administration during pregnancy, have been reported and include:

CNS (hydrocephalus, hydranecephaly, microcephaly, posterior fossa abnormalities, cranial nerve dysfunction, cerebellar malformation); craniofacial (anotia, microtia, low set ears, small or absent external auditory canals, microphthalmia, facial dysmorphia, cleft palate); cardiac (septal defects, aortic arch abnormalities, tetralogy of Fallot); thymus gland abnormalities; and parathyroid hormone deficiency. Cases of IQ scores less than 85 with or without other abnormalities have been reported.

Pregnancy Tests: Female patients of childbearing potential must not be given CLARUS until pregnancy is excluded. The patient must have two negative pregnancy tests before starting CLARUS therapy with the first pregnancy test conducted at initial assessment when the patient is qualified for CLARUS therapy by the physician. A second pregnancy test must be performed within 11 days prior to starting CLARUS treatment. CLARUS treatment should start on the second or third day of the next normal menstrual period following this negative pregnancy test.

It is mandatory that all female patients of childbearing potential treated with CLARUS have regular monthly pregnancy tests during treatment and one month after the discontinuation of treatment. The dates and results of pregnancy tests should be documented. These pregnancy tests will:

a. Serve primarily to reinforce to the patient the necessity of avoiding pregnancy.
b. In the event of accidental pregnancy, provide the physician and patient an immediate opportunity to discuss the serious risk to the fetus from this exposure to isotretinoin and the desirability of continuing the pregnancy in view of the potential teratogenic effect of isotretinoin (see Contraindications).

Contraception: Effective contraception must be used for at least one month before starting CLARUS treatment, during treatment and for at least one month following the discontinuation of CLARUS treatment. It is recommended that two reliable forms of contraception be used simultaneously. At least 1 of these forms of contraception must be a primary form, unless the patient has undergone a hysterectomy. Effective forms of contraception include: tubal ligation, partner's vasectomy, intrauterine devices, birth control pills, and topical/injectable/insertable hormonal birth control products. Barrier forms of contraception include diaphragms, latex condoms, and cervical caps; each must be used with a spermicide. Any birth control method can fail. Therefore, it is critically important that women of childbearing potential use 2 effective forms of contraception simultaneously (see Drug Interactions, Drug-Drug Interactions).

Pregnancy occurring during treatment with isotretinoin and for one month after its discontinuation, carries the risk of fetal malformation and the increased risk of spontaneous abortion (see Contraindications). Isotretinoin, treatment must be stopped and the patient should be fully counselled on the serious risk to the fetus should they become pregnant while undergoing treatment. If pregnancy does occur during this time the physician and patient should discuss the desirability of continuing the pregnancy.

Nursing Women: It is not known whether isotretinoin is excreted in human milk. As isotretinoin is highly lipophilic, the passage of the drug in human milk is very likely. Because of the potential for adverse effects, women should not breast-feed if they are receiving isotretinoin (see Contraindications).

Pediatrics: The long term safety of isotretinoin, in prepubertal children **(<12 years of age)**, has not been established.

In studies with isotretinoin adverse reactions reported in pediatric patients ages 12 to 17 years were similar to those described in adults except for the increased incidence of back pain and arthralgia (both of which were sometimes severe) and myalgia in pediatric patients (see Adverse Reactions).

Pediatric patients and their caregivers should be informed that approximately 29% (104/358) of pediatric patients treated with isotretinoin developed back pain. Back pain was severe in 13.5% (14/104) of the cases and occurred at a higher frequency in female patients than male patients. Arthralgias were experienced in 22% (79/358) of pediatric patients. Arthralgias were severe in 7.6% (6/79) of patients. Appropriate evaluation of the musculoskeletal system should be done in patients who present with these symptoms during or after a course of CLARUS. Consideration should be given to discontinuation of CLARUS if any significant abnormality is found.

Geriatrics (>65 years of age): Clinical studies of isotretinoin did not include sufficient numbers of subjects aged 65 years and over to determine whether they respond differently from younger subjects.

Special Patient Groups: In high risk patients (with diabetes, obesity, alcoholism or lipid metabolism disorder) undergoing treatment with isotretinoin, more frequent checks of serum values for lipids (see Warnings and Precautions, Endocrine and Metabolism and Hepatic/Biliary/Pancreatic) and/or blood glucose may be necessary.

Male Patients: The available data suggest that the level of maternal exposure from the semen of the patients receiving isotretinoin is not of a sufficient magnitude to be associated with the teratogenic effects of isotretinoin. The threshold dose of isotretinoin exposure causing birth defects is not known. Postmarketing reports through 20 years include 4 with isolated defects compatible with features of retinoid exposed fetus; however 2 of these reports were incomplete, and 2 had other possible explanations for the defects observed.

Male patients should be reminded that they must not share their medication with anyone, particularly not females.

Isotretinoin, in therapeutic dosages, does not affect the number, motility and morphology of sperm.

Both male and female patients should be given a copy of the Information for the Patient.

Monitoring and Laboratory Tests: Pregnancy Tests: The patient should have two negative pregnancy tests (β-hCG in urine or serum) before starting CLARUS therapy with the first pregnancy test conducted at initial assessment when the patient is qualified for CLARUS therapy by the physician. The patient then should have a second pregnancy test with a sensitivity of at least 25 mIU/mL with a negative result, performed in a licensed laboratory, within 11 days prior to initiating therapy. The patient has had two or three days of the next normal menstrual period before CLARUS therapy is initiated. **Pregnancy test must be repeated monthly for pregnancy detection** during CLARUS treatment and at one month after discontinuation of treatment. The dates and results of the pregnancy tests should be documented.

Signs of Depression: sad mood, hopelessness, feeling of guilt, worthlessness or helplessness, loss of pleasure or interest in activities, fatigue, difficulty concentrating, changes in sleep pattern, change in weight or appetite, suicidal thoughts or attempts, restlessness, irritability, acting on dangerous impulses, and persistent physical symptoms unresponsive to treatment If symptoms of depression develop or worsen during treatment with CLARUS, the drug should be discontinued promptly and the patient referred for appropriate psychiatric treatment.

The following tests are required before starting CLARUS, at first month, then as clinically indicated:

- Serum blood lipid determinations (under fasting conditions) should be performed before CLARUS is given and then at intervals (one month after the start of therapy) until the lipid response to CLARUS is established (which usually occurs within four weeks), and also at the end of treatment.
- Complete blood count and differential: for early detection of leukopenia, neutropenia, thrombocytopenia and anemia.
- Liver function tests: Increases in about 15% of ALT, AST, ALP baseline levels have been reported. Liver function tests should be monitored before treatment and at regular intervals during treatment (one month after the start of treatment and at least three month intervals thereafter) unless more frequent monitoring is clinically indicated.
- Blood glucose levels: all patients and in particular patients with known or suspected diabetes should have periodic blood sugar determinations.

ADVERSE REACTIONS: Adverse Drug Reaction Overview: The adverse reactions listed below reflect the experience from clinical studies of Isotretinoin, and the post-marketing experience. The relationship of some of these events to Isotretinoin therapy is unknown.

Many of the side effects and adverse reactions seen or expected in patients receiving Isotretinoin are similar to those described in patients taking high doses of vitamin A.

Clinical Trial and Post-Market Adverse Drug Reactions: Dose-Relationship and Duration: Cheilitis and hypertriglyceridemia are usually dose related.

Adverse reactions were generally reversible when therapy was discontinued; however, some have persisted after cessation of therapy.

The most common side-effects are mucocutaneous or dermatologic. The common side effects include: cheilitis (96%), facial erythema/dermatitis (55%), dry nose (51%), desquamation (50%), pruritus (30%), dry skin (22%), conjunctivitis (19%), alopecia (13%), irritation of the eyes (11%), rash (<10%). Dryness of the nasal mucosa and pharynx may be associated with mild epistaxis and hoarseness, respectively. Mild-to-moderate conjunctivitis may be alleviated by use of an ophthalmic ointment. In rare cases, hair loss persisted after treatment was completed.

Approximately 13% of patients experience joint pain during treatment.

Peeling of palms and soles, skin infections, increased susceptibility to sunburn, nonspecific urogenital symptoms, nonspecific gastrointestinal symptoms, headache, fatigue occured in approximately 5% of patients.

Body as a Whole: weight loss, anemia, lymphadenopathy, vasculitis including Wegener's granulomatosis, allergic vasculitis, allergic responses, and systemic hypersensitivity.

Cardiovascular: edema, transient pain in the chest, palpitations, tachycardia, vascular thrombotic disease, stroke.

Endocrine and Metabolism: new cases of diabetes (see Warning and Precautions, Endocrine and Metabolism).

Gastrointestinal: nausea, severe diarrhea, mild gastrointestinal bleeding, rectal bleeding, abdominal pain, inflammatory bowel disease (including regional ileitis, colitis and hemorrhage) (see Warnings and Precautions, Gastrointestinal).

Hearing Disorders: tinnitus, impaired hearing at certain frequencies.

Hepatic/Biliary/Pancreatic: Patients treated with isotretinoin especially those with high triglyceride levels are at risk of developing pancreatitis. Rare cases of fatal pancreatitis and several cases of clinical hepatitis have been reported (see Warnings and Precautions, Hepatic/Biliary/Pancreatic).

Mucocutaneous and Dermatologic: flushing, changes in skin pigment, urticaria, bruising, disseminated herpes simplex, hair problems (other than thinning), hirsutism, erythema nodosum, paronychia, nail dystrophy, pyogenic granuloma, bleeding and inflammation of the gums, acne fulminans, exanthema, sweating, increased formation of granulation tissue, photoallergic/photosensitizing reactions, skin fragility. Acne flare occurs at the start of treatment and persists for several weeks.

Musculoskeletal: arthritis, muscle pain (myalgia; elevations of serum CPK values), arthralgia, calcification of ligaments, tendon and tendinitis, reduced bone density, back pain, epiphyses, premature fusion, hyperostosis (see Warnings and Precautions, Musculoskeletal, Hyperostosis).

There have been rare postmarketing reports of rhabdomyolysis, some associated with strenuous physical activity. However, there is insufficient information to suggest an association between treatment with isotretinoin and the development of rhabdomyolysis.

Neurologic: seizures, dizziness, nervousness, drowsiness, malaise, weakness, insomnia, lethargy, paresthesia, benign intracranial hypertension (see Warnings and Precautions, Serious Warnings and Precautions, Neurologic).

Ophthalmologic: optic neuritis, photophobia, eye lid inflammation, lenticular cataracts, keratitis, blurred vision, blepharitis, conjunctivitis, papilledema as sign of benign intracranial hypertension and colour vision disturbances. Dry eyes and/or decreased tolerance to contact lenses have also been reported during therapy. In some instances these conditions have persisted after cessation of therapy.

Of 72 patients who had normal pre-treatment ophthalmological examinations, five developed corneal opacities while taking isotretinoin (all five patients had a disorder of keratinization). Corneal opacities have also been reported in nodular and/or inflammatory acne patients treated with isotretinoin (see Warnings and Precautions, Ophthalmologic). Decrease in night vision has been reported and in rare instances has persisted (see Warnings and Precautions, Ophthalmologic). Cataracts and visual disturbances have also been reported.

Psychiatric Disorders: Depression, psychotic symptoms and, rarely, suicide attempts, suicide, and aggressive and/or violent behaviours (see Warnings and Precautions, Psychiatric). Depression has been reported during and after therapy. In some of these patients, depression has subsided with discontinuation of therapy and recurred when isotretinoin therapy was reintroduced. Emotional instability has been reported with isotretinoin.

Respiratory: respiratory infections.

Bronchospasm has been rarely reported; sometimes in patients with pre-history of asthma.

Reproductive System: abnormal menses.

Urinary System: glomerulonephritis.

Laboratory Abnormalities: Isotretinoin therapy induces changes in serum lipids in a significant number of treated subjects. These changes consisted of: elevation of serum triglycerides (25% of patients), mild to moderate decrease in serum high density lipoprotein (HDL) (16% of patients), and minimal elevations of serum cholesterol (7% of patients). Abnormalities of serum triglycerides, HDL and cholesterol were reversible upon cessation of isotretinoin therapy.

A rise in serum levels of liver enzymes may occur, especially with higher dosages. Although the changes have usually been within the normal range, and may return to baseline levels despite continued treatment, significant increases have occurred in a few cases, necessitating dosage reduction or discontinuation of isotretinoin (see Warnings and Precautions, Hepatic/Biliary/Pancreatic). An elevated erythrocyte sedimentation rate may also occur (40% of patients).

Other less commonly reported laboratory abnormalities were: Elevated fasting blood sugar, elevated CPK, and hyperuricemia. Decreases in red blood cell parameters, decreases in white blood cell counts, elevated sedimentation rates, elevated platelet counts, thrombocytopenia and anemia. White blood cells in the urine, proteinuria, and red blood cells in the urine.

DRUG INTERACTIONS: Drug-Drug Interactions: Tetracyclines: Rare cases of benign intracranial hypertension 'pseudotumor cerebri' have been reported after use of isotretinoin and/or tetracyclines. Therefore, concomitant treatment with tetracyclines must be avoided (see Warnings and Precautions, Serious Warnings and Precautions, Neurologic).

Vitamin A: Because of the relationship of isotretinoin to vitamin A, patients should be advised against taking vitamin supplements containing vitamin A, to avoid additive toxic effects.

Phenytoin: Isotretinoin has not been shown to alter the pharmacokinetics of phenytoin in a study in seven healthy volunteers. These results are consistent with the in vitro finding that neither isotretinoin nor its metabolites induce or inhibit the activity of the CYP 2C9 human hepatic P450 enzyme. Phenytoin is known to cause osteomalacia. No formal clinical studies have been conducted to assess if there is an interactive effect on bone loss between phenytoin and isotretinoin. Therefore, caution should be exercised when using these drugs together.

Norethindrone/Ethinyl Estradiol: In a study of 31 premenopausal women with severe recalcitrant nodular acne receiving OrthoNovum 7/7/7 Tablets as an oral contraceptive agent, isotretinoin at the recommended dose of 1 mg/kg/day, did not induce clinically relevant changes in the pharmacokinetics of ethinyl estradiol and norethindrone and in the serum levels of progesterone, follicle-stimulating hormone (FSH) and luteinizing hormone (LH). A drug interaction that decreases effectiveness of hormonal contraceptives has not been entirely ruled out for isotretinoin.

Microdosed progesterone preparations (minipills) are not a suitable method of contraception during CLARUS therapy.

Systemic Corticosteroids: Systemic corticosteroids are known to cause osteoporosis. No formal clinical studies have been conducted to assess if there is an interactive effect on bone loss between systemic corticosteroids and isotretinoin. Therefore, caution should be exercised when using these drugs together.

Drug-Food Interactions: Due to its lipophilic properties, absorption of isotretinoin is increased when taken with food. Therefore, the recommended dose is to be taken with food (see Dosage and Administration, Recommended Dose and Dosage Adjustment).

Drug-Herb Interactions: St. John's Wort: Isotretinoin use is associated with depression in some patients (see Warnings and Precautions, Serious Warnings and Precautions, Psychiatric and Adverse Reactions, Psychiatric Disorders). Patients should be prospectively cautioned not to self-medicate with the herbal supplement St. John's Wort because a possible interaction has been suggested with hormonal contraceptives based on reports of breakthrough bleeding on oral contraceptives shortly after starting St. John's Wort. Pregnancies have been reported by users of combined hormonal contraceptives who also used some form of St. John's Wort.

DOSAGE AND ADMINISTRATION: Dosing Considerations: The therapeutic response to isotretinoin is dose-related and varies between patients. This necessitates individual adjustment of dosage according to the response of the condition and the patient's tolerance of the drug. In most cases, complete or near-complete suppression of acne is achieved with a single 12 to 16 week course of therapy. If a second course of therapy is needed, it can be initiated eight or more weeks after completion of the first course, since experience has shown that patients may continue to improve while off the drug.

Recommended Dose and Dosage Adjustment: Initial Therapy: The initial dose of CLARUS should be individualized according to the patient's weight and severity of the disease.

In general, patients initially should receive isotretinoin 0.5 mg/kg body weight daily for a period of two to four weeks, when their responsiveness to the drug will usually be apparent. It should be noted that transient exacerbation of acne is occasionally seen during this initial period. The daily dosage should be taken with food in the nearest number of whole capsules, either as a single dose or in two divided doses during the day, whichever is more convenient.

Maintenance Therapy: Maintenance dose should be adjusted between 0.1 and 1 mg/kg body weight daily and, in exceptional instances, up to 2 mg/kg body weight daily, depending upon individual patient response and tolerance to the drug.

A complete course of therapy consists of 12-16 weeks of CLARUS administration.

Patients may show additional improvement for up to several months after a course of isotretinoin has been completed. With effective treatment, appearance of new lesions will not normally be evident for a period of at least three to six months.

OVERDOSAGE:

In the event of acute isotretinoin overdose evacuation of the stomach should be considered during the first few hours after this overdose. Signs and symptoms of acute overdose have been associated with headache, vomiting, facial flushing, cheilitis, abdominal pain, dizziness and ataxia. To date, all symptoms have quickly resolved without apparent residual effects and usually without treatment. Elevated intracranial pressure has been reported with patients receiving therapeutic doses of isotretinoin. Patients with a CLARUS overdose should be monitored closely for signs of increased intracranial pressure. Signs of hypervitaminosis A could appear in cases of overdose.

Limited data exists on the pharmacokinetic characteristics of isotretinoin in an overdose situation. Following the oral administration of single 80, 160, 240 and 340 mg doses to 12 healthy male subjects C_{max} was 366, 820, 1056 and 981 ng/mL, and $t_{½}$ was 13.6, 14.1, 14.4 and 16.5 hours for isotretinoin, respectively. Twenty-three compromised cancer patients received weekly oral doses of 200 (3 patients); 400 (7 patients); 660 (2 patients); 1000 (3 patients); 1400 (6 patients) and 1800 (1 patient) mg/m^2. Normal body surface area for healthy subjects is 1.73 m^2. After the first dose, C_{max} was 1.5, 3.8, 3.5, 2.5, 2.7 and 4.6 µg/mL, and $t_{½}$ was 45, 9.1, 14.5, 57, 13.1 and 6.1 hours for isotretinoin, respectively. The absorption of isotretinoin appears to be a saturable process.

Since it is difficult to extrapolate from the results of these studies to the overdose situation, the following precautions should be taken with all female patients of childbearing potential who have taken an overdose of CLARUS.

1. At the time of the overdose, a pregnancy test must be performed and a blood sample collected for the determination of isotretinoin and metabolite concentrations.
2. One complete menstrual cycle after the overdose, a second pregnancy test must be performed and a second blood sample collected for the determination of isotretinoin and metabolite concentrations.
3. Effective contraception must be used for at least one complete menstrual cycle after the overdose and continued longer, if necessary until isotretinoin and its metabolites are no longer measurable in the blood.

Patients who present with a positive pregnancy test at the time of the overdose, one complete menstrual cycle after the overdose, or while isotretinoin or metabolite blood concentrations are measurable, should be fully counselled on the serious risk to the fetus from this exposure to isotretinoin and the physician and patient should discuss the desirability of continuing the pregnancy. (See Contraindications, Warnings and Precautions, Special Populations, Pregnant Women.)

Canadian Regional Poison Information Centres have been advised on the proper collection and handling of isotretinoin blood samples and also on the laboratory(s) equipped to assay these samples.

For management of a suspected drug overdose, contact your **regional Poison Control Centre**. See the *CPS* Directory section for a list of Poison Control Centres.

ACTION AND CLINICAL PHARMACOLOGY: Mechanism of Action: The mechanism of action of isotretinoin is unknown. Vitamin A is important for functional integrity of the skin and is known to affect the keratinization process. In acne patients, improvement occurs in association with a reduction in sebum secretion. The decrease in sebum secretion is temporary and is related to either the dose or duration of isotretinoin administration and reflects a reduction in sebaceous gland size and an inhibition of sebaceous gland differentiation.

Pharmacokinetics: Absorption: Following oral administration of 80 mg, peak plasma concentrations ranged from 167 to 459 ng/mL (mean 256 ng/mL) with a mean time to peak of 3.2 hours in volunteers, while in acne patients peak plasma concentrations ranged from 98 to 535 ng/mL (mean 262 ng/mL) with a mean time to peak of 2.9 hours.

When isotretinoin is taken with food, the bioavailability is doubled relative to fasting conditions (see Dosage and Administration).

Distribution: Isotretinoin is 99.9% protein bound in human plasma, almost exclusively to albumin.

Metabolism: The major metabolite identified in blood and urine was 4-oxo-isotretinoin. Tretinoin and 4-oxo-tretinoin were also observed. The apparent half-life for elimination of the 4-oxo-isotretinoin ranged from 11 to 50 hours, with a mean of 28 hours. Following 80 mg of isotretinoin administered orally, maximum plasma concentrations of the 4-oxo-isotretinoin was 87 to 399 ng/mL and maxima were observed between 6 and 20 hours. The blood concentration of the major metabolite generally exceeded that of isotretinoin after 6 hours. The data suggest that both isotretinoin and the major metabolite are excreted in the bile and reabsorbed. The mean minimum steady-state blood concentrations of isotretinoin were 160 ng/mL in 10 patients receiving 40 mg twice daily doses. After single and multiple doses, the mean ratio of areas under the curves of 4-oxo-isotretinoin to isotretinoin was between 3 and 3.5.

Comparative Bioavailability: A blinded, randomized, single-dose, 2-way crossover, relative bioavailability study was conducted in healthy volunteers to compare CLARUS 40 mg soft gelatin capsules and Accutane Roche 40 mg soft gelatin capsules under fed conditions. The pharmacokinetic data is summarized in Table 1.

Table 1: CLARUS

Table of Comparative Bioavailability Data

Fed Isotretinoin (2×40 mg) From Measured Data Geometric Mean Arithmetic Mean (CV %)				
Parameter	**Test CLARUS**	**Reference Accutane Roche[a]**	**% Ratio of Geometric Means**	**95% Confidence Interval**
AUC_T (ng·h/mL)	10 228.66 10 397.5 (18.0%)	11 257.18 11 455.8 (18.5%)	90.9%	87.3–94.6%
AUC_{INF} (ng·h/mL)	10 591.93 10 772.1 (18.2%)	11 647.46 11 856.6 (18.7%)	90.9%	87.4–94.6%
C_{max} (ng/mL)	1134.17 1221.5 (36.5%)	1260.06 1374.81 (38.6%)	90.0%	81.7–99.2%
T_{max}[b] (h)	4.406 (36.8%)	5.129 (60.1%)		
$T_{½}$[b] (h)	15.75 (16.9%)	15.55 (18.7%)		

[a] Accutane Roche soft gelatin capsules manufactured by Hoffmann-LaRoche Limited/Limitée (Canada) were purchased in Canada.
[b] Expressed as arithmetic mean (CV%) only.

A blinded, randomized, single-dose, 2-way crossover, relative bioavailability study was conducted in healthy volunteers to compare CLARUS 40 mg soft gelatin capsules and Accutane Roche 40 mg soft gelatin capsules under fasting conditions. The pharmacokinetic data is summarized in Table 2.

Table 2: CLARUS

Table of Comparative Bioavailability Data

Fasted Isotretinoin (2×40 mg) From Measured Data Geometric Mean Arithmetic Mean (CV %)				
Parameter	**Test CLARUS**	**Reference Accutane Roche[a]**	**% Ratio of Geometric Means**	**95% Confidence Interval**
AUC_T (ng·h/mL)	4247.97 4481.4 (33.7%)	4412.22 4636.2 (31.2%)	96.3%	86.3–107.5%
AUC_{INF} (ng·h/mL)	4567.88 4812.5 (33.2%)	4819.48 5037.7 (30.2%)	94.8%	85.5–105.1%
C_{max} (ng/mL)	390.98 407.35 (27.4%)	386.46 407.63 (32.4%)	101.2%	90.6–113.0%
T_{max}[b] (h)	3.892 (103.0%)	3.208 (51.8%)		
$T_{½}$[b] (h)	20.06 (21.3%)	20.76 (40.9%)		

[a] Accutane Roche soft gelatin capsules manufactured by Hoffmann-LaRoche Limited/Limitée (Canada) were purchased in Canada.
[b] Expressed as arithmetic mean (CV%) only.

Excretion: The mean terminal elimination half-life of isotretinoin in patients with acne has a mean value of 19 hours. Following oral administration of ^{14}C-isotretinoin ^{14}C activity in blood declined with a mean half-life of 90 hours. Approximately equal amounts of radioactivity were recovered in the urine and feces, with 65-83% of the dose recovered.

Special Populations and Conditions: Pediatrics: The pharmacokinetics of isotretinoin were evaluated after single and multiple doses in 38 pediatric patients (12 to 15 years) and 19 adult patients (≥18 years) who received isotretinoin for the treatment of severe recalcitrant nodular acne. In both age groups, 4-oxo-isotretinoin was the major metabolite; tretinoin and 4-oxo-tretinoin were also observed. The dose-normalized pharmacokinetic parameters for isotretinoin following single and multiple doses are summarized in Table 3 for pediatric patients. There were no statistically significant differences in the pharmacokinetics of isotretinoin between pediatric and adult patients.

Table 3: CLARUS

Pharmacokinetic Parameters of Isotretinoin Following Single and Multiple Dose Administration in Pediatric Patients, 12 to 15 Years of Age Mean (± SD), N38[a]

Parameter	Isotretinoin (Single Dose)	Isotretinoin (Steady-State)
C_{max} (ng/mL)	573.25 (278.79)	731.98 (361.86)
$AUC_{(0-12)}$ (ng·hr/mL)	3033.37 (1394.17)	5082.00 (2184.23)
$AUC_{(0-24)}$ (ng·hr/mL)	6003.81 (2885.67)	—

(cont'd)

Table 3: CLARUS *(cont'd)*

Pharmacokinetic Parameters of Isotretinoin Following Single and Multiple Dose Administration in Pediatric Patients, 12 to 15 Years of Age Mean (± SD), N38[a]

Parameter	Isotretinoin (Single Dose)	Isotretinoin (Steady-State)
T_{max} (hr)[b]	6.00 (1.00–24.60)	4.00 (0–12.00)
Css_{min} (ng/mL)	—	352.32 (184.44)
$T_{½}$ (hr)	—	15.69 (5.12)
CL/F (L/hr)	—	17.96 (6.27)

[a] The single and multiple dose data in this table were obtained following a non-standardized meal (non high-fat meal).
[b] Median (range).

In pediatric patients (12 to 15 years), the mean±SD elimination half-lives ($t_{½}$) of isotretinoin and 4-oxo-isotretinoin were 15.7±5.1 hours and 23.1±5.7 hours, respectively. The accumulation ratios of isotretinoin ranged from 0.46 to 3.65 for pediatric patients.

STORAGE AND STABILITY: CLARUS (isotretinoin) 10 mg and 40 mg capsules: Store at 15-30°C. Protect from exposure to light.

Keep in a safe place out of the reach of children.

SPECIAL HANDLING INSTRUCTIONS: There are no special handling instructions for CLARUS (isotretinoin) capsules.

INFORMATION FOR THE PATIENT: Published in e-CPS, available by subscription at www.e-cps.ca.

DOSAGE FORMS, COMPOSITION AND PACKAGING: 10 mg: Each oval capsule with a yellow to orange paste fill and a reddish brown opaque gelatin shell, printed with black ink "I" logo on one side, contains: isotretinoin 10 mg. Nonmedicinal ingredients: ammonium hydroxide, beeswax yellow, gelatin, glycerin, hydrogenated vegetable oil, polyethylene glycol, polyvinyl acetate phthalate, propylene glycol, red iron oxide, soybean oil, synthetic black iron oxide and titanium dioxide. Blister packages of 30.
40 mg: Each oval capsule with a yellow to orange paste fill and an orange brown opaque gelatin shell, printed with black ink "I40" logo on one side, contains: isotretinoin 40 mg. Nonmedicinal ingredients: ammonium hydroxide, beeswax yellow, gelatin, glycerin, hydrogenated vegetable oil, polyethylene glycol, polyvinyl acetate phthalate, propylene glycol, red iron oxide, soybean oil, synthetic black iron oxide, titanium dioxide and yellow iron oxide. Blister packages of 30.

(Shown in Product Identification Section)

The reader is invited to consult CPhA's monograph **Bisphosphonates: Oral.**

Clasteon®

clodronate disodium

Bone Metabolism Regulator

Sepracor

Date of Preparation: November 25, 2004
Date of Revision: April 14, 2009

SUMMARY PRODUCT INFORMATION:

Route of Administration	Dosage Form/ Strength	Clinically Relevant Nonmedicinal Ingredients
Oral	Capsule/400 mg	Gelatin For a complete listing see Dosage Forms, Composition and Packaging.
Intravenous (i.v.)	Concentrate for i.v. infusion	Disodium hydrogen carbonate For a complete listing see Dosage Forms, Composition and Packaging.

INDICATIONS AND CLINICAL USE: CLASTEON (clodronate disodium) is indicated:

- as an adjunct in the management of osteolysis resulting from bone metastases of malignant tumors.
- for the management of hypercalcemia of malignancy.

Prior to treatment with clodronate disodium, renal excretion of excess calcium should be promoted by restoration and maintenance of adequate fluid balance and urine output.

In responsive patients, intravenous infusion of clodronate disodium inhibits osteoclastic activity and bone resorption by decreasing the flux of calcium from the bones and thus reducing the calcium level in the blood.

Clodronate disodium may be administered as a higher single infusion dose or a lower dose for multiple infusion use. Both methods have been shown to be effective.

Treatment with oral clodronate disodium following intravenous infusion has been found to prolong the duration of action (see Dosage and Administration).

CONTRAINDICATIONS:

- Renal functional impairment (serum creatinine exceeding 440 µmol/L (5.0 mg/dL).
- Patients who are hypersensitive to clodronate disodium or other bisphosphonates, or to any ingredient in the formulation or component of the container. For a complete listing, see Dosage Forms, Composition and Packaging.
- Severe inflammation of the gastrointestinal tract.
- Pregnancy and lactation.

WARNINGS AND PRECAUTIONS:

Serious Warnings and Precautions

- CLASTEON (clodronate disodium) should **not** be given as a bolus injection since severe local reactions and thrombophlebitis may occur as the result of high local concentrations. The rapid bolus injection may also precipitate acute renal failure.

General: The recommended daily dose of CLASTEON i.v. concentrate for intravenous infusion should always be diluted and administered as a slow intravenous infusion over a minimum 2-hour period (during multiple infusion use) or a minimum 4-hour period (during single infusion use) (see Dosage and Administration).

CLASTEON should not be given together with other bisphosphonates since the combined effects of these agents are unknown.

CLASTEON should not be mixed with calcium-containing intravenous infusions.

Endocrine and Metabolism and Fluid Balance: Hypercalcemia causes a reversible tubular defect in the kidney that results in the loss of urinary concentrating ability and polyuria, both of which promote dehydration. Hypovolemia in patients with hypercalcemia can diminish glomerular filtration and lead to progressive renal insufficiency.

Most hypercalcemic patients are significantly dehydrated at initial presentation and restoration of intravascular volume is an important initial measure.

The cornerstone of initial treatment is vigorous hydration with isotonic saline (0.9%). It is essential to institute hydration to replenish extracellular fluid volume and restore normal glomerular filtration, as well as sodium diuresis to promote calcium excretion even after hydration status has been corrected.

The rate of administration of isotonic saline should be determined primarily by the severity of the hypercalcemia, the degree of dehydration, and the cardiovascular status of the patient. In general, at least 3 L/day should be administered initially and hydration continued until normocalcaemia has been achieved. Urine output must be maintained to avoid possible fluid overload. As many patients with hypercalcemia have other electrolyte abnormalities at presentation, appropriate attention must be given to maintaining electrolyte balance. For example, for hypokalemia, which may be further aggravated by aggressive diuresis, supplementation may be required. The development of hypernatremia during rehydration has been reported, especially in obtunded patients, and may complicate management.

Hypocalcemia: Infusion of clodronate disodium may present a risk of hypocalcemia.

The drug may chelate blood calcium during therapy, this may contribute to hypocalcemia.

In most cases, plasma calcium concentrations remain within the normal range during the administration of recommended doses of clodronate disodium. When plasma calcium falls into the hypocalcemic range, the patient may remain asymptomatic.

In these cases intravenous administration should be stopped or the oral dose should be decreased. In severe or symptomatic cases of hypocalcemia, oral or parenteral calcium supplementation may be required.

Serum Phosphate: Hyperphosphatemia has not been reported during clodronate disodium therapy in hypercalcemic patients. However, transient hypophosphatemia can occur following therapy with clodronate disodium.

Hyperparathyroidism: Clodronate disodium has not been shown to affect the renal handling of calcium and/or the action of plasma parathyroid hormone (PTH) on this process. A transitory increase in PTH has been reported in certain subjects.

Musculoskeletal: Osteonecrosis of the jaw (ONJ) has been reported in patients with cancer receiving treatment regimens including bisphosphonates. Many of these patients were also receiving chemotherapy and corticosteroids. The majority of reported cases have been associated with dental procedures such as tooth extraction. Many had signs of local infection including osteomyelitis.

A dental examination with appropriate preventative dentistry should be considered prior to treatment with bisphosphonates in patients with concomitant risk factors (e.g. cancer, chemotherapy, head and neck radiotherapy, corticosteroids, poor oral hygiene).

While on treatment, these patients should avoid invasive dental procedures if possible. For patients who develop ONJ while on bisphosphonate therapy, dental surgery may exacerbate the condition. For patients requiring dental procedures, there are no data available to suggest whether discontinuation of bisphosphonate treatment reduces the risk of ONJ. Clinical judgment of the treating physician should guide the management plan of each patient based on individual benefit/risk assessment.

Renal: Administration of clodronate disodium may aggravate renal function in some patients. Therefore, appropriate monitoring of renal function during and after intravenous infusion is required. The effect of the drug on the renal function of patients with serum creatinine in excess of 220 µmol/L (2.5 mg/dL) has not been studied in controlled trials. In such situations dose reduction should be considered or the drug should be withheld (see Warnings and Precautions, Monitoring and Laboratory Tests).

If during therapy there is deterioration of renal function, the intravenous solution should be stopped.

Special Populations: Pregnant Women: The safety and efficacy of CLASTEON in pregnancy has not been established (see Contraindications).

Nursing Women: There is not clinical experience with CLASTEON in lactating women and it is not known whether CLASTEON passes into breast milk (see Contraindications).

Pediatrics: The safety and efficacy of CLASTEON in children has not been established.

Monitoring and Laboratory Tests: Serum calcium levels should be monitored throughout treatment with clodronate disodium.

Corrected (adjusted) serum calcium values should be calculated using established algorithms, such as:

Ca_{adj}	=	Ca_t-0.71 (A-A_m)
Ca_{adj}	=	adjusted calcium concentration (mg/100 mL)
Ca_t	=	total calcium concentration (mg/100 mL)
A	=	albumin concentration (g/100 mL)
A_m	=	mean normal albumin concentration for the given laboratory (g/100 mL)

Alternative: corrected calcium (mg/dL) = measured calcium + [4.0-albumin (g/dL)] × 0.8

Appropriate monitoring of hepatic function and hematological parameters, including white cell count is advised.

Additionally, serum creatinine and blood urea nitrogen should be monitored in patients with known or suspected renal insufficiency.

ADVERSE REACTIONS: Adverse Drug Reaction Overview: Gastrointestinal symptoms such as nausea, vomiting, anorexia and diarrhea are the most frequent adverse events reported during clodronate disodium therapy, particularly with the oral form. A reduction in dosage, a change to i.v. clodronate disodium or a temporary interruption of therapy may assist in the management of patients where these symptoms are relevant.

Clinical Trial Adverse Drug Reactions: Because clinical trials are conducted under very specific conditions the adverse reaction rates observed in the clinical trials may not reflect the rates observed in practice and should not be compared to the rates in the clinical trials of another drug. Adverse drug reaction information from clinical trials is useful for identifying drug-related adverse events and for approximating rates.

Listed in Table 1 are the crude incidence rates for the most common adverse events reported during therapy with CLASTEON 400 mg capsules and CLASTEON i.v. (concentrate for intravenous infusion).

Table 1: CLASTEON

Most Common Adverse Events Reported During Therapy

Adverse Event	Oral (N=390) % (N)	I.V. (N=188) % (N)
Digestive System		
Vomiting	—	3.6 (14)
Nausea	3.1 (12)	1.1 (2)
Diarrhea	1.8 (7)	0.5 (1)
Anorexia	1.0 (4)	—
Metabolic and Nutritional		
Hypocalcemia	1.5 (6)	—
Creatinine Increased	1.3 (5)	—
ALT Increased	0.3 (1)	—
Cardiovascular System		
Heart Failure	1.3 (5)	—
Respiratory System		
Pneumonia	1.3 (5)	—

(cont'd)

Table 1: CLASTEON *(cont'd)*

Most Common Adverse Events Reported During Therapy

Adverse Event	Oral (N=390) % (N)	I.V. (N=188) % (N)
Musculoskeletal System		
Spontaneous Fracture	1.0 (4)	—

Cardiovascular: Adverse events affecting the cardiovascular system were all assessed as unrelated to clodronate disodium therapy since alternative causalities were evident (e.g. heart failure prior to clodronate disodium therapy).

Endocrine and Metabolism: Adverse events affecting the calcium homeostasis leading to hypocalcemia were all assessed as possible or probable and reflect the calcium lowering properties of clodronate disodium.

Immune: Patient surveillance encompassing about 2700 patient-years treated with clodronate disodium detected five cases of acute non-lymphocytic leukemia or myelodysplasia in patients without multiple myeloma, and two cases in patients with multiple myeloma (two patients with multiple myeloma also developed non-lymphocytic leukemia while receiving placebo). The causal relationship to clodronate disodium or to the underlying disease has not been established. Appropriate monitoring of hematological parameters, including white cell count is still advised.

Hypersensitivity reactions, including angioedema, urticaria, rash and/or pruritus, in association with oral or parenteral clodronate disodium, have been reported in two patients.

Musculoskeletal: Adverse events reported as spontaneous fractures were all assessed as unrelated to clodronate disodium therapy since alternative causalities were evident (e.g. deficient immune state in patients suffering from advanced malignant diseases).

Respiratory: Adverse events affecting the respiratory system were all assessed as unrelated to clodronate disodium therapy since alternative causalities were evident (e.g. pneumonia).

A case of a bronchospastic reaction in a female patient suffering from an acetylsalicylic acid-sensitive asthma bronchiole has been reported after administration of i.v. clodronate disodium.

Abnormal Hematologic and Clinical Chemistry Findings: Hypercalcemia of malignancy is frequently associated with abnormal elevation in serum creatinine and BUN. Transient increases in serum creatinine were observed during clodronate disodium therapy. Although in some cases a causal relationship could not be excluded with certainty, the assessment of causality is difficult since in longstanding hypercalcemia, an impairment in renal function, possibly due to the nephrocalcinosis, can reasonably be expected. Careful monitoring of renal function is advised. Transient proteinuria and oliguria have also been reported in few cases immediately following single infusion use of i.v. clodronate disodium.

A causal relationship between clodronate disodium and liver function abnormalities, i.e. increased liver enzymes (ALT, AP, LDH) is also difficult to assess. Pre-existing liver metastases and abnormal liver function values often exist prior to therapy with clodronate disodium. Causal relationship, however, cannot be excluded with certainty in some patients. Careful monitoring of liver function values is advised.

Post-Market Adverse Drug Reactions: Cases of osteonecrosis (primarily involving the jaws) have been reported in patients treated with bisphosphonates. The majority of the reported cases are in cancer patients attendant to a dental procedure. Osteonecrosis of the jaw has multiple well documented risk factors including a diagnosis of cancer, concomitant therapies (e.g. chemotherapy, radiotherapy, corticosteroids) and co-morbid conditions (e.g. anemia, coagulopathies, infection, pre-existing oral disease).

Although causality cannot be determined, it is prudent to avoid dental surgery as recovery may be prolonged (see Warnings and Precautions, Musculoskeletal).

DRUG INTERACTIONS: Overview: Compatibility with i.v. solutions: CLASTEON should not be mixed with calcium-containing intravenous infusions. CLASTEON i.v. is a concentrate for intravenous infusion which **must** be diluted before use. The only recommended diluents are 0.9% w/v sodium chloride injection, USP or 5% w/v dextrose, USP. A single (1) 10 mL ampoule (for multiple infusion use) or five (5) 10 mL ampoules (for single infusion use) of CLASTEON i.v. (300 mg/10 mL) should be added aseptically to 500 mL of 0.9% w/v sodium chloride injection, USP or 5% w/v dextrose, USP. No other drugs or nutrients may be added (see Dosage and Administration).

Drug-Drug Interactions: The use of clodronate disodium with other agents indicated for reduction of calcium such as corticosteroids, phosphate, calcitonin, mithramycin, loop-diuretics may result in increased hypocalcemic effect depending on tumour type and pathophysiological situation.

Concurrent use of antacids or any drug containing calcium, iron, magnesium or aluminum may prevent absorption of oral clodronate disodium.

Concomitant use of clodronate disodium with mithramycin and thiazides is not recommended.

Concomitant use of i.v. clodronate disodium and aminoglycosides can result in an increased incidence of hypocalcemia.

Concomitant use of clodronate disodium and NSAIDs may promote renal dysfunction. However, a synergistic action has not been established.

Drug-Food Interactions: Interactions with food have not been established.

Drug-Herb Interactions: Interactions with herbal products have not been established.

Drug-Laboratory Test Interactions: Since clodronate disodium binds to bone, CLASTEON may interfere with bone scintigraphy examinations.

DOSAGE AND ADMINISTRATION: Dosing Considerations: CLASTEON should not be mixed with calcium-containing intravenous infusions.

Recommended Dose and Dosage Adjustment: CLASTEON i.v. (concentrate for intravenous infusion): Single Infusion: Recommended dosage: The contents of five (5) 10 mL ampoules is administered by slow intravenous infusion over a period of not less than 4 hours.

Multiple Infusions: Recommended dosage: The contents of one (1) 10 mL ampoule is administered as a single daily dose over a period of 2 to 6 hours (see Administration).

Oral CLASTEON: Recommended dosage: The oral recommended daily maintenance dose following intravenous therapy is in the range of 1600 mg (4 capsules) to 2400 mg (6 capsules) given in single or two divided doses. Maximal recommended daily dose is 3200 mg (8 capsules).

Oral doses higher than 3200 mg daily have not been evaluated but would be likely to increase the frequency of adverse intestinal effects.

Dosage should be reduced in patients with severe renal impairment (see Contraindications, Warnings and Precautions).

Administration: CLASTEON i.v. (concentrate for intravenous infusion): CLASTEON i.v. may be administered either as a single infusion or as multiple infusions.

CLASTEON (clodronate disodium) for infusion is available as a concentrated preparation which must be diluted before use. The only recommended diluents are 0.9% w/v sodium chloride injection, USP or 5% w/v dextrose, USP.

Paravenous infiltration should be avoided. Local reactions may occur.

Single Infusion: Administration: Five (5) 10 mL ampoules of CLASTEON i.v. concentrate for intravenous infusion (300 mg/10 mL) is diluted aseptically with 500 mL of 0.9% w/v sodium chloride injections, USP or 5% w/v dextrose, USP and administered by slow intravenous infusion over a period of not less than 4 hours. As with any other highly concentrated i.v. solution there exists a potential for injection site symptoms if extravenous infiltration occurs. The infusion should be monitored closely to avoid infiltration. Prior to infusion of a single 1500 mg dose, it is important to establish and maintain full hydration with oral or i.v. fluids. Note: Other diluents should not be used. No other drugs or nutrients may be added.

Multiple Infusions: Administration: One (1) 10 mL ampoule of CLASTEON i.v. concentrate for intravenous infusion (300 mg/10 mL) is diluted aseptically with 500 mL of 0.9% w/v sodium chloride injection, USP or 5% w/v dextrose, USP and administered by slow intravenous infusion over a period of 2 to 6 hours. Slow infusion is important for safety. In patients with hypercalcemia it is recommended that oral or intravenous fluids be administered to establish or maintain full hydration.

Protect the diluted solution from temperatures below 15°C and above 30°C. The reconstituted solution of CLASTEON i.v. should be administered within 12 hours of preparation by slow intravenous infusion over a period of 2 to 6 hours.

Note: Other diluents should not be used. No other drugs or nutrients may be added.

Since the duration of treatment is adjusted in accordance with patient response, daily determination of serum calcium levels must be carried out. Duration of treatment by multiple intravenous infusions should not exceed 10 days.

Response: In most cases, elevated serum calcium levels can be reduced to normal within 2 to 5 days, which ever method of infusion is used. Following normalization, treatment should be continued with CLASTEON (clodronate disodium) 400 mg capsules in order to maintain normocalcemia. Should the serum calcium level rise again during oral treatment, the intravenous infusion can be reintroduced.

Prior to using clodronate disodium (single or multiple infusions) it is important to establish and maintain full hydration with oral or intravenous fluids.

Oral CLASTEON: Administration: CLASTEON (clodronate disodium) 400 mg blue and white gelatin capsules should be administered whole with copious fluids, but not with milk. The patient should not eat one hour before or after CLASTEON intake.

The duration of treatment is normally 6 months. Treatment, however, can be extended beyond 6 months depending on the course of the disease. Similarly it may be necessary to restart treatment after an interruption.

Retreatment: No formalized studies have been carried out with respect to retreatment. Clinical experience shows that patients with re-increased serum calcium after termination of therapy with clodronate disodium or during oral administration may be retreated either with a higher oral dosage (up to 3200 mg/day) or with the i.v. infusion preparation as a single infusion (1500 mg/day) or multiple infusions (300 mg/day). Oral or i.v. treatment should be chosen dependant on the severity of hypercalcemia.

It is recommended that appropriate monitoring of renal function with serum creatinine and/or blood urea nitrogen be carried out during treatment. Serum calcium and phosphate should be monitored periodically. Appropriate monitoring of hepatic function and hematological parameters, including white cell count is advised.

OVERDOSAGE:

There is a lack of documented experience on acute overdosing with clodronate disodium. An overdose of the intravenous preparation could provoke renal damage. Renal function should be monitored. Overdosage may result in hypocalcemia. Careful monitoring for several days for signs and symptoms of hypocalcemia is recommended in cases where the dose given was too high in relation to initial serum calcium (see Warnings and Precautions, Monitoring and Laboratory Tests). Oral or parenteral calcium supplementation may be required to restore plasma calcium levels.

Gastric lavage may be used to remove unabsorbed drug following acute oral overdosage.

> For management of a suspected drug overdose, CPhA recommends that you contact your **regional Poison Control Centre**. See the *CPS* Directory section for a list of Poison Control Centres.

ACTION AND CLINICAL PHARMACOLOGY: Mechanism of Action: CLASTEON (clodronate disodium) belongs to the class of bisphosphonates which act primarily on bone. This tissue specificity is due to the high affinity of bisphosphonates for calcium phosphate crystals. Clodronate disodium forms complexes with the hydroxyapatite of bone, altering the crystalline structure in such a way that dissolution of the crystals is inhibited.

The major effect of clodronate disodium is to inhibit osteoclast-mediated bone resorption without an inhibitory effect on mineralization. In responsive patients, inhibition of abnormal bone resorption by clodronate disodium leads to the management of osteolytic bone metastases and, if present, reduction of hypercalcemia.

Pharmacodynamics: In patients with bone metastases, clodronate prevents the progression of bone destruction. Prevention of the progression and dissemination of existing metastases, as well as the formation of new skeletal metastases has been demonstrated both by scintigraphy and by radiography. In normocalcemic patients, the anti-osteolytic action of clodronate disodium is also clearly shown in reduced urinary calcium and hydroxyproline excretion. During and also after intravenous administration of clodronate disodium, the elevated serum calcium decreases, in some rare instances to hypocalcemic levels.

Several variables interfere with a precise assessment of the duration of the effect. Variations in the tumour load, in the amount and type of osteolytic mediators produced by the tumour cells, concomitant anticancer therapy and the renal handling of calcium can influence the duration of action.

In hypercalcemic patients, after successful treatment patients remain normocalcemic for some days up to several weeks. In general they become hypercalcemic again within 2-3 weeks after termination of therapy with clodronate disodium.

Clodronate disodium is not metabolized and is excreted unchanged by the kidneys. In calcium homeostasis the kidneys have a prominent role. Skeletal osteolysis may be accompanied by the pathogenesis of hypercalcemia and renal dysfunction may occur. At the time of diagnosis most hypercalcemic patients are significantly dehydrated.

The antagonistic effects of calcium on the action of antidiuretic hormone impair the renal concentration mechanisms resulting in polyuria and excessive fluid loss. Hydration status is further compromised by reduction of oral fluid intake due to nausea, vomiting and mental status. Prior to initiation of therapy with clodronate disodium, the state of negative fluid balance requires vigorous and adequate hydration with isotonic saline (0.9% w/v).

Normalization of blood calcium levels by clodronate disodium in adequately hydrated patients may also normalize suppressed plasma parathyroid hormone (PTH) levels and decrease urinary calcium, hydroxyproline and phosphate excretion.

Pharmacokinetics: Clodronate disodium is rapidly cleared from the blood. The mean value for plasma half-life after oral administration of clodronate disodium is 5.6 h. About 20% of the quantity absorbed is bound to bone. Since no biotransformation occurs, the drug is exclusively cleared by the kidneys at a rate of about 80 mL/min., when kidney function is normal. As with all bisphosphonates, the intestinal absorption and bioavailability of clodronate disodium after oral administration is low (1-3%).

After i.v. dose, clodronate disodium exhibits a plasma concentration profile which fits a two-compartment model with a $t_{½α}$ approximately 0.3 h and a $t_{½β}$ approximately 2 h, and terminal elimination phase with $t_{½}$ approximately 13 h. The latter accounts for 10-15% of renal excretion. Total clearance is about 110 mL/min. and renal clearance is approximately 90 mL/min. Volume of distribution is approximately 20 L.

The clinical effect of clodronate disodium is based on its concentration at the site of action, i.e. in bone tissue. Its half-life is dependent on the rate of skeletal turnover. When the bound substance is released from bone tissue during bone resorption, high local concentrations develop at the site of osteolysis, which has a direct action on the bone-resorbing osteoclasts.

STORAGE AND STABILITY: CLASTEON (clodronate disodium) i.v. (concentrate for intravenous infusion) and blue and white gelatin capsules should be stored at room temperature (15-30°C). Protect from high humidity.

Storage of Diluted Solution: Protect the diluted solution from temperatures below 15°C and above 30°C. The reconstituted solution of CLASTEON i.v. should be administered within 12 hours of preparation by slow intravenous infusion over a period of 2 to 6 hours.

INFORMATION FOR THE PATIENT: Published in e-CPS, available by subscription at www.e-cps.ca.

DOSAGE FORMS, COMPOSITION AND PACKAGING: Capsules: Each blue and white gelatin capsule contains: clodronate disodium 400 mg. Nonmedicinal ingredients: gelatin, indigotin, magnesium stearate, maize starch, sodium starch glycolate, talc and titanium oxide. Blister packs of 120 capsules per box. Boxes of 120 capsules contain 12 blister strips (10 capsules/blister strip).

Concentrate for Intravenous Infusion: Each 10 mL sterile ampoule contains: clodronate disodium 300 mg. Nonmedicinal ingredients: disodium hydrogen carbonate. Boxes of 5 ampoules.

Clavulin® Ⓟ

amoxicillin—clavulanic acid

Antibiotic—β-lactamase Inhibitor

GlaxoSmithKline

Date of Revision: May 18, 2010

PHARMACOLOGY: Amoxicillin exerts a bactericidal action against sensitive organisms during the stage of active multiplication, through the inhibition of the biosynthesis of bacterial cell wall mucopeptides. Clavulanic acid inhibits specific β-lactamases of some microorganisms and allows amoxicillin to inhibit amoxicillin (ampicillin)-resistant organisms which produce clavulanic acid sensitive β-lactamases.

INDICATIONS: For the treatment of the following infections when caused by CLAVULIN-susceptible strains of the designated bacteria: Upper respiratory tract infections when caused by β-lactamase producing strains of *S. aureus*. Sinusitis when caused by β-lactamase producing strains of *H. influenzae* or *M. (B.) catarrhalis*. Otitis media when caused by β-lactamase producing strains of *H. influenzae* or *M. (B.) catarrhalis*. Lower respiratory tract infections when caused by β-lactamase producing strains of *H. influenzae, K. pneumoniae, S. aureus* or *M. (B.) catarrhalis*. Skin and soft tissue infections when caused by β-lactamase producing strains of *S. aureus*. Urinary tract infections when caused by β-lactamase producing strains of *E. coli, P. mirabilis* or Klebsiella species.

While CLAVULIN is indicated only for the conditions listed above, infections caused by ampicillin (amoxicillin) susceptible organisms are also amenable to CLAVULIN treatment due to its amoxicillin content. Furthermore, mixed infections caused by organisms susceptible to ampicillin (amoxicillin) and β-lactamase producing organisms susceptible to CLAVULIN should not require the addition of another antibiotic.

Appropriate culture and susceptibility studies should be performed to identify the causative organism(s) and determine its (their) susceptibility to CLAVULIN. However, when there is reason to believe an infection may involve any of the β-lactamase producing organisms listed above, therapy may be instituted prior to obtaining the results from bacteriological and susceptibility studies. Once these results are known, therapy should be adjusted if appropriate.

CONTRAINDICATIONS: In patients with a history of hypersensitivity to the penicillin, or cephalosporin group of β-lactams.

In patients where infectious mononucleosis is either suspected or confirmed.

In patients with a previous history of CLAVULIN-associated jaundice/hepatic dysfunction.

WARNINGS: Serious and occasionally fatal hypersensitivity reactions (anaphylaxis and angioedema) have been reported in patients on penicillin therapy, including CLAVULIN. Although these reactions are more frequent following parenteral therapy, they have occurred in patients receiving penicillins orally. These reactions are more apt to occur in individuals with a history of sensitivity to multiple allergens. There have been reports of individuals with a history of cephalosporin hypersensitivity who have experienced severe reactions when treated with penicillins. Before initiating therapy with CLAVULIN, careful inquiry should be made concerning previous hypersensitivity reactions to penicillins, cephalosporins, or other allergens.

If an allergic reaction occurs, the administration of CLAVULIN should be discontinued and appropriate therapy should be instituted. Serious anaphylactoid reactions require immediate emergency treatment with epinephrine. Oxygen, i.v. steroids, and airway management, including intubation, should also be used as indicated.

Abnormal prolongation of prothrombin time (increased international normalized ratio (INR)) has been reported in patients receiving CLAVULIN and oral anticoagulants. Appropriate monitoring should be undertaken when anticoagulants are prescribed concurrently. Adjustments in the dose of oral anticoagulants may be necessary to maintain the desired level of anticoagulation.

CLAVULIN should be used with caution in patients with evidence of hepatic dysfunction. Hepatic toxicity associated with the use of CLAVULIN is usually reversible. On rare occasions, deaths have been reported (less than 1 death reported per estimated 4 million prescriptions worldwide). These have generally been cases associated with serious underlying diseases or concomitant medications (see Contraindications and Adverse Effects, Liver).

In patients with reduced urine output, crystalluria has been observed very rarely, predominantly with parenteral therapy. During the administration of high doses of amoxicillin, it is advisable to maintain adequate fluid intake and urinary output in order to reduce the possibility of amoxicillin crystalluria (see Overdose).

PRECAUTIONS: General: Periodic assessment of renal, hepatic, and hematopoietic function should be made during prolonged therapy with CLAVULIN.

The possibility of superinfections with mycotic or bacterial pathogens should be kept in mind during therapy with CLAVULIN. If superinfection should occur (usually involving Aerobacter, Pseudomonas, or Candida), the administration of CLAVULIN should be discontinued and appropriate therapy instituted.

The occurrence of a morbilliform rash following the use of ampicillin in patients with infectious mononucleosis is well documented. This reaction has also been reported following the use of amoxicillin. A similar reaction would also be expected with CLAVULIN.

Prolonged use may also occasionally result in overgrowth of non-susceptible organisms.

CLAVULIN Suspensions, which contain aspartame, should be used with caution in patients with phenylketonuria.

C. difficile-associated Disease: *C. difficile*-associated disease (CDAD) has been reported with the use of many antibacterial agents, including CLAVULIN. CDAD may range in severity from mild diarrhea to fatal colitis. It is important to consider this diagnosis in patients who present with diarrhea, or symptoms of colitis, pseudomembranous colitis, toxic megacolon, or perforation of colon subsequent to the administration of any antibacterial agent.

CDAD has been reported to occur over 2 months after the administration of antibacterial agents.

Treatment with antibacterial agents may alter the normal flora of the colon and may permit overgrowth of *C. difficile*. *C. difficile* produces toxins A and B, which contribute to the development of CDAD. CDAD may cause significant morbidity and mortality. CDAD can be refractory to antimicrobial therapy.

If the diagnosis of CDAD is suspected or confirmed, appropriate therapeutic measures should be initiated. Mild cases of CDAD usually respond to discontinuation of antibacterial agents not directed against *C. difficile*. In moderate to severe cases, consideration should be given to management with fluids and electrolytes, protein supplementation, and treatment with an antibacterial agent clinically effective against *C. difficile*. Surgical evaluation should be instituted as clinically indicated, as surgical intervention may be required in certain severe cases (see Adverse Effects).

Renal: CLAVULIN is excreted mostly by the kidney. There are insufficient data to make specific dosage recommendations for patients with renal dysfunction. However, either a reduction in dose level or an extension in dose interval in proportion to the degree of loss of renal function will be needed.

Pregnancy: In a single study in women with preterm, premature rupture of the fetal membranes (pPROM), it was reported that prophylactic treatment with CLAVULIN may be associated with an increased risk of necrotising enterocolitis in neonates. Use should be avoided in pregnancy, unless considered essential by the physician.

Lactation: Penicillins (including ampicillin) have been shown to be excreted in human breast milk. It is not known whether clavulanic acid is excreted in breast milk. Caution should be exercised if CLAVULIN is to be administered to a nursing mother.

Drug Interactions: In common with other broad spectrum antibiotics, amoxicillin-clavulanate may reduce the efficacy of combined oral contraceptives by altering the gut-flora to result in lower estrogen reabsorption. Concomitant use of probenecid is not recommended, and may result in increased and prolonged blood levels of amoxicillin, but not of clavulanic acid.

Increases in prothrombin time, INR or bleeding have been reported in patients maintained on coumarin anticoagulants, such as acenocoumarol and warfarin and then coadministered amoxicillin or CLAVULIN. If coadministration is necessary, the prothrombin time or INR should be carefully monitored upon antibiotic addition or withdrawal.

Children: Because of incompletely developed renal function in neonates and young infants, the elimination of amoxicillin may be delayed. Dosing of CLAVULIN should be modified in pediatric patients younger than 12 weeks (3 months) (see Dosage, Children).

In infants 12 weeks (3 months) of age or older and in children, b.i.d. use of the CLAVULIN 200 and 400 mg formulations is recommended because of a significantly reduced incidence of diarrhea with the b.i.d. regimen (see Adverse Effects).

ADVERSE EFFECTS: The following adverse reactions have been observed during therapy with CLAVULIN.

Gastrointestinal: Diarrhea has been reported very commonly in adults and commonly in children. Nausea and vomiting have been reported commonly in adults and children. Abdominal cramps, flatulence, constipation, anorexia, colic pain, acid stomach, intestinal candidiasis, antibiotic-associated colitis (including pseudomembranous colitis and haemorrhagic colitis) have been reported rarely. Mucocutaneous candidiasis has been reported commonly. If gastrointestinal reactions are evident, they may be reduced by taking CLAVULIN at the start of the meal.

A US-Canadian clinical trial compared a 10-day CLAVULIN b.i.d. regimen (45/6.4 mg/kg/day q12h) with a 10-day CLAVULIN t.i.d. regimen (40/10 mg/kg/day q8h) in 575 patients with acute otitis media, aged 2 months to 12 years. The incidence of diarrhea was significantly lower in patients who received the b.i.d. regimen compared to patients who received the t.i.d. regimen (9.6% vs 26.7%; p<0.001). Significantly fewer patients who received the b.i.d. regimen withdrew due to diarrhea compared to patients receiving the t.i.d. regimen (2.8% vs 7.6%; p=0.009). The incidence of related/possibly related diaper rash was also lower in patients who received the b.i.d. regimen compared to patients who received the t.i.d. regimen (3.1% vs 6.6%; p=0.054).

Data from 2 pivotal studies in 1191 patients treated for either lower respiratory tract infections or complicated urinary tract infections compared a regimen of 875 mg CLAVULIN tablets every 12 hours with 500 mg CLAVULIN tablets dosed every 8 hours.

The most frequently reported adverse event was diarrhea; incidence rates were similar (14.9% and 14.3% respectively) for the 875 mg every 12 hours and 500 mg every 8 hours dosing regimens. However, there was a statistically significant difference in rates of moderate/severe diarrhea between the regimens: 3.4% for 875 mg every 12 hours dosing vs 5.9% for the 500 mg every 8 hours dosing.

Hypersensitivity: Erythematous maculopapular rash, urticaria, anaphylaxis, hypersensitivity vasculitis and pruritus. A morbilliform rash in patients with mononucleosis. Rarely erythema multiforme and Stevens-Johnson syndrome have been reported. Other reactions, including angioedema, toxic epidermal necrolysis and exfoliative dermatitis, and acute generalized exanthematous pustulosis (AGEP) as in the case of other β-lactam antibiotics, have been seen rarely. Interstitial nephritis can occur rarely.

Note: Urticaria, other skin rashes, and serum sickness-like reactions may be controlled with antihistamines and if necessary systemic corticosteroids. Whenever such reactions occur, CLAVULIN should be discontinued, unless, in the opinion of the physician, the condition being treated is life-threatening and amenable only to CLAVULIN therapy.

Liver: Transient hepatitis and cholestatic jaundice have been reported rarely. These events have been noted with other penicillins and cephalosporins. The hepatic events associated with CLAVULIN may be severe, and occur predominantly in males and elderly patients and may be associated with prolonged treatment. These events have been very rarely reported in children. Signs and symptoms usually occur during or shortly after treatment, but in some cases may not become apparent until several weeks after treatment has ceased. The hepatic events are usually reversible. However, in extremely rare circumstances, deaths have been reported. These have almost always been cases associated with serious underlying disease or concomitant medications. Moderate rises in AST, alkaline phosphatase, lactic dehydrogenase, and/or ALT have been noted in patients treated with ampicillin class antibiotics. The significance of these findings is unknown.

Hemic and Lymphatic Systems: As with other β-lactams, anemia, hemolytic anemia, thrombocytopenia, thrombocytopenic purpura, eosinophilia, leukopenia, lymphocytopenia, basophilia, slight increase in platelets, neutropenia and agranulocytosis have been reported rarely during therapy with the penicillins. These reactions are usually reversible on discontinuation of therapy and are believed to be hypersensitivity phenomena. Prolongation of bleeding time and prolongation of prothrombin time have also been reported.

Central Nervous Systems Effects: Convulsions may occur with impaired renal function or in those receiving high doses.

Renal and Urinary Tract Disorders: Very rare: crystalluria and interstitial nephritis (see Overdose, Symptoms and Treatment).

Other: vaginitis, headache, bad taste, dizziness, malaise, glossitis, black hairy tongue and stomatitis. Tooth discoloration has been reported very rarely in children and adults. Good oral hygiene may help to prevent tooth discoloration as it can often be removed by brushing.

OVERDOSE:

Symptoms: Many patients have been asymptomatic following overdosage or have experienced primarily gastrointestinal symptoms including stomach and abdominal pain, vomiting, and diarrhea. Rash, hyperactivity, or drowsiness have also been observed in a small number of patients. Amoxicillin crystalluria, in some cases leading to renal failure, has been observed (see Warnings for use).

Treatment: In the case of overdosage, discontinue CLAVULIN, treat symptomatically, and institute supportive measures as required. If gastrointestinal symptoms and disturbance of the fluid and electrolyte balances are evident, they may be treated symptomatically. CLAVULIN can be removed from the circulation by hemodialysis. If the overdosage is very recent and there is no contraindication, an attempt at emesis or other means of removal of drug from the stomach may be performed. A prospective study of 51 pediatric patients at a poison centre suggested that overdosages of less than 250 mg/kg of amoxicillin are not associated with significant clinical symptoms and do not require gastric emptying. Interstitial nephritis resulting in oliguric renal failure has been reported in a small number of patients after overdosage with amoxicillin. Renal impairment appears to be reversible with cessation of drug administration. High blood levels may occur more readily in patients with impaired renal function because of decreased renal clearance of both amoxicillin and clavulanate. Both amoxicillin and clavulanate are removed from the circulation by hemodialysis.

> For management of a suspected drug overdose, contact your **regional Poison Control Centre**. See the *CPS* Directory section for a list of Poison Control Centres.

DOSAGE: While CLAVULIN can be given without regard to meals, absorption of clavulanic acid when taken with food is greater relative to the fasted state. Dosing in the fasted or fed state has minimal effect on the pharmacokinetics of amoxicillin. The safety and efficacy of CLAVULIN have been established in clinical trials where CLAVULIN was taken without regard to meals.

Adults: The usual adult dose is 1 CLAVULIN 500 mg tablet every 12 hours. For more severe infections and infections of the lower respiratory tract, the dose should be 1 CLAVULIN 875 mg tablet every 12 hours or 1 CLAVULIN 500 mg tablet every 8 hours.

Children: Based on the amoxicillin component, CLAVULIN should be dosed as in Table 1 in patients aged 12 weeks (3 months) and older.

Table 1: CLAVULIN

Dosage for Children Aged 12 Weeks (3 months) and Older

Infection	Severity	Dosing Regimen b.i.d.[a]	Dosing Regimen t.i.d.
Urinary Tract; Upper Respiratory Tract; Skin and Soft Tissue	Mild to moderate	25 mg/kg/day in divided doses every 12 hours	20 mg/kg/day in divided doses every 8 hours
	Severe	45 mg/kg/day in divided doses every 12 hours	40 mg/kg/day in divided doses every 8 hours
Lower Respiratory Tract; Sinusitis		45 mg/kg/day in divided doses every 12 hours	40 mg/kg/day in divided doses every 8 hours
Otitis Media[b]			40 mg/kg/day in divided doses every 8 hours

[a] The b.i.d. regimen is recommended as it is associated with significantly less diarrhea.
[b] Duration of therapy studied and recommended for acute otitis media is 10 days.

The normal duration of treatment was 7 to 10 days. However, in general, treatment should be continued for a minimum of 48 to 72 hours beyond the time that the patient becomes asymptomatic or evidence of bacterial eradication has been obtained. It is recommended that there be at least 10 days treatment for any infection caused by β-hemolytic streptococci to prevent the occurrence of acute rheumatic fever or glomerulonephritis.

Neonates and children aged <12 weeks (3 months): Due to incompletely developed renal function affecting elimination of amoxicillin in this age group, the recommended dose of CLAVULIN is 30 mg/kg/day divided every 12 hours, based on the amoxicillin component. Clavulanate elimination is unaltered in this age group. Experience with the 200 mg/5 mL formulation in this age group is limited and, thus, use of the 125 mg/5 mL oral suspension is recommended.

The children's dosage should not exceed that recommended for adults. Children weighing more than 38 kg should be dosed according to the adult recommendations.

Table 2 may be used as a guide to determine the dosage of oral suspension (CLAVULIN-125F or CLAVULIN-250F) according to body weight.

Table 2: CLAVULIN

Pediatric Dosage Schedule for CLAVULIN-125F and CLAVULIN-250F Oral Suspensions

Body Weight (kg)	20 mg/kg/day dosing regimen[a]: Total Daily Dose[b] (mg)	20 mg/kg/day: Volume (mL) of Reconstituted Oral Suspension Every 8 Hours — CLAVULIN-125F	20 mg/kg/day: Volume (mL) of Reconstituted Oral Suspension Every 8 Hours — CLAVULIN-250F	40 mg/kg/day dosing regimen[a]: Total Daily Dose[b] (mg)	40 mg/kg/day: Volume (mL) of Reconstituted Oral Suspension Every 8 Hours — CLAVULIN-125F	40 mg/kg/day: Volume (mL) of Reconstituted Oral Suspension Every 8 Hours — CLAVULIN-250F
5	125	1.3	0.7	250	2.7	1.3
7	175	1.9	0.9	350	3.7	1.9
10	250	2.7	1.3	500	5.3	2.7
12	300	3.2	1.6	600	6.4	3.2
14	350	3.7	1.9	700	7.5	3.7
16	400	4.3	2.1	800	8.5	4.3
18	450	4.8	2.4	900	9.6	4.8
20	500	5.3	2.7	1000	10.7	5.3
25	625	6.7	3.3	1250	13.3	6.7
30	750	8.0	4.0	1500	16.0	8.0
35	875	9.3	4.7	1750	18.7	9.3
38	950	10.1	5.1	1900	20.3	10.1

(cont'd)

Table 2: CLAVULIN *(cont'd)*

Pediatric Dosage Schedule for CLAVULIN-125F and CLAVULIN-250F Oral Suspensions

[a] Based on amoxicillin component.
[b] Dosages are expressed in terms of amoxicillin plus clavulanic acid. These 2 ingredients are in a ratio of 4:1 in both oral suspensions, CLAVULIN-125F and CLAVULIN-250F.

20 mL of reconstituted CLAVULIN-125F oral suspension or 10 mL of reconstituted CLAVULIN-250F oral suspension are equivalent to 1 CLAVULIN-500F tablet.

Table 3 may be used as a guide to determine the dosage of oral suspension (CLAVULIN-200 or CLAVULIN-400) according to body weight.

Table 3: CLAVULIN

Pediatric Dosage Schedule for CLAVULIN-200 and CLAVULIN-400 Oral Suspensions

Body Weight (kg)	25 mg/kg/day dosing regimen[a]: Total Daily Dose[b] (mg)	25 mg/kg/day: Volume (mL) of Reconstituted Oral Suspension Every 12 Hours — CLAVULIN-200	25 mg/kg/day: Volume (mL) of Reconstituted Oral Suspension Every 12 Hours — CLAVULIN-400	45 mg/kg/day dosing regimen[a]: Total Daily Dose[b] (mg)	45 mg/kg/day: Volume (mL) of Reconstituted Oral Suspension Every 12 Hours — CLAVULIN-200	45 mg/kg/day: Volume (mL) of Reconstituted Oral Suspension Every 12 Hours — CLAVULIN-400
5	143	1.6	0.8	257	2.8	1.4
7	200	2.2	1.1	360	3.9	2.0
10	286	3.1	1.6	514	5.6	2.8
12	343	3.8	1.9	617	6.8	3.4
14	400	4.4	2.2	720	7.9	3.9
16	458	5.0	2.5	822	9.0	4.5
18	515	5.6	2.8	925	10.1	5.1
20	572	6.3	3.1	1028	11.3	5.6
25	715	7.8	3.9	1285	14.1	7.0
30	858	9.4	4.7	1542	16.9	8.4
35	1001	11.0	5.5	1799	19.7	9.8
38	1087	11.9	5.9	1953	21.4	10.7

[a] Based on amoxicillin component.
[b] Dosages are expressed in terms of amoxicillin plus clavulanic acid. These 2 ingredients are in a ratio of 7:1 in both oral suspensions, CLAVULIN-200 and CLAVULIN-400.

A calibrated dropper should be used to measure the appropriate volume for dosing.

Reconstitution: Reconstitute powder for oral suspension with purified water.

CLAVULIN-125F Powder for Oral Suspension: The approximate average concentration after reconstitution is 125 mg of amoxicillin (as the trihydrate) and 31.25 mg of clavulanic acid (as the potassium salt) per 5 mL. See Table 4.

Table 4: CLAVULIN

Reconstitution—CLAVULIN-125F

Bottle Size	Volume to Be Added
100 mL	92 mL

CLAVULIN-200 Powder for Oral Suspension: The approximate average concentration after reconstitution is 200 mg of amoxicillin (as the trihydrate) and 28.5 mg of clavulanic acid (as the potassium salt) per 5 mL. See Table 5.

Table 5: CLAVULIN

Reconstitution—CLAVULIN-200

Bottle Size	Volume to Be Added
70 mL	64 mL

CLAVULIN-250F Powder for Oral Suspension: The approximate average concentration after reconstitution is 250 mg of amoxicillin (as the trihydrate) and 62.5 mg of clavulanic acid (as the potassium salt) per 5 mL. See Table 6.

Table 6: CLAVULIN
Reconstitution—CLAVULIN-250F

Bottle Size	Volume to Be Added
100 mL	90 mL

CLAVULIN-400 Powder for Oral Suspension: The approximate average concentration after reconstitution is 400 mg of amoxicillin (as the trihydrate) and 57 mg of clavulanic acid (as the potassium salt) per 5 mL. See Table 7.

Table 7: CLAVULIN
Reconstitution—CLAVULIN-400

Bottle Size	Volume to Be Added
70 mL	62 mL

Shake vigorously.

Stability and Storage: **Oral Suspensions:** Store powder in a dry place at room temperature (15 to 25°C). Use the powder only if its appearance is white to off-white.

The reconstituted CLAVULIN-125F and CLAVULIN-250F oral suspension should be stored under refrigeration and should be used within 10 days.

The reconstituted CLAVULIN-200 and CLAVULIN-400 oral suspension should be stored under refrigeration and should be used within 7 days.

Keep bottle tightly closed at all times.

Tablets: Store in a dry place at room temperature (15 to 25°C).

SUPPLIED: Suspension: CLAVULIN-125F: Each 5 mL of reconstituted suspension contains: amoxicillin 125 mg as the trihydrate and clavulanic acid 31.25 mg as the potassium salt (in a ratio of 4:1). Nonmedicinal ingredients: aspartame, colloidal silica, flavors (golden syrup dry, orange dry 1, orange dry 2, raspberry dry), hydroxypropyl methylcellulose, silicon dioxide, succinic acid and xanthan gum. Bottles of 100.

CLAVULIN-200: Each 5 mL of reconstituted suspension contains amoxicillin 200 mg as the trihydrate and clavulanic acid 28.5 mg as the potassium salt (in a ratio of 7:1). Nonmedicinal ingredients: aspartame, colloidal silica, flavors (golden syrup dry, orange dry 1, orange dry 2, raspberry dry), hydroxypropyl methylcellulose, silicon dioxide, succinic acid and xanthan gum. Bottles of 70 mL.

CLAVULIN-250F: Each 5 mL of reconstituted suspension contains: amoxicillin 250 mg as the trihydrate and clavulanic acid 62.5 mg as the potassium salt (in a ratio of 4:1). Nonmedicinal ingredients: aspartame, colloidal silica, flavors (golden syrup dry, orange dry 1, orange dry 2, raspberry dry), hydroxypropyl methylcellulose, silicon dioxide, succinic acid and xanthan gum. Bottles of 100.

CLAVULIN-400: Each 5 mL of reconstituted suspension contains: amoxicillin 400 mg as the trihydrate and clavulanic acid 57 mg as the potassium salt (in a ratio of 7:1). Nonmedicinal ingredients: aspartame, colloidal silica, flavors (golden syrup dry, orange dry 1, orange dry 2, raspberry dry), hydroxypropyl methylcellulose, silicon dioxide, succinic acid and xanthan gum. Bottles of 70 mL.

Tablets: CLAVULIN-500F: Each white to off white oval film-coated tablet, scored and debossed with 'AC' on only one side, and plain on the other, contains: amoxicillin 500 mg as the trihydrate and clavulanic acid 125 mg as the potassium salt (in a ratio of 4:1). Nonmedicinal ingredients: colloidal silica, dimethicone 500, hydroxypropyl methylcellulose (methocel E5), hydroxypropyl methylcellulose (methocel E15), magnesium stearate, microcrystalline cellulose, polyethylene glycol 4000, polyethylene glycol 6000, sodium starch glycolate and titanium dioxide. Bottles of 100. Blister packs of 20.

CLAVULIN-875: Each white to off white, capsule-shaped tablet, debossed with 'AC' on both sides, and a scoreline on only one side, contains: amoxicillin 875 mg as the trihydrate and clavulanic acid 125 mg as the potassium salt (in a ratio of 7:1). Nonmedicinal ingredients: colloidal silica, dimethicone 500, hydroxypropyl methylcellulose (methocel E5), hydroxypropyl methylcellulose (methocel E15), magnesium stearate, microcrystalline cellulose, polyethylene glycol 4000, polyethylene glycol 6000, sodium starch glycolate and titanium dioxide. Bottles of 60. Blister packs of 20.

(Shown in Product Identification Section)

Climara® Ⓟ
estradiol-17β
Estrogen

Bayer

Date of Revision: March 7, 2007

SUMMARY PRODUCT INFORMATION:

Route of Administration	Dosage Form/ Strength	Clinically Relevant Nonmedicinal Ingredients
Topical	Transdermal system/ 0.025 mg/day 0.05 mg/day 0.075 mg/day 0.1 mg/day	Acrylate copolymer (consisting of isooctyl acrylate, acrylamide, vinyl acetate copolymer), ethyl oleate, glyceryl monolaurate, isopropyl myristate For a complete listing see Dosage Forms, Composition and Packaging.

INDICATIONS AND CLINICAL USE: Climara (estradiol hemihydrate transdermal system) is indicated for:

- the relief of menopausal and postmenopausal symptoms occurring in naturally or surgically induced estrogen deficiency states.

Climara 50, 75 and 100 are indicated for:

- the prevention of osteoporosis in naturally occurring or surgically induced estrogen-deficiency states. In post-menopausal women already diagnosed as having osteoporosis and vertebral fractures, treatment with Climara may retard further bone loss.

Climara 25 is not indicated for the prevention of osteoporosis.

When Climara is prescribed solely for the prevention of postmenopausal osteoporosis, it is to be considered in light of other available therapies. Adequate diet, calcium and vitamin D intake, cessation of smoking as well as regular physical weight bearing exercise are required in addition to the administration of Climara.

Climara should be prescribed with an appropriate dosage of a progestin for women with intact uteri, in order to prevent endometrial hyperplasia/carcinoma.

CONTRAINDICATIONS: Climara (estradiol hemihydrate transdermal system) should not be used in individuals with any of the following conditions:

- Hypersensitivity to this drug or to any ingredient in the formulation or component of the container. For a complete listing, see Dosage Forms, Composition and Packaging.
- Liver dysfunction or disease as long as liver function tests have failed to return to normal.
- Known or suspected estrogen-dependent malignant neoplasia (e.g. endometrial cancer).
- Endometrial hyperplasia.
- Known, suspected, or past history of breast cancer.
- Undiagnosed abnormal genital bleeding.
- Known or suspected pregnancy or lactation.
- Active or past history of arterial thromboembolic disease (e.g. stroke, myocardial infarction, coronary heart disease).
- Active or past history of confirmed venous thromboembolism (such as deep vein thrombosis or pulmonary embolism) or active thrombophlebitis.
- Partial or complete loss of vision due to ophthalmic vascular disease.
- Presence or history of liver tumours (benign or malignant)

WARNINGS AND PRECAUTIONS:

Serious Warnings and Precautions

The Women's Health Initiative (WHI) trial examined the health benefits and risks of oral combined estrogen plus progestin therapy (n=16 608) and oral estrogen-alone therapy (n=10,739) in postmenopausal women aged 50 to 79 years.

The estrogen plus progestin arm of the WHI trial (mean age 63.3 years) indicated an increased risk of myocardial infarction (MI), stroke, invasive breast cancer, pulmonary emboli and deep vein thrombosis in postmenopausal women receiving treatment with combined conjugated equine estrogens (CEE, 0.625 mg/day) and medroxyprogesterone acetate (MPA, 2.5 mg/day) for 5.2 years compared to those receiving placebo.

The estrogen-alone arm of the WHI trial (mean age 63.6 years) indicated an increased risk of stroke and deep vein thrombosis in hysterectomized women treated with CEE-alone (0.625 mg/day) for 6.8 years compared to those receiving placebo.

Other doses of oral conjugated estrogens with medroxyprogesterone acetate, and other combinations and dosage forms of estrogens and progestins were not studied in the WHI clinical trials and, in the absence of comparable data, these risks should be assumed to be similar.

Therefore, the following should be given serious consideration at the time of prescribing:

- Estrogens with or without progestins **should not** be prescribed for primary or secondary prevention of cardiovascular diseases.
- Estrogens with or without progestins should be prescribed at **the lowest effective dose** for the approved indication.
- Estrogens with or without progestins should be prescribed for **the shortest period** possible for the approved indication.
- For the prevention of osteoporosis, Climara (estradiol hemihydrate transdermal system) should be considered in light of other available therapies.

General: The effects of Climara on the ability to drive and use machines have not been studied.

Carcinogenesis and Mutagenesis: Breast Cancer: Available epidemiological data indicate that the use of combined estrogen plus progestin by postmenopausal women is associated with an increased risk of invasive breast cancer.

In the estrogen plus progestin arm of the WHI trial, among 10 000 women over a one year period, there were:

- 8 more cases of invasive breast cancer (38 on combined HRT versus 30 on placebo).

The WHI study also reported that the invasive breast cancers diagnosed in the estrogen plus progestin group were similar in histology but were larger (mean [SD], 1.7 cm [1.1] vs 1.5 cm [0.9], respectively; P=0.04) and were at a more advanced stage compared with those diagnosed in the placebo group. The percentage of women with abnormal mammograms (recommendations for short-interval follow-up, a suspicious abnormality, or highly suggestive of malignancy) was significantly higher in the estrogen plus progestin group versus the placebo group. This difference appeared at year one and persisted in each year thereafter.

In the estrogen-alone arm of the WHI trial, there was no statistically significant difference in the rate of invasive breast cancer in hysterectomized women treated with conjugated equine estrogens versus women treated with placebo.

It is recommended that estrogens not be given to women with existing breast cancer or those with a previous history of the disease (see Contraindications).

There is a need for caution in prescribing estrogens for women with known risk factors associated with the development of breast cancer, such as strong family history of breast cancer (first degree relative) or who present a breast condition with an increased risk (abnormal mammograms and/or atypical hyperplasia at breast biopsy).

Other known risk factors for the development of breast cancer such as nulliparity, obesity, early menarche, late age at first full term pregnancy and at menopause should also be evaluated.

It is recommended that women undergo mammography prior to the start of HRT treatment and at regular intervals during treatment, as deemed appropriate by the treating physician and according to the perceived risks for each patient. HRT increases the density of mammographic images which may adversely affect the radiological detection of breast cancer in some cases.

The overall benefits and possible risks of hormone replacement therapy should be fully considered and discussed with patients. It is important that the modest increased risk of being diagnosed with breast cancer after 4 years of treatment with combined estrogen plus progestin HRT (as reported in the results of the WHI trial) be discussed with the patient and weighed against its known benefits.

Instructions for regular self-examination of the breasts should be included in this counselling.

Endometrial Hyperplasia and Endometrial Carcinoma: Estrogen-only HRT increases the risk of endometrial hyperplasia if taken by women with intact uteri.

Estrogen should be prescribed with an appropriate dosage of progestin for women with intact uteri in order to prevent endometrial hyperplasia/carcinoma.

Clinical surveillance of all women taking estrogen/progestin combinations is important. Adequate diagnostic measures, including endometrial sampling when indicated, should be undertaken to rule out malignancy in all cases of undiagnosed persistent or recurring abnormal vaginal bleeding.

Cardiovascular: The results of the Heart and Estrogen/progestin Replacement Studies (HERS and HERS II) and the Women's Health Initiative (WHI) trial indicate that the use of estrogen plus progestin is associated with an increased risk of coronary heart disease (CHD) in postmenopausal women. The results of the WHI trial indicate that the use of estrogen-alone and estrogen plus progestin is associated with an increased risk of stroke in postmenopausal women.

WHI trial findings: In the combined estrogen plus progestin arm of the WHI trial, among 10 000 women over a one-year period, there were:

- 8 more cases of stroke (29 on combined HRT versus 21 on placebo)
- 7 more cases of CHD (37 on combined HRT versus 30 on placebo).

In the estrogen-alone arm of the WHI trial of women with prior hysterectomy, among 10 000 women over a one year period, there were/was:

- 12 more cases of stroke (44 on estrogen-alone therapy versus 32 on placebo)
- no statistically significant difference in the rate of CHD.

HERS and HERS II findings: In the Heart and Estrogen/progestin Replacement Study (HERS) of postmenopausal women with documented heart disease (n=2763, average age 66.7 years), a randomized placebo-controlled clinical trial of secondary prevention of coronary heart disease (CHD), treatment with 0.625 mg/day oral conjugated equine estrogen (CEE) plus 2.5 mg medroxyprogesterone acetate (MPA) demonstrated no cardiovascular benefit. Specifically, during an average follow-up of 4.1 years, treatment with CEE plus MPA did not reduce the overall rate of CHD events in postmenopausal women with established coronary heart disease. There were more CHD events in the hormone treated group than in the placebo group in year 1, but not during the subsequent years.

From the original HERS trial, 2321 women consented to participate in an open label extension of HERS known as HERS II. Average follow-up in HERS II was an additional 2.7 years, for a total of 6.8 years overall. After 6.8 years, hormone therapy did not reduce the risk of cardiovascular events in women with CHD.

Blood Pressure: Women using hormone replacement therapy sometimes experience increased blood pressure. Blood pressure should be monitored with HRT use. Elevation of blood pressure in previously normotensive or hypertensive patients should be investigated and HRT may have to be discontinued.

Ear/Nose/Throat: Estrogens should be used with caution in patients with otosclerosis.

Endocrine and Metabolism: Glucose and Lipid Metabolism: A worsening of glucose tolerance and lipid metabolism have been observed in a significant percentage of peri- and post-menopausal patients. Therefore, diabetic patients or those with a predisposition to diabetes should be observed closely to detect any alterations in carbohydrate or lipid metabolism, especially in triglyceride blood levels.

Women with familial hyperlipidemias need special surveillance. Lipid-lowering measures are recommended additionally, before treatment is started.

Women with porphyria need special surveillance.

Calcium and Phosphorus Metabolism: Because the prolonged use of estrogens influences the metabolism of calcium and phosphorus, estrogens should be used with caution in patients with metabolic and malignant bone diseases associated with hypercalcemia and in patients with renal insufficiency.

Hypothyroidism: Patients who require thyroid hormone replacement therapy and who are also taking estrogen should have their thyroid function monitored regularly to assure that thyroid hormone levels remain in an acceptable range (see Drug Interactions, Drug-Laboratory Test Interactions).

Genitourinary: Vaginal Bleeding: Abnormal vaginal bleeding, due to its prolongation, irregularity or heaviness, occurring during therapy should prompt appropriate diagnostic measures to rule out the possibility of uterine malignancy and the treatment should be re-evaluated.

Uterine Leiomyomata: Pre-existing uterine leiomyomata may increase in size during estrogen use. Growth, pain or tenderness of uterine leiomyomata requires discontinuation of medication and appropriate investigation.
Endometriosis: Symptoms and physical findings associated with a previous diagnosis of endometriosis may reappear or become aggravated with estrogen use.
Hematologic: Venous Thromboembolism: Available epidemiological data indicate that use of estrogen with or without progestin by postmenopausal women is associated with an increased risk of developing venous thromboembolism (VTE).

In the estrogen plus progestin arm of the WHI trial, among 10 000 women on combined HRT over a one-year period, there were 18 more cases of venous thromboembolism, including 8 more cases of pulmonary embolism.

In the estrogen-alone arm of the WHI trial, among 10 000 women on estrogen therapy over a one year period, there were 7 more cases of venous thromboembolism, although there was no statistically significant difference in the rate of pulmonary embolism.

Generally recognized risk factors for VTE include a personal history, a family history (the occurrence of VTE in a direct relative at a relatively early age may indicate genetic predisposition), severe obesity (body mass index >30 kg/m^2) and systemic lupus erythematosus. The risk of VTE also increases with age and smoking.

The risk of VTE may be temporarily increased with prolonged immobilization, major surgery or trauma. In women on HRT, attention should be given to prophylactic measures to prevent VTE following surgery. Also, patients with varicose veins should be closely supervised. The physician should be alert to the earliest manifestations of thrombotic disorders (thrombophlebitis, retinal thrombosis, cerebral embolism and pulmonary embolism). If these occur or are suspected, hormone therapy should be discontinued immediately, given the risks of long-term disability or fatality.

If feasible, estrogens should be discontinued at least 4 weeks before major surgery which may be associated with an increased risk of thromboembolism, or during periods of prolonged immobilization.
Hepatic/Biliary/Pancreatic: Gallbladder Disease: A 2- to 4-fold increase in the risk of gallbladder disease requiring surgery in women receiving postmenopausal estrogens has been reported.
Jaundice: Caution is advised in patients with a history of liver and/or biliary disorders. If cholestatic jaundice develops, or if there is a recurrence of cholestatic pruritis which first occurred during pregnancy or during previous use of sex steroids, the treatment should be discontinued and appropriate investigations carried out.
Liver Function Tests: Liver function tests should be done periodically in subjects who are suspected of having hepatic disease. For information on endocrine and liver function tests, see Monitoring and Laboratory Tests.
Hepatic Tumours: Benign hepatic adenomas have been associated with the use of combined estrogen and progestin oral contraceptives. Although benign and rare, these tumours may rupture and cause death from intra-abdominal hemorrhage. Such lesions have not yet been reported in association with other estrogen or progestin preparations, but they should be considered if abdominal pain and tenderness, abdominal mass, or hypovolemic shock occurs in patients receiving estrogen. Hepatocellular carcinoma has also been reported in women taking estrogen-containing oral contraceptives. The causal relationship of this malignancy to these drugs is not known.
Immune: Angioedema: Exogenous estrogens may induce or exacerbate symptoms of angioedema, in particular in women with hereditary angioedema.
Neurologic: Cerebrovascular Insufficiency: Patients who develop visual disturbances, classical migraine, transient aphasia, paralysis or loss of consciousness should discontinue medication.

Patients with a previous history of classical migraine and who develop a recurrence or worsening of migraine symptoms should be reevaluated.
Dementia: Available epidemiological data indicate that the use of combined estrogen plus progestin in women age 65 and over may increase the risk of developing probable dementia.

The Women's Health Initiative Memory Study (WHIMS), a clinical substudy of the WHI, was designed to assess whether postmenopausal hormone replacement therapy (oral estrogen plus progestin or oral estrogen-alone) reduces the risk of dementia in women aged 65 and over (age range 65-79 years) and free of dementia at baseline.
In the estrogen plus progestin arm of the WHIMS (n=4532), women with intact uteri were treated with daily 0.625 mg conjugated equine estrogens (CEE) plus 2.5 mg medroxyprogesterone acetate (MPA) or placebo for an average of 4.05 years. The results, when extrapolated to 10 000 women treated over a one-year period showed:
- 23 more cases of probable dementia (45 on combined HRT versus 22 on placebo).

In the estrogen-alone arm of the WHIMS (n=2947), women with prior hysterectomy were treated with daily 0.625 mg CEE or placebo for an average of 5.21 years. The results, when extrapolated to 10 000 women treated over a one year period showed:
- 12 more cases of probable dementia (37 on estrogen-alone versus 25 on placebo) although this difference did not reach statistical significance.

When data from the estrogen plus progestin arm of the WHIMS and the estrogen-alone arm of the WHIMS were combined, as per the original WHIMS protocol, in 10 000 women over a one-year period, there were:
- 18 more cases of probable dementia (41 on estrogen plus progestin or estrogen-alone versus 23 on placebo).

Epilepsy: Particular caution is indicated in women with epilepsy, as HRT may cause an exacerbation of this condition.
Renal: Fluid Retention: Estrogens may cause fluid retention. Therefore, particular caution is indicated in cardiac or renal dysfunction, or asthma. If, in any of the above-mentioned conditions, a worsening of the underlying disease is diagnosed or suspected during treatment, the benefits and risks of treatment should be reassessed based on the individual case.
Skin: Persistent erythema or pruritis at the application site may occur.

Estrogens should be used with caution in patients with chloasma, or a history or chloasma gravidarum.
Dermatologic Sensitivity: Contact sensitization is known to occur with topical applications. Although it is extremely rare, patients who develop contact sensitization to any component of the patch should be warned that a severe hypersensitivity reaction may occur with continuing exposure to the causative agent.
Special Populations: Estrogens should be used with caution in patients with chorea minor.
Pregnant Women: If pregnancy occurs during medication with Climara, treatment should be withdrawn immediately.
Monitoring and Laboratory Tests: Before Climara is administered, the patient should have a complete physical examination, including a blood pressure determination. Breasts and pelvic organs should be appropriately examined and a Papanicolaou smear should be performed. Endometrial biopsy should be done only when indicated. Baseline tests should include mammography, measurement of blood glucose, calcium, triglycerides and cholesterol, and liver function tests.

The first follow-up examination should be done within three to six months after initiation of treatment to assess response to treatment. Thereafter, examinations should be made at intervals of at least once a year. Appropriate investigations should be arranged at regular intervals as determined by the physician.

The importance of regular self-examination of the breasts should be discussed with the patient.

Liver function tests should be done periodically in subjects who are suspected of having hepatic disease.
ADVERSE REACTIONS: Adverse Drug Reaction Overview: See Warnings and Precautions regarding the potential for induction of malignant neoplasms and adverse effects similar to those of oral contraceptives.
The following adverse reactions have been reported with estrogen/progestin combination in general:
Blood and Lymphatic System Disorders: Altered coagulation tests (see Drug Interactions, Drug-Laboratory Test Interactions).
Cardiac Disorders: palpitations; increase in blood pressure (see Warnings and Precautions); coronary thrombosis.
Endocrine Disorders: increased blood sugar levels; decreased glucose tolerance.
Eye Disorders: neuro-ocular lesions (e.g retinal thrombosis, optic neuritis); visual disturbances; steepening of the corneal curvature; intolerance to contact lenses.
Gastrointestinal Disorders: nausea; vomiting; abdominal discomfort (cramps, pressure, pain, bloating).
General Disorders and Administration Site Conditions: fatigue; changes in appetite; changes in body weight; change in libido.
Hepatobiliary Disorders: gallbladder disorder; asymptomatic impaired liver function; cholestatic jaundice.
Immune System Disorders: Exogenous estrogens may induce or exacerbate symptoms of angioedema, in particular in women with hereditary angioedema.
Musculoskeletal and Connective Tissue Disorders: Musculoskeletal pain including leg pain not related to thromboembolic disease (usually transient, lasting 3-6 weeks) may occur.
Nervous System Disorders: aggravation of migraine episodes; headaches; dizziness; neuritis.
Psychiatric Disorders: mental depression; nervousness; irritability.
Renal and Urinary Disorders: cystitis; dysuria; sodium retention; edema.
Reproductive System and Breast Disorders: breakthrough bleeding; spotting; change in menstrual flow; dysmenorrhea; vaginal itching/discharge; dyspareunia; endometrial hyperplasia; pre-menstrual-like syndrome; reactivation of endometriosis; changes in cervical erosion and amount of cervical secretion; breast swelling and tenderness.
Skin and Subcutaneous Tissue Disorders: chloasma or melasma, which may persist when drug is discontinued; erythema multiforme; erythema nodosum; haemorrhagic eruption; loss of scalp hair; hirsutism and acne.
Vascular Disorders: isolated cases of: thrombophlebitis; thromboembolic disorders.

Clinical Trial Adverse Drug Reactions: Because clinical trials are conducted under very specific conditions, the adverse reaction rates observed in the clinical trials may not reflect the rates observed in practice and should not be compared to the rates in the clinical trials of another drug. Adverse drug reaction information from clinical trials is useful for identifying drug-related adverse events and for approximating rates. See Table 1.

Table 1: Climara

Adverse Events Occurring at Rate of ≥1% Reported in Climara Phase III Clinical Trials[a] R-838T-010, R-838T-011 in the Indication: Relief of Menopausal Symptoms

	Incidence (%)			
Reported Adverse Event	**Climara 50 (n=201)**	**Climara 100 (n=194)**	**Premarin[b] (n=136)**	**Placebo Patch (n=72)**
Cardiac Disorders				
Syncope	1.0	0.0	0.0	1.4
Palpitation	1.0	1.5	1.3	1.5
Ear and Labyrinth Disorders				
Earache	2.0	1.0	2.2	0.0
Tinnitus	0.5	1.0	0.7	0.0
Eye Disorders				
Vision abnormal	2.0	0.5	0.7	1.4
Gastrointestinal Disorders				
Abdominal pain	10.9	16.0	14.7	8.3
Nausea	5.5	6.2	4.4	2.8
Vomiting	3.0	8.2	11.8	5.6
Flatulence	3.5	6.7	3.7	1.4
Constipation	3.0	2.6	0.0	1.4
Dyspepsia	2.0	1.0	0.0	0.0
Hemorrhoids	0.0	1.0	0.0	1.4
General Disorders and Administration Site Conditions				
Edema	12.9	10.3	5.1	5.6
Pain	8.5	10.8	2.9	6.9
Malaise	5.0	2.6	4.4	6.9
Rigors	3.0	3.1	1.5	0.0
Fatigue	2.0	1.5	3.7	0.0
Chest pain	1.0	2.1	0.7	5.6
Immune System Disorders				
Allergic reactions	2.5	0.5	2.2	0.0
Infections and Infestations				
Infection viral	10.0	8.8	10.3	9.7
Infection fungal	4.0	2.6	1.5	1.4
Infection bacterial	1.0	1.5	0.0	0.0
Infection	1.5	0.5	0.0	1.4
Herpes zoster	1.0	0.5	0.0	0.0
Investigations				
Weight increase	3.0	3.1	1.5	0.0
Musculoskeletal and Connective Tissue Disorders				
Back pain	8.0	9.3	3.7	5.6
Arthralgia	5.5	4.6	2.2	2.8
Myalgia	2.0	2.1	2.2	1.4
Leg cramps	0.5	2.6	4.4	0.0
Arthritis	1.0	1.5	0.0	0.0
Arthrosis	1.5	0.5	1.5	0.0
Fracture, accidental	0.0	2.1	1.5	0.0
Myostasis	1.0	0.0	0.0	0.0
Nervous System Disorders				

(cont'd)

Table 1: Climara *(cont'd)*

Adverse Events Occurring at Rate of ≥1% Reported in Climara Phase III Clinical Trials[a] R-838T-010, R-838T-011 in the Indication: Relief of Menopausal Symptoms

	Incidence (%)			
Reported Adverse Event	**Climara 50 (n=201)**	**Climara 100 (n=194)**	**Premarin[b] (n=136)**	**Placebo Patch (n=72)**
Headache	17.9	13.4	22.8	9.7
Dizziness	3.0	2.6	2.9	2.8
Hyperesthesia	2.0	1.0	2.2	1.4
Sweating increased	2.0	0.0	0.0	0.0
Psychiatric Disorders				
Depression	5.5	8.2	6.6	0.0
Insomnia	2.5	2.1	0.7	0.0
Anxiety	2.0	2.1	2.2	0.0
Nervousness	2.0	1.0	0.0	1.4
Somnolence	0.0	1.5	0.0	0.0
Amnesia	0.0	1.0	0.0	0.0
Renal and Urinary Disorders				
Urinary tract infection	3.0	3.1	0.7	1.4
Polyuria	0.5	1.0	1.5	2.8
Dysuria	0.5	1.0	0.0	1.4
Cystitis	1.0	0.0	0.7	1.4
Urinary incontinence	1.0	0.0	0.0	0.0
Reproductive System and Breast Disorders				
Breast pain	8.0	28.9	13.2	4.2
Leukorrhea	6.5	7.2	2.9	1.4
Vaginitis	4.0	5.2	2.2	0.0
Pelvic pain	1.0	3.6	2.9	2.8
Breast malformation	0.5	1.5	0.7	0.0
Vaginal disorder	1.0	1.0	0.0	0.0
Respiratory, Thoracic and Mediastinal Disorders				
Upper respiratory tract infection	16.9	17.0	26.5	8.3
Pharyngitis	3.0	7.2	5.1	2.8
Rhinitis	4.0	5.7	2.9	1.4
Sinusitis	4.0	5.2	5.9	2.8
Coughing	2.0	2.6	2.9	0.0
Bronchitis	3.0	1.0	0.7	0.0
Respiratory disorder	1.0	0.5	0.7	0.0
Laryngitis	1.0	0.0	0.0	0.0
Skin and Subcutaneous Tissue Disorders				
Dermatitis	4.0	5.7	3.7	4.2
Pruritus	6.0	3.1	3.7	5.6
Rash	2.5	0.5	0.7	4.2
Urticaria	1.5	0.5	0.0	1.4
Sweating increased	1.0	0.0	0.0	0.0
Acne	0.5	1.0	2.9	1.4
Rash, etythematous	0.0	1.5	0.7	0.0
Rash, pustular	0.0	1.0	0.0	0.0
Skin cold and clammy	0.5	1.0	0.0	0.0
Vascular Disorders				
Hypertension	1.0	3.1	0.0	0.0

(cont'd)

Table 1: Climara *(cont'd)*

Adverse Events Occurring at Rate of ≥1% Reported in Climara Phase III Clinical Trials[a] R-838T-010, R-838T-011 in the Indication: Relief of Menopausal Symptoms

[a] Both clinical trials R-838T-010 and R-838T-011 were double-blind, randomized, parallel, active- and placebo-controlled, multiple-dose (3×3 week treatment cycles, separated by 1 week washout) studies.

[b] 0.625 mg conjugated estrogen tablets, administered daily.

The most commonly reported adverse event reported in Climara (estradiol hemihydrate transdermal system) clinical trials R-838T-010 and R-838T-011 were abdominal pain (10.9% for Climara 50, 16.0% for Climara 100, 14.7% for Premarin, 8.3% for placebo), viral infection (10.0% for Climara 50, 8.8% for Climara 100, 10.3% for Premarin, 9.7% for placebo), edema (12.9% for Climara 50, 10.3% for Climara 100, 5.1% for Premarin, 5.6% for placebo), headache (17.9% for Climara 50, 13.4% for Climara 100, 22.8% for Premarin, 9.7% for placebo), breast pain (8.0% for Climara 50, 28.9% for Climara 100, 13.2% for Premarin, 4.2% for placebo) and upper respiratory tract infection (16.9% for Climara 50, 17.0% for Climara 100, 26.5% for Premarin, 8.3% for placebo). The overall rate of discontinuation due to skin irritation at the application site was 6.8% (7.9% for the Climara 50 system and 5.3% for the Climara 100 system) compared to 11.5% for the placebo system.

In a further randomized, controlled, two year clinical trial (Study 308-3B) comparing Climara with placebo, the overall rate of application site reactions with Climara was 28.7%, compared to 17.4% for the placebo system; the dropout rate due to application site reactions during the period was 4.7% (6 out of 129 subjects), compared to 0% for the placebo system.

Overall, the most commonly reported adverse reaction to Climara in clinical trials was breast pain and skin irritation at the application site.

Post-Market Adverse Drug Reactions: Adverse events occurring post-market with Climara are consistent with those reported during clinical trials.

If adverse symptoms persist, the prescription of HRT should be re-considered.

DRUG INTERACTIONS: Overview: Estrogens may diminish the effectiveness of anticoagulant, antidiabetic and antihypertensive agents.

Preparations inducing liver enzymes (e.g., barbiturates, hydantoins, carbamazepine, meprobamate, phenylbutazone or rifampicin) may interfere with the activity of orally administered estrogens. The extent of interference with transdermally administered estradiol-17β is not known.

Drug-Drug Interactions: Estrogens are metabolized partially by cytochrome P450 (CYP 3A4). Therefore, inducers or inhibitors of CYP 3A4 may affect estrogen drug metabolism. Inducers of CYP 3A4 such as phenobarbital, carbamazepine and rifampicin may reduce plasma concentrations of estrogens, possibly resulting in a decrease in therapeutic effect and/or changes in the uterine bleeding profile. Inhibitors of CYP 3A4 such as erythromycin, clarithromycin, ketoconazole, itraconazole, ritonavir and grapefruit juice may increase plasma concentrations of estrogens and may result in side effects.

Drug-Food Interactions: Grapefruit juice is an inhibitor of cytochrome P450 (CYP 3A4) and could therefore increase plasma concentrations of estrogens, which might result in side effects.

Drug-Herb Interactions: It was found that some herbal products (e.g. St. John's wort) which are available as over-the-counter (OTC) products might interfere with steroid metabolism and therefore alter the efficacy and safety of estrogen/progestin products.

Physicians and other health care providers should be made aware of other non-prescription products concomitantly used by the patient, including herbal and natural products obtained from the widely spread health stores.

Drug-Laboratory Test Interactions: The results of certain endocrine, adrenal, renal and liver function tests may be affected by estrogen-containing products:

- increased prothrombin time and partial thromboplastin time; increased levels of fibrinogen and fibrinogen activity; increased coagulation factors VII, VIII, IX, X; increased norepinephrine-induced platelet aggregability; decreased antithrombin III;
- increased thyroxine-binding globulin (TBG), leading to increased circulating total thyroid hormone (T4) as measured by column or radioimmunoassay; T3 resin uptake is decreased, reflecting the elevated TBG; free T4 concentration is unaltered;
- other binding proteins may be elevated in serum i.e., corticosteroid binding globulin (CBG), sex-hormone binding globulin (SHBG), leading to increased circulating corticosteroids and sex steroids respectively; free or biologically active hormone concentrations are unchanged;
- impaired glucose tolerance;
- increased serum triglycerides and phospholipids concentration;

With transdermally administered estradiol-17β, no effect on fibrinogen, antithrombin III, TBG, CBG or SHBG nor decreases in serum triglycerides have been observed.

The results of the above laboratory tests should not be considered reliable unless therapy has been discontinued for two to four weeks.

The pathologist should be informed that the patient is receiving hormone replacement therapy when relevant specimens are submitted.

Drug-Lifestyle Interactions: Acute alcohol ingestion during use of HRT may lead to elevations in circulating estradiol levels.

DOSAGE AND ADMINISTRATION: Dosing Considerations: Climara (estradiol hemihydrate transdermal system) should be prescribed with an appropriate dosage of a progestin for women with intact uteri in order to prevent endometrial hyperplasia/carcinoma. Progestin therapy is not required as part of hormone replacement therapy in women who have had a previous hysterectomy.

Use of estrogen, alone or in combination with a progestin, should be limited to the shortest duration consistent with treatment goals and risks for the individual woman. Patients should be re-evaluated periodically as clinically appropriate (e.g., 3- to 6-month intervals) to determine if treatment is still necessary. For women who have intact uteri, adequate diagnostic measures, such as endometrial sampling, when indicated, should be undertaken to rule out malignancy in cases of undiagnosed persistent or recurring abnormal vaginal bleeding.

Recommended Dose and Dosage Adjustment: Climara should be applied once a week and worn on a continuous basis for 7 days. It should be removed and a new one applied after 7 days. Only one patch should be worn at any one time during the 7-day dosing interval.

Initiation of Therapy: Four Climara systems are available: Climara 25 (0.025 mg/day), Climara 50 (0.05 mg/day), Climara 75 (0.075 mg/day) and Climara 100 (0.1 mg/day). Treatment is usually initiated with Climara 50 applied to the skin once weekly. The dose should be adjusted as necessary to control symptoms.

Clinical response at the lowest effective dose should be the guide for establishing administration of Climara. The necessity for hormone replacement therapy for menopausal symptoms should be re-assessed periodically. Attempts to taper or discontinue the medication should be made at 3- to 6-month intervals.

For the prevention of osteoporosis, Climara 50 (0.05 mg/day) is the minimum dose approved. The choice of which dose to use should be made on the basis of individual considerations such as the age of the patient, other risk factors for osteoporosis and response to therapy as assessed by biochemical markers.

Missed Dose: If the patient forgets to apply the patch, then she should be counseled to apply a new patch and continue with her regular treatment schedule.

Administration: Patch Application: The physician should discuss the most appropriate placement of the patch with the patient. Immediately after removal of a patch from the pouch and removal of the protective liner, the adhesive side of the Climara patch should be placed on a clean, dry area of intact skin. The area selected should not be oily, damaged or irritated, and not exposed to the sun. The site selected should also be one at which little wrinkling of the skin occurs during movement of the body, preferably the buttocks, lower abdomen or hip. The patch may also be placed on the side or lower back. The patch should be placed consistently on the same area of the body with each application (e.g., either the buttocks, lower abdomen, hip, side or lower back). Experience to date has shown that less irritation of the skin occurs on the buttocks than on other sites of application. Therefore, it is advisable to apply Climara to the buttocks. The waistline should be avoided, since tight clothing may dislodge the patch. The patch should be pressed firmly in place with the palm of the hand, making sure there is good contact, especially around the edges.

In the event that a patch should fall off, a new one should be applied and the original treatment schedule should be continued. Patches should not be applied to the same skin site twice in succession.

Climara must not be applied to the breasts in order to avoid potentially harmful effects on the breast tissue.

OVERDOSAGE:
Symptoms: Overdosage with transdermal application of estradiol is unlikely. Numerous reports of ingestion of large doses of estrogen products and estrogen-containing oral contraceptives by young children have not revealed acute serious ill effects. Overdosage with estrogen may cause nausea, breast discomfort, fluid retention, bloating or vaginal bleeding in women.
Treatment: Symptomatic treatment should be given and the Climara patch(es) should be removed.

For management of a suspected drug overdose, CPhA recommends that you contact your **regional Poison Control Centre**. See the *CPS* Directory section for a list of Poison Control Centres.

ACTION AND CLINICAL PHARMACOLOGY: Mechanism of Action: Climara (estradiol hemihydrate transdermal system) is composed of a translucent polyethylene film with an acrylate adhesive matrix containing estradiol-17β. Upon application to intact skin, Climara provides continuous systemic delivery of estrogen by releasing estradiol-17β, the major estrogenic hormone secreted by the human ovary.
Pharmacodynamics: Estradiol-17β is the predominant estrogen produced by the ovaries in premenopausal women. Administration of transdermal estradiol to postmenopausal women elevates plasma estradiol concentrations into the range observed in premenopausal women at the early to mid-follicular stage. As a result of the increased plasma estradiol concentrations, plasma concentrations of follicle-stimulating hormone and luteinizing hormone are decreased and vaginal cytology is converted to a pattern resembling that found in premenopausal women, with improvement of the maturation and karyopyknotic indices. Estrogens are effective in reducing the number and intensity of hot flushes associated with menopause and in the prevention of osteoporosis.
Pharmacokinetics: Absorption: Climara provides controlled delivery of approximately 0.025, 0.05, 0.075 or 0.1 mg of estradiol per day into the systemic circulation, depending on the strength of the system.
Distribution and Metabolism: When given orally, estrogens and their esters are extensively metabolized by the liver (first-pass effect) and circulate primarily as estrone sulfate, with smaller amounts of other conjugated and unconjugated weaker estrogens. This results in limited oral potency.

In contrast, because the skin metabolizes estradiol only to a small extent, the transdermal administration of estradiol produces therapeutic serum levels of estradiol with lower circulating levels of estrone and estrone conjugates. Climara maintains the favourable estradiol/estrone ratio associated with transdermal application, which is comparable to that observed in premenopausal women during the early follicular phase.

Transdermal administration of estradiol offers some advantages over oral administration. It avoids the hepatic "first-pass" effect thereby minimizing interpatient and intrapatient variations due to variable hepatic metabolism. Transdermal administration avoids gastrointestinal intolerance associated with oral administration of estrogens.

Consistent serum estradiol concentrations are maintained with Climara over a one-week application interval. Linear pharmacokinetics have been demonstrated for Climara. On average, Climara 100 maintained mean steady state serum estradiol levels of 70 pg/mL and Climara 50 maintained mean steady-state serum estradiol levels of approximately 35 pg/mL.

Climara does not produce an estrogen accumulation following multiple one-week applications.
Excretion: Because estradiol has a short half-life (0.3 to 2 hours after parenteral administration), transdermal administration allows a rapid decline in blood levels after Climara is removed.
Estrogen Pharmacology: Independent of the route of administration, estrogen exerts a dose-dependent stimulating effect on mitosis and proliferation of the endometrium. Unopposed estrogen increases the frequency of endometrial hyperplasia and thus the risk of endometrial carcinoma. In order to avoid endometrial hyperplasia the sequential administration of an appropriate dosage of progestin is recommended during long-term therapy in women with intact uteri.

STORAGE AND STABILITY: Store between 15 and 30°C. Store in sealed pouch. Apply immediately upon removal from the protective pouch.

Keep out of the reach of children before and after use.

INFORMATION FOR THE PATIENT: Published in e-CPS, available by subscription at www.e-cps.ca.

DOSAGE FORMS, COMPOSITION AND PACKAGING: The Climara system is composed of 2 layers: (1) a translucent polyethylene film and (2) an acrylate adhesive matrix containing estradiol hemihydrate, Ph. Eur. A protective polyester liner is attached to the adhesive surface and must be removed before the system can be used.
Climara 25: Each translucent 6.5 cm² system contains: estradiol hemihydrate 2.04 mg Ph. Eur. (equivalent to 2 mg estradiol-17β), and provides controlled delivery of estradiol-17β 0.025 mg/day to the patient. Nonmedicinal ingredients: acrylate copolymer (acrylamide, isooctyl acrylate, vinyl acetate copolymer), ethyl oleate, glyceryl monolaurate and isopropyl myristate. Packages of 4.
Climara 50: Each translucent 12.5 cm² system contains: estradiol hemihydrate 3.9 mg Ph. Eur. (equivalent to 3.8 mg estradiol-17β), and provides controlled delivery of estradiol-17β 0.05 mg/day to the patient. Nonmedicinal ingredients: acrylate copolymer (acrylamide, isooctyl acrylate, vinyl acetate copolymer), ethyl oleate, glyceryl monolaurate and isopropyl myristate. Packages of 4.
Climara 75: Each translucent 18.75 cm² system contains: estradiol hemihydrate 5.85 mg Ph. Eur. (equivalent to 5.7 mg estradiol-17β), and provides controlled delivery of estradiol-17β 0.075 mg/day to the patient. Nonmedicinal ingredients: acrylate copolymer (acrylamide, isooctyl acrylate, vinyl acetate copolymer), ethyl oleate, glyceryl monolaurate and isopropyl myristate. Packages of 4.
Climara 100: Each translucent 25 cm² system contains: estradiol hemihydrate 7.8 mg Ph. Eur. (equivalent to 7.6 mg estradiol-17β), and provides controlled delivery of estradiol-17β 0.1 mg/day to the patient. Nonmedicinal ingredients: acrylate copolymer (acrylamide, isooctyl acrylate, vinyl acetate copolymer), ethyl oleate, glyceryl monolaurate and isopropyl myristate. Packages of 4.

(Shown in Product Identification Section)

Climara Pro® ℞

estradiol-17β—levonorgestrel
Estrogen—Progestin

Bayer

Date of Revision: June 27, 2008

Warning
As the Women's Health Initiative (WHI) study results indicated increased risk of myocardial infarction (MI), stroke, invasive breast cancer, pulmonary emboli and deep venous thrombosis in postmenopausal women receiving treatment with combined conjugated equine estrogens and medroxyprogesterone acetate compared to those receiving placebo tablets, the following should be highly considered:

- Estrogens with or without progestins **should not** be prescribed for primary or secondary prevention of cardiovascular diseases.
- Estrogens with or without progestins should be prescribed at **the lowest effective dose** for the approved indication.
- Estrogens with or without progestins should be prescribed for **the shortest period** possible for the recognized indication.

PHARMACOLOGY: CLIMARA PRO (estradiol/levonorgestrel transdermal system) is a transdermal system containing estradiol-17β (estrogen) and levonorgestrel (progestin) intended for continuous administration as hormone replacement therapy. Following once-weekly application to intact skin, CLIMARA PRO provides continuous, controlled delivery of estradiol-17β and levonorgestrel to the systemic circulation.
Clinical Pharmacology of Estrogens: Endogenous estrogens are largely responsible for the development and maintenance of the female reproductive system and secondary sexual characteristics. Although circulating estrogens exist in a dynamic equilibrium of metabolic interconversions, estradiol-17β is the principal intracellular human estrogen and is substantially more potent than its metabolites, estrone and estriol, at the receptor level.

The primary source of estrogen in normally cycling adult women is the ovarian follicle, which secretes 70 to 500 µg of estradiol daily, depending on the phase of the menstrual cycle. After menopause, most endogenous estrogen is produced by conversion of androstenedione, secreted by the adrenal cortex, to estrone by peripheral tissues. Thus, estrone and the sulfate conjugated form, estrone sulfate, are the most abundant circulating estrogens in postmenopausal women.

Estrogens act through binding to nuclear receptors in estrogen-responsive tissues. To date, two estrogen receptors have been identified. These vary in proportion from tissue to tissue.

Circulating estrogens modulate the pituitary secretion of the gonadotropins, luteinizing hormone (LH) and follicle stimulating hormone (FSH) through a negative feedback mechanism. Administration of transdermal estradiol to postmenopausal women elevates plasma estradiol concentrations into the range observed in premenopausal women at the early to mid-follicular stage. As a result of the increased plasma estradiol concentrations, plasma concentrations of FSH and LH are decreased and vaginal cytology is converted to a pattern resembling that found in premenopausal women, with improvement of the maturation and karyopyknotic indices.

Loss of ovarian estradiol-17β production after menopause can result in instability of thermoregulation, causing hot flushes associated with sleep disturbance and excessive sweating. Estrogen replacement therapy is effective in reducing the number and intensity of hot flushes associated with menopause.
Clinical Pharmacology of Progestins: Levonorgestrel is a 19-nortestosterone derivative with potent progestogenic effects, but no significant estrogenic activity. It has been established that the inclusion of either cyclic or continuous administration of a progestin, such as levonorgestrel, in hormone replacement therapy inhibits endometrial proliferation induced by estrogen. This inhibition of endometrial proliferation is associated with a reduction in risk of endometrial hyperplasia and the attendant risk of carcinoma in women with intact uteri. Progestin compounds enhance cellular differentiation and generally oppose the actions of estrogens by decreasing estrogen receptor levels, increasing local metabolism of estrogens to less active metabolites, or inducing gene products that blunt cellular responses to estrogen.
Pharmacokinetics: When given orally, estrogens and their esters are extensively metabolized by the liver (first pass effect) and circulate primarily as estrone sulfate, with smaller amounts of other conjugated and unconjugated weaker estrogens. This results in limited oral potency.

In contrast, because the skin metabolizes estradiol only to a small extent, the transdermal administration of estradiol produces therapeutic serum levels of estradiol with lower circulating levels of estrone and estrone conjugates. CLIMARA PRO maintains the favourable estradiol/estrone ratio associated with transdermal application, which is comparable to that observed in premenopausal women during the early follicular phase.

Transdermal administration of estradiol offers several advantages over oral administration. It avoids the hepatic "first pass" effect thereby minimizing interpatient and intrapatient variations due to variable hepatic metabolism. Transdermal administration also avoids gastrointestinal intolerance associated with oral administration of estrogens.
Absorption: Administration of CLIMARA PRO to postmenopausal women produces mean maximum estradiol concentrations in serum in about 2 to 2.5 days. Estradiol concentrations equivalent to the normal ranges observed at the early follicular phase in premenopausal women are achieved within 12-24 hours after the first application, and are sustained for the entire patch wear period. A summary of estradiol, estrone and levonorgestrel pharmacokinetic parameters after CLIMARA PRO single and multiple applications is shown in Table 1 and Table 2.

Table 1: CLIMARA PRO

Summary of Mean (±SD) Pharmacokinetic Parameters Following a Single Application of CLIMARA PRO in 24 Healthy Postmenopausal Women

Parameter	Units	Estradiol	Estrone	Levonorgestrel
C_{max}	pg/mL	54.3±18.9	43.9±14.9	138±51.8
T_{max}[a]	hours	42	84	90
AUC	pg·h/mL	6340±1740	6890±2520	22 900±8860

[a] T_{max} is expressed as the median value.

Table 2: CLIMARA PRO

Summary of Mean (±SD) Pharmacokinetic Parameters (Week 4) Following Four Consecutive Weekly Applications of CLIMARA PRO in 44 Healthy Postmenopausal Women

Parameter	Units	Estradiol	Estrone	Levonorgestrel
C_{max}	pg/mL	50.7±28.6	81.6±252	194±111
T_{max}[a]	hours	36	48	48
C_{min}	pg/mL	33.8±28.7	72.5±253	153±69.6
AUC	pg·h/mL	6002±1919	7642±10 518	27 948±16 426

[a] T_{max} is expressed as the median value.

At steady state, CLIMARA PRO maintains an average serum estradiol concentration of about 36 pg/mL during the application period, as depicted in Figure 1.

Figure 1: CLIMARA PRO

Mean Estradiol Concentration Profile (Week 4) Following Four Consecutive Weekly Applications of CLIMARA PRO

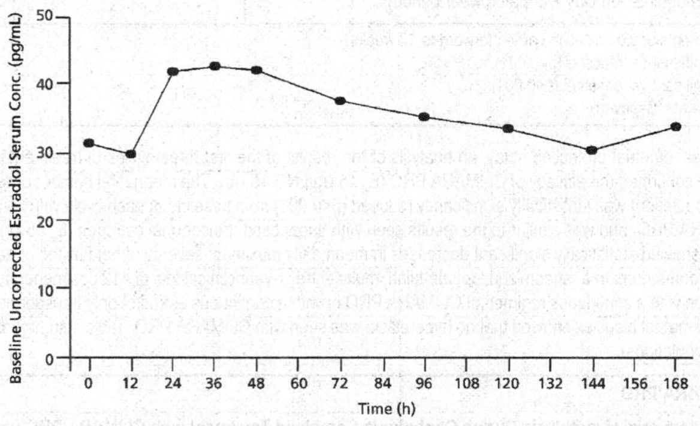

Following the application of CLIMARA PRO, levonorgestrel concentrations reach a maximum in about 3 days. At steady state, CLIMARA PRO maintains an average serum levonorgestrel concentration of about 166 pg/mL during the application period, as depicted in Figure 2.
Distribution: The distribution of exogenous estrogens is similar to that of endogenous estrogens. Estrogens are widely distributed in the body and are generally found in higher concentrations in the sex hormone target organs. Estrogens circulate in the blood largely bound to sex hormone binding globulin (SHBG) and albumin. In a multiple dose study with CLIMARA PRO, about 57-58% of estradiol was bound nonspecifically to serum albumin and about 40-41% to SHBG. The fraction of unbound estradiol in blood was less than 2%.

Levonorgestrel in serum is bound to both SHBG and albumin. In a multiple dose study with CLIMARA PRO, less than 2% of levonorgestrel was found to circulate in blood unbound. Approximately 77-79% was strongly bound to SHBG and 19-22% to albumin.
Metabolism: The biotransformation of transdermally administered estradiol is the same as that of the endogenous hormone. Estradiol is mainly metabolized in the liver but also extrahepatically, e.g., in the gut, kidney, skeletal muscles and target organs. These processes involve the formation of estrone, estriol, catecholestrogens and sulfate and glucuronide conjugates of these

compounds, which are all distinctly less estrogenic or even nonestrogenic. After transdermal administration, the metabolism of estradiol to estrone and conjugates remains within the physiological range as seen during the early follicular phase in the reproductive period, indicated by an estradiol/estrone serum level ratio of approximately 1.

The most important metabolic pathway for levonorgestrel occurs in the reduction of the △4- and the 3-oxo group as well as hydroxylations at positions 2α, 1β and 16β, followed by conjugation. Most of the metabolites that circulate in the blood are sulfates of 3α, 5β-tetrahydro-levonorgestrel, while excretion occurs predominantly in the form of glucuronides. Some of the parent levonorgestrel also circulates as the 17β-sulfate.

Figure 2: CLIMARA PRO

Mean Levonorgestrel Concentration Profile (Week 4) Following Four Consecutive Weekly Applications of CLIMARA PRO

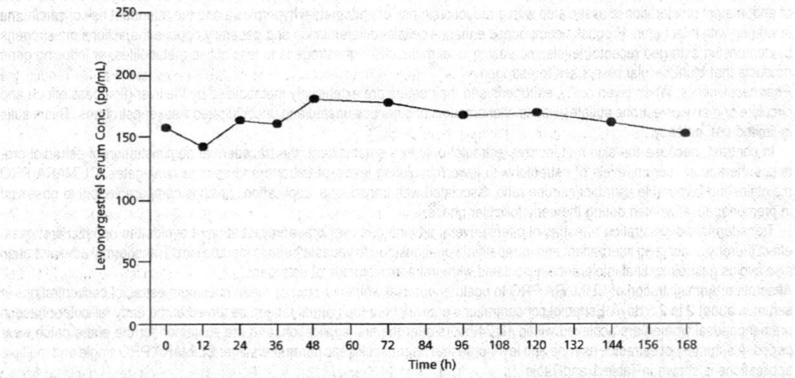

Excretion: Estradiol, estrone and estriol are excreted in the urine along with glucuronide and sulfate conjugates. Following patch removal, serum estradiol concentrations decline rapidly with a mean terminal half-life of 3.0±0.67 hours.

Levonorgestrel and its metabolites are primarily excreted in the urine. Mean (±SD) terminal half-life for levonorgestrel was determined to be 28±6.4 hours.

Pivotal Clinical Trials: Although different strengths of levonorgestrel were tested, for the purpose of endometrial protection against hyperplasia, the 45 µg estradiol/15 µg levonorgestrel transdermal system has been determined to deliver enough levonorgestrel to obtain adequate protection against endometrial hyperplasia, and the higher strengths are therefore not justified.

Effect on Vasomotor Symptoms: The efficacy of a 45 µg estradiol/30 µg levonorgestrel (E_2 45 µg/LNG 30 µg) transdermal system in the relief of vasomotor symptoms in postmenopausal women was demonstrated in a double-blind, randomized, placebo-controlled trial. The system was administered continuously for three 28-day cycles, with a new system applied weekly. The mean weekly number of hot flushes (primary efficacy variable) was statistically significantly reduced from baseline at Weeks 4, 8 and 12 and at All Endpoints as compared to baseline (intent-to-treat population). Pairwise comparisons showed statistically significant differences for the E_2 45 µg/LNG 30 µg group versus the placebo group at all timepoints. The severity of hot flushes was evaluated by analysis of mean decrease from baseline in daily maximum severity on Days 1, 2, 3, 4, 5, 6 and 7 of each cycle. The E_2 45 µg/LNG 30 µg group had statistically significant decreases in severity from baseline at all timepoints. CLIMARA PRO (E_2 45 µg/LNG 15 µg) and the E_2 45 µg/LNG 30 µg strength used in this study have been shown to be bioequivalent in terms of estradiol delivery.

Table 3: CLIMARA PRO

Mean Changes in Weekly Number and Daily Maximum Severity of Hot Flushes at All Endpoints[a] (Vasomotor Symptoms study)

	E_2 45 µg/LNG 30 µg (n=92)	Placebo (n=88)
Mean weekly number of hot flushes at baseline	88.17	93.83
Mean weekly number of hot flushes at All Endpoints	16.22	54.64
Mean change from baseline in weekly number of hot flushes at All Endpoints	−72.02[b,c]	−37.74
Mean daily maximum severity of hot flushes at baseline (on Day 7 of run-in period)	2.9	2.84
Mean change from baseline in mean daily maximum severity[d] of hot flushes at All Endpoints (on Day 7 of patch wear period)	−2.12[b,c]	−0.61

[a] Final evaluation on study medication carried forward to 12 weeks.
[b] Statistically significant vs. placebo (p<0.001).
[c] Statistically significant vs. baseline (p<0.001).
[d] 1=mild, 2=moderate, 3=severe.

In the 1-year endometrial protection study, an analysis of the results of the first three cycles of treatment in a symptomatic subset of women confirmed the efficacy of CLIMARA PRO (E_2 45 µg/LNG 15 µg). The mean total number of weekly hot flushes (intent-to-treat population) was statistically significantly reduced (p<0.001) from baseline at each cycle with continuous administration of CLIMARA PRO, and was similar to the results seen with unopposed transdermal estrogen (E_2 45 µg). The CLIMARA PRO group also showed statistically significant decreases in mean daily maximum severity of hot flushes at each cycle.

Effects on the Endometrium: In a randomized, double-blind, multicentre, 1-year clinical trial of 412 postmenopausal women (with intact uteri) treated with a continuous regimen of CLIMARA PRO or with a continuous estradiol-only transdermal system, results of evaluable endometrial biopsies showed that no hyperplasia was seen with CLIMARA PRO. Table 4 summarizes these results (intent-to-treat populations).

Table 4: CLIMARA PRO *(cont'd)*

Incidence of Endometrial Hyperplasia During Continuous Combined Treatment with CLIMARA PRO (Intent-to-Treat Population)

	CLIMARA PRO (E_2 45µg/LNG 15 µg) (n=210)	Estradiol (E_2 45 µg) (n=201)
No. of patients with biopsies at ≥6 months[a]	124	139
No. of patients with biopsies at 1 year[b]	102	110
No. (%) of patients with hyperplasia[c]	0 (0%)	19 (17.3%)
95% Confidence Interval	0–3.55%	9.75–24.79%
p-value[d]	<0.001	

[a] Defined as ≥180 days of treatment.
[b] Defined as ≥323 days of treatment.
[c] Includes hyperplasia occurring at any time after initiation of treatment as a proportion of patients with biopsies at one year.
[d] P-value for comparison to unopposed estradiol dose using the Fisher Exact test. P-values were adjusted by the method of Bonferroni: p<0.0167.

Effects on Uterine Bleeding or Spotting: The effects of CLIMARA PRO on uterine bleeding or spotting were evaluated in the 1-year endometrial protection trial. Results are shown in Figure 3.

Figure 3: CLIMARA PRO

Cumulative Proportion of Subjects at Each Cycle with No Bleeding/Spotting Through the End of Cycle 13. Last Observation Carried Forward.

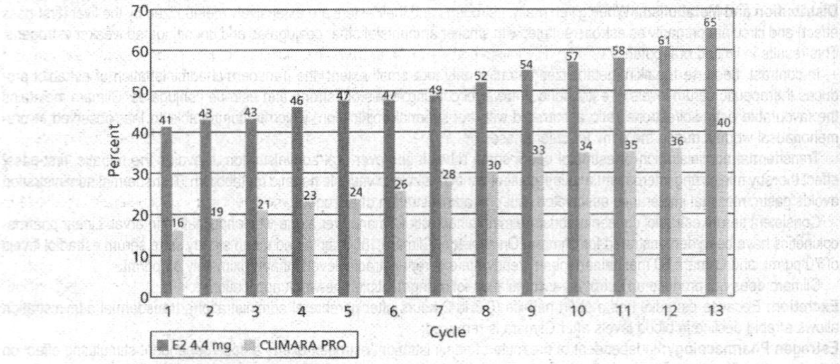

Percent based upon number of subjects at each cycle with data.
Last non-missing cycle carried forward through cycle 13.
Bleeding associated with endometrial biopsies not included.

Effect on Lipids: In the 1-year endometrial protection trial, CLIMARA PRO significantly (p<0.001) decreased total cholesterol and triglycerides compared to continuous transdermal estradiol alone. Furthermore, CLIMARA PRO maintained the favourable effects of estradiol on low density lipoprotein cholesterol (LDL-C). As observed with other progestin-containing therapies, CLIMARA PRO decreased the favourable effects of estradiol on high density lipoprotein cholesterol (HDL-C).

Table 5: CLIMARA PRO

Mean % Change from Baseline Lipid Profile: Values After 1 Year of Treatment

Lipid Parameter	Estradiol 45 µg (n=204) %	CLIMARA PRO (E_2 45 µg/LNG 15 µg) (n=212) %
Total cholesterol	−1.5	−6.5
Triglycerides	1.2	−18.5
LDL-C	−3.2	−5.6
HDL-C	1.6	−4.3

Effect on Coagulation Parameters: Effects on coagulation parameters were assessed following one year of treatment with E_2 45 µg/LNG 30 µg (n=23) and E_2 45 µg/LNG 40 µg (n=26) transdermal systems. No clinically signfiicant changes were observed for fibrinogen and thrombin-antithrombin III complex (TAT).

INDICATIONS: CLIMARA PRO (estradiol/levonorgestrel transdermal system) is indicated for the relief of menopausal and postmenopausal symptoms occurring in naturally or surgically induced estrogen deficiency states.

CLIMARA PRO is recommended for use only in patients with an intact uterus since the regimen includes a progestin whose role is to prevent endometrial hyperplasia.

CONTRAINDICATIONS: Estrogen/progestin combinations are contraindicated in patients with any of the following conditions: Active hepatic dysfunction or disease, especially of the obstructive type. Personal history of known or suspected estrogen/progestin-dependent neoplasia, such as breast or endometrial cancer. Endometrial hyperplasia. Undiagnosed abnormal genital bleeding. Known or suspected pregnancy. Lactation. Active or past history of arterial thromboembolic disease (e.g., stroke, myocardial infarction, coronary heart disease). Classical migraine. Active or past history of confirmed venous thromboembolism (such as deep venous thrombosis or pulmonary embolism) or active thrombophlebitis. Partial or complete loss of vision due to ophthalmic vascular disease. Known or suspected hypersensitivity to any component of the product.

WARNINGS: See Boxed Warning.

Cardiovascular Disorders: Available epidemiological data indicate that use of estrogen with or without progestin is associated with an increased risk of stroke and coronary heart disease. The WHI trial results concluded that there are more risks than benefits among women using combined Hormone Replacement Therapy (HRT), compared to the group using placebo. In 10 000 women on combined HRT (conjugated equine estrogens/medroxyprogesterone acetate) over a one year period, there were seven more cases of coronary heart disease (37 on combined HRT versus 30 on placebo) and eight more cases of stroke (29 vs 21).

In the Heart and Estrogen/progestin Replacement Study (HERS) of postmenopausal women with documented heart disease (n=2763, average age 66.7 years), a randomized placebo-controlled clinical trial of secondary prevention of coronary heart disease (CHD), treatment with 0.625 mg/day oral conjugated equine estrogen (CEE) plus 2.5 mg medroxyprogesterone acetate (MPA) demonstrated no cardiovascular benefit. Specifically, during an average follow-up of 4.1 years, treatment with CEE plus MPA did not reduce the overall rate of CHD events in postmenopausal women with established coronary heart disease. There were more CHD events in the hormone-treated group than in the placebo group in year 1, but not during the subsequent years.

From the original HERS trial, 2321 women consented to participate in an open label extension of HERS, known as HERS II. Average follow-up in HERS II was an additional 2.7 years, for a total of 6.8 years overall. After 6.8 years, hormone therapy did not reduce the risk of cardiovascular events in women with CHD.

Breast Cancer: Current epidemiological data indicate that the use of combined HRT is associated with an increased risk of invasive breast cancer. The WHI trial results concluded that there are more risks than benefits among women using combined HRT (conjugated equine estrogens/medroxyprogesterone acetate), compared to the group using placebo. In 10 000 women on combined HRT over a one year period, there were eight more cases of invasive breast cancer (38 on combined HRT versus 30 on placebo).

The WHI study reported that the invasive breast cancers diagnosed in the estrogen plus progestin group were similar in histology but were larger (mean [SD] 1.7 cm [1.1] vs. 1.5 cm [0.9], respectively; p=0.04) and were at a more advanced stage compared with those diagnosed in the placebo group. The WHI trial also reported that the percentage of women with abnormal mammograms (recommendations for short-interval follow-up, a suspicious abnormality or highly suggestive of malignancy) was significantly higher in the estrogen plus progestin group versus the placebo group. This difference appeared at year one and persisted in each year thereafter.

It is recommended that estrogens not be given to women with existing breast cancer or those with a previous history of the disease. There is a need for caution in prescribing estrogens for women with known risk factors associated with the development of breast cancer, such as strong family history of breast cancer (first degree relative) or who present a breast condition with an increased risk (abnormal mammograms and/or atypical hyperplasia at breast biopsy). Other known risk factors for the development of breast cancer such as nulliparity, obesity, early menarche, late age at first full term pregnancy and at menopause should also be evaluated.

It is recommended that women undergo mammography prior to the start of HRT treatment and at regular intervals during treatment, as deemed appropriate by the treating physician and according to the perceived risks for each patient.

The overall benefits and possible risks of hormone replacement therapy should be fully considered and discussed with patients. It is important that the modest increased risk of being diagnosed with breast cancer after 4 years of treatment with HRT (as reported in the results of the WHI trial) be discussed with the patient and weighed against its known benefits.

Instructions for regular self-examination of the breasts should be included in this counselling.

Venous Thromboembolism: Recent epidemiological data indicate that use of estrogen with or without progestin is associated with an increased risk of developing venous thromboembolism (VTE). The WHI trial results concluded that there are more risks than benefits among women using combined HRT (conjugated equine estrogens/medroxyprogesterone acetate), compared to the group using placebo. In 10 000 women on combined HRT over a period of one year, there were eighteen more cases of total blood clots in the lungs and legs (34 on combined HRT versus 16 on placebo).

Generally recognized risk factors for VTE include a personal history, a family history (the occurrence of VTE in a direct relative at a relatively early age may indicate genetic predisposition) and severe obesity (body mass index >30 kg/m²). The risk of VTE also increases with age and smoking.

The risk of VTE may be temporarily increased with prolonged immobilization, major elective surgery or posttraumatic surgery, or major trauma (if feasible, HRT should be discontinued at least 4 weeks before major surgery which may be associated with an increased risk of thromboembolism, or during periods of prolonged immobilization). In women on HRT, attention should be given to prophylactic measures to prevent VTE following surgery. Also, patients with varicose veins should be closely supervised. The physician should be alert to the earliest manifestations of thrombotic disorders (thrombophlebitis, retinal thrombosis, cerebral embolism and pulmonary embolism). If these occur or are suspected, hormone therapy should be discontinued immediately.

Endometrial Hyperplasia and Endometrial Carcinoma: There is evidence from several studies that estrogens, unopposed by progestins, increase the risk of endometrial carcinoma in postmenopausal women. CLIMARA PRO (estradiol/levonorgestrel transdermal system) provides plasma levonorgestrel levels within the therapeutic range necessary to counteract the effects of estradiol on the endometrium. In a 1-year clinical study conducted in 840 postmenopausal women with intact uteri, no cases of endometrial hyperplasia were reported in women using CLIMARA PRO (n=210) (see Pharmacology, Pivotal Clinical Trials, Effects on the Endometrium).

Clinical surveillance of all women taking estrogen/progestin combinations is important. Adequate diagnostic measures, including endometrial sampling when indicated, should be undertaken to rule out malignancy in all cases of undiagnosed persistent or recurrent abnormal vaginal bleeding.

Gallbladder Disease : A 2- to 4-fold increase in the risk of gallbladder disease requiring surgery in women receiving postmenopausal estrogens has been reported.

Dementia: Current epidemiological evidence indicates that the use of combined HRT is associated with a significantly increased risk of developing probable dementia. The Women's Health Initiative Memory Study, a clinical substudy of the WHI, followed 4532 postmenopausal women age 65 and over and free of dementia at baseline. There was a reported two-fold increase in the relative risk of developing probable dementia after an average follow-up of 4.05 years in the group treated with daily 0.625 mg conjugated equine estrogen plus 2.5 mg medroxyprogesterone versus those treated with placebo (hazard ratio [HR] 2.05, 95% confidence interval [CI], 1.21-3.48). This increased risk would result in an additional 23 cases of dementia per 10 000 women per year (45 vs 22 per 10 000 person-years; p=0.01).

Contact Sensitization : Contact sensitization is known to occur with topical applications. Although it is extremely rare, patients who develop contact sensitization to any component of the patch should be warned that a severe hypersensitivity reaction may occur with continuing exposure to the causative agent.

PRECAUTIONS: Before CLIMARA PRO (estradiol/levonorgestrel transdermal system) is administered, the patient should have a complete physical examination, including a blood pressure determination. Breasts and pelvic organs should be appropriately examined and a Papanicolaou smear should be performed. Endometrial biopsy should be done when indicated. Baseline tests should include mammography, measurement of blood glucose, calcium, triglycerides and cholesterol, and liver function tests.

The first follow-up examination should be done within three to six months after initiation of treatment to assess medical response to treatment. Thereafter, examinations should be made at intervals of at least once a year and should include at least those procedures outlined above. **It is important that patients are encouraged to practice frequent self-examination of the breasts.**

Abnormal vaginal bleeding, due to its prolongation, irregularity or heaviness, occurring during therapy should prompt diagnostic measures like hysteroscopy, endometrial biopsy or curettage to rule out the possibility of uterine malignancy, and the treatment should be re-evaluated.

Pre-existing uterine leiomyoma may increase in size during estrogen use. Growth, pain or tenderness of uterine leiomyoma requires discontinuation of medication.

Symptoms and physical findings associated with a previous diagnosis of endometriosis may reappear or become aggravated with estrogen use.

Caution is advised in patients with a history of estrogen-related jaundice and pruritus. If cholestatic jaundice develops during treatment, the treatment should be discontinued and appropriate investigations carried out.

Patients who develop visual disturbances, classical migraine, transient aphasia, paralysis or loss of consciousness should discontinue medication.

If feasible, HRT should be discontinued at least 4 weeks before major surgery which may be associated with an increased risk of thromboembolism, or during periods of prolonged immobilization.

Women using HRT sometimes experience increased blood pressure. Blood pressure should be monitored with HRT use. Elevation of blood pressure in previously normotensive or hypertensive patients should be investigated and HRT may have to be discontinued.

Estrogens may cause fluid retention. Therefore, particular caution is indicated in cardiac or renal dysfunction, epilepsy or asthma. Treatment should be stopped if there is an increase in epileptic seizures. If, in any of the above-mentioned conditions, a worsening of the underlying disease is diagnosed or suspected during treatment, the benefits and risks of treatment should be reassessed based on the individual case.

Because the prolonged use of estrogens influences the metabolism of calcium and phosphorus, estrogens should be used with caution in patients with metabolic and malignant bone diseases associated with hypercalcemia and in patients with renal insufficiency.

Exogenous estrogens may induce/exacerbate symptoms of angioedema, in particular in women with hereditary angioedema. Discontinuation of this medication should be considered.

A worsening of glucose tolerance and lipid metabolism have been observed in a significant percentage of peri- and postmenopausal patients. Therefore, diabetic patients or those with a predisposition to diabetes should be observed closely to detect any alterations in carbohydrate or lipid metabolism, especially in triglyceride blood levels.

If any surgical procedures are performed, the pathologist should be advised of the patient's therapy when specimens are sent for examination.

Women with familial hypertriglyceridemia or porphyria need special surveillance. Lipid-lowering measures are recommended additionally, before treatment is started.

Liver function tests should be done periodically in subjects who are suspected of having hepatic disease. For information on endocrine and liver function tests, see Laboratory Tests. When liver or endocrine tests are indicated, the laboratory should be advised of the patient's therapy before specimens are forwarded.

Drug Interactions: Estrogens may diminish the effectiveness of anticoagulant, antidiabetic and antihypertensive agents.

Preparations inducing liver enzymes (e.g., barbiturates, hydantoins, carbamazepine, meprobamates, phenylbutazone or rifampicin) may interfere with the activity of orally administered estrogens. The extent of interference with transdermally administered estradiol and levonorgestrel is not known.

The following section contains information on drug interactions with ethinyl estradiol-containing products (specifically, oral contraceptives) that have been reported in the public literature. It is unknown whether such interactions occur with drug products containing other types of estrogens.

The metabolism of ethinyl estradiol is increased by rifampin and anticonvulsants such as phenobarbital, phenytoin and carbamazepine. Coadministration of troglitazone and certain ethinyl estradiol containing drug products (e.g., oral contraceptives containing ethinyl estradiol) reduce the plasma concentrations of ethinyl estradiol by 30 percent.

Ascorbic acid and acetaminophen may increase AUC and/or plasma concentrations of ethinyl estradiol. Coadministration of atorvastatin and certain ethinyl estradiol containing drug products (e.g., oral contraceptives containing ethinyl estradiol) increase AUC values for ethinyl estradiol by 20 percent.

Clinical pharmacokinetic studies have not demonstrated any consistent effect of antibiotics (other than rifampin) on plasma concentrations of synthetic steroids.

Drug products containing ethinyl estradiol may inhibit the metabolism of other compounds. Increased plasma concentrations of cyclosporin, prednisolone and theophylline have been reported with concomitant administration of certain drugs containing ethinyl estradiol (e.g., oral contraceptives containing ethinyl estradiol). In addition, these drugs containing ethinyl estradiol may induce the conjugation of other compounds.

Decreased plasma concentrations of acetaminophen and increased clearance of temazepam, salicylic acid, morphine and clofibric acid have been noted when these drugs were administered with certain ethinyl estradiol containing drug products (e.g., oral contraceptives containing ethinyl estradiol).

Concomitant administration of aminoglutethimide with medroxyprogesterone acetate (MPA) may significantly reduce the bioavailability of MPA.

It was found that some herbal products (e.g., St. John's wort) which are available as OTC products might affect metabolism, and therefore, efficacy and safety of estrogen/progestin products.

Physicians and other health care providers should be aware of other non-prescription products concomitantly used by the patient, including herbal and natural products obtained from the widely spread health stores.

Laboratory Tests: The results of certain endocrine and liver function tests may be affected by estrogen-containing products: increased sulfobromophthalein retention; increased prothrombin time and partial thromboplastin time; increased levels of fibrinogen and fibrinogen activity; increased coagulation factors VII, VIII, IX, X; increased norepinephrine-induced platelet aggregability; decreased antithrombin III; increased thyroxine-binding globulin (TBG), leading to increased circulating total thyroid hormone (T_4) as measured by column or radioimmunoassay; free T_3 resin uptake is decreased, reflecting the elevated TBG; free T_4 concentration is unaltered; other binding proteins may be elevated in serum, i.e., corticosteroid binding globulin (CBG), sex hormone-binding globulin (SHBG), leading to increased circulating corticosteroids and sex steroids respectively; free or biologically active hormone concentrations are unchanged; reduced response to the METOPIRONE test; impaired glucose tolerance; reduced serum folate concentration; increased serum triglyceride and phospholipid concentration.

Following four consecutive weekly applications of CLIMARA PRO mean (±SD) SHBG concentrations (C_{min}) declined from a predose value of 47.5 (25.8) to 41.2 (22.4) nmol/L at week 4.

Although different strengths of levonorgestrel were tested, for the purpose of endometrial protection against hyperplasia, the 45 µg estradiol/15 µg levonorgestrel transdermal system has been determined to deliver enough levonorgestrel to obtain adequate protection against endometrial hyperplasia, and the higher strengths are therefore not justified. In a 1-year clinical trial conducted with 45 µg estradiol/30 µg levonorgestrel and 45 µg estradiol/40 µg levonorgestrel transdermal systems, there were no clinically significant changes in fibrinogen or thrombin-antithrombin III complex values in either treatment group. In a 4-week clinical trial conducted with 45 µg estradiol/30 µg levonorgestrel and 45 µg estradiol/40 µg levonorgestrel transdermal systems, mean serum levels of SHBG and CBG at week 4 were decreased by about 20% in comparison to their respective baseline values, while no differences were observed in protein binding of either estradiol or levonorgestrel between weeks 1 and 4.

The results of the above laboratory tests should not be considered reliable unless therapy has been discontinued for two to four weeks. The pathologist should be informed that the patient is receiving estrogen/progestin therapy when relevant specimens are submitted.

ADVERSE EFFECTS: See Warnings and Precautions regarding potential induction of malignant neoplasms and adverse effects similar to those of oral contraceptives.

The most commonly reported adverse reaction to CLIMARA PRO (estradiol/levonorgestrel transdermal system) in clinical trials was skin irritation at the application site. In controlled clinical trials, discontinuation due to application site reaction occurred in 1.5% of subjects receiving CLIMARA PRO for up to 3 cycles (vs. 3.2% of placebo subjects) and in 8.3% of subjects receiving CLIMARA PRO for up to 13 cycles.

The following adverse reactions have been reported with estrogen/progestin combinations in general:

Gastrointestinal: nausea; vomiting; abdominal discomfort (cramps, pressure, pain); bloating; gallbladder disorder; asymptomatic impaired liver function; cholestatic jaundice.

Genito-urinary: breakthrough bleeding; spotting; change in menstrual flow; dysmenorrhea; vaginal itching/discharge; dyspareunia; dysuria; endometrial hyperplasia; premenstrual-like syndrome; reactivation of endometriosis; cystitis; changes in cervical erosion and amount of cervical secretion.

Skin: exogenous estrogens may induce or exacerbate symptoms of angioedema, in particular in women with hereditary angioedema; chloasma or melasma, which may persist when drug is discontinued; erythema multiforme; erythema nodosum; hemorrhagic eruption; loss of scalp hair; hirsutism and acne.

Endocrine: breast swelling and tenderness; increased blood sugar levels; decreased glucose tolerance; sodium retention.

Cardiovascular/Hematologic: palpitations; isolated cases of thrombophlebitis, thromboembolic disorders; exacerbations of varicose veins; increase in blood pressure (see Warnings and Precautions); coronary thrombosis; altered coagulation tests (see Precautions, Laboratory Tests).

Central Nervous System: aggravation of migraine episodes; headaches; mental depression; nervousness; dizziness; fatigue; irritability; neuro-ocular lesions (e.g., retinal thrombosis, optic neuritis).

Ophthalmic: visual disturbances; steepening of the corneal curvature; intolerance to contact lenses; neuro-ocular lesions (see Central Nervous System above).

Miscellaneous: changes in appetite; changes in body weight; edema; neuritis; changes in libido; musculoskeletal pain, including leg pain not related to thromboembolic disease (usually transient, lasting 3-6 weeks) may occur.

If adverse symptoms persist, the prescription of HRT should be re-considered.

OVERDOSE:

Symptoms: Numerous reports of ingestion of large doses of estrogen products and estrogen-containing oral contraceptives by young children have not revealed acute serious ill effects. Overdosage with estrogen may cause nausea, breast discomfort, fluid retention, bloating or vaginal bleeding in women.

Progestin overdosage has been characterized by depressed mood, tiredness, acne and hirsutism.

Treatment: In the event of a possible overdose, the system(s) should be removed immediately and symptomatic treatment should be given.

> For management of a suspected drug overdose, CPhA recommends that you contact your **regional Poison Control Centre**. See the *CPS* Directory section for a list of Poison Control Centres.

DOSAGE: Combination estrogen/progestin regimens are indicated for women with an intact uterus. CLIMARA PRO (estradiol/levonorgestrel transdermal system) delivers 45 µg estradiol and 15 µg levonorgestrel per day, and is worn continuously on the abdomen or buttocks. A new system should be applied once a week during each 28-day cycle. Irregular uterine bleeding may occur, particularly in the first 6 months, but generally decreases with time, and eventually may lead to an amenorrheic state.

Patients should be reevaluated within 3 to 6 months after initiation of treatment, to assess response to treatment.

Initiation of Therapy: Women not currently using continuous estrogen or combination estrogen/progestin therapy may start therapy with CLIMARA PRO at any time. However, women currently using continuous estrogen or combination estrogen/progestin therapy should complete the current cycle of therapy before initiating CLIMARA PRO therapy. Women often experience bleeding at the completion of the cycle. The first day of this bleeding would be an appropriate time to begin CLIMARA PRO therapy.

Patch Application: The physician should discuss the most appropriate placement of the patch with the patient. Immediately after removal of a patch from the pouch and removal of one-half of the protective liner, the adhesive side of the CLIMARA PRO patch should be placed on a clean, dry area of intact skin, and the remaining one-half of the protective liner peeled off. The area selected should not be oily, damaged or irritated, and not exposed to the sun. The area selected should also be one at which little wrinkling of the skin occurs during movement of the body, preferably the buttocks, lower abdomen or hip. The patch may also be placed on the side or lower back. The patch should be placed consistently on the same area of the body with each application (e.g., either the buttocks, lower abdomen, hip, side or lower back). Experience to date has shown that less irritation of the skin occurs on the buttocks than on other sites of application. Therefore, it is advisable to apply CLIMARA PRO to the buttocks. The waistline should be avoided, since tight clothing may dislodge the patch. The patch should be pressed firmly in place with the palm of the hand, making sure there is good contact, especially around the edges. In the event that a patch should fall off, it can be reapplied. If it fails to adhere then a new patch should be applied. In either case, the original treatment schedule should be continued. Patches should not be applied to the same skin site twice in succession. **CLIMARA PRO must not be applied to the breasts to avoid potentially harmful effects on the breast tissue.**

INFORMATION FOR THE PATIENT: Published in e-CPS, available by subscription at www.e-cps.ca.

SUPPLIED: The CLIMARA PRO system is composed of 3 layers. Proceeding from the visible surface towards the surface attached to the skin, these layers are (1) a translucent polyethylene backing film, (2) an acrylate adhesive matrix containing estradiol and levonorgestrel, and (3) a protective liner of either siliconized or fluoropolymer-coated polyester film. The protective liner is attached to the adhesive surface and must be removed before the system can be used.

Each translucent system contains: estradiol hemihydrate 4.55 mg (equivalent to 4.40 mg of estradiol-17β) and levonorgestrel 1.39 mg and provides controlled delivery of estradiol-17β 45 µg/day and levonorgestrel 15 µg/day to the patient. Nonmedicinal ingredients: acrylate copolymer adhesive and polyvinylpyrrolidone/vinyl acetate copolymer. Packages of 4. Store between 15 and 30°C in sealed pouch. Do not refrigerate or freeze. Apply immediately upon removal from the protective pouch. **Keep out of the reach of children and pets before and after use.**

(Shown in Product Identification Section)

Clindamycin Injection USP

clindamycin phosphate

Antibiotic

Sandoz

SUPPLIED: Each mL of sterile solution contains: clindamycin (as phosphate) 150 mg, disodium edetate 0.5 mg, sodium hydroxide and/or hydrochloric acid to adjust pH and water for injection. Preservative-free. Single-use vials of 2, 4 and 6 mL, boxes of 10. Pharmacy bulk vials of 60 and 120 mL, boxes of 1. Discard unused portion. Store between 15 and 30°C.

Clindasol®

clindamycin phosphate

Antibiotic

Stiefel, a GSK company

Date of Preparation: October 25, 2000
Date of Revision: December 14, 2005

PHARMACOLOGY: Clindamycin phosphate is a water soluble ester from which the phosphate radical must be cleaved before it possesses antibiotic activity. In vivo clindamycin phosphate is hydrolysed into active clindamycin probably by the action of phosphatases contained in the skin.

Clindamycin is an inhibitor of protein synthesis which exerts its action at the ribosomal level. The primary effect is inhibition of initiation of the peptide chain synthesis by binding to the 50S subunit of ribosomes and blocking the access of transfer RNA to the bacterial ribosomal/messenger RNA complex. Susceptible micro organisms are thus unable to synthesize essential proteins.

Clindamycin has been shown to have in vivo activity against isolates of *P. acnes*. This may account for its usefulness in the treatment of acne vulgaris. Studies have shown that a significantly greater reduction in the number of inflammatory lesions occurred in patients treated with topical clindamycin phosphate 1% compared to patients treated with the vehicle. The mean free clindamycin content of comedones extracted from subjects who used topical 1% clindamycin phosphate solution for a period of four weeks 0.6 µg/mg.

Clindamycin is metabolized in the liver to both bio-active and inactive metabolites which are excreted in the urine. About 10% of active clindamycin is excreted unaltered in the urine and only small quantities were found in the faeces. The clindamycin phosphate ester is virtually undetectable in serum one hour after intravenous administration but can still be detected three hours following intramuscular dosage. The half life of clindamycin phosphate is between 1.5 and 2 hours.

INDICATIONS: CLINDASOL (clindamycin phosphate) cream with sunscreens is indicated in the treatment of acne vulgaris.

CONTRAINDICATIONS: CLINDASOL (clindamycin phosphate) cream with sunscreens is contraindicated in persons who have shown hypersensitivity to clindamycin especially its phosphate ester, lincomycin, Parsol MCX, Parsol 1789 or to any of the ingredients contained in CLINDASOL.

CLINDASOL is also contraindicated in patients with a history of previous regional enteritis, ulcerative colitis, spastic colitis or any other form of chronic or recurrent diarrhea.

WARNINGS: CLINDASOL (clindamycin phosphate) cream with sunscreens is intended for external use only. Orally and parenterally administered clindamycin has been associated with severe colitis which may result in patient death. Use of the topical formulation of clindamycin results in absorption of the antibiotic from the skin surface. Diarrhea, bloody diarrhea, and colitis (including pseudomembranous colitis) have been reported with the use of topical and systemic clindamycin.

Studies indicate that a toxin(s) produced by clostridia is one primary cause of antibiotic-associated pseudomembranous colitis. The colitis is usually characterized by severe persistent diarrhea and severe abdominal cramps and may be associated with the passage of blood and mucous. Endoscopic examination may reveal pseudomembranous colitis. Stool culture for *C. difficile* and stool assay for *C. difficile* toxin may be helpful diagnostically. **When significant diarrhea occurs, the drug should be discontinued. Large bowel endoscopy should be considered to establish a definitive diagnosis in cases of severe diarrhea.**

Diarrhea, colitis, and pseudomembranous colitis have been observed to begin up to several weeks following cessation of oral and parenteral therapy with clindamycin.

PRECAUTIONS: The use of preparations containing antibiotics such as CLINDASOL (clindamycin phosphate) cream with sunscreens may be associated with overgrowth of antibiotic resistant microorganisms including those initially sensitive to the drug. If this should occur, therapy should be discontinued and appropriate measures taken. A cross-resistance between erythromycin and clindamycin has rarely been reported.

Pregnancy: The safety of CLINDASOL during pregnancy has not been established. Clindamycin readily crosses the placental barrier.

Lactation: It is not known if clindamycin when topically applied is excreted in human milk. Oral and parenteral clindamycin is excreted in human milk. Consequently, caution should be exercised whenever CLINDASOL is given to a nursing mother.

ADVERSE EFFECTS: Adverse reactions reported with CLINDASOL (clindamycin phosphate) cream with sunscreens included symptoms of mild to moderate skin irritation such as burning or itching, peeling or dryness, oiliness, erythema and stinging on application. Oiliness was the most frequently encountered side effect.

Cases of diarrhea, bloody diarrhea and colitis (including, rarely, pseudomembranous colitis) have been reported as adverse reactions in patients treated with topical formulation of clindamycin.

Oral and parenteral clindamycin have been associated with gastrointestinal side effects such as nausea, vomiting and diarrhea. Clindamycin associated diarrhea occurs in two forms: mild to moderate short lived diarrhea which may recover spontaneously either during or after stopping the treatment and pseudomembranous colitis where persistent profuse watery diarrhea occurs associated with typical histological changes in the colon and presence of a specific toxin produced by some strains of *C. difficile* bacteria. This latter form of diarrhea has occasionally been associated with blood and mucus in the stools.

Short lived diarrhea which recovered spontaneously either during or after stopping the treatment was observed in 2.2% of the patients using CLINDASOL. There were no cases of pseudomembranous colitis.

OVERDOSE:

Symptoms: No cases of overdosage have been reported with CLINDASOL (clindamycin phosphate) cream with sunscreens. It would be expected that, should overdosage occur, gastrointestinal side effects including abdominal pain, nausea, vomiting and diarrhea might occur.

Treatment: No specific antidote is available. Perform simple gastric lavage. Treatment should be symptomatic.

For management of a suspected drug overdose, CPhA recommends that you contact your **regional Poison Control Centre**. See the *CPS* Directory section for a list of Poison Control Centres.

DOSAGE: CLINDASOL (clindamycin phosphate) cream with sunscreens should be applied twice daily to areas affected by acne. These areas should be washed first with a mild soap, rinsed well, and patted dry, followed by application of the cream in a gentle rubbing motion, using fingertips to apply the medication. Wash hands thoroughly after application. Care should be taken to avoid eyes, nostrils, mouth, and other mucous membranes. The method of application to affected areas only may not lead to a full sun protection (SPF 15). The patient should be instructed to use a regular sunscreen for areas not covered by CLINDASOL.

INFORMATION FOR THE PATIENT: Published in e-CPS, available by subscription at www.e-cps.ca.

SUPPLIED: Each tube contains: clindamycin phosphate (equivalent to 1% w/w clindamycin) in a cream base with 7.5% Parsol MCX and 2% Parsol 1789 (SPF15). Nonmedicinal ingredients: carbomer 934, D.C. fluid Nos. 556 and 344, diisopropyl adipate, elefac I-205, germaben II, glycerin, light mineral oil, polysorbate 60, purified water, sorbitan monostearate, sodium hydroxide and stearyl alcohol. Tubes of 25 g. Store at 15-30°C. Avoid freezing.

Clindets®

clindamycin phosphate

Topical Antibiotic

Stiefel, a GSK company

PHARMACOLOGY: Although clindamycin phosphate is inactive in vitro, rapid in vivo hydrolysis converts this compound to the active antibiotic clindamycin. Like other macrolides, clindamycin inhibits bacterial protein synthesis by binding to the 50S subunit of ribosomes. Clindamycin in vitro inhibits *P. acnes*.

Bacterial resistance may develop to macrolides, such as clindamycin, especially when used alone and cross resistance between macrolides has been demonstrated. Following multiple topical applications of clindamycin phosphate at a concentration equivalent to 10 mg per mL in an isopropyl alcohol and water solution, very low levels of clindamycin are present in the serum (0-3 ng/mL) and less than 0.2% of the dose is recovered in urine as clindamycin.

INDICATIONS: CLINDETS (clindamycin phosphate pledget) is indicated in the treatment of moderate acne vulgaris.

CONTRAINDICATIONS: CLINDETS (clindamycin phosphate pledget) is contraindicated in individuals with a history of hypersensitivity to preparations containing clindamycin or lincomycin, or any other component of the preparation, a history of regional enteritis or ulcerative colitis, or a history of antibiotic-associated colitis.

WARNINGS: For external use only. Not for ophthalmic use. Avoid contact with eyes and mucous membranes. The solution contains isopropyl alcohol, therefore, in the event of accidental contact with sensitive surfaces (eyes, abraded skin, mucous membranes), bathe with copious amounts of cool tap water.

Orally and parenterally administered clindamycin has been associated with severe colitis which may result in patient death. Use of the topical formulation of clindamycin results in absorption of the antibiotic from the skin surface. Diarrhea, bloody diarrhea, and colitis (including pseudomembranous colitis) have been reported with the use of topical and systemic clindamycin.

Studies indicate that a toxin(s) produced by clostridia is one primary cause of antibiotic-associated pseudomembranous colitis. The colitis is usually characterized by severe persistent diarrhea and severe abdominal cramps and may be associated with the passage of blood and mucous. Endoscopic examination may reveal pseudomembranous colitis. Stool culture for *C. difficile* and stool assay for *C. difficile* toxin may be helpful diagnostically. **When significant diarrhea occurs, the drug should be discontinued. Large bowel endoscopy should be considered to establish a definitive diagnosis in cases of severe diarrhea.**

Diarrhea, colitis, and pseudomembranous colitis have been observed to begin up to several weeks following cessation of oral and parenteral therapy with clindamycin.

PRECAUTIONS: General: The use of preparations containing antibiotics such as clindamycin may be associated with overgrowth of antibiotic resistant microorganisms including those initially sensitive to the drug. If this should occur, therapy should be discontinued and appropriate measures taken. A cross-resistance between erythromycin and clindamycin has been reported.

Pregnancy: **No adequate or controlled reproduction studies have been conducted with clindamycin in pregnant women. Animal reproduction studies have not been conducted with CLINDETS (clindamycin phosphate pledget) and it is not known whether CLINDETS can cause fetal harm when administered to pregnant women or can affect reproduction capacity. CLINDETS should not be given to a pregnant woman unless the potential benefits to the mother outweigh the possible risks to the foetus.**

Reproduction studies have been performed in rats and mice using subcutaneous and oral doses of clindamycin ranging from 100 to 600 mg/kg/day and have revealed no evidence of impaired fertility or harm to the fetus due to clindamycin. Conclusions from such animal studies may not always be predictive of the effects on human reproduction.

Lactation: **It is not known whether clindamycin is excreted in human milk following the topical use of CLINDETS. However, orally and parenterally administered, clindamycin have been reported to appear in breast milk. Because of the potential for serious adverse reactions in nursing infants, a decision should be made whether to discontinue nursing or to discontinue the drug, taking into account the potential benefits to the mother and the potential risks to the infant.**

Children: **Safety and effectiveness in the pediatric population under the age of 12 have not been established.**

Drug Interactions: Clindamycin has been shown to have neuromuscular blocking properties that may enhance the action of other neuromuscular blocking agents. Therefore, it should be used with caution in patients receiving such agents.

ADVERSE EFFECTS: In an 11-week placebo controlled study with CLINDETS (clindamycin phosphate pledget), local tolerance in acne patients was assessed by observing the incidence and change in underlying erythema, peeling and burning. With CLINDETS occurrences were mild and self resolving. These results are summarized in Table 1.

Table 1: CLINDETS

Patients With Worsening Signs or Symptoms of Acne

		Local Tolerance[a]			
		Number of Patients with Worsening Score			
Signs and Symptoms	**Treatment**	**Week 2**	**Week 5**	**Week 8**	**Week 11**
Erythema	CLINDETS	1 (1.4%)[b]	2 (2.8%)	0	0
	Vehicle	1 (1.4%)	2 (2.9%)	0	0
Peeling	CLINDETS	2 (2.7%)	2 (2.8%)	1 (1.4%)	0
	Vehicle	1 (1.4%)	3 (4.3%)	0	0
Burning	CLINDETS	4 (5.5%)	1 (1.4%)	2 (2.7%)	1 (1.4%)
	Vehicle	4 (5.6%)	4 (5.7%)	0	0

[a] Change from Baseline of Signs and Symptoms.
[b] () represents % of patients.

Overall tolerance in the study was considered excellent in 97% of the patients receiving CLINDETS.

In the literature, dryness and itching have also often been associated with the use of alcoholic topical clindamycin solutions.

Orally and parenterally administered clindamycin have also been associated, in the literature, with severe potentially fatal colitis. Cases of diarrhea, bloody diarrhea and colitis (including, rarely, pseudomembranous colitis) have been infrequently reported as adverse reactions in patients treated with topical clindamycin (see Warnings). Abdominal pain and gastrointestinal disturbances as well as gram-negative folliculitis have also been reported in association with the use of topical formulations of clindamycin.

OVERDOSE:

Symptoms: Topically applied clindamycin phosphate formulations can be absorbed in sufficient amounts to produce systemic effects (see Warnings). If the medication is applied excessively, topical irritation can be expected (see Adverse Effects). No cases of overdosage have been reported with CLINDETS (clindamycin phosphate pledget).

Treatment: Topical overuse of CLINDETS, should be treated symptomatically.

> For management of a suspected drug overdose, CPhA recommends that you contact your **regional Poison Control Centre**. See the *CPS* Directory section for a list of Poison Control Centres.

DOSAGE: CLINDETS (clindamycin phosphate pledget) should be applied twice daily, once in the morning and once before bedtime, to areas affected by acne. The area to be treated should be washed first with a mild soap or cleanser, rinsed well and patted dry. A thin film of medication should be applied avoiding the eyes and mouth. Each pledget should be removed from the foil immediately before use, used only once and then discarded.

INFORMATION FOR THE PATIENT: Published in e-CPS, available by subscription at www.e-cps.ca.

SUPPLIED: Each CLINDETS pledget applicator contains: approximately 1 mL of 1% clindamycin (as phosphate) topical solution in a vehicle of isopropyl alcohol 52% v/v, propylene glycol, and purified water. Containers of 60 pledgets. Store below 30°C. Keep from freezing.

Clindoxyl® Ⓟ

clindamycin phosphate—benzoyl peroxide

Topical Acne Therapy

Stiefel, a GSK company

Date of Revision: July 28, 2010

PHARMACOLOGY: Clindamycin Phosphate: Although clindamycin phosphate is inactive in vitro, rapid in vivo hydrolysis converts this compound to the active antibiotic clindamycin. Like other macrolides, clindamycin inhibits bacterial protein synthesis by binding to the 50S subunit of ribosomes. Clindamycin in vitro inhibits *P. acnes*.

Bacterial resistance may develop to macrolides, such as clindamycin, especially when used alone and cross resistance between macrolides has been demonstrated. Following multiple topical applications of clindamycin phosphate at a concentration equivalent to 10 mg per mL in an isopropyl alcohol and water solution, very low levels of clindamycin are present in the serum (0-3 ng/mL) and less than 0.2% of the dose is recovered in urine as clindamycin.

Benzoyl Peroxide: The effectiveness of benzoyl peroxide in the treatment of acne vulgaris is primarily attributable to its antibacterial activity, especially with respect to *P. acnes*, the predominant organism in sebaceous follicles and comedones. The antibacterial activity of this compound is presumably due to the release of active or free-radical oxygen capable of oxidizing bacterial proteins. This action, combined with mild keratolytic effect, is believed to be responsible for its usefulness in acne. *P. acnes* resistance has not been reported with benzoyl peroxide. In acne patients treated topically with benzoyl peroxide, resolution of the acne usually coincides with the reduction in the level of *P. acnes* and free fatty acids. Benzoyl peroxide has been shown to be absorbed by the skin, where it is metabolized to benzoic acid and then excreted as benzoate in the urine.

INDICATIONS: CLINDOXYL Gel (clindamycin phosphate and benzoyl peroxide) is indicated in the topical treatment of moderate acne vulgaris characterised by the presence of comedones, papules and pustules. CLINDOXYL Gel is not indicated for the treatment of cystic acne.

CONTRAINDICATIONS: CLINDOXYL Gel (clindamycin phosphate and benzoyl peroxide) is contraindicated in individuals with a history of hypersensitivity to preparations containing clindamycin or lincomycin, benzoyl peroxide, or any other component of the preparation, a history of regional enteritis or ulcerative colitis, or a history of antibiotic-associated colitis.

WARNINGS: For external use only. Not for ophthalmic use. Avoid contact with eyes and mucous membranes. In the event of accidental contact with sensitive surfaces (eyes, abraded skin, mucous membranes), bathe with copious amounts of cool tap water.

Clostridium-Difficile-Associated Disease (CDAD): Use of topical formulation of clindamycin results in absorption of clindamycin from the skin surface. *C. difficile*-associated disease (CDAD) has been reported with the use of topical, oral and parenteral administration of clindamycin. CDAD may range in severity from mild diarrhea to fatal colitis. It is important to consider this diagnosis in patients who present with diarrhea, or symptoms of colitis, pseudomembranous colitis, toxic mega colon, or perforation of colon subsequent to the administration of any antibacterial agent. CDAD has been reported to occur 2 months after the administration of antibacterial agents.

Treatment with antibacterial agents may alter the normal flora of the colon and may permit overgrowth of *C. difficile*. *C. difficile* produces toxins A and B, which contribute to the development of CDAD. CDAD may cause significant morbidity and mortality.

If the diagnosis of CDAD is suspected or confirmed, appropriate therapeutic measures should be initiated. Mild cases of CDAD usually respond to discontinuation of antibacterial agents not directed against *C. difficile*. In moderate to severe cases, consideration should be given to management with fluids and electrolytes, protein supplementation, and treatment with an antibacterial agent clinically effective against *C. difficile*. Surgical evaluation should be instituted as clinically indicated, as surgical intervention may be required in certain severe cases. See Adverse Effects.

PRECAUTIONS: General: Concomitant topical acne treatments are not recommended because a possible cumulative irritancy effect may occur, especially with peeling, or abrasive agents. If severe irritation develops, discontinue use and institute appropriate therapy.

Pregnancy: **Animal reproductive studies have not been performed with benzoyl peroxide. Reproductive studies have been performed in rats and mice using subcutaneous and oral doses of clindamycin ranging from 100 to 600 mg/kg/day and have revealed no evidence of impaired fertility or harm to the fetus due to clindamycin.**

Animal reproduction studies have not been conducted with CLINDOXYL Gel (clindamycin phosphate and benzoyl peroxide). It is not known whether CLINDOXYL Gel can cause fetal harm when administered to a pregnant woman or can affect reproduction capacity. CLINDOXYL Gel should not be given to a pregnant woman unless the potential benefits to the mother outweigh the possible risks to the fetus.

Lactation: **It is not known whether benzoyl peroxide or clindamycin are excreted in human milk following the topical use of CLINDOXYL Gel. However, orally and parenterally administered clindamycin have been reported to appear in breast milk. Because of the potential for serious adverse reactions in nursing infants, a decision should be made whether to discontinue nursing or to discontinue the drug, taking into account the potential benefits to the mother and the potential risks to the infant.**

Children: **Safety and effectiveness in the pediatric population under the age of 12 have not been established.**

Drug Interactions: Clindamycin has been shown to have neuromuscular blocking properties that may enhance the action of other neuromuscular blocking agents. Therefore, it should be used with caution in patients receiving such agents. Benzoyl peroxide inactivates tretinoin when used concomitantly.

ADVERSE EFFECTS: In controlled clinical trials where a total of 172 patients received CLINDOXYL Gel (clindamycin phosphate and benzoyl peroxide), the reported adverse events considered to have a relationship to CLINDOXYL Gel were comprised mainly of reactions at the site of application such as peeling (16.3%), erythema (7.6%), dryness (7.0%), burning (2.3%) and pruritus (1.7%). Mild paraesthesia and worsening of acne were noted in one patient each.

Orally and parenterally administered clindamycin has been associated with severe colitis which may end fatally.

Cases of diarrhea, bloody diarrhea and colitis (including, rarely, pseudomembranous colitis) have been infrequently reported as adverse reactions in patients treated with topical clindamycin (see Warnings). Abdominal pain and gastrointestinal disturbances as well as gram-negative folliculitis have also been reported in association with the use of topical formulations of clindamycin.

Post-Market Adverse Drug Reactions: Anaphylaxis, as well as allergic reactions leading to hospitalization, application site hypersensitivity, application site swelling and swelling of the face including angioedema.

OVERDOSE:

Symptoms: Topically applied clindamycin phosphate formulations can be absorbed in sufficient amounts to produce systemic effects (see Warnings). If medication is applied excessively, marked redness and peeling may occur. There are no reports of human ingestion overdosage with CLINDOXYL Gel (clindamycin phosphate and benzoyl peroxide).

Treatment: Excessive application of CLINDOXYL Gel may cause increased skin irritation from the benzoyl peroxide and gastrointestinal side effects, including abdominal pain, nausea, vomiting and diarrhea, due to systemic absorption of clindamycin phosphate from CLINDOXYL Gel. In the case of symptoms resulting from excessive application of CLINDOXYL Gel, CLINDOXYL Gel should be discontinued for several days before resuming therapy.

In the event of accidental ingestion of CLINDOXYL Gel, the same gastrointestinal side effects as those expected with topical clindamycin are expected (see Warnings). No specific antidote is available. In such cases, CLINDOXYL Gel should be discontinued. Activated charcoal may be administered to aid in the removal of unabsorbed CLINDOXYL Gel.

> For management of a suspected drug overdose, contact your regional Poison Control Centre. See the *CPS* Directory section for a list of Poison Control Centres.

DOSAGE: CLINDOXYL Gel (clindamycin phosphate and benzoyl peroxide) should be applied to affected areas once daily before bed time, after the skin has been thoroughly washed, rinsed with warm water and gently patted dry.

INFORMATION FOR THE PATIENT: Published in e-CPS, available by subscription at www.e-cps.ca.

SUPPLIED: Each g of gel contains: clindamycin phosphate equivalent to 1% (10 mg) clindamycin in combination with 5% (50 mg) benzoyl peroxide in a base consisting of carbomer 940, dimethicone, disodium lauryl sulfosuccinate, edetate disodium, glycerin, hydrated silica, methylparaben, poloxamer, purified water and sodium hydroxide. Tubes of 45 g. Sample tubes of 5 g. Prior to dispensing, CLINDOXYL Gel should be stored in a cold environment, preferably in a refrigerator between 2 and 8°C. Do not freeze.

To the Pharmacist: Dispense with a 120 day expiration date and specify "Store at room temperature (15-25°C). Keep tube tightly closed. Keep out of the reach of children".

Clobazam Ⓝ

CPhA Monograph

see *Benzodiazepines*

Clobetasol Ⓟ

CPhA Monograph

see *Corticosteroids: Topical*

Clobetasone

CPhA Monograph

see *Corticosteroids: Topical*

> The reader is invited to consult CPhA's monograph **Corticosteroids: Topical**.

Clobex™ Lotion Ⓟ

clobetasol propionate

Topical Corticosteroid

Galderma

Date of Preparation: July 26, 2004

PHARMACOLOGY: Clobex (clobetasol propionate) is a super-high potency topical corticosteroid. Clobex Lotion (clobetasol propionate lotion, 0.05%) contains clobetasol propionate, a synthetic fluorinated corticosteroid for topical dermatological use. Corticosteroids constitute a class of primarily synthetic steroids used topically as anti-inflammatory and antipruritic agents. Clobetasol, an analogue of prednisolone, has a high degree of glucocorticoid activity and a slight degree of mineralocorticoid activity. Studies performed with clobetasol propionate lotion, 0.05% indicate that it is in the very high range of potency as compared with other topical corticosteroids.

Mechanism of Action: Like other topical corticosteroids, Clobex Lotion has anti-inflammatory, antipruritic, and vasoconstrictive properties. The mechanism of the anti-inflammatory activity of topical steroids in general is unclear. However, corticosteroids are thought to act by induction of phospholipase A_2 inhibitory proteins, collectively called lipocortins. It is postulated that these proteins control the biosynthesis of potent mediators of inflammation such as prostaglandins and leukotrienes by inhibiting the release of their common precursor, arachidonic acid. Arachidonic acid is released from membrane phospholipids by phospholipase A_2.

Pharmacokinetics: The extent of percutaneous absorption of topical corticosteroids is determined by many factors, including the vehicle, the integrity of the epidermal barrier and occlusion. Topical corticosteroids can be absorbed from normal intact skin. Inflammation and other disease processes in the skin may increase percutaneous absorption.

There is no human data regarding the distribution of corticosteroids to body organs following topical application. Nevertheless, once absorbed through the skin, topical corticosteroids are handled through pharmacokinetic pathways similar to systemically administered corticosteroids. Due to the fact that circulating levels are usually below the level of detection, the use of pharmacodynamic endpoints for assessing the systemic exposure of topical corticosteroids is necessary. They are metabolized primarily in the liver and are then excreted by the kidneys. In addition, some corticosteroids and their metabolites are also excreted in the bile.

Clobex Lotion is in the super-high range of potency as compared with other topical corticosteroids in vasoconstrictor studies.

INDICATIONS: Clobex Lotion (clobetasol propionate lotion, 0.05%) is a super-high potency corticosteroid with the potential to suppress the HPA axis.

Clobex Lotion is indicated for the treatment of corticosteroid-responsive dermatoses where an anti-inflammatory or anti-pruritic activity is required for the topical management of these conditions.

Treatment should be limited to 2 consecutive weeks, not to exceed 50 g (50 mL) per week, and be applied to no more than 10% of the body surface area. Use should be restricted to those 18 years or older.

In the treatment of moderate to severe plaque-type psoriasis that has not sufficiently improved after the initial 2 weeks, Clobex Lotion can be used for up to 2 additional weeks. Any additional benefits of extending treatment should be weighed against the risk of HPA axis suppression.

Patients should be instructed to use Clobex Lotion for the minimum amount of time necessary.

CONTRAINDICATIONS: Clobex Lotion (clobetasol propionate lotion, 0.05%) is contraindicated in patients who are hypersensitive to clobetasol propionate, to other corticosteroids, or to any ingredient in this preparation.

Treatment with topical corticosteroids is not indicated in patients with untreated tubercular, bacterial and fungal infections involving the skin, and in certain viral diseases such as herpes simplex, chickenpox, and vaccinia.

WARNINGS: Use in those under 18 years of age is not recommended.

In the treatment of moderate to severe plaque-type psoriasis, Clobex Lotion (clobetasol propionate lotion, 0.05%) applied to no more than 10% of the body surface area can be used up to 4 consecutive weeks (when dosing for more than 2 weeks, any additional benefits of extending treatment should be weighed against the risk of HPA suppression).

Patients should be instructed to use Clobex Lotion for the minimum amount of time necessary to achieve the desired results (see Precautions).

PRECAUTIONS: General: Systemic absorption of topical corticosteroids has caused reversible adrenal suppression with the potential for glucocorticosteroid insufficiency after withdrawal of treatment. Manifestations of Cushing's syndrome, hyperglycemia, and glucosuria can also be produced in some patients by systemic absorption of topical corticosteroids while on treatment.

Conditions which increase systemic absorption include the application of the more potent steroids, use over large surface areas, prolonged use, and the addition of occlusive dressings. Therefore, patients applying a topical steroid to a large surface area or to areas under occlusion should be evaluated periodically for evidence of adrenal suppression (see Laboratory Tests). If adrenal suppression is noted, an attempt should be made to withdraw the drug, to reduce the frequency of application, or to substitute a less potent steroid. Recovery of HPA axis function is generally prompt upon discontinuation of topical corticosteroids. Infrequently, signs and symptoms of glucocorticosteroid insufficiency may occur requiring supplemental systemic corticosteroids. For information on systemic supplementation, see prescribing information for those products.

Clobex Lotion is a super-high potency topical corticosteroid that has been shown in two adult studies to suppress the HPA axis at the lowest doses tested.

In total, 8 of 10 evaluable patients with moderate to severe plaque psoriasis experienced adrenal suppression following 4 weeks of Clobex Lotion treatment (treatment beyond 4 weeks is not recommended in moderate to severe plaque psoriasis). In follow-up testing, 1 of 2 subjects remained suppressed after 8 days.

Furthermore, 5 of 9 evaluable patients with moderate to severe atopic dermatitis experienced adrenal suppression following two weeks of Clobex Lotion treatment (treatment beyond 2 consecutive weeks is not recommended in moderate to severe atopic dermatitis). Of the 3 subjects that had follow-up testing, 1 subject failed to recover adrenal function 7 days post treatment. The proportion of subjects suppressed may be underestimated because the adrenal glands were stimulated weekly with cosyntropin in these studies.

The potential increase in systemic exposure does not correlate with any proven benefit, but may lead to an increased potential for hypothalamic-pituitary-adrenal (HPA) suppression. Patients with acute illness or injury may have increased morbidity and mortality with intermittent HPA axis suppression. Patients should be advised to use Clobex Lotion for the minimum amount of time necessary to achieve the desired results.

Clobex Lotion should not be used on lesions close to the eye because of the risk of increased intraocular pressure, glaucoma, and cataracts. Clobex Lotion should not be used under occlusion or on limbs with impaired circulation. Clobex Lotion should not be used on the face, groin or axilla.

If irritation develops, Clobex Lotion should be discontinued and appropriate therapy instituted. Allergic contact dermatitis with corticosteroids is usually diagnosed by a failure to heal rather than noting a clinical exacerbation, as with most products not containing a corticosteroid.

In the presence of fungal infections, an appropriate antifungal treatment should be instituted and Clobex Lotion should be discontinued until the fungal infection is cured. In the presence of a bacterial infection, an appropriate antibacterial agent should be instituted. If a favorable response does not occur promptly, Clobex Lotion should be discontinued until the bacterial infection is adequately controlled.

Laboratory Tests: The following tests may be helpful in evaluating patients for HPA axis suppression:

- ACTH stimulation test
- AM plasma cortisol test
- Urinary free cortisol test

Pregnancy: There are no adequate and well-controlled studies of the teratogenic potential of clobetasol propionate in pregnant women. Clobex Lotion should be used during pregnancy only if its benefit justifies the potential risk to the fetus.

Lactation: Systemically administered corticosteroids appear in human milk and could suppress growth, interfere with endogenous corticosteroid production, or cause other untoward effects. It is not known whether topical administration of corticosteroids could result in sufficient systemic absorption to produce detectable quantities in breast milk. Because many drugs are excreted in human milk, caution should be exercised when Clobex Lotion is administered to a nursing woman.

Pediatrics: Safety and effectiveness of Clobex Lotion in pediatric patients have not been established and its use in pediatric patients under 18 years of age is not recommended.

Because of a higher ratio of skin surface area to body mass, pediatric patients may absorb a higher percentage of topically applied corticosteroids and therefore may be at a greater risk than adults of HPA axis suppression and Cushing's syndrome. They are therefore also at greater risk of glucocorticosteroid insufficiency during and/or after withdrawal of treatment. Adverse effects including striae have been reported with inappropriate use of topical corticosteroids in infants and children.

HPA axis suppression, Cushing's syndrome, linear growth retardation, delayed weight gain, and intracranial hypertension have been reported in children receiving topical corticosteroids. Manifestations of adrenal suppression in children include low plasma cortisol levels and absence of response to ACTH stimulation. Manifestations of intracranial hypertension include bulging fontanelles, headaches, and bilateral papilledema.

The HPA axis suppression potential of Clobex Lotion has been studied in adolescents (12 to 17 years of age) with moderate to severe atopic dermatitis covering a minimum of 20% of the total body surface area. In total, 14 patients were evaluated for HPA axis function and for safety. Patients were treated twice daily for 2 weeks with Clobex Lotion. After 2 weeks of therapy, 9 out of 14 subjects had suppression of their HPA axis and two weeks after stopping therapy 1 out of 4 continued to have suppression of the HPA axis. None of the patients who developed HPA axis suppression had concomitant clinical signs of adrenal suppression and none of them were discontinued from the study for reasons related to the safety or tolerability of Clobex Lotion.

Geriatrics: Clinical studies of Clobex Lotion did not include sufficient numbers of patients aged 65 and over to determine whether they respond differently than younger patients. In general, dose selection for an elderly patient should be made with caution, usually starting at the low end of the dosing range, reflecting the greater frequency of decreased hepatic, renal or cardiac function, and of concomitant disease or other drug therapy.

Carcinogenesis, Mutagenesis, and Reproduction: Long term animal studies have not been performed to evaluate the carcinogenic potential of clobetasol propionate. Clobetasol propionate did not produce any increase in chromosomal aberrations in Chinese hamster ovary cells in vitro in the presence or absence of metabolic activation. Clobetasol propionate was also negative in the micronucleus test in mice after oral administration. Studies of the effect of Clobex Lotion on fertility have not been performed.

ADVERSE EFFECTS: In controlled clinical trials with Clobex Lotion (clobetasol propionate lotion, 0.05%), the following adverse reactions have been reported: burning/stinging, skin dryness, irritation, erythema, folliculitis, pruritus, skin atrophy, and telangiectasia.

The incidence of local adverse reactions reported in the trials with Clobex Lotion was 1% or less, with the exception of telangiectasia (3.2%) and skin atrophy (4.2%). Similar rates of local adverse reactions were reported in the comparator groups (two formulations of clobetasol propionate cream). Most adverse events were rated as mild to moderate and they are not affected by age, race or gender. No serious drug-related adverse events were reported during any of the clinical trials. See Table 1.

Table 1: Clobex Lotion

Adverse Events

	Phase II/III Studies—Number of Subjects (%)	
	Clobex Lotion	**Lotion Vehicle**
Patients with Psoriasis	188	62
Patients with Atopic Dermatitis	121	33
Total Number of Patients	309	95
Subjects w/Adverse Events	49 (15.9%)	9 (9.5%)
Subjects w/Drug-Related[a] Adverse Events	13 (4.2%)	5 (5.3%)
Dermatological	13 (4.2%)	4 (4.2%)
Non-dermatological	0	1 (1.1%)
Adverse Events with incidence >1%		
No. of Subjects with Increases in Skin Atrophy Scores (%)		
Psoriasis	7 (3.7)	0
Atopic Dermatitis	6 (4.9)	0
Totals	13 (4.2)	0
No. of Subjects with Increases in Telangiectasia Scores (%)		
Psoriasis	6 (3.2)	0
Atopic Dermatitis	4 (3.3)	0
Totals	10 (3.2)	0

[a] Possibly, probably, definitely related.

In controlled clinical trials with other internationally marketed topical clobetasol propionate formulations (creams), burning/stinging, folliculitis, cracking and fissuring of the skin, numbness of the fingers, tenderness of the elbow, skin atrophy and telangiectasia have been reported. Cushing's syndrome has been reported in infants and adults as a result of prolonged use of other topical clobetasol propionate formulations.

The following additional local adverse reactions have been reported with topical corticosteroids. They may occur more frequently with the use of occlusive dressings, use over a prolonged period of time, use over large surface areas and use of super-high potency corticosteroids, such as clobetasol propionate. These reactions are listed in an approximate decreasing order of occurrence: irritation, dryness, itching, burning, local irritation, folliculitis, acneiform eruptions, hypopigmentation, perioral dermatitis, allergic contact dermatitis, skin atrophy, atrophy of subcutaneous tissues, telangiectasia, hypertrichosis, change in pigmentation, secondary infection, striae and miliaria. If applied to the face, acne rosacea or perioral dermatitis can occur. When occlusive dressings are used, pustules, milaria, folliculitis and pyoderma may occur. In rare instances, treatment of psoriasis with systemic or very potent topical corticosteroids (or their withdrawal) is thought to have provoked the pustular form of the disease.

Systemic absorption of topical corticosteroids has produced reversible adrenal suppression, manifestations of Cushing's syndrome, hyperglycemia and glucosuria.

OVERDOSE:

Symptoms: Topically applied Clobex Lotion (clobetasol propionate lotion, 0.05%) can be absorbed in sufficient amounts to produce systemic effects (see Precautions). In case of chronic overdosage or misuse, features of hypercortism may appear.

Treatment: Recovery of the HPA axis is usually prompt and complete following discontinuation; however, if symptoms of adrenal insufficiency occur, supplemental oral steroid therapy may be initiated and tapered off gradually.

For management of a suspected drug overdose, CPhA recommends that you contact your **regional Poison Control Centre**. See the *CPS* Directory section for a list of Poison Control Centres.

DOSAGE: Clobex Lotion (clobetasol propionate lotion, 0.05%) should be applied to the affected skin areas twice daily and rubbed in gently and completely (see Indications).

Clobex Lotion contains a super-high potency topical corticosteroid; therefore, treatment should be limited to:

- 2 consecutive weeks for the relief of the inflammatory and pruritic manifestations of corticosteroid-responsive dermatoses,
- 4 consecutive weeks in the treatment of moderate to severe plaque-type psoriasis.

The total dosage should not exceed 50 g (50 mL) per week or be used on more than 10% of body surface area because of the potential for the drug to suppress the hypothalamic-pituitary-adrenal (HPA) axis.

Therapy should be discontinued when control has been achieved. If no improvement is seen within two weeks, reassessment of diagnosis may be necessary.

Use is not recommended in patients under 18 years of age since it has not been studied sufficiently and also due to numerically high rates of HPA axis suppression in this age group.

Unless directed by physician, Clobex Lotion should not be used with occlusive dressings.

INFORMATION FOR THE PATIENT: Published in e-CPS, available by subscription at www.e-cps.ca.

SUPPLIED: Each g of lotion contains: clobetasol propionate USP 0.5 mg. Nonmedicinal ingredients: carbomer 1342, hydroxypropylmethyl cellulose, mineral oil, polyoxyethylene glycol 300 isostearate, propylene glycol, purified water and sodium hydroxide. Bottles of 120 mL. Store at controlled room temperature (15-30°C). Do not freeze.

The reader is invited to consult CPhA's monograph **Corticosteroids: Topical**.

Clobex™ Shampoo

clobetasol propionate

Topical Corticosteroid

Galderma

Date of Preparation: July 26, 2004
Date of Revision: December 9, 2004

PHARMACOLOGY: Mechanism of Action: Clobex (clobetasol propionate) is a super-high potency topical corticosteroid. Like other topical corticosteroids, Clobex Shampoo (clobetasol propionate shampoo, 0.05%) has anti-inflammatory, antipruritic, and vasoconstrictive properties. The mechanism of the anti-inflammatory activity of the topical steroids, in general, is unclear. However, corticosteroids are thought to act by the induction of phospholipase A_2 inhibitory proteins, collectively called lipocortins. It is postulated that these proteins control the biosynthesis of potent mediators of inflammation such as prostaglandins and leukotrienes by inhibiting the release of their common precursor, arachidonic acid. Arachidonic acid is released from membrane phospholipids by phospholipase A_2.

Pharmacokinetics: The extent of percutaneous absorption of topical corticosteroids is determined by many factors, including the vehicle, the integrity of the epidermal barrier and the use of occlusive dressings. Topical corticosteroids can be absorbed from normal intact skin while inflammation and/or other disease processes in the skin may increase percutaneous absorption.

Once absorbed through the skin, topical corticosteroids are handled through pharmacokinetic pathways similar to systemically administered corticosteroids. Due to the fact that circulating levels are well below the level of detection, the use of pharmacodynamic endpoints for assessing the systemic exposure of topical corticosteroids is necessary. They are metabolized, primarily in the liver, and are then excreted by the kidneys. In addition, some corticosteroids, including clobetasol propionate and its metabolites, are also excreted in the bile.

INDICATIONS: Clobex Shampoo (clobetasol propionate shampoo, 0.05%) is a super-high potent topical corticosteroid formulation indicated for the relief of the inflammatory and pruritic manifestations of moderate to severe forms of scalp psoriasis in subjects 18 years of age and older.

Treatment should be limited to 4 consecutive weeks because of the potential for the drug to suppress the hypothalamic-pituitary-adrenal (HPA) axis. The total dose should not exceed 50 g (50 mL) per week (see Dosage).

Patients should be instructed to use Clobex Shampoo for the minimum time period necessary to achieve the desired results (see Precautions).

Use in patients under 18 years of age is not recommended.

There were insufficient numbers of non-Caucasian patients in the studies evaluating the safety and efficacy of Clobex Shampoo to determine whether they responded differently than Caucasian patients with regards to efficacy and safety.

CONTRAINDICATIONS: Clobex Shampoo (clobetasol propionate shampoo, 0.05%) is contraindicated in patients who are hypersensitive to clobetasol propionate, to other corticosteroids, or to any ingredient in this preparation. Clobetasol propionate is also contraindicated in dermatoses in children under one year of age, including dermatitis.

Clobex Shampoo should not be used in bacterial/fungal infections, tuberculosis of the skin, syphilitic skin infections, chicken pox, eruptions following vaccinations, and viral diseases of the skin in general. This preparation is also contraindicated in the treatment of rosacea, acne vulgaris, perioral dermatitis or perianal and genital pruritis.

WARNINGS: Clobex Shampoo should not be used under occlusive dressing, over extensive areas, or on the face, axillae and scrotum, as sufficient absorption may occur giving rise to adrenal suppression and other systemic effects.

PRECAUTIONS: General: Systemic absorption of topical corticosteroids can produce reversible hypothalamic-pituitary-adrenal (HPA) axis suppression with the potential for glucocorticosteroid insufficiency after withdrawal of treatment. Manifestations of Cushing's syndrome, hyperglycemia, and glucosuria can also be produced in some patients by systemic absorption of topical corticosteroids while on treatment.

The effect of Clobex Shampoo (clobetasol propionate, 0.05%) on HPA axis suppression was evaluated in one study in adolescents 12 to 17 years of age. In this study, 5 of 12 evaluable subjects developed suppression of their HPA axis following 4 weeks of treatment with Clobex Shampoo applied once daily.

Conditions which increase systemic absorption include the application of the more potent corticosteroids, use over large surface areas, prolonged use, and the addition of occlusive dressings. Therefore, patients applying a topical steroid to a large surface area or to areas under occlusion should be evaluated periodically for evidence of HPA axis suppression. This may be done by using the ACTH stimulation, A.M. plasma cortisol, and urinary free cortisol tests. If HPA axis suppression is noted, an attempt should be made to withdraw the drug, to reduce the frequency of application, or to substitute a less potent steroid. Recovery of HPA axis function is generally prompt and complete upon discontinuation of topical corticosteroids. Infrequently, signs and symptoms of glucocorticosteroid insufficiency may occur, requiring supplemental systemic corticosteroids. For information on systemic supplementation, see prescribing information for those products.

If irritation develops, Clobex Shampoo (clobetasol propionate shampoo, 0.05%) should be discontinued and appropriate therapy instituted. Allergic contact dermatitis with corticosteroids is usually diagnosed by observing a failure to heal rather than noting a clinical exacerbation, as with most topical products not containing corticosteroids. Such an observation should be corroborated with appropriate diagnostic patch testing.

In the presence of dermatological infections, the use of an appropriate antifungal or antibacterial agent should be instituted. If a favorable response does not occur promptly, use of Clobex Shampoo should be discontinued until the infection has been adequately controlled.

Although Clobex Shampoo is intended for the topical treatment of moderate to severe scalp psoriasis, it should be noted that certain areas of the body, such as the face, groin, and axillae, are more prone to atrophic changes than other areas of the body following treatment with corticosteroids. Clobex Shampoo should not be used on the groin or axillae. Avoid any contact of the drug product with the facial skin, eyes and lips. In case of contact, rinse thoroughly with water all parts of the body that came in contact with the shampoo.

Suitable precautions should be taken when using topical corticosteroids in patients with stasis dermatitis and other skin diseases with impaired circulation.

Geriatrics: Clinical studies of Clobetasol Propionate Shampoo, 0.05%, did not include sufficient numbers of patients aged 65 years and over to determine whether they respond differently than younger patients. In general, dose selection for an elderly patient should be made with caution, usually starting at the low end of the dosing range, reflecting the greater frequency of decreased hepatic, renal or cardiac function, and of concomitant disease or other drug therapy.

Pediatrics: Safety and effectiveness of Clobex Shampoo have been established in patients 18 years and older. Insufficient data have been obtained in patients under the age of 18 years. Because of a higher ratio of skin surface area to body mass, pediatric patients are at a greater risk than adults of HPA axis suppression and Cushing's syndrome when they are treated with topical corticosteroids. They are therefore also at greater risk of adrenal insufficiency during and/or after withdrawal of treatment. Adverse effects including striae have been reported with inappropriate use of topical corticosteroids in infants and children. Therefore, use is not recommended in patients under the age of 18 years.

HPA axis suppression, Cushing's syndrome, linear growth retardation, delayed weight gain, and intracranial hypertension have been reported in children receiving topical corticosteroids. Manifestations of adrenal suppression in children include low plasma cortisol levels and an absence of response to ACTH stimulation. Manifestations of intracranial hypertension include bulging fontanelles, headaches, and bilateral papilledema.

Pregnancy: Corticosteroids have been shown to be teratogenic in laboratory animals when administered systemically at relatively low dosage levels. Some corticosteroids have been shown to be teratogenic after dermal application in laboratory animals. A teratogenicity study of clobetasol propionate in rats using the dermal route resulted in dose related material toxicity and fetal effects from 0.05 to 0.5 mg/kg/day. These doses are approximately 0.1 to 1.0 times, respectively, the maximum human topical dose of clobetasol propionate from Clobex Shampoo. Abnormalities seen included low fetal weights, umbilical herniation, cleft palate, reduced skeletal ossification, and other skeletal abnormalities. Clobetasol propionate administered to rats subcutaneously at a dose of 0.1 mg/kg from day 17 of gestation to day 21 postpartum was associated with prolongation of gestation, decreased number of offspring, increased perinatal mortality of offspring, delayed eye opening and delayed hair appearance in surviving offspring. Some increase in offspring perinatal mortality was also observed at a dose of 0.05 mg/kg. Doses of 0.05 and 0.1 mg/kg are approximately 0.1 and 0.2 fold the maximum human topical dose of clobetasol propionate from Clobex Shampoo.

There have been no adequate and well controlled studies in pregnant women. Clobex Shampoo should be used during pregnancy only if the potential benefit justifies the potential risk to the fetus.

Lactation: Systemically administered corticosteroids appear in human milk and could suppress growth, interfere with endogenous corticosteroid production, or cause other untoward effects. It is not known whether topical administration of corticosteroids could result in sufficient systemic absorption to produce detectable quantities in human milk. Because many drugs are excreted in human milk, caution should be exercised when Clobex Shampoo is administered to a nursing woman.

Carcinogenesis, Mutagenesis, and Reproduction: Long term animal studies have not been performed to evaluate the carcinogenic potential of clobetasol propionate. Clobetasol propionate did not produce any increase in chromosomal aberrations in Chinese hamster ovary cells in vitro in the presence or absence of metabolic activation. Clobetasol propionate was also negative in the micronucleus test in mice after oral administration. Studies of the effect of Clobex Shampoo on fertility have not been performed.

Laboratory Tests: The following tests may be helpful in evaluating patients for HPA axis suppression:

- ACTH stimulation test
- A.M. plasma cortisol test
- Urinary free cortisol test

Information to Be Provided to the Patient: Patients using topical corticosteroids should receive the following information and instructions:

1. This medication is to be used as directed by the physician and should not be used longer than the prescribed time period. Patients should not use more than 50 g (50 mL) per week of clobetasol propionate shampoo 0.05%. It is for external use only. Avoid contact with the eyes.
2. Patients should be advised to inform subsequent physicians of the prior use of corticosteroids.
3. This medication should not be used for any disorder other than that for which it was prescribed.
4. The scalp area should not be covered while the medication is on the scalp (e.g., shower cap, bathing cap) so as to be occlusive unless directed by the physician.
5. Patients should report to their physician any signs of local adverse reactions.
6. As with other corticosteroids, therapy should be discontinued when control is achieved. If no improvement is seen within 4 weeks, contact the physician.
7. Patients should wash their hands after applying the medication.
8. Patients should inform their physician(s) that they are using Clobex Shampoo if surgery is contemplated.

For additional information, see Information for the Patient.

ADVERSE EFFECTS: A total of 214 (23.8%) of the 900 subjects in the safety population reported at least one AE during the nine Phase II and III studies. Out of the total 558 subjects exposed to Clobex Shampoo (clobetasol propionate shampoo, 0.05%), 129 (23.1%) experienced at least one adverse event. These AEs were mainly dermatological (49 subjects, 8.8%), leading to discontinuation in 6 subjects and were considered to be related to the drug for 40 subjects. Dermatological events consisted mainly of skin discomfort (4.7%), pruritus (0.5%) and urticaria (0.5%). These are functional symptoms without clinically visible signs of intolerance. Clinically visible skin irritation was reported only for three subjects (0.5%). No cases of contact allergy were reported. Few of the AEs classically described with corticosteroid therapy were recorded: six subjects (1.1%) reported acne or folliculitis or infected skin.

The most frequently occurring non dermatological adverse events were pharyngitis (2.2%), headache (1.8%), injury/accident (1.4%), flu syndrome (1.1%), tooth disease (1.1%), gastro-enteritis (1.1%). All other adverse events occurred with a frequency less than 1%.

Adverse events leading to discontinuation of therapy were mostly dermatological. Six subjects in the Clobex Shampoo group discontinued therapy. Of the 6 subjects, 5 had dermatological events and 2 had non-dermatological events (one subject had one dermatological and one non-dermatological events).

Systemic absorption of topical corticosteroids has produced reversible HPA axis suppression, manifestations of Cushing's syndrome, hyperglycemia, and glucosuria in some patients.

The following additional local adverse reactions have been reported with topical corticosteroids, and they may occur more frequently with the use of occlusive dressings, especially with higher potency corticosteroids. These reactions are listed in approximately decreasing order of occurrence: burning, itching, irritation, dryness, folliculitis, hypertrichosis, acneiform eruptions, hypopigmentation, perioral dermatitis, allergic contact dermatitis, maceration of the skin, secondary infection, skin atrophy, striae, and miliaria. In addition, there are reports of the development of pustular psoriasis from chronic plaque psoriasis following reduction or discontinuation of potent topical corticosteroid products.

See Table 1 for a summary of adverse events in the safety population of 558 patients for Clobex Shampoo and 127 patients in the Vehicle Shampoo group.

Table 1: Clobex Shampoo

Summary of Adverse Events by Body System and Detail of Events with Frequency of 1% or More in Clobex Shampoo Group

Body System[a] Costart Term[b]	Clobex Shampoo (N=558)	Vehicle Shampoo (N=127)
Total Number of AE(s)	166	69
Total Number of Subjects with AE(s)[c]	129 (23.1%)	40 (31.5%)
Skin and Appendages	**49 (8.8%)**	**28 (22.0%)**
Discomfort Skin	26 (4.7%)	16 (12.6%)
Body as a Whole	**33 (5.9%)**	**12 (9.4%)**
Headache	10 (1.8%)	1 (0.8%)
Injury/Accident	8 (1.4%)	3 (2.4%)
Flu Syndrome	6 (1.1%)	3 (2.4%)
Respiratory System	**20 (3.6%)**	**6 (4.7%)**
Pharyngitis	12 (2.2%)	4 (3.1%)
Digestive System	**(2.9%)**	**4 (3.1%)**
Tooth Disease	6 (1.1%)	0 (0.0%)
Gastroenteritis	6 (1.1%)	0 (0.0%)
Urogenital System	**9 (1.6%)**	**1 (0.8%)**
Hemic and Lymphatic System	**4 (0.7%)**	**0 (0.0%)**
Metabolic and Nutritional Disorder	**4 (0.7%)**	**1 (0.8%)**
Nervous System	**4 (0.7%)**	**2 (1.6%)**
Cardiovascular System	**3 (0.5%)**	**0 (0.0%)**
Musculoskeletal System	**3 (0.5%)**	**1 (0.8%)**
Special Senses	**2 (0.4%)**	**1 (0.8%)**

[a] A subject was counted once per body system even if more than one occurrence of the event was experienced within the body system.

[b] A subject was counted once per COSTART term even if more than one occurrence of the event was experienced within the COSTART term.

[c] A subject was counted once even if the subject experienced more than one occurrence of the event during the study.

OVERDOSE:

Symptoms: In the event of overdose, systemic absorption of topical corticosteroids can produce reversible HPA axis suppression with the potential for glucocorticosteroid insufficiency after withdrawal from treatment. (See Precautions.)

For management of a suspected drug overdose, CPhA recommends that you contact your **regional Poison Control Centre**. See the *CPS* Directory section for a list of Poison Control Centres.

DOSAGE: Clobex Shampoo (clobetasol propionate) should be applied in a thin film to the affected areas of the scalp once a day. The product should be applied on dry scalp and left in place for 15 minutes before lathering and rinsing.

Move the hair away from the scalp so that one of the affected areas is exposed. Position the bottle over the lesion. Apply a small amount of the shampoo directly onto the lesion, letting the product naturally flow from the bottle (gently squeeze the bottle), avoiding any contact of the product with the facial skin, eyes or lips. In case of contact, rinse thoroughly with water. Spread the product so that the entire lesion is covered with a thin uniform film. Massage gently into the lesion and repeat for additional lesion(s). Wash your hands after applying Clobex Shampoo.

Leave the shampoo in place for 15 minutes. Add water, lather and rinse thoroughly all parts of the scalp and body that came in contact with the shampoo (e.g., hands, face, neck and shoulders). Avoid contact with eyes and lips. Minimize contact to non-affected areas of the body. Although no additional shampoo is necessary to cleanse your hair, you may use a non medicated shampoo if desired.

Clobex Shampoo is a super-high potent topical corticosteroid formulation. Treatment should be limited to 4 consecutive weeks. The maximum amount of clobetasol propionate shampoo 0.05% to be used per week is 50 g (50 mL).

As with other corticosteroids, therapy should be discontinued when control is achieved. If no improvement is seen within 4 weeks, reassessment of diagnosis may be necessary.

Use in pediatric patients under 18 years of age is not recommended.

Clobex Shampoo should not be used with occlusive dressings unless directed by a physician.

INFORMATION FOR THE PATIENT: Published in e-CPS, available by subscription at www.e-cps.ca.

SUPPLIED: Each bottle contains: clobetasol propionate, 0.05%, USP, in a shampoo base consisting of alcohol 10%, citric acid monohydrate, coco-betaine, polyquaternium-10, purified water, sodium citrate dihydrate and sodium laureth sulfate. Bottles of 118 mL. Keep tightly closed. Store at controlled room temperature 15-30°C.

Clobex™ Spray ℞

clobetasol propionate

Topical Corticosteroid

Galderma

Date of Preparation: September 14, 2007

SUMMARY PRODUCT INFORMATION:

Route of Administration	Dosage Form/ Strength	Clinically Relevant Nonmedicinal Ingredients
Topical (spray)	Solution, 0.05% w/w	Alcohol For a complete listing see Dosage Forms, Composition and Packaging.

INDICATIONS AND CLINICAL USE: Clobex Spray (clobetasol propionate solution), 0.05% is indicated for:
- the treatment of moderate to severe plaque psoriasis.

Clobex Spray (clobetasol propionate solution), 0.05% is not indicated for long-term use. Patients should be instructed to use Clobex Spray for the minimum amount of time necessary. Intermittent use has not been studied.

Clobex Spray is a super-high potent topical corticosteroid formulation, indicated for use in the treatment of subjects 18 years of age and older. Treatment should be limited to a maximum of four consecutive weeks, and the total dose per week should not exceed 50 mL (50 g) per week (see Dosage and Administration).

Geriatrics (>65 years of age): Limited data are available. See Warnings and Precautions.

Pediatrics (<18 years of age): No data are available.

CONTRAINDICATIONS:
- Patients who are hypersensitive to clobetasol propionate, to corticosteroids, or to any ingredient in the formulation or component of the container. For a complete listing, see Dosage Forms, Composition and Packaging.
- Patients with untreated tubercular, bacterial, or fungal infections involving the skin, and in certain viral diseases such as herpes simplex, chickenpox, and vaccinia.

WARNINGS AND PRECAUTIONS: General: Use in those under 18 years of age is not recommended.

Clobex Spray (clobetasol propionate solution), 0.05% should not be used under occlusive dressing, over extensive areas, or on the face, axillae, or scrotum, as sufficient absorption may occur to give rise to adrenal suppression and other systemic effects.

In the presence of fungal infections, an appropriate antifungal treatment should be instituted and Clobex Spray, 0.05% should be discontinued until the fungal infection is cured. In the presence of a bacterial infection, an appropriate antibacterial agent should be instituted. If a favorable response does not occur promptly, Clobex Spray, 0.05% should be discontinued until the bacterial infection is adequately controlled.

Endocrine and Metabolism: Systemic absorption of topical corticosteroids has caused reversible adrenal suppression with the potential for glucocorticosteroid insufficiency after withdrawal of treatment. Manifestations of Cushing's syndrome, hyperglycemia, and glucosuria can also be produced in some patients by systemic absorption of topical corticosteroids while on treatment.

Conditions which increase systemic absorption include the application of the more potent steroids, use over large surface areas, prolonged use, and the addition of occlusive dressings. Therefore, patients applying a topical steroid to a large surface area or to areas under occlusion should be evaluated periodically for evidence of adrenal suppression (see Monitoring and Laboratory Tests). If adrenal suppression is noted, an attempt should be made to withdraw the drug, to reduce the frequency of application, or to substitute a less potent steroid. Recovery of HPA axis function is generally prompt upon discontinuation of topical corticosteroids. Infrequently, signs and symptoms of glucocorticosteroid insufficiency may occur, requiring supplemental systemic corticosteroids. For information on systemic supplementation, see the Prescribing Information for those products.

Two studies were conducted to evaluate the effect of twice daily applications of Clobex Spray, 0.05% on HPA axis function in adults with plaque psoriasis covering at least 20% of their body. Study duration was two or four weeks. In the first study four of 14 (29%) patients displayed adrenal suppression after four weeks of use. In the second study, four of 19 (21%) of patients in the two week treatment group and four of 17 (24%) of patients in the four week treatment group displayed adrenal suppression. Suppression was transient, and all patients had returned to normal within 15-16 days of therapy cessation.

Ophthalmologic: Clobex Spray, 0.05% should not be used on plaques close to the eye because of the risk of increased intraocular pressure, glaucoma, and cataracts.

Sensitivity/Resistance: If irritation develops, Clobex Spray, 0.05% should be discontinued and appropriate therapy instituted. Allergic contact dermatitis with corticosteroids is usually diagnosed by a failure to heal rather than by noting a clinical exacerbation, as is the case with most products not containing a corticosteroid.

Special Populations: Pregnant Women: There are no adequate and well-controlled studies of the teratogenic potential of clobetasol propionate in pregnant women. Clobex Spray, 0.05% should be used during pregnancy only if its benefit justifies the potential risk to the fetus. The extent of exposure during the clinical trials with Clobex Spray, 0.05% was very limited (one case).

Nursing Women: Systemically administered corticosteroids appear in human milk and could suppress growth, interfere with endogenous corticosteroid production, or cause other untoward effects. It is not known whether topical administration of corticosteroids could result in sufficient systemic absorption to produce detectable quantities in human milk. Because many drugs are excreted in human milk, caution should be exercised when Clobex Spray, 0.05% is administered to a nursing woman.

Pediatrics (<18 years of age): Safety and effectiveness of Clobex Spray, 0.05% have been established in patients 18 years and older. Insufficient data have been obtained in patients under the age of 18 years. Because of a higher ratio of skin surface area to body mass, pediatric patients are at a greater risk than adults for HPA axis suppression and Cushing's syndrome when they are treated with topical corticosteroids. They are therefore also at greater risk of adrenal insufficiency during and/or after withdrawal of treatment. Adverse effects including striae have been reported with inappropriate use of topical corticosteroids in infants and children. Therefore, use is not recommended in patients under the age of 18 years.

HPA axis suppression, Cushing's syndrome, linear growth retardation, delayed weight gain, and intracranial hypertension have been reported in children receiving topical corticosteroids. Manifestations of adrenal suppression in children include low plasma cortisol levels and an absence of response to ACTH stimulation. Manifestations of intracranial hypertension include bulging fontanelles, headaches, and bilateral papilledema.

Geriatrics (>65 years of age): Clinical studies of Clobex Spray, 0.05%, did not include sufficient numbers of patients aged 65 years and over to determine whether they respond differently than younger patients. In general, dose selection for an elderly patient should be made with caution reflecting the greater frequency of decreased hepatic, renal or cardiac function, and of concomitant disease or other drug therapy.

Monitoring and Laboratory Tests: The following tests may be helpful in evaluating patients for HPA axis suppression:
- ACTH stimulation test
- A.M. plasma cortisol test
- Urinary free cortisol test

ADVERSE REACTIONS: Adverse Drug Reaction Overview: The most common adverse reaction reported with Clobex Spray (clobetasol propionate solution), 0.05% is burning at the application site. Other common adverse reactions are local site effects as well, including pruritus, dryness, pain, hyperpigmentation around resolving plaque, irritation, and atrophy. Most local adverse events were rated as mild to moderate and were not affected by age, race or gender.

One serious, unexpected adverse event, designated as possibly related to treatment by the clinical investigator, was reported during the clinical trial programme with Clobex Spray, 0.05%. This severe event was reported as paranoid delusions in a subject with a seven-year history of intermittent methamphetamine use. Although the event was thought to be related to methamphetamine use by the treating psychiatrist, the possibility of a treatment relationship to clobetasol propionate solution (i.e., spray) could not be absolutely ruled out by the investigator.

Systemic absorption of topical corticosteroids has produced reversible HPA axis suppression, manifestations of Cushing's syndrome, hyperglycemia, and glucosuria in some patients.

The following additional local adverse reactions have been reported with topical corticosteroids in general, and they may occur more frequently with the use of occlusive dressings, use over a prolonged period of time, or use over large surface areas, especially with higher potency corticosteroids, including clobetasol propionate. These reactions are listed in an approximate decreasing order of occurrence: irritation, dryness, itching, burning, local irritation, folliculitis, acneiform eruptions, hypopigmentation, perioral dermatitis, allergic contact dermatitis, skin atrophy, atrophy of subcutaneous tissues, telangiectasia, hypertrichosis, change in pigmentation, secondary infection, striae and miliaria. If applied to the face, acne rosacea or perioral dermatitis can occur. When occlusive dressings are used, pustules, milaria, folliculitis and pyoderma may occur. In rare instances, treatment of psoriasis with systemic or very potent topical corticosteroids (or their withdrawal) is thought to have provoked the pustular form of the disease.

Clinical Trial Adverse Drug Reactions: Because clinical trials are conducted under very specific conditions the adverse reaction rates observed in the clinical trials may not reflect the rates observed in practice and should not be compared to the rates in the clinical trials of another drug. Adverse drug reaction information from clinical trials is useful for identifying drug-related adverse events and for approximating rates.

The data presented in Table 1 include the combined data from two multicentre, randomized, blinded, vehicle-controlled studies conducted in patients 18 years of age or older, with moderate to severe plaque psoriasis. Clobex Spray, 0.05% or Spray Vehicle were applied twice daily to affected areas until healing, or for a maximum of four weeks.

Table 1: Clobex Spray

Treatment Related Adverse Events (At Least Possibly Related) Occurring at a Frequency of ≥1% of Subjects in at Least One Group (Clinical Studies TI01-01008 and TI01-01010 Combined)

	Clobex Spray, 0.05% n=120 (%)	Spray Vehicle n=120 (%)
General Disorders and Administration Site Conditions		
Application site atrophy	0 (0%)	1 (1%)
Application site burning	47 (39%)	55 (46%)
Application site pruritus	3 (3%)	3 (3%)
Application site dryness	2 (2%)	0 (0%)
Application site irritation	1 (1%)	0 (0%)
Application site pain	1 (1%)	2 (2%)
Application site pigmentation changes	1 (1%)	0 (0%)
Oedema peripheral	0 (0%)	1 (1%)
Sensation of pressure	0 (0%)	1 (1%)
Musculoskeletal and Connective Tissue Disorders		
Pain in extremity	0 (0%)	1 (1%)
Skin and Subcutaneous Tissue Disorders		
Eczema asteatotic	2 (2%)	0 (0%)
Psoriasis aggravated	0 (0%)	1 (1%)

Abnormal Hematologic and Clinical Chemistry Findings: One subject treated for four weeks with Clobex Spray 0.05% experienced an elevated WBC, which was designated by the investigator as possibly related to treatment.

DRUG INTERACTIONS: Overview: To date, there have not been any documented interactions with Clobex Spray (clobetasol propionate solution), 0.05%.

Drug-Drug Interactions: Interactions with other drugs have not been established.

Drug-Food Interactions: Interactions with food have not been established. However, given the topical route of administration, such interactions seem unlikely.

Drug-Herb Interactions: Interactions with herbal products have not been established.

Drug-Laboratory Test Interactions: Interactions with laboratory tests have not been established.

DOSAGE AND ADMINISTRATION: Dosing Considerations:
- treatment should be limited to adult patients, aged 18 years of age and older

Recommended Dose and Dosage Adjustment: Clobex Spray (clobetasol propionate solution), 0.05% should be applied to the affected skin areas twice daily and rubbed in gently and completely.

Treatment with Clobex Spray, 0.05% should be limited to four weeks. Treatment beyond two weeks should be limited to localized lesions of moderate to severe plaque psoriasis that have not sufficiently improved after the initial two weeks of treatment with Clobex Spray, 0.05%.

Total dosage of the product should not exceed 50 mL per week because of the potential for the drug to suppress the hypothalamic-pituitary-adrenal (HPA) axis. Therapy should be discontinued when control has been achieved. If no improvement is seen within two weeks, reassessment of diagnosis may be necessary.

Clobex Spray (clobetasol propionate solution), 0.05% is not indicated for long-term use. Patients should be instructed to use Clobex Spray for the minimum amount of time necessary. Intermittent use has not been studied.

Clobex Spray, 0.05% should not be used with occlusive dressings.

Missed Dose: In the event of a missed dose, Clobex Spray, 0.05% should be applied as soon as possible after the missed dose is remembered. If this is close to the scheduled application time for the next dose, the subject should wait and apply the next scheduled dose. The usual schedule should be resumed thereafter.

Administration: Clobex Spray, 0.05% should be applied to the affected skin areas twice daily and rubbed in gently and completely.

OVERDOSAGE:
In the event of overdose, systemic absorption of topical corticosteroids can produce reversible HPA axis suppression with the potential for glucocorticosteroid insufficiency after withdrawal from treatment. (See Warnings and Precautions.)

> For management of a suspected drug overdose, CPhA recommends that you contact your **regional Poison Control Centre**. See the *CPS* Directory section for a list of Poison Control Centres.

ACTION AND CLINICAL PHARMACOLOGY: Mechanism of Action: Clobetasol propionate is a super-high potency topical corticosteroid. Like other topical corticosteroids, clobetasol propionate has anti-inflammatory, antipruritic, and vasoconstrictive properties. The mechanism of the anti-inflammatory activity of the topical steroids, in general, is unclear. However, corticosteroids are thought to act by the induction of phospholipase A_2 inhibitory proteins, collectively called lipocortins. It is postulated that these proteins control the biosynthesis of potent mediators of inflammation such as prostaglandins and leukotrienes by inhibiting the release of their common precursor, arachidonic acid. Arachidonic acid is released from membrane phospholipids by phospholipase A_2.

Pharmacodynamics: The vasoconstriction capacity of Clobex Spray (clobetasol propionate solution), 0.05% is comparable to that of cream formulations of clobetasol propionate and superior to that of amcinonide cream, 0.1%.

Pharmacokinetics: The extent of percutaneous absorption of topical corticosteroids is determined by many factors, including the vehicle, the integrity of the epidermal barrier and the use of occlusive dressings. Topical corticosteroids can be absorbed from normal intact skin while inflammation and/or other disease processes in the skin may increase percutaneous absorption.

Once absorbed through the skin, topical corticosteroids are handled through pharmacokinetic pathways similar to systemically administered corticosteroids. They are metabolized, primarily in the liver, and are then excreted by the kidneys. In addition, some corticosteroids, including clobetasol propionate and its metabolites, are also excreted in the bile.

STORAGE AND STABILITY: Store at room temperature (15-30°C). Do not refrigerate. Keep tightly closed. Product is flammable, and should be kept away from heat or open flame. Keep in a safe place out of the reach of children.

INFORMATION FOR THE PATIENT: Published in e-CPS, available by subscription at www.e-cps.ca.

DOSAGE FORMS, COMPOSITION AND PACKAGING: Each g contains: clobetasol propionate 0.5 mg. Nonmedicinal ingredients: alcohol, isopropyl myristate, sodium lauryl sulphate and undecylenic acid. Each 59 mL bottle is accompanied by a spray pump which is to be attached by the pharmacist prior to dispensing the product. Each spray from the pump delivers approximately 0.16 mL. Botttles of 59 mL (50 g).

Clodronate ℞

CPhA Monograph

see *Bisphosphonates: Oral*

Clolar® ℞

clofarabine

Antineoplastic Agent

Genzyme

Date of Preparation: July 16, 2009

SUMMARY PRODUCT INFORMATION:

Route of Administration	Dosage Form/ Strength	Clinically Relevant Nonmedicinal Ingredients
Intravenous infusion	Injection/1 mg/mL	Not applicable For a complete listing see Dosage Forms, Composition and Packaging.

INDICATIONS AND CLINICAL USE: Clolar (clofarabine) is indicated for the treatment of pediatric patients 1 to 21 years old with relapsed or refractory acute lymphoblastic leukemia after at least two prior regimens. This use is based on the induction of complete responses. Approval is based on objective response rates. No survival advantage has been demonstrated and palliative benefit was not evaluated.

CONTRAINDICATIONS:

- Hypersensitivity to clofarabine or any of the excipients (see Dosage Forms, Composition and Packaging).
- Symptomatic central nervous system involvement.
- History of serious heart, liver, kidney or pancreas disease (see Adverse Reactions).
- Severe hepatic impairment (defined as elevated transaminases (AST and/or ALT) >5×ULN, and/or elevated bilirubin >3×ULN) or severe renal insufficiency (defined as creatinine clearance <30 mL/min).

WARNINGS AND PRECAUTIONS:

Serious Warnings and Precautions

Clolar (clofarabine) must be administered under the supervision of a physician qualified in the use of antineoplastic agents. Clolar is associated with:

- Tumor Lysis Syndrome, (TLS)
- Systemic Inflammatory Response Syndrome (SIRS)/Capillary Leak Syndrome (see Warnings and Precautions below)

General: Clolar should be administered under the supervision of a qualified physician experienced in the use of antineoplastic therapy.

Dehydration/Hypotension: As with other chemotherapeutic agents, patients receiving Clolar may experience vomiting and diarrhea; they should therefore be advised regarding appropriate measures to avoid dehydration. Patients should be instructed to seek medical advice if they experience symptoms of dizziness, lightheadedness, fainting spells, or decreased urine output. Clolar administration should be stopped if the patient develops hypotension for any reason during the 5 days of administration. If hypotension is transient and resolves without pharmacological intervention, Clolar treatment can be re-instituted with a dose reduction (see Dosage and Administration).

Hematologic: Obtain complete blood counts and platelet counts at regular intervals during Clolar therapy. Suppression of bone marrow function should be anticipated. Severe bone marrow suppression, including neutropenia, anemia, and thrombocytopenia, has been observed in patients treated with Clolar. At initiation of treatment, most patients in the clinical studies had hematological impairment as a manifestation of leukemia.

These patients are at risk of prolonged neutropenia when treated with Clolar. For all subsequent courses, recovery of absolute neutrophil count (ANC) to $>0.5 \times 10^9/L$ prior to restarting therapy is recommended. In clinical trials, no dose reductions were permitted for hematological toxicities, including thrombocytopenia, except for neutropenia ($\leq 0.5 \times 10^9/L$) lasting for more than 28 days (see Dosage and Administration). Patients with prolonged neutropenia (ANC $\leq 0.5 \times 10^9/L$ for >28 days) should undergo a bone marrow examination to exclude progressive disease.

Hepatic/Biliary/Pancreatic: Clolar has not been studied in patients with hepatic impairment (serum billirubin >1.5×ULN plus ALT and AST >5×ULN). In patients with mild to moderate hepatic impairment Clolar should be used with the greatest caution. Avoid concomitant use of medications known to induce hepatic toxicity. (See Adverse Reactions, Dosage and Administration.)

Patients who have previously received a hematopoietic stem cell transplant (HSCT) may be at higher risk for hepatotoxicity suggestive of veno-occlusive disease (VOD) following treatment with clofarabine when used in combination (etoposide and cyclophosphamide). Severe hepatotoxic events have been reported in an ongoing Phase 1/2 combination study of clofarabine in pediatric patients with relapsed or refractory acute leukemia.

Hyperuricemia (Tumor Lysis): Administration of Clolar may result in a rapid destruction of peripheral leukemia cells that may lead to tumor lysis syndrome. Evaluate and monitor patients undergoing treatment for signs and symptoms of tumor lysis syndrome. Provide intravenous infusion fluids throughout the five days of Clolar administration to reduce the effects of tumor lysis and other adverse events. The initiation of measures to prevent tumor lysis syndrome (such as the administration of alkalinized intravenous fluids, allopurinol and/or other uric acid-lowering agents) may be considered prior to clofarabine administration. Institutional guidelines should be followed in regards to the dosing and schedule of administration of these agents.

Systemic Inflammatory Response Syndrome (SIRS) and Capillary Leak Syndrome: Evaluate and monitor patients undergoing treatment with Clolar for signs and symptoms of cytokine release (e.g., tachypnea, tachycardia, hypotension, pulmonary edema) that could progress to systemic inflammatory response syndrome (SIRS), capillary leak syndrome and multi-organ dysfunction. Discontinue Clolar immediately in the event of clinically significant signs or symptoms of SIRS or capillary leak syndrome, either of which can be fatal, and consider use of steroids, diuretics, and albumin. Re-institute Clolar when the patient is stable see Dosage and Administration. The use of prophylactic steroids may be of benefit in preventing signs and symptoms of cytokine release (see Dosage and Administration).

Immune: The use of Clolar is likely to increase the risk of infection, including severe sepsis, as a result of bone marrow suppression. Because of the pre-existing immunocompromised condition of these patients and prolonged neutropenia that can result from treatment with Clolar, patients are at increased risk for severe opportunistic infections.

Renal: Clolar has not been studied in patients with renal dysfunction (serum creatinine ≥2 ULN) and it is predominantly excreted via the kidney. Therefore, Clolar should be used with caution in patients with mild to moderate renal insufficiency. Avoid drugs with known renal toxicity during the 5 days of Clolar administration (see Drug Interactions, Dosage and Administration).

Sexual Function/Reproduction: Fertility studies with clofarabine have not been performed in animals. Degenerative effects on reproductive organs in the general toxicity studies suggest a potential effect on male and female fertility. The effect of Clolar treatment on human fertility is unknown.

Carcinogenesis and Mutagenesis: Carcinogenicity studies have not been conducted. Clofarabine was clastogenic in mammalian cells in the in vitro chromosomal aberration assay and in the in vivo micronucleus assay in rats. Clofarabine was not mutagenic in bacteria (Ames assay).

Special Populations: Pregnant Women: Clolar may cause fetal harm when administered to a pregnant woman.

Clofarabine was teratogenic in rats and rabbits at doses much lower than recommended human dose.

There are no adequate and well-controlled studies in pregnant women using clofarabine. If this drug is used during pregnancy, or if the patient becomes pregnant while taking this drug, the patient should be apprised of the potential hazard to the fetus.

Women of childbearing potential should be advised to avoid becoming pregnant while receiving treatment with clofarabine. All patients should be advised to use effective contraceptive measures to prevent pregnancy.

Nursing Women: It is not known whether clofarabine or its metabolites are excreted in human milk. The excretion of clofarabine in milk has not been studied in animals. Because of the potential for serious adverse reactions in nursing infants, women treated with clofarabine should not nurse. Female patients should be advised to discontinue breast-feeding during treatment with Clolar.

Pediatrics (1-21 years of age): Safety and effectiveness have been established in pediatric patients 1 to 21 years old with relapsed or refractory acute lymphoblastic leukemia.

Geriatrics (>65 years of age): Safety and effectiveness of Clolar has not been established in geriatric patients aged 65 and older.

Adults (>21 and <65 years of age): Safety and effectiveness have not been established in adults. One study was performed in highly refractory and/or relapsed adult patients with hematologic malignancies. The Phase 2 dose of Clolar was determined to be 40 mg/m²/day administered as a 1- to 2-hour IV infusion daily × 5 every 28 days.

Monitoring and Laboratory Tests: The following parameters should be closely monitored in patients undergoing treatment with Clolar:

- Complete blood cells and platelets counts on Days 1, 3, and 5 of each cycle. Repeat 1 to 2 times weekly, as clinically indicated (more frequently in patients who develop cytopenia) thereafter.
- **Bone Marrow Aspiration and/or Biopsy:** prior to each cycle. If the bone marrow has not recovered and there is no evidence of leukemia, a bone marrow aspiration and/or biopsy should be repeated within 14 days.
- Renal and hepatic function daily during the 5 days of Clolar administration
- Respiratory status, blood pressure, fluid balance and weight at least daily for the 5 days of Clolar administration and at regular intervals throughout the entire treatment cycle
- Uric acid, potassium, phosphate, signs and symptoms of TLS, SIRS/capillary leak syndrome (see Warnings and Precautions)

Close monitoring of patients taking medications known to affect blood pressure or cardiac function during administration of Clolar is advised (see Drug Interactions).

ADVERSE REACTIONS: Adverse Drug Reaction Overview: The most frequent Adverse Events (AE) observed were hematologic toxicities and infections resulting from the immunosuppressive effect of clofarabine. Other significant groups of AEs observed for clofarabine are found in the hepatobiliary, renal, and gastrointestinal organ systems. In addition, tumor lysis syndrome, capillary leak syndrome or SIRS have been reported. The most common toxicities observed during exposure to clofarabine were gastrointestinal system AEs (including vomiting, nausea, and diarrhea), adverse hematologic effects (including anemia, leukopenia, thrombocytopenia, neutropenia, and febrile neutropenia), and infection. It should be noted that a large number of the adverse effects were already present in many of the patients at baseline.

Clinical Trial Adverse Drug Reactions: Open-label Single Arm Studies: Phase I Study ID99-383 (ALL/AML), Phase II CLO212 (ALL) and CLO222 (AML): The data described below reflect exposure to Clolar (clofarabine) in 115 pediatric patients with relapsed or refractory ALL (70) or AML (45).

One hundred and fifteen (115) of the pediatric patients treated in clinical trials received at least 1 infusion of Clolar at 52 mg/m². The data for these patients were combined into an integrated database. The patients in the integrated database participated in the 3 clinical trials presented (CLO-212, N=61 ALL, CLO-222, N=41 AML and ID99-383N=13). Treatment cycle comprised a 5-day course of Clolar 52 mg/m²/day followed by the recovery period of approximately 2 to 6 weeks from the starting day of the previous cycle (see Dosage and Administration).

The median number of cycles was 2. The median cumulative amount of Clolar received by pediatric patients during all cycles was 540 mg.

The most common adverse reactions with Clolar are: nausea, vomiting, diarrhea, febrile neutropenia, headache, rash, pruritus, pyrexia, fatigue, palmar-plantar erythrodysesthesia syndrome, anxiety, flushing, and mucosal inflammation. Of 29 deaths on-study within 30 days of the last Clolar dose, 19 were disease related 7 were multifactorial (both disease and Clolar-related) and 3 were possibly Clolar-related by investigator.

Table 1 lists adverse reactions by System Organ Class, including severe or life-threatening events (NCI CTC grade 3 or grade 4), reported in ≥ 5% of the 115 patients in the 52 mg/m²/day dose group (pooled analysis of pediatric patients with ALL and AML). More detailed information and follow-up of certain events is given below.

Table 2 lists the incidence of treatment emergent laboratory abnormalities after Clolar administration at 52 mg/m² among pediatric patients with ALL and AML (n=115).

Table 1: Clolar

Most Commonly Reported (≥ 5% Overall) Adverse Reactions by System Organ Class Regardless of Causality (N=115 pooled analysis)

		ALL/AML (N=115)		Worst NCI Common Terminology Criteria Grade[a]					
				3		4		5	
System Organ Class[a]	Preferred Term[a]	N	%	N	%	N	%	N	%
Blood and Lymphatic System Disorders	Febrile neutropenia	63	54.8	59	51.3	3	2.6	—	—
	Neutropenia	11	9.6	3	2.6	8	7.0	—	—
Cardiac Disorders	Pericardial effusion	9	7.8	—	—	1	0.9	—	—
	Tachycardia	40	34.8	6	5.2	—	—	—	—
Gastrointestinal Disorders	Abdominal pain	40	34.8	8	7.0	—	—	—	—
	Abdominal pain upper	9	7.8	1	0.9	—	—	—	—
	Diarrhea	64	55.7	14	12.2	—	—	—	—
	Gingival bleeding	16	13.9	7	6.1	1	0.9	—	—
	Mouth hemorrhage	6	5.2	2	1.7	—	—	—	—
	Nausea	84	73.0	16	13.9	1	0.9	—	—
	Oral mucosal petechiae	6	5.2	4	3.5	—	—	—	—
	Proctalgia	9	7.8	2	1.7	—	—	—	—
	Stomatitis	8	7.0	1	0.9	—	—	—	—
	Vomiting	90	78.3	9	7.8	1	0.9	—	—

(cont'd)

Table 1: Clolar *(cont'd)*

Most Commonly Reported (≥ 5% Overall) Adverse Reactions by System Organ Class Regardless of Causality (N=115 pooled analysis)

		ALL/AML (N=115)		Worst NCI Common Terminology Criteria Grade[a]					
				3		4		5	
System Organ Class[a]	Preferred Term[a]	N	%	N	%	N	%	N	%
General Disorders and Administration Site Conditions	Asthenia	12	10.4	1	0.9	1	0.9	—	—
	Chills	39	33.9	3	2.6	—	—	—	—
	Fatigue	39	33.9	3	2.6	2	1.7	—	—
	Irritability	11	9.6	1	0.9	—	—	—	—
	Mucosal inflammation	18	15.7	2	1.7	—	—	—	—
	Edema	14	12.2	2	1.7	—	—	—	—
	Pain	17	14.8	7	6.1	1	0.9	—	—
	Pyrexia	45	39.1	16	13.9	—	—	—	—
Hepatobiliary Disorder	Jaundice	9	7.8	2	1.7	—	—	—	—
Infections and Infestations	Bacteremia	10	8.7	10	8.7	—	—	—	—
	Candidiasis	8	7.0	1	0.9	—	—	—	—
	Catheter related infection	14	12.2	13	11.3	—	—	—	—
	Cellulitis	9	7.8	7	6.1	—	—	—	—
	Clostridium colitis	8	7.0	6	5.2	—	—	—	—
	Herpes simplex	11	9.6	6	5.2	—	—	—	—
	Herpes zoster	8	7.0	6	5.2	—	—	—	—
	Oral candidiasis	13	11.3	2	1.7	—	—	—	—
	Pneumonia	11	9.6	6	5.2	1	0.9	1	0.9
	Sepsis	11	9.6	5	4.4	2	1.7	4	3.5
	Septic shock	8	7.0	1	0.9	2	1.7	5	4.4
	Staphylococcal bacteremia	7	6.1	5	4.4	1	0.9	—	—
	Staphylococcal sepsis	6	5.2	5	4.4	1	0.9	—	—
	Upper respiratory tract infection	6	5.2	1	0.9	—	—	—	—
Metabolism and Nutrition Disorders	Anorexia	34	29.6	6	5.2	8	7.0	—	—
Musculoskeletal and Connective Tissue Disorders	Arthralgia	10	8.7	3	2.6	—	—	—	—
	Back pain	12	10.4	3	2.6	—	—	—	—
	Bone pain	11	9.6	3	2.6	—	—	—	—
	Myalgia	16	13.9	—	—	—	—	—	—
	Pain in extremity	34	29.6	6	5.2	—	—	—	—
Neoplasms Benign, Malignant and Unspecified (incl cysts and polyps)	Tumor lysis syndrome	7	6.1	7	6.1	—	—	—	—
Nervous System Disorders	Headache	49	42.6	6	5.2	—	—	—	—
	Lethargy	12	10.4	1	0.9	—	—	—	—
	Somnolence	11	9.6	1	0.9	—	—	—	—
Psychiatric Disorders	Agitation	6	5.2	1	0.9	—	—	—	—
	Anxiety	24	20.9	2	1.7	—	—	—	—
Renal and Urinary Disorders	Hematuria	15	13.0	2	1.7	—	—	—	—
Respiratory, Thoracic and Mediastinal Disorders	Dyspnea	15	13.0	6	5.2	2	1.7	—	—
	Epistaxis	31	27.0	15	13.0	—	—	—	—
	Pleural effusion	14	12.2	4	3.5	2	1.7	—	—
	Respiratory distress	12	10.4	5	4.4	4	3.5	1	0.9
	Tachypnea	10	8.7	4	3.5	1	0.9	—	—
Skin and Subcutaneous Tissue Disorders	Erythema	13	11.3	—	—	—	—	—	—
	Palmar-plantar erythrodysaesthesia syndrome	18	15.7	8	7.0	—	—	—	—
	Petechiae	30	26.1	7	6.1	—	—	—	—
	Pruritus	49	42.6	1	0.9	—	—	—	—
	Rash	44	38.3	8	7.0	—	—	—	—
	Rash pruritic	9	7.8	—	—	—	—	—	—
Vascular Disorders	Flushing	22	19.1	—	—	—	—	—	—
	Hypertension	15	13.0	6	5.2	—	—	—	—
	Hypotension	33	28.7	13	11.3	9	7.8	—	—

[a] Patients with more than one preferred term within a SOC are counted only once in the SOC totals. Patients with more than one occurrence of the same preferred term are counted only once within that term and at the highest severity grade.

Table 2: Clolar

Incidence of Treatment Emergent Laboratory Abnormalities After Clolar Administration

Parameter	Any Grade	Grade 3 or Higher
Hematology		
Anemia (N=114)	95 (83.3%)	86 (75.4%)
Leukopenia (N=114)	100 (87.7%)	100 (87.7%)
Lymphopenia (N=113)	93 (82.3%)	93 (82.3%)
Neutropenia (N=113)	72 (63.7%)	72 (63.7%)
Thrombocytopenia (N=114)	92 (80.7%)	91 (79.8%)
Elevated Creatinine (N=115)	57 (49.5%)	9 (7.8%)
Elevated AST (N=100)	74 (74.0%)	36 (36.0%)
Elevated ALT (N=113)	91 (80.5%)	49 (43.4%)
Elevated Total Bilirubin (N=114)	51 (44.7%)	15 (13.2%)

Table 3: Clolar

BIOV-111 Study Most Commonly Reported (≥5% Overall) Adverse Events by System Organ Class Regardless of Causality (N=71)*

		ALL/AML (N=71)		Worst NCI Common Terminology Criteria Grade[a]					
				3		4		5	
System Organ Class[a]	Preferred Term[a]	N	%	N	%	N	%	N	%
Blood and Lymphatic System Disorders	Anemia	5	7.0	3	4.2	1	1.4	—	—
	Febrile neutropenia	37	52.1	31	43.7	5	7.0	—	—
	Neutropenia	7	9.9	3	4.2	4	5.6	—	—
	Thrombocytopenia	6	8.5	—	—	6	8.5	—	—
Cardiac Disorders	Tachycardia	5	7.0	—	—	—	—	1	1.4
Ear and Labyrinth Disorders	Ear pain	4	5.6	—	—	—	—	—	—
Gastrointestinal Disorders	Abdominal pain	26	36.6	6	8.5	—	—	—	—
	Constipation	10	14.1	—	—	—	—	—	—
	Diarrhea	27	38.0	5	7.0	1	1.4	—	—
	Nausea	37	52.1	5	7.0	—	—	—	—
	Vomiting	52	73.2	3	4.2	—	—	—	—

(cont'd)

Table 3: Clolar *(cont'd)*

BIOV-111 Study Most Commonly Reported (≥5% Overall) Adverse Events by System Organ Class Regardless of Causality (N=71)*

System Organ Class[a]	Preferred Term[a]	ALL/AML (N=71)		Worst NCI Common Terminology Criteria Grade[a] 3		4		5	
		N	%	N	%	N	%	N	%
General Disorders and Administration Site Conditions	Asthenia	6	8.5	2	2.8	—	—	—	—
	Chills	5	7.0	—	—	—	—	—	—
	Fatigue	11	15.5	—	—	—	—	—	—
	Mucosal inflammation	13	18.3	4	5.6	—	—	—	—
	Pain	7	9.9	4	5.6	—	—	—	—
	Pyrexia	38	53.5	9	12.7	1	1.4	—	—
Immune System Disorders	Hypersensitivity	7	9.9	4	5.6	—	—	—	—
Infections and Infestations	Bronchopulmonary aspergillosis	4	5.6	2	2.8	1	1.4	1	1.4
	Herpes zoster	5	7.0	1	1.4	—	—	—	—
	Sepsis	7	9.9	3	4.2	2	2.8	1	1.4
Investigations	Alanine aminotransferase increased	5	7.0	4	5.6	—	—	—	—
	Aspartate aminotransferase increased	4	5.6	1	1.4	1	1.4	—	—
	Platelet count decreased	5	7.0	—	—	4	5.6	—	—
	Weight decreased	6	8.5	—	—	—	—	—	—
Metabolism and Nutrition Disorders	Anorexia	11	15.5	3	4.2	—	—	—	—
Musculoskeletal and Connective Tissue Disorders	Arthralgia	6	8.5	4	5.6	—	—	—	—
	Back pain	8	11.3	1	1.4	—	—	—	—
	Bone pain	12	16.9	6	8.5	—	—	—	—
	Musculoskeletal pain	5	7.0	2	2.8	—	—	—	—
	Pain in extremity	18	25.4	3	4.2	—	—	—	—
Neoplasms Benign, Malignant and Unspecified (incl cysts and polyps)	Malignant neoplasm progression	13	18.3	—	—	—	—	13	18.3
Nervous Systems Disorders	Convulsion	6	8.5	2	2.8	—	—	—	—
	Headache	30	42.3	7	9.9	—	—	—	—
Psychiatric Disorders	Anxiety	7	9.9	3	4.2	—	—	—	—
	Depression	6	8.5	2	2.8	—	—	—	—
	Mood altered	7	9.9	1	1.4	—	—	—	—
Respiratory, Thoracic and Mediastinal Disorders	Cough	13	18.3	—	—	—	—	—	—
	Dyspnea	4	5.6	1	1.4	—	—	—	—
	Epistaxis	10	14.1	3	4.2	—	—	—	—
	Pharyngolaryngeal pain	5	7.0	—	—	—	—	—	—
Skin and Subcutaneous Tissue Disorders	Erythema	4	5.6	—	—	—	—	—	—
	Palmar-plantar erythrodysesthesia syndrome	5	7.0	4	5.6	—	—	—	—
	Petechiae	4	5.6	—	—	—	—	—	—
	Pruritus	20	28.2	1	1.4	—	—	—	—
	Rash	27	38.0	4	5.6	—	—	—	—
Vascular Disorders	Flushing	5	7.0	—	—	—	—	—	—
	Hypertension	8	11.3	2	2.8	—	—	—	—
	Hypotension	10	14.1	—	—	—	—	2	2.8

[a] Patients with more than one preferred term within a SOC are counted only once in the SOC totals. Patients with more than one occurrence of the same preferred term are counted only once within that term and at the highest severity grade.

Less Common Clinical Trial Adverse Drug Reactions (1-4%): The following less common adverse reactions have been reported in 1-4% of the 115 pediatric patients with ALL or AML:
Gastrointestinal Disorders: caecitis.
General Disorders: SIRS.
Hepatobiliary Disorders: hyperbilirubinemia, jaundice, VOD.
Immune System Disorders: hypersensitivity.
Infections and Infestations: bacterial infection, Enterococcal bacteremia, Escherichia bacteremia, Escherichia sepsis, fungal infection, fungal sepsis, gastroenteritis adenovirus, infection, influenza, Parainfluenzae virus infection, pneumonia fungal, pneumonia primary atypical, Respiratory syncytial virus infection, sinusitis, staphylococcal infection.
Investigations: blood creatinine increased.
Psychiatric Disorders: mental status change.
Respiratory, Thoracic and Mediastinal Disorders: pulmonary edema.
Vascular Disorders: capillary leak syndrome.

Uncommon occurrences of Stevens-Johnson Syndrome (SJS) and toxic epidermal necrolysis (TEN) have been reported in patients who were receiving or had recently been treated with other medications (e.g. allopurinol or antibiotics) known to cause these syndromes.

Open-label Single Arm Phase II BIOV-111 Study: In an additional pediatric ALL study, "A phase II, open-label study of clofarabine in pediatric patients with refractory/relapsed acute lymphoblastic leukemia" (BIOV-111 Study) 71 patients received Clolar. Of these 65 patients received at least on full course of Clolar and 32 received at least two full courses at the recommended dose of 52 mg/m^2 daily × 5 days. Small numbers of patients (6, 4, 1) started third, fourth and sixth courses, respectively.

There were 43/71 (61%) in this study who experienced severe or life-threatening events (NCI CTC grade 3 or grade 4) adverse reactions related to Clolar. The most common event was febrile neutropenia (43.7%).

The most frequent AEs (incidence of >50%) were vomiting in 52 (73.2%) patients, headache in 40 (56.3%) patients, pyrexia in 38 (53.5%) patients, and nausea and febrile neutropenia each in 37 (52.1%) patients. Sixty-two out of 71 (87.3%) patients died during the course of the study; 42 of these deaths occurred >30 days after the last dose of Clolar. Seven (9.9%) deaths were considered to be Clolar related in this study.

Table 3 lists adverse reactions by System Organ Class, including severe or life-threatening events (NCI CTC grade 3 or grade 4), reported in ≥5% of the 71 patients.

The following sections provide more detailed information regarding the incidence of the most commonly occurring adverse events and/or laboratory abnormalities observed in all the pediatric clinical studies mentioned above:

Hematologic Toxicity: In the integrated safety population (n=115), the most frequently reported hematologic adverse reactions in pediatric patients included febrile neutropenia (55%) and neutropenia (10%). One (1) report of grade 4 bone marrow depression, and 1 report of grade 4 thrombocytopenia were considered related to study drug.

In the BIOV-111 Study more than 90% of patients experienced Grade 3 or 4 leukopenia, lymphopenia, neutropenia or thrombocytopenia.

Infection: In the integrated safety population (n=115), at baseline, 48% of the pediatric ALL and AML patients had 1 or more concurrent infections. A total of 83% of patients experienced at least 1 infection after Clolar treatment, including fungal, viral and bacterial infections.

Infections occurred in 25.4% of patients on the BIOV-111 Study.

Hepatic: The liver is a potential target organ of Clolar, and in the integrated safety population (n=115), 25% of patients experienced at least one hepato-biliary disorders adverse event. Grade 3 or 4 elevated aspartate aminotransferase (AST) occurred in 36% of patients and grade 3 or 4 elevated alanine aminotransferase (ALT) occurred in 43% of patients. Grade 3 or 4 elevated bilirubin occurred in 13% of patients, with 2 events reported as grade 4 hyperbilirubinemia (2%), one of which resulted in treatment discontinuation, one patient had multi-organ failure and died. One report (1%) of veno-occlusive disease (VOD) was considered related to study drug.

For patients with follow-up data, elevations in AST and ALT were transient and typically ≤15 days duration. The majority of AST and ALT elevations occurred within 10 days of Clolar administration and returned to ≤ grade 2 within 15 days while the majority of bilirubin elevations returned to ≤ grade 2 within 10 days. Eight patients had grade 3 or 4 elevations in serum bilirubin at the last time point measured, these patients died due to sepsis and/or multi-organ failure.

In the BIOV-111 Study elevated ALT (60.9%) was the most common chemistry abnormality, while other liver function abnormalities (AST increased: 41.1%; total bilirubin increased: 7.6%) also occurred at lower frequencies.

Renal: In the integrated safety population (n=115), a total of 53% (61/115) of patients experienced the onset or worsening of elevated creatinine. Grade 3 or 4 elevated creatinine occurred in 8% of patients. Nephrotoxic medications, tumor lysis, and tumor lysis with hyperuricemia may contribute to renal toxicity. Hematuria was observed in 13% of patients overall. This event likely reflects thrombocytopenia that is a pre-existing condition in these patients.

In the BIOV-111 Study, elevated creatinine occurred in 8.9% of patients. Renal failure and renal impairment were each reported in 2 (2.8%) patients and considered to be Clolar-related in 1 (1.4%) patient each.

Systemic Inflammatory Response Syndrome (SIRS)/Capillary Leak Syndrome: In the integrated safety population (n=115), other concurrent medical conditions, including sepsis, disease progression and/or prior therapies may also have contributed to the incidence of capillary leak syndrome.

There were no cases of SIRS or Capillary leak syndrome in the BIOV-111 Study.

Gastrointestinal Disorders: In the integrated safety population (n=115), gastrointestinal disorders were the most frequently affected system organ class with 97% of patients overall experiencing at least one AE in this class. Vomiting (78%) was the most frequent adverse event, followed by nausea (73%), diarrhea (56%), and abdominal pain (35%), constipation (17%), and gingival bleeding (14%).

In the BIOV-111 Study, 78.9% of patients experienced gastrointestinal disorders. Among patients with gastrointestinal disorders, vomiting, nausea, diarrhea , abdominal pain, and anorexia occurred in 66.2%, 47.9% ,26.8%, 21.1% and 41.1%, respectively.

Cardiovascular: In the integrated safety population (n=115), the most frequently reported cardiac disorder was tachycardia (35%), which was, however, already present in 35% of patients at study entry. Most of the cardiac adverse events were reported in the first 2 cycles of Clolar treatment. Pericardial effusion was a finding in these patients on post-treatment studies, [9/115 (8%)]. The effusion was almost always minimal to small and in no cases had hemodynamic significance.

In the BIOV-111 Study, 7/71 patients (9.9%) experienced cardiac disorders. Preferred Terms (PTs) for adverse events in this System Organ Class (SOC) include, tachycardia, LV dysfunction, sinus arrhythmia, and cardiac failure.

Post-Market Adverse Drug Reactions: The following list of post market adverse reactions is based on one or more of the following factors: (1) seriousness of the reaction, (2) reported frequency of the reaction, or (3) strength of causal connection to Clolar.

- Blood and Lymphatic System Disorders: bone marrow failure and pancytopenia.
- Cardiac: pericardial effusion and tachycardia.
- Gastrointestinal Disorders: cecitis, colitis.
- General Disorders: mucosal inflammation, SIRS.
- Hepatobiliary Disorders: hepatic function abnormal, hepatotoxicity, and hyperbilirubinemia. Serious hepatotoxic events of VOD have been reported in patients who had previous HSCT and who received conditioning regimens that included busulfan, melphalan, and/or the combination of cyclophosphamide and total body irradiation.
- Immune System Disorders: hypersensitivity.
- Infections and Infestations:
  Systemic: sepsis: neutropenic sepsis, bacterial (Streptococcus, Enterococcus, Klebsiella), fungal (Candida), bacteremia (Streptococcus).
  Respiratory: bronchopulmonary fungal (Aspergillus) infection, lung abscess, bacterial pneumonia (Klebsiella), lower respiratory tract infection, respiratory tract infection fungal.
  GI: tonsillitis, hepatosplenic fungal infection (Candida), *C. difficile* colitis.
  Neurological: brain abscess, central nervous system infection.
  Musculoskeletal: necrotizing fasciitis.
  Skin: bacterial wound infection (Staphylococcus).
  Unspecified: CMV, Fusarium, Pseudomonas, central line infection, vaginal cellulitis, Herpes simplex, Herpes zoster.
- Nervous System Disorders: syncope.
- Psychiatric Disorders: confusional state, agitation, mental status changes.

DRUG INTERACTIONS: Interactions with other drugs have not been established. However, the concomitant use of medicinal products that have been associated with hepatic and/or renal toxicity should be avoided wherever possible. Patients taking medicinal products known to affect blood pressure or cardiac function should be closely monitored during treatment with clofarabine.

Clofarabine is not detectably metabolized by the cytochrome P450 (CYP) enzyme system. In vitro studies, clofarabine was not a substrate and did not significantly inhibit 5 human CYP isoforms (1A2, 2C9, 2C19, 2D6 and 3A4) or induce 2 of these isoforms (1A2 and 3A4). Thus, clofarabine is not expected to affect the metabolism of active substances which are known substrates for these enzymes.

Clofarabine is predominantly excreted via the kidneys; renal clearance is higher than glomerular filtration rates. Studies of the mechanisms of clearance in isolated rat kidney are consistent with elimination of clofarabine by a combination of filtration, tubular secretion and reabsorption. In this model, co-infusion with cimetidine reduced clearance of clofarabine, an effect that was confirmed in vivo in the rat. Hence, the concomitant use of drugs that have been associated with renal toxicity and those eliminated by tubular secretion or reabsorption should be avoided particularly during the 5 day clofarabine administration period.

There are no known clinically significant interactions of Clolar with other medications or laboratory tests. No formal drug/laboratory test interaction studies have been conducted with Clolar (clofarabine).

DOSAGE AND ADMINISTRATION: Recommended Concomitant Medications:

- Provide IV infusion fluids throughout the 5 days of Clolar (clofarabine) administration to reduce the effects of tumor lysis and other adverse events. Consider prophylactic anti-emetic medications as Clolar is moderately emetogenic. The use of prophylactic steroids (e.g., 100 mg/m² hydrocortisone on Days 1 through 3) may be of benefit in preventing signs or symptoms of SIRS or capillary leak (e.g., hypotension, tachycardia, tachypnea, and pulmonary edema).
- The administration of alkalinized intravenous fluids, allopurinol and/or other uric acid-lowering agents may be considered prior to clofarabine administration to prevent tumor lysis syndrome. Institutional guidelines should be followed in regards to the dosing and schedule of administration of these agents.

Recommended Dose and Dosage Adjustment: Dosing Schedule and Administration:

- The pediatric (ages 1-21) dose of 52 mg/m² of body surface area is administered by intravenous infusion over 2 hours daily for 5 consecutive days.
- Treatment cycle comprises a 5-day course of Clolar followed by the recovery period of 2 to 6 weeks (median 4 weeks) from the starting day of the previous cycle.
- The cycles are repeated following recovery or return to baseline organ function. In clinical trials in pediatric acute leukemias, the median duration of a cycle was 28 days (range of 12-55 days).
- The majority of patients who respond to Clolar achieve a response after 1 or 2 treatment cycles. Therefore the potential benefit and risks associated with continued therapy in patients who do not show hematological or clinical improvement after 2 treatment cycles should be assessed by treating physicians.
- Close monitoring of fluid status, and renal and hepatic function during the 5 days of Clolar administration is advised (see Warnings and Precautions).
- Close monitoring of patients taking medications known to affect blood pressure or cardiac function during administration of Clolar is advised.

Dose Modifications and Reinitiation of Therapy:

- Hematologic Toxicity
  - Administer subsequent cycles no sooner than 14 days from the starting day of the previous cycle provided the patient's ANC is ≥0.75×10⁹/L.
  - If a patient experiences a Grade 4 neutropenia (ANC <0.5×10⁹/L) lasting ≥4 weeks, reduce dose by 25% for the next cycle.
- Non-hematologic Toxicity
  - Withhold Clolar if a patient develops a clinically significant infection, until the infection is clinically resolved and then restart at the full dose.
  - Withhold Clolar if a Grade 3 non-infectious non-hematologic toxicity (excluding transient elevations in serum transaminases and/or serum bilirubin and/or nausea/vomiting that was controlled by antiemetic therapy) occurs. Re-institute Clolar administration at a 25% dose reduction when resolution or return to baseline.
  - Discontinue Clolar administration if a Grade 4 non-infectious non-hematologic toxicity occurs.
  - Discontinue Clolar administration if a patient shows early signs or symptoms of SIRS or capillary leak (e.g., hypotension, tachycardia, tachypnea, and pulmonary edema) and provide appropriate supportive measures. Re-institute Clolar when the patient is stable, generally with a 25% dose reduction.
  - Clolar administration should be stopped if the patient develops hypotension for any reason during the 5 days of administration. If hypotension is transient and resolves without pharmacological intervention, Clolar treatment can be re-initiated generally with a 25% dose reduction.
  - Discontinue Clolar administration if substantial increases in creatinine or bilirubin are noted. Re-institute Clolar when the patient is stable and organ function has returned to baseline, possibly with a 25% dose reduction. If hyperuricemia is anticipated (tumor lysis), prophylactically administer allopurinol or other uric acid lowering medications. Institutional guidelines should be followed in regards to the dosing and schedule of administration of these agents.
  - Use in patients with hepatic and renal dysfunction: Clolar has not been studied in patients with renal or hepatic dysfunction. Its use in such patients should be undertaken only with the greatest caution.

Administration: Clolar should be filtered through a sterile 0.2 µm syringe filter and then diluted with 5% Dextrose Injection, USP, or 0.9% Sodium Chloride Injection, USP, prior to intravenous (IV) infusion to a final concentration between 0.15 mg/mL and 0.4 mg/mL. Use diluted preparation immediately.

Do not administer any other medications through the same intravenous line.

As with all parenteral drug products, Clolar injection and diluted IV infusion should be inspected visually for clarity, haziness, particulate matter or precipitate and leakage prior to administration. Solution showing discoloration, haziness, precipitate, particulate, or leakage should not be used. Discard unused portion.

OVERDOSAGE:

There were no known overdoses of Clolar (clofarabine). The highest daily dose administered to a human to date (on a mg/m² basis) has been 70 mg/m²/day × 5 days (2 pediatric ALL patients). The toxicities in these 2 patients included grade 4 hyperbilirubinemia, grade 2 and 3 vomiting, and grade 3 maculopapular rash.

For management of a suspected drug overdose, CPhA recommends that you contact your regional Poison Control Centre. See the *CPS* Directory section for a list of Poison Control Centres.

ACTION AND CLINICAL PHARMACOLOGY: Mechanism of Action: Clofarabine is transported into target cells by both diffusion and facilitated diffusion. Intracellular clofarabine is mono-phosphorylated by deoxycytidine kinase (dCK) and then serially phosphorylated by other kinases to form clofarabine triphosphate, the active moiety. Clofarabine has high affinity for the dCK, which is equal or exceeds that of deoxycytidine, the natural substrate. Clofarabine is a prodrug and exerts its activity through active metabolites. Clofarabine triphosphate inhibits DNA synthesis via: (1) reduction of deoxynucleotide triphosphate pools by inhibiting ribonucleotide reductase; (2) by competitive inhibition of DNA polymerase alpha (IC50=3.9 µM), and (3) by terminating DNA chain elongation. In addition, the triphosphate induces apoptosis through the disruption of mitochondrial membrane integrity with the release of cytochrome C and other pro-apoptotic factors. Clofarabine monophosphate has been shown to inhibit DNA repair through incorporation into the DNA chain during the repair process.

Pharmacodynamics: Based on its cellular mechanism of action, clofarabine is expected to demonstrate anticancer activity and also produce adverse effects such as damage to rapidly proliferating tissues (e.g. bone marrow, lymphoid tissue and the gastrointestinal tract).

The inhibitory effect of clofarabine on DNA synthesis in leukemia blast cells was observed in 4 pediatric patients who received doses of 11.25, 15, 40, or 52 mg/m². Generally, DNA synthesis declined rapidly after each infusion with a 10 to 50% recovery 24 hours later. The recovery of DNA synthesis appeared to be inversely related to clofarabine dose. Doses less than 52 mg/m² MTD) showed breakthrough DNA synthesis prior to the second infusion. At the MTD, the inhibition of DNA synthesis was maintained throughout the therapy cycle. Administration of 52 mg/m² clofarabine resulted in dramatic and rapid reduction in peripheral leukemia cells in 94% (31/33) of pediatric ALL patients (33/61) who had measurable absolute blast count at baseline. No relationship between clofarabine or clofarabine triphosphate exposure and either efficacy or toxicity has been established in this population.

A dose-dependent inhibition of DNA synthesis was also reported in adult patients with acute leukemia treated with clofarabine. The pretreatment capacity of mononuclear cells to synthesize DNA was compared to their capacities after 3 to 4 days of therapy. At a dose of 22.5 mg/m²/day, a 60% decrease in DNA synthesis was observed. At 30 mg/m²/day, the DNA synthesis inhibition was almost complete, but not sustainable. And only at 55 mg/m²/day the complete sustainable DNA synthesis inhibition was achieved. The decrease in DNA synthesis was accompanied by a decrease in white blood cell (WBC) counts. For the 12 adult patients at the MTD of 40 mg/m²/day, the WBC count at pre-treatment ranged from 1000 to 78 000/µL with a blast percentage of 80 to 97%. After 5 days of therapy, WBC counts declined a median of 97% (range 68-99%).

* The average of the daily values.

The anti-cancer activity of clofarabine appeared to be dose and schedule dependent, and greater antitumor activity was associated with more frequent administration.

Pharmacokinetics: Population pharmacokinetics of clofarabine were studied in 32 patients (M/F 18/14). Of these, 17 patients had ALL and 15 had AML. Patients aged between 2.9 to 17.8 years old (median 11.8 years old) were predominantly Caucasian (n=15) with an equal number of Blacks and Hispanics (n=6). Of the remaining patients, 1 was Asian and 4 were classified as other. Patient's average weight was 45.0 kg (range 15.6 to 129.9 kg). Body surface area averaged 1.32 m² (range 0.65 to 2.58 m²). All patients received a dose adjusted by BSA of 52 mg/m². Total doses administered ranged from 12.3 to 134 mg/day. The PK was best described by a 2-compartment model. In this analysis, weight was the most important predictor for all primary pharmacokinetic parameters. Sex, disease type, and race were not predictive of clofarabine pharmacokinetics. Although WBC negatively correlated with C_{max}, this effect did not appear clinically relevant to individualize a patient's dosage regimen based on their WBC count. C_{max} was inversely proportional to patient's weight, and therefore, small children may have a higher C_{max} at the end of infusion than a typical 40 kg child given the same dose of clofarabine per m². Accordingly, longer infusion times should be considered in children weighing <20 kg.

Pharmacokinetics parameters of clofarabine were estimated in 22 ALL patients (M/F: 12/10) with mean age of 12.3 years old, weight of 48.1 kg, and BSA of 1.38 m². All patients received 52 mg/m² clofarabine daily. Clofarabine was administered by IV infusion over 2-hours for 5 consecutive days.

Pharmacokinetic parameters were estimated on Day 1 and on Day 5 of Cycle 1, as well as at steady-state, (Typical*). Plasma clofarabine concentrations were generally maximal by the end of infusion. Little accumulation in plasma was observed by the end of a 5-day cycle. See Table 4.

Table 4: Clolar

Pharmacokinetics in Pediatric Patients with Relapsed/refractory ALL Following IV Administration of Clofarabine at 52 mg/m² on Day 1, Day 5 and Typical Across Days

	C_{max} (ng/mL)	$t_{½\,\alpha}$ (h)	$t_{½\,\beta}$ (h)	$AUC_{0\text{-}inf}$ (ng·h/mL)	Clearance (L/h)	Volume of distribution (L)
Day 1						
Mean	452.9	0.434	6.2	2480	34.0	195
SD	186.7	0.171	3.7	1290	15.8	118.2
Day 5						
Mean	600.6	0.43	4.3	2379	33.0	145
SD	280.7	0.186	1.3	995	13.4	80.3
Typical[a]						
Mean		0.432	5.3	2451	31.8	173.4
SD	N/A	0.172	1.5	828	13.3	87.4

[a] The average of the daily values.

Distribution: Only 47% of clofarabine is bound to human plasma proteins, predominantly to albumin. Clofarabine shows high tissue distribution. There is no evidence that intracellular uptake of clofarabine is cell specific.

Metabolism: Clofarabine is not detectably metabolized by the cytochrome P450 (CYP) enzyme system. Clofarabine undergoes step-wise intracellular phosphorylation. The in vitro studies suggest that once clofarabine triphosphate is formed it remains trapped in the cell until incorporated into DNA. There is very little to no metabolism of the triphosphate. The metabolic pathways of clofarabine in humans were not characterized. The pharmacokinetics of the active metabolite, clofarabine triphosphate, were not estimated in any studies. The triphosphate concentrations were measured in peripheral mononuclear cells of 10 pediatric patients with acute leukemia. Sustainable intracellular clofarabine triphosphate concentrations (mean of 15.7 µM, range 2.9 to 42.3 µM) were rapidly achieved and maintained over 24 hours with no indication that triphosphate concentrations declined.

Excretion: The mean clofarabine renal clearance was 15.1 L/h (90% CI: 11.1 to 20.6 L/h) with an observed minimum and maximum of 1.34 and 55.0 L/h, respectively.

Approximately 60% of clofarabine dose is eliminated by renal excretion as unchanged drug within 24 hours after dosing. Clofarabine renal clearance rates appear to be much higher than glomerular filtration rates suggesting filtration and tubular secretion as kidney elimination mechanism. Studies in the isolated perfused rat model suggest that the human Organic Cation Transporter Type 2 (hOCT2) may be the transporter responsible for tubular secretion. The pathways of non-renal elimination of the 40% of the administered dose remain unknown.

Although the pharmacokinetics of clofarabine have not been studied in patients with severe renal dysfunction, given the percent of dose excreted in urine as unchanged clofarabine, it is recommended that clofarabine should not be administered in this sub-population.

STORAGE AND STABILITY: Vials containing undiluted Clolar (clofarabine) should be stored at 25°C; excursions permitted to 15-30°C.

Diluted admixtures must be used immediately.

SPECIAL HANDLING INSTRUCTIONS: Caution should be used during handling, preparation and disposal of Clolar (clofarabine). Use of gloves and other protective clothing to prevent skin contact is recommended. Proper aseptic technique should be used.

Guidelines on the proper handling and disposal of anticancer drugs should be consulted.

INFORMATION FOR THE PATIENT: Published in e-CPS, available by subscription at www.e-cps.ca.

DOSAGE FORMS, COMPOSITION AND PACKAGING: Each mL of sterile solution for injection contains: clofarabine 1 mg. The 20 mL vial contains 20 mg clofarabine formulated in 20 mL unbuffered normal saline (comprised of Water for Injection, USP, and Sodium Chloride, USP). Single-use vials of 20 mL, single-pack cartons.

Clomid® Pr

clomiphene citrate

Ovulatory Agent

sanofi-aventis

Date of Revision: July 31, 2009

PHARMACOLOGY: Clomiphene is an orally-administered, nonsteroidal agent which may induce ovulation in anovulatory women in appropriately selected cases. The ovulatory response to cyclic clomiphene therapy appears to be mediated through increased output of pituitary gonadotropins, which in turn stimulate the maturation and endocrine activity of the ovarian follicle and the subsequent development and function of the corpus luteum. The role of the pituitary is indicated by increased urinary excretion of gonadotropins and by the response of the ovary, as manifested by increased urinary estrogen excretion. Antagonism of competitive inhibition of endogenous estrogen may play a role in the action of clomiphene on the pituitary.

Clomiphene is a drug of considerable pharmacologic potency. Its administration should be preceded by careful evaluation and selection of the patient, and must be accompanied by close attention to the timing of the dose. With conservative selection and management of the patient, clomiphene has been demonstrated to be a useful therapy for the anovulatory patient.

Based on studies with ^{14}C-labeled clomiphene, the drug is readily absorbed orally in humans, and is excreted principally in the feces. Cumulative excretion of the ^{14}C-label averaged 51% of the oral dose after 5 days in 6 subjects, with mean urinary excretion of 8% and mean fecal excretion of 42%; less than 1% per day was excreted in fecal and urine samples collected from 31 to 53 days after ^{14}C-labeled clomiphene administration. Since C-14 appeared in the feces 6 weeks after administration, available data suggested that the remaining drug/metabolites were being slowly excreted from a sequestered enterohepatic recirculation pool. After i.v. administration, 37% was excreted in 5 days.

INDICATIONS: For induction of ovulation in patients with persistent ovulatory dysfunction who desire pregnancy. The work-up and treatment of candidates for clomiphene therapy should be supervised by physicians experienced in management of gynecologic or endocrine disorders. Patients should be chosen for therapy with clomiphene only after careful diagnostic evaluation. The work-up of the patient must begin with a careful and detailed history of menstrual and reproductive function, and a complete physical examination. It should be followed by a selective and careful laboratory investigation based on historical and physical findings.

Clomiphene is indicated only in patients who meet the criteria or have been assessed as described below:

Exclusion of pregnancy: If any doubt exists as to the presence of early pregnancy, clomiphene therapy should be withheld until a diagnosis of pregnancy has been excluded.

Assessment of abnormal or excessive bleeding: Patients with abnormal or excessive bleeding should have particularly careful evaluation prior to clomiphene therapy. It is most important to ensure that neoplastic lesions are not overlooked (see also Contraindications).

Exclusion of presence or history of liver dysfunction: Clinical evaluation of liver function should always precede clomiphene therapy (see also Contraindications).

Exclusion of presence of ovarian cyst: Clomiphene should not be used in patients with ovarian enlargement except those with polycystic ovary syndrome. Pelvic examination is necessary prior to the first and each subsequent course of clomiphene treatment in order to rule out the presence of an ovarian cyst (see also Contraindications).

Confirmed ovulatory dysfunction: The diagnosis of ovulatory dysfunction should be established by such standard techniques as basal body temperature curves, serial vaginal smears, cervical mucus, endometrial biopsy, and pregnanediol determination.

Exclusion of primary pituitary or ovarian failure: Appropriate diagnostic measures should be undertaken to exclude primary pituitary failure or primary ovarian failure. Intact pituitary and ovaries are required for successful therapy. Ovulatory dysfunction in the presence of abnormally high levels of pituitary gonadotropins is indicative of ovarian failure, and patients in this category cannot be expected to respond to clomiphene.

Assessment of estrogen levels: Adequacy of endogenous estrogen, as estimated by vaginal smears, cervical mucus, endometrial biopsy, or urinary estrogen determination, furnishes a measure of ovarian function and indirectly of pituitary function. Bleeding after progesterone administration (progesterone alone, not combined with estrogen) furnishes evidence of an adequate level of endogenous estrogen. A good level of endogenous estrogen provides a favorable prognosis for treatment with clomiphene. A reduced estrogen level, although less favorable, does not always preclude successful therapy.

Exclusion of mechanical impediments to conception: Mechanical impediments to conception, such as tubal obstruction, should be excluded or adequately treated, before undertaking clomiphene therapy.

Exclusion of medical impediments to pregnancy: When disorders such as diabetes, adrenal disease, or thyroid disease are identified during the investigation, specific treatment should be undertaken and subfertility therapy reconsidered only after the underlying disorder has been adequately treated. Clomiphene cannot be expected to substitute for specific therapy of these conditions.

Exclusion of male factor infertility: The husband's potential fertility should be ascertained by semen analysis and other indicated examination. There are no adequate or well-controlled studies that demonstrate the effectiveness of clomiphene in the treatment of male infertility. In addition, testicular tumors and gynecomastia have been reported in males using clomiphene. The cause and effect relationship between reports of testicular tumors and the administration of clomiphene is not known.

CONTRAINDICATIONS: *Pregnancy:* Clomiphene should not be administered during pregnancy. Although no causative evidence of a deleterious effect of clomiphene therapy on the human fetus has been established, such evidence in regard to the rat and the rabbit has been presented (see Precautions). **To avoid inadvertent clomiphene administration during early pregnancy, careful pelvic examination must be done prior to each course of therapy, the basal body temperature must be recorded throughout all treatment cycles, and the patient should be carefully observed to determine whether ovulation occurs.** If the basal body temperature following clomiphene is biphasic and is not followed by menses, the patient should be examined carefully for the presence of an ovarian cyst and should have a pregnancy test. The next course of therapy should be delayed until the possibility of pregnancy has been excluded.

Liver Disease: Clomiphene therapy is contraindicated in patients with liver disease or a history of liver dysfunction.

Hormone-dependent Tumors or Abnormal Uterine Bleeding: Clomiphene is contraindicated in patients with hormone-dependent tumors and in patients with abnormal uterine bleeding of undetermined origin. Clomiphene is not indicated for the management of menstrual disorders.

Ovarian Cyst: Clomiphene should not be given in the presence of an ovarian cyst, except polycystic ovary, since further enlargement of the cyst may occur. Patients should be evaluated for the presence of ovarian cyst prior to each course of treatment.

Hypersensitivity: Clomiphene is contraindicated in patients with a known hypersensitivity or allergy to clomiphene or any of its ingredients.

WARNINGS: Ovarian Hyperstimulation Syndrome During Clomiphene Therapy: Ovarian Hyperstimulation Syndrome (OHSS) has been reported in patients receiving clomiphene therapy alone or in combination with gonadotropins.

OHSS is a medical event distinct from uncomplicated ovarian enlargement. The early warning signs of OHSS are abdominal pain and distention, nausea, vomiting, diarrhea, and weight gain. Elevated urinary steroid levels, varying degrees of electrolyte imbalance, hypovolemia, hemoconcentration, and hypoproteinemia may occur. Transient liver function test abnormalities suggestive of hepatic dysfunction, which may be accompanied by morphologic changes on liver biopsy, have been reported in association with OHSS. The clinical signs of this syndrome in severe cases can include gross ovarian enlargement, gastrointestinal symptoms, ascites, dyspnea, oliguria, and pleural effusion.

Rare cases of severe forms of OHSS have been reported in patients receiving clomiphene therapy alone or in combination with gonadotropins where the following symptoms have occurred: pericardial effusion, anasarca, hydrothorax, acute abdomen, renal failure, pulmonary edema, hypotension, intraperitoneal and ovarian hemorrhage, deep venous thrombosis, torsion of the ovary and acute respiratory distress. Death due to hypovolemic shock, hemoconcentration or thromboembolism has occurred. If conception results, rapid progression to the severe form of the syndrome may occur.

In order to minimize the hazard associated with the occasional abnormal ovarian enlargement associated with clomiphene (see Adverse Effects), the lowest dose consistent with expectation of good results should be used. Maximal enlargement of the ovary, whether physiologic or abnormal, may not occur until several days after discontinuation of the recommended dose of clomiphene. Some patients with polycystic ovary syndrome who are unusually sensitive to gonadotropin may have an exaggerated response to usual doses of clomiphene. Therefore, patients with polycystic ovary syndrome should be started on the lowest recommended dose and shortest treatment duration for the first course of therapy (see Dosage).

The patient should be advised of the possibility of ovarian cyst formation and should be instructed to return for repeat pelvic examination between 2 and 3 weeks after starting each course of treatment. The patient should inform the physician of any abdominal or pelvic pain, weight gain, discomfort or distention after taking clomiphene.

The patient who complains of abdominal or pelvic pain after receiving clomiphene should be examined because of the possible presence of an ovarian cyst or other cause. Due to fragility of enlarged ovaries in severe cases, abdominal and pelvic examination should be performed with care.

If abnormal enlargement of the ovary occurs, additional clomiphene therapy should not be given until the ovaries have returned to pretreatment size, and the dosage or duration of the next course should be reduced. Ovarian enlargement and cyst formation associated with clomiphene therapy regress spontaneously within a few days or weeks after discontinuing treatment. **Unless surgical indication for laparotomy exists, such cystic enlargement should always be managed conservatively.**

Occupational Hazards: Visual Symptoms: Patients should be advised that blurring or other visual symptoms such as spots or flashes (scintillating scotomata) may occasionally occur during therapy or shortly after therapy with clomiphene. Patients should be warned that visual symptoms may render such activities as driving a car or operating machinery more hazardous than usual, particularly under conditions of variable lighting. These visual disturbances are usually reversible; however, cases of prolonged visual disturbance have been reported even after clomiphene discontinuation. The visual disturbances may be irreversible, especially with increased dosage or duration of therapy. The significance of these visual symptoms is not yet understood (see Adverse Effects). If the patient has any visual symptoms, treatment should be discontinued and complete ophthalmologic evaluation carried out.

PRECAUTIONS: Diagnosis Prior to Clomiphene Therapy: Careful attention should be given to diagnosis in candidates for clomiphene therapy. Complete pelvic examination including cervical cytology is mandatory prior to treatment, and pelvic examination should be repeated before each subsequent course.

Patients in later reproductive life have a greater tendency to endometrial carcinoma as well as a higher incidence of anovulatory disorders. Dilatation and curettage should always be done for diagnosis before starting clomiphene therapy in such patients. If abnormal bleeding is present, full diagnostic measures are mandatory (see also Contraindications and Warnings).

Uterine Fibroids: Caution should be exercised when using clomiphene in patients with uterine fibroids due to the potential for further enlargement of the fibroids.

Pregnancy: (See also Contraindications and Adverse Effects, Birth Defects).

Teratogenic/Nonteratogenic Effects: The overall incidence of reported birth anomalies from pregnancies associated with maternal clomiphene ingestion during clinical studies was within the range of that reported for the general population.

Pregnancy Wastage: The experience from patients of all diagnoses during clinical investigation of clomiphene shows a pregnancy (single and multiple) wastage or fetal loss rate of 21.4% (abortion rate of 19.0%), ectopic pregnancies 1.18%, hydatidiform mole 0.17%, fetal papyraceous 0.04%, and pregnancies with one or more stillbirths 1.01%.

Multiple Pregnancy: The incidence of multiple pregnancy (including triplets, quadruplets and quintuplets) has been increased up to tenfold when conception takes place during a cycle in which clomiphene therapy is given. During the clinical investigation studies, the incidence of multiple pregnancy was 7.9% (186 of 2369 clomiphene associated pregnancies on which outcome was reported). Among these 2369 pregnancies, 165 (6.9%) were twin, 11 (0.5%) triplet, 7 (0.3%) quadruplet, and 3 (0.13%) quintuplet. Of the 165 twin pregnancies for which sufficient information was available, the ratio of monozygotic to dizygotic twins was 1:5. The patient and her husband should be advised of the frequency and potential hazards of multiple pregnancy before starting treatment.

Ectopic Pregnancy: There is an increased chance of ectopic pregnancy (including tubal and ovarian sites) in women who conceive following clomiphene therapy.

Lactation: It is not known whether clomiphene is excreted in human milk. Clomiphene may reduce lactation.

Carcinogenicity: Prolonged use of clomiphene may increase the risk of developing a borderline or invasive ovarian tumor.

Mutagenicity: Mutagenic potential of clomiphene has not been evaluated.

ADVERSE EFFECTS: Clinical Trials: Overview: At recommended dosage, side effects are not prominent and infrequently interfere with treatment. Side effects tend to be dose related, occurring more frequently at the higher doses and longer duration of treatment courses used in some earlier studies. The more common side effects include hot flashes, abdominal discomfort (distention, bloating, pain, or soreness), ovarian enlargement, and visual blurring. The vasomotor symptoms resembling menopausal "hot flashes" are not usually severe and disappear promptly after treatment is discontinued. Abdominal symptoms may be most often related to ovulatory (mittelschmerz) or premenstrual phenomena, or to ovarian enlargement.

Other less frequently reported symptoms during clomiphene therapy have included nausea or vomiting, constipation, diarrhea, increased nervous tension, depression, fatigue, dizziness or lightheadedness, insomnia, headache, breast soreness, heavier menses, intermenstrual spotting, urticaria or allergic dermatitis, weight gain, and increased urinary frequency or volume. Moderate, reversible hair loss has been reported in a few patients, primarily on prolonged continuous therapy.

Birth Defects: From 2339 completed pregnancies associated with clomiphene administration, 58 birth defects have been reported. They have been reported in 4 conceptions in the abortion/stillbirth category, 14 of 353 infants from multiple pregnancies, and 39 of 1676 infants from single pregnancies. Three live-born infants failed to survive.

Reported defects were congenital heart lesions (8 infants), Down's syndrome (5 infants), club foot (4 infants), congenital gut lesions (4 infants), hypospadias (3 infants), microcephaly (2 infants), harelip and cleft palate (2 infants), congenital hip (2 infants), hemangioma (2 infants), undescended testes (2 infants), polydactyly (both of twins), conjoined twins with teratomatous malformation, patent ductus arteriosus, amaurosis (blindness), arteriovenous fistula, inguinal hernia, umbilical hernia, syndactyly, pectus excavatum, myopathy, dermoid cyst of scalp, omphalocele, spina bifida occulta, icthyosis, persistent lingual frenulum, and 7 infants with multiple somatic defects.

Eight of the entire group of 58 infants were born to 7 of 153 mothers who received a course of clomiphene during the first 6 weeks after conception.

An interval of 4, 4, and 10 months respectively elapsed between the last clomiphene therapy and conception in 3 mothers. In a 4th mother conception occurred during a subsequent ovulation induced by gonadotropin therapy.

Gastrointestinal System: Sulfobromophthalein (BSP) retention of greater than 5% has been reported in 32 of 141 patients in whom it was measured, including 5 of 43 patients who received approximately the dose of clomiphene now recommended. Retention was usually minimal unless associated with prolonged continuous clomiphene administration or with apparently unrelated liver disease. In some patients, pre-existing BSP retention decreased even though clomiphene therapy was continued. Other liver function tests were usually normal. In a later study in which patients were given 6 consecutive monthly courses of clomiphene (100 mg daily for 3 days) or matching placebo, BSP tests were done on 94 patients. Values in excess of 5% retention were recorded in 11 patients, 6 of whom had received drug and 5 placebo. One patient developed jaundice on the 19th day of treatment (50 mg/day); liver biopsy revealed bile stasis without evidence of hepatitis. A male prison subject who received 200 mg daily for 77 days developed the clinical picture of infectious hepatitis; his cellmate was discovered to have had infectious hepatitis 4 months earlier.

Genitourinary System: At recommended dosage, abnormal ovarian enlargement (see also Warnings) is infrequent, although the usual cyclic variation in ovarian size may be exaggerated. Similarly, cyclic ovarian pain (mittelschmerz) may be accentuated. With higher or prolonged dosage, more frequent ovarian enlargement and cyst formation (usually luteal) may occur, and the luteal phase of the cycle may be prolonged. Rare instances of massive ovarian enlargement are on record. Southam and Janovski described such an instance in a patient with polycystic ovary syndrome whose clomiphene therapy consisted of 100 mg daily for 14 days. Abnormal ovarian enlargement usually regresses spontaneously, and while laparotomy was performed on several such patients, investigators believe most of these patients should have been treated conservatively.

Multiple pregnancies, (see also Precautions), including simultaneous intrauterine and extrauterine pregnancies, ovarian hemorrhage, tubal pregnancy, uterine hemorrhage have been reported.

Laboratory: Clomiphene has not been reported to cause significant abnormality in the hematologic or renal systems, in protein bound iodine, or in serum cholesterol. Analysis by gas liquid chromatography (GLC) of serum sterols from patients on prolonged, continuous administration of clomiphene yields a peak compatible with an elevated level of desmosterol. This peak is indicative of an interference with cholesterol synthesis. However, the serum sterol GLC pattern from patients receiving recommended doses of clomiphene is not significantly altered.

Special Senses: Visual symptoms (see also Warnings for further recommendations) described usually as "blurring" or spots or flashes (scintillating scotomata) increase in incidence with increasing total dose. These symptoms appear to be due to intensification and prolongation of after-images. Symptoms often first appear or are accentuated with exposure to a more brightly lit environment. Ophthalmologically definable scotoma, photophobia, diplopia, phosphenes, and reduced visual acuity have been reported. There are rare reports of cataracts and optic neuritis. These visual disturbances are usually reversible; however, cases of prolonged visual disturbance have been reported even after clomiphene discontinuation. The visual disturbances may be irreversible, especially with increased dosage or duration of therapy.

While measured visual acuity has not generally been affected, one patient taking 200 mg daily developed visual blurring on the 7th day of treatment, which progressed to severe diminution of visual acuity by the 10th day. No other abnormality was found and the visual acuity returned to normal on the 3rd day after treatment was stopped. Another patient treated during clinical studies developed scotomata during prolonged clomiphene administration, which disappeared on placebo. Monolateral exophthalmos associated with laboratory evidence of hyperthyroidism was observed in 1 patient concomitant with completion of the 3rd course of clomiphene.

In a 34-year-old patient who had taken 3 courses of clomiphene, slit-lamp microscopic examination showed a mild amount of posterior cortical subcapsular opacity in each eye. Ophthalmoscopic examination revealed normal findings. The ocular diagnosis was posterior cortical senile cataracts.

Tumors/Neoplasms: Ovarian cancer has been reported in a very small number of infertile women who have been treated with fertility drugs. A causal relationship between treatment with fertility drugs and ovarian cancer has not been established.

Postmarketing Surveillance: Other than the adverse events reported above, the following adverse events were reported in postmarketing surveillance data.

Birth Defects: The following fetal abnormalities have also been reported: delayed development; abnormal bone development including skeletal malformations of the skull, face, nasal passages, jaw, hand, limb (ectromelia including amelia, hemimelia, and phocomelia), foot and joints; tissue malformations including imperforate anus, tracheosophageal fistula, diaphragmatic hernia, renal agenesis and dysgenesis, and malformations of the eye and lens (cataract), ear, lung, heart (ventricular septal defect and tetralogy of Fallot), and genitalia; as well as dwarfism, deafness, mental retardation, chromosomal disorders, and neural tube defects (including anencephaly).

Body as a Whole: fever, tinnitus and weakness have also been reported.

Cardiovascular: arrhythmia, chest pain, edema, hypertension, palpitation, phlebitis, pulmonary embolism, shortness of breath, tachycardia, thrombophlebitis.

Central Nervous System: Migraine headache, paresthesia, stroke and syncope have been reported. Seizures have been observed rarely with clomiphene therapy.

Dermatologic: rash, urticaria, acne, allergic reaction, erythema, erythema multiforme, erythema nodosum, hypertrichosis, pruritus.
Genitourinary: There are reports of new cases of endometriosis and exacerbation of pre-existing endometriosis during clomiphene therapy.
Hepatic: transaminases increased, hepatitis.
Musculoskeletal: arthralgia, back pain, myalgia.
Other: Leukocytosis and thyroid disorder have also been reported.
Psychiatric: Anxiety, irritability, mood changes, and psychosis have also been reported.
Special Senses: Abnormal accomodation, eye pain, macular edema, photopsia, posterior vitreous detachment, retinal hemorrhage, retinal thrombosis, retinal vascular spasm, and temporary loss of vision.
Tumors/Neoplasms: Liver (hepatic hemangiosarcoma, liver cell adenoma, hepatocellular carcinoma); breast (fibrocystic disease, breast carcinoma); endometrium (endometrial carcinoma); nervous system (astrocytoma, pituitary tumor, prolactinoma, neurofibromatosis, glioblastoma multiforme, brain abscess); trophoblastic (hydatidiform mole, choriocarcinoma); miscellaneous (melanoma, myeloma, perianal cysts, renal cell carcinoma, Hodgkin's lymphoma, tongue carcinoma, bladder carcinoma); and neoplasms of offspring (neuroectodermal tumor, thyroid tumor, hepatoblastoma, lymphocytic leukemia).

Isolated reports have been received on the occurrence of endocrine-related or dependent tumors/neoplasms or their aggravation.

OVERDOSE:

Treatment: There is no known antidote but gastric lavage and other appropriate supportive measures should be performed.

> For management of a suspected drug overdose, CPhA recommends that you contact your **regional Poison Control Centre**. See the *CPS* Directory section for a list of Poison Control Centres.

DOSAGE: General Considerations: The work-up and treatment of candidates for clomiphene therapy should be supervised by physicians experienced in management of gynecologic or endocrine disorders. Patients should be chosen for therapy with clomiphene only after careful diagnostic evaluation (see Indications). The plan of therapy should be outlined in advance. Impediments to achieving the goal of therapy must be excluded or adequately treated before beginning clomiphene. Many patients will respond to 50 mg daily for 5 days (see Recommended Dosage). In the determination of a recommended starting dose schedule, efficacy must be balanced against potential side effects. For example, the data available so far suggest that ovulation and pregnancy are slightly more attainable on 100 mg/day for 5 days than on 50 mg/day for 5 days. As the dosage is increased, however, ovarian overstimulation and other side effects may be expected to increase. Furthermore, although the data do not yet establish a relationship between dosage and multiple births, it would seem reasonable on pharmacologic grounds that such a relationship does exist.

For these reasons, it would seem prudent to begin the treatment of the usual patient with a lower dose, 50 mg daily for 5 days, and to increase the dose only in those patients who do not respond to the 1st course (see Recommended Dosage). Special care in dosage is particularly recommended if unusual sensitivity to pituitary gonadotropin is suspected, such as in patients with polycystic ovary syndrome.

Recommended Dosage: The recommended dose for the 1st course of clomiphene is 50 mg (1 tablet) daily for 5 days. Therapy may be started at any time in the patient who has had no recent uterine bleeding. If progestin-induced bleeding is planned, or if spontaneous uterine bleeding occurs prior to therapy, the regimen of 50 mg daily for 5 days should be started on or about the 5th day of the cycle. When ovulation occurs at this dosage, there is no advantage to increasing the dose in subsequent cycles of treatment.

If ovulation appears not to have occurred after the 1st course of therapy, a 2nd course of 100 mg daily (two 50 mg tablets given as a single daily dose) for 5 days should be given. This course may be started as early as 30 days after the previous one. **Increasing the dosage or duration of therapy beyond 100 mg/day for 5 days should never be undertaken.**

The majority of patients who are going to respond will respond to the 1st course of therapy, and 3 courses should constitute an adequate therapeutic trial. If ovulatory menses have not yet occurred, the diagnosis should be re-evaluated. Treatment beyond this is not recommended in the patient who does not exhibit evidence of ovulation.

Pregnancy: The importance of properly timed coitus cannot be over-emphasized. In most patients, ovulation appears to occur from 6 to 12 days after completion of therapy. For regularity of cyclic ovulatory response it is also important that each course of clomiphene be started on or about the 5th cycle day, once ovulation has been established. In common with other therapeutic modalities, clomiphene therapy follows the rule of diminishing returns, such that likelihood of conception diminishes with each succeeding course of therapy. If pregnancy has not been achieved after 3 ovulatory responses to clomiphene, further treatment is not recommended. Patients should be advised of the possibility of multiple pregnancy and its potential hazards if conception occurs during a cycle in which clomiphene is given.

Long-term Cyclic Therapy Not Recommended: Since the relative safety of long-term cyclic therapy has not yet been conclusively demonstrated, and since the majority of patients will ovulate following 3 courses, long-term cyclic therapy is not recommended, i.e., beyond a total of about 6 cycles (including 3 ovulatory cycles).

SUPPLIED: Each white, rounded, flat-faced, beveled-edged, compressed tablet, scored on one side with "Clomid" debossed above score and "50" debossed below score, other side plain, contains: clomiphene citrate USP 50 mg. Nonmedicinal ingredients: cornstarch, lactose monohydrate, magnesium stearate, pregelatinized starch and sucrose. Energy: 4.5 kJ (1.1 kcal)/tablet. Unit pack boxes of 50 (5×10 blister packed). Protect from light and moisture.

(Shown in Product Identification Section)

Clonazepam

CPhA Monograph

see *Benzodiazepines*

Clopixol®

zuclopenthixol dihydrochloride

Antipsychotic

Lundbeck

Clopixol-Acuphase®

zuclopenthixol acetate

Antipsychotic

Lundbeck

Clopixol® Depot

zuclopenthixol decanoate

Antipsychotic

Lundbeck

Date of Revision: January 23, 2009

SUMMARY PRODUCT INFORMATION:

Route of Administration	Dosage Form/ Strength	All Nonmedicinal Ingredients
Oral	Tablet/10 mg, 25 mg	castor oil (hydrogenated), copovidone, ferric oxide, glycerol, hypromellose, lactose, macrogol 6000, magnesium stearate, microcrystalline cellulose, potato starch, talc, titanium dioxide
Intramuscular injection	Acuphase/50 mg/mL	medium-chain triglycerides
	Depot/200 mg/mL	medium-chain triglycerides

INDICATIONS AND CLINICAL USE: Clopixol (zuclopenthixol dihydrochloride), Clopixol-Acuphase (zuclopenthixol acetate) and Clopixol Depot (zuclopenthixol decanoate) are indicated for:

- the management of the manifestations of schizophrenia.

Clopixol (zuclopenthixol dihydrochloride) may be used during initial treatment and for maintenance treatment. Clopixol-Acuphase (zuclopenthixol acetate) is intended for the initial treatment of acute psychotic episodes or exacerbation of psychosis associated with schizophrenia. Clopixol Depot (zuclopenthixol decanoate) is intended for maintenance treatment.

Geriatrics (>65 years of age): The pharmacokinetics, safety, and efficacy of zuclopenthixol in elderly patients with schizophrenia have not been systematically evaluated in clinical trials. Caution should thus be exercised in dose selection for an elderly patient, recognizing the more frequent hepatic, renal and cardiac dysfunctions in this population.

Pediatrics (<18 years): The safety and efficacy of zuclopenthixol in children under the age of 18 years have not been established, therefore its use is not recommended.

CONTRAINDICATIONS:

- Acute alcohol, barbiturate or opiate intoxication.
- CNS depression due to any cause, comatose states, suspected or established subcortical brain damage or circulatory collapse.
- Patients with known hypersensitivity to thioxanthenes, zuclopenthixol or to any ingredient in the formulation or component of the container. For a complete listing, see Dosage Forms, Composition and Packaging.

WARNINGS AND PRECAUTIONS:

> **Serious Warnings and Precautions**
> - Neuroleptic malignant syndrome (NMS) is a rare, sometimes fatal, neurological disorder that has been reported in association with antipsychotic drugs including zuclopenthixol (see Warnings and Precautions, Neurologic and Adverse Reactions).

General: Occupational Hazards Sedative Effects: Since sedation is known to occur with zuclopenthixol, patients should be cautioned against performing activities requiring a high degree of mental alertness and physical coordination (such as driving a car or operating machinery) until the effect of the drug is determined.

Antiemetic Effects: An antiemetic effect of zuclopenthixol has been observed in animals. Since this effect may also occur in man, zuclopenthixol may mask signs of toxicity due to overdosage of other drugs, or may mask symptoms of disease such as brain tumor or intestinal obstruction.

Cardiovascular: Cardiovascular Disease: Caution should be used when using zuclopenthixol in patients with advanced cardiovascular disease or in those at risk of developing conduction abnormalities.

Cerebrovascular Accidents: An approximately 3-fold increase risk of cerebrovascular adverse events has been seen in randomized placebo controlled clinical trials in the dementia population with some atypical antipsychotics. The mechanism for this increased risk is not known. An increased risk cannot be excluded for other antipsychotics or other patient populations. Zuclopenthixol should be used with caution in patients with risk factors for stroke.

Cardiotoxicity: As with other drugs belonging to the therapeutic class of antipsychotics, zuclopenthixol may cause QT prolongation. Persistently prolonged QT intervals may increase the risk of malignant arrhythmias. Therefore, zuclopenthixol should be used with caution in susceptible individuals (with hypokalemia, hypomagnesia or genetic predisposition) and in patients with a history of cardiovascular disorders, e.g. QT prolongation, significant bradycardia (<50 beats per minute), a recent acute myocardial infarction, uncompensated heart failure, or cardiac arrhythmia. Concomitant treatment with other antipsychotics should be avoided.

Increases in the QT interval related to antipsychotic treatment may be exacerbated by the co-administration of other drugs known to significantly increase the QT interval. Co-administration of such drugs should be avoided (see Drug Interactions).

Endocrine and Metabolism: Endocrine Effects: Antipsychotic drugs elevate prolactin levels with the effect persisting during chronic administration. Since tissue culture experiments indicate that approximately one third of human breast cancers are prolactin dependent in vitro, zuclopenthixol should only be administered to patients with previously detected breast cancer if the benefits outweigh the potential risks. Caution should also be exercised when considering zuclopenthixol treatment in patients with pituitary tumors. Possible manifestations associated with elevated prolactin levels are amenorrhea, galactorrhea, and menorrhagia (see Adverse Reactions).

Chronic administration of zuclopenthixol (30 mg/kg/day for two years) in rats resulted in small, but significant, increases in the incidence of thyroid parafollicular carcinomas and, in females, of mammary adenocarcinomas and of pancreatic islet cell adenomas and carcinomas. An increase in the incidence of mammary adenocarcinomas is a common finding for D_2 antagonists which increase prolactin secretion when administered to rats. An increase in the incidence of pancreatic islet cell tumors has been observed for some other D_2 antagonists. The physiological differences between rats and humans with regard to prolactin make the clinical significance of these findings unclear, but it is accepted as not predicting an oncogenic risk in patients.

Hepatic/Biliary/Pancreatic: Impaired Liver Function: The use of zuclopenthixol in patients with impaired liver function has not been studied. As zuclopenthixol is extensively metabolized by the liver and primarily excreted in the bile (see Action and Clinical Pharmacology, Pharmacokinetics), caution should be exercised in dose selection for patients with this condition.

Neurologic: Neuroleptic Malignant Syndrome: Neuroleptic Malignant Syndrome (NMS) is characterized by hyperthermia, muscle rigidity, altered consciousness, and signs of autonomic instability including irregular blood pressure, tachycardia, cardiac arrhythmias and diaphoresis. Additional signs may include greatly elevated creatine phosphokinase, myoglobinuria and acute renal failure.

The management of NMS should include immediate discontinuation of all antipsychotic drugs including zuclopenthixol, intensive monitoring of symptoms, and treatment of any associated medical problems. There is no general agreement about specific pharmacological treatment for NMS. If a patient requires antipsychotic drug treatment after recovery from NMS, the reintroduction of therapy should be carefully considered, since recurrence of NMS has been reported.

Anticholinergic Effects: Zuclopenthixol may potentiate anticholinergic effects of concurrent medications. See Ophthalmologic for more details.

Patients with Parkinson's Disease: Zuclopenthixol should be used with caution in patients with Parkinsonism, as it is known that dopamine antagonists such as zuclopenthixol, can cause a deterioration of the disease.

Seizures: Zuclopenthixol should be used with caution in patients with a history of convulsive disorders, as drugs of this class are known to lower seizure threshold.

Tardive Dyskinesia: Is a potentially irreversible neurological syndrome associated with the use of antipsychotic drugs, including zuclopenthixol (see Adverse Reactions). It is characterized by stereotypical, repetitive, involuntary movements of the jaw, tongue and in some cases, the extremities. Tardive dyskinesia occurs more frequently in elderly patients. However, patients of any age can be affected. The risk of developing tardive dyskinesia and the chance of it becoming irreversible are believed to increase as the duration of treatment and the cumulative dose of antipsychotic drugs increase. However, the syndrome can develop, although less commonly, after relatively brief periods of treatment at low doses. Tardive dyskinesia may remit, partially or completely, if antipsychotic drug treatment is withdrawn. Antipsychotic drug treatment itself, however, may suppress the signs and symptoms of tardive dyskinesia, thereby masking the underlying process.

In view of these considerations, zuclopenthixol should be prescribed in a manner that is most likely to minimize the risk of tardive dyskinesia. The lowest effective dose and the shortest duration of treatment should be used, and treatment should be discontinued at the earliest opportunity, or if a satisfactory response cannot be obtained. If the signs and symptoms of tardive dyskinesia appear during treatment, discontinuation of zuclopenthixol should be considered.

Ophthalmologic: Anticholinergic Effects: Although its anticholinergic effects are weak, zuclopenthixol use should be avoided in patients who are known to have, or suspected of having narrow angle glaucoma.

Photosensitivity Reactions: Photosensitivity reactions, pigmentary retinopathy and lenticular and corneal deposits have been reported with related drugs. Lens opacity has been reported rarely with zuclopenthixol.
Renal: Impaired Renal Function: The use of zuclopenthixol in patients with impaired renal function has not been studied. Caution should thus be exercised in dose selection for patients with this condition.
Special Populations: Pregnant Women: The safe use of zuclopenthixol during pregnancy has not been established. Zuclopenthixol was not teratogenic in either rats or rabbits, however, increases in the number of stillbirths, reduced pup survival and delayed development of pups were seen in rats. The clinical significance of these findings is unclear. It has been shown that zuclopenthixol crosses the placenta of mice. Zuclopenthixol should not be administered during pregnancy unless the expected benefit to the patient outweighs the potential risk to the fetus.
Nursing Women: Zuclopenthixol is excreted in human milk with an average milk/serum concentration ratio of approximately 0.3. The safe use of zuclopenthixol during lactation has not been established.
Pediatrics (<18 years): The safety and efficacy of zuclopenthixol in children under the age of 18 years have not been established, therefore its use is not recommended.
Geriatrics (>65 years of age): The pharmacokinetics, safety, and efficacy of zuclopenthixol in elderly patients with schizophrenia have not been systematically evaluated in clinical trials. Caution should thus be exercised in dose selection for an elderly patient, recognizing the more frequent hepatic, renal and cardiac dysfunctions in this population.
ADVERSE REACTIONS: Clinical Trial Adverse Drug Reactions: Because clinical trials are conducted under very specific conditions the adverse reaction rates observed in the clinical trials may not reflect the rates observed in practice and should not be compared to the rates in the clinical trials of another drug. Adverse drug reaction information from clinical trials is useful for identifying drug-related adverse events and for approximating rates.

Adverse events were recorded in controlled and uncontrolled European and Canadian clinical trials in which 1922 patients were treated with either Clopixol tablets (zuclopenthixol dihydrochloride), Clopixol-Acuphase (zuclopenthixol acetate) or Clopixol Depot (zuclopenthixol decanoate).

The majority of adverse events are dose dependent. The frequency and severity are most pronounced in the early phase of treatment and decline during continued treatment.

The most common adverse events reported were drowsiness, fatigue, dizziness, and extrapyramidal symptoms. See Table 1.

Table 1: Clopixol

Treatment Emergent Adverse Events Reported with Clopixol at a Frequency of >1% from the Combined European and Canadian Clinical Trial Database

	Number of Patients (Percentage of Patients)		
	Clopixol Dosage Form		
Adverse Event[a]	**Tablet (n=523)**	**Acuphase (n=588)**	**Depot (n=811)**
Body as a Whole			
Asthenia/Fatigue	79 (15.1)	46 (7.8)[b]	111 (13.7)[b]
Malaise	12 (2.3)	—	—
Pain	9 (1.7)	—	—
Paleness	6 (1.1)	—	—
Syncope	6 (1.2)	—	5 (0.6)
Psychiatric			
Somnolence/Drowsiness	169 (32.3)[b]	95 (16.2)[b,c]	159 (19.6)[b]
Anxiety/Nervousness	88 (16.9)	24 (4.1)	70 (8.6)
Insomnia	85 (16.2)	27 (4.6)[b]	84 (10.4)[b]
Agitation	52 (9.9)	7 (1.2)[b]	11 (1.4)
Depression	41 (7.8)	18 (3.1)	59 (7.3)
Concentration Impaired	40 (7.6)	15 (2.6)	32 (3.9)[b]
Anorexia	20 (3.8)	—	12 (1.5)
Hallucination	18 (3.4)	—	—
Apathy	17 (3.2)	14 (2.4)	7 (0.9)
Confusion	14 (2.7)	1 (0.2)	3 (0.4)
Amnesia	13 (2.5)	12 (2.0)	13 (1.6)
Dreaming Abnormal	12 (2.3)	12 (2.0)	12 (1.5)
Appetite Increased	5 (1.0)	1 (0.2)	18 (2.2)
Neurological			
Hypertonia	98 (18.7)	150 (25.5)	37 (4.6)
Tremor	98 (18.7)	122 (20.7)[b]	68 (8.4)
Hyperkinesia (Akathisia)	71 (13.6)[b]	94 (16.0)[b]	107 (13.2)
Extrapyramidal Disorder	68 (13.0)	3 (0.5)	97 (12.0)
Dizziness	59 (11.3)	121 (20.6)	55 (6.8)[b]
Hypokinesia	39 (7.4)[b]	122 (20.7)[b]	82 (10.1)
Vertigo	27 (5.2)	6 (1.0)	16 (2.0)
Headache	26 (5.0)	8 (1.4)	43 (5.3)[b]
Dystonia	25 (4.8)	83 (14.1)	56 (6.9)
Dyskinesia Tardive	15 (2.9)	1 (0.2)	7 (0.9)

(cont'd)

Table 1: Clopixol *(cont'd)*

Treatment Emergent Adverse Events Reported with Clopixol at a Frequency of >1% from the Combined European and Canadian Clinical Trial Database

	Number of Patients (Percentage of Patients)		
	Clopixol Dosage Form		
Adverse Event[a]	**Tablet (n=523)**	**Acuphase (n=588)**	**Depot (n=811)**
Gait Abnormal	11 (2.1)	—	6 (0.7)
Neurological Disorder NOS	9 (1.7)	—	1 (0.1)
Paresthesia	6 (1.1)	18 (3.1)	15 (1.8)
Dyskinesia	—	1 (0.2)	10 (1.2)
Gastrointestinal			
Mouth Dry	79 (15.1)	148 (25.2)	106 (13.1)[b]
Constipation	41 (7.8)	4 (0.7)[b]	51 (6.3)[b]
Salivation Increased	40 (7.6)	58 (9.9)	52 (6.4)
Vomiting	17 (3.2)	6 (1.0)	17 (2.1)
GI Disorder NOS	15 (2.9)	1 (0.2)	10 (1.2)
Nausea	10 (1.9)	4 (0.7)	11 (1.4)
Diarrhea	4 (0.8)	4 (0.7)	9 (1.1)
Dyspepsia	—	—	10 (1.2)
Cardiovascular			
Tachycardia	19 (3.6)	58 (9.9)	21 (2.6)
Postural Hypotension	13 (2.5)	2 (0.2)	—
Arterial Hypotension	9 (1.7)	—	—
Palpitation	7 (1.3)	—	15 (1.8)
Musculoskeletal System			
Myalgia	—	—	10 (1.2)
Skin and Appendages			
Sweating Increased	16 (3.0)	7 (1.2)	47 (5.8)[b]
Pruritus	—	1 (0.2)	17 (2.1)
Seborrhea	8 (1.5)	—	2 (0.2)
Skin Disorder	7 (1.3)	—	—
Metabolic and Nutritional			
Weight Increase	20 (3.8)	—	17 (2.1)
Weight Decrease	17 (3.2)	—	14 (1.7)
Thirst	5 (1.0)	—	17 (2.1)[b]
Vision			
Accommodation Abnormal	29 (5.5)	65 (11.0)	33 (4.1)
Vision Abnormal	19 (3.6)	—	17 (2.1)[b]
Urinary			
Micturition Disorder	16 (3.0)	3 (0.5)	26 (3.2)
Reproductive			
Libido Decreased	17 (3.2)	1 (0.2)	11 (1.4)
Menstrual Disorder	5 (2.2)	—	12 (4.3)[b]
Ejaculation Failure	1 (0.4)	1 (0.3)	8 (1.8)[b]
Anorgasmia Female	1 (0.4)	—	3 (1.1)

[a] The incidence of adverse events is not directly comparable across formulations, as distinct clinical trials were conducted for each dosage form. Trial duration varied considerably between formulations (i.e., 2-12 weeks for Tablets; 3-9 days for Acuphase; and 4-52 weeks for Depot).
[b] Incidence in Canadian studies at least 10 percentage points higher than the combined European and Canadian incidence.
[c] Somnolence was not rated as an adverse event in many European Acuphase trials, as sedation was considered a therapeutic effect. Therefore, the incidence of this event is considered under-represented for the Acuphase formulation.

Less Common Clinical Trial Adverse Drug Reactions (≤1%): Adverse events reported in clinical trials, occurring at rates of 1% or less, are provided in the summary below for all three formulations together:
Body as a Whole: allergic reaction, application site disorder, arthritis, back pain, chest pain, precordial chest pain, conjunctivitis, faintness, fever, hot flushes, toothache.
Cardiovascular: hypotension.
Gastrointestinal: abdominal pain, dysphagia, gastric ulcer, glossitis, meteorism.

Hematological: purpura.
Neurological: acute dyskinesia, ataxia, convulsions, hyperreflexia, hypotonia, migraine, oculogyric crisis, speech disorder.
Psychiatric: drug dependence, excitability, irritability, increased libido, melancholia, paroniria.
Reproductive: erectile dysfunction, galactorrhea, gynecomastia, dry vagina.
Respiratory: dyspnea, nasal congestion, pharyngitis, rhinitis.
Skin and Appendages: dermatitis, photosensitivity reaction, abnormal pigmentation, rash, erythematous rash, psoriasiform rash.
Special Senses: mydriasis, hyperacusis, tinnitus.
Urinary: polyuria, urinary incontinence, urinary infection, urinary retention.
Post-Market Adverse Drug Reactions: Adverse events not listed above that have been reported since Clopixol was introduced on the market are provided below.
Blood and Lymphatic System Disorders: thrombocytopenia, leukopenia, neutropenia, agranulocytosis.
Cardiac Disorders: As with other drugs belonging to the therapeutic class of antipsychotics, rare cases of QT prolongation, ventricular arrhythmias, ventricular fibrillation, ventricular tachycardia, Torsade de Pointes and sudden unexplained death have been reported with zuclopenthixol.
Endocrine Disorders: hyperprolactinaemia.
General Disorders: hypothermia. Peripheral edema has occasionally been reported.
Hepato-biliary Disorders: cholestatic hepatitis, jaundice.

Alterations in liver function, particularly increased bilirubin levels have occasionally been reported. Transient increases in ALT and ALP values may also occur.
Immune System Disorders: anaphylactic reaction.
Metabolism and Nutrition Disorders: hyperglycaemia, impaired glucose tolerance, hyperlipidaemia.
Musculoskeletal and Connective Tissue Disorders: muscle rigidity, trismus, torticollis.
Nervous System Disorders: parkinsonism, Neuroleptic Malignant Syndrome (NMS).
Reproductive System Disorders: priapism.

DRUG INTERACTIONS: Overview: Zuclopenthixol enhances the sedative response to alcohol and the effects of barbiturates and other CNS depressants. It should not be administered with high doses of hypnotics due to the possibility of potentiation.

Zuclopenthixol should not be given concomitantly with guanethidine or similar acting compounds, since antipsychotic drugs such as zuclopenthixol may block the antihypertensive effect of these compounds.

Many antipsychotic and tricyclic antidepressant drugs may mutually inhibit the metabolism of each other.

Concomitant use of metoclopramide increases the risk of extrapyramidal symptoms.

Zuclopenthixol may antagonize the effects of levodopa and dopamine agonists.

The routine prophylactic use of antiparkinsonian drugs is not recommended. Antiparkinsonian drugs do not alleviate tardive dyskinesia and may aggravate it. Reduction in dosage or, if possible, discontinuation of zuclopenthixol therapy is recommended. If akathisia persists, a benzodiazepine or propranolol may be useful.

Since zuclopenthixol is partly metabolised by CYP2D6 concomitant use of drugs known to inhibit this enzyme may lead to decreased clearance of zuclopenthixol.

Drugs Known to Increase the QT Interval: Increases in the QT interval related to antipsychotic treatment may be exacerbated by the co-administration of other drugs known to significantly increase the QT interval. Co-administration of such drugs should be avoided. Relevant classes include:

- Class Ia and III antiarrhythmics (e.g. quinidine, amiodarone, sotalol)
- Some antipsychotics (e.g. thioridazine)
- Some macrolides (e.g. erythromycin)
- Some quinolone antibiotics (e.g. moxifloxacin)

The above list is not exhaustive and other individual drugs known to significantly increase QT interval (e.g. lithium) should be avoided.

Drugs known to cause electrolyte disturbances such as thiazide diuretics (hypokalemia) and drugs known to increase the plasma concentration of zuclopenthixol should also be used with caution as they may increase the risk of QT prolongation and malignant arrhythmias.

DOSAGE AND ADMINISTRATION:

Dosing Considerations: Clopixol Tablets (zuclopenthixol dihydrochloride): Dosage should be individualized according to the patient's condition. In general, small doses should be used initially and increased until an optimal response is obtained.

Clopixol-Acuphase (zuclopenthixol acetate): Clopixol-Acuphase is intended for use during acute psychotic episodes or exacerbation of psychosis associated with schizophrenia, when compliance with oral medication may be unreliable. Clopixol-Acuphase has an onset of action within 2-4 hours, and a duration of action of 2-3 days following a single intramuscular injection. Significant dose-dependent sedation occurs within 2 hours of injection, usually reaching a maximum after 8 hours. Tolerance to the sedative effect may develop with repeated injection. Maximum serum concentrations of zuclopenthixol are reached, on average, 24 to 48 hours after injection.

Clopixol-Acuphase is not intended for long-term use, and the duration of treatment should not exceed two weeks. The maximum cumulative dosage should not exceed 400 mg, and the number of injections should not exceed four.

Following treatment with Clopixol-Acuphase, antipsychotic therapy, when indicated, should be continued with either oral or long-acting injectable antipsychotic medications such as Clopixol tablets or Clopixol Depot (zuclopenthixol decanoate), respectively.

Clopixol-Acuphase is administered by deep intramuscular injection into the upper outer quadrant of the gluteal region. Injection volumes exceeding 2 ml should be distributed between 2 injection sites. Local tolerability is good.

Clopixol Depot (zuclopenthixol decanoate): Clopixol Depot is intended for maintenance treatment of chronic schizophrenia in patients who have been stabilized with oral or other short-acting medication, and who might benefit from transfer to long-acting injectable therapy.

Clopixol Depot is administered by deep intramuscular injection into the upper outer quadrant of the gluteal region. Injection volumes exceeding 2 mL should be distributed between 2 injection sites. Local tolerability is good.

Co-injection of Clopixol-Acuphase and Clopixol Depot: For patients with exacerbation of chronic psychoses, Clopixol-Acuphase and Clopixol Depot can be mixed in a syringe and given as one injection (co-injection). Since Clopixol-Acuphase and Clopixol Depot are dissolved in the same vehicle, mixing will not affect the pharmacokinetics of either formulation and will allow the administration of an acute and maintenance dose with one injection. **Clopixol-Acuphase cannot be mixed with other antipsychotic depot formulations.** Subsequent doses of Clopixol Depot and the interval between injections should be adjusted according to the patient's response.

Recommended Dose and Dosage Adjustment: Clopixol Tablets: When initiating treatment with Clopixol tablets, it is recommended that the drug be given in divided doses (BID or TID). During the maintenance phase of treatment Clopixol tablets may be given as a single nighttime dose.

For acute psychosis, the usual starting dose is 10-50 mg/day, which may be increased by 10-20 mg every 2-3 days, according to the patient's response. The usual therapeutic range is 20 mg to 60 mg daily. However, as with other antipsychotic drugs, some patients may require lower, while others may require higher dosage in order to obtain optimal benefit. Daily dosage higher than 100 mg is not recommended. For maintenance therapy, dosage should be reduced to the lowest level compatible with symptom control. The usual maintenance dose is 20-40 mg/day.

Clopixol-Acuphase: Dosage should be individually adjusted according to the patient's condition. The usual dose is 50-150 mg (1-3 mL) administered intramuscularly and repeated if necessary, at intervals of 2-3 days. Some patients may need an additional injection 1 or 2 days after the **first** injection.

Due to the delay in reaching peak zuclopenthixol blood levels and maximum pharmacologic effect, close supervision is required in order to minimize the risk of over-medication or insufficient suppression of psychotic symptoms.

The maximum cumulative dosage should not exceed 400 mg, and the number of injections should not exceed four.

Table 2 and Table 3 provide guidelines for dosage form conversion. Clopixol tablets should usually be started 2 to 3 days after the last injection of Clopixol-Acuphase. If Clopixol Depot is used for maintenance, it can be given concomitantly with the last injection of Clopixol-Acuphase (see Dosage and Administration, Recommended Dose and Dose Adjustment, Dose Adjustment with Co-injection of Clopixol-Acuphase and Clopixol Depot).

Clopixol Depot: Close supervision is required during the period following initiation of Clopixol Depot treatment, in order to minimize the risk of over-medication or insufficient suppression of psychotic symptoms. Supplemental oral antipsychotic medication may be required in diminishing dosage during this period.

The usual maintenance dose is 150-300 mg intramuscularly, every 2-4 weeks. Some patients may require higher or lower doses, or shorter intervals between doses.

During treatment with Clopixol Depot, the patient should be maintained at the lowest dose level compatible with adequate symptom control.

Table 4 provides guidelines for conversion from Clopixol tablets to Clopixol Depot.

Table 2: Clopixol

Suggested Dose to be Used When Transferring Patients from Clopixol-Acuphase to Clopixol Tablets

Clopixol-Acuphase Dose	Clopixol Tablet Dose[a]
50 mg	20 mg daily
100 mg	40 mg daily
150 mg	60 mg daily

[a] Initial total daily dose usually given in divided dosages (see Dosage and Administration, Recommended Dose and Dose Adjustment, Clopixol Tablets).

Table 3: Clopixol

Suggested Dose to be Used When Transferring Patients from Clopixol-Acuphase to Clopixol Depot

Clopixol-Acuphase Dose	Clopixol Depot Dose[a]
50 mg	100 mg Q2 weekly
100 mg	200 mg Q2 weekly
150 mg	300 mg Q2 weekly

[a] See Dosage and Administration, Recommended Dose and Dose Adjustment, Clopixol Depot.

Table 4: Clopixol

Suggested Dose to be Used When Transferring Patients from Clopixol Tablets to Clopixol Depot

Clopixol Tablet Dose	Clopixol Depot Dose[a]
Up to 20 mg daily	100 mg Q2 weekly
25 mg to 40 mg daily	200 mg Q2 weekly
50 mg to 75 mg daily	300 mg Q2 weekly
More than 75 mg daily	400 mg Q2 weekly

[a] See Dosage and Administration, Recommended Dose and Dose Adjustment, Clopixol Depot.

Dose Adjustment with Co-injection of Clopixol-Acuphase and Clopixol Depot: See Dosage and Administration, Dosing Considerations, Co-injection of Clopixol-Acuphase and Clopixol Depot.

Use in the Elderly: The use of zuclopenthixol in elderly patients with schizophrenia has not been systematically evaluated. Caution should thus be exercised in dose selection for an elderly patient, recognizing the more frequent hepatic, renal and cardiac dysfunctions in this population.

Impaired Liver Function: The use of zuclopenthixol in patients with impaired liver function has not been studied. As zuclopenthixol is extensively metabolized by the liver and primarily excreted in the bile (see Action and Clinical Pharmacology, Pharmacokinetics), caution should be exercised in dose selection for patients with this condition.

Impaired Renal Function: The use of zuclopenthixol in patients with impaired renal function has not been studied. Caution should be exercised in dose selection for patients with this condition.

Missed Dose: Clopixol Tablets: A missed dose should be taken at the next scheduled dose. Doses should not be doubled.

Discontinued Dose: Clopixol Tablets: Abrupt discontinuation of zuclopenthixol may be accompanied by withdrawal symptoms. The most common symptoms are nausea, vomiting, anorexia, diarrhoea, rhinorrhoea, sweating, myalgias, paraesthesias, insomnia, restlessness, anxiety, and agitation. Patients may also experience vertigo, alternate feelings of warmth and coldness, and tremor. Symptoms generally begin within 1 to 4 days of withdrawal and abate within 7 to 14 days.

OVERDOSAGE:

The symptoms are likely to be somnolence, coma, extrapyramidal symptoms, convulsions, hypotension, QT prolongation, Torsade de Pointes, cardiac arrest, ventricular arrhythmias, shock, or hyper- or hypothermia.

There is no specific antidote for zuclopenthixol. Treatment should be symptomatic and supportive. Gastric lavage (after intubation, if the patient is unconscious) and administration of activated charcoal should be considered. Measures aimed at supporting the respiratory and cardiovascular systems should be instituted. Hypotension and circulatory collapse may be counteracted by use of IV fluids. **Adrenaline (epinephrine) must not be used as a further lowering of blood pressure may result.** In cases of severe extrapyramidal reactions, antiparkinsonian medication should be administered. Close monitoring and medical supervision should continue until the patient recovers.

In managing overdose, the physician should consider the possibility of multiple drug involvement.

For management of a suspected drug overdose, CPhA recommends that you contact your **regional Poison Control Centre**. See the *CPS* Directory section for a list of Poison Control Centres.

ACTION AND CLINICAL PHARMACOLOGY: Pharmacodynamics: Zuclopenthixol, a thioxanthene derivative, has high affinity for both dopamine D_1 receptors and dopamine D_2 receptors. Zuclopenthixol also has high affinity for α_1-adrenergic and 5-HT_2 receptors. It has weaker histamine H_1 receptor blocking activity, and even lower affinity for muscarinic cholinergic and α_2-adrenergic receptors.

Pharmacokinetics: The pharmacokinetics of zuclopenthixol appear to be linear over the dosage range studied. A strong correlation exists between dose and steady state serum level, and between dose and area under the serum concentration time curve. The apparent volume of distribution is 20 L/kg. Protein binding is approximately 98%.

Clopixol-Acuphase (zuclopenthixol acetate) and Clopixol Depot (zuclopenthixol decanoate) are long-acting forms of zuclopenthixol that have been made more lipophilic by esterification with acetic and decanoic acid, respectively. Both esters of zuclopenthixol are dissolved in medium-chain triglycerides and when injected intramuscularly, diffuse slowly from the oil depot to the body water phase where they are rapidly hydrolyzed to the active substance, zuclopenthixol. Once hydrolyzed, zuclopenthixol is distributed, metabolized, and excreted as described.

Absorption: Clopixol Tablets (zuclopenthixol dihydrochloride): Maximum serum concentrations of zuclopenthixol are reached in approximately 4 hours (range 2-12 hours) following administration. The elimination half-life is approximately 20 hours (range 12-28 hours). The mean steady state serum level of zuclopenthixol corresponding to a daily 20 mg dose of zuclopenthixol dihydrochloride is about 13 ng/mL (33 nmol/L).

Clopixol-Acuphase: Maximum serum concentrations of zuclopenthixol are reached, on average, 24 to 48 hours after intramuscular injection, followed by a gradual decline. Average maximum serum concentration of zuclopenthixol corresponding to a 100 mg intramuscular dose of zuclopenthixol acetate is 41 ng/mL (102 nmol/L). Three days after injection, serum levels are approximately one-third the maximum.

Clopixol Depot: Maximum serum concentrations of zuclopenthixol are reached 3 to 7 days following intramuscular injection. The serum concentration time curve declines exponentially with a half-life of 19 days, reflecting the rate of release from the oil depot. Zuclopenthixol decanoate, when given at a dose of 200 mg every 2 weeks, results, on average, in a steady state zuclopenthixol serum concentration of approximately 10 ng/mL (25 nmol/L), when measured immediately prior to the next injection.

Metabolism: The metabolism of zuclopenthixol is mainly by sulfoxidation, side chain N-dealkylation and glucuronic acid conjugation. The metabolites are devoid of pharmacological activity.

Excretion: Zuclopenthixol is excreted mainly in feces with about 10% excreted in the urine. Approximately 0.1% of a dose is excreted unchanged in the urine. The systemic clearance is approximately 0.9 L/min.

Based on the above characteristics for elimination it is reasonable to assume that reduced kidney function is likely not to have much influence on the serum levels of parent drug.

STORAGE AND STABILITY: Clopixol tablets (zuclopenthixol dihydrochloride) should be stored between 15 and 25°C.

Clopixol-Acuphase (zuclopenthixol acetate) is provided in single-dose ampoules which should be stored between 15 and 25°C, and protected from light. Discard unused portion.

Clopixol Depot (zuclopenthixol decanoate) is provided in single-dose ampoules which should be stored between 15 and 25°C, and protected from light. Discard unused portion.

INFORMATION FOR THE PATIENT: Published in e-CPS, available by subscription at www.e-cps.ca.

DOSAGE FORMS, COMPOSITION AND PACKAGING: Clopixol: 10 mg: Each light red-brown, round, biconvex, film-coated tablet contains: zuclopenthixol 10 mg as zuclopenthixol dihydrochloride. Nonmedicinal ingredients: castor oil, copovidone, ferric oxide, glycerol, hypromellose, lactose, macrogol 6000, magnesium stearate, microcrystalline cellulose, potato starch, talc and titanium dioxide. Bottles of 100.

25 mg: Each red-brown, round, biconvex, film-coated tablet contains: zuclopenthixol 25 mg as zuclopenthixol dihydrochloride. Nonmedicinal ingredients: castor oil, copovidone, ferric oxide, glycerol, hypromellose, lactose, macrogol 6000, magnesium stearate, microcrystalline cellulose, potato starch, talc and titanium dioxide. Bottles of 100.

Clopixol-Acuphase: Each mL contains: zuclopenthixol acetate 50 mg (equivalent to zuclopenthixol 45.25 mg/mL) in medium-chain triglycerides. Colorless glass ampoules of 1 mL, packages of 5.

Clopixol Depot: Each mL contains: zuclopenthixol decanoate 200 mg (equivalent to zuclopenthixol 144.4 mg/mL) in medium-chain triglycerides. Colorless glass ampoules of 1 mL, packages of 10. Colorless vials of 10 mL.

(Shown in Product Identification Section)

Clorazepate

CPhA Monograph

see *Benzodiazepines*

Clotrimaderm

clotrimazole

Antifungal

Taro

SUPPLIED: Topical Cream 1%: Each g contains: clotrimazole 10 mg in a vanishing cream base consisting of cetostearyl alcohol, cetyl esters wax, 2-octyldodecanol, polysorbate 60, purified water, sorbitan monostearate and, as preservative, benzyl alcohol (1%). Tubes of 20, 30 and 50 g. Jars of 500 g.

Vaginal Cream: 1%: Each g contains: clotrimazole 10 mg in a vanishing cream base consisting of cetostearyl alcohol, cetyl esters wax, 2-octyldodecanol, polysorbate 60, purified water, sorbitan monostearate and, as preservative, benzyl alcohol (1%). Each carton contains: one 50 g tube of cream with 6 disposable plastic applicators and patient instructions. 50 g of vaginal cream is sufficient for 6 intravaginal applications with additional cream for extravaginal use if required.

2%: Each g contains: clotrimazole 20 mg in a vanishing cream base consisting of cetostearyl alcohol, cetyl esters wax, 2-octyldodecanol, polysorbate 60, purified water, sorbitan monostearate and, as preservative, benzyl alcohol (1%). Each carton contains: one 25 g tube of cream with 3 disposable plastic applicators and patient instructions. 25 g of vaginal cream is sufficient for 3 intravaginal applications with additional cream for extravaginal use if required.

Store at room temperature (15-30°C).

Cloxacillin

Antibacterial

CPhA Monograph

Date of Preparation: November 2005
Date of Revision: March 2009

This monograph has been compiled by CPhA and reviewed by experts. It may contain information different from that found in Health Canada-approved Product Monographs. The reader is referred to the *CPS* Editorial Policy for more information.

SUMMARY PRODUCT INFORMATION:

Route of Administration	Dosage Form	Product Strength
Oral	Capsule	250 mg, 500 mg
	Suspension	125 mg/5 mL
Parenteral	Dry powder vial for reconstitution	500 mg, 1 g, 2 g

INDICATIONS AND CLINICAL USE:

- Cloxacillin is indicated for treatment of bacterial infections caused by susceptible strains of penicillinase-producing staphylococci. It is considered a drug of choice for the treatment of endocarditis, osteomyelitis, pneumonia, sepsis and skin and soft-tissue infections caused by methicillin-sensitive *S. aureus* (MSSA). The oral route should not be used initially to administer cloxacillin in the treatment of severe, life-threatening infections as it is poorly absorbed.

CONTRAINDICATIONS:

- Patients who are hypersensitive to cloxacillin, to any ingredient in the formulation or component of the container, or to any penicillin.

WARNINGS AND PRECAUTIONS:

- The oral route should not be relied upon to treat severe infections or in the presence of conditions that may impair absorption (e.g., nausea/vomiting, intestinal hypomotility).
- The use of antibacterial agents can result in overgrowth of nonsusceptible organisms, such as *C. difficile* or *C. albicans*. The possibility of *C. difficile* infection should be considered in patients presenting with diarrhea during or following therapy with cloxacillin.
- Serious and occasionally fatal hypersensitivity reactions have been reported in patients receiving penicillins. Although anaphylaxis is more frequent following parenteral therapy, it has occurred in patients taking oral penicillins. These reactions are more likely to occur in individuals with a history of sensitivity to multiple allergens.

Special Populations: Pregnant Women: Although cloxacillin has not been proven to be safe in pregnancy, it is generally considered to pose no significant teratogenic risk.

Nursing Women: Based on the knowledge that some penicillins are excreted in breast milk, it should be expected that cloxacillin is as well. Although possible effects on a nursing infant include alteration of the gut flora (potentially resulting in oral thrush or diarrhea), obscured diagnosis of fever and hypersensitivity reactions, cloxacillin is generally considered to be compatible with breast-feeding.

Pediatrics (birth to 16 years old): Plasma levels and the elimination half-life of cloxacillin are higher in neonates. Recommended dosing intervals are longer for this age group (see Table 5).

ADVERSE REACTIONS: More Common Adverse Drug Reactions (≥1%): See Table 1.

Table 1: Cloxacillin

More Common Adverse Drug Reactions (≥1%)

Body System	Effect
Gastrointestinal	Nausea, vomiting, epigastric discomfort, flatulence, loose stools.
Local	Phlebitis with iv administration.

Less Common Adverse Drug Reactions (<1%): Gastrointestinal: *C. difficile*-associated diarrhea and pseudomembranous colitis have been reported rarely. Other uncommon GI effects include black or hairy tongue and oral lesions such as stomatitis or glossitis.

Hematologic: Rarely: transient neutropenia, leukopenia, granulocytopenia, thrombocytopenia; more commonly associated with high-dose parenteral administration but can occur with oral therapy.

Hepatic: elevated liver enzymes; cholestatic jaundice.

Hypersensitivity: rash, fever, chills, pruritus, serum-sickness, anaphylaxis.

Renal: interstitial nephritis (rare).

DRUG INTERACTIONS: Drug-Drug Interactions: See Table 2.

Table 2: Cloxacillin

Drug-Drug Interactions

Interacting Drug	Effect	Clinical Comment
Aminoglycosides	Concurrent administration with penicillins has resulted in inactivation of aminoglycosides.	Do not mix parenteral aminoglycosides and penicillins in the same iv solution.
Methotrexate	Competition for excretion sites in the renal tubules may cause elevated methotrexate concentrations, increasing the risk of toxicity.	Monitor for methotrexate toxicity. Measure methotrexate concentrations twice a week for at least the first 2 weeks in patients receiving low-dose oral methotrexate. May need a dosage adjustment for methotrexate during therapy with cloxacillin. Avoid cloxacillin immediately before and during iv methotrexate treatment.
Oral contraceptives	Theoretically antibacterial agents may suppress intestinal flora that provide hydrolytic enzymes essential for enterohepatic recirculation of estrogens, resulting in decreased contraceptive effectiveness.	Possible contraceptive failure. An additional form of birth control may be considered to avoid a theoretical slight increased risk of pregnancy.
Tetracyclines (e.g., doxycycline, minocycline, tetracycline)	Pharmacologic and therapeutic action of penicillins could be reduced.	Avoid concomitant use.
Warfarin	Effects of warfarin may be increased, resulting in an increased risk of bleeding.	INR should be closely monitored upon addition and withdrawal of cloxacillin. INR should also be reassessed periodically during therapy since an adjustment in the warfarin dose may be necessary to maintain an effective level of anticoagulation.

Drug-Food Interactions: Food decreases the extent of absorption of cloxacillin and therefore may reduce its antimicrobial effectiveness. Administer cloxacillin on an empty stomach (1 hour before or 2 hours after meals) to enhance its absorption.

Drug-Laboratory Interactions: Cloxacillin may interfere with or cause false-positive results in test methods used to determine urinary or serum proteins.

Cloxacillin may cause decreased results in serum aminoglycoside assays due to chemical inactivation. Samples should be frozen until assay can be performed.

DOSAGE AND ADMINISTRATION: Recommended Dose and Dosage Adjustment: Adults: See Table 3.

Geriatrics: See adult dosing.

Pediatrics: See Table 4 and Table 5.

OVERDOSAGE:

For management of a suspected drug overdose, CPhA recommends that you contact your **regional Poison Control Centre.** See the *CPS* Directory section for a list of Poison Control Centres.

ACTION AND CLINICAL PHARMACOLOGY: Mechanism of action: Cloxacillin is a semi-synthetic isoxazolyl penicillin developed for use against penicillinase-producing staphylococci. It is also active against many streptococci but is less active than natural penicillins in penicillin-sensitive strains. Like other β-lactams it exerts its bactericidal effect by inhibition of cell wall peptidoglycan synthesis.

Table 3: Cloxacillin

Dose in Adult Patients

Indication	Route	Usual Dose	Duration of Treatment	Detailed Information
Bacterial infections caused by susceptible strains of penicillinase-producing staphylococci.	Oral	250–500 mg Q6H	Varies according to severity of infection and patient response. Treatment of severe staphylococcal infections should be continued for at least 14 days. Duration of treatment of osteomyelitis is usually for a total of 6 weeks, including initial parenteral therapy.	Take 1 hour before or 2 hours after meals
As above	IV/IM	1–2 g iv Q6H; severe infections (e.g., endocarditis, meningitis): up to 2 g iv Q4H	As above	Phlebitis or thrombophlebitis can occur with iv administration.

Table 4: Cloxacillin

Dose in Infants and Children (>1 month, <20 kg; over 20 kg refer to adult dosing)

Indication	Route	Usual Dose	Duration of Treatment	Detailed Information
Bacterial infections caused by susceptible strains of penicillinase-producing staphylococci	Oral	50–100 mg/kg daily divided Q6H, to a maximum of 4 g/day	See Table 3	Administer 1 hour before or 2 hours after meals. Shake suspension well before use.
As above	IV/IM	50–100 mg/kg daily divided Q6H, to a maximum of 4 g/day. Severe infections: 150–200 mg/kg daily divided Q6H to a maximum of 12 g/day	See Table 3	Phlebitis or thrombophlebitis can occur with iv administration.

Table 5: Cloxacillin

Dose in Neonates (≤1 month)

Indication	Body Weight	Age	Usual Dose/Route	Duration of Treatment
Meningitis	<2 kg	≤7 days	100 mg/kg daily iv divided Q12H	See Table 3
		>7 days	150 mg/kg daily iv divided Q8H	
	≥2 kg	≤7 days	150 mg/kg daily iv divided Q8H	
		>7 days	200 mg/kg daily iv divided Q6H	
Other infections	<2 kg	≤7 days	50 mg/kg daily po/iv divided Q12H	See Table 3
		>7 days	75 mg/kg daily po/iv divided Q8H	
	≥2 kg	≤7 days	75 mg/kg daily po/iv divided Q8H	
		>7 days	100 mg/kg daily po/iv divided Q6H	

Pharmacokinetics: Cloxacillin is rapidly but incompletely absorbed from the gastrointestinal tract. Food decreases both the rate and extent of absorption and it is therefore best taken 1 hour before or 2 hours after food. Peak plasma levels are attained approximately 1 hour after oral dosing. Cloxacillin is highly protein bound (>90%). It is widely distributed in body fluids except in the CSF where minimal concentrations are reached unless the meninges are inflamed. Elimination is via renal and hepatic mechanisms. The elimination half-life is reported to be 0.4 to 0.8 hours and increases to 0.8 to 2.3 hours in severe renal impairment; dosage adjustment is not necessary. Cloxacillin is not appreciably removed by hemodialysis.

STORAGE AND STABILITY: Reconstituted oral solution should be stored in the refrigerator.

Clozaril® Pr

clozapine

Antipsychotic

Novartis Pharmaceuticals

Date of Preparation: March 20, 1991
Date of Revision: July 16, 2010

PHARMACOLOGY: CLOZARIL (clozapine), a dibenzodiazepine derivative, is an atypical antipsychotic drug because its profile of binding to dopamine receptors and its effects on various dopamine-mediated behaviors differ from those exhibited by conventional antipsychotics. In contrast to conventional antipsychotics, clozapine produces little or no prolactin elevation. Clozapine exerts potent anticholinergic, adrenolytic, antihistaminic and antiserotoninergic activity.

Controlled clinical trials indicate that clozapine improves both positive and negative symptoms.

Patients on rare occasions may report an intensification of dream activity during clozapine therapy. Rapid eye movement (REM) sleep was found to be increased to 85% of the total sleep time. In these patients, the onset of REM sleep occurred almost immediately after falling asleep.

As is true of more typical antipsychotic drugs, clinical EEG studies have shown that clozapine increases delta and theta activity and slows dominant alpha frequencies. Enhanced synchronization occurs, and sharp wave activity and spike and wave complexes may also develop.

Pharmacokinetics: The absorption of orally administered clozapine is 90 to 95%. Food does not affect either the rate or the extent of absorption. Clozapine is subject to first-pass metabolism, resulting in an absolute bioavailability of 50 to 60%.

Plasma concentrations show large inter-individual differences, with peak concentrations occurring approximately 2.5 hours (range: 1 to 6 hours) after dosing. In a dose range of 37.5 mg b.i.d. to 150 mg b.i.d., the area under the curve (AUC) and the peak plasma concentration (C_{max}) increase linearly in a dose-related fashion.

Clozapine is approximately 95% bound to plasma proteins. The elimination of clozapine is biphasic with a mean terminal half-life of 12 hours (range: 6 to 30 hours, calculated from 3 steady-state in vivo studies). After single doses of 75 mg, the mean terminal half-life was 7.9 hours; it increased to 14.2 hours when steady-state conditions were reached by administering daily doses of 75 mg for at least 7 days. Clozapine is almost completely metabolized prior to excretion. Only trace amounts of unchanged drug are detected in the urine and feces. Approximately 50% of the administered dose is excreted as metabolites in the urine and 30% in the feces.

Recent studies suggest that there is a significant correlation between clozapine plasma levels and clinical response. The concentrations of clozapine, and its major metabolite norclozapine, were significantly higher in responders than in nonresponders although the mean doses of clozapine did not differ between the 2 groups. Of the main metabolites, only norclozapine was found to be active. In patients who responded to treatment, plasma clozapine levels reached at least 350 to 370 ng/mL.

Clinical Trial Data on Suicidal Behaviour (InterSePT Study): The International Suicide Prevention Study (InterSePT) Study ABA 451 was a prospective, open-label randomized, international, parallel-group comparison of CLOZARIL vs. Zyprexa (olanzapine) of two years duration, with approximately 490 patients per treatment group.

Trial Design: Patients were diagnosed with schizophrenia or schizoaffective disorder using DSM-IV criteria, and meeting at least one of the following criteria in order to be deemed at high risk for suicide: a) a suicide attempt, or hospitalization to prevent an attempt, within the last three years; or b) moderate to severe suicidal ideation with either a depressive component or command hallucinations, within the last week. One fourth (27%) of the patient population was considered "treatment-resistant".

Due to the high-risk nature of the study population, the principle investigators (PIs) were permitted to treat patients as they judged necessary, including concomitant medications, non-drug treatments, and hospitalizations. Both the PIs and the patients were aware of the treatment group assignment.

Efficacy Measures: The primary efficacy measure was time to the first occurrence of either a Type I or Type II event.

The unblinded PIs were responsible for identifying Type I events: a suicide attempt, or the judgement of need for hospitalization/increased surveillance to prevent an attempt. In the case of the Type I events, all relevant information from the PIs was blinded and forwarded to a blinded group of experts (the Suicide Monitoring Board) for final confirmation of each potential Type I event. Blinded psychiatrists, who assessed the patients at pre-determined intervals, were responsible for identifying Type II events: "much worsening" or "very much worsening" from baseline in the Clinical Global Impression of Severity of Suicidality-Blinded Psychiatrist (CGI-SS-BP) scale.

Results: Analysis using the Cox's proportional hazard regression model demonstrates that within the context of the InterSePT trial there was a 26% reduced risk for a suicide attempt or hospitalization to prevent suicide (Type 1 event) for CLOZARIL-treated patients compared to Zyprexa treated-patients (p=0.02, hazard ratio 0.74 [95% C.I.:0.57,0.96].

Factors that preclude regulatory endorsement of an indication for CLOZARIL for the risk of recurrent suicidal behaviour in patients with schizophrenia or schizoaffective disorder:

1. The heavy reliance of the endpoints on clinical judgement, when combined with the fact that the principle investigators were not blinded to the treatment group, creates the potential for bias in the results.
2. Separate indications for the domain of recurrent suicidal behaviour versus that of psychosis require a conclusion that the two domains are independent; currently, there is insufficient evidence to allow such a conclusion.
3. The usual concerns with generalizability of study results to individual patients in clinical practice are magnified in this therapeutic area. Given that schizophrenia is associated with long-term increased risk of suicide, the two year duration of the study limits generalizability. Many patients in this study had multiple suicide risk factors; the variable and dynamic nature of risk and protective factors, and the unpredictability of interaction with unique life circumstances also limit generalizability, as do the unusual efforts made in the study to prevent a suicide attempt, including frequent patient-clinician contact.
4. Because decisions about concomitant treatment were made by unblinded PIs, the post-hoc finding that the CLOZARIL group received significantly less psychotropic medication than did the ZYPREXA group is not readily interpretable.
5. This is the sole prospective randomized trial.

Conclusion: Under the currently approved Canadian indication, CLOZARIL is already available to a substantial percentage of psychotic patients at risk of suicide, given the frequency of tolerability issues and the fact that a complete response to an antipsychotic is rare. The InterSePT study is a source of further information with regards to these patients.

While the InterSePT results are hypothesis-generating, they fail to provide sufficient evidence to support the safety and efficacy of the use of CLOZARIL in patients who are naive to anti-psychotics, or have schizoaffective disorder.

INDICATIONS: CLOZARIL (clozapine) is indicated in the management of symptoms of treatment-resistant schizophrenia. In controlled clinical trials, clozapine was found to improve both positive and negative symptoms.

Due to the significant risk of agranulocytosis and seizure associated with its use, clozapine should be limited to treatment-resistant schizophrenic patients who are non-responsive to, or intolerant of, conventional antipsychotic drugs. Non-responsiveness is defined as the lack of satisfactory clinical response, despite treatment with appropriate courses of at least 2 marketed chemically-unrelated antipsychotic drugs. Intolerance is defined as the inability to achieve adequate benefit with conventional antipsychotic drugs because of dose-limiting, intolerable adverse effects.

Because of the significant risk of agranulocytosis and seizure, events which both present a continuing risk over time, the extended treatment of patients failing to show an acceptable level of clinical response to clozapine should ordinarily be avoided. In addition, the need for continuing treatment in patients exhibiting beneficial clinical responses should be periodically re-evaluated.

Clozapine can be used only if regular hematological examinations can be guaranteed, as specified under Warnings and Dosage.

CLOZARIL is available only through a distribution system CSAN that ensures: weekly or every-2-week hematological testing prior to the dispensing of the next period's supply of CLOZARIL (see Warnings).

This requires:

- registration of the patient, their current location, treating physician, testing laboratory and dispensing pharmacist in the CSAN system.
- maintenance of a national Novartis Pharmaceuticals Canada Inc. -specific database that enables the monitoring of the hematological results of all patients on CLOZARIL and provides timely feedback (within 24 hours of receipt of the blood test results) to the treating physician and dispensing pharmacist/or pharmacy.
- the ability to identify patients who have been assigned "Non-rechallengeable Status" (see Warnings). This requires that Novartis both provide to, and obtain from, all other approved suppliers* of clozapine, the Non-rechallengeable Status/Hematological Status of all patients (see Dosage). Novartis must be able to provide this information within 24 hours of receiving a written request.

Physicians should not prescribe CLOZARIL until the non-rechallengeable status and the hematological status of the patient has been verified.

For the distribution system to be effective, treating physicians must ensure that the hematological testing is performed at the required frequency (see Warnings) and that arrangements are made for the hematological results are sent to CSAN.

Physicians may obtain details on the CSAN distribution system by calling a toll-free phone number (1-800-267-2726).

Other Monitoring and Distribution Systems: Between 1991 and 2003, clozapine was distributed by a single manufacturer, and patients were monitored by this manufacturer's specific registry and distribution system. The introduction of clozapine from other manufactures has now resulted in the establishment of manufacturer-specific registry and distribution systems.

In order to ensure the safe use and continued monitoring of all patients taking clozapine, the physician must have obtained consent from the patient for the potential sharing of hematological and other safety data between clozapine registries.

Patients may not be switched from one brand of clozapine to another without the completion of a new registry-specific patient registration form signed by the prescribing physician.

If a patient is switched from one brand of clozapine to another, the frequency of hematological monitoring may continue unaltered unless a change is clinically indicated.

CONTRAINDICATIONS: CLOZARIL (clozapine) is contraindicated in patients with myeloproliferative disorders, a history of toxic or idiosyncratic agranulocytosis or severe granulocytopenia (with the exception of granulocytopenia/agranulocytosis from previous chemotherapy). [Clozapine should not be used simultaneously with other agents known to suppress bone marrow function.]

CLOZARIL is also contraindicated in patients with active liver disease associated with nausea, anorexia, or jaundice; progressive liver disease; hepatic failure.

Other contraindications include severe CNS depression or comatose states, severe renal or cardiac disease (e.g., myocarditis), paralytic ileus, uncontrolled epilepsy, and previous hypersensitivity to clozapine or any other components of CLOZARIL.

CLOZARIL is also contraindicated in patients unable to undergo blood tests.

WARNINGS: Elderly Patients with Dementia: Elderly patients with dementia treated with atypical antipsychotic drugs are at an increased risk of death compared to placebo. Analyses of thirteen placebo-controlled trials with various atypical antipsychotics (modal duration of 10 weeks) in these patients showed a mean 1.6 fold increase in the death rate in the drug treated patients. Although the causes of death were varied, most of the deaths appeared to be either cardiovascular (e.g., heart failure, sudden death) or infectious (e.g., pneumonia) in nature. CLOZARIL has not been studied in elderly patients with dementia and therefore no such data were included in this analysis.

CLOZARIL (clozapine) is not recommended in elderly patients with dementia (see Precautions, Geriatrics, Use in Geriatric Patients with Dementia).

Agranulocytosis: Because of the significant risk of granulocytopenia and agranulocytosis, a potentially life-threatening adverse event (see below), CLOZARIL (clozapine) should be reserved for use in the treatment of schizophrenic patients who fail to show an acceptable response to adequate courses of conventional antipsychotic drug treatment, either because of insufficient effectiveness or the inability to achieve an effective dose due to intolerable adverse effects.

Patients must have a normal white blood cell (WBC) count and differential count prior to starting clozapine therapy. Subsequently, a WBC count and differential count must be carried out at least weekly for the first 26 weeks of treatment with clozapine and at least at 2-week intervals thereafter†. Monitoring must continue for as long as the patient is on the drug. Furthermore, monitoring should occur at least weekly for a period of 4 weeks following discontinuation of clozapine therapy, irrespective of the cause of discontinuation.

* "approved supplier" is a manufacturer who holds a valid Notice of Compliance (NOC) for clozapine.

† The change from a weekly to a "once every 2 weeks" schedule should be evaluated on an individual patient basis after 26 weeks of treatment. This decision should be made based upon the clinical judgment of the treating physician, and if he/she deems it appropriate, a consulting hematologist, as well as the patient's willingness to pursue a given frequency of blood monitoring. In turn, the clinical evaluation should take into consideration possible factors that would place the patient in a higher risk group, as well as the hematological profile of the patient during the first 26 weeks of treatment.

CLOZARIL is available only through a distribution system (CSAN) that requires weekly or every-2-week hematological testing prior to the dispensing of the next period's supply of CLOZARIL (see Indications).

> Granulocytopenia (defined as a granulocyte count of less than 1.5×10^9/L) and agranulocytosis (defined as a granulocyte count of less than 0.5×10^9/L, including polys+bands) have been shown to occur in association with CLOZARIL use at an incidence of 3% and 0.7%, respectively. These incidences are derived from post-marketing data as per June 1993, covering over 60 000 patients treated with CLOZARIL for up to 3 years in the USA, Canada and U.K. Approximately 88% of the cases of agranulocytosis have occurred during the first 26 weeks of therapy.
>
> A fatality rate of 32% for clozapine-induced agranulocytosis had been reported in association with CLOZARIL use as of December 31, 1989. However, more than half of these deaths occurred before 1977, prior to the recognition of the risk of agranulocytosis and the need for routine blood monitoring. From February 1990 to August 21, 1997, among approximately 150 409 patients treated with CLOZARIL in the USA, 585 new cases of agranulocytosis have been reported, of which 19 (3.2%) had a fatal outcome.
>
> Fatalities occurring in association with clozapine-induced granulocytopenia/agranulocytosis have generally resulted from infections due to compromised immune system responses.
>
> Therefore, patients should be advised to report immediately the appearance of lethargy, weakness, fever, sore throat, flu-like complaints or any other signs of infection.
>
> All patients must be screened to ensure that they do not have a history of neutropenia/agranulocytosis associated with clozapine use (i.e., are not in the Non-rechallengeable databases of any of the current approved suppliers of clozapine).
>
> CLOZARIL treatment should be initiated and carried out according to the following guidelines:
>
> - Treatment should not be initiated if the WBC count is less than 3.5×10^9/L and/or the absolute neutrophil count (ANC) is less than 2.0×10^9/L, or if the patient has a history of a myeloproliferative disorder, or toxic or idiosyncratic agranulocytosis or severe granulocytopenia (with the exception of granulocytopenia/agranulocytosis from previous chemotherapy).
> - Independently of the frequency of their blood monitoring regimen (weekly or at 2-week intervals), patients should be evaluated immediately and WBC and differential counts checked at least **twice weekly** if after the initiation of treatment:
>   i) the total WBC count falls to between 2.0×10^9/L and 3.5×10^9/L,
>   ii) the ANC falls to between 1.5×10^9/L and 2.0×10^9/L,
>   iii) a single fall or sum of falls in WBC count of 3.0×10^9/L or more is measured in the last 4 weeks, reaching a value below 4.0×10^9/L,
>   iv) a single fall or sum of falls in ANC of 1.5×10^9/L or more is measured in the last 4 weeks, reaching a value below 2.5×10^9/L,
>   and/or
>   v) flu-like complaints or other symptoms appear which might suggest infection.
>
> In the event of a fall in total WBC to below 2.0×10^9/L or in ANC to below 1.5×10^9/L, CLOZARIL therapy must be immediately withheld and the patient closely monitored. **The patient is to be assigned "Non-rechallengeable" status upon confirmation of fall in WBC and neutrophil counts. CLOZARIL therapy must not be resumed.** Particular attention should be paid to any flu-like complaints or other symptoms which might suggest infection. If the patient should develop a further fall in the WBC count to below 1.0×10^9/L, or a decrease in ANC to below 0.5×10^9/L, it is recommended that patients be placed in protective isolation with close observation and be watched for signs of infection by their physician. Should evidence of infection develop, the appropriate cultures should be performed and an appropriate antibiotic regimen instituted.

The development of granulocytopenia and agranulocytosis does not appear to be dose dependent, nor is duration of treatment a reliable predictor. Approximately 88% of the cases have occurred in the first 26 weeks of treatment, but some cases have developed after years of clozapine use. The incidence of neutropenia and agranulocytosis associated with the use of clozapine increases as a function of age. Experience in the U.S. (approximately 58 000 patients, as per June 1993) reveals that patients over 50 years old would present an approximately 2 to 3 times higher incidence of agranulocytosis when compared with the overall incidence in patients treated with clozapine.

Patients who have shown hematopoietic reactions to other medications may also be more likely to demonstrate such reactions with clozapine. A disproportionate number of the U.S. cases of agranulocytosis occurred in patients of Jewish origin compared to the overall proportion of such patients exposed to the drug in pre-marketing clinical experience in the U.S.

Agranulocytosis associated with other antipsychotic drugs has been reported to occur with a greater frequency in patients who are cachectic or have a serious underlying medical illness.

Cardiotoxicity: Important safety information regarding a constellation of cardiovascular events reported in patients treated with clozapine.

> **Cardiovascular Toxicity:**
>
> **Analysis of safety databases suggests that the use of clozapine is associated with an increased risk of myocarditis especially during, but not limited to, the first month of therapy. Myocarditis has been reported in patients 19 years of age and older, at dosages within the approved dosage range and during titration of clozapine. In Canada, there have been 9 reported cases of myocarditis. Of these, three have been fatal. Given the estimated 15 600 Canadian clozapine-treated patients as of August 2001, this represents an estimated incidence of 0.06% for all reports of myocarditis (or 1/1667 patients) and 0.02% for myocarditis fatalities (or 1/5200).**
>
> **Pericarditis, pericardial effusion and cardiomyopathy have also been reported in association with clozapine use, as have heart failure, myocardial infarction and mitral insufficiency; these reports include fatalities.**
>
> **In patients who develop persistent tachycardia at rest accompanied by other signs and symptoms of heart failure (e.g. chest pain, tachypnoea (shortness of breath), or arrhythmias), the possibility of myocarditis, cardiomyopathy and/or other cardiovascular dysfunction must be considered. Other symptoms which may be present in addition to the above include fatigue, flu-like symptoms, fever that is otherwise unexplained, hypotension and/or raised jugular venous pressure.**
>
> **The occurrence of such signs and symptoms necessitates an urgent diagnostic evaluation for myocarditis, cardiomyopathy and/or other cardiovascular dysfunction by a cardiologist. Patients with a family history of heart failure should have a cardiac evaluation prior to commencing treatment; clozapine is contraindicated in patients with severe cardiac disease.**
>
> **In patients in whom myocarditis is suspected, clozapine treatment should be promptly discontinued. Patients with clozapine-induced myocarditis should not be re-exposed to clozapine.**
>
> **If cardiomyopathy and/or other cardiovascular dysfunction is diagnosed, discontinuation of clozapine, based on clinical grounds, should be considered.**

Background Information For Cardiotoxicity Boxed Warning (as of early 2002): A) Myocarditis, pericarditis and pericardial effusion: Canadian Reports: In Canada, a total of 16 post-marketing surveillance spontaneous reports of myocarditis/pericarditis/pericardial effusion have been received by Health Canada since marketing in 1991 (see also boxed warning regarding myocarditis cases). Information additional to the Boxed Warning: the age range was 19-37 years; the shortest known clozapine treatment duration was 2 weeks.

International Reports: Reporting incidences for myocarditis can be reliably calculated from the four countries with CLOZARIL national registries (USA, United Kingdom, Canada, Australia). The lowest rate is reported in the U.S. (1/20 000 person years) and the highest in Australia (1/800 person years). Of these 81 cases, 37% were fatal, with 80% of fatal cases showing evidence of myocarditis at autopsy. When all international reports of myocarditis are included (n=213 cases), the myocarditis rate is 1/14 000 patient years; 23% of cases had a fatal outcome and 85% occurred within the first two months of initiation of clozapine therapy. Recurrences of myocarditis upon rechallenge with clozapine have been documented.

Another analysis of clozapine and myocarditis revealed that 70% of patients were under 50 years of age; thus, clozapine-associated myocarditis can occur in younger patients. Dosages were mostly in accordance with current labelled dosage recommendations, with a third of patients taking less than therapeutic doses; this likely reflects the occurrence of myocarditis during dose titration.

There are also reports of pericarditis/pericardial effusion, some of which have been fatal. Eosinophilia has been co-reported in some cases, which may indicate that the carditis is a hypersensitivity reaction to clozapine; however, it is not known whether eosinophilia is a reliable predictor of carditis.

B) Cardiomyopathy/heart failure/mitral insufficiency: Canadian Reports: In Canada, 7 cases of cardiomyopathy and 3 cases of heart failure/mitral insufficiency have been reported to Health Canada, with individual cases reported to have concomitant myo/endo-carditis. The age range is 19-55 years; Two of the reports of heart failure are known to have been fatal (61y male, 46y male).

International Reports: A total of 178 cardiomyopathy reports (18% fatal), have been received by Novartis. Analysis of the reports revealed that four times as many men as women were diagnosed with cardiomyopathy. About 80% of the cases occurred in patients under the age of 50; the incidence rate of spontaneous reports of cardiomyopathy for this age range was greater in clozapine-treated patients than in the general population in established international market economies.

Diagnosis was confirmed (by echocardiography or autopsy) in 44% of the cases. Typically, the clozapine dose was within therapeutic range, with the duration of treatment more than 6 months in 65% of the patients. There was no other apparent cause of the cardiomyopathy in about 50% of all reported cases of cardiomyopathy and in 28% of fatalities including history, concomitant medications, comorbidities), with an average age of approximately 37 years. Terms most commonly co-reported with cardiomyopathy were: congestive heart failure (21%), heart rate and rhythm disorders (10%), cardiomegaly (8%). In the 4 cases where follow-up was reported after withdrawal of clozapine, there was improvement of the cardiomyopathy.

C) Myocardial infarction: In Canada, 30 reports of myocardial infarction in patients receiving clozapine have been received by Health Canada with 50% of cases known to be fatal.

Other Adverse Cardiovascular and Respiratory Effects: CLOZARIL should be used with caution in patients with known cardiovascular and/or pulmonary disease, particularly in those with cardiac arrhythmias and conduction disturbances, and the recommendation for gradual titration of dose should be carefully observed.

Orthostatic hypotension, with or without syncope, can occur during CLOZARIL treatment and may represent a continuing risk in some patients. Rarely (approximately 1 case per 3 000 patients in the United States), collapse can be profound and can be accompanied by respiratory and/or cardiac arrest. Orthostatic hypotension is more likely to occur during initial titration in association with rapid dose escalation and may even occur on first dose. In one report, initial doses as low as 12.5 mg were associated with collapse and respiratory arrest. When restarting patients who have had even a brief interval of CLOZARIL (clozapine), i.e. 2 days or more since the last dose, it is recommended that treatment be reinitiated with one-half of a 25 mg tablet (12.5 mg) once or twice daily (see Dosage).

Cases of collapse/respiratory arrest/cardiac arrest during initial clozapine treatment occurred in patients administered clozapine by itself and in patients administered clozapine in combination with benzodiazepines or other psychotropic drugs. Although it has not been established that there is an interaction between CLOZARIL (clozapine) and benzodiazepines or other psychotropics, caution is advised when clozapine is initiated in patients taking a benzodiazepine or any other psychotropic drug.

Tachycardia, which may be sustained, has been observed in approximately 25% of patients taking CLOZARIL with patients having an average increase in pulse rate of 10 to 15 bpm. The sustained tachycardia is not simply a reflex response to hypotension and is present in all positions monitored. Tachycardia may be due to the anticholinergic effect of CLOZARIL and its ability to elevate plasma norepinephrine. Either tachycardia or hypotension may pose a serious risk for an individual with compromised cardiovascular function.

A minority of CLOZARIL-treated patients experience ECG repolarization changes similar to those seen with other antipsychotic drugs, including S-T segment depression and flattening or inversion of T waves. The clinical significance of these changes is unclear. However, in clinical trials with clozapine, several patients experienced significant cardiac events, including ischemic changes, myocardial infarction, arrhythmias, and sudden death. In addition, there have been post-marketing reports of congestive heart failure. Causality assessment was difficult in many of these cases due to serious preexisting cardiac disease and plausible alternative causes. Rare instances of sudden, unexplained death have been reported in psychiatric patients, with or without associated antipsychotic drug treatment, and the relationship of these events to antipsychotic drug use is unknown.

As with other antipsychotics, caution is advised in patients with known cardiovascular disease, a family history of QT prolongation, or when CLOZARIL is prescribed with medicines known to increase the QTc interval.

Seizures: Caution should be used in administering CLOZARIL to patients having a history of seizures or other predisposing factors.

Seizures have been estimated to occur in association with CLOZARIL use at a cumulative incidence at 1 year of approximately 5%, based on the occurrence of 1 or more seizures in the patients exposed to CLOZARIL during clinical trials in the U.S. Dose appears to be an important predictor of seizure. At doses below 300 mg/day, seizure risk is comparable to that of other antipsychotic drugs (about 1 to 2%). At higher doses, seizure risk rises accordingly, reaching 5% at doses of 600 to 900 mg/day. Because of the risk of seizure associated with CLOZARIL use, patients should be advised not to engage in any activity where sudden loss of consciousness could cause serious risk to themselves or others (e.g., driving, operating machinery, swimming, climbing, etc.).

Neuroleptic Malignant Syndrome: A potentially fatal symptom complex sometimes referred to as neuroleptic malignant syndrome (NMS) has been reported in association with antipsychotic drugs. Cases of NMS have been reported in patients treated with clozapine, most of which have included the concomitant use of lithium or other CNS-active agents.

Clinical manifestations of NMS are hyperpyrexia, muscle rigidity, altered mental status (including catatonic signs) and evidence of autonomic instability (irregular pulse or blood pressure, tachycardia, diaphoresis and cardiac dysrhythmias). Additional signs may include elevated creatine phosphokinase, myoglobinuria (rhabdomyolysis), and acute renal failure.

The diagnostic evaluation of patients with this syndrome is complicated. In arriving at a diagnosis, it is important to identify cases where the clinical presentation includes both serious medical illness (e.g., pneumonia, systemic infection, etc.) and untreated or inadequately treated extrapyramidal signs and symptoms (EPS). Other important considerations in the differential diagnosis include central anticholinergic toxicity, heat stroke, drug fever and primary CNS pathology.

The management of NMS should include: 1) immediate discontinuation of antipsychotic drugs and other drugs not essential to concurrent therapy; 2) intensive symptomatic treatment and medical monitoring; and 3) treatment of any concomitant serious medical problems for which specific treatments are available. There is no general agreement about specific pharmacological treatment regimens for uncomplicated NMS.

If a patient requires antipsychotic drug treatment after recovery from NMS, the potential reintroduction of drug therapy should be carefully considered. The patient should be carefully monitored, since recurrences of NMS have been reported.

Tardive Dyskinesia: A syndrome consisting of potentially irreversible, involuntary, dyskinetic movements may develop in patients treated with conventional antipsychotic drugs. Although the prevalence of tardive dyskinesia with conventional antipsychotics appears to be highest among the elderly, especially elderly women, it is impossible to rely upon prevalence estimates to predict, at the beginning of treatment, which patients are likely to develop the syndrome.

Both the risk of developing tardive dyskinesia and the likelihood that it will become irreversible are believed to increase as the duration of treatment and the total cumulative dose of antipsychotic drugs administered to the patient increase. However, the syndrome can develop, although much less commonly, after relatively brief treatment periods at low doses. There is no known treatment for established cases of tardive dyskinesia, although the syndrome may remit, partially or completely, if antipsychotic drug treatment is withdrawn. Antipsychotic drug treatment itself, however, may suppress (or partially suppress) the signs and symptoms of tardive dyskinesia and thereby may possibly mask the underlying process. The effect that symptom suppression has upon the long-term course of the syndrome is unknown.

There are several reasons for predicting that CLOZARIL may be different from other antipsychotic drugs in its potential for inducing tardive dyskinesia. These include the preclinical finding that it has a relatively weak dopamine receptor blocking effect and the clinical finding that it is associated with a low incidence of extrapyramidal symptoms. Very rarely tardive dyskinesia has been reported in patients on clozapine who had been previously treated with other antipsychotic agents, so that a causal relationship cannot be established. Nevertheless, it cannot be concluded, without more extended experience, that CLOZARIL will not induce this syndrome.

Given this consideration, CLOZARIL should be prescribed in a manner that is most likely to minimize the risk of the occurrence of tardive dyskinesia. As with any antipsychotic drug, chronic CLOZARIL use should be reserved for patients who appear to be obtaining substantial benefit from the drug. In such patients, the smallest dose and the shortest duration of treatment should be sought. The need for continued treatment should be reassessed periodically.

Patients in whom tardive dyskinesia developed with other neuroleptics have improved on clozapine.

If signs and symptoms of tardive dyskinesia appear in a patient on CLOZARIL, drug discontinuation should be considered. However, some patients may require treatment with CLOZARIL despite the presence of the syndrome.

PRECAUTIONS: Because of the significant risk of agranulocytosis and seizure, events which both present a continuing risk over time, the extended treatment of patients failing to show an acceptable level of clinical response to CLOZARIL (clozapine) should ordinarily be avoided. In addition, the need for continuing treatment in patients exhibiting beneficial clinical responses should be reassessed periodically.

Patients with a history of primary bone marrow disorders may be treated only if the benefit outweighs the risk. They should be carefully evaluated by a hematologist prior to starting CLOZARIL.

Patients who have low WBC counts because of benign ethnic neutropenia should be given special consideration and may be started on CLOZARIL after agreement of a hematologist.

Fever: During CLOZARIL therapy, patients may experience transient temperature elevations above 38°C with the peak incidence within the first 3 weeks of treatment. This fever is generally benign and self-limiting; however, on occasion there may be an associated increase or decrease in the white blood cell count. Patients should be carefully evaluated to rule out the possibility of an underlying infectious process or the development of blood dyscrasia. In the presence of high fever, the possibility of neuroleptic malignant syndrome must be considered (see Warnings). Fever that is otherwise unexplained can accompany myocarditis (see Warnings).

Occupational Hazards: Interference with Cognitive and Motor Performance: Because of the potential for initial sedation, CLOZARIL may impair mental and/or physical abilities especially during the first few days of therapy. The recommendation for gradual dose escalation should be carefully adhered to and patients should be cautioned about activities requiring alertness (e.g., driving, operating machinery, swimming, climbing, etc.) [see Dosage].

Drug Interactions: CLOZARIL may enhance the central effects of alcohol, MAO inhibitors, CNS depressants including narcotics, antihistamines and benzodiazepines, as well as the effects of anticholinergic and antihypertensive agents.

Caution is advised with patients who are receiving (or have recently received) benzodiazepines or other psychotropic drugs, as these patients may have an increased risk of circulatory collapse accompanied by respiratory and/or cardiac arrest.

Owing to its anti-alpha-adrenergic properties, CLOZARIL may reduce the blood pressure increasing effect of norepinephrine or other predominantly alpha-adrenergic agents and reverse the pressor effect of epinephrine.

CLOZARIL should not be used with other agents, such as carbamazepine, having a known potential to suppress bone marrow function. In particular, the concomitant use of long-acting depot antipsychotic drugs should be avoided because these medications, which may have the potential to be myelosuppressive, cannot be rapidly removed from the body.

Concomitant use of valproic acid with CLOZARIL may alter the plasma levels of clozapine. Rare but serious reports of seizures, including onset of seizures in nonepileptic patients, and isolated cases of delirium where CLOZARIL was co-administered with valproic acid have been reported. These effects are possibly due to a pharmacodynamic interaction, the mechanism of which has not been determined.

As with other antipsychotics, caution should be exercised when CLOZARIL is prescribed with medicines known to increase the QTc interval, or causing electrolyte imbalance.

Clozapine is a substrate for many CYP 450 isoenzymes, in particular 1A2 and 3A4. Caution is called for in patients receiving concomitant treatment with other drugs which are either inhibitors or inducers of these enzymes.

Concomitant administration of drugs known to inhibit the activity of cytochrome P450 isozymes may increase the plasma levels of clozapine:

- Drugs known to inhibit the activity of the major isozymes involved in the metabolism of clozapine and with reported interactions include, cimetidine (2D6, 3A4), and erythromycin (3A4). Other potent inhibitors of CYP3A, such as azole antimycotics and protease inhibitors, could potentially also increase clozapine plasma concentrations; however, no interactions have been reported to date.
- Substantial elevation of the plasma concentration of clozapine has been reported in patients receiving the drug in combination with fluvoxamine (1A2). Smaller elevations in clozapine plasma concentrations have also been reported in patients receiving the drug in combination with other selective serotonin re-uptake inhibitors (SSRIs) such as paroxetine, sertraline, fluoxetine and citalopram (possibly a weak inhibitor of CYP1A2 and possibly the least likely among SSRIs to cause a clinically significant interaction with clozapine).
- The plasma concentration of clozapine is increased by caffeine (1A2) intake and decreased by nearly 50% following a 5-day caffeine-free period.

No clinically relevant interactions have been observed thus far with tricyclic antidepressants, phenothiazines or type 1_C anti-arrhythmics, known to bind to cytochrome P450 2D6.

Concomitant administration of drugs known to induce cytochrome P450 enzymes may decrease the plasma levels of clozapine:

- Drugs known to induce the activity of 3A4 and with reported interactions with clozapine include, for instance, carbamazepine, phenytoin and rifampin.
- Known inducers of 1A2 include, for instance, omeprazole and cigarette smoking. In cases of sudden smoking cessation, the plasma clozapine concentration may be increased, thus leading to an increase in adverse effects.

Anticholinergic Activity: CLOZARIL has potent anticholinergic effects, which may produce undesirable effects throughout the body. Great care should be exercised in using the drug in the presence of prostatic enlargement, narrow-angle glaucoma or paralytic ileus. Probably on account of its anticholinergic properties, CLOZARIL has been associated with varying degrees of impairment of intestinal peristalsis, ranging from constipation to intestinal obstruction, fecal impaction and paralytic ileus. On rare occasions, these cases have been fatal.

Deep Vein Thrombosis and Pulmonary Embolism: Deep vein thrombosis has been observed in association with CLOZARIL. Since CLOZARIL may cause sedation and weight gain, thereby increasing the risk of thromboembolism, immobilization of patients should be avoided.

Whether pulmonary embolism can be attributed to CLOZARIL or some characteristic(s) of its users is not clear. However, the possibility of pulmonary embolism should be considered in patients receiving CLOZARIL who present with deep vein thrombosis, acute dyspnea, chest pain, or other respiratory symptoms.

Eosinophilia: In the event of eosinophilia, it is recommended to discontinue CLOZARIL if the eosinophil count rises above 3.0×10^9/L, and to re-start therapy only after the eosinophil count has fallen below 1.0×10^9/L. Eosinophilia has been co-reported in some cases of myocarditis and thus such cardiovascular adverse events associated with clozapine use may represent hypersensitivity reactions to clozapine. Patients with both eosinophilia and clozapine-induced myocarditis should not be re-exposed to clozapine.

Thrombocytopenia: In the event of thrombocytopenia, it is recommended to discontinue CLOZARIL therapy if the platelet count falls below 50.0×10^9/L.

Hepatitis: Patients with stable pre-existing liver disorders may receive CLOZARIL , but need regular liver function test. In patients in whom, during CLOZARIL treatment, symptoms of possible liver dysfunction such as nausea, vomiting and/or anorexia develop, liver function tests should be performed immediately. If the elevation of these values is clinically relevant or if symptoms of jaundice occur, treatment with CLOZARIL must be discontinued. It may be resumed (see Dosage: Re-Initiation of Treatment in Patients Previously Discontinued) only when the liver function tests have returned to normal values. In such cases, liver function should be closely monitored after the re-introduction of the drug.

Hyperglycemia: On rare occasions, severe hyperglycemia, sometimes leading to ketoacidosis/hyperosmolar coma including some fatal cases, has been reported during CLOZARIL treatment in patients with no prior history of hyperglycemia. While a causal relationship to clozapine use has not been definitely established, glucose levels returned to normal in most patients after discontinuation of CLOZARIL and rechallenge produced a recurrence of hyperglycemia in a few cases. The effect of clozapine on glucose metabolism in patients with diabetes mellitus has not been studied. Impaired glucose tolerance, severe hyperglycemia, ketoacidosis and hyperosmolar coma have been reported in patients with no prior history of hyperglycaemia. In patient receiving CLOZARIL who developed symptom of hyperglycaemia, such as polydipsia, polyuria, polyphagia or weakness discontinuation should be considered.

There is a risk of altering the metabolic balance resulting in slight impairment of glucose homeostasis and a possibility of unmasking a pre-diabetic condition or aggravating pre-existing diabetes.

Assessment of the relationship between atypical antipsychotic use and glucose abnormalities is complicated by the possibility of an increased background risk of diabetes mellitus in patients with schizophrenia and the increasing incidence of diabetes mellitus in the general population. Given these confounders, the relationship between atypical antipsychotic use and hyperglycemia-related adverse events is not completely understood. However, epidemiological studies suggest an increased risk of treatment-emergent hyperglycemia-related adverse events in patients treated with the atypical antipsychotics. Precise risk estimates for hyperglycemia-related adverse events in patients treated with atypical antipsychotics are not available.

Any patient treated with atypical antipsychotics should be monitored for symptoms of hyperglycemia including polydipsia, polyuria, polyphagia, and weakness. Patients who develop symptoms of hyperglycemia during treatment with atypical antipsychotics should undergo fasting blood glucose testing. In some cases, hyperglycemia has resolved when the atypical antipsychotic was discontinued; however, some patients required continuation of anti-diabetic treatment despite discontinuation of the suspect drug. Patients with risk factors for diabetes mellitus (e.g., obesity, family history of diabetes) who are starting treatment with atypical antipsychotics should undergo fasting blood glucose testing at the beginning of treatment and periodically during treatment. Patients with an established diagnosis of diabetes mellitus who are started on atypical antipsychotics should be monitored regularly for worsening of glucose control.

Dysphagia: Esophageal dysmotility and aspiration have been associated with antipsychotic drug use. Aspiration pneumonia is a common cause of morbidity and mortality in elderly patients, in particular those with advanced Alzheimer's dementia. CLOZARIL and other antipsychotic drugs should be used cautiously in patients at risk for aspiration pneumonia.

Use in Patients with Concomitant Illness: Clinical experience with CLOZARIL in patients with concomitant systemic diseases is limited. Nevertheless, caution is advised when using CLOZARIL in patients with hepatic, renal or cardiac disease. For severe cases, see Contraindications.

Pregnancy: Reproduction studies, performed in rats and rabbits at doses of approximately 2 to 4 times the human dose, have revealed no evidence of impaired fertility or harm to the fetus due to clozapine. However, there has not been any adequate and well-controlled studies in pregnant women. Because animal reproduction studies are not always predictive of human response and in view of the desirability of keeping the administration of all drugs to a minimum during pregnancy, CLOZARIL should be used only if the benefits clearly outweigh the risks.

Lactation: Animal studies suggest that clozapine may be excreted in breast milk and have an effect on the nursing infant. Therefore, women receiving CLOZARIL should not breast-feed.

Women of Childbearing Potential: Some female patients treated with antipsychotics other than CLOZARIL may become amenorrheic. A return to normal menstruation may occur as a result of switching from other antipsychotics to CLOZARIL. Adequate contraceptive measures must therefore be ensured in women of childbearing potential.

Children: Safety and efficacy in children below age 18 have not been established.

Geriatrics: Use in Geriatric Patients with Dementia: Overall Mortality: Elderly patients with dementia treated with atypical antipsychotic drugs are at an increased risk of death compared to placebo. CLOZARIL has not been studied in elderly patients with dementia. Clozaril (clozapine) is not recommended for the treatment of patients with dementia (see Warnings).

Orthostatic hypotension can occur with CLOZARIL treatment and there have been rare reports of tachycardia, which may be sustained, in patients taking clozapine. Elderly patients, particularly those with compromised cardiovascular function, may be more susceptible to these effects.

Elderly patients may also be particularly susceptible to the anticholinergic effects of clozapine such as urinary retention and constipation.

Information to Be Provided to the Patient: Physicians are advised to discuss the following issues with patients (and/or their guardians) for whom they prescribe CLOZARIL:

- Patients who are to receive CLOZARIL should be warned about the significant risk of developing agranulocytosis, a potentially life-threatening adverse event. They should be informed that regular blood tests are required to monitor for the occurrence of agranulocytosis, and that CLOZARIL tablets will be made available only through a special program designed to ensure the required blood monitoring. They should also be informed that weekly blood tests will be required for the first 26 weeks of their treatment with clozapine and that, following this initial higher risk period, they could be allowed to change to a "once every 2 weeks" schedule, provided that their clinical condition is permitting such a change in monitoring regimen. Patients should be advised to report immediately the appearance of lethargy, weakness, fever, sore throat, malaise, mucous membrane ulceration or other possible signs of infection. Particular attention should be paid to any flu-like complaints or other symptoms that might suggest infection.
- Patients should be advised to contact their physician immediately if they develop persistent tachycardia (rapid heart rate) at rest accompanied by other signs and symptoms of heart failure (e.g. chest pain, shortness of breath, swelling of the ankles and feet, or arrhythmias (abnormal heart rhythms). Other symptoms which may be present in addition to the above include fatigue, flu-like symptoms, fever that is otherwise unexplained, hypotension (low blood pressure) and/or raised jugular venous pressure (bulging neck veins when sitting or standing). Patients are advised to contact their physician before discontinuing any medication.
- Patients should be informed of the significant risk of seizure during CLOZARIL treatment and should be advised to avoid activities that require alertness (e.g., driving, operating machinery, swimming, climbing, etc.).
- Patients should be advised of the risk of orthostatic hypotension, especially during the period of initial dose titration.
- Patients should be informed that if they stop taking CLOZARIL for 2 days or more, they should not restart their medication at the same dosage, but should contact their physician for dosage instructions.
- Patients should notify their physician if they are taking, or plan to take, any prescription or over-the-counter drugs or alcohol.
- Patients should notify their physician if they become pregnant or intend to become pregnant during therapy.
- Patients should not breast-feed an infant if they are taking CLOZARIL.

ADVERSE EFFECTS: The most serious adverse reactions experienced with CLOZARIL (clozapine) are agranulocytosis, seizure, cardiovascular effects and fever (see Warnings and Precautions). The most common side effects are drowsiness, hypersalivation, tachycardia and sedation.

Adverse Reactions Associated with Discontinuation of Treatment: Sixteen percent of 1080 patients who received (clozapine) in premarketing clinical trials discontinued treatment due to an adverse event, including both those that could be reasonably attributed to (clozapine) treatment and those that might more appropriately be considered intercurrent illness. The more common events considered to be causes of discontinuation included: CNS, primarily drowsiness/sedation, seizures, dizziness/syncope; cardiovascular, primarily tachycardia, hypotension and ECG changes; gastrointestinal, primarily nausea/vomiting; hematologic, primarily leukopenia/granulocytopenia/agranulocytosis; and fever. None of the events enumerated accounts for more than 1.7% of all discontinuations attributed to adverse clinical events.

Commonly Observed Adverse Reactions: Adverse events observed in association with the use of (clozapine) in clinical trials at an incidence of greater than 5% were: central nervous system complaints, including drowsiness/sedation, dizziness/vertigo, headache and tremor; autonomic nervous system complaints, including salivation, sweating, dry mouth and visual disturbances; cardiovascular findings, including tachycardia, hypotension and syncope; and gastrointestinal complaints, including constipation and nausea; and fever. Complaints of drowsiness/sedation tend to subside with continued therapy or dose reduction. Salivation may be profuse, especially during sleep, but may be diminished with dose reduction.

Incidence in Clinical Trials: Table 1 enumerates adverse events that occurred at a frequency of 1% or greater among (clozapine) patients who participated in clinical trials. These rates are not adjusted for duration of exposure.

Table 1: CLOZARIL

Treatment-emergent Adverse Experience Incidence Among Patients Taking Clozapine in Clinical Trials (N=842) (Percentage of Patients Reporting)

Body System Adverse Event [a]	Percent
CNS	
Drowsiness/Sedation	39
Dizziness/Vertigo	19
Headache	7
Tremor	6
Syncope	6
Disturbed Sleep/Nightmares	4
Restlessness	4
Hypokinesia/Akinesia	4
Agitation	4
Seizures (convulsions)	3[b]
Rigidity	3
Akathisia	3
Confusion	3
Fatigue	2

(cont'd)

Table 1: CLOZARIL *(cont'd)*

Treatment-emergent Adverse Experience Incidence Among Patients Taking Clozapine in Clinical Trials (N=842) (Percentage of Patients Reporting)

Body System Adverse Event [a]	Percent
Insomnia	2
Hyperkinesia	1
Weakness	1
Lethargy	1
Ataxia	1
Slurred Speech	1
Depression	1
Epileptiform Movements/Myoclonic Jerks	1
Anxiety	1
Cardiovascular	
Tachycardia	25[b]
Hypotension	9
Hypertension	4
Chest Pain/Angina	1
ECG Change/Cardiac Abnormality	1
Gastrointestinal	
Constipation	14
Nausea	5
Abdominal Discomfort/Heartburn	4
Nausea/Vomiting	3
Vomiting	3
Diarrhea	2
Liver Test Abnormality	1
Anorexia	1
Urogenital	
Urinary Abnormalities	2
Incontinence	1
Abnormal Ejaculation	1
Urinary Urgency/Frequency	1
Urinary Retention	1
Autonomic Nervous System	
Salivation	31
Sweating	6
Dry Mouth	6
Visual Disturbances	5
Integumentary (Skin)	
Rash	2
Musculoskeletal	
Muscle Weakness	1
Pain (back, neck, legs)	1
Muscle Spasm	1
Muscle Pain, Ache	1
Respiratory	
Throat Discomfort	1
Dyspnea, Shortness of breath	1
Nasal Congestion	1
Hemic/Lymphatic	

(cont'd)

Table 1: CLOZARIL *(cont'd)*

Treatment-emergent Adverse Experience Incidence Among Patients Taking Clozapine in Clinical Trials (N=842) (Percentage of Patients Reporting)

Body System Adverse Event [a]	Percent
Leukopenia/Decreased WBC/Neutropenia	3
Agranulocytosis	1[b]
Eosinophilia	1
Miscellaneous	
Fever	5
Weight Gain	4
Tongue Numb/Sore	1

[a] Events reported by at least 1% of clozapine patients are included.
[b] Rate based on population of approximately 1700 exposed during premarket clinical evaluation of clozapine.

Adverse Events Observed During the InterSePT Study: Adverse events reported during the InterSePT study were consistent with the known safety profiles for clozapine and olanzapine. The 10 most frequently reported adverse events in the CLOZARIL treatment group were: salivary hypersecretion, somnolence, weight increase, anxiety, depression, dizziness (excluding vertigo), psychotic disorder, suicidal ideation, constipation, and insomnia.

Other Events Observed During the Premarketing Evaluation of CLOZARIL (clozapine): This section reports additional, less frequent adverse events which occurred among the patients taking clozapine in clinical trials. Various adverse events were reported as part of the total experience in these clinical studies; a causal relationship to clozapine treatment cannot be determined in the absence of appropriate controls in some of the studies. Table 1 enumerates adverse events that occurred at a frequency of at least 1% of patients treated with clozapine. The list below includes all additional adverse experiences reported as being temporally associated with the use of the drug which occurred at a frequency less than 1%, enumerated by organ system.

Central Nervous System: loss of speech, amentia, tics, poor coordination, delusions/hallucinations, involuntary movement, dysphemia (stuttering), dysarthria, amnesia/memory loss, histrionic movements, libido increase or decrease, paranoia, shakiness, Parkinsonism, and irritability.

Cardiovascular: edema, palpitations, phlebitis/thrombophlebitis, cyanosis, premature ventricular contraction, bradycardia, and nose bleed; ischemic changes, arrhythmias, myocardial infarction, and sudden death.

Gastrointestinal: abdominal distention, gastroenteritis, rectal bleeding, nervous stomach, abnormal stools, hematemesis, gastric ulcer, bitter taste, and eructation.

Urogenital: dysmenorrhea, impotence, breast pain/discomfort, and vaginal itch/infection.

Autonomic Nervous System: numbness, polydypsia, hot flashes, dry throat, and mydriasis.

Integumentary (Skin): pruritus, pallor, eczema, erythema, bruise, dermatitis, petechiae, and urticaria.

Musculoskeletal: twitching and joint pain.

Respiratory: coughing, pneumonia/pneumonia-like symptoms, rhinorrhea, hyperventilation, wheezing, bronchitis, laryngitis, and sneezing.

Hemic and Lymphatic System: anemia and leukocytosis.

Miscellaneous: chills/chills with fever, malaise, appetite increase, ear disorder, hypothermia, eyelid disorder, bloodshot eyes, and nystagmus.

Postmarketing Clinical Experience: Postmarketing experience has shown an adverse experience profile similar to that presented above. Voluntary reports of adverse events temporally associated with clozapine not mentioned above that have been received since market introduction and that may have no causal relationship with the drug include the following:

Central Nervous System: delirium; EEG abnormal; exacerbation of psychosis; myoclonus; overdose; paresthesia; possible mild cataplexy; and status epilepticus.

Cardiovascular: analysis of safety databases suggests that the use of clozapine is associated with an increased risk of myocarditis especially during, but not limited to, the first month of therapy (see Warnings); atrial or ventricular fibrillation, periorbital edema, pericarditis, pericardial effusion, cardiomyopathy, heart failure, mitral insufficiency and myocardial infarction. Very rare events of ventricular tachycardia, cardiac arrest and QT prolongation which may be associated with torsades de pointes have been observed.

Gastrointestinal: acute pancreatitis; dysphagia; fecal impaction; intestinal obstruction/paralytic ileus; and salivary gland swelling.

Hepatobiliary System: cholestasis; hepatitis; jaundice.

Hepatic System: cholestasis.

Urogenital: acute interstitial nephritis and priapism.

Integumentary (Skin): hypersensitivity reactions: photosensitivity, vasculitis, erythema multiforme, and Stevens-Johnson syndrome.

Metabolic and Nutritional Disorders: hyperglycemia, ketoacidosis/hyperosmolar coma, hyperuricemia, hyponatremia, weight loss, impaired glucose tolerance, diabetes aggravated, hypercholesterolemia, and hypertriglyceridemia.

Musculoskeletal: myasthenic syndrome and rhabdomyolysis.

Respiratory: aspiration, pleural effusion and respiratory arrest.

Hemic and Lymphatic System: deep vein thrombosis; elevated hemoglobin/hematocrit; ESR increased; pulmonary embolism; sepsis; thrombocytosis; thrombocytopenia; and thrombocythaemia.

Vision Disorders: narrow angle glaucoma.

Miscellaneous: CPK elevation.

OVERDOSE:

Symptoms: The signs and symptoms associated with clozapine overdose are: drowsiness, lethargy, coma, areflexia, confusion, agitation, delirium, hyperreflexia, convulsions, hypersalivation, mydriasis, blurred vision, thermolability, tachycardia, hypotension, collapse, cardiac arrhythmias, heart block, respiratory depression or failure, hallucinations, extrapyramidal symptoms, aspiration pneumonia and dyspnea.

In cases of acute intentional or accidental clozapine overdosage, for which information on the outcome is available, to date the mortality is about 12%. Most of the fatalities were associated with cardiac failure or pneumonia caused by aspiration and occurred at doses above 2000 mg. There have been reports of patients recovering from an overdose in excess of 10 000 mg. However, in a few adult individuals, primarily those not previously exposed to clozapine, the ingestion of doses as low as 400 mg led to life-threatening comatose conditions and, in 1 case, to death. In young children, the intake of 50 to 200 mg resulted in strong sedation or coma without being lethal.

Treatment: Establish and maintain an airway; ensure adequate oxygenation and ventilation. Perform gastric lavage and/or the administration of activated charcoal within the first 6 hours after the ingestion of the drug. Activated charcoal, which may be used with sorbitol, may be as or more effective than emesis or lavage, and should be considered in treating overdosage. Cardiac and vital signs monitoring is recommended along with general symptomatic and supportive measures. Surveillance should be continued for several days because of the risk of delayed effects. Avoid epinephrine when treating hypotension, and quinidine and procainamide when treating cardiac arrhythmia.

There are no specific antidotes for CLOZARIL. Forced diuresis, dialysis, hemoperfusion and exchange transfusion are unlikely to be of benefit.

In managing overdosage, the physician should consider the possibility of multiple drug involvement.

For management of a suspected drug overdose, contact your regional Poison Control Centre. See the *CPS* Directory section for a list of Poison Control Centres.

DOSAGE: CLOZARIL (clozapine) treatment must be initiated on an in-patient basis or in an out-patient setting where medical supervision is available and vital signs can be monitored for a minimum of 6 to 8 hours after the initial 2 to 3 doses.

When treatment is initiated in out-patients, special caution is advised in patients who are receiving benzodiazepines or other psychotropic drugs as these patients may have an increased risk of circulatory collapse accompanied by respiratory and/or cardiac arrest (see Precautions, Drug Interactions). Extra caution is advised in patients with cardiovascular disease or a history of seizures (see Warnings).

CLOZARIL is restricted to patients who have a normal white blood cell (WBC) count and differential cell (DC) count and in whom a WBC count and DC count can be carried out at least weekly for the first 26 weeks of treatment with clozapine and at least at 2-week intervals thereafter‡. Monitoring must continue for as long as the patient is on the drug, as well as for at least 4 weeks after discontinuation of treatment.

CLOZARIL is available only through a distribution system that requires weekly or every-2-week hematological testing prior to the delivery of the next period's supply of medication (see Indications).

Novartis will provide the Non-rechallengeable Status/Hematological Status of patients to the requesting approved suppliers* of clozapine within 24 hours of receipt of a written request (see Indications).

The dosage of clozapine must be adjusted individually. For each patient the lowest effective dose should be used.

Other Monitoring and Distribution Systems: The introduction of clozapine from other manufacturers has resulted in the establishment of manufacturer-specific registry and distribution systems.

In order to ensure the safe use and continued monitoring of all patients taking clozapine, the physician must have obtained consent from the patient for the potential sharing of hematological and other safety data between clozapine registries.

Patients may not be switched from one brand of clozapine to another without the completion of a new registry-specific patient registration form signed by the prescribing physician.

If a patient is switched from one brand of clozapine to another, the frequency of hematological monitoring may continue unaltered unless a change is clinically indicated.

Initial Dose: On the first day, CLOZARIL (clozapine) should be given at a 12.5 mg dose (one-half of a 25 mg tablet) once or twice, followed by one or two 25 mg tablets on the second day. If well tolerated, the dosage may be increased in daily increments of 25 to 50 mg, achieving a target dose of 300 to 450 mg/day by the end of 2 weeks. Subsequent dosage increases should be made no more than once or twice weekly, in increments not to exceed 100 mg. Cautious titration and a divided dosage schedule are necessary to minimize the risks of hypotension, seizure and sedation.

Switching from Previous Neuroleptics: When CLOZARIL therapy is initiated in a patient undergoing oral neuroleptic therapy, it is generally recommended that the other neuroleptic should first be discontinued by tapering the dosage downwards. Once the neuroleptic is completely discontinued for at least 24 hours, CLOZARIL treatment can be started as described above. It is generally recommended that CLOZARIL should not be used in combination with other neuroleptics.

Therapeutic Dose Range: In most patients, antipsychotic efficacy can be expected within the therapeutic range of 300 to 600 mg/day in divided doses. The total daily dose may be divided unevenly, with the larger portion at bedtime.

Since improvement may be gradual, continued therapeutic response can be expected beyond the first month of treatment.

Maximum Dose: Occasionally, patients may require doses higher than 600 mg/day to obtain an acceptable therapeutic response. Because of the possibility of increased adverse reactions (particularly seizures) at daily doses of 600 mg and higher, the decision to treat in the range of 600 to 900 mg/day must be taken prudently. Patients must be given adequate time to respond to a given dose level before escalation to a higher dose is contemplated. **The maximum dose of 900 mg/day should not be exceeded.**

Maintenance Dose: After achieving maximum therapeutic benefit, many patients can be maintained effectively at lower doses. Careful downward titration is recommended to the level of 150 to 300 mg/day in divided doses. At daily doses not exceeding 200 mg, a single administration in the evening may be appropriate.

Discontinuation of Therapy: In the event of planned termination of CLOZARIL therapy, gradual reduction in dose is recommended over a 1 to 2 week period. However, should a patient's medical condition require abrupt discontinuation (e.g., severe leukopenia, cardiovascular toxicity), the patient should be carefully observed for the recurrence of psychotic symptoms and symptoms related to cholinergic rebound such as headache, nausea, vomiting and diarrhea.

Re-initiation of Treatment in Patients Previously Discontinued: CLOZARIL therapy must not be resumed in:

- **Patients who have been discontinued from treatment due to neutropenia (ANC<1.5x10⁹/L) or severe leukopenia (WBC <2.0x10⁹/L, i.e. Non-rechallengeable Status).**
- **Patients with clozapine-induced myocarditis.**

When restarting patients who have had even a brief interval off CLOZARIL, i.e., 2 days or more since the last dose, it is recommended that treatment be re-initiated with 12.5 mg (one half of a 25 mg tablet) once or twice on the first day (see Dosage for hematological testing conditions). If that dose is well tolerated, it may be feasible to titrate patients back to a therapeutic dose more quickly than is recommended for initial treatment.

Certain additional precautions seem prudent when re-initiating treatment. The mechanisms underlying some of the CLOZARIL-induced adverse reactions are unknown. It is conceivable that re-exposure of a patient might enhance the risk of an untoward event's occurrence and increase its severity. Such phenomena, for example, occur when immune mediated mechanisms are responsible. Therefore, any patient who has previously experienced respiratory or cardiac arrest with initial dosing, but was then able to be successfully titrated to a therapeutic dose, should be re-titrated with extreme caution after even 24 hours of discontinuation.

INFORMATION FOR THE PATIENT: Published in e-CPS, available by subscription at www.e-cps.ca.

SUPPLIED: 25 mg: Each round, pale yellow, uncoated, easy to break, scored tablet, embossed "CLOZARIL" on one side and "25 mg" on the other, contains: clozapine 25 mg. Nonmedicinal ingredients: colloidal silicon dioxide, lactose, magnesium stearate, povidone, starch and talc. Bottles of 100. Store below 30°C.

100 mg: Each round, pale yellow, uncoated, easy to break, scored tablet, embossed "CLOZARIL" on one side and "100 mg" on the other, contains: clozapine 100 mg. Nonmedicinal ingredients: colloidal silicon dioxide, lactose, magnesium stearate, povidone, starch and talc. Bottles of 100. Store below 30°C.

CLOZARIL is available only through a distribution system that requires weekly or every-2 week hematological testing prior to the delivery of the next period's supply of medication (see Indications).

(Shown in Product Identification Section)

CoActifed® Expectorant Ⓝ

triprolidine HCl—pseudoephedrine HCl—guaifenesin—codeine phosphate

Antihistamine—Decongestant—Expectorant—Antitussive

GlaxoSmithKline

CoActifed® Syrup Ⓝ

triprolidine HCl—pseudoephedrine HCl—codeine phosphate

Antihistamine—Decongestant—Antitussive

GlaxoSmithKline

CoActifed® Tablets Ⓝ

triprolidine HCl—pseudoephedrine HCl—codeine phosphate

Antihistamine—Decongestant—Antitussive

GlaxoSmithKline

Date of Revision: April 24, 2009

‡ The change from a weekly to a "once every 2 weeks" schedule should be evaluated on an individual patient basis after 26 weeks of treatment. This decision should be made based upon the clinical judgment of the treating physician, and if he/she deems it appropriate, a consulting hematologist, as well as the patient's willingness to pursue a given frequency of blood monitoring. In turn, the clinical evaluation should take into consideration possible factors that would place the patient in a higher risk group, as well as the hematological profile of the patient during the first 26 weeks of treatment. Weekly hematological testing should be resumed for an additional 6 weeks if therapy is disrupted for more than 3 days. If clozapine is interrupted for 4 weeks or longer, weekly monitoring is required for an additional 26 weeks.

* "approved supplier" is a manufacturer who holds a valid Notice of Compliance (NOC) for clozapine.

INDICATIONS: CoActifed Expectorant: To facilitate expectoration and control cough associated with inflamed mucosa and tenacious sputum.

CoActifed Syrup and Tablets: The treatment of cough associated with inflamed mucosa.

CONTRAINDICATIONS: CoActifed should not be used in newborn or premature infants.

CoActifed is contraindicated in individuals with known hypersensitivity to: codeine phosphate or other opioids; triprolidine HCl, or other antihistamines of similar chemical structure; sympathomimetic amines including pseudoephedrine; guaifenesin; any of the excipients.

CoActifed should not be administered to patients receiving MAO inhibitors or who have taken any within the preceding 2 weeks. The concomitant use of pseudoephedrine and this type of product may cause a rise in blood pressure. In addition, the concomitant use of a codeine-containing product and MAOIs can occasionally result in symptoms such as hyperpyrexia, arrhythmia, myoclonus or coma.

Antihistamines should not be used to treat lower respiratory tract symptoms, including asthma.

CoActifed must not be administered to patients with chronic or persistent cough, such as occurs with asthma, smoking or emphysema, or where cough is accompanied by excessive secretions.

Codeine, in common with other centrally acting antitussive agents, must not be given to subjects in or at risk of developing respiratory failure.

CoActifed is contraindicated in individuals with severe hypertension or severe coronary artery disease.

CoActifed is contraindicated in individuals with severe hepatic impairment, as it may precipitate hepatic encephalopathy.

CoActifed is contraindicated in patients with moderate to severe renal impairment (glomerular filtration rate less than 20 mL/min).

CoActifed is contraindicated in patients with pheochromocytoma.

CoActifed is contraindicated in patients with head injury or raised intracranial pressure, since further depression of respiration will increase cerebral edema.

CoActifed is contraindicated in all but the mildest forms of ulcerative colitis, since in common with other opioid analgesics, codeine may precipitate toxic dilatation or spasm of the colon.

WARNINGS: CoActifed should be used with considerable caution in patients with increased intraocular pressure (narrow angle glaucoma), stenosing peptic ulcer, pyloroduodenal obstruction, symptomatic prostatic hypertrophy, bladder neck obstruction, mild to moderate hypertension, diabetes mellitus, ischemic heart disease and hyperthyroidism.

In the presence of head injury or other intracranial lesions, the respiratory depressant effects of codeine and other opioids may be markedly enhanced, as well as their capacity for elevating cerebrospinal fluid pressure. Opioids also produce other CNS effects, such as drowsiness, that may further obscure the clinical course of patients with head injuries.

Codeine or other opioids may obscure signs on which to judge the diagnosis or clinical course of patients with acute abdominal conditions.

PRECAUTIONS: General: Before prescribing medication to suppress or modify cough, it is important to ascertain that the underlying cause of the cough is identified, that modification of the cough does not increase the risk of clinical or physiologic complications, and that appropriate therapy for the primary disease is provided.

In young children, the respiratory centre is especially susceptible to the depressant action of opioid cough suppressants. Benefit-to-risk ratio should be carefully considered, especially in children with respiratory embarrassment (e.g., croup). Estimation of dosage relative to the child's age and weight is of great importance.

CoActifed should be prescribed with caution for certain special risk patients such as the elderly and debilitated, for those with severe impairment of hepatic or renal function, gallbladder disease or gallstones, respiratory impairment, cardiac arrhythmias, history of bronchial asthma, prostate hypertrophy or urethral stricture, and in patients known to be taking other antitussive, antihistamine or decongestant medications.

Patients' self-medication habits should be assessed. CoActifed should not be used by patients intolerant to sympathomimetics used for the relief of nasal or sinus congestion. Such drugs include ephedrine, epinephrine, phenylpropanolamine and phenylephrine. Symptoms of intolerance include drowsiness, dizziness, weakness, difficulty in breathing, tenseness, muscle tremors or palpitations.

Although codeine may be habit-forming when used over long periods or in high doses, studies indicate that addiction to codeine is extremely uncommon and requires very high parenteral doses. Nevertheless, patients should take the drug only for as long, in the amounts, and as frequently as prescribed.

Large doses of codeine may cause the release of significant quantities of histamine, which may be associated with hypotension, cutaneous vasodilation, urticaria and, more rarely, bronchoconstriction.

Although there are no objective data, users of CoActifed should avoid the concomitant use of alcohol and other centrally acting sedatives (see Drug Interactions).

Occupational Hazards: CoActifed may cause drowsiness and impair performance in tests of auditory vigilance. There is individual variation in response to antihistamines.

Patients should be warned about engaging in activities requiring mental alertness such as driving a car, or operating dangerous machinery or hazardous appliances, until they are reasonably certain that CoActifed does not adversely affect their performance.

Drug Interactions: Because of its pseudoephedrine content, CoActifed may partially reverse the hypotensive action of drugs which interfere with sympathetic activity including bretylium, guanethidine, methyldopa, and alpha- and beta-adrenergic blocking agents.

Concomitant use of CoActifed with tricyclic antidepressants, sympathomimetic agents (such as decongestants, appetite suppressants and amphetamine-like psychostimulants), or with MAOIs, which interfere with the catabolism of sympathomimetic amines, may cause a rise in blood pressure.

Although there are no objective data, users of CoActifed should avoid the concomitant use of alcohol or other centrally acting sedatives. Patients receiving other opioid analgesics, antipsychotics, tricyclic antidepressants, anxiolytics, hypnotics or other CNS depressants concomitantly with CoActifed may exhibit increased sedation and an enhanced effect on respiratory function.

Codeine, like other opioids, may antagonise the effects of metoclopramide on gastrointestinal motility.

Codeine, like other opioids, may delay the absorption of the antiarrhythmic agent mexiletine. A larger oral loading dose of the antiarrhythmic may be required.

Laboratory Tests: If urine is collected within 24 hours of a dose of CoActifed Expectorant, a metabolite of guaifenesin may cause a color interference with laboratory determinations of urinary 5-hydroxyindoleacetic acid (5-HIAA) and vanillylmandelic acid (VMA).

Pregnancy: CoActifed should be given to a pregnant woman only if clearly needed and caution should be exercised. CoActifed should not be given to women during the last trimester of pregnancy, since codeine may cause withdrawal symptoms in the neonate.

Administration of opioids during labor may produce gastric stasis and increase the risk of vomiting and aspiration pneumonia in the mother.

No clinical data on exposed pregnancies are available for CoActifed. Animal studies with pseudoephedrine and triprolidine do not indicate direct or indirect harmful effects on embryofetal development. There is insufficient information available to determine the effects of guaifenesin.

Lactation: The use of CoActifed in nursing mothers is not recommended unless the expected benefit to the mother is greater than any possible risk to the infant.

The components of CoActifed are excreted in breast milk in small amounts, but the significance of their combined effects on the nursing infant is unknown.

In nursing mothers who are ultra-rapid metabolisers of codeine, higher than expected serum and breast milk morphine levels can occur. Morphine toxicity in babies can cause excessive somnolence, hypotonia and difficulty breast-feeding or breathing. In severe cases, respiratory depression and death can occur. The lowest effective dose should be used for the shortest possible time. Nursing mothers should be informed about carefully monitoring the infant during treatment for any sign and symptoms of morphine toxicity such as increased drowsiness or sedation, difficulty breast-feeding, breathing difficulties, and decreased tone, and seeking immediate medical care if such symptoms or signs are noticed.

Geriatrics: Although there have been no specific studies of CoActifed in this group of patients, it may be anticipated that the elderly may be more susceptible to adverse effects. Therefore, reduced dosage and careful monitoring are advised, particularly in cases where there is impairment of renal, hepatic or mental status (see Contraindications and Dosage).

Children: CoActifed may elicit either mild stimulation or mild sedation. In infants and children, the ingredients, in overdosage, may produce hallucinations, convulsions and death. Symptoms of toxicity in children may include fixed dilated pupils, flushed face, dry mouth, fever, excitation, hallucinations, ataxia, incoordination, athetosis, tonic clonic convulsions, and postictal depression.

Patients with Special Diseases and Conditions: Hepatic Insufficiency: Experience with the use of the product suggests that normal adult dosage is appropriate in the presence of mild to moderate hepatic impairment, although it may be prudent to exercise caution (see Dosage; for severe hepatic impairment, see Contraindications).

There have been no specific studies of CoActifed, triprolidine, pseudoephedrine, codeine, or guaifenesin in hepatic impairment.

Renal Insufficiency: Caution should be exercised when administering CoActifed to patients with mild to moderate renal impairment, particularly if accompanied by cardiovascular disease (see Contraindications).

There have been no specific studies of CoActifed, triprolidine, codeine, or guaifenesin in renally impaired patients.

ADVERSE EFFECTS: In some patients, drowsiness, dizziness, dry mouth, nausea, and vomiting or mild stimulation may occur (see also Precautions, Children).

Triprolidine: Triprolidine may cause drowsiness. Skin rashes, with or without irritation, have occasionally been reported. Dryness of the mouth, nose and throat may occur. Tachycardia may also occur.

Pseudoephedrine: Symptoms of CNS excitation may occur, including sleep disturbance and, rarely, hallucinations. Skin rashes, with or without irritation, have occasionally been reported with pseudoephedrine. Urinary retention has been reported occasionally in men receiving pseudoephedrine; prostatic enlargement could have been an important predisposing factor.

Codeine: In therapeutic doses, codeine is less likely than morphine to produce adverse effects. The most common adverse effects noted with codeine include nausea, vomiting and constipation. Micturition may be difficult. Dry mouth, vertigo, lightheadedness, tachycardia, rash and urticaria also occur. These effects occur more commonly in ambulant patients than those at rest in bed. Therapeutic doses of codeine occasionally induce hallucinations. Symptoms of CNS depression may also occur.

Guaifenesin: Gastrointestinal discomfort has occasionally been reported with guaifenesin.

OVERDOSE:

Symptoms: In addition to the undesirable effects seen with recommended doses, overdosage with codeine can cause transient euphoria, drowsiness, dizziness, weariness, diminution of sensibility, loss of sensation, vomiting, transient excitement in children and occasionally in adults, miosis progressing to nonreactive pinpoint pupils, itching sometimes with skin rashes and urticaria, and clammy skin with mottled cyanosis. In more severe cases, muscular relaxation with depressed or absent superficial and deep reflexes and a positive Babinski sign may appear. Marked slowing of the respiratory rate with inadequate pulmonary ventilation and consequent cyanosis may occur. Terminal signs include shock, pulmonary edema, hypostatic or aspiration pneumonia and respiratory arrest, with death occurring within 6 to 12 hours following ingestion.

Overdoses of antihistamines may cause hallucinations, convulsions, or possibly death, especially in infants and children. Antihistamines are more likely to cause dizziness, sedation and hypotension in elderly patients. Overdosage with triprolidine may produce reactions varying from depression to stimulation of the CNS; the latter is particularly likely in children. Atropine-like signs and symptoms (dry mouth, fixed dilated pupils, flushing, tachycardia, hallucinations, convulsions, urinary retention, cardiac arrhythmias and coma) may occur.

Overdosage with pseudoephedrine can cause excessive CNS stimulation, resulting in excitement, nervousness, anxiety, tremor, restlessness and insomnia. Other effects include tachycardia, hypertension, pallor, mydriasis, hyperglycemia and urinary retention. Severe overdosage may cause tachypnea or hyperpnea, hallucinations, hypertensive crisis, convulsions or delirium, but in some individuals there may be CNS depression with somnolence, stupor or respiratory depression. Arrhythmias (including ventricular fibrillation) may lead to hypotension and circulatory collapse. Severe hypokalemia can occur, probably due to compartmental shift rather than depletion of potassium. No organ damage or significant metabolic derangement is associated with pseudoephedrine overdosage.

Treatment: Therapy, if instituted within 4 hours of overdosage, is aimed at reducing further absorption of the drug. In the conscious patient, vomiting should be induced even though it may have occurred spontaneously. If vomiting cannot be induced, gastric lavage is indicated. Adequate precautions must be taken to protect against aspiration, especially in infants and children. Charcoal slurry or other suitable agents should be instilled into the stomach after vomiting or lavage. Saline cathartics or milk of magnesia may be of additional benefit.

In the unconscious patient, the airway should be secured with a cuffed endotracheal tube before attempting to evacuate the gastric contents. Intensive supportive and nursing care is indicated, as for any comatose patient. If breathing is significantly impaired, maintenance of an adequate airway and mechanical support of respiration is the most effective means of providing adequate oxygenation.

Hypotension is an early sign of impending cardiovascular collapse and should be treated vigorously.

Do not use CNS stimulants. Convulsions should be controlled by careful administration of diazepam or short-acting barbiturate, repeated as necessary. Physostigmine may be also considered for use in controlling centrally-mediated convulsions.

Ice packs and cooling sponge baths, not alcohol, can aid in reducing the fever commonly seen in children.

For codeine, continuous stimulation that arouses, but does not exhaust, the patient is useful in preventing coma. Continuous or intermittent oxygen therapy is usually indicated, while naloxone is useful as a codeine antidote. Close nursing care is essential.

Saline cathartics, such as milk of magnesia, help to dilute the concentration of the drugs in the bowel by draining water into the gut, thereby hastening drug elimination.

Adrenergic receptor blocking agents are antidotes to pseudoephedrine. In practice, the most useful is the beta-blocker propranolol, which is indicated when there are signs of cardiac toxicity.

There are no specific antidotes to triprolidine. Histamine should not be given.

Pseudoephedrine and codeine are theoretically dialyzable, but the procedures have not been clinically established.

In severe cases of overdosage, it is essential to monitor both the heart (by ECG) and plasma electrolytes, and to give i.v. potassium as indicated by these continuous controls. Vasopressors may be used to treat hypotension, and excessive CNS stimulation may be counteracted with parenteral diazepam. Stimulants should not be used.

> For management of a suspected drug overdose, contact your **regional Poison Control Centre**. See the *CPS* Directory section for a list of Poison Control Centres.

DOSAGE: Dosage should be individualized according to the needs and response of the patient.

Do not exceed 4 doses in 24 hours.

Adults and Children 12 Years and Over: 1 tablet **or** 10 mL syrup, 3 or 4 times a day, to be taken orally.

Children Aged 6 to 11 Years: 1/2 tablet **or** 5 mL syrup, 3 or 4 times a day, to be taken orally.

Children Aged 2 to 5 Years: 1/4 tablet **or** 2.5 mL syrup, 3 or 4 times a day, to be taken orally.

Children Under 2 Years of Age: CoActifed is not recommended for children under 2 years of age.

Geriatrics: Although there have been no specific studies of CoActifed in this group of patients, it may be anticipated that the elderly may be more susceptible to adverse effects. Therefore, reduced dosage and careful monitoring is advised, particularly in cases where there is impairment of renal, hepatic or mental status (see Contraindications and Dosage).

Patients with Special Diseases and Conditions: Hepatic Insufficiency: Experience with the use of the product suggests that normal adult dosage is appropriate in the presence of mild to moderate hepatic impairment, although it may be prudent to exercise caution (see Dosage; for severe hepatic impairment, see Contraindications).

There have been no specific studies of CoActifed, triprolidine, pseudoephedrine, codeine, or guaifenesin in hepatic impairment.

Renal Insufficiency: Caution should be exercised when administering CoActifed to patients with mild to moderate renal impairment, particularly if accompanied by cardiovascular disease (see Contraindications).

There have been no specific studies of CoActifed, triprolidine, pseudoephedrine, codeine, or guaifenesin in renally impaired patients.

INFORMATION FOR THE PATIENT: Published in e-CPS, available by subscription at www.e-cps.ca.

SUPPLIED: Expectorant: Each 5 mL of clear, orange, syrupy liquid with a mixed fruit odor contains: triprolidine HCl 2 mg, pseudoephedrine HCl 30 mg, guaifenesin 100 mg and codeine phosphate 10 mg. Nonmedicinal ingredients: flavour, glycerin, methylparaben, sodium benzoate, sucrose and yellow colourant. Alcohol-free. Bottles of 100 mL and 2 L. Store between 15 to 30°C. Protect from light. Do not refrigerate.

Syrup: Each 5 mL of clear, dark red syrupy liquid contains: triprolidine HCl 2 mg, pseudoephedrine HCl 30 mg and codeine phosphate 10 mg. Nonmedicinal ingredients: flavour, glycerin, methylparaben, red colourant, sodium benzoate and sucrose. Alcohol-free. Bottles of 100 mL and 2 L. Store between 15 to 30°C. Protect from light.

Tablets: Each white to off-white, biconvex tablet, code number WELLCOME P4B on same side as score mark, contains: triprolidine HCl 4 mg, pseudoephedrine HCl 60 mg and codeine phosphate 20 mg. Nonmedicinal ingredients: corn starch, gelatin, lactose, magnesium stearate, starch and yellow colourant. Each tablet is equivalent to 10 mL of syrup. If tablet is broken in half, it reveals a yellow core. Tartrazine-free. Bottles of 50. Store between 15 to 30°C. Protect from light. Keep dry.

(Shown in Product Identification Section)

> The reader is invited to consult CPhA's monograph **Bisphosphonates: Oral**.

CO Alendronate

alendronate sodium

Bone Metabolism Regulator

Cobalt

SUPPLIED: 40 mg: Each white to off-white, arc triangle tablet, embossed "AN" over "40" on one side and ">" on the other, contains: alendronate sodium 40 mg. Nonmedicinal ingredients: croscarmellose sodium, lactose monohydrate, magnesium stearate and microcrystalline cellulose. Gluten-free. Blister strips of 30. Store at room temperature (15-30°C).

70 mg: Each white to off-white, oval tablet, embossed "AN70" on one side and ">" on the other, contains: alendronate sodium 70 mg. Nonmedicinal ingredients: croscarmellose sodium, lactose monohydrate, magnesium stearate and microcrystalline cellulose. Gluten-free. Blister strips of 4. Store at room temperature (15-30°C).

Coal Tar

Antipsoriasis—Antiseborrheic

CPhA Monograph

Date of Preparation: October 2005
Date of Revision: May 2009

> This monograph has been compiled by CPhA and reviewed by experts. It may contain information different from that found in Health Canada-approved Product Monographs. The reader is referred to the *CPS* Editorial Policy for more information.

SUMMARY PRODUCT INFORMATION:

Route of Administration	Dosage Form	Product Strength
Topical	Cream	0.55%, 4%
	Emulsion	1%, 2%
	Gel	1.25%, 8%, 10%
	Liquid	0.5%, 0.66%, 2%, 2.5%, 10%, 20%
	Lotion	1%, 4%, 40.8%
	Ointment	2%
	Shampoo	0.05–10% (various concentrations)
	Soap	0.5%

INDICATIONS AND CLINICAL USE: Topical treatment with coal tar is used for controlling the itching, redness, and scaling associated with psoriatic plaques. Coal tar is generally added to treatment regimens when other topical therapies (e.g., corticosteroids, vitamin D derivatives) are insufficient. It may be also used as second line therapy in combination with ultraviolet B (UVB) phototherapy, known as the Goeckerman regimen.

Coal tar has been used topically for the following dermatologic conditions: atopic dermatitis, dandruff, seborrheic dermatitis, chronic exudative or lichenoid dermatitis.

CONTRAINDICATIONS: Contraindicated in patients who are hypersensitive to coal tar preparations, or to any ingredient used in specific formulations. Coal tar is also contraindicated in patients with acutely inflamed or broken skin, pustular psoriasis and in the presence of any skin infections.

WARNINGS AND PRECAUTIONS: General: Coal tar is intended for external use only.

Coal tar should not be used near the eyes. If contact occurs, the affected eye should be thoroughly rinsed with water.

Coal tar should not be applied around the genital, groin or rectal area (see Carcinogenesis and Mutagenesis).

Coal tar is messy and odorous and can stain clothing and skin. Preparations can discolour blond or grey hair to a yellowish tint. Use of modified formulations of coal tar (e.g., liquor carbonis detergens, coal tar distillate, coal tar extract) has mitigated but not eliminated its aesthetic disadvantages.

To avoid falls patients should be warned that coal tar preparations can make the bathtub slippery.

Carcinogenesis and Mutagenesis: A review of the literature found a small number of reported cases of skin cancer attributable to coal tar between 1900-1966. Most of these cases occurred in the anogenital region, prompting the recommendation that coal tar not be applied around the genital, groin or rectal area. Studies in occupational settings have shown an increased risk of non-melanoma skin cancer after chronic exposure to coal tar. The limited available evidence does not conclusively show an increased incidence of cancer with dermatological use of coal tar. However, the need for further studies to determine the risk is widely recognized and some countries and states have banned the dermatological use of coal tar due to limited evidence of efficacy and concern about carcinogenicity.

Sensitivity/Resistance: Hypersensitive patients may experience a pustular eruption or keratocystic response.

Skin: Skin irritation may develop or increase during therapy and such concerns should be directed to a physician.

Treated areas should not be exposed to sunlight or sunlamps for at least 24 hours after application (unless otherwise directed by physician) because of photosensitivity reactions.

Coal tar preparations should not be used in patients with unstable forms of psoriasis because of a risk of precipitating erythrodermic psoriasis (a severe generalized form of the condition that can lead to total body exfoliation).

Special Populations: Pregnant Women: The teratogenicity risk in pregnant women is not certain. Advise women to carefully consider the potential benefits versus risks of therapy before undergoing treatment.

Nursing Women: The potential for absorption or distribution of coal tar into milk is uncertain. Because of a risk of carcinogenicity to nursing infants, advise women to discontinue nursing or the use of coal tar depending on the importance of the coal tar treatment.

ADVERSE REACTIONS: Skin: When used long-term, coal tar may produce dermatitis. Irritation caused by coal tar appears to worsen with increasing concentration. Strong preparations may induce a pain-free but chronic folliculitis, also known as tar acne, which generally subsides when coal tar use is discontinued. This folliculitis may also be avoided by not covering treated areas, not using coal tar for extended treatment periods and not applying coal tar to hairy areas. Exposure to UV light should be avoided because of potential photosensitivity reactions. It is possible to become sunburnt when UVA penetrates glass. Other adverse reactions include erythema, stinging, atrophy, pigmentation, cutaneous horns, tar warts and keratoacanthomas.

DRUG INTERACTIONS: There are no known drug interactions. However, coal tar should be used cautiously with drugs that have known photosensitivity or phototoxic potential.

DOSAGE AND ADMINISTRATION: Coal tar is applied topically to the scalp as a shampoo or to the skin as a variety of formulations including lotion or bath. Liquor carbonis detergens (LCD) is a 20% coal tar tincture used to formulate esthetically acceptable tar products.

Pediatrics: Typical dosages are the same as for adults.

Bath: About 60–90 mL of a 5–20% solution should be added to lukewarm bath water and mixed. Patients should be directed to soak for 5–20 minutes before patting skin dry. The preparation should be used every 1–3 days.

Shampoo: Coal tar should be applied to wet hair and massaged with firm strokes, rinsed thoroughly and repeated. The formulation should be used twice weekly for the first 2 weeks, then once weekly (application may be more frequent if needed). For scalp psoriasis, a small amount of coal tar solution or tar oil bath may be applied to the lesions. Application should be 3–12 hours before a shampoo.

Skin Application: The preparation should be applied topically to the affected area 1–4 times daily. Once-daily application should be at bedtime. Coal tar should be massaged into the skin. Any excess amount should be removed with tissues. The frequency of application may be decreased to 2–3 times weekly as the condition improves. For thick scales, coal tar should be used with salicylic acid and applied several times daily. Hair follicles can become inflamed if coal tar is massaged into skin with a circular motion. Coal tar should be applied with linear motions. Application should be in the direction that hair lies flat.

OVERDOSAGE:

> For management of a suspected drug overdose, CPhA recommends that you contact your **regional Poison Control Centre**. See the *CPS* Directory section for a list of Poison Control Centres.

ACTION AND CLINICAL PHARMACOLOGY: Coal tar reportedly has anti-proliferative, anti-inflammatory, vasoconstrictive, astringent, anti-pruritic and weak antiseptic properties.

The precise mechanism of action is unknown; however, a possible explanation includes the inhibition of mitosis through the suppression of DNA synthesis, resulting in a decrease in the overall thickness of cells in the stratum corneum and stratum germinativum. Coal tars used in soaps and shampoos may also work by penetrating the skin and removing the scales associated with psoriasis.

STORAGE AND STABILITY: Store in airtight containers and keep away from cold. Follow manufacturer's directions for individual products.

SPECIAL HANDLING INSTRUCTIONS: Because of carcinogenic potential, some recommend that chemical gloves be worn during extemporaneous preparation of coal tar formulations.

> The reader is invited to consult CPhA's monograph **Calcium Channel Blockers**.

CO Amlodipine Pr

amlodipine besylate

Antihypertensive—Antianginal

Cobalt

SUPPLIED: 2.5 mg: Each white to off-white, diamond shaped tablet with "AM 2" on one side and "Σ" on the other side, contains: amlodipine besylate 2.5 mg. Nonmedicinal ingredients: calcium hydrogen phosphate dihydrate, magnesium stearate, microcrystalline cellulose and sodium starch glycolate. HDPE bottles of 100. Store at 15-30°C. Protect from light and moisture.

5 mg: Each white to off-white, elongated octagon shaped tablet with "AM| 5" on one side and "Σ" on the other side, contains: amlodipine besylate 5 mg. Nonmedicinal ingredients: calcium hydrogen phosphate dihydrate, magnesium stearate, microcrystalline cellulose and sodium starch glycolate. HDPE bottles of 100 and 500. Store at 15-30°C. Protect from light and moisture.

10 mg: Each white to off-white, elongated octagon shaped tablet with "AM 10" on one side and "Σ" on the other side, contains: amlodipine besylate 10 mg. Nonmedicinal ingredients: calcium hydrogen phosphate dihydrate, magnesium stearate, microcrystalline cellulose and sodium starch glycolate. HDPE bottles of 100 and 500. Store at 15-30°C. Protect from light and moisture.

Coated Aspirin®

ASA

Analgesic—Anti-inflammatory—Antipyretic—Platelet Aggregation Inhibitor

Bayer Consumer Care

PHARMACOLOGY: ASA interferes with the production of prostaglandins in various organs and tissues through acetylation of the enzyme cyclo-oxygenase. Prostaglandins are themselves powerful irritants and produce headaches and pain on injection in man. Prostaglandins also appear to sensitize pain receptors to other noxious substances such as histamine and bradykinin. By preventing the synthesis and release of prostaglandins in inflammation, ASA may avert the sensitization of pain receptors.

The antipyretic activity of ASA is due to its ability to interfere with the production of prostaglandin E_1 in the brain. Prostaglandin E_1 is one of the most powerful pyretic agents known.

The inhibition of platelet aggregation by ASA is due to its ability to interfere with the production of thromboxane A_2 within the platelet. Thromboxane A_2 is largely responsible for the aggregating properties of platelets.

When ASA is taken orally, it is rapidly absorbed from the stomach and proximal small intestine. The gastric mucosa is permeable to the nonionized form of ASA, which passes through the stomach wall by a passive diffusion process.

Optimum absorption of salicylate in the human stomach occurs in the pH range of 2.15 to 4.10. Absorption in the small intestine occurs at a significantly faster rate than in the stomach. After an oral dose of 650 mg ASPIRIN, the plasma acetylsalicylate concentration in man usually reaches a level between 0.6 and 1.0 mg% within 20 minutes after ingestion and drops to 0.2 mg% within an hour. Within the same period of time, half or more of the ingested dose is hydrolyzed to salicylic acid by esterases in the gastrointestinal mucosa and the liver, the total plasma salicylate concentration reaching a peak between 1 or 2 hours after ingestion, averaging between 3 and 7 mg%. Many factors influence the speed of absorption of ASA in a particular individual at a given time; tablet disintegration, solubility, particle size, gastric emptying time, psychological state, physical condition, nature and quantity of gastric contents, etc., all affect absorption.

Distribution of salicylate throughout most body fluids and tissues proceeds at a rapid rate after absorption. Aside from the plasma itself, fluids which have been found to contain substantial amounts of salicylate after oral ingestion include spinal, peritoneal and synovial fluids, saliva and milk. Tissues containing high concentrations of the drug are the kidney, liver, heart and lungs. Concentrations in the brain are usually low, and are minimal in feces, bile and sweat.

The drug readily crosses the placental barrier. At clinical concentrations, from 50% to 90% of the salicylate is bound to plasma proteins especially albumin, while ASA itself is bound to only a very limited extent. However, ASA has the capacity of acetylating various proteins, hormones, DNA, platelets and hemoglobin, which at least partly explains its wide-ranging pharmacological actions.

The liver appears to be the principal site for salicylate metabolism, although other tissues may also be involved. The three chief metabolic products of salicylic acid are salicyluric acid, the ether or phenolic glucuronide and the ester or acyl glucuronide. A small fraction is also converted to gentisic acid and other hydroxybenzoic acids. The half-life of ASA in the circulation is from 13 to 19 minutes so that the blood level drops quickly after absorption is complete. However, the half-life of the salicylate ranges between 3.5 and 4.5 hours, which means that 50% of the ingested dose leaves the circulation within that time.

Excretion of salicylates occurs principally via the kidney, through a combination of glomerular filtration and tubular excretion, in the form of free salicylic acid, salicyluric acid, as well as phenolic and acyl glucuronides. Salicylate can be detected in the urine shortly after its ingestion but the full dose requires up to 48 hours for complete elimination. The rate of excretion of free salicylate is extremely variable, reported recovery rates in human urine ranging from 10% to 85%, depending largely on urinary pH. In general, it can be stated that acid urine facilitates reabsorption of salicylate by renal tubules, while alkaline urine promotes excretion of the drug.

INDICATIONS: The relief of pain, fever and inflammation of a variety of conditions such as influenza, common cold, low back and neck pain, dysmenorrhea, headache, toothache, sprains and strains, myositis, neuralgia, synovitis, arthritis, bursitis, burns, injuries, following surgical and dental procedures.

ASPIRIN 81 mg is indicated for the following uses, based on its platelet aggregation inhibitory properties:

For reducing the risk of vascular mortality in patients with a suspected acute myocardial infarction.

For reducing the risk of a **first** non-fatal myocardial infarction in individuals deemed to be at sufficient risk of such an event by their physician. There is no evidence for a reduction in the risk of a **first** fatal myocardial infarction.

ASPIRIN does not reduce the risk of either cardiovascular mortality of **first** strokes, fatal or non-fatal.

The decrease in the risk of **first** non-fatal myocardial infarction must be assessed against a much smaller but not insignificant increase in risk of haemorrhagic stroke as well as gastrointestinal bleeding.

For reducing the risk of morbidity and death in patients with unstable angina and in those with previous myocardial infarction.

For reducing the risk of transient ischemic attacks (TIA) and for secondary prevention of atherothrombotic cerebral infarction.

CONTRAINDICATIONS: Salicylate sensitivity, active peptic ulcer.

WARNINGS: ASA is one of the most frequent causes of accidental poisonings in toddlers and infants. Tablets should be kept well out of the reach of children.

A possible association between Reye's syndrome and the use of salicylates has been suggested but not established. Reye's syndrome has also occurred in many patients not exposed to salicylates. However, caution is advised when prescribing salicylate-containing medications for children and teenagers with influenza or chickenpox.

PRECAUTIONS: Salicylates should be administered cautiously to patients with asthma and other allergic conditions, a history of gastrointestinal ulcerations, bleeding tendencies, significant anemia or hypoprothrombinemia.

Patients taking ASA daily are at an increased risk of developing gastrointestinal bleeding following the ingestion of alcohol.

Caution is necessary when salicylates and anticoagulants are prescribed concurrently, as salicylates can depress the concentration of prothrombin in the plasma.

Diabetics receiving concurrent salicylate and hypoglycemic therapy should be monitored closely: reduction of the sulfonylurea hypoglycemic drug dosage may be necessary; insulin requirements may change.

Pregnancy: High doses (3 g daily) of ASA during pregnancy may lengthen the gestation and parturition time.

Salicylates can produce changes in thyroid function tests.

Sodium excretion produced by spironolactone may be decreased by salicylate administration.

Salicylates in large doses are uricosuric agents, smaller amounts may depress uric acid clearance and thus decrease the uricosuric effects of other drugs.

Salicylates also retard the renal elimination of methotrexate.

Salicylates may alter valproic acid (VPA) metabolism and may displace VPA from protein binding sites, possibly intensifying the effects of VPA. Caution is recommended when VPA is administered concomitantly with salicylates.

ADVERSE EFFECTS: Gastrointestinal: (the frequency and severity of these adverse effects are dose related) nausea, vomiting, diarrhea, gastrointestinal bleeding and/or ulceration, dyspepsia, heartburn.

Ear: tinnitus, vertigo, hearing loss.

Hematologic: leukopenia, thrombocytopenia, purpura, anemia.

Dermatologic and Hypersensitivity: urticaria, angioedema, pruritus, skin eruptions, asthma, anaphylaxis.

Miscellaneous: mental confusion, drowsiness, sweating, thirst.

OVERDOSE:

Symptoms: In mild overdosage these may include rapid and deep breathing, nausea, vomiting, vertigo, tinnitus, flushing, sweating, thirst and tachycardia. In more severe cases, acid-base disturbances including respiratory alkalosis and metabolic acidosis can occur. Severe cases may show fever, hemorrhage, excitement, confusion, convulsions or coma and respiratory failure.

Treatment: Treatment consists of prevention and management of acid-base and fluid and electrolyte disturbances. Renal clearance is increased by increasing urine flow and by alkaline diuresis but care must be taken in this approach to not further aggravate metabolic acidosis and hypokalemia. Acidemia should be prevented by administration of adequate sodium-containing fluids and sodium bicarbonate. Hypoglycemia is an occasional accompaniment of salicylate overdosage and can be managed by glucose solutions. If a hemorrhagic diathesis is evident, give vitamin K. Hemodialysis may be useful in complex acid base disturbances particularly in the presence of abnormal renal function.

> For management of a suspected drug overdose, CPhA recommends that you contact your **regional Poison Control Centre**. See the *CPS* Directory section for a list of Poison Control Centres.

DOSAGE: Analgesic and Antipyretic: Adults: 1 to 2 tablets (325 to 650 mg) orally every 4 hours.

Children under 12: 10 to 15 mg/kg every 6 hours, not to exceed total daily dose of 2.4 g.

Anti-inflammatory: Adults: 3 tablets (975 mg) 4 to 6 times a day, up to 30 tablets daily, may be required for optimal anti-inflammatory effect. A blood level between 15 and 30 mg/100 mL is in the desirable therapeutic range.

Children: 60 to 125 mg/kg daily in 4 to 6 divided doses.

Platelet Aggregation Inhibitor: Suspected Acute Myocardial Infarction: An initial dose of at least 160-162.5 mg chewed or crushed to ensure rapid absorption as soon as a myocardial infarction is suspected. The same dose should be given as maintenance over the next 30 days. After 30 days, consider further therapy based on dosage and administration for prevention of recurrent MI (see Prior Myocardial Infarction below).

Prevention of a First Non-fatal Myocardial Infarction: 80-325 mg once daily, according to the individual needs of the patient, as determined by the physician.

Prior Myocardial Infarction or Unstable Angina Pectoris: 80-325 mg daily according to the individual needs of the patient, as determined by the physician.

Transient Ischemic Attack (TIA) and Secondary Prevention of Atherothrombotic Cerebral Infarction: 80-325 mg daily according to the individual needs of the patient, as determined by the physician.

SUPPLIED: ASPIRIN Arthritis Pain Relief Caplets, 325 mg: Each pale yellow, enteric-coated caplet, with BAYER 325 in brown ink on one side, contains: ASA 325 mg. Nonmedicinal ingredients: black and brown iron oxides, carnauba wax, corn starch, D&C Yellow #10, D&C Yellow #7, hypromellose, methacrylic acid copolymer, polysorbate 80, powdered cellulose, sodium lauryl sulphate, talc, titanium dioxide, triacetin and triethyl citrate. Bottles of 50, 100 and 200.

ASPIRIN Arthritis Pain Relief, Extra Strength Caplets, 500 mg: Each pale yellow, enteric-coated caplet, with BAYER 500 in brown ink on one side, contains: ASA 500 mg. Nonmedicinal ingredients: black and brown iron oxides, carnauba wax, corn starch, D&C Yellow #10, D&C Yellow #7, hypromellose, methacrylic acid copolymer, polysorbate 80, powdered cellulose, sodium lauryl sulphate, talc, titanium dioxide, triacetin and triethyl citrate. Bottles of 100.

ASPIRIN 81 mg: Each pale blue, enteric-coated tablet, with 81 in dark blue ink on one side, contains: ASA 81 mg. Nonmedicinal ingredients: carnauba wax, corn starch, croscarmellose sodium, FD&C Blue #1, FD&C Blue #2, hypromellose, lactose monohydrate, methacrylic acid copolymer, microcrystalline cellulose, polysorbate 80, powdered cellulose, propylene glycol, shellac, sodium lauryl sulphate, starch, titanium dioxide and triacetin. Bottles of 30, 120 and 180.

(Shown in Product Identification Section)

CO Atenolol Pr

atenolol

Beta-adrenergic Receptor Blocking Agent

Cobalt

SUPPLIED: 50 mg: Each white to off-white, round, flat faced, beveled-edge tablet, marked with "Σ" on one side and scored with "AN" over "50" on the other side, contains: atenolol 50 mg. Nonmedicinal ingredients: magnesium stearate, microcrystalline cellulose, povidone and sodium starch glycolate. Gluten-free. Blister strips of 10 tablets, packages of 30 tablets. Bottles of 30, 100 and 500. Store at 15-30°C, protect from light and moisture.

100 mg: Each white to off-white, round, flat faced, beveled-edge tablet, marked with "Σ" on one side and scored with "AN" over "100" on the other side, contains: atenolol 100 mg. Nonmedicinal ingredients: magnesium stearate, microcrystalline cellulose, povidone and sodium starch glycolate. Gluten-free. Blister strips of 10 tablets, packages of 30 tablets. Bottles of 30, 100 and 500. Store at 15-30°C, protect from light and moisture.

> The reader is invited to consult CPhA's monograph **HMG-CoA Reductase Inhibitors**.

CO Atorvastatin Pr
atorvastatin calcium
Lipid Metabolism Regulator

Cobalt

SUPPLIED: 10 mg: Each white, elliptical, film-coated tablet, coded "10" on one side and "GD" on the other contains: atorvastatin 10 mg. Nonmedicinal ingredients: calcium carbonate, candelilla wax, croscarmellose sodium, hydroxypropyl cellulose, hydroxypropyl methylcellulose, lactose monohydrate, magnesium stearate, microcrystalline cellulose, polyethylene glycol, polysorbate 80, simethicone emulsion, talc and titanium dioxide. Bottles of 90 and 500. Store at controlled room temperature 15 to 30°C.

20 mg: Each white, elliptical, film-coated tablet, coded "20" on one side and "GD" on the other contains: atorvastatin 20 mg. Nonmedicinal ingredients: calcium carbonate, candelilla wax, croscarmellose sodium, hydroxypropyl cellulose, hydroxypropyl methylcellulose, lactose monohydrate, magnesium stearate, microcrystalline cellulose, polyethylene glycol, polysorbate 80, simethicone emulsion, talc and titanium dioxide. Bottles of 90 and 500. Store at controlled room temperature 15 to 30°C.

40 mg: Each white, elliptical, film-coated tablet, coded "40" on one side and "GD" on the other contains: atorvastatin 40 mg. Nonmedicinal ingredients: calcium carbonate, candelilla wax, croscarmellose sodium, hydroxypropyl cellulose, hydroxypropyl methylcellulose, lactose monohydrate, magnesium stearate, microcrystalline cellulose, polyethylene glycol, polysorbate 80, simethicone emulsion, talc, and titanium dioxide. Bottles of 90 and 500. Store at controlled room temperature 15 to 30°C.

80 mg: Each white, elliptical, film-coated tablet, coded "80" on one side and "GD" on the other contains: atorvastatin 80 mg. Nonmedicinal ingredients: calcium carbonate, croscarmellose sodium, hydroxypropyl cellulose, hydroxypropyl methylcellulose, lactose monohydrate, magnesium stearate, microcrystalline cellulose, polyethylene glycol, polysorbate 80, simethicone emulsion, talc, and titanium dioxide. Bottles of 90 and 500. Store at controlled room temperature 15 to 30°C.

CO Azithromycin Pr
azithromycin monohydrate
Antibiotic

Cobalt

SUPPLIED: 250 mg: Each pink, film-coated, capsular-shaped tablet, embossed "Σ>" on the upper face, and "AT 250" on the lower face, contains: azithromycin monohydrate equivalent to 250 mg of azithromycin. Nonmedicinal ingredients: Carmoisine (Azorubine) Aluminum Lake, dibasic calcium phosphate anhydrous, lecithin (soya), magnesium stearate, Ponceau 4R Aluminum Lake, pregelatinized starch, sodium croscarmellose, Quinoline Yellow Lake, sodium lauryl sulphate, talc, titanium dioxide and xanthum gum. Blister strips of 6. HDPE bottles of 30 and 100.

600 mg: Each white to off-white, film-coated, oval, biconvex tablet, with "Σ>" on the upper face, and "AT.600" on the lower face, contains: azithromycin monohydrate equivalent to 600 mg of azithromycin. Nonmedicinal ingredients: dibasic calcium phosphate anhydrous, lecithin (soya), magnesium stearate, pregelatinized starch, sodium croscarmellose, sodium lauryl sulphate, titanium dioxide, talc and xanthum gum. Blister strips of 6.

CO Bicalutamide Pr
bicalutamide
Nonsteroidal Antiandrogen

Cobalt

SUPPLIED: Each white, film-coated tablet, marked with "L" on one side and "RG" on the other side, contains: bicalutamide 50 mg. Nonmedicinal ingredients: colloidal anhydrous silica, lactose monohydrate, magnesium stearate, providone and sodium starch glycolate; coating: hypromellose, lactose monohydrate, polyethylene glycol, titanium dioxide and triacetin. Blister strips of 10 tablets, 30 tablets per package. Bottles of 100 tablets.

CO Cabergoline Pr
cabergoline
Dopamine Receptor Agonist

Cobalt

SUPPLIED: Each white to off-white, capsule-shaped tablet with "C|5" on one side and "Σ>" partial bisect "Σ>" on the other side contains: cabergoline 0.5 mg. Nonmedicinal ingredients: lactose and leucine. HDPE bottles of 8. Store at room temperature (15 to 30°C).

Cocaine Hydrochloride Topical Solution Ⓝ
cocaine HCl
Local Anesthetic—Vasoconstrictor

Sandoz

SUPPLIED: 4%: Each mL of sterile buffered aqueous solution contains: cocaine hydrochloride 4% (40 mg). Nonmedicinal ingredients: benzalkonium chloride 0.01% as a preservative. Vials of 5 mL, boxes of 5. Store between 15 and 30°C.

10%: Each mL of sterile buffered aqueous solution contains: cocaine hydrochloride 10% (100 mg). Nonmedicinal ingredients: benzalkonium chloride 0.01% as a preservative. Vials of 5 mL, boxes of 5. Store between 15 and 30°C.

> The reader is invited to consult CPhA's monograph **ACE Inhibitors**.

CO Cilazapril Pr
cilazapril monohydrate
Angiotensin Converting Enzyme Inhibitor

Cobalt

SUPPLIED: 2.5 mg: Each pinkish-brown, film-coated, oval-shaped, biconvex tablet with "CL|2" on one side and "Σ>" on the other side yellow, contains: cilazapril monohydrate 2.5 mg. Nonmedicinal ingredients: corn starch, hypromellose, iron oxide red, iron oxide yellow, lactose monohydrate, PEG 3350, polyvinyl alcohol, sodium stearyl fumarate and titanium dioxide. HDPE bottles of 100. Store at room temperature (15-30°C).

5 mg: Each reddish-brown, film-coated, oval-shaped, biconvex tablet with "CL|3" on one side and "Σ>" on the other side, contains: cilazapril monohydrate 5 mg. Nonmedicinal ingredients: corn starch, hypromellose, iron oxide red, lactose monohydrate, PEG 3350, polyvinyl alcohol, sodium stearyl fumarate and talc. HDPE bottles of 100. Store at room temperature (15-30°C).

> The reader is invited to consult CPhA's monograph **Fluoroquinolones**.

CO Ciprofloxacin Pr
ciprofloxacin HCl
Antibacterial

Cobalt

SUPPLIED: 250 mg: Each white to off-white round, biconvex, film-coated tablet, embossed "CR 250" on one side and "Σ>" on the other side, contains: ciprofloxacin HCl equivalent to ciprofloxacin 250 mg. Nonmedicinal ingredients: colloidal silicon dioxide, cornstarch, crospovidone, magnesium stearate, microcrystalline cellulose, polyethylene glycol, polyvinyl alcohol, pregelatinized cornstarch, purified water, talc and titanium dioxide. Gluten-free. Bottles of 100. Store between 15 and 30°C.

500 mg: Each white to off-white, capsule shaped, biconvex, film-coated tablet, embossed "CR 500" on one side and "Σ>" on the other side, contains: ciprofloxacin HCl equivalent to ciprofloxacin 500 mg. Nonmedicinal ingredients: colloidal silicon dioxide, cornstarch, crospovidone, magnesium stearate, microcrystalline cellulose, polyethylene glycol, polyvinyl alcohol, pregelatinized cornstarch, purified water, talc and titanium dioxide. Gluten-free. Bottles of 100. Store between 15 and 30°C.

750 mg: Each white to off-white , capsule shaped, biconvex, film-coated tablet, embossed "CR 750" on one side and "Σ>" on the other side, contains: ciprofloxacin HCl equivalent to ciprofloxacin 750 mg. Nonmedicinal ingredients: colloidal silicon dioxide, cornstarch, crospovidone, magnesium stearate, microcrystalline cellulose, polyethylene glycol, polyvinyl alcohol, pregelatinized cornstarch, purified water, talc and titanium dioxide. Gluten-free. Bottles of 50. Store between 15 and 30°C.

> The reader is invited to consult CPhA's monograph **Selective Serotonin Reuptake Inhibitors**.

CO Citalopram Pr
citalopram HBr
Antidepressant

Cobalt

SUPPLIED: 20 mg: Each oval, white, scored, film-coated tablet, marked "C | A" on one side and "Σ>" on the other, contains: citalopram 20 mg (as citalopram HBr). Nonmedicinal ingredients: corn starch, crospovidone, lactose monohydrate, magnesium stearate, microcrystalline cellulose PH101, povidone and purified water; film coating: hypromellose, lactose monohydrate, polyethylene glycol and titanium dioxide. Gluten-free. Bottles of 100 and 250. Blister packages of 30. Store in a dry place at room temperature between 15 and 30°C.

40 mg: Each oval, white, scored, film-coated tablet, marked "C | 40" on one side and "Σ>" on the other, contains: citalopram 40 mg (as citalopram HBr). Nonmedicinal ingredients: corn starch, crospovidone, lactose monohydrate, magnesium stearate, microcrystalline cellulose PH101, povidone and purified water; film coating: hypromellose, lactose monohydrate, polyethylene glycol and titanium dioxide. Gluten-free. Bottles of 100. Blister packages of 30. Store in a dry place at room temperature between 15 and 30°C.

CO Clomipramine Pr
clomipramine HCl
Antidepressant—Antiobsessional

Cobalt

SUPPLIED: 10 mg: Each cream-colored, triangular, sugar-coated tablet, contains: clomipramine HCl equivalent to clomipramine 10 mg. Nonmedicinal ingredients: cellulose compounds, corn starch, gelatin, glycerin, iron oxide, lactose, magnesium stearate, polyethylene glycol, polyvinylpyrrolidone, sucrose, talc and titanium dioxide. Gluten-free. Bottles of 100. Protect from heat (store between 2 and 30°C). Keep out of reach of children.

25 mg: Each cream-colored, round, biconvex, sugar-coated tablet branded GEIGY on one side and FH on the other side in black, contains: clomipramine HCl equivalent to clomipramine 25 mg. Nonmedicinal ingredients: cellulose compounds, colloidal silicon dioxide, corn starch, glycerin, iron oxide, lactose, magnesium stearate, polyethylene glycol, polyvinylpyrrolidone, stearic acid, sucrose, talc and titanium dioxide. Gluten-free. Bottles of 100. Protect from heat (store between 2 and 30°C). Keep out of reach of children.

50 mg: Each white, round, beveled edge, film-coated tablet engraved GEIGY on one side and LP on the other side, contains: clomipramine HCl equivalent to clomipramine 50 mg. Nonmedicinal ingredients: cellulose compounds, colloidal silicon dioxide, lactose, magnesium stearate, polysorbates, talc and titanium dioxide. Gluten-free. Bottles of 100. Protect from heat (store between 2 and 30°C). Keep out of reach of children.

CO Clonazepam TC
clonazepam
Anticonvulsant

Cobalt

SUPPLIED: 0.5 mg: Each round, biconvex, orange tablet, scored on one side and embossed C31 on the other side, contains: clonazepam 0.5 mg. Nonmedicinal ingredients: colour (FD&C & D&C), FD&C Yellow #6 lake 15%; FD&C Blue #2 aluminum lake 12% and D&C Yellow #10 Aluminum Lake 17%, lactose, NF, magnesium stearate, NF and pregelatinized starch, NF. Bottles of 100 and 500.

1 mg: Each round, biconvex, green tablet, scored on one side and embossed C32 on the other side, contains: clonazepam 1 mg. Nonmedicinal ingredients: colour (FD&C & D&C), FD&C Yellow #6 lake 15%; FD&C Blue #2 aluminum lake 12% and D&C Yellow #10 Aluminum Lake 17%, lactose, NF, magnesium stearate, NF and pregelatinized starch, NF. Bottles of 100.

2 mg: Each round, biconvex, white tablet, scored on one side and embossed C33 on the other side, contains: clonazepam 2 mg. Nonmedicinal ingredients: colour (FD&C & D&C), FD&C Yellow #6 lake 15%; FD&C Blue #2 aluminum lake 12% and D&C Yellow #10 Aluminum Lake 17%, lactose, NF, magnesium stearate, NF and pregelatinized starch, NF. Bottles of 100 and 500.

Codeine Ⓝ
CPhA Monograph

see *Opioids*

Codéine Ⓝ
codeine phosphate
Analgesic—Antitussive

Trianon

SUPPLIED: 15 mg: Each white tablet, scored on one side and engraved with "CT15" on the other side, contains: codeine phosphate 15 mg. Nonmedicinal ingredients: cellulose, colloidal silicon dioxide, croscarmellose, lactose and magnesium stearate. Alcohol-, gluten-, sulfite- and tartrazine-free. Bottles of 100.
30 mg: Each white tablet, scored on one side and engraved with "CT30" on the other side, contains: codeine phosphate 30 mg. Nonmedicinal ingredients: cellulose, colloidal silicon dioxide, croscarmellose, lactose and magnesium stearate. Alcohol-, gluten-, sulfite- and tartrazine-free. Bottles of 100.

Codeine Contin® Ⓝ
codeine monohydrate—codeine sulfate trihydrate
Opioid Analgesic

Purdue Pharma

Date of Revision: August 25, 2009

PHARMACOLOGY: Codeine is an opioid analgesic which exerts an agonist effect at specific, saturable opioid receptors in the CNS and other tissues. In man, codeine produces a variety of effects including analgesia, constipation from decreased gastrointestinal motility, suppression of the cough reflex, respiratory depression from reduced responsiveness of the respiratory center to CO_2, nausea and vomiting via stimulation of the CTZ, changes in mood including euphoria and dysphoria, sedation, mental clouding, miosis and alterations of the endocrine and autonomic nervous systems.

Orally administered codeine is approximately 60% as potent as intramuscular codeine in terms of total analgesia. The relative potency of I.M. codeine phosphate is approximately 1/12 that of I.M. morphine sulfate and orally, 200 mg of codeine phosphate is equivalent to 20-30 mg of morphine sulfate during chronic dosing.

The analgesic efficacy of Codeine Contin (codeine controlled release tablets) has been evaluated in multiple dose studies in patients with cancer pain and chronic non-malignant pain. In a dose-response study in cancer patients, Codeine Contin 150 mg every 12 hours provided approximately equivalent analgesia to 600 mg acetaminophen plus 60 mg codeine every 6 hours. In patients with cancer pain and chronic non-malignant pain receiving q4h p.r.n. acetaminophen plus codeine, Codeine Contin (100, 150 or 200 mg every 12 hours) produced improved pain control and reduced consumption of supplementary acetaminophen plus codeine. In patients with chronic low back pain, Codeine Contin (100 mg every 12 hours), supplemented with p.r.n. plain acetaminophen, produced lower pain scores and less fluctuation in pain throughout the day than p.r.n. acetaminophen plus codeine.

Pharmacokinetics: Codeine is readily absorbed from the gastrointestinal tract and has an oral bioavailability of 53%, relative to the intramuscular route. Codeine is rapidly distributed from blood to body tissues, passes the blood-brain barrier and is found in fetal tissue and breast milk. Codeine is metabolized in the liver to morphine and norcodeine, each representing about 10% of the administered dose of codeine. Urinary excretion products are free and glucuronide-conjugated codeine (about 70%), free and conjugated morphine (about 10%), normorphine (under 4%) and hydrocodone (<1%). The remainder of the dose appears in the feces.

The conversion of codeine to morphine by CYP2D6 has a high degree of variability in humans. About 5-10 percent of Caucasians and 1 percent of Asians exhibit the poor metabolizer phenotype. However a range of CYP2D6 activity levels, including very efficient metabolizers of codeine, have been documented. Given the higher potency of morphine relative to codeine, CYP2D6 activity levels have been associated with outcomes from codeine administration that range from an absence of effect to responses with the potential of serious medical consequences.

Codeine Contin is absorbed to an equivalent extent as immediate-release tablet or liquid formulations of codeine. In single dose studies in fasting, healthy volunteers, the maximum plasma codeine concentration (C_{max}) is approximately 56% of that from immediate-release formulations and is achieved approximately 2.6 times later—at 3.3 hours post-dosing. In steady-state studies in healthy volunteers, both the extent of absorption and maximum plasma codeine concentrations are equivalent to those from immediate release formulations at the same total daily dose. In the presence of food, the extent of absorption of Codeine Contin is not significantly increased but peak concentrations are somewhat delayed, occurring at 3.9-4.5 hours post-dose.

INDICATIONS: Codeine Contin (codeine controlled release tablets) are indicated for the relief of mild to moderate pain requiring the prolonged use of an opioid analgesic preparation.

CONTRAINDICATIONS: Codeine Contin (codeine controlled release tablets) should not be given to patients with: hypersensitivity to opioid analgesics; acute asthma or other obstructive airway disease and acute respiratory depression; cor pulmonale; acute alcoholism; delirium tremens; severe CNS depression; convulsive disorders; increased cerebrospinal or intracranial pressure; head injury; suspected surgical abdomen; concomitant MAO inhibitors (or within 14 days of such therapy).

WARNINGS: Codeine Contin (codeine controlled release tablets) should be swallowed whole, and should not be chewed, dissolved or crushed. Taking broken, chewed, dissolved or crushed tablets could lead to the rapid release and absorption of a potentially fatal dose of codeine. All strengths may be halved, except 50 mg. The half tablets should also be swallowed intact.

Patients should be instructed not to give Codeine Contin to anyone other than for whom it was prescribed, as such, inappropriate use may have severe medical consequences, including death.

Patients should be cautioned not to consume alcohol while taking Codeine Contin, as it may increase the chance of experiencing dangerous side effects.

Codeine Contin should be used with caution preoperatively and within the first 24 hours postoperatively.

Abuse of Opioid Formulations: Codeine Contin consists of a polymer matrix intended for oral use only. Abuse can lead to overdose and death. This risk is increased when the tablets are crushed, broken, dissolved or chewed, and with concurrent consumption of alcohol or other CNS depressants. With parenteral abuse, the tablet excipients, especially talc, can be expected to result in local tissue necrosis, infection, pulmonary granulomas, and increased risk of endocarditis and valvular heart injury.

Drug Dependence: As with other opioids, tolerance and physical dependence may develop upon repeated administration of codeine and there is potential for development of psychological dependence. Codeine Contin (codeine controlled release tablets) should therefore be prescribed and handled with the degree of caution appropriate to the use of a drug with abuse potential. Drug abuse is not usually a problem in patients with pain in whom codeine is appropriately indicated. Withdrawal symptoms may occur following abrupt discontinuation of codeine therapy or upon administration of an opioid antagonist. Therefore, patients on prolonged therapy should be withdrawn gradually from the drug if it is no longer required for pain control.

CNS Depression: Codeine should be used only with caution and in reduced dosage during concomitant administration of other opioid analgesics, general anaesthetics, phenothiazines and other tranquilizers, sedative-hypnotics, tricyclic antidepressants and other CNS depressants (including alcohol). Respiratory depression, hypotension and profound sedation or coma may result.

Severe pain antagonizes the subjective and respiratory depressant actions of opioid analgesics. Should pain suddenly subside, these effects may rapidly become manifest. Patients who are scheduled for cordotomy or other interruption of pain transmission pathways should not receive Codeine Contin within 24 hours of the procedure.

Pregnancy: Animal studies with a number of opioids, including codeine, have indicated the possibility of teratogenic effects. In humans, it is not known whether codeine can cause fetal harm when administered during pregnancy or can affect reproductive capacity. Since codeine crosses the placental barrier, Codeine Contin should be given to pregnant patients only when the anticipated benefits outweigh the risks to the fetus. Dependence and withdrawal signs have been reported in newborns whose mothers took opiates regularly during pregnancy. These signs include irritability, excessive crying, tremors, hyperreflexia, fever, vomiting and diarrhea. Signs usually appear during the first few days of life.

PRECAUTIONS: Respiratory Depression: Codeine should be used with extreme caution in patients with substantially decreased respiratory reserve, pre-existing respiratory depression, hypoxia or hypercapnia. Such patients are often less sensitive to the stimulatory effects of carbon dioxide on the respiratory center and the respiratory depressant effects of codeine may reduce respiratory drive to the point of apnea.

Head Injury: The respiratory depressant effects of codeine, and the capacity to elevate cerebrospinal fluid pressure, may be greatly increased in the presence of an already elevated intracranial pressure produced by trauma. Also, codeine may produce confusion, miosis, vomiting and other side effects which obscure the clinical course of patients with head injury. In such patients, codeine must be used with extreme caution and only if it is judged essential.

Hypotension: Codeine administration may result in severe hypotension in patients whose ability to maintain adequate blood pressure is compromised by reduced blood volume, or concurrent administration of such drugs as phenothiazines or certain anaesthetics.

Acute Abdominal Conditions: Codeine has been shown to decrease bowel motility. Codeine may obscure the diagnosis or clinical course of patients with acute abdominal conditions.

Special Risk Groups: Codeine should be administered with caution, and in reduced dosages, to elderly or debilitated patients, to patients with severely reduced hepatic or renal function, and in patients with Addison's disease, hypothyroidism, prostatic hypertrophy or urethral stricture.

Labor/Delivery: Codeine crosses the placental barrier and its administration during labor can produce respiratory depression in the neonate. If the mother has received narcotic analgesics during labour, newborn infants should be observed closely for signs of respiratory depression. Resuscitation may be required.

Lactation: In nursing mothers who are ultra-rapid metabolizers of codeine, higher than expected serum and breast milk morphine levels can occur. Morphine toxicity in babies can cause excessive somnolence, hypotonia and difficulty breastfeeding or breathing. In severe cases, respiratory depression and death can occur. The lowest effective dose should be used for the shortest possible time. Nursing mothers should be informed about carefully monitoring the infant during treatment for any sign and symptoms of morphine toxicity such as increased drowsiness or sedation, difficulty breastfeeding, breathing difficulties, and decreased tone, and seek immediate medical care if such symptoms or signs are noticed.

Occupational Hazards: Driving and Operating Dangerous Machinery: Codeine may impair the mental and/or physical abilities needed for certain potentially hazardous activities such as driving a car or operating machinery. Patients should be cautioned accordingly.

Drug Interactions: Patients should also be cautioned about the combined effects of codeine with other CNS depressants, including other opioids, phenothiazines, sedative/hypnotics and alcohol. The analgesic effect of codeine is potentiated by amphetamines, chlorpromazine and methocarbamol. CNS depressants, such as other opioids, anaesthetics, sedatives, hypnotics, barbiturates, phenothiazines, chloral hydrate and glutethimide may enhance the depressant effect of codeine. Monoamine oxidase inhibitors (including procarbazine hydrochloride) should not be taken within two weeks of use. Pyrazolidone antihistamines, beta-blockers and alcohol may also enhance the depressant effect of codeine. When combined therapy is contemplated, the dose of one or both agents should be reduced.

"In Vitro" Dissolution Studies of Interaction with Alcohol: Increasing concentrations of alcohol in the dissolution medium, resulted in a slight decrease in the rate of release of codeine from Codeine Contin tablets.

Mixed agonist/antagonist opioid analgesics (i.e., pentazocine, nalbuphine, butorphanol, and buprenorphine) should be administered with caution to a patient who has received or is receiving a course of therapy with a pure opioid agonist analgesic such as codeine. In this situation, mixed agonist/antagonist analgesics may reduce the analgesic effect of codeine and/or may precipitate withdrawal symptoms in these patients.

Codeine may increase the anticoagulant activity of coumarin and other anticoagulants.

ADVERSE EFFECTS: Adverse effects of Codeine Contin (codeine controlled release tablets) are similar to those of other opioid analgesics and represent an extension of pharmacological effects of the drug class. The major hazards associated with codeine, are respiratory and central nervous system depression and, to a lesser degree, circulatory depression.

The most frequently observed adverse effects are sedation, nausea, vomiting, constipation, light-headedness, dizziness, and sweating.

Sedation: Sedation is a common side effect of opioid analgesics, especially in opioid naive individuals. Sedation may also occur partly because patients often recuperate from prolonged fatigue after the relief of persistent pain. Most patients develop tolerance to the sedative effects of opioids within three to five days and, if the sedation is not severe, will not require any treatment except reassurance. If excessive sedation persists beyond a few days, the dose of the opioid should be reduced and alternate causes investigated. Some of these are: concurrent CNS depressant medication, hepatic or renal dysfunction, brain metastases, hypercalcemia and respiratory failure. If it is necessary to reduce the dose, it can be carefully increased again after three or four days if it is obvious that the pain is not being well controlled. Dizziness and unsteadiness may be caused by postural hypotension, particularly in elderly or debilitated patients, and may be alleviated if the patient lies down.

Nausea and Vomiting: Nausea is a common side effect on initiation of therapy with opioid analgesics and is thought to occur by activation of the chemoreceptor trigger zone, stimulation of the vestibular apparatus and through delayed gastric emptying. The prevalence of nausea declines following continued treatment with opioid analgesics. When instituting therapy with an opioid for chronic pain, the routine prescription of an antiemetic should be considered. In the cancer patient, investigation of nausea should include such causes as constipation, bowel obstruction, uremia, hypercalcemia, hepatomegaly, tumor invasion of celiac plexus and concurrent use of drugs with emetogenic properties. Persistent nausea which does not respond to dosage reduction may be caused by opioid-induced gastric stasis and may be accompanied by other symptoms including anorexia, early satiety, vomiting and abdominal fullness. These symptoms respond to chronic treatment with gastrointestinal prokinetic agents.

Constipation: Practically all patients become constipated while taking opioids on a chronic basis. In some patients, particularly the elderly or bedridden, fecal impaction may result. It is essential to caution the patients in this regard and to institute an appropriate regimen of bowel management at the start of prolonged opioid therapy. Stimulant laxatives, stool softeners and other appropriate measures should be used as required.

Less Frequently Observed with Opioid Analgesics: General and CNS: agitation, alterations of mood (nervousness, apprehension, depression, floating feelings, dreams), blurred vision, diplopia and miosis, dysphoria, euphoria, headache, insomnia, increased intracranial pressure, muscle rigidity, muscle tremor, nystagmus, paresthesia, transient hallucinations and disorientation, tremors, uncoordinated muscle movements, visual disturbances and weakness.

Cardiovascular: bradycardia, chills, faintness, flushing of the face, hypertension, hypotension, palpitation, syncope and tachycardia.

Respiratory: bronchospasm and laryngospasm.

Gastrointestinal: anorexia, biliary tract spasm, cramps, diarrhea, dry mouth and taste alterations.

Genitourinary: antidiuretic effects, urinary retention or hesitancy.

Dermatologic: diaphoresis, other skin rashes, pruritus and urticaria.

Withdrawal (Abstinence) Syndrome: Physical dependence with or without psychological dependence tends to occur with chronic administration of opioids. An abstinence syndrome may be precipitated when opioid administration is discontinued or opioid antagonists administered. The following withdrawal symptoms may be observed after opioids are discontinued: body aches, diarrhea, gooseflesh, loss of appetite, nausea, nervousness or restlessness, runny nose, sneezing, tremors or shivering, stomach cramps, tachycardia, trouble with sleeping, unusual increase in sweating, unexplained fever, weakness and yawning. In patients who are appropriately treated with opioid analgesics and who undergo gradual withdrawal from the drug, these symptoms are usually mild.

OVERDOSE:

Symptoms: Serious overdosage with opioids may be characterized by respiratory depression (a decrease in respiratory rate and/or tidal volume, Cheyne-Stokes respiration, cyanosis), extreme somnolence progressing to stupor or coma, skeletal muscle flaccidity, cold and clammy skin, and sometimes bradycardia and hypotension. In severe overdosage, apnea, circulatory collapse, cardiac arrest and death may occur.

Treatment: Primary attention should be given to the establishment of adequate respiratory exchange through the provision of a patent airway and controlled or assisted ventilation. The opioid antagonist naloxone hydrochloride is a specific antidote against respiratory depression due to overdosage or as a result of unusual sensitivity to opioids. An appropriate dose of the antagonist should therefore be administered, preferably by the intravenous route. The usual initial i.v. adult dose of naloxone is 0.4 mg or higher. Concomitant efforts at respiratory resuscitation should be carried out. Since the duration of action of opioids, particularly sustained release formulations, may exceed that of the antagonist, the patient should be under continued surveillance and doses of the antagonist should be repeated as needed to maintain adequate respiration.

An antagonist should not be administered in the absence of clinically significant respiratory or cardiovascular depression. Oxygen, intravenous fluids, vasopressors and other supportive measures should be used as indicated.

In individuals physically dependent on opioids, the administration of the usual dose of opioid antagonist will precipitate an acute withdrawal syndrome. The severity of this syndrome will depend on the degree of physical dependence and the dose of antagonist administered. The use of opioid antagonists in such individuals should be avoided if possible. If an opioid antagonist must be used to treat serious respiratory depression in the physically dependent patient, the antagonist should be administered with extreme care by using dosage titration, commencing with 10 to 20% of the usual recommended initial dose.

Evacuation of gastric contents may be useful in removing unabsorbed drug, particularly when a sustained release formulation has been taken.

For management of a suspected drug overdose, contact your **regional Poison Control Centre**. See the *CPS* Directory section for a list of Poison Control Centres.

DOSAGE: Codeine Contin tablets should be swallowed whole and should not be chewed, dissolved or crushed. Taking broken, chewed, dissolved or crushed tablets could lead to rapid release and absorption of a potentially fatal dose of codeine. All strengths may be halved, except 50 mg. The half tablets should also be swallowed intact.

Adults: Individual dosing requirements vary considerably based on each patient's age, weight, severity and cause of pain, and medical and analgesic history.

Doses of Codeine Contin (codeine controlled release tablets) are expressed as codeine base. Codeine phosphate formulations contain approximately 75% codeine base. Patients currently receiving oral immediate release formulations of plain codeine phosphate may be transferred to Codeine Contin at an approximately 25% lower total daily codeine dosage, equally divided into two 12 hourly Codeine Contin doses.

For patients who are currently receiving analgesic combinations of codeine phosphate and acetaminophen or A.S.A., Table 1 provides a guide to the recommended initial and maintenance doses of Codeine Contin.

Table 1: Codeine Contin

Conversion from Acetaminophen (or ASA) Plus Codeine Phosphate Combinations

Number of 30 mg Codeine Combination Tablets Per Day	Initial Dose of Codeine Contin	Maintenance Dose of Codeine Contin
4–6	50 mg q12h	100 mg q12h
7–9	100 mg q12h	150 mg q12h
10–12	150 mg q12h	200 mg q12h
>12	200 mg q12h	as needed (maximum 300 mg q12h)

Patients with pain who are not currently receiving other opioid analgesics, or who are receiving fewer than four tablets per day of a codeine combination preparation, should be initiated at a dose of 50 mg Codeine Contin every 12 hours and the dose titrated as needed.

For patients who are receiving an alternate opioid, the "oral codeine phosphate equivalent" of the analgesic presently being used should be determined. Having determined the total daily dosage of the present analgesic, Table 2 can be used to calculate the approximate daily oral codeine phosphate dosage that should provide equivalent analgesia. An approximately 25% lower dose of Codeine Contin should then be prescribed, equally divided into two 12 hourly doses.

Dose Titration: Dose titration is the key to success with opioid analgesic therapy. **Proper optimization of doses scaled to the relief of the patient's pain should aim at regular administration of the lowest dose of controlled release codeine (Codeine Contin) which will achieve the overall treatment goal of satisfactory pain relief with acceptable side effects.**

Dosage adjustments should be based on the patient's clinical response. In patients receiving Codeine Contin chronically, the dose should be titrated at intervals of 48 hours to that which provides satisfactory pain relief without unmanageable side effects. Doses of Codeine Contin above 300 mg q12h have not been extensively studied, and above these levels it is preferable that patients be transferred to an opioid such as morphine, which is recommended for severe pain. Codeine Contin is designed to allow 12 hourly dosing.

If breakthrough pain repeatedly occurs at the end of the dosing interval it is generally an indication for a dosage increase rather than more frequent administration of controlled release codeine (Codeine Contin).

Adjustment or Reduction of Dosage: Following successful relief of pain, periodic attempts to reduce the opioid dose should be made. Smaller doses or complete discontinuation may become feasible due to a change in the patient's condition or mental state. If treatment discontinuation is required, the dose of opioid may be decreased as follows: one-half of the previous daily dose given q12h for the first two days, followed thereafter by a 25% reduction every two days.

Opioid analgesics may only be partially effective in relieving dysesthetic pain, postherpetic neuralgia, stabbing pains, activity-related pain and some forms of headache. That is not to say that patients suffering from some of these forms of chronic pain should not be given an adequate trial of opioid analgesics, but it may be necessary to refer such patients at an early time to other forms of pain therapy.

Management of Breakthrough Pain: For patients whose dose has been titrated to the recommended maintenance dose, without attainment of adequate analgesia, the total daily dose may be increased, unless precluded by side effects. If breakthrough pain persists despite appropriate adjustments of Codeine Contin dose, plain acetaminophen may be given (325-650 mg q4-6h p.r.n. to a maximum of 4000 mg/24 hours). If immediate release codeine phosphate preparations or acetaminophen plus codeine phosphate combination analgesics (q4-6h p.r.n.) are used for breakthrough pain, the doses of codeine phosphate* are 15, 30, 45, 60, 90 mg for patients receiving Codeine Contin 100, 200, 300, 400, 600 mg/day, respectively.

Table 2: Codeine Contin

Opioid Analgesics: Approximate Analgesic Equivalences[a]

Drug	Equivalent Dose (mg)[b] (compared to morphine 10 mg IM)		Duration of Action (hours)
	Parenteral	Oral	
Strong Opioid Agonists			
Morphine	10	60[c]	3–4
Oxycodone	15	30[d]	2–4
Hydromorphone	1.5	7.5	2–4
Anileridine	25	75	2–3
Levorphanol	2	4	4–8
Meperidine[f]	75	300	1–3
Oxymorphone	1.5	5 (rectal)	3–4
Methadone[e]	—	—	—
Heroin	5–8	10–15	3–4
Weak Opioid Agonists			
Codeine	120	200	3–4

* (Based on a rescue dose of codeine base which should not exceed 1/8 of the daily dose of Codeine Contin.)

(cont'd)

Table 2: Codeine Contin *(cont'd)*

Opioid Analgesics: Approximate Analgesic Equivalences[a]

Drug	Equivalent Dose (mg)[b] (compared to morphine 10 mg IM)		Duration of Action (hours)
	Parenteral	Oral	
Propoxyphene	50	100	2–4
Mixed Agonist-Antagonists[g]			
Pentazocine[f]	60	180	3–4
Nalbuphine	10	—	3–6
Butorphanol	2	—	3–4

a References:
Expert Advisory Committee on the Management of Severe Chronic Pain in Cancer Patients, Health and Welfare Canada. Cancer pain: A monograph on the management of cancer pain. Ministry of Supplies and Services Canada, 1987. Cat. No. H42-2/5-1984E.
Foley KM. The treatment of cancer pain. N Engl J Med 1985;313(2):84-95.
Aronoff GM, Evans WO. Pharmacological management of chronic pain: A review. In: Aronoff GM, editor. Evaluation and treatment of chronic pain. 2nd ed. Baltimore (MD): Williams and Wilkins; 1992. p. 359-68.
Cherny NI, Portenoy RK. Practical issues in the management of cancer pain. In: Wall PD, Melzack R, editors. Textbook of pain. 3rd ed. New York: Churchill Livingstone; 1994. p. 1437-67.

b **Most of the data were derived from single-dose, acute pain studies and should be considered an approximation for selection of doses when treating chronic pain.**

c **For acute pain, the oral or rectal dose of morphine is six times the injectable dose. However, for chronic dosing, clinical experience indicates that this ratio is 2-3: 1 (i.e., 20-30 mg of oral or rectal morphine is equivalent to 10 mg of parenteral morphine).**

d Based on single entity oral oxycodone in acute pain.

e Extremely variable equianalgesic dose. Patients should undergo individualized titration starting at an equivalent to 1/10 of the morphine dose.

f Not recommended for the management of chronic pain.

g Mixed agonist-antagonists can precipitate withdrawal in patients on pure opioid agonists.

INFORMATION FOR THE PATIENT: Published in e-CPS, available by subscription at www.e-cps.ca.

SUPPLIED: 50 mg: Each blue, round, film-coated tablet, with PF printed on one side and CC 50 on the other side, contains: codeine monohydrate 26.5 mg and codeine sulfate trihydrate 31.35 mg (each equivalent to codeine anhydrous 25 mg). Nonmedicinal ingredients: hydroxyethyl cellulose, lactose, magnesium stearate, stearyl alcohol and talc; film coating: Opadry Blue Y-5-10544: FD&C Blue No. 2 Aluminum Lake, hydroxypropyl cellulose, hydroxypropyl methylcellulose, polyethylene glycol and titanium dioxide. Opaque, plastic bottles of 50. Store at room temperature (15-30°C).

100 mg: Each yellow, round, scored, film-coated tablet, with PF imprinted on one side and CC 100 on the other side, contains: codeine monohydrate 53 mg and codeine sulfate trihydrate 62.7 mg (each equivalent to codeine anhydrous 50 mg). Nonmedicinal ingredients: hydroxyethyl cellulose, lactose, magnesium stearate, stearyl alcohol and talc; film coating: Opadry Yellow Y-5-2036: D&C Yellow No. 10 Aluminum Lake, FD&C Yellow No. 5 Aluminum Lake, hydroxypropyl cellulose, hydroxypropyl methylcellulose, polyethylene glycol and titanium dioxide. Opaque, plastic bottles of 50. Store at room temperature (15-30°C).

150 mg: Each red, round, scored, film-coated tablet, with PF imprinted on one side and CC 150 on the other side, contains: codeine monohydrate 79.5 mg and codeine sulfate trihydrate 94.1 mg (each equivalent to codeine anhydrous 75 mg). Nonmedicinal ingredients: hydroxyethyl cellulose, lactose, magnesium stearate, stearyl alcohol and talc; film coating: Opadry Red Y-5-1842: FD&C Yellow No. 6 Aluminum Lake, FD&C Red No. 40 Aluminum Lake, hydroxypropyl cellulose, hydroxypropyl methylcellulose, polyethylene glycol and titanium dioxide. Opaque, plastic bottles of 50. Store at room temperature (15-30°C).

200 mg: Each orange, caplet-shaped, scored, film-coated tablet, with PF imprinted on one side and CC 200 on the other side, contains: codeine monohydrate 106 mg and codeine sulfate trihydrate 125.4 mg (each equivalent to codeine anhydrous 100 mg). Nonmedicinal ingredients: hydroxyethyl cellulose, lactose, magnesium stearate, stearyl alcohol and talc; film coating: Opadry Orange Y-5-2467: FD&C Yellow No. 6 Aluminum Lake, hydroxypropyl cellulose, hydroxypropyl methylcellulose, polyethylene glycol and titanium dioxide. Opaque, plastic bottles of 50. Store at room temperature (15-30°C).

(Shown in Product Identification Section)

The reader is invited to consult CPhA's monograph **ACE Inhibitors.**

CO Enalapril Ⓟ

enalapril maleate

Angiotensin Converting Enzyme Inhibitor

Cobalt

SUPPLIED: 2.5 mg: Each white to off-white, oval-shaped, biconvex tablet with "EL|25" on one side and "Σ|Σ" on the other side, contains: enalapril maleate 2.5 mg. Nonmedicinal ingredients: lactose monohydrate, magnesium stearate (vegetable grade), maize starch, pregelatinized maize starch and sodium bicarbonate. Blisters of 30. HDPE bottles of 100 and 500. The splitting of CO EnalapriL tablets is not advised. Store at controlled room temperature between 15-30°C. Keep container tightly closed. Protect from moisture.

Note: 100 and 500 tablet bottle: discard remaining tablets six months after opening bottle.

5 mg: Each white to off-white, rounded triangle-shaped, biconvex tablet with "EL|5" on one side and "Σ" on the other side, contains: enalapril maleate 5 mg. Nonmedicinal ingredients: lactose monohydrate, magnesium stearate (vegetable grade), maize starch, pregelatinized maize starch and sodium bicarbonate. Blisters of 30. HDPE bottles of 100 and 500. The splitting of CO EnalapriL tablets is not advised. Store at controlled room temperature between 15-30°C. Keep container tightly closed. Protect from moisture.

Note: 100 and 500 tablet bottle: discard remaining tablets six months after opening bottle.

10 mg: Each peach, rounded triangle-shaped, biconvex tablet with "EL|10" on one side and "Σ" on the other side, contains: enalapril maleate 10 mg. Nonmedicinal ingredients: iron oxide red, lactose monohydrate, magnesium stearate (vegetable grade), maize starch, pregelatinized maize starch and sodium bicarbonate. Blisters of 30. HDPE bottles of 100 and 500. The splitting of CO EnalapriL tablets is not advised. Store at controlled room temperature between 15-30°C. Keep container tightly closed. Protect from moisture.

Note: 100 and 500 tablet bottle: discard remaining tablets six months after opening bottle.

20 mg: Each salmon, rounded triangular-shaped, biconvex tablet with "EL|20" on one side and "Σ" on the other side, contains: enalapril maleate 20 mg. Nonmedicinal ingredients: iron oxide red, iron oxide yellow, lactose monohydrate, magnesium stearate (vegetable grade), maize starch, pregelatinized maize starch and sodium bicarbonate. Blisters of 30. HDPE bottles of 100 and 500. The splitting of CO EnalapriL tablets is not advised. Store at controlled room temperature between 15-30°C. Keep container tightly closed. Protect from moisture.

Note: 100 and 500 tablet bottle: discard remaining tablets six months after opening bottle.

The reader is invited to consult CPhA's monograph **Bisphosphonates: Oral**.

CO Etidrocal Pr

etidronate disodium—calcium carbonate

Bone Metabolism Regulator

Cobalt

SUPPLIED: The CO Etidrocal 90-day therapy is supplied in a unit-of-use dispensing system that consists of patient informations and the therapy tablets on five blister cards.

Etidronate Disodium: The first blister card contains a 14-day supply of 14 tablets. Each off-white, capsule-shaped, scored tablet, embossed "ED4" on one side and "Σ>" on the other, contains: etidronate disodium 400 mg. Nonmedicinal ingredients: magnesium stearate, microcrystalline cellulose, pregelatinized starch and starch (corn). Store at controlled room temperature (15-30°C) protected from light and moisture.

Calcium Carbonate : The remaining four blister cards contain a 76-day supply of 76 tablets. Each blue, biconvex, plain-faced, oblong, film-coated tablet, contains: calcium carbonate 1250 mg, each providing 500 mg elemental calcium. Nonmedicinal ingredients: acacia, carnauba wax, FD&C Blue No. 2 Aluminum Lake, maltodextrin, magnesium stearate, microcrystalline cellulose, polyethylene glycol, polyvinyl alcohol, sodium croscarmellose, talc and titanium dioxide. Store at controlled room temperature (15-30°C) protected from light and moisture.

The CO Etidrocal packaging is designed to provide important benefits to patients. The separately blister-packed tablets and the patient information help patients to comply with the cyclical regimen. Dispense only in the original packaging to help patients avoid co-ingestion of calcium carbonate and etidronate disodium, which will interfere with absorption of etidronate.

The reader is invited to consult CPhA's monograph **Bisphosphonates: Oral**.

CO Etidronate Pr

etidronate disodium

Bone Metabolism Regulator—Antipagetic Agent—Antihypercalcemic Agent

Cobalt

SUPPLIED: Each off-white, rectangular-shaped tablet, embossed "ED 2" on one side and "Σ>" on the other, contains etidronate disodium 200 mg. Nonmedicinal ingredients: magnesium stearate, maize starch, microcrystalline cellulose and pregelatinized maize starch. Gluten-free. Bottles of 100. Store at room temperature (15-30°C).

CO Famciclovir Pr

famciclovir

Antiviral Agent

Cobalt

SUPPLIED: 125 mg: Each white to off-white, film-coated, round biconvex tablet with "FC" on one side and "Σ>" on the other, contains: famciclovir 125 mg. Nonmedicinal ingredients: hydroxypropyl cellulose, magnesium stearate, microcrystalline cellulose, polyethylene glycol, polyvinyl alcohol, sodium starch glycolate, talc and titanium dioxide. HDPE bottles of 30, 100 and 500. Aluminum foil-PVC/PVDC unit dose blister packages. Store between 15 and 30°C. Protect from light.

250 mg: Each white to off-white, film-coated, round biconvex tablet with "FC" on one side and "Σ>" on the other, contains: famciclovir 250 mg. Nonmedicinal ingredients: hydroxypropyl cellulose, magnesium stearate, microcrystalline cellulose, polyethylene glycol, polyvinyl alcohol, sodium starch glycolate, talc and titanium dioxide. HDPE bottles of 30, 100 and 500. Aluminum foil-PVC/PVDC unit dose blister packages. Store between 15 and 30°C. Protect from light.

500 mg: Each white to off-white, film-coated, capsule-shaped, biconvex tablet with "FC500" on one side and "Σ>" on the other, contains: famciclovir 500 mg. Nonmedicinal ingredients: hydroxypropyl cellulose, magnesium stearate, microcrystalline cellulose, polyethylene glycol, polyvinyl alcohol, sodium starch glycolate, talc and titanium dioxide. HDPE bottles of 30, 100 and 500. Aluminum foil-PVC/PVDC unit dose blister packages. Store between 15 and 30°C. Protect from light.

CO Fluconazole Pr

fluconazole

Antifungal

Cobalt

SUPPLIED: 50 mg: Each pink, trapezoidal shaped tablet, embossed with "Σ>" on one side and "50" on the other side, contains: fluconazole 50 mg. Nonmedicinal ingredients: croscarmellose sodium, dicalcium phosphate anhydrous, FD&C Red No. 40 aluminum lake, magnesium stearate, microcrystalline cellulose and povidone. HDPE bottles of 50. Store between 15 and 30°C.

100 mg: Each pink, trapezoidal shaped tablet, embossed with "Σ>" on one side and "100" on the other side, contains: fluconazole 100 mg. Nonmedicinal ingredients: croscarmellose sodium, dicalcium phosphate anhydrous, FD&C Red No. 40 aluminum lake, magnesium stearate, microcrystalline cellulose and povidone. HDPE bottles of 50. Store between 15 and 30°C.

150 mg: Each hard, white gelatin capsule, the body has "FZ 150" and the cap has "Σ>", both printed in black, contains: fluconazole 150 mg. Nonmedicinal ingredients: colloidal silicon dioxide, lactose, magnesium stearate, maize starch and sodium lauryl sulphate; capsule shell: gelatin and titanium dioxide. Unit dose blister (PVC) packs of 1. Store between 15 and 30°C.

The reader is invited to consult CPhA's monograph **Selective Serotonin Reuptake Inhibitors**.

CO Fluoxetine Pr

fluoxetine HCl

Antidepressant—Antiobsessional—Antibulimic

Cobalt

SUPPLIED: 10 mg: Each green and gray capsule, printed with R on cap and "10" on body, contains: fluoxetine HCl equivalent to fluoxetine 10 mg. Nonmedicinal ingredients: FD&C Blue No. 2, FD&C Red No. 40 on an aluminum substrate and pregelatinized starch; capsule shell: black iron oxide, D&C Yellow No. 10, FD&C Yellow No. 6, FD&C Blue No. 1, gelatin and titanium dioxide. Gluten-free. Bottles of 100.

20 mg: Each green and white capsule, printed with R on cap and "20" on body, contains: fluoxetine HCl equivalent to fluoxetine 20 mg. Nonmedicinal ingredients: FD&C Blue No. 2 and FD&C Red No. 40 on an aluminum substrate and pregelatinized starch; capsule shell: D&C Yellow No. 10, FD&C Blue No. 1, FD&C Yellow No. 6, gelatin and titanium dioxide. Gluten-free. Bottles of 100 and 500.

Store between 15 and 25°C. Keep tightly closed. Protect from light.

The reader is invited to consult CPhA's monograph **Selective Serotonin Reuptake Inhibitors**.

CO Fluvoxamine Pr

fluvoxamine maleate

Antidepressant—Antiobsessional

Cobalt

SUPPLIED: 50 mg: Each white, round-shaped, deep scored, film-coated 50 mg tablet, debossed "FV" over "50" on one side and "Σ>" on the other, contains: fluvoxamine maleate 50 mg. Nonmedicinal ingredients: mannitol powder, microcrystalline cellulose, Opadry II white (polydextrose, titanium dioxide, hydroxypropyl methylcellulose 2910, polyethylene glycol 400, carnauba wax, and iron oxide yellow), pregelatinized starch, sodium starch glycolate and sodium stearyl fumarate. Gluten-free. Bottles of 100. Preserve in well-closed containers. Store at controlled room temperature (15-30°C).

100 mg: Each white, elliptical-shaped, film-coated 100 mg tablet, debossed "FV" over "100" on one side and "Σ>" on the other, contains: fluvoxamine maleate 100 mg. Nonmedicinal ingredients: mannitol powder, microcrystalline cellulose, Opadry II white (polydextrose, titanium dioxide, hydroxypropyl methylcellulose 2910, polyethylene glycol 400, carnauba wax, and iron oxide yellow), pregelatinized starch, sodium starch glycolate and sodium stearyl fumarate. Gluten-free. Bottles of 100. Preserve in well-closed containers. Store at controlled room temperature (15-30°C).

CO Gabapentin Pr

gabapentin

Antiepileptic

Cobalt

SUPPLIED: 100 mg: Each hard gelatin CONI-SNAP capsule, with white opaque body and cap printed with "GA100" on one side and ">" on the other, contains: gabapentin 100 mg. Nonmedicinal ingredients: gelatin, lactose, maize starch, red iron oxide, talc, titanium dioxide and yellow iron oxide. Gluten-free. Bottles of 100 and 500. Store at controlled room temperatures, 15-30°C.

300 mg: Hard gelatin CONI-SNAP capsule, with yellow opaque body and cap printed with "GA300" on one side and ">" on the other, contains: gabapentin 300 mg. Nonmedicinal ingredients: gelatin, lactose, maize starch, red iron oxide, talc, titanium dioxide and yellow iron oxide. Gluten-free. Bottles of 100 and 500. Store at controlled room temperatures, 15-30°C.

400 mg: Hard gelatin CONI-SNAP capsule, with orange opaque body and cap printed with "GA400" on one side and ">" on the other, contains: gabapentin 400 mg. Nonmedicinal ingredients: gelatin, lactose, maize starch, red iron oxide, talc, titanium dioxide and yellow iron oxide. Gluten-free. Bottles of 100 and 500. Store at controlled room temperatures, 15-30°C.

Colace®

docusate sodium

Stool Softener

WellSpring

INDICATIONS: The management of constipation due to hard stools, in painful anorectal conditions, in cardiac and other conditions in which maximum ease of passage is desirable to avoid difficult or painful defecation, and when peristaltic stimulants are contraindicated.

CONTRAINDICATIONS: Presence of abdominal pain, nausea, fever or vomiting.

WARNINGS: No data supplied by the manufacturer.

PRECAUTIONS: Do not administer concomitantly with mineral oil: increased absorption of the oil may result. Frequent or prolonged use may result in dependence on laxatives. Do not administer docusate within 2 hours of another medicine, because the desired effect of the other medication may be reduced.

ADVERSE EFFECTS: No data supplied by the manufacturer.

OVERDOSE:
No data supplied by the manufacturer.

For management of a suspected drug overdose, CPhA recommends that you contact your **regional Poison Control Centre**. See the *CPS* Directory section for a list of Poison Control Centres.

DOSAGE: Adults and older children: 100 to 200 mg; 0 to 3 years: as prescribed by physician; 3 to 6 years: 20 to 60 mg; 6 to 12 years: 40 to 120 mg. May be given in divided dosage with water. Retention enema: 5 mL of drops (50 mg) to 90 mL enema fluid. Flushing enema: 1 mL of drops (10 mg) to 100 mL enema fluid. To counteract barium constipation: add 10 to 20 mL (100 to 200 mg) to the barium mixture before administration or prescribe 100 to 200 mg as capsules after fluoroscopy. Give syrup or drops in 120 mL of milk or fruit juice or in infant formula, to mask bitter taste.

SUPPLIED: Capsules: Each maroon capsule contains: docusate sodium USP 100 mg. Sodium: <1 mmol (5.17 mg). Bottles of 60 and 100.

Drops: Each mL of solution contains: docusate sodium USP 10 mg (1%). Sodium: <1 mmol (0.65 mg)/mL. Dropper bottles of 30 mL.

Syrup: Each 5 mL of syrup contains: docusate sodium USP 20 mg. Also contains ethyl alcohol 0.03 mL/5 mL. Energy: 50 kJ (12 kcal)/5 mL. Sodium: <1 mmol (3.7 mg)/5 mL. Bottles of 250 mL.

Colchicine-Odan™ Pr

colchicine

Gout Therapy

Odan

SUPPLIED: 0.6 mg: Each yellow scored tablet, engraved O/0.6, contains: colchicine USP 0.6 mg (600 µg). Nonmedicinal ingredients: D&C Yellow No. 10, FD&C Yellow No. 6, magnesium stearate, polyvinylpyrrolidone, sodium starch glycolate and sucrose. Alcohol-, gluten-, paraben-, lactose-, sulfite- and tartrazine-free. White plastic bottles of 100, 500 and 1000.

1 mg: Each pink, scored tablet, engraved O/1.0, contains: colchicine USP 1 mg. Nonmedicinal ingredients: FD&C Red No. 40, magnesium stearate, polyvinylpyrrolidone, sodium starch glycolate and sucrose. Alcohol-, gluten-, paraben-, lactose-, sulfite- and tartrazine-free. White plastic bottles of 100.

Colchicine: Oral

Gout Therapy

CPhA Monograph

Date of Revision: September 2010

This monograph has been compiled by CPhA and reviewed by experts. It may contain information different from that found in Health Canada-approved Product Monographs. The reader is referred to the *CPS* Editorial Policy for more information.

SUMMARY PRODUCT INFORMATION:

Route of Administration	Dosage Form	Strength
Oral	Tablet	0.6 mg, 1 mg

PHARMACOLOGY: Although its exact mode of action in the relief of gout is not completely understood, colchicine is known to decrease the inflammatory response to urate crystal deposition by inhibiting migration of leukocytes, to interfere with urate deposition by decreasing lactic acid production by leukocytes, to interfere with kinin formation and to diminish phagocytosis and the subsequent anti-inflammatory response. The anti-inflammatory effect of colchicine is relatively selective for acute gouty arthritis. It is neither an analgesic nor a uricosuric and will not prevent progression to chronic gouty arthritis. It does have a prophylactic, suppressive effect that helps to reduce the incidence of acute attacks and to relieve the residual pain and mild discomfort that patients with gout occasionally experience.

Pharmacokinetics: Colchicine is rapidly absorbed from the gastrointestinal tract. Food does not affect the rate but slightly decreases the extent of absorption. Peak concentrations occur in 0.5 to 2 hours. The drug and its metabolites are distributed in leukocytes, kidneys, liver, spleen and the intestinal tract. The plasma half-life after a single 1 mg oral dose is about 4.4 hours. The half-life in leukocytes is approximately 60 hours. It is approximately 50% protein bound. Colchicine is metabolized in the liver mainly by CYP3A4 demethylation and excreted primarily in the feces, with 10 to 20% eliminated unchanged in the urine. Severe renal disease may result in a longer elimination half-life.

INDICATIONS: Health Canada-approved uses include:

- treatment of acute gout and prophylaxis of recurrent attacks
- prevention of acute attacks of familial Mediterranean fever (FMF)

Although colchicine is highly effective, the higher dosages traditionally used in acute gout can be associated with considerable toxicity, i.e., severe diarrhea may occur before relief of pain or clinical response. Lower dosage regimens offer comparable efficacy and a better safety profile.

Colchicine is often used during the initial months of uricosuric or allopurinol therapy, to suppress acute attacks.

Uses without Health Canada approval include treatment of amyloidoses, pericarditis and severe recurrent aphthous stomatitis. There is insufficient evidence to either support or refute the efficacy of colchicine in the treatment of hepatic cirrhosis [*Cochrane Database Syst Rev* 2005;(2):CD002148], primary biliary cirrhosis [*Cochrane Database Syst Rev* 2004;(2):CD004481] and Behçet's syndrome [*Cochrane Database Syst Rev* 2000;(2):CD001084].

CONTRAINDICATIONS: Blood dyscrasias; active peptic ulcer; serious gastrointestinal, renal, hepatic or cardiac disease; known hypersensitivity to colchicine; concurrent use with strong CYP3A4 or P-glycoprotein (P-gp) inhibitors in patients with renal or hepatic impairment (see Drug Interactions).

WARNINGS: Concomitant use of CYP3A4 or P-glycoprotein (P-gp) inhibitors with colchicine may cause severe toxicity, even at therapeutic colchicine doses. Fatalities have been reported with the combined use of colchicine and clarithromycin. These two drugs should not be used concurrently in elderly patients and/or those with renal or hepatic impairment. Patients requiring concomitant therapy with colchicine and an interacting drug (see Drug Interactions) should be monitored for signs of colchicine toxicity.

PRECAUTIONS: Colchicine should be used with caution in geriatric or debilitated patients and those with cardiac, renal or gastrointestinal disease. Blood dyscrasias (pancytopenia, granulocytopenia, thrombocytopenia, leukopenia, aplastic anemia, myelosuppression) have been reported with therapeutic doses; periodic blood counts should be performed during long-term therapy.

Rhabdomyolysis and neuromuscular toxicity may occur with chronic colchicine use. Elderly patients, those with impaired renal function and those taking antilipemic agents (fibrates, HMG Co-A reductase inhibitors) or cyclosporine may be at increased risk (see Drug Interactions).

Drug Interactions: Drugs that can inhibit P-glycoprotein (P-gp) and/or CYP3A4 (see Table 1): Severe colchicine toxicity, which may be characterized by myopathy, pancytopenia and multiple organ failure is possible due to increased colchicine concentrations. The risk may be increased in patients with pre-existing renal or hepatic dysfunction. Fatalities have been reported when colchicine and clarithromycin (a CYP3A4 and P-gp inhibitor) were used concomitantly. Combinations of colchicine and drugs inhibiting CYP3A4 or the P-gp transport system are best avoided; if used, the colchicine dose should be decreased while monitoring the patient. Azithromycin does not interact with colchicine.

Alcohol: Because alcohol can increase uric acid levels it may decrease the efficacy of prophylactic gout medication. Alcohol combined with colchicine may also increase GI toxicity.

Pregnancy: Colchicine crosses the placenta; fetal plasma levels are reported to be approximately 15% of the mother's levels. Cell division in animals and plants can be arrested by colchicine. In mice and hamsters it has produced teratogenic effects and has adversely affected spermatogenesis in animals and humans. Cases of Down syndrome have been reported in babies born to parents receiving colchicine but healthy infants have also been born to parents treated with colchicine. There have been reports of azoospermia in men receiving colchicine.

Table 1: Colchicine: Oral

Drug-Drug Interactions

Interacting Drug	Effect	Comments
CYP3A4 inhibitors, strong: • atazanavir, indinavir, nelfinavir, ritonavir, saquinavir • clarithromycin, telithromycin • itraconazole, ketoconazole	Inhibits colchicine metabolism, which may result in a significant increase in levels. Clarithromycin inhibits both CYP3A4 and P-glycoprotein. Fatalities have been reported with concomitant administration of colchicine and clarithromycin.	Avoid combination in patients with renal or hepatic dysfunction. In others, decrease colchicine dose: For acute gout, give 0.6 mg first dose, followed by 0.3 mg 1 h later. Repeat courses may be given no earlier than 3 days later. For familial Mediterranean fever (FMF), do not exceed 0.6 mg daily (may be given as 0.3 mg bid).
CYP3A4 inhibitors, moderate: • diltiazem, verapamil • erythromycin • fluconazole • fosamprenavir • grapefruit and grapefruit juice	Inhibits colchicine metabolism, which may result in a significant increase in levels. Neuromuscular toxicity has been reported when colchicine was administered with diltiazem and verapamil.	Avoid combination in patients with renal or hepatic dysfunction. In others, decrease colchicine dose: For acute gout, give 1.2 mg (one dose only). Do not give a dose 1 h later. Repeat courses may be given no earlier than 3 days later. For FMF, do not exceed 1.2 mg daily (may be given as 0.6 mg bid). Avoid consuming grapefruit or grapefruit juice.

(cont'd)

Table 1: Colchicine: Oral *(cont'd)*

Drug-Drug Interactions

Interacting Drug	Effect	Comments
Cyclosporine	Inhibits P-glycoprotein, which may result in significantly increased colchicine levels. The addition of cyclosporine to the medication regimens of renal transplant patients previously stabilized on colchicine has resulted in gastrointestinal, hepatorenal and neuromuscular toxicity.	Decrease colchicine dose: For acute gout, give 0.6 mg (one dose only). Repeat courses may be given no earlier than 3 days later. For FMF, do not exceed 0.6 mg daily (may be given as 0.3 mg bid). Closely observe patients for signs of an interaction if these drugs are used concomitantly.
Digoxin	Rhabdomyolysis has been reported.	Digitalis glycosides are substrates of P-glycoprotein.
Lipid-lowering drugs • fibrates (bezafibrate, fenofibrate, gemfibrozil) • HMG Co-A reductase inhibitors (atorvastatin, fluvastatin, pravastatin, simvastatin)	Combination with colchicine may result in myopathy and rhabdomyolysis.	Monitor patients carefully, especially during initial therapy, for signs and symptoms of myotoxicity, e.g., muscle pain, weakness, or tenderness.
Nonsteroidal anti-inflammatory drugs (NSAIDs)	The combination of NSAIDs and colchicine may cause additive GI toxicity and increase the risk of bleeding.	
Vitamin B_{12}	Colchicine has been shown to induce reversible malabsorption of vitamin B_{12}, apparently by altering the function of ileal mucosa.	

While colchicine should be avoided in pregnancy if possible, in women with familial Mediterranean fever, discontinuation may be detrimental. These patients may elect to continue therapy with colchicine during pregnancy in order to reduce the risk of adverse outcomes from amyloid-related nephropathy.

Amniocentesis or detailed fetal ultrasound may be recommended in cases of colchicine exposure during pregnancy.

Lactation: Colchicine is distributed into human milk. A limited number of case reports are available, but colchicine is considered by the American Academy of Pediatrics to be compatible with breastfeeding.

Children: Open-label studies have shown that colchicine is effective in the prophylaxis of familial Mediterranean fever attacks, and the amyloidosis associated with this condition, in children and adolescents. Growth does not appear to be affected by the drug.

ADVERSE EFFECTS: Adverse reactions to colchicine appear to be dose-related. Diarrhea is the most common adverse effect. Other prominent symptoms related to the gastrointestinal tract include cramping, nausea, vomiting and abdominal pain and may be particularly troublesome in the presence of peptic ulcer or spastic colon. If these symptoms appear, colchicine should be discontinued immediately as they are early signs of toxicity.

Hypersensitivity to colchicine is a very rare but possible occurrence.

When given for a prolonged period, colchicine may cause bone marrow depression and agranulocytosis, thrombocytopenia or aplastic anemia. Periodic blood counts should be performed during long-term therapy. Peripheral neuritis or neuropathy, myopathy, hair loss, vesicular dermatitis, anuria, reversible azoospermia, renal damage, hematuria and a malabsorption syndrome with steatorrhea have also been reported with prolonged administration.

Patients with renal insufficiency may be at increased risk for neuromyopathy, with possible myotonia, that resolves when colchicine is discontinued.

OVERDOSAGE:

Colchicine poisoning frequently results in severe, delayed toxicity, and large doses may be fatal. Deaths have been reported with as little as 7 mg, though individuals have survived larger doses. The average lethal dose is estimated to be 65 mg.

Symptoms: Symptoms are usually delayed regardless of the route of administration. This asymptomatic period usually lasts 3 to 6 h (range 2 to 12 h). Serious toxicity has been observed following topical administration to mucous membranes.

Colchicine toxicity can affect any organ system. The first symptoms to appear are usually gastrointestinal—nausea, vomiting, abdominal pain and diarrhea. Diarrhea may be severe and may be bloody due to hemorrhagic gastroenteritis. Paralytic ileus may develop. Electrolyte abnormalities are common and are largely due to gastrointestinal toxicity. Burning sensations of the throat, stomach and skin may occur. Extensive vascular damage may result in shock, and a resulting oliguric renal failure is common. Bone marrow suppression and hematologic abnormalities may occur. Fever is common. Rhabdomyolysis, profound muscular weakness or an ascending paralysis may develop. The patient usually remains conscious. However, delirium and seizures may occur. Death is usually the result of respiratory failure, cardiovascular collapse or sepsis secondary to bone marrow failure. Transient, delayed alopecia is common in survivors.

Treatment: Given the severity of colchicine overdose, gastric lavage may be considered in the unusual case where a patient presents within one to two hours of ingestion of a large amount of colchicine and vomiting has not yet occurred. Gastric lavage should not be routinely performed, and the physician should be comfortable with the procedure. Consultation with a Poison Control Centre is advised.

Activated charcoal should be administered even in cases of delayed presentation because colchicine undergoes enterohepatic circulation.

Symptomatic and supportive treatment is the mainstay of patient management. Maintain ventilation and fluid and electrolyte balance. Monitor patient's vital signs, serum electrolytes, CBC and urine output. ECG, blood gases, renal and hepatic function should also be monitored in severe cases. Hypotension may occur and should be treated with fluid replacement and patient positioning. If these measures fail, vasopressors may be necessary. Opioid analgesics may be used to relieve abdominal pain, but the patient should be monitored closely for ileus. Hemodialysis is not helpful.

There is some evidence that granulocyte colony-stimulating factor may be helpful in treating bone marrow suppression and related hematologic abnormalities.

For management of a suspected drug overdose, CPhA recommends that you contact your **regional Poison Control Centre**. See the *CPS* Directory section for a list of Poison Control Centres.

DOSAGE: Acute Gouty Arthritis: Colchicine therapy must be initiated at the first warning of an acute attack; a delay of a few hours impairs its effectiveness. Traditional high-dose regimens for acute gout very commonly lead to gastrointestinal side effects; lower doses have been shown to offer comparable efficacy and a more acceptable safety profile [*Arthritis Rheum* 2010;62(4):1060-8].

Adults: 1.2 mg as a single dose at the first sign of an acute gout flare, followed by 0.6 mg 1 hour later (total of 1.8 mg). To prevent cumulative toxicity, a second course of therapy should not be initiated before 3 days have elapsed since treating the previous attack.

Prophylaxis of Recurrent Gouty Arthritis: 0.6 mg once or twice daily. Lower doses or alternate day administration should be used if renal function is decreased (see Renal Impairment).

Prophylaxis of Familial Mediterranean Fever: Adults: 1 to 2 mg daily divided into 1 or 2 doses. If patients experience significant GI side effects the dose may be reduced to 0.6 mg daily. Children: ≤5 years of age: 0.5 mg or less per day; 5–10 years of age: 1 mg/day; >10 years of age: 1.5 mg/day in 2 to 3 divided doses. Doses may be increased or decreased in increments of 0.25 mg up to a total maximum of 2 mg daily. An alternate regimen may be used: Adults and Children >12 years of age: 1.2 to 2.4 mg per day. Children: 4–6 years of age: 0.3 to 1.8 mg/day; 6–12 years of age: 0.9 to 1.8 mg/day. Colchicine may be given once daily or in 2 divided doses, and the dose adjusted in increments of 0.3 mg daily.

The following dosage reductions have been suggested when CYP3A4 or P-glycoprotein inhibitors are co-administered with colchicine or within 14 days prior to initiation of colchicine therapy (see Drug Interactions).

Co-administration with Strong CYP3A4 Inhibitors: Acute Gout Flares: 0.6 mg as a single dose, followed by 0.3 mg 1 hour later (total of 0.9 mg). Do not repeat for at least 3 days. Prophylaxis of Acute Gout Attacks: 0.3 mg once daily or every 2 days. Familial Mediterranean Fever: Do not exceed 0.6 mg daily (may give 0.3 mg twice daily).

Co-administration with Moderate CYP3A4 Inhibitors: Acute Gout Flares: one dose of 1.2 mg only. Do not repeat for at least 3 days. Prophylaxis of Acute Gout Attacks: 0.3 mg once or twice daily. Familial Mediterranean Fever: Do not exceed 1.2 mg daily (may give 0.6 mg twice daily).

Co-administration of P-gp Inhibitors: Acute Gout Flares: one dose of 0.6 mg only. Do not repeat for at least 3 days. Prophylaxis of Acute Gout Attacks: 0.3 mg once daily or every 2 days. Familial Mediterranean Fever: Do not exceed 0.6 mg daily (may give 0.3 mg twice daily).

Pericarditis: For secondary prophylaxis of recurrent pericarditis (not an approved use in Canada), 1 mg twice daily for one day, then 0.5 mg twice daily (with concomitant ASA) has been studied [*Circulation* 2005;112(13):2012-6].

Renal Impairment: Dose should be decreased by up to 50% in patients with creatinine clearance of 10 to 50 mL/minute and by 75% in patients with creatinine clearance of <10 mL/minute. Avoid prolonged colchicine use if creatinine clearance is <50 mL/minute.

Hepatic Impairment: Use low doses. Monitor carefully for adverse effects.

COLD-FX®

North American ginseng (Panax quinquefolius)

Natural Health Product

Afexa Life Sciences

INDICATIONS: Recommended Use or Purpose: Helps reduce the frequency, duration and severity of cold and flu symptoms by boosting the immune system.

CONTRAINDICATIONS/WARNINGS/PRECAUTIONS: Individuals requiring anticoagulant therapy such as warfarin should avoid use of COLD-FX. Do not use if pregnant or breastfeeding. Not recommended for individuals with impaired liver or renal function. Do not exceed the recommended daily dose. Individuals with known allergies to ginseng should avoid use of COLD-FX.

OVERDOSE:

For management of a suspected drug overdose, CPhA recommends that you contact your **regional Poison Control Centre**. See the *CPS* Directory section for a list of Poison Control Centres.

DOSAGE: Recommended Dose: Adults and children (12 years and older): 200 to 300 mg, 2 times per day.

SUPPLIED: 200 mg: Each white capsule is certified to contain: 200 mg of CVT-E002, a proprietary ChemBioPrint (CBP) product containing greater than 80% poly-furanosyl-pyranosyl-saccharides extracted by an aqueous method from Panax quinquefolius (North American ginseng, root). As a ChemBioPrint product, proprietary standardization technology has been used to identify and isolate the active ingredient (CVT-E002) and ensure consistency from batch to batch. CVT-E002 is scientifically proven to provide health benefits by enhancing the immune system's viral-fighting Natural Killer cells and macrophages. Nonmedicinal ingredients: gelatin. Security sealed bottles of 46, 60, 80, 150 and 225. Store at room temperature. Shelf-life of five years.

300 mg: Each white and blue capsule is certified to contain: 300 mg of CVT-E002, a proprietary ChemBioPrint (CBP) product containing greater than 80% poly-furanosyl-pyranosyl-saccharides extracted by an aqueous method from Panax quinquefolius (North American ginseng, root). As a ChemBioPrint product, proprietary standardization technology has been used to identify and isolate the active ingredient (CVT-E002) and ensure consistency from batch to batch. CVT-E002 is scientifically proven to provide health benefits by enhancing the immune system's viral-fighting Natural Killer cells and macrophages. Nonmedicinal ingredients: gelatin. Security sealed bottles of 45, 100 and 168. Store at room temperature. Shelf-life of five years.

(Shown in Product Identification Section)

Colestid® ℞

colestipol HCl

Oral Antihypercholesterolemic

Pfizer

PHARMACOLOGY: Colestipol is hygroscopic, water insoluble, and it is neither hydrolyzed by digestive enzymes nor is it absorbed. Colestipol binds with bile acids in the intestine forming a complex that is excreted in the feces. This nonsystemic action results in a continuous, partial removal of bile acids from the enterohepatic circulation preventing their reabsorption. This increased fecal loss of bile acids due to colestipol administration leads to an increased oxidation of cholesterol to bile acids. This results in an increase in the number of hepatic low density lipoprotein (LDL) receptors, and consequently an increased uptake of LDL and a decrease in serum/plasma beta lipoprotein or total and LDL cholesterol levels. Although colestipol produces an increase in the hepatic synthesis of cholesterol in man, serum cholesterol levels fall.

INDICATIONS: As adjunctive therapy to diet and exercise for the reduction of elevated serum cholesterol in patients with primary hypercholesterolemia (elevated low density lipoproteins). Such a reduction of serum cholesterol may reduce the risks of atherosclerotic coronary artery disease and myocardial infarction. In patients with combined hypercholesterolemia and hypertriglyceridemia, colestipol may be useful in lowering elevated cholesterol but is not indicated where hypertriglyceridemia is the abnormality of most concern.

Patients should be placed on a standard cholesterol-lowering diet at least equivalent to the American Heart Association (AHA) Step 1 Diet, which should be continued during treatment. If appropriate, a programme of weight control and physical exercise should be implemented.

CONTRAINDICATIONS: In patients with complete biliary obstruction where bile is not secreted into the intestine.

In individuals who have shown hypersensitivity to any of the components of the products.

In addition, the orange granules are contraindicated in phenylketonurics as each 7.5 g contains 18.2 mg phenylalanine.

WARNINGS: The granules and orange granules should never be taken in its dry form. Esophageal spasm or respiratory distress can result from attempting to swallow the granules dry. The granules and orange granules should always be mixed with water, beverages, cereals, soups or other foods with sufficient fluid for mixing.

PRECAUTIONS: Studies have suggested that control of elevated cholesterol and triglycerides may not lessen the danger of cardiovascular related mortality, although the incidence of nonfatal myocardial infarctions is decreased.

Before instituting therapy with colestipol, diseases contributing to increased serum cholesterol such as hypothyroidism, diabetes mellitus, nephrotic syndrome, dysproteinemias and obstructive liver disease should be ruled out or specifically treated. In addition, the current medications of the patient should be reviewed for their potential to increase serum LDL-C or total cholesterol.

It should be verified that an elevated LDL-C is responsible for the high total cholesterol level, especially in those patients with marked elevations of HDL-C and elevations of triglyceride over 4.5 mmol/L (400 mg/100 mL). An LDL-C level may be estimated using the following formula:

$$\text{LDL-C} = \text{total cholesterol} - \text{HDL-C} - \frac{\text{triglyceride}}{2.19}$$

All units are in mmol/L. The accuracy of this approximation falls when triglycerides are greater than 4.5 mmol/L. Patients with triglyceride levels above 4.5 mmol/L should not be considered for initial therapy with colestipol alone. Instead, the use of colestipol given in combination with another lipid lowering agent like a fibrate or niacin would be more beneficial.

When used as the sole therapy, colestipol does not improve hypertriglyceridemia and in fact may elevate serum triglycerides. This elevation is generally transient, but may sometimes persist. If a significant rise in triglyceride level occurs, consideration should be given to dose reduction, drug discontinuation or combination therapy with another lipid lowering agent.

Appropriate use of serum lipid profiles (with LDL-C and triglyceride levels) at regular intervals is advised so that therapeutic effect can be determined.

Colestipol may produce or worsen pre-existing constipation. In patients with pre-existing constipation, the starting dose should be 5 g colestipol granules, or 2 g colestipol tablets, given once or twice daily. Increased fluid and fiber intake is encouraged to alleviate the constipation. A stool softener may be added if needed. If the initial dose is well tolerated, the dosage may be increased (by daily increments of 5 g colestipol granules or 2 to 4 g colestipol tablets) at monthly intervals. If the constipation worsens or the desired therapeutic response is not achieved at the maximum recommended dose, then combination lipid-lowering therapy or alternate therapy should be considered. Particular effort should be made to avoid constipation in patients with symptomatic coronary artery disease. Constipation may aggravate hemorrhoids.

Since colestipol is a chloride form of an anion exchange resin, there is a possibility that prolonged use may lead to the development of hyperchloremic acidosis.

Carcinogenesis and Mutagenesis: In studies conducted in rats in which cholestyramine resin (a bile acid sequestering agent similar to colestipol) was used as a tool to investigate the role of various intestinal factors, such as fat, bile salts and microbial flora, in the development of intestinal tumors induced by potent carcinogens, the incidence of such tumors was observed to be greater in cholestyramine resin treated rats than in control rats. The relevance of this laboratory observation from studies in rats with cholestyramine resin to the clinical use of colestipol is not known. When colestipol was administered in the diet to rats for 18 months, there was no evidence of any drug related intestinal tumor formation. In the Ames assay, colestipol was not mutagenic.

Pregnancy: The use of colestipol in pregnancy or lactation or by women of childbearing potential requires that the benefits of drug therapy be weighed against the possible hazards to the mother and the child. Safety for use in pregnant women has not been established.

Lactation: See Pregnancy.

Children: The use of colestipol in children is limited. Clinical trials conducted in children with the granules have usually employed doses of 5 to 20 g/day. The National Cholesterol Education Program (NCEP) Expert Panel recommends drug therapy be considered in children 10 years or older, who have previously undergone an adequate trial of diet therapy but still have unacceptably high serum cholesterol levels. In certain situations where a young child has extremely high serum cholesterol levels, drug treatment may even be initiated before 10 years of age. If the child is started on drug therapy, a carefully assessed diet therapy should also be continued in order to obtain optimal results.

However, the safety of using the tablets in patients under the age of 18 years has not been established.

Because bile acid sequestrants may interfere with the absorption of fat-soluble vitamins, appropriate monitoring of growth and development is essential if colestipol is used in children.

Geriatrics: Appropriate studies on the relationship of age to the effects of colestipol have not been performed in the geriatric population. However, patients over 60 years of age may be more likely to experience gastrointestinal side effects, as well as adverse nutritional effects.

Effect on Vitamin Absorption: Due to the action of colestipol in sequestering bile acids, colestipol may theoretically interfere with normal fat absorption and thus may reduce the absorption of folic acid and fat soluble vitamins A, D and K. In general, supplementation of vitamins A, D and K is not needed unless a deficiency is shown to exist.

Chronic use of colestipol has been rarely associated with an increased bleeding tendency due to hypoprothrombinemia resulting from vitamin K deficiency. This deficiency can be corrected with oral vitamin K.

Drug Interactions: (See Pharmacology.) Since colestipol is an anion-exchange resin, it may have a strong affinity for anions other than the bile acids. Colestipol does not bind in vivo with an affinity and to an extent that results in clinically significant drug-drug interactions with all anionic compounds or weak acids. Clinically relevant reductions in bioavailability have been found for several weakly acid drugs (summarized below). However, other weakly acid (anionic) drugs have been studied and found not to be affected by colestipol coadministration. The drugs that are affected by coadministration of colestipol vary widely in pharmacologic effect and mechanisms, in magnitude of doses, and in physicochemical characteristics. Therefore, it is not possible to predict a priori whether or not coadministration with colestipol will interfere with absorption. Unless a particular drug has been studied, it should be assumed that concomitantly administered drugs have the potential for interacting with colestipol. **Since colestipol may bind other drugs given concurrently, patients should take other drugs at least 1 hour before or 4 hours after colestipol (or at as great an interval as possible) to avoid impeding their absorption.**

Interactions between colestipol and drugs can be divided into 2 major categories: substantially decreased bioavailability (defined as a decrease of >20%), and little or no effect on bioavailability (defined as a decrease of <20%).

Drug Interactions with Other Lipid-Lowering Drugs: Fibric Acid Derivatives: Based upon the definitions above, colestipol reduced the bioavailability of gemfibrozil (C_{max} reduced 27%, AUC reduced 30%) when both drugs were administered together; this interaction was avoided by dosing gemfibrozil either 2 hours before or after colestipol. Colestipol had little or no effect on the bioavailability of clofibrate and fenofibrate.

Niacin (nicotinic acid): Niacin plasma concentrations were highly variable among subjects due in part to rapid absorption and elimination of niacin. The median C_{max} and AUC were 35 and 48% lower when niacin was given with colestipol, but were not statistically significantly different from a niacin alone treatment. Concomitant multiple dosing of colestipol and niacin had minimal effect on niacin absorption. The interaction between colestipol and niacin does not appear to be clinically significant as evidenced by the additive efficacy of combination colestipol and niacin.

Other Classes of Lipid-lowering Drugs: Colestipol drug interaction studies have not been conducted with HMG-CoA reductase inhibitors (i.e. lovastatin, simvastatin, etc.) or with probucol. However, clinical studies indicate that the cholesterol-lowering effects of colestipol and HMG-CoA reductase inhibitors are additive; therefore, a clinically significant drug interaction is unlikely. Other drug interaction studies have been conducted with cholestyramine (another bile acid sequestrant) and various HMG-CoA reductase inhibitors. Cholestyramine significantly reduced the bioavailability of fluvastatin and pravastatin when the HMG-CoA reductase inhibitor was given 1 hour before and up to 4 hours after the cholestyramine dose. However, in clinical studies cholestyramine and HMG0-CoA reductase inhibitors had additive cholesterol-lowering effects. The relevance of these cholestyramine drug interaction findings to colestipol is unknown.

Drug Interactions with Other Drugs: Antibiotics: When coadministered, colestipol significantly reduced the bioavailability of penicillin G (C_{max} reduced 79%, AUC reduced 84%) and tetracycline (C_{max} reduced 52% and AUC reduced 59%). Colestipol had little effect on clindamycin bioavailability.

Anticoagulants: Colestipol had little effect on the bioavailability of warfarin sodium or phenprocoumon.

Anticonvulsants: Colestipol had little or no effect on the bioavailability of phenytoin or carbamazepine.

Antihypertensives: Repeated doses of colestipol given prior to a single dose of propranolol have been reported to decrease propranolol absorption. However, in a follow-up study involving healthy volunteers, single dose administration of colestipol and propranolol, twice a day administration for 5 doses of both agents, did not affect the extent of propranolol absorption, but had a small yet statistically significant effect on its rate of absorption. The time to reach maximum concentration was delayed approximately 30 minutes. Therefore, patients on propranolol should be observed when colestipol either added or deleted from a therapeutic regimen. The effects on the absorption of other beta-blockers have not been determined. Colestipol had little effect on the bioavailability of methyldopa.

Anti-inflammatory Agents: Colestipol had little effect on the bioavailability of ASA.

Cardiac Glycosides: Particular caution should be exercised with digitalis preparations because there are conflicting results about the effects of colestipol on the bioavailability of digoxin and digitoxin in clinical and animal studies. In a single-dose, crossover study in healthy volunteers, the C_{max} and AUC of digoxin did not differ when digoxin was coadministered with colestipol vs. when digoxin was given alone (C_{max} was 118% and AUC was 97% of the values determined with digoxin alone). Since the potential for binding of digoxin and digitoxin to colestipol may exist, the serum digoxin and digitoxin levels should be monitored during periods of administration or discontinuation of colestipol.

Diuretics: Colestipol significantly lowered the bioavailability of hydrochlorothiazide (C_{max} reduced 14%, 24 hour urinary excretion reduced 31%), chlorothiazide (urinary excretion reduced 58%) and furosemide (C_{max} reduced 86%, AUC reduced 79%).

Hypoglycemic Agents: Colestipol had little effect on the bioavailability of tolbutamide.

Nonmedicinal Ingredients: 1) Colloidal Silicon Dioxide: The granules and the tablets contain Colloidal Silicon Dioxide that can adversely influence patients with irritable bowel syndrome, diverticulosis and diverticulitis. 2) Aspartame: The orange granules contain aspartame. Phenylketonurics are sensitive to the phenylalanine in aspartame.

ADVERSE EFFECTS: The most frequently encountered adverse effects in clinical trials with colestipol are gastrointestinal. Constipation is the major single complaint and at times is severe and occasionally accompanied by fecal impaction. Hemorrhoids may be aggravated. Most instances of constipation are mild, transient and controlled with standard treatment. See Precautions for recommendation on how to minimize constipation side effect. Predisposing factors for most complaints of constipation are high dose and increasing age (more than 60 years of age).

Less frequent gastrointestinal complaints are abdominal discomfort (abdominal pain and cramping), bloating, flatulence, indigestion, heartburn, nausea, vomiting, diarrhea and loose stools.

Peptic ulceration, gastrointestinal irritation and bleeding, cholecystitis and cholelithiasis have been rarely reported and are not necessarily drug related. Bleeding hemorrhoids and blood in the stool have been infrequently reported.

Other rarely reported adverse reactions include rash, urticaria, dermatitis, muscle and joint pains, arthritis, headache, dizziness, anxiety, vertigo, drowsiness, anorexia, fatigue, weakness, and shortness of breath.

Transient and modest elevations of AST, ALT and serum alkaline phosphatase were infrequently observed in patients treated with colestipol.

During initial registration studies for the granules, adverse reactions occurring at a frequency of 0.1% or more are listed by body system as follows:
Gastrointestinal: (10%): constipation; (1 to 5%): abdominal pain and distention, belching, flatulence, nausea, vomiting, diarrhea; (0.1 to 1%): peptic ulceration, gastrointestinal irritation and bleeding, cholecystitis, cholelithiasis.
Hypersensitivity: (0.1 to 1%): urticaria, dermatitis.
Musculoskeletal: (0.1 to 1%): muscle and joint pains, arthritis.
Neurologic: (0.1 to 1%): headache, dizziness, anxiety, vertigo, drowsiness.
Miscellaneous: (0.1 to 1%): anorexia, fatigue, weakness, shortness of breath.

OVERDOSE:

Symptoms: Overdosage with colestipol has not been reported. Should overdosage occur, the chief potential harm would be obstruction of the gastrointestinal tract. The location of such potential obstruction, the degree of obstruction and the presence or absence of normal gut motility would determine treatment.

Treatment: See Symptoms.

For management of a suspected drug overdose, CPhA recommends that you contact your **regional Poison Control Centre**. See the *CPS* Directory section for a list of Poison Control Centres.

DOSAGE: Treatment for elevated serum cholesterol levels should begin with dietary therapy. Patients should be placed on a standard cholesterol-lowering diet at least equivalent to the American Heart Association (AHA) Step 1 Diet, which should be continued during treatment. If appropriate, a programme of weight control and physical exercise should be implemented. A minimum of 6 months of dietary therapy and counselling should usually be undertaken before initiating drug therapy. Shorter periods can be considered in patients with severe elevations of LDL-C (greater than 225 mg/100 mL or 5.85 mmol/L) or with definite coronary heart disease. Drug therapy should be added to dietary therapy and not substituted for it.
Granules and Orange Granules: Adults: Recommended in doses of 5 to 30 g/day of colestipol given once or in divided doses. Initiation of therapy is recommended at 5 g either once or twice a day, with daily increments of 5 g no more frequently than at 1 month intervals.
Tablets: Adults: Recommended in doses of 2 to 16 g/day given once or in divided doses. Initiation of therapy is recommended at 2 g either once or twice a day. Dosage increments of 2 g once or twice daily may be instituted no more frequently than at 1 month intervals.

Serum cholesterol (total, fractionated and triglyceride levels) should be monitored periodically. Consideration should be given to reducing the dosage of colestipol if serum cholesterol levels fall below the targeted range, such as that recommended by the Second Report of the U.S. National Cholesterol Education Program (NCEP). If the desired serum cholesterol levels are not obtained at maximal colestipol doses with good compliance and acceptable side effects, combination lipid lowering therapy or alternate treatment should be considered.

According to the U.S. NCEP Expert Panel, children 10 years and older can be considered for drug therapy after an adequate trial of diet therapy alone is unsuccessful. If drug therapy is initiated, diet therapy should be continued in order to make the entire treatment regimen as effective as possible. The dose of colestipol used is not related to the body weight of the child but to the levels of total and LDL cholesterol after an adequate trial of diet therapy. Initially start the child on the lowest dose of the granules or orange granules. If needed, this dose is increased gradually over time in order to achieve the required total and LDL cholesterol levels. Breakfast and dinner are preferred times for the administration of this medication to children (see Precautions, Children).
Preparation: The granules and orange granules should always be taken mixed in a liquid such as water or a beverage; or in foods such as cereals, soups, yogurt, pudding, cottage cheese or pulpy fruits.

To avoid accidental inhalation or esophageal distress, the granules and orange granules should not be taken in their dry form.
With beverages: 1. Add the prescribed amount of granules or orange granules to a glass (100 mL or more) of water, milk, flavored drink, juice (orange, tomato, pineapple, etc.), or carbonated beverage. A heavy or pulpy juice may minimize complaints relative to consistency. An unsweetened juice may improve palatability. 2. Stir the mixture until the medication is completely suspended. The granules and orange granules will **not** dissolve in the liquid. 3. After drinking the mixture, rinse the glass with a small amount of additional beverage to make sure all the medicine is taken.
With cereals, soups and fruits: The granules or orange granules may be taken with milk in hot or regular breakfast cereals, or in soups with a high fluid content. It may also be added to fruits that are pulpy such as crushed pineapple, pears, peaches, or fruit cocktail.

The tablets should be swallowed whole. Do not cut, chew or crush the tablets. The prescribed amount of tablets can be taken with water or any other appropriate fluid based on patient preference. The tablets should be taken with meals.

INFORMATION FOR THE PATIENT: Published in e-CPS, available by subscription at www.e-cps.ca.

SUPPLIED: Granules: Each packet contains: colestipol 5 g. Nonmedicinal ingredients: Colloidal Silicon Dioxide. Cartons of 30 foil packets.
Orange Granules: Each packet contains: 7.5 g orange granules equivalent to 5 g colestipol. Nonmedicinal ingredients: aspartame (phenylalanine 18.2 mg/7.5 g granules), artificial flavor, beta carotene, citric acid, glycerin, maltol, mannitol, methylcellulose, natural flavor. Cartons of 30 foil packets.
Tablets: Each light yellow, film-coated tablet contains: colestipol HCl 1 g. Nonmedicinal ingredients: carnauba wax, cellulose acetate phthalate, colloidal silicon dioxide, magnesium stearate, hypromellose, povidone and triacetin. The tablets contain no calories. Bottles of 120.

Store at controlled room temperature (15 to 30°C). Protect from moisture and humidity.

(Shown in Product Identification Section)

CO Levetiracetam [Pr]
levetiracetam
Antiepileptic

Cobalt

SUPPLIED: 250 mg: Each blue, oval-shaped tablet, with "LE 250" on one side and "⊳" on the other side, contains: levetiracetam 250 mg. Nonmedicinal ingredients: colloidal silicon dioxide, cornstarch, FD&C Blue #1, FD & C Blue #2, FD & C Red #40, FD & C Yellow #6, macrogol, magnesium stearate, polyvinyl alcohol - part hydrolysed, povidone, purified talc, talc and titanium dioxide. Bottles of 100.
500 mg: Each yellow, oval-shaped tablet, with "LE 500" on one side and "⊳" on the other side, contains: levetiracetam 500 mg. Nonmedicinal ingredients: colloidal silicon dioxide, cornstarch, D&C Yellow #10 Aluminum Lake, FD&C Blue #2, FD & C Red #40, iron oxide yellow, macrogol, magnesium stearate, polyvinyl alcohol - part hydrolysed, povidone, purified talc, talc and titanium dioxide. Bottles of 100 and 500.
750 mg: Each orange, oval-shaped tablet, with "LE 750" on one side and "⊳" on the other side, contains: levetiracetam 750 mg. Nonmedicinal ingredients: colloidal silicon dioxide, cornstarch, D&C Yellow #10 Aluminum Lake, FD & C Blue #2, FD&C Yellow #6, macrogol, magnesium stearate, polyvinyl alcohol - part hydrolysed, povidone, purified talc, talc and titanium dioxide. Bottles of 100.

The reader is invited to consult CPhA's monograph **Fluoroquinolones**.

CO Levofloxacin [Pr]
levofloxacin
Antibacterial

Cobalt

SUPPLIED: 250 mg: Each pink, film-coated, oval-shaped, biconvex tablet, with "LO 250" on one side and "⊳" on the other, contains: levofloxacin 250 mg (as levofloxacin hemihydrate). Nonmedicinal ingredients: colloidal anhydrous silica, crospovidone, hydroxypropylcellulose, microcrystalline cellulose and sodium stearyl fumarate; film-coating: FD&C blue #1, FD&C red #40, FD&C yellow #6, iron oxide red, polyethylene glycol, polyvinyl alcohol, talc and titanium dioxide. HDPE bottles of 50 and 100. Store at room temperature (15-30°C) in well-closed containers.
500 mg: Each peach-coloured, film-coated, oval-shaped, biconvex tablet, with "LO 500" on one side and "⊳" on the other, contains: levofloxacin 500 mg (as levofloxacin hemihydrate). Nonmedicinal ingredients: colloidal anhydrous silica, crospovidone, hydroxypropylcellulose, microcrystalline cellulose and sodium stearyl fumarate; film-coating: iron oxide black, iron oxide red, iron oxide yellow, polyethylene glycol, polyvinyl alcohol, talc and titanium dioxide. HDPE bottles of 50 and 100. Store at room temperature (15-30°C) in well-closed containers.
750: Each white to off-white, film-coated, oval-shaped, biconvex tablet, with "LO 750" on one side and "⊳" on the other, contains: levofloxacin 750 mg (as levofloxacin hemihydrate). Nonmedicinal ingredients: colloidal anhydrous silica, crospovidone, hydroxypropylcellulose, microcrystalline cellulose and sodium stearyl fumarate; film coating: polyethylene glycol, polyvinyl alcohol, titanium oxide and talc. HDPE bottles of 50 and 100. Store at room temperature (15-30°C) in well-closed containers.

The reader is invited to consult CPhA's monograph **ACE Inhibitors**.

CO Lisinopril [Pr]
lisinopril
Angiotensin Converting Enzyme Inhibitor

Cobalt

SUPPLIED: 5 mg: Each pink, round, biconvex tablet marked "L" scoreline "5" on one side and "⊳" on the other side contains: lisinopril 5 mg. Nonmedicinal ingredients: calcium hydrogen phosphate dihydrate, colloidal anhydrous silica, magnesium stearate, maize starch, mannitol, pregelatinized starch and red iron oxide. Blisters of 30. HDPE bottles of 100 and 500. Store at 15-30°C.
10 mg: Each pink, round, biconvex tablet marked "L" scoreline "10" on one side and "⊳" on the other side contains: lisinopril 10 mg. Nonmedicinal ingredients: calcium hydrogen phosphate dihydrate, colloidal anhydrous silica, magnesium stearate, maize starch, mannitol, pregelatinized starch and red iron oxide. Blisters of 30. HDPE bottles of 100 and 500. Store at 15-30°C.
20 mg: Each pink, round, biconvex tablet with "L" scoreline "20" on one side and "⊳" on the other side contains: lisinopril 20 mg. Nonmedicinal ingredients: calcium hydrogen phosphate dihydrate, colloidal anhydrous silica, magnesium stearate, maize starch, mannitol, pregelatinized starch and red iron oxide. Blisters of 30. HDPE bottles of 100 and 500. Store at 15-30°C.

Colistimethate for Injection U.S.P. [Pr]
sodium colistimethate
Antibiotic

SteriMax

SUPPLIED: Each vial of sterile, lyophilized powder contains: sodium colistimethate equivalent to 150 mg of colistimethate base. Reconstituted solution provides sodium colistimethate equivalent to 75 mg colistin base per mL. Single unit cartons. Store sterile dry powder under controlled room temperature (15-30°C).

The reader is invited to consult CPhA's monograph **HMG-CoA Reductase Inhibitors**.

CO Lovastatin [Pr]
lovastatin
Lipid Metabolism Regulator

Cobalt

SUPPLIED: 20 mg: Each blue, octagonal, flat-faced, bevelled-edge, scored tablet, engraved with "LS" over "20" on one side and "⊳" on the other side, contains: lovastatin 20 mg. Nonmedicinal ingredients: butylated hydroxyanisole, D&C Yellow No. 10, Indigo Carmine 20 mg, Indigo Carmine 40 mg, lactose, magnesium stearate, microcrystalline cellulose and pregelatinized maize starch. Gluten-free. Bottles of 100 and 500. Unit dose blisters of 30. Keep container tightly closed and store at 15-30°C. Protect from light.
40 mg: Each green, octagonal, flat-faced, bevelled-edge, scored tablet, engraved with "LS" over "40" on one side and "⊳" on the other side, contains: lovastatin 40 mg. Nonmedicinal ingredients: butylated hydroxyanisole, D&C Yellow No. 10, Indigo Carmine 20 mg, Indigo Carmine 40 mg, lactose, magnesium stearate, microcrystalline cellulose and pregelatinized maize starch. Gluten-free. Bottles of 100. Unit dose blisters of 30. Keep container tightly closed and store at 15-30°C. Protect from light.

Colyte®
polyethylene glycol—electrolytes
Colon Electrolyte Lavage Preparation

PendoPharm

SUPPLIED: Each disposable 4 L jug contains: 240 g polyethylene glycol 3350, sodium chloride 5.84 g, potassium chloride 2.98 g, sodium bicarbonate 6.72 g, sodium sulfate 22.72 g. Colyte also contains Magnasweet, pineapple flavour and sodium saccharin.

When reconstituted with water, final 4-litres solution contains 125 mEq/L sodium, 10 mEq/L potassium, 20 mEq/L bicarbonate, 80 mEq/L sulfate, 35 mEq/L chloride and 17.9 mEq/L polyethylene glycol 3350. The reconstituted solution is isosmotic and has a mild fruit flavour.

Reconstituted solution should be used within 48 hours after mixing if stored at room temperature. If kept refrigerated at 2-8°C, use within 30 days. Discard unused portion.

Combantrin®
pyrantel pamoate
Anthelmintic

McNeil Consumer Healthcare

Date of Revision: June 2, 2008

PHARMACOLOGY: Pyrantel exerts its anthelmintic effect by interfering with the neuromuscular function of the parasite. It is also a cholinesterase inhibitor and a ganglionic stimulant.

The anthelmintic activity of pyrantel has been demonstrated in several animal models. These tests carried out in mice and dogs showed the compound to be effective against intestinal nematodes representative of those found in humans, such as pinworms, large roundworms and hookworms. It is poorly absorbed by the intestinal mucosa so that its activity is confined to the lumen of the bowel. In the dog, the peak plasma levels were low and similarly the tissue levels were low. Less than 15% is excreted via the urine, the major proportion of the dose being excreted in the feces.

INDICATIONS: For the treatment of infection with any of the following gastrointestinal parasites when these are present either alone or as a mixed infection. *Enterobius vermicularis* (threadworm, pinworm) *Ascaris lumbricoides* (roundworm), *Ancylostoma duodenale* (hookworm), *Necator americanus* (hookworm), *Trichostrongylus colubriformis* and *T. orientalis*.

Pyrantel should be used for the treatment of infection with one or more of these parasites in both adults and children. It is well tolerated and will not stain the oral mucosa upon ingestion or the clothing by fecal contamination. The presence of an infection with any of the 5 parasites in one member of a family or group of persons in close proximity may indicate unidentified infection in other members. In these circumstances, pyrantel administration to all the family or group members is recommended. (Rigorous cleaning of living quarters and clothing to destroy helminthic ova will help prevent reinfection.)

CONTRAINDICATIONS: In patients who are hypersensitive to the drug or to any of the components of the product.

WARNINGS: *Pregnancy:* Animal reproductive studies have not resulted in any teratogenic effects, but pyrantel has not been studied in the pregnant patient. It should not be used in pregnant women, unless, in the judgment of the physician, it is deemed essential for the welfare of the patient.

Lactation: It is not known whether pyrantel is excreted in breast milk; nursing should be discontinued if use of this drug is deemed essential.

Children: Pyrantel should not be used in children under the age of 1 year because safety in this age group has not been established.

PRECAUTIONS: Should be used with caution in patients with pre-existing hepatic dysfunction, as minor transient elevations of AST have occurred in a small percentage of patients.

Occupational Hazards: The effect of pyrantel on the ability to drive and operate heavy machinery has not been studied. There is no evidence to suggest that pyrantel pamoate may affect these abilities.

ADVERSE EFFECTS: Pyrantel is well tolerated. The infrequent side effects consist for the most part of vomiting and diarrhea. Headache, insomnia, irritability, drowsiness, dizziness, anorexia, abdominal cramps, nausea and rash have seldom been reported. While adverse reactions have been few at the recommended therapeutic dose of 11 mg/kg, they become considerably more frequent at higher dose concentrations without significant gain in therapeutic effect. No significant changes in total blood count, urinalysis, AST, ALT, alkaline phosphatase and BUN have been observed.

OVERDOSE:

Symptoms: Because of its low rate of absorption, plasma concentrations are low. The probable effects of overdosage would include autonomic dysfunction, muscle spasm, twitches and weakness, prostration and ultimately asphyxia due to muscular paralysis.

Treatment: No specific antidote is known. Early gastric lavage and measures to support respiration and blood pressure may be advisable.

For management of a suspected drug overdose, CPhA recommends that you contact your **regional Poison Control Centre**. See the *CPS* Directory section for a list of Poison Control Centres.

DOSAGE: Pyrantel base should be administered in a single oral dose determined on the basis of body weight, i.e., 11 mg/kg. Treatment of pinworm and roundworm: See Table 1.

Table 1: Combantrin

Treatment of Pinworm and Roundworm

Patient Weight	Dosage	Oral Suspension	Tablets
(over 1 year old and)			
11 kg or less	125 mg	2.5 mL	1 tablet
12–23 kg	250 mg	5 mL	2 tablets
24–45 kg	500 mg	10 mL	4 tablets
46–68 kg	750 mg	15 mL	6 tablets
69 kg and over	1000 mg	20 mL	8 tablets

Treatment of Hookworm: The same dosage as in Table 1 given once daily for 3 days.

Pyrantel may be administered without regard to ingestion of food or time of day, and purging is not necessary prior to or during therapy. On rare occasions a second dose has been necessary to eradicate pinworm or roundworm infection. Pyrantel may be taken with milk or fruit juice. The presence of an infection of Enterobius in one patient may indicate unidentified infections in other members of the family. Pyrantel pamoate treatment for all family members is recommended. Rigorous cleaning of living quarters and clothing to destroy helminthic ova and strict attention to personal hygiene will help prevent reinfection. It will not stain the oral mucosa upon ingestion or the clothing by fecal contamination.

Children: Use in infants under 1 year is not recommended because safety in this age group has not been established.

INFORMATION FOR THE PATIENT: Published in e-CPS, available by subscription at www.e-cps.ca.

SUPPLIED: Suspension: Each mL of caramel-flavored suspension contains: pyrantel pamoate 144 mg equivalent to 50 mg of pyrantel base. Nonmedicinal ingredients: citric acid, flavor, glycerin, lecithin, magnesium aluminum silicate, polysorbate, povidone, simethicone, sodium benzoate, sorbitol and water. Tartrazine-free. Amber glass bottles of 45 mL. The suspension must be kept in the amber glass container to protect from light.

Tablets: Each round, pale orange, scored tablet, contains: pyrantel pamoate 360 mg equivalent to 125 mg of pyrantel base. Nonmedicinal ingredients: alginic acid, cornstarch, FD&C Yellow #6, magnesium stearate and sodium lauryl sulfate. Tartrazine-free. Amber plastic blister packages of 12. Tablets must be kept in the amber blister package to protect from light.

Store between 15 and 30°C.

Combigan® ℞
brimonidine tartrate—timolol maleate
Elevated Intraocular Pressure Therapy

Allergan

Date of Preparation: November 25, 2003
Date of Revision: August 21, 2007

SUMMARY PRODUCT INFORMATION:

Route of Administration	Dosage Form/ Strength	Clinically Relevant Nonmedicinal Ingredients
Ophthalmic	Solution, 0.2% brimonidine tartrate/timolol 0.5% as timolol maleate	Contains 0.005% benzalkonium chloride as preservative For a complete listing see Dosage Forms, Composition and Packaging.

INDICATIONS AND CLINICAL USE: COMBIGAN (brimonidine tartrate 0.2%/timolol maleate as timolol 0.5%) ophthalmic solution is indicated for the control of intraocular pressure in patients with chronic open-angle glaucoma or ocular hypertension who are insufficiently responsive to IOP reducing monotherapy **and** when the use of COMBIGAN is considered appropriate.

COMBIGAN is also indicated for reduction of long term fluctuation in IOP. In addition to controlling IOP, COMBIGAN reduces long term variability, or fluctuation, in IOP. Together, reductions in IOP and in IOP fluctuation are expected to slow the progression of visual field loss in patients with glaucoma.

Diabetics: Results from pivotal trials indicate that the mean change from baseline IOP was significantly lower ($p < 0.001$) with COMBIGAN than with either brimonidine tartrate alone or timolol maleate alone for both patients with diabetes and those without diabetes. See Warnings and Precautions for considerations during use in this population.

Patients Using Systemic Beta-blockers: Results from pivotal trials indicate that the mean change from baseline IOP was significantly lower ($p < 0.001$) with COMBIGAN than with either brimonidine tartrate alone or timolol maleate alone for both patients treated with systemic beta-blockers and those who were not. Topical beta-blockers are known to be less effective in patients on systemic beta-blockers. See Drug Interactions. This analysis shows that this is not the case with COMBIGAN, despite having timolol as one of the ingredients.

Geriatrics (>65 years of age): Based on evidence from clinical studies and experience, use in the geriatric population is not associated with any differences in safety or effectiveness. Use as is for adult patients.

Pediatrics (<18 years of age): Not recommended for paediatric use. The safety and efficacy of COMBIGAN in paediatric patients have not been established in clinical trials.

CONTRAINDICATIONS: Note: COMBIGAN is a combination of brimonidine tartrate 0.2% and timolol 0.5% as timolol maleate. When COMBIGAN is prescribed, the relevant Product Monographs for brimonidine tartrate and/or timolol maleate should be consulted.

- Patients who are hypersensitive to brimonidine tartrate, timolol maleate or to any ingredient in the formulation or component of the container. For a complete listing, see Dosage Forms, Composition and Packaging.
- Patients with bronchial asthma or a history of bronchial asthma; severe chronic obstructive pulmonary disease
- Patients with sinus bradycardia; second- or third-degree atrioventricular block; overt cardiac failure; cardiogenic shock
- Patients receiving monoamine oxidase (MAO) inhibitor therapy

WARNINGS AND PRECAUTIONS: General: Note: COMBIGAN is a combination of brimonidine tartrate 0.2% and timolol 0.5% as timolol maleate. When COMBIGAN is prescribed, the relevant Product Monographs for brimonidine tartrate and/or timolol maleate should be consulted.

For topical ophthalmic use only.

If signs of serious reactions or hypersensitivity occur, discontinue use of this preparation.

As with many topically applied ophthalmic drugs, this drug is absorbed systemically. The same adverse reactions found with systemic administration of beta-adrenergic blocking agents may occur with topical administration of COMBIGAN (brimonidine tartrate 0.2%/timolol maleate as timolol 0.5%) ophthalmic solution. For example, severe respiratory reactions and cardiac reactions, including death due to bronchospasm in patients with asthma, and rarely death in association with cardiac failure, have been reported following systemic or ophthalmic administration of timolol maleate. See Contraindications.

Cardiovascular: Because of the timolol maleate component, cardiac failure should be adequately controlled before beginning therapy with COMBIGAN. In patients with a history of severe cardiac disease, signs of cardiac failure should be watched for and pulse rates should be checked.

Caution should be exercised in treating patients with severe cardiovascular disease.

Use with caution in patients with cerebral or coronary insufficiency, Raynaud's phenomenon, orthostatic hypotension or thromboangiitis obliterans.

Because of potential effects of beta-adrenergic blocking agents on blood pressure and pulse, these agents should be used with caution in patients with cerebrovascular insufficiency. If signs or symptoms suggesting reduced cerebral blood flow develop following initiation of therapy with COMBIGAN, alternative therapy should be considered.

Endocrine and Metabolism: Beta-adrenergic blocking agents should be administered with caution in patients subject to spontaneous hypoglycaemia or to diabetic patients (especially those with labile diabetes) who are receiving insulin or oral hypoglycaemia agents. Beta-adrenergic receptor blocking agents may mask the signs and symptoms of acute hypoglycaemia.

Beta-adrenergic blocking agents may mask certain clinical signs of hyperthyroidism (e.g., tachycardia). Patients suspected of developing thyrotoxicosis should be managed carefully to avoid abrupt withdrawal of beta-adrenergic blocking agents that might precipitate a thyroid storm.

Hepatic/Biliary/Pancreatic: COMBIGAN has not been studied in patients with hepatic impairment; caution should be exercised in treating such patients.

Musculoskeletal: Beta-adrenergic blockade has been reported to increase muscle weakness consistent with certain myasthenic symptoms (e.g., diplopia, ptosis and generalized weakness). Timolol maleate has been reported rarely to increase muscle weakness in some patients with myasthenia gravis or myasthenic symptoms.

Ophthalmologic: COMBIGAN should not be used alone in the treatment of acute angle-closure glaucoma.

COMBIGAN contains the preservative benzalkonium chloride, which may be deposited in soft contact lenses; therefore, COMBIGAN should not be administered while wearing these lenses. The lenses should be removed before application of the drops and not be reinserted earlier than 15 minutes after use.

Choroidal detachment after filtration procedures has been reported with administration of aqueous suppressant therapy (e.g., timolol maleate, acetazolamide). Management of eyes with chronic or recurrent choroidal detachment should include stopping all forms of aqueous suppressant therapy and treating endogenous inflammation vigorously.

There have been reports of bacterial keratitis associated with the use of multiple dose containers of topical ophthalmic products. These containers had been inadvertently contaminated by patients who, in most cases, had a concurrent corneal disease or a disruption of the ocular epithelial surface.

Peri-Operative Considerations: The necessity or desirability of withdrawal of beta-adrenergic blocking agents prior to major surgery is controversial. If necessary during surgery, the effects of beta-adrenergic blocking agents may be reversed by sufficient doses of such agonists as isoproterenol, dopamine, dobutamine or levarterenol.

Psychiatric: COMBIGAN should be used with caution in patients with depression.

Renal: COMBIGAN has not been studied in patients with renal impairment; caution should be exercised in treating such patients. In patients with severe renal impairment on dialysis, treatment with timolol maleate has been associated with pronounced hypotension.

Sensitivity/Resistance: Because of the brimonidine tartrate component COMBIGAN should be used with caution in patients with known hypersensitivity to other alpha-adrenoceptor agonists.

While taking beta-blockers, patients with a history of atopy or a history of severe anaphylactic reaction to a variety of allergens may be more reactive to repeated accidental, diagnostic, or therapeutic challenge with such allergens. These patients may be unresponsive to the usual doses of epinephrine used to treat anaphylactic reactions since timolol maleate may blunt the beta agonist effect of epinephrine. In such cases, alternatives to epinephrine should be considered.

Special Populations: Pregnant Women: There are no adequate and well-controlled studies of COMBIGAN in pregnant women. Because animal reproduction studies are not always predictive of human response, COMBIGAN should be used during pregnancy only if the potential benefit to the mother justifies the potential risk to the fetus.

There has been no experience with exposure during pregnancy in clinical trials.

Nursing Women: Timolol maleate has been detected in human milk following oral and ophthalmic drug administration. It is not known whether brimonidine tartrate is excreted in human milk, although in animal studies, brimonidine tartrate has been shown to be excreted in breast milk. Because of the potential for serious adverse reactions from timolol maleate or brimonidine tartrate in nursing infants, a decision should be made whether to discontinue nursing or to discontinue the drug, taking into account the importance of the drug to the mother.

Pediatrics (<18 years of age): The use of COMBIGAN in pediatric patients is currently not recommended. Several serious adverse reactions have been reported in association with the administration of brimonidine tartrate ophthalmic solution 0.2% to infants in the age range of 28 days to 3 months. (See Adverse Reactions.)

Monitoring and Laboratory Tests: Patients prescribed IOP-lowering medication should be routinely monitored for IOP.

Occupational Hazards: COMBIGAN, as with other similar medications, can potentially cause fatigue and/or drowsiness in some patients. Patients who engage in hazardous activities should be cautioned of the potential for a decrease in mental alertness.

ADVERSE REACTIONS: Adverse Drug Reaction Overview: Based on 12 month clinical data, the most commonly reported adverse drug reactions were conjunctival hyperaemia (approximately 15% of patients) and burning sensation in the eye (approximately 11% of patients). The majority of cases were mild and led to discontinuation rates of only 3.4% and 0.5% respectively.

Clinical Trial Adverse Drug Reactions: Because clinical trials are conducted under very specific conditions the adverse reaction rates observed in the clinical trials may not reflect the rates observed in practice and should not be compared to the rates in the clinical trials of another drug. Adverse drug reaction information from clinical trials is useful for identifying drug-related adverse events and for approximating rates.

In clinical trials, COMBIGAN (brimonidine tartrate 0.2%/timolol maleate as timolol 0.5%) ophthalmic solution was safe and well tolerated and had an acceptable safety profile. No adverse reactions unique to the combination product have been observed. All adverse reactions have been previously reported for brimonidine tartrate 0.2% or timolol maleate as timolol 0.5%, though at different incidences.

In two clinical studies including 385 patients treated with COMBIGAN for up to 12 months, treatment-related adverse events reported (pooled analysis) occurring at >1% with COMBIGAN are presented in Table 1.

Table 1: COMBIGAN

Treatment Related Adverse Events Occurring at >1% with COMBIGAN

Body System Preferred Term[a]	Combination N=385	Brimonidine Tartrate N=382	Timolol Maleate N=392
Body as a Whole			
Asthenia	8 (2.1%)	16 (4.2%)	3 (0.8%)
Headache	4 (1.0%)	13 (3.4%)[b]	4 (1.0%)
Digestive			
Oral dryness	8 (2.1%)	35 (9.2%)[b]	2 (0.5%)
Nervous			
Somnolence	6 (1.6%)	14 (3.7%)	2 (0.5%)
Special Senses (Ocular)			
Conjunctival hyperemia	56 (14.5%)	87 (22.8%)[b]	29 (7.4%)[c]
Burning sensation in eye	42 (10.9%)	28 (7.3%)	53 (13.5%)
Stinging sensation eye	24 (6.2%)	11 (2.9%)[c]	26 (6.6%)
Eye pruritus	21 (5.5%)	42 (11.0%)[b]	11 (2.8%)
Allergic conjunctivitis	20 (5.2%)	36 (9.4%)[b]	1 (0.3%)[c]
Conjunctival folliculosis	19 (4.9%)	35 (9.2%)[b]	7 (1.8%)[c]
Visual disturbance (blurred vision)	14 (3.6%)	16 (4.2%)	12 (3.1%)
Epiphora	12 (3.1%)	19 (5.0%)	5 (1.3%)
Eye dryness	12 (3.1%)	13 (3.4%)	4 (1.0%)[c]
Superficial punctate keratitis	12 (3.1%)	5 (1.3%)	4 (1.0%)[c]
Erythema eyelid	11 (2.9%)	12 (3.1%)	4 (1.0%)
Blepharitis	11 (2.9%)	11 (2.9%)	2 (0.5%)[c]
Eye discharge	10 (2.6%)	7 (1.8%)	3 (0.8%)[c]
Eyelid edema	10 (2.6%)	6 (1.6%)	2 (0.5%)[c]
Corneal erosion	10 (2.6%)	5 (1.3%)	11 (2.8%)
Eye pain	6 (1.6%)	10 (2.6%)	6 (1.5%)
Foreign body sensation	5 (1.3%)	17 (4.5%)[b]	7 (1.8%)

[a] Body system and preferred terms from Allergan's modified COSTART dictionary.
[b] Incidence with the Combination was significantly lower than with monotherapy (p ≤0.05.)
[c] Incidence with the Combination was significantly higher than with monotherapy (p ≤0.05).

Less Common Clinical Trial Adverse Drug Reactions (<1%): Cardiovascular: congestive heart failure, palpitations.
Gastrointestinal: taste perversion.
Nervous: dizziness, syncope.
Respiratory: rhinitis, nasal dryness.
Skin: allergic contact dermatitis.
Special Senses (ocular): visual acuity worsened, conjunctival oedema, follicular conjunctivitis, allergic belpharitis, conjunctivitis, vitreous floater, asthenopia, photophobia, papillary hypertrophy, eyelid pain, conjunctival blanching, corneal oedema, corneal infiltrates, vitreous detachment.
Abnormal Hematologic and Clinical Chemistry Findings: Common: Liver function tests abnormal.
Post-Market Adverse Drug Reactions: To date, there has not been any serious, unexpected adverse drug reactions related to treatment with COMBIGAN during post-marketing use.

Additional adverse events that have been reported with one of the components and may be potential adverse reactions for COMBIGAN are:

Brimonidine Tartrate: Adverse events reported in ≥1% and <8% of patients receiving ALPHAGAN (brimonidine tartrate) ophthalmic solution 0.2% include: Dizziness, upper respiratory symptoms, gastrointestinal symptoms, abnormal taste, nasal dryness, photophobia, tearing, conjunctival edema, conjunctival blanching, conjunctival papillae, and abnormal vision.

Several serious adverse reactions have been reported in association with the administration of brimonidine tartrate ophthalmic solution 0.2% to infants in the age range of 28 days to 3 months. These reactions included: bradycardia, hypotension, hypothermia, hypotonia, apnea, dyspnoea, hypoventilation, cyanosis and lethargy resulting in hospitalisation. Upon discontinuation of brimonidine tartrate 0.2% the infants recovered without sequelae.

For other detailed information, please consult the Product Monograph for brimonidine tartrate.

Timolol Maleate: Adverse events reported with timolol maleate include: Cardiovascular: Aggravation or precipitation of certain cardiovascular, pulmonary, and other disorders presumably related to effects of systemic beta-blockade (see Contraindications, Warnings and Precautions), including bradycardia; arrhythmia; hypotension; syncope; heart block; cerebrovascular accident; cerebral ischemia; palpitation; cardiac arrest; edema; claudication; Raynaud's phenomenon; cold hands and feet; congestive heart failure. Endocrine: masked symptoms of hypoglycaemia in insulindependent diabetics. Respiratory: bronchospasm (predominantly in patients with pre-existing bronchospastic disease); respiratory failure; dyspnea; cough. Body as a whole: chest pain; fatigue. Nervous System/Psychiatric: increase in signs and symptoms of myasthenia gravis; paresthesia; insomnia; nightmares; memory loss. Skin: alopecia; psoriasiform rash or exacerbation of psoriasis. Hypersensitivity: signs and symptoms of allergic reactions including angioedema, urticaria, localized and generalized rash. Immunologic: systemic lupus erythematous. Digestive: nausea; diarrhea, dyspepsia. Special Senses: decreased corneal sensitivity; visual disturbances including refractive changes (due to withdrawal of miotic therapy in some cases); diplopia; ptosis; choroidal detachment following filtration surgery; tinnitus. Urogenital: decreased libido, Peyronie's disease.

Causal Relationship Unknown: The following adverse reactions have been reported but a causal relationship to therapy with timolol maleate has not been established: aphakic cystoid macular edema, nasal congestion, anorexia, CNS effects (e.g., behavioral changes including confusion, hallucinations, anxiety, disorientation, nervousness, somnolence, and other psychic disturbances), hypertension, retroperitoneal fibrosis and pseudopemphigoid.

Timolol Maleate (systemic formulation): Adverse reactions reported in clinical experience with oral timolol maleate may be considered potential side effects of ophthalmic timolol maleate.

Clinically important changes in standard laboratory parameters were rarely associated with the administration of systemic timolol maleate. Slight increases in blood urea nitrogen, serum potassium and uric acid and triglycerides, and slight decreases in hemoglobin and hematocrit and HDL-cholesterol occurred, but were not progressive or associated with clinical manifestations.

For other detailed information, please consult the Product Monograph for timolol maleate.

DRUG INTERACTIONS: Antihypertensives/Cardiac Glycosides: Because of the brimonidine tartrate 0.2% component, COMBIGAN (brimonidine tartrate 0.2%/timolol maleate as timolol 0.5%) ophthalmic solution may reduce pulse and blood pressure. Caution in the concomitant use of drugs such as antihypertensives and/or cardiac glycosides is advised.

Beta-adrenergic Blockers: Patients who are receiving a beta-adrenergic blocking agent orally and COMBIGAN should be observed for potential additive effects of beta-blockade, both systemically and on intraocular pressure. The concomitant use of two topical beta-adrenergic blocking agents is not recommended.

Calcium Channel Blockers or Catecholamine-depleting Drugs: Close observation of the patient is recommended when timolol maleate is administered to patients receiving oral calcium channel blockers, catecholamine-depleting drugs such as reserpine, or beta-adrenergic blocking agents. The potential exists for additive effects and the production of hypotension, atrioventricular conduction disturbances, left ventricular failure and/or marked bradycardia.

CNS Depressants: Although specific drug interaction studies have not been conducted with COMBIGAN, the possibility of an additive or potentiating effect with CNS depressants (alcohol, barbiturates, opiates, sedatives, or anesthetics) should be considered.

Epinephrine: Mydriasis resulting from concomitant use of timolol maleate and epinephrine has been reported occasionally.

Quinidine: Potentiated systemic beta-blockade (e.g., decreased heart rate) has been reported during combined treatment with quinidine and timolol maleate, possibly because quinidine inhibits the metabolism of timolol maleate via the P-450 enzyme, CYP2D6.

Clonidine: Oral beta-adrenergic blocking agents may exacerbate the rebound hypertension which can follow the withdrawal of clonidine. There have been no reports of exacerbation of rebound hypertension with ophthalmic timolol maleate.

Tricyclic Antidepressants: Tricyclic antidepressants have been reported to blunt the hypotensive effect of systemic clonidine. It is not known whether the concurrent use of these agents with COMBIGAN can lead to an interference in IOP lowering effect.

No data are available on the level of circulating catecholamines after COMBIGAN is instilled. Caution, however, is advised in patients taking tricyclic antidepressants which can affect the metabolism and uptake of circulating amines.

Drug-Food Interactions: Interactions with food have not been established.
Drug-Herb Interactions: Interactions with herbal products have not been established.
Drug-Laboratory Test Interactions: Interactions with laboratory tests have not been established.
Drug-Lifestyle Interactions: Although specific drug interaction studies have not been conducted with COMBIGAN, the possibility of an additive or potentiating effect with CNS depressants such as alcohol exists.

DOSAGE AND ADMINISTRATION: Recommended Dose and Dosage Adjustment: The recommended dose is one drop of COMBIGAN (brimonidine tartrate 0.2%/timolol maleate as timolol 0.5%) ophthalmic solution in the affected eye(s) twice daily (doses taken approximately 12 hours apart).

Missed Dose: A missed dose should be applied as soon as the patient remembers. The regular dosing schedule should then be resumed with the next dose.

Administration: As with any eye drops, it is recommended that the lachrymal sac be compressed at the medial canthus (punctual occlusion) for one minute, to reduce possible systemic absorption. This should be performed immediately following the instillation of each drop.

If more than one topical ophthalmic product is to be used, the different products should be instilled at least 10 minutes apart.

The preservative in COMBIGAN, benzalkonium chloride, may be absorbed by soft (hydrophilic) contact lenses. Patients wearing soft contact lenses should be instructed to wait at least 15 minutes after instilling COMBIGAN to insert soft contact lenses.

Patients should be instructed to avoid allowing the tip of the dispensing container to contact the eye or surrounding structures. If handled improperly, ocular solutions can become contaminated by common bacteria known to cause ocular infections. Serious damage to the eye and subsequent loss of vision may result from using contaminated solutions.

OVERDOSAGE:
No data are available on overdoses with COMBIGAN (brimonidine tartrate 0.2%/timolol maleate as timolol 0.5%) ophthalmic solution in humans.

There have been reports of inadvertent overdoses with timolol maleate ophthalmic solution resulting in systemic effects similar to those seen with systemic beta-adrenergic blocking agents such as dizziness, headache, shortness of breath, bradycardia, bronchospasm, and cardiac arrest.

Treatment of an oral overdose includes supportive and symptomatic therapy; a patent airway should be maintained. Evacuation of the stomach should be considered during the first few hours after an overdose.

A study of patients with renal failure showed that timolol maleate did not dialyze readily.

Specific therapeutic measures for the treatment of overdose with timolol maleate are reproduced below for ease of reference:

Gastric Lavage: If ingested.

Symptomatic Bradycardia: Use atropine sulfate intravenously in a dosage of 0.25 to 2 mg to induce vagal blockade. If bradycardia persists, intravenous isoproterenol hydrochloride should be administered cautiously. In refractory cases the use of a transvenous cardiac pacemaker may be considered.

Hypotension: Use sympathomimetic pressor drug therapy, such as dopamine, dobutamine or levarterenol. In refractory cases the use of glucagon hydrochloride has been reported to be useful.

Bronchospasm: Use isoproterenol hydrochloride. Additional therapy with aminophylline may be considered.

Acute Cardiac Failure: Conventional therapy with digitalis, diuretics and oxygen should be instituted immediately. In refractory cases the use of intravenous aminophylline is suggested. This may be followed if necessary by glucagon hydrochloride which has been reported to be useful.

Heart Block (second or third degree): Use isoproterenol hydrochloride or a transvenous cardiac pacemaker.

For management of a suspected drug overdose, CPhA recommends that you contact your **regional Poison Control Centre**. See the *CPS* Directory section for a list of Poison Control Centres.

ACTION AND CLINICAL PHARMACOLOGY: Mechanism of Action: COMBIGAN (brimonidine tartrate 0.2%/timolol maleate as timolol 0.5%) ophthalmic solution reduces intraocular pressure (IOP) by reducing aqueous humor production and increasing uveoscleral outflow.

COMBIGAN is a combination product containing brimonidine tartrate and timolol maleate. Individually, each of these components is used to control IOP in humans.

Brimonidine tartrate is a relatively selective alpha adrenergic receptor agonist that in radioligand binding assays and in functional assays, is approximately 1000 times more selective for the alpha-2 adrenoceptor than the alpha-1 adrenoceptor. This selectivity results in the absence of vasoconstriction in microvessels associated with human retinal xenografts.

Fluorophotometric studies in animals and humans suggest that brimonidine tartrate has a dual mechanism of action. Brimonidine tartrate lowers IOP by reducing aqueous humor production and increasing uveoscleral outflow.

Timolol maleate is a general beta-adrenergic receptor blocking agent that combines reversibly with a part of the cell membrane, the beta-adrenergic receptor, and thus inhibits the usual biological response that would occur with stimulation of that receptor. This specific competitive antagonism blocks stimulation of the beta-adrenergic receptors by catecholamines having beta-adrenergic stimulating (agonist) activity, whether these originate from an endogenous or exogenous source. Reversal of this blockade can be accomplished by increasing the concentration of agonist, which will restore the usual biologic response.

The precise mechanism of action of timolol maleate in lowering intraocular pressure is not clearly established at this time, although a fluorescein study and tonography studies indicate that its predominant action may be related to reduced aqueous humor formation.

Both brimonidine tartrate and timolol maleate have a rapid onset of action, with the peak ocular hypotensive effect occurring at approximately two hours post-dosing for brimonidine tartrate and one to two hours for timolol maleate. The duration of effect is 12 hours or greater for brimonidine tartrate and 24 hours for timolol maleate.

Pharmacodynamics: The topical administration of brimonidine tartrate 0.2% ophthalmic solution decreases intraocular pressure (IOP) with minimal effect on cardiovascular parameters. Brimonidine tartrate 0.2% has no effect on pulmonary function or exercise-induced tachycardia. The cardiovascular effects of brimonidine tartrate 0.2% during exercise in normal volunteers were found to be limited to a slight suppression of systolic blood pressure, which was clinically insignificant, during the recovery period following a treadmill test.

Timolol maleate is a non-cardioselective beta-adrenergic receptor blocking agent that does not have significant intrinsic sympathomimetic, direct myocardial depressant, or local anesthetic (membrane-stabilizing) activity.

Pharmacokinetics: Absorption: Plasma brimonidine tartrate and timolol maleate concentrations were determined in 16 healthy subjects dosed with COMBIGAN, ALPHAGAN (brimonidine tartrate) ophthalmic solution 0.2%, or TIMOPTIC (timolol maleate) ophthalmic solution USP 0.5%, each BID for seven days in a three-period, complete crossover study. There were no statistically significant differences in brimonidine tartrate or timolol maleate AUC between COMBIGAN and the respective monotherapy treatments. Mean plasma brimonidine tartrate C_{max} values from the COMBIGAN and ALPHAGAN 0.2% groups were 0.0327±0.0150 (N=15) and 0.0347±0.0226 ng/mL (N=16), respectively, indicating no apparent difference. Mean plasma timolol maleate C_{max} values from the COMBIGAN and TIMOPTIC USP 0.5% treatment groups were 0.406±0.216 (N=15) and 0.507±0.269 ng/mL (N=14), respectively. Although the C_{max} of timolol maleate was approximately 20% lower in the COMBIGAN treatment, the difference was not statistically significant (p=0.088).

Therapeutic drug monitoring was conducted in the two Phase 3 trials. Brimonidine tartrate and timolol maleate plasma concentrations from the COMBIGAN BID group were 15-49% lower than their respective monotherapy values. In the case of brimonidine tartrate, the difference appears to be due to BID dosing for COMBIGAN and TID dosing for ALPHAGAN.

The lower timolol maleate plasma concentrations seen with COMBIGAN, as compared to timolol maleate 0.5%, appear to be related to a slower absorption of timolol maleate, which may be due to a difference in the benzalkonium concentrations rather than a drug-drug (brimonidine tartrate-timolol maleate) interaction.

Orally administered timolol maleate is rapidly and nearly completely absorbed (~90% availability). The apparent elimination half-life of timolol maleate in plasma is 4 hours. The half-life is essentially unchanged in patients with moderate renal insufficiency.

Metabolism: Timolol maleate is partially metabolized by the liver and timolol maleate and its metabolites are excreted by the kidney. Timolol maleate is not extensively bound to plasma proteins (~60%). After oral dosing, timolol maleate is subject to moderate first-pass metabolism (~50%). Only a small amount of unchanged drug appears in the urine, along with its metabolites after oral dosing.

Excretion: In humans, brimonidine tartrate is eliminated rapidly via extensive systemic metabolism; there is no marked systemic accumulation after multiple dosing. It is metabolized primarily by the liver. Urinary excretion is the major route of elimination of the drug and its metabolites. Approximately 87% of an orally-administered radioactive dose was eliminated within 120 hours, with 74% found in the urine in the first 96 hours.

STORAGE AND STABILITY: COMBIGAN (brimonidine tartrate 0.2%/timolol maleate as timolol 0.5%) ophthalmic solution should be stored at room temperature (15 to 25°C). Protect from light.

Keep in a safe place out of the reach of children.

SPECIAL HANDLING INSTRUCTIONS: Avoid allowing the tip of the dispensing container to contact the eye or surrounding structures.

Ocular solutions, if handled improperly or if the tip of the dispensing container contacts the eye or surrounding structures, can be contaminated by common bacteria known to cause ocular infections. Serious damage to the eye and subsequent loss of vision may result from using contaminated solutions.

INFORMATION FOR THE PATIENT: Published in e-CPS, available by subscription at www.e-cps.ca.

DOSAGE FORMS, COMPOSITION AND PACKAGING: Each mL of ophthalmic solution contains: brimonidine tartrate 2 mg (0.2%) and timolol maleate 5 mg (0.5 %). Nonmedicinal ingredients: benzalkonium chloride 0.005% as preservative, purified water, sodium phosphate, monobasic monohydrate and sodium phosphate, dibasic heptahydrate. Hydrochloric acid and/or sodium hydroxide may be added to adjust pH. White, opaque plastic dropper bottles of 2.5, 5 and 10 mL.

Combivent® UDV Ⓟ

ipratropium bromide—salbutamol sulfate

Bronchodilator

Boehringer Ingelheim

Date of Revision: August 14, 2009

SUMMARY PRODUCT INFORMATION:

Route of Administration	Dosage Form/Strength	All Nonmedicinal Ingredients
Inhalation	Solution Each unit dose vial contains 0.50 mg of ipratropium bromide (as ipratropium bromide monohydrate) and 2.5 mg salbutamol (as salbutamol sulphate) in 2.5 mL.	Sodium chloride, hydrochloric acid and purified water For a complete listing see Dosage Forms, Composition and Packaging.

INDICATIONS AND CLINICAL USE: COMBIVENT UDV (ipratropium bromide and salbutamol sulfate) Inhalation Solution is indicated for the management of bronchospasm in patients suffering from chronic obstructive pulmonary disease (COPD) who require regular treatment with both ipratropium and salbutamol.

Pediatrics (<12 years of age): The efficacy and safety in children under 12 years has not been established.

CONTRAINDICATIONS:

- COMBIVENT UDV is contraindicated in patients with cardiac tachyarrhythmias, hypertrophic obstructive cardiomyopathy and in patients with a history of hypersensitivity to any of its components or to atropine or its derivatives.

WARNINGS AND PRECAUTIONS: General: The unit dose vials are intended only for inhalation with suitable nebulizing devices and should not be taken orally or administered parenterally.

Patients must be instructed in the correct use of COMBIVENT UDV and warned not to allow the solution or mist to enter the eyes. Acute angle glaucoma has been reported rarely when nebulized solutions of ipratropium bromide have been used in conjunction with $beta_2$-agonist bronchodilators. Protection of the eyes appears to prevent any increase in intraocular pressure and patients who may be susceptible to glaucoma should be warned specifically on the need for ocular protection.

Eye pain or discomfort, blurred vision, visual halos or coloured images in association with red eyes from conjunctival congestion and corneal edema may be signs of acute narrow-angle glaucoma. Should any combination of these symptoms develop, treatment with miotic drops should be initiated and specialist advice sought immediately.

Care should be taken with patients suffering from cardiovascular disorders, especially coronary insufficiency, recent myocardial infarction, severe organic heart or vascular disorders, cardiac arrhythmias and hypertension; in patients with convulsive disorders, diabetes mellitus, hyperthyroidism, phaeochromocytoma, risk of narrow-angle glaucoma, prostatic hypertrophy or bladder-neck obstruction and in patients who are usually responsive to sympathomimetic amines. Fatalities have been reported following excessive use of inhaled sympathomimetic amines, the exact cause of which is unknown.

In the following conditions COMBIVENT UDV should only be used after careful risk/benefit assessment: hypertrophic obstructive cardiomyopathy, tachyarrhythmia, inadequately controlled diabetes mellitus, recent myocardial infarction and/or severe organic heart or vascular disorders, hyperthyroidism, pheochromocytoma, risk of narrow-angle glaucoma, prostatic hypertrophy, urinary retention, or bladder-neck obstruction.

The patient should be instructed to consult a doctor immediately in the event of acute, rapidly worsening dyspnea. In addition, the patient should be warned to seek medical advice should a reduced response become apparent.

The concomitant use of COMBIVENT UDV with other sympathomimetic agents is not recommended since such combined use may lead to deleterious cardiovascular effects.

Carcinogenesis and Mutagenesis: Animal data only.

Cardiovascular: Special care and supervision are required in patients with idiopathic hypertrophic subvalvular aortic stenosis, in whom an increase in the pressure gradient between the left ventricle and the aorta may occur, causing increased strain on the left ventricle.

Patients with underlying severe heart disease (e.g. ischaemic heart disease, tachyarrhythmia or severe heart failure) who are receiving COMBIVENT UDV for respiratory disease should be warned to seek medical advice if they experience chest pain or other symptoms of worsening heart disease. There is some evidence from post-marketing data and published literature of rare occurrences of myocardial ischaemia associated with salbutamol, one of the components of COMBIVENT UDV.

Hematologic: In common with other beta-adrenergic agents, salbutamol can induce reversible metabolic changes; these are more pronounced during infusions of the drug and include hyperglycemia and hypokalemia.

Potentially serious hypokalemia may result from $beta_2$-agonist therapy, mainly from parenteral and nebulized administration.

Particular caution is advised in acute severe asthma as hypokalemia may be potentiated by concomitant treatment with xanthine derivatives, steroids and diuretics: the adverse effects of hypokalemia may be exacerbated by hypoxia.

Hypokalemia will increase the susceptibility of digitalis-treated patients to cardiac arrhythmias. It is recommended that serum potassium levels be monitored in such situations. Large doses of intravenous salbutamol have been reported to aggravate pre-existing diabetes mellitus and may precipitate ketoacidosis. The relevance of these observations to the use of COMBIVENT UDV is unknown.

Immune: Immediate hypersensitivity reactions may occur after administration of salbutamol, as demonstrated by rare cases of urticaria, angioedema, rash, bronchospasm, anaphylaxis, and oropharyngeal edema.

Ophthalmologic: Care should be taken to ensure that the nebulizer mask fits the patient's face properly and that nebulized solution does not escape into the eyes. In patients with glaucoma or narrow anterior chambers, the administration by nebulizer of a combined ATROVENT/$beta_2$-agonist solution should be avoided unless measures (eg., use of swimming goggles or use of a nebulizer with a mouthpiece) are taken to ensure that nebulized solution does not reach the eye. There have been isolated reports of ocular complications (ie., mydriasis, increased intraocular pressure, narrow angle closure glaucoma, eye pain) when nebulized ipratropium bromide either alone or in combination with an adrenergic $beta_2$-agonist solution has escaped into the eyes. Eye pain or discomfort, blurred vision, visual halos or coloured images in association with red eyes from conjunctival congestion and corneal edema may be signs of acute narrow-angle glaucoma. In the event that glaucoma is precipitated or worsened, treatment should include standard measures for this condition (i.e. treatment with miotic drops should be initiated and specialist advice sought immediately.

Respiratory: Some patients receiving $beta_2$-adrenergic agonist have been reported to have developed severe paradoxical bronchospasm which has been life threatening.

Patients with cystic fibrosis may be more prone to gastrointestinal motility disturbances.

Special Populations: Pregnant Women: Salbutamol, a component of COMBIVENT UDV, has been shown to be teratogenic in mice when given in doses corresponding to 14 times the human aerosol dose; 5 times the human inhalation dose, 0.2 times the maximum human (child weighing 21 kg) oral dose; and 0.4 times the maximum human oral dose and at doses corresponding to the human nebulization dose.

The safety of COMBIVENT UDV in pregnancy has not been established. The benefits of using COMBIVENT UDV when pregnancy is present or suspected must be weighed against possible hazards caused to the fetus.

It has been reported that high doses of salbutamol, administered intravenously, inhibits uterine contractions. Although this effect is extremely unlikely as a consequence of the use of inhaled formulations, it should be kept in mind.

Oral salbutamol has been shown to delay preterm labour in some reports. There are presently no well-controlled studies which demonstrated that it will stop preterm labour or prevent labour at term. Therefore, cautious use of COMBIVENT UDV is required in pregnant patients when it is given for relief of bronchospasm so as to avoid interference with uterine contractility.

Nursing Women: It is not known whether the components of COMBIVENT UDV (ipratropium bromide and salbutamol) are excreted in human milk. As salbutamol is probably secreted in breast milk and because of the potential for tumorigenicity shown for salbutamol in animal studies, a decision should be made whether to discontinue nursing or to discontinue the drug, taking into account the importance of the drug to the mother. It is not known whether salbutamol in breast milk has a harmful effect on the neonate. No specific studies have been conducted on the excretion of ipratropium bromide in breast milk. The benefits of COMBIVENT UDV use during lactation should therefore be weighed against possible effects on the infant.

Pediatrics (<12 years of age): The efficacy and safety in children under 12 years has not been established.

ADVERSE REACTIONS: Adverse Drug Reaction Overview: Adverse reaction information concerning COMBIVENT UDV (ipratropium bromide and salbutamol sulfate) is derived from a total of 1070 COPD patients randomized and treated with either COMBIVENT UDV (222 patients); ipratropium bromide + salbutamol sulfate (100 patients); ipratropium bromide (327 patients) or salbutamol sulfate (421 patients).

Adverse reactions, judged by the investigator to be possibly related to drug treatment, as well as adverse events occurring in one or more patients in any group in the controlled clinical trials, appear in Table 1 and Table 2.

Clinical Trial Adverse Drug Reactions: Because clinical trials are conducted under very specific conditions the adverse reaction rates observed in the clinical trials may not reflect the rates observed in practice and should not be compared to the rates in the clinical trials of another drug. Adverse drug reaction information from clinical trials is useful for identifying drug-related adverse events and for approximating rates.

Table 1: COMBIVENT UDV

Number (Percent) of Patients with Adverse Reactions Occurring in 1% or More of Patients by Treatment Group, Body System and Preferred Term

	COMBIVENT UDV N (%)	Ipratropium + Salbutamol N (%)	Ipratropium N (%)	Salbutamol N (%)
Total Treated	222 (100)	100 (100)	327 (100)	421 (100)
Total with any possible related event	24 (10.8)	15 (15.0)	34 (10.4)	47 (11.2)
Cardiac Disorders				
Hypertension	0	1 (1.0)	0	1 (0.2)
Gastrointestinal Disorders				
Mouth (dry)	4 (1.8)	3 (3.0)	7 (2.1)	9 (2.1)
Nausea	0	0	3 (0.9)	5 (1.2)

(cont'd)

Table 1: COMBIVENT UDV *(cont'd)*

Number (Percent) of Patients with Adverse Reactions Occurring in 1% or More of Patients by Treatment Group, Body System and Preferred Term

	COMBIVENT UDV N (%)	Ipratropium + Salbutamol N (%)	Ipratropium N (%)	Salbutamol N (%)
Nervous System Disorders				
Headache	2 (0.9)	4 (4.0)	3 (0.9)	7 (1.7)
Dizziness	1 (0.5)	2 (2.0)	0	3 (0.7)
Dysphonia	3 (1.4)	0	1 (0.3)	1 (0.2)
Nervousness	1 (0.5)	1 (1.0)	0	8 (1.9)
Respiratory, Thoracic and Mediastinal Disorders				
Coughing	2 (0.9)	2 (2.0)	6 (1.8)	1 (0.2)
Skin and Subcutaneous Tissue Disorders				
Rash	0	1 (1.0)	0	2 (0.5)
Special Senses Other				
Taste perversion	1 (0.5)	2 (2.0)	0	2 (0.5)

Table 2: COMBIVENT UDV

Number (Percent) of Patients with Adverse Events[a] by Treatment Group, Body System and Preferred Term

	COMBIVENT UDV N (%)	Ipratropium + Salbutamol N (%)	Ipratropium N (%)	Salbutamol N (%)
Total Treated	222	100	327	421
Total with any possible related event	24 (10.8)	15 (15.0)	34 (10.4)	47 (11.2)
Body as a Whole (General)				
Rigors	0	0	1 (0.3)	1 (0.2)
Body odour	0	0	0	1 (0.2)
Fatigue	0	0	1 (0.3)	2 (0.5)
Hot flashes	1 (0.5)	0	0	0
Oedema (legs)	1 (0.5)	0	0	0
Back pain	0	0	0	1 (0.2)
Influenza-like symptoms	0	0	1 (0.3)	0
Chest pain	0	0	1 (0.3)	0
Pain	0	0	1 (0.3)	0
Cardiovascular				
Cardiac failure	0	0	0	1 (0.2)
Syncope	0	0	0	1 (0.2)
Central and Peripheral Nervous System				
Somnolence	1 (0.5)	0	2 (0.6)	0
Confusion				1 (0.2)
Paraesthesia	0	0	1 (0.3)	1 (0.2)
Hypoaesthesia	0	0	1 (0.3)	1 (0.2)
Insomnia	0	0	1 (0.3)	1 (0.2)
Gastrointestinal System				
Diarrhoea	0	0	0	1 (0.2)
Anorexia	0	0	0	1 (0.2)
Flatulence	0	0	0	1 (0.2)
Stomatitis ulcerative	0	0	0	1 (0.2)
Saliva (increased)	0	0	1 (0.3)	0
Psychiatric				
Agitation	1 (0.5)		0	0
Amnesia	0	0	0	1 (0.2)
Anxiety	0	0	0	1 (0.2)
Depression	0	0	1 (0.3)	0
Resistance Mechanism				
Moniliasis	1 (0.5)	0	0	0
Respiratory System—Lower				
Dyspnoea	2 (0.9)	0	6 (1.8)	8 (1.9)
Bronchitis	0	0	1 (0.3)	7 (1.7)
Sputum (increased)	1 (0.5)	0	2 (0.6)	3 (0.7)
Haemoptysis	0	0	0	1 (0.2)
Respiratory System—Upper				
Rhinitis	0	0	3 (0.9)	0
Pharyngitis	2 (0.9)	0	4 (1.2)	3 (0.7)
Special Senses Other				
Taste perversion	1 (0.5)	2 (2.0)	0	2 (0.5)
Vision Disorders				
Conjunctivitis	1 (0.5)	0	0	0

(cont'd)

[a] Not considered to have a causal relationship to treatment.

Less Common Clinical Trial Adverse Drug Reactions (<1%): Eye Disorders: vision (abnormal), eye pain.
Cardiac Disorders: arrhythmia, palpitation, tachycardia, ECG abnormal specific.
Musculoskeletal and Connective Tissue Disorders: myalgia.
Nervous System Disorders: tremor.
Resistance Mechanism Disorders: infection (fungal).
Respiratory, Thoracic and Mediastinal Disorders: bronchospasm.
Skin and Subcutaneous Tissue Disorders: sweating increased, pruritus, urticaria.
Urinary System Disorders: micturation frequency, dysuria, urinary retention.

Additional adverse reactions reported during treatment with COMBIVENT UDV include hypertension, nervousness, tachycardia, tremor, palpitations, and urinary retention especially in susceptible patients.

Additional adverse events observed during treatment with COMBIVENT UDV include fatigue, abdominal pain, dyspepsia, sinusitis, and dysuria.

Post-Market Adverse Drug Reactions: World-wide safety data, including post-marketing data, spontaneous reports, literature reports, and reports from clinical trials list below the most frequent undesirable effects of COMBIVENT UDV according to system organ class.

Cardiac Disorders: atrial fibrillation, myocardial ischaemia, palpitations, arrhythmia, tachycardia, blood pressure diastolic decreased, blood pressure systolic increased.
Eye Disorders: angle closure glaucoma, eye pain, intraocular pressure increased, mydriasis, vision blurred. (There have been isolated reports of ocular complications with symptoms mentioned above when aerosolised ipratropium bromide either alone or in combination with an adrenergic beta$_2$-agonist, has escaped into the eyes).
Gastrointestinal Disorders: oedema mouth, dry mouth, nausea, gastrointestinal motility disorder, vomiting.
General Disorders and Administration Site Conditions: asthenia.
Immune System Disorders: anaphylactic reaction, hypersensitivity.
Metabolism and Nutrition Disorders: hypokalaemia.
Musculoskeletal and Connective Tissue Disorders: muscle spasms (fine tremor of skeletal muscles), myalgia, muscular weakness.
Nervous System Disorders: dizziness, headache, tremor.
Psychiatric Disorders: psychological alterations (mental disorder), nervousness.
Renal and Urinary Disorders: urinary retention.
Respiratory, Thoracic and Mediastinal Disorders: bronchospasm, cough, dysphonia, laryngospasm, local (throat) irritation, pharyngeal oedema.
Skin and Subcutaneous Tissue Disorders: angioedema, hyperhidrosis, rash, urticaria, skin reaction.

Literature reports regarding adverse events associated with the use of ipratropium bromide or salbutamol inhalation solution singly or in combination include, cases of taste perversion, bronchitis, angina, lightheadedness, drowsiness, insomnia, vertigo, CNS stimulation, weakness (asthenia), itching, flushing, alopecia, gastrointestinal distress, vomiting, diarrhea, edema, constipation and urinary difficulty have been reported.

DRUG INTERACTIONS:

> It is strongly recommended not to mix COMBIVENT UDV solution with other drugs in the same nebulizer.

Overview: In patients receiving other anticholinergic drugs, COMBIVENT UDV should be used with caution because of possible additive effects.

Xanthine derivatives and beta$_2$-adrenergic agents may enhance the effect of COMBIVENT UDV.

Beta-agonist induced hypokalaemia may be increased by concomitant treatment with xanthine derivatives, glucocorticosteroids, and diuretics. This should be taken into account particularly in patients with severe airway obstruction.

Hypokalaemia may result in an increased susceptibility to arrhythmias in patients receiving digoxin. It is recommended that serum potassium levels are monitored in such situations.

Other sympathomimetic bronchodilators or epinephrine should not be used concomitantly with COMBIVENT Inhalation Solution. If additional adrenergic drugs are to be administered by any route, they should be used with caution to avoid deleterious cardiovascular effects. Such concomitant use must be individualized and not given on a routine basis. If regular co-administration is required then alternative therapy must be considered.

COMBIVENT UDV should be administered with extreme caution to patients being treated with monoamine oxidase inhibitors or tricyclic antidepressants because the action of salbutamol on the vascular system may be potentiated.

Beta-receptor blocking agents and salbutamol inhibit the effect of each other.

Inhalation of halogenated hydrocarbon anaesthetics such as halothane, trichloroethylene and enflurane may increase the susceptibility to the cardiovascular effects of beta-agonists.

DOSAGE AND ADMINISTRATION: Dosing Considerations: COMBIVENT UDV (ipratropium bromide/salbutamol sulfate) dosage should be individualized, and patient response should be monitored to determine the requirement for more than a single bronchodilator by the prescribing physician on an ongoing basis.

Counselling on smoking cessation should be the first step in treating patients with chronic bronchitis who smoke. Smoking cessation produces symptomatic benefits and has been shown to confer a survival advantage by slowing or stopping the progression of chronic bronchitis and emphysema.

Recommended Dose and Dosage Adjustment: Adults and Children Over 12 Years: COPD: COMBIVENT UDV in UDV's may be administered from a suitable nebulizer or an intermittent positive pressure ventilator. The recommended dosage is 1 UDV vial (0.50 mg ipratropium bromide (as ipratropium monohydrate) and 2.5 mg salbutamol (as salbutamol sulphate) in 2.5 mL) three or four times daily.

Dilution Instructions: If necessary, before use, doses may be diluted to a total nebulization volume of 3-5 mL with preservative free 0.9% sterile sodium chloride solution and used immediately. Discard any unused solution. Nebulize over 10-15 minutes at gas flow of 6-10L/min. Repeat every six hours as necessary.

OVERDOSAGE:

The effects of overdosage are expected to be related primarily to salbutamol because acute overdosage with ipratropium bromide is unlikely since ipratropium bromide is not well absorbed systemically after aerosol or oral administration. Expected symptoms of overdosage with ipratropium bromide (such as dry mouth, visual accomodation disturbances) are mild and transient in nature. However, should signs of serious anticholinergic toxicity appear, cholinesterase inhibitors may be considered.

The expected symptoms with overdosage are those of excessive beta-adrenergic stimulation, such as: tachycardia, palpitations, tremor, cardiac arrhythmia, hypokalemia, hypertension, hypotension, widening of pulse pressure, anginal pain, flushing and, in extreme cases, sudden death.

Administration of sedatives, tranquillizers or in severe cases, intensive therapy may be appropriate for the treatment of overdosage. To antagonize the effect of salbutamol, the judicious use of a cardioselective beta-adrenergic blocking agent, (eg. metoprolol, atenolol), may be considered, bearing in mind the danger of inducing an asthmatic attack. Serum potassium levels should be monitored.

> For management of a suspected drug overdose, contact your regional Poison Control Centre. See the *CPS* Directory section for a list of Poison Control Centres.

ACTION AND CLINICAL PHARMACOLOGY: Mechanism of Action: COMBIVENT UDV is a combination of the anticholinergic bronchodilator, ipratropium bromide, and the beta$_2$-adrenergic bronchodilator, salbutamol sulfate.

Ipratropium bromide is a quaternary ammonium derivative of atropine and is an anticholinergic drug which has bronchodilator properties. On inhalation, the onset of action is noted within 5 to 15 minutes, with a peak response between 1 and 2 hours, lasting about 2 additional hours, with subsequent decline from the peak. Bronchodilation is still evident 8 hours after inhalation.

Salbutamol produces bronchodilation through stimulation of beta$_2$-adrenergic receptors in bronchial smooth muscle, thereby causing relaxation of muscle fibres. This action is manifested by an increase in pulmonary function as demonstrated by spirometric measurements. A measurable decrease in airway resistance is typically observed 5 to 15 minutes after inhalation of salbutamol. The maximum improvement in pulmonary function usually occurs after 60 to 90 minutes, and significant bronchodilator activity has been observed to persist from 3 to 6 hours.

Pharmacodynamics: Ipratropium Bromide: Large, single inhaled doses of ipratropium bromide have been given to man without any signs of toxicity. After the administration of 400 µg to 10 normal subjects, no changes were detected in pulse rate, blood pressure, intra ocular pressure, salivary secretion, visual accommodation or electrocardiograms. Likewise, in a similar study no change in pulse rate or salivary secretion were seen when cumulative doses up to 1.2 mg were administered by inhalation to normal volunteers.

Special studies utilizing normal therapeutic doses in asthmatic and chronic bronchitic patients, again have not revealed any systemic anticholinergic effects.

In one study, 14 patients were treated for 45 days with either ipratropium bromide 40 µg q.i.d. or ipratropium bromide 40 µg q.i.d. plus oral fenoterol 5 mg q.i.d. No changes in visual acuity, intra ocular pressure, pupil size or accommodation of vision occurred. Micturition function studies in 20 male patients showed no differences in urinary flow, total flow time and time until maximum flow between placebo and ipratropium bromide 40 µg t.i.d administered for 3 days.

A wide variety of challenge studies has been conducted using ipratropium bromide as a protective agent. In pharmacologically induced bronchospasm, ipratropium bromide, in clinical doses, was very effective against methacholine and acetylcholine, moderately effective against propranolol but had no effect against histamine or serotonin. Studies in exercise induced bronchospasm have yielded variable results. Some investigations have indicated that ipratropium bromide has little or no effect but other studies have shown that some patients, at least, were protected against bronchospasm induced by exercise. Likewise, the protection against cold air induced bronchospasm has been variable.

The Lung Health Study: The Lung Health Study was a randomized multi centre clinical trial carried out from October 1986 to April 1994 in North America. It was designed to test the effectiveness of intervention-smoking cessation and bronchodilator administration in smokers aged 35-60 years who have mild obstructive pulmonary disease. The main outcome or end point was the rate of change and cumulative change in FEV$_1$ over a 5-year period.

A total of 5887 male and female smokers, aged 35 to 60 years, with spirometric signs of early chronic obstructive pulmonary disease were recruited. Participants were randomized to one of the following groups: (1) smoking intervention plus bronchodilator, (2) smoking intervention plus placebo, or (3) no intervention.

Smoking intervention consisted of an intensive 12-session smoking cessation program combining behaviour modification and use of nicotine gum, with continuing 5-year maintenance program to minimize relapse. Two puffs ipratropium bromide was prescribed three times daily from a metered-dose inhaler.

The results showed that participants in the two smoking intervention groups showed significantly smaller declines in FEV$_1$ than did those in the control group. Most of this difference occurred during the first year following entry into the study and was attributable to smoking cessation, with those who achieved sustained smoking cessation experiencing the largest benefit. The benefit associated with the use of the ipratropium bromide vanished after the ipratropium bromide was discontinued at the end of the study.

In summary the results showed that smoking intervention reduced the rate of decline in FEV$_1$ in middle aged smokers with mild airways obstruction who remained non-smokers throughout the 5 years. The other intervention, administration of ipratropium bromide, did not alter the rate of decline in lung function. There was a small one time improvement in lung function associated with the onset of ipratropium use, but this disappeared rapidly when ipratropium use was discontinued at the end of the study. Otherwise, the regular use of ipratropium bromide had no effect on the rate of decline of lung function over 5 years in patients studied.

Salbutamol: In controlled clinical trials, the onset of improvement in pulmonary function was within 15 minutes, as determined by both maximum mid-expiratory flow rate (MMEF) and FEV$_1$. MMEF measurements also showed that near maximum improvement in pulmonary function generally occurs within 60 to 90 minutes following two inhalations of salbutamol and that clinically significant improvement generally continues for three to four hours in most patients. In clinical trials some patients with asthma showed a therapeutic response (defined as maintaining FEV$_1$ values 15% or more above baseline) that was still apparent at six hours. Continued effectiveness of salbutamol was demonstrated over a 13-week period in these same trials.

In clinical studies, two inhalations of salbutamol taken approximately 15 minutes before exercise prevented exercise-induced bronchospasm, as demonstrated by the maintenance of FEV$_1$ within 80% of baseline values in the majority of patients. One of these studies also evaluated the duration of the prophylactic effect to repeated exercise challenges which was evident at four hours in the majority of patients and at six hours in approximately one third of the patients.

The ability of salbutamol to produce bronchodilation in humans has been demonstrated in many spirometric and plethysmographic studies. Following a challenge with acetylcholine aerosol, in a study examining the effects of salbutamol in airway resistance following challenge testing in 12 patients, the mean airway resistance increased 250%. After salbutamol aerosol (200 µg), the mean airway resistance decreased to 78% of the initial value.

Challenges with grass pollen or house dust aerosols in five and eight patients, respectively, increased activity resistance 265% and 255%, respectively. Administration of salbutamol decreased airway resistance to initial levels.

Controlled clinical studies and other clinical experience have shown that inhaled salbutamol, like other beta-adrenergic agonist drugs, can produce a significant cardiovascular effect in some patients, as measured by pulse rate, blood pressure, symptoms, and/or ECG changes. Fatalities have been reported following excessive use of inhaled sympathomimetic agents, the exact cause of which is unknown.

When salbutamol was administered as a metered-dose inhaler preparation to six normal volunteers, at doses of three or seven inhalations of 100 µg, it was observed that three inhalations of salbutamol did not alter serum potassium while seven inhalations resulted in a decrease in serum potassium from 4.4 to 3.8 mEq/L. Thus, the recommended dose of salbutamol aerosol (two inhalations) would not be expected to alter serum potassium levels.

Prolonged use of salbutamol Inhalation Aerosol in most patients caused no significant changes in ECG pattern, blood sugar, liver and kidney functions and hematological values.

The hemodynamic effects of intravenous salbutamol were studied in patients with mitral valve disease. At the dose of 1 µg/kg, salbutamol reduced mean aortic pressure by 7 mmHg, increased the cardiac output by 0.6 L/minute and reduced systemic vascular resistance by 7 units. It caused no change in left ventricular ejection time. At the dose of 2 µg/kg, salbutamol increased the mean oxygen uptake by 21 mL/minute, narrowing the mean arteriovenous oxygen difference by 10 mL/minute. Salbutamol has no effect on the pulmonary ventilation/perfusion ratio; therefore, unlike isoprenaline, it does not increase hypoxia during acute asthmatic attacks.

Pharmacokinetics: Ipratropium Bromide: Ipratropium bromide is absorbed quickly after oral inhalation of a nominal dose of 40 µg administered from a pressurized metered dose inhaler. The peak plasma concentration (mean C_{max}=32 pg/mL) is reached within 5 minutes after inhalation. The therapeutic effect of ipratropium bromide is produced by a local action in the airways. Therefore time courses of bronchodilation and systemic pharmacokinetics do not run in parallel. The plasma concentration-versus-time curve was similar to that seen after oral administration, likely reflecting the large fraction of inhaled dose which is deposited on the pharyngeal mucosa and swallowed.

Intravenous administration of 1.0 mg in man showed a rapid distribution into tissues (half-life of an alpha phase approximately five minutes), and a terminal half-life (beta phase) of 3-4 hours. Plasma concentrations after inhaled ipratropium bromide were about 1000 times lower than equipotent oral or intravenous doses (15 and 0.15 mg, respectively).

Up to 8 metabolites of ipratropium bromide have been detected in man, dog and rat. In man, about 70% of the drug is excreted unchanged after i.v. administration and only one metabolite exceeds 10% of the total radioactivity. The elimination occurs primarily via the kidneys with less than 10% of the total i.v. dose excreted via the biliary or fecal route. After oral or inhaled doses, however, up to 90% of the dose is detectable in the feces, suggesting poor absorption. Thirty-nine percent of the active ingredient is excreted renally after intravenous administration, 4.4%-13.1% after inhalation from a metered dose inhaler is excreted as unchanged compound in urine.

In a crossover pharmacokinetic study in 12 healthy male volunteers comparing the pattern of absorption and excretion of a single-dose of COMBIVENT UDV to the two active components individually, the co-nebulization of ipratropium bromide and salbutamol sulfate does not potentiate the systemic absorptions of either component.

Salbutamol: After inhalation of recommended doses of salbutamol, plasma drug levels are very low. When 100 µg of tritiated salbutamol aerosol was administered to two normal volunteers, plasma levels of drug-radioactivity were insignificant at 10, 20 and 30 minutes following inhalation. The plasma concentration of salbutamol may be even less as the amount of plasma drug-radioactivity does not differentiate salbutamol from its principal metabolite, a sulfate ester. In a separate study, plasma salbutamol levels ranged from less than 0.5 mg/mL to 1.6 mg/mL in ten asthmatic children one hour after inhalation of 200 µg of salbutamol.

Approximately 10% of an inhaled salbutamol dose is deposited in the lungs. Eighty-five percent of the remaining salbutamol administered from a metered-dose inhaler is swallowed; however, since the dose is low (100 to 200 µg), the absolute amount swallowed is too small to be of clinical significance. Salbutamol is only weakly bound to plasma proteins. Results of animal studies indicate that following systemic administration, salbutamol does not cross the blood-brain barrier but does cross the placenta using an in vitro perfused isolated human placenta model. It has been found that between 2% and 3% of salbutamol was transferred from the maternal side to the fetal side of the placenta.

Salbutamol is metabolized in the liver. The principal metabolite in humans is salbutamol-o-sulfate, which has negligible pharmacologic activity. Salbutamol may also be metabolized by oxidative deamination and/or conjugation with glucuronide.

Salbutamol is longer acting than isoprenaline in most patients by any route of administration because it is not a substrate for the cellular uptake processes for catecholamines nor for catechol-o-methyl transferase. Salbutamol and its metabolites are excreted in the urine (>80%) and the feces (5% to 10%). Plasma levels are insignificant after administration of aerosolized salbutamol; the plasma half-life ranges from 3.8 to 7.1 hours.

STORAGE AND STABILITY: Unopened unit dose vials of COMBIVENT UDV should be stored at controlled room temperature (between 15 and 25°C) and protected from light and heat. Do not use if solution is discoloured. Keep out of reach of children.

INFORMATION FOR THE PATIENT: Published in e-CPS, available by subscription at www.e-cps.ca.

DOSAGE FORMS, COMPOSITION AND PACKAGING: Each unit dose vial contains: ipratropium bromide (as ipratropium bromide monohydrate) 0.50 mg and salbutamol 2.5 mg (as salbutamol sulphate) in a 2.5 mL isotonic preservative-free solution for inhalation. Nonmedicinal ingredients: hydrochloric acid, purified water and sodium chloride. Plastic single dose vials of 2.5 mL, strips of 10. Each UDV strip is packaged in an aluminium/ low density polyethylene (LDPE) pouch.

Combivir® Ⓟ

lamivudine—zidovudine

Antiretroviral Agent

ViiV Healthcare ULC

Date of Revision: April 23, 2010

SUMMARY PRODUCT INFORMATION:

Route of Administration	Dosage Form/ Strength	Clinically Relevant Nonmedicinal Ingredients
Oral	Tablets/150 mg lamivudine and 300 mg zidovudine	None For a complete listing see Dosage Forms, Composition and Packaging.

INDICATIONS AND CLINICAL USE: COMBIVIR (lamivudine and zidovudine) is indicated for:

- the treatment of HIV-infection when therapy is warranted.

The clinical trial data obtained with COMBIVIR is limited. See Action and Clinical Pharmacology, Pharmacokinetics for information on bioequivalence.

CONTRAINDICATIONS:

- COMBIVIR (lamivudine and zidovudine) is contraindicated in patients with previously demonstrated clinically significant hypersensitivity to any of the components of the product. For a complete listing see Dosage Forms, Composition and Packaging. The coadministration of COMBIVIR with 3TC or RETROVIR (AZT) is not recommended.
- Due to the active ingredient zidovudine, COMBIVIR is contraindicated in patients with abnormally low neutrophil counts (<0.75×10⁹/L) or abnormally low haemoglobin levels (<7.5 g/dL or 4.65 mmol/L).

WARNINGS AND PRECAUTIONS:

> **Serious Warnings and Precautions**
> - **Lactic Acidosis and Severe Hepatomegaly with Steatosis:** Lactic acidosis and severe hepatomegaly with steatosis, including fatal cases, have been reported with the use of nucleoside analogues alone or in combination, including COMBIVIR and other antiretrovirals. A majority of these cases have been in women. Obesity and prolonged nucleoside exposure may be risk factors. However, cases have also been reported in patients with no known risk factors. Treatment with COMBIVIR should be suspended in any patient who develops clinical or laboratory findings suggestive of lactic acidosis or pronounced hepatotoxicity (which may include hepatomegaly and steatosis even in the absence of marked transaminase elevations).
> - **Post-Treatment Exacerbation of Hepatitis:** It is recommended that all patients with HIV be tested for the presence of chronic hepatitis B virus (HBV) before initiating antiretroviral therapy. COMBIVIR is not indicated for the treatment of chronic HBV infection and the safety and efficacy of COMBIVIR have not been established in patients coinfected with HBV and HIV. Exacerbations of hepatitis B have been reported in patients after the discontinuation of antiretroviral therapy. Patients coinfected with HIV and HBV should be closely monitored with both clinical and laboratory follow-up for at least several months after stopping treatment with COMBIVIR.
> - **Pancreatitis in Pediatric Patients:** In pediatric patients with a history of prior antiretroviral nucleoside exposure, a history of pancreatitis, or other significant risk factors for the development of pancreatitis, COMBIVIR should be used with caution. Treatment with COMBIVIR should be stopped immediately if clinical signs, symptoms, or laboratory abnormalities suggestive of pancreatitis occur (see Adverse Reactions).

General: The incidence of adverse reactions appears to increase with disease progression and patients should be monitored carefully, especially as disease progression occurs.

The complete prescribing information for all agents being considered for use with COMBIVIR (lamivudine and zidovudine) should be consulted before combination therapy with COMBIVIR is initiated.

Patients should be cautioned about the concomitant use of self-administered medications.

Serious Adverse Reactions: Zidovudine: Several serious adverse events have been reported with use of zidovudine in clinical practice. Reports of pancreatitis, sensitization reactions (including anaphylaxis in one patient), vasculitis, and seizures have been rare. These adverse events, except for sensitization, have also been associated with HIV disease. Changes in skin and nail pigmentation have been associated with the use of zidovudine.

Lamivudine: Several serious adverse events have been reported with use of lamivudine in clinical practice. Reports of anaphylaxis, rhabdomyolysis and peripheral neuropathy have been rare (<1 in 1000) (see Drug Interactions).

Patients receiving COMBIVIR or any other antiretroviral therapy may continue to develop opportunistic infections and other complications of HIV infection. Therefore, patients should remain under close observation by physicians experienced in the treatment of patients with HIV-associated diseases.

Patients should be advised that current antiretroviral therapy, including COMBIVIR, has not been proven to prevent the risk of transmission of HIV to others through sexual contact or blood contamination. Appropriate precautions should continue to be taken.

It is recommended that the dose of lamivudine be reduced for adults with body weight below 50 kg therefore; a patient may be on a reduced dose of lamivudine and a standard dose of zidovudine and would not be a candidate for the use of COMBIVIR tablets. See complete prescribing information for 3TC and RETROVIR (AZT) for dosage adjustment.

Endocrine and Metabolism: Fat Redistribution: Redistribution/accumulation of body fat including central obesity, dorsocervical fat enlargement ("buffalo hump"), peripheral wasting, facial wasting, breast enlargement, and "cushingoid appearance" have been observed in patients receiving antiretroviral therapy. The mechanism and long-term consequences of these events are currently unknown. A causal relationship has not been established.

Hematologic: Very rare occurrences of pure red cell aplasia have been reported with lamivudine or zidovudine use. Discontinuation of lamivudine and/or zidovudine has resulted in normalization of hematologic parameters in patients with suspected lamivudine or zidovudine-induced pure red cell aplasia.

Anemia, neutropenia and leucopenia (usually secondary to neutropenia) can be expected to occur in patients receiving zidovudine. These occurred more frequently at higher zidovudine dosages (1200 to 1500 mg/day), in patients with advanced HIV disease and in those who had poor marrow reserve prior to treatment (see Adverse Reactions). Hematological parameters should therefore be carefully monitored (see Contraindications) in patients receiving COMBIVIR.

These hematological effects are not usually observed before four to six weeks therapy. For patients with advanced symptomatic HIV disease, it is generally recommended that blood tests are performed at least every two weeks for the first three months of therapy and at least monthly thereafter. In patients with early HIV disease hematological adverse reactions are infrequent. Depending on the overall condition of the patient, blood tests may be performed less often, for example every one to three months.

Bone Marrow Suppression: COMBIVIR should be used with extreme caution in patients who have bone marrow compromise evidenced by granulocyte count <1000 cells/mm^3 or haemoglobin <9.5 g/dL. In patients with advanced symptomatic disease, anemia and granulocytopenia were the most significant adverse events observed (see Adverse Reactions). There have been reports of pancytopenia associated with the use of zidovudine, which was reversible in most instances after discontinuation of the drug.

Additionally dosage adjustment of zidovudine may be required if severe anemia or myelosuppression occurs during treatment with COMBIVIR, or in patients with pre-existing bone marrow compromise for example haemoglobin less than 9 g/dL (5.59 mmol/l) or neutrophil count less than 1.0×10^9/L. As dosage adjustment of COMBIVIR is not possible separate preparations of zidovudine and lamivudine should be used (see Contraindications).

Hepatic/Biliary/Pancreatic: Lactic Acidosis/Severe Hepatomegaly with Steatosis: Lactic acidosis and severe hepatomegaly with steatosis, including fatal cases, have been reported with the use of antiretroviral nucleoside analogues either alone or in combination, including lamivudine and zidovudine. A majority of these cases have been in women.

Clinical features which may be indicative of the development of lactic acidosis include generalized weakness, anorexia and sudden unexplained weight loss, gastrointestinal symptoms and respiratory symptoms (dyspnea and tachypnea).

Caution should be exercised when administering COMBIVIR to any patient, and particularly to those with known risk factors for liver disease. Treatment with COMBIVIR should be suspended in any patient who develops clinical or laboratory findings suggestive of lactic acidosis or hepatotoxicity (which may include hepatomegaly and steatosis even in the absence of marked transaminase elevations).

Cases of pancreatitis have occurred rarely in patients treated with lamivudine and zidovudine. However it is not clear whether these cases were due to treatment with the medicinal products or to the underlying HIV disease. Pancreatitis must be considered whenever a patient develops abdominal pain, nausea, vomiting or elevated biochemical markers. Discontinue use of COMBIVIR until diagnosis of pancreatitis is excluded.

Coadministration of zidovudine with other drugs metabolized by glucuronidation should be avoided because the toxicity of either drug may be potentiated (see Drug Interactions).

Patients Co-infected with Hepatitis B virus: Clinical trials and marketed use of lamivudine, have shown that some patients with chronic hepatitis B virus (HBV) disease may experience clinical or laboratory evidence of recurrent hepatitis upon discontinuation of lamivudine, which may have more severe consequences in patients with decompensated liver disease. If COMBIVIR is discontinued in a patient with HIV and HBV coinfection, periodic monitoring of both liver function tests and markers of HBV replication should be considered.

Patients Co-infected with Hepatitis C Virus: Exacerbation of anaemia due to ribavirin has been reported when zidovudine is part of the regimen used to treat HIV although the exact mechanism remains to be elucidated. Therefore, the coadministration of ribavirin and zidovudine is not advised and consideration should be given to replacing zidovudine in a combination ART regimen if this is already established. This would be particularly important in patients with a known history of zidovudine induced anemia.

Use with Interferon- and Ribavirin-Based Regimens: In vitro studies have shown ribavirin can reduce the phosphorylation of pyrimidine nucleoside analogues such as lamivudine and zidovudine. Although no evidence of a pharmacokinetic or pharmacodynamic interaction (e.g., loss of HIV/HCV virologic suppression) was seen when ribavirin was coadministered with lamivudine or zidovudine in HIV/HCV co-infected patients, **hepatic decompensation (some fatal) has occurred in HIV/HCV co-infected patients receiving combination antiretroviral therapy for HIV and interferon alfa with or without ribavirin.** Patients receiving interferon alfa with or without ribavirin and COMBIVIR should be closely monitored for treatment-associated toxicities, especially hepatic decompensation, neutropenia, and anemia. Discontinuation of COMBIVIR should be considered as medically appropriate. Dose reduction or discontinuation of interferon alfa, ribavirin, or both should also be considered if worsening clinical toxicities are observed, including hepatic decompensation (e.g., Child Pugh >6) (see the complete prescribing information for interferon and ribavirin).

Immune: Immune Reconstitution: During the initial phase of treatment, patients responding to antiretroviral therapy may develop an inflammatory response to indolent or residual opportunistic infections (such as MAC, CMV, PCP, and TB), which may necessitate further evaluation and treatment.

Ophthalmologic: Myopathy: Myopathy and myositis with pathological changes similar to those produced by HIV disease have been associated with prolonged use of zidovudine and may occur with COMBIVIR therapy.

Renal: Patients with impaired renal function may be at a greater risk of toxicity from COMBIVIR due to decreased renal clearance of the drug. Therefore a dosage adjustment of lamivudine and zidovudine may be necessary. It is recommended that COMBIVIR not be used in patients with reduced renal function (creatinine clearance ≤50 mL/min). For these patients, it is recommended that 3TC (lamivudine) and RETROVIR (AZT) (zidovudine) be administered. The individual Product Monographs for 3TC (lamivudine) and RETROVIR (AZT) (zidovudine) should be consulted for appropriate dosage adjustments.

Special Populations: Pregnant Women: There are no adequate and well-controlled studies of COMBIVIR in pregnant women.

Consistent with passive transmission of the drug across the placenta, lamivudine concentrations in infant serum at birth were similar to those in maternal and cord serum.

A randomized, double-blind, placebo-controlled trial was conducted in HIV-infected pregnant women to determine the utility of zidovudine for the prevention of maternal-fetal HIV-transmission. Congenital abnormalities occurred with similar frequency between infants born to mothers who received zidovudine and infants born to mothers who received placebo. Abnormalities were either problems in embryogenesis (prior to 14 weeks) or were recognized on ultrasound before or immediately after initiation of study drug.

The long-term consequences of in utero and infant exposure to zidovudine are unknown. The long-term effects of early or short-term use of zidovudine in pregnant women are also unknown.

There have been reports of mild, transient elevations in serum lactate levels, which may be due to mitochondrial dysfunction, in neonates and infants exposed in utero or peri-partum to nucleoside reverse transcriptase inhibitors (NRTIs). The clinical relevance of transient elevations in serum lactate is unknown. There have also been very rare reports of developmental delay, seizures and other neurological disease. However, a causal relationship between these events and NRTI exposure in utero or peri-partum has not been established. These findings do not affect current recommendations to use antiretroviral therapy in pregnant women to prevent vertical transmission of HIV.

Reproductive studies with lamivudine in animals have not shown evidence of teratogenicity, and showed no effect on male or female fertility. Lamivudine induced early embryolethality when lamivudine was administered to pregnant rabbits at exposure levels comparable to those achieved in man.

Because animal reproduction studies are not always predictive of the human response, COMBIVIR should be used during pregnancy only if the potential benefit outweighs any possible risk. Administration of COMBIVIR during the first three months of pregnancy is not recommended unless the benefit outweighs the risk.

Antiretroviral Pregnancy Registry: To monitor maternal-fetal outcomes of pregnant women exposed to COMBIVIR, an Antiretroviral Pregnancy Registry has been established. Physicians are encouraged to register patients by calling ViiV Healthcare ULC's Drug Safety Department (1-877-393-8448).

Nursing Women: It is recommended that HIV infected women do not breastfeed their infants in order to avoid transmission of HIV. Both lamivudine and zidovudine are excreted in human milk at similar concentrations to those found in serum. Since lamivudine, zidovudine and HIV virus pass into breast milk it is recommended that mothers taking COMBIVIR do not breastfeed their infants.

Following oral administration, lamivudine was excreted in breast milk at similar concentrations to those found in serum. It is recommended that mothers taking lamivudine do not breastfeed to avoid risking postnatal transmission of HIV infection and potential adverse effects from lamivudine in nursing infants.

Zidovudine is excreted in human milk. After administration of a single dose of 200 mg zidovudine to 13 HIV-infected women, the mean concentration of zidovudine was similar in human milk and serum. Mothers should be instructed to discontinue nursing if they are receiving COMBIVIR.

Pediatrics: There are no data on the use of COMBIVIR in pediatric patients.

COMBIVIR is not recommended in children less than 12 years of age, as appropriate dose reduction for the weight of the child cannot be made (see Dosage and Administration).

ADVERSE REACTIONS: Clinical Trial Adverse Drug Reactions: Because clinical trials are conducted under very specific conditions the adverse reaction rates observed in the clinical trials may not reflect the rates observed in practice and should not be compared to the rates in the clinical trials of another drug. Adverse drug reaction information from clinical trials is useful for identifying drug-related adverse events and for approximating rates.

In a human bioequivalence trial, the clinical adverse events associated with COMBIVIR (lamivudine and zidovudine) in 24 subjects were similar when compared to 3TC 150 mg plus RETROVIR (AZT) 300 mg administered as separate tablets. All reported adverse events were mild in intensity. The most frequently reported adverse events after single-dose administration were headache or dizziness (seven events in six subjects) and nausea (four events in four subjects). Other reported adverse events included pruritus, skin lesion, visual disturbance, rhinorrhea, and phlebitis (one event in one subject, each). Ten events in seven subjects were assessed by the investigator as possibly or probably drug related and included headache, nausea, phlebitis, and disturbance of vision.

The safety of chronic dosing with COMBIVIR has not been assessed but is not expected to be different from the safety profiles of 3TC and RETROVIR (AZT) administered concurrently as separate formulations. In four randomized, controlled trials of 3TC 300 mg per day plus RETROVIR (AZT) 600 mg per day, the following selected clinical adverse events were observed (see Table 1).

Table 1: COMBIVIR

Selected Clinical Adverse Events (≥5% Frequency) in 4 Controlled Clinical Trials with 3TC 300 mg/day and RETROVIR (AZT) 600 mg/day

Adverse Event	3TC Plus RETROVIR (AZT) (n=251) (%)
Body as a Whole	
Headache	35
Malaise and Fatigue	27
Fever or Chills	10
Digestive	
Nausea	33
Diarrhea	18
Nausea and Vomiting	13
Anorexia and/or Decreased Appetite	10
Abdominal Pain	9
Abdominal Cramps	6
Dyspepsia	5
Nervous System	
Neuropathy	12
Insomnia and Other Sleep Disorders	11
Dizziness	10
Depressive Disorders	9
Respiratory	
Nasal Signs and Symptoms	20
Cough	18
Skin	
Skin Rashes	9
Musculoskeletal	
Musculoskeletal Pain	12
Myalgia	8

(cont'd)

Table 1: COMBIVIR *(cont'd)*

Selected Clinical Adverse Events (≥5% Frequency) in 4 Controlled Clinical Trials with 3TC 300 mg/day and RETROVIR (AZT) 600 mg/day

Adverse Event	3TC Plus RETROVIR (AZT) (n=251) (%)
Arthralgia	5

Other clinical adverse events reported in controlled clinical trials in association with 3TC (lamivudine) 150 mg b.i.d. plus zidovudine 600 mg per day in at least 1% of patients were:

Gastrointestinal: abdominal discomfort and pain (3%), abdominal distension (3%), dyspepsia (2%), gastrointestinal discomfort and pain (3%), gastrointestinal gas (4%), hyposalivation (2%), oral ulceration (1%).
Musculoskeletal: muscle atrophy/weakness/tiredness (1%), muscle pain (2%).
Neurological: mood disorders (1%), sleep disorders (4%), taste disturbances (1%).
Other: breathing disorders (2%), general signs and symptoms (1%), pain (2%), sexual function disturbances (1%), temperature regulation disturbance (1%).
Skin: pruritus (1%), skin rashes (1%), sweating (1%).

Pancreatitis was observed in three of the 656 adult patients (<0.5%) who received 3TC in controlled clinical trials.

Selected laboratory abnormalities observed during therapy are listed in Table 2.

Table 2: COMBIVIR

Frequencies of Selected Laboratory Abnormalities Among Adults in 4 Controlled Clinical Trials of 3TC 300 mg/day Plus RETROVIR (AZT) 600 mg/day[a]

Test (Abnormal Level)	3TC Plus RETROVIR (AZT) % (n)
Neutropenia (ANC <750/mm^3)	7.2 (237)
Anemia (Hgb <8.0 g/dL)	2.9 (241)
Thrombocytopenia (platelets <50 000/mm^3)	0.4 (240)
ALT (>5.0×ULN)	3.7 (241)
AST (>5.0×ULN)	1.7 (241)
Bilirubin (>2.5×ULN)	0.8 (241)
Amylase (>2.0×ULN)	4.2 (72)

[a] Frequencies of these laboratory abnormalities were higher in patients with mild laboratory abnormalities at baseline.
Legend: ULN=upper limit of normal; ANC=absolute neutrophil count; n=number of patients assessed.

Post-Market Adverse Drug Reactions: The following events have been identified during post-approval use of 3TC and/or RETROVIR (AZT) alone or in combination with other antiretroviral therapy in clinical practice. Because they are reported voluntarily from a population of unknown size, estimates of frequency cannot be made. These events have been chosen for inclusion due to either their seriousness, frequency of reporting, causal connection to 3TC and/or RETROVIR (AZT), or a combination of these factors.

Body as a Whole: redistribution/accumulation of body fat (see Warnings and Precautions, Fat Redistribution).
Cardiovascular: cardiac arrest, cardiac failure, cardiomegaly, cardiomyopathy, cerebrovascular accident, hypertension, hypotension, intracranial hemorrhage, orthostatic hypotension, palpitation(s), syncope, tachycardia, vasculitis, vasodilation.
Endocrine and Metabolic: acidosis, anorexia, dehydration, gynecomastia, hypercholesterolemia, hyperglycemia, hyperlactataemia, hyperlipidemia, hyperuricemia, hypoglycemia, hyponatremia, inappropriate antidiuretic hormone secretion, increased appetite, increased CPK, increased LDH, increased serum iron, lactic acidosis and hepatic steatosis (see Warnings and Precautions), weight loss.
Eye: conjunctivitis, retinitis, visual field defect.
Gastrointestinal: abdominal distention, ascites, bleeding gums, constipation, diarrhea, discolouration of tongue, dyspepsia, dysphagia, edema of the tongue, esophagitis, esophageal ulcer, flatulence, gastritis, gastrointestinal hemorrhage, mouth ulcer, nausea and vomiting, oral mucosa pigmentation, peptic ulcer, rectal hemorrhage, rises in serum amylase, sialoadenitis, stomatitis.
General: abdominal pain, allergic reaction, anaphylaxis, back pain, Candida infection, chills, chest pain, death, edema of face, edema of extremities, fatigue, fever, flu syndrome, hypertonia, hypotonia, malaise, pain, pallor, sepsis, weakness.
Hemic and Lymphatic: abnormalities of red cells, abnormalities of white cells, agranulocytosis, anemia, aplastic anemia, bone marrow depression, eosinophilia, hemolysis, impaired red cell maturation, leukocytosis, leukopenia, lymphadenopathy, lymphocytosis, lymphoma, methemoglobinemia, neutropenia, pancytopenia, pure red cell aplasia, sarcoma, splenomegaly, thrombocytopenia, thrombotic thrombocytopenic purpura.
Hepatobiliary Tract and Pancreas: cholestatic jaundice, fatty liver, hepatic impairment, hepatic failure, hepatitis, hepatomegaly, hyperbilirubinemia, increased aminotransferase levels, increased amylase, jaundice, pancreatitis.
Musculoskeletal: amyotrophy, arthralgia, muscle disorders including rarely rhabdomyolysis, myositis, tremor, twitch, myalgia, hemarthrosis, leg cramps.
Nervous: aggressive behavior, agitation, amnesia, anxiety, ataxia, confusion, convulsions, delusions, dementia, depression, dizziness, dystonic movement(s), emotional lability, encephalitis, facial palsy, hallucinations, headache, hypoesthesia, insomnia, loss of mental acuity, meningitis, myasthenia, nervousness, mania, paresthesia, paranoia, peripheral neuritis, peripheral neuropathy, personality disorder, psychotic disorders, somnolence, tremor, vertigo.
Reproductive: amenorrhea, decreased libido, gynaecomastia impotence, intermenstrual bleeding.
Respiratory: apnea, cough, dyspnea, epistaxis, hyperventilation, influenza, pharyngitis, pneumonia, rhinitis, sinusitis.
Skin: acne, alopecia, changes in skin and nail pigmentation, dryness of skin, erythema multiforme, exfoliative dermatitis, hair colour change, hirsutism, hyperpigmentation, maculopapular lesions, nail disorders, photosensitivity, pruritus, rash, rubelliform rash, Stevens-Johnson syndrome, sweating, urticaria, vesiculobullous rash.
Special Senses: ageusia, amblyopia, hearing loss, photophobia, taste disturbance, speech disorder, tinnitus.
Urogenital: albuminuria, dysuria, hematuria, increased creatinine levels, polyuria, renal dysfunction, renal failure, urinary frequency.

DRUG INTERACTIONS: Overview: As COMBIVIR contains lamivudine and zidovudine, any interactions that have been identified with these agents individually may occur with COMBIVIR.

Zidovudine plasma levels are not significantly altered when coadministered with lamivudine. Zidovudine had no effect on the pharmacokinetics of lamivudine (see Action and Clinical Pharmacology).

The possibility of interactions with other drugs administered concurrently should be considered, particularly when the main route of elimination is renal.

Drug-Drug Interactions: See Table 3.

DOSAGE AND ADMINISTRATION: Recommended Dose and Dosage Adjustment: The recommended oral dose of COMBIVIR (lamivudine and zidovudine) for adults and adolescents who are at least 12 years old is one tablet (containing 150 mg of lamivudine and 300 mg zidovudine) twice daily.

Dose Adjustment: It is recommended that separate doses of lamivudine (as 3TC) and zidovudine [as RETROVIR (AZT)] be administered to patients with reduced renal function (see Warnings and Precautions), pediatric patients below 12 years of age, patients with low body weights (less than 50 kg) or patients requiring dosing adjustments due to adverse events. See complete prescribing information for 3TC and RETROVIR (AZT) for dosage adjustments.

Missed Dose: If you forget to take your medicine, take it as soon as you remember. Then continue as before.

OVERDOSAGE:
There is no known antidote for COMBIVIR (lamivudine and zidovudine).

If overdosage occurs the patient should be monitored, and standard supportive treatment applied as required. Although no data is available, administration of activated charcoal may be used to aid in removal of unabsorbed drug. Because a negligible amount of lamivudine was removed via (4-hour) hemodialysis, continuous ambulatory peritoneal dialysis, and automated peritoneal dialysis, it is not known if continuous hemodialysis would provide clinical benefit in a lamivudine overdose event. Hemodialysis and peritoneal dialysis appear to have a negligible effect on the removal of zidovudine while elimination of its primary metabolite, GZDV is enhanced.

Limited data are available on the consequences of ingestion of acute overdoses in humans. No fatalities occurred, and the patient recovered. No specific signs or symptoms have been identified following such overdose.

One case of acute overdose in an adult ingesting 6 g of lamivudine was reported; there were no clinical signs or symptoms noted and hematologic tests remained normal. One other adult patient in error ingested lamivudine 1200 mg per day plus zidovudine 1200 mg per day for approximately 2 weeks; he had a Grade 3 decrease in absolute neutrophil count that resolved upon reduction of doses of lamivudine and zidovudine. In Phase I studies, lamivudine was administered at doses up to 20 mg/kg per day (i.e., approximately five times the usual recommended dose in adults) without serious consequences.

Cases of acute overdose of zidovudine in both children and adults have been reported with doses up to 50 g. The only consistent finding in these cases of overdose was spontaneous or induced nausea and vomiting. Hematologic changes were transient and not severe. Some patients experienced nonspecific CNS symptoms such as headache, dizziness, drowsiness, lethargy, and confusion. One report of a grand mal seizure possibly attributable to zidovudine occurred in a 35-year-old male 3 hours after ingesting 36 grams of zidovudine. No other cause could be identified. All patients recovered without permanent sequelae.

Table 3: COMBIVIR

Established or Potential Drug-Drug Interactions

Proper Name	Effect	Clinical Comment
Atovaquone	Zidovudine does not appear to affect the pharmacokinetics of atovaquone.	Pharmacokinetic data have shown that atovaquone appears to decrease the rate of metabolism of zidovudine to its glucuronide metabolite (steady state AUC of zidovudine was increased by 33% and peak plasma concentration of the glucuronide was decreased by 19%). At zidovudine dosages of 500 or 600 mg/day it would seem unlikely that a three week, concomitant course of atovaquone for the treatment of acute PCP would result in an increased incidence of adverse reactions attributable to higher plasma concentrations of zidovudine. Extra care should be taken in monitoring patients receiving prolonged atovaquone therapy.
Bone Marrow Suppressive Agents/ Cytotoxic Agents	Coadministration may increase risk of hematologic toxicity.	Coadministration of zidovudine with drugs that are cytotoxic or which interfere with RBC/WBC number or function (e.g. dapsone, flucytosine, vincristine, vinblastine, or adriamycin) may increase the risk of hematologic toxicity.
Clarithromycin	Clarithromycin tablets reduce the absorption of zidovudine.	This can be avoided by separating the administration of zidovudine and clarithromycin by at least two hours.
Fluconazole	Fluconazole interferes with the oral clearance and metabolism of zidovudine.	Preliminary data suggest that fluconazole interferes with the oral clearance and metabolism of zidovudine. In a pharmacokinetic interaction study in which 12 HIV-positive men received zidovudine alone and in combination with fluconazole, increases in the mean peak serum concentration (79%), AUC (70%) and half-life (38%) were observed at steady state. The clinical significance of this interaction is unknown.
Ganciclovir	Coadministration increases the risk of hematologic toxicities in some patients with advanced HIV disease.	Use of zidovudine in combination with ganciclovir increases the risk of hematologic toxicities in some patients with advanced HIV disease. Should the use of this combination become necessary in the treatment of patients with HIV disease, dose reduction or interruption of one or both agents may be necessary to minimize hematologic toxicity. Hematologic parameters, including hemoglobin, hematocrit, and white blood cell count with differential, should be monitored frequently in all patients receiving this combination.
Interferon-alpha	Hematologic toxicities have been seen when zidovudine is used concomitantly with interferon-alpha.	As with the concomitant use of RETROVIR (AZT) and ganciclovir, dose reduction or interruption of one or both agents may be necessary, and hematologic parameters should be monitored frequently.
Methadone	Plasma levels of zidovudine can be elevated in some patients while remaining unchanged in others.	In a pharmacokinetic study of 9 HIV-positive patients receiving methadone-maintenance (30 to 90 mg daily) concurrent with 200 mg of zidovudine every 4 hours, no changes were observed in the pharmacokinetics of methadone upon initiation of therapy with zidovudine and after 14 days of treatment with zidovudine. No adjustments in methadone-maintenance requirements were reported. However, plasma levels of zidovudine were elevated in some patients while remaining unchanged in others. The exact mechanism and clinical significance of these data are unknown.
Phenytoin	A decrease in oral zidovudine clearance.	Phenytoin plasma levels have been reported to be low in some patients receiving zidovudine, while in one case a high level was documented. However, in a pharmacokinetic interaction study in which 12 HIV-positive volunteers received a single 300 mg phenytoin dose alone and during steady-state zidovudine conditions (200 mg every 4 hours), no change in phenytoin kinetics was observed. Although not designed to optimally assess the effect of phenytoin on zidovudine kinetics, a 30% decrease in oral zidovudine clearance was observed with phenytoin. Phenytoin concentrations should be carefully monitored in patients receiving COMBIVIR and Phenytoin.

(cont'd)

Table 3: COMBIVIR *(cont'd)*
Established or Potential Drug-Drug Interactions

Proper Name	Effect	Clinical Comment
Probenecid	May increase zidovudine levels.	Limited data suggest that probenecid may increase zidovudine levels by inhibiting glucuronidation and/or reducing renal excretion of zidovudine. Some patients who have used zidovudine concomitantly with probenecid have developed flu-like symptoms consisting of myalgia, malaise, and/or fever and maculopapular rash.
Ribavarin	Coadministration of ribavirin and zidovudine may lead to increased ribavirin levels and increased risk of anemia.	Preliminary data suggest that the use of ribavirin and zidovudine lead to increased ribavirin levels and increased risk of anemia. The use of ribavirin concomitantly with zidovudine in the treatment of HIV/Hep C co-infected patients is not advised. Consideration should be given to replacing zidovudine in a combination ART regimen if this is already established.
Stavudine	Zidovudine may inhibit intracellular phosphorylation of stavudine	Zidovudine may inhibit the intracellular phosphorylation of stavudine when the two medicinal products are used concurrently. Stavudine is therefore not recommended to be used in combination with zidovudine.
Trimethoprim, a constituent of co-trimoxazole	Administration of trimethoprim, a constituent of co-trimoxazole causes a 40% increase in lamivudine plasma levels.	However, unless the patient has renal impairment, no dosage adjustment of lamivudine is necessary. Lamivudine has no effect on the pharmacokinetics of co-trimoxazole. Administration of co-trimoxazole with the lamivudine/zidovudine combination in patients with renal impairment should be carefully assessed.
Valproic Acid	Increase in zidovudine AUC and a decrease in the plasma GZDV AUC.	The concomitant administration of valproic acid 250 mg (n=5) or 500 mg (n=1) every 8 hours and zidovudine 100 mg orally every 8 hours for 4 days to 6 HIV-infected, asymptomatic male volunteers resulted in a 79%±61% (mean±SD) increase in the plasma zidovudine AUC and a 22%±10% decrease in the plasma GZDV AUC as compared to the administration of zidovudine in the absence of valproic acid. The GZDV/zidovudine urinary excretion ratio decreased 58%±12%. Because no change in the zidovudine plasma half-life occurred, these results suggest that valproic acid may increase the oral bioavailability of zidovudine through inhibition of first-pass metabolism. Although the clinical signification of this interaction is unknown, patients should be monitored more closely for a possible increase in zidovudine-related adverse effects. The effect of zidovudine on the pharmacokinetics of valproic acid was not evaluated.
Zalcitabine	Lamivudine may inhibit the intracellular phosphorylation of zalcitabine when the two medicinal products are used concurrently.	COMBIVIR is therefore not recommended to be used in combination with zalcitabine.
Other Agents		Preliminary data from a drug interaction study (n=10) suggest that coadministration of 200 mg RETROVIR (AZT) and 600 mg rifampin decreases the area under the plasma concentration curve of zidovudine by an average of 48%±34%. However, the effect of once daily dosing of rifampin on multiple daily doses of RETROVIR (AZT) is unknown.

(cont'd)

Table 3: COMBIVIR *(cont'd)*
Established or Potential Drug-Drug Interactions

Proper Name	Effect	Clinical Comment
Miscellaneous		Other medicinal products, including but not limited to, acetylsalicylic acid, codeine, morphine, methadone, indomethacin, ketoprofen, naproxen, oxazepam, lorazepam, cimetidine, clofibrate, dapsone and isoprinosine, may alter the metabolism of zidovudine by competitively inhibiting glucuronidation or directly inhibiting hepatic microsomal metabolism. Careful thought should be given to the possibilities of interactions before using such medicinal products particularly for chronic therapy, in combination with COMBIVIR. Concomitant treatment, especially acute therapy, with potentially nephrotoxic or myelosuppressive medicinal products (for example systemic pentamidine, dapsone, pyrimethamine, co-trimoxazole, amphotericin, flucytosine, ganciclovir, interferon, vincristine, vinblastine and doxorubicin) may also increase the risk of adverse reactions to zidovudine. If concomitant therapy with COMBIVIR and any of these medicinal products is necessary then extra care should be taken in monitoring renal function and hematological parameters and, if required, the dosage of one or more agents should be reduced.

For management of a suspected drug overdose, contact your regional Poison Control Centre. See the *CPS* Directory section for a list of Poison Control Centres.

ACTION AND CLINICAL PHARMACOLOGY: Mechanism of Action: Lamivudine and zidovudine are potent, selective inhibitors of HIV-1 and HIV-2 replication in vitro. Lamivudine is the (-) enantiomer of a dideoxy analogue of cytidine. Zidovudine is a thymidine analogue in which the 3'-hydroxy (-OH) group is replaced by an azido (-N3) group. Intracellularly, lamivudine and zidovudine are phosphorylated to their active 5'-triphosphate metabolites, lamivudine triphosphate (L-TP) and zidovudine triphosphate (ZDV-TP). In vitro L-TP has an intracellular half-life of approximately 10.5 to 15.5 hours. The principal mode of action of L-TP and ZDV-TP is inhibition of HIV reverse transcription (RT) via viral DNA chain termination. L-TP is a weak inhibitor of mammalian α, β, and γ-DNA polymerases. ZDV-TP is a weak inhibitor of the cellular DNA polymerase-α and mitochondrial polymerase-γ and has been reported to be incorporated into the DNA of cells in culture.

Pharmacokinetics: The single-dose pharmacokinetic properties of COMBIVIR (lamivudine and zidovudine) have been studied in 24 healthy adult subjects in a single-centre, open label, randomized, three-way crossover study to evaluate the bioequivalence between COMBIVIR and the 150 mg 3TC tablet and the 300 mg RETROVIR (AZT) tablet given simultaneously. COMBIVIR was bioequivalent to one 3TC tablet (150 mg) plus one RETROVIR (AZT) tablet (300 mg) when administered to fasting subjects. A summary of the results is provided in Table 4.

The pharmacokinetic properties of lamivudine have been studied in asymptomatic, HIV-infected adult patients after administration of single oral, multiple oral and intravenous (IV) doses ranging from 0.25 to 10 mg/kg. After oral administration of 2 mg/kg, the peak plasma lamivudine concentration (C_{max}) was 1.5±0.5 µg/mL (mean±S.D.) and half-life was 2.6±0.5 hours. There were no significant differences in half-life across the range of single doses (0.25 to 8 mg/kg). The area under the plasma concentration versus time curve (AUC) and C_{max} increased in proportion to dose over the range from 0.25 to 10 mg/kg.

Lamivudine is well absorbed from the gut, and the bioavailability of oral lamivudine in adults is normally between 80 and 85%. Following oral administration, the mean time (t_{max}) to maximal serum concentrations (C_{max}) is about an hour.

Pharmacokinetic studies of RETROVIR (AZT) following intravenous dosing in adults indicate dose-independent kinetics over the range of 1 to 5 mg/kg with a mean zidovudine half-life of 1.1 hours. Zidovudine is rapidly metabolized in the liver to 3'-azido-3'-deoxy-5'-O-β-D- glucopyranuronosylthymidine (GZDV, formerly called GAZT), and both are rapidly eliminated by the kidney. A second metabolite, 3'-amino-3'-deoxythymidine (AMT) has been identified in the plasma following single dose intravenous administration of zidovudine.

After oral dosing in adults, zidovudine is rapidly absorbed from the gastrointestinal tract with peak serum concentrations occurring within 0.5 to 1.5 hours, with an average oral bioavailability of 65%.

STORAGE AND STABILITY: COMBIVIR (lamivudine and zidovudine) tablets should be stored between 2 and 30°C.

SPECIAL HANDLING INSTRUCTIONS: Not applicable.

INFORMATION FOR THE PATIENT: Published in e-CPS, available by subscription at www.e-cps.ca.

DOSAGE FORMS, COMPOSITION AND PACKAGING: Each white to off-white, capsule-shaped, film-coated tablet, scored, embossed "GX FC3" on both sides, contains: lamivudine 150 mg and zidovudine 300 mg. Nonmedicinal ingredients: colloidal silicon dioxide, hydroxypropyl methylcellulose, magnesium stearate, microcrystalline cellulose, polyethylene glycol, polysorbate 80, sodium starch glycolate and titanium dioxide. HDPE bottles of 60.

(Shown in Product Identification Section)

Table 4: COMBIVIR
Summary Table of Measured Comparative Bioavailability Data for COMBIVIR (Lamivudine and Zidovudine) Tablets

	Geometric Mean and Arithmetic Mean (CV)									
	Treatment A Combined 150 mg Lamivudine and Zidovudine 300 mg Fasted		Treatment B 3TC 150 mg Tablet + RETROVIR (AZT) 300 mg Tablet Fasted		Treatment C Combined 150 mg Lamivudine and Zidovudine 300 mg Fed		Ratio of Geometric Means A:B (%) (CI)		Ratio of Geometric Means C:A (%) (CI)	
	ZDV	LAM	ZDV	LAM	ZDV	LAM	ZDV	LAM	ZDV	LAM
AUC_{last} (ng·h/mL)	2266.80 2365.63 (29.60)	5747.93 5896.06 (21.45)	2296.02 2357.09 (23.22)	5931.51 6131.41 (26.37)	2029.33 1810.16 (31.21)	5683.12 5167.96 (18.67)	0.99 (0.91–1.07)	0.97 (0.92–1.03)	0.90 (0.83–0.97)	0.99 (0.93–1.05)
AUC_{∞} (ng·h/mL)	2299.44 2398.16 (29.43)	6004.95 6137.56 (20.11)	2329.36 2390.88 (23.13)	6185.54 6374.20 (25.22)	2061.10 2147.63 (30.95)	5932.26 6035.41 (19.23)	0.99 (0.91–1.07)	0.97 (0.92–1.02)	0.90 (0.83–0.97)	0.99 (0.94–1.04)
C_{max} (ng/mL)	1827.27 2008.27 (40.33)	1536.96 1620.28 (32.07)	1883.15 1992.64 (31.92)	1634.32 1742.22 (35.37)	1000.26 1139.24 (51.59)	1311.73 1367.59 (29.53)	0.97 (0.82–1.15)	0.94 (0.84–1.06)	0.55 (0.46–0.65)	0.85 (0.76–0.96)
T_{max} (h)	0.50[a] 0.57 (80.32)	0.75[a] 0.91 (53.16)	0.50[a] 0.58 (58.83)	1.00[a] 0.91 (40.51)	1.00[a] 1.07 (61.26)	1.50[a] 1.86 (50.81)	N/A	N/A	N/A	N/A
$T_{1/2}$ (h)	1.48 1.50 (15.73)	9.66 9.98 (27.85)	1.43 1.45 (16.24)	9.52 9.79 (24.71)	1.48 1.53 (26.78)	9.80 10.52 (50.61)	N/A	N/A	N/A	N/A

[a] Median.
Legend: ZDV=zidovudine; LAM=lamivudine; NA=not applicable.

CO Meloxicam 🄿

meloxicam

Anti-inflammatory—Analgesic

Cobalt

SUPPLIED: 7.5 mg: Each light yellow, round, bevelled-edged, biconvex tablet, with "Σ>" on one side and "ML" over "7.5" on the other, contains: meloxicam 7.5 mg. Nonmedicinal ingredients: colloidal silicon dioxide (Cab-O-Sil M5), crospovidone (polyplasdone XL), lactose monohydrate (Impalpable #312), magnesium stearate, microcrystalline cellulose (Vivapur type 102), povidone (plasdone) and sodium citrate (dihydrate). Gluten-free. Bottles of 100. Unit dose blisters (3×10 tablets) of 30. Store in a dry place at controlled room temperature (15-30°C), safely out of the reach of children.

15 mg: Each light yellow, round, convex and bevelled-edged tablet, with "Σ>" on one side and "ML" over "15" on the other, contains: meloxicam 15 mg. Nonmedicinal ingredients: colloidal silicon dioxide (Cab-O-Sil M5), crospovidone (polyplasdone XL), lactose monohydrate (Impalpable #312), magnesium stearate, microcrystalline cellulose (Vivapur type 102), povidone (plasdone) and sodium citrate (dihydrate). Gluten-free. Bottles of 100. Unit dose blisters (3×10 tablets) of 30. Store in a dry place at controlled room temperature (15-30°C), safely out of the reach of children.

CO Memantine 🄿

memantine HCl

N-methyl-D-aspartate (NMDA) Receptor Antagonist

Cobalt

SUPPLIED: Each white to off-white, film-coated, peanut-shaped, biconvex tablet with "MT | 10" on one side and "Σ>|Σ>" on the other side, contains: memantine hydrochloride 10 mg. Nonmedicinal ingredients: lactose monohydrate, magnesium stearate and microcrystalline cellulose; film coating: hydroxypropyl methylcellulose, lactose monohydrate, polyethylene glycol and titanium dioxide. HDPE bottles of 100. Unit dose blister packs of 30 (blister strip of 10 tablets). Store in a dry place at room temperature between 15 and 30°C.

CO Metformin Coated 🄿

metformin HCl

Oral Antihyperglycemic Agent

Cobalt

SUPPLIED: 500 mg: Each white to off-white, round, film-coated, biconvex tablet, with "Σ>" on one side and "M" over "M" on the other, contains: metformin HCl 500 mg. Nonmedicinal ingredients: crospovidone, magnesium stearate, polyethyleneglycol, polyvinyl alcohol, povidone, talc and titanium dioxide. Bottles of 100 and 500. Store at room temperature (15-30°C) in well closed containers.

850 mg: Each white to off-white, film-coated, capsule-shaped tablet, with "Σ>" on one side and "850" on the other, contains: metformin HCl 850 mg. Nonmedicinal ingredients: crospovidone, magnesium stearate, polyethyleneglycol, polyvinyl alcohol, povidone, talc and titanium dioxide. Bottles of 100 and 500. Store at room temperature (15-30°C) in well closed containers.

Comtan® 🄿

entacapone

Adjunct to Levodopa and DDC Inhibitor—COMT-Inhibitor

Novartis Pharmaceuticals

Date of Preparation: April 23, 2001
Date of Revision: December 24, 2008

PHARMACOLOGY: Entacapone is a reversible, selective and mainly peripherally acting inhibitor of catechol-O-methyltransferase (COMT). Entacapone has no antiparkinsonian effect of its own and is designed for concomitant administration with levodopa preparations.

COMT catalyzes the transfer of the methyl group of S-adenosyl-L-methionine to the phenolic group of substrates that contain a cathecol structure. Physiological substrates of COMT include dopa, catecholamines (dopamine, norepinephrine, epinephrine) and their hydroxylated metabolites. In the presence of a decarboxylase inhibitor, COMT becomes the major enzyme which is responsible for the metabolism of levodopa to 3-methoxy-4-hydroxy-1-phenylalanine (3-OMD).

The mechanism of action of entacapone is believed to be related to its ability to inhibit COMT and thereby alter the plasma pharmacokinetics of levodopa. When administered with levodopa and a dopa decarboxylase (DDC) inhibitor (carbidopa or benserazide), entacapone decreases the degradation of levodopa in the peripheral tissues further by inhibiting the metabolism of levodopa to 3-OMD through the COMT pathway. This leads to more sustained plasma concentrations of levodopa. It is believed that at a given frequency of levodopa administration, these more sustained plasma levels of levodopa result in more constant dopaminergic stimulation in the brain leading to greater effects on the signs and symptoms of Parkinson's disease. The higher levodopa levels also lead to increased levodopa adverse effects, sometimes requiring a decrease in the dose of levodopa.

In animals, while entacapone enters the CNS to a minimal extent, it has been shown to inhibit central COMT activity. In humans, entacapone inhibits the COMT enzyme in peripheral tissues. The effects of entacapone on central COMT activity in humans have not been studied.

Pharmacodynamics: Effect of Entacapone on Erythrocyte COMT Activity: Studies in healthy volunteers and patients with Parkinson's disease have shown that entacapone dose-dependently and reversibly inhibits human erythrocyte COMT activity after oral administration. Following single doses of 200 and 800 mg of entacapone, maximal inhibition of erythrocyte COMT activity was 64% and 82%, respectively.

Effect of Entacapone on the Pharmacokinetics of Levodopa and its Metabolites: When 200 mg of entacapone is administered together with levodopa/carbidopa, it increases the area under the curve (AUC) of levodopa by approximately 35% and the elimination half-life of levodopa is prolonged from 1.3 to 2.4 hours. In general, the average peak levodopa plasma concentration and the time of its occurrence (T_{max} of 1 h) are unaffected. The onset of effect occurs after the first administration and is maintained during long-term treatment.

In a dose-response study in patients with Parkinson's disease, the maximal effect was obtained with a single dose of 200 mg entacapone. Doses of entacapone greater than 200 mg did not further improve the bioavailability of levodopa.

Studies in healthy volunteers and in patients with Parkinson's disease show that entacapone dose-dependently decreases the formation of 3-OMD from levodopa. The chronic use of entacapone (200 mg, 3 to 10 times daily) in patients with Parkinson's disease, decreases the AUC of 3-OMD by 42 to 61%.

Pharmacokinetics: Entacapone pharmacokinetics are linear over a dose range of 5 to 200 mg. A slight non linearity in AUC was seen at doses greater than or equal to 400 mg in a single dose, dose-response, study in patients with Parkinson's disease. The pharmacokinetics of entacapone are independent of levodopa/DDC coadministration.

Absorption: There are large intra- and interindividual variations in the absorption of entacapone.

Entacapone is rapidly absorbed from the gastrointestinal tract, reaching peak concentrations (C_{max}) in the plasma in approximately 1 hour. The drug has an extensive first-pass metabolism with bioavailability of about 35% following oral administration of a 200 mg dose. C_{max}, after a single 200 mg dose of entacapone, is approximately 1.2 µg/mL. Food does not affect the absorption of entacapone to any significant extent.

Distribution and Protein Binding: The volume of distribution of entacapone at steady state after i.v. injection is small (20 L). Entacapone does not distribute widely into tissues due to its high plasma protein binding. Based on in vitro studies, the plasma protein binding of entacapone is 98% over the concentration range of 0.4 to 50 µg/mL. Entacapone binds mainly to serum albumin.

Metabolism/Elimination: Entacapone undergoes extensive metabolism, mainly in the liver. The main metabolic pathway of entacapone in humans is the isomerization to the cis-isomer, followed by direct glucuronidation of the parent and cis-isomer; the glucuronide conjugate is inactive.

The elimination of entacapone occurs mainly by non-renal metabolic pathways. It is estimated that 80 to 90% of the dose is excreted in feces, although this has not been confirmed in man. Approximately 10 to 20% is excreted in urine. Only traces of entacapone are found as unchanged drug in urine. The major part (95%) of the drug excreted in urine is conjugated with glucuronic acid. Of the metabolites found in urine only about 1% have been formed through oxidation.

The total body clearance of entacapone, after i.v. administration, is about 800 mL/min. It is eliminated with a short elimination half-life; the half-life for β-phase being about 0.5 hours and for the γ-phase about 2.5 hours. The β-phase is predominant, and the γ-phase accounts for approximately 8% of the plasma-time-concentration curve (AUC) following i.v. administration.

Hepatic Impairment: The metabolism of the drug is slowed in patients with mild to moderate (Child-Pugh grading Class A and B) hepatic insufficiency caused by cirrhotic disease. In these patients, the AUC and C_{max} values were approximately 2-fold greater than those in demographically matched healthy volunteers. As there are no clinical trial data to establish a safe and effective dosing regimen for hepatically impaired patients, entacapone should not be administered to patients with hepatic impairment (see Contraindications).

Renal Impairment: The pharmacokinetics of entacapone were evaluated in healthy volunteers and in patients with moderately (Cl_{cr} 0.60 to 0.89 mL/s/1.73 m^2) and severely (Cl_{cr} 0.20 to 0.44 mL/s/1.73 m^2) impaired renal function. After a single oral dose of 200 mg, the pharmacokinetics of entacapone were not significantly changed in patients with moderate to severe renal insufficiency.

Age, Gender and Race: Entacapone pharmacokinetics are independent of age. No formal gender studies have been conducted. Racial representation in clinical trials was largely limited to Caucasians (there were only 4 blacks in one U.S. trial and no Asians in any of the clinical trials); no conclusions can therefore be reached about the effect of entacapone on groups other than Caucasian.

Studies Assessing Potential Drug Interactions: Effect of Entacapone on the Metabolism of Other Drugs: Protein Binding: Entacapone is highly protein bound (98%). In vitro studies have shown that entacapone, at therapeutic concentrations, does not displace drugs of which a large proportion is bound to plasma proteins (e.g., warfarin, salicylic acid, phenylbutazone, and diazepam). On the other hand, entacapone is not markedly displaced by any of these drugs at therapeutic concentrations.

Clinical Trials: The effectiveness of entacapone as an adjunct to levodopa/DDC therapy in the treatment of Parkinson's disease was demonstrated in 3 separate 24-week randomized, placebo-controlled, double-blind, multicenter studies in 676 patients with mild to moderate Parkinson's disease (average Hoen and Yahr score: 1.5 to 3). In 2 of these studies (Nordic Study and North American "SEESAW" Study), the patients' disease was "fluctuating", i.e., was characterized by documented periods of "On" (periods with relatively good functioning) and "Off" (periods of relatively poor functioning), despite optimum levodopa therapy. In the third trial (German-Austrian "CELOMEN" Study) patients were not required to have been experiencing fluctuations. On average, the patients evaluated had been treated with levodopa/DDC inhibitor therapy for 8.3 years and 86% were treated with other antiparkinsonian medication (dopamine agonists, selegiline, amantadine, anticholinergics) in addition to a levodopa/DDC inhibitor.

In the 2 studies in patients with Parkinson's disease with documented episodes of end-of-dose motor fluctuations despite optimal levodopa therapy, patients were randomized to receive placebo (n=188) or 200 mg entacapone (n=188) with each daily dose of levodopa/dopa decarboxylase inhibitor (carbidopa or benserazide; average 4 to 6 doses/day). The formal double-blind portion of both trials was 6 months. Patients recorded the time spent in the "On" and "Off" states in home diaries periodically throughout the duration of the trial. In the Nordic Study the primary outcome measure was the total mean time spent in the "On" state during an 18-hour diary recorded day, in the North American "SEESAW" study, the primary outcome measure was the proportion of awake time spent over 24 hours in the "On" state.

In addition to the primary outcome measure, as secondary measures, the amount of time spent in the "Off" state was evaluated and patients were also evaluated in subparts of the Unified Parkinson's disease Rating Scale (UPDRS), an investigator's and patient's global assessment of clinical condition, a 7-point subjective scale designed to assess global functioning in Parkinson's disease and for change in daily levodopa/DDC dose. Results for the primary efficacy measure for these 2 studies are shown in Table 1.

Table 1: Comtan

Primary Outcome Measures: Hours of Awake Time "On" (Nordic Study); Percent of Awake Time "On" (North American "SEESAW" Study)

	Nordic Study		
	Placebo (n=86) Mean (±SD)	**Entacapone (n=85) Mean (±SD)**	**Difference**
Baseline[a]	9.2±2.5	9.3±2.2	
Week 8–24[a,b]	9.4±2.6	10.7±2.2	1 h 20 min (8.3%) $CI_{95\%}$ 45 min, 1 h 56 min
	North American "SEESAW" Study		
	Placebo (n=102)	**Entacapone (n=103)**	**Difference**
Baseline[c]	60.8±14.0	60.0±15.2	
Week 8–24[c,d]	62.8±16.8	66.8±14.5	4.5% (0 h 35 min) $CI_{95\%}$ 0.93%, 7.97%

[a] Daily "On" time (h).
[b] Values represent the average of weeks 8, 16 and 24, by protocol-defined outcome measure.
[c] Proportion "On" time %.
[d] Values represent the average of weeks 8, 16 and 24, by protocol defined outcome measure.
Legend: SD=Standard Deviation.

Effects on "On" time did not differ by age, weight, disease severity at baseline, levodopa dose and concurrent treatment with dopamine agonists or selegiline.

Corresponding significant decreases in "Off" time were also noted. Change from baseline in hours of awake time "Off" in the Nordic Study were: −1.3 hours for the entacapone group; 0 hours for the placebo group and in the North American "SEESAW" Study were: −1.2 hours for the entacapone group; −0.3 for the placebo group.

Withdrawal of Entacapone: In the North American "SEESAW" Study, abrupt withdrawal of entacapone, without alteration of the dose of levodopa/carbidopa, resulted in significant worsening of fluctuations, compared to placebo. In some cases, symptoms were slightly worse at baseline, but returned to approximately baseline severity within 2 weeks following levodopa dose increase on average by 80 mg. In the Nordic Study, similarly, a significant worsening of Parkinsonian symptoms were observed after entacapone withdrawal, as assessed 2 weeks after drug withdrawal. At this phase the symptoms were approximately baseline severity following levodopa dose increase by about 50 mg.

In the third placebo-controlled trial (Austrian-German "CELOMEN" Study), as in the other 2 trials, patients were randomized to receive 200 mg entacapone or placebo with each dose of levodopa/dopa decarboxylase inhibitor (up to 10 times daily). The CELOMEN study was primarily designed as a safety trial. Measures of effectiveness in this study were the UPDRS Parts II and III and total daily "On" time (see Table 2).

INDICATIONS: As an adjunct to levodopa/carbidopa or levodopa/benserazide preparations to treat patients with idiopathic Parkinson's disease who experience the signs and symptoms of end-of-dose "wearing-off" (see Pharmacology, Clinical Trials).

Entacapone's effectiveness has not been systematically evaluated in patient's with idiopathic Parkinson's disease who do not experience end-of-dose "wearing-off".

Since entacapone is to be used in combination with a levodopa/dopa-decarboxylase inhibitor, the prescribing information for levodopa/carbidopa and levodopa/benserazide are also applicable when entacapone is added to the treatment regimen.

CONTRAINDICATIONS: In patients with hypersensitivity to entacapone or to any of the excipients.

Entacapone should not be given concomitantly with nonselective MAOIs (e.g., phenelzine and tranylcypromine). The combination of selective MAO-A and selective MAO-B inhibitors is equivalent to nonselective MAO-inhibition; therefore, they should not both be given concomitantly with entacapone and levodopa preparations. Nonselective MAOIs must be discontinued at least 2 weeks prior to initiating therapy with entacapone.

Table 2: Comtan

Outcome Measures: UPDRS and Hours of Awake Time "On" (Austrian-German "CELOMEN" Study)

UPDRS ADL[a]			
	Placebo (n=104) Mean (±SD)	**Entacapone (n=191) Mean (±SD)**	**Difference**
Baseline	12.0±5.8	12.4±6.1	
Week 24	12.4±6.5	11.1±6.3	−1.35 $CI_{95\%}$ −2.54, −0.16
UPDRS MOTOR[a]			
	Placebo (n=102)	**Entacapone (n=190)**	**Difference**
Baseline	24.1±12.1	24.9±12.9	
Week 24	24.3±12.9	21.7±12.1	−2.83 $CI_{95\%}$ −4.95, −0.71
Hours of Awake Time "On" (Home diary)[b]			
	Placebo (n=60)	**Entacapone (n=114)**	**Difference**
Baseline	10.1±2.5	10.2±2.6	
Week 24	10.6±3.0	11.8±2.7	1.08 $CI_{95\%}$ 0.13, 2.03

[a] Total population; score change at endpoint.
[b] Fluctuating population, with 5-10 doses
Legend: SD=Standard Deviation.

Selective MAO-B inhibitors should not be used at higher than recommended doses (e.g., selegiline 10 mg/day) when coadministered with entacapone (see Precautions, Drug Interactions, Selegiline).

Entacapone is contraindicated in patients with a previous history of Neuroleptic Malignant Syndrome (NMS) and/or nontraumatic rhabdomyolysis.

Entacapone is contraindicated in patients with liver impairment.

Entacapone is contraindicated in patients with pheochromocytoma due to the increased risk of hypertensive crisis.

WARNINGS: Sudden Onset of Sleep: Patients receiving treatment with entacapone in combination with levodopa/decarboxylase inhibitor and/or other dopaminergic agents have reported suddenly falling asleep while engaged in activities of daily living, including the driving of a car, which sometimes resulted in accidents. Although some of the patients reported somnolence while treated with levodopa/dopa decarboxylase inhibitor and entacapone, others perceived that they had no warning signs, such as excessive drowsiness, and believed that they were alert immediately prior to the event.

Physicians should alert patients of the reported cases of sudden onset of sleep, bearing in mind that these events are **not** limited to initiation of therapy. Patients should also be advised that sudden onset of sleep has occurred without warning signs and should be specifically asked about factors that may increase the risk with entacapone used in combination with levodopa/decarboxylase inhibitor, such as concomitant medications or the presence of sleep disorders. Given the reported cases of somnolence and sudden onset of sleep (not necessarily preceded by somnolence), physicians should caution patients about the risk of operating hazardous machinery, including driving motor vehicles, while taking entacapone in combination with levodopa/decarboxylase inhibitor. If drowsiness or sudden onset of sleep should occur, patients should be informed to refrain from driving or operating machines and to immediately contact their physician.

Episodes of falling asleep while engaged in activities of daily living have also been reported in patients taking other dopaminergic agents, therefore, symptoms may not be alleviated by substituting these products.

While dose reduction clearly reduces the degree of somnolence, there is insufficient information to establish that dose reduction will eliminate episodes of falling asleep while engaged in activities of daily living.

Currently, the precise cause of this event is unknown. It is known that many Parkinson's disease patients experience alterations in sleep architecture, which results in excessive daytime sleepiness or spontaneous dozing, and that dopaminergic agents can also induce sleepiness.

Drugs Metabolized by Catechol-O-Methyltransferase (COMT): When a single 400 mg dose of entacapone was given together with intravenous isoprenaline (isoproterenol) and epinephrine without coadministered levodopa/dopa decarboxylase inhibitor, the overall mean maximal changes in heart rate during infusion were about 50% and 80% higher than with placebo, for isoprenaline and epinephrine, respectively.

Therefore, drugs known to be metabolized by COMT, such as isoproterenol, epinephrine, norepinephrine, dopamine, dobutamine, α-methyldopa, apomorphine, isoetherine and bitolterol should be administered with caution in patients receiving entacapone regardless of the route of administration (including inhalation), as their interaction may result in increased heart rates, possibly arrhythmias, and excessive changes in blood pressure.

Ventricular tachycardia was noted in a 32-year-old healthy male volunteer in an interaction study after epinephrine infusion and oral entacapone administration. Treatment with propranolol was required. A causal relationship to entacapone administration appears probable but cannot be attributed with certainty.

Abnormal Weight Decrease: In isolated cases, combined progressive anorexia, asthenia and weight decrease within a relatively short period of time have been reported prior to elevations in liver enzymes and serious hepatic adverse events. For patients who experience progressive anorexia, asthenia and weight decrease within a relatively short period of time, a general medical evaluation including assessment of liver function should be considered.

PRECAUTIONS: Skin: Melanoma: Epidemiological studies have shown that patients with Parkinson's disease have a higher risk (2- to approximately 6-fold higher) of developing melanoma than the general population. Whether the increased risk observed was due to Parkinson's disease or other factors, such as drugs used to treat Parkinson's disease, is unclear. For the reasons stated above, patients and healthcare providers are advised to monitor for melanomas frequently and on a regular basis when using entacapone for **any** indication. Ideally, periodic skin examinations should be performed by appropriately qualified individuals (e.g., dermatologists).

General: Entacapone enhances the effects of levodopa. Therefore, to reduce levodopa-related dopaminergic adverse reactions, e.g. dyskinesias, nausea, vomiting and hallucinations, it may be necessary to adjust the levodopa dosage within the first days to first weeks following the initiation of entacapone treatment.

Entacapone has no antiparkinsonian effect of its own and therefore should only be used as an adjunct to levodopa/carbidopa or levodopa/benserazide treatment. The warnings and precautions given for levodopa/carbidopa and levodopa/benserazide treatment should therefore be taken into account when entacapone is used.

If entacapone treatment is discontinued, it is necessary to adjust the dosing of other parkinsonian treatments, especially levodopa, to achieve a sufficient level of control of the parkinsonian symptoms (see Dosage).

Neuroleptic Malignant Syndrome: A symptom complex resembling the neuroleptic malignant syndrome (NMS), characterized by elevated temperature, muscular rigidity, altered consciousness (e.g., agitation, confusion, coma), autonomic instability (tachycardia, labile blood pressure) and elevated CPK has been reported in association with the rapid dose reduction, or withdrawal of, or changes in antiparkinsonian therapy. In individual cases, only some of these symptoms and/or findings may be evident. This syndrome should be considered in the differential diagnosis for any patient who develops a high fever or severe rigidity.

Cases with similar signs and symptoms have been reported in association with entacapone therapy, especially following abrupt reduction or discontinuation of entacapone and other dopaminergic medications. The complicated nature of these cases makes it difficult to determine what role, if any, entacapone may have played in their pathogenesis. No cases have been reported following abrupt withdrawal or dose reduction of entacapone treatment during clinical studies.

Prescribers should exercise caution when discontinuing entacapone treatment. When considered necessary, withdrawal should proceed slowly. If a decision is made to discontinue treatment with entacapone, recommendations include monitoring the patient closely and adjusting other dopaminergic treatments as needed. If signs and/or symptoms occur despite a slow withdrawal of entacapone, an increase in levodopa dosage may be necessary. Tapering entacapone has not been systematically evaluated.

Rhabdomyolysis: Rhabdomyolysis secondary to severe dyskinesias or Neuroleptic Malignant Syndrome (NMS) has been observed rarely in patients with Parkinson's disease. Very rare cases of rhabdomyolysis have been reported with entacapone treatment.

Symptoms associated with rhabdomyolysis can include muscle pain, muscle tenderness and weakness, bruising, elevated temperature, urinary retention, confusion, and elevated CPK. Acute renal failure is serious complication associated rhabdomyolysis and has been reported in some cases of rhabdomyolysis that have occurred during entacapone treatment.

Orthostatic Hypotension/Syncope: Entacapone may aggravate levodopa-induced orthostatic hypotension. Entacapone should be given with caution to patients who are treated with drugs which may cause orthostatic hypotension. In controlled clinical trials approximately 1.2% of patients who received 200 mg entacapone and 0.8% of patients treated with placebo reported at least 1 episode of syncope. Reports of syncope were generally more frequent in patients in both treatment groups who had an episode of documented hypotension.

Diarrhea and Weight Decrease: In clinical trials, diarrhea was reported as an adverse event in 60 of 603 (10%) and 16 of 400 (4%) of patients treated with 200 mg of entacapone and placebo, respectively. In patients treated with entacapone, diarrhea was generally mild to moderate in severity (8.6%) but was reported as severe in 1.3%. Diarrhea resulted in withdrawal in 10 of 603 (1.7%) patients (1.2% with mild to moderate diarrhea and 0.3% with severe diarrhea). Diarrhea generally resolved after discontinuation of entacapone. Two patients with diarrhea required hospitalization. Typically, diarrhea presents within 4 to 12 weeks after entacapone is started, but it may appear as early as the first week and as late as many months after the initiation of treatment.

For patients experiencing diarrhea, close monitoring of weight is recommended in order to assess the need for treatment discontinuation to avoid excessive weight loss. Some patients who experienced diarrhea and weight loss during entacapone treatment were subsequently diagnosed with colitis, following colonoscopy and biopsy (see Adverse Effects, Post-Introduction Reports).

For patients who experience progressive anorexia, asthenia and weight decrease within a relatively short period of time, a general medical evaluation including assessment of liver function should be considered.

Patients with Fructose Intolerance: Comtan tablets contain sucrose. Therefore, patients with rare hereditary problems of fructose intolerance, glucose-galactose malabsorption or sucrase-isomaltase insufficiency should not take this medicine.

Dyskinesia: Entacapone may potentiate the dopaminergic side effects of levodopa and may cause and/or exacerbate pre-existing dyskinesia. Although decreasing the dose of levodopa may ameliorate this side effect, many patients in controlled trials continued to experience frequent dyskinesias despite a reduction in their dose of levodopa. The rates of withdrawal for dyskinesia were 1.5% and 0.8% for 200 mg of entacapone and placebo, respectively.

Psychiatric: Behavioral Changes: Pathological gambling, increased libido and hypersexuality have been reported in Parkinson's disease patients treated with dopamine agonists and other dopaminergic treatments such as entacapone in combination with levodopa, and were generally reversible upon dose reduction or treatment discontinuation (see Adverse Effects).

Hallucinations: Dopaminergic therapy in Parkinson's disease patients has been associated with hallucinations. In clinical trials, hallucinations developed in approximately 4% of patients treated with 200 mg of entacapone or placebo. Hallucinations led to drug discontinuation and premature withdrawal from clinical trials in 0.8% and 0% of patients treated with 200 mg of entacapone and placebo, respectively. Hallucinations led to hospitalization in 1% and 0.3% of patients in the 200 mg of entacapone and placebo groups, respectively.

Fibrotic Complications: Cases of retroperitoneal fibrosis, pulmonary infiltrates, pleural effusion, and pleural thickening have been reported in some patients treated with ergot derived dopaminergic agents. These complications may resolve when the drug is discontinued, but complete resolution does not always occur. Although these adverse events are believed to be related to the ergoline structure of these compounds, it is unknown whether other, non-ergot derived drugs (e.g., entacapone) that increase dopaminergic activity can cause them. It should be noted that the expected incidence of fibrotic complications is so low that even if entacapone caused these complications at rates similar to those attributable to other dopaminergic therapies, it is unlikely that it would have been detected in a cohort of the size exposed to entacapone. Four cases of pulmonary fibrosis were reported during clinical development of entacapone; 3 of these patients were also treated with pergolide and 1 with bromocriptine. The duration of treatment with entacapone ranged from 7 to 17 months.

Urine, Sweat and Saliva Discolouration: Entacapone may cause a harmless intensification in the color of the patient's urine to brownish-orange. Entacapone may also cause darkening of sweat and saliva.

Occupational Hazards: Psychomotor Performance: Entacapone together with levodopa may cause dizziness and symptomatic orthostatism. Therefore, patients should be cautioned about operating machinery, including automobiles, until they are reasonably certain that the drug treatment does not affect them adversely.

Entacapone in association with levodopa may have major influence on the ability to drive and use machines. Patients being treated with entacapone in association with levodopa and presenting with somnolence and/or sudden sleep onset episodes must be instructed to refrain from driving or engaging in activities where impaired alertness may put themselves or others at risk of serious injury or death (e.g. operating machines) until such recurrent episodes have resolved (see Warnings, Sudden Onset of Sleep).

Special Populations: Hepatic Impairment: The metabolism of entacapone is slowed in patients with mild to moderate (Child-Pugh grading Class A and B) hepatic insufficiency caused by cirrhotic disease. In these patients, the AUC and C_{max} values were approximately two-fold greater than those in demographically-matched healthy volunteers. As there are no clinical trial data to establish a safe and effective dosing regimen for hepatically impaired patients, entacapone should be not be administered to patients with hepatic impairment (see Contraindications).

Renal Impairment: The pharmacokinetics of entacapone were not significantly changed in patients with moderate to severe renal insufficiency and there is no need for dose adjustment (see Pharmacology, Pharmacokinetics). There is no experience with entacapone in patients receiving dialysis.

Pregnancy : There are no studies or clinical experience of the use of entacapone in pregnant women. Use of entacapone in women of child-bearing potential requires that the anticipated benefits of the drug be weighed against possible hazards to mother and child.

Lactation: Studies in rats have shown that entacapone is excreted in milk.

It is not known whether entacapone is excreted in human milk. Since the safety of entacapone in infants is unknown, women should not breast-feed during treatment with entacapone.

Children: The safety and efficacy of entacapone in pediatric patients has not been established and use in patients below the age of 18 is not recommended.

Carcinogenesis, Mutagenesis, Impairment of Fertility: Carcinogenesis: Two-year carcinogenicity studies have been conducted in the mouse at dosages up to 600 mg/kg/day and in the rat at dosages up to 400 mg/kg/day. In the rat, the only drug-related finding was an increased incidence of renal tubular adenomas and carcinomas noted in males at doses of 400 mg/kg/day. Plasma exposures (AUC) associated with this dose were approximately 20 times higher than estimated plasma exposures of humans receiving the maximum recommended daily dose of entacapone (8×200 mg=1600 mg). In the mouse study, there was a high incidence of premature mortality in animals receiving the highest dose of entacapone (600 mg/kg/day, corresponding to 2 times the maximum recommended human dose on a mg/m² basis). Thus, the mouse study does not allow adequate assessment of carcinogenicity. Although no treatment related tumors were observed in animals receiving lower doses, the carcinogenic potential of entacapone has not been fully evaluated. The carcinogenic potential of entacapone in combination with levodopa/DDC has not been studied.

Mutagenesis: Entacapone was mutagenic and clastogenic in the in vitro mouse lymphoma/thymidine kinase assay in the presence and absence of metabolic activation, and was clastogenic in cultured human lymphocytes in the presence of metabolic activation. Entacapone, either alone or in combination with levodopa-carbidopa (Sinemet), was not clastogenic in the in vivo mouse micronucleus test or mutagenic in the bacterial reverse mutation assay (Ames test).

Teratogenicity: Reproduction studies have been performed in rats and rabbits at doses up to 1000 mg/kg/day and 300 mg/kg/day, respectively, of entacapone. Increased incidence of fetal variations were evident in litters from rats treated at the highest dose in the absence of overt maternal toxicity. The maternal plasma drug exposure (AUC) associated with this dose was approximately 34 times the estimated plasma exposure in humans receiving the maximal recommended dose of 8×200 mg (1600 mg/day). Increased frequencies of abortion and late/total resorptions and decreased fetal weights were observed in litters of rabbits treated with maternotoxic doses of 100 mg/kg/day (plasma AUC 0.4 times those in humans receiving the maximal recommended daily dose) or greater. There was no evidence of teratogenicity in these studies.

However, when entacapone was administered to female rats prior to mating and during early gestation, an increased incidence of fetal eye anomalies (macrophthalmia, microphthalmia, anophthalmia) was observed in litters of dams treated with doses of 160 mg/kg/day (plasma AUCs 7 times those in humans receiving the maximal recommended daily dose) or greater, in the absence of maternal toxicity. Administration of up to 700 mg/kg/day (plasma AUCs 28 times those in humans receiving the maximal recommended daily dose) to female rats during the later part of gestation and throughout lactation produced no evidence of developmental impairments in the offspring.

Entacapone is always given concomitantly with levodopa/dopa-decarboxylase inhibitor, which is known to cause visceral and skeletal malformations in rabbits. Although the teratogenicity of entacapone was assessed in animals, the teratogenic potential of entacapone in combination with levodopa/carbidopa was not assessed.

Impairment of Fertility: No effect on fertility was observed in male and female rats treated with up to 700 mg/kg/day of entacapone (exposure achieved approximately 28 times higher than that in man after the maximum recommended daily dose of 8×200 mg/day).

Drug Interactions: Protein Binding: Entacapone is highly protein bound (98%). In vitro studies have shown that entacapone, at therapeutic concentrations, does not displace drugs of which a large proportion is bound to plasma proteins (e.g., warfarin, salicylic acid, phenylbutazone and diazepam). Entacapone is not markedly displaced by any of these drugs at therapeutic concentrations (see Pharmacology).

Drugs Metabolized by Cytochrome P450: Data from in vitro studies using human liver microsomal preparations indicate that entacapone inhibits cytochrome P450 2C9 (IC50 ~4 μM).

Other P450 isoenzymes (CYP1A2, CYP2A6, CYP2D6, CYP2E1, CYP3A and CYP2C19) were inhibited only by very high concentrations of entacapone (IC50 from 200 to greater than 1000 μM). The highest concentration of entacapone achieved with an oral 200 mg dose is approximately 5 μM and is not expected to inhibit these enzymes.

Drugs Metabolized by Cytochrome P450 (CYP2C9): Entacapone has been shown to inhibit the activity of cytochrome P450 2C9 in vitro and may potentially interfere with drugs whose metabolism is dependent on this isoenzyme, such as S-warfarin. However, in an interaction study in healthy volunteers, entacapone did not change the plasma levels of S-warfarin, while the AUC for R-warfarin increased on average by 18% [CI90 11-26%]. The INR values increased on average by 13% [CI90 6-19%]. Thus, control of INR is recommended when entacapone treatment is initiated for patients receiving warfarin.

Drugs Metabolized by the Catechol-O-Methyltransferase (COMT): The experience of the clinical use of entacapone with medicinal products that are metabolized by COMT (e.g. catechol-structured compounds: rimiterole, isoprenaline, adrenaline, noradrenaline, dopamine, dobutamine, alpha-methyldopa, apomorphine, and paroxetine) is still limited (see Warnings). Regardless of their route of administration, including inhalation, drugs known to be metabolized by COMT should be used with caution in patients treated concomitantly with entacapone, as their interaction may result in increased heart rates, possible arrhythmias and excessive changes in blood pressure (see Warnings).

Non-selective MAO Inhibitors: Entacapone should not be given concomitantly with non-selective monoamine oxidase (MAO) inhibitors (e.g. phenelzine and tranylcypromine). The combination of selective MAO-A and selective MAO-B inhibitors is equivalent to non-selective MAO-inhibition, therefore, they should not both be given concomitantly with entacapone and levodopa preparations. Non-selective MAO inhibitors must be discontinued at least two weeks prior to initiating therapy with entacapone (see Contraindications).

Selegiline: In 2 multiple-dose interaction studies in patients with Parkinson's disease, no interactions between entacapone and selegiline (10 mg) were observed in the presence of coadministered levodopa/dopa decarboxylase inhibitor. More than 400 parkinsonian patients in phase 2 and 3 studies used selegiline in combination with entacapone and levodopa/DDC inhibitor without any apparent interactions (also see Contraindications).

Tricyclic Antidepressants and Noradrenaline Re-uptake Inhibitors: In a single-dose study in healthy volunteers, no interactions between entacapone and imipramine were observed in the absence of coadministration of levodopa/dopa decarboxylase inhibitor.

The potential for interactions between entacapone and tricyclic antidepressants or noradrenaline re-uptake inhibitors has not been systematically evaluated in patients with Parkinson's disease. The experience on the clinical use of entacapone with tricyclic antidepressants and noradrenaline reuptake inhibitors (desipramine, maprotiline and venlafaxine) is limited. Therefore, patients should be carefully monitored when entacapone is administered in combination with these drugs.

Dopa Decarboxylase Inhibitors: Carbidopa: No interaction of entacapone with carbidopa were observed with the recommended dosage regimen; however, high single doses (in excess of 400 mg of entacapone) may decrease the bioavailability of carbidopa. Benserazide: Pharmacokinetic interaction studies with benserazide have not been conducted.

Entacapone increases the bioavailability of levodopa from standard levodopa/benserazide preparations 5 to 10% more than from standard levodopa/carbidopa preparations. Consequently, undesirable dopaminergic effects may be more frequent when entacapone is added to levodopa/benserazide treatment. A larger reduction of the levodopa dose may be required when entacapone treatment is initiated in patients receiving levodopa/benserazide (see Dosage).

Drugs Interfering with Biliary Excretion: As most entacapone excretion is via the bile, caution should be exercised when drugs known to interfere with biliary excretion, glucuronidation, and intestinal beta-glucuronidase are given concurrently with entacapone. These include probenicid, cholestyramine, and some antibiotics (e.g., erythromycin, rifampin, ampicillin and chloramphenicol).

Iron: Similar to levodopa, entacapone may impair the absorption of iron from the gastrointestinal tract. Therefore, entacapone and iron-containing supplements or multivitamins should be ingested at least 2 to 3 hours apart.

Hormone Levels: Levodopa is known to depress prolactin secretion and increase growth hormone levels. Treatment with entacapone coadministered with levodopa/dopa decarboxylase inhibitor does not change these effects.

Laboratory Tests: Entacapone is a chelator of iron. The impact of entacapone on the body's iron stores is unknown; however, a tendency towards decreased serum iron concentrations was noted in a clinical trial. In a controlled clinical study serum ferritin levels (as marker of iron deficiency and subclinical anemia) were not changed with entacapone compared to placebo after 1 year of treatment and there was no difference in the rates of anemia or decreased hemoglobin levels.

The laboratory tests required during extended levodopa therapy should be normally conducted also during entacapone treatment.

ADVERSE EFFECTS: A total of 1450 patients with Parkinson's disease received entacapone during the pre-marketing clinical trials. Approximately 14% of the 603 patients given entacapone in the double-blind placebo-controlled trials discontinued treatment due to adverse events compared to 9% of the 400 patients who received placebo. The most frequent causes of discontinuation in decreasing order for entacapone vs placebo are: psychiatric reasons (2% vs 1%), diarrhea (2% vs 0%), dyskinesia/hyperkinesia (2% vs 1%), nausea (2% vs 1%), abdominal pain (1% vs 0%), and aggravation of Parkinson's disease symptoms (1% vs 1%).

Incidence of Adverse Events in Placebo Controlled Trials: The most frequently observed adverse events reported with entacapone were dyskinesias/hyperkinesia (29%/10%), nausea (14%), abnormal urine (intensification of the color of urine, 13%), diarrhea (10%), dizziness (10%) and abdominal pain (9%). Dyskinesia, nausea and abdominal pain, may be more common with higher doses (>1400 mg/day) than with lower doses of entacapone.

Adverse events related to the treatment with entacapone are usually mild to moderate in severity, leading only rarely to discontinuation of the treatment (see Table 3).

Table 3: Comtan

Adverse Events, Irrespective of Causal Relationship to Study Drug, Occurring in ≥1% of Comtan Patients During Controlled Phase 3 Studies

Adverse Events by Body System	Comtan N=603 % of Patients	Placebo N=400 % of Patients
Autonomic Nervous System Disorders		
Hypotension Postural	4.3	4.0
Body as a Whole–General Disorders		
Fatigue	6.1	3.5
Pain	6.0	4.5
Back Pain	5.0	3.0
Sweating Increased	3.6	3.0
Asthenia	1.8	1.3
Weight Decrease	1.7	0.5
Fever	1.3	0.5
Syncope	1.0	0.8
Central and Peripheral Nervous System Disorders		
Dyskinesia	25.2	14.8
Hyperkinesia	9.5	5.0
Hypokinesia	8.6	7.5
Dizziness	7.5	6.0
Ataxia	1.2	0.5
Speech Disorder	1.2	0.8
Gastrointestinal System Disorders		
Nausea	13.8	7.5
Diarrhea	10.0	4.0
Abdominal Pain	8.1	4.5
Constipation	6.3	4.3
Vomiting	4.0	1.0
Dry Mouth	3.0	0.3
Dyspepsia	2.3	0.8
Flatulence	1.5	0.3
Anorexia	1.5	1.3
Gastrointestinal Disorders	1.0	0.3
Gastritis	1.0	0.3
Musculoskeletal System Disorders		
Arthralgia	1.8	1.5
Platelet, Bleeding and Clotting Disorders		
Purpura	1.5	0.8
Psychiatric Disorders		
Hallucinations	4.1	4.0
Paroniria	2.2	1.8
Anxiety	2.0	1.3
Agitation	1.7	0.3
Confusion	1.7	1.5
Somnolence	1.7	0.3
Amnesia	1.3	0.8
Sleep Disorder	1.3	0.8
Reproductive Disorders, Male		
Prostatic Disorder	1.0	0.3
Resistance Mechanism Disorders		
Infection Bacterial	1.3	0.0
Respiratory System Disorders		
Dyspnea	2.7	1.3
Bronchitis	1.2	1.0
Skin and Appendages Disorders		
Rash	3.6	3.0
Special Senses Other, Disorders		

(cont'd)

Table 3: Comtan *(cont'd)*

Adverse Events, Irrespective of Causal Relationship to Study Drug, Occurring in ≥1% of Comtan Patients During Controlled Phase 3 Studies

Adverse Events by Body System	Comtan N=603 % of Patients	Placebo N=400 % of Patients
Taste Perversion	1.0	0.3
Urinary System Disorders		
Urine Abnormal	9.5	0.0
Cystitis	1.2	0.5

Adverse Events Reported in <1% of Patients Treated With Entacapone in Phase 3 Trials:
Body as a Whole, General: malaise, hot flushes, temperature changed sensation, aspiration, edema generalized, carpal tunnel syndrome, leg pain.
Cardiovascular, General: hypertension, heart valve disorders.
Central and Peripheral Nervous Systems: hypoesthesia, muscle contractions involuntary, eye abnormality, hypotonia.
Endocrine: hyperthyroidism.
Gastrointestinal: gastroenteritis, esophagitis, tooth disorder, saliva increased, dysphagia, feces discolored, diverticulitis, change in bowel habits, fecal abnormality.
Heart Rate And Rhythm: extrasystoles, bradycardia, bundle branch block, fibrillation atrial.
Liver and Biliary: gamma-glutamyl-transferase increased, cholelithiasis, bilirubinemia, cholangitis.
Metabolic and Nutritional: hyperglycemia, hypoglycemia, phosphatase alkaline increased, hypercholesterolemia.
Musculoskeletal: bursitis, arthritis, tendinitis.
Myo-, Endo-, Pericardial and Valve: angina pectoris.
Platelet, Bleeding and Clotting: epistaxis, thrombocytopenia.
Psychiatric: nervousness, thinking abnormal, concentration impaired, dreaming abnormal, delusion, paranoid reaction.
Reproductive, Female: breast fibroadenosis.
Reproductive, Male: impotence, sexual function abnormal.
Resistance Mechanism: herpes simplex.
Respiratory: pneumonia, pharyngitis, sinusitis.
Secondary Terms-Events: inflicted injury.
Skin and Appendages: pruritus, skin disorder, dermatitis, eczema, dermatitis fungal.
Special Senses, Others: taste loss.
Urinary: urinary incontinence, hematuria, albuminuria, dysuria, nocturia, renal pain.
Vascular (Extracardiac): skin cold clammy, claudication intermittent.
Vision: diplopia, conjunctivitis, cataract, photopsia.
White Cell and Reticuloendothelial System: leukopenia.

The following adverse events were reported only once but are considered clinically important: hepatic function abnormal, hepatic enzymes increased (>3 times ULN), cholecystitis and allergic reaction.

Laboratory Findings: Slight decreases in hemoglobin, erythrocyte count and hematocrit have been reported during entacapone treatment. The underlying mechanism may involve decreased absorption of iron from the gastrointestinal tract. During long-term treatment (6 months) with entacapone a clinically significant decrease in hemoglobin has been observed in 1.5% of patients.

Post-Introduction Reports: Voluntary reports of adverse events that have been received since market introduction that are not listed above, are listed in Table 4. Because these reactions are reported voluntarily from a population of uncertain size, it is not always possible to reliably estimate their frequency or establish a causal relationship to drug exposure.

Table 4: Comtan

Comtan Post-Market Spontaneous Adverse Event Reports

Adverse Event	Frequency			
	Common (≥1%)	Uncommon (<1% and ≥0.1%)	Rare (<0.1% and ≥0.01%)	Very Rare (<0.01%)
Liver and Biliary System Disorders				
Hepatitis with mainly cholestatic features				X
Clinically significant increases in liver enzymes			X	
Central and Peripheral Nervous System Disorders				
Neuroleptic Malignant Syndrome				X
Gastrointestinal Disorders				
Colitis				X
Musculoskeletal System Disorders				
Rhabdomyolysis				X
Skin and Appendage Disorders				
Erythematous/maculopapular rash			X	
Urticaria				X
Skin, hair, beard and nail discolorations				X

Isolated cases of hepatic failure and severe, serious skin reactions resembling erythema multiforme and toxic epidermal necrolysis have been reported in patients treated with entacapone.

Patients treated with entacapone in combination with levodopa/dopa decarboxylase inhibitor have very rarely reported falling asleep while engaged in activities of daily living, including operation of motor vehicles, which has sometimes resulted in accidents (see Warnings).

Pathological (compulsive) gambling has been reported in post-market data, including those in the literature, for antiparkinson drugs. Parkinson's disease patients treated with dopamine agonists and other dopaminergic treatments such as entacapone in combination with levodopa, especially at high doses, have been reported as exhibiting signs of pathological gambling, increased libido and hypersexuality. Pathological gambling, increased libido and hypersexuality were generally reversible upon reduction of the dose or treatment discontinuation.

OVERDOSE:

Symptoms: The COMT inhibition by entacapone is dose-dependent; a massive overdose of entacapone may, therefore, produce a 100% inhibition of COMT enzyme in man, and thereby prevent the metabolism of endogenous and exogenous catechols. The post-marketing data includes isolated cases of accidental and intentional overdose in which the reported highest daily dose of entacapone has been 16,000 mg. The acute symptoms and signs in these cases of overdose included confusion, mydriasis, decreased activity, somnolence, hypotonia, skin discolouration and urticaria.

Treatment: Hospitalization is advised and general supportive care is indicated. Management is symptomatic; there is no known antidote to entacapone. The drug is rapidly absorbed and eliminated with a short mean residence time. There is no experience with dialysis or hemoperfusion, and these procedures are unlikely to be of benefit, because entacapone is highly bound to plasma proteins. An immediate gastric lavage and repeated doses of charcoal over time may hasten the elimination of entacapone by decreasing the absorption/reabsorption of entacapone from the gastrointestinal tract. The adequacy of the respiratory and circulatory systems should be carefully observed and appropriate supportive measures employed. In managing overdosage, the possibility of interaction among drugs, especially catechol-structured drugs, should be borne in mind.

For management of a suspected drug overdose, contact your **regional Poison Control Centre**. See the *CPS* Directory section for a list of Poison Control Centres.

DOSAGE: Method of Administration: Entacapone has no antiparkinsonian effect of its own and therefore should always be administered simultaneously with each levodopa/carbidopa or levodopa/benserazide dose. The efficacy of entacapone as an adjunct to controlled-release levodopa/dopa-decarboxylase inhibitor preparations has not been established.

Entacapone is taken orally with or without food (see Pharmacology).

Dosage: The recommended dose of entacapone is one 200 mg tablet administered concomitantly with each levodopa/carbidopa or levodopa/benserazide dose up to 8 times daily (1600 mg/day).

Because entacapone enhances the bioavailability and therefore the central effects of levodopa, it may be necessary to adjust the dosage of levodopa during the initial days to weeks of entacapone therapy in order to reduce levodopa-related dopaminergic adverse reactions, e.g., dyskinesias, nausea, vomiting and hallucinations. In some cases, it may be necessary to reduce the daily dosages of levodopa by about 10 to 30%. This can be achieved through either reducing the dose of the levodopa preparation itself, or by extending the interval between doses, according to the clinical condition of the patient.

In clinical trials, the majority of patients required a decrease in daily levodopa dose if their daily dose of levodopa had been greater than or equal to 800 mg, or if patients had moderate or severe dyskinesias before beginning treatment. The average reduction in daily levodopa dose for patients in clinical trials requiring levodopa dose reduction was about 25% (more than 58% of patients with levodopa doses above 800 mg daily required such a reduction).

Entacapone increases the bioavailability of levodopa from standard levodopa/benserazide preparations slightly (5 to 10%) more than from standard levodopa/carbidopa preparations. Therefore, patients who are taking standard levodopa/benserazide preparations may need a larger reduction of levodopa dose when entacapone is initiated.

Impaired Hepatic Function: As there is no clinical trial data to establish a safe and effective dosing regimen for hepatically impaired patients, entacapone should be not be administered to patients with hepatic impairment (see Contraindications).

Impaired Renal Function: No dose adjustment of entacapone is necessary in patients with moderate to severe renal insufficiency. There is no experience with entacapone in patients receiving dialysis therapy.

Elderly: No dose adjustment is required in elderly patients.

Discontinuation of Entacapone: Rapid withdrawal or abrupt reduction in the entacapone dose could lead to emergence of signs and symptoms of Parkinson's disease (see Pharmacology, Clinical Trials) and may lead to a symptom complex resembling neuroleptic malignant syndrome (see Precautions, Neuroleptic Malignant Syndrome). This syndrome should be considered in the differential diagnosis for any patient who develops high fever or severe rigidity. If a decision is made to discontinue treatment with entacapone, patients should be monitored closely and other dopaminergic treatments should be adjusted as needed. Although tapering entacapone has not been systematically evaluated, it seems prudent to withdraw patients slowly if the decision to discontinue treatment is made.

INFORMATION FOR THE PATIENT: Published in e-CPS, available by subscription at www.e-cps.ca.

SUPPLIED: Each brownish-orange, unscored, oval-shaped, film-coated tablet, embossed with "COMTAN" on one side, contains: entacapone 200 mg. Nonmedicinal ingredients: core: croscarmellose sodium, hydrogenated vegetable oil, magnesium stearate, mannitol and microcrystalline cellulose; coating: glycerol 85%, hydroxypropylmethyl cellulose, magnesium stearate, polysorbate 80, red iron oxide, sucrose, titanium dioxide and yellow iron oxide. Bottles of 100. Store at room temperature (15 and 30°C). Must be kept out of the reach and sight of children.

(Shown in Product Identification Section)

Concerta® Ⓒ

methylphenidate HCl

CNS Stimulant

Janssen-Ortho

Date of Preparation: June 18, 2003
Date of Revision: July 20, 2010

SUMMARY PRODUCT INFORMATION:

Route of Administration	Dosage Form/Strength	Nonmedicinal Ingredients
Oral	Extended-release tablet 18 mg, 27 mg, 36 mg and 54 mg	Butylated hydroxytoluene, carnauba wax, cellulose acetate, hypromellose, lactose, phosphoric acid, poloxamer, polyethylene glycol, polyethylene oxides, povidone, propylene glycol, sodium chloride, stearic acid, succinic acid, synthetic iron oxides, titanium dioxide and triacetin

INDICATIONS AND CLINICAL USE: CONCERTA (methylphenidate hydrochloride) is indicated for the treatment of Attention Deficit Hyperactivity Disorder (ADHD) in:

- **Children (6-12 years of age)**
- **Adolescents (13-18 years of age)**
- **Adults (>18 years of age)**

Pediatrics (<6 years of age): CONCERTA should not be used in children under six years, since safety and efficacy in this age group have not been established.

Geriatrics (>65 years of age): No data available.

A diagnosis of ADHD (DSM-IV) implies the presence of hyperactive-impulsive or inattentive symptoms that caused impairment and that were present before age 7 years. The symptoms must be persistent, must be more severe than is typically observed in individuals at a comparable level of development, must cause clinically significant impairment, e.g., in social, academic, or occupational functioning, and must be present in 2 or more settings, e.g., school (or work) and at home. The symptoms must not be better accounted for by another mental disorder. For the Inattentive Type, at least 6 of the following symptoms must have persisted for at least 6 months: lack of attention to details/careless mistakes, lack of sustained attention, poor listener, failure to follow through on tasks, poor organization, avoids tasks requiring sustained mental effort, loses things, easily distracted, forgetful. For the Hyperactive-Impulsive Type, at least 6 of the following symptoms must have persisted for at least 6 months: fidgeting/squirming, leaving seat, inappropriate running/climbing, difficulty with quiet activities, "on the go," excessive talking, blurting answers, can't wait turn, intrusive. For a Combined Type diagnosis, both inattentive and hyperactive-impulsive criteria must be met.

Special Diagnostic Considerations: The specific etiology of ADHD is unknown, and there is no single diagnostic test. Adequate diagnosis requires the use not only of medical but of special psychological, educational, and social resources. Learning may or may not be impaired. The diagnosis must be based upon a complete history and evaluation of the patient and not solely on the presence of the required number of DSM-IV characteristics.

Need for Comprehensive Treatment Program: CONCERTA is indicated as an integral part of a total treatment program for ADHD that may include other measures (psychological, educational, social) for patients with this syndrome. Drug treatment may not be indicated for all patients with this syndrome. Drug treatment is not intended for use in the patient who exhibits symptoms secondary to environmental factors and/or other primary psychiatric disorders, including psychosis. Appropriate educational placement is essential in children and adolescents with this diagnosis and psychosocial intervention is often helpful. When remedial measures alone are insufficient, the decision to prescribe drug treatment medication will depend upon the physician's assessment of the chronicity and severity of the patient's symptoms.

Long-Term Use: The effectiveness of CONCERTA for long-term use, i.e., for more than 4 weeks in children and adolescents or 5 weeks in adults, has not been systematically evaluated in placebo-controlled trials. Therefore, the physician who elects to use CONCERTA for extended periods should periodically re-evaluate the long-term usefulness of the drug for the individual patient (see Dosage and Administration).

CONTRAINDICATIONS:

- Anxiety, tension, agitation, thyrotoxicosis, advanced arteriosclerosis, symptomatic cardiovascular disease, moderate to severe hypertension or glaucoma.
- Patients who are hypersensitive to methylphenidate or to any ingredient in the formulation or component of the container. For a complete listing, see Dosage Forms, Composition and Packaging.
- Patients with motor tics or with a family history or diagnosis of Tourette's syndrome (verbal tics) (see Adverse Reactions).
- During treatment with monoamine oxidase inhibitors, and also within a minimum of 14 days following discontinuation of a monoamine oxidase inhibitor (hypertensive crises may result) (see Drug Interactions, Drug-Drug Interactions).

WARNINGS AND PRECAUTIONS:

Serious Warnings and Precautions
- **Drug Dependence** (see Dependence/Tolerance)

General: CONCERTA is intended for oral use only. In dogs, the intravenous injection of the pulverized CONCERTA tablets resulted in death.

Sudden Death and Pre-Existing Structural Cardiac Abnormalities or Other Serious Heart Problems: Children and Adolescents: Sudden death has been reported in association with stimulant drugs used for ADHD treatment at usual doses in children and adolescents with structural cardiac abnormalities or other serious cardiac problems. Although some serious heart problems alone carry an increased risk of sudden death, CONCERTA generally should not be used in children, adolescents, or adults with known structural cardiac abnormalities, cardiomyopathy, serious heart rhythm abnormalities, or other serious cardiac problems that may place them at increased vulnerability to the sympathomimetic effects of a stimulant drug.

Adults: Sudden deaths, stroke, and myocardial infarction have been reported in adults taking stimulant drugs at usual doses for ADHD. Although the role of stimulants in these adult cases is also unknown, adults have a greater likelihood than children of having serious structural cardiac abnormalities, cardiomyopathy, serious heart rhythm abnormalities, coronary artery disease, or other serious cardiac problems. Adults with such abnormalities should also generally not be treated with stimulant drugs (see Contraindications).

General: Children: Theoretically there exists a pharmacological potential for all ADHD drugs to increase the risk of sudden/cardiac death. Although confirmation of an incremental risk for sudden/cardiac death arising from treatment with ADHD medications is lacking, prescribers should consider this potential risk.

All drugs with sympathomimetic effects prescribed in the management of ADHD should be used with caution in patients who: a) are involved in strenuous exercise or activities b) use other sympathomimetic ADHD drugs or c) have a family history of sudden/cardiac death. Prior to the initiation of treatment with sympathomimetic medications, a personal and family history (including assessment for a family history of sudden death or ventricular arrhythmia) and physical exam should be obtained to assess for the presence of cardiac disease. In patients with relevant risk factors and based on the clinician's judgment, further cardiovascular evaluation may be considered (e.g., electrocardiogram and echocardiogram). Patients who develop symptoms such as exertional chest pain, unexplained syncope, or other symptoms suggestive of cardiac disease during ADHD treatment should undergo a prompt cardiac evaluation.

Fatigue: CONCERTA should not be used for the prevention or treatment of normal fatigue states.

Information to Be Provided to the Patient: Patients should be informed that CONCERTA should be swallowed whole with the aid of liquids. Tablets should not be chewed, divided, or crushed. The medication is contained within a non-absorbable shell designed to release the drug at a controlled rate. The tablet shell, along with insoluble core components, is eliminated from the body; patients should not be concerned if they occasionally notice in their stool something that looks like a tablet. Patient information is provided in Information for the Patient. To assure safe and effective use of CONCERTA, the information and instructions provided in Information for the Patient should be discussed with patients.

Cardiovascular: Pre-Existing Cardiovascular and Cerebral Vascular Conditions: CNS stimulants should be used with caution in patients with a pre-existing cardiovascular or cerebrovascular condition, taking into account risk predictors for these conditions. Patients should be screened for pre-existing or underlying cardiovascular or cerebrovascular conditions before initiation of treatment with CONCERTA and monitored for new conditions of the heart or brain during the course of treatment.

Hypertension and Other Cardiovascular Conditions: CONCERTA should be used cautiously in patients with mild hypertension and other cardiovascular conditions. Blood pressure should be monitored at appropriate intervals in patients receiving CONCERTA, especially in patients with hypertension. In the laboratory classroom clinical trials in children (Studies 1 and 2), both CONCERTA and methylphenidate t.i.d. increased resting pulse by an average of 2-6 beats per minute (bpm) and produced average increases of systolic blood pressure (SBP) and diastolic blood pressure (DBP) of approximately 1-4 mm Hg during the day, relative to placebo. In the double-blind, placebo-controlled study in adults (Study 5), changes in mean DBP and SBP were observed with CONCERTA doses up to 72 mg. A statistically significant ($p<0.05$) mean increase in standing DBP and SBP versus baseline was reached at Week 1 in the 72 mg CONCERTA dose group (mean increase of 2.0 mm Hg for standing DBP and 4.0 mm Hg for standing and supine SBP) but not at later time points. A statistically significant increase in pulse was observed for all CONCERTA dose groups (18 mg, 36 mg and 72 mg) versus baseline (range of mean increase of 2.0-10.6 bpm). Therefore, caution is advised in treating patients whose underlying medical conditions might be compromised by increases in blood pressure or heart rate, e.g., those with pre-existing hypertension, heart failure or recent myocardial infarction.

Dependence/Tolerance: Drug Dependence: CONCERTA should be given cautiously to patients with a history of drug dependence or alcoholism. Chronic abusive use can lead to marked tolerance and psychological dependence with varying degrees of abnormal behaviour. Frank psychotic episodes can occur, especially with parenteral abuse (see Dosage and Administration, Administration). Careful supervision is required during withdrawal from abuse since severe depression may occur. Withdrawal following chronic therapeutic use may unmask symptoms of an underlying disorder that may require follow-up.

Endocrine and Metabolism: Long-Term Suppression of Growth: Sufficient data on the safety of long-term use of methylphenidate in children are not yet available. Although a causal relationship has not been established, suppression of growth (i.e. weight gain and/or height) has been reported with the long-term use of stimulants in children. Therefore, patients requiring long-term therapy should be carefully monitored. Patients who are not growing or gaining weight as expected should have their treatment interrupted.

Gastrointestinal: Potential for Gastrointestinal Obstruction: Because the CONCERTA tablet does not appreciably change in shape in the gastrointestinal tract, CONCERTA should not be administered to patients with pre-existing gastrointestinal narrowing (pathologic or iatrogenic, such as small bowel inflammatory disease, "short gut" syndrome due to adhesions or decreased transit time, past history of peritonitis, cystic fibrosis, chronic intestinal pseudo-obstruction, or Meckel's diverticulum). There have been rare reports of obstructive symptoms in patients with known strictures in association with the ingestion of other drugs in nondeformable controlled-release formulations. There have been very rare reports of obstructive symptoms associated with the use of CONCERTA in patients without known gastrointestinal stricture. Due to the controlled-release design, CONCERTA tablets should only be used in patients who are able to swallow the tablets whole (see Dosage and Administration, Administration).

Neurologic: Seizures: There is some clinical evidence that methylphenidate may lower the convulsive threshold in patients with a prior history of seizures, in patients with prior EEG abnormalities in the absence of seizures, and, very rarely, in the absence of history of seizures and no prior EEG evidence of seizures. In the presence of seizures or suspected seizures, the drug should be discontinued.

Effects on Ability to Drive and Use Machines: Stimulants may impair the ability of the patient to operate potentially hazardous machinery or vehicles. Patients should be cautioned accordingly until they are reasonably certain that CONCERTA does not adversely affect their ability to engage in such activities.

Ophthalmologic: Visual Disturbance: Symptoms of visual disturbances have been encountered in rare cases. Difficulties with accommodation and blurring of vision have been reported.

Psychiatric: Pre-Existing Psychosis: Administration of stimulants may exacerbate symptoms of behaviour disturbance and thought disorder in patients with a pre-existing psychotic disorder.

Bipolar Illness: Particular care should be taken in using stimulants to treat ADHD in patients with comorbid bipolar disorder because of concern for possible induction of a mixed/manic episode in such patients. Prior to initiating treatment with a stimulant, patients with comorbid depressive symptoms should be adequately screened to determine if they are at risk for bipolar disorder; such screening should include a detailed psychiatric history, including a family history of suicide, bipolar disorder, and depression.

Emergence of New Psychotic or Manic Symptoms: Treatment emergent psychotic or manic symptoms, e.g., hallucinations, delusional thinking, or mania in children and adolescents without a prior history of psychotic illness or mania can be caused by stimulants at usual doses. If such symptoms occur, consideration should be given to a possible causal role of the stimulant, and discontinuation of treatment may be appropriate. In a pooled analysis of multiple short-term, placebo-controlled studies, such symptoms occurred in about 0.1% (4 patients with events out of 3482 exposed to methylphenidate or amphetamine for several weeks at usual doses) of stimulant-treated patients compared to 0 in placebo-treated patients.

Aggression: Aggressive behaviour or hostility is often observed in children and adolescents with ADHD, and has been reported in clinical trials and the postmarketing experience of some medications indicated for the treatment of ADHD. Although there is no systematic evidence that stimulants cause aggressive behaviour or hostility, patients beginning treatment for ADHD should be monitored for the appearance of or worsening of aggressive behaviour or hostility.

Special Populations: Pregnant Women: Methylphenidate hydrochloride has been shown to have teratogenic effects in rabbits when given in doses of 200 mg/kg/day, which is approximately 100 times and 40 times the maximum recommended human dose on a mg/kg and mg/m² basis, respectively.

A reproduction study in rats revealed no evidence of harm to the fetus at oral doses up to 30 mg/kg/day, approximately 15-fold and 3-fold the maximum recommended human dose of CONCERTA on a mg/kg and mg/m² basis, respectively. The approximate plasma exposure to methylphenidate plus its main metabolite alpha-phenyl-2-piperidine acetic acid (PPAA) in pregnant rats was 2 times that seen in trials in volunteers and patients with the maximum recommended dose of CONCERTA based on the AUC.

There are no adequate and well-controlled studies in pregnant women. CONCERTA should be used during pregnancy only if the potential benefit justifies the potential risk to the fetus.

Nursing Women: A study conducted in rats indicated that the distribution profiles of methylphenidate in milk and plasma are similar. It is not known whether methylphenidate is excreted in human milk. Because many drugs are excreted in human milk, CONCERTA methylphenidate hydrochloride should not be administered to a nursing woman unless the anticipated benefits to the mother outweigh the potential hazards to the infant.

Pediatrics (<6 years of age): CONCERTA should not be used in children under six years, since safety and efficacy in this age group have not been established. Long-term effects of methylphenidate in children have not been well established (see Warnings and Precautions, Endocrine and Metabolism).

Monitoring and Laboratory Tests: Periodic laboratory tests are advised during prolonged therapy. The tests should include, but not be limited to, haematological parameters, including complete blood count, differential and platelet counts, and liver enzymes.

ADVERSE REACTIONS: Clinical Trial Adverse Drug Reactions: Because clinical trials are conducted under very specific conditions the adverse reaction rates observed in the clinical trials may not reflect the rates observed in practice and should not be compared to the rates in the clinical trials of another drug. Adverse drug reaction information from clinical trials is useful for identifying drug-related adverse events and for approximating rates.

The development program for CONCERTA included exposures in a total of 2227 participants in clinical trials. The patients in these studies received CONCERTA 18, 36, 54 or 72 mg/day. Children, adolescents, and adults with ADHD were evaluated in five placebo-controlled clinical studies (Studies 1, 2, and 3 in children; Study 4 in adolescents; Study 5 in adults), three open-label clinical trials and two open-label extensions. A limited number of adolescents and adults received CONCERTA 72 mg/day or 90 mg/day, respectively. Adverse reactions were assessed by collecting adverse events, results of physical examinations, vital signs, weights, laboratory analyses, and ECGs.

Adverse events during exposure were obtained primarily by general inquiry and recorded by clinical investigators using terminology of their own choosing. Consequently, it is not possible to provide a meaningful estimate of the proportion of individuals experiencing adverse events without first grouping similar types of events into a smaller number of standardized event categories. In the tables and listings that follow, COSTART terminology has been used to classify reported adverse events, except for Study 5 in adults, where MedDRA terminology was used.

The stated frequencies of adverse events represent the proportion of individuals who experienced, at least once, a treatment-emergent adverse event of the type listed. An event was considered treatment emergent if it occurred for the first time or worsened while receiving therapy following baseline evaluation.

Adverse Events Leading to Discontinuation of Treatment: In a 4-week placebo-controlled, parallel-group trial (Study 3), one patient treated with CONCERTA (0.9%; 1/106), one methylphenidate t.i.d.-treated patient (0.9%; 1/107), and one placebo-treated patient (1.0%; 1/99) discontinued due to an adverse event (sadness, emotional lability, and increase in tics, respectively).

In the 2-week placebo-controlled phase of a trial in adolescents (Study 4), no patients treated with CONCERTA (0%; 0/87) and 1 placebo-treated patient (1.1%; 1/90) discontinued due to an adverse event (increased mood irritability).

In the 5-week placebo-controlled phase of a trial in adults (Study 5), 0% (0/96) of the patients in the placebo group, 1.0% (1/101) of the patients in the CONCERTA 18 mg dose group, 2.9% (3/102) of the patients in the CONCERTA 36 mg dose group and 7.8% (8/102) of the patients in the CONCERTA 72 mg dose group discontinued due to an adverse event.

In two open-label, long-term safety trials (Studies 6 and 7), one study up to 27 months in children aged 6 to 13 and one study up to 9 months in child, adolescent and adult patients treated with CONCERTA, 6.7% (101/1514) of patients discontinued due to adverse events. Those events leading to discontinuation of CONCERTA, with an incidence of >0.5%, included: insomnia (1.5%), twitching (tics, 1.0%), nervousness (0.7%), emotional lability (0.7%), abdominal pain (0.7%), and anorexia (0.7%).

Adverse Events Occurring in Patients Treated with CONCERTA: Table 1 enumerates, for the 4-week placebo-controlled, parallel-group trial in children with ADHD at CONCERTA doses of 18, 36, or 54 mg q.d., the incidence of treatment-emergent adverse events. The table includes only those events that occurred in 1% or more of patients treated with CONCERTA, methylphenidate hydrochloride and placebo-treated patients.

Table 2 lists the incidence of treatment-emergent adverse events for a 2-week placebo- controlled trial (Study 4) in adolescents with ADHD at CONCERTA doses of 18, 36, 54 or 72 mg/day.

Table 3 lists the incidence of treatment-emergent adverse events for a 5-week placebo-controlled trial (Study 5) in adults with ADHD at CONCERTA doses of 18, 36, or 72 mg/day.

Adverse Events Occurring in Long-Term Safety Trials: CONCERTA was evaluated in two long-term open-label studies (n=1514) up to 27 months. The adverse event profile seen is similar to that observed in shorter term trials. COSTART terminology is used to classify reported adverse experiences. The experiences are classified within body system categories and grouped by frequency. See Table 4.

Tics: During two long-term, open-label studies, the overall incidence of tics (twitching) in children was 4.3% (48/1109 subjects). In one study, the incidence of tics rose from 3% at baseline to 5% after one month. The incidence remained the same during the rest of the study. Treatment period was up to 27 months with mean treatment duration of 10.3 months.

In a long-term study of up to 9 months of treatment, the incidence of tics was 0.4% (1/269) in adolescents and 0.7% (1/136) in adults.

Post-Market Adverse Drug Reactions: Adverse events reported since market introduction in patients taking CONCERTA include palpitations, cardiac arrhythmia, sudden cardiac death, suicide, suicide ideation, suicide attempt, exfoliative dermatitis, Stevens-Johnson Syndrome, emerging psychosis, seizure, dyskinesia, pancreatitis, aplastic anaemia, serum sickness, hypoglycaemia, abnormal liver function tests (e.g., transaminase elevation), leukopenia, thrombocytopenia, transient pancytopenia, difficulties in visual accommodation, blurred vision. The causal relationship between CONCERTA and the emergence of these events has not been established.

Adverse Events with Other Methylphenidate Hydrochloride Products: Nervousness and insomnia are the most common adverse reactions reported with other methylphenidate products. Other reactions include hypersensitivity (including skin rash, urticaria, fever, arthralgia, exfoliative dermatitis, erythema multiforme with histopathological findings of necrotizing vasculitis, and thrombocytopenic purpura); anorexia; nausea; dizziness; headache; dyskinesia; drowsiness; blood pressure and pulse changes, both up and down; tachycardia; angina; abdominal pain; weight loss during prolonged therapy. There have been rare reports of Tourette's syndrome. Toxic psychosis has been reported. Although a definite causal relationship has not been established, the following have been reported in patients taking this drug: instances of abnormal liver function, e.g., hepatic coma; isolated cases of cerebral arteritis and/or occlusion; leukopenia and/or anaemia; transient depressed mood; a few instances of scalp hair loss. Very rare reports of neuroleptic malignant syndrome (NMS) have been received, and in most of these, patients were concurrently receiving therapies associated with NMS. In a single report, a ten-year-old boy who had been taking methylphenidate for approximately 18 months experienced an NMS-like event within 45 minutes of ingesting his first dose of venlafaxine. It is uncertain whether this case represented a drug-drug interaction, a response to either drug alone, or some other cause.

Table 1: CONCERTA

Incidence (%) of Treatment-Emergent Events[a] in a 4-Week Placebo-Controlled Clinical Trial of CONCERTA in Children

Body System	Preferred Term[b]	CONCERTA q.d. (n=106)	Methylphenidate Hydrochloride t.i.d. (n=107)	Placebo (n=99)
General	Headache	14	6	10
	Abdominal pain	7	6	1
	Aggravation reaction	2	2	2
Digestive	Vomiting	4	2	3
	Anorexia	4	0	0
Nervous	Insomnia	4	1	1
	Dizziness	2	0	0
Respiratory	Upper respiratory tract infection	8	7	5
	Cough increased	4	8	2
	Pharyngitis	4	4	3
	Sinusitis	3	1	0

[a] Events, regardless of causality, for which the incidence for patients treated with CONCERTA was at least 1%. Incidence greater than 1% has been rounded to the nearest whole number.
[b] COSTART terms.

Table 2: CONCERTA

Incidence (%) of Treatment-Emergent Events[a] in a 2-Week Placebo-Controlled Clinical Trial of CONCERTA in Adolescents

Body System	Preferred Term[b]	CONCERTA q.d. (n=87)	Placebo (n=90)
General	Abdominal pain	2	2
	Accidental injury	6	3
	Allergic reaction	1	0
	Asthenia	2	2
	Chest pain	1	0
	Fever	3	0
	Flu syndrome	1	0
	Headache	9	8
	Infection	1	6
	Pain	1	1
Digestive	Anorexia	2	0
	Diarrhoea	2	0
	Dyspepsia	1	0
	Gastrointestinal disorder	1	0
	Increased appetite	1	0
	Nausea	1	2
	Tooth caries	1	0
	Vomiting	3	0
Musculoskeletal	Myalgia	1	0
Nervous	Agitation	1	0
	Anxiety	1	0
	Dizziness	1	0
	Insomnia	4	0
	Neurosis	1	1
	Tremor	1	0
Respiratory	Pharyngitis	2	1
	Rhinitis	3	2
Urogenital	Dysmenorrhoea	2	0

[a] Events, regardless of causality, for which the incidence for patients treated with CONCERTA was at least 1%. Incidence has been rounded to the nearest whole number.
[b] COSTART terms.

Table 3: CONCERTA

Incidence (%) of Treatment-Emergent Events[a] in a 5-Week Placebo-Controlled Clinical Trial of CONCERTA in Adults

Body System	Preferred Term[b]	CONCERTA			Placebo
		18 mg q.d. (n=101)	36 mg q.d. (n=102)	72 mg q.d. (n=102)	q.d. (n=96)
Cardiac Disorders	Palpitations	2	5	5	0
	Tachycardia	4	5	8	0
Ear and Labyrinth Disorders	Vertigo	2	3	2	0
Gastrointestinal Disorders	Abdominal pain upper	4	2	2	5
	Diarrhea	3	1	4	5
	Dry mouth	8	7	21	2
	Hemorrhoids	0	0	4	0
	Nausea	8	16	15	4
General Disorders and Administration Site Conditions	Fatigue	4	4	6	6
Infectious and Infestations	Influenza	4	2	2	3
	Nasopharyngitis	7	8	4	9
Investigations	Weight decreased	3	8	11	5
Metabolism and Nutrition Disorders	Decreased appetite	20	22	34	7
Nervous System Disorders	Confusional state	0	3	1	0
	Dizziness	6	10	9	7
	Headache	26	21	17	18
	Initial insomnia	3	2	5	2
	Insomnia	12	12	17	7
	Migraine	0	1	3	3
	Paresthesia	3	1	1	0
	Tremor	1	1	7	1
Psychiatric Disorders	Aggression	2	3	2	1
	Agitation	0	1	3	1
	Anxiety	3	5	8	1
	Attention deficit/hyperactivity disorder	0	0	4	0
	Depressed mood	6	3	5	1
	Depression	0	3	4	1
	Irritability	4	4	9	1
	Nervousness	0	3	8	1
	Restlessness	0	2	6	0
	Tension	0	3	0	0
Respiratory, Thoracic and Mediastinal Disorders	Pharyngolaryngeal pain	2	0	4	1
Skin and Subcutaneous Tissue Disorders	Hyperhidrosis	5	3	8	1
Vascular Disorders	Hypertension	0	1	4	4

[a] Events, regardless of causality, for which the incidence in any CONCERTA dosage group was at least 2%. Incidence has been rounded to the nearest whole number.
[b] MedDRA Terms.

DRUG INTERACTIONS: Overview: Alcohol may exacerbate the CNS adverse effect of psychoactive drugs. Therefore, patients undergoing CONCERTA therapy should be advised to avoid alcohol during treatment.

Because of possible increases in blood pressure and heart rate, CONCERTA should be used cautiously with drugs with similar pharmacological actions.

Drug-Drug Interactions: Inhibition of Drug Metabolism by Methylphenidate: Human pharmacologic studies have shown that methylphenidate may inhibit the metabolism of coumarin anticoagulants (e.g., warfarin), anticonvulsants (e.g., phenobarbital, phenytoin, primidone) and some antidepressants (tricyclics and selective serotonin reuptake inhibitors). Downward dose adjustment of these drugs may be required when given concomitantly with methylphenidate. It may be necessary to adjust the dosage and monitor plasma drug concentrations (or, in the case of coumarin, coagulation times) when initiating or discontinuing concomitant methylphenidate.

Monoamine Oxidase Inhibitors: Methylphenidate is contraindicated during treatment with monoamine oxidase inhibitors, and also within a minimum of 14 days following discontinuation of a monoamine oxidase inhibitor (hypertensive crises may result). The same precautions apply to CONCERTA (see Contraindications).

Clonidine: Serious adverse events have been reported in concomitant use with clonidine, although no causality for the combination has been established. The safety of using methylphenidate in combination with clonidine or other centrally acting alpha-2 agonists has not been systematically evaluated.
Drug-Food Interactions: There are no known food interactions with CONCERTA.
Drug-Herb Interactions: Interactions with herbal products have not been established.
Drug-Laboratory Test Interactions: Interactions with laboratory tests have not been established.

Table 4: CONCERTA

Adverse Events Occurring in Long-Term Safety Trials

Frequency	**Very Frequent**	**Frequent**		**Less Frequent**
Body System	**>10%–<50%**	**5–10%**	**<5% and ≥1%**	**<1%**
Body as a Whole	headache	accidental injury, abdominal pain, fever	flu syndrome, allergic reaction, infection, aggravation reaction, pain, extremity pain, back pain	surgery procedure, accidental overdose, chest pain, cyst, infection fungal, photosensitivity reaction, malaise, asthenia, neck pain
Cardiovascular System			hypertension	cardiovascular disorder, tachycardia, migraine
Digestive System		anorexia, vomiting	gastroenteritis, diarrhea, nausea, dyspepsia	rectal disorder, gastritis, increased appetite, nausea and vomiting, periodontal abscess, tongue disorder, tooth disorder, constipation
Endocrine System				diabetes mellitus
Hemic and Lymphatic Systems				ecchymosis, petechia, lymphadenopathy
Metabolic and Nutritional System			weight loss	dehydration
Musculoskeletal System			myalgia	arthralgia, leg cramps
Nervous System	insomnia		twitching, nervousness, emotional lability, anxiety, depression, somnolence, hostility, dizziness	apathy, neurosis, hallucinations, speech disorder, sleep disorder, tremor, thinking abnormal, abnormal dreams
Respiratory System	upper respiratory tract infection	pharyngitis, cough increased, rhinitis	sinusitis, respiratory disorder, asthma, bronchitis, epistaxis	dyspnea, pneumonia, voice alterations, laryngitis
Skin System			rash, contact dermatitis	pustular rash, urticaria, eczema, pruritus, skin benign neoplasm, acne, alopecia, nail disorder, psoriasis, herpes simplex
Special Senses		otitis media	conjunctivitis	ear disorder, diplopia, ear pain
Urogenital System				albuminuria, urinary frequency, urinary tract infection, urinary urgency

DOSAGE AND ADMINISTRATION: Dosing Considerations: CONCERTA should be administered starting at the lowest possible dose. Dosage should then be individually and slowly adjusted, to the lowest effective dosage, since individual patient response to CONCERTA varies widely.

CONCERTA should not be used in patients with symptomatic cardiovascular disease and should generally not be used in patients with known structural cardiac abnormalities (see Contraindications and Warnings and Precautions).

Children: Theoretically there exists a pharmacological potential for all ADHD drugs to increase the risk of sudden/cardiac death. Although confirmation of an incremental risk for sudden/cardiac death arising from treatment with ADHD medications is lacking, prescribers should consider this potential risk.

All drugs with sympathomimetic effects prescribed in the management of ADHD should be used with caution in patients who: a) are involved in strenuous exercise or activities b) use other sympathomimetic ADHD drugs or c) have a family history of sudden/cardiac death. Prior to the initiation of treatment with sympathomimetic medications, a personal and family history (including assessment for a family history of sudden death or ventricular arrhythmia) and physical exam should be obtained to assess for the presence of cardiac disease. In patients with relevant risk factors and based on the clinician's judgment, further cardiovascular evaluation may be considered (e.g., electrocardiogram and echocardiogram). Patients who develop symptoms such as exertional chest pain, unexplained syncope, or other symptoms suggestive of cardiac disease during ADHD treatment should undergo a prompt cardiac evaluation. Patients who are considered to need extended treatment with CONCERTA should undergo periodic evaluation of their cardiovascular status (see Warnings and Precautions).

Recommended Dose and Dosage Adjustment: General: CONCERTA should be administered orally once daily in the morning, with or without food. For patients new to methylphenidate, the starting dose for CONCERTA should be 18 mg daily. For patients currently on a methylphenidate-based product, see the conversion in Table 5.

Initial Dose Selection: Patients New to Methylphenidate: The recommended **starting** dose of CONCERTA for patients who are not currently taking methylphenidate, or for patients who are on stimulants other than methylphenidate, is 18 mg once daily.

Table 5: CONCERTA

Recommended Starting Dose and Maximum Dosage of CONCERTA for Patients New to Methylphenidate

Patient Age	**Recommended Starting Dose**	**Maximum Dosage**
Children (6–12 years of age)	18 mg/day	54 mg/day
Adolescents (13–18 years of age)	18 mg/day	54 mg/day
Adults (>18 years of age)	18 mg/day	72 mg/day

A limited number of adolescents have been treated with CONCERTA 72 mg/day in the open-label extension of Study 4 (n=62). A limited number of adults have been treated with doses up to 90 mg/day in the open-label extension of Study 5 (n=41).

Patients Currently Using Methylphenidate Hydrochloride: The recommended **conversion** dose of CONCERTA for patients who are currently taking methylphenidate hydrochloride b.i.d., t.i.d., or sustained-release (SR) at doses of 10 to 60 mg/day is provided in Table 6. Dosing recommendations are based on current dose regimen and clinical judgment.

Table 6: CONCERTA

Recommended Dose Conversion from Methylphenidate Hydrochloride Regimens to CONCERTA

Previous Methylphenidate Hydrochloride Daily Dose	**Recommended CONCERTA Initial Dose**
5 mg methylphenidate hydrochloride b.i.d./t.i.d. or 20 mg methylphenidate hydrochloride SR	18 mg q. a.m.
10 mg methylphenidate hydrochloride b.i.d./t.i.d. or 40 mg methylphenidate hydrochloride SR	36 mg q. a.m.
15 mg methylphenidate hydrochloride b.i.d./t.i.d. or 60 mg methylphenidate hydrochloride SR	54 mg q. a.m.

A dosage strength of 27 mg is available for physicians who wish to prescribe between the 18 mg and 36 mg dosages.

Dose Titration: Dosage should be individualized according to the needs and responses of the patient. Based on an assessment of clinical benefit and tolerability, doses may be adjusted at weekly intervals for patients who have not achieved an optimal response.

Maintenance/Extended Treatment: There is no evidence available from controlled trials to indicate how long the patient with ADHD should be treated with CONCERTA. It is generally agreed that pharmacological treatment of ADHD may be needed for extended periods. The physician who elects to use CONCERTA for extended periods in patients with ADHD should periodically re-evaluate the long-term usefulness of the drug for the individual patient with trials off medication to assess the patient's functioning without pharmacotherapy.

Dose Reduction and Discontinuation: If paradoxical aggravation of symptoms or other adverse events occur, the dosage should be reduced or, if necessary, the drug should be discontinued.

If improvement is not observed after appropriate dosage adjustment over a one-month period, the drug should be discontinued.

Administration: CONCERTA tablets must be swallowed whole with liquids, and must not be chewed, divided or crushed. In dogs, the intravenous injection of the pulverized CONCERTA tablets resulted in death. The medication is contained within a non-absorbable shell designed to release the drug at a controlled rate. The tablet shell, along with insoluble core components, is eliminated from the body; patients should not be concerned if they occasionally notice something that looks like a tablet in their stool.

OVERDOSAGE:

Signs and Symptoms: Signs and symptoms of CONCERTA overdosage, resulting principally from overstimulation of the CNS and from excessive sympathomimetic effects, may include the following: vomiting, agitation, muscle twitching, convulsion, grand mal convulsions, confusional state, hallucination (auditory and/or visual), hyperhidrosis, headache, pyrexia, tachycardia, palpitations, heart rate increased, sinus arrhythmias, hypertension, mydriasis and dry mouth.

Recommended Treatment: Treatment consists of appropriate supportive measures. The patient must be protected against self-injury and against external stimuli that would aggravate the overstimulation already present. Gastric contents may be evacuated by gastric lavage as indicated. Before performing gastric lavage, control agitation and seizures (if present) and protect the airway. Other measures to detoxify the gut include administration of activated charcoal and a cathartic. Intensive care must be provided to maintain adequate circulation and respiratory exchange; external cooling procedures may be required for pyrexia.

Efficacy of peritoneal dialysis or extracorporeal hemodialysis for CONCERTA overdosage has not been established. The prolonged release of methylphenidate from CONCERTA tablets should be considered when treating patients with overdose. Alcohol may induce the production of ethylphenidate. The amount of ethylphenidate production is proportional to the blood alcohol concentration (see Drug Interactions, Overview). As with the management of all overdosage, the possibility of multiple drug ingestion, including alcohol, should be considered.

For management of a suspected drug overdose, contact your regional Poison Control Centre. See the *CPS* Directory section for a list of Poison Control Centres.

ACTION AND CLINICAL PHARMACOLOGY: Mechanism of Action: Methylphenidate hydrochloride is a central nervous system (CNS) stimulant. The mechanism of action on the CNS is not completely understood, but methylphenidate is thought to block the reuptake of dopamine and norepinephrine into the presynaptic neuron and increase the release of these monoamines into the extraneuronal space.

Pharmacodynamics: Methylphenidate is a racemic mixture comprised of the d- and l-isomers. The d-isomer is pharmacologically active; the l-isomer has little pharmacologic activity. Following administration of CONCERTA methylphenidate hydrochloride, plasma concentrations of the l-isomer were approximately 1/40th the plasma concentrations of the d-isomer.

Pharmacokinetics: Absorption: Methylphenidate is readily absorbed. Following oral administration of CONCERTA, plasma methylphenidate concentrations reach an initial maximum at about 1 hour followed by gradual ascending concentrations over the next 5 to 9 hours. Mean times to reach peak plasma concentrations across all doses of CONCERTA occurred between 6 to 10 hours. CONCERTA once daily (q.d.) minimizes the fluctuations between peak and trough concentrations associated with multiple doses of immediate-release methylphenidate treatments (see Figure 1). The relative bioavailability of CONCERTA q.d. and methylphenidate three times a day (t.i.d.) in adults is comparable.

Figure 1: CONCERTA

Mean Methylphenidate Plasma Concentrations in 36 Fasted Adults, Following a Single Dose of CONCERTA 18 mg q.d. and Immediate-Release Methylphenidate Hydrochloride 5 mg t.i.d. Administered Every 4 Hours

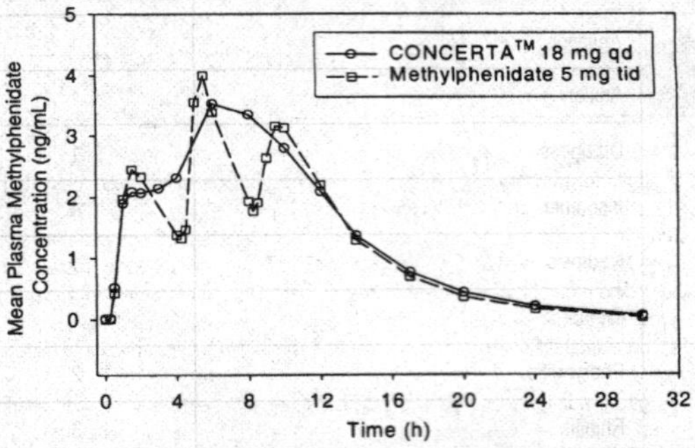

Children (Single Dose): The mean pharmacokinetic parameters in 13 children 7-12 years of age following administration of CONCERTA 18, 36 or 54 mg are summarized in Table 7.

Adolescents (Steady-State): The pharmacokinetics of methylphenidate were evaluated in adolescents 13-16 years of age with ADHD following steady-state dosing with CONCERTA 36 mg, 54 mg, or 72 mg. The mean pharmacokinetic parameters are summarized in Table 8.

Adults: The mean single dose pharmacokinetic parameters in 36 healthy adults following the administration of CONCERTA 18 mg q.d. and methylphenidate hydrochloride 5 mg t.i.d. are summarized in Table 9.

The mean single dose and steady-state pharmacokinetic parameters in 25 healthy adults following the administration of CONCERTA 54 and 72 mg q.d. are summarized in Table 10.

Table 7: CONCERTA

Pharmacokinetic Parameters in Children after Single Dosing (Mean±SD)

Parameters	CONCERTA 18 mg (n=3)	CONCERTA 36 mg (n=7)	CONCERTA 54 mg (n=3)
C_{max} (ng/mL)	6.0±1.3	11.3±2.6	15.0±3.8
T_{max} (h)	9.4±0.02	8.1±1.1	9.1±2.5
$AUC_{0-11.5}$ (ng·h/mL)[a]	50.4±7.8	87.7±18.2	121.5± 37.3

[a] Limited blood sampling.

Table 8: CONCERTA

Pharmacokinetic Parameters in Adolescents at Steady-State (Mean±SD)

Parameters	CONCERTA 36 mg (n=10)	CONCERTA 54 mg (n=8)	CONCERTA 72 mg[a] (n=6)
C_{max} (ng/mL)	9.9±5.5	12.8±3.4	17.8±4.5
T_{max} (h)	7.0±2.1	6.8±1.7	7.0±1.8
AUC_{inf} (ng·h/mL)	112±55.9	141±34.3	186±33.9
$t_{½}$ (h)	4.3±2.0	3.6±0.5	3.5±0.5

[a] Not recommended. In the clinical study, only 62 adolescents received CONCERTA at this dose level.

Table 9: CONCERTA

Pharmacokinetic Parameters in Adult Subjects after Single Dosing (Mean±SD)

Parameters	CONCERTA (18 mg q.d.) (n=36)	Methylphenidate Hydrochloride (5 mg t.i.d.) (n=35)
C_{max} (ng/mL)	3.7±1.0	4.2±1.0
T_{max} (h)	6.8±1.8	6.5±1.8
AUC_{inf} (ng·h/mL)	41.8±13.9	38.0±11.0
$T_{½}$ (h)	3.5±0.4	3.0±0.5

Table 10: CONCERTA

Pharmacokinetic Parameters in Adult Subjects Following Single Dose and at Steady-State (Mean±SD)

Parameters	CONCERTA 54 mg (n=25)	CONCERTA 72 mg (n=25)
Single Dose		
C_{max} (ng/mL)	12.03±3.54	17.12±5.80
T_{max}[a] (h)	6 (1–10)	6 (5–10)
AUC_{inf} (ng·h/mL)	130±32.4	196±65.7
$t_{½}$ (h)	3.58±0.629	3.57±0.617
Steady State		
C_{max} (ng/mL)	12.45±2.84	16.12±4.60
T_{max}[a] (h)	6 (1–10)	6 (5–8)
AUC_{tau} (ng·h/mL)	139±33.6[b]	185±49.0
$t_{½}$ (h)	3.60±0.844	3.63±0.49

[a] Median and range are listed.
[b] N=24.

Distribution: Plasma methylphenidate concentrations in adults decline bi-exponentially following oral administration. The half-life of methylphenidate in adults following oral administration of CONCERTA was approximately 3.5 h. In humans, 15±5% of methylphenidate in the blood is bound to plasma proteins.
Metabolism and Excretion: In humans, methylphenidate is metabolized primarily by de-esterification to PPAA, which has little pharmacologic activity. In adults the metabolism of CONCERTA q.d., as evaluated by metabolism to PPAA, is similar to that of methylphenidate t.i.d. The metabolism of single and repeated q.d. doses of CONCERTA is similar. After oral dosing of radio-labelled methylphenidate in humans, about 90% of the radioactivity was recovered in urine. The main urinary metabolite was PPAA, accounting for approximately 80% of the dose (see Action and Clinical Pharmacology, Special Populations and Conditions, Renal Insufficiency).
Dose Proportionality: Following administration of CONCERTA in single doses of 18, 36, and 54 mg/day to healthy adults, C_{max} and $AUC_{(0-inf)}$ of d-methylphenidate were proportional to dose, whereas l-methylphenidate C_{max} and $AUC_{(0-inf)}$ increased disproportionately with respect to dose. Following administration of CONCERTA, plasma concentrations of the l-isomer were approximately 1/40th the plasma concentrations of the d-isomer.

In a multiple-dose study in adolescent ADHD patients aged 13 to 16 administered their prescribed dose (18 to 72 mg/day) of CONCERTA, mean C_{max} and AUC_{tau} of d- and total methylphenidate increased proportionally with respect to dose.
Food Effects: In patients, there were no differences in either the pharmacokinetics or the pharmacodynamic performance of CONCERTA when administered after a high fat breakfast. There is no evidence of dose dumping in the presence or absence of food.
Special Populations and Conditions: Gender: In healthy adults, the mean dose-adjusted $AUC_{(0-inf)}$ values for CONCERTA were 36.7 ng·h/mL in men and 37.1 ng·h/mL in women, with no differences noted between the two groups.

Race: In adults receiving CONCERTA tablets, dose-adjusted $AUC_{(0-inf)}$ was consistent across ethnic groups; however, the sample size may have been insufficient to detect ethnic variations in pharmacokinetics.
Age: The pharmacokinetics of CONCERTA have not been studied in children less than 6 years of age, and CONCERTA should not be used in this patient population. There are no data available for the use of CONCERTA in patients over 65 years of age.
Hepatic Insufficiency: CONCERTA has not been studied in patients with hepatic insufficiency.
Renal Insufficiency: There is very limited experience with the use of methylphenidate in patients with renal insufficiency. Renal clearance is not significant for methylphenidate elimination, but the main methylphenidate metabolic product, PPAA, is predominantly (80%) cleared through the urine.
STORAGE AND STABILITY: Store at controlled room temperature (15-30°C). Protect from moisture.
INFORMATION FOR THE PATIENT: Published in e-CPS, available by subscription at www.e-cps.ca.
DOSAGE FORMS, COMPOSITION AND PACKAGING: 18 mg: Each yellow, capsule-shaped, extended-release tablet, 5.3 mm in diameter and 12.0 mm in length, printed with "alza 18", contains: methylphenidate HCl 18 mg. Nonmedicinal ingredients: butylated hydroxytoluene, carnauba wax, cellulose acetate, hypromellose, lactose, phosphoric acid, poloxamer, polyethylene glycol, polyethylene oxides, povidone, propylene glycol, sodium chloride, stearic acid, succinic acid, synthetic iron oxides, titanium dioxide and triacetin. Bottles of 100.
27 mg: Each gray, capsule-shaped, extended-release tablet, 5.3 mm in diameter and 12.2 mm in length, printed with "alza 27", contains: methylphenidate HCl 27 mg. Nonmedicinal ingredients: butylated hydroxytoluene, carnauba wax, cellulose acetate, hypromellose, lactose, phosphoric acid, poloxamer, polyethylene glycol, polyethylene oxides, povidone, propylene glycol, sodium chloride, stearic acid, succinic acid, synthetic iron oxides, titanium dioxide and triacetin. Bottles of 100.
36 mg: Each white, capsule-shaped, extended-release tablet, 6.8 mm in diameter and 15.0 mm in length, printed with "alza 36", contains: methylphenidate HCl 36 mg. Nonmedicinal ingredients: butylated hydroxytoluene, carnauba wax, cellulose acetate, hypromellose, lactose, phosphoric acid, poloxamer, polyethylene glycol, polyethylene oxides, povidone, propylene glycol, sodium chloride, stearic acid, succinic acid, synthetic iron oxides, titanium dioxide and triacetin. Bottles of 100.
54 mg: Each brownish-red, capsule-shaped, extended-release tablet, 6.8 mm in diameter and 15.4 mm in length, printed with "alza 54", contains: methylphenidate HCl 54 mg. Nonmedicinal ingredients: butylated hydroxytoluene, carnauba wax, cellulose acetate, hypromellose, lactose, phosphoric acid, poloxamer, polyethylene glycol, polyethylene oxides, povidone, propylene glycol, sodium chloride, stearic acid, succinic acid, synthetic iron oxides, titanium dioxide and triacetin. Bottles of 100.
System Components and Performance: CONCERTA tablets use osmotic pressure to deliver methylphenidate hydrochloride at a controlled rate. The system, which resembles a conventional tablet in appearance, comprises an osmotically active trilayer core surrounded by a semipermeable membrane with an immediate-release drug overcoat.

The trilayer core is composed of two drug layers containing the drug and excipients, and a push layer containing osmotically active components. There is a precision-laser drilled orifice on the drug-layer end of the tablet. In an aqueous environment, such as the gastrointestinal tract, the drug overcoat, which consists of 22% of the drug dose, dissolves within one hour, providing an initial dose of methylphenidate. Water permeates through the membrane into the tablet core. As the osmotically active polymer excipients expand, methylphenidate is released through the orifice. The membrane controls the rate at which water enters the tablet core, which in turn controls drug delivery. Furthermore, the drug release rate from the system increases with time over a period of 6-7 hours due to the drug-concentration gradient incorporated into the two drug layers of CONCERTA. The biologically inert components of the tablet remain intact during gastrointestinal transit and are eliminated in the stool as a tablet shell along with insoluble core components. It is possible that CONCERTA extended-release tablets may be visible on abdominal x-rays under certain circumstances, especially when digitally enhancing techniques are utilized.

(Shown in Product Identification Section)

Condyline™ Ⓟ
podofilox
Antimitotic

Canderm Pharma

PHARMACOLOGY: Necrosis of visible tissue is observed following treatment of genital warts with podofilox. The exact mechanism of action is unknown.

Podofilox is believed to exert its antimitotic effect by binding to tubulin, at a site close to but not identical to the binding site of colchicine; it is thought that this antimitotic effect causes necrosis of wart tissue, the observed clinical effect. In addition, podofilox is known to interfere with nucleoside transport which may also contribute to its action. Crude podophyllum resin, from which podofilox is extracted, has been shown to produce mitotic arrest and necrosis of wart tissue.
INDICATIONS: For the topical treatment of external genital warts (Condylomata acuminata) confined to the penile and vulvar regions. The effectiveness of podofilox in the treatment of perianal or mucous membrane warts has not been established.
CONTRAINDICATIONS: Patients who develop hypersensitivity to podofilox or intolerance to any component of the formulation. Podofilox **should not** be applied to open wounds. The consumption of alcoholic beverages for several hours after treatment is to be avoided.
WARNINGS: Podofilox is intended for topical use only.

Podofilox is a potent vesicant and is to be used only as directed by a physician. Extreme care should be taken to avoid contact with the eye, tongue or any mucosal tissue of the genital area (including vagina, cervix, anus or perianus). If contact with the eyes occurs, flush immediately with copious amounts of water and see a doctor immediately.
PRECAUTIONS: Diagnosis: Although Condylomata (genital warts) have a characteristic appearance, histopathologic confirmatory tests should be obtained if there is any question of the diagnosis. Differential diagnosis from squamous cell carcinoma (so called "Bowenoid papulosis") is of particular concern. Squamous cell carcinoma may also be associated with human papillomavirus but **should not** be treated with podofilox.
General: Podofilox may not prevent either the recurrence of previously resolved warts or the development of new warts at sites remote from the treatment site. The recommended method of application, frequency of application and duration of usage should not be exceeded (see Dosage).

The use of large volumes, greater than 0.25 mL per application or 0.5 mL/day, should be avoided. This can best be accomplished by limiting the treatment area to less than 10 cm² and instructing the patient in the proper application of the product.

Genital warts may be contagious and the patient should be instructed to abstain from sexual intercourse. If this is not possible, a latex condom must be used until the infected partner is declared cured by the physician.

The patient should be instructed that if the product is accidentally spilled on undiseased skin, it should be wiped off at once and the exposed skin washed vigorously with warm soapy water and rinsed thoroughly. This product should not be used if the growth or surrounding tissue is inflamed or irritated. Self-treatment of genital warts with surface areas greater than 10 cm² should not be permitted. The patient should be cautioned against applying the drug to lesions other than warts.
Information to Be Provided to the Patient: The patient should be provided with a Patient Information leaflet when a Condyline prescription is filled.
Long-term Safety: Reports of lifetime carcinogenicity studies in rodents with podofilox, the drug substance, are not available. In general, podofilox was not shown to be carcinogenic in published animal studies. There are published reports that, in the mouse studies, crude podophyllin resin (containing podofilox) applied topically to the cervix produced changes resembling carcinoma in situ. These changes were reversible at 5 weeks after cessation of treatment. In another published study, epidermal carcinoma of the vagina and cervix was found in 1 out of 18 mice following 120 applications of podophyllin, applied twice weekly over a 15-month treatment period.

Podofilox was not mutagenic in the Ames plate reverse mutation assay, either with or without metabolic activation, at concentrations up to 5 mg/plate. There was no evidence of potential oncogenicity in the BALB/3T3 cell transformation assay. Results from the mouse micronucleus in vivo assay using podofilox 0.5% solution in concentrations up to 25 mg/kg indicate that podofilox should be considered a potential clastogen (a chemical that induces disruption and breakage of chromosomes).

Daily topical application of podofilox at doses up to the equivalent of 0.2 mg/kg (5 times the recommended maximum human dose) to rats throughout gametogenesis, mating, gestation, parturition and lactation for 2 generations demonstrated no impairment of fertility.
Pregnancy: There are no adequate and well-controlled studies in pregnant women. Podofilox should be used in pregnancy only if the potential benefit justifies the potential risk to the fetus.
Lactation: It is not known whether this drug is excreted in human milk. Because of the potential for serious adverse reactions in nursing infants from podofilox, a decision should be made whether to discontinue nursing or to discontinue the drug, taking into account the importance of the drug to the mother.
Children: Safety and effectiveness in children have not been established.

Patients with Special Diseases and Conditions: Podofilox should not be used in diabetics or people with poor blood circulation. Podofilox should not be applied on moles, birthmarks or unusual warts with hair growing from them. Podofilox should not be used on tissue which was recently exposed to laser surgery or cryosurgery.

ADVERSE EFFECTS: In clinical trials the following have been shown to be the most common local adverse events which were reported at some time during treatment: inflammation 67%, burning 62%, erosion 59%, pain 49%, other, e.g., bleeding, itching, dizziness, insomnia 21%.

These reactions may be greater in the occluded prepuce of the uncircumcised male patient.

OVERDOSE:

Symptoms: Topical: In cases of tingling, burning or extreme tenderness, soak the area in cold water for 10 minutes; repeat as required for the relief of pain. A mild analgesic, e.g. ASA with codeine or acetaminophen with codeine may be beneficial for pain management in some cases. Adjuvant topical anti-inflammatory therapy e.g. hydrocortisone acetate, can be advantageous for alleviation of local discomfort.

Systemic: Topically applied podofilox may be absorbed systemically. It may cause systemic toxicity after oral ingestion. Neurotoxic reactions are observed after oral doses exceeding 0.5 mg podofilox per kg body weight. For an adult this dose corresponds to the equivalent of the content of 2 bottles of 3.5 mL Condyline.

Systemic toxicity may lead to prolonged peripheral neuropathy. Initial symptoms are weakness, drowsiness, dizziness, diarrhea and general indisposition. A later symptom may be coma with the risk of respiratory failure, ileus, vascular crisis and death.

Treatment: Treatment of overdosage is principally symptomatic and supportive therapy.

Hemoperfusion through coal filter and symptomatic treatment may prevent a fatal outcome. Possible toxic effects of the bone marrow (e.g. leukocytosis, pancytosis) are generally transitory.

For management of a suspected drug overdose, CPhA recommends that you contact your **regional Poison Control Centre**. See the *CPS* Directory section for a list of Poison Control Centres.

DOSAGE: Apply twice daily, morning and evening (every 12 hours) for 3 consecutive days followed by 4 days without treatment. The use of podofilox twice a day for 3 days constitutes a treatment cycle. Treatment cycles should be repeated up to 4 times until there is no visible wart tissue. **If there is incomplete response after 4 treatment cycles, alternative treatment should be considered.**

Podofilox is applied to the warts with a cotton tipped applicator supplied with the drug. The wetted applicator should be touched to the wart to be treated, applying the minimum amount of solution necessary to cover the lesion. **Treatment should be limited to less than 10 cm² of wart tissue and to no more than 500 µg of the solution per day.**

To ensure that only the genital warts are treated and properly applied, the physician performs the first application for the patient as an office procedure. The patient is shown how to minimize contact with the surrounding healthy tissue and the use of a hand mirror which may help, when he/she applies the solution at home. There is no evidence to suggest that more frequent application will increase efficacy, but this would be expected to increase the rate of local adverse reactions and systemic absorption.

Before applying the medication, the area to be treated should be gently washed with soap and water and gently patted dry. If an area in the occluded prepuce (under the foreskin) is being treated, care should be taken to allow the solution to dry before letting the foreskin return to its normal position. Avoid contact with clothing until the solution has dried. After each treatment, the used applicator should be properly and safely disposed of in a garbage can, out of reach of children, and the patient should wash his/her hands. It is recommended that the area not be washed following application of podofilox as is the practice with traditional podophyllum resin preparations.

INFORMATION FOR THE PATIENT: Published in e-CPS, available by subscription at www.e-cps.ca.

SUPPLIED: Each mL of topical solution contains: podofilox 0.5%. Amber glass bottles of 3.5 mL with plastic child-resistant cap. Package includes cotton-tipped applicators. Store at controlled room temperature (15 to 30°C), away from light and heat, in a tightly closed container.

The reader is invited to consult CPhA's monograph **Fluoroquinolones**.

CO Norfloxacin ℞

norfloxacin

Antibacterial

Cobalt

SUPPLIED: Each white, coated, oval, convex tablet, embossed with "N" breakline "O" on one side and "Σ>" on the other side, contains norfloxacin 400 mg. Nonmedicinal ingredients: croscarmellose sodium, magnesium stearate and microcrystalline cellulose; film coating: polyvinyl alcohol, soya lecithin, talc, titanium dioxide and xanthan gum. HDPE bottles of 100.

Conray® 30

iothalamate meglumine

Radiopaque Medium

tyco Healthcare

Conray® 43

iothalamate meglumine

Radiopaque Medium

tyco Healthcare

Conray® 60

iothalamate meglumine

Radiopaque Medium

tyco Healthcare

Date of Revision: July 02, 2002

PHARMACOLOGY: Following intravascular injection, Conray is rapidly transported through the circulatory system to the kidneys and is excreted unchanged in the urine by glomerular filtration. Renal accumulation is sufficiently rapid that maximum radiographic density in the calyces and pelves occurs in most instances about 3 to 8 minutes after injection. In patients with impaired renal function, diagnostic opacification frequently is achieved only after prolonged periods.

Angiography may be performed following intravascular injection of Conray which will permit visualization until significant hemodilution occurs.

The biliary system, pancreatic duct or joint spaces may be visualized by injecting the contrast medium directly into the region to be studied.

Injectable iodinated contrast agents are excreted either through the kidneys or through the liver. These 2 excretory pathways are not mutually exclusive, but the main route of excretion seems to be related to the affinity of the contrast medium for serum albumin. Iothalamate salts are poorly bound to serum albumin, and are excreted mainly through the kidneys.

The liver and small intestine provide the major alternate route of excretion. In patients with severe renal impairment, the excretion of this contrast medium through the gallbladder and into the small intestine sharply increases.

Pregnancy: Iothalamate salts cross the placental barrier in humans; and are excreted unchanged in human milk.

Lactation: See Pregnancy.

Computerized Tomography of the Head: When Conray 30, Conray 43 or Conray 60 is used for contrast enhancement in computed tomographic brain scanning, the degree of enhancement is directly related to the amount of iodine administered. Rapid infusion of the entire dose amount yields peak blood iodine concentrations immediately following the infusion, which fall rapidly over the next 5 to 10 minutes. This can be accounted for by the dilution in the vascular and extracellular fluid compartments which causes an initial sharp fall in plasma concentration. Equilibration with the extracellular compartments is reached by about 10 minutes; thereafter, the fall becomes exponential. With respect to tumors, maximum contrast enhancement frequently occurs at a time following peak blood iodine concentration. This delay in maximum contrast enhancement can range from 5 to 40 minutes, depending on the peak iodine levels achieved and the cell type and vascularity of the tumor. This lag suggests that the contrast enhancement of the image is at least in part dependent on the passage of iodine through the defective blood-brain barrier and on its accumulation within the lesion and outside the blood pool. The image enhancement of nontumoral lesions, such as arteriovenous malformations and aneurysms, is probably dependent on the iodine content of the circulating blood pool. Studies indicate that equilibrated blood iodine levels of 100 mg% are required in most cases to achieve adequate contrast enhancement. This can be accomplished by the infusion of approximately 30 to 40 g of iodine (100 to 150 mL of Conray 60 or 200 to 300 mL of Conray 30).

In brain scanning, the contrast medium does not accumulate in normal brain tissue due to the presence of the "blood brain barrier". The increase in X-ray absorption in the normal brain is due to the presence of the contrast agent within the blood pool. A break in the blood brain barrier, such as occurs in malignant tumors of the brain, allows accumulation of the contrast medium within the interstitial tumor tissue; adjacent normal brain tissue does not contain the contrast medium. When used for cranial computerized angiotomography, rapid bolus injection and/or infusion combined with rapid CT scanning will provide clear delineation of the cerebral vessels.

Computerized Tomography of the Body: In non-neural tissues (during CT of the body), Conray diffuses rapidly from the vascular to the extravascular space. Increase in X-ray absorption is related to blood flow, concentration of the contrast medium and extraction of the contrast medium by interstitial tissue since no barrier exists; contrast enhancement is thus due to the relative differences in extravascular diffusion between normal and abnormal tissue, quite different from that in the brain.

Enhancement of CT with Conray 60 may be of benefit in establishing diagnoses of certain lesions in some sites with greater assurance than is possible with unenhanced CT and in supplying additional features of the lesions. In other cases, the contrast medium may allow visualization of lesions not seen with CT alone or may help to define suspicious lesions seen with unenhanced CT.

The pharmacokinetics of Conray in normal and abnormal tissue has been shown to be variable. Contrast enhancement appears to be greatest within 30 to 90 seconds after bolus administration, thus greatest enhancement can be detected by a series of consecutive 2- to 3-second scans ("Dynamic CT Scanning") during this time period. Dynamic scanning may improve enhancement and diagnostic assessment of tumors and other lesions such as an abscess, occasionally revealing more extensive disease. A cyst, or similar nonvascularized lesions may be distinguished from vascularized solid lesions by comparing enhanced and unenhanced scans; the vascularized lesions would show an increase. The latter might be benign, malignant or normal, but it is unlikely that it would be a cyst, hematoma or other nonvascularized lesion.

Venography: Venography may be performed with Conray 43 or Conray 60 following injection into an appropriate vein and will permit visualization until sufficient hemodilution occurs.

INDICATIONS: Conray 30: For use in i.v. infusion urography and for contrast enhancement in computerized tomography of the brain.

Conray 43: For use in lower extremity venography, i.v. infusion urography and for the i.v. contrast enhancement in computerized tomography of the brain.

Conray 60: For use in excretory urography, cerebral angiography, peripheral arteriography, venography, arthrography, direct cholangiography, endoscopic retrograde cholangiopancreatography, i.v. contrast enhancement in computed tomography and digital subtraction angiography.

CONTRAINDICATIONS: Known hypersensitivity to salts of iothalamic acid and in patients with anuria or severe oliguria. Arthrography should not be performed if infection is present in or near the joint.

Percutaneous transhepatic cholangiography is contraindicated in patients with coagulation defects and prolonged prothrombin times until normal, or near normal, coagulation is achieved.

Endoscopic retrograde cholangiography is contraindicated during an acute attack of pancreatitis or during clinically evident cholangitis. The procedure is also contraindicated in patients in whom endoscopic examination is prohibited.

Conray must not be used for myelography or for injection into cysts and sinuses that might communicate with the subarachnoid space.

Conray should not be used for the enhancement of CT brain images in patients suspected of having cranial subarachnoid hemorrhage.

WARNINGS: Ionic iodinated contrast media inhibit blood coagulation more than nonionic contrast media. Nonetheless, it is necessary to avoid prolonged contact of blood with syringes containing all contrast media.

Serious, rarely fatal, thromboembolic events causing myocardial infarction and stroke have been reported during angiographic procedures with both ionic and nonionic contrast media. Therefore, meticulous intravascular administration technique is necessary, particularly during angiographic procedures, to minimize thromboembolic events. Numerous factors, including length of procedure, number of injections, catheter and syringe material, underlying disease state, and concomitant medications may contribute to the development of thromboembolic events. For these reasons meticulous angiographic techniques are recommended including close attention to keeping guidewires, catheters and all angiographic equipment free of blood, use of manifold systems and/or 3-way stopcocks, frequent catheter flushing and heparinized saline solutions, and minimizing the length of the procedure. The use of plastic syringes in place of glass syringes has been reported to decrease but not eliminate the likelihood of in vitro clotting.

Serious or fatal reactions have been associated with the administration of iodine containing radiopaque media. It is of utmost importance to be completely prepared to treat any contrast medium reaction.

A definite risk exists in the use of intravascular contrast agents in patients who are known to have multiple myeloma. In some instances anuria has developed resulting in progressive uremia, renal failure and eventually death. Although neither the contrast agent nor dehydration has separately proved to be the cause of anuria in myeloma, it has been speculated that the combination of both may be causative factors. The risk in myelomatous patients is not an absolute contraindication to the procedure; however, partial dehydration in the preparation of these patients for the examination is not recommended since this may predispose to precipitation of myeloma protein in the renal tubules. No form of therapy, including dialysis, has been successful in reversing the effect. Myeloma, which occurs most commonly in persons over 40, should be considered before instituting intravascular administration of contrast agents.

Administration of radiopaque materials to patients known or suspected to have pheochromocytoma should be performed with extreme caution. If, in the opinion of the physician, the possible benefits of such procedures outweigh the considered risks, the procedures may be performed; however, the amount of radiopaque medium injected should be kept to an absolute minimum. The blood pressure should be assessed throughout the procedure, and measures for treatment of a hypertensive crisis should be available.

Contrast media have been shown to promote the phenomenon of sickling in individuals who are homozygous for sickle cell disease when the material is injected i.v. or intra-arterially.

Conray must not be used for myelography or for injection into cysts and sinuses that might communicate with the subarachnoid space.

In computed tomography of the brain, it has been reported that in low density lesions false negative results may be produced following contrast media administration, i.e., contrast media may obscure low density lesions. Steps should be taken to insure that patients undergoing computed tomography have received no injections of water-soluble contrast media at least 24 hours prior to examination. It is recommended that a computed tomographic brain scan always be obtained prior to the administration of Conray.

PRECAUTIONS: General: All procedures utilizing contrast media carry a definite risk of producing adverse reactions. While most reactions may be minor, life-threatening and fatal reactions may occur without warning. The risk-benefit factor should always be carefully evaluated before such a procedure is undertaken. At all times a fully equipped emergency cart, or equivalent supplies and equipment, and personnel competent in recognizing and treating adverse reactions of all severity or situations which may arise as a result of the procedure, should be immediately available. Since severe delayed reactions have been known to occur, emergency facilities and competent personnel should be available for at least 30 to 60 minutes after administration.

Diagnostic procedures which involve the use of iodinated intravascular contrast agents should be carried out under the direction of personnel skilled and experienced in the particular procedure to be performed.

The possibility of an idiosyncratic reaction in patients who have previously received a contrast medium without ill effect should always be considered. Prior to the injection of any contrast medium, the patient should be questioned to obtain a medical history with emphasis on allergy and hypersensitivity. A positive history of bronchial asthma or allergy, a family history of allergy, or a previous reaction or hypersensitivity to a contrast agent may imply a greater than usual risk. Such a history, by suggesting histamine sensitivity and consequently proneness to reactions, may be more accurate than pretesting in predicting the potential for reaction, although not necessarily the severity or type of reaction in the individual case. A positive history of this type does not arbitrarily contraindicate the use of a contrast agent, when a diagnostic procedure is thought essential, but does call for caution. Premedication with antihistamines or corticosteroids to avoid or minimize the possible allergic reactions in such patients should be considered. Under no circumstance should the antihistamine or the corticosteroid be mixed in the same syringe with the contrast medium because of chemical incompatibility.

In order to screen patients for allergy potential, various pretesting procedures have been developed; however, specific literature reports indicate that none of these provocative test procedures can be relied upon to predict severe or fatal reactions. The pretest most often performed is the slow i.v. injection of 0.5 to 1.0 mL of the radiopaque medium prior to the injection of the full dose. The absence of a reaction to the test dose does not preclude the possibility of a reaction to the full dose. In some instances, reactions to the test dose itself may be extremely severe; therefore, close observation of the patient and facilities for emergency treatment are indicated.

Partial dehydration prior to the examination should be avoided in patients with chronic renal disease, multiple myeloma, diabetes and in infants and small children.

In patients with advanced renal disease, iodinated contrast media should be used with caution, and only when the need for the examination dictates, since excretion of the medium may be impaired. Patients with combined renal and hepatic disease and those with severe hypertension or congestive heart failure may present an additional risk. Renal failure has been reported in patients with liver dysfunction who were given an oral cholecystographic agent, followed by an intravascular iodinated radiopaque agent and also in patients with occult renal disease, notably diabetics and hypertensives.

Administration of Conray should, therefore, be postponed in any patient with a known or suspected hepatic or biliary disorder who has recently taken cholecystographic contrast agent.

Caution should be exercised in performing contrast medium studies in patients with endotoxemia and/or those with elevated body temperatures.

Reports of thyroid storm occurring following the intravascular use of iodinated radiopaque agents in patients with hyperthyroidism or with an autonomously functioning thyroid nodule, suggest that this additional risk be evaluated in such patients before use of this drug.

Iodine-containing contrast agents may alter the results of thyroid function tests which depend on iodine estimation, e.g., PBI and radioactive iodine uptake studies. Such tests, if indicated, should be performed prior to the administration of this preparation.

Pregnancy: Reproduction studies with various concentrations of iothalamate sodium, iothalamate meglumine or a combination of both have been performed in mice, rats, and rabbits, and have revealed no evidence of impaired fertility or harm to the fetus.

There are no well controlled studies in pregnant women, but marketing experience does not include any positive evidence of adverse effects on the fetus. Although there is no clearly defined risk, such experience cannot exclude the possibility of infrequent or subtle damage to the fetus. Conray should be used in pregnant women only when clearly needed.

Lactation: It is not known whether this drug is excreted in human milk. As a general rule, nursing should not be undertaken or continued following administration of this drug since many drugs are excreted in human milk.

Precautions for specific procedures receive comment under that procedure in the Dosage section.

ADVERSE EFFECTS: General: Adverse reactions accompanying the use of iodine-containing intravascular contrast agents are usually mild and transient, although severe and life-threatening reactions, including fatalities, have occurred. Because of the possibility of severe reactions to both the procedure and radiopaque medium, appropriate emergency facilities and well trained personnel should be available to treat both types. These emergency facilities and personnel should remain available for 30 to 60 minutes following the procedure since severe delayed reactions have been reported.

The following adverse reactions have been observed in conjunction with the use of iodine-containing intravascular contrast agents.

The most frequent reactions are nausea, vomiting, facial flush and a feeling of body warmth. These are usually of brief duration. Other reactions include the following:

Allergic: dermal manifestations of urticaria with or without pruritus, erythema and maculopapular rash, dry mouth, sweating, conjunctival symptoms, facial, peripheral and angioneurotic edema. Symptoms relating to the respiratory system include sneezing, nasal stuffiness, coughing, choking, dyspnea, chest tightness and wheezing, which may be initial manifestations of more severe and infrequent reactions including asthmatic attack, laryngospasm and bronchospasm with or without edema, pulmonary edema, apnea and cyanosis. Rarely, these allergic type reactions can progress into anaphylactic shock with loss of consciousness and coma and severe cardiovascular disturbances.

Cardiovascular: generalized vasodilatation, flushing and venospasm. Occasionally, thrombosis or, rarely, thrombophlebitis. Red blood cell clumping and agglutination, crenation and interference in clot formation. Extremely rare cases of disseminated intravascular coagulation resulting in death have been reported. Severe cardiovascular responses include rare cases of hypotensive shock, coronary insufficiency, cardiac arrhythmia, fibrillation and arrest. These severe reactions are usually reversible with prompt and appropriate management; however, fatalities have occurred.

Technique: extravasation with burning pain, hematomas, ecchymosis and tissue necrosis, paresthesia or numbness, vascular constriction due to injection rate, thrombosis and thrombophlebitis, perforation and dissection of blood vessels, dislodgement of atheromatous plaques, injury to neighboring organs.

Neurological: spasm, convulsions, aphasia, syncope, paresis, paralysis resulting from spinal cord injury and pathology associated with the syndrome of transverse myelitis, visual field losses which are usually transient, but may be permanent, coma and death.

Other: headache, trembling, shaking, chills without fever and lightheadedness. Temporary renal shutdown or other nephropathy.

(Adverse reactions to specific procedures receive comment under that procedure in the Dosage section.)

Treatment of Adverse Effects to Contrast Media: Contrast media should be administered only by physicians thoroughly familiar with the emergency treatment of all adverse reactions to contrast media. The assistance of other trained personnel such as cardiologists, internists and anesthetists is required in the management of severe reactions.

A guideline for the treatment of adverse reactions is presented below. This outline is not intended to be a complete manual on the treatment of adverse reactions to contrast media or on cardiopulmonary resuscitation. The physician should refer to the appropriate texts on the subject.

It is also realized that institutions or individual practitioners will already have appropriate systems in effect and that circumstances may dictate the use of additional or different measures.

Minor Allergic Reactions: (if considered necessary) The i.v. or i.m. administration of an antihistamine such as diphenhydramine HCl 25 to 50 mg is generally sufficient (contraindicated in epileptics). The resulting drowsiness makes it imperative to ensure that out-patients do not drive or go home unaccompanied.

Major or Life-threatening Reactions: A major reaction may be manifested by signs and symptoms of cardiovascular collapse, severe respiratory difficulty and nervous system dysfunction. Convulsions, coma and cardiorespiratory arrest may ensue.

The following measures should be considered: Start emergency therapy immediately—carefully monitoring vital signs. Have emergency resuscitation team summoned—do not leave patient unattended. Ensure patent airway—guard against aspiration. Commence artificial respiration if patient is not breathing. Administer oxygen if necessary. Start external cardiac massage in the event of cardiac arrest. Establish route for i.v. medication by starting infusion of appropriate solution (5% dextrose in water). Judiciously administer specific drug therapy as indicated by the type and severity of the reaction. Careful monitoring is mandatory to detect adverse reactions of all drugs administered: a) soluble hydrocortisone 500 to 1 000 mg i.v. for all acute allergic-anaphylactic reactions. b) epinephrine 1:1 000 solution (in the presence of anoxia it may cause ventricular fibrillation): i) 0.2 to 0.4 mL s.c. for severe allergic reactions. ii) in extreme emergency 0.1 mL/min, appropriately diluted, may be given i.v. until desired effect is obtained. Do not exceed 0.4 mL. iii) in case of cardiac arrest 0.1 to 0.2 mL appropriately diluted may be given intracardially. c) in hypotension (carefully monitoring blood pressure): i) phenylephrine HCl 0.1 to 0.5 mg appropriately diluted slowly i.v. or by slow infusion or ii) levarterenol bitartrate 4 mL of 0.2% solution in 1 000 mL of 5% dextrose by slow drip infusion. d) sodium bicarbonate 5%; 50 mL i.v. every 10 minutes as needed to combat post-arrest acidosis. e) Atropine 0.4 to 0.6 mg i.v. to increase heart rate in sinus bradycardia. May reverse 2nd or 3rd degree block. f) to control convulsions: i) pentobarbital sodium 50 mg in fractional doses slowly i.v. (contraindicated if cyanosis is present) or ii) Diazepam 5 to 10 mg slowly i.v. titrating the dose to the response of the patient. Defibrillation, administration of antiarrhythmics and additional emergency measures and drugs may be required. Transfer patient to intensive care unit when feasible for further monitoring and treatment.

OVERDOSE:

Symptoms: Overdosage may occur. The adverse effects of overdosage are life-threatening and affect mainly the pulmonary and cardiovascular system. The symptoms may include cyanosis, bradycardia, acidosis, pulmonary hemorrhage, convulsions, coma and cardiac arrest.

Treatment: Treatment of an overdose is directed toward the support of all vital functions and prompt institution of specific therapy. Iothalamate salts are dialyzable.

For management of a suspected drug overdose, CPhA recommends that you contact your **regional Poison Control Centre**. See the *CPS* Directory section for a list of Poison Control Centres.

DOSAGE: **I.V. Infusion Urography:** (Conray 30, Conray 43): I.V. infusion urography enhances the potential for more diagnostic information in those patients in whom the usual i.v. pyelography technique has not provided satisfactory visualization, or in those patients in whom there is reason to believe the usual i.v. pyelography technique will not provide satisfactory visualization. If renal function is not seriously impaired, the infusion urography technique usually provides satisfactory visualization of an unobstructed urinary tract, including nephrogram and cystogram. Additional advantages are the lack of necessity for dehydration of the patients and compression techniques.

Patient Preparation: For urography study, appropriate preparation of the patient is important for optimal visualization. A low residue diet is recommended on the day preceding the examination. Dehydration is not indicated for the performance of infusion urography. Patients should be maintained in an optimal state of hydration prior to the procedure. Unless contraindicated, a laxative may be given the evening before examination.

A preliminary radiograph usually is made prior to infusion of the contrast agent.

Precautions: A definite risk is involved in i.v. infusion urography in patients known to have chronic renal disease or multiple myeloma. This risk is not a contraindication to the procedure. However, partial dehydration in preparation of these patients is not recommended.

In addition to the general precautions previously described, infants and small children should not have any fluid restrictions prior to i.v. infusion urography. Injections of Conray represent an osmotic load which, if superimposed on increased serum osmolality due to partial dehydration, may magnify hypertonic dehydration. I.V. infusion urography in diabetic patients may involve increased risks and partial dehydration in these patients is not recommended (see also Precautions, General).

Patients with severely impaired renal function should be maintained in an appropriate state of hydration before the procedure. The increased osmotic load associated with i.v. infusion urography should be considered in patients with congestive heart failure.

Adverse Reactions: (see Adverse Effects, General).

Dosage: It is advisable that Conray be at or close to body temperature when infused.

Conray 30: The recommended dose for adults, older children and infants is 2 to 4 mL/kg with a maximum not exceeding 300 mL in adults and a proportionally smaller amount in children according to age and weight.

The solution is injected through an appropriate i.v. needle at a rate of approximately 50 mL/min. Any appropriate i.v. administration set may be used observing the usual precautions for maintaining sterility and safety in administration. Films are usually taken at 5-minute intervals following the initiation of the infusion for a total of 20 minutes.

In patients with impaired renal function, diagnostic opacification frequently is achieved only after prolonged periods. In these individuals, periodic film obtained up to 24 hours after infusion might yield useful information.

Special procedures such as nephrotomography and cystography are best accomplished within 30 minutes of the conclusion of the infusion.

Conray 43: The usual dose in adults and children is 2 to 3 mL/kg by i.v. administration, not to exceed a total dose of 200 mL in adults and a proportionally smaller amount in children according to age and weight.

The solution is infused at a rate of approximately 40 to 50 mL/min. Other infusion details are as for Conray 30.

Contrast Enhancement of Computed Tomographic (CT) Brain Imaging: Tumors: Conray may be useful to enhance the demonstration of the presence and extent of certain malignancies such as: gliomas including malignant gliomas, glioblastomas, astrocytomas, oligodendrogliomas and gangliomas; ependymomas, medulloblastomas; meningiomas; neuromas, pinealomas; pituitary adenomas; craniopharyngiomas; germinomas; and metastatic lesions.

The usefulness of contrast enhancement for the investigation of the retrobulbar space and in cases of low grade or infiltrative glioma has not been demonstrated.

Maximum contrast enhancement frequently occurs at a time following peak blood iodine concentration. This delay in maximum contrast enhancement can range from 5 to 40 minutes, depending on the peak blood iodine concentration achieved (total dose and rate of administration) and the cell type of the tumor.

In cases where lesions have calcified, there is less likelihood of enhancement. Following therapy, tumors may show decreased or no enhancement.

Non-neoplastic Conditions: The use of Conray may be beneficial in the image enhancement of non-neoplastic lesions. Cerebral infarctions of recent onset may be better visualized with the contrast enhancement while some infarctions are obscured if contrast media are used. The use of Conray resulted in contrast enhancement in 60% of cerebral infarctions studied from 1 to 4 weeks from the onset of symptoms.

Sites of active infection may also be enhanced following contrast medium administration.

Arteriovenous malformations and aneurysms usually show contrast enhancement. In the case of these vascular lesions, the enhancement is probably dependent on the iodine content of the circulating blood pool.

Hematomas and intraparenchymal bleeders seldom demonstrate any contrast enhancement. However, in case of intraparenchymal clot, for which there is no obvious clinical explanation, contrast medium administration may be helpful in ruling out the possibility of associated arteriovenous malformation.

The opacification of the inferior vermis following contrast medium administration has resulted in false positive diagnosis in a number of normal studies.

Patient Preparation: No special patient preparation is required for contrast enhancement of CT brain scanning. However, it is advisable to ensure that patients are well hydrated prior to examination.

Warning: Convulsions have occurred in patients with primary or metastatic cerebral lesions following the administration of iodine containing radiopaque media for the contrast enhancement of CT brain images.

Dosage: Conray 60: Usual Dose: Computed Tomography of the Brain: The recommended dose of Conray 60 for adults and children is 1 to 2 mL/kg of body weight, not exceeding 150 mL in adults and proportionally smaller amount in children according to age and weight. In most cases, scanning may be performed immediately after completion of administration; however when fast scanning equipment (less than 1 minute) is used consideration should be given to waiting approximately 5 minutes to allow for maximum contrast enhancement of the neoplasm (tumor).

Conray 43: Usual Dose: The usual dose in adults and children is 2 to 3 mL/kg by i.v. administration, not to exceed a total dose of 200 mL in adults and a proportionally smaller amount in children according to age and weight. In most cases, scanning may be performed immediately after completion of administration; however when fast scanning equipment (less than 1 minute) is used consideration should be given to waiting approximately 5 minutes to allow for maximum contrast enhancement.

Conray 30: Usual Dose: The recommended dose for adults and children is 2 to 4 mL/kg, not exceeding 300 mL in adults and proportionately smaller amount in children according to age and weight. The dose should be infused as rapidly as possible through any well vented i.v. administration set and needle, observing the usual precautions for maintaining sterility.

Cranial Computed Angiotomography: Conray 60 may be administered by i.v. bolus injection, or by bolus injection followed by rapid infusion.

For bolus injection, the usual dose in adults and children is 1 mL/kg at an injection rate of 2 mL/s with scanning begun immediately after administration.

This dose may be repeated as necessary. The total dose per procedure should not exceed 200 mL in adults and in children the total dose is reduced in approximate proportion to age and body weight.

In adults, when the rapid, high dose combination bolus and infusion technique is used, a 50 mL bolus injection followed by a rapid infusion of 150 mL may be given or a 100 mL bolus injection followed by a rapid infusion of 100 mL may be used. Scanning is begun immediately after the bolus administration. In children, the dose is reduced in approximate proportion to age and body weight.

Computed Tomography of the Body: Conray 60 may be administered when necessary to visualize vessels and organs in patients undergoing CT of the chest, abdomen and pelvis.

Because unenhanced scanning may provide adequate information in the individual patient, the decision to employ contrast enhancement, which may be associated with additional risk and increased radiation exposure, should be based upon a careful evaluation of clinical, other radiological and unenhanced CT findings.

Continuous or multiple scans separated by intervals of 1 to 3 seconds during the first 30 to 90 seconds postinjection of the contrast medium (dynamic CT scanning) provide enhancement of diagnostic significance. Subsets of patients in whom delayed body CT scans might be helpful have not been identified. Inconsistent results have been reported and abnormal and normal tissues are usually isodense during the time frame used for delayed CT scanning. The risks of such indiscriminate use of contrast media are well known and such use is not recommended. At present, consistent results have been documented using dynamic CT techniques only.

Precautions: In addition to the general precautions previously described, it should be noted that patient motion, including respiration, can markedly effect image quality, therefore, patient cooperation is essential. The use of an intravascular contrast medium can obscure tumors in patients undergoing CT evaluation of the liver resulting in a false negative diagnosis (see Pharmacology).

Patient Preparation: No special patient preparation is required for contrast enhancement in computerized tomography. However, it is advisable to insure that patients are well hydrated prior to examination.

In patients undergoing abdominal or pelvic examination, opacification of the bowel may be valuable in scan interpretation.

Usual Dosage: Conray 60 may be administered by bolus injection, by rapid infusion or by a combination of both.

For vascular opacification, a bolus injection of 25 to 50 mL may be used, repeated as necessary. When prolonged arterial or venous phase enhancement is required and for the enhancement of specific lesions, a rapid infusion of 150 mL may be used. In some instances, a 100 to 150 mL infusion may be employed to define the area of interest followed by bolus injections of 20 to 50 mL to clarify selected scans.

Excretory Urography: (Conray 60): Following i.v. injection, Conray is rapidly excreted by the kidneys. Conray may be visualized in the renal parenchyma 30 seconds following bolus injection. Maximum radiographic density of the calyces and pelves occurs in most instances about 3 to 8 minutes after injection. In patients with severe renal impairment, contrast visualization may be substantially delayed, or opacification may not occur at all.

Patient Preparation: Appropriate preparation of the patient is important for optimal visualization. A low residue diet is recommended for the day preceding the examination and a laxative is given the evening before the examination, unless contraindicated. A preliminary radiograph is usually made prior to the injection of the contrast agent.

Precautions: In addition to the general precautions previously described, infants and small children should not have any fluid restrictions prior to excretory urography. Injections of Conray represent an osmotic load which, if superimposed on increased serum osmolality due to partial dehydration, may magnify hypertonic dehydration. Therefore, patients' state of dehydration should be evaluated prior to and following this procedure and adjusted if necessary.

A definite risk is involved in excretory urography in patients known to have chronic renal disease, multiple myeloma or diabetes. This risk is not a contraindication to the procedure (see Warnings and Precautions, General Concerning Preparatory Dehydration).

Adverse Reactions: see Adverse Effects, General.

Usual Dosage: (Conray 60): Adults: The usual dose is 30 to 60 mL. Children 14 years of age and over, of average weight, may receive the adult dose.

The total dose is normally injected within 30 to 90 seconds. The higher dosage may be indicated to achieve optimum results in instances where poor visualization may be anticipated. When nephrograms and/or sequential urograms are desired, the total dose should be rapidly injected, normally within 15 to 30 seconds. The dosage for children is reduced in proportion to age and body weight. The following approximate schedule is recommended for infants and children based on a dosage of about 0.5 mL/kg of body weight: Under 6 months of age: 5 mL, 6 to 12 months: 8 mL, 1 to 2 years: 10 mL, 2 to 5 years: 12 mL, 5 to 8 years: 15 mL, 8 to 12 years: 18 mL, 12 to 14 years: 20 to 30 mL.

Cerebral Angiography: Conray 60 may be used to visualize the cerebral vasculature by any of the accepted techniques, including digital subtraction angiography.

Patient Preparation: Cerebral angiography is normally performed with local or general anesthesia (see Precautions, General). Premedication may be employed as indicated.

A preliminary radiograph is usually made prior to injection of the contrast agent.

Precautions: In addition to the general precautions previously described, cerebral angiography should be performed with special caution in patients with advanced arteriosclerosis, severe hypertension, cardiac decompensation, senility, recent cerebral thrombosis or embolism and migraine.

Adverse Reactions: In addition to the general adverse reactions previously described, the major sources of cerebral arteriographic adverse reactions appear to be related to repeated injections of the contrast material, administration of doses higher than those recommended, the presence of occlusive atherosclerotic vascular disease and the method and technique of injection.

Adverse reactions are normally mild and transient. A feeling of warmth in the face and neck is frequently experienced. Infrequently, a more severe burning discomfort is observed.

Serious neurological reactions that have been associated with cerebral angiography include stroke, amnesia, respiratory difficulties, hemiparesis, visual field loss, aphasia, convulsions, hypotension, bradycardia, coma and death.

Usual Dosage: The usual dosage employed varies with the site and method of injection and the age, condition and weight of the patient. In adults carotid and vertebral angiography, by either the percutaneous needle or catheter methods, is usually performed with a single rapid injection of 6 to 10 mL. Additional injections are made as indicated. Retrograde brachial cerebral angiography, in adults, is usually performed with a single rapid injection of 35 to 50 mL into the right brachial artery. Other dosages may be employed depending upon the vessel injected and the procedure followed. The dose for children is reduced in approximate proportion to age and body weight.

The use of an arterial digital subtraction technique allows the dose (concentration and/or volume) of the contrast material to be reduced by approximately 50% and permits less selective arterial catheterization.

Peripheral Arteriography and Venography: (Conray 60): Conray may be injected to visualize the arterial and venous peripheral circulation. Arteriograms of the upper and lower extremities may be obtained by any of the established techniques. Most frequently a percutaneous injection is made into the brachial artery in the arm or the femoral artery in the leg. Venograms are obtained by injection into an appropriate vein in the upper and lower extremity.

Patient Preparation: The procedure is normally performed with local or general anesthesia (see Precautions, General). Premedication may be employed as indicated. A preliminary radiograph is usually made prior to the injection of the contrast agent.

Precautions: In addition to the general precautions previously described, moderate decreases in blood pressure occur frequently with intra-arterial (brachial) injections. This change is usually transient and requires no treatment; however, the blood pressure should be monitored for approximately 10 minutes following injection. Special care is required when venography is performed in patients with suspected thrombosis, phlebitis, severe ischemic disease, local infection or a totally obstructed venous system. In the presence of venous stasis, vein irrigation with normal saline should be considered following the procedure.

Adverse Reactions: In addition to the general adverse reactions previously described, hemorrhage and thrombosis have occurred at the puncture site of the percutaneous injection.

Brachial plexus injury has been reported following axillary artery injection. Thrombophlebitis, syncope and very rare cases of gangrene have been reported following venography.

Usual Dosage: Peripheral Arteriography: In adults a single rapid injection of 20 to 40 mL is normally sufficient to visualize the entire extremity. The dose for children is reduced in proportion to body weight.

The use of an arterial digital subtraction technique allows the dose (concentration and/or volume) of the contrast material to be reduced by approximately 50% and permits less selective arterial catheterization.

Venography: The usual dose of Conray 60 for adults is a single rapid injection of 20 to 40 mL. The dose for children is reduced in proportion to body weight.

The usual dose of Conray 43 is 30 mL single dose up to a cumulative total dose of 125 mL per lower extremity, depending on the technique used. The dose for children is reduced in proportion to body weight. Following the procedure the venous system should be flushed with either 5% dextrose in water (D5W) or normal saline (Sodium Chloride Injection U.S.P.), or the contrast medium should be removed by leg massage and/or leg elevation.

Arthrography: (Conray 60): Precautions: In addition to the general precautions previously described, strict aseptic technique is required to prevent the introduction of infection. Fluoroscopic control should be used to ensure proper introduction of the needle into the synovial space and prevent extracapsular injection. Aspiration of excessive synovial fluid will reduce the pain on injection and prevent the rapid dilution of the contrast agent. It is important that undue pressures not be exerted during the injection.

Adverse Reactions: In addition to the general adverse reactions previously described, arthrography may induce joint pain or discomfort which is usually mild and transient but occasionally may be severe and persist for 24 to 48 hours following the procedure. Effusion requiring aspiration may occur in patients with rheumatoid arthritis.

Usual Dosage: Arthrography is usually performed under local anesthesia. The amount of contrast agent required is solely dependent on the size of the joint to be injected and the technique employed.

The following dosage schedule for normal adult joints should serve only as a guide since joints may require more or less contrast medium for optimal visualization. Dosage should be reduced for children in proportion to body weight. Knee, hip: 5 to 15 mL. Shoulder, ankle: 5 to 10 mL. Other: 1 to 4 mL.

Passive or active manipulation is used to disperse the medium throughout the joint space.

The lower volumes of contrast medium are usually employed for double contrast examinations. Following the injection of the contrast medium 50 to 100 mL of either filtered room air or carbon dioxide is introduced for examination of the knee and lesser volumes for other joints.

Direct Cholangiography: (Conray 60): Precautions: In addition to the general precautions previously described, percutaneous transhepatic cholangiography should only be attempted when compatible blood for potential transfusions is in readiness and emergency surgical facilities are available.

The patient should be carefully monitored for at least 24 hours to ensure prompt detection of bile leakage and hemorrhage. Appropriate premedication of the patient is recommended and drugs which are cholespastic, such as morphine, should be avoided. Respiratory movements should be controlled during introduction of the needle.

Adverse Reactions: In addition to the general adverse reactions previously described, adverse reactions may often be attributed to injection pressure or excessive volume of the medium resulting in overdistention of the ducts and producing local pain.

Some of the medium may enter the pancreatic duct which may result in pancreatic irritation. Occasionally, nausea, vomiting, fever, and tachycardia have been observed. Pancholangitis resulting in liver abscess or septicemia has been reported.

In percutaneous transhepatic cholangiography, some discomfort is common, but severe pain is unusual. Complications of the procedure are often serious and have been reported in 4 to 5% of patients. These reactions have included bile leakage and biliary peritonitis, gallbladder perforation, internal bleeding (sometimes massive), blood-bile fistula resulting in septicemia involving gram-negative organisms, and tension pneumothorax from inadvertent puncture of the diaphragm or lung. Bile leakage is more likely to occur in patients with obstructions that cause unrelieved high biliary pressure.

Dosage: It is advisable that Conray 60 be at or close to body temperature when injected. The injection is made slowly without undue pressure, taking the necessary precautions to avoid the introduction of bubbles.

Operative Cholangiography: The usual dose is 10 mL but as much as 25 mL may be needed depending upon the caliber of the ducts. If desired, the contrast agent may be diluted 1:1 with Sodium Chloride Injection U.S.P. using strict aseptic procedures. Following surgical exploration of the ductal system, repeat studies may be performed before closure of the abdomen, using the same dose as before.

Postoperative Cholangiography: Postoperatively, under fluoroscopic control, the ductal system may be examined by injection of the contrast agent through an in-place T-tube. These delayed cholangiograms are usually made from the fifth to the tenth postoperative day prior to removal of the T-tube. The usual dose is the same as for operative cholangiography.

Percutaneous Transhepatic Cholangiography: This procedure is recommended for carefully selected patients only for the diagnosis of jaundice in suspected extrahepatic biliary obstruction. The procedure is only employed where oral or i.v. cholangiography and other procedures have failed to provide the necessary information. In obstructed cases, percutaneous transhepatic cholangiography is used to determine the cause and site of obstruction to help plan surgery. The technique may also be of value in avoiding laparotomy in poor risk jaundice patients since failure to enter a duct by an experienced physician is considered to be suggestive evidence against obstructive jaundice. Careful attention to technique is essential for the success and safety of the procedure. The procedure is performed under fluoroscopic control; local anesthesia following analgesic premedication is usually employed.

Depending upon the caliber of the biliary tree, a dose of 10 to 40 mL is generally sufficient to opacify the entire ductal system. If desired, the contrast agent may be diluted 1:1 with Sodium Chloride Injection U.S.P. using strict aseptic procedures.

As the needle is advanced or withdrawn, a bile duct may be located by frequent aspiration for bile or mucus. Before the dose is administered, as much bile as possible is aspirated. The injection may be repeated for exposures in different planes and repositioning of the patient, if necessary, should be done with care. If a duct is not readily located by aspiration, successive small doses of 1 to 2 mL of the medium are injected into the liver as the needle is gradually withdrawn, until a duct is visualized by X-ray. If no duct can be located after 3 or 4 attempts, the procedure should be terminated. Inability to enter a duct by a person experienced in the technique is generally considered to be suggestive evidence against obstructive disease.

Endoscopic Retrograde Cholangiopancreatography: (Conray 60): Endoscopic retrograde cholangiopancreatography (ERCP) is indicated in carefully selected patients with known or suspected pancreatic or biliary tract disease when other diagnostic procedures have failed to provide the necessary diagnostic information. Prior to the development of ERCP, X-ray examination of the pancreatic ducts could only be obtained at laparotomy.

Precautions: In addition to the general precautions previously described, endoscopic retrograde cholangiopancreatography should only be performed by personnel skilled and experienced with the procedure, and careful attention to technique is essential for the success and safety of the procedure. Fluoroscopy is mandatory during injection to prevent over distention of the duct systems.

Filling of the pancreatic parenchyma must be avoided. Retrograde injection of contrast media beyond a significant stenosis or obstruction is not recommended, since this is considered to increase the risk of ascending infection. ERCP should not be performed in patients with a positive test for Hepatitis Associated Antigen, since fiberscopes cannot be sterilized and there is a real possibility of transmitting viral hepatitis to successive patients.

Adverse Reactions: In addition to the general adverse reactions previously described, adverse reactions that have occurred and attributable to either the procedure or contrast agent include nausea, vomiting, fever, severe abdominal pain, duodenal wall intravasation, septicemia, pancreatitis, and perforation of the common bile duct associated with pathology. Frequently, elevation of serum amylase is observed following an ERCP procedure.

Dosage: The procedure is usually performed following pharyngeal anesthesia and analgesic or sedative premedication. Duodenal motility may be controlled in patients with active duodenal peristalsis with an appropriate antiperistaltic agent.

The contrast medium should be injected slowly without undue pressure under fluoroscopic control employing the minimal dose that is adequate to visualize the common bile duct, the pancreatic duct, or both duct systems. When both systems are filled simultaneously, overfilling of the pancreas is a potential risk. The dosage will vary greatly depending on the pathological findings and can range from 10 to 40 mL for visualization of the common bile duct, and from 2 to 10 mL for visualization of the pancreatic duct. Following the procedure, the patient should be kept under close observation for 24 hours.

Intravenous Digital Subtraction Angiography: (Conray 60): I.V. digital subtraction angiography (IV DSA) is a radiographic modality which allows dynamic imaging of the arterial system following i.v. injection of iodinated X-ray contrast media through the use of image intensification, enhancement of the iodine signal and digital processing of the image data. Temporal subtraction of the images obtained during the "first arterial pass" of the injected contrast medium injection yield images which are devoid of bone and soft tissue.

Areas that have been examined by i.v. DSA are the heart, including coronary by-pass grafts; the pulmonary arteries; the arteries of the brachiophalic circulation; the aortic arch; the abdominal aorta and its major branches including the celiac, mesenterics and renal arteries; the iliac arteries; and the arteries of the extremities.

Patient Preparation: No special patient preparation is required for i.v. digital subtraction angiography. However, it is advisable to ensure that patients are well hydrated prior to examination.

Warnings: Convulsions have occurred in patients with primary or metastatic cerebral lesions following the administration of iodine containing radiopaque media for the contrast enhancement of CT brain images.

Patients with diabetes mellitus and impaired renal function are considered to be at greater risk to develop acute renal failure following the injection of large doses of contrast media for contrast enhancement in CT scanning.

Precautions: In addition to the general precautions previously described, the risks associated with IV DSA are those usually attendant with catheter procedures and include intramural injections, vessel dissection or rupture and tissue extravasation. Small test injections of contrast medium made under fluoroscopic observation to ensure the catheter tip is properly positioned, and in the case of peripheral placement that the vein is of adequate size, will reduce the potential for intramural injections, vessel dissection or tissue extravasation occurring.

Patient motion, including respiration and swallowing, can result in marked image degradation yielding nondiagnostic studies. Therefore, patient cooperation is essential.

Adverse Reactions: see section on Adverse Effects, General.

Usual Dosage: Conray 60 may be injected either centrally, into the superior or inferior vena cava, or peripherally into an appropriate arm vein. For central injections, catheters may be introduced at the antecubital fossa into either the basilic or cephalic vein or at the leg into the femoral vein and advanced to the distal segment of the corresponding vena cava. For peripheral injections, the catheter is introduced at the antecubital fossa into an appropriate size arm vein. In order to reduce the potential for extravasation during peripheral injection, a catheter of approximately 20 cm in length should be employed.

Depending on the area to be imaged, the usual adult dose range is 20 to 60 mL. Injections may be repeated as necessary.

Central catheter injections are usually made with a power injection rate of between 10 and 30 mL/s. When making peripheral injections, rates of 12 to 20 mL/s should be used, depending on the size of the vein. Also, since contrast medium may remain in the arm vein for an extended period following injection, it may be advisable to flush the vein, immediately following injection, with an appropriate volume (20 to 25 mL) or 5% Dextrose in water or normal saline.

Administration: It is advisable that sterile Conray product in vials, bottles or in Ultraject syringes be at or close to body temperature when infused.

SUPPLIED: Conray 30: Each mL of sterile aqueous solution contains: iothalamate meglumine 300 mg (organically bound iodine 14.15%-141 mg/mL). Nonmedicinal ingredients: edetate calcium disodium and monobasic sodium phosphate. Conray 30 has an osmolarity of approximately 750 mOsm/L (0.75 mOsm/mL) and is, therefore, hypertonic under conditions of use and is supplied in containers from which the air has been displaced by nitrogen. Bottles of 150 mL containing 100 mL (partial fill), boxes of 12. Bottles of 150 mL, boxes of 12. Infusion bottles of 300 mL, packages of 12.

Conray 43: Each mL of sterile aqueous solution contains: iothalamate meglumine 430 mg (organically bound iodine 20.2%-202 mg/mL). Nonmedicinal ingredients: edetate calcium disodium and monobasic sodium phosphate. Conray 43 has an osmolarity of approximately 800 mOsm/L (0.80 mOsm/mL) and is, therefore, hypertonic under conditions of use and is supplied in containers from which the air has been displaced by nitrogen. Conray 43 has a specific gravity of 1,22 at 25°C and a viscosity of 3 cps at 25°C and 2 cps at 37°C. Vials of 50 mL, packages of 50. Bottles of 150 mL containing 100 mL (partial fill), boxes of 12. Bottles of 200 mL and 250 mL, packages of 12.

Conray 60: Each mL of sterile aqueous solution contains: iothalamate meglumine 600 mg (organically bound iodine 28.2%-282 mg/mL). Nonmedicinal ingredients: edetate calcium disodium and monobasic sodium phosphate. Conray 60 has an osmolarity of approximately 1 000 mOsm/L (1.0 mOsm/mL) and is, therefore, hypertonic under conditions of use and is supplied in containers from which the air has been displaced by nitrogen. Conray 60 has a specific gravity of 1,32 at 25°C and a viscosity of 6 cps at 25°C and 4 cps at 37°C. Vials of 20, 30 and 50 mL, packages of 50. Bottles of 150 and 200 mL, packages of 12. Bottles of 150 mL containing 100 mL (partial fill), packages of 12. Ultraject prefilled syringes of 50 mL (hand held), boxes of 20.

Store between 15 and 30°C. Protect from light. Protect from freezing. Crystallization does not occur at normal room temperatures. Discard unused portion.

CO Olanzapine ℞

olanzapine

Antipsychotic

Cobalt

SUPPLIED: 2.5 mg: Each white to off-white, film-coated, round, biconvex tablet with "ON" on one side and "Σ" on the other side, contains: olanzapine 2.5 mg. Nonmedicinal ingredients: crospovidone, hydroxypropyl cellulose, lactose monohydrate, low substituted hydroxypropyl cellulose, magnesium stearate and microcrystalline cellulose; film coating: lecithin, polyvinyl alcohol, talc, titanium dioxide and xanthan gum. HDPE bottles of 100 and 500. Store between 15-30°C. Protect from light and moisture.

5 mg: Each white to off-white, film-coated, round, biconvex tablet with "ON/5" on one side and "Σ" on the other side, contains: olanzapine 5 mg. Nonmedicinal ingredients: crospovidone, hydroxypropyl cellulose, lactose monohydrate, low substituted hydroxypropyl cellulose, magnesium stearate and microcrystalline cellulose; film coating: lecithin, polyvinyl alcohol, talc, titanium dioxide and xanthan gum. HDPE bottles of 100 and 500. Store between 15-30°C. Protect from light and moisture.

7.5 mg: Each white to off-white, film-coated, round, biconvex tablet with "ON/7.5" on one side and "Σ" on the other side, contains: olanzapine 7.5 mg. Nonmedicinal ingredients: crospovidone, hydroxypropyl cellulose, lactose monohydrate, low substituted hydroxypropyl cellulose, magnesium stearate and microcrystalline cellulose; film coating: lecithin, polyvinyl alcohol, talc, titanium dioxide and xanthan gum. HDPE bottles of 100 and 500. Store between 15-30°C. Protect from light and moisture.

10 mg: Each white to off-white, film-coated, round, biconvex tablet with "ON/10" on one side and "Σ" on the other side, contains: olanzapine 10 mg. Nonmedicinal ingredients: crospovidone, hydroxypropyl cellulose, lactose monohydrate, low substituted hydroxypropyl cellulose, magnesium stearate and microcrystalline cellulose; film coating: lecithin, polyvinyl alcohol, talc, titanium dioxide and xanthan gum. HDPE bottles of 100 and 500. Store between 15-30°C. Protect from light and moisture.

15 mg: Each blue, film-coated, oval-shaped, biconvex tablet with "ON15" on one side and "Σ" on the other side, contains: olanzapine 15 mg. Nonmedicinal ingredients: crospovidone, hydroxypropyl cellulose, lactose monohydrate, low substituted hydroxypropyl cellulose, magnesium stearate and microcrystalline cellulose; film coating: FD&C Blue #2, FD&C Red #40, FD&C Yellow #6, lecithin, polyvinyl alcohol, talc, titanium dioxide and xanthan gum. HDPE bottles of 100 and 500. Store between 15-30°C. Protect from light and moisture.

20 mg: Each pink, film-coated, oval-shaped, biconvex tablet with "ON20" on one side and "Σ" on the other side, contains: olanzapine 20 mg. Nonmedicinal ingredients: crospovidone, hydroxypropyl cellulose, lactose monohydrate, low substituted hydroxypropyl cellulose, magnesium stearate and microcrystalline cellulose; film coating: FD&C Blue #2, FD&C Red #40, FD&C Yellow #6, lecithin, polyvinyl alcohol, talc, titanium dioxide and xanthan gum. HDPE bottles of 100 and 500. Store between 15-30°C. Protect from light and moisture.

CO Olanzapine ODT ℞

olanzapine

Antipsychotic

Cobalt

SUPPLIED: 5 mg: Each yellow, round, flat faced bevel edged tablet, with '01' on one side and "Σ" on the other side, contains: olanzapine 5 mg. Nonmedicinal ingredients: aspartame, colloidal anhydrous silica, crospovidone, mannitol, sodium stearyl fumarate and sorbitol crystalline. Unit dose blister cartons of 30. Store between 15-30°C. Protect from light and moisture.

10 mg: Each yellow, round, flat faced bevel edged tablet, with '02' on one side and "Σ" on the other side, contains: olanzapine 10 mg. Nonmedicinal ingredients: aspartame, colloidal anhydrous silica, crospovidone, mannitol, sodium stearyl fumarate and sorbitol crystalline. Unit dose blister cartons of 30. Store between 15-30°C. Protect from light and moisture.

15 mg: Each yellow, round, flat faced bevel edged tablet, with '03' on one side and "Σ" on the other side, contains: olanzapine 15 mg. Nonmedicinal ingredients: aspartame, colloidal anhydrous silica, crospovidone, mannitol, sodium stearyl fumarate and sorbitol crystalline. Unit dose blister cartons of 30. Store between 15-30°C. Protect from light and moisture.

20 mg: Each yellow, round, flat faced bevel edged tablet, with '04' on one side and "Σ" on the other side, contains: olanzapine 20 mg. Nonmedicinal ingredients: aspartame, colloidal anhydrous silica, crospovidone, mannitol, sodium stearyl fumarate and sorbitol crystalline. Unit dose blister cartons of 30. Store between 15-30°C. Protect from light and moisture.

CO Ondansetron ℞

ondansetron HCl dihydrate

Antiemetic

Cobalt

SUPPLIED: 4 mg: Each yellow, film-coated, oval, biconvex tablet, with "OD4" and "Σ" on the other side, contains: ondansetron 4 mg (as ondansetron hydrochloride dihydrate). Nonmedicinal ingredients: corn starch, lactose monohydrate, magnesium stearate and microcrystalline cellulose; film-coating: hypromellose, iron oxide yellow, polyethylene glycol and titanium dioxide. Unit dose blister cartons of 10 tablets. Store at room temperature (15-30°C).

8 mg: Each yellow, film-coated, oval, biconvex tablet, with "OD8" and "Σ" on the other side, contains: ondansetron 8 mg (as ondansetron hydrochloride dihydrate). Nonmedicinal ingredients: corn starch, lactose monohydrate, magnesium stearate and microcrystalline cellulose; film-coating: hypromellose, iron oxide yellow, polyethylene glycol and titanium dioxide. Unit dose blister cartons of 10 tablets. Store at room temperature (15-30°C).

CO Pantoprazole ℞

pantoprazole sodium

H+, K+-ATPase Inhibitor

Cobalt

SUPPLIED: Each yellow, round, biconvex, enteric-coated tablet, printed with "PA 784" in black on one side, contains: pantoprazole sodium 40 mg. Nonmedicinal ingredients: colloidal anhydrous silica, crospovidone, hydroxypropylmethyl-cellulose, magnesium stearate, mannitol, sodium lauryl sulphate and talc; coatings: glycerol monostearate, iron oxide yellow, lecithin (soya), methacrylic acid–ethyl acrylate copolymer, polysorbate 80, polyvinyl alcohol–partially hydrolysed, titanium dioxide, talc, triethyl citrate, quinoline yellow aluminum lake and xanthan gum. Bottles of 100. Keep at room temperature (15 to 30°C).

The reader is invited to consult CPhA's monograph **Selective Serotonin Reuptake Inhibitors**.

CO Paroxetine ℞

paroxetine

Antidepressant—Antiobsessional—Antipanic—Anxiolytic Agent—Social Phobia (Social Anxiety Disorder) Therapy—Post-traumatic Stress Disorder Therapy

Cobalt

SUPPLIED: 10 mg: Each yellow, film-coated, oval, biconvex tablet, with "PX 10" on one side and "Σ" on the other side, contains: paroxetine 10 mg. Nonmedicinal ingredients: magnesium stearate, mannitol, microcrystalline cellulose and sodium starch glycolate; film-coating: basic butylated methacrylate copolymer, lecithin, polyvinyl alcohol-partially hydrolyzed, talc, titanium dioxide, xanthan gum, and one or more of the following coloring components: FD&C blue #2, FD&C red #30, iron oxide red and iron oxide yellow. Gluten-free. Bottles of 100. Store at 15-30°C.

20 mg: Each pink, film-coated, oval, biconvex tablet, with "PX" scoreline "20" on one side and "Σ" on the other side, contains: paroxetine 20 mg. Nonmedicinal ingredients: magnesium stearate, mannitol, microcrystalline cellulose and sodium starch glycolate; film-coating: basic butylated methacrylate copolymer, lecithin, polyvinyl alcohol-partially hydrolyzed, talc, titanium dioxide, xanthan gum, and one or more of the following coloring components: FD&C blue #2, FD&C red #30, iron oxide red and iron oxide yellow. Gluten-free. HDPE bottles of 30, 100 and 500. Store at 15-30°C.

30 mg: Each blue, film-coated, oval, biconvex tablet, with "PX30" on one side and "Σ" on the other side, contains: paroxetine 30 mg. Nonmedicinal ingredients: magnesium stearate, mannitol, microcrystalline cellulose and sodium starch glycolate; film-coating: basic butylated methacrylate copolymer, lecithin, polyvinyl alcohol-partially hydrolyzed, talc, titanium dioxide, xanthan gum, and one or more of the following coloring components: FD&C blue #2, FD&C red #30, iron oxide red and iron oxide yellow. Gluten-free. HDPE bottles of 30 and 100. Store at 15-30°C.

Copaxone® ℞

glatiramer acetate

Immunomodulator

Teva Canada Innovation

Date of Preparation: August 28, 1997
Date of Revision: April 2, 2010

SUMMARY PRODUCT INFORMATION:

Route of Administration	Dosage Form/Strength	Nonmedicinal Ingredients
SC	20 mg/1 mL Pre-filled syringes and lyophilized vials	40 mg mannitol in sterile water for injection

INDICATIONS AND CLINICAL USE: COPAXONE is indicated for:

- Treatment of ambulatory patients with Relapsing Remitting Multiple Sclerosis (RRMS)
  - To decrease the frequency of clinical exacerbations
  - To reduce the number and volume of active brain lesions identified on Magnetic Resonance Imaging (MRI) scans.
- Treatment of patients who have experienced a single demyelinating event, accompanied by abnormal MRI scans and are considered to be at risk of developing Clinically Definite MS (CDMS), after alternative diagnoses are excluded:
  - To delay the onset of definite MS;
  - To decrease the number and volume of active brain lesions and overall disease burden (as identified by MRI scans).

The safety and efficacy of COPAXONE in chronic progressive MS have not been established.

Geriatrics (>65 years of age): COPAXONE has not been studied in the elderly (>65 years old).

Pediatrics (<18 years of age): The safety and effectiveness of COPAXONE have not been established in individuals below 18 years of age.

CONTRAINDICATIONS:

- COPAXONE (glatiramer acetate) is contraindicated in patients with known hypersensitivity to glatiramer acetate or mannitol.

WARNINGS AND PRECAUTIONS: The only recommended route of administration of COPAXONE (glatiramer acetate) injection is the subcutaneous route. COPAXONE should not be administered by the intravenous route.

Cardiovascular: Symptoms of Potentially Cardiac Origin: Approximately 13% of COPAXONE patients in the multicenter controlled trials (compared to 5% of placebo patients) experienced at least one episode of what was described as transient chest pain (see Adverse Reactions, Adverse Drug Reaction Overview, Chest Pain). While some of these episodes occurred in the context of the Immediate Post-Injection Reaction (see Adverse Reactions, Adverse Drug Reaction Overview, Immediate Post-Injection Reaction), many did not. The pathogenesis of this symptom is unknown. Patients in controlled clinical trials were free of significant cardiovascular problems (New York Heart Association Class I and II) and thus the risks associated with COPAXONE treatment for Multiple Sclerosis patients with comorbid cardiovascular disease are unknown.

COPAXONE has been associated with an Immediate Post-Injection Reaction consisting of a constellation of symptoms appearing immediately after injection that could include flushing, chest pain, palpitations, anxiety, dyspnea, constriction of the throat and urticaria (see Adverse Reactions, Adverse Drug Reaction Overview, Immediate Post-Injection Reaction).

COPAXONE has not been studied in patients with a history of severe anaphylactoid reactions, obstructive pulmonary disease or asthma, nor in patients under treatment for either of these two latter conditions. Particular caution is therefore advised regarding the use of COPAXONE in such patients.

Anaphylactoid reactions associated with the use of COPAXONE have been reported in rare instances (<1/1000) during the post-marketing period. Some cases required treatment with epinephrine and other appropriate medical treatment.

General: Patients should be instructed in self-injection techniques to assure the safe administration of COPAXONE (glatiramer acetate), including a careful review (see Information for the Patient). The first injection should be performed under the supervision of an appropriately qualified health care professional. Patient understanding and use of aseptic self-injection techniques and procedures should be periodically re-evaluated. Patients should be cautioned against the re-use of needles or syringes and instructed in safe disposal procedures. A puncture-resistant container for disposal of used needles and syringes should be used by the patient. Patients should be instructed on the safe disposal of full containers.

Localized Adverse Reactions Associated with Subcutaneous Use: At injection sites, localized lipoatrophy and, rarely, injection site skin necrosis have been reported during clinical trials and postmarketing experience. Lipoatrophy may occur after treatment onset (sometimes as early as several months) and may be permanent. There is no known therapy for lipoatrophy. To assist in possibly minimizing these events the patient should be advised to follow proper injection technique and to rotate injection areas and sites on a daily basis (see Information for the Patient).

Immune: Considerations Involving the Use of a Product Capable of Modifying Immune Responses: COPAXONE is an antigenic substance and thus it is possible that detrimental host responses can occur with its use. Whether COPAXONE can alter normal human immune responses, such as the recognition of foreign antigens is unknown. It is therefore possible that treatment with COPAXONE may undermine the body's defenses against infections and tumor surveillance. Systematic assessments of these risks have not been done. Continued alteration of cellular immunity due to chronic treatment with glatiramer acetate might result in untoward effects.

Glatiramer acetate-reactive antibodies are formed in practically all patients exposed to daily treatment with the recommended dose. Studies in both the rat and monkey have suggested that immune complexes are deposited in the renal glomeruli. Furthermore, in a controlled clinical trial of 125 RRMS patients given glatiramer acetate 20 mg for 2 years, serum IgG levels reached at least 3 times baseline values in 80% of patients by 3 months of initiation of treatment. By 12 months of treatment, however, 30% of patients still had IgG levels at least 3 times baseline values, and 90% had levels above baseline by 12 months. The antibodies are exclusively of the IgG subtype—and predominantly of the IgG-1 subtype. No IgE type antibodies could be detected in any of the 94 sera tested.

Nevertheless, anaphylaxis can be associated with the administration of almost any foreign substance and, therefore, this risk cannot be excluded.

Carcinogenesis and Mutagenesis: Preclinical studies to assess the carcinogenic potential of glatiramer acetate in mice and rats do not suggest any evidence of carcinogenic potential related to glatiramer acetate administered subcutaneously at dose levels of up to 30 mg/kg/day in rats and 60 mg/kg/day in mice. The relevance of these findings for humans is unknown (see Warnings and Precautions, Immune, Considerations Involving the Use of a Product Capable of Modifying Immune Responses).

Renal: The pharmacokinetics of COPAXONE in patients with impaired renal function have not been determined.

Special Populations: Pregnant Women: There are no adequate and well-controlled studies in pregnant women. No evidence of reproductive toxicity was observed in preclinical studies. Because animal reproduction studies are not always predictive of human response, this drug should be used during pregnancy only if clearly needed. During pre- marketing clinical trials with COPAXONE, seven women conceived while being treated with the active drug. One case was lost to follow-up. Three of the patients electively discontinued pregnancy. Three patients stopped treatment 1, 1.5 and 2 months after learning they were pregnant; all delivered healthy babies.

Nursing Women: It is not known whether this drug is excreted in human milk. Because many drugs are excreted in human milk, treating a nursing woman with COPAXONE should only be considered after careful risk/benefit assessment and be used with caution.

Pediatrics (<18 years of age): The safety and effectiveness of COPAXONE have not been established in individuals below 18 years of age.

Geriatrics (>65 years of age): COPAXONE has not been studied in the elderly (>65 years old).

Monitoring and Laboratory Tests: Data collected pre- and post-market do not suggest the need for routine laboratory monitoring.

ADVERSE REACTIONS: Adverse Drug Reaction Overview: In the 4 placebo-controlled clinical trials, the most commonly observed adverse events associated with the use of COPAXONE occurring at an incidence of at least 10% and at least 1.5 times higher than in placebo treated patients were: injection site reactions, vasodilatation, rash, dyspnea and chest pain.

In the placebo-controlled clinical trials approximately 5% discontinued treatment due to an adverse event compared to 1% for placebo treated patients. The adverse events most commonly associated with discontinuation were (in order of descending frequency): injection site reactions, dyspnea, urticaria, vasodilatation and hypersensitivity. Treatment discontinuation due to a serious adverse event considered by investigators to be related to COPAXONE treatment included a case of life-threatening serum sickness.

Immediate Post-Injection Reaction: Approximately 14% of Multiple Sclerosis patients exposed to COPAXONE in the 4 placebo-controlled studies reported a post-injection reaction immediately following subcutaneous injection of COPAXONE compared to 2% for placebo treated patients. An immediate post-injection reaction is a constellation of symptoms occurring immediately after injection that includes at least two of the following: flushing, chest pain, palpitations, anxiety, dyspnea, constriction of the throat and urticaria (individual symptoms are listed separately in Table 1). These symptoms were invariably transient, self-limited, did not require specific treatment and in general, arose several months after initiation of treatment, although they may occur earlier in the course of treatment. A given patient may experience one or several episodes of these symptoms during treatment with COPAXONE. Whether these episodes are mediated by an immunologic or non-immunologic mechanism, and whether several similar episodes seen in a given patient have identical mechanisms is unknown. In fact, whether or not this constellation of symptoms actually represents a specific syndrome is unknown. During the post-marketing period, there have been reports of patients with similar symptoms who received emergency medical care (see Warnings and Precautions, Cardiovascular, Symptoms of Potentially Cardiac Origin).

Chest Pain: Approximately 13% of glatiramer acetate patients in the 4 placebo-controlled studies (compared to 5% of placebo patients) experienced at least one episode of what was described as transient chest pain. While some of these episodes occurred in the context of the Immediate Post-Injection Reaction described above, many did not. The temporal relationship of the chest pain to an injection of glatiramer acetate was not always known, although the pain was transient (usually lasting only a few minutes), often unassociated with other symptoms, and appeared to have no important clinical sequelae. Some patients experienced more than one such episode, and episodes usually began at least 1 month after the initiation of treatment. The pathogenesis of this symptom is unknown. Patients in clinical trials were free of significant cardiovascular disease (New York Heart Association Class I or II); therefore, the risks associated with glatiramer acetate treatment for Multiple Sclerosis patients with comorbid cardiovascular disease are unknown (see Warnings and Precautions, Cardiovascular, Symptoms of Potentially Cardiac Origin).

Clinical Trial Adverse Drug Reactions: Because clinical trials are conducted under very specific conditions the adverse reaction rates observed in the clinical trials may not reflect the rates observed in practice and should not be compared to the rates in the clinical trials of another drug. Adverse drug reaction information from clinical trials is useful for identifying drug-related adverse events and for approximating rates.

The adverse reaction data in this section is derived from 4 pivotal, double-blind, placebo-controlled clinical trials which were conducted during premarketing and postmarketing periods in a total of 512 patients treated with glatiramer acetate and 509 patients treated with placebo for up to 36 months. Three trials were conducted in RRMS. The fourth trial was in patients presenting with a first clinical event and MRI features suggestive of MS and included 243 patients treated with glatiramer acetate and 238 patients treated with placebo.

All adverse events were recorded by the clinical investigators, using terminology of their own choosing. To provide a meaningful estimate of the proportion of individuals having adverse events, similar types of events were grouped into standardized categories using MedDRA dictionary terminology.

Table 1 lists treatment-emergent signs and symptoms that occurred in at least 2% of patients treated with glatiramer acetate in the placebo-controlled trials. These signs and symptoms were numerically more common in patients treated with glatiramer acetate than in patients treated with placebo.

Table 1: COPAXONE

Controlled Trials: Incidence of Glatiramer Acetate Adverse Reactions ≥2% and More Frequent than Placebo

MedDRA Version 10.0		GA 20 mg (N=512) % of Patients	Placebo (N=509) % of Patients
Blood and Lymphatic System Disorders	Lymphadenopathy	7.2	2.9
Cardiac Disorders	Palpitations	7.6	3.3
	Tachycardia	4.7	1.6
Eye Disorders	Eye Disorder	3.3	1.2
	Diplopia	2.9	1.8
Gastrointestinal Disorders	Nausea	14.5	10.4
	Vomiting	7.4	4.3
	Constipation	7.0	6.3
	Dyspepsia	6.6	6.5
	Dysphagia	2.3	1.2
	Faecal Incontinence	2.3	2.0

(cont'd)

Table 1: COPAXONE *(cont'd)*

Controlled Trials: Incidence of Glatiramer Acetate Adverse Reactions ≥2% and More Frequent than Placebo

MedDRA Version 10.0		GA 20 mg (N=512) % of Patients	Placebo (N=509) % of Patients
General Disorders and Administration Site Conditions	Injection Site Erythema	46.1	10.6
	Injection Site Pain	36.3	17.1
	Injection Site Mass	25.8	5.9
	Injection Site Pruritus	24.4	2.8
	Asthenia	23.8	23.2
	Injection Site Edema	20.9	4.5
	Pain	18.9	16.7
	Chest Pain	12.5	4.9
	Injection Site Inflammation	8.2	1.6
	Injection Site Reaction	8.2	1.4
	Pyrexia	6.4	5.7
	Injection Site Hypersensitivity	4.1	0.0
	Local Reaction	3.7	1.4
	Face Edema	3.3	0.6
	Edema Peripheral	3.3	2.4
	Chills	2.9	0.4
	Injection Site Atrophy[a]	2.0	0.0
	Injection Site Fibrosis	2.0	0.6
Immune System Disorders	Hypersensitivity	3.3	1.8
Infections and Infestations	Infection	31.8	30.8
	Influenza	15.4	14.5
	Rhinitis	7.4	5.9
	Bronchitis	6.4	5.7
	Gastroenteritis	6.3	4.3
	Vaginal Candidiasis	4.9	2.6
	Otitis Media	3.7	2.9
	Herpes Simplex	2.5	1.8
	Tooth Abscess	2.3	2.2
Metabolism and Nutrition Disorders	Weight Increased	2.9	0.8
	Anorexia	2.3	2.2
Musculoskeletal and Connective Tissue Disorders	Back Pain	13.5	11.2
	Arthralgia	10.4	9.4
	Neck Pain	4.5	3.9
Nervous System Disorders	Headache	30.9	29.1
	Hypertonia	7.8	7.3
	Tremor	4.1	1.8
	Migraine	3.7	2.4
	Syncope	3.1	1.8
Psychiatric Disorders	Depression	13.1	12.0
	Anxiety	11.1	8.8
	Nervousness	2.3	1.0
Renal and Urinary Disorders	Micturition Urgency	5.1	4.3
	Pollakiuria	4.7	4.5
Respiratory, Thoracic and Mediastinal Disorders	Dyspnoea	13.3	2.8
	Cough	6.6	5.3

(cont'd)

Table 1: COPAXONE *(cont'd)*

Controlled Trials: Incidence of Glatiramer Acetate Adverse Reactions ≥2% and More Frequent than Placebo

MedDRA Version 10.0		GA 20 mg (N=512) % of Patients	Placebo (N=509) % of Patients
Skin and Subcutaneous Tissue Disorders	Rash	13.7	9.0
	Hyperhidrosis	6.6	4.7
	Pruritus	5.1	4.3
	Ecchymosis	3.5	3.3
	Urticaria	3.1	1.6
	Skin Disorder	2.9	0.8
Vascular Disorders	Vasodilatation	18.0	4.7

[a] "Injection site atrophy" comprises terms relating to localized lipoatrophy at injection site.

Data on adverse events occurring in the controlled clinical trials were analyzed to evaluate gender related differences. No clinically significant differences were identified. In these clinical trials 96% of patients were Caucasian. This percentage reflects the higher representation of Caucasian in the MS population, even though it does not reflect the exact world racial distribution among MS patients. In addition, the vast majority of patients treated with COPAXONE were between the ages of 18 and 45. Consequently, inadequate data are available to perform an analysis of the incidence of adverse events related to clinically relevant age subgroups.

Laboratory analyses were performed on all patients participating in the clinical program for COPAXONE. Clinically significant changes in laboratory values for hematology, chemistry, and urinalysis were similar for both COPAXONE and placebo groups in blinded clinical trials. No patient receiving COPAXONE withdrew from any placebo-controlled trial due to abnormal laboratory findings which were assessed as possibly related to glatiramer acetate.

Other Adverse Events Observed During All Clinical Trials: In the pre- marketing clinical trials, approximately 900 individuals have received at least one dose of COPAXONE (glatiramer acetate) in controlled and uncontrolled clinical trials. Total patient exposure to COPAXONE in clinical trials ranged from 6 months (693 patients) to 2 years (306 patients), with a subset of patients continuing to 10 years (n=108) and some patients to an average of 13.6 years (n=100) in open-label extensions at a daily dose of 20 mg.

During these trials, all adverse events were recorded by clinical investigators using terminology of their own choosing. To provide a meaningful estimate of the proportion of individuals having adverse events, similar types of events were grouped into a smaller number of standardized categories using COSTART II dictionary terminology. All reported events that occurred at least twice and potentially important events occurring once, are included except those already listed in the previous table, those too general to be informative, trivial events, and other events which occurred in at least 2% of treated patients and were present at equal or greater rates in the placebo group.

Events are further classified within body system categories and enumerated in order of decreasing frequency using the following definitions: **Frequent** adverse events are defined as those occurring in at least 1/100 patients; **infrequent** adverse events are those occurring in 1/100 to 1/1000 patients.

Body as a Whole: Frequent: injection site edema, injection site atrophy, abscess and injection site hypersensitivity. Infrequent: injection site hematoma, injection site fibrosis, moon face, cellulitis, generalized edema, hernia, injection site abscess, serum sickness, suicide attempt, injection site hypertrophy, injection site melanosis, lipoma, and photosensitivity reaction.

Cardiovascular: Frequent: hypertension. Infrequent: hypotension, midsystolic click, systolic murmur, atrial fibrillation, bradycardia, fourth heart sound, postural hypotension and varicose veins.

Digestive: Infrequent: dry mouth, stomatitis, burning sensation on tongue, cholecystitis, colitis, esophageal ulcer, esophagitis, gastrointestinal carcinoma, gum hemorrhage, hepatomegaly, increased appetite, melena, mouth ulceration, pancreas disorder, pancreatitis, rectal hemorrhage, tenesmus, tongue discoloration and duodenal ulcer.

Endocrine: Infrequent: goiter, hyperthyroidism, and hypothyroidism.

Gastrointestinal: Frequent: bowel urgency, oral moniliasis, salivary gland enlargement, tooth caries, and ulcerative stomatitis.

Hemic and Lymphatic: Infrequent: leukopenia, anemia, cyanosis, eosinophilia, hematemesis, lymphedema, pancytopenia, and splenomegaly.

Metabolic and Nutritional: Infrequent: weight loss, alcohol intolerance, Cushing's syndrome, gout, abnormal healing, and xanthoma.

Musculoskeletal: Infrequent: arthritis, muscle atrophy, bone pain, bursitis, kidney pain, muscle disorder, myopathy, osteomyelitis, tendon pain, and tenosynovitis.

Nervous: Frequent: abnormal dreams, emotional lability and stupor. Infrequent: aphasia, ataxia, convulsion, circumoral paresthesia, depersonalization, hallucinations, hostility, hypokinesia, coma, concentration disorder, facial paralysis, decreased libido, manic reaction, memory impairment, myoclonus, neuralgia, paranoid reaction, paraplegia, psychotic depression and transient stupor.

Respiratory: Frequent: hyperventilation, hay-fever. Infrequent: asthma, pneumonia, epistaxis, hypoventilation, and voice alteration.

Skin and Appendages: Frequent: eczema, herpes zoster, pustular rash, skin atrophy and warts. Infrequent: dry skin, skin hypertrophy, dermatitis, furunculosis, psoriasis, angioedema, contact dermatitis, erythema nodosum, fungal dermatitis, maculopapular rash, pigmentation, benign skin neoplasm, skin carcinoma, skin striae, and vesiculobullous rash.

Special Senses: Frequent: visual field defect. Infrequent: dry eyes, otitis externa, ptosis, cataract, corneal ulcer, mydriasis, optic neuritis, photophobia, and taste loss.

Urogenital: Frequent: amenorrhea, hematuria, impotence, menorrhagia, suspicious Papanicolaou smear, urinary frequency and vaginal hemorrhage. Infrequent: vaginitis, flank pain (kidney), abortion, breast engorgement, breast enlargement, breast pain, carcinoma cervix in situ, fibrocystic breast, kidney calculus, nocturia, ovarian cyst, priapism, pyelonephritis, abnormal sexual function, and urethritis.

Post-Market Adverse Drug Reactions: Adverse Events Reported Post-Marketing and Not Previously Noted in Clinical Trials: Post-marketing experience has shown an adverse event profile similar to that presented above. Reports of adverse reactions occurring under treatment with COPAXONE (glatiramer acetate) in either ongoing phases of clinical trials or from spontaneous reports, that have been received since market introduction and that may have or not have causal relationship to the drug include the following:

Body as a Whole: sepsis, SLE syndrome, hydrocephalus, enlarged abdomen, injection site hypersensitivity, allergic reaction, anaphylactoid reaction, bacterial infection, fever, infection.

Cardiovascular: thrombosis, peripheral vascular disease, pericardial effusion, myocardial infarct, deep thrombophlebitis, coronary occlusion, congestive heart failure, cardiomyopathy, cardiomegaly, arrhythmia, angina pectoris, tachycardia.

Digestive: tongue edema, stomach ulcer hemorrhage, liver function abnormality, liver damage, hepatitis, eructation, cirrhosis of the liver, cholelithiasis, diarrhea, gastrointestinal disorder.

Hemic and Lymphatic: thrombocytopenia, lymphoma-like reaction, acute leukemia.

Metabolic and Nutritional: hypercholesteremia.

Musculoskeletal: rheumatoid arthritis, generalized spasm.

Nervous: myelitis, meningitis, CNS neoplasm, cerebrovascular accident, brain edema, abnormal dreams, aphasia, convulsion, neuralgia, anxiety, foot drop, nervousness, speech disorder, vertigo.

Respiratory: pulmonary embolus, pleural effusion, carcinoma of lung, hay fever, laryngismus.

Skin and Appendages: herpes simplex, pruritus, rash, urticaria.

Special Senses: glaucoma, blindness, visual field defect.

Urogenital: urogenital neoplasm, urine abnormality, ovarian carcinoma, nephrosis, kidney failure, breast carcinoma, bladder carcinoma, urinary frequency.

Localized Adverse Reactions Associated with Subcutaneous Use: At injection sites, localized lipoatrophy and, rarely, injection site skin necrosis have been reported during postmarketing experience. Lipoatrophy may occur after treatment onset (sometimes as early as several months) and may be permanent. There is no known therapy for lipoatrophy. To assist in possibly minimizing these events the patient should be advised to follow proper injection technique and to rotate injection areas and sites on a daily basis (see Information for the Patient).

DRUG INTERACTIONS: Interactions between COPAXONE and other drugs have not been fully evaluated. Results from existing clinical trials do not suggest any significant interactions of COPAXONE with therapies commonly used in MS patients. This includes the concurrent use of corticosteroids for up to 28 days. COPAXONE has not been formally evaluated in combination with Interferon beta. However, 246 patients who failed on or who did not tolerate therapy with Interferon beta and were later treated with COPAXONE within the framework of an open clinical-trial did not report any serious or unexpected adverse events thought to be related to treatment.

DOSAGE AND ADMINISTRATION: Dosing Considerations: COPAXONE should only be prescribed by (or following consultation with) clinicians who are experienced in the diagnosis and management of Multiple Sclerosis.

The only recommended route of administration of COPAXONE (glatiramer acetate) injection is the subcutaneous route. COPAXONE should not be administered by the intravenous route.

Recommended Dose and Dosage Adjustment: The recommended dose of COPAXONE (glatiramer acetate for injection or glatiramer acetate injection) for the treatment of Clinically Isolated Syndrome and Relapsing Remitting MS is a daily injection of 20 mg given subcutaneously.

Administration: Reconstitution: Single-Use Vials of Lyophilized Powder: To reconstitute lyophilized COPAXONE for injection, use a sterile syringe and adapter to transfer 1.1 mL of the diluent supplied, Sterile Water for Injection, into the COPAXONE vial. Gently swirl the vial of COPAXONE and let stand at room temperature until the solid material is completely dissolved. Inspect the reconstituted product visually and discard or return the product to the pharmacist before use if it contains particulate matter. Use within 8 hours after reconstitution. Withdraw 1.0 mL of the solution into a sterile syringe. Remove the adapter, connect a 27-gauge needle and inject the solution subcutaneously. Sites for self-injection include arms, stomach (abdomen), buttocks, and thighs. A vial is suitable for single use only; unused portions should be discarded (see Information for the Patient, Reconstituted product). The reconstituted solution should not be left longer than 8 hours at room temperature.

COPAXONE should be reconstituted only with the provided diluent, Sterile Water for Injection.

Vial Size	Volume of Diluent to be Added	Volume to be Injected	Nominal Concentration per mL
2 mL	1.1 mL	1.0 mL	20 mg

For the pre-filled syringe of COPAXONE, please see Information for the Patient—pre-filled syringe for instructions on the preparation and injection of COPAXONE.

OVERDOSAGE:

Overdose with COPAXONE has been reported in three patients. One patient injected four doses (80 mg total) of COPAXONE at once. No sequelae were noted. Two other patients, a 28-year old male and a 37-year old female, were given 3 injections of 20 mg of COPAXONE at one half hour intervals by error. Neither patient evidenced any change in blood pressure, heart rate, or temperature. Telephone follow-up several hours later produced no report of adverse experiences from either patient. The maximum COPAXONE dose reported in an overdose case is 80 mg glatiramer acetate injection.

For management of a suspected drug overdose, CPhA recommends that you contact your **regional Poison Control Centre**. See the *CPS* Directory section for a list of Poison Control Centres.

ACTION AND CLINICAL PHARMACOLOGY: Mechanism of Action: COPAXONE (glatiramer acetate) is a sterile, lyophilized mixture of synthetic polypeptides containing four naturally occurring amino acids: L-glutamic acid, L-alanine, L-tyrosine and L-lysine with an average molar fraction of 0.141, 0.427, 0.095 and 0.338, respectively.

The mechanism(s) by which glatiramer acetate exerts its effect on Multiple Sclerosis (MS) is (are) not fully elucidated. However, it is thought to act by modifying immune processes that are currently believed to be responsible for the pathogenesis of MS. This hypothesis is supported by findings of studies that have been carried out to explore the pathogenesis of experimental autoimmune encephalomyelitis (EAE), a condition induced in animals that is generally accepted as an experimental model of MS.

Studies in animals and in vitro systems suggest that upon its administration glatiramer acetate specific suppressor T cells are induced and activated in the periphery.

Because the immunological profile of glatiramer acetate remains to be fully elucidated, concerns exist about its potential to alter naturally occurring immune responses (see Warnings and Precautions).

Pharmacokinetics: Results obtained in pharmacokinetic studies performed in humans (healthy volunteers) and animals support the assumption that a substantial fraction of the therapeutic dose delivered to patients subcutaneously is hydrolyzed locally. Nevertheless, larger fragments of glatiramer acetate can be recognized by glatiramer acetate reactive antibodies. Some fraction of the injected material, either intact or partially hydrolyzed, is presumed to enter the lymphatic circulation, enabling it to reach regional lymph nodes, and some, may enter the systemic circulation intact.

STORAGE AND STABILITY: Pre-filled Syringes: The pre-filled syringes of COPAXONE should be refrigerated immediately upon receipt (2-8°C). **Do not freeze.**

If you cannot have refrigerator storage, pre-filled syringes of COPAXONE can be stored at room temperature (15-30°C) for up to 1 month. Do not store pre-filled syringes at room temperature for longer than 1 month. Note: this drug is light sensitive, do not expose to light when not injecting. Each pre-filled syringe is for single use only.

Single-Use Vials of Lyophilized Powder: Vials of lyophilized COPAXONE should be stored under refrigeration (2- 8°C). COPAXONE may also be stored at room temperature (15-30°C) for up to 14 days. The vials of diluent (Sterile Water for Injection) should be stored at room temperature.

Reconstituted solution: The reconstituted solution should not be left longer than 8 hours at room temperature before administration. A vial is suitable for single use only; unused portions should be discarded.

INFORMATION FOR THE PATIENT: Published in e-CPS, available by subscription at www.e-cps.ca.

DOSAGE FORMS, COMPOSITION AND PACKAGING: Pre-filled Syringes: Each pre-filled syringe contains: a sterile solution equivalent with the glatiramer acetate reconstituted solution i.e., 20 ng/mL glatiramer acetate and 40 mg mannitol in sterile water for injection. Single-use pre-filled glass syringes of 1 mL, packs of 30 with 33 alcohol preps (swabs).

Single-Use Vials of Lyophilized Powder: A sterile, lyophilized drug product, intended for subcutaneous injection following reconstitution with Sterile Water for Injection. Each vial of lyophilized drug product contains: 20 mg glatiramer acetate, plus a 2 mg overage to allow for losses in reconstitution and transfer, and 40 mg mannitol, packaged in single use 2 mL amber vials. Each vial of Sterile Water for Injection contains 1.1 mL of Sterile Water for Injection plus a 0.35 mL overage to allow for losses in reconstitution and transfer. Packs of 32 amber vials of sterile lyophilized material for subcutaneous injection. The diluent (Sterile Water for Injection) is supplied in packs of 32 clear vials and is located in the Self Injection Administration Package.

(Shown in Product Identification Section)

Cophylac® Ⓝ

normethadone HCl—p-hydroxyephedrine HCl

Antitussive

Valeo Pharma

Date of Revision: October 12, 2005

INDICATIONS: The treatment of cough associated with inflamed mucosa, which does not respond to products of lesser potency.

CONTRAINDICATIONS: Do not administer to patients receiving MAO inhibitors.

PRECAUTIONS: Before prescribing medication to suppress or modify cough, it is important to ascertain that the underlying cause of the cough is identified, that modification of the cough does not increase the risk of clinical or physiologic complications, and that appropriate therapy for the primary disease is provided.

In young children the respiratory centre is especially susceptible to the depressant action of narcotic cough suppressants. Benefit to risk ratio should be carefully considered especially in children with respiratory embarrassment, e.g. croup. Estimation of dosage relative to the child's age and weight is of great importance.

Pregnancy: Since normethadone crosses the placental barrier, its use in pregnancy is not recommended.

As normethadone may inhibit peristalsis, patients with chronic constipation should be given Cophylac only after weighing the potential therapeutic benefit against the hazards involved.

Contains normethadone. May be habit forming.

OVERDOSE:

Symptoms: An overdose of 4 mL (approx. 90 drops) taken within 4 to 5 hours has produced transient nausea, cold sweat, and tachycardia in one reported case. Should 33% or more of one bottle be ingested, paralysis of the respiratory centre may result.

Treatment: Naloxone HCl.

> For management of a suspected drug overdose, CPhA recommends that you contact your **regional Poison Control Centre**. See the *CPS* Directory section for a list of Poison Control Centres.

DOSAGE: Adults and children over 14 years, 15 drops twice daily; children 3 to 14 years, 5 to 10 drops twice daily; children under 3 years, 2 to 5 drops twice daily.

Drops are dispensed by inverting the drop dispensing bottle. May be taken plain, with sugar or in any beverage, preferably after breakfast and at bedtime.

SUPPLIED: Each mL of sugar-free solution contains: normethadone HCl 10 mg (1%) and p-hydroxyephedrine HCl 20 mg (2%). Nonmedicinal ingredients: citric acid anhydrous, glycerin, lemon oil, methylparaben and purified water. Energy: 3.3 kJ (0.8 kcal). Tartrazine-free. Dispensing bottles of 15 mL.

CO Pioglitazone

pioglitazone HCl

Antidiabetic—Insulin Resistance Reducing Agent

Cobalt

SUPPLIED: 15 mg: Each white, round, flat-faced, bevel-edged tablet with "15" embossed on one side, contains: pioglitazone HCl equivalent to pioglitazone 15 mg. Nonmedicinal ingredients: carmellose calcium, hydroxypropyl cellulose, lactose monohydrate and magnesium stearate. HDPE bottles of 100. Store between 15 and 30°C. Keep container tightly closed and protect from moisture and humidity.

30 mg: Each white, round, flat-faced, bevel-edged tablet with "30" embossed on one side, contains: pioglitazone HCl equivalent to pioglitazone 30 mg. Nonmedicinal ingredients: carmellose calcium, hydroxypropyl cellulose, lactose monohydrate and magnesium stearate. HDPE bottles of 100. Store between 15 and 30°C. Keep container tightly closed and protect from moisture and humidity.

45 mg: Each white, round, flat-faced, bevel-edged tablet with "45" embossed on one side, contains: pioglitazone HCl equivalent to pioglitazone 45 mg. Nonmedicinal ingredients: carmellose calcium, hydroxypropyl cellulose, lactose monohydrate and magnesium stearate. HDPE bottles of 100. Store between 15 and 30°C. Keep container tightly closed and protect from moisture and humidity.

CO Pramipexole

pramipexole dihydrochloride

Antiparkinsonian Agent—Dopamine Agonist

Cobalt

SUPPLIED: 0.25 mg: Each white to off-white, oval, flat-faced, bevel-edged tablet with "PM2|PM2" on one side and "Σ|Σ" on the other side, contains: pramipexole dihydrochloride monohydrate 0.25 mg. Nonmedicinal ingredients: collodial silicon dioxide, magnesium stearate, mannitol, povidone and starch (corn). HDPE bottles of 100 and 1000. Store at room temperature (15 to 25°C). Protect from light and moisture.

0.5 mg: Each white to off-white, oval, flat-faced, bevel-edged tablet with "PM3|PM3" on one side and "Σ|Σ" on the other side, contains: pramipexole dihydrochloride monohydrate 0.5 mg. Nonmedicinal ingredients: collodial silicon dioxide, magnesium stearate, mannitol, povidone and starch (corn). HDPE bottles of 100 and 1000. Store at room temperature (15 to 25°C). Protect from light and moisture.

1 mg: Each white to off-white, round, flat-faced, bevel-edged tablet with "PM4/PM4" one side and "Σ/Σ" on the other side, contains: pramipexole dihydrochloride monohydrate 1 mg. Nonmedicinal ingredients: collodial silicon dioxide, magnesium stearate, mannitol, povidone and starch (corn). HDPE bottles of 100 and 1000. Store at room temperature (15 to 25°C). Protect from light and moisture.

1.5 mg: Each white to off-white, round, flat-faced, bevel-edged tablet with "PM5/PM5" one side and "Σ/Σ" on the other side, contains: pramipexole dihydrochloride monohydrate 1.5 mg. Nonmedicinal ingredients: collodial silicon dioxide, magnesium stearate, mannitol, povidone and starch (corn). HDPE bottles of 100 and 1000. Store at room temperature (15 to 25°C). Protect from light and moisture.

> The reader is invited to consult CPhA's monograph **HMG-CoA Reductase Inhibitors**.

CO Pravastatin

pravastatin sodium

Lipid Metabolism Regulator

Cobalt

SUPPLIED: 10 mg: Each pink to peach, rounded, rectangular-shaped, biconvex tablet, with "Σ" on one side and "PV" over "10" on the other side, contains: pravastatin sodium 10 mg. Nonmedicinal ingredients: croscarmellose sodium, lactose monohydrate, magnesium aluminium silicate, magnesium stearate, microcrystalline cellulose, povidone, Red 30 Iron Oxide and talc. Gluten-free. Bottles of 30 and 100. Store at room temperature (15-30°C). Protect from moisture and light.

20 mg: Each yellow, rounded, rectangular-shaped, biconvex tablet, with "Σ" on one side and "PV" over "20" on the other side, contains: pravastatin sodium 20 mg. Nonmedicinal ingredients: croscarmellose sodium, lactose monohydrate, magnesium aluminium silicate, magnesium stearate, microcrystalline cellulose, povidone, talc and Yellow 10 Iron Oxide. Gluten-free. Bottles of 30, 100 and 500. Unit dose blisters of 30. Store at room temperature (15-30°C). Protect from moisture and light.

40 mg: Each green, rounded, rectangular-shaped, biconvex tablet, with "Σ" on one side and "PV" over 40 on the other side, contains: pravastatin sodium 40 mg. Nonmedicinal ingredients: croscarmellose sodium, lactose monohydrate, Lake Blend Green, magnesium aluminium silicate, magnesium stearate, microcrystalline cellulose, povidone and talc. Gluten-free. Bottles of 30 and 100. Unit dose blisters of 30. Store at room temperature (15-30°C). Protect from moisture and light.

CO Quetiapine

quetiapine fumarate

Antipsychotic

Cobalt

SUPPLIED: 25 mg: Each peach, film-coated, round, biconvex tablet with "QT" on one side and "Σ" on the other, contains: quetiapine fumarate equivalent to quetiapine 25 mg. Nonmedicinal ingredients: calcium hydrogen phosphate dihydrate, lactose monohydrate, magnesium stearate, microcrystalline cellulose, povidone and sodium starch glycolate; film coating: FD&C blue #2, FD&C red #40, FD&C yellow #6, polyethylene glycol 3350, polyvinyl alcohol, talc and titanium dioxide. HDPE bottles of 100 and 500. Store at room temperature (between 15-30°C) and well out of the reach of children. Protect from light.

100 mg: Each yellow, film-coated, round, biconvex tablet with "QT/100" on one side and "Σ" on the other, contains: quetiapine fumarate equivalent to quetiapine 100 mg. Nonmedicinal ingredients: calcium hydrogen phosphate dihydrate, lactose monohydrate, magnesium stearate, microcrystalline cellulose, povidone and sodium starch glycolate; film coating: iron oxide yellow, polyethylene glycol 3350, polyvinyl alcohol, talc and titanium dioxide. HDPE bottles of 100 and 500. Store at room temperature (between 15-30°C) and well out of the reach of children. Protect from light.

200 mg: Each white to off-white, film-coated, round, biconvex tablet with "QT/200" on one side and "Σ" on the other, contains: quetiapine fumarate equivalent to quetiapine 200 mg. Nonmedicinal ingredients: calcium hydrogen phosphate dihydrate, lactose monohydrate, magnesium stearate, microcrystalline cellulose, povidone and sodium starch glycolate; film coating: polyethylene glycol 3350, polyvinyl alcohol, talc and titanium dioxide. HDPE bottles of 100 and 500. Store at room temperature (between 15-30°C) and well out of the reach of children. Protect from light.

300 mg: Each white to off-white, film-coated, capsule-shaped, biconvex tablet with "QT/300" on one side and "Σ" on the other, contains: quetiapine fumarate equivalent to quetiapine 300 mg. Nonmedicinal ingredients: calcium hydrogen phosphate dihydrate, lactose monohydrate, magnesium stearate, microcrystalline cellulose, povidone and sodium starch glycolate; film coating: polyethylene glycol 3350, polyvinyl alcohol, talc and titanium dioxide. HDPE bottles of 100 and 500. Store at room temperature (between 15-30°C) and well out of the reach of children. Protect from light.

> The reader is invited to consult CPhA's monograph **ACE Inhibitors**.

CO Ramipril

ramipril

Angiotensin Converting Enzyme Inhibitor

Cobalt

SUPPLIED: 1.25 mg: Each hard gelatin capsule with white opaque body and yellow opaque cap, the body has "RP 1.25" and the cap has "Σ" both printed in black contains: ramipril 1.25 mg. Nonmedicinal ingredients: black ink; capsule shell: pre-gelatinized starch, titanium dioxide and yellow iron oxide. Cartons of 30 (2×foil/foil blister strips of 15 capsules). HDPE bottles of 100 and 500. Store between 15 and 25°C. Protect from heat and humidity.

2.5 mg: Each hard gelatin capsule with white opaque body and orange opaque cap, the body has "RP 2.5" and the cap has "Σ" both printed in black contains: ramipril 2.5 mg. Nonmedicinal ingredients: black ink, D&C Red #28 and FD&C Red #40; capsule shell: pre-gelatinized starch, titanium dioxide and yellow iron oxide. Cartons of 30 (2×foil/foil blister strips of 15 capsules). HDPE bottles of 100 and 500. Store between 15 and 25°C. Protect from heat and humidity.

5 mg: Each hard gelatin capsule with white opaque body and red opaque cap, the body has "RP 5" and the cap has "Σ" both printed in black contains: ramipril 5 mg. Nonmedicinal ingredients: black ink, D&C Red #28, D&C Yellow #10, FD&C Blue #1 and FD&C Red #40; capsule shell: pre-gelatinized starch and titanium dioxide. Cartons of 30 (2×foil/foil blister strips of 15 capsules). HDPE bottles of 100 and 500. Store between 15 and 25°C. Protect from heat and humidity.

10 mg: Each hard gelatin capsule with white opaque body and blue opaque cap, the body has "RP 10" and the cap has "Σ" both printed in black contains: ramipril 10 mg. Nonmedicinal ingredients: black ink, black iron oxide, D&C Red #28, FD&C Blue #1 and FD&C Red #40; capsule shell: pre-gelatinized starch and titanium dioxide. Cartons of 30 (2×foil/foil blister strips of 15 capsules). HDPE bottles of 100 and 500. Store between 15 and 25°C. Protect from heat and humidity.

CO Ranitidine

ranitidine HCl

Histamine H2-Receptor Antagonist

Cobalt

SUPPLIED: 150 mg: Each white to off-white, round, biconvex, film-coated tablet, with "Σ" on one side and 150 on the other, contains: ranitidine HCl 168 mg (ranitidine 150 mg free base). Nonmedicinal ingredients: croscarmellose sodium, magnesium stearate and microcrystalline cellulose; film-coating suspension: hydroxypropyl methylcellulose, polydextrose, polyethylene glycol, titanium dioxide and triethyl citrate. Gluten-free. Bottles of 60, 100 and 500. Unit dose blisters of 60. Store between 15 and 30°C. Protect from light and moisture.

300 mg: Each white to off-white, capsule-shaped, film-coated tablet, with "Σ" on one side and 300 on the other, contains: ranitidine HCl 336 mg (ranitidine 300 mg free base). Nonmedicinal ingredients: croscarmellose sodium, magnesium stearate and microcrystalline cellulose; film-coating suspension: hydroxypropyl methylcellulose, polydextrose, polyethylene glycol, titanium dioxide and triethyl citrate. Gluten-free. Bottles of 100. Unit dose blisters of 30. Store between 15 and 30°C. Protect from light and moisture.

Cordarone®

amiodarone HCl

Antiarrhythmic

Pfizer

Date of Revision: April 28, 2010

SUMMARY PRODUCT INFORMATION:

Route of Administration	Dosage Form/ Strength	Clinically Relevant Nonmedicinal Ingredients
Oral	CORDARONE (Amiodarone Hydrochloride Tablets) 200 mg	None For a complete listing see Dosage Forms, Composition and Packaging.

INDICATIONS AND CLINICAL USE:

> No antiarrhythmic drug has been shown to reduce the incidence of sudden death in patients with asymptomatic ventricular arrhythmias. Most antiarrhythmic drugs have the potential to cause dangerous arrhythmias; some have been shown to be associated with an increased incidence of sudden death. In light of the above, physicians should carefully consider the risks and benefits of antiarrhythmic therapy for all patients with ventricular arrhythmias.

Because the life-threatening nature of arrhythmias treated, potential interaction with prior therapy, and potential exacerbation of arrhythmia, initiation of therapy with CORDARONE should be carried out in the hospital.

CORDARONE should be used only by physicians familiar with and with access to (directly or referral) the use of all available modalities for treating recurrent life-threatening ventricular arrhythmias, and who have access to appropriate monitoring facilities, including in-hospital and ambulatory continuous electrocardiographic monitoring and electrophysiologic technique.

Oral CORDARONE: Because of its potential for life-threatening side effects and the substantial management difficulties associated with its oral use, CORDARONE is indicated only for the treatment of patients with the following documented life-threatening, recurrent ventricular arrhythmias when these have not responded to documented adequate doses of other available antiarrhythmics, or when alternative agents could not be tolerated.

1. Hemodynamically unstable ventricular tachycardia (VT).
2. Recurrent ventricular fibrillation (VF).

As is the case for other antiarrhythmic agents, there is no evidence from controlled clinical trials that the use of CORDARONE (amiodarone HCl) tablets favourably affects survival.

Geriatrics (>65 years of age): Clinical studies of CORDARONE tablets did not include sufficient number of subjects aged 65 years and over to determine whether they respond differently from younger subjects. Other reported clinical experience has not identified differences in responses between the elderly and younger patients. In general, dose selection for an elderly patient should be cautious, usually starting at the low end of the dosing range, reflecting the greater frequency of decreased hepatic, renal, or cardiac function, and of concomitant disease or other drug therapy.

Pediatrics (<18 years of age) : The safety and efficacy of amiodarone in children have not been established; therefore, its use in children is not recommended.

CONTRAINDICATIONS: CORDARONE (amiodarone HCl) is contraindicated in patients with known hypersensitivity to any of the components of oral CORDARONE (tablets) including iodine, and in patients with cardiogenic shock. It is contraindicated in severe sinus-node dysfunction, causing bradycardia; second- or third-degree V block, and when episodes of bradycardia have caused syncope (except when used in conjunction with a pacemaker). In addition oral CORDARONE is contraindicated in patients with evidence of hepatitis (see Warnings and Precautions, Hepatic/Biliary/Pancreatic), thyroid dysfunction (see Warnings and Precautions, Endocrine and Metabolism, Thyrotoxicosis) or pulmonary interstitial abnormalities (see Warnings and Precautions, Respiratory, Pulmonary Toxicity).

WARNINGS AND PRECAUTIONS:

CORDARONE is intended for use only in patients with the indicated life-threatening arrhythmias because its use is accompanied by substantial toxicity.

CORDARONE has several potentially fatal toxicities, the most important of which is pulmonary toxicity (hypersensitivity pneumonitis or interstitial/alveolar pneumonitis) that has resulted in clinically manifest disease at rates as high as 10 to 17% in some series of patients with ventricular arrhythmias given doses around 400 mg/day, and as abnormal diffusion capacity without symptoms in a much higher percentage of patients. Pulmonary toxicity has been fatal about 10% of the time. Liver injury is common with CORDARONE, but is usually mild and evidenced only by abnormal liver enzymes. Overt liver disease can occur, however, and has been fatal in a few cases. Like other antiarrhythmics, CORDARONE can exacerbate the arrhythmia, e.g., by making the arrhythmia less well tolerated or more difficult to reverse. This has occurred in 2 to 5% of patients in various series, and significant heart block or sinus bradycardia has been seen in 2 to 5%. All of these events should be manageable in the proper clinical setting in most cases. Although the frequency of such proarrhythmic events does not appear greater with CORDARONE than with many other agents used in this population, the effects are prolonged when they occur.

Even in patients at high risk of arrhythmic death, in whom the toxicity of CORDARONE is an acceptable risk, CORDARONE poses major management problems that could be life-threatening in a population at risk of sudden death, so that every effort should be made to utilize alternative agents first.

The difficulty of using CORDARONE effectively and safely itself poses a significant risk to patients. Patients with the indicated arrhythmias must be hospitalized while the loading dose of CORDARONE is given, and a response generally requires at least one week, usually two or more. Because absorption and elimination are variable, maintenance-dose selection is difficult, and it is not unusual to require dosage decrease or discontinuation of treatment. In a retrospective survey of 192 patients with ventricular tachyarrhythmias, 84 required dose reduction and 18 required at least temporary discontinuation because of adverse effects, and several series have reported 15 to 20% overall frequencies of discontinuation due to adverse reactions. The time at which a previously controlled life-threatening arrhythmia will recur after discontinuation or dose adjustment is unpredictable, ranging from weeks to months. The patient is obviously at great risk during this time and may need prolonged hospitalization. Attempts to substitute other antiarrhythmic agents when CORDARONE must be stopped will be made difficult by the gradually, but unpredictably, changing amiodarone body burden. A similar problem exists when CORDARONE is not effective; it still poses the risk of an interaction with whatever subsequent treatment is tried.

General: Oral CORDARONE (amiodarone HCl): Mortality: The results of the Cardiac Arrhythmia Suppression Trial (CAST) in post myocardial infarction patients with asymptomatic non-life threatening ventricular arrhythmias who had a myocardial infarction more than six days but less than two years previously showed a significant increase in mortality and non-fatal cardiac arrest rate in patients treated with encainide or flecainide (56/730) compared with a matched placebo treatment group (22/725). CAST was continued using a revised protocol with moricizine and placebo treatment groups only. The trial was prematurely terminated because of the trend towards an increase in mortality in the moricizine-treated group.

The applicability of these results to other populations or other antiarrhythmic agents is uncertain, but at present, it is prudent to consider these results when using any antiarrhythmic agent.

CORDARONE therapy was evaluated in two multicenter, randomized, double-blind, placebo-controlled trials involving 1202 (Canadian Amiodarone Myocardial Infarction Arrhythmia Trial; CAMIAT) and 1486 (European Myocardial Infarction Amiodarone Trial; EMIAT) post-MI patients followed for up to 2 years. Patients in CAMIAT qualified with ventricular arrhythmias, and those randomized to amiodarone received weight- and response-adjusted doses of 200 to 400 mg/day. Patients in EMIAT qualified with ejection fraction <40%, and those randomized to amiodarone received fixed doses of 200 mg/day. Both studies had weeks-long loading dose schedules. Intent-to-treat all-cause mortality results were as follows:

	Placebo		Amiodarone		Relative Risk	
	N	Deaths	N	Deaths		95 % CI
EMIAT	743	102	743	103	0.99	0.76–1.31
CAMIAT	596	68	606	57	0.88	0.58–1.16

These data are consistent with the results of a pooled analysis of 13 smaller, controlled studies involving patients with structural heart disease (including myocardial infarction) where total mortality was reduced by only 13% (odds ratio 0.87, [95% confidence interval 0.75 to 0.99] p=0.03) based on classic fixed effects meta-analysis.

Patients with life-threatening arrhythmias may experience serious adverse events during their treatment and therefore should be properly monitored. CORDARONE (amiodarone HCl) should be administered only by physicians who are experienced in the treatment of life-threatening arrhythmias, who are thoroughly familiar with the risks and benefits of CORDARONE therapy, and who have access to facilities adequate for monitoring the effectiveness and adverse events of treatment (see Indications and Clinical Use).

Loading Phase: The higher doses of **oral** CORDARONE used in the loading phase may sometimes be associated with adverse effects such as nausea or tremor. The nausea may respond to dividing the total dose into two or three fractions taken with meals, or by decreasing the total daily dose. The tremor may respond to dose reduction as well.

Carcinogenesis and Mutagenesis: Oral CORDARONE caused a statistically significant, dose-related increase in the incidence of thyroid tumors (follicular adenoma and/or carcinoma) in rats. The incidence of thyroid tumors in rats was greater than the incidence in controls even at the lowest dose level tested, i.e., 5 mg/kg/day (approximately 0.08 times the maximum recommended human maintenance dose*).

Mutagenicity studies conducted with amiodarone HCl (Ames, micronucleus, and lysogenic induction tests) were negative.

* 600 mg in a 50 kg patient (dose compared on a body surface area basis).

In a study which amiodarone HCl was orally administered to male and female rats, beginning 9 weeks prior to mating, reduced fertility was observed at a dose level of 90 mg/kg/day (approximately 1.4 times the maximum recommended human maintenance dose*)

Cardiovascular: Proarrhythmia/QT Interval Prolongation: Amiodarone may cause a worsening of the existing arrhythmias or precipitate a new arrhythmia. Amiodarone causes prolongation of the QT interval. Proarrhythmia, primarily torsades de pointes, has been associated with prolongation of the QTc interval to 500 ms or greater. Proarrhythmia has been reported (2 to 5%) with oral CORDARONE, especially in the presence of concomitant antiarrhythmic therapy and has included new-onset VF, incessant VT, increased resistance to cardioversion, and paroxysmal polymorphic VT associated with QT prolongation "torsades de pointes". Although QTc prolongation occurred frequently in patients receiving I.V. amiodarone, torsades de pointes or new-onset VF occurred infrequently (less than 2% of all patients treated with I.V. amiodarone in controlled clinical trials). Patients should be monitored carefully for QTc prolongation during amiodarone therapy. Combination of amiodarone with other antiarrhythmic therapy that prolongs the QTc should be reserved for patients with life-threatening ventricular arrhythmias who are incompletely responsive to a single agent. The need to co-administer amiodarone with any other drug known to prolong the QTc interval must be based on a careful assessment of the potential risks and benefits of doing so for each patient.

Fluoroquinolones, macrolide antibiotics, and azoles are known to cause QTc prolongation. There have been reports of QTc prolongation, with or without torsades de pointes, in patients taking amiodarone when fluoroquinolones, macrolide antibiotics, or azoles were administered concomitantly.

A careful assessment of the potential risks and benefits of administering oral CORDARONE must be made in patients with thyroid dysfunction due to the possibility of arrhythmia breakthrough or exacerbation of arrhythmia in these patients. For patients receiving I.V. amiodarone, death may result.

Even in patients at high risk of arrhythmic death, in whom the toxicity of amiodarone is an acceptable risk, amiodarone poses major management problems that could be life-threatening in a population at risk of sudden death, so that every effort should be made to utilize alternative agents first

The difficulty of using amiodarone effectively and safely poses a significant risk to patients. Patients with the indicated arrhythmias must be hospitalized while the loading dose of amiodarone is given, and a response generally requires at least one week, usually two or more. Because absorption and elimination are variable, maintenance-dose selection is difficult, and it is not unusual to require dosage decrease or discontinuation of treatment. In a retrospective survey of 192 patients with ventricular tachyarrhythmias, 84 required dose reduction and 18 required at least temporary discontinuation because of adverse effects, and several series have reported 15 to 20% overall frequencies of discontinuation due to adverse reactions. The time at which a previously controlled life-threatening arrhythmia will recur after discontinuation or dose adjustment is unpredictable, ranging from weeks to months. The patient is obviously at great risk during this time and may need prolonged hospitalization. Attempts to substitute other antiarrhythmic agents when amiodarone must be stopped will be made difficult by the gradually, but unpredictably, changing amiodarone body burden. A similar problem exists when amiodarone is not effective; it still poses the risk of an interaction with whatever subsequent treatment is tried.

Bradycardia and AV Block: In patients treated with **oral** CORDARONE, symptomatic bradycardia or sinus arrest with suppression of escape foci occurs in approximately 2 to 4% of patients. Bradycardia was reported as an adverse drug reaction in 4.9% of patients receiving I.V. amiodarone for life-threatening VT/VF in clinical trials. AV block was reported as an adverse drug reaction in 1.4% of patients receiving I.V. amiodarone. There was no dose-related increase in bradycardia or AV block in these studies.

In patients who develop symptomatic bradycardia while taking **oral** CORDARONE, dose reduction or discontinuation, and possibly pacing, may be considered. Due to the large body load of amiodarone that accumulates with chronic dose administration, and the long half-life of the drug, serum concentrations decline slowly after dose reduction or discontinuation.

Intravenous Amiodarone: Hypotension: Hypotension is the most common adverse event seen with I.V. amiodarone therapy: it is uncommon (<1%) during oral CORDARONE therapy. In clinical trials, treatment-emergent, drug-related hypotension was reported as an adverse effect in 288 (16%) of 1836 patients treated with I.V. amiodarone. Clinically significant hypotension during infusions was seen most often in the first several hours of treatment and was not dose related, but appeared to be related to the rate of infusion. Hypotension necessitating temporary discontinuation of I.V. amiodarone therapy was reported in 3% of the 814 patients, with permanent discontinuation required in an additional 2% of the 814 patients. In some cases, hypotension may be refractory resulting in fatal outcome.

Oral CORDARONE: Cardiac Disorders: Oral CORDARONE should be used with caution in patients with latent or manifest heart failure because this condition may be worsened by its administration. In these cases, **oral** CORDARONE should be given with appropriate concurrent therapy.

Oral CORDARONE therapy may be considered in the treatment of patients with Wolff-Parkinson-White (WPW) syndrome, atrial flutter, or atrial fibrillation, when these conditions are complicated by life-threatening ventricular tachyarrhythmias. In such cases, care is required since the effect of **oral** CORDARONE in these conditions does not appear to be uniform. Electrophysiologic studies may be of value in the selection of these patients who may respond to **oral** CORDARONE, particularly in WPW syndrome.

Implantable Cardiac Devices: In patients with implanted defibrillators or pacemakers, chronic administration of antiarrhythmic drugs affects pacing or defibrillating thresholds. Therefore, at the inception of and during amiodarone treatment, pacing and defibrillation thresholds should be assessed.

Endocrine and Metabolism: Thyrotoxicosis: Cordarone-induced hyperthyroidism may result in thyrotoxicosis and/or the possibility of arrhythmia breakthrough or aggravation. There have been reports of death associated with amiodarone-induced thyrotoxicosis. If any new signs of arrhythmia appear, the possibility of hyperthyroidism should be considered (also see Thyroid Abnormalities and Dysfunction).

Thyroid Abnormalities and Dysfunction: CORDARONE inhibits peripheral conversion of thyroxine (T_4) to triiodothyronine (T_3) and may cause increased thyroxine levels, decreased T_3 levels, and increased levels of inactive reverse T_3 (rT_3) in clinically euthyroid patients. It is also a potential source of large amounts of inorganic iodine. **Both hyper- and hypothyroidism may occur during, or soon after treatment with oral CORDARONE.** Because of its release of inorganic iodine, or perhaps for other reasons, CORDARONE can cause either hypothyroidism or hyperthyroidism. Thyroid function should be monitored prior to treatment and periodically thereafter, particularly in elderly patients, and in any patient with a history of thyroid nodules, goiter, or other thyroid dysfunction. Because of the slow elimination of amiodarone and its metabolites, high plasma iodide levels, altered thyroid function, and abnormal thyroid-function tests may persist for several weeks or even months following CORDARONE withdrawal.

Hypothyroidism has been reported in 2 to 4% of patients in most series, but in 8 to 10% in some series. This condition may be identified by relevant clinical symptoms and particularly by elevated serum TSH levels. In some clinically hypothyroid amiodarone-treated patients, free thyroxine index values may be normal. Hypothyroidism is best managed by amiodarone dose reduction and/or thyroid hormone supplement. However, therapy must be individualized, and it may be necessary to discontinue CORDARONE tablets in some patients.

Hyperthyroidism occurs in about 2% of patients receiving CORDARONE, but the incidence may be higher among patients with prior inadequate dietary iodine intake. Amiodarone-induced hyperthyroidism usually poses a greater hazard to the patient than hypothyroidism because of the possibility of arrhythmia breakthrough or aggravation, which may result in death. There have been reports of death associated with amiodarone-induced thyrotoxicosis. In fact, **if any new signs of arrhythmia appear, the possibility of hyperthyroidism should be considered.** Hyperthyroidism is best identified by relevant clinical symptoms and signs, accompanied usually by abnormally elevated levels of serum T_3 RIA, and further elevations of serum T_4, and a subnormal serum TSH level (using a sufficiently sensitive TSH assay). The finding of a flat TSH response to TRH is confirmatory of hyperthyroidism and may be sought in equivocal cases. Since arrhythmia breakthroughs may accompany amiodarone-induced hyperthyroidism, aggressive medical treatment is indicated, including, if possible, dose reduction or withdrawal of CORDARONE.

The institution of antithyroid drugs, beta-adrenergic blockers and/or temporary corticosteroid therapy may be necessary. The action of antithyroid drugs may be especially delayed in amiodarone-induced thyrotoxicosis because of substantial quantities of preformed thyroid hormones stored in the gland. There have been reports of death associated with amiodarone-induced thyrotoxicosis. Radioactive iodine therapy is contraindicated because of the low radioiodine uptake associated with amiodarone-induced hyperthyroidism. Experience with thyroid surgery in this setting is extremely limited, and this form of therapy could induce thyroid storm. Amiodarone-induced hyperthyroidism may be followed by a transient period of hypothyroidism.

There have been postmarketing reports of thyroid nodules/thyroid cancer in patients treated with amiodarone. In some instances hyperthyroidism was also present.

In a rat carcinogenicity study, at doses of 5, 16 and 50 mg/kg/day, amiodarone produced statistically significant dose-related changes in the thyroid gland, including follicular adenomas and carcinomas. The significance of these changes for the long-term use of CORDARONE in humans is unknown.

Neonatal Hypo- or Hyperthyroidism: CORDARONE (amiodarone HCl) can cause fetal harm when administered to a pregnant woman. Although amiodarone use during pregnancy is uncommon, there have been a small number of published reports of congenital goiter/hypothyroidism and hyperthyroidism associated with its oral administration. If CORDARONE is used during pregnancy, or if the patient becomes pregnant while taking CORDARONE, the patient should be apprised of the potential hazard to the fetus.

In general, CORDARONE should be used during pregnancy only if the potential benefit to the mother justifies the unknown risk to the fetus.

In pregnant rats and rabbits, amiodarone HCl in dose of 25 mg/kg/day (approximately 0.4 and 0.9 times, respectively, the maximum recommended human maintenance dose*) had no adverse effects on the fetus. In the rabbit, 75 mg/kg/day (approximately 2.7 times the maximum recommended human maintenance dose*) caused abortions in greater than 90% of the animals. In the rat, doses of 50 mg/kg/day or more were associated with slight displacement of the testes and an increased incidence of incomplete ossification of some skull and digital bones; at 100 mg/kg/day or more, fetal body weights were reduced; at 200 mg/kg/day, there was an increased incidence of fetal resorption. (These doses in the rat are approximately 0.8, 1.6 and 3.2 times the maximum recommended human maintenance dose.*) Adverse effects on fetal growth and survival also were noted in one of two strains of mice at a dose of 5 mg/kg/day (approximately 0.04 times the maximum recommended human maintenance dose*).

Gastrointestinal: Certain gastrointestinal reactions (e.g., nausea, vomiting, constipation, and bad taste) occur frequently at the initiation of therapy when high doses are used. These may disappear on reduction of the dose.

Hepatic/Biliary/Pancreatic: Liver Enzyme Elevations: In patients with life-threatening arrhythmias, the potential risk of hepatic injury should be weighed against the potential benefit of amiodarone therapy. However, patients receiving oral CORDARONE should be monitored carefully for evidence of progressive hepatic injury.

Elevations of blood hepatic enzyme values—alanine aminotransferase (ALT), aspartate aminotransferase (AST), and gamma-glutamyl transferase (GGT)—are seen commonly in patients with immediately life-threatening VT/VF. Interpreting elevated AST activity can be difficult because the values may be elevated in patients with recent myocardial infarction, congestive heart failure, and in those who have received multiple electrical defibrillations.

If the increase in hepatic enzyme levels exceeds three times normal or double in a patient with elevated baseline, discontinuation of CORDARONE should be considered.

Asymptomatic elevations of liver enzymes (AST and ALT) are frequently associated with the use of **oral** CORDARONE. The mechanism whereby this hepatic effect occurs has not been defined. Phospholipidosis and fibrosis of the liver resembling alcoholic hepatitis or cirrhosis, accompanied by only a mild elevation of hepatic enzymes, have been reported in association with the use of **oral** CORDARONE. Rises in hepatic enzymes, especially when associated with clinical signs and symptoms of hepatitis, or with asymptomatic hepatomegaly, may indicate a liver scan and, if needed, a liver biopsy with ultrastructural study. If serum enzyme levels increase significantly, or persist over time, consideration should be given to discontinuation or reducing the dose of amiodarone. Hepatic failure has been a rare cause of death in patients treated with **oral** CORDARONE.

Approximately 54% of patients receiving I.V. amiodarone in clinical studies had baseline elevations in liver enzyme values, and 13% had clinically significant elevations. In 81% of patients with baseline and on-therapy data available, the liver enzyme elevations either improved during therapy or remained at baseline levels. Baseline abnormalities in hepatic enzymes are not a contraindication to treatment.

Rare cases of fatal hepatocellular necrosis after treatment with I.V. amiodarone have been reported. Two patients, one 28 and the other 60 years of age, received an initial infusion of 1500 mg over 5 hours, a rate much higher than recommended. Both patients developed hepatic and renal failure within 24 hours after the start of I.V. amiodarone treatment and died on day 14 and day 4, respectively. Because these episodes of hepatic necrosis may have been due to the rapid rate of infusion and hypotension is related to the rate of infusion, **the initial rate of infusion should be monitored closely and should not exceed that recommended.**

Neurologic: Nervous System Disorders: Chronic administration of **oral** CORDARONE in rare instances may lead to the development of peripheral neuropathy that may resolve when CORDARONE is discontinued, but this resolution has been slow and incomplete.

Ophthalmologic: Loss of Vision: Cases of optic neuropathy and/or optic neuritis, usually resulting in visual impairment, have been reported in patients treated with amiodarone. In some cases, visual impairment has progressed to permanent blindness. Optic neuropathy and/or neuritis may occur at any time following initiation of therapy. A causal relationship to the drug has not been clearly established. If symptoms of visual impairment appear, such as changes in visual acuity and decreases in peripheral vision, prompt ophthalmic examination is recommended. Appearance of optic neuropathy and/or neuritis calls for re-evaluation of amiodarone therapy. The risks and complications of antiarrhythmic therapy with CORDARONE must be weighed against its benefits in patients whose lives are threatened by cardiac arrhythmias. Regular ophthalmic examination, including fundoscopy and slit-lamp examination, is recommended during administration of CORDARONE (see Adverse Reactions, Ophthalmological Abnormalities).

Ocular Abnormalities (Corneal Microdeposits): Corneal micro-deposits appear in the majority of adults treated with CORDARONE, they are usually discernible only by slit-lamp examination, but give rise to symptoms such as visual halos or blurred vision in as many as 10% of patients. Corneal microdeposits are reversible upon reduction of dose or termination of treatment. Asymptomatic microdeposits alone are not a reason to reduce dose or discontinue treatment (see Adverse Reactions, Ophthalmological Abnormalities).

Peri-Operative Considerations: Surgery: Occurrences of adult respiratory syndrome (ARDS) and low cardiac output syndrome have been reported postoperatively in patients receiving **oral** CORDARONE therapy who have undergone either cardiac or noncardiac surgery. An intraaortic balloon pump augmentation has been required in some patients with the low cardiac output syndrome at discontinuation of cardiopulmonary bypass. In the case of ARDS, although patients usually respond well to vigorous respiratory therapy, in rare instances the outcome has been fatal. A number of patients who developed ARDS were subjected to a high concentration of oxygen in the inspired air; this could have been a factor in the respiratory complications. Until further studies have been performed, it is recommended that FiO_2 and the determinants of oxygen delivery to the tissues (e.g., SaO_2, PaO_2) be closely monitored in patients on CORDARONE. Caution should also be exercised in considering CORDARONE patients for surgery in the presence of preoperative pulmonary dysfunction. However, as amiodarone has a very long half-life, withdrawal before surgery implies delaying operations by several weeks and putting patients at increased risk of malignant dysrhythmias. The ARDS in these cases has rarely been fatal.

Hypotension independent of, or associated with, discontinuation of cardiopulmonary bypass following open-heart surgery has been reported. Blood vessels may respond poorly to adrenoreceptor agonists. Atropine-resistant bradycardia and complete heart block have also been reported in patients being weaned from cardiopulmonary bypass.

Corneal Refractive Surgery: Patients should be advised that most manufacturers of corneal refractive laser surgery devices contraindicate that procedure in patients taking amiodarone.

Volatile Anaesthetic Agents: Close peri-operative monitoring is recommended in patients undergoing general anaesthesia who are on amiodarone therapy as they may be more sensitive to the myocardial depressant and conduction effects of halogenated inhalation anaesthetics.

Respiratory: Intravenous and Oral Amiodarone: Pulmonary Toxicity: There have been post-marketing reports of acute-onset (days to weeks) pulmonary injury in patients treated with oral Cordarone with or without initial I.V. therapy. Findings have included pulmonary infiltrates and/or mass on X-ray, pulmonary alveolar hemorrhage, pleural effusion, bronchospasm, wheezing, fever, dyspnea, cough, hemoptysis, and hypoxia. Some cases have progressed to respiratory failure and/or death.

One of the most serious complications resulting from **oral** CORDARONE therapy is pulmonary toxicity, characterized by pneumonitis. Clinical symptoms include cough, progressive dyspnea, accompanied by functional, radiographic, gallium-scan, weight loss, weakness, and pathological data consistent with pulmonary toxicity. On chest x-ray, there is a diffuse interstitial pattern lung involvement frequently with patchy alveolar infiltrates, particularly in the upper lobe. Predicting which patient will develop pulmonary toxicity has been difficult (see Contraindications). Pulmonary toxicity can appear abruptly either early or late during therapy and it commonly mimics viral or bacterial infection or worsening congestive heart failure. The relationship of pulmonary toxicity to duration of therapy, maintenance dose, and total dose is unclear. The majority of patients have recovered with this management, although some fatalities have occurred. Therefore, when CORDARONE therapy is initiated, a baseline chest X ray and pulmonary-function tests, including diffusion capacity, should be performed. The patient should return for a history, physical exam, and chest X-ray every 3 to 6 months.

Pulmonary toxicity secondary to amiodarone seems to result from either indirect or direct toxicity as represented by hypersensitivity pneumonitis (including eosinophilic pneumonia) or interstitial/alveolar pneumonitis, respectively at rates as high as 10-17% in patients with ventricular arrhythmias given doses around 400 mg/day. Pulmonary toxicity has been fatal about 10% of the time.

Recent reports suggest that the use of lower loading and maintenance doses of amiodarone are associated with a decreased incidence of amiodarone-induced pulmonary toxicity.

Hypersensitivity pneumonitis usually appears earlier in the course of therapy, and rechallenging these patients with amiodarone results in a more rapid recurrence of greater severity. Bronchoalveolar lavage is the procedure of choice to confirm this diagnosis, which can be made when a T suppressor/cytotoxic (CD8-positive) lymphocytosis is noted. Steroid therapy should be instituted and amiodarone therapy discontinued in these patients.

Interstitial/alveolar pneumonitis may result from the release of oxygen radicals and/or phospholipidosis and is characterized by findings of diffuse alveolar damage, interstitial pneumonitis or fibrosis in lung biopsy specimens. Phospholipidosis (foamy cells, foamy macrophages), due to inhibition of phospholipase, will be present in most cases of amiodarone-induced pulmonary toxicity; however, these changes also are present in approximately 50% of all patients on amiodarone therapy. These cells should be used as markers of therapy, but not as evidence of toxicity. A diagnosis of amiodarone-induced interstitial/alveolar pneumonitis should lead, at a minimum, to dose reduction or, preferably to withdrawal of the amiodarone to establish reversibility, especially if other acceptable antiarrhythmic therapies are available. Where these measures have been instituted, a reduction in symptoms of amiodarone-induced pulmonary toxicity was usually noted within the first week, and a clinical improvement was greatest in the first two to three weeks. Chest X ray changes usually resolve within two to four months. According to some experts steroids may prove beneficial. Prednisone in doses of 40 to 60 mg/day or equivalent doses of other steroids have been given and tapered over the course of several weeks depending upon the condition of the patient. In some cases rechallenge with amiodarone at a lower dose has not resulted in return of toxicity.

In a patient receiving CORDARONE (amiodarone HCl), any new respiratory symptoms should suggest the possibility of pulmonary toxicity, and the history, physical exam, chest X ray, and pulmonary-function tests (with diffusion capacity) should be repeated and evaluated. A 15% decrease in diffusion capacity has a high sensitivity but only a moderate specificity for pulmonary toxicity; as the decrease in diffusion capacity approaches 30%, the sensitivity decreases but the specificity increases. A gallium-scan also may be performed as part of the diagnostic workup.

Fatalities, secondary to pulmonary toxicity, have occurred in approximately 10% of cases. However, in patients with life-threatening arrhythmias, discontinuation of CORDARONE therapy due to suspected drug-induced pulmonary toxicity should be undertaken with caution, as the most common cause of death in these patients is sudden cardiac death. Therefore, every effort should be made to rule out other causes of respiratory impairment (i.e., congestive heart failure with Swan-Ganz catheterization if necessary, respiratory infection, pulmonary embolism, malignancy etc.) before discontinuing CORDARONE in these patients. In addition, bronchoalveolar lavage, transbronchial lung biopsy and/or open lung biopsy may be necessary to confirm the diagnosis, especially in those cases where no acceptable alternative therapy is available.

If a diagnosis of amiodarone-induced hypersensitivity pneumonitis is made, CORDARONE should be discontinued, and treatment with steroids should be instituted. If a diagnosis of amiodarone-induced interstitial/alveolar pneumonitis is made, steroid therapy should be instituted and, preferably, CORDARONE discontinued or, at a minimum, reduced in dosage. Some cases of amiodarone-induced interstitial/alveolar pneumonitis may resolve following a reduction in CORDARONE dosage in conjunction with the administration of steroids. In some patients, rechallenge at a lower dose has not resulted in return of interstitial/alveolar pneumonitis; however, in some patients (perhaps because of severe alveolar damage) the pulmonary lesions have not been reversible.

Only 1 of more than 1000 patients treated with I.V. amiodarone in clinical studies developed pulmonary fibrosis. For that patient, the condition was diagnosed 3 months after treatment with I.V. amiodarone, during which time she had received **oral** amiodarone. I.V. amiodarone therapy should be discontinued if a diagnosis of pulmonary fibrosis is made.

During clinical studies of I.V. amiodarone, 2% of patients were reported to have adult respiratory distress syndrome (ARDS). ARDS is a disorder characterized by bilateral, diffuse pulmonary infiltrates with pulmonary edema and varying degrees of respiratory insufficiency. The clinical and radiographic picture can arise after a variety of lung injuries, such as those resulting from trauma, shock, prolonged cardiopulmonary resuscitation, and aspiration pneumonia, conditions present in many of the patients enrolled in the clinical studies. It is not possible to determine what role, if any, I.V. amiodarone played in causing or exacerbating the pulmonary disorder in those patients.

Sexual Function/Reproduction: Urogenital System Disorders: Oral amiodarone-induced epididymitis has been observed in some patients. This form of epididymitis is rare, benign, self-limited, and requires no treatment. Physicians should be aware of it to protect their patients from unnecessary invasive urologic examinations and antibiotic therapy.

Skin: Dermatologic Disorders/Photosensitivity: Oral CORDARONE induces photosensitization in about 10% of patients. Sunscreen preparations or protective clothing may afford some protection to individual patients experiencing photosensitization. Blue-grey discoloration of exposed skin has been reported during long-term treatment. With discontinuation of therapy, the pigmentation regresses slowly over a period of up to several years. The risk may be increased in patients of fair complexion or those with excessive sun exposure, and may be related to cumulative dose and duration of therapy.

Special Populations: Pregnant Women: Amiodarone has been shown to be embryotoxic in some animal species. In three different human case reports, both the parent drug and its DEA metabolite have been shown to pass through the placenta, quantitatively ranging between 10 and 50% of human maternal serum concentrations. Although amiodarone use during pregnancy is uncommon, there have been a small number of published reports of congenital goiter/hypothyroidism and hyperthyroidism. Therefore, amiodarone should be used during pregnancy only if the potential benefit to the mother justifies the risk to the fetus.

In addition to causing infrequent congenital goiter/hypothyroidism and hyperthyroidism (see Warnings and Precautions, Endocrine and Metabolism, Neonatal Hypo- or Hyperthyroidism), amiodarone has caused a variety of adverse effects in animals.

In a reproductive study in which amiodarone was given intravenously to rabbits at dosages of 5, 10, or 25 mg/kg per day (about 0.1, 0.3, and 0.7 times the maximum recommended human dose [MRHD] on a body surface area basis), maternal deaths occurred in all groups, including controls. Embryotoxicity (as manifested by fewer full-term fetuses and increased resorptions with concomitantly lower litter weights) occurred at dosages of 10 mg/kg and above. No evidence of embryotoxicity was observed at 5 mg/kg and no teratogenicity was observed at any dosages.

In a teratology study in which amiodarone was administered by continuous i.v. infusion to rats at dosages of 25, 50, or 100 mg/kg per day (about 0.4, 0.7, and 1.4 times the MRHD when compared on a body surface area basis), maternal toxicity (as evidenced by reduced weight gain and food consumption) and embryotoxicity (as evidenced by increased resorptions, decreased live litter size, reduced body weights, and retarded sternum and metacarpal ossification) were observed in the 100 mg/kg group. Intravenous amiodarone should be used during pregnancy only if the potential benefit to the mother justifies the risk to the fetus.

Use During Labour and Delivery: It is not known whether the use of amiodarone during labour or delivery has any immediate or delayed adverse effects. Preclinical studies in rodents have not shown any effect on the duration of gestation or on parturition.

Nursing Women: Amiodarone and its DEA metabolite are excreted in human milk, suggesting that breast-feeding could expose the nursing infant to a significant dose of the drug. Nursing offspring of lactating rats administered amiodarone have demonstrated reduced viability and reduced body weight gains. The risk of exposing the infant to amiodarone should be weighed against the potential benefit of arrhythmia suppression in the mother. The mother should be advised to discontinue nursing.

Pediatrics (<18 years of age): The safety and efficacy of amiodarone in children have not been established; therefore, its use in children is not recommended.

Geriatrics (> 65 years of age): Clinical studies of CORDARONE tablets did not include sufficient number of subjects aged 65 years and over to determine whether they respond differently from younger subjects. Other reported clinical experience has not identified differences in responses between the elderly and younger patients. In general, dose selection for an elderly patient should be cautious, usually starting at the low end of the dosing range, reflecting the greater frequency of decreased hepatic, renal, or cardiac function, and of concomitant disease or other drug therapy.

Monitoring and Laboratory Tests: CORDARONE should be used only by physicians familiar with and with access to (directly or referral) the use of all available modalities for treating recurrent life-threatening ventricular arrhythmias, and who have access to appropriate monitoring facilities, including in-hospital and ambulatory continuous electrocardiographic monitoring and electrophysiologic technique.

In addition, the following should be considered and/or monitored for patient on amiodarone:

Oral Amiodarone: Electrolyte Disturbances : Since antiarrhythmic drugs may be ineffective or may be arrhythmogenic in any patient with potassium or magnesium deficiency, patients with hypokalemia or hypomagnesemia should have the condition corrected before instituting CORDARONE tablets therapy (amiodarone HCl), since these disorders can exaggerate the degree of QTc prolongation and increase the potential for torsades de pointes. Special attention should be given to electrolyte and acid-base in patients experiencing severe or prolonged diarrhea or in patients receiving concomitant diuretics. Use caution when co-administering CORDARONE with drugs which may induce hypokalemia and/or hypomagnesemia.

Thyroid Function: Thyroid function should be monitored prior to treatment and periodically thereafter, particularly in elderly patients, and in any patient with a history of thyroid nodules, goiter, or other thyroid dysfunction. Because of the slow elimination of amiodarone and its metabolites, high plasma iodide levels, altered thyroid function, and abnormal thyroid-function tests may persist for several weeks or even months following CORDARONE withdrawal.

Liver Enzyme Elevations: In patients with life-threatening arrhythmias, the potential risk of hepatic injury should be weighed against the potential benefit of amiodarone therapy. However, patients receiving oral CORDARONE should be monitored carefully for evidence of progressive hepatic injury.

QTc Prolongation: Patients should be monitored carefully for QTc prolongation during amiodarone therapy.

Surgery: It is recommended that FiO_2 and the determinants of oxygen delivery to the tissues (e.g., SaO_2, PaO_2) be closely monitored in patients on CORDARONE.

Elderly: During chronic treatment with oral amiodarone, close monitoring may be prudent for elderly patients.

Ventricular Dysfunction: During chronic treatment with oral amiodarone, close monitoring may be prudent for patients with severe left ventricular dysfunction.

Monitoring Effectiveness: Predicting the effectiveness of any antiarrhythmic agent in long-term prevention of recurrent ventricular tachycardia and ventricular fibrillation is difficult and controversial, with highly qualified investigators recommending use of ambulatory monitoring, programmed electrical stimulation with various stimulation regimens, or a combination of these, to assess response. There is no present consensus on many aspects of how best to assess effectiveness, but there is a reasonable consensus on some aspects:

1. If a patient with a history of cardiac arrest does not manifest a hemodynamically unstable arrhythmia during electrocardiographic monitoring prior to treatment, assessment of the effectiveness of CORDARONE requires some provocative approach, either exercise or programmed electrical stimulation (PES).
2. Whether provocation is also needed in patients who do manifest their life-threatening arrhythmia spontaneously is not settled, but there are reasons to consider PES or other provocation in such patients. In the fraction of patients whose PES-inducible arrhythmia can be made noninducible by CORDARONE (a fraction that has varied widely in various series from less than 10% to almost 40%, perhaps due to different stimulation criteria), the prognosis has been almost uniformly excellent, with very low recurrence (ventricular tachycardia or sudden death) rates. More controversial is the meaning of continued inducibility. There has been an impression that continued inducibility in CORDARONE patients may not foretell a poor prognosis but, in fact, many observers have found greater recurrence rates in patients who remain inducible than in those who do not. A number of criteria have been proposed, however, for identifying patients who remain inducible but who seem likely nonetheless to do well on CORDARONE. These criteria include increased difficulty of induction (more stimuli or more rapid stimuli), which has been reported to predict a lower rate of recurrence, and ability to tolerate the induced ventricular tachycardia without severe symptoms, a finding that has been reported to correlate with better survival but not with lower recurrence rates. While these criteria require confirmation and further study in general, **easier** inducibility or **poorer** tolerance of the induced arrhythmia should suggest consideration of a need to revise treatment.

Several predictors of success not based on PES have also been suggested, including complete elimination of all nonsustained ventricular tachycardia on ambulatory monitoring and very low premature ventricular-beat rates (less than 1 VPB/1000 normal beats).

While these issues remain unsettled for CORDARONE, as for other agents, the prescriber of CORDARONE should have access to (direct or through referral), and familiarity with, the full range of evaluatory procedures used in the care of patients with life-threatening arrhythmias.

It is difficult to describe the effectiveness rates of CORDARONE, as these depend on the specific arrhythmia treated, the success criteria used, the underlying cardiac disease of the patient, the number of drugs tried before resorting to CORDARONE, the duration of follow-up, the dose of CORDARONE, the use of additional antiarrhythmic agents, and many other factors. As CORDARONE has been studied principally in patients with refractory life-threatening ventricular arrhythmias, in whom drug therapy must be selected on the basis of response and cannot be assigned arbitrarily, randomized comparisons with other agents or placebo have not been possible. Reports of series of treated patients with a history of cardiac arrest and mean follow-up of one year or more have given mortality (due to arrhythmia) rates that were highly variable, ranging from less than 5 to over 30%, with most series in the range of 10 to 15%. Overall arrhythmia-recurrence rates (fatal and nonfatal) also were highly variable (and, as noted above, depended on response to PES and other measures), and depend on whether patients who do not seem to respond initially are included. In most cases, considering only patients who seemed to respond well enough to be placed on long-term treatment, recurrence rates have ranged from 20 to 40% in series with a mean follow-up of a year or more.

ADVERSE REACTIONS: Adverse Drug Reaction Overview: Oral CORDARONE (amiodarone HCl): Because of the extensive distribution of amiodarone in body tissues, and the prolonged time required for its elimination from the body following discontinuation of long-term therapy, the relationship between adverse reactions and dosage and duration of therapy, has not been fully established. For some adverse reactions—for example, corneal microdeposits—a relationship to dosage and duration of therapy has been established, so that corneal deposits are reversible with dose-reduction or with discontinuation of therapy. However, for other adverse reactions—for example, fibrosing alveolitis or peripheral neuropathy—the dose relationship and the reversibility of the adverse reaction have not been established. Certain gastrointestinal reactions (e.g., nausea, vomiting, constipation, and bad taste) and central nervous system reactions (e.g., fatigue, headaches, vertigo, nightmares, and sleeplessness) occur frequently at the initiation of therapy when high doses are used. These may disappear on reduction of the dose. The time and dose relationship of adverse events are under continued study.

The most serious and potentially life-threatening adverse effects associated with the use of CORDARONE are pulmonary fibrosis, the aggravation of arrhythmias, and cirrhotic hepatitis. Published data reflecting the North American experience with chronic **oral** CORDARONE therapy suggest that amiodarone-associated adverse drug reactions are very common, having occurred in approximately 75% of patients taking 400 mg or more per day; these adverse events have led to the discontinuation of amiodarone treatment in 7 to 18% of patients. The adverse reactions most frequently requiring discontinuation of CORDARONE have included pulmonary infiltrates or fibrosis, paroxysmal ventricular tachycardia, congestive heart failure, and elevation of liver enzymes. Other symptoms causing discontinuations less often have included visual disturbances, solar dermatitis, blue skin discoloration, hyperthyroidism, and hypothyroidism.

Clinical Trial Adverse Drug Reactions: Because clinical trials are conducted under very specific conditions the adverse reaction rates observed in the clinical trials may not reflect the rates observed in practice and should not be compared to the rates in the clinical trials of another drug. Adverse drug reaction information from clinical trials is useful for identifying drug-related adverse events and for approximating rates.

Please see Table 1 (oral Cordarone) and Table 2 (intravenous amiodarone).

Commonly Observed Adverse Reactions: Intravenous Amiodarone: In a total of 1836 patients in controlled and uncontrolled clinical trials, 14% of patients received I.V. amiodarone for up to 1 week, 5% received it for up to 2 weeks, 2% received it for up to 3 weeks, and 1% received it for more than 3 weeks, without an increased incidence of serious adverse events. The mean duration of therapy in these studies was 5.6 days.

Overall, treatment was discontinued in 9% of the patients because of adverse events. The most common serious adverse events leading to discontinuation of I.V. amiodarone therapy were ventricular tachycardia (2%), hypotension (2%), cardiac arrest (asystole/cardiac arrest/electromechanical dissociation) (1%), and cardiogenic shock (1%).

The following adverse events are based upon retrospective multicentre analysis of 241 patients treated at various doses of amiodarone for 2 to 1515 days (mean duration: 441.3 days).

Table 2 lists the most common (incidence ≥1%) adverse drug reactions during I.V. amiodarone therapy that were collected from controlled and open-label clinical trials involving 1836 patients with hemodynamically unstable VT or VF.

Table 1: CORDARONE

Incidence of Adverse Events in Patients Receiving Oral Cordarone

Body System	Incidence % n=241	Adverse Event
Gastrointestinal	10–33	Nausea, vomiting
	4–9	Constipation, anorexia
	1–3	Abdominal pain, dyspepsia, diarrhea, abnormal taste, dry mouth
Dermatologic	4–9	Solar dermatitis/photosensitivity
	1–3	Blue skin discolouration, rash
	<1	Alopecia, onycholysis
Neurologic	4–9	Malaise/fatigue, tremor/abnormal involuntary movements, lack of coordination, abnormal gait/ataxia, dizziness, paresthesias
	1–3	Decreased libido/impotence, insomnia and other sleep disturbances, headache, cognitive disturbances and disorders of alertness, general weakness, peripheral motor and sensory neuropathies
	<1	Tinnitus

(cont'd)

Table 1: CORDARONE *(cont'd)*

Incidence of Adverse Events in Patients Receiving Oral Cordarone

Body System	Incidence % n=241	Adverse Event
Opthalmologic	10–33	Corneal microdeposits
	4–9	Visual disturbances
	up to 2	Optic neuropathology with visual impairment/decreased acuity[a]
Hepatic	4–9	Hepatomegaly, abnormal liver function test results
	1–3	Non-specific hepatic disorders
Respiratory	4–9	Pulmonary inflammation or fibrosis
Cardiovascular	1–3	Congestive heart failure, cardiac arrhythmias, SA node dysfunction
	<1	Hypotension, cardiac conduction abnormalities
Thyroid	1–3	Hyperthyroidism, hypothyroidism
	<1	Goiter
Other	1–3	Flushing, coagulation abnormalities
	<1	Spontaneous ecchymosis, epididymitis

[a] Based on one retrospective study from 1981 to June 1986 at the Mayo Clinic, up to 2% optic neuropath with visual impairment/decreased acuity.

Table 2: CORDARONE

Summary Tabulation of Adverse Drug Reactions in Patients Receiving Cordarone I.V. Amiodarone in Controlled and Open-Label Studies (≥1% Incidence)

Study Event	Controlled Trials (N=814)	Open-Label Trials (N=1022)	Total Incidence (N=1836)
Any Adverse Reactions	412 (50.6%)	384 (37.5%)	796 (43.3%)
Body as a Whole	54 (6.6%)	32 (3.1%)	86 (4.6%)
Fever	24 (2.9%)	13 (1.2%)	37 (2.0%)
Cardiovascular System	308 (37.8%)	264 (25.8%)	572 (31.1%)
Atrial Fibrillation	15 (1.8%)	9 (<1)	24 (1.3%)
AV Block	14 (1.5%)	12 (1.2%)	26 (1.4%)
Bradycardia	49 (6.0%)	41 (4.0%)	90 (4.9%)
Congestive Heart Failure	18 (2.2%)	21 (2.0%)	39 (2.1%)
Heart Arrest	29 (3.5%)	26 (2.5%)	55 (2.9%)
Hypotension	165 (20.2%)	123 (12.0%)	288 (15.6%)
Nodal Arrhythmia	15 (1.8%)	15 (1.4%)	30 (1.6%)
QT Interval Prolonged	15 (1.8%)	4 (<1%)	19 (1.0%)
Shock	13 (1.5%)	12 (1.1%)	25 (1.3%)
Ventricular Fibrillation	12 (1.4%)	13 (1.2%)	25 (1.3%)
Ventricular Tachycardia	15 (1.8%)	30 (2.9%)	45 (2.4%)
Digestive System	102 (12.5%)	97 (9.4%)	199 (10.8%)
Diarrhea	8 (<1%)	12 (1.1%)	20 (1.0%)
Liver Function Tests Abnormal	35 (4.2%)	29 (2.8%)	64 (3.4%)
Nausea	29 (3.5%)	43 (4.2%)	72 (3.9%)
Vomiting	16 (1.9%)	17 (1.6%)	33 (1.7%)
Hemic and Lymphatic System	34 (4.1%)	34 (3.3%)	68 (3.7%)
Thrombocytopenia	14 (1.7%)	16 (1.5%)	30 (1.6%)
Metabolic and Nutritional	56 (6.8%)	49 (4.7%)	105 (5.7%)
AST Increased	14 (1.7%)	6 (<1%)	20 (1.0%)
ALT Increased	14 (1.7%)	5 (<1%)	19 (1.0%)
Nervous System	46 (5.6%)	38 (3.7%)	84 (4.5%)
Respiratory System	54 (6.6%)	61 (5.9%)	115 (6.2%)
Lung Edema	6 (<1%)	15 (1.4%)	21 (1.1%)
Respiratory Disorder	11 (1.3%)	8 (<1%)	19 (1.0%)
Urogenital System	27 (3.3%)	30 (2.9%)	57 (3.1%)

(cont'd)

Table 2: CORDARONE *(cont'd)*

Summary Tabulation of Adverse Drug Reactions in Patients Receiving Cordarone I.V. Amiodarone in Controlled and Open-Label Studies (≥1% Incidence)

Study Event	Controlled Trials (N=814)	Open-Label Trials (N=1022)	Total Incidence (N=1836)
Kidney Function Abnormal	8 (<1%)	16 (1.5%)	24 (1.3%)

Ophthalmological Abnormalities: Corneal microdeposits are apparent upon slit-lamp examination in virtually all adult patients who have taken amiodarone for longer than 6 months. These deposits may give rise to symptoms such as visual halos or blurred vision (see Warnings and Precautions). Other reported amiodarone-associated abnormalities have included photophobia corneal degeneration, papilledema, photosensitivity, eye discomfort, dry eyes, scotoma, lens opacities, and macular degeneration, optic neuropathy and/or optic neuritis, in some cases progressing to permanent blindness (See Warnings and Precautions, Ophthalmologic).

Neurological Abnormalities: Occurring in 20 to 40% of patients, these common problems have included ataxia, tremor, fatigue, dizziness, weakness, sleep disorders, headaches, cognitive disorders, disturbances of alertness, peripheral motor and sensory neuropathies, proximal muscle weakness, impotence (see Warnings And Precautions, Neurologic) and pseudotumor cerebri. There have been spontaneous reports of demyelinating polyneuropathy.

Pulmonary Abnormalities: In some studies symptomatic pulmonary disease has been detected at rates as high as 10 to 15%, whereas asymptomatic abnormalities of pulmonary diffusion capacity have been demonstrated at greater than twice that incidence. Pulmonary toxicity has been fatal about 10% of the time (see Warnings and Precautions, Respiratory).

Cardiovascular Abnormalities: Exacerbation of arrhythmia has had a reported incidence of about 2 to 5% in most series (new ventricular fibrillation, incessant ventricular tachycardia, increased resistance to cardioversion, and paroxysmal polymorphic ventricular tachycardia (torsades de pointes). In addition, symptomatic bradycardia or sinus arrest with suppression of escape foci has occurred in 2 to 4% of patients. Congestive heart failure has occurred in approximately 3% of patients. Second degree AV block and left bundle branch block (LBBB) have occurred in less than 1% of patients, vasculitis and angioedema have also been reported. Hypotension independent of - as well as associated with - discontinuation of cardiopulmonary bypass following open heart surgery has also been reported (see Warnings and Precautions, Cardiovascular).

Gastrointestinal Abnormalities: Complaints of this nature have occurred in about 25% of patients and have included nausea, vomiting, constipation, anorexia, abnormal taste and smell, abnormal salivation, dyspepsia, abdominal pain, and diarrhoea (see Warnings and Precautions, Gastrointestinal).

Hepatic Abnormalities: Abnormal elevations of serum levels of enzymes associated with hepatic dysfunction have occurred in approximately 15% of patients. Symptomatic hepatitis has occurred in less than 1% of patients, and cholestatic hepatitis and cirrhosis have been reported (see Warnings and Precautions, Hepatic/Biliary/Pancreatic). The frequency of rare serious liver injury, abnormal liver-function tests, hepatitis, cholestatic hepatitis and cirrhosis is undetermined. Overt liver disease can occur however, and has been fatal in a few cases.

Dermatologic Abnormalities: These have occurred in approximately 15% of patients, with photosensitivity (10% of patients) being the most common. Blue-grey skin pigmentation has been reported in 2 to 3% of patients. Hair loss (alopecia) has been observed in up to 4% of patients. Other amiodarone-associated phenomena reported with less than 1% incidence have included non-specific skin eruptions, pruritus, acquired keratoderma, hyperhidrosis, onycholysis, generalized pustular psoriasis, vasculitis and polyserositis, and toxic epidermal necrolysis (sometimes fatal) (see Warnings and Precautions, Skin, Dermatologic Disorders/Photosensitivity).

Thyroid Abnormalities: Amiodarone-associated hypothyroidism has been reported in 2 to 4% of patients in most series but in 8 to 10% of patients with other series: hyperthyroidism has been reported in 1 to 3% of patients (see Warnings and Precautions, Endocrine and Metabolism, Thyrotoxicosis).

Post-Market Adverse Drug Reactions: CORDARONE INTRAVENOUS is no longer marketed.

In post-marketing surveillance, hypotension (sometimes fatal), sinus arrest, anaphylactic/anaphylactoid reaction (including shock), angioedema, urticaria, eosinophilic pneumonia, hepatitis, cholestatic hepatitis, cirrhosis, pancreatitis, renal impairment, renal insufficiency, acute renal failure, bronchospasm, possibly fatal respiratory disorders (including distress, failure, arrest, and ARDS), bronchiolitis obliterans organizing pneumonia (possibly fatal), fever, dyspnea, cough, hemoptysis, wheezing, hypoxia, pulmonary infiltrates and/or mass, pulmonary alveolar hemorrhage, pleural effusion, pleuritis, pseudotumor cerebri, syndrome of inappropriate antidiuretic hormone secretion (SIADH), thyroid nodules/thyroid cancer, toxic epidermal necrolysis (sometimes fatal), erythema multiforme, Stevens-Johnson syndrome, exfoliative dermatitis, eczema, skin cancer, vasculitis, pruritus, hemolytic anemia, aplastic anemia, pancytopenia, neutropenia, thrombocytopenia, agranulocytosis, granuloma, myopathy, muscle weakness, rhabdomyolysis, demyelinating polyneuropathy, hallucination, confusional state, disorientation, delirium, epididymitis, and impotence, also have been reported in patients receiving amiodarone.

Women receiving amiodarone have been reported to be at greater risk of experiencing torsade de pointes.

Also, in patients receiving recommended dosages, there have been postmarketing reports of the following injection site reactions: pain, erythema, edema, pigment changes, venous thrombosis, phlebitis, thrombophlebitis, cellulitis, necrosis, and skin sloughing (see Dosage and Administration).

DRUG INTERACTIONS: Drug-Drug Interactions: See Table 3 and Table 4.

Table 3: CORDARONE

Summary of Drug Interactions with Amiodarone

Drugs Whose Effects May Be Increased By Amiodarone	
Concomitant Drug	**Interaction**
Warfarin	Increases prothrombin time.
Digoxin	**Oral** amiodarone, increases digoxin serum concentration by 70% after one day. May reach toxic levels with resultant clinical toxicity.
Digitalis	With **oral** amiodarone, the need for digitalis therapy should be reviewed and the dose reduced by approximately 50% or discontinued. If digitalis treatment is continued, serum levels should be closely monitored and patients observed for clinical evidence of toxicity. These precautions probably should apply to digitoxin administration as well.
Quinidine	Increases quinidine serum concentration by 33% after two days. Quinidine dose should be reduced by 1/3 when administered with amiodarone.
Procainamide	Increases plasma concentrations of procainamide and n-acetyl procainamide by 55% and 33%, respectively if taken for less than 7 days. Procainamide dose should be reduced by 1/3 when administered with amiodarone.
Flecainide	Plasma levels of flecainide have been reported to increase in the presence of oral amiodarone; because of this, the dosage of flecainide should be adjusted when these drugs are administered concomitantly.
Lidocaine	**Oral:** Sinus bradycardia was observed in a patient receiving oral amiodarone who was given lidocaine for local anaesthesia. **I.V.:** Seizure associated with increased lidocaine concentrations was observed in one patient.
Phenytoin	Increases phenytoin serum concentration.
Disopyramide	Increases QT prolongation which could cause arrhythmia.

(cont'd)

Table 3: CORDARONE *(cont'd)*

Summary of Drug Interactions with Amiodarone

Drugs Whose Effects May Be Increased By Amiodarone	
Concomitant Drug	**Interaction**
Fentanyl	May cause hypotension, bradycardia, decreased cardiac output.
Cyclosporine	Administered in combination with **oral** amiodarone, produces persistently elevated plasma concentrations of cyclosporine resulting in elevated creatinine, despite reduction in dose of cyclosporine.
Fluoroquinolones, Macrolide Antibiotics, Azoles	Are known to cause QTc prolongation. There have been reports of QTc prolongation, with or without torsades de pointes, in patients taking amiodarone when fluoroquinolones, macrolide antibiotics, or azoles were administered concomitantly.

Table 4: CORDARONE

Summary of Drug Interactions With Amiodarone

Drugs That May Interfere with the Actions of Amiodarone	
Concomitant Drug	**Interaction**
Cholestyramine	Increases enterohepatic recirculation of amiodarone and may reduce serum levels and $t_{½}$.
Cimetidine	Increases serum amiodarone levels.
Phenytoin	Decreases serum amiodarone levels.

Volatile Anaesthetic Agents: Close perioperative monitoring is recommended in patients undergoing general anaesthesia who are on amiodarone therapy as they may be more sensitive to the myocardial depressant and conduction effect of halogenated inhalation anaesthetics.

Beta Blockers: Amiodarone should be used with caution in patients receiving β-receptor blocking agents (e.g., propranolol, a CYP3A4 inhibitor) because of the possible potentiation of bradycardia, sinus arrest, and AV block. If necessary, amiodarone can continue to be used after insertion of a pacemaker in patients with severe bradycardia or sinus arrest.

Calcium Channel Antagonists: Amiodarone should be used with caution in patients receiving calcium channel antagonists (e.g., verapamil, a CYP3A4 substrate, and diltiazem, a CYP3A4 inhibitor) because of the possible potentiation of bradycardia, sinus arrest, and AV block. If necessary, amiodarone can continue to be used after insertion of a pacemaker in patients with severe bradycardia or sinus arrest.

Anticoagulants: Potentiation of warfarin-type (CYP2C9 and CYP3A4 substrate) anticoagulant response is almost always seen in patients receiving amiodarone and can result in serious or fatal bleeding. Since the concomitant administration of warfarin with amiodarone increases the prothrombin time by 100% after 3 to 4 days, the dose of warfarin should be reduced by one-third to one-half, and prothombin times should be monitored closely.

Clopidogrel, an inactive thienopyridine prodrug, is metabolized in the liver by CYP3A4 to an active metabolite. A potential interaction between clopidogrel and amiodarone resulting in ineffective inhibition of platelet aggregation has been reported.

Antidepressants: Trazodone, an antidepressant, is metabolized primarily by CYP3A4. QT interval prolongation and torsade de pointes have been reported with the co-administration of trazodone and amiodarone.

Drugs Affecting Cardiac Conduction: Hemodynamic and electrophysiologic interactions have also been observed after concomitant administration with propranolol, diltiazem, and verapamil.

Antiarrhythmics: In general, combination of amiodarone with other antiarrhythmic therapy should be reserved for patients with life-threatening ventricular arrhythmias who are incompletely responsive to a single agent or incompletely responsive to amiodarone. During transfer to amiodarone the dose levels of previously administered agents should be reduced by 30 to 50% several days after the addition of amiodarone, when arrhythmia suppression should be beginning.

The continued need for the other antiarrhythmic agent should be reviewed after the effects of amiodarone have been established, and discontinuation ordinarily should be attempted. If the treatment is continued, these patients should be particularly carefully monitored for adverse effects, especially conduction disturbances and exacerbation of tachyarrhythmias, as amiodarone is continued. In amiodarone-treated patients who require additional antiarrhythmic therapy, the initial dose of such agents should be approximately half of the usual recommended dose.

Interactions via Cytochrome P450 System: Amiodarone is metabolized to desethylamiodarone by the cytochrome P450 (CYP450) enzyme group, specifically cytochrome P450 3A4 (CYP3A4) and CYP2C8. The CYP3A4 isoenzyme is present in both the liver and intestines (see Action and Clinical Pharmacology, Pharmacokinetics). Amiodarone is a substrate and an inhibitor of CYP3A4 and a substrate of p-glycoprotein. Therefore, amiodarone has the potential for interactions with drugs or substances that may be substrates, inhibitors or inducers of CYP3A4 and substrates of p-glycoprotein. While only a limited number of in vivo drug-drug interactions with amiodarone have been reported, chiefly with the **oral** formulation, the potential for other interactions should be anticipated. This is especially important for drugs associated with serious toxicity, such as other antiarrhythmics. If such drugs are needed, their dose should be reassessed and, where appropriate, plasma concentration measured. In view of the long and variable half-life of amiodarone, potential for drug interactions exists not only with concomitant medication but also with drugs administered after discontinuation of amiodarone.

Examples of Drugs that May Have Serum Concentrations Increased By Amiodarone: Amiodarone inhibits p-glycoprotein and certain CYP450 enzymes (enzyme inhibition). This can result in unexpectedly high plasma levels of other drugs which are metabolized by those CYP450 enzymes or are substrates of p-glycoprotein and may lead to toxic effects. Reported examples of this interaction include the following:

HMG-CoA Reductase Inhibitors: HMG-CoA reductase inhibitors that are CYP3A4 substrates (including simvastatin and atorvastatin) in combination with amiodarone have been associated with reports of myopathy/rhabdomyolysis.

Immunosuppressives: Oral amiodarone administered in combination with Cyclosporine (CYP3A4 substrate) has been reported to produce persistently elevated plasma concentrations of cyclosporine resulting in elevated creatinine, despite reduction in dose of cyclosporine. Combination of amiodarone with other antiarrhythmic therapy should be reserved for patients with life-threatening ventricular arrhythmias who are incompletely responsive to a single agent or incompletely responsive to amiodarone. During transfer to amiodarone the dose levels of previously administered agents should be reduced by 30 to 50% several days after the addition of amiodarone, when arrhythmia suppression should be beginning. The continued need for the other antiarrhythmic agent should be reviewed after the effects of amiodarone have been established, and discontinuation ordinarily should be attempted. If the treatment is continued, these patients should be particularly carefully monitored for adverse effects, especially conduction disturbances and exacerbation of tachyarrhythmias, as amiodarone is continued. In amiodarone-treated patients who require additional antiarrhythmic therapy, the initial dose of such agents should be approximately half of the usual recommended dose.

Antihypertensives: Amiodarone should be used with caution in patients receiving -receptor blocking agents (e.g., propranolol, a CYP3A4 inhibitor) or calcium channel antagonists (e.g., verapamil, a CYP3A4 substrate, and diltiazem, a CYP3A4 inhibitor) because of the possible potentiation of bradycardia, sinus arrest, and AV block; if necessary, amiodarone can continue to be used after insertion of a pacemaker in patients with severe bradycardia or sinus arrest.

Anticoagulants: Potentiation of warfarin-type (CYP2C9 and CYP3A4 substrate) anticoagulant response is almost always seen in patients receiving amiodarone and can result in serious or fatal bleeding. Since the concomitant administration of warfarin with amiodarone increases the prothrombin time by 100% after 3 to 4 days, the dose of the anticoagulant should be reduced by one-third to one-half, and prothrombin times should be monitored closely.

Since amiodarone is a substrate for CYP3A4 and CYP2C8, drugs/substances that inhibit these isoenzymes may decrease the metabolism and increase serum concentrations of amiodarone, with the potential for toxic effects. Reported examples include the following:

Protease Inhibitors: Protease inhibitors are known to inhibit CYP3A4 to varying degrees. Inhibition of CYP3A4 by indinavir has been reported to result in increased serum concentrations of amiodarone. Monitoring for amiodarone toxicity and serial measurement of amiodarone serum concentration during concomitant protein inhibitor therapy should be considered.

Histamine H1 antagonists: Loratadine, a non-sedating antihistaminic, is metabolized primarily by CYP3A4. QT interval prolongation and torsade de pointes have been reported with the co-administration of loratadine and amiodarone.

Other Drugs: Dextromethorphan is a substrate for both CYP2D6 and CYP3A4. Amiodarone inhibits CYP2D6.

Some drugs/substances are known to accelerate the metabolism of amiodarone by stimulating the synthesis of CYP3A4 (enzyme induction). This may lead to low amiodarone serum levels and potential decrease in efficacy. Reported examples of this interaction include the following:

Antibiotics: Rifampin is a potent inducer of CYP3A4. Administration of rifampin concomitantly with oral amiodarone has been shown to result in decreases in serum concentrations of amiodarone and desethylamiodarone.

In addition to the interactions noted above, chronic (>2 weeks) **oral** CORDARONE administration impairs metabolism of phenytoin, dextromethorphan, and methotrexate.

Drug-Food Interactions: Grapefruit Juice: Grapefruit juice inhibits CYP3A4-mediated metabolism of **oral** amiodarone in the intestinal mucosa, resulting in significant increased plasma levels of amiodarone (C_{max} and AUC increased by 84% and 50%, respectively); therefore, grapefruit juice should not be taken during treatment with **oral** amiodarone. Therefore, this information should be considered when changing from intravenous amiodarone to **oral** amiodarone.

Drug-Herb Interactions: St. John's Wort: St. John's Wort (Hypericum perforatum) induces CYP3A4. Since amiodarone is a substrate for CYP3A4, there is the potential that the use of St. John's Wort in patients receiving amiodarone could result in reduced amiodarone levels.

DOSAGE AND ADMINISTRATION: Dosing Considerations: Oral CORDARONE (amiodarone HCl): General Considerations: BECAUSE OF THE UNIQUE PHARMACOKINETIC PROPERTIES, DIFFICULT DOSING SCHEDULE, AND SEVERITY OF SIDE EFFECTS IF PATIENTS ARE IMPROPERLY MONITORED, CORDARONE (AMIODARONE HCL) THERAPY SHOULD BE INITIATED IN HOSPITAL AND CONTINUED IN A MONITORED ENVIRONMENT UNTIL ADEQUATE CONTROL OF THE ARRHYTHMIA HAS OCCURRED. PATIENTS TREATED WITH CORDARONE SHOULD BE UNDER THE SUPERVISION OF A CARDIOLOGIST OR A PHYSICIAN WITH EQUIVALENT EXPERIENCE IN CARDIOLOGY WHO IS EXPERIENCED IN THE TREATMENT OF LIFE-THREATENING ARRHYTHMIAS, WHO IS THOROUGHLY FAMILIAR WITH THE RISK AND BENEFIT OF CORDARONE THERAPY, AND WHO HAS ACCESS TO LABORATORY FACILITIES CAPABLE OF ADEQUATELY MONITORING EFFECTIVENESS AND SIDE EFFECTS OF TREATMENT. DOSE ADMINISTRATION MUST BE INDIVIDUALIZED, PARTICULARLY TAKING INTO ACCOUNT CONCOMITANT ANTIARRHYTHMIC THERAPY.

The dosage schedule for CORDARONE (amiodarone HCl) is still somewhat controversial, probably in part due to its poor absorption, unusually long elimination half-life, and huge volume of distribution. Extensive tissue stores of amiodarone hydrochloride must be established before the effects on the heart of **oral** dose administration are apparent. Intersubject variability as well as differences in dosage regimens and methods of assessment have made it difficult to precisely define the time of onset of initial and maximal antiarrhythmic effect in an individual patient. In order to ensure that an antiarrhythmic effect will be observed without waiting several months, loading doses are required. A uniform, optimal dosage schedule for administration of CORDARONE has not been determined. Because of the food effect on the absorption of CORDARONE, administration of CORDARONE should be consistent with regard to meals. (see Action and Clinical Pharmacology, Pharmacokinetics). Amiodarone's antiarrhythmic effect after oral administration may be noted in as early as 3 days (72 hours) but more often takes 1 to 3 weeks.

Because of the slow rate of elimination of amiodarone, its antiarrhythmic effects may persist for weeks or months after its discontinuation, but the time of arrhythmia recurrence is variable and unpredictable. In general, when the drug is resumed after recurrence of the arrhythmia, control is established more rapidly relative to the initial response, possibly because tissue stores were not wholly depleted at the time of recurrence.

The combination of CORDARONE with other antiarrhythmic therapy should be reserved for patients with life-threatening arrhythmias who are unresponsive to adequate doses of a single agent (see Drug Interactions).

Recommended Dose and Dosage Adjustment: Adult Dosage: Ventricular Arrhythmias: Loading Dose: Loading doses of 800 to 1600 mg/day are required for 1 to 3 weeks (occasionally longer) until therapeutic response occurs. (Administration of CORDARONE in divided doses at meals is suggested for total daily doses of 1000 mg or higher, when gastrointestinal intolerance occurs). If side effects become excessive, the dose should be reduced.

Since grapefruit juice is known to inhibit CYP3A4-mediated metabolism of oral amiodarone in the intestinal mucosa, resulting in significant increased plasma levels of amiodarone, grapefruit juice should not be taken during treatment with oral amiodarone (see Drug Interactions).

Maintenance Dose: When adequate arrhythmia control has been achieved, or if adverse drug reactions become prominent, the CORDARONE dose should be reduced to 600 to 800 mg/day for one month and then to the maintenance dose, usually 200 to 400 mg/day (occasionally 600 mg/day). CORDARONE may be administered as a single daily dose, or in patients with severe gastrointestinal intolerance, as a b.i.d. dose. In each patient, the chronic maintenance dose should be determined according to antiarrhythmic effect as assessed by symptoms, Holter recordings, and/or programmed electrical stimulation, and by patient tolerance. Plasma concentrations may be helpful in evaluating nonresponsiveness or unexpectedly severe toxicity.

The lowest effective dose should be used to prevent the occurrence of adverse drug reactions. In all instances, the physician must be guided by the severity of the individual patient's arrhythmia and response to therapy. When dose adjustments are necessary, the patient should be closely monitored for an extended period of time because of the long and variable half-life of amiodarone and the difficulty in predicting the time required to attain a new steady-state level of drug. Dosage suggestions are summarized in Table 5.

Table 5: CORDARONE

Oral Cordarone Dosage for Ventricular Arrhythmia Suppression

Loading Dose (Daily)	Adjustment and Maintenance Dose (Daily)	
1–3 weeks	1 month	usual maintenance
800–1600 mg	600–800 mg	200–400 mg (some 600 mg)

Elderly Patients: In general, dose selection for an elderly patient should be cautious, usually starting at the low end of the dosing range, reflecting the greater frequency of decreased hepatic, renal, or cardiac function, and of concomitant disease or other drug therapy.

Administration: CORDARONE may be administered as a single daily dose, or in patients with severe gastrointestinal intolerance, as a b.i.d. dose.

Food increases the rate and extent of absorption of amiodarone. Because of the food effect on the absorption of CORDARONE, administration of CORDARONE should be consistent with regard to meals.

Administration of CORDARONE in divided doses at meals is suggested for total daily doses of 1000 mg or higher, when gastrointestinal intolerance occurs. If side effects become excessive, the dose should be reduced.

OVERDOSAGE:

There have been cases, some fatal, of CORDARONE overdose. Overdose may lead to severe bradycardia and to conduction disturbances with the appearance of an idioventricular rhythm, particularly in elderly patients or patients on digitalis therapy.

One report of the acute ingestion of a single 8 g dose of **oral** CORDARONE by a healthy 20 year old female has been reported. At first assessment, the patient was conscious and profuse perspiration and a slight tachycardia were the only abnormal findings on clinical observation. Slight bradycardia was observed during the second and third day; thereafter, QT interval and heart rate returned to normal. No clinical adverse events were documented over the subsequent 3 month monitoring period.

The acute oral LD_{50} of amiodarone HCl in mice and rats is greater than 3000 mg/kg.

Intravenous Amiodarone: There have been cases, some fatal, of amiodarone overdose. Effects of an inadvertent overdose of I.V. amiodarone include hypotension, cardiogenic shock, bradycardia, AV block, and hepatotoxicity. Hypotension and cardiogenic shock should be treated by slowing the infusion rate or with standard therapy: vasopressor drugs, positive inotropic agents and volume expansion. Bradycardia and AV block may require temporary pacing. Hepatic enzyme concentrations should be monitored closely. Neither amiodarone nor DEA is dialyzable.

Overdosage Management: If an overdose should occur, gastric lavage or induced emesis should be employed to reduce absorption, in addition to general supportive measures. The patient's cardiac rhythm and blood pressure should be monitored, and if clinically significant bradycardia ensues, a β-adrenergic agonist or a temporary pacemaker should be used. Hypotension with inadequate tissue perfusion should be treated with positive inotropic and/or vasopressor agents. Neither amiodarone nor its metabolite is dialyzable.

For management of a suspected drug overdose, CPhA recommends that you contact your **regional Poison Control Centre**. See the *CPS* Directory section for a list of Poison Control Centres.

ACTION AND CLINICAL PHARMACOLOGY: Mechanism of Action: CORDARONE (amiodarone HCl) is generally considered a class III antiarrhythmic drug, but it possesses electrophysiologic characteristics of all four Vaughan Williams classes. Like Class I drugs, amiodarone blocks sodium channels at rapid pacing frequencies, and like Class II drugs, it exerts antisympathetic activity. One of its main effects, with prolonged administration, is to lengthen the cardiac action potential, a Class III effect. The negative chronotropic effect of amiodarone in nodal tissues is similar to the effect of Class IV drugs. In addition to blocking sodium channels, amiodarone blocks myocardial potassium channels, which contributes to slowing of conduction and prolongation of refractoriness (class III effect). The antisympathetic action and block of calcium and potassium channels are responsible for the negative dromotropic effects on the sinus node and for the slowing of conduction and prolongation of refractoriness in the atrioventricular (AV) node.

Additionally, amiodarone has vasodilatory action that can decrease cardiac workload and consequently myocardial oxygen consumption.

A comparison of the electrophysiologic effects of oral and intravenous (I.V.) amiodarone is shown in Table 6.

Table 6: CORDARONE

Effects of Oral and Intravenous Amiodarone on Electrophysiologic Parameters

Formulation	SCL	QRS	QTc	AH	HV	ERP RA	ERP RV	ERP AVN
Oral	↑	↔	↑	↑	↔	↑	↑	↑
Intravenous	↔	↔	↔	↑	↔	↔	↔	↑

Legend: ↔ No change; SCL=sinus cycle length; QRS=a measure of intraventricular conduction; QTc=corrected QT, a measure of repolarization; AH=atrial His, a measure of intranodal conduction; HV=His ventricular, a measure of infranodal conduction; ERP=effective refractory period; RA=right atrium; RV=right ventricle; AVN=atrioventricular node.

At higher doses (>10 mg/kg) of I.V. amiodarone, prolongation of the ERP RV and modest prolongation of the QRS have been seen. These differences between oral and intravenous focused on the AV node, causing an intranodal conduction delay and increased nodal refractoriness due to calcium channel blockade (Class IV activity) and β-adrenoreceptor antagonism (Class II activity).

Pharmacodynamics: Amiodarone has been reported to produce negative inotropic and vasodilating effects in animals and humans. After long-term treatment with **oral** amiodarone in a dose range of 200 to 600 mg/day, patients with decreased left ventricular ejection fraction (LVEF) show no significant change in mean LVEF. Hypotension is uncommon (<1%) during chronic **oral** amiodarone therapy. In clinical studies of patients with refractory ventricular fibrillation (VF) or hemodynamically unstable ventricular tachycardia (VT), drug-related hypotension occurred in 15.6% of 1836 patients treated with I.V. amiodarone. No correlations were seen between the baseline ejection fraction and the occurrence of clinically significant hypotension during infusion of I.V. amiodarone.

Pharmacokinetics: Absorption: The absorption of **oral** amiodarone is slow and variable, with peak serum amiodarone concentrations being attained at 3 to 12 hours after administration. Absorption may continue for up to 15 hours after **oral** ingestion. There is extensive intersubject variation: mean **oral** bioavailability is approximately 50% (mean range, 33 to 65%). First-pass metabolism in the gut wall and liver appears to be an important factor in determining the systemic availability of the drug. The mean terminal half-life after steady-state administration is approximately 53 days and has been found in one study (n=8) to range from 26 to 107 days. Since at least 3 to 4 half-lives are needed to approach steady-state concentrations, loading doses must be administered at the onset of oral amiodarone therapy. In the absence of a loading-dose period, steady-state plasma concentrations, at constant oral dosing, would therefore be reached between 130 and 535 days, with an average of 265 days. For the metabolite, the mean plasma-elimination half-life was approximately 61 days. These data probably reflect an initial elimination of drug from well-perfused tissue (the 2.5- to 10- day half-life phase), followed by a terminal phase representing extremely slow elimination from poorly perfused tissue compartments such as fat.

Food increases the rate and extent of absorption of amiodarone. The effects of food upon the bioavailability of amiodarone have been studied in thirty healthy subjects who received a single 600 mg dose both immediately after consuming a meal and following an overnight fast. The area under the plasma concentration-time curve (AUC) and the peak plasma concentration (C_{max}) of amiodarone increase by as much as 2.4 and 3.8 times, respectively, in the presence of food. Food also increased the rate of absorption, decreasing the time to peak plasma concentration (T_{max}) by 37%.

Distribution: Amiodarone has a very high apparent volume of distribution (approximately 5000 L) with an extensive accumulation in tissues, especially adipose tissues, and in highly perfused organs such as liver, lung, spleen, heart and kidney. One major metabolite of amiodarone, desethylamiodarone, has been identified, but the pharmacological activity of this metabolite is not known in humans. During chronic treatment, the plasma ratio of metabolite to parent compound approximates 1.

Amiodarone exhibits complex disposition characteristics after intravenous administration. Peak serum concentrations after single 5 mg/kg 15-minute intravenous infusions in healthy subjects range between 5 and 41 mg/L. Peak concentrations after 150 mg supplemental infusions in patients with ventricular fibrillation (VF) or hemodynamically unstable ventricular tachycardia (VT) range between 7 and 26 mg/L. Due to rapid disposition, serum concentrations decline to 10% of peak values within 30 to 45 minutes after the end of the infusion. In clinical trials, after 48 hours of continued infusions (125, 500, or 1000 mg/day) plus supplemental (150 mg) infusions (for recurrent arrhythmias), amiodarone mean serum concentrations between 0.7 to 1.4 mg/L were observed (n=260).

Metabolism: Amiodarone is eliminated primarily by hepatic metabolism and biliary excretion. Desethylamiodarone (DEA) is the major active metabolite of amiodarone. At the usual amiodarone daily maintenance dose of 400 mg, mean steady-state DEA/amiodarone ratios ranged from 0.61 to 0.93. High-dose oral amiodarone loading in patients yielded 24-hour DEA/amiodarone ratios of 0.083 to 0.19. High-dose intravenous loading yielded a mean 24-hour DEA/amiodarone ratio of 0.041. No data are presently available on the activity of DEA in humans, but animal studies have shown that it has significant electrophysiologic and antiarrhythmic properties. The major enzyme responsible for the N-deethylation to DEA is believed to be cytochrome P450 3A4. Large interindividual variability in CYP-450 3A4 activity may explain the variable systemic availability of amiodarone. DEA is highly lipophilic and has a very large apparent volume of distribution, showing a higher concentration than amiodarone in all tissue except fat at steady-state. Myocardial concentrations of DEA are approximately 3- to 4.5-fold greater than those of amiodarone during long-term **oral** amiodarone therapy. However, after either acute oral or acute intravenous administration, both mean serum and mean myocardial DEA concentrations are quite low compared to those of amiodarone.

Excretion: Amiodarone is eliminated primarily by hepatic metabolism and biliary excretion. There is negligible excretion of amiodarone or DEA in urine. Neither amiodarone nor DEA is dialyzable. Amiodarone and DEA cross the placenta and both appear in breast milk.

Table 7 summarizes the mean ranges of pharmacokinetic parameters of amiodarone reported in single dose I.V. (5 mg/kg over 15 min) and oral (400 or 600 mg) studies of healthy subjects and in in vitro (protein binding) studies. Pharmacokinetics were similar in males and females.

Table 7: CORDARONE

Amiodarone Pharmacokinetic Profile

Drug	Clearance (mL/h/kg)	V_C (L/kg)	V_{SS} (L/kg)	$t_{1/2}$ (days)	Protein Binding	F_{oral} (%)
Amiodarone	90–158	0.2	40–84	20–47	>0.96	33–65
Desethylamiodarone	197–290	—	68–168	≥ AMI $t_{1/2}$	—	—

Notes: V_C and V_{SS} denote the central and steady-state volumes of distribution from i.v. studies; F_{oral} is systemic availability of amiodarone. "—" denotes not available. AMI is Amiodarone. $t_{1/2}$=terminal phase elimination half-life. Desethylamiodarone clearance and volume involve an unknown biotransformation factor.

There is no well-established relationship between drug concentration and therapeutic response for long-term oral use. Steady-state amiodarone concentrations of 1 to 2.5 mg/L, however, have been effective with minimal toxicity following chronic **oral** amiodarone.

Special Populations and Conditions: Pediatrics: The safety and efficacy of amiodarone in children have not been established; therefore, its use in children is not recommended.

Geriatrics: Clinical studies of CORDARONE tablets did not include sufficient number of subjects aged 65 years and over to determine whether they respond differently from younger subjects.

Other reported clinical experience has not identified differences in responses between the elderly and younger patients. In general, dose selection for an elderly patient should be cautious, usually starting at the low end of the dosing range, reflecting the greater frequency of decreased hepatic, renal, or cardiac function, and of concomitant disease or other drug therapy.

Gender: No data on dosage adjustment is available for the oral formulation. Based on a single-dose clinical trial with the intravenous formulation, no gender-based dosage adjustment is required. Recommendations regarding gender-based dosage adjustment are based on intravenous data, and may not be representative of the oral formulation.

Hepatic Insufficiency: No data on dosage adjustment is available for the oral formulation. Based on a single-dose clinical trial with the intravenous formulation, no dosage adjustment is required for patients with hepatic impairment, although these patients should be monitored closely. Recommendations regarding dosage adjustment for patients with hepatic impairment are based on intravenous data, and may not be representative of the oral formulation (see Warnings and Precautions, Hepatic/Biliary/Pancreatic).

Renal Insufficiency: No data on dosage adjustment is available for the oral formulation. Based on a single-dose clinical trial with the intravenous formulation, no dosage adjustment is required for patients with renal dysfunction, end-stage renal disease or dialysis. Recommendations regarding dosage adjustment for patients with renal dysfunction, end-stage renal disease or dialysis are based on intravenous data, and may not be representative of the oral formulation.

Genetic Polymorphism: No data on dosage adjustment available.

Race: No data on dosage adjustment available.

STORAGE AND STABILITY: Keep bottle tightly closed. Store at controlled room temperature, 15 to 30°C. Protect from light.

SPECIAL HANDLING INSTRUCTIONS: None.

INFORMATION FOR THE PATIENT: Published in e-CPS, available by subscription at www.e-cps.ca.

DOSAGE FORMS, COMPOSITION AND PACKAGING: Each round, flat, pink tablet, with a raised "C" and marked "200" on one side with the reverse side scored, contains: amiodarone HCl 200 mg. Nonmedicinal ingredients: colloidal silicon dioxide, cornstarch, FD&C Red No. 40 Lake, lactose, magnesium stearate and povidone. Bottles of 100.

(Shown in Product Identification Section)

CO Risperidone ℞

risperidone

Antipsychotic

Cobalt

SUPPLIED: 0.25 mg: Each yellow, film-coated, capsule-shaped, biconvex tablet, embossed "R" on one side and "Σ>" on the other side, contains: risperidone 0.25 mg. Nonmedicinal ingredients: colloidal silicon dioxide, cornstarch, lactose monohydrate, magnesium stearate, microcrystalline cellulose, polyethylene glycol, polyvinyl alcohol, talc and titanium dioxide. HDPE bottles of 100.

0.5 mg: Each brownish-red, film-coated, capsule-shaped, biconvex tablet, embossed "R|R" on one side and "Σ>" on the other side, contains: risperidone 0.5 mg. Nonmedicinal ingredients: colloidal silicon dioxide, cornstarch, lactose monohydrate, magnesium stearate, microcrystalline cellulose, polyethylene glycol, polyvinyl alcohol, talc and titanium dioxide. HDPE bottles of 100.

1 mg: Each white to off-white, film-coated, capsule-shaped, biconvex tablet, embossed "R1" on one side and "Σ>" on the other side, contains: risperidone 1 mg. Nonmedicinal ingredients: colloidal silicon dioxide, cornstarch, lactose monohydrate, magnesium stearate, microcrystalline cellulose, polyethylene glycol, polyvinyl alcohol, talc and titanium dioxide. Blisters of 10, cartons of 60. HDPE botttles of 500.

2 mg: Each tan, film-coated, capsule-shaped, biconvex tablet, embossed "R|2" on one side and "Σ>" on the other side, contains: risperidone 2 mg. Nonmedicinal ingredients: colloidal silicon dioxide, cornstarch, lactose monohydrate, magnesium stearate, microcrystalline cellulose, polyethylene glycol, polyvinyl alcohol, talc and titanium dioxide. Blisters of 10, cartons of 60. HDPE bottles of 500.

3 mg: Each yellow, film-coated, capsule-shaped, biconvex tablet, embossed "R|3" on one side and "Σ>" on the other side, contains: risperidone 3 mg. Nonmedicinal ingredients: colloidal silicon dioxide, cornstarch, lactose monohydrate, magnesium stearate, microcrystalline cellulose, polyethylene glycol, polyvinyl alcohol, talc and titanium dioxide. Blisters of 10, cartons of 60. HDPE bottles of 250.

4 mg: Each green, film-coated, capsule-shaped, biconvex tablet, embossed "R|4" on one side and "Σ>" on the other side, contains: risperidone 4 mg.Nonmedicinal ingredients: colloidal silicon dioxide, cornstarch, lactose monohydrate, magnesium stearate, microcrystalline cellulose, polyethylene glycol, polyvinyl alcohol, talc and titanium dioxide. HDPE bottles of 60.

CO Ropinirole ℞

ropinirole HCl

Antiparkinsonian Agent—Dopamine Agonist

Cobalt

SUPPLIED: 0.25 mg: Each white to off white, film-coated, raised pentagon-shaped tablet with "RI/25" on one side and "Σ>" on the other side, contains: ropinirole 0.25 mg as ropinirole hydrochloride. Nonmedicinal ingredients: croscarmellose sodium, lactose monohydrate, magnesium stearate and microcrystalline cellulose; coating: polyethylene glycol, polyvinyl alcohol (part hydrolyzed), talc and titanium dioxide. HDPE bottles of 100. Store between 15 to 30°C. Protect from light and moisture. Close container tightly after each use.

1 mg: Each green, film-coated, raised pentagon-shaped tablet with "RI/1" on one side and "Σ>" on the other side, contains: ropinirole 1 mg as ropinirole hydrochloride. Nonmedicinal ingredients: croscarmellose sodium, lactose monohydrate, magnesium stearate and microcrystalline cellulose; coating: FD&C Blue #2, iron oxide yellow, polyethylene glycol, polyvinyl alcohol (part hydrolyzed), talc and titanium dioxide. HDPE bottles of 100. Store between 15 to 30°C. Protect from light and moisture. Close container tightly after each use.

2 mg: Each pink, film-coated, raised pentagon-shaped tablet with "RI/2" on one side and "Σ>" on the other side, contains: ropinirole 2 mg as ropinirole hydrochloride. Nonmedicinal ingredients: croscarmellose sodium, lactose monohydrate, magnesium stearate and microcrystalline cellulose; coating: FD&C Blue #2, FD&C Yellow #6, iron oxide yellow, polyethylene glycol, polyvinyl alcohol (part hydrolyzed), talc and titanium dioxide. HDPE bottles of 100. Store between 15 to 30°C. Protect from light and moisture. Close container tightly after each use.

5 mg: Each blue, film-coated, raised pentagon-shaped tablet with "RI/5" on one side and "Σ>" on the other side, contains: ropinirole 5 mg as ropinirole hydrochloride. Nonmedicinal ingredients: croscarmellose sodium, lactose monohydrate, magnesium stearate and microcrystalline cellulose; coating: iron oxide black, iron oxide red, iron oxide yellow, polyethylene glycol, polyvinyl alcohol (part hydrolyzed), talc and titanium dioxide. HDPE bottles of 100. Store between 15 to 30°C. Protect from light and moisture. Close container tightly after each use.

Cortef® Tablets ℞

hydrocortisone

Corticosteroid

Pfizer

PHARMACOLOGY: Hydrocortisone (cortisol) is a corticosteroid secreted by the adrenal cortex. In physiologic doses, it is administered to replace deficient endogenous hormones. In larger (pharmacologic) doses, hydrocortisone decreases inflammation and suppresses the immune response. It stimulates erythroid cells of the bone marrow, prolongs survival time of erythrocytes and platelets, and produces neutrophilia and eosinopenia. Hydrocortisone promotes protein catabolism, gluconeogenesis, and redistribution of fat from peripheral to central areas of the body. It reduces intestinal absorption and increases renal excretion of calcium.

In pharmacologic doses, systemically administered glucocorticoids suppress release of corticotropin from the pituitary. The degree and duration of hypothalamic-pituitary-adrenal (HPA) axis suppression produced is highly variable among patients and depends on the dose, frequency and time of administration, and duration of therapy. If suppressive doses are administered for prolonged periods, the adrenal cortex atrophies and patients develop cushingoid features and respond to stress like patients with primary adrenocortical insufficiency. The duration of anti-inflammatory activity approximately equals the duration of HPA-axis suppression. In one study, the duration of HPA-axis suppression after a single oral dose of hydrocortisone 250 mg was 1.25 to 1.5 days.

Hydrocortisone is extensively bound to the plasma proteins, corticosteroid binding globulin (transcortin) and albumin. With physiologic concentrations, it is bound primarily to transcortin and only 5 to 10% of cortisol in plasma is unbound.

Hydrocortisone is metabolized in most tissues, but primarily in the liver to biologically inactive compounds. The half-life of hydrocortisone may be prolonged in patients with hypothyroidism. Inactive metabolites are excreted by the kidneys, primarily as glucuronides and sulfates, but also as unconjugated products. Negligible amounts are excreted in bile.

INDICATIONS: Endocrine Disorders: Primary or secondary adrenocortical insufficiency (hydrocortisone or cortisone is the first choice; synthetic analogs may be used in conjunction with mineralocorticoids where applicable; in infancy, mineralocorticoid supplementation is of particular importance); congenital adrenal hyperplasia; nonsuppurative thyroiditis; hypercalcemia associated with cancer.

Nonendocrine Disorders: Rheumatic Disorders: As adjunctive therapy for short-term administration (to tide the patient over an acute episode or exacerbation) in: psoriatic arthritis, rheumatoid arthritis, including juvenile rheumatoid arthritis (selected cases may require low dose maintenance therapy), ankylosing spondylitis, acute and subacute bursitis, acute non-specific tenosynovitis, acute gouty arthritis, post-traumatic osteoarthritis, synovitis of osteoarthritis, epicondylitis.

Collagen Diseases: During an exacerbation or as maintenance therapy in selected cases of systemic lupus erythematosus, acute rheumatic carditis, systemic dermatomyositis (polymyositis).

Dermatologic Diseases: pemphigus, bullous dermatitis herpetiformis, severe erythema multiforme (Stevens-Johnson syndrome), exfoliative dermatitis, mycosis fungoides, severe psoriasis and severe seborrheic dermatitis.

Allergic States: Control of severe or incapacitating allergic conditions intractable to adequate trials of conventional treatment: seasonal or perennial allergic rhinitis, bronchial asthma, contact dermatitis, atopic dermatitis, serum sickness and drug hypersensitivity reactions.

Ophthalmic Diseases: Severe acute and chronic allergic and inflammatory processes involving the eye and its adnexa such as: allergic conjunctivitis, keratitis, allergic corneal marginal ulcers, herpes zoster ophthalmicus, iritis and iridocyclitis, chorioretinitis, anterior segment inflammation, diffuse posterior uveitis and choroiditis, optic neuritis, sympathetic ophthalmia.

Respiratory Diseases: Symptomatic sarcoidosis, Löffler's syndrome not manageable by other means, berylliosis, fulminating or disseminated pulmonary tuberculosis when used concurrently with appropriate antituberculous chemotherapy, aspiration pneumonitis.

Hematologic Disorders: Idiopathic thrombocytopenic purpura in adults, secondary thrombocytopenia in adults, acquired (autoimmune) hemolytic anemia, erythroblastopenia (RBC anemia), congenital (erythroid) hypoplastic anemia.

Neoplastic Diseases: For palliative management of: leukemias and lymphomas in adults, acute leukemia of childhood.

Edematous States: To induce a diuresis or remission of proteinuria in the nephrotic syndrome, without uremia, of the idiopathic type or that due to lupus erythematosus.

Gastrointestinal Diseases: To tide the patient over a critical period of the disease in: ulcerative colitis, regional enteritis.

Central Nervous System: Acute exacerbations of multiple sclerosis.

Miscellaneous: Tuberculous meningitis with subarachnoid block or impending block when used concurrently with appropriate antituberculous chemotherapy, trichinosis with neurologic or myocardial involvement.

CONTRAINDICATIONS: Systemic fungal infections and known hypersensitivity to hydrocortisone or components of the tablet.

WARNINGS: In patients on corticosteroid therapy subjected to unusual stress, increased dosage of rapidly acting corticosteroids before, during and after the stressful situation is indicated.

Corticosteroids may mask some signs of infection, and new infections may appear during their use. There may be decreased resistance and inability to localize infection when corticosteroids are used. Infections with any pathogen including viral, bacterial, fungal, protozoan or helminthic infections, in any location in the body, may be associated with the use of corticosteroids alone or in combination with other immunosuppressive agents that affect cellular immunity, humoral immunity, or neutrophil function. These infections may be mild, but can be severe and at times fatal. With increasing doses of corticosteroids, the rate of occurrence of infectious complications increases.

Persons who are on drugs which suppress the immune system are more susceptible to infections than healthy individuals. Chickenpox and measles, for example, can have a more serious or even fatal course in nonimmune children or adults on corticosteroids. In such children or adults who have not had these diseases, particular care should be taken to avoid exposure. How the dose, route and duration of corticosteroid administration affects the risk of developing a disseminated infection is not known. The contribution of the underlying disease and/or prior corticosteroid treatment to the risk is also not known. If exposed to chickenpox, prophylaxis with varicella zoster immune globulin (VZIG) may be indicated. If exposed to measles, prophylaxis with pooled i.m. immunoglobulin (IG) may be indicated. If chickenpox develops, treatment with antiviral agents may be considered. Similarly, corticosteroids should be used with great care in patients with known or suspected Strongyloides (threadworm) infestation. In such patients, corticosteroid-induced immunosuppression may lead to Strongyloides hyperinfection and dissemination with widespread larval migration often accompanied by severe enterocolitis and potentially fatal gram-negative septicemia.

Prolonged use of corticosteroids may produce posterior subcapsular cataracts, glaucoma with possible damage to the optic nerves, and may enhance the establishment of secondary ocular infections due to fungi or viruses.

Allergic reactions (e.g., angioedema) may occur.

Average and large doses of hydrocortisone or cortisone can cause elevation of blood pressure, salt and water retention, and increased excretion of potassium. These effects are less likely to occur with the synthetic derivatives except when used in large doses. Dietary salt restriction and potassium supplementation may be necessary. All corticosteroids increase calcium excretion.

Administration of live or live, attenuated vaccines is contraindicated in patients receiving immunosuppressive doses of corticosteroids. Killed or inactivated vaccines may be administered to patients receiving immunosuppressive doses of corticosteroids. However the response to such vaccines may be diminished. Indicated immunization procedures may be undertaken in patients receiving non-immunosuppressive doses of corticosteroids.

The use of hydrocortisone in active tuberculosis should be restricted to those cases of fulminating or disseminated tuberculosis in which the corticosteroid is used for the management of the disease in conjunction with an appropriate antituberculous regimen.

If corticosteroids are indicated in patients with latent tuberculosis or tuberculin reactivity, close observation is necessary as reactivation of the disease may occur. During prolonged corticosteroid therapy, these patients should receive chemoprophylaxis.

There is no universal agreement on whether corticosteroids per se are responsible for peptic ulcers encountered during therapy; however, glucocorticoid therapy may mask the symptoms of peptic ulcer so that perforation or hemorrhage may occur without significant pain.

Osteoporosis is a common but infrequently recognized adverse effect associated with a long-term use of large doses of glucocorticoid.

Growth may be suppressed in children receiving long-term daily, divided dose glucocorticoid therapy and use of such regimen should be restricted to the most urgent indications. Alternate day glucocorticoid therapy usually avoids or minimizes this side effect.

Host defenses are impaired in patients receiving large doses of glucocorticoids and this effect increases susceptibility to fungus infections as well as bacterial and viral infections.

Pregnancy: Some animal studies have shown that corticosteroids, when administered to the mother at high doses, may cause fetal malformations. Adequate human reproduction studies have not been done with corticosteroids. Therefore, the use of this drug in pregnancy, nursing mothers or women of childbearing potential requires that the benefits of the drug be carefully weighed against the potential risk to the mother and embryo or fetus. Since there is inadequate evidence of safety in human pregnancy, this drug should be used in pregnancy only if clearly needed.

Corticosteroids readily cross the placenta. Infants born of mothers who have received substantial doses of corticosteroids during pregnancy must be carefully observed and evaluated for signs of adrenal insufficiency. There are no known effects of corticosteroids on labour and delivery. Corticosteroids are excreted in breast milk.

Lactation: See Pregnancy.

PRECAUTIONS: Drug induced secondary adrenocortical insufficiency may be minimized by gradual reduction of dosage. This type of relative insufficiency may persist for months after discontinuation of therapy; therefore, in any situation of stress occurring during that period, hormone therapy should be reinstituted. Since mineralocorticoid secretion may be impaired, salt and/or a mineralocorticoid should be administered concurrently.

There is an enhanced effect of corticosteroids on patients with hypothyroidism and in those with cirrhosis.

Corticosteroids should be used cautiously in patients with ocular herpes simplex because of possible corneal perforation.

The lowest possible dose of corticosteroid should be used to control the condition under treatment and when reduction in dosage is possible, the reduction should be gradual.

Psychic derangements may appear when corticosteroids are used, ranging from euphoria, insomnia, mood swings, personality changes and severe depression to frank psychotic manifestations. Also, existing emotional instability or psychotic tendencies may be aggravated by corticosteroids.

ASA and nonsteroidal anti-inflammatory agents should be used cautiously in conjunction with corticosteroids in patients with hypoprothrombinemia.

Corticosteroids should be used with caution in nonspecific ulcerative colitis, if there is a probability of impending perforation, abscess or other pyogenic infection; diverticulitis; fresh intestinal anastomoses; active or latent peptic ulcer; renal insufficiency; hypertension; osteoporosis; or myasthenia gravis.

Because complications of treatment with glucocorticoids are dependent on the size of the dose and the duration of treatment, a risk/benefit decision must be made in each individual case as to dose and duration of treatment and as to whether daily or intermittent therapy should be used.

Convulsions have been reported with concurrent use of methylprednisolone and cyclosporine. Since concurrent administration of these agents results in a mutual inhibition of metabolism, it is possible that convulsions and other adverse events associated with the individual use of either drug may be more apt to occur.

Drug Interactions: The pharmacokinetic interactions listed below are potentially clinically important. Drugs that induce hepatic enzymes such as phenobarbital, phenytoin and rifampin may increase the clearance of corticosteroids and may require increases in corticosteroid dose to achieve the desired response. Drugs such as troleandomycin and ketoconazole may inhibit the metabolism of corticosteroids and thus decrease their clearance. Therefore, the dose of corticosteroid should be titrated to avoid steroid toxicity. Corticosteroids may increase the clearance of chronic high dose ASA. This could lead to decreased salicylate serum levels or increase the risk of salicylate toxicity when the corticosteroid is withdrawn. ASA should be used cautiously in conjunction with corticosteroids in patients suffering from hypothrombinemia. The effect of corticosteroids on oral anticoagulants is variable. There are reports of enhanced as well as diminished effects of anticoagulants when given concurrently with corticosteroids. Therefore, coagulation indices should be monitored to maintain the desired anticoagulant effect.

Information to Be Provided to the Patient: Persons who are on immunosuppressant doses of corticosteroids should be warned to avoid exposure to chickenpox or measles. Patients should also be advised that if they are exposed medical advice should be sought without delay.

ADVERSE EFFECTS: Note: The following are typical for all systemic corticosteroids. Their inclusion in this list does not necessarily indicate that the specific event has been observed with this particular formulation.

Fluid and Electrolyte Disturbances: sodium retention; fluid retention; congestive heart failure in susceptible patients; potassium loss, hypokalemic alkalosis; hypertension.

Musculoskeletal: steroid myopathy; muscle weakness; osteoporosis; pathologic fractures; vertebral compression fractures, aseptic necrosis of femoral and humeral heads, loss of muscle mass, tendon rupture, particular of the Achilles.

Gastrointestinal: peptic ulcer with possible perforation and hemorrhage; pancreatitis; abdominal distention; ulcerative esophagitis; increases in AST, ALT and alkaline phosphatase have been observed following corticosteroid treatment. These changes are usually small, not associated with any clinical significance.

Dermatologic: impaired wound healing; petechiae and ecchymoses; thin fragile skin; increased sweating, facial erythema may suppress reactions to skin tests.

Metabolic: negative nitrogen balance due to protein catabolism.

Neurological: increased intracranial pressure; pseudotumor cerebri; psychic derangements and seizures; convulsions, vertigo and headache.

Endocrine: menstrual irregularities; development of cushingoid state; suppression of pituitary-adrenal axis particularly at times of stress as in trauma, surgery or illness; decreased carbohydrate tolerance; manifestations of latent diabetes mellitus; increased requirements for insulin or oral hypoglycemic agents in diabetes; suppression of growth in children.

Ophthalmic: posterior subcapsular cataracts; increased intraocular pressure; exophthalmos glaucoma.

Immune System: masking of infections; latent infections becoming active; opportunistic infections; hypersensitivity reactions including anaphylaxis; may suppress reactions to skin tests.

OVERDOSE:

No data supplied by the manufacturer.

For management of a suspected drug overdose, CPhA recommends that you contact your **regional Poison Control Centre**. See the *CPS* Directory section for a list of Poison Control Centres.

DOSAGE: The initial dosage may vary from 20 to 240 mg of hydrocortisone per day depending on the specific disease entity being treated. In situations of less severity, lower doses will generally suffice, while in selected patients higher initial doses may be required. The initial dosage should be maintained or adjusted until a satisfactory response is noted. If after a reasonable period of time there is a lack of satisfactory clinical response, hydrocortisone should be discontinued and the patient transferred to another appropriate therapy.

It should be emphasized that dosage requirements are variable and must be individualized on the basis of the disease under treatment and the response of the patient.

After a favorable response is noted, the proper maintenance dosage should be determined by decreasing the initial drug dosage in small decrements at appropriate time intervals until the lowest dosage which will maintain an adequate clinical response is reached. It should be kept in mind that constant monitoring is needed in regard to drug dosage. Included in the situations which may make dosage adjustments necessary are changes in clinical status secondary to remissions or exacerbations in the disease process, the patient's individual drug responsiveness, and the effect of patient exposure to stressful situations not directly related to the disease entity under treatment; in this latter situation it may be necessary to increase the dosage of hydrocortisone for a period of time consistent with the patient's condition.

SUPPLIED: 10 mg: Each white, round, scored, compressed tablet, engraved "Cortef 10", contains: hydrocortisone 10 mg. Nonmedicinal ingredients: calcium stearate, cornstarch, lactose, mineral oil, sorbic acid, sucrose. Sodium: <1 mmol. Gluten- and tartrazine-free. Bottles of 100.

20 mg: Each white, round, scored, compressed tablet, engraved "Cortef 20", contains: hydrocortisone 20 mg. Nonmedicinal ingredients: calcium stearate, cornstarch, lactose, mineral oil, sorbic acid, sucrose. Sodium: <1 mmol. Gluten- and tartrazine-free. Bottles of 100.

Store between 15 and 30°C.

(Shown in Product Identification Section)

Cortenema® Pr

hydrocortisone

Glucocorticoid

Axcan Pharma

INDICATIONS: An adjunct in the treatment of nonspecific inflammatory diseases involving the rectum, sigmoid and left colon such as idiopathic ulcerative colitis, ulcerative proctitis, regional enteritis (granulomatous colitis) with left side involvement, proctitis, proctocolitis, and radiation proctitis.

CONTRAINDICATIONS: Local contraindications to the use of intrarectal steroids include obstruction, abscess, perforation, peritonitis, fresh intestinal anastomoses, extensive fistulas and sinus tracts.

Active tuberculosis (active, latent or nonpositively healed), ocular herpes simplex, and acute psychosis are usually considered absolute contraindications to the use of corticosteroids.

Relative contraindications include active peptic ulcer, acute glomerulonephritis, myasthenia gravis, osteoporosis, diverticulitis, thrombophlebitis, psychic disturbances, pregnancy, diabetes, hyperthyroidism, acute coronary disease, hypertension, limited cardiac reserve, and local or systemic infections, including fungal, viral or exanthematous diseases. Where these conditions exist, the expected benefits from hydrocortisone retention enema must be weighed against the risks involved in its use.

If there is no evidence of clinical or proctologic improvement within 2 or 3 weeks after starting hydrocortisone retention enema therapy, discontinue the drug.

WARNINGS: No data supplied by the manufacturer.

PRECAUTIONS: Hydrocortisone retention enema should be administered with caution in patients with severe ulcerative disease because these patients are predisposed to perforation of the bowel wall. In the advanced stages of chronic ulcerative colitis, where there is loss of mucosa, and thickening and fibrosis of the bowel wall, steroid therapy theoretically might hasten deterioration, although this has not been proved with steroids in actual practice.

In severe cases, such as acute fulminating ulcerative colitis, where surgery is imminent, in the absence of marked clinical improvement, it is hazardous to wait more than a few days for a satisfactory response to medical treatment.

Of particular importance is the complication of adrenal insufficiency caused by suppression of the adrenal cortex by glucocorticoids, especially after prolonged therapy. It is therefore important that therapy be withdrawn gradually. If the patient is subjected to unusual stress, while on therapy or up to a year after discontinuation of steroids, adequate supportive measures and increased or reinstated systemic steroid therapy are indicated.

In the case of surgery, these measures should be continued throughout the pre- and the postoperative recovery periods, bearing in mind the possible deleterious effects of corticosteroids on fresh intestinal anastomoses. Steroid therapy might impair the prognosis in surgery by increasing the hazard of infection. If infection is suspected, appropriate antibiotic therapy must be administered, usually in doses larger than those customarily employed.

General precautions common to all corticosteroids therapy should be observed during treatment with hydrocortisone retention enema, including those pertaining to growth suppression in children during prolonged use.

Patients should be kept under close observation, for, as with all drugs, rare individuals may react unfavorably under certain conditions.

If severe reactions or idiosyncrasies occur, steroids should be discontinued immediately and appropriate measures instituted.

Pregnancy: If it is necessary to use hydrocortisone retention enema in pregnant patients, the infants of these mothers should be closely observed following delivery for signs of hypoadrenalism and appropriate measures, including administration of corticosteroids, should be instituted if such signs are seen.

Corticosteroid therapy may cause hyperacidity or peptic ulcer, and may aggravate diabetes mellitus or precipitate manifestations of latent diabetes mellitus.

When hydrocortisone retention enema is used in the presence of glaucoma, intraocular pressure should be measured frequently and optic nerve heads and visual fields observed.

Patients should be advised to inform subsequent physicians of the prior use of corticosteroids.

ADVERSE EFFECTS: Hydrocortisone retention enema may produce adverse effects known to occur with other forms of hydrocortisone therapy. These include moon face, buffalo hump, fluid retention, excessive appetite and weight gain, abnormal fat deposits, mental symptoms, hypertrichosis, acne, striae, ecchymosis, increased sweating, pigmentation, dry scaly skin, thinning scalp hair, thrombophlebitis, decreased resistance to infection, negative nitrogen balance with delayed bone and wound healing, menstrual disorders, neuropathy, peptic ulcer, decreased glucose tolerance, hypopotassemia, adrenal insufficiency, necrotizing angiitis, hypertension, pancreatitis and increased intraocular pressure.

In children, suppression of growth may occur. Increased intracranial pressure may occur and possibly account for headache, insomnia and fatigue. Subcapsular cataracts may result from prolonged usage. Long-term use of all corticosteroids results in catabolic effects characterized by negative protein and calcium balance. Osteoporosis, spontaneous fractures and aseptic necrosis of the hip and humerus may occur as part of this catabolic phenomenon.

Where hypokalemia and the other symptoms associated with fluid and electrolyte imbalance call for potassium supplementation and salt-poor or salt-free diets, these may be instituted and are compatible with the diet requirements for ulcerative colitis.

OVERDOSE:

Treatment: No known antidote but gastric lavage should be performed.

For management of a suspected drug overdose, CPhA recommends that you contact your **regional Poison Control Centre**. See the *CPS* Directory section for a list of Poison Control Centres.

DOSAGE: The usual dose is one 60 mL enema (100 mg hydrocortisone) daily for 2 or 3 weeks, and every second day thereafter, administered intrarectally in the evening before retiring. Every effort should be made to retain the medication at least 1 hour, and preferably all night. This may be facilitated by prior sedation and/or antidiarrheal medication. Certain cases may require 2 doses a day (30 or 60 mL) until alleviation of symptoms allows better retention. If clinical or proctologic improvement fail to occur within 2 or 3 weeks, hydrocortisone retention enema therapy should be discontinued.

For administration by retention enema, instruct the patient to lie on his left side during instillation of the medication. Shake the bottle vigorously to resuspend the insoluble portion of hydrocortisone. Expose the lubricated tip by removal of the protective sheath, grasping the bottle at the neck where it is most rigid. Carefully, insert the lubricated tip into the rectum in the direction of the sacrum. Slowly express the contents by compressing the container. After instillation, the patient should remain in the same position (on left side) for at least 30 minutes, to allow distribution of the medication in the colon. The 60 mL hydrocortisone retention enema may be expected to distribute throughout the descending colon and rectum.

The duration of treatment is dependent on the degree of response. If a satisfactory response is to be obtained, it usually occurs within 5 to 7 days, as evidenced by a marked reduction of clinical symptoms. Improvement in the appearance of the mucosa, gauged by barium enemas and sigmoidoscopic examinations, may lag somewhat behind clinical improvement.

The usual duration of therapy is 2 weeks.

Minimal control of symptoms is an insufficient basis for the prolonged use of CORTENEMA. If there is no clinical or proctologic response within 2 or 3 weeks, or if the patient's condition worsens, discontinue the drug.

Because of hydrocortisone absorption, proper precautions against unwanted systemic reactions or side effects should be observed. Symptomatic improvement, evidenced by decreased diarrhea, weight gain, improved appetite, lessened fever, and decrease in leukocytosis, may be misleading and should not be used as the sole criterion in judging efficacy. Actual sigmoidoscopic examination and x-ray visualization are most reliable. Since steroids can inhibit wound healing, enema or drip therapy should not be employed in the immediate or early postoperative period following ileorectostomy.

SUPPLIED: Each single-dose unit contains: hydrocortisone USP 100 mg in 60 mL of an aqueous suspension. Nonmedicinal ingredients: carboxypolymethylene, polysorbate 80, methylparaben, purified water and sodium hydroxide. Lactose-, sulfite- and tartrazine-free. Boxes of 7.

Corticosteroids: Eye Ear Nose ℞

beclomethasone dipropionate
betamethasone sodium phosphate
budesonide
dexamethasone
dexamethasone sodium phosphate
flumethasone pivalate
flunisolide
fluorometholone
fluorometholone acetate
fluticasone propionate
hydrocortisone
mometasone furoate
prednisolone
prednisolone acetate
prednisolone sodium phosphate
rimexolone
triamcinolone acetonide

CPhA Monograph

Date of Revision: November 2004

> This monograph has been compiled by CPhA and reviewed by experts. It may contain information different from that found in Health Canada-approved Product Monographs. The reader is referred to the *CPS* Editorial Policy for more information.

PHARMACOLOGY: Corticosteroids are used to inhibit the inflammatory response of the eye, nasal mucosa or external ear canal to irritating agents of a mechanical, chemical or immunological nature. They reduce edema, fibrin deposition, capillary dilation, leukocyte migration, capillary proliferation, deposition of collagen and scar formation. Used intranasally, corticosteroids inhibit IgE and mast cell-mediated early phase allergic reactions and migration of inflammatory cells into the nasal tissue. Corticosteroids complex with specific cytoplasmic receptors and these complexes stimulate the transcription of mRNA and protein synthesis of enzymes responsible for the anti-inflammatory effect. Topical ophthalmic corticosteroids may cause a rise in intraocular pressure by decreasing the outflow of aqueous humor.

The relative potency of corticosteroids depends on the molecular structure, concentration and release of the drug from the vehicle. Modifications of the chemical structure such as introducing a fluorine atom, an acetonide group or omission or esterification of a hydroxyl group may increase the anti-inflammatory potency of the molecule; however, other properties of the molecule may be affected. For example, adding fluorine to topical ophthalmic drops reduces their corneal penetration which decreases their clinical efficacy in anterior chamber inflammations.

Pharmacokinetics: Corticosteroids applied to the eye are absorbed into the cornea, aqueous humor, iris, choroid, ciliary body and retina. Dosages used ophthalmically are less than those used systemically. As a result, clinically significant systemic absorption usually does not occur at recommended doses.

When administered intranasally, beclomethasone, fluticasone, flunisolide, budesonide and triamcinolone may be absorbed and produce systemic effects; however, adrenal suppression has not been observed with these drugs even when used at recommended doses for prolonged periods of time.

INDICATIONS: Eye: May be used in the treatment of corticosteroid responsive inflammatory conditions of the anterior segment of the eye and its adnexa such as: iridocyclitis; lid allergy; nonpurulent conjunctivitis including vernal, allergic or catarrhal; herpes zoster ophthalmicus (not to be used in herpes simplex infections); corneal, conjunctival or scleral injury caused by foreign body penetration; aseptic burns (thermal, radiation or chemical); superficial keratitis including punctate epithelial lesions (Thygeson type) and phlyctenular keratoconjunctivitis; deep keratitis including interstitial and parenchymatous keratitis; acne rosacea; sclerosing keratitis; mild acute iritis; anterior uveitis; post-operative inflammation following ocular surgery; recurrent marginal ulceration whether endogenous or allergic and nonpurulent blepharitis including catarrhal and allergic.

Corticosteroids are also used in conjunction with antimicrobials in some cases where bacterial infection or a risk of ocular bacterial infection exists.

Acute disorders respond more favorably than chronic disorders. In stubborn cases of anterior segment eye disease, systemic adrenocortical therapy may be required. When the deeper ocular structures are involved, systemic therapy is necessary.

Ear: Dexamethasone is indicated for the treatment of corticosteroid responsive inflammatory conditions of the external ear canal such as localized neurodermatitis, seborrheic dermatitis, eczema and diffuse otitis externa. It is not to be used if the ear drum is perforated.

Other products are found in combination with antimicrobials and can, in addition, be used in some cases of bacterial otitis externa.

Nasal: Beclomethasone, flunisolide, fluticasone and triamcinolone are used for the treatment of perennial and seasonal rhinitis unresponsive to conventional treatment. Budesonide is used in the above conditions as well as for non-allergic and vasomotor rhinitis. Beclomethasone and budesonide are also indicated for the treatment of nasal polyps to prevent their return after surgery or to prevent their increase in size.

CONTRAINDICATIONS: Topical corticosteroids are contraindicated in patients with a history of hypersensitivity to any of the ingredients of these preparations. Cross-allergenicity among corticosteroids has been demonstrated.

Eye: Topical corticosteroids are contraindicated in: epithelial herpes simplex keratitis, vaccinia, varicella and most other viral diseases of the cornea and conjunctiva (see Indications and Warnings); infectious tuberculous lesions of the eye and fungal diseases of ocular structures; uncomplicated removal of a corneal foreign body; acute purulent untreated infections of the conjunctiva and lids which may be masked or enhanced by the presence of a corticosteroid.

Ear: Topical corticosteroids are contraindicated in tuberculous, fungal or viral lesions and acute untreated purulent bacterial infections. The absence or perforation of the ear drum is a contraindication.

Nasal: Topical corticosteroids are contraindicated in active or quiescent tuberculosis of the respiratory tract or untreated bacterial, fungal or viral infections. The intranasal use of budesonide or flunisolide is contraindicated in children under 6 years of age.

WARNINGS: Infections may be masked or enhanced and new infections may appear during corticosteroid use due to suppression of the immune response. If an infection develops, appropriate therapy should be initiated and the corticosteroid may need to be stopped. If the infection does not respond promptly to therapy or worsens, the corticosteroid should be discontinued.

Eye: Prolonged ophthalmic use may result in increased intraocular pressure in some individuals. If these products are used for 10 days or longer, intraocular pressure should be monitored. In diseases causing thinning of the cornea or sclera, perforation has been known to occur with the use of topical preparations containing corticosteroids. Protracted use of topical corticosteroids in the eye may result in the development of posterior subcapsular cataracts.

Although corticosteroids are contraindicated in acute viral infection of the cornea caused by herpes simplex, there may be occasion to employ steroids in the healing stage to prevent scarring; however, this must only be done with great caution and close observation, usually under the care of an ophthalmologist. In patients with a history of herpetic infection of the cornea, reactivation of the disease may occur with use of topical ophthalmic corticosteroids. Use of steroids after cataract surgery may delay healing and increase the incidence of filtering blebs.

Nasal: Adrenal insufficiency (even death) may occur when patients are transferred from long-term oral corticosteroid therapy to orally or nasally inhaled preparations. Withdrawal of the oral corticosteroid should be achieved very gradually, after the initiation of inhaled therapy. Symptoms of adrenal insufficiency include weakness, hyperpigmentation of skin and mucous membranes, weight loss, anorexia, nausea, vomiting and hypotension.

Flunisolide is not recommended for patients with a history of recurrent nasal bleeding.

Pregnancy: Ophthalmic, otic or nasal application of corticosteroids results in minimal systemic absorption and has not been associated with increased risk of fetal malformations.

Lactation: Corticosteroids are secreted into human milk; however, the minimal systemic absorption following ophthalmic, otic or intranasal administration limits the amount of corticosteroid that could potentially be secreted into the milk. Ophthalmic, otic or nasal application of corticosteroids is generally considered to be compatible with breast-feeding.

PRECAUTIONS: Patients should be advised to inform their physician of any prior use of corticosteroids. Under most circumstances, treatment with corticosteroids should not be stopped abruptly but tapered off gradually.

There may be an enhanced effect of corticosteroids in patients with hypothyroidism or cirrhosis.

ASA should be used cautiously in conjunction with corticosteroids in patients with hypoprothrombinemia.

Eye: During long-term use of preparations containing corticosteroids, the possibility of fungal infection must be considered, especially in the presence of a persistent corneal ulceration that fails to respond to conventional therapy.

If irritation occurs, the possibility of hypersensitivity to a component of the preparation should be considered.

If redness, irritation, swelling or pain persists, the product should be discontinued and the physician notified. Patients should be advised regarding the use of contact lenses while on therapy. The use of ophthalmic corticosteroids with contact lenses will increase the risk of infection.

To avoid possible contamination, the tip of the dropper or ointment tube should not touch any surface, including the eye. Contamination of the eye dropper tip can cause serious damage including bacterial keratitis and loss of vision.

An abnormally heavy challenge of summer allergens may, in certain instances, necessitate appropriate additional therapy, particularly to control eye symptoms. Treatment of seasonal rhinitis should, if possible, start before the exposure to allergens.

Patients should be informed that the full effect of triamcinolone acetate and fluticasone is not achieved until after 2 or 3 days of treatment have been completed.

Studies in asthmatic patients have shown that the combined administration of alternate-day prednisone systemic treatment and orally inhaled beclomethasone dipropionate increases the likelihood of HPA axis suppression compared to a therapeutic dose of either drug alone. Patients on alternate-day prednisone therapy should use beclomethasone nasal spray with caution due to the increased likelihood of HPA axis suppression.

Long-term Effects: During long-term therapy, HPA axis function and hematological status should be assessed.

Patients using a nasal spray over several months or longer should be examined for possible changes in nasal mucosa. It has been suggested that aiming the spray away from the septum may reduce the risk of long-term damage to the septum.

The potential for the occurrence of atrophic rhinitis and/or pharyngeal candidiasis should be kept in mind.

Inhibitory Effect on Wound Healing: Because of inhibitory effect of corticosteroids on wound healing, patients who have experienced recent nasal septal ulcer, nasal surgery or trauma should use a nasal corticosteroid with caution until healing has occurred. Rare instances of nasal septum perforation have been reported.

Effect on Infections: Infections may be masked or enhanced and new infections may appear during corticosteroid use due to suppression of the immune response (see Warnings).

Fluorocarbon Propellants: May be hazardous if deliberately abused. Inhalation of high concentrations of aerosol sprays has brought about cardiovascular toxic effects and even death, especially under conditions of hypoxia. Aerosols are safe when used properly and with adequate ventilation, but excessive use should be avoided.

Drug Interactions: Cushing's syndrome and adrenal suppression have been reported with the concurrent use of ritonavir (a potent CYP3A4 inhibitor) and fluticasone (a substrate of CYP3A4). Other corticosteroids metabolized by CYP3A4 (e.g., budesonide) could potentially be affected in a similar manner by ritonavir or other inhibitors of CYP3A4 (e.g., ketaconazole).

Children: Due to limited clinical data in this age group, the use of intranasal corticosteroids in children under 6 years of age is not recommended.

ADVERSE EFFECTS: Eye: Increased intraocular pressure may occur. The extent is dependent upon the frequency and duration of use as well as the type and concentration of the corticosteroid. Dexamethasone is most likely to increase intraocular pressure. Fluorometholone and rimexolone are least likely to increase intraocular pressure and may be preferred in long-term use. Ocular hypertension may occur after 1 to 6 weeks of therapy. This is reversible over a period of weeks after discontinuing the medication.

Glaucoma optic nerve damage, posterior subcapsular cataract formation and delayed wound healing have been reported, as well as mydriasis, defects in visual acuity and visual fields, loss of accommodation and ptosis. Topical application may cause discomfort, burning, stinging of the eye and lacrimation in some patients.

Fungal infections of the cornea are particulary likely to develop with long-term application of corticosteroids.

In those diseases causing thinning of the cornea, perforation has occurred with the use of topical steroids.

Ear: Stinging and burning have been reported rarely when the medication has gained access to the middle ear.

Nasal: In general, side effects have been primarily associated with the nasal mucosa and are consistent with what one would expect from applying a topical medication to an already inflamed membrane. The commonly reported adverse effects are irritation and dryness. Less common are headache, nasal bleeding, nasal stinging, crusting, sore throat, cough, fatigue, nausea, dizziness, loss of sense of taste or smell, stuffy nose, and stomach pains. In rare cases, skin reactions such as urticaria, rash or dermatitis occur. Rarely, ulcerations of the mucous membranes and nasal septal perforation have been reported. Aiming the spray away from the septum may decrease the risk of damage to the septum. One suggested method to achieve this is to use the right hand to spray the left nostril, and vice versa.

When patients are transferred to nasal preparations from a systemic steroid, allergic conditions such as asthma or eczema may be unmasked. With beclomethasone, sneezing attacks directly after use occur in about 10% of aerosol users and 4% of those using aqueous suspension. After the sneezing has stopped, the patient should clear their nose and repeat the dose.

OVERDOSE:

Symptoms: Eye: Overdosage in the use of topical ophthalmic corticosteroids is a remote possibility. Discontinue medication when heavy or protracted use is suspected. Excessive prolonged use may suppress HPA axis function resulting in secondary adrenal insufficiency.

Nasal: Acute overdosing is unlikely in view of the total amount of active ingredient present. However, when used chronically in excessive doses or in conjunction with other corticosteroid formulations, systemic corticosteroid effects such as hypercorticism and adrenal suppression may appear. If such changes occur, the dosage should be discontinued slowly consistent with accepted procedures for discontinuation of chronic steroid therapy.

The restoration of HPA axis function may be slow during periods of pronounced physical stress. Supplementation with systemic steroids may be advisable.

> For management of a suspected drug overdose, CPhA recommends that you contact your **regional Poison Control Centre**. See the *CPS* Directory section for a list of Poison Control Centres.

DOSAGE: For proper dosage and administration of the drug and to attain maximum improvement, patients must be instructed by the physician or other health care professional in the correct use of these preparations. The patient should contact the physician if symptoms do not improve, if the condition worsens or if sneezing or nasal irritation occurs with the use of intranasal preparations.

Eye: For use in the eye, corticosteroids are available as sterile solutions, suspensions and ointments. Solutions and suspensions are preferable for daytime use as they are less likely to impair vision. For inflammatory conditions of the eyelid and for nighttime use, ointments are preferred because they provide longer contact time. Dexamethasone, fluorometholone, prednisolone and rimexolone are available as single entity products. Hydrocortisone, betamethasone and dexamethasone are available in combination with anti-infectives.

To avoid possible contamination, the tip of the dropper or ointment tube should not touch any surface, including the eye. Ophthalmic suspensions should be shaken well before each use.

Ear: For use in the ear, corticosteroids are available as solutions and suspensions. Dexomethasone is available as a single entity product. Betamethasone and flumethasone are available in combination with anti-infectives. To decrease the buildup of debris in the ear canal, suspensions should be used sparingly. For administration of solutions or suspensions, the patient should lie with the affected ear upward and then the drops should be instilled. This position should be maintained for 5 minutes to facilitate penetration of the drops into the ear canal. This procedure may be repeated if necessary for the opposite ear.

Patients should avoid contamination of the dropper with material from the eye, ear, fingers or other sources in order to maintain the sterility of the product.

Nasal: For intranasal use corticosteroids are available as nasal aerosols, solutions or suspensions. Available products include beclomethasone, budesonide, flunisolide, mometasone and triamcinolone. The therapeutic effects of corticosteroids, unlike those of decongestants, are not immediate. Because the therapeutic benefit depends on regular use, patients must be instructed to administer the nasal inhalations at regular intervals as prescribed and not on an as-needed basis to treat acute symptoms.

Careful attention must be given to patients previously treated for prolonged periods with systemic corticosteroids when those patients are transferred to a nasal spray (see Warnings). Initially, the corticosteroid nasal spray and the systemic corticosteroid must be given concomitantly, while the dose of the latter is gradually decreased. Many withdrawal or tapering regimens have been described. Factors such as the dose and duration of systemic therapy and the underlying health of the patient should be considered when determining the withdrawal schedule.

In the presence of excessive nasal mucous secretion or edema of the nasal mucosa, the drug may fail to reach the site of action. In such cases, a nasal decongestant may be used 5 to 15 minutes prior to the corticosteroid for the first 2 to 3 days of therapy.

It has been suggested that using the right hand to spray the left nostril and vice versa may decrease the risk of side effects such as nosebleeds by helping to aim the spray away from the septum.

The reader is referred to individual product monographs for more specific dosing information.

Corticosteroids: Inhaled ℞

beclomethasone dipropionate
budesonide
ciclesonide
fluticasone propionate

CPhA Monograph

Date of Revision: November 2008

This monograph has been compiled by CPhA and reviewed by experts. It may contain information different from that found in Health Canada-approved Product Monographs. The reader is referred to the *CPS* Editorial Policy for more information.

SUMMARY PRODUCT INFORMATION:

Drug	Route of Administration	Dosage Form	Strength
Single Entity			
Beclomethasone dipropionate	Inhaled	Pressurized metered-dose inhaler (pMDI)	50 µg/inhalation 100 µg/inhalation
Budesonide	Inhaled	Dry powder inhaler (DPI)—turbuhaler	100 µg/inhalation 200 µg/inhalation 400 µg/inhalation
Budesonide	Inhaled	Nebules	0.125 mg/mL, 0.25 mg/mL, 0.5 mg/mL
Ciclesonide	Inhaled	Pressurized metered-dose inhaler (pMDI)	100 µg/inhalation 200 µg/inhalation
Fluticasone propionate	Inhaled	Dry powder inhaler (DPI)—diskus	50 µg/inhalation 100 µg/inhalation 250 µg/inhalation 500 µg/inhalation
Fluticasone propionate	Inhaled	Pressurized metered-dose inhaler (pMDI)	50 µg/inhalation 125 µg/inhalation 250 µg/inhalation
Combination			
Budesonide/ formoterol fumarate dihydrate	Inhaled	Dry powder inhaler (DPI)—turbuhaler	budesonide 100 µg plus formoterol 6 µg/inhalation budesonide 200 µg plus formoterol 6 µg/inhalation
Fluticasone propionate/ salmeterol	Inhaled	Pressurized metered-dose inhaler (pMDI)	fluticasone propionate 125 µg plus salmeterol 25 µg/inhalation fluticasone propionate 250 µg plus salmeterol 25 µg/inhalation
Fluticasone propionate/ salmeterol	Inhaled	Dry powder inhaler (DPI)—diskus	fluticasone propionate 100 µg plus salmeterol 50 µg/inhalation fluticasone propionate 250 µg plus salmeterol 50 µg/inhalation fluticasone propionate 500 µg plus salmeterol 50 µg/inhalation

PHARMACOLOGY: Inhaled corticosteroid (ICS) therapy is the cornerstone of asthma management and has a role in select patients with chronic obstructive pulmonary disease (COPD). These agents relieve persistent symptoms, improve lung function and reduce the morbidity associated with asthma. Benefits are usually seen in a few weeks, with most benefit seen within several months.

The most important action of ICS is thought to be inhibition of gene transcription of the cytokines implicated in airway inflammation. Gene transcription is interrupted through the formation of glucocorticoid-receptor complexes, which occurs after the lipophilic drug rapidly enters the airway cell. At the cellular level, corticosteroids may have direct inhibitory effects on cells involved in airway inflammation, including mast cells, macrophages, T-lymphocytes, eosinophils and epithelial cells. They may also inhibit plasma exudation and mucus secretion in inflamed airways.

Long-term treatment with ICS in children and adults with asthma lowers the sensitivity and maximal narrowing of the airway in response to spasmogens, lessens airway hyperresponsiveness to histamine, cholinergic agonists and allergens, and reduces responsiveness to exercise, cold air, fog, adenosine, bradykinin and irritants such as sulfur dioxide and metabisulfites. Although treatment suppresses inflammation, it may not reverse the persistent structural changes underlying the disease.

Pharmacokinetics: ICS are commercially available in many different formulations including delivery devices such as pressurized metered dose inhalers (pMDIs) with hydrofluoroalkane (HFA) propellants, various types of breath-actuated dry powder inhalers (DPIs) and solutions for nebulization. Spacer devices can be used with pMDIs to aid the coordination of administration, reduce variability in lung deposition, reduce systemic bioavailability by minimizing oral deposition and significantly reducing side effects such as thrush and dysphonia.

As of 2005, all pMDIs are CFC-free.

The relative lung deposition of ICS is dependent on many factors: physicochemical properties of the corticosteroid molecule such as lipophilicity, rate of dissolution, receptor binding affinity and receptor binding half-life; patient factors such as age, degree of airway obstruction, inhaler technique and concurrent therapy; delivery device and use of a spacer. A portion of an inhaled dose that does not reach the respiratory tract is deposited in the oropharynx and swallowed.

Ideally, an ICS should have high lipophilicity and topical potency, low oral bioavailability and be rapidly inactivated and/or cleared after systemic absorption. These properties confer maximal topical efficacy with minimal risk of systemic effects. Table 1 compares some of the properties of ICS.

INDICATIONS AND CLINICAL USE: ICS are used for:

- Prophylactic management of corticosteroid-responsive bronchial asthma.
- Combination of budesonide and formoterol is indicated for maintenance and rescue therapy for asthma in adults and children ≥12 years.
- Reducing frequency and severity of acute exacerbations of COPD, improving health status and improving on spirometry measurements when given as a combination of ICS plus long-acting beta$_2$-agonist, and tiotropium in patients with moderate to severe COPD with frequent exacerbations (>1 per year). The combination of ICS plus long-acting beta$_2$-agonist may also be given to patients with moderate to severe COPD who have infrequent exacerbations (<1 per year) but who have persistent symptoms despite therapy with long-acting beta$_2$-agonist and tiotropium. Optimal bronchodilation is necessary before adding ICS. ICS may be a useful add-on for patients who are short of breath despite optimal bronchodilation. ICS monotherapy is not recommended in COPD. [*Can Respir J*2007;14(Suppl B):5B-32B]
- Nebulized budesonide is also used in the management of croup.

CONTRAINDICATIONS: The product monographs of the various ICS list the following as contraindications:

- Patients with a history of hypersensitivity to any ingredients in the preparations
- Primary treatment of status asthmaticus or acute episodes of asthma
- Active or quiescent pulmonary tuberculosis, untreated fungal, bacterial or viral infections of the respiratory system

ICS, however, have been used to reduce airway inflammation especially in patients with cystic fibrosis with or without asthma. In addition, ICS have been used to treat allergic bronchopulmonary mycosis.

Several manufacturers of ICS list bronchiectasis as a contraindication; however, expert clinicians may disagree. [*Chest* 2008;134:815-823]. Therapy with ICS may reduce inflammation in patients with bronchiectasis [*Am J Respir Crit Care Med* 1998;158:723-727].

WARNINGS: ICS are not effective in relieving acute asthmatic attacks.

Switching from systemic to ICS therapy must be done gradually and monitored closely, to prevent life-threatening exacerbations of asthma or acute adrenal insufficiency. Rarely, deaths have occurred during and after switching from systemic to ICS therapy. Recovery of hypothalamic-pituitary-adrenocortical (HPA) function following systemic corticosteroid therapy can take up to 12 months. During this time, patients are at increased risk of: acute adrenal insufficiency during exposure to trauma, surgery or infection; corticosteroid withdrawal symptoms such as joint and muscle pain or depression; acute exacerbation of allergic conditions such as rhinitis or eczema that were suppressed during systemic corticosteroid therapy. Patients who have been switched to ICS therapy may require the administration of systemic corticosteroid therapy when exposed to trauma, surgery or infection, particularly gastroenteritis.

PRECAUTIONS: ICS should not be discontinued abruptly. The dose should be gradually tapered prior to discontinuation.

Patients should be advised to inform all treating physicians of their past and/or present use of corticosteroids.

Drug Interactions: There are reports of Cushing's syndrome and adrenal suppression resulting from the concurrent use of ICS that are substrates of CYP3A4 (e.g., budesonide, ciclesonide, fluticasone) with inhibitors of CYP3A4 (e.g., itraconazole, ketoconazole, nelfinavir, ritonavir).

Pregnant Women: To avoid adverse perinatal outcomes such as low birth weight and preeclampsia associated with uncontrolled asthma in pregnancy, aggressive asthma management may be necessary. The use of ICS in pregnant women has not been associated with an increased risk of fetal malformations or other adverse fetal outcomes. The use of the lowest dose of ICS that maintains optimal asthma control is recommended.

Table 1: Corticosteroids: Inhaled
Pharmacokinetics

Drug	Relative Binding Affinity[a]	Receptor Binding Half-life (hours)	Blanching Potency[b]	Systemic Bioavailability (%)	Metabolism in Liver	Plasma Half-life (hours)
Beclomethasone dipropionate (BDP)	0.4	See BMP	600	<5	BDP metabolized to more active BMP, which then undergoes rapid transformation.	0.5
Beclomethasone monopropionate (BMP)	13.5	7.5	450	NA	See above.	2.7
Budesonide	9.4	5.1	980	11	Extensive first-pass.	2.8
Ciclesonide	0.12	NA	NA	<0.5	Extensive first-pass. Ciclesonide metabolized to active metabolite, des-ciclesonide, in the lungs. Active metabolite undergoes transformation in the liver.	0.7
Des-ciclesonide	12.0	NA	NA	<1	See above.	3.5
Fluticasone propionate	18.0	10.5	1200	<1	Extensive first-pass and high systemic clearance mediated by CYP3A4 in gut and liver.	>14

[a] To human glucocorticoid receptors in vitro; Dexamethasone=1.
[b] Effect on human skin indicating relative topical potency; Dexamethasone=1.

Nursing Women: ICS are generally considered to be compatible with breastfeeding.

Pediatrics: Growth velocity may be reduced in children using ICS, even in the absence of evidence of HPA-axis suppression. This is usually seen during the first year of use. No impact on final adult height has been found to date. Growth velocity may also be reduced in chronic untreated asthma. Periodic monitoring of growth is recommended.

The use of ICS has not been associated with an increased risk of fractures in children.

Special Diseases and Conditions: Systemic effects of corticosteroids may be enhanced in patients with advanced liver cirrhosis, and in those with hypothyroidism. In hypoprothrombinemia, ASA should be used cautiously in conjunction with corticosteroids. In patients with glaucoma or who are at risk of glaucoma (e.g., elderly, positive family history) the intraocular pressure should be measured at the beginning of therapy and periodically thereafter.

ADVERSE EFFECTS: Adrenal Insufficiency: The risk of clinically significant adrenal suppression with the use of ICS is thought to be low but is increased with higher doses or with combined systemic and inhaled therapy.

Dermatology: Prolonged use of ICS therapy has been associated with a dose-related increase in the risk of skin thinning/bruising. Women may be at an increased risk of bruising.

Fungal Infections: Increased colonization of the oropharynx with *C. albicans* is common in patients using ICS. Actual infection is much less common, occurring in about 5 to 15% of patients. Studies have shown that the incidence is related to both the magnitude and frequency of dosing. To decrease the risk of oral candidiasis, advise the patient to rinse mouth well after each inhalation and consider using spacer devices. Institute antifungal therapy if active thrush present.

Growth: See Precautions, Pediatrics.

Ocular: Prolonged use of ICS therapy has been associated with a dose-related increase in the incidence of posterior subcapsular and nuclear cataract formation. There also appears to be an association between increased intraocular pressure or glaucoma and ICS use in patients with a family history of glaucoma. This increased risk appears to be dose-related. Monitor intraocular pressure in patients with personal or family history of glaucoma and who require ICS, especially high doses, soon after starting therapy and periodically thereafter. The influence of factors such as choice of corticosteroid, inhalation technique, type of delivery device, concurrent use of other antiasthmatic drugs or individual patient susceptibility on cataract formation, increased intraocular pressure or glaucoma is not yet known.

Osteoporosis: Decreases in bone density have been demonstrated with long-term use of high doses of ICS. The exact dose of ICS that negatively impacts bone mineral density and therefore fracture risk is not known. Monitor bone mineral density in patients who require high doses of ICS especially in those with coexisting risk factors for osteoporosis. Patients with COPD may be at an increased risk for osteoporosis and osteopenia.

Respiratory: Bronchospasm, coughing and/or wheezing may occur in some patients following oral inhalation of corticosteroids. It may be a reaction to excipients in the formulation or to materials like rubber or metal in the delivery device. This may be prevented in some patients by using an inhaled bronchodilator a few minutes before the ICS. Pneumonia is seen at an increased rate in patients on combination therapy (i.e., ICS plus long-acting beta$_2$-agonist) relative to monotherapy with long-acting beta$_2$-agonist. Predictable complications of pneumonia, such as death and hospitalization rate, may not be increased.

Other: Dysphonia (hoarseness, temporary or permanent change in voice) and throat irritation are not uncommon. Consider obtaining informed consent if used by professional singers. Dermatitis involving the perioral skin can occur, more commonly with the use of face masks or nebulizers. To reduce the risk of perioral dermatitis, wash the face after each treatment.

OVERDOSE:

> For management of a suspected drug overdose, CPhA recommends that you contact your **regional Poison Control Centre**. See the *CPS* Directory section for a list of Poison Control Centres.

DOSAGE: ICS are available in many different dosage forms including pMDIs which may be used with or without a spacer device, breath-actuated DPIs or solutions for use with nebulizers. Nebulization via face mask may be an inefficient delivery system for ICS as it is associated with facial and oropharyngeal deposition. Spacer devices with face mask are available for use with pMDIs in younger children (e.g., <5 years). Each method of administration offers certain advantages and disadvantages which may influence the choice of delivery system for a particular patient. For example, breath-actuated DPIs are generally considered unsuitable for children <5 years. Spacers with a mouthpiece maximize lung deposition and can be used in conjunction with pMDIs in patients with poor coordination. The minimum dose that adequately controls symptoms and maintains lung function should be targeted. Review inhaler technique at each visit.

Table 2 lists the estimated equivalent doses of ICS.

Table 2: Corticosteroids: Inhaled

Estimated Equivalent Dosages in Adults

Drug	Dose (μg/day) Low	Medium	High
Beclomethasone dipropionate pMDI[a]	≤250	251–500	>500
Budesonide DPI[b]	≤400	401–800	>800
Budesonide WN[c]	≤1000	1001–2000	>2000
Ciclesonide pMDI[a]	≤200	201–400	>400
Fluticasone propionate pMDI[a] or DPI[b]	≤250	251–500	>500

[a] Pressurized metered dose inhaler.
[b] Dry powder inhalation device.
[c] Wet nebulization.

Asthma: Table 3 and Table 4 list doses for adults and children, respectively.

Table 3: Corticosteroids: Inhaled

Dose in Adults for Asthma

Drug	Dose
Beclomethasone dipropionate	pMDI: 100–800 μg daily divided BID
Budesonide	DPI: 400–2400 μg daily divided BID Nebules: 1–2 mg/dose; dose is individualized
Ciclesonide	pMDI: 100–800 μg daily; max 800 μg daily divided BID
Fluticasone propionate	pMDI & DPI: 200–1000 μg daily divided BID; may ↑ to 1000 μg BID

Table 4: Corticosteroids: Inhaled

Dose in Pediatrics for Asthma

Drug	Dose
Beclomethasone dipropionate	pMDI: 5–11 y: 100–200 μg daily divided BID ≥12 y: 100–800 μg daily divided BID
Budesonide	DPI: 6–12 y: 200–400 μg daily divided BID >12 y: 400–2400 μg daily divided BID Nebules: 1–2 mg/dose BID; dose is individualized. 3 mo–12 y: 0.25–0.5 mg BID, can ↑ to 1 mg BID
Ciclesonide	pMDI: ≥12 y: 100–800 μg daily; max 800 μg daily divided BID
Fluticasone propionate	pMDI: 12 mo–4 y: 200 μg daily divided BID via pediatric spacer device with a face mask pMDI & DPI: 4–16 y: 100–400 μg daily divided BID pMDI & DPI: ≥16 y: 200–1000 μg daily divided BID

(cont'd)

The combination of budesonide and formoterol is indicated for maintenance and for rescue therapy in adults and children ≥12 years. Patients using a combination product of budesonide and formoterol for maintenance therapy can use additional doses of this product as needed, in response to symptoms. A maximum of 6 inhalations is recommended on a single occasion; the total daily dose should not exceed 8 inhalations.

The transfer of corticosteroid-dependent asthmatic patients from oral to ICS therapy requires special care because of the slow recovery of HPA function. Asthma should be stable before considering the transfer. Initially, the maintenance dose of systemic steroid and the inhaled steroid should be given concurrently. After 1 week, the dose of systemic steroid should be very gradually decreased. Many withdrawal or tapering regimens have been described. Factors such as dose and duration of oral therapy and overall health of the patient should be considered when determining the withdrawal schedule. During dose tapering, some patients may experience symptoms of steroid withdrawal despite maintenance or even improvement of respiratory function. These patients should be encouraged to continue with the inhaler and be monitored closely for signs of adrenal insufficiency (see Warnings). If such signs occur, the systemic steroid dose should be increased temporarily; further withdrawal will have to be done more slowly. In patients being transferred, consideration must be given to supplementation with systemic steroids during periods of stress or severe asthmatic attacks. Some patients cannot completely discontinue oral steroids. In these cases, a minimum maintenance oral dose should be given concurrently with the inhaled steroid. Consider compliance assessment, trigger avoidance, addition of long-acting beta$_2$-agonist, addition of a leukotriene antagonist and anti-IgE therapy.

Once asthma is under control, inhaled steroids should be given twice daily in order to improve compliance. The schedule should be increased to 4 times/day for patients with more severe asthma. Once daily dosing may be sufficient for patients with mild asthma.

Patients must be instructed regarding the correct use of inhalation devices to ensure that the drug reaches the target areas within the lung. The use of a spacer device should be encouraged in patients who have difficulty coordinating the use of pMDIs and in patients who require high doses, to minimize thrush and dysphonia by decreasing oral deposition. Patients using DPI devices must be capable of generating the required inspiratory flow rate to mobilize the powder into the lungs. Rinsing the mouth and gargling with water after each inhalation is helpful in preventing oral candidiasis and reducing systemic bioavailability.

It must be stressed to patients that ICS are to be used at regular intervals as prescribed and are not intended for treatment of an acute asthmatic attack.

All asthmatic patients should have a written action plan that provides explicit treatment directives for management of flare-ups.

Croup: Single dose of budesonide 2 mg by nebulization.

Corticosteroids: Systemic Ⓟ

betamethasone sodium phosphate
cortisone acetate
dexamethasone
dexamethasone sodium phosphate
fludrocortisone acetate
hydrocortisone
hydrocortisone sodium succinate
methylprednisolone
methylprednisolone acetate
methylprednisolone sodium succinate
prednisolone
prednisolone acetate
prednisolone sodium phosphate
prednisone
triamcinolone
triamcinolone acetonide
triamcinolone diacetate

CPhA Monograph

Date of Revision: September 2006

> This monograph has been compiled by CPhA and reviewed by experts. It may contain information different from that found in Health Canada-approved Product Monographs. The reader is referred to the *CPS* Editorial Policy for more information.

PHARMACOLOGY: This monograph deals with the systemic use of corticosteroids by the oral, iv and im routes. It does not address local (e.g., intra-articular) use of corticosteroids.

Corticosteroids are synthetic analogues of hormones secreted by the adrenal cortex. They possess anti-inflammatory (glucocorticoid) and/or salt-retaining (mineralocorticoid) properties to varying degrees (see Table 1). Glucocorticoids affect almost all body systems and cause varied metabolic effects. They promote protein catabolism, gluconeogenesis, and redistribution of fat from peripheral to central areas of the body. They reduce intestinal absorption and increase renal excretion of calcium. Mineralocorticoids affect electrolyte and fluid balance by acting on the distal renal tubule to promote sodium reabsorption and potassium and hydrogen excretion.

The mechanism of action of corticosteroids is not fully understood. Glucocorticoids decrease inflammation through multiple mechanisms, including stabilization of leukocyte lysosomal membranes, inhibition of macrophage accumulation in inflamed areas, and reduction of capillary permeability. They suppress the body's immune responses through mechanisms such as reduction of activity and volume of the lymphatic system, decreased immunoglobulin and complement concentrations as well as decreased passage of immune complexes through basement membranes. They also stimulate the erythroid cells of bone marrow and lengthen the survival time of erythrocytes and platelets. The mechanism of action for the antiemetic effect of corticosteroids is not well established.

Pharmacokinetics: Most glucocorticoids in the form of free alcohols, ketones or acetates are readily absorbed when administered orally. With im administration, the rate of absorption of the lipid soluble acetate and acetonide esters is much slower than that of the water soluble sodium phosphate and sodium succinate salts. A water soluble corticosteroid salt should be administered iv to achieve a rapid onset of action.

In animal studies, most glucocorticoids have been shown to be removed rapidly from blood and distributed to muscles, liver, skin, intestine and kidneys. They bind to plasma proteins to varying extents. Because only unbound drug is pharmacologically active, patients with low serum albumin concentrations may be more susceptible to the effects of glucocorticoids than patients with normal serum albumin concentrations. Glucocorticoids cross the placenta and may be distributed into breast milk.

Cortisone and prednisone are reduced to their pharmacologically active forms, hydrocortisone and prednisolone respectively. These active compounds are then metabolized, primarily in the liver, to biologically inactive compounds. Inactive metabolites, primarily glucuronides and sulfates, are excreted by the kidneys. Small amounts of unmetabolized drug are excreted in urine and bile.

Table 1: Corticosteroids: Systemic

Comparative Properties

Drug	Biologic Half-Life (hours)	Equivalent Anti-inflammatory Dose (mg)[a]	Relative Mineralo-corticoid Potency
Glucocorticoids:			
Short-acting	8 to 12		
Cortisone		25	2
Hydrocortisone		20	2
Intermediate-acting	18 to 36		
Methylprednisolone		4	0
Prednisolone		5	1
Prednisone		5	1
Triamcinolone		4	0
Long-acting	36 to 54		
Betamethasone		0.6	0
Dexamethasone		0.75	0
Mineralocorticoid:			
Fludrocortisone	12 to 24	10	125

[a] Equivalent doses are approximations and may not apply to all diseases or routes of administration. Duration of HPA axis suppression and degree of mineralocorticoid activities must be considered separately.

INDICATIONS: Endocrine Disorders: Primary or secondary adrenocortical insufficiency (hydrocortisone or cortisone is the first choice; synthetic analogues may be used in conjunction with mineralocorticoids where applicable; in infancy, mineralocorticoid supplementation is of particular importance), congenital adrenal hyperplasia, nonsuppurative thyroiditis, hypercalcemia associated with some forms of cancer. Used parenterally in acute adrenal cortical insufficiency (hydrocortisone or cortisone is the drug of choice), preoperatively or in the event of serious trauma or illness with known adrenal insufficiency or when adrenal cortical reserve is doubtful, shock unresponsive to conventional therapy if adrenal cortical insufficiency exists or is suspected.

Rheumatic Disorders and Collagen Diseases: As adjunctive therapy for short-term administration (for acute episode or exacerbation) in: psoriatic and rheumatoid arthritis (selected cases may require low dose maintenance therapy), ankylosing spondylitis, acute and subacute bursitis, acute nonspecific tenosynovitis, acute gouty arthritis; for exacerbation or maintenance therapy in selected cases of systemic lupus erythematosus, acute rheumatic carditis, systemic dermatomyositis, polymyositis, polymyalgia rheumatica, giant-cell arteritis.

Dermatologic Diseases: Blistering immune diseases such as pemphigus vulgaris, bullous pemphigoid and acute severe contact dermatitis; widespread and recalcitrant atopic dermatitis; other inflammatory skin diseases such as lichen planus, vasculitis or acne fulminans.

Allergic Conditions: For short-term administration in the control of severe or incapacitating allergic conditions intractable to adequate trials of conventional treatment such as seasonal or perennial allergic rhinitis, bronchial asthma, contact dermatitis, atopic dermatitis, serum sickness and drug hypersensitivity reactions. Parenteral therapy is indicated for urticarial transfusion reactions, angioedema and anaphylaxis (epinephrine is the drug of choice).

Ophthalmic Diseases: severe acute and chronic allergic and inflammatory processes involving the eye and its adnexa such as allergic conjunctivitis, keratitis, allergic corneal marginal ulcers, herpes zoster ophthalmicus (but not herpes simplex), iritis and iridocyclitis, chorioretinitis, anterior segment inflammation, diffuse posterior uveitis and choroiditis, optic neuritis, retrobulbar neuritis, sympathetic ophthalmia.

Respiratory Diseases: moderate to severe croup, symptomatic sarcoidosis, Löffler's syndrome not manageable by other means, berylliosis, fulminating or disseminated pulmonary tuberculosis when concurrently accompanied by appropriate antituberculous chemotherapy, aspiration pneumonitis, acute exacerbations of chronic obstructive pulmonary disease, diffuse interstitial pulmonary fibrosis (Hamman-Rich syndrome), adjunctive therapy in the treatment of selected cases of *Pneumocystis jiroveci* pneumonia (PJP) in patients with HIV.

Hematological Disorders: idiopathic thrombocytopenia purpura and secondary thrombocytopenia in adults, acquired (autoimmune) hemolytic anemia, aplastic crisis, congenital (erythroid) hypoplastic anemia.

Neoplastic Diseases: leukemias and lymphomas in adults, acute leukemia of childhood.

Edematous States: to induce diuresis or remission of proteinuria in the nephrotic syndrome (without uremia) of the idiopathic type or that due to lupus erythematosus.

Gastrointestinal Diseases: as adjunctive therapy in the treatment of ulcerative colitis and regional enteritis (Crohn's disease).

Nervous System: acute exacerbations of multiple sclerosis. Dexamethasone may be used to treat patients with cerebral edema associated with primary or metastatic brain tumors, neurosurgery, pseudotumor cerebri and cerebral vascular accident (acute stroke) excluding intracerebral hemorrhage. Dexamethasone may also be used in the preoperative preparation of patients with increased intracranial pressure secondary to brain tumors or for palliation of patients with inoperable or recurrent brain neoplasms.

Organ Transplants: used in high dose concurrently with other immunosuppressive drugs to prevent rejection of transplanted organs and to prevent and treat graft versus host disease after bone marrow transplant.

Miscellaneous: tuberculosis meningitis with subarachnoid block or impending block when concurrently accompanied by appropriate antituberculous chemotherapy; acute bacterial meningitis; trichinosis with neurologic or myocardial involvement; postoperative dental inflammatory reactions; prevention of chemotherapy-associated nausea and vomiting. Recent guidelines suggest that corticosteroids are indicated in selected patients in septic shock (e.g., patients with relative adrenal insufficiency who require vasopressors to maintain adequate blood pressure). Dexamethasone is also used in the diagnostic testing of adrenocortical hyperfunction and antenatal prophylaxis of neonatal respiratory distress.

CONTRAINDICATIONS: Hypersensitivity to the product and its constituents; systemic fungal infections; administration of live virus vaccines in patients receiving immunosuppressive corticosteroid doses.

WARNINGS: Adrenal Suppression: Following prolonged therapy, abrupt discontinuation may result in a withdrawal syndrome and secondary adrenocortical insufficiency. Symptoms of adrenal insufficiency resulting from rapid withdrawal include: nausea, fatigue, anorexia, dyspnea, hypotension, hypoglycemia, myalgia, fever, malaise, arthralgia, dizziness, desquamation of skin and fainting. This type of relative insufficiency may persist for up to a year after discontinuation of therapy; therefore, in any stressful situation occurring during that period, reinstitute hormone therapy. If the patient is receiving corticosteroids already, the dosage may have to be increased. Since mineralocorticoid secretion may be impaired, salt and/or a mineralocorticoid may be needed.

Fluid and Electrolyte Balance: Average and large doses of hydrocortisone or cortisone can cause elevation of blood pressure, salt and water retention and increased potassium excretion. These effects are less likely to occur with the synthetic derivatives (except fludrocortisone) unless these are used in large doses. Dietary salt restriction and potassium supplementation may be necessary. All corticosteroids increase calcium excretion.

Gastrointestinal Effects: The association between peptic ulceration and corticosteroid therapy remains controversial. However, corticosteroid therapy may mask the symptoms of peptic ulcer. Perforation or hemorrhage may occur without significant pain.

Corticosteroids should be used with caution in patients with diverticulitis, fresh intestinal anastomoses, active or latent peptic ulcer and in nonspecific ulcerative colitis, if there is a probability of impending perforation, abscess or other pyogenic infection.

Hypersensitivity: Rare instances of anaphylactoid reactions have occurred in patients receiving parenteral corticosteroid therapy. Appropriate precautionary measures should be taken prior to parenteral administration, especially when the patient has a history of allergy to any drug. Some corticosteroid products contain tartrazine and sodium bisulfite, both of which may cause severe allergic reactions in susceptible individuals.

Immunosuppression: Immunization procedures should generally not be undertaken in patients receiving systemic corticosteroids, especially those on high doses, because of possible neurological complications and a lack of antibody response. Immunization procedures may be undertaken in patients who are receiving corticosteroids as replacement therapy. Corticosteroids may suppress reactions to patch tests.

Infections: When subjected to unusual stress, patients on corticosteroid therapy require increased dosage of rapidly-acting corticosteroids before, during and after the stressful situation.

Corticosteroids should only be used in active tuberculosis in cases of fulminating disseminated tuberculosis for the management of the disease in conjunction with an appropriate antituberculous regimen. If corticosteroids are indicated in patients with latent tuberculosis or tuberculin reactivity, close observation is necessary as reactivation of the disease may occur. During prolonged corticosteroid therapy, these patients should receive chemoprophylaxis.

Corticosteroids may mask some signs of infection, and new infections may appear during their use. There may be decreased resistance and inability to localize infection when corticosteroids are used. If corticosteroids have to be used in the presence of bacterial infections, institute appropriate anti-infective therapy. Patients exposed to certain infections (e.g., measles, chickenpox) should seek medical advice.

Corticosteroids may activate latent amebiasis. Amebiasis should be ruled out before giving corticosteroids to a patient who has spent time in the tropics or has unexplained diarrhea.

Ocular Effects: Corticosteroids should be used cautiously in patients with ocular herpes simplex because of possible corneal ulceration and perforation. Prolonged use of corticosteroids may produce posterior subcapsular cataracts, glaucoma with possible damage to the optic nerves and may enhance the establishment of secondary ocular infections due to fungi or viruses.

Renal Function Impairment: Edema may occur in the presence of renal disease with a fixed or decreased glomerular filtration rate. Caution is advised when corticosteroids are used in patients with renal insufficiency, acute glomerulonephritis and chronic nephritis.

PRECAUTIONS: Because complications of treatment with corticosteroids are dependent on the dosage regimen, a risk/benefit decision must be made in each individual case with respect to dose and duration of treatment and whether daily or intermittent therapy should be used. The lowest effective corticosteroid dose should be used to control the condition under treatment. Patients on long-term corticosteroid therapy who are subjected to unusual stress such as injury or surgery may require an increased dosage of corticosteroid during and after the stress.

When corticosteroids are used in myasthenia gravis, hospitalization with careful observation is recommended because a transient worsening of symptoms, possibly leading to respiratory distress, may precede clinical improvement.

Corticosteroid therapy can cause mental or mood disturbances including hypomania, mania, depression and psychosis. These reactions appear to be dose-related and more commonly seen in the first few weeks of therapy, but are sometimes seen following sharp decreases in corticosteroid dosage or during pulse therapy. Existing mood instability or psychotic tendencies may be aggravated by corticosteroids.

Avascular or aseptic necrosis of the femoral or humeral head has been associated with long-term corticosteroid treatment; however, it has also occurred in patients receiving high dose, short-term therapy. This adverse effect is more likely to occur in patients with a predisposing illness such as rheumatoid arthritis or systemic lupus erythematosis.

Systemic corticosteroid therapy has been associated with loss of bone density and osteoporosis, which are reversible after discontinuation of the corticosteroid. Adults chronically taking systemic corticosteroids should maintain an intake of at least 1500 mg of calcium and 800 IU of vitamin D daily, either through diet or supplementation, to prevent corticosteroid-induced osteoporosis. Some oral bisphosphonates are used to treat or prevent corticosteroid-induced osteoporosis and should be prescribed to patients at risk. (see Bisphosphonates: Oral, CPhA Monograph).

There is an enhanced effect of corticosteroids on patients with hypothyroidism and in those with cirrhosis.

ASA and nonsteroidal anti-inflammatory agents should be used cautiously in conjunction with corticosteroids in patients with hypoprothrombinemia.

To minimize the likelihood and severity of dermal atrophy, corticosteroids should not be injected sc. Injections into the deltoid area or repeat injections into any one site should also be avoided.

Pregnancy: The use of systemic corticosteroids in pregnant women has not been associated with an increased incidence of major fetal malformations. However, the incidence of oral cleft may be increased. Monitoring of neonates for signs of expected physiologic effects of exogenous corticosteroids is recommended, especially if high doses were used during pregnancy.

Lactation: The extent of corticosteroid excretion in breast milk is thought to be clinically insignificant. The use of systemic corticosteroid therapy is generally considered to be compatible with breast-feeding. Caution is advised if extremely high doses are used.

Children: Avoid prolonged therapy with systemic corticosteroids in infants and children if possible since corticosteroids may suppress growth. If deemed essential to institute chronic therapy, consider alternate day therapy to minimize this side effect. Growth and development should be closely monitored.

Drug Interactions: See Table 2.

Table 2: Corticosteroids: Systemic

Corticosteroid Drug Interactions

Drug(s) Involved	Description of Interaction	Action Required
Anticholinesterase agents (e.g., neostigmine, pyridostigmine)	Corticosteroids antagonize the effect of anticholinesterase agents, resulting in severe weakness in patients with myasthenia gravis.	Withdraw anticholinesterase medication if possible at least 24 hours prior to initiation of corticosteroid therapy.
Antidiabetic agents, including insulin	Corticosteroids may increase blood glucose concentrations.	Monitor blood glucose concentrations. Dose of antidiabetic agent may need to be increased.
Cyclosporine	Corticosteroid clearance may be decreased and plasma concentrations of cyclosporine may be increased through mutual inhibition of metabolism. Seizures have been reported in patients receiving high dose corticosteroid and cyclosporine concurrently.	Monitor cyclosporine levels closely; adjust dose of both medications if required.
Digoxin	Corticosteroid-induced potassium loss may potentiate digoxin toxicity.	Monitor serum potassium.
Estrogens	Corticosteroid clearance may be decreased.	Decrease corticosteroid dose if required.

(cont'd)

Table 2: Corticosteroids: Systemic *(cont'd)*

Corticosteroid Drug Interactions

Drug(s) Involved	Description of Interaction	Action Required
Hepatic microsomal enzyme inducers (e.g., barbiturates, phenytoin, rifampin)	Corticosteroid clearance may be increased through enzyme induction.	Increase corticosteroid dose if required.
Hepatic microsomal enzyme inhibitors (e.g., erythromycin, ketoconazole)	Corticosteroid clearance may be decreased through enzyme inhibition.	Decrease corticosteroid dose if required.
Isoniazid	Corticosteroids may increase hepatic metabolism and/or excretion of isoniazid.	Increase isoniazid dose if required.
Oral anticoagulants	Corticosteroids may increase or decrease anticoagulant action.	Monitor INR and adjust anticoagulant dose if required.
Potassium-depleting diuretics (e.g., thiazides, furosemide, ethacrynic acid)	Corticosteroid potassium-wasting effect is enhanced.	Monitor serum potassium and add supplement if required.
Nonsteroidal anti-inflammatory drugs (NSAIDs)	ASA: Corticosteroids may increase renal clearance of salicylate, resulting in either a decrease in salicylate efficacy, or salicylate toxicity when corticosteroid dose is decreased or discontinued.	Monitor salicylate level.
	All NSAIDs (including low-dose ASA): Concomitant use may increase the risk of peptic ulceration.	Avoid concurrent administration. If deemed necessary, monitor closely for gastrointestinal side effects and consider prophylaxis with misoprostol or a proton pump inhibitor.
Vaccines or toxoids	Corticosteroids inhibit antibody response resulting in enhanced toxicity from or diminished response to vaccines or toxoids.	Avoid use of vaccines or toxoids in patients receiving immunosuppressive doses of corticosteroids (see Warnings).

Drug-Laboratory Test Interactions: Corticosteroids may decrease I^{131} uptake and produce false negative results in the nitroblue tetrazolium test for systemic bacterial infection.

ADVERSE EFFECTS: Cardiovascular: thromboembolism; fat embolism; hypercholesterolemia; accelerated atherosclerosis; cardiac arrhythmias or ECG changes due to potassium deficiency; syncope; aggravation of hypertension; myocardial rupture following recent MI; reports of cardiac arrhythmias, fatal arrest or circulatory collapse following rapid administration of iv methylprednisolone greater than 0.5 g given over a period of less than 10 minutes.

Dermatologic: impaired wound healing; thin fragile skin; petechiae and ecchymoses; facial erythema; striae; hirsutism; acneiform eruptions; suppressed reactions to skin tests; hypersensitivity reactions such as allergic dermatitis, urticaria, angioneurotic edema.

Endocrine: decreased carbohydrate tolerance; hyperglycemia; glycosuria; increased requirements for oral hypoglycemics or insulin in diabetes; manifestations of latent diabetes mellitus; menstrual irregularities; development of cushingoid state; suppression of growth in children; secondary adrenocortical and pituitary unresponsiveness, particularly in times of stress, as in trauma, surgery or illness; increased sweating.

Fluid and Electrolyte Disturbances: sodium retention; fluid retention; congestive heart failure in susceptible patients; potassium loss; hypokalemic alkalosis; hypertension; hypocalcemia.

Gastrointestinal: nausea, vomiting, anorexia which may result in weight loss; increased appetite which may result in weight gain; diarrhea or constipation, abdominal distention, pancreatitis, gastric irritation and ulcerative esophagitis; peptic ulcer with possible perforation and hemorrhage; perforation of the small and large bowel, particularly in inflammatory bowel disease.

Hematologic: leukocytosis, thrombocytopenia, lymphopenia.

Hypersensitivity Reactions: Anaphylactic and hypersensitivity reactions occur occasionally and, depending on their severity, may be treated with antihistamines with or without epinephrine. General supportive measures should also be employed.

Metabolic: negative nitrogen balance due to protein catabolism.

Musculoskeletal: aseptic necrosis of femoral and humeral heads; muscle weakness; steroid myopathy; loss of muscle mass; osteoporosis; spontaneous fractures including vertebral compression fractures and pathologic fractures of long bones.

Neurological: seizures; increased intracranial pressure with papilledema (pseudotumor cerebri) in association with withdrawal of corticosteroid therapy; neuritis; paresthesias.

Ophthalmic: increased intraocular pressure; glaucoma; exophthalmos; posterior subcapsular cataracts.

Psychologic: hallucinations; psychosis; euphoria; mood changes.

Other: necrotizing angiitis, thrombophlebitis; aggravation or masking of infections; insomnia; anaphylactoid reactions. Burning or tingling of the perineal area may occur after iv injection of corticosteroids. Parenteral corticosteroid therapy has also produced hypo- or hyperpigmentation, scarring, induration, delayed pain or soreness, subcutaneous and cutaneous atrophy and sterile abscesses.

OVERDOSE:

> For management of a suspected drug overdose, CPhA recommends that you contact your **regional Poison Control Centre**. See the *CPS* Directory section for a list of Poison Control Centres.

DOSAGE: Because injections of slightly soluble corticosteroids may produce atrophy at the site of injection, im injections of these products should be made deeply into gluteal muscle; repeated im injections at the same site should be avoided and these products should not be administered sc.

Dosage ranges for corticosteroids are extremely wide and patient responses are quite variable. Dosage should be individualized according to the diagnosis, severity, prognosis, probable duration of disease, patient response and tolerance. For infants and children, the recommended dosage should be governed by the same considerations rather than by strict adherence to the ratio indicated by age or body weight.

Dosages used in various conditions are considered either physiologic (amount of corticosteroid normally secreted by the adrenal cortex daily) or pharmacologic (anything greater). See Table 3. Refer to Table 1 for equivalent doses for other corticosteroids.

Table 3: Corticosteroids: Systemic

Oral Prednisone Dosage (Adult)

Type of Dosage Range	Approximate Daily Dose
Physiologic	5 mg
Pharmacologic	
Maintenance or Low Dose	5 to 15 mg
Moderate Dose	0.5 mg/kg
High Dose	1 to 3 mg/kg
Massive Dose	15 to 30 mg/kg

(cont'd)

Table 3: Corticosteroids: Systemic *(cont'd)*

Dosage should be decreased or discontinued gradually when the drug has been administered for more than a few weeks to minimize the risk of adrenal insufficiency, as adrenal suppression has occurred after as little as 2 weeks of corticosteroid therapy. A number of different regimens for tapering corticosteroid therapy have been described. It has been suggested that the dosage be reduced by the equivalent of 2.5 to 5 mg of prednisone every 3 days to 2 weeks. An increase in dose followed by a more gradual withdrawal may be necessary if the disease flares up during tapering.

In the management of acute disorders, corticosteroid dosage should be sufficient to ensure that symptoms are controlled quickly, and treatment should be discontinued as soon as possible. In acute conditions where prompt relief is imperative, large doses are permissible and may be mandatory for a short period.

In chronic conditions requiring long-term therapy, use the lowest dosage that provides adequate but not necessarily complete relief. If a high dosage for prolonged periods is considered essential, observe patients closely for signs that might necessitate reduction in dosage or discontinuance of the drug. Chronic conditions are subject to periods of remission. When such periods occur, consider discontinuing corticosteroids gradually. Continued supervision of the patient after cessation of corticosteroids is essential since there may be a reappearance of severe manifestations of the disease.

Alternate day therapy in which a single dose is administered every other morning is considered by many clinicians to be the dosage regimen of choice for long-term corticosteroid treatment of most conditions; however, this remains controversial. Morning administration of the corticosteroid simulates the natural circadian rhythm of corticosteroid secretion which is high in the morning and low in the evening. This regimen provides relief of symptoms while minimizing adrenal suppression, cushingoid state, withdrawal symptoms and growth suppression in children. Intermediate-acting agents should be used for alternate day therapy (see Table 1). Dexamethasone is not suitable for every other day dosing to minimize adrenal suppression due to its long duration of effect.

The reader is referred to individual product monographs for more specific dosing information.

Corticosteroids: Topical Pr

amcinonide
betamethasone dipropionate
betamethasone sodium phosphate
betamethasone valerate
budesonide
clobetasol 17-propionate
clobetasone 17-butyrate
desonide
desoximetasone
diflucortolone valerate
flumethasone
fluocinolone acetonide
fluocinonide
halobetasol propionate
hydrocortisone
hydrocortisone 17-valerate
methylprednisolone acetate
mometasone furoate
prednicarbate
triamcinolone acetonide

CPhA Monograph

Date of Revision: November 2007

> This monograph has been compiled by CPhA and reviewed by experts. It may contain information different from that found in Health Canada-approved Product Monographs. The reader is referred to the *CPS* Editorial Policy for more information.

SUMMARY PRODUCT INFORMATION:

Drug[a]	Dosage Form	Strength
Amcinonide	Cream	0.1%
	Lotion	0.1%
	Ointment	0.1%
Betamethasone dipropionate	Cream	0.05%
	Lotion	0.05%
	Ointment	0.05%
Betamethasone sodium phosphate	Enema	5 mg/100 mL
Betamethasone valerate	Cream	0.05%, 0.1%
	Lotion	0.05%, 0.1%
	Ointment	0.05%, 0.1%
Budesonide	Enema	0.02 mg/mL

Drug[a]	Dosage Form	Strength
Clobetasol 17-propionate	Cream	0.05%
	Lotion	0.05%
	Ointment	0.05%
	Shampoo	0.05%
	Solution	0.05%
Clobetasone 17-butyrate[b]	Cream	0.05%
Desonide	Cream	0.05%
	Lotion	0.05%
	Ointment	0.05%
Desoximetasone	Cream	0.05%, 0.25%
	Gel	0.05%
	Ointment	0.25%
Diflucortolone valerate	Cream	0.1%
	Ointment	0.1%
Flumethasone pivalate	No single-entity products available	
Fluocinolone acetonide	Shampoo	0.01%
	Solution	0.01%
Fluocinonide	Cream	0.05%
	Gel	0.05%
	Ointment	0.05%
Halobetasol propionate	Cream	0.05%
	Ointment	0.05%
Hydrocortisone[b]	Cream	0.5%, 1%, 2%, 2.5%
	Enema suspension	100 mg/60 mL
	Liquid	2.5%
	Lotion	1%, 2.5%
	Ointment	0.5%, 1%
	Rectal aerosol	10%
Hydrocortisone 17-valerate	Cream	0.2%
	Ointment	0.2%
Methylprednisolone acetate	No single-entity products available	
Mometasone furoate	Cream	0.1%
	Lotion	0.1%
	Ointment	0.1%
Prednicarbate	Cream	0.1%
	Ointment	0.1%
Triamcinolone acetonide	Cream	0.1%, 0.5%
	Ointment	0.1%
	Paste	0.1%

[a] This table contains single-entity topical corticosteroid products only.

[b] Clobetasone 17-butyrate 0.05% and hydrocortisone 0.5% are available without a prescription.

PHARMACOLOGY: Topical corticosteroids are synthetic derivatives of cortisone which are effective when applied locally to control many types of inflammatory, allergic and pruritic dermatoses. Certain modifications to the chemical structure of hydrocortisone increase the anti-inflammatory potency of the molecule (see Table 1). For example, introduction of fluorine atoms into the molecule enhances anti-inflammatory activity. The more potent topical corticosteroids are generally more effective and more likely to cause adverse effects than less potent preparations.

Topically applied corticosteroids are thought to act by controlling the rate of synthesis of proteins. The overall effect of corticosteroids is a catabolic one. Topical corticosteroids inhibit the migration of macrophages and leukocytes into treated areas by reversing vascular dilation and permeability. With repeated administration to the same site, 3 times daily for 4 to 5 days, tolerance to the anti-inflammatory effects of the drug may occur. Withdrawal of the drug for 2 to 4 days should restore the response; however, tolerance will recur once application is restarted. Many dermatologic disorders respond equally well to low-potency corticosteroids such as hydrocortisone, although for severe acute dermatoses a more potent preparation may be preferred initially. Some dermatoses may require occlusion of the drug under a plastic film or intralesional administration.

Pharmacokinetics: Following topical application to normal skin, corticosteroids are minimally absorbed. Only small amounts of drug reach the dermis and are then absorbed into the systemic circulation. Absorption is greater when corticosteroids are applied to certain areas of the body, including the scalp, face, eyelid, axilla and scrotum. Absorption will also be increased if the epidermis is damaged by disease or inflammation or by the use of different vehicles or occlusive dressings. Continued absorption of corticosteroids may occur, even after washing, due to retention of the drug in the stratum corneum.

Following rectal administration or application of corticosteroids to the mucosa of the genitourinary tract, significant systemic absorption may occur. As much as 30 to 90% of hydrocortisone may be absorbed when administered as a retention enema. Absorption will be further increased if the mucosa is inflamed. Hypothalamic pituitary adrenal (HPA) axis suppression may occur.

Table 1: Corticosteroids: Topical

Comparative Potencies

Weak
Hydrocortisone
Hydrocortisone acetate
Methylprednisolone
Methylprednisolone acetate

Moderately Potent
Clobetasone 17-butyrate
Desonide
Flumethasone pivalate
Hydrocortisone valerate
Prednicarbate
Triamcinolone acetonide

Potent
Amcinonide
Betamethasone valerate
Desoximetasone
Diflucortolone valerate
Fluocinolone acetonide
Fluocinonide
Mometasone furoate

Very Potent
Betamethasone dipropionate
Clobetasol 17-propionate
Halobetasol propionate

INDICATIONS: Topical therapy of corticosteroid responsive acute and chronic skin eruptions, where an anti-inflammatory, anti-allergenic and antipruritic activity is required in the topical management of these conditions.

Corticosteroid enemas are used as adjunctive therapy in the management of certain inflammatory diseases involving the rectum, or sigmoid and left colon.

CONTRAINDICATIONS: Untreated tubercular, bacterial and fungal infections involving the skin, and in certain viral diseases such as herpes simplex, chickenpox, and vaccinia; hypersensitivity to any of the components of the product. Individual products may contain nonmedicinal ingredients causing hypersensitivity in some patients, e.g., the manufacturer of prednicarbate warns the product is contraindicated in individuals sensitive to wool/lanolin since the emollient cream contains wool alcohols ointment and wool wax alcohols.

WARNINGS: If used under an occlusive dressing, particularly over extensive areas, or on the face, scalp, axilla(e), scrotum or when applied to the genitourinary tract or when administered rectally, sufficient absorption may take place to give rise to adrenal suppression and other systemic effects. Fluorinated corticosteroids in particular should be used with caution on the face.

PRECAUTIONS: Topical corticosteroids (particularly the potent ones) should be used with caution on lesions close to the eye because systemic absorption may cause increased intraocular pressure, glaucoma or cataracts.

Tolerance to the vasoconstrictive effects of topical corticosteroids may occur with repeated administration (see Pharmacology).

Although hypersensitivity reactions have been rare with topically applied steroid products, the drug should be discontinued and appropriate therapy initiated if there are signs of reaction.

Prolonged use of topical corticosteroid products may produce atrophy of the skin and of subcutaneous tissues particularly on flexor surfaces and on the face. If this is noted, discontinue the use of the product.

In cases of infections of the skin, appropriate anti-infective agents should be used in primary therapy. In selected cases, the topical corticosteroid product may be used as an adjunct to control inflammation, erythema, and itching.

Topical corticosteroids should be used with caution in patients with stasis dermatitis and other skin diseases associated with impaired circulation. They should also be used with caution in patients receiving other immunosuppressants.

If a symptomatic response is not noted within a few days to a week, the local applications of corticosteroid should be discontinued and the patient re-evaluated. During the use of topical corticosteroids secondary infections may occur.

Under certain circumstances such as prolonged use, application over a large area of the body, use of an occlusive dressing, administration by retention enema, use in children or infants or use of a potent agent, adverse systemic corticosteroid effects may occur. If long-term therapy is anticipated, measures such as interrupting treatment periodically or treating one body area at a time may help to minimize the risk of adverse systemic effects. When long-term rectal use is discontinued, it must be tapered gradually.

Patients should be advised to inform current and subsequent physicians of the prior use of corticosteroids.

Occlusive dressings should not be applied if there is an elevation of body temperature.

Pregnancy: The use of topical corticosteroids is generally considered to be compatible with pregnancy.

Lactation: The use of topical corticosteroids is generally considered to be compatible with lactation.

Children: Pediatric patients have a higher skin surface to body weight ratio than adults and may absorb a higher percentage of topically applied corticosteroids. This may translate into a greater susceptibility to topical corticosteroid-induced HPA axis suppression and to exogenous corticosteroid effects. Caregivers should be reminded that diapers or plastic pants could constitute occlusive dressings when topical corticosteroids are applied in the diaper area.

HPA axis suppression, Cushing's syndrome, linear growth retardation, delayed weight gain, and intracranial hypertension have been reported in children receiving topical corticosteroids. Manifestations of adrenal suppression in children include low plasma cortisol levels and absence of response to ACTH stimulation. Manifestations of intracranial hypertension include bulging fontanelle, headaches and bilateral papilledema.

ADVERSE EFFECTS: The following local adverse reactions have been reported with the use of topical corticosteroids: dryness, itching, burning, local irritation, striae, skin atrophy, atrophy of subcutaneous tissues, telangiectasia, hypertrichosis, change in pigmentation and secondary infection. It should be noted that infection can be masked by the anti-inflammatory action of topical corticosteroids. If applied to the face, acne rosacea or perioral dermatitis can occur. When occlusive dressings are used, pustules, miliaria, folliculitis and pyoderma may occur. Contact sensitivity to a particular dressing material or adhesive may occur occasionally.

In rare instances, treatment of psoriasis with systemic or very potent topical corticosteroids (or their withdrawal) is thought to have provoked the pustular form of the disease.

Adrenal suppression has also been reported following topical corticosteroid therapy. Conditions that may increase systemic adsorption include use of the more potent steroids, use over a prolonged period of time, use over a large surface area and use with an occlusive dressing.

OVERDOSAGE:

Symptoms: Overdosage is very unlikely to occur. However, in the case of chronic overdosage or misuse, the features of hypercorticism may appear.

Treatment: Recovery of the HPA axis is usually prompt and complete following discontinuation of the topical steroid; however, if symptoms of adrenal insufficiency occur, supplemental oral steroid therapy may be initiated and tapered off gradually.

For management of a suspected drug overdose, CPhA recommends that you contact your **regional Poison Control Centre**. See the *CPS* Directory section for a list of Poison Control Centres.

DOSAGE: Generally, the least potent effective agent should be used. Ointments may be preferred for dry, scaly lesions. Creams, which are more acceptable cosmetically, are used for most inflammatory lesions. In hairy areas, a lotion or a liquefying vehicle such as a gel may permit better skin contact than creams or ointments. Some, but not all, topical corticosteroids are formulated in bases free of sensitizing agents. Apply the corticosteroid preparation sparingly to the clean affected skin area(s) either with gentle massage or use under occlusive dressings, as prescribed. Once control is achieved, reduce frequency of application.

Areas of increased permeability (scrotum, axilla, eyelids, scalp and face) respond better than areas such as the forearm, knee, elbow, palm and sole.

Frequency of application has traditionally been 3 to 4 times daily. Because of the repository effect of topical corticosteroids, less frequent applications (1 to 2 times per day) are equally effective.

For instillation of retention enemas, the patient should lie on the left side during administration and for 30 minutes after. The enema should be retained for at least 1 hour and preferably overnight. Various dosage regimens are used, depending on the indication, severity of symptoms and individual response.

The reader is referred to individual product monographs for more specific dosing information, as well as specific Precautions and Contraindications.

The reader is invited to consult CPhA's monograph **Corticosteroids: Topical.**

Cortifoam ℞

hydrocortisone acetate

Rectal Anti-Inflammatory Corticosteroid Foam

Paladin

SUPPLIED: An aerosol container with a special rectal applicator. Each applicatorful delivers approximately 900 mg of foam containing approximately 80 mg of hydrocortisone as 90 mg of hydrocortisone acetate. Nonmedicinal ingredients: cetyl alcohol, ethoxylated stearyl alcohol, methylparaben, polyoxyethylene-10 stearyl ether, propylparaben, propylene glycol, triethanolamine, water and inert propellants isobutane and propane. The 15 g aerosol container will deliver approximately 14 applications. Contents of the container are under pressure and are flammable. Do not use in the presence of an open flame or spark. Do not puncture or incinerate the aerosol container. Store at room temperature, not over 50°C.

Cortisone ℞

CPhA Monograph

see *Corticosteroids: Systemic*

Cortisone Acetate ℞

cortisone acetate

Corticosteroid

Valeant

PHARMACOLOGY: Corticosteroids diffuse across cell membranes and build complexes with specific cytoplasmic receptors. These complexes then enter the cell nucleus, bind to DNA, and stimulate transcription of messenger RNA (mRNA) and subsequent protein synthesis of various enzymes thought to be ultimately responsible for two categories of effects (glucocorticoid effects and mineralocorticoid effects) of systemic corticosteroids. However, these agents may suppress transcription of mRNA in some cells (e.g., lymphocytes).

Glucocorticoid effects are anti-inflammatory and immunosuppressant effects. **Mineralocorticoid effects** influence the water and electrolyte balance.

INDICATIONS: Corticosteroids are indicated in the management of disorders responsive to adrenocortical hormone therapy such as:

Endocrine Disorders: primary or secondary adrenocortical insufficiency (hydrocortisone or cortisone is the first choice; synthetic analogs may be used in conjunction with mineralocorticoids where applicable; in infancy, mineralocorticoid supplementation is of particular importance); congenital adrenal hyperplasia; nonsuppurative thyroiditis; hypercalcemia associated with cancer.

Rheumatic Disorders: as adjunctive therapy for short-term administration (to support the patient in an acute episode or exacerbation) in psoriatic arthritis, rheumatoid arthritis (selected cases may require low-dose maintenance therapy), ankylosing spondylitis, acute and subacute bursitis, acute gouty arthritis.

Collagen Diseases: during an exacerbation or as maintenance therapy in selected cases of systemic lupus erythematosus or acute rheumatic carditis.

Dermatologic Diseases: pemphigus, bullous dermatitis herpetiformis, severe erythema multiforme (Steven-Johnson Syndrome), exfoliative dermatitis, mycosis fungoides, severe psoriasis.

Allergic States: control of severe or incapacitating allergic conditions intractable to adequate trials of conventional treatment: seasonal or perennial allergic rhinitis, bronchial asthma, contact dermatitis, atopic dermatitis, serum sickness, angio-edema and urticaria.

Ophthalmic Diseases: severe acute and chronic allergic and inflammatory processes involving the eye and its adnexa such as allergic conjunctivitis, keratitis, allergic corneal marginal ulcers, herpes zoster ophthalmicus (but not herpes simplex), iritis and iridocyclitis, chorioretinitis, anterior segment inflammation, diffuse posterior uveitis and choroiditis, optic neuritis, sympathetic ophthalmia.

Respiratory Diseases: symptomatic sarcoidosis, Loeffler's syndrome not manageable by other means, berylliosis, fulminating or disseminated pulmonary tuberculosis when concurrently accompanied by appropriate antituberculous chemotherapy, pulmonary emphysema where bronchospasm or bronchial edema plays a significant role, diffuse interstitial pulmonary fibrosis (Hamman-Rich syndrome).

Hematological Disorders: idiopathic and secondary thrombocytopenia in adults, acquired (autoimmune) hemolytic anemia, erythroblastopenia (RBC anemia), congenital (erythroid) hypoplastic anemia.

Neoplastic Diseases: for palliative management of leukemias and lymphomas in adults and acute leukemia of childhood.

Edematous States: to induce a diuresis or remission of proteinuria in the nephrotic syndrome, without uremia, of the idiopathic type or that due to lupus erythematosus. In conjunction with diuretic agents, to induce a diuresis in cirrhosis of the liver with refractory ascites and/or congestive heart failure.

Gastrointestinal Diseases: to support the patient over an acute period of the disease including ulcerative colitis, regional enteritis, intractable sprue.

Miscellaneous: tuberculous meningitis with subarachnoid block or impending block when concurrently accompanied by appropriate antituberculous chemotherapy, systemic dermatomyositis (polymyositis), dental postoperative inflammatory reactions.

CONTRAINDICATIONS: Tuberculosis, whether active or healed, is usually an absolute contraindication to steroid therapy. However, cortisone may be a life-saving measure to control the acute toxicity of overwhelming infection. It must be accompanied by specific antituberculosis therapy. Should other infections exist, cortisone may be employed if the condition indicating its use is sufficiently severe. Appropriate antibiotic therapy must be given as well, usually in substantially larger doses than customary.

Ocular herpes simplex and acute psychoses also are usually absolute contraindications to steroid therapy.

Relative contraindications are diverticulitis; fresh intestinal anastomosis; active or latent peptic ulcer; renal insufficiency; hypertension; thromboembolic tendencies; osteoporosis; diabetes mellitus; psychotic tendencies; acute or chronic infections including fungus and viral diseases; especially chickenpox and vaccinia; myasthenia gravis; and diminished cardiac reserve or congestive heart failure other than that due to acute rheumatic carditis.

Pregnancy: Pregnancy is a relative contraindication to corticosteroid therapy, particularly during the first trimester, because fetal abnormalities have been observed in experimental animals. If it is necessary to give corticosteroids during pregnancy, the newborn infant should be watched closely for signs of hypoadrenalism and appropriate therapy should be instituted if such signs are present.

When any of these conditions exist, the risks of corticosteroid therapy must be weighed against the possible benefits.

Intrasynovial and soft tissue injections should not be made into infected areas.

WARNINGS: No data supplied by the manufacturer.

PRECAUTIONS: Cortisone should be given only with full cognizance of the characteristic activity of, and the varied responses to adrenocortical hormones.

Average and large doses can cause elevation of blood pressure, salt and water retention, and increased potassium and calcium excretion. Dietary salt restriction and potassium supplementation may be necessary.

Salt and water retention is frequently followed by spontaneous diuresis on continued administration of cortisone. In some instances, however, salt and water retention may be pronounced and occasionally may develop suddenly. Rarely, congestive heart failure, peripheral or pulmonary edema, ascites, or increased arterial pressure may develop if therapy is continued despite signs of fluid retention.

Hypokalemia can be detected early in the course of treatment by paying careful attention to the patient's symptoms and, if necessary, by doing an electrocardiogram, and by determining the CO2 combining power, and blood potassium and chloride levels. It may possibly be avoided by a low sodium, high potassium diet.

If any changes indicating metabolic alkalosis are noted, cortisone should be reduced or stopped, and potassium chloride administered. Diuretics may provoke a further dangerous loss of potassium.

Potassium salts must be avoided or undertaken with great caution in the presence of renal impairment or cardiac decompensation.

Although hypokalemia is a relatively uncommon complication, it may occur quite suddenly. For this reason, if electrocardiography is not feasible, the prophylactic administration of 2 to 4 g daily of potassium chloride is advisable with larger maintenance doses, e.g., 80 mg per day.

Important: It is of importance to keep in mind that the tissues may be low in potassium even when blood potassium levels appear to be adequate.

Since spontaneous remission of some diseases, such as rheumatoid arthritis, may occur during pregnancy, every effort should be made to avoid hormone treatment in pregnancy.

Corticosteroids may mask the signs of infection and enhance dissemination of the infecting organism. All patients receiving these substances should be watched for evidence of intercurrent infection. Should infection occur, vigorous, appropriate anti-infective therapy should be initiated. Abrupt cessation of steroids should be avoided if possible because of the danger of superimposing adrenocortical insufficiency on the infectious process.

Prolonged hormone therapy usually causes a reduction in the activity and size of the adrenal cortex. Relative adrenocortical insufficiency upon discontinuation of therapy may be avoided by gradual reduction of dosage. A potentially critical degree of insufficiency may persist asymptomatically, however, for some time even after gradual discontinuation. Therefore, if a patient is subjected to significant stress, such as surgery, trauma, or serious illness, while being treated or within 1 year (occasionally up to 2 years) after treatment has been terminated, hormone therapy should be augmented or reinstituted and continued for the duration of the stress and immediately following it. Since mineralocorticoid secretion may be impaired, salt and/or desoxycorticosterone may be required conjunctively. It is preferable to use a soluble hormone preparation during immediate preoperative and postoperative periods.

Corticosteroid therapy may cause hyperacidity or peptic ulcer. Therefore, an ulcer regimen including an antacid is recommended as a prophylactic measure during prolonged therapy. Since appearance of peptic ulcer may be asymptomatic until perforation or hemorrhage occurs, X-rays should be taken when treatment is prolonged or when there is gastric distress, and when changes are noted an ulcer regimen is recommended.

Cortisone, like other glucocorticoids, may aggravate diabetes mellitus so that higher insulin dosage may become necessary, or it may precipitate manifestations of latent diabetes mellitus.

When systemic adrenocorticosteroid preparations are used in the presence of glaucoma, intraocular pressure should be measured frequently and optic nerve heads and visual fields observed.

Continued supervision of the patient after cessation of corticosteroids is essential, since there may be a sudden reappearance of severe manifestations of the disease for which the patient was treated.

Steroids may increase or decrease motility and number of spermatozoa in some patients. Diphenylhydantoin may enhance the rate of metabolism and clearance of corticosteroids, and this may increase steroid dosage requirements.

ADVERSE EFFECTS: Fluid and Electrolyte Disturbances: sodium retention; fluid retention; congestive heart failure in susceptible patients; potassium loss; hypokalemic alkalosis; hypertension.

Musculoskeletal: muscle weakness; steroid myopathy; loss of muscle mass; osteoporosis; vertebral compression fractures; aseptic necrosis of femoral and humeral heads; pathologic fractures of long bones.

Gastrointestinal: peptic ulcer with possible perforation and hemorrhage; pancreatitis; abdominal distention; ulcerative esophagitis.

Dermatologic: impaired wound healing; thin fragile skin; petechiae and ecchymoses; facial erythema; increased sweating; may suppress reactions to skin tests.

Neurologic: convulsions; increased intracranial pressure with papilledema (pseudo-tumor cerebri) usually after treatment; vertigo; headache.

Endocrine: menstrual irregularities; development of Cushingoid state; suppression of growth in children; secondary adrenocortical and pituitary unresponsiveness, particularly in times of stress, as in trauma, surgery or illness; decreased carbohydrate tolerance; manifestations of latent diabetes mellitus; increased requirements for insulin or oral hypoglycemic agents in diabetes.

Ophthalmic: posterior subcapsular cataracts; increased intraocular pressure; glaucoma, exophthalmus.

Metabolic: negative nitrogen balance due to protein catabolism.

Others: hypersensitivity, thromboembolism.

OVERDOSE:

No data supplied by the manufacturer.

For management of a suspected drug overdose, CPhA recommends that you contact your **regional Poison Control Centre**. See the *CPS* Directory section for a list of Poison Control Centres.

DOSAGE: In chronic, nonfatal diseases (e.g., rheumatoid arthritis, chronic bronchial asthma, ulcerative colitis, sprue), it is recommended that therapy be initiated with a low dose of 25 mg to 50 mg per day which is gradually increased to the smallest amount that gives the desired degree of symptomatic relief. When adequate suppression of symptoms is achieved, dosage should be maintained at the minimum amount capable of providing sufficient relief without excessive hormonal effects. This amount may be as low as 25 mg per day.

In acute, nonfatal diseases (e.g., severe seasonal asthma, self-limiting ocular and dermatologic disorders), dosage ranges between 75 mg and 150 mg per day. In some patients higher doses are necessary. Since these conditions are self-limiting in their course, prolonged maintenance therapy is not necessary.

In chronic potentially fatal diseases (e.g., disseminated lupus erythematosus, pemphigus, sarcoidosis, nephrotic syndrome), the recommended initial dosage ranges from 75 mg to 150 mg per day. In some patients, higher doses are necessary. As soon as adequate relief is obtained, reduce dosage gradually to the minimum effective level.

When the disease is acute and life-threatening (e.g., acute rheumatic fever, crisis of disseminated lupus erythematosus, severe allergic reactions), the initial dosage is between 125 mg and 300 mg a day, administered in at least 4 divided doses. This dosage may have to be increased in some patients to establish control. As soon as control is attained, reduce dosage to minimum effective level. When extremely rapid onset of action is desired, one of the soluble adrenocortical hormone preparations may be administered intravenously for the first 2 or 3 doses. In severe allergic reactions, epinephrine is the first drug of choice. Cortisone is useful either concurrently or as supplementary therapy.

In dental surgical conditions, 25 mg to 50 mg 3 times daily, starting several hours before operation and continuing for no longer than 2 or 3 days postoperatively may give protection from the inflammatory reaction incidental to oral surgery procedures.

In chronic adrenocortical insufficiency (e.g., Addison's disease, postadrenalectomy), 10 to 25 mg per day or occasionally more, with 4 to 6 g of sodium chloride or 1 to 3 mg of desoxycorticosterone acetate. When immediate support is mandatory, one of the soluble adrenocortical hormone preparations, which may be effective within minutes after parenteral administration can be lifesaving.

In crises, intercurrent infections, surgical procedures, or other significantly stressful conditions, 100 to 300 mg or more daily until unusual stress no longer exists and normal food intake is restored. In these conditions, oral administration is preferable to intramuscular.

SUPPLIED: Each white, round, biconvex tablet, scored on one side and embossed "ICN C23" on the other side, contains: cortisone acetate USP 25 mg. Nonmedicinal ingredients: cornstarch, croscarmellose sodium NF, lactose NF, magnesium stearate NF, and talc USP. Bottles of 100.

Cortisporin® Ointment Pr

neomycin sulfate—polymyxin B sulfate—bacitracin zinc—hydrocortisone

Anti-inflammatory—Antibacterial

GlaxoSmithKline

PHARMACOLOGY: Corticosteroids suppress the inflammatory response to a variety of agents and they may delay healing. Since corticosteroids may inhibit the body's defense mechanism against infection, a concomitant antimicrobial drug may be used when this inhibition is considered to be clinically significant in a particular case.

The anti-infective components in the combination are included to provide action against specific organisms susceptible to them. Polymyxin B sulfate and neomycin sulfate together are considered active against the following microorganisms: *S. aureus*, *E. coli*, *H. influenzae*, Klebsiella-Enterobacter species, Neisseria species and *P. aeruginosa*. This product does not provide adequate coverage against *S. marcescens* and streptococci, including *S. pneumoniae*.

When used topically, bacitracin zinc, polymyxin B sulfate and neomycin sulfate are rarely irritating and are not absorbed systemically in significant amounts through intact skin or mucous membrane, but the possibility of significant absorption exists when extensive raw areas are being treated. The incidence of skin sensitization to this combination has been shown to be low on normal skin. Since these antibiotics are seldom used systemically, the patient is spared sensitization to those antibiotics which might later be required systemically.

Hydrocortisone is partially absorbed through intact skin and this absorption is enhanced when the skin is broken or occluded. The relative potency of corticosteroids depends on the molecular structure, concentration, and release from the vehicle.

INDICATIONS: For the treatment of inflammation of the anterior segment of the eye and skin infections and inflammation.

Not for use in the eyes.

CONTRAINDICATIONS: The ointment should not be used to treat otitis externa in the presence of a perforated tympanic membrane because of the risk of ototoxicity.

Only the sterile ophthalmic 3.5 g tube is for use in the eyes and not the regular topical ointment.

The use of Cortisporin ointment is contraindicated in patients who have demonstrated allergic hypersensitivity to any of the components of the preparation or to cross-sensitizing substances such as aminoglycosides and other related antibiotics.

The presence of pre-existing nerve deafness is a contraindication to the use of Cortisporin ointment in circumstances in which significant systemic absorption could occur.

Due to the known ototoxic and nephrotoxic potential of neomycin sulfate, the use of Cortisporin in large quantities or on large areas for prolonged periods of time is not recommended in circumstances where significant systemic absorption may occur.

Viral, tuberculous, primary bacterial and fungal infections of the skin are contraindications to the use of Cortisporin ointment.

A possibility of increased neomycin absorption exists in very young children, thus Cortisporin ointment is not recommended for use in neonates and infants (up to 2 years). In neonates and infants, absorption by immature skin may be enhanced and renal function may be immature.

WARNINGS: The concurrent use of other aminoglycoside antibiotics is not recommended in circumstances where significant systemic absorption of neomycin sulfate following topical application could occur.

Neomycin sulfate may cause cutaneous sensitization. A precise incidence of hypersensitivity reactions (primarily skin rash) due to topical neomycin is not known.

When using neomycin-containing products to control secondary infection in the chronic dermatoses, such as chronic otitis externa or stasis dermatitis, it should be borne in mind that the skin in these conditions is more liable than is normal skin to become sensitized to many substances including neomycin.

The manifestation of sensitization to neomycin is usually a low-grade reddening with swelling, dry scaling and itching; it may be manifested simply as a failure to heal. Periodic examination for such signs is advisable, and the patient should be told to discontinue the product if they are observed. These symptoms regress quickly on withdrawing the medication. Neomycin-containing applications should be avoided for the patient thereafter.

Following significant systemic absorption: aminoglycosides such as neomycin can cause irreversible ototoxicity; neomycin sulfate, polymyxin B sulfate and bacitracin zinc have nephrotoxic potential; polymyxin B sulfate has neurotoxic potential.

PRECAUTIONS: General: As with any antibiotic preparation, prolonged use may result in the overgrowth of nonsusceptible organisms, including fungi. The possibility of persistent fungal infections of the cornea and ear should be considered after prolonged steroid dosing. Appropriate measures should be taken if this occurs.

The use of Cortisporin ointment should not be continued for more than 7 days in the absence of any clinical improvement. If the infection is not improved after 1 week, cultures and susceptibility tests should be repeated to verify the identity of the organism and to determine whether therapy should be changed.

Allergic cross-reactions may occur which could prevent the use of any or all of the aminoglycoside antibiotics for the treatment of future infections.

Hydrocortisone may mask the allergic effects produced by any component of Cortisporin ointment.

Signs and symptoms of exogenous hyperadrenocorticism, including adrenal suppression, can occur with the use of topical corticosteroids. Systemic absorption of topically applied steroids will be increased if extensive body suface areas are treated or if occlusive dressings are used. Under these circumstances, suitable precautions should be taken when long-term use is anticipated.

Geriatrics: Cortisporin ointment is suitable for use in elderly patients. Caution should be exercised in cases where a decrease in renal function exists and significant systemic absorption of neomycin sulfate may occur (see Dosage).

Children: Cortisporin ointment is suitable for use in children (2 years and over) at the same dose as adults. A possibility of increased absorption exists in very young children, thus Cortisporin ointment is not recommended for use in neonates and infants (<2 years) (see Contraindications and Dosage).

Pregnancy: There is little information to demonstrate the possible effect of topically applied neomycin in pregnancy. However, neomycin present in maternal blood can cross the placenta and may give rise to a theoretical risk of fetal toxicity, thus use of Cortisporin ointment is not recommended in pregnancy.

Lactation: There is little information to demonstrate the possible effect of topically applied neomycin in lactation. Thus use of Cortisporin ointment is not recommended in nursing mothers.

Patients with Special Diseases and Conditions: In renal impairment, the plasma clearance of neomycin is reduced (see Dosage).

Drug Interactions: Following significant systemic absorption, both neomycin sulfate and polymyxin B sulfate can intensify and prolong the respiratory depressant effects of neuromuscular blocking agents. However, the neuromuscular blocking activity of neomycin sulfate and polymyxin B sulfate is unlikely to present a hazard during use of Cortisporin ointment.

Laboratory Tests: Systemic effects of excessive levels of hydrocortisone may include a reduction in the number of circulating eosinophils and a decrease in urinary excretion of 17-hydroxycorticosteroids.

Carcinogenicity: Long-term studies in animals (rats, rabbits, mice) showed no evidence of carcinogenicity attributable to oral administration of corticosteroids.

ADVERSE EFFECTS: Adverse reactions have occurred with topical use of antibiotic combinations containing neomycin and polymyxin B. Exact incidence figures are not available since no denominator of treated patients is available. The reaction occurring most often is allergic sensitization. In one clinical study, using a 20% neomycin patch, neomycin-induced allergic skin reactions occurred in 2 of 2175 (0.09%) individuals in the general population. In another study, the incidence was found to be approximately 1%.

Neomycin occasionally causes skin sensitization. There is, however, an increased incidence of hypersensitivity to neomycin sulfate in certain selected groups of patients in dermatological practice, in particular venous stasis eczema and ulceration, and chronic otitis externa.

Allergic hypersensitivity to neomycin following topical use may manifest itself as an eczematous exacerbation with reddening, scaling, swelling and itching of the affected skin, or as a failure of the lesion to heal.

Allergic hypersensitivity reactions following the topical administration of bacitracin zinc, hydrocortisone and polymyxin B sulfate are rare events.

Anaphylactic reactions following the topical application of bacitracin zinc have been reported, but are rare events.

Topically applied hydrocortisone may produce skin atrophy such as telangiectasiae and striae. However, this effect only occurs following prolonged use, high dosage, occlusion of the topical site (for example by plastic or by natural occlusion as in the groin), and particularly applies to infants and young children. The possibility of systemic adverse effects when steroid preparations are used over larger areas or for a long period of time also exists.

The following local adverse reactions have been reported with topical corticosteroids, especially under occlusive dressings: burning, itching, irritation, dryness, folliculitis, hypertrichosis, acneiform eruptions, hypopigmentation, perioral dermatitis, allergic contact dermatitis, maceration of the skin, secondary infection, skin atrophy, striae and miliaria.

OVERDOSE:

No information is available concerning accidental ingestion of Cortisporin ointment.

Symptoms: No specific symptoms or signs have been associated with excessive use of Cortisporin ointment. However, consideration should be given to significant systemic absorption (see Contraindications, Warnings, and Precautions).

Treatment: Use of the product should be stopped and the patient's general status, hearing acuity, renal and neuromuscular functions should be monitored.

Blood levels of neomycin sulfate and bacitracin zinc should also be determined, and hemodialysis may reduce the serum level of neomycin sulfate.

> For management of a suspected drug overdose, CPhA recommends that you contact your **regional Poison Control Centre**. See the *CPS* Directory section for a list of Poison Control Centres.

DOSAGE: Prior to treatment, remove any debris such as pus, crusts, etc. from the affected area.

Treatment should not be continued for more than 7 days without medical supervision.

Dilution of Cortisporin ointment is not recommended; reduction of the antibiotic concentrations may reduce their therapeutic efficacy.

Adults: Apply a thin film of ointment to the affected area 2 to 4 times per day, depending on the clinical condition.

Children: Cortisporin ointment is suitable for use in children (2 years and over) at the same dose as adults. A possibility of increased absorption exists in very young children, thus Cortisporin ointment is not recommended for use in neonates and infants (<2 years) (see Contraindications and Precautions).

Geriatrics: Cortisporin ointment is suitable for use in elderly patients. Caution should be exercised in cases where a decrease in renal function exists and significant systemic absorption of neomycin sulfate may occur (see Warnings, and Precautions sections).

Dosage in Renal Impairment: Dosage should be reduced in patients with reduced renal function (see Warnings and Precautions).

SUPPLIED: Each g of ointment contains: polymyxin B sulfate 5000 units, bacitracin zinc 400 units, neomycin sulfate 5 mg and hydrocortisone 10 mg in a low melting point petrolatum base. Tubes of 15 g. Store between 15 and 25°C.

Cortisporin® Otic Solution Sterile Pr

neomycin sulfate—polymyxin B sulfate—hydrocortisone

Anti-inflammatory—Antibacterial

GlaxoSmithKline

PHARMACOLOGY: Corticosteroids suppress the inflammatory response to a variety of agents and they may delay healing. Since corticosteroids may inhibit the body's defense mechanism against infection, a concomitant antimicrobial drug may be used when this inhibition is considered to be clinically significant in a particular case.

The anti-infective components in the combination are included to provide action against specific organisms susceptible to them. Polymyxin B sulfate and neomycin sulfate together are considered active against the following microorganisms: *S. aureus*, *E. coli*, *H. influenzae*, Klebsiella-Enterobacter species, Neisseria species and *P. aeruginosa*. This product does not provide adequate coverage against *S. marcescens* and streptococci, including *S. pneumoniae*.

When used topically, polymyxin B sulfate and neomycin sulfate are rarely irritating and are not absorbed systemically in significant amounts through intact skin or mucous membrane, but the possibility of significant absorption exists when extensive raw areas are being treated. The incidence of skin sensitization to this combination has been shown to be low on normal skin. Since these antibiotics are seldom used systemically, the patient is spared sensitization to those antibiotics which might later be required systemically.

Hydrocortisone is partially absorbed through intact skin and this absorption is enhanced when the skin is broken or occluded. The relative potency of corticosteroids depends on the molecular structure, concentration, and release from the vehicle.

INDICATIONS: For the treatment of superficial bacterial infections of the external auditory canal caused by organisms susceptible to the action of the antibiotics.

CONTRAINDICATIONS: Not for use in the eyes.

The use of Cortisporin otic solution is contraindicated in patients in whom perforation of the tympanic membrane is known or suspected, because of the possibility of ototoxicity caused by neomycin.

Due to the known ototoxic and nephrotoxic potential of neomycin sulfate, the use of Cortisporin otic solution in large quantities or on large areas for prolonged periods of time is not recommended in circumstances where significant systemic absorption may occur.

The use of Cortisporin otic solution is contraindicated in patients who have demonstrated allergic hypersensitivity to any of the components of the preparation or to cross-sensitizing substances such as aminoglycosides and other related antibiotics. The use of Cortisporin otic solution is contraindicated in the presence of untreated Herpes simplex, Herpes zoster and fungal infections, and in vaccinia and varicella infections.

A possibility of increased neomycin absorption exists in very young children, thus Cortisporin otic solution is not recommended for use in neonates and infants (up to 2 years). In neonates and infants, absorption by immature skin may be enhanced and renal function may be immature.

WARNINGS: Neomycin sulfate may cause cutaneous sensitization. A precise incidence of hypersensitivity reactions (primarily skin rash) due to topical neomycin is not known.

When using neomycin-containing products to control secondary infection in the chronic dermatoses, such as chronic otitis externa or stasis dermatitis, it should be borne in mind that the skin in these conditions is more liable than is normal skin to become sensitized to many substances including neomycin.

The manifestation of sensitization to neomycin is usually a low-grade reddening with swelling, dry scaling and itching; it may be manifested simply as a failure to heal. Periodic examination for such signs is advisable, and the patient should be told to discontinue the product if they are observed. These symptoms regress quickly on withdrawing the medication. Neomycin-containing applications should be avoided for the patient thereafter.

Following significant systemic absorption: aminoglycosides such as neomycin can cause irreversible ototoxicity; neomycin sulfate and polymyxin B sulfate have nephrotoxic potential; polymyxin B sulfate has neurotoxic potential.

This product contains potassium metabisulfite, a sulfite that may cause allergic-type reactions including anaphylactic symptoms and life-threatening or less severe asthmatic episodes in certain susceptible people. The overall prevalence of sulfite sensitivity in the general population is unknown and probably low. Sulfite sensitivity is seen more frequently in asthmatic than in nonasthmatic people.

PRECAUTIONS: General: As with any antibiotic preparation, prolonged use may result in the overgrowth of nonsusceptible organisms, including fungi. The possibility of persistent fungal infections of the ear should be considered after prolonged steroid dosing. Appropriate measures should be taken if this occurs.

The use of Cortisporin otic solution should not be continued for more than 7 days without medical supervision. If the infection is not improved after 1 week, cultures and susceptibility tests should be repeated to verify the identity of the organism and to determine whether therapy should be changed.

Allergic cross-reactions may occur which could prevent the use of any or all of the aminoglycoside antibiotics for the treatment of future infections.

Hydrocortisone may mask the allergic effects produced by any component of Cortisporin otic solution.

All topically active corticosteroids possess the potential to suppress the pituitary-adrenal axis following systemic absorption. Development of adverse systemic effects due to the hydrocortisone component of Cortisporin otic solution is considered to be unlikely, but the recommended dosage should not be exceeded.

Cortisporin otic solution should only be used in the ear and is not suitable for use in the eyes.

Geriatrics: Cortisporin otic solution is suitable for use in elderly patients. Caution should be exercised in cases where a decrease in renal function exists and significant systemic absorption of neomycin sulfate may occur (see Dosage).

Children: Cortisporin otic solution is suitable for use in children (2 years and over) at the same dose as adults. A possibility of increased absorption exists in very young children, thus Cortisporin otic solution is not recommended for use in neonates and infants (<2 years) (see Contraindications, Warnings, and Dosage).

Pregnancy: There is little information to demonstrate the possible effect of topically applied neomycin in pregnancy. However, neomycin present in maternal blood can cross the placenta and may give rise to a theoretical risk of fetal toxicity, thus use of Cortisporin otic solution is not recommended in pregnancy.

Lactation: There is little information to demonstrate the possible effect of topically applied neomycin in lactation. Thus use of Cortisporin otic solution is not recommended in nursing mothers.
Patients with Special Diseases and Conditions: In renal impairment, the plasma clearance of neomycin is reduced (see Dosage).
Drug Interactions: Following significant systemic absorption, both neomycin sulfate and polymyxin B sulfate can intensify and prolong the respiratory depressant effects of neuromuscular blocking agents. However, the neuromuscular blocking activity of neomycin sulfate and polymyxin B sulfate is unlikely to present a hazard during use of Cortisporin otic solution.
Laboratory Tests: Systemic effects of excessive levels of hydrocortisone may include a reduction in the number of circulating eosinophils and a decrease in urinary excretion of 17-hydroxycorticosteroids.
Carcinogenicity: Long-term studies in animals (rats, rabbits, mice) showed no evidence of carcinogenicity attributable to oral administration of corticosteroids.
Information to Be Provided to the Patient: Avoid contaminating the dropper with material from the ear, fingers, or other source. This caution is necessary if the sterility of the drops is to be preserved.
If sensitization or irritation occurs, discontinue use immediately and contact your physician.
Do not use in the eyes.

ADVERSE EFFECTS: Adverse reactions have occurred with topical use of antibiotic combinations containing neomycin and polymyxin B. Exact incidence figures are not available since no denominator of treated patients is available. The reaction occurring most often is allergic sensitization. In one clinical study, using a 20% neomycin patch, neomycin-induced allergic skin reactions occurred in 2 of 2175 (0.09%) individuals in the general population. In another study, the incidence was found to be approximately 1%.
Ototoxicity and nephrotoxicity have also been reported (see Warnings).
Neomycin occasionally causes skin sensitization. There is, however, an increased incidence of hypersensivity to neomycin sulfate in certain selected groups of patients in dermatological practice, particularly those with venous stasis eczema and ulceration, and chronic otitis externa.
Allergic hypersensitivity to neomycin following topical use may manifest itself as an eczematous exacerbation with reddening, scaling, swelling and itching of the affected skin, or as a failure of the lesion to heal.
Allergic hypersensitivity reactions following the topical administration of hydrocortisone and polymyxin B sulfate are rare events.
The following local adverse reactions have been reported with topical corticosteroids, especially under occlusive dressings: burning, itching, irritation, dryness, folliculitis, hypertrichosis, acneiform eruptions, hypopigmentation, perioral dermatitis, allergic contact dermatitis, maceration of the skin, secondary infection, skin atrophy, striae and miliaria.
Stinging and burning have been reported when this product has gained access to the middle ear.

OVERDOSE:

Symptoms: No specific symptoms or signs have been associated with excessive use of Cortisporin otic solution. However, consideration should be given to significant systemic absorption (see Contraindications, Warnings, and Precautions).
Treatment: Use of the product should be stopped and the patient's general status, hearing acuity, renal and neuromuscular functions should be monitored.
Blood levels of neomycin sulfate and polymyxin B sulfate should be determined. Hemodialysis may reduce the serum level of neomycin sulfate.

For management of a suspected drug overdose, CPhA recommends that you contact your **regional Poison Control Centre**. See the *CPS* Directory section for a list of Poison Control Centres.

DOSAGE: The external auditory meatus and canal should be cleansed and dried with a sterile cotton applicator.
Soap should not be used for cleansing of the external auditory meatus and canal as it may inactivate the antibiotics.
The patient should lie with the affected ear upward and Cortisporin otic solution instilled. This position should be maintained for 5 minutes to facilitate penetration of the drops into the ear canal.
Repeat, if necessary for the opposite ear.
Alternatively, a cotton gauze may be inserted into the external auditory canal and then saturated with Cortisporin otic solution. This wick should be kept moist by adding further solution every 4 hours. The wick should be replaced at least once every 24 hours.
Treatment should not be continued for more than 7 days without medical supervision.
Adults: Four drops of the solution should be instilled into the affected ear 3 or 4 times daily.
Children: Cortisporin otic solution is suitable for use in children (2 years and over) at the same dose as adults. A possibility of increased absorption exists in very young children, thus Cortisporin otic solution is not recommended for use in neonates and infants (<2 years) (see Contraindications, Warnings, and Precautions).
Geriatrics: Cortisporin otic solution is suitable for use in elderly patients. Caution should be exercised in cases where a decrease in renal function exists and significant systemic absorption of neomycin sulfate may occur (see Contraindications, Warnings, and Precautions).
Use in Renal Impairment: Dosage should be reduced in patients with reduced renal function (see Warnings and Precautions).

SUPPLIED: Each mL of sterile otic solution contains: polymyxin B sulfate 10 000 units, neomycin sulfate equivalent to 3.5 mg neomycin base, and hydrocortisone 10 mg (1%). Nonmedicinal ingredients: cupric sulfate, glycerin, potassium metabisulfite and propylene glycol. Bottles of 10 mL with sterilized dropper. Protect from light. Store at 15 to 25°C.

The reader is invited to consult CPhA's monograph **Corticosteroids: Topical**.

Cortoderm
hydrocortisone
Topical Corticosteroid
Taro

SUPPLIED: 0.5%: Each g of soft emollient ointment contains: hydrocortisone 0.5%. Nonmedicinal ingredients: fractionated coconut oil, methylparaben, propylparaben and white petrolatum. Tubes of 15 g. Store at room temperature (15-30°C).
1%℞: Each g of soft emollient ointment contains: hydrocortisone 1%. Nonmedicinal ingredients: fractionated coconut oil, methylparaben, propylparaben and white petrolatum. Jars of 454 g. Store at room temperature (15-30°C).

Cortrosyn® ℞
cosyntropin
Adrenocorticotropic Hormone
Amphastar

PHARMACOLOGY: The pharmacologic profile of cosyntropin is similar to that of purified natural ACTH, it has been established that 250 µg of cosyntropin will stimulate the adrenal cortex maximally and to the same extent as 25 units of natural ACTH. These clinical observations confirm earlier animal and assay studies establishing the 1:100 ratio. This dose of cosyntropin will produce maximal secretion of 17-OH corticosteroids, 17-ketosteroids and/or 17-ketogenic steroids. Aldosterone secretion is increased also to some degree.
The extra adrenal effects which natural ACTH and cosyntropin have in common include increased melanotropic activity, increased growth hormone secretion and an adipokinetic effect. These are considered to be without physiological or clinical significance.
Severe hypofunction of the pituitary-adrenal axis is usually associated with subnormal plasma cortisol values but a low basal concentration is not per se evidence of adrenal insufficiency and does not suffice to make the diagnosis. Many patients with proven insufficiency, will have normal basal concentrations and will develop signs of insufficiency only when stressed. For this reason, the only criterion which should be used in establishing the diagnosis is the failure to respond to adequate corticotropin stimulation as provided by 250 µg of cosyntropin. When presumptive adrenal insufficiency is diagnosed by a negative cosyntropin test, further studies are indicated to determine if it is primary or secondary.
Primary adrenal insufficiency (Addison's disease) is the result of an intrinsic disease process, such as tuberculosis, within the gland. The production of adrenocortical hormones is deficient despite high ACTH concentrations (feedback mechanism). Secondary or relative insufficiency arises as the result of defective production of ACTH leading in turn to disuse atrophy of the adrenal cortex. It is commonly seen, for example, as a result of corticosteroid therapy, Sheehan's syndrome and pituitary tumors or ablation.
The differentiation of both types is based on the premise that a primarily defective gland cannot be stimulated by ACTH whereas a secondarily defective gland is potentially functional and will respond to adequate stimulation with ACTH. Patients selected for further study as the result of a negative cosyntropin test should be given a 3 or 4 day course of treatment with purified cortrophin gel and then retested. Suggested doses are 40 USP units twice daily for 4 days or 60 USP units twice daily for 3 days. Under these conditions little or no increase in plasma cortisol concentrations will be seen in Addison's disease whereas higher or even normal concentrations will be seen in cases with secondary adrenal insufficiency.

INDICATIONS: A diagnostic agent in the screening of patients presumed to have adrenocortical insufficiency. Because of its rapid effect on the adrenal cortex it is now possible to perform a 30 minute test of adrenal function (plasma cortisol response) as an office or outpatient procedure, using only 2 venipunctures (see Dosage).

CONTRAINDICATIONS: A history of a previous adverse reaction to cosyntropin.

WARNINGS: No data supplied by the manufacturer.

PRECAUTIONS: *Pregnancy:* When pregnancy is present or suspected, weigh the benefits of using cosyntropin against the possible hazards to the fetus.
It is not advisable to add cosyntropin, a synthetic polypeptide, to blood and plasma transfusions, because prolonged interaction with enzymes present in these fluids may cause breakdown of the polypeptide.
Allergic reactions may occur in response to cosyntropin. Marked redness and pain at the injection site, urticaria, pruritus, severe malaise or dyspnea may occur.
Severe anaphylactic reactions usually can be avoided by discontinuing the use of the drug at the earliest sign of local or systemic hypersensitivity. In the rare event of a serious incident occurring despite these precautions, initiate the following emergency measures as treatment for shock: i.v. injection of epinephrine HCl 100 to 800 µg and high doses of an i.v. corticosteroid, should be administered immediately. Because of the possibility of an allergic reaction occurring the injections should be given under medical supervision and the patient kept under observation for about 1 hour. Self-injection by patients is not recommended. Should prodromal signs occur, further use of cosyntropin should be stopped. Repeat administration may increase the risk of hypersensitivity. Patients should be instructed to inform subsequent physicians of previous use of corticotropic hormones.

ADVERSE EFFECTS: Cosyntropin is intended for short-term use. Adverse reactions other than a rare hypersensitivity reaction are not anticipated. To date, only 9 such reactions have been reported in the literature and in each instance the patient had a pre-existing allergic disease and/or a previous reaction to natural ACTH.

OVERDOSE:
No data supplied by the manufacturer.

For management of a suspected drug overdose, CPhA recommends that you contact your **regional Poison Control Centre**. See the *CPS* Directory section for a list of Poison Control Centres.

DOSAGE: Cosyntropin may be administered i.m. or as a direct i.v. injection when used as a rapid screening test of adrenal function. It may also be given as an i.v. infusion over a 4 to 8 hour period to provide a greater stimulus to the adrenal glands. Doses of 250 to 750 µg have been used in clinical studies and a maximal response noted with the smallest dose.
A suggested method for a rapid screening test of adrenal function is as follows: A control blood sample is taken and 250 µg of cosyntropin, dissolved in sterile saline, is then injected intramuscularly. A second blood sample is collected exactly 30 minutes later and the plasma cortisol response is then determined. In children, aged 2 years or less, a dose of 125 µg will often suffice.
The usual normal response in most cases is an approximate doubling of the basal concentration, provided that this does not exceed the normal range. Patients taking inadvertent doses of hydrocortisone on the test day and women taking estrogen containing drugs may exhibit abnormally high basal plasma cortisol concentrations. A paradoxical response may be noted in the former group as seen in a decrease in plasma cortisol values following a stimulating dose of cosyntropin. In the latter group only a normal incremental response is to be expected. Many patients with normal adrenal function, however, do not respond to the expected degree so that the following criteria have been established to denote a normal response:

1. The control plasma cortisol concentration should exceed 5 µg/100 mL.
2. The 30 minute concentration should show an increment of at least 7 µg/100 mL above the basal concentration.
3. The 30 minute concentration should exceed 18 µg/100 mL.

These criteria also apply when the drug is injected i.v. in 2 to 5 mL of saline over a 2 minute period.
Plasma cortisol concentrations usually peak about 45 to 60 minutes after an injection of cosyntropin and some prefer the 60 minute interval for testing for this reason. While it is true that the 60 minute values are usually higher than the 30 minute values, the difference may not be significant enough in most cases to outweigh the disadvantage of a longer testing period. If the 60 minute test period is used, the criterion for a normal response is an approximate doubling of the basal plasma cortisol value.
When given as an i.v. infusion, 250 µg may be added to glucose or saline solutions and given at the rate of approximately 40 µg/hour over a 6 hour period. It should not be added to blood or plasma as it is apt to be inactivated by enzymes.
Adrenal response may be measured in the usual manner by determining urinary steroid excretion before and after treatment or by measuring plasma cortisol concentrations before and at the end of the infusion. The latter is preferable because urinary steroid excretion does not always accurately reflect the adrenal or plasma cortisol response to ACTH.
Patients receiving hydrocortisone should omit their pretest doses on the day selected for testing. The test may be performed at anytime during the day but, because of the physiological diurnal variation of plasma cortisol, the criteria listed above cannot apply. It has been shown that basal plasma cortisol concentrations and the post-cosyntropin increment exhibit diurnal changes. However, the 30 minute plasma cortisol concentration remains unchanged throughout the day so that only this single criterion should be used.

SUPPLIED: Each vial contains: cosyntropin 250 µg (as a lyophilized powder). Nonmedicinal ingredients: glacial acetic acid, mannitol and sodium chloride. Each ampul of diluent contains: 1 mL of sodium chloride 0.9 % injection. Boxes of 10 vials and 10 ampuls. Store at 15 to 30°C. Cortrosyn is intended as a single dose injection and contains no antimicrobial preservative. Any unused portion should be discarded.

Corvert ℞
ibutilide fumarate
Antiarrhythmic Agent
Pfizer

Date of Preparation: September 10, 2003

PHARMACOLOGY: CORVERT (ibutilide fumarate injection) is an antiarrhythmic drug with predominantly class III (cardiac action potential prolongation) properties according to the Vaughan Williams Classification.
Ibutilide fumarate prolongs action potential duration in isolated adult cardiac myocytes and increases both atrial and ventricular refractoriness in vivo, i.e. class III electrophysiologic effects. Voltage clamp studies indicate that ibutilide at nanomolar concentrations, delays repolarisation by activation of a slow, inward current (predominantly sodium), rather than by blocking outward potassium currents, which is the mechanism by which most other class III antiarrhythmics act. These effects lead to prolongation of atrial and ventricular action potential duration and refractoriness, the predominant electrophysiologic properties of ibutilide in humans that are thought to be the basis for its antiarrhythmic effect.
Pharmacodynamics: Electrophysiologic Effects: Ibutilide produces mild slowing of the sinus rate and atrioventricular conduction. Ibutilide produces no clinically significant effect on QRS duration at the recommended dosage. Ibutilide produces dose-related prolongation of the QT interval, which is thought to be associated with its antiarrhythmic activity. However, there is no established relationship between plasma concentration and antiarrhythmic activity. In studies in healthy volunteers, intravenous infusions of ibutilide resulted in prolongation of the QT interval that was directly correlated with ibutilide plasma concentration during and after

10-minute and 8-hour infusions. There is a steep relationship between plasma concentration of ibutilide and QT prolongation and the maximum effect on QT interval is a function of both the dose of ibutilide and the infusion rate. Prolongation in QT interval is similar in women and men.

Hemodynamic Effects: A study of hemodynamic function in patients stratified for ejection fractions (above or below 35%) demonstrated no clinically significant effects on cardiac output, mean pulmonary arterial pressure, or capillary wedge pressure at doses of ibutilide up to 0.03 mg/kg.

Pharmacokinetics: The pharmacokinetics of ibutilide in patients with atrial flutter or atrial fibrillation are similar regardless of the type of arrhythmia, age, sex, left ventricular ejection fraction, occurrence of polymorphic ventricular tachycardia, or the concomitant use of digoxin, calcium channel blockers, or beta-blockers.

Ibutilide pharmacokinetics is highly variable among subjects but it is linear with respect to the dose over a range of 0.01 mg/kg to 0.10 mg/kg.

After intravenous infusion, ibutilide plasma concentrations rapidly decrease in a tri-exponential fashion. It is cleared rapidly and highly distributed extravascularly as evidenced by the short distribution half-life and large volume of distribution. Drug distribution is one of the primary mechanisms responsible for termination of pharmacological effect. The initial distribution half-life is short (1.5 minutes) and the elimination half-life averages 6 hours (range from 2 to 12 hours).

Ibutilide has a high systemic plasma clearance (approximately 29 mL/min/kg) that approximates liver blood flow. Total body clearance is primarily due to hepatic metabolism. It has a large steady-state volume of distribution (approximately 11 L/kg) and moderate degree of protein binding (approximately 40%).

Eight metabolites of ibutilide were detected in metabolic profiling of urine. These metabolites are thought to be formed primarily by ω-oxidation followed by sequential β-oxidation of the heptyl side chain of ibutilide. Only the initial metabolite of the primary pathway (ω-oxidation) possesses class III electrophysiologic properties similar to ibutilide in an in vitro isolated rabbit myocardium model. Plasma concentrations of this metabolite are <1% of the C_{max} of ibutilide concentrations and, therefore, it is assumed not to contribute to overall pharmacologic effect.

In healthy male volunteers, about 82% of a 0.01 mg/kg dose of [^{14}C] ibutilide was excreted in the urine (about 7% of the dose as unchanged ibutilide) within 4 days of dosing, and the remainder (19%) was recovered in the faeces within 7 days of dosing.

The enantiomers of ibutilide have pharmacokinetic properties similar to each other and there is no evidence that one enantiomer is safer than the other or the racemate. Substantial racemization of one isomer to the other has not been observed.

INDICATIONS: CORVERT (ibutilide fumarate injection) is indicated for the rapid conversion of atrial fibrillation or atrial flutter to sinus rhythm. CORVERT should be considered an alternative to electric cardioversion.

Patients with atrial arrhythmias of longer duration are less likely to respond to CORVERT. The effectiveness of CORVERT has not been determined in patients with arrhythmias of more than 90 days in duration.

Life-threatening Arrhythmias-Appropriate Treatment Environment: CORVERT can cause potentially fatal arrhythmias, particularly sustained polymorphic ventricular tachycardia, usually in association with QT prolongation, but sometimes without documented QT prolongation. In placebo-controlled clinical studies, possibly causally related sustained polymorphic ventricular tachycardia, which required cardioversion, occurred in 3.2% (7/218) of the patients with atrial flutter and 1.5% (4/340) of those with atrial fibrillation. None of the patients who received placebo in the placebo-controlled clinical studies experienced sustained polymorphic ventricular tachycardia (see Warnings, Proarrhythmia, Adverse Effects and Pharmacology). These arrhythmias can be reversed if treated promptly (see Warnings, Proarrhythmia).

It is essential that CORVERT be administered in a setting of continuous ECG monitoring and by personnel trained in identification and treatment of acute ventricular arrhythmias, particularly polymorphic ventricular tachycardia.

Patients with atrial fibrillation lasting more than 2 to 3 days must be adequately anticoagulated, generally for at least 2 weeks.

Choice of Patients: Patients with chronic atrial fibrillation have a strong tendency to revert after conversion to sinus rhythm, and treatments to maintain sinus rhythm carry risks.

Therefore, patients to be treated with CORVERT should be carefully selected such that the expected benefits of maintaining sinus rhythm outweigh the immediate risks of CORVERT and the risks of maintenance therapy, and such that CORVERT is likely to offer an advantage compared with alternative management.

CONTRAINDICATIONS: CORVERT (ibutilide fumarate injection) is contraindicated in patients who have previously demonstrated hypersensitivity to ibutilide or any of the other product components.

WARNINGS: Proarrhythmia: Like other antiarrhythmic agents, CORVERT (ibutilide fumarate injection) can induce or worsen ventricular arrhythmias, which, in some patients, might have potentially fatal consequences. Torsades de pointes, a polymorphic ventricular tachycardia (VT) that develops in the setting of QT interval prolongation, might occur because of the effect CORVERT has on cardiac repolarization. However, CORVERT can also cause polymorphic VT in the absence of excessive prolongation of the QT interval. In general, with drugs that prolong the QT interval, the risk of torsades de pointes is thought to increase progressively as the QT interval is prolonged, and this risk may be increased with bradycardia, a varying heart rate, or hypokalemia. In clinical trials, patients with atrial fibrillation or atrial flutter having QTc interval >440 msec or serum potassium ≤4.0 mM/L were excluded. Although change in QTc was directly related to ibutilide dosage, there was no clear relationship between risk of serious proarrhythmias and dose in clinical studies. This might have been due to the small number of events observed.

Because proarrhythmic events must be anticipated, CORVERT, as with other class III agents, is not recommended for patients with QTc intervals >440 msec.

Before treatment with CORVERT, hypokalemia and hypomagnesemia should be corrected to reduce the potential for proarrhythmia. Patients should be closely monitored for at least 4 hours following infusion or until QTc has returned to baseline. Longer monitoring is required if any arrhythmic activity is noted. Management of polymorphic VT includes discontinuation of CORVERT, correction of electrolyte abnormalities, (especially potassium and magnesium), and overdrive cardiac pacing, and electrical cardioversion or defibrillation. Pharmacologic therapies include magnesium sulfate infusions. Treatment of polymorphic VT with antiarrhythmics generally should be avoided.

During three placebo-controlled clinical trials involving patients treated with CORVERT (see Adverse Effects), 3.2% of 218 patients with atrial flutter and 1.2% of 340 patients with atrial fibrillation developed ibutilide-related sustained polymorphic VT requiring cardioversion; 7.8% of 218 patients with atrial flutter and 1.5% of 340 patients with atrial fibrillation experienced ibutilide-related nonsustained polymorphic VT. In the placebo-controlled clinical trial in post cardiac surgery patients, none of 77 patients with atrial flutter and 1.4% of 141 patients with atrial fibrillation experienced ibutilide-related sustained polymorphic VT; none of 141 patients with atrial flutter and 0.7% of 141 patients with atrial fibrillation experienced non-sustained polymorphic VT. In clinical trials, many initial episodes of polymorphic VT occurred during or soon after the infusion was stopped but generally within 40 minutes from the beginning of treatment. However, there were instances of recurrent polymorphic VT that occurred about 3 hours after the initial infusion of ibutilide.

Sustained monomorphic VT occurred in 0.2% of the patients, and nonsustained monomorphic VT occurred in 5.5% of patients in the four placebo-controlled studies. All patients with proarrhythmias in the controlled trials recovered with or without interventions. All patients with sustained VT received interventions, mainly DC shocks or intravenous magnesium sulfate.

Patients with a history of congestive heart failure (CHF) or low ejection fraction had a higher incidence of sustained polymorphic ventricular tachycardia (VT) than those without these underlying conditions (see Precautions).

Skilled personnel and proper equipment, such as cardiac monitoring equipment, a cardioverter/defibrillator, intracardiac pacing facilities, and medication for treatment of sustained ventricular tachycardias, including polymorphic ventricular tachycardia, must be available during and after administration of CORVERT (see Dosage).

Heart Block: Nine (1.5%) CORVERT-treated patients experienced reversible heart block: five had first degree, three had second degree and one had complete heart block.

PRECAUTIONS: Congestive Heart failure: CORVERT (ibutilide fumarate) caused a higher incidence of polymorphic VT in patients who had a history of congestive heart failure or low ejection fraction than those without these underlying conditions.

Torsade de Pointes: CORVERT is not recommended in patients with a history of polymorphic ventricular tachycardias (e.g., torsades de pointes).

Use in Patients with Hepatic Dysfunction: The safety, efficacy and pharmacokinetics of CORVERT have not been formally studied in patients with hepatic dysfunction. However, there are no changes in dosing recommendations for patients with hepatic dysfunction based on the following considerations: 1) CORVERT is indicated only for intravenous therapy of short duration (≤30 minutes). CORVERT is dosed to a known, well-defined pharmacologic action (termination of arrhythmia), the occurrence of specific adverse events or to a maximum of two 10-minute infusions (see Dosage). 2) The hepatic metabolic clearance of ibutilide is perfusion-rate limited and independent of hepatic function, as measured by serum alanine aminotransferase and aspartate aminotransferase. 3) Drug distribution appears to be one of the primary mechanisms responsible for termination of the pharmacologic effect.

Nevertheless, patients with impaired hepatic function should be closely monitored for more than the 4-hour period generally recommended.

Use in Patients with Renal Dysfunction: The safety, efficacy and pharmacokinetics of CORVERT have not been formally studied in patients with renal dysfunction. However, it is unlikely that dosage adjustment would be necessary because less than 10% of the dose of CORVERT is excreted unchanged in the urine and the metabolites of CORVERT do not contribute to overall pharmacologic effect. In patients who were treated with CORVERT, the clearance of ibutilide was independent of renal function as measured by estimated creatinine clearance (from a range 21 to 140 mL/min). No dosing changes are recommended.

Geriatrics: The mean age of patients in clinical trials was 65. No age-related differences were observed in pharmacokinetic, efficacy, or safety parameters for patients less than 65 compared to patients 65 years and older. Therefore, no changes in dosage are recommended for the elderly.

Children: Clinical trials with CORVERT did not include patients under the age of 18 years and, therefore, Safety and effectiveness of CORVERT in pediatric patients have not been established.

Pregnancy: CORVERT was teratogenic and embryocidal in reproduction studies in rats at oral doses 16 times the recommended clinical dose when corrected for oral bioavailability. Therefore, the potential risk to the fetus must be considered when anticipating treatment of pregnant women or women of child-bearing potential.

Lactation: The excretion of ibutilide into breast milk has not been studied; therefore, breast feeding is not recommended during therapy with CORVERT.

Carcinogenesis, Mutagenesis, Impairment of Fertility: No animal studies have been conducted to determine the carcinogenic potential of CORVERT; however, it was not genotoxic in a battery of assays (Ames assay, mammalian cell forward gene mutation, unscheduled DNA synthesis assay, and mouse micronucleus assay). Similarly, no drug related effects on fertility or mating were noted in a reproductive study in rats in which ibutilide was administered orally to both sexes up to doses of 20 mg/kg/day. On a mg/m² basis, corrected for 3% bioavailability, the highest dose tested was approximately four times the maximum recommended human dose.

Drug Interactions: No specific or formal drug interaction studies have been conducted.

Antiarrhythmics: Class Ia antiarrhythmic drugs (Vaughan Williams classification), such as disopyramide, quinidine, and procainamide, and other class III drugs, such as amiodarone and sotalol, should not be given concomitantly with CORVERT or within 4 hours post-infusion because of their potential to prolong refractoriness. These antiarrhythmics may be administered 4 hours after the CORVERT dosing.

Drugs that Prolong the QT Interval: The potential for proarrhythmia may increase with the administration of CORVERT to patients who are being treated with drugs that prolong the QT interval. These include psychoactive drugs such as phenothiazines, tricyclic antidepressants, tetracyclic antidepressants, and pimozide; antihistamine drugs (eg., terfenadine, astemizole); antimicrobials (eg., erythromycin particularly intravenously); antimalarials (eg., halofantrine); gastrointestinal prokinetic drugs (eg., cisapride).

Digoxin: Supraventricular arrhythmias might mask the cardiotoxicity associated with excessive digoxin levels. Therefore, it is advisable to be particularly cautious in patients whose plasma digoxin levels are above or suspected to be above the usual therapeutic range. Concomitant treatment with digoxin did not affect either serum digoxin levels or the pharmacokinetics of ibutilide in clinical trials.

Calcium Channel Blocking Agents: Concomitant treatment with calcium channel blocking agents did not affect the pharmacokinetics of ibutilide in clinical trials.

Beta Adrenergic Blocking Agents: Concomitant treatment with beta adrenergic blocking agents did not affect the pharmacokinetics of ibutilide in clinical trials.

ADVERSE EFFECTS: CORVERT (ibutilide fumarate injection) has been evaluated for safety in 1085 patients with atrial flutter or atrial fibrillation. Approximately half of these patients received two 10-minute infusions of ibutilide 1 mg at a 10-minute interval. Seven hundred and seventy six of these patients were treated with CORVERT in placebo-controlled trials. In these placebo-controlled studies, adverse events regardless of causality were reported in 319 of 776 (41.1%) of the ibutilide-treated patients compared to 76 of 254 (29.9%) of the patients on placebo (see Table 1). This difference is accounted mainly by the significantly greater incidence of cardiovascular adverse events observed in ibutilide-treated patients and the majority of cardiovascular adverse events were ventricular tachyarrhythmias. (See Table 1.)

In placebo-controlled studies, the rate of discontinuation of patients on ibutilide due to adverse events, regardless of causality was 5% (39 of 776 patients) compared to 0% (0 of 254 patients) on placebo.

The main reasons for premature discontinuation of CORVERT treatment were the emergence of ventricular extrasystoles (6 of 776 patients; 0.8%), non-sustained monomorphic ventricular tachycardia (7 of 776 patients; 0.9%), non-sustained polymorphic ventricular tachycardia (14 of 776 patients; 1.8%), sustained polymorphic ventricular tachycardia (7 of 776 patients; 0.9%) and QT segment prolongation (6 of 776 patients; 0.8%).

The following serious or severe adverse events that occurred in the placebo-controlled trials, for which a causal relationship with ibutilide could not be excluded, were: non-sustained polymorphic ventricular tachycardia (7 of 776 patients), sustained polymorphic ventricular tachycardia (14 of 776 patients), sustained monomorphic ventricular tachycardia (2 of 776 patients), supraventricular tachycardia (1 of 776 patients), heart arrest (3 of 776 patients), ventricular extrasystoles (1 of 776 patients), bigeminy (1 of 776 patients), cerebrovascular accident (3 of 776 patients), atrioventricular block (2 of 776 patients), hypotension (3 of 776 patients) and dizziness (1 of 776 patients).

In the placebo controlled trials, the most common adverse events with an incidence of ≥1%, but also with an incidence equal or greater than placebo, regardless of causal relationship to ibutilide, were: See Table 1.

Table 1: CORVERT

Adverse Events with an Incidence ≥1% and ≥ Placebo

Adverse Event	Placebo N=254	Ibutilide N=776
Cardiovascular		
Chest pain	1.2%	2.6%
Bradycardia	0.8%	1.4%
Extrasystoles, ventricular	0.8%	3.7%
Hypotension	0.8%	2.6%
Non-sustained monomorphic ventricular tachycardia	0.4%	3.4%
Non-sustained polymorphic ventricular tachycardia	0.4%	3.5%
Sinus bradycardia	0.8%	1.2%
Sustained polymorphic ventricular tachycardia	—	1.8%
Heart Arrest	—	1.0%
Other Body Systems		
Headache	3.1%	4.1%
Procedural non-surgical event	1.2%	1.9%
Nausea	3.1%	4.8%
Dizziness	1.6%	1.8%
Diarrhea	1.6%	1.8%

Proarrhythmias: Proarrhythmias causally related to CORVERT observed in the placebo-controlled trials in patients with atrial fibrillation (AFIB) and atrial flutter (AFL) are shown in Table 2 and Table 3.

Table 2: CORVERT

Percent and Number of Patients with Proarrhythmias Possibly Causally Related to Ibutilide (n/N=number of patients with proarrhythmias over the total number of patients with AFIB or AFL) in Three Placebo-controlled Trials

	Patients with AFIB % (n/N)	Patients with AFL % (n/N)
All proarrhythmias[a]	14/340 (4.1%)	35/218 (16.0%)
Non-sustained and sustained polymorphic VT	9/340 (2.7%)	24/218 (11.0%)
Sustained polymorphic VT	4/340 (1.2%)	7/218 (3.2%)

[a] Include non-sustained and sustained monomorphic and polymorphic VT but not premature beats or couplets.

Table 3: CORVERT

Percent and Number of Patients with Proarrhythmias Possibly Causally Related to Ibutilide (n/N=number of patients with proarrhythmias over the total number of patients with AFIB or AFL) in the Placebo-controlled trial (#017) in Patients with Atrial Fibrillation or Flutter Following Coronary Artery Bypass Graft or Valvular Surgery

	Patients with AFIB % (n/N)	Patients with AFL % (n/N)
All proarrhythmias[a]	8/141 (5.7%)	0/77 (0%)
Non-sustained and sustained polymorphic VT	3/141 (2.1%)	0/77 (0%)
Sustained polymorphic VT	2/141 (1.4%)	0/77 (0%)

[a] Include non-sustained and sustained monomorphic and polymorphic VT but not premature beats or couplets.

Other adverse events in the placebo-controlled trials not necessarily causally related to ibutilide with an incidence greater than placebo and between 0.3 to 1% are: **(incidence ibutilide, incidence placebo)** constipation (0.9%, 0.4%), urinary tract infection (0.9%, 0.8%), first degree AV block (0.9%, 0.4%), bundle branch block (0.9%, 0%), supraventricular tachycardia (0.8%, 0%), QT segment prolongation (0.8%, 0%), confusion (0.8%, 0.4%), hypertension (0.6%, 0%), nodal arrhythmia (0.6%, 0%), fatigue (0.5%, 0.4%), bigeminy (0.5%, 0%), leukocytosis (0.4%, 0%), leg cramps (0.4%, 0%), insomnia (0.4%, 0%), atrial fibrillation (0.4%, 0%), second degree AV block (0.4%, 0%), abdominal cramp (0.3%, 0%), asthenia (0.3%, 0%), arthralgia (0.3%, 0%), myalgia (0.3%, 0%), tremor (0.3%, 0%), pruritis (0.3%, 0%), abnormal vision (0.3%, 0%), precordial chest pain (0.3%, 0%), generalized edema (0.3%, 0%), trauma (0.3%, 0%), hematoma (0.3%, 0%), phlebitis (0.3%, 0%), acute kidney failure (0.3%, 0%), dysuria (0.3%, 0%), angina pectoris (0.3%, 0%), ventricular arrhythmia (0.3%, 0%).

Laboratory Abnormalities: The clinically relevant laboratory abnormalities observed in the placebo-controlled trials of CORVERT included elevated liver function tests (ALT, AST), elevated BUN, elevated creatine kinase, elevated creatinine, either elevated or low serum electrolytes (magnesium, sodium, potassium), low haemoglobin and abnormal platelet or white blood cell counts.

OVERDOSE:

Symptoms: In the clinical trials with CORVERT (ibutilide fumarate injection), four patients were unintentionally overdosed. The largest dose was 3.4 mg administered over 15 minutes. One patient developed increased ventricular ectopy and monomorphic ventricular tachycardia, another patient developed third degree A-V block and nonsustained polymorphic VT, and two patients had no medical event reports. Based on known pharmacology, the clinical effects of an overdosage with ibutilide could be an exaggeration of the expected prolongation of repolarization seen at usual clinical doses.

Treatment: Medical events (eg, proarrhythmia, A-V block) that occur after the overdosage should be treated with measures appropriate for that condition (see Warnings, Proarrhythmia).

For management of a suspected drug overdose, CPhA recommends that you contact your **regional Poison Control Centre**. See the *CPS* Directory section for a list of Poison Control Centres.

DOSAGE: The recommended dose of ibutilide is outlined in Table 4. Infusion of CORVERT (ibutilide fumarate injection) should be stopped as soon as the presenting arrhythmia is terminated, or if sustained or nonsustained ventricular tachycardia, or marked prolongation of QT or QTc occurs.

Table 4: CORVERT

Recommended Dose of CORVERT

Patient Weight	Initial Intravenous Infusion (over 10 minutes)	Second Intravenous Infusion
≥60 kg	1 mg ibutilide fumarate (One 10-mL vial)	If the arrhythmia does not terminate within 10 minutes after the end of the initial infusion, a second 10 minute infusion of equal strength may be administered.
<60 kg	0.01 mg/kg ibutilide fumarate (0.1 mL/kg)	

Table 5: CORVERT

Recommended Dose of CORVERT in Post Cardiac Surgery Patients

Patient Weight	Initial Intravenous Infusion (over 10 minutes)	Second Intravenous Infusion
≥60 kg	0.5 mg ibutilide fumarate (5 mL of 0.1 mg/mL solution)	If the arrhythmia does not terminate within 10 minutes after the end of the initial infusion, a second 10 minute infusion of equal strength may be administered
<60 kg	0.005 mg/kg ibutilide fumarate (0.05 mL/kg)	

In a study in patients with atrial fibrillation or flutter after valvular or CABG surgery, one or two intravenous infusions of 0.5 mg (0.005 mg/kg per dose for patients weighing less than 60 kg) was effective in terminating atrial fibrillation or atrial flutter and did not induce serious proarrhythmias unlike two 10-minute infusions of 1 mg.

More rapid infusion is not recommended. CORVERT may be administered undiluted or diluted (see Dilution).

Doses in addition to the second infusion are not recommended because of the risk of adverse events associated with QT interval prolongation.

If new arrhythmias develop or the original arrhythmia worsens during administration of CORVERT, the infusion should be stopped immediately.

Patients should be observed with continuous ECG monitoring for at least 4 hours following infusion or until QTc has returned to baseline. Longer monitoring is required if any arrhythmic activity is noted or in patients with clinically manifest liver dysfunction. Skilled personnel and proper equipment, such as a cardioverter/defibrillator, and medication for treatment of sustained ventricular tachycardia, including polymorphic ventricular tachycardia, must be available during administration of CORVERT and subsequent monitoring of the patient (see Warnings, Proarrhythmia).

Dilution: CORVERT may be administered undiluted or diluted in 50 mL of diluent. CORVERT may be added to 0.9% Sodium Chloride or 5% Dextrose Injection before infusion. The contents of one 10 mL vial (0.1 mg/mL ibutilide fumarate) may be added to a 50 mL infusion bag to form an admixture of 0.017 mg/mL ibutilide fumarate. Parenteral drug products should be inspected visually for particulate matter and discoloration prior to administration.

Compatibility: The following diluents are compatible with CORVERT: 5% Dextrose, 0.9% Sodium Chloride.

The following intravenous solution containers are compatible with admixtures of CORVERT: polyvinyl chloride plastic bags, polyolefin bags.

Stability: Admixtures of CORVERT, with the compatible diluents, should be used immediately after mixing. Protect from light.

SUPPLIED: Each mL of isotonic, clear, colourless, sterile aqueous solution contains: ibutilide fumarate 0.1 mg which is equivalent to 0.087 mg ibutilide (free base). Nonmedicinal ingredients: sodium acetate trihydrate, sodium chloride and sodium hydroxide solution or hydrochloric acid solution and water for injection. pH: approx. 4.6. Single use 10 mL clear glass vials with a pink flip-top. Store the product at controlled room temperature (15 to 30°C). Keep the product in its original carton until used. Protect from light.

As with all parenteral drug products, intravenous admixtures should be inspected visually for clarity, particulate matter, precipitate, discolouration and leakage prior to administration, whenever solution and container permit. Solutions showing haziness, particulate matter, precipitate, discolouration or leakage should not be used. Discard unused portion.

The reader is invited to consult CPhA's monograph **Selective Serotonin Reuptake Inhibitors**.

CO Sertraline

sertraline HCl

Antidepressant—Antipanic—Antiobsessional Agent

Cobalt

SUPPLIED: 25 mg: Each hard gelatin capsule, with yellow opaque body with "SL 25" printed in black and yellow opaque cap with " " printed in black, contains: sertraline 25 mg. Nonmedicinal ingredients: dibasic calcium phosphate anhydrous, magnesium stearate, microcrystalline cellulose and sodium starch glycolate; capsule shell: D&C Yellow #10, FD&C Yellow #6, gelatin and titanium dioxide. Tartrazine-free. Bottles of 100. Store at room temperature between 15 to 30°C.

50 mg: Each hard gelatin capsule, with white opaque body with "SL 50" printed in black and yellow opaque cap with " " printed in black, contains: sertraline 50 mg. Nonmedicinal ingredients: dibasic calcium phosphate anhydrous, magnesium stearate, microcrystalline cellulose and sodium starch glycolate; capsule shell: D&C Yellow #10, FD&C Yellow #6, gelatin and titanium dioxide. Tartrazine-free. Bottles of 100 and 250. Store at room temperature between 15 to 30°C.

100 mg: Each hard gelatin capsule with orange opaque body with "SL 100" printed in black and orange opaque cap with " " printed in black, contains: sertraline 100 mg. Nonmedicinal ingredients: dibasic calcium phosphate anhydrous, magnesium stearate, microcrystalline cellulose and sodium starch glycolate; capsule shell: D&C Yellow #10, FD&C Red #40, gelatin and titanium dioxide. Tartrazine-free. Bottles of 100 and 250. Store at room temperature between 15 to 30°C.

The reader is invited to consult CPhA's monograph **HMG-CoA Reductase Inhibitors**.

CO Simvastatin

simvastatin

Lipid Metabolism Regulator

Cobalt

SUPPLIED: 5 mg: Each cream, shield-shaped tablet for oral administration, with "SV 5" on one side and " " on the other side, contains: simvastatin 5 mg. Nonmedicinal ingredients: ascorbic acid, butylated hydroxyanisole, citric acid, lactose monohydrate, magnesium stearate, microcrystalline cellulose, pregelatinized starch and talc; tablet coating: hydroxypropylmethylcellulose, iron oxide yellow, polydextrose, polyethyleneglycol, titanium dioxide and triacetin. Gluten-free. Bottles of 100. Store at room temperature (15-30°C).

10 mg: Each pink, shield-shaped tablet for oral administration, with "SV 10" on one side and " " on the other side, contains: simvastatin 10 mg. Nonmedicinal ingredients: ascorbic acid, butylated hydroxyanisole, citric acid, lactose monohydrate, magnesium stearate, microcrystalline cellulose, pregelatinized starch and talc; tablet coating: hydroxypropylmethylcellulose, iron oxide red, polydextrose, polyethyleneglycol, titanium dioxide and triacetin. Gluten-free. Unit dose blisters of 30. Bottles of 100 and 500. Store at room temperature (15-30°C).

20 mg: Each tan, shield-shaped tablet for oral administration, with "SV 20" on one side and " " on the other side, contains: simvastatin 20 mg. Nonmedicinal ingredients: ascorbic acid, butylated hydroxyanisole, citric acid, lactose monohydrate, magnesium stearate, microcrystalline cellulose, pregelatinized starch and talc; tablet coating: hydroxypropylmethylcellulose, iron oxide red, iron oxide yellow, polydextrose, polyethyleneglycol, titanium dioxide and triacetin. Gluten-free. Unit dose blisters of 30. Bottles of 100 and 500. Store at room temperature (15-30°C).

40 mg: Each pink, shield-shaped tablet for oral administration, with "SV 40" on one side and " " on the other side, contains: simvastatin 40 mg. Nonmedicinal ingredients: ascorbic acid, butylated hydroxyanisole, citric acid, lactose monohydrate, magnesium stearate, microcrystalline cellulose, pregelatinized starch and talc; tablet coating: hydroxypropylmethylcellulose, iron oxide red, lactose monohydrate, titanium dioxide and triacetin. Gluten-free. Unit dose blisters of 30. Bottles of 100 and 500. Store at room temperature (15-30°C).

80 mg: Each pink, capsule-shaped tablet for oral administration, with "SV 80" on one side and " " on the other side, contains: simvastatin 80 mg. Nonmedicinal ingredients: ascorbic acid, butylated hydroxyanisole, citric acid, lactose monohydrate, magnesium stearate, microcrystalline cellulose, pregelatinized starch and talc; tablet coating: FD&C Red #40, hydroxypropylmethylcellulose, polydextrose, polyethyleneglycol, titanium dioxide and triacetin. Gluten-free. Unit dose blisters of 30. Bottles of 100. Store at room temperature (15-30°C).

Cosopt®

dorzolamide HCl—timolol maleate

Elevated Intraocular Pressure Therapy

Merck Frosst

Date of Revision: April 21, 2010

SUMMARY PRODUCT INFORMATION:

Route of Administration	Dosage Form/ Strength	Clinically Relevant Nonmedicinal Ingredients
Ophthalmic	Solution, each mL contains dorzolamide 20 mg and timolol 5 mg	For a complete listing see Dosage Forms, Composition and Packaging.

INDICATIONS AND CLINICAL USE: COSOPT (dorzolamide hydrochloride and timolol maleate) and COSOPT preservative-free formulation (without benzalkonium chloride as the preservative) are indicated in the treatment of elevated intraocular pressure (IOP) in patients with:

- ocular hypertension

• open-angle glaucoma
when concomitant therapy is appropriate.

COSOPT preservative-free formulation is indicated in patients who may be sensitive to a preservative, or for whom the use of a preservative-free formulation is otherwise advisable. **A comparative clinical trial of 3 months duration has been performed with COSOPT preservative-free formulation and COSOPT (with preservative) in adult patients. The results have indicated that the efficacy and safety profile of these two formulations appear to be equivalent. No studies were conducted in special populations (pediatric, kidney or liver diseases, etc.). For details please also refer to Dosage and Administration.**

CONTRAINDICATIONS: Hypersensitivity to any component of this product. For a complete listing see Dosage Forms, Composition and Packaging.

Bronchospasm, including bronchial asthma or a history of bronchial asthma, or chronic obstructive pulmonary disease.

Sinus bradycardia, second or third degree atrioventricular block, overt cardiac failure, cardiogenic shock.

COSOPT (dorzolamide hydrochloride and timolol maleate) has not been studied in patients with severe renal impairment (CrCl <0.5 mL/s). Because dorzolamide hydrochloride and its metabolite are excreted predominantly by the kidney, COSOPT is not recommended in such patients.

There is a potential for an additive effect with the known systemic effects of carbonic anhydrase inhibition in patients receiving an oral carbonic anhydrase inhibitor and topical carbonic anhydrase inhibitors concomitantly. The concomitant administration of COSOPT and oral carbonic anhydrase inhibitors has not been studied and is not recommended.

WARNINGS AND PRECAUTIONS: General: As with other topically-applied ophthalmic agents, the active substances may be absorbed systemically. Dorzolamide is a sulfonamide and timolol is a beta-blocker. Therefore, the same types of adverse reactions found with systemic administration of sulfonamides or beta-blockers may occur with topical administration, including severe reactions such as Stevens-Johnson syndrome and toxic epidermal necrolysis.

If signs of serious reactions or hypersensitivity occur, discontinue use of this preparation.

The management of patients with acute angle-closure glaucoma requires therapeutic interventions in addition to ocular hypotensive agents. COSOPT has not been studied in patients with acute angle-closure glaucoma.

Beta-adrenergic blocking agents should be administered with caution in patients subject to spontaneous hypoglycemia or to diabetic patients (especially those with labile diabetes) who are receiving insulin or oral hypoglycemic agents. Beta-adrenergic blocking agents may mask the signs and symptoms of acute hypoglycemia.

Because of the timolol maleate component, cardiac failure should be adequately controlled before beginning therapy with COSOPT (dorzolamide hydrochloride and timolol maleate). In patients with a history of severe cardiac disease, signs of cardiac failure should be watched for and pulse rates should be checked.

Respiratory reactions and cardiac reactions, including death due to bronchospasm in patients with asthma and rarely death in association with cardiac failure, have been reported following administration of timolol maleate ophthalmic solution.

Cardiovascular: Major Surgery: The necessity or desirability of withdrawal of beta-adrenergic blocking agents prior to major surgery is controversial. If necessary during surgery, the effects of beta-adrenergic blocking agents may be reversed by sufficient doses of such agonists as isoproterenol, dopamine, dobutamine or levarterenol.

Endocrine and Metabolism: Thyrotoxicosis: Beta-adrenergic blocking agents may mask certain clinical signs of hyperthyroidism (e.g., tachycardia). Patients suspected of developing thyrotoxicosis should be managed carefully to avoid abrupt withdrawal of beta-adrenergic blocking agents which might precipitate a thyroid storm.

Immune: Immunology and Hypersensitivity: In clinical studies, local ocular adverse effects, primarily conjunctivitis and eyelid reactions, were reported with chronic administration of dorzolamide hydrochloride ophthalmic solution. Some of these reactions had the clinical appearance and course of an allergic-type reaction that resolved upon discontinuation of drug therapy. Similar reactions have been reported with COSOPT (dorzolamide hydrochloride and timolol maleate). If such reactions are observed, discontinuation of treatment with COSOPT should be considered.

While taking beta-blockers, patients with a history of atopy or a history of severe anaphylactic reaction to a variety of allergens may be more reactive to accidental, diagnostic, or therapeutic repeated challenge with such allergens. Such patients may be unresponsive to the usual doses of epinephrine used to treat anaphylactic reactions.

Neurologic: Muscle Weakness: Beta-adrenergic blockade has been reported to increase muscle weakness consistent with certain myasthenic symptoms (e.g., diplopia, ptosis and generalized weakness). Timolol has been reported rarely to increase muscle weakness in some patients with myasthenic symptoms.

Cerebrovascular Insufficiency: Because of potential effects of beta-adrenergic blocking agents relative to blood pressure and pulse, these agents should be used with caution in patients with cerebrovascular insufficiency. If signs or symptoms suggesting reduced cerebral blood flow develop following initiation of therapy with COSOPT, alternative therapy should be considered.

Ophthalmologic: Corneal Edema: There is an increased risk of developing irreversible corneal edema in a subset of glaucoma patients with endothelial abnormalities including cellular density and/or morphology. In this group of patients evaluation of the cornea, with particular attention to the corneal endothelium, is recommended prior and during treatment with COSOPT.

Corneal Edema and Irreversible Corneal Decompensation: Corneal edema and irreversible corneal decompensation has been reported in patients with pre-existing chronic corneal defects and/or a history of intraocular surgery while using dorzolamide. COSOPT should be used with caution in such patients.

Contact Lenses: COSOPT contains the preservative benzalkonium chloride, which may be deposited in soft contact lenses; therefore, COSOPT should not be administered while wearing these lenses. The lenses should be removed before application of the drops and not be reinserted earlier than 15 minutes after use. COSOPT preservative-free formulation does not contain the preservative benzalkonium chloride.

Choroidal Detachment: Choroidal detachment has been reported with administration of aqueous suppressant therapy (e.g., timolol, acetazolamide) after filtration procedures. Management of eyes with chronic or recurrent choroidal detachment should include stopping all forms of aqueous suppressant therapy and treating endogenous inflammation vigorously.

Hepatic: COSOPT has not been studied in patients with hepatic impairment and therefore should be used with caution in such patients.

Special Populations: Pregnant Women: There are no adequate and well-controlled studies in pregnant women. COSOPT should be used during pregnancy only if the potential benefit justifies the potential risk to the fetus.

Nursing Women: It is not known whether dorzolamide hydrochloride is excreted in human milk. Timolol maleate does appear in human milk. Because of the potential for serious adverse reactions on the nursing infant, a decision should be made whether to discontinue nursing or discontinue the drug, taking into account the importance of the drug to the mother.

In a study of dorzolamide hydrochloride in lactating rats, decreases in body weight gain of 5 to 7% in offspring at an oral dose of 7.5 mg/kg/day (94 times the maximum recommended human ophthalmic dose) were seen during lactation. A slight delay in postnatal development (incisor eruption, vaginal canalization and eye openings), secondary to lower fetal body weight, was noted at 7.5 mg/kg/day (94 times the maximum recommended human ophthalmic dose).

Pediatrics: Safety and effectiveness in children have not been established.

Geriatrics (>65 years of age): Of the total number of patients in clinical studies of COSOPT, 49% were 65 years of age and over, while 13% were 75 years of age and over. No overall differences in effectiveness or safety were observed between these patients and younger patients, but greater sensitivity of some older individuals cannot be ruled out.

In a clinical study comparing COSOPT preservative-free formulation and COSOPT, 26% of all patients were over the age of 65, while 11% were 75 years of age and over. No overall differences in effectiveness or safety were observed between these patients and younger patients.

Monitoring and Laboratory Tests: COSOPT was not associated with clinically meaningful electrolyte disturbances.

ADVERSE REACTIONS: Adverse Drug Reaction Overview: Adverse reactions that have been seen with one of the components and may be potential adverse reactions of COSOPT are:

Dorzolamide Hydrochloride: Headache; eyelid inflammation; eyelid crusting; eyelid irritation; asthenia/fatigue; iridocyclitis; rash; dizziness; paraesthesia; superficial punctate keratitis, transient myopia (which resolved upon discontinuation of therapy); signs and symptoms of local reactions including palpebral reactions and systemic allergic reactions including angioedema, bronchospasm, urticaria, epistaxis and pruritus; throat irritation, dry mouth.

Timolol Maleate (topical formulation): Signs and symptoms of ocular irritation, including conjunctivitis, blepharitis, keratitis, and decreased corneal sensitivity, dry eyes; visual disturbances, including refractive changes (due to withdrawal of miotic therapy in some cases), diplopia, and ptosis; choroidal detachment following filtration surgery, tinnitus; aggravation or precipitation of certain cardiovascular pulmonary and other disorders presumably related to effects of systemic beta-blockade has been reported (see Contraindications and Warnings and Precautions). These include bradycardia; arrhythmia; hypotension; syncope; heart block; cerebrovascular accident; cerebral ischemia; palpitation; cardiac arrest, edema, claudication, Raynaud's phenomenon, cold hands and feet; congestive heart failure, and in insulin-dependent diabetics masked symptoms of hypoglycemia have been reported rarely. In clinical trials, slight reduction of the resting heart rate in some patients; bronchospasm (predominantly in patients with pre-existing bronchospastic disease); cough; headache; asthenia; fatigue; chest pain; alopecia; psoriasiform rash or exacerbation of psoriasis; signs and symptoms of allergic reactions including anaphylaxis angioedema, urticaria, localized and generalized rash; dizziness; increase in signs and symptoms of myasthenia gravis; insomnia; nightmares; memory loss; paresthesia; diarrhea, dyspepsia, dry mouth; decreased libido, Peyronie's disease; systemic lupus erythematous.

Timolol Maleate (systemic formulation): Adverse reactions reported in clinical experience with oral timolol maleate may be considered potential side effects of ophthalmic timolol maleate.

Clinical Trial Adverse Drug Reactions: In clinical studies, COSOPT (dorzolamide hydrochloride and timolol maleate) was generally well tolerated; no adverse experiences peculiar to this combination drug have been observed. Adverse experiences have been limited to those that were reported previously with dorzolamide hydrochloride and/or timolol maleate. In general, common adverse experiences were mild and did not cause discontinuation.

During clinical studies of up to 15 months duration, 1035 patients were treated with COSOPT. Approximately 2.4% of all patients discontinued therapy with COSOPT because of local ocular adverse reactions. Approximately 1.2% of all patients discontinued because of local adverse reactions suggestive of allergy or hypersensitivity.

The most frequently reported drug-related adverse effects were: ocular burning and stinging (10.7%), taste perversion (5.8%), corneal erosion (2.0%), conjunctival injection (1.8%), blurred vision (1.4%), tearing (1.0%), and ocular itching. Urolithiasis was reported rarely (0.9%).

In an active treatment-controlled clinical study of 3 months duration, 131 patients received COSOPT preservative-free formulation. Approximately 3.1% of patients receiving COSOPT preservative-free formulation discontinued therapy due to adverse experiences. Approximately 0.8% of all patients receiving COSOPT preservative-free formulation discontinued therapy because of adverse reactions suggestive of allergy and/or hypersensitivity.

The most frequently reported drug related adverse effects for COSOPT preservative-free formulation were ocular burning and stinging (16%) and taste perversion (3.1%).

Post-Market Adverse Drug Reactions: The following adverse reactions have been reported in post-marketing experience: dyspnea, respiratory failure, contact dermatitis, bradycardia, heart block, choroidal detachment following filtration surgery, nausea, corneal edema in glaucoma patients with endothelial abnormalities including cellular density and/or morphology, Stevens-Johnson syndrome, and toxic epidermal necrolysis.

DRUG INTERACTIONS: Overview: Specific drug interaction studies have not been performed with COSOPT.

In clinical studies, COSOPT was used concomitantly with the following systemic medications without evidence of adverse interactions: ACE-inhibitors, calcium channel blockers, diuretics, non-steroidal anti-inflammatory drugs includingacetylsalicylic acid, and hormones (e.g., estrogen, insulin, thyroxine). However, the potential for interactions with any drug should be considered.

Drug-Drug Interactions: The following drug interactions have been associated either with the components of COSOPT or with other beta-blockers or sulfonamides.

Acid-base Disturbances: The dorzolamide component of COSOPT is a carbonic anhydrase inhibitor and although administered topically, is absorbed systemically. In clinical studies, dorzolamide hydrochloride ophthalmic solution was not associated with acid-base disturbances. However, these disturbances have been reported with oral carbonic anhydrase inhibitors and have, in some instances, resulted in drug interactions (e.g., toxicity associated with high-dose salicylate therapy). Therefore, the potential for such drug interactions should be considered in patients receiving COSOPT.

Calcium Channel Blockers or Catecholamine-depleting Drugs: The potential exists for additive effects and production of hypotension, atrioventricular conduction disturbances, left ventricular failure and/or marked bradycardia when timolol maleate ophthalmic solution is administered together with oral calcium channel blockers, catecholamine-depleting drugs or beta-adrenergic blocking agents.

Quinidine: Potentiated systemic beta-blockade (e.g., decreased heart rate, depression) has been reported during combined treatment with CYP2D6 inhibitors (e.g. quinidine, SSRIs) and timolol.

Clonidine: Oral β-adrenergic blocking agents may exacerbate the rebound hypertension which can follow the withdrawal of clonidine. If the two drugs are coadministered, the β-adrenergic blocking agent should be withdrawn several days before the gradual withdrawal of clonidine. If replacing clonidine by β-blocker therapy, the introduction of β-adrenergic blocking agents should be delayed for several days after clonidine administration has stopped.

Beta-adrenergic Blockers: Patients who are already receiving a beta-adrenergic blocking agent systemically and who are given COSOPT should be observed for a potential additive effect either on the intraocular pressure or on the known systemic effects of beta-blockade. The concomitant use of two topical beta-adrenergic blocking agents is not recommended.

Epinephrine: Although COSOPT used alone has little or no effect on pupil size, mydriasis resulting from concomitant use of timolol maleate and epinephrine has been reported occasionally.

Drug-Laboratory Test Interactions: Clinically important changes in standard laboratory parameters were rarely associated with the administration of systemic timolol maleate. Slight increases in blood urea nitrogen, serum potassium and serum uric acid and triglycerides, and slight decreases in hemoglobin and hematocrit and HDL-cholesterol occurred, but were not progressive or associated with clinical manifestations.

Drug-Lifestyle Interactions: Effects on the Ability to Drive and Use Machines: There are side effects of COSOPT that may affect some patients' ability to drive and use machines. (See Drug Interactions and Adverse Reactions.)

DOSAGE AND ADMINISTRATION: Recommended Dose and Dosage Adjustment: The dose is one drop of COSOPT (dorzolamide hydrochloride and timolol maleate) or COSOPT preservative-free formulation ophthalmic solution in the affected eye(s) two times daily.

A comparative clinical trial of 3 months duration has been performed with COSOPT preservative-free formulation and COSOPT (with preservative) in adult patients. The results have indicated that the efficacy and safety profile of these two formulations appear to be equivalent. No studies were conducted in special populations (pediatric, kidney or liver diseases, etc.).

When substituting COSOPT for another ophthalmic antiglaucoma agent(s), discontinue the other agent(s) after proper dosing on one day, and start COSOPT on the next day.

If more than one topical ophthalmic drug is being used, the drugs should be administered at least ten minutes apart.

Missed Dose: If a dose is missed, it should be applied as soon as possible. However, if it is almost time for the next dose, the missed dose should be skipped and the next dose should be taken as usual.

OVERDOSAGE:

No data are available with regard to human overdosage by accidental or deliberate ingestion of COSOPT (dorzolamide hydrochloride and timolol maleate).

There have been reports of inadvertent overdosage with timolol maleate ophthalmic solution resulting in systemic effects similar to those seen with systemic beta-adrenergic blocking agents such as dizziness, headache, shortness of breath, bradycardia, bronchospasm, and cardiac arrest. The most common signs and symptoms to be expected with overdosage of dorzolamide are electrolyte imbalance, development of an acidotic state, and possibly central nervous system effects (see Adverse Reactions).

Treatment should be symptomatic and supportive. Serum electrolyte levels (particularly potassium) and blood pH levels should be monitored. Studies have shown that timolol does not dialyze readily.

Specific Therapeutic Measures for the treatment of overdosage with timolol maleate are reproduced below for ease of reference.

Gastric Lavage: If ingested.

Symptomatic Bradycardia: Use atropine sulfate intravenously in a dosage of 0.25 to 2 mg to induce vagal blockade. If bradycardia persists, intravenous isoproterenol hydrochloride should be administered cautiously. In refractory cases the use of a transvenous cardiac pacemaker may be considered.

Hypotension: Use sympathomimetic pressor drug therapy, such as dopamine, dobutamine or levarterenol. In refractory cases the use of glucagon hydrochloride has been reported to be useful.

Bronchospasm: Use isoproterenol hydrochloride. Additional therapy with aminophylline may be considered.

Acute Cardiac Failure: Conventional therapy with digitalis, diuretics and oxygen should be instituted immediately. In refractory cases the use of intravenous aminophylline is suggested. This may be followed if necessary by glucagon hydrochloride which has been reported to be useful.

Heart Block (second or third degree): Use isoproterenol hydrochloride or a transvenous cardiac pacemaker.

For management of a suspected drug overdose, contact your regional Poison Control Centre. See the *CPS* Directory section for a list of Poison Control Centres.

ACTION AND CLINICAL PHARMACOLOGY: Mechanism of Action: COSOPT (dorzolamide hydrochloride and timolol maleate) is the first combination of dorzolamide hydrochloride and timolol maleate. Each of these two components decreases elevated intraocular pressure by reducing aqueous humor secretion, but does so by a different mechanism of action.

Dorzolamide hydrochloride is a potent inhibitor of human carbonic anhydrase II. Inhibition of carbonic anhydrase in the ciliary processes of the eye decreases aqueous humor secretion, presumably by slowing the formation of bicarbonate ions with subsequent reduction in sodium and fluid transport. Timolol maleate is a nonselective beta-adrenergic receptor blocking agent that does not have significant intrinsic sympathomimetic, direct myocardial depressant, or local anesthetic (membrane-stabilizing) activity. The combined effect of these two agents results in additional intraocular pressure reduction compared to either component administered alone.

Following topical administration, COSOPT reduces elevated intraocular pressure, whether or not associated with glaucoma. Elevated intraocular pressure is a major risk factor in the pathogenesis of optic nerve damage and glaucomatous visual field loss. The higher the level of intraocular pressure, the greater the likelihood of glaucomatous visual field loss and optic nerve damage. COSOPT reduces intraocular pressure without the common side effects of miotics such as night blindness, accommodative spasm and pupillary constriction.

Pharmacokinetics: Dorzolamide Hydrochloride: Unlike oral carbonic anhydrase inhibitors, topically-applied dorzolamide hydrochloride exerts its effects at substantially low doses and therefore with less systemic exposure.

When applied topically, dorzolamide reaches the systemic circulation. To assess the potential for systemic carbonic anhydrase inhibition following topical administration, drug and metabolite concentrations in RBCs and plasma and carbonic anhydrase inhibition in RBCs were measured. Dorzolamide accumulates in RBCs during chronic dosing as a result of selective binding to CA-II while extremely low concentrations of free drug in plasma are maintained. The parent drug forms a single N-desethyl metabolite that inhibits CA-II less potently than the parent drug but also inhibits a less active isoenzyme (CA-I). The metabolite also accumulates in RBCs where it binds primarily to CA-I. Dorzolamide binds moderately to plasma proteins (approximately 33%). Dorzolamide is excreted unchanged in the urine; the metabolite is also excreted in urine. After dosing ends, dorzolamide washes out of RBCs in a non-linear manner, resulting in a rapid decline of drug concentration initially, followed by a slower elimination phase with a half-life of about four months.

To simulate the maximum systemic exposure after long term topical ocular administration, dorzolamide was given orally to eight healthy subjects for up to 20 weeks. The oral dose of 4 mg/day closely approximates the maximum amount of dorzolamide delivered by topical ocular administration of dorzolamide hydrochloride 2% t.i.d. Dorzolamide and metabolite reached steady state by 4 and 13 weeks, respectively, and the following observations were noted:

- In plasma, concentrations of dorzolamide and metabolite were generally below the assay limit of quantitation (15 nM) indicating almost no free drug or metabolite;
- In RBCs, dorzolamide concentrations approached the binding capacity of CA-II (20-25 μM) and metabolite concentrations approached 12-15 μM, well below the binding capacity of CA-I (125-155 μM);
- In RBCs, inhibition of CA-II activity and total carbonic anhydrase activity was below the degree of inhibition anticipated to be necessary for a pharmacological effect on renal function and respiration.

Timolol Maleate: Timolol maleate is a general beta-adrenergic receptor blocking agent that does not have intrinsic sympathomimetic, direct myocardial depressant or local anesthetic (membrane-stabilizing) activity.

Timolol maleate combines reversibly with a part of the cell membrane, the beta-adrenergic receptor, and thus inhibits the usual biologic response that would occur with stimulation of that receptor. This specific competitive antagonism blocks stimulation of the beta-adrenergic receptors by catecholamines having beta-adrenergic stimulating (agonist) activity, whether these originate from an endogenous or exogenous source. Reversal of this blockade can be accomplished by increasing the concentration of the agonist, which will restore the usual biologic response.

Timolol maleate (S(-) enantiomer) is significantly metabolized after oral and ophthalmic administration. The drug and the metabolites (hydroxyethylamino, hydroxyethylglycolamino derivatives and a third minor metabolite that results from the hydroxylation of a terminal methyl group on the tertiary butylamino moiety) are excreted primarily via the kidney. Based on correlation with debrisoquine metabolism, timolol metabolism is mediated primarily by cytochrome P-450 2D6. Dorzolamide is eliminated primarily by urinary excretion as unchanged drug. The metabolic pathway utilized by dorzolamide (cytochrome P-450 2C9, 2C19, and 3A4) is different from that utilized by timolol. In vitro studies using human liver microsomes have shown that dorzolamide at concentrations up to 200 μM does not affect the metabolism of timolol. Therefore, there is little potential for altered systemic exposure to either drug when administered in combination. Timolol is moderately (<60%) bound to plasma proteins.

In a study of plasma drug concentration in six subjects, the systemic exposure to timolol was determined following twice daily topical administration of timolol maleate ophthalmic solution 0.5%. The mean peak plasma concentration following morning dosing was 0.46 ng/mL and following afternoon dosing was 0.35 ng/mL.

By comparison to plasma concentration (10 to 20 ng/mL) following oral 5 mg dose, it was estimated that timolol was approximately 50% bioavailable systemically following intraocular administration.

STORAGE AND STABILITY: COSOPT Ophthalmic Solution: Store at 15-25°C. Protect from light.
COSOPT preservative-free formulation Ophthalmic Solution: Store at 15-25°C. Protect from light. Store in protective foil pouch.

INFORMATION FOR THE PATIENT: Published in e-CPS, available by subscription at www.e-cps.ca.

DOSAGE FORMS, COMPOSITION AND PACKAGING: COSOPT: Each mL of clear, colorless to nearly colorless, slightly viscous, sterile, isotonic, buffered, aqueous ophthalmic solution contains: dorzolamide 20 mg (equivalent to dorzolamide HCl 22.3 mg) and timolol 5 mg (equivalent to timolol maleate 6.83 mg). Nonmedicinal ingredients: benzalkonium chloride (0.0075%) (as preservative), hydroxyethyl cellulose, mannitol, sodium citrate, sodium hydroxide and water for injection. Translucent, high-density polyethylene Ocumeter Plus ophthalmic dispensers of 10 mL, with a sealed controlled drop tip, a flexible fluted side area which is depressed to dispense the drops and a 2-piece cap assembly. The opaque, white, 2-piece cap mechanism punctures the dropper tip seal upon initial use, then locks to provide a single cap during the usage period. Tamper evidence is provided by a safety tip on the container label.
COSOPT, Preservative-Free: For patients who may be sensitive to the preservative benzalkonium chloride or when use of a preservative-free topical medication is advisable, a formulation of COSOPT without the preservative benzalkonium chloride is available. Each mL of clear, colorless to nearly colorless, slightly viscous, sterile, isotonic, buffered, aqueous ophthalmic solution contains: dorzolamide 20 mg (equivalent to dorzolamide HCl 22.3 mg) and timolol 5 mg (equivalent to timolol maleate 6.83 mg). Nonmedicinal ingredients: hydroxyethyl cellulose, mannitol, sodium citrate, sodium hydroxide and water for injection. Packages of 15 individual fill volume translucent, low density polyethylene (without additives) unit dose pipettes of 0.2 mL, aluminum foil pouches of 4.

CO Sotalol Pr
sotalol HCl
Antiarrhythmic

Cobalt

SUPPLIED: 80 mg: Each light blue, capsule-shaped tablet, embossed "ICN-S31" contains: sotalol HCl 80 mg. Nonmedicinal ingredients: colloidal silicon dioxide, FD&C blue #2 Aluminium Lake, lactose monohydrate, magnesium stearate and microcrystalline cellulose. Bottles of 100.
160 mg: Each light blue, capsule-shaped tablet, embossed "ICN-S32" contains: sotalol HCl 160 mg. Nonmedicinal ingredients: colloidal silicon dioxide, FD&C blue #2 Aluminium Lake, lactose monohydrate, magnesium stearate and microcrystalline cellulose. Bottles of 100.

CO Sumatriptan Pr
sumatriptan succinate
Migraine Therapy

Cobalt

SUPPLIED: 25 mg: Each white to off-white, round biconvex tablet, with "Σ>" on one side and "SA" over "25" on the other, contains: sumatriptan succinate 25 mg. Nonmedicinal ingredients: croscarmellose sodium, lactose, magnesium stearate and microcrystalline cellulose. Blister packages of 6.
50 mg: Each white to off-white, triangular shaped biconvex tablet, with "Σ>" on one side and "SA" over "50" on the other, contains: sumatriptan succinate 50 mg. Nonmedicinal ingredients: croscarmellose sodium, lactose, magnesium stearate and microcrystalline cellulose. Blister packages of 6.
100 mg: Each pink, triangular shaped biconvex tablet, with "Σ>" on one side and "SA" over "100" on the other, contains: sumatriptan succinate 100 mg. Nonmedicinal ingredients: croscarmellose sodium, lactose, magnesium stearate, microcrystalline cellulose and Red 30 iron oxide. Blister packages of 6.

Cotazym®
pancrelipase
Enzymes—Digestant

Schering-Plough

INDICATIONS: Pancreatic enzyme replacement therapy in established pancreatic insufficiency where pancreatic enzymes are absent from or present in insufficient amount in the intestine: pancreatectomy, chronic pancreatitis, cystic fibrosis, steatorrhea and other malabsorption syndromes in which fat digestion is inadequate because of deficiency of pancreatic enzymes.

CONTRAINDICATIONS: Allergy to porcine protein.

WARNINGS: In the event that capsules are opened for sprinkling the powder on food or drink or for any other reason, care should be taken so that powder is not spilled on hands or inhaled since it may prove irritating to the skin or mucous membranes. These warnings are particularly applicable to allergic persons.

PRECAUTIONS: A proper balance between fat, protein and starch intake must be maintained to avoid temporary indigestion. Use with caution in patients sensitive to pork protein.

ADVERSE EFFECTS: As with any pancreatic extract, hyperuricosuria or hyperuricaemia due to the purine content of the product may occur at very high dosage.

OVERDOSE:

> For management of a suspected drug overdose, CPhA recommends that you contact your **regional Poison Control Centre**. See the *CPS* Directory section for a list of Poison Control Centres.

DOSAGE: The capsules should be taken orally with each meal or snack. Average dose: 1 to 3 capsules with each meal and 1 capsule with each snack as directed by physician. They can either be swallowed whole, preferably with some fluid, or can be opened and the contents sprinkled on food or drink.

SUPPLIED: Cotazym: Each clear capsule contains: lipase activity of 8000 USP units, amylase activity of 30 000 USP units, protease activity of 30 000 USP units. Nonmedicinal ingredients: gelatin, magnesium stearate, opacode S-1-4126 (print ink), precipitated calcium carbonate, pregelatinized starch, silicon dioxide, sodium lauryl sulfate and talc. Tartrazine-free. Bottles of 100 and 1000.
Cotazym-65 B: Each white capsule contains: lipase activity of 8000 USP units, amylase activity of 30 000 USP units, protease activity of 30 000 USP units, mixed conjugated bile salts 65 mg, cellulase 2 mg. Nonmedicinal ingredients: colloidal silicon dioxide, gelatin, magnesium stearate, opacode S-1-4126 (print ink), precipitated calcium carbonate, silicon dioxide, sodium lauryl sulfate and titanium dioxide. Tartrazine-free. Bottles of 100.
Cotazym ECS 4: Each clear pink capsule with enteric coated microspheres contains: lipase 4000 USP units, amylase 11 000 USP units and protease 11 000 USP units. Nonmedicinal ingredients: cellulose acetate phthalate, colloidal silicon dioxide, cornstarch, diethyl phthalate, gelatin, opacode S-1-4126 (print ink), providone, propylene glycol monostearate, silicon dioxide, sodium lauryl sulfate, sucrose and talc. Tartrazine-free. Bottles of 100.
Cotazym ECS 8: Each clear capsule with enteric coated microspheres contains: lipase 8000 USP units, amylase 30 000 USP units and protease 30 000 USP units. Nonmedicinal ingredients: cellulose acetate phthalate, colloidal silicon dioxide, cornstarch, diethyl phthalate, gelatin, opacode S-1-4126 (print ink), povidone, propylene glycol, propylene glycol monostearate, silicon dioxide, sodium lauryl sulfate, sucrose and talc. Tartrazine-free. Bottles of 100 and 500.
Cotazym ECS 20: Each orange capsule with enteric coated microspheres contains: lipase 20 000 USP units, amylase 55 000 USP units and protease 55 000 USP units. Nonmedicinal ingredients: cellulose acetate phthalate, colloidal silicon dioxide, cornstarch, D&C Yellow No. 10, diethyl phthalate, FD&C Red No. 40, gelatin, opacode S-1-4126 (print ink), povidone, propylene glycol, propylene glycol monostearate, silicon dioxide, sodium lauryl sulfate, sucrose and talc. Tartrazine-free. Bottles of 100.

(Shown in Product Identification Section)

CO Temazepam T/C
temazepam
Hypnotic

Cobalt

SUPPLIED: 15 mg: Each maroon and flesh, size 3 hard shell gelatin capsule, printed "Σ>" on the cap and "TZ 15" on the body in white, contains: temazepam 15 mg. Nonmedicinal ingredients: colloidal silicon dioxide, D&C Red #28, D&C Yellow #10, FD&C Blue #1, gelatin, lactose, magnesium stearate, sodium lauryl sulfate and titanium dioxide. The agents used to polish the capsules are: canner special salt, Tween 60 and alcohol. Gluten-free. Bottles of 100. Store at controlled room temperature (15-30°C). Protect from moisture and light.
30 mg: Each maroon and blue, size 3 hard shell gelatin capsule, printed "Σ>" on the cap and "TZ 30" on the body in white, contains: temazepam 30 mg. Nonmedicinal ingredients: colloidal silicon dioxide, D&C Red #28, FD&C Blue #1, gelatin, lactose, magnesium stearate, sodium lauryl sulfate and titanium dioxide. The agents used to polish the capsules are: canner special salt, Tween 60 and alcohol. Gluten-free. Bottles of 100. Store at controlled room temperature (15-30°C). Protect from moisture and light.

CO Terbinafine Pr
terbinafine HCl
Antifungal

Cobalt

SUPPLIED: Each white to off-white, round tablet, with a score line on one side and a "T" on the other side, contains: terbinafine 250 mg, present as the hydrochloride salt. Nonmedicinal ingredients: colloidal anhydrous silica, hydroxypropylmethyl cellulose, magnesium stearate, microcrystalline cellulose and sodium starch glycolate. Gluten-free. Bottles of 100. Blister strips of 30. Store at temperatures between 15 and 30°C. Protect from light.

CO Topiramate Pr
topiramate
Antiepileptic—Migraine Prophylaxis

Cobalt

SUPPLIED: 25 mg: Each white to off-white, round, biconvex, film-coated tablet with "Σ>" on one side and "25" on the other side, contains: topiramate 25 mg. Nonmedicinal ingredients: hydroxypropyl methyl cellulose, lactose, magnesium stearate, microcrystalline cellulose, PEG 400, polysorbate 80, pregelatinized starch, sodium starch glycolate and titanium dioxide. HDPE bottles of 100. Store at room temperature between 15 to 30°C.

100 mg: Each yellow, round, biconvex, film-coated tablet with "Σ" on one side and "100" on the other side, contains: topiramate 100 mg. Nonmedicinal ingredients: hydroxypropyl methyl cellulose, iron oxide red, iron oxide yellow, lactose, magnesium stearate, microcrystalline cellulose, PEG 400, polysorbate 80, pregelatinized starch, sodium starch glycolate and titanium dioxide. HDPE bottles of 100. Store at room temperature between 15 to 30°C.

200 mg: Each pink, round, biconvex, film-coated tablet with "Σ" on one side and "200" on the other side, contains: topiramate 200 mg. Nonmedicinal ingredients: hydroxypropyl methyl cellulose, iron oxide red, iron oxide yellow, lactose, magnesium stearate, microcrystalline cellulose, PEG 400, polysorbate 80, pregelatinized starch, sodium starch glycolate and titanium dioxide. HDPE bottles of 100. Store at room temperature between 15 to 30°C.

Cotrimoxazole 🄿

CPhA Monograph

see *Sulfamethoxazole-Trimethoprim*

Coumadin® 🄿

warfarin sodium

Anticoagulant

Bristol-Myers Squibb

Date of Revision: March 11, 2008

PHARMACOLOGY: COUMADIN (warfarin sodium) and other coumarin anticoagulants act by inhibiting the synthesis of vitamin K dependent clotting factors, which include Factors II, VII, IX and X, and the anticoagulant proteins C and S. Half-lives of these clotting factors are as follows: Factor II - 60 hours, VII - 4 to 6 hours, IX - 24 hours, and X - 48 to 72 hours. The half-lives of proteins C and S are approximately 8 hours and 30 hours, respectively. The resultant in vivo effect is a sequential depression of Factors VII, IX, X and II. Vitamin K is an essential cofactor for the post ribosomal synthesis of the vitamin K dependent clotting factors. The vitamin promotes the biosynthesis of g-carboxyglutamic acid residues in the proteins which are essential for biological activity. Warfarin is thought to interfere with clotting factor synthesis by inhibition of the regeneration of vitamin K_1 epoxide. The degree of depression is dependent upon the dosage administered. Therapeutic doses of warfarin decrease the total amount of the active form of each vitamin K dependent clotting factor made by the liver by approximately 30 to 50%.

An anticoagulation effect generally occurs within 24 hours after drug administration. However, peak anticoagulant effect may be delayed 72 to 96 hours. The duration of action of a single dose of racemic warfarin is 2 to 5 days. The effects of COUMADIN may become more pronounced as effects of daily maintenance doses overlap. Anticoagulants have no direct effect on an established thrombus, nor do they reverse ischemic tissue damage. However, once a thrombus has occurred, the goal of anticoagulant treatment is to prevent further extension of the formed clot and prevent secondary thromboembolic complications which may result in serious and possibly fatal sequelae.

The administration of COUMADIN via the i.v. route should provide the patient with the same concentration of an equal oral dose, but maximum plasma concentration will be reached earlier. However, the full anticoagulant effect of a dose of warfarin may not be achieved until 72 to 96 hours after dosing, indicating that the administration of i.v. COUMADIN should not provide any increased biological effect or earlier onset of action.

Pharmacokinetics: COUMADIN is a racemic mixture of the R- and S-enantiomers. The S-enantiomer exhibits 2 to 5 times more anticoagulant activity than the R-enantiomer in humans, but generally has a more rapid clearance. It is important that all warfarin sodium products provide the same ratio of enantiomers as that which is present in COUMADIN.

Absorption: COUMADIN is essentially completely absorbed after oral administration with peak concentration generally attained within the first 4 hours. Studies using warfarin sodium indicate the rate but not the extent of absorption of the drug is decreased by the presence of food in the GI tract. Warfarin is also absorbed percutaneously. Individuals differ in the rate at which they absorb warfarin.

Distribution: There are no differences in the apparent volumes of distribution after i.v. and oral administration of single doses of warfarin solution. Warfarin distributes into a relatively small apparent volume of distribution of about 0.14 L/kg. A distribution phase lasting 6 to 12 hours is distinguishable after rapid i.v. or oral administration of an aqueous solution. Using a one compartment model, and assuming complete bioavailability, estimates of the volumes of distribution of R- and S-warfarin are similar to each other and to that of the racemate. Warfarin is distributed to the liver, lungs, spleen, kidney, and crosses the placenta. Concentrations in fetal plasma approach the maternal values, but warfarin has not been found in human milk (see Warnings, Lactation). Approximately 99% of the drug is bound to plasma proteins.

Metabolism: Individual patients vary greatly in the rate at which they metabolize warfarin. The elimination of warfarin is almost entirely by metabolism. COUMADIN is stereoselectively metabolized by hepatic microsomal enzymes (cytochrome P450) to inactive hydroxylated metabolites (predominant route) and by reductases to reduced metabolites (warfarin alcohols). The warfarin alcohols have minimal anticoagulant activity. The metabolites are principally excreted into the urine; and to a lesser extent into the bile. The metabolites of warfarin that have been identified include dehydrowarfarin, 2 diastereoisomer alcohols, 4'-, 6-, 7-, 8- and 10-hydroxywarfarin. Numerous cytochrome P450 isozymes may be involved in the metabolism of warfarin, including CYP 2C9, 2C19, 2C8, 2C18, 1A2 and 3A4. CYP2C9 is likely to be the principal isozyme modulating anticoagulant activity in clinical use. This enzyme constitutes the primary pathway for the metabolism of S-warfarin, the more potent enantiomer found in racemic mixtures of warfarin. Its complete inhibition in vivo may be expected to result in lower maintenance dose requirement of warfarin. Individuals with allelic polymorphisms of CYP2C9 have been identified and have been shown to have lower maintenance dose requirements of warfarin and increased risk of overanticoagulation.

The S-enantiomer of warfarin is mainly metabolized to 7-hydroxywarfarin by CYP2C9, a polymorphic enzyme. The variant alleles CYP2C9*2 and CYP2C9*3 result in decreased in vitro CYP2C9 enzymatic 7-hydroxylation of S-warfarin. The frequencies of these alleles in Caucasians are approximately 11% and 7% for CYP2C9*2 and CYP2C9*3, respectively. Patients with one or more of these variant CYP2C9 alleles have decreased S-warfarin clearance (Table 1).

Table 1: COUMADIN

Relationship Between S-Warfarin Clearance and CYP2C9 Genotype in Caucasian Patients

CYP2C9 Genotype	N	S-Warfarin Clearance/Lean Body Weight (mL/min/kg) Mean (SD)[a]
*1/*1	118	0.065 (0.025)[b]
*1/*2 or *1/*3	59	0.041 (0.021)[b]
*2/*2, *2/*3 or *3/*3	11	0.020 (0.011)[b]
Total	188	

[a] SD=standard deviation.
[b] p<0.001. Pairwise comparisons indicated significant differences among all 3 genotypes.

Other CYP2C9 alleles associated with reduced enzymatic activity occur at lower frequencies, including *5, *6, and *11 alleles in populations of African ancestry and *5, *9 and *11 alleles in Caucasians.

Pharmacogenomics: A meta-analysis of 9 qualified studies including 2775 patients (99% Caucasian) was performed to examine the clinical outcomes associated with CYP2C9 gene variants in warfarin-treated patients. In this meta-analysis, 3 studies assessed bleeding risks and 8 studies assessed daily dose requirements. The analysis suggested an increased bleeding risk for patients carrying either the CYP2C9*2 or CYP2C9*3 alleles. Patients carrying at least one copy of the CYP2C9*2 allele required a mean daily warfarin dose that was 17% less than the mean daily dose for patients homozygous for the CYP2C9*1 allele. For patients carrying at least one copy of the CYP2C9*3 allele, the mean daily warfarin dose was 37% less than the mean daily dose for patients homozygous for the CYP2C9*1 allele.

In an observational study, the risk of achieving INR >3 during the first 3 weeks of warfarin therapy was determined in 219 Swedish patients retrospectively grouped by CYP2C9 genotype. The relative risk of over anticoagulation as measured by INR >3 during the first 2 weeks of therapy was approximately doubled for those patients classified as *2 or *3 compared to patients who were homozygous for the *1 allele.

Warfarin reduces the regeneration of vitamin K from vitamin K epoxide in the vitamin K cycle, through inhibition of vitamin K epoxide reductase (VKOR), a multiprotein enzyme complex. Certain single nucleotide polymorphisms in the VKORC1 gene (especially the -1639G>A allele) have been associated with lower dose requirements for warfarin. In 201 Caucasian patients treated with stable warfarin doses, genetic variations in the VKORC1 gene were associated with lower warfarin doses. In this study, about 30% of the variance in warfarin dose could be attributed to variations in the VKORC1 gene alone; about 40% of the variance in warfarin dose could be attributed to variations in VKORC1 and CYP2C9 genes combined. About 55% of the variability in warfarin dose could be explained by the combination of VKORC1 and CYP2C9 genotypes, age, height, body weight, interacting drugs, and indication for warfarin therapy in Caucasian patients. Similar observations have been reported in Asian patients.

Elimination: The terminal half-life of warfarin after a single dose is approximately 1 week; however, the effective half-life ranges from 20 to 60 hours, with a mean of about 40 hours. The clearance of R-warfarin is generally half that of S-warfarin, thus as the volumes of distribution are similar, the half-life of R-warfarin is longer than that of S-warfarin. The half-life of R-warfarin ranges from 37 to 89 hours, while that of S-warfarin ranges from 21 to 43 hours. Studies with radiolabeled drug have demonstrated that up to 92% of the orally administered dose is recovered in urine. Very little warfarin is excreted unchanged in urine. Urinary excretion is in the form of metabolites.

Geriatrics: Patients 60 years or older appear to exhibit greater than expected PT/INR response to the anticoagulation effects of warfarin. The cause of this increased sensitivity in this age group is not known. This increased anticoagulant effect of warfarin may be due to a combination of pharmacokinetic and pharmacodynamic factors. Racemic warfarin clearance may be unchanged or reduced with increasing age. Limited information suggests that there is no difference in the clearance of S-warfarin in the elderly, compared to that seen in young subjects. However, there may be a slight decrease in the clearance of R-warfarin in the elderly, compared to the young. Therefore, as patient age increases, a lower dose of warfarin is usually required to produce a therapeutic level of anticoagulation.

Renal Impairment: Renal clearance is considered to be a minor determinant of anticoagulant response to warfarin. No dosage adjustment is necessary for patients with renal failure.

Hepatic Impairment: Hepatic dysfunction can potentiate the response to warfarin through impaired synthesis of clotting factors and decreased metabolism of warfarin.

INDICATIONS: COUMADIN (warfarin sodium) is indicated for the prophylaxis and/or treatment of venous thrombosis and its extension, pulmonary embolism, atrial fibrillation with embolization, and as an adjunct in the prophylaxis of systemic embolism after myocardial infarction, including stroke and reinfarction.

The following are some of the more common clinical disorders which may be associated with or predispose patients to the above indications: thrombophlebitis, congestive heart failure, surgical procedure or trauma associated with a high risk of thromboembolism, myocardial infarction, cerebral embolism.

It may also be useful as an adjunct in the treatment of transient cerebral ischemic attacks due to intravascular clotting.

CONTRAINDICATIONS: Anticoagulation is contraindicated in any localized or general physical condition or personal circumstances in which the hazard of hemorrhage might be greater than the potential clinical benefits of anticoagulation, such as:

Pregnancy: COUMADIN (warfarin sodium) is contraindicated in pregnancy because the drug passes through the placental barrier and may cause fatal hemorrhage to the fetus in utero. Women of childbearing potential must take precautions not to become pregnant while on COUMADIN therapy. Furthermore, there have been reports of birth malformations in children born to mothers who have been treated with warfarin during pregnancy.

Embryopathy characterized by nasal hypoplasia with or without stippled epiphyses (chondrodysplasia punctata) has been reported in pregnant women exposed to warfarin during the first trimester. CNS abnormalities also have been reported, including dorsal midline dysplasia characterized by agenesis of the corpus callosum, Dandy-Walker malformation, and midline cerebellar atrophy. Ventral midline dysplasia, characterized by optic atrophy, and eye abnormalities have been observed. Mental retardation, blindness, and other CNS abnormalities have been reported in association with second and third trimester exposure. Although rare, teratogenic reports following in utero exposure to warfarin include urinary tract anomalies such as single kidney, asplenia, anencephaly, spina bifida, cranial nerve palsy, hydrocephalus, cardiac defects and congenital heart disease, polydactyly, deformities of toes, diaphragmatic hernia, corneal leukoma, cleft palate, cleft lip, schizencephaly, and microcephaly.

Spontaneous abortion and still birth are known to occur and a higher risk of fetal mortality is associated with the use of warfarin. Low birth weight and growth retardation have also been reported.

Women of childbearing potential who are candidates for anticoagulant therapy should be carefully evaluated and the indications critically reviewed with the patient. If the patient becomes pregnant while taking this drug, she should be apprised of the potential risks to the fetus, and the possibility of termination of the pregnancy should be discussed in the light of those risks.

Hemorrhagic Tendencies or Blood Dyscrasias: Recent or contemplated surgery of: central nervous system, eye, traumatic surgery resulting in large open surfaces.

Bleeding tendencies associated with active ulceration or overt bleeding of: gastrointestinal, genitourinary or respiratory tracts, cerebrovascular hemorrhage, aneurysms—cerebral, dissecting aorta, pericarditis and pericardial effusions, bacterial endocarditis.

Threatened abortion, eclampsia and pre-eclampsia.

Inadequate laboratory facilities.

Unsupervised patients with senility, alcoholism, or psychosis or other lack of patient cooperation.

Spinal puncture and other diagnostic or therapeutic procedures with potential for uncontrollable bleeding.

Miscellaneous: major regional, lumbar block anesthesia, malignant hypertension and known hypersensitivity to warfarin or to any other components of COUMADIN.

WARNINGS:

Warning: Bleeding Risk: Warfarin sodium can cause major or fatal bleeding. Bleeding is more likely to occur during the starting period and with a higher dose (resulting in a higher INR). Risk factors for bleeding include high intensity of anticoagulation (INR >4.0), age ≥65, highly variable INRs, history of gastrointestinal bleeding, hypertension, cerebrovascular disease, serious heart disease, anemia, malignancy, trauma, renal insufficiency, concomitant drugs (see Precautions), and long duration of warfarin therapy. Regular monitoring of INR should be performed on all treated patients. Those at high risk of bleeding may benefit from more frequent INR monitoring, careful dose adjustment to desired INR, and a shorter duration of therapy. Patients should be instructed about prevention measures to minimize risk of bleeding and to report immediately to physicians signs and symptoms of bleeding. (See Information for the Patient.)

Hemorrhage: The most serious risks associated with anticoagulant therapy with COUMADIN (warfarin sodium) are hemorrhage in any tissue or organ (see Warning Box) and, less frequently (<0.1%), necrosis and/or gangrene of skin and other tissues. The risk of hemorrhage is related to the level of intensity and the duration of anticoagulant therapy. Hemorrhage and necrosis have in some cases been reported to result in death or permanent disability. Necrosis appears to be associated with local thrombosis and usually appears within a few days of the start of anticoagulant therapy. In severe cases of necrosis, treatment through débridement or amputation of the affected tissue, limb, breast or penis has been reported. Careful diagnosis is required to determine whether necrosis is caused by an underlying disease. Warfarin therapy should be discontinued when warfarin is suspected to be the cause of developing necrosis and heparin therapy may be considered for anticoagulation. Although various treatments have been attempted, no treatment for necrosis has been considered uniformly effective. See below for information on predisposing conditions. These and other risks associated with anticoagulant therapy must be weighed against the risk of thrombosis or embolization in untreated cases.

It cannot be emphasized too strongly that treatment of each patient is a highly individualized matter. COUMADIN, a narrow therapeutic range (index) drug, may be affected by factors such as other drugs and dietary Vitamin K. Dosage should be controlled by periodic determinations of prothrombin times (PT) ratio/International Normalized Ratio (INR) or other suitable coagulation tests. Determinations of whole blood clotting and bleeding times are not effective measures for control of therapy. Heparin prolongs the one-stage PT. When heparin and COUMADIN are administered concomitantly, refer to Dosage, Conversion from Heparin Therapy for recommendations.

Caution should be observed when COUMADIN is administered in any situation or in the presence of any predisposing condition where added risk of hemorrhage, necrosis and/or gangrene is present.

Anticoagulation therapy with COUMADIN may enhance the release of atheromatous plaque emboli, thereby increasing the risk of complications from systemic cholesterol microembolization, including the "purple toe syndrome". Discontinuation of COUMADIN therapy is recommended when such phenomena are observed. While the "purple toe syndrome" is reported to be reversible, other complications of microembolization may not be reversible.

Systemic atheroemboli and cholesterol microemboli can present with a variety of signs and symptoms including purple toe syndrome, livedo reticularis, rash, gangrene, abrupt and intense pain in the leg, foot, or toes, foot ulcers, myalgia, penile gangrene, abdominal pain, flank or back pain, hematuria, renal insufficiency, hypertension, cerebral ischemia, spinal cord infarction, pancreatitis, symptoms simulating polyarteritis, or any other sequelae of vascular compromise due to embolic occlusion. The most commonly involved visceral organs are the kidneys followed by the pancreas, spleen, and liver. Some cases have progressed to necrosis or death.

Purple toe syndrome is a complication of oral anticoagulation characterized by a dark, purplish or mottled color of the toes, usually occurring between 3 to 10 weeks, or later, after the initiation of therapy with warfarin or related compounds. Major features of this syndrome include purple color of plantar surfaces and sides of the toes that blanches on moderate pressure and fades with elevation of the legs; pain and tenderness of the toes; waxing and waning of the color over time. While the purple toe syndrome is reported to be reversible, some cases progress to gangrene or necrosis which may require débridement of the affected area, or may lead to amputation.

A severe elevation (>50 seconds) in activated partial thromboplastin time (aPTT) with a PT ratio/INR in the desired range has been identified as an indication of increased risk of postoperative hemorrhage. This has been noted in patients undergoing elective hip surgery receiving warfarin alone.

Administration of anticoagulants in the following conditions will be based upon clinical judgment in which the risks of anticoagulant therapy are weighed against the risk of thrombosis or embolization in untreated cases. The following may be associated with these increased risks:

Severe to moderate hepatic or renal insufficiency.

Infectious diseases or disturbances of intestinal flora, such as sprue or as seen with antibiotic use.

Trauma which may result in internal bleeding.

Surgery or trauma resulting in large exposed raw surfaces.

Indwelling catheters.

Severe to moderate hypertension.

Hereditary or acquired deficiencies of protein C or its cofactor, protein S, have been associated with tissue necrosis following warfarin administration. Not all patients with these conditions develop necrosis, and tissue necrosis occurs in patients without these deficiencies. Inherited resistance to activated protein C has been described in many patients with venous thromboembolic disorders but has not yet been evaluated as a risk factor for tissue necrosis. The risk associated with these conditions, both for recurrent thrombosis and for adverse reactions, is difficult to evaluate since it does not appear to be the same for everyone. Decisions about testing and therapy must be made on an individual basis. It has been reported that concomitant anticoagulation therapy with heparin for 5 to 7 days during initiation of therapy with COUMADIN may minimize the incidence of tissue necrosis. Warfarin therapy should be discontinued when warfarin is suspected to be the cause of developing necrosis and heparin therapy may be considered for anticoagulation.

Diseases affecting the microvasculature or microcirculation, such as polycythemia vera, vasculitis, and severe diabetes.

Heparin-induced Thrombocytopenia: COUMADIN should be used with caution in patients with heparin-induced thrombocytopenia and deep vein thrombosis. Cases of venous limb ischemia, necrosis, and gangrene have occurred in patients when heparin treatment was discontinued and warfarin therapy was started or continued especially when large initiation doses were used. In some patients sequelae have included amputation of the involved area and/or death. The use of alternative anticoagulant therapy should be considered in patients with heparin-induced thrombocytopenia and deep vein thrombosis.

Lactation: Based on very limited published data, warfarin has not been detected in the breast milk of mothers treated with warfarin. The same limited published data reports that breast-fed infants, whose mothers were treated with warfarin, had prolonged prothrombin times. The decision to breast-feed should be undertaken only after careful consideration of the available alternatives. Women who are breast-feeding and anticoagulated with warfarin should be very carefully monitored so that recommended INR values are not exceeded. It is prudent to perform coagulation tests on infants at risk for bleeding before advising women taking warfarin to breast-feed. Effects in premature infants have not been evaluated.

Miscellaneous: Minor and severe allergic/hypersensitivity reactions and anaphylactic reactions have been reported.

In patients with acquired or inherited warfarin resistance, decreased therapeutic responses to COUMADIN have been reported. Exaggerated therapeutic responses have been reported in other patients.

Patients with congestive heart failure may become more responsive to COUMADIN, thereby requiring more frequent laboratory monitoring, and reduced doses of COUMADIN.

Concomitant use of anticoagulants with streptokinase or urokinase is not recommended and may be hazardous. (Please note recommendations accompanying these preparations.)

PRECAUTIONS: Periodic determination of PT ratio/INR or other suitable coagulation test is essential (see Dosage, Laboratory Control).

Numerous factors, alone or in combination, including travel, changes in diet, environment, physical state or medication, or the use of natural medicines, may influence the patient's response to anticoagulants. It is generally good practice to monitor the patient's response with additional PT ratio/INR determinations in the period immediately after discharge from the hospital, and whenever other medications, including natural medicines, are initiated, discontinued or taken irregularly. Table 2 and Table 3 provide a listing of factors, alone or in combination, which may effect the PT. However, other factors may also affect the anticoagulant response and the tables are provided for your reference only.

Drugs may interact with COUMADIN (warfarin sodium) through pharmacodynamic or pharmacokinetic mechanisms. Pharmacodynamic mechanisms for drug interactions with COUMADIN are synergism (impaired hemostasis, reduced clotting factor synthesis), competitive antagonism (vitamin K), and altered physiologic control loop for vitamin K metabolism (hereditary resistance). Pharmacokinetic mechanisms for drug interactions with COUMADIN are mainly enzyme induction, enzyme inhibition, and reduced plasma protein binding. It is important to note that some drugs may interact by more than one mechanism.

Because a patient may be exposed to a combination of listed factors, the net effect of COUMADIN on PT ratio/INR responses may be unpredictable. More frequent PT/INR monitoring is therefore advisable.

I.M. injections of concomitant medications should be confined to the upper extremities which permits easy access for manual compression, inspections for bleeding and use of pressure bandages.

Drug Interactions: The complete in vivo inhibition of the CYP2C9 isozyme may be expected to result in lower maintenance dose requirement of warfarin. Individuals with allelic polymorphisms of CYP2C9 have been identified and have been shown to have lower maintenance dose requirements of warfarin and increased risk of overanticoagulation. Acquired or inherited warfarin resistance should be suspected if large daily doses of COUMADIN are required to maintain a patient's PT ratio/INR within a normal therapeutic range.

Medications of unknown interaction with coumarins are best regarded with caution. When these medications are started or stopped, more frequent PT ratio/INR monitoring is advisable. Coumarins may also affect the action of other drugs. Hypoglycemic agents (chlorpropamide and tolbutamide) and anticonvulsants (phenytoin and phenobarbital) may accumulate in the body as a result of interference with either their metabolism or excretion.

It has been reported that concomitant administration of warfarin and ticlopidine may be associated with cholestatic hepatitis.

Close monitoring of patients receiving NSAIDs is recommended to be certain that no change in anticoagulation dosage is required. In addition to specific drug interactions that might affect prothrombin time, NSAIDs can inhibit platelet aggregation, and can cause GI bleeding, peptic ulceration and/or perforation.

Table 2: COUMADIN

The Following Factors, Alone or in Combination, May Be Responsible for Increased PT Ratio or INR, or Increased Risk of Bleeding

Endogenous Factors		
blood dyscrasias	elevated temperature	hyperthyroidism
cancer	hepatic disorders:	poor nutritional state
collagen vascular disease	infectious hepatitis	steatorrhea
congestive heart failure	jaundice	vitamin K deficiency
diarrhea		

Exogenous Factors: Potential drug interactions with COUMADIN are listed below by drug class and by specific drugs

(cont'd)

Table 2: COUMADIN *(cont'd)*

The Following Factors, Alone or in Combination, May Be Responsible for Increased PT Ratio or INR, or Increased Risk of Bleeding

Classes of Drugs		
5-lipoxygenase Inhibitors	Antiplatelet Drugs/Effects	MAO Inhibitors
Adrenergic Stimulants, central	Antithyroid Drugs[a]	Narcotics, prolonged
Alcohol Abuse Reduction	Beta-Adrenergic Blockers	Natural Medicines
Preparations	Cholelitholytic Agents	Nonsteroidal Anti-Inflammatory
Analgesics	Diabetes Agents, oral	Agents
Anesthetics, inhalation	Diuretics[a]	COX-2 Inhibitors
Antiandrogens	Gastric Acidity and Peptic Ulcer	Nonselective NSAIDs
Antiarrhythmics[a]	Agents[a]	Psychostimulants
Antibiotics[a]	Gastrointestinal, ulcerative colitis	Pyrazolones
Aminoglycosides (oral)	agents	Salicylates
Cephalosporins, parenteral	Gastrointestinal, prokinetic agents	Selective Serotonin Reuptake
Macrolides	Gout Treatment Agents	Inhibitors
Penicillins, i.v., high dose	Hemorrheologic Agents	Steroids, adrenocortical[a]
Quinolones (fluoroquinolones)	Hepatotoxic Drugs	Steroids, anabolic (17-Alkyl
Sulfonamides, long acting	Hyperglycemic Agents	Testosterone Derivatives)
Tetracyclines	Hypertensive Emergency Agents	Thrombolytics
Anticoagulants	Hypnotics[a]	Thyroid Drugs
Anticonvulsants[a]	Leukotriene Receptor Antagonists	Tuberculosis Agents[a]
Antidepressants[a]	Lipid Lowering Agents[a]	Uricosuric Agents
Antifungal Medications,	Bile Acid-Binding Resins[a]	Vaccines
Intravaginal, systemic[a]	Fibrates	Vitamins[a]
Antimalarial Agents	HMG-CoA Reductase Inhibitors[a]	
Antineoplastics[a]		
Antiparasitic/Antimicrobials		

Specific Drugs Reported		
acetaminophen	fenoprofen	omeprazole
alcohol[a]	fluconazole	oxaprozin
allopurinol	fluorouracil	oxymetholone
aminosalicylic acid	fluoxetine	pantoprazole
amiodarone HCl	flutamide	paroxetine
argatroban	fluvastatin	penicillin G, i.v.
ASA	fluvoxamine	pentoxifylline
azithromycin	gatifloxacin	phenylbutazone
bivalirudin	gefitinib	phenytoin[a]
capecitabine	gemfibrozil	piperacillin
cefamandole	glucagon	piroxicam
cefazolin	halothane	prednisone[a]
cefoperazone	heparin	propafenone
cefotetan	ibuprofen	propoxyphene
cefoxitin	ifosfamide	propranolol
ceftriaxone	indomethacin	propylthiouracil[a]
celecoxib	influenza virus vaccine	quinidine
chenodiol	itraconazole	quinine
chloramphenicol	ketoprofen	rabeprazole
chloral hydrate[a]	ketorolac	ranitidine[a],
chlorpropamide	lansoprazole	rofecoxib
cholestyramine[a]	lepirudin	sertraline
cimetidine	levamisole	simvastatin
ciprofloxacin	levofloxacin	stanozolol
cisapride	levothyroxine	streptokinase
clarithromycin	liothyronine	sulfamethizole
clofibrate	lovastatin	sulfamethoxazole
COUMADIN overdose	mefenamic acid	sulfinpyrazone
cyclophosphamide[a]	methimazole[a]	sulfisoxazole
danazol	methyldopa	sulindac
danshen (Chinese herb)	methylphenidate	tamoxifen
dextran	methylsalicylate ointment (topical)	tetracycline
dextrothyroxine	metronidazole	thyroid
diazoxide	miconazole (intravaginal, oral,	ticarcillin
diclofenac	systemic[a])	ticlopidine
dicumarol	moricizine HCl[a]	tissue plasminogen activator (t-PA)
diflunisal	moxifloxacin	tolbutamide
disulfiram	nalidixic acid	tramadol
doxycycline	naproxen	trimethoprim/sulfamethoxazole
erythromycin	neomycin	urokinase
esomeprazole	norfloxacin	valproate
ethacrynic acid	ofloxacin	vitamin E
ezetimibe	olsalazine	zafirlukast
fenofibrate		

Also: Other medications affecting blood elements which may modify hemostasis dietary deficiencies; prolonged hot weather; unreliable PT determinations.

[a] Increased and decreased PT ratio/INR responses have been reported.

Natural Medicines (Including Herbals and Botanicals): **Caution should be exercised when natural medicines are taken concomitantly with COUMADIN.** Few adequate, well-controlled studies exist evaluating the potential for metabolic and/or pharmacologic interactions between natural medicines and COUMADIN. Due to a lack of manufacturing standardization with natural medicines, the amount of active ingredients may vary. This could further confound the ability to assess potential interactions and effects on anticoagulants. It is good practice to monitor the patient's response with additional PT/INR determinations when initiating or discontinuing natural medicines.

Specific natural medicines reported to affect COUMADIN therapy include the following:

- Bromelains, danshen, dong quai (Angelica sinensis), garlic, Ginkgo biloba, ginseng and cranberry products are associated most often with an **increase** in the effects of COUMADIN. However, the effects of ginseng can be variable (increased or decreased effect of COUMADIN) and the combination should be avoided or more careful monitoring is warranted.
- Coenzyme Q_{10} (ubidecarenone) and St. John's wort are associated most often with a **decrease** in the effects of COUMADIN.

Some natural medicines may cause bleeding events when taken alone (e.g., garlic and Ginkgo biloba) and may have anticoagulant, antiplatelet, and/or fibrinolytic properties. These effects would be expected to be additive to the anticoagulant effects of COUMADIN. Conversely, other natural medicines may have coagulant properties when taken alone or may decrease the effects of COUMADIN.

Table 3: COUMADIN

The Following Factors Alone or in Combination, May Be Responsible for Decreased PT Ratio or INR, or Increased Potential Risk of Thromboembolic Events

Endogenous Factors		
edema hereditary coumarin resistance	hyperlipemia hypothyroidism	nephrotic syndrome
Exogenous Factors: Potential drug interactions with COUMADIN are listed below by drug class and by specific drugs		
Classes of Drugs		
Adrenal Cortical Steroid Inhibitors Antacids Antianxiety Agents Antiarrhythmics[a] Antibiotics[a] Anticonvulsants[a] Antidepressants[a] Antifungal Medications, systemic[a] Antihistamines Antineoplastics[a]	Antipsychotic Medications Antithyroid Drugs[a] Barbiturates Diuretics[a] Enteral Nutritional Supplements Gastric Acidity and Peptic Ulcer Agents[a] Hypnotics[a] Immunosuppressives	Lipid Lowering Agents Bile Acid-Binding Resins[a] HMG-CoA Reductase Inhibitors[a] Natural Medicines Oral Contraceptives, estrogen containing Selective Estrogen Receptor Modulators Steroids, adrenocortical[a] Tuberculosis Agents[a] Vitamins[a]
Specific Drugs Reported		
alcohol[a] aminoglutethimide amobarbital atorvastatin azathioprine butabarbital butalbital carbamazepine chloral hydrate[a] chlordiazepoxide chlorthalidone cholestyramine[a] corticotropin cortisone COUMADIN underdosage	cyclophosphamide[a] dicloxacillin ethchlorvynol glutethimide griseofulvin haloperidol meprobamate 6-mercaptopurine methimazole[a] moricizine HCl[a] nafcillin paraldehyde pentobarbital phenobarbital	phenytoin[a] prednisone[a] primidone propylthiouracil[a] raloxifene ranitidine[a] rifampin secobarbital spironolactone sucralfate trazodone vitamin C (high dose) vitamin K
Also: diet high in vitamin K, unreliable PT determinations		

[a] Increased and decreased PT ratio/INR responses have been reported.

Some natural medicines that may affect coagulation are listed in Table 4 for reference; however, this list should not be considered all-inclusive. Many natural medicines have several common names and scientific names.

Table 4: COUMADIN

Natural Medicines that May Affect Coagulation

Natural Medicines That Contain Coumarins with Potential Anticoagulant Effects	
Agrimony[c] (Argimonia eupatoria) Alfalfa (Medicago sativa) Aniseed (Pimpinella anisum) Arnica Asa Foetida (Asafetida) Bogbean[a] (Menyanthis folium) Peumus Boldo Buchu (Barosmae boldo) Paprika (Capsicum) Cassia[c] Celery (Apium graveolens) Chamomile, German and Roman (Anthemis nobilis) Dandelion[c] (Taraxacum officinale) Dong Quai (Angelica sinensis) Fenugreek (Trigonella foenumgraecum) Horse Chestnut (Aesculus hippocastanum)	Horseradish (Cochleria armoracia) Licorice[c] (Glycyrrhiza globra) Meadowsweet[a] (Spiraea ulmaria) Nettle (Urtica dioica) Parsley (Carum petroselinum) Passion Flower (Passiflora edulis) Prickley Ash, Northern (Zanthoxylum americanum) Quassia (Amara) Red Clover (Trifolium pratense) Sweet Clover (Melilotus officinalis) Sweet Woodruff (Galii odorati herba) Tonka Beans (Dipteryx odorata) Wild Carrot (Daucus carota) Wild Lettuce (Lactuca virosa)
Miscellaneous Natural Medicines with Anticoagulant Properties	
Bladder Wrack (Fucus vesiculosus)	Pau d'arco (Tabebuia avellanedae)
Natural Medicines that Contain Salicylate and/or Have Antiplatelet Properties	
Agrimony[c] (Argimonia eupatoria) Aloe Gel Aspen (Populus tremuloides) Black Cohosh (Cimicifuga racemosa) Black Haw (Viburnum prunifolium) Bogbean[a] Cassia[c] Clove (Eugenia caryophyllus) Dandelion[c] Feverfew (Chrysanthenum parthenum) Garlic[d] (Tremuloides) German Sarsaparilla (Corex arenaria)	Ginger Ginko Biloba Ginseng (Panax)[d] Licorice[c] Meadowsweet[a] Onion[d] (Allium cepa) Policosanol Poplar (Populi gemma) Senega (Polygala) Tamarind (Tamarindus Indica) Willow (Salix nigra) Wintergreen (Gaultheria procumbens)
Natural Medicines with Fibrinolytic Properties	
Bromelains (Bromelainum) Capsicum[b] Garlic[d]	Ginseng (Panax)[d] Inositol Nicotinate Onion[d]
Natural Medicines with Coagulant Properties	

(cont'd)

Table 4: COUMADIN *(cont'd)*

Natural Medicines that May Affect Coagulation

Goldenseal (Chrysanthenum)	Mistletoe (Viscum album) Yarrow (Achillea millefolium)

[a] Contains coumarins and salicylate.
[b] Contains coumarins and has fibrinolytic properties.
[c] Contains coumarins and has antiplatelet properties.
[d] Has antiplatelet and fibrinolytic properties.

Considerations for Increased Bleeding Risk: COUMADIN is a narrow therapeutic range (index) drug, and additional caution should be observed when warfarin sodium is administered to certain patients. Reported risk factors for bleeding include high intensity of anticoagulation (INR >4.0), age ≥65, highly variable INRs, history of gastrointestinal bleeding, hypertension, cerebrovascular disease, serious heart disease, anemia, malignancy, trauma, renal insufficiency, concomitant drugs (see Precautions) and long duration of warfarin therapy. Identification of risk factors for bleeding and certain genetic variations in CYP2CP and VKORC1 in a patient may increase the need for more frequent INR monitoring and the use of lower warfarin doses (see Pharmacology, Metabolism and Dosage). Bleeding is more likely to occur during the starting period and with a higher dose of COUMADIN (resulting in a higher INR).

Intramuscular (I.M.) injections of concomitant medications should be confined to the upper extremities which permits easy access for manual compression, inspections for bleeding and use of pressure bandages.

Caution should be observed when COUMADIN (or warfarin) is administered concomitantly with nonsteroidal anti-inflammatory drugs (NSAIDs), including aspirin, to be certain that no change in anticoagulation dosage is required. In addition to specific drug interactions that might affect PT/INR, NSAIDs, including aspirin, can inhibit platelet aggregation, and can cause gastrointestinal bleeding, peptic ulceration and/or perforation.

Geriatrics and/or Debilitated Patients: Patients 60 years or older appear to exhibit greater than expected PT/INR response to the anticoagulant effects of warfarin (see Pharmacology, Geriatrics). COUMADIN is contraindicated in any unsupervised patient with senility. Caution should be exercised with administration of warfarin sodium to elderly and/or debilitated patients in any situation or physical condition where added risk of hemorrhage is present. Low initiation and maintenance doses of COUMADIN are recommended in the elderly (see Dosage).

Pregnancy: See Contraindications.

Children: Safety and effectiveness in children below 18 years of age have not been established in randomized, controlled clinical trials. However, the use of COUMADIN in pediatric patients has been documented for the prevention and treatment of thromboembolic events. Difficulty achieving and maintaining therapeutic PT ratio/INR ranges in the pediatric patient has been reported. More frequent PT ratio/INR determinations are recommended because of possible changing warfarin requirements.

ADVERSE EFFECTS: Potential adverse reactions to COUMADIN may include:

- Fatal or nonfatal hemorrhage from any tissue or organ. This is a consequence of the anticoagulant effect. The signs, and symptoms, and severity will vary according to the location and degree or extent of the bleeding. Hemorrhagic complications may present as paralysis; paresthesia; headache, chest, abdomen, joint, muscle or other pain; dizziness; shortness of breath, difficult breathing or swallowing; unexplained swelling; weakness; hypotension; or unexplained shock. Therefore, the possibility of hemorrhage should be considered in evaluating the condition of any anticoagulated patient with complaints which do not indicate an obvious diagnosis. Bleeding during anticoagulant therapy does not always correlate with PT ratio/INR (see Overdose, Symptoms and Treatment).
- Bleeding which occurs when the PT ratio/INR is within the therapeutic range warrants diagnostic investigation, since it may unmask a previously unsuspected lesion, e.g., tumor, ulcer, etc.
- Necrosis of skin and other tissues (see Warnings).
- Adverse reactions reported infrequently include:

Body as a Whole: hypersensitivity/allergic reactions, pain, edema, asthenia, fever, headache, fatigue, lethargy, malaise, anemia, pallor.

Central and Peripheral Nervous Systems: dizziness, cold intolerance, coma, loss of consciousness, syncope and paresthesia, including feeling cold and chills.

Gastrointestinal: nausea, diarrhea, abdominal pain, including cramping, flatulence/bloating, vomiting.

Liver and Biliary: elevated liver enzymes, hepatitis, jaundice, cholestatic hepatic injury.

Skin and Appendages: alopecia, rash, pruritus, urticaria, dermatitis, including bullous eruptions.

Vascular, Extracardiac: angina syndrome, chest pain, systemic cholesterol microembolization, purple toe syndrome, vasculitis.

Special Senses: taste perversion.

Rare events of tracheal or tracheobronchial calcification have been reported in association with long-term warfarin therapy. The clinical significance of this event is unknown.

Priapism has been associated with anticoagulant administration, however, a causal relationship has not been established.

OVERDOSE:

Symptoms: Suspected or overt abnormal bleeding (e.g., appearance of blood in stools or urine, hematuria, excessive menstrual bleeding, melena, petechiae, excessive bruising or persistent oozing from superficial injuries) are early manifestations of anticoagulation beyond a safe and satisfactory level.

Treatment: Excessive anticoagulation, with or without bleeding, may be controlled by discontinuing COUMADIN therapy and if necessary, by administration of oral or parenteral vitamin K_1. (Please see recommendations accompanying vitamin K_1 preparations prior to use.)

Such use of vitamin K_1 reduces responses to subsequent COUMADIN therapy. Patients may return to a pretreatment thrombotic status following the rapid reversal of a prolonged PT. Resumption of warfarin administration reverses the effect of vitamin K_1, and a therapeutic PT can again be obtained by careful dosage adjustment. If rapid anticoagulation is indicated, heparin may be preferable for initial therapy.

If minor bleeding progresses to major bleeding, give 5 to 25 mg (rarely up to 50 mg) parenteral vitamin K_1. In emergency situations of severe hemorrhage, clotting factors can be returned to normal by administering 200 to 500 mL of whole blood or fresh frozen plasma, or by giving commercial Factor IX complex.

A risk of hepatitis and other viral diseases is associated with the use of these blood products; Factor IX complex is also associated with an increased risk of thrombosis. Therefore, these preparations should be used only in exceptional or life-threatening bleeding episodes secondary to COUMADIN overdosage.

Purified Factor IX preparations should not be used because they cannot increase the levels of prothrombin, Factor VII and Factor X, which are also depressed along with the levels of Factor IX as a result of COUMADIN treatment. Packed red blood cells may also be given if significant blood loss has occurred. Infusions of blood or plasma should be monitored carefully to avoid precipitating pulmonary edema in elderly patients or patients with heart disease.

> For management of a suspected drug overdose, CPhA recommends that you contact your **regional Poison Control Centre**. See the *CPS* Directory section for a list of Poison Control Centres.

DOSAGE: Administration: The administration and dosage of COUMADIN (warfarin sodium) must be individualized according to the patient's responsiveness to the drug. The dosage should be adjusted according to results of the patient's PT ratio/INR. Measurement of warfarin induced effects on PT can vary substantially due to the sensitivity of different thromboplastin reagents.

Early clinical studies of oral anticoagulants, which formed the basis for recommended therapeutic ranges of 1.5 to 2.5 times control PT, used sensitive human brain thromboplastin. When using the less sensitive rabbit brain thromboplastins commonly employed in PT assays today, adjustments must be made to the targeted PT range that reflect this decrease in sensitivity.

The best available information supports the following recommendations for dosing of COUMADIN:

Venous Thromboembolism (including deep venous thrombosis [DVT] and pulmonary embolism [PE]): For patients with a first episode of DVT or PE secondary to a transient (reversible) risk factor, treatment with warfarin for 3 months is generally recommended. For patients with a first episode of idiopathic DVT or PE, warfarin is generally recommended for at least 6 to 12 months. For patients with two or more episodes of documented DVT or PE, indefinite treatment with warfarin is suggested. For patients with specific risk factors (e.g. documented antiphospholipid antibodies), please refer to current treatment guidelines for recommended duration of treatment.

The dose of warfarin should be adjusted to maintain a target INR of 2.5 (INR range, 2.0 to 3.0) for all treatment durations.

Atrial Fibrillation: Five recent clinical trials evaluated the effects of warfarin in patients with non-valvular atrial fibrillation (AF). Findings of these studies revealed that the effects of warfarin in reducing thromboembolic events including stroke were similar at either moderately high INR (2.0-4.5) or low INR (1.4-3.0). There was a significant reduction in minor bleeds at the low INR. There are no adequate and well-controlled studies in populations with atrial fibrillation and valvular heart disease. Although clinical studies have used a wide range of warfarin dosing, a more recent study suggests that in patients with atrial fibrillation, anticoagulant prophylaxis is effective at INRs of 2.0 to 3.0. The study also shows that the risk of thromboembolic stroke may increase substantially at INR's less than 2.0. INR value should not exceed 4.0, to reduce the risk of anticoagulant-related bleeding.

Similar data from clinical studies in valvular atrial fibrillation patients are not available. The trials in non-valvular atrial fibrillation support the recommendation that an INR of 2.0-3.0 be used for long term warfarin therapy in appropriate AF patients. In cases where the risk of thromboembolism is great, such as in patients with recurrent systemic embolism, a higher INR may be required. An INR ratio of greater than 4.0 appears to provide no additional therapeutic benefit in most patients and is associated with a higher risk of bleeding. In AF patients undergoing elective cardioversion, anticoagulant therapy should be given for three weeks before cardioversion and continued until normal sinus rhythm has been maintained for four weeks.

Oral anticoagulation is recommended in patients with persistent or paroxysmal atrial fibrillation without valvular disease but at high risk of embolic stroke, i.e., having any of the following features: prior ischemic stroke, transient ischemic attack, or systemic embolism; age >75 years; moderately or severely impaired left ventricular systolic function or congestive heart failure, history of hypertension, or diabetes mellitus. For patients at lower risk, individualized treatment is required. For patients with atrial fibrillation and valvular heart disease, especially mitral valve stenosis, anticoagulation is recommended. For patients with atrial fibrillation and prosthetic heart valves, anticoagulation is required, with the target INR generally increased, with or without aspirin added, depending of risk factors related to the replaced valve or inherent to the patient.

Post-Myocardial Infarction: For most patients following myocardial infarction and not at high risk, antithrombotic treatment should consist of aspirin alone. In patients with acute coronary syndrome that were revascularised by percutaneous coronary intervention (PCI), clopidogrel is usually added. For high-risk patients with myocardial infarction (MI), including those with a large anterior MI, significant heart failure, intracardiac thrombus visible on echocardiography, or those with a history of a thromboembolic event, therapy with combined moderate-intensity warfarin (INR 2.0 to 3.0) plus low-dose aspirin (100 mg/day) for 3 months following myocardial infarction should be considered.

Laboratory Control: The Prothrombin Time (PT) should be determined daily after the administration of the initial dose until International Normalized Ratio (INR) results stabilize in the therapeutic range. Intervals between subsequent INR determinations should be based upon the physician's judgment of the patient's reliability and response to COUMADIN in order to maintain the individual within the therapeutic range. Acceptable intervals for INR determinations are normally within the range of one to four weeks after a stable dosage has been determined.

To ensure adequate control, it is recommended that additional PT tests be done when other warfarin products are interchanged with warfarin sodium tablets, as well as whenever other medications are initiated, discontinued, or taken irregularly (see Precautions). Safety and efficacy of warfarin therapy can be improved by increasing the quality of laboratory control. Reports suggest that in usual care monitoring, patients are in therapeutic range only 33%-64% of the time. Time in therapeutic range is significantly greater (56%-93%) in patients managed by anticoagulation clinics.

In switching to another warfarin product, particular emphasis needs to be placed on INR control. INR outside of the therapeutic range may result in serious clinical consequences: lack of efficacy leading to thromboembolic stroke or myocardial infarction, if INR values are low, and intracranial bleeding if they are high.

Initial Dosage: The dosing of COUMADIN must be individualized according to the patient's sensitivity to the drug as indicated by the PT/INR. Use of a large loading dose may increase the incidence of hemorrhagic and other complications, does not offer more rapid protection against thrombi formation, and is not recommended. It is recommended that COUMADIN therapy be initiated with a dose of 2 to 5 mg per day with dosage adjustments based on the results of PT/INR determinations. The lower initiation doses should be considered for patients with certain genetic variations in CYP2C9 and VKORC1 enzymes as well as for elderly and/or debilitated patients and patients with potential to exhibit greater than expected PT/INR responses to COUMADIN. Elderly and Asian patients may require lower initiation and maintenance doses of COUMADIN (see Precautions).

Maintenance: Most patients are satisfactorily maintained at a dose of 2 to 10 mg daily. Flexibility of dosage is provided by breaking scored tablets in half. The individual dose and interval should be gauged by the patient's prothrombin response.

Duration of Therapy: The duration of therapy in each patient should be individualized. In general, anticoagulant therapy should be continued until the danger of thrombosis and embolism has passed.

Missed Dose: The anticoagulant effect of COUMADIN persists beyond 24 hours. If the patient forgets to take the prescribed dose of COUMADIN at the scheduled time, the dose should be taken as soon as possible on the same day. The patient should not take the missed dose by doubling the daily dose to make up for missed doses, but should refer back to his or her physician.

Treatment during Dentistry and Surgery: The management of patients who undergo dental and surgical procedures requires close liaison between attending physicians, surgeons and dentists. PT ratio/INR determination is recommended just prior to any dental or surgical procedure. In patients undergoing minimal invasive procedures who must be anticoagulated prior to, during, or immediately following these procedures, adjusting the dosage of COUMADIN to maintain the PT ratio/INR at the low end of the therapeutic range, may safely allow for continued anticoagulation. The operative site should be sufficiently limited and accessible to permit the effective use of local procedures for haemostasis. Under these conditions, dental and surgical procedures may be performed without undue risk of haemorrhage. Some dental or surgical procedures may necessitate the interruption of COUMADIN therapy. When discontinuing COUMADIN even for a short period of time, the benefits and risks should be strongly considered.

Conversion from Heparin Therapy: Since the anticoagulant effect of COUMADIN is delayed, heparin is preferred initially for rapid anticoagulation. Conversion to COUMADIN may begin concomitantly with heparin therapy or may be delayed 3 to 6 days. To ensure continuous anticoagulation, it is advisable to continue full dose heparin therapy and that COUMADIN therapy be overlapped with heparin for 4 to 5 days, until COUMADIN has produced the desired therapeutic response as determined by PT ratio/INR. When COUMADIN has produced the desired PT ratio/INR or prothrombin activity, heparin may be discontinued.

COUMADIN may increase the aPTT test, even in the absence of heparin. During initial therapy with COUMADIN, the interference with heparin anticoagulation is of minimal clinical significance.

As heparin may affect the PT, patients receiving both heparin and COUMADIN should have blood drawn for PT ratio/INR determination, at least: 5 hours after the last i.v. bolus dose of heparin; or 4 hours after cessation of a continuous i.v. infusion of heparin; or 24 hours after last s.c. heparin injection.

INFORMATION FOR THE PATIENT: Published in e-CPS, available by subscription at www.e-cps.ca.

SUPPLIED: 1 mg: Each pink, round, biconvex tablet, one side bisected and imprinted with "COUMADIN" and "1", and the other side blank, contains: crystalline warfarin sodium 1 mg. Nonmedicinal ingredients: D&C Red No. 6 Barium Lake, lactose anhydrous, magnesium stearate and pregelatinized tapioca starch. Bottles of 100, 250 and 1000. Protect from light. Store at room temperature (15 to 30°C). Dispense in a tight, light-resistant container as defined in the USP.

2 mg: Each lavender, round, biconvex tablet, one side bisected and imprinted with "COUMADIN" and "2", and the other side blank, contains: crystalline warfarin sodium 2 mg. Nonmedicinal ingredients: FD&C Blue No. 2 Aluminum Lake, FD&C Red No. 40 Aluminum Lake, lactose anhydrous, magnesium stearate and pregelatinized tapioca starch. Bottles of 100, 250 and 1000. Protect from light. Store at room temperature (15 to 30°C). Dispense in a tight, light-resistant container as defined in the USP.

2.5 mg: Each green, round, biconvex tablet, one side bisected and imprinted with "COUMADIN" and "2 ½", and the other side blank, contains crystalline warfarin sodium 2.5 mg. Nonmedicinal ingredients: D&C Yellow No. 10 Aluminum Lake, FD&C Blue No. 1 Aluminum Lake, lactose anhydrous, magnesium stearate and pregelatinized tapioca starch. Bottles of 100 and 250. Protect from light. Store at room temperature (15 to 30°C). Dispense in a tight, light-resistant container as defined in the USP.

3 mg: Each tan, round, biconvex tablet, one side bisected and imprinted with "COUMADIN" and "3", and the other side blank, contains crystalline warfarin sodium 3 mg. Nonmedicinal ingredients: FD&C Blue No. 2 Aluminum Lake, FD&C Red No. 40 Aluminum Lake, FD&C Yellow No. 6 Aluminum Lake, lactose anhydrous, magnesium stearate and pregelatinized tapioca starch. Bottles of 100 and 250. Protect from light. Store at room temperature (15 to 30°C). Dispense in a tight, light-resistant container as defined in the USP.

4 mg: Each blue, round, biconvex tablet, one side bisected and imprinted with "COUMADIN" and "4", and the other side blank, contains: crystalline warfarin sodium 4 mg. Nonmedicinal ingredients: FD&C Blue #1 Aluminum Lake, lactose anhydrous, magnesium stearate and pregelatinized tapioca starch. Bottles of 100 and 250. Protect from light. Store at room temperature (15 to 30°C). Dispense in a tight, light-resistant container as defined in the USP.

5 mg: Each peach, round, biconvex tablet, one side bisected and imprinted with "COUMADIN" and "5", and the other side blank, contains: crystalline warfarin sodium 5 mg. Nonmedicinal ingredients: FD&C Yellow No. 6 Aluminum Lake, lactose anhydrous, magnesium stearate and pregelatinized tapioca starch. Bottles of 100, 250 and 1000. Protect from light. Store at room temperature (15 to 30°C). Dispense in a tight, light-resistant container as defined in the USP.

6 mg: Each teal, round, biconvex tablet, one side bisected and imprinted with "COUMADIN" and "6", and the other side blank, contains: crystalline warfarin sodium 6 mg. Nonmedicinal ingredients: FD&C Blue No. 1 Aluminum Lake, FD&C Yellow No. 6 Aluminum Lake, lactose anhydrous, magnesium stearate and pregelatinized tapioca starch. Bottles of 100. Protect from light. Store at room temperature (15 to 30°C). Dispense in a tight, light-resistant container as defined in the USP.

10 mg: Each white, round, biconvex tablet, one side bisected and imprinted with "COUMADIN" and "10", and the other side blank, contains: crystalline warfarin sodium 10 mg. Nonmedicinal ingredients: lactose anhydrous, magnesium stearate and pregelatinized tapioca starch. Dye-free. Bottles of 100. Protect from light. Store at room temperature (15 to 30°C). Dispense in a tight, light-resistant container as defined in the USP.

(Shown in Product Identification Section)

CO Valacyclovir

valacyclovir HCl

Antiviral Agent

Cobalt

SUPPLIED: Each blue, capsule shaped, film-coated tablet with "VA500" on one side and "Σ>" on the other contains: valacyclovir 500 mg (as valacyclovir hydrochloride). Nonmedicinal Ingredients: crospovidone, FD&C Blue #2, FD&C Red #40, FD&C Yellow #6, magnesium stearate, microcrystalline cellulose, polyethylene glycol, polyvinyl alcohol, povidone, talc and titanium dioxide. HDPE bottles of 100. Store between 15 and 30°C and protect from light.

CO Venlafaxine XR

venlafaxine HCl

Antidepressant—Anxiolytic

Cobalt

SUPPLIED: 37.5 mg: Each extended release, hard gelatin capsule with peach opaque body and gray opaque cap, the body has "VXR 37.5" and the cap has "Σ>" both printed in red, contains: venlafaxine HCl 37.5 mg. Nonmedicinal ingredients: colloidal silicon dioxide, copovidone, ethyl cellulose, magnesium stearate, microcrystalline cellulose, povidone and talc; capsule shell: gelatin. HDPE bottles of 100 and 500. Store at room temperature (15-30°C), in a dry place.

75 mg: Each extended release, hard gelatin capsule with peach opaque body and cap, the body has "VXR 75" and the cap has "Σ>" both printed in red, contains: venlafaxine HCl 75 mg. Nonmedicinal ingredients: colloidal silicon dioxide, copovidone, ethyl cellulose, magnesium stearate, microcrystalline cellulose, povidone and talc; capsule shell: gelatin. HDPE bottles of 100 and 500. Store at room temperature (15-30°C), in a dry place.

150 mg: Each extended release, hard gelatin capsule with dark orange opaque body and cap, the body has "VXR 150" and the cap has "Σ>" both printed in white, contains: venlafaxine HCl 150 mg. Nonmedicinal ingredients: colloidal silicon dioxide, copovidone, ethyl cellulose, magnesium stearate, microcrystalline cellulose, povidone and talc; capsule shell: gelatin. HDPE bottles of 100 and 500. Store at room temperature (15-30°C), in a dry place.

The reader is invited to consult CPhA's monograph **ACE Inhibitors**.

Coversyl®

perindopril erbumine

Angiotensin Converting Enzyme Inhibitor

Servier

Date of Preparation: June 6, 1994
Date of Revision: April 21, 2010

SUMMARY PRODUCT INFORMATION:

Route of Administration	Dosage Form/ Strength	Clinically Relevant Nonmedicinal Ingredients
Oral	Tablet 2 mg, 4 mg and 8 mg	Lactose For a complete listing see Dosage Forms, Composition and Packaging.

INDICATIONS AND CLINICAL USE: COVERSYL (perindopril erbumine) is indicated for:

- The treatment of mild to moderate essential hypertension. It may be used alone or in association with other drugs, particularly thiazide diuretics.

  The safety and efficacy of COVERSYL in renovascular hypertension have not been established and therefore, its use in this condition is not recommended.

  The safety and efficacy of concurrent use of COVERSYL with antihypertensive agents other than thiazide diuretics have not been established.
- The treatment of mild to moderate congestive heart failure, generally as adjunctive therapy to diuretics, and where appropriate a digitalis glycoside. Treatment should be initiated under close medical supervision. The safety and efficacy of COVERSYL has not been demonstrated for New York Heart Association Category IV patients.
- The reduction of cardiovascular risk in patients with hypertension or post-myocardial infarction and stable coronary disease.

  COVERSYL has been demonstrated to reduce the risk of cardiovascular death, non-fatal myocardial infarction, and cardiac arrest in mild or moderately hypertensive patients with stable coronary artery disease, or in patients with a previous (>3 months ago) myocardial infarction and stable coronary artery disease, when administered as an add-on to conventional treatment, such as platelet inhibitors, beta blockers, lipid-lowering agents, nitrates, calcium channel blockers or diuretics.

Geriatrics (>65 years of age): Although clinical experience has not identified significant differences in response between the elderly (>65 years) and younger patients, greater sensitivity of some older individuals cannot be ruled out.

Pediatrics: The safety and effectiveness of COVERSYL in children have not been established. Its use in this age group, therefore, is not recommended.

General: In using COVERSYL, consideration should be given to the risk of angioedema (see Warnings and Precautions).

When using COVERSYL Tablets, consideration should be given to the fact that other angiotensin converting enzyme inhibitors have caused agranulocytosis, particularly in patients with renal impairment or collagen vascular disease (see Warnings and Precautions).

CONTRAINDICATIONS: COVERSYL (perindopril erbumine) is contraindicated in:

- Patients who are hypersensitive to this drug or to any ingredient in the formulation. For a complete listing, see Dosage Forms, Composition and Packaging.
- Patients with a history of angioedema related to previous treatment with an angiotensin converting enzyme inhibitor.

WARNINGS AND PRECAUTIONS:

Serious Warnings and Precautions
When used in pregnancy, angiotensin converting enzyme (ACE) inhibitors can cause injury or even death of the developing fetus. When pregnancy is detected, COVERSYL should be discontinued as soon as possible.

Cardiovascular: Hypotension: COVERSYL can cause symptomatic hypotension. COVERSYL Tablets have been associated with hypotension in 0.3% of uncomplicated hypertensive patients in U.S. placebo-controlled trials. Symptoms related to orthostatic hypotension were reported in another 0.8% of patients. It is more likely to occur after the first or second dose or when the dose was increased and in patients who are volume depleted by diuretic therapy, dietary salt restriction, dialysis, diarrhoea, or vomiting or with impaired renal function. Volume and/or salt depletion should be corrected before initiation of therapy with COVERSYL (see Dosage and Administration). In patients with ischemic heart or cerebrovascular disease and/or severe congestive heart failure, with or without associated renal insufficiency, ACE inhibitors may cause an excessive fall in blood pressure which could result in syncope, a myocardial infarction, neurological deficits, oliguria and/or progressive azotemia and, rarely, in acute renal failure and/or death (see Adverse Reactions). In all high-risk patients it is advisable to initiate treatment with COVERSYL 2 mg.

Because of the potential fall in blood pressure in these patients, therapy with COVERSYL should be started under very close medical supervision. Such patients should be followed closely for the first two weeks of treatment and whenever the dose of COVERSYL and/or diuretic is increased.

In controlled studies versus placebo and other ACE inhibitors, the first administration of 2 mg of COVERSYL in patients with mild-moderate heart failure was not associated with any significant reduction in blood pressure as compared to placebo (see Actions and Clinical Pharmacology, Pharmacodynamics).

In patients with severe congestive heart failure, with or without associated renal insufficiency, excessive hypotension can be associated with oliguria and/or progressive azotemia and, rarely, with acute renal failure and/or death.

If hypotension occurs, the patient should be placed in a supine position and, if necessary, receive an intravenous infusion of 0.9% sodium chloride. A transient hypotensive response is not a contraindication to further doses which usually can be given without difficulty once the blood pressure has increased after volume expansion. However, lower doses of COVERSYL and/or reduced concomitant diuretic therapy should be considered.

Aortic Stenosis/Hypertrophic Cardiomyopathy: As with other ACE inhibitors, COVERSYL should be given with caution to patients with mitral valve stenosis and obstruction in the outflow of the left ventricle such as aortic stenosis or hypertrophic cardiomyopathy. There is concern on theoretical grounds that patients with aortic stenosis might be at particular risk of decreased coronary perfusion when treated with vasodilators including ACE inhibitors because they do not develop as much afterload reduction. Vasodilators may tend to drop diastolic pressure, and hence coronary pressure, without producing the concomitant reduction in myocardial oxygen demand that normally accompanies vasodilation.

Hematologic: Neutropenia/Agranulocytosis/Thrombocytopenia/Anaemia: Neutropenia/agranulocytosis, thrombocytopenia and anaemia have been reported in patients receiving ACE inhibitors. In patients with normal renal function and no other complicating factors, neutropenia occurs rarely. Perindopril should be used with extreme caution in patients with collagen vascular disease such as systemic lupus erythematosus or scleroderma, and those on multiple drug therapy with agents known to be nephrotoxic or myelosuppressive (immunosuppressant therapy, treatment with allopurinol or procainamide), or a combination of these complicating factors, especially if there is pre-existing impaired renal function. Some of these patients developed serious infections, which in a few instances did not respond to intensive antibiotic therapy. If perindopril is used in such patients, periodic monitoring of white blood cell counts is advised and patients should be instructed to report any sign of infection.

Hepatic/Biliary/Pancreatic: Hepatic Failure: Rarely, ACE inhibitors have been associated with a syndrome that starts with cholestatic jaundice and progresses to fulminant hepatic necrosis and (sometimes) death. The mechanism of this syndrome is not understood. Patients receiving ACE inhibitors who develop jaundice or marked elevations of hepatic enzymes should discontinue the ACE inhibitor and receive appropriate medical follow-up.

Immune: Anaphylactoid Reactions During Membrane Exposure (Hemodialysis Patients): Anaphylactoid reactions have been reported in patients dialyzed with high-flux membranes (e.g. polyacrylonitrile [PAN]) and treated concomitantly with an ACE inhibitor. Dialysis should be stopped immediately if symptoms such as nausea, abdominal cramps, burning, angioedema, shortness of breath and severe hypotension occur. Symptoms are not relieved by antihistamines. In these patients, consideration should be given to using a different type of dialysis membrane or a different class of antihypertensive agents.

Anaphylactoid Reactions During LDL Apheresis: Rarely, patients receiving ACE inhibitors during low density lipoprotein apheresis with dextran sulfate absorption have experienced life-threatening anaphylactoid reactions. These reactions were avoided by temporarily withholding the ACE inhibitor therapy prior to each apheresis.

Anaphylactoid Reactions During Desensitization: There have been isolated reports of patients experiencing sustained, life-threatening anaphylactoid reactions while receiving ACE inhibitors during desensitization treatment with hymenoptera (bees, wasps) venom. In the same patients, these reactions have been avoided when ACE inhibitors were temporarily withheld for at least 24 hours, but they reappeared upon inadvertent rechallenge.

Peri-Operative Considerations: ACE inhibitors may augment the hypotensive effects of anaesthetics and analgesics. In patients undergoing major surgery or during anaesthesia with agents that produce hypotension, COVERSYL will block the angiotensin II formation that could otherwise occur secondary to compensatory renin release. If hypotension occurs and is considered to be due to this mechanism, it can be corrected by volume expansion.

Renal: Impaired Renal Function: As a consequence of inhibiting the renin-angiotensin-aldosterone system, changes in renal function may be anticipated in susceptible individuals.

In cases of renal impairment (creatinine clearance <60 mL/min) the initial perindopril dosage should be adjusted according to the patient's creatinine clearance and then as a function of the patient's response to treatment. Routine monitoring of potassium and creatinine are part of normal medical practice for these patients.

Hypertensive Patients with Congestive Heart Failure: In patients with severe congestive heart failure, where renal function may depend on the activity of the renin-angiotensin-aldosterone system, treatment with ACE inhibitors, including COVERSYL Tablets, may be associated with oliguria and/or progressive azotemia, and rarely with acute renal failure and/or death.

In patients with symptomatic heart failure, hypotension following the initiation of therapy with ACE inhibitors may lead to some further impairment in renal function. Acute renal failure, usually reversible, has been reported in this situation.

Hypertensive Patients with Renal Artery Stenosis: In clinical trials in hypertensive patients with unilateral or bilateral renal artery stenosis, increases in blood urea nitrogen and serum creatinine were observed in 20% of patients. Experience with ACE inhibitors suggests that these increases are usually reversible upon discontinuation of the drug. In such patients, renal function should be monitored during the first few weeks of therapy. ACE inhibitors should be avoided in patients with known or suspected renal artery stenosis. When an ACE inhibitor is given to a patient with stenosis of the renal artery supplying a solitary kidney, or bilateral artery stenosis, acute renal insufficiency may occur. ACE inhibition may also cause a decrease in renal function in patients with stenosis of the artery supplying a transplanted kidney. It is believed that renal artery stenosis reduces the pressure in the afferent glomerular arteriole, and transglomerular hydrostatic pressure is then maintained by angiotensin II-induced constriction of the efferent arteriole. When an ACE inhibitor is given, the efferent arteriole relaxes, glomerular filtration falls, and renal failure may result. The thrombotic occlusion of a stenosed renal artery can be precipitated by ACE inhibitors.

Some hypertensive patients without apparent pre-existing renal vascular disease have developed increases in blood urea nitrogen and serum creatinine, usually minor and transient. These increases are more likely to occur in patients treated concomitantly with a diuretic and in patients with pre-existing renal impairment. Reduction of dosages of COVERSYL Tablets, the diuretic or both may be required. In some cases, discontinuation of either or both drugs may be necessary. Evaluation of hypertensive patients should always include an assessment of renal function (see Dosage and Administration). If deterioration in renal function has occurred after treatment with one ACE inhibitor, then it is likely to be precipitated by another and in these patients usage of another class of antihypertensive agent would be preferable. Patients with unilateral renal artery disease present a special problem as deterioration of function may not be apparent from measurement of blood urea and serum creatinine.

Proteinuria: Some ACE inhibitors have been associated with the occurrence (up to 0.7%) of proteinuria (<1 gram/24 hours) and/or decline in renal function in patients with one or more of the following characteristics: old age, pre-existing renal disease, concomitant treatment with potassium-sparing diuretics or high doses of other diuretics, limited cardiac reserve, or treatment with a non-steroidal anti-inflammatory drug.

Perindoprilat, the active form of perindopril, is dialysable with a clearance of 70 mL/min.

Hyperkalemia and Potassium-Sparing Diuretics, Potassium Supplements or Potassium-Containing Salt Substitutes: In clinical trials, hyperkalemia (serum potassium >5.5 mEq/L) occurred in approximately 2.2% of the hypertensive patients compared to 1.4% in placebo (see Adverse Reactions). In most cases, these were isolated values which resolved despite continued therapy. In controlled studies, no patient discontinued therapy due to hyperkalemia.

Risk factors for development of hyperkalemia may include renal impairment, diabetes mellitus, elderly patients and the concomitant use of potassium-sparing diuretics, potassium supplements, potassium-containing salt substitutes or other drugs associated with increases in serum potassium (e.g. heparin) which should be used cautiously, if at all, with COVERSYL Tablets (see Drug Interactions). In some patients hyponatremia may co-exist with hyperkalemia. If concomitant use of the above-mentioned agents is deemed appropriate, regular monitoring of serum potassium and urea is recommended.

Respiratory: Cough: A dry, persistent cough, which usually disappears only after withdrawal or lowering of the dose of COVERSYL has been reported. Such possibility should be considered as part of the differential diagnosis of the cough.

The cough is often worse when lying down or at night, and has been reported more frequently in women (who account for 2/3 of the reported cases). Patients who cough may have increased bronchial reactivity compared with those who do not. The observed higher frequency of this side-effect in non-smokers may be due to a higher level of tolerance of smokers to cough.

The cough is most likely due to stimulation of the pulmonary cough reflex by kinins (bradykinin) and/or prostaglandins, which accumulate because of ACE inhibition. Once a patient has developed intolerable cough, an attempt may be made to switch the patient to another ACE inhibitor; the reaction may recur but this is not invariably the case. A change to another class of drugs may be required in severe cases.

Sensitivity/Resistance: Due to the presence of lactose, patients with hereditary problems of galactose intolerance, glucose-galactose malabsorption or the Lapp lactose deficiency should not take this medicinal product.

Skin: Head and Neck Angioedema: Life-threatening angioedema has been reported with ACE inhibitors. The overall incidence is approximately 0.1-0.2%. The aetiology is thought to be non-immunogenic and may be related to accentuated bradykinin activity. Usually, the angioedema is non-pitting edema of the skin mucous membrane and subcutaneous tissue.

Angioedema involving the face, extremities, lips, tongue, glottis and/or larynx has been reported in patients treated with ACE inhibitors, including COVERSYL (perindopril) Tablets. Angioedema associated with laryngeal involvement may be fatal. If laryngeal stridor or angioedema of the face, tongue, or glottis occurs, COVERSYL should be discontinued immediately, the patient treated appropriately in accordance with accepted medical care, and carefully observed until the swelling disappears. In instances where swelling is confined to the face and lips, the condition generally resolves without treatment, although antihistamines may be useful in relieving symptoms. Where there is involvement of the tongue, glottis or larynx, angioedema may be fatal due to airway obstruction, appropriate therapy (including but not limited to 0.3 to 0.5 mL of subcutaneous epinephrine solution 1:1000 and oxygen) should be administered promptly (see Adverse Reactions).

Treatment of progressive angioedema should be aggressive. Failing a rapid response to medical therapy, mechanical methods to secure an airway should be undertaken before massive edema complicates oral or nasal intubation.

Patients who respond to medical treatment should be observed carefully for a possible rebound phenomenon.

The onset of angioedema associated with use of ACE inhibitors may be delayed for weeks or months.

Patients may have multiple episodes of angioedema with long symptom-free intervals.

Angioedema may occur with or without urticaria.

The incidence of angioedema during ACE inhibitor therapy has been reported to be higher in black than in non-black patients.

There are reports that switching a patient to another ACE inhibitor could be followed by a recurrence of angioedema. Because of the potential severity of this rare event, another ACE inhibitor should not be used in patients with a history of angioedema (see Contraindications).

Patients with a history of angioedema unrelated to ACE inhibitor therapy may be at increased risk of angioedema while receiving an ACE inhibitor (see Contraindications).

Intestinal Angioedema: Intestinal angioedema has been reported in patients treated with ACE inhibitors. These patients presented with abdominal pain (with or without nausea or vomiting); in some cases there was no prior history of facial angioedema and C-1 esterase levels were normal. Angioedema was diagnosed by procedures including abdominal CT scan or ultrasound, or at surgery, and symptoms resolved after stopping the ACE inhibitor. Intestinal angioedema should be included in the differential diagnosis of patients on ACE inhibitors presenting with abdominal pain.

Dermatological Reactions: Dermatological reactions characterised by maculo-papular pruritic rashes and sometimes photosensitivity has been reported with another ACE inhibitor. Rare and sometimes severe skin reactions (lichenoid eruptions, psoriasis, pemphigus like rash, rosacea, Stevens-Johnson syndrome, etc.) have occurred.

Patients who develop a cutaneous reaction with one ACE inhibitor might not when switched to another drug of the same class, but there are reports of cross-reactivity.

Taste Disturbances (Dysgeusia): Taste disturbances were reported to be common (prevalence up to 12.5%) with high doses of another ACE inhibitor.

Taste disturbance with ACE inhibitors have been described as suppression of taste or a metallic sensation in the mouth. Any dysgeusia usually occurs in the first weeks of treatment and may disappear in most cases within 1-3 months.

Special Populations: Pregnant Women: ACE inhibitors can cause fetal and neonatal morbidity and mortality when administered to pregnant women. When pregnancy is detected, COVERSYL should be discontinued as soon as possible.

The use of ACE inhibitors during the second and third trimesters of pregnancy has been associated with fetal and neonatal injury including hypotension, neonatal skull hypoplasia, anuria, reversible or irreversible renal failure, and death.

Oligohydramnios has also been reported, presumably resulting from decreased fetal renal function, associated with fetal limb contractures, craniofacial deformation, and hypoplastic lung development.

Prematurity, and patent ductus arteriosus and other structural cardiac malformations, as well as neurologic malformations, have also been reported following exposure in the first trimester of pregnancy.

Infants with a history of in utero exposure to ACE inhibitors should be closely observed for hypotension, oliguria, and hyperkalemia. If oliguria occurs, attention should be directed toward support of blood pressure and renal perfusion. Exchange transfusion or dialysis may be required as a means of reversing hypotension and/or substituting for impaired renal function; however, limited experience with those procedures has not been associated with significant clinical benefit.

Perindoprilat, the active form of perindopril, can be removed from the body by hemodialysis (see Actions and Clinical Pharmacology, Pharmacokinetics and Metabolism; Special Populations and Conditions, Renal Insufficiency).

Nursing Women: The presence of concentrations of ACE inhibitor have been reported in human milk. Use of ACE inhibitors is not recommended during breast-feeding.

Pediatrics: The safety and effectiveness of COVERSYL in children have not been established. Its use in this age group, therefore, is not recommended.

Geriatrics (>65 years of age): Although clinical experience has not identified significant differences in response between the elderly (>65 years) and younger patients, greater sensitivity of some older individuals cannot be ruled out.

Renal insufficiency is commonly observed in elderly people. Care should therefore be taken when prescribing COVERSYL to elderly patients. The initial dose of COVERSYL in the elderly should always be 2 mg daily and patients should be monitored closely during the initial stages of treatment (see Dosage and Administration).

In a study of 91 elderly patients with a mean age of 71.9 years, a 6% increase in serum potassium occurred in the first month of treatment and subsequently remained stable. There was no change in the group in blood urea, creatinine or creatinine clearance.

Particular care should be taken in elderly patients with congestive heart failure who have renal and/or hepatic insufficiency.

Diabetic Patients: In diabetic patients treated with oral antidiabetic agents or insulin, glycemic control should be closely monitored during the first month of treatment with an ACE inhibitor.

Patients with Impaired Liver Function: Hepatitis (hepatocellular and/or cholestatic), elevations of liver enzymes and/or serum bilirubin have occurred during therapy with ACE inhibitors, in patients with or without pre-existing liver abnormalities. In most cases, the changes were reversed upon discontinuation of the drug.

Elevations of liver enzymes and/or serum bilirubin have been reported with COVERSYL (see Adverse Reactions). Should the patient receiving COVERSYL experience any unexplained symptoms, particularly during the first weeks or months of treatment, it is recommended that a full set of liver function tests and any other necessary investigation be carried out. Discontinuation of COVERSYL should be considered when appropriate.

COVERSYL should be used with particular caution in patients with pre-existing liver abnormalities. In such patients, baseline liver function tests should be obtained before administration of the drug and close monitoring of response and metabolic effects should apply.

Monitoring and Laboratory Tests: Not applicable.

ADVERSE REACTIONS: Adverse Drug Reaction Overview: COVERSYL (perindopril erbumine) has been evaluated for safety in approximately 3000 hypertensive patients, of which, 1216 patients, 181 of which were elderly, participated in controlled clinical trials. COVERSYL has been evaluated for long-term safety in approximately 1000 patients treated for one year or more. In heart failure trials, 167 patients were treated with perindopril in 3-month placebo-controlled trials and long-term safety was assessed in 513 patients treated for 6 months or more, of which 352 have been followed for at least one year.

The Most Serious and Important Post-Marketing Adverse Drug Reactions Were: Blood and Lymphatic System Disorders: haemoglobin decreased and haematocrit decreased. Thrombocytopenia, leukopenia/neutropenia, agranulocytosis or pancytopenia, haemolytic anemia in patients with a congenital deficiency of G-6PDH.

Cardiac Disorders, Possibly Secondary to Excessive Hypotension: angina pectoris, arrhythmia, myocardial infarction, palpitations.

Respiratory/Thoracic and Mediastinal Disorders: bronchospasm, eosinophilic pneumonia.

Gastrointestinal Disorders: pancreatitis.

Hepato-Biliary Disorders: cytolytic hepatitis, cholestatic hepatitis.

Skin and Subcutaneous Tissue Disorders: angioneurotic oedema (face, extremities, lips, mucous membranes, tongue, glottis and/or larynx, erythema multiforme.

Renal and Urinary Disorders: renal insufficiency, acute renal failure.

Musculoskeletal, Connective Tissue Disorders: oedema.

Reproductive System and Breast Disorders: erectile dysfunction.

Vascular Disorders: cerebrovascular accident, peripheral vascular disorder (impaired peripheral circulation).

The most severe adverse drug reactions occurring in hypertensive patients treated with perindopril are angioneurotic oedema and renal insufficiency. Myocardial infarction and cerebrovascular accident occurred possibly secondary to excessive hypotension in high-risk patients (see Warnings and Precautions, Cardiovascular).

During the long-term safety assessment in heart failure patients, the severe adverse events occurring with the highest frequency were angina pectoris and orthostatic hypotension.

The Most Frequent Post-Marketing Adverse Drug Reactions (Incidence ≥1%-<10%) Are:

Nervous System Disorders: headache, dizziness, paresthesia, dysgeusia.

Eye Disorders: vision disturbance.

Ear and Labyrinth Disorders: vertigo, ear infection, tinnitus.

Vascular Disorders: hypotension.

Respiratory/Thoracic and Mediastinal Disorders: cough, dyspnoea.

Gastrointestinal Disorders: nausea, vomiting, abdominal pain (including–upper), diarrhoea, constipation.

General Disorders and Administration Site Conditions: asthenia, dyspepsia, pyrexia.

Infections and Infestations: sinusitis, viral infection.

Musculoskeletal, Connective Tissue and Bone Disorders: muscle cramps, pain in extremity, back pain, hypertonia.

Renal and Urinary Disorders: proteinuria.

Adverse drug reactions that most commonly result in premature discontinuation of therapy are cough (0.5%), headache (0.5%), dizziness (0.5%) and asthenia (0.4%).

Withdrawals: In total 56 of 1275 patients studied (4.4%) stopped treatment because of adverse reactions. In a specific study of 632 patients, 36 (5.7%) patients withdrew because of adverse events. A plausible or probable relationship with COVERSYL treatment were considered to exist in 19 (3%) cases.

Clinical Trial Adverse Drug Reactions: Because clinical trials are conducted under very specific conditions the adverse reaction rates observed in the clinical trials may not reflect the rates observed in practice and should not be compared to the rates in the clinical trials of another drug. Adverse drug reaction information from clinical trials is useful for identifying drug-related adverse events and for approximating rates.

Perindopril has been evaluated for safety in approximately 3400 patients with hypertension in U.S. and foreign clinical trials.

In an open-labelled European study of about 47 000 patients with essential hypertension, seen in everyday medical practice, and treated for one year with COVERSYL, with or without multiple other medications, the most frequently observed adverse events were: cough 9.7%, digestive symptoms 2.0%, fatigue 1.8%, headache 1.4% and dizziness 1.4%. In total, 5.1% of patients in this study withdrew due to adverse events, 3.2% due to cough.

The data presented below are based on results from the 1417 COVERSYL-treated patients who participated in the U.S. clinical trials. Over 220 of these patients were treated with COVERSYL for at least one year.

Among 1012 patients in placebo-controlled U.S. trials, Table 1 presents adverse events that occurred in ≥1% of the patients and that were more common for perindopril than placebo by at least 1%. Depending on the specific adverse event, approximately 30 to 70% of the common complaints were considered possibly or probably related to treatment.

Table 1: COVERSYL

Drug-Related Adverse Experience Reported in ≥1% of Patients Treated for Hypertension (%)

	All Adverse Events		Possibly- or Probably-Related Adverse Events	
	Perindopril n=789	**Placebo n=223**	**Perindopril n=789**	**Placebo n=223**
Cough	12.0	4.5	6.0	1.8
Back pain	5.8	3.1	0.0	0.0
Sinusitis	5.2	3.6	0.6	0.0
Viral infection	3.4	1.6	0.3	0.0
Upper extremity pain	2.8	1.4	0.2	0.0
Hypertonia	2.7	1.4	0.2	0.0
Dyspepsia	1.9	0.9	0.3	0.0
Fever	1.5	0.5	0.3	0.0
Proteinuria	1.5	0.5	1.0	0.5
Ear infection	1.3	0.0	0.0	0.0
Palpitation	1.1	0.0	0.9	0.0

The most frequent adverse events which occurred in North-American placebo-controlled trials with COVERSYL monotherapy in hypertension (n=630) were: headache (26.0%), cough (13.0%), asthenia (8.7%), dizziness (8.6%), upper respiratory infection (7.9%), back pain (6.8%), diarrhoea (4.6%) and edema (4.3%). Discontinuation of therapy because of adverse events was required in 6.9% of the patients.

The incidence of premature discontinuation of therapy due to adverse events in the placebo-controlled U.S clinical trials was 6.5% in patients treated with perindopril and 6.7% in patients treated with placebo. The most common causes of premature discontinuation were cough, headache, asthenia and dizziness. Of these, cough was the reason for withdrawal in 1.3% of perindopril and 0.4% of placebo patients. While dizziness was not reported more frequently in the perindopril group (8.2%) than in the placebo group (8.5%), it was clearly increased with dose, suggesting a causal relationship with perindopril.

Other commonly reported complaints (1% or greater), regardless of causality, include: headache (23.8%), upper respiratory infection (8.6%), asthenia (7.9%), rhinitis (4.8%), low extremity pain (4.7%), diarrhea (4.3%), edema (3.9%), pharyngitis (3.3%), urinary tract infection (2.8%), abdominal pain (2.7%), sleep disorder (2.5%), chest pain (2.4%), injury, paresthesia, nausea, rash (each 2.3%), seasonal allergy, depression (each 2.0%), abnormal ECG (1.8%); ALT increase (1.7%), tinnitus, vomiting (each 1.5%), neck pain, male sexual dysfunction (each 1.4%), triglyceride increase, somnolence (each 1.3%), joint pain, nervousness, myalgia, menstrual disorder (each 1.1%), flatulence and arthritis (each 1.0%), but none of those was more frequent by at least 1% on perindopril than on placebo.

The most severe adverse reactions occurring in all hypertensive patients treated with perindopril in controlled clinical trials were: angioedema (0.1%), orthostatic hypotension (0.4%) and syncope (0.6%). Myocardial infarction and cerebrovascular accident occurred possibly secondary to excessive hypotension in high risk patients (see Warnings and Precautions). During the long-term safety assessment in heart failure patients, the severe adverse events occurring with the highest frequency were anginal pain (2.5%) and orthostatic hypotension (2.3%).

In heart failure trials, safety has been evaluated in 167 patients treated with perindopril in 3-month placebo-controlled trials and long-term safety was assessed in 513 patients treated for 6 months or more. Table 2 presents adverse events that occurred in ≥1% of the 167 patients treated with perindopril during the double-blind period lasting three months, as compared to the same adverse events occurring in the 170 patients receiving a placebo.

In the double-blind phase of the placebo-controlled trials in heart failure, the most frequent adverse events were: asthenia (6.6%), dizziness (6.0%), abdominal pain/gastralgia (4.2%), skin disorders (4.2%), nausea/vomiting (3.6%) and headache (3.0%), palpitations (2.4%) and muscle cramps (2.4%). Discontinuation of therapy due to adverse events was required in 5.4% of the 167 patients with perindopril, as compared to 4.7% of the 170 patients who received a placebo.

Perindopril has been evaluated for safety in the EUROPA trial. This was a double-blind, placebo-controlled study in 12 218 patients with stable coronary artery disease (CAD), the majority of which had hypertension and/or had survived a previous heart attack. The overall rate of discontinuation was 22.8% (1391/6110 patients) and 20.7% (1266/6108 patients) in the perindopril and in the placebo groups, respectively. The most common reasons for discontinuation that were more frequent on COVERSYL than placebo were cough, drug intolerance, hypotension and kidney failure.

Table 2: COVERSYL

Drug-Related Adverse Experience Reported in ≥1% of Patients Treated for Congestive Heart Failure (%)

	Perindopril n=167	**Placebo n=170**
Asthenia	6.6	5.3
Dizziness	6.0	6.5
Skin disorder	4.2	2.4
Nausea	3.6	1.2
Abdominal pain upper	3.6	2.9
Headache	3.0	2.4
Palpitations	2.4	1.8
Muscular cramps	2.4	0.0
Cough	1.8	0.6
Chest pain—cardiac	1.8	0.0
Dyspnoea	1.8	2.4
Diarrhoea	1.8	1.8
Mood altered and sleep disturbance	1.8	2.9
Oedema	1.2	1.8
Sweating	1.2	0.6
Erectile dysfunction	1.2	0.6

Mortality in EUROPA Trial: There were no significant differences in numbers of deaths between the groups (375 in the perindopril group and 420 deaths in the control group). However, ten patients died during the open run-in period of the study, of whom 7 from cardiovascular causes, including stroke. A total of 795 patients (out of 12 230; 6.5%) died during the study, 464 of the 795 died (58%) from a cardiovascular cause.

Serious Adverse Drug Reactions in EUROPA Trial: During the open run-in period, 12 patients experienced serious ADRs attributed to perindopril: 7 episodes of hypotension, 3 episodes of syncope, 2 cases of non-fatal angioedema and one sudden death. During the double-blind treatment period, 28 patients experienced serious ADRs: 16 patients in the perindopril group experienced 24 events, and 12 patients in the placebo group had 17 events. Hypotension was the most frequent (6 episodes in the perindopril group and 3 in the placebo group), followed by angioedema of the face and/or tongue (3 and 0), syncope, (3 and 3), chest pain, angina (3 and 1), and brachycardia, arrythmia (2 and 0). All other serious ADRs occurred once in either of the treatment groups.

Atrial cardioversion, on the other hand, occurred significantly more frequently in the perindopril group: 0.5% (n=42) vs 0.3% (n=17) in the control group.

Less Common Clinical Trial Adverse Drug Reactions (<1%): Adverse events, irrespective of causal relationship to the drug, which occurred in less than 1.0% of hypertensive and heart failure patients treated with COVERSYL in clinical trials, are listed as follows:

Blood and Lymphatic System Disorders: haemolytic anaemia, leucopenia including neutropenia, thrombocytopenia, ecchymosis, haematoma.

Cardiac Disorders: syncope, arrhythmia, ventricular extrasystole, conduction disorder, cardiac murmur, palpitations, bradycardia, myocardial infarction.

Ear and Labyrinth Disorders: vertigo, ear pain, tinnitus.

Eye Disorders: visual disturbance, lacrimation increased, conjunctivitis.

Gastrointestinal Disorders: constipation, dry mouth, flatulence, haematemesis, G.I. haemorrhage, stomatitis, diarrhoea, vomiting, dyspepsia.

General Disorders and Administration Site Conditions: chest pain, pyrexia, malaise, pain, peripheral oedema, thirst, feeling cold and hot, rigors.

Immune System Disorders: anaphylactic reaction, angioneurotic oedema (head, neck, face, extremities, lips, tongue, glottis and/or larynx).

Infections and Infestations: herpes simplex, peritoneal infection (mesenteric infarction, 1 patient), bronchitis, pharyngitis, pneumonia, rhinitis, sinusitis, skin infection, tinea infection, gastroenteritis, vaginitis.

Metabolism and Nutrition Disorders: anorexia, increased appetite, gout.

Musculoskeletal and Connective Tissue Disorders: neck pain, oedema, arthralgia, arthritis, bone pain, myalgia, myasthenia, sciatalgia, hypertonia/muscle cramps, back (lumbar) pain.

Nervous System Disorders: hyperkinesia, amnesia, cerebrovascular accident (0.2%), cognitive disorders, memory impairment, perceptual distortion, somnolence, speech disorder, tremor, dysgeusia, migraine.

Psychiatric Disorders: abnormal dreams, agitation, confusional state, depression, mood altered, nervousness, illusion, sleep disturbance, libido disorder, anxiety, psychosexual disorder.

Renal and Urinary Disorders: haematuria, nephrolithiasis, nocturia, oliguria, polyuria, pollakiuria, urinary incontinence, urinary retention, fluid retention, renal insufficiency, flank pain.

Reproductive System and Breast Disorders: menstrual disorder, scrotal oedema, erectile dysfunction.

Respiratory, Thoracic and Mediastinal Disorders: asthma, bronchospasm, dyspnoea, pulmonary fibrosis, throat irritation, rhinorrhoea, epistaxis, postnasal drip, hoarseness, sneezing.

Skin and Subcutaneous Tissue Disorders: alopecia, erythema, dry skin, skin disorder, dermatitis, pemphigus, pruritus, purpura, rash, Steven-Johnson syndrome, hyperhidrosis, toxic skin eruption, urticaria, mucous membrane disorder.

Vascular Disorders: hypotension, orthostatic hypotension, peripheral coldness, intermittent claudication, vasodilation, flushing, peripheral vascular disorder (impaired peripheral circulation, swollen legs).

Laboratory: Increases in blood urea and plasma creatinine, hyperkalemia may occur especially in the presence of renal insufficiency, severe heart failure and renovascular hypertension. Elevation of liver enzymes (ALT: 1.6% COVERSYL vs 0.9% placebo, AST: 0.5% COVERSYL vs 0.4% placebo have been observed in U.S. placebo-controlled clinical trials), serum bilirubin, cholesterol increase, hematuria, and glucose increase.

Abnormal Hematologic and Clinical Chemistry Findings: Serum Electrolytes: In clinical trials, hyperkalemia (serum potassium >5.5 mEq/L) occurred in approximately 2.2% of the hypertensive patients compared to 1.4% in placebo (see Warnings and Precautions, Renal).

Blood Urea Nitrogen/Serum Creatinine: Elevations of BUN or serum creatinine (BUN >40 mg/dl; serum creatinine >2.5 mg/dl) have been observed, respectively, in 0.2% and 0.3% of patients treated with COVERSYL monotherapy. Decreases in serum sodium and increases in serum creatinine occurred more frequently in patients on concomitant diuretics than in those treated with COVERSYL alone.

Hematology: Small decreases in hemoglobin and hematocrit occurred in hypertensive patients treated with COVERSYL, but were rarely of clinical importance. In controlled clinical trials, no patient was discontinued from therapy due to the development of anemia.

Liver Function: Elevations of liver enzymes and/or serum bilirubin have been observed (see Warnings and Precautions, Special Populations).

Potential Adverse Effects Reported with ACE Inhibitors: Other medically important adverse effects reported with other available ACE inhibitors include cardiac arrest, eosinophilic pneumonitis, neutropenia/agranulocytosis, pancytopenia, anemia (including hemolytic and aplastic), thrombocytopenia, acute renal failure, nephritis, hepatic failure, jaundice (hepatocellular or cholestatic), symptomatic hyponatremia, bullous pemphigus, acute pancreatitis, exfoliative dermatitis and a syndrome which may include: arthralgia/arthritis, vasculitis, serositis, myalgia, fever, rash or other dermatologic manifestations, a positive ANA, leukocytosis, eosinophilia or an elevated ESR. Many of these adverse effects have also been reported for perindopril.

Post-Market Adverse Drug Reactions: Four general practice post-marketing surveillance studies in 98 010 hypertensive patients were performed in France and Australia. The most frequent adverse events, which occurred in these studies, were cough (more than 5%) and gastrointestinal symptoms, fatigue, dizziness, headache (between 1 and 5%).

Post-marketing experience with all ACE inhibitors suggests that exposure in utero may be associated with hypotension and decreased renal perfusion in the fetus. ACE inhibitors have also been associated with fetal death in utero. No ACE inhibitor should be used in pregnancy.

For a complete report of Post-marketing Adverse Drug Reactions, please refer to Adverse Drug Reaction Overview for the most serious and important adverse drug reactions and the most frequent adverse drug reactions (incidence ≥1%-<10%).

DRUG INTERACTIONS: Overview: Like for other ACE inhibitors, perindoprilat binding to ACE is characterised by its high affinity but low capacity, leading to a dose dependence of the free fraction.

The influence of the binding to ACE in the terminal phase of the ACE inhibitors is well known. The value of Kd has an influence on the terminal half-life, thus on the estimation of the extrapolated AUC. Since the K_d and bound concentrations have a major impact only in the lower range of concentrations, the binding of perindoprilat to ACE should have a minor impact on steady state in therapeutic conditions.

For perindopril, the dose has no influence on the primary PK parameters and AUC increased proportionally with dose.

Drug-Drug Interactions: See Table 3.

Drug-Food Interactions: The presence of food in the gastrointestinal tract does not affect the rate or extent of perindopril absorption. However, the extent of biotransformation of perindopril to perindoprilat is reduced, resulting in a decrease of perindoprilat bioavailability by 35%. Due to the saturable nature of ACE inhibition, the pharmacodynamic effect, as measured by the area under the plasma ACE inhibition-time curve, is reduced by approximately 15%. Therefore it is recommended that COVERSYL is taken before a meal.

Drug-Herb Interactions: Interactions with herbal products have not been established.

Drug-Laboratory Test Interactions: Interactions with laboratory products/methods have not been established.

Drug-Lifestyle Interactions: Lifestyle interactions have not been established.

Table 3: COVERSYL

Established or Potential Drug-Drug Interactions

Proper Name	Ref	Effect	Clinical Comment
Agents affecting sympathetic activity	CT C	Beta adrenergic blocking drugs add further antihypertensive effect to COVERSYL.	Agents affecting sympathetic activity (e.g. ganglionic blocking agents or adrenergic neuron blocking agents) may be used with caution.
Agents causing renin release	CT C	The antihypertensive effect of COVERSYL is augmented by antihypertensive agents that cause renin release (e.g. diuretics).	
Agents increasing serum potassium	CT	Since COVERSYL decreases aldosterone production, elevation of serum potassium may occur.	Potassium-sparing diuretics such as spironolactone, triamterene or amiloride, or potassium supplements or other drugs capable of increasing serum potassium (indomethacin, heparin, cyclosporine and others) should be given only for documented hypokalemia and with caution and frequent monitoring of serum potassium, since they may lead to a significant increase in serum potassium. Salt substitutes which contain potassium should also be used with caution.
Antihypertensive agents and vasodilators		Concomitant use of these agents may increase the hypotensive effects of perindopril. Concomitant use with nitroglycerin and other nitrates, or other vasodilators, may further reduce blood pressure.	
Antidiabetic agents		Epidemiological studies have suggested that concomitant administration of ACE inhibitors and antidiabetic medicines (insulins, oral hypoglycaemic agents) may cause an increased blood-glucose lowering effect with risk of hypoglycaemia.	This phenomenon appeared to be more likely to occur during the first weeks of combined treatment and in patients with renal impairment.
Concomitant diuretic therapy	C	Patients concomitantly taking ACE inhibitors and diuretics, and especially those in whom diuretic therapy was recently instituted may occasionally experience an excessive reduction of blood pressure after initiation of therapy.	The possibility of hypotensive effects after the first dose of COVERSYL can be minimized by either discontinuing the diuretic or increasing the salt intake prior to initiation of treatment with COVERSYL. If it is not possible to discontinue the diuretic, the starting dose of COVERSYL can be reduced, and the patient should be closely observed for several hours following the initial dose and until blood pressure has stabilized. The rate and extent of perindopril absorption and elimination are not affected by concomitant diuretics. The bioavailability of perindoprilat was reduced by diuretics, however, and this was associated with a decrease in plasma ACE inhibition (see Warnings and Precautions and Dosage and Administration).

(cont'd)

Table 3: COVERSYL *(cont'd)*

Established or Potential Drug-Drug Interactions

Proper Name	Ref	Effect	Clinical Comment
Digoxin	C	A pharmacokinetic study has shown no effect on plasma digoxin concentration when coadministered with COVERSYL but an effect of digoxin on the plasma concentration of perindopril/perindoprilat has not been excluded.	
Gentamicin		Animal data have suggested the possibility of interaction between perindopril and gentamicin. However, this has not been investigated in human studies.	Coadministration of both drugs should proceed with caution.
Lithium	C	Increased serum lithium levels and symptoms of lithium toxicity have been reported in patients receiving concomitant lithium and ACE inhibitor therapy.	These drugs should be coadministered with caution and frequent monitoring of serum lithium levels is recommended. If a diuretic is also used, the risk of lithium toxicity may be further increased.
Non-steroidal anti-inflammatory drugs (NSAIDs) including aspirin ≥3 g/day		The administration of a NSAID may reduce the antihypertensive effect of ACE inhibitors. NSAIDs also exert an additive effect on the increase in serum potassium and may result in a deterioration of renal function.	These effects are usually reversible. Rarely, acute renal failure may occur, especially in patients with compromised renal function such as those who are elderly or dehydrated.
Tricyclic antidepressants/antipsychotic/anesthetics		Concomitant use of certain anesthetics, tricyclic antidepressants and antipsychotics with ACE inhibitors may result in further reduction of blood pressure.	

Legend: C=Case Study; CT=Clinical Trial; T=Theoretical.

DOSAGE AND ADMINISTRATION: Dosing Considerations: Dosage of COVERSYL (perindopril erbumine) must be individualized and adjustment is required in the elderly, and in case of renal impairment.

Recommended Dose and Dosage Adjustment: Hypertension: Initiation of therapy requires consideration of recent antihypertensive drug treatment, the extent of blood pressure elevation and salt restriction. The dosage of other antihypertensive agents being used with COVERSYL may need to be adjusted. The presence of food in the gastrointestinal tract reduces the bioavailability of perindoprilat.

Monotherapy: The recommended initial dose of COVERSYL, in patients not on diuretics, is 4 mg once daily. Dosage should be adjusted according to blood pressure response, generally at intervals of at least 2 weeks. The usual maintenance dose is 4 to 8 mg daily administered in a single daily dose. No additional blood pressure lowering effects were achieved with doses greater than 8 mg daily.

In some patients treated once daily, the antihypertensive effect may diminish towards the end of the dosing interval. This can be evaluated by measuring blood pressure just prior to dosing to determine whether satisfactory control is maintained for 24 hours. If it is not, either twice daily administration with the same total daily dose, or an increase in dose should be considered. If blood pressure is not controlled with COVERSYL alone, a diuretic may be added. After the addition of a diuretic, it may be possible to reduce the dose of COVERSYL.

Concomitant Diuretic Therapy: Symptomatic hypotension occasionally may occur following the initial dose of COVERSYL and is more likely in patients who are currently being treated with a diuretic. The diuretic should, if possible, be discontinued for two or three days before beginning therapy with COVERSYL to reduce the likelihood of hypotension (see Warnings and Precautions). If the diuretic cannot be discontinued, an initial dose of 2 mg COVERSYL should be used with careful medical supervision for several hours and until blood pressure has stabilized. The dosage of COVERSYL should subsequently be titrated to the optimal response.

Congestive Heart Failure: COVERSYL is generally used in conjunction with a diuretic and, where appropriate, a digitalis glycoside in patients with congestive heart failure. Therapy should be initiated under close medical supervision. Blood pressure and renal function should be monitored, both before and during treatment with perindopril because severe hypotension and, more rarely, consequent renal failure have been reported (see Warnings and Precautions).

Initiation of therapy requires consideration of recent diuretic therapy and the possibility of severe salt/volume depletion. If possible, the dose of diuretic should be reduced before beginning treatment. Serum potassium should also be monitored (see Drug Interactions, Drug-Drug Interactions).

The recommended initial dose is 2 mg once daily taken in the morning under close medical supervision. The dose may, in most instances, be increased to 4 mg once daily (once blood pressure acceptability has been demonstrated). The usual effective dose in clinical trials was 4 mg/day administered as a single dose. Dose titration may be performed over a 2- to 4-week period.

Reduction of Cardiovascular Risk in Hypertension or Post-Myocardial Infarction: In patients with hypertension and stable coronary artery disease or in post-myocardial infarction patients with coronary artery disease, COVERSYL (perindopril erbumine) Tablets should be given at an initial dose of 4 mg once daily for 2 weeks, and then increased as tolerated, to a maintenance dose of 8 mg once daily, preferably to be taken early in the morning. In elderly patients (>70 years), COVERSYL Tablets should be given as a 2 mg dose once daily in the first week, followed by 4 mg once daily in the second week and 8 mg once daily for maintenance dose if tolerated.

The Elderly: In the elderly, treatment should begin with a 2 mg dose in the morning. If necessary, after one month of treatment this dose can be increased to 4 mg daily given in one or two divided doses.

Renal Impairment: In case of renal impairment, the dosage of COVERSYL must be adjusted. The following dosages are recommended:

Creatinine Clearance	Recommended Dosage
Between 30 and 60 mL/min	2 mg per day
Between 15 and 30 mL/min	2 mg every other day
<15 mL/min	2 mg on the day of dialysis

In these patients, normal medical follow up includes periodic control of potassium and creatinine.

Missed Dose: If a dose is missed, a double dose should not be taken, but just carry on with the next dose at the normal time.

Administration: It is recommended that COVERSYL is taken once daily in the morning before a meal.

OVERDOSAGE:

Limited data are available regarding overdosage of COVERSYL (perindopril erbumine) in humans. The most likely clinical manifestation would be symptoms attributable to severe hypotension. In the case of overdosage, gastric washout and intravenous infusion of a normal saline solution are recommended.

However, of the two cases reported in the perindopril clinical trials, one (dosage unknown) required ventilation assistance and the other developed hypothermia, circulatory arrest, and subsequently died, following ingestion of up to 180 mg of COVERSYL (perindopril erbumine). Thus, intervention in COVERSYL overdosage may require vigorous support.

COVERSYL can be removed by hemodialysis, with clearances of about 52 mL/min for perindopril and 67 mL/min for perindoprilat, the active metabolite (see Actions and Clinical Pharmacology, Special Populations and Conditions, Renal Insufficiency).

For management of a suspected drug overdose, CPhA recommends that you contact your **regional Poison Control Centre**. See the *CPS* Directory section for a list of Poison Control Centres.

ACTION AND CLINICAL PHARMACOLOGY: Mechanism of Action: COVERSYL (perindopril erbumine) is a nonsulphydryl angiotensin converting enzyme (ACE) inhibitor, which is used in the treatment of hypertension and mild to moderate congestive heart failure.

Following oral administration, COVERSYL is rapidly hydrolysed to perindoprilat, its principal active metabolite.

Angiotensin-converting enzyme catalyses the conversion of angiotensin I to the vasoconstrictor substance, angiotensin II. Angiotensin II also stimulates aldosterone secretion by the adrenal cortex. Inhibition of ACE activity leads to decreased levels of angiotensin II, thereby resulting in decreased vasoconstriction and decreased aldosterone secretion. The latter change may result in a small increase in serum potassium (see Warnings and Precautions, Hyperkalemia and Potassium-Sparing Diuretics, Potassium Supplements or Potassium-Containing Salt Substitutes). Decreased levels of angiotensin II and the accompanying lack of negative feedback on renal renin secretion results in increases in plasma renin activity.

ACE is identical to kininase II. Thus, perindopril erbumine administration may interfere with the degradation of the vasodepressor peptide bradykinin. It is not known whether this effect contributes to the therapeutic activity of COVERSYL.

The mechanism through which COVERSYL lowers blood pressure appears to result primarily from suppression of the renin-angiotensin-aldosterone system.

Pharmacodynamics: In most patients with mild to moderate essential hypertension, administration of 4 to 8 mg daily of COVERSYL results in a reduction of both supine and standing blood pressure with little or no effect on heart rate. Antihypertensive activity commences within one hour with peak effects usually achieved by 4 to 6 hours after dosing. At recommended doses given once daily, antihypertensive effects persist over 24 hours. The blood pressure reductions observed at trough plasma concentration were 75-100% of peak effects. When once and twice daily dosing were compared, the twice daily regimen was slightly superior, but by no more than about 0.5 to 1.0 mmHg. Abrupt withdrawal of COVERSYL has not been associated with a rapid increase in blood pressure. In studies carried out in patients with mild to moderate essential hypertension, the reduction in blood pressure was accompanied by a reduction in peripheral resistance with no change in glomerular filtration rate. When COVERSYL is given together with thiazide-type diuretics, the antihypertensive effects are additive.

In uncontrolled studies in patients with insulin-dependent diabetes, COVERSYL did not appear to affect glycemic control. In long term use in this population, no effect on urinary protein excretion was seen.

Administration of COVERSYL to patients with congestive heart failure reduces cardiac work by a decrease in preload and afterload. Clinical trials have demonstrated that perindopril decreases left and right ventricular filling pressures, reduces total peripheral vascular resistance, increases cardiac output with an improved cardiac index, and increases muscular regional blood flow. The exercise tolerance of these patients is improved and is associated with an improvement of clinical symptomatology. At the recommended doses, the hemodynamic effects are maintained throughout the 24-hour dosing interval in most patients.

In controlled studies versus placebo and other ACE inhibitors, the first administration of 2 mg of COVERSYL in patients with mild-moderate heart failure was not associated with any significant reduction in blood pressure as compared to placebo.

The efficacy of COVERSYL (perindopril erbumine) in reduction of cardiovascular risk in hypertension or post-myocardial infarction was based on one mortality/morbidity study (EUROPA trial).

Pharmacokinetics: Perindopril erbumine is a nonsulphydryl angiotensin converting enzyme (ACE) inhibitor. Following oral administration, perindopril erbumine is rapidly hydrolysed to perindoprilat, its active metabolite. The clearance of perindoprilat and other metabolites is primarily by the renal pathway. See Table 4 and Table 5.

Table 4: COVERSYL

Summary of Perindopril and Perindoprilat Pharmacokinetic Parameters Following Repeated Oral Administrations of Three Doses of Perindopril Erbumine Salt in Healthy Male Volunteers (C_{max}-$T_{½}$-AUC)

		C_{max} (ng/mL)	$T_{½,L}$ (h)	AUC (ng·h/mL)
2 mg of perindopril erbumine	Perindopril	20±4.9	0.41±0.07	23±3.9
	Perindoprilat	4.9±1.2	ND	72±15
4 mg of perindopril erbumine	Perindopril	36±11	0.47±0.13	47±8.0
	Perindoprilat	11.0±3.4	ND	122±27
8 mg of perindopril erbumine	Perindopril	83±27	0.41±0.06	94±16
	Perindoprilat	22±6.5	ND	212±38

Legend: ND: not determined.

Table 5: COVERSYL

Summary of Perindopril and Perindoprilat Pharmacokinetic Parameters: Population Pharmacokinetics Combined Analysis (Clearance, Central Volume and Peripheral Volume)

	Clearance (mL/min)	Central Volume (L)	Peripheral Volume (L)
Perindopril	367	13	7.2
Perindoprilat	167	32	93

Absorption: After oral administration, perindopril erbumine is rapidly absorbed with peak plasma concentrations occurring at about one hour, with a bioavailability of 65 to 70%.

Following absorption, perindopril is converted into perindoprilat, its active metabolite, with a mean bioavailability of about 20%. Peak plasma concentration of perindoprilat is attained within 4 to 7 hours and corresponding peak pharmacodynamic activity occurs at about 6 hours.

The presence of food in the gastrointestinal tract does not affect the rate or extent of perindopril absorption. However, the extent of biotransformation of perindopril to perindoprilat is reduced, resulting in a decrease of perindoprilat bioavailability by 35%. Due to the saturable nature of ACE inhibition, the pharmacodynamic effect, as measured by the area under the plasma ACE inhibition-time curve, is reduced by approximately 15%.

Distribution: Perindoprilat is not extensively bound to plasma proteins, this being only 10 to 20%, but the binding is concentration dependent due to the saturable binding of perindoprilat to the circulating angiotensin-converting enzyme. The volume of distribution is approximately 0.2 L/kg for unbound perindoprilat.

Metabolism: Perindopril is extensively metabolised following oral administration, with only 4 to 12% of the dose recovered unchanged in the urine. Six metabolites have been identified. They include perindoprilat, the active form, and five others that do not possess appreciable therapeutic activity. These are comprised of perindopril glucuronide, perindoprilat glucuronide, a perindopril lactam, and two perindoprilat lactams.

The two main circulating metabolites of perindopril are perindoprilat and perindoprilat glucuronide.

The two pathways identified and quantified for perindoprilat formation are the pre-systemic (first pass effect) and systemic hydrolysis of perindopril. Perindopril is indeed sensitive to a pre-systemic first-past effect, accounting for 62% of the perindoprilat formation. The systemic hydrolysis of perindopril into perindoprilat accounts for the remaining 38% left.

Excretion: The clearance of perindoprilat and other metabolites is primarily by the renal pathway.

The systemic clearance of perindopril (367 mL/min) can be split into 39% leading to perindoprilat formation and 61% to renal excretion or other biotransformations. The terminal plasma half-life of perindopril is very short (1.2 h), thus leading to no accumulation with a once daily oral dosing regimen. The terminal plasma half-life of unbound perindoprilat is 17 hours. The apparent terminal plasma half-life of perindoprilat (total concentrations) is much longer (30-120 hours) due to the very slow dissociation of perindoprilat from ACE binding sites. With on-going administration of perindopril, steady state plasma levels of perindoprilat are obtained in 3-6 days and perindoprilat accumulates 1.5-2.0 folds.

Special Populations and Conditions: Pediatrics: The safety and effectiveness of COVERSYL in children have not been established. Its use in this age group, therefore, is not recommended.

Geriatrics: In a pharmacokinetic study with single dose administration, mean peak plasma concentrations of perindoprilat were significantly higher in elderly healthy volunteers (32.5 ng/mL) than in younger volunteers (13.5 ng/mL) due to both higher bioavailability and reduced renal clearance in this group.

Single and multiple dose pharmacokinetics of perindopril were evaluated in a study of elderly hypertensive patients (72 to 91 years of age), C_{max} and AUC were found to be approximately two-fold higher than in healthy younger subjects. The higher concentrations of perindoprilat observed in these patients were reflected in greater ACE inhibition (see Warnings and Precautions, Geriatrics (>65 years of age) and Dosage and Administration, Recommended Dose and Dosage Adjustment).

Gender: The effectiveness of COVERSYL was not influenced by sex.

Race: The blood pressure lowering effects of angiotensin converting enzyme (ACE) inhibitors generally are lower in black persons than Caucasian patients. The cardiovascular benefits of ACE inhibitors, in terms of risk reduction in coronary artery disease, have not been extensively studied in blacks.

Hepatic Insufficiency: The bioavailability of perindoprilat is increased in patients with impaired hepatic function. Plasma concentrations in patients with hepatic impairment were about 50% higher than those observed in healthy subjects or hypertensive patients with normal liver function.

Renal Insufficiency: In patients with renal insufficiency, perindoprilat AUC increases with decreasing renal function. At creatinine clearances of 30-80 mL/min, AUC is about double that of 100 mL/min. When creatinine clearance drops below 30 mL/min, AUC increases more markedly. Therefore the dosage of COVERSYL should be adjusted in patients with a creatinine clearance below 30 mL/min.

Perindopril, and its active metabolite perindoprilat, are dialysable. In a limited number of patients studied, perindopril hemodialysis clearance ranged from 41.7 to 76.7 mL/min (mean 52.0 mL/min). Perindoprilat hemodialysis clearance ranged from 37.4 to 91.0 mL/min (mean 67.2 mL/min).

Heart Failure: Patients with heart failure have reduced perindoprilat clearance, which may result in a dose interval AUC that is increased up to 40% which should lead to an initial reduction of perindopril dosage.

Genetic Polymorphism: Pharmacokinetics differences due to genetic polymorphism have not been studied.

STORAGE AND STABILITY: Store at room temperature (15-30°C). Protect from elevated humidity.

SPECIAL HANDLING INSTRUCTIONS: No special requirements.

INFORMATION FOR THE PATIENT: Published in e-CPS, available by subscription at www.e-cps.ca.

DOSAGE FORMS, COMPOSITION AND PACKAGING: 2 mg: Each white, round, film-coated, biconvex tablet contains: perindopril erbumine 2 mg. Nonmedicinal ingredients: hydrophobic colloidal silica, lactose monohydrate, magnesium stearate and microcrystalline cellulose. Blister packs of 30. Bottles of 100.

4 mg: Each light green, rod shaped, film-coated tablet, engraved with on one face and scored on both edges contains: perindopril erbumine 4 mg. Nonmedicinal ingredients: chlorophyllin (E141ii) aluminium lake, hydrophobic colloidal silica, lactose monohydrate, magnesium stearate and microcrystalline cellulose. Blister packs of 30. Bottles of 100.

8 mg: Each green, round, film-coated, biconvex tablet, engraved with on one face and on the other contains: perindopril erbumine 8 mg. Nonmedicinal ingredients: chlorophyllin (E141ii) aluminium lake, hydrophobic colloidal silica, lactose monohydrate, magnesium stearate and microcrystalline cellulose. Blister packs of 30. Bottles of 100.

(Shown in Product Identification Section)

Coversyl® Plus LD ℞

perindopril erbumine—indapamide

Angiotensin Converting Enzyme Inhibitor—Diuretic

Servier

Coversyl® Plus ℞

perindopril erbumine—indapamide

Angiotensin Converting Enzyme Inhibitor—Diuretic

Servier

Coversyl® Plus HD ℞

perindopril erbumine—indapamide

Angiotensin Converting Enzyme Inhibitor—Diuretic

Servier

Date of Preparation: October 4, 2002
Date of Revision: April 21, 2010

SUMMARY PRODUCT INFORMATION:

Route of Administration	Dosage Form/ Strength	All Nonmedicinal Ingredients
Oral	Tablet 2 mg/0.625 mg, 4 mg/1.25 mg, 8 mg/2.5 mg	Hydrophobic colloidal silica, lactose monohydrate, magnesium stearate and microcrystalline cellulose

INDICATIONS AND CLINICAL USE: COVERSYL PLUS LD (perindopril erbumine/indapamide) is indicated for the initial treatment of mild to moderate essential hypertension.

COVERSYL PLUS (perindopril erbumine/indapamide) and COVERSYL PLUS HD (perindopril erbumine/indapamide) are indicated in the treatment of mild to moderate essential hypertension in patients for whom combination therapy is appropriate.

COVERSYL PLUS and COVERSYL PLUS HD are not indicated for initial therapy. Patients in whom perindopril and indapamide are initiated simultaneously can develop symptomatic hypotension (see Drug Interactions, Drug-Drug Interactions, Concomitant ACE Inhibitor and Diuretic Therapy).

Patients should be titrated on the individual drugs. If the fixed combination represents the dosage determined by this titration, the use of COVERSYL PLUS or COVERSYL PLUS HD may prove to be more convenient in the management of patients. If during maintenance therapy dosage adjustment is necessary, it is advisable to use individual drugs.

The safety and efficacy of COVERSYL PLUS LD/COVERSYL PLUS/COVERSYL PLUS HD in renovascular hypertension and in congestive heart failure have not been established and therefore, their use in this condition is not recommended.

General: In using COVERSYL PLUS LD/COVERSYL PLUS/COVERSYL PLUS HD, consideration should be given to the risk of angioedema (see Warnings and Precautions).

Geriatrics (>65 years of age): Although the blood pressure response and safety profile of COVERSYL PLUS LD/COVERSYL PLUS/COVERSYL PLUS HD in patients over 65 years old were comparable to those of the younger adult patients, greater sensitivity of some elderly patients cannot be ruled out.

Pediatrics: The safety and effectiveness of COVERSYL PLUS LD/COVERSYL PLUS/COVERSYL PLUS HD in children have not been established. Its use in this age group, therefore, is not recommended.

CONTRAINDICATIONS: COVERSYL PLUS HD (perindopril erbumine/indapamide) is contraindicated in moderate renal impairment (creatinine clearance 30-60 mL/min).

COVERSYL PLUS LD/COVERSYL PLUS/COVERSYL PLUS HD (perindopril erbumine/indapamide) are contraindicated:
- in patients with a history of hypersensitivity to any component of these products, and to other sulfonamide derivatives,
- in patients with hereditary/idiopathic angioedema or a history of angioedema related to previous treatment with an angiotensin converting enzyme inhibitor,
- during the second and third trimesters of pregnancy,
- during breast-feeding,
- severe renal impairment (creatinine clearance <30 mL/min),
- hypokalemia,
- severe hepatic impairment,
- hepatic encephalopathy,
- in combination with non-antiarrhythmic agents causing torsade de pointes (see Drug Interactions, Drug-Drug Interactions).

WARNINGS AND PRECAUTIONS:

Serious Warnings and Precautions
When used in pregnancy, angiotensin converting enzyme (ACE) inhibitors can cause injury or even death of the developing fetus. When pregnancy is detected, COVERSYL PLUS LD/COVERSYL PLUS/COVERSYL PLUS HD should be discontinued as soon as possible.

General: Head and Neck Angioedema: Life-threatening angioedema has been reported with ACE inhibitors. The overall incidence is approximately 0.1-0.2%. The aetiology is thought to be non-immunogenic and may be related to accentuated bradykinin activity. Usually, the angioedema is non-pitting edema of the skin mucuous membrane and subcutaneous tissue.

Angioedema involving the face, extremities, lips, tongue, glottis and/or larynx has been reported in patients treated with ACE inhibitors, including perindopril. Angioedema associated with laryngeal involvement may be fatal. If laryngeal stridor or angioedema of the face, tongue, or glottis occurs, COVERSYL PLUS LD/COVERSYL PLUS/COVERSYL PLUS HD should be discontinued immediately, the patient treated appropriately in accordance with accepted medical care, and carefully observed until the swelling disappears. In instances where swelling is confined to the face and lips, the condition generally resolves without treatment, although antihistamines may be useful in relieving symptoms.

Where there is involvement of the tongue, glottis or larynx, angioedema may be fatal due to airway obstruction, appropriate therapy (including but not limited to 0.3 to 0.5 mL of subcutaneous epinephrine solution 1:1000 and oxygen) should be administered promptly (see Adverse Reactions).

Treatment of progressive angioedema should be aggressive. Failing a rapid response to medical therapy, mechanical methods to secure an airway should be undertaken before massive oedema complicates oral or nasal intubation.

Patients who respond to medical treatment should be observed carefully for a possible rebound phenomenon.

The onset of angioedema associated with use of ACE inhibitors may be delayed for weeks or months.

Patients may have multiple episodes of angioedema with long symptom-free intervals.

Angioedema may occur with or without urticaria.

The incidence of angioedema during ACE inhibitor therapy has been reported to be higher in black than in non-black patients.

There are reports that switching a patient to another ACE inhibitor could be followed by a recurrence of angioedema. Because of the potential severity of this rare event, another ACE inhibitor should not be used in patients with a history of angioedema (see Contraindications).

Patients with a history of angioedema unrelated to ACE inhibitor therapy may be at increased risk of angioedema while receiving an ACE inhibitor (see Contraindications).

Intestinal Angioedema: Intestinal angioedema has been reported in patients treated with ACE inhibitors. These patients presented with abdominal pain (with or without nausea or vomiting); in some cases there was no prior history of facial angioedema and C-1 esterase levels were normal.

Angioedema was diagnosed by procedures including abdominal CT scan or ultrasound, or at surgery, and symptoms resolved after stopping the ACE inhibitor. Intestinal angioedema should be included in the differential diagnosis of patients on ACE inhibitors presenting with abdominal pain.

Cardiovascular: Hypotension: Perindopril can cause symptomatic hypotension. Perindopril has been associated with hypotension in 0.3% of uncomplicated hypertensive patients in U.S. placebo-controlled trials. Symptoms related to orthostatic hypotension were reported in another 0.8% of patients. It is more likely to occur after the first or second dose or when the dose was increased and in patients who are volume depleted by diuretic therapy, dietary salt restriction, dialysis, diarrhoea, vomiting or with impaired renal function. Volume and/or salt depletion should be corrected before initiation of therapy with perindopril (see Dosage and Administration). In patients with ischemic heart or cerebrovascular disease and/or severe congestive heart failure, with or without associated renal insufficiency, ACE inhibitors may cause an excessive fall in blood pressure which could result in syncope, myocardial infarction, neurological deficits, oliguria and/or progressive azotemia and, rarely, in acute renal failure and/or death (see Adverse Reactions).

Because of the potential fall in blood pressure in these patients therapy with COVERSYL PLUS LD/COVERSYL PLUS/COVERSYL PLUS HD should be started under very close medical supervision. Such patients should be followed closely for the first two weeks of treatment.

If hypotension occurs, the patient should be placed in a supine position and, if necessary, receive an intravenous infusion of 0.9% sodium chloride. A transient hypotensive response is not a contraindication to further doses which usually can be given without difficulty once the blood pressure has increased after volume expansion. If hypotension recurs, treatment with COVERSYL PLUS LD/COVERSYL PLUS/COVERSYL PLUS HD should be discontinued.

Aortic Stenosis/Hyperthrophic Cardiomyopathy: As with other ACE inhibitors, COVERSYL PLUS LD/COVERSYL PLUS/COVERSYL PLUS HD should be given with caution to patients with mitral valve stenosis and obstruction in the outflow of the left ventricle such as aortic stenosis or hypertrophic cardiomyopathy. There is concern on theoretical grounds that patients with aortic stenosis might be at particular risk of decreased coronary perfusion when treated with vasodilators including ACE inhibitors because they do not develop as much afterload reduction. Vasodilators may tend to drop diastolic pressure, and hence coronary pressure, without producing the concomitant reduction in myocardial oxygen demand that normally accompanies vasodilation.

Hematologic: Neutropenia/Agranulocytosis/Thrombocytopenia/Anaemia: Neutropenia/agranulocytosis, thrombocytopenia and anaemia have been reported in patients receiving ACE inhibitors. In patients with normal renal function and no other complicating factors, neutropenia occurs rarely. Perindopril should be used with extreme caution in patients with collagen vascular disease such as systemic lupus erythematosus or scleroderma, and those on multiple drug therapy with agents known to be nephrotoxic or myelosuppressive (immunosuppressant therapy, treatment with allopurinol or procainamide), or a combination of these complicating factors, especially if there is pre-existing impaired renal function. Some of these patients developed serious infections, which in a few instances did not respond to intensive antibiotic therapy. If perindopril is used in such patients, periodic monitoring of white blood cell counts is advised and patients should be instructed to report any sign of infection.

Hepatic/Biliary/Pancreatic: Hepatic Failure: Rarely, ACE inhibitors have been associated with a syndrome that starts with cholestatic jaundice and progresses to fulminant hepatic necrosis and (sometimes) death. The mechanism of this syndrome is not understood. Patients receiving ACE inhibitors who develop jaundice or marked elevations of hepatic enzymes should discontinue the ACE inhibitor and receive appropriate medical follow-up.

Impaired Liver Function: Hepatitis (hepatocellular and/or cholestatic), elevations of liver enzymes and/or serum bilirubin have occurred during therapy with ACE inhibitors, in patients with or without pre-existing liver abnormalities. In most cases, the changes were reversed upon discontinuation of the drug.

Elevations of liver enzymes and/or serum bilirubin have been reported with perindopril (see Adverse Reactions). Should the patient receiving COVERSYL PLUS LD/COVERSYL PLUS/COVERSYL PLUS HD experience any unexplained symptoms, particularly during the first weeks or months of treatment, it is recommended that a full set of liver function tests and any other necessary investigation be carried out. Discontinuation of COVERSYL PLUS LD/COVERSYL PLUS/COVERSYL PLUS HD should be considered when appropriate.

COVERSYL PLUS LD/COVERSYL PLUS/COVERSYL PLUS HD should be used with particular caution in patients with pre-existing liver abnormalities. In such patients, baseline liver function tests should be obtained before administration of the drug and close monitoring of response and metabolic effects should apply.

COVERSYL PLUS LD/COVERSYL PLUS/COVERSYL PLUS HD are contraindicated in patients with severe hepatic impairment since diuretics may induce metabolic alkalosis in cases of potassium depletion which may precipitate episodes of hepatic encephalopathy (see Contraindications).

Immune: Anaphylactoid Reactions during Membrane Exposure (hemodialysis patients): Anaphylactoid reactions have been reported in patients dialyzed with high-flux membranes (e.g. polyacrylonitrile [PAN]) and treated concomitantly with an ACE inhibitor. Dialysis should be stopped immediately if symptoms such as nausea, abdominal cramps, burning, angioedema, shortness of breath and severe hypotension occur. Symptoms are not relieved by antihistamines. In these patients, consideration should be given to using a different type of dialysis membrane or a different class of antihypertensive agent.

Anaphylactoid Reactions during LDL Apheresis: Rarely, patients receiving ACE inhibitors during low density lipoprotein apheresis with dextran sulphate absorption have experienced life-threatening anaphylactoid reactions. These reactions were avoided by temporarily withholding the ACE inhibitor therapy prior to each apheresis.

Anaphylactoid Reactions during Desensitization: There have been isolated reports of patients experiencing sustained, life-threatening anaphylactoid reactions while receiving ACE inhibitors during desensitization treatment with hymenoptera (bees, wasps) venom. In the same patients, these reactions have been avoided when ACE inhibitors were temporarily withheld for at least 24 hours, but they reappeared upon inadvertent rechallenge.

Metabolism: Calcium excretion is decreased by diuretics pharmacologically related to indapamide. After six to eight weeks of indapamide 1.25 mg treatment and in long-term studies of hypertensive patients with higher doses of indapamide, however, serum concentrations of calcium increased only slightly with indapamide. Prolonged treatment with drugs pharmacologically related to indapamide may in rare instances be associated with hypercalcemia and hypophosphatemia secondary to physiologic changes in the parathyroid gland; however, the common complications of hyperparathyroidism, such as renal lithiasis, bone resorption, and peptic ulcer, have not been seen. Treatment should be discontinued before tests for parathyroid function are performed. Like the thiazides, indapamide may decrease serum PBI levels without signs of thyroid disturbance.

The antihypertensive effect of the drug may be enhanced in the patient postsympathectomy.

Other Metabolic Parameters: Blood urea nitrogen, uric acid, and glucose levels should also be assessed during therapy.

Hyperuricemia may occur during administration of indapamide. Rarely gout has been reported. Blood uric acid levels should be monitored, particularly in patients with a history of gout who should continue to receive appropriate treatment.

Due to the presence of lactose, patients with hereditary problems of galactose intolerance, glucose-galactose malabsorption or the Lapp lactose deficiency should not take this medicinal product.

Peri-Operative Considerations: ACE inhibitors may augment the hypotensive effects of anaesthetics and analgesics. In patients undergoing major surgery or during anaesthesia with agents that produce hypotension, perindopril may block the angiotensin II formation that could otherwise occur secondary to compensatory renin release. If hypotension occurs and is considered to be due to this mechanism, it can be corrected by volume expansion.

Renal: Impaired Renal Function: As a consequence of inhibiting the renin-angiotensin-aldosterone system, changes in renal function may be anticipated in susceptible individuals.

Use of COVERSYL PLUS LD/COVERSYL PLUS/COVERSYL PLUS HD should include appropriate assessment of renal function.

In patients with severe renal impairment (creatinine clearance <30 mL/min), all dosages are contraindicated (see Contraindications).

In patients with moderate renal impairment (creatinine clearance 30-60 mL/min), COVERSYL PLUS HD is contraindicated (see Contraindications), and the initial dosage of COVERSYL PLUS LD/COVERSYL PLUS should be adjusted according to the patient's creatinine clearance and then as a function of the patient's response to treatment. Routine monitoring of potassium and creatinine are part of normal medical practice for these patients.

In patients whose renal function may depend on the activity of the renin-angiotensin-aldosterone system, such as patients with bilateral renal artery stenosis, unilateral renal artery stenosis to a solitary kidney, or severe congestive heart failure, treatment with agents that inhibit this system has been associated with oliguria, progressive azotemia, and rarely, acute renal failure and/or death. In susceptible patients, concomitant diuretic use may further increase risk.

Hypertensive Patients with Renal Artery Stenosis: In clinical trials in hypertensive patients with unilateral or bilateral renal artery stenosis, increases in blood urea nitrogen and serum creatinine were observed in 20% of patients. Experience with ACE inhibitors suggests that these increases are usually reversible upon discontinuation of the drug. In such patients, renal function should be monitored during the first few weeks of therapy. ACE inhibitors should be avoided in patients with known or suspected renal artery stenosis. When an ACE inhibitor is given to a patient with stenosis of the renal artery supplying a solitary kidney, or bilateral artery stenosis, acute renal insufficiency may occur. ACE inhibition may also cause a decrease in renal function in patients with stenosis of the artery supplying a transplanted kidney. It is believed that renal artery stenosis reduces the pressure in the afferent glomerular arteriole, and transglomerular hydrostatic pressure is then maintained by angiotensin II–induced constriction of the efferent arteriole. When an ACE inhibitor is given, the efferent arteriole relaxes, glomerular filtration falls, and renal failure may result. The thrombotic occlusion of a stenosed renal artery can be precipitated by ACE inhibitors.

Some hypertensive patients without apparent pre-existing renal vascular disease have developed increases in blood urea nitrogen and serum creatinine, usually minor and transient. These increases are more likely to occur in patients treated concomitantly with a diuretic and in patients with pre-existing renal impairment. Reduction of dosages of perindopril, the diuretic or both may be required. In some cases, discontinuation of either or both drugs may be necessary. Evaluation of hypertensive patients should always include an assessment of renal function (see Dosage and Administration). If deterioration in renal function has occurred after treatment with one ACE inhibitor, then it is likely to be precipitated by another and in these patients usage of another class of antihypertensive agent would be preferable. Patients with unilateral renal artery disease present a special problem as deterioration of function may not be apparent from measurement of blood urea and serum creatinine.

Proteinuria: Some ACE inhibitors have been associated with the occurrence (up to 0.7%) of proteinuria (<1 gram/24 hours) and/or decline in renal function in patients with one or more of the following characteristics: old age, pre-existing renal disease, concomitant treatment with potassium-sparing diuretics or high doses of other diuretics, limited cardiac reserve, or treatment with a non-steroidal anti-inflammatory drug.

Perindoprilat, the active form of perindopril, is dialysable with a clearance of 70 mL/min.

Fluid and Electrolyte Imbalance: Electrolyte changes observed with indapamide may be severe. The recommended maximum daily dose of 2.5 mg/day should not be exceeded.

Hypokalemia may occur with consequent weakness, cramps and cardiac dysrhythmias. Hypokalemia is a particular hazard in digitalized patients; dangerous or fatal cardiac arrhythmias may be precipitated. Hypokalemia occurs commonly with diuretics; electrolyte monitoring is essential particularly in patients who would be at increased risk from hypokalemia, such as patients with cardiac arrhythmias or those who are receiving concomitant cardiac glycosides.

Patients with renal insufficiency receiving COVERSYL PLUS LD/COVERSYL PLUS/COVERSYL PLUS HD should be carefully monitored. If increased azotemia and oliguria occur during treatment, COVERSYL PLUS LD/COVERSYL PLUS/COVERSYL PLUS HD should be discontinued.

Patients receiving indapamide should be carefully observed for signs and symptoms of electrolyte imbalance, namely hypokalemia, hyponatremia and hypochloremia, and their serum electrolytes should be closely monitored. Hypokalemia will be more common in association with concomitant steroid or ACTH therapy and with inadequate electrolyte intake. The serum potassium should be determined at regular intervals and potassium supplementation instituted when indicated.

The signs of electrolyte imbalance are: dryness of the mouth, thirst, weakness, lethargy, drowsiness, restlessness, muscle pains or cramps, muscle fatigue, hypotension, oliguria, gastrointestinal disturbances such as nausea and vomiting, tachycardia and ECG changes.

Potassium Balance: Hypokalemia: In clinical trials with the perindopril/indapamide combination, hypokalemia (serum potassium <3.4 mmol/L) occurred in an apparent dose-related fashion. Potassium supplementation should be given.

Hyperkalemia: In clinical trials with perindopril/indapamide combination, hyperkalemia (serum potassium >5.5 mmol/L) occurred in approximately 1% of hypertensive patients. In most cases, these were isolated values which resolved despite continued therapy. Risk factors for development of hyperkalemia may include renal insufficiency, diabetes mellitus, and the concomitant use of potassium-sparing diuretics, potassium supplements, potassium—containing salt substitutes or other drugs associated with increases in serum potassium (e.g. heparin) (see Drug Interactions, Drug-Drug Interactions).

Respiratory: Cough: A dry persistent irritating cough, which usually disappears only after withdrawal or lowering of the dose of perindopril has been reported. Such possibility should be considered as part of the differential diagnosis of the cough.

The cough is often worse when lying down or at night, and has been reported more frequently in women (who account for 2/3 of the reported cases). Patients who cough may have increased bronchial reactivity compared with those who do not. The observed higher frequency of this side-effect in non-smokers may be due to a higher level of tolerance of smokers to cough.

The cough is most likely due to stimulation of the pulmonary cough reflex by kinins (bradykinin) and/or prostaglandins, which accumulate because of ACE inhibition. Once a patient has developed intolerable cough, an attempt may be made to switch the patient to another ACE inhibitor; the reaction may recur but this is not invariably the case. A change to another class of drugs may be required in severe cases.

Skin: Dermatological Reactions: Dermatological reactions characterised by maculo-papular pruritic rashes and sometimes photosensitivity have been reported with ACE inhibitors. Rare and sometimes severe skin reactions (lichenoid eruptions, psoriasis, pemphigus like rash, rosacea, Stevens-Johnson syndrome, etc) have occurred.

Patients who develop a cutaneous reaction with one ACE inhibitor might not when switched to another drug of the same class, but there are reports of cross-reactivity.

Severe dermatological adverse reactions, some accompanied by systemic manifestations, have been rarely reported with the use of indapamide. In the majority of cases, the condition subsided within 14 days following discontinuation of indapamide therapy (see Adverse Reactions).

Lupus Erythematosus: Sulfonamide derivatives have been reported to exacerbate or activate systemic lupus erythematosus. These possibilities should be kept in mind with the use of indapamide although no case has been reported to date.

Taste Disturbances (dysgeusia): Taste disturbances were reported to be common (prevalence up to 12.5%) with high doses of an ACE inhibitor.

Taste disturbance with ACE inhibitors have been described as suppression of taste or a metallic sensation in the mouth. Any dysgeusia usually occurs in the first weeks of treatment and may disappear in most cases within 1-3 months.

Special Populations: Pregnant Women: The use of ACE inhibitors is not recommended during the first trimester of pregnancy. The use of ACE inhibitors is contraindicated during the second and third trimesters of pregnancy (see Contraindications).

ACE inhibitors can cause fetal and neonatal morbidity and mortality when administered to pregnant women. When pregnancy is detected, COVERSYL PLUS LD/COVERSYL PLUS/COVERSYL PLUS HD should be discontinued as soon as possible.

The use of ACE inhibitors during the second and third trimesters of pregnancy has been associated with fetal and neonatal injury including hypotension, neonatal skull hypoplasia, anuria, reversible or irreversible renal failure, and death.

Oligohydramnios has also been reported, presumably resulting from decreased fetal renal function, associated with fetal limb contractures, craniofacial deformation, and hypoplastic lung development.

Prematurity and patent ductus arteriosus and other structural cardiac malformations, as well as neurologic malformations, have also been reported following exposure in the first trimester of pregnancy.

Infants with a history of in utero exposure to ACE inhibitors should be closely observed for hypotension, oliguria, and hyperkalemia. If oliguria occurs, attention should be directed toward support of blood pressure and renal perfusion. Exchange transfusion or dialysis may be required as a means of reversing hypotension and/or substituting for impaired renal function; however, limited experience with those procedures has not been associated with significant clinical benefit. Perindoprilat, the active form of perindopril, can be removed from the body by hemodialysis (see Action and Clinical Pharmacology, Special Populations and Conditions, Renal Insufficiency).

Nursing Women: The presence of concentrations of ACE inhibitor have been reported in human milk. Use of COVERSYL PLUS LD/COVERSYL PLUS/COVERSYL PLUS HD is contraindicated during breast-feeding (see Contraindications).

Diabetic Patients: In diabetic patients treated with oral antidiabetic agents or insulin, glycemic control should be closely monitored during the first month of treatment with an ACE inhibitor.

Pediatrics: The safety and effectiveness of COVERSYL PLUS LD/COVERSYL PLUS/COVERSYL PLUS HD in children have not been established. Its use in this age group, therefore, is not recommended.

Geriatrics (>65 years of age): Although the blood pressure response and safety profile of COVERSYL PLUS LD/COVERSYL PLUS/COVERSYL PLUS HD in patients over 65 years old were comparable to those of the younger adult patients, greater sensitivity of some elderly patients cannot be ruled out.

Monitoring and Laboratory Tests: Not applicable.

ADVERSE REACTIONS: Adverse Drug Reaction Overview: COVERSYL PLUS LD has been evaluated for safety in 1974 patients, (of which 1898 participated in controlled clinical trials). Long-term safety was assessed in 745 patients, of which 659 were treated for three months, 597 for six months and 385 for one year or longer.

COVERSYL PLUS has been evaluated for safety in 1029 patients in controlled clinical trials. Long-term safety was assessed in 492 patients, of which 444 were treated for three months, 420 for six months and 245 for one year or longer.

COVERSYL PLUS HD has been evaluated for safety in 199 patients in controlled clinical trials. Long-term safety was assessed in 137 patients in two 52-week trials for a mean duration of exposure of 6 ½ months.

Clinical Trial Adverse Drug Reactions: Because clinical trials are conducted under very specific conditions the adverse reaction rates observed in the clinical trials may not reflect the rates observed in practice and should not be compared to the rates in the clinical trials of another drug. Adverse drug reaction information from clinical trials is useful for identifying drug-related adverse events and for approximating rates.

In controlled trials, the overall incidence of adverse events reported with COVERSYL PLUS LD/COVERSYL PLUS was comparable to placebo. The overall incidence of adverse events reported with COVERSYL PLUS HD were comparable to COVERSYL PLUS. Adverse events have generally been mild and transient and have not required discontinuation of therapy.

The most frequent clinical adverse drug reactions reported in patients treated with COVERSYL PLUS LD were: cough (3.7%), headache (1.8%), asthenia (1.3%), dizziness (0.9%) and nausea/vomiting (0.8%).

The most frequent clinical adverse drug reactions reported in patients treated with COVERSYL PLUS were: cough (3.0%), headache (2.1%), asthenia (1.6%), nausea/vomiting (1.5%) and dizziness (1.2%).

The most frequent clinical adverse drug reactions reported in patients treated with COVERSYL PLUS HD in the two long-term trials (137 patients) were: cough (3.9%) and headache (1.7%).

The most serious adverse drug reactions were isolated cases of: worsening of heart failure due to atrial fibrillation, hyperglycaemia with renal failure, loss of consciousness, renal colic and transient cerebral ischemia.

Discontinuation of therapy due to adverse drug reactions was required in 2.3% of patients treated with COVERSYL PLUS LD and in 2.5% of patients treated with COVERSYL PLUS, versus 1.5% of patients treated with placebo, mainly because of cough, headache and nausea/vomiting, in 0.5%, 0.4%, and 0.4% respectively under COVERSYL PLUS LD and in 0.6%, 0.5% and 0.4% of patients treated with COVERSYL PLUS.

Adverse events that have been reported in at least 1.0% of hypertensive patients treated with one tablet daily of COVERSYL PLUS LD or COVERSYL PLUS in short-term controlled trials are listed by body system in Table 1. Their occurrence was always low and they correspond to those which have been previously reported with perindopril and indapamide when used separately for the treatment of hypertension.

Table 1: COVERSYL PLUS LD/COVERSYL PLUS

Drug-related Adverse Experience Reported in ≥1% of Patients (%)

Adverse Drug Reaction	COVERSYL PLUS LD (n=789) %	COVERSYL PLUS (n=1029) %	Placebo (n=717) %
Body as a Whole			
Asthenia	1.0	1.9	2.0
Gastrointestinal			
Dyspepsia	0.5	1.1	0.6
Nausea, vomiting	0.1	1.5	0.4
Musculoskeletal			
Joint pain	1.1	0.4	0.6
Nervous			
Headache	2.5	3.7	5.7
Dizziness	1.3	1.6	0.6
Respiratory			
Cough	5.4	3.4	2.1
Rhinopharyngitis	1.8	0.1	1.5
Upper respiratory influenzal infection	0.9	1.5	1.4
Bronchitis	1.0	0.7	0.7

Adverse events that have been reported in at least 1.0% of hypertensive patients treated with COVERSYL PLUS HD correspond to those which have been previously reported with COVERSYL PLUS and with perindopril and indapamide when used separately for the treatment of hypertension.

In a long-term study including 492 patients (444 were treated for three months, 420 for six months and 245 for one year or longer), the nature and frequency of adverse events were similar to those listed in Table 1.

The safety profile of COVERSYL PLUS LD in patients over 65 years old was comparable to that in the younger adult patients; this was demonstrated in a specific 3-month placebo-controlled study involving 193 patients treated with COVERSYL PLUS LD,and in a sub-population analysis on 618 elderly patients who received COVERSYL PLUS LD in all short-term studies combined, and confirmed in a one-year follow-up study on 253 elderly patients (215 were treated for three months, 177 for six months and 140 for one year or longer).

The safety profile of COVERSYL PLUS in patients over 65 years old was comparable to that in the younger adult patients; this was demonstrated in a sub-population analysis on 197 elderly patients who received COVERSYL PLUS in all short term studies combined, and in a sub-population analysis on 87 elderly patients who received COVERSYL PLUS in a one year study.

The safety profile of COVERSYL PLUS HD in patients over 65 years old was comparable to that in the younger adult patients; this was demonstrated in a sub-population analysis in the elderly patients who received COVERSYL PLUS HD in the short-term and the two long-term studies.

Less Common Clinical Trial Adverse Drug Reactions (<1%): Adverse events that have been reported in less than 1.0% of patients treated with COVERSYL PLUS LD/COVERSYL PLUS/COVERSYL PLUS HD in controlled clinical trials include the following:

Body as a Whole: bloating, chest pain, oedema, epistaxis, malaise, pallor and flushing, poisoning, pyrexia, tetany, weight loss.

Cardiovascular: abnormal ECG, angina pectoris, heart rate and rhythm disorders, hypertension, orthostatic hypotension, palpitations, Raynaud's syndrome, syncope and collapse, tachycardia; venous insufficiency.

Dermatological: contact dermatitis, dermatomycosis, eczema, herpes zoster, local infection of skin/subcutaneous tissues, pruritus, rash.

Ear/Nose/Throat: coryza, impacted cerumen, otitis media, laryngitis, pharyngitis, rhinitis, sinusitis, tonsillitis, tinnitus, tracheitis, upper respiratory tract infections.

Gastrointestinal: abdominal pain, colitis, constipation, diarrhoea, esophageal reflux, esophagitis, functional digestive disorders, gastritis, gastroduodenitis, infective and non-infective gastroenteritis, intestinal infection, nausea, periapical abscess, salivary secretion disturbance, vomiting.

Genitourinary: dysuria, enuresis, female genital neoplasm, penis disorders, polyuria, prostate hyperplasia, urinary frequency, urinary tract infection, cystitis, ureamia.

Hematological: blood creatinine increased.

Metabolic and Nutritional: gout, liver and biliary system disorders.

Musculoskeletal: backache, cervicalgia, cervicobrachial syndrome, enthesopathy of elbow region, injury, pain in limb, symptoms referable to limbs, lumbago, muscle/ligament/fascia disorders, localized osteoarthrosis, periarthritis/fibrositis of shoulder, sciatica, sprains of ankle/knee/leg.

Neurologic: anxiety, depression, drowsiness, fall, migraine, nervousness, sleep disturbance, somnolence, peripheral vertigo, smell and taste disturbances, skin sensation disturbances.

Ophthalmologic: conjunctivitis, visual disturbances.

Respiratory: allergic rhinitis, asthma, pharynx diseases, respiratory insufficiency.

Sexual Function: frigidity, impotence.

Abnormal Hematologic and Clinical Chemistry Findings: Serum Electrolytes: The administration of perindopril inhibits the renin-angiotensin-aldosterone axis and tends to reduce the potassium loss caused by indapamide.

During 12-week studies, 1.8% of patients treated with one tablet daily of COVERSYL PLUS LD and 3.9% of patients treated with one tablet daily of COVERSYL PLUS had at least one potassium level below 3.4 mmol/L (versus 0.3% in placebo-treated patients). These percentages were statistically significantly lower than in patients treated with indapamide alone at the usual therapeutic dose of 1.25 mg. The mean reduction of potassium level with one tablet of COVERSYL PLUS LD was 0.10 mmol/L and 0.20 mmol/L with one tablet of COVERSYL PLUS (versus 0.03 mmol/L under placebo).

During the 52-week studies, the maximum mean reduction of potassium level with COVERSYL PLUS HD was of 0.16 mmol/L (versus 0.11 mmol/L under COVERSYL PLUS and versus 0.07 mmol/L with COVERSYL PLUS LD).

The incidence of potassium levels below 3.4 mmol/L during long-term treatment was not significantly different from that observed during short-term studies and the probability to have potassium levels below this limit did not depend on the extent of exposure.

Of the 137 patients treated with COVERSYL PLUS HD in two 52-week trials, 9 (6.6%) presented with an emergent hypokalemia (see Warnings and Precautions).

Increases in potassium levels above 5.5 mmol/L occurred in 0.8% of patients treated with one tablet daily of COVERSYL PLUS LD and 1.0% of patients treated with one tablet daily of COVERSYL PLUS (versus 0.7% under placebo) (see Warnings and Precautions).

Similar percentages of potassium levels variations were observed in elderly patients.

Blood Urea/Serum Creatinine Levels: Elevations of blood urea (>10 mmol/L) or serum creatinine (>160 µmol/L) have been observed in 3.5% and 0.5% of patients treated with one tablet daily of COVERSYL PLUS LD and in 2.3% and 0.3% of patients treated with one tablet daily of COVERSYL PLUS (versus 1.5% and 0.14% under placebo), respectively. The mean increases in blood urea levels and serum creatinine levels were 0.4 mmol/L and 1.1 µmol/L in patients treated with one tablet of COVERSYL PLUS LD, 0.5 mmol/L and 2.1 µmol/L in patients treated with one tablet daily of COVERSYL PLUS (versus 0.1 mmol/L and 0.9 µmol/L under placebo), respectively. The serum creatinine level was stable in patients with mild to moderate renal failure after 12 weeks of treatment.

Mean increases in blood urea levels and serum creatinine have been observed in patients treated with COVERSYL PLUS HD, larger than the increases seen under COVERSYL PLUS.

Blood Uric Acid: Increases of uric acid level (>600 µmol/L) have been observed in 0.7% of patients treated with one tablet daily of COVERSYL PLUS LD and in 0.5% of patients treated with one tablet daily of COVERSYL PLUS (versus 0.1% under placebo). Uric acid level remained stable during the long-term studies including patients treated for up to one year.

As under COVERSYL PLUS, increases of uric acid level have been observed in patients treated with COVERSYL PLUS HD.

Calcium: Calcium excretion is decreased by diuretics pharmacologically related to indapamide (see Warnings and Precautions). Serum concentrations of calcium increased only slightly with indapamide.

Hematology: Minor decreases in haemoglobin (mean decrease of approximately 1 g/L) occurred in hypertensive patients treated with COVERSYL PLUS LD or COVERSYL PLUS (versus 0.1 g/L under placebo), but were rarely of clinical importance. In clinical trials, hematocrit was unaffected by treatment and no patients discontinued therapy due to anemia.

Minor changes in haemoglobin occurred in hypertensive patients treated with COVERSYL PLUS HD, but were not of clinical relevance.

In clinical trials, haematocrit was mostly unaffected by treatment.

Liver Function: Rarely, elevations of liver enzymes have been reported (see Warnings and Precautions).

Post-Market Adverse Drug Reactions: Among the less common suspected adverse reactions reported, the following have been published in the medical literature and/or are potentially serious: anemia, agranulocytosis, neutropenia, thrombocytopenia; fever, confusion; cataract, acute myopia, optic neuritis; ventricular arrhythmia, torsade de pointes, stroke, orthostatic hypotension, myocardial infarction; eosinophilic pneumonia; hepatitis; pancreatitis; Stevens-Johnson syndrome, bullous eruption, photosensitivity, erythroderma, purpura, epidermal necrolysis, erythema multiforme, angioedema, vasculitis, hypersensitivity; interstitial nephritis, renal failure; metabolic alkalosis, dehydration, hypokalemia, hyponatremia, hyperosmolar coma, lithium toxicity, rhabdomyolysis.

DRUG INTERACTIONS: Overview: The combined use of perindopril and indapamide in COVERSYL PLUS LD, COVERSYL PLUS or COVERSYL PLUS HD does not expose to any additional interactions with concomitant drugs other than those known for each of these components.

Drug-Drug Interactions: See Table 2.

Table 2: COVERSYL PLUS LD/COVERSYL PLUS/COVERSYL PLUS HD

Established or Potential Concomitant Drug-Drug Interactions

Proper name	Ref	Effect	Clinical Comment
Agents affecting sympathetic activity	CT C	Beta adrenergic blocking drugs add further antihypertensive effect to perindopril.	Agents affecting sympathetic activity (e.g. ganglionic blocking agents or adrenergic neuron blocking agents) may be used with caution. Beta adrenergic blocking drugs add further antihypertensive effect to perindopril/indapamide.
Agents causing renin release	CT C	The antihypertensive effect of perindopril is augmented by antihypertensive agents that cause renin release (e.g. diuretics).	
Agents increasing serum potassium	CT	Since perindopril decreases aldosterone production, elevation of serum potassium may occur.	Potassium-sparing diuretics such as spironolactone, triamterene or amiloride, or potassium supplements should be given only for documented hypokalemia and with caution and frequent monitoring of serum potassium, since they may lead to a significant increase in serum potassium. Salt substitutes which contain potassium should also be used with caution.
Alcohol, barbiturates, narcotics		In the presence of indapamide, potentiation of orthostatic hypotension may occur.	
Antihypertensive agents and vasodilators		Concomitant use of these agents may increase the hypotensive effects of perindopril. Concomitant use with nitroglycerin and other nitrates, or other vasodilators, may further reduce blood pressure.	
Antidiabetic agents		Epidemiological studies have suggested that concomitant administration of ACE inhibitors and antidiabetic medicines (insulins, oral hypoglycaemic agents) may cause an increased blood-glucose lowering effect with risk of hypoglycaemia.	This phenomenon appeared to be more likely to occur during the first weeks of combined treatment and in patients with renal impairment.
Concomitant ACE inhibitor and diuretic therapy		Patients concomitantly taking ACE inhibitors and diuretics, and especially those in whom diuretic therapy was recently instituted, may occasionally experience an excessive reduction of blood pressure after initiation of therapy.	The possibility of hypotensive effects after the first dose of perindopril/indapamide can be minimized by either increasing the salt intake prior to initiation of treatment or reducing the starting dose of the combination. In this case, the patient should be closely observed for several hours following the initial dose and until blood pressure has stabilized (see Warnings and Precautions and Dosage and Administration).
Digoxin	C	A pharmacokinetic study has shown no effect on plasma digoxin concentration when coadministered with perindopril but an effect of digoxin on the plasma concentration of perindopril/perindoprilat has not been excluded.	
Gentamicin		Animal data have suggested the possibility of interaction between perindopril and gentamicin. However, this has not been investigated in human studies.	Coadministration of both drugs should proceed with caution.
Insulin		Although indapamide exerts minimal effect on glucose metabolism, insulin requirements may be affected in diabetics and hyperglycemia and glycosuria may occur in patients with latent diabetes.	
Lithium	C	Increased serum lithium levels and symptoms of lithium toxicity have been reported in patients receiving concomitant lithium and ACE inhibitor therapy. If a diuretic is also used, it may further increase the risk of lithium toxicity.	Perindopril/indapamide should be coadministered with caution and frequent monitoring of serum lithium levels is recommended.

(cont'd)

Table 2: COVERSYL PLUS LD/COVERSYL PLUS/COVERSYL PLUS HD *(cont'd)*

Established or Potential Concomitant Drug-Drug Interactions

Proper name	Ref	Effect	Clinical Comment
Non-steroidal anti-inflammatory drugs (NSAIDs) including aspirin ≥3 g/day		The administration of a NSAID may reduce the antihypertensive effect of ACE inhibitors. NSAIDs also exert an additive effect on the increase in serum potassium and may result in a deterioration of renal function.	These effects are usually reversible. Rarely, acute renal failure may occur, especially in patients with compromised renal function such as those who are elderly or dehydrated.
Tricyclic antidepressants/Antipsychotic/Anesthetics		Concomitant use of certain anesthetics, tricyclic antidepressants and antipsychotics with ACE inhibitors may result in further reduction of blood pressure.	
Gold salts	CT	Nitritoid reactions (symptoms include facial flushing, nausea, vomiting and hypotension) have been reported rarely in patients on therapy with injectable gold (sodium aurothiomalate) and concomitant ACE inhibitor therapy including perindopril.	
Clofibrate	C	Synergetic effect of clofibrate with indapamide leading to hyponatremia, hypokalemia, hypoosmolarity, nausea and progressive loss of consciousness.	
- Class IA antiarrhythmic agents (quinidine, hydroquinidine, disopyramide); - Class III antiarrhythmic agents (amiodarone, dofetilide, ibutilide, bretylium, sotalol); - Some neuroleptics (chlorpromazine, cyamemazine, levomepromazine, thioridazine, trifluoperazine), - Benzamides (amisulpride, sulpiride, tiapride), - Butyrophenones (droperidol, haloperidol), - Other neuroleptics (pimozide); - Other substances such as bepridil, cisapride, diphemanil, IV erythromycin, halofantrine, mizolastine, moxifloxacin, pentamidine, sparfloxacin, IV vincamine, methadone, astemizole, terfenadine.	C	Torsade de pointes caused by excessive hypokalemia	Perindopril/indapamide should not be administered with medicinal products that induce torsade de pointes (see Contraindications).

Legend: C=Case Study; CT=Clinical Trial; T=Theoretical.

Drug-Food Interactions: The presence of food in the gastrointestinal tract does not affect the rate or extent of perindopril absorption. However the extent of biotransformation of perindopril to perindoprilat is reduced resulting in a decrease of perindoprilat bioavailability by 35%. Therefore it is recommended that COVERSYL PLUS LD/COVERSYL PLUS/COVERSYL PLUS HD are taken before a meal.

Drug-Herb Interactions: Interactions with herbal products have not been established.

Drug-Laboratory Test Interactions: Interactions with laboratory products/methods have not been established.

Drug-Lifestyle Interactions: Lifestyle interactions have not been established.

DOSAGE AND ADMINISTRATION: Dosing Considerations: Dosage of COVERSYL PLUS LD/COVERSYL PLUS/COVERSYL PLUS HD (perindopril erbumine/indapamide) must be individualized and adjustment is required in the elderly, and in case of renal impairment. COVERSYL PLUS/COVERSYL PLUS HD are not for initial therapy and the dose should be determined by titration of the individual components.

Recommended Dose and Dosage Adjustment: Initiation of therapy requires consideration of recent antihypertensive drug treatment, the extent of blood pressure elevation and salt restriction. The dosage of other antihypertensive agents being used with COVERSYL PLUS LD/COVERSYL PLUS/COVERSYL PLUS HD may need to be adjusted. The presence of food in the gastrointestinal tract reduces the bioavailability of perindoprilat.

One COVERSYL PLUS LD (perindopril erbumine/indapamide) tablet per day as a single dose, to be taken orally, preferably in the morning. In case of uncontrolled blood pressure the dose may be increased to two tablets of COVERSYL PLUS LD as a single dose or one tablet of COVERSYL PLUS.

Once the patient has been successfully titrated with the individual components, one tablet per day of COVERSYL PLUS or COVERSYL PLUS HD may be substituted if the titrated doses and dosing schedule can be achieved by the fixed combination (see Indications and Clinical Use and Warnings and Precautions).

Geriatrics: Treatment should be initiated after considering blood pressure response and renal function.

Renal Impairment: In patients with severe renal impairment (creatinine clearance below 30 mL/min), all dosages are contraindicated (see Contraindications).

In patients with moderate renal impairment (creatinine clearance 30-60 mL/min), COVERSYL PLUS HD is contraindicated (see Contraindications) and it is recommended to start treatment with COVERSYL PLUS LD/COVERSYL PLUS with the adequate dosage of the combination of the individual components. Caution should be exercised especially in the elderly patients as greater sensitivity in the elderly cannot be ruled out.

In patients with creatinine clearance greater than or equal to 60 mL/min, no dose modification is required.

Usual medical follow-up will include frequent monitoring of creatinine and potassium levels.

In patients whose renal function may depend on the activity of the renin-angiotensin-aldosterone system, such as patients with bilateral renal artery stenosis, unilateral renal artery stenosis to a solitary kidney, or severe congestive heart failure, treatment with agents that inhibit this system has been associated with oliguria, progressive azotemia, and rarely, acute renal failure and/or death. In susceptible patients, concomitant diuretic use may further increase risk (see Warnings and Precautions).

Missed Dose: If a dose is missed, a double dose should not be taken, but just carry on with the next dose at the normal time.

Administration: It is recommended that COVERSYL PLUS LD/COVERSYL PLUS/COVERSYL PLUS HD be taken once daily, preferably in the morning before a meal (see Drug Interactions, Drug-Food Interactions).

OVERDOSAGE:
The most likely adverse event in case of COVERSYL PLUS LD/COVERSYL PLUS/COVERSYL PLUS HD overdose is hypotension with nausea, vomiting, cramps, dizziness, sleepiness, mental confusion, polyuria or oliguria which may progress to anuria. Electrolytes and water disturbances may occur.

The first measure to be taken consists in rapidly eliminating ingested COVERSYL PLUS LD/COVERSYL PLUS/COVERSYL PLUS HD by gastric lavage and/or administration of activated charcoal. Fluid and electrolyte balance should then be restored.

If marked hypotension is produced, this can be treated by placing the patient in a supine position with the head lower than the rest of the body. If necessary an IV infusion of 0.9% sodium chloride may be given, or any other method of volume expansion may be used.

Perindoprilat, the active form of perindopril, can be dialysed (see Actions and Clinical Pharmacology, Pharmacokinetics).

> For management of a suspected drug overdose, contact your regional Poison Control Centre. See the *CPS* Directory section for a list of Poison Control Centres.

ACTION AND CLINICAL PHARMACOLOGY: Mechanism of Action: COVERSYL PLUS LD/COVERSYL PLUS/COVERSYL PLUS HD (perindopril erbumine/indapamide) are a combination of perindopril erbumine, an angiotensin converting enzyme (ACE) inhibitor, and indapamide, a chlorosulphamoyl diuretic.

In COVERSYL PLUS LD, the ACE inhibitor component is half the usual dose used for monotherapy and the diuretic component is four times lower than the highest dose recommended for monotherapy.

In COVERSYL PLUS, the ACE inhibitor component is the usual dose used for monotherapy and the diuretic component is half the highest dose recommended for monotherapy.

In COVERSYL PLUS HD, the ACE inhibitor and the diuretic components are at the highest doses recommended for monotherapy.

The pharmacological properties are derived from those of each of the components taken separately, in addition to those due to the additive synergistic action of the two products when combined.

COVERSYL PLUS LD/COVERSYL PLUS/COVERSYL PLUS HD exert a dose-dependent antihypertensive effect on diastolic and systolic arterial pressure whilst supine or standing in hypertensive patients regardless of age. This antihypertensive effect lasts for 24 hours. The reduction in blood pressure is obtained in less than one month without tachyphylaxis; stopping treatment has no rebound effects. During clinical trials, the concomitant administration of perindopril and indapamide produced antihypertensive effects of a synergistic nature in relation to each of the products administered alone.

Perindopril Erbumine: Perindopril is a nonsulphydryl angiotensin converting enzyme (ACE) inhibitor which is used in the treatment of hypertension.

Following oral administration, perindopril is rapidly hydrolysed to perindoprilat, its principal active metabolite.

Angiotensin-converting enzyme catalyses the conversion of angiotensin I to the vasoconstrictor substance, angiotensin II. Angiotensin II also stimulates aldosterone secretion by the adrenal cortex. Inhibition of ACE activity leads to decreased levels of angiotensin II, thereby resulting in decreased vasoconstriction and decreased aldosterone secretion. The latter change may result in a small increase in serum potassium (see Warnings and Precautions). Decreased levels of angiotensin II and the accompanying lack of negative feedback on renal renin secretion results in increases in plasma renin activity.

Perindopril administration may interfere with the degradation of the vasodepressor peptide bradykinin. It is not known whether this effect contributes to the therapeutic activity of perindopril.

The mechanism through which perindopril lowers blood pressure appears to result primarily from suppression of the renin-angiotensin-aldosterone system.

Indapamide: Indapamide is a diuretic antihypertensive agent. The mechanism whereby indapamide exerts its action in the control of hypertension is not completely elucidated: both renal and extrarenal actions may be involved. The renal site of action is the proximal part of the distal tubule and the ascending part of Henle's loop. Sodium and chloride ions are excreted in approximately equivalent amounts. The increased delivery of sodium to the distal tubular exchange site results in increased potassium excretion and hypokalemia.

Pharmacodynamics: In most patients with mild to moderate essential hypertension, administration of 4 to 8 mg daily of perindopril results in a reduction of both supine and standing blood pressure with little or no effect on heart rate. Antihypertensive activity commences within one hour with peak effects usually achieved by 4 to 6 hours after dosing. At recommended doses given once daily, antihypertensive effects persist over 24 hours. The blood pressure reductions observed at trough plasma concentration were 75-100% of peak effects. When once and twice daily dosing were compared, the twice daily regimen was slightly superior, but by no more than about 0.5 to 1.0 mmHg. Abrupt withdrawal of perindopril has not been associated with a rapid increase in blood pressure. In studies carried out in patients with mild to moderate essential hypertension, the reduction in blood pressure was accompanied by a reduction in peripheral resistance with no change in glomerular filtration rate. When perindopril is given together with thiazide-type diuretics, the antihypertensive effects are additive.

In uncontrolled studies in patients with insulin-dependent diabetes, perindopril did not appear to affect glycemic control. In long term use in this population, no effect on urinary protein excretion was seen.

Pharmacokinetics: The coadministration of perindopril and indapamide in healthy volunteers and hypertensive patients does not change their pharmacokinetic properties by comparison to separate administration. The bioequivalence between one tablet of COVERSYL PLUS and one tablet of perindopril 4 mg plus one tablet of indapamide 1.25 mg has been demonstrated as well as the similarity between one tablet of COVERSYL PLUS and one tablet of COVERSYL PLUS HD.

After repeated administration in elderly patients (69 to 97 years of age) and in patients with various degrees of renal failure, AUC of both indapamide and perindoprilat increased with renal failure, whereas C_{max} and AUC of indapamide only increased with age (1.5- to 2-fold factor). The AUC ratio between indapamide and perindoprilat was not significantly affected by age and by creatinine clearance >30 mL/min.

Perindopril Erbumine: Absorption: After oral administration, perindopril is rapidly absorbed with peak plasma concentrations occurring at about one hour, with a bioavailability of 65 to 70%.

Following absorption, perindopril is converted into perindoprilat, its active metabolite, with a mean bioavailability of about 20%. Peak plasma concentration of perindoprilat is attained within 4 to 7 hours and corresponding peak pharmacodynamic activity occurs at about 6 hours.

The presence of food in the gastrointestinal tract does not affect the rate or extent of perindopril absorption after oral administration of perindopril erbumine. However the extent of biotransformation of perindopril to perindoprilat is reduced resulting in a decrease of perindoprilat bioavailability by 35%. Due to the saturable nature of ACE inhibition, the pharmacodynamic effect, as measured by the area under the plasma ACE inhibition-time curve, is reduced by approximately 15%.

Distribution: Perindoprilat is not extensively bound to plasma proteins, this being only 10 to 20%, but the binding is concentration dependent due to the saturable binding of perindoprilat to the circulating angiotensin-converting enzyme. The volume of distribution is approximately 0.2 L/kg for unbound perindoprilat.

Metabolism: Perindopril is extensively metabolised following oral administration, with only 4 to 12% of the dose recovered unchanged in the urine. Six metabolites have been identified. They include perindoprilat, the active form, and five others that do not possess appreciable therapeutic activity. These are comprised of perindopril glucuronide, perindoprilat glucuronides, a perindopril lactam, and two perindoprilat lactams.

The two main circulating metabolites of perindopril are perindoprilat and perindoprilat glucuronide.

The two pathways identified and quantified for perindoprilat formation are the pre-systemic (first pass effect) and systemic hydrolysis of perindopril. Perindopril is indeed sensitive to a pre-systemic first-past effect, accounting for 62% of the perindoprilat formation. The systemic hydrolysis of perindopril into perindoprilat accounts for the remaining 38% left.

Excretion: The clearance of perindoprilat and other metabolites is primarily by the renal pathway.

The systemic clearance of perindopril (367 mL/min) can be split into 39% leading to perindoprilat formation and 61% to renal excretion or other biotransformations. The terminal plasma half-life of perindopril is very short (1.2 h), thus leading to no accumulation with a once daily oral dosing regimen. The terminal plasma half-life of unbound perindoprilat is 17 hours. The apparent terminal plasma half-life of perindoprilat (total concentrations) is much longer (30-120 hours) due to the very slow dissociation of perindoprilat from ACE binding sites.

With chronic administration of perindopril, steady state plasma levels of perindoprilat are reached in 3-6 days, during which perindoprilat accumulates 1.5 to 2.0 fold.

Indapamide: Absorption: Indapamide is rapidly and completely absorbed after oral administration.

Distribution: Peak blood levels are obtained after 1 to 2 hours. Indapamide is concentrated in the erythrocytes and is 79% bound to plasma proteins and to erythrocytes. It is taken up by the vascular wall in smooth vascular muscle according to its high lipid solubility.

Metabolism: Indapamide is metabolized to a marked degree, with approximately 5% of the total dose being recovered as unchanged drug in the urine within 48 hours after administration.

Excretion: Seventy per cent of a single oral dose of indapamide is eliminated by the kidneys and 23% is excreted in feces. The decrease in plasma concentrations of indapamide is biphasic with a terminal half life between 14 and 25 hours.

Special Populations and Conditions: Pediatrics: The safety and effectiveness of COVERSYL PLUS LD/COVERSYL PLUS/COVERSYL PLUS HD in children have not been established. Its use in this age group, therefore, is not recommended.

Geriatrics (>65 years of age): In a pharmacokinetic study with single dose administration, mean peak plasma concentrations of perindoprilat were significantly higher in elderly healthy volunteers (32.5 ng/mL) than in younger volunteers (13.5 ng/mL) due to both higher bioavailability and reduced renal clearance in this group.

Single and multiple dose pharmacokinetics of perindopril were evaluated in a study of elderly hypertensive patients (72 to 91 years of age), C_{max} and AUC were found to be approximately two-fold higher than in healthy younger subjects. The higher concentrations of perindoprilat observed in these patients were reflected in greater ACE inhibition (see Warnings and Precautions, Geriatrics (>65 years of age), and Dosage and Administration, Geriatrics).

Gender: The effectiveness of COVERSYL PLUS LD/COVERSYL PLUS/COVERSYL PLUS HD was not influenced by gender.

Race: The blood pressure lowering effects of angiotensin converting enzyme (ACE) inhibitors generally are lower in black patients than in non-blacks.

Hepatic Insufficiency: The bioavailability of perindoprilat is increased in patients with impaired hepatic function. Plasma concentrations in patients with hepatic impairment were about 50% higher than those observed in healthy subjects or hypertensive patients with normal liver function.

COVERSYL PLUS LD/COVERSYL PLUS/COVERSYL PLUS HD are contraindicated in patients with severe hepatic impairment.

Renal Insufficiency: In patients with renal insufficiency, perindoprilat AUC increases with decreasing renal function. At creatinine clearances of 30-80 mL/min, AUC is about double that of 100 mL/min. When creatinine clearance drops below 30 mL/min, AUC increases more markedly.

In patients with severe renal impairment (creatinine clearance below 30 mL/min), all dosages are contraindicated (see Contraindications and Dosage and Administration).

In patients with moderate renal impairment (creatinine clearance 30-60 mL/min), COVERSYL PLUS HD is contraindicated (see Contraindications and Dosage and Administration) and it is recommended to start treatment with COVERSYL PLUS LD/COVERSYL PLUS with the adequate dosage of the combination of the individual components. Caution should be exercised especially in the elderly patients as greater sensitivity in the elderly cannot be ruled out (see Contraindications and Dosage and Administration).

In patients with creatinine clearance greater than or equal to 60 mL/min, no dose modification is required (see Dosage and Administration).

Usual medical follow-up will include frequent monitoring of creatinine and potassium levels.

Perindopril, and its active metabolite perindoprilat, are dialysable. In a limited number of patients studied, perindopril hemodialysis clearance ranged from 41.7 to 76.7 mL/min (mean 52.0 mL/min). Perindoprilat hemodialysis clearance ranged from 37.4 to 91.0 mL/min (mean 67.2 mL/min) (see Warnings and Precautions and Dosage and Administration).

Heart Failure: Patients with heart failure have reduced perindoprilat clearance, which may result in a dose interval AUC that is increased up to 40%, which should lead to an initial reduction of perindopril dosage.

Genetic Polymorphism: Pharmacokinetics differences due to genetic polymorphism have not been studied.

STORAGE AND STABILITY: Store at room temperature (15-30°C).

SPECIAL HANDLING INSTRUCTIONS: No special requirements.

INFORMATION FOR THE PATIENT: Published in e-CPS, available by subscription at www.e-cps.ca.

DOSAGE FORMS, COMPOSITION AND PACKAGING: Coversyl Plus LD: Each white, rod-shaped scored tablet, contains: perindopril erbumine 2 mg and indapamide 0.625 mg. Nonmedicinal ingredients: hydrophobic colloidal silica, lactose monohydrate, magnesium stearate and microcrystalline cellulose. Blister packs of 30.

Coversyl Plus: Each white, rod-shaped tablet, contains: perindopril erbumine 4 mg and indapamide 1.25 mg. Nonmedicinal ingredients: hydrophobic colloidal silica, lactose monohydrate, magnesium stearate and microcrystalline cellulose. Blister packs of 30. Bottles of 100.

Coversyl Plus HD: Each white, round tablet, contains: perindopril erbumine 8 mg and indapamide 2.5 mg. Nonmedicinal ingredients: hydrophobic colloidal silica, lactose monohydrate, magnesium stearate and microcrystalline cellulose. Blister packs of 30.

(Shown in Product Identification Section)

Cozaar® Pr
losartan potassium
Angiotensin II Receptor Antagonist

Merck Frosst

Date of Revision: December 22, 2009

SUMMARY PRODUCT INFORMATION:

Route of Administration	Dosage Form/Strength	Nonmedicinal Ingredients
Oral	Tablet 25 mg, 50 mg, 100 mg	Corn starch, hydroxypropyl cellulose, hydroxypropyl methylcellulose, lactose, magnesium stearate, microcrystalline cellulose, titanium dioxide, carnauba wax and potassium. See Dosage Forms, Composition and Packaging.

INDICATIONS AND CLINICAL USE: Hypertension: COZAAR (losartan potassium) is indicated for the treatment of essential hypertension. COZAAR is also indicated in patients with essential hypertension and left ventricular hypertrophy.

COZAAR may be used alone or concomitantly with thiazide diuretics.

A great majority of patients with severe hypertension in controlled clinical trials required combination therapy. COZAAR has been used concomitantly with beta-blockers and calcium channel blockers, but the data on such use are limited.

The safety and efficacy of concurrent use with angiotensin converting enzyme inhibitors have not been established.

Type 2 Diabetic Patients with Proteinuria and Hypertension: COZAAR is also indicated to delay the progression of renal disease as measured by the occurrence of doubling of serum creatinine, and end stage renal disease, and to reduce proteinuria.

Geriatrics (≥65 years of age): In clinical studies, there was no age-related difference in the efficacy or safety profile of losartan (see Warnings and Precautions).

Pediatrics (6-16 years of age): Antihypertensive effects of COZAAR have been demonstrated in hypertensive pediatric patients aged 6 to 16 years. Use of COZAAR in these age groups is supported by evidence from adequate and well-controlled studies of COZAAR in pediatric patients (see Contraindications, Warnings and Precautions, Action and Clinical Pharmacology).

CONTRAINDICATIONS:

- Patients who are hypersensitive to this drug or to any ingredient in the formulation. For a complete listing, see Dosage Forms, Composition and Packaging.

WARNINGS AND PRECAUTIONS:

> **Serious Warnings and Precautions**
> **When used in pregnancy, angiotensin receptor (AT_1) blockers (ARB) can cause injury or even death of the developing fetus. When pregnancy is detected, COZAAR should be discontinued as soon as possible (see Warnings and Precautions, Special Populations).**

Carcinogenesis and Mutagenesis: There is no evidence of carcinogenesis and mutagenesis associated with losartan.

Cardiovascular: Hypotension: Occasionally, symptomatic hypotension has occurred after administration of losartan, in some cases after the first dose. It is more likely to occur in patients who are volume-depleted by diuretic therapy, dietary salt restriction, dialysis, diarrhea, or vomiting. In these patients, because of the potential fall in blood pressure, therapy should be started under close medical supervision. Similar considerations apply to patients with ischemic heart or cerebrovascular disease, in whom an excessive fall in blood pressure could result in myocardial infarction or cerebrovascular accident.

Valvular Stenosis: There is concern on theoretical grounds that patients with aortic stenosis might be at particular risk of decreased coronary perfusion when treated with vasodilators because they do not develop as much afterload reduction.

Hepatic/Biliary/Pancreatic: Hepatic Impairment: Based on pharmacokinetic data which demonstrate significantly increased plasma concentrations of losartan and its active metabolite in cirrhotic patients after administration of COZAAR, a lower dose should be considered for patients with hepatic impairment, or a history of hepatic impairment (see Dosage and Administration).

Renal: Renal Impairment: As a consequence of inhibiting the renin-angiotensin-aldosterone system, changes in renal function have been reported in susceptible individuals. In patients whose renal function may depend on the activity of the renin-angiotensin-aldosterone system, such as patients with bilateral renal artery stenosis, unilateral renal artery stenosis to a solitary kidney, or severe congestive heart failure, treatment with agents that inhibit this system has been associated with oliguria, progressive azotemia, and rarely, acute renal failure and/or death. In susceptible patients, concomitant diuretic use may further increase risk.

Use of losartan should include appropriate assessment of renal function.

Hyperkalemia: In a clinical study conducted in patients with type 2 diabetes with proteinuria and hypertension, the incidence of hyperkalemia was higher in the group treated with COZAAR (9.9%) as compared to the placebo group (3.4%), however, few patients discontinued therapy due to hyperkalemia. Careful monitoring of serum potassium is recommended (see Adverse Reactions, Abnormal Hematologic and Clinical Chemistry Findings).

Sensitivity/Resistance: Hypersensitivity: Anaphylactic reactions, angioedema (involving swelling of the larynx and glottis causing airway obstruction and/or swelling of the face, lips, and/or tongue and pharynx, requiring intubation/tracheotomy in some cases) have been reported rarely in patients treated with losartan; some of these patients previously experienced angioedema with ACE inhibitors. Vasculitis, including Henoch-Schoenlein purpura, has been reported rarely.

Special Populations: Pregnant Women: Drugs that act directly on the renin-angiotensin-aldosterone-system (RAAS) can cause fetal and neonatal morbidity and death when administered to pregnant women. When pregnancy is detected, COZAAR should be discontinued as soon as possible.

The use of ARB is not recommended during pregnancy. Epidemiological evidence regarding the risk of teratogenicity following exposure to angiotensin converting enzyme inhibitors (another class of therapeutic products interfering with the RAAS) during the first trimester of pregnancy has not been conclusive; however a small increase in risk cannot be excluded. Given the current evidence available on the risk with ARB, similar risks may exist for this class of drugs. Patients planning pregnancy should be changed to alternative antihypertensive treatments which have an established safety profile for use in pregnancy. When pregnancy is diagnosed, treatment with angiotensin II antagonists should be stopped immediately, and, if appropriate, alternative therapy should be started.

The use of ARBs during the second and third trimesters is known to induce human fetotoxicity (decreased renal function; oligohydramnios, skull ossification retardation) and neonatal toxicity (renal failure, hypotension, hyperkalemia).

Infants with a history of in utero exposure to ARBs should be closely observed for hypotension, oliguria, and hyperkalemia. If oliguria occurs, attention should be directed toward support of blood pressure and renal perfusion. Exchange transfusion or dialysis may be required as means of reversing hypotension and/or substituting for impaired renal function; however, limited experience with those procedures has not been associated with significant clinical benefit. Neither losartan nor the active metabolite can be removed by hemodialysis.

Animal Data: Losartan potassium has been shown to produce adverse effects in rat fetuses and neonates, which include decreased body weight, mortality and/or renal toxicity. Significant levels of losartan and its active metabolite were shown to be present in rat milk. Based on pharmacokinetic assessments, these findings are attributed to drug exposure in late gestation and during lactation.

Nursing Women: It is not known whether losartan or its active metabolite are excreted in human milk, but significant levels of both of these compounds have been found in the milk of lactating rats. Because many drugs are excreted in human milk, and because of their potential for affecting the nursing infant adversely, a decision should be made whether to discontinue nursing or discontinue the drug, taking into account the importance of the drug to the mother.

Geriatrics (≥65 years of age): No overall differences in safety were observed between elderly and younger patients, but appropriate caution should nevertheless be used when prescribing to elderly, as increased vulnerability to drug effect is possible in this patient population. This conclusion is based on 391 of 2085 (19%) patients, 65 years and over who received losartan monotherapy in controlled trials for hypertension. This was also the finding in a controlled clinical study in type 2 diabetic patients with proteinuria and hypertension with 248 (33%) of patients 65 years of age and over and in a controlled clinical study in hypertensive patients with left ventricular hypertrophy with 2857 (62%) of patients 65 years of age and over.

Pediatrics: The antihypertensive effect has been demonstrated in a dose-response study of a limited duration of three weeks, after which half of the patients continued on assigned dosage up to six weeks. Blood pressure declines were maintained in the two highest dose groups.

Renal Impairment: There are no data on the effect of COZAAR on blood pressure in pediatric patients under the age of six years and neonate, or in pediatric patients with glomerular filtration rate <30 mL/min/1.73m².

As a consequence of inhibiting the renin-angiotensin-aldosterone system, changes in renal function have been reported in susceptible individuals. In patients whose renal function may depend on the activity of the renin-angiotensin-aldosterone system, such as patients with bilateral renal artery stenosis, unilateral renal artery stenosis to a solitary kidney, or severe congestive heart failure, treatment with agents that inhibit this system has been associated with oliguria, progressive azotemia, and rarely, acute renal failure and/or death. In susceptible patients, concomitant diuretic use may further increase risk.

Use of losartan should include appropriate assessment of renal function.

Hepatic Impairment: There are no data on the effect of COZAAR in pediatric patients with hepatic impairments. Long-term safety has been studied in pediatric patients, as an extension of 6 months of the above cited dose-response study.

The pharmacokinetics of losartan have been investigated in 50 hypertensive pediatric patients >1 month to <16 years of age following once daily oral administration of approximately 0.54 to 0.77 mg/kg of losartan (mean doses). The active metabolite is formed from losartan in all age groups. Pharmacokinetics of losartan and its active metabolite are generally similar across the studied age groups and consistent with pharmacokinetic historic data in adults (see Adverse Reactions).

Race: In the LIFE study, Afro-American Black patients treated with atenolol were at lower risk of experiencing the primary composite endpoint and stroke compared with Afro-American Black patients treated with COZAAR. Based on the LIFE study, the benefits of COZAAR on the primary composite endpoint and stroke compared to atenolol do not apply to Afro-American Black patients with hypertension and left ventricular hypertrophy although both treatment regimens effectively lowered blood pressure in these patients.

Monitoring and Laboratory Tests: Not applicable.

ADVERSE REACTIONS: Adverse Drug Reaction Overview: COZAAR has been evaluated for safety in more than 3300 patients treated for essential hypertension. Of these, 2085 were treated with losartan monotherapy in controlled clinical trials.

In open studies, over 1200 patients were treated with losartan for more than 6 months, and over 800 for more than one year.

In controlled clinical trials, discontinuation of therapy due to clinical adverse experiences occurred in 2.3% and 3.7% of patients treated with COZAAR and placebo, respectively.

The following potentially serious adverse reactions have been reported rarely with losartan in controlled clinical trials: syncope, hypotension.

No relevant differences between the adverse experience profile for pediatric patients and the previously reported for adult patients were identified.

Clinical Trial Adverse Drug Reactions: Because clinical trials are conducted under very specific conditions the adverse reaction rates observed in the clinical trials may not reflect the rates observed in practice and should not be compared to the rates in the clinical trials of another drug. Adverse drug reaction information from clinical trials is useful for identifying drug-related adverse events and for approximating rates.

In these double-blind controlled clinical trials, the following adverse reactions reported with COZAAR occurred in ≥1% of patients, regardless of drug relationship: see Table 1.

Table 1: COZAAR

Adverse Reactions that Occurred in ≥1% of Patients

	COZAAR (n=2085) %	Placebo (n=535) %
Body as a Whole		
Asthenia/Fatigue	3.8	3.9
Edema/Swelling	1.7	1.9
Abdominal Pain	1.7	1.7
Chest Pain	1.1	2.6
Cardiovascular		
Palpitation	1.0	0.4
Tachycardia	1.0	1.7
Digestive		
Diarrhea	1.9	1.9
Dyspepsia	1.1	1.5
Nausea	1.8	2.8
Musculoskeletal		
Back Pain	1.6	1.1
Muscle Cramps	1.0	1.1
Nervous/Psychiatric		
Dizziness	4.1	2.4
Headache	14.1	17.2
Insomnia	1.1	0.7
Respiratory		
Cough	3.1	2.6
Nasal Congestion	1.3	1.1
Pharyngitis	1.5	2.6
Sinus Disorder	1.0	1.3
Upper Respiratory Infection	6.5	5.6

In these controlled clinical trials for essential hypertension, dizziness was the only adverse experience, occurring in more than 1% of cases, that was reported as drug-related, and that occurred at a greater incidence in losartan-treated (2.4%) than placebo-treated (1.3%) patients.

COZAAR was generally well tolerated in a controlled clinical trial in type 2 diabetic patients with proteinuria and hypertension. The most common drug-related side effects were asthenia/fatigue, dizziness, hypotension and hyperkalemia (see Warnings and Precautions). In hypertensive patients with left ventricular hypertrophy, the most common drug-related side effects were dizziness, asthenia/fatigue, and vertigo.

Less Common Clinical Trial Adverse Drug Reactions (<1%): In double-blind, controlled clinical trials for essential hypertension, the following adverse reactions were reported with COZAAR at an occurrence rate of less than 1%, regardless of drug relationship: orthostatic effects, somnolence, vertigo, epistaxis, tinnitus, constipation, malaise, rash.

Abnormal Hematologic and Clinical Chemistry Findings: In controlled clinical trials for essential hypertension, clinically important changes in standard laboratory parameters were rarely associated with administration of COZAAR.

Liver Function Tests: In double-blind hypertensive trials, elevations of AST and ALT occurred in 1.1% and 1.9% of patients treated with losartan monotherapy and in 0.8% and 1.3% of patients treated with placebo, respectively. When AST or ALT elevations ≥2×upper limit of normal were compared, the frequency was similar to that seen in placebo.

Hyperkalemia: In controlled clinical trials for essential hypertension, hyperkalemia (serum potassium >5.5 mEq/L) occurred in 1.5% of patients treated with COZAAR.

In a clinical study conducted in type 2 diabetic patients with proteinuria and hypertension, 9.9% of patients treated with COZAAR and 3.4% of patients treated with placebo developed hyperkalemia (see Warnings and Precautions, Renal, Hyperkalemia).

Creatinine, Blood Urea Nitrogen: Minor increases in blood urea nitrogen (BUN) or serum creatinine were observed in less than 0.1 percent of patients with essential hypertension treated with COZAAR alone. No patient discontinued taking COZAAR alone due to increased BUN or serum creatinine.

Hemoglobin and Hematocrit: Small decreases in hemoglobin and hematocrit (mean decreases of approximately 0.11 g percent and 0.09 volume percent, respectively) occurred frequently in patients treated with COZAAR alone, but were rarely of clinical importance. In controlled clinical trials no patients were discontinued due to anemia. Discontinuation of losartan treatment due to anemia was reported with post-marketing use of losartan.

In clinical trials, the following were noted to occur with an incidence of <1%, regardless of drug relationship: thrombocytopenia, eosinophilia.

Post-Market Adverse Drug Reactions: Other adverse reactions reported rarely in open-label studies or post-marketing use in patients with essential hypertension, regardless of drug relationship, include anemia, thrombocytopenia (reported rarely), hepatitis, liver function tests abnormalities, vomiting, drug induced cough, asthenia, diarrhea, migraine, dysgeusia, arthralgia, pruritus, erythroderma, taste disorder, urticaria, malaise, erectile dysfunction/impotence and photosensitivity. Cases of muscle pain, muscle weakness, myositis and rhabdomyolysis have been reported in patients receiving angiotensin II receptor blockers.

Anaphylactic reactions, angioedema (involving swelling of the larynx and glottis causing airway obstruction and/or swelling of the face, lips, and/or tongue and pharynx, requiring intubation/tracheotomy in some cases) have been reported rarely in patients treated with losartan; some of these patients previously experienced angioedema with ACE inhibitors. Vasculitis, including Henoch-Schoenlein purpura, has been reported rarely.

DRUG INTERACTIONS: Drug-Drug Interactions: Diuretics: Patients on diuretics, and especially those in whom diuretic therapy was recently instituted, may occasionally experience an excessive reduction of blood pressure after initiation of therapy with COZAAR. The possibility of symptomatic hypotension with the use of COZAAR can be minimized by discontinuing the diuretic prior to initiation of treatment and/or lowering the initial dose of losartan (see Warnings and Precautions, Cardiovascular, Hypotension and Dosage and Administration). No drug interaction of clinical significance has been identified with thiazide diuretics.

Agents Increasing Serum Potassium: Concomitant use of potassium-sparing diuretics (e.g., spironolactone, triamterene, amiloride), potassium supplements, or salt substitutes containing potassium may lead to increases in serum potassium.

Since COZAAR decreases the production of aldosterone, potassium-sparing diuretics or potassium supplements should be given only for documented hypokalemia and with frequent monitoring of serum potassium. Potassium-containing salt substitutes should also be used with caution.

Lithium Salts: As with other drugs which affect the excretion of sodium, lithium excretion may be reduced. Therefore, serum lithium levels should be monitored carefully if lithium salts are to be co-administered with angiotensin II receptor antagonists.

Digitalis: In 9 healthy volunteers, when a single oral dose of 0.5 mg digoxin was administered to patients receiving losartan for 11 days, digoxin AUC and digoxin C_{max} ratios, relative to placebo, were found to be 1.06 (90% C.I. 0.98-1.14) and 1.12 (90% C.I. 0.97-1.28), respectively. The effect of losartan on steady-state pharmacokinetics of cardiac glycosides is not known.
Warfarin: Losartan administered for 7 days did not affect the pharmacokinetics or pharmacodynamic activity of a single dose of warfarin. The effect of losartan on steady-state pharmacokinetics of warfarin is not known.
Drugs Affecting Cytochrome P450 System: Rifampin, an inducer of drug metabolism, decreases the concentrations of the active metabolite of losartan. In humans, two inhibitors of P450 3A4 have been studied. Ketoconazole did not affect the conversion of losartan to the active metabolite after intravenous administration of losartan, and erythromycin had no clinically significant effect after oral losartan administration. Fluconazole, an inhibitor of P450 2C9, decreased active metabolite concentration. The pharmacodynamic consequences of concomitant use of losartan and inhibitors of P450 2C9 have not been examined.

When losartan was administered to 10 healthy male volunteers as a single dose in steady-state conditions of phenobarbital, a cytochrome P450 inducer, losartan AUC, relative to baseline, was 0.80 (90% C.I. 0.72-0.88), while AUC of the active metabolite, E-3174, was 0.80 (90% C.I. 0.78-0.82).

When losartan was administered to 8 healthy male volunteers as a single dose in steady-state conditions of cimetidine, a cytochrome P450 inhibitor, losartan AUC, relative to baseline, was 1.18 (90% C.I. 1.10-1.27), while AUC of the active metabolite, E-3174, was 1.00 (90% C.I. 0.92-1.08).
Non-Steroidal Anti-Inflammatory Drugs Including Cyclooxygenase-2 Inhibitors: Non-steroidal anti-inflammatory drugs (NSAIDs) including indomethacin and selective cyclooxygenase-2 inhibitors (COX-2 inhibitors) may reduce the effect of diuretics and other antihypertensive drugs. Therefore, the antihypertensive effect of angiotensin II receptor antagonists or ACE inhibitors may be attenuated by NSAIDs including selective COX-2 inhibitors.

In some patients with compromised renal fonction (e.g., elderly patients or patients who are volume-depleted, including those on diuretic therapy) who are being treated with NSAIDS, including selective COX-2 inhibitors, the co-administration of angiotensin II receptor antagonists or ACE inhibitors may result in a further deterioration of renal function. Cases of acute renal failure, usually reversible, have been reported. Therefore, this combination should be administered with caution in this patient population.
Drug-Food Interactions: COZAAR may be administered with or without food.
Drug-Herb Interactions: Interactions with herbal products have not been established.
Drug-Laboratory Test Interactions: Interactions with laboratory tests have not been established.

DOSAGE AND ADMINISTRATION: Recommended Dose and Dosage Adjustment: COZAAR may be administered with or without food, however it should be taken consistently with respect to food intake at about the same time every day.
Hypertension: The dosage of COZAAR must be individualized.

Initiation of therapy requires consideration of recent antihypertensive drug treatment, the extent of blood pressure elevation, salt restriction, and other pertinent clinical factors. The dosage of other antihypertensive agents used with COZAAR may need to be adjusted.
Monotherapy: The usual starting dose of COZAAR is 50 mg once daily.

Dosage should be adjusted according to blood pressure response. The maximal antihypertensive effect is attained 3-6 weeks after initiation of therapy.

The usual dose range for COZAAR is 50 to 100 mg once daily. A dose of 100 mg daily should not be exceeded, as no additional antihypertensive effect is obtained with higher doses.

In most patients taking COZAAR 50 mg once daily, the antihypertensive effect is maintained. In some patients treated once daily, the antihypertensive effect may diminish toward the end of the dosing interval. This can be evaluated by measuring the blood pressure just prior to dosing to determine whether satisfactory control is being maintained for 24 hours. If it is not, either twice daily administration with the same total daily dosage, or an increase in the dose should be considered. If blood pressure is not adequately controlled with COZAAR alone, a non-potassium-sparing diuretic may be administered concomitantly.

For patients with volume-depletion, a starting dose of 25 mg once daily should be considered (see Warnings and Precautions, Cardiovascular, Hypotension and Drug Interactions).
Concomitant Diuretic Therapy: In patients receiving diuretics, COZAAR therapy should be initiated with caution, since these patients may be volume-depleted and thus more likely to experience hypotension following initiation of additional antihypertensive therapy. Whenever possible, all diuretics should be discontinued two to three days prior to the administration of COZAAR, to reduce the likelihood of hypotension (see Warnings and Precautions, Cardiovascular, Hypotension and Drug Interactions). If this is not possible because of the patient's condition, COZAAR should be administered with caution and the blood pressure monitored closely. Thereafter, the dosage should be adjusted according to the individual response of the patient.
Type 2 Diabetic Patients with Proteinuria and Hypertension: The usual starting dose is 50 mg once daily. The dose may be increased to 100 mg once daily based on blood pressure response. COZAAR may be administered with other antihypertensive agents (e.g., diuretics, calcium channel blockers, alpha- or beta-blockers, and centrally acting agents) as well as with insulin and other commonly used hypoglycemic agents (e.g., sulfonylureas, glitazones and glucosidase inhibitors).
Geriatrics (≥65 years of age): No initial dosage adjustment is necessary for most elderly patients. However, appropriate monitoring of these patients is recommended.
Pediatrics (6-16 years of age): For patients who can swallow tablets, the recommended dose is 25 mg once daily in patients ≥20 to <50 kg. The dose can be increased to a maximum of 50 mg once daily. In patients >50 kg, the starting dose is 50 mg once daily. The dose can be increased to a maximum of 100 mg once daily.

Dosage should be adjusted to blood pressure response.

In pediatric patients who are intravascularly volume depleted, these conditions should be corrected prior to administration of COZAAR.

COZAAR is not recommended in pediatric patients with glomerular filtration rate <30 mL/min/1.73 m², in pediatric patients with hepatic impairment, or in neonates as no data are available.
Renal Impairment: No initial dosage adjustment is usually necessary for patients with renal impairment, including those requiring hemodialysis. However, appropriate monitoring of these patients is recommended.
Hepatic Impairment: An initial dosage of 25 mg should be considered for patients with hepatic impairment, or a history of hepatic impairment (see Warnings and Precautions, Hepatic/Biliary/Pancreatic, Hepatic Impairment).
Missed Dose: If a dose is missed, an extra dose should not be taken. The usual schedule must be resumed.

OVERDOSAGE:
Limited data are available in regard to overdosage with COZAAR in humans. The most likely manifestation of overdosage would be hypotension and/or tachycardia. If symptomatic hypotension should occur, supportive treatment should be instituted.

Neither losartan nor the active metabolite can be removed by hemodialysis.

> For management of a suspected drug overdose, contact your regional Poison Control Centre. See the *CPS* Directory section for a list of Poison Control Centres.

ACTION AND CLINICAL PHARMACOLOGY: Mechanism of Action: COZAAR antagonizes angiotensin II by blocking the angiotensin type one (AT_1) receptor.

Angiotensin II is the primary vasoactive hormone of the renin-angiotensin system. Its effects include vasoconstriction and the stimulation of aldosterone secretion by the adrenal cortex.

Losartan, and its active metabolite, E-3174, block the vasoconstrictor and aldosterone-secreting effects of angiotensin II by selectively blocking the binding of angiotensin II to AT_1 receptors found in many tissues, including vascular smooth muscle. A second type of angiotensin II receptor has been identified as the AT_2 receptor, but it plays no known role in cardiovascular homeostasis to date. Both losartan and its active metabolite do not exhibit any agonist activity at the AT_1 receptor, and have much greater affinity, in the order of 1000-fold, for the AT_1 receptor than for the AT_2 receptor. In vitro binding studies indicate that losartan itself is a reversible, competitive antagonist at the AT_1 receptor, while the active metabolite is 10 to 40 times more potent than losartan, and is a reversible, non-competitive antagonist of the AT_1 receptor.

Neither losartan nor its active metabolite inhibits angiotensin converting enzyme (ACE), also known as kininase II, the enzyme that converts angiotensin I to angiotensin II and degrades bradykinin, nor do they bind to or block other hormone receptors or ion channels known to be important in cardiovascular regulation.
Pharmacodynamics: Losartan inhibits the pressor effect of angiotensin II. A dose of 100 mg inhibits this effect by about 85% at peak, with 25-40% inhibition persisting for 24 hours. Removal of the negative feedback of angiotensin II causes a 2-3 fold rise in plasma renin activity, and a consequent rise in angiotensin II plasma concentration, in hypertensive patients.

Maximum blood pressure lowering, following oral administration of a single dose of losartan, as seen in hypertensive patients, occurs at about 6 hours.

In losartan-treated patients during controlled trials, there was no meaningful change in heart rate.

There is no apparent rebound effect after abrupt withdrawal of losartan therapy.

Black hypertensive patients show a smaller average blood pressure response to losartan monotherapy than other hypertensive patients.
Pharmacokinetics:

Table 2: COZAAR

Pharmacokinetic Parameters in Hypertensive Adults Following Multiple Dosing

	Adults Given 50 mg Once Daily for 7 days n=12	
	Parent	**Active Metabolite**
$AUC_{0\text{-}24hr}$[a] (ng·hr/mL)	442±173	1685±452
C_{max} (ng/mL)[a]	224±82	212±73
$t_{1/2}$ (hr)[b]	2.1±0.70	7.4±2.4
T_{max} (hr)[c]	0.9	3.5
Cl_r (mL/min)[a]	56±23	20±3

[a] Mean±standard deviation.
[b] Harmonic mean±standard deviation.
[c] Median.

Absorption: Following oral administration, losartan is well absorbed, with systemic bioavailability of losartan approximately 33%. About 14% of an orally-administered dose of losartan is converted to the active metabolite, although about 1% of subjects did not convert losartan efficiently to the active metabolite.

Mean peak concentrations of losartan occur at about one hour, and that of its active metabolite at about 3-4 hours. Although maximum plasma concentrations of losartan and its active metabolite are approximately equal, the AUC of the metabolite is about 4 times greater than that of losartan.
Distribution: Both losartan and its active metabolite are highly bound to plasma proteins, primarily albumin, with plasma free fractions of 1.3% and 0.2% respectively. Plasma protein binding is constant over the concentration range achieved with recommended doses. Studies in rats indicate that losartan crosses the blood-brain barrier poorly, if at all.

The volume of distribution of losartan is about 34 L, and that of the active metabolite is about 12 L.
Metabolism: Losartan is an orally active agent that undergoes substantial first-pass metabolism by cytochrome P450 enzymes. It is converted, in part, to an active carboxylic acid metabolite, E-3174, that is responsible for most of the angiotensin II receptor antagonism that follows oral losartan administration.

Various losartan metabolites have been identified in human plasma and urine. In addition to the active carboxylic acid metabolite, E-3174, several inactive metabolites are formed. In vitro studies indicate that the cytochrome P450 isoenzymes 2C9 and 3A4 are involved in the biotransformation of losartan to its metabolites.
Excretion: The terminal half-life of losartan itself is about 2 hours, and that of the active metabolite, about 6-9 hours. The pharmacokinetics of losartan and this metabolite are linear with oral losartan doses up to 200 mg and do not change over time. Neither losartan nor its metabolite accumulate in plasma upon repeated once-daily administration.

Total plasma clearance of losartan is about 600 mL/min, with about 75 mL/min accounted for by renal clearance. Total plasma clearance of the active metabolite is about 50 mL/min, with about 25 mL/min accounted for by renal clearance. Both biliary and urinary excretion contribute substantially to the elimination of losartan and its metabolites.

Following oral ^{14}C-labeled losartan, about 35% of radioactivity is recovered in the urine and about 60% in the feces. Following an intravenous dose of ^{14}C-labeled losartan, about 45% of radioactivity is recovered in the urine and 50% in the feces.
Pediatrics: The pharmacokinetics of losartan and its active metabolite were generally similar across the studied age groups and historical pharmacokinetic data in adults.

Table 3: COZAAR

Pharmacokinetic Parameters in Hypertensive Infants and Toddlers (Group I; 3-23 months), Preschool Children (Group II; 2-5 years), School-Age Children (Group III; 6-11 years), and Adolescents (Group IV; 12-15 years) Following Multiple Dosing

	Parent	Active Metabolite
$AUC_{0\text{-}24\ hr}$ observed (ng·hr/mL)[a]		
Group I (n=9)	244.5±175.7	1456.5±1422.7
Group II (n=12)[d]	314.5±177.8	950.9±498.0
Group III (n=11)	251.0±265.6	1163.6±1017.5
Group IV (n=14)	303.1±123.6	1589.9±996.2
$AUC_{0\text{-}24\ hr}$ per 0.7 mg/kg[a]		
Group I (n=9)	246.1±154.0	1466.3±1 498.8
Group II (n=13)	305.2±164.9	933.2±510.5
Group III (n=11)	232.6±199.4	1078.0±783.4
Group IV (n=14)	405.4±120.3	2126.8±1 082.4
C_{max} observed (ng/mL)[a]		
Group I (n=9)	66.6±103.6	146.9±179.5
Group II (n=12)[d]	89.8±96.5	91.5±75.2
Group III (n=11)	98.7±94.5	139.1±148.1
Group IV (n=14)	105.1±112.3	188.2±91.2
C_{max} per 0.7 mg/kg[a]		
Group I (n=9)	67.0±92.8	147.9±190.6
Group II (n=13)	89.5±88.3	92.0±77.6
Group III (n=11)	91.4±81.7	128.8±112.1
Group IV (n=14)	140.6±90.5	251.7±118.2

(cont'd)

Table 3: COZAAR *(cont'd)*

Pharmacokinetic Parameters in Hypertensive Infants and Toddlers (Group I; 3-23 months), Preschool Children (Group II; 2-5 years), School-Age Children (Group III; 6-11 years), and Adolescents (Group IV; 12-15 years) Following Multiple Dosing

	Parent	Active Metabolite
T_{max} (hr)[c]		
Group I (n=9)	1.05±1.38	5.53±2.0
Group II (n=13)	1.07±1.43	6.01±1.5
Group III (n=11)	2.03±1.79	4.46±2.1
Group IV (n=14)	1.54±1.27	5.00±1.0
Half-Life (hr)[b]		
Group I (n=9)	1.93±0.44	4.83±1.1
Group II (n=13)	2.37±1.24	5.59±1.1
Group III (n=11)	2.18±1.50	5.37±1.4
Group IV (n=14)	2.41±1.84	5.72±1.0

a Geometric Mean±Standard Deviation.
b Harmonic Mean±Standard Deviation.
c Median±Standard Deviation.
d n=12: excludes AN 4051 who received 2.5 times the intended dose.

A pharmacokinetic study was performed to estimate plasma and urine pharmacokinetic parameters of losartan and its active metabolite, E-3174, in infants and toddlers, preschool children, school-age children, and adolescents.

The pharmacokinetics of losartan and its active metabolite, E-3174, in this study were comparable in all age groups studied. Differences in some parameters were statistically significant, especially for the active metabolite, E-3174, when the preschool children were compared with adolescents. Importantly, the youngest patients were comparable with older pediatric patients, and the active metabolite, E-3174, was formed from losartan in all age groups studied.

STORAGE AND STABILITY: Store at room temperature (15-30°C). Keep container tightly closed. Protect from light.

INFORMATION FOR THE PATIENT: Published in e-CPS, available by subscription at www.e-cps.ca.

DOSAGE FORMS, COMPOSITION AND PACKAGING: 25 mg: Each white, oval-shaped, unscored, film-coated tablet, with code 951 on one side and plain on the other, contains: losartan potassium 25 mg. Nonmedicinal ingredients: carnauba wax, corn starch, hydroxypropyl cellulose, hydroxypropyl methylcellulose, lactose, magnesium stearate, microcrystalline cellulose and titanium dioxide. Potassium: 2.12 mg (<1 mmol). Bottles of 100.

50 mg: Each white, oval-shaped, film-coated tablet, with code 952 on one side and scored on the other, contains: losartan potassium 50 mg. The splitting of COZAAR 50 mg tablets is not advised. Nonmedicinal ingredients: carnauba wax, corn starch, hydroxypropyl cellulose, hydroxypropyl methylcellulose, lactose, magnesium stearate, microcrystalline cellulose and titanium dioxide. Potassium: 4.24 mg (<1 mmol). Blister packages of 30. Bottles of 100.

100 mg: Each white, teardrop-shaped, unscored, film-coated tablet, with code 960 on one side and plain on the other, contains: losartan potassium 100 mg. Nonmedicinal ingredients: carnauba wax, corn starch, hydroxypropyl cellulose, hydroxypropyl methylcellulose, lactose, magnesium stearate, microcrystalline cellulose and titanium dioxide. Potassium: 8.48 mg (<1 mmol). Blister packages of 30. Bottles of 100.

(Shown in Product Identification Section)

CO Zopiclone

zopiclone

Hypnotic

Cobalt

SUPPLIED: 5 mg: Each white to off-white, round tablet, with "Z5"on one side and "Σ>" on the other side, contains: zopiclone 5 mg. Nonmedicinal ingredients: calcium hydrogen phosphate, HPMC 2910/hypromellose 6cP, lactose monohydrate, macrogol/PEG 3000, magnesium stearate, potato starch dried, silicon dioxide, sodium starch glycolate, titanium dioxide and triacetine/glycerol triacetate. Bottles of 100.

7.5 mg: Each blue, oval tablet, with "Z 7.5" on one side and "Σ>" on the other side, contains: zopiclone 7.5 mg. Nonmedicinal ingredients: calcium hydrogen phosphate, FD&C Blue #1/Billiant Blue FCF Aluminum Lake, macrogol/PEG 3350, magnesium stearate, polyvinyl alcohol (partially hydrolyzed), potato starch dried, silicon dioxide, sodium starch glycolate, talc and titanium dioxide. Bottles of 100 and 500.

Creon 5 Minimicrospheres®

pancreatic enzymes

Digestant

Abbott Products

Creon 10 Minimicrospheres®

pancreatic enzymes

Digestant

Abbott Products

Creon 25 Minimicrospheres®

pancreatic enzymes

Digestant

Abbott Products

Date of Preparation: August 3, 2001
Date of Revision: April 15, 2008

INDICATIONS: For replacement therapy where digestion is not adequate due to pancreatic exocrine insufficiency as in cystic fibrosis, chronic pancreatitis, steatorrhoea, post pancreatectomy, post gastrointestinal bypass surgery (e.g., gastroenterostomy) and ductal obstruction from neoplasm.

CONTRAINDICATIONS: Patients with known hypersensitivity to porcine proteins, pancreatic enzymes, or to any excipients. Do not use during the early stages of acute pancreatitis.

WARNINGS: Rarely, cases of hyperuricosuria and hyperuricaemia have been reported with very high doses of pancreatin.

Perianal irritation, and rarely, inflammation, could occur when large doses are used.

PRECAUTIONS: See Warnings.

Pregnancy: There are no adequate data from the use of CREON MINIMICROSPHERES in pregnant women. Animal studies are insufficient with respect to effects on pregnancy and embryonal/foetal development, parturition and postnatal development. The potential risk for humans is unknown. CREON MINIMICROSPHERES should not be used during pregnancy or lactation unless clearly necessary.

Lactation: See Pregnancy.

Drug Interactions: There have been no reports of interactions with other drugs or other forms of interaction.

Occupational Hazards: Effects on Ability to Drive and Use Machines: There is no evidence that CREON has any effect on the ability to drive or operate machines.

ADVERSE EFFECTS: Adverse effects from pancreatin products are rare. In pooled data from clinical trials, the overall incidence of adverse drug reactions reported with pancreatin was the same as with placebo.

Gastrointestinal Disorders: abdominal discomfort/pain (common), constipation (uncommon), abnormal stool (uncommon), diarrhea (uncommon), and nausea/vomiting (uncommon) have been reported, but are also often symptoms of the diseases treated. With high doses perianal irritation/inflammation have also been reported.

Strictures of the ileo-caecum and large bowel (fibrosing colonopathy) and colitis have been reported in patients with cystic fibrosis taking high doses of pancreatin preparations. Case control studies did not reveal evidence of an association between Creon and the appearance of fibrosing colonopathy. As a precaution, unusual abdominal symptoms or changes in abdominal symptoms should be reviewed to exclude the possibility of colonic damage, especially if the patient is taking in excess of 10 000 units of lipase/kg/day.

Metabolism and Nutritional: With high doses, cases of hyperuricosuria and hyperuricaemia have been reported.

Skin and Subcutaneous Tissue Disorders: Allergic or hypersensitivity reactions of the skin were reported (uncommon).

OVERDOSE:

Symptoms: Extremely high doses of pancreatin have been reported to be associated with hyperuricosuria and hyperuricaemia.

Treatment: Most cases of overdose respond to supportive measures, including stopping enzyme therapy and ensuring adequate rehydration.

For management of a suspected drug overdose, CPhA recommends that you contact your **regional Poison Control Centre**. See the *CPS* Directory section for a list of Poison Control Centres.

DOSAGE: CREON 5 MINIMICROSPHERES: Initially, two to four capsules with each meal and two to four capsules with each snack.

CREON 10 MINIMICROSPHERES: Initially, one or two capsules with each meal and one capsule with each snack.

CREON 25 MINIMICROSPHERES: Initially, one capsule with each meal and one capsule with each snack.

Dosage increases, if required, should be added slowly, with careful monitoring of response and symptomatology.

It is important to ensure adequate hydration of patients at all times during dosing with pancreatic enzymes.

The capsules should be swallowed whole. Where swallowing the capsules is difficult, they may be opened and the minimicrospheres taken with soft food or fluid. Any mixture of the minimicrospheres with food or liquids should be used immediately and not stored; otherwise dissolution of the enteric coating may occur.

To protect the enteric coating, the minimicrospheres must not be crushed or chewed.

The product should not be administered after the expiry date printed on the package.

SUPPLIED: CREON 5 MINIMICROSPHERES: Each opaque, blue/orange hard gelatin capsule, imprinted in white with SOLVAY and 1205, contains: buff-colored enteric-coated minimicrospheres of pancreatin corresponding to: 5000 USP units of lipase, 16 600 USP units of amylase and 18 750 USP units proteases. Nonmedicinal ingredients: dibutylphthalate, dimethicone 1000, FD&C Blue #2, gelatin, hydroxypropyl methylcellulose phthalate, red iron oxide, yellow iron oxide, light mineral oil, polyethylene glycol 4000 and titanium dioxide. Gluten-, lactose- and tartrazine-free. Bottles of 100. Store in tightly closed, light resistant container at controlled room temperature (15 to 30°C). Protect from moisture. Do not refrigerate. Keep out of reach of children.

CREON 10 MINIMICROSPHERES: Each opaque, brown/colorless-transparent, hard gelatin capsule, imprinted in white with SOLVAY and 1210, contains: buff-colored enteric-coated minimicrospheres of pancreatin corresponding to 10 000 USP units of lipase, 33 200 USP units of amylase and 37 500 USP units of proteases. Nonmedicinal ingredients: dibutylphthalate, dimethicone 1000, gelatin, hydroxypropyl methylcellulose, phthalate, black iron oxide, red iron oxide, yellow iron oxide, light mineral oil, polyethylene glycol 4000 and titanium dioxide. Gluten-, lactose- and tartrazine-free. Bottles of 100. Store in tightly closed, light resistant container at controlled room temperature (15 to 30°C). Protect from moisture. Do not refrigerate. Keep out of reach of children.

CREON 25 MINIMICROSPHERES: Each opaque, orange/colorless-transparent hard gelatin capsule, contains: buff-colored enteric-coated minimicrospheres of pancreatin corresponding to: 25 000 USP units of lipase, 74 000 USP units of amylase and 62 500 USP units of proteases. Nonmedicinal ingredients: dibutylphthalate, dimethicone 1000, gelatin, red iron oxide, yellow iron oxide, macrogol 4000, methylhydroxypropylcellulose phthalate, paraffinum perliquidum and titanium dioxide. Gluten-, lactose- and tartrazine-free. Bottles of 100. Store in tightly closed, light resistant container at controlled room temperature (15 to 30°C). Protect from moisture. Do not refrigerate. Keep out of reach of children.

(Shown in Product Identification Section)

The reader is invited to consult CPhA's monograph **HMG-CoA Reductase Inhibitors**.

Crestor®

rosuvastatin calcium

Lipid Metabolism Regulator

AstraZeneca

Date of Preparation: February 10, 2003
Date of Revision: April 28, 2010

SUMMARY PRODUCT INFORMATION:

Route of Administration	Dosage Form/Strength	All Nonmedicinal Ingredients
Oral	Tablets: 5, 10, 20 and 40 mg	Calcium phosphate, crospovidone, glycerol triacetate, hydroxypropyl methylcellulose, lactose monohydrate, magnesium stearate, microcrystalline cellulose, ferric oxide red, ferric oxide yellow, titanium dioxide

INDICATIONS AND CLINICAL USE: Hypercholesterolemia: Adults: CRESTOR (rosuvastatin calcium) is indicated as an adjunct to diet, at least equivalent to the Adult Treatment Panel III (ATP III TLC diet), for the reduction of elevated total cholesterol (Total-C), LDL-C, ApoB, the Total-C/HDL-C ratio and triglycerides (TG) and for increasing HDL-C; in hyperlipidemic and dyslipidemic conditions, when response to diet and exercise alone has been inadequate including:

- Primary hypercholesterolemia (Type IIa including heterozygous familial hypercholesterolemia and severe non-familial hypercholesterolemia)
- Combined (mixed) dyslipidemia (Type IIb)
- Homozygous familial hypercholesterolemia where CRESTOR is used either alone or as an adjunct to diet and other lipid lowering treatments such as apheresis.

Pediatrics (10-17 years of age): CRESTOR is indicated as an adjunct to diet for the reduction of elevated total cholesterol (Total-C), LDL-C and ApoB in boys and girls who are at least one year post-menarche, 10 to 17 years of age with heterozygous familial hypercholesterolemia, when response to diet alone has been inadequate.

Prevention of Major Cardiovascular Events: In adult patients without documented history of cardiovascular or cerebrovascular events, but with at least two conventional risk factors for cardiovascular disease, CRESTOR is indicated to:

- Reduce the risk of nonfatal myocardial infarction
- Reduce the risk of nonfatal stroke
- Reduce the risk of coronary artery revascularization

CONTRAINDICATIONS: CRESTOR (rosuvastatin calcium) is contraindicated:

- In patients who are hypersensitive to any component of this medication (see Dosage Forms, Composition and Packaging).
- In patients with active liver disease or unexplained persistent elevations of serum transaminases exceeding 3 times the upper limit of normal (see Warnings and Precautions).
- In pregnant and nursing women.

Cholesterol and other products of cholesterol biosynthesis are essential components for fetal development (including synthesis of steroids and cell membranes). CRESTOR should be administered to women of childbearing age only when such patients are highly unlikely to conceive and have been informed of the possible harm. If the patient becomes pregnant while taking CRESTOR, the drug should be discontinued immediately and the patient apprised of the potential harm to the fetus. Atherosclerosis being a chronic process, discontinuation of lipid metabolism regulating drugs during pregnancy should have little impact on the outcome of long-term therapy of primary hypercholesterolemia (see Warnings and Precautions, Special Populations, Pregnant Women, Nursing Women).

- In patients using concomitant cyclosporine (see Drug Interactions).

CRESTOR **40 mg is contraindicated** in:

- Asian patients
- Patients with pre-disposing factors for myopathy/rhabdomyolysis such as:
  - Personal or family history of hereditary muscular disorders
  - Previous history of muscle toxicity with another HMG-CoA reductase inhibitor
  - Concomitant use of a fibrate or niacin
  - Severe hepatic impairment
  - Severe renal impairment (CrCl <30 mL/min/1.73 m²) (see Dosage and Administration, Patients with Renal Impairment)
  - Hypothyroidism
  - Alcohol abuse
  - Situations where an increase in rosuvastatin plasma levels may occur.

WARNINGS AND PRECAUTIONS: General: Before instituting therapy with CRESTOR (rosuvastatin calcium), an attempt should be made to control hypercholesterolemia with appropriate diet, exercise, weight reduction in overweight patients and to treat other underlying medical problems and associated cardiovascular risk factors. The patient should be advised to inform subsequent physicians of the prior use of CRESTOR or any other lipid-lowering agent.

Cardiovascular: Co-enzyme Q_{10} (ubiquinone): Ubiquinone levels were not measured in CRESTOR clinical trials. Significant decreases in circulating ubiquinone levels in patients treated with other statins have been observed. The clinical significance of a potential long-term statin-induced deficiency of ubiquinone has not been established. It has been reported that a decrease in myocardial ubiquinone levels could lead to impaired cardiac function in patients with borderline congestive heart failure.

Endocrine and Metabolism: Endocrine Function: HMG-CoA reductase inhibitors interfere with cholesterol synthesis and lower cholesterol levels and, as such, might theoretically blunt adrenal or gonadal steroid hormone production. Rosuvastatin demonstrated no effect upon nonstimulated cortisol levels and no effect on thyroid metabolism as assessed by TSH plasma concentration. In CRESTOR-treated patients, there was no impairment of adrenocortical reserve and no reduction in plasma cortisol concentrations. Clinical studies with other HMG-CoA reductase inhibitors have suggested that these agents do not reduce plasma testosterone concentration. The effects of HMG-CoA reductase inhibitors on male fertility have not been studied. The effects, if any, on the pituitary-gonadal axis in premenopausal women are unknown.

Patients treated with rosuvastatin who develop clinical evidence of endocrine dysfunction should be evaluated appropriately. Caution should be exercised if an HMG-CoA reductase inhibitor or other agent used to lower cholesterol levels is administered to patients receiving other drugs (e.g. ketoconazole, spironolactone or cimetidine) that may decrease the levels of endogenous steroid hormones.

Plasma Glucose: In the JUPITER trial, rosuvastatin 20 mg was observed to increase plasma glucose levels, which were sufficient to shift some prediabetic subjects to the diabetes mellitus status (see Adverse Reactions).

Lipoprotein (a): In some patients, the beneficial effect of lowered total cholesterol and LDL-C levels may be partly blunted by a concomitant increase in the Lipoprotein(a) [Lp(a)] concentrations. Present knowledge suggests the importance of high Lp(a) levels as an emerging risk factor for coronary heart disease. It is thus desirable to maintain and reinforce lifestyle changes in high risk patients placed on rosuvastatin therapy.

Hepatic/Biliary/Pancreatic: Hepatic Effects: CRESTOR is contraindicated in patients with active liver disease or unexplained persistent elevations of serum transaminases exceeding 3 times the upper limit of normal.

As with other HMG-CoA reductase inhibitors, it is recommended that a liver function test be carried out prior to, and 3 months following, the initiation of CRESTOR or if the patient is titrated to the dose of 40 mg. CRESTOR should be discontinued or the dose reduced if the level of transaminases is greater than 3 times the upper limit of normal.

CRESTOR, as well as other HMG-CoA reductase inhibitors should be used with caution in patients who consume substantial quantities of alcohol and/or have a past history of liver disease.

As with other HMG-CoA reductase inhibitors, a dose-related increase in transaminases has been observed in a small number of patients taking rosuvastatin (<0.5%); the majority of cases were mild, asymptomatic and transient.

Hepatic Impairment: In subjects with varying degrees of hepatic impairment there was no evidence of increased exposure to rosuvastatin other than in 2 subjects with the most severe liver disease (Child-Pugh scores of 8 and 9). In these subjects, systemic exposure was increased by at least 2-fold compared to subjects with lower Child-Pugh scores (see Dosage and Administration, Patients with Hepatic Impairment).

Muscle Effects: Rare cases of rhabdomyolysis with acute renal failure secondary to myoglobinuria, have been reported with CRESTOR and with other HMG-CoA reductase inhibitors.

Effects on skeletal muscle such as myalgia, myopathy and, rarely, rhabdomyolysis have been reported in patients treated with CRESTOR at all doses and in particular with the 40 mg dose.

Myopathy, defined as muscle pain or muscle weakness in conjunction with increases in creatine kinase (CK) values to greater than ten times the upper limit of normal, should be considered in any patient with diffuse myalgias, muscle tenderness or weakness and/or marked elevation of CK. Patients should be advised to report promptly any unexplained muscle pain, tenderness or weakness, particularly if associated with malaise or fever. Patients who develop any signs or symptoms suggestive of myopathy should have their CK levels measured. CRESTOR therapy should be discontinued if markedly elevated CK levels (>10×ULN) are measured or myopathy is diagnosed or suspected.

Pre-disposing Factors for Myopathy/Rhabdomyolysis: CRESTOR, as with other HMG-CoA reductase inhibitors, should be prescribed with caution in patients with pre-disposing factors for myopathy/rhabdomyolysis. Such factors include: personal or family history of hereditary muscular disorders; previous history of muscle toxicity with another HMG-CoA reductase inhibitor; concomitant use of a fibrate or niacin; hypothyroidism; alcohol abuse; excessive physical exercise; age >70 years; renal impairment; hepatic impairment; diabetes with hepatic fatty change; surgery and trauma; frailty; situations where an increase in plasma levels of rosuvastatin may occur.

In CRESTOR trials there was no evidence of increased skeletal muscle effects when CRESTOR was dosed with concomitant therapy such as fibric acid derivatives (including fenofibrate and gemfibrozil), nicotinic acid, azole antifungals and macrolide antibiotics. However, an increase in the incidence of myositis and myopathy has been seen in patients receiving other HMG-CoA reductase inhibitors together with these medicines.

CRESTOR therapy should be temporarily withheld or discontinued in any patient with an acute serious condition suggestive of myopathy or predisposing to the development of rhabdomyolysis (e.g. sepsis, hypotension, major surgery, trauma, severe metabolic endocrine and electrolyte disorders, or uncontrolled seizures).

Renal: Renal Impairment: Subjects with severe renal impairment (CrCl <30 mL/min/1.73 m²) had a 3-fold increase in plasma concentration of rosuvastatin compared to healthy volunteers and, therefore, CRESTOR 40 mg is contraindicated in these patients (see Contraindications, and Dosage and Administration, Patients with Renal Impairment).

In subjects with varying degrees of renal impairment, mild to moderate renal disease had little influence on plasma concentrations of rosuvastatin.

During the clinical development program, dipstick-positive proteinuria and microscopic hematuria were observed among rosuvastatin-treated patients, predominantly in patients dosed above the recommended dose range (i.e. 80 mg). Abnormal urinalysis testing (dipstick-positive proteinuria) has been seen in patients taking CRESTOR and other HMG-CoA reductase inhibitors. This finding was more frequent in patients taking 40 mg when compared to lower doses of rosuvastatin or comparator statins. Shifts in urine protein from none or trace to ++ (dipstick) or more were seen in <1% of patients at some time during treatment with 10 and 20 mg, and in approximately 3% of patients treated with 40 mg. The protein detected was mostly tubular in origin. In most cases, proteinuria was generally transient and it decreased or disappeared spontaneously on continued therapy. It has not been shown to be predictive of acute or progressive renal disease.

Nevertheless, a dose reduction may be considered for patients with unexplained persistent proteinuria during routine testing.

Sensitivity/Resistance: Hypersensitivity: An apparent hypersensitivity syndrome has been reported rarely with other HMG-CoA reductase inhibitors. This has included one or more of the following features: anaphylaxis, angioedema, lupus erythematous-like syndrome, polymyalgia rheumatica, vasculitis, purpura, thrombocytopenia, leukopenia, hemolytic anemia, positive antinuclear antibody (ANA), erythrocyte sedimentation rate (ESR) increase, eosinophilia, arthritis, arthralgia, urticaria, asthenia, photosensitivity, fever, chills, flushing, malaise, dyspnea, toxic epidermal necrolysis and erythema multiforme including Stevens-Johnson syndrome. Treatment should be discontinued if hypersensitivity is suspected (see Contraindications).

Special Populations: Pregnant Women: CRESTOR is contraindicated during pregnancy (see Contraindications).

Nursing Women: It is not known whether rosuvastatin is excreted in human milk. Because of the potential for adverse reactions in nursing infants, women taking CRESTOR should not breast-feed (see Contraindications).

Pediatrics (10-17 years of age): Elevations in serum creatine phosphokinase (CK) >10×ULN were observed more frequently in pediatric patients treated with CRESTOR compared with placebo. CK elevation >10×ULN (with or without muscle symptoms) was more frequent with increasing CRESTOR dose (see Adverse Reactions, Pediatrics (10-17 years of age)).

The evaluation of linear growth (height), weight, BMI (body mass index), and secondary characteristics of sexual maturation by Tanner staging in boys and girls who are at least one year post-menarche (10 to 17 years of age) with heterozygous familial hypercholesterolemia treated with CRESTOR was limited to a one-year period. Although endocrinology function, such as hormone disturbances, was not assessed, CRESTOR had no detectable effect on growth or sexual maturation. The effects on menstrual cycle were not assessed. CRESTOR doses greater than 20 mg have not been studied in this patient population (see Adverse Reactions, Pediatrics (10-17 years of age) and Dosage and Administration, Pediatrics (10-17 years of age)).

Adolescent females should be counselled on appropriate contraceptive methods while on CRESTOR therapy (see Contraindications and Warnings and Precautions, Special Populations, Pregnant Women).

Treatment experience with CRESTOR in pediatric patients (aged 8 years and above) with homozygous familial hypercholesterolemia is limited to 8 patients.

Geriatrics (≥65 years of age): There were no clinically significant pharmacokinetic differences between young and elderly patients (≥65 years) (see Dosage and Administration, Use in Elderly). However, elderly patients may be more susceptible to myopathy (see Warnings and Precautions, Muscle Effects, Pre-disposing Factors for Myopathy/Rhabdomyolysis).

Race: Results of pharmacokinetic studies, including a large study conducted in North America, have demonstrated an approximate 2-fold elevation in median exposure in Asian subjects (having either Filipino, Chinese, Japanese, Korean, Vietnamese or Asian-Indian origin) when compared with a Caucasian control group. This increase should be considered when making rosuvastatin dosing decisions for Asian patients and the dose of 40 mg is contraindicated in these patients (see Action and Clinical Pharmacology, Pharmacokinetics, Special Populations and Conditions, Contraindications and Dosage and Administration, Race).

ADVERSE REACTIONS: Adverse Drug Reaction Overview: CRESTOR (rosuvastatin calcium) is generally well tolerated. The adverse events seen with CRESTOR are generally mild and transient.

CRESTOR clinical trial experience is extensive, involving 9800 patients treated with CRESTOR in placebo controlled trials and 9855 patients treated with CRESTOR in active controlled clinical trials. Discontinuation of therapy due to adverse events occurred in 2.6% of patients receiving CRESTOR and 1.8% of patients receiving placebo. The most frequently reported adverse events at an incidence ≥1% and at a rate greater than placebo were arthralgia, upper abdominal pain and ALT increase. Adverse events observed or reported in short- and long-term trials are as follows.

Clinical Trial Adverse Drug Reactions: Because clinical trials are conducted under very specific conditions the adverse drug reaction rates observed in the clinical trials may not reflect the rates observed in practice and should not be compared to the rates in the clinical trials of another drug. Adverse drug reaction information from clinical trials is useful for identifying drug-related adverse events and for approximating rates.

Adults: Short-term Controlled Trials: Short-term controlled trials involved 1290 patients within placebo-controlled trials of 6 to 16 weeks' duration (768 of which were treated with rosuvastatin) and 11641 patients within placebo and active controlled clinical trials of 6 to 52 weeks duration (5319 of which were treated with rosuvastatin). In all controlled clinical trials, 3.2% of patients were withdrawn from CRESTOR therapy due to adverse events. This withdrawal rate was comparable to that reported in placebo-controlled studies.

Associated adverse events occurring at an incidence ≥1% in patients participating in placebo-controlled clinical studies of rosuvastatin, are shown in Table 1.

Table 1: CRESTOR

Number (%) of Subjects with Associated Adverse Events Occurring with ≥1% Incidence in any Treatment Group: Placebo Controlled Pool

Body System/ Adverse Event	Placebo (%) (N=367)	Total Rosuvastatin (%) (N=768)
Whole Body		
Abdominal Pain	2.2	1.7
Asthenia	0.5	1.3
Headache	2.2	1.4
Digestive		
Constipation	1.4	1.0
Diarrhea	1.6	1.3
Dyspepsia	1.9	0.7
Flatulence	2.7	1.8
Nausea	1.6	2.2
Musculoskeletal		
Myalgia	0.5	1.6
Nervous System		
Dizziness	1.6	0.5
Insomnia	1.9	0.4

Long-term Controlled Morbidity and Mortality Trials: In the Justification for the Use of Statins in Primary Prevention: An Intervention Trial Evaluating Rosuvastatin (JUPITER) study involving 17 802 participants treated with CRESTOR 20 mg once daily (n=8901) or placebo (n=8901), CRESTOR 20 mg was generally well tolerated. Subjects were followed for a mean duration of 2 years.

Discontinuation of therapy due to an adverse event occurred in 5.6% of subjects treated with CRESTOR and 5.5% of subjects treated with placebo. The most common adverse events that led to discontinuation from the study were: myalgia, arthralgia, abdominal pain and constipation. The associated adverse reaction reported in ≥1% of patients and at a rate greater than or equal to placebo was myalgia (2.4 % CRESTOR, 2.0 % placebo).

Treatment emergent adverse events regardless of causality occurring at an incidence ≥1% and at a rate greater than placebo in patients participating in the JUPITER trial are shown in Table 2.

Table 2: CRESTOR

Number (%) of Subjects with Treatment Emergent Adverse Events Regardless of Causality Occurring with ≥1% Incidence and > than Placebo: JUPITER

Body System/Adverse Event	Placebo (%) (N=8901)	Total Rosuvastatin 20 mg (%) (N=8901)
Blood		
Anemia	2.1	2.2
Cardiac		
Palpitations	0.9	1.0
Gastrointestinal		
Diarrhea	4.6	4.7
Constipation	3.0	3.3
Nausea	2.3	2.4
General Disorders		
Edema peripheral	3.0	3.7
Fatigue	3.5	3.7
Hepatobiliary		
Cholelithiasis	0.9	1.0
Infections		
Urinary tract	8.6	8.7
Nasopharyngitis	7.2	7.6
Bronchitis	7.1	7.2
Sinusitis	3.7	4.0
Influenza	3.6	4.0
Lower Respiratory tract	2.7	2.9
Gastroenteritis	1.7	1.9
Herpes zoster	1.4	1.6
Injury		
Contusion	1.4	1.7
Investigation		
ALT increased	1.0	1.4
Blood glucose increased	0.7	1.0
Metabolism		
Diabetes mellitus	2.5	3.0
Musculoskeletal		
Back pain	6.9	7.6
Myalgia	6.6	7.6
Arthritis	5.6	5.8
Arthralgia	3.2	3.8
Muscle spasms	3.2	3.6
Osteoarthritis	1.4	1.8
Bursitis	1.3	1.5
Neck pain	1.0	1.1
Osteoporosis	0.8	1.0
Neoplasms		
Basal cell carcinoma	0.9	1.0
Psychiatric		
Insomnia	2.3	2.5
Renal		
Hematuria	2.0	2.4
Proteinuria	1.3	1.4

(cont'd)

Table 2: CRESTOR *(cont'd)*

Number (%) of Subjects with Treatment Emergent Adverse Events Regardless of Causality Occurring with ≥1% Incidence and > than Placebo: JUPITER

Body System/Adverse Event	Placebo (%) (N=8901)	Total Rosuvastatin 20 mg (%) (N=8901)
Respiratory		
Epistaxis	0.8	1.0

Less Common Clinical Trial Adverse Drug Reactions (<1%): The frequency of adverse events in all clinical trials and considered possibly, probably or definitely drug related are as follows:

Uncommon (≥0.1% and <1%): pruritus, rash, urticaria, arthralgia, muscle weakness, arthritis, constipation, nausea, dyspepsia, gastroesophageal reflux disease, ALT increase, creatine phosphokinase increase, hepatic enzyme increase, creatinine increase, paraesthesia, tremor, general pain, proteinuria, sinusitis, insomnia, abnormal hepatic function, vertigo, diabetes mellitus.

Rare (≥0.01% and <0.1%): myopathy (including myositis), rhabdomyolysis, and hypersensitivity reactions including angioedema.

The following additional adverse events were reported in controlled clinical trials, regardless of causality: accidental injury, back and chest pain, flu syndrome, infection, urinary tract infection, diarrhea, flatulence, gastroenteritis, hypertonia, bronchitis, increased cough, rhinitis and pharyngitis.

In long-term controlled clinical trials CRESTOR was shown to have no harmful effect on the ocular lens.

Abnormal Hematologic and Clinical Chemistry Findings: As with other HMG-CoA reductase inhibitors, a dose-related increase in liver transaminases and CK has been observed in a small number of patients taking rosuvastatin (see Warnings and Precautions, Hepatic/Biliary/Pancreatic).

Abnormal urinalysis testing (dipstick-positive proteinuria) has been seen in a small number of patients taking CRESTOR and other HMG-CoA reductase inhibitors. The protein detected was mostly tubular in origin. In most cases, proteinuria decreases or disappears spontaneously on continued therapy and is not predictive of acute or progressive renal disease (see Warnings and Precautions, Renal).

In the JUPITER trial, occurrences of diabetes mellitus as a pre-specified secondary outcome were reported more frequently in the CRESTOR-treated patients (2.8%) than in placebo (2.3%) and a slight increase in the number of subjects whose fasting glucose levels increased to ≥5.6 mmol/L (126 mg/dL) was observed in subjects treated with CRESTOR. There was a 0.1% increase in mean HbA1c with CRESTOR compared to placebo. A causal relationship with statins and diabetes mellitus has not been definitely established.

Pediatrics (10-17 years of age): The safety profile of CRESTOR in pediatric patients (boys and girls who are at least one year post-menarche, 10-17 years of age with heterozygous familial hypercholesterolemia) is similar to adults although CK elevations >10×ULN (with or without muscle symptoms) were observed more frequently in a clinical trial of pediatric patients.

CRESTOR was evaluated in a multicentre double-blind, placebo-controlled study of pediatric patients with heterozygous familial hypercholesterolemia. During the 12-week double-blind phase (n=176), patients were randomized to CRESTOR 5 mg, 10 mg or 20 mg or placebo. Four of 130 (3.0%) pediatric patients treated with CRESTOR (2 treated with 10 mg and 2 treated with 20 mg) had increased CK >10×ULN compared to 0 of 46 patients on placebo.

Myopathy was reported in 2 patients receiving CRESTOR, one on 10 mg and one on 20 mg. During the 40-week open label titration-to-goal phase of the study (n=173), 122 of 173 patients were titrated to CRESTOR 20 mg; 4 of the 173 (2.3%) pediatric patients treated with CRESTOR 20 mg had increased CK >10×ULN (with or without muscle symptoms). All patients with CK elevations either continued treatment or resumed treatment after an interruption.

Myalgia was reported in 4 of the 130 (3.0%) pediatric patients treated with CRESTOR (1 treated with 5 mg, 1 treated with 10 mg and 2 treated with 20 mg) compared with 0 of 46 on placebo in the 12-week double-blind phase. In the 40-week open label titration-to-goal phase, myalgia was reported in 5 of 173 (2.9%) pediatric patients treated with CRESTOR.

Mean change in ALT and AST values from baseline were slightly higher in the CRESTOR group versus placebo; however, were not considered to be clinically significant. One patient, experienced an ALT elevation >3×ULN which returned to normal subsequent to an interruption in treatment.

Two adverse events of depression were reported in pediatric patients treated with CRESTOR 20 mg, one of which was determined to be causally related to treatment by the investigator.

Not all adverse reactions that have been identified in the adult populations have been observed in the clinical trials of pediatric patients. However, the same warnings and precautions for use and adverse events in adults also apply to pediatric patients (see Warnings and Precautions and Adverse Reactions).

Post-Market Adverse Drug Reactions: In addition to the events reported above, the following adverse events have been reported during post-marketing experience with CRESTOR, regardless of causality assessment.

Skeletal Muscle Effects: Very rare: arthralgia.

It has been observed that as with other HMG-CoA reductase inhibitors, the reporting rate for rhabdomyolysis in post-marketing use is higher at the highest marketed dose (see Warnings and Precautions, Muscle Effects).

Hepatobiliary Disorders: Very rare: jaundice, hepatitis.

Nervous System Disorders: Very rare: memory loss.

Other: Rare: pancreatitis; Very rare: gynecomastia.

DRUG INTERACTIONS: Overview: In CRESTOR (rosuvastatin calcium) clinical trials there was no evidence of increased skeletal muscle effects when rosuvastatin was dosed with any concomitant therapy. However, CRESTOR and other HMG-CoA reductase inhibitors may cause dose-related increases in serum transaminases and CK levels. An increase in the incidence of myositis and myopathy has been seen in patients receiving other HMG-CoA reductase inhibitors with cyclosporine, fibric acid derivatives (including gemfibrozil), nicotinic acid, azole antifungals and macrolide antibiotics.

Cytochrome P450 Inhibitors: In vitro and in vivo data indicate that rosuvastatin has no clinically significant cytochrome P450 interactions (as substrate, inhibitor or inducer). Consequently, there is little potential for drug-drug interactions upon coadministration with agents that are metabolised by cytochrome P450. Rosuvastatin clearance is not dependent on metabolism by cytochrome P450 3A4 to a clinically significant extent. This has been confirmed in studies with known cytochrome P450 3A4 inhibitors (ketoconazole, erythromycin, itraconazole).

Concomitant Therapy with Other Lipid Metabolism Regulators: Coadministration of fenofibrate and CRESTOR 10 mg did not lead to a clinically significant change in the plasma concentrations of either drug. In addition, neither myopathy nor marked CK elevations (>10×ULN) were observed in a study of 128 patients who received CRESTOR 10, 20 and 40 mg plus extended-release niacin or in a second study of 103 patients who received CRESTOR 5 and 10 mg plus fenofibrate. Based on the above data, no pharmacokinetic or pharmacodynamic interaction was observed. No data is available with other fibrates.

Based on post-marketing surveillance, gemfibrozil, fenofibrate, other fibrates and lipid lowering doses of niacin (nicotinic acid) may increase the risk of myopathy when given concomitantly with HMG-CoA reductase inhibitors, probably because they can produce myopathy when given alone (see Warnings and Precautions, Muscle Effects, Pre-disposing Factors for Myopathy/Rhabdomyolysis). Therefore, combined drug therapy should be approached with caution.

Protease Inhibitors: Lopinavir/Ritonavir: In a pharmacokinetic study, coadministration of CRESTOR and a combination product of two protease inhibitors (400 mg lopinavir/100 mg ritonavir) in healthy volunteers was associated with an approximately 2-fold and 5-fold increase in rosuvastatin steady-state $AUC_{(0-24)}$ and C_{max} respectively.

Increased systemic exposure to rosuvastatin has been observed in subjects receiving CRESTOR with various protease inhibitors in combination with ritonavir. Consideration should be given both to the benefit of lipid lowering by the use of CRESTOR in HIV patients receiving protease inhibitors and the potential for increased rosuvastatin plasma concentrations when initiating and up-titrating CRESTOR doses in patients treated with protease inhibitors (see Warnings and Precautions, Muscle Effects, Pre-disposing Factors for Myopathy/Rhabdomyolysis).

Concomitant Therapies Without Clinically Significant Interactions: Bile Acid Sequestrants: CRESTOR can be used in combination with bile acid sequestrant (e.g. cholestyramine).

Ketoconazole: Coadministration of ketoconazole with CRESTOR resulted in no change in plasma concentrations of rosuvastatin.

Erythromycin: Coadministration of erythromycin with CRESTOR resulted in small decreases in plasma concentrations of rosuvastatin. These reductions were not considered clinically significant.

Itraconazole: Coadministration of itraconazole with CRESTOR resulted in a 28% increase in the AUC of rosuvastatin. This small increase was not considered clinically significant.

Fluconazole: Coadministration of fluconazole with CRESTOR resulted in a 14% increase in the AUC of rosuvastatin. This small increase was not considered clinically significant.

Digoxin: Coadministration of digoxin and CRESTOR did not lead to any clinically significant interactions.

Other Drugs: Although specific interaction studies were not performed, CRESTOR has been studied in over 5300 patients in clinical trials. Many patients were receiving a variety of medications including antihypertensive agents (beta-adrenergic blocking agents, calcium channel blockers, angiotensin-converting enzyme inhibitors, angiotensin receptor blockers and diuretics), antidiabetic agents (biguanides, sulfonylureas, alpha glucosidase inhibitors and thiazolidinediones) and hormone replacement therapy without evidence of clinically significant adverse interactions.

Drug-Drug Interactions: The drugs listed in Table 3 are based on either drug interaction case reports or studies or potential interactions due to the expected magnitude and seriousness of the interaction (i.e. those identified as contraindicated).

Table 3: CRESTOR

Established or Potential Drug-Drug Interactions

Proper Name	Effect	Clinical Comment
Gemfibrozil	Coadministration of a single rosuvastatin dose (10 mg) to healthy volunteers on gemfibrozil (600 mg bid) resulted in a 2.2- and 1.9-fold increase in mean C_{max} and mean AUC of rosuvastatin respectively.	Patients taking this combination should not exceed a dose of CRESTOR 20 mg once daily and the concomitant use of CRESTOR 40 mg once daily is contraindicated.
Coumarin Anticoagulants	As with other HMG-CoA reductase inhibitors, coadministration of CRESTOR and coumarin (e.g. warfarin) may result in a rise in International Normalized Ratio (INR) compared to coumarin alone. In healthy subjects, the co administration of rosuvastatin 40 mg (10 days) and warfarin 25 mg (single dose) produced a higher mean $_{max}$INR and AUC-INR than achieved with warfarin alone. Coadministration of CRESTOR 10 and 80 mg to patients on stable warfarin therapy resulted in clinically significant rises in INR (>4, baseline 2-3). The mechanism for this effect is unknown, but is likely due to a pharmacodynamic interaction with warfarin rather than a pharmacokinetic interaction as no relevant differences in the pharmacokinetics of either drug were observed.	In patients taking coumarin, monitoring of INR is recommended at initiation or cessation of therapy with rosuvastatin or following dose adjustment. Rosuvastatin therapy has not been associated with bleeding or changes in INR in patients not taking anticoagulants.
Antacids	Simultaneous dosing of CRESTOR with an antacid suspension containing aluminium and magnesium hydroxide resulted in a decrease of rosuvastatin plasma concentration by approximately 50%.	The clinical relevance of this interaction has not been studied. However, the effect was mitigated when the antacid was dosed 2 hours after CRESTOR. This interaction should not be clinically relevant in patients using this type of antacid infrequently. A frequent antacid user should be instructed to take CRESTOR at a time of day when they are less likely to need the antacid.
Oral Contraceptives	When CRESTOR 40 mg was coadministered with a representative oral contraceptive (ethinyl estradiol [35 µg] and norgestrel [180 µg on days 1 to 7, 215 µg on days 8 to 15, and 250 µg on days 16 to 21]) no reduction in contraceptive efficacy was observed. An increase in plasma concentrations (AUC) of ethinyl estradiol (26%) and norgestrel (34%) occurred.	These increased plasma levels should be considered when selecting oral contraceptive doses.
Immunosuppressants (Including Cyclosporine)	CRESTOR 10 and 20 mg were administered to cardiac transplant patients (at least 6 months post-transplant) whose concomitant medication included cyclosporine, prednisone and azathioprine. Results showed that cyclosporine pharmacokinetics were not affected by rosuvastatin. However, cyclosporine did increase the systemic exposure of rosuvastatin by 11-fold (C_{max}) and 7-fold ($AUC_{[0-24]}$) compared with historical data in healthy individuals.	The concomitant use of CRESTOR and cyclosporine is contraindicated (see Contraindications).

Drug-drug interaction studies have not been performed in pediatric patients (boys and girls who are at least one year post-menarche, 10 to 17 years of age) with heterozygous familial hypercholesterolemia.

Drug-Food Interactions: CRESTOR can be taken with or without food (see Dosage and Administration).

DOSAGE AND ADMINISTRATION: Patients should be placed on a standard cholesterol-lowering diet (at least equivalent to the Adult Treatment Panel III (ATP III TLC diet)) before receiving CRESTOR (rosuvastatin calcium), and should continue on this diet during treatment with CRESTOR. If appropriate, a program of weight control and physical exercise should be implemented.

Prior to initiating therapy with CRESTOR, secondary causes for elevations in plasma lipid levels should be excluded. A lipid profile should also be performed.

CRESTOR may be taken in the morning or evening, with or without food.

Recommended Dose and Dosage Adjustment: Adults: Hypercholesterolemia: The dose range of CRESTOR is 5 to 40 mg orally once a day. The recommended starting dose of CRESTOR in most patients is 10 mg orally once daily. The majority of patients are controlled at the 10 mg dose. If necessary, dose adjustment can be made at 2-4 week intervals. The maximum response is usually achieved within 2-4 weeks and is maintained during chronic therapy.

Initiation of therapy with CRESTOR 5 mg once daily may be considered for patients requiring less aggressive LDL-C reductions or who have predisposing factors for myopathy (see Warnings and Precautions, Muscle Effects).

Patients who are switched to CRESTOR from treatment with another HMG-CoA reductase inhibitor should be started on 10 mg even if they were on a high dose of the previous HMG-CoA reductase inhibitor. A switch dose of 20 mg may be considered for patients with severe hypercholesterolemia.

For patients with severe hypercholesterolemia (including those with familial hypercholesterolemia), a 20 mg start dose may be considered. These patients should be carefully followed.

A dose of 40 mg once daily should only be used in patients with severe hypercholesterolemia who do not achieve the desired effect on 20 mg and have no predisposing factors for myopathy/rhabdomyolysis (see Contraindications). Consultation with a specialist is recommended when initiating CRESTOR 40 mg dose.

The dosage of CRESTOR should be individualized according to baseline LDL-C, total C/HDL-C ratio and/or TG levels to achieve the recommended desired lipid values at the lowest possible dose.

Prevention of Major Cardiovascular Events: A dose of 20 mg once daily has been found to reduce the risk of major cardiovascular events.

Dosing Considerations in Special Populations: Patients with Hepatic Impairment: The usual dose range applies in patients with mild to moderate hepatic impairment. Increased systemic exposure has been observed in patients with severe hepatic impairment and, therefore, in these patients the dose of CRESTOR should not exceed 20 mg once daily (see Contraindications, and Warnings and Precautions, Hepatic/Biliary/Pancreatic, Hepatic Impairment).

Patients with Renal Impairment: The usual dose range applies in patients with mild to moderate renal impairment. Increased systemic exposure to rosuvastatin has been observed in patients with severe renal impairment. For patients with severe renal impairment (creatinine clearance <30 mL/min/1.73 m²) the starting dose of CRESTOR should be 5 mg and not exceed 10 mg once daily (see Contraindications, and Warnings and Precautions, Renal, Renal Impairment).

Race: The initial dose of CRESTOR, in Asian patients, should be 5 mg once daily. The potential for increases in systemic exposure must be considered when making treatment decisions. The maximum dose should not exceed CRESTOR 20 mg once daily (see Contraindications, and Warnings and Precautions, Special Populations, Race).

Pediatrics (10-17 years of age): In pediatric patients with heterozygous familial hypercholesterolemia the recommended starting dose of CRESTOR is 5 mg taken orally once daily. The CRESTOR dose should be individualized according to baseline LDL-C levels and the recommended goal of therapy. The maximum daily dose in this patient population is 10 mg.

The safety and efficacy of CRESTOR doses greater than 20 mg have not been studied in this population.

Treatment experience with CRESTOR in pediatric patients (aged 8 years and above) with homozygous familial hypercholesterolemia is limited to 8 patients. Use in this patient population should be supervised by specialists (see Warnings and Precautions, Special Populations, Pediatrics (10-17 years of age)).

Use in Elderly: No dose adjustment is necessary in the elderly (see Warnings and Precautions, Special Populations, Geriatrics (≥65 years of age).

Concomitant Therapy: See Warnings and Precautions, and Drug Interactions.

OVERDOSAGE:

There is no specific treatment in the event of over dosage. Should an overdose occur, the patient should be treated symptomatically and supportive measures instituted as required. Hemodialysis does not significantly enhance clearance of rosuvastatin.

> For management of a suspected drug overdose, contact your regional Poison Control Centre. See the *CPS* Directory section for a list of Poison Control Centres.

ACTION AND CLINICAL PHARMACOLOGY: Mechanism of Action: CRESTOR (rosuvastatin calcium) is a synthetic, enantiomerically pure lipid-lowering agent. It is a selective, potent and competitive inhibitor of 3-hydroxy-3-methylglutaryl-coenzyme A (HMG-CoA) reductase. This enzyme catalyses the conversion of HMG-CoA to mevalonate, which is an early and rate-limiting step in cholesterol biosynthesis.

Studies have shown that CRESTOR lowers plasma cholesterol and lipoprotein levels by inhibiting HMG-CoA reductase and cholesterol synthesis in the liver by increasing the number of hepatic Low Density Lipoprotein (LDL) receptors on the cell-surface for enhanced uptake and catabolism of LDL. Additionally, CRESTOR inhibits the hepatic synthesis of Very Low Density Lipoprotein (VLDL), thereby reducing the total number of VLDL and LDL particles.

Pharmacodynamics: Epidemiologic, clinical and experimental studies have established that high LDL-C, low HDL-C and high plasma TG promote human atherosclerosis and are risk factors for developing cardiovascular disease. Some studies have also shown that the total-C/HDL-C ratio is the best predictor of coronary artery disease. In contrast, increased levels of HDL-C are associated with decreased cardiovascular risk. Drug therapies that reduce levels of LDL-C or decrease TG while simultaneously increasing HDL-C have demonstrated reductions in rates of cardiovascular mortality and morbidity.

Pharmacokinetics: Absorption: CRESTOR is administered orally following which rosuvastatin, the active moiety, is rapidly absorbed, reaching peak plasma concentration 3 to 5 hours after dosing.

Both peak concentration (C_{max}) and area under the plasma concentration-time curve (AUC) increase in proportion to rosuvastatin dose. The absolute bioavailability of rosuvastatin is approximately 20% and there is no accumulation on repeated dosing. CRESTOR may be given with or without food. Administration in the morning or evening did not affect the rate and extent of absorption nor the ability of rosuvastatin to reduce LDL-C.

Distribution: Rosuvastatin undergoes first pass extraction in the liver, which is the primary site of cholesterol synthesis and LDL-C clearance. The mean volume of distribution at steady state of rosuvastatin is approximately 134 L. Rosuvastatin is approximately 90% bound to plasma proteins, mostly albumin. This binding is reversible and independent of plasma concentrations.

Metabolism: Rosuvastatin is not extensively metabolised with approximately 10% of a radiolabeled dose recovered as metabolite. The major metabolite is N-desmethyl rosuvastatin, which is formed principally by cytochrome P450 2C9, and in in vitro studies has demonstrated to have approximately one-half the HMG-CoA reductase inhibitory activity of rosuvastatin. The parent compound accounts for greater than 87% of the circulating active HMG-CoA reductase inhibitor activity.

Excretion: Following an oral dose, rosuvastatin and its metabolites are primarily excreted in the faeces (90%) with the remainder being excreted in the urine. Fecal recovery represents absorbed drug, metabolites in the bile and unabsorbed drug. The elimination half-life ($t_{1/2}$) of rosuvastatin is approximately 19 hours and does not increase with increasing doses.

Special Populations and Conditions: Pediatrics (10-17 years of age): There was no clinically relevant effect of age or sex on the pharmacokinetics of rosuvastatin in adults. The pharmacokinetics of rosuvastatin in pediatric patients 10 to 17 years of age with heterozygous familial hypercholesterolemia was similar to that of adult volunteers. Following single dose administration of CRESTOR 10 mg, the C_{max} values in two studies of healthy adult volunteers were 5.8 ng/mL (n=12) and 3.8 ng/mL (n=18) compared to 6.3 ng/mL (n=6) in pediatric patients with heterozygous familial hypercholesterolemia. The $AUC_{(0-t)}$ values in healthy adult volunteers were 45.9 ng·h/mL (n=12) and 31.6 ng·h/mL (n=18) compared to 52.2 ng·h/mL in pediatric patients with heterozygous familial hypercholesterolemia.

Race: A population pharmacokinetic analysis revealed no clinically relevant differences in pharmacokinetics among Caucasian, Hispanic and Black or Afro-Caribbean groups. However, pharmacokinetic studies with rosuvastatin, including one conducted in North America, have demonstrated an approximate 2-fold elevation in median exposure (AUC and C_{max}) in Asian subjects when compared with a Caucasian control group (see Contraindications and Warnings and Precautions, Special Populations, Race and Dosage and Administration, Race).

Primary Dysbetalipoproteinemia (Fredrickson Type III hyperlipoproteinemia): In a randomized, multicenter, double-blind crossover study, 32 patients (27 with ε2/ε2 genotype and 4 with apo E mutation [Arg145Cys]) with dysbetalipoproteinemia (Fredrickson Type III) received CRESTOR 10 or 20 mg daily for 6 weeks. CRESTOR 10 and 20 mg reduced non-HDL-C (primary end point) by 48% (95% CI: 45.6, 56.7) and 56% (95% CI: 48.5, 61.4), respectively. CRESTOR 10 and 20 mg respectively, also reduced Total-C (43% and 48%), TG (40% and 43%), VLDL-C+IDL-C (47% and 56%), LDL-C (54% and 57%), Remnant Lipoprotein Cholesterol (56% and 65%), Apo E (43% and 43%) and increased HDL-C (10% and 11%). The effect of CRESTOR on morbidity and mortality in this patient population has not been studied.

STORAGE AND STABILITY: Store between 15 and 30°C.

INFORMATION FOR THE PATIENT: Published in e-CPS, available by subscription at www.e-cps.ca.

DOSAGE FORMS, COMPOSITION AND PACKAGING: 5 mg: Each yellow, round, biconvex, film-coated tablet, printed "5" and "ZD4522" on one side, contains: rosuvastatin 5 mg as rosuvastatin calcium. Nonmedicinal ingredients: calcium phosphate, crospovidone, ferric oxide red, ferric oxide yellow, glycerol triacetate, hydroxypropyl methylcellulose, lactose monohydrate, microcrystalline cellulose, magnesium stearate and titanium dioxide. Blisters of 2×15 tablets. High-density polyethylene (HDPE) bottles of 90.

10 mg: Each pink, round, biconvex, film-coated tablet, printed "10" and "ZD4522" on one side, contains: rosuvastatin 10 mg as rosuvastatin calcium. Nonmedicinal ingredients: calcium phosphate, crospovidone, ferric oxide red, ferric oxide yellow, glycerol triacetate, hydroxypropyl methylcellulose, lactose monohydrate, microcrystalline cellulose, magnesium stearate and titanium dioxide. Blisters of 2×15 tablets. High-density polyethylene (HDPE) bottles of 90.

20 mg: Each pink, round, biconvex, film-coated tablet, printed "20" and "ZD4522" on one side, contains: rosuvastatin 20 mg as rosuvastatin calcium. Nonmedicinal ingredients: calcium phosphate, crospovidone, ferric oxide red, ferric oxide yellow, glycerol triacetate, hydroxypropyl methylcellulose, lactose monohydrate, microcrystalline cellulose, magnesium stearate and titanium dioxide. Blisters of 2×15 tablets. High-density polyethylene (HDPE) bottles of 90.

40 mg: Each pink, oval, biconvex, film-coated tablet, printed "40" on one side and "ZD4522" on the other, contains: rosuvastatin 40 mg as rosuvastatin calcium. Nonmedicinal ingredients: calcium phosphate, crospovidone, ferric oxide red, ferric oxide yellow, glycerol triacetate, hydroxypropyl methylcellulose, lactose monohydrate, microcrystalline cellulose, magnesium stearate and titanium dioxide. Blisters of 2×15 tablets. High-density polyethylene (HDPE) bottles of 30.

(Shown in Product Identification Section)

Crinone® ℞
progesterone
Progestin

EMD Canada

Date of Revision: May 2008

PHARMACOLOGY: CRINONE (progesterone gel) is a bioadhesive vaginal gel containing micronized progesterone in a diluted emulsion system. The carrier vehicle is a oil-in-water emulsion containing the water swellable, but insoluble polymer, polycarbophil. Physically, CRINONE has the appearance of a soft, white to off-white gel packed in single-use applicators designed for vaginal administration.

Progesterone is a naturally occurring steroid that is secreted by the ovary, placenta, and adrenal gland. In the presence of adequate estrogen progesterone transforms a proliferative endometrium into a secretory endometrium. Progesterone is essential for the development of decidual tissue, and the effect of progesterone on the differentiation of glandular epithelia and stroma has been extensively studied. Progesterone is necessary to increase endometrial receptivity for implantation of an embryo. Once an embryo is implanted, progesterone acts to maintain the pregnancy. Normal or near-normal endometrial responses to oral estradiol and intramuscular progesterone have been noted in functionally agonadal women through the sixth decade of life. Progesterone administration decreases the circulatory level of gonadotropins.

The release of progesterone from CRINONE 8% has been investigated in vitro.

Results indicate that approximately 65% of the progesterone is released from the gel within 24 hours, 87% is released at 48 hours, and 96% is released by 72 hours.

The pharmacokinetics of CRINONE are rate-limited by absorption rather than by elimination. Due to CRINONE's bioadhesive and sustained release properties, progesterone absorption is prolonged with an absorption half-life of approximately 25-50 hours, and an elimination half-life of 5-20 minutes.

The bioavailability of progesterone in CRINONE was determined relative to progesterone administered orally and vaginally. In a parallel group study, 18 healthy, estrogenized postmenopausal women received single doses of either 90 mg progesterone vaginally in CRINONE 8%, 100 mg progesterone orally in a capsule, or 100 mg progesterone vaginally in a capsule. After CRINONE 8% administration, the mean area under the plasma concentration curve (AUC) was 157.83 ng≅h/mL indicating a similar relative bioavailability to the vaginal capsule (247.41 ng≅h/mL) and more than 20 times higher than the bioavailability of the oral capsule (6.74 ng≅h/mL). These data suggested that when progesterone is given orally, up to 95% of the dose is eliminated by first-pass metabolism. The mean plasma concentrations following oral progesterone capsules and vaginal CRINONE administration were 1.04 and 3.49 ng/mL at 2 hours postdose (C_{max} for oral capsules), and 0 and 8.15 ng/mL at 8 hours (C_{max} for CRINONE), respectively. The variability in bioavailability was lower with CRINONE than with the capsule administered vaginally, indicating a more consistent delivery of progesterone.

The pharmacokinetics of CRINONE 90 mg administered twice daily for 12 days were studied in 10 healthy, estrogenized postmenopausal women. The average peak serum concentration achieved was 14.6 ng/mL four hours after administration. The average steady-state concentration was 11.6 ng/mL. Steady state was achieved within the first 24 hours after initialization of treatment. Upon attainment of steady-state, the disposition of progesterone administered by CRINONE suggests zero order release and absorption kinetics.

CRINONE 90 mg was applied twice daily in 50 women without ovarian function undergoing estrogen/CRINONE physiologic hormone replacement cycles designed for an Assisted Reproductive Technology (ART) procedure. Endometrial biopsies performed on Day 25-27 were histologically in-phase, consistent in morphological evaluation to natural luteal phase biopsy specimens at comparable time intervals. In this study, CRINONE was administered beginning the evening of Day 14 through Day 27 of the replacement cycle and continued if a pregnancy occurred, for about 10-12 weeks. Clinical pregnancies occurred in 48% of the women treated with CRINONE as part of their regimen.

In clinical pharmacodynamic studies, vaginal application of CRINONE containing 45 mg, 90 mg or 180 mg of progesterone every other day for a total of 6 or 7 applications resulted in mean steady state plasma progesterone concentrations of 1-4 ng/mL. CRINONE was administered in these studies from Day 15 through Day 25 of a replacement cycle. Despite the relatively low plasma progesterone concentrations, CRINONE induced a secretory transformation of the endometrium in 35 of the 36 women studied. The apparent discrepancy between the low plasma progesterone concentrations and the pronounced endometrial effects observed in these studies suggest a preferential distribution of transvaginally administered progesterone or a First Uterine-Pass Effect.

INDICATIONS: CRINONE (Progesterone gel) 8% is indicated for luteal phase support in induced cycles such as In Vitro Fertilization (IVF) cycles including in oocyte donation recipient.

CONTRAINDICATIONS: CRINONE (Progesterone gel) should not be used in individuals with any of the following conditions: undiagnosed vaginal bleeding, liver dysfunction or disease, known or suspected malignancy of the breast or genital organs, known or suspected progesterone-dependent neoplasia, known sensitivity to CRINONE (progesterone or any of the other ingredients), missed abortion, thrombophlebitis, thromboembolic disorders, cerebral apoplexy or patients with a history of these conditions, acute porphyria.

WARNINGS: The physician should be alert to the earliest manifestations of thrombotic disorders (thrombophlebitis, cerebrovascular disorders, pulmonary embolism, and retinal thrombosis). Should any of these occur or be suspected, the drug should be discontinued immediately. Patients who have risk factors for thrombotic disorders should be kept under careful observation.

Treatment should be discontinued if the results of liver function tests become abnormal or if cholestatic jaundice appears.

Progesterone and progestins have been used to prevent miscarriage in women with a history of recurrent spontaneous pregnancy losses. No adequate evidence is available to show that they are effective for this purpose.

As with all prescription drugs, this medicine should be kept out of the reach of children.

PRECAUTIONS: General: The pretreatment physical examination should include special reference to breast and pelvic organs, as well as Papanicolaou smear.

Because progestins may cause some degree of fluid retention, conditions which might be influenced by this factor (e.g., epilepsy, migraine, asthma, cardiac or renal dysfunction) require careful observation.

The pathologist should be advised of progesterone therapy when relevant specimens are submitted.

In cases of breakthrough bleeding, as in all cases of irregular bleeding per vagina, nonfunctional causes should be considered. In cases of undiagnosed vaginal bleeding, adequate diagnostic measures should be undertaken.

Patients who have a history of psychic depression should be carefully observed and the drug discontinued if the depression recurs to a serious degree.

A decrease in glucose tolerance has been observed in a small number of patients on oestrogen-progestin combination drugs. The mechanism of this decrease is not known. For this reason, diabetic patients should be carefully observed while receiving progestin therapy.

Lactation: CRINONE should not be used during lactation. While CRINONE is administered vaginally, detectable amounts of other orally administered progesterone have been identified in the milk of mothers receiving progesterone. The possible effects of progesterone on the nursing infant have not been determined.

Pregnancy: In case of corpus luteum deficiency, CRINONE can be used during the first trimester of pregnancy. CRINONE has been used to successfully support embryo implantation and maintain pregnancies through its use as part of ART treatment regimens. In fifty patients receiving donor oocyte transfer procedures, clinical pregnancies occurred in 48% of those receiving CRINONE. One woman had an elective termination of pregnancy at 19 weeks due to congenital malformations. Other deliveries resulted in normal newborns. CRINONE has been used in the luteal phase support of patients undergoing in vitro fertilization (IVF) procedures. In a clinical study, 139 patients received CRINONE (90 mg) once daily beginning on the day of embryo transfer and continuing through Day 30 post-transfer. The IVF success rates for pregnancies at Day 90 (26% of those transferred) and deliveries (23% of those transferred) were similar to success rates observed in larger IVF studies. Of the 47 newborns delivered, one suffered from a teratoma associated with a cleft palate and another from respiratory distress syndrome. Forty-four newborns were normal and one was lost to follow-up. The resulting rate of malformations was similar to that reported in the literature for pregnancies following IVF procedures as in normal pregnancies.

Drug Interactions: Although no drug interaction with other drugs have been reported, CRINONE is not recommended for use concurrently with other local vaginal preparations. If other local intravaginal therapy is to be used concurrently, there should be at least a 6 hour period before or after CRINONE administration.

Children: Safety and effectiveness in females before menarche have not been established. As CRINONE is indicated for use in women who are post-menarcheal, pediatric use is not applicable.

ADVERSE EFFECTS: In a multiple-dose study in a total of 57 women with ovarian failure undergoing a donor oocyte transfer procedure, the most frequently reported treatment emergent adverse reactions (in decreasing order) were cramps (non-specific) (16%), breast tenderness (14%), headache (12%), pain (7%), bloating (7%), nausea (7%) and vaginal discharge (7%). An increase (7%) of drowsiness frequency has been reported in a study on regular IVF.

In addition, intermenstrual bleeding (spotting), vaginal irritation and other mild application site reactions have been reported post-marketing. For adverse reactions identified during post-marketing surveillance, quantification of frequency has not been attempted, but it is most likely uncommon to very rare.

OVERDOSE:

Symptoms: There have been no reports of overdosage with CRINONE (progesterone gel). Acute overdosage is unlikely with this product due to the concentration-dependent, rate-limited absorption of progesterone by the vaginal epithelium and the controlled release characteristics of the formulation.

Treatment: In the case of overdosage, however, discontinue CRINONE, treat the patient symptomatically, and institute supportive measures.

> For management of a suspected drug overdose, CPhA recommends that you contact your **regional Poison Control Centre**. See the *CPS* Directory section for a list of Poison Control Centres.

DOSAGE: From the day of embryo transfer, one application of 1.125 g CRINONE 8% Vaginal Gel (90 mg progesterone) should be taken intravaginally once or twice daily. Most women will respond to 90 mg once daily. However, some women may need 90 mg twice daily. If pregnancy occurs treatment may continue for up to 10-12 weeks.

INFORMATION FOR THE PATIENT: Published in e-CPS, available by subscription at www.e-cps.ca.

SUPPLIED: Each single-use, one piece, disposable, white polyethylene vaginal applicator with a twist-off top, contains: progesterone 90 mg (8%). Each applicator contains 1.45 g of gel and delivers 1.125 g of gel. Nonmedicinal ingredients: carbomer 974P, glycerin, hydrogenated palm oil glyceride, light liquid paraffin, polycarbophil, purified water, sodium hydroxide and sorbic acid. Single-use vaginal applicator of 1.45 g in cartons, boxes of 6 and 18. Store at room temperature (15 to 25°C). Avoid exposure to extreme heat or cold.

Crixivan® ℞
indinavir sulfate
HIV Protease Inhibitor

Merck Frosst

Date of Revision: March 27, 2009

SUMMARY PRODUCT INFORMATION:

Route of Administration	Dosage Form/ Strength	Clinically Relevant Nonmedicinal Ingredients
Oral	Capsules/200 mg and 400 mg as indinavir	Anhydrous lactose For a complete listing see Dosage Forms, Composition and Packaging.

INDICATIONS AND CLINICAL USE: CRIXIVAN (indinavir sulfate) in combination with other antiretroviral agents is indicated for the treatment of HIV-1 infection.

Clinical studies with indinavir sulfate in adults demonstrated:

- reduced risk of progression to an AIDS-defining illness or death;
- durable reduction in serum viral RNA;
- durable increase in CD4 cell counts.

CONTRAINDICATIONS:

- CRIXIVAN is contraindicated in patients with clinically significant hypersensitivity to any of its ingredients. For a complete listing, see Dosage Forms, Composition and Packaging.
- Coadministration of indinavir sulfate is contraindicated with drugs that are highly dependent on CYP3A for clearance and for which elevated plasma concentrations are associated with serious and/or life-threatening events (i.e. cardiac arrhythmias, prolonged sedation). These drugs are listed in Table 1.

Table 1: CRIXIVAN

Drugs That Are Contraindicated with Indinavir Sulfate

Drug Class	Drugs Within Class That Are Contraindicated with Indinavir Sulfate
Antiarrhythmics	amiodarone
Ergot derivatives	dihydroergotamine, ergonovine, ergotamine, methylergonovine
GI motility agents	cisapride (no longer marketed in Canada)
Neuroleptics	pimozide
Sedative/hypnotics	alprazolam, midazolam[a], triazolam

[a] Administered orally (for parenterally administered midazolam, see Drug Interactions).

WARNINGS AND PRECAUTIONS: Coadministration of CRIXIVAN, a CYP3A4 inhibitor, with calcium channel blockers, trazodone and other drugs metabolized by CYP3A4, may result in increased plasma concentrations of these drugs which could increase or prolong their therapeutic and adverse effects.

The potential exists for interaction between indinavir sulfate and other P450 (CYP3A4) substrates which have not been studied (see Contraindications, Table 1, Drug Interactions, and Action and Clinical Pharmacology, Pharmacokinetics).

Lactose Intolerance: CRIXIVAN contains lactose and is not recommended for patients with rare hereditary problems of galactose intolerance, the Lapp lactase deficiency or glucose-galactose malabsorption (for a complete listing of excipients, see Dosage Forms, Composition and Packaging).

Endocrine and Metabolism: Hyperglycemia: There have been reports of new onset diabetes mellitus or hyperglycemia, or exacerbation of pre-existing diabetes mellitus occurring in HIV-infected patients receiving protease inhibitor therapy. Many of these reports occurred in patients with confounding medical conditions, some of which required therapy with agents that have been associated with the development of diabetes mellitus or hyperglycemia. Some patients required either initiation or dose adjustments of insulin or oral hypoglycemic agents for treatment of these events. In some cases diabetic ketoacidosis has occurred.

In the majority of cases, treatment with protease inhibitors was continued while in some cases treatment was either discontinued or interrupted. In some patients, hyperglycemia persisted after the protease inhibitor was withdrawn, whether or not diabetes was reported at baseline. A causal relationship between protease inhibitor therapy and these events has not been established.

Redistribution/Accumulation of Body Fat: Redistribution/accumulation of body fat including central obesity, dorsocervical fat enlargement (buffalo hump), peripheral wasting, breast enlargement, facial wasting, and "cushingoid appearance" have been observed in patients receiving antiretroviral therapy. The mechanism and long-term consequences of these events are currently unknown. A causal relationship has not been established.

Genitourinary: Nephrolithiasis/Urolithiasis and Tubulointerstitial Nephritis: Nephrolithiasis/urolithiasis has occurred with CRIXIVAN therapy in patients. The cumulative frequency of nephrolithiasis events increases with increasing exposure to CRIXIVAN; however, the risk over time remains relatively constant. In some cases, nephrolithiasis has been associated with renal insufficiency or acute renal failure. In the majority of these cases, renal insufficiency and acute renal failure were reversible. If signs and symptoms of nephrolithiasis, including flank pain with or without hematuria (including microscopic hematuria), occur, temporary interruption of therapy (e.g., 1-3 days) during the acute episode of nephrolithiasis or discontinuation of therapy may be considered. **Adequate hydration is recommended (at least 1.5 L a day) in all patients treated with indinavir sulfate (see Adverse Reactions, Nephrolithiasis/Urolithiasis and Dosage and Administration).**

During post-marketing surveillance of patients treated with indinavir, rare reports of interstitial nephritis with medullary calcification and cortical atrophy have been observed in patients with asymptomatic severy leukocyturia (>100 cells/high power field). Asymptomatic severe leukocyturia could indicate the presence of renal damage (e.g., tubulointerstitial nephritis) and further evaluation may be warranted. Change in the management of these patients may be necessary to prevent progression of renal damage. The regular use of microscopic urinalyses may add significantly to the safe management of individuals on indinavir treatment.

Hematologic: Hyperbilirubinemia: Indirect hyperbilirubinemia has occurred frequently during treatment with CRIXIVAN and has infrequently been associated with increases in serum transaminases (see Adverse Reactions). However, because of the theoretical potential for the compound to exacerbate the physiologic hyperbilirubinemia seen in human neonates, careful consideration must be given to the use of indinavir sulfate in pregnant women at the time of delivery (see Pregnant Women).

Hemolytic Anemia: Acute hemolytic anemia, including cases resulting in death, has been reported in patients treated with CRIXIVAN. Once a diagnosis is apparent, appropriate measures for the treatment of hemolytic anemia should be instituted, including discontinuation of indinavir sulfate.

Bleeding in Hemophiliacs: There have been reports of increased bleeding including spontaneous skin hematomas and hemarthrosis in patients with Hemophilia Type A and Type B treated with protease inhibitors. In some patients, additional Factor VIII was given. In many of the reported cases, treatment with protease inhibitors was continued or re-introduced. There is no proven relationship between protease inhibitors and such bleeding, however, the frequency of bleeding episodes should be closely monitored in patients on indinavir sulfate.

Hepatic/Biliary/Pancreatic: Hepatitis: Hepatitis including cases resulting in hepatic failure and death has been reported in patients treated with CRIXIVAN. Because the majority of these patients had confounding medical conditions and/or were receiving concomitant therapy(ies), a causal relationship between CRIXIVAN and these events has not been established.

Patients with Hepatic Insufficiency Due to Cirrhosis: In these patients, the dosage of indinavir sulfate should be lowered because of decreased metabolism of the drug (see Dosage and Administration, Hepatic Insufficiency Due to Cirrhosis).

Immune: Immune Reconstitution: During the initial phase of treatment, patients responding to antiretroviral therapy may develop an inflammatory response to indolent or residual opportunistic infections (such as MAC, CMV, PCP and TB), which may necessitate further evaluation and treatment.

Neurologic: CNS penetration of indinavir sulfate has not been established.

Renal: Patients with renal insufficiency have not been studied.

Drug Interactions: (see Drug Interactions).

HMG-CoA Reductase Inhibitors (statins): HMG-CoA reductase inhibitors (statins) may interact with protease inhibitors and increase the risk of myopathy, including rhabdomyolysis. Concomitant use of CRIXIVAN with lovastatin, simvastatin, or rosuvastatin is not recommended. Caution should be exercised if HIV protease inhibitors, including CRIXIVAN, are used concurrently with atorvastatin. The interaction of CRIXIVAN with pravastatin or fluvastatin is not known. The risk of myopathy including rhabdomyolysis may be increased when HIV protease inhibitors, including CRIXIVAN, are used in combination with these statin drugs (see Drug Interactions, Table 4).

Other Drugs Metabolized by CYP3A4: Coadministration of CRIXIVAN, a CYP3A4 inhibitor, with calcium channel blockers, trazodone and other drugs metabolized by CYP3A4, may result in increased plasma concentrations of these drugs which could increase or prolong their therapeutic and adverse effects (see Drug Interactions, Table 5).

Rifampin: Rifampin is a potent inducer of P450 (CYP3A4) which markedly diminishes plasma concentrations of indinavir. Therefore, CRIXIVAN and rifampin should not be coadministered (see Drug Interactions, Table 4).

Other drugs that induce CYP3A4 less potently than rifampin, such as phenobarbital, phenytoin, carbamazepine, and dexamethasone should be used cautiously together with indinavir sulfate since they could also diminish plasma concentrations of indinavir sulfate.

St. John's Wort (H. perforatum): Coadministration of CRIXIVAN and St. John's wort has been shown to substantially decrease indinavir concentrations and may lead to loss of virologic response and possible resistance to CRIXIVAN or to the class of protease inhibitors (see Drug Interactions, Table 4).

PDE5 Inhibitors (sildenafil, tadalafil, vardenafil): Particular caution should be used when prescribing PDE5 inhibitors in patients receiving protease inhibitors, including indinavir. Coadministration of protease inhibitors with sildenafil, tadalafil, or vardenafil (PDE5 inhibitors) is expected to substantially increase the plasma concentrations of these compounds and may result in an increase in PDE5 inhibitors-associated adverse events, including hypotension, visual changes, and priapism (see Drug Interactions, Table 5; Information for the Patient, and the complete prescribing information for sildenafil, tadalafil or vardenafil for recommended dosage adjustments).

Special Populations: Pregnant Women: There are no adequate and well controlled studies in pregnant patients. Indinavir sulfate may be used during pregnancy only if the potential benefit justifies the potential risk to the fetus. Given substantially lower antepartum exposures that have been observed in a small study of HIV-infected pregnant patients and the limited data in this patient population, indinavir use is not recommended in HIV-infected pregnant patients (see Action and Clinical Pharmacology, Special Populations and Conditions, Pregnant Women).

In Rhesus monkeys, administration of indinavir sulfate to neonates caused a mild exacerbation of the transient physiologic hyperbilirubinemia seen in this species after birth. Administration of indinavir sulfate to pregnant Rhesus monkeys during the third trimester did not cause a similar exacerbation in neonates; however, only limited placental transfer of indinavir sulfate occurred.

Antiviral Pregnancy Registry: To monitor maternal-fetal outcomes of pregnant patients exposed to CRIXIVAN, an Antiretroviral Pregnancy Registry has been established. Physicians are encouraged to register patients by calling 910-256-0238 (in the U.S. and Canada, call 1-800-258-4263).

Nursing Women: It is not known whether this drug is excreted in human milk. Because many drugs are excreted in human milk, and because of the potential for adverse reactions from indinavir sulfate in nursing infants, mothers should be instructed to discontinue nursing if they are receiving indinavir sulfate. In addition, it is advisable for HIV-infected women not to breast-feed to avoid post-natal transmission of HIV to a child who may not be infected.

Pediatrics: A dose of 500 mg/m² every 8 hours has been studied in uncontrolled studies of 70 children, 3 to 18 years of age. The pharmacokinetic profiles of indinavir at this dose were not comparable to profiles previously observed in adults receiving the recommended dose of 800 mg every 8 hours. Viral suppression was observed in some of the 21 patients who were followed on a regimen of indinavir 500 mg/m² in combination with D4T and 3TC through 24 weeks. However, a substantially higher rate of nephrolithiasis/urolithiasis was reported when compared to adult historical data (see Warnings and Precautions, Nephrolithiasis/Urolithiasis and Tubulointerstitial Nephritis).

In clinical trials with CRIXIVAN, asymptomatic pyuria of unknown etiology was noted in 10.9% (6/55) of pediatric patients 3 years of age and older who received CRIXIVAN at the dose of 500 mg/m² every 8 hours. Some of these events were associated with mild elevation of serum creatinine.

Geriatrics: Safety and effectiveness in elderly patients have not been established.

ADVERSE REACTIONS: Nephrolithiasis/Urolithiasis: In clinical trials with CRIXIVAN, nephrolithiasis, including flank pain with or without hematuria (including microscopic hematuria), has been reported in approximately 9.8% (252/2577) of patients receiving CRIXIVAN at the recommended dose compared to 2.2% in the control arms. In general these events were not associated with renal dysfunction and resolved with hydration and temporary interruption of therapy (e.g., 1-3 days). The cumulative frequency of nephrolithiasis events increases with increasing exposure to CRIXIVAN; however, the risk over time remains relatively constant (see Warnings and Precautions and Dosage and Administration).

Hyperbilirubinemia: Asymptomatic hyperbilirubinemia [total bilirubin ≥42.75 µmol/L (≥2.5 mg/dL)], reported predominantly as elevated indirect bilirubin, has occurred in approximately 14% of patients treated with indinavir sulfate. In <1% this was associated with elevations in ALT or AST.

Hyperbilirubinemia and nephrolithiasis occurred more frequently at doses exceeding 2.4 g/day.

Clinical Trial Adverse Drug Reactions: Because clinical trials are conducted under very specific conditions the adverse reaction rates observed in the clinical trials may not reflect the rates observed in practice and should not be compared to the rates in the clinical trials of another drug. Adverse drug reaction information from clinical trials is useful for identifying drug-related adverse events and for approximating rates.

In controlled clinical trials conducted worldwide, indinavir sulfate was administered alone or in combination with other antiretroviral agents (zidovudine, didanosine, and/or lamivudine) and was found to be generally well tolerated. Indinavir sulfate did not alter the type, frequency, or severity of known major toxicities associated with the use of zidovudine, didanosine, or lamivudine.

Study 028, a double-blind, multicenter, randomized, clinical endpoint trial compared the effects of indinavir sulfate plus zidovudine with those of indinavir sulfate alone or zidovudine alone on the progression to an AIDS-defining illness (ADI) or death, and on surrogate marker responses. The median length of follow-up was 56 weeks with a maximum of 97 weeks.

Study ACTG 320 was a multicenter, randomized, double-blind clinical endpoint trial to compare the effect of indinavir sulfate in combination with zidovudine (or stavudine) and lamivudine with that of zidovudine (or stavudine) plus lamivudine on the progression to an AIDS-defining illness (ADI) or death. The median length of follow-up was 38 weeks with a maximum of 52 weeks.

Drug-related clinical adverse reactions of moderate or severe intensity in ≥2% of patients treated with indinavir sulfate alone, indinavir sulfate in combination with zidovudine, or zidovudine alone are presented in Table 2.

Table 2: CRIXIVAN

Clinical Adverse Experiences Reported in ≥2% of Patients

	Study 028 Considered Drug-Related and of Moderate or Severe Intensity			Study ACTG 320 of Unknown Drug Relationship and of Severe or Life-Threatening Intensity	
Adverse Experience	**CRIXIVAN % (n=332)**	**CRIXIVAN plus Zidovudine % (n=332)**	**Zidovudine % (n=332)**	**CRIXIVAN plus Zidovudine plus Lamivudine % (n=571)**	**Zidovudine plus Lamivudine % (n=575)**
Body as a Whole					
Abdominal pain	16.6	16.0	12.0	1.9	0.7
Asthenia/fatigue	2.1	4.2	3.6	2.4	4.5
Fever	1.5	1.5	2.1	3.8	3.0
Malaise	2.1	2.7	1.8	0	0
Digestive System					
Nausea	11.7	31.9	19.6	2.8	1.4
Diarrhea	3.3	3.0	2.4	0.9	1.2
Vomiting	8.4	17.8	9.0	1.4	1.4
Acid regurgitation	2.7	5.4	1.8	0.4	0
Anorexia	2.7	5.4	3.0	0.5	0.2
Appetite increase	2.1	1.5	1.2	0	0
Dyspepsia	1.5	2.7	0.9	0	0
Jaundice	1.5	2.1	0.3	0	0
Hemic and Lymphatic Systems					
Anemia	0.6	1.2	2.1	2.4	3.5
Musculoskeletal System					
Back pain	8.4	4.5	1.5	0.9	0.7
Nervous System/Psychiatric					
Headache	5.4	9.6	6.0	2.4	2.8
Dizziness	3.0	3.9	0.9	0.5	0.7
Somnolence	2.4	3.3	3.3	0	0
Skin and Skin Appendages					
Pruritus	4.2	2.4	1.8	0.5	0
Rash	1.2	0.6	2.4	1.1	0.5
Respiratory System					
Cough	1.5	0.3	0.6	1.6	1.0
Difficulty breathing/ dyspnea/shortness of breath	0	0.6	0.3	1.8	1.0
Urogenital System					
Nephrolithiasis/ urolithiasis[a]	8.7	7.8	2.1	2.6	0.3
Dysuria	1.5	2.4	0.3	0.4	0.2
Special Senses					
Taste perversion	2.7	8.4	1.2	0.2	0

[a] Including renal colic, and flank pain with and without hematuria.

In Phase I and II controlled trials, the following adverse reactions were reported significantly more frequently by those randomized to the arms containing indinavir sulfate than by those randomized to nucleoside analogues: rash, upper respiratory infection, dry skin, pharyngitis, taste perversion.

Adverse reactions occurring in less than 2% of patients receiving indinavir sulfate in Phase II/Phase III studies and considered at least possibly related or of unknown relationship to treatment and of at least moderate intensity are listed below by body system.

Body as a Whole/Site Unspecified: abdominal distention, chest pain, chills, fever, flank pain, flu-like illness, fungal infection, malaise, pain, syncope, redistribution/accumulation of body fat (see Warnings and Precautions, Redistribution/Accumulation of Body Fat).

Cardiovascular System: cardiovascular disorder, palpitation.

Digestive System: acid regurgitation, anorexia, aphthous stomatitis, cheilitis, cholecystitis, cholestasis, constipation, dry mouth, dyspepsia, eructation, flatulence, gastritis, gingivitis, glossodynia, gingival hemorrhage, increased appetite, infectious gastroenteritis, jaundice, liver cirrhosis.
Hemic and Lymphatic Systems: anemia, lymphadenopathy, spleen disorder, bleeding in hemophiliacs (see Warnings and Precautions).
Metabolic/Nutritional/Immune: food allergy.
Musculoskeletal System: arthralgia, back pain, leg pain, myalgia, muscle cramps, muscle weakness, musculoskeletal pain, shoulder pain, stiffness.
Nervous System and Psychiatric: agitation, anxiety, anxiety disorder, bruxism, decreased mental acuity, depression, dizziness, dream abnormality, dysesthesia, excitement, fasciculation, hypesthesia, nervousness, neuralgia, neurotic disorder, paresthesia, peripheral neuropathy, sleep disorder, somnolence, tremor, vertigo.
Respiratory System: cough, dyspnea, halitosis, pharyngeal hyperemia, pharyngitis, pneumonia, rales/rhonchi, respiratory failure, sinus disorder, sinusitis, upper respiratory infection.
Skin and Skin Appendages: body odor, contact dermatitis, dermatitis, dry skin, flushing, folliculitis, herpes simplex, herpes zoster, night sweats, pruritus, seborrhea, skin disorder, skin infection, sweating, urticaria.
Special Senses: accommodation disorder, blurred vision, eye pain, eye swelling, orbital edema, taste disorder.
Urogenital System: dysuria, hematuria, hydronephrosis, nocturia, premenstrual syndrome, proteinuria, renal colic, urinary frequency, urinary tract infection, urine abnormality, urine sediment abnormality, urolithiasis.
Abnormal Hematologic and Clinical Chemistry Findings: The most frequently occurring selected laboratory adverse experiences (incidence ≥5%) considered to be possibly, probably, or definitely drug-related by the study investigator in the group treated with indinavir sulfate alone, were changes in ALT, AST, indirect serum bilirubin, total serum bilirubin, and urine protein. Only 1% of patients discontinued treatment due to these laboratory adverse experiences, when treated with indinavir sulfate alone or in combination with other antiretroviral agents. With the exception of hyperbilirubinemia, the incidences of these adverse events with indinavir sulfate monotherapy were lower than in the groups treated with indinavir sulfate in combination with other antiretroviral agents. Similar incidences in drug-related laboratory adverse experiences of changes in ALT, AST, and urine protein were observed in the group treated with zidovudine alone.

Presented in Table 3 are selected laboratory abnormalities reported in patients treated with indinavir sulfate alone, indinavir sulfate in combination with zidovudine, or zidovudine alone in Phase III clinical trials (Studies 028 and ACTG 320).

Table 3: CRIXIVAN

Selected Laboratory Abnormalities of Severe or Life-Threatening Intensity Reported in Studies 028 and ACTG 320

	Study 028			Study ACTG 320	
	CRIXIVAN % (n=329)	CRIXIVAN plus Zidovudine % (n=320)	Zidovudine % (n=330)	CRIXIVAN plus Zidovudine plus Lamivudine % (n=571)	Zidovudine plus Lamivudine % (n=575)
Hematology					
Decreased hemoglobin <7.0 g/dL	0.6	0.9	3.3	2.4	3.5
Decreased platelet count <50×10³/mm³	0.9	0.9	1.8	0.2	0.9
Decreased neutrophils <0.75×10³/mm³	2.4	2.2	6.7	5.1	14.6
Blood Chemistry					
Increased ALT >500% ULN[a]	4.9	4.1	3.0	2.6	2.6
Increased AST >500% ULN	3.7	2.8	2.7	3.3	2.8
Total serum bilirubin >250% ULN	11.9	9.7	0.6	6.1	1.4
Increased serum amylase >200% ULN	2.1	1.9	1.8	0.9	0.3
Increased glucose >250 mg/dL	0.9	0.9	0.6	1.6	1.9
Increased creatinine >300% ULN	0	0	0.6	0.2	0

[a] Upper limit of the normal range.

Post-Market Adverse Drug Reactions: The following additional adverse experiences have been reported in post-marketed experience without regard to causality.
Body as a Whole/Site Unspecified: redistribution/accumulation of body fat in areas such as the back of the neck, abdomen, and retro-peritoneum (see Warnings and Precautions, Redistribution/Accumulation of Body Fat).
Cardiovascular System: cardiovascular disorders including myocardial infarction and angina pectoris.
Digestive System: liver function abnormalities, hepatitis including reports of hepatic failure (see Warnings and Precautions, Hepatitis); pancreatitis.
Endocrine/Metabolic: new onset diabetes mellitus or hyperglycemia, or exacerbation of pre-existing diabetes mellitus (see Warnings and Precautions).
Hematologic: increased spontaneous bleeding in patients with hemophilia (see Warnings and Precautions), thrombocytopenia, anemia including acute hemolytic anemia (see Warnings and Precautions).
Hypersensitivity: angioedema, anaphylaxis, vasculitis.
Nervous System/Psychiatric: oral paresthesia.
Skin and Skin Appendages: alopecia, hyperpigmentation, urticaria, rash including erythema multiforme and Stevens-Johnson syndrome; ingrown toenails and/or paronychia.
Urogenital System: nephrolithiasis/urolithiasis, generally without renal dysfunction; however, there have been reports of nephrolithiasis/urolithiasis with renal dysfunction including acute renal failure; pyelonephritis; renal insufficiency; renal failure; leukocyturia; crystalluria; and interstitial nephritis sometimes with indinavir crystal deposits, in some patients, the interstitial nephritis did not resolve following discontinuation of CRIXIVAN.

The following additional laboratory experiences have been reported: increased serum triglycerides; increased serum cholesterol.

DRUG INTERACTIONS:

Serious Drug Interactions
Indinavir sulfate should not be administered concurrently with the following:

- **alprazolam,**
- **amiodarone,**
- **cisapride** (no longer marketed in Canada),
- **ergot derivatives,**
- **oral midazolam,**
- **pimozide,**
- **triazolam**

Competition for P450 (CYP3A4) by indinavir sulfate could result in inhibition of the metabolism of these drugs and create the potential for serious and/or life-threatening events (i.e., cardiac arrhythmias, prolonged sedation). The potential exists for interaction between indinavir sulfate and other P450 (CYP3A4) substrates which have not been studied.

Overview: (See Contraindications.) Overview: Indinavir is an inhibitor of the cytochrome P450 isoform CYP3A4. Coadministration of CRIXIVAN and a drug primarily metabolized by CYP3A4 may result in increased plasma concentrations of the other drug, which could increase or prolong its therapeutic and adverse effects (see Contraindications, Warnings and Precautions). Based on in vitro data in human liver microsomes, indinavir does not inhibit CYP1A2, CYP2C9, CYP2E1 and CYP2B6. However, indinavir may be a weak inhibitor of CYP2D6.

Indinavir is metabolized by CYP3A4. Drugs that induce CYP3A4 activity would be expected to increase the clearance of indinavir, resulting in lowered plasma concentrations of indinavir. Coadministration of CRIXIVAN and other drugs that inhibit CYP3A4 may decrease the clearance of indinavir and may result in increased plasma concentrations of indinavir.
Drug-Drug Interactions: The drugs listed in Table 4 are based on either drug interaction case reports or studies, or potential interactions due to the expected magnitude and seriousness of the interaction (i.e. those identified as contraindicated).

Table 4: CRIXIVAN

Drugs That Should Not Be Coadministered with CRIXIVAN

Drug Class: Drug Name	Clinical Comment
Antiarrhythmics: amiodarone	**Contraindicated** due to potential for serious and/or life-threatening reactions such as cardiac arrhythmias.
Ergot derivatives: dihydroergotamine, ergonovine, ergotamine, methylergonovine	**Contraindicated** due to potential for serious and/or life-threatening reactions such as acute ergot toxicity characterized by peripheral vasospasm and ischemia of the extremities and other tissues.
Sedative/hypnotics: oral midazolam, triazolam, alprazolam	**Contraindicated** due to potential for serious and/or life-threatening reactions such as prolonged or increased sedation or respiratory depression (for parenterally administered midazolam, see Drug Interactions, Table 5).
GI motility agents: cisapride[a]	**Contraindicated** due to potential for serious and/or life-threatening reactions such as cardiac arrhythmias.
Neuroleptic: pimozide	**Contraindicated** due to potential for serious and/or life-threatening reactions such as cardiac arrhythmias.
Herbal products: St. John's wort (Hypericum perforatum)	May lead to loss of virologic response and possible resistance to CRIXIVAN or to the class of protease inhibitors.
Antimycobacterial: rifampin	May lead to loss of virologic response and possible resistance to CRIXIVAN or to the class of protease inhibitors or other coadministered antiretroviral agents. Rifampin is a potent inducer of P450 (CYP3A4) which markedly diminishes plasma concentrations of indinavir sulfate. Therefore, CRIXIVAN and rifampin should not be coadministered (see Warnings and Precautions). Specific drug interaction studies were performed with indinavir sulfate and the following drugs: clarithromycin, fluconazole, isoniazid, methadone, norethindrone/ethinyl estradiol 1/35, trimethoprim/sulfamethoxazole, zidovudine, zidovudine/lamivudine. No clinically significant interactions were observed with these drugs.
HMG-CoA reductase inhibitors (statins): lovastatin, simvastatin, rosuvastatin	Potential for serious reactions such as risk of myopathy including rhabdomyolysis. Concomitant use of CRIXIVAN with lovastatin, simvastatin or rosuvastatin is not recommended. Caution should be exercised if HIV protease inhibitors, including CRIXIVAN, are used concurrently with atorvastatin. The interaction of CRIXIVAN with pravastatin or fluvastatin is not known. The risk of myopathy including rhabdomyolysis may be increased when HIV protease inhibitors, including CRIXIVAN, are used in combination with these statin drugs (see Warnings and Precautions, Drug Interactions, HMG-CoA Reductase Inhibitors (statins)).
Protease inhibitor: atazanavir	Both CRIXIVAN and atazanavir are associated with indirect (unconjugated) hyperbilirubinemia. Combinations of these drugs have not been studied and coadministration of CRIXIVAN and atazanavir is not recommended.

[a] Cisapride is no longer marketed in Canada.

Table 5: CRIXIVAN

Established and Other Potentially Significant Drug Interactions: Alteration in Dose or Regimen May Be Recommended Based on Drug Interaction Studies or Predicted Interaction (see also Action and Clinical Pharmacology for magnitude of interaction, Warnings and Precautions, and Dosage and Administration)

Concomitant Drug Class: Drug Name	Effect on Concentration of Indinavir or Concomitant Drug	Clinical Comment
	HIV-Antiviral Agents	
Non-nucleoside reverse transcriptase inhibitor: delavirdine	↑ indinavir	Due to an increase in indinavir plasma concentrations (preliminary results), a dosage reduction of indinavir should be considered when CRIXIVAN and delavirdine are coadministered (see Dosage and Administration, Concomitant Therapy, Delavirdine).

(cont'd)

Table 5: CRIXIVAN *(cont'd)*

Established and Other Potentially Significant Drug Interactions: Alteration in Dose or Regimen May Be Recommended Based on Drug Interaction Studies or Predicted Interaction (see also Action and Clinical Pharmacology for magnitude of interaction, Warnings and Precautions, and Dosage and Administration)

Concomitant Drug Class: Drug Name	Effect on Concentration of Indinavir or Concomitant Drug	Clinical Comment
Non-nucleoside reverse transcriptase inhibitor: efavirenz	↓ indinavir	The optimal dose of indinavir, when given in combination with efavirenz is not known. Increasing the indinavir dose to 1000 mg every 8 hours does not compensate for the increased indinavir metabolism due to efavirenz. When indinavir at an increased dose (1000 mg every 8 hours) was given with efavirenz (600 mg once daily) in uninfected volunteers, the indinavir AUC and C_{min} were decreased by approximately 33-46% and 39-57%, respectively, compared to when indinavir was given alone at the standard dose (800 mg every 8 hours).
Nucleoside reverse transcriptase inhibitor: didanosine	interaction has not been evaluated	A normal (acidic) gastric pH may be necessary for optimum absorption of indinavir whereas acid rapidly degrades didanosine which is formulated with buffering agents to increase the pH. Indinavir and didanosine formulations containing buffer should be administered at least one hour apart on an empty stomach. Antiretroviral activity was unaltered when didanosine was administered 3 hours after treatment with indinavir.
Nucleoside reverse transcriptase inhibitor: enteric-coated didanosine	interaction has not been evaluated	There is no drug-drug interaction between enteric coated didanosine and indinavir; these two products can be given together.
HIV protease inhibitor: ritonavir	↑ indinavir ↑ ritonavir	In cases of coadministration of ritonavir and indinavir (dosed at 800 mg twice daily), caution is warranted as the risk of nephrolithiasis can be increased. Appropriate hydration is recommended.
Other Agents		
Antifungal: itraconazole	↑ indinavir	Itraconazole is an inhibitor of CYP3A4 that increases plasma concentrations of indinavir. Therefore, a dose reduction of indinavir is recommended when CRIXIVAN and itraconazole are coadministered (see Dosage and Administration, Concomitant Therapy, Itraconazole).
Antifungal: ketoconazole	↑ indinavir	Ketoconazole is an inhibitor of CYP3A4 that increases plasma concentrations of indinavir. Therefore, a dose reduction of indinavir is recommended when CRIXIVAN and ketoconazole are coadministered (see Dosage and Administration, Concomitant Therapy, Ketoconazole).
Antidepressant: venlafaxine	↓ indinavir ↔ venlafaxine	Venlafaxine decreases indinavir plasma concentrations. Indinavir did not affect the plasma concentrations of venlafaxine and active metabolite O-desmethyl-venlafaxine. The clinical significance of this finding is unknown.
Antimycobacterial: rifabutin	↓ indinavir ↑ rifabutin	When rifabutin and CRIXIVAN are coadministered, there is an increase in the plasma concentration of rifabutin and a decrease in the plasma concentration of indinavir. A dose reduction of rifabutin and a dose increase of CRIXIVAN are necessary when rifabutin is coadministered with CRIXIVAN. The suggested dose adjustments are expected to result in rifabutin concentrations at least 50% higher than typically observed when rifabutin is administered alone at its usual dose (300 mg/day) and indinavir concentrations which may be slightly less than typically observed when indinavir is administered alone at its usual dose (800 mg every 8 hours) (see Dosage and Administration, Concomitant Therapy, Rifabutin).
PDE5 inhibitor (phosphodiesterase type 5 inhibitors): sildenafil tadalafil vardenafil	↑ sildenafil concentration ↑ tadalafil concentration ↑ vardenafil concentration	Particular caution should be used when prescribing sildenafil in patients receiving protease inhibitors, including indinavir. Coadministration of protease inhibitors with sildenafil is expected to substantially increase sildenafil concentrations and may result in an increase in sildenafil-associated adverse events, including hypotension, visual changes, and priapism (see Warnings and Precautions). Tadalafil dose should not exceed a maximum of 10 mg in a 72-hour period in patients receiving concomitant indinavir therapy. Vardenafil dose should not exceed a maximum of 2.5 mg in a 24-hour period in patients receiving concomitant indinavir therapy.
Drugs metabolized by CYP3A4	↑ calcium channel blockers ↑ trazodone ↑ other drugs metabolized by CYP3A4	Coadministration of CRIXIVAN, a CYP3A4 inhibitor, with calcium channel blockers, trazodone and other drugs metabolized by CYP3A4, may result in increased plasma concentrations of these drugs which could increase or prolong their therapeutic and adverse effects. The potential exists for interaction between indinavir sulfate and other P450 (CYP3A4) substrates which have not been studied (e.g., mefloquine).
Other drugs that induce CYP3A4	↓ indinavir	Other drugs that induce CYP3A4 less potently than rifampin, such as phenobarbital, phenytoin, carbamazepine, and dexamethasone should be used cautiously together with indinavir sulfate since they could also diminish plasma concentrations of indinavir sulfate.

(cont'd)

Table 5: CRIXIVAN *(cont'd)*

Established and Other Potentially Significant Drug Interactions: Alteration in Dose or Regimen May Be Recommended Based on Drug Interaction Studies or Predicted Interaction (see also Action and Clinical Pharmacology for magnitude of interaction, Warnings and Precautions, and Dosage and Administration)

Concomitant Drug Class: Drug Name	Effect on Concentration of Indinavir or Concomitant Drug	Clinical Comment
Sedative/hypnotics: midazolam	↑ midazolam	Midazolam is extensively metabolized by CYP3A4. Coadministration with CRIXIVAN may cause a large increase in the concentration of this benzodiazepine. No drug interaction study has been performed for the coadministration of CRIXIVAN with benzodiazepines. Based on data from other CYP3A4 inhibitors, plasma concentrations of midazolam are expected to be significantly higher when midazolam is given orally. Therefore CRIXIVAN should not be coadministered with orally administered midazolam (see Contraindications), whereas caution should be used with coadministration of CRIXIVAN and parenteral midazolam. Data from concomitant use of parenteral midazolam with other protease inhibitors suggest a possible 3-4 fold increase in midazolam plasma levels. If CRIXIVAN is coadministered with parenteral midazolam, it should be done in an intensive care unit (ICU) or similar setting which ensures close clinical monitoring and appropriate medical management in case of respiratory depression and/or prolonged sedation. Based on a drug interaction study between saquinavir and midazolam, there is a potential for midazolam overexposure due to the inhibitor effects of CRIXIVAN on CYP3A4. Dosage reduction for midazolam should be considered, especially if more than a single dose of midazolam is administered.

Legend: ↑=increase; ↓=decrease; ↔=no change.

Drug-Food Interactions: Ingestion of CRIXIVAN with a meal high in calories, fat, and protein reduces the absorption of CRIXIVAN. For optimal absorption, CRIXIVAN should be administered without food but with water 1 hour before or 2 hours after a meal (see Dosage and Administration).

Drug-Herb Interactions: St. John's Wort (H. perforatum): Coadministration of CRIXIVAN and St. John's wort has been shown to substantially decrease indinavir concentrations and may lead to loss of virologic response and possible resistance to CRIXIVAN or to the class of protease inhibitors (see Warnings and Precautions).

Drug-Laboratory Test Interactions: Interactions with laboratory tests have not been established.

DOSAGE AND ADMINISTRATION:

Recommended Dose and Dosage Adjustment: Adults: The recommended dosage of CRIXIVAN is 800 mg orally every 8 hours. **Therapy with INDINAVIR sulfate must be initiated at the recommended dose of 2.4 g/day.**

Since CRIXIVAN must be taken at intervals of 8 hours, a schedule convenient for the patient should be developed. For optimal absorption, indinavir sulfate should be administered without food but with water, 1 hour before or 2 hours after a meal. Alternatively, indinavir sulfate may be administered with other liquids such as skim milk, juice, coffee, or tea, or a light meal (e.g., dry toast with jelly, apple juice, and coffee with skim milk and sugar or corn flakes, skim milk and sugar).

To ensure adequate hydration, it is recommended that adults drink at least 1.5 liters (approximately 48 ounces) of liquids during the course of 24 hours.

In addition to adequate hydration, medical management of patients who experience nephrolithiasis may include temporary interruption of therapy (e.g., 1-3 days) during the acute episode of nephrolithiasis or discontinuation of therapy.

Concomitant Therapy: Delavirdine: Dose reduction of CRIXIVAN to 600 mg every 8 hours should be considered when administering delavirdine 400 mg three times a day (see Warnings and Precautions, Drug Interactions).

Itraconazole: Dose reduction of CRIXIVAN to 600 mg every 8 hours is recommended when administering itraconazole 200 mg twice daily concurrently (see Warnings and Precautions, Drug Interactions).

Ketoconazole: Dose reduction of CRIXIVAN to 600 mg every 8 hours is recommended when administering ketoconazole concurrently (see Warnings and Precautions, Drug Interactions).

Rifabutin: Dose reduction of rifabutin to half the standard dose (consult the manufacturer's product circular for rifabutin) and a dose increase of CRIXIVAN to 1000 mg every 8 hours are recommended when rifabutin and CRIXIVAN are coadministered (see Warnings and Precautions, Drug Interactions).

Other: Hepatic Insufficiency Due to Cirrhosis: Dose reduction of indinavir sulfate to 600 mg every 8 hours should be considered in patients with mild-to-moderate hepatic insufficiency due to cirrhosis.

Missed Dose: If a dose is missed by more than 2 hours, do not take it later in the day. Simply continue to follow the usual schedule.

OVERDOSAGE:

There have been reports of human overdosage with CRIXIVAN. The most commonly reported symptoms were gastrointestinal (e.g., nausea, vomiting, diarrhea) and renal (e.g., nephrolithiasis/urolithiasis, flank pain, hematuria).

It is not known whether indinavir sulfate is dialyzable by peritoneal dialysis or hemodialysis.

There is no specific antidote for overdose with CRIXIVAN. Treatment of overdose with CRIXIVAN consists of general supportive measures including monitoring of vital signs and observation of the clinical status of the patient. Administration of activated charcoal may be used to aid in removal of unabsorbed active substance.

> For management of a suspected drug overdose, contact your **regional Poison Control Centre**. See the *CPS* Directory section for a list of Poison Control Centres.

ACTION AND CLINICAL PHARMACOLOGY: Mechanism of Action: CRIXIVAN is a selective protease inhibitor active against the Human Immunodeficiency Virus (HIV-1).

HIV protease is an enzyme required for the proteolytic cleavage of the viral polyprotein precursors into the individual functional proteins found in infectious HIV. Indinavir sulfate binds to the protease active site and inhibits the activity of the enzyme. This inhibition prevents cleavage of the viral polyproteins resulting in the formation of immature non-infectious viral particles.

Antiretroviral Potency: The relationship between in vitro susceptibility of HIV to indinavir sulfate and inhibition of HIV replication in humans has not been established. The in vitro activity of indinavir sulfate was assessed in cell lines of lymphoblastic and monocytic origin and in peripheral blood lymphocytes. HIV variants used to infect the different cell types include laboratory-adapted variants, primary clinical isolates and clinical isolates resistant to nucleoside analogue and nonnucleoside inhibitors of the HIV reverse transcriptase. The IC_{95} (95% inhibitory concentration) of indinavir sulfate in these test systems was in the range of 25 to 100 nM. In drug combination studies with the nucleoside analogues zidovudine and didanosine, as well as with an investigational nonnucleoside (L-697,661), indinavir sulfate showed synergistic activity in cell culture.

Virus Mutations: Isolates of HIV with reduced susceptibility to the drug have been recovered from some patients treated with indinavir sulfate. Viral resistance was correlated with the accumulation of mutations that resulted in the expression of amino acid substitutions in the viral protease. Eleven amino acid residue positions, at which substitutions are associated with resistance, have been identified. Resistance was mediated by the co-expression of multiple and variable substitutions at these positions. In general, higher levels of resistance were associated with the co-expression of greater numbers of substitutions.

Cross-resistance between indinavir sulfate and HIV reverse transcriptase inhibitors is unlikely because the enzyme targets involved are different. Cross-resistance was noted between indinavir sulfate and the protease inhibitor ritonavir. Varying degrees of cross-resistance have been observed between indinavir sulfate and other HIV-protease inhibitors.

Pharmacokinetics: See Table 6.

Table 6: CRIXIVAN

Summary of Indinavir's Pharmacokinetic Parameters in Adult Patients

Regimen	$AUC_{0\text{-}8h}$ (nM· hour±SD)	C_{max} (nM±SD)	C_{8h} (nM±SD)	n[a]
Adult patients, 800 mg every 8 hrs	30 691±11 407	12 617±4037	251±178	16

[a] n=number of subjects.
Lgend : SD=standard deviation.

Absorption: Pharmacokinetic parameters of indinavir are summarized in Table 6. In adult patients, indinavir was rapidly absorbed in the fasted state with a time to peak plasma concentration (T_{max}) of 0.8±0.3 hours (mean±S.D.) (n=11). A greater than dose-proportional increase in indinavir plasma concentrations was observed over the 200-1000 mg dose range. Between 800 mg and 1000 mg dose levels, the deviation from dose-proportionality is less pronounced.

Administration of indinavir with a meal high in calories, fat, and protein (784 kcal, 48.6 g fat, 31.3 g protein) resulted in a 77%±8% reduction in AUC and an 84%±7% reduction in C_{max} (n=10). Administration with lighter meals (e.g., a meal of dry toast with jelly, apple juice, and coffee with skim milk and sugar or a meal of corn flakes, skim milk and sugar) resulted in little or no change in AUC, C_{max} or trough concentration (see Dosage and Administration).

Distribution: Indinavir was approximately 60% bound to human plasma proteins over a concentration range of 81 nM to 16 300 nM.

Metabolism: Following a 400 mg dose of ^{14}C-indinavir sulfate, 83±1% (n=4) and 19±3% (n=6) of the total radioactivity was recovered in feces and urine, respectively; radioactivity due to parent drug in feces and urine was 19.1% and 9.4%, respectively. Seven metabolites have been identified, one glucuronide conjugate and six oxidative metabolites. In vitro studies indicate that cytochrome P450 (CYP3A4) is the major enzyme responsible for formation of the oxidative metabolites.

Excretion: Less than 20% of indinavir is excreted unchanged in the urine. Mean urinary excretion of unchanged drug was 10.4±4.9% (n=10) and 12.0±4.9% (n=10) following a single 700 mg and 1000 mg dose, respectively. Indinavir was rapidly eliminated with a half-life of 1.8±0.4 hours (n=10). Significant accumulation was not observed after multiple dosing at 800 mg every 8 hours.

Special Populations and Conditions: Gender: The effect of gender on the pharmacokinetics of indinavir was evaluated in 10 HIV seropositive women who received indinavir 800 mg every 8 hours with zidovudine 200 mg every 8 hours and lamivudine 150 mg twice a day for one week. Indinavir pharmacokinetic parameters in these women were compared to those in HIV seropositive men (pooled historical control data). The mean percentage decrease in $AUC_{0\text{-}8h}$, C_{max} and C_{8h} for females relative to males was 13%, 13%, and 22%, respectively. The clinical significance of these gender differences in the pharmacokinetics of indinavir is not known.

Race: Pharmacokinetics of indinavir appear to be comparable in Caucasians and Blacks based on pharmacokinetic studies including 42 Caucasians (26 HIV-positive) and 16 Blacks (4 HIV-positive).

Hepatic Insufficiency: Patients with mild-to-moderate hepatic insufficiency and clinical evidence of cirrhosis had evidence of decreased metabolism of indinavir resulting in approximately 60% higher mean AUC following a single 400 mg dose (n=12). The half-life of indinavir increased to 2.8±0.5 hours. Indinavir pharmacokinetics have not been studied in patients with severe hepatic insufficiency (see Dosage and Administration, Hepatic Insufficiency Due to Cirrhosis).

Renal Insufficiency: The pharmacokinetics of indinavir have not been studied in patients with renal insufficiency.

For information on pharmacokinetic drug-drug interactions, see Drug Interactions, Overview.

Pregnant Women: A CRIXIVAN dose of 800 mg every 8 hours (with zidovudine 200 mg every 8 hours and lamivudine 150 mg twice a day) has been studied in 16 HIV-infected pregnant patients at 14 to 28 weeks of gestation at enrollment (study PACTG 358). Given the substantially lower antepartum exposures observed and the limited data in this patient population, indinavir use is not recommended in HIV-infected pregnant patients (see Warnings and Precautions, Special Populations, Pregnant Women).

Absorption of orally administered indinavir sulfate is rapid. Peak plasma concentration occurs within 1 hour and is not dose dependent. The oral absorption of a 400 mg dose of indinavir sulfate is reduced by 78% when administered with a standard meal high in calories, fat and protein contents. Indinavir sulfate has a relatively short half-life of 1.8 hours. There is very little drug accumulation following either an 8 hour or 6 hour dosing regimen over the clinical dose range.

Indinavir is widely distributed in the body and is approximately 60% bound to human plasma proteins. Less than 20% of indinavir is excreted unchanged in the urine. Following a single 400 mg dose of indinavir sulfate, patients with mild-to-moderate hepatic insufficiency and clinical evidence of cirrhosis had a mean AUC which was found to be higher by approximately 60% compared to that in healthy subjects and the half-life increased to approximately 2.8 hours, a reflection of reduced metabolism.

Therapy with indinavir sulfate should be initiated at the full recommended dose to increase suppression of viral replication and therefore inhibit the emergence of resistant virus (see Dosage and Administration). No titration is necessary upon initiating therapy.

STORAGE AND STABILITY: Store in a tightly closed container at room temperature (15-30°C). Protect from moisture. CRIXIVAN capsules are sensitive to moisture. CRIXIVAN should be dispensed and stored in the original container. The desiccant should remain in the original bottle.

INFORMATION FOR THE PATIENT: Published in e-CPS, available by subscription at www.e-cps.ca.

DOSAGE FORMS, COMPOSITION AND PACKAGING: 200 mg: Each white, semi-translucent capsule, coded CRIXIVAN™ 200 mg in blue, contains: indinavir 200 mg (as a sulfate salt ethanolate). Nonmedicinal ingredients: anhydrous lactose 74.8 mg (as a diluent) and magnesium stearate (as a lubricant); empty capsule shell: gelatin, silicon dioxide, sodium lauryl sulfate and titanium dioxide. Bottles of 360, with desiccant.

400 mg: Each white, semi-translucent capsule, coded CRIXIVAN™ 400 mg in green, contains: indinavir 400 mg (as a sulfate salt ethanolate). Nonmedicinal ingredients: anhydrous lactose 149.6 mg (as a diluent) and magnesium stearate (as a lubricant); empty capsule shell: gelatin, silicon dioxide, sodium lauryl sulfate and titanium dioxide. Bottles of 180, with desiccant.

(Shown in Product Identification Section)

Cromolyn
sodium cromoglycate
Seasonal Conjunctivitis Prophylaxis—Antiallergic

PendoPharm

SUPPLIED: Each drop of sterile ophthalmic solution contains: approximately 0.04 mL of the 2% (w/v) solution or sodium cromoglycate 0.8 mg. Nonmedicinal ingredients: benzalkonium chloride, edetate disodium and purified water. Plastic dropper bottles of 5, 10 and 12.5 mL. Store between 15-30°C.

The reader is invited to consult CPhA's monograph **Selective Serotonin Reuptake Inhibitors**.

CTP 30 Ⓟ
citalopram HBr
Antidepressant

Sepracor

SUPPLIED: Each white to off-white, film-coated tablet with "C/30" on one side and "Σ>" on the other side contains: citalopram hydrobromide equivalent to citalopram 30 mg. Nonmedicinal ingredients: corn (maize) starch, crospovidone, lactose monohydrate, magnesium stearate, microcrystalline cellulose PH101, Opadry White OY-LS-28908, povidone and purified water; film coating: hypromellose, lactose monohydrate, polyethylene glycol and titanium dioxide. Blisters of 30. Store in a dry place at room temperature.

Cubicin® Ⓟ
daptomycin
Antibacterial

Sepracor

Date of Revision: March 8, 2010

SUMMARY PRODUCT INFORMATION:

Route of Administration	Dosage Form/ Strength	Clinically Relevant Nonmedicinal Ingredients
Intravenous	10 mL vial, 500 mg/vial	Sodium hydroxide For a complete listing see Dosage Forms, Composition and Packaging.

INDICATIONS AND CLINICAL USE: CUBICIN (daptomycin for injection) is indicated for the following infections in adults:

Complicated skin and skin structure infections (cSSSI) caused by susceptible strains of the following Gram-positive microorganisms: *S. aureus* (including methicillin-resistant strains), *S. pyogenes* and *S. agalactiae*.

Combination therapy may be clinically indicated if the documented or presumed pathogens include Gram-negative and/or anaerobic organisms. Skin and soft tissues infections are considered complicated when they involve deeper skin structures, such as fascia or muscle layers, require significant surgical intervention or arise in the presence of significant co-morbidity.

***S. aureus* bloodstream infections (bacteremia) including those with right-sided *S. aureus* infective endocarditis (native valve)** caused by methicillin-susceptible and methicillin-resistant strains.

Patients with prosthetic valves, meningitis, known osteomyelitis, polymicrobial bloodstream infections or with intravascular foreign material not planned for removal within 4 days of dosing (except vascular stents in place for >6 months or permanent pacemakers) were **not** enrolled in clinical trials.

The efficacy of CUBICIN in patients with left-sided infective endocarditis due to *S. aureus* has **not** been demonstrated. The clinical trial of daptomycin in patients with *S. aureus* bloodstream infections included limited data from patients with left-sided infective endocarditis; outcomes in these patients were poor.

Combination therapy may be clinically indicated if the documented or presumed pathogens include Gram-negative and/or anaerobic organisms.

CUBICIN is **not** indicated for the treatment of pneumonia.

Patients with persisting or relapsing *S. aureus* infection or poor clinical response should have repeat blood cultures. Appropriate surgical intervention (e.g., debridement, removal of prosthetic devices, valve replacement surgery) and/or consideration of a change in antibiotic regimen may be required.

CONTRAINDICATIONS: CUBICIN (daptomycin for injection) is contraindicated in patients with known hypersensitivity to daptomycin.

WARNINGS AND PRECAUTIONS: General: The use of antibiotics may promote the overgrowth of non-susceptible organisms. Should superinfection occur during therapy, appropriate measures should be taken.

Prescribing CUBICIN (daptomycin for injection) in the absence of a proven or strongly suspected bacterial infection is unlikely to provide benefit to the patient and increases the risk of the development of drug-resistant bacteria.

CUBICIN is inactive against Gram-negative bacteria.

Because daptomycin activity is inhibited in the presence of pulmonary surfactant, CUBICIN is **not** indicated for use in pneumonia.

The safety and efficacy of CUBICIN has **not** been established in patients with co-morbidities of meningitis, musculopathies, neuropathies or severe renal impairment.

Immune: Hypersensitivity: Anaphylaxis and hypersensitivity reactions (including pruritus, hives, shortness of breath, difficulty swallowing, truncal erythema and pulmonary eosinophilia) have been reported with CUBICIN use. If an allergic reaction occurs, administration of CUBICIN should be discontinued and appropriate therapy should be initiated.

Persisting or Relapsing *S. aureus* Infection: Patients with persisting or relapsing *S. aureus* infection or poor clinical response should have repeat blood cultures. If a culture is positive for *S. aureus*, MIC susceptibility testing of the isolate should be performed using a standardized procedure, as well as diagnostic evaluation to rule out sequestered foci of infection. Appropriate surgical intervention (e.g., debridement, removal of prosthetic devices, valve replacement surgery) and/or consideration of a change in antibiotic regimen may be required.

In the *S. aureus* bacteremia/*S. aureus* infective endocarditis (SAB/SAIE) trial, failure of treatment due to persisting or relapsing *S. aureus* infections was assessed in 19/120 (15.8%) CUBICIN-treated patients [12 with methicillin-resistant *S. aureus* (MRSA) and 7 with methicillin-susceptible *S. aureus* (MSSA)] and 11/115 (9.6%) comparator-treated patients (9 with MRSA treated with vancomycin and 2 with MSSA treated with anti-staphylococcal semi-synthetic penicillin). Among all failures, 6 CUBICIN-treated patients and 1 vancomycin-treated patient developed increasing MICs (reduced susceptibility) on or following therapy. Most patients who failed due to persisting or relapsing *S. aureus* infection had deep-seated infection and did not receive necessary surgical intervention.

Musculoskeletal: Myopathy and Creatine Phosphokinase (CPK): Myopathy (muscular pains, weakness, and/or rhabdomyolysis) associated with creatine phosphokinase (CPK) elevations has been observed with the use of daptomycin in human and animal studies and during post-marketing use (see Adverse Reactions).

Therefore, in patients receiving CUBICIN it is recommended that:

- Patients should be monitored regularly for any signs and symptoms that might represent myopathy including muscle pain or weakness, particularly in the distal extremities.
- Any patient who develops unexplained muscle pain, tenderness, weakness or cramps should have CPK levels monitored every 2 days.
- Plasma CPK levels should be measured at baseline and at least once weekly during therapy in all patients.
- Patients who develop unexplained elevations in CPK should be monitored more frequently than once weekly.
- Consideration should be given prior to initiation of CUBICIN therapy in patients with increased baseline CPK as these patients may be at increased risk of further increases of CPK during CUBICIN therapy. If CUBICIN is given, these patients should be monitored more frequently than once weekly.
- CPK should be measured more frequently than once weekly in patients who are at higher risk of developing myopathy. These patients include but are not limited to those with renal insufficiency, and those who recently received or are currently taking other medications known to be associated with myopathy (e.g., HMG-CoA reductase inhibitors).

CUBICIN should be discontinued in patients with unexplained signs and symptoms of myopathy in conjunction with CPK elevation >1000 U/L (approximately 5 times ULN), or in patients without reported symptoms who have marked elevations in CPK (≥10 times ULN). In addition, consideration should be given to temporarily suspending agents associated with rhabdomyolysis, such as HMG-CoA reductase inhibitors, in patients receiving CUBICIN.

In Phase 3 complicated skin and skin structure infection trials (cSSSI) of CUBICIN, at a dose of 4 mg/kg, elevations in serum CPK were reported as clinical adverse events in 15/534 (2.8%) CUBICIN-treated patients, compared to 10/558 (1.8%) comparator-treated patients.

In the *S. aureus* bacteremia/*S. aureus* infective endocarditis (SAB/SAIE) trial, at a dose of 6 mg/kg, elevations in CPK were reported as clinical adverse events in 8/120 (6.7%) of CUBICIN-treated patients, compared to 1/116 (<1%) of the comparator-treated patients. There were a total of 11 patients who experienced CPK elevations to above 500 U/L (2.5 times ULN). Of these 11 patients, 5 had recent prior or concomitant treatment with an HMG-CoA reductase inhibitor. Three (2.6%) CUBICIN-treated patients, including 1 with trauma associated with heroin overdose, 1 with spinal cord compression and 1 with concomitant HMG-CoA reductase inhibitor, had an elevation in CPK >500 U/L with associated musculoskeletal symptoms. None of the patients in the comparator group had an elevation of CPK >500 U/L with associated musculoskeletal symptoms.

In a Phase 1 study in healthy volunteers examining doses up to 12 mg/kg q24h of CUBICIN for 14 days, no skeletal muscle effects or CPK elevations were observed.

Skeletal muscle effects associated with CUBICIN were observed in animals.

Neurologic: Neuropathy: Patients should be monitored for signs and symptoms of neuropathy during therapy with CUBICIN.

Direct effects on the central nervous system have not been investigated.

In a small number of patients in Phase 1 and Phase 2 studies at doses up to 6 mg/kg, administration of CUBICIN was associated with decreases in nerve conduction velocity and with adverse events (e.g., paresthesias, Bell's palsy) possibly reflective of peripheral or cranial neuropathy. In the *S. aureus* bacteremia/*S. aureus* infective endocarditis (SAB/SAIE) trial, a total of 11/120

(9.2%) CUBICIN-treated patients had treatment-emergent adverse events related to the peripheral nervous system. All of the events were classified as mild to moderate in severity, most were of short duration and resolved during continued treatment with CUBICIN or were likely due to an alternative etiology.

In a Phase 1 study in healthy volunteers examining doses up to 12 mg/kg q24h of CUBICIN for 14 days, no evidence of peripheral nerve conduction deficits or symptoms of peripheral neuropathy were observed.

In animals, effects of CUBICIN on peripheral nerve were observed.

Renal: The safety and efficacy of CUBICIN in patients with severe renal insufficiency (creatinine clearance <30 mL/min) have not been established. **CUBICIN should only be considered for use in patients with severe renal impairment when the expected clinical benefit outweighs the potential risk and there are no further available therapeutic options.** In these patients, a dose adjustment is required (see Dosage and Administration, Patients with Renal Impairment). Response to treatment, renal function and creatine phosphokinase (CPK) should be closely monitored.

No dose adjustment is required in patients with mild to moderate renal impairment (creatinine clearance ≥30 mL/min). However, due to limited clinical experience, response to treatment, renal function and creatine phosphokinase (CPK) should be closely monitored in all patients with some degree of renal insufficiency (creatinine clearance <80 mL/min).

Consideration should be given to monitoring renal function in patients treated with CUBICIN. Renal insufficiency has been reported during treatment with CUBICIN although the relationship to daptomycin remains unclear (see Adverse Reactions).

Caution is advised prior to commencing therapy with CUBICIN in patients who already have some degree of renal insufficiency (creatinine clearance <80 mL/min).

Regular monitoring of renal function is advised during the concomitant administration of potentially nephrotoxic agents, regardless of the patient's underlying renal function.

In the *S. aureus* bacteremia/*S. aureus* infective endocarditis (SAB/SAIE) trial, at a dose of CUBICIN 6 mg/kg/day, a lower clinical success rate and an increase in serious adverse events were seen in patients with moderately impaired renal function (creatinine clearance 30 to <50 mL/min).

Carcinogenesis and Mutagenesis: Long-term carcinogenicity studies in animals have not been conducted to evaluate the carcinogenic potential of daptomycin. However, neither mutagenic nor clastogenic potential was found in a battery of genotoxicity tests.

Gastrointestinal: *Clostridium difficile*-associated Disease : *C. difficile*-associated disease (CDAD) has been reported with the use of many antibacterial agents, including CUBICIN. CDAD may range in severity from mild diarrhea to fatal colitis. It is important to consider this diagnosis in patients who present with diarrhea, or symptoms of colitis, pseudomembranous colitis, toxic megacolon, or perforation of the colon subsequent to the administration of any antibacterial agent. CDAD has been reported to occur over 2 months after the administration of antibacterial agents.

Treatment with antibacterial agents may alter the normal flora of the colon and may permit overgrowth of *C. difficile*. *C. difficile* produces toxins A and B which contribute to the development of CDAD. CDAD may cause significant morbidity and mortality. CDAD can be refractory to antimicrobial therapy.

If the diagnosis of CDAD is suspected or confirmed, appropriate therapeutic measures should be initiated. Mild cases of CDAD usually respond to discontinuation of antibacterial agents not directed against *C. difficile*. In moderate to severe cases, consideration should be given to management with fluids and electrolytes, protein supplementation, and treatment with an antibacterial agent clinically effective against *C. difficile*. Surgical evaluation should be instituted as clinically indicated, as surgical intervention may be required in certain severe cases (see Adverse Reactions).

Respiratory: In Phase 3 studies of community-acquired pneumonia, the death rate and rates of serious cardiorespiratory adverse events were higher in CUBICIN-treated patients than in comparator-treated patients. These differences were due to lack of therapeutic effectiveness of CUBICIN in the treatment of community-acquired pneumonia in patients experiencing these adverse events (see Indications and Clinical Use). Daptomycin's activity in vitro is inhibited by the presence of pulmonary surfactant.

Special Populations: Pregnant Women: No clinical studies have been performed in pregnant women. CUBICIN should not be used during pregnancy unless clearly necessary and the benefits to the mother outweigh the potential risks to the fetus. Animal studies have not demonstrated harmful effects with respect to pregnancy, embryonal/fetal development, parturition or postnatal development.

Nursing Women: It is not known if daptomycin is excreted in human milk. Breastfeeding should be discontinued during treatment with CUBICIN.

Pediatrics (<18 years of age): The safety and efficacy of CUBICIN in patients under the age of 18 have not been established.

Geriatrics (>65 years of age): In the Phase 3 clinical studies, lower clinical success rates were seen in patients ≥65 years of age compared to those <65 years of age. In addition, treatment-emergent adverse events were more common in patients ≥65 years old than in patients <65 years of age. Of the 534 patients treated with CUBICIN in Phase 3 controlled clinical trials of complicated skin and skin structure infection (cSSSI), 27.0% were 65 years of age or older and 12.4% were 75 years or older. Of the 120 patients treated with CUBICIN in the Phase 3 *S. aureus* bacteremia/*S. aureus* infective endocarditis (SAB/SAIE) controlled clinical trial, 25.0% were 65 years of age or older and 15.8% were 75 years or older.

Monitoring and Laboratory Tests: Creatine Phosphokinase (CPK): Patients should be monitored regularly for any signs and symptoms that might represent myopathy including muscle pain or weakness, particularly in the distal extremities. Any patient who develops unexplained muscle pain, tenderness, weakness or cramps should have CPK levels monitored every 2 days.

Plasma CPK levels should be measured at baseline and at least once weekly during CUBICIN therapy in all patients. Patients who develop unexplained elevations in CPK should be monitored more frequently than once weekly. Consideration should be given prior to initiation of CUBICIN therapy in patients with increased baseline CPK as these patients may be at increased risk of further increases of CPK during CUBICIN therapy. If CUBICIN is given, these patients should be monitored more frequently than once weekly.

CPK should be measured more frequently than once weekly in patients who are at higher risk of developing myopathy. These patients include but are not limited to those with renal insufficiency, and those who recently received or are currently taking other medications known to be associated with myopathy (e.g., HMG-CoA reductase inhibitors) [see Warnings and Precautions, Musculoskeletal, Myopathy and Creatine Phosphokinase (CPK)].

Renal: Consideration should be given to monitoring renal function in patients treated with CUBICIN.

In patients with renal insufficiency (creatinine clearance <80 mL/min) response to treatment, renal function and creatine phosphokinase (CPK) should be closely monitored.

The safety and efficacy of CUBICIN in patients with severe renal insufficiency (creatinine clearance <30 mL/min) have not been established.

Neuropathy: Patients should be monitored for signs and symptoms of neuropathy during therapy with CUBICIN.

Warfarin: As experience with the concomitant administration of CUBICIN and warfarin is limited, anticoagulant activity in patients receiving CUBICIN and warfarin should be monitored for the first several days after initiating therapy with CUBICIN.

ADVERSE REACTIONS: Adverse Drug Reaction Overview: Clinical studies enrolled 1667 patients treated with CUBICIN and 1319 treated with comparator. Overall, at least one adverse event was reported by 51.3% of CUBICIN-treated subjects and by 52.5% of comparator-treated subjects in two Phase 3, double-blind, controlled complicated skin and skin structure infection (cSSSI) trials. In the randomized, comparative, open-label *S. aureus* bacteremia/*S. aureus* infective endocarditis (SAB/SAIE) trial, the majority of patients experienced at least one treatment emergent adverse event during the study, including 95.8% and 94.8% of patients in the CUBICIN and comparator groups, respectively. The majority of adverse events reported in the Phase 1, 2 and 3 clinical studies were described as mild or moderate in intensity.

In the cSSSI trials, CUBICIN was discontinued in 15/534 (2.8%) patients due to an adverse event while comparator was discontinued in 17/558 (3.0%) patients. In the SAB/SAIE trial, CUBICIN was discontinued in 20/120 (16.7%) patients due to an adverse event while comparator was discontinued in 21/116 (18.1%) patients.

The most frequent adverse events observed in the cSSSI trials were: constipation, nausea, injection site reactions, headache and diarrhea. In the SAB/SAIE trial, the most frequent adverse events were: diarrhea, vomiting, constipation and nausea.

The safety data for the administration of daptomycin via 2-minute intravenous injection are derived from two pharmacokinetic studies in healthy volunteers. Based on these study results, both methods of daptomycin administration, the 2-minute intravenous injection and the 30-minute intravenous infusion, had a similar safety and tolerability profile. There was no relevant difference in local tolerability or in the nature and frequency of adverse reactions.

Clinical Trial Adverse Drug Reactions: Because clinical trials are conducted under very specific conditions the adverse reaction rates observed in the clinical trials may not reflect the rates observed in practice and should not be compared to the rates in the clinical trials of another drug. Adverse drug reaction information from clinical trials is useful for identifying drug-related adverse events and for approximating rates.

Complicated Skin and Skin Structure Infection (cSSSI) Trials: Most Common Clinical Trial Adverse Drug Reactions in Two Phase 3 cSSSI Studies: The rates of the most common treatment emergent adverse events irrespective of causality, organized by body system, observed in the cSSSI clinical trials are displayed in Table 1.

Additional adverse events that occurred in <1 to 2% of patients in either CUBICIN (4 mg/kg) or comparator treatment groups in the cSSSI studies are as follows: edema, cellulitis, hypoglycemia, elevated alkaline phosphatase, cough, back pain, abdominal pain, hypokalemia, hyperglycemia, decreased appetite, anxiety, chest pain, sore throat, cardiac failure, confusion and Candida infections. These events occurred at rates ranging from 0.2 to 1.7% in CUBICIN-treated patients and at rates of 0.4 to 1.8% in comparator-treated patients.

Table 1: CUBICIN

Incidence (%) of Treatment Emergent Adverse Events Irrespective of Causality that Occurred in ≥2% of Patients in Either CUBICIN or Comparator Treatment Groups in the Phase 3 cSSSI Studies[a] (Population: Safety[b])

Adverse Event	CUBICIN 4 mg/kg (N=534) %	Comparator[c] (N=558) %
Gastrointestinal Disorders		
Constipation	6.2	6.8
Nausea	5.8	9.5
Diarrhea	5.2	4.3
Vomiting	3.2	3.8
Dyspepsia	0.9	2.5
General Disorders		
Injection Site Reactions	5.8	7.7
Fever	1.9	2.5
Nervous System Disorders		
Headache	5.4	5.4
Insomnia	4.5	5.4
Dizziness	2.2	2.0
Skin/Subcutaneous Disorders		
Rash	4.3	3.8
Pruritus	2.8	3.8
Diagnostic Investigations		
Abnormal Liver Function Tests	3.0	1.6
Elevated CPK	2.8	1.8
Infections		
Fungal Infections	2.6	3.2
Urinary Tract Infections	2.4	0.5
Vascular Disorders		
Hypotension	2.4	1.4
Hypertension	1.1	2.0
Renal/Urinary Disorders		
Renal Failure	2.2	2.7
Blood/Lymphatic Disorders		
Anemia	2.1	2.3
Respiratory Disorders		
Dyspnea	2.1	1.6
Musculoskeletal Disorders		
Limb Pain	1.5	2.0
Arthralgia	0.9	2.2

a This table includes Adverse Events from both cSSSI Phase 3 trials. The first trial was conducted in the U.S. and South Africa, the second in Europe, South Africa, Australia and Israel.

b Safety population includes all subjects who received at least one dose of CUBICIN or comparator according to treatment actually received during the trials.

c Comparators included vancomycin (1 g IV q12h), which was used in patients with known or suspected penicillin allergy or with methicillin-resistant *S. aureus* infection, and anti-staphylococcal semi-synthetic penicillin (i.e. nafcillin, oxacillin, cloxacillin, flucloxacillin 4-12 g/day IV), which were selected based on the standard therapy in each country.

The most common possibly or probably drug-related treatment emergent adverse events organized by body system, observed in the cSSSI trials are displayed in Table 2.

Less Common Clinical Trial Adverse Drug Reactions (<1%) in Two Phase 3 cSSSI Studies: Additional drug-related adverse events (possibly or probably related) that occurred in <1% of patients receiving CUBICIN in the complicated skin and skin structure infection (cSSSI) trials are as follows:

Body as a Whole: fatigue, weakness, rigors, discomfort, jitteriness, flushing, hypersensitivity.

Blood/Lymphatic System: leukocytosis, thrombocytopenia, thrombocytosis, eosinophilia, increased international normalized ratio (INR).

Table 2: CUBICIN

Incidence (%) of Possibly or Probably Drug-Related Treatment Emergent Adverse Events Occurring in ≥1% of Patients in Either CUBICIN or Comparator Treatment Groups in the Phase 3 cSSSI Studies (Population: Safety)

Adverse Event	CUBICIN 4 mg/kg (N=534) %	Comparator (N=558) %
Gastrointestinal Disorders		
Nausea	2.2	3.4
Investigations		
Blood Creatine Phosphokinase Increased	2.1	1.4

Cardiovascular System: supraventricular arrhythmia.
Dermatologic System: eczema.
Digestive System: abdominal distension, flatulence, stomatitis, jaundice, increased serum lactate dehydrogenase.
Metabolic/Nutritional System: hypomagnesemia, increased serum bicarbonate, electrolyte disturbance.
Musculoskeletal System: myalgia, muscle cramps, muscle weakness, osteomyelitis.
Nervous System: vertigo, mental status change, paraesthesia.
Special Senses: taste disturbance, eye irritation.
Abnormal Hematologic and Clinical Chemistry Findings in Two Phase 3 cSSSI Studies: In the two Phase 3 comparator-controlled complicated skin and skin structure (cSSSI) studies, there was no clinically or statistically significant difference (p<0.05) in the incidence of creatine phosphokinase (CPK) elevations between patients treated with CUBICIN and those treated with comparator. CPK elevations in both groups were generally related to medical conditions, for example, skin and skin structure infection, surgical procedures, or intramuscular injections; and were not associated with muscle symptoms.

Table 3 summarizes the CPK shifts from Baseline through End of Treatment in the cSSSI trials.

Table 3: CUBICIN

Incidence (%) of Creatine Phosphokinase (CPK) Elevations From Baseline Through End of Treatment in either CUBICIN or Comparator Treatment Groups in Phase 3 cSSSI Studies

	All Patients				Patients with Normal CPK at Baseline			
	CUBICIN (N=430)		Comparator (N=459)		CUBICIN (N=374)		Comparator (N=392)	
Change	**%**	**N**	**%**	**N**	**%**	**N**	**%**	**N**
No Increase	90.7	390	91.1	418	91.2	341	91.1	357
Maximum Value								
>1×ULN[a]	9.3	40	8.9	41	8.8	33	8.9	35
>2×ULN	4.9	21	4.8	22	3.7	14	3.1	12
>4×ULN	1.4	6	1.5	7	1.1	4	1.0	4
>5×ULN	1.4	6	0.4	2	1.1	4	0.0	0
>10×ULN	0.5	2	0.2	1	0.2	1	0.0	0

[a] ULN (Upper Limit of Normal) is defined as 200 U/L.

In the cSSSI studies, 0.2% of patients treated with CUBICIN had symptoms of muscle pain or weakness associated with CPK elevations to greater than 4 times the upper limit of normal. The symptoms resolved within 3 days and CPK returned to normal within 7 to 10 days after discontinuing treatment [see Warnings and Precautions, Musculoskeletal, Myopathy and Creatine Phosphokinase (CPK)].

S. aureus **Bacteremia/*****S. aureus*** **Infective Endocarditis (SAB/SAIE) Trial: Most Common Clinical Trial Adverse Drug Reactions in the SAB/SAIE Trial:** The rates of the most common treatment emergent adverse events irrespective of causality and organized by body system observed in the *S. aureus* bacteremia/*S. aureus* infective endocarditis (SAB/SAIE) trial are displayed in Table 4.

Table 4: CUBICIN

Incidence (%) of Treatment Emergent Adverse Events Irrespective of Causality that Occurred in ≥5% of Patients in CUBICIN or Comparator Treatment Groups in the SAB/SAIE Study (Population: Safety[a])

Adverse Events	CUBICIN 6 mg/kg (N=120) %	Comparator[b] (N=116) %
Infections and Infestations	54.2	48.3
Urinary Tract Infection NOS[c]	6.7	9.5
Osteomyelitis NOS	5.8	6.0
Sepsis NOS	5.0	2.6
Bacteremia	5.0	0
Pneumonia NOS	3.3	7.8
Gastrointestinal Disorders	**50.0**	**58.6**
Diarrhea NOS	11.7	18.1
Vomiting NOS	11.7	12.9
Constipation	10.8	12.1
Nausea	10.0	19.8
Abdominal Pain NOS	5.8	3.4
Dyspepsia	4.2	6.9

(cont'd)

Table 4: CUBICIN *(cont'd)*

Incidence (%) of Treatment Emergent Adverse Events Irrespective of Causality that Occurred in ≥5% of Patients in CUBICIN or Comparator Treatment Groups in the SAB/SAIE Study (Population: Safety[a])

Adverse Events	CUBICIN 6 mg/kg (N=120) %	Comparator[b] (N=116) %
Loose stools	4.2	5.2
Gastrointestinal Hemorrhage NOS	1.7	5.2
General Disorders and Administration Site Conditions	**44.2**	**59.5**
Edema Peripheral	6.7	13.8
Pyrexia	6.7	8.6
Chest Pain	6.7	6.0
Edema NOS	6.7	4.3
Asthenia	5.0	5.2
Injection Site Erythema	2.5	6.0
Respiratory, Thoracic and Mediastinal Disorders	**31.7**	**37.1**
Pharyngolaryngeal Pain	8.3	1.7
Pleural Effusion	5.8	6.9
Cough	3.3	6.0
Dyspnea	3.3	5.2
Skin and Subcutaneous Tissue Disorders	**30.0**	**34.5**
Rash NOS	6.7	8.6
Pruritus	5.8	5.2
Erythema	5.0	5.2
Sweating Increased	5.0	0
Musculoskeletal and Connective Tissue Disorders	**29.2**	**36.2**
Pain in Extremity	9.2	9.5
Back Pain	6.7	8.6
Arthralgia	3.3	11.2
Psychiatric Disorders	**29.2**	**24.1**
Insomnia	9.2	6.9
Anxiety	5.0	5.2
Nervous System Disorders	**26.7**	**27.6**
Headache	6.7	10.3
Dizziness	5.8	6.0
Investigations	**25.0**	**28.4**
Blood Creatine Phosphokinase Increased	6.7	<1
Blood and Lymphatic System Disorders	**24.2**	**20.7**
Anemia NOS	12.5	15.5
Metabolism and Nutrition Disorders	**21.7**	**32.8**
Hypokalemia	9.2	12.9
Hyperkalemia	5.0	8.6
Vascular Disorders	**17.5**	**17.2**
Hypertension NOS	5.8	2.6
Hypotension NOS	5.0	7.8
Injury, Poisoning and Procedural Complications	**15.8**	**15.5**
Renal and Urinary Disorders	**15.0**	**22.4**
Renal Failure NOS	3.3	9.5
Renal Failure Acute	3.3	6.0
Cardiac Disorders	**11.7**	**15.5**
Reproductive System and Breast Disorders	**5.0**	**6.9**

(cont'd)

Table 4: CUBICIN *(cont'd)*

Incidence (%) of Treatment Emergent Adverse Events Irrespective of Causality that Occurred in ≥5% of Patients in CUBICIN or Comparator Treatment Groups in the SAB/SAIE Study (Population: Safety[a])

Adverse Events	CUBICIN 6 mg/kg (N=120) %	Comparator[b] (N=116) %
Eye Disorders	4.2	8.6

[a] Safety population includes all subjects who received at least one dose of CUBICIN or comparator according to treatment actually received during the trials.
[b] Comparator: vancomycin (1 g IV q12h), which was used in patients with known or suspected penicillin allergy or with methicillin-resistant *S. aureus*, or anti-staphylococcal semi-synthetic penicillins (i.e., nafcillin, oxacillin, cloxacillin, flucloxacillin; 2 g IV q4h), which were selected based on the standard therapy in each country, each with initial synergistic gentamicin.
[c] NOS: Not Otherwise Specified.
Note: p-values by body system were as follows: infections p=0.435; gastrointestinal p=0.194; general and administration site p=0.020; respiratory, thoracic, mediastinal p=0.412; skin and subcutaneous tissue p=0.488; musculoskeletal and connective tissue p=0.269; psychiatric p=0.462; nervous system p=0.885; investigations p=0.560; blood and lymphatic system p=0.537; metabolism and nutrition p=0.059; vascular p>0.999; injury, poisoning p>0.999; renal and urinary p=0.181; cardiac disorders p=0.449; reproductive system p=0.591; eye disorders p=0.189.

The most common possibly or probably drug-related treatment emergent adverse events, organized by body system, observed in the SAB/SAIE trial are displayed in Table 5.

Table 5: CUBICIN

Incidence (%) of Possibly or Probably Drug-Related Treatment Emergent Adverse Events Occurring in ≥1% of Patients in Either CUBICIN or Comparator Treatment Groups in the Phase 3 SAB/SAIE Study (Population: Safety)

Adverse Events	CUBICIN 6 mg/kg (N=120) %	Comparator (N=116) %
Investigations		
Blood Creatine Phosphokinase (CPK) Increased	5.0	0
Blood Phosphorus Increased	2.5	<1
Blood Alkaline Phosphatase Increased	1.7	0
International Normalized Ratio Increased	1.7	0
Liver Function Test Abnormal	1.7	<1
Blood Creatinine Increased	0	2.6
Gastrointestinal Disorders		
Loose Stools	3.3	1.7
Dyspepsia	2.5	<1
Diarrhea NOS	1.7	9.5
Nausea	1.7	5.2
Vomiting	<1	1.7
Skin and Subcutaneous Tissue Disorders		
Rash NOS	2.5	2.6
Renal and Urinary Disorders		
Renal Failure NOS	1.7	6.0
Renal Impairment NOS	<1	1.7
Renal Failure Acute	0	2.6
Infections and Infestations		
Candidal Infection NOS	1.7	0
Vaginal Candidiasis	1.7	0
General Disorders and Administration Site Conditions		
Chest Pain	1.7	0
Pyrexia	0	2.6
Blood and Lymphatic System Disorders		
Eosinophilia	1.7	0
Nervous System Disorders		
Dysgeusia	0	2.6
Vascular Disorders		
Hypotension NOS	0	2.6
Musculoskeletal and Connective Tissue Disorders		
Arthralgia	0	1.7
Weakness in Extremity	1.7	0

Less Common Clinical Trial Adverse Drug Reactions in the SAB/SAIE Trial (<1%): The following events, not included above in Table 5, were reported as possibly or probably drug-related in the *S. aureus* bacteremia/*S. aureus* infective endocarditis (SAB/SAIE) CUBICIN-treated group:
Blood and Lymphatic System Disorders: lymphadenopathy, thrombocythemia, thrombocytopenia.
Cardiac Disorders: atrial fibrillation, atrial flutter, cardiac arrest.
Ear and Labyrinth Disorders: tinnitus.
Eye Disorders: vision blurred.
Gastrointestinal Disorders: dry mouth, epigastric discomfort, gingival pain, hypoesthesia oral.
Infections and Infestations: fungemia, oral candidiasis, urinary tract infection fungal.
Investigations: alanine aminotransferase increased, aspartate aminotransferase increased, prothrombin time prolonged.
Metabolism and Nutrition Disorders: appetite decreased NOS.
Musculoskeletal and Connective Tissue Disorders: myalgia.
Nervous System Disorders: dyskinesia, paresthesia.
Psychiatric Disorders: hallucination NOS.
Renal and Urinary Disorders: proteinuria, renal impairment NOS.
Skin and Subcutaneous Tissue Disorders: heat rash, pruritus generalized, rash vesicular.
Abnormal Hematologic and Clinical Chemistry Findings in the SAB/SAIE Trial: In the *S. aureus* bacteremia/*S. aureus* infective endocarditis (SAB/SAIE) trial, a total of 11 CUBICIN patients (9.2%) had treatment-emergent elevations in creatine phosphokinase (CPK) to >500 U/L, including 4 patients with elevations >10×ULN. Three of these 11 patients had CPK levels return to the normal range during continued CUBICIN treatment, 6 had values return to the normal range during follow-up, 1 had values returning toward baseline at the last assessment, and 1 did not have follow-up values reported. Six of the 11 patients with treatment-emergent CPK elevations >500 U/L had medical or surgical reasons for the elevated CPK. Three patients discontinued CUBICIN due to CPK elevation. Table 6 presents the incidence of CPK elevations from baseline in all patients and in patients with normal CPK levels through the end of treatment with CUBICIN and comparator in the SAB/SAIE trial.

Table 6: CUBICIN

Incidence (%) of Creatine Phosphokinase (CPK) Elevations From Baseline through End of Treatment in either CUBICIN or Comparator Treatment Groups in the SAB/SAIE Study

	All Patients				Patients with Normal CPK at Baseline			
	CUBICIN (N=116)		Comparator (N=111)		CUBICIN (N=92)		Comparator (N=96)	
Change	%	N	%	N	%	N	%	N
No Increase	75.9	88	87.4	97	75	69	87.5	84
Maximum Value								
>1×ULN[a]	24.1	28	12.6	14	25	23	12.5	12
>2×ULN	13.8	16	6.3	7	12	11	5.2	5
>4×ULN	8.6	10	0.9	1	7.6	7	0	0
>5×ULN	6.9	8	0.9	1	5.4	5	0	0
>10×ULN	3.4	4	0.9	1	2.2	2	0	0

[a] ULN (Upper Limit of Normal) is laboratory specific.
Note: CPK evaluations through 3 days post-treatment are included in the analysis.

There was more renal dysfunction in comparator-treated patients than in CUBICIN-treated patients. The incidence of decreased renal function, defined as the proportion of patients with a creatinine clearance level <50 mL/min if baseline clearance was ≥50 mL/min or with a decrease of ≥10 mL/min if baseline clearance was <50 mL/min, is shown in Table 7.

Table 7: CUBICIN

Incidence of Decreased Renal Function Based on Creatinine Clearance Levels

Study Interval	CUBICIN 6 mg/kg (N=120) n/N (%)	Comparator[a] (N=116) n/N (%)
Days 2 to 4	2/96 (2.1)	6/90 (6.7)
Days 2 to 7	6/115 (5.2)	16/113 (14.2)
Days 2 to End of Study	13/118 (11.0)	30/114 (26.3)

[a] Comparator: vancomycin (1 g IV q12h) or anti-staphylococcal semi-synthetic penicillin (i.e. nafcillin, oxacillin, cloxacillin, flucloxacillin; 2 g IV q4h), each with initial low-dose gentamicin.

Post-Market Adverse Drug Reactions: The following adverse reactions have been reported with CUBICIN in worldwide post-marketing experience. Because these events are reported voluntarily from a population of unknown size, estimates of frequency cannot be made and causal relationship cannot be precisely established.
Immune System Disorders: anaphylaxis; hypersensitivity reactions, including pruritus, hives, shortness of breath, difficulty swallowing, truncal erythema and pulmonary eosinophilia.
Musculoskeletal System: rhabdomyolysis; some reports involved patients treated concurrently with CUBICIN and HMG-CoA reductase inhibitors.
Neurologic: one case of coma post-anaesthesia/surgery.

DRUG INTERACTIONS: Overview: There is limited experience regarding concomitant administration of CUBICIN (daptomycin for injection) with other medicinal products that may trigger myopathy. However, some cases of marked rises in creatine phosphokinase (CPK) levels and cases of rhabdomyolysis occurred in patients taking one of these medications at the same time as CUBICIN. It is recommended that other medications associated with myopathy should, if possible, be temporarily discontinued during treatment with CUBICIN unless the benefits of concomitant administration outweigh the risk. If co-administration cannot be avoided, CPK levels should be measured more frequently than once weekly and patients should be closely monitored for any signs or symptoms that might represent myopathy.

Daptomycin is primarily cleared by renal filtration and, therefore, plasma levels may be increased during co-administration with medicinal products that reduce renal filtration (e.g., NSAIDs and COX-2 inhibitors). In addition, there is a potential for a pharmacodynamic interaction to occur during co-administration due to additive renal effects. Therefore, caution is advised when CUBICIN is co-administered with any other medicinal product known to reduce renal filtration.
Drug-Drug Interactions: Drug-drug interaction studies were performed with CUBICIN and other drugs that are likely to either be co-administered or associated with overlapping toxicity as shown in Table 8.
Drug-Food Interactions: Interactions with food have not been established.
Drug-Herb Interactions: Interactions with herbal products have not been established.
Drug-Laboratory Test Interactions: Clinically relevant plasma levels of daptomycin have been observed to cause a significant concentration-dependent false prolongation of prothrombin time (PT) and elevation of International Normalized Ratio (INR) when certain recombinant thromboplastin reagents are utilized for the assay. The possibility of an erroneously elevated PT/INR result due to interaction with a recombinant thromboplastin reagent may be minimized by drawing specimens for PT or INR testing near the time of trough plasma concentrations of daptomycin.

If confronted with an abnormally high PT/INR result in a patient being treated with CUBICIN, consideration should be given for evaluating PT/INR utilizing alternative methods.

Table 8: CUBICIN

Established or Potential Drug-Drug Interactions with CUBICIN

Drug Name	Ref	Effect	Clinical Comment
Aztreonam	CT	In a study in which 15 healthy adult subjects received a single dose of CUBICIN 6 mg/kg IV, aztreonam 1 g IV, and both in combination, the C_{max} and $AUC_{0-\infty}$ of daptomycin were not significantly altered by aztreonam; the C_{max} and $AUC_{0-\infty}$ of aztreonam were also not significantly altered by CUBICIN.	No dosage adjustment of either antibiotic is warranted when co-administered.
HMG-CoA Reductase Inhibitors	CT	In 20 healthy subjects on a stable daily dose of oral simvastatin 40 mg, administration of CUBICIN 4 mg/kg IV q24h for 14 days (N=10) was not associated with a higher incidence of adverse events than subjects receiving placebo once daily (N=10).	Inhibitors of HMG-CoA reductase may cause myopathy, which is manifested as muscle pain or weakness associated with elevated levels of CPK. Experience with co-administration of HMG-CoA reductase inhibitors and CUBICIN in patients is limited, therefore, consideration should be given to temporarily suspending use of HMG-CoA reductase inhibitors in patients receiving CUBICIN (see Warnings and Precautions, Musculoskeletal).
Probenecid	CT	Concomitant administration of oral probenecid (500 mg four times daily) and a single dose of CUBICIN 4 mg/kg IV did not significantly alter the C_{max} and $AUC_{0-\infty}$ of daptomycin.	No dosage adjustment of CUBICIN is warranted when CUBICIN is co-administered with probenecid.
Tobramycin	CT	In a study in which 6 healthy adult males received a single dose of CUBICIN 2 mg/kg IV, tobramycin 1 mg/kg IV, and both in combination, the mean C_{max} and $AUC_{0-\infty}$ of daptomycin increased 12.7% and 8.7%, respectively, when administered with tobramycin. The mean C_{max} and $AUC_{0-\infty}$ of tobramycin decreased 10.7% and 6.6%, respectively, when administered with CUBICIN. These differences were not statistically significant.	The interaction between CUBICIN and tobramycin with a clinical dose of CUBICIN is unknown. Caution is warranted when CUBICIN is co-administered with tobramycin.
	Non-Clinical	In rats, mild skeletal muscle degeneration and/or regeneration was observed with 20 mg/kg IV CUBICIN when administered alone. During concurrent administration with tobramycin 10 mg/kg SC b.i.d., mild skeletal muscle changes were observed with 5 mg/kg IV CUBICIN. Tobramycin may have a weak potentiating effect on muscle damage caused by CUBICIN.	
Warfarin	CT	In 16 healthy subjects, concomitant administration of CUBICIN 6 mg/kg IV q24h for 5 days followed by a single oral dose of warfarin (25 mg) had no significant effect on the pharmacokinetics of either drug and did not significantly alter the INR (International Normalized Ratio).	As experience with the concomitant administration of CUBICIN and warfarin is limited, anticoagulant activity in patients receiving CUBICIN and warfarin should be monitored for the first several days after initiating therapy with CUBICIN.
Gentamicin	Non-Clinical	An increase in nephrotoxicity was apparent upon combination treatment with daptomycin 30 mg/kg/day IV and a high dose of gentamicin (30 mg/kg/day IM) in dogs. No meaningful difference in nephrotoxicity was observed in animals receiving daptomycin in combination with a more clinically relevant dose of gentamicin (9 mg/kg/day IM).	Concurrent administration of daptomycin and clinical levels of gentamicin is unlikely to alter the nephrotoxic potential of gentamicin in humans. However, caution should be used when administering the combination to renally impaired patients.

Legend: CT=Clinical Trial.

DOSAGE AND ADMINISTRATION: Complicated Skin and Skin Structure Infections: CUBICIN (daptomycin for injection) 4 mg/kg should be administered intravenously in 0.9% sodium chloride injection, USP once every 24 hours for 7 to 14 days, either by injection over a 2 minute period or by infusion over a 30 minute period.

***S. aureus* Bloodstream Infections (Bacteremia) Including Those with Right-Sided *S. aureus* Infective Endocarditis (Native Valve):** CUBICIN 6 mg/kg should be administered intravenously in 0.9% sodium chloride injection, USP once every 24 hours, either by injection over a 2 minute period or by infusion over a 30 minute period. Duration of treatment should be based on the treating physician's working diagnosis. In the clinical trial, duration ranged from 10 days to 42 days with an option for an additional 14 days. There are limited safety data for the use of CUBICIN for more than 28 days.

Clinical studies in patients employed infusion of daptomycin over 30 minutes. There is no clinical experience in patients with the administration of daptomycin as an injection over 2 minutes. This mode of administration was only studied in healthy subjects. However, when compared with the same doses given as intravenous infusions over 30 minutes there were no clinically important differences in the pharmacokinetics and safety profile of daptomycin (see also Adverse Reactions, Adverse Drug Reaction Overview and Action And Clinical Pharmacology, Pharmacokinetics).

Dosing Considerations: General:

- CUBICIN should not be dosed more frequently than once a day. In Phase 1 and 2 clinical studies, creatine phosphokinase (CPK) elevations appeared to be more frequent when CUBICIN was dosed more frequently than once daily.
- Clinical studies have shown that dosing adjustments based on age alone, gender, race or obesity are not required (see Action and Clinical Pharmacology, Special Populations and Conditions).
- Appropriate specimens for microbiological examination should be obtained in order to isolate and identify the causative pathogens and to determine their susceptibility to daptomycin. Empiric therapy may be initiated while awaiting test results. Antimicrobial therapy should be adjusted as needed based upon test results.
- To reduce the development of drug-resistant bacteria and maintain the effectiveness of CUBICIN and other antibacterial drugs, CUBICIN should be used only to treat infections that are proven or strongly suspected to be caused by susceptible bacteria. When culture and susceptibility information are available, they should be considered in selecting or modifying antibacterial therapy. In the absence of such data, local epidemiology and susceptibility patterns may contribute to the empiric selection of therapy.

The recommended dosing schedule for adult patients including those with creatinine clearance ≥30 mL/min is presented in Table 9.

Table 9: CUBICIN

Recommended Dosage of CUBICIN (daptomycin for injection) in Adult Patients Including Those with Creatinine Clearance ≥30 mL/min

Creatinine Clearance	Indication	Dosage Regimen	Duration
≥30 mL/min	Complicated Skin and Skin Structure Infections	4 mg/kg once every 24 hours	7 to 14 days
	S. aureus Bloodstream Infections (Bacteremia) including those with Right-Sided *S. aureus* Infective Endocarditis (Native Valve)	6 mg/kg once every 24 hours	10 to 42 days with an option for an additional 14 days

Patients with Renal Impairment: Daptomycin is eliminated primarily by the kidney.

No dose adjustment is required in patients whose creatinine clearance is ≥30 mL/min (see Table 9).

Patients with Creatinine Clearance <30 mL/min: CUBICIN should only be used in patients whose creatinine clearance is <30 mL/min when it is considered that the expected clinical benefit outweighs the potential risk and for whom there are no further therapeutic options.

Clinical efficacy and safety of CUBICIN have not been established in patients with severe renal impairment (creatinine clearance <30 mL/min).

The dose interval adjustment guidance presented below in Table 10 is based on pharmacokinetic modeling data.

Response to treatment, renal function and creatine phosphokinase (CPK) should be closely monitored in these patients.

Whenever possible, CUBICIN should be administered following the completion of dialysis on dialysis days. The use of high-flux dialysis membranes during 4 hours of hemodialysis may increase the percentage of dose removed compared with low-flux membranes.

Table 10: CUBICIN

Dosage Adjustment of CUBICIN (daptomycin for injection) in Adult Patients with Severe Renal Impairment (creatinine clearance <30 mL/min)

Creatinine Clearance	Indication	Dosage Regimen	Duration
<30 mL/min	Complicated Skin and Skin Structure Infections	4 mg/kg once every 48 hours	7 to 14 days
	S. aureus Bloodstream Infections (Bacteremia) including those with Right-Sided *S. aureus* Infective Endocarditis (Native Valve)	6 mg/kg once every 48 hours	10 to 42 days with an option for an additional 14 days

Patients with Hepatic Insufficiency: No dose adjustment is necessary when administering CUBICIN to patients with mild or moderate hepatic insufficiency (Child-Pugh Class B). No data are available in patients with severe hepatic insufficiency (Child-Pugh Class C).

Reconstitution: CUBICIN is supplied in single-use vials containing 500 mg daptomycin as a sterile, lyophilized powder. The contents of a CUBICIN 500 mg vial should be reconstituted with 10 mL of 0.9% sodium chloride for injection to 50 mg/mL. Since no preservative or bacteriostatic agent is present in the product, aseptic technique must be used in preparation of the product.

Procedure:

- Prior to reconstitution, remove the CUBICIN vials from refrigeration and allow the product to sit at room temperature for a few minutes. CUBICIN vials do not need to be warmed to room temperature prior to reconstitution.
- Remove the polypropylene flip-off cap from the CUBICIN vial to expose the central portions of the rubber stoppers. Gently tap vial twice on counter to settle/loosen the lyophilized powder cake.
- Using a syringe, slowly transfer the diluent through the center of the rubber stopper into the CUBICIN vial, pointing the transfer needle toward the wall of the vial to prevent excessive foaming. Ensure that the complete daptomycin product is wetted by gently rotating the vial.
- Allow the product to sit undisturbed for approximately 10 minutes at room temperature.
- Gently swirl the CUBICIN vial until a clear, fully reconstituted solution is obtained. This typically takes from 5 to 15 minutes.
- **Avoid vigorous shaking to prevent foaming of the product during reconstitution.**

The reconstituted solution should be checked carefully to ensure that the product is in solution and visually inspected for the absence of particulates prior to use. Freshly reconstituted solutions of CUBICIN range in colour from pale yellow to light brown.

For IV injection over a period of 2 minutes : Reconstitute CUBICIN, as directed above, to a concentration of 50 mg/mL with 0.9% Sodium Chloride for Injection.

For IV infusion over a period of 30 minutes: Reconstitute CUBICIN, as directed above, to a concentration of 50 mg/mL with 0.9% Sodium Chloride for Injection. Further dilute using aseptic technique with additional 0.9% Sodium Chloride to a final concentration in the range of 2.5 to 20 mg/mL (typically 10 mg/mL).

Vial Size	Nominal Concentration of Reconstituted Solution	Approximate Available Volume of Reconstituted Solution	Volume of Additional Diluent	Total Volume of Solution for Infusion	Nominal Concentration of Solution for Infusion
500 mg	50 mg/mL	10 mL	15 mL	25 mL	20 mg/mL
500 mg	50 mg/mL	10 mL	40 mL	50 mL	10 mg/mL
500 mg	50 mg/mL	10 mL	190 mL	200 mL	2.5 mg/mL

Because CUBICIN does not contain any preservative or bacteriostatic agent, aseptic technique must be used during preparation for administration and the product should be used promptly. If the reconstituted product is not used immediately, it must be refrigerated at 2 to 8°C. It is recommended that the solution be used within 72 hours due to the possibility of microbial contamination during reconstitution (see also Storage and Stability).

CUBICIN vials are for single-use only.

Compatible Intravenous Solutions: CUBICIN is compatible with 0.9% sodium chloride injection and lactated Ringer's injection. CUBICIN is not compatible with glucose (dextrose) containing diluents. Because only limited data are available on the compatibility of CUBICIN with other IV substances, additives or other medications should not be added to CUBICIN single-use vials or infused simultaneously through the same IV line. If the same IV line is used for sequential infusion of several different drugs, the line should be flushed with a compatible infusion solution before and after infusion with CUBICIN.

As with all parenteral drug products, intravenous admixtures should be inspected visually for clarity, particulate matter, precipitate, discoloration and leakage prior to administration, whenever solution and container permit. Solutions showing haziness, particulate matter, precipitate, discoloration or leakage should not be used. Discard unused portion.

OVERDOSAGE:

In the event of overdosage, supportive care is advised with maintenance of glomerular filtration. CUBICIN is slowly cleared from the body by hemodialysis (approximately 15% recovered over 4 hours) or peritoneal dialysis (approximately 11% recovered over 48 hours). The use of high-flux membranes during 4 hours of hemodialysis may increase the percentage of dose removed, as evidenced by the larger decrease in the pre- to post-dose concentrations (41%) compared with low-flux membranes (5 to 7%).

A 58-year old male with a history of multiple sclerosis, diabetes and hypertension was administered an accidental single dose of CUBICIN 3 g (43 mg/kg). Twenty-four hours later symptoms of orofacial movements, lip smacking and shoulder shrugging were observed and diagnosed as dyskinesia. CUBICIN was discontinued and the patient was treated with benztropine and lorazepam. The events resolved and therapy was restarted without further incident.

For management of a suspected drug overdose, contact your regional Poison Control Centre. See the *CPS* Directory section for a list of Poison Control Centres.

ACTION AND CLINICAL PHARMACOLOGY: Mechanism of Action: CUBICIN (daptomycin for injection) is a cyclic lipopeptide antibacterial agent. Daptomycin binds to Gram-positive bacterial membranes in a calcium-dependant manner and causes a rapid depolarization of membrane potential. This loss of membrane potential causes inhibition of protein, DNA, and RNA synthesis, which results in bacterial cell death. Activity of daptomycin is dependent on the presence of physiological levels of free calcium ions (50 µg/mL).

Resistance: Cases of daptomycin resistance have been reported in staphylococci in clinical trials and during post-marketing use.

Pharmacokinetics: The mean pharmacokinetic parameters of CUBICIN at steady-state following IV administration of 4 to 12 mg/kg q24h to healthy young adults are summarized in Table 11.

Table 11: CUBICIN

Mean CUBICIN Pharmacokinetic Parameters in Healthy Volunteers at Steady-State

Dose[b] (mg/kg)	N	Pharmacokinetic Parameters[a] Mean (Standard Deviation)					
		[c]$AUC_{0\text{-}24}$ (µg·h/mL)	$t_{1/2}$ (h)	V_{ss} (L/kg)	CL_T (mL/h/kg)	[c]C_{max} (µg/mL)	[c]C_{min} (µg/mL)
4	6	494 (75)	8.1 (1.0)	0.096 (0.009)	8.3 (1.3)	57.8 (3.0)	5.9 (1.6)
6	6	632 (78)	7.9 (1.0)	0.101 (0.007)	9.1 (1.5)	93.9 (6.0)	6.7 (1.6)
8	6	858 (213)	8.3 (2.2)	0.101 (0.013)	9.0 (3.0)	123.3 (16.0)	10.3 (5.5)
10	9	1039 (178)	7.9 (0.6)	0.098 (0.017)	8.8 (2.2)	141.1 (24.0)	12.9 (2.9)
12	9	1277 (253)	7.7 (1.1)	0.097 (0.018)	9.0 (2.8)	183.7 (25.0)	13.7 (5.2)

a $AUC_{0\text{-}24}$: area under the concentration-time curve from 0 to 24 hours; $t_{½}$: terminal elimination half-life, V_{ss}: volume of distribution at steady-state; CL_T: plasma clearance; C_{max}: maximum plasma concentration (total drug).
b Doses of CUBICIN in excess of 6 mg/kg have not been approved.
c Values relate to total drug in plasma (free+protein bound).

Absorption: Daptomycin pharmacokinetics were generally linear and time-independent at doses of 4 to 12 mg/kg q24h. Steady-state trough concentrations were achieved by the third daily dose. The mean (standard deviation) steady-state trough concentrations attained following administration of 4, 6, 8, 10 and 12 mg/kg q24h were 5.9 (1.6), 6.7 (1.6), 10.3 (5.5), 12.9 (2.9) and 13.7 (5.2) µg/mL, respectively. The mean AUC and C_{min} (minimum plasma concentration) of daptomycin during once-daily dosing with 6, 8, 10 and 12 mg/kg were dose proportional; however, the mean C_{max} (maximum plasma concentration) was slightly less than dose proportional. Total clearance was unchanged across 4 to 12 mg/kg q24h.

Daptomycin administered as a 2-minute intravenous injection also exhibited dose proportional pharmacokinetics in the approved therapeutic dose range of 4 to 6 mg/kg. Comparable exposure (AUC and C_{max}) was demonstrated in healthy subjects following administration of daptomycin as a 30-minute intravenous infusion or as a 2-minute intravenous injection.

Following IV administration of CUBICIN to healthy volunteers over a 2-minute period at doses of 4 and 6 mg/kg, the mean (SD) steady-state $AUC_{0\text{-tau}}$ values were 475 (71) and 701 (82) µg·h/mL, respectively. The mean (SD) steady-state C_{max} values were 63 (11) and 92 (18) µg/mL, respectively.

Distribution: Daptomycin is reversibly bound to human plasma proteins, primarily to serum albumin, in a concentration-independent manner. The overall mean binding at doses from 4 to 12 mg/kg ranged from 90 to 93%. The apparent volume of distribution (V_d) of daptomycin at steady-state in healthy adult subjects was low, approximately 0.1 L/kg at doses of 4 to 12 mg/kg, consistent with distribution primarily within the extracellular space.

Daptomycin penetrates into skin blister fluid and reaches a mean C_{max} of 27.6 µg/mL (mean $t_{½}$=17.3 hrs).

In clinical studies, mean serum protein binding in subjects with creatinine clearance (CL_{CR}) ≥30 mL/min was comparable to that observed in healthy subjects with normal renal function. However, there was a trend toward decreasing serum protein binding among subjects with CL_{CR} <30 mL/min (87.6%), including hemodialysis patients (85.9%) and continuous ambulatory peritoneal dialysis patients (83.5%). The protein binding of daptomycin in subjects with moderate hepatic impairment (Child-Pugh B) was similar to healthy adult subjects.

Metabolism: In vitro studies with human hepatocytes indicate that daptomycin does not inhibit or induce the activities of the following human cytochrome P450 (CYP) isoforms: 1A2, 2A6, 2C9, 2C19, 2D6, 2E1, and 3A4. In in vitro studies, daptomycin was not detectably metabolized by human liver microsomes. It is unlikely that daptomycin will inhibit or induce the metabolism of drugs metabolized by the CYP system.

In a separate study, no metabolites were observed in plasma on Day 1 following administration of daptomycin at 6 mg/kg to healthy subjects. Inactive metabolites have been detected in urine, as determined by the difference in total radioactivity concentrations and microbiologically active concentrations. Minor amounts of 3 oxidative metabolites and one unidentified compound were detected in urine. The site of metabolism has not been identified.

Excretion: Daptomycin is excreted primarily by the kidney. In a mass balance study of 5 healthy subjects using radiolabelled daptomycin, approximately 78% of the administered dose was recovered from urine based on total radioactivity (approximately 52% of the dose based on microbiologically active concentrations) and 5.7% of the dose was recovered from feces (collected for up to nine days) based on total radioactivity.

Due to limited clinical experience, response to treatment, renal function and creatine phosphokinase (CPK) should be closely monitored in all patients with some degree of renal insufficiency (CL_{CR} <80 mL/min) (see Dosage and Administration).

Special Populations and Conditions: Pediatrics: The pharmacokinetics of CUBICIN in pediatric populations (<18 years of age) have not been established.

Geriatrics: The pharmacokinetics of CUBICIN were evaluated in 12 healthy elderly subjects (≥75 years of age) and 11 healthy young matched controls (18 to 30 years of age). Following administration of a single 4 mg/kg IV dose, the mean total clearance of daptomycin was reduced approximately 35% and the mean $AUC_{0\text{-}\infty}$ increased approximately 58% in elderly subjects compared to young healthy subjects. There were no differences in C_{max}. No dosage adjustment is warranted for elderly patients with normal renal function based on age alone.

Gender: No clinically significant gender-related differences in CUBICIN pharmacokinetics have been observed. No dosage adjustment is warranted based on gender when administering CUBICIN.

Hepatic Insufficiency: The pharmacokinetics of CUBICIN were evaluated in 10 subjects with moderate hepatic impairment (Child-Pugh Class B) and compared with healthy volunteers (N=9) matched for gender, age, and weight. The pharmacokinetics of CUBICIN were not altered in subjects with moderate hepatic impairment. No dosage adjustment is warranted when administering CUBICIN to patients with mild to moderate hepatic impairment. The pharmacokinetics of CUBICIN in patients with severe hepatic insufficiency have not been evaluated.

Renal Insufficiency in Complicated Skin and Skin Structure Infections (cSSSI): Population derived pharmacokinetic parameters were determined for patients with cSSSI and healthy non-infected subjects with varying degrees of renal function (N=282). Following the administration of a single 4 mg/kg IV dose of CUBICIN, the plasma clearance (CL_T) was reduced and the systemic exposure ($AUC_{0\text{-}\infty}$) was increased with decreasing renal function (see Table 12). The mean $AUC_{0\text{-}\infty}$ was not markedly different for subjects and patients with creatinine clearance (CL_{CR}) 30-80 mL/min as compared to those with normal renal function (CL_{CR} >80 mL/min). The mean $AUC_{0\text{-}\infty}$ for subjects and patients with CL_{CR} <30 mL/min was approximately 2-times higher than that observed in individuals with normal renal function. For subjects on hemodialysis (dosed post-dialysis)/continuous ambulatory peritoneal dialysis, the mean $AUC_{0\text{-}\infty}$ was 3-times higher than that observed in individuals with normal renal function. The mean C_{max} ranged from 59.6 to 69.6 µg/mL in subjects with CL_{CR} ≥30 mL/min while those with CL_{CR} <30 mL/min ranged from 41.1 to 57.7 µg/mL. In non-infected adult subjects undergoing dialysis, approximately 15% and 11% of the administered dose was removed by 4 hours of hemodialysis and 48 hours of continuous ambulatory peritoneal dialysis, respectively. In patients with renal insufficiency, both renal function and creatine phosphokinase (CPK) should be monitored more frequently. CUBICIN should be administered following the completion of hemodialysis on hemodialysis days (see Dosage and Administration).

Table 12: CUBICIN

CUBICIN Population Pharmacokinetic Parameters Following a Single 30-Minute IV Infusion of 4 mg/kg to Patients with Complicated Skin and Skin Structure Infections (cSSSI) and Healthy Volunteers with Varying Degrees of Renal Function

Renal Function	N	Pharmacokinetic Parameters Mean (Standard Deviation)			
		$AUC_{0\text{-}\infty}$ (µg·h/mL)	$t_{1/2}$ (h)	V_{ss} (L/kg)	CL_T (mL/h/kg)
Normal (CL_{CR} >80 mL/min)	165	417 (155)	9.39 (4.74)	0.13 (0.05)	10.9 (4.0)
Mild Renal Impairment (CL_{CR} 50–80 mL/min)	64	466 (177)	10.75 (8.36)	0.12 (0.05)	9.9 (4.0)
Moderate Renal Impairment (CL_{CR} 30–<50 mL/min)	24	560 (258)	14.70 (10.50)	0.15 (0.06)	8.5 (3.4)
Severe Renal Impairment (CL_{CR} <30 mL/min)	8	925 (467)	27.83 (14.85)	0.20 (0.15)	5.9 (3.9)
Hemodialysis and CAPD	21	1244 (374)	29.81 (6.13)	0.15 (0.04)	3.7 (1.9)

Legend: CL_{CR}: creatinine clearance estimated using the Cockcroft-Gault equation with actual body weight; V_{ss}: volume of distribution at steady-state; CAPD: continuous ambulatory peritoneal dialysis.

Renal Insufficiency in the *S. aureus* Bacteremia/*S. aureus* Infective Endocarditis (SAB/SAIE) Trial: A second population analysis was conducted to determine pharmacokinetic parameters at steady-state in SAB/SAIE patients (see Table 13). Patients (N=108) received 6 mg/kg q24h and were stratified by varying degrees of renal function. Plasma clearance (CL_T) decreased with decreasing renal function, whereas AUC and C_{min} increased with decreasing renal function. Mean AUC increased 1.6-fold while mean C_{min} increased 2.8-fold in patients with moderate renal impairment compared to those with CL_{CR} >80 mL/min. In the two patients with CL_{CR} <30 mL/min, pharmacokinetic parameters were similar to those with moderate renal impairment. Mean C_{max} values ranged from 80 to 114 µg/mL in patients with moderate to mild renal impairment and were similar to those of normal subjects. In SAB/SAIE patients, the overall mean volume of distribution at steady-state (V_{ss}) was 0.16 L/kg and was greater than that in non-infected subjects (0.1 L/kg), but similar to cSSSI patients. In non-infected adult subjects undergoing dialysis, approximately 15% and 11% of the administered dose was removed by 4 hours of hemodialysis (N=6) and 48 hours of continuous ambulatory peritoneal dialysis [CAPD (N=5)], respectively. In patients with renal insufficiency, both renal function and CPK should be monitored more frequently. CUBICIN should be administered following the completion of hemodialysis on hemodialysis days (see Dosage and Administration).

Table 13: CUBICIN

CUBICIN Population Pharmacokinetic Parameters at Steady-State in SAB/SAIE Patients Dosed with 6 mg/kg with Varying Degrees of Renal Function

Renal Function	N	Pharmacokinetic Parameters Mean (Standard Deviation)[a]					
		$AUC_{0\text{-}24}$ (µg·h/mL)	$t_{1/2}$ (h)	V_{ss} (L/kg)	CL_T (mL/h/kg)	C_{max} (µg/mL)	C_{min} (µg/mL)
Normal CL_{CR}[b] >80 L/min	62	545 (296)	9.0 (2.86)	0.15 (0.07)	13.2 (5.0)	108 (143)	6.9 (3.5)
Mild Impairment CL_{CR} 50–80 mL/min	29	637 (215)	12.0 (2.26)	0.17 (0.04)	10.5 (3.5)	80 (41)	12.4 (5.6)
Moderate Impairment CL_{CR} 30–<50 mL/min	15	868 (349)	16.1 (3.62)	0.17 (0.05)	8.2 (3.6)	114 (124)	19.0 (9.0)
Severe Impairment CL_{CR} <30 mL/min	2	1050, 892	25.8, 16.0	0.20, 0.15	5.7, 6.7	97, 83	25.4, 21.4

a Mean (SD) values are presented except Severe Impairment where N=2.
b Creatinine clearance was estimated using the Cockcroft-Gault equation with actual body weight.

A 41% reduction in CUBICIN plasma concentration was achieved using high-flux dialysis membranes, and a 5 to 7% reduction was achieved using low-flux dialysis membranes.

Obesity: The pharmacokinetics of CUBICIN were evaluated in 6 moderately obese [Body Mass Index (BMI) 25 to 39.9 kg/m²] and 6 extremely obese (BMI ≥40 kg/m²) subjects and controls matched for age, sex, and renal function. Following administration of a single 4 mg/kg IV dose based on total body weight, the plasma clearance of CUBICIN normalized to total body weight was approximately 15% lower in moderately obese subjects and 23% lower in extremely obese subjects compared with non-obese controls. The $AUC_{0\text{-}\infty}$ of CUBICIN increased approximately 30% in moderately obese and 31% in extremely obese subjects compared with non-obese controls. In the complicated skin and skin structure infection trials (cSSSI), 8 patients >150 kg received CUBICIN 4 mg/kg. The highest total dose exposure occurred in one patient weighing 238.6 kg (total exposure 20 900 mg daptomycin over 21 days). No dosage adjustment of CUBICIN is warranted in obese patients based solely on weight.

STORAGE AND STABILITY: Store vials containing lyophillized powder at 2 to 8°C.

Chemical and physical in-use stability on the reconstituted solution in the vial, or infusion solutions, has been demonstrated for 12 hours at 25°C and up to 10 days if stored under refrigeration (2 to 8°C), under normal lighting conditions. However, because CUBICIN does not contain any preservative or bacteriostatic agent, aseptic technique must be used during preparation for administration and the product should be used promptly. If the reconstituted product is not used immediately, it must be refrigerated at 2 to 8°C. It is recommended that the solution be used within 72 hours due to the possibility of microbial contamination during reconstitution. Avoid excessive heat.

The combined time (vial and infusion bag) at room temperature, up to 25°C, should not exceed 12 hours. The combined time (vial and infusion bag) at 2-8°C should not exceed 10 days.

SPECIAL HANDLING INSTRUCTIONS: For information on reconstitution, see Dosage and Administration.

INFORMATION FOR THE PATIENT: Published in e-CPS, available by subscription at www.e-cps.ca.

DOSAGE FORMS, COMPOSITION AND PACKAGING: Each vial of a pale yellow to light brown lyophilized cake, contains: daptomycin 500 mg. May also contain sodium hydroxide used to adjust pH in trace amounts. Single-use vials of 10 mL, packages of 10.

Cuprimine® Pr

penicillamine

Chelating Agent

Aton Pharma

Date of Revision: November 13, 2007

PHARMACOLOGY: As a chelating agent, penicillamine removes copper and lead from the body. In copper chelation, from in vitro studies which indicate that one atom of copper combines with two molecules of penicillamine, it would appear that one gram of penicillamine should be followed by the excretion of about 200 milligrams of copper; however, the actual amount excreted is about one percent of this. The manner in which lead is chelated is not known. It may be bound in the same way as copper.

Penicillamine also reduces excess cystine excretion in cystinuria. This is done, at least in part, by disulfide interchange between penicillamine and cystine, resulting in formation of penicillamine-cysteine disulfide, a substance that is much more soluble than cystine and is excreted readily.

Penicillamine interferes with the formation of cross-links between tropocollagen molecules and cleaves them when newly formed.

The mechanism of action of penicillamine in rheumatoid arthritis is unknown although it appears to suppress disease activity. Unlike cytotoxic immunosuppressants, penicillamine markedly lowers IgM rheumatoid factor but produces no significant depression in absolute levels of serum immunoglobulins. Also, unlike cytotoxic immunosuppressants which act on both, penicillamine in vitro depresses T-cell activity but not B-cell activity.

In vitro, penicillamine dissociates macroglobulins (rheumatoid factor) although the relationship of the activity to its effect in rheumatoid arthritis is not known.

INDICATIONS AND CLINICAL USE:

Cuprimine (penicillamine capsules, USP) is indicated for: treatment of Wilson's disease, chronic lead poisoning, cystinuria, and in patients with severe, active rheumatoid arthritis who have failed to respond to an adequate trial of conventional therapy.

Available evidence suggests that Cuprimine is not of value in ankylosing spondylitis. Because of the severe toxicity of this agent, penicillamine should never be used casually.

Wilson's Disease: Treatment has two objectives:

1. to minimize dietary intake and absorption of copper.
2. to promote excretion of copper deposited in tissues.

For the second objective, a copper chelating agent is used. Penicillamine is the only one of these agents that is orally effective.

In symptomatic patients, this treatment usually produces marked neurologic improvement, fading of Kayser-Fleisher rings, and gradual amelioration of hepatic dysfunction and psychic disturbances.

Clinical experience to date suggests that life is prolonged with the above regimen.

Noticeable improvement may not occur for one to three months. Occasionally, neurologic symptoms become worse during the initiation of therapy with Cuprimine. Despite this, the drug should not be discontinued permanently. Although temporary interruption may result in clinical improvement of the neurological symptoms, it carries an increased risk of developing a sensitivity reaction upon resumption of therapy (see Warnings and Precautions).

Treatment of asymptomatic patients has been carried out for over ten years. Symptoms and signs of the disease appear to be prevented indefinitely if daily treatment with Cuprimine can be continued.

Chronic Lead Poisoning: Cuprimine should be considered adjunctive to rigorous control of environmental exposure to lead.

When used in children with chronic lead poisoning, Cuprimine should be used only if the children are asymptomatic, have blood lead levels between 50 and 80 µg/deciliter (1 dL=100 mL) whole blood, and:

a. have an erythrocyte protoporphyrin level greater than 400 to 500 µg/dL erythrocytes, as determined by a standard free erythrocyte protoporphyrin method (bearing in mind that values differ according to the method used).
b. excrete excessive amounts of δ-aminolevulinic acid (normal=up to 2 mg/m²/day), or of coproporphyrin (normal = 2 µg/kg/day), or both.

When using Cuprimine to treat chronic lead poisoning in children, it is essential that whole blood lead levels be determined periodically during treatment.

Cuprimine is recommended for use in adults with chronic lead poisoning.

Cystinuria: Conventional treatment is directed at keeping urinary cystine diluted enough to prevent stone formation, keeping the urine alkaline enough to dissolve as much cystine as possible, and minimizing cystine production by a diet low in methionine (the major dietary precursor of cystine). Patients must drink enough fluid to keep urine specific gravity below 1.010, take enough alkali to keep urinary pH at 7.5 to 8, and maintain a diet low in methionine. This diet is not recommended in growing children and probably is contraindicated in pregnancy because of its low protein content (see Warnings and Precautions).

When these measures are inadequate to control recurrent stone formation, Cuprimine may be used as additional therapy. When patients refuse to adhere to conventional treatment, Cuprimine may be a useful substitute. It is capable of keeping cystine excretion to near normal values, thereby hindering stone formation and the serious consequences of pyelonephritis and impaired renal function that develop in some patients.

Bartter and colleagues depict the process by which penicillamine interacts with cystine to form penicillamine-cysteine mixed disulfide as:

$$\text{CSSC} + \text{PS'} \leftrightarrow \text{CS'} + \text{CSSP}$$

$$\text{PSSP} + \text{CS'} \leftrightarrow \text{PS'} + \text{CSSP}$$

$$\text{CSSC} + \text{PSSP} \leftrightarrow 2\ \text{CSSP}$$

CSSC=cystine. CS'=deprotonated cysteine. PSSP=penicillamine. PS'=deprotonated penicillamine sulfhydryl. CSSP=penicillamine-cysteine mixed disulfide.

In this process, it is assumed that the deprotonated form of penicillamine, PS', is the active factor in bringing about the disulfide interchange.

Rheumatoid Arthritis: Because Cuprimine can cause severe adverse reactions; its use in rheumatoid arthritis should be restricted to patients who have severe, active disease and who have failed to respond to an adequate trial of conventional therapy. Even then benefit-to-risk ratio should be carefully considered. Other measures, such as rest, physiotherapy, salicylates, and corticosteroids, may need to be used in conjunction with Cuprimine (see Warnings and Precautions).

Geriatrics: Clinical studies of Cuprimine are limited in subjects aged 65 and over; they did not include sufficient numbers of elderly subjects aged 65 and over to adequately determine whether they respond differently from younger subjects. Review of reported clinical trials with penicillamine in the elderly (>65 years of age) showed a statistically significant increase in the frequency of minor and serious skin rash and serious abnormality of taste than in younger patients in 1 clinical trial. In general, dose selection for an elderly patient should be cautious, starting at the low end of the dosing range, reflecting the greater frequency of decreased hepatic, renal or cardiac function, and of concomitant disease or other drugs.

This drug is known to be substantially excreted by the kidney, and the risk of toxic reactions to this drug may be greater in patients with impaired renal function. Because elderly patients are more likely to have decreased renal function, care should be taken in dose selection, and careful monitoring of renal function is recommended.

Pediatrics: See Warnings and Precautions, Pediatrics (<18 years of age).

CONTRAINDICATIONS: Patients who are hypersensitive to this drug or to any ingredient in the formulation. For a complete listing, see Dosage Forms, Composition and Packaging.

Pregnancy: Exceptions to this contraindication include the treatment of Wilson's disease or certain cases of cystinuria (see Warnings and Precautions).

Lactation: Although breast milk studies have not been reported in animals or humans, mothers on therapy with penicillamine should not nurse their infants.

Patients with a history of penicillamine-related aplastic anemia or agranulocytosis should not be restarted on penicillamine (see Warnings and Precautions and Adverse Reactions).

Because of its potential for causing renal damage, penicillamine should not be administered to rheumatoid arthritis patients with a history or other evidence of renal insufficiency.

Cuprimine (penicillamine capsules, USP) should not be given with chronic lead poisoning when there is x-ray evidence of lead-containing substances in the gastrointestinal tract. Treatment with the drug may be instituted after the gastrointestinal tract has been cleared of these substances. Studies in animals suggest that Cuprimine may be ineffective, and possibly hazardous, if excessive oral ingestion of lead continues during administration of the drug.

Penicillamine should not be used in patients who are receiving gold therapy, antimalarial or cytotoxic drugs, oxyphenbutazone or phenylbutazone because these drugs are also associated with similar serious hematologic and renal adverse reactions. Patients who have had gold salt therapy discontinued due to a major toxic reaction may be at greater risk of serious adverse reactions with penicillamine but not necessarily of the same type.

WARNINGS AND PRECAUTIONS: General: The use of penicillamine has been associated with fatalities due to certain diseases such as aplastic anemia, agranulocytosis, thrombocytopenia, Goodpasture's syndrome, and myasthenia gravis.

Because of the potential for serious hematological and renal adverse reactions to occur at any time, routine urinalysis, white and differential blood cell count, hemoglobin determination, and direct platelet count must be done every two weeks for at least the first six months of penicillamine therapy and monthly thereafter. Patients should be instructed to report promptly the development of signs and symptoms of granulocytopenia and/or thrombocytopenia such as fever, sore throat, chills, bruising or bleeding. The above laboratory studies should then be promptly repeated.

Leukopenia and thrombocytopenia have been reported to occur in up to five percent of patients during penicillamine therapy. Leukopenia is of the granulocytic series and may or may not be associated with an increase in eosinophils. A confirmed reduction in WBC below 3500 mandates discontinuance of penicillamine therapy. Thrombocytopenia may be on an idiosyncratic basis, with decreased or absent megakaryocytes in the marrow, when it is part of an aplastic anemia. In other cases the thrombocytopenia is presumably on an immune basis since the number of megakaryocytes in the marrow has been reported to be normal or sometimes increased. The development of a platelet count below 100 000, even in the absence of clinical bleeding, requires at least temporary cessation of penicillamine therapy. A progressive fall in either platelet count or WBC in three successive determinations, even though values are still within the normal range, likewise requires at least temporary cessation.

Carcinogenesis and Mutagenesis: Long-term animal carcinogenicity studies have not been done with penicillamine. There is a report that five of ten autoimmune disease-prone NZB hybrid mice developed lymphocytic leukemia after 6 months' intraperitoneal treatment with a dose of 400 mg/kg penicillamine 5 days per week.

Endocrine and Metabolism: Because of their dietary restrictions, patients with Wilson's disease and cystinuria should be given 25 mg/day of pyridoxine during therapy, since penicillamine increases the requirement for this vitamin. Patients also may receive benefit from a multivitamin preparation, although there is no evidence that deficiency of any vitamin other than pyridoxine is associated with penicillamine. In Wilson's disease, multivitamin preparations must be copper-free.

Rheumatoid arthritis patients whose nutrition is impaired should also be given a daily supplement of pyridoxine. Mineral supplements should not be given, since they may block the response to penicillamine.

Iron deficiency may develop, especially in children and in menstruating women. In Wilson's disease, this may be a result of adding the effects of the low copper diet, which is probably also low in iron, and the penicillamine to the effects of blood loss or growth. In cystinuria, a low methionine diet may contribute to iron deficiency, since it is necessarily low in protein. If necessary, iron may be given in short courses, but a period of two hours should elapse between administration of penicillamine and iron, since orally administered iron has been shown to reduce the effects of penicillamine.

Gastrointestinal: Hypogeusia (a blunting or diminution in taste perception) has occurred in some patients. This may last two to three months or more and may develop into a total loss of taste; however, it is usually self-limited despite continued penicillamine treatment. Such taste impairment is rare in patients with Wilson's disease.

Some patients may develop oral ulcerations which in some cases have the appearance of aphthous stomatitis. The stomatitis usually recurs on rechallenge but often clears on a lower dosage. Although rare, cheilosis, glossitis and gingivostomatitis have also been reported. These oral lesions are frequently dose-related and may preclude further increase in penicillamine dosage or require discontinuation of the drug.

Genitourinary: Rheumatoid arthritis patients who develop moderate degrees of proteinuria may be continued cautiously on penicillamine therapy, provided that quantitative 24-hour urinary protein determinations are obtained at intervals of one to two weeks. Penicillamine dosage should not be increased under these circumstances. Proteinuria which exceeds 1 g/24 hours, or proteinuria which is progressively increasing, requires either discontinuance of the drug or a reduction in the dosage. In some patients, proteinuria has been reported to clear following reduction in dosage.

In patients with Wilson's disease or cystinuria the risks of continued penicillamine therapy in patients manifesting potentially serious urinary abnormalities must be weighed against the expected therapeutic benefits.

When penicillamine is used in cystinuria, an annual x-ray for renal stones is advised. Cystine stones form rapidly, sometimes in six months.

Up to one year or more may be required for any urinary abnormalities to disappear after penicillamine has been discontinued. Goodpasture's syndrome has occurred rarely. The development of abnormal urinary findings associated with hemoptysis and pulmonary infiltrates on x-ray requires immediate cessation of penicillamine.

Proteinuria and/or hematuria may develop during therapy and may be warning signs of membranous glomerulopathy which can progress to a nephrotic syndrome. Close observation of these patients is essential. In some patients the proteinuria disappears with continued therapy; in others, penicillamine must be discontinued. When a patient develops proteinuria or hematuria the physician must ascertain whether it is a sign of drug-induced glomerulopathy or is unrelated to penicillamine.

In rheumatoid arthritis patients penicillamine should be discontinued if unexplained gross hematuria or persistent microscopic hematuria develops.

Hepatic/Biliary/Pancreatic: Because of rare reports of intrahepatic cholestasis and toxic hepatitis, liver function tests are recommended every six months for the duration of therapy.

Immune: Should drug fever occur in patients receiving penicillamine, stop the drug. In patients with Wilson's disease, trientine hydrochloride (where available) or zinc compounds such as zinc sulfate may be tried. In patients with cystinuria, in whom these alternative agents are inappropriate, penicillamine should be temporarily discontinued until the reaction subsides. Then penicillamine should be reinstituted with a small dose that is gradually increased until the desired dosage is attained. Systemic steroid therapy may be necessary, and is usually helpful, in such patients in whom toxic reactions develop a second or third time.

In the case of drug fever in rheumatoid arthritis patients, because other treatments are available, penicillamine should be discontinued and another therapeutic alternative tried since experience indicates that the febrile reaction will recur in a very high percentage of patients upon re-administration of penicillamine.

Most of the various forms of pemphigus have occurred during treatment with penicillamine. Pemphigus vulgaris and pemphigus foliaceus are reported most frequently, usually as a late complication of therapy. The seborrhea-like characteristics of pemphigus foliaceus may obscure an early diagnosis. When pemphigus is suspected, Cuprimine (penicillamine capsules, USP) should be discontinued. Treatment has consisted of high doses of corticosteroids alone or, in some cases, concomitantly with an immunosuppressant. Treatment may be required for only a few weeks or months, but may need to be continued for more than a year.

Some patients may experience drug fever, a marked febrile response to penicillamine, usually in the second to third week following initiation of therapy. Drug fever may sometimes be accompanied by a macular cutaneous eruption.

The skin and mucous membranes should be observed for allergic reactions. Early and late rashes have occurred. Early rash occurs during the first few months of treatment and is more common. It is usually a generalized pruritic, erythematous, maculopapular or morbilliform rash and resembles the allergic rash seen with other drugs. Early rash usually disappears within days after stopping penicillamine and seldom recurs when the drug is restarted at a lower dosage. Pruritus and early rash may often be controlled by the concomitant administration of antihistamines. Less commonly, a late rash may be seen, usually after six months or more of treatment, and requires discontinuation of penicillamine. It is usually on the trunk, is accompanied by intense pruritus, and is usually unresponsive to topical corticosteroid therapy. Late rash may take weeks to disappear after penicillamine is stopped and usually recurs if the drug is restarted.

The appearance of a drug eruption accompanied by fever, arthralgia, lymphadenopathy or other allergic manifestations usually requires discontinuation of penicillamine.

Certain patients will develop a positive antinuclear antibody (ANA) test and some of these may show a lupus erythematosus-like syndrome similar to drug-induced lupus associated with other drugs. The lupus erythematosus-like syndrome is not associated with the hypocomplementemia and may be present without nephropathy. The development of a positive ANA test does not mandate discontinuance of the drug; however, the physician should be alerted to the possibility that a lupus erythematosus-like syndrome may develop in the future.

Neurologic: Onset of new neurologic symptoms has been reported with Cuprimine (see Adverse Reactions). Occasionally, neurologic symptoms become worse during initiation of therapy with Cuprimine (see Indications and Clinical Use). Myasthenic syndrome sometimes progressing to myasthenia gravis has been reported. Ptosis and diplopia, with weakness of the extraocular muscles, are often early signs of myasthenia. In the majority of cases, symptoms of myasthenia have receded after withdrawal of penicillamine.

Peri-Operative Considerations: The effects of penicillamine on collagen and elastin make it advisable to consider a reduction in dosage to 250 mg/day, when surgery is contemplated. Reinstitution of full therapy should be delayed until wound healing is complete.

Respiratory: Obliterative bronchiolitis has been reported rarely. The patient should be cautioned to reportimmediately pulmonary symptoms such as exertional dyspnea, unexplained cough or wheezing. Pulmonary function studies should be considered at that time.

Sensitivity/Resistance: Once instituted for Wilson's disease or cystinuria, treatment with penicillamine should, as a rule, be continued on a daily basis. Interruptions for even a few days have been followed by sensitivity reactions after reinstitution of therapy.

Patients who are allergic to penicillin may theoretically have cross-sensitivity to penicillamine. The possibility of reactions from contamination of penicillamine by trace amounts of penicillin, has been eliminated now that penicillamine is being produced synthetically rather than as a degradation product of penicillin.

Skin: Penicillamine causes an increase in the amount of soluble collagen. In the rat this results in inhibition of normal healing and also a decrease in tensile strength of intact skin. In man this may be the cause of increased skin friability at sites especially subject to pressure or trauma, such as shoulders, elbows, knees, toes, and buttocks. Extravasations of blood may occur and may appear as purpuric areas, with external bleeding if the skin is broken, or as vesicles containing dark blood. Neither type is progressive. There is no apparent association with bleeding elsewhere in the body and no associated coagulation defect has been found. Therapy with penicillamine may be continued in the presence of these lesions. They may not recur if dosage is reduced.

Other reported effects probably due to the action of penicillamine on collagen are excessive wrinkling of the skin and development of small, white papules at venipuncture and surgical sites.

Special Populations: *Pregnant Women:* Penicillamine has been shown to be teratogenic in rats when given in doses 6 times higher than the highest dose recommended for human use. Skeletal defects, cleft palates and fetal toxicity (resorptions) have been reported. There is a report that a woman with rheumatoid arthritis treated with less than one gram a day of penicillamine during pregnancy gave birth (cesarean delivery) to an infant with growth retardation, flattened face with broad nasal bridge, low set ears, short neck with loose skin folds, and unusually lax body skin.

There are no controlled studies on the use of penicillamine in pregnant women. Although normal outcomes have been reported, characteristic congenital cutis laxa and associated birth defects have been reported in infants born of mothers who received therapy with penicillamine during pregnancy. Penicillamine should be used in women of childbearing potential only when the expected benefits outweigh the possible hazards. Women on therapy with penicillamine who are of childbearing potential should be apprised of this risk and followed closely for early recognition of pregnancy.

Wilson's Disease: Reported experience shows that continued treatment with penicillamine throughout pregnancy protects the mother against relapse of the Wilson's disease, and that discontinuation of penicillamine has deleterious effects on the mother.

If penicillamine is administered during pregnancy to patients with Wilson's disease, it is recommended that the daily dosage be limited to 1 g. If cesarean section is planned, the daily dosage should be limited to 250 mg during the last six weeks of pregnancy and postoperatively until wound healing is complete.

Cystinuria: If possible, penicillamine should not be given during pregnancy to women with cystinuria (see Contraindications). There are reports of women with cystinuria on therapy with penicillamine who gave birth to infants with generalized connective tissue defects who died following abdominal surgery. If stones continue to form in these patients, the benefits of therapy to the mothers must be evaluated against the risk to the fetus.

Nursing Women: See Contraindications.

Pediatrics (<18 years of age): The efficacy of Cuprimine in juvenile rheumatoid arthritis has not been established.

Geriatrics: See Indications and Clinical Use and Post-Market Adverse Drug Reactions (since May 2003).

ADVERSE REACTIONS: Adverse Drug Reaction Overview: Penicillamine is a drug with a high incidence of untoward reactions, some of which are potentially fatal. Therefore, it is mandatory that patients receiving penicillamine therapy remain under close medical supervision throughout the period of drug administration (see Warnings and Precautions).

Clinical Trial Adverse Drug Reactions: Because clinical trials are conducted under very specific conditions the adverse reaction rates observed in the clinical trials may not reflect the rates observed in practice and should not be compared to the rates in the clinical trials of another drug. Adverse drug reaction information from clinical trials is useful for identifying drug-related adverse events and for approximating rates.

Reported incidences (%) for the most commonly occurring adverse reactions in rheumatoid arthritis patients are noted, based on 17 representative clinical trials reported in the literature (1270 patients).

Allergic: Generalized pruritus, early and late rashes (5%), pemphigoid-type reactions, and drug eruptions which may be accompanied by fever, arthralgia, or lymphadenopathy have occurred (see Warnings and Precautions). Some patients may show a lupus erythematosus-like syndrome similar to drug-induced lupus produced by other pharmacological agents (see Warnings and Precautions). Urticaria and exfoliative dermatitis have occurred. Thyroiditis has been reported; hypoglycemia in association with anti-insulin antibodies has been reported. These reactions are extremely rare. Some patients may develop a migratory polyarthralgia, often with objective synovitis (see Dosage and Administration).

Gastrointestinal: Anorexia, epigastric pain, nausea, vomiting, or occasional diarrhea may occur (17%).

Isolated cases of reactivated peptic ulcer have occurred, as have hepatic dysfunction and pancreatitis. Intrahepatic cholestasis and toxic hepatitis have been reported rarely. There have been a few reports of increased serum alkaline phosphatase, lactic dehydrogenase, and positive cephalin flocculation and thymol turbidity tests.

Some patients may report a blunting, diminution, or total loss of taste perception (12%); or may develop oral ulcerations. Although rare, cheilosis, glossitis, and gingivostomatitis have been reported (see Warnings and Precautions).

Gastrointestinal side effects are usually reversible following cessation of therapy.

Hematological: Penicillamine can cause bone marrow depression (see Warnings and Precautions). Leukopenia (2%) and thrombocytopenia (4%) have occurred. Fatalities have been reported as a result of thrombocytopenia, agranulocytosis, aplastic anemia, and sideroblastic anemia.

Thrombotic thrombocytopenic purpura, hemolytic anemia, red cell aplasia, monocytosis, leukocytosis, eosinophilia, and thrombocytosis have also been reported.

Renal: Patients on penicillamine therapy may develop proteinuria (6%) and/or hematuria which, in some, may progress to the development of the nephrotic syndrome as a result of an immune complex membranous glomerulopathy (see Warnings and Precautions).

Central Nervous System: Tinnitus, optic neuritis and peripheral sensory and motor neuropathies (including polyradiculoneuropathy, i.e., Guillain-Barré Syndrome) have been reported. Muscular weakness may or may not occur with the peripheral neuropathies. Visual and psychic disturbances; mental disorders; and agitation and anxiety have been reported.

Neuromuscular: Myasthenia gravis (see Warnings and Precautions); dystonia. Side effects that have been reported rarely include thrombophlebitis; hyperpyrexia (see Warnings and Precautions); falling hair or alopecia; lichen planus; (see Warnings and Precautions); polymyositis; dermatomyositis; mammary hyperplasia; elastosis perforans serpiginosa; toxic epidermal necrolysis; anetoderma (cutaneous macular atrophy); and Goodpasture's syndrome, a severe and ultimately fatal glomerulonephritis associated with intra-alveolar hemorrhage (see Warnings and Precautions). Fatal renal vasculitis, has also been reported. Allergic alveolitis, obliterative bronchiolitis, interstitial pneumonitis and pulmonary fibrosis have been reported in patients with severe rheumatoid arthritis, some of whom were receiving penicillamine. Bronchial asthma also has been reported.

Increased skin friability, excessive wrinkling of skin, and development of small white papules at venipuncture and surgical sites have been reported (see Warnings and Precautions).

The chelating action of the drug may cause increased excretion of other heavy metals such as zinc and mercury and lead.

Post-Market Adverse Drug Reactions (since May 2003): The following adverse reactions have been reported in post-marketing experience since May 2003:

- Hepatobiliary disorders: hepatic failure.
- Renal and urinary disorders: renal failure.
- Vascular disorders: vasculitis.
- Skin and Subcutaneous disorders: yellow nail syndrome.

Geriatrics: In post-marketing surveillance, the most frequently reported serious adverse events seen in geriatric patients (≥65 years of age) were related to taste abnormalities, skin and subcutaneous tissue disorders and blood and lymphatic system disorders, including anemia, bone marrow failure, and thrombocytopenia. The frequency of these adverse events in the elderly is greater than in younger patients.

DRUG INTERACTIONS: Drug-Drug Interactions: Cuprimine should not be used in patients who are receiving gold therapy, antimalarial or cytotoxic drugs, oxyphenbutazone, or phenylbutazone (see Contraindications). Other measures, such as salicylates, other non-steroidal anti-inflammatory drugs, or systemic corticosteroids, may be continued when penicillamine is initiated. After improvement commences, analgesic and anti-inflammatory drugs may be slowly discontinued as symptoms permit. Steroid withdrawal must be done gradually, and many months of treatment with Cuprimine may be required before steroids can be completely eliminated.

Drug-Food Interactions: See Dosage and Administration.

Drug-Herb Interactions: Interactions with herbal products have not been established.

Drug-Laboratory Test Interactions: Penicillamine may cause alteration of the biodistribution of technetium Tc-99m gluceptate.

DOSAGE AND ADMINISTRATION: Dosing Considerations: Physicians planning to use penicillamine should thoroughly familiarize themselves with its toxicity, special dosage considerations, and therapeutic benefits. Penicillamine should never be used casually. Each patient should remain constantly under the close supervision of the physician. Patients should be warned to report promptly any symptoms suggesting toxicity.

Recommended Dose and Dosage Adjustment: In all patients receiving penicillamine, it is important that Cuprimine (penicillamine capsules, USP) be given on an empty stomach, at least one hour before meals or two hours after meals, and at least one hour apart from any other drug, food, or milk. This permits maximum absorption and reduces the likelihood of inactivation by metal binding.

Wilson's Disease: Optimal dosage can be determined by measurement of urinary copper excretion and the determination of free copper in the serum. The urine must be collected in copper-free glassware, and should be quantitatively analyzed for copper before, and soon after, initiation of therapy with Cuprimine.

Determination of 24-hour urinary copper excretion is a greatest value in the first week of therapy with penicillamine. In the absence of any drug reaction, a dose between 0.75 and 1.5 g that results in an initial 24-hour cupruresis of over 2 mg should be continued for about three months, by which time the most reliable method of monitoring maintenance treatment is the determination of free copper in the serum. This equals the difference between quantitatively determined total copper and ceruloplasmin-copper. Adequately treated patients will usually have less than 10 µg free copper/dL of serum. It is seldom necessary to exceed a dosage of 2 g/day. If the patient is intolerant to therapy with Cuprimine, alternative treatment is trientine hydrochloride (where available) or zinc compounds such as zinc sulfate.

In patients who cannot tolerate as much as 1 g/day initially, initiating dosage with 250 mg/day, and increasing gradually to the requisite amount, gives closer control of the effects of the drug and may help to reduce the incidence of adverse reactions.

Chronic Lead Poisoning: Cuprimine should be given when the gastrointestinal tract is empty of lead - containing substances. It may be given to children by dissolving the contents of the capsules no longer than five minutes before administration in a small amount of chilled purée de fruits or fruit juice.

For **children**, the recommended dosage is 30 to 40 mg/kg/day, or 600 to 750 mg/m²/day, not to exceed 750 mg a day. Cuprimine may be given to children as a single dose or in two divided doses at least two hours before meals. Treatment should be continued until blood lead levels remain below 40 µg/dL whole blood for two consecutive months and at least one of the following is achieved:

a. erythrocyte protoporphyrin level decreases to less than three to five times the average normal level
b. excretion of δ-aminolevulinic acid decreases to upper limit of normal
c. excretion of coproporphyrin decreases to upper limit of normal.

For **adults**, the recommended dosage is 900 to 1500 mg a day, in three divided doses for one to two weeks, followed by 750 mg a day in divided doses until blood lead levels are reduced to 60 µg/dL, or until urinary lead excretion remains below 500 µg/L for two consecutive months. All doses should be given at least two hours before meals.

Cystinuria: It is recommended that Cuprimine be used along with conventional therapy. By reducing urinary cystine, it decreases crystalluria and stone formation. In some instances, it has been reported to decrease the size of, and even to dissolve, stones already formed.

The usual dosage of Cuprimine in the treatment of cystinuria is 2 g/day for adults, with a range of 1 to 4 g/day. For children, dosage can be based on 30 mg/kg/day. The total daily amount should be divided into four doses. If four equal doses are not feasible, give the larger portion at bedtime. If adverse reactions necessitate a reduction in dosage, it is important to retain the bedtime dose.

Initiating dosage with 250 mg/day, and increasing gradually to the requisite amount, gives closer control of the effects of the drug and may help to reduce the incidence of adverse reactions.

In addition to taking Cuprimine, patients should drink copiously. It is especially important to drink about a pint (½ liter) of fluid at bedtime and another pint (½ liter) once during the night when urine is more concentrated and more acid than during the day. The greater the fluid intake, the lower the required dosage of Cuprimine.

Dosage must be individualized to an amount that limits cystine excretion to 100-200 mg/day in those with no history of stones, and below 100 mg in those who have had stone formation and/or pain. Thus, in determining dosage, the inherent tubular defect, the patient's size, age and rate of growth, and his diet and water intake all must be taken into consideration.

The standard nitroprusside cyanide test has been reported useful as a qualitative measure of the effective dose. Add 2 mL of freshly prepared 5% sodium cyanide to 5 mL of a 24-hour aliquot of protein-free urine and let stand ten minutes. Add 5 drops of freshly prepared 5% sodium nitroprusside and mix. Cystine will turn the mixture magenta. If the result is negative, it can be assumed that cystine excretion is less than 100 mg/g creatinine.

Although penicillamine is rarely excreted unchanged, it also will turn the mixture magenta. If there is any question as to which substance is causing the reaction, a ferric chloride test can be done to eliminate doubt: Add 3% ferric chloride dropwise to the urine. Penicillamine will turn the urine an immediate and quickly fading blue. Cystine will not produce any change in appearance.

Rheumatoid Arthritis: In rheumatoid arthritis, the onset of therapeutic response to Cuprimine may not be seen for two or three months. In those patients who respond, however, the first evidence of suppression of symptoms such as pain, tenderness, and swelling is generally apparent within three months. The optimum duration of therapy has not been determined. If remissions occur, they may last from months to years, but usually require continued treatment.

In patients with rheumatoid arthritis, it is important that Cuprimine be given on an empty stomach, at least one hour before meals and at least one hour apart from any other drug, food, or milk. This permits maximum absorption and reduces the likelihood of inactivation by metal binding.

When treatment with Cuprimine has been interrupted because of adverse reactions or other reasons, the drug should be reintroduced cautiously by starting with a lower dosage and increasing slowly.

Initial Therapy: The recommended dosage regimen in rheumatoid arthritis begins with a single daily dose of 250 mg which is thereafter increased at one to three month intervals, by 250 mg/day, as patient response and tolerance indicates. If a satisfactory remission of symptoms is achieved, the dose associated with the remission should be continued (see Maintenance Therapy). If there is no improvement and there are no signs of potentially serious toxicity after two to three months of treatment with doses of 500-750 mg/day, increases of 250 mg/day at two to three month intervals may be continued until a satisfactory remission occurs (see Maintenance Therapy) or signs of toxicity develop (see Warnings and Precautions). If there is no discernible improvement after three to four months of treatment with 1000 to 1500 mg of penicillamine/day, it may be assumed the patient will not respond and Cuprimine should be discontinued.

Maintenance Therapy: The maintenance dosage of Cuprimine must be individualized, and may require adjustment during the course of treatment. Many patients respond satisfactorily to a dosage within the 500-750 mg/day range. Some need less.

Changes in maintenance dosage levels may not be reflected clinically or in the erythrocyte sedimentation rate for two to three months after each dosage adjustment.

Some patients will subsequently require an increase in the maintenance dosage to achieve maximal disease suppression. In those patients who do respond, but who evidence incomplete suppression of their disease after the first six to nine months of treatment, the daily dosage of Cuprimine may be increased by 250 mg/day at three-month intervals. It is unusual in current practice to employ a dosage in excess of 1 g/day, but up to 1.5 g/day has sometimes been required.

Management of Exacerbation: During the course of treatment some patients may experience an exacerbation of disease activity following an initial good response. These may be self-limited and can subside within twelve weeks. They are usually controlled by the addition of nonsteroidal anti-inflammatory drugs, and only if the patient has demonstrated a true "escape" phenomenon (as evidenced by failure of the flare to subside within this time period) should an increase in the maintenance dose ordinarily be considered.

In the rheumatoid patient, migratory polyarthralgia due to penicillamine is extremely difficult to differentiate from an exacerbation of the rheumatoid arthritis. Discontinuance or a substantial reduction in dosage of Cuprimine for up to several weeks will usually determine which of these processes is responsible for the arthralgia.

Duration of Therapy: The optimum duration of therapy with Cuprimine in rheumatoid arthritis has not been determined. If the patient has been in remission for six months or more, a gradual, stepwise dosage reduction in decrements of 250 mg/day at approximately three month intervals may be attempted.

Dosage Frequency: Based on clinical experience, dosages up to 500 mg/day can be given as a single daily dose. Dosages in excess of 500 mg/day should be administered in divided doses.

Missed Dose: If a tablet is missed at its usual time, an extra dose should not be taken. The next dose should be taken as usual.

OVERDOSAGE:
Symptoms: There are no known instances of acute poisoning with penicillamine. In therapeutic doses, however, it may cause a wide variety of adverse reactions. Penicillamine may cause acute sensitivity reactions early in therapy. Cross sensitivity with penicillin may exist.
Treatment: In general, treatment is symptomatic.
Allergic Reactions: Discontinue penicillamine promptly and treat the patient with glucocorticoids, followed by reinstitution of penicillamine in small doses that are increased gradually to the desired amount.
Iron and Pyridoxine Deficiencies: Iron and pyridoxine supplementation.
Impairment of Taste: 5-10 mg of copper a day can be administered as 5-10 drops of a 4% solution of $CuSO_4\ 5H_2O$ in fruit juice twice a day. (Do not give copper to patients with Wilson's disease.)

> For management of a suspected drug overdose, contact your **regional Poison Control Centre**. See the *CPS* Directory section for a list of Poison Control Centres.

STORAGE AND STABILITY: Keep container tightly closed.

DOSAGE FORMS, COMPOSITION AND PACKAGING: Each capsule with an ivory opaque cap and an ivory opaque body imprinted radially with MSD 602 and CUPRIMINE respectively, contains: penicillamine 250 mg. Nonmedicinal ingredients: D&C Yellow 10, gelatin, lactose, magnesium stearate and titanium dioxide. Bottles of 100.

Cyanocobalamin

CPhA Monograph

see *Vitamin B12*

Cyclen® Ⓟ

norgestimate—ethinyl estradiol
Oral Contraceptive

Janssen-Ortho

Date of Preparation: July 6, 1992
Date of Revision: January 13, 2010

PHARMACOLOGY: The primary mechanism of action is an inhibition of ovulation. Additionally, other effects caused by the treatment (e.g., alteration of the endometrium and the thickening of the cervical mucus) appear to interfere with implantation and conception.

INDICATIONS: Conception control.

CONTRAINDICATIONS: History of/or actual thrombophlebitis or thromboembolic disorders; known thrombophilic conditions; history of/or actual cerebrovascular disorders; history of/or actual myocardial infarction or coronary arterial disease; active liver disease or history of/or actual benign or malignant liver tumors; known or suspected carcinoma of the breast; known or suspected estrogen-dependent neoplasia; undiagnosed abnormal vaginal bleeding; any ocular lesion arising from ophthalmic vascular disease, such as partial or complete loss of vision or defect in visual fields; when pregnancy is suspected or diagnosed; valvular heart disease with complications; persistent blood pressure values ≥160 mm Hg systolic or ≥100 mm Hg diastolic; diabetes with vascular involvement; cholestatic jaundice or history of jaundice of pregnancy; migraine with focal aura; hypersensitivity to any component of this product.

WARNINGS: Predisposing Factors For Coronary Artery Disease: Cigarette smoking increases the risk of serious cardiovascular side effects and mortality. Birth control pills increase this risk, especially with increasing age. Convincing data are available to support an upper age limit of 35 years for oral contraceptive use by women who smoke.

Other women who are independently at high risk for cardiovascular disease include those with diabetes, hypertension (persistent blood pressure values ≥140 mm Hg systolic or ≥90 mm Hg diastolic), abnormal lipid profile, or a family history of these. Whether oral contraceptives accentuate this risk is unclear.

In low-risk, non-smoking women of any age, the benefits of oral contraceptive use outweigh the possible cardiovascular risks associated with low-dose formulations. Consequently, oral contraceptives may be prescribed for these women up to the age of menopause.

> Cigarette smoking increases the risk of serious adverse effects on the heart and blood vessels. This risk increases with age and becomes significant in oral contraceptive users over 35 years of age. Women should be counselled not to smoke.

Venous and Arterial Thrombosis and Thromboembolism: Venous thrombosis and thromboembolism: Epidemiological studies have shown that the incidence of venous thromboembolism (VTE) in users of oral contraceptives with low estrogen content (<50 µg ethinyl estradiol) ranges from about 20 to 40 cases per 100 000 women-years, but this risk estimate varies according to the progestogen. This compares with 5 to 10 cases per 100 000 women-years for non-users.

The use of any combined oral contraceptive carries an increased risk of VTE compared with no use. The excess risk of VTE is highest during the first year a woman ever uses a combined oral contraceptive. The increased risk is less than the risk of VTE associated with pregnancy, which is estimated as 60 cases per 100 000 pregnancies. VTE is fatal in 1-2% of cases.

Other generalized risk factors for venous thromboembolism include but are not limited to a personal history, a family history (the occurrence of VTE in a direct relative at a relatively early age may indicate genetic predisposition), severe obesity (body mass index >30 kg/m²) and systemic lupus erythematosus. The risk of VTE also increases with age and smoking. The risk of VTE may be temporarily increased with prolonged immobilization, major surgery, or trauma. Also, patients with varicose veins and leg cast should be closely supervised.

If a hereditary or acquired predisposition for venous thromboembolism is suspected, the woman should be referred to a specialist for advice before deciding on any combination oral contraceptives (COC) use.

Arterial thrombosis and thromboembolism: The use of COCs increases the risk of arterial thrombotic and thromboembolic events. Reported events include myocardial infarction and cerebrovascular events (ischemic and hemorrhagic stroke, transient ischemic attack).

The risk of arterial thrombotic and thromboembolic events is further increased in women with underlying risk factors. Caution must be exercised when prescribing COCs for women with risk factors for arterial thrombotic and thromboembolic events.

Discontinue medication at the earliest manifestation of the following:

A. Thromboembolic and cardiovascular disorders such as: thrombophlebitis, pulmonary embolism, cerebrovascular disorders, myocardial ischemia, mesenteric thrombosis and retinal thrombosis.
B. Conditions that predispose to venous stasis and to vascular thrombosis (e.g., immobilization after accidents or confinement to bed during long-term illness). Other non-hormonal methods of contraception should be used until regular activities are resumed. For use of oral contraceptives when surgery is contemplated, see Precautions.
C. Visual defects—partial or complete.
D. Papilledema, or ophthalmic vascular lesions.
E. Severe headache of unknown etiology or worsening of pre-existing migraine headache.

PRECAUTIONS: Physical Examination and Follow-up: Before oral contraceptives are used, a thorough history and physical examination should be performed, including a blood pressure determination. Breasts, liver, extremities and pelvic organs should be examined. A Papanicolaou smear should be taken if the patient has been sexually active.

The first follow-up visit should be 3 months after oral contraceptives are prescribed. Thereafter, examinations should be performed at least once a year or more frequently if indicated. At each annual visit, examination should include those procedures that were done at the initial visit as outlined above or per recommendations of the Canadian Workshop on Screening for Cancer of the Cervix. Their suggestion was that, for women who had 2 consecutive negative Pap smears, screening could be continued every 3 years up to the age of 69.

Pregnancy: Oral contraceptives should not be taken by pregnant women. However, if conception accidentally occurs while taking the pill, there is no conclusive evidence that the estrogen and progestin contained in the oral contraceptive will damage the developing child.

Lactation: In breast-feeding women, the use of oral contraceptives results in the hormonal components being excreted in breast milk and may reduce its quantity and quality. If the use of oral contraceptives is initiated after the establishment of lactation, there does not appear to be any effect on the quantity and quality of the milk. There is no evidence that low-dose oral contraceptives are harmful to the nursing infant.

Hepatic Function: Patients who have had jaundice, including a history of cholestatic jaundice during pregnancy, should be given oral contraceptives with great care and under close observation.

The development of severe generalized pruritus or icterus requires that the medication be withdrawn until the problem is resolved.

If a patient develops jaundice that proves to be cholestatic in type, the use of oral contraceptives should not be resumed. In patients taking oral contraceptives, changes in the composition of the bile may occur and an increased incidence of gallstones has been reported.

Hepatic nodules (adenoma and focal nodular hyperplasia) have been reported, particularly in long-term users of oral contraceptives. Although these lesions are extremely rare, they have caused fatal intra-abdominal hemorrhage and should be considered in women with an abdominal mass, acute abdominal pain, or evidence of intra-abdominal bleeding.

Hypertension: Patients with essential hypertension whose blood pressure (BP) is well controlled may be given oral contraceptives but only under close supervision. If a significant persistent elevation of blood pressure in previously normotensive or hypertensive subjects occurs at any time during the administration of the drug, cessation of medication is necessary and an alternate method of contraception should be prescribed (see Contraindications).

Migraine and Headache: The onset or exacerbation of migraine or the development of headache of a new pattern, that is recurrent, persistent or severe, requires discontinuation of oral contraceptives and evaluation of the cause.

Diabetes: Current low-dose oral contraceptives exert minimal impact on glucose metabolism. Diabetic patients, or those with a family history of diabetes, should be observed closely to detect any worsening of carbohydrate metabolism. Patients predisposed to diabetes who can be kept under close supervision may be given oral contraceptives. Young diabetic patients whose disease is of recent origin, well-controlled, and not associated with hypertension or other signs of vascular disease such as ocular fundal changes, should be monitored more frequently while using oral contraceptives.

Ocular Disease: Patients who are pregnant or are taking oral contraceptives may experience corneal edema that may cause visual disturbances and changes in tolerance to contact lenses, especially of the rigid type. Soft contact lenses usually do not cause disturbances. If visual changes or alterations in tolerance to contact lenses occur, temporary or permanent cessation of wear may be advised.

Breasts: Increasing age and a strong family history are the most significant risk factors for the development of breast cancer. Other established risk factors include obesity, nulliparity and late age at first full-term pregnancy. The identified groups of women that may be at increased risk of developing breast cancer before menopause are long-term users of oral contraceptives (more than 8 years) and starters at early age. In a few women, the use of oral contraceptives may accelerate the growth of an existing but undiagnosed breast cancer. Since any potential increased risk related to oral contraceptive use is small, there is no reason to change prescribing habits at present.

Women receiving oral contraceptives should be instructed in self-examination of their breasts. Their physicians should be notified whenever any masses are detected. A yearly clinical breast examination is also recommended because, if a breast cancer should develop, estrogen-containing drugs may cause a rapid progression.

Vaginal Bleeding: Persistent irregular vaginal bleeding requires assessment to exclude underlying pathology.

Fibroids: Patients with fibroids (leiomyomata) should be carefully observed. Sudden enlargement, pain or tenderness requires discontinuance of the use of oral contraceptives.

Emotional Disorders: Patients with a history of emotional disturbances, especially the depressive type, may be more prone to have a recurrence of depression while taking oral contraceptives. In cases of a serious recurrence, a trial of an alternative method of contraception should be made which may help to clarify the possible relationship. Women with premenstrual syndrome (PMS) may have a varied response to oral contraceptives, ranging from symptomatic improvement to worsening of the condition.

Laboratory Tests: Results of laboratory tests should be interpreted in light of the fact that the patient is on oral contraceptives. The following laboratory tests are modified.

A. Liver Function Tests: Bromsulphthalein Retention Test (BSP): moderate increase; AST and GGT: minor increase; alkaline phosphatase: variable increase; serum bilirubin: increased, particularly in conditions predisposing to or associated with hyperbilirubinemia.
B. Coagulation Tests: Factors II, VII, IX, X, XII and XIII: increased; Factor VIII: mild increase; platelet aggregation and adhesiveness: mild increase in response to common aggregating agents; fibrinogen: increased; plasminogen: mild increase; antithrombin III: mild decrease; prothrombin time: increased.
C. Thyroid Function Tests: Protein-bound Iodine (PBI): increased; Total Serum Thyroxine (T_4): increased; Thyroid Stimulating Hormone (TSH): unchanged; T_3 resin-uptake: decreased.
D. Adrenocortical Function Tests: plasma cortisol: increased.
E. Miscellaneous Tests: serum folate: occasionally decreased; glucose tolerance test: variable increase with return to normal after 6 to 12 months; insulin response: mild to moderate increase; C-Peptide response: mild to moderate increase.

Tissue Specimens: Pathologists should be advised of oral contraceptive therapy when specimens obtained from surgical procedures and Pap smears are submitted for examination.

Return to Fertility: After discontinuing oral contraceptive therapy, the patient should delay pregnancy until at least 1 normal spontaneous menstrual cycle has occurred in order to date the pregnancy. An alternative contraceptive method should be used during this time.

Amenorrhea: Women having a history of oligomenorrhea, secondary amenorrhea, or irregular cycles may remain anovulatory or become amenorrheic following discontinuation of estrogen-progestin combination therapy.

Amenorrhea, especially if associated with breast secretion, that continues for 6 months or more after withdrawal, warrants a careful assessment of hypothalamic-pituitary function.

Thromboembolic Complications—Post-surgery: There is an increased risk of thromboembolic complications in oral contraceptive users after major surgery. If feasible, oral contraceptives should be discontinued and an alternative method substituted at least 1 month prior to **major** elective surgery. Oral contraceptive use should not be resumed until the first menstrual period after hospital discharge following surgery.

Drug Interactions: The concurrent administration of oral contraceptives with other drugs may result in an altered response to either agent (see Table 1 and Table 2). Reduced effectiveness of the oral contraceptive, should it occur, is more likely with the low-dose formulations.

It is important to ascertain all drugs that a patient is taking, both prescription and nonprescription, including herbal preparations/remedies, before oral contraceptives are prescribed.

Changes in Contraceptive Effectiveness Associated With Co-Administration of Other Drugs: If a woman on hormonal contraceptives takes a drug or herbal product that induces enzymes, including CYP3A4, that metabolize contraceptive hormones, she should be counselled to use additional contraception or a different method of contraception. Drugs or herbal products that induce such enzymes may decrease the plasma concentrations of contraceptive hormones, and may decrease the effectiveness of hormonal contraceptives or increase breakthrough bleeding. Some drugs or herbal products that may decrease the effectiveness of hormonal contraceptives include:*

- modafinil
- oxcarbazepine
- St. John's wort
- topiramate

HIV protease inhibitors and non-nucleoside reverse transcriptase inhibitors: Significant changes (increase or decrease) in the plasma levels of the estrogen and progestin have been noted in some cases of co-administration of HIV protease inhibitors and non-nucleoside reverse transcriptase inhibitors.

Antibiotics: There have been reports of pregnancy while taking hormonal contraceptives and antibiotics, but clinical pharmacokinetic studies have not shown consistent effects of antibiotics on plasma concentrations of synthetic steroids.

Increase in Plasma Hormone Levels Associated With Co-Administered Drugs: Some drugs and grapefruit juice may increase the plasma levels of ethinyl estradiol if co-administered. Examples include:

- acetaminophen
- ascorbic acid
- CYP3A4 inhibitors (including itraconazole, ketoconazole, voriconazole and fluconazole)
- grapefruit juice

* Additional drugs are listed in Table I.

- HMG-CoA reductase inhibitors (including atorvastatin and rosuvastatin)

Changes in Plasma Levels of Co-Administered Drugs: Combination hormonal contraceptives may also affect the pharmacokinetics of some other drugs if used concomitantly. Examples of drugs whose plasma levels may be increased (due to CYP inhibition) include:†

- omeprazole
- voriconazole

Examples of drugs whose plasma levels may be decreased (due to induction of glucuronidation) include:†

- morphine
- salicyclic acid
- temazepam

Physicians are advised to consult the labelling of concurrently used drugs to obtain further information about interactions with hormonal contraceptives or the potential for enzyme alterations.

Refer to Oral Contraceptives 1994 (Chapter 8), Health Canada, for other possible drug interactions with OCs.

Table 1: CYCLEN

Drugs That May Decrease the Efficacy of Oral Contraceptives

Class of Compound	Drug	Proposed Mechanism	Suggested Management
Anticonvulsants	Carbamazepine Ethosuximide Phenobarbital Phenytoin Primidone	Induction of hepatic microsomal enzymes: Rapid metabolism of estrogen and increased binding of progestin and ethinyl estradiol to SHBG.	Use higher dose OCs (50 µg ethinyl estradiol), another drug or another method.
Antibiotics	Ampicillin Cotrimoxazole Penicillin	Enterohepatic circulation disturbance, intestinal hurry.	For short course, use additional method or use another drug. For long course, use another method.
	Rifampin	Increased metabolism of progestins. Suspected acceleration of estrogen metabolism.	Use another method.
	Chloramphenicol, Metronidazole, Neomycin, Nitrofurantoin, Sulfonamides, Tetracyclines	Induction of hepatic microsomal enzymes. Also disturbance of enterohepatic circulation.	For short course, use additional method or use another drug. For long course, use another method.
	Troleandomycin	May retard metabolism of OCs, increasing the risk of cholestatic jaundice.	
Antifungals	Griseofulvin	Stimulation of hepatic metabolism of contraceptive steroids may occur.	Use another method.
Cholesterol-lowering Agent	Cholestyramine	May result in hastened elimination and impaired effectiveness.	
Sedatives and Hypnotics	Benzodiazepines, Barbiturates, Chloral hydrate, Glutethimide, Meprobamate	Induction of hepatic microsomal enzymes.	For short course, use additional method or another drug. For long course, use another method or higher dose OCs.
Antacids		Decreased intestinal absorption of progestins.	Dose 2 hours apart.
Other Drugs	Phenylbutazone, Antihistamines, Analgesics, Antimigraine preparations, Vitamin E	Reduced OC efficacy has been reported. Remains to be confirmed.	
	Bosentan	Induction of hepatic microsomal enzymes.	Consider switching to a non-hormonal contraceptive method or adding a barrier method to oral contraceptive therapy.

Table 2: CYCLEN

Modification of Other Drug Action by Oral Contraceptives

Class of Compound	Drug	Modification of Drug Action	Suggested Management
Alcohol		Possible increased levels of ethanol or acetaldehyde.	Use with caution.
Alpha-II Adrenoreceptor Agents	Clonidine	Sedation effect increased.	Use with caution.
Anticoagulants	All	OCs increase clotting factors, decrease efficacy. However, OCs may potentiate action in some patients.	Use another method.

† Additional drugs are listed in Table II.

(cont'd)

Table 2: CYCLEN *(cont'd)*

Modification of Other Drug Action by Oral Contraceptives

Class of Compound	Drug	Modification of Drug Action	Suggested Management
Anticonvulsants	All	Fluid retention may increase risk of seizures.	Use another method.
	Lamotrigine	Significantly decreased lamotrigine levels (due to induction of lamotrigine glucuronidation) may lead to breakthrough seizures.	Adjust dose of drug if necessary.
Antidiabetic Drugs	Oral hypoglycemics and insulin	OCs may impair glucose tolerance and increase blood glucose.	Use low-dose estrogen and progestin OC or another method. Monitor blood glucose.
Antihypertensive Agents	Guanethidine and methyldopa	Estrogen component causes sodium retention, progestin has no effect.	Use low-dose estrogen OC or use another method.
	Beta-blockers	Increased drug effect (decreased metabolism).	Adjust dose of drug if necessary. Monitor cardiovascular status.
Antipyretics	Acetaminophen	Increased metabolism and renal clearance.	Dose of drug may have to be increased.
	Antipyrine	Impaired metabolism.	Decrease dose of drug.
	ASA	Effects of ASA may be decreased by the short-term use of OCs.	Patients on chronic ASA therapy may require an increase in ASA dosage.
Aminocaproic Acid		Theoretically, a hypercoagulable state may occur because OCs augment clotting factors.	Avoid concomitant use.
Betamimetic Agents	Isoproterenol	Estrogen causes decreased response to these drugs.	Adjust dose of drug as necessary. Discontinuing OCs can result in excessive drug activity.
Caffeine		The actions of caffeine may be enhanced as OCs may impair the hepatic metabolism of caffeine.	Use with caution.
Corticosteroids	Prednisone Prednisolone	Markedly increased serum levels.	Possible need for decrease in dose.
Cyclosporine		May lead to an increase in cyclosporine levels and hepatotoxicity.	Monitor hepatic function. The cyclosporine dose may have to be decreased.
Folic Acid		OCs have been reported to impair folate metabolism.	May need to increase dietary intake, or supplement.
Meperidine		Possible increased analgesia and CNS depression due to decreased metabolism of meperidine.	Use combination with caution.
Phenothiazine Tranquilizers	All phenothiazines, Reserpine and similar drugs	Estrogen potentiates the hyperprolactinemia effect of these drugs.	Use other drugs or lower dose OCs. If galactorrhea or hyperprolactinemia occurs, use other method.
Sedatives and Hypnotics	Chlordiazepoxide, Lorazepam, Oxazepam, Diazepam	Increased effect (increased metabolism).	Use with caution.
Theophylline	All	Decreased oxidation, leading to possible toxicity.	Use with caution. Monitor theophylline levels.
Tricyclic Antidepressants	Clomipramine (possibly others)	Increased side effects, i.e., depression.	Use with caution.
Vitamin B_{12}		OCs have been reported to reduce serum levels of Vitamin B_{12}.	May need to increase dietary intake, or supplement.

Non-contraceptive Benefits of Oral Contraceptives: Several health advantages other than contraception have been reported.

1. Combination oral contraceptives reduce the incidence of cancer of the endometrium and ovaries.
2. Oral contraceptives reduce the likelihood of developing benign breast disease and, as a result, decrease the incidence of breast biopsies.
3. Oral contraceptives reduce the likelihood of development of functional ovarian cysts.
4. Pill users have less menstrual blood loss and have more regular cycles, thereby reducing the chance of developing iron-deficiency anemia.
5. The use of oral contraceptives may decrease the severity of dysmenorrhea and premenstrual syndrome, and may improve acne vulgaris, hirsutism, and other androgen-mediated disorders.
6. Oral contraceptives decrease the incidence of acute pelvic inflammatory disease and, thereby, reduce as well the incidence of ectopic pregnancy.
7. Oral contraceptives have potential beneficial effects on endometriosis.

Oral contraceptives **do not protect** against sexually transmitted diseases (STDs) including HIV/AIDS. For protection against STDs, it is advisable to use latex condoms **in combination with** oral contraceptives.

ADVERSE EFFECTS: An increased risk of the following serious adverse reactions has been associated with the use of oral contraceptives: thrombophlebitis and venous thrombosis with or without embolism; arterial thromboembolism; pulmonary embolism; mesenteric thrombosis; neuro-ocular lesions (e.g., retinal thrombosis); myocardial infarction; cerebral thrombosis; cerebral hemorrhage; hypertension; benign hepatic tumors; gallbladder disease.

The following adverse reactions also have been reported in patients receiving oral contraceptives: nausea and vomiting, usually the most common adverse reaction, occurs in approximately 10% or less of patients during the first cycle. Other reactions, as a general rule, are seen less frequently or only occasionally, as follows:

Cardiovascular System: edema, slight rise of blood pressure.

Genital Tract: breakthrough bleeding, spotting, change in menstrual flow, dysmenorrhea, amenorrhea during and after treatment, vaginal candidiasis, premenstrual-like syndrome, temporary infertility after discontinuance of treatment, vaginitis, endocervical hyperplasias, increase in cervical erosion and secretion.

Neoplasms: malignant hepatic tumors, cervical cancer, increase in size of uterine leiomyomata, breast cancer.

Breast: pain, tenderness, enlargement, and secretion, possible diminution in lactation when given immediately postpartum.

Skin and Subcutaneous Tissue: chloasma or melasma which may persist, rash (allergic), hirsutism, loss of scalp hair, erythema multiforme, erythema nodosum, Raynaud's phenomenon, hemorrhagic eruption, porphyria, acne, seborrhea, pemphigoid (herpes gestationis), urticaria, angioedema.

CNS: migraine, depression, headache, nervousness, dizziness, changes in libido, chorea.

Metabolic: reduced tolerance to carbohydrates, change in weight (increase or decrease), changes in appetite.

Gastro-intestinal Tract: gastrointestinal symptoms (such as abdominal cramps and bloating), colitis, pancreatitis.

Hepatobiliary: cholestatic jaundice, Budd-Chiari syndrome.

Eyes: intolerance to contact lenses, change in corneal curvature (steepening), cataracts, optic neuritis, retinal thrombosis.

Urinary: impaired renal function, hemolytic uremic syndrome, cystitis-like syndrome.

Others: rhinitis, auditory disturbances.

OVERDOSE:

Treatment: In case of overdosage or accidental ingestion by children, the physician should observe the patient closely although generally no treatment is required. Gastric lavage may be utilized if considered necessary. Overdosage may cause nausea and vomiting and withdrawal bleeding may occur in females. There are no antidotes and treatment should be symptomatic.

For management of a suspected drug overdose, contact your regional Poison Control Centre. See the *CPS* Directory section for a list of Poison Control Centres.

DOSAGE: **Information for the Patient on How to Take the Birth Control Pill:**

1. **Read these directions:**
   - before you start taking your pills, and
   - any time you are not sure what to do.
2. **Look at your pill pack** to see if it has 21 or 28 pills:
   - **21-Pill Pack:** 21 active pills (with hormones) taken daily for 3 weeks, and then take no pills for 1 week or
   - **28-Pill Pack:** 21 active pills (with hormones) taken daily for 3 weeks, and then 7 "reminder" pills (no hormones) taken daily for 1 week.

   Also check the pill pack for instructions on (1) where to start and (2) directions to take pills (see package insert for illustrations).
3. You may wish to use a second method of birth control (e.g., latex condoms and spermicidal foam or gel) for the first 7 days of the first cycle of pill use. This will provide a back-up in case pills are forgotten while you are getting used to taking them.
4. **When receiving any medical treatment, be sure to tell your doctor that you are using birth control pills.**
5. **Many women have spotting or light bleeding or may feel sick to their stomach during the first 3 months on the pill.** If you do feel sick, do not stop taking the pill. The problem will usually go away. If it does not go away, check with your doctor or clinic.
6. **Missing pills also can cause some spotting or light bleeding,** even if you make up the missed pills. You also could feel a little sick to your stomach on the days you take 2 pills to make up for missed pills.
7. **If you miss pills at any time, you could get pregnant. The greatest risks for pregnancy are:**
   - when you start a pack late, or
   - when you miss pills at the beginning or at the very end of the pack.
8. **Always be sure you have ready:**
   - **another kind of birth control** (such as latex condoms and spermicidal foam or gel) to use as a back-up in case you miss pills, and
   - **an extra, full pack of pills.**
9. **If you experience vomiting or diarrhea, or if you take certain medicines,** such as antibiotics, your pills may not work as well. Use a back-up method, such as latex condoms and spermicidal foam or gel, until you can check with your doctor or clinic.
10. **If you forget more than 1 pill 2 months in a row,** talk to your doctor or clinic about how to make pill-taking easier or about using another method of birth control.
11. **If your questions are not answered here, call your doctor or clinic.**

When to start the first pack of pills: Be sure to read these instructions:

- before you start taking your pills, and
- any time you are not sure what to do.

Decide with your doctor or clinic what is the best day for you to start taking your first pack of pills. Your pills may be either a 21-day or a 28-day type.

Directions for 21-Day and 28-Day Pill Packs:

1. **The first day of your menstrual period (bleeding) is Day 1 of your cycle.** The pills may be started up to Day 6 of your cycle. Your starting day will be chosen in discussion with your doctor. You will **always** begin taking your pill on this day of the week. Your doctor may advise you to start taking the pills on Day 1, on Day 5, or on the first Sunday after your period begins. If your period starts on Sunday, start that same day.
2. **If you are using a:**

   21-Day Pill Pack: With this type of birth control pill, you are on pills for 21 days and off pills for 7 days. You must not be off the pills for more than 7 days in a row.

   Take 1 pill at approximately the same time every day for 21 days; **do not take a pill for 7 days**. Start a new pack on the 8th day. You will probably have a period during the 7 days off the pill. (This bleeding may be lighter and shorter than your usual period.)

   28-Day Pill Pack: With this type of birth control pill, you take 21 pills that contain hormones and 7 pills that contain no hormones.

   Take 1 pill at approximately the same time every day for 28 days. Begin a new pack the next day, **not missing any days on the pills.** Your period should occur during the last 7 days of using that pill pack.

Instructions for using your Discreet package for both 21-day and 28-day packs. Follow these instructions carefully.

1. **For Day 1 start:** Label the Discreet Package by selecting the day label that starts with Day 1 of your menstrual period (the first day of menstruation is Day 1). For example, if your first day of menstruation is Tuesday, attach the day label that begins with **TUE** in the space provided.

   or

   For Day 5 start: Label the Discreet Package by selecting the day label that starts with the day that is 5 days after your period begins. (Count 5 days **including** the first day of menstruation.) For example, if your first day of menstruation is Saturday, place the day label that starts with **WED** in the space provided.

   or

   For Sunday start: No day label is required. The Discreet Package is printed for a Sunday start. (The first Sunday **after** your period begins, or, if your period starts on Sunday, start that **same day**.)
2. Place the day label in the space where you see the words "Place day label here". Having the Discreet Package labelled with the days of the week will help remind you to take your pill every day.
3. To begin taking your pills, start with the pill inside the red circle (where you see the word **START**). This pill should correspond to the day of the week that you are taking your first pill. To remove the pill, push through the back of the Discreet Package.
4. On the following day, take the next pill in the same row, always proceeding from left to right (→). Each row will always begin on the same day of the week.

What to do during the month:

1. **Take a pill at approximately the same time every day until the pack is empty.**
   - Try to associate taking your pill with some regular activity such as eating a meal or going to bed.
   - Do not skip pills even if you have bleeding between monthly periods or feel sick to your stomach (nausea).
   - Do not skip pills even if you do not have sex very often.
2. **When you finish a pack:**
   - **21 pills: Wait 7 days** to start the next pack. You will have your period during that week.
   - **28 pills:** Start the next pack **on the next day**. Take 1 pill every day. Do not wait any days between packs.

What to do if you miss pills: Table 3 outlines the actions you should take if you miss 1 or more of your birth control pills. Match the number of pills missed with the appropriate starting time for your type of pill pack.

Table 3: CYCLEN

What to Do If You Miss Pills

Sunday Start	Other Than Sunday Start
Miss 1 pill	**Miss 1 pill**
Take it as soon as you remember, and take the next pill at the usual time. This means that you might take 2 pills in one day.	Take it as soon as you remember, and take the next pill at the usual time. This means that you might take 2 pills in one day.
Miss 2 pills in a row	**Miss 2 pills in a row**
First 2 Weeks: 1. Take 2 pills the day you remember and 2 pills the next day. 2. Then take 1 pill a day until you finish the pack. 3. Use a back-up method of birth control if you have sex in the 7 days after you miss the pills. **Third Week:** 1. Keep taking 1 pill a day until Sunday. 2. On Sunday, safely discard the rest of the pack and start a new pack that day. 3. Use a back-up method of birth control if you have sex in the 7 days after you miss the pills. 4. You may not have a period this month. **If you miss 2 periods in a row, call your doctor or clinic.**	**First 2 Weeks:** 1. Take 2 pills the day you remember and 2 pills the next day. 2. Then take 1 pill a day until you finish the pack. 3. Use a back-up method of birth control if you have sex in the 7 days after you miss the pills. **Third Week:** 1. Safely dispose of the rest of the pill pack and start a new pack that same day. 2. Use a back-up method of birth control if you have sex in the 7 days after you miss the pills. 3. You may not have a period this month. **If you miss 2 periods in a row, call your doctor or clinic.**
Miss 3 or more pills in a row	**Miss 3 or more pills in a row**
Any Time in the Cycle: 1. Keep taking 1 pill a day until Sunday. 2. On Sunday, safely discard the rest of the pack and start a new pack that day. 3. Use a back-up method of birth control if you have sex in the 7 days after you miss the pills. 4. You may not have a period this month. **If you miss 2 periods in a row, call your doctor or clinic.**	**Any Time in the Cycle:** 1. Safely dispose of the rest of the pill pack and start a new pack that same day. 2. Use a back-up method of birth control if you have sex in the 7 days after you miss the pills. 3. You may not have a period this month. **If you miss 2 periods in a row, call your doctor or clinic.**

Note: 28-Day Pack: If you forget any of the 7 "reminder" pills (without hormones) in Week 4, just safely dispose of the pills you missed. Then keep taking 1 pill each day until the pack is empty. You do not need to use a back-up method.

Always be sure you have on hand:

- a back-up method of birth control (such as latex condoms and spermicidal foam or gel) in case you miss pills, and
- an extra full pack of pills.

If you forget more than 1 pill 2 months in a row, talk to your doctor or clinic. Talk about ways to make pill-taking easier or about using another method of birth control.

INFORMATION FOR THE PATIENT: Published in e-CPS, available by subscription at www.e-cps.ca.

SUPPLIED: Each blue tablet contains: norgestimate 0.25 mg and ethinyl estradiol 0.035 mg. In the 28-day regimen, the green tablets contain inert ingredients. Nonmedicinal ingredients: Blue tablets: FD&C Blue No. 2 Aluminum lake, lactose, magnesium stearate and starch. Green tablets: D&C Yellow No. 10 Aluminum lake, FD&C Blue No. 2 Aluminum lake, lactose, magnesium stearate, microcrystalline cellulose and starch. Available in 21-day (21 blue tablets) or 28-day (21 blue tablets and 7 green tablets) Discreet Packages. Store between 15 and 25°C. Leave contents in protective packaging until time of use.

(Shown in Product Identification Section)

Cyclobenzaprine

Skeletal Muscle Relaxant

CPhA Monograph

Date of Preparation: July 2006
Date of Revision: October 2010

This monograph has been compiled by CPhA and reviewed by experts. It may contain information different from that found in Health Canada-approved Product Monographs. The reader is referred to the *CPS* Editorial Policy for more information.

SUMMARY PRODUCT INFORMATION:

Route of Administration	Dosage Form	Strength
Oral	Tablet	10 mg

INDICATIONS AND CLINICAL USE: Health Canada approved indications: Cyclobenzaprine is indicated for the short term (≤3 weeks) treatment of muscle spasm associated with acute musculoskeletal conditions. Cyclobenzaprine is not effective for the treatment of spasticity associated with cerebral or spinal cord disease, including cerebral palsy in children.

Uses without Health Canada approval:

- Fibromyalgia
- Acute neck or back pain. In a 7-day study of adult patients with acute neck or back pain, cyclobenzaprine alone (5 mg three times daily) was as effective as cyclobenzaprine (5 mg three times daily) plus ibuprofen (400 mg or 800 mg three times daily).

Geriatrics: Cyclobenzaprine has anticholinergic and CNS depressant effects. The drug should be used with caution in elderly patients who may be more susceptible to these and other adverse effects of the drug.

Pediatrics: The safety and efficacy of cyclobenzaprine has not been established in children aged less than 15 years.

CONTRAINDICATIONS:

- Patients who are hypersensitive to cyclobenzaprine or to any ingredient in the formulation.

- Use of monoamine oxidase inhibitors, including use of these drugs within the preceding 14 days.
- Acute recovery phase of myocardial infarction.
- Patients with a history of cardiac arrhythmias, heart block or conduction disturbances, or heart failure.
- Hyperthyroidism.

WARNINGS AND PRECAUTIONS:

Serious Warnings and Precautions
Cyclobenzaprine is structurally similar to tricyclic antidepressants and has a similar adverse event profile including central nervous system disorders and cardiac conduction abnormalities.

General: Cyclobenzaprine has anticholinergic effects that may precipitate or exacerbate the following conditions: urinary retention, angle-closure glaucoma, increased intraocular pressure.

The anticholinergic effects of cyclobenzaprine may be additive to those of other agents.

Plasma concentrations are increased in the elderly and in those with mild hepatic impairment.

Neurologic: Cyclobenzaprine may enhance the effects of central nervous system depressants such as alcohol, barbiturates and benzodiazepines.

Special Populations: Pregnant Women: There is no evidence of harm to the fetus in animal studies. The drug should be used in pregnancy only if clearly needed.

Nursing Women: It is not known whether cyclobenzaprine is excreted in human breast milk. Some closely related tricyclic antidepressants are excreted in breast milk; therefore, caution is advised when considering use of this agent in women who are breastfeeding.

Geriatrics: Plasma levels of cyclobenzaprine are elevated in elderly people. Moreover, older individuals may be more susceptible to anticholinergic and CNS adverse events than younger individuals. For these reasons, initiate therapy at lower doses; elderly patients should be closely supervised during treatment with cyclobenzaprine.

Occupational Hazards: Cyclobenzaprine may impair mental or physical abilities required to operate machinery or drive a motor vehicle, particularly if taken with alcohol or drugs with CNS depressant properties.

ADVERSE REACTIONS: Adverse Drug Reactions Overview: Cyclobenzaprine is structurally related to tricyclic antidepressants, and may cause adverse effects similar to these compounds. CNS depressant and anticholinergic effects are the most commonly seen adverse effects associated with cyclobenzaprine.

More Common Adverse Drug Reactions: See Table 1.

Table 1: Cyclobenzaprine

More Common Adverse Drug Reactions (≥10%)

Body System	Effect	Clinical Comment
CNS	Drowsiness/fatigue, dizziness	Advise patients that their ability to perform tasks requiring mental or physical alertness (e.g., driving) may be impaired by cyclobenzaprine.
Gastrointestinal	Dry mouth	Advise patients that chewing sugar-free gum or sucking on sugar-free hard candies may help alleviate dry mouth.

Less Common Adverse Drug Reactions: Cardiovascular: arrhythmia, edema, heart block, hypo- or hypertension, myocardial infarction, stroke, syncope, tachycardia, vasodilation.

Central Nervous System: agitation, anxiety, confusion, convulsions, decreased mental acuity, depressed mood, diplopia, disorientation, dysarthria, hallucinations, headache, hypertonia, insomnia, irritability, malaise, nervousness, paresthesias, psychosis, seizures, tinnitus, vertigo.

Dermatologic: alopecia, rash, sweating, photosensitivity.

Endocrine and Metabolism: elevated or decreased blood sugar, SIADH, weight gain, weight loss.

Gastrointestinal: abdominal pain, acid reflux, ageusia, anorexia, constipation, diarrhea, dyspepsia, flatulence, gastritis, gastrointestinal pain, nausea, paralytic ileus, stomatitis, unpleasant taste.

Genitourinary: urinary frequency, urinary retention.

Hematologic: bone marrow suppression, eosinophilia, leukopenia, thrombocytopenia, purpura.

Hepatic: hepatitis (jaundice, cholestasis, elevated transaminases).

Immune: anaphylaxis, angioedema, pruritus, facial edema, urticaria.

Musculoskeletal: local weakness, myalgia.

Neurologic: abnormal gait, ataxia, tremors, Bell's palsy, extrapyramidal symptoms.

Ophthalmologic: blurred vision.

Sexual Function/Reproduction: decreased or increased libido, impotence.

DRUG INTERACTIONS:

Serious Drug Interactions
Cyclobenzaprine may precipitate an acute life-threatening reaction if administered together with or within 14 days of administration of a monoamine oxidase inhibitor.

Drug-Drug Interactions: Cyclobenzaprine is metabolized by CYP1A2, CYP3A4 and CYP2D6. Concomitant therapy with drugs known to inhibit or induce these isoenzymes may enhance or diminish the effects of cyclobenzaprine. See Table 2.

Table 2: Cyclobenzaprine

Drug-Drug Interactions

Interacting Drug	Effect	Clinical Comment
Anticholinergic agents	Cyclobenzaprine has anticholinergic effects which are considered additive to those induced by other drugs.	Avoid concurrent use if possible, particularly in elderly patients who are more susceptible to anticholinergic effects.
CNS Depressants	Cyclobenzaprine may enhance the effects of alcohol, antidepressants, barbiturates, benzodiazepines, hypnotics, opioids and other medications causing CNS depression.	Advise patients of increased risk of sedation and CNS impairment; monitor for these effects. Avoid alcohol.
Droperidol	There is one case report of QTc prolongation in a patient receiving cyclobenzaprine and droperidol together with fluoxetine.	Avoid concurrent use; if combination used, monitor for evidence of QTc prolongation.
Fluoxetine	Fluoxetine may elevate serum levels of cyclobenzaprine. The suspected mechanism is inhibition of CYP2D6-mediated metabolism of cyclobenzaprine.	Avoid concurrent use. If used together monitor patients for side effects of cyclobenzaprine.

(cont'd)

Table 2: Cyclobenzaprine *(cont'd)*

Drug-Drug Interactions

Interacting Drug	Effect	Clinical Comment
Guanethidine	Cyclobenzaprine, which is structurally similar to tricyclic antidepressants, may block the antihypertensive action of guanethidine and similar compounds.	Avoid concurrent use. Use an alternative antihypertensive medication if treatment is required in a patient taking cyclobenzaprine.
Monoamine oxidase inhibitors	Cyclobenzaprine may provoke a life-threatening interaction in patients taking monoamine oxidase inhibitors. Hyperpyretic crises, severe convulsions and deaths have been reported.	Concurrent use is contraindicated.
Serotonergic agents (e.g., SNRIs, SSRIs, triptans)	Cases of serotonin syndrome have been reported when cyclobenzaprine was used with escitalopram and with duloxetine. Therapy with other serotonergic drugs may increase the risk of serotonin syndrome.	Symptoms may include mental status changes (e.g., agitation), autonomic effects (e.g., diaphoresis, hyperthermia, tachycardia), vomiting, diarrhea, tremor, muscle rigidity, hyperreflexia.
Tramadol	Cyclobenzaprine, which is structurally similar to tricyclic antidepressants, may increase the risk of seizures in patients taking tramadol.	Avoid concurrent use.

DOSAGE AND ADMINISTRATION: Dosing Considerations: In Canada, cyclobenzaprine is available only as a 10 mg tablet; however, clinical studies have shown that a dose of 5 mg three times daily is as effective as 10 mg three times daily, and that the lower dose produces less sedation [*Clin Ther* 2003;25:1056-73]. Splitting tablets may result in increased variation in the administered dose, although the potential lower risk of adverse events may be preferred, especially in elderly patients.

Recommended Dose and Dosage Adjustment: Adults: See Table 3.

Table 3: Cyclobenzaprine

Dose in Adult Patients

Indication	Route	Initial Dose	Maximum Dose	Duration of Therapy	Clinical Comment
Acute musculoskeletal spasm	oral	5–10 mg three times daily	30 mg/day	2–3 weeks	In elderly patients and those with mild hepatic dysfunction a dose of 5 mg three times daily is recommended.
Fibromyalgia (a use without Health Canada approval)	oral	10 mg at bedtime	40 mg/day		May divide higher doses between morning and evening (e.g., 10 mg QAM and 20–30 mg QHS)

Pediatric Patients: Dosage and safety in children less than 15 years of age have not been established.

Hepatic Impairment: In patients with mild hepatic impairment the AUC and C_{max} of cyclobenzaprine were approximately double those in healthy volunteers. For this reason, cyclobenzaprine should be used with caution in patients with mild hepatic impairment; consider initiating therapy at a lower dose and/or less frequent dosing in these patients. Monitor patients for signs of cyclobenzaprine excess (e.g., sedation). Avoid use of the drug in patients with moderate to severe hepatic impairment.

OVERDOSAGE:

Signs and Symptoms: Cyclobenzaprine is extremely toxic in overdose.

Symptoms of overdose may vary in severity depending on factors such as the amount of drug absorbed, the interval between drug ingestion and the start of treatment and the age of the patient.

Cyclobenzaprine overdose shares many similarities with overdose of tricyclic antidepressants (TCAs), and deaths, while rare, may occur. Toxicity most commonly occurs within two hours of ingestion. The onset of symptoms is frequently precipitous, with the rapid development of neurologic and cardiac manifestations in patients who appear otherwise well. Central nervous system involvement stems from the sedative and anticholinergic properties of the drug with manifestations ranging from somnolence to confusion, agitated delirium and coma. Peripheral anticholinergic signs (e.g., constipation, dry mucous membranes, mydriasis, urinary retention and, occasionally, adynamic ileus) may also be present. Patients may have elevated body temperatures, in part related to impaired dissipation of heat. Myoclonus, twitching, hyperreflexia, hypertonicity, nystagmus and parkinsonism can occur rarely. Seizures have been reported in some patients.

Serious cardiovascular abnormalities can occur with large overdoses and mimic those of TCA overdose. Sinus tachycardia is common, but is not a reliable predictor of serious toxicity. Other possible cardiac disturbances include QT interval prolongation and ECG manifestations of sodium channel blockade (widening of the QRS complex and a dominant terminal 40-msec of the QRS complex in a lead VR). Hypotension and bradycardia, when present, suggest either a co-ingestant or severe (and possibly preterminal) cyclobenzaprine toxicity.

Accidental ingestion in children should be regarded as serious.

Recommended Management: Adults and children in whom overdose is suspected should be evaluated in hospital without delay. A regional poison centre should be consulted to assist in the management of patients with serious toxicity. Asymptomatic cases of overdose without ECG abnormalities should be monitored for a minimum of 6 hours. Protect the patient's airway, and support ventilation and perfusion. Treatment should be designed to ensure maintenance of the vital functions and careful monitoring of ECG, blood gases, serum electrolytes and acid-base balance. Secure intravenous access.

Hypotension should be promptly corrected using crystalloid and direct-acting pressors such as norepinephrine, if necessary. Sodium bicarbonate may be helpful in patients with a widened QRS interval (>100-120 msec), particularly those with myocardial depression.

Typically, 1 to 2 mmol/kg of sodium bicarbonate (1 to 3 ampoules containing 50 mmol/50 mL for an average adult) can be given for QRS widening >100 msec, or ventricular arrhythmias, which may reflect myocardial fast sodium channel antagonism. The blood pH should be maintained in the range of 7.45 to 7.55, and the use of sodium bicarbonate should be reconsidered in patients with hypokalemia, heart failure or volume overload states.

Most patients will require potassium supplementation. Hyperventilation has also been used to alkalinize the blood.

Ventricular arrhythmias refractory to bicarbonate may respond to lidocaine. Quinidine, procainamide and other type 1A or 1C antiarrhythmic agents should not be used because they may exacerbate arrhythmias and conduction slowing due to the overdose. Overdrive pacing should be considered in patients whose arrhythmias are not responding to drug therapy.

Forced diuresis, peritoneal dialysis and hemodialysis are ineffective in the removal of cyclobenzaprine. Hyperpyrexia, if severe, should be controlled by evaporative cooling.

If seizures occur, anticonvulsants (preferably i.v. lorazepam or diazepam) should be administered. Although most seizures are short-lived, barbiturates and other measures should be employed for refractory cases. Phenytoin is not recommended for the treatment of seizures resulting from cyclobenzaprine overdose. Start artificial ventilation if the patient fails to respond rapidly to anticonvulsants. Seizures aggravate hypoxia and acidosis and may precipitate cardiac arrhythmias and arrest, so they must be promptly controlled.

Flumazenil is contraindicated in any patient with an altered level of consciousness who has or may have taken a cyclic antidepressant, as it may precipitate seizures, even in cases of mixed overdoses in which the patient is known to have taken benzodiazepines. Patients with significant central anticholinergic features and no ECG evidence of sodium channel toxicity may benefit from the judicious use of physostigmine, a short-acting cholinesterase inhibitor (available through the Special Access Programme, see Appendix 2). This should generally be done only after consultation with a regional poison centre.

For management of a suspected drug overdose, CPhA recommends that you contact your **regional Poison Control Centre**. See the *CPS* Directory section for a list of Poison Control Centres.

ACTION AND CLINICAL PHARMACOLOGY: Mechanism of Action: Cyclobenzaprine is structurally related to the tricyclic antidepressants and, in common with this class of agents, cyclobenzaprine potentiates the effect of norepinephrine, has central and peripheral anticholinergic effects, including increasing heart rate, and also causes sedation.

With respect to the muscle relaxant properties of the drug, these appear to result from effects at the level of the brain stem that result in a net reduction in tonic somatic motor activity in both the alpha and gamma systems. Cyclobenzaprine does not act directly on skeletal muscle cells or at the level of the neuromuscular junction. Cyclobenzaprine relieves muscle spasm of local origin and is ineffective in muscle spasm due to central nervous system disease.

Pharmacokinetics: Adults: Absorption: The mean oral bioavailability of cyclobenzaprine is estimated to range from 33% to 55%.

Distribution: Plasma concentrations increased in proportion to dose in healthy volunteers receiving 2.5 to 10 mg three times daily. Upon multiple dose administration the plasma levels increased approximately four-fold relative to single-dose studies. At steady state, the mean peak plasma concentrations in 18 volunteers receiving 10 mg three times daily was 25.9 ng/mL (range 12.8 to 46.1 ng/mL).

Cyclobenzaprine is highly bound to plasma proteins in circulation and undergoes enterohepatic recirculation.

Metabolism: Cyclobenzaprine undergoes extensive hepatic metabolism in humans. The results of in vitro studies with human microsomes suggest that CYP3A4, CYP1A2 and to a lesser extent CYP2D6, are involved in the production of cyclobenzaprine N-demethylation. The drug also undergoes N+ glucuronidation, and more than 10% of an administered dose is excreted as the quaternary ammonium-linked glucuronide metabolite.

Excretion: Plasma clearance of cyclobenzaprine in healthy volunteers was approximately 689 mL/min. The terminal elimination half-life of the drug was estimated to be approximately 18 hours in healthy volunteers (range 8 to 37 hours). Only a small portion of an administered dose is excreted unchanged in urine.

Special Populations: Geriatrics: Steady state plasma concentrations in elderly subjects were approximately two-fold greater than those in healthy young volunteers.

Gender: There is little difference in steady state plasma concentrations between males and females.

The reader is invited to consult CPhA's monograph **Corticosteroids: Topical**.

Cyclocort®
amcinonide
Topical Corticosteroid

Stiefel, a GSK company

INDICATIONS: The relief of inflammatory manifestations of acute and chronic corticosteroid-responsive dermatoses, such as atopic dermatitis, contact and eczematous dermatoses, psoriasis and neurodermatitis.

Topical corticosteroid therapy, although responsible for remissions of dermatoses, especially of allergic origin, cannot be expected to prevent recurrence. In the case of contact or allergic dermatitis, it is important to investigate causal factors and to remove the offending material or allergen.

CONTRAINDICATIONS: Fungal diseases of the skin, untreated bacterial infections, tuberculosis of the skin, certain viral diseases such as herpes simplex, vaccinia and varicella. Hypersensitivity to any of the product's components. Not for ophthalmic use.

PRECAUTIONS: *Pregnancy:* The safety of topical corticosteroids during pregnancy or lactation has not been established. Weigh the potential benefit of topical corticosteroids, if used during pregnancy or lactation, against possible hazard to the fetus or the infant being nursed.

Lactation: See Pregnancy.

Significant systemic absorption may occur when corticosteroids are applied over large areas of the body, especially under occlusive dressings. To minimize this possibility, when long-term therapy is anticipated, interrupt treatment periodically, or treat one area of the body at a time. Avoid contact with the eyes.

Although hypersensitivity reactions have been rare with topically applied corticosteroids, discontinue the cream and initiate appropriate therapy if there are signs of sensitivity.

The use of topical corticosteroids on infected areas should be attended with caution and careful observation, bearing in mind the potential spreading of infection and the possible advisability of discontinuing corticosteroid therapy and/or initiating antibacterial measures. If a symptomatic response is not noted within a few days to a week, discontinue the local application until the infection is brought under control.

Advise patients to inform subsequent physicians of the prior use of corticosteroids.

Occlusive dressings should not be applied if there is an elevation of body temperature.

Prolonged use of topical corticosteroids may produce atrophy of the skin and of s.c. tissues, particularly on flexor surfaces and on the face. If this is noted, discontinue the use of topical corticosteroids.

Topical corticosteroids should be used with caution in patients with stasis dermatitis and other skin diseases associated with impaired circulation.

ADVERSE EFFECTS: When occlusive dressings are used, pustules, miliaria, folliculitis, and pyoderma may occur. The following adverse skin reactions have been reported with the use of topical steroids: dryness, itching, burning, local irritation, striae, skin atrophy, atrophy of s.c. tissues, telangiectasia, hypertrichosis, change in pigmentation, and secondary infection. Adrenal suppression also has been reported following topical corticosteroid therapy. Posterior subcapsular cataracts have been reported following systemic use of corticosteroids.

OVERDOSE:

For management of a suspected drug overdose, CPhA recommends that you contact your **regional Poison Control Centre**. See the *CPS* Directory section for a list of Poison Control Centres.

DOSAGE: Apply to affected area 2 or 3 times daily and rub in gently. Application twice a day is usually sufficient.

SUPPLIED: Cream: Each tube contains: amcinonide (a fluorinated corticosteroid) 0.1%, compounded with emulsifying wax, isopropyl palmitate, glycerin, sorbitol solution, lactic acid, purified water and benzyl alcohol 2.0%. Lanolin-, propylene glycol-, tartrazine- and urea-free. Tubes of 15, 30 and 60 g.

Lotion: Each bottle contains: amcinonide 0.1%, emulsifying wax, isopropyl palmitate, glycerin, sorbitol solution, lactic acid, purified water, and benzyl alcohol 1.0%. Lanolin-, propylene glycol-, tartrazine- and urea-free. Bottles of 20 and 60 mL.

Ointment: Each tube contains: amcinonide 0.1%, emulsifying wax, benzyl alcohol 2.0%, TENOX II, and white petrolatum. Tartrazine-free. Tubes of 15, 30 and 60 g.

Cyclogyl®
cyclopentolate HCl
Cycloplegic—Mydriatic—Anticholinergic

Alcon

SUPPLIED: Each dispenser contains: cyclopentolate HCl 1% preserved with benzalkonium chloride. Nonmedicinal ingredients: boric acid, edetate disodium, hydrochloric acid, potassium chloride, purified water and sodium carbonate. Drop-Tainer dispensers of 15 mL.

Cyclomen®
danazol
Pituitary Gonadotropin Inhibitor

sanofi-aventis

Date of Revision: February 3, 2010

PHARMACOLOGY: In women of reproductive age, the primary mode of action of danazol is believed to be by suppression of the pituitary-ovarian axis, and inhibition of the output of gonadotropins from the pituitary-gland.

Other mechanisms of action currently postulated to explain its effects are: inhibition of midcycle FSH and LH surges; inhibition of enzymes required for gonadal hormone synthesis; and competitive binding of danazol to steroid receptors at target organs.

Danazol may also inhibit cyclic AMP accumulation in granulosa and luteal cells in response to gonadotropic hormones. A wide range of actions on plasma proteins including increasing prothrombin, plasminogen, antithrombin III, alpha-2-macroglobulin, C1 esterase inhibitor, erythropoietin and reducing fibrinogen, thyroid binding and sex hormone-binding globulins has been observed. Danazol increases the proportion and concentration of testosterone carried unbound in the plasma.

In postmenopausal women, danazol suppresses FSH and LH levels. It has a weak dose-related androgenic activity. Danazol is a weak androgen but antiandrogenic, progestogenic, antiprogestogenic, estrogenic and antiestrogenic actions have also been observed.

Following oral administration in healthy adult females, danazol displays dose-dependent absorption, which approaches linearity over the dosage range 100 to 400 mg twice daily in multiple dosing. Absorption is affected by prandial state, being approximately doubled if danazol is taken just after, compared with 2 hours before, a meal. The principal metabolites of danazol appear to be ethisterone and 17-hydroxymethylethisterone. The mean plasma elimination half-life of danazol is in the order of 24 hours.

Bioavailability studies indicate that blood levels do not increase proportionally with increases in the administered dose. When the dose is doubled, the increase in plasma levels is only about 35 to 40%.

When used for the treatment of endometriosis, danazol alters the endometrium so that it becomes inactive and atrophic. Danazol produces marked regression of ectopic endometrial tissue. Pre- and post-medication laparoscopy was done on 96 subjects. Complete or partial resolution of ectopic endometrial sites was found in 85 out of 88 patients (97%) receiving 800 mg danazol daily and in 6 out of 8 patients receiving 600 mg. This regression is due to the suppression of ovarian function which results in anovulation and associated amenorrhea. Changes in vaginal cytology and cervical mucus reflect the suppressive effect of danazol on gonadal steroid actions and were found in 75% of 116 patients.

After institution of therapy with danazol, patients (generally) have one additional menstrual period and then become anovulatory and amenorrheic, though some patients have occasional spotting or bleeding for the duration of treatment. In cases where it has been examined, this bleeding was associated with an atrophic endometrium. On regimens of 200 to 600 mg daily for 3 to 6 months, highly effective relief of the signs and symptoms of endometriosis was obtained. Complete or partial relief of dysmenorrhea occurred in 94% (290/309) of patients, of pelvic pain in 85% (276/322), of dyspareunia in 84% (134/160) and of induration of the cul-de-sac in 79% (217/274). Dysmenorrhea and pelvic pain are usually relieved within the first few weeks after initiation of therapy; relief of dyspareunia and induration of the cul-de-sac take somewhat longer.

Generally, the action of danazol on hormonal regulation is reversible. Ovulation and predictable cyclical bleeding usually return within 60 to 90 days when danazol therapy is discontinued. Discontinuation results in a rebound in FSH and LH secretion with consequent increase in fecundity.

In the treatment of fibrocystic breast disease, the mode of action of danazol on the breasts is not known. Therapy with this drug lasting up to 6 months, however, results in relief of pain, tenderness and various degrees of regression of nodularity. An alteration or improvement of the pathological process at the tissue level has not been demonstrated.

Oligomenorrhea and amenorrhea occur in a dose-dependent manner in most patients. Generally, however, the action of danazol on hormonal regulation is reversible and normal menstrual patterns return within 2 months following discontinuation of therapy.

INDICATIONS: Endometriosis: Danazol is indicated for the treatment of endometriosis associated symptoms and/or to reduce the extent of endometriotic foci. Danazol may be used either in conjunction with surgery or, as sole hormonal therapy, in patients not responding to other treatments.

Fibrocystic Breast Disease: The symptomatic relief of severe pain and tenderness associated with fibrocystic disease of the breast. Danazol should be used in those patients who do not obtain adequate relief through other therapeutic measures or in whom such measures are otherwise inadvisable.

Carcinoma of the breast should be excluded prior to commencing treatment.

The treatment course should be limited to three to six months maximum.

CONTRAINDICATIONS: In patients presenting with undiagnosed abnormal genital bleeding; genital neoplasia; markedly impaired hepatic, renal or cardiac function; pregnancy; lactation (breast-feeding); porphyria—danazol can induce ALA synthetase activity and should not be used in patients with known or suspected acute intermittent porphyria; known hypersensitivity to danazol or to any ingredient in the formulation (for a complete list, see Supplied section); androgen-dependent tumor; active thrombosis or thromboembolic disease and history of such events.

WARNINGS: *Pregnancy:* Danazol may cause fetal harm when administered to a pregnant woman. Exposure to danazol in utero may result in androgenic effects on the female fetus, comprising to date clitoral hypertrophy, labial fusion, urogenital sinus defect, vaginal atresia, and ambiguous genitalia. A sensitive test (e.g., beta subunit test if available) capable of determining early pregnancy is recommended immediately prior to start of therapy. Additionally, danazol should be initiated during menstruation and an effective non-hormonal method of contraception should be used during therapy. If a patient becomes pregnant while taking danazol, administration of the drug should be discontinued and the patient should be apprised of the potential risk to the fetus.

Lactation: Danazol has the theoretical potential for androgenic effects in breast-fed infants and therefore either danazol therapy or breast-feeding should be discontinued.

Before initiating therapy of fibrocystic breast disease with danazol, carcinoma of the breast should be excluded.

Nodularity, pain and tenderness due to fibrocystic breast disease may prevent recognition of underlying carcinoma before treatment is begun. As evidenced during clinical trials with danazol, breast pain and tenderness are usually significantly relieved by the first month of treatment and eliminated in 2 to 3 months. Regression of nodularity may require up to 6 months of uninterrupted therapy. Therefore, if any nodule persists or enlarges during treatment, carcinoma should be considered and ruled out.

Attempts should be made to determine the lowest clinically effective dose. In view of the fact that some cases of endometriosis may be resistant to one specific form of hormone therapy and responsive to another, danazol may prove to be of benefit in such cases. There are some limited data in support of the use of danazol in therapy-resistant cases of this type.

Cyclomen should be stopped if any clinically significant adverse event arises, and particularly if there is evidence of: virilization. Patients should be watched closely for signs of virilization. Some of these, in rare cases (such as deepening of voice, clitoral hypertrophy and more than minimal hirsutism), may not be reversible. In these cases, cessation of therapy should be considered in order to prevent further progression due to the risk of irreversible androgenic effects; papilledema, headache, visual disturbances or other signs or symptoms of raised intracranial pressure; jaundice or other indication of significant hepatic disturbance; thrombosis or thromboembolism.

It should be stressed to the patient that danazol treatment involves considerable alterations of hormone levels which may be evidenced by such side effects as the occurrence of acne, weight gain, irregular menstrual patterns or amenorrhea, signs of virilization and that recurrence of the initial symptoms may occur following cessation of therapy.

Experience with danazol greater than 6 months is limited. While a course of therapy may need to be repeated, care should be observed, as no safety data are available in relation to repeated courses of treatment over time. Therapy with other steroids alkylated at the 17 position has been associated with serious toxicity (cholestatic jaundice, peliosis hepatis, benign hepatic adenoma, malignant hepatic tumors). The physician therefore should be alerted to the possibility that similar toxicity may develop during therapy with danazol, especially when administration is continued beyond recommended time periods. Peliosis hepatitis and hepatic adenoma may be silent until complicated by acute potentially life-threatening intra-abdominal hemorrhage.

Data, from two case-control epidemiological studies, were pooled to examine the relationship between endometriosis, endometriosis treatments and ovarian cancer. These preliminary results suggest that the use of danazol might increase the baseline risk of ovarian cancer in endometriosis-treated patients.

Extremely rare cases of serious adverse events and death have been reported in individual patients who were taking danazol; however, a causal relation to the administration of danazol has neither been confirmed nor refuted. These included one case of acute leukemia, one fatal case of primary liver carcinoma, and a few cases of peliosis, hepatomas and the association of danazol with several cases of benign hepatic adenoma, malignant hepatic tumors, benign intracranial hypertension (pseudotumor cerebri), thromboembolism, thrombotic and thrombophlebitic events, including sagittal sinus thrombosis and life-threatening or fatal strokes.

PRECAUTIONS: In view of its pharmacology, known interactions and side effects, particular care should be observed in using danazol in those with hepatic or renal disease; hypertension or other cardiovascular disease; any state which may be exacerbated by fluid retention; diabetes mellitus; polycythemia; epilepsy; lipoprotein disorder; a history of thrombosis or thromboembolic disease; a history of marked or persistent androgenic reaction to previous gonadal steroid therapy; migraine (see below for further precautions on several of these conditions).

The treatment course should be limited to three to six months maximum.

Danazol may cause erratic results in thyroid function tests. Patients who are taking danazol have shown the uncommon combination of low or low-normal serum thyroxine, much reduced thyroxine binding globulin and normal free thyroxine index. In men and women a dose of 600 mg danazol daily for 15 days has been shown to have no significant effect on basal levels of TSH or on its response to thyrotropin-releasing hormone.

The finding of normal thyroid-stimulating hormone levels and free thyroxine index during danazol therapy indicates that patients are euthyroid. It is believed that the abnormality of thyroid function tests is due to an androgen-like reduction in thyroxine-binding globulin rather than a true decrease in thyroid function or interference with the pituitary-thyroid axis.

Changes in plasma levels of several other proteins have been observed during danazol administration. Pre-albumin, C_1-esterase inhibitor, haptoglobins, transferrin, antithrombin III, prothrombin and plasminogen were all shown to increase following administration of danazol. The concentrations of T_4-binding globulin, pregnancy zone protein and sex hormone-binding globulin decreased to one-third or less on administration of danazol. Uptake of T_3 was increased. The plasma estradiol content fell correspondingly. The clinical significance of these changes has not yet been determined.

A temporary alteration of lipoproteins in the form of decreased high density lipoproteins and possibly increased low density lipoproteins has been reported in some patients during danazol therapy. Prescribers should consider the possible risk of atherosclerosis and coronary artery disease versus the benefit of therapy.

Since hepatic and hematologic dysfunction has been reported in patients treated with danazol, periodic liver function tests and hematological tests should be performed (see Adverse Effects).

For repeated courses of treatment, biannual hepatic ultrasonography is recommended.

Fatal cases of fulminant hepatitis have been reported in 3 patients while on danazol therapy. One of these patients was shown to have an infection with hepatitis B virus while the symptoms and clinical course of the other 2 patients were consistent with non A-non B hepatitis.

If faced with continuing abnormalities of biochemical tests and/or their corresponding clinical manifestations, the possible risks should be carefully weighed against the potential benefits and discontinuation of danazol treatment should be considered.

It may be prudent to continue non-hormonal contraception after danazol treatment for fibrocystic breast disease until a menstrual period that is normal in amount of flow and duration has occurred.

Drug Interactions: Danazol may potentiate the effects of coumarin-type anticoagulants. In cases where such drugs are given concurrently with danazol, careful attention to and, if necessary, readjustment of their dosages is recommended.

Danazol can increase the plasma level of carbamazepine and may affect responsiveness to this agent and to phenytoin. A similar interaction with phenobarbital is likely.

Plasma concentrations of cyclosporine and tacrolimus, administered concurrently with danazol may be higher than expected, leading to an increase of the renal toxicity of these drugs. Elevated plasma glucagon levels have been reported in a few patients receiving danazol; diabetic patients on insulin or oral hypoglycemic agents may need to have the dosage of those agents increased appropriately in order to maintain euglycemia as danazol can cause insulin resistance.

Danazol can diminish the effectiveness of antihypertensive agents and likely interact with gonadal steroid therapy.

Danazol can increase the calcemic response to alpha calcidol in primary hypoparathyroidism.

Alteration in values for laboratory tests may occur during danazol therapy, including CPK, glucose tolerance, glucagon, thyroid-binding globulin, sex hormone binding globulin, other plasma proteins, lipid and lipoproteins and urinary 17-ketosteroids.

Statins: The risk of myopathy and rhabdomyolysis is increased by concomitant administration of danazol with statins metabolized by CYP3A4 such as simvastatin, atorvastatin and lovastatin.

Pregnancy: See Contraindications and Warnings.

Lactation: See Contraindications and Warnings.

Children: Safety and effectiveness in children have not been established.

Occupational Hazards: Ability to Drive and Use Machines: Danazol is unlikely to affect the ability to drive or use machines.

ADVERSE EFFECTS: Any of the following adverse effects can occur in patients receiving danazol: acne, edema (facial), mild hirsutism, decrease in breast size, deepening of the voice, oiliness of the skin or hair, weight gain, seborrhea, and rarely, clitoral hypertrophy.

Also hypoestrogenic manifestations such as flushing, sweating, vaginitis including itching, dryness, burning and vaginal bleeding, nervousness and emotional lability have been reported.

Hepatic dysfunction, as evidenced by reversible elevated serum enzymes has been reported. Cholestatic jaundice has been reported rarely. It is recommended that patients receiving danazol be monitored for hepatic dysfunction by laboratory tests and clinical observation (see Precautions). Rare occurrences of benign hepatic adenomata, malignant hepatic tumor and peliosis hepatis have also been observed with long-term use (>6 months). Rare cases of pancreatitis have been reported.

Although the following reactions have also been reported, a causal relationship to the administration of danazol has neither been confirmed nor refuted:

Allergic: urticaria, pruritus, rarely nasal congestion.

Skin and Mucous Membranes: rashes (maculopapular, vesicular, papular, purpuric, petechial), acne, hyperpigmentation, hair loss, inflammatory erythematous nodules, altered skin pigmentation, exfoliative dermatitis, erythema multiforme, Stevens-Johnson syndrome and rarely sun sensitivity.

Gastrointestinal: nausea, vomiting, constipation, gastroenteritis and rarely pancreatitis.

Genitourinary: hematuria, prolonged post-therapy amenorrhea, disturbance of the menstrual cycle, intermenstrual spotting and/or prolonged anovulation.

Musculoskeletal: muscle cramps or spasms sometimes with elevation of creatine phosphokinase levels, muscle or joint pain, joint lock-up, joint swelling, pain in back, neck or extremities, fasciculation, limb pain and rarely carpal tunnel syndrome.

Cardiovascular: exacerbation of hypertension, palpitation, tachycardia; thrombotic events have also been observed, including sagittal sinus and cerebrovascular thrombosis as well as arterial thrombosis; cases of myocardial infarction have been reported.

CNS: headache, nervousness and emotional lability, dizziness and fainting, vertigo, depression, fatigue, paresthesias, chills, visual disturbances including visual hallucination followed by seizure, papilledema, retrobulbar neuritis, and rarely benign intracranial hypertension (pseudotumor cerebri), anxiety, sleep disorders, tremor, weakness, changes in appetite (including increased appetite), aggravation of epilepsy, provocation of migraine and Guillain-Barré syndrome.

Ophthalmic: visual disturbances such as blurring of vision, difficulty in focusing, difficulty in wearing contact lenses and need for temporary alteration in refractive correction.

Hematologic: an increase in red cell and platelet count, thrombocytopenia, leukopenia and rarely eosinophilia, splenic peliosis, leukocytosis or polycythemia, thrombophlebitis.

Other: hyperglucagonemia, increased insulin requirements in diabetic patients, decreased HDL cholesterol affecting all subfractions, increased LDL cholesterol levels with variable changes in total cholesterol, decrease in apolipoproteins A1 and A11 (the clinical significance of these changes is not established), induction of aminolevulinic acid (ALA) synthetase, changes in libido, elevation in blood pressure, and rarely nipple discharge, cataracts, bleeding gums, fever, pelvic pain, epigastric and pleuritic pain, interstitial pneumonitis. Also, very rarely, reduction of spermatogenesis.

OVERDOSE:

Treatment: Available evidence suggests that acute overdosage would be unlikely to give rise to immediate serious reaction. Nonetheless, consideration should be given to removal of the drug by emesis or stomach pump, or to reduce the absorption of the drug by activated charcoal, and the patient should be kept under observation in case of any delayed reactions.

> For management of a suspected drug overdose, contact your **regional Poison Control Centre**. See the *CPS* Directory section for a list of Poison Control Centres.

DOSAGE: Danazol is for oral administration only.

Danazol should be given as a continuous course, dosage being adjusted according to the severity of the condition and the patient's response. A reduction in dosage once a satisfactory response has been achieved may prove possible.

Therapy should begin during menstruation. Otherwise, appropriate tests should be performed to ensure that the patient is not pregnant while on danazol therapy. An effective non-hormonal method of contraception should be used during the complete course of treatment. Regular menstrual patterns, irregular menstrual patterns and amenorrhea each occur in approximately one-third of patients treated with 100 mg danazol. Irregular menstrual patterns and amenorrhea are observed more frequently with higher doses.

The treatment course should be limited to three to six months maximum.

Endometriosis: Clinical effectiveness has been achieved with total daily doses of danazol ranging from 200 to 800 mg in 2 to 4 divided doses and administered without interruption for 3 to 6 months.

If at the lower doses, an anovulatory and amenorrheic state is not achieved and if the symptomatology is not relieved in 30 to 60 days, the dose should be increased. In patients with severe presenting symptomatology, the usual starting dose is 800 mg daily. The maximum recommended daily dose is 800 mg. It is essential that therapy continue uninterrupted for 3 to 6 months. Shorter courses of therapy have been used as adjuncts to surgery. After termination of therapy, if symptoms recur, treatment can be reinstated.

Fibrocystic Breast Disease: The total daily dose of danazol ranges from 100 to 400 mg in two divided doses, depending on patient response. Pain and tenderness usually respond to treatment after 30 to 40 days. Nodularity usually does not begin to regress until 60 to 90 days after initiation of therapy. Treatment should continue uninterrupted until complete disappearance of symptoms or for 6 months, whichever occurs first. Clinical studies have demonstrated that approximately 50% of patients may show evidence of recurrence of symptoms within 1 year. In this event, treatment may be reinstated.

INFORMATION FOR THE PATIENT: Published in e-CPS, available by subscription at www.e-cps.ca.

SUPPLIED: 50 mg: Each hard pink gelatin capsule, with "D50" on the cap and on the body contains: danazol 50 mg. Nonmedicinal ingredients: gelatin, lactose monohydrate, magnesium stearate, maize starch, red iron oxide, talc and titanium dioxide. Energy:<8 kJ (2 kcal). Bisulfite-, gluten-, sucrose- and tartrazine-free. Blisters of 100.

100 mg: Each hard bicolor (grey cap/white body) gelatin capsule, with "D100" on the cap and on the body contains: danazol 100 mg. Nonmedicinal ingredients: black iron oxide, gelatin, lactose monohydrate, magnesium stearate, maize starch, talc and titanium dioxide. Energy:<8 kJ (2 kcal). Bisulfite-, gluten-, sucrose- and tartrazine-free. Blisters of 100.

200 mg: Each hard white gelatin capsule, with "D200" on the cap and on the body contains: danazol 200 mg. Nonmedicinal ingredients: gelatin, lactose monohydrate, magnesium stearate, maize starch, talc and titanium dioxide. Energy:<8 kJ (2 kcal). Bisulfite-, gluten-, sucrose- and tartrazine-free. Blisters of 100.

(Shown in Product Identification Section)

Cyclopentolate ℞

Cycloplegic—Mydriatic—Anticholinergic

CPhA Monograph

Date of Revision: November 2006

> This monograph has been compiled by CPhA and reviewed by experts. It may contain information different from that found in Health Canada-approved Product Monographs. The reader is referred to the *CPS* Editorial Policy for more information.

PHARMACOLOGY: Cyclopentolate is an anticholinergic agent that induces relaxation of the sphincter of the iris and the ciliary muscles. When applied topically to the eyes, it causes a rapid, intense cycloplegic and mydriatic effect that is maximal in 15 to 60 minutes; recovery usually occurs within 24 hours. The cycloplegic and mydriatic effects are slower in onset and longer in duration in patients who have heavily pigmented irides.

INDICATIONS: Cyclopentolate is used mainly to produce mydriasis and cycloplegia for diagnostic purposes.

CONTRAINDICATIONS: Cyclopentolate is contraindicated in patients with angle-closure glaucoma or in patients with shallow anterior chambers (see Warnings).

Cyclopentolate should not be used in patients, especially children, who have previously experienced a severe systemic reaction to the drug, or in patients with hypersensitivity to any component of a cyclopentolate formulation.

WARNINGS: Cyclopentolate may cause increased intraocular pressure. Angle-closure glaucoma may be induced by cyclopentolate in patients with higher susceptibility to increased intraocular pressure including the elderly and individuals with shallow anterior chambers.

Very rarely, some patients with open-angle glaucoma may experience abrupt elevations in intraocular pressure.

The use of cyclopentolate in patients with higher susceptibility to increased intraocular pressure should be preceded by complete ocular examination, including measurement of intraocular pressure.

PRECAUTIONS: Cyclopentolate may cause an increase in intraocular pressure which if sustained, can potentially lead to irreversible loss of vision (see Warnings). The drug should be discontinued and the physician consulted immediately if eye pain, rapid pulse or dizziness occurs.

Patients may require the use of dark glasses following the application of cyclopentolate, due to photophobia associated with mydriasis.

Patients should be advised to avoid driving or performing hazardous tasks if blurred vision occurs, and to contact their physician if blurred vision and photophobia continue for more than 48 hours after discontinuing cyclopentolate.

Systemic absorption of topical cyclopentolate from the nasal mucosal surfaces may result in systemic adverse effects. This is particularly the case in children, who are most susceptible to the drug's adverse effects. If signs of systemic toxicity appear, such as dry mouth, tachycardia or dizziness, the dosage schedule should be reduced or the drug discontinued.

Children: Infants and young children and children with blond hair or blue eyes may be especially sensitive to the effects of cyclopentolate, increasing the chance of side effects during treatment. Use of cyclopentolate in children has been associated with psychotic reactions and behavioral disturbances.

Drug Interactions: Anticholinergic agents, such as cyclopentolate, antagonize miosis and ciliary body contraction induced by cholinesterase inhibitors and cholinergic agonists.

ADVERSE EFFECTS: Blinding acute angle-closure glaucoma and raised intraocular pressure may occur during cyclopentolate therapy. The mydriasis may be reduced by the intraocular application of pilocarpine.

Transient burning sensation of the eye is more likely with the 1% than the 0.5% solution.

Systemic effects, resulting from excessive absorption from mucosal surfaces or from ingestion of the drug, may include xerostomia, flushing, tachycardia and urinary retention. More severe systemic effects are tachypnea, scarlatiniform rash, delirium, psychosis, fever, stupor, coma, respiratory failure and death.

OVERDOSE:

Symptoms: Tachycardia, dizziness, dry mouth, behavioral disturbances, decreased coordination or drowsiness.

Treatment: In most cases of topical exposure, patients recover without specific therapy. If drops are accidentally ingested, more pronounced anticholinergic effects may occur. Treatment is supportive and symptomatic. A single dose of activated charcoal may be administered in cases of recent ingestion.

> For management of a suspected drug overdose, CPhA recommends that you contact your **regional Poison Control Centre**. See the *CPS* Directory section for a list of Poison Control Centres.

DOSAGE: To produce mydriasis and cycloplegia for diagnostic purposes, in adults and children over 1 year: 1 drop of 0.5% or 1% solution instilled in the eye(s), followed by a second drop 5 minutes later, if necessary. Drops should be administered 40 to 50 minutes prior to the procedure. To minimize systemic absorption, finger pressure should be applied to the lacrimal sac for 2 to 3 minutes following administration. Alternatively, the eyelids should be kept closed for 2 to 5 minutes following instillation.

Patients with heavily pigmented irides may require larger doses.

Complete recovery from mydriasis and cycloplegia should occur within 24 hours.

CyEstra-35 Pr

cyproterone acetate—ethinyl estradiol

Acne Treatment for Women

Pharmascience

SUPPLIED: Each yellow, film-coated, biconvex tablet, contains: cyproterone acetate 2 mg and ethinyl estradiol 0.035 mg. Nonmedicinal ingredients: cornstarch, D&C Yellow #10, hydroxypropyl methylcellulose, magnesium stearate, povidone, propylene glycol, talc and titanium dioxide. Blister packs of 21. Store at room temperature (15-30°C).

Cyklokapron® Pr

tranexamic acid

Antifibrinolytic

Pfizer

PHARMACOLOGY: Tranexamic acid produces an antifibrinolytic effect by competitively inhibiting the activation of plasminogen to plasmin. It is also a weak noncompetitive inhibitor of plasmin. These properties make possible its clinical use as an antifibrinolytic in the treatment of both general and local fibrinolytic hemorrhages. It has an action mechanism similar to, but about 10 times more potent in vitro than that of epsilon aminocaproic acid (EACA).

Absorption from the human gastrointestinal tract is not complete (40%).

Tranexamic acid binds considerably more strongly than EACA to both the strong and weak sites in the plasminogen molecule in a ratio corresponding to the difference in potency between the compounds. The pharmacological significance of the binding to these different sites has not yet been evaluated.

Tranexamic acid does not bind to serum albumin. The plasma protein binding seems to be fully accounted for by its binding to plasminogen and appears to be negligible at therapeutic plasma levels of 5 to 10 mg/L.

Possible routes of biotransformation are acetylation or deamination followed by oxidation or reduction. After oral administration approximately 50% of the parent compound, 2% of the deaminated dicarboxylic acid, and 0.5% of the acetylated product are excreted.

Tranexamic acid is eliminated by glomerular filtration, excretion being about 30% at 1 hour, 55% at 3 hours and 90% at 24 hours after i.v. administration of 10 mg/kg body weight. After oral administration of 10 to 15 mg/kg body weight excretion was 1% at 1 hour, 7% at 3 hours and 39% at 24 hours.

I.V. administration of 10 mg/kg body weight gave plasma concentrations of 18.3 µg, 9.6 µg and 5 µg/mL 1, 3 and 5 hours after the injection.

When administered 36 to 48 hours before surgery in 4 doses of 10 to 20 mg/kg body weight an antifibrinolytically active concentration (10 µg/mL) of tranexamic acid remained up to 17 hours in the tissues investigated, and up to 7 to 8 hours in the serum.

Tranexamic acid crosses the placenta. After an i.v. injection of 10 mg/kg the concentration can rise to about 30 µg/mL of fetal serum.

Tranexamic acid also passes over into the breast milk during lactation in concentrations 1/100 of the corresponding serum levels.

After both oral and i.v. administration tranexamic acid passes into the semen and inhibits its fibrinolytic activity, but without affecting the motility of the spermatozoa.

The ability of tranexamic acid to cross the blood-brain barrier has been demonstrated when administered to patients with ruptured intracranial aneurysms.

Tranexamic acid diffuses rapidly to the joint fluid and to the synovial membrane. In the joint fluid, the same concentration was obtained as in the serum. The biological half-life in the joint fluid was about 3 hours.

Three hours after a single oral dose of 25 mg/kg body weight the peak serum level was 15.4 g/L and the aqueous humour level was 1.6 g/L.

INDICATIONS: Hereditary angioneurotic edema. Increased local fibrinolysis when the diagnosis is indicative of hyperfibrinolysis, as with conization of the cervix, dental extraction in patients with coagulopathies (in conjunction with antihemophilic factor), epistaxis, hyphema, and menorrhagia (hypermenorrhea).

CONTRAINDICATIONS: Patients with a history or risk of thrombosis should not be given tranexamic acid, unless at the same time it is possible to give treatment with anticoagulants. The preparation should not be given to patients with acquired disturbances of color vision. If disturbances of color vision arise during the course of treatment the administration of the preparation should be discontinued.

Patients with active thromboembolic disease, such as deep vein thrombosis, pulmonary embolism and cerebral thrombosis.

Patients with subarachnoid haemorrhage: the limited clinical experience shows that a reduced risk for re-bleeding is offset by an increase in the rate of cerebral ischaemia.

Hypersensitivity to tranexamic acid or any of the ingredients.

WARNINGS: For patients who are to be treated for several weeks with tranexamic acid an ophthalmic checkup is advisable (sharpness of vision, color vision, fundus, field of vision, etc.). If possible, before treatment is initiated and regularly during treatments.

Patients with irregular menstrual bleeding should not use tranexamic acid until the cause of the irregularity has been established.

If menstrual bleeding is not adequately reduced by tranexamic acid, an alternative treatment should be considered.

Patients with a high risk for thrombosis (a previous thromboembolic event and a family history of thromboembolic disease) should use tranexamic acid only if there is a strong medical indication and under strict medical supervision.

Patients with disseminated intravascular coagulation (DIC), who require treatment with tranexamic acid, must be under the strict supervision of a physician experienced in treating this disorder.

Pregnancy: The safety of tranexamic acid during pregnancy has not yet been established. No harmful effects have been reported.

A woman with fibrinolytic bleeding in the fourth month of pregnancy was treated with tranexamic acid for a total of 64 days. The total dose was 256 g. The delivery occurred spontaneously in the 30th week of pregnancy and was normal in all other respects. The infant was healthy.

In a case of threatened placental abruption that was prevented by giving tranexamic acid, the patient had already lost 2 children in connection with placental abruption. In the 26th week of her third pregnancy bleeding occurred, indicating abruption. Pathological proteolysis with predominant activation of the fibrinolytic system was established. Between the 26th and 33rd week of pregnancy about 250 g of tranexamic acid were given, both i.v. and orally. The bleeding was arrested and a healthy child was delivered by Caesarean section.

Tranexamic acid crosses over to the fetus. After an i.v. injection of 10 mg/kg the concentration can reach a level of about 30 µg/mL fetal serum. Fibrinolytic activity is very high in neonates. It is not known for certain whether a reduction of this activity during the first hours of life is harmful. Kullander and Nilsson who have wide experience with tranexamic acid in connection with childbirth have observed no negative effect on the infants.

Tranexamic acid therapy is not indicated in hematuria caused by diseases of the renal parenchyma. Intravascular precipitation of fibrin frequently occurs in these conditions and may aggravate the disease. In addition, in cases of massive renal hemorrhage of any cause, antifibrinolytic therapy carries the risk of clot retention in the renal pelvis.

PRECAUTIONS: Care should be taken in cases of renal insufficiency due to the risk of accumulation, and where there is pronounced hematuria from the upper urinary tract, since in isolated cases obstacles to passage have been observed in the tract.

Lactation: Tranexamic acid is secreted in the mother's milk at a concentration only a hundredth of the corresponding serum levels. The investigators are of the opinion that tranexamic acid can be given during lactation without risk to the child.

Children: Clinical experience with tranexamic acid in menorrhagic children under 15 years of age is not available.

Drug Interactions: Clinically important interactions have not been observed with tranexamic acid tablets. Because of the absence of interaction studies, simultaneous treatment with anticoagulants must take place under the strict supervision of a physician experienced in this field.

ADVERSE EFFECTS: Gastrointestinal symptoms (nausea, vomiting, diarrhea) occur but disappear when the dose is reduced. Isolated cases of dizziness or reduced blood pressure have been reported. Allergic skin reactions have been reported less commonly.

To be observed by reason of experimental findings in animals: in the dog, retinal changes have been observed after long-term administration of large doses of tranexamic acid and in the cat, after i.v. injection of 250 mg/kg body weight/day for 14 days. Such changes have not been obtained in the rat, where the maximum tolerated dose has been administered. No retinal changes have been reported or observed at ophthalmic checkups of patients treated with tranexamic acid for several weeks or months.

Post-market Surveillance: Rare cases of adverse events have been reported with the use of tranexamic acid; thromboembolic events, impaired colour vision or other visual disturbances and dizziness. Hypotension may occur after fast injection.

OVERDOSE:

Symptoms: There is no known case of overdosage of tranexamic acid in humans. Symptoms may be nausea, diarrhoea, dizziness, headache, vomiting orthostatic symptoms and hypotension.

Treatment: Initiate vomiting, institution of gastric lavage, charcoal therapy, and symptomatic treatment. Maintain adequate diuresis.

It has been seen that 37 g of tranexamic acid caused mild intoxication in a 17-year-old after gastric lavage.

> For management of a suspected drug overdose, CPhA recommends that you contact your **regional Poison Control Centre**. See the *CPS* Directory section for a list of Poison Control Centres.

DOSAGE: Conization of the cervix: 2 to 3 tablets every 8 to 12 hours, 12 days postoperatively.

Epistaxis: 2 to 3 tablets every 8 to 12 hours for 10 days.

Hyphema: 2 to 3 tablets every 8 to 12 hours for 7 days.

Dental surgery in patients with coagulopathies: 2 hours before the operation, Factor VIII and Factor IX should be given as well as tranexamic acid, 25 mg orally or 10 mg i.v/kg body weight. After the operation, 25 mg/kg of tranexamic acid is given orally 3 to 4 times a day for 6 to 8 days. After the operation the patient does not generally require further substitution therapy.

Tranexamic acid solution for injection is administered intravenously by slow i.v. injection over a period of at least 5 minutes. For i.v. infusion, the tranexamic acid solution for injection may be mixed with electrolyte solutions, carbohydrate solutions, Aminosol and dextran solutions. Heparin may be added to tranexamic acid solution for injection. Tranexamic acid solution for injection should not be mixed with blood and infusion solutions containing penicillin.

Menorrhagia (hypermenorrhea): 2 to 3 tablets 3 to 4 times a day for several days. Tranexamic acid treatment should only be started when copious bleeding has begun.

Hereditary Angioneurotic Edema: Some patients can sense the onset of attacks and are best treated intermittently with 2 to 3 tablets 2 to 3 times a day for several days. Others should be treated continuously with this dose.

Children: Dosage should be calculated according to body weight at 25 mg/kg, 2 to 3 times a day.

Patients with Impaired Renal Function: In patients with serum creatine concentrations of 120 to 250 µmol/L, 15 mg orally or 10 mg i.v. tranexamic acid/kg body weight twice daily. At serum creatine levels of 250 to 500 µmol/L the dosage should be 15 mg orally or 10 mg i.v./kg body weight at 24 hourly intervals, and at serum creatine levels of 500 µmol/L or more, the same dose should be given at intervals of 48 hours between doses.

SUPPLIED: Injection: Each ampul contains: tranexamic acid BP 100 mg/mL. Ampuls of 5 and 10 mL. Packages of 10.
Tablets: Each white, film-coated, capsule-shaped tablet, with CY engraved in arcs, contains: tranexamic acid 500 mg. Tartrazine-free. Bottles of 100.

Store at room temperature between 15 and 30°C.

(Shown in Product Identification Section)

Cymbalta® Pr

duloxetine HCl

Antidepressant—Anxiolytic—Analgesic

Lilly

Date of Revision: January 15, 2010

SUMMARY PRODUCT INFORMATION:

Route of Administration	Dosage Form/Strength	All Nonmedicinal Ingredients
Oral	Delayed-release capsule/ 30 mg and 60 mg	FD&C Blue No. 2, gelatin, hydroxypropyl methylcellulose, hydroxypropyl methylcellulose acetate succinate, sodium lauryl sulfate, sucrose, sugar spheres, talc, titanium dioxide, triethyl citrate, yellow iron oxide (60 mg capsule only)

INDICATIONS AND CLINICAL USE: Adults: Major Depressive Disorder: CYMBALTA (duloxetine hydrochloride) is indicated for the symptomatic relief of major depressive disorder (MDD).

The efficacy of CYMBALTA in maintaining an antidepressant response for up to 6 months in patients who have shown initial treatment response following 12 weeks of open label acute treatment was demonstrated in a placebo-controlled trial.

The efficacy of CYMBALTA in hospitalized patients with MDD has not been studied.

Generalized Anxiety Disorder: CYMBALTA is indicated for the symptomatic relief of anxiety causing clinically significant distress in patients with generalized anxiety disorder (GAD).

The efficacy of CYMBALTA in maintaining anxiolytic response for up to 6 months in patients with GAD was demonstrated in a long-term placebo-controlled trial in patients who had initially responded to CYMBALTA during a 6-month open-label phase.

Neuropathic Pain Associated with Diabetic Peripheral Neuropathy: CYMBALTA is indicated for the management of neuropathic pain associated with diabetic peripheral neuropathy (DPN).

Fibromyalgia: CYMBALTA is indicated for the management of pain associated with fibromyalgia (FM).

Long-Term Use of CYMBALTA: The effectiveness of CYMBALTA in long-term use (i.e. more than 6 months in patients with MDD, and 12 weeks in patients with DPN or FM) has not been systematically evaluated in controlled clinical trials. The physician who elects to use CYMBALTA for extended periods in any indication should periodically re-evaluate the long-term usefulness of the drug for the individual patient.

Geriatrics (≥65 years of age): Pharmacokinetic results suggest no overall differences between these subjects and younger subjects. Other reported clinical experience has not identified differences in responses between the elderly and younger patients, but greater sensitivity of some older individuals cannot be ruled out (see Warnings and Precautions, Special Populations, Geriatrics (≥65 years of age) and Action and Clinical Pharmacology, Special Populations and Conditions).

Pediatrics (<18 years of age): The safety and efficacy of CYMBALTA in paediatric patients (<18 years of age) have not been established and its use in this patient population is not indicated. See Warnings and Precautions, General, Potential Association with Behavioural And Emotional Changes, Including Self-Harm; see also Dosage and Administration.

CONTRAINDICATIONS: Hypersensitivity: CYMBALTA (duloxetine hydrochloride) is contraindicated in patients with a known hypersensitivity to the drug or the other components of the product.

Monoamine Oxidase Inhibitors (MAOIs): CYMBALTA should not be used concomitantly with a monoamine oxidase inhibitor (MAOI), including linezolid, an antibiotic which is a non-selective reversible MAOI or within at least 14 days of discontinuing treatment with an MAOI. Based on the half-life of duloxetine, at least 5 days should be allowed after stopping CYMBALTA before starting an MAOI (see Warnings and Precautions, General, Monoamine Oxidase Inhibitors (MAOI)).

Hepatic Impairment: CYMBALTA is contraindicated in patients with any liver disease resulting in hepatic impairment (see Warnings and Precautions, General, Hepatic Impairment; and Dosage and Administration, Dosage for Patients with Hepatic Impairment).

Uncontrolled Narrow-Angle Glaucoma: In clinical trials, CYMBALTA was associated with an increased risk of mydriasis; therefore, its use should be avoided in patients with uncontrolled narrow-angle glaucoma (see Warnings and Precautions, General, Controlled Narrow-Angle Glaucoma).

Severe Renal Impairment: CYMBALTA is contraindicated in patients with severe renal impairment (i.e. creatinine clearance <30 mL/min) or end-stage renal disease (see Warnings and Precautions, Renal).

Thioridazine: Concomitant use of CYMBALTA and thioridazine is contraindicated (see Warnings and Precautions, General, Thioridazine).

CYP1A2 Inhibitors: CYMBALTA should not be used concomitantly with potent CYP1A2 inhibitors (e.g. fluvoxamine) and some quinolone antibiotics (e.g. ciprofloxacin, or enoxacine) (see Drug Interactions).

WARNINGS AND PRECAUTIONS: General: Potential Association with Behavioural And Emotional Changes, Including Self-Harm: Pediatrics: Placebo-Controlled Clinical Trial Data:

- **Recent analyses of placebo-controlled clinical trial safety databases from selective serotonin reuptake inhibitors (SSRIs) and other newer antidepressants suggest that use of these drugs in patients under the age of 18 may be associated with behavioural and emotional changes, including an increased risk of suicidal ideation and behaviour over that of placebo.**
- **The small denominators in the clinical trials database, as well as the variability in placebo rates, preclude reliable conclusions on the relative safety profiles among these drugs.**

Adults and Pediatrics: Additional Data:

- **There are clinical trial and post-marketing reports with SSRIs and other newer antidepressants, in both pediatrics and adults, of severe agitation-type adverse events coupled with self-harm or harm to others. The agitation-type events include: akathisia, agitation, disinhibition, emotional lability, hostility, aggression, and depersonalization. In some cases, the events occurred within several weeks of starting treatment.**

Rigorous clinical monitoring for suicidal ideation or other indicators of potential for suicidal behaviour is advised in patients of all ages. This includes monitoring for agitation-type emotional and behavioural changes.

Discontinuation Symptoms: Patients currently taking SSRIs or newer antidepressants should not be discontinued abruptly, due to risk of discontinuation symptoms. At the time that a medical decision is made to discontinue an SSRI or other newer antidepressant drug, a gradual reduction in the dose rather than an abrupt cessation is recommended (see Warnings and Precautions, Dependence, Discontinuation of Treatment; Adverse Reactions, Adverse Events Following Discontinuation of Treatment; and Dosage and Administration, Discontinuation of Treatment).

Monoamine Oxidase Inhibitors (MAOI): In patients receiving a serotonin reuptake inhibitor in combination with a MAOI, there have been reports of serious, sometimes fatal, reactions including hyperthermia, rigidity, myoclonus, autonomic instability with possible rapid fluctuations of vital signs, and mental status changes that include extreme agitation progressing to delirium and coma. These reactions have also been reported in patients who have recently discontinued serotonin reuptake inhibitors and are then started on a MAOI. Some cases presented with features resembling neuroleptic malignant syndrome. The effects of combined use of CYMBALTA (duloxetine hydrochloride) and MAOIs have not been evaluated in humans or animals. Therefore, because CYMBALTA is an inhibitor of both serotonin and norepinephrine reuptake, it is recommended that CYMBALTA not be used in combination with a MAOI (including linezolid, an antibiotic which is a non-selective reversible MAOI), or within at least 14 days of discontinuing treatment with a MAOI. Based on the half-life of duloxetine, at least 5 days should be allowed after stopping CYMBALTA before starting a MAOI (see Contraindications, Monoamine Oxidase Inhibitors (MAOIs); and Drug Interactions).

Hepatic Impairment: Patients with clinically evident hepatic impairment have decreased duloxetine metabolism and elimination. After a single non-therapeutic (20 mg) dose of CYMBALTA, 6 cirrhotic patients with moderate liver impairment (Child-Pugh Class B) had a mean plasma duloxetine clearance about 15% that of age- and gender-matched healthy subjects, with a 5-fold increase in mean exposure (AUC). Although C_{max} was similar to normals in the cirrhotic patients, the half-life was about 3 times longer. CYMBALTA is contraindicated in patients with any liver disease resulting in hepatic impairment (see Contraindications, Hepatic Impairment; Action and Clinical Pharmacology, Hepatic Insufficiency; and Dosage and Administration, Dosage for Patients with Hepatic Impairment).

Hepatotoxicity: CYMBALTA increases the risk of elevation of serum aminotransferase levels. In clinical trials, the median time to detection of the aminotransferase elevation was about two months. In these patients, these were usually transient and self-limiting with continued use, or resolved upon discontinuation of CYMBALTA. Liver aminotransferase elevations resulted in the discontinuation of 0.3% (73/23 983) of CYMBALTA-treated patients.

In placebo-controlled trials in MDD, elevations of alanine aminotransferase (ALT) to >3 times the upper limit of normal occurred in 0.4% (8/1902) of CYMBALTA-treated patients and in 0.2% (2/1200) of placebo-treated patients. In placebo-controlled trials in DPN, elevations of ALT to >3 times the upper limit of normal occurred in 2% (13/662) of CYMBALTA-treated patients and in 0% (0/281) of placebo-treated patients.

In the full cohort of placebo-controlled trials in any indication, elevation of ALT >3 times the upper limit of normal occurred in 1.1% (75/6871) of CYMBALTA-treated patients compared with 0.3% (13/5036) of placebo-treated patients. In placebo-controlled studies using a fixed-dose design, there was evidence of a dose-response relationship for ALT and AST elevation of >3 times the upper limit of normal and >5 times the upper limit of normal.

Postmarketing reports have described cases of hepatitis with abdominal pain, hepatomegaly and elevation of transaminase levels to more than twenty times the upper limit of normal with or without jaundice, reflecting a mixed or hepatocellular pattern of liver injury. Cases of cholestatic jaundice with minimal elevation of transaminase levels have also been reported (see Adverse Reactions, Post-Market Adverse Drug Reactions, Hepatic).

The combination of aminotransferase elevations and elevated bilirubin, without evidence of cholestasis, is generally recognized as an important predictor of severe liver injury. In clinical trials, 7 CYMBALTA patients had elevations of aminotransferase and bilirubin, but 5 of 7 also had elevation of alkaline phosphatase, suggesting an obstructive process; in 3 of these 7 patients, there was evidence of heavy alcohol use and this may have contributed to the abnormalities seen. Two placebo-treated patients also had aminotransferase elevations with elevated bilirubin.

Post-marketing reports indicate that elevated aminotransferase, bilirubin, and alkaline phosphatase have occurred in patients with chronic liver disease or cirrhosis. Severe elevations of liver enzymes (>10 times the upper limit of normal) or liver injury with a cholestatic or mixed pattern have been rarely reported, in some cases associated with excessive alcohol use or pre-existing liver disease. Because it is possible that duloxetine and alcohol may interact to cause liver injury or that duloxetine may aggravate pre-existing liver disease, CYMBALTA should ordinarily not be prescribed to patients with substantial alcohol use (see Special Populations, Use In Patients with Substantial Alcohol Use). CYMBALTA should not be used in patients with any liver disease resulting in hepatic impairment (see Contraindications, Hepatic Impairment). CYMBALTA should be used with caution in patients treated with other drugs associated with hepatic injury (see Adverse Reactions, Post-Market Adverse Drug Reactions, Hepatic).

Physicians should be aware of the signs and symptoms of liver damage (e.g. pruritus, dark urine, jaundice, right upper quadrant tenderness, or unexplained "flu-like" symptoms) and should investigate such symptoms promptly. CYMBALTA should be discontinued and should not be restarted in patients with jaundice.

Controlled Narrow-Angle Glaucoma: In clinical trials, CYMBALTA was associated with an increased risk of mydriasis; therefore it should be used cautiously in patients with controlled narrow-angle glaucoma (see Contraindications, Uncontrolled Narrow-Angle Glaucoma).

Thioridazine: Thioridazine administration alone produces prolongation of the QTc interval, which is associated with serious ventricular arrhythmias, such as torsades de pointes-type arrhythmias, and sudden death. This effect appears to be dose-related.

An in vivo study suggests that drugs which inhibit P4502D6, including certain SSRIs such as paroxetine, fluoxetine, and fluvoxamine, will elevate plasma levels of thioridazine. Therefore, as CYMBALTA is a moderate inhibitor of CYP2D6 and increases the AUC and C_{max} of drugs metabolized by CYP2D6, CYMBALTA should not be used in combination with thioridazine. See Contraindications and Drug Interactions.

Inhibitors of CYP1A2: Because CYP1A2 is involved in duloxetine metabolism, the potential exists for increased concentrations of duloxetine when co-administered with a CYP1A2 inhibitor. Fluvoxamine (100 mg QD), a potent inhibitor of CYP1A2, decreased the apparent plasma clearance of duloxetine by about 77%. CYMBALTA should not be used concomitantly with potent CYP1A2 inhibitors (e.g. fluvoxamine) and some quinolone antibiotics (e.g. ciprofloxacin, or enoxacine). See Contraindications and Drug Interactions.

Sucrose: CYMBALTA capsules contain sucrose. Patients with rare hereditary problems of fructose intolerance, glucose-galactose malabsorption or sucrose-isomaltase insufficiency should not take this medicine.

Cardiovascular: Blood Pressure and Heart Rate: CYMBALTA has been associated with an increase in blood pressure and clinically significant hypertension in some patients. This may be due to the noradrenergic effect of duloxetine.

In clinical trials across indications, relative to placebo, CYMBALTA treatment was associated with a mean increase of approximately 1 mm Hg in both systolic and diastolic blood pressure. There was no significant difference in the frequency of sustained (3 consecutive visits) elevated blood pressure (see Adverse Reactions, Vital Sign Changes).

There was no significant difference between treatment groups in the rate of discontinuation due to elevated blood pressure.

CYMBALTA treatment, for up to 26 weeks in placebo-controlled trials typically caused a small mean increase in heart rate compared to placebo of up to 3-4 beats per minute.

Cases of hypertensive crisis have been reported very rarely with CYMBALTA, especially in patients with pre-existing hypertension. CYMBALTA should be used with caution in patients with uncontrolled hypertension as it may expose them to hypertensive crisis (see Adverse Reactions, Post-Market Adverse Drug Reactions).

Blood pressure and heart rate should be evaluated prior to initiating treatment and periodically measured throughout treatment, especially in patients with known hypertension and/or other cardiac disease. CYMBALTA should be used with caution in patients whose conditions could be compromised by an increased heart rate or by an increase in blood pressure. Caution should also be exercised when CYMBALTA is used with drugs that may impair its metabolism (see Drug Interactions). For patients who experience a sustained increase in blood pressure while receiving CYMBALTA either dose reduction or gradual discontinuation should be considered.

Electrocardiogram Changes: CYMBALTA has not been systematically evaluated in patients with a recent history of myocardial infarction or unstable heart disease. Patients with these diagnoses were generally excluded from clinical studies during the product's pre-marketing testing. However, electrocardiograms of 321 patients who received CYMBALTA in MDD placebo-controlled clinical trials and 728 patients who received CYMBALTA in DPN placebo-controlled clinical trials were evaluated; CYMBALTA was not associated with the development of clinically significant ECG abnormalities (see Adverse Reactions, Electrocardiogram Changes). Additionally a clinical pharmacology study was conducted to assess the safety of duloxetine at the highest tolerable level of exposure of duloxetine (200 mg BID) and to measure QT interval. QT interval at doses up to 200 mg BID was not prolonged (see Action and Clinical Pharmacology, Clinical Safety Pharmacology).

In MDD and DPN placebo-controlled clinical trials, CYMBALTA-treated patients did not develop abnormal ECGs at a rate different from that in placebo-treated patients (see Adverse Reactions, Electrocardiogram Changes).

Concomitant Illness: Clinical experience with CYMBALTA in patients with concomitant systemic illnesses is limited. Caution is advisable when using CYMBALTA in patients with diseases or conditions that produce altered metabolism or hemodynamic responses. For example, caution should be exercised in using CYMBALTA in patients with conditions that slow gastric emptying (e.g., some patients with diabetic gastroparesis) (see Drug Interactions, Potential for Interaction with Drugs that Affect Gastric Acidity).

Dependence/Tolerance: Dependence Liability: In animal studies, duloxetine did not demonstrate stimulant or barbiturate-like (depressant) abuse potential. Duloxetine did produce reductions in activity in rodents and monkeys. In drug dependence studies, duloxetine did not demonstrate any dependence-producing potential in monkeys or rats.

While CYMBALTA has not been systematically studied in humans for its potential for abuse, there was no indication of drug-seeking behaviour in the clinical trials. However, it is not possible to predict on the basis of pre-marketing experience the extent to which a CNS active drug will be misused, diverted, and/or abused once marketed. Consequently, physicians should carefully evaluate patients for a history of drug abuse and follow such patients closely, observing them for signs of misuse or abuse of CYMBALTA (e.g. development of tolerance, incrementation of dose, drug-seeking behaviour).

Discontinuation of Treatment: Discontinuation symptoms have been systematically evaluated in patients taking CYMBALTA. Following abrupt or tapered discontinuation in placebo-controlled clinical trials, the following symptoms occurred at a rate greater than or equal to 1% and at a significantly higher rate in CYMBALTA-treated patients compared with those discontinuing from placebo: dizziness, nausea, headache, paresthesia, vomiting, irritability, nightmare, fatigue, insomnia, diarrhoea, anxiety, hyperhidrosis, and vertigo.

Patients should be monitored for these symptoms when discontinuing treatment with CYMBALTA. A gradual reduction in the dose rather than abrupt cessation is recommended whenever possible. If intolerable symptoms occur following a decrease in the dose or upon discontinuation of treatment, dose titration should be managed on the basis of the patient's clinical response (see Adverse Reactions, Adverse Events Following Discontinuation of Treatment; and Dosage and Administration, Discontinuation of Treatment).

Endocrine and Metabolism: Glucose Regulation: In DPN trials, CYMBALTA treatment worsened glycemic control in some diabetic patients. In three clinical trials of CYMBALTA for the management of pain associated with DPN, the mean duration of diabetes was approximately 12 years, the mean baseline fasting blood glucose was 9.8 mmol/L (176 mg/dL), and the mean baseline hemoglobin A1c (HbA_{1c}) was 7.8%. In the 12-week acute treatment phase of these studies, CYMBALTA was associated with a small increase in mean fasting blood glucose as compared to placebo. In the extension phase of these studies, which lasted up to 52 weeks, mean fasting blood glucose increased by 0.67 mmol/L (12 mg/dL) in the CYMBALTA group and decreased by 0.64 mmol/L (11.5 mg/dL) in the routine care group, which was statistically significantly different. HbA_{1c} increased by 0.5% in the CYMBALTA group and by 0.2% in the routine care groups.

Hematologic: Abnormal Bleeding: There have been reports of bleeding abnormalities with selective serotonin reuptake inhibitors (SSRIs) and serotonin/norepinephrine reuptake inhibitors (SNRIs), including very rare cases of ecchymoses and gastrointestinal bleeding reported with CYMBALTA (see Adverse Reactions, Post-Market Adverse Drug Reactions). While a causal relationship to CYMBALTA has not been established, impaired platelet aggregation may result from platelet serotonin depletion and contribute to such occurrences. Skin and other mucous membrane bleedings have been reported following treatment with CYMBALTA. Thus, caution is advised in patients taking anticoagulants (e.g. warfarin) and/or medicinal products known to affect platelet function (e.g. nonsteroidal anti-inflammatories and ASA), and in patients with known tendency for bleeding or those with predisposing conditions.

Hyponatremia: Hyponatremia may occur as a result of treatment with SSRIs and SNRIs, including CYMBALTA. In many cases, this hyponatremia appears to be the result of the syndrome of inappropriate antidiuretic hormone secretion (SIADH). Cases with serum sodium lower than 110 mmol/L have been reported and appeared to be reversible when CYMBALTA was discontinued. Elderly patients may be at greater risk of developing hyponatremia with SSRIs and SNRIs. Also, patients taking diuretics or who are otherwise volume depleted may be at greater risk. Discontinuation of CYMBALTA should be considered in patients with symptomatic hyponatremia and appropriate medical intervention should be instituted.

Signs and symptoms of hyponatremia include headache, difficulty concentrating, memory impairment, confusion, weakness, and unsteadiness, which may lead to falls. More severe and/or acute cases have been associated with hallucination, syncope, seizure, coma, respiratory arrest, and death (see Adverse Reactions, Post-Market Adverse Drug Reactions).

Neurologic: Seizures: Although anticonvulsant effects of duloxetine have been observed in animal studies, CYMBALTA has not been systematically evaluated in patients with a seizure disorder. These patients were excluded from clinical studies during the product's premarketing testing. In placebo-controlled clinical trials across all indications, seizures/convulsions occurred in 0.03% (3/9445) of patients treated with duloxetine and 0.01% (1/6770) of patients treated with placebo. As with other CNS active drugs, CYMBALTA should be used with caution in patients with a history of a seizure disorder.

Serotonin Syndrome/Neuroleptic Malignant Syndrome: On rare occasions serotonin syndrome or neuroleptic malignant syndrome-like events have occurred in association with treatment with SSRIs, particularly when given in combination with other serotonergic and/or neuroleptic drugs. Serotonin syndrome symptoms may include mental status changes (e.g., confusion, irritability, extreme agitation progressing to delirium and coma), autonomic instability with rapid fluctuations of vital signs (e.g., tachycardia, labile blood pressure, hyperthermia), neuromuscular aberrations (e.g., rigidity, myoclonus, hyperreflexia, incoordination) and/or gastrointestinal symptoms (e.g., nausea, vomiting, diarrhea). As these syndromes may result in potentially life-threatening conditions, treatment with CYMBALTA should be discontinued if such events occur and supportive symptomatic treatment should be initiated. CYMBALTA should not be used in combination with MAOIs (including linezolid, an antibiotic which is a non-selective reversible MAOI) or serotonin-precursors (such as L-tryptophan, oxitriptan) and should be used with caution in combination with other serotonergic drugs (triptans, certain tricyclic antidepressants, lithium, tramadol, St. John's Wort) due to the risk of serotonergic syndrome (see Contraindications and Drug Interactions).

Triptans ($5HT_1$ Agonists): Cases of life-threatening serotonin syndrome have been reported during combined use of selective serotonin reuptake inhibitors (SSRIs)/serotonin norepinephrine reuptake inhibitors (SNRIs) and triptans. If concomitant treatment with CYMBALTA and a triptan is clinically warranted, careful observation of the patient is advised, particularly during treatment initiation and dose increases. See Warnings and Precautions, Serotonin Syndrome/Neuroleptic Malignant Syndrome, and Drug Interactions, Triptans ($5HT_1$ Agonists).

Effects on the Ability to Drive and Use Machines: Any psychoactive drug may impair judgment, thinking, or motor skills. CYMBALTA may be associated with undesirable effects such as sedation and dizziness. Therefore, patients should be cautioned about operating hazardous machinery, including automobiles, until they are reasonably certain that CYMBALTA therapy does not affect their ability to engage in such activities.

Psychiatric: Suicide: The possibility of a suicide attempt is inherent in MDD and other psychiatric disorders and may persist until significant remission occurs.

As with other drugs with similar pharmacological action (inhibitor of serotonin reuptake [SSRI] or inhibitor of serotonin and norepinephrine reuptake [SNRI]), isolated cases of suicidal ideation and suicidal behaviours have been reported during CYMBALTA therapy or early after treatment discontinuation.

Close supervision of high-risk patients should accompany initial drug therapy. Prescriptions should be written for the smallest quantity consistent with good patient management, in order to reduce the risk of overdose (see Warnings and Precautions, General, Potential Association with Behavioural And Emotional Changes, Including Self-Harm; Adverse Reactions, Adverse Events Following Discontinuation of Treatment; and Dosage and Administration, Discontinuation of Treatment).

Because of the well established comorbidity between depression and other psychiatric disorders, the same precautions observed when treating patients with depression should be observed when treating patients with other psychiatric disorders (see Warnings and Precautions, General, Potential Association with Behavioural And Emotional Changes, Including Self-Harm).

Physicians should encourage patients to report any distressing thoughts or feelings at any time.

Activation of Mania/Hypomania: In placebo-controlled trials in patients with MDD, activation of mania or hypomania was reported in 0.1% (2/2489) of CYMBALTA-treated patients and 0.1% (1/1625) of placebo-treated patients. No activation of mania or hypomania was reported in DPN, GAD or FM placebo-controlled trials. Activation of mania/hypomania has been reported in a small proportion of patients with mood disorders who were treated with other marketed drugs effective in the treatment of MDD. As with similar CNS active drugs, CYMBALTA should be used cautiously in patients with a history of mania.

A major depressive episode may be the initial presentation of bipolar disorder. Patients with bipolar disorder may be at an increased risk of experiencing manic episodes when treated with antidepressants alone. Therefore, the decision to initiate symptomatic treatment of depression should be made only after patients have been adequately assessed to determine if they are at risk for bipolar disorder.

Renal: Increased plasma concentrations of duloxetine occur in patients with end-stage renal disease (requiring dialysis). For this reason CYMBALTA is not recommended for patients with end-stage renal disease or severe renal impairment (see Action and Clinical Pharmacology, Renal Insufficiency; and Dosage and Administration, Dosage for Patients with Renal Impairment).

Sexual Function/Reproduction: Refer to Adverse Reactions, Sexual Function.

Special Populations: Pregnant Women: Safe use of CYMBALTA during pregnancy has not been established. Therefore, CYMBALTA should not be administered to pregnant women or those intending to become pregnant, unless, in the opinion of the treating physician, the expected benefits to the patient markedly outweigh the possible hazards to the fetus.

Nonteratogenic Effects: Post-marketing reports indicate that some neonates exposed to SSRIs or newer antidepressants late in the third trimester have developed complications requiring prolonged hospitalization, respiratory support, and tube feeding. Such complications can arise immediately upon delivery. Reported clinical findings have included respiratory distress, cyanosis, apnea, seizures, temperature instability, feeding difficulty, vomiting, hypoglycemia, hypotonia, hypertonia, hyperreflexia, tremor, jitteriness, irritability, and constant crying. These features are consistent with either a direct toxic effect of SSRIs and other newer antidepressants or, possibly, a drug discontinuation syndrome. It should be noted that, in some cases, the clinical picture is consistent with serotonin syndrome (see Contraindications, Monoamine Oxidase Inhibitors (MAOIs)). When treating a pregnant woman with CYMBALTA during the third trimester, the physician should carefully consider the potential risks and benefits of treatment (see Dosage and Administration, Treatment of Pregnant Women During the Third Trimester).

There are no adequate and well-controlled studies in pregnant women. In animal reproductive studies, duloxetine has been shown to have adverse effects on embryo/fetal and post-natal development. Because animal reproduction studies are not always predictive of human response, this drug should be used during pregnancy only if the potential benefit justifies the potential risk to the fetus.

Patients should be advised to notify their physician if they become pregnant or intend to become pregnant during therapy.

Labour and Delivery: The effect of duloxetine on labour and delivery in humans is unknown. However, because duloxetine and/or its metabolites cross the placenta in rats and because of the possibility that duloxetine and/or its metabolites may have adverse effects on the newborn, duloxetine should be used during labour and delivery only if the potential benefit justifies the potential risk to the fetus.

Nursing Women: Duloxetine is excreted into the milk of lactating women. The estimated daily infant dose on a mg/kg basis is approximately 0.14% of the maternal dose. Because the safety of duloxetine in infants is not known, nursing while on CYMBALTA is not recommended.

Patients should be advised to notify their physician if they are breast-feeding.

Pediatrics (<18 years of age): The safety and efficacy of CYMBALTA in paediatric patients (<18 years of age) have not been established and its use in this patient population is not indicated. See Warnings and Precautions, General, Potential Association with Behavioural And Emotional Changes, Including Self-Harm. See also Dosage and Administration, Dosage for Pediatric Patients; and Indications and Clinical Use, Pediatrics (<18 years of age).

Geriatrics (≥65 years of age): Of the 2418 CYMBALTA-treated patients in the MDD clinical studies 5.9% (143) were 65 years of age or over. Of the 1429 CYMBALTA-treated patients in the DPN studies, 31.9% (456) were 65 years of age or over. Of the 1226 CYMBALTA-treated patients in FM studies, 7.9% (97) were 65 years of age or over. No overall differences in safety or effectiveness were observed between these subjects and younger subjects, and other reported clinical experience has not identified differences in responses between the elderly and younger patients, but greater sensitivity of some older individuals cannot be ruled out.

Use In Patients with Substantial Alcohol Use: Use of CYMBALTA in patients who consume substantial amounts of alcohol may be associated with severe liver injury. Isolated cases of liver failure, including fatal cases, have been reported. CYMBALTA should only be used in exceptional circumstances and with extreme caution in these patients (see Warnings and Precautions, Hepatotoxicity, and Adverse Reactions, Post-Market Adverse Drug Reactions, Hepatic).

Monitoring and Laboratory Tests: No specific laboratory tests are recommended.

ADVERSE REACTIONS: Adverse Drug Reaction Overview: Major Depressive Disorder: CYMBALTA (duloxetine hydrochloride) has been evaluated for safety in 2418 patients diagnosed with MDD who participated in multiple-dose pre-marketing trials, representing 1099 patient-years of exposure. Among these 2418 CYMBALTA-treated patients, 1139 patients participated in eight 8- or 9-week, placebo-controlled trials at doses ranging from 40 to 120 mg/day, while the remaining 1279 patients were followed for up to 1-year in an open-label safety study using flexible doses between 80 and 120 mg/day. Two placebo-controlled studies with doses of 80 and 120 mg/day had 6-month maintenance extensions. Of these 2418 patients, 993 CYMBALTA-treated patients were exposed for at least 180 days and 445 CYMBALTA-treated patients were exposed for at least 1 year. Adverse reactions were assessed by collecting adverse events, results of physical examinations, vital signs, weights, laboratory analyses, and ECGs.

Generalized Anxiety Disorder: CYMBALTA has also been evaluated for safety in 1797 patients with GAD. Most patients in the acute placebo-controlled studies received CYMBALTA 60 mg QD or 120 mg QD as their final dose.

Neuropathic Pain Associated with DPN: CYMBALTA has also been evaluated for safety in 1429 patients with neuropathic pain associated with DPN representing 894.13 patient-years of exposure. Among these 1429 CYMBALTA-treated patients, 800 patients participated in three 12- to 13-week, placebo-controlled trials at doses ranging from 20 to 120 mg/day. An additional 449 patients were enrolled in an open-label safety study using 120 mg/day for a duration of 6 months (87 patients continued on to an open-label extension phase for an additional 24 weeks). Another 57 patients, originally treated with placebo, were exposed to CYMBALTA for up to 12 months at 60 mg twice daily in an extension phase. Among these 1429 patients, 881 had ≥6 months of exposure to CYMBALTA, and 515 had greater than 12 months of exposure.

Fibromyalgia: CYMBALTA has also been evaluated for safety in 1236 patients with fibromyalgia. In placebo-controlled trials, 369 patients received CYMBALTA 60 mg QD (120.08 patient-years), 221 patients received CYMBALTA 120 mg QD (102.18 patient-years), and 220 patients received CYMBALTA 60 mg BID (36.49 patient-years) as a maximum dose.

Clinical Trial Adverse Drug Reactions: The data in the following tables and text cannot be used to predict the incidence of side effects in the course of usual medical practice where patient characteristics and other factors differ from those that prevailed in the clinical trials. Similarly, the cited frequencies cannot be compared with data obtained from other clinical investigations involving different treatments, uses, or investigators. The cited data provide the prescribing physician with some basis for estimating the relative contribution of drug and non-drug factors to the adverse event incidence in the population studied.

Adverse Events Reported as Reasons for Discontinuation of Treatment: Placebo-Controlled MDD Trials: Approximately 10% of the 1139 patients who received CYMBALTA in acute placebo-controlled trials discontinued treatment due to an adverse event, compared with 4% of the 777 patients receiving placebo. Nausea (CYMBALTA 1.4%, placebo 0.1%) was the only common adverse event reported as reason for discontinuation and considered to be drug-related (i.e., discontinuation occurring in at least 1% of the CYMBALTA-treated patients and at a rate of at least twice that of placebo).

Placebo-Controlled GAD Trials: Approximately 14% of the 910 patients who received CYMBALTA in acute placebo-controlled trials for GAD discontinued treatment due to an adverse event, compared with 5.3% of the 665 patients receiving placebo. Nausea (CYMBALTA 3.3%, placebo 0.5%) and dizziness (CYMBALTA 1.0%, placebo 0.5%) were the common adverse events reported as reasons for discontinuation and considered to be drug-related (as defined under MDD Trials, above).

Placebo-Controlled Trials for Neuropathic Pain Associated with DPN: Approximately 12% of the 800 patients who received CYMBALTA in acute placebo-controlled trials discontinued treatment due to an adverse event, compared with 5% of the 339 patients receiving placebo. Nausea (CYMBALTA 3.0%, placebo 0.3%), dizziness (CYMBALTA 1.1%, placebo 0.3%), and somnolence (CYMBALTA 1.2%, placebo 0%) were the common adverse events reported as reasons for discontinuation and considered to be drug-related (as defined under MDD Trials, above).

Placebo-Controlled FM Trials: Approximately 19% of the 876 patients who received CYMBALTA in placebo-controlled trials for FM discontinued treatment due to an adverse event, compared with 11.8% of the 535 patients receiving placebo. Nausea (CYMBALTA 1.9%, placebo 0.7%), fatigue (CYMBALTA 1.3%, placebo 0.2%) and somnolence (CYMBALTA 1.5%, placebo 0%) were the common adverse events reported as reasons for discontinuation and considered to be drug-related (as defined under MDD Trials, above).

Adverse Events Following Discontinuation of Treatment: Discontinuation symptoms have been systematically evaluated in patients taking CYMBALTA. Following abrupt or tapered discontinuation in placebo-controlled clinical trials, the following symptoms occurred at a rate greater than or equal to 1% and at a significantly higher rate in CYMBALTA-treated patients compared with those discontinuing from placebo: dizziness, nausea, headache, paresthesia, vomiting, irritability, nightmare, fatigue, insomnia, diarrhea, anxiety, hyperhidrosis, and vertigo. Although these events are generally self-limiting, some have been reported to be severe. (See Warnings and Precautions, Discontinuation of Treatment and Dosage and Administration.)

Adverse Events Occurring Among CYMBALTA-Treated Patients in Placebo-Controlled Major Depressive Disorder (MDD) Trials: Table 1 lists the incidence of treatment-emergent adverse events that occurred in 2% or more of patients treated with CYMBALTA in the acute phase of MDD placebo-controlled trials and with an incidence greater than placebo. The most commonly observed adverse events in CYMBALTA-treated MDD patients (incidence 5% or greater and at least twice the incidence in placebo patients) were: nausea, dry mouth, constipation, decreased appetite, fatigue, somnolence, and increased sweating. MedDRA terminology has been used to classify reported adverse events.

Table 1: CYMBALTA

Treatment-Emergent Adverse Events Incidence in the Acute Phase of MDD Placebo-Controlled Trials[a]

System Organ Class/Adverse Event	Percentage of Patients Reporting Event	
	Placebo (N=777)	CYMBALTA (N=1139)
Gastrointestinal Disorders		
Nausea	7	20
Dry mouth	6	15
Constipation	4	11
Diarrhea	6	8
Vomiting	3	5
Metabolism and Nutrition Disorders		
Appetite decreased[b]	2	8
General Disorders		
Fatigue	4	8
Investigations		
Weight decreased	1	2
Nervous System Disorders		
Dizziness	5	9
Somnolence	3	7
Tremor	1	3
Skin and Subcutaneous Tissue Disorders		
Sweating increased	2	6
Vascular Disorders		
Hot flushes	1	2
Eye Disorders		
Vision blurred	1	4
Psychiatric Disorders		
Anxiety	2	3
Insomnia[c]	6	11
Libido decreased	1	3
Anorgasmia	1	3
Reproductive System		
Erectile dysfunction[d,e]	1	4
Ejaculation delayed[d]	1	3
Ejaculation dysfunction[d,e]	1	3

[a] Events reported by at least 2% of patients treated with CYMBALTA and more often than with placebo. The following events were reported by at least 2% of patients treated with CYMBALTA for MDD and had an incidence equal to or less than placebo: upper abdominal pain, palpitations, dyspepsia, back pain, arthralgia, headache, pharyngitis, cough, nasopharyngitis, and upper respiratory tract infection.
[b] Term includes anorexia.
[c] Term includes middle insomnia.
[d] Male patients only.
[e] Term includes ejaculation disorder and ejaculation failure.

Adverse events seen in men and women were generally similar except for effects on sexual function (see Adverse Reactions, Sexual Function). Clinical studies of CYMBALTA did not suggest a difference in adverse event rates in people over or under 65 years of age. There were too few non-Caucasian patients studied to determine if these patients responded differently from Caucasian patients.

Adverse Events Occurring Among CYMBALTA-Treated Patients in Placebo-Controlled Generalized Anxiety Disorder (GAD) Trials: Table 2 lists the incidence of treatment-emergent adverse events that occurred in ≥2% of patients treated with CYMBALTA in the GAD acute placebo-controlled trials and with an incidence greater than placebo. The most commonly observed adverse events in CYMBALTA-treated GAD patients (incidence 5% or greater and at least twice the incidence in placebo patients) included nausea, dizziness, dry mouth, fatigue, constipation, somnolence and increased sweating.

Dose Dependency of Adverse Events in GAD: Adverse events that occurred in the duloxetine 120 mg/day group at an incidence rate that was 5% or greater, and approximately twice that of the duloxetine 60 mg/day group included the following: increased sweating (15.3% vs. 8.3%), diarrhea (7.6% vs. 3.0%), and vomiting (6.5% vs. 3.0%).

Adverse Events Occurring Among CYMBALTA-Treated Patients in Placebo-Controlled Trials of Pain Associated with Diabetic Peripheral Neuropathy (DPN): Table 3 lists the incidence of treatment-emergent adverse events that occurred in 2% or more of patients treated with CYMBALTA in the acute phase (12-week) of DPN placebo-controlled trials (doses of 20 to 120 mg/day) and with an incidence greater than placebo. The most commonly observed adverse events in CYMBALTA-treated DPN patients (incidence of 5% or greater and at least twice the incidence in placebo patients) were: nausea, constipation, dry mouth, vomiting, fatigue, decreased appetite, somnolence, erectile dysfunction, and hyperhidrosis. MedDRA terminology has been used to classify reported adverse events.

Table 2: CYMBALTA

Treatment-Emergent Adverse Events Incidence in the Acute Phase of GAD Placebo-Controlled Trials[a]

	Percentage of Patients Reporting Event	
System Organ Class/Adverse Event	**Placebo (N=665)**	**CYMBALTA (N=910)**
Gastrointestinal Disorders		
Nausea	10	34
Dry mouth	4	12
Constipation	4	10
Diarrhea	6	8
Vomiting	3	5
Metabolism and Nutrition Disorders		
Appetite decreased[b]	1	4
General Disorders		
Fatigue	4	11
Investigations		
Weight decreased	1	4
Nervous System Disorders		
Dizziness	8	14
Somnolence	2	8
Tremor	1	4
Skin and Subcutaneous Tissue Disorders		
Sweating increased	2	7
Vascular Disorders		
Hot flushes	1	2
Eye Disorders		
Vision blurred	1	4
Psychiatric Disorders		
Anxiety	1	2
Insomnia[c]	4	8
Libido decreased	1	5
Respiratory, Thoracic and Mediastinal Disorder		
Yawning	0	3
Reproductive System		
Erectile dysfunction[d,e]	0	2

[a] Events reported by at least 2% of patients treated with CYMBALTA and more often than with placebo.
[b] Term includes anorexia.
[c] Term includes middle insomnia.
[d] Male patients only.
[e] Term includes ejaculation disorder and ejaculation failure.

Table 3: CYMBALTA

Treatment-Emergent Adverse Events Incidence in the Acute Phase of Neuropathic Pain Associated with DPN Placebo-Controlled Trials[b]

	Percentage of Patients Reporting Event			
System Organ Class/Adverse Event	**CYMBALTA 60 QD N=344**	**CYMBALTA 60 BID N=341**	**CYMBALTA Total[a] N=800**	**Placebo N=339**
Gastrointestinal Disorders				
Nausea	24	27	24	9
Diarrhea	11	7	10	7
Constipation	8	12	9	2
Dry mouth	6	10	8	3
Vomiting	5	6	6	3
Dyspepsia[c]	4	4	4	2
General Disorders and Administration Site Conditions				
Fatigue[d]	12	16	12	6
Abdominal pain[e]	5	2	4	2
Infections and Infestations				
Nasopharyngitis	5	7	6	5
Influenza[f]	3	2	3	3
Metabolism and Nutrition Disorders				
Decreased appetite[g]	7	14	10	1
Musculoskeletal and Connective Tissue Disorders				
Back pain	5	2	4	3
Muscle spasm	3	3	3	2
Nervous System Disorders				
Somnolence[h]	17	21	17	5
Headache	12	11	12	9
Dizziness	11	13	11	6
Paraesthesia[h]	2	2	2	1
Psychiatric Disorders				
Insomnia[j]	8	10	9	5
Agitation[k]	3	3	3	1
Renal and Urinary Disorders				
Pollakiuria	1	3	2	1
Reproductive System and Breast Disorder				
Erectile dysfunction[l]	2	8	5	0
Respiratory, Thoracic and Mediastinal Disorders				
Cough[m]	3	4	4	4
Pharyngolaryngeal pain	1	4	3	2
Skin and Subcutaneous Tissue Disorders				
Sweating increased	8	10	9	2

(cont'd)

[a] Includes all doses used in DPN studies (i.e. 20 mg QD, 60 mg QD and 60 mg BID).
[b] Events reported by at least 2% of patients treated with CYMBALTA and more often than placebo. The following events were reported by at least 2% of patients treated with CYMBALTA for DPNP and had an incidence equal to or less than placebo: pain in extremity, upper respiratory tract infection, arthralgia, cough, influenza, pruritus, musculoskeletal pain (includes myalgia and neck pain), and edema peripheral.
[c] Includes stomach discomfort.
[d] Also includes asthenia.
[e] Includes abdominal pain upper, abdominal pain lower, abdominal tenderness, abdominal discomfort, and gastrointestinal pain.
[f] 2.8% of patients treated with CYMBALTA; 2.7% of patients who received placebo.
[g] Includes anorexia.
[h] Includes hypersomnia, sedation.
[i] Includes hypoesthesia, hypoesthesia facial, and paresthesia oral.
[j] Also includes middle insomnia, early morning awakening, and initial insomnia.
[k] Also includes feeling jittery, nervousness, restlessness, tension, and psychomotor agitation.
[l] Male patients only. (CYMBALTA 60 mg QD, N=201; CYMBALTA 60 mg BID, N=190; all CYMBALTA, N=466; placebo, N=181).
[m] 3.9% of patients treated with CYMBALTA; 3.8% of patients who received placebo.

Adverse Events Occurring Among CYMBALTA-Treated Patients in Placebo-Controlled Fibromyalgia (FM) Trials: Table 4 lists the incidence of treatment-emergent adverse events (TEAEs) that occurred in ≥2% of patients treated with CYMBALTA in the fibromyalgia (FM) placebo-controlled trials and with an incidence greater than placebo. The following TEAEs had an incidence in the CYMBALTA treatment group ≥5.0% and were significantly more frequent with CYMBALTA than with placebo: nausea, headache, dry mouth, insomnia, fatigue, constipation, diarrhoea, dizziness, somnolence, hyperhidrosis, and decreased appetite.

Dose Dependency of Adverse Events in Fibromyalgia: In one fibromyalgia study the most common adverse events that occurred in the duloxetine 120 mg QD group at an incidence rate that was 5% or greater, and approximately twice that of the duloxetine 60 mg/day group included the following: constipation (21.1% vs. 10.0%; p=.01) and somnolence (15.0% vs. 7.3%, p=.043).

In another fibromyalgia study somnolence was the most common adverse event that occurred in the duloxetine 60 mg BID group at an incidence rate that was 5% or greater, and approximately twice that of the duloxetine 60 mg QD group (12.1% vs. 5.1%, p=.064).

Other Adverse Events: Urinary Hesitation: CYMBALTA is in a class of drugs known to affect urethral resistance during the filling stage of the bladder. In placebo-controlled clinical trials in patients with MDD and DPN, urinary hesitation on voiding was reported in <1% of female patients and approximately 1% of male patients. If symptoms of urinary hesitation develop during treatment with CYMBALTA, consideration should be given to the possibility that they might be drug-related.

Laboratory Changes: CYMBALTA treatment in placebo-controlled clinical trials across indications was associated with small mean increases from baseline to endpoint in ALT, AST, CPK, and alkaline phosphatase; infrequent, transient, abnormal values were observed for these analytes in CYMBALTA-treated patients, compared with placebo-treated patients (see Warnings and Precautions, Hepatotoxicity).

Table 4: CYMBALTA

Treatment-Emergent Adverse Events Incidence in the FM Placebo-Controlled Trials[a]

System Organ Class/Adverse Reaction	Percentage of Patients Reporting Reaction	
	Placebo (N=535)	CYMBALTA (N=876)
Cardiac Disorders		
Palpitations	2	2
Eye Disorders		
Vision blurred	1	2
Gastrointestinal Disorders		
Nausea	11	29
Dry mouth	5	18
Constipation	4	15
Diarrhea	8	12
Dyspepsia	3	5
General Disorders and Administration Site Conditions		
Fatigue[c]	8	15
Immune System Disorders		
Seasonal allergy	2	3
Infections and Infestations		
Upper respiratory tract infection	6	7
Urinary tract infection	3	3
Influenza	2	2
Gastroenteritis viral	2	2
Investigations		
Weight increased	1	2
Metabolism and Nutrition Disorders		
Decreased appetite[d]	2	11
Musculoskeletal and Connective Tissue Disorders		
Musculoskeletal pain	4	5
Muscle spasms	3	4
Nervous System Disorders		
Headache	12	20
Dizziness	7	11
Somnolence[e]	3	11
Tremor	1	4
Paraesthesia	4	4
Migraine	3	3
Dysgeusia	1	3
Psychiatric Disorders		
Insomnia[f]	10	16
Agitation[g]	2	6
Sleep disorder	2	3
Abnormal dreams[h]	1	3
Orgasm abnormal[i]	<1	3
Libido decreased[j]	<1	2
Reproductive System and Breast Disorders		
Ejaculation disorder[b,k]	0	4
Penis disorder[b]	0	2

(cont'd)

Table 4: CYMBALTA *(cont'd)*

Treatment-Emergent Adverse Events Incidence in the FM Placebo-Controlled Trials[a]

System Organ Class/Adverse Reaction	Percentage of Patients Reporting Reaction	
	Placebo (N=535)	CYMBALTA (N=876)
Respiratory, Thoracic, and Mediastinal Disorders		
Cough	3	4
Pharyngolaryngeal pain	3	3
Skin and Subcutaneous Tissue Disorders		
Hyperhidrosis	1	7
Rash	2	4
Pruritus	2	3
Vascular Disorders		
Hot flush	2	3

a Events reported by at least 2% of patients treated with CYMBALTA and more often than with placebo. The following events were reported by at least 2% of patients treated with CYMBALTA for FM and had an incidence equal to or less than placebo: nasopharyngitis, back pain, sinusitis, anxiety, arthralgia, depression, pain in extremity, vomiting, pain, abdominal pain, bronchitis, abdominal pain upper.
b Male patients only (N=46 duloxetine-treated patients versus 26 placebo patients).
c Also includes asthenia.
d Also includes anorexia.
e Also includes hypersomnia and sedation.
f Also includes middle insomnia, early morning awakening, and initial insomnia.
g Also includes feeling jittery, nervousness, restlessness, tension, and psychomotor agitation.
h Also includes nightmare.
i Also includes anorgasmia.
j Also includes loss of libido.
k Also includes ejaculation failure and ejaculation dysfunction.

Vital Sign Changes: In placebo-controlled clinical trials across all indications, CYMBALTA treatment was associated with mean increases of approximately 1 mm Hg in both systolic and diastolic blood pressure compared with placebo (see Warnings and Precautions, Cardiovascular)

CYMBALTA treatment, for up to 9 weeks in MDD placebo-controlled clinical trials of 40 to 120 mg daily doses in patients diagnosed with MDD was associated with increases in systolic blood pressure, averaging 2 mm Hg systolic and 0.5 mm Hg diastolic compared with placebo.

In placebo-controlled clinical trials in patients with DPN, mean changes in systolic blood pressure for CYMBALTA-treated patients were not statistically nor clinically significantly different from those who received placebo. However, a statistically significant difference was observed between CYMBALTA- and placebo-treated patients in diastolic blood pressure. Both the CYMBALTA and the placebo treatment groups had a decrease in diastolic blood pressure from baseline to endpoint, but the decrease in placebo group was 1.6 mm Hg greater.

In the FM placebo-controlled clinical trials, CYMBALTA-treated patients experienced a mean increase from baseline to endpoint in systolic (0.91 mm Hg, p=.003) and diastolic blood pressure (1.04 mm Hg, p<.001) compared with placebo-treated patients (−1.58 mm Hg and −1.17 mm Hg, respectively).

Sustained elevations of either systolic or diastolic blood pressure were also measured in placebo-controlled studies. A patient had a sustained elevation in systolic blood pressure if the value was ≥140 mm Hg with an increase ≥10 mm Hg from baseline for three consecutive visits. A patient had a sustained elevation in diastolic blood pressure if the value was ≥90 mm Hg with an increase of ≥10 mm Hg from baseline for three consecutive visits. A patient had sustained elevation in blood pressure if the criterion for sustained elevation in systolic blood pressure or diastolic blood pressure was met.

In MDD placebo-controlled trials, the incidence for sustained elevation in systolic or diastolic blood pressure was not significantly different between CYMBALTA-treated patients (1.3%, 14/1116) and placebo-treated patients (0.8%, 6/757).

In GAD placebo-controlled trials, the incidence for sustained elevation in systolic or diastolic blood pressure was not significantly different between CYMBALTA-treated patients (1.0%, 9/881) and placebo-treated patients (0.9%, 6/653).

In DPN placebo-controlled trials, the incidence for sustained elevation in systolic and diastolic blood pressure was not significantly different between CYMBALTA-treated patients (2.2% systolic BP and 0.9% diastolic BP) and placebo-treated patients (2.4% systolic BP and 1.2% diastolic BP).

When alternative criteria for blood pressure elevation were substituted (alternative criteria was a systolic blood pressure of 130 mm Hg or greater and an increase from baseline of ≥10 mm Hg; alternative diastolic blood pressure criteria was a diastolic blood pressure of ≥85 mm Hg and an increase from baseline of ≥10 mm Hg), the results remained essentially the same and without statistical significance.

In FM placebo-controlled trials, the incidence for sustained elevation in systolic and diastolic blood pressure was not significantly different between CYMBALTA-treated patients (1.3% systolic BP and 0.7% diastolic BP) and placebo-treated patients (1.1% systolic BP and 0.2% diastolic BP).

In both MDD and DPN placebo-controlled studies, there was no significant difference between treatment groups in the frequency of elevated blood pressure as a reason for discontinuation.

CYMBALTA treatment, for up to 26 weeks in placebo-controlled trials, typically caused a small increase in heart rate compared with placebo of up to 3-4 beats per minute.

Weight Changes: CYMBALTA had minimal effect on weight. In MDD and GAD placebo-controlled clinical trials, patients treated with CYMBALTA for up to 9 weeks experienced a mean weight loss of approximately 0.5 kg, compared with a mean weight gain of approximately 0.35 kg in placebo-treated patients. This represents a small but significant decrease in weight compared with placebo-treated patients. Long-term trials over 52 weeks in duration demonstrated a mean weight gain of 2.4 kg (5.3 lbs) but this was not clinically significant.

In 3 placebo-controlled DPN clinical trials, patients treated with CYMBALTA for up to 13 weeks experienced a mean weight loss of 0.92 kg, compared with a mean weight gain of 0.16 kg in placebo-treated patients. In long-term trials of up to 52 weeks in duration, the mean decrease in weight was 0.35 kg for CYMBALTA-treated patients.

In FM studies, patients treated with CYMBALTA for up to 26-weeks experienced a mean weight loss of approximately 0.4 kg compared with a mean weight gain of approximately 0.3 kg in placebo-treated patients. In one long-term FM 60-week uncontrolled study, (195 patients completed the study) CYMBALTA patients had a mean weight increase of 0.7 kg.

Electrocardiogram Changes: Electrocardiograms were obtained from CYMBALTA-treated patients and placebo-treated patients in clinical trials across all indications. No clinically significant differences were observed for QTc, QT, PR, and QRS intervals between CYMBALTA-treated and placebo-treated patients. There were no differences in clinically meaningful QTcF elevations between CYMBALTA and placebo.

Additionally a clinical pharmacology study was conducted to assess the safety of duloxetine at the highest tolerable level of exposure of duloxetine (200 mg BID) and to measure QT interval. QT interval at doses up to 200 mg BID was not prolonged (see Action and Clinical Pharmacology, Clinical Safety Pharmacology).

Glucose Regulation: In DPN trials, CYMBALTA treatment worsened glycemic control in some diabetic patients. In three clinical trials of CYMBALTA for the management of pain associated with DPN, the mean duration of diabetes was approximately 12 years, the mean baseline fasting blood glucose was 9.8 mmol/L (176 mg/dL), and the mean baseline hemoglobin A_{1c} (HbA_{1c}) was 7.8%. In the 12-week acute treatment phase of these studies, CYMBALTA was associated with a small increase in mean fasting blood glucose as compared to placebo. In the extension phase of these studies, which lasted up to 52 weeks, mean fasting blood glucose increased by 0.67 mmol/L (12 mg/dL) in the CYMBALTA group and decreased by 0.64 mmol/L (11.5 mg/dL) in the routine care group, which was statistically different. HbA1c increased by 0.5% in the CYMBALTA group and by 0.2% in the routine care groups.

Sexual Function: Although changes in sexual desire, sexual performance, and sexual satisfaction often occur as manifestations of a psychiatric disorder, they may also be a consequence of pharmacologic treatment. Reliable estimates of the incidence and severity of untoward experiences involving sexual desire, performance, and satisfaction are difficult to obtain, however, in part because patients and physicians may be reluctant to discuss them. Table 5 displays the incidence of sexual side effects spontaneously reported by at least 2% of either male or female patients taking CYMBALTA in MDD placebo-controlled trials.

Table 5: CYMBALTA

Treatment-Emergent Sexual Dysfunction-Related Adverse Events Incidence in MDD Placebo-Controlled Trials[a]

Adverse Event	Percentage of Patients Reporting Event			
	% Male Patients		% Female Patients	
	CYMBALTA (N=378)	Placebo (N=247)	CYMBALTA (N=761)	Placebo (N=530)
Orgasm abnormal[b]	4	1	2	0
Ejaculatory dysfunction[c]	3	1	NA	NA
Libido decreased	6	2	1	0
Erectile dysfunction	4	1	NA	NA
Ejaculation delayed	3	1	NA	NA

[a] Events reported by at least 2% of patients treated with CYMBALTA and more often than with placebo.
[b] Term includes anorgasmia.
[c] Term includes ejaculation disorder and ejaculation failure.
Legend: NA=not applicable.

Other Adverse Reactions Observed During the Premarketing and Postmarketing Clinical Trial Evaluation of Duloxetine: The following is a list of treatment-emergent adverse reactions reported by patients treated with duloxetine in clinical trials. In clinical trials across all indications, 27 229 patients were treated with duloxetine. Of these, 29% (7886) took duloxetine for at least 6 months, and 13.3% (3614) for at least one year. The following listing is not intended to include reactions (1) already listed in previous tables or elsewhere in labelling, (2) for which a drug cause was remote, (3) which were so general as to be uninformative, (4) which were not considered to have significant clinical implications, or (5) which occurred at a rate equal to or less than placebo. Reactions are categorized by body system according to the following definitions: common adverse reactions are those occurring in at least 1/100 patients; uncommon adverse reactions are those occurring in 1/100 to 1/1000 patients; rare reactions are those occurring in fewer than 1/1000 patients.
Cardiac Disorders: Common: palpitations. Uncommon: myocardial infarction, tachycardia.
Ear and Labyrinth Disorders: Common: vertigo. Uncommon: ear pain, tinnitus.
Endocrine Disorders: Rare: hypothyroidism.
Eye Disorders: Uncommon: diplopia, visual disturbance, mydriasis.
Gastrointestinal Disorders: Common: flatulence. Uncommon: eructation, gastritis, halitosis, stomatitis, gastroenteritis. Rare: gastric ulcer, melena.
General Disorders and Administration Site Conditions: Common: chills (includes rigors). Uncommon: feeling abnormal, feeling hot and/or cold, malaise, thirst. Rare: gait disturbance.
Infections and Infestations: Uncommon: laryngitis.
Investigations: Uncommon: weight increased, blood cholesterol increased.
Metabolism and Nutrition Disorders: Uncommon: dehydration, hyperlipidemia. Rare: dyslipidemia.
Musculoskeletal and Connective Tissue Disorders: Common: musculoskeletal pain. Uncommon: muscle tightness (includes musculoskeletal stiffness), muscle twitching.
Nervous System Disorders: Common: dysgeusia, lethargy, parasthesia/hypoesthesia. Uncommon: disturbance in attention, dyskinesia, myoclonus, poor quality sleep. Rare: dysarthria.
Psychiatric Disorders: Common: abnormal dreams (includes nightmares), sleep disorder. Uncommon: apathy, bruxism, disorientation (includes confusional state), irritability, mood swings, suicide attempt. Rare: completed suicide.
Renal and Urinary Disorders: Uncommon: dysuria, micturition urgency, nocturia, polyuria, urine flow decreased, urine odour abnormal.
Reproductive System and Breast Disorders: Common: anorgasmia/orgasm abnormal. Uncommon: menopausal symptoms, sexual dysfunction.
Respiratory, Thoracic and Mediastinal Disorders: Uncommon: throat tightness.
Skin and Subcutaneous Tissue Disorders: Uncommon: cold sweat, dermatitis contact, increased tendency to bruise, night sweats, photosensitivity reaction. Rare: ecchymosis.
Vascular Disorders: Common: flushing (includes hot flush). Uncommon: peripheral coldness, orthostatic hypotension.
Post-Market Adverse Drug Reactions: Hepatic: Post-marketing surveillance has identified reports of hepatic injury, including hepatocellular, pure cholestatic and mixed injury ranging from mild elevations in laboratory values to more severe clinical signs and symptoms of liver injury. Isolated cases of liver failure, including fatal cases, have been reported. Most of these cases have been reported in patients with past or current medical and other risk factors for liver injury, including alcohol abuse, hepatitis, or exposure to drugs with known adverse effects on the liver and it is unclear to what extent duloxetine may have played a contributing role (see Contraindications and Warnings and Precautions, Hepatotoxicity).
Hyponatremia: Hyponatremia may occur as a result of treatment with SSRIs and SNRIs, including CYMBALTA. In many cases, this hyponatremia appears to be the result of the syndrome of inappropriate antidiuretic hormone secretion (SIADH). Cases with serum sodium lower than 110 mmol/L have been reported and appeared to be reversible when CYMBALTA was discontinued. Elderly patients may be at greater risk of developing hyponatremia with SSRIs and SNRIs. Also, patients taking diuretics or who are otherwise volume depleted may be at greater risk. Discontinuation of CYMBALTA should be considered in patients with symptomatic hyponatremia and appropriate medical intervention should be instituted.

Signs and symptoms of hyponatremia include headache, difficulty concentrating, memory impairment, confusion, weakness, and unsteadiness, which may lead to falls. More severe and/or acute cases have been associated with hallucination, syncope, seizure, coma, respiratory arrest, and death (see Warnings and Precautions).

Since the first global approval of CYMBALTA on 03 August 2004 through 02 May 2009, it is estimated that over 21 million patients have been treated with CYMBALTA worldwide, accounting for over 7 million patient-years of therapy.

Table 6 is based on post-market spontaneous adverse event reports. The percentages shown are calculated by dividing the number of adverse events reported to the company by the estimated number of patients exposed to the drug during the same time period. A causal relationship between CYMBALTA and the emergence of these events has not been clearly established.

Table 6: CYMBALTA

Post-Market Spontaneous Adverse Event Reports for All Indications

Adverse Event	Frequency			
	Common ≥1%	Uncommon <1% and ≥0.1%	Rare <0.1% and ≥0.01%	Very Rare <0.01%
Blood Disorders				
Thrombocytopenia				X
Cardiac Disorders				
Supraventricular arrhythmia				X

(cont'd)

Table 6: CYMBALTA *(cont'd)*

Post-Market Spontaneous Adverse Event Reports for All Indications

Adverse Event	Frequency			
	Common ≥1%	Uncommon <1% and ≥0.1%	Rare <0.1% and ≥0.01%	Very Rare <0.01%
Ear and Labyrinth Disorders				
Tinnitus upon treatment discontinuation				X
Endocrine Disorders				
Syndrome of Inappropriate Antidiuretic Hormone (SIADH)				X
Eye Disorders				
Glaucoma				X
Gastrointestinal Disorders				
Gastrointestinal bleeding				X
Hematochezia			X	
Hepatobiliary Disorders				
Hepatitis				X
Jaundice				X
Immune System Disorders				
Anaphylactic reaction				X
Hypersensitivity				X
Investigations				
Alanine aminotransferase increased				X
Alkaline phosphatase increased				X
Aspartate aminotransferase increased				X
Bilirubin increased				X
Metabolism and Nutritional Disorders				
Hyponatremia				X
Hyperglycemia (reported especially in diabetic patients)				X
Musculoskeletal and Connective Tissue Disorders				
Muscle spasm				X
Trismus				X
Nervous System Disorders				
Extrapyramidal disorder				X
Restless leg syndrome				X
Serotonin syndrome				X
Seizures				X
Seizures upon treatment discontinuation				X
Psychiatric Disorders				
Hallucinations			X	
Mania				X
Aggression and anger (particularly early in treatment or after treatment discontinuation)				X
Renal and Urinary Disorders				
Urinary retention			X	
Reproductive System and Breast Disorders				
Gynecological bleeding				X
Skin and Subcutaneous Tissue Disorders				
Rash			X	
Angioneurotic edema				X
Contusion				X
Ecchymosis				X

(cont'd)

Table 6: CYMBALTA *(cont'd)*

Post-Market Spontaneous Adverse Event Reports for All Indications

Adverse Event	Frequency			
	Common ≥1%	Uncommon <1% and ≥0.1%	Rare <0.1% and ≥0.01%	Very Rare <0.01%
Erythema multiforme				X
Stevens-Johnson Syndrome				X
Urticaria				X
Vascular Disorders				
Orthostatic hypotension (especially at initiation of treatment)				X
Syncope (especially at initiation of treatment)				X
Hypertensive crisis				X

DRUG INTERACTIONS:

> **Serious Drug Interactions**
> **Monoamine Oxidase Inhibitors, Linezolid, Fluvoxamine, Ciprofloxacin, Enoxacine, Thioridazine: See Contraindications.**

Overview: Patients should be advised to inform their physicians if they are taking, or plan to take, any prescription or over-the-counter medications.

Drug-Drug Interactions: Potential for Other Drugs to Affect Duloxetine: Both CYP1A2 and CYP2D6 are responsible for duloxetine metabolism.

Inhibitors of CYP1A2: When duloxetine 60 mg was co-administered with fluvoxamine 100 mg, a potent CYP1A2 inhibitor, to male subjects (n=14) duloxetine AUC was increased by approximately 6-fold, the C_{max} was increased about 2.5-fold, and duloxetine $t_{½}$ was increased by approximately 3-fold. CYMBALTA (duloxetine hydrochloride) should not be used concomitantly with potent CYP1A2 inhibitors (e.g. fluvoxamine) and some quinolone antibiotics (e.g. ciprofloxacin, or enoxacine).

Inhibitors of CYP2D6: Because CYP2D6 is involved in duloxetine metabolism, concomitant use of duloxetine with potent inhibitors of CYP2D6 would be expected to, and does, result in higher concentrations (on average 60%) of duloxetine. Paroxetine (20 mg QD) increased duloxetine (40 mg QD) AUC and C_{max} by 60%. Caution is advised if administering duloxetine with inhibitors of CYP2D6 (e.g., SSRIs).

Dual Inhibition of CYP1A2 and CYP2D6: Concomitant administration of duloxetine 40 mg BID with fluvoxamine 100 mg, a potent CYP1A2 inhibitor, to CYP2D6 poor metabolizer subjects (n=14) resulted in a 6-fold increase in duloxetine AUC and C_{max}.

Potential for Duloxetine to Affect Other Drugs: Drugs Metabolized by CYP2D6: Duloxetine is a moderate inhibitor of CYP2D6. When duloxetine (60 mg BID) was co-administered with a single 50-mg dose of desipramine, a CYP2D6 substrate, the AUC of desipramine increased 3-fold. The co-administration of duloxetine (40 mg BID) increased steady-state AUC of tolterodine (2 mg BID) by 71% but did not affect the pharmacokinetics of the 5-hydroxyl metabolite. Therefore, caution should be used if duloxetine is co-administered with medications that are predominately metabolized by the CYP2D6 system and which have a narrow therapeutic index such as antiarrhythmics (e.g. flecainide and encainide) (see Drug Interactions, Tricyclic Antidepressants (TCA)).

Drugs Metabolized by CYP1A2: In vitro drug interaction studies demonstrate that duloxetine does not induce catalytic activity associated with the CYP1A2 isoform. Therefore, an increase in the metabolism of CYP1A2 substrates (e.g., theophylline and caffeine) resulting from induction is not anticipated, although clinical studies of induction have not been performed. Duloxetine has been shown to be a potential inhibitor of the CYP1A2 isoform in in vitro studies. However, in a clinical study, the pharmacokinetics of theophylline, a CYP1A2 substrate, were not significantly affected by co-administration with duloxetine (60 mg BID). These results suggest that duloxetine is unlikely to have a clinically significant effect on the metabolism of CYP1A2 substrates.

Drugs Metabolized by CYP2C9: Results of in vitro studies demonstrate that duloxetine does not inhibit the enzyme activity of CYP2C9. Therefore, inhibition in metabolism of CYP2C9 substrates is not anticipated, although clinical studies have not been performed.

Drugs Metabolized by CYP3A: Results of in vitro studies demonstrate that duloxetine does not inhibit or induce the catalytic activity of CYP3A. Therefore, an increase or decrease in the metabolism of CYP3A substrates (e.g., oral contraceptives and other steroidal agents) resulting from induction or inhibition is not anticipated, although clinical studies have not been performed.

Drugs Metabolized by CYP2C19: Results of in vitro studies demonstrate that duloxetine does not inhibit CYP2C19 activity at therapeutic concentrations. Inhibition of the metabolism of CYP2C19 substrates is therefore not anticipated, although clinical studies have not been performed.

CNS Drugs: Caution is advised when CYMBALTA is taken in combination with other centrally acting drugs and substances, especially those with a similar mechanism of action, including alcohol. Concomitant use of other drugs with serotonergic activity (e.g., SNRIs, SSRIs, triptans, or tramadol) may result in serotonin syndrome.

Drugs Highly Bound to Plasma Protein: Duloxetine is highly bound to plasma proteins (>90%). Therefore, administration of CYMBALTA to a patient taking another drug that is highly protein bound may cause increased free concentrations of either drug.

Electroconvulsive Therapy (ECT): There are no clinical studies of the combined use of electroconvulsive therapy and duloxetine.

Benzodiazepines: Lorazepam: Under steady-state conditions, duloxetine (60 mg Q 12 hours) had no effect on lorazepam (2 mg Q 12 hours) pharmacokinetics and lorazepam had no effect on duloxetine pharmacokinetics. The combination of duloxetine and lorazepam resulted in increased sedation compared with lorazepam alone.

Temazepam: Under steady-state conditions, duloxetine (60 mg qhs) had no effect on temazepam (2 mg qhs) kinetics and temazepam had no effect on duloxetine pharmacokinetics.

Monoamine Oxidase Inhibitors: See Contraindications, Monoamine Oxidase Inhibitors (MAOIs) and Warnings and Precautions, Monoamine Oxidase Inhibitors (MAOI).

Serotonergic Drugs: Based on the mechanism of action of duloxetine and the potential for serotonin syndrome, caution is advised when CYMBALTA is co-administered with other drugs or agents that may affect the serotonergic neurotransmitter systems, such as tryptophan, triptans, serotonin reuptake inhibitors, lithium, tramadol, or St. John's Wort (see Warnings and Precautions, Serotonin Syndrome/Neuroleptic Malignant Syndrome).

Triptans (5HT$_1$ Agonists): Cases of life-threatening serotonin syndrome have been reported during combined use of selective serotonin reuptake inhibitors (SSRIs)/serotonin norepinephrine reuptake inhibitors (SNRIs) and triptans. If concomitant treatment with CYMBALTA and a triptan is clinically warranted, careful observation of the patient is advised, particularly during treatment initiation and dose increases (see Warnings and Precautions, Serotonin Syndrome/Neuroleptic Malignant Syndrome).

Tricyclic Antidepressants (TCA): Caution is advised in the co-administration of tricyclic antidepressants (TCAs) (e.g. amitriptyline, desipramine, nortriptyline) with duloxetine, because duloxetine may inhibit TCA metabolism. Plasma TCA concentrations may need to be monitored and the dose of the TCA may need to be reduced if a TCA is co-administered with duloxetine (see Drug Interactions, Drugs Metabolized by CYP2D6).

Warfarin: Increases in INR have been reported when duloxetine was co-administered with warfarin.

Potential for Interaction with Drugs that Affect Gastric Acidity: CYMBALTA has an enteric coating that resists dissolution until reaching a segment of the gastrointestinal tract where the pH exceeds 5.5. In extremely acidic conditions, CYMBALTA, unprotected by the enteric coating, may undergo hydrolysis to form naphthol. Caution is advised in using CYMBALTA in patients with conditions that may slow gastric emptying (e.g. some patients with diabetic gastroparesis). Drugs that raise the gastrointestinal pH may lead to an earlier release of duloxetine. However, co-administration of CYMBALTA with aluminum- and magnesium-containing antacids (51 mEq) or CYMBALTA with famotidine, had no significant effect on the rate or extent of duloxetine absorption after administration of a 40-mg oral dose. It is unknown whether the concomitant administration of proton pump inhibitors affects duloxetine absorption.

Drug-Food Interactions: Food delays the time for duloxetine to reach peak concentration from 6 to 10 hours and it marginally decreases the extent of absorption (approximately 11%) (see Action and Clinical Pharmacology). However food does not affect the C_{max} of duloxetine. CYMBALTA may be taken with or without food.

Drug-Herb Interactions: In common with other SSRIs and SNRIs, pharmacodynamic interactions between duloxetine and the herbal remedy St. John's Wort may occur and may result in an increase in undesirable effects. Interactions with other herbal products have not been established.

Drug-Laboratory Test Interactions: Interactions with laboratory tests have not been established.

Drug-Lifestyle Interactions: Smoking: Duloxetine bioavailability appears to be about 34% lower in smokers than in nonsmokers, although dosage modifications are not routinely recommended.

Alcohol: Although duloxetine does not increase the impairment of mental and motor skills caused by alcohol, the concomitant use of duloxetine and substantial amounts of alcohol is not recommended.

In the CYMBALTA clinical trials database, three CYMBALTA-treated patients had liver injury as manifested by ALT and total bilirubin elevations, with evidence of cholestasis. Substantial inter-current ethanol use was present in each of these cases, and this may have contributed to the abnormalities seen (see Warnings and Precautions, Hepatotoxicity).

DOSAGE AND ADMINISTRATION: Dosing Considerations: CYMBALTA (duloxetine hydrochloride) is not indicated for use in children under 18 years of age (see Warnings and Precautions, General, Potential Association with Behavioural And Emotional Changes, Including Self-Harm).

CYMBALTA may be administered with or without food; however, **food may help reduce the incidence of initial nausea**. Results from a well-controlled dose comparison study (N=647) have demonstrated that patients taking CYMBALTA 60 mg/day with food experienced similar rates of nausea as patients treated with CYMBALTA 30 mg/day with or without food.

CYMBALTA should be swallowed whole and should not be chewed or crushed, nor should the contents be sprinkled on food or mixed with liquids. All of these might affect the enteric coating.

Recommended Dose and Dosage Adjustment: Adults: Major Depressive Disorder: The recommended dose is 60 mg once daily. A lower starting dose of 30 mg may be considered for tolerability reasons in some patients, with a target dose of 60 mg/day within 1-2 weeks. Therapeutic response is usually seen after 1-4 weeks of treatment. There was no evidence that doses greater than 60 mg/day conferred additional benefits.

Generalized Anxiety Disorder: The recommended starting dose is 60 mg once daily. A lower starting dose of 30 mg may be considered for tolerability reasons in some patients, with a target dose of 60 mg/day within 1-2 weeks. Therapeutic response is usually seen after 1-4 weeks of treatment. While a 120 mg once daily dose was shown to be effective, there is no evidence that doses greater than 60 mg/day confer additional benefit and the higher dose is less well tolerated. The safety of doses above 120 mg once daily has not been evaluated.

Neuropathic Pain Associated with Diabetic Peripheral Neuropathy: The recommended dose is 60 mg once daily. A lower starting dose of 30 mg may be considered for tolerability reasons in some patients, with a target dose of 60 mg/day within 1-2 weeks. Efficacy of CYMBALTA has been demonstrated within the first week.

Some patients may benefit from dosages above the recommended 60 mg once daily up to a maximum dose of 120 mg per day. While a 120 mg/day dose was shown to be safe and effective, there is no evidence that doses higher than 60 mg confer additional significant benefit, and the higher dose is less well tolerated (see Adverse Events, Table 3). Doses above 120 mg have not been evaluated and are not recommended.

Fibromyalgia: The recommended dose is 60 mg once daily. A lower starting dose of 30 mg may be considered for tolerability reasons in some patients, with a target dose of 60 mg/day within 1-2 weeks. Some patients may respond within the first week. There is no evidence that doses greater than 60 mg/day (e.g., 120 mg/day) confer additional benefit. Additionally, patients who do not respond to 60 mg/day may not respond to 120 mg/day. Furthermore, doses higher than 60 mg/day are associated with more severe and frequent rate of adverse reactions (see Adverse Reactions). The safety of doses above 120 mg once daily has not been evaluated.

Maintenance/Continuation/Extended Treatment: Major Depressive Disorder: It is generally agreed that acute episodes of major depression require several months or longer of sustained pharmacologic therapy beyond response to the acute episode. There is insufficient evidence available to answer the question of how long a patient should continue to be treated with CYMBALTA for MDD. Patients should be periodically reassessed to determine the need for maintenance treatment and the appropriate dose for such treatment.

Generalized Anxiety Disorder: During long-term therapy, the dosage should be maintained at the lowest effective level and patients should be periodically re-assessed to determine the need to continue treatment.

Fibromyalgia and Neuropathic Pain Associated with Diabetic Peripheral Neuropathy: The effectiveness of CYMBALTA in long-term use (i.e. more than 12 weeks in patients with DPN or FM) has not been systematically evaluated in controlled clinical trials. The physician who elects to use CYMBALTA for extended periods in the treatment of DPN or fibromyalgia should periodically re-evaluate the long-term usefulness of the drug for the individual patient.

General Considerations for Dosing in Special Populations: Dosage for Patients with Renal Impairment: CYMBALTA is not recommended for patients with end-stage renal disease (requiring dialysis) or in severe renal impairment (estimated creatinine clearance <30 mL/min) (see Contraindications, Severe Renal Impairment; Warnings and Precautions, Renal and Action and Clinical Pharmacology).

Dosage for Patients with Hepatic Impairment: CYMBALTA should not be used in patients with any liver disease resulting in hepatic impairment (see Contraindications, Warnings and Precautions and Action and Clinical Pharmacology).

Dosage for Elderly Patients: No dose adjustment is recommended for elderly patients on the basis of age. Caution should be exercised in treating the elderly. Pharmacokinetic results suggest no overall differences between these subjects and younger subjects. Other reported clinical experience has not identified differences in responses between the elderly and younger patients, but greater sensitivity of some older individuals cannot be ruled out. When individualizing the dosage, extra care should be taken when increasing the dose.

Dosage for Pediatric Patients: The safety and efficacy of CYMBALTA in paediatric patients (<18 years of age) have not been established and its use in this patient population is not indicated (see Warnings and Precautions, General, Potential Association with Behavioural And Emotional Changes, Including Self-Harm).

Treatment of Pregnant Women During the Third Trimester: Post-marketing reports indicate that some neonates exposed to SSRIs or other newer antidepressants late in the third trimester have developed complications requiring prolonged hospitalization, respiratory support, and tube feeding (see Warnings and Precautions, Special Populations, Pregnant Women). When treating pregnant women with CYMBALTA during the third trimester, the physician should carefully consider the potential risks and benefits of treatment. The physician may consider tapering CYMBALTA in the third trimester.

Discontinuation of Treatment: When discontinuing CYMBALTA after more than 1 week of therapy, it is recommended that the dose be tapered to minimize the risk of discontinuation symptoms (see Warnings And Precautions, General, Discontinuation Symptoms; Warnings and Precautions, Dependance, Discontinuation of Treatment; and Adverse Reactions, Adverse Events Following Discontinuation of Treatment). If intolerable symptoms occur following a decrease in the dose or upon discontinuation of treatment, then resuming the previously prescribed dose may be considered. Subsequently, the physician may continue decreasing the dose but at a more gradual rate.

Switching Patients to or from a Monoamine Oxidase Inhibitor: At least 14 days should elapse between discontinuation of an MAOI and initiation of therapy with CYMBALTA. In addition, at least 5 days should be allowed after stopping CYMBALTA before starting an MAOI (see Contraindications, Monoamine Oxidase Inhibitors (MAOIs) and Warnings and Precautions, General, Monoamine Oxidase Inhibitors (MAOI)).

OVERDOSAGE:

Human Experience: In clinical trials, cases of acute ingestions above 3000 mg, alone or in combination with other drugs, were reported, with none being fatal. However, in post marketing experience fatal outcomes have been reported for acute overdoses, primarily with mixed overdoses, but also with duloxetine only, at doses as low as approximately 1000 mg. Signs and symptoms of overdose (duloxetine alone or with mixed drugs) included somnolence, serotonin syndrome, seizures, vomiting, and tachycardia.

Animal Experience: In animal studies, the major signs of overdose toxicity related to the central nervous and gastrointestinal systems. These included central nervous system effects such as tremors, clonic convulsions, ataxia, emesis, and decreased appetite.

Management of Overdose: No specific antidote is known, but if serotonin syndrome ensues, specific treatment (such as with cyproheptadine and/or temperature control) may be considered. An airway should be established. Monitoring of cardiac and vital signs is recommended, along with appropriate symptomatic and supportive measures. Gastric lavage may be indicated if performed soon after ingestion or in symptomatic patients. Activated charcoal may be useful in limiting absorption. Duloxetine has a large volume of distribution and forced diuresis, hemoperfusion, and exchange perfusion are unlikely to be beneficial.

In managing overdose, consider the possibility of multiple drug involvement. A specific caution involves patients who are taking or have recently taken duloxetine and might ingest excessive quantities of a tricyclic antidepressant. In such a case, accumulation of the parent tricyclic and/or its active metabolite may increase the possibility of clinically significant sequelae and extend the time needed for close medical observation (see Drug Interactions).

> For management of a suspected drug overdose, CPhA recommends that you contact your regional Poison Control Centre. See the *CPS* Directory section for a list of Poison Control Centres.

ACTION AND CLINICAL PHARMACOLOGY: Mechanism of Action: CYMBALTA (duloxetine hydrochloride) is a serotonin and norepinephrine reuptake inhibitor, and weakly inhibits dopamine uptake with no significant affinity for histaminergic, dopaminergic, cholinergic, and adrenergic receptors. Duloxetine is also a potent in vitro inhibitor of transporter binding, with 5-HT and transporter NE inhibition constants (Ki) of 0.8 and 7.5 nM, respectively. Duloxetine dose-dependently increased extracellular levels of serotonin and norepinephrine in various brain areas of animals. It is chemically unrelated to other SNRIs, tricyclic, tetracyclic, or other available drugs effective in the treatment of MDD.

Pharmacodynamics: The effectiveness of duloxetine in the treatment of MDD is presumed to be linked to its inhibition of central nervous system (CNS) neuronal uptake of serotonin and norepinephrine, and a resultant increase in serotonin and norepinephrine neurotransmission. The pain inhibitory action of duloxetine is believed to be a result of potentiation of descending inhibitory pain pathways within the central nervous system. Studies at clinically relevant doses in humans (i.e., 40-60 mg BID) have shown that duloxetine decreases 5-hydroxytryptamine concentration in the blood and decreases the urinary excretion of norepinephrine and its metabolites, consistent with blockade of serotonin and norepinephrine uptake processes, respectively. Duloxetine undergoes extensive metabolism; however, the major circulating metabolites have not been shown to contribute significantly to the pharmacologic activity of duloxetine. Neurochemical and behavioural studies in laboratory animals showed an enhancement of both serotonin and norepinephrine neurotransmission in the CNS. Responses consistent with enhanced serotonergic and noradrenergic neurotransmission include lowered food intake, body weight, and alcohol intake. Duloxetine also normalized pain thresholds in several preclinical models of neuropathic [L5/L6 spinal nerve ligation model and partial sciatic nerve ligation model] and inflammatory pain [carrageenan model and acetic-acid induced writhing model] and attenuated pain behaviour in a model of persistent pain [formalin model, late phase] at doses that are consistent with in vivo blockade of 5HT and NE reuptake sites].

Duloxetine's affinity for dopamine uptake sites is low. Nevertheless, animal studies have shown increases in extracellular levels of dopamine in prefrontal cortex in addition to increases in norepinephrine and serotonin levels. This is presumed to be associated with the known propensity of cortical norepinephrine transporters to take up dopamine as well as norepinephrine, rather than an effect on dopamine transporters themselves.

Pharmacokinetics: Absorption: In humans, orally administered duloxetine hydrochloride is well absorbed, with maximal plasma concentrations (C_{max}) of duloxetine occurring 6 hours post dose. Food does not affect the C_{max} of duloxetine. However, food delays the time to reach peak concentration from 6 to 10 hours and it marginally decreases the extent of absorption (approximately 11%). Duloxetine plasma exposure increases in proportion to dose for doses up to 60 mg twice a day. Steady-state plasma concentrations are typically achieved after 3 days of dosing. Based upon AUC, multiple once daily doses of 60 mg produce steady-state concentrations that are approximately 1.5 times higher than that predicted from a 60 mg single dose. Average minimum and maximum steady-state concentrations for the 60 mg QD dose are 27.0 and 89.5 ng/mL, respectively. There is no clinically important difference in the pharmacokinetic parameters of morning and evening doses.

Distribution: The apparent volume of distribution ranges from 701 to 3800 L (5th to 95th percentile, mean of 1640 L). Duloxetine is highly bound (>90%) to proteins in human plasma, binding primarily to albumin and α1-acid glycoprotein. Plasma protein binding of duloxetine is not affected by renal or hepatic impairment.

Metabolism: Biotransformation and disposition of duloxetine in humans have been determined following oral administration of ^{14}C-labelled duloxetine. Integrated over time, duloxetine comprises about 3% of the total radiolabelled material in the plasma, indicating that it undergoes extensive metabolism to numerous metabolites. The major biotransformation pathways for duloxetine involve oxidation of the naphthyl ring followed by conjugation and further oxidation. Both CYP2D6 and CYP1A2 catalyze the formation of 2 major metabolites found in plasma and urine (glucuronide conjugate of 4-hydroxy duloxetine, and the sulfate conjugate of 5-hydroxy, 6-methoxy duloxetine). The major circulating metabolites are not pharmacologically active.

Excretion: The elimination half-life of duloxetine ranges from 8.1 to 17.4 hours (5th to 95th percentile, mean of 12.1 hours) and the apparent plasma clearance ranges from 33 to 261 L/hr (5th to 95th percentile, mean of 101 L/hr). Apparent plasma clearance of duloxetine does not differ between once daily and twice daily dosing. Only trace (<1% of the dose) amounts of unchanged duloxetine are present in the urine following single dose administration of ^{14}C-labelled duloxetine. The majority (72%) of the duloxetine dose is recovered in the urine as metabolites of duloxetine and approximately 19% is recovered in the feces.

Special Populations and Conditions: Pediatrics: Safety and efficacy in pediatric patients have not been established.

Geriatrics: The pharmacokinetics of duloxetine after a single dose of 40 mg were evaluated in 12 healthy elderly females (65 to 77 years) and 12 healthy middle-age females (32 to 50 years). There was no difference in the C_{max}, but the AUC of duloxetine was 24% higher and the half-life 4.3 hours longer in the elderly females. Pharmacokinetic results suggest no overall differences between these subjects and younger subjects. Other reported clinical experience has not identified differences in responses between the elderly and younger patients, but greater sensitivity of some older individuals cannot be ruled out. Dosage adjustment based on the age of the patient is not necessary (see Dosage and Administration, Dosage for Elderly Patients).

Gender: In clinical pharmacology studies, the mean apparent clearance of duloxetine was 9 to 55% lower in females as compared with males. In these studies, duloxetine half-life was similar between males and females. A similar effect of gender on the apparent plasma clearance was identified in patients with MDD. Since exposure in males and females spans a similar range, these differences in average clearance values do not appear to be clinically significant. Dosage adjustment based on gender is not necessary.

Race: No specific pharmacokinetic study was conducted to investigate the effects of race. Due to large interpatient variability, clinically significant differences in drug level exposure among ethnic groups are not likely.

Hepatic Insufficiency: Patients with clinically evident hepatic impairment have decreased duloxetine metabolism and elimination. After a single, non-therapeutic (20 mg) dose of CYMBALTA, 6 cirrhotic patients with moderate liver impairment (Child-Pugh Class B) had a mean plasma duloxetine clearance about 15% that of age- and gender-matched healthy subjects, with a 5-fold increase in mean exposure (AUC). Although C_{max} was similar to normals in the cirrhotic patients, the half-life was about 3 times longer. CYMBALTA is contraindicated in patients with any liver disease resulting in hepatic impairment (see Contraindications, Hepatic Impairment; Warnings and Precautions, Hepatic Impairment; and Dosage and Administration, Dosage for Patients with Hepatic Impairment).

Renal Insufficiency: Duloxetine C_{max} and AUC values were approximately 2-fold higher in patients with end stage renal disease (ESRD) receiving chronic intermittent hemodialysis, compared with subjects with normal renal function. In contrast, the elimination half-life was similar in both groups. Studies have not been conducted in patients with a moderate degree of renal dysfunction. Population PK analyses suggest that mild renal dysfunction has no significant effect on duloxetine apparent clearance. CYMBALTA is not recommended for patients with end-stage renal disease or severe renal impairment (see Contraindications; Warnings and Precautions, Renal; and Dosage and Administration, Dosage for Patients with Renal Impairment).

Smoking Status: Duloxetine bioavailability appears to be about 34% lower in smokers than in nonsmokers, although dosage modifications are not routinely recommended.

Clinical Safety Pharmacology: Effect on QTc Interval: A clinical pharmacology study was conducted to assess the safety of duloxetine at the highest tolerable level of exposure of duloxetine and measure QT interval. Of the 117 subjects enrolled, 84 were available for statistical analysis at the maximum dosage of 200 mg BID, and 91 on placebo. Seventy subjects (approximately 60%) completed the entire protocol. Compared with placebo, the mean change in the QTcF interval decreased at each time point with duloxetine 200 mg BID, ranging between −3.0 and −6.4 msec. The upper limit of the two-sided 90% confidence intervals was less than 5 msec at each time point, indicating no clinically relevant increase in the QTcF interval. Similar results were found with the covariance approach and the individual correction method.

No individual QTcF exceeded 470 msec on either duloxetine or placebo, and only 2 subjects had a categorical QTcF increase >30 msec at either 160 mg BID or 200 mg BID dosages (n=84), compared with 6 subjects (n=97) at placebo. Furthermore, no subject had a maximal QTc interval greater than 450 msec based on the average of replicate QTcF and QTcI values on day four of duloxetine 200 mg BID. The ability to detect relevant changes in QTc intervals in this study was confirmed by observing significant differences in the QTc interval at two time points (mean change in QTcF=6.7 msec at 2 hours, p<0.0001 and 2.7 msec at 6 hours, p=0.0186) with moxifloxacin as compared with placebo. QT interval at doses up to 200 mg BID were not prolonged.

STORAGE AND STABILITY: Store between 15 and 30°C.

INFORMATION FOR THE PATIENT: Published in e-CPS, available by subscription at www.e-cps.ca.

DOSAGE FORMS, COMPOSITION AND PACKAGING: 30 mg: Each opaque white body and opaque blue cap, delayed-release capsule, imprinted "30 mg" on the body and "9543" on the cap contains: duloxetine HCl 30 mg. Nonmedicinal ingredients: FD&C Blue No. 2, gelatin, hydroxypropyl methylcellulose, hydroxypropyl methylcellulose acetate succinate, sodium lauryl sulfate, sucrose, sugar spheres, talc, titanium dioxide and triethyl citrate. Blisters of 7 and 28.

60 mg: Each opaque green body and opaque blue cap, delayed-release capsule, imprinted "60 mg" on the body and "9542" on the cap contains: duloxetine HCl 60 mg. Nonmedicinal ingredients: FD&C Blue No. 2, gelatin, hydroxypropyl methylcellulose, hydroxypropyl methylcellulose acetate succinate, sodium lauryl sulfate, sucrose, sugar spheres, talc, titanium dioxide, triethyl citrate and yellow iron oxide. Blisters of 7 and 28.

(Shown in Product Identification Section)

Cysto-Conray® II

iothalamate meglumine

Radiopaque Medium

tyco Healthcare

Date of Revision: June 20, 2002

DESCRIPTION: Retrograde instillation opacifies selected segments of the urinary tract, permitting fluoroscopic and radiographic visualization of structures such as the urethra, bladder, ureters and pelvico-calyceal system.

INDICATIONS: Use in retrograde cystography and cystourethrography. Cysto-Conray is also indicated for use in retrograde pyelography.

CONTRAINDICATIONS: In patients with a known hypersensitivity to salts of iothalamic acid, the use of this preparation is contraindicated as intravasation may lead to hypersensitivity reactions and anaphylactic shock. However, a history of sensitivity to iodine per se or to other contrast media is not an absolute contraindication to the use of Cysto-Conray II, but calls for extreme caution in administration.

Obstruction and acute or severe infection of the urinary tract are generally regarded as contraindications to instrumentation and to the retrograde instillation of contrast material; do not inject by intravascular, s.c. or i.m. routes.

WARNINGS: A history of allergy, bronchial asthma, sensitivity to other iodine-containing compounds or a previous reaction to a contrast agent warrant special attention and may predict the likelihood of an allergic reaction.

Severe irritation of the urinary tract and hemorrhagic cystitis may occur following prolonged exposure to contrast media. It is imperative that the urinary bladder be emptied at the completion of the diagnostic procedures.

Pregnancy: The safe use of these preparations during pregnancy has not been established. Exposures of the abdomen and pelvis to radiation during pregnancy, especially in the first trimester, should be avoided, unless in the judgment of the physician the expected benefits to the mother outweigh the risk to the developing fetus.

PRECAUTIONS: Diagnostic procedures which involve the use of radiopaque contrast media should be carried out under the direction of appropriately trained personnel. Appropriate facilities should be available for coping with emergencies which may arise.

For sensitivity testing 0.1 mL of the contrast medium may be injected intradermally. The patient should be observed for local and general hypersensitivity reaction for 15 to 30 minutes.

Sensitivity testing cannot be relied upon to predict severe reactions.

An impending reaction is often indicated by apprehension, respiratory difficulty, faintness, sneezing, itching, vomiting or urticaria. In some instances, reactions to the test dose may be delayed.

Since iodine-containing contrast agents may alter the results of thyroid function tests, such tests, if indicated, should be performed prior to the administration of this preparation.

ADVERSE EFFECTS: Irritation of the bladder or ureter, common to some degree to all contrast media administered for retrograde urographic procedures, may occasionally occur. Hemorrhagic cystitis may result. As with all contrast media, intravasation may lead to hypersensitivity reactions such as a sense of warmth, flushing, sneezing, sweating, chills, fever, urticaria, laryngeal edema, bronchospasm, hypertension, hypotension, cardiac arrhythmias, cardiac arrest and anaphylactic shock.

Treatment of Adverse Effects: Contrast media should be administered only by physicians thoroughly familiar with the emergency treatment of all adverse reactions to contrast media. The assistance of other trained personnel such as cardiologists, internists and anesthetists is required in the management of severe reactions.

OVERDOSE:
No data supplied by the manufacturer.

> For management of a suspected drug overdose, CPhA recommends that you contact your **regional Poison Control Centre**. See the *CPS* Directory section for a list of Poison Control Centres.

DOSAGE: Patient Preparation: Unless contraindicated, an appropriate laxative is given the night before the examination. The bladder should be emptied before the contrast agent is instilled.

Radiographic Technique: The radiographic procedure normally employed for cystography and for cystourethrography should be employed. A preliminary radiograph is recommended before the contrast agent is administered.

Administration: Sterile catheterization is essential. Cysto-Conray II may be introduced by gravity flow using an appropriate venoclysis set or by syringe. Excessive pressure should be avoided with any method of administration.

Adults: Retrograde Cystography and Cystourethrography: The desired concentration will vary depending on the patient's size and age and also with the technique and equipment used. Sufficient volume of contrast medium is administered to adequately fill the urinary bladder. The volume of solution required will vary depending upon the individual patient. Adults usually require a volume in the range of 200 to 400 mL.

Children: Children require a volume in proportion to their body size. The usual dose ranges from 30 to 300 mL. Until further experience has been gained, the use of Cysto-Conray II for retrograde pyelography in children is not recommended.

SUPPLIED: Each mL of sterile aqueous solution contains: iothalamate meglumine 172 mg (iodine 8.1%), edetate calcium disodium 0.110 mg as a stabilizer and sodium biphosphate 0.115 mg as a buffer. Bottles of 200 mL fill/250 mL, boxes of 12; bottles of 500 mL, boxes of 12.

Cysto-Conray II is hypertonic under conditions of use and is supplied in containers from which the air has been displaced by nitrogen.

Store between 15 to 30°C. Protect from light. Protect from freezing. Discard unused portion.

Cytarabine Injection Ⓟ

cytarabine

Antileukemic

Hospira

SUPPLIED: Each mL of sterile aqueous solution contains: cytarabine 100 mg. Nonmedicinal ingredients: none. May contain hydrochloric acid or sodium hydroxide as pH adjusters. Preservative-free. Single use vials of 1 mL, cartons of 5. Single use vials of 10 and 20 mL, cartons of 1. Store between 15 and 25°C. Protect from light. Discard unused portion.

CytoGam®

cytomegalovirus immune globulin intravenous (human)

Passive Immunizing Agent

CSL Behring

Date of Preparation: May 8, 2007

PHARMACOLOGY: CytoGam, Cytomegalovirus Immune Globulin Intravenous (Human) (CMV-IGIV), contains IgG antibodies representative of the large number of normal persons who contributed to the plasma pools from which the product was derived. The globulin contains a relatively high concentration of antibodies directed against Cytomegalovirus (CMV). In the case of persons who may be exposed to CMV, CytoGam can raise the relevant antibodies to levels sufficient to attenuate or reduce the incidence of serious CMV disease.

In two separate clinical trials, CytoGam was shown to provide effective prophylaxis in renal transplant recipients at risk for primary CMV disease. In the first randomized trial, the incidence of virologically confirmed CMV-associated syndromes was reduced from 60% in controls (n=35) to 21% in recipients of CMV immune globulin (n=24) (P <0.01); marked leukopenia was reduced from 37% in controls to 4% in globulin recipients (P <0.01); and fungal or parasitic superinfections were not seen in globulin recipients but occurred in 20% of controls (P=0.05). Serious CMV disease was reduced from 46% to 13%. There was a concomitant but not statistically significant reduction in the incidence of CMV pneumonia (17% of controls as compared with 4% of globulin recipients). There was no effect on rates of viral isolation or seroconversion although the rate of viremia was less in CytoGam recipients. In a subsequent non-randomized trial in renal transplant recipients (n=36), the incidence of virologically confirmed CMV-associated syndrome was reduced to 36% in the globulin recipients in comparison to a 60% incidence in control patients (n=35) in the randomized trial. The rates of CMV-associated pneumonia, CMV-associated hepatitis, and concomitant fungal and parasitic superinfection were similar to those in the first trial.

INDICATIONS: Cytomegalovirus Immune Globulin Intravenous (Human) is indicated for the attenuation of primary (1°) Cytomegalovirus disease associated with kidney transplantation. Specifically, the product is indicated for kidney transplant recipients who are seronegative for CMV and who receive a kidney from a CMV seropositive donor. In a population of seronegative recipients of seropositive kidneys approximately 75% of the untreated recipients would be expected to develop CMV disease. Clinical studies have shown a 50% reduction in 1° CMV disease in renal transplant patients given Cytomegalovirus Immune Globulin Intravenous (Human).

CONTRAINDICATIONS: CytoGam, Cytomegalovirus Immune Globulin Intravenous (Human), should not be used in individuals with a history of a prior severe reaction associated with the administration of this or other human immunoglobulin preparations. Persons with selective immunoglobulin A deficiency have the potential for developing antibodies to immunoglobulin A and could have anaphylactic reactions to subsequent administration of blood products that contain immunoglobulin A, including CytoGam.

WARNINGS: CytoGam, Cytomegalovirus Immune Globulin Intravenous (Human) is made from human plasma and, like other plasma products, carries the possibility for transmission of blood-borne viral agents, and theoretically, the Creutzfeldt-Jakob disease (CJD) agent. The risk of transmission of recognized blood-borne viruses is considered to be low because of the viral inactivation and removal properties in the Cohn-Oncley cold ethanol precipitation procedure used for purification of immune globulin products. Until 1993, cold ethanol manufactured immune globulins licensed in the United States had not been documented to transmit any viral agent. However, during a brief period in late 1993 to early 1994, intravenous immune globulin made by one U.S. manufacturer was associated with transmission of Hepatitis C virus. To further guard against possible transmission of blood-borne viruses, including Hepatitis C, CMV-IGIV is treated with a solvent detergent viral inactivation procedure known to inactivate a wide spectrum of lipid enveloped viruses, including HIV-1, HIV-2, Hepatitis B, and Hepatitis C. However, because new blood-borne viruses may yet emerge, some of which may not be inactivated by the manufacturing process or by solvent detergent treatment, CMV-IGIV, like any other blood product, should be given only if a benefit is expected.

Immune Globulin Intravenous (Human) products have been reported to be associated with renal dysfunction, acute renal failure, osmotic nephrosis and death. Patients predisposed to acute renal failure include patients with any degree of pre-existing renal insufficiency, diabetes mellitus, age greater than 65, volume depletion, sepsis, paraproteinemia or patients receiving known nephrotoxic drugs. Especially in such patients, IGIV products should be administered at the minimum concentrations available and the minimum rate of infusion practical. While these reports of renal dysfunction and acute renal failure have been associated with the use of many IGIV products, those containing sucrose as a stabilizer (and given at daily doses of 350 mg/kg or greater) account for a disproportionate share of the total number. CytoGam contains sucrose as a stabilizer. See Precautions and Dosage for important information intended to reduce the risk of acute renal failure.

During administration, the patient's vital signs should be monitored continuously and careful observation made for any symptoms throughout the infusion. Epinephrine should be available for the treatment of an acute anaphylactic reaction (see Precautions).

PRECAUTIONS: General: CytoGam does not contain a preservative. The vial should be entered only once for administration purposes and the infusion should begin within 6 hours. The infusion schedule should be adhered to closely (see Infusion section). Do not use if the solution is turbid.

Although systemic allergic reactions are rare (see Adverse Effects), epinephrine and diphenhydramine should be available for treatment of acute allergic symptoms. If hypotension or anaphylaxis occur, the administration of the immunoglobulin should be discontinued immediately and an antidote should be given as noted above.

Renal Function: Assure that patients are not volume depleted prior to the initiation of IGIV. Periodic monitoring of renal function tests and urine output is particularly important in patients judged to have a potential increased risk for developing acute renal failure. Renal function, including the measurement of blood urea nitrogen (BUN) or serum creatinine should be assessed prior to the initial infusion of CytoGam and again at appropriate intervals thereafter. If renal function deteriorates, discontinuation of the product should be considered. For patients judged to be at risk for developing renal dysfunction, it may be prudent to reduce the amount of product infused per unit time. The recommended rate of Cytogam infusion for prophylaxis of CMV disease in kidney transplant patients should **not exceed** 60 mg Ig/kg/hr (see Dosage).

Aseptic Meningitis Syndrome: An aseptic meningitis syndrome (AMS) has been reported to occur infrequently in association with Immune Globulin Intravenous (Human) (IGIV) treatment. The syndrome usually begins within several hours to two days following IGIV treatment. It is characterized by symptoms and signs including severe headache, nuchal rigidity, drowsiness, fever, photophobia, painful eye movements, and nausea and vomiting. Cerebrospinal fluid studies are frequently positive with pleocytosis up to several thousand cells/mm^3, predominantly from the granulocytic series, and elevated protein levels up to several hundred mg/dL. Patients exhibiting such symptoms and signs should receive a thorough neurological examination, including CSF studies, to rule out other causes of meningitis. AMS may occur more frequently in association with high dose (2 g/kg) IGIV treatment. Discontinuation of IGIV treatment has resulted in remission of AMS within several days without sequelae.

Hemolysis: Immune Globulin Intravenous (Human) (IGIV) products can contain blood group antibodies which may act as hemolysins and induce in vivo coating of red blood cells with immunoglobulin, causing a positive direct antiglobulin reaction and, rarely, hemolysis. Hemolytic anemia can develop subsequent to IGIV therapy due to enhanced RBC sequestration (see Adverse Effects). IGIV recipients should be monitored for clinical signs and symptoms of hemolysis (see Laboratory Tests).

Transfusion-Related Acute Lung Injury (TRALI): There have been reports of noncardiogenic pulmonary edema [Transfusion-Related Acute Lung Injury (TRALI)] in patients administered IGIV. TRALI is characterized by severe respiratory distress, pulmonary edema, hypoxemia, normal left ventricular function, and fever and typically occurs within 1-6 hours after transfusion. Patients with TRALI may be managed using oxygen therapy with adequate ventilatory support.

IGIV recipients should be monitored for pulmonary adverse reactions. If TRALI is suspected, appropriate tests should be performed for the presence of anti-neutrophil antibodies in both the product and patient serum (see Laboratory Tests).

Thrombotic Events: Thrombotic events have been reported in association with IGIV (see Adverse Effects). Patients at risk may include those with a history of atherosclerosis, multiple cardiovascular risk factors, advanced age, impaired cardiac output, and/or known or suspected hyperviscosity. The potential risks and benefits of IGIV should be weighed against those of alternative therapies for all patients for whom IGIV administration is being considered. Baseline assessment of blood viscosity should be considered in patients at risk for hyperviscosity, including those with cryoglobulins, fasting chylomicronemia/ markedly high triacylglycerols (triglycerides), or monoclonal gammopathies (see Laboratory Tests).

Laboratory Tests: If signs and/or symptoms of hemolysis are present after IGIV infusion, appropriate confirmatory laboratory testing should be done (see Precautions).

If TRALI is suspected, appropriate tests should be performed for the presence of anti-neutrophil antibodies in both the product and patient serum (see Precautions).

Because of the potentially increased risk of thrombosis, baseline assessment of blood viscosity should be considered in patients at risk for hyperviscosity, including those with cryoglobulins, fasting chylomicronemia/markedly high triacylglycerols (triglycerides), or monoclonal gammopathies (see Precautions).

Drug Interactions: Antibodies present in immune globulin preparations may interfere with the immune response to live virus vaccines such as measles, mumps, and rubella; therefore, vaccination with live virus vaccines should be deferred until approximately three months after administration of CytoGam. If such vaccinations were given shortly after CytoGam, a revaccination may be necessary. Admixtures of CytoGam with other drugs have not been evaluated. It is recommended that CytoGam be administered separately from other drugs or medications which the patient may be receiving (see Dosage).

Pregnancy: Category C: Animal reproduction studies have not been conducted with Cytomegalovirus Immune Globulin Intravenous (Human). It is also not known whether Cytomegalovirus Immune Globulin Intravenous (Human) can cause fetal harm when administered to a pregnant woman or can affect reproduction capacity. Cytomegalovirus Immune Globulin Intravenous (Human) should be given to a pregnant woman only if clearly needed.

ADVERSE EFFECTS: Minor reactions such as flushing, chills, muscle cramps, back pain, fever, nausea, vomiting, arthralgia, and wheezing were the most frequent adverse reactions observed during the clinical trials of CytoGam, Cytomegalovirus Immune Globulin Intravenous (Human). The incidence of these reactions during the clinical trials was less than 6.0% of all infusions and were most often related to infusion rates. If a patient develops a minor side effect, slow the rate immediately or temporarily interrupt the infusion.

Increases in serum creatinine and blood urea nitrogen (BUN) have been observed as soon as one to two days following IGIV infusion. Progression to oliguria or anuria requiring dialysis has been observed. Types of severe renal adverse events that have been seen following IGIV therapy include acute renal failure, acute tubular necrosis, proximal tubular nephropathy and osmotic nephrosis.

Severe reactions such as angioneurotic edema and anaphylactic shock, although not observed during clinical trials, are a possibility. Clinical anaphylaxis may occur even when the patient is not known to be sensitized to immune globulin products. A reaction may be related to the rate of infusion; therefore, carefully adhere to the infusion rates as outlined under Dosage. If anaphylaxis or drop in blood pressure occurs, discontinue infusion and use antidote such as diphenhydramine and adrenalin.

Postmarketing: In addition to adverse events reported during clinical trials, the following events have been reported during the post-approval use of Cytogam: Acute Respiratory Distress Syndrome (ARDS), cyanosis, pulmonary edema, dyspnea, cardiac arrest, circulatory collapse, hypotension, convulsions, bullous dermatitis, hemolysis, hepatic failure, and abdominal pain.

In addition to the adverse reactions seen with the use of CytoGam, the following adverse reactions have been identified and reported during the post-approval use of IGIV products:

Respiratory: apnea, Transfusion Associated Lung Injury (TRALI), hypoxemia, bronchospasm.

Cardiovascular: thromboembolism.

Neurological: coma, loss of consciousness, tremor.

Integumentary: Stevens-Johnson syndrome, epidermolysis, erythema multiforme.

Hematologic: pancytopenia, leukopenia, positive direct antiglobulin (Coombs) test.

Because postmarketing reporting of these reactions is voluntary and the at-risk populations are of uncertain size, it is not always possible to reliably estimate the frequency of the reaction or establish a causal relationship to exposure to the product. Such is also the case with literature reports authored independently.

OVERDOSE:

Although little data are available, clinical experience with other immunoglobulin preparations suggests that the major manifestations would be those related to volume overload.

For management of a suspected drug overdose, CPhA recommends that you contact your **regional Poison Control Centre**. See the *CPS* Directory section for a list of Poison Control Centres.

DOSAGE: The maximum recommended total dosage per infusion is 150 mg Ig/kg, administered according to the following schedule: Within 72 hours of transplant: 150 mg/kg; 2 weeks post transplant: 100 mg/kg; 4 weeks post transplant: 100 mg/kg; 6 weeks post transplant: 100 mg/kg; 8 weeks post transplant: 100 mg/kg; 12 weeks post transplant: 50 mg/kg; 16 weeks post transplant: 50 mg/kg.

Preparation for Administration: Remove the tab portion of the vial cap and clean the rubber stopper with 70% alcohol or equivalent. **Do not shake vial; avoid foaming.**

Parenteral drug products should be inspected visually for particulate matter and discoloration prior to administration whenever solution and container permit. Infuse the solution only if it is colorless, free of particulate matter and not turbid. CytoGam, Cytomegalovirus Immune Globulin Intravenous (Human), does not contain a preservative. The vial should be entered only once for administration purposes.

Infusion should begin within 6 hours after entering the vial and should be complete within 12 hours of entering the vial. Vital signs should be taken pre-infusion, mid-way and post-infusion as well as before any rate increase. CytoGam should be administered through an intravenous line using an administration set that contains an in-line filter (pore size 15 μm) and a constant infusion pump (i.e., IVAC pump or equivalent). A smaller in-line filter (0.2 μm) is also acceptable. Pre-dilution of CytoGam before infusion is not recommended. CytoGam should be administered through a separate intravenous line. If this is not possible, CytoGam may be "piggybacked" into a pre-existing line if that line contains either Sodium Chloride, Injection, USP, or one of the following dextrose solutions (with or without NaCl added): 2.5% dextrose in water, 5% dextrose in water, 10% dextrose in water, 20% dextrose in water. If a pre-existing line must be used, the CytoGam should not be diluted more than 1:2 with any of the above-named solutions. Admixtures of CytoGam with any other solutions have not been evaluated.

Initial Dose: Administer intravenously at 15 mg Ig per kg body weight per hour. If no adverse reactions occur after 30 minutes, the rate may be increased to 30 mg Ig/kg/hr; if no adverse reactions occur after a subsequent 30 minutes, then the infusion may be increased to 60 mg Ig/kg/hr (volume not to exceed 75 mL/hour). **Do not exceed this rate of administration.** The patient should be monitored closely during and after each rate change.

Subsequent Doses: Administer at 15 mg Ig/kg/hr for 15 minutes. If no adverse reactions occur, increase to 30 mg Ig/kg/hr for 15 minutes and then increase to a **maximum rate of 60 mg Ig/kg/hr** (volume not to exceed 75 mL/hour). **Do not exceed this rate of administration.** The patient should be monitored closely during each rate change.

CytoGam should be used with caution in patients with pre-existing renal insufficiency and in patients judged to be at increased risk of developing renal insufficiency (including, but not limited to those with diabetes mellitus, age greater than 65, volume depletion, paraproteinemia, sepsis and patients receiving known nephrotoxic drugs). In these cases especially, it is important to assure that patients are not volume depleted prior to CytoGam infusion. While most cases of renal insufficiency have occurred in patients receiving total doses of 350 mg Ig/kg or greater, no prospective data are presently available to identify a maximum safe dose, concentration or rate of infusion in patients determined to be at increased risk of acute renal failure. In the absence of prospective data, recommended doses should not be exceeded and the concentration and infusion rate selected should be the minimum practicable.

Potential adverse reactions are: flushing, chills, muscle cramps, back pain, fever, nausea, vomiting, wheezing, drop in blood pressure. Minor adverse reactions have been infusion rate related—if the patient develops a minor side effect (i.e., nausea, back pain, flushing), slow the rate or temporarily interrupt the infusion. If anaphylaxis or drop in blood pressure occurs, **discontinue infusion** and use antidote such as diphenhydramine and adrenalin.

To prevent the transmission of hepatitis viruses or other infectious agents from one person to another, sterile disposable syringes and needles should be used. The syringes and needles should not be reused.

SUPPLIED: CytoGam, Cytomegalovirus Immune Globulin Intravenous (Human), is an immunoglobulin G (IgG) product containing a standardized amount of antibody to Cytomegalovirus (CMV). CytoGam is formulated in final vial as a sterile liquid. The globulin is stabilized with 5% sucrose and 1% Albumin (Human). CytoGam contains no preservative. The purified immunoglobulin is derived from pooled adult human plasma selected for high titers of antibody for Cytomegalovirus (CMV). Source material for fractionation may be obtained from another U.S. licensed manufacturer. Pooled plasma was fractionated by ethanol precipitation of the proteins according to Cohn Methods 6 and 9, modified to yield a product suitable for intravenous administration.

A widely utilized solvent-detergent viral inactivation process is also used. Certain manufacturing operations may be performed by other firms. Each milliliter contains: 50±10 mg of immunoglobulin, primarily IgG, and trace amounts of IgA and IgM; 50 mg of sucrose; 10 mg of Albumin (Human). The sodium content is 20-30 mEq per liter; i.e. 1.0-1.5 mEq per 50 mL. The solution should appear colorless and translucent. Cytogam is supplied in a single use vial and therefore, any product remaining after administration should be discarded.

Each single use vial contains: 2500 mg±500 mg of immunoglobulin. Store between 2-8°C and use within 6 hours after entering the vial. The product is stable up to the expiration date which is stamped on the outer carton and vial label. It should not be used after that date.

Cytomel®
liothyronine sodium
Hypothyroidism Therapy

King Pharmaceuticals

PHARMACOLOGY: Action: There are two principal naturally occurring thyroid hormones, L-tetraiodothyronine (T_4, levothyroxine, L-thyroxine) and L-triiodothyronine (T_3, liothyronine).

The mechanisms by which thyroid hormones exert their physiologic actions are not well understood. It is generally believed that they exert most if not all of their actions through control of protein synthesis.

At moderate concentrations, thyroid hormones increase the synthesis of RNA and protein, followed by an increase in basal metabolic rate (BMR). They stimulate oxidative enzyme systems generally, and enhance the release of free fatty acids from adipose tissue. They also increase the intestinal absorption and peripheral utilization of glucose.

At higher concentrations, thyroid hormones decrease protein synthesis, uncouple oxidative phosphorylation and increase the breakdown of glycogen, lipids and protein.

Clinical Pharmacology: Cytomel brand of liothyronine is the synthetic levo form of triiodothyronine, with all pharmacologic activities of the natural substance. Its onset of action is rapid, occurring within a few hours. Maximum pharmacological response occurs within two or three days, providing early clinical response.

Following oral administration, about 95% of the dose of liothyronine is absorbed from the gastrointestinal tract in 4 hours. Liothyronine, not firmly bound to serum protein, is readily available to body tissues. Its biologic half-life is about 2.5 days.

Liothyronine has a rapid cut-off of activity, which permits quick dosage adjustment and facilitates control of the effects of overdosage, should they occur.

INDICATIONS: Cytomel is indicated in conditions of inadequate endogenous thyroid production. These include: hypothyroidism (all gradations from frank myxedema to mild hypofunction, cretinism, male infertility due to hypothyroidism); simple (nontoxic) goiter (liothyronine may be tried therapeutically in an attempt to reduce the size of such a goiter, the rationale being that suppression of pituitary thyroid stimulating hormone (TSH) removes at least one of the growth-promoting factors.

Liothyronine may be used in the T_3 suppression test to differentiate suspected hyperthyroidism from euthyroidism (see Special Instruction under Dosage).

Cytomel can be used in patients allergic to desiccated thyroid or thyroid extract derived from pork or beef.

Pregnancy: Thyroid hormones do not readily cross the placental barrier. The clinical experience to date does not indicate any adverse effect on fetuses when thyroid hormones are administered to pregnant women. On the basis of current knowledge, thyroid replacement therapy to hypothyroid women should not be discontinued during pregnancy.

Lactation: See Precautions.

Children: Pregnant mothers provide little or no thyroid hormone to the fetus. The incidence of congenital hypothyroidism is relatively high (1:4000) and the hypothyroid fetus would not derive any benefit from the small amounts of hormone crossing the placental barrier. Treatment should be initiated immediately upon diagnosis and maintained for life, unless transient hypothyroidism is suspected, in which case therapy may be interrupted for two to eight weeks after the age of three years to reassess the condition. Cessation of therapy is justified in patients who have maintained a normal TSH level during those two to eight weeks.

CONTRAINDICATIONS: Uncorrected adrenal insufficiency.

WARNINGS: The use of Cytomel or other thyroid preparations in the therapy of obesity is unjustified. In euthyroid patients, doses within the range of daily hormonal requirements are ineffective for weight reduction. Larger doses may produce serious or even life-threatening manifestations of toxicity, particularly when given in association with sympathomimetic amines such as those used for anorectic effects.

PRECAUTIONS: Since Cytomel is a metabolic stimulant, it is not recommended for use in patients in whom the integrity of the cardiovascular system, particularly the coronary arteries, is suspect. These include patients with angina pectoris, ischemic states, and the elderly (in whom there is a greater likelihood of occult cardiac disease). However, if it is used in such patients, caution should be exercised and the dosage should never be more than 5 µg daily. If dosage is increased, it should be in increments of no more than 5 µg daily at 2-week intervals.

Myxedematous patients are very sensitive to thyroid substances; dosage should be started at a very low level and increased gradually.

Morphologic hypogonadism and nephrosis should be ruled out before the drug is administrated. If hypopituitarism is present, the adrenal deficiency must be corrected before Cytomel therapy is started.

Severe and prolonged hypothyroidism can lead to a decreased level of adrenocortical activity commensurate with the lowered metabolic state. When thyroid replacement therapy is administered, the metabolism increases at a greater rate than adrenocortical activity. This can precipitate adrenocortical insufficiency. Therefore, in severe and prolonged hypothyroidism, supplemental adrenocortical steroids may be necessary.

Thyroid hormone therapy aggravates the symptoms of patients with concomitant diabetes mellitus, diabetes insipidus or adrenal cortical insufficiency, requiring appropriate adjustments of the various therapeutic measures directed at these concomitant endocrine diseases.

In rare instances, the administration of thyroid hormone may precipitate a hyperthyroid state or may aggravate existing hyperthyroidism.

Children: In infants, excessive doses of thyroid hormone preparations may produce craniosynostosis.

Lactation: Thyroid hormones are excreted in human milk in minimal amounts which are not associated with serious adverse reactions. Thyroid hormones do not have a known tumorigenic potential. Nevertheless, caution should be exercised when thyroid is administered to a nursing woman.

Drug Interactions: Oral Anticoagulants: Thyroid hormones appear to increase catabolism of vitamin K-dependent clotting factors. Patients stabilized on oral anticoagulants may require dosage adjustment, through close monitoring of prothrombin time, when thyroid hormone therapy is started. No special precautions appear to be necessary when oral anticoagulant therapy is begun in a patient already stabilized on maintenance thyroid therapy.

Catecholamines: Thyroid hormones increase the adrenergic effect of catecholamines such as epinephrine and norepinephrine. Therefore, injection of these agents into patients receiving thyroid preparations increases the risk of precipitating coronary insufficiency, especially in patients with coronary artery disease. Careful observation is required.

Cholestyramine: Cholestyramine binds orally administered thyroid hormones in the intestine, impairing their absorption. In vitro studies indicate that the binding is not easily overcome. Therefore, 4 to 5 hours should elapse between administration of cholestyramine and thyroid hormones.

Digitalis: Thyroid preparations may potentiate the toxic effects of digitalis. Thyroid hormonal replacement increases metabolic rate, which requires an increase in digitalis dosage.

Estrogen, Oral Contraceptives: Estrogens tend to increase serum thyroxine-binding globulin (TBG) and may require, depending on the level of thyroid gland function, adjustment of (supplemental or replacement) thyroid hormone dosage.

Insulin or Oral Hypoglycemics: Initiating thyroid replacement therapy may require increases in insulin or oral hypoglycemic requirements. The effects seen are poorly understood and depend upon a variety of factors such as dose and type of thyroid preparations and endocrine status of the patient.

Ketamine: When administered to patients on a thyroid preparation, this parenteral anesthetic may cause hypertension and tachycardia. Use with caution and be prepared to treat hypertension, if necessary.

Tricyclic Antidepressant: Use of thyroid products with imipramine and other tricyclic antidepressants may increase receptor sensitivity and enhance antidepressant activity; transient cardiac arrhythmias have been observed. Thyroid hormone activity may also be enhanced.

Laboratory Test Interactions: Since liothyronine is not as firmly bound to serum protein as thyroxine, the PBI usually remains at levels below normal during full replacement therapy. As with all thyroid preparations, thyroid gland function reflected by I^{131} uptake may be depressed by Cytomel, particularly when dosage exceeds 75 µg daily. This effect disappears rapidly, and useful I^{131} thyroid uptake values may be obtained usually within 2 weeks following discontinuance of the drug.

The following drugs or moieties are known to interfere with laboratory tests performed in patients on thyroid hormone therapy: androgens, corticosteroids, estrogens and estrogen-containing oral contraceptives, iodine-containing preparations and salicylates.

ADVERSE EFFECTS: Overdosage will produce signs and symptoms of hyperthyroidism such as headache, excessive sweating, nervousness, cardiac arrhythmias, angina pectoris, and menstrual irregularities (see Overdose). Medication should be interrupted until symptoms disappear, then resume in smaller doses. Therapy can usually be resumed after 1 or 2 days.

Rare instances of allergic skin reactions have been reported.

OVERDOSE:

Symptoms: Headache, irritability, nervousness, sweating, tachycardia, increased bowel motility and menstrual irregularities. Because of liothyronine's rapid cut-off of activity, such symptoms will generally disappear within a few days after dosage is reduced. Angina pectoris or congestive heart failure may be induced or aggravated.

Shock may also develop. Massive overdosage may result in symptoms resembling thyroid storm. Chronic excessive dosage will produce the signs and symptoms of hyperthyroidism.

Treatment: General supportive measures. Sedation if indicated. If tachycardia is present, reserpine may be helpful. Measures should be instituted to control shock if present, such as intravenous fluids, oxygen. Intravenous hydrocortisone should be considered for the treatment of unrecognized adrenal insufficiency.

> For management of a suspected drug overdose, CPhA recommends that you contact your **regional Poison Control Centre**. See the *CPS* Directory section for a list of Poison Control Centres.

DOSAGE: Optimum dosage is usually determined by the patient's clinical response. Confirmatory tests include: RAI T_3 Resin Uptake, T_3-I^{131} Red Cell Uptake, BMR and the Achilles Tendon Reflex test. Comparatively small doses (as little as 5 µg daily) may be fully effective in some cases; however, in other instances, a satisfactory clinical response may not be achieved until recommended dosage levels have been exceeded. Daily doses up to 150 µg are sometimes well tolerated and may be optimal in a few resistant patients.

It is not necessary to divide daily maintenance doses. Although liothyronine has a rapid cut-off, its metabolic effects persist for a few days following discontinuance.

Mild Hypothyroidism: Recommended starting dosage is 25 µg daily. Daily dosage then may be increased by 12.5 or 25 µg every 1 or 2 weeks. Usual maintenance dosage is 25 to 75 µg daily. Smaller doses may be fully effective in some patients, while 100 µg may be required in others.

Myxedema: Myxedematous patients are very sensitive to thyroid substances; dosage should be started at a very low level and increased gradually. Recommended starting dose is 5 µg daily. This may be increased by 5 or 10 µg daily every 1 or 2 weeks. Usual maintenance dosage is 50 to 100 µg daily.

Cretinism: Since the mother provides little or no thyroid hormone to the fetus, infants with thyroid dysfunction will require replacement therapy from birth. Treatment should be initiated as early as possible to avoid permanent physical and mental changes. Recommended starting dosage is 5 µg daily, with a 5 µg increment every 3 to 4 days until the desired response is achieved. Infants a few months old may require only 20 µg daily for maintenance. At 1 year, 50 µg daily may be required. Above 3 years, full adult dosage may be necessary.

Male Infertility due to Hypothyroidism: Recommended starting dosage is 5 µg daily. Based on sperm count and motility, daily dosage may be increased by 5 or 10 µg every 2 to 4 weeks. Daily dosage will usually not exceed 25 µg and rarely should dosage exceed 50 µg daily in this indication.

Simple (non-toxic) Goiter: Recommended starting dosage is 5 µg daily. This dosage my be increased by 5 to 10 µg daily every 1 to 2 weeks. When 25 µg daily is reached, dosage may be increased every week or two by 12.5 or 25 µg. Usual maintenance dosage is 75 µg daily.

In the elderly or in children, therapy should be started with 5 µg daily and increased only by 5 µg increments at the recommended intervals.

When switching a patient to Cytomel from thyroid, L-thyroxine or thyroglobulin, discontinue the other medication, initiate Cytomel at a low dosage, and increase gradually according to the patient's response. When selecting a starting dosage, bear in mind that this drug has a rapid onset of action, and that residual effects of the other thyroid preparation may persist for the first several weeks of therapy.

Special Instruction for T_3 Suppression Test: When I^{131} thyroid uptake is in the borderline high range, administer 75 to 100 µg of Cytomel daily for 7 days, then repeat I^{131} thyroid uptake test. In the hyperthyroid patient, 24-hour I^{131} thyroid uptake will not be affected significantly. In the euthyroid patient, 24-hour I^{131} thyroid uptake will drop to less than 20%.

SUPPLIED: 5 µg: Each round, flat-faced, bevel-edged, white, compressed tablet, debossed with KPI on one side and 115 on the other side, contains: liothyronine 5 µg (present as liothyronine sodium 5.18 µg). Nonmedicinal ingredients: calcium sulfate, gelatin, starch, stearic acid, sucrose and talc. Bottles of 100.

25 µg: Each round, flat-faced, bevel-edged, white, compressed tablet, debossed with KPI 116 on one side and scored on the other side, contains: 25 µg (present as liothyronine sodium 25.9 µg). Nonmedicinal ingredients: calcium sulfate, gelatin, starch, stearic acid, sucrose and talc. Bottles of 100.

25 µg of liothyronine is equivalent to approximately 65 mg of desiccated thyroid or thyroglobulin and 0.1 mg of L-thyroxine.

Cytosar®
cytarabine
Antileukemic

Pfizer

> **Caution:** CYTOSAR (cytarabine) is a potent drug and should be used only by physicians experienced with cancer therapeutic drugs (see Warnings and Precautions). Hematologic, renal and hepatic evaluations must be done at regular intervals.

PHARMACOLOGY: CYTOSAR (cytarabine) is metabolized by deoxycytidine kinase and other nucleotide kinases to the nucleotide triphosphate, an effective inhibitor of DNA polymerase; it is inactivated by pyrimidine nucleoside deaminase which converts it to the nontoxic uracil derivative. It appears that the balance of kinase and deaminase levels may be an important factor in determining sensitivity or resistance of the cell to cytarabine.

CYTOSAR is rapidly metabolized and is not effective orally; less than 20% of the orally administered dose is absorbed from the gastrointestinal tract.

Following rapid intravenous injection of CYTOSAR, the disappearance from plasma is biphasic. There is an initial distributive phase with a half-life of about 10 minutes, followed by a second elimination phase with a half-life of about 1 to 3 hours. After the distributive phase, over 80% of plasma radioactivity can be accounted for by the inactive metabolite 1-β-D-arabinofuranosyluracid (ara-U). Within 24 hours about 80% of the administered radioactivity can be recovered in the urine, approximately 90% of which is excreted as ara-U.

After subcutaneous or intramuscular administration of CYTOSAR, peak plasma levels of radioactivity are achieved about 20 to 60 minutes after injection and are considerably lower than those after intravenous administration.

Cerebrospinal fluid levels of cytarabine are low in comparison to plasma levels after single intravenous injection. However, in one patient in whom cerebrospinal levels were examined after 2 hours of constant intravenous infusion, levels approached 40% of the steady-state plasma level. With intrathecal administration, levels of cytarabine in the cerebrospinal fluid declined with a first order half-life of about 2 hours. Because cerebrospinal fluid levels of deaminase are low, little conversion to ara-U was observed.

INDICATIONS: CYTOSAR (cytarabine) is indicated primarily for induction and maintenance of remission in acute leukemia in children and adults.

It has been found useful in the treatment of acute myelocytic leukemia, chronic myelocytic leukemia (blast phase), acute lymphocytic leukemia and erythroleukemia. CYTOSAR may be used alone or in combination with other antineoplastic agents; the best results are obtained with combination therapy.

Children with non-Hodgkin's lymphoma have benefited from a combination drug program (LSA_2L_2) that included CYTOSAR.

CYTOSAR has been used intrathecally in newly diagnosed children with acute lymphocytic leukemia as well as in the treatment of meningeal leukemia.

CYTOSAR, in high dose 2 to 3 g/m² as an i.v. infusion over 1 to 3 hours given every 12 hours for 2 to 6 days with or without additional cancer chemotherapeutic agents, has been shown to be effective in the treatment of poor-risk leukemia, refractory leukemia, and relapsed acute leukemia.

Remissions induced by CYTOSAR not followed by maintenance treatment have been brief.

Acute Myelocytic Leukemia: Table 1 and Table 2 outline the results of treatment with CYTOSAR alone and in combination with other chemotherapeutic agents, in the treatment of acute myelocytic leukemia in adults and children.

The treatment regimens outlined in the tables should not be compared for efficacy. These were independent studies with a number of variables involved, such as patient population, duration of disease, and previous treatment.

The responsiveness and course of childhood acute myelocytic leukemia (AML) appear to be different from that in adults. Numerous studies show response rates to be higher in children than in adults with similar treatment schedules. Experience indicates that at least with induction and initial drug responsiveness, childhood AML appears to be more similar to childhood acute lymphocytic leukemia (ALL) than to its adult variant.

Table 1: CYTOSAR

Acute Myelocytic Leukemia—Remission Induction: Adults

Drug Dosage Schedule[a]	No. Patients Evaluated	Complete Remissions	Investigator
CYTOSAR Single-Dose Therapy			
(Infusion)			
10 mg/m² 12 h/day	12	2 (17%)	Ellison (1968)
30 mg/m² 12 h/day	41	10 (24%)	
10 mg/m² 24 h/day	9	2 (22%)	
30 mg/m² 24 h/day	36	2 (6%)	
(Infusion)			
200 mg/m² 24 h/5 days	36	9 (25%)	Bodey (1969)
10 mg/m² i.v. injection initially, then infusions of 30 mg/m²/12 h or 60 mg/m²/day for 4 days	49	21 (43%)	Goodell (1970)
(Infusion Therapy)			
800 mg/m²/2 days	53	12 (23%)	Southwest Oncology Group (1974)
1000 mg/m²/5 days	60	24 (40%)	
100 mg/m²/day 1 h infusion	49	7 (14%)	Carey (1975)
5–12.5 mg/kg/12 h infusion following i.v. synchronizing dose[b]	5	5 (100%)	Lampkin (1976)
Combined Therapy			
CYTOSAR—doxorubicin	41	30 (73%)	Preisler (1979)
CYTOSAR—thioguanine—daunorubicin	28	22 (79%)	Gale (1977)
CYTOSAR—doxorubicin—vincristine—prednisolone	35	23 (66%)	Weinstein (1980)
CYTOSAR—daunorubicin—thioguanine—prednisone—vincristine	139	84 (60%)	Glucksberg (1981)
CYTOSAR—daunorubicin	21	14 (67%)	Cassileth (1977)
High Dose Therapy			
CYTOSAR	7	6 (86%)	Lister (1983)
CYTOSAR	21	12 (57%)	Herzig (1983)
CYTOSAR	11	8 (73%)	Preisler (1983)
CYTOSAR—doxorubicin	14	7 (50%)	Willemze (1982)
CYTOSAR—asparaginase	13	9 (69%)	Capizzi (1983)

[a] Unless otherwise stated, all doses given until drug effect-modifications then based on hematologic reasons. See references available from manufacturer.
[b] Highly experimental—requires ability to study mitotic indices.

Table 2: CYTOSAR

Acute Myelocytic Leukemia—Remission Induction: Children (21 and under)

Drug Therapy	No. Patients Evaluated	Complete Remissions	Investigator
CYTOSAR (5–12.5 mg/kg following i.v. synchronizing dose[a])	16	12 (75%)	Lampkin (1976)
CYTOSAR, vincristine, doxorubicin, prednisolone	48	35 (73%)	Weinstein (1980)
CYTOSAR, thioguanine, doxorubicin	11	8 (72%)	Hagbin (1975)
CYTOSAR, thioguanine	47	20 (43%)	Pizzo (1976)
CYTOSAR, cyclophosphamide	12	7 (58%)	Pizzo (1976)

[a] Highly experimental—requires ability to study mitotic indices.

Acute Lymphocytic Leukemia: CYTOSAR has been used in the treatment of acute lymphocytic leukemia in both adults and children. When CYTOSAR was used with other antineoplastic agents as part of a total therapy program, results were equal to or better than reported with such programs which did not include CYTOSAR. Used singly, or in combination with other agents, CYTOSAR has also been effective in treating patients who had relapsed on other therapy. Table 3 and Table 4 summarize the results obtained in previously treated patients. Since these are independent studies with such variables as patient population, duration of disease and previous treatment, results shown should not be used for comparing the efficacy of the outlined treatment programs.

Intrathecal Use in Meningeal Leukemia: CYTOSAR has been used intrathecally in acute leukemia in doses ranging from 5 to 75 mg/m² of body surface area. The frequency of administration varied from once a day for 4 days to once every 4 days. The most frequently used dose was 30 mg/m² every 4 days until cerebrospinal fluid findings were normal, followed by one additional treatment. The dosage schedule is usually governed by the type and severity of CNS manifestations and the response to previous therapy.

Table 3: CYTOSAR

Acute Lymphocytic Leukemia—Remission Induction—Previously Treated Patients, Adults and Children

Drug Therapy	No. Patients Evaluated	Complete Remissions	Response	Investigator
CYTOSAR 3–5 mg/kg/day (i.v. injection)	43	2 (5%)	15 (35%)	Howard (1968)
CYTOSAR—asparaginase	9	8 (89%)	8 (89%)	McElwain (1969)
CYTOSAR—cyclophosphamide	11	7 (64%)	9 (82%)	Bodey (1970)
CYTOSAR—prednisone	83	—	(49%)	Nesbitt (1970)
CYTOSAR 150–200 mg/m²/5 days (infusion)	34	1 (3%)	4 (12%)	Wang (1970)
CYTOSAR—L-asparaginase—prednisone—vincristine—doxorubicin	91	72 (79%)	—	Klemperer (1978)
CYTOSAR—L-asparaginase—prednisone—vincristine—doxorubicin	55	42 (76%)	—	Klemperer (1978)
CYTOSAR—asparaginase	22	13 (59%)	15 (68%)	Ortega (1972)
CYTOSAR—thioguanine	19	9 (47%)	9 (47%)	Bryan (1974)

Table 4: CYTOSAR

Acute Lymphocytic Leukemia—Remission Induction—Previously Treated Patients, Adults and Children

	No. Patients Evaluated	Complete Remissions	Investigator
High-dose Therapy			
CYTOSAR	8	3 (38%)	Rohatinar (1983)
CYTOSAR—doxorubicin	3	2 (67%)	Willemze (1982)
CYTOSAR—asparaginase	10	3 (30%)	Capizzi (1983)

CYTOSAR has been used intrathecally with Solu-Cortef sterile powder and methotrexate, both as prophylaxis in newly diagnosed children with acute lymphocytic leukemia, as well as in the treatment of meningeal leukemia. Sullivan has reported that prophylactic triple therapy has prevented late CNS disease and given overall cure and survival rates similar to those seen in patients in whom CNS radiation and intrathecal methotrexate was used as initial CNS prophylaxis. The dose of CYTOSAR was 30 mg/m², Solu-Cortef 15 mg/m², and methotrexate 15 mg/m². The physician should be familiar with this report before initiation of the regimen.

Prophylactic triple therapy following the successful treatment of the acute meningeal episode may be useful. The physician should familiarize himself with the current literature before instituting such a program. Focal leukemic involvement of the CNS may not respond to intrathecal CYTOSAR and may better be treated with radiotherapy.

If used intrathecally, do not use a diluent containing benzyl alcohol. Reconstitute with preservative-free saline and use immediately.

Non-Hodgkin's Lymphoma in Children: CYTOSAR has been used as part of a multi-drug program (LSA_2L_2) to treat non-Hodgkin's lymphoma in children.

CONTRAINDICATIONS: Patients who are hypersensitive to the drug.

WARNINGS: For induction therapy, patients should be treated in a facility with laboratory and supportive resources sufficient to monitor drug tolerance and protect and maintain a patient compromised by drug toxicity. The main toxic effect of CYTOSAR is bone marrow suppression with leukopenia, thrombocytopenia and anemia. Less serious toxicity includes nausea, vomiting, diarrhea and abdominal pain, oral ulceration, and hepatic dysfunction.

The physician must judge possible benefit to the patient against known toxic effects of this drug in considering the advisability of therapy with CYTOSAR. Before making this judgment or beginning treatment, the physician should be familiar with the following text.

CYTOSAR (cytarabine) is a potent bone marrow suppressant. Therapy should be started cautiously in patients with pre-existing drug-induced bone marrow suppression. Patients receiving this drug must be under close medical supervision and during induction therapy, should have leukocyte and platelet counts performed daily. Bone marrow examinations should be performed frequently after blasts have disappeared from the peripheral blood. Facilities should be available for management of complications (possibly fatal) of bone marrow suppression (infection resulting from granulocytopenia and other impaired body defenses, and hemorrhage secondary to thrombocytopenia). One case of anaphylaxis that resulted in acute cardiopulmonary arrest and required resuscitation has been reported. This occurred immediately after the intravenous administration of CYTOSAR.

Severe and at times fatal, CNS, GI and pulmonary toxicity (different from that seen with conventional therapy regimens of CYTOSAR) has been reported following high dose schedules (2 to 3 g/m²) of CYTOSAR. These reactions include reversible corneal toxicity and hemorrhagic conjunctivitis, which may be prevented or diminished by prophylaxis with a local corticosteroid eye drop; cerebral and cerebellar dysfunction including personality changes, somnolence and coma, usually reversible; severe gastrointestinal ulceration, including pneumatosis cystoides intestinalis, leading to peritonitis; sepsis and liver abscess; and pulmonary edema; liver damage with increased hyperbilirubinemia; bowel necrosis; and necrotizing colitis. Two patients treated with conventional doses of CYTOSAR sterile powder and daunomycin developed abdominal tenderness (peritonitis) and guaiac positive colitis. Both patients responded to nonoperative medical management. Both patients exhibited neutropenia and thrombocytopenia and were receiving numerous other drugs. The authors recommend careful, conservative management in patients receiving CYTOSAR who appear to have a surgical abdomen, but in whom a definitive surgical diagnosis cannot be made. Two patients with childhood acute myelogenous leukemia who received intrathecal and intravenous CYTOSAR at conventional doses, in addition to a number of other concomitantly administered drugs, developed delayed progressive ascending paralysis resulting in death in one of the two patients.

Rarely, severe skin rash, leading to desquamation has been reported. Complete alopecia is more commonly seen with high-dose therapy than with standard CYTOSAR treatment programs.

If high-dose therapy is used, do not use a diluent containing benzyl alcohol. Benzyl alcohol is contained in the diluent for this product. Benzyl alcohol has been reported to be associated with a fatal "Gasping Syndrome" in premature infants.

An increase in cardiomyopathy with subsequent death has been reported following experimental high dose CYTOSAR and cyclophosphamide therapy when used for bone marrow transplant preparation. This may be schedule dependent.

A syndrome of sudden respiratory distress, rapidly progressing to pulmonary edema and radiographically pronounced cardiomegaly has been reported following experimental high dose CYTOSAR therapy used for the treatment of relapsed leukemia from one institution in 16/72 patients. In one case, the outcome was fatal.

Acute pancreatitis has been reported to occur in patients being treated with CYTOSAR in combination with other drugs.

Carcinogenesis, Mutagenesis, Impairment of Fertility: Extensive chromosomal damage, including chromatoid breaks, have been produced by cytarabine and malignant transformation of rodent cells in culture has been reported.

Pregnancy: CYTOSAR is known to be teratogenic in some animal species. Use of this drug in women who are or who may become pregnant should be undertaken only after due consideration of potential benefit and potential hazard to both mother and child. Women of childbearing potential should be advised to avoid becoming pregnant.

A review of the literature has shown 32 reported cases where CYTOSAR was given during pregnancy, either alone or in combination with other cytotoxic agents. Eighteen normal infants were delivered. Four of these had first trimester exposure. Five infants were premature or of low birth weight. Twelve of the 18 normal infants were followed up at ages ranging from 6 weeks to 7 years, and showed no abnormalities. One apparently normal infant died at 90 days of gastroenteritis.

Two cases of congenital abnormalities have been reported, one with upper and lower distal limb defects, and the other with extremity and ear deformities. Both of these cases had first trimester exposure.

There were 7 infants with various problems in the neonatal period, including pancytopenia; transient depression of WBC, hematocrit or platelets; electrolyte abnormalities; transient eosinophilia; and one case of increased IgM levels and hyperpyrexia possibly due to sepsis. Six of the 7 infants were also premature. The child with pancytopenia died at 21 days of sepsis.

Therapeutic abortions were done in 5 cases. Four fetuses were grossly normal, but one had an enlarged spleen and another showed Trisomy C chromosome abnormality in the chorionic tissue.

Because of the potential for abnormalities with cytotoxic therapy, particularly during the first trimester, a patient who is or who becomes pregnant while on CYTOSAR should be apprised of the potential risk to the fetus and the advisability of pregnancy continuation. There is a definite, but considerably reduced risk if therapy is initiated during the second or third trimester. Although normal infants have been delivered to patients treated in all three trimesters of pregnancy, follow-up of such infants would be advisable.

Lactation: It is not known whether this drug is excreted in human milk. Because many drugs are excreted in human milk and because of the potential for serious adverse reactions in nursing infants from cytarabine, a decision should be made whether to discontinue nursing or to discontinue the drug, taking into account the importance of the drug to the mother.

PRECAUTIONS: Patients receiving CYTOSAR (cytarabine) must be monitored closely. Frequent platelet and leukocyte counts and bone marrow examinations are mandatory. Consider suspending or modifying therapy when drug-induced marrow depression has resulted in a platelet count under 50 000 or a polymorphonuclear granulocyte count under 1000/mm^3. Counts of formed elements in the peripheral blood may continue to fall after the drug is stopped and reach lowest values after drug-free intervals of 12 to 24 days. When indicated, restart therapy when definite signs of marrow recovery appear (on successive bone marrow studies). Patients whose drug is withheld until "normal" peripheral blood values are attained, may escape from control.

When large intravenous doses are given quickly, patients are frequently nauseated and may vomit for several hours post injection. This problem tends to be less severe when the drug is infused.

The human liver apparently detoxifies a substantial fraction of an administered cytarabine dose. In particular, patients with renal or hepatic function impairment may have a higher likelihood of CNS toxicity after high-dose treatment with CYTOSAR. Use the drug with caution and at reduced dose in patients whose liver function is poor.

Periodic checks of bone marrow, liver and kidney function should be performed in patients receiving CYTOSAR.

Children: The safety of the drug for use in infants is not established.

Like other cytotoxic drugs, CYTOSAR may induce hyperuricemia secondary to rapid lysis of neoplastic cells. The clinician should monitor the patient's blood uric acid level and be prepared to use such supportive and pharmacologic measurements as might be necessary to control this problem.

ADVERSE EFFECTS: Because CYTOSAR (cytarabine) is a bone marrow suppressant, anemia, leukopenia, thrombocytopenia, megaloblastosis, and reduced reticulocytes can be expected as a result of its administration. The severity of these reactions are dose and schedule dependent. Cellular changes in the morphology of bone marrows and peripheral smears can be expected.

Following 5 day constant infusions or acute injections of 50 mg/m^2 to 600 mg/m^2, white cell depression follows a biphasic course. Regardless of initial count, dosage level, or schedule, there is an initial fall starting the first 24 hours with a nadir at days 7 to 9. This is followed by a brief rise which peaks around the twelfth day. A second and deeper fall reaches nadir at days 15 to 24. Then there is a rapid rise to above baseline in the next 10 days. Platelet depression is noticeable at 5 days with a peak depression occurring between days 12 to 15. Thereupon, a rapid rise to above baseline occurs in the next 10 days.

Infectious Complications: Infection: Viral, bacterial, fungal, parasitic, or saprophytic infections, in any location on the body, may be associated with the use of CYTOSAR alone or in combination with other immunosuppressive agents following immunosuppressive doses that affect cellular or humoral immunity. These infections may be mild, but can be severe and at times fatal.

The Cytarabine Syndrome: A cytarabine syndrome has been described by Castleberry. It is characterized by fever, myalgia, bone pain, occasionally chest pain, maculopapular rash, conjunctivitis and malaise. It usually occurs 6 to 12 hours following drug administration. Corticosteroids have been shown to be beneficial in treating or preventing this syndrome. If the symptoms of the syndrome are deemed treatable, corticosteroids should be contemplated as well as continuation of therapy with CYTOSAR.

The following additional adverse reactions have been reported with the use of CYTOSAR: anorexia, nausea, vomiting, diarrhea, oral and anal inflammation or ulceration, rash, hepatic dysfunction, fever and thrombophlebitis. Nausea and vomiting are most frequent following rapid intravenous injection. Less frequent adverse reactions are bleeding (all sites), sepsis, pneumonia, cellulitis at injection site, skin ulceration, urinary retention, renal dysfunction, neuritis, neural toxicity, sore throat, esophageal ulceration, esophagitis, chest pain, pericarditis, bowel necrosis, abdominal pain, freckling, jaundice, conjunctivitis (may occur with rash), dizziness, alopecia, anaphylaxis, allergic edema, pruritus, shortness of breath, urticaria and headache.

High-Dose Therapy: Severe and at times fatal CNS, GI and pulmonary toxicity (different from that seen with conventional therapy regimens of CYTOSAR) has been reported following high dose schedules (2 to 3 g/m^2 every 12 hours for 12 doses). These reactions include reversible corneal toxicity and hemorrhagic conjunctivitis, which may be prevented or diminished by prophylaxis with a local corticosteroid eyedrop; cerebral and cerebellar dysfunction including personality changes, somnolence and coma, usually reversible; severe gastrointestinal ulceration, including pneumatosis cystoides intestinalis leading to peritonitis; sepsis and liver abscess; and pulmonary edema; liver damage with increased bilirubin; bowel necrosis; and necrotizing colitis.

Two patients with adult acute non-lymphocytic leukemia developed peripheral motor and sensory neuropathies after consolidation with high-dose CYTOSAR, daunorubicin, and asparaginase. Patients treated with high-dose CYTOSAR should be observed for neuropathy since dose schedule alterations may be needed to avoid irreversible neurologic disorders.

Ten patients treated with experimental intermediate doses of CYTOSAR(1 g/m^2) with and without other chemotherapeutic agents (meta-AMSA, daunorubicin, VP 16) developed a diffuse interstitial pneumonitis without clear cause that may have been related to the CYTOSAR.

Rarely, severe skin rash leading to desquamation has been reported. Complete alopecia is more commonly seen with high dose therapy than with standard CYTOSAR treatment programs. If high dose therapy is used, do not use a diluent containing benzyl alcohol.

CYTOSAR given intrathecally may cause systemic toxicity and careful monitoring of the hemopoietic system is indicated. Modification of other anti-leukemia therapy may be necessary. Major toxicity is rare. The most frequently reported reactions after intrathecal administration were nausea, vomiting and fever; these reactions are mild and self-limiting. Paraplegia has been reported. Necrotizing leukoencephalopathy occurred in 5 children; these patients had also been treated with intrathecal methotrexate and hydrocortisone, as well as by CNS radiation. Isolated neurotoxicity has been reported. Blindness occurred in 2 patients in remission whose treatment had consisted of combination systemic chemotherapy, prophylactic CNS radiation and intrathecal CYTOSAR. When CYTOSAR is administered both intrathecally and intravenously within a few days, there is an increased risk of spinal cord toxicity, however, in serious life-threatening disease, concurrent use of intravenous and intrathecal CYTOSAR is left to the discretion of the treating physician.

Corneal toxicity consisting of ocular pain, tearing, foreign-body sensation, photophobia and blurred vision have been reported.

One case of anaphylaxis that resulted in acute cardiopulmonary arrest and required resuscitation has been reported. This occurred immediately after the intravenous administration of CYTOSAR.

OVERDOSE:

Symptoms: Chronic overdosage may cause serious bone marrow suppression. Daily hematological evaluation should be performed to prevent overdosage. Nausea and vomiting, although a general side effect of the drug, may be an additional warning of overdosage. Severe hemorrhage into the gastrointestinal tract may indicate overdosage as may severe generalized infections.

Doses exceeding recommended dosage schedules have been used clinically and have been tolerated. The major toxicity with the use of 3 g/m^{2}intravenous infusion over 1 hour every 12 hours for 12 doses and 3 g/m^2 continuous infusion for 4 days, other than reversible bone marrow suppression has been reversible corneal, cerebral and cerebellar dysfunction. Doses of 4.5 g/m^2 intravenous infusion over 1 hour every 12 hours for 12 doses has caused an unacceptable increase in irreversible toxicity and death.

Treatment:

There is no antidote for CYTOSAR (cytarabine) overdosage.

Discontinuation of the drug and supportive therapy are of course indicated. Transfusions of platelets should be given if there is any sign of hemorrhage. Patients should be carefully observed for intercurrent infection and if such appears they should be rapidly and rigorously treated with appropriate antibiotic therapy.

For management of a suspected drug overdose, CPhA recommends that you contact your **regional Poison Control Centre**. See the *CPS* Directory section for a list of Poison Control Centres.

DOSAGE: **Caution:** The following precautionary measures are recommended in proceeding with the preparation and handling of cytotoxic agents such as CYTOSAR (cytarabine):

1. The procedure should be carried out in a vertical laminar flow hood (Biological Safety Cabinet—Class II).
2. Personnel should wear: PVC gloves, safety glasses, disposable gowns and masks.
3. All needles, syringes, vials, and other materials which have come in contact with CYTOSAR should be segregated and destroyed by incineration (sealed containers may explode). If incineration is not available, neutralization should be carried out using 5% sodium hypochlorite, or 5% sodium thiosulfate.
4. Personnel regularly involved in the preparation and handling of CYTOSAR should have biannual hematologic examinations.

CYTOSAR is not active orally. The schedule and method of administration varies with the program of therapy to be used. CYTOSAR may be given by intravenous infusion, injection/subcutaneously or intrathecally. Thrombophlebitis has occurred at the site of drug injection or infusion in some patients, and rarely patients have noted pain and inflammation at subcutaneous injection sites. In most instances, however, the drug has been well tolerated.

Patients can tolerate higher total doses when they receive the drug by rapid intravenous injection as compared with slow infusion. This phenomenon is related to the drug's rapid inactivation and brief exposure of susceptible normal and neoplastic cells to significant levels after rapid injection. Normal and neoplastic cells seem to respond to somewhat parallel fashion to these different modes of administration and no clear-cut clinical advantage has been demonstrated for either.

Clinical experience accumulated to date suggests that success with CYTOSAR is dependent more on adeptness in modifying day-to-day dosage to obtain maximum leukemic cell kill with tolerable toxicity than on the basic treatment schedule chosen at the outset of therapy. Toxicity necessitating dosage alteration almost always occurs.

Relatively constant plasma levels can be achieved by continuous intravenous infusion.

In many chemotherapeutic programs, CYTOSAR is used in combination with other cytotoxic drugs. The addition of these cytotoxic drugs has necessitated changes and dose alterations. The dosage schedules for combination therapy outlined below have been reported in the literature.

Dosage Schedules: Acute Myelocytic Leukemia: Induction remission: Adults: CYTOSAR 200 mg/m^2 daily by continuous infusion for 5 days (120 hours). Total dose 1000 mg/m^2. This course is repeated approximately every 2 weeks. Modifications must be made based on hematologic response.

Meningeal Leukemia: Intrathecal Use: (see Indications and Warnings).

High-dose Chemotherapy: Before instituting a program of high dose chemotherapy, the physician should be familiar with the literature, adverse reactions, precautions, contraindications, and warnings applicable to all the drugs involved in the program: CYTOSAR: 2 g/m^2 infused over 3 hours every 12 hours×12 doses (Days 1 to 6). 3 g/m^2 infused over 1 hour every 12 hours×12 doses (Days 1 to 6). 3 g/m^2 infused over 75 minutes every 12 hours×12 doses (Days 1 to 6).

CYTOSAR—Doxorubicin: CYTOSAR: 3 g/m^2 infused over 2 hours every 12 hours×12 doses (Days 1 to 6). Doxorubicin: 30 mg/m^2 i.v. on Days 6 and 7.

CYTOSAR—Asparaginase: CYTOSAR: 3 g/m^2 infused over 3 hours at 0 hours, 12 hours, 24 hours, and 36 hours. At 42 hours, 6 000 units/m^2 of asparaginase i.m. (Days 1 and 2); repeat same schedules Days 8 and 9.

Combined Chemotherapy: Before instituting a program of combined chemotherapy, the physician should be familiar with the literature, adverse reactions, precautions, contraindications, and warnings applicable to all the drugs involved in the program.

CYTOSAR—Doxorubicin: CYTOSAR 100 mg/m^2/day, continuous i.v. infusion (Days 1 to 10). Doxorubicin: 30 mg/m^2/day, i.v. infusion of 30 minutes (Days 1 to 3).

Additional (complete or modified) courses as necessary at 2 to 4 week intervals if leukemia is persistent.

CYTOSAR—Thioguanine—Daunorubicin: CYTOSAR: 100 mg/m^2, i.v. infusion over 30 minutes every 12 hours (Days 1 to 7). Thioguanine: 100 mg/m^2, orally every 12 hours (Days 1 to 7). Daunorubicin: 60 mg/m^2/day, i.v. infusion (Days 5 to 7).

Additional (complete or modified) courses as necessary at 2 to 4 week intervals if leukemia is persistent.

CYTOSAR—Doxorubicin—Vincristine—Prednisone: CYTOSAR: 100 mg/m^2/day, continuous i.v. infusion (Days 1 to 7). Doxorubicin: 30 mg/m^2/day, i.v. infusion (Days 1 to 3). Vincristine: 1.5 mg/m^2/day, i.v. infusion (Days 1 and 5). Prednisone: 40 mg/m^2/day, i.v. infusion every 12 hours (Days 1 to 5).

Additional (complete or modified) courses as necessary at 2 to 4 week intervals if leukemia is persistent.

CYTOSAR—Daunorubicin—Thioguanine—Prednisone— Vincristine: CYTOSAR: 100 mg/m^2/day, i.v. infusion (Days 1 to 10). Daunorubicin: 70 mg/m^2/day, i.v. infusion (Days 1 to 3). Thioguanine: 100 mg/m^2, orally every 12 hours (Days 1 to 7). Prednisone: 40 mg/m^2/day, orally (Days 1 to 7). Vincristine: 1 mg/m^2/day, i.v. infusion (Days 1 and 7).

Additional (complete or modified) courses as necessary at 2 to 4 week intervals if leukemia is persistent.

CYTOSAR—Daunorubicin: CYTOSAR: 100 mg/m^2/day, continuous i.v. infusion (Days 1 to 7). Daunorubicin: 45 mg/m^2/day, i.v. push (Days 1 to 3).

Additional (complete or modified) courses as necessary at 2 to 4 week intervals if leukemia is persistent.

Acute Myelocytic Leukemia: Maintenance: Adults: Maintenance programs are modifications of induction programs and, in general, use similar schedules of drug therapy as were used during induction. Most programs have a greater time spacing between courses of therapy during remission maintenance.

Acute Myelocytic Leukemia: Induction and Maintenance: In Children: Numerous studies have shown that childhood AML responds better than adult AML given similar regimens. Where the adult dosage is stated in terms of body weight or surface area, the children's dosage may be calculated on the same basis. When specified amounts of a drug are indicated for the adult dosage, these should be adjusted for children on the basis of such factors as age, body weight or body surface area.

Acute Lymphocytic Leukemia: In general, dosage schedules are similar to those used in acute myelocytic leukemia with some modifications. For dosage recommendations see referenced literature in Table 3 and Table 4 under Indications.

Non-Hodgkin's Lymphoma in Children: CYTOSAR has been used as part of a multidrug program (LSA_2L_2) to treat non-Hodgkin's lymphoma in children.

LSA_2-L_2 Protocol: Woolner N, Burchenal JH, Lieberman PH, et al: Non-Hodgkin's Lymphoma in Children—A Comparative Study of Two Modalities of Therapy. Cancer 37:123-134,1976.

Induction Phase: Day 1. Cyclophosphamide 1 200 mg/m^2 single push injection. Day 3 to 31. Prednisone 60 mg/m^2 orally divided into 3 daily doses. Day 3, 10, 17, 24. Vincristine 1.5 to 2.25 mg/m^2 i.v. Day 5, 27, 30. Spinal tap and intrathecal injection of methotrexate 6.25 mg/m^2. Day 12, 13. Daunomycin 60 mg/m^2 i.v.

At the end of induction (last dose of intrathecal methotrexate) patient rests for 3 to 5 days before consolidation.

Consolidation Phase: Day 34 or 36, daily i.v. injections of cytosine arabinoside (Ara-C) 150 mg/m^2 for a total of 15 injections are given. (Injections are given from Monday through Friday.) Thioguanine 75 mg/m^2 is given orally, 8 to 12 hours after the injection of Ara-C. If the white blood count is 1500 or more and the platelet count 150 000 or more on the 5th day of Ara-C, the patient continues to receive the same dosage of thioguanine over the weekend. However, both are discontinued temporarily when there is evidence of marrow depression; this usually occurs after the initial seventh to tenth doses of the combination and ordinarily recovers within 7 to 10 days. Hence, the patients may receive more than 15 doses of thioguanine orally, but receive only 15 doses of i.v. cytosine arabinoside (Ara-C). This first phase of the consolidation takes an average of 30 to 35 days. The second phase of the consolidation should be started immediately after completion of the 15 doses of Ara-C; it entails daily i.v. administration of L asparaginase, 60 000 U/m^2 for a total of 12 injections, excluding weekends.

Two days after the last injection of the L-asparaginase, 2 more intrathecal injections of methotrexate are given 2 days apart. Three days after the last intrathecal methotrexate, BCNU (1, 3-Bis (2 chloroethyl 1-1-nitrosourea)) 60 mg/m^2 is given i.v., which completes the consolidation. The average duration of the induction and consolidation is 85 to 100 days.

Maintenance Phase: The maintenance period consists of 5 cycles of 5 days each and is started 3 to 4 days after completion of consolidation.

Cycle I: Oral thioguanine 300 mg/m^2 for 4 consecutive days: i.v. cyclophosphamide 600 mg/m^2 on the 5th day. Rest 7 to 10 days.

Cycle II: Oral hydroxyurea 2 400 mg/m^2 for 4 consecutive days: i.v. daunomycin 45 mg/m^2 on the 5th day. Rest 7 to 10 days.

Cycle III: Oral methotrexate 10 mg/m^2 for 4 consecutive days: i.v. BCNU 60 mg/m^2 on the 5th day. Rest 7 to 10 days.

Cycle IV: I.V. Ara-C 150 mg/m^2 for 4 consecutive days: i.v. vincristine 1.5 mg/m^2 on day 5. Rest 7 to 10 days.

Cycle V: Two doses of intrathecal methotrexate 6.25 mg/m^2 2 to 3 days apart. Rest 7 to 10 days and restart with Cycle I.

Dosage Modification: The dosage of CYTOSAR must be modified or suspended when signs of serious hematologic depression appear. In general, consider discontinuing the drug if the patient has less than 50 000 platelets or 1000 polymorphonuclear granulocytes/mm^3 in his peripheral blood. These guidelines may be modified depending on signs of toxicity in other systems and on the rapidity of fall in formed blood elements. Restart the drug when there are signs of marrow recovery and the above platelet and granulocyte levels have been attained. Withholding therapy until the patient's blood values are normal may result in escape of the patient's disease from control by the drug.

Intrathecal Use in Meningeal Leukemia: CYTOSAR has been used intrathecally in acute leukemia in doses ranging from 5 mg/m^2 to 75 mg/m^2 of body surface area. The frequency of administration varied from once a day for 4 days to once every 4 days. The most frequently used dose was 30 mg/m^2 every 4 days until cerebrospinal fluid findings were normal, followed by one additional treatment. The dosage schedule is usually governed by the type and severity of CNS manifestations and the response to previous therapy.

CYTOSAR has been used intrathecally with Solu-Cortef sterile powder and methotrexate, both as prophylaxis in newly diagnosed children with acute lymphocytic leukemia, as well as in the treatment of meningeal leukemia. Sullivan has reported that prophylactic triple therapy has prevented late CNS disease and given overall cure and survival rates similar to those seen in patients in whom CNS radiation and intrathecal methotrexate was used as initial CNS prophylaxis. The dose of CYTOSAR was 30 mg/m², Solu-Cortef 15 mg/m², and methotrexate 15 mg/m². The physician should be familiar with this report before initiation of the regimen.

Prophylactic triple therapy following the successful treatment of the acute meningeal episode may be useful. The physician should familiarize himself with the current literature before instituting such a program.

CYTOSAR given intrathecally may cause systemic toxicity and careful monitoring of the hemopoietic system is indicated. Modification of the antileukemia therapy may be necessary. Major toxicity is rare. The most frequently reported reactions after intrathecal administration were nausea, vomiting and fever; these reactions are mild and self-limiting. Paraplegia has been reported. Necrotizing leukoencephalopathy occurred in 5 children; these patients had also been treated with intrathecal methotrexate and hydrocortisone, as well as by CNS radiation. Isolated neurotoxicity has been reported. Blindness occurred in 2 patients in remission whose treatment had consisted of combination systemic chemotherapy, prophylactic CNS radiation and intrathecal CYTOSAR.

Focal leukemic involvement of the CNS may not respond to intrathecal CYTOSAR and may better be treated with radiotherapy.

Intrathecal Use: If solutions are used intrathecally, do not use a diluent containing benzyl alcohol. Reconstitute with preservative-free 0.9% Sodium Chloride for Injection. Use immediately.

High-dose Use: Do not use diluent containing benzyl alcohol.

Chemical Stability and Compatibility: CYTOSAR is compatible for 24 hours at 5°C with Lactated Ringers, Dextrose 5% in Water, 0.9% Sodium Chloride, Dextrose 5% in Water in 0.9% Sodium Chloride.

CYTOSAR 0.8 mg/mL and sodium cephalothin 1.0 mg/mL are chemically stable for 8 hours in dextrose 5% in water.

CYTOSAR 0.4 mg/mL and prednisolone sodium phosphate 0.2 mg/mL are compatible in dextrose 5% in water for 8 hours.

CYTOSAR 16 µg/mL and vincristine sulfate 4 µg/mL are compatible in dextrose 5% in water for 8 hours.

CYTOSAR has been known to be physically incompatible with heparin, insulin, methotrexate, 5-fluorouracil, penicillin G, and Solu-Medrol.

As with all i.v. admixtures, dilution should be made just prior to administration and the resulting unpreserved solution used within 24 hours.

Reconstitution: CYTOSAR sterile powder may be reconstituted with the following diluents: 0.9% Sodium Chloride for injection, Dextrose 5% in Water, Sterile Water for Injection, Bacteriostatic Water for Injection. pH of reconstituted solution is approximately 5. Solutions reconstituted without a preservative should be used immediately. Solutions reconstituted with Bacteriostatic Water for Injection with Benzyl Alcohol 0.9% (for multidose use) may be stored at controlled room temperature (15 to 30°C) for 48 hours. Discard any solution in which a slight haze develops.

When reconstituted with a diluent the following concentrations result as shown in Table 5.

Table 5: CYTOSAR

Reconstitution

Vial Size	Volume of Diluent to be Added to Vial	Nominal Concentration
100 mg	5 mL	20 mg/mL
1 g	10 mL	100 mg/mL

SUPPLIED: 100 mg: Each vial of freeze-dried preparation contains: cytarabine 100 mg. Vials of 5 mL, packs of 5.
1 g: Each vial of freeze-dried preparation contains: cytarabine 1 g. Single vials.
Storage Recommendations Sterile powder: Store at controlled room temperature (15-30°C).

Cytovene® Pr

ganciclovir sodium

Antiviral Agent

Roche

Date of Revision: May 29, 2008

SUMMARY PRODUCT INFORMATION:

Route of Administration	Dosage Form/ Strength	Clinically Relevant Nonmedicinal Ingredients
Intravenous	Ganciclovir, 50 mg/mL when reconstituted	For a complete listing see Dosage Forms, Composition and Packaging.

INDICATIONS AND CLINICAL USE: CYTOVENE (ganciclovir sodium for injection) is indicated for the treatment of CMV retinitis in immunocompromised patients, including patients with acquired immunodeficiency syndrome (AIDS), iatrogenic suppression secondary to organ transplantation or those administered chemotherapy for neoplasia. CYTOVENE is also indicated for the prevention of CMV disease in transplant recipients at risk for CMV disease.

The diagnosis of CMV retinitis is primarily an ophthalmologic one and should be made by indirect ophthalmoscopy. Other conditions in the differential diagnosis of CMV retinitis include candidiasis, toxoplasmosis, histoplasmosis, retinal scars, and cotton wool spots, any of which may produce a retinal appearance similar to CMV. For this reason it is essential that the diagnosis of CMV be established by an ophthalmologist familiar with the retinal presentation of these conditions. The diagnosis of CMV retinitis may be aided by culture of CMV from urine, blood, throat, or other sites, but a negative CMV culture does not rule out CMV retinitis.

Geriatrics: No studies on the efficacy or safety of CYTOVENE specifically in elderly patients have been conducted. Since elderly individuals may have reduced renal function, CYTOVENE should be administered to the elderly patients with care and with special consideration of their renal status (see Dosage and Administration, Renal Impairment).

Pediatrics: The safety and efficacy of CYTOVENE in children has not been established. The use of CYTOVENE warrants extreme caution due to the probability of long-term carcinogenicity and reproductive toxicity. Administration to children should be undertaken only after careful evaluation and only of the potential benefits of treatment outweigh these considerable risks.

CONTRAINDICATIONS: CYTOVENE (ganciclovir sodium for injection) is contraindicated in patients who are hypersensitive to ganciclovir, valganciclovir or to any component of the product.

Due to the similarity of the chemical structure of CYTOVENE and that of acyclovir and valacyclovir, a cross-hypersensitivity reaction between these drugs is possible.

WARNINGS AND PRECAUTIONS:

Serious Warnings and Precautions

The clinical toxicity of CYTOVENE (ganciclovir sodium for injection) includes granulocytopenia, anemia and thrombocytopenia. In animal and in vitro studies, ganciclovir was mutagenic, teratogenic, carcinogenic and caused aspermatogenesis; therefore it should be considered a potential teratogen and carcinogen in humans.

CYTOVENE is indicated for use only in immunocompromised patients, where the potential benefit outweighs the risks stated herein.

The safety and efficacy of CYTOVENE have not been evaluated for congenital or neonatal CMV disease, nor for treatment of CMV infection in non-immunocompromised individuals (see Indications and Clinical Use).

General: In clinical studies with CYTOVENE, the maximum single dose studied has been 6 mg/kg infused intravenously over one hour. Larger doses have resulted in increased toxicity. It is likely that more rapid infusions would also result in increased toxicity.

Administration of CYTOVENE should be accompanied by adequate hydration. Since ganciclovir is excreted by the kidneys, normal clearance depends on adequate renal function. **If renal function is impaired, dosage adjustments are required.** Such adjustments should be based on measured or estimated creatinine clearance values (see Dosage and Administration, Renal Impairment).

For patients on hemodialysis (CrCl <10 mL/min) it is recommended that intravenous ganciclovir be used (see Dosage and Administration, Renal Impairment).

Hemodialysis reduces plasma concentrations of ganciclovir by approximately 50% (see Dosage and Administration, Hemodialysis).

Carcinogenesis and Mutagenesis: Ganciclovir caused point mutations and chromosomal damage in mammalian cells in vitro and in vivo, but did not cause point mutations in bacterial or yeast cells, dominant lethality in mice, or morphologically transformed cells in vitro.

In a study conducted over 18 months, ganciclovir was carcinogenic in the mouse after oral doses of 20 and 1000 mg/kg/day (approximately 0.1× and 1.4×, respectively, based on area under the plasma concentration curve [AUC] comparisons). The principally affected tissues at the dose of 1000 mg/kg/day were the preputial gland in males, forestomach (nonglandular mucosa) in males and females, and reproductive tissues and liver in females. At dose of 20 mg/kg/day, slightly increased tumor incidences occurred in the preputial and harderian glands in males, forestomach in males and females, and liver in females. All ganciclovir-induced tumours were of epithelial or vascular origin except for histiocytic sarcoma of the liver. No carcinogenic effect occurred at 1 mg/kg/day (estimated as 0.01× the human dose based on AUC comparison). The preputial and clitoral glands, forestomach and harderian glands of mice have no human counterpart. CYTOVENE should be considered a potential carcinogen in humans.

Hematologic: CYTOVENE should not be administered if the absolute neutrophil count is less than 500 cells/µL or the platelet count is less than 25 000 cells/µL or the hemoglobin is less than 80 g/L. Severe leukopenia, neutropenia, anemia, thrombocytopenia, pancytopenia, bone marrow depression and aplastic anemia have been observed in patients treated with CYTOVENE. The frequency and severity of these events vary widely in different patient populations (see Warnings and Precautions, Monitoring and Laboratory Tests; Dosage and Administration, Patients with Severe Leukopenia, Neutropenia, Anemia, Thrombocytopenia and/or Pancytopenia; Adverse Reactions). CYTOVENE should therefore, be used with caution in patients with pre-existing cytopenias, or with a history of cytopenic reactions to other drugs, chemicals, or irradiation.

Neutropenia: Neutropenia typically occurs during the first or second week of induction therapy and prior to administration of a total cumulative dose of 200 mg/kg of CYTOVENE but may occur at any time during treatment. Evidence of recovery of cell counts usually occurs within 3 to 7 days after discontinuing the drug. Colony stimulating factors have been shown to increase neutrophil and white blood cell counts in patients receiving CYTOVENE for treatment of CMV retinitis.

Thrombocytopenia: Thrombocytopenia (platelet count of less than 50 000 cells/µL) was observed in patients treated with CYTOVENE. Immunodeficient patients without AIDS were more likely to develop lowered platelet counts than those with AIDS. Patients with initial platelet counts less than 100 000 cells/µL were also at increased risk of this toxicity of CYTOVENE.

Renal: It is possible that probenecid, as well as other drugs which inhibit renal tubular secretion or resorption, may reduce renal clearance of ganciclovir and could increase its plasma half-life.

Use in Patients with Renal Impairment: CYTOVENE should be used with caution in patients with impaired renal function. Both the plasma half-life of ganciclovir as well as peak plasma levels are increased in patients with elevated serum creatinine levels.

Patients Undergoing Hemodialysis: Hemodialysis reduces plasma concentrations of ganciclovir by approximately 50% after i.v. administration (see Dosage and Administration, Hemodialysis).

Sexual Function/Reproduction: Animal data indicate that administration of ganciclovir caused inhibition of spermatogenesis and subsequent infertility, which were reversible at lower doses and irreversible at higher doses (see Warnings and Precautions, Carcinogenesis and Mutagenesis). Although clinical data have not yet been obtained regarding this effect, **it is considered probable that CYTOVENE at the recommended doses may cause temporary or permanent inhibition of spermatogenesis in humans. Animal data also indicate that suppression of fertility in females may occur.**

Because of the mutagenic and teratogenic potential of ganciclovir, women of childbearing potential should be advised to use effective contraception during treatment with CYTOVENE. Similarly men should be advised to practice barrier contraception during and for at least 90 days following treatment with CYTOVENE (see Warnings and Precautions, Carcinogenesis and Mutagenesis).

CYTOVENE is considered to be a potential teratogen and carcinogen in humans with the potential to cause birth defects and cancers (see Special Handling Instructions).

Female mice exhibited decreased fertility, decreased mating behaviour, and increased embryolethality after daily intravenous doses of 90 mg/kg (approximately 1.7× the mean drug exposure in humans following the dose of 5 mg/kg, based on AUC comparisons).

In male mice, fertility was decreased after daily intravenous doses of ≥2 mg/kg and daily oral doses of ≥10 mg/kg. These effects were reversible after daily intravenous doses of 2 mg/kg and daily oral doses of 10 mg/kg, but were irreversible or incompletely reversible after daily intravenous doses of 10 mg/kg and daily oral doses of 100 or 1000 mg/kg. Ganciclovir has also caused hypospermatogenesis in rats after daily oral doses of ≥100 mg/kg and in dogs after daily intravenous and oral doses of ≥0.4 mg/kg and 0.2 mg/kg, respectively.

Ganciclovir has been shown to be embryotoxic in rabbits and mice following intravenous administration, and teratogenic in rabbits. Fetal resorptions were present in at least 85% of rabbits and mice administered 60 mg/kg/day and 108 mg/kg/day (2× the human exposure based on AUC comparisons), respectively. Effects observed in rabbits included: fetal growth retardation, embryolethality, teratogenicity and/or maternal toxicity. Teratogenic changes included cleft palate, anophthalmia/microphthalmia, aplastic organs (kidney and pancreas), hydrocephaly and brachygnathia. In mice, effects observed were maternal/fetal toxicity and embryolethality.

Daily intravenous doses of 90 mg/kg ganciclovir administered to female mice prior to mating, during gestation, and during lactation caused hypoplasia of the testes and seminal vesicles in the month old male offspring, as well as pathologic changes in the nonglandular region of the stomach. The drug exposure in mice as estimated by the AUC was approximately 1.7× the human AUC.

Skin: Initially reconstituted solutions of CYTOVENE have a high pH (ph 11). Despite further dilution in intravenous fluids, phlebitis and/or pain may occur at the site of intravenous infusion. Care must be taken to infuse solutions containing CYTOVENE only into veins with adequate blood flow to permit rapid dilution and distribution (see Dosage and Administration).

Special Populations: Animal data indicate that administration of ganciclovir caused inhibition of spermatogenesis and subsequent infertility, which were reversible at lower doses and irreversible at higher doses (see Warnings and Precautions, Sexual Function/Reproduction). Although clinical data have not yet been obtained regarding this effect, **it is considered probable that CYTOVENE at the recommended doses may cause temporary or permanent inhibition of spermatogenesis in humans. Animal data also indicate that suppression of fertility in females may occur.**

Because of the mutagenic and teratogenic potential of ganciclovir, women of childbearing potential should be advised to use effective contraception during treatment with CYTOVENE. Similarly men should be advised to practice barrier contraception during and for at least 90 days following treatment with CYTOVENE (see Warnings and Precautions, Sexual Function/Reproduction).

CYTOVENE is considered to be a potential teratogen and carcinogen in humans with the potential to cause birth defects and cancers (see Special Handling Instructions).

Pregnant Women: The safety of CYTOVENE for use in human pregnancy has not been established. The use of CYTOVENE should be avoided in pregnant woman unless the benefit to the mother outweighs the potential risk to the fetus.

Data obtained using an ex vivo human placental model show that ganciclovir crosses the placenta and that simple diffusion is the most likely mechanism of transfer. The transfer was not saturable over a concentration range of 1 to 10 mg/mL and occurred by passive diffusion.

Nursing Women: It is not known if ganciclovir is excreted in human milk. Since many drugs are, and, because carcinogenic and teratogenic effects occurred in animals treated with ganciclovir, the possibility of serious adverse reactions from ganciclovir in nursing infants is considered likely. CYTOVENE should not be given to breastfeeding mothers. Mothers should be instructed to discontinue the drug or discontinue nursing if they are receiving CYTOVENE.

Pediatrics: The safety and efficacy of CYTOVENE in children has not been established. The use of CYTOVENE warrants extreme caution due to the probability of long-term carcinogenicity and reproductive toxicity. Administration to children should be undertaken only after careful evaluation and only if the potential benefits of treatment outweigh these considerable risks.

There has been very limited clinical experience using CYTOVENE for the treatment of CMV retinitis in patients under the age of 12 years.

The safety and efficacy of CYTOVENE have not been evaluated for congenital or neonatal CMV disease, nor for treatment of CMV infection in non-immunocompromised individuals (see Indications and Clinical Use).

Geriatrics: No studies on the efficacy or safety of CYTOVENE specifically in elderly patients have been conducted. Since elderly individuals may have reduced renal function, CYTOVENE should be administered to the elderly patients with care and will special consideration of their renal status (see Dosage and Administration, Renal Impairment).

Use in Patients with Renal Impairment: CYTOVENE should be used with caution in patients with impaired renal function. Both the plasma half-life of ganciclovir as well as peak plasma levels are increased in patients with elevated serum creatinine levels.

Patients Undergoing Hemodialysis: Hemodialysis reduces plasma concentrations of ganciclovir by approximately 50% after i.v. administration (see Dosage and Administration, Hemodialysis).

Patients with HIV and CMV Retinitis: CYTOVENE is not a cure for CMV retinitis, and immunocompromised patients may continue to experience progression of retinitis during or following treatment. Patients should be advised to have ophthalmologic follow-up examinations at a minimum of every 4 to 6 weeks while being treated with CYTOVENE. Some patients will require more frequent follow-up.

Patients with HIV may be receiving zidovudine (ZDV); patients should be counselled that as zidovudine and CYTOVENE each have the potential to cause neutropenia and anemia, some patients may not tolerate concomitant therapy (see Drug Interactions).

Transplant Recipients: Transplant recipients should be counselled regarding the high frequency of impaired renal function in transplant recipients who received CYTOVENE in controlled clinical trials, particularly in patients receiving concomitant administration of nephrotoxic agents such as cyclosporine and amphotericin B. Although the specific mechanism of this toxicity, which is most cases was reversible, has not been determined, the higher rate of renal impairment in patients receiving CYTOVENE compared with those who received placebo in the same trials may indicate that CYTOVENE played a significant role.

Monitoring and Laboratory Tests: Due to the frequency of neutropenia, anemia or thrombocytopenia observed in patients receiving CYTOVENE (see Adverse Reactions), it is recommended that complete blood counts and platelet counts be performed frequently, especially in patients in whom CYTOVENE or other nucleoside analogs have previously resulted in leukopenia, or in whom pretreatment neutrophil counts are less than 1000 cells/μL at the beginning of treatment. In patients with severe leukopenia, neutropenia, anemia and/or thrombocytopenia, it is recommended that treatment with hematopoietic growth factors and/or dose interruption be considered (see Dosage and Administration, Patient Monitoring, Reduction of Dose).

Because dosing modifications based on creatinine clearance are required in patients with renal impairment and because of the incidence of increased serum creatinine levels observed in transplant recipients treated with CYTOVENE, patients should have serum creatinine or creatinine clearance monitored carefully (see Adverse Reactions, renal adverse events and Dosage and Administration, Patient Monitoring).

ADVERSE REACTIONS: Clinical Trial Adverse Drug Reactions: Because clinical trials are conducted under very specific conditions the adverse reaction rates observed in the clinical trials may not reflect the rates observed in practice and should not be compared to the rates in the clinical trials of another drug. Adverse drug reaction information from clinical trials is useful for identifying drug-related adverse events and for approximating rates.

Adverse events that occurred during clinical trials of CYTOVENE (ganciclovir sodium for injection) are summarized below, according to the participating study subject population.

Adverse events seen in studies using CYTOVENE might also occur in studies using ganciclovir capsules, and vice versa.

HIV-1 Infected Subjects: The safety of CYTOVENE in HIV-1 infected patients was studied in several clinical trials. The pooled safety information of the use of CYTOVENE for the treatment of CMV disease in HIV infected patients in six clinical trials is displayed below. The data is shown in comparison to the control arm (oral placebo plus intravitreal ganciclovir implant) of one of these studies. Clinical adverse events, which occurred in ≥2% of patients taking intravenous ganciclovir, regardless of causal relationship or seriousness, however at a greater frequency than in the control arm, are summarized in Table 1.

Table 1: CYTOVENE

Percentage of Patients with Adverse Events Occurring in ≥2% of All Patients Receiving Intravenous Ganciclovir

Body Systems Adverse Events	Intravenous Ganciclovir N=412 %	Control N=119 %
Hemic and Lymphatic System		
Neutropenia	25.7	11.8
Anemia	19.7	16.8
Thrombocytopenia	6.6	5.0
Leukopenia	3.2	0.8
Lymphadenopathy	2.9	1.7
Gastrointestinal System		
Diarrhea	26.5	24.4
Nausea	—	21.8
Vomiting	—	12.6
Abdominal pain	9.0	7.6
Flatulence	—	1.7
Loose stools	—	1.7
Dysphagia	2.7	1.7
Esophageal candidiasis	2.2	1.7
Body as a Whole		
Pyrexia	35.9	35.3
Headache	18.7	16.0
Candida	10.4	4.2
Injection site infection	8.0	0.8
Sepsis	6.1	3.4
Sepsis secondary	5.8	—
Anorexia	4.9	—
Mycobacterium avium complex	4.9	4.2
Pain	4.6	2.5
Chest pain	4.4	3.4
Malaise	—	0.8
Asthenia	—	0.8
Blood culture positive	3.2	1.7
Injection site inflammation	2.2	—
Central and Peripheral Nervous Systems		
Confusion	—	2.5
Hypoesthesia	3.2	1.7
Anxiety	2.4	1.7
Skin and Appendages		
Pruritus	3.2	2.5
Respiratory System		
Cough	16.0	15.1
P. carinii pneumonia	7.3	2.5
Productive cough	3.6	2.5
Upper respiratory tract infection	—	0.8
Lower respiratory tract infection	—	1.7
Sinus congestion	3.4	2.5
Metabolic and Nutritional Disorders		
Blood alkaline phosphatase increased	4.4	4.2
Blood creatinine increased	3.2	1.7
Musculoskeletal System		
Arthralgia	2.4	1.7

Retinal Detachment: Retinal detachment has been observed in subjects with CMV retinitis both before and after initiation of therapy with CYTOVENE. The relationship of retinal detachment to therapy with CYTOVENE is unknown. Retinal detachment occurred in 11% of patients treated with CYTOVENE and in 8% of patients treated with ganciclovir capsules. Patients with CMV retinitis should have frequent ophthalmologic evaluations to monitor the status of their retinitis and to detect any other retinal pathology.

Laboratory abnormalities reported from three clinical trials in HIV infected patients taking oral or intravenous ganciclovir as maintenance treatment for CMV retinitis are listed in Table 2. Three hundred twenty-six patients receiving ganciclovir capsules and 179 patients receiving CYTOVENE (ganciclovir sodium for injection) were eligible for the laboratory abnormality analysis.

Table 2: CYTOVENE

Laboratory Data: Minimum ANC, Hemoglobin, and Platelets and Maximum Serum Creatinine Values During Treatment with CYTOVENE (ganciclovir sodium for injection) and Ganciclovir Capsules in Three Controlled Clinical Trials[a]

	% of subjects Oral Ganciclovir Capsules[b] (3000 mg/day) (n=326)	% of subjects Intravenous Solution[c] 5 mg/kg/day (n=179)
Neutropenia [n(%)]		
ANC/μL		
<500	18.4	25.1
500 to <750	16.6	14.3
750 to <1000	19.1	26.3
Anemia [n(%)]		
Hemoglobin g/dL		
< 6.5	1.6	4.6
6.5 to <8.0	10.0	16.0
8.0 to <9.5	24.7	25.7
Thrombocytopenia		
Platelets/μL		
<25 000	1.3	2.9
25 000 to <50 000	8.1	5.1
50 000–<100 000	20.0	22.9
Serum Creatinine (SeCr)		

(cont'd)

Table 2: CYTOVENE *(cont'd)*

Laboratory Data: Minimum ANC, Hemoglobin, and Platelets and Maximum Serum Creatinine Values During Treatment with CYTOVENE (ganciclovir sodium for injection) and Ganciclovir Capsules in Three Controlled Clinical Trials[a]

	% of subjects Oral Ganciclovir Capsules[b] (3000 mg/day) (n=326)	% of subjects Intravenous Solution[c] 5 mg/kg/day (n=179)
SeCr mg/dL		
≥2.5	0.9	1.7
≥1.5 to <2.5	12.2	13.9

[a] Data from Study ICM 1653, Study ICM 1774, and Study AVI034 pooled.
[b] Mean time on therapy=103 days, including allowed reinduction treatment periods.
[c] Mean time on therapy=91 days, including allowed reinduction treatment periods.

Overall, patients treated with CYTOVENE (ganciclovir sodium for injection) experienced lower minimum ANCs and hemoglobin levels, consistent with more neutropenia and anemia, compared with those who received ganciclovir capsules; P=0.024 for neutropenia; P=0.027 for anemia.

For the majority of subjects, maximum serum creatinine levels were less than 1.5 mg/dL and no difference was noted between CYTOVENE and ganciclovir capsule for the occurrence of renal impairment. Serum creatinine elevations ≥2.5 mg/dL occurred in <2% of all subjects and no significant differences were noted in the time from the start of maintenance to the occurrence of elevations in serum creatinine values.

Transplant Recipients: Several clinical trials have investigated intravenous ganciclovir for the treatment or prevention of CMV disease in transplant patients.

Summarized below are clinical adverse events, which occurred in ≥5% of patients taking i.v. ganciclovir in three pooled bone marrow studies, regardless of causal relationship or seriousness. Adverse events which occurred in a higher frequency in the placebo/observational control arm compared to the i.v. ganciclovir arm, have not been included in Table 3.

Table 3: CYTOVENE

Adverse Events Occurring in ≥5% of Patients Taking iv Ganciclovir

Body System Adverse Event	Bone Marrow Transplant Patients (ICM 1308, 1570 and 1689) I.V. Ganciclovir (N=122) %	Placebo/Observational Control (N=120) %
Hemic and Lymphatic System		
Pancytopenia	31	25
Leukopenia	20	7
Body as a Whole		
Headache	15	13
Mucous membrane disorder	14	13
Pyrexia	11	8
Rigors	5	4
Sepsis	7	2
Anorexia	7	5
Face edema	5	2
Gastrointestinal System		
Diarrhea	24	23
Nausea	20	19
Dyspepsia	8	6
Abdominal distension	8	6
Metabolic and Nutritional Disorders		
Blood creatinine increased	16	13
Hepatic function abnormal	11	10
Blood magnesium decreased	11	10
Hypocalcemia	9	8
Hypokalemia	9	8
Central and Peripheral Nervous Systems		
Tremor	8	7
Confusion	5	3
Skin and Appendages		
Dermatitis exfoliative	10	9
Respiratory System		
Rhinitis	9	5
Dyspnea	6	4
Cardiovascular System		
Tachycardia	16	15
Hypotension	11	7
Urogenital System		
Hematuria present	16	13
Special Senses		
Eye hemorrhage	5	3
Musculoskeletal System		
Myalgia	5	3

Clinical adverse events, which occurred in ≥5% of patients taking i.v. ganciclovir in a placebo controlled heart transplant study (ICM 1496), regardless of causal relationship or seriousness, but which occurred in a higher frequency in the i.v. ganciclovir arm (N=76) compared to the placebo arm (N=73), are listed below.

Body as a Whole: headache (18%), infection (18%).
Metabolic and Nutritional Disorders: edema (9%).
Central and Peripheral Nervous Systems: confusion (5%), peripheral neuropathy (7%).
Respiratory System: pleural effusion (5%).
Cardiovascular System: hypertension (20%).
Urogenital System: renal impairment (14%), renal failure (12%).

Less Common Clinical Trial Adverse Drug Reactions (<1%): Relevant adverse events, which are not listed above, as they did not fulfil the criteria for inclusion into any of the tables of previous sections are given below.
Body as a Whole: cachexia, dehydration, fatigue, injection site abscess, injection site edema, injection site hemorrhage, injection site pain, injection site thrombosis, malaise, photosensitivity reaction.
Gastrointestinal System: pancreatitis, gastrointestinal disorder, gastrointestinal hemorrhage, eructation, esophagitis, fecal incontinence, gastritis, mouth ulceration, tongue disorder.
Hemic and Lymphatic System: aplastic anemia, bone marrow depression, eosinophilia, splenomegaly.
Central and Peripheral Nervous Systems: hallucinations, psychotic disorder, euphoric mood, emotional disturbance, hyperkinetic syndrome, myoclonic jerks, abnormal dreams, agitation, amnesia, ataxia, coma, convulsion, dry mouth, hypertonia, libido decreased, nervousness, somnolence, thinking abnormal.
Skin and Appendages: dermatitis, acne, alopecia, dry skin, herpes simplex, urticaria.
Special Senses: retinal detachment, vision abnormal, earache, blindness, deafness, eye pain, glaucoma, tinnitus, vitreous disorder.
Metabolic and Nutritional Disorders: blood creatine phosphokinase increased, blood glucose decreased, blood lactic dehydrogenase increased.
Cardiovascular System: arrhythmia (including ventricular arrhythmia), thrombophlebitis deep, phlebitis, migraine.
Urogenital System: impotence, urinary frequency.
Musculoskeletal System: myasthenic syndrome.
Infections: events related to bone marrow depression and immune system compromise such as local and systemic infections and sepsis.
Bleeding Complications: potentially life-threatening bleeding associated with thrombocytopenia.
Hepatic System: hepatitis, jaundice.
Abnormal Hematologic and Clinical Chemistry Findings: Laboratory data from three controlled clinical trials of CYTOVENE (ganciclovir sodium for injection) for the prevention of CMV disease in transplant recipients are summarized in Table 4.

Table 4: CYTOVENE

Laboratory Data: Neutropenia and Thrombocytopenia in Trials for the Prevention of CMV Disease in Transplant Recipients

	CYTOVENE Intravenous[c]			
	Heart Allograft[a]		Bone Marrow Allograft[b]	
Subjects (number)	CYTOVENE n=76 %	Placebo n=73 %	CYTOVENE n=57 %	Placebo n=55 %
Neutropenia (ANC/µL)				
<500	4	3	12	6
500–1000	3	8	29	17
Thrombocytopenia (platelets/µL)				
<25 000	3	1	32	28
25 000– 50 000	5	3	25	37

[a] Study ICM 1496: Mean duration of treatment=28 days.
[b] Studies ICM 1570 and ICM 1689: Mean duration of treatment=45 days.
[c] Ganciclovir sodium for injection

Table 5 shows the frequency of elevated serum creatinine values in these controlled clinical trials.

(cont'd)

Table 5: CYTOVENE

Laboratory Data: Elevated Serum Creatinine Values in Trials for the Prevention of CMV Disease in Transplant Recipients

Maximum Serum Creatinine Levels	CYTOVENE Intravenous[a]					
	Heart Allograft		Bone Marrow Allograft			
	ICM 1496		ICM 1570		ICM 1689	
	CYTOVENE (N=76) %	Placebo (n=73) %	CYTOVENE (n=20) %	Control (n=20) %	CYTOVENE (n=37) %	Placebo (n=35) %
Serum Creatinine (≥2.5 mg/dL)	18	4	20	0	0	0
Serum Creatinine (≥1.5–<2.5 mg/dL)	58	69	50	35	43	44

[a] Ganciclovir sodium for injection.

Patients receiving CYTOVENE had elevated serum creatinine levels when compared to those receiving placebo. Most patients in these studies also received cyclosporine. The mechanism of impairment of renal function is not known. However, careful monitoring of renal function during therapy with CYTOVENE is essential, especially for those patients receiving concomitant agents that may cause nephrotoxicity.

Post-Market Adverse Drug Reactions: The following adverse events have been reported since the marketing introduction of CYTOVENE and are not listed under adverse reactions above. Because they are reported voluntarily from a population of unknown size, estimates of frequency cannot be made. These events have been chosen for inclusion due to either the seriousness frequency of reporting, the apparent causal connection, or a combination of these factors:

Acidosis, allergic reaction, anaphylactic reaction, arthritis, bronchospasm, cardiac arrest, cardiac conduction abnormality, cataracts, cholelithiasis, cholestasis, congenital anomaly, dry eyes, dysesthesia, dysphasia, elevated triglyceride levels, exfoliative dermatitis, extrapyramidal reaction, facial palsy, hallucinations, hemolytic anemia, hemolytic-uremic syndrome, hepatic failure, hepatitis, hypercalcemia, hyponatremia inappropriate serum ADH, infertility, intestinal ulceration, intracranial hypertension, irritability, ischemia, loss of memory, loss of sense of smell, myelopathy, peripheral oculomotor nerve paralysis, pulmonary fibrosis, renal tubular disorder, rhabdomyolysis, Stevens-Johnson syndrome, stroke, testicular hypotrophy, Torsades de Pointes, vasculitis, ventricular tachycardia.

Adverse events from post-marketing spontaneous reports with ganciclovir that were reported in HIV infected or other immunocompromised patients such as transplant recipients, which are not mentioned in any section above, and for which a causal relationship can not be excluded, are: anaphylaxis, decreased fertility in males.

Adverse events that have been reported during the post-marketing period are consistent with those seen in clinical trials with ganciclovir.

DRUG INTERACTIONS: Ganciclovir: Binding of ganciclovir to plasma proteins is only about 1%-2%, and drug interactions involving binding site displacement are not anticipated.

Probenecid: At a dose of 1000 mg of ganciclovir capsules every 8 hours, ganciclovir serum concentrations increased 45% in the presence of probenecid, 500 mg every 6 hours. Renal clearance of ganciclovir decreased 22%, which is consistent with an interaction involving competition for renal tubular secretion. Patients taking probenecid and ganciclovir capsules should be closely monitored for ganciclovir toxicity.

Zidovudine: At a dose of 1000 mg of ganciclovir capsules every 8 hours, there was a trend for decreased ganciclovir AUC in the presence of zidovudine, 100 mg every 4 hours (18%), but the decrease was not statistically significant. There was a statistically significant increase in AUC for zidovudine (15%) in the presence of ganciclovir.

Since both zidovudine and ganciclovir have the potential to cause neutropenia and anemia, many patients will not tolerate combination therapy with these two drugs at full dosage strength. However, studies with CYTOVENE for the treatment of CMV retinitis in AIDS showed no difference in the rate of severe neutropenia (ANC $<0.5\times10^9$ cells/L) or of severe anemia (hemoglobin <8.0 g/dL), with or without concomitant zidovudine.

Didanosine: At an oral dose of 1000 mg of ganciclovir capsules every 8 hours, the steady state AUC_{0-12} for didanosine, 200 mg every 12 hours, increased approximately 80% when didanosine was administered 2 hours prior to or concurrently with administration of ganciclovir capsules. Decreased steady state AUC (23%) was observed for ganciclovir in the presence of didanosine when the drug was administered 2 hours prior to administration of ganciclovir capsules, but AUC was not affected by the presence of didanosine when the two drugs were administered simultaneously. There were no significant changes in renal clearance for either drug.

When the standard CYTOVENE induction dose (5 mg/kg infused over 1 hour every 12 hours) was coadministered with didanosine at a dose of 200 mg orally every 12 hours, the steady state didanosine AUC_{0-12} increased 70±40% (range, 3 to 121%, n=11) and C_{max} increased 49±48% (range, −28 to 125%). In a separate study, when the standard CYTOVENE maintenance dose (5 mg/kg infused over 1 hour every 24 hours) was coadministered with didanosine at a dose of 200 mg orally every 12 hours, didanosine AUC_{0-12} increased 50±26% (range, 22 to 110%, n=11) and C_{max} increased 36±36% (range, −27 to 94%) over the first didanosine dosing interval. Didanosine plasma concentrations (AUC_{12-24}) were unchanged during the dosing intervals when CYTOVENE was not coadministered. Ganciclovir pharmacokinetics were not affected by didanosine. In neither study were there significant changes in the renal clearance of either drug.

This increase in didanosine plasma concentration cannot be explained by competition for renal tubular secretion, as there was an increase in the percentage of didanosine dose excreted. This increase could arise from either increased bioavailability or decreased metabolism. However, given the increase in didanosine plasma concentrations in the presence of ganciclovir, patients should be closely monitored for didanosine toxicity.

Didanosine has been associated with pancreatitis. In three controlled trials, pancreatitis was reported in 2% of patients taking didanosine and CYTOVENE. The rates of pancreatitis were similar in the intravenous solution and capsule groups.

Other than laboratory abnormalities, concomitant treatment with zidovudine, didanosine, or zalcitabine did not appear to affect the type or frequency of reported adverse events, with the exception of moderately increased rates of diarrhea. Among patients taking CYTOVENE, the diarrhea rates were 51% and 49% respectively with didanosine versus 39% and 35% respectively, without didanosine.

Zalcitabine: Zalcitabine increased the AUC_{0-8} of oral ganciclovir by 13%. There were no statistically significant changes in any of the other pharmacokinetic parameters assessed. Additionally, there were no clinically relevant changes in zalcitabine pharmacokinetics in the presence of oral ganciclovir although a small increase in the elimination rate constant was observed.

Stavudine: No statistically significant pharmacokinetic interaction was observed when stavudine and oral ganciclovir were given in combination.

Trimethoprim: Trimethoprim statistically significantly decreased the renal clearance of oral ganciclovir by 16.3% and this was associated with a statistically significant decrease in the terminal elimination rate and corresponding increase in half-life by 15%. However, these changes are unlikely to be clinically significant, as AUC_{0-8} and C_{max} were unaffected. The only statistically significant change in trimethoprim pharmacokinetic parameters when coadministered with ganciclovir was an increase in C_{min}. However, this is unlikely to be of clinical significance and no dose adjustment is recommended.

Cyclosporin: There was no evidence that introduction of ganciclovir affects the pharmacokinetics of cyclosporin based on the comparison of cyclosporin trough concentrations. However, there was some evidence of increases in the maximum serum creatinine value observed following initiation of ganciclovir therapy.

Imipenem-cilastatin: Generalized convulsions have been reported in patients who received CYTOVENE (ganciclovir sodium for injection) and imipenem-cilastatin. These drugs should not be used concomitantly unless the potential benefits outweigh the risks.

Mycophenolate Mofetil: Following single-dose administration to twelve stable renal transplant patients, no pharmacokinetic interaction was observed between mycophenolate mofetil (1.5 g) and CYTOVENE (5 mg/kg). Mean (±SD) ganciclovir AUC and C_{max} were 54.3 (±19.0) µg·h/mL and 11.5 (±1.8) µg/mL, respectively after coadministration of the two drugs, compared to 51.0 (±17.0) µg·h/mL and 10.6 (±2.0) µg/mL, respectively after administration of CYTOVENE alone. The mean (±SD) AUC and C_{max} of MPA (active metabolite of mycophenolate) after coadministration were 80.9 (±21.6) µg·h/mL and 27.8 (±13.9) µg/mL, respectively compared to values of 80.3 (±16.4) µg·h/mL and 30.9 (±11.2) µg/mL, respectively after administration of mycophenolate mofetil alone. However, based on the known effects of renal impairment on the pharmacokinetics of ganciclovir and mycophenolate, it is anticipated that coadministration of these agents (which have the potential to compete for mechanisms of renal tubular secretion) will result in increases in ganciclovir concentration and MPAG (inactive metabolite of mycophenolate). In patients with renal impairment in which ganciclovir and mycophenolate are coadministered, the dose recommendations for ganciclovir should be observed and patients monitored carefully.

Other Medications: It is possible that drugs that inhibit replication of rapidly dividing cell populations such as bone marrow, spermatogonia, and germinal layers of skin and gastrointestinal mucosa, may have additive toxicity when administered concomitantly with CYTOVENE. In addition, toxicity may be enhanced when ganciclovir is coadministered with other drugs known to be associated with renal impairment. Therefore, drugs known to be myelosuppressive or associated with renal impairment such as dapsone, pentamidine, flucytosine, vincristine, vinblastine, adriamycin, amphotericin B, trimethoprim/sulfamethoxazole combinations or other nucleoside analogues, or hydroxyurea, should be considered for concomitant use with CYTOVENE only if the potential benefits are judged to outweigh the risks.

Allograft recipients treated with CYTOVENE in three controlled clinical studies also received a variety of concomitant medications, including amphotericin B, azathioprine, cyclosporine, muromonab-CD3 (OKT3), and/or prednisone. Increases in serum creatinine were observed in patients treated with CYTOVENE plus either cyclosporine or amphotericin B, drugs with known potential for nephrotoxicity (see Adverse Reactions). In a retrospective analysis of 93 liver allograft recipients receiving ganciclovir (5 mg/kg infused over 1 hour every 12 hours) and oral cyclosporine (at therapeutic doses), there was no evidence of an effect on cyclosporine whole blood concentrations.

DOSAGE AND ADMINISTRATION: Dosing Considerations: Do not administer CYTOVENE (ganciclovir sodium for injection) by rapid or bolus intravenous injection. The toxicity of ganciclovir may be increased as a result of excessive plasma levels.

Intramuscular or subcutaneous injection may result in severe tissue irritation due to the high pH (approximately 11) of CYTOVENE solutions.

Recommended Dose and Dosage Adjustment: The recommended dose for CYTOVENE (ganciclovir sodium for injection) should not be exceeded. The recommended infusion rate for CYTOVENE solution should not be exceeded.

Because of individual patient variations in the clinical response of CMV disease and the sensitivity to the myelosuppressive effects of CYTOVENE, the treatment of each patient with CYTOVENE should be individualized on a case by case basis. Changes in dose should be based on regular clinical evaluations as well as on regular hematologic monitoring.

For Treatment of CMV Retinitis: Induction Treatment: The recommended dose of CYTOVENE for patients with normal renal function is 5 mg/kg every 12 hours for 14 to 21 days, given as a constant intravenous infusion over one hour.

Maintenance Treatment: Following the induction treatment, the recommended dose of CYTOVENE is 5 mg/kg given as an intravenous infusion over one hour once per day for seven days each week, or 6 mg/kg once per day for five days each week.

For patients who experience progression of CMV retinitis while receiving maintenance treatment with CYTOVENE, reinduction treatment using the twice daily regimen of CYTOVENE is recommended.

For the Prevention of CMV Disease in Transplant Recipients: The recommended initial dose for patients with normal renal function is 5 mg/kg (given intravenously at a constant rate over 1 hour) every 12 hours for 7 to 14 days, followed by either 5 mg/kg once per day if on a seven-day weekly regimen, or 6 mg/kg once per day if on a five-day weekly regimen.

The duration of treatment with CYTOVENE in transplant recipients is dependent upon the duration and degree of immunosuppression. In controlled clinical trials in bone marrow allograft recipients, treatment with CYTOVENE was continued until day 100 to 120 post-transplantation. CMV disease occurred in several patients who discontinued treatment with CYTOVENE prematurely. In heart allograft recipients, the onset of newly diagnosed CMV disease occurred after treatment with CYTOVENE was stopped at day 28 post-transplant, suggesting that continued dosing may be necessary to prevent late occurrence of CMV disease in this patient population.

Patients with Severe Leukopenia, Neutropenia, Anemia, Thrombocytopenia and/or Pancytopenia: Severe leukopenia, neutropenia, anemia, thrombocytopenia, bone marrow depression and aplastic anemia have been observed in patients treated with ganciclovir. Therapy should not be initiated if the absolute neutrophil count is less than 500 cells /µL or the platelet count is less than 25 000/µL or the hemoglobin is less than 80 g/L (see Warnings and Precautions,Hematologic; Warnings and Precautions, Monitoring and Laboratory Tests; and Adverse Reactions).

Patient Monitoring: Due to the frequency of leukopenia, granulocytopenia (neutropenia), anemia, thrombocytopenia, pancytopenia, bone marrow depression, and aplastic anemia in patients receiving ganciclovir (see Adverse Reactions), it is recommended that complete blood counts and platelet counts be performed frequently, especially in patients in whom ganciclovir or other nucleoside analogues have previously resulted in cytopenia, or in whom neutrophil counts are less than 1000 cells/µL at the beginning of treatment. Patients should have serum creatinine or creatinine clearance values followed carefully to allow for dosage adjustments in renally impaired patients (see Dosage and Administration, Recommended Dose and Dosage Adjustment, Renal Impairment).

Reduction of Dose: Dosage reductions in renally impaired patients are required for CYTOVENE (see Renal Impairment). Dosage reductions should also be considered for patients with neutropenia, anemia and/or thrombocytopenia. CYTOVENE should not be administered in patients with severe neutropenia (ANC less than 500/µL) or severe thrombocytopenia (platelets less than 25 000/µL) or severe anemia (hemoglobin less than 80 g/L).

Renal Impairment: For patients with impairment of renal function (see Warnings and Precautions), refer to Table 6 for recommended doses of CYTOVENE and adjust the dosing interval as indicated.

Table 6: CYTOVENE

Induction and Maintenance Doses of CYTOVENE (Ganciclovir Sodium for Injection) in Renal Impairment

Creatinine Clearance[a] (mL/min)	Induction Dose (mg/kg)	Dosing Interval (hours)	Maintenance Dose (mg/kg)	Dosing Interval (hours)
≥70	5.0	12	5.0	24
50 to 69	2.5	12	2.5	24
25 to 49	2.5	24	1.25	24
10 to 24	1.25	24	0.625	24
<10	1.25	3 times per week, following hemodialysis	0.625	3 times per week, following hemodialysis

[a] Creatinine clearance can be related to serum creatinine by the formulae below:

$$\text{Creatinine clearance for males} = \frac{(140-\text{age [years]})\times(\text{body weight [kg]})}{(72)\times(0.011\times\text{serum creatinine [µmol/L]})}$$

Creatinine clearance for females = 0.85×male value

Creatinine Clearance in SI units (mL/S)=0.01667×value obtained from the above formula in traditional units (mL/min).

Hemodialysis: Dosing for patients undergoing hemodialysis should not exceed 1.25 mg/kg three times per week, following each hemodialysis session. CYTOVENE should be given shortly after completion of the hemodialysis session, since hemodialysis has been shown to reduce plasma levels by approximately 50%.

Administration: Infusion concentrations greater than 10 mg/mL are not recommended. Do not administer CYTOVENE by rapid or bolus intravenous injection. It should be given by constant intravenous infusion over 1 hour.

Reconstitution: Reconstitution of Sterile Lyophilized Powder: Reconstitute by injecting sterile water for injection into the vial. See Table 7.

Table 7: CYTOVENE

Reconstitution

Vial Size	Volume of Diluent to be Added to Vial	Approximate Available Volume	Nominal Concentration per mL
500 mg	10 mL	10.29 mL	50 mg/mL

Shake well, until dissolved.

Do not use bacteriostatic water for injection containing parabens, since these are incompatible with ganciclovir sodium sterile powder and may cause precipitation.

The reconstituted solution should be inspected for particulate matter or discolouration prior to proceeding with admixture preparation.

Admixture Preparation: The reconstituted solution is further diluted in one of the solutions listed below for intravenous infusion.

Solutions for Intravenous Infusion: Normal saline, dextrose 5% in water, Ringer's injection, lactated Ringer's injection.

OVERDOSAGE:

Overdosage with CYTOVENE (ganciclovir sodium for injection) has been reported in both adults and children below 2 years of age. In two cases of overdosage in adults, no adverse events were reported after patients received either one dose of 3500 mg or 7 doses of 11 mg/kg over a 3 day period. Similarly, the following overdoses in pediatric patients did not result in adverse events: a single dose of 500 mg (72.5 mg/kg) followed by 48 hours of peritoneal dialysis (4 month-old), single dose of approximately 60 mg/kg followed by exchange transfusion (18 month-old), two doses of 500 mg instead of 31 mg (21 month-old).

Reports of overdoses with intravenous ganciclovir have been received from clinical trials and during post-marketing experience. In some of these cases no adverse events were reported. The majority of patients experienced one or more of the following adverse events:

Hematological Toxicity: pancytopenia, bone marrow depression, medullary aplasia, leukopenia, neutropenia, granulocytopenia.

Hepatotoxicity: hepatitis, liver function disorder.

Renal Toxicity: worsening of hematuria in a patient with pre-existing renal impairment, acute renal failure, elevated creatinine.

Gastrointestinal Toxicity: abdominal pain, diarrhea, vomiting.

Neurotoxicity: generalized tremor, convulsion.

In addition, one adult received 0.4 mL (instead of 0.1 mL) CYTOVENE by intravitreal injection, and experienced temporary loss of vision and central retinal artery occlusion secondary to increased intraocular pressure related to the injected fluid volume.

Overdose Experience with Valganciclovir: One adult developed fatal bone marrow depression (medullary aplasia) after several days of dosing that was at least 10-fold greater than recommended for the patients degree of renal impairment (decreased creatinine clearance).

Treatment: Hemodialysis may be useful in reducing serum concentrations, given that it reduces plasma concentrations of ganciclovir by approximately 50% (see Dosage and Administration, Hemodialysis). Adequate hydration should be maintained. The use of hematopoietic growth factors should be considered.

> For management of a suspected drug overdose, please contact your **regional Poison Control Centre**. See the *CPS* Directory section for a list of Poison Control Centres.

ACTION AND CLINICAL PHARMACOLOGY: Mechanism of Action: CYTOVENE (ganciclovir sodium for injection) is a synthetic nucleoside analogue of guanine which inhibits the replication of herpes viruses both in vitro and in vivo.

Intracellular ganciclovir is phosphorylated to ganciclovir monophosphate by a cellular deoxyguanosine kinase. Further phosphorylation occurs by several cellular kinases to produce ganciclovir triphosphate. It has been shown in vitro that the levels of ganciclovir triphosphate are as much as 100-fold greater in CMV-infected cells than non-infected cells. Thus, there is a preferential phosphorylation of ganciclovir in virus-infected cells. In virus-infected cells, ganciclovir triphosphate is metabolized slowly, with 60 to 70% remaining intracellularly 18 hours after removal of ganciclovir from the extracellular fluid. The antiviral activity of ganciclovir is the result of inhibition of viral DNA synthesis by two modes: (1) ganciclovir triphosphate competitively inhibits dGTP incorporation into DNA by DNA polymerase and (2) incorporation of ganciclovir triphosphate into viral DNA causes subsequent termination or very limited viral DNA elongation.

Ganciclovir inhibits mammalian cell proliferation in vitro at concentrations from 10 to 60 µg/mL, with bone marrow colony forming cells being most sensitive (IC50 of 10 µg/mL).

Pharmacokinetics: The pharmacokinetics of CYTOVENE have been evaluated in immunocompromised patients with serious CMV disease. In patients with normal renal function, the plasma half-life was 2.9±1.3 hours. Dose independent kinetics were demonstrated over the range of 1.6 to 5.0 mg/kg. Renal excretion through both glomerular filtration and active tubular secretion is the major route of elimination of ganciclovir (see Warnings and Precautions, Use in Patients with Renal Impairment). At the end of a one-hour intravenous infusion of 5 mg/kg CYTOVENE (ganciclovir sodium for injection), total ganciclovir area under the serum concentration vs. time curve (AUC) ranged between 22.1±3.2 (n=16) and 26.8±6.1 µg·hr/mL(n=16) and maximum serum concentration (C_{max}) ranged between 8.27±1.02 (n=16) and 9.0±1.4 µg/mL (n=16).

STORAGE AND STABILITY: Stability and Storage Recommendations: CYTOVENE (ganciclovir sodium for injection): Store at room temperature (15-30°C), avoid excessive heat above 40°C. The reconstituted solution in the vial may be stored at room temperature up to 12 hours and should not be refrigerated.

CYTOVENE, when reconstituted with sterile water for injection, further diluted with 0.9% sodium chloride injection, and stored refrigerated at 5°C in polyvinyl chloride (PVC) bags, remain physically and chemically stable for 14 days. **However, because CYTOVENE is reconstituted with nonbacteriostatic sterile water, it is recommended that the infusion solution be used within 24 hours of dilution to reduce the risk of bacterial contamination.** The reconstituted and further diluted solutions should be stored under refrigeration. Freezing is not recommended.

SPECIAL HANDLING INSTRUCTIONS: Caution should be exercised in the handling and preparation of CYTOVENE (ganciclovir sodium for injection). Avoid ingestion, inhalation or direct contact with the skin and mucous membranes. CYTOVENE should be considered a potential teratogen and carcinogen in humans. CYTOVENE solutions are alkaline (pH approximately 11). The use of latex gloves and safety glasses is recommended to avoid exposure in case of breakage of the vial or other accidental spillage. If the solution contacts the skin or mucous membranes, wash thoroughly with soap and water; rinse eyes for at least 15 minutes with plain water.

Several guidelines for the handling and disposal of hazardous pharmaceuticals (including cytotoxic drugs) are available (e.g. CSHP, 1991). Disposal of CYTOVENE should follow provincial, municipal, and local hospital guidelines or requirements.

INFORMATION FOR THE PATIENT: Published in e-CPS, available by subscription at www.e-cps.ca.

DOSAGE FORMS, COMPOSITION AND PACKAGING: Each 10 mL clear glass vial of sterile powder contains: ganciclovir sodium equivalent to ganciclovir 500 mg. Sodium: 46 mg (2 mEq).

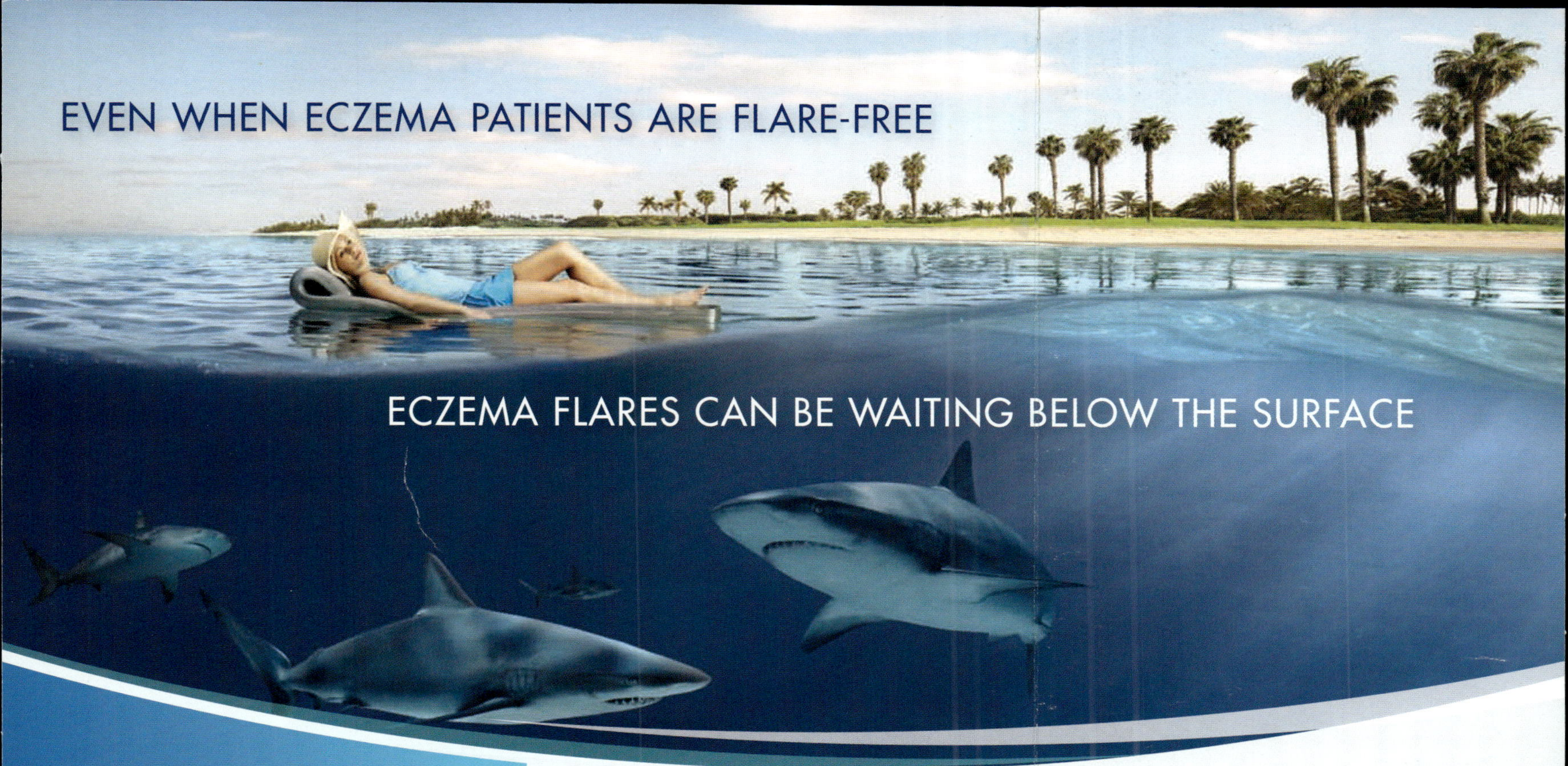

NEW INDICATION

PROTOPIC: The **First and Only** TCI Indicated for Maintenance Therapy to **Prevent Flares** and **Prolong Flare-Free Intervals** in Patients with Moderate to Severe Atopic Dermatitis Who are:

- Experiencing a high frequency of flares (i.e., occurring ≥ 5 times per year) and
- Who have had an initial response (i.e., lesions cleared, almost cleared or mildly affected) with up to 6 weeks of treatment with twice daily Protopic

Twice-Weekly 0.1% Protopic Maintenance Therapy (n=80)	MONTH 1, MONTH 2, MONTH 3, MONTH 4, MONTH 5	**142*** DAYS TO FIRST FLARE ($p<0.001$)
Twice-Weekly Vehicle Maintenance Therapy (n=73)	MONTH 1	**15*** DAYS TO FIRST FLARE

***Median time to first disease exacerbation (DE) requiring substantial intervention in adult patients.**

TWICE-WEEKLY PROTOPIC. DEMONSTRATED TO HELP PREVENT ECZEMA FLARES.[1]

Protopic® (tacrolimus ointment), both 0.03% and 0.1% for adults and only 0.03% for children aged 2 to 15 years, is indicated as a second-line therapy for short and long-term intermittent treatment of moderate to severe atopic dermatitis in non-immunocompromised patients, in whom the use of conventional therapies are deemed inadvisable because of potential risks, or who are not adequately responsive to or intolerant of conventional therapies.

If signs and symptoms of atopic dermatitis do not improve within 6 weeks of twice-daily treatment, Protopic treatment should be discontinued and patients should be re-examined by their healthcare provider and their diagnosis be confirmed. There should be 2 to 3 days between twice-weekly maintenance applications of Protopic. After 12 months, a review of the patient's condition should be conducted by the physician and a decision taken whether to continue maintenance treatment in the absence of safety data for maintenance treatment beyond 12 months.

Long-term safety of topical calcineurin inhibitors has not been established. Although a causal relationship has not been established, rare cases of skin malignancy and lymphoma have been reported in patients treated with topical calcineurin inhibitors, including Protopic ointment 0.1% and 0.03%. Therefore, continuous long-term use of topical calcineurin inhibitors including Protopic ointment 0.1% and 0.03% should be avoided, and application limited to areas of involvement with atopic dermatitis. Protopic ointment is not indicated in children less than 2 years of age. Only 0.03% Protopic ointment is indicated for use in children 2-15 years of age.

The use of Protopic may cause local symptoms of short duration, such as skin burning (burning sensation, stinging, soreness) or pruritus. Localized symptoms are most common during the first few days of Protopic application and typically resolve as the lesions of atopic dermatitis heal. The nature and incidence of adverse events for maintenance therapy were consistent with the established safety profile of Protopic. The most common adverse events reported in Protopic maintenance clinical trials were application-site pruritus (17.5%, 15.4%), nasopharyngitis (13.8%, 38.5%) and headache (11.3%, 5.1%) in adult and pediatric patients who received 0.1% Protopic and 0.03% Protopic, respectively.

There may also be an increased risk of varicella zoster virus infection, herpes simplex virus infection, or eczema herpeticum.

In clinical studies, cases of lymphadenopathy were usually related to infections and resolved with antibiotic therapy. Patients who develop lymphadenopathy should be monitored to ensure that it resolves.

Patients should be advised to minimize or avoid natural or artificial sunlight exposure.

Protopic has not been studied for its efficacy and safety in the treatment of clinically infected atopic dermatitis.

Please see Product Monograph for more information.

TCI=Topical Calcineurin Inhibitor.

astellas

PAAB Member R&D

Pr Protopic®
(tacrolimus 0.03%, 0.1% ointment)

New twice-weekly maintenance treatment to prevent eczema flares

D
E

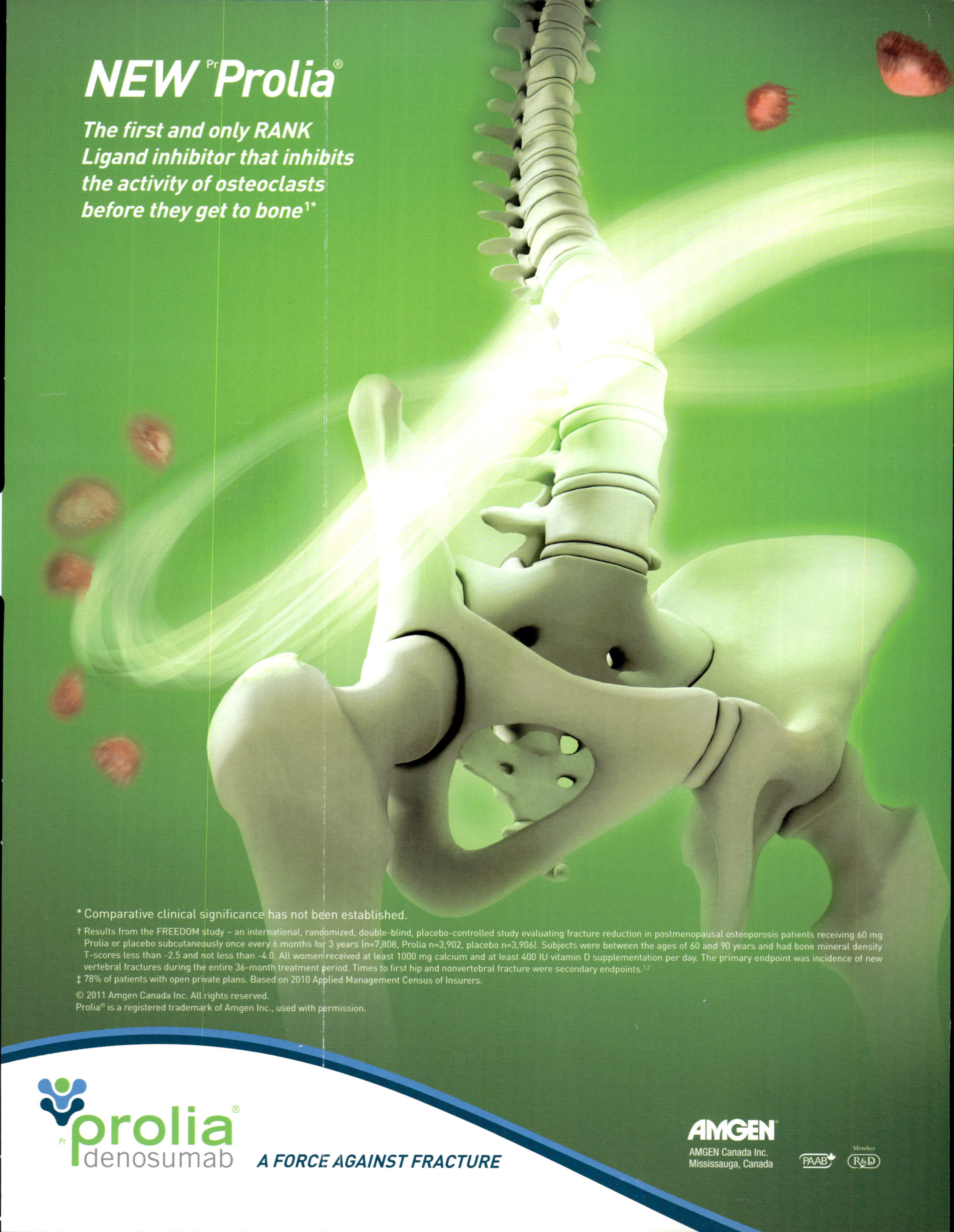
NEW Pr Prolia®
The first and only RANK Ligand inhibitor that inhibits the activity of osteoclasts before they get to bone[1*]
* Comparative clinical significance has not been established.
† Results from the FREEDOM study – an international, randomized, double-blind, placebo-controlled study evaluating fracture reduction in postmenopausal osteoporosis patients receiving 60 mg Prolia or placebo subcutaneously once every 6 months for 3 years (n=7,808, Prolia n=3,902, placebo n=3,906). Subjects were between the ages of 60 and 90 years and had bone mineral density T-scores less than -2.5 and not less than -4.0. All women received at least 1000 mg calcium and at least 400 IU vitamin D supplementation per day. The primary endpoint was incidence of new vertebral fractures during the entire 36-month treatment period. Times to first hip and nonvertebral fracture were secondary endpoints.[1,2]
‡ 78% of patients with open private plans. Based on 2010 Applied Management Census of Insurers.
© 2011 Amgen Canada Inc. All rights reserved.
Prolia® is a registered trademark of Amgen Inc., used with permission.
Pr prolia® denosumab
A FORCE AGAINST FRACTURE
AMGEN
AMGEN Canada Inc.
Mississauga, Canada
PAAB
Member R&D
D
E

Demonstrated powerful fracture risk reduction at all measured sites throughout the skeleton: hip, vertebral and nonvertebral[1,2†]

N Engl J Med: FREEDOM Study Results (Prolia n=3,902, placebo n=3,906)

Reduction in risk of new vertebral fractures[1,2]	Reduction in risk of hip fractures[1,2]	Reduction in risk of nonvertebral fractures[1,2]
68%	40%	20%
$p<0.0001$, absolute risk reduction **4.8%**	$p=0.04$, absolute risk reduction **0.3%**	$p=0.01$, absolute risk reduction **1.5%**

Significant increases in bone mineral density at all measured sites vs. placebo ($p<0.0001$): lumbar spine (8.8%), total hip (6.4%), femoral neck (5.2%) and trochanter (8.3%)[1†]

Prolia has a proven safety profile and is generally well tolerated[1]

- The incidence of adverse events and serious adverse events in patients taking Prolia was comparable to that of patients taking placebo (adverse events: Prolia and placebo 93%, $p=0.91$) (serious adverse events: Prolia 25.8%, placebo 25.1%, $p=0.61$).[1]
- The three most common adverse events in patients taking Prolia vs. placebo, respectively, were back pain (34.7% vs. 34.6%), arthralgia (20.2% vs. 20.2%) and hypertension (15.8% vs. 16.4%). The three most common serious adverse events, respectively, were osteoarthritis (1.6% vs. 2.0%), atrial fibrillation (0.9% vs. 0.9%) and pneumonia (0.9% vs. 0.9%).[1]
- Serious infections leading to hospitalization were reported more frequently in the Prolia (4.1%) group than in the placebo (3.4%) group.[1]

60 mg prefilled syringe dosed every six months as a 1 mL subcutaneous injection[1]

Prolia is covered by the majority of Private Open Drug Plans‡

Prolia is indicated for the treatment of postmenopausal women with osteoporosis at high risk for fracture, defined as a history of osteoporotic fracture, or multiple risk factors for fracture; or patients who have failed or are intolerant to other available osteoporosis therapy. In postmenopausal women with osteoporosis, Prolia reduces the incidence of vertebral, nonvertebral and hip fractures.[1] Prolia is contraindicated in patients with hypocalcemia or who are hypersensitive to the drug or any component of the product. For a complete listing, see the dosage forms, composition and packaging section of the Product Monograph.[1] The safety and efficacy of Prolia have not been studied in pediatric populations. Prolia is not indicated for use in pediatric patients.[1]

Prolia is indicated only for women who are postmenopausal and is not recommended for women who could become pregnant or who are nursing.[1]Adequate intake of calcium and vitamin D is important in all patients including patients with severe renal impairment or receiving dialysis.[1]

Physicians should note the following warnings and precautions:

Correct hypocalcemia with calcium and vitamin D prior to initiating Prolia. Monitor calcium levels in patients predisposed to hypocalcemia. Patients should be advised to seek prompt medical attention if they develop signs or symptoms of hypocalcemia (e.g. paresthesias or muscle spasms).[1]

Overall skin infections leading to hospitalization were reported more frequently in the Prolia (0.4%) group than in the placebo (<0.1%) group. These cases were predominantly cellulitis. Patients should be advised to seek prompt medical attention if signs or symptoms of cellulitis and erysipelas develop and physicians should assess the need for continued Prolia therapy. Consider the benefit/risk profile in patients taking immunosuppressant agents before treating with Prolia.[1]

In the FREEDOM trial, epidermal and dermal adverse events (e.g. dermatitis, eczema and rash) occurred at a significantly higher rate in the Prolia (10.8%) group compared to the placebo (8.2%) group. Consider discontinuing Prolia if severe symptoms develop.[1]

Osteonecrosis of the jaw (ONJ) has been reported in patients treated with Prolia or bisphosphonates. A dental examination with appropriate preventative dentistry should be considered in patients with risk factors for ONJ. If ONJ occurs during treatment, guide the management plan of each patient based on individual benefit/risk evaluation.[1]

Treatment with Prolia resulted in significant suppression of bone remodelling. The significance of these findings and the effect of long-term treatment with Prolia are unknown. Monitor patients for ONJ, atypical fractures and delayed fracture healing.[1]

Please see Product Monograph for complete Warnings and Precautions, Dosage and Administration. Physicians should become fully familiarized with the efficacy/safety profile of Prolia and the full content of the Product Monograph prior to prescribing the drug.

References: 1. Prolia Product Monograph. Amgen Canada Inc., August 6, 2010. **2.** Cummings SR, *et al.* Denosumab for prevention of fractures in postmenopausal women with osteoporosis. *N Engl J Med* 2009;361(8):756-65.

D

Dacarbazine For Injection BP ℞
dacarbazine
Antineoplastic

Hospira

SUPPLIED: Each vial of sterile lyophilized powder for reconstitution contains: dacarbazine 600 mg. Nonmedicinal ingredients: citric acid, mannitol and sodium hydroxide or citric acid (as pH adjuster). Single use amber glass vials of 100 mL. Store at 2 to 8°C. Protect from light.

Daily Complete™
multiple vitamins and minerals
Vitamin-Mineral Supplement

Awareness Corporation/dba AwarenessLife

SUPPLIED: One cupfull (30 mL) contains: vitamin complex: vitamin A acetate 10 000 IU, vitamin D 400 IU, vitamin E (dl & d-a-tocopherol) 30 IU, vitamin C 150 mg; B-vitamins in a base of brown rice concentrate: vitamin B_1 (thiamine HCl) 6 mg, vitamin B_2 (riboflavin 5'phosphate) 4.25 mg, niacinamide 20 mg, vitamin B_6 (pyridoxine HCl) 5 mg, folic acid 0.4 mg, vitamin B_{12} 100 µg, biotin 120 µg, pantothenic acid (panthenol) 10 mg; plant-sourced minerals chelates: potassium (citrate, HVP: Hydrolyzed Vegetable Chelates) 100 mg, zinc (HVP chelate) 15 mg, selenium (selenite) 80 µg, chromium (chloride) 50 µg. Nonmedicinal ingredients: macro mineral complex: calcium (gluconate) 28 mg, magnesium (gluconate, citrate) 6 mg; botanical polyphenol complex: polyphenols, proanthocyanidins, bioflavonoids from green tea, grape seed, pine bark and grape skin; proprietary sea vegetable complex: sea lettuce, wild Atlantic nori, bladderwrack, dulse, whole leaf rockweed (Norwegian kelp), whole leaf kelp, irish moss; whole food green complex: wheat grass, barley grass, dunallella salina red algae (source of b-carotene), pectin apple fiber, sprouted barley malt, brown rice bran (source of B-vitamins), bee pollen, Nova Scotia dulse, fructooligosaccharides, oat grass, rye grass, spirulina, chorella; essential fatty acid complex: glycerine, soy lecithin (providing soy phosphatides), sorbitol fatty acid esters, cold pressed flax oil (source of omega 3 fatty acids, cold pressed borage oil, cold pressed evening primrose oil; fruit and vegetable concentrate: whole juice concentrates (apricot, mango, apple, tangerine, cranberry, lime, beets, green bell peppers, parsley), carotenoid concentrate (carrot, peach, yellow squash, cantaloupe, red pepper, tomatoe), flavonoid concentrate (orange, lemon, celery, grapefruit), phenolic acid concentrate (red grape, strawberry, cherry, pear), cruciferous/ thioally concentrate (broccoli, cabbage, cauliflower, brussel sprouts, mustard greens), lutein concentrate (spinach, kale, asparagus, alfalfa), isoflavone concentrate (sources of genistein, daidzein); proprietary herbal extracts 1:1 of the following: lemon balm (Melissa officinalis), bioflavonoids, marigold flower (Calendula off.), cinnamon bark (Cinnamomum cassia), echinacea root (Echinacea angustifolia), liquorice root (Glycyrrhiza glabra), yebra maté leaves ext. (Ilex paraguariensis), alfalfa leaves (Medicago sativa), peppermint leaves (Mentha piperita), saw palmetto berries (Serenoa serrulata), dandelion root (Taraxacum off.), red clover flower (Trifolium pratense), nettle herbs (Urtica dioica), ginger root (Zingiber off.), ginseng root (Panax ginseng), astragalus root (Astragalus membranaceus), cayenne fruit ext. (Capsium minimum), aloes (Aloe barbadensis), celery fruit (Apium Graveolens), oats (Avena Sativa), chamomille flowers (Chamomilla), Cina., Cocculus Indicus, gentian (Gentiana lutea), helonias root (Chamaelirium luteum), dioica, goldenseal (Hydrastis canadensis), horehound (Marrubium vulgare), passion flower (Passiflora incarta), sarsparilla (Smilax), Senega officinale, sepia, skullcap (Scutellaria lateriflora), valerian (Valeriana officinalis), wild yam (Dioscorea), macca (Lepidium meyenii), biberry fruit (Myrtilli fructus), aloes extract (Aloe barbadensis), Iceland moss (Centraria islandica), naturals colors and flavors.

No animal ingredients, artificial flavors, colors, dairy, or sweeteners. Bottles of 886 mL. Shake well before use. Refrigerate after opening. Store at 15-30°C. Keep out of reach of children.

(Shown in Product Identification Section)

Dairy Free®
lactase
Lactose Digestant

SteriMax

SUPPLIED: Regular Strength: Each white, round, biconvex tablet contains: 3000 FCC lactase units of β-D-galactosidase derived from *A. oryzae*. Nonmedicinal ingredients: cellulose, colloidal silicon dioxide, magnesium stearate and povidone. Bottles of 100. Store at room temperature, away from heat.

Extra Strength: Each white, round, scored, biconvex tablet contains: 4500 FCC lactase units of β-D-galactosidase derived from *A. oryzae*. Nonmedicinal ingredients: cellulose, colloidal silicon dioxide, magnesium stearate and povidone. Bottles of 80. Store at room temperature, away from heat.

Dalacin® C ℞
clindamycin HCl
Antibiotic

Pfizer

Date of Revision: May 30, 2008

PHARMACOLOGY: Clindamycin exerts its antibacterial effect by causing cessation of protein synthesis and also causing a reduction in the rate of synthesis of nucleic acids.

The mechanism of action of clindamycin in combination with primaquine on *P. carinii* is not known.

Pharmacokinetics: Absorption: Clindamycin is rapidly and almost completely absorbed from the gastrointestinal tract in man and peak serum levels are seen in about 45 minutes. The average peak serum level following a single 150 mg dose in adults is 2.74 µg/mL. Therapeutically effective average levels of 0.73 µg/mL are found at 6 hours after a 150 mg dose.

The absorption of clindamycin is not appreciably affected by food intake. Peak serum levels following a single 250 mg oral dose of clindamycin with the patient in the fasting state were 3.1 µg/mL at 45 minutes whereas the same dose administered with food gave a peak level of 2.4 µg/mL. A 250 mg dose administered 1 hour after food gave a peak level of 2.8 µg/mL but this peak did not occur until 2 hours after administration of the medication. A 250 mg dose with the patient in a fasting state and with food administered 1 hour after the medication resulted in peak levels of 3.1 µg/mL at 1.5 hours.

Excretion: The 48-hour urinary excretion of clindamycin in adults following a single dose of 150 mg represented 10.9% of the administered dose (range 4.8 to 12.8%). These measurements were made by bio-assay and both the percent recovered and the urinary concentration are quite variable. The urinary concentration following a single 50 mg dose of clindamycin in the first 24 hours ranged from 8 to 25 µg/mL of urine.

Fecal excretion of clindamycin has also been determined. Patients on a 3-week study when administered 1 g of clindamycin/day had an average of 283 µg/g of stool. Patients on lincomycin 2 g/day under the same conditions showed 3980 µg/g of stool. In single-dose studies following administration of 250 mg of clindamycin, only 2.7% of the dose was excreted in the feces in 48 to 96 hours.

Tissue Penetration: In 3 patients following the administration of 150 mg of clindamycin, serum levels reached 2.25 µg/mL in 2 hours and declined to 1.5 µg/mL at 4 hours. During this period antibiotic synovial fluid levels were 1 µg/mL at 2 hours and remained unchanged for the next and last 2 hours of observation.

Various other body fluids and tissues were also assayed for clindamycin at the same time and the results of these assays and serum levels are recorded in Table 1.

Table 1: Dalacin C

Fluid/Tissue Levels

Specimen	No. of Specimens	Average Serum Level µg/mL	Average Fluid Level µg/mL	Tissue Level µg/mL
Pancreatic Fluid (C6-264)	4	1.15	45.1	
Bile (C6-264)	19	3.35	52.45	
Gall Bladder (C6-24)	16	0.81		4.33
Liver (C6-265)	1	42.35		3.80
Kidney (C6-265)	1	1.50		9.07
Bone (C4-390)	2	2.44		9.91

Clindamycin does not cross the blood-brain barrier even in the presence of inflamed meninges.

INDICATIONS: Dalacin C (Clindamycin Hydrochloride) is indicated in the treatment of serious infections due to sensitive anaerobic bacteria, such as Bacteroides species, Peptostreptococcus, anaerobic streptococci, Clostridium species and microaerophilic streptococci.

Clindamycin is also indicated in serious infections due to sensitive gram-positive aerobic organisms (staphylococci, including penicillinase-producing staphylococci, streptococci and pneumococci) when the patient is intolerant of, or the organism resistant to other appropriate antibiotics.

Clindamycin is indicated for the treatment of the *P. carinii* pneumonia in patients with AIDS. Clindamycin in combination with primaquine may be used in patients who are intolerant to, or fail to respond to conventional therapy.

Clindamycin is indicated for prophylaxis against alpha-hemolytic (viridans group) Streptococci before dental, oral and upper respiratory tract surgery.

a) The prophylaxis of bacterial endocarditis in patients allergic to penicillin with any of the following conditions: congenital cardiac malformations, rheumatic and other acquired valvular dysfunction, prosthetic heart valves, previous history of bacterial endocarditis, hypertrophic cardiomyopathy, surgically constructed systemic-pulmonary shunts, mitral valve prolapse with valvular regurgitation or mitral valve prolapse without regurgitation but associated with thickening and/or redundancy of the valve leaflets.

b) Patients taking oral penicillin for prevention or recurrence of rheumatic fever should be given another agent such as clindamycin, for prevention of bacterial endocarditis.

CONTRAINDICATIONS: Dalacin C (Clindamycin Hydrochloride) is contraindicated in patients previously found to be sensitive to clindamycin or lincomycin or to any component of the formulation.

Until further clinical experience is obtained clindamycin is not indicated in the newborn (infant below 30 days of age).

WARNINGS: *C. difficile*-associated disease (CDAD) has been reported with use of many antibacterial agents, including clindamycin hydrochloride capsules. CDAD may range in severity from mild diarrhea to fatal colitis. It is important to consider this diagnosis in patients who present with diarrhea, or symptoms of colitis, pseudomembranous colitis, toxic megacolon, or perforation of colon subsequent to the administration of any antibacterial agent. CDAD has been reported to occur over 2 months after the administration of antibacterial agents.

Treatment with antibacterial agents may alter the normal flora of the colon and may permit overgrowth of *C. difficile*. *C. difficile* produces toxins A and B, which contribute to the development of CDAD. CDAD may cause significant morbidity and mortality. CDAD can be refractory to antimicrobial therapy.

If the diagnosis of CDAD is suspected or confirmed, appropriate therapeutic measures should be initiated. Mild cases of CDAD usually respond to discontinuation of antibacterial agents not directed against *C. difficile*. In moderate to severe cases, consideration should be given to management with fluids and electrolytes, protein supplementation, and treatment with an antibacterial agent clinically effective against *C. difficile*. Surgical evaluation should be instituted as clinically indicated, as surgical intervention may be required in certain severe cases (see Adverse Effects).

In patients with G-6-PD deficiency, the combination of clindamycin with primaquine may cause hemolytic reactions; reference should also be made to the primaquine product monograph for other possible risk groups for other hematologic reactions.

PRECAUTIONS: General: Clindamycin should be prescribed with caution in atopic individuals and in individuals with a history of gastrointestinal disease, particularly colitis.

Clindamycin does not diffuse adequately into CSF and thus should not be used in the treatment of meningitis.

The use of antibiotics occasionally results in overgrowth of nonsusceptible organisms—particularly yeasts. Should superinfections occur, appropriate measures should be taken as dictated by the clinical situation.

As with all antibiotics, perform culture and sensitivity studies in conjunction with drug therapy.

Periodic liver and kidney function tests and blood counts should be performed during prolonged therapy.

Routine blood examinations should be done during therapy with primaquine to monitor potential hematologic toxicities.

Clindamycin dose modification may not be necessary in patients with renal disease. The serum half-life of clindamycin is increased slightly in patients with markedly reduced renal function.

In patients with moderate to severe liver disease, prolongation of the half-life of clindamycin has been found. However, it was postulated from studies that when given every 8 hours, accumulation of clindamycin should rarely occur. Therefore, dosage reduction in liver disease is not generally considered necessary. Periodic liver enzyme determinations should be made when treating patients with severe liver disease.

Geriatrics: Experience has demonstrated that antibiotic-associated colitis may occur more frequently and with increased severity among elderly (>60 years) and debilitated patients.

Pregnancy: Reproduction studies have been performed in rats and mice using s.c. and oral doses of clindamycin ranging from 20 to 600 mg/kg/day and have revealed no evidence of impaired fertility or harm to the fetus due to clindamycin. In one mouse strain, cleft palates were observed in treated fetuses; this response was not produced in other mouse strains or in other species, and therefore may be a strain specific effect.

Safety for use in pregnancy has not been established.

Clindamycin crosses the placenta in humans. After multiple doses, amniotic fluid concentrations were approximately 30% of maternal blood concentrations. Clindamycin was widely distributed in fetal tissues with the highest concentration found in the liver. Clindamycin should not be used in pregnancy unless clearly needed.

Lactation: Clindamycin has been reported to appear in human breast milk in the range of 0.7 to 3.8 µg/mL at doses of 150 mg orally to 600 mg i.v. Because of the potential for adverse reactions in neonates, a decision should be made whether to discontinue nursing or not administer clindamycin after taking into account the importance of the drug to the mother.

Drug Interactions: Antagonism has been demonstrated between clindamycin and erythromycin in vitro. Because of a possible clinical significance, the two drugs should not be administered concurrently.

Clindamycin has been shown to have neuromuscular blocking properties that may enhance the action of other neuromuscular blocking agents. Therefore, it should be used with caution in patients receiving such agents.

ADVERSE EFFECTS: Gastrointestinal: abdominal pain, nausea, vomiting, diarrhea, colitis, esophagitis and esophageal ulcer. *C. difficile*-associated disease (CDAD) has been observed and may manifest as a range of symptoms varying from watery diarrhea to fatal colitis, the onset of which may occur during or after antibacterial treatment (see Warnings).
Hypersensitivity Reactions: Maculopapular rash and urticaria have been observed during drug therapy. Generalized mild to moderate morbilliform-like skin rashes are the most frequently reported reactions. Rare instances of erythema multiforme, some resembling Stevens-Johnson syndrome, have been associated with clindamycin. A few cases of anaphylactoid reactions have been reported.
Liver: Jaundice and abnormalities in liver function tests have been observed during clindamycin therapy.
Skin and Mucous Membranes: Pruritus, vaginitis and rare instances of exfoliative and vesiculobullous dermatitis have been reported. Rare cases of toxic epidermal necrolysis have been reported during post-marketing surveillance.
Hematopoietic: Transient neutropenia (leukopenia) and eosinophilia have been reported. Reports of agranulocytosis and thrombocytopenia have been made. No direct etiologic relationship to concurrent clindamycin therapy could be made in any of these instances. However, in clindamycin/primaquine combination studies, serious hematologic toxicities (grade III, grade IV neutropenia or anemia, platelet counts <50×10^9/L, or methemoglobin levels of 15% or greater) have been observed.
Renal: Although no direct relationship of clindamycin to renal damage has been established, renal dysfunction as evidenced by azotemia, oliguria and/or proteinuria has been observed in rare instances.
Musculoskeletal: Rare instances of polyarthritis have been reported.
Nervous System: Dysgeusia has been reported during post-marketing surveillance.

OVERDOSE:

Symptoms: No cases of overdosage have been reported. It would be expected, however, that should overdosage occur, gastrointestinal side effects including abdominal pain, nausea, vomiting and diarrhea might be seen. During clinical trials, one 3-year-old child was given 100 mg/kg of clindamycin for 5 days and showed mild abdominal pain and diarrhea. One 13-year-old patient was given 75 mg/kg for 5 days with no side effects. In both cases laboratory values remained normal.
Treatment: Hemodialysis and peritoneal dialysis are not effective means of removing the compound from the blood. No specific antidote is known.

> For management of a suspected drug overdose, contact your **regional Poison Control Centre**. See the *CPS* Directory section for a list of Poison Control Centres.

DOSAGE: Adults: 150 mg every 6 hours; moderately severe infections: 300 mg every 6 hours; severe infections: 450 mg every 6 hours. Children (over 1 month of age): One of the following two dosage ranges should be selected depending on the severity of the infection: 8 to 16 mg/kg/day divided into 3 or 4 equal doses or 16 to 20 mg/kg/day divided into 3 or 4 equal doses.
P. carinii pneumonia in patients with AIDS: Clindamycin 300 to 450 mg may be given orally every 6 hours in combination with 15 to 30 mg of primaquine for 21 days. Alternatively, clindamycin phosphate 600 to 900 mg (i.v.) may be given every 6 hours or 900 mg (i.v.) every 8 hours in combination with an oral daily dose of 15 to 30 mg of primaquine. If patients should develop serious hematologic adverse effects, reducing the dosage regimen of primaquine and/or clindamycin capsule should be considered.
Absorption of clindamycin is not appreciably modified by ingestion of food and the capsules may be taken with meals.
To avoid the possibility of esophageal irritation, clindamycin capsules should be taken with a full glass of water.
For prevention of endocarditis: Adults: 300 mg orally 1 hour before procedure; then 150 mg 6 hours after initial dose.
Children: 10 mg/kg (not to exceed adult dose) orally 1 hour before procedure; then 5 mg/kg 6 hours after initial dose.
Note: With β-hemolytic streptococcal infections, treatment should continue for at least 10 days to diminish the likelihood of subsequent rheumatic fever or glomerulonephritis.
Elderly: Pharmacokinetic studies with clindamycin have shown no clinically important differences between young and elderly subjects with normal hepatic function and normal (age-adjusted) renal function after oral or intravenous administration. Therefore, dosage adjustments are not necessary in the elderly with normal hepatic function and normal (age-adjusted) renal function.

SUPPLIED: 150 mg: Each hard gelatin capsule with maroon cap and lavender body, branded "Upjohn 225", contains: clindamycin HCl hydrate equivalent to 150 mg of clindamycin base. Nonmedicinal ingredients: cornstarch, lactose, magnesium stearate and talc. Sodium: <1 mmol (0.3 mg). Gluten-free. Bottles of 100 and 500.
300 mg: Each hard gelatin capsule with light blue cap and body branded, "Upjohn 395" contains: clindamycin HCl hydrate equivalent to 300 mg of clindamycin base. Nonmedicinal ingredients: cornstarch, lactose, magnesium stearate and talc. Sodium: <1 mmol. Gluten-free. Bottles of 100.
Store at controlled room temperature (15 to 30°C).

(Shown in Product Identification Section)

Dalacin® C Flavored Granules ℞

clindamycin palmitate HCl

Antibiotic

Pfizer

Date of Revision: May 30, 2008

PHARMACOLOGY: Clindamycin palmitate HCl is a water soluble palmitic acid ester of clindamycin. The intact ester is essentially inactive as an antibacterial agent. Chemical or enzymatic hydrolysis of clindamycin palmitate HCl is necessary to obtain the antibiotic activity of the clindamycin base. Clindamycin base exerts its antibacterial effect by causing cessation of protein synthesis and also by causing a reduction in the rate of synthesis of nucleic acids.
INDICATIONS: The treatment of serious infections due to sensitive anaerobic bacteria, such as Bacteroides species, Peptostreptococcus, anaerobic streptococci, Clostridium species and microaerophilic streptococci.
Also indicated in serious infections due to sensitive gram-positive organisms (staphylococci, including penicillinase-producing staphylococci, streptococci and pneumococci) when the patient is intolerant of, or the organism resistant to other appropriate antibiotics.
Clindamycin palmitate is indicated for prophylaxis against alpha-hemolytic (viridans group) Streptococci before dental, oral and upper respiratory tract surgery.
a) The prophylaxis of bacterial endocarditis in patients allergic to penicillin with any of the following conditions: congenital cardiac malformations, rheumatic and other acquired valvular dysfunction, prosthetic heart valves, previous history of bacterial endocarditis, hypertrophic cardiomyopathy, surgically constructed systemic-pulmonary shunts, mitral valve prolapse with valvular regurgitation or mitral valve prolapse without regurgitation but associated with thickening and/or redundancy of the valve leaflets.
b) Patients taking oral penicillin for prevention or recurrence of rheumatic fever should be given another agent such as clindamycin, for prevention of bacterial endocarditis.
CONTRAINDICATIONS: In patients previously found to be sensitive to clindamycin or lincomycin or to any component of the formulation.
Until further clinical experience is obtained, clindamycin palmitate is not indicated in the newborn (infant below 30 days of age).
WARNINGS: *C. difficile*-associated disease (CDAD) has been reported with use of many antibacterial agents, including clindamycin palmitate. CDAD may range in severity from mild diarrhea to fatal colitis. It is important to consider this diagnosis in patients who present with diarrhea, or symptoms of colitis, pseudomembranous colitis, toxic megacolon, or perforation of colon subsequent to the administration of any antibacterial agent. CDAD has been reported to occur over 2 months after the administration of antibacterial agents.
Treatment with antibacterial agents may alter the normal flora of the colon and may permit overgrowth of *C. difficile*. *C. difficile* produces toxins A and B, which contribute to the development of CDAD. CDAD may cause significant morbidity and mortality. CDAD can be refractory to antimicrobial therapy.
If the diagnosis of CDAD is suspected or confirmed, appropriate therapeutic measures should be initiated. Mild cases of CDAD usually respond to discontinuation of antibacterial agents not directed against *C. difficile*. In moderate to severe cases, consideration should be given to management with fluids and electrolytes, protein supplementation, and treatment with an antibacterial agent clinically effective against *C. difficile*. Surgical evaluation should be instituted as clinically indicated, as surgical intervention may be required in certain severe cases (see Adverse Effects)
In patients with G-6-PD deficiency, the combination of clindamycin with primaquine may cause hemolytic reactions; reference should also be made to the primaquine product monograph for other possible risk groups for other hematologic reactions.

PRECAUTIONS: General: Clindamycin palmitate should be prescribed with caution in atopic individuals and in individuals with a history of gastrointestinal disease, particularly colitis.
Clindamycin palmitate does not diffuse adequately into CSF and thus should not be used in the treatment of meningitis.
The use of antibiotics occasionally results in overgrowth of nonsusceptible organisms—particularly yeasts. Should superinfections occur, appropriate measures should be taken as dictated by the clinical situation.
As with all antibiotics, perform culture and sensitivity studies in conjunction with drug therapy.
Periodic liver and kidney function tests and blood counts should be performed during prolonged therapy.
Clindamycin palmitate dose modification may not be necessary in patients with renal disease. The serum half-life of clindamycin is increased slightly in patients with markedly reduced renal function.
In patients with moderate to severe liver disease, prolongation of the half-life of clindamycin has been found. However, it was postulated from studies that, when given every 8 hours, accumulation of clindamycin should rarely occur. Therefore, dosage reduction in liver disease is not generally considered necessary. Periodic liver enzyme determinations should be made when treating patients with severe liver disease.
Geriatrics: Experience has demonstrated that antibiotic-associated colitis may occur more frequently and with increased severity among elderly (>60 years) and debilitated patients.
Pregnancy: Reproduction studies have been performed in rats and mice using s.c. and oral doses of clindamycin ranging from 20 to 600 mg/kg/day and have revealed no evidence of impaired fertility or harm to the fetus due to clindamycin. In one mouse strain, cleft palates were observed in treated fetuses; this response was not produced in other mouse strains or in other species, and therefore may be a strain-specific effect.
Safety for use in pregnancy has not been established.
Clindamycin crosses the placenta in humans. After multiple doses, amniotic fluid concentrations were approximately 30% of maternal blood concentrations. Clindamycin was widely distributed in fetal tissues with the highest concentration found in liver. Clindamycin should not be used in pregnancy unless clearly needed.
Lactation: Clindamycin has been reported to appear in human breast milk in the range of 0.7 to 3.8 μg/mL at doses of 150 mg orally to 600 mg i.v. Because of the potential for adverse reactions in neonates, a decision should be made whether to discontinue nursing or to not administer clindamycin after taking into account the importance of the drug to the mother.
Drug Interactions: Antagonism has been demonstrated between clindamycin and erythromycin in vitro. Because of a possible clinical significance, the two drugs should not be administered concurrently.
Clindamycin has been shown to have neuromuscular blocking properties that may enhance the action of other neuromuscular blocking agents. Therefore, it should be used with caution in patients receiving such agents.

ADVERSE EFFECTS: Gastrointestinal: abdominal pain, nausea, vomiting, diarrhea, colitis, esophagitis and esophageal ulcer. *C. difficile*-associated disease (CDAD) has been observed and may manifest as a range of symptoms varying from watery diarrhea to fatal colitis, the onset of which may occur during or after antibacterial treatment (see Warnings).
Hypersensitivity Reactions: Maculopapular rash and urticaria have been observed during drug therapy. Generalized mild to moderate morbilliform-like skin rashes are the most frequently reported reactions. Rare instances of erythema multiforme, some resembling Stevens-Johnson syndrome, have been associated with clindamycin. A few cases of anaphylactoid reactions have been reported.
Liver: Jaundice and abnormalities in liver function tests have been observed during clindamycin therapy.
Skin and Mucous Membranes: Pruritus, vaginitis and rare instances of exfoliative and vesiculobullous dermatitis have been reported. Rare cases of toxic epidermal necrolysis have been reported during post-marketing surveillance.
Hematopoietic: Transient neutropenia (leukopenia) and eosinophilia have been reported. Reports of agranulocytosis and thrombocytopenia have been made. No direct etiologic relationship to concurrent clindamycin therapy could be made in any of these instances.
Renal: Although no direct relationship of clindamycin to renal damage has been established, renal dysfunction as evidenced by azotemia, oliguria and/or proteinuria has been observed in rare instances.
Musculoskeletal: Rare instances of polyarthritis have been reported.
Nervous System: Dysgeusia has been reported during post-marketing surveillance.

OVERDOSE:

Symptoms: No cases of overdosage have been reported. It would be expected, however, that should overdosage occur, gastrointestinal side effects including abdominal pain, nausea, vomiting and diarrhea might be seen. During clinical trials, one 3 year old child was given 100 mg/kg of clindamycin for 5 days and showed mild abdominal pain and diarrhea. One 13 year old patient was given 75 mg/kg for 5 days with no side effects. In both cases laboratory values remained normal. In a study in normal adult volunteers up to 1800 mg/day for 21 days of clindamycin palmitate was given with only a change in the consistency and frequency of stools reported as well as 3 rashes, 2 cases of nausea and 1 case of dizziness.
Treatment: Hemodialysis and peritoneal dialysis are not effective means of removing the compound from the blood.

> For management of a suspected drug overdose, contact your **regional Poison Control Centre**. See the *CPS* Directory section for a list of Poison Control Centres.

DOSAGE: Children (over 1 month of age): One of the following three dosage ranges should be selected depending on the severity of the infection: 8 to 12 mg/kg/day divided into 3 or 4 equal doses. 13 to 16 mg/kg/day divided into 3 or 4 equal doses. 17 to 25 mg/kg/day divided into 3 or 4 equal doses (see Table 1).

Table 1: Dalacin C Flavored Granules

Dosage Ranges

Weight (kg)	8–12 mg/kg/day	13–16 mg/kg/day	17–25 mg/kg/day
10–18.2	37.5 mg q 6 h	75 mg q 8 h	75 mg q 6 h
18.2–25	75 mg q 8 h	75 mg q 6 h	150 mg q8 h
25–34	75 mg q 6 h	150 mg q 8 h	150 mg q 6 h
34–45.4	150 mg q 8 h	150 mg q 6 h	300 mg q 8 h
45.5 and over-use adult dosage	150 mg q 6 h	300 mg q 6 h	450 mg q 6 h

Note: In cases of β-hemolytic streptococcal infections, treatment should continue for at least 10 days to diminish the likelihood of subsequent rheumatic fever or glomerulonephritis.
For Prevention of Endocarditis: Adults: 300 mg orally 1 hour before procedure; then 150 mg 6 hours after initial dose.
Children: 10 mg/kg (not to exceed adult dose) orally 1 hour before procedure; then 5 mg/kg 6 hours after initial dose.
Elderly: Pharmacokinetic studies with clindamycin have shown no clinically important differences between young and elderly subjects with normal hepatic function and normal (age-adjusted) renal function after oral or intravenous administration. Therefore, dosage adjustments are not necessary in the elderly with normal hepatic function and normal (age-adjusted) renal function.

SUPPLIED: After reconstitution with 75 mL demineralized or distilled water, each 5 mL of solution contains: clindamycin palmitate HCl equivalent to 75 mg clindamycin base. Nonmedicinal ingredients: artificial cherry flavor, ethyl paraben, methylene chloride, Pluronic F68, polymethylsiloxane and sucrose. Energy: 25.1 kJ (6 kcal)/5 mL. Sodium: trace. Gluten-free. Bottles of 100 mL. Store at controlled room temperature (20-25°C).
Note: Do not refrigerate the reconstituted solution since under conditions of low temperature, the solution may thicken and is difficult to pour. The reconstituted solution is stable at room temperature for 14 days.

> **New CPhA monographs in 2011 include bisoprolol, dantrolene and propafenone. Consult the CPhA Monographs Index in the front pages of the *CPS* to obtain a complete list.**

Dalacin® C Phosphate Sterile Solution ℞

clindamycin phosphate

Antibiotic

Pfizer

Date of Revision: May 30, 2008

PHARMACOLOGY: Following parenteral administration, biologically inactive clindamycin phosphate is rapidly hydrolyzed in plasma to active clindamycin. Clindamycin exerts its antibacterial effect by binding to the 50 S ribosomal subunit of susceptible bacteria, causing a reduction in the rate of synthesis of nucleic acid, and cessation of protein synthesis.

Clindamycin is primarily bacteriostatic, but may be bactericidal at high concentrations. The mechanism of action of clindamycin in combination with primaquine on *P. carinii* is not known.

Pharmacokinetics: See Table 1. Clindamycin is distributed into body fluids and tissues including bone, synovial fluid, bile and pleural fluid. Significant levels of clindamycin are not reached in cerebrospinal fluid even in the presence of inflamed meninges. Clindamycin readily crosses the placenta and is distributed into breast milk. The half-life of clindamycin phosphate is 3.5 to 4.5 hours. Approximately 10% of the microbiologically active form is excreted in the urine and about 4% in the feces. The remainder is excreted as biologically inactive metabolites.

Table 1: Dalacin C Phosphate Sterile Solution

Average Peak Serum Concentrations After Dosing with Clindamycin Phosphate

Clindamycin Phosphate Dosage Regimen	Clindamycin µg/mL	Clindamycin Phosphate µg/mL
Healthy Adult Male (Post Equilibrium)		
300 mg i.v. in 10 min, q8h	7	15
600 mg i.v. in 20 min, q8h	10	23
900 mg i.v. in 30 min, q12h	11	29
1200 mg i.v. in 45 min, q12h	14	49
300 mg i.m. q8h	6	3
600 mg i.m. q12h[a]	9	3
Children (first dose)[a]		
5–7 mg/kg i.v. in 1 hour	10	
3–5 mg/kg i.m.	4	
5–7 mg/kg i.m.	8	

[a] Data in this group from patients being treated for infection.

INDICATIONS: For the treatment of serious infections due to susceptible anaerobic bacteria, such as Bacteroides species, Peptostreptococcus, anaerobic streptococci, Clostridium species and microaerophilic streptococci.

Also indicated for the treatment of serious infections due to susceptible strains of gram-positive aerobic bacteria (staphylococci, including penicillinase-producing staphylococci, streptococci and pneumococci) as well as in the treatment of *C. trachomatis*, when the patient is intolerant of, or the organism resistant to other appropriate antibiotics.

Because of the risk of *C. difficile*-associated disease (CDAD) as described in the Warnings section, before selecting clindamycin the physician should consider the nature of the infection and the suitability of alternative therapy.

Clindamycin phosphate is indicated for the treatment of the following serious infections when caused by susceptible strains of the designated organisms in the conditions listed below:

Lower respiratory infections including pneumonia, empyema, and lung abscess when caused by anaerobes, *S. pneumoniae*, other streptococci (except *E. faecalis*) and *S. aureus*.

Skin and skin structure infections including cellulitis, abscesses, and wound infections when caused by *S. pyogenes*, *S. aureus* and anaerobes.

Gynecological infections including endometritis, pelvic cellulitis, vaginal cuff infections, nongonococcal tubo-ovarian abscess, salpingitis, and pelvic inflammatory disease when caused by susceptible anaerobes or *C. trachomatis*. Clindamycin should be given in conjunction with an antibiotic of appropriate gram-negative aerobic spectrum.

Intra-abdominal infections including peritonitis and abdominal abscess when caused by susceptible anaerobes. Clindamycin should be given in conjunction with an antibiotic of appropriate gram-negative aerobic spectrum.

Septicemia caused by *S. aureus*, streptococci (except *E. faecalis*) and susceptible anaerobes, where the bactericidal efficacy of clindamycin against the infecting organism has been determined in vitro at achievable serum levels.

Bone and joint infections including osteomyelitis and septic arthritis when caused by sensitive strains of *S. aureus* and anaerobes.

P. carinii pneumonia in patients with AIDS. Clindamycin in combination with primaquine may be used in patients who are intolerant to, or fail to respond to conventional therapy.

Note: Clindamycin phosphate is not indicated in the treatment of meningitis since it penetrates poorly into cerebrospinal fluid, even in the presence of inflamed meninges.

Bacteriologic studies should be performed to determine the causative organisms and their susceptibility to clindamycin.

Indicated surgical procedures and drainage should be performed in conjunction with antibiotic therapy.

CONTRAINDICATIONS: In patients with a known hypersensitivity to preparations containing clindamycin or lincomycin or to any component of the formulation.

WARNINGS: *C. difficile*-associated disease (CDAD) has been reported with use of many antibacterial agents, including clindamycin phosphate. CDAD may range in severity from mild diarrhea to fatal colitis. It is important to consider this diagnosis in patients who present with diarrhea, or symptoms of colitis, pseudomembranous colitis, toxic megacolon, or perforation of colon subsequent to the administration of any antibacterial agent. CDAD has been reported to occur over 2 months after the administration of antibacterial agents.

Treatment with antibacterial agents may alter the normal flora of the colon and may permit overgrowth of *C. difficile*. *C. difficile* produces toxins A and B, which contribute to the development of CDAD. CDAD may cause significant morbidity and mortality. CDAD can be refractory to antimicrobial therapy.

If the diagnosis of CDAD is suspected or confirmed, appropriate therapeutic measures should be initiated. Mild cases of CDAD usually respond to discontinuation of antibacterial agents not directed against *C. difficile*. In moderate to severe cases, consideration should be given to management with fluids and electrolytes, protein supplementation, and treatment with an antibacterial agent clinically effective against *C. difficile*. Surgical evaluation should be instituted as clinically indicated, as surgical intervention may be required in certain severe cases (see Adverse Effects)

In patients with G-6-PD deficiency, the combination of clindamycin with primaquine may cause hemolytic reactions; reference should also be made to the primaquine product monograph for other possible risk groups for other hematologic reactions.

Clindamycin phosphate contains benzyl alcohol. Benzyl alcohol has been reported to be associated with a fatal "Gasping Syndrome" in premature infants.

PRECAUTIONS: General: Clindamycin phosphate should be prescribed with caution in atopic individuals and in individuals with a history of gastrointestinal disease particularly colitis.

Clindamycin phosphate does not diffuse adequately into cerebrospinal fluid and thus should not be used in the treatment of meningitis.

Clindamycin phosphate must be diluted for i.v. administration. It should not be injected undiluted as an i.v. bolus (see Dosage).

The use of antibiotics occasionally results in overgrowth of nonsusceptible organisms, particularly yeasts. Should superinfections occur, appropriate measures should be taken as dictated by the clinical situation.

Periodic liver and kidney function tests and blood counts should be performed during prolonged therapy.

Routine blood examinations should be done during therapy with primaquine to monitor potential hematologic toxicities.

Clindamycin phosphate dose modification may not be necessary in patients with renal disease. The serum half-life of clindamycin is increased slightly in patients with markedly reduced renal function.

In patients with moderate to severe liver disease, prolongation of the half-life of clindamycin has been found however, it was postulated from studies that when given every 8 hours, accumulation of clindamycin should rarely occur. Therefore, dosage reduction in liver disease is not generally considered necessary. Periodic liver enzyme determinations should be made when treating patients with severe liver disease (see Pharmacology).

Geriatrics: Experience has demonstrated that antibiotic-associated colitis may occur more frequently and with increased severity among elderly (>60 years) and debilitated patients.

Pregnancy: Reproduction studies have been performed in rats and mice using s.c. and oral doses of clindamycin ranging from 20 to 600 mg/kg/day and have revealed no evidence of impaired fertility or harm to the fetus due to clindamycin. In 1 mouse strain, cleft palates were observed in treated fetuses; this response was not produced in other mouse strains or in other species, and therefore may be a strain-specific effect.

Safety for use in pregnancy has not been established.

Clindamycin crosses the placenta in humans. After multiple doses, amniotic fluid concentrations were approximately 30% of maternal blood concentrations. Clindamycin was widely distributed in fetal tissues with the highest concentration found in the liver. Clindamycin should not be used in pregnancy unless clearly needed.

Lactation: Clindamycin has been reported to appear in breast milk in the range of 0.7 to 3.8 µg/mL at doses of 150 mg orally to 600 mg i.v. Because of the potential for adverse reactions in neonates, a decision should be made whether to discontinue nursing or to not administer clindamycin after taking into account the importance of the drug to the mother.

Drug Interactions: Antagonism has been demonstrated between clindamycin and erythromycin in vitro. Because of a possible clinical significance, the two drugs should not be administered concurrently.

Clindamycin has been shown to have neuromuscular blocking properties that may enhance the action of other neuromuscular blocking agents. Therefore, it should be used with caution in patients receiving such agents.

ADVERSE EFFECTS: Gastrointestinal: abdominal pain, nausea, vomiting, diarrhea, colitis. *C. difficile*-associated disease (CDAD) has been observed and may manifest as a range of symptoms varying from watery diarrhea to fatal colitis, the onset of which may occur during or after antibacterial treatment (see Warnings).

Hypersensitivity Reactions: Maculopapular rash and urticaria have been observed during drug therapy. Generalized mild to moderate morbilliform-like skin rashes are the most frequently reported reactions. Rare instances of erythema multiforme, some resembling Stevens-Johnson syndrome, have been associated with clindamycin. A few cases of anaphylactoid reactions have been reported.

Liver: Jaundice and abnormalities in liver function tests have been observed during clindamycin therapy.

Skin and Mucous Membranes: Pruritus, vaginitis and rare instances of exfoliative and vesiculobullous dermatitis have been reported. Rare cases of toxic epidermal necrolysis have been reported during post-marketing surveillance.

Hematopoietic: Transient neutropenia (leukopenia) and eosinophilia have been reported. Reports of agranulocytosis and thrombocytopenia have been made. No direct etiologic relationship to concurrent clindamycin therapy could be made in any of these instances. However, in clindamycin/primaquine combination studies, serious hematologic toxicities (grade III, grade IV neutropenia or anemia, platelet counts $<50 \times 10^9$/L, or methemoglobin levels of 15% or greater) have been observed.

Cardiovascular: Rare instances of cardiopulmonary arrest and hypotension have been reported following too rapid i.v. administration (see Dosage).

Renal: Although no direct relationship of clindamycin to renal damage has been established, renal dysfunction as evidenced by azotemia, oliguria and/or proteinuria has been observed in rare instances.

Musculoskeletal: Rare instances of polyarthritis have been reported.

Local Reactions: Local irritation, pain, abscess formation have been seen with i.m. injection. Thrombophlebitis has been reported with i.v. injection. These reactions can be minimized by deep i.m. injection and avoidance of indwelling i.v. catheters.

Nervous System: dysgeusia.

OVERDOSE:

Symptoms: Reported cases of overdosage have occurred very infrequently. The majority of these reports have involved infants and young children ranging in age from 1 day to 3 years. In this age group, doses as high as 2.4 g have been used i.v. in 36 hours without observation of adverse reactions.

Treatment: Hemodialysis and peritoneal dialysis are not effective in removing clindamycin from the serum. No specific antidote is known.

> For management of a suspected drug overdose, contact your **regional Poison Control Centre**. See the *CPS* Directory section for a list of Poison Control Centres.

DOSAGE: **Note:** If diarrhea occurs during treatment, this antibiotic should be discontinued (see Warnings).

Dosage and route of administration should be determined by the severity of the infection, the condition of the patient and the susceptibility of the causative microorganisms.

In cases of β hemolytic streptococcal infections, treatment should be continued for at least 10 days.

Adults (I.M. or I.V. Administration): The usual daily adult dosage for infections of the intra-abdominal area, female pelvis, and other complicated or serious infections is 2400 to 2700 mg given in 2, 3 or 4 equal doses. Less complicated infections may respond to lower doses such as 1200 to 1800 mg/day administered in 3 or 4 equal doses.

Doses of up to 4800 mg daily have been used without adverse effects. Single i.m. doses of greater than 600 mg are not recommended.

Pelvic Inflammatory Disease: 900 mg (i.v.) every 8 hours plus an antibiotic with appropriate gram-negative aerobic spectrum administered i.v. Treatment with i.v. drugs should continue for at least 48 hours after the patient demonstrates significant clinical improvement. Then continue with appropriate oral therapy to complete 10 to 14 days total therapy.

P. carinii pneumonia in patients with AIDS: 600 to 900 mg (i.v.) every 6 hours or 900 mg (i.v.) every 8 hours in combination with oral daily dose of 15 to 30 mg of primaquine. Alternatively, clindamycin HCl 300 to 450 mg may be given orally every 6 hours in combination with 15 to 30 mg of primaquine for 21 days. If patients should develop serious hematologic adverse effects, reducing the dosage regimen of primaquine and/or clindamycin phosphate should be considered.

Children over 1 month of age (I.M. or I.V. Administration): 20 to 40 mg/kg/day in 3 or 4 equal doses. The higher doses would be used for more severe infections.

Neonates under 1 month of age (I.M. or I.V. Administration): 10 to 20 mg/kg/day in 3 or 4 equal doses. The lower dosage may be adequate for small prematures. See Table 2.

Table 2: Dalacin C Phosphate Sterile Solution

Dosage—Neonates Under One Month of Age

Weight	Age	Dose	Route
<2 kg	0–7 days	5 mg/kg q12h	i.v.
<2 kg	8–30 days	5 mg/kg q8h	i.v.
≥2 kg	0–7 days	5 mg/kg q8h	i.v.
≥2 kg	8–30 days	5 mg/kg q6h	i.v.

Note: Clindamycin phosphate injections should be administered with caution to newborn infants less than 30 days of age. This product contains benzyl alcohol which has been associated with a fatal gasping syndrome in infants.

Dilution and Infusion Rates: Clindamycin phosphate must be diluted prior to i.v. administration (see Preparation for I.V. Use for a listing of infusion solutions). The concentration in diluent for infusion should not exceed 18 mg/mL. Infusion rates should **not exceed 30 mg/min** as indicated in Table 3.

Table 3: Dalacin C Phosphate Sterile Solution
Dilution and Infusion Rates

Dose (mg)	Diluent (mL)	Time (min)
300	50	10
600	50	20
900	100	30
1200	100	45

Administration of more than 1200 mg in a single 1 hour infusion is not recommended.

Alternatively, the drug may be administered in the form of a single rapid infusion of the first dose followed by continuous i.v. infusion as in Table 4.

Table 4: Dalacin C Phosphate Sterile Solution
Maintenance of Serum Levels

To Maintain Serum Clindamycin Levels	Rapid Infusion Rate	Maintenance Infusion Rate
Above 4 µg/mL	10 mg/min for 30 min	0.75 mg/min
Above 5 µg/mL	15 mg/min for 30 min	1 mg/min
Above 6 µg/mL	20 mg/min for 30 min	1.25 mg/min

Elderly: Pharmacokinetic studies with clindamycin have shown no clinically important differences between young and elderly subjects with normal hepatic function and normal (age-adjusted) renal function after oral or intravenous administration. Therefore, dosage adjustments are not necessary in the elderly with normal hepatic function and normal (age-adjusted) renal function.

Parenteral Products: All parenteral products should be visually inspected for haziness, particulate matter, discoloration and leakage prior to administration.

Preparation for I.V. Use: Clindamycin phosphate was found to be compatible over a period of 24 hours when 4 mL (600 mg) of clindamycin phosphate was diluted with 1000 mL of the following commonly used infusion solutions: Sodium chloride injection, Dextrose 5% in water, Dextrose 5% in saline, Dextrose 5% in Ringer's Solution, Dextrose 5% in half-strength saline plus 40 mEq potassium chloride, Dextrose 2½% in Lactated Ringer's Solution (Hartmann's Solution).

Compatibility with Other Products: Clindamycin phosphate was not stable when added to Dextrose 5% in water plus vitamins. **Although clindamycin phosphate is compatible with Dextrose 5% in water, it is not recommended that clindamycin phosphate be mixed with any infusion solutions containing B vitamins.**

Clindamycin phosphate has been shown to be compatible with gentamicin sulfate, tobramycin sulfate and amikacin sulfate. However, a precipitate has been observed when clindamycin phosphate and gentamicin are drawn undiluted into the same syringe before subsequent dilution. This precipitate appears to be a zinc-clindamycin complex which results from the zinc content of some gentamicin products. The particle size of the insoluble material is very small and disappears when the admixture is shaken. To avoid this problem, do not mix clindamycin phosphate and gentamicin sulfate prior to dilution. Rather, dilute one drug or the other, agitate the solution and then add the second antibiotic.

Incompatibility with Other Products: When combined with clindamycin phosphate in an infusion solution, ampicillin, phenytoin sodium, barbiturates, aminophyllin, calcium gluconate, magnesium sulfate, ceftriaxone sodium, and ciprofloxacin are each physically incompatible with clindamycin phosphate.

SUPPLIED: Each mL of sterile solution contains: clindamycin phosphate equivalent to 150 mg of clindamycin base, benzyl alcohol 9 mg, disodium edetate 0.5 mg and water for injection q.s. When necessary, the pH is adjusted with sodium hydroxide and/or hydrochloric acid to maintain a pH range of 5.5 to 7.0. Vials of 2, 4 and 6 mL. Pharmacy bulk vials of 60 mL. **The availability of the pharmacy bulk vial is limited to hospitals with a pharmacy based i.v. admixture program. The pharmacy bulk vial is intended for single puncture, multiple dispensing for i.v. use only.** Store at controlled room temperature (15 to 30°C).

Dalacin® T Topical Solution Ⓟ
clindamycin phosphate
Antibiotic

Pfizer

Date of Revision: June 16, 2009

PHARMACOLOGY: Clindamycin phosphate is inactive in vitro but in vivo hydrolysis converts this compound to the antibacterially active clindamycin. Clindamycin has been shown to have in vitro activity against isolates of *P. acnes* which may account for its usefulness in acne. Clindamycin activity has been demonstrated in serum, urine and in comedonal extracts from acne patients.

The mean concentration of antibiotic activity in extracted comedones after application of clindamycin topical solution for 4 weeks was 597 µg/g of comedonal material (range 60 to 1490). Clindamycin in vitro inhibits *P. acnes* cultures tested.

INDICATIONS: For the treatment of acne vulgaris.

CONTRAINDICATIONS: In individuals with a history of hypersensitivity to preparations containing clindamycin or lincomycin, a history of inflammatory bowel disease (including regional enteritis and ulcerative colitis), or a history of antibiotic-associated colitis.

WARNINGS: Gastrointestinal: *C. difficile*-associated disease: *C. difficile*-associated disease (CDAD) has been reported with use of many antibacterial agents, including DALACIN T (clindamycin phosphate topical solution USP 1%). CDAD may range in severity from mild diarrhea to fatal colitis. It is important to consider this diagnosis in patients who present with diarrhea, or symptoms of colitis, pseudomembranous colitis, toxic megacolon, or perforation of colon subsequent to the administration of any antibacterial agent. CDAD has been reported to occur over 2 months after the administration of antibacterial agents.

Treatment with antibacterial agents may alter the normal flora of the colon and may permit overgrowth of *C. difficile. C. difficile* produces toxins A and B, which contribute to the development of CDAD. CDAD may cause significant morbidity and mortality. CDAD can be refractory to antimicrobial therapy.

If the diagnosis of CDAD is suspected or confirmed, appropriate therapeutic measures should be initiated. Mild cases of CDAD usually respond to discontinuation of antibacterial agents not directed against *C. difficile*. In moderate to severe cases, consideration should be given to management with fluids and electrolytes, protein supplementation, and treatment with an antibacterial agent clinically effective against *C. difficile*. Surgical evaluation should be instituted as clinically indicated, as surgical intervention may be required in certain severe cases (see Adverse Effects).

PRECAUTIONS: Clindamycin topical solution contains an alcohol base which will cause burning and irritation of the eye. In the event of accidental contact with sensitive surfaces (eye, abraded skin, mucous membranes), bathe with copious amounts of cool tap water.

The solution has an unpleasant taste and caution should be exercised when applying medication around the mouth.

Clindamycin phosphate should be prescribed with caution in atopic individuals.

Pregnancy: Safety for use in pregnancy has not been established.

Lactation: It is not known whether clindamycin when topically applied is excreted in human milk. However, oral and parenteral clindamycin have been reported to appear in breast milk and therefore, nursing should not be undertaken while a patient is on the drug.

Drug Interactions: Antagonism has been demonstrated between clindamycin and erythromycin in vitro. Because of a possible clinical significance, the two drugs should not be administered concurrently. Clindamycin (oral and parenterally administered) has been shown to have neuromuscular blocking properties that may enhance the action of other neuromuscular blocking agents. Therefore, Dalacin T should be used with caution in patients receiving such agents.

ADVERSE EFFECTS: In a large U.S. postmarketing surveillance study among 1298 patients treated only with topical clindamycin phosphate solution, skin dryness/irritation, diarrhea or gastrointestinal symptoms were the most commonly reported medical events. Of those, 258 (19.9%) reported 1 or more of the following dermatological events: dry skin, acne worse, rash/redness, peeling, discoloration, urticaria, irritation, itching, new acne, sunburn and contact dermatitis. Among patients treated with oral antibiotics only, or no antibiotics, the percentage of patients reporting dermatologic event(s) was 20.8% and 25.4% respectively.

The following new gastrointestinal problems were reported in this surveillance study by 18.7% of the clindamycin treated patients, 22.9% of the oral antibiotic treated patients, and 18.4% of the patients with no antibiotic exposure: abdominal pain/cramps, nausea, flu/virus, indigestion, gas/bloating, "nervous" stomach, ulcers, vomiting and colon problems (not colitis).

Cases of diarrhea, bloody diarrhea and colitis (including pseudomembranous colitis) have been reported as adverse reactions in patients treated with topical formulations of clindamycin. Diarrhea was reported by 55 of the 1298 (5%) clindamycin patients, compared to 3.9% of control patients. (See Warnings, Gastrointestinal, CDAD.)

In addition to the above, the following side effects have also been occasionally reported during drug treatment with clindamycin topical solution: oily skin and gram-negative folliculitis.

OVERDOSE:
Topically applied clindamycin can be absorbed in sufficient amounts to produce systemic effects.

> For management of a suspected drug overdose, contact your **regional Poison Control Centre**. See the *CPS* Directory section for a list of Poison Control Centres.

DOSAGE: Apply a thin film of topical solution twice daily to the clean and dry skin in the area to be treated. Patients responding to clindamycin topical solution should show improvement in 8 weeks. Treatment beyond 12 weeks may call for evaluation by the physician.

INFORMATION FOR THE PATIENT: Published in e-CPS, available by subscription at www.e-cps.ca.

SUPPLIED: Each mL of topical solution contains: clindamycin phosphate equivalent to clindamycin 10 mg. Nonmedicinal ingredients: isopropyl alcohol 50% v/v, propylene glycol and purified water. When needed, the pH of the solution is adjusted with hydrochloric acid and/or sodium hydroxide. Bottles of 30 and 60 mL. A dab-o-matic applicator and cap is provided external to each bottle for placement into the bottle. To assist the patient, the pharmacist may assemble the bottle upon dispensing as follows: remove cap from bottle and discard, firmly press applicator into bottle, seal firmly by tightening domed-cap. Store in an upright fashion. Store at controlled room temperature (15 to 30°C).

Dalacin® Vaginal Cream Ⓟ
clindamycin phosphate
Antibacterial

Paladin

SUPPLIED: Each g of semi-solid white cream contains: clindamycin 20 mg (as clindamycin phosphate). Each full applicator (one dose) contains: clindamycin 100 mg (as clindamycin phosphate) in 5 g of cream. Nonmedicinal ingredients: benzyl alcohol, cetostearyl alcohol, cetyl palmitate, mineral oil, polysorbate 60, propylene glycol, purified water, sorbitan monostearate and stearic acid. Collapsible laminate tubes of 40 g with 7 disposable applicators for intravaginal use. Store at controlled room temperature (15 to 30°C). Protect from freezing.

Dalmacol Ⓝ
hydrocodone bitartrate—etafedrine HCl—sodium citrate—doxylamine succinate
Antihistaminic—Antitussive—Decongestant

Riva

SUPPLIED: Each mL contains: hydrocodone bitartrate 0.33 mg, etafedrine HCl 3.33 mg, sodium citrate 40 mg and doxylamine succinate 1.2 mg. Nonmedicinal ingredients: alcohol, aromate, FD&C yellow, glycerin, propylparaben, sorbitol and sucrose. Bottles of 500 mL and 2 L.

Dalteparin Ⓟ

CPhA Monograph

see *Heparins: Low Molecular Weight*

Dantrolene Ⓟ
Skeletal Muscle Relaxant

CPhA Monograph

Date of Preparation: October 2010

> This monograph has been compiled by CPhA and reviewed by experts. It may contain information different from that found in Health Canada-approved Product Monographs. The reader is referred to the *CPS* Editorial Policy for more information.

SUMMARY PRODUCT INFORMATION:

Route of Administration	Dosage Form	Strength
Oral	Capsule	25 mg, 100 mg
Intravenous	Powder	20 mg/vial

INDICATIONS AND CLINICAL USE: Health Canada-approved Indications Include:

Injectable:
- Treatment of malignant hyperthermia

Oral:
- Management of chronic spasticity of skeletal muscle from nonrheumatic causes (e.g., spinal cord injury, cerebral palsy, multiple sclerosis and stroke)
- Step-down therapy for post-crisis management in patients with malignant hyperthermia who have been stabilized with iv dantrolene
- Preoperative management of patients known to be susceptible to malignant hyperthermia

Uses Without Health Canada Approval: Dantrolene has been used for the treatment of neuroleptic malignant syndrome.

CONTRAINDICATIONS:
- Patients who are hypersensitive to dantrolene or to any ingredient in the formulation or component of the container.
- Patients with hepatitis, cirrhosis or other active liver disease.
- Cases where spasticity is needed to sustain posture/balance, or when spasticity is used to obtain or maintain increased body function.

WARNINGS AND PRECAUTIONS:

> **Serious Warnings and Precautions**
> Fatal hepatitis has occurred rarely in patients taking dantrolene (see Hepatic/Biliary/Pancreatic).

Carcinogenesis and Mutagenesis: One case of fatal lymphocytic lymphoma in a patient taking dantrolene for 3 years has been reported [*Postgrad Med J* 1980;56(654):261-2].
Cardiovascular: Dantrolene should be used with caution in patients with impaired myocardial function due to muscle-weakening effects of dantrolene.
Hepatic/Biliary/Pancreatic: Dose-dependent fatal and nonfatal hepatitis have been reported, even during a short course of therapy. Consider discontinuing dantrolene if liver enzymes are elevated or if symptoms of hepatotoxicity occur, such as discoloured stool, pruritus, jaundice, anorexia, nausea and vomiting. The risk of hepatotoxicity is higher in females, patients older than 35 years and patients concomitantly taking other hepatotoxic agents. Use the lowest effective dose, and discontinue therapy if no benefit is observed within 45 days. Liver function (e.g., ALT, AST) should be periodically monitored.
Musculoskeletal: Dantrolene may cause excessive muscle weakness, leading to decreased grip strength or leg muscle weakness. Dantrolene should be used with caution in patients using rehabilitation devices such as wheelchairs, crutches, braces, walkers, canes. Discontinue dantrolene if weakness persists and interferes with use of the device.
Respiratory: Dantrolene should be used with caution in patients with impaired lung function, especially that of obstructive nature. Pleural effusion has been reported in patients taking dantrolene.
Special Populations: Pregnant Women: Dantrolene crosses placenta. There are reports of dantrolene use shortly before delivery in approximately 20 women at risk for malignant hyperthermia (MH), with no reported fetal or neonatal adverse effects; however, safety of prophylactic use during pregnancy has not been established. When surgery is required in at-risk women, avoid use of anesthetics that could trigger MH, monitor carefully during delivery and be prepared to treat MH if it occurs.
Nursing Women: Dantrolene is excreted in breast milk. Safety of dantrolene use during breastfeeding has not been established. The half-life of dantrolene in breast milk is 9 hours. It has been suggested that breastfeeding be discontinued during dantrolene therapy and until 2 days after the last dose, to minimize exposure to the nursing infant.
Pediatrics: Dantrolene has been used in children for spasticity, malignant hyperthermia and neuroleptic malignant syndrome. Its use is generally not recommended in children younger than 5 years.
Monitoring and Laboratory Tests: Elevations of serum AST and ALT have been noted (see Adverse Reactions).
Occupational Hazards: Patients should be warned about the potential impairment of mental or physical abilities required to operate machinery or drive a motor vehicle, particularly if dantrolene is taken with alcohol or drugs with CNS depressant properties.

ADVERSE REACTIONS: More Common Adverse Drug Reactions (≥1%): Table 1 lists the more common adverse effects of dantrolene.

Table 1: Dantrolene

More Common Adverse Drug Reactions (≥1%)

Body System	Effect	Clinical Comment
CNS	Drowsiness, dizziness	May be avoided by starting with a low dose and titrating as needed.
Liver	Increased transaminase levels (1.8%)	Monitor liver function periodically.
Gastrointestinal	Diarrhea	Severe diarrhea may require discontinuation of therapy.
Others	Malaise, fatigue	

Less Common Adverse Drug Reactions (<1%): Cardiovascular: tachycardia, erratic blood pressure, phlebitis, heart failure.
Central Nervous System: chills, fever, speech disturbances, seizures, headache, lightheadedness, mental depression, confusion, nervousness.
Allergic/Dermatologic: rash, pruritus, urticaria, eczematoid eruption, abnormal hair growth, sweating.
Gastrointestinal: constipation, anorexia, gastric irritation, gastric bleeding, abdominal cramps, dysphagia, nausea, vomiting, taste alterations.
Genitourinary: urinary frequency or retention, crystalluria, urinary incontinence, nocturia, dysuria, hematuria.
Hematologic: lymphocytic lymphoma, aplastic anemia, leucopenia, thrombocytopenia.
Hepatic/Biliary/Pancreatic: hepatitis, liver failure.
Musculoskeletal: myalgia, backache, muscle weakness.
Ophthalmologic: excessive tearing, diplopia, blurred vision.
Respiratory: respiratory depression, feeling of suffocation, pleural effusion with pericarditis, pulmonary edema.

DRUG INTERACTIONS: Drug-Drug Interactions: See Table 2.

Table 2: Dantrolene

Drug-Drug Interactions

Interacting Drug	Effect	Clinical Comment
Calcium channel blockers	Intravenous dantrolene may cause hyperkalemia and myocardial depression in malignant hyperthermia-susceptible patients taking calcium channel blockers.	Avoid concurrent use. Calcium channel blockers should not be used to manage malignant hyperthermia-associated arrhythmias.
CNS depressants (e.g., alcohol, benzodiazepines, barbiturates, opioids, phenothiazines)	Additive CNS depressant effects (e.g., sedation).	If used concurrently, monitor for additive CNS depressant effects.
Methotrexate	Dantrolene may increase plasma levels of methotrexate, probably due to altered renal excretion and protein binding of methotrexate.	Avoid concurrent use. If used together monitor methotrexate levels and signs of methotrexate toxicity (e.g., hepatotoxicity, renal failure, thrombocytopenia and mucositis).

DOSAGE AND ADMINISTRATION: See Table 3 and Table 4.

Recommended Dose and Dosage Adjustment: Adults: See Table 3.
Pediatrics: See Table 4.
Administration: For iv injection, reconstitute vials with sterile water 60 mL (without a bacteriostatic agent). Reconstituted solution may be administered over 5 minutes or diluted further in normal saline or dextrose 5% solution for intermittent infusion.

OVERDOSAGE:

> For management of a suspected drug overdose, CPhA recommends that you contact your **regional Poison Control Centre**. See the *CPS* Directory section for a list of Poison Control Centres.

ACTION AND CLINICAL PHARMACOLOGY: Mechanism of Action: Dantrolene is a hydantoin derivative that is structurally and pharmacologically different from other skeletal muscle relaxants. Dantrolene inhibits the release of calcium from sarcoplasmic reticulum by limiting the activation of skeletal muscle ryanodine receptors. In therapeutic doses, dantrolene has little effect on cardiac and smooth muscle. In patients with spasticity, dantrolene directly inhibits skeletal muscle contractility and reduces muscle tension by 40-70%, with no observed electromyographic changes. Dantrolene also induces CNS depression, causing drowsiness, dizziness and weakness, but without affecting neuromuscular transmission.

Dantrolene does not cause total paralysis due to its limited magnitude of activity.

Pharmacokinetics: Adults: Absorption: Dantrolene is slowly and incompletely (35-70%) absorbed after oral administration. Peak serum concentrations are achieved within 4-6 hours following oral administration. Pharmacologic effect peaks at 1.5 to 3 hours. Dantrolene has a half-life of 8.7 hours after oral administration. Duration of action following oral administration is 6 to 18 hours.

Dantrolene has a half-life of 5 hours after intravenous administration.

Distribution: Dantrolene is extensively bound to plasma proteins, especially albumin.
Metabolism: Dantrolene is rapidly metabolized in the liver via hydroxylation, N-reduction and acetylation. Major metabolites are 5-hydroxy (active, less potent than parent compound) and acetamido (inactive) analogs.
Excretion: Approximately 20% of the oral dose is renally excreted as metabolites (primarily as 5-hydroxyl and acetylated analogs) and unchanged dantrolene.
Special Populations: Pediatrics: The half-life of dantrolene is 20 hours in neonates. In children 2-7 years of age the half-life after intravenous administration is 10 hours.

STORAGE AND STABILITY: Sterile dry powder vials should be stored at room temperature (between 20 and 25°C). Reconstituted solution should be stored at room temperature (between 15 and 30°C) and must be used within 6 hours after reconstitution.

Table 3: Dantrolene

Dose in Adult Patients

Indication	Route	Initial Dose	Dose Titration	Usual Dose	Maximum Dose	Duration of Therapy	Clinical Comment
Spasticity, chronic	Oral	25 mg once daily	Increase daily dose by 25 mg at 4–7 day intervals as needed		400 mg/day in 3–4 divided doses		Dose should be individualized. Discontinue if no benefit after 45 days, to avoid hepatotoxicity.
Malignant hyperthermia, initial treatment[a]	IV	2.5 mg/kg	Repeat as needed until signs of malignant hyperthermia are reversed; occasionally a cumulative dose >10 mg/kg is required (up to 30 mg/kg)	2.5 mg/kg	Cumulative dose of 30 mg/kg		Individual doses administered by rapid iv injection. To manage malignant hyperthermia, prompt recognition of the condition, interruption of the surgery, cessation of the offending drug and external cooling are also necessary.[a]
Malignant hyperthermia, post-crisis management	IV			1 mg/kg Q6H		1–3 days	Use when oral administration is not suitable.
	Oral			1–2 mg/kg QID		1–3 days	
Neuroleptic malignant syndrome, treatment (Not an approved use in Canada)	IV	1 mg/kg	May repeat dose as needed to maximum cumulative iv dose of 10 mg/kg		Cumulative dose of 10 mg/kg		Once maximum cumulative iv dose is reached, switch to oral dantrolene 1–2 mg/kg QID

[a] Malignant hyperthermia crisis management protocol is available on the Malignant Hyperthermia Association of the United States (MHAUS) website at medical.mhaus.org/.

Table 4: Dantrolene

Dose in Pediatric Patients

Indication	Route	Age/Weight	Initial Dose	Dose Titration	Usual Dose	Maximum Dose	Clinical Comment
Spasticity, chronic	Oral	5–12 y	0.5 mg/kg once daily	Increase daily dose by 0.5 mg/kg at 4–7 day intervals as needed.	2 mg/kg TID	400 mg/day in 3–4 divided doses	
Malignant hyperthermia	IV, Oral	≥5 y	See adult dosing in Table 3.	See adult dosing in Table 3.	See adult dosing in Table 3.	See adult dosing in Table 3.	See adult dosing in Table 3.

Dapsone ℞
dapsone
Antibacterial Sulfone

Jacobus

INDICATIONS: Leprosy, dermatitis herpetiformis, actinomycotic mycetoma.

CONTRAINDICATIONS: Sulfones are contraindicated in patients with advanced amyloidosis of the kidneys.

PRECAUTIONS: Dapsone should be used with caution in patients with cardiac, pulmonary, hepatic or renal disease. Routine hematologic analyses should be carried out during long-term therapy with sulfones, because of the danger of hemolytic anemia. The hemolytic effect of sulfones may be exaggerated in glucose-6-phosphate dehydrogenase deficient individuals.

Drug Interactions: Rifampicin has been reported to increase the plasma clearance of Dapsone, and probenecid has been reported to increase excretion of Dapsone. Administration of Dapsone with chloroquine and/or primaquine may lead to an increase of methemoglobin levels in individuals predisposed to methemoglobinemia.

Pregnancy: The sulfone drugs are generally contra-indicated in pregnancy and therefore the use of Dapsone during pregnancy should be avoided unless, in the judgement of a physician, potential benefit outweighs the risk. Dapsone in high doses has been reported to be carcinogenic in rats and mice, but negative in salmonella mutagenicity assays. The relevance of this finding to human exposure is unclear.

Lactation: Dapsone is excreted in breast milk in therapeutic amounts. Sulfones may cause hemolytic anemia in glucose-6-phosphate dehydrogenase deficient neonates.

Reaction States: Leprosy patients receiving effective chemotherapy may suffer episodes of acute or chronic inflammation. Generally, anti-leprosy chemotherapy should be continued unchanged but these reactions must be adequately treated since they may result in crippling deformity.

Non Lepromatous Lepra Reactions: Complications may include severe peripheral neuritis with accompanying cutaneous sensory loss and paralysis. In the management of acute neuritis corticosteroids may be considered.

Lepromatous Lepra Reactions: Complications may include neuritis, an increase in muscle weakness, lymphadenitis, iridocyclitis, orchitis and more rarely nephritis and large-joint arthritis. In the management of these reactions, corticosteroids, and clofazimine may be considered.

ADVERSE EFFECTS: Most adverse reactions are dose-related and uncommon at dosages up to 100 mg daily. They include anorexia, nausea, vomiting, headache, dizziness, tachycardia, nervousness, insomnia and skin disorders. Agranulocytosis, peripheral neuritis and psychosis have also been reported. Varying degrees of dose-related hemolysis and methoglobinemia occur in most individuals given more than 200 mg daily. Dosages up to 100 mg daily are unlikely to cause hemolysis, but individuals with glucose-6-dehydrogenase deficiency may be affected by dosages above 50 mg daily. Rare reactions include the "Dapsone syndrome" and hypoalbuminemia.

The "Dapsone syndrome" is hypersensitivity reactions which develop rarely and tend to occur during the first 6 weeks of therapy. Symptoms may include fever, eosinophilia, mononucleosis, lymphadenopathy, leukopenia, jaundice with hepatitis, and exanthematous skin eruptions which may progress to exfoliative dermatitis, toxic epidermal necrolysis, or Stevens-Johnson syndrome. Although patients usually improve if Dapsone is withdrawn fatalities have occurred. Fixed drug eruptions occur in dark-skinned people. Although agranulocytosis has been reported rarely for Dapsone when used alone, reports have been more common when the drug has been used with other agents in the prophylaxis of malaria. Other miscellaneous reactions such as peripheral neuropathy, nephrotic syndrome and renal papillary necrosis have been reported.

OVERDOSE:
In cases of severe overdosage the stomach should be emptied by aspiration and lavage. There is no specific antidote and therefore treatment should be symptomatic e.g. intravenous methylene blue 1-2 mg/kg bodyweight, intravenous ascorbic acid 0.5-1 g and oxygen for the methemoglobinemia plus general supportive measures. The repeated administration of activated charcoal has been reported to increase the elimination rate of Dapsone and its metabolite following overdosage.

For management of a suspected drug overdose, CPhA recommends that you contact your **regional Poison Control Centre**. See the *CPS* Directory section for a list of Poison Control Centres.

DOSAGE: Leprosy: Adults: The standard dose is 100 mg daily (1-2 mg/kg bodyweight).

Children: Dosage should be adjusted according to bodyweight.

The modern treatment of leprosy involves the use of multiple drug regimens to avoid the development of resistant strains. The World Health Organization has made the following recommendations for standard adult treatment regimens (with dosage adjustments according to bodyweight):

Multibacillary Leprosy: rifampicin 600 mg once-monthly, supervised; dapsone 100 mg daily, self-administered; clofazimine 300 mg once-monthly, supervised and 50 mg daily, self administered.

Paucibacillary Leprosy: rifampicin 600 mg once a month for 6 months, supervised; dapsone 100 mg daily for 6 months, self-administered.

Further information on treatment regimens is contained in "Chemotherapy of Leprosy for Control Programmes" W.H.O. Technical Report Series 675(1982).

Dermatitis Herpetiformis: Adults: The usual maintenance dosage is 50 to 100 mg daily, but as little as 50 mg weekly may be adequate. Dosage of up to 300 mg daily may be considered, but efforts should be made to reduce this to a minimal maintenance dosage as soon as possible.

Actinomycotic Mycetoma: Adults: Published reports suggest that a dose of 100 mg should be given twice daily and continued for some months after the clinical symptoms have disappeared.

SUPPLIED: Each round, scored tablet, debossed "100" above and "101" below the score and on the obverse "Jacobus", contains: dapsone 100 mg. Nonmedicinal ingredients: corn starch, colloidal silicon dioxide, magnesium stearate and microcrystalline cellulose. Light, child-resistant bottles of 100. Store at room temperature protected from light.

Daraprim® ℞
pyrimethamine
Antimalarial

GlaxoSmithKline

PHARMACOLOGY: Pyrimethamine is an antiparasitic agent of the diaminopyrimidine type. It is a folic acid antagonist and the rationale for its therapeutic action is based on the differential requirement between host and parasite for nucleic acid precursors involved in growth. It competitively inhibits the dihydrofolate reductase enzyme with an affinity far greater for the protozoal than for the human enzyme. This activity is highly selective against plasmodia and *T. gondii*. Pyrimethamine does not destroy gametocytes, but arrests sporogony in the mosquito.

Pharmacokinetics: Pyrimethamine is rapidly absorbed from the gastrointestinal tract after administration. Time to peak plasma concentrations is reached in 2 to 4 hours in healthy volunteers. Peak plasma concentrations vary widely between individuals and range from 260 to 1411 ng/mL after daily doses of 25 mg. Plasma levels of pyrimethamine in patients with AIDS can vary by a factor of 4 following the same oral dose.

Pyrimethamine has a volume of distribution of about 2 L/kg. About 87% of the drug binds to plasma proteins. Pyrimethamine has been shown to reach the CSF achieving concentrations that were approximately one fifth of those in blood from patients with AIDS given daily doses.

Pyrimethamine is predominantly metabolized by the liver. The mean elimination half-life is 85 hours (ranging from 35 to 175 hours). Total body clearance can range between 20 and 28 mL/h/kg. Pyrimethamine is slowly excreted in urine; following a single 50 mg dose only 23% was recovered from the urine over one week, while 16 to 32% of a 100 mg dose was excreted over 40 days.

INDICATIONS: Treatment of Acute Malaria: Fast-acting schizonticides (e.g., chloroquine or quinine) are indicated and preferable for the treatment of acute attacks. However, conjoint use of pyrimethamine will initiate transmission control and suppressive cure.

Treatment of Toxoplasmosis: Pyrimethamine is also indicated for the treatment of toxoplasmosis. For this purpose the drug should be used conjointly with a sulfonamide, since synergism exists with this combination.

CONTRAINDICATIONS: In patients with a history of hypersensitivity to pyrimethamine or any component of the preparation.

WARNINGS: No data supplied by the manufacturer.

PRECAUTIONS: General: The coadministration of a folate supplement is necessary for treatment of toxoplasmosis. In the treatment of toxoplasmosis, all patients receiving pyrimethamine should be given a folate supplement to reduce the risk of bone marrow depression. Whenever possible folinic acid should be administered; or alternatively, folic acid may be given. Full blood counts should be carried out weekly during therapy and for a further 2 weeks after treatment is stopped. Should signs of folate deficiency develop, treatment must be discontinued and high doses of folinic acid administered.

Pyrimethamine may exacerbate folate deficiency in subjects predisposed to this condition through disease or malnutrition. Accordingly, a folinic acid supplement should be given to such individuals. In patients with megaloblastic anemia due to folate deficiency the risks versus benefits of administering pyrimethamine require careful consideration.

Caution should be exercised in administering pyrimethamine to patients with a history of seizures; large loading doses should be avoided in such patients (see Adverse Effects and Dosage).

When a sulfonamide is given in combination, an adequate fluid intake should be ensured to minimize the risk of crystalluria.

Since pyrimethamine is administered with a sulfonamide for the conditions indicated the general precautions applicable to sulfonamides should be observed.

The dosage of pyrimethamine required for the treatment of toxoplasmosis is 10 to 20 times the recommended antimalarial dosage and approaches the toxic level. If signs of folic acid deficiency develop (see Adverse Effects) reduce the dosage or discontinue the drug according to the response of the patient. Folinic acid may be administered in a dosage of 5 to 15 mg orally, i.v. or i.m. daily for 3 days, or as required to produce a return of depressed platelet or white blood cell counts to safe levels.

Warn patients to keep pyrimethamine out of the reach of children since accidental ingestion has led to fatality.

Pregnancy: Pyrimethamine in combination with sulfonamide has been used for many years in the treatment of malaria and toxoplasmosis during pregnancy. Both these infections carry a high risk to the fetus. Pyrimethamine crosses the placenta and, although there is a theoretical risk of fetal abnormalities from all folate inhibitors given during pregnancy, there have been no reports that have shown with any certainty that pyrimethamine is associated with human teratogenicity. Nevertheless, caution should be exercised in the administration of pyrimethamine.

Pregnant women receiving pyrimethamine must be given a concurrent folic acid supplement.

Malaria: At the recommended treatment doses, pyrimethamine is not contraindicated during pregnancy.

Toxoplasmosis: When pyrimethamine is used for the treatment of toxoplasmosis, the risks associated with the administration must be balanced against the danger of abortion or fetal malformation due to the infection.

Treatment during pregnancy is indicated in the presence of confirmed placental or fetal infection or when the mother is at risk of serious sequelae. However, in view of the theoretical risk of fetal abnormality arising from the use of pyrimethamine in early pregnancy, its use in combination therapy should be restricted to the second and third trimesters. Alternative therapy is therefore advised in the early stages of pregnancy.

Pyrimethamine, like other folic acid antagonists, may in large doses produce teratogenic effects in laboratory animals.

In patients receiving high dosage, as for the treatment of toxoplasmosis, full blood counts should be carried out weekly. In patients with convulsive disorders a smaller "starting" dose (for toxoplasmosis) is recommended to avoid the potential nervous system toxicity of pyrimethamine.

Lactation: Pyrimethamine enters human breast milk. It has been estimated that over a 9-day period an average weight infant would receive about 45% of the dose ingested by the mother. In view of the high doses of pyrimethamine and concurrent sulfonamides needed in toxoplasmosis treatment, breast-feeding should be avoided for the duration of treatment.

Patients with Special Diseases and Conditions: Pyrimethamine should be used with caution in patients with hepatic or renal disorders.

Renal Impairment: The kidney is not the major route of excretion of pyrimethamine and excretion is not significantly altered in patients with renal failure. There are, however, no substantial data on the use of pyrimethamine in renally impaired subjects. Since pyrimethamine is coadministered with a sulfonamide, care should be taken to avoid accumulation of the sulfonamide in renally impaired patients.

Hepatic Impairment: The liver is the main route for metabolism of pyrimethamine. Data on the use of pyrimethamine in patients with liver disease are limited. Pyrimethamine in combination with sulphonamides has been used effectively to treat toxoplasmosis in a patient with mild hepatic disease. Pyrimethamine was also successfully used to treat malaria in 2 patients who also had concurrent hepatitis infections. There are no general recommendations for dosage reductions for liver-impaired states but consideration should be given to dose adjustments for individual cases.

Pyrimethamine may exacerbate folate deficiency due to innate disease or malnutrition.

Drug Interactions: The high protein binding exhibited by pyrimethamine may prevent protein binding by other compounds (e.g., quinine or warfarin). This could affect the efficacy or toxicity of the concomitant drug depending on the levels of unbound drug.

The concurrent administration of lorazepam and pyrimethamine may induce hepatotoxicity.

Pyrimethamine, by its mode of action, may further depress folate metabolism in patients receiving treatment with other folate inhibitors, or agents associated with myelosuppression, including cotrimoxazole, trimethoprim, proguanil, zidovudine, or cytostatic agents (e.g., methotrexate). Cases of fatal bone marrow aplasia have been associated with the administration of daunorubicin, cytosine arabinoside and pyrimethamine to individuals suffering from acute myeloid leukemia. When used prophylactically, megaloblastic anemia has been reported occasionally in individuals who took pyrimethamine in excess of 25 mg weekly concurrently with a trimethoprim/ sulfonamide combination.

Convulsions have occurred after concurrent administration of methotrexate and pyrimethamine to children with leukemia affecting the CNS. Also, seizures have occasionally been reported when pyrimethamine was used in combination with other antimalarial drugs.

In vitro data suggest that antacid salts and the antidiarrheal agent kaolin reduce the absorption of pyrimethamine.

ADVERSE EFFECTS: Since a concurrent sulfonamide is to be taken with pyrimethamine for the indications listed, the relevant prescribing information for the sulfonamide should be consulted for sulfonamide-associated adverse events.

Nausea, colic, vomiting and diarrhea are common during early toxoplasmosis treatment and have also occasionally occurred in association with malaria treatment.

At the 75 mg dose used in malaria treatment, disorders of cardiac rhythm and hematuria have occurred which may have been associated to some extent with the nature of the infection.

Insomnia has been reported when pyrimethamine has been given at weekly doses above those recommended.

There have been rare instances of pneumonia with cellular and eosinophilic pulmonary infiltration when pyrimethamine was taken once weekly in association with sulfadoxine.

Daily therapeutic doses of pyrimethamine have been shown to depress hematopoiesis in some 25 to 50% of patients. The likelihood of inducing leukopenia, anemia or thrombocytopenia is reduced by concurrent administration of folinic acid.

Pancytopenia responsive to folate treatments, has been reported very rarely in patients with probable pre-existing folate deficiency. Fatalities have occurred in the absence of folate treatment.

Less common side effects are headache, giddiness, dryness of mouth and throat, fever, malaise, depression, rash and other skin disorders, including dermatitis and abnormal skin pigmentation.

There have been isolated reports of hyperphenylalaninemia in neonates treated for congenital toxoplasmosis.

Buccal ulceration has been reported in association with pyrimethamine. Circulatory collapse has also been reported but only in patients treated with higher doses than recommended.

Precipitation of a grand mal seizure in one patient predisposed to epilepsy has been reported, but the clinical significance has not been defined.

OVERDOSE:

Symptoms: Vomiting and convulsions occur in cases of severe, acute overdoses. Ataxia, tremor and respiratory depression can also occur.

Chronic excess doses can result in bone marrow depression (e.g., megaloblastic anemia, leukopenia, thrombocytopenia) resulting from folic acid deficiency.

Other reported symptoms have included cyanosis and tachycardia.

Treatment: Routine supportive treatment including maintenance of a clear airway and control of convulsions.

Adequate fluids should be given to ensure optimal diuresis.

Gastric lavage may be of value only if instituted within 2 hours of ingestion in view of the rapid absorption of pyrimethamine.

Fresh blood transfusions to counteract blood dyscrasias should be available.

To counteract possible folate deficiency, folinic acid, 9 to 15 mg daily, should be given until the signs of toxicity have subsided. There may be a delay of 7 to 10 days before the leukopenic side effects become evident; therefore, folinic acid therapy should be continued for the period at risk.

For management of a suspected drug overdose, CPhA recommends that you contact your **regional Poison Control Centre**. See the *CPS* Directory section for a list of Poison Control Centres.

DOSAGE: Treatment of Acute Malaria: Use pyrimethamine in areas where only susceptible plasmodia exist. The drug is not recommended alone in the treatment of acute attacks of malaria in nonimmune persons. Fast-acting schizonticides (chloroquine or quinine) are indicated for treatment of acute attacks. However, conjoint pyrimethamine dosage of 25 mg daily for 2 days will initiate transmission control and suppressive cure.

Should circumstances arise wherein pyrimethamine must be used alone in semi-immune persons, the adult dosage for an acute attack is 50 mg daily for 2 days; children 4 to 10 years old may be given 25 mg daily for 2 days.

Pyrimethamine should be given concurrently with sulfalene, sulfadoxine or another long-acting sulfonamide.

Adults and children over 14 years: As a single dose, 50 to 75 mg pyrimethamine with 1 to 1.5 g sulfalene or sulfadoxine; children 9 to 14 years: As a single dose, 50 mg pyrimethamine with 1 g sulfalene or sulfadoxine; children 4 to 8 years: As a single dose, 25 mg pyrimethamine with 500 mg sulfalene or sulfadoxine; children under 4 years: As a single dose, 12.5 mg pyrimethamine with 250 mg sulfalene or sulfadoxine.

Treatment of Toxoplasmosis: Pyrimethamine should be given concurrently with sulfadiazine or another appropriate sulfonamide (see Precautions).

Adults and children over 6 years: An initial dose of 50 mg pyrimethamine followed by 25 mg pyrimethamine daily given with 150 mg/kg (maximum 4 g) sulfadiazine daily in 4 divided doses; children 2 to 6 years: An initial dose of 25 mg pyrimethamine followed by 12.5 mg pyrimethamine daily given with 150 mg/kg (maximum 2 g) sulfadiazine daily in 4 divided doses; children 10 months to 2 years: 12.5 mg pyrimethamine daily given with 150 mg/kg (maximum 1.5 g) sulfadiazine daily in 4 divided doses; infants 3 to 9 months: 6.25 mg pyrimethamine daily given with 100 mg/kg (maximum 1 g) sulfadiazine daily in 4 divided doses; infants under 3 months: 6.25 mg pyrimethamine on alternate days given with 100 mg/kg (maximum 750 mg) sulfadiazine given in 4 divided doses on alternate days.

The risk of administering sulfadiazine or other sulfonamides to neonates should be weighed against their therapeutic benefit. Treatment should be continued for 3 to 6 weeks. If further therapy is indicated a period of 2 weeks should elapse between treatments.

SUPPLIED: Each white, biconvex tablet, with code number DARAPRIM A3A on same side as score mark, contains: pyrimethamine USP 25 mg. Also contains cornstarch, lactose and potato starch. Bottles of 50. Store between 15 to 30°C and keep dry.

(Shown in Product Identification Section)

Darvon-N® Ⓝ
propoxyphene napsylate
Analgesic

Paladin

SUPPLIED: Each size 3 gelatin capsule with a pink body and cap, imprinted with Paladin and the Identicode H64, contains: propoxyphene napsylate 100 mg. Nonmedicinal ingredients: dimethicone and starch. Tartrazine-free. Bottles of 100.

Daypro® Ⓟ
oxaprozin
Anti-inflammatory—Analgesic

Pfizer

PHARMACOLOGY: Oxaprozin is a nonsteroidal anti-inflammatory agent with analgesic and antipyretic properties. The modes of action of oxaprozin, like that of other nonsteroidal anti-inflammatory agents, are not fully established. It is known, however, that it does inhibit prostaglandin synthesis.

Pharmacokinetics: Oxaprozin is almost completely absorbed from the gastrointestinal tract, with peak plasma levels attained 2 to 4 hours after administration. The mean peak plasma concentration (C_{max}) is approximately 120 µg/mL with a single dose of 1200 mg and approximately 190 µg/mL at steady-state. At therapeutic levels, more than 99% of oxaprozin is bound to plasma proteins, mostly albumin. The mean biological half-life in humans is approximately 50 hours. Total body clearance of oxaprozin rises from 2.5 mL/h/kg after a single 1200 mg dose to 5 mL/h/kg at steady-state. The apparent volume of distribution rises from 180 to 300 mL/kg from single dose to steady-state. These increases are due to nonlinear protein binding. One study demonstrated that food had no effect on the extent of absorption of oral doses of oxaprozin in healthy subjects, whereas the rate of absorption was slightly slower. No abnormal drug accumulation occurred in patients treated with multiple doses (1200 mg/day) for up to 6 months.

A dual metabolism has been identified for oxaprozin. Approximately 60% of the drug is oxidized to hydroxyoxaprozin I or II and approximately 30% is glucuronidated to form oxaprozin acyl glucuronide. These inactive metabolic products are excreted in the feces (one third) and in the urine (two thirds). About 30% of an oral dose is recovered as conjugates in urine.

Less than 5% is recovered as oxaprozin. Biliary excretion in cholecystectomized humans accounts for 5% of the drug in 5 days. Oxaprozin does not induce its own metabolism.

Oxaprozin disposition during steady-state conditions is not affected by either subject age or sex. However the volume of distribution declined with increasing age (see Dosage).

The pharmacokinetics of oxaprozin in patients with impaired renal function, patients maintained on hemodialysis, and healthy subjects were evaluated following a single 600 mg oral dose. Total body clearance and elimination half-life did not differ substantially among the 3 groups. In a multiple dose study of subjects and patients with normal albumin levels, who were undergoing hemodialysis, total body clearance and volume of distribution of unbound drug were higher in patients undergoing hemodialysis. Total oxaprozin levels were not affected and there was no evidence of accumulation in subjects or renally impaired patients. Caution should be used when oxaprozin is given to patients with renal impairment (see Dosage).

One study compared the pharmacokinetics of a single dose of oxaprozin in patients with cirrhosis. Elimination half-life, and clearance of unbound drug were unchanged.

The elimination half-life, volume of distribution, and total body clearance of unbound oxaprozin following a single dose were similar for patients with congestive heart failure as compared to healthy subjects.

The effects of therapeutic doses of oxaprozin (1200 mg) and ASA (3900 mg) on the gastric mucosa and fecal blood were studied in healthy subjects. Oxaprozin produced significantly less submucosal hemorrhage or bleeding than did ASA in a 10-day crossover study utilizing gastroscopic evaluation of the gastric mucosa. The average amount of fecal blood loss that was induced by oxaprozin during a 2 week study using ^{51}Cr-labelled autologous red blood cells was similar to that caused by placebo during the second week, but was significantly greater during the first week. The fecal blood loss induced by oxaprozin was significantly less than that caused by ASA throughout the 2-week study.

The effects of oxaprozin on renal function were studied in normal subjects and in patients with impaired renal function. In clearance studies of normal subjects during sustained water diuresis, oxaprozin caused no acute reduction in glomerular filtration rate (GFR), had no effect on overall sodium clearance, and had no long-term effect on serum creatinine, blood urea nitrogen, or serum potassium. In renally impaired patients with a GFR below 30 to 40 mL/min and in patients undergoing hemodialysis, oxaprozin was distributed more extensively because of a reduction in binding to plasma proteins. The mean biological half-life was not altered by renal disease, although urinary excretion of both oxaprozin and its conjugates was greatly reduced. A multiple-dose study in patients undergoing hemodialysis demonstrated no impairment of total or unbound clearance in the disease state.

INDICATIONS: For acute and chronic use in the relief of the signs and symptoms of rheumatoid arthritis and osteoarthritis.

CONTRAINDICATIONS: The following are contraindications to the use of oxaprozin: Active peptic ulcer, a history of recurrent ulceration or active inflammatory disease of the gastrointestinal system. Known or suspected hypersensitivity to the drug, its components, or other NSAIDs. The potential for cross-reactivity between different NSAIDs must be kept in mind. Oxaprozin should not be used in patients with the complete or partial syndrome of nasal polyps, or in whom asthma, anaphylaxis, urticaria, rhinitis, or other allergic manifestations are precipitated by ASA or other nonsteroidal anti-inflammatory agents. Fatal anaphylactoid reactions have occurred in such individuals. As well, individuals with the above medical problems are at risk of a severe reaction even if they have taken NSAIDs in the past without any adverse effects. Significant hepatic impairment or active liver disease. Severely impaired or deteriorating renal function (creatinine clearance <30 mL/min or <0.5 mL/s). Individuals with lesser degrees of renal impairment are at risk of deterioration of their renal function when prescribed NSAIDs and must be monitored. Oxaprozin is not recommended for use with other NSAIDs because of the absence of any evidence demonstrating synergistic benefits and the potential for additive side effects.

WARNINGS: Gastrointestinal System: Serious gastrointestinal toxicity, such as peptic ulceration, perforation and gastrointestinal bleeding, **sometimes severe and occasionally fatal**, can occur at any time, with or without symptoms in patients treated with NSAIDs, including oxaprozin.

Minor upper gastrointestinal problems, such as dyspepsia, are common, usually developing early in therapy. Physicians should remain alert for ulceration and bleeding in patients treated with NSAIDs, even in the absence of previous gastrointestinal tract symptoms.

In patients observed in clinical trials of such agents, symptomatic upper gastrointestinal ulcers, gross bleeding, or perforation appear to occur in approximately 1% of patients treated for 3 to 6 months and in about 2 to 4% of patients treated for 1 year. The risk continues beyond 1 year and possibly increases.

The incidence of these complications increases with increasing dose.

Oxaprozin should be given under close medical supervision to patients prone to gastrointestinal tract irritation, particularly those with a history of peptic ulcer, diverticulosis or other inflammatory disease of the gastrointestinal tract, such as ulcerative colitis and Crohn's disease. In these cases the physician must weigh the benefits of treatment against the possible hazards.

Physicians should inform patients about the signs and/or symptoms of serious gastrointestinal toxicity and instruct them to contact a physician immediately if they experience persistent dyspepsia or other symptoms or signs suggestive of gastrointestinal ulceration or bleeding.

Because serious gastrointestinal tract ulceration and bleeding can occur without warning symptoms, physicians should follow chronically treated patients by checking their hemoglobin periodically and by being vigilant for the signs and symptoms of ulceration and bleeding and should inform the patients of the importance of this follow-up.

If ulceration is suspected or confirmed, or if gastrointestinal bleeding occurs, oxaprozin should be discontinued immediately, appropriate treatment instituted and the patient monitored closely.

No studies, to date, have identified any group of patients **not** at risk of developing ulceration and bleeding. A prior history of serious gastrointestinal events and other factors such as excess alcohol intake, smoking, age, female gender and concomitant oral steroid and anticoagulant use have been associated with increased risk.

Studies to date show that all NSAIDs can cause gastrointestinal tract adverse events. Although existing data does not clearly identify differences in risk between various NSAIDs, this may be shown in the future.

Geriatrics: Patients older than 65 years and frail or debilitated patients are most susceptible to a variety of adverse reactions from NSAIDs; the incidence of these adverse reactions increases with dose and duration of treatment. In addition, these patients are less tolerant to ulceration and bleeding. Most reports of fatal gastrointestinal events are in this population. Older patients are also at risk of lower esophageal ulceration and bleeding.

For such patients, consideration should be given to a starting dose lower than the one usually recommended, with individual adjustment when necessary, and under close supervision (see Precautions).

Cross-sensitivity: Patients sensitive to any one of the NSAIDs may be sensitive to any of the other NSAIDs also.

Aseptic Meningitis: In occasional cases, with some NSAIDs, the symptoms of aseptic meningitis (stiff neck, severe headaches, nausea and vomiting, fever or clouding of consciousness) have been observed. Patients with autoimmune disorders (systemic lupus erythematosus, mixed connective tissues diseases, etc.) seem to be predisposed. Therefore, in such patients, the physician must be vigilant to the development of this complication.

Pregnancy: The use of oxaprozin during pregnancy is not recommended as its safety in this condition has not been established. Oxaprozin should be used during pregnancy only if the benefit justifies the potential risk to the fetus and/or mother.

Lactation: Oxaprozin is not recommended for use in nursing mothers, since many NSAIDs have been shown to be partially excreted in breast milk. Oxaprozin has been found in the milk of lactating rats.

Children: Oxaprozin is not recommended for use in patients less than 18 years of age.

PRECAUTIONS: Gastrointestinal System: There is no definitive evidence that the concomitant administration of sucralfate, histamine H_2-receptor antagonists and/or antacids will either prevent the occurrence of gastrointestinal side effects or allow the continuation of oxaprozin therapy when and if these adverse reactions appear.

Renal Function: Long-term administration of NSAIDs to animals has resulted in renal papillary necrosis and other abnormal renal pathology. In humans, there have been reports of acute interstitial nephritis with hematuria, proteinuria, and occasionally nephrotic syndrome.

A second form of renal toxicity has been seen in patients with prerenal conditions leading to the reduction in renal blood flow or blood volume, where the renal prostaglandins have a supportive role in the maintenance of renal perfusion. In these patients, administration of a NSAID may cause a dose-dependent reduction in prostaglandin formation and may precipitate overt renal decompensation.

Patients at greater risk of this reaction are those with impaired renal function, heart failure, liver dysfunction, those taking diuretics, and the elderly. Discontinuation of nonsteroidal anti-inflammatory therapy is usually followed by recovery to the pretreatment state.

Oxaprozin and its metabolites are eliminated primarily by the kidneys, therefore, the drug should be used with great caution in patients with impaired renal function. In these cases, utilization of lower doses of oxaprozin should be considered and patients carefully monitored.

During long-term therapy, kidney function should be monitored periodically.

Genitourinary Tract: Some NSAIDs are known to cause persistent urinary symptoms (bladder pain, dysuria, urinary frequency), hematuria or cystitis. The onset of these symptoms may occur at any time after the initiation of therapy with a NSAID. Some cases have become severe on continued treatment. Should urinary symptoms occur, treatment with oxaprozin **must be stopped immediately** to obtain recovery. This should be done before any urological investigations or treatments are carried out.

Hepatic Function: As with other NSAIDs, borderline elevations of one or more liver function tests may occur in up to 15% of patients. These abnormalities may progress, may remain essentially unchanged, or may be transient with continued therapy. A patient with symptoms and/or signs suggesting liver dysfunction, or in whom an abnormal liver test has occurred, should be evaluated for evidence of the development of more severe hepatic reaction while on therapy with this drug. Severe hepatic reactions including jaundice and cases of fatal hepatitis have been reported with NSAIDs.

Although such reactions are rare, if abnormal liver tests persist or worsen, if clinical signs and symptoms consistent with liver disease develop, or if systemic manifestations occur (e.g., eosinophilia, rash, etc.), this drug should be discontinued.

During long-term therapy, liver function tests should be monitored periodically. If there is a need to prescribe this drug in the presence of impaired liver function, it must be done under strict observation.

Fluid and Electrolyte Balance: Fluid retention and edema have been observed in patients treated with oxaprozin. Therefore, as with many other NSAIDs, the possibility of precipitating congestive heart failure in elderly patients or those with compromised cardiac function should be born in mind. Oxaprozin should be used with caution in patients with heart failure, hypertension or other conditions predisposing to fluid retention.

With nonsteroidal anti-inflammatory treatment, there is a potential risk of hyperkalemia particularly in patients with conditions such as diabetes mellitus or renal failure; elderly patients; or in patients receiving concomitant therapy with beta-adrenergic blockers, angiotensin-converting enzyme inhibitors or some diuretics.

Serum electrolytes should be monitored periodically during long-term therapy, especially in those patients who are at risk.

Hematology: Drugs inhibiting prostaglandin biosynthesis do interfere with platelet function to varying degrees; therefore, patients who may be adversely affected by such an action should be carefully observed when oxaprozin is administered.

Blood dyscrasias (such as neutropenia, leukopenia, thrombocytopenia, aplastic anemia and agranulocytosis) associated with the use of NSAIDs are rare, but could occur with severe consequences.

Anemia may occur in patients receiving oxaprozin or other NSAIDs. This may be due to fluid retention, gastrointestinal blood loss, or an incompletely described effect upon erythrogenesis. Patients on long-term treatment with oxaprozin should have their hemoglobin or hematocrit values determined at appropriate intervals as determined by the clinical situation.

Infection: In common with other anti-inflammatory drugs, oxaprozin may mask the usual signs of infection.

Ophthalmology: Blurred and/or diminished vision has been reported with the use of oxaprozin and other NSAIDs. If such symptoms develop, this drug should be discontinued and an ophthalmologic examination performed; ophthalmologic examination should be carried out at periodic intervals in any patient receiving this drug for an extended period of time.

Occupational Hazards: CNS: Some patients may experience drowsiness, dizziness, vertigo, insomnia or depression with the use of oxaprozin. If patients experience these side effects, they should exercise caution in carrying out activities that require alertness.

Drug Interactions: ASA or other NSAIDs: The use of oxaprozin in addition to any other NSAID, including those over the counter ones (such as ASA and ibuprofen) is not recommended due to the possibility of additive side effects. Studies in man have shown that such combined administration produces decreased protein-binding of oxaprozin, with a reduced biological half-life, and increased clearance of oxaprozin.

Because of the long biological half-life of oxaprozin (approximately 50 hours), a clinical study of patients with rheumatoid arthritis was conducted to determine its interactions with ASA, naproxen, ibuprofen, and tolmetin sodium after therapy with oxaprozin was discontinued and the other drugs were started. In the same manner, patients with osteoarthritis were studied for interactions between oxaprozin and ASA, naproxen, ibuprofen and indomethacin. No clinically detectable interactions were found.

Acetaminophen: The coadministration of oxaprozin and acetaminophen resulted in no statistically significant changes in pharmacokinetic parameters in single- and/or multiple-dose studies.

Antacids: The coadministration of oxaprozin and antacids resulted in no statistically significant changes in pharmacokinetic parameters in single- and/or multiple-dose studies.

Anticoagulants: Numerous studies have shown that the concomitant use of NSAIDs and anticoagulants increases the risk of gastrointestinal adverse events such as ulceration and bleeding.

Because prostaglandins play an important role in hemostatis, and NSAIDs affect platelet function, concurrent therapy of oxaprozin with warfarin requires close monitoring to be certain that no change in anticoagulant dosage is necessary.

Concomitant warfarin and oxaprozin therapy did not produce further alterations of prothrombin times or a variety of other clotting factors when administered to normal subjects. Patients stabilized on phenprocoumon showed significant potentiation of the anticoagulation effect after 2.5 weeks of oxaprozin therapy. The values returned to pretreatment levels within 1 week after stopping oxaprozin.

Gold Salts, Antimalarial Agents, Corticosteroids: Oxaprozin may be used in combination with gold salts, antimalarial agents, or corticosteroids in the treatment of rheumatoid arthritis in adults.

In patients who received concomitant antimalarial therapy, a significantly higher incidence of muscular cramps/aching/pain, gastrointestinal bleeding, vision disorders and edema of the lower extremities was found. In patients who received concomitant gold therapy, a significantly higher incidence of sedation, skin disorders and E.N.T. disorders or symptoms was found.

Numerous studies have shown that the concomitant use of NSAIDs and oral glucocorticoids increases the risk of gastrointestinal side effects such as ulceration and bleeding. This is especially the case in older (>65 years old) individuals. In patients who received concomitant steroid therapy, significantly higher incidences of constipation, dyspepsia and alteration in taste were found.

Cimetidine/Ranitidine: Concomitant administration of cimetidine or ranitidine results in a clinically insignificant reduction of oxaprozin clearance. This does not require dosage adjustment.

Conjugated Estrogens: No interaction was observed when oxaprozin was administered concomitantly with conjugated estrogens.

Antihypertensives: Some NSAIDs have been reported to reduce the effects of antihypertensive agents. Hypertensive patients treated with the beta-adrenergic blocker, metoprolol, showed a small and transient increase in systolic blood pressure after 2 weeks on oxaprozin, with a return to baseline values at 4 weeks of therapy.

ACE-inhibitors: While oxaprozin does alter the pharmacokinetics of enalapril and its active metabolite enalaprilat, coadministration of oxaprozin to hypertensive patients did not produce significant changes in blood pressure values. However, reports suggest that NSAIDs may diminish the antihypertensive effect of ACE-inhibitors. This interaction should be given consideration in patients taking NSAIDs concomitantly with ACE-inhibitors.

Diuretics: NSAIDs have been shown to interfere with the action of thiazide diuretics and potassium-sparing diuretics.

Lithium: NSAIDs have been reported to increase steady-state plasma lithium concentrations. It is recommended that these concentrations be monitored when initiating, adjusting and discontinuing drug treatment.

Methotrexate: Coadministration of oxaprozin with methotrexate results in approximately a 36% decrease in oral plasma clearance of methotrexate. A reduction in methotrexate dosage may be considered due to the potential for increased methotrexate toxicity associated with the increased exposure.

Glyburide: While oxaprozin does alter the pharmacokinetics of glyburide, coadministration of oxaprozin to type II non-insulin dependent diabetic patients did not affect the area under the glucose concentration curve nor the magnitude or duration of control. However, it is advisable to monitor patients' blood glucose in the beginning phase of glyburide and oxaprozin cotherapy.

Other Drug Interactions: No drug interaction data are available for oxaprozin and the co-administration of the following products: alcohol, aminoglycosides, bone marrow depressants, butemide, cholestyramine, colchicine, cyclosporine, digoxin, indapamide, insulin, nephrotoxic agents, potassium supplements, probenecid, valproic acid, zidovudine.

Clinical Laboratory Test Interactions: False-positive urine immunoassay screening tests for benzodiazepines have been reported in patients taking oxaprozin. This is due to lack of specificity of the screening tests. False-positive test results may be expected for several days following discontinuation of oxaprozin therapy. Confirmatory tests, such as gas chromatography/mass spectrometry, will distinguish oxaprozin from benzodiazepines.

ADVERSE EFFECTS: The most common adverse reactions encountered with NSAIDs are gastrointestinal, of which peptic ulcer, with or without bleeding, is the most severe. Fatalities have occurred, particularly in the elderly.

Adverse reaction data were derived from patients who received oxaprozin in multidose, controlled, and open-label clinical trials, and from worldwide marketing experience. Rates for events occurring in more than 1% of patients, and for most of the less common events, are based on 2253 patients who took 1200 to 1800 mg oxaprozin/day in clinical trials. Of these, 1721 were treated for at least 1 month, 971 for at least 3 months, and 366 for more than 1 year. Rates for rarer events and for events reported from worldwide marketing experience are difficult to estimate accurately and are only listed as less than 1%.

Listed below are the adverse events and their incidences in the first month of use in clinical trials. Most of the events were seen by this time for common adverse reactions. However, the cumulative incidence can be expected to rise with continued therapy, and some events, such as gastrointestinal bleeding seem to occur at a constant or possibly increasing rising rate over time.

The most frequently reported adverse reactions were related to the gastrointestinal tract. They were nausea (8%) and dyspepsia (8%).

Incidence greater than 1%: In clinical trials the following adverse reactions occurred at an incidence greater than 1% and are probably related to treatment. Reactions occurring in 3 to 9% of patients treated with oxaprozin are indicated by an asterisk (*); those reactions occurring in less than 3% of patients are unmarked.

Gastrointestinal: abdominal pain/distress, anorexia, constipation*, diarrhea*, dyspepsia*, flatulence, nausea*, vomiting.

Central Nervous System: CNS inhibition (depression, sedation, somnolence, or confusion), disturbance of sleep.

Dermatologic: rash*.

Special Senses: tinnitus.

Urogenital: dysuria or frequency.

Incidence less than 1%: Probable causal relationship: The following adverse reactions were reported in clinical trials or from worldwide marketing experience at an incidence of less than 1%. Those reactions reported only from worldwide marketing experience are in *italics*. The probability of a causal relationship exists between the drug and these adverse reactions.

Gastrointestinal: peptic ulceration and/or gastrointestinal bleeding, liver function abnormalities including *hepatitis*, stomatitis, hemorrhoidal or rectal bleeding, *pancreatitis*.

Allergic: drug hypersensitivity reactions including anaphylaxis and *serum sickness*.

Central Nervous System: weakness, malaise.

Dermatologic: pruritus, urticaria, photosensitivity, *pseudoporphyria, exfoliative dermatitis, erythema multiforme, Stevens-Johnson syndrome, toxic epidermal necrolysis (Lyell's syndrome)*.

Cardiovascular: edema, blood pressure changes.

Special Senses: blurred vision, conjunctivitis.

Hematologic: anemia, thrombocytopenia, leukopenia, ecchymoses, *agranulocytosis, pancytopenia*.

Metabolic: weight gain, weight loss.

Respiratory: symptoms of upper respiratory tract infection.

Urogenital: *acute interstitial nephritis, nephrotic syndrome*, hematuria, renal insufficiency, *acute renal failure*, decreased menstrual flow.

Causal relationship unknown: The following adverse reactions occurred at an incidence of less than 1% in clinical trials, or were suggested from marketing experience, under circumstances where a causal relationship could not be definitely established. They are listed as alerting information for the physician.

Gastrointestinal: alteration in taste.

Dermatologic: alopecia.

Cardiovascular: palpitations.

Special Senses: hearing decrease.

Respiratory: sinusitis, pulmonary infections.

Urogenital: increase in menstrual flow.

OVERDOSE:

Symptoms: The symptoms of overdosage may include: lethargy, drowsiness, nausea, vomiting, and epigastric pain.

Treatment: In the event of overdosage, the stomach should be emptied by inducing vomiting or by gastric lavage. The patient should be carefully observed and given symptomatic and supportive treatment for as long as necessary.

For management of a suspected drug overdose, CPhA recommends that you contact your **regional Poison Control Centre**. See the *CPS* Directory section for a list of Poison Control Centres.

DOSAGE: In a clinical study in which healthy volunteers were administered oxaprozin after a meal, the extent of absorption was unchanged while the rate of absorption was slightly delayed. Oxaprozin may be administered orally once or twice daily with food or milk, and dosage adjusted for optimal response as described below.

Rheumatoid Arthritis: The initial therapy is 1200 mg once daily. This may be decreased or increased depending on the patient's response. The maximum daily dose should not exceed 1800 mg, or 26 mg/kg, whichever is less. Doses larger than 1200 mg/day should be reserved for patients who weigh more than 50 kg, have normal renal and hepatic function, are at low risk of peptic ulcer and whose severity of disease justifies maximal therapy. Physicians should ensure that patients are tolerating lower doses before advancing to the larger doses.

The 1800 mg dose should be divided into 2 doses (1200 mg in the morning and 600 mg in the evening).

Osteoarthritis: The initial therapy is 1200 mg once daily. This may be decreased to 600 mg once daily depending on the patient's response.

For patients of low body weight or with milder disease, an initial dose of 600 mg once daily may be appropriate.

Note: Consideration should be given to reducing the starting dose in elderly patients. In patients with moderate to severe renal impairment, and in those on hemodialysis, a maximum daily dosage of 600 mg administered under careful monitoring is recommended.

INFORMATION FOR THE PATIENT: Published in e-CPS, available by subscription at www.e-cps.ca.

SUPPLIED: Each white, film-coated, capsule-shaped, scored caplet, with "DAYPRO" debossed on one side and "1381" on the other side, contains: oxaprozin 600 mg. Nonmedicinal ingredients: cellulose, cornstarch, hypromellose, magnesium stearate, methylcellulose, polacrilin potassium, polyethylene glycol and titanium dioxide. HDPE bottles with plastic caps of 100. Store at 15 to 25°C. Protect from light. Keep bottles tightly closed.

(Shown in Product Identification Section)

DDAVP® Injection Ⓟ

desmopressin acetate

Antidiuretic Hormone Analogue—Antihemorrhagic

Ferring

PHARMACOLOGY: Desmopressin is a synthetic structural analogue of the natural human hormone, arginine vasopressin. As such, it exerts its action on the reabsorption of water in the renal tubule.

It also causes a transient increase in all components of the Factor VIII complex and plasminogen activator. These are released very rapidly from their endothelial cell storage sites. Moreover, it may have a direct effect on the vessel wall, with increased platelet spreading and adhesion at injury sites. The duration of action is from 8 to 12 hours. A second dose given before endothelial cell stores are replenished will not have as great an effect as the initial dose. Responses as great as the initial one usually are seen if 48 hours or more have elapsed between doses.

INDICATIONS: Antidiuretic hormone replacement therapy in the treatment of central diabetes insipidus, primary and secondary.

Hemophilia A: For patients with hemophilia A with Factor VIII levels greater than 5%. It will often maintain hemostasis in patients with hemophilia A during surgical procedures and postoperatively, when administered 45 minutes prior the scheduled procedure. It will also stop bleeding in hemophilia A patients with episodes of spontaneous or trauma-induced injuries such as hemarthroses, i.m. hematomas or mucosal bleeding.

In certain clinical situations, it may be justified to try desmopressin in patients with Factor VIII levels between 2 and 5%, however, these patients should be carefully monitored.

Desmopressin is **not indicated for the treatment of hemophilia B** because it has no effect on Factor IX levels.

Desmopressin should not be given to patients with Factor VIII antibodies.

Von Willebrand's Disease (Type 1): For patients with mild to moderate classic von Willebrand's disease (Type 1) with Factor VIII levels greater than 5%. Desmopressin will often maintain hemostasis in patients with mild to moderate von Willebrand's disease during surgical procedures and postoperatively when administered 45 minutes prior to the scheduled procedure.

Desmopressin will usually stop bleeding in mild to moderate von Willebrand's disease patients with episodes of spontaneous or trauma-induced injuries such as hemarthroses, i.m. hematomas or mucosal bleeding.

Those von Willebrand's disease patients who are least likely to respond are those with severe homozygous von Willebrand's disease with Factor VIII coagulant activity, Factor VIII antigen and von Willebrand's factor (ristocetin cofactor) activities less than 1%. Other patients may respond in a variable fashion depending on the type of molecular defect they have.

Bleeding time and Factor VIII coagulant activity, Factor VIII antigen and von Willebrand's factor activities should be checked during administration of desmopressin to ensure that adequate levels are being achieved.

Desmopressin is **not indicated for the treatment of severe classic Type 1 von Willebrand's Disease and Type II B** and when there is evidence of an abnormal molecular form of Factor VIII antigen (see Warnings).

CONTRAINDICATIONS: Hypersensitivity to desmopressin.

Desmopressin should not be used to treat patients with Type II B von Willebrand's Disease, since severe thrombocytopenia may be induced.

WARNINGS: When used for bleeding disorders, desmopressin is for **i.v. use only, by infusion**. Patients who do not have need of antidiuretic hormone for its antidiuretic effect, in particular those who are young or elderly, should be cautioned to ingest only enough fluid to satisfy thirst, in order to decrease potential occurrence of water intoxication and hyponatremia.

Desmopressin must be used with caution in patients prone to vascular headaches, patients with coronary insufficiency and hypertensive cardiovascular diseases, because of possible change in blood pressure and tachycardia. Very occasionally, injection of desmopressin has produced local erythema, swelling or burning pain, along course of vein.

Desmopressin has no therapeutic effect in Glanzmann's thrombasthenia.

Tachyphylaxis may develop with repeated use.

Lack of therapeutic effect has been noted in patients who have been febrile or otherwise stressed' for several days. Whenever possible, therapeutic efficacy (i.e. Factor VIII response in hemophilia and bleeding time correction in other disorders) should be established in individual patients prior to use and followed throughout the course of treatment. The coincident use of antifibrinolytic agents to counteract desmopressin-induced plasminogen activator release has been recommended; however, benefit has not been clearly established.

Desmopressin has no therapeutic effect in renal diabetes insipidus.

PRECAUTIONS: Use desmopressin with caution in patients with coronary arterial insufficiency and/or hypertensive cardiovascular disease because of possible tachycardia, and changes in blood pressure. Severe allergic reactions have **not** been reported with desmopressin. It is not known whether antibodies to desmopressin acetate are produced after repeated injections.

Hemophilia A: Laboratory tests for assessing patient status include levels of Factor VIII coagulant, Factor VIII antigen and Factor VIII ristocetin cofactor (von Willebrand factor) as well as activated partial thromboplastin time. Factor VIII coagulant activity should be determined before giving desmopressin for hemostasis. If Factor VIII coagulant activity is present at less than 5% of normal, desmopressin should not be relied upon alone.

Hemophilia B: Desmopressin should not be used for these patients, because it has no effect on Factor IX levels.

Von Willebrand's Disease: Laboratory tests for assessing patient status include levels of Factor VIII coagulant, Factor VIII antigen and Factor VIII ristocetin cofactor (von Willebrand factor). The skin bleeding time may be helpful in following these patients and should always be assessed pre-operatively.

Diabetes Insipidus: In the control of diabetes insipidus, use the lowest effective dose and assess dosage periodically.

Do not administer desmopressin to dehydrated patients until water balance has been adequately restored.

Laboratory tests for monitoring the patient include urine volume and osmolality. In some cases, plasma osmolality may be required.

Pregnancy: Reproduction studies performed in rats and rabbits with s.c. doses up to 12.5 times the human dose when used for Factor VIII stimulation and 125 times the human dose when used in diabetes insipidus have revealed no evidence of harm to the fetus due to desmopressin. There are several publications of management of diabetes insipidus in pregnant women with no harm to the fetus reported; however, there are no adequate and well controlled studies in pregnant women. Published reports stress that, as opposed to preparations containing the natural hormones, desmopressin in antidiuretic doses has no uterotonic action, but the physician will have to weigh possible therapeutic advantages against possible danger in each case.

Lactation: It is not known whether this drug is excreted in human milk. Because many drugs are excreted in human milk, caution should be exercised when desmopressin is administered to a nursing woman.
Children: Observe children closely for possible hyponatremia and water intoxication due to overingestion of fluids.
Desmopressin should not be used in infants younger than 3 months in the treatment of hemophilia A or von Willebrand's disease.

ADVERSE EFFECTS: Infrequently, desmopressin has produced transient headache, nausea, mild abdominal cramps and vulvar pain. Facial flushing, tachycardia, mild hypotension (fall in systolic and diastolic blood pressure by approximately 15 torr) have also been reported, and decreased urine output for 6 to 8 hours commonly observed. See Warnings for the possibility of water intoxication and hyponatremia.
Very occasionally, injection of desmopressin has produced local erythema, swelling or burning pain, along course of vein.
Drug Interactions: Although the pressor activity of desmopressin is very low compared with the antidiuretic activity, the use of desmopressin doses as large as 0.3 μg/kg with other pressor agents, should be done only with careful patient monitoring.
Clofibrate, chlorpropamide and carbamazepine may potentiate the antidiuretic activity of desmopressin while demeclocycline, lithium and norepinephrine may decrease its activity.

OVERDOSE:
Symptoms: Headaches, abdominal cramps and nausea (see Adverse Effects).
Treatment: No specific antidote. Reduce dosage and frequency of administration or withdraw the drug according to severity of the condition.
Water intoxication responds rapidly to diuretic therapy (e.g. furosemide) and appropriate replacement fluid support, without interference with hemostatic effects.

For management of a suspected drug overdose, CPhA recommends that you contact your **regional Poison Control Centre**. See the *CPS* Directory section for a list of Poison Control Centres.

DOSAGE: Hemophilia A and von Willebrand's Disease Type I: Desmopressin is administered as an i.v. infusion. Children: 0.3 μg/kg. Adults: 0.3 μg/kg (maximum dose 20 μg).
Dilution for Infusion: Diluted in sterile physiological saline and infused slowly over 20 to 30 minutes. In adults and children weighing more than 10 kg: 50 mL of diluent is used; in children weighing 10 kg or less, 10 mL of diluent is used. Side effects may be decreased by slow infusion. Blood pressure and pulse rate should be monitored during infusion. (If desmopressin is used preoperatively, it should be administered 30 minutes prior to the scheduled procedure.) The peak effect is obtained in 1 hour after administration. Response is immediate for bleeding time reduction.
The necessity for repeat administration of desmopressin or use of any blood products for hemostasis should be determined by laboratory response as well as the clinical condition of the patient. The tendency toward tachyphylaxis (lessening of response) with repeated administration, given more frequently than every 48 hours should be considered in treating each patient.
Parenteral drug products should be inspected visually for particulate matter and discoloration prior to administration whenever solution and container permit.
Diabetes Insipidus: Diagnosis of Central Diabetes Insipidus: Central diabetes insipidus may be demonstrated by the inability to produce urine osmolality above 175 mOsm/kg with dehydration severe enough to cause a loss of greater than 2% of body weight. The patient responding to 5 units of arginine vasopressin given s.c. after dehydration confirms the diagnosis of central diabetes insipidus.
Parenteral Application: Desmopressin may be administered s.c., i.m. or i.v. In the majority of adults 1 to 4 μg once daily will provide satisfactory control of the diabetes insipidus. In children a dose of 0.4 μg once a day may be used. The dose should be drawn up from the ampul at a fraction of a mL, using an insulin syringe and not prepared by dilution.
Desmopressin dosage must be determined for each patient and adjusted according to the pattern of response. Response should be estimated by 2 parameters: adequate duration of sleep and adequate, not excessive, water turnover.
To institute desmopressin therapy, patients should be withdrawn from previous medication and allowed to establish a baseline polyuria and polydipsia. The stable polyuria is used as a baseline to determine the magnitude and duration of the response to medication. In less severe cases, prior water loading may be desirable to establish a vigorous flow of urine. When the urine osmolality reaches a plateau at the low level (in most cases, less than 100 mOsm/kg), the first dose of desmopressin is administered intranasally or parenterally. A urine sample is obtained after 2 hours and hourly thereafter following desmopressin administration. Samples are measured for volume and osmolality. When the patient has reached the previous baseline urine osmolality and urine flow, the drug effect has ceased and the next desmopressin dose is administered. The cycle is then repeated until the patient has reached a stable condition.
I.V., I.M. or S.C.: Children: 0.1 mL (0.4 μg) once daily. Adults: 0.25 to 1 mL (1 to 4 μg) once daily.
One mL (4 μg) of desmopressin solution has an antidiuretic activity of about 16 IU.; 1 μg of desmopressin is equivalent to 4 IU.
For patients who have been controlled on intranasal desmopressin and who must be switched to the injection form, either because of poor intranasal absorption, or because of the need for surgery, the comparable antidiuretic dose of the injection is explained below.
Intranasal administration requires a higher dosage than i.v. administration since only 10% of intranasally administered drug will be absorbed. The intranasal dosage that is required is therefore 10 times larger than the i.v. dose; thus an approximate parenteral dosage of 1/10 that of the intranasal is required and should be adjusted for each patient individually, to obtain an adequate diurnal rhythm of water turnover.
Instructions for Opening Ampuls: 1) Hold ampul with blue dot pointing upwards. Shake or tap ampul to empty the tip. 2) With blue dot pointing upwards, snap off tip by forcing it downwards.

SUPPLIED: Each mL contains: desmopressin acetate 4 μg (equivalent to 3.6 μg free base) in an isotonic sterile and pyrogen-free water solution, for i.v., i.m. or s.c. administration. Clear glass ampuls of 1 mL, with a brown identification ring and a blue dot indicating the cut area. Cartons of 10. Store at about 4°C in a refrigerator. Do not freeze. Store away from light.

DDAVP® Melt Pr
desmopressin acetate
Antidiuretic

Ferring

Date of Preparation: March 2, 2005
Date of Revision: May 5, 2009

SUMMARY PRODUCT INFORMATION:

Route of Administration	Dosage Form/ Strength	Clinically Relevant Nonmedicinal Ingredients
Sublingual	Oral Disintegrating Tablets 60 μg, 120 μg, 240 μg	Gelatin, mannitol, citric acid

INDICATIONS AND CLINICAL USE: DDAVP MELT is indicated for:
- treatment of central diabetes insipidus
- treatment of primary nocturnal enuresis

Central Diabetes Insipidus: DDAVP MELT (60 μg, 120 μg and 240 μg desmopressin) is indicated for the management of vasopressin sensitive central diabetes insipidus, and for the control of temporary polyuria and polydipsia following head trauma, hypophysectomy or surgery in the pituitary region.
Primary Nocturnal Enuresis: DDAVP MELT (60 μg, 120 μg and 240 μg desmopressin) is indicated in the management of nocturnal enuresis in patients 5 years of age and older who have normal ability to concentrate urine. DDAVP MELT should be used in conjunction with non-medicinal therapy, such as motivational counselling and bladder exercises.

CONTRAINDICATIONS: Hypersensitivity to desmopressin or any of the tablet constituents. Because of the risk of platelet aggregation and thrombocytopenia, the drug should not be used in patients with type IIB or platelet-type (pseudo) von Willebrand's disease.
Known hyponatremia, severe liver disease, nephrosis or any other condition associated with impaired water excretion, cardiac insufficiency, chronic renal insufficiency, congestive heart failure, habitual or psychogenic polydypsia.
Patients with existing medical conditions, which lead to sodium losing states such as nausea, bulimia, anorexia nervosa, chronic vomiting, diarrhoea and adrenocortical insufficiency as well as salt losing nephropathies, should only be prescribed DDAVP under close medical supervision and with extreme caution.

WARNINGS AND PRECAUTIONS: General: In general, by adequate treatment with DDAVP MELT, thirst is automatically reduced. However, there is potential risk of water intoxication if, during treatment, excessive liquid is consumed. Fluid intake should be adjusted to reduce possibility of water intoxication and hyponatremia especially in the very young and elderly patients (see Dosage and Administration). Particular attention should be paid to the risk of extreme decrease in plasma osmolality and resulting seizures in young children. It is advisable that patients, and especially the parents of child patients, be cautioned about this.
In patients with water and/or electrolyte balance disorder [such as systemic infections, fever, and Syndrome of Inappropriate Antidiuretic Hormone secretion (SIADH)], and in patients with high intra-cranial pressure, it is also necessary that extra care be exercised with liquid intake. Desmopressin should not be administered to dehydrated patients until water balance has been adequately restored.
Desmopressin is not effective in controlling polyuria caused by renal disease, nephrogenic diabetes insipidus, psychogenic diabetes insipidus, hypokalemia or hypercalcemia.
Cardiovascular: Desmopressin acetate administered intranasally at high dosage (40 μg or more) has occasionally produced a slight elevation of blood pressure, which disappeared with a reduction in dosage. The drug should be used with caution in patients with coronary artery insufficiency and/or hypertensive cardiovascular disease because of possible tachycardia and changes in blood pressure.
Genitourinary: Severe bladder dysfunction and outlet obstruction should be considered before starting treatment.
Respiratory: Desmopressin should be used with caution in patients with cystic fibrosis because these patients are prone to hyponatremia.
Special Populations: General: Children and geriatric patients should be closely observed for possible water retention due to over-ingestion of fluids. When fluid intake is not excessive, there is little danger of water intoxication and hyponatremia. Fluid intake should be carefully adjusted to prevent over-hydration.
Pregnant Women: No controlled studies in pregnant women have been carried out. However, as with all medication used during pregnancy, the physician should weigh possible therapeutic advantages against potential risks in each case.
Data on a limited number (n=53) of exposed pregnancies in women with diabetes insipidus indicate no adverse effects of desmopressin on pregnancy or on the health of the fetus or newborn child. To date, no other relevant epidemiological data are available. Animal studies do not indicate direct or indirect harmful effects with respect to pregnancy, embryonal/fetal development, parturition or postnatal development.
Nursing Women: There have been no controlled studies in nursing mothers. Results from analysis of milk from nursing mothers receiving high doses of desmopressin (300 μg intranasal), indicate that the amounts of desmopressin that may be transferred to the child are considerably less than the amounts required to influence diuresis.
Pediatrics: Desmopressin has been used in children with diabetes insipidus. The dose must be individually adjusted to the patient with attention in the very young to the danger of an extreme decrease of plasma osmolality with resulting convulsions. Dosage in infants younger than 3 months has not been established. Dosage should start at 60 μg or less. Use of desmopressin in infants and children will require careful fluid intake restriction to prevent possible hyponatremia and water intoxication.
Monitoring and Laboratory Tests: Diagnosis of Central Diabetes Insipidus: Central diabetes insipidus may be demonstrated by the inability to produce urine of osmolality above 175 mOsm/kg with dehydration severe enough to cause a loss of greater than 2% of body weight.
Patients are selected for therapy by establishing a diagnosis by means of a water deprivation test, the hypertonic saline infusion test, and/or response to 5 units arginine vasopressin given subcutaneously after dehydration. Continued response to desmopressin acetate is monitored by urine volume and osmolality. In cases of severe dehydration, plasma osmolality determination may be required.
Special Conditions/Diseases: Desmopressin should be used with caution in patients with cystic fibrosis because these patients are prone to hyponatremia.
Treatment with desmopressin should be interrupted during acute inter-current illnesses characterised by fluid and/or electrolyte imbalance (such as systemic infections, fever, and gastroenteritis).

ADVERSE REACTIONS: Clinical Trial Adverse Drug Reactions: Because clinical trials are conducted under very specific conditions the adverse reaction rates observed in the clinical trials may not reflect the rates observed in practice and should not be compared to the rates in the clinical trials of another drug. Adverse drug reaction information from clinical trials is useful for identifying drug-related adverse events and for approximating rates.
Five pharmacokinetic and pharmacodynamic (PK/PD) studies were conducted. Four studies enrolled healthy volunteers and one study was conducted in children with primary nocturnal enuresis (PNE). Comparison of the methodologies of the five studies is presented in Table 1.

Table 1: DDAVP MELT
Study Design of the Pharmacokinetic and Pharmacodynamic Studies

Study No.	Type of Study	Formulation & Dosage	Number, Age & Sex of Patients
Study 1	Single-center, open-label, randomized, balanced, 4-way cross-over study	DDAVP MELT 200, 400, 800 μg sublingually Desmopressin 2 μg IV	24 healthy male volunteers (18–55 years)
Study 2	Open-label, randomized, 2-period cross-over study	DDAVP MELT 240 μg sublingually DDAVP Tablets 2×200 μg orally	14 male and 14 female healthy volunteers (18–55 years)
Study 3	Single-center, open-label, randomized, balanced, 6-sequence, 3-period cross-over study	DDAVP MELT 60, 120, 240 μg sublingually	15 male and 10 female healthy volunteers (18–55 years)
Study 4	Single-center, open-label, replicated, randomized, 2-sequence, 4-period, cross-over study	DDAVP MELT 240 μg sublingually DDAVP tablets 2×200 μg orally	32 male and 33 female healthy volunteers (18–55 years)
Study 5	Double-blind, randomized, placebo-controlled, parallel group study	DDAVP MELT 30, 60, 120, 240, 360, 480 μg sublingually Placebo sublingually	64 males and 20 females with PNE (6–12 years) 72 DDAVP MELT 12 Placebo

A total of 214 subjects were treated with DDAVP MELT in the PK/PD studies. Of these, 172 were also administered DDAVP tablets: 28 in Study 2, 65 in Study 4 and 79 patients in the open-label part of Study 5. Twenty-four (24) subjects were also administered desmopressin intravenously. One hundred and forty two subjects were healthy volunteers and 72 were PNE children.
Sixty-one subjects (29%) of the 214 subjects exposed to desmopressin from DDAVP MELT reported 96 adverse events, all of which were mild to moderate in intensity.
Sixty-five subjects (38%) of the 172 subjects exposed to desmopressin from DDAVP Tablets reported 82 adverse events, all of which were mild to moderate in intensity.
The most frequently reported adverse events (>3%) in subjects in the PK/PD studies are presented by body system in Table 2 for the Safety Population (received at least one dose of study medication) of each study.

Table 2: DDAVP MELT

Number of Subjects Reporting AEs in the PK/PD Studies (Frequency >3%)

	DDAVP MELT		DDAVP Tablets	
Adverse Event	No.	%	No.	%
No. Subjects Exposed	214	—	172	—
No. Subjects with Adverse Events	61	29	65	38
No. Adverse Events	96	—	82	—
Nervous System				
Headache	26	12.1	27	15.7
Gastrointestinal				
Nausea	7	3.3	5	2.9

The most commonly reported adverse events in the PK/PD studies were headache and nausea. Overall, numbers of adverse events reported were low, and were generally reported with similar frequency between the DDAVP MELT and DDAVP Tablets, desmopressin i.v. and/or placebo.

Headache, nausea and vomiting are known adverse drug reactions to desmopressin, and may be signs and symptoms of water retention and hyponatremia which are recognized sequelae of unrestricted fluid intake during desmopressin administration.

Infrequently, high doses of desmopressin have produced transient headache and nausea. Nasal congestion, rhinitis, flushing, and mild abdominal cramps have been reported. These symptoms disappeared with reduction in dosage.

Treatment without concomitant reduction of fluid intake may lead to water retention/hyponatremia with or without accompanying warning signs or symptoms (headache, nausea/vomiting, weight gain and in severe cases convulsions).

Serum AST levels were elevated in 4/16 patients, 6 months after commencing oral desmopressin acetate therapy (200 to 600 µg/day). Two of these patients had exhibited baseline levels of AST that were above the normal range and all four patients had normal AST levels on repeat test at 9 months, even though desmopressin acetate administration continued. The possibility that desmopressin acetate has an adverse effect on serum enzymes is therefore remote.

Primary nocturnal enuresis & diabetes insipidus:

Common (>1/100)	General: headache Gastrointestinal: abdominal pain, nausea
Very Rare (<1/10 000)	Hyponatremia

Post-Market Adverse Drug Reactions (DDAVP Tablet): Very rare cases of emotional disturbances in children have been reported. Isolated cases of allergic skin reactions and more severe general allergic reactions have been reported.

DRUG INTERACTIONS: Overview: Clofibrate, chlorpropamide and carbamazepine may potentiate the antidiuretic activity of desmopressin while demeclocycline, lithium and norepinephrine may decrease its activity.

Although the pressor activity of desmopressin acetate is very low compared with the antidiuretic activity, use of large doses of desmopressin with other pressor agents should be done only with careful patient monitoring.

Concomitant treatment with drugs which are known to induce SIADH, e.g. tricyclic antidepressants, selective serotonin reuptake inhibitors, chlorpromazine and carbamazepine, may cause an additive antidiuretic effect leading to an increased risk of water intoxication.

Concomitant use of non-steroidal anti-inflammatory drugs (NSAIDs) including Cox-2 inhibitors may induce water retention and hyponatremia.

Concomitant treatment with opiates such as loperamide may result in a 3-fold increase of plasma desmopressin concentrations, which may lead to water retention and hyponatremia. Although not investigated, other drugs slowing intestinal transport might have the same effect.

Drug-Food Interactions: It has been previously shown that intake of a standardized meal with DDAVP Tablets has no effect on pharmacodynamic parameters (urine production and osmolality) despite some pharmacokinetic influence. The fact that DDAVP MELT is absorbed initially in the oral mucosa, pharynx and oesophagus implies that it is even less likely that food intake will influence its absorption. Therefore, it is very unlikely that any clinically significant drug-food interaction exists with sublingual administration of DDAVP MELT.

DOSAGE AND ADMINISTRATION: Dosing Considerations: Central Diabetes Insipidus: DDAVP MELT dosage must be determined for each patient and adjusted according to the pattern of response, but the total daily sublingual dose normally lies in the range of 120 µg to 720 µg. Response should be estimated by adequate duration of sleep and adequate, not excessive, water turnover and maintenance of urine osmolality at levels of 400 mOsmol/kg or greater.

To institute desmopressin therapy, patients should be withdrawn from previous medication and allowed to establish a baseline polyuria and polydipsia. The stable polyuria is used as a baseline to determine the magnitude and duration of the response to medication. In less severe cases, prior water loading may be desirable to establish a vigorous flow of urine. When the urine osmolality reaches a plateau at the low level (in most cases, less than 100 mOsm/kg), the first oral dose (e.g. 60 µg) of desmopressin is administered. A urine sample is obtained after two hours and hourly thereafter; urine volume is measured and urine osmolality determined. When the patient has reached the previous baseline urine osmolality and urine flow, the drug effect has ceased and the next desmopressin dose is administered. The cycle is then repeated until the patient has reached a stable condition.

Dosage must be individualized. A suitable starting dose for adults and children is 60 µg three times daily administered sublingually. This dosage regimen should then be adjusted in accordance with the patient's response in order to ensure an optimum dose.

In children, the evening dose is usually 2×higher than the morning and midday dose to ensure sufficient antidiuresis during sleep. This is generally not a requirement for adult patients, presumably because adults sleep for shorter periods of time.

For the majority of patients, the maintenance dose is 60 µg to 120 µg sublingually three times daily.

Lack of therapeutic response to oral desmopressin may be noted in some patients even at the maximum recommended dosage. These patients should be switched to the intranasal or injectable dosage form of desmopressin.

In the control of diabetes insipidus, the lowest effective dose should be used and the effective dosage, as determined by urine volume and osmolality and in some cases, plasma osmolality, should be assessed periodically.

In the event of signs of water retention/hyponatremia treatment should be interrupted and the dose should be adjusted.

Primary Nocturnal Enuresis: The dosage of DDAVP MELT must be determined for each individual patient and adjusted according to response. The recommended initial dose is 120 µg 1 hour before bedtime. If the patient experiences a wet night after three days on an initial dose of 120 µg increase the dose by 120 µg. The dose may be titrated up to 360 µg to achieve the desired response.

The physician should be consulted if enuresis persists at the maximal dose of 360 µg. A restricted fluid intake is recommended a few hours before administration, especially one hour before bedtime. As most children sleep between 8 to 12 hours, further restriction is not required. In the event that the child wakes up during the night, liquid intake should be restricted.

In the event of signs of water retention and/or hyponatremia (headache, nausea/vomiting, weight gain, and in severe cases, convulsions) treatment should be interrupted until the patient has fully recovered. When restarting treatment, strict fluid restriction should be enforced.

DDAVP MELT is intended for treatment periods of up to three months. The need for continued treatment should be reassessed by means of period of at least one week without DDAVP MELT If the patient is still wetting the bed, then reintroduce DDAVP MELT at the same dosage prior to discontinuing treatment for another three months and reassess.

Recommended Dose and Dosage Adjustment: Central Diabetes Insipidus: The recommended initial dose in adults and children is 60 µg three times daily administered sublingually. This dosage regimen should then be adjusted in accordance with the patient's response. The recommended daily dose range is 120-720 µg divided equally into 2 or 3 doses a day.

Missed Dose: If the patient misses a dose, the patient should be advised to take the missed dose as soon as possible. However if it is almost time for the next dose, the patient should be advised to skip the missed dose, to return to the regular dosing schedule and to **not** double dose.

Primary Nocturnal Enuresis: The recommended initial dose is 120 µg at bedtime administered sublingually. If this dose is not sufficiently effective, the dose may be increased up to 360 µg sublingually. The maximum recommended dose is 360 µg per day.

Missed Dose: If the patient misses a dose, the patient should be advised not to take the missed dose.

Administration: Restricted fluid intake is recommended a few hours before administration, especially one hour before, and until the next morning (at least 8 hours) after administration.

OVERDOSAGE:

Overdosage of desmopressin acetate may lead to an increased duration of action. This will increase the risk of fluid retention and symptoms which include headaches, abdominal cramps, nausea, and facial flushing. There is no known antidote. Dosage and frequency of administration should be reduced, or the drug withdrawn, according to severity of the condition.

If hyponatremia occurs following medication or excessive fluid intake, treatment should be discontinued and fluid intake restricted until serum sodium is normalized. In most cases this is sufficient. In cases with severe symptoms, [e.g., those associated with the central nervous system (CNS) such as unconsciousness], admission to hospital and a slow normalization of serum sodium is required to avoid additional complications. Intensive fluid intake regulation may be required in these cases.

Water retention can be controlled by decreasing the dosage of desmopressin; severe water retention caused by over dosage maybe treated with a diuretic such as furosemide.

> For management of a suspected drug overdose, CPhA recommends that you contact your **regional Poison Control Centre**. See the *CPS* Directory section for a list of Poison Control Centres.

ACTION AND CLINICAL PHARMACOLOGY: Mechanism of Action: Desmopressin is a synthetic structural analogue of the antidiuretic hormone, arginine vasopressin, which alters the permeability of the renal tubule to increase resorption of water. The increase in the permeability of both the distal tubules and collecting ducts appears to be mediated by a stimulation of the adenylcyclase activity in the renal tubules.

The bioavailability of orally ingested desmopressin has been found to be approximately 0.08%, sufficient to induce an antidiuresis (urine osmolality greater than 400 mOsm/kg) lasting 7 to 9 hours in healthy subjects and in patients with diabetes insipidus.

Recent clinical studies of the pharmacokinetics and pharmacodynamics of desmopressin showed that desmopressin has a longer antidiuretic action than previously reported. Plasma desmopressin concentrations from healthy volunteers were analysed using a new and sensitive bioassay with a low limit of quantification (LLOQ) of 0.8 ng/L. Desmopressin in-vivo potency was found to be 1.64 ng/L based on urine osmolality of 200 mOsm/kg. Given the new sensitive assay and the high variability in absorption, the pharmacological antidiuretic effects of desmopressin can be expected to last from 6 hours up to 14 hours.

Onset of action, as determined by decreased urine volume and increased urine osmolality, is within one hour. Mean maximum plasma concentrations in the range 6.57-16.6 pg/mL (0.2 mg dose) to 31.4-51.6 pg/mL (0.4 mg dose) are reached within 2 hours (t_{max} 0.75-1.9 hours). The oral mean terminal half-life varies between 2.0 and 3.2 hours. Intra- and inter-individual variability of about 30% in absorption of desmopressin is apparent. However, the plasma levels obtained are well above the amount required for a maximal antidiuretic effect, even for a prolonged period.

In both adults and children, there is a log linear relationship between desmopressin acetate doses and maximal urine osmolality and duration of antidiuresis within the dose range 12.5 to 400 µg. Measurements of plasma desmopressin concentrations after peroral desmopressin administration show a linear relationship between amounts of desmopressin absorbed and dose, but with great inter-individual differences.

Pharmacodynamics: Clinical studies have demonstrated that peroral administration of desmopressin is active in eliciting an antidiuretic effect in humans, be they normal subjects, or adults and children suffering from central diabetes insipidus (CDI) of various etiologies, or from nocturnal enuresis. The synthetic analogue exhibits a greater antidiuretic potency, as well as a longer half-life and duration of action, as compared to endogenous antidiuretic hormone.

When administered as a solution (20-200 µg per 50 mL water), desmopressin acetate produced a dose dependent effect both on the magnitude and the duration of the antidiuretic response as determined by measurements of urine osmolality, urine volume and free water clearance. Administration of desmopressin acetate through a duodenal tube caused similar antidiuretic effects, indicating that the intact peptide can be absorbed from the gastrointestinal mucosa. Onset of action was approximately one hour.

Desmopressin acetate does not directly affect urinary sodium or potassium excretion, or serum sodium, potassium, or creatinine concentrations. It does not stimulate uterine contractions, adrenocorticotropic hormone release or increase plasma cortisol concentrations.

Currently available information indicates that although absorption of desmopressin is low after oral administration, sufficient quantities are available to be clinically effective. The only recognized pharmacodynamic actions detected after orally administered desmopressin are reduction in urine flow and increase in urine osmolality. A number of studies have examined dose, and concentration-effect relationships of desmopressin with respect to its antidiuretic effects. Some studies show clear dose- and concentration-effect relationships, while others do not.

Recently performed pharmacokinetic/pharmacodynamic modelling indicated that the EC_{50} of desmopressin for antidiuretic effects is in the range of 1-2 pg/mL.

Two studies have been conducted to investigate the anti-diuretic effectiveness of five low doses of desmopressin (30, 60, 125, 250 and 500 ng), and placebo, in healthy volunteers and in subjects with pituitary diabetes insipidus. The drug was administered as an intravenous infusion in order to minimize the variation associated with oral delivery. The studies were designed to provide information about the PK/PD relationship of low doses of desmopressin and the duration of anti-diuretic action of these doses.

The studies showed that antidiuresis can be achieved in healthy volunteers and patients with pituitary diabetes insipidus at intravenous doses as low as 60 ng. No placebo effect was seen, and there was very little response at 30 ng. In both studies a clear response relationship was observed between desmopressin dose and duration of antidiuretic effect, at all cut-off levels of osmolality. The dose response curve did not plateau in the dose range tested (0-500 ng). Analysis of the PK data showed that an increase in AUC was observed with increasing doses of desmopressin, and based on AUC and AUC_t there was no evidence against dose linearity over the dose range 125-500 ng.

In healthy volunteers at the 250 ng i.v. dose, the median duration of anti-diuretic action was 5.36 hours (range: 0.75-10.64 hours) when using 200 mOsm/kg as cut-off, and 3.94 hours (range: 0-7.56 hours) using 400 mOsm/kg as cut-off.

In patients with pituitary diabetes insipidus the mean duration of action for the cut off level of 200 mOsm/kg was 3.45 hours for 60 ng, 6.15 hours for 125 ng, 9.5 hours for 250 ng and 13.3 hours for 500 ng, and for the cut off level of 400 mOsm/kg the corresponding values were 3.88 hours, 8.33 hours and 11 hours.

In vitro human liver microsome metabolism of desmopressin has shown that no significant amount is metabolised in the liver, and thus human liver metabolism in vivo is not likely to occur. Furthermore, no in vitro inhibition of human Cytochrome P450 enzymes could be demonstrated.

Desmopressin did not show any effect on any of the nine Cytochrome P450 subtypes. In vivo drug-drug interactions based on activation or inhibition of Cytochrome P450 are therefore very unlikely.

Pharmacokinetics: Human pharmacokinetic studies have been conducted on desmopressin using the oral and intravenous formulations.

Absorption: Due to the rapid disintegration of DDAVP MELT, desmopressin is immediately available for absorption via the membranes of the mouth, followed by the pharynx, the oesophagus and the stomach. This larger absorption surface likely contributes to a higher bioavailability as compared to DDAVP Tablets.

A comparative bioavailability study was conducted between MINIRIN tablet and DDAVP Melt. The study was an open-labelled, randomised, two period cross-over study in 28 non-smoking healthy male (n=14) and female volunteers (n=14). The subjects were 18 to 55 years of age and were enrolled at a single centre. All subjects completed the study. Each subject, in a randomised order, was administered 240 µg of DDAVP Melt and 2×0.2 mg MINIRIN tablets. Subjects were admitted to the study centre about 12 hours pre-dosing. The subjects remained at the study site at least 24 hours post-dose. A light meal was served 4 hours after administration of the study medication. The total fluid intake in the 24 hours after administration was limited to 1.5 litres and distributed evenly. The subjects were asked not to drink two hours prior to and four hour post dosing in order to normalise the buccal mucosa, before administration of the sublingual tablet. Between the doses there was a washout period of seven days. Blood samples were drawn in both treatment periods to provide a reliable estimate of the rate and extent of absorption of desmopressin. Blood samples for plasma concentration of desmopressin were collected according to the following schedule: pre-dose (i.e. 0-30 minutes pre-dosing), 15, 30 min 1, 1.5, 2, 3, 4, 6, 8, 9, 10, 11, 12, 13 and 14 hours after dosing. Desmopressin plasma concentrations were determined by a validated RIA method. The relative oral bioavailability of desmopressin in the DDAVP Melt relative to MINIRIN tablet was 1.52. Thus, an increase oral bioavailability from the DDAVP Melt compared to MINIRIN tablet was observed. A summary of the pharmacokinetic parameters for both products are summarized in Table 3.

Table 3: DDAVP MELT

Summary Table of the Comparative Bioavailability Data

Parameter	Desmopressin (1×240 μg DDAVP MELT Versus 2×200 μg MINIRIN) From Measured Data, Uncorrected for Potency Geometric Mean Arithmetic Mean (CV %)			
	Test[a] DDAVP MELT	Reference[b] MINIRIN	% Ratio of Geometric Means	90 % Confidence Interval
AUC_T (pg·h/mL)	73.2 85.7 (61.9%)	71.8 84.3 (57.0%)	102%	86–121%
AUC_I (pg·h/mL)	79.0 91.5 (59.0%)	77.2 89.8 (54.6%)	102%	87–121%
C_{max} (pg/mL)	18.0 21.1 (59.5%)	20.8 26.1 (59.8%)	87%	73–103%
[c]T_{max} (h)	1.5 (0.5–4.0)	1.0 (0.5–3.0)		
[c]$T_{1/2}$ (h)	3.19 (1.51–5.25)	3.17 (1.60–5.59)		

[a] DDAVP MELT Tablets (Ferring Inc, Canada).
[b] MINIRIN Tablets (Ferring Pharmaceuticals, Denmark).
[c] Expressed as the median and (range).

It is known that the efficacy of desmopressin is not influenced by C_{max}, but by total exposure over time, i.e. AUC. Until recently, information about the actual dynamic effects in target populations has been limited. In children with PNE, little has been known about the actual plasma levels of desmopressin required to obtain a maximal antidiuretic effect for a relevant time period.

The required kinetic parameters of desmopressin that match clinical experience are now understood in one of the target populations for desmopressin. It is evident that that an AUC_{inf} of 50-100 pg·h /mL desmopressin is sufficient to give a duration of antidiuretic action in PNE children of 7-11 hours with a cut-off level of 125 mOsm/kg (see Figure 1). This corresponds to a dose in the range of 120-360 μg.

Figure 1: DDAVP MELT

Relationship Between $AUC_{inf\ of\ desmopressin}$ and Duration of Action (cut-off 125 mOsm/kg)

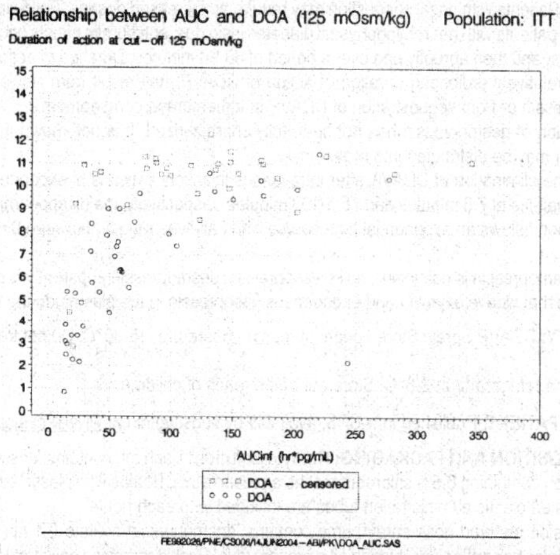

Linearity (dose proportional pharmacokinetics) was established for DDAVP MELT for dose levels from 60 μg and up to 240 μg (see Table 4).

Table 4: DDAVP MELT

Deduced Pharmacokinetic Parameters from Dose Proportionality Study of DDAVP MELT

Parameter	60 μg Dose	120 μg Dose	240 μg Dose
AUC_I (pg·h/mL)	20.0 21.6 (40.7%)	36.4 39.3 (40.8%)	67.7 79.6 (57.9%)
C_{max} (pg/mL)	3.81 4.03 (34.1%)	8.03 9.58 (62.4%)	15.0 19.0 (83.6%)
Dose Normalized AUC_I	0.333 0.360 (40.7%)	0.303 0.328 (40.8%)	0.282 0.332 (57.9%)
Dose Normalized C_{max}	0.064 0.067 (34.1%)	0.067 0.080 (62.4%)	0.063 0.079 (83.6%)

The inserted numbers are geometric mean and arithmetic mean and (CV %).

Table 5: DDAVP MELT

Correlation Between DDAVP Tablets and DDAVP MELT

DDAVP Tablets	DDAVP Tablets	DDAVP MELT	DDAVP MELT
Desmopressin acetate	Desmopressin free base	Desmopressin free base	Desmopressin acetate
0.1 mg	89 μg	60 μg	Approx. 67 μg[a]
0.2 mg	178 μg	120 μg	Approx. 135 μg[a]
0.4 mg	356 μg	240 μg	Approx. 270 μg[a]

[a] Calculated for comparative purposes.

The pharmacokinetic parameters (AUC and C_{max}) obtained in children were comparable to those obtained in adults. After the oral administration of 240 μg to children and 240 μg to adults, the AUC was found to be 99.8 and 79 pg/mL×hr, respectively; the C_{max} was 16.9 and 18 pg/mL, respectively.

Distribution: The distribution of desmopressin has not been fully characterized. It is not known if desmopressin crosses the placenta. The drug may be distributed into milk. The metabolic fate of desmopressin is unknown. Unlike vasopressin, desmopressin apparently is not degraded by aminopeptidases or other peptidases that cleave oxytocin and endogenous vasopressin.

Metabolism: In vitro human liver microsome metabolism of desmopressin has shown that no significant amount is metabolised in the liver, and thus human liver metabolism in vivo is not likely to occur. Furthermore, no in vitro inhibition of human Cytochrome P450 enzymes could be demonstrated.

Desmopressin did not show any effect on any of the nine Cytochrome P450 subtypes. In vivo drug-drug interactions based on activation or inhibition of Cytochrome P450 are therefore very unlikely.

Excretion: Urinary clearance in 6 hydrated volunteers was calculated to be 0.514 mL/min/kg body weight and the amount of peptide excreted in the urine during the 6-hour observation period constituted 16.4% of the amount absorbed from the intestine over the same period of time. Urinary clearance for desmopressin is thus smaller than reported for vasopressin.

STORAGE AND STABILITY: DDAVP MELT should be stored in the original package in a dry place at a temperature between 15 to 25°C. DDAVP MELT are stable for 24 months.

SPECIAL HANDLING INSTRUCTIONS: No special requirement.

INFORMATION FOR THE PATIENT: Published in e-CPS, available by subscription at www.e-cps.ca.

DOSAGE FORMS, COMPOSITION AND PACKAGING: 60 μg : Each white, round, oral disintegrating tablet, marked with a drop shape figure on one side contains: desmopressin acetate equivalent to desmopressin 60 μg. Nonmedicinal ingredients: citric acid, gelatin and mannitol. Blister packs of 10 tablets, boxes of 30 tablets.

120 μg: Each white, round, oral disintegrating tablet, marked with two drop shape figures on one side contains: desmopressin acetate equivalent to desmopressin 120 μg. Nonmedicinal ingredients: citric acid, gelatin and mannitol. Blister packs of 10 tablets, boxes of 30 tablets.

240 μg: Each white, round, oral disintegrating tablet, marked with three drop shape figures on one side contains: desmopressin acetate equivalent to desmopressin 240 μg. Nonmedicinal ingredients: citric acid, gelatin and mannitol. Blister packs of 10 tablets, boxes of 30 tablets.

DDAVP® Spray ℞

desmopressin acetate

Antidiuretic

Ferring

DDAVP® Rhinyle Nasal Solution ℞

desmopressin acetate

Antidiuretic

Ferring

Date of Revision: June 19, 2008

SUMMARY PRODUCT INFORMATION:

Route of Administration	Dosage Form/ Strength	Clinically Relevant Nonmedicinal Ingredients
Intranasal	Spray 10 μg/metered dose	DDAVP Spray: sodium chloride, citric acid monohydrate, disodium hydrogen phosphate dihydrate, benzalkonium chloride
	Solution 0.1 mg/mL	DDAVP Rhinyle: sodium chloride, hydrochloric acid, chlorobutanol For a complete listing see Dosage Forms, Composition and Packaging.

INDICATIONS AND CLINICAL USE: Diabetes Insipidus: DDAVP (desmopressin acetate) is indicated for the management of vasopressin sensitive central diabetes insipidus and for the control of temporary polyuria and polydipsia following head trauma, hypophysectomy or surgery in the pituitary region.

CONTRAINDICATIONS:

- Hypersensitivity to desmopressin acetate or to any of the constituents.
- Type IIB or platelet-type (pseudo) von Willebrand's disease.
- Habitual or psychogenic polydipsia.
- Cardiac insufficiency or other conditions requiring treatment with diuretics.
- Moderate or severe renal insufficiency.
- Known hyponatremia.
- Primary Nocturnal Enuresis (PNE).

Worldwide post-marketing data indicate a higher incidence of hyponatremia in patients being treated with the desmopressin intranasal formulations compared to the oral formulations (DDAVP Tablet and DDAVP Melt). Since safer formulations are available, intranasal formulations are contraindicated for use in primary nocturnal enuresis.

WARNINGS AND PRECAUTIONS: Hyponatremia is the most important adverse event reported for desmopressin, resulting from water retention caused by the potent antidiuretic effect of desmopressin. Desmopressin may lead to water intoxication and/or hyponatremia. Unless properly diagnosed and treated, hyponatremia can be fatal. Therefore, fluid restriction is recommended and should be discussed with the patient and/or guardian. Careful medical supervision is required.

For intranasal use only. DDAVP (desmopressin acetate) is not effective in controlling polyuria caused by renal disease, nephrogenic diabetes insipidus, psychogenic diabetes insipidus, hypokalemia or hypercalcemia.

Fluid intake or desmopressin dosage should be adjusted in order to reduce the possibility of water retention and hyponatremia especially in very young and elderly patients or when significant daily variables occur such as hot climate conditions, intense exercise or other situations where increased water intake can be expected (see Dosage and Administration). Particular attention should be paid to the risk of an extreme decrease in plasma osmolality and resulting seizures in young children. Should prodromal symptoms (headache, nausea and vomiting) which may herald impending hyponatraemia occur, treatment should be discontinued immediately and the patient should seek medical assessment.

Changes in the nasal mucosa resulting from rhinitis, scarring, edema or other disease may cause erratic, unreliable absorption in which case intranasal desmopressin should not be used. In the case of temporary rhinitis, consideration should be given to using an injectable form of desmopressin, until the nasal mucosa returns to normal.

General: Desmopressin acetate at high dosage (40 μg or more) has very occasionally produced a slight elevation of blood pressure, which disappeared with a reduction in dosage. The drug should be used with caution in patients with coronary artery insufficiency and/or hypertensive cardiovascular disease because of possible tachycardia and changes in blood pressure.

In the control of diabetes insipidus, the lowest effective dose should be used and the effective dosage, as determined by urine volume and osmolality and, in some cases, plasma osmolality, should be assessed periodically.

Desmopressin should not be administered to dehydrated patients until water balance has been adequately restored.

Desmopressin should be used with caution in patients with conditions associated with fluid and electrolyte imbalance such as cystic fibrosis, heart failure and renal disorders because these patients are prone to hyponatremia. Desmopressin should also be used with caution in patients at risk for increased intracranial pressure.

Children and geriatric patients should be closely observed for possible water retention due to over-ingestion of fluids. When fluid intake is not excessive, there is little danger of water intoxication and hyponatremia with the usual intranasal doses of desmopressin used to control diabetes insipidus. Fluid intake should be carefully adjusted to prevent overhydration.

There are reports of changes in response over time, usually when the drug has been administered for periods longer than 6 months. Some patients may show decreased responsiveness, others a shortened duration of effect. There is no evidence that this effect is due to the development of binding antibodies, but may be due to local inactivation of the peptide.

There is some evidence from post-marketing data for the occurrence of severe hyponatremia in association with the nasal spray formulation of desmopressin, when it is used in the treatment of cranial diabetes insipidus.

Special Populations: Pregnant Women: Reproductive studies performed in rats and rabbits have revealed no evidence of harm to the fetus by desmopressin. The use of desmopressin in pregnant women with no harm to the fetus has been reported. However, no controlled studies in pregnant women have been carried out.

One investigator has reported three cases of malformations in children born to mothers suffering from diabetes insipidus and receiving desmopressin during pregnancy. However, several other published reports comprising more than 120 cases showed that women treated with desmopressin during pregnancy have given birth to normal children. Furthermore, a review of a very large data set identifying 29 children who were exposed to desmopressin during the entire pregnancy showed no increase in the malformation rate in the children born. Unlike preparations containing the natural hormone, DDAVP in antidiuretic doses has no uterotonic action, but the physician should weigh possible therapeutic advantages against potential risks in each case.

Nursing Women: There have been no controlled studies in nursing mothers. A single study on a post-partum woman demonstrated a marked change in maternal plasma desmopressin level following an intranasal dose of 10 µg, but little desmopressin was detectable in breast milk.

Pediatrics: DDAVP (desmopressin acetate) has been used in children with diabetes insipidus. The dose must be individually adjusted to the patient with attention in the very young to the danger of an extreme decrease of plasma osmolality with resulting convulsions. Dosage in infants younger than 3 months has not been established. Dose should start at 5 µg or less. Use of desmopressin in infants and children will require careful fluid intake restriction to prevent possible hyponatremia and water intoxication.

Geriatrics: Older patients may be more sensitive to the antidiuretic effect of the usual adult dose of DDAVP. Patients over the age of 65 should be closely observed for possible water retention due to over-ingestion of fluids. Fluid intake should be carefully adjusted to prevent over-hydration.

Monitoring and Laboratory Tests: Diagnosis of Central Diabetes Insipidus: Central diabetes insipidus may be demonstrated by the inability to produce urine of osmolality above 175 mOsm/kg with dehydration severe enough to cause a loss of greater than 2% of body weight.

Patients are selected for therapy by establishing a diagnosis by means of a water deprivation test, the hypertonic saline infusion test, and/or response to 5 units arginine vasopressin given s.c. after dehydration. Continued response to DDAVP can be monitored by urine volume and osmolality. In cases of severe dehydration, plasma osmolality determination may be required.

ADVERSE REACTIONS: Adverse Drug Reaction Overview: Infrequently, high doses of desmopressin have produced transient headache and nausea. Nasal congestion, rhinitis, flushing, and mild abdominal cramps have been reported. These symptoms disappeared with reduction in dosage. Side effects reported from controlled clinical trials involving 638 subjects included headache (2%), rhinitis (1%), nasal discomfort (1%), epistaxis (1%) and abdominal pain (1%). Other effects, reported at a frequency of less than 1%, included dizziness, chills, wheezing, rash, edema of face and hands, nausea, constipation, anorexia, increased appetite, conjunctivitis and after taste in the mouth. These symptoms disappeared with reduction of dosage or withdrawal of drug. Adverse effects rarely necessitated discontinuance of the drug.

Treatment without concomitant reduction of fluid intake may lead to water retention/hyponatremia with accompanying signs and symptoms (headache, nausea/vomiting, decreased serum sodium, weight gain, and in serious cases, convulsions.

Very rare cases of emotional disturbances in children have been reported. Isolated cases of allergic skin reactions and more serious general allergic reactions have been reported.

Post-Market Adverse Drug Reactions: Hyponatremia has been reported at an approximate rate of 5 cases per 10 million doses from worldwide post marketing experience in patients treated with DDAVP intranasal formulations. The reported rate for DDAVP oral formulations worldwide is considerably less at about 1 case per 10 million doses. Patients are recommended to take the oral formulations (e.g., DDAVP Melt) which are available for children with PNE. Desmopressin is a potent antidiuretic, which may lead to water intoxication and/or hyponatremia. Unless properly diagnosed and treated, hyponatremia can be fatal. Therefore, fluid restriction is recommended and should be discussed with the patient and/or guardian. Careful medical supervision is required.

DRUG INTERACTIONS: Overview: Clofibrate, chlorpropamide and carbamazepine may potentiate the antidiuretic activity of desmopressin leading to an increased risk of water retention/hyponatremia, while demeclocycline, lithium and norepinephrine may decrease its activity. Indomethacin increases the urine concentrating effect of desmopressin without influencing the duration. The effect is probably without any clinical significance.

Although the pressor activity of desmopressin is very low compared with the antidiuretic activity, use of large doses of desmopressin with other pressor agents should be done only with careful patient monitoring.

The selective serotonin reuptake inhibitors (SSRIs, venlafaxine and citalopram), and the neuroleptic risperidone have been associated with water intoxication and hyponatremia in rare cases.

DOSAGE AND ADMINISTRATION: Central Diabetes Insipidus: Central diabetes insipidus may be demonstrated by the inability to produce urine of osmolality above 175 mOsm/kg with dehydration severe enough to cause a loss of greater than 2% of body weight (see Warnings and Precautions, Monitoring and Laboratory Tests).

Dosing Considerations: Dosage must be individualized but clinical experience has shown that the average daily dose for adults is 10 µg to 40 µg DDAVP (desmopressin acetate) and for children 3 months to 12 years of age, 5 µg to 30 µg. This may be given as a single dose or divided into two or three doses. About one third of patients can be treated with a single daily dose. Geriatric patients may be more sensitive to the antidiuretic effect of the usual adult dose of DDAVP.

Dosage in children with central diabetes insipidus up to 3 months of age has not been established.

DDAVP Spray is not indicated for use in children with Primary Nocturnal Enuresis (PNE).

Recommended Dose: Children (3 months to 12 years): The usual dose range is 5 µg to 30 µg daily either as a single dose or divided into two doses. About 1/3 of patients can be controlled by a single dose daily dose of DDAVP administered intranasally.

DDAVP Spray pump can only deliver 0.1 mL (10 µg) or multiples of 0.1 mL. In those children who require less than 10 µg, the rhinyle presentation should be used. In some patients, better control of polyuria is attained with smaller doses given at 6 to 8 hour intervals.

DDAVP Spray should be used in children who only require a single dose of 10 µg or more. The spray pump must be primed prior to use. To prime pump, press down four times. The bottle will now deliver 10 µg of drug.

Adult: Average daily dose is 10 µg to 40 µg. Most adults require 20 µg daily, administered in two divided doses (in the morning and the evening). Initially, therapy should be directed to control nocturia with a single evening dose. Response to therapy can be measured by the volume and frequency of urination and duration of uninterrupted sleep. The dosage of DDAVP should be adjusted according to the diurnal pattern of response, with the morning and evening doses being adjusted separately. Patients being switched from parenteral to intranasal administration generally require 10 times their maintenance intravenous dose intranasally. In order to minimize the risk of hyponatremia, the following should be considered a part of individualized dosage titration:

- Desmopressin should be given with caution and the dosage adjusted as necessary during acute illness, febrile episodes, hot days and other conditions with increased water intake.

To institute therapy with DDAVP, patients should be withdrawn from previous medication and allowed to establish a baseline polyuria to permit determination of the magnitude and duration of the response to medication. In less severe cases, prior water loading may be desirable to establish a vigorous flow of urine. When the urine osmolality reaches a plateau at low level (in most cases, less than 100 mOsm/kg), the first dose of DDAVP (10 µg) is administered intranasally. A urine sample is obtained after two hours and hourly thereafter following DDAVP administration. Urine volume and osmolality are measured. When the patient has reached the previous baseline urine osmolality and urine flow, the drug effect has ceased and the next dose of DDAVP is administered. The cycle is then repeated until the patient has reached a stable condition.

In the event of signs of water retention/hyponatremia, treatment should be interrupted and the dose should be adjusted.

OVERDOSAGE:

Overdose symptoms include headaches, abdominal cramps, nausea, and facial flushing.There is no known antidote. However, the following general recommendations can be provided. Asymptomatic hyponatremia is treated by discontinuing the desmopressin treatment and fluid restriction. Infusion of isotonic or hypertonic sodium chloride may be added in cases with symptoms. When the water retention is severe (convulsions and unconsciousness) treatment with furosemide should be added.

For management of a suspected drug overdose, contact your **regional Poison Control Centre**. See the *CPS* Directory section for a list of Poison Control Centres.

ACTION AND CLINICAL PHARMACOLOGY: Mechanism of Action: Desmopressin is a synthetic structural analogue of the antidiuretic hormone, arginine vasopressin, which alters the permeability of the renal tubule to increase resorption of water.The increase in the permeability of both the distal tubules and collecting ducts appears to be mediated by a stimulation of the adenylcyclase activity in the renal tubules.

Approximately 10 to 20% of the dose of desmopressin solution administered intranasally is absorbed through the nasal mucosa. Antidiuretic effects occur within 1 hour, peak in 1 to 5 hours, persist for 8 to 20 hours and then abruptly end over a period of 60 to 90 minutes. Duration of action varies greatly among individuals and is dependent upon the rate of absorption from the nasal mucosa, persistence in plasma, and effect on renal tubules.

Pharmacodynamics: Maximum urine concentration was studied in 10 healthy adults (24 to 37 years of age) after administration of 20, 40 and 80 µg DDAVP intranasally with one week between each administration. Maximum effect on urine osmolality occurred between 3 and 5 hours (Figure 1), and the 20 µg dose was as effective as the higher doses. There were no side effects and mean body weight increase during the 24 hours after DDAVP administration did not exceed 0.5 kg after any dose.

The use of DDAVP (desmopressin acetate) in patients with an established diagnosis of central diabetes insipidus will result in a reduction in urinary output with concomitant increase in urine osmolality and decrease in plasma osmolality. This will allow the resumption of a more normal lifestyle with a decrease in urinary frequency.

Figure 1: DDAVP Spray/DDAVP Rhinyle Nasal
Urine Osmolality After Various Doses of DDAVP Given Intranasally (mean±SD)

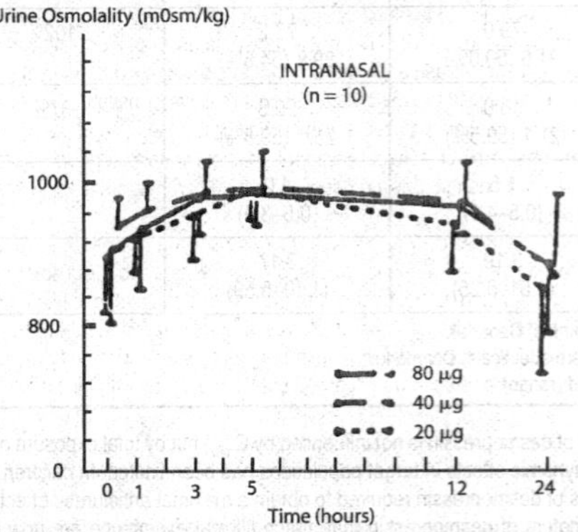

DDAVP does not directly affect urinary sodium or potassium excretion, or serum sodium, potassium, or creatinine concentrations. DDAVP does not stimulate uterine contractions, adrenocorticotropic hormone release or increase plasma cortisol concentrations. In children, intranasal administration of DDAVP has no effect on growth hormone, prolactin, or luteinizing hormone concentration. Intranasal doses of 20 µg of DDAVP have no effect on blood pressure or pulse rate, but mean arterial pressure may increase as much as 15 mm Hg with doses of 40 µg or more.

Pharmacokinetics: Absorption: Following intranasal administration of DDAVP, approximately 10-20% of a dose is absorbed through the nasal mucosa. Patients with nasal congestion may require an increased dosage. Following intranasal administration of usual doses of DDAVP in patients with neurohypophyseal diabetes insipidus, antidiuretic effects occur within 1 hour, peak in 1-5 hours, persist for 8-20 hours, and then abruptly end over a period of 60-90 minutes. Duration of action varies among individuals with a specific dose. The relatively prolonged duration of action of DDAVP may result from slower enzymatic inactivation of desmopressin than vasopressin or from sequestration of DDAVP in a membrane compartment.

Distribution: The distribution of desmopressin has not been fully characterized. It is not known if desmopressin crosses the placenta. Some of the drug may be distributed into breast milk.

Excretion: In contrast to the elimination of DDAVP after intravenous injection, which is bi-exponential with a rapid first phase and slower second phase half-life of 7.8 minutes and 75.5-103 minutes, respectively, the disappearance of DDAVP from plasma after intranasal administration follows an exponential time course with half-lives ranging between 0.4 to 4 hours after intranasal application.

The metabolic fate of desmopressin is unknown. Unlike vasopressin, desmopressin apparently is not degraded by aminopeptidases or other peptidases that cleave oxytocin and endogenous vasopressin in the plasma during late pregnancy.

STORAGE AND STABILITY: DDAVP Spray: Store upright at room temperature, 15-30°C. Do not freeze. Store out of the reach of children.

DDAVP Rhinyle: Keep in the refrigerator at 2-8°C. Store out of the reach of children.

INFORMATION FOR THE PATIENT: Published in e-CPS, available by subscription at www.e-cps.ca.

DOSAGE FORMS, COMPOSITION AND PACKAGING: Rhinyle Solution: Each mL contains: desmopressin acetate 0.1 mg in an isotonic, aqueous solution containing 0.5% chlorobutanol as a preservative. Bottles with plastic administration tube (Rhinyle). Two precalibrated and marked plastic administration tubes are included with each bottle.

Spray: Each pre-compression metered dose spray pump contains: desmopressin acetate 0.1 mg/mL in a buffered, isotonic, aqueous solution. Also contains benzalkonium chloride as a preservative. Each depression delivers desmopressin acetate 10 µg. Spray bottles of 2.5 mL containing 25 doses and 5 mL containing 50 doses.

DDAVP® Tablets Ⓡ

desmopressin acetate

Antidiuretic

Ferring

Date of Preparation: August 26, 2005
Date of Revision: November 10, 2005

SUMMARY PRODUCT INFORMATION:

Route of Administration	Dosage Form/ Strength	Clinically Relevant Nonmedicinal Ingredients
Oral	Tablet 0.1 mg, 0.2 mg	Lactose, potato starch, povidone, magnesium stearate For a complete listing see Dosage Forms, Composition and Packaging.

INDICATIONS AND CLINICAL USE: DDAVP Tablets is indicated for:

- treatment of central diabetes insipidus
- treatment of nocturnal enuresis

Central Diabetes Insipidus: DDAVP Tablets (0.1 and 0.2 mg desmopressin acetate) are indicated for the management of vasopressin sensitive central diabetes insipidus, and for the control of temporary polyuria and polydipsia following head trauma, hypophysectomy or surgery in the pituitary region.

Nocturnal Enuresis: DDAVP Tablets (0.1 and 0.2 mg desmopressin acetate) are indicated in the management of nocturnal enuresis in patients 5 years of age and older who have normal ability to concentrate urine. DDAVP Tablets should be used in conjunction with non-medicinal therapy, such as motivational counselling and bladder exercises.

CONTRAINDICATIONS: Hypersensitivity to desmopressin acetate or any of the tablet's constituents. Because of the risk of platelet aggregation and thrombocytopenia, the drug should not be used in patients with type IIB or platelet-type (pseudo) von Willebrand's disease.

Known hyponatremia, severe liver disease, nephrosis or any other condition associated with impaired water excretion, cardiac insufficiency, chronic renal insufficiency, congestive heart failure, habitual or psychogenic polydypsia.

Patients with existing medical conditions, which lead to sodium losing states such as nausea, bulimia, anorexia nervosa, chronic vomiting, diarrhoea and adrenocortical insufficiency as well as salt losing nephropathies, should only be prescribed DDAVP under close medical supervision and with extreme caution.

WARNINGS AND PRECAUTIONS: General: In general, by adequate treatment with DDAVP, thirst is automatically reduced. However, there is potential risk of water intoxication, if during treatment, excessive liquid is consumed. It is advisable that patients, and especially the parents of child patients, be cautioned about this.

In patients with water and/or electrolyte balance disorder [such as systemic infections, fever, and Syndrome of Inappropriate Antidiuretic Hormone secretion (SIADH)], and in patients with high intra-cranial pressure, it is also necessary that extra care be exercised with liquid intake.

Desmopressin acetate is not effective in controlling polyuria caused by renal disease, nephrogenic diabetes insipidus, psychogenic diabetes insipidus, hypokalemia or hypercalcemia.

Fluid intake should be adjusted to reduce the possibility of water intoxication and hyponatremia especially in the very young and elderly patients (see Dosage and Administration). Particular attention should be paid to the risk of an extreme decrease in plasma osmolality and resulting seizures in young children.

Intranasal formulation of desmopressin acetate at high dosage (40 µg or more) has occasionally produced a slight elevation of blood pressure, which disappeared with a reduction in dosage. The drug should be used with caution in patients with coronary artery insufficiency and/or hypertensive cardiovascular disease because of possible tachycardia and changes in blood pressure.

Lack of therapeutic response to oral desmopressin may be noted in some patients even at the maximum recommended dosage. These patients should be switched to the intranasal or injectable dosage form of desmopressin.

In the control of diabetes insipidus, the lowest effective dose should be used and the effective dosage, as determined by urine volume and osmolality and in some cases, plasma osmolality, should be assessed periodically.

Desmopressin should not be administered to dehydrated patients until water balance has been adequately restored.

Desmopressin should be used with caution in patients with cystic fibrosis because these patients are prone to hyponatremia.

Children and geriatric patients should be closely observed for possible water retention due to over ingestion of fluids. When fluid intake is not excessive, there is little danger of water intoxication and hyponatremia. Fluid intake should be carefully adjusted to prevent overhydration.

There are reports of changes in response over time, usually when the drug has been administered for periods longer than 6 months. Some patients may show decreased responsiveness, others a shortened duration of effect. There is no evidence that this effect is due to the development of binding antibodies, but may be due to local inactivation of the peptide.

Special Populations: Pregnant Women: Reproductive studies performed in rats and rabbits have revealed no evidence of harm to fetus by desmopressin. The use of desmopressin acetate in pregnant women with no harm to the fetus has been reported.

No controlled studies in pregnant women have been carried out. However, as with all medication used during pregnancy, the physician should weigh possible therapeutic advantages against potential risks in each case.

Nursing Women: There have been no controlled studies in nursing mothers. A single study on a post-partum woman demonstrated a marked change in maternal plasma desmopressin acetate level following an intranasal dose of 10 µg, but little desmopressin was detectable in breast milk.

Pediatrics: Desmopressin acetate has been used in children with diabetes insipidus. The dose must be individually adjusted to the patient with attention in the very young to the danger of an extreme decrease of plasma osmolality with resulting convulsions. Dosage in infants younger than 3 months has not been established. Dose should start at 100 µg or less. Use of desmopressin acetate in infants and children will require careful fluid intake restriction to prevent possible hyponatremia and water intoxication.

Monitoring and Laboratory Tests: Diagnosis of Central Diabetes Insipidus: Central diabetes insipidus may be demonstrated by the inability to produce urine of osmolality above 175 mOsm/kg with dehydration severe enough to cause a loss of greater than 2% of body weight.

Patients are selected for therapy by establishing a diagnosis by means of a water deprivation test, the hypertonic saline infusion test, and/or response to 5 units arginine vasopressin given s.c. after dehydration. Continued response to desmopressin acetate is monitored by urine volume and osmolality. In cases of severe dehydration, plasma osmolality determination may be required.

ADVERSE REACTIONS: Infrequently, high doses of desmopressin have produced transient headache and nausea. Nasal congestion, rhinitis, flushing, and mild abdominal cramps have been reported. These symptoms disappeared with reduction in dosage.

Side effects reported from controlled clinical trials involving 638 subjects included headache (2%), and rhinitis (1%), nasal discomfort (1%), epistaxis (1%) and abdominal pain (1%). Other effects, reported at a frequency of less than 1% included dizziness, chills, wheezing, rash, edema of face and hands, nausea, constipation, anorexia, increased appetite, conjunctivitis and after taste in the mouth. These symptoms disappeared with reduction of dosage or withdrawal of drug. Adverse effects rarely necessitate discontinuance of the drug.

Serum AST levels were elevated in 4/16 patients 6 months after commencing oral desmopressin acetate therapy (200 to 600 µg/day). Two of these patients had exhibited baseline levels of AST that were above the normal range and all four patients had normal AST levels on repeat test at 9 months, even though desmopressin acetate administration continued. The possibility that desmopressin acetate has an adverse effect on serum enzymes is therefore remote.

DRUG INTERACTIONS: Clofibrate, chlorpropamide and carbamazepine may potentiate the antidiuretic activity of desmopressin while demeclocycline, lithium and norepinephrine may decrease its activity.

Although the pressor activity of desmopressin acetate is very low compared with the anti-diuretic activity, use of large doses of desmopressin with other pressor agents should be done only with careful patient monitoring.

Concomitant treatment with drugs which are known to induce SIADH, e.g. tricyclic antidepressants, selective serotonine reuptake inhibitors, chlorpromazine and carbamazepine, may cause an additive antidiuretic effect leading to an increased risk of water intoxication.

Concomitant use of non-steroidal anti-inflammatory drugs (NSAIDs) including Cox-2 inhibitors such as Celebrex may induce water retention and hyponatremia.

Concomitant treatment with opiates such as loperamide may result in a 3-fold increase of plasma desmopressin concentrations, which may lead to water retention and hyponatremia. Although not investigated, other drugs slowing intestinal transport might have the same effect.

Intake of a standardised meal with oral desmopressin resulted in significant decreased bioavailability compared to fasting. This is hypothesised to be due to reduced absorption from the gastrointestinal tract. However no effect on dynamics (urine production or osmolality) was observed.

DOSAGE AND ADMINISTRATION: Central Diabetes Insipidus: DDAVP dosage must be determined for each patient and adjusted according to the pattern of response. Response should be estimated by adequate duration of sleep and adequate, not excessive, water turnover and maintenance of urine osmolality at levels of 400 mOsmol/kg or greater.

To institute desmopressin therapy, patients should be withdrawn from previous medication and allowed to establish a baseline polyuria and polydipsia. The stable polyuria is used as a baseline to determine the magnitude and duration of the response to medication. In less severe cases, prior water loading may be desirable to establish a vigorous flow of urine. When the urine osmolality reaches a plateau at the low level (in most cases, less than 100 mOsm/kg), the first oral dose e.g., 100 µg) of desmopressin is administered. A urine sample is obtained after two hours and hourly thereafter; urine volume is measured and urine osmolality determined. When the patient has reached the previous baseline urine osmolality and urine flow, the drug effect has ceased and the next desmopressin dose is administered. The cycle is then repeated until the patient has reached a stable condition.

Dosage must be individualized. A suitable starting dose for adults and children is 100 µg (0.1 mg desmopressin acetate) three times daily. This dosage regimen should then be adjusted in accordance with the patient's response in order to ensure an optimum dose. For patients who have been controlled on intranasal desmopressin and who are to be switched to the oral form, the oral dose producing comparable antidiuresis is about 10-20 times greater than the established intranasal dose. Geriatric patients may be more sensitive to the antidiuretic effect of the usual adult dose of desmopressin acetate.

In children, the evening dose is usually 2× higher than the morning and midday dose to ensure sufficient antidiuresis during sleep. This is generally not a requirement for adult patients, presumably because adults sleep for shorter periods of time.

The maximum recommended dosage for both adults and children is 1.2 mg per day (400 µg t.i.d.). Although there is no evidence that potentially serious adverse reactions would occur at daily doses greater than 1.2 mg, a maximum of 1.2 mg is being recommended at the present time since clinical experiences with daily dosages exceeding 1.2 mg is limited. The lowest effective dosage should be given. Rarely, during long term use, patients may develop tolerance to the drug and require cautious increase in dosage to achieve adequate therapeutic response.

Primary Nocturnal Enuresis: The dosage of DDAVP Tablets must be determined for each individual patient and adjusted according to response. Patients previously on intranasal DDAVP therapy can begin tablet therapy the night following (24 hours after) the last intranasal dose. The recommended initial dose is 0.2 mg 1 hour before bedtime. The dose may be titrated up to 0.6 mg to achieve the desired response using the following dosage plan. If the patient experiences a wet night after three days on an initial dose of 0.2 mg (1×0.2 mg tablet), increase the dose by 0.2 mg. The dose may be increased by 0.2 mg increments, in the manner described (every 3 days), to a maximal dose of 0.6 mg. The physician should be consulted if enuresis persists at the maximal dose. A restricted fluid intake is recommended a few hours before administration, especially one hour before bedtime. As most children sleep between 8 to 12 hours, further restriction is not required. In the event that the child wakes up during the night, liquid intake should be restricted.

OVERDOSAGE:

Overdose symptoms include headaches, abdominal cramps, nausea, and facial flushing. There is no known antidote. Dosage and frequency of administration should be reduced, or the drug withdrawn, according to severity of the condition.

Water retention can be controlled by decreasing the dosage of desmopressin; severe water retention caused by overdosage may be treated with a diuretic such as furosemide.

> For management of a suspected drug overdose, CPhA recommends that you contact your **regional Poison Control Centre**. See the *CPS* Directory section for a list of Poison Control Centres.

ACTION AND CLINICAL PHARMACOLOGY: Desmopressin acetate is a synthetic structural analogue of the antidiuretic hormone, arginine vasopressin, which alters the permeability of the renal tubule to increase resorption of water. The increase in the permeability of both the distal tubules and collecting ducts appears to be mediated by a stimulation of the adenylcyclase activity in the renal tubules.

Although the bioavailability of orally ingested desmopressin is low, reported as being about 1 to 5%, it is sufficient to induce an antidiuresis (urine osmolality greater than 400 mOsm/kg) lasting 7 to 9 hours in healthy subjects and in patients with diabetes insipidus. Recent clinical studies of the pharmacokinetics and pharmacodynamics of desmopressin showed that desmopressin has a longer antidiuretic action than previously reported. Plasma desmopressin concentrations from healthy volunteers were analysed using a new and sensitive bioassay with a low limit of quantification (LLOQ) of 0.8 ng/L. Desmopressin in-vivo potency was found to be 1.64 ng/L based on urine osmolality of 200 mOsm/kg. Given the high variability in absorption, the pharmacological antidiuretic effects of desmopressin can be expected to last from 6 hours up to 14 hours.

Onset of action, as determined by decreased urine volume and increased urine osmolality, is within one hour. In both adults and children, there is a log linear relationship between desmopressin acetate doses and maximal urine osmolality and duration of antidiuresis within the dose range 12.5 to 400 µg. Measurements of plasma desmopressin concentrations after peroral desmopressin acetate administration show a linear relationship between amounts of desmopressin acetate absorbed and dose, but with great interindividual differences.

Pharmacodynamics: Clinical studies have demonstrated that peroral administration of desmopressin acetate is active in eliciting an antidiuretic effects in humans, be they normal subjects, or adults and children suffering from central diabetes insipidus (CDI) of various etiologies, or from nocturnal enuresis. The synthetic analogue exhibits a greater antidiuretic potency, as well as a longer half-life and duration of action, as compared to endogenous antidiuretic hormone.

When administered as a solution (20-200 µg per 50 mL water), desmopressin acetate produced a dose dependent effect both on the magnitude and the duration of the antidiuretic response as determined by measurements of urine osmolality, urine volume and free water clearance. Administration of desmopressin acetate through a duodenal tube caused similar antidiuretic effects, indicating that the intact peptide can be absorbed from the gastrointestinal mucosa. Onset of action was approximately 1 hour. (See Figure 1.)

Figure 1: DDAVP Tablets

Urine Osmolality (Top Panel), Urine Volume (Mid Panel) and Free Water Clearance (Lower Panel) During 15 Minute Periods in Hydrated Human Volunteers Following Peroral Administration of 20, 40 and 200 µg of Desmopressin Acetate. Mean±Sem, N=5 for Each Dose

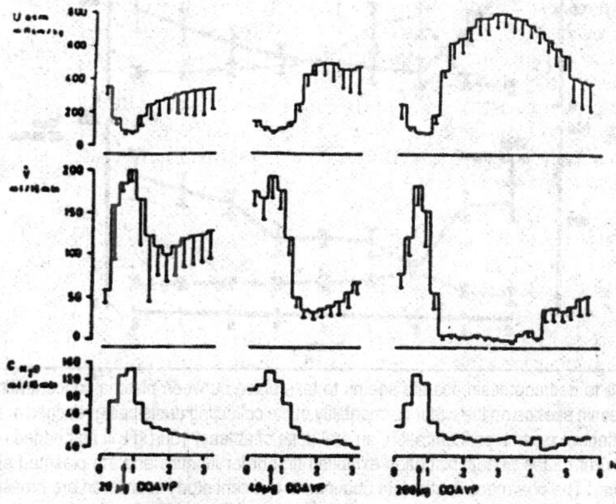

The effect of desmopressin acetate tablets was similar to that of the desmopressin solution but with an apparently slightly longer duration of action; each patient required a slightly different daily regimen for satisfactory control of water balance. The average daily PO dose, 300 µg (range of 200-350 µg), was 11× that of the mean previous intranasal dose (27 µg, range of 10 to 40 µg), with dosing frequency being more often t.i.d. (in 8/9 patients) rather than the more usual b.i.d. intranasal regimen.

Urine osmolality increased rapidly during the second hour and in a similar manner following either intranasal doses of 10 or 20 µg or peroral doses of 200 or 400 µg desmopressin acetate. The onset of action tends to coincide with the appearance of desmopressin in the plasma (15 min) and plasma levels, which reached maximal values 1-2 hours after 100-200 µg desmopressin acetate was administered orally, remained fairly constant over the six-hour observation period.

There are no differences in terms of magnitude and duration of the response between the two routes of administration, with free water clearance remaining negative for approximately 7 to 8 hours. When the criterion for a good antidiuretic effect was set at a urine osmolality of greater than 400 mOsmol/kg, the mean (±SD) duration of the antidiuretic effect, in hours, was 7.4±3.0 and 9.0±3.2 after 10 and 20 µg IN, respectively, and 7.2±3.3 and 8.8±2.3 after 200 and 400 µg PO, respectively. Large interindividual differences in duration of the antidiuretic effect (i.e., 5-24 hours) following intranasal application of 20 µg desmopressin acetate have also been reported in earlier studies.

The data recorded from urine volume and osmolality measurements showed no statistically significant difference between fasting and non-fasting healthy subjects in response to 100 and 200 µg desmopressin acetate tablets; no effects on blood pressure 1 or 3 hours after desmopressin acetate administration were seen.

Intranasal desmopressin acetate (10-25 µg) in children had a more marked and prolonged antidiuretic effect compared to the response obtained with 50 and 100 µg oral doses in the same children. This difference is not surprising in view of the greater peptidase activity in GI secretions.

Desmopressin acetate does not directly affect urinary sodium or potassium excretion, or serum sodium, potassium, or creatinine concentrations. It does not stimulate uterine contractions, adrenocorticotropic hormone release or increase plasma cortisol concentrations. (See Figure 2.)

Pharmacokinetics: The results of pharmacokinetic studies conducted with oral desmopressin acetate are summarized in Table 1. The most striking feature of the pharmacokinetic data was the large intra- and interindividual differences noted in all of the studies.

Dose-response relationships and pharmacokinetic profile of orally administered desmopressin acetate were similar in normal subjects and in adults and children with CDI. In all studies, both the magnitude of the plasma peak concentration and the AUC were dose dependent. Time to peak plasma concentration and the plasma half-life were not affected by the size of the dose.

Plasma desmopressin levels increased in a dose-dependent fashion and its disappearance from plasma followed an exponential time course, with half-life of 86 to 142 minutes. In contrast, the elimination of desmopressin after IV injection is biexponential with rapid first phase and slower second phase half-lives of 7.8 minutes and 75.5-103 minutes, respectively. Because of the great inter-individual differences, the dose-response curves of the different patients show different slopes.

Linear regression analysis suggests that the lowest dose of peroral desmopressin acetate having a biological effect is approximately 10 µg and that a significant antidiuretic effect (i.e., urine volume less than 2 mL/min) would be obtained with a peroral desmopressin acetate dose of 40 µg; doubling this dose would increase the duration of the antidiuresis approximately 4.5 hours. These results are in accordance with those reported by Moses et al. following SC administration of desmopressin acetate.

Table 1: DDAVP Tablets

Summary of Pharmacokinetic Parameters in Normal Subjects (NS) and Patients with Central Diabetes Insipidus (CDI). Numbers in brackets indicate the number of subject/patients from which the parameter was derived

Dose (µg)	AUC (ng/L·h) (N)				C_{max} (µg/L) (N)				T_{max} (min) (N)				$T_{½}$ (hour) (N)			
	A	B	C	D	A	B	C	D	A	B	C	D	A	B	C	D
50 NS	10.2 (2)	—	—	—	1.9 (5)	1.7 (5)	—	—	96 (5)	60	—	—	3.1 (2)	1.4 (5)	—	—
100 NS	14.4 (5)	—	—	—	3.6 (5)	3.2 (5)	—	—	96 (5)	60	—	—	1.9 (5)	1.9 (5)	—	—
200 NS	39.8 (3)	—	—	—	7.1 (4)	7.0 (4)	—	—	90 (4)	120	—	—	2.0 (3)	2.4 (4)	—	—
12.5 CDI	—	—	—	—	—	—	3.5 (3)	—	—	—	53 (3)	—	—	—	—	—
25 CDI	—	—	15.1 (5)	—	—	—	5.3 (5)	—	—	—	96 (5)	—	—	—	2.3 (5)	—
50 CDI	—	—	11.4 (2)	—	—	—	7.3 (3)	—	—	—	84 (3)	—	—	—	2.3 (2)	—
100 CDI	—	—	25.9 (4)	—	—	—	9.2 (4)	—	—	—	53 (4)	—	—	—	1.8 (4)	—
200 CDI	27.1 (5)	—	129 (5)	148 (7)	7.8 (6)	7 (7)	34 (4)	33 (7)	70 (6)	60	54 (5)	48 (7)	2.5 (5)	2.1 (7)	2.6 (5)	3 (7)
400 CDI	—	—	162 (4)	246 (7)	—	—	56 (4)	104 (7)	—	—	50 (4)	49 (7)	—	—	1.9 (4)	2.5 (7)

Figure 2: DDAVP Tablets

Mean (±SEM) Urine Flow Rate (Solid Lines) and Urinary Osmolality (Dotted Lines) in Four Water-Loaded Children with CDI After 50 and 100 µg Oral Desmopressin Acetate and 10–25 µg Intranasal Desmopressin Acetate

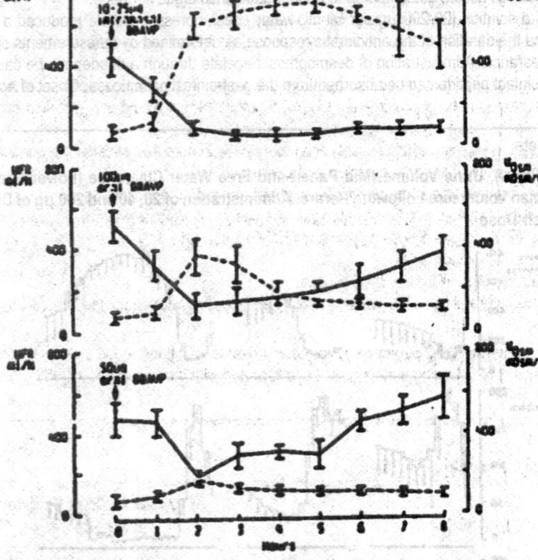

Figure 3: DDAVP Tablets

Relationship Between Intranasal and Oral Dosing Were Seen with Any of the Desmopressin Doses Administered

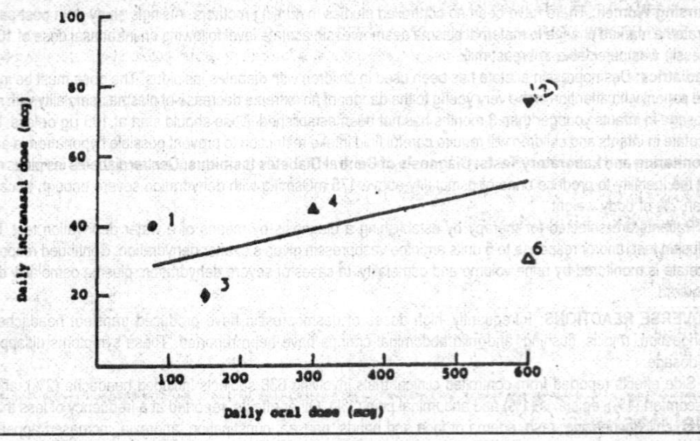

A graded renal response to desmopressin acetate seems to take place between plasma concentrations of 1 to 5 ng/L with maximal effect of desmopressin acetate on the water permeability of the collecting ducts being reached at plasma concentrations of 4-5 ng/L. To obtain an effective plasma concentration, an oral dose of at least 100 µg will be needed in most cases.

Both the intranasal and oral routes of administration exhibited first order kinetics and the plasma half-life was not different after oral or intranasal dosing. The pharmacokinetic data obtained in a recent study in children are presented in Table 2.

Table 2: DDAVP Tablets

Pharmacokinetics of Typical Therapeutic Doses of Oral and Intranasal Desmopressin in CDI Patients

Test	Unit	10 µg IN	20 µg IN	200 µg PO	400 µg PO
AUC (0-infinity)	ng/L/h	135±116	226±187	148±152	246±367
C_{max}	ng/L	41.4±31.6	75.6±70.3	33.2±30.7	103.9±176.4
T_{max}	min	41±23	39±14	48±21	49±19
$t_{½}$	hours	2.52±1.39	4.19±2.84	2.96±2.04	2.47±2.92
K_{el}	h^{-1}	0.35±0.16	0.23±0.11	0.34±0.22	0.47±0.27
Max osm	mOsm/kg	756±201	828±198	733±156	809±77
Time to max osm	min	253±111	373±126	315±127	345±77

The distribution of desmopressin has not been fully characterized. It is not known if desmopressin crosses the placenta. The drug may be distributed into milk. The metabolic fate of desmopressin is unknown. Unlike vasopressin, desmopressin apparently is not degraded by aminopeptidases or other peptidases that cleave oxytocin and endogenous vasopressin in the plasma during late pregnancy.

Urinary clearance in 6 hydrated volunteers was calculated to be 0.514 mL/min/kg body weight and the amount of peptide excreted in the urine during the 6-hour observation period constituted 16.4% of the amount absorbed from the intestine over the same period of time. Urinary clearance for desmopressin is thus smaller than that reported for vasopressin.

Comparisons of Routes of Administration: Peroral desmopressin acetate offers an effective alternative to intranasal administration in the treatment of central diabetes insipidus and nocturnal enuresis. In one study, five out of six patients with CDI of varying etiology who were effectively treated with intranasal desmopressin acetate therapy (mean daily dose=37 µg, range: 15-75 µg) were well-controlled with mean daily doses of 345 µg desmopressin acetate PO (range: 75-900 µg). The ratio of PO/IN dose was therefore approximately 10 in this study. As with intranasal application, patient dosage requirements varied and a dose range rather than a standard dose is usually necessary to control diabetes insipidus in a given patient population. However, a significant (p<0.01) correlation between the previous intranasal dose and the effective oral daily dose can generally be established both in adults (see Figure 3) and children (see Figure 4).

Figure 4: DDAVP Tablets

Correlation Between Intranasal and Oral Doses of Desmopressin Acetate in Seven Pediatric Cases. Coefficient of Correlation r=0.79 (p<0.01)

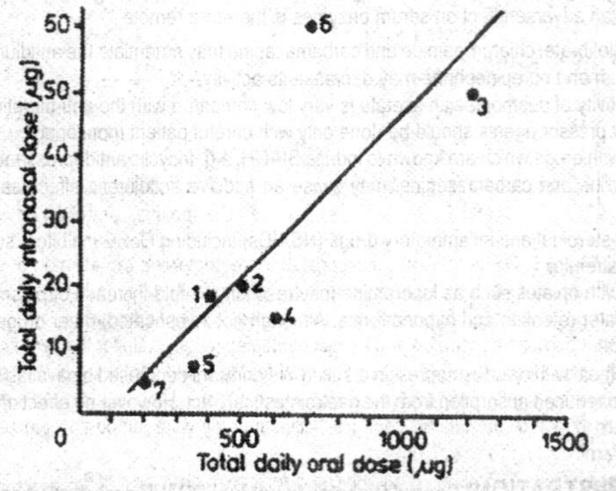

Other long term studies of 6 to 18 months duration have variously reported IN/PO dose ratios as being 1:14, 1:15, 1:20, and 1:40. In CDI patients, the intranasal dose was 25× greater than an equipotent intravenous dose and the peroral dose is approximately 10 to 20× the previous intranasal dose. Thus, the ratio between equipotent doses of IV, IN and PO administered desmopressin acetate seems to be, in general, 1:25:300.

In a recently conducted study, healthy subjects were water loaded to suppress endogenous vasopressin levels. The aim of the study was to investigate the antidiuretic effectiveness of five low doses of desmopressin and placebo. Due to wide inter- and intra-individual variations seen with the oral route, an intravenous infusion study was designed to minimize the variations. The study provided information about the pharmacokinetic and pharmacodynamic (PK/PD) relationship of low doses of desmopressin levels and their duration of antidiuretic action. Combining this new insight into the correlation between plasma desmopressin levels and antidiuretic effects of desmopressin with plasma concentration-time profiles after oral administration of desmopressin, showed that desmopressin is a potent compound with EC_{50} value of 1.6 ng/L. Thus desmopressin can be expected to have a continued effect even at a very low plasma level of 1 ng/L. After oral administration, an effect lasting from 6 to 14 hours can be expected.

Seventy two over-hydrated non smoking male subjects participated in a phase I study investigating the antidiuretic effect and pharmacokinetics of 30, 60, 125, 250 and 500 ng desmopressin and placebo infused intravenously at a constant rate for two hours. A clear positive dose-response slope was seen between duration of antidiuretic action (primary endpoint) and dose of desmopressin (placebo included as zero), independent of the cut-off level (either 200 mOsm/kg or 400 mOsm/kg. No placebo response was seen, and very limited response was seen with 30 ng desmopressin. An increase in duration of antidiuretic action (DOA) with increasing dose of desmopressin was statistically significant for most pairwise comparisons. In the 250 ng and 500 ng desmopressin groups the median duration of anti-diuretic action was 5.36 hours (range: 0.75-10.64 hours) and 8.00 hours (range: 4.45-11.66 hours), respectively, when using 200 mOsm/kg as cut-off, while it was 3.94 hours (range: 0-7.56 hours) and 6.27 hours (range: 4.35-8.28 hours), respectively, when using 400 mOsm/kg as cut-off. The dose-response curve for the DOA did not flatten out within the dose range of 0-500 ng desmopressin for either cut-off (200 or 400 mOsm/kg), i.e. the plateau of the curve was not observed. This indicates that further increase in dosage (>500 ng) may increase duration of antidiuretic action. Linear relationship between DOA and log (dose) among the dose range of 30-500 ng desmopressin was observed independent of cut-off level (either 200mOsm/kg or 400mOsm/kg).

No serious adverse events were seen with any of the desmopressin doses administered.

The analysis of other pharmacodynamic endpoints (maximum osmolality, AUC 0-6 hour for osmolality, AUC 0-6 hour for absolute change from dosing in osmolality) showed a clear positive dose-response relationship. The median maximum osmolality in the placebo group was 80 mOsm/kg (range: 55-183 mOsm/kg), while median maximum osmolality was 830 mOsm/kg (range: 762-1052 mOsm/kg) in the 500 ng desmopressin group.

Twenty-eight non-smoking healthy (n=14 male and n=14 female) subjects took part in a single-centre, open-labelled, randomised, study investigating the antidiuretic effect and pharmacokinetics of a 400 µg dose of desmopressin, taken as two of the currently marketed 200 µg tablets. Blood samples for plasma concentrations of desmopressin were collected according to the following schedule: pre-dose (i.e. 0-30 minutes pre-dosing), 15, 30 min 1, 1.5, 2, 3, 4, 6, 8, 9, 10, 11, 12, 13 and 14 hours after dosing. The concentration of desmopressin in plasma was determined by a validated RIA method. The lower limit of quantification (LLOQ) of the assay was 0.8 ng/L. After administration of DDAVP tablets, the geometric mean t_{max} was observed at 1.0 hour after dosing, the geometric mean value for C_{max} was 20.8 (CV =60%) ng/L, the geometric mean value for AUC_t was 71.8 (CV=57%) (h·ng/L), and the geometric value for AUC was 77.2 (CV=55%) (h·ng/L).

Sixty four percent (64%) of the subjects had plasma desmopressin concentration above 1 ng/L at 12 hours post dose. No safety concerns were observed.

Pediatric Considerations: As was the case with adults, peroral desmopressin acetate proved to be as effective as the intranasal administration of desmopressin acetate and was preferred by the patients. The pharmacodynamic activity is also similar. Doses as small as 12.5 µg have an effect on diuresis and urine osmolality but therapeutic doses start at above 100 µg; 200 µg peroral desmopressin acetate produces antidiuresis varying from 8 to 12.5 h. As with adults, more frequent oral administration (t.i.d. vs. b.i.d.) often resulted in a better clinical response.

Bioavailability: Any cleavage of peptide bonds or reduction of the disulfide bridge of desmopressin leads to biological inactivation. The antidiuretic effect observed after peroral administration indicates that the desmopressin molecule is absorbed into the systemic circulation in intact chemical form.

Transmucosal absorption of the peptide takes place over a considerable period of time. Using a value of 2.2 mL/min/kg body weight for the metabolic clearance of desmopressin obtained during infusion of desmopressin acetate in humans, it was calculated that the bioavailability of desmopressin acetate during the first 6 hours after administration of the drug was 11.3% for the intranasal route as compared to 1.0 and 0.7% for the oral route at doses of 100 and 200 µg respectively. This value is lower than that calculated for children in which the relative bioavailability of the oral route of administration compared to the intranasal route was found to be approximately 5%.

STORAGE AND STABILITY: DDAVP Tablets should be stored between 15-25°C in a dry place.

INFORMATION FOR THE PATIENT: Published in e-CPS, available by subscription at www.e-cps.ca.

DOSAGE FORMS, COMPOSITION AND PACKAGING: 0.1 mg: Each white, uncoated tablet contains: desmopressin acetate 0.1 mg. Nonmedicinal ingredients: lactose monohydrate, magnesium stearate, potato starch and povidone. Bottles of 30 and 100.

0.2 mg: Each white, uncoated tablet contains: desmopressin acetate 0.2 mg. Nonmedicinal ingredients: lactose monohydrate, magnesium stearate, potato starch and povidone. Bottles of 30 and 100.

Dehydrated Alcohol Injection USP

dehydrated ethyl alcohol

Analgesic

Sandoz

SUPPLIED: Each mL of solution 100% v/v contains: dehydrated ethyl alcohol 0.789 g. Vials of 10 mL, boxes of 5. Store between 15 and 30°C. Protect from freezing.

Delatestryl® Ⓒ

testosterone enanthate

Androgen

Theramed

Date of Preparation: June 14, 2007

SUMMARY PRODUCT INFORMATION:

Route of Administration	Dosage Form/ Strength	Clinically Relevant Nonmedicinal Ingredients
Intramuscular Injection	Solution for injection/200 mg/mL	For a complete listing see Dosage Forms, Composition and Packaging.

INDICATIONS AND CLINICAL USE: DELATESTRYL is indicated for testosterone replacement therapy in adult males for conditions associated with a deficiency or absence of endogenous testosterone (hypogonadism).

DELATESTRYL (testosterone enanthate) should not be used to treat non-specific symptoms suggestive of hypogonadism if testosterone deficiency has not been demonstrated and if other etiologies responsible for the symptoms have not been excluded. Testosterone deficiency should be clearly demonstrated by clinical features and confirmed by two separate biochemical assays (morning testosterone) before initiating therapy with any testosterone replacement, including DELATESTRYL treatment.

Geriatrics (>65 years of age): There are limited controlled clinical study data supporting the use of DELATESTRYL in the geriatric population (see Warnings and Precautions).

Pediatrics (<18 years of age): DELATESTRYL is not indicated for use in children <18 years of age since safety and efficacy have not been established in this patient population (see Warnings and Precautions, Special Populations).

CONTRAINDICATIONS:

- DELATESTRYL is not indicated for use in women.
- Androgens are contraindicated in men with known or suspected carcinoma of the prostate or breast.
- DELATESTRYL should not be used in patients with known hypersensitivity to any of its ingredients, including testosterone USP that is chemically synthesized from soy. For a complete listing, see Dosage Forms, Composition and Packaging.

WARNINGS AND PRECAUTIONS: General: There is very limited data from clinical trials with DELATESTRYL in the geriatric male (>65 years of age) to support the efficacy and safety of prolonged use. Impacts to prostate and cardiovascular event rates and patient important outcomes are unknown.

DELATESTRYL should not be used to attempt to improve body composition, bone and muscle mass, increase lean body mass and decrease total fat mass. Efficacy and safety have not been established. Serious long term deleterious health issues may arise.

DELATESTRYL has not been shown to be safe and effective for the enhancement of athletic performance. Because of the potential risk of serious adverse health effects, this drug should not be used for such purpose.

If testosterone deficiency has not been established, testosterone replacement therapy should not be used for the treatment of sexual dysfunction.

Testosterone replacement therapy is not a treatment for male infertility.

Special Populations: Pediatrics (<18 years of age): Androgen therapy should be used cautiously in males with hypogonadism causing delayed puberty. Androgens can accelerate bone maturation without producing compensatory gain in linear growth. This adverse effect may result in compromised adult stature. The younger the child is the greater risk of compromising final mature height. The effect of androgens on bone maturation should be monitored closely by assessing bone age of the wrist and hand on a regular basis.

Geriatrics (>65 years of age): There are very limited controlled clinical study data supporting the use of testosterone in the geriatric population and virtually no controlled clinical studies on subjects 75 years and over.

Geriatric patients treated with androgens may be at an increased risk for the development of prostatic hyperplasia and prostatic carcinoma.

Geriatric patients and other patients with clinical or demographic characteristics that are recognized to be associated with an increased risk of prostate cancer should be evaluated for the presence of prostate cancer prior to initiation of testosterone replacement therapy.

In men receiving testosterone replacement therapy, surveillance for prostate cancer should be consistent with current practices for eugonadal men.

Carcinogenesis: Prostatic: Geriatric patients treated with androgens may be at an increased risk for the development of prostatic hyperplasia and prostatic carcinoma (see Special Populations, Geriatrics (>65 years of age)).

Breast: Patients using long-term androgen therapy may be at an increased risk for the development of breast cancer.

Hepatic: Prolonged use of high doses of orally active 17-alpha-alkyl androgens (e.g., methyltestosterone) has been associated with serious hepatic adverse effects (peliosis hepatis, hepatic neoplasms, cholestatic hepatitis, and jaundice). Peliosis hepatis can be a life-threatening or fatal complication. Long-term therapy with testosterone enanthate, which elevates blood levels for prolonged periods, has produced multiple hepatic adenomas.

Skeletal: Patients with skeletal metastases are at a risk of exacerbating hypercalcemia/hypercalciuria with concomitant androgen therapy.

Cardiovascular: Testosterone may increase blood pressure and should be used with caution in patients with hypertension.

Edema, with or without congestive heart failure, may be a serious complication in patients with pre-existing cardiac, renal or hepatic disease. Diuretic therapy may be required, in addition to discontinuation of the drug.

Dependence/Tolerance: DELATESTRYL contains testosterone, a Schedule G controlled substance, as defined by the Food and Drugs Act.

Endocrine and Metabolism: Androgens have been shown to alter glucose tolerance tests. Diabetics should be followed carefully and the insulin or oral hypoglycemic dosage adjusted accordingly (see Drug Interactions, Drug-Drug Interactions).

Hypercalciuria/hypercalcemia (caused by malignant tumors) may be exacerbated by androgen treatment. Androgens should be used with caution in cancer patients at risk of hypercalcemia (and associated hypercalciuria). Regular monitoring of serum calcium concentrations is recommended in patients at risk of hypercalciuria/hypercalcemia.

Hypercalcemia may occur in immobilized patients. If this occurs, the drug should be discontinued.

Hematologic: Hemoglobin and hematocrit levels should be checked periodically (to detect polycythemia) in patients on long-term androgen therapy (see Monitoring and Laboratory Tests).

Alkylated derivatives of testosterone such as methandrostenolone, have been reported to decrease the anticoagulant requirement of patients receiving oral anticoagulants (e.g. warfarin). Patients receiving oral anticoagulants therapy require close monitoring, especially when androgens are started or stopped (see Drug Interactions, Drug-Drug Interactions).

Respiratory: The treatment of hypogonadal men with testosterone may potentiate sleep apnea, particularly for those with risk factors such as obesity or chronic lung diseases.

Sexual Function/Reproduction: Gynecomastia may frequently develop and occasionally persist in patients being treated for hypogonadism.

Priapism or excessive sexual stimulation may develop.

Oligospermia may occur after prolonged administration or excessive dosage.

Inflammation and pain at the site of intramuscular injection may occur.

Monitoring and Laboratory Tests: The patient should be monitored (including serum testosterone levels) on a regular basis to ensure adequate response to treatment.

Currently there is no consensus about age specific testosterone levels. The normal serum testosterone level for young eugonadal men is generally accepted to be approximately 10.4-34.6 nmol/L (300-1000 ng/dL). It should be taken into account that physiological testosterone levels (mean and range) decrease with increasing age.

The following laboratory tests, performed routinely, are recommended to ensure that adverse experience possibly caused by or related to testosterone replacement therapy is detected and addressed:

- hemoglobin and hematocrit levels should be checked periodically (to detect polycythemia);
- liver function tests; to detect hepatotoxicity associated with the use of 17-alpha-alkylated androgens;
- prostate specific antigen (PSA), Digital Rectal Examination (DRE), especially if the patient presents with progressive difficulty with urination or a change in voiding habits;
- lipid profile, total cholesterol, LDL, HDL, and triglycerides;
- diabetics should be followed carefully and the insulin or oral hypoglycemic dosage adjusted accordingly (see Drug Interactions, Drug-Drug Interactions).

ADVERSE REACTIONS: Adverse Drug Reaction Overview: Adverse reactions to DELATESTRYL are similar in nature to reactions to other androgens. The following events have been reported with the use of DELATESTRYL in clinical practice (see Table 1).

Table 1: DELATESTRYL
Adverse Reactions to DELATESTRYL

MedDRA System Organ Class (SOC)	Adverse Drug Reaction Preferred Term
Blood and the Lymphatic System Disorders	Leucopenia; haemostasis: bleeding in patients on concomitant anticoagulant therapy
General Disorders and Administration Site Conditions	Injection site inflammation
Nervous System Disorders	Insomnia
Psychiatric Disorders	Increased libido, decreased libido, habituation (dependence)
Renal and Urinary Disorders	Bladder irritability
Reproductive System and Breast Disorders	Testicular atrophy, oligospermia, impotence, priapism, gynecomastia, epididymitis
Skin and Subcutaneous Tissue Disorders	Urticaria, rash, vesiculo-bullous rash, acne

Clinical Trial Adverse Drug Reactions: Clinical safety and efficacy of DELATESTRYL (testosterone enanthate injection) is supported by clinical use with Canadian patients since 1956.

Post-Market Adverse Drug Reactions: In addition to those adverse events reported during clinical trials, the following adverse reactions have been identified during post-marketing use of DELATESTRYL and known reactions of testosterone treatment in general. Because these reactions are reported voluntarily from a population of uncertain size, it is not always possible to reliably estimate their frequency or establish a causal relationship to drug exposure. See Table 2.

Table 2: DELATESTRYL
Adverse Drug Reactions from Post-Marketing Experience of DELATESTRYL and Known Adverse Drug Reactions of General Testosterone Treatment

MedDRA System Organ Class (SOC)	Adverse Drug Reaction
Blood and the Lymphatic System Disorders	Polycythemia, erythropoiesis abnormal
Endocrine Disorders	Abnormal accelerated growth (growth accelerated)
Gastrointestinal Disorders	Nausea, vomiting, diarrhea, abdominal pain, gastrointestinal bleeding
General Disorders and Administration Site Conditions	Edema, malaise, fatigue, application site burning, application site induration, application site rash, application site dermatitis, application site blister, application site erythema

(cont'd)

Table 2: DELATESTRYL *(cont'd)*

Adverse Drug Reactions from Post-Marketing Experience of DELATESTRYL and Known Adverse Drug Reactions of General Testosterone Treatment

MedDRA System Organ Class (SOC)	Adverse Drug Reaction
Hepatobiliary Disorders	Hepatic neoplasms, peliosis hepatis
Immune System Disorders	Allergic reaction, hypersensitivity reaction
Investigations	Weight increase, fluctuating testosterone levels, testosterone decreased, abnormal liver function tests (e.g. elevated GGTP), lipid abnormalities
Metabolism and Nutrition Disorders	Increased appetite, electrolyte changes (nitrogen, potassium, phosphorus, sodium), urine calcium decrease, glucose tolerance impaired, elevated cholesterol
Musculoskeletal and Connective Tissue Disorders	Myalgia, arthralgia
Nervous System Disorders	Insomnia, headache, dizziness
Psychiatric Disorders	Personality disorder, confusion, anger, aggression, depression, anxiety, decreased libido, cognitive disturbance
Renal and Urinary Disorders	Dysuria, hematuria, incontinence, bladder irritability
Reproductive System and Breast Disorders	Prostate carcinoma, enlarged prostate (benign), free prostate-specific antigen increased, testicular atrophy, epididymitis, oligospermia, priapism, impotence, precocious puberty, gynecomastia, mastodynia
Respiratory, Thoracic and Mediastinal Disorders	Dyspnea, sleep apnea
Skin and Subcutaneous Tissue Disorders	Pruritus, rash, urticaria, vesiculo-bullous rash, seborrhea, acne, alopecia, male pattern baldness, hirsutism
Vascular Disorders	Hypertension

DRUG INTERACTIONS: Drug-Drug Interactions: Insulin: In diabetic patients, the metabolic effects of androgens may decrease blood glucose and, therefore, insulin requirements.

Propranolol: In a published pharmacokinetic study of an injectable testosterone product, administration of testosterone cypionate led to an increased clearance of propranolol in the majority of men tested. It is unknown if this would apply to DELATESTRYL.

Corticosteroids: The concurrent administration of testosterone with ACTH or corticosteroids may enhance edema formation; thus these drugs should be administered cautiously particularly in patients with cardiac, renal or hepatic disease.

Anticoagulants: Androgens may increase sensitivity to oral anticoagulants. Dosage of the anticoagulant may require reduction in order to maintain satisfactory therapeutic hypoprothrombinemia.

Drug-Food Interactions: Interactions with food have not been established.

Drug-Herb Interactions: It was found that some herbal products (e.g. St. John's wort) which are available as over-the-counter (OTC) products might interfere with steroid metabolism and therefore may decrease plasma testosterone levels.

Drug-Laboratory Test Interactions: Androgens may decrease levels of thyroxine-binding globulin, resulting in decreased total T_4 serum levels and increased resin uptake of T_3 and T_4. Free thyroid hormone levels remain unchanged, and there is no clinical evidence of thyroid dysfunction.

DOSAGE AND ADMINISTRATION: Dosing Considerations: Dosage and duration of therapy with DELATESTRYL (Testosterone Enanthate Injection) will depend on age, diagnosis, patient's response to treatment, and appearance of adverse effects. When properly given, injections of DELATESTRYL are well tolerated.

In general, total doses above 400 mg per month are not required because of the prolonged action of the preparation. Injections more frequently than every two weeks are rarely indicated.

Recommended Dose and Dosage Adjustment: For replacement in hypogonadal male, the usual dose is 100-400 mg every four weeks.

The AACE Hypogonadism Task Force suggested the following regimen of parenteral testosterone preparations in treatment of hypogonadism in adult male patients:

DELATESTRYL (testosterone enanthate) and testosterone cypionate are long-acting testosterone esters suspended in oil to prolong absorption. Peak levels occur about 72 hours after intramuscular injection and are followed by a slow decline during the subsequent 1 to 2 weeks.

For complete androgen replacement, the regimen should be between 50 and 100 mg of testosterone enanthate administered intramuscularly every 7 to 10 days, which will achieve relatively normal levels of testosterone throughout the time interval between injections. Longer time intervals are more convenient but are associated with greater fluctuations in testosterone levels. Higher doses of testosterone produce longer-term effects but also higher peak levels and wider swings between peak and nadir circulating testosterone levels; the result is fluctuating symptoms in many patients.

The use of 100 to 150 mg of testosterone every 2 weeks is a reasonable compromise. Use of 300 mg injections every 3 weeks is associated with wider fluctuations of testosterone levels and is generally inadequate to ensure a consistent clinical response. With use of these longer-interval regimens, many men will have pronounced symptoms during the week preceding the next injection. In such instances, a smaller dose at closer intervals should be tried.

As a guide, testosterone levels should be above the lower limit of normal, in the range of 250 to 300 ng/dL, just before the next injection. Excessive peak levels and side effects should also be monitored and used to adjust the dosing regimens.

When full androgen replacement is not required, patients should receive lower doses of testosterone. One such category includes adult male patients with prepubertal onset of hypogonadism who are going through puberty for the first time during therapy and who often may require psychologic counseling, especially when a spouse is involved as well. In these patients, testosterone therapy should be initiated at 50 mg every 3 to 4 weeks and then gradually increased during subsequent months, as tolerated, up to full replacement within 1 year. Men with appreciable benign prostatic hypertrophy who have hypogonadism and symptoms may be given 50 to 100 mg of testosterone every 2 weeks as an initial regimen and maintained on this dosage with careful monitoring of urinary symptoms and prostate examinations; therapy can be withdrawn if necessary.

Attaining full virilization in the patient with hypogonadism may take as long as 3 to 4 years. Follow-up intervals should be between 4 and 6 months to monitor progress, review compliance, and determine whether any complications or psychologic adjustment problems are present.

Administration: Care should be taken to inject the preparation deeply into the gluteal muscle following the usual precautions for intramuscular administration.

Note: Use of a wet needle or wet syringe may cause the solution to become cloudy; however this does not affect the potency of the material.

Missed Dose: A missed dose should be administered as soon as possible. However, if it is almost time for the next regularly scheduled dose, then the missed dose should be skipped and next one should be taken as directed.

OVERDOSAGE:

Symptoms of a testosterone overdose are not known. No specific antidote is available. Symptomatic and supportive treatment should be given.

For management of a suspected drug overdose, CPhA recommends that you contact your **regional Poison Control Centre**. See the *CPS* Directory section for a list of Poison Control Centres.

ACTION AND CLINICAL PHARMACOLOGY: Pharmacodynamics: Testosterone and Hypogonadism: Testosterone and dihydrotestosterone (DHT), endogenous androgens, are responsible for normal growth and development of male sex organs and for maintenance of secondary sex characteristics. These effects include the growth and maturation of the prostate, seminal vesicles, penis, and scrotum; the development of male hair distribution, such as facial, pubic, chest, and axillary hair; laryngeal enlargement; vocal cord thickening; alterations in body musculature; and fat distribution.

Male hypogonadism results from insufficient secretion of testosterone and is characterized by low serum testosterone concentrations. Symptoms associated with male hypogonadism include decreased sexual desire with or without impotence, fatigue and loss of energy, mood depression, regression of secondary sexual characteristics, and osteoporosis. Hypogonadism is a risk factor for osteoporosis in men.

General Androgen Effects: Drugs in the androgen class also promote retention of nitrogen, sodium, potassium, phosphorus, and decreased urinary excretion of calcium.

Androgens have been reported to increase protein anabolism and decrease protein catabolism. Nitrogen balance is improved only when there is sufficient intake of calories and protein. Androgens have been reported to stimulate the production of red blood cells by enhancing erythropoietin production.

Androgens are responsible for the growth spurt of adolescence and for the eventual termination of linear growth brought about by fusion of the epiphyseal growth centers. In children, exogenous androgens accelerate linear growth rates but may cause a disproportionate advancement in bone maturation. Use over long periods may result in fusion of the epiphyseal growth centers and termination of the growth process.

During exogenous administration of androgens, endogenous testosterone release may be inhibited through feedback inhibition of pituitary luteinizing hormone (LH). At large doses of exogenous androgens, spermatogenesis may also be suppressed through feedback inhibition of pituitary follicle-stimulating hormone (FSH).

Pharmacokinetics: DELATESTRYL is a sterile, long acting preparation of an esterified derivative of the naturally occurring androgenic hormone, testosterone. Testosterone esters are less polar than free testosterone. Testosterone esters in oil injected intramuscularly are absorbed slowly from the lipid phase; thus testosterone enanthate can be given at intervals of two to four weeks.

Absorption: One study was performed to provide comparison of the serum testosterone levels achieved by injection of testosterone enanthate or testosterone cypionate in equivalent doses. Testosterone enanthate (194 mg) and testosterone cypionate (200 mg) were injected so that the amount of unesterified testosterone was the same in both preparations (140 mg). The serum testosterone levels were identical after both preparations. The concentrations increased sharply, reaching maximal levels three times above basal on days one and two after injection, and decreased gradually thereafter, so that basal levels were reached on day ten. In an earlier study, the same authors were investigating serum testosterone and LH concentrations in normal and hypogonadal men after injection of 250 mg of testosterone enanthate. Increasing the dose of injected testosterone enanthate from 194 mg to 250 mg did not influence the maximal concentration but rather the duration of the effect.

Distribution: Circulating testosterone is chiefly bound in the serum to sex hormone-binding globulin (SHBG) and albumin. The albumin-bound fraction of testosterone easily dissociates from albumin and is presumed to be bioactive. The portion of testosterone bound to SHBG is not considered biologically active. Approximately 40% of testosterone in plasma is bound to SHBG, 2% remains unbound (free) and the rest is bound to albumin and other proteins. The amount of SHBG in the serum and the total testosterone level will determine the distribution of bioactive and nonbioactive androgen.

Metabolism: There is considerable variation in the half-life of testosterone as reported in the literature, ranging from ten to 100 minutes.

Testosterone is metabolized to various 17-keto steroids through two different pathways. The major active metabolites of testosterone are estradiol and dihydrotestosterone (DHT). Testosterone is metabolized to DHT by steroid 5α reductase located in the skin, liver, and urogenital tract of the male. Estradiol is formed by an aromatase enzyme complex in the brain, fat, and testes. DHT binds with greater affinity to SHBG than does testosterone. In many tissues, the activity of testosterone depends on its reduction to DHT, which binds to cytosol receptor proteins. The steroid-receptor complex is transported to the nucleus where it initiates transcription and cellular changes related to androgen action. In reproductive tissues, DHT is further metabolized to 3-α and 3-β androstanediol.

Excretion: About 90% of a dose of testosterone given intramuscularly is excreted in the urine as glucuronic and sulfuric acid conjugates of testosterone and its metabolites; about 6% of dose is excreted in the feces, mostly in the unconjugated form. Inactivation of testosterone occurs primarily in the liver.

STORAGE AND STABILITY: Store at controlled room temperature between 15 and 30°C.

INFORMATION FOR THE PATIENT: Published in e-CPS, available by subscription at www.e-cps.ca.

DOSAGE FORMS, COMPOSITION AND PACKAGING: Each mL of sterile solution contains: testosterone enanthate 200 mg formulated in sesame oil with 0.5% chlorobutanol as preservative. Glass vials of 5 mL, sealed with latex free stoppers.

Demerol® Tablets Ⓝ

pethidine HCl

Analgesic

sanofi-aventis

SUPPLIED: Each white tablet with stylized W on one side, scored on the other with D above and 35 below, contains: meperidine HCl 50 mg. Nonmedicinal ingredients: calcium phosphate (dibasic, dihydrate), calcium sulfate, (dihydrate), cornstarch, stearic acid and talc. Energy: 0.2 kJ (0.06 kcal). Gluten-, lactose-, sucrose- and tartrazine-free. Bottles of 100 and 1000.

(Shown in Product Identification Section)

Demulen® 30 🅁

ethynodiol diacetate—ethinyl estradiol

Oral Contraceptive

Pfizer

PHARMACOLOGY: Estrogen-progestogen combinations act primarily through the mechanism of gonadotropin suppression due to the estrogenic and progestational activity of their components. Although the primary mechanism of action is inhibition of ovulation, alterations in the cervical mucus and the endometrium may also contribute to effectiveness.

INDICATIONS: Prevention of pregnancy.

CONTRAINDICATIONS: History of or actual thrombophlebitis or thromboembolic disorders; history of or actual cerebrovascular disorders; history of or actual myocardial infarction or coronary arterial disease; active liver disease or history of or actual benign or malignant liver tumors; history of or known or suspected carcinoma of the breast; history of or known or suspected estrogen-dependent neoplasia; undiagnosed abnormal vaginal bleeding; any ocular lesion arising from ophthalmic vascular disease, such as partial or complete loss of vision or defect in visual fields; when pregnancy is suspected or diagnosed.

WARNINGS: Predisposing Factors for Coronary Artery Disease: Cigarette smoking increases the risk of serious cardiovascular side effects and mortality. Birth control pills increase this risk, especially with increasing age. Convincing data are available to support an upper age limit of 35 years for oral contraceptive use by women who smoke.

Other women who are independently at high risk for cardiovascular disease include those with diabetes, hypertension, abnormal lipid profile, or a family history of these. Whether oral contraceptives accentuate this risk is unclear.

In low risk, non-smoking women of any age, the benefits of oral contraceptive use outweigh the possible cardiovascular risks associated with low dose formulations. Consequently, oral contraceptives may be prescribed for these women up to the age of menopause.

Cigarette smoking increases the risk of serious adverse effects on the heart and blood vessels. This risk increases with age and becomes significant in oral contraceptive users over 35 years of age. Women should be counselled not to smoke.

Discontinue medication at the earliest manifestation of the following:

A. Thromboembolic and cardiovascular disorders such as: thrombophlebitis, pulmonary embolism, cerebrovascular disorders, myocardial ischemia, mesenteric thrombosis, and retinal thrombosis.

B. Conditions that predispose to venous stasis and to vascular thrombosis, e.g., immobilization after accidents or confinement to bed during long-term illness. Other non-hormonal methods of contraception should be used until regular activities are resumed. For use of oral contraceptives when surgery is contemplated, see Precautions.
C. Visual defects, partial or complete.
D. Papilledema or ophthalmic vascular lesions.
E. Severe headache of unknown etiology or worsening of pre-existing migraine headache.

PRECAUTIONS: Physical Examination and Follow-up: Before oral contraceptives are used, a thorough history and physical examination should be performed, including a blood pressure determination. Breasts, liver, extremities and pelvic organs should be examined and a Papanicolaou smear should be taken if the patient has been sexually active.

The first follow-up visit should be done 3 months after oral contraceptives are prescribed. Thereafter, examinations should be performed at least once a year or more frequently if indicated. At each annual visit, examination should include those procedures that were done at the initial visit as outlined above or per recommendations of the Canadian Workshop on Screening for Cancer of the Cervix. Their suggestion was that, for women who had 2 consecutive negative Pap smears, screening could be continued every 3 years up to the age of 69.

Pregnancy: Fetal abnormalities have been reported to occur in the offspring of women who have taken estrogen-progestogen combinations in early pregnancy. Rule out pregnancy as soon as it is suspected.

Lactation: The use of oral contraceptives during the period a mother is breast-feeding her infant may not be advisable. The hormonal components are excreted in breast milk and may reduce its quantity and quality. The long-term effects on the developing child are not known.

Hepatic Function: Patients who have had jaundice including a history of cholestatic jaundice during pregnancy should be given oral contraceptives with great care and under close observation.

The development of severe generalized pruritus or icterus requires that the medication be withdrawn until the problem is resolved.

If a patient develops jaundice that proves to be cholestatic in type, the use of oral contraceptives should not be resumed. In patients taking oral contraceptives, changes in the composition of the bile may occur and an increased incidence of gallstones has been reported.

Hepatic nodules have been reported to be associated with use of oral contraceptives, particularly in long-term users of oral contraceptives. These nodules include benign hepatic adenomas, focal nodular hyperplasia and other hepatic lesions. In addition, hepatocellular carcinoma has been reported. Although these lesions are extremely rare, they have caused fatal intra-abdominal hemorrhage and should be considered in women presenting with an abdominal mass, acute abdominal pain, or evidence of intra-abdominal bleeding.

Hypertension: Patients with essential hypertension whose blood pressure is well-controlled may be given oral contraceptives but only under close supervision. If a significant elevation of blood pressure in previously normotensive or hypertensive subjects occurs at any time during the administration of the drug, cessation of medication is necessary.

Migraine and Headache: The onset or exacerbation of migraine or the development of headache of a new pattern which is recurrent, persistent or severe, requires discontinuation of oral contraceptives and evaluation of the cause.

Diabetes: Current low-dose oral contraceptives exert minimal impact on glucose metabolism. Diabetic patients, or those with a family history of diabetes, should be observed closely to detect any worsening of carbohydrate metabolism. Patients predisposed to diabetes who can be kept under close supervision may be given oral contraceptives. Young diabetic patients whose disease is of recent origin, well-controlled, and not associated with hypertension or other signs of vascular disease such as ocular fundal changes, should be monitored more frequently while using oral contraceptives.

Ocular Disease: Patients who are pregnant or are taking oral contraceptives, may experience corneal edema that may cause visual disturbances and changes in tolerance to contact lenses, especially of the rigid type. Soft contact lenses usually do not cause disturbances. If visual changes or alterations in tolerance to contact lenses occur, temporary or permanent cessation of wear may be advised.

Breasts: Increasing age and a strong family history are the most significant risk factors for the development of breast cancer. Other established risk factors include obesity, nulliparity and late age at first full-term pregnancy. The identified groups of women that may be at increased risk of developing breast cancer before menopause are long-term users of oral contraceptives (more than 8 years) and starters at early age. In a few women, the use of oral contraceptives may accelerate the growth of an existing but undiagnosed breast cancer. Since any potential increased risk related to oral contraceptive use is small, there is no reason to change prescribing habits at present.

Women receiving oral contraceptives should be instructed in self-examination of their breasts. Their physicians should be notified whenever any masses are detected. A yearly clinical breast examination is also recommended because, if a breast cancer should develop, drugs that contain estrogen may cause a rapid progression.

Vaginal Bleeding: Persistent irregular vaginal bleeding requires assessment to exclude underlying pathology.

Fibroids: Patients with fibroids (leiomyomata) should be carefully observed. Sudden enlargement, pain, or tenderness requires discontinuation of the use of oral contraceptives.

Emotional Disorders: Patients with a history of emotional disturbances, especially the depressive type, may be more prone to have a recurrence of depression while taking oral contraceptives. In cases of a serious recurrence, a trial of an alternate method of contraception should be made which may help to clarify the possible relationship. Women with premenstrual syndrome (PMS) may have a varied response to oral contraceptives, ranging from symptomatic improvement to worsening of the condition.

Metabolic and Endocrine Diseases: In metabolic or endocrine diseases and when metabolism of calcium and phosphorus is abnormal, careful clinical evaluation should precede medication and a regular follow-up is recommended.

Connective Tissue Disease: The use of oral contraceptives in some women has been associated with positive lupus erythematosus cell tests and with clinical lupus erythematosus. In some instances exacerbation of rheumatoid arthritis and synovitis have been observed.

Laboratory Tests: Results of laboratory tests should be interpreted in light of the fact that the patient is on oral contraceptives. The laboratory tests listed below are modified.
A. Liver function tests: Aspartate serum transaminase (AST): variously reported elevations. Alkaline phosphatase and gamma glutamine transaminase (GGT): slightly elevated.
B. Coagulation tests: Minimal elevation of test values reported for such parameters as Factors VII, VIII, IX and X. Increased platelet aggregation, decreased antithrombin III.
C. Thyroid function tests: Protein binding of thyroxine is increased as indicated by increased total serum thyroxine concentrations and decreased T_3 resin uptake.
D. Lipoproteins: Small changes of unproven clinical significance may occur in lipoprotein cholesterol fractions.
E. Gonadotropins: LH and FSH levels are suppressed by the use of oral contraceptives. Wait 2 weeks after discontinuing the use of oral contraceptives before measurements are made.

Tissue Specimens: Pathologists should be advised of oral contraceptive therapy when specimens obtained from surgical procedures and Pap smears are submitted for examination.

Return to Fertility: After discontinuing oral contraceptive therapy, the patient should delay pregnancy until at least one normal spontaneous cycle has occurred in order to date the pregnancy. An alternate contraceptive method should be used during this time.

Amenorrhea: Women having a history of oligomenorrhea, secondary amenorrhea, or irregular cycles may remain anovulatory or become amenorrheic following discontinuation of estrogen-progestin combination therapy.

Amenorrhea, especially if associated with breast secretion, that continues for 6 months or more after withdrawal, warrants a careful assessment of hypothalamic-pituitary function.

Thromboembolic Complications—Post-surgery: There is an increased risk of post-surgery thromboembolic complications in oral contraceptive users, after major surgery. If feasible, oral contraceptives should be discontinued and an alternative method substituted at least 1 month prior to **major** elective surgery. Oral contraceptives should not be resumed until the first menstrual period after hospital discharge following surgery.

Drug Interactions: The concurrent administration of oral contraceptives with other drugs may result in an altered response to either agent. Reduced effectiveness of the oral contraceptive, should it occur, is more likely with the low dose formulations. It is important to ascertain all drugs that a patient is taking, both prescription and nonprescription, before oral contraceptives are prescribed.

Refer to the revised 1994 Report on Oral Contraceptives, Health Canada, for possible drug interactions with oral contraceptives.

Noncontraceptive Benefits of Oral Contraceptives: Several health advantages other than contraception have been reported.

Effects on Menses: Increased menstrual cycle regularity; decreased menstrual blood loss; decreased incidence of iron deficiency anemia secondary to reduced menstrual blood loss; decreased incidence of dysmenorrhea.

Effects Related to Ovulation Inhibition: Decreased incidence of functional ovarian cysts; decreased incidence of ectopic pregnancy.

Effects on Other Organs of the Reproductive Tract: Decreased incidence of acute salpingitis; decreased incidence of endometrial cancer (50%); decreased incidence of ovarian cancer (40%); potential beneficial effects on endometriosis; improvement of acne vulgaris, hirsutism, and other androgen-mediated disorders.

Effects on Breasts: Decreased incidence of benign breast disease (fibroadenomas and fibrocystic breast disease); decreased incidence of breast biopsies.

The non-contraceptive benefits of oral contraceptives should be considered in addition to the efficacy of these preparations when counselling patients regarding contraceptive method selection.

> Oral contraceptives **do not protect** against sexually transmitted diseases including HIV/AIDS. For protection against STDs, it is advisable to use latex condoms **in combination with** oral contraceptives.

ADVERSE EFFECTS: An increased risk of the following serious adverse reactions has been associated with the use of oral contraceptives: thrombophlebitis; pulmonary embolism; mesenteric thrombosis; neuro-ocular lesions (e.g., retinal thrombosis); myocardial infarction; cerebral thrombosis; cerebral hemorrhage; hypertension; benign hepatic tumors; gallbladder disease.

The following adverse reactions also have been reported in patients receiving oral contraceptives: nausea and vomiting, usually the most common adverse reaction, occurs in approximately 10% or less of patients during the first cycle. Other reactions, as a general rule, are seen less frequently or only occasionally.

Other adverse reactions: gastrointestinal symptoms (such as abdominal cramps and bloating); breakthrough bleeding; spotting; change in menstrual flow; dysmenorrhea; amenorrhea during and after treatment; infertility after discontinuance of treatment; edema; chloasma or melasma which may persist; breast changes: tenderness, enlargement, and secretion; change in weight (increase or decrease); endocervical hyperplasias; possible diminution in lactation when given immediately post-partum; cholestatic jaundice; migraine; increase in size of uterine leiomyomata; rash (allergic); mental depression; reduced tolerance to carbohydrates; vaginal candidiasis; premenstrual-like syndrome; intolerance to contact lenses; change in corneal curvature (steepening); cataracts; optic neuritis; retinal thrombosis; changes in libido; chorea; changes in appetite; cystitis-like syndrome; rhinitis; headache; nervousness; dizziness; hirsutism; loss of scalp hair; erythema multiforme; erythema nodosum; hemorrhagic eruption; vaginitis; porphyria; impaired renal function; Raynaud's phenomenon; auditory disturbances; hemolytic uremic syndrome; pancreatitis; arterial thromboembolism.

OVERDOSE:

Symptoms: Numerous cases of the ingestion, by children, of estrogen-progestogen combinations have been reported. Although mild nausea may occur, there appears to be no other reaction.

Treatment: Treatment should be limited to a laxative such as citrate of magnesia with the aim of removing unabsorbed material as rapidly as possible.

> For management of a suspected drug overdose, CPhA recommends that you contact your **regional Poison Control Centre**. See the *CPS* Directory section for a list of Poison Control Centres.

DOSAGE: Information for the Patient on How to Take the Birth Control Pill:

1. **Read these directions:**
   - before you start taking your pills, and
   - any time you are not sure what to do.
2. **Look at your pill pack** to see if it has 21 or 28 pills:
   - 21-Pill Pack: 21 active pills (with hormones) taken daily for 3 weeks, and then no pills taken for 1 week

   or
   - 28-Pill Pack: 21 active pills (with hormones) taken daily for 3 weeks, and then 7 "reminder" pills (no hormones) taken daily for 1 week.

   Also check the pill pack for instructions on (1) where to start and (2) directions to take pills (see package insert for illustrations).
3. It is recommended that you use a second method of birth control (e.g., latex condoms and spermicidal foam or gel) for the first 7 days of the first cycle of pill use. This will provide a backup in case pills are forgotten while you are getting used to taking them.
4. **When receiving any medical treatment, be sure to tell your doctor that you are using birth control pills.**
5. **Many women have spotting or light bleeding, or may feel sick to their stomach during the first 3 months on the pill.** If you do feel sick, do not stop taking the pill. The problem will usually go away. If it does not go away, check with your doctor or clinic.
6. **Missing pills also can cause some spotting or light bleeding**, even if you make up the missed pills. You also could feel a little sick to your stomach on the days you take 2 pills to make up for missed pills.
7. **If you miss pills at any time, you could get pregnant. The greatest risks for pregnancy are:**
   - when you start a pack late, or
   - when you miss pills at the beginning or at the very end of the pack.
8. **Always be sure you have ready:**
   - **another kind of birth control** (such as latex condoms and spermicidal foam or gel) to use as a backup in case you miss pills, and
   - an extra, full pack of pills.
9. **If you experience vomiting or diarrhea, or if you take certain medicines**, such as antibiotics, your pills may not work as well. Use a backup method, such as latex condoms and spermicidal foam or gel, until you can check with your doctor or clinic.
10. **If you forget more than 1 pill 2 months in a row**, talk to your doctor or clinic about how to make pill-taking easier or about using another method of birth control.
11. **If your questions are not answered here, call your doctor or clinic.**

When to start the first pack of pills: Be sure to read these instructions:
- before you start taking your pills, and
- any time you are not sure what to do.

Decide with your doctor or clinic what is the best day for you to start taking your first pack of pills. Your pills may be either a 21-day or a 28-day type.

A. 21-Day Combination: With this type of birth control pill, you are on pills for 21 days and off pills for 7 days. You must not be off the pills for more than 7 days in a row.
1. **The first day of your menstrual period (bleeding) is Day 1 of your cycle.** Your doctor may advise you to start taking the pills on Day 1, on Day 5, or on the first Sunday after your period begins. If your period starts on Sunday, start that same day.
2. Take 1 pill at approximately the same time every day for 21 days; **then take no pills for 7 days**. Start a new pack on the 8th day. You will probably have a period during the 7 days off the pill. (This bleeding may be lighter and shorter than your usual period.)

B. 28-Day Combination: With this type of birth control pill, you take 21 pills which contain hormones and 7 pills which contain no hormones.
1. **The first day of your menstrual period (bleeding) is Day 1 of your cycle.** Your doctor may advise you to start taking the pills on Day 1, on Day 5, or on the first Sunday after your period begins. If your period starts on Sunday, start that same day.
2. Take 1 pill at approximately the same time every day for 28 days. Begin a new pack the next day, **not missing any days on the pills**. Your period should occur during the last 7 days of using that pill pack.

What to do during the month:
1. **Take a pill at approximately the same time every day until the pack is empty.**
   - Try to associate taking your pill with some regular activity like eating a meal or going to bed.
   - Do not skip pills even if you have bleeding between monthly periods or feel sick to your stomach (nausea).
   - Do not skip pills even if you do not have sex very often.
2. **When you finish a pack:**
   - **21 pills: Wait 7 days** to start the next pack. You will have your period during that week.
   - **28 pills:** Start the next pack **on the next day**. Take 1 pill every day. Do not wait any days between packs.

What to do if you miss pills: Table 1 outlines the actions you should take if you miss 1 or more of your birth control pills. Match the number of pills missed with the appropriate starting time for your type of pill pack.

Table 1: Demulen 30
What to Do if Pills are Missed

Sunday Start	Other than Sunday Start
Miss 1 pill	**Miss 1 pill**
Take it as soon as you remember, and take the next pill at the usual time. This means that you might take 2 pills in 1 day.	Take it as soon as you remember, and take the next pill at the usual time. This means that you might take 2 pills in 1 day.
Miss 2 pills in a row	**Miss 2 pills in a row**
First 2 weeks: 1. Take 2 pills the day you remember and 2 pills the next day. 2. Then take 1 pill a day until you finish the pack. 3. Use a backup method of birth control if you have sex in the 7 days after you miss the pills. **Third week:** 1. Keep taking 1 pill a day until Sunday. 2. On Sunday, safely discard the rest of the pack and start a new pack that day. 3. Use a backup method of birth control if you have sex in the 7 days after you miss the pills. 4. You may not have a period this month. **If you miss 2 periods in a row, call your doctor or clinic.**	**First 2 weeks:** 1. Take 2 pills the day you remember and 2 pills the next day. 2. Then take 1 pill a day until you finish the pack. 3. Use a backup method of birth control if you have sex in the 7 days after you miss the pills. **Third week:** 1. Safely dispose of the rest of the pill pack and start a new pack that same day. 2. Use a back-up method of birth control if you have sex in the 7 days after you miss the pills. 3. You may not have a period this month. **If you miss 2 periods in a row, call your doctor or clinic.**
Miss 3 or more pills in a row	**Miss 3 or more pills in a row**
Anytime in the cycle: 1. Keep taking 1 pill a day until Sunday. 2. On Sunday, safely discard the rest of the pack and start a new pack that day. 3. Use a backup method of birth control if you have sex in the 7 days after you miss the pills. 4. You may not have a period this month. **If you miss 2 periods in a row, call your doctor or clinic.**	**Anytime in the cycle:** 1. Safely dispose of the rest of the pill pack and start a new pack that same day. 2. Use a backup method of birth control if you have sex in the 7 days after you miss the pills. 3. You may not have a period this month. **If you miss 2 periods in a row, call your doctor or clinic.**

Note: 28-Day Pack: If you forget any of the 7 "reminder" pills (without hormones) in Week 4, just safely dispose of the pills you missed. Then keep taking 1 pill each day until the pack is empty. You do not need to use a backup method.

Always be sure you have on hand:

- a backup method of birth control (such as latex condoms and spermicidal foam or gel) in case you miss pills, and
- an extra, full pack of pills.

If **you forget more than 1 pill 2 months in a row, talk to your doctor or clinic** about ways to make pill-taking easier or about using another method of birth control.

Dosage: A. **21-Day Pack:** With this type of birth control pill, the patient is 21 days on pills with 7 days off pills. The patient must not be off the pills for more than 7 days in a row.

1. **The first day of the patient's menstrual period (bleeding) is day 1 of a cycle.** The doctor may advise the patient to start taking the pills on Day 1, on Day 5, or on the first Sunday after a period begins. If a period starts on Sunday, the patient starts that same day.
2. The pack must be labelled correctly before starting. The pack is pre-printed with a Sunday starting day. If the patient is starting on a day other than a Sunday, she should use the Flexi-start sticker labels provided. The patient peels off the label with the chosen starting day and applies it over the pre-printed days on top of the card.
3. The patient takes 1 pill at approximately the same time every day for 21 days; **then she takes no pills for 7 days**. She starts a new pack on the 8th day. She will probably have a period during the 7 days off the pill. (This bleeding may be lighter and shorter than a usual period.)

B. **28-Day Pack:** With this type of birth control pill, the patient takes 21 pills which contain hormones and 7 pills which contain no hormones.

1. **The first day of the patient's menstrual period (bleeding) is day 1 of a cycle.** The doctor may advise the patient to start taking the pills on Day 1, on Day 5, or on the first Sunday after a period begins. If a period starts on Sunday, the patient starts that same day.
2. The pack must be labelled correctly before starting. The pack is pre-printed with a Sunday starting day. If the patient is starting on a day other than a Sunday, she should use the Flexi-start sticker labels provided. The patient peels off the label with the chosen starting day and applies it over the pre-printed days on top of the card.
3. The patient takes 1 pill at approximately the same time every day for 28 days. She begins a new pack the next day, **not missing any days on the pills.** The patient's period should occur during the last 7 days of using that pill pack.

What to do during the month:

1. **The patient takes a pill at approximately the same time every day until the pack is empty.**
   - The patient should try to associate taking the pill with some regular activity like eating a meal or going to bed.
   - The patient must not skip pills even if she has bleeding between monthly periods or feels sick to her stomach (nausea).
   - The patient must not skip pills even if she does not have sex very often.
2. **When a pack is finished:**
   - **21 Pills: The patient must wait 7 days** to start the next pack. A period will begin during that week.
   - **28 Pills:** The patient starts the next pack **on the next day**. She takes 1 pill every day. She does not wait any days between packs.

INFORMATION FOR THE PATIENT: Published in e-CPS, available by subscription at www.e-cps.ca.

SUPPLIED: Each white, circular, biconvex, film-coated tablet, 6 mm in diameter, impressed SEARLE 930 on one side, contains: ethynodiol diacetate 2 mg and ethinyl estradiol 0.03 mg. Inert peach-colored tablets are impressed "SEARLE" on one side and "P" on the other. Nonmedicinal ingredients: Active tablets: cornstarch, ethylcellulose, hydroxypropylcellulose, lactose, magnesium stearate, polyvidone, sodium acid phosphate, sodium phosphate dibasic anhydrous and titanium dioxide. Placebo tablets: FD&C Yellow No. 6 Lake, lactose, lactose monohydrate, magnesium stearate and microcrystalline cellulose. Dispensers of 21 (21 active tablets) and 28 (21 active and 7 inert tablets) days. Store below 25°C.

(Shown in Product Identification Section)

Depakene® Ⓟ
valproic acid
Anticonvulsant
Abbott

SUPPLIED: Capsules: Each orange-colored, soft gelatin capsule contains: valproic acid 250 mg. Nonmedicinal ingredients: corn oil, ethyl vanillin, FD&C yellow no. 6, gelatin, glycerin, methylparaben, propylparaben and titanium dioxide. Alcohol-, gluten-, lactose-, sucrose-, sulfite- and tartrazine-free. Bottles of 100.

Syrup: Each 5 mL of red syrup contains: the equivalent of 250 mg valproic acid, as the sodium salt. Nonmedicinal ingredients: artificial flavor, FD&C red no. 40, glycerin, hydrochloric acid, methylparaben, propylparaben, sodium hydroxide, sorbitol, sucrose and vanillin. Energy: 74.8 kJ (17.9 kcal/5 mL). Alcohol-, gluten-, lactose-, sulfite- and tartrazine-free. Bottles of 480 mL.

Store between 15 and 25°C.

(Shown in Product Identification Section)

Depo-Medrol® Ⓟ
methylprednisolone acetate
Glucocorticoid
Pfizer

PHARMACOLOGY: Depo-Medrol is a sterile aqueous suspension of the **synthetic** glucocorticoid methylprednisolone acetate. It has a strong and prolonged anti-inflammatory, immunosuppressive and anti-allergic activity. Depo-Medrol can be administered i.m. for a prolonged systemic activity, as well as in situ for a local treatment. The prolonged activity of Depo-Medrol is explained by the slow release of the active substance.

INDICATIONS: I.M.: When oral therapy is not feasible and the strength, dosage form, and route of administration of the drug reasonably lend the preparation to the treatment of the condition, the i.m. use of methylprednisolone is indicated as follows:

Endocrine Disorders: Primary or secondary adrenocortical insufficiency (hydrocortisone or cortisone is the drug of choice, synthetic analogs may be used in conjunction with mineralocorticoids where applicable; in infancy, mineralocorticoid supplementation is of particular importance). Acute adrenocortical insufficiency (hydrocortisone or cortisone is the drug of choice; mineralocorticoid supplementation may be necessary, particularly when synthetic analogs are used). Congenital adrenal hyperplasia, hypercalcemia associated with cancer, nonsuppurative thyroiditis.

Rheumatic Disorders: As adjunctive therapy for short-term administration (to tide the patient over an acute episode or exacerbation) in: post-traumatic osteoarthritis, synovitis of osteoarthritis, rheumatoid arthritis, including juvenile rheumatoid arthritis (selected cases may require low dose maintenance therapy), acute and subacute bursitis, epicondylitis, acute nonspecific tenosynovitis, acute gouty arthritis, psoriatic arthritis, ankylosing spondylitis.

Collagen Diseases: During an exacerbation or as maintenance therapy in selected cases of: systemic lupus erythematosus, systemic dermatomyositis (polymyositis), acute rheumatic carditis.

Dermatologic Diseases: Pemphigus, severe erythema multiforme (Stevens-Johnson syndrome), exfoliative dermatitis, bullous dermatitis herpetiformis, severe seborrheic dermatitis, severe psoriasis, mycosis fungoides.

Allergic States: Control of severe or incapacitating allergic conditions intractable to adequate trials of conventional treatment in: bronchial asthma, contact dermatitis, atopic dermatitis, serum sickness, seasonal or perennial allergic rhinitis, drug hypersensitivity reactions, urticarial transfusion reactions, acute noninfectious laryngeal edema (epinephrine is the drug of first choice).

Ophthalmic Diseases: Severe acute and chronic allergic and inflammatory processes involving the eye, such as: herpes zoster ophthalmicus, iritis, iridocyclitis, chorioretinitis, diffuse posterior uveitis, optic neuritis, drug hypersensitivity reactions, anterior segment inflammation, allergic conjunctivitis, allergic corneal marginal ulcers, keratitis.

Gastrointestinal Diseases: To tide the patient over a critical period of the disease in: ulcerative colitis (systemic therapy), regional enteritis (systemic therapy).

Respiratory Diseases: Symptomatic sarcoidosis, berylliosis, fulminating or disseminated pulmonary tuberculosis when used concurrently with appropriate antituberculous chemotherapy, Löeffler's syndrome not manageable by other means, aspiration pneumonitis.

Hematologic Disorders: Acquired (autoimmune) hemolytic anemia, secondary thrombocytopenia in adults, erythroblastopenia (RBC anemia), congenital (erythroid) hypoplastic anemia.

Neoplastic Diseases: For palliative management of: leukemias and lymphomas in adults, acute leukemia of childhood.

Edematous States: To induce diuresis or remission of proteinuria in the nephrotic syndrome, without uremia, of the idiopathic type or that due to lupus erythematosus.

Central Nervous System: Acute exacerbations of multiple sclerosis.

Miscellaneous: Tuberculous meningitis with subarachnoid block or impending block when used concurrently with appropriate antituberculous chemotherapy, trichinosis with neurologic or myocardial involvement.

Intra-Synovial or Soft Tissue Administration (including periarticular and intrabursal): **See Warnings**. Indicated as adjunctive therapy for short-term administration (to tide the patient over an acute episode or exacerbation) in: synovitis of osteoarthritis, rheumatoid arthritis, acute and subacute bursitis, acute gouty arthritis, epicondylitis, acute nonspecific tenosynovitis, post-traumatic osteoarthritis.

Intralesional Administration: Indicated for intralesional use in the following conditions: keloids, localized hypertrophic infiltrated, inflammatory lesions of: lichen planus, psoriatic plaques, granuloma annulare, and lichen simplex chronicus (neurodermatitis), discoid lupus erythematosus, necrobiosis lipoidica diabeticorum, alopecia areata.

May also be useful in cystic tumors of an aponeurosis or tendon (ganglia).

CONTRAINDICATIONS: Intrathecal administration. I.V. administration. Systemic fungal infections. Known hypersensitivity to the product and its constituents.

WARNINGS: Benzyl Alcohol Formulation (20 mg/mL-5 mL vial, 40 mg/mL-2 and 5 mL vial, 80 mg/mL-5 mL vial): Multidose use of Depo-Medrol from a single vial requires special care to avoid contamination. Although initially sterile, any multidose use of vials may lead to contamination unless strict aseptic technique is observed. Particular care, such as use of disposable sterile syringes and needles is necessary. Multidose use of Depo-Medrol from vials is not recommended for intrasynovial injection.

This product contains benzyl alcohol which is potentially toxic when administered locally to neural tissue.

Depo-Medrol should not be used in premature infants, because the formulation contains benzyl alcohol. Benzyl alcohol has been reported to be associated with fatal "gasping syndrome" in premature infants.

Myristyl Gamma Picolinium Chloride Formulation (40 mg/mL-1 mL vial, 80 mg/mL-1 mL vial): This product is not suitable for multidose use. Following administration of the desired dose, any remaining suspension should be discarded.

General Warnings: While crystals of adrenal steroids in the dermis suppress inflammatory reactions, their presence may cause disintegration of the cellular elements and physiochemical changes in the ground substance of the connective tissue. The resultant infrequently occurring dermal and/or subdermal changes may form depressions in the skin at the injection site. The degree to which this reaction occurs will vary with the amount of adrenal steroid injected. Regeneration is usually complete within a few months or after all crystals of the adrenal steroid have been absorbed.

In order to minimize the incidence of dermal and subdermal atrophy, care must be exercised not to exceed recommended doses in injections. Multiple small injections into the area of the lesion should be made whenever possible. The technique of intrasynovial and i.m. injections should include precautions against injection or leakage into the dermis. Injection into the deltoid muscle should be avoided because of a high incidence of s.c. atrophy.

Depo-Medrol should not be administered by any route other than those listed under Indications. It is critical that, during administration of methylprednisolone, appropriate technique be used and care taken to assure proper placement of drug.

Administration by other than indicated routes has been associated with reports of serious medical events including: arachnoiditis, meningitis, paraparesis/paraplegia, sensory disturbances, bowel/bladder dysfunction, seizures, visual impairment including blindness, ocular and periocular inflammation, and residue or slough at injection site.

In patients on corticosteroid therapy subjected to any unusual stress, increased dosage of rapidly acting corticosteroids before, during, and after the stressful situation is indicated.

Corticosteroids may mask some signs of infection, and new infections may appear during their use. There may be decreased resistance and inability to localize infection when corticosteroids are used. Infections with any pathogen including viral, bacterial, fungal, protozoan or helminthic infections, in any location in the body, may be associated with the use of corticosteroids alone or in combination with other immunosuppressive agents that affect cellular immunity, humoral immunity, or neutrophil function. These infections may be mild, but can be severe and at times fatal. With increasing doses of corticosteroids, the rate of occurrence of infectious complication increases. Do not use intra-articularly, intrabursally, or for intratendinous administration for local effect in the presence of acute infection.

Prolonged use of corticosteroids may produce posterior subcapsular cataracts, glaucoma with possible damage to the optic nerves, and may enhance the establishment of secondary ocular infections due to fungi or viruses.

Growth may be suppressed in children receiving long-term, daily-divided dose glucocorticoid therapy. The use of such a regimen should be restricted to those most serious indications.

Administration of live or live, attenuated vaccines is contra-indicated in patients receiving immunosuppressive doses of corticosteroids. Killed or inactivated vaccines may be administered to patients receiving immunosuppressive doses of corticosteroids. However, the response to such vaccines may be diminished. Indicated immunization procedures may be undertaken in patients receiving nonimmunosuppressive doses of corticosteroids. While on corticosteroid therapy patients should not be vaccinated against smallpox. Other immunization procedures should not be undertaken in patients who are on corticosteroids especially in high doses, because of the possible hazards of neurological complications and lack of antibody response.

The use of methylprednisolone in active tuberculosis should be restricted to those cases of fulminating or disseminated tuberculosis in which the corticosteroid is used for the management of the disease in conjunction with appropriate antituberculous regimen.

If corticosteroids are indicated in patients with latent tuberculosis or tuberculin reactivity, close observation is necessary as reactivation of the disease may occur. During prolonged corticosteroid therapy, these patients should receive chemoprophylaxis.

Because rare instances of anaphylactoid reactions have occurred in patients receiving parenteral corticosteroid therapy, appropriate precautionary measures should be taken prior to administration, especially when the patient has a history of allergy to any drug.

Allergic skin reactions have been reported apparently related to the excipients in the formulation. Rarely has skin testing demonstrated a reaction to methylprednisolone acetate, per se.

Average and large doses of cortisone or hydrocortisone can cause elevation of blood pressure, salt and water retention, and increased excretion of potassium. These effects are less likely to occur with the synthetic derivatives except when used in large doses. Dietary salt restriction and potassium supplementation may be necessary. All corticosteroids increase calcium excretion.

Pregnancy: Some animal studies have shown that corticosteroids, when administered to the mother at high doses, may cause fetal malformations. Adequate human reproductive studies have not been done with corticosteroids. Therefore, the use of this drug in pregnancy, nursing mothers, or women of childbearing potential requires that the benefits of the drug be carefully weighed against the potential risk to the mother and embryo or fetus. Since there is inadequate evidence of safety in human pregnancy, this drug should be used in pregnancy only if clearly needed.

Corticosteroids readily cross the placenta. Infants born of mothers who have received substantial doses of corticosteroids during pregnancy must be carefully observed and evaluated for signs of adrenal insufficiency. There are no known effects of corticosteroids on labor and delivery. Corticosteroids are excreted in breast milk.

Lactation: See Pregnancy.

PRECAUTIONS: Drug induced secondary adrenocortical insufficiency may be minimized by gradual reduction of dosage. This type of relative insufficiency may persist for months after discontinuation of therapy, therefore, in any situation of stress occurring during that period, hormone therapy should be reinstituted. Since mineralocorticoid secretion may be impaired, salt and/or a mineralocorticoid should be administered concurrently.

There is an enhanced effect of corticosteroids in patients with hypothyroidism and in those with cirrhosis.

ASA should be used cautiously in conjunction with corticosteroids in hypoprothrombinemia.

Growth and development of infants and children on prolonged corticosteroid therapy should be carefully followed.

When multidose vials are used, special care to prevent contamination of the contents is essential. There is some evidence that benzalkonium chloride is not an adequate antiseptic for sterilizing multidose vials. A povidone-iodine solution or similar product is recommended to cleanse the vial top prior to aspiration of contents (see Warnings).

Corticosteroids should be used cautiously in patients with ocular herpes simplex for fear of corneal perforation.

The lowest possible dose of corticosteroid should be used to control the condition under treatment, and when reduction in dosage is possible, the reduction must be gradual.

Psychic derangements may appear when corticosteroids are used, ranging from euphoria, insomnia, mood swings, personality changes, and severe depression to frank psychotic manifestations. Also, existing emotional instability or psychotic tendencies may be aggravated by corticosteroids.

Corticosteroids should be used with caution in nonspecific ulcerative colitis, if there is a probability of impending perforation, abscess or other pyogenic infection. Caution must also be used in diverticulitis, fresh intestinal anastomoses, active or latent peptic ulcer, renal insufficiency, hypertension, osteoporosis, and myasthenia gravis, when steroids are used as direct or adjunctive therapy.

The following additional precautions apply for parenteral corticosteroids: Intra-synovial injection of a corticosteroid may produce systemic as well as local effects.

Appropriate examination of any joint fluid present is necessary to exclude a septic process.

A marked increase in pain accompanied by local swelling, further restriction of joint motion, fever, and malaise are suggestive of septic arthritis. If this complication occurs and the diagnosis of sepsis is confirmed, appropriate antimicrobial therapy should be instituted.

Local injection of a steroid into a previously infected joint is to be avoided.

Corticosteroids should not be injected into unstable joints.

Sterile technique is necessary to prevent infections or contamination.

The slower rate of absorption by i.m. administration should be recognized.

Although controlled clinical trials have shown corticosteroids to be effective in speeding the resolution of acute exacerbations of multiple sclerosis, they do not show that corticosteroids affect the ultimate outcome or natural history of the disease. The studies do show that relatively high doses of corticosteroids are necessary to demonstrate a significant effect (see Dosage).

Since complications of treatment with glucocorticoids are dependent on the size of the dose and the duration of treatment, a risk/benefit decision must be made in each individual case as to dose and duration of treatment, and as to whether daily or intermittent therapy should be used.

Kaposi's sarcoma has been reported to occur in patients receiving corticosteroid therapy. Discontinuation of corticosteroids may result in clinical remission.

Carcinogenesis, Mutagenesis, Impairment of Fertility: No evidence exists showing that corticosteroids are carcinogenic, mutagenic or impair fertility.

Drug Interactions: The pharmacokinetic interactions listed below are potentially clinically important. Mutual inhibition of metabolism occurs with concurrent use of cyclosporine and methylprednisolone, therefore it is possible that adverse events associated with the individual use of either drug may be more apt to occur. Convulsions have been reported with concurrent use of methylprednisolone and cyclosporine.

Drugs that induce hepatic enzymes such as phenobarbital, phenytoin and rifampin may increase the clearance of methylprednisolone and may require increase in methylprednisolone dose to achieve the desired response.

Drugs such as troleandomycin and ketoconazole may inhibit the metabolism of methylprednisolone and thus decrease its clearance. Therefore the dose of methylprednisolone should be titrated to avoid steroid toxicity.

Methylprednisolone may increase the clearance of chronic high dose ASA. This could lead to a decrease in salicylate serum levels or increase the risk of salicylate toxicity when methylprednisolone is withdrawn. ASA should be used cautiously in conjunction with corticosteroids in patients suffering from hypoprothrombinemia.

The effect of methylprednisolone on oral anticoagulants is variable. There are reports of enhanced as well as diminished effects of anticoagulant when given concurrently with corticosteroids. Therefore coagulation indices should be monitored to maintain the desired anticoagulant effect.

ADVERSE EFFECTS: Fluid and Electrolyte Disturbances: sodium retention, fluid retention, congestive heart failure in susceptible patients, potassium loss, hypokalemic alkalosis, hypertension.

Musculoskeletal: muscle weakness, steroid myopathy, osteoporosis, vertebral compression fractures, aseptic necrosis of femoral and humeral heads, pathologic fracture of long bones, tendon rupture—particularly of the Achilles tendon.

Gastrointestinal: peptic ulcer with possible subsequent perforation and hemorrhage, pancreatitis, gastric hemorrhage, esophagitis, perforation of the bowel.

Increases in ALT, AST and alkaline phosphatase have been observed following corticosteroid treatment. These changes are usually small, not associated with any clinical syndrome and are reversible upon discontinuation.

Dermatologic: impaired wound healing, thin fragile skin, petechiae and ecchymoses.

Neurological: increased intracranial pressure (pseudotumor cerebri), psychic derangements, seizures.

Endocrine: menstrual irregularities, development of Cushingoid state, suppression of growth in children, decreased carbohydrate tolerance, manifestations of latent diabetes mellitus, increased requirements for insulin or oral hypoglycemic agents in diabetes, suppression of pituitary-adrenal axis.

Ophthalmic: posterior subcapsular cataracts, increased intraocular pressure, glaucoma, exophthalmos.

Metabolic: negative nitrogen balance due to protein catabolism.

Immune System: masking infections, latent infections becoming active, opportunistic infections, hypersensitivity reactions including anaphylaxis, may suppress reactions to skin tests.

The following additional adverse reactions are related to parenteral corticosteroid therapy: rare instances of blindness associated with intralesional therapy around the face and head, anaphylactic reaction or allergic reactions, hyperpigmentation or hypopigmentation, s.c. and cutaneous atrophy, sterile abscess, postinjection flare—following intra-synovial use, Charcot-like arthropathy. Injection site infections can occur following nonsterile technique.

OVERDOSE:

Symptoms: There is no clinical syndrome of acute overdosage with methylprednisolone. Repeated frequent doses (daily or several times/week) over a protracted period may result in a Cushingoid state.

> For management of a suspected drug overdose, CPhA recommends that you contact your **regional Poison Control Centre**. See the *CPS* Directory section for a list of Poison Control Centres.

DOSAGE: Because of possible physical incompatibilities, methylprednisolone should not be diluted or mixed with other solutions. Parenteral suspensions should be inspected visually for foreign particulate matter and discoloration prior to administration whenever drug product and container permit.

Administration for Local Effect: Therapy with methylprednisolone does not obviate the need for the conventional measures usually employed. Although this method of treatment will ameliorate symptoms, it is in no sense a cure and the hormone has no effect on the cause of the inflammation.

Rheumatoid and Osteoarthritis: The dose for intra-articular administration depends upon the size of the joint and varies with the severity of the condition in the individual patient. In chronic cases, injections may be repeated at intervals ranging from 1 to 5 or more weeks depending upon the degree of relief obtained from the initial injection. The doses in Table 1 are given as a general guide.

Procedure: It is recommended that the anatomy of the joint involved be reviewed before attempting intra-articular injection. In order to obtain the full anti-inflammatory effect, it is important that the injection be made into the synovial space. Employing the same sterile technique as for a lumbar puncture, a sterile 20 to 24 gauge needle (on a dry syringe) is quickly inserted into the synovial cavity. Procaine infiltration is elective. The aspiration of only a few drops of joint fluid proves the joint space has been entered by the needle. The injection site for each joint is determined by that location where the synovial cavity is most superficial and most free of large vessels and nerves. With the needle in place, the aspirating syringe is removed and replaced by a second syringe containing the desired amount of methylprednisolone. The plunger is then pulled outward slightly to aspirate synovial fluid and to make sure the needle is still in the synovial space. After the injection, the joint is moved gently a few times to aid mixing of the synovial fluid and the suspension. The site is covered with a small sterile dressing.

Table 1: Depo-Medrol

Dosage—Rheumatoid and Osteoarthritis

Size of Joint	Examples	Range of Dosage
Large	knees ankles shoulders	20 to 80 mg
Medium	elbows wrists	10 to 40 mg
Small	metacarpophalangeal interphalangeal sternoclavicular acromioclavicular	4 to 10 mg

Suitable sites for intra-articular injection are the knee, ankle, wrist, elbow, shoulder, phalangeal, and hip joints. Since difficulty is occasionally encountered in entering the hip joint, precautions should be taken to avoid any large blood vessels in the area. Joints not suitable for injection are those that are anatomically inaccessible such as the spinal joints and those like the sacroiliac joints that are devoid of synovial space. Treatment failures are most frequently the result of failure to enter the joint space. Little or no benefit follows injection into surrounding tissue. If failures occur when injections into the synovial spaces are certain, as determined by aspiration of fluid, repeated injections are usually futile. Local therapy does not alter the underlying disease process, and whenever possible comprehensive therapy including physiotherapy and orthopedic correction should be employed.

Following intra-articular steroid therapy, care should be taken to avoid overuse of joints in which symptomatic benefit has been obtained. Negligence in this matter may permit an increase in joint deterioration that will more than offset the beneficial effects of the steroid.

Unstable joints should not be injected. Repeated intra-articular injection may in some cases result in instability of the joint. X-ray follow-up is suggested in selected cases to detect deterioration.

If a local anesthetic is used prior to the injection of methylprednisolone, the anesthetic package insert should be read carefully and all the precautions observed.

Bursitis: The area around the injection site is prepared in a sterile way and a wheal at the site made with 1% procaine HCl solution. A 20 to 24 gauge needle attached to a dry syringe is inserted into the bursa and the fluid aspirated. The needle is left in place and the aspirating syringe changed for a small syringe containing the desired dose. After injection, the needle is withdrawn and a small dressing applied.

Miscellaneous: Ganglion, Tendinitis, Epicondylitis: In the treatment of conditions such as tendinitis or tenosynovitis, care should be taken, following application of a suitable antiseptic to the overlying skin, to inject the suspension into the tendon sheath rather than into the substance of the tendon. The tendon may be readily palpated when placed on a stretch. When treating conditions such as epicondylitis, the area of greatest tenderness should be outlined carefully and the suspension infiltrated into the area. For ganglia of the tendon sheaths, the suspension is injected directly into the cyst. In many cases, a single injection causes a marked decrease in the size of the cystic tumor and may effect disappearance.

The usual sterile precautions should be observed, of course, with each injection.

The dose in the treatment of the various conditions of the tendinous or bursal structures listed above varies with the condition being treated and ranges from 4 to 30 mg. In recurrent or chronic conditions, repeated injections may be necessary.

Injections for Local Effect in Dermatologic Conditions: Following cleansing with an appropriate antiseptic such as 70% alcohol, 20 to 60 mg of the suspension is injected into the lesion. It may be necessary to distribute doses ranging from 20 to 40 mg by repeated local injections in the case of large lesions. Care should be taken to avoid injection of sufficient material to cause blanching since this may be followed by a small slough. One to four injections are usually employed, the intervals between injections varying with the type of lesion being treated and the duration of improvement produced by the initial injection.

When multidose vials are used, special care to prevent contamination of the contents is essential (see Warnings).

Administration for Systemic Effect: The i.m. dosage will vary with the condition being treated. When a prolonged effect is desired, the weekly dose may be calculated by multiplying the daily oral dose by 7 and given as a single i.m. injection.

Dosage must be individualized according to the severity of the disease and response of the patient. For infants and children, the recommended dosage will have to be reduced, but dosage should be governed by the severity of the condition rather than by strict adherence to the ratio indicated by age or body weight.

Hormone therapy is an adjunct to, and not a replacement for, conventional therapy. Dosage must be decreased or discontinued gradually when the drug has been administered for more than a few days. The severity, prognosis and expected duration of the disease and the reaction of the patient to medication are primary factors in determining dosage. If a period of spontaneous remission occurs in a chronic condition, treatment should be discontinued. Routine laboratory studies, such as urinalysis, 2-hour postprandial blood sugar, determination of blood pressure and body weight, and a chest x-ray should be made at regular intervals during prolonged therapy. Upper gastrointestinal x-rays are desirable in patients with an ulcer history or significant dyspepsia.

In patients with the adrenogenital syndrome, a single i.m. injection of 40 mg every 2 weeks may be adequate. For maintenance of patients with rheumatoid arthritis, the weekly i.m. dose will vary from 40 to 120 mg. The usual dosage for patients with dermatologic lesions benefited by systemic corticoid therapy is 40 to 120 mg methylprednisolone administered i.m. at weekly intervals for 1 to 4 weeks. In acute severe dermatitis due to poison ivy, relief may result within 8 to 12 hours following i.m. administration of a single dose of 80 to 120 mg. In chronic contact dermatitis, repeated injections at 5 to 10 day intervals may be necessary. In seborrheic dermatitis, a weekly dose of 80 mg may be adequate to control the condition.

Following i.m. administration of 80 to 120 mg to asthmatic patients, relief may result within 6 to 48 hours and persist for several days to 2 weeks. Similarly in patients with allergic rhinitis (hay fever) an i.m. dose of 80 to 120 mg may be followed by relief of coryzal symptoms within 6 hours persisting for several days to 3 weeks.

If signs of stress are associated with the condition being treated, the dosage of the suspension should be increased. If a rapid hormonal effect of maximum intensity is required, the i.v. administration of highly soluble methylprednisolone sodium succinate is indicated.

Multiple Sclerosis: In treatment of acute exacerbations of multiple sclerosis daily doses of 200 mg of prednisolone for a week followed by 80 mg every other day for 1 month have been shown to be effective (4 mg of methylprednisolone is equivalent to 5 mg of prednisolone).

SUPPLIED: Multidose Vials: 20 mg: Each mL of sterile suspension contains: methylprednisolone acetate 20 mg. Nonmedicinal ingredients: dibasic sodium phosphate, monobasic sodium phosphate, polyethylene glycol, polysorbate 80, sodium chloride to adjust tonicity and benzyl alcohol as a preservative. When necessary, pH was adjusted with sodium hydroxide and/or hydrochloric acid. Vials of 5 mL, cartons of 1.

40 mg: Each mL of sterile suspension contains: methylprednisolone acetate 40 mg. Nonmedicinal ingredients: dibasic sodium phosphate, monobasic sodium phosphate, polyethylene glycol, polysorbate 80, sodium chloride to adjust tonicity and benzyl alcohol as a preservative. When necessary, pH was adjusted with sodium hydroxide and/or hydrochloric acid. Vials of 2 and 5 mL, cartons of 5.

80 mg: Each mL of sterile suspension contains: methylprednisolone acetate 80 mg. Nonmedicinal ingredients: dibasic sodium phosphate, monobasic sodium phosphate, polyethylene glycol, polysorbate 80, sodium chloride to adjust tonicity and benzyl alcohol as a preservative. When necessary, pH was adjusted with sodium hydroxide and/or hydrochloric acid. Vials of 5 mL, cartons of 1.

Single Use Vials: 40 mg: Each mL of sterile suspension contains: methylprednisolone acetate 40 mg. Nonmedicinal ingredients: myristyl gamma picolinium chloride (MGPC), polyethylene glycol and sodium chloride to adjust the tonicity. When necessary, pH was adjusted with sodium hydroxide and/or hydrochloric acid. Vials of 1 mL, cartons of 10.

80 mg: Each mL of sterile suspension contains: methylprednisolone acetate 80 mg. Nonmedicinal ingredients: myristyl gamma picolinium chloride (MGPC), polyethylene glycol and sodium chloride to adjust the tonicity. When necessary, pH was adjusted with sodium hydroxide and/or hydrochloric acid. Vials of 1 mL, cartons of 5.

The pH of the finished product remains within the USP specified range i.e., 3.5 to 7.0. Store at room temperature between 15 and 30°C. Protect from freezing.

Depo-Medrol® with Lidocaine ℞

methylprednisolone acetate—lidocaine HCl

Glucocorticoid with Local Anesthetic

Pfizer

PHARMACOLOGY: Methylprednisolone is an anti-inflammatory steroid. Estimates of the relative potencies of methylprednisolone and prednisolone range from 1.13 to 2.1 with an average of 1.5. In general the required daily dose of methylprednisolone can be estimated to be two-thirds (or 0.7) the required daily dose of prednisolone. While the effect of parenterally administered methylprednisolone acetate is prolonged, it has the same metabolic and anti-inflammatory actions as orally administered drug.

Cortisol and its synthetic analogues, such as methylprednisolone acetate, exert their action locally by preventing or suppressing the development of local heat, redness, swelling and tenderness by which inflammation is recognized at the gross level of observation. At the microscopic level, such compounds inhibit not only the early phenomena of the inflammatory process (edema, fibrin deposition, capillary dilatation, migration of phagocytes into the inflamed area and phagocytic activity), but also the later manifestations (capillary proliferation, fibroblast proliferation, deposition of collagen and still later cicatrization). These compounds inhibit inflammatory response whether the inciting agent is mechanical, chemical or immunological.

Lidocaine is a potent local anesthetic agent widely used both for topical and injection anaesthesia. Lidocaine prevents both the generation and the conduction of the nerve impulse. Its main site of action is the cell membrane, and there is seemingly little action of physiological importance on the axoplasm. The exact mechanism whereby a local anesthetic influences the permeability of the membrane is unknown. As a general rule, small nerve fibres are more susceptible to the action of local anesthetics than are large fibres.

INDICATIONS: For intra-synovial or soft tissue administration (including periarticular and intrabursal): See Warnings.

Depo-Medrol with Lidocaine is indicated as adjunctive therapy for short-term administration (to tide the patient over an acute episode or exacerbation) in: synovitis of osteoarthritis, rheumatoid arthritis, acute and subacute bursitis, acute gouty arthritis, epicondylitis, acute nonspecific tenosynovitis, post-traumatic osteoarthritis.

Depo-Medrol with Lidocaine may also be useful in cystic tumors of an aponeurosis or tendon (ganglia).

CONTRAINDICATIONS: Not for i.v. use or intrathecal administration. Contraindicated in systemic fungal infections and patients with known hypersensitivity to components of the Depo-Medrol, lidocaine or other local anesthetics of the amide type.

WARNINGS: This product contains benzyl alcohol which is potentially toxic when administered locally to neural tissue.

Multidose use of Depo-Medrol with Lidocaine from a single vial requires special care to avoid contamination. Although initially sterile, any multidose use of vials may lead to contamination unless strict aseptic technique is observed. Particular care, such as use of disposable sterile syringes and needles is necessary.

While crystals of adrenal steroids in the dermis suppress inflammatory reactions, their presence may cause disintegration of the cellular elements and physicochemical changes in the ground substance of the connective tissue. The resultant infrequently occurring dermal and/or subdermal changes may form depressions in the skin at the injection site. The degree to which this reaction occurs will vary with the amount of adrenal steroid injected. Regeneration is usually complete within a few months or after all crystals of the adrenal steroid have been absorbed.

In order to minimize the incidence of dermal and subdermal atrophy, care must be exercised not to exceed recommended doses in injections. Multiple small injections into the area of the lesion should be made whenever possible. The technique of intra-articular injection should include precautions against injection or leakage into the dermis.

Depo-Medrol with Lidocaine should not be administered by any route other than those listed under Indications. It is critical that, during administration of this drug appropriate technique be used and care taken to assure proper placement of drug.

Administration by other than indicated routes has been associated with reports of serious medical events including: arachnoiditis, meningitis, paraparesis/paraplegia, sensory disturbances, bowel/bladder dysfunction, seizures, visual impairment including blindness, ocular and periocular inflammation, and residue or slough at injection site. Appropriate measures must be taken to avoid intravascular injection.

In patients on corticosteroid therapy subjected to any unusual stress, increased dosage of rapidly acting corticosteroids before, during, and after the stressful situation is indicated.

Corticosteroids may mask some signs of infection, and new infections may appear during their use. There may be decreased resistance and inability to localize infection when corticosteroids are used. Infections with any pathogen including viral, bacterial, fungal, protozoan or helminthic infections, in any location in the body, may be associated with the use of corticosteroids alone or in combination with other immunosuppressive agents that affect cellular immunity, humoral immunity, or neutrophil function. These infections may be mild, but can be severe and at times fatal. With increasing doses of corticosteroids, the rate of occurrence of infectious complication increases. Do not use intra-synovially, intrabursally, or for intratendinous administration for local effect in the presence of acute infection.

Prolonged use of corticosteroids may produce posterior sub-capsular cataracts, glaucoma with possible damage to the optic nerves, and may enhance the establishment of secondary ocular infections due to fungi or viruses.

If corticosteroids are indicated in patients with latent tuberculosis or tuberculin reactivity, close observation is necessary as reactivation of the disease may occur. During prolonged corticosteroid therapy, these patients should receive chemoprophylaxis.

Because rare instances of anaphylactoid reactions have occurred in patients receiving parenteral corticosteroid therapy, appropriate percautionary measures should be taken prior to administration, especially when the patients have a history of allergy to any drug.

Allergic skin reactions have been reported apparently related to the excipients in the formulation (see Supplied). Rarely has skin testing demonstrated a reaction to methylprednisolone acetate, per se.

Pregnancy: Some animal studies have shown that corticosteroids, when administered to the mother at high doses, may cause fetal malformations. Adequate human reproductive studies have not been done with corticosteroids or with Lidocaine. Therefore, the use of this drug in pregnancy, nursing mothers, or women of child bearing potential requires that the benefits of the drug be carefully weighed against the potential risk to the mother and embryo or fetus. Since there is inadequate evidence of safety in human pregnancy, this drug should be used in pregnancy only if clearly needed.

Labor and Delivery: Corticosteroids and lidocaine readily cross the placenta. Infants born of mothers who have received substantial doses of corticosteroids during pregnancy must be carefully observed and evaluated for signs of adrenal insufficiency. There are no known effects of corticosteroids on labor and delivery. The use of local anesthetics such as lidocaine during labor and delivery may be associated with adverse effects on mother and fetus.

Lactation: Corticosteroids are excreted in breast milk. It is not known whether lidocaine is excreted in breast milk.

Children: Growth may be suppressed in children receiving long-term, daily-divided dose glucocorticoid therapy. The use of such a regimen should be restricted to those most serious indications.

Administration of live or live, attenuated vaccines is contra-indicated in patients receiving immunosuppressive doses of corticosteroids. Killed or inactivated vaccines may be administered to patients receiving immunosuppressive doses of corticosteroids. However the response to such vaccines may be diminished. Indicated immunization procedures may be undertaken in patients receiving nonimmunosuppressive doses of corticosteroids.

PRECAUTIONS: When multidose vials are used, special care to prevent contamination of the contents is essential. There is some evidence that benzalkonium chloride is not an adequate antiseptic for sterilizing multidose vials. A povidone-iodine solution or similar product is recommended to cleanse the vial top prior to aspiration of contents (see Warnings).

Corticosteroids should be used cautiously in patients with ocular herpes simplex for fear of corneal perforation.

Psychic derangements may appear when corticosteroids are used, ranging from euphoria, insomnia, mood swings, personality changes, and severe depression to frank psychotic manifestations. Also, existing emotional instability or psychotic tendencies may be aggravated by corticosteroids.

Corticosteroids should be used with caution in nonspecific ulcerative colitis, if there is a probability of impending perforation, abscess or other pyogenic infection. Caution must also be used in diverticulitis, fresh intestinal anastomoses, active or latent peptic ulcer, renal insufficiency, hypertension, osteoporosis, and myasthenia gravis, when steroids are used as direct or adjunctive therapy.

The following additional precautions apply for parenteral corticosteroids: Intrasynovial injection of a corticosteroid may produce systemic as well as local effects. No additional benefit derives from the i.m. administration of Depo-Medrol with Lidocaine. Where parenteral corticosteroid therapy for sustained systemic effect is desired, plain Depo-Medrol should be used.

Appropriate examination of any joint fluid present is necessary to exclude a septic process.

A marked increase in pain accompanied by local swelling, further restriction of joint motion, fever, and malaise are suggestive of septic arthritis. If this complication occurs and the diagnosis of sepsis is confirmed, appropriate antimicrobial therapy should be instituted.

Local injection of a steroid into a previously infected joint is to be avoided.

Corticosteroids should not be injected into unstable joints.

Sterile technique is necessary to prevent infections or contamination.

Since complications of treatment with glucocorticoids are dependent on the size of the dose and the duration of treatment, a risk/benefit decision must be made in each individual case as to dose and duration of treatment.

This product contains benzyl alcohol. Benzyl alcohol has been reported to be associated with a fatal "gasping syndrome" in premature infants.

Kaposi's sarcoma has been reported to occur in patients receiving corticosteroid therapy. Discontinuation of corticosteroids may result in clinical remission.

Carcinogenesis, Mutagenesis, Impairment of Fertility: No evidence exists showing that corticosteroids are carcinogenic, mutagenic or impair fertility.

Drug Interactions: The pharmacokinetic interactions listed below are potentially clinically important. Mutual inhibition of metabolism occurs with concurrent use of cyclosporine and methylprednisolone, therefore, it is possible that adverse events associated with the individual use of either drug may be more apt to occur. Convulsions have been reported with concurrent use of methylprednisolone and cyclosporine.

Drugs that induce hepatic enzymes such as phenobarbital, phenytoin and rifampin may increase the clearance of methylprednisolone and may require increase in methylprednisolone dose to achieve the desired response.

Drugs such as troleandomycin and ketoconazole may inhibit the metabolism of methylprednisolone and thus decrease its clearance. Therefore, the dose of methylprednisolone should be titrated to avoid steroid toxicity.

Methylprednisolone may increase the clearance of chronic high dose ASA. This could lead to a decrease in salicylate serum levels or increase the risk of salicylate toxicity when methylprednisolone is withdrawn. ASA should be used cautiously in conjunction with corticosteroids in patients suffering from hypoprothrombinemia.

The effect of methylprednisolone on oral anticoagulants is variable. There are reports of enhanced as well as diminished effects of anticoagulant when given concurrently with corticosteroids. Therefore, coagulation indices should be monitored to maintain the desired anticoagulant effect.

ADVERSE EFFECTS: Depo-Medrol: Note: The following are typical for all systemic corticosteroids. Their inclusion in this list does not necessarily indicate the specific event has been observed with this particular formulation.

Fluid and electrolyte disturbances: sodium retention, fluid retention, congestive heart failure in susceptible patients, potassium loss, hypokalemic alkalosis, hypertension.

Musculoskeletal: muscle weakness, steroid myopathy, osteoporosis, vertebral compresssion fractures, aseptic necrosis of femoral and humeral heads, pathologic fractures, tendon rupture—particularly of the Achilles tendon.

Gastrointestinal: peptic ulcer with possible subsequent perforation and hemorrhage, pancreatitis, gastrointestinal hemorrhage, esophagitis, perforation of the bowel.

Increases in ALT, AST and alkaline phosphatase have been observed following corticosteroid treatment. These changes are usually small, not associated with any clinical syndrome and are reversible upon discontinuation.

Dermatologic: impaired wound healing, thin fragile skin, petechiae and ecchymoses.

Neurological: increased intracranial pressure, pseudotumor cerebri, psychic derangements, seizures.

Endocrine: menstrual irregularities, development of Cushingoid state, suppression of growth in children, suppression of pituitary-adrenal axis, decreased carbohydrate tolerance, manifestations of latent diabetes mellitus, increased requirements for insulin or oral hypoglycemic agents in diabetics.

Ophthalmic: posterior subcapsular cataracts, increased intraocular pressure, exophthalmos.

Metabolic: negative nitrogen balance due to protein catabolism.

Immune System: masking of infections, latent infections becoming active, opportunistic infections, hypersensitivity reactions including anaphylaxis, may suppress reactions to skin tests.

Lidocaine: CNS: lightheadedness, nervousness, apprehension, euphoria, confusion, dizziness, drowsiness, tinnitus, blurred or double vision, vomiting, sensation of heat or cold, numbness, twitching, tremors, convulsions, loss of consciousness, respiratory depression, respiratory arrest.

Cardiovascular: bradycardia, hypotension, cardiovascular collapse, cardiac arrest.

Allergic Reactions: cutaneous lesions, urticaria, edema, anaphylactic reactions.

OVERDOSE:

Symptoms: There is no clinical syndrome of acute overdosage with Depo-Medrol with Lidocaine.

Repeated frequent doses (daily or several times per week) over a protracted period may result in a Cushingoid state, and other complications of chronic steroid therapy.

For management of a suspected drug overdose, CPhA recommends that you contact your **regional Poison Control Centre**. See the *CPS* Directory section for a list of Poison Control Centres.

DOSAGE: Because of possible physical incompatibilities, Depo-Medrol with Lidocaine should not be diluted or mixed with other solutions. Parenteral suspensions should be inspected visually for foreign particulate matter and discoloration prior to administration whenever drug product and container permit.

Administration for local effect: Therapy with Depo-Medrol with Lidocaine does not obviate the need for the conventional measures usually employed. Although this method of treatment will ameliorate symptoms, it is in no sense a cure and the hormone has no effect on the cause of the inflammation.

Rheumatoid and Osteoarthritis: The dose for intra-articular administration depends upon the size of the joint and varies with the severity of the condition in the individual patient. In chronic cases, injections may be repeated at intervals ranging from 1 to 5 or more weeks depending upon the degree of relief obtained from the initial injection. The doses in Table 1 are given as a general guide.

Procedure: It is recommended that the anatomy of the joint involved be reviewed before attempting intra-articular injection. In order to obtain the full anti-inflammatory effect, it is important that the injection be made into the synovial space. Employing the same sterile technique as for a lumbar puncture, a sterile 20 to 24 gauge needle (on a dry syringe) is quickly inserted into the synovial cavity. Procaine infiltration is elective. The aspiration of only a few drops of joint fluid proves the joint space has been entered by the needle. The injection site for each joint is determined by that location where the synovial cavity is most superficial and most free of large vessels and nerves. With the needle in place, the aspirating syringe is removed and replaced by a second syringe containing the desired amount of Depo-Medrol with Lidocaine. The plunger is then pulled outward slightly to aspirate synovial fluid and to make sure the needle is still in the synovial space. After injection, the joint is moved gently a few times to aid mixing of synovial fluid and the suspension. The site is covered with a small sterile dressing.

Suitable sites for intra-articular injection are the knee, ankle, wrist, elbow, shoulder, phalangeal, and hip joints. Since difficulty is not occasionally encountered in entering the hip joint, precautions should be taken to avoid any large blood vessels in the area. Joints not suitable for injection are those that are anatomically inaccessible such as the spinal joints and those like the sacroiliac joints that are devoid of synovial space. Treatment failures are most frequently the result of failure to enter the joint space. Little or no benefit follows injection into surrounding tissue. If failures occur when injections into the synovial spaces are certain, as determined by aspiration of fluid, repeated injections are usually futile. Local therapy does not alter the underlying disease process, and whenever possible comprehensive therapy including physiotherapy and orthopedic correction should be employed.

Following intra-articular steroid therapy, care should be taken to avoid overuse of joints in which symptomatic benefit has been obtained. Negligence in this matter may permit an increase in joint deterioration that will more than offset the beneficial effects of the steroid.

Unstable joints should not be injected. Repeated intra-articular injection may in some cases result in instability of the joint. X-ray follow-up is suggested in selected cases to detect deterioration.

If a local anesthetic is used prior to injection of Depo-Medrol with Lidocaine, the anesthetic package insert should be read carefully and all the precautions observed.

Table 1: Depo-Medrol with Lidocaine
Dosage—Rheumatoid and Osteoarthritis

Size of Joint	Examples	Range of Dosage (methylprednisolone acetate)
Large	knees ankles shoulders	20 to 80 mg
Medium	elbows wrists	10 to 40 mg
Small	metacarpophalangeal interphalangeal sternoclavicular acromioclavicular	4 to 10 mg

Bursitis: The area around the injection site is prepared in a sterile way and a wheal at the site made with 1% procaine HCl solution. A 20 to 24 gauge needle attached to a dry syringe is inserted into the bursa and the fluid aspirated. The needle is left in place and the aspirating syringe changed for a small syringe containing the desired dose. After injection, the needle is withdrawn and a small dressing applied.

Miscellaneous: Ganglion, Tendinitis, Epicondylitis: In the treatment of conditions such as tendinitis or tenosynovitis, care should be taken, following application of a suitable antiseptic to the overlying skin, to inject the suspension into the tendon sheath rather than into the substance of the tendon. The tendon may be readily palpated when placed on a stretch. When treating conditions such as epicondylitis, the area of greatest tenderness should be outlined carefully and the suspension infiltrated into the area. For ganglia of the tendon sheaths, the suspension is injected directly into the cyst.

The usual sterile precautions should be observed, of course, with each injection.

The dose in the treatment of the various conditions of the tendinous or bursal structures listed above varies with the condition being treated and ranges from 4 to 30 mg. In recurrent of chronic conditions, repeated injections may be necessary.

When multidose vials are used, special care to prevent contamination of the contents is essential (see Warnings).

SUPPLIED: Each mL contains: methylprednisolone acetate 40 mg and lidocaine HCl 10 mg. Nonmedicinal ingredients: benzyl alcohol, polyethylene glycol, sodium chloride and myristyl-gamma-picolinium chloride in water for injection q.s. When necessary, pH was adjusted with sodium hydroxide and/or hydrochloric acid. Gluten-free. Vials of 1, 2 and 5 mL. Store at room temperature between 15 to 30°C. Protect from freezing.

Depo-Provera® ℞

medroxyprogesterone acetate

Progestogen

Pfizer

Date of Revision: July 11, 2006

SUMMARY PRODUCT INFORMATION:

Route of Administration	Dosage Form/ Strength	Clinically Relevant Nonmedicinal Ingredients
Intramuscular	Sterile aqueous suspensions 50 mg/mL and 150 mg/mL	None are clinically relevant. For a complete listing see Dosage Forms, Composition and Packaging.

INDICATIONS AND CLINICAL USE: DEPO-PROVERA is indicated for:
- conception control (prevention of pregnancy)
- treatment of endometriosis

DEPO-PROVERA should be used as a birth control method or endometrial treatment **only** if other treatments have been considered to be unsuitable or unacceptable and should be used for the shortest period of time possible. The risks and benefits of treatment should be carefully reevaluated on a regular basis in all users of this drug.

Although there are no studies addressing whether calcium and vitamin D may lessen bone mineral density (BMD) loss in women using DEPO-PROVERA, all patients should have adequate calcium and vitamin D intake. Cessation of smoking and regular weight bearing exercise should be discussed with all patients.

CONTRAINDICATIONS: Not for intravenous use.

DEPO-PROVERA (medroxyprogesterone acetate) is contraindicated in women with:
- Known or suspected pregnancy or as a diagnostic test for pregnancy
- Undiagnosed vaginal and/or urinary tract bleeding
- Known or suspected carcinoma of the breast
- Undiagnosed breast pathology
- Known or suspected progestin-dependent neoplasia
- History of or actual thrombophlebitis or thromboembolic disorders
- History of or actual cerebrovascular disorders including cerebral apoplexy
- History of or actual myocardial infarction or coronary artery disease
- Presence of severe or multiple risk factor(s) for arterial or venous thrombosis:
  - Severe hypertension (persistent values of ≥160/100 mm Hg)
  - Hereditary or acquired predisposition for venous or arterial thrombosis, such as activated protein C(APC-) resistance, antithrombin-III-deficiency, protein C deficiency, protein S deficiency, hyperhomocysteinaemia and antiphospholipid-antibodies (anticardiolipin antibodies, lupus anticoagulant)
  - Severe dyslipoproteinemia
  - Heavy smoking (>15 cigarettes per day) and over age 35
  - Diabetes mellitus with vascular involvement
- Any ocular lesion arising from ophthalmic vascular disease, such as partial or complete loss of vision or defect in visual fields
- Current or history of migraine with focal aura
- Active liver disease or history of or actual benign or malignant liver tumours
- Hypersensitivity to this drug or to any ingredient in the formulation or component of the container. For a complete listing, see Dosage Forms, Composition and Packaging.

DEPO-PROVERA should not be used before menarche.

WARNINGS AND PRECAUTIONS:

> **Serious Warnings and Precautions**
> The use of DEPO-PROVERA has been associated with loss of bone mineral density (BMD) which may not be completely reversible. Loss of bone mineral density is greater with increasing duration of use.
> It is unknown if the use of DEPO-PROVERA during adolescence or early adulthood, a critical period of bone accretion, will reduce peak bone mass and increase the risk for osteoporotic fracture in later life.
> DEPO-PROVERA should be used as a birth control method or endometrial treatment **only** if other treatments have been considered to be unsuitable or unacceptable and should be used for the shortest period of time possible. The risks and benefits of treatment should be carefully reevaluated on a regular basis in all users of this drug.
> Cigarette smoking increases the risk of serious adverse effects on the heart and blood vessels. Women should be counseled not to smoke.
> This product **does not protect** against sexually transmitted diseases (STDs) including HIV/AIDS. For protection against STDs it is advisable to use latex condoms.

General: Discontinue medication at the earliest manifestation of:

A. **Thromboembolic and cardiovascular disorders** such as thrombophlebitis, pulmonary embolism, cerebrovascular disorders, myocardial ischemia, mesenteric thrombosis and retinal thrombosis;
B. **Conditions that predispose to venous stasis and vascular thrombosis**, such as immobilization after accidents or confinement to bed during long-term illness. Other non-hormonal methods of contraception should be used until regular activities are resumed. For use of hormonal contraceptives when surgery is contemplated, see Peri-Operative Considerations:
C. **Visual defects-partial or complete**
D. **Papilledema or ophthalmic (retinal) vascular lesions**
E. **Severe headache of unknown etiology or worsening of pre-existing migraine headache.**

Carcinogenesis and Mutagenesis: Long-term, case-controlled surveillance of users of DEPO-PROVERA found slight or no increased overall risk of breast cancer and no overall increased risk of ovarian, liver, or cervical cancer and a prolonged, protective effect of reducing the risk of endometrial cancer in the population of users.

Breast Cancer: The World Health Organization Study, a component of a pooled analysis, showed an increased RR of 2.19 (95% CI 1.23 to 3.89) of breast cancer associated with the use of DEPO-PROVERA in women whose first exposure to drug was within the previous 4 years and who were under 35 years of age. However, the overall RR for women who have ever used DEPO-PROVERA was only 1.2 (95% CI 0.96 to 1.52).

[**Note:** A RR of 1.0 indicates neither an increased nor a decreased risk of cancer associated with the use of the drug, relative to no use of the drug. In the case of the subpopulation with a RR of 2.19, the 95% CI is fairly wide and does not include the value of 1.0, thus inferring an increased risk of breast cancer in the defined subgroup relative to nonusers. The value of 2.19 means that women whose first exposure to drug was within the previous 4 years and who are under 35 years of age have a 2.19-fold (95% CI 1.23 to 3.89-fold) increased risk of breast cancer relative to nonusers. The National Cancer Institute reports an average annual incidence rate for breast cancer for US women, all races, age 30 to 34 years of 26.7 per 100 000. A RR of 2.19, thus, increases the possible risk from 26.7 to 58.5 cases per 100 000 women. The attributable risk, thus, is 31.8 per 100 000 women per year.]

Women receiving DEPO-PROVERA should be counselled regarding the importance of breast self-examination. Clinical breast examination should be performed at regular intervals.

Cervical Cancer: A statistically insignificant increase in RR estimates of invasive squamous-cell cervical cancer has been associated with the use of DEPO-PROVERA in women who were first exposed before the age of 35 years (RR 1.22 to 1.28 and 95% CI 0.93 to 1.70). The overall, nonsignificant relative rate of invasive squamous-cell cervical cancer in women who ever used DEPO-PROVERA was estimated to be 1.11 (95% CI 0.96 to 1.29). No trends in risk with duration of use or times since initial or most recent exposure were observed.

Cardiovascular: Thromboembolic Disorders: Before prescribing DEPO-PROVERA, the physician should be alert to the earliest manifestations of thrombotic disorders (thrombophlebitis, cerebrovascular disorders, pulmonary embolism, and retinal thrombosis). Should any of these occur or be suspected, the drug should be discontinued immediately.

Predisposing Factors for Coronary Artery Disease: Cigarette smoking increases the risk of serious cardiovascular side effects and mortality. Convincing data are available to support an upper age limit of 35 years for hormonal contraceptive use by women who smoke.

Other women who are independently at high risk for cardiovascular disease include those who suffer from or have a family history of diabetes, hypertension or an abnormal lipid profile. Whether hormonal contraceptives accentuate this risk is unclear.

There have been post-market reports of cardiovascular events, including heart attack and stroke (e.g. medullary infarction in a heavy smoker) in women using DEPO-PROVERA (see Adverse Reactions, Post-Market Adverse Drug Reactions). Generally, it is not clear if the risk of cardiovascular events is different for users of DEPO-PROVERA than for non-users.

Hypertension: Patients with essential hypertension whose blood pressure is well controlled may be given hormonal contraceptives but only under close supervision. If a significant elevation of blood pressure in previously normotensive or hypertensive subjects occurs at any time during the administration of the drug, cessation of medication is necessary (see also Contraindications).

Endocrine and Metabolism: Loss of Bone Mineral Density : Use of DEPO-PROVERA reduces serum estrogen levels and is associated with significant loss of BMD as bone metabolism accommodates to a lower estrogen level. This loss of BMD is of particular concern during adolescence and early adulthood, a critical period of bone accretion. Bone loss is greater with increasing duration of use and may not be completely reversible. It is unknown if the use of DEPO-PROVERA by younger women will reduce peak bone mass and increase the risk for osteoporotic fractures in later life. A study to assess the reversibility of loss of BMD in adolescent females is ongoing.

BMD should be monitored in women using DEPO-PROVERA for longer than 2 years, or earlier as clinically appropriate. In adolescent females, interpretation of BMD results should take into account patient age and skeletal maturity. If a clinically significant decrease in BMD is detected, treatment with DEPO-PROVERA should be reconsidered.

Use of DEPO-PROVERA should be considered a risk factor for osteoporosis. The use of DEPO-PROVERA should be considered in light of a patient's possible other risk factors for osteoporosis (including metabolic bone disease, chronic alcohol and/or tobacco use, anorexia nervosa, strong family history of osteoporosis or chronic use of drugs that can reduce bone mass such as anticonvulsants or corticosteroids).

BMD Changes in Adult Women: In a controlled, open-label, non-randomized clinical study (DEPO-PROVERA n=248, placebo n=360), adult women using DEPO-PROVERA (150 mg IM) for up to 5 years for contraception showed spine and hip mean BMD decreases of 5-6%, compared to no significant change in BMD in the control group. The decline in BMD was more pronounced during the first 2 years of use, with smaller declines in subsequent years. Mean changes in lumbar spine BMD of −2.86%, −4.11%, −4.89%, −4.93% and −5.38% after 1, 2, 3, 4 and 5 years, respectively, were observed. Mean decreases in BMD of the total hip and femoral neck were similar. Table 1 shows the extent of recovery of BMD for women who received one or more DEPO-PROVERA injections during Years 1 through 5.

Table 1: DEPO-PROVERA

Mean Percent Change from Baseline in BMD in Adults by Skeletal Site and Cohort (ITT Population[a])

Time in Study	Lumbar Spine		Total Hip		Femoral Neck	
	DEPO-PROVERA[b]	Control[c]	DEPO-PROVERA[b]	Control[c]	DEPO-PROVERA[b]	Control[c]
1 year	n=135 −2.86%	n=253 0.22%	n=88 −1.56%	n=125 0.95%	n=137 −2.85%	n=254 0.28%
2 years	n=94 −4.11%	n=197 0.29%	n=57 −3.06%	n=94 0.69%	n=95 −3.99%	n=195 −0.22%
3 years	n=71 −4.89%	n=159 0.31%	n=42 −3.89%	n=77 −0.06%	n=72 −4.80%	n=159 −0.23%

(cont'd)

Table 1: DEPO-PROVERA *(cont'd)*

Mean Percent Change from Baseline in BMD in Adults by Skeletal Site and Cohort (ITT Population[a])

Time in Study	Lumbar Spine		Total Hip		Femoral Neck	
	DEPO-PROVERA[b]	Control[c]	DEPO-PROVERA[b]	Control[c]	DEPO-PROVERA[b]	Control[c]
4 years	n=59 −4.93%	n=137 0.35%	n=31 −4.52%	n=70 −0.02%	n=58 −5.90%	n=138 −0.53%
5 years	n=33 −5.38%	n=105 0.43%	n=21 −5.16%	n=65 0.19%	n=34 −6.12%	n=106 −0.27%
Post-therapy[d] Year 1	n=45 −2.42%	n=87 0.28%	n=31 −0.70%	n=54 0.65%	n=45 −3.04%	n=86 −0.27%
Post-therapy[d] Year 2	n=41 −1.19%	n=66 0.47%	n=25 −0.20%	n=43 0.84%	n=42 −3.11%	n=69 −0.36%

[a] Intent-to-treat population consisted of patients who enrolled in the study and had BMD measured at screening/baseline and at least one post-baseline time point.
[b] DMPA group consisted of women who received one or more DMPA injections during Years 1 through 5.
[c] The control group consisted of women who did not use DEPO-PROVERA prior to the indicated time point.
[d] Women who took one or more doses of DEPO-PROVERA, and then stopped treatment, entered the Post-therapy phase of the study; BMD results from such subjects would no longer be reported in the on-therapy section of the Table. For Control women, results from Years 6 and 7 are shown in the Post-therapy section.

After stopping use of DEPO-PROVERA (150 mg IM), there was partial recovery of BMD toward baseline values during the 2-year post-therapy period. A longer duration of treatment was associated with a less complete BMD recovery observed during the 2-year, post-therapy period.

BMD Changes in Adolescent Females (12-18 years): Preliminary results from an ongoing, open-label, self-selected, non-randomized clinical study of DEPO-PROVERA injectable (150 mg IM every 12 weeks for up to 5 years) in adolescent females (12-18 years) for contraception (DEPO-PROVERA n=177, Control n=237), also showed that DEPO-PROVERA use was associated with a significant decline in BMD from baseline (Table 2). In contrast, most adolescent girls will significantly increase bone density during this period of growth following menarche.

Table 2: DEPO-PROVERA

Mean Percent Changes from Baseline Bone Mineral Density (BMD) and Bone Mineral Content (BMC) for Adolescents on DEPO-PROVERA (Regular Users) and Unmatched, Untreated Controls

Visit	DEPO-PROVERA[a,c]		Unmatched Controls[b,c]	
	n	Mean % (SD)	n	Mean % (SD)
Total Hip BMD				
Week 60	113	−2.72 (3.18)	206	1.31 (2.70)
Week 120	79	−5.29 (3.40)	154	2.00 (4.19)
Week 240	34	−6.91 (4.93)	100	1.83 (5.50)
Femoral Neck BMD				
Week 60	113	−2.91 (4.23)	206	1.74 (3.57)
Week 120	79	−5.49 (4.62)	154	2.70 (5.07)
Week 240	34	−6.53 (5.89)	101	2.14 (6.64)
Lumbar Spine BMD				
Week 60	114	−2.44 (2.67)	206	3.13 (3.22)
Week 120	80	−2.64 (3.67)	154	4.87 (4.99)
Week 240	35	−2.76 (4.84)	102	6.27 (6.80)
Whole Body BMC				
Week 60	115	0.86 (3.52)	207	3.95 (4.20)
Week 120	81	1.34 (4.61)	154	6.91 (6.69)
Week 240	34	3.76 (7.28)	101	9.60 (8.69)
Total Hip BMC				
Week 60	113	−1.54 (4.23)	206	2.65 (3.67)
Week 120	79	−4.03 (4.71)	154	3.88 (5.49)
Week 240	34	−5.61 (6.75)	100	3.29 (6.61)
Femoral Neck BMC				
Week 60	113	−2.70 (5.26)	206	2.73 (4.81)
Week 120	79	−4.42 (5.92)	154	3.97 (6.77)
Week 240	34	−5.42 (7.23)	101	3.52 (9.11)
Lumbar Spine BMC				
Week 60	114	−2.67 (3.90)	206	5.38 (5.26)
Week 120	80	−2.05 (5.33)	154	8.97 (8.43)

(cont'd)

Table 2: DEPO-PROVERA *(cont'd)*

Mean Percent Changes from Baseline Bone Mineral Density (BMD) and Bone Mineral Content (BMC) for Adolescents on DEPO-PROVERA (Regular Users) and Unmatched, Untreated Controls

Visit	DEPO-PROVERA[a,c]		Unmatched Controls[b,c]	
	n	Mean % (SD)	n	Mean % (SD)
Week 240	35	−1.00 (7.27)	102	11.85 (12.20)

[a] DEPO-PROVERA group consists of "regular users" who received at least 4 injections of DEPO-PROVERA prior to Week 60; 8 injections prior to Week 120; 16 injections prior to Week 240.
[b] Control group consists of subjects who did not receive any DEPO-PROVERA prior to the time of the result; in some cases, control subjects chose to start DEPO-PROVERA after that point but were subsequently excluded from the control group.
[c] Treatment and control subjects were not matched for age, gynecologic age or race.

Preliminary data from a small number of adolescents have shown only partial recovery of BMD during the 2-year, post-use observation period. Follow-up bone measurements for the treatment-free period are ongoing. The Product Monograph will be updated once final results are available.

In addition to BMD results, Table 2 also shows the % changes (vs baseline) in Bone Mineral Content (BMC). Whole body BMC is a measure of the overall mineral content of the skeleton. Unlike the adult skeleton, that of the adolescent is growing in size. Therefore, while examination of BMD changes is generally sufficient for understanding the adult subject, both BMD and BMC should be assessed together in the adolescent. The results in Table 2 indicate that adolescents who chose DEPO-PROVERA increased whole body BMC at a slower rate than adolescents who initially chose abstinence or non-hormonal contraception and may have elected non-DEPO-PROVERA hormonal contraception (e.g., oral contraceptives) after the initial visit. BMC measurements of the specific skeletal sites (total hip, femoral neck and lumbar spine) in adolescents taking DEPO-PROVERA showed decreases that are similar in magnitude to the decreases in BMD seen at those sites. Preliminary results obtained from all users of DEPO-PROVERA (defined as adolescents who took one or more doses of DEPO-PROVERA, and then stopped the treatment) show that BMC increases during the 2 year post-use observation period after treatment is stopped. The full extent of BMC recovery has not been defined and follow-up measurements for the treatment-free period are on-going. The Product Monograph will be updated once final results are available.

In post-marketing experience, there have been cases of osteoporosis including osteoporotic fractures reported in patients taking DEPO-PROVERA. Patient age ranged from 16 years to 48 years (see Adverse Reactions, Post-Market Adverse Drug Reactions).

Adrenocortical Function: Clinical suppression of adrenocortical functions has not been observed at low dose levels used for contraception (ovulation suppression).

Carbohydrate Metabolism: A decrease in glucose tolerance has been observed in some women receiving DEPO-PROVERA. The mechanisms of this decrease are obscure. For this reason, diabetic women should be carefully observed while receiving DEPO-PROVERA.

Fluid Retention: Since progestogens may cause some degree of fluid retention, conditions that might be influenced by this factor, such as migraine, asthma, or cardiac or renal dysfunction, require careful observation.

Weight Changes: Weight gain may be associated with the use of DEPO-PROVERA (see Adverse Reactions). The majority of studies report a mean weight gain of 5.4 lbs (2.5 kg) at the end of 1 year, but only 2% of women discontinued treatment due to excessive weight gain (see Adverse Reactions, Clinical Trial Adverse Drug Reactions, Weight Gain Experience). Many studies indicate that weight gain occurs mainly in the first year of use, however, others do report a slow and continuing increase which may reach a mean of 8 lbs (3.6 kg) by the end of 2 years. Some 20 to 40 percent of DEPO-PROVERA users actually lose weight during treatment.

Genitourinary: Irregular Menstrual Patterns: Disruption of menstrual patterns is common following the administration of DEPO-PROVERA. This includes irregular or unpredictable bleeding or spotting, or rarely heavy or continuous bleeding. If undiagnosed vaginal bleeding occurs, or if abnormal bleeding persists or is severe, appropriate investigation should be instituted to rule out the possibility of organic pathology, and appropriate treatment instituted if necessary.

As women continue to use DEPO-PROVERA, fewer experience irregular bleeding patterns and more experience amenorrhea. By month 12, amenorrhea was reported by 55% of women, and by month 24, amenorrhea was reported by 68% of women using DEPO-PROVERA.

Because of the prolonged effect following intramuscular injection of DEPO-PROVERA, re-establishment of menstruation may be delayed and difficult to predict. For this reason, DEPO-PROVERA is not recommended for treatment of secondary amenorrhea or functional uterine bleeding. For these conditions, oral progestogen therapy is recommended.

Hematologic: There have been post-market reports of arterial and venous thromboembolism (VTE) in women using DEPO-PROVERA (see Adverse Reactions, Post-Market Adverse Drug Reactions). Generally, it is not clear if the risk of arterial and venous thromboembolism is different for users of DEPO-PROVERA than for non-users.

Generalized risk factors for venous thromboembolism include a personal history, a family history (the occurrence of VTE in a direct relative at a relatively early age may indicate genetic predisposition), severe obesity (body mass index >30 kg/m^2) and systemic lupus erythematosus. The risk of VTE also increases with age and smoking. The risk of VTE may be temporarily increased with prolonged immobilization, major surgery or trauma.

Hepatic/Biliary/Pancreatic: Liver function tests should be performed periodically in women who are suspected of, or who are at risk of, having hepatic disease. The physician should be alert to the earliest manifestations of impaired liver function. Should this occur or be suspected, the treatment should not be continued. The woman's status should be re-evaluated at appropriate intervals. If jaundice develops, consideration should be given to discontinue the drug.

Patients who have had jaundice, including a history of cholestatic jaundice during pregnancy or during use of oral contraceptives should be given hormonal contraceptives only with great care and under close observation.

Immune: Anaphylactic Reactions: Anaphylactic and anaphylactoid reactions have occasionally been reported in women treated with DEPO-PROVERA. If an anaphylactic reaction occurs, appropriate therapy should be instituted. Serious anaphylactic reactions require emergency medical treatment.

Neurologic: CNS Disorders and Convulsions: There have been few reported cases of convulsions in patients who were treated with DEPO-PROVERA. Association with DEPO-PROVERA use or pre-existing conditions is not clear. Women with known seizure disorders, including epilepsy, require careful observation.

Migraine and Headache: The onset or exacerbation of migraine or the development of headaches with a new pattern that is recurrent, persistent or severe requires discontinuation of hormonal contraceptives and evaluation of the cause.

Women with migraine headache who take hormonal contraceptives may be at increased risk of stroke (see Contraindications).

Ophthalmologic: Ocular Disorders: Discontinue medication pending examination, if there is sudden partial or complete loss of vision, or if there is a sudden onset of proptosis, diplopia or migraine. If examination reveals papilledema or retinal vascular lesions, medication should be withdrawn.

Peri-Operative Considerations: If feasible, hormonal contraceptives should be discontinued and an alternative method substituted at least four weeks prior to elective surgery of a type associated with an increase in risk of thromboembolism and during prolonged immobilization. Hormonal contraceptives should not be resumed until the first menstrual period after hospital discharge following surgery or following prolonged immobilization.

Psychiatric: Women who have a history of mental depression should be carefully observed and this drug discontinued if serious depression re-occurs. Some women may complain of premenstrual like depression while on DEPO-PROVERA therapy

Sexual Function/Reproduction: Return of Fertility: There is no evidence that DEPO-PROVERA causes infertility. A large study of return of fertility shows that women conceived 9 months on average after the last injection, or 5.5 months after discontinuing (discontinuance is assumed to be 15 weeks after the last injection). In addition, the number of users who had conceived within 2 years of discontinuing their method of contraception (92% of DEPO-PROVERA users had conceived within 2 years after discontinuing compared with 93% for users of the IUD and 95% for users of oral contraceptives) were comparable. Discuss this information with women who intend to conceive in the next 1 to 2 years.

In some cases, women have not become pregnant after stopping injections of DEPO-PROVERA. It is not known whether DEPO-PROVERA or other factors resulted in a change in the ability to conceive. Many reasons exist for such changes, including increased age and the onset of menopause. The infertility rate in the normal population is 7%.

Figure 1: DEPO-PROVERA

Cumulative Conception Rates for Women Discontinuing Use of an IUD, Oral Contraceptives, or DEPO-PROVERA in Order to Become Pregnant

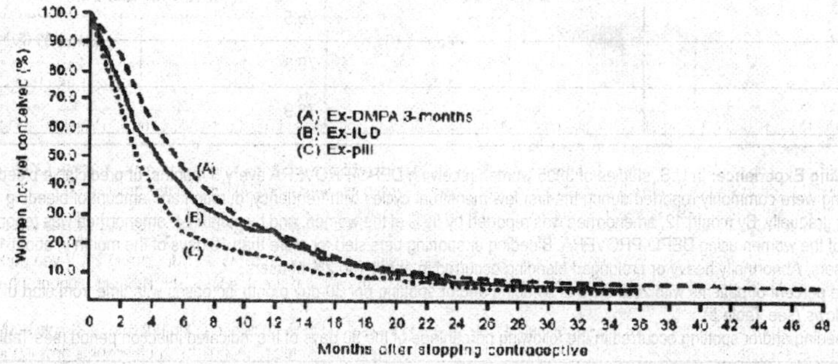

Ectopic Pregnancy: Physicians should investigate the possibility of an ectopic pregnancy among women using DEPO-PROVERA who complain of severe abdominal pain.

Special Populations: Pregnant Women: To increase assurance that the woman is not pregnant at the time of the first administration, it is recommended that the first injection be given only within the first 5 days of the onset of a normal menstrual period or, only within the first 5 days post-partum if not breast-feeding (see Dosage and Administration).

Infants from unexpected pregnancies that occurred 1 to 2 months after injection of DEPO-PROVERA may be at an increased risk of low birth weight, which, in turn, is associated with an increased risk of neonatal death. The attributable risk is low because such pregnancies are uncommon.

A significant increase in incidence of polysyndactyly and chromosomal anomalies was observed among infants of users of DEPO-PROVERA, the former being most pronounced in women under 30 years of age. The unrelated nature of these defects, the lack of confirmation from other studies, the distant preconceptual exposure to DEPO-PROVERA and the chance effects due to multiple statistical comparisons, make a causal association unlikely.

Children exposed to medroxyprogesterone acetate in utero and followed to adolescence, showed no evidence of any adverse effects on their health including their physical, intellectual, sexual, or social development.

Several reports suggest an association between intra-uterine exposure to progestational drugs in the first trimester of pregnancy and genital abnormalities in male and female fetuses. The risk of hypospadias (5 to 8 per 1000 male births in the general population) may be approximately doubled with exposure to these drugs. Although there are insufficient data to quantify the risk to exposed female fetuses, some of these drugs induce mild virilization of the external genitalia of the female fetus. Because of these changes, it is prudent to avoid the use of progestogens during the first trimester of pregnancy.

Nursing Women: Detectable amounts of progestogen have been identified in the milk of mothers receiving DEPO-PROVERA. Two studies have indicated that the maximum amount of medroxyprogesterone acetate (MPA) which might be ingested by a breast-feeding infant whose mother is receiving DEPO-PROVERA for contraception would be 1.0 to 1.5 µg/day (or 0.0015 mg/day, 0.045 mg/month, 0.27 mg over 6 months which is about 0.05 mg/kg over 6 months for a 5.5 kg baby). If absorption properties between adult and infant are comparable, this amount would be too low to suppress pituitary function in the infant. No adverse effects related to lactation itself or infant growth were reported in studies where DEPO-PROVERA was started 1-4 days, 7 days or within 6 weeks postpartum.

In nursing mothers treated with DEPO-PROVERA, milk composition, quality and amount are not adversely affected.

To date, no adverse effects have been observed in children whose mothers were using DEPO-PROVERA while lactating. A study of children exposed to MPA with median observation periods of 14-16 years, indicated no incidence of adverse effects on physical growth, mental growth and development of general health status. However, the long-term effects on the child are not fully understood. It is recommended that DEPO-PROVERA not be administered until 6 weeks postpartum in women who are breast feeding to avoid risk of exposure of the neonate to steroid hormones. The physician and woman should discuss the risks of pregnancy versus the risks to the child, if DEPO-PROVERA is used during lactation, to determine the most appropriate course of action for the individual woman.

Pediatrics: DEPO-PROVERA should not be used before menarche (see Contraindications).

Other: In the perimenopausal population, age constitutes no absolute limiting factor, although treatment with a progestogen may mask the onset of the climacteric.

Monitoring and Laboratory Tests: Before DEPO-PROVERA is used, a thorough history and physical examination should be performed, including a blood pressure determination. Breasts, liver, extremities and pelvic organs should be examined. A Papanicolaou smear should be taken if the patient has been sexually active. The first follow-up visit should be three months after the initiation of therapy. Thereafter, examinations should be performed at least once a year, or more frequently if indicated. Women with a strong family history of breast cancer or who have breast nodules should be monitored with particular care. At each visit, examination should include those procedures that were done at the initial visit, as outlined above or as per the recommendations of the Canadian Task force on the Periodic Health Examination.

Bone mineral density (BMD) should be monitored in women using DEPO-PROVERA for longer than 2 years, or earlier as clinically appropriate. In adolescent females, interpretation of BMD results should take into account patient age and skeletal maturity. If a clinically significant decrease in BMD is detected, treatment with DEPO-PROVERA should be reconsidered (see Warnings and Precautions, Loss of Bone Mineral Density).

For Conception Control: Counseling: It is very important that adequate explanations of the long-term nature of DEPO-PROVERA as a contraceptive be given to each woman prior to her first injection. The possible side effects including BMD changes, changes in menstrual cycle and the relatively slow return of fertility should be emphasized. Every effort should be made to ensure that each woman receives such counseling as to enable her to understand fully these explanations and the possible consequences. A detailed Patient Information leaflet that describes the actions, benefits, risks and adverse effects of this contraceptive should be made available to each woman before she makes the decision to use DEPO-PROVERA for conception control.

ADVERSE REACTIONS: Adverse Drug Reaction Overview: The following adverse reactions have been associated with the use of DEPO-PROVERA (medroxyprogesterone acetate):

A. **Irregular Menstrual Patterns:** The most common adverse reactions associated with the use of DEPO-PROVERA for contraception is the disruption of menstrual patterns. This includes irregular or unpredictable bleeding or spotting, or rarely heavy or continuous bleeding.

B. **Non-Menstrual Adverse Reactions:** Other than menstrual changes, weight gain, headache and abdominal discomfort are the most common side effects.

In a few instances there have been undesirable sequelae at the site of injection, such as a residual lump, change in colour of the skin or a sterile abscess.

Anaphylactic and anaphylactoid reactions have been reported on rare occasions.

Clinical Trial Adverse Drug Reactions: Because clinical trials are conducted under very specific conditions the adverse reaction rates observed in the clinical trials may not reflect the rates observed in practice and should not be compared to the rates in the clinical trials of another drug. Adverse drug reaction information from clinical trials is useful for identifying drug-related adverse events and for approximating rates.

In clinical studies of 3905 women receiving DEPO-PROVERA every 3 months, there were a total of 8467 side effect reports. Headache, abdominal distress, nervousness, dizziness and decreased libido were reported in greater than 5.0 percent of study patients. Thrombophlebitis was reported by 4 women (0.10%).

Total Adverse Reaction Experience: Table 3 contains a list of reported side effects, the number of times each side effect was reported and the number and percent of patients who reported each side effect. Table 4 contains the number of side effects reported by month and the number of side effect reports per 100 patients "exposed" by month.

According to Table 4, 1135 (13.40%) of the total 8467 side effect reports were reported during the first injection period (90 days); during the first two injection periods (first 180 days) 2070 (24.45%) were reported; 2826 (33.38%) were reported during the first three injection periods (first 270 days); and 3536 (41.75%) were reported during the first four injection periods (first 360 days). The number of patients not reporting any side effects was 2117 (54.2%).

Table 3: DEPO-PROVERA

DEPO-PROVERA Every 90 Days Side Effects

Symptom	No. of Times Reported	No. of Women Reporting	Percent of Women (3905)
Headache	2187	682	17.46
Abdominal Distress	990	463	11.85
Nervousness	1143	451	11.55
Dizziness	411	232	5.94
Decreased Libido	541	225	5.76
Asthenia	321	177	4.53
Limb Pain and Varicose Vein Pain	311	152	3.89
Nausea	209	138	3.53
Vaginal Discharge	178	120	3.07
Breast Swelling and Tenderness	188	114	2.92
Bloating	170	94	2.41
Edema Peripheral	170	87	2.22
Backache	131	87	2.22
Dysmenorrhea	95	69	1.77
Depression	100	62	1.59
Acne	72	48	1.23
Pruritus Vulvae	67	48	1.23
No Hair Growth, Alopecia	108	46	1.18
Rash	78	41	1.05
Hot Flash	51	40	1.02
Insomnia	54	38	0.97
Genitourinary Infection	45	34	0.87
Eye Discomfort	45	33	0.85
Anorexia	37	29	0.74
Increased Appetite	37	28	0.72
Chest Pain	33	28	0.72
Dysuria	39	28	0.72
Diarrhea	28	25	0.64
Heartburn	26	23	0.59
Galactorrhea	40	22	0.56
Pruritus	28	22	0.56
D&C for Bleeding	21	21	0.54
Pain	25	19	0.49
Somnolence Drowsiness	23	19	0.49
Dyspareunia	21	17	0.43
Dyspnea	30	17	0.43
Abdominal Swelling	25	17	0.43
Allergic Reactions	21	15	0.38
Chloasma	26	13	0.33
Vomiting	16	12	0.31
Constipation	19	11	0.28
Tachycardia	11	10	0.26
Liver disorders NOS, altered liver function	14	10	0.26
Hirsutism	13	10	0.26
Frequency Urination	11	10	0.26

(cont'd)

Table 3: DEPO-PROVERA *(cont'd)*

DEPO-PROVERA Every 90 Days Side Effects

Symptom	No. of Times Reported	No. of Women Reporting	Percent of Women (3905)
Paraesthesia, Sensory Disturbances	13	9	0.23

Table 4: DEPO-PROVERA

DEPO-PROVERA Every 90 Days—Side Effects (by Month)

Month	# Pts Entering/Mnth	# Reports	# Reports/100 Patients
1	3905	355	9.09
2	3670	373	10.16
3	3571	407	11.40
4	3294	290	8.80
5	3084	283	9.18
6	3004	362	12.05
7	2792	249	8.91
8	2634	218	8.28
9	2579	289	11.22
10	2419	224	9.26
11	2299	220	9.57
12	2253	266	11.81
15	1872	212	11.32
18	1659	225	13.56
21	1485	198	13.33
24	1344	194	14.43
27	1180	155	13.14
30	1037	124	11.96
33	927	127	13.70
36	827	128	15.48
39	722	112	15.51
42	664	99	14.91
45	573	84	14.66
48	474	45	9.49
51	412	52	12.62
54	350	46	13.14
57	305	44	14.43
60	263	23	8.75
63	227	19	8.37
66	201	20	9.95
69	184	17	9.24
72	157	17	10.83
75	118	12	9.32
78	91	16	17.58
81	49	3	6.12
84	1	0	0.00

Table 5: DEPO-PROVERA

Percent of Patients with Zero Days of Bleeding and/or Spotting

Month	Percent Having Zero Bleeding and/or Spotting
3	29.3
12	54.6
24	67.7
36	73.8
48	75.5
60	79.3
72	78.9

Bleeding Experience: In U.S. studies of 3905 women receiving DEPO-PROVERA every 3 months, unpredictable bleeding or spotting were commonly reported during the first few menstrual cycles with frequency, duration and amount of bleeding diminishing gradually. By month 12, amenorrhea was reported by 55% of the women, and by month 24, amenorrhea was reported by 68% of the women using DEPO-PROVERA. Bleeding or spotting persisted for more than 10 days of the month in about 12% of the users. Abnormally heavy or prolonged bleeding occurred in about 1 to 2% of users.

The percent of patients with zero days of bleeding and/or spotting per 30-day month increases with time from start of study, as follows (see Table 5).

Bleeding and/or spotting occurred in the following percentage of the 90 days of the indicated injection period (see Table 6).

Table 6: DEPO-PROVERA

Percent of Days with Bleeding and/or Spotting

Injection Period	Months	Percent of Days with Bleeding and/or Spotting
First	1–3	25.7
Fourth	10–12	11.8
Eighth	22–24	6.8
Twelfth	34–36	4.8
Sixteenth	46–48	4.3
Twentieth	58–60	4.1
Twenty-fourth	70–72	4.3

One hundred and ninety four (194) patients reported no bleeding or spotting from first injection to the end of their participation in the study. The median number of days of no spotting or bleeding for these 194 women was 120 days. The minimum number of days of no spotting or bleeding was 30 and the maximum was 1674 days.

Thirteen (13) patients reported bleeding and/or spotting every day from first injection to the end of their participation in the study.

Weight Gain Experience: The U.S. studies of 3905 women receiving DEPO-PROVERA every 3 months report a mean weight gain of 5.4 lbs (2.5 kg) at the end of 1 year, but only 2% of women discontinued treatment due to excessive weight gain. Many studies indicate that weight gain occurs mainly in the first year of use, however, others report a slow and continuing increase which may reach a mean of 8 lbs (3.6 kg) by the end of 2 years. However, some 20 to 40 percent of DEPO-PROVERA users actually lose weight during treatment.

A much higher proportion of patients had an increase as had a decrease of more than 15 pounds. The mean body weight changes from baseline (in pounds) were as follows (see Table 7).

Table 7: DEPO-PROVERA

Mean Body Weight Changes from Baseline (in Pounds)

Month	Weight Increase (pounds)	n
12	5.4	1644
24	8.1	960
36	11.3	567
48	13.8	282
60	14.1	150
72	16.5	109

Laboratory Assay Results: Laboratory assays were performed on a sample of women, rather than on all women. There were no clinically significant changes in any of the hematology, urine or serum chemistry variables that were monitored.

The number of women having had an initial Pap smear taken is 2052. Ten (10) patients dropped from the study due to a Grade IV Pap smear, while 4 patients dropped out due to a Grade III Pap smear.

Non-Menstrual Adverse Reactions: The occurrence rates for non-menstrual adverse reactions reported in U.S. studies of 3905 women receiving DEPO-PROVERA every 3 months are listed in Table 8. 2253 women were in the study for 12 months or more; 827 women were in the study for 36 months or more. The total number of patient-months of experience was 82 384. A total of 2117 of the 3905 women (54%) reported no side effects.

Table 8: DEPO-PROVERA

Occurrence Rates for Non-menstrual Adverse Reactions Reported in U.S. Studies of 3905 Women Receiving DEPO-PROVERA Every 3 Months

System Organ Class	Event
General Disorders and Administration Site Conditions	Asthenia (5%) Peripheral edema (2%) The following adverse events occurred in less than 1% of patients: Axillary swelling, pain, chills, excessive thirst, fever, pain at injection site.
Blood and Lymphatic System Disorders	The following adverse events occurred in less than 1% of patients: Anemia, blood dyscrasia.
Cardiac Disorders	Chest pain, tachycardia (0.2–1.0%)
Eye Disorders	Eye discomfort (0.2–1.0%)

(cont'd)

Table 8: DEPO-PROVERA *(cont'd)*

Occurrence Rates for Non-menstrual Adverse Reactions Reported in U.S. Studies of 3905 Women Receiving DEPO-PROVERA Every 3 Months

System Organ Class	Event
Gastrointestinal Disorders	Abdominal distress (12%) Nausea (4%) Bloating (2%) Anorexia, increased appetite, diarrhea, heartburn, abdominal swelling, vomiting, constipation (0.2–1.0%) The following adverse events occurred in less than 1% of patients: Gastrointestinal disturbances, rectal bleeding.
Hepatobiliary Disorders	Liver disorders NOS, altered liver function (0.2–1.0%) The following adverse event occurred in less than 1% of patients: Jaundice.
Immune System Disorders	Allergic reactions (0.2–1.0%)
Infections and Infestations	Genitourinary infection (0.2–1.0%)
Musculoskeletal and Connective Tissue Disorders	Backache (2%) Limb pain (4%) Leg cramps, arthralgia (1–5%) The following adverse events occurred in less than 1% of patients: Osteoporosis.
Neoplasms Benign, Malignant and Unspecified (incl cysts and polyps)	The following adverse events occurred in less than 1% of patients: Breast cancer, cervical cancer.
Nervous System Disorders	Headache (17%) Dizziness (6%) Somnolence or drowsiness, paraesthesia, sensory disturbances (0.2–1.0%) The following adverse events occurred in less than 1% of patients: Syncope, convulsions, paralysis, facial palsy.
Pregnancy, Puerperium and Perinatal Conditions	The following adverse events occurred in less than 1% of patients: Unexpected pregnancy, sensation of pregnancy.
Psychiatric Disorders	Nervousness (12%) Decreased libido (6%) Depression (2%) Anorgasmia (1-5%) Insomnia (0.2–1.0%) The following adverse event occurred in less than 1% of patients: Increased libido.
Renal and Urinary Disorders	Dysuria, urinary frequency (0.2–1.0%)
Reproductive System and Breast Disorders	Breast swelling/tenderness (3%) Vaginal discharge (3%) Leukorrhoea (1–5%) Pelvic pain (1–5%) Vaginitis (1–5%) Dysmenorrhea (2%) Pruritus vulvae (1%) Galactorrhea, bleeding requiring D&C, dyspareunia (0.2–1.0%) The following adverse events occurred in less than 1% of patients: Changes in breast size, breast lumps or nipple bleeding, prevention of lactation, vaginal cysts, lack of return to fertility, uterine hyperplasia.
Respiratory, Thoracic and Mediastinal Disorders	Dyspnea (0.2–1.0%) The following adverse events occurred in less than 1% of patients: Asthma, hoarseness, pulmonary embolus.
Skin and Subcutaneous Tissue Disorders	Acne, alopecia, rash (1%) Hirsutism, pruritus (0.2–1%) Hives (0.2–1.0%) The following adverse events occurred in less than 1% of patients: Melasma, chloasma, scleroderma, excessive sweating, body odour, dry skin.
Vascular Disorders	Hot flashes (1%) The following adverse events occurred in less than 1% of patients: Varicose veins, thrombophlebitis, deep vein thrombosis.

Post-Market Adverse Drug Reactions: In post-marketing experience, there have been cases of osteoporosis including osteoporotic fractures reported in patients taking DEPO-PROVERA. Patient age ranged from 16 years to 48 years. Other adverse events reported during post-marketing experience, regardless of causality and frequency, are listed below. It should be noted that the nature of post-marketing surveillance makes it difficult to determine if a reported event was actually caused by DEPO-PROVERA.

Blood and Lymphatic System Disorders: hemolytic anemia, hemorrhagic disorder, sickle cell crisis, splenic infarction, thrombocytopenia, thrombotic thrombocytopenic purpura.

Cardiac Disorders: bradycardia, myocardial infarction, palpitations, pericarditis, possible exacerbation of prolonged QT interval syndrome (with fatal outcome), supraventricular tachycardia.

Congenital and Familial/Genetic Disorders: acute porphyria, in cases of failure of contraception: Trisomy 21, Trisomy 16, Turner's syndrome.

Ear and Labyrinth Disorders: change in hearing, tinnitus, vertigo.

Endocrine Disorders: adrenal dysfunction NOS, Cushingoid, estrogen deficiency, hyperthyroidism, hypoglycemia, hypopituitarism, hypothyroidism, thyroiditis.

Eye Disorders: macular edema, optic ischemic neuropathy, optic neuritis, papilloedema, ptosis, retinal vein occlusion, vision loss, visual changes.

Gastrointestinal Disorders: acute pancreatitis, dysphagia, intestinal infarction, mouth ulceration, oral mucosal blistering, salivary gland enlargement.

General Disorders and Administration Site Conditions: fatigue, injection site reactions (including swelling, rash, ulcer, necrosis, edema, infection, abscess), malaise, sudden infant death syndrome (exposure-in-utero).

Hepatobiliary Disorders: cholangitis, cholelithiasis, gallbladder disorder, hepatitis, hepatomegaly, obstructive jaundice, hepatic failure (with fatal outcome).

Injury, Poisoning, and Procedural Complications: exposure in utero: abnormal genitalia, anencephaly, cleft palate, congenital adenomatoid malformation, congenital diaphragmatic hernia, congenital heart defects, congenital megacolon, ear malformation NOS, esophageal atresia, hydrocephalus, hypospadias, limb deformity, microcephaly, polydactyly, single umbilical artery, skull malformation, spina bifida, Talipes, tracheoesophageal fistula.

Immune System Disorders: anaphylactic reaction (with fatal outcome in rare cases), hypersensitivity.

Infections and Infestations: salpingitis, sepsis, vulval abscess.

Investigations: coagulation Factor X decreased, decreased blood folate, decreased blood pressure, decreased estrogen, decreased testosterone, elevated blood creatinine, hypernatremia, hypokalemia, increased alanine aminotransferase, increased alkaline phosphatase, increased blood pressure, increased creatine phosphokinase, increased triglycerides, leukocytosis, weight decreased.

Metabolism and Nutrition Disorders: cachexia, excessive thirst.

Musculoskeletal, Connective Tissue and Bone Disorders: joint swelling, muscle weakness, myalgia, osteonecrosis.

Neoplasms Benign, Malignant and Unspecified: acute leukemia, benign breast neoplasm, benign hydatidiform mole, fibroadenoma of breast, Hodgkin's disease, kidney neoplasm, malignant melanoma, meningioma, neurofibroma, ovarian cancer, squamous cell carcinoma of the cervix, uterine leiomyoma.

Nervous System Disorders: amnesia, anosmia, ataxia, balance disorder, benign intracranial hypertension, cerebral hemorrhage, cerebral ischemia/infarct, cerebral venous thrombosis, cerebrovascular accident, confusion, dysarthria, dysgeusia, memory loss, migraine, myoclonus, Parkinsonism, seizures, speech disorder, stroke (with fatal outcome), third nerve palsy, transient ischemic attack, tremor.

Pregnancy, Puerperium and Perinatal Conditions: exposure-in-utero: antepartum hemorrhage, blighted ovum, ectopic pregnancy, fetal hydrops, intrauterine growth retardation, missed abortion, polyhydramnios, prematurity, spontaneous abortion, stillbirth.

Psychiatric Disorders: acute psychosis, agitation, anxiety, attention deficit/hyperactivity disorder, dysphemia, eating disorder, irritability, mood swings, paranoia, suicidality.

Renal and Urinary Disorders: interstitial nephritis, nephrolithiasis, nephrotic syndrome, proteinuria, renal infarct, urinary retention.

Reproductive System and Breast Disorders: cervical dysplasia, fibrocystic breast disease, menorrhagia, ovarian cyst, premature menopause, uterine cyst, vaginal dysplasia, vaginal mucosal blistering.

Respiratory, Thoracic and Mediastinal Disorders: acute respiratory distress syndrome, bronchospasm, epistaxis, laryngeal edema, laryngospasm, oropharyngeal swelling.

Skin and Subcutaneous Tissue Disorders: angioedema, erythema multiforme, erythema nodosum, facial edema, porphyria aggravated.

Vascular Disorders: arterial thrombosis, embolism, Henoch-Schonlein purpura, postural hypotension, venous thrombosis (including rare cases with fatal outcome).

DRUG INTERACTIONS: Overview: Aminoglutethimide: Aminoglutethimide administered concomitantly with DEPO-PROVERA (medroxyprogesterone acetate) may significantly depress the serum concentration of medroxyprogesterone acetate. Users of DEPO-PROVERA should be warned of the possibility of decreased efficacy with the use of this or any related drugs.

Rifampin: Rifampin can increase the metabolism of exogenously administered progestational agents. Norethindrone has specifically been affected; a reduction of plasma concentrations has occurred. The extent to which rifampin may alter the metabolism of other progestogens remains to be determined; the possibility of an interaction should be considered.

Drug-Drug Interactions: The results of one study indicated that intramuscularly administered medroxyprogesterone acetate may induce or activate the CYP3A4 enzyme system, leading to an increased metabolism of many CYP3A4 substrates.

Drug-Food Interactions: Interactions with food have not been established.

Drug-Herb Interactions: Interactions with herbal products have not been established.

Drug-Laboratory Test Interactions: Certain endocrine and possibly liver function tests may be affected by treatment with DEPO-PROVERA. Therefore, if such tests are abnormal in a woman taking DEPO-PROVERA, it is recommended that they be repeated 6 to 12 months after the drug has been withdrawn.

The clinical chemist or pathologist should be advised of progestogen therapy when a woman's blood or tissue specimens are submitted for laboratory diagnosis or biochemical analysis.

The following laboratory tests may be affected by the use of DEPO-PROVERA: (a) Gonadotropin levels—inhibition of the midcycle LH surge; (b) Plasma progesterone levels—inhibition of ovulation and thus the postovulatory rise of progesterone; (c) Plasma estrogen levels—do not exceed early-to-mid-proliferative phase levels; (d) Plasma cortisol levels—not significantly affected by the dose used for contraception; (e) Glucose tolerance test—occasionally some degree of glucose intolerance may develop; (f) Plasma lipid concentrations—decrease in high density lipoprotein cholesterol (HDL-C) in some studies. The clinical relevance of this has yet to be determined; (g) Urinary pregnanediol levels. (Note: DEPO-PROVERA does not interfere with the assay of human chorionic gonadotropin (HCG) either chemically or pharmacologically.)

DOSAGE AND ADMINISTRATION: Recommended Dose and Dosage Adjustment: Conception Control (prevention of pregnancy): The recommended dose for contraception is 150 mg of DEPO-PROVERA (medroxyprogesterone acetate) every 3 months, administered by deep intramuscular injection. To increase assurance that the woman is not pregnant at the time of the first administration, it is recommended that this injection be given **only** within the 5 five days of the onset of a normal menstrual period or, **only** within the first 5 days post-partum if not breast-feeding. If the woman has chosen to breast-feed, discuss the risks of pregnancy and possible risks of DEPO-PROVERA to determine the most appropriate course of action for the individual woman (see Warnings and Precautions).

If administered within the first 5 days after the onset of a normal menstrual period, DEPO-PROVERA is effective from the day of injection. When DEPO-PROVERA is given later in the menstrual cycle it may not be effective for the first 3 to 4 weeks after the injection and another method of contraception (non-hormonal) should be used during this time.

After miscarriage or first trimester therapeutic abortion, the injection is normally given within 5 days of the procedure and no extra precautions are required. After a late (second trimester) abortion, some further delay is recommended to reduce the risk of heavy and prolonged bleeding, therefore, the first injection should not be given until 4 weeks after the procedure.

The woman must return every 10 to 13 weeks for a repeat injection to maintain contraceptive effectiveness. **Intervals between injections must not exceed 13 weeks (3 months).**

Endometriosis: The recommended dose of DEPO-PROVERA is 50 mg weekly or 100 mg every 2 weeks intramuscularly for at least 6 months. It should be noted that return of ovulation may be delayed following this therapy due to the depot properties of the drug (see Warnings and Precautions).

Use in Children: DEPO-PROVERA should not be used before menarche (see Contraindications and Warnings and Precautions).

See Warnings and Precautions, Loss of Bone Mineral Density for available data for adolescent females (12-18 years).

Missed Dose: If an injection is not given within 13 weeks a pregnancy test should be done before any further treatment with DEPO-PROVERA.

Administration: DEPO-PROVERA is intended for **intramuscular administration only**. Immediately before use, the sterile aqueous suspension should be vigorously shaken to assure that the dose being administered represents a uniform suspension.

OVERDOSAGE:

Overdosage may result in a period of amenorrhea of a variable length and may be followed by irregular menses for several cycles. Very high doses of DEPO-PROVERA (500 mg daily or more) have been associated with corticoid-like activity and with Cushingoid symptoms (e.g. moon facies and blood pressure elevation). There is no known therapy for overdosage.

> For management of a suspected drug overdose, CPhA recommends that you contact your **regional Poison Control Centre**. See the *CPS* Directory section for a list of Poison Control Centres.

ACTION AND CLINICAL PHARMACOLOGY: Pharmacodynamics: DEPO-PROVERA (medroxyprogesterone acetate) is a long-acting progestational steroid (progestogen) derived from a natural source (soybeans). Its long duration of action is a result of slow absorption from the injection site. DEPO-PROVERA does not contain estrogen.

For conception control, DEPO-PROVERA inhibits the secretion of gonadotropins which, in turn, prevents follicular maturation and ovulation, and results in endometrial thinning. Additional progestational effects that may contribute to the contraceptive effectiveness of DEPO-PROVERA include the transformation and maintenance of an endometrium hostile to implantation, and thickening of cervical mucus making sperm penetration of the cervix more difficult.

DEPO-PROVERA administered parenterally to women with adequate endogenous estrogen transforms proliferative endometrium into secretory endometrium.

Endometriosis is an estrogen-dependent disorder in women of reproductive age that is characterized by the presence of endometrial-like tissue (glands and stoma) outside the uterine lining. The putative mechanisms of action of DEPO-PROVERA in the treatment of endometriosis is by inhibition of gonadotropin production, induction of decidualization followed by atrophy of endometriotic implants, prevention of follicular maturation and ovulation and decrease in circulating estrogen levels.

Pharmacokinetics: (See Table 9.)

Table 9: DEPO-PROVERA

Summary of Medroxyprogesterone Acetate Suspension for Injection's Pharmacokinetic Parameters in an Adult Women Population

	C_{max}	$t_{½}$ (h)	$AUC_{0-\infty}$	Clearance	Volume of distribution
Single 150 mg i.m.	1–7 ng/mL	≈1000	NA[a]	1600–4000 L/day	20±3 L

[a] Not available.

Absorption: Following intramuscular administration, MPA is slowly released from the injection site, resulting in low, but persistent levels of drug and drug-related materials in the circulation. On average, the time required to obtain a maximum concentration of MPA in the circulation is between 4 and 20 days. Following a single 150 mg IM dose of DEPO-PROVERA, medroxyprogesterone acetate (MPA) concentrations, measured by an extracted radioimmunoassay procedure, increase for approximately 3 weeks to reach peak plasma concentrations of 1 to 7 ng/mL.

Circulating levels of MPA can be detected for as long as 7 to 9 months. Increasing the injection volume of medroxyprogesterone acetate produces an increased rate of absorption and higher serum levels; however, extent of absorption is not affected.

Distribution: Medroxyprogesterone acetate is approximately 90 to 95 percent protein bound. Volume of distribution is reported as 20±3 L. It crosses the blood-brain barrier and is secreted in breast milk.

Metabolism: The principal metabolite of medroxyprogesterone acetate that has been identified is a 6α-methyl-6β, 17α, 21-trihydroxy-4-pregnene-3, 20-dione-17-acetate, which is excreted in the urine. Numerous other metabolites of medroxyprogesterone acetate have been reported; however, these have not been well quantified. Metabolism may be influenced by the route of administration as well as the physical state of the drug.

Excretion: The terminal half-life of MPA is approximately 30 to 60 hours. The elimination half-life following intramuscular administration is approximately 6 weeks, reflecting the prolonged absorption of the drug from the intramuscular injection site. The levels then decrease exponentially until they become undetectable (<100 pg/mL) between 120 to 200 days following injection. Plasma clearance is reported as approximately 1600-4000 L per day. Medroxyprogesterone acetate (as the glucuronide conjugate) is primarily excreted in the feces, via biliary secretion.

Special Populations and Conditions: Hepatic Insufficiency: The effect of hepatic disease on the pharmacokinetics of DEPO-PROVERA is unknown.

Renal Insufficiency: The effect of renal disease on the pharmacokinetics of DEPO-PROVERA is unknown.

STORAGE AND STABILITY: Protect from freezing. Store at controlled room temperature 15 to 30°C. Shake well before using. Keep out of reach of children.

INFORMATION FOR THE PATIENT: Published in e-CPS, available by subscription at www.e-cps.ca.

DOSAGE FORMS, COMPOSITION AND PACKAGING: 50 mg/mL: Each mL contains: medroxyprogesterone acetate 50 mg. Nonmedicinal ingredients: hydrochloric acid, methylparaben, polyethylene glycol, polysorbate, propylparaben, sodium chloride, sodium hydroxide and water for injection. Vials of 5 mL, boxes of 1. Single use only.

150 mg/mL: Each mL contains: medroxyprogesterone acetate 150 mg. Nonmedicinal ingredients: hydrochloric acid, methylparaben, polyethylene glycol, polysorbate, propylparaben, sodium chloride, sodium hydroxide and water for injection. Vials of 1 mL, boxes of 1, 5 and 25.

Depo-Testosterone ©

testosterone cypionate

Androgen

Pfizer

PHARMACOLOGY: Qualitatively similar to testosterone and its esters in physiologic activity, testosterone cypionate has the advantage of prolonged effect. In hypogonadal males, the effect of a single injection of 200 to 400 mg of testosterone cypionate was observed to be maintained for 2 to 4 weeks, which is 2 to 4 times longer than the effect produced by a comparable dose of testosterone propionate.

INDICATIONS: Male: Eunuchism, eunuchoidism, deficiency after castration. Male climacteric symptoms when these are secondary to androgen deficiency. Oligospermia.

Male or Female: Postmenopausal or senile osteoporosis. Androgens are without value as primary therapy, but may be of value as adjunctive therapy. Equal or greater consideration should be given to diet, calcium balance, physiotherapy, and good general health-promoting measures.

CONTRAINDICATIONS: In patients with prostatic carcinoma, severe cardiorenal disease and severe persistent hypercalcemia. *Pregnancy:* Since it may cause masculinization of the female fetus, testosterone cypionate is also contraindicated during pregnancy.

WARNINGS: No data supplied by the manufacturer.

PRECAUTIONS: Since androgens, in general, tend to promote retention of sodium and water, patients receiving testosterone cypionate—in particular, elderly patients—should be observed for edema. Hypercalcemia may occur, particularly in immobilized patients; use of testosterone cypionate should be discontinued as soon as hypercalcemia is detected.

ADVERSE EFFECTS: In the male, excessive doses or prolonged administration of testosterone cypionate may cause inhibition of testicular function resultant oligospermia and decreased ejaculation volume. Gynecomastia has been reported in males treated with testosterone, but this complication usually disappears upon cessation of therapy. In young boys, androgens should be used with caution to avoid precocious sexual development and premature epiphyseal closure.

In the female, large doses of testosterone cypionate may produce masculinization with signs such as hirsutism, deepening of the voice, enlargement of the clitoris, acne, increased libido and menstrual irregularities. With the exception of the voice change, these effects tend to disappear following cessation of therapy.

OVERDOSE:

No data supplied by the manufacturer.

> For management of a suspected drug overdose, CPhA recommends that you contact your **regional Poison Control Centre**. See the *CPS* Directory section for a list of Poison Control Centres.

DOSAGE: Sterile solution of testosterone cypionate is for i.m. use only. Dosage will vary depending upon the individual, the condition being treated, its severity, and prior androgen therapy. Because of the protracted action of testosterone cypionate, injections more frequently than every 2 weeks are seldom required.

Eunuchism, Eunuchoidism: For complete replacement in eunuchs and eunuchoid patients, the usual dose of testosterone cypionate is 200 to 400 mg injected at intervals of 3 to 4 weeks. It is usually preferable to begin treatment with full therapeutic doses, which are later adjusted to individual requirements. Priapism is a sign of excessive dosage and is an indication for temporary withdrawal of androgen therapy.

Impotence due to Testicular Deficiency, Male Climacteric. Testosterone cypionate may be given every 3 to 4 weeks in doses ranging from 200 to 400 mg.

Oligospermia: To stimulate spermatogenesis when trial androgen therapy is indicated in subfertile males with oligospermia, recommended dosage of testosterone cypionate is: (1) 100 to 200 mg every 3 to 6 weeks for development and maintenance of testicular function; or (2) 200 mg each week for 6 to 10 weeks for suppression which may then be followed by rebound spermatogenesis following discontinuance of the injection.

Anabolic Effect, Osteoporosis: The dosage of testosterone cypionate for anabolic effect should be adjusted according to age, sex, and the condition of the individual patient. In the majority of cases, the dose will range from 200 to 400 mg injected every 3 to 4 weeks. In addition, an adequate diet should be provided and prolonged immobilization avoided whenever possible.

SUPPLIED: Each mL contains: testosterone cypionate 100 mg. Nonmedicinal ingredients: benzyl alcohol and benzyl benzoate in cottonseed oil. Vials of 10 mL. Store at room temperature (15 to 30°C). Warming and shaking the vial should redissolve any crystals that may have formed during storage at temperatures lower than recommended.

Dequadin® Preparations

dequalinium chloride

Antibacterial—Antifungal

WellSpring

INDICATIONS: For the treatment of mouth and throat infections.

CONTRAINDICATIONS: Dequalinium chloride sensitivity.

WARNINGS: No data supplied by the manufacturer.

PRECAUTIONS: If irritation persists or sensitization occurs, discontinue use and consult a physician.

ADVERSE EFFECTS: Allergic reactions have been reported rarely.

OVERDOSE:

No data supplied by the manufacturer.

> For management of a suspected drug overdose, CPhA recommends that you contact your **regional Poison Control Centre**. See the *CPS* Directory section for a list of Poison Control Centres.

DOSAGE: Lozenges: Adults and children 2 years of age and older: One lozenge to be dissolved slowly in the mouth, may be repeated every 2 hours as needed.

Oral Paint: Apply freely to infected area, every 2 or 3 hours or as directed by the physician.

SUPPLIED: Lozenges: Each lozenge contains: dequalinium chloride 0.25 mg in a flavored sucrose base. Available in orange and cherry flavors. Energy: 18.0 kJ (4.29 kcal). Sodium: <1 mmol (0.273 mg). Gluten- and tartrazine-free. Blisters of 16.

Oral Paint: Each bottle contains: dequalinium chloride 0.5% w/v in a propylene glycol base. Also contains alcohol 3.0% v/v. Cartoned bottles of 25 mL.

Dermalac™

lactic acid

Alpha-Hydroxy Acid (AHA) Preparation

TaroPharma

SUPPLIED: Cream: Each g contains: neutralized lactic acid 12% w/w. Nonmedicinal ingredients: ammonium hydroxide, cetyl alcohol, glycerin, glyceryl monostearate, lactic acid, laureth-4, light mineral oil, magnesium aluminum silicate, methylcellulose, methylparaben, polyoxyethylene 100 stearate, polyoxyl 40 stearate, propylene glycol, propylparaben and purified water. Tubes of 60 and 140 g.

Lotion: Each g contains: neutralized lactic acid 12% w/w. Nonmedicinal ingredients: ammonium hydroxide, cetyl alcohol, glycerin, glyceryl monostearate, lactic acid, laureth-4, light mineral oil, magnesium aluminum silicate, methylcellulose, methylparaben, polyoxyethylene 100 stearate, polyoxyl 40 stearate, propylene glycol, propylparaben and purified water. Bottles of 225 mL.

Store at room temperature (15 to 30°C). Protect from light.

Derma-Smoothe/FS® Ⓟ

fluocinolone acetonide

Topical Oil

Hill

SUPPLIED: Each bottle contains: fluocinolone acetonide 0.1 mg USP (0.01%). Nonmedicinal ingredients: balsam pine, cream fragrance, isopropyl myristate, mineral oil, oleth-2 and refined peanut oil. Bottles of 118 mL.

Dermatix® Ultra

cyclopentasiloxane— polysilicone-11—phenyl trimethicone—dimethicone—polymethylsilsesquioxane—tetrahexyldecyl ascorbate

Scar Management

Valeant

DESCRIPTION: Dermatix Ultra is a topical silicone gel that is transparent, dries quickly and helps maintain the skin's moisture balance, while aiding the management of damaged skin surfaces resulting from surgery, burns, acne scarring, laser resurfacing and other injuries.

Silicone gel has been shown to flatten, soften and smooth scars, relieve the itching and discomfort of scars as well as reduce the redness and discoloration associated with scars.

Dermatix Ultra formula utilizes four major silicone components exclusively formulated to balance benefits with patients comfort. It also contains a Vitamin C-ester which is a lipid-soluble, non-acidic, and stable form known for its powerful anti-oxidant effect.

INDICATIONS: Dermatix Ultra is used for the treatment and prevention of keloids and hypertrophic scars (such as those resulting from general surgical procedures, trauma wounds, burns, cosmetic procedures and acne), after the wound has healed and the skin surface is intact.

WARNINGS:

- Dermatix Ultra should not be applied to open or fresh wounds.
- Dermatix Ultra should not be placed in contact with mucous membranes, or applied too close to the eyes.
- Dermatix Ultra should not be applied over antibiotic skin preparations or other skin treatments and/or products.

Note: Dermatix Ultra should be applied to clean, dry skin only.

ADVERSE EFFECTS: Rarely, the gel may cause redness, pain or irritation to the skin. If you are concerned about these or any other unwanted effects, consult your pharmacist or doctor.

OVERDOSE:

> For management of a suspected drug overdose, CPhA recommends that you contact your **regional Poison Control Centre**. See the *CPS* Directory section for a list of Poison Control Centres.

DOSAGE: Dermatix Ultra gel is easily applied to all areas of the skin, including the face, joints and flexures, and dries rapidly to form an invisible "sheet".

Wash the affected area and pat dry. Gently massage a small amount of Dermatix Ultra into the scar. If you apply too much gently wipe away any excess with a tissue in order to avoid staining of clothing. Apply twice daily in the morning and evening. Once dry, Dermatix Ultra may be covered with cosmetic blush.

Note: Dermatix Ultra can also be used on children.

SUPPLIED: Each 15 g tube of topical silicone gel contains: cyclopentasiloxane (and) polysilicone-11, phenyl trimethicone (and) polysilicone-11, dimethicone, polymethylsilsesquioxane, tetrahexyldecyl ascorbate. Store below 25°C. Keep gel away from the heat. Keep out of reach of children.

The reader is invited to consult CPhA's monograph **Corticosteroids: Topical**.

Dermatop® ℞
prednicarbate
Topical Corticosteroid

sanofi-aventis

Date of Revision: September 25, 2008

PHARMACOLOGY: Prednicarbate is a mid-potency, nonfluorinated topical corticosteroid. Topical corticosteroids are synthetic derivatives of cortisone which are effective when applied locally to control many types of inflammatory, allergic and pruritic dermatoses. The mechanism of anti-inflammatory activity of topical corticosteroids is unclear. However, corticosteroids are thought to induce phospholipase A2 inhibitor proteins, preventing arachidonic acid release and the biosynthesis of potent mediators of inflammation.

INDICATIONS: For the relief of the inflammatory and pruritic manifestations of acute and chronic corticosteroid-responsive dermatoses. The emollient cream formulation has been shown to be safe and effective in infants and children.

CONTRAINDICATIONS: In those patients with a history of hypersensitivity to any of the components of the preparation. Dermatop emollient cream contains wool alcohols ointment and wool wax alcohols and is contraindicated in individuals hypersensitive to wool/lanolin. Prednicarbate should not be used to treat bacterial/fungal skin infections, tuberculosis of the skin, syphilitic skin infections, chickenpox, eruptions following vaccinations and viral diseases of the skin in general. Prednicarbate is not for ophthalmic use.

WARNINGS: When used under occlusive dressing, over extensive areas, or on the face, scalp, axillae and scrotum, sufficient absorption of the topical corticosteroid may occur giving rise to adrenal suppression and other systemic effects.

PRECAUTIONS: General: Systemic absorption of topical corticosteroids can produce reversible hypothalamic-pituitary-adrenal (HPA) axis suppression. Manifestations of Cushing's syndrome, hyperglycemia, and glucosuria can also be produced in some patients by systemic absorption of topical corticosteroids.

Prednicarbate applied to human skin at 30 g daily for 7 days did not produce an indication of systemic effects on the HPA axis. Conditions which augment systemic absorption include application of the more potent steroids, use over large surface areas, prolonged use, occlusive dressings. Patients receiving a large dose of potent topical steroids to a large surface area or under an occlusive dressing should be evaluated periodically for evidence of HPA axis suppression. This may be done using ACTH stimulation test or other recognized, validated test. If HPA axis suppression is noted, an attempt should be made to withdraw the drug, to reduce the frequency of application, or to substitute a less potent steroid. Recovery of HPA axis is generally prompt and complete upon discontinuation of the drug. Infrequently, signs and symptoms of steroid withdrawal may occur requiring supplemental systemic corticosteroids. Occlusive dressings should not be applied if body temperature is elevated.

To minimize systemic absorption when long-term therapy or large surface area for treatment is likely, periodic interruption of treatment or treatment of one area of the body at a time should be considered.

Children may be more susceptible to systemic toxicity from equivalent dosing due to larger skin surface to body mass ratios (see Children).

If concomitant skin infections are present or develop, an appropriate antifungal or antibacterial agent should be used. If a favorable response does not occur promptly, use of prednicarbate should be discontinued until the infection has been adequately controlled.

If irritation develops, prednicarbate should be discontinued and appropriate therapy instituted. Allergic contact dermatitis from corticosteroids is usually diagnosed by observing "failure to heal" rather than clinical exacerbations as with most topical products not containing corticosteroids. Such an observation should be corroborated with appropriate diagnostic patch testing.

Suitable precautions should be taken when using topical corticosteroids in patients with stasis dermatitis and other skin diseases associated with impaired circulation.

Topical corticosteroids, particularly the more potent ones, should be used with caution on lesions close to the eye because systemic absorption may cause increased intraocular pressure, glaucoma or cataracts.

Prolonged use of topical corticosteroid preparations may produce stria or atrophy of the skin or s.c. tissue. Topical corticosteroids should be used with caution on lesions of the face, groin and axillae as these areas are more prone to atrophic changes than other areas of the body. Frequent observation is important if these areas are to be treated. If skin atrophy is observed, treatment should be discontinued.

Patients should be advised to inform subsequent physicians of the prior use of corticosteroids.

Dermatop contains a paraffin, which can cause leaking or breaking of latex condoms. Contact between Dermatop and latex condoms must therefore be avoided.

Pregnancy: Corticosteroids are generally teratogenic in laboratory animals when administered systemically at relatively low dosage. Prednicarbate has been shown to be teratogenic and embryotoxic in rats and rabbits when administered s.c.

There are no adequate and well-controlled studies in pregnant women on teratogenic effects of prednicarbate. Prednicarbate should be used in pregnancy only if the potential benefit justifies the potential risk to the fetus, particularly in the first trimester of pregnancy. Drugs of this class should not be used extensively on pregnant patients, in large amounts, or for prolonged periods of time. Infants born of mothers who have received substantial doses of corticosteroids during pregnancy should be carefully observed for hypoadrenalism.

Lactation: Systemically administered corticosteroids are secreted into human milk, and could suppress growth, interfere with endogenous corticosteroid production or cause untoward effects. Caution should be exercised when prednicarbate is administered to a nursing mother.

Children: Prednicarbate cream has been shown to be safe and effective in children and infants, and is indicated in this population. A systemic tolerance study using this formulation in patients from 4 to 143 months (mean age=5 years), found no effects on HPA axis function when it was used to treat at least 20% of their total body surface for 21 consecutive days.

The safety and effectiveness of prednicarbate ointment in children and infants have not been established. Because of the higher ratio of skin surface area to body mass, children are at a greater risk than adults for HPA axis suppression when treated with topical corticosteroids. They are also at a greater risk of glucocorticosteroid insufficiency after withdrawal of treatment and of Cushing's syndrome while on treatment. Adverse effects including striae have been reported with use of topical corticosteroids in infants and children. HPA axis suppression, Cushing's syndrome and intracranial hypertension have been reported in children receiving topical corticosteroids. Manifestations of adrenal suppression in children include: linear growth retardation, delayed weight gain, low plasma cortisol and absence of response to ACTH stimulation. Manifestations of intracranial hypertension include bulging fontanelles, headaches and bilateral papilloedema.

Administration of topical corticosteroids to children should be limited to the latest amount compatible with an effective therapeutic regimen. Chronic corticosteroid therapy may interfere with the growth and development of children.

Prednicarbate cream should not be used in the treatment of diaper dermatitis.

Carcinogenesis, Mutagenicity, Reproduction: Long-term animal studies have not been performed to evaluate the carcinogenic potential of prednicarbate. Prednicarbate was not mutagenic in the Salmonella reversion test (Ames test) over a wide range of concentrations in the presence and absence of S-9 microsomal fraction. It was not clastogenic in the mouse micronucleus test when mice were administered doses ranging from 1 to 160 mg/kg of the drug.

Prednicarbate was tested for effects on reproduction. In a study of the effect of prednicarbate on fertility, pregnancy and postnatal development in rats, no effect was noted on the fertility or pregnancy of parent animals or postnatal development of the offspring after administration of up to 0.20 mg/kg/day of prednicarbate s.c. A 0.8 mg/kg/day dose produced slight growth retardation of fetuses and placentas.

Prednicarbate has been shown to be teratogenic and embryotoxic in Wistar rats and Himalayan rabbits when administered s.c. during gestation at doses of 2.24 mg/kg/day and 0.018 to 0.056 mg/kg/day respectively during organogenesis.

In the rats, slightly retarded fetal development and an incidence of thickened and wavy ribs higher than the spontaneous rate were noted. In rabbits, increased liver weights and a slight increase in the fetal intrauterine death rate were observed. The fetuses that were delivered exhibited reduced placental weight, increased frequency of cleft palate, ossification disorders in the sternum, omphalocele, and anomalous posture of the forelimbs.

ADVERSE EFFECTS: In controlled clinical trials in adults, the total incidence of adverse reactions associated with the use of prednicarbate ointment was low (1.6%). These adverse reactions were moderate to severe and are listed in decreasing order of occurrence as follows: pruritus (0.6%), burning (0.3%), drying, scaling and cracking of the skin accompanied by pain (0.3%), and irritant dermatitis with increased pruritus (0.3%).

A similar frequency of adverse reactions (1.8%) was associated with the use of prednicarbate cream in controlled clinical trials with patients aged 12 to 86 years. These adverse reactions were usually mild to moderate in severity and listed in decreasing order of occurrence are as follows: pruritus (0.9%), edema (0.4%), burning sensation (0.4%) and rash (0.4%).

In pediatric studies with patients ranging in age from 2 months to 12 years, the frequency of adverse reactions seen with prednicarbate cream was 5.1%. This was similar to the frequency observed with 1% hydrocortisone cream in the same study (7.8%). Adverse reactions associated with the use of prednicarbate cream were usually mild in severity and are listed in decreasing order of occurrence as follows: application site reaction (2.8%), skin disorder (1.1%), infection (0.6%) and rash (0.6%).

In a controlled study in pediatric patients with atopic dermatitis, mild signs of atrophy were observed in 3 (3%) of the prednicarbate treated subjects (mild telangiectasia and thinness, mild loss of elasticity, mild shininess) and 1 (1%) of the hydrocortisone treated subjects (mild shininess). In an uncontrolled study in a similar patient population, mild signs of atrophy developed in 5 patients (8%) with 2 patients exhibiting more than 1 sign. Two patients (3%) developed shininess, and 2 patients (3%) developed thinness. Three patients were observed with mild telangiectasia. It is unknown whether prior use of topical corticosteroids was a contributing factor in the development of telangiectasia in 2 of the patients.

The following local adverse reactions have been reported infrequently with topical corticosteroids, but may occur more frequently with the use of occlusive dressings. These reactions are listed in an approximate decreasing order of frequency: burning, itching, irritation, dryness, folliculitus, hypertrichosis, acneiform eruptions, hypopigmentation, perioral dermatitis, allergic contact dermatitis, maceration of the skin, secondary infection, skin atrophy, striae, miliaria. In addition, there are reports of the development of pustular psoriasis from chronic plaque psoriasis following reduction or discontinuation of potent topical steroid products.

Adrenal suppression has been reported following topical corticosteroid therapy. Posterior subcapsular cataracts have been reported following systemic use of corticosteroids.

OVERDOSE:

Treatment: No specific antidote to prednicarbate is available and treatment should be symptomatic. Topically applied prednicarbate can be absorbed systemically. Percutaneous absorption is enhanced when large amounts of corticosteroids are applied, when used under occlusive dressing or when used chronically. Toxic effects of hypercorticism and adrenal suppression may appear. Should toxic effects occur, the dosage of prednicarbate should be discontinued slowly, consistent with accepted procedures for discontinuation of chronic steroid therapy. The restoration of hypothalmic-pituitary axis may be slow during periods of pronounced physical stress (severe infections, trauma, surgery); a supplement with systemic steroids may need to be considered. Toxic effects may include ecchymosis of skin, peptic ulceration, hypertension, aggravation of infection, hirsutism, acne, edema and muscle weakness due to protein depletion. Treatment of a patient with systemic toxic manifestations consists of assuring and maintaining a patent airway and supporting ventilation using oxygen and assisted or controlled respiration as required. This usually will be sufficient in the management of most reactions. Should circulatory depression occur, vasopressors such as ephedrine and i.v. fluids may be used. Should a convulsion persist despite oxygen therapy, small increments of an ultra-short acting barbiturate (pentobarbital or secobarbital) may be given i.v. Allergic reactions are characterized by cutaneous lesions, urticaria, edema or anaphylactoid reactions.

For management of a suspected drug overdose, CPhA recommends that you contact your **regional Poison Control Centre**. See the *CPS* Directory section for a list of Poison Control Centres.

DOSAGE: Apply a thin film of prednicarbate to affected areas of skin twice daily. Rub in gently and completely.

Therapy should be limited to 2 weeks. If a symptomatic response is not noted within a few days to a week, the local applications of corticosteroid should be discontinued and the patient re-evaluated. Therapy should be discontinued as soon as lesions heal. Prednicarbate should not be used with occlusive dressings unless directed by the physician.

Prednicarbate emollient cream 0.1% may be used with caution in pediatric patients 1 year of age or older. Prednicarbate emollient cream 0.1% should not be applied in the diaper area if the child still requires diapers or plastic pants as these garments may constitute occlusive dressing.

INFORMATION FOR THE PATIENT: Published in e-CPS, available by subscription at www.e-cps.ca.

SUPPLIED: Emollient Cream: Each tube contains: prednicarbate 0.1%. Nonmedicinal ingredients: benzyl alcohol, edetate sodium, isopropyl myristate, lactic acid, purified water, wool alcohols ointment and wool wax alcohols. Tubes of 20 and 60 g.
Ointment: Each tube contains: prednicarbate 0.1%. Nonmedicinal ingredients: butylated hydroxyanisole, citric acid, glycerin, glyceryl monoleate/dioleate, propylene glycol, 2-octyldodecanol and white petrolatum. Tubes of 60 g.
Store between 15 and 30°C.

DermOtic® Oil Ear Drops ℞
fluocinolone acetonide
Anti-inflammatory—Antipruritic—Vasoconstricting Agent

Hill

SUPPLIED: Each bottle contains: fluocinolone acetonide 0.1 mg USP (0.01%). Nonmedicinal ingredients: balsam pine fragrance, cream fragrance, isopropyl alcohol, isopropyl myristate, mineral oil, oleth-2 and refined peanut oil. Bottles of 20 mL with dropper.

The reader is invited to consult CPhA's monograph **Corticosteroids: Topical**.

Dermovate® ℞
clobetasol 17-propionate
Topical Corticosteroid

TaroPharma

SUPPLIED: Cream 0.05%: Each g contains: clobetasol 17-propionate 0.5 mg. Nonmedicinal ingredients: cetyl alcohol, chlorocresol, citric acid, glyceryl monostearate, glyceryl stearate/PEG 100 stearate, propylene glycol, purified water, stearyl alcohol, sodium citrate and white wax. Tubes of 15 and 50 g.
Ointment 0.05%: Each g contains: clobetasol 17-propionate 0.5 mg. Nonmedicinal ingredients: propylene glycol, sorbitan sesquioleate and white petrolatum. Tubes of 15 and 50 g.
Topical Solution 0.05%: Each g contains: clobetasol 17-propionate 0.5 mg. Nonmedicinal ingredients: carbomer 934P, isopropyl alcohol, purified water and sodium hydroxide for pH adjustment. Bottles of 60 mL.
Store at room temperature (15 to 30°C).

SYMBOLS:
℞ = Prescription required
Ⓒ = Controlled Drug
Ⓝ = Narcotic
T/C = Targeted Controlled Substance

Desferal® Pr

deferoxamine mesylate

Iron and Aluminum Chelating Agent

Novartis Pharmaceuticals

Date of Preparation: December 20, 1972
Date of Revision: May 7, 2010

SUMMARY PRODUCT INFORMATION:

Route of Administration	Dosage Form/ Strength	Clinically Relevant Nonmedicinal Ingredients
Parenteral	Lyophilized powder in vials, 500 mg and 2 g	None. For a complete listing see Dosage Forms, Composition and Packaging.

INDICATIONS AND CLINICAL USE: DESFERAL (deferoxamine mesylate) is indicated for:

- Acute iron intoxication.
- Chronic iron overload due to transfusion-dependent anemias.
- Diagnosis of aluminum overload (DESFERAL (deferoxamine mesylate) infusion test).
- Chronic aluminum overload in patients with End-Stage Renal Failure (ESRF) under maintenance dialysis.

In cases of acute iron intoxication, DESFERAL is an adjunct to, and not a substitute for, standard therapeutic measures which may include:

- Induction of emesis.
- Gastric lavage.
- Maintenance of clear airways.
- Control of peripheral vascular failure.
- Correction of acidosis.

Geriatrics (≥65 years of age): Clinical Studies of DESFERAL did not include sufficient numbers of subjects aged 65 years and over to determine whether they respond differently from the younger subjects. Post marketing reports suggest a possible trend for an increased risk of eye disorders in the geriatric population, specifically the occurrence of color blindness, maculopathy, and scotoma. However, it is unclear if these eye disorders were dose related. Although the number of reports was very small, certain elderly patients may be predisposed to eye disorders when taking DESFERAL. Post marketing reports also suggest that there may be an increased risk of deafness and hearing loss in the geriatric population (see Adverse Reactions). In general, dose selection for an elderly patient should be cautious, usually starting at the low end of the dosing range, reflecting the greater frequency of decreased hepatic, renal, or cardiac function, and of concomitant disease or other drug therapy.

Pediatrics (<16 years of age): High doses of DESFERAL and concomitant low ferritin levels during the treatment of chronic iron overload in children, have been associated with growth retardation. After reduction of the DESFERAL dose, growth velocity may resume to pre-treatment levels in some patients.

Pediatric patients receiving DESFERAL should be monitored for body weight and longitudinal growth every three months.

CONTRAINDICATIONS: Patients who are hypersensitive to deferoxamine mesylate or component of the container, except where desensitization is successful. For a complete listing, see Dosage Forms, Composition and Packaging.

WARNINGS AND PRECAUTIONS: General: Therapy with DESFERAL should be initiated and maintained by physician experienced in the treatment of chronic iron overload due to blood transfusions.

It should be noted that some of the signs and symptoms reported as adverse effects may in fact be manifestations of the underlying disease (iron and/or aluminum overload).

As with all medicines, DESFERAL should be kept out of reach of children.

Ear/Nose/Throat: There have been reports of hearing loss and audiometric abnormalities occurring in patients receiving DESFERAL treatment, particularly where the doses used were higher than those recommended and/or where the serum ferritin levels were low. The hearing loss returned to normal in several cases when the drug was discontinued. However in some cases, a residual effect remained. Renal failure patients receiving maintenance dialysis having low ferritin levels may be particularly prone to adverse reactions.

When low-dose therapy is used the risk of adverse reactions is reduced. If disturbances of hearing occur, treatment with DESFERAL should be discontinued in order to further the chances that disturbances of hearing will prove reversible. If treatment with DESFERAL is subsequently resumed using a reduced dosage, auditory examination/testing should be performed at more frequent intervals. It is always important to reconsider the benefit/risk ratio when DESFERAL treatment is resumed after the occurrence of an adverse reaction.

Endocrine and Metabolism: DESFERAL may lower blood sugar, serum calcium, and serum sodium, and increase blood coagulability. Therefore, these parameters should be monitored during therapy, if possible.

Infections and Infestations: In patients suffering from iron overload it has been reported that infections (including septicemia), especially with *Y. enterocolitica* and *Y. pseudotuberculosis*, may be promoted by DESFERAL (deferoxamine mesylate). If a patient under treatment with DESFERAL develops fever accompanied by acute enteritis/enterocolitis, diffuse abdominal pain, or pharyngitis the treatment should be temporarily withdrawn, appropriate bacteriological tests performed, and suitable antibiotic therapy instituted at once. **This therapy should include special coverage for Yersinia organisms.** After the infection has cleared, treatment with DESFERAL can be resumed.

In patients undergoing maintenance hemodialysis while receiving DESFERAL for aluminum and/or iron overload, rare cases of mucormycosis have been reported, a severe fungal infection that can be fatal. DESFERAL abolishes the fungistatic effect of serum and increased the in vitro growth of the fungus by potentiating iron uptake by the fungus. If any of the suspected signs or symptoms are observed, DESFERAL treatment should be discontinued, mycological tests performed and appropriate treatment instituted immediately. Mucormycosis may also occur in dialysis patients who are not receiving DESFERAL therapy, indicating that other factors, e.g. a compromised immune system, may play a role in the development of this infection.

Neurologic: In patients with aluminum-related encephalopathy, high doses of DESFERAL may exacerbate neurological dysfunction (convulsion), probably due to an increase in circulating aluminum. DESFERAL may also precipitate the onset of dialysis dementia. Pretreatment with clonazepam is reported to provide protection against such neurological deterioration. In addition, aluminum overload treatment may decrease serum calcium and aggravate hyperparathyroidism.

Ophthalmologic: There have been reports of visual disturbances occurring in patients receiving DESFERAL treatment, particularly where the doses used were higher than those recommended and/or where the serum ferritin levels were low. The visual disturbances returned to normal in several cases when the drug was discontinued. However in some cases, a residual effect remained. Renal failure patients receiving maintenance dialysis having low ferritin levels may be particularly prone to adverse reactions.

Visual symptoms have been reported after single doses of DESFERAL.

During chronic toxicity tests in dogs, high doses of DESFERAL (>200 mg/kg daily) were associated with cataracts. However, cataracts have rarely been observed in humans who receive DESFERAL over prolonged periods.

When low-dose therapy is used the risk of adverse reactions is reduced. If disturbances of vision occur, treatment with DESFERAL should be discontinued in order to further the chances that disturbances of vision will prove reversible. If treatment with DESFERAL is subsequently resumed using a reduced dosage, ophthalmological examination/testing should be performed at more frequent intervals. It is always important to reconsider the benefit/risk ratio when DESFERAL treatment is resumed after the occurrence of an adverse reaction.

Renal: In patients with severe renal failure, caution is indicated as the DESFERAL-metal complexes are excreted mainly via the kidneys. Elimination of chelated iron and aluminum can be increased by dialysis.

Isolated cases of acute renal failure have been reported (see Adverse Reactions).

Respiratory: Respiratory distress syndrome has been reported in patients with acute iron intoxication and also in thalassemic patients treated with excessively high doses of intravenous DESFERAL for more than one day. The daily dose should not exceed 80 mg/kg up to a maximum of 6 grams. Treatment should be terminated at the first signs of respiratory complications (see Dosage and Administration).

Sensitivity/Resistance: Patients may develop sensitivity reactions (see Contraindications).

Skin: Flushing of the skin, urticaria, hypotension, and shock have occurred in a few patients following the rapid intravenous injection of DESFERAL (deferoxamine mesylate). Treatment by intravenous route should **not** exceed 15 mg/kg/h.

Special Populations: Pregnant Women: In animal experiments, deferoxamine mesylate has proven teratogenic. Women of childbearing potential with chronic iron and/or aluminum overload should not receive DESFERAL unless the use of an effective form of contraception, established before treatment, is continued throughout treatment and for at least the first month after treatment. Those patients reported to have received DESFERAL therapy during pregnancy have born children without any malformations. However, during pregnancy, particularly in the first trimester, DESFERAL should only be used if the hazard of acute iron intoxication is considered to be greater than the potential teratogenic hazard of DESFERAL.

Nursing Women: It is not known whether deferoxamine mesylate passes into the breast milk. Therefore, mothers receiving DESFERAL should not breast feed their infants.

Pediatrics (<16 years of age): Pediatric patients receiving DESFERAL should be monitored for body weight and longitudinal growth every three months.

High doses of DESFERAL and concomitant low ferritin levels during the treatment of chronic iron overload in children, have been associated with growth retardation. After reduction of the DESFERAL dose, growth velocity may resume to pre-treatment levels in some patients.

Geriatrics (>65 years of age): Clinical Studies of DESFERAL did not include sufficient numbers of subjects aged 65 years and over to determine whether they respond differently from the younger subjects. Post marketing reports suggest a possible trend for an increased risk of eye disorders in the geriatric population, specifically the occurrence of color blindness, maculopathy, and scotoma. However, it is unclear if these eye disorders were dose related. Although the number of reports was very small, certain elderly patients may be predisposed to eye disorders when taking DESFERAL. Post marketing reports also suggest that there may be an increased risk of deafness and hearing loss in the geriatric population (see Adverse Reactions). In general, dose selection for an elderly patient should be cautious, usually starting at the low end of the dosing range, reflecting the greater frequency of decreased hepatic, renal, or cardiac function, and of concomitant disease or other drug therapy.

Monitoring and Laboratory Tests: Complete ophthalmological examination, audiological testing and studies of visual evoked potential should be carried out before the start of long-term DESFERAL treatment as well as at regular intervals preferably every 3 months, during the time that DESFERAL treatment is continued.

The following parameters (blood sugar, serum calcium, serum sodium, and increase blood coagulability) should be monitored during therapy, if possible.

Pediatric patients receiving DESFERAL should be monitored for body weight and longitudinal growth every three months.

ADVERSE REACTIONS: Adverse Drug Reaction Overview: Some of the signs and symptoms reported as adverse effects may also be manifestations of the underlying disease (iron and/or aluminum overload).

Clinical Trial Adverse Drug Reactions: Because clinical trials are conducted under very specific conditions the adverse reaction rates observed in the clinical trials may not reflect the rates observed in practice and should not be compared to the rates in the clinical trials of another drug. Adverse drug reaction information from clinical trials is useful for identifying drug-related adverse events and for approximating rates.

Adverse reactions (Table 1 and section Less Common Clinical Trial Adverse Drug Reactions (<1%)) are ranked under the heading of frequency estimate, the most frequent first, using the following convention: very common (≥1/10); common (≥1/100 to <1/10); uncommon (≥1/1000 to <1/100); rare (≥1/10 000 to <1/1000); very rare (<1/10 000) including isolated reports. Within each frequency grouping, adverse reactions are ranked in order of decreasing seriousness.

The following unwanted effects have been observed: See Table 1.

Table 1: DESFERAL

Unwanted Effects

Nervous System	
Common	Headache
Gastrointestinal	
Common	Nausea
Skin and Subcutaneous Tissue	
Common	Urticaria
Musculoskeletal and Connective Tissue	
Very common	Arthralgia, myalgia
Common	Growth retardation and bone disorder (e.g. metaphyseal dysplasia) in higher doses and young children (see Warnings and Precautions and Special Remarks below)
General and Administration Site	
Very common	Injection site reaction including pain, swelling, infiltration, erythema, pruritus, eschar, crust (see Special Remarks below)
Common	Pyrexia

Special Remarks: Musculoskeletal and Connective Tissue Disorders: Growth retardation and bone disorder (e.g. metaphyseal dysplasia) are common with doses of above 60 mg/kg, especially those who begin iron chelation in the first three years of life. With doses of 40 mg/kg or less, the risk is considerably reduced.

General Disorders and Administration Site Conditions: At the injection site, reactions including pain, swelling, infiltration, erythema, pruritus, and eschar/crust are very common, vesicles, local edema and burning uncommon reactions. The local manifestations may be accompanied by systemic reactions like arthralgia/myalgia (very common), headache (common), urticaria (common), nausea (common), pyrexia (common), vomiting (uncommon), abdominal pain (uncommon) or asthma (uncommon).

Less Common Clinical Trial Adverse Drug Reactions (<1%): Blood and Lymphatic System: Very rare: blood disorder (incl. thrombocytopenia), leucopenia.

Ear and Labyrinth: Uncommon: deafness neurosensory, tinnitus (see Warnings and Precautions and Special Remarks below).

Eye: Rare: loss of vision, scotoma, retinal degeneration, optic neuritis, cataracts, visual acuity decreased, blurred vision, night blindness, visual field defects, chromatopsia (impairment of colour vision), corneal opacities (see Warnings and Precautions and Special Remarks below).

Gastrointestinal: Uncommon: vomiting, abdominal pain. Very rare: diarrhea.

General and Administration Site: Uncommon: injection site reaction including vesicles, edema, burning.

Immune System: Very rare: anaphylactic reaction, anaphylactic shock, angioneurotic oedema.

Infections and Infestations: Rare: mucormycosis (see Warnings and Precautions). Very rare: gastroenteritis Yersinia (see Warnings and Precautions).

Musculoskeletal and Connective Tissue: Very rare: bone pain. Unknown: muscle spasms.

Nervous System: Very rare: neurological disturbances, dizziness, precipitation or exacerbation of aluminium-related dialysis encephalopathy, neuropathy peripheral, paraesthesia (see Warnings and Precautions).

Unknown: convulsion.

Renal and Urinary: Unknown: acute renal failure, renal tubular disorder, blood creatinine increased.

Respiratory, Thoracic and Mediastinal: Uncommon: asthma. Very rare: acute respiratory distress, lung infiltration (see Warnings and Precautions).

Skin and Subcutaneous Tissue: Very rare: rash generalized.

Vascular: Rare: hypotension (if precautions for administration are not adhered to).

Special Remarks: Ear and Labyrinth Disorders: Deafness neurosensory and tinnitus are uncommon if doses are kept within guidelines and if doses are reduced when ferritin levels fall (ratio of the mean daily dose of Desferal divided by the serum ferritin should be below 0.025).

Eye Disorders: The various eye disorders are rare, except if high doses are given (see Warnings and Precautions).

Hepatic Impairment: Rare cases of hepatic impairment have been reported in patients who have been treated with DESFERAL, however a causality with the drug is not established.

Rare cases of increased transaminases have been reported in patients who have been treated with DESFERAL, however a causality with the drug is not established.
Nervous System Disorders: Convulsion has been mainly reported in dialyzed patients with aluminum overload.

DRUG INTERACTIONS: Drug-Drug Interactions: Concomitant use of Prochlorperazine: Concurrent treatment with DESFERAL and prochlorperazine, a phenothiazine derivative, may lead to temporary impairment of consciousness.
Concomitant Use of Vitamin C: Where an iron-overload is associated with ascorbic acid deficiency, oral administration of Vitamin C in the standard dosage (150-250 mg daily) may serve to enhance excretion of the iron complex in response to DESFERAL. Larger doses of Vitamin C fail to produce an additional effect.

In patients with severe chronic iron overload receiving combined treatment of DESFERAL with high doses of Vitamin C (more than 500 mg daily) impairment of cardiac function may be experienced; the impaired cardiac function proved reversible when the Vitamin C was withdrawn. Cardiac impairment results from high doses of Vitamin C which increases the labile iron within the tissues to toxic levels.

The following precautions should be taken when DESFERAL and Vitamin C are to be used concomitantly:
- Vitamin C supplements should not be given to patients with cardiac failure.
- Cardiac function should be monitored before commencing and during the combined therapy of DESFERAL and Vitamin C.
- Vitamin C therapy should be initiated only after an initial month of regular DESFERAL therapy.
- Vitamin C therapy should be given only if patient is receiving DESFERAL regularly (ideally soon after setting up the pump).
- Daily doses of approximately 200 mg of Vitamin C in adults, 100 mg of Vitamin C in older children and 50 mg of Vitamin C in children under 10 years, should not be exceeded.

Concomitant use of Erythropoietin: There is evidence that aluminum intoxication causes reduced erythropoiesis. In dialysis patients with iron and/or aluminum overload receiving DESFERAL and erythropoietin, it is important to adjust the dosage of the latter when necessary. Regular monitoring of iron stores should also be conducted. Gallium-67-imaging results may be distorted due to rapid urinary excretion of DESFERAL-bound Gallium-67. Discontinuing DESFERAL treatment 48 hours prior to scintigraphy is recommended.

DOSAGE AND ADMINISTRATION: Dosing Considerations: DESFERAL (deferoxamine mesylate) **should only be given parenterally. The dose should not exceed 6 grams in a twenty-four hour period.** Although DESFERAL can be given by intramuscular injection, in most cases it exerts a considerably greater effect when administered by continuous infusion either intravenously (especially in cases of acute iron intoxication) or subcutaneously (especially in patients with chronic iron overload).
Recommended Dose and Dosage Adjustment: Acute Iron Intoxication: DESFERAL is an adjunct to standard measures generally used in treating acute iron intoxication, which may include induction of emesis, gastric lavage, maintenance of clear airways, control of peripheral vascular failure, and correction of acidosis.

Treatment should be adapted to the severity of the intoxication, with reference to serum iron (SI) and total iron binding capacity (TIBC) which should be regularly monitored. In addition, the total amount of iron ingested and remaining in the gastrointestinal tract should be taken into account.

DESFERAL should be instituted I.V. or I.M. in:

a. All patients with SI >TIBC (>500 µg/dL or 89.5 µmol/L),
b. Any patient with SI >350 µg/dL or 62.6 µmol/L (if TIBC is unavailable) and evidence of free iron, or
c. Any patient where SI is not readily available and the patient demonstrates the signs and symptoms of iron intoxication.
   Note: Leukocytosis (WBC >15 000/mm^3), hyperglycemia (blood sugar >150 mg/dL) or diarrhea strongly suggest SI will be in the toxic range.

Intravenous Infusion: The intravenous route should be used when the patient is hypotensive, in shock or major clinical findings are present. In general, provided infusion lines can be readily established and maintained, and SI levels and TIBC can be readily monitored, intravenous infusion is the preferred route of administration. Infusion rates should be adapted to the severity of intoxication. The rate of infusion should not exceed 15 mg/kg/h and should be reduced as soon as the situation permits, usually after 4 to 6 hours such that the total intravenous dose does not exceed 80 mg/kg up to a maximum of 6 grams in 24 hours. Respiratory distress syndrome has been reported following intravenous administration of excessive doses of DESFERAL. Treatment should be interrupted if signs of toxicity occur.
Intramuscular Route: The intramuscular route may be used when the patient is normotensive. When administering DESFERAL in children by the intramuscular route, initially inject 90 mg/kg. This may be followed by 45 mg/kg every four to twelve hours, as necessary, up to a maximum of 6 grams per 24 hours. **In children, the maximum single injection should not exceed 1 gram (2 grams in adults).** Attention should be given to volume of solution injected and in small children, two injection sites may be required.

Duration of treatment with DESFERAL by either route will depend on the patient's condition and should be based on the SI levels and TIBC.

The effectiveness of treatment is dependent on an adequate output of urine in order to ensure that the iron complex ferrioxamine is excreted from the body. If oliguria or anuria develop, peritoneal dialysis or hemodialysis may become necessary to remove the ferrioxamine.
Chronic Iron Overload: The daily dose of DESFERAL in children and adults should be tailored to the iron burden of the individual patient as reflected by serum ferritin levels and 24-hour urinary iron excretion. These levels should be monitored daily initially and thereafter at longer intervals (but not less than once every 2 weeks).

Intravenous infusions usually prove somewhat more effective than subcutaneous infusions, but the latter are particularly suitable for ambulant patients.

For subcutaneous infusions, a portable light-weight infusion pump is a practical, effective means of promoting sustained and substantial net urinary iron excretion. The usual needle used is a 25-gauge or 27-gauge, butterfly type, placed in the subcutaneous tissues of the anterior abdominal wall.

For the purpose of infusion treatment the average daily dose range is 1-4 g (20-60 mg/kg depending upon iron load) administered S.C. or I.V. over a period of approximately 12 hours. In some cases it is possible to achieve a further increase in iron excretion by infusing the same daily dose over a 24-hour period. When administered S.C. by pump, DESFERAL should be given 4 to 7 times per week depending on the severity of the iron overload. Patients with serum ferritin levels less than 2000 ng/mL require approximately 25 mg/kg/day. Doses of 35 mg/kg/day are required when serum ferritin levels are in the range of 2000 ng/mL to 3000 ng/mL. Higher doses should be administered only if tests the benefits outweigh the risks associated with repeated high daily doses.

For intramuscular treatment when more effective subcutaneous infusions are not feasible, the average initial dose is 0.5-1 g daily, given in 1-2 injections. The maintenance dose will depend on the patient's iron excretion rate.

Since the iron excretion rates obtained with the above-mentioned modes of administration vary from patient to patient, one should first determine which route and dosage will yield the best results for the individual.
Diagnosis of Aluminum Overload: Use in Adults with ESRF: Serum aluminum levels should be determined before and after DESFERAL administration. The DESFERAL Infusion Test is recommended in patients with serum aluminum levels exceeding 60 ng/mL (2.22 µmol/L) associated with serum ferritin levels above 100 ng/mL. A blood sample is taken just prior to a hemodialysis session to determine the baseline serum aluminum level. A 5 mg/kg dose of DESFERAL is given as a single, slow I.V. infusion at an infusion rate not exceeding 15 mg/kg/h, ideally during post-dialysis to avoid loss of free drug. An acceptable compromise is during the last 60 minutes of the hemodialysis session. A continuous increase in serum aluminum during the 24-48 hour period following administration is suggestive of aluminum overload. The Test is considered positive if the serum aluminum levels increase above baseline by more than 150 ng/mL (5.55 µmol/L) when a second blood sample is taken at the start of the next hemodialysis session.

The diagnostic capability of the DESFERAL Infusion Test is greatly enhanced if performed in conjunction with histological and biochemical examination of a bone biopsy.
Use in Children with ESRF: Little clinical experience has been gained to date on use of DESFERAL in aluminum-overloaded children, the condition being rare in the very young. Dosage should be adapted from the adult dose at the discretion of the physician and adjusted for body-weight (15-20 mg/kg).
Chronic Aluminum Overload in Patients with ESRF: The precise dosage should be individually determined and adapted during the course of treatment.

DESFERAL should be used in the treatment of patients having symptoms or evidence of organ dysfunction due to aluminum overload. In addition, treatment should be considered in symptomatic patients if serum aluminum levels are consistently above 60 ng/mL (2.22 µmol/L) and are associated with a positive DESFERAL Infusion Test (see above), particularly if bone biopsy findings present evidence of aluminum-related bone disease. DESFERAL should be given once weekly at a 5 mg/kg dose administered as a slow intravenous infusion not exceeding 15 mg/kg/h infusion rate, ideally during post-dialysis to avoid loss of free drug. An acceptable compromise is during the last 60 minutes of the hemodialysis session.

After completing the first 3-month course of DESFERAL treatment, followed by a 4 week wash out period, the DESFERAL Infusion Test should be performed. If two successive performed at 1-month intervals yield an increase in serum aluminum levels of less than 75 ng/mL (2.78 µmol/L) above baseline, further treatment is not recommended.

Patients on Continuous Ambulatory or Cyclic Peritoneal Dialysis: A 5 mg/kg dose once per week prior to the final daily exchange. The intraperitoneal route is recommended in these patients, however, DESFERAL is equally effective when administered I.M., by slow I.V., or S.C. infusion. The mode of administration should be individually determined and the dosage adapted during the course of therapy.
Administration: Reconstitution of Lyophilized Vials: The sterile lyophilized powder in each vial should be reconstituted under aseptic conditions just prior to dilution, only with Sterile Water for Injection. DESFERAL is dissolved by adding 5 mL of sterile water for injection to each 500 mg vial or 20 mL of sterile water for injection to each 2 g vial. The DESFERAL solution should appear clear and colorless to slightly yellow at the recommended concentration of 10%.

The final volume of the reconstituted Lyophilized Vial is greater than the specified volume of Sterile Water for injection.
Dilution of Reconstituted Solution for I.V. Infusion: Reconstituted solutions that have been prepared with Sterile Water for Injection can be further diluted with physiological saline (0.9%), glucose in water or Ringer's lactate for infusion prior to infusion. The use of freshly prepared diluted solutions is recommended. Reconstituted solutions and solutions further diluted for infusion should be used or discarded within 24 hours from reconstitution when protected from heat (i.e., store below 23°C) due to the possibility of microbial contamination during preparation. Discard any infusion solution found to have particulate matter or discoloration.

For clinical situations requiring a smaller volume of solution (e.g., I.M injection) the reconstitution Table 2 below is to be considered.

Table 2: DESFERAL
Reconstitution Table

Vial Size	Volume of Diluent to be Added to Vial	Approximate Available Volume	Nominal Concentration per mL
500 mg	2 mL	2.38 mL	210 mg/mL
2 g	8 mL	9.52 mL	210 mg/mL

This concentration may produce a stronger yellow-colored solution. The drug should be completely dissolved before the solution is withdrawn.
Incompatibilities: Heparin injectable solution or physiological saline (0.9%) should not be used to reconstitute the vials of lyophilized powder.

OVERDOSAGE:
Since DESFERAL (deferoxamine mesylate) is available only for parenteral administration, acute intoxication is unlikely to occur.

Rapid intravenous injection of DESFERAL exceeding 15 mg/kg/h has produced flushing of the skin, urticaria, hypotension and shock (see Warnings and Precautions).

Tachycardia, hypotension and gastrointestinal symptoms have occasionally developed in patients who received overdoses of DESFERAL.

Inadvertent I.V. administration of an overdose of DESFERAL may be associated with acute but transient vision loss, aphasia, agitation, headache, nausea, bradycardia and hypotension.

Respiratory distress syndrome including death has been reported following intravenous administration of excessive doses of DESFERAL (see Warnings and Precautions).

High doses of DESFERAL for the treatment of chronic iron and/or aluminum overload have resulted in visual disturbances and hearing loss (see Warnings and Precautions).
Treatment: There is no specific antidote. Signs and symptoms of overdosage may be eliminated by reducing the dosage or interrupting treatment. DESFERAL is dialyzable.

For management of a suspected drug overdose, CPhA recommends that you contact your regional Poison Control Centre. See the *CPS* Directory section for a list of Poison Control Centres.

ACTION AND CLINICAL PHARMACOLOGY: Mechanism of Action: DESFERAL (deferoxamine mesylate) is a chelating agent which forms complexes predominantly with trivalent iron and aluminum ions; it is thus of value in the treatment of acute/chronic iron intoxication, and also chronic aluminum overload in dialysis patients with end-stage renal failure (ESRF).

DESFERAL complexes with iron to form ferrioxamine, a stable chelate, which cannot take part in further chemical reactions. It can also mobilize and chelate tissue-bound aluminum, forming an aluminoxamine complex. Both complexes—ferrioxamine and aluminoxamine—are freely soluble in water and are readily excreted through the kidneys. Excreted ferrioxamine gives the urine a characteristic reddish colour. Some of the DESFERAL-metal complexes are also excreted in feces.

Theoretically chelation occurs on a 1:1 molar basis, hence 100 parts by weight of DESFERAL can bind approximately 8.5 and 4.1 parts by weight of trivalent iron and aluminum respectively.

Although primarily effective in raising iron and aluminum excretion, DESFERAL may also cause a slight increase in the excretion of sodium and calcium.
Pharmacodynamics: DESFERAL (deferoxamine mesylate) is a chelating agent which forms complexes predominantly with trivalent iron and aluminum ions: the complex formation constants are 10^{31} and 10^{25} respectively. Affinity for divalent ions such as iron, copper, zinc and calcium is substantially lower (complex formation constants $\leq 10^{14}$). It has little influence on the excretion of trace elements.

Following parenteral administration of DESFERAL, tissue iron and aluminum are mobilized resulting in a sharp rise in serum iron and/or aluminum concentration(s).

DESFERAL chelates iron, either free or bound in ferritin and hemosiderin, forming the complex ferrioxamine. DESFERAL can also mobilize and chelate tissue-bound aluminum forming an aluminoxamine complex. Since both ferrioxamine and aluminoxamine are completely excreted, DESFERAL promotes iron and aluminum excretion in the urine and feces, thereby reducing pathological iron and/or aluminum deposits in the organs.

Clinical studies have shown that ascorbic acid, when taken orally at least 3 days before DESFERAL is given, considerably enhances (by an average of 96%) the iron excretion. This action of ascorbic acid is probably due to its reducing property which facilitates the mobilization of iron from ferritin by producing a dissociable pool of ferrous ions that are then available for binding to transferrin or a chelating agent such as deferoxamine. DESFERAL is not capable of removing iron from the bone marrow or from the erythrocytes.
Pharmacokinetics: Absorption: DESFERAL is very poorly absorbed orally but well absorbed by the intramuscular and subcutaneous routes.
Distribution: The serum protein-binding rate is less than 10%. It is distributed throughout all body fluids.
Metabolism: Metabolites were isolated and identified from the urine of patients being treated for iron overload. The metabolism reactions to occur were transamination and oxidation yielding an acid metabolite, beta-oxidation also yielding an acid metabolite, decarboxylation and N-hydroxylation yielding natural metabolites.
Excretion: It is excreted through the kidneys by glomerular filtration and tubular secretion.

In healthy subjects and in patients with transfusion-induced iron overload, plasma concentrations of between 80 and 130 µmol/L were recorded 3 minutes after an intravenous injection of deferoxamine (10 mg/kg), these concentrations falling to one-half within 5-10 minutes and thereafter declining more slowly. This rapid fall in the concentration is due not only to distribution and excretion of the active substance but also both to formation of the iron complex ferrioxamine (which commences within a few minutes and the extent of which depends on the individual's iron status) and to metabolic transformation.

During continuous subcutaneous or intravenous infusion of deferoxamine (100 mg/kg in 24 mL sterile water at a rate of 1 mL per hour), the plasma concentrations of deferoxamine and ferrioxamine in healthy subjects rose—depending on the subject's individual iron status (serum ferritin concentration)—to a plateau after 6 or, more frequently, after 12 hours, i.e. to maximum levels of 20 µmol/L for deferoxamine and 2.75 µmol/L for ferrioxamine. The corresponding values in patients were 8.3 µmol/L for deferoxamine and 12.9 µmol/L for ferrioxamine. The 48-hour urinary excretion averaged 118 µmol in the healthy subjects and 836 µmol in the patients. In patients with hemochromatosis, the increase in iron excretion occurring in response to deferoxamine was roughly just as high in the feces as in the urine.

Within 12 hours after deferoxamine had been administered to 20 volunteers, 33.1% of the dose was excreted in the urine (the bulk of it in the first 3 hours) in the form of deferoxamine and ferrioxamine and the remainder in the form of metabolites; the corresponding figure in a patient with hemochromatosis was 60.5% of the dose. There are reported cases where deferoxamine was diluted with water and given by mouth or stomach tube after gastric aspiration and lavage in the treatment of acute iron overload. The aqueous deferoxamine solution was left in the stomach to bind unabsorbed iron in the gastrointestinal tract to prevent further absorption. Note however, that the efficacy of oral deferoxamine for this purpose is not clearly established.

In ESRF dialysis patients who received 40 mg/kg DESFERAL infused I.V. over 1 hour, plasma concentration at the end of infusion was 152 µmol/L (85.2 µg/mL) when the infusion was given between dialysis sessions. Plasma concentrations of DESFERAL were between 13 and 27% lower when the infusion was administered during dialysis. In all cases, concentrations of ferrioxamine were approximately 7.0 µmol/L (4.3 µg/mL); and for aluminoxamine 2.0-3.0 µmol/L (1.2-1.8 µg/mL). After infusion was discontinued, plasma concentration of DESFERAL decreased rapidly with a half life of 20 minutes. A smaller fraction of the dose was eliminated with a longer half life of 14 hours. The plasma concentrations of aluminoxamine continued to increase for up to 48 hours after infusion and reached values of approximately 7.0 µmol/L (4.0 µg/mL). Following dialysis the plasma concentration of aluminoxamine dropped to 2.2 µmol/L (1.3 µg/mL).

During peritoneal dialysis DESFERAL is absorbed if administered in the dialysis fluid.

STORAGE AND STABILITY: Protect vials from heat (store below 25°C).

INFORMATION FOR THE PATIENT: Published in e-CPS, available by subscription at www.e-cps.ca.

DOSAGE FORMS, COMPOSITION AND PACKAGING: 500 mg: Each vial of white to practically white sterile lyophilized powder contains: deferoxamine mesylate 500 mg. Nonmedicinal ingredients: none. Vials of 7.5 mL, cartons of 10. Protect vials from heat (store below 25°C).

2 g: Each vial of white to practically white sterile lyophilized powder contains: deferoxamine mesylate 2 g. Nonmedicinal ingredients: none. Vials of 50 mL, cartons of 1. Protect vials from heat (store below 25°C).

Desferrioxamine Mesilate for Injection BP Ⓟ

desferrioxamine mesilate

Iron and Aluminum Chelating Agent

Hospira

SUPPLIED: 500 mg: Each vial of lyophilized powder for reconstitution contains: desferrioxamine mesilate 500 mg. Nonmedicinal ingredients: none. Single use vials, cartons of 10. Store between 15 and 25°C. Protect from light. Discard unused portion.

2 g: Each vial of lyophilized powder for reconstitution contains: desferrioxamine mesilate 2 g. Nonmedicinal ingredients: none. Single use vials, cartons of 1. Store between 15 and 25°C. Protect from light. Discard unused portion.

Desipramine Ⓟ

Antidepressant—Analgesic

CPhA Monograph

Date of Preparation: October 2009

This monograph has been compiled by CPhA and reviewed by experts. It may contain information different from that found in Health Canada-approved Product Monographs. The reader is referred to the *CPS* Editorial Policy for more information.

SUMMARY PRODUCT INFORMATION:

Route of Administration	Dosage Form	Strength
Oral	Tablet	10 mg, 25 mg, 50 mg, 75 mg, 100 mg

INDICATIONS AND CLINICAL USE: Desipramine is indicated for:
- treatment of major depressive disorder.

Desipramine has also been used:
- as an atypical analgesic agent in the management of chronic peripheral neuropathic pain or other chronic pain conditions.
- in the management of abdominal pain associated with diarrhea-predominant irritable bowel syndrome (IBS). In constipation-predominant IBS, use of desipramine may exacerbate symptoms.
- as a second-line agent in the management of anxiety disorders (e.g., panic disorder, generalized anxiety disorder).
- as a second- or third-line agent in the treatment of attention deficit hyperactivity disorder (ADHD).

CONTRAINDICATIONS:
- Patients who are hypersensitive to desipramine or to any ingredient in the formulation or component of the container.
- Cross-sensitivity between desipramine and other tricyclic antidepressants (TCAs) is possible.
- Desipramine should not be used in conjunction with or within 14 days after monoamine oxidase inhibitor use.
- Desipramine is contraindicated for use in heart block or during the acute recovery period following myocardial infarction.

WARNINGS AND PRECAUTIONS: Cardiovascular: Use with caution in patients with cardiovascular disease; desipramine has been associated with conduction defects, arrhythmia, stroke and acute myocardial infarction. Desipramine may also cause orthostatic hypotension.

Endocrine and Metabolism: Use with caution in patients with diabetes mellitus as desipramine may decrease insulin sensitivity and cause hyperglycemia. Use of desipramine in patients who are hyperthyroid may result in cardiovascular toxicity including arrhythmias.

Gastrointestinal: Use with caution in patients with decreased gastrointestinal motility and paralytic ileus due to the potential anticholinergic effects of desipramine.

Genitourinary: Use with caution in patients with urinary retention, benign prostatic hyperplasia as potential anticholinergic effects of desipramine may aggravate symptoms.

Hematologic: Desipramine has been rarely associated with bone marrow suppression, which may be of concern if a patient presents with signs of serious infection.

Hepatic/Biliary/Pancreatic: Use with caution in patients with hepatic impairment as desipramine is metabolized in the liver by cytochrome P450 isozymes.

Neurologic: Use with caution in patients with a history of seizure disorder as desipramine may lower seizure threshold.

Ophthalmologic: Use with caution in patients with angle closure glaucoma as the condition may be exacerbated by potential anticholinergic effects of desipramine.

Peri-Operative Considerations: Perioperative use of desipramine may increase the risk of cardiovascular events, including hypertensive episodes. Discontinue therapy several days prior to elective surgery whenever possible.

Periprocedural Considerations: Concurrent use of desipramine may increase risks associated with electroconvulsive therapy.

Psychiatric: Use of desipramine may unmask bipolar disorder and may increase the risk of rapid cycling or precipitate a shift to mania/hypomania in patients with bipolar disorder.

Self Harm: The potential for suicidality must always be considered in depressed patients. Use of antidepressants, especially during periods of therapy initiation and dosage adjustment, may result in behavioural and/or emotional changes that place patients at increased risk of suicidal ideation and attempt. Patients should be monitored closely for any signs of worsening condition.

Withdrawal: Desipramine should not be abruptly discontinued in patients receiving high doses for prolonged periods, as doing so may result in withdrawal symptoms such as insomnia, gastrointestinal symptoms (anorexia, nausea or vomiting), flu-like symptoms (e.g., fever, malaise, fatigue, myalgias or weakness), anxiety, agitation, hypomania, mania, akathisia, delirium, dizziness, tremor, muscle twitching, and rarely, dyskinesia. Rebound depression has been reported and may occur in patients who take antidepressants for indications other than depression. These usually occur within 1 to 3 days of discontinuation, are mild and self-limiting and resolve within 2 weeks. Very rarely, cardiac disturbances have also occurred.

Special Populations: Pregnant Women: There is insufficient evidence to draw definite conclusions about the safety of desipramine use during pregnancy. Though no reports link desipramine to teratogenicity, tricyclic antidepressants do cross the placenta. Transient withdrawal symptoms such as cyanosis, tachycardia, diaphoresis, weight loss, colic and irritability have been reported in neonates whose mothers took desipramine during pregnancy. The potential risks to the fetus should be weighed against the risks to mother and fetus of untreated maternal depression. Among tricyclic antidepressants, desipramine may be more favorable during pregnancy because of its lower propensity to cause anticholinergic effects and orthostatic hypotension.

Nursing Women: Despite the detection of low levels of desipramine in breast milk, there have been no reports of adverse events. When levels were measured, there was no evidence of drug in infants' serum or any clinical signs of toxicity, especially in infants older than 2 months. Observe infants for any changes in behavior such as drowsiness or difficulty breast feeding.

Pediatrics: Cases of collapse and/or sudden death have been reported in children receiving desipramine for the treatment of ADHD and depression, but a causal relationship has not been established. Desipramine should be used in children and adolescents only by physicians experienced in the use of such agents in the pediatric population and with full consideration of the associated risks and potential benefits.

Geriatrics: Use with caution in elderly patients as they are more susceptible to sedative and anticholinergic effects and which can increase the risk of falls and confusion/cognitive impairment. See Table 4 for dosing recommendations.

Occupational Hazards: Patients should be cautioned regarding potential impairment of their mental and/or physical acuity which may affect their ability to safely operate a vehicle or perform other potentially hazardous tasks.

ADVERSE REACTIONS: More Common Adverse Drug Reactions (≥1%): Table 1 lists the more common adverse effects of desipramine.

Table 1: Desipramine

More Common Adverse Drug Reactions (≥1%)

Body System	Effect
Anticholinergic	Dry mouth and/or eyes Blurred vision Constipation Mild tremors Urinary retention Sweating
Cardiovascular	Tachycardia Orthostatic hypotension Arrhythmias
CNS	Asthenia Drowsiness Excitement Fatigue Hypomania Insomnia Sedation Weakness Headache Lethargy
Dermatologic	Dermatitis Rash
Endocrine and Metabolism	Weight gain
Gastrointestinal	Abdominal cramps Nausea Vomiting
Genitourinary	Sexual dysfunction (e.g., decreased libido, erectile or ejaculatory dysfunction, anorgasmia)

Less Common Adverse Drug Reactions (<1%): Cardiovascular: edema, flushing, heart block, myocardial infarction, stroke.
Central Nervous System: agitation, anxiety, ataxia, confusion, delirium, disorientation, drug fever, hallucinations, incoordination, nervousness, numbness, paresthesias of the extremities, parkinsonian syndrome, restlessness, seizures.
Dermatologic: alopecia, itching, petechiae, photosensitivity, urticaria, skin pigmentation.
Ear/Nose/Throat: tinnitus.
Endocrine and Metabolism: breast enlargement and galactorrhea in women, gynecomastia in men, hyperglycemia, and syndrome of inappropriate antidiuretic hormone (SIADH).
Gastrointestinal: anorexia; black tongue; decreased lower esophageal sphincter tone may cause GE reflux/heartburn; diarrhea, stomatitis, unpleasant taste.
Genitourinary: dysuria, polyuria, urinary retention.
Hematologic: agranulocytosis, eosinophilia, purpura, thrombocytopenia.
Hepatic/Biliary/Pancreatic: altered liver function, cholestatic jaundice, hepatitis, elevated liver function tests, increased pancreatic enzymes.
Ophthalmologic: increased intraocular pressure, loss of focusing ability of eye.

DRUG INTERACTIONS: Overview: Desipramine is hepatically metabolized by the cytochrome (CYP) isozymes system. The major metabolic pathway is CYP2D6, with minor involvement of CYP1A2. Desipramine may also inhibit CYP2D6, CYP2C19 and CYP2E1 activity. Any drug that is a substrate, inducer or inhibitor of these CYP isozymes may interact with desipramine.

Drug-Drug Interactions: Drug-drug interactions involving desipramine are listed in Table 2.

Table 2: Desipramine

Drug-Drug Interactions

Interacting Drug	Effect	Clinical Comment
CNS depressants (e.g., benzodiazepines, ethanol, opioids)	Additive CNS depressant effects (e.g., sedation)	Caution patients about potential effects and monitor appropriately.
Drugs that prolong the QTc-interval (e.g., amiodarone, chlorpromazine, clarithromycin, domperidone, erythromycin, haloperidol, methadone, pimozide, quinidine, quinine, sotalol, ziprasidone)	Increased risk of QTc prolongation	Consider therapy modification; obtain ECG early in therapy.
Direct-acting alpha/beta agonists (e.g., epinephrine, norepinephrine)	Concurrent use of desipramine and these agents may enhance their vasopressor effect	Consider therapy modification.
Serotonergic drugs (e.g., buspirone, irreversible MAOIs such as phenelzine and tranylcypromine, reversible MAOIs such as moclobemide and selegiline, sibutramine, SSRIs, tramadol)	Increased risk of serotonin syndrome	Avoid combination.
Strong inhibitors of CYP2D6 (e.g., chlorpromazine, fluoxetine, haloperidol, paroxetine, quinidine, terbinafine)	Increased toxicity of desipramine	Consider therapy modification or lower dose of desipramine.

Drug-Food Interactions: A high-fibre diet may decrease desipramine absorption, resulting in reduced serum levels.

Drug-Herb Interactions: Concurrent use of valerian or St. John's wort with desipramine should be avoided as it may result in additive serotonergic effects and/or sedation; St. John's wort can also increase the metabolism and decrease the effectiveness of desipramine, possibly through hepatic enzyme induction.

DOSAGE AND ADMINISTRATION: Dosing Considerations:

- Administration of the entire daily dose at bedtime may reduce daytime sedation.
- Patients who experience insomnia and stimulation from the drug may find it optimal to take the entire daily dose in the morning.
- Desipramine therapy should not be terminated abruptly in patients who have received high doses for prolonged periods (see Warnings and Precautions, Withdrawal).

Recommended Dose and Dosage Adjustment: Adults: See Table 3.

Table 3: Desipramine

Dose in Adult Patients

Indication	Initial Dose	Dose Titration	Usual Dose	Maximum Dose
Depression or anxiety[a]	75 mg/day in divided doses	Increase gradually; dose can be increased every 3 to 7 days	100–200 mg/day	300 mg/day
Irritable bowel syndrome[a]	10 to 50 mg QHS	Start low and titrate as needed; dose can be increased every 3 to 7 days	10 to 150 mg QHS	
Neuropathic pain[a]	25 mg QHS	Increase by 25 mg daily every 3 to 7 days as tolerated	50–150 mg/day	150 mg/day
Urge incontinence[a]	10 mg QHS	Increase gradually as needed; dose can be increased every 3 to 7 days	10–100 mg QHS	100 mg/day

[a] Not an approved indication in Canada.

Geriatrics: Due to the increased risk of orthostatic hypotension and possible increased sensitivity to anticholinergic effects in the geriatric population, desipramine is usually given to older patients in reduced doses. See Table 4.

Table 4: Desipramine

Dose in Geriatric Patients

Indication	Initial Dose	Dose Titration	Usual Dose	Maximum Dose
Depression or anxiety[a]	10 to 25 mg/day	Increase by 10 to 25 mg every 3 to 7 days if tolerated	75 to 100 mg/day	150 mg/day

[a] Not an approved indication in Canada.

Pediatrics: See Table 5.

Table 5: Desipramine

Dose in Pediatric Patients

Indication	Age/Weight	Initial Dose	Dose Titration	Usual Dose	Maximum Dose
ADHD[a]	6 to 12 years	10–20 mg/day in 3–4 divided doses	6–12 y: gradually increase every 3 to 7 days up to 20–30 mg/day in divided doses if needed	20–30 mg/day in divided doses	150 mg/day
	Adolescents >12 y	30 to 50 mg/day in 3 to 4 divided doses	Gradually increase (every 3 to 7 days) up to 100 mg/day in single or divided doses as needed	50–100 mg/day	150 mg/day

[a] Not an approved indication in Canada. See Warnings and Precautions, Special Populations.

Dose in Adult Patients with Renal Impairment: Dosage adjustments are generally not required for patients with renal impairment.

Dose in Dialysis: No dosage supplementation is required following hemodialysis.

OVERDOSAGE:

Signs and Symptoms: Desipramine and other TCAs are extremely toxic in overdose. Consultation with a Poison Control Centre is recommended. See the *CPS* Directory for contact numbers.

Cardiac arrhythmias and CNS involvement pose the greatest threat and may occur suddenly even when initial symptoms appear to be mild. The toxic dose is variable but, in general, acute ingestion of 10 to 20 mg/kg may result in serious toxicity and may be lethal. TCA overdose has one of the highest mortality rates of any type of ingestion. Toxicity most commonly begins within 2 hours of ingestion. The onset of symptoms is frequently precipitous, with patients progressing from wakeful, interactive state to having severe CNS and cardiac involvement within a matter of minutes.

Peripheral anticholinergic symptoms may include urinary retention, dry mucous membranes, mydriasis, constipation and occasionally adynamic ileus (diminished or absent peristalsis/bowel sounds). Patients may also be hyperpyrexic. CNS signs and symptoms can be highly variable and may range from somnolence to agitation, irritability, confusion, delirium, and hallucinations. In severe cases, patients may display extreme drowsiness, areflexia, respiratory depression and coma. Patients may occasionally become hypothermic. Seizures are common and may precipitate cardiac toxicity.

Cardiac irregularities are frequent and generally dose-dependent. Sinus tachycardia is common; its presence is not a reliable predictor of serious toxicity, and its absence does not ensure a benign clinical course. An effect on cardiac conduction similar to that of quinidine may be seen with slowing of conduction, widening of QRS complex, rightward shift in the axis of the terminal 40 milliseconds of the QRS complex, prolongation of the PR and QT intervals, right bundle branch and AV block, ventricular tachyarrhythmias (including torsades de pointes and fibrillation), and death. Prolongation of the QRS duration to more than 0.1 seconds is generally associated with more severe toxicity. Bradycardia may be seen in severely poisoned patients. Hypotension is common and may be severe, resulting from vasodilation, central and peripheral alpha-adrenergic blockade, and myocardial depression. Metabolic and/or respiratory acidosis may occur secondary to seizures, poor tissue perfusion, respiratory depression or poor gas exchange. In an otherwise healthy young person, prolonged resuscitation may be required.

Recommended Management: All cases of accidental pediatric exposure or adult overdose should be monitored at a health care facility. Asymptomatic cases without ECG abnormalities should be monitored for a minimum of 6 hours. Plasma concentrations of desipramine are of little use and should not guide management of the patient. In managing overdose, consider the possibility of multiple drug overdose, interactions among drugs and altered pharmacokinetics, including delayed absorption. Protect the patient's airway and support ventilation and perfusion. Closely monitor and maintain patient's vital signs, ECG, blood gases, serum electrolytes, and acid-base balance. Minimize external stimulation to reduce the risk of seizures.

Consultation with a regional poison centre is advisable in all patients with TCA overdose. Activated charcoal (1 gram per kilogram) may reduce absorption of drug from the gastrointestinal tract, and should be considered in patients who present within 2 hours of ingestion. This can be given through nasogastric tube if necessary. Although it should not be routinely performed, gastric lavage may be considered in the unusual case where a patient presents within 30 to 60 minutes of massive TCA overdose, but only on the advice of a Poison Control Centre. If performed, gastric lavage should be followed by administration of activated charcoal. If the patient has a decreased level of consciousness, consideration should be given to placement of endotracheal tube with cuff inflated before beginning the lavage procedure, to lessen the likelihood of aspiration of gastric contents.

Hypotension should be promptly corrected. If hypotension does not respond to a rapid isotonic fluid bolus and the patient has a widened QRS interval (>0.1 seconds), sodium bicarbonate boluses should be administered at a dose of 1 to 2 mmol/kg (an average adult would typically receive 1 to 3 ampoules of 50 mmol/50 mL). If hypotension still hasn't responded, vasopressors should be employed, with a direct-acting agonist such as norepinephrine being the drug of choice.

Widened QRS intervals (>0.14 seconds) and ventricular arrhythmias should be treated with iv sodium bicarbonate. An iv bolus of 1 to 2 mmol/kg (typically 1 to 3 ampoules of 50 mmol/50 mL) should be administered and repeated if necessary to achieve a serum pH of 7.45 to 7.55. Maintain the pH between 7.45 and 7.55. Do not exceed pH 7.6. Monitor for hypokalemia and fluid overload. Hyperventilation may also be used to maintain alkalemia.

Ventricular arrhythmias refractory to sodium bicarbonate may respond to lidocaine. Quinidine, procainamide and other type IA or IC antiarrhythmics should not be used because they may exacerbate arrhythmias and conduction slowing due to the overdosage. Overdrive pacing should be considered in patients whose arrhythmias are not responsive to drug therapy.

In patients with severe/refractory toxicity, consideration should be given to the use of intravenous lipid emulsion. Consult a toxicologist.

Seizures should be aggressively treated with iv benzodiazepines such as lorazepam or diazepam. If this is unsuccessful, barbiturates and other measures should be employed as for status epilepticus. However, phenytoin is no longer recommended in the treatment of TCA-induced seizures.

Diuresis, hemoperfusion and dialysis are not helpful in TCA overdose.

Flumazenil is contraindicated in any patient with an altered level of consciousness who has or may have taken a TCA or any drug that can cause seizures or arrhythmias, as it may precipitate seizures or even cardiac arrest. This is true even in cases of mixed overdose where the patient is known to have coingested benzodiazepines.

For management of a suspected drug overdose, CPhA recommends that you contact your **regional Poison Control Centre**. See the *CPS* Directory section for a list of Poison Control Centres.

ACTION AND CLINICAL PHARMACOLOGY: Mechanism of Action: Desipramine is a secondary amine tricyclic antidepressant. Desipramine blocks the reuptake of and prolongs the synaptic effects of norepinephrine, with a high degree of neurotransmitter selectivity. It has some effect on serotonin reuptake as well.

Pharmacokinetics: Adults: Absorption: Desipramine is well absorbed from the GI tract, and undergoes extensive first-pass metabolism. Peak plasma concentrations occur 4-6 hours after oral administration.

Distribution: Desipramine is 73 to 92% bound to plasma protein.

Metabolism: Desipramine is hepatically metabolized by CYP2D6 (major) and CYP1A2 (minor) to its pharmacologically active metabolite, 2-hydroxydesipramine. Desipramine may also inhibit CYP2D6, CYP2C19 and CYP2E1 activity.

Excretion: The elimination half-life of desipramine is 7 to 60 hours, with 70% of excretion occurring renally. The elimination half life is prolonged in the elderly and slow metabolizers. Desipramine is not removed by hemodialysis.

Special Populations: Geriatrics: The half-life of desipramine was slightly prolonged in studies of elderly males.

STORAGE AND STABILITY: Desipramine should be stored in airtight containers at room temperature (preferably at less than 30°C), and protected from excessive heat.

The reader is invited to consult CPhA's monograph **Corticosteroids: Topical**.

Desocort® Ⓟ

desonide

Topical Corticosteroid

Galderma

PHARMACOLOGY: Desonide, like all topical corticosteroids, exhibits anti-inflammatory, antipruritic and vasoconstrictive actions.

INDICATIONS: For the relief of the inflammatory and pruritic manifestations of corticosteroid-responsive dermatoses.

CONTRAINDICATIONS: Tuberculous, fungal and most viral lesions of the skin (including herpes simplex, vaccinia and varicella). Hypersensitivity to any of the components. Not for ophthalmic use.

WARNINGS: No data supplied by the manufacturer.

PRECAUTIONS: General: Systemic absorption of topical corticosteroids has produced reversible hypothalamic-pituitary-adrenal (HPA) axis suppression, manifestations of Cushing's syndrome, hyperglycemia and glucosuria in some patients.

Conditions which augment systemic absorption include the application of the more potent steroids, use over large surface areas, prolonged use, and the addition of occlusive dressings.

Therefore, patients receiving a large dose of a potent topical steroid applied to a large surface area or under an occlusive dressing should be evaluated periodically for evidence of HPA axis suppression by using the urinary free cortisol and ACTH stimulation tests. If HPA axis suppression is noted, an attempt should be made to withdraw the drug, to reduce the frequency of application, or to substitute a less potent steroid.

Recovery of HPA axis function is generally prompt and complete upon discontinuation of the drug. Infrequently, signs and symptoms of steroid withdrawal may occur, requiring supplemental systemic corticosteroids.

Children may absorb proportionally larger amounts of topical corticosteroids and thus be more susceptible to systemic toxicity (see Children).

If irritation develops, topical corticosteroids should be discontinued and appropriate therapy instituted.

In the presence of dermatological infections, the use of an appropriate antifungal or antibacterial agent should be instituted. If a favorable response does not occur promptly, the corticosteroid should be discontinued until the infection has been adequately controlled.

Laboratory Tests: The following tests may be helpful in evaluating the HPA axis suppression: urinary free cortisol test and ACTH stimulation test.

Carcinogenesis, Mutagenesis, and Impairment of Fertility: Long-term animal studies have not been performed to evaluate the carcinogenic potential or the effect on fertility of desonide.

Pregnancy: Corticosteroids are generally teratogenic in laboratory animals when administered systemically at relatively low dosage levels. Desonide has been shown to be teratogenic after dermal application in laboratory animals at doses similar to recommended human dose. There are not adequate and well-controlled studies in pregnant women on teratogenic effects from topically applied corticosteroids. Therefore, topical corticosteroids should be used during pregnancy only if the potential benefit justifies the potential risk to the fetus. Drugs of this class should not be used extensively on pregnant patients, in large amounts or for prolonged periods of time.

Lactation: It is not known whether topical administration of corticosteroids could result in sufficient systemic absorption to produce detectable quantities in breast milk. Systemically administered corticosteroids are secreted into breast milk. Caution should be exercised when topical corticosteroids are administered to a nursing woman.

Children: Pediatric patients may demonstrate greater susceptibility to topical corticosteroid-induced HPA axis suppression and Cushing's syndrome than mature patients because of a larger skin surface area to body weight ratio.

Hypothalamic-pituitary-adrenal (HPA) axis suppression, Cushing's syndrome and intracranial hypertension have been reported in children receiving topical corticosteroids. Manifestations of adrenal suppression in children include linear growth retardation, delayed weight gain, low plasma cortisol levels and absence of response to ACTH stimulation. Manifestations of intracranial hypertension include bulging fontanelles, headaches and bilateral papilledema.

Administration of topical corticosteroids to children should be limited to the least amount compatible with an effective therapeutic regimen. Chronic corticosteroid therapy may interfere with the growth and development of children.

ADVERSE EFFECTS: The following local adverse reactions are reported infrequently with topical corticosteroids, but may occur more frequently with the use of occlusive dressings. These reactions are listed in an approximate decreasing order of occurrence: burning, itching, irritation, dryness, folliculitis, hypertrichosis, acneiform eruptions, hypo-pigmentation, perioral dermatitis, allergic contact dermatitis, maceration of the skin, secondary infection, skin atrophy, striae and miliaria.

OVERDOSE:

Topically applied corticosteroids can be absorbed in sufficient amounts to produce systemic effects (see Precautions).

For management of a suspected drug overdose, CPhA recommends that you contact your **regional Poison Control Centre**. See the *CPS* Directory section for a list of Poison Control Centres.

DOSAGE: Lotion: Shake well before using. Apply a small amount to affected areas 2 or 3 times daily.
Ointment: Apply a small amount to affected areas 2 to 3 times daily.

Occlusive dressings may be used for the management of psoriasis or recalcitrant conditions.

If an infection develops, the use of occlusive dressings should be discontinued and appropriate antimicrobial therapy instituted.

SUPPLIED: Lotion: Each bottle contains: desonide 0.05% in a water base lotion. Nonmedicinal ingredients: cetyl alcohol, glyceryl stearate SE, methyl paraben, mineral oil, propyl paraben, propylene glycol, purified water, sodium lauryl sulfate, sorbitan monostearate, stearyl alcohol and tetrasodium EDTA. May contain sodium hydroxide and/or citric acid to adjust pH. Bottles of 60 and 120 mL. Store at room temperature (15 to 30°C).
Ointment: Each tube contains: desonide 0.05%. Nonmedicinal ingredients: mineral oil and polyethylene. Tubes of 15 and 60 g. Store at room temperature (15 to 30°C).

Desonide Ⓟ

CPhA Monograph

see *Corticosteroids: Topical*

Desoximetasone Ⓟ

CPhA Monograph

see *Corticosteroids: Topical*

Desyrel® Ⓟ

trazodone HCl

Antidepressant

Bristol-Myers Squibb

Desyrel® Dividose Ⓟ

trazodone HCl

Antidepressant

Bristol-Myers Squibb

Date of Preparation: June 29, 1979
Date of Revision: October 29, 2004

PHARMACOLOGY: Trazodone is a psychoactive compound with sedative and antidepressant properties. Its mechanism of action in humans is not clear.
Pharmacokinetics: Absorption: Trazodone is well absorbed after oral administration with peak plasma levels obtained within 0.5 to 2 hours after ingestion. Absorption is somewhat delayed and enhanced by food. Trazodone is 89-95% protein bound in vitro at concentrations attained with therapeutic doses.
Metabolism: In vitro studies in human liver microsomes show that trazodone is metabolized to an active metabolite, m-chlorophenylpiperazine (mCPP) by cytochrome P450 3A4 (CYP3A4). Other metabolic pathways that may be involved in metabolism of trazodone have not been well characterized.
Elimination: Approximately 60-70% of ^{14}C-labelled trazodone was found to be excreted in the urine within two days and 9-29% in feces over 60-100 hours.

In some patients DESYREL may accumulate in the plasma.

Drug Interactions: (See also Precautions, Drug Interactions.) In vitro drug metabolism studies reveal that trazodone is a substrate of the cytochrome P450 3A4 (CYP3A4) enzyme and trazodone metabolism can be inhibited by the CYP3A4 inhibitors ketoconazole, ritonavir, and indinavir. The effect of short-term administration of ritonavir (200 mg twice daily, 4 doses) on the pharmacokinetics of a single dose of trazodone (50 mg) has been studied in 10 healthy subjects. The C_{max} of trazodone increased by 34%, the AUC increased 2.4-fold, the half-life increased by 2.2-fold, and the clearance decreased by 52%. Adverse effects including nausea, hypotension, and syncope were observed when ritonavir and trazodone were co-administered.

Carbamazepine induces CYP3A4. Following co-administration of carbamazepine 400 mg/day with trazodone 100 mg to 300 mg daily, carbamazepine reduced plasma concentrations of trazodone (as well as mCPP) by 76 and 60%, respectively, compared to pre-carbamazepine values.

INDICATIONS: DESYREL (trazodone hydrochloride) is of value in the symptomatic relief of depressive illness.

CONTRAINDICATIONS: Known hypersensitivity to trazodone.

WARNINGS: Trazodone has been associated with the occurrence of priapism. In approximately 33% of the cases reported, surgical intervention was required and, in a portion of these cases, permanent impairment of erectile function or impotence resulted. Male patients with prolonged or inappropriate erections should immediately discontinue the drug and consult their physician. If the condition persists for more than 24 hours, it would be advisable for the treating physician to consult a urologist or appropriate specialist in order to decide on a management approach.

Caution should be used when administering DESYREL to patients with cardiac disease, and such patients should be closely monitored, since antidepressant drugs (including DESYREL) have been associated with the occurrence of cardiac arrhythmias. Recent clinical studies in patients with pre-existing cardiac disease indicate that DESYREL (trazodone hydrochloride) may be arrhythmogenic in some patients in that population. Arrhythmias identified include isolated PVCs, ventricular couplets, and in 2 patients short episodes (3 to 4 beats) of ventricular tachycardia. There have also been several postmarketing reports of arrhythmias in DESYREL-treated patients who have pre-existing cardiac disease and in some patients who did not have pre-existing cardiac disease. DESYREL is not recommended for use during the initial recovery phase of myocardial infarction.

PRECAUTIONS: General: The possibility of suicide in depressed patients remains during treatment and until significant remission occurs. Therefore, the number of tablets prescribed at any one time should take into account this possibility, and patients with suicide ideation should never have access to large quantities of trazodone.

Episodes of grand mal seizures have been reported in a small number of patients. The majority of these patients were already receiving anticonvulsant therapy for a previously diagnosed seizure disorder.

Occupational Hazards: Safety of Driving: Since DESYREL (trazodone hydrochloride) may impair the mental and/or physical abilities required for performance of potentially hazardous tasks, such as operating an automobile or machinery, the patient should be cautioned not to engage in such activities while impaired.

Drug Interactions: In vitro drug metabolism studies suggest that there is a potential for drug interactions when trazodone is given with CYP3A4 inhibitors. Ritonavir, a potent CYP3A4 inhibitor, increased the C_{max}, AUC, and elimination half-life, and decreased clearance of trazodone after administration of ritonavir twice daily for 2 days. Adverse effects including nausea, hypotension, and syncope were observed when ritonavir and trazodone were co-administered. It is likely that ketoconazole, indinavir, and other CYP3A4 inhibitors such as itraconazole or nefazodone may lead to substantial increases in trazodone plasma concentrations with the potential for adverse effects. If trazodone is used with a potent CYP3A4 inhibitor, a lower dose of trazodone should be considered.

Carbamazepine reduced plasma concentrations of trazodone when co-administered. Patients should be closely monitored to see if there is a need for an increased dose of trazodone when taking both drugs.

Trazodone may enhance the response to alcohol and the effects of barbiturates and other CNS depressants and patients should be cautioned accordingly.

Increased serum digoxin and phenytoin levels have been reported to occur in patients receiving DESYREL concurrently with either of those 2 drugs. Little is known about the interaction between DESYREL and general anesthetics; therefore, prior to elective surgery, DESYREL should be discontinued for as long as clinically feasible.

Because it is not known whether an interaction will occur between DESYREL and MAO inhibitors, administration of DESYREL should be initiated very cautiously with gradual increase in dosage as required, if an MAO inhibitor is given concomitantly or has been discontinued shortly before medication with DESYREL is instituted.

DESYREL may cause hypotension including orthostatic hypotension and syncope; caution is required if it is given to patients receiving antihypertensive drugs and an adjustment in the dose of the antihypertensive medication may be required.

Because of the absence of experience, concurrent administration of electro-shock therapy should be avoided.

There have been reports of increased and decreased prothrombin time occurring in warfarinized patients who take DESYREL.

Pregnancy: Since the safety and use of DESYREL in pregnant women has not been established, it should not be used in women of childbearing potential unless, in the opinion of the physician, the expected benefits justify the potential risk to the fetus.
Lactation: Since DESYREL and/or its metabolites have been detected in the milk of lactating animals, it should not be administered to nursing mothers unless the potential benefits justify the possible risks to the child.
Children: The safety and effectiveness of DESYREL in children below the age of 18 have not been established.
Laboratory Tests: It is recommended that white blood cell and differential counts should be performed in patients who develop sore throat, fever, or other signs of infection or blood dyscrasia and DESYREL should be discontinued if the white blood cell or absolute neutrophil count falls below normal.
Hyperprolactinemia and Breast Tumors: There is sufficient experimental evidence to conclude that chronic administration of those psychotropic drugs, such as trazodone, which increase prolactin secretion has the potential to induce mammary neoplasms in rodents under appropriate conditions. Tissue culture experiments indicate that approximately 33% of human breast cancers are prolactin dependent in vitro, a factor of potential importance if the prescription of these drugs is contemplated in a patient with a previously detected breast cancer.

Although disturbances such as galactorrhea, amenorrhea, gynecomastia and impotence have been reported, the clinical significance of elevated serum prolactin levels or increased secretion and turnover are unknown for most patients. Neither clinical studies nor epidemiological studies conducted to date, however, have shown an association between chronic administration of these drugs and mammary tumorigenesis: available evidence is considered too limited to be conclusive at this time.

ADVERSE EFFECTS: The most common adverse reactions encountered are drowsiness, nausea/vomiting, headache and dry mouth. Adverse reactions reported include the following:
Behavioural: drowsiness, fatigue, lethargy, retardation, lightheadedness, dizziness, difficulty in concentration, confusion, impaired memory, disorientation, excitement, agitation, anxiety, tension, nervousness, restlessness, insomnia, nightmares, anger, hostility and, rarely, hypomania, visual distortions, hallucinations, delusions and paranoia.
Neurologic: tremor, headache, ataxia, akathisia, muscle stiffness, slurred speech, retarded speech, vertigo, tinnitus, tingling of extremities, paresthesia, weakness, grand mal seizures (see Precautions), and, rarely impaired speech, muscle twitching, numbness, dystonia and involuntary movements.
Autonomic: dry mouth, blurred vision, diplopia, miosis, nasal congestion, constipation, sweating, urinary retention, increased urinary frequency and incontinence.
Cardiovascular: orthostatic hypotension, hypertension, tachycardia, palpitations, shortness of breath, apnea, syncope, arrhythmias, prolonged P-R interval, atrial fibrillation, bradycardia, ventricular ectopic activity (including ventricular tachycardia), myocardial infarction, cardiac arrest and conduction block.
Gastrointestinal: nausea, vomiting, diarrhea, gastrointestinal discomfort, anorexia, increased appetite.
Endocrine: priapism (see Warnings), decrease and, more rarely, increase in libido, weight gain and loss, and rarely, menstrual irregularities, retrograde ejaculation and inhibition of ejaculation.
Allergic or Toxic: skin rash, itching, edema, and, rarely, hemolytic anemia, methemoglobinemia, liver enzyme alterations, obstructive jaundice, leukocytoblastic vasculitis, purpuric maculopapular eruptions, photosensitivity and fever.
Miscellaneous: aching joints and muscles, peculiar taste, hypersalivation, chest pain, hematuria, red, tired and itchy eyes.

OVERDOSE:

Symptoms: Overdosage of DESYREL (trazodone hydrochloride) may cause an increase in incidence or severity of any of the reported adverse reactions, e.g. hypotension and excessive sedation. In one known suicide attempt, the patient presented with symptoms of drowsiness and weakness 3 hours after ingesting 7.5 g (12.5 times the maximum daily dose) of trazodone. Recovery was uneventful. Death by deliberate or accidental overdosage with trazodone alone has not been reported.

Treatment: There is no specific antidote for trazodone. Management of overdosage should, therefore, be symptomatic and supportive. Any patient suspected of having taken an overdosage should be admitted to hospital as soon as possible and the stomach emptied by gastric lavage. Forced diuresis may be useful in facilitating elimination of the drug.

For management of a suspected drug overdose, CPhA recommends that you contact your **regional Poison Control Centre**. See the *CPS* Directory section for a list of Poison Control Centres.

DOSAGE: Dosage should be initiated at a low level and increased gradually noting carefully the clinical response and any evidence of intolerance. It should be kept in mind that there may be a lag in the therapeutic response. Increasing the dosage rapidly does not normally shorten this latent period and may increase the incidence of side effects.
Adults: The recommended initial dose is 150 to 200 mg daily, in 2 or 3 divided doses. DESYREL (trazodone hydrochloride) should be taken shortly after a meal or light snack in order to reduce the incidence of adverse reactions. The initial dose may be increased according to tolerance and response by increments of 50 mg, usually up to 300 mg daily in divided doses. In some patients, doses up to 400 mg daily and rarely up to 600 mg daily in hospitalized patients, may be required. Occurrence of drowsiness may require the administration of a major portion of the daily dose at bedtime or a reduction of dosage.

Once an adequate response has been achieved, the dosage may be gradually reduced, with adjustment depending on therapeutic response. During prolonged maintenance therapy the dosage should be kept at the lowest effective level.
Geriatrics: If used in the elderly, doses not exceeding one-half the recommended adult dosage should be used, with adjustments made depending on tolerance and response.
Pediatrics: Because safety and effectiveness in children have not been established DESYREL is not recommended in the pediatric age group.

SUPPLIED: DESYREL: 50 mg: Each orange, round, biconvex tablet, engraved with "DESYREL" and "BL" around the periphery on one side and with a bisect bar on the other side, contains: trazodone HCl 50 mg. Nonmedicinal ingredients: cornstarch, dibasic calcium phosphate, FD&C yellow No. 6 aluminum lake, lactose monohydrate, magnesium stearate, microcrystalline cellulose, povidone and sodium starch glycolate. Bottles of 100 and 250.
100 mg: Each white to off-white, round, biconvex tablet engraved with "DESYREL" and "BL" around the periphery on one side and with a bisect bar on the other side, contains: trazodone HCl 100 mg. Nonmedicinal ingredients: cornstarch, dibasic calcium phosphate, lactose monohydrate, magnesium stearate, microcrystalline cellulose, povidone and sodium starch glycolate. Bottles of 100.
DESYREL DIVIDOSE: Each orange, rectangular, flat-faced, bevel-edged tablet, with bisect/trisect scoring, engraved on one side with a "BL" logo on the left segment, a blank center segment, and a "BL" logo on the right segment, the other side engraved with a "50" on each segment contains: trazodone HCl 150 mg. Nonmedicinal ingredients: FD&C yellow No. 6 aluminum lake, magnesium stearate, microcrystalline cellulose, pregelatinized starch and stearic acid. Bottles of 100.

The DIVIDOSE 150 mg tablet design makes dosage adjustments easy. Each tablet can be broken accurately to provide any of the following dosages: 50 mg (one-third of a tablet); 75 mg (one-half of a tablet); 100 mg (two-thirds of a tablet); 150 mg (the entire tablet). Instructions: To break a DIVIDOSE tablet accurately and easily, hold the tablet between your thumbs and index fingers close to the appropriate tablet score (groove). Then with the tablet score facing you, apply pressure and snap the tablet segments apart.

(Shown in Product Identification Section)

Detrol® Ⓟ

tolterodine L-tartrate

Anticholinergic—Antispasmodic

Pfizer

Date of Revision: February 10, 2010

SUMMARY PRODUCT INFORMATION:

Route of Administration	Dosage Form/ Strength	Clinically Relevant Nonmedicinal Ingredients
Oral	Tablet 1 mg, 2 mg	Colloidal anhydrous silica, calcium hydrogen phosphate dihydrate, hypromellose, magnesium stearate, cellulose microcrystalline, sodium starch glycolate (pH 3.0-5.0), stearic acid and titanium dioxide.

INDICATIONS AND CLINICAL USE: DETROL (tolterodine L-tartrate tablets) is indicated for:

- the symptomatic management of patients with an overactive bladder with symptoms of urinary frequency, urgency, or urge incontinence, or any combination of these symptoms (see Warnings and Precautions).

Geriatrics (≥65 years of age): No overall differences were observed in safety between older (patients ≥65 years) and younger patients (patients <65 years) on tolterodine immediate release tablets; and therefore, no dosage adjustment for elderly patients is recommended (see Warnings and Precautions, Special Populations).

CONTRAINDICATIONS: DETROL (tolterodine L-tartrate tablets) is contraindicated in patients with:

- urinary retention,
- gastric retention,
- uncontrolled narrow angle glaucoma,
- a known hypersensitivity to this drug or to any ingredient in the formulation or component of the container (see Dosage Forms, Composition and Packaging).

WARNINGS AND PRECAUTIONS: Gastrointestinal and Genitourinary: Patients at Risk of Urinary Retention and Gastric Retention: DETROL (tolterodine L-tartrate tablets) should be administered with caution to patients with clinically significant bladder outflow obstruction because of the risk of urinary retention, to patients at risk of decreased gastrointestinal motility, and to patients with gastrointestinal obstructive disorders, such as pyloric stenosis, because of the risk of gastric retention (see Contraindications).

Cardiovascular: Patients with Congenital or Acquired QT Prolongation: In a clinical QT study, the QT prolonging effect of two times the highest labeled dose of tolterodine (8 mg/day in divided doses, given as DETROL immediate release tablets) was 50% to 60% less than that of the active control moxifloxacin (400 mg) at its labeled dose. At the recommended therapeutic dose (4 mg daily) of DETROL (tolterodine L-tartrate tablets), the effect was lower.

The clinical relevance of these findings will depend on individual patient risk factors and susceptibilities present. Particular care should be exercised in patients who are at an increased risk of experiencing torsades de pointes during treatment with QT/QTc-prolonging drugs. This especially holds true in patients with abnormally long baseline QT/QTc intervals or when taking potent CYP3A4 inhibitors (see Drug Interactions, Drug-Drug Interactions, Dosage and Administration).

In the general population, the risk factors for torsades de pointes include, but are not limited to, the following: female; elderly (65 years); genetic variants affecting cardiac ion channels or regulatory proteins, especially congenital long QT syndrome; family history of sudden cardiac death at <50 years; cardiac disease (e.g., myocardial ischemia or infarction, congestive heart failure, left ventricular hypertrophy, cardiomyopathy); demonstrated history of arrhythmias (especially ventricular arrhythmias, atrial fibrillation, or recent conversion from atrial fibrillation); bradycardia (<50 beats per minute); acute neurological events (e.g., intracranial or subarachnoid haemorrhage, stroke, intracranial trauma; electrolyte disturbances (e.g., hypokalemia, hypomoagnesemia, hypocalcemia); nutritional deficits (e.g., eating disorders, extreme diets); diabetes mellitus; autonomic neuropathy; hepatic or renal dysfunction if relevant to the elimination of the drug.

Approximately 7% of Caucasians are poor metabolizers of CYP2D6 substrates. A pharmacokinetic/pharmacodynamic model estimated that QTc interval increases in poor metabolizers treated with tolterodine 2 mg BID are comparable to those observed in extensive metabolizers receiving 4 mg BID.

Discontinuation of the drug should be considered if symptoms suggestive of arrhythmia occur.

Hepatic/Biliary/Pancreatic: Patients with impaired hepatic function and patients with renal impairment should not receive doses of DETROL greater than 1 mg, twice daily.

Neurologic: DETROL should be used with caution in patients with myasthenia gravis.

Ophthalmologic: Controlled Narrow Angle Glaucoma: DETROL should be used with caution in patients being treated for narrow angle glaucoma.

Special Populations: Pregnant Women: Studies in mice have shown that at doses of 30 to 40 mg/kg/day, tolterodine caused embryolethality, reduced fetal weight, and increased incidence of fetal abnormalities (cleft palate, digital abnormalities, intraabdominal hemorrhage, various skeletal abnormalities, primarily reduced ossification in mice). At these doses, AUC values were about 20- to 25-fold higher than in humans. At doses of 20 mg/kg/day (AUC value was about 15-fold higher than in humans), no anomalies or malformations were seen in mice. There are no studies of tolterodine in pregnant women. Therefore, DETROL (tolterodine L-tartrate tablets) should be used during pregnancy only if the potential benefit for the mother justifies the potential risk for the fetus. Women of childbearing potential should be considered for treatment only if using adequate contraception.

Nursing Women: Tolterodine is excreted into the milk in mice. It is not known whether tolterodine is excreted in human milk. Because many drugs are excreted into human milk, administration of DETROL should be avoided during nursing.

Pediatrics: The safety and effectiveness of DETROL in pediatric patients have not been established.

Geriatrics (65-91 years of age): Of the 1120 patients who were treated in the four, phase III, 12-week clinical studies of DETROL, 474 (42%) were 65 to 91 years of age. No overall differences in safety were observed between the older and younger patients.

Monitoring and Laboratory Tests: Monitoring of the QT/QTc interval and/or serum electrolyte levels may be appropriate in high risk patients who are being treated with DETROL, such as: patients with known congenital or acquired QT/QTc prolongation or electrolyte disturbances; patients with impaired hepatic or renal function or other comorbid conditions that may increase tolterodine exposure or cause QT/QTc prolongation; patients who are taking drugs that have been associated with QT/QTc prolongation and/or torsades de pointes such as Class IA (e.g., quinidine, procainamide) or Class III (e.g., amiodarone, sotalol) antiarrhythmic medications or those taking potent CYP3A4 inhibitors.

(See Warnings and Precautions, Cardiovascular; Drug Interactions, Drug-Drug Interactions and Dosage and Administration.)

Discontinuation of the drug should be considered if symptoms suggestive of arrhythmia occur or if the QT/QTc interval becomes markedly prolonged.

Information to Be Provided to the Patient: The ability to drive and use machinery may be negatively affected. Patients should be advised to exercise caution.

ADVERSE REACTIONS: Adverse Drug Reaction Overview: The clinical trial program for DETROL (tolterodine L-tartrate tablets) comprised 2398 patients who were treated with either DETROL (N=1619), oxybutynin (N=349), or placebo (N=430). No differences in the safety profile of tolterodine were identified based on age, gender, race, or metabolism.

A total of 1120 patients were treated in four, phase III, 12-week, controlled clinical studies with either DETROL, 2 mg twice daily (N=474), DETROL 1 mg twice daily (N=121), oxybutynin 5 mg three times daily (N=349), or placebo (N=176). The percentage of patients reporting any adverse event in the 12 week studies was similar for DETROL 2 mg twice daily (75.5%), DETROL 1 mg twice daily (74.4%), and placebo (77.8%). The overall incidence rates for these treatment groups were lower than that reported for oxybutynin 5 mg three times daily (93.1%); these rates were significantly less for DETROL 2 mg and placebo compared with oxybutynin (P<0.0001). The incidence of serious adverse events was similar among treatment groups (DETROL 1 and 2 mg twice daily, 3.7%; oxybutynin 5 mg three times daily, 3.7%; placebo, 3.4%).

Dry mouth was the most frequently reported adverse event across all treatment groups. However, the incidence was significantly less for patients treated with either dose of DETROL or placebo compared with oxybutynin 5 mg three times daily (P=0.001). Dry mouth, constipation, abnormal vision (accommodation abnormalities), urinary retention, and xerophthalmia are all expected side effects of antimuscarinic agents.

Clinical Trial Adverse Drug Reactions: Because clinical trials are conducted under very specific conditions the adverse reaction rates observed in the clinical trials may not reflect the rates observed in practice and should not be compared to the rates in the clinical trials of another drug. Adverse drug reaction information from clinical trials is useful for identifying drug-related adverse events and for approximating rates.

Table 1 lists all adverse events that occurred in ≥5% of patients in either of the tolterodine treatment groups in the 12-week studies.

Table 1: DETROL

Incidence of Adverse Events that Occurred in ≥5% Tolterodine-treated Patients (1 or 2 mg BID) in the 12-week Controlled Clinical Studies

	Placebo		Tolterodine 1 mg BID		Tolterodine 2 mg BID		Oxybutynin 5 mg TID	
Number Treated	176		121		474		349	
Reported AE n (%)	137	(77.8)	90	(74.4)	358	(75.5)	325	(93.1)
Adverse Event by Body System	n	%	n	%	n	%	n	%
Autonomic Nervous System								
Mouth Dry	28	(15.9)	29	(24.0)	187	(39.5)	273	(78.2)
Palpitation	5	(2.8)	8	(6.6)	2	(0.4)	8	(2.3)
General								
Headache	13	(7.4)	8	(6.6)	52	(11.0)	24	(6.9)
Fatigue	13	(7.4)	9	(7.4)	32	(6.8)	16	(4.6)
Central/Peripheral Nervous Systems								
Vertigo/Dizziness	16	(9.1)	11	(9.1)	42	(8.9)	30	(8.6)
Gastrointestinal								
Abdominal Pain	11	(6.3)	7	(5.8)	36	(7.6)	22	(6.3)
Constipation	8	(4.5)	7	(5.8)	31	(6.5)	33	(9.5)
Dyspepsia	3	(1.7)	2	(1.7)	28	(5.9)	39	(11.2)
Diarrhea	11	(6.3)	7	(5.8)	19	(4.0)	18	(5.2)
Respiratory								
Upper Respiratory Tract Infection	16	(9.1)	3	(2.5)	28	(5.9)	11	(3.2)
Sinusitis	10	(5.7)	7	(5.8)	5	(1.1)	8	(2.3)
Urinary								
Urinary Tract Infection	13	(7.4)	6	(5.0)	26	(5.5)	27	(7.7)

Other adverse events observed in patients during the 12-week clinical trials were chest pain (3.4%), somnolence (3.0%), dysuria (2.5%), bronchitis (2.1%), dry skin (1.7%), increased weight (1.3%), and flatulence (1.3%).

Less Common Clinical Trial Adverse Drug Reactions (<1%): Central and Peripheral Nervous Systems: confusion.

Gastrointestinal: gastroesophageal reflux.

Skin/Appendages: flushed skin, and allergic reactions.

Post-Market Adverse Drug Reactions: The following events have been reported in association with tolterodine use in clinical practice: anaphylactoid reactions (including angioedema), tachycardia, palpitations, peripheral edema, and hallucinations, disorientation, memory impairment, and diarrhea.

Cholinesterase Inhibitors: Worsening of symptoms of dementia (e.g., confusion, disorientation, delusion) have been reported after tolterodine therapy was initiated in patients taking cholinesterase inhibitors for the treatment of dementia.

DRUG INTERACTIONS: Overview: Concomitant medication with other drugs that possess antimuscarinic properties may result in more pronounced therapeutic and/or adverse effects. Conversely, the therapeutic effect of tolterodine may be reduced by concomitant administration of muscarinic receptor agonists.

Drug-Drug Interactions: Effects of Other Drugs on DETROL: Drugs Which Prolong the QT/QTc Interval: Drugs that have been associated with QT/QTc interval prolongation and/or torsades de pointes include, but are not limited to, the examples in the following list. Chemical/pharmacological classes are listed if some, although not necessarily all, class members have been implicated in QT/QTc prolongation and/or torsades de pointes: antiarrhythmics (class IA, e.g., quinidine, procainamide, disopyramide; class III, e.g., amiodarone, sotalol, ibutilide; class IC, e.g., flecainide, propafenone); antipsychotics (e.g., thioridazine, chlorpromazine, pimozide, haloperidol, droperidol); antidepressants (e.g., amitriptyline, imipramine, maprotiline, fluoxetine, venlafaxine); opioids (e.g., methadone); antibacterials (e.g., erythromycin, clarithromycin, telithromycin, moxifloxacin, gatifloxacin); antimalarials (e.g., quinine); pentamidine; azole antifungals (e.g., ketoconazole, fluconazole, voriconazole); gastrointestinal drugs (e.g., domperidone, dolasetron, ondansetron); B_2-adrenoreceptor agonist (salmeterol, formoterol); tacrolimus.

This list of potentially interacting drugs is not comprehensive. Prior to initiating drug treatment in the presence of concomitant medications, physicians should consult current scientific literature for information on the ability of newly approved drugs to prolong the QT/QTc interval, inhibit the metabolizing enzyme or transporter, or cause electrolyte disturbances, as well for older drugs for which these effects have recently been established (see Warnings and Precautions).

Cytochrome P450 3A4 Inhibitors: Patients treated with ketoconazole or other potent CYP3A4 inhibitors such as other azole antifungals (e.g., itraconazole, miconazole) or macrolide antibiotics (e.g., erythromycin, clarithromycin) or cyclosporine or vinblastine, should not receive doses of DETROL (tolterodine L-tartrate tablets) greater than 1 mg twice daily.

Fluoxetine: Fluoxetine, a potent inhibitor of P450 2D6, inhibits significantly the metabolism of tolterodine in extensive metabolizers. The sum of unbound serum concentrations of tolterodine and the 5-hydroxymethyl derivative (DD 01) is 25% higher when the two drugs are administered concomitantly. No dose adjustment is required.

Effects of DETROL on Other Drugs: Other Drugs Metabolized by P450 2D6: The potential effect of tolterodine on the pharmacokinetics of drugs that are metabolized by P450 2D6 (such as flecainide, vinblastine, carbamazepine, tricyclic antidepressants) has not been formally evaluated.

Diuretics: Coadministration of diuretics (such as indapamide, hydrochlorothiazide, triamterene, bendroflumethiazide, chlorothiazide, methylchlorothiazide, or furosemide) with DETROL (2 mg, twice daily) did not cause any adverse ECG effects, however, in the presence of diuretics causing hypokalemia, and, concomitant medications known or suspected to cause adverse ECG effects (such as QT/QTC prolongation), the physician is advised to exercise caution and advise the patient about the signs and symptoms of cardiac arrhythmia.

Oral Contraceptives: Clinical drug interaction studies have shown that there are no known interactions between tolterodine and oral contraceptives (ethinyl estradiol/levonorgestrel).

Warfarin: Clinical drug interaction studies have shown that there are no known interactions between tolterodine and warfarin.

Drug-Food Interactions: Food intake does not result in clinically relevant changes in the pharmacokinetic profile.

Drug-Herb Interactions: Interaction with herbal products has not been established.

Drug-Laboratory Test Interactions: Interactions between tolterodine and laboratory tests have not been studied.

Patient Counselling: Patients should be informed that antimuscarinic agents such as DETROL (tolterodine L-tartrate tablets) may produce blurred vision or dizziness.

DOSAGE AND ADMINISTRATION: Dosing Considerations: Dosing of DETROL (tolterodine L-tartrate tablets) may be affected by the following:
- individual response and tolerability
- impaired hepatic function and renal impairment
- potent CYP3A4 inhibitors

(See Warnings and Precautions and Dosage and Administration, Recommended Dose and Dosage Adjustment.)

Recommended Dose and Dosage Adjustment: The initial recommended dose of DETROL (tolterodine L-tartrate tablets) is 2 mg twice daily. The dose may be reduced to 1 mg twice daily based on individual response and tolerability. For patients with impaired hepatic function and patients with renal impairment, the recommended dose is 1 mg twice daily (see Warnings and Precautions). No dosage adjustment for elderly patients (≥65 years of age) is recommended (see Warnings and Precautions, Special Populations).

Patients treated with potent CYP3A4 inhibitors should **not** receive doses of DETROL greater than 1 mg twice daily (see Warnings and Precautions).

The maximum recommended daily dose of 4 mg should not be exceeded.

Administration: Administration of DETROL (tolterodine L-tartrate tablets) at the recommended dosage, for a minimum of two weeks may be required before relief of overactive bladder can be expected/detected. Further improvement is seen after 8 weeks. DETROL can be taken with food.

OVERDOSAGE:
The highest dose of tolterodine tartrate given to human volunteers was 12.8 mg as single dose. The most severe adverse events observed were accommodation disturbances and micturition difficulties. One case of overdose has been reported prior to the marketing of DETROL (tolterodine L-tartrate tablets) that involved a 27-month-old child who ingested 5 to 7 tablets of DETROL 2 mg. He was hospitalized overnight with symptoms of dry mouth and was treated with a suspension of activated charcoal. The child recovered fully.

Management of Overdosage: Treatment of overdosage with DETROL should consist of gastric lavage and activated charcoal. Treatments for symptoms are recommended as follows. For severe central anticholinergic effects (hallucinations, severe excitation), an anticholinesterase agent, such as physostigmine, may be used. If excitation and convulsions occur, administer an anticonvulsant, such as diazepam. Patients with respiratory insufficiency should be given respiratory assistance. If respiratory arrest occurs, patients should be given artificial respiration. Patients with tachycardia may be treated with a beta-blocker, and those with urinary retention may be catheterized. Patients with troublesome mydriasis may be placed in a dark room or treated with pilocarpine eye drops, or both. ECG should be monitored. In clinical trials of normal volunteers, QT interval prolongation was observed with tolterodine immediate release at doses of 8 mg (4 mg BID). The risk of torsades de pointes with a QT/QTc-prolonging drug is usually dose-dependent. It is recommended that continuous ECG monitoring may be appropriate in cases of overdose with DETROL (or DETROL LA). Concomitant therapy should be immediately reviewed and stopped if potential for drug-drug interaction and exacerbation of the QT prolongation effect is possible (see Warnings and Precautions and Drug Interactions, Drug-Drug Interactions).

> For management of a suspected drug overdose, CPhA recommends that you contact your **regional Poison Control Centre**. See the *CPS* Directory section for a list of Poison Control Centres.

ACTION AND CLINICAL PHARMACOLOGY: Mechanism of Action: Tolterodine L-tartrate, is a competitive muscarinic receptor antagonist, which has been shown to inhibit carbachol-induced contraction of isolated bladder preparations from rats, guinea pigs, and man. Tolterodine L-tartrate (henceforth referred to as tolterodine) inhibits contractions of the detrusor muscle from the guinea pig, and electrically induced contractions of human detrusor muscle from stable and overactive bladders ex vivo. Tolterodine is significantly more active in inhibiting acetylcholine-induced urinary bladder contractions than electrically induced salivation in the anesthetized cat.

Pharmacodynamics: Tolterodine has a pronounced effect on bladder function in healthy volunteers. The main effects following a 6.4 mg single dose of tolterodine were an increase in residual urine, reflecting an incomplete emptying of the bladder, and a decrease in detrusor pressure. These findings are consistent with antimuscarinic action on the lower urinary tract.

In patients with an overactive bladder who received recommended therapeutic doses of tolterodine, urodynamic measurements have shown that tolterodine increased the volume at first contraction and maximum cystometric capacity.

Tolterodine is converted to a pharmacologically active 5-hydroxymethyl metabolite (DD 01) by the isozyme cytochrome P450 2D6 (debrisoquine hydroxylase). This metabolite exhibits an antimuscarinic profile similar to that of tolterodine, both in vitro and in vivo. In view of the antimuscarinic activity of DD 01 and pharmacokinetic data from both humans and animals, it has been concluded that this metabolite contributes significantly to the therapeutic effect in extensive metabolizers (see Metabolism).

Pharmacokinetics: Absorption: In a study of ^{14}C-tolterodine in healthy volunteers who received a 5 mg oral dose, at least 77% of the radiolabeled dose was absorbed. Tolterodine is rapidly absorbed, and maximum serum concentrations (C_{max}) typically occur within 1 to 2 hours after dose administration. The pharmacokinetics of tolterodine, based on C_{max} and area under the concentration time curve (AUC) determinations, are dose proportional over the range of 1 to 4 mg. Food intake does not result in clinically relevant changes in the pharmacokinetic profile.

Distribution: Tolterodine is highly bound to plasma proteins, primarily α 1-acid glycoprotein. Unbound concentrations of tolterodine average 3.7%±0.13% over the concentration range achieved in clinical studies. The 5-hydroxymethyl metabolite (DD 01) is not extensively protein bound, with unbound fraction concentrations averaging 36%±4.0%. The blood to serum ratio of tolterodine and DD 01 averages 0.6 and 0.8, respectively, indicating that these compounds do not distribute extensively into erythrocytes. The volume of distribution of tolterodine following administration of a 1.28 mg intravenous dose is 113±26.7 L.

Metabolism: Tolterodine is extensively metabolized by the liver following oral dosing, and is converted to DD 01 by the isozyme cytochrome P450 2D6. Further metabolism leads to formation of the 5-carboxylic acid and N-dealkylated 5-carboxylic acid metabolites which account for 51%±14% and 29%±6.3% of the metabolites recovered in the urine respectively.

The potential effect of tolterodine on the pharmacokinetics of other drugs also metabolized by P450 2D6, such as tricyclic antidepressants, some antiarrhythmics and selective serotonin reuptake inhibitors, and neuroleptics has not been formally evaluated.

Variability in Metabolism: A subset (about 7%) of the population is devoid of the drug metabolizing isoenzyme cytochrome P450 2D6, the enzyme responsible for the formation of DD 01. The identified pathway of metabolism for these individuals, referred to as "poor metabolizers" (PMs), is dealkylation via cytochrome P450 3A4 to N-dealkylated tolterodine. The remainder of the population is referred to as "extensive metabolizers" (EMs). Since tolterodine and DD 01 have similar antimuscarinic effects, the net activity of DETROL is expected to be similar in EMs and PMs.

Excretion: Following administration of a 5 mg oral dose of ^{14}C-tolterodine solution to healthy volunteers, 77% of radioactivity was recovered in urine and 17% was recovered in feces in 7 days. Less than 1% (<2.5% in poor metabolizers) of the dose was recovered in urine and feces as intact tolterodine; 5% to 14% (<1% in poor metabolizers) was recovered as DD 01 within the first 24 hours. This is consistent with the apparent half life of tolterodine: 1.9 to 3.7 hours.

Special Populations and Conditions: Age: No overall differences were observed in safety between older and younger patients on tolterodine in Phase III, 12 week, controlled clinical studies; and therefore, no dosage adjustment for elderly patients is recommended.

Gender: There are no sex dependent differences in the pharmacokinetic profile of tolterodine or DD 01.

Race: Pharmacokinetic differences due to race have not been identified.

Hepatic Insufficiency: Subjects with hepatic cirrhosis exhibit higher serum concentrations and longer half-lives of tolterodine and DD 01 compared to young healthy subjects given the same dose.

Renal Insufficiency: Potential pharmacologic effects and also the toxicological significance of metabolite levels should be taken into account if exposing subjects with renal impairment (GFR <30 mL/min) to repeated doses of tolterodine.

STORAGE AND STABILITY: Store at room temperature 15 to 30°C.

SPECIAL HANDLING INSTRUCTIONS: Not applicable.

INFORMATION FOR THE PATIENT: Published in e-CPS, available by subscription at www.e-cps.ca.

DOSAGE FORMS, COMPOSITION AND PACKAGING: 1 mg: Each white, round, biconvex, film-coated tablet, engraved with arcs above and below the letters "TO", contains: tolterodine L-tartrate 1 mg. Nonmedicinal ingredients: calcium hydrogen phosphate dihydrate, cellulose microcrystalline, colloidal anhydrous silica, hypromellose, magnesium stearate, sodium starch glycolate (pH 3.0-5.0), stearic acid and titanium dioxide. Bottles of 60 and 500.

2 mg: Each white, round, biconvex, film-coated tablet, engraved with arcs above and below the letters "DT", contains: tolterodine L-tartrate 2 mg. Nonmedicinal ingredients: calcium hydrogen phosphate dihydrate, cellulose microcrystalline, colloidal anhydrous silica, hypromellose, magnesium stearate, sodium starch glycolate (pH 3.0-5.0), stearic acid and titanium dioxide. Bottles of 60 and 500.

(Shown in Product Identification Section)

Detrol LA™ Ⓟ

tolterodine L-tartrate

Anticholinergic—Antispasmodic

Pfizer

Date of Revision: February 10, 2010

SUMMARY PRODUCT INFORMATION:

Route of Administration	Dosage Form/ Strength	Clinically Relevant Nonmedicinal Ingredients
Oral	Extended release capsules 2 mg, 4 mg	Starch, sucrose, hypromellose, ethylcellulose, ammonium hydroxide, medium chain triglycerides, oleic acid, gelatin and FD&C Blue 2. The 2 mg capsules also contain yellow iron oxide. Both capsule strengths are imprinted with a pharmaceutical grade ink, Opacode White S-1-7085 that contains shellac glaze, titanium dioxide, ammonium hydroxide, propylene glycol and simethicone.

INDICATIONS AND CLINICAL USE: DETROL LA (tolterodine L-tartrate extended release capsules) is indicated for:
- the symptomatic management of patients with an overactive bladder with symptoms of urinary frequency, urgency, or urge incontinence, or any combination of these symptoms (see Warnings and Precautions).

Geriatrics (≥ 65 years of age): No overall differences were observed in safety between older (patients ≥65 years) and younger patients (patients <65 years) on tolterodine extended release capsules; and therefore, no dosage adjustment for elderly patients is recommended (see Warnings and Precautions, Special Populations).

CONTRAINDICATIONS: DETROL LA (tolterodine L-tartrate extended release capsules) is contraindicated in patients with:
- urinary retention,
- gastric retention,
- uncontrolled narrow angle glaucoma,
- a known hypersensitivity to this drug or to any ingredient in the formulation or component of the container.

WARNINGS AND PRECAUTIONS: Cardiovascular: Patients with Congenital or Acquired QT Prolongation: In a clinical QT study, the QT prolonging effect of two times the highest labeled dose of tolterodine (8 mg/per day in divided doses, given as DETROL immediate release tablets) was 50% to 60% less than that of the active control moxifloxacin (400 mg) at its labeled dose. At the recommended therapeutic dose (4 mg daily) of DETROL (tolterodine L-tartrate tablets), the effect was lower. Since the QT prolongation effect is in linear relationship with exposure, any QT effect of DETROL LA (tolterodine L-tartrate extended release capsules) would also be expected to be similarly lower. This study, however, was not designed to make direct statistical comparisons between drugs, tolterodine formulations, or dose levels.

The clinical relevance of these findings will depend on individual patient risk factors and susceptibilities present. Particular care should be exercised in patients who are at an increased risk of experiencing torsade de pointes during treatment with QT/QTc-prolonging drugs. This especially holds true in patients with abnormally long baseline QT/QTc intervals or when taking potent CYP3A4 inhibitors (see Drug Interactions, Drug-Drug Interactions and Dosage and Administration).

In the general population, the risk factors for torsade de pointes include, but are not limited to, the following: female; elderly (65 years); genetic variants affecting cardiac ion channels or regulatory proteins, especially congenital long QT syndrome; family history of sudden cardiac death at <50 years; cardiac disease (e.g., myocardial ischemia or infarction, congestive heart failure, left ventricular hypertrophy, cardiomyopathy); demonstrated history of arrhythmias (especially ventricular arrhythmias, atrial fibrillation, or recent conversion from atrial fibrillation); bradycardia (<50 beats per minute); acute neurological events (e.g., intracranial or subarachnoid haemorrhage, stroke, intracranial trauma; electrolyte disturbances (e.g., hypokalemia, hypomagnesemia, hypocalcemia); nutritional deficits (e.g., eating disorders, extreme diets); diabetes mellitus; autonomic neuropathy; hepatic or renal dysfunction if relevant to the elimination of the drug.

Approximately 7% of Caucasians are poor metabolizers of CYP2D6 substrates. A pharmacokinetic/pharmacodynamic model estimated that QTc interval increases in poor metabolizers treated with tolterodine 2 mg BID are comparable to those observed in extensive metabolizers receiving 4 mg BID.

Discontinuation of the drug should be considered if symptoms suggestive of arrhythmia occur.

Gastrointestinal and Genitourinary: Patients at Risk of Urinary Retention and Gastric Retention: DETROL LA (tolterodine L-tartrate extended release capsules) should be administered with caution to patients with clinically significant bladder outflow obstruction because of the risk of urinary retention, to patients at risk of decreased gastrointestinal motility, and to patients with gastrointestinal obstructive disorders, such as pyloric stenosis, because of the risk of gastric retention (see Contraindications).

Hepatic/Biliary/Pancreatic/Renal: Patients with impaired hepatic function and patients with renal impairment should not receive doses of DETROL LA greater than 2 mg daily.

Neurologic: DETROL LA should be used with caution in patients with myasthenia gravis.

Ophthalmologic: Controlled Narrow Angle Glaucoma: DETROL LA should be used with caution in patients being treated for narrow angle glaucoma.

Special Populations: Pregnant Women: Studies in mice have shown that at doses of 30 to 40 mg/kg/day, tolterodine caused embryolethality, reduced fetal weight, and increased incidence of fetal abnormalities (cleft palate, digital abnormalities, intra-abdominal hemorrhage, various skeletal abnormalities, primarily reduced ossification in mice). At these doses, AUC values were about 20- to 25-fold higher than in humans. At doses of 20 mg/kg/day (AUC value was about 15-fold higher than in humans), no anomalies or malformations were seen in mice. There are no studies of tolterodine in pregnant women. Therefore, DETROL LA should be used during pregnancy only if the potential benefit for the mother justifies the potential risk for the fetus. Women of childbearing potential should be considered for treatment only if using adequate contraception.

Nursing Women: Tolterodine is excreted into the milk in mice. It is not known whether tolterodine is excreted in human milk. Because many drugs are excreted into human milk, administration of DETROL LA should be avoided during nursing.

Pediatrics: The safety and effectiveness of DETROL LA in pediatric patients have not been established.

Geriatrics (65-93 years of age): Of the 1120 patients who were treated in the four, phase III, 12-week clinical studies of DETROL, 474 (42%) were 65 to 91 years of age. No overall differences in safety were observed between the older and younger patients.

Of the 1526 patients who were treated in the 12-week clinical study comparing DETROL LA and tolterodine immediate release tablets versus placebo, 642 (42%) were 65 to 93 years of age. No overall differences in safety were observed between the older and younger patients.

Monitoring and Laboratory Tests: Monitoring of the QT/QTc interval and/or serum electrolyte levels may be appropriate in high risk patients who are being treated with DETROL LA, such as: patients with known congenital or acquired QT/QTc prolongation or electrolyte disturbances; patients with impaired hepatic or renal function or other comorbid conditions that may increase tolterodine exposure or cause QT/QTc prolongation; patients who are taking drugs that have been associated with QT/QTc prolongation and/or torsade de pointes such as Class IA (e.g., quinidine, procainamide) or Class III (e.g., amiodarone, sotalol) antiarrhythmic medications, or those taking potent CYP3A4 inhibitors.

(See Warnings and Precautions, Cardiovascular, Drug Interactions, Drug-Drug Interactions and Dosage and Administration.)

Discontinuation of the drug should be considered if symptoms suggestive of arrhythmia occur or if the QT/QTc interval becomes markedly prolonged.

Information to Be Provided to the Patient: The ability to drive and use machinery may be negatively affected. Patients should be advised to exercise caution.

ADVERSE REACTIONS: Adverse Drug Reaction Overview: In a large randomized, multicenter, double-blind, 12-week study, patients treated with DETROL LA (tolterodine L-tartrate extended release capsules), 4 mg once daily (N=505), tolterodine immediate release tablets, 2 mg twice daily (N=512), or placebo (N=507), were evaluated for safety.

DETROL LA, 4 mg once daily, was generally well tolerated, with an overall incidence of adverse events comparable to tolterodine immediate release tablets, 2 mg twice daily, and placebo. Dry mouth was the most frequently reported adverse event for patients treated with DETROL LA occurring in 23.4% of patients treated with DETROL LA, 30.5% in patients treated with tolterodine immediate release tablets and 7.7% of placebo-treated patients. The overall dry mouth rate for patients taking DETROL LA, in this single pivotal trial, was 23% lower than for tolterodine immediate release tablets (P<0.02) (see Table 1).

Table 1: DETROL LA

Adverse Events Considered to Be Related to Treatment with DETROL LA, Tolterodine Immediate Release Tablets, Versus Placebo

	DETROL LA (tolterodine extended release capsules)	Tolterodine immediate release tablets	Placebo
Dry Mouth	23.4%	30.5%	7.7%
Abdominal Pain	3.8%	2.5%	1.6%
Dyspepsia	3.0%	3.1%	1.4%
Dizziness/Vertigo	2.2%	1.8%	1.0%
Fatigue	2.2%	1.2%	0.8%
Sinusitis	1.8%	0.6%	0.6%
Abnormal Vision	1.2%	0.8%	0.4%
Dysuria	1.0%	1.6%	0.2%

Dry mouth, constipation, abnormal vision (accommodation abnormalities), urinary retention, and dry eyes are expected side effects of antimuscarinic agents.

The frequency of discontinuation due to adverse events was highest during the first 4 weeks of treatment. Similar percentages of patients treated with DETROL LA, tolterodine immediate release tablets or placebo, discontinued treatment due to adverse events; the most common adverse events associated with discontinuation were dry mouth (1.6%), headache (1.0%), and constipation (0.7%).

Clinical Trial Adverse Drug Reactions: Because clinical trials are conducted under very specific conditions the adverse reaction rates observed in the clinical trials may not reflect the rates observed in practice and should not be compared to the rates in the clinical trials of another drug. Adverse drug reaction information from clinical trials is useful for identifying drug-related adverse events and for approximating rates.

Table 2 lists the adverse events reported in ≥5% or more of patients treated with DETROL LA, 4 mg once daily, in the 12-week study. The adverse events were reported regardless of causality.

Table 2: DETROL LA

Incidence (%) of Adverse Events that Occurred in ≥5% of Patients Treated with DETROL LA and Tolterodine Immediate Release Tablets in a 12-week Controlled Clinical Trial

	DETROL LA (tolterodine extended release capsules) 4 mg Once Daily N=505	Placebo N=507	Tolterodine immediate release tablets 2 mg twice daily N=512
% Patients Reporting Serious Events	1.4	3.6	2.3
% Patients Discontinuing due to Adverse Events	5.3	6.5	5.4
Dry mouth	23.4	7.7	30.5
Headache	6.3	4.5	3.7
Constipation	5.9	4.3	6.6

Less Common Clinical Trial Adverse Drug Reactions (1% to <5%): Other events reported by 1% to <5% of patients treated with DETROL LA and numerically greater than those reported for patients receiving placebo are listed in order of descending frequency: abdominal pain, dry eyes, urinary tract infection, dyspepsia, upper respiratory tract infection, somnolence, dizziness, fatigue, flatulence, sinusitis, edema, pain, abnormal vision, and dysuria.

Over 400 patients treated for up to 6 months with DETROL LA, 4 mg once daily, had an overall incidence and adverse event profile similar to those patients treated with DETROL LA for 12 weeks.

Post-Market Adverse Drug Reactions: The following events have been reported in association with tolterodine use in clinical practice: anaphylactoid reactions (including angioedema), tachycardia, palpitations, peripheral edema, hallucinations, disorientation, memory impairment, and diarrhea.

Cholinesterase Inhibitors: Worsening of symptoms of dementia (e.g. confusion, disorientation, delusion) have been reported after tolterodine therapy was initiated in patients taking cholinesterase inhibitors for the treatment of dementia.

DRUG INTERACTIONS: Overview: Concomitant medication with other drugs that possess antimuscarinic properties may result in more pronounced therapeutic and/or adverse effects. Conversely, the therapeutic effect of tolterodine may be reduced by concomitant administration of muscarinic receptor agonists.

Drug-Drug Interactions: Effects of Other Drugs on DETROL LA: Drugs Which Prolong the QT/QTc Interval: Drugs that have been associated with QT/QTc interval prolongation and/or torsade de pointes include, but are not limited to, the examples in the following list. Chemical/pharmacological classes are listed if some, although not necessarily all, class members have been implicated in QT/QTc prolongation and/or torsade de pointes: antiarrhythmics (Class IA, e.g., quinidine, procainamide, disopyramide; Class III, e.g., amiodarone, sotalol, ibutilide; Class IC, e.g., flecainide, propafenone); antipsychotics (e.g., thioridazine, chlorpromazine, pimozide, haloperidol, droperidol); antidepressants (e.g., amitriptyline, imipramine, maprotiline, fluoxetine, venlafaxine); opioids (e.g., methadone); antibacterials (e.g., erythromycin, clarithromycin, telithromycin, moxifloxacin, gatifloxacin); antimalarials (e.g., quinine); pentamidine; azole antifungals (e.g., ketoconazole, fluconazole, voriconazole); gastrointestinal drugs (e.g., domperidone, dolasetron, ondasetron); B_2-adrenoreceptor agonist (salmeterol, formoterol); tacrolimus.

This list of potentially interacting drugs is not comprehensive. Prior to initiating drug treatment in the presence of concomitant medications, physicians should consult current scientific literature for information on the ability of newly approved drugs to prolong the QT/QTc interval, inhibit the metabolizing enzyme or transporter, or cause electrolyte disturbances, as well for older drugs for which these effects have recently been established (see Warnings and Precautions).

Cytochrome P450 3A4 inhibitors: Patients treated with ketoconazole or other potent CYP3A4 inhibitors such as other azole antifungals (e.g., itraconazole, miconazole) or macrolide antibiotics (e.g., erythromycin, clarithromycin) or cyclosporine or vinblastine, should not receive doses of DETROL LA (tolterodine L-tartrate extended release capsules) greater than 2 mg daily.

Fluoxetine: Fluoxetine, a potent inhibitor of P450 2D6, inhibits significantly the metabolism of tolterodine in extensive metabolizers. The sum of unbound serum concentrations of tolterodine and the 5 hydroxymethyl derivative (DD 01) is 25% higher when the two drugs are administered concomitantly. No dose adjustment is required.

Effects of DETROL LA on Other Drugs: Other Drugs Metabolized by P450 2D6: The potential effect of tolterodine on the pharmacokinetics of drugs that are metabolized by P450 2D6 (such as flecainide, vinblastine, carbamazepine, tricyclic antidepressants) has not been formally evaluated.

Diuretics: Coadministration of diuretics (such as indapamide, hydrochlorothiazide, triamterene, bendroflumethiazide, chlorothiazide, methylchlorothiazide, or furosemide) with DETROL (2 mg, twice daily) did not cause any adverse ECG effects, however, in the presence of diuretics causing hypokalemia, and, concomitant medications known or suspected to cause adverse ECG effects (such as QT/QTC prolongation), the physician is advised to exercise caution and advise the patient about the signs and symptoms of cardiac arrhythmia.

Oral Contraceptives: Clinical drug interaction studies have shown that there are no known interactions between tolterodine immediate release tablets and oral contraceptives (ethinyl estradiol/levonorgestrel).

Warfarin: Clinical drug interaction studies have shown that there are no known interactions between tolterodine immediate release tablets and warfarin.

Drug-Food Interactions: Food intake does not result in clinically relevant changes in the pharmacokinetic profile of either the tolterodine immediate release tablets or extended release capsules.

Drug-Herb Interactions: Interaction with herbal products has not been established.

Drug-Laboratory Test Interactions: Interactions between tolterodine and laboratory tests have not been studied.

Patient Counselling: Patients should be informed that antimuscarinic agents such as DETROL LA (tolterodine L-tartrate extended release capsules) may produce blurred vision or dizziness.

DOSAGE AND ADMINISTRATION: Dosing Considerations: Dosing of DETROL LA (tolterodine L-tartrate extended release capsules) may be affected by the following:

- individual response and tolerability
- impaired hepatic function and renal impairment
- potent CYP3A4 inhibitors

(See Warnings and Precautions and Dosage and Administration, Recommended Dose and Dosage Adjustment.)

Recommended Dose and Dosage Adjustment: The initial recommended maximum dose of DETROL LA (tolterodine L-tartrate extended release capsules) is 4 mg once daily. The dose may be reduced to 2 mg once daily based on individual response and tolerability. However, limited efficacy data are available for DETROL LA 2 mg once daily. For patients with impaired hepatic function and patients with renal impairment, the recommended dose is 2 mg once daily (see Warnings and Precautions). No dosage adjustment for elderly patients (≥ 65 years of age) is recommended (see Warnings and Precautions, Special Populations).

Patients treated with potent CYP3A4 inhibitors should not receive doses of DETROL LA greater than 2 mg once daily (see Warnings and Precautions).

The maximum recommended daily dose of 4 mg should not be exceeded.

Administration: DETROL LA can be taken with food. It should be swallowed whole.

OVERDOSAGE:

The highest dose of tolterodine tartrate given to human volunteers was 12.8 mg as single dose. The most severe adverse events observed were accommodation disturbances and micturition difficulties. One case of overdose has been reported prior to the marketing of the tolterodine immediate release tablets that involved a 27-month-old child who ingested 5 to 7 tablets of tolterodine immediate release 2 mg. He was hospitalized overnight with symptoms of dry mouth and was treated with a suspension of activated charcoal. The child recovered fully.

Management of Overdosage: Treatment of overdosage with DETROL LA (tolterodine L-tartrate extended release capsules) should consist of gastric lavage and activated charcoal. Treatments for symptoms are recommended as follows. For severe central anticholinergic effects (hallucinations, severe excitation), an anticholinesterase agent, such as physostigmine, may be used. If excitation and convulsions occur, administer an anticonvulsant, such as diazepam. Patients with respiratory insufficiency should be given respiratory assistance. If respiratory arrest occurs, patients should be given artificial respiration. Patients with tachycardia may be treated with a beta-blocker, and those with urinary retention may be catheterized. Patients with troublesome mydriasis may be placed in a dark room or treated with pilocarpine eye drops, or both. ECG should be monitored. In clinical trials of normal volunteers, QT interval prolongation was observed with tolterodine immediate release at doses of 8 mg (4 mg BID). The risk of torsade de pointes with a QT/QTc-prolonging drug is usually dose-dependent. It is recommended that continuous ECG monitoring may be appropriate in cases of overdose with Detrol (or Detrol LA). Concomitant therapy should be immediately reviewed and stopped if potential for drug-drug interaction and exacerbation of the QT prolongation effect is possible (see Warnings and Precautions, Drug Interactions, Drug-Drug Interactions).

For management of a suspected drug overdose, CPhA recommends that you contact your **regional Poison Control Centre**. See the *CPS* Directory section for a list of Poison Control Centres.

ACTION AND CLINICAL PHARMACOLOGY: Mechanism of Action: Tolterodine L-tartrate, is a competitive muscarinic receptor antagonist, which has been shown to inhibit carbachol-induced contraction of isolated bladder preparations from rats, guinea pigs, and man. Tolterodine L tartrate (henceforth referred to as tolterodine) inhibits contractions of the detrusor muscle from the guinea pig, and electrically induced contractions of human detrusor muscle from stable and overactive bladders ex vivo. Tolterodine is significantly more active in inhibiting acetylcholine-induced urinary bladder contractions than electrically induced salivation in the anesthetized cat.

Pharmacodynamics: Tolterodine has a pronounced effect on bladder function in healthy volunteers. The main effects following a 6.4 mg single dose of tolterodine were an increase in residual urine, reflecting an incomplete emptying of the bladder, and a decrease in detrusor pressure. These findings are consistent with antimuscarinic action on the lower urinary tract.

In patients with an overactive bladder who received recommended therapeutic doses of the tolterodine immediate release tablets, urodynamic measurements have shown that tolterodine increased the volume at first contraction and maximum cystometric capacity.

Tolterodine is converted to a pharmacologically active 5-hydroxymethyl metabolite (DD 01) by the isozyme cytochrome P450 2D6 (debrisoquine hydroxylase). This metabolite exhibits an antimuscarinic profile similar to that of tolterodine, both in vitro and in vivo. In view of the antimuscarinic activity of DD 01 and pharmacokinetic data from both humans and animals, it has been concluded that this metabolite contributes significantly to the therapeutic effect in extensive metabolizers (see Metabolism).

A dose-effect relationship was established in a Phase II study for the tolterodine extended release capsule (002) for mean residual volume per micturition during 12 hours. The dose of the tolterodine extended release capsule that has the same effect as the tolterodine immediate release tablets, 2 mg twice daily, was estimated to be 4.7 mg (3.7 mg after correction for relative exposure to the active moiety). A dose-effect relationship was also observed for the inhibition of salivation.

Pharmacokinetics: Absorption: In a study of ^{14}C tolterodine in healthy volunteers who received a 5 mg oral dose, at least 77% of the radiolabeled dose was absorbed. Tolterodine immediate release tablets are rapidly absorbed, and maximum serum concentrations (C_{max}) occur within 1 to 2 hours after dose administration. The pharmacokinetics of tolterodine immediate release tablets, based on C_{max} and area under the concentration time curve (AUC) determinations, are dose proportional over the range of 1 to 4 mg. Based on the sum of unbound serum concentrations of tolterodine and DD 01, the AUC of tolterodine extended release capsules, 4 mg once daily, is equivalent to tolterodine immediate release tablets, 2 mg twice daily. C_{max} and C_{min} levels of the extended release capsule are about 75% and 150% of the immediate release tablet, respectively, with maximum serum concentrations observed 2 to 6 hours after dose administration. Food intake does not result in clinically relevant changes in the pharmacokinetic profile of either the tolterodine immediate release tablets or extended release capsules.

Distribution: Tolterodine is highly bound to plasma proteins, primarily α 1-acid glycoprotein. Unbound concentrations of tolterodine average 3.7%±0.13% over the concentration range achieved in clinical studies. The 5-hydroxymethyl metabolite (DD 01) is not extensively protein bound, with unbound fraction concentrations averaging 36%±4.0%. The blood to serum ratio of tolterodine and DD 01 averages 0.6 and 0.8, respectively, indicating that these compounds do not distribute extensively into erythrocytes. The volume of distribution of tolterodine following administration of a 1.28 mg intravenous dose is 113±26.7 L.

Metabolism: Tolterodine is extensively metabolized by the liver following oral dosing, and is converted to DD 01 by the isozyme cytochrome P450 2D6. Further metabolism leads to formation of the 5 carboxylic acid and N dealkylated 5 carboxylic acid metabolites which account for 51%±14% and 29%±6.3% of the metabolites recovered in the urine respectively.

The potential effect of tolterodine on the pharmacokinetics of other drugs also metabolized by P450 2D6, such as tricyclic antidepressants, some antiarrhythmics and selective serotonin reuptake inhibitors, and neuroleptics has not been formally evaluated.

Variability in Metabolism: A subset (about 7%) of the population is devoid of the drug metabolizing isoenzyme cytochrome P450 2D6, the enzyme responsible for the formation of DD 01. The identified pathway of metabolism for these individuals, referred to as "poor metabolizers" (PMs), is dealkylation via cytochrome P450 3A4 to N dealkylated tolterodine. The remainder of the population is referred to as "extensive metabolizers" (EMs). Pharmacokinetic studies revealed that tolterodine is metabolized at a slower rate in PMs than in EMs. Since tolterodine and DD 01 have similar antimuscarinic effects, the net activity of DETROL LA is expected to be similar in EMs and PMs.

Excretion: Following administration of a 5 mg oral dose of ^{14}C-tolterodine solution to healthy volunteers, 77% of radioactivity was recovered in urine and 17% was recovered in feces in 7 days. Less than 1% (<2.5% in poor metabolizers) of the dose was recovered in urine and feces as intact tolterodine; 5% to 14% (<1% in poor metabolizers) was recovered as DD 01 within the first 24 hours. This is consistent with the apparent half life of tolterodine: 1.9 to 3.7 hours. The levels of the serum metabolites other than DD 01 determined in four poor metabolizers and four extensive metabolizers, were comparable for the tolterodine extended release capsule and immediate release tablet.
Special Populations and Conditions: Age: No overall differences were observed in safety between older and younger patients on tolterodine immediate release tablets in Phase III, 12 week, controlled clinical studies; and therefore, no dosage adjustment for elderly patients is recommended.
Gender: There are no sex dependent differences in the pharmacokinetic profile of tolterodine or DD 01.
Race: Pharmacokinetic differences due to race have not been identified.
Hepatic Insufficiency: Subjects with hepatic cirrhosis exhibit higher serum concentrations and longer half-lives of tolterodine and DD 01 compared to young healthy subjects given the same dose.
Renal Insufficiency: Potential pharmacologic effects and also the toxicological significance of metabolite levels should be taken into account if exposing subjects with renal impairment (GFR <30 mL/min) to repeated doses of tolterodine.

STORAGE AND STABILITY: Store at room temperature 15 to 30°C. Protect from light.

SPECIAL HANDLING INSTRUCTIONS: Not applicable.

INFORMATION FOR THE PATIENT: Published in e-CPS, available by subscription at www.e-cps.ca.

DOSAGE FORMS, COMPOSITION AND PACKAGING: 2 mg: Each blue-green extended release capsule, with symbol and "2" printed in white ink, contains: tolterodine L-tartrate 2 mg. Nonmedicinal ingredients: ammonium hydroxide, ethylcellulose, FD&C Blue 2, gelatin, hypromellose, medium chain triglycerides, oleic acid, Opacode White S-1-7085 (shellac glaze, titanium dioxide, ammonium hydroxide, propylene glycol and simethicone), starch, sucrose and yellow iron oxide. Bottles of 30 and 90.
4 mg: Each blue extended release capsule, with symbol and "4" printed in white ink, contains: tolterodine L-tartrate 4 mg. Nonmedicinal ingredients: ammonium hydroxide, ethylcellulose, FD&C Blue 2, gelatin, hypromellose, medium chain triglycerides, oleic acid, Opacode White S-1-7085 (shellac glaze, titanium dioxide, ammonium hydroxide, propylene glycol and simethicone), starch and sucrose. Bottles of 30 and 90.

(Shown in Product Identification Section)

Dexamethasone

CPhA Monograph

see *Corticosteroids: Eye Ear Nose*

see *Corticosteroids: Systemic*

Dexamethasone Sodium Phosphate Injection USP

dexamethasone sodium phosphate
Corticosteroid

Sandoz

SUPPLIED: 4 mg/mL: Each mL contains: dexamethasone sodium phosphate equivalent to dexamethasone phosphate 4 mg. Nonmedicinal ingredients: creatinine, methylparaben, propylparaben, sodium citrate·$2H_2O$, sodium hydroxide to adjust pH, sodium metabisulfite and water for injection. Multidose vials of 5 mL, boxes of 1 and 10. Do not autoclave. Store between 15 and 30°C. Protect from light.
10 mg/mL: Each mL contains: dexamethasone sodium phosphate equivalent to dexamethasone phosphate 10 mg. Nonmedicinal ingredients: anhydrous citric acid and/or sodium hydroxide to adjust pH, creatinine, sodium citrate·$2H_2O$ and water for injection. Preservative- and sulfite-free. Single use vials of 1 mL, boxes of 10. Discard unused portion. Store between 15 and 30°C. Protect from light. Do not autoclave.

Dexasone®

dexamethasone
Corticosteroid

Valeant

SUPPLIED: 0.5 mg: Each oval, yellow, scored tablet, imprinted ICN D11 contains: dexamethasone USP 0.5 mg. Nonmedicinal ingredients: cornstarch, colloidal silicon dioxide, lactose, magnesium stearate, microcrystalline cellulose and sodium starch glycolate. Bottles of 100.
0.75 mg: Each oval, pale blue, scored tablet, imprinted ICN D12 contains: dexamethasone USP 0.75 mg. Nonmedicinal ingredients: cornstarch, colloidal silicon dioxide, lactose, magnesium stearate, microcrystalline cellulose and sodium starch glycolate. Bottles of 100.
4 mg: Each oval, pale green, scored tablet, imprinted ICN D13 contains: dexamethasone USP 4 mg. Nonmedicinal ingredients: cornstarch, colloidal silicon dioxide, lactose, magnesium stearate, microcrystalline cellulose and sodium starch glycolate. Bottles of 100.

Dexedrine® Ⓒ

dextroamphetamine sulfate
Sympathomimetic

Paladin

Date of Revision: February 2, 2009

PHARMACOLOGY: Dextroamphetamine (dexamphetamine, d-amphetamine) sulfate is a sympathomimetic agent with indirect effects on adrenergic receptors. It has alpha-and beta-adrenergic activity. It has actions qualitatively similar to those of amphetamine sulfate but is approximately twice as potent. It has a marked stimulant effect on the CNS, particularly the cerebral cortex and the respiratory and vasomotor centres.

Dextroamphetamine sulfate causes a lessening of fatigue, an increase in mental activity, an elevation of mood, and a general feeling of well-being. However, its indiscriminate use in attempts to increase capacity for work or to overcome fatigue is undesirable. At high doses, it produces a euphoria which, upon abrupt withdrawal of the drug, reverts to severe depression and lethargy.

The mechanism by which amphetamines produce mental and behavioral effects in children is not conclusively established.

INDICATIONS: In the adjunctive treatment of: Narcolepsy.
Attention Deficit Hyperactivity Disorder (ADHD): A diagnosis of ADHD (DSM-IV) implies the presence of hyperactive-impulsive or inattentive symptoms that caused impairment and that were present before age 7 years. The symptoms must be persistent, must be more severe than is typically observed in individuals at a comparable level of development, must cause clinically significant impairment, e.g., in social, academic, or occupational functioning, and must be present in 2 or more settings, e.g., school (or work) and at home. The symptoms must not be better accounted for by another mental disorder. For the Inattentive Type, at least 6 of the following symptoms must have persisted for at least 6 months: lack of attention to details/careless mistakes, lack of sustained attention, poor listener, failure to follow through on tasks, poor organization, avoids tasks requiring sustained mental effort, loses things, easily distracted, forgetful. For the Hyperactive-Impulsive Type, at least 6 of the following symptoms must have persisted for at least 6 months: fidgeting/squirming, leaving seat, inappropriate running/climbing, difficulty with quiet activities, "on the go," excessive talking, blurting answers, can't wait turn, intrusive. For a Combined Type diagnosis, both inattentive and hyperactive-impulsive criteria must be met.
Special Diagnostic Considerations: The specific aetiology of ADHD is unknown, and there is no single diagnostic test. Adequate diagnosis requires the use not only of medical but of special psychological, educational, and social resources. Learning may or may not be impaired. The diagnosis must be based upon a complete history and evaluation of the patient and not solely on the presence of the required number of DSM-IV characteristics.
Need for Comprehensive Treatment Program: Dextroamphetamine is indicated as an integral part of a total treatment program for ADHD that may include other measures (psychological, educational, social) for patients with this syndrome. Drug treatment may not be indicated for all patients with this syndrome. Drug treatment is not intended for use in the patient who exhibits symptoms secondary to environmental factors and/or other primary psychiatric disorders, including psychosis. Appropriate educational placement is essential in children and adolescents with this diagnosis and psychosocial intervention is often helpful. When remedial measures alone are insufficient, the decision to prescribe drug treatment medication will depend upon the physician's assessment of the chronicity and severity of the patient's symptoms.

CONTRAINDICATIONS: Advanced arteriosclerosis, symptomatic cardiovascular disease, moderate to severe hypertension, hyperthyroidism, hypersensitivity or idiosyncrasy to sympathomimetic amines, agitated states, history of drug abuse, glaucoma, anxiety, tension, patients with known hypersensitivity to dextroamphetamine or to any ingredient in the formulation or component of the container, patients with motor tics or with a family history of diagnosis of Tourette's Syndrome (verbal tics), concomitant treatment with MAO inhibitors.

During administration or within 14 days following the withdrawal of MAOI, administration of dextroamphetamine may cause hypertensive crises.

WARNINGS: Sudden Death and Pre-existing Structural Cardiac Abnormalities: Children and Adolescents: Sudden death has been reported in association with stimulant drugs used for ADHD treatment at usual doses in children and adolescents with structural cardiac abnormalities or other serious heart problems.

Although some serious heart problems alone carry an increased risk of sudden death, stimulant products generally should not be used in children or adolescents with known serious structural cardiac abnormalities, cardiomyopathy, serious heart rhythm abnormalities, or other serious cardiac problems that may place them at increased vulnerability to the sympathomimetic effects of a stimulant drug.
Adults: Sudden deaths, stroke, and myocardial infarction have been reported in adults taking stimulant drugs at usual doses for ADHD. Although the role of stimulants in these adult cases is also unknown, adults have a greater likelihood than children of having serious structural cardiac abnormalities, cardiomyopathy, serious heart rhythm abnormalities, coronary artery disease, or other serious cardiac problems. Adults with such abnormalities should also generally not be treated with stimulant drugs (see Contraindications).
General: Theoretically there exists a pharmacological potential for all ADHD drugs to increase the risk of sudden/cardiac death. Although confirmation of an incremental risk for adverse cardiac events arising from treatment with ADHD medications is lacking, prescribers should consider this potential risk.
Hypertension and Other Cardiovascular Conditions: Stimulant medications cause a modest increase in average blood pressure (about 2-4 mmHg) and average heart rate (about 3-6 bpm), and individuals may have larger increases. While the mean changes alone would not be expected to have short-term consequences, all patients should be monitored for larger changes in heart rate and blood pressure. Caution is indicated in treating patients whose underlying medical conditions might be compromised by increases in blood pressure or heart rate, e.g., those with pre-existing hypertension, heart failure, recent myocardial infarction, or ventricular arrhythmia (see Contraindications).
Assessing Cardiovascular Status in Patients being Treated with Stimulant Medications: Children, adolescents, or adults who are being considered for treatment with stimulant medications should have a careful history (including assessment for a family history of sudden death or ventricular arrhythmia) and physical exam to assess for the presence of cardiac disease, and should receive further cardiac evaluation if findings suggest such disease (e.g., electrocardiogram and echocardiogram). Patients who develop symptoms such as exertional chest pain, unexplained syncope, or other symptoms suggestive of cardiac disease during stimulant treatment should undergo a prompt cardiac evaluation. All drugs with sympathomimetic effects prescribed in the management of ADHD should be used with caution in patients who: a) are involved in strenuous exercise or activities b) use other stimulants or c) have a family history of sudden/cardiac death.
Psychiatric Adverse Events: Pre-Existing Psychosis: Administration of stimulants may exacerbate symptoms of behavior disturbance and thought disorder in patients with a pre-existing psychotic disorder.
Bipolar Illness: Particular care should be taken in using stimulants to treat ADHD in patients with comorbid bipolar disorder because of concern for possible induction of a mixed/manic episode in such patients. Prior to initiating treatment with a stimulant, patients with comorbid depressive symptoms should be adequately screened to determine if they are at risk for bipolar disorder; such screening should include a detailed psychiatric history, including a family history of suicide, bipolar disorder, and depression.
Emergence of New Psychotic or Manic Symptoms: Treatment emergent psychotic or manic symptoms, e.g., hallucinations, delusional thinking, or mania in children and adolescents without a prior history of psychotic illness or mania can be caused by stimulants at usual doses. If such symptoms occur, consideration should be given to a possible causal role of the stimulant, and discontinuation of treatment may be appropriate. In a pooled analysis of multiple short-term, placebo-controlled studies, such symptoms occurred in about 0.1% (4 patients with events out of 3482 exposed to methylphenidate or amphetamine for several weeks at usual doses) of stimulant-treated patients compared to 0 in placebo-treated patients.
Aggression: Aggressive behavior or hostility is often observed in children and adolescents with ADHD, and has been reported in clinical trials and the postmarketing experience of some medications indicated for the treatment of ADHD. Although there is no systematic evidence that stimulants cause aggressive behavior or hostility, patients beginning treatment for ADHD should be monitored for the appearance of or worsening of aggressive behavior or hostility.
Long-Term Suppression of Growth: Careful follow-up of weight and height in children ages 7 to 10 years who were randomized to either methylphenidate or non-medication treatment groups over 14 months, as well as in naturalistic subgroups of newly methylphenidate-treated and non-medication treated children over 36 months (to the ages of 10 to 13 years), suggests that consistently medicated children (i.e., treatment for 7 days per week throughout the year) have a temporary slowing in growth rate (on average, a total of about 2 cm less growth in height and 2.7 kg less growth in weight over 3 years), without evidence of growth rebound during this period of development. Published data are inadequate to determine whether chronic use of amphetamines may cause a similar suppression of growth, however, it is anticipated that they likely have this effect as well. Therefore, growth should be monitored during treatment with stimulants, and patients who are not growing or gaining height or weight as expected may need to have their treatment interrupted.
Seizures: There is some clinical evidence that stimulants may lower the convulsive threshold in patients with prior history of seizures, in patients with prior EEG abnormalities in absence of seizures, and, very rarely, in patients without a history of seizures and no prior EEG evidence of seizures. In the presence of seizures, the drug should be discontinued.
Visual Disturbances: Difficulties with accommodation and blurring of vision have been reported with stimulant treatment.

Amphetamines have been subject to extensive abuse. Tolerance, extreme psychological dependence, and severe social disability can occur. Patients have been reported to increase their dosage to many times the recommended level. The smallest possible amount of the drug should be prescribed or dispensed at one time.

PRECAUTIONS: Occupational Hazards: Amphetamines may mask extreme fatigue, which can impair the ability to perform potentially hazardous activities such as operating machinery or driving motor vehicles; patients should be cautioned accordingly.

Amphetamines may alter insulin requirements in diabetes mellitus, and may decrease the hypotensive effect of guanethidine.

DEXEDRINE tablets contain tartrazine (FD&C yellow #5), which can cause allergic type reactions (including bronchial asthma) in susceptible individuals, especially people with a history of allergy to ASA. Cross-sensitivity to salicylates and tartrazine is frequently seen.

The possibility of tolerance and psychological dependence, particularly with excessive use, should be kept in mind. Therefore, care should be used in the selection of candidates for dextroamphetamine therapy. Should psychological dependence occur, discontinue medication. Abrupt cessation following prolonged high dosage administration may result in extreme fatigue and mental depression. Changes have also been noted on the sleep EEG.

Manifestations of chronic intoxication with amphetamines include severe dermatoses, marked insomnia, irritability, hyperactivity, and personality changes. The most severe manifestation of chronic intoxication is psychosis, often clinically indistinguishable from schizophrenia.
Children: Amphetamines are not recommended for use in Attention-Deficit Hyperactivity Disorder in children under 6 years of age.

Long-term effects of amphetamines in children have not been well established.

Chronic administration of amphetamines may be associated with growth inhibition; growth should be monitored during treatment.

Clinical experience suggests that in psychotic children, administration of amphetamines may exacerbate symptoms of behavior disturbance and thought disorder.

The presence of tics or Tourette's syndrome should be ruled out before administering amphetamines to children.
Drug Interactions: Caution should be exercised when co-prescribing amphetamines and other drugs, since clinically significant interactions with a number of drugs have been reported. In some instances, potentiation of CNS and cardiac effects could be life threatening. Dosages should be closely monitored.

Known interactions with amphetamines are as follows: Synergistic Interactions: tricyclic antidepressants, MAO inhibitors, meperidine, norepinephrine, phenobarbital, phenytoin, propoxyphene, acetazolamide, thiazides, gastrointestinal and urinary alkalinizing agents.
Antagonistic Interactions: adrenergic blockers, antihistamines, antihypertensives, chlorpromazine, ethosuximide, guanethidine, haloperidol, lithium carbonate, methenamine, Veratrum alkaloids, gastrointestinal and urinary acidifying agents.
Pregnancy: Safe use in pregnancy has not been established. Infants born to mothers dependent on amphetamines have an increased risk of premature delivery and low birth weight. Also, these infants may experience symptoms of withdrawal, as manifested by dysphoria, agitation and significant lassitude. Reproductive studies in mammals, at high multiples of the human dose, have suggested an embryotoxic and a teratogenic potential. Use of amphetamines by women who are or who may become pregnant, and especially those in the first trimester of pregnancy, requires that the potential benefit be weighed against the possible hazard to mother and child.
Lactation: Amphetamines are excreted in human milk. Mothers taking dextroamphetamine should be advised to refrain from nursing.
Laboratory Test Interactions: Amphetamines can elevate plasma corticosteroid levels, particularly in the evening, and may interfere with urinary steroid determinations.

ADVERSE EFFECTS: Cardiovascular: palpitations, tachycardia, elevation of blood pressure. There have been isolated reports of cardiomyopathy associated with chronic amphetamine use.
Central Nervous System: overstimulation, restlessness, dizziness, euphoria or dysphoria, dyskinesia, headache, insomnia, exacerbation of motor and phonic tics, Tourette's syndrome, tremor; rarely, psychotic episodes at recommended doses.
Gastrointestinal: dryness of the mouth, unpleasant taste, loss of appetite, diarrhea, constipation, other gastrointestinal disturbances, anorexia and weight loss.
Allergic: urticaria.
Other: impotence, changes in libido.
Post-marketing: sudden/cardiac death.

OVERDOSE:
The toxic dose of amphetamine varies widely according to the degree of tolerance present. Blood levels are, therefore, of little value in assessing the severity of the overdose; this assessment must depend almost entirely on clinical signs.
Symptoms: Dilated and reactive pupils, shallow rapid respiration, rhabdomyolysis, hyperpyrexia, fever, chills, sweating, hyperactive tendon reflexes. Other symptoms are:

Central effects may include restlessness, tremor, aggressiveness, anxiety, confusion, delirium, hallucinations, panic attacks and even suicidal or homicidal tendencies. The stimulant effect is usually followed by depression, lethargy, exhaustion.

Cardiovascular effects may include anginal pain, extrasystoles and other arrhythmias, flushing, headache, hypertension or hypotension, pallor, palpitations, tachycardia. Circulatory collapse and syncope may occur.

Gastrointestinal effects include nausea, vomiting, diarrhea, abdominal cramps.

Fatal poisoning is usually preceded by convulsions and coma.

Treatment: Treatment is essentially symptomatic and supportive. In addition to the usual measures (including emesis, gastric lavage, catharsis), sedatives should be given when indicated. Oral or parenteral barbiturates are generally used for this purpose. To provide a basal level of sedation, one or more doses of sodium amobarbital may be given by mouth or, if necessary, by i.m. injection. This may be repeated as often as necessary and in quantities sufficient to control the symptoms.

Sedation may also be accomplished with chlorpromazine: in children 1 mg/kg body weight i.m. and in adults 100 mg i.m., repeated at half-hourly intervals if necessary. If the amphetamine has been taken with a barbiturate, as is often the case, the chlorpromazine dosage should be halved.
Note: It has been stated that the effects of amphetamines are best treated with haloperidol (Med Lett 1983 Sep 16;25:87), a dopamine antagonist with minimal anticholinergic side effects. Haloperidol, however, possesses central antiemetic properties; it may prolong the hypnotic action of barbiturates and may potentiate the effects of alcohol and other CNS depressant drugs; it may lower the convulsion threshold.

In general, the hypertension which may result from massive overdose of dextroamphetamine does not require treatment. A gradual drop in blood pressure will usually result when sufficient sedation has been administered. Phentolamine may be used to decrease blood pressure and hyperthermia. In the presence of severe hypotension, the usual procedures employed for shock should be instituted.

Acidification of the urine enhances excretion. Experience with forced diuresis, hemodialysis, peritoneal dialysis or charcoal hemoperfusion is inadequate to permit recommendations in this regard.

Since much of the Spansule capsule medication is coated for gradual release, therapy directed at reversing the effects of the ingested drug and at supporting the patient should be continued for as long as overdosage symptoms remain. Saline cathartics are useful for hastening the evacuation of pellets that have not already released medication.

For management of a suspected drug overdose, CPhA recommends that you contact your **regional Poison Control Centre**. See the *CPS* Directory section for a list of Poison Control Centres.

DOSAGE: Dosing Considerations: Dextroamphetamine should be administered starting at the lowest possible dose. Dosage should then be individually and slowly adjusted, to the lowest effective dosage, since individual patient response to dextroamphetamine varies widely. Time of administration should receive special attention—particularly with the Spansule capsule form—because of possible insomnia. Late evening medication should be avoided.

Dextroamphetamine should not be used in patients with symptomatic cardiovascular disease and should generally not be used in patients with known structural cardiac abnormalities (see Contraindications and Warnings).

Theoretically there exists a pharmacological potential for all ADHD drugs to increase the risk of sudden/cardiac death. Although confirmation of an incremental risk for adverse cardiac events arising from treatment with ADHD medications is lacking, prescribers should consider this potential risk.

All drugs with sympathomimetic effects prescribed in the management of ADHD should be used with caution in patients who: a) are involved in strenuous exercise or activities b) use stimulants or c) have a family history of sudden/cardiac death. Prior to the initiation of treatments, a personal and family history should be obtained. In patients with relevant risk factors and based on the clinician's judgment, further cardiovascular evaluation may be considered.

Patients who are considered to need extended treatment with dextroamphetamine should undergo periodic evaluation of their cardiovascular status (see Warnings).
Narcolepsy: Daily dosage may range from 5 to 60 mg, depending on individual patient response.
Suggested initial dosage for patients aged 6 to 12: Start with 5 mg daily; daily dosage may be raised in increments of 5 mg at weekly intervals until optimal response is obtained.
In patients 12 years of age and older: start with 10 mg daily; Daily dosage may be raised in increments of 10 mg at weekly intervals until optimal response is obtained.

If bothersome adverse reactions appear (e.g., insomnia or anorexia), dosage should be reduced. Spansule capsules may be used for once-a-day dosage wherever appropriate. With tablets, give first dose on awakening; additional doses (1 or 2) at intervals of 4 to 6 hours.
Attention-deficit Hyperactivity Disorder in Children: Daily dosage may range from 2.5 to 40 mg, although some older children may require more than 40 mg daily for optimal response. If bothersome adverse reactions appear (e.g., insomnia or anorexia), dosage should be reduced. Spansule capsules may be used for once-a-day dosage wherever appropriate. With tablets, give first dose on awakening; additional doses (1 or 2) at intervals of 4 to 6 hours.

Not recommended for this use in children under 6 years of age.

In children 6 years of age or older, start with 5 mg once or twice daily; daily dosage may be raised in increments of 5 mg at weekly intervals, until optimal response is obtained. Only in rare cases will it be necessary to exceed a total of 40 mg/day.

Most children suffering from Attention-Deficit Hyperactivity Disorder require medication for several years, although once symptoms have been controlled, it may be possible to reduce dosage or to interrupt drug therapy during the summer months and at other times when the child is under less stress. During periods of interrupted drug therapy, behavioral symptoms should be assessed to determine whether their recurrence is sufficient to justify the resumption of treatment.

INFORMATION FOR THE PATIENT: Published in e-CPS, available by subscription at www.e-cps.ca.

SUPPLIED: Spansules: 10 mg: Each brown-capped, natural colored body taper-end capsule, with 2 shades of orange pellets, monogrammed "3513" on the cap with "10 mg" and "SB" on the body in white ink, contains: dextroamphetamine sulfate 10 mg, and releases a therapeutic dose promptly with the remaining dose being delivered gradually and without interruption to sustain the effects for 10 to 12 hours. Nonmedicinal ingredients: cetyl alcohol, D&C Yellow No. 10, dibutyl sebacate, ethylcellulose, FD&C Blue No. 1, FD&C Blue No. 1 Aluminum Lake, FD&C Red No. 40, FD&C Yellow No. 6, gelatin, hydroxypropyl methylcellulose, propylene glycol, povidone, silicon dioxide, sodium lauryl sulfate, sugar spheres and trace amounts of other inactive ingredients. Energy: 3.72 kJ (0.88 kcal). Bottles of 100.
15 mg: Each brown-capped, natural colored body taper-end capsule, with 2 shades of orange pellets, monogrammed "3514" on the cap with "15 mg" and "SB" on the body in white ink, contains: dextroamphetamine sulfate 15 mg, and releases a therapeutic dose promptly with the remaining dose being delivered gradually and without interruption to sustain the effect for 10 to 12 hours. Nonmedicinal ingredients: cetyl alcohol, D&C Yellow No. 10, dibutyl sebacate, ethylcellulose, FD&C Blue No. 1, FD&C Blue No. 1 Aluminum Lake, FD&C Red No. 40, FD&C Yellow No. 6, gelatin, hydroxypropyl methylcellulose, propylene glycol, povidone, silicon dioxide, sodium lauryl sulfate, sugar spheres and trace amounts of other inactive ingredients. Energy: 4.78 kJ (1.14 kcal). Bottles of 100.
Tablets: Each orange, round-cornered, equilaterally triangular shaped, scored, compressed tablet, engraved "SKF E19", contains: dextroamphetamine sulfate 5 mg. Nonmedicinal ingredients: calcium sulfate, gelatin, lactose, FD&C Yellow No. 5 (tartrazine), FD&C Yellow No. 6, starch, stearic acid, sucrose and talc. Energy: 1.46 kJ (0.35 kcal). Bottles of 100.

(Shown in Product Identification Section)

Dexilant™ Ⓟ

dexlansoprazole

H+, K+-ATPase Inhibitor

Takeda Canada

Date of Preparation: July 21, 2010
SUMMARY PRODUCT INFORMATION:

Route of Administration	Dosage Form/ Strength	Clinically Relevant Nonmedicinal Ingredients
Oral	Capsule 30 mg, 60 mg	None For a complete listing see Dosage Forms, Composition and Packaging.

INDICATIONS AND CLINICAL USE: DEXILANT is indicated for the following in adults 18 years of age and older:
Healing of Erosive Esophagitis: DEXILANT is indicated for healing of all grades of erosive esophagitis for up to 8 weeks.
Maintenance of Healed Erosive Esophagitis: DEXILANT is indicated for maintaining healing of erosive esophagitis for up to 6 months.
Symptomatic Non-Erosive Gastroesophageal Reflux Disease: DEXILANT is indicated for the treatment of heartburn associated with symptomatic non-erosive gastroesophageal reflux disease (GERD) for 4 weeks.
Geriatrics (>65 years of age): No dosage adjustment is necessary for elderly patients.
Pediatrics (<18 years of age): Safety and effectiveness of DEXILANT in pediatric patients have not been established.
CONTRAINDICATIONS: Patients who are hypersensitive to this drug or to any ingredient in the formulation. For a complete listing, see Dosage Forms, Composition and Packaging.

DEXILANT should not be concomitantly administered with atazanavir (see Drug Interactions, Drugs with pH-Dependent Absorption Pharmacokinetics).
WARNINGS AND PRECAUTIONS: General: Symptomatic response with DEXILANT does not preclude the presence of gastric malignancy.

Pseudomembranous colitis has been reported with nearly all antibacterial agents, including clarithromycin and amoxicillin, and may range in severity from mild to life threatening. Therefore, it is important to consider this diagnosis in patients who present with diarrhea subsequent to the administration of antibacterial agents.

Treatment with antibacterial agents alters the normal flora of the colon and may permit overgrowth of Clostridia. Studies indicate that a toxin produced by *C. difficile* is a primary cause of "antibiotic-associated colitis".

After the diagnosis of pseudomembranous colitis has been established, therapeutic measures should be initiated. Mild cases of pseudomembranous colitis usually respond to discontinuation of the drug alone. In moderate to severe cases, consideration should be given to management with fluids and electrolytes, protein supplementation, and treatment with an antibacterial drug clinically effective against *C. difficile* colitis.

Decreased gastric acidity due to any means, including proton pump inhibitors, increases gastric counts of bacteria normally present in the gastrointestinal tract. Treatment with proton pump inhibitors may lead to slightly increased risk of gastrointestinal infections such as Salmonella and Campylobacter and possibly *C. difficile*.
Carcinogenesis and Mutagenesis: Dexlansoprazole was positive in the Ames test for mutagenicity in bacteria. In an in vitro chromosome aberration test using Chinese hamster lung cells, dexlansoprazole was considered positive based on equivocal data in which the percentage of cells with aberrant chromosomes increased slightly but did not reach the preset criteria for a positive response. Dexlansoprazole was negative in the in vivo mouse micronucleus test.

Lansoprazole is a racemic mixture of R- and S-enantiomers. Following administration of lansoprazole in humans and animals, the major component circulating in plasma is dexlansoprazole, the R-enantiomer of lansoprazole. Therefore, the carcinogenic potential of dexlansoprazole was assessed using existing lansoprazole studies. Lansoprazole treatment for 2-years was associated with hyperplasia and neoplasms (carcinoids) of enterochromaffin-like cells (ECL cells) in the stomach of conventional rats and mice. These proliferations are related to prolonged hypergastrinemia secondary to gastric acid suppression. Benign tumors of the testis (interstitial cell adenomas in rats and rete testis adenomas in mice) were secondary to an inhibitory effect on testosterone synthesis at high doses in these species. Hepatocellular adenomas and carcinomas were increased in the livers of mice related to induction of CYP enzymes leading to increased liver weights.
Genitourinary: Testicular interstitial cell adenoma occurred in 1 of 30 rats treated with 50 mg/kg/day of lansoprazole (13 times the recommended human dose based on body surface area) in a one-year toxicity study.

These changes are associated with endocrine alterations which have not been, to date, observed in humans.
Special Populations: Pregnant Women: There are no adequate or well-controlled studies in pregnant women with DEXILANT. Exposure in clinical trials was very limited. DEXILANT should not be administered to pregnant women unless the expected benefits outweigh the potential risks.
Nursing Women: It is not known whether dexlansoprazole is excreted in human milk. However, lansoprazole (the racemate) and its metabolites are excreted in the milk of rats. As many drugs are excreted in human milk, DEXILANT should not be given to nursing mothers unless its use is considered essential.
Pediatrics (<18 years of age): Safety and effectiveness of DEXILANT in pediatric patients have not been established.
Geriatrics (>65 years of age): In clinical studies of DEXILANT, 11% of patients were aged 65 years and over. No overall differences in safety or effectiveness were observed between these patients and younger patients. No dosage adjustment is necessary for elderly patients. See Action and Clinical Pharmacology, Special Populations and Conditions.
Hepatic Impairment: No dosage adjustment is necessary for patients with mild hepatic impairment (Child-Pugh Class A). A maximum daily dose of 30 mg should be considered for patients with moderate hepatic impairment (Child-Pugh Class B). No studies have been conducted in patients with severe hepatic impairment. See Action and Clinical Pharmacology, Special Populations and Conditions.
Renal Impairment: No dosage adjustment is necessary for patients with renal impairment. See Action and Clinical Pharmacology, Special Populations and Conditions.
ADVERSE REACTIONS: Clinical Trial Adverse Drug Reactions: Because clinical trials are conducted under very specific conditions the adverse reaction rates observed in the clinical trials may not reflect the rates observed in practice and should not be compared to the rates in the clinical trials of another drug. Adverse drug reaction information from clinical trials is useful for identifying drug-related adverse events and for approximating rates.

The safety of DEXILANT was evaluated in 4548 patients in controlled and uncontrolled clinical studies (30 mg, 60 mg, and 90 mg), including 863 patients treated for at least 6 months and 282 patients treated for one year. Patients ranged in age from 18 to 90 years (median age 48 years), with 54% female, 85% Caucasian, 8% Black, 4% Asian and 3% other races. Six randomized controlled clinical trials were conducted for the treatment of erosive esophagitis, maintenance of healed erosive esophagitis, and symptomatic GERD, which included 896 patients on placebo, 2621 patients on DEXILANT 30 mg or 60 mg and 1363 patients on lansoprazole 30 mg.

The following adverse events were reported to have a possible or definite treatment-relationship to DEXILANT in 1% or more of the treated patients in placebo and positive-controlled clinical trials (Table 1 and Table 2, respectively). Numbers in parentheses indicate the percentage of the adverse events reported.

Table 1: DEXILANT

Incidence of Possibly or Definitely Treatment-Related Adverse Events in Placebo Controlled Studies

Body System Adverse Event	Placebo (N=896) n (%)	DEXILANT 30 mg and 60 mg (N=1399) n (%)
Gastrointestinal Disorders		
Diarrhea	17 (1.9)	52 (3.7)
Abdominal Pain	14 (1.6)	37 (2.6)
Nausea	16 (1.8)	31 (2.2)
Flatulence	5 (0.6)	25 (1.8)
Constipation	9 (1.0)	15 (1.1)
Nervous System Disorders		
Headache	21 (2.3)	31 (2.2)

Table 2: DEXILANT

Incidence of Possibly or Definitely Treatment-Related Adverse Events in Active Controlled Clinical Trials

Body System Adverse Event	DEXILANT 60 mg (N=2621) n (%)	Lansoprazole 30 mg (N=1363) n (%)
Gastrointestinal Disorders		
Diarrhea	44 (3.2)	28 (2.1)
Abdominal pain	21 (1.5)	19 (1.4)
Nausea	14 (1.0)	18 (1.3)
Nervous System Disorders		
Headache	16 (1.2)	19 (1.4)

In placebo-controlled studies, gastrointestinal adverse reactions other than constipation occurred at a higher incidence for DEXILANT than placebo. In active-controlled studies, diarrhea occurred at a higher incidence for DEXILANT than lansoprazole. The incidence of other common adverse reactions for DEXILANT were similar to or lower than placebo or lansoprazole.

Less Common Clinical Trial Adverse Drug Reactions (<1%): Other adverse reactions that were reported for DEXILANT (30 mg, 60 mg or 90 mg) in controlled studies at an incidence of less than 1% are listed below by body system:

Blood and Lymphatic System Disorders: anemia, lymphadenopathy.

Cardiac Disorders: acute myocardial infarction, angina, arrhythmia, bradycardia, edema, palpitations, tachycardia.

Ear and Labyrinth Disorders: ear pain, tinnitus, vertigo.

Endocrine Disorders: goiter.

Eye Disorders: eye irritation, eye swelling.

Gastrointestinal Disorders: abdominal discomfort, abdominal tenderness, abnormal feces, anal discomfort, Barrett's esophagus, bezoar, bowel sounds abnormal, breath odor, colitis microscopic, colonic polyp, dry mouth, duodenitis, dyspepsia, dysphagia, enteritis, eructation, esophagitis, gastric polyp, gastritis, gastroenteritis, gastrointestinal disorders, gastrointestinal hypermotility disorders, GERD, GI ulcers and perforation, hematemesis, hematochezia, hemorrhoids, impaired gastric emptying, irritable bowel syndrome, mucus stools, oral mucosal blistering, painful defecation, paresthesia oral, proctitis, rectal hemorrhage, vomiting.

General Disorders and Administration Site Conditions: adverse drug reaction, asthenia, chest pain, chills, feeling abnormal, inflammation, mucosal inflammation, nodule, pain, pyrexia.

Hepatobiliary Disorders: biliary colic, cholelithiasis, hepatomegaly.

Immune System Disorders: hypersensitivity.

Infections and Infestations: candida infections, influenza, nasopharyngitis, oral herpes, pharyngitis, sinusitis, upper respiratory tract infection, viral infection, vulvo-vaginal infection.

Injury, Poisoning and Procedural Complications: overdose, procedural pain, sunburn.

Laboratory Investigations: ALP increased, ALT increased, AST increased, bilirubin decreased/increased, blood creatinine increased, blood gastrin increased, blood glucose increased, blood potassium increased, liver function test abnormal, platelet count decreased, total protein increased, weight increased.

Metabolism and Nutrition Disorders: appetite changes, hypercalcemia, hypokalemia.

Musculoskeletal and Connective Tissue Disorders: arthralgia, arthritis, muscle cramps, musculoskeletal pain, myalgia.

Nervous System Disorders: altered taste, convulsion, dizziness, memory impairment, migraine, paresthesia, psychomotor hyperactivity, tremor, trigeminal neuralgia.

Psychiatric Disorders: abnormal dreams, anxiety, depression, insomnia, libido changes.

Renal and Urinary Disorders: dysuria, micturition urgency.

Reproductive System and Breast Disorders: dysmenorrhea, dyspareunia, menorrhagia, menstrual disorder.

Respiratory, Thoracic and Mediastinal Disorders: aspiration, asthma, bronchitis, cough, dyspnoea, hiccups, hyperventilation, respiratory tract congestion, sore throat.

Skin and Subcutaneous Tissue Disorders: acne, dermatitis, erythema, pruritus, rash, skin lesion, urticaria.

Vascular Disorders: deep vein thrombosis, hot flush, hypertension.

Additional adverse reactions that were reported for DEXILANT (60 mg or 90 mg) in a long-term uncontrolled study included: anaphylaxis, auditory hallucination, B-cell lymphoma, bursitis, central obesity, cholecystitis acute, decreased hemoglobin, dehydration, diabetes mellitus, dysphonia, epistaxis, folliculitis, gout, herpes zoster, hyperglycemia, hyperlipidemia, hypothyroidism, increased neutrophils, MCHC decreased, neutropenia, oral soft tissue disorder, rectal tenesmus, restless legs syndrome, somnolence, thrombocythemia, tonsillitis.

Post-Market Adverse Drug Reactions: Adverse reactions have been identified during post-marketing surveillance of DEXILANT. As these reactions are reported voluntarily from a population of uncertain size, it is not always possible to reliably estimate their frequency or establish a causal relationship to drug exposure.

Eye Disorders: blurred vision.

Gastrointestinal Disorders: oral edema.

General Disorders and Administration Site Conditions: facial edema.

Immune System Disorders: anaphylactic shock (requiring emergency intervention), Stevens-Johnson syndrome, toxic epidermal necrolysis (some fatal).

Respiratory, Thoracic and Mediastinal Disorders: pharyngeal edema, throat tightness.

Skin and Subcutaneous Tissue Disorders: generalized rash, leucocytoclastic vasculitis.

DRUG INTERACTIONS: Drug-Drug Interactions: Drugs with pH-Dependent Absorption Pharmacokinetics: DEXILANT causes inhibition of gastric acid secretion. DEXILANT is likely to substantially decrease the systemic concentrations of the HIV protease inhibitor atazanavir, which is dependent upon the presence of gastric acid for absorption, and may result in a loss of therapeutic effect of atazanavir and the development of HIV resistance. Therefore, DEXILANT should not be co-administered with atazanavir.

It is theoretically possible that DEXILANT may interfere with the absorption of other drugs where gastric pH is an important determinant of oral bioavailability (e.g., ampicillin esters, digoxin, iron salts, ketoconazole).

Cytochrome P450 Interactions: DEXILANT is metabolized, in part, by CYP2C19 and CYP3A4 (see Action and Clinical Pharmacology, Metabolism).

In vitro studies have shown that DEXILANT is not likely to inhibit CYP isoforms 1A1, 1A2, 2A6, 2B6, 2C8, 2C9, 2C19, 2D6, 2E1 or 3A4. As such, no clinically relevant interactions with drugs metabolized by these CYP enzymes would be expected. Furthermore, clinical drug-drug interaction studies have shown that DEXILANT does not affect the pharmacokinetics of diazepam, phenytoin, or theophylline.

Warfarin: In a study of 20 healthy subjects, co-administration of DEXILANT 90 mg once daily for 11 days with a single 25 mg oral dose of warfarin on day 6 did not result in any significant differences in the pharmacokinetics of warfarin or INR compared to administration of warfarin with placebo. However, there have been reports of increased INR and prothrombin time in patients receiving proton pump inhibitors (PPIs) and warfarin concomitantly. Patients treated with PPIs and warfarin concomitantly may need to be monitored for increases in INR and prothrombin time.

Concomitant Use of Antacids with DEXILANT: No formal drug-drug interaction studies were conducted with DEXILANT and antacids. Drug-drug interactions studies were performed with the racemate lansoprazole and antacids. Simultaneous administration of lansoprazole with aluminum and magnesium hydroxide or magaldrate results in lower peak plasma levels, but does not significantly reduce bioavailability. Antacids may be used concomitantly if required. In clinical trials, antacids were administered concomitantly with lansoprazole delayed-release capsules. In a single-dose crossover study when 30 mg of lansoprazole was administered concomitantly with one gram of sucralfate in healthy volunteers, absorption of lansoprazole was delayed and its bioavailability was reduced. The value of lansoprazole AUC was reduced by 17% and that for C_{max} was reduced by 21%. In a similar study when 30 mg of lansoprazole was administered concomitantly with 2 grams of sucralfate, lansoprazole AUC and C_{max} were reduced by 32% and 55%, respectively. When lansoprazole dosing occurred 30 minutes prior to sucralfate administration, C_{max} was reduced by only 28% and there was no statistically significant difference in lansoprazole AUC. Therefore, lansoprazole should be administered at least 30 minutes prior to sucralfate. It would be expected that similar results would be seen with DEXILANT.

Theophylline: Although a study of the use of concomitant theophylline and dexlansoprazole did not reveal any changes in the pharmacokinetics or pharmacodynamics of theophylline, individual patients should monitor their theophylline level while taking the two drugs concomitantly.

Tacrolimus: Concomitant administration of dexlansoprazole and tacrolimus may increase whole blood levels of tacrolimus, especially in transplant patients who are intermediate or poor metabolizers of CYP2C19.

Clopidogrel: Cytochrome P450 2C19 (CYP2C19) is responsible for the metabolism of clopidogrel to its active metabolite. Although in vitro metabolism studies have demonstrated that PPIs inhibit hepatic CYP2C19, the level of inhibition varies among PPIs, and it is unknown as to the amount other PPIs may interfere with clopidogrel. Various clinical drug-drug interaction studies have demonstrated that dexlansoprazole does not affect the pharmacokinetics of diazepam, phenytoin or R-warfarin, drugs that are metabolized by CYP2C19.

Drug-Food Interactions: DEXILANT can be taken without regard to food or timing of food (see Action and Clinical Pharmacology).

Drug-Herb Interactions: Interactions with herbal products have not been established.

Drug-Laboratory Test Interactions: Interactions with laboratory tests have not been established.

DOSAGE AND ADMINISTRATION: **Recommended Dose and Dosage Adjustment:** See Table 3.

Table 3: DEXILANT

Recommended Dose and Dosage Adjustment

Indication	Recommended Dose	Frequency
Healing of Erosive Esophagitis	60 mg	Once daily for up to 8 weeks
Maintenance of Healed Erosive Esophagitis	30 mg[a]	Once daily[b]
Symptomatic Non-Erosive Gastroesophageal Reflux Disease (GERD)	30 mg	Once daily for 4 weeks

[a] In patients who had moderate or severe erosive esophagitis, a maintenance dose of 60 mg may be used.
[b] Controlled studies did not extend beyond 6 months.

No dosage adjustment for DEXILANT is necessary for patients with mild hepatic impairment (Child-Pugh Class A). DEXILANT 30 mg should be considered for patients with moderate hepatic impairment (Child-Pugh Class B). No studies have been conducted in patients with severe hepatic impairment (Child-Pugh Class C).

No dosage adjustment is necessary for elderly patients or for patients with renal impairment.

Missed Dose: If a capsule is missed at its usual time, it should be taken as soon as possible. But if it is too close to the time of the next dose, only the prescribed dose should be taken at the appointed time. A double dose should not be taken.

Administration: DEXILANT can be taken without regard to food or the timing of food.

DEXILANT should be swallowed whole with plenty of water.

- Alternatively, DEXILANT capsules can be opened and administered as follows:
  - Open capsule;
  - Sprinkle intact granules on one tablespoon of applesauce;
  - Swallow immediately.

OVERDOSAGE:

There have been no reports of significant overdose of DEXILANT. Dexlansoprazole is not expected to be removed from the circulation by hemodialysis.

For management of a suspected drug overdose, contact your regional Poison Control Centre. See the *CPS* Directory section for a list of Poison Control Centres.

ACTION AND CLINICAL PHARMACOLOGY: Mechanism of Action: DEXILANT is a PPI that suppresses gastric acid secretion by specific inhibition of the (H^+, K^+)-ATPase in the gastric parietal cell. By acting specifically on the proton pump, DEXILANT blocks the final step of acid production.

Pharmacodynamics: Antisecretory Activity: The effects of DEXILANT 60 mg (n=20) or lansoprazole 30 mg (n=23) once daily for five days on 24-hour intragastric pH were assessed in healthy subjects in a multiple-dose crossover study. The results are summarized in Table 4.

Table 4: DEXILANT

Effect on 24-Hour Intragastric pH on Day 5 After Administration of DEXILANT or Lansoprazole

DEXILANT 60 mg	Lansoprazole 30 mg
Mean Intragastric pH	
4.55[a]	4.13

(cont'd)

Table 4: DEXILANT *(cont'd)*

Effect on 24-Hour Intragastric pH on Day 5 After Administration of DEXILANT or Lansoprazole

DEXILANT 60 mg	Lansoprazole 30 mg
% Time Intragastric pH >4 (hours)	
71[a] (17 hours)	60 (14 hours)

[a] p value ≤0.05 versus lansoprazole.

Pharmacokinetics: The formulation of DEXILANT utilizing Dual Delayed Release technology results in a dexlansoprazole plasma concentration-time profile with two distinct peaks; the first peak occurs 1 to 2 hours after administration, followed by a second peak within 4 to 5 hours (see Figure 1).

Figure 1: DEXILANT

Mean Plasma Dexlansoprazole Concentration – Time Profile Following Oral Administration of 60 mg DEXILANT or 30 mg Lansoprazole Once Daily for 5 Days in Healthy Subjects

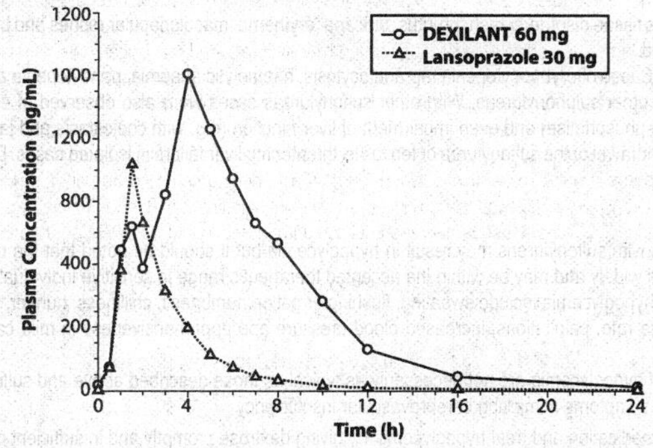

Dexlansoprazole is eliminated with a half-life of approximately 1 to 2 hours in healthy subjects (see Table 5) and in patients with symptomatic GERD. No accumulation of dexlansoprazole occurs after multiple, once daily doses of DEXILANT 30 mg or 60 mg.

Table 5: DEXILANT

Mean (CV %) Pharmacokinetic Parameters for Healthy Subjects on Day 5 After Administration of DEXILANT

Dose (mg)	C_{max} (ng/mL)	AUC_{24} (ng·h/mL)	$t_{½}$[a] (h)	CL/F (L/h)	V_z/F
30 mg	658 (40%) (N=44)	3275 (47%) (N=43)	1.49 (N=43)	11.4 (48%) (N=43)	25.7 (49%) (N=43)
60 mg	1397 (51%) (N=79)	6529 (60%) (N=73)	1.54 (N=73)	11.6 (46%) (N=41)	33.8 (89%) (N=41)

[a] Harmonic mean.

Absorption: After oral administration of DEXILANT 30 mg or 60 mg to healthy subjects , mean C_{max} and AUC values of dexlansoprazole increased approximately dose proportionally (see Figure 2).

Figure 2: DEXILANT

Mean Plasma Dexlansoprazole Concentration – Time Profile Following Oral Administration of DEXILANT on Day 5 in Healthy Subjects

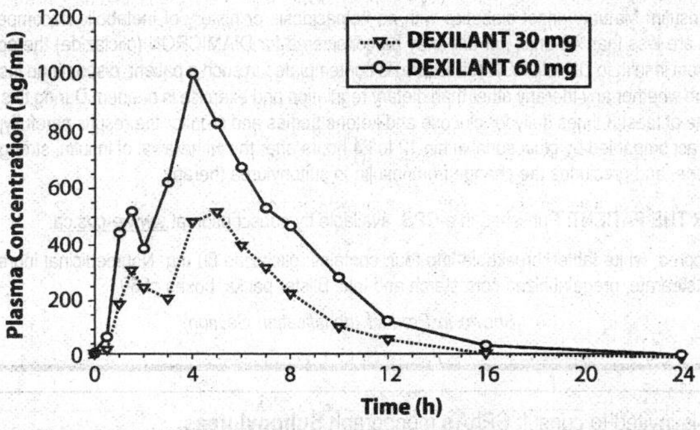

Distribution: Plasma protein binding of dexlansoprazole ranged from 96.1% to 98.8% in healthy subjects and was independent of concentration from 0.01 to 20 µg/mL. The apparent volume of distribution (Vz/F) after multiple doses in symptomatic GERD patients was 40.3 L.

Metabolism: Dexlansoprazole is extensively metabolized in the liver by oxidation, reduction, and subsequent formation of sulfate, glucuronide and glutathione conjugates to inactive metabolites. Oxidative metabolites are formed by the cytochrome P450 (CYP) enzyme system including hydroxylation mainly by CYP2C19, and oxidation to the sulfone by CYP3A4.

CYP2C19 is a polymorphic liver enzyme which exhibits three phenotypes in the metabolism of CYP2C19 substrates; extensive metabolizers (*1/*1), intermediate metabolizers (*1/mutant) and poor metabolizers (mutant/mutant). Systemic exposure of dexlansoprazole is generally higher in intermediate and poor metabolizers. Dexlansoprazole is the major circulating component in plasma, regardless of CYP2C19 metabolizer status. In CYP2C19 intermediate and extensive metabolizers, the major plasma metabolites are 5-hydroxy dexlansoprazole and its glucuronide conjugate, while in CYP2C19 poor metabolizers dexlansoprazole sulfone is the major plasma metabolite.

Excretion: Following the administration of DEXILANT, no unchanged dexlansoprazole is excreted in urine. Following the administration of [^{14}C]dexlansoprazole to 6 healthy male subjects, approximately 50.7% (standard deviation (SD): 9.0%) of the administered radioactivity was excreted in urine and 47.6% (SD: 7.3%) in the feces. Apparent clearance (CL/F) in healthy subjects was 11.4 to 11.6 L/h, respectively, after 5-days of 30 or 60 mg once daily administration.

Effect of Food: DEXILANT can be taken without regard to food or the timing of food. In food-effect studies in healthy subjects receiving DEXILANT, increases in C_{max} ranged from 12% to 55% and increases in AUC ranged from 9% to 37% under various fed conditions compared to fasting. However, no relevant differences with regard to intragastric pH were observed. An additional study showed that administration of 60 mg DEXILANT prior to consumption of breakfast, lunch, dinner or an evening snack did not have an effect on dexlansoprazole exposure, or a clinically relevant effect on 24-hour intragastric pH control.

Special Populations and Conditions: Pediatrics: The pharmacokinetics of dexlansoprazole in patients under the age of 18 years have not been studied.

Geriatrics: In a study of 12 male and 12 female healthy subjects who received a single oral dose of DEXILANT 60 mg, the terminal elimination half-life of dexlansoprazole was statistically significantly longer in geriatric subjects compared to younger subjects (2.23 and 1.5 hours, respectively). In addition, dexlansoprazole exhibited higher systemic exposure (AUC) in geriatric subjects (34.5% higher) than younger subjects. These differences were not clinically relevant. No dosage adjustment is necessary in geriatric patients (see Warnings and Precautions and Dosage and Administration).

Gender: In a study of 12 male and 12 female healthy subjects who received a single oral dose of DEXILANT 60 mg, females had higher systemic exposure (AUC) (42.8% higher) than males. No dosage adjustment is necessary in patients based on gender.

Hepatic Insufficiency: In a study of 12 patients with moderately impaired hepatic function who received a single oral dose of DEXILANT 60 mg, plasma exposure (AUC) of bound and unbound dexlansoprazole in the hepatic impairment group was approximately 2 times greater compared to subjects with normal hepatic function. This difference in exposure was not due to a difference in protein binding between the two liver function groups. No adjustment for DEXILANT is necessary for patients with mild hepatic impairment (Child-Pugh Class A). DEXILANT 30 mg should be considered for patients with moderate hepatic impairment (Child-Pugh Class B). No studies have been conducted in patients with severe hepatic impairment (Child-Pugh Class C) (see Warnings and Precautions).

Renal Insufficiency: Dexlansoprazole is extensively metabolized in the liver to inactive metabolites, and no parent drug is recovered in the urine following an oral dose of dexlansoprazole. Therefore, the pharmacokinetics of dexlansoprazole are not expected to be altered in patients with renal impairment, and no studies were conducted in subjects with renal impairment (see Warnings and Precautions).

STORAGE AND STABILITY: Store at room temperature (15 to 30°C).

SPECIAL HANDLING INSTRUCTIONS:

INFORMATION FOR THE PATIENT: Published in e-CPS, available by subscription at www.e-cps.ca.

DOSAGE FORMS, COMPOSITION AND PACKAGING: DEXILANT is supplied as a dual delayed release formulation in capsules for oral administration using Dual Delayed Release technology. The capsules contain dexlansoprazole in a mixture of two types of enteric-coated granules with different pH-dependent dissolution profiles. One type of granule is designed to release dexlansoprazole after the granules reach the proximal small intestine; the second type of granule is designed to release dexlansoprazole in the distal region of the small intestine, generally several hours later.

30 mg: Each opaque, blue and gray delayed release capsule, with TAP and "30" imprinted on the capsule contains: dexlansoprazole 30 mg. Nonmedicinal ingredients: colloidal silicon dioxide, hydroxypropyl cellulose, hypromellose 2910, low-substituted hydroxypropyl cellulose, magnesium carbonate, methacrylic acid copolymer, polyethylene glycol 8000, polysorbate 80, sucrose, sugar spheres, talc, titanium dioxide and triethyl citrate; capsule shell: black ferric oxide, carrageenan, FD&C Blue No. 2 aluminum lake, hypromellose, potassium chloride and titanium dioxide. High-density polyethylene (HDPE) bottles of 90.

60 mg: Each opaque, blue delayed release capsule, with TAP and "60" imprinted on the capsule contains: dexlansoprazole 60 mg. Nonmedicinal ingredients: colloidal silicon dioxide, hydroxypropyl cellulose, hypromellose 2910, low-substituted hydroxypropyl cellulose, magnesium carbonate, methacrylic acid copolymer, polyethylene glycol 8000, polysorbate 80, sucrose, sugar spheres, talc, titanium dioxide and triethyl citrate; capsule shell: carrageenan, FD&C Blue No. 2 aluminum lake, hypromellose, potassium chloride and titanium dioxide. High-density polyethylene (HDPE) bottles of 90.

Dextropropoxyphene Ⓝ

CPhA Monograph

see *Opioids*

Diabeta® Ⓟ

glyburide

Oral Hypoglycemic

sanofi-aventis

SUPPLIED: 2.5 mg: Each compressed white, flat round beveled tablet with code letter "LB" above and "G" below the breakline on one side and plain on the other, contains: glyburide 2.5 mg. Nonmedicinal ingredients: colloidal anhydrous silica, lactose monohydrate, magnesium stearate, starch (corn starch and pre-gelatinized corn starch) and talc. Cartons of 30 (2×15 blister pack).

5 mg: Each white, biplane, oblong tablet with a score line on both sides, "LDI" engraved on each side of the score-line and inverted, the other face plain, contains: glyburide 5 mg. Nonmedicinal ingredients: colloidal anhydrous silica, lactose monohydrate, magnesium stearate, starch (corn starch and pre-gelatinized corn starch). Cartons of 30 (2×15 blister pack). HDPE bottles of 300.

(Shown in Product Identification Section)

The reader is invited to consult CPhA's monograph **Sulfonylureas**.

Diamicron® Ⓟ

gliclazide

Hypoglycemic Sulfonylurea—Oral Hypoglycemic Agent

Servier

Date of Preparation: December 1989
Date of Revision: January 15, 2009

PHARMACOLOGY: DIAMICRON (gliclazide) is an hypoglycemic agent of the sulfonylurea group.

The hypoglycemic action of DIAMICRON (gliclazide) is related to an improvement in insulin secretion from the functioning beta cells of the pancreas. It potentiates the insulin release, improves the dynamics of insulin.

Hemobiological properties of DIAMICRON (gliclazide) have been observed in pharmacology studies. These are attributed to gliclazide action on the platelet behaviour, prostaglandin equilibrium and fibrinolysis.

Gliclazide is rapidly absorbed from the gastro-intestinal tract and the plasma peak of gliclazide occurs between 4 and 6 hours. In man it is highly bound to plasma proteins, about 94%. The mean elimination half-life in man approximates 10.4 hours.

Following oral administration the unchanged gliclazide in plasma is extensively metabolized with little of the unchanged compound (<1%) appearing in the urine.

Gliclazide metabolites and conjugates are primarily eliminated via kidneys: 60 to 70%, and about 10 to 20% via faeces.

Some five principal metabolites have been identified in urine, essentially oxidized and hydroxylated derivatives, some as glucuronic acid conjugates.

INDICATIONS: Control of hyperglycemia in gliclazide responsive diabetes mellitus of stable, mild, non-ketosis prone, maturity onset or adult type which cannot be controlled by proper dietary management and exercise, or when insulin therapy is not appropriate.

CONTRAINDICATIONS: Known hypersensitivity or allergy to gliclazide, other sulfonylureas, sulfonamides, or to any of the excipients of this product (for a complete listing, see Supplied). Unstable and/or insulin dependent diabetes mellitus, particularly juvenile diabetes, diabetic ketoacidosis, diabetic pre-coma and coma. During stress conditions such as serious infection, trauma or surgery. In the presence of liver disease or renal impairment. Treatment with miconazole via systemic route or oromucosal gel (see Drug Interactions). Pregnancy and lactation (see Precautions, Pregnancy and Lactation).

WARNINGS: The use of DIAMICRON (gliclazide) will not prevent the development of complications peculiar to diabetes mellitus.

Use of DIAMICRON (gliclazide) must be considered as treatment in addition to proper dietary regimen and not as substitute for diet.

The efficacy of gliclazide, in reducing glucose to the desired level decreases over a long period of time in many patients: this may be due to progression in the severity of the diabetes, or to a reduced response to treatment. If a loss of adequate blood glucose-lowering response to DIAMICRON (gliclazide) is detected, the drug should be discontinued.

PRECAUTIONS: Patient Selection and Follow-up: Careful selection of patients is important. It is imperative that there be rigid attention to diet, careful adjustment of dosage and instruction of the patient on hypoglycemic reactions, their recognition, remedies and control as well as regular, thorough medical follow-up.

Since the effects of oral hypoglycemic agents on the vascular changes and other long-term sequelae of diabetes mellitus are not fully known, patients receiving such drugs must be closely observed for both short- and long-term complications. Periodic assessment of cardiovascular, ophthalmic, renal and hepatic status is advisable.

In patients stabilized on gliclazide therapy, loss of blood sugar control may occur in cases of acute intercurrent disease or in stressful situations such as trauma or surgery. Under these conditions, discontinuation of DIAMICRON (gliclazide) and administration of insulin should be considered.

Hematologic: Treatment of patients with glucose-6-phosphate dehydrogenase (G6PD)-deficiency with sulfonylurea agents can lead to haemolytic anaemia. Since DIAMICRON belongs to the class of sulfonylurea agents, caution should be used in patients with G6PD-deficiency and a non-sulfonylurea alternative should be considered.

Hepatic: The metabolism and excretion of sulfonylureas including DIAMICRON 80 mg may be slowed in patients with impaired hepatic function (see Monitoring and Laboratory Tests).

Renal: The metabolism and excretion of sulfonylureas including DIAMICRON may be slowed in patients with impaired renal function. If hypoglycemia should occur in such patients, it may be prolonged and appropriate management should be instituted (see Monitoring and Laboratory Tests).

Peri-Operative Considerations: In patients stabilized on gliclazide therapy, loss of blood sugar control may occur in cases of acute intercurrent disease or in stressful situations such as trauma or surgery. Under these conditions, discontinuation of DIAMICRON and administration of insulin should be considered.

Hypoglycemic Reactions: As with other sulfonylurea drugs, manifestations of hypoglycemia including dizziness, lack of energy, drowsiness, headache and sweating have been observed and weakness, nervousness, shakiness and paresthesia have also been reported. Severe hypoglycemia can be induced by all sulfonylurea drugs. Particularly susceptible are elderly subjects, patients with impaired hepatic or renal function, those who are debilitated or malnourished and patients with primary or secondary adrenal insufficiency. Hypoglycemia is more likely to occur when caloric intake is inadequate or after strenuous or prolonged physical exercise. Some cases may be severe and prolonged. Hospitalisation may be necessary and glucose administration may need to be continued for several days. Hypoglycemia may be difficult to recognize in elderly patients and in patients receiving beta-blockers.

Possible other symptoms of hypoglycaemia are: intense hunger, lassitude, sleep disorders, agitation, aggression, poor concentration, reduced awareness and slowed reactions, depression, confusion, visual and speech disorders, aphasia, paresis, sensory disorders, feeling of powerlessness, loss of self-control, delirium, convulsions, shallow respiration, bradycardia, drowsiness and loss of consciousness, possibly resulting in coma and lethal outcome. In addition, signs of adrenergic counter-regulation may be observed: clammy skin, anxiety, tachycardia, hypertension, palpitations, angina pectoris and cardiac arrhythmia.

Usually, hypoglycaemic symptoms disappear after intake of carbohydrates (sugar). However, artificial sweeteners have no effect. Experience with other sulphonylureas shows that hypoglycaemia can recur even when measures prove effective initially. If a hypoglycaemic episode is severe or prolonged, and even if it is temporarily controlled by intake of sugar, immediate medical treatment or even hospitalisation are required.

Treatment with DIAMICRON can have effects on ability to drive and use machines. Patients should be made aware of the symptoms of hypoglycaemia and should be careful if driving or operating machinery, especially at the beginning of treatment.

Other factors which increase the risk of hypoglycemia are: overdose of DIAMICRON, certain endocrine disorders (thyroid disorders, hypopituitarism and adrenal insufficiency) as well as withdrawal of prolonged and/or high dose corticosteroid therapy, severe vascular disease (severe coronary heart disease, severe carotid impairment, diffuse vascular disease) and concomitant administration of certain medicines (see Drug Interactions).

Drug Interactions: As a result of drug interaction, hypoglycemia may be potentiated when a sulfonylurea is used concurrently with agents such as: long-acting sulfonamides, tuberculostatics, clarithromycin, phenylbutazone, clofibrate, monoamine oxidase inhibitors, coumarin derivatives, salicylates, non-steroidal anti-inflammatory agents, probenecid, beta-blockers, miconazole (see Contraindications), azole antifungal agents (oral and parenteral preparations), H2-receptor antagonists, disopyramide and angiotensin converting enzyme inhibitors. In addition, hypoglycaemia is potentiated when gliclazide is used in combination with other antidiabetic agents (insulin, alpha gluclosidase inhibitors, biguanides) which is not indicated.

Certain drugs tend to induce hyperglycemia and may lead to loss of control of blood sugar control. These include diuretics (thiazides, furosemide), corticosteroids and tetracosactrin, danazol, chlorpromazine, ritodrine/ salbutamol/ terbutaline (IV), oral contraceptives (estrogen plus progestogen) and nicotinic acid in pharmacologic doses.

Barbiturates should be used with caution in patients receiving an oral hypoglycemic agent since they may reduce the hypoglycemic effect.

Combination with anticoagulant therapy (warfarin and other) must be taken into account because sulfonulureas may lead to potentiation of anticoagulation during concomitant treatment. Adjustment of the anticoagulant dosage may be necessary.

Intolerance to alcohol (disulfiram-like reaction: flushing, sensation of warmth, giddiness, nausea and occasionally tachycardia) may occur in patients treated with sulfonylurea. This reaction can be prevented by avoiding the use of alcohol. Alcohol increases the hypoglycaemic reaction (by inhibiting compensatory reactions) that can lead to the onset of hypoglycaemic coma. Avoid alcohol or medicines containing alcohol.

Pregnancy: Gliclazide is contraindicated in pregnancy. It is recommended that insulin be used during pregnancy in diabetic women (see Contraindications).

Uncontrolled diabetes (gestational or not) is associated with a higher incidence of congenital abnormalities and perinatal mortality. Blood glucose control should be optimal around the time of conception to reduce the risk of congenital malformations.

Lactation: The product is contra-indicated in breast-feeding mothers. Some sulfonylurea drugs are excreted in human milk although it is not known whether DIAMICRON (gliclazide) is one of them. Because the potential for hypoglycemia in nursing infants may exist, the product is contra-indicated in breast-feeding mothers (see Contraindications).

Children: Safety and effectiveness in children have not been established. DIAMICRON is therefore not recommended for use in children and adolescents.

Geriatrics: Efficacy and tolerance of DIAMICRON, prescribed using the same therapeutic regimen in subjects over 65 years, has been confirmed in clinical trials. Severe hypoglycemia can be induced by all sulfonylurea drugs, particularly susceptible are elderly subjects.

Monitoring and Laboratory Tests: Measurement of glycated haemoglobin levels (or fasting venous plasma glucose) is recommended in assessing blood glucose control. Blood glucose self-monitoring is also recommended.

Blood glucose control in a patient receiving antidiabetic treatment may be affected by fever and infection or surgical intervention. Closed monitoring is required in these patients. In some cases, it may be necessary to administer insulin.

Hepatic function should be assessed before initiating therapy and the liver function should be assessed periodically in patients with impaired hepatic function.

In patients with impaired renal function, blood and urine glucose should be regularly monitored. Measurements of glycated hemoglobin levels are recommended.

Elderly patients (malnourished, with impaired hepatic, renal, or adrenal function) will require periodic monitoring and special care.

ADVERSE EFFECTS: In clinical trials involving about 2000 patients treated with DIAMICRON (gliclazide), the overall incidence of adverse reaction was 10.5%; this necessitated the discontinuation of therapy in 1.2% of patients.

Adverse Drug Reaction Overview: The most frequently reported adverse drug reactions during long-term studies and post-market experience are hypoglycaemia (see Warnings and Precautions) and gastrointestinal disturbances (including abdominal pain, nausea, vomiting, dyspepsia, diarrhea, constipation).

Hypoglycemia: (See Precautions.) Weakness, nervousness, shakiness and paresthesia have been reported. Severe hypoglycemia which mimics acute CNS disorders may occur. Hepatic and/or renal disease, malnutrition, debility, advanced age, alcoholism, adrenal or pituitary insufficiency may be predisposing factors.

Gastrointestinal: Nausea, vomiting, diarrhea, epigastric fullness and gastric irritation can be observed. These reactions are generally dose-related and may disappear when the dose is reduced.

Hepatobiliary: With other sulfonylureas cases were also observed of elevated liver enzyme levels (AST, ALT, alkaline phosphatise) and even impairment of liver function (e.g. with cholestasis and jaundice) and hepatitis which regressed after withdrawal of the sulfonylurea or led to life-threatening liver failure in isolated cases. Rare cases of jaundice have been reported. Discontinue treatment if cholestatic jaundice appears.

Dermatological: Allergic reactions such as pruritus, erythema, urticaria and morbilliform or maculopapular rash have been reported. These reactions may persist during treatment, which must then be interrupted. Cases of cutanea porphyria tarda and of photosensitivity have also been described with sulfonylurea drugs.

Hematological: As with all hypoglycemic sulfonylurea drugs, a few rare cases have been reported of leukopenia, erythrocytopenia agranulocytosis, thrombocytopenia, haemolytic anemia, pancytopenia and allergic vasculitis.

Metabolic: Cases of hepatic porphyria and disulfiram-like reactions have been described with sulfonylurea drugs. Clinical experience to date has shown that DIAMICRON (gliclazide) has a low incidence of disulfiram type reactions.

Cardiovascular: arteritis, cardiac failure, cerebrovascular disorder, coronary artery disorder, epistaxis, hypotension, myocardial infarction, oedema legs, palpitation, tachycardia, thrombophlebitis, vein disorder.

Endocrine: A decrease in the uptake of radioactive iodine by the thyroid gland has been reported with other sulfonylurea drugs. This has not been shown with DIAMICRON (gliclazide) during a study involving 15 patients.

Laboratory Tests: The pattern of laboratory tests abnormalities observed with DIAMICRON (gliclazide) was similar to that for other sulfonylureas. Occasional mild to moderate elevations of AST, LDH and creatinine and decrease in natremia have been observed. These abnormalities frequently encountered with treated or untreated diabetic patients are rarely associated with clinical symptoms and generally not considered to be drug related.

Post-Market Adverse Drug Reactions: In post-marketing experience with gliclazide, the most frequently reported adverse drug reaction is hypoglycaemia.

The most serious adverse drug reactions reported with gliclazide are hypoglycaemic coma, pancytopenia, thrombocytopenia, hepatitis, cholestatic jaundice, pyrexia, and skin reactions (pruritus and rash).

Gastrointestinal disturbances, including abdominal pain, nausea, vomiting, dyspepsia, diarrhea and constipation have been reported.

Skin and subcutaneous tissue disorders, rash, pruritus, urticaria, erythema, maculopapular rashes and bullous reactions have been more rarely reported.

Class Attribution Effects: Cases of erythrocytopenia, agranulocytosis, haemolytic anaemia, pancytopenia and allergic vasculitis, have been described for other sulphonylureas. With other sulfonylureas cases were also observed of elevated liver enzyme levels (AST, ALT, alkaline phosphatise) and even impairment of liver function (e.g. with cholestasis and jaundice) and hepatitis which regressed after withdrawal of the sulfonylurea or led to life-threatening liver failure in isolated cases. Discontinue treatment if cholestatic jaundice appears.

OVERDOSE:

Symptoms: Overdosage with sulfonylureas may result in hypoglycemia but it should be noted that the dosage which causes such hypoglycemia varies widely and may be within the accepted therapeutic range in sensitive individuals.

The manifestations of hypoglycemia include sweating, flushing or pallor, numbness, chilliness, hunger, trembling, headache, dizziness, increased pulse rate, palpitations, increased blood pressure and apprehensiveness in mild cases. In more severe cases, coma appears.

However, symptoms of hypoglycemia are not necessarily as typical as those described above and sulfonylureas may cause insidious development of symptoms mimicking cerebrovascular insufficiency.

Treatment: Discontinue medication and treat hypoglycemia by giving dextrose promptly and in sufficient quantity.

Some sulfonylurea-induced hypoglycemias may be refractory to treatment and susceptible to relapse especially in elderly or malnourished patients. Continuous dextrose infusions for hours or days have been necessary.

Strict monitoring should be continued until the doctor is sure that the patient is out of danger.

Severe hypoglycaemic reactions, with coma, convulsions or other neurological disorders are possible and must be treated as a medical emergency, requiring immediate hospitalisation. If hypoglycaemic coma is diagnosed or suspected, the patient should be given a rapid I.V. injection of 50 mL of concentrated glucose solution (20 to 30 %). This should be followed by continuous infusion of a more dilute glucose solution (10 %) at a rate that will maintain blood glucose levels above 1 g/L. Patients should be monitored closely and, depending on the patient's condition after this time, the doctor will decide if further monitoring is necessary.

Dialysis is of no benefit to patients due to the strong binding of gliclazide to proteins.

> For management of a suspected drug overdose, CPhA recommends that you contact your **regional Poison Control Centre**. See the *CPS* Directory section for a list of Poison Control Centres.

DOSAGE: Determination of the proper dosage for DIAMICRON (gliclazide) for each patient should be made on the basis of frequent determinations of blood glucose during dose titration and throughout maintenance.

The recommended daily dosage of DIAMICRON (gliclazide) is 80 to 320 mg (1 to 4 tablets). Dosage of 160 mg and above should be divided into two equal parts for twice a day administration. DIAMICRON should be taken preferentially with meals.

The recommended starting dose of DIAMICRON (gliclazide) is 2 tablets per day (160 mg) taken as one tablet twice a day with meals. The total daily dose should not exceed 320 milligrams.

In patients where on initial trial the maximal recommended dose fails to lower blood glucose adequately, the drug should be discontinued. During the course of therapy a loss of effectiveness may occur.

It is advisable to ascertain the contribution of the drug in control of the blood glucose by discontinuing the medication semi-annually or at least annually with careful monitoring of the patient. If the need for the drug is not evident, the drug should not be resumed. In some diabetic subjects, short-term administration periods of the drug may be sufficient during periods of transient loss of blood sugar controls.

Patients Receiving Insulin: Maturity onset diabetics with no ketoacidosis or history of metabolic decompensation and whose insulin requirements are less than 40 units per day may be considered for DIAMICRON (gliclazide) therapy after cessation of insulin. If a change from insulin to DIAMICRON (gliclazide) is contemplated in such a patient, discontinue insulin for a period of 2 or 3 days to determine whether any therapy other than dietary regulation and exercise is needed. During this insulin free interval, test the patient's urine at least 3 times daily for glucose and ketone bodies and monitor the results carefully. The appearance of significant ketonuria accompanied by glucosuria within 12 to 24 hours after the withdrawal of insulin, strongly suggests that the patient is ketosis prone, and precludes the change from insulin to sulfonylurea therapy.

INFORMATION FOR THE PATIENT: Published in e-CPS, available by subscription at www.e-cps.ca.

SUPPLIED: Each scored, white tablet, breakable into four, contains: gliclazide 80 mg. Nonmedicinal ingredients: corn starch, lactose, magnesium stearate, pregelatinized corn starch and talc. Blister packs, boxes of 60.

(Shown in Product Identification Section)

> The reader is invited to consult CPhA's monograph **Sulfonylureas**.

Diamicron® MR Ⓟ

gliclazide

Hypoglycemic Sulfonylurea—Oral Antidiabetic Agent

Servier

Date of Preparation: November 14, 2000
Date of Revision: January 15, 2009

SUMMARY PRODUCT INFORMATION:

Route of Administration	Dosage Form/ Strength	Clinically Relevant Nonmedicinal Ingredients
Oral	Tablet 30 mg	For a complete listing see Dosage Forms, Composition and Packaging.

INDICATIONS AND CLINICAL USE: DIAMICRON MR 30 mg is indicated for:

- Control of hyperglycemia in gliclazide responsive diabetes mellitus of stable, mild, non-ketosis prone, maturity onset or adult type which cannot be controlled by proper dietary management and exercise, or when insulin therapy is not appropriate.

Geriatrics (≥65 years of age): The efficacy and tolerance of DIAMICRON MR 30 mg, prescribed using the same therapeutic regimen in subjects over 65 years, has been confirmed in clinical trials. The dosage will therefore be identical to that recommended for adults under the age of 65 years.

Pediatrics (<18 years of age): Safety and effectiveness of DIAMICRON MR 30 mg in children have not been established. DIAMICRON MR 30 mg is therefore not recommended for use in children and adolescents.

CONTRAINDICATIONS: DIAMICRON MR 30 mg is contraindicated in patients with:

- Known hypersensitivity or allergy to gliclazide, other sulfonylureas, sulfonamides, or to any of the excipients of this product (For a complete listing see Dosage Forms, Composition and Packaging).
- Unstable and/or insulin-dependent diabetes mellitus, particularly juvenile diabetes, diabetic ketoacidosis, diabetic pre-coma and coma.
- During stress conditions such as serious infection, trauma or surgery. In the presence of severe liver disease or renal impairment (see Warnings and Precautions).
- Treatment with miconazole via systemic route or oromucosal gel (see Drug-Drug Interactions).
- Pregnancy and lactation (see Warnings and Precautions, Special Population, Pregnant Women and Nursing Women).

WARNINGS AND PRECAUTIONS: General: Use of DIAMICRON MR 30 mg must be considered as treatment in addition to proper dietary regimen and not as substitute for diet.

Careful selection of patients is important. It is imperative that there be rigid attention to diet, careful adjustment of dosage and instruction of the patient on hypoglycemic reactions, their recognition, remedies and control as well as regular, thorough medical follow-up.

Since the effects of oral hypoglycemic agents on the vascular changes and other long-term sequelae of diabetes mellitus are not fully known, patients receiving such drugs must be closely observed for both short- and long-term complications. Periodic assessment of cardiovascular, ophthalmic, renal and hepatic status is advisable.

DIAMICRON MR 30 mg use is not recommended with medications containing alcohol, phenylbutazone (systemic route) and danazol and precautions are required when used with chlorpromazine, glucocorticoids, ritodrine, salbutamol, terbutaline and anticoagulant therapy (see Drug-Drug Interactions).

Endocrine and Metabolism: Hypoglycemic Reactions: As with other sulfonylurea drugs, manifestations of hypoglycemia including dizziness, lack of energy, drowsiness, headache and sweating have been observed and weakness, nervousness, shakiness and paresthesia have also been reported. All sulfonylurea drugs can induce severe hypoglycemia. Particularly susceptible are elderly subjects, patients with impaired hepatic or renal function, those who are debilitated or malnourished and patients with primary or secondary adrenal insufficiency. Some cases may be severe and prolonged. Hospitalization may be necessary and glucose administration may need to be continued for several days. Hypoglycemia may be difficult to recognize in elderly patients and in patients receiving beta-blockers.

Possible other symptoms of hypoglycaemia are: intense hunger, nausea, vomiting, lassitude, sleep disorders, agitation, aggression, poor concentration, reduced awareness and slowed reactions, depression, confusion, visual and speech disorders, aphasia, tremor, paresis, sensory disorders, feeling of powerlessness, loss of self-control, delirium, convulsions, shallow respiration, bradycardia, drowsiness and loss of consciousness, possibly resulting in coma and lethal outcome. In addition, signs of adrenergic counter-regulation may be observed: clammy skin, anxiety, tachycardia, hypertension, palpitations, angina pectoris and cardiac arrhythmia.

This treatment should only be prescribed if the patient is likely to have a regular food intake (including breakfast). It is important to have a regular carbohydrate intake due to the increased risk of hypoglycemia if a meal is taken late, if an inadequate amount of food is consumed or if the food is low in carbohydrate. Hypoglycemia is more likely to occur during periods of low-calorie diet, following prolonged or strenuous exercise, following alcohol intake or during the administration of a combination of hypoglycemic agents.

Usually, hypoglycemic symptoms disappear after intake of carbohydrates (sugar). However, artificial sweeteners have no effect. Experience with other sulphonylureas shows that hypoglycemia can recur even when measures prove effective initially.

If a hypoglycemic episode is severe or prolonged, and even if it is temporarily controlled by intake of sugar, immediate medical treatment or even hospitalization are required.

Other factors which increase the risk of hypoglycemia are: overdose of DIAMICRON MR 30 mg, certain endocrine disorders (thyroid disorders, hypopituitarism and adrenal insufficiency) as well as withdrawal of prolonged and/or high dose corticosteroid therapy, severe vascular disease (severe coronary heart disease, severe carotid impairment, diffuse vascular disease) and concomitant administration of certain medicines (see Drug-Drug Interactions).

Poor Blood Glucose Control: The efficacy of gliclazide, in reducing glucose to the desired level decreases over a long period of time in many patients: this may be due to progression in the severity of the diabetes, or to a reduced response to treatment. This phenomenon is known as secondary failure and should be distinguished from primary failure, when the drug is ineffective when prescribed as first-line treatment. Adequate dose adjustment and compliance with dietary measures should be considered before classifying the patient as secondary failure. If a loss of adequate blood glucose-lowering response to DIAMICRON MR 30 mg is detected, the drug should be discontinued.

Hematologic: Treatment of patients with glucose-6-phosphate dehydrogenase (G6PD)-deficiency with sulfonylurea agents can lead to haemolytic anaemia. Since DIAMICRON MR 30 mg belongs to the class of sulfonylurea agents, caution should be used in patients with G6PD-deficiency and a non-sulfonylurea alternative should be considered.

Hepatic/Biliary/Pancreatic: The metabolism and excretion of sulfonylureas including DIAMICRON MR 30 mg may be slowed in patients with impaired hepatic function (see Monitoring and Laboratory Tests).

Peri-Operative Considerations: In patients stabilized on gliclazide therapy, loss of blood sugar control may occur in cases of acute intercurrent disease or in stressful situations such as trauma or surgery. Under these conditions, discontinuation of DIAMICRON MR 30 mg (gliclazide) and administration of insulin should be considered.

Renal: The metabolism and excretion of sulfonylureas including DIAMICRON MR 30 mg may be slowed in patients with impaired renal function. If hypoglycemia should occur in such patients, it may be prolonged and appropriate management should be instituted (see Monitoring and Laboratory Tests).

Special Populations: Pregnant Women: Gliclazide is contraindicated in pregnancy. It is recommended that insulin be used during pregnancy in diabetic women (see Contraindications).

Uncontrolled diabetes (gestational or not) is associated with a higher incidence of congenital abnormalities and perinatal mortality. Blood glucose control should be optimal around the time of conception to reduce the risk of congenital malformations.

Nursing Women: The product is contraindicated in breast-feeding mothers because the potential for hypoglycemia in nursing infants may exist. Some sulfonylurea drugs are excreted in human milk although it is not known whether gliclazide is one of them (see Contraindications).

Pediatrics (<18 years of age): Safety and effectiveness of DIAMICRON MR 30 mg in children have not been established. DIAMICRON MR 30 mg is therefore not recommended for use in children and adolescents.

Geriatrics (≥65 years of age): Efficacy and tolerance of DIAMICRON MR 30 mg, prescribed using the same therapeutic regimen in subjects over 65 years, has been confirmed in clinical trials.

Severe hypoglycemia can be induced by all sulfonylurea drugs, particularly susceptible are elderly subjects.

Monitoring and Laboratory Tests: Measurement of glycated haemoglobin levels (or fasting venous plasma glucose) is recommended in assessing blood glucose control. Blood glucose self-monitoring is also recommended.

Blood glucose control in a patient receiving antidiabetic treatment may be affected by fever and infection or surgical intervention. Closed monitoring is required in these patients. In some cases, it may be necessary to administer insulin.

Hepatic function should be assessed before initiating therapy and the liver function should be assessed periodically in patients with impaired hepatic function.

In patients with impaired renal function, blood and urine glucose should be regularly monitored. Measurements of glycated hemoglobin levels are recommended.

Elderly patients (malnourished, with impaired hepatic, renal, or adrenal function) will require periodic monitoring and special care.

ADVERSE REACTIONS: Adverse Drug Reaction Overview: DIAMICRON MR 30 mg (gliclazide) has been evaluated for safety in controlled clinical trials in 955 patients, of which 728 were treated in long-term studies for up to 10 months, in comparison with gliclazide 80 mg tablets.

The most frequent adverse drug reactions are hypoglycaemia and gastrointestinal disturbances (including abdominal pain, nausea, vomiting, dyspepsia, diarrhea, constipation).

Serious adverse drug reactions that resulted in hospitalization during clinical trials were malaise, acute renal failure, and thrombophlebitis.

Clinical Trial Adverse Drug Reactions: Because clinical trials are conducted under very specific conditions the adverse reaction rates observed in the clinical trials may not reflect the rates observed in practice and should not be compared to the rates in the clinical trials of another drug. Adverse drug reaction information from clinical trials is useful for identifying drug-related adverse events and for approximating rates.

Hypoglycemia: (See Warnings and Precautions.) Severe hypoglycemia which mimics acute CNS disorders may occur. Hepatic and/or renal disease, malnutrition, debility, advanced age, alcoholism, adrenal or pituitary insufficiency may be predisposing factors.

In long-term studies, the percentage of patients experiencing hypoglycemic episodes was similar between patients treated with DIAMICRON MR 30 mg (11.6%) and those treated with gliclazide 80 mg tablets (11.1%). However, the number of hypoglycemic episodes for 100 patient-months was lower in the DIAMICRON MR 30 mg group (3.5) than in the gliclazide 80 mg tablets group (4.8).

Analysis in elderly patients (over 65 years old) showed that this population experienced, overall, less hypoglycemia than the whole population with a prevalence of hypoglycemic episodes lower in the DIAMICRON MR 30 mg group (2.6 hypoglycemic episodes for 100 patient-months) than in the gliclazide 80 mg tablets group (4.1).

Other Adverse Events: Adverse events reported during controlled clinical trials with DIAMICRON MR 30 mg were those expected in the population of interest, a population whose underlying disease is recognized atheromatous risk factor. Adverse events that have been reported in at least 1.0% of diabetic patients in long-term controlled studies, whatever their relationship to treatment, are listed by body system in Table 1. The most frequent adverse events were unspecific of the disease as respiratory infections or back pain.

Table 1: DIAMICRON MR

Adverse Events Reported in ≥1% of Type 2 Diabetic Patients in Long-Term Controlled Studies with DIAMICRON MR 30 mg vs Gliclazide 80 mg

	DIAMICRON MR 30 mg (n=728) %	Gliclazide 80 mg Tablets (n=734) %
Resistance Mechanism		
Infection Viral	7.7	5.6
Otitis media	1.1	0.8
Respiratory		
Rhinitis	4.4	4.6
Bronchitis	4.4	4.6
Pharyngitis	4.3	3.5
Upper Respiratory Infection	3.3	3.7
Coughing	2.1	2.0
Pneumonia	1.5	1.4
Sinusitis	1.5	1.1
Musculoskeletal		
Back Pain	5.2	4.1
Arthralgia	3.0	3.5
Arthrosis	2.2	2.2
Arthritis	1.4	2.3
Tendinitis	1.1	1.0
Myalgia	2.3	1.5
Secondary Term		
Inflicted Injury	4.3	4.5
Body as a Whole		
Headache	3.8	4.6
Asthenia	2.2	2.6
Cardiovascular		
Hypertension	3.2	3.7
Angina Pectoris	2.1	2.2
Oedema legs	1.2	1.4
Urinary		
Urinary Tract Infections	2.6	3.0
Gastrointestinal		
Diarrhea	2.5	2.0
Constipation	1.6	1.2
Gastritis	1.2	0.5
Gastroenteritis	1.1	1.5
Nausea	1.1	0.7
Abdominal pain	1.1	1.4
Central and Peripheral Nervous Systems		
Dizziness	2.2	2.3

(cont'd)

Table 1: DIAMICRON MR *(cont'd)*

Adverse Events Reported in ≥1% of Type 2 Diabetic Patients in Long-Term Controlled Studies with DIAMICRON MR 30 mg vs Gliclazide 80 mg

	DIAMICRON MR 30 mg (n=728) %	Gliclazide 80 mg Tablets (n=734) %
Neuralgia	1.2	0.7
Metabolism and Nutrition		
Hypoglycemia	11.6	11.1
Hyperglycemia	1.9	2.2
Lipid metabolism disorder	1.4	0.5
Hyperlipaemia	1.0	0.8
Skin and Appendages Disorders		
Dermatitis	1.6	1.2
Rash	1.0	1.2
Skin disorder	1.9	2.0
Pruritus	1.0	0.4
Vision Disorders		
Conjunctivitis	1.0	0.8
Psychiatric Disorders		
Depression	1.9	1.2
Insomnia	1.1	2.0

Analysis of adverse events in sub-populations led to similar pattern as in the whole population and showed that sex, age and renal insufficiency had no significant influence on the safety profile of 30 mg.

Less Common Clinical Trial Adverse Drug Reactions (<1%): Adverse events other than those already specifically mentioned in this product monograph and that have been reported with DIAMICRON MR 30 mg during long-term studies in more than one patient and/or that have been previously reported with gliclazide 80 mg tablets or with other sulfonylurea drugs include the following (drug relationship has not been proved for all cases):

Body as a Whole: allergy, carpal tunnel syndrome, chest pain, fever, infection, fungal infection, leg pain, malaise, pain, weight increase.

Cardiovascular: arteritis, cardiac failure, cerebrovascular disorder, coronary artery disorder, epistaxis, hypotension, myocardial infarction, palpitation, tachycardia, thrombophlebitis, vein disorder.

Central, Peripheral Nervous Systems: anxiety, confusion, depression, insomnia, nervousness, neuropathy.

Endocrine: hypothyroidism. A decrease in the uptake of radioactive iodine by the thyroid gland has been reported with other sulfonylurea drugs. This has not been shown with gliclazide 80 mg tablets during a study involving 15 patients.

Gastrointestinal: abdominal pain, anal fissure, appetite increased, colitis, duodenal ulcer, epigastric fullness, faecal incontinence, flatulence, gastric irritation, gastroesophageal reflux, GI neoplasm benign, hemorrhoids, melena, dry mouth, oesophagitis, saliva increased, tooth ache, tooth disorder, vomiting. These reactions are generally dose-related and may disappear when the dose is reduced.

Hearing and Vestibular: hearing decreased, tinnitus.

Liver and Biliary: increased liver enzymes, hepatitis, hepatomegaly.

Metabolic and Nutritional: gout, glycosuria, hypercholesterolemia, hypertriglyceridemia, thirst. Cases of hepatic porphyria and disulfiram-like reactions have been described with sulfonylurea drugs. Clinical experience to date has shown that gliclazide 80 mg tablets has a low incidence of disulfiram type reactions.

Musculoskeletal: arthropathy, bursitis, hernia congenital, skeletal pain, spine malformation.

Reproductive: balanoposthitis, benign female breast neoplasm, impotence, mastitis, menstrual disorder, prostatic disorder, vaginitis.

Respiratory: asthma, dyspnea, tracheitis.

Skin and Appendages: fungal dermatitis, eczema, erythema, hyperkeratosis, maculopapular or morbiliform rash, nail disorder, onychomycosis, pruritus, dry skin, skin ulceration, urticaria. These reactions may persist during treatment, which must be then interrupted. Cases of porphyria tarda and of photosensitivity have also been described with sulfonylurea drugs.

Urinary: albuminuria, cystitis, nocturia, polyuria, renal calculus, renal cyst.

Vision: cataract, conjunctival haemorrhage, diplopia, glaucoma, abnormal lacrimation, retinal disorder, abnormal vision, vitreous disorder, xerophthalmia.

Abnormal Hematologic and Clinical Chemistry Findings: The pattern of laboratory tests abnormalities previously observed with gliclazide 80 mg tablets was similar to that for other sulfonylureas. Occasional mild to moderate elevations of hepatic enzymes, LDH and creatinine and decrease in natremia have been observed. These abnormalities frequently encountered with treated or untreated diabetic patients are rarely associated with clinical symptoms and generally not considered to be drug related. As with all hypoglycemic sulfonylurea drugs, a few rare cases of leukopenia, agranulocytosis, thrombocytopenia and anemia have been reported with gliclazide 80 mg tablets. No laboratory tests abnormalities other than those already reported with gliclazide 80 mg tablets have been observed during controlled clinical trials performed on DIAMICRON MR 30 mg.

Post-Market Adverse Drug Reactions: In post-marketing experience with DIAMICRON MR 30 mg, gastrointestinal disturbance, including abdominal pain, nausea, vomiting, dyspepsia, diarrhea and constipation have been reported. Skin and subcutaneous tissue disorders, rash, pruritus, urticaria, erythema, maculopapular rashes and bullous reactions have been more rarely reported.

The most serious adverse drug reactions reported with gliclazide are hypoglycaemic coma, pancytopenia, thrombocytopenia, hepatitis, cholestatic jaundice, pyrexia, pancreatitis acute and skin reactions (pruritus and rash).

Class Attribution Effects: Cases of erythrocytopenia, agranulocytosis, haemolytic anaemia, pancytopenia and allergic vasculitis, have been described for other sulphonylureas.

With other sulfonylureas cases were also observed of elevated liver enzyme levels (AST, ALT, alkaline phosphatise) and even impairment of liver function (e.g. with cholestasis and jaundice) and hepatitis which regressed after withdrawal of the sulfonylurea or led to life-threatening liver failure in isolated cases. Discontinue treatment if cholestatic jaundice appears.

DRUG INTERACTIONS: Overview: As a result of drug interaction, hypoglycemia may be potentiated when a sulfonylurea is used concurrently with agents such as: long-acting sulfonamides, tuberculostatics, NSAIDs, fibrates, monoamine oxidase inhibitors, salicylates, probenecid, beta-blockers, azole antifungal agents (oral and parenteral preparations), H_2 receptor antagonists, angiotensin converting enzyme inhibitors and clarithromycin. In addition, hypoglycemia is potentiated when gliclazide is used in combination with other antidiabetic agents (insulin, alpha glucosidase inhibitors, biguanides) which is not indicated.

Certain drugs tend to induce hyperglycemia and may lead to loss of blood sugar control. These include diuretics (thiazides, furosemide), corticosteroids, oral contraceptives (estrogen plus progestogen), chlorpromazine, ritodrine, salbutamol, terbutaline and nicotinic acid in pharmacologic doses.

Barbiturates should be used with caution in patients receiving an oral hypoglycemic agent since they may reduce the hypoglycemic effect.

Sulfonylureas may potentiate the action of anticoagulants. Adjustment of the anticoagulant dose may be necessary.

Drug-Drug Interactions: See Table 2.

Table 2: DIAMICRON MR

Established or Potential Drug-Drug Interactions

Gliclazide	Reference	Effect	Clinical Comment
Miconazole (systemic route, oromucosal gel)	C	Increases the risk of hypoglycaemia	**Contra-indicated combination.** Increases the hypoglycaemic effect with possible onset of hypoglycaemic symptoms, or even coma.
Phenylbutazone (systemic route)	C	Increases the risk of hypoglycaemia	**Combination is not recommended.** Increases the hypoglycaemic effect of sulphonylureas (displaces their binding to plasma proteins and/or reduces their elimination). It is preferable to use a different anti-inflammatory agent, or else to warn the patient and emphasise the importance of self-monitoring. Where necessary, adjust the dose during and after treatment with the anti-inflammatory agent.
Other antidiabetic agents (insulins, acarbose, biguanides)	C	Increases the risk of hypoglycaemia	**Combinations requiring precautions for use.** Potentiation of the blood glucose lowering effect and thus, in some instances, hypoglycaemia may occur.
Beta-blockers	C	Increases the risk of hypoglycaemia	**Combinations requiring precautions for use.** Potentiation of the blood glucose lowering effect and thus, in some instances, hypoglycaemia may occur.
Fluconazole	C	Increases the risk of hypoglycaemia	**Combinations requiring precautions for use.** Potentiation of the blood glucose lowering effect and thus, in some instances, hypoglycaemia may occur.
Angiotensin converting enzyme inhibitors	C	Increases the risk of hypoglycaemia	**Combinations requiring precautions for use.** Potentiation of the blood glucose lowering effect and thus, in some instances, hypoglycaemia may occur.
H_2-receptor antagonists	C	Increases the risk of hypoglycaemia	**Combinations requiring precautions for use.** Potentiation of the blood glucose lowering effect and thus, in some instances, hypoglycaemia may occur.
MAOIs	C	Increases the risk of hypoglycaemia	**Combinations requiring precautions for use.** Potentiation of the blood glucose lowering effect and thus, in some instances, hypoglycaemia may occur.
Sulfonamides	C	Increases the risk of hypoglycaemia	**Combinations requiring precautions for use.** Potentiation of the blood glucose lowering effect and thus, in some instances, hypoglycaemia may occur.
Nonsteroidal anti-inflammatory agents	C	Increases the risk of hypoglycaemia	**Combinations requiring precautions for use.** Potentiation of the blood glucose lowering effect and thus, in some instances, hypoglycaemia may occur.
Clarithromycin	T	Increases the risk of hypoglycaemia	**Combinations requiring precautions for use.** May potentiate the hypoglycemic action of sulfonylurea agents.
Danazol	C	Causes an increase in blood glucose levels	**Combination is not recommended because of diabetogenic effect of danazol.** If the use of this active substance cannot be avoided, warn the patient and emphasise the importance of urine and blood glucose monitoring. It may be necessary to adjust the dose of the antidiabetic agent during and after treatment with danazol.
Chlorpromazine (neuroleptic agent)	C	Causes an increase in blood glucose levels	**Combination requiring precautions during use.** High doses (>100 mg per day of chlorpromazine) increase blood glucose levels (reduced insulin release). Warn the patient and emphasise the importance of blood glucose monitoring. It may be necessary to adjust the dose of the antidiabetic active substance during and after treatment with the neuroleptic agent.
Glucocorticoids (systemic and local route: intra-articular, cutaneous and rectal preparations) and tetracosactrin	C	Causes an increase in blood glucose levels	**Combination requiring precautions during use.** Increase in blood glucose levels with possible ketosis (reduced tolerance to carbohydrates due to glucocorticoids). Warn the patient and emphasise the importance of blood glucose monitoring, particularly at the start of treatment. It may be necessary to adjust the dose of the antidiabetic active substance during and after treatment with glucocorticoids.
Ritodrine, salbutamol, terbutaline: (I.V.)	C	Causes an increase in blood glucose levels	**Combination requiring precautions during use.** Increased blood glucose levels due to beta-2 agonist effects. Emphasise the importance of monitoring blood glucose levels. If necessary, switch to insulin.
Anticoagulant therapy (Warfarin and other)	C	Potentiation of anticoagulation	**Combination which must be taken into account.** Sulfonylureas may lead to potentiation of anticoagulation during concurrent treatment. Adjustment of the anticoagulant may be necessary.
Drugs containing alcohol	C	Increases the risk of hypoglycaemia	Intolerance to alcohol (disulfiram-like reaction: flushing, sensation of warmth, giddiness, nausea and occasionally tachycardia) may occur in patients treated with sulfonylurea.

Legend: C=Case Study; CT=Clinical Trial; T=Theoretical.

Drug-Food Interactions: There are no established drug-food interactions.

Drug-Herb Interactions: Interactions with herbal products have not been established.

Drug-Laboratory Test Interactions: Interactions with laboratory tests have not been established.

Drug-Lifestyle Interactions: This treatment should only be prescribed if the patient is likely to have a regular food intake (including breakfast). It is important to have a regular carbohydrate intake due to the increased risk of hypoglycemia if a meal is taken late, if an inadequate amount of food is consumed or if the food is low in carbohydrate. Hypoglycemia is more likely to occur during periods of low-calorie diet and following prolonged or strenuous exercise.

Intolerance to alcohol (disulfiram-like reaction: flushing, sensation of warmth, giddiness, nausea and occasionally tachycardia) may occur in patients treated with sulfonylurea. Alcohol increases the hypoglycaemic reaction (by inhibiting compensatory reactions) that can lead to the onset of hypoglycaemic coma. Avoid alcohol or medicines containing alcohol.

Treatment with DIAMICRON MR 30 mg can have effects on ability to drive and use machines. Patients should be made aware of the symptoms of hypoglycaemia and should be careful if driving or operating machinery, especially at the beginning of treatment.

DOSAGE AND ADMINISTRATION: Dosing Considerations: Determination of the proper dosage for DIAMICRON MR 30 mg for each patient should be made on the basis of frequent determinations of blood glucose during dose titration and throughout maintenance.

The daily dose of DIAMICRON MR 30 mg may vary from 30 to 120 mg (1 to 4 tablets), once daily.

Recommended Dose and Dosage Adjustment: The recommended starting dose of DIAMICRON MR 30 mg is 1 tablet per day (30 mg), even in elderly patients (over 65 years old).

A single daily dose provides effective blood glucose control. The single daily dose may be between one and three, or even four, tablets. The daily dose should not exceed 120 mg.

Dose adjustment should be carried out in steps of 30 mg, according to the blood glucose response. Each step should last for at least two weeks.

Administration: It is recommended that the medication be taken at breakfast time. The tablets should be swallowed whole and must not be chewed or crushed.

- Previously untreated patients should commence with a dose of 30 mg and will benefit from dose adjustment until the appropriate dose is reached.
- DIAMICRON MR 30 mg can replace gliclazide 80 mg immediate release tablets (Diamicron 80 mg).
- DIAMICRON MR 30 mg can replace an antidiabetic treatment without any transitional period. If a patient is switched from a hypoglycemic sulfonylurea with a prolonged half-life (i.e. chlorpropamide) he/she should be carefully monitored (for 1 to 2 weeks) in order to avoid hypoglycemia due to possible residual effects of the previous therapy.

It is advisable to ascertain the contribution of the drug in control of the blood glucose level by discontinuing the medication semi-annually or at least annually with careful monitoring of the patient. If the need for the drug is not evident, the drug should not be resumed. In some diabetic subjects, short-term administration periods of the drug may be sufficient during periods of transient loss of blood sugar controls.

Geriatrics: The efficacy and tolerance of DIAMICRON MR 30 mg, prescribed using the same therapeutic regimen in subjects over 65 years, has been confirmed in clinical trials. The dosage will therefore be identical to that recommended for adults under the age of 65 years.

Renal Insufficiency: The efficacy and tolerance of DIAMICRON MR 30 mg, prescribed using the same therapeutic regimen in subjects with mild to moderate renal failure (creatinine clearance of between 15 and 80 mL/min), has been confirmed in clinical trials. The dosage will therefore be identical to that in subjects with normal renal function.

Patients Receiving Insulin: Maturity onset diabetics with no ketoacidosis or history of metabolic decompensation and whose insulin requirements are less than 40 units per day may be considered for DIAMICRON MR 30 mg therapy after cessation of insulin.

If a change from insulin to DIAMICRON MR 30 mg is contemplated in such a patient, discontinue insulin for a period of 2 or 3 days to determine whether any therapy other than dietary regulation and exercise is needed. During this insulin-free interval, test the patient's urine at least 3 times daily for glucose and ketone bodies and monitor the results carefully. The appearance of significant ketonuria accompanied by glucosuria within 12 to 24 hours after the withdrawal of insulin, strongly suggests that the patient is ketosis prone, and precludes the change from insulin to sulfonylurea therapy.

Missed Dose: If a dose is forgotten, the dose taken on the next day should not be increased.

OVERDOSAGE:

Symptoms: Overdosage with sulfonylureas may result in hypoglycemia but it should be noted that the dosage which causes such hypoglycemia varies widely and may be within the accepted therapeutic range in sensitive individuals. The manifestations of hypoglycemia include sweating, flushing or pallor, numbness, chilliness, hunger, trembling, headache, dizziness, increased pulse rate, palpitations, increased blood pressure and apprehensiveness in mild cases. In more severe cases, coma appears.

However, symptoms of hypoglycemia are not necessarily as typical as those described above and sulfonylureas may cause insidious development of symptoms mimicking cerebrovascular insufficiency.

Treatment of Overdosage: Discontinue medication and treat hypoglycemia by giving dextrose promptly and in sufficient quantity. Some sulfonylurea-induced hypoglycemias may be refractory to treatment and susceptible to relapse especially in elderly or malnourished patients. Continuous dextrose infusions for hours or days have been necessary. Strict monitoring should be continued until the doctor is sure that the patient is out of danger.

Severe hypoglycaemic reactions, with coma, convulsions or other neurological disorders are possible and must be treated as a medical emergency, requiring immediate hospitalization. If hypoglycaemic coma is diagnosed or suspected, the patient should be given a rapid I.V. injection of 50 mL of concentrated glucose solution (20 to 30%). This should be followed by continuous infusion of a more dilute glucose solution (10%) at a rate that will maintain blood glucose levels above 1 g/L. Patients should be monitored closely and, depending on the patient's condition after this time, the doctor will decide if further monitoring is necessary.

Dialysis is of no benefit to patients due to the strong binding of gliclazide to proteins.

> For management of a suspected drug overdose, contact your **regional Poison Control Centre**. See the *CPS* Directory section for a list of Poison Control Centres.

ACTION AND CLINICAL PHARMACOLOGY: Mechanism of Action: DIAMICRON MR 30 mg (gliclazide) is a hypoglycemic agent of the sulfonylurea group. The hypoglycemic action of DIAMICRON MR 30 mg is related to an improvement in insulin secretion from the functioning beta cells of the pancreas. It potentiates the insulin release, improves the dynamics of insulin. Increase in postprandial insulin and Cpeptide secretion persists after two years of treatment. Gliclazide has extra-pancreatic actions. These metabolic actions are accompanied by hemovascular effects. However, the mechanism of action regarding these effects is still poorly understood. The clinical significance of these effects has not been established.

Effects on insulin release. In type 2 diabetics, gliclazide restores the first peak of insulin secretion in response to glucose and increases the second phase of insulin secretion. A significant increase in insulin response is seen in response to stimulation induced by a meal or glucose.

Extra-pancreatic effects. It has been demonstrated that gliclazide increases peripheral insulin sensitivity: In muscle: the action of insulin on glucose uptake, measured during an euglycemic hyperinsulinemic clamp is significantly increased (+35%), due to an improvement in peripheral sensitivity to insulin. This leads to an improvement in diabetes control. Gliclazide acts mainly by potentiating insulin action on muscle glycogen synthetase. Moreover, results of studies on the muscle are consistent with a post-transcriptional action of gliclazide on GLUT4 glucose carriers; In the liver: studies on glucose turnover show that gliclazide decreases hepatic glucose production, leading to an improvement in fasting blood glucose levels.

Hemovascular effects. Gliclazide decreases microthrombosis by two mechanisms which may be involved in complications of diabetes: A partial inhibition of platelet aggregation and adhesion, with a decrease in the markers of platelet activation (beta thromboglobulin, thromboxane B2); A restoration of the vascular endothelium fibrinolytic activity with an increase in t-PA activity.

Antioxidant effects. A controlled clinical study in diabetics has confirmed the antioxidant effects of gliclazide, that were already demonstrated in clinical pharmacology: reduction in plasma levels of lipid peroxides, increase in the activity of erythrocyte superoxide dismutase.

Pharmacodynamics: Hypoglycemic Activity: The main mechanism of action of gliclazide consists in an increase in the insulin secretory potential of pancreatic beta-cells in a situation of hyperglycemia. This effect of gliclazide on insulin secretion is maintained during long-term treatment in type 2 diabetic patients. It was observed that the administration of gliclazide was followed by: a consistent and significant decrease in fasting blood glucose; a more than 1% decrease in mean glycated hemoglobin; an inhibition by 12 to 27% of the rise in blood glucose after a standard meal or an oral glucose load.

A slight and transitory increase in mean fasting plasma insulin levels was occasionally observed with gliclazide treatment.

Regarding the biphasic nature of insulin secretion, the first peak, that is severely blunted in type 2 diabetes, is improved during gliclazide treatment.

In addition to the effect of gliclazide on the secretion of insulin, extrapancreatic effects have also been evidenced. Gliclazide improves peripheral sensitivity to insulin and increases glucose utilization rate: with euglycemic hyperinsulinemic clamps in obese and non-obese type 2 diabetic patients, it has been shown that gliclazide, after 3 months of treatment, increases the disappearance rate and metabolic clearance of glucose at the highest insulin infusion rates (100 and 300 mU/kg/h); in comparison to diet treatment, gliclazide also enhances insulin-stimulated glucose metabolism after 8 weeks of treatment by potentiating insulin action on skeletal muscle glycogen synthetase.

Studies on glucose turnover have also shown that basal hepatic glucose production, measured by tracer methodology, was markedly reduced (28-50%) after 3 months of treatment.

Hemovascular Activity: Gliclazide possesses anti-platelet properties which are independent of its antidiabetic action, and improves the fibrinolytic potential in diabetic patients: numerous studies have shown inhibitory effects of gliclazide on platelet aggregation and hyperadhesiveness. A statistically significant 22% decrease in collagen-induced platelet aggregation has been observed after 3 and 6 months of treatment with gliclazide in 15 patients previously well controlled under glibenclamide. A concentration-dependent inhibition of PAF-induced platelet aggregation has also been reported with gliclazide in vitro in platelet-rich plasma from healthy subjects and type 2 diabetic patients. Finally, a consistent decrease in markers of platelet activation (e.g. beta thromboglobuline and thromboxane B2 levels) has been observed with gliclazide whether glycemic control improved or not; change to gliclazide of patients treated since several years by chlorpropamide is followed by normalisation of the t-PA activity, sustained over 24-48 months. This has been confirmed by 2 studies in type 1 and glibenclamide-treated type 2 diabetics: in both, the addition of gliclazide to insulin or the switch to this sulfonylurea were followed by significant increase in t-PA and in the activity of the intrinsic fibrinolytic system.

Antioxidant Activity: Gliclazide is a strong free radical scavenging agent, an effect demonstrated both in vitro and in patient. In 17 type 2 diabetic patients switched to gliclazide and seen at regular intervals during a 36-week period, peroxidized lipids and oxidized damaged IgG decreased significantly. These effects of gliclazide on the oxidative stress have been confirmed in a double-blind study in diabetic patients. Highly significant and sustained decrease in peroxidized lipid levels and increase in erythrocyte superoxide dismutase activity were obtained with gliclazide, but not with glibenclamide.

Pharmacokinetics: The initial development of gliclazide led to the marketing of two different formulations of 80 mg tablets worldwide, with only one formulation being registered in each country. Although the two formulations differed substantially in their pharmacokinetic performance in vivo, there was no evidence that they were different in their efficiency and safety in type 2 diabetic patients, thus suggesting that gliclazide does not exert its effect in a dose-dependent manner but by virtue of a threshold plasma drug concentration. Both formulations of gliclazide are prescribed in the dose range 80-320 mg per day, tablets being taken once to 3-times daily. Individual dose requirements vary between patients, which most likely reflect the inter-individual variability in pharmacokinetic characteristics in addition to differences in diabetes severity. Also the noted variability in prescribed average dose between countries may partly be explained by differences in the marketed pharmaceutical formulation. It was therefore essential to develop a new standardized pharmaceutical formulation for worldwide use, presenting optimal and consistent release characteristics. Furthermore, it was thought that a medication suitable for once-daily administration would be desirable. These considerations led to the development of a new modified release formulation of gliclazide, DIAMICRON MR 30 mg.

Gliclazide is slowly and completely absorbed from the gastro-intestinal tract and plasma levels increase progressively, resulting in a plateau-shaped curve from the sixth to the twelfth hour after administration of DIAMICRON MR 30 mg. Intra-individual variability is low. Food intake does not affect the rate and extent of absorption. The relationship between the dose administered and the area under the concentration curve as a function of time is linear. In man it is highly bound to plasma proteins, about 95%. The mean elimination half life in man approximates 16 hours. A single daily dose of DIAMICRON MR 30 mg maintains effective gliclazide plasma concentrations over 24 hours. No clinically significant modifications in the pharmacokinetic parameters have been observed in elderly patients.

Following oral administration the unchanged gliclazide in plasma is extensively metabolized with little of the unchanged compound (<1%) appearing in the urine. No active metabolites have been detected in plasma. Gliclazide metabolites and conjugates are primarily eliminated via kidneys 60 to 70%, and about 10 to 20% via feces. Six principal metabolites have been identified in urine, essentially oxidized and hydroxylated derivatives, and two glucuronoconjugates.

Absorption: The absorption of gliclazide from DIAMICRON MR 30 mg tablets is slow and complete (mean absolute bioavailability of 97%) and is not affected by simultaneous food intake. Plasma concentrations rise gradually and the maximum concentration is usually reached after about 6 hours, with a plateau maintained for another 4 to 6 hours.

Distribution: The volume of distribution is relatively small, which can partially be explained by high protein binding (about 95%).

Metabolism: Although more than 90% of unchanged gliclazide is found in plasma following administration, this is intensively metabolized with little of the unchanged compound (<1%) found in urine. Six principal metabolites have been found in urine, essentially oxidized and hydroxylated derivatives, and two glucuronoconjugates. No active metabolites have been detected in plasma. The principal metabolic pathways of gliclazide may be summarized as shown hereafter.

Excretion: Gliclazide is essentially eliminated via the urine: 60 to 70% as against 10 to 20% via feces. The mean elimination half life is 16 h (range 12-20 h).

Linear kinetics were observed with DIAMICRON MR 30 mg in the dose range up to 90 mg.

Special Populations and Conditions: Pediatrics: Safety and effectiveness of DIAMICRON MR 30 mg in children have not been established. DIAMICRON MR 30 mg is therefore not recommended for use in children and adolescents.

Gender: No significant relationship was found between any of the pharmacokinetic parameters and the covariables gender, body weight and creatinine clearance.

STORAGE AND STABILITY: DIAMICRON MR 30 mg should be stored at room temperature (15-30°C).

INFORMATION FOR THE PATIENT: Published in e-CPS, available by subscription at www.e-cps.ca.

DOSAGE FORMS, COMPOSITION AND PACKAGING: Each white, oblong, modified release tablet, engraved on both faces, "DIA 30" on one face and on the other, contains: gliclazide 30 mg. Nonmedicinal ingredients: anhydrous colloidal silica, calcium hydrogen phosphate dihydrate, hypromellose, magnesium stearate and maltodextrin. Boxes of 60 (containing 2 blister strips of 30).

(Shown in Product Identification Section)

Diane®-35

cyproterone acetate—ethinyl estradiol

Acne Therapy

Bayer

Date of Revision: October 2, 2008

PHARMACOLOGY: DIANE-35 (cyproterone acetate and ethinyl estradiol) is a combination antiandrogen-estrogen for use in the treatment of androgen-dependent dermatological conditions in females.

Cyproterone acetate is a steroid compound with potent antiandrogenic, progestogenic and antigonadotrophic activity. It exerts its antiandrogenic effect by blocking androgen receptors. It also reduces androgen synthesis by a negative feedback effect on the hypothalamo-pituitary-ovarian systems. The estrogen component (ethinyl estradiol) of DIANE-35 increases levels of sex hormone binding globulin (SHBG) and thus reduces the free circulating plasma levels of androgens. Cyproterone acetate has no tendency to reduce SHBG levels.

If used alone in women, cyproterone acetate leads to menstrual cycle disturbances which are avoided when combined with ethinyl estradiol. When DIANE-35 is administered in a cyclic manner it has the added effect of preventing ovulation and possible conception.

The components of DIANE-35 are rapidly absorbed after oral administration. Due to the long terminal half-life of cyproterone acetate, a 4-fold increase in plasma levels occurs after 6 to 12 days of daily dosing. Long-term therapy (36 months) with DIANE-35 did not have a significant influence on lipid metabolism. A trend to increased plasma cholesterol and triglyceride levels was observed. There was a slight decrease in low density lipoprotein (LDL) with a simultaneous increase in high density lipoprotein (HDL).

INDICATIONS: DIANE-35 (cyproterone acetate and ethinyl estradiol) is indicated for the treatment of women with severe acne, unresponsive to oral antibiotic and other available treatments, with associated symptoms of androgenization, including seborrhea and mild hirsutism.

Note: DIANE-35 should not be prescribed for the purpose of contraception alone. However, when taken as recommended (see Dosage), DIANE-35 will provide reliable contraception in patients treated for the above clinical conditions. If patient compliance is uncertain and contraception is necessary, then a supplementary non-hormonal contraceptive method should be considered.

> 1. DIANE-35, as with all estrogen/progestogen combinations, is contraindicated in women with thrombophlebitis, thromboembolic disorders, or a history of these conditions.
> 2. DIANE-35 users appear to have an **elevated risk of venous thromboembolic events** compared to users of combination oral contraceptives in some published studies. Estrogen and/or progestogen should not be taken during treatment with DIANE-35.
> 3. DIANE-35 should **not** be prescribed for the purpose of contraception alone.
> 4. During treatment with DIANE-35, other oral contraceptives should not be used.
> 5. DIANE-35 should be discontinued 3 to 4 cycles after signs have completely resolved.

CONTRAINDICATIONS:
1. History of or actual thrombophlebitis or thromboembolic disorders;
2. History of or actual cerebrovascular disorders;
3. History of or actual myocardial infarction or coronary arterial disease;
4. Active liver disease;
5. Previous or existing liver tumours (benign or malignant);
6. History of cholestatic jaundice;
7. Known or suspected carcinoma of the breast;
8. Known or suspected estrogen-dependent neoplasia;
9. Undiagnosed abnormal vaginal bleeding;
10. Any ocular lesion arising from ophthalmic vascular disease, such as partial or complete loss of vision or defect in visual fields;
11. When pregnancy is suspected or diagnosed;
12. Severe diabetes with vascular changes;
13. A history of otosclerosis with deterioration during pregnancy;
14. Known or suspected hypersensitivity to any of the components of DIANE-35.

WARNINGS: Predisposing Factors for Coronary Artery Diseases: Cigarette smoking increases the risk of serious cardiovascular side effects and mortality. In women with predisposing factors for coronary artery disease (such as cigarette smoking, hypertension, hypercholesterolemia, obesity, diabetes, and increasing age) the use of estrogen/progestogen combinations have been reported as an additional risk factor.

After the age of 35 years, estrogen/progestogen combinations should be considered only in exceptional circumstances and when the risk/benefit ratio has been carefully weighed by both the patient and the physician.

> Cigarette smoking increases the risk of serious adverse effects on the heart and blood vessels from the use of DIANE-35. This risk increases with age and heavy smoking (15 or more cigarettes per day) and is more marked in women over 35 years of age. Women who use this medication should not smoke.

DIANE-35, like all estrogen/progestogen combinations, is associated with an increased risk of venous thromboembolism (VTE) compared with no use.

Based on a review of the published literature, cases of non-fatal VTE ranging in incidence from 1.2 to 9.9 events per 10 000 women-years have been observed in users of DIANE-35 (Spitzer 2003). As context, the incidence of VTE in non-users of any oral contraceptive is estimated to be 0.5 to 1 event per 10 000 women-years, and increases to 4 events per 10 000 women-years in long-term users of low estrogen content (<50 µg ethinyl estradiol) combination oral contraceptives. These event rates are rare, but still justify caution in the use of DIANE-35.

Since market introduction in 1998 to 2003, Health Canada has received 11 reports of VTE (deep vein thrombosis, pulmonary embolism, and stroke) equivalent to a reporting rate of 0.33 events per 10 000 women-years. One of these cases involved a death. It should be noted that reporting rates determined on the basis of spontaneously reported post-marketing adverse events are generally presumed to underestimate the risks associated with drug treatments.

Women with androgen-related conditions (eg, severe acne or hirsutism) may have an inherently increased cardiovascular risk.

The excess risk of VTE is highest during the first year a woman ever uses a combination estrogen/progestogen combination.

Estrogen/progestogen combinations may cause an increase in plasma lipoproteins and should be administered with caution to women known to have pre-existent hyperlipoproteinemia. Lipid profiles should be determined regularly in these patients.

The combination of obesity, hypertension, and diabetes is particularly hazardous to women who are taking DIANE-35. Should this triad of conditions develop, the patient should be placed on an alternate form of therapy for acne.

Discontinue Medication at the Earliest Manifestation of the Following:

A. Thromboembolic and cardiovascular disorders such as thrombophlebitis, pulmonary embolism, cerebrovascular disorders, myocardial ischemia, mesenteric thrombosis and retinal thrombosis.
B. Conditions that predispose to venous stasis and to vascular thrombosis (eg, immobilization after accidents or confinement to bed during long-term illness). Non-hormonal treatment for acne should be used until regular activities are resumed. For use of DIANE-35 when surgery is contemplated, see Precautions.
C. Visual defects—partial or complete
D. Papilledema, or ophthalmic vascular lesions
E. Severe headache of unknown etiology, or worsening of pre-existing migraine headache
F. Onset of jaundice or hepatitis
G. Itching of the whole body
H. Significant rise in blood pressure
I. Onset of severe depression
J. Severe upper abdominal pain or liver enlargement

Pregnancy: Fetal abnormalities have been reported to occur in the offspring of women who have taken estrogen/progestogen combinations in early pregnancy. Rule out pregnancy as soon as it is suspected.

Lactation: The use of estrogen/progestogen combinations during the period a mother is breast-feeding her infant may not be advisable. The hormonal components are excreted in breast milk and may reduce its quantity and quality. The long-term effects on the developing child are not known.

This drug may cause fluid retention. Conditions such as epilepsy, asthma, and cardiac or renal dysfunction require careful observation.

Recognized first-line tests of genotoxicity gave negative results when conducted with cyproterone acetate. However, further tests showed that cyproterone acetate was capable of producing adducts with DNA (and an increase in DNA repair activity) in liver cells from rats and monkeys and also in freshly isolated human hepatocytes. The DNA-adduct level in dog liver cells was extremely low. This DNA-adduct formation occurred at systemic exposures that might be expected to occur in the recommended dose regimens for cyproterone acetate. One in vivo consequence of cyproterone acetate treatment was the increased incidence of focal, possibly pre-neoplastic, liver lesions in which cellular enzymes were altered in female rats.

The relevance of these findings does not appear to be clinically significant based on the results of a multicentre international liver tumour case control study which demonstrated that there is no evidence of an increased risk of hepatocellular carcinoma associated with contraceptive steroids containing cyproterone acetate, even after long-term use.

PRECAUTIONS: Physical Examination and Follow-up: Before estrogen/progestogen combinations are used, a thorough history and physical examination should be performed including a blood pressure determination. Breasts, liver, extremities, abdomen and pelvic organs should be examined. A Papanicolaou smear should be taken if the patient has been sexually active and a urinalysis should be done.

The first follow-up visit should be done 3 months after the initial prescription. Thereafter, examinations should be performed at regular intervals during treatment and more frequently for those patients at greater risk for adverse effects.

Hepatic Function: If there is a clear-cut history of cholestatic jaundice, especially if it occurred during pregnancy, other methods of treatment should be prescribed. The development of severe generalized pruritus or icterus requires that the medication be withdrawn until the problem is resolved. If a patient develops jaundice that proves to be cholestatic in type, therapy should not be resumed. In patients taking estrogen/progestogen combinations, changes in the composition of the bile may occur and an increased incidence of gallstones has been reported. Hepatic nodules (adenoma and focal nodular hyperplasia) have been reported, particularly in long-term users of estrogen/progestogen combinations. Although these lesions are uncommon, they have caused fatal intra-abdominal hemorrhage and should be considered in women presenting with an abdominal mass, acute abdominal pain, or evidence of intra-abdominal bleeding.

Hypertension: Patients with essential hypertension whose blood pressure is well controlled may be given the drug but only under close supervision. If a significant elevation of blood pressure in previously normotensive or hypertensive subjects occurs at any time during the administration of the drug, cessation of medication is necessary.

Migraine and Headache: The onset or exacerbation of migraine or the development of headache of a new pattern which is recurrent, persistent, or severe, requires discontinuation of medication and evaluation of the cause.

Diabetes: Diabetic patients, or those with a family history of diabetes, should be observed closely to detect any alterations in carbohydrate metabolism. Patients predisposed to diabetes who can be kept under close supervision may be given estrogen/progestogen combinations under strict medical supervision. Young diabetic patients whose disease is of recent origin, well-controlled, and not associated with hypertension or other signs of vascular disease such as ocular fundal changes, should be closely observed.

Metabolic and Endocrine Diseases: In metabolic or endocrine diseases and when metabolism of calcium and phosphorus is abnormal, careful clinical evaluation should precede medication and a regular follow-up is recommended.

Ocular Disease: Progressive astigmatic error, possibly leading to keratoconus, has been noted in some myopic women receiving drugs of the estrogen/progestogen class. In women who developed myopia at or near puberty, and in whom myopia stabilized in adult life, estrogen/progestogen combinations after some 6 months of use have increased the refractive error 2 to 3 fold. Women with a family history of myopic astigmatism or keratoconus who are using such therapy may experience rapid advancement of the ocular disorder.

Contact lens wearers who develop visual changes or changes in lens tolerance should be assessed by an ophthalmologist and temporary or permanent cessation of wear considered.

Connective Tissue Disease: The use of estrogen/progestogen combinations in some women has been associated with positive lupus erythematous cell tests and with clinical lupus erythematosus. In some instances exacerbation of rheumatoid arthritis and synovitis have been observed.

Breasts: Increasing age and a strong family history are the most significant risk factors for the development of breast cancer. Other established risk factors include obesity, nulliparity, and late age for first full-term pregnancy. The identified groups of women that may be at increased risk of developing breast cancer before menopause are long-term users of estrogen/progestogen combinations (more than eight years) and starters at early age.

Special judgment should be used in prescribing such medications for women with fibrocystic disease of the breast.

Women receiving such medications should be instructed in self-examination of their breasts. Their physicians should be notified whenever any masses are detected. A yearly clinical breast examination is also recommended, because, if a breast cancer should develop, drugs that contain estrogen may cause a rapid progression if the malignancy is hormone-dependant.

Vaginal Bleeding: Persistent irregular vaginal bleeding requires special diagnostic judgment to exclude the possibility of pregnancy or neoplasm.

Fibroids: Patients with fibroids (leiomyomata) should be carefully observed. Sudden enlargement, pain or tenderness requires discontinuation of the use of the medication.

Age: In general, women in the later reproductive years gradually assume an increasing risk of circulatory and metabolic complications which become more prominent at 35 years of age. In view of this, closer observation, shorter duration of estrogen/progestogen combination use and avoidance of cigarette smoking is advisable. Alternatively, adoption of other means of therapy should be considered for this age group.

Estrogen/progestogen combinations may mask the onset of climacteric.

Emotional Disorders: Patients with a history of emotional disturbances, especially the depressive type, are more prone to have a recurrence of depression while taking estrogen/progestogen combinations. In cases of a serious recurrence, a trial of an alternate method of therapy should be made which may help to clarify the possible relationship. Women with premenstrual syndrome (PMS) may have a varied response to estrogen/progestogen combinations, ranging from symptomatic improvement to worsening of the condition.

Laboratory Tests: Results of laboratory tests should be interpreted in light of the fact that the patient is taking estrogen/progestogen therapy. The following laboratory tests could be modified.

A. Liver Function Tests: Aspartate serum transaminase (AST): variously reported elevations. Alkaline phosphatase and gamma glutamine transaminase (GGT): slightly elevated.
B. Coagulation Tests: Minimal elevation of test values reported for such parameters as prothrombin and Factors VII, VIII, IX and X.
C. Thyroid Function Tests: Protein binding of thyroxine is increased as indicated by increased total serum thyroxine concentrations and decreased T_3 resin uptake.
D. Lipoproteins: Small changes of unproven clinical significance may occur in lipoprotein cholesterol fractions.
E. Gonadotropins: LH and FSH levels are suppressed by the use of estrogen/progestogen therapy. Wait 2 weeks after discontinuing the use of estrogen/progestogen therapy before measurements are made.

Tissue Specimens: Pathologists should be advised of estrogen/progestogen therapy when specimens obtained from surgical procedures and Papanicolaou smears are submitted for examination.

Return to Fertility: After discontinuing therapy, the patient should delay pregnancy until at least one normal spontaneous cycle has occurred in order to date the pregnancy. The patient should be instructed to use a non-hormonal method of contraception during this time period.

Amenorrhea: Women having a history of oligomenorrhea, secondary amenorrhea, or irregular cycles may remain anovulatory or become amenorrheic following discontinuation of estrogen/progestogen combination therapy.

Amenorrhea, especially if associated with breast secretion, that continues for 6 months or more after withdrawal, warrants a careful assessment of hypothalamic-pituitary function.

Thromboembolic Complications—Post-surgery: There is an increased risk of thromboembolic complications in estrogen/progestogen combination users after major surgery. If feasible, such drugs should be discontinued and a non-hormonal method of treatment substituted at least one month prior to **major** elective surgery. Such medication should not be resumed until the first menstrual period after hospital discharge following surgery.

Drug Interactions: The concurrent administration of estrogen/progestogen combinations with other drugs may result in an altered response to either agent. Estrogen/progestogen combinations like DIANE-35 may affect the metabolism of certain other drugs. Accordingly, plasma and tissue concentrations may either increase (eg, cyclosporine) or decrease (eg, lamotrigine) (see Table 1 and Table 2). It is important to ascertain all drugs that a patient is taking, both prescription and non-prescription, before estrogen/progestogen therapy is prescribed.

Pregnancy: Estrogen/progestogen combinations should not be taken by pregnant women. Rule out pregnancy before treatment is begun. Because of the anti-androgenic action of DIANE-35, feminization of male fetuses has occurred in animal studies and may possibly occur in humans.

Immune: Exogenous estrogens may induce or exacerbate symptoms of angioedema, in particular in women with hereditary angioedema. Discontinuation of this medication should be considered.

Table 1: DIANE-35

Drugs Which May Decrease the Therapeutic Effect of DIANE-35 and Increase the Incidence of Breakthrough Bleeding

Class of Compound	Drug	Proposed Mechanism
Anticonvulsants	Carbamazepine Ethosuximide Phenobarbital Phenytoin Primidone Lamotrigine	Induction of hepatic microsomal enzymes. Rapid metabolism of estrogen and increased binding of progestin and ethinyl estradiol to SHBG.
Antibiotics	Ampicillin Cotrimoxazole Penicillin (V)	Enterohepatic circulation disturbance, intestinal hurry.
	Rifampin	Increased metabolism of progestins. Suspected acceleration of estrogen metabolism.
	Chloramphenicol Metronidazole Neomycin Nitrofurantoin Sulfonamides Tetracyclines	Induction of hepatic microsomal enzymes. Also disturbance of enterohepatic circulation.
	Troleandomycin	May retard metabolism of DIANE-35, increasing the risk of cholestatic jaundice.
Antifungals	Griseofulvin	Stimulation of hepatic metabolism of DIANE-35 may occur.
Cholesterol Lowering Agents	Clofibrate	Reduces elevated serum triglycerides and cholesterol; this reduces DIANE-35 efficacy.

(cont'd)

Table 1: DIANE-35 *(cont'd)*

Drugs Which May Decrease the Therapeutic Effect of DIANE-35 and Increase the Incidence of Breakthrough Bleeding

Class of Compound	Drug	Proposed Mechanism
Sedatives and Hypnotics	Benzodiazepines Barbiturates Chloral hydrate Glutethimide Meprobamate	Induction of hepatic microsomal enzymes.
Antacids		Decreased intestinal absorption of progestins[a].
Other Drugs	Phenylbutazone Antihistamines Analgesics Antimigraine preparations Vitamin E	Reduced efficacy has been reported with estrogen/progestogen combinations. Remains to be confirmed.
HIV Protease Inhibitors	Ritonavir	Induction of hepatic microsomal enzymes.
Non-nucleoside Reverse Transcriptase Inhibitors	Nevirapine	Induction of hepatic microsomal enzymes.

[a] Dose two hours apart.

Table 2: DIANE-35

Modification of Other Drug Action by Estrogen/Progestogen Combinations

Class of Compound	Drug	Modification of Drug Action	Suggested Management
Alcohol		Possible increased levels of ethanol or acetaldehyde.	Use with caution.
Alpha-II adrenoreceptor agents	Clonidine	Sedation effect increased.	Use with caution.
Anticoagulants	All	Estrogen/progestogen combinations increase clotting factors, decrease efficacy. However, estrogen/progestogen combinations may potentiate action in some patients.	Use another treatment for acne.
Anticonvulsants	All	Fluid retention may increase risk of seizures.	Use another treatment for acne.
Antidiabetic drugs	Oral hypoglycemics and insulin	Estrogen/progestogen combinations may impair glucose tolerance and increase blood glucose.	Monitor blood glucose. Use another treatment for acne.
Antihypertensive agents	Guanethidine and methyldopa	Estrogen component causes sodium retention, progestin has no effect.	Use another treatment for acne.
	Beta-blockers	Increased drug effect (decreased metabolism).	Monitor cardiovascular status.
Antipyretics	Acetaminophen	Increased metabolism and renal clearance.	
	Antipyrine	Impaired metabolism.	
	ASA	Effects of ASA may be decreased by the short-term use of estrogen/progestogen combinations.	Patients on chronic ASA therapy may require an increase in ASA dosage.
Aminocaproic acid		Theoretically, a hypercoagulable state may occur because estrogen/progestogen combinations augment clotting factors.	Avoid concomitant use.
Betamimetic agents	Isoproterenol	Estrogen causes decreased response to these drugs.	Discontinuing estrogen/ progestogen combinations can result in excessive drug activity.
Caffeine		The actions of caffeine may be enhanced as estrogen/ progestogen combinations may impair the hepatic metabolism of caffeine.	Use with caution.
Cholesterol lowering agents	Clofibrate	Their action may be antagonized by estrogen/progestogen combinations. Estrogen/ progestogen combinations may also increase metabolism of clofibrate.	May need to increase dose of clofibrate.
Corticosteroids	Prednisone	Markedly increased serum levels.	Use another treatment for acne.
Cyclosporine		May lead to an increase in cyclosporine levels and hepatotoxicity.	Monitor hepatic function. The cyclosporine dose may have to be decreased.
Folic acid		Estrogen/progestogen combinations have been reported to impair folate metabolism.	May need to increase dietary intake, or supplement.
Meperidine		Possible increased analgesia and CNS depression due to decreased metabolism of meperidine.	Use combination with caution.

(cont'd)

Table 2: DIANE-35 *(cont'd)*

Modification of Other Drug Action by Estrogen/Progestogen Combinations

Class of Compound	Drug	Modification of Drug Action	Suggested Management
Phenothiazine tranquilizers	All phenothiazines, reserpine and similar drugs	Estrogen potentiates the hyperprolactinemia effect of these drugs.	Use other drugs or lower dose estrogen/ progestogen combinations. If galactorrhea or hyperprolactinemia occurs, use other method.
Sedatives and hypnotics	Chlordiazepoxide Lorazepam Oxazepam Diazepam	Increased effect (increased metabolism).	Use with caution.
Theophylline	All	Decreased oxidation, leading to possible toxicity.	Use with caution. Monitor theophylline levels.
Tricyclic antidepressants	Clomipramine (possibly others)	Increased side effects: ie, depression.	Use with caution.
Vitamin B_{12}		Estrogen/progestogen combinations have been reported to reduce serum levels of Vitamin B_{12}.	May need to increase dietary intake, or supplement.

Several of the anti-HIV protease inhibitors (eg, ritonavir) and non-nucleoside reverse transcriptase inhibitors (eg, nevirapine) have been studied with coadministration of estrogen/progestogen combinations; significant changes (increase and decrease) in the mean AUC of the estrogen and progestogen and the potential to affect hepatic metabolism have been noted in some cases. The efficacy and safety of estrogen/progestogen combination products may be affected. Healthcare providers should refer to the label of the individual anti-HIV protease inhibitor for further drug-drug interaction information.

No formal drug-drug interaction studies have been conducted with DIANE-35.

Vitamin C (ascorbic acid) with estrogen/progestogen combinations has been reported to result in a significant rise in plasma ethinyl estradiol levels.

ADVERSE EFFECTS: General: An increased risk of the following serious adverse reactions has been associated with the use of estrogen/progestogen combinations: thrombophlebitis; arterial thromboembolism; pulmonary embolism; mesenteric thrombosis; neuro-ocular lesions (eg, retinal thrombosis and optic neuritis); myocardial infarction; cerebral thrombosis; cerebral hemorrhage; hypertension; hepatic tumours; gallbladder disease; congenital anomalies.

The following adverse reactions also have been reported in patients receiving estrogen/progestogen combinations: nausea and vomiting, usually the most common adverse reaction, occurs in approximately 10 per cent or fewer of patients during the first cycle. Other reactions, as a general rule, are seen less frequently or only occasionally, as follows: gastrointestinal symptoms (such as abdominal cramps and bloating); breakthrough bleeding; spotting; change in menstrual flow; dysmenorrhea; amenorrhea during and after treatment; temporary infertility after discontinuation of treatment; edema; chloasma or melasma which may persist; breast changes (tenderness, enlargement, secretion); change in weight (increase or decrease); change in cervical erosion and secretion; endocervical hyperplasias; possible diminution in lactation when given immediately postpartum; cholestatic jaundice; migraine; increase in size of uterine leiomyomata; rash (allergic); mental depression; reduced tolerance to carbohydrates; vaginal candidiasis; premenstrual-like syndrome; intolerance to contact lenses; change in corneal curvature (steepening); cataracts; optic neuritis; retinal thrombosis; changes in libido; chorea; changes in appetite; cystitis-like syndrome; rhinitis; headache; nervousness; dizziness; hirsutism; loss of scalp hair; erythema multiforme; erythema nodosum; hemorrhagic eruption; vaginitis; porphyria; impaired renal function; Raynaud's phenomenon; auditory disturbances; hemolytic uremic syndrome; pancreatitis.

Exogenous estrogens may induce or exacerbate symptoms of angioedema, in particular, in women with hereditary angioedema.

Product Specific Adverse Reactions: DIANE-35 (cyproterone acetate and ethinyl estradiol) was generally well tolerated in studies involving 1563 women who were treated for periods of 6 to 36 cycles. The most frequently reported complaint was dysmenorrhea (10.2%) which decreased over time in a manner characteristic of treatment with estrogen/progestogen combinations. Other effects reported were also similar in nature and frequency to those reported with estrogen/progestogen combinations (see Table 3).

Table 3: DIANE-35

Product Specific Adverse Reactions

Adverse Events	No. of Cycles[a]	% Frequency
Dysmenorrhea	23 426	10.2
Breast tension/tenderness	23 814	6.5
Headache	23 810	5.2
Nervousness	23 827	4.4
Chloasma	23 112	4.2
Depressed mood	23 829	3.4
Decreased libido	23 821	3.1
Varicosities	23 829	2.9
Nausea	23 822	1.9
Edema	23 118	1.7
Dizziness	23 340	1.1

[a] Number of cycles evaluated.

Serious post-marketing adverse reactions reported with DIANE-35 include deep venous thrombosis, venous thrombosis with pulmonary embolism, arterial emboli involving the extremities and the spleen, cerebral ischemic vascular accident, cerebral venous thrombosis, sinus thrombosis, retinal vein thrombosis, hypertensive crisis, migraine, pancreatitis focal nodular hyperplasia of the liver, subcapsular liver hematoma, liver adenoma, hepatocellular carcinoma, primary bile duct carcinoma, hepatitis, liver dystrophy, cholangitis, pseudo-membranous colitis, cholestasis, abdominal pain, epileptic seizures, cerebral tumor symptoms, acute brachiofacial paresis, acute hydrocephalus, manic syndrome, hyperpathia, anaphylactoid reactions, ascites, diabetes mellitus, acute leukemia and breast cancer.

The following non-serious adverse reactions, listed according to body system, have been reported postmarketing:

Cardiovascular System: headaches, migraine, superficial phlebitis, palpitations, flushing.

Gastrointestinal System: focal nodular hyperplasia, liver tumor, hepatitis, jaundice, hepatomegaly without abnormal liver tests, nausea, diarrhea, flatulence, stomatitis, salivary gland swelling.

Genitourinary System: menstrual disorder, ovarian cyst, myoma, cervix dysplasia, vaginitis, urinary tract infection, premature birth, abortion, missed abortion and placenta insufficiency.

Metabolism: abnormal liver enzymes, hyperthyroidism, hyperprolactinemia.

Nervous System: depression, decreased libido, nervousness, insomnia, somnolence, confusion, hypesthesia, paresthesia, seizures (in patients with a history of epilepsy), visual disturbances, symptoms of conjunctival irritation, hearing disorder.

Skin: alopecia, acne, chloasma, exanthema, erythema nodosum, striae, neurodermitis, skin allergy, urticaria, facial edema, pruritus, photosensitivity, pigmentation, dry skin, Herpes zoster, cellulitis, subcutaneous lumps, eczema, livedo, blue spots.

OVERDOSE:

Treatment: There have been no reports of overdose with DIANE-35 (cyproterone acetate and ethinyl estradiol). There are no specific antidotes and treatment should be symptomatic, based on the knowledge of the pharmacological action of the constituents.

> For management of a suspected drug overdose, CPhA recommends that you contact your **regional Poison Control Centre**. See the *CPS* Directory section for a list of Poison Control Centres.

DOSAGE: DIANE-35 (cyproterone acetate and ethinyl estradiol) should not be prescribed for the purpose of contraception alone. If patient compliance is uncertain and contraception is necessary, then a supplementary non-hormonal contraceptive method should be considered.

DIANE-35 is supplied in blister pack units consisting of 21 tablets; each tablet containing 2 mg cyproterone acetate and 0.035 mg ethinyl estradiol.

Each cycle consists of 21 days on medication and a 7-day interval without medication (3 weeks on, 1 week off).

First Treatment Course: The patient is instructed to take 1 tablet daily for 21 consecutive days beginning on day 1 of her menstrual cycle. (For the first cycle only the first day of menstrual flow is considered Day 1.) The tablets are then discontinued for 7 days (1 week). Withdrawal bleeding should usually occur during the period that the patient is off the tablets. The first cycle will be somewhat shorter than usual, whereas all following cycles will last four weeks.

Subsequent Courses: The patient begins her next and all subsequent 21-day course of tablets (following the same 21 days on, 7 days off) on the same day of the week that she began her first course. She begins taking her tablets 7 days after discontinuation, regardless of whether or not withdrawal bleeding is still in progress.

Treatment should be continued for several months, since improvement may not be observed with 4 or 5 cycles. DIANE-35 should be discontinued 3 to 4 cycles after signs have completely resolved.

Pregnancy should be ruled out before continuing treatment with DIANE-35 in patients who have missed a menstrual period. If pregnancy is suspected, medication should be discontinued.

Special Notes on Administration: It is recommended that DIANE-35 tablets be taken at the same time each day. Irregular tablet-taking, vomiting or intestinal affections with diarrhea, very rare individual metabolic disturbances or prolonged simultaneous use of certain medical preparations can affect the contraceptive action (see Precautions, Drug Interactions).

If spotting or breakthrough bleeding occurs during the 3 weeks in which DIANE-35 is being taken, the patient is instructed to continue taking the medication. This type of bleeding usually is transient and without significance. However if the bleeding is persistent or prolonged, the patient is advised to consult her physician.

In exceptional cases, menstruation may fail to occur during the 7-day tablet-free interval. The patient is advised not to resume tablet-taking and to consult her physician.

Although the occurrence of pregnancy is highly unlikely if the tablets are taken according to directions, the possibility of pregnancy should be ruled out before continuing treatment with DIANE-35 in patients who have missed a period of withdrawal bleeding. The patient should consult her physician and in the meantime, a supplementary non-hormonal method of contraception should be employed.

If the patient forgets to take a tablet at the usual time, the tablet may be taken within the next 12 hours. If more than 12 hours have elapsed from the time of usual administration, the patient must discard the missed tablet and continue to take the remaining tablets in the pack at the usual time in order to avoid a premature withdrawal bleeding during this cycle. A supplementary non-hormonal method of contraception must be employed until the pack is empty to prevent pregnancy which would necessitate immediate discontinuation of DIANE-35 treatment.

Use of the Blister Pack: The patient should be instructed to take the first tablet from the blister pack out of the section marked with the corresponding day of the week (for example "MO" for Monday), and swallow it whole with some liquid. The patient should be instructed to take the tablet at the same time each day.

INFORMATION FOR THE PATIENT: Published in e-CPS, available by subscription at www.e-cps.ca.

SUPPLIED: Each beige, round, biconvex, sugar-coated tablet contains: cyproterone acetate 2 mg and ethinyl estradiol 0.035 mg. Nonmedicinal ingredients: cornstarch, lactose, magnesium stearate, povidone and talc; tablet coating: calcium carbonate, ferric oxide yellow, glycerol, polyethylene glycol, povidone, sucrose, talc, titanium dioxide and wax. Blister pack units of 21. Store at room temperature (15 to 25°C).

(Shown in Product Identification Section)

Diastat® C

diazepam

Benzodiazepine Anticonvulsant

Valeant

Date of Revision: October 15, 2008

SUMMARY PRODUCT INFORMATION:

Route of Administration	Dosage Form/ Strength	Clinically Relevant Nonmedicinal Ingredients
Rectal	Gel 5 mg/mL	Ethyl alcohol (10%) For a complete listing see Dosage Forms, Composition and Packaging.

INDICATIONS AND CLINICAL USE: DIASTAT (diazepam gel) is indicated for the management of selected, refractory, patients with epilepsy, on stable regimens of AEDs, who require intermittent use of diazepam to control bouts of increased seizure activity.

These bouts are defined as a form of severe seizures variously referred to as recurrent, serial, cluster or crescendo seizures. These clusters are a predictable component of the patient's seizure disorder that are historically distinct from the patient's other seizures in either type, frequency, severity or duration and have an onset that is easily recognized by the family and physician. The clusters have a consistent component, such as an aura, prodrome or characteristic single or multiple seizures, that is predictably and temporally linked to subsequent seizures. Patients typically demonstrate recovery between these seizures. As is the case with all seizure classifications, there is a common pattern of seizure presentation and there are clearly different features for every individual.

DIASTAT is intended for use by caregivers to treat patients in the home setting, as well as in hospitals, emergency and urgent care units and residential institutions.

Geriatrics (>60 years of age): Evidence from clinical studies and experience suggests that use in the geriatric population may be associated with differences in safety or effectiveness. A brief discussion can be found in the appropriate sections (see Dosage and Administration; Action and Clinical Pharmacology and Warnings and Precautions).

Pediatrics (<2 years of age): Evidence from clinical experience suggests that use in the infant pediatric population is associated with differences in safety. A brief discussion can be found in the appropriate sections (see Dosage and Administration; Action and Clinical Pharmacology and Warnings and Precautions).

CONTRAINDICATIONS:

- Patients who are hypersensitive to this drug or to any ingredient in the formulation or component of the container. For a complete listing, see Dosage Forms, Composition and Packaging.
- DIASTAT (diazepam gel) is contraindicated in patients with a known hypersensitivity to diazepam. DIASTAT (diazepam gel) may be used in patients with open angle glaucoma who are receiving appropriate therapy but is contraindicated in acute narrow angle glaucoma.

WARNINGS AND PRECAUTIONS: General: DIASTAT should only be administered by caregivers who in the opinion of the prescribing physician: 1) are able to distinguish the distinct cluster of seizures (and/or the events presumed to herald their onset) from the patient's ordinary seizure activity, 2) have been instructed and judged to be competent to administer the treatment rectally, 3) understand explicitly which seizure manifestations may or may not be treated with DIASTAT, and 4) are able to monitor the clinical response and recognize when that response is such that immediate professional medical evaluation is required.

Carcinogenesis and Mutagenesis: Only animal data are available.

The data currently available are inadequate to determine the mutagenic potential of diazepam.

Dependence/Tolerance: Although diazepam can produce drug dependence, it is expected that DIASTAT has minimal potential for abuse. It is recommended that patients be treated with DIASTAT no more frequently than every five days and no more than five times per month.

Addiction-prone individuals (such as drug addicts or alcoholics) should be under careful surveillance when receiving diazepam or other psychotropic agents because of the predisposition of such patients to habituation and dependence.

Abrupt discontinuation of diazepam following chronic daily use has resulted in withdrawal symptoms, similar in character to those noted with barbiturates and alcohol (convulsions, tremor, abdominal and muscle cramps, vomiting and sweating). The more severe withdrawal symptoms have usually been limited to those patients who had received excessive doses over an extended period of time. Generally milder withdrawal symptoms (e.g., dysphoria and insomnia) have been reported following abrupt discontinuation of benzodiazepines taken continuously at therapeutic levels for several months.

DIASTAT is not recommended for chronic, daily use as an anticonvulsant because of the potential for development of tolerance to diazepam. Chronic daily use of diazepam may increase the frequency and/or severity of grand mal seizures, requiring an increase in the dosage of standard anticonvulsant medication. In such cases, abrupt withdrawal of chronic diazepam may also be associated with a temporary increase in the frequency and/or severity of seizures.

Hepatic/Biliary/Pancreatic: Precautions in treating patients with impaired hepatic function should be observed because patients with severely impaired hepatic function may be unable to biotransform diazepam to inactive metabolites.

Neurologic: CNS Depression: Occupational Hazards: As is true of most preparations containing central nervous system (CNS)-acting drugs, patients should be cautioned against engaging in hazardous occupations requiring complete mental alertness, such as operating machinery, driving a motor vehicle or riding a bicycle following use of DIASTAT (diazepam gel).

Concomitant Use of Other CNS Depressants: Since diazepam has a CNS-depressant effect, patients should be advised against the simultaneous use of alcohol or other CNS-depressants during DIASTAT therapy.

Use in Patients with Petit Mal Status: Tonic status epilepticus has been precipitated in patients treated with intravenous diazepam for petit mal status or petit mal variant status.

Use in Patients with Neurologic Damage: DIASTAT should be used with caution in patients with neurologic damage.

Renal: Metabolites of diazepam are excreted by the kidney; to avoid their excess accumulation, caution should be exercised in the administration to patients with compromised kidney function.

Respiratory: DIASTAT should be used with caution in patients with compromised respiratory function related to a concurrent disease process (e.g., asthma, pneumonia).

Special Populations: Pregnant Women: In humans, measurable amounts of diazepam have been found in maternal and cord blood, indicating placental transfer of the drug. Diazepam has been shown to be teratogenic in mice and hamsters when given orally in doses that are more than 140 times the highest DIASTAT treatment dose. Cleft palates and resorptions are the most common and consistently reported form of developmental toxicity produced in laboratory animals by high doses (>100 mg/kg) of diazepam during gestation. There are no adequate and well-controlled studies of diazepam in pregnant women. However, benzodiazepines have been associated with an increased risk of congenital malformations after first trimester exposure. Hypotonia, lethargy, hypothermia, respiratory and suckling difficulties have been reported in infants whose mothers received benzodiazepines during labor. Children born to mothers receiving benzodiazepines on a regular basis late in pregnancy may be at some risk of experiencing withdrawal symptoms during the postnatal period. DIASTAT should be used during pregnancy only if the potential benefit justifies the potential risk to the fetus.

It is important to note that anticonvulsant drugs should not be discontinued in patients in whom the drug is administered to prevent seizures because of the strong possibility of precipitating status epilepticus with attendant hypoxia and threat to life. In individual cases where the severity and frequency of the seizure disorder are such that the removal of medication does not pose a serious threat to the patient, discontinuation of the drug may be considered prior to and during pregnancy, although it cannot be said with any confidence that even mild seizures do not pose some hazards to the developing embryo or fetus.

Patients should be advised to notify their physician if they become pregnant or intend to become pregnant during therapy with DIASTAT.

Nursing Women: Diazepam is excreted in human milk; therefore, DIASTAT should not be administered to nursing women.

Pediatrics (<2 years of age): Clinical studies have not been conducted to establish the efficacy and safety of DIASTAT in children under 2 years of age. Prolonged CNS depression has been observed in neonates treated with diazepam, apparently due to an inability to biotransform diazepam into inactive metabolites. Therefore, DIASTAT is not recommended for use in children under 6 months of age.

Geriatrics (>60 years of age): The effects of DIASTAT in patients over 60 years of age have not been well characterized. In elderly patients, DIASTAT should be used with caution due to an increase in half-life with a corresponding decrease in the clearance of free diazepam. It is also recommended that the dosage be adjusted downward to reduce the likelihood of ataxia or oversedation.

ADVERSE REACTIONS: Adverse Drug Reaction Overview: The most frequent adverse event (AE) reported to be related to DIASTAT (diazepam gel) in the 2 double-blind, placebo-controlled studies was somnolence (23%). Less frequent AEs were dizziness, headache, pain, diarrhea, euphoria, incoordination and nervousness, which occurred in approximately 2-5% of patients. In addition, ataxia (8%), asthenia (4%), hiccup (2%) and vertigo (2%) were reported in open-label studies. There were no differences in the pattern of AEs in children and adults.

Clinical Trial Adverse Drug Reactions: Because clinical trials are conducted under very specific conditions the adverse reaction rates observed in the clinical trials may not reflect the rates observed in practice and should not be compared to the rates in the clinical trials of another drug. Adverse drug reaction information from clinical trials is useful for identifying drug-related adverse events and for approximating rates.

DIASTAT AE data were collected from double-blind, placebo-controlled studies and open-label studies. The majority of AEs were mild to moderate in severity and transient in nature. See Table 1.

The following infrequent AEs were not seen with DIASTAT but have been reported previously with diazepam use: depression, slurred speech, syncope, constipation, changes in libido, urinary retention, bradycardia, cardiovascular collapse, nystagmus, urticaria, neutropenia and jaundice.

Paradoxical reactions such as acute hyperexcited states, anxiety, hallucinations, increased muscle spasticity, insomnia, rage, sleep disturbances and stimulation have been reported with diazepam; should these occur, use of DIASTAT should be discontinued.

Less Common Clinical Trial Adverse Drug Events (<1%): Body as a Whole: asthenia, infection.

Cardiovascular: palpitation.

Digestive: dyspepsia, dysphagia, fecal incontinence, nausea.

Hemic and Lymphatic: anemia, cyanosis, ecchymosis, lymphadenopathy, thromboplastin decreased.

Metabolic and Nutritional: acidosis, dehydration, peripheral edema.

Nervous: agitation, grand mal convulsion, hyperkinesia, increased salivation, stupor, tremor, twitching.

Respiratory: cough increased, pneumonia, sinusitis.

Skin and Appendages: pruritus, skin discoloration, sweating.

Special Senses: mydriasis.

Urogenital: kidney failure, urinary incontinence, urinary tract infection.

Other AEs Occurring Less Frequently (<2%) and Reported to be Related to DIASTAT in Clinical Studies: Body as a Whole: abdominal pain, accidental injury, accidental overdose, back pain, chills, fever, infection.

Cardiovascular: hypotension, pallor, postural hypotension, vasodilation.

Digestive: abnormal stools, anorexia, diarrhea, dysphagia, increased salivation, nausea, nausea and vomiting, rectal disorder, rectal hemorrhage, tenesmus, thirst, vomiting.

Hemic and Lymphatic: prothrombin time increased.

Musculoskeletal: myasthenia.

Nervous: agitation, amnesia, confusion, convulsion, dysarthria, emotional lability, euphoria, hyperkinesia, hypokinesia, hypotonia, incoordination, increased salivation, insomnia, movement disorder, nervousness, speech disorder, stupor, thinking abnormal, tremor, twitching.

Respiratory: cough increased, hypoventilation, hypoxia.

Skin and Appendages: pruritus, rash.

Special Senses: abnormal vision, amblyopia, diplopia, mydriasis, taste perversion.

Urogenital: urinary incontinence.

Table 1: DIASTAT

Number and Percent of Patients with Adverse Events for Combined Data from the Controlled Studies (AN094-001, AN094-003) (Adverse events with a frequency of ≥1%). Intent-to-Treat Population

	DIASTAT (n=101)		Placebo (n=104)	
	All n (%)	Related[a] n (%)	All n (%)	Related[a] n (%)
Body as a Whole	**12 (12)**	**7 (7)**	**14 (13)**	**9 (9)**
Abdominal Pain	2 (2)	1 (<1)	2 (2)	1 (<1)
Fever	0 (0)	0 (0)	4 (4)	2 (2)
Headache	5 (5)	2 (2)	4 (4)	3 (3)
Pain[b]	3 (3)	3 (3)	4 (4)	3 (3)
Cardiovascular	**2 (2)**	**2 (2)**	**1 (<1)**	**1 (<1)**
Vasodilatation	2 (2)	2 (2)	0 (0)	0 (0)
Digestive	**6 (6)**	**4 (4)**	**8 (8)**	**6 (6)**
Anorexia	1 (<1)	1 (<1)	2 (2)	2 (2)
Diarrhea	4 (4)	2 (2)	1 (<1)	0 (0)
Vomiting	1 (<1)	1 (<1)	2 (2)	2 (2)
Hemic and Lymphatic[c]	**2 (2)**	**0 (0)**	**3 (3)**	**1 (<1)**
Metabolic and Nutritional[c]	**0 (0)**	**0 (0)**	**3 (3)**	**1 (<1)**
Nervous	**32 (32)**	**29 (29)**	**16 (15)**	**13 (13)**
Ataxia	3 (3)	1 (<1)	1 (<1)	1 (<1)
Convulsion	1 (<1)	1 (<1)	3 (3)	0 (0)
Dizziness	3 (3)	3 (3)	2 (2)	2 (2)
Euphoria	3 (3)	3 (3)	0 (0)	0 (0)
Incoordination	3 (3)	3 (3)	0 (0)	0 (0)
Nervousness	2 (2)	2 (2)	2 (2)	2 (2)
Somnolence	23 (23)	23 (23)	8 (8)	8 (8)
Other Body System	**1 (<1)**	**1 (<1)**	**2 (2)**	**2 (2)**
Other	1 (<1)	1 (<1)	2 (2)	2 (2)
Respiratory	**4 (4)**	**0 (0)**	**3 (3)**	**2 (2)**
Asthma	2 (2)	0 (0)	0 (0)	0 (0)
Rhinitis	2 (2)	0 (0)	2 (2)	2 (2)
Skin and Appendages	**5 (5)**	**3 (3)**	**1 (<1)**	**0 (0)**
Rash	3 (3)	2 (2)	0 (0)	0 (0)
Special Senses	**1 (<1)**	**1 (<1)**	**2 (2)**	**0 (0)**
Otitis Media	0 (0)	0 (0)	2 (2)	0 (0)
Urogenital[c]	**1 (<1)**	**0 (0)**	**2 (2)**	**0 (0)**

[a] Related means the adverse event was definitely, probably, or possibly related to the study drug.
[b] Pain includes rectal symptoms such as rectal burning, discomfort, that code to "pain".
[c] Individual adverse events in these categories were less than 1% and therefore are not included in this table.

DRUG INTERACTIONS: Overview: Effects of Other Drugs on the Metabolism of Diazepam: There have been no clinical studies or reports in the literature to evaluate the interaction of rectally administered diazepam with other drugs. As with all drugs, the potential for interaction by a variety of mechanisms is a possibility.

In vitro studies using human liver preparations suggest that CYP2C19 and CYP3A4 are the principal isozymes involved in the initial oxidative metabolism of diazepam. Therefore, potential drug-drug interactions may occur when diazepam is given concurrently with agents that affect CYP2C19 (e.g., cimetidine, quinidine, tranylcypromine, rifampicin) or CYP3A4 (e.g., ketoconazole, clotrimazole, carbamazepine, phenytoin, dexamethasone and phenobarbital) activity.

The clearance of diazepam and certain other benzodiazepines can be delayed in association with cimetidine administration. The clinical significance of this is unclear.

If DIASTAT is to be combined with other psychotropic agents or other CNS depressants, careful consideration should be given to the pharmacology of the agents to be employed—particularly with known compounds which may potentiate the action of diazepam, such as phenothiazines, narcotics, barbiturates, MAO inhibitors and other antidepressants.

When diazepam is used simultaneously with alcohol or other CNS depressants, the potential for a synergistic CNS-depressant effect must be considered. Valproate is known to potentiate the CNS-depressant effects of diazepam; therefore, DIASTAT should be used with caution in patients expected to have high plasma concentrations of valproic acid.

Effects of Diazepam on the Metabolism of Other Drugs: There are no reports as to which isozymes could be inhibited or induced by diazepam. But, based on the fact that diazepam is a substrate for CYP2C19 and CYP3A4, it is possible that diazepam may interfere with the metabolism of drugs which are substrates for CYP2C19, (e.g. omeprazole, propranolol, and imipramine) and CYP3A4 (e.g. cyclosporine, paclitaxel, terfenadine, theophylline and warfarin) leading to a potential drug-drug interaction.

Drug-Food Interactions: Interactions with food have not been established.

Drug-Herb Interactions: Interactions with herbal products have not been established.

Drug-Laboratory Interactions: Interactions with laboratory tests have not been established.

DOSAGE AND ADMINISTRATION: Dosing Considerations:

- In elderly and debilitated patients, it is recommended that the dosage be adjusted downward to reduce the likelihood of ataxia or oversedation.
- The prescribed dose of study medication should be adjusted by the physician periodically to reflect changes in the patient's age or weight. It is recommended that dosage be reviewed at 6 month intervals.

Recommended Dose and Dosage Adjustment: Calculating Prescribed Dose: The DIASTAT (diazepam gel) dose should be individualized for maximum beneficial effect. The target dose of DIASTAT is 0.2-0.5 mg/kg depending on age. See Table 2 for specific recommendations.

Table 2: DIASTAT

Dosing Recommendations

Age (years)	Target Dose
2 through 5	0.5 mg/kg
6 through 11	0.3 mg/kg
12 and older	0.2 mg/kg

Because DIASTAT is provided in fixed, unit-doses of 5, 10, 15 and 20 mg, the prescribed dose is obtained by rounding upward to the next available dose. Table 3 provides acceptable weight ranges for each dose and age category, such that patients will receive between 90% and 180% of the calculated target dose. The safety of this strategy has been established in clinical trials.

Table 3: DIASTAT

Acceptable Weight Ranges for Each Dose and Age Category

2–5 Years 0.5 mg/kg		6–11 Years 0.3 mg/kg		12+ Years 0.2 mg/kg	
Weight (kg)	**Dose (mg)**	**Weight (kg)**	**Dose (mg)**	**Weight (kg)**	**Dose (mg)**
6 to 11	5	10 to 18	5	14 to 27	5
12 to 22	10	19 to 37	10	28 to 50	10
23 to 33	15	38 to 55	15	51 to 75	15
34 to 44	20	56 to 74	20	76 to 111	20

A 2.5 mg dose is available for use as a supplemental dose. This dose may be prescribed at the discretion of the physician for patients who require more precise dose titration than is achieved using on of the 4 standard doses provided. The 2.5 mg dose may also be used as a partial replacement dose for patients who may expel a portion of the first dose.

Additional Dose: If a single dose does not adequately treat the episode, the physician may wish to prescribe 2 doses of DIASTAT. The second dose may be given 4-12 hours after the first dose if seizures persist, are known to reoccur, or if the patient is known to have especially refractory seizures.

Treatment Frequency: It is recommended that patients be treated with DIASTAT no more frequently than every five days and no more than five times per month. If a patient requires more frequent administration of DIASTAT for seizure control, the patient's treatment regimen may require reevaluation by the physician.

Administration: See Warnings and Precautions for general considerations.

OVERDOSAGE:

In the DIASTAT (diazepam gel) clinical trials, the practice was to dose patients up to twice the target dose (see Dosage and Administration). Two patients received more than twice the target dose and reported no AEs.

Previous reports of diazepam overdosage have shown that manifestations of diazepam overdosage include somnolence, confusion, coma, and diminished reflexes. Respiration, pulse and blood pressure should be monitored, as in all cases of drug overdosage, although, in general, these effects have been minimal. General supportive measures should be employed, along with intravenous fluids, and an adequate airway maintained. Hypotension may be combated by the use of levarterenol or metaraminol. Dialysis is of limited value.

For management of a suspected drug overdose, CPhA recommends that you contact your **regional Poison Control Centre**. See the *CPS* Directory section for a list of Poison Control Centres.

ACTION AND CLINICAL PHARMACOLOGY: Mechanism of Action: Animal and in vitro studies indicate that diazepam acts to suppress seizures through an allosteric influence on the γ-aminobutyric acid (GABA) receptors of the A-type ($GABA_A$). GABA acts at this receptor to open the membrane channel allowing chloride ions to flow into neurons. Entry of chloride ions causes an inhibitory potential that reduces the ability of neurons to depolarize to the threshold potential necessary to produce action potentials. Excessive depolarization of neurons is implicated in the generation and spread of seizures.

The benzodiazepine binding site is associated with the $GABA_A$ receptor. Diazepam binds to this site and enhances the actions of GABA by causing GABA to bind more tightly to the $GABA_A$ receptor, increasing the opening of the chloride channel and increasing the chloride ion influx into the neuron. At doses in the lower therapeutic range, diazepam decreases the spread of seizures from the active site or focus by increasing inhibition in the surrounding neurons. At high therapeutic doses, diazepam may suppress seizures originating at the active focus as well.

Pharmacokinetics: Absorption and Distribution: The absorption, distribution, metabolism and excretion of diazepam are well characterized. Protein binding is high, ranging from 96.8%-98.6%. After DIASTAT (diazepam gel) administration, the absorption of diazepam from the rectum is rapid with an absolute bioavailability of 90.4% relative to an intravenous dose. Figure 1 shows diazepam plasma levels following rectal administration of 15 mg diazepam as DIASTAT and intravenous administration of 7.5 mg diazepam. Following rectal dosing, diazepam plasma levels reach 200 ng/mL within 15 minutes, reaching peak plasma concentrations within 1.5 hours. Intravenous dosing results in a quicker rise in plasma levels followed quickly by a fall as diazepam is sequestered in muscle and fat. Following rectal dosing, absorptive and redistribution phases overlap and therapeutic levels of diazepam are maintained for at least 4 hours without having the high peak concentrations of intravenous diazepam, which are often associated with adverse events. The time to maximum plasma concentration (T_{max}) following rectal administration is not different in children and adults given doses normalized to body weight.

Figure 1: DIASTAT

Diazepam Plasma Levels Following Rectal Administration vs I.V. Administration

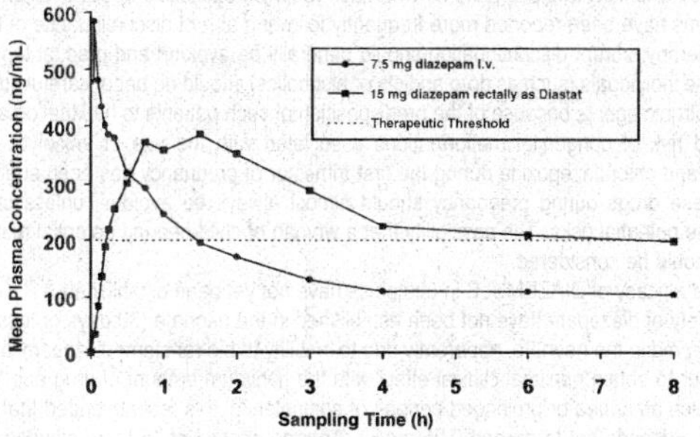

Metabolism: It has been reported in the literature that diazepam is extensively metabolized to one major active metabolite (desmethyldiazepam) and two minor active metabolites, 3-hydroxydiazepam (temazepam) and 3-hydroxy-N-diazepam (oxazepam) in plasma. At therapeutic doses, desmethyldiazepam is found in plasma at concentrations equivalent to those of diazepam while oxazepam and temazepam are not usually detectable. The metabolism of diazepam is primarily hepatic and involves demethylation (involving primarily CYP2C19 and CYP3A4) and 3-hydroxylation (involving primarily CYP3A4), followed by glucuronidation. The marked inter-individual variability in the clearance of diazepam reported in the literature is probably attributable to variability of CYP2C19 (which is known to exhibit genetic polymorphism; about 3-5% of Caucasians have little or no activity and are "poor metabolizers") and CYP3A4. No inhibition was demonstrated in the presence of inhibitors selective for CYP2A6, CYP2C9, CYP2D6, CYP2E1, or CYP1A2, indicating that these enzymes are not significantly involved in metabolism of diazepam.

The primary metabolite of diazepam following a single dose is desmethyldiazepam in both children and adults.

Excretion: The elimination kinetics of diazepam are similar following rectal and intravenous administration.

Special Populations and Conditions: Pediatrics: Clinical studies have not been conducted to establish the efficacy and safety of DIASTAT in children under 2 years of age. Prolonged CNS depression has been observed in neonates treated with diazepam, apparently due to an inability to biotransform diazepam into inactive metabolites. Therefore, DIASTAT is not recommended for use in children under 6 months of age.

Geriatrics: The effects of DIASTAT (diazepam gel) in patients over 60 years of age have not been well characterized. In elderly patients, DIASTAT should be used with caution due to an increase in half-life with a corresponding decrease in the clearance of free diazepam.

Hepatic Insufficiency: Precautions in treating patients with impaired hepatic function should be observed because patients with severely impaired hepatic function may be unable to biotransform diazepam to inactive metabolites.

Renal Insufficiency: Metabolites of diazepam are excreted by the kidney; to avoid their excess accumulation, caution should be exercised in the administration to patients with compromised kidney function.

STORAGE AND STABILITY: Store at controlled room temperature 15-30°C.

INFORMATION FOR THE PATIENT: Published in e-CPS, available by subscription at www.e-cps.ca.

DOSAGE FORMS, COMPOSITION AND PACKAGING: Each rectal delivery system of clear to slightly yellow, non-sterile gel, with a pH between 6.5 to 7.2, contains: diazepam 5 mg/mL. Nonmedicinal ingredients: benzoic acid, benzyl alcohol (1.5%), ethyl alcohol (10%), hydroxypropyl methylcellulose, propylene glycol, sodium benzoate and water. Prefilled, unit dose, rectal delivery systems, including a plastic applicator with a flexible, molded tip available in 2 lengths, designated for convenience as Pediatric, Universal or Adult. Rectal tip size of 4.4 cm for doses of 5 mg (pediatric). Rectal tip size of 4.4 cm for doses of 10 mg (universal). Rectal tip size of 6 cm for doses of 15 mg (adults). Each package contains 2 rectal delivery systems, 2 packets of lubricating jelly and instructions for use.

Diazemuls® ℞

diazepam

Anxiolytic—Sedative

Pfizer

Date of Preparation: February 20, 2007

PHARMACOLOGY: DIAZEMULS is an injectable emulsion of diazepam, a drug with known anxiolytic-sedative and muscle relaxant properties. Diazepam has been found useful for short-term symptomatic relief of excessive anxiety and tension in patients with anxiety neurosis, although anxiety and tension associated with the stresses of everyday life usually do not require treatment with anxiolytic drugs.

Diazepam must first be released from the oil phase of the DIAZEMULS emulsion before it can exert a therapeutic effect. In fact, peak blood levels of diazepam are reached only after 15 minutes following i.v. injection of DIAZEMULS, and after 2 hours following i.m. administration. Subsequent to a rapid distribution phase, diazepam undergoes a longer elimination phase, which varies with age, from approximately 20 hours at age 20 to approximately 80 hours at age 80.

Diazepam is metabolized in the liver to N desmethyl-diazepam, and to some extent to N-methyl-oxazepam, which in turn is metabolized to oxazepam. Although these metabolites are pharmacologically active, only N-desmethyl-diazepam is formed in sufficient quantity to produce significant clinical effects. The desmethyl metabolite has an elimination half-life of 50 to 120 hours.

Diazepam and its metabolites are excreted mainly in the urine, as glucoronides or sulfates.

Diazepam crosses the placenta and is secreted in breast milk. It is approximately 98% bound to plasma proteins.

INDICATIONS: DIAZEMULS (diazepam injectable emulsion) is indicated when an injectable preparation of diazepam is required. It has been found useful: to alleviate the symptoms of acute alcohol withdrawal, such as acute agitation, tremor, impending or acute delirium tremens and hallucinosis; as an adjunct prior to endoscopic procedures if apprehension, anxiety or acute stress reactions are present, and to diminish the patients recall of the procedures (see Warnings); for the relief of muscle spasm in cerebral palsy, athetosis and stiff man syndrome; as premedication for relief of anxiety states prior to surgical procedures (i.m. route) or cardioversion (i.v. route).

CONTRAINDICATIONS: Patients with known hypersensitivity to diazepam or the components of the emulsion vehicle (see Supplied); myasthenia gravis; acute narrow angle glaucoma, and open angle glaucoma unless patients are receiving appropriate therapy.

WARNINGS: DIAZEMULS should not be administered to patients in shock or coma. There have been rare reports of apnea or cardiac arrest, usually following i.v. administration, especially in elderly or very ill patients and in those with limited pulmonary reserve. Resuscitative equipment including that necessary to support respiration should therefore be readily available. Since lingual obstruction of the airway may occur, particularly in children and in the elderly, caution is required to maintain a free airway in patients receiving DIAZEMULS injection.

Rapid injection or the use of veins with too small a lumen carries the risk of thrombophlebitis. I.V. injection should therefore be directly into a large lumen vessel, such as an antecubital vein, and the drug should be administered slowly, at the rate of no more than 5 mg (1 mL/min). Extreme care should be taken to avoid intra-arterial administration or extravasation.

When used i.v., DIAZEMULS should be injected directly into the vein without prior dilution or mixing with other products or solutions (see Dosage).

Concomitant use of barbiturates, alcohol or other CNS depressants increases depression with increased risk of apnea. When diazepam is used in a patient taking narcotic analgesics, the dosage of the narcotic should be reduced by at least one-third and administered in small increments. In some instances, the use of a narcotic may not be necessary. DIAZEMULS should not be administered to patients with acute alcoholic intoxication with depression of vital signs.

Occupational Hazards: Patients receiving DIAZEMULS should be cautioned against engaging in hazardous occupations requiring complete mental alertness, such as operating machinery or driving a motor vehicle.

Physical and Psychological Dependence: Withdrawal symptoms similar to those noted with barbiturates and alcohol may occur following abrupt discontinuance of diazepam (convulsions, tremor, abdominal and muscle cramps, vomiting and sweating). Severe symptoms are usually limited to those patients who have received excessive doses over an extended period of time. Milder withdrawal symptoms have been reported more frequently following abrupt discontinuance of benzodiazepines. Consequently, after extended therapy, abrupt discontinuation should generally be avoided and gradual tapering in dosage followed. Particularly addiction-prone individuals (such as drug addicts or alcoholics) should be under careful surveillance when receiving diazepam or other psychotropic agents because of the predisposition of such patients to habituation and dependence.

Pregnancy: An increased risk of congenital malformations associated with the use of anxiolytic-sedative drugs including diazepam, meprobamate and chlordiazepoxide during the first trimester of pregnancy has been suggested in several studies. Therefore, the use of these drugs during pregnancy should almost always be avoided, unless the expected benefits are considered to outweigh the potential risks. The possibility that a woman of child-bearing potential may be pregnant at the time of institution of therapy should be considered.

Obstetrics: The safety and efficacy of DIAZEMULS in obstetrics have not yet been established.

Children: Efficacy and safety of diazepam have not been established in the neonate (30 days or less of age). Prolonged CNS depression has been observed in the neonate, apparently due to inability to biotransform diazepam into inactive metabolites.

In pediatric use, in order to obtain maximal clinical effect with the minimum amount of drug and thus to reduce the risk of hazardous side effects, such as apnea or prolonged periods of somnolence, it is recommended that the drug be given slowly over a 3 minute period in a dosage not to exceed 0.25 mg/kg. After an interval of 15 to 30 minutes the initial dosage can be cautiously repeated. If, however, relief of symptoms is not obtained after a third administration, adjunctive therapy appropriate to the condition being treated should be considered.

PRECAUTIONS: Geriatrics: Elderly and debilitated patients and those with organic brain disorders have been found to be very prone to CNS depression following even low doses of diazepam. DIAZEMULS (diazepam injectable emulsion) should be used in those patients with caution and in low doses to preclude development of ataxia, sedation and other possible adverse effects.

Emotional Disorders: DIAZEMULS is not recommended in the treatment of psychotic or severely depressed patients. Precautions are indicated for severely depressed patients or those who show evidence of impending depression, particularly in the recognition that suicidal tendencies may be present and protective measures may be necessary.

Since excitement and other paradoxical reactions may result from use of the drug in psychotic patients, diazepam should not be used in ambulatory patients suspected of having psychotic tendencies.

Use before Bronchoscopy and Laryngoscopy: Since there are insufficient data available to establish the safety of DIAZEMULS prior to bronchoscopy and laryngoscopy, its use is not recommended.

Use before Gastroscopy, Esophagoscopy, Cardioversion and Surgical Procedures: DIAZEMULS should be used only under conditions in which safeguards are available should laryngospasm and circulatory or respiratory depression occur.

Since an increase in cough reflex and laryngospasm may occur with peroral endoscopic procedures, the use of a topical anesthetic agent and the availability of necessary counter measures are recommended.

Concurrent use of narcotics and barbiturates with DIAZEMULS may produce a potentiation of effect and, when such combinations are used, appropriate reduction of dosage is required.

Impaired Renal and Hepatic Function: The usual precautions in treating patients with impaired hepatic function should be observed. Since metabolites of diazepam are excreted by the kidney, in order to avoid their excess accumulation, caution should be exercised in the administration of the drug to patients with compromised kidney function.

Potentiation of Drug Effects: Careful consideration should be given if diazepam is to be used concomitantly with other psychotropic agents such as phenothiazines, barbiturates, MAO inhibitors and other antidepressants, since the pharmacological action of these agents may potentiate the action of diazepam.

Due to the possible potentiation of effects and the occurrence of adverse reactions, patients should be advised to abstain from CNS depressant drugs during treatment with diazepam.

The clearance of diazepam and of certain other benzodiazepines can be delayed when used in association with cimetidine.

Parenteral diazepam has produced hypotension or muscular weakness in some patients, particularly when used with barbiturates, narcotics and alcohol.

General: **After administration of diazepam, ambulation should be delayed until complete alertness is restored.**

ADVERSE EFFECTS: Evidence suggests that there is a lower incidence of local reactions when DIAZEMULS (diazepam injectable emulsion) is used. Side effects most commonly reported are drowsiness, fatigue and ataxia. Other adverse reactions less frequently reported include:

Central Nervous System: confusion, depression, dysarthria, headache, hypoactivity, slurred speech, syncope, tremor, vertigo and floppy infant syndrome.

Gastrointestinal: constipation, nausea.

Urogenital: incontinence, changes in libido, urinary retention.

Cardiovascular: bradycardia, cardiovascular collapse, hypotension, venous thrombosis and phlebitis at site of injection.

Ophthalmological: blurred vision, diplopia, nystagmus.

Dermatological: urticaria, skin rash.

Other: hiccups, changes in salivation, neutropenia, jaundice. Paradoxical reactions such as acute hyperexcited states, anxiety, hallucinations, increased muscle spasticity, insomnia, rage, sleep disturbances and stimulation have been reported; should these occur, use of the drug should be discontinued. Minor changes in EEG patterns, usually low-voltage fast activity, have been observed in patients during and after DIAZEMULS therapy and are of no known significance.

In peroral endoscopic procedures, coughing, depressed respiration, dyspnea, hyperventilation, laryngospasm and pain in throat or chest have been reported.

Because of isolated reports of neutropenia and jaundice, periodic blood counts and liver function tests are advisable during long-term therapy.

OVERDOSE:

Symptoms: Manifestations of diazepam overdosage include somnolence, confusion, coma, and diminished reflexes.

Treatment: Respiration, pulse and blood pressure should be monitored, as in all cases of drug overdosage, although, in general, these effects have been minimal unless overdose is extreme. General supportive measures should be employed, along with i.v. fluids, and an adequate airway maintained. Hypotension may be combatted by the use of levarterenol. Dialysis is of limited value.

> For management of a suspected drug overdose, CPhA recommends that you contact your **regional Poison Control Centre**. See the *CPS* Directory section for a list of Poison Control Centres.

DOSAGE: Dosage should be individualized for maximal beneficial effect. The usual recommended dose in older children and adults ranges from 2 to 20 mg i.m. or i.v., depending on the indication and/or the severity of the condition (see subsection Dosage for specific indications). In acute conditions, the injection may be repeated within 1 hour, although an interval of 3 to 4 hours is usually satisfactory.

When a continuing drug effect is required, lower doses (usually 2 to 5 mg) with small increments if necessary, should be used in elderly or debilitated patients and when other sedative drugs are administered (see Warnings and Adverse Effects).

For dosage in pediatric use, see subsection Dosage and Warnings.

Because of its delayed action, DIAZEMULS (diazepam injectable emulsion) is not recommended for the management of status epilepticus.

I.V. Use: DIAZEMULS should be injected slowly, taking at least 1 minute for each 5 mg (1 mL) administered. Extreme care should be taken to avoid intra-arterial administration or extravasation (see Warnings, particularly for use in children).

When i.v. use is indicated, facilities for respiratory assistance should be readily available.

When used i.v., DIAZEMULS should be injected directly into the vein without prior dilution or mixing with other products or solutions. DIAZEMULS may, however, be mixed or diluted with Intralipid, but such an admixture should be used within 6 hours. If it is not feasible to administer DIAZEMULS directly i.v., it may be injected slowly through the infusion tubing as close as possible to the vein insertion.

DIAZEMULS has been shown to be incompatible with morphine and glycopyrrolate. Mixing or further diluting DIAZEMULS with products or solutions other than its own emulsion base (Intralipid) may de-stabilize the emulsion. Although such an effect may not be recognizable on visual inspection, it could give rise to potentially serious adverse reactions. Polyethylene-lined or glass infusion sets and polyethylene/polypropylene plastic syringes are recommended for use with DIAZEMULS. Do not use infusion sets containing polyvinylchloride.

I.M. Use: DIAZEMULS should be injected deeply into the muscle.

Dosage: Adults: Acute anxiety or tension states related to stressful conditions or non-psychotic emotional disorders when parenteral administration is required. Depending on severity, 2 to 10 mg, i.m. or i.v. Repeat in 3 to 4 hours, if necessary.

Acute alcohol withdrawal: As an aid in symptomatic relief of acute agitation, tremor, impending or acute delirium tremens and hallucinosis. Initially 10 mg i.m. or i.v., then 5 to 10 mg in 3 to 4 hours, if necessary.

Minor surgical procedures including esophagoscopy and gastroscopy: as an adjunct in relieving anxiety states that may be present before these procedures. Approximately 5 to 10 mg, i.m. or i.v., as required, about 30 minutes prior to procedures.

For the relief of muscle spasm in cerebral palsy, athetosis and stiff man syndrome. Initially, 5 to 10 mg i.m. or i.v., then 5 to 10 mg in 3 to 4 hours, if necessary.

Pre-operative medication for the relief of anxiety states. If premedications other than atropine sulfate, scopolamine hydrobromide, meperidine or fentanyl citrate are desired, they must be administered in separate syringes. Extreme caution must be exercised in patients with chronic lung disease or unstable cardiovascular status. 10 mg i.m. or i.v. 1 to 2 hours before surgery.

Cardioversion: to relieve anxiety and tension and to reduce recall of procedure. 5 to 10 mg, i.v., within 10 to 20 minutes prior to procedure.

Children: See Warnings. Dosage not to exceed 0.25 mg/kg slowly over a 3 minute period.

Geriatrics and Debilitated: See Precautions. 2 to 5 mg, i.m. or i.v.

Once the acute symptomatology has been properly controlled with DIAZEMULS (diazepam injectable emulsion), the patient may be placed on oral therapy with diazepam if further treatment is required.

SUPPLIED: Each mL contains: diazepam 5 mg, dissolved in the oil phase of an oil/water emulsion compounded with purified soybean oil 150 mg, acetylated monoglycerides 50 mg, purified egg phospholipids 12 mg, glycerol anhydrous 22 mg and sodium hydroxide to adjust pH to approximately 8. DIAZEMULS is a sterile formulation and contains no preservatives. It is intended for i.v. or i.m. use only. Ampuls of 2 mL, packages of 10. Store at 15 to 25°C. Do not freeze.

Diazepam

CPhA Monograph

see Benzodiazepines

Diazepam Injection USP

diazepam

Anxiolytic—Sedative

Sandoz

SUPPLIED: Each mL contains: diazepam 5 mg. Nonmedicinal ingredients: dehydrated alcohol (10%), benzoic acid, benzyl alcohol (1.5%) as preservative, propylene glycol, sodium hydroxide to adjust pH and water for injection. Ampuls of 2 mL, boxes of 10. Store between 15 and 30°C.

Dicetel®

pinaverium bromide

Gastrointestinal Calcium Antagonist

Abbott Products

Date of Preparation: July 19, 2010

PHARMACOLOGY: Dicetel (pinaverium bromide) is a calcium antagonist which inhibits the calcium influx by blocking the voltage-dependent calcium channel at the smooth muscle cell level. It possesses a high degree of selectivity for the intestinal smooth muscle.

Many studies showed that pinaverium bromide induces a relaxation of the gastrointestinal and biliary tracts and mainly of the colon, an inhibition of the motor colonic response to food and/or pharmacological stimulations, implying the action of the drug in irritable bowel syndrome.

INDICATIONS: For the treatment and relief of symptoms associated with irritable bowel syndrome (IBS): abdominal pain, bowel disturbances and intestinal discomfort.

It is also indicated for the treatment of symptoms related to functional disorders of the biliary tract.

CONTRAINDICATIONS: In patients with known hypersensitivity to Dicetel or any of the excipients.

No other contraindications have been identified at this time.

WARNINGS: Contact of Dicetel (pinaverium bromide) with the esophageal mucosa may be irritating. Therefore, it is strongly recommended that the tablet be taken with a glass of water during mealtime. The tablet must be swallowed without being chewed or sucked. If more than 3 tablets are prescribed per day, the additional tablet(s) should be taken concurrently with a glass of water and a snack.

PRECAUTIONS: Dicetel (pinaverium bromide) should not be administered for the relief of motility dysfunction due to underlying organic disease.

Patients with rare hereditary problems of galactose intolerance, the Lapp lactase deficiency or glucose-galactose malabsorption should not take this medication.

Pregnancy: No clinical data on exposed pregnancies are available. Animal studies are insufficient with respect to effects on pregnancy, embryonal/ fetal development, parturition and/or postnatal development. The potential risk for humans is unknown. The safety of Dicetel during pregnancy has not been established. Consequently, in the pregnant patient, this drug should only be administered if, in the judgement of the physician, its use is essential to the welfare of the patient.

Furthermore, the presence of bromine should be taken into account. Theoretically, administration of pinaverium bromide at the end of the pregnancy can affect the new-born neurologically (hypotony, sedation). No such cases however have been reported with Dicetel.

Lactation: There is insufficient information on the excretion of Dicetel in human or animal breast milk. Physico-chemical and available pharmacodynamic/toxicological data on Dicetel point to excretions in breast milk and a risk to the suckling infant cannot be excluded. Dicetel should not be used during breast-feeding.

ADVERSE EFFECTS: Minor adverse events were reported and listed as mild and moderate. They were mainly minor digestive disorders that may be related to the disease, such as epigastric pain and/or fullness (0.8%), nausea (0.5%), constipation (0.4%), heartburn (0.3%), distention (0.3%) and diarrhea (0.2%).

Other Systems: headache (0.3%), dryness of the mouth (0.3%), drowsiness (0.2%), vertigo (0.2%) and skin allergy (0.2%).

There have been spontaneous reports of systemic hypersensitivity reactions involving the subcutaneous tissue and other organ systems of the body such as angioedema and anaphylactic shock.

OVERDOSE:

Symptoms: In man, apart from diarrhea and/or flatulence, Dicetel (pinaverium bromide) induced no undesirable effects in daily dosages of up to 1200 mg.

Treatment: No cases of overdosage of Dicetel have been reported to date. No specific antidote is known. However, if overdosage occurs, gastric lavage is recommended and symptomatic treatment initiated if deemed necessary.

> For management of a suspected drug overdose, CPhA recommends that you contact your **regional Poison Control Centre**. See the *CPS* Directory section for a list of Poison Control Centres.

DOSAGE: The usual adult dosage is 50 mg 3 times a day (total daily dose of 150 mg). The dosage may be increased up to a maximum of 100 mg taken 3 times a day (maximum total daily dose of 300 mg).

It is recommended that the tablet be taken with a glass of water during meals or snacks. The tablet should not be swallowed when in the lying position or just before bedtime.

The duration of treatment depends on the disorders for which Dicetel is given.

INFORMATION FOR THE PATIENT: Published in e-CPS, available by subscription at www.e-cps.ca.

SUPPLIED: 50 mg: Each orange-colored, circular-shaped, film-coated tablet, with a slightly convex surface, engraved with "S" on one side and "50" on the reverse side, contains: pinaverium bromide 50 mg. Nonmedicinal ingredients: in the core: hydrophobic anhydrous silica, magnesium stearate, microcrystalline cellulose, modified cornstarch, modified lactose and talc; film coating: basic butylated methacrylate copolymer, Sepisperse Dry 3203 (hydroxypropyl methylcellulose, microcrystalline cellulose, anatase titanium dioxide, sunset yellow (aluminium lake)), sodium laurylsulfate, stearic acid and talc. Blister packs, boxes of 100 tablets. Store at room temperature (15 to 30°C) in the dispensing box to protect from light.

100 mg: Each orange-colored, circular-shaped, film-coated tablet, with a slightly convex surface, engraved with "S" on one side and "100" on the reverse side, contains: pinaverium bromide 100 mg. Nonmedicinal ingredients: in the core: hydrophobic anhydrous silica, magnesium stearate, microcrystalline cellulose, modified cornstarch, modified lactose and talc; film coating: basic butylated methacrylate copolymer, Sepisperse Dry 3203 (hydroxypropyl methylcellulose, microcrystalline cellulose, anatase titanium dioxide, sunset yellow (aluminium lake)), sodium laurylsulfate, stearic acid and talc. Blister packs, boxes of 100 tablets. Store at room temperature (15 to 30°C) in the dispensing box to protect from light.

(Shown in Product Identification Section)

Diclectin®

doxylamine succinate—pyridoxine HCl

Antinauseant against Nausea and Vomiting of Pregnancy

Duchesnay

Date of Revision: July 25, 2008

SUMMARY PRODUCT INFORMATION:

Route of Administration	Dosage Form/ Strength	Clinically Relevant Nonmedicinal Ingredients
Oral	Tablet, 10 mg/10 mg	None

INDICATIONS AND CLINICAL USE: Diclectin (doxylamine succinate and pyridoxine hydrochloride) is indicated in cases of nausea and vomiting of pregnancy.

CONTRAINDICATIONS: Patients who are hypersensitive to doxylamine succinate or pyridoxine hydrochloride.

WARNINGS AND PRECAUTIONS: General: Due to the anticholinergic properties of antihistamines, caution should be used when Diclectin is taken concurrently with other medications or alcohol.

Carcinogenesis and Mutagenesis: A case-control investigation was performed by the Inter-Regional Epidemiological Study of Childhood Cancer (IRESCC) to analyze the incidence of childhood cancer in relation to the maternal consumption of doxylamine succinate, dicyclomine hydrochloride and pyridoxine hydrochloride. Dicyclomine hydrochloride was a component of the earlier formulations intended for nausea and vomiting of pregnancy that has since been removed due to a lack of evidence of contribution to efficacy.

Data were derived from interview reports and medical records of 555 mothers of children (under 15 years of age) with cancer and 1110 mothers of matched control children. Maternal ingestion of the antiemetic drug during the index pregnancy was not associated with increasing the risk of childhood malignant disease. No dose-response relationship was evident.

Dependence/Tolerance: There is no information to indicate that abuse or dependency occurs with the concentration of doxylamine succinate and pyridoxine hydrochloride found in Diclectin.

Special Populations: Pregnant Women—Category A: Diclectin is intended for use in pregnant women. There has been a vast clinical experience (>30 million pregnancies worldwide) regarding the use of a combination of doxylamine succinate, pyridoxine hydrochloride with or without dicyclomine hydrochloride in this population.

Diclectin has been the subject of many epidemiological studies (cohort, case control and meta-analyses) designed to detect possible teratogenicity. Two separate meta-analyses have been conducted that have assessed pregnancy outcome following the use of a combination of doxylamine succinate, pyridoxine hydrochloride with or without dicyclomine hydrochloride during the first trimester. McKeigue et al. conducted a meta-analysis of 16 cohort and 11 case-control studies published between 1963 and 1991. No increased risk for malformations was found in first trimester exposures to doxylamine succinate and pyridoxine hydrochloride, with or without dicyclomine hydrochloride. A second meta-analysis, conducted by Einarson et al. incorporated 12 cohort and 5 case-control studies. No statistically significant relationships were found between first trimester use of the combination doxylamine succinate, pyridoxine hydrochloride with or without dicyclomine hydrochloride and fetal abnormalities.

In 1989, a report on the safety of Diclectin for use in the management of nausea and vomiting of pregnancy was prepared by a panel of experts for the Special Advisory Committee on Reproductive Physiology to the Health Protection Branch of Health Canada. The Motherisk Program at the Hospital for Sick Children systematically reviewed the literature to develop an evidence-based algorithm on the safety and efficacy of treatments for nausea and vomiting of pregnancy. Doxylamine succinate combined with pyridoxine hydrochloride (Diclectin) is listed as first line therapy on this algorithm. Similarly, the 2002 Society of Obstetricians and Gynaecologists of Canada (SOGC) Clinical Practice Guidelines on the management of nausea and vomiting of pregnancy recommend that this formulation be the standard of care, since it has the greatest evidence to support its safety and efficacy.

Atanackovic et al. evaluated the safety of higher than standard doses of Diclectin in 225 pregnant women with Nausea and Vomiting of Pregnancy (NVP) in an observational, prospective study. A total of 123 women received standard doses of up to 4 tablets a day and 102 women received a higher than standard dose ("supradose") of 5 to 12 tablets/day. Despite a twice larger mean maximal dose of Diclectin, women receiving the supradose did not report more prevalent adverse effects while taking Diclectin. The lack of any major malformation with the supradose strongly suggests that the higher dose is not teratogenic. It was concluded that supradoses of 5 to 12 tablets daily did not appear to affect the incidence of maternal adverse effects or pregnancy outcome.

Baseline Risk: The background baseline risk of major malformations for all pregnancies is approximately 1-3%. This is the risk of having a child with a birth defect when no teratogenic exposure occurs in pregnancy. This underlying risk may be increased due to maternal age, medical or family history, or exposures to certain drugs, chemicals or levels of radiation known to cause birth defects. Published data clearly shows that Diclectin use in pregnancy does not increase a woman's baseline risk of having a child with a major malformation. Diclectin has the highest safety rating in Briggs: "Category A". No other prescription drug has been more extensively studied for safety in pregnancy.

Nursing Women: There are no published reports describing the use of Diclectin during lactation. However, the passage of doxylamine succinate into breast milk can be expected. Effects on a nursing infant, if any, are unknown, but sedative and other antihistamine actions are a potential concern. Pyridoxine hydrochloride is excreted into breast milk, but in the doses provided in Diclectin, presents no risk to a nursing infant.

Occupational Hazards: Diclectin may have a minor to moderate influence on the ability to drive and use machines. Because of potential drowsiness, Diclectin should be prescribed with caution for patients who must drive automobiles or operate machinery.

ADVERSE REACTIONS: Adverse Drug Reaction Overview: The most common adverse reaction associated with doxylamine succinate is drowsiness. Other adverse drug reactions associated with doxylamine succinate may include: vertigo, nervousness, epigastric pain, headache, palpitation, diarrhea, disorientation, irritability, convulsions, urinary retention or insomnia.

Pyridoxine is a vitamin that is generally recognized as having no adverse effects.

Clinical Trial Adverse Drug Reactions: Because clinical trials are conducted under very specific conditions the adverse reaction rates observed in the clinical trials may not reflect the rates observed in practice and should not be compared to the rates in the clinical trials of another drug. Adverse drug reaction information from clinical trials is useful for identifying drug-related adverse events and for approximating rates.

In a randomized, double-blind, multi-center study in 2308 women with nausea and vomiting of pregnancy, various combinations of doxylamine succinate, dicyclomine hydrochloride and pyridoxine hydrochloride (each at 10 mg) were compared with placebo in an 8-way study design. The incidence of adverse reactions was 8.7% in the doxylamine/pyridoxine group versus 11.2% in the placebo group. In the doxylamine/pyridoxine group the most common adverse reactions were drowsiness (15/265, 5.7%), dizziness (3/265, 1.1%), fatigue or lethargy (2/265, 0.75%), gastric irritation, heartburn or indigestion (2/265, 0.75%) and headache (2/265, 0.75%). Corresponding values for the placebo group were drowsiness 8/269 (3%) dizziness 2/269 (0.75%), fatigue or lethargy 3/269 (1.1%), gastric irritation, heartburn or indigestion 0/269 (0%) and headache 4/269 (1.5%).

In a double-blind comparison study of placebo and combination drug product (doxylamine succinate, dicyclomine hydrochloride and pyridoxine hydrochloride) in 81 patients 18 adverse events were reported (22.2%). In the active group 12 side effects were reported (29.2%) versus 6 (15%) in the placebo group. Feelings of weakness were reported by 2/41 (5%) in the active group versus 0% in the placebo group, tiredness by 2/41 (5%) in the active versus 2/40 (5%) in the placebo group and drowsiness by 3/41 (7%) in the active versus 1/40 (2.5%) in the placebo group. Also reported were: lack of energy, constipation, furry sensation in mouth, wind and headache.

Atanackovic et al., 2001 evaluated the safety of higher than standard doses of Diclectin in 225 pregnant women with nausea and vomiting of pregnancy in an observational, prospective study. A total of 123 women received standard doses of up to 4 tablets a day and 102 women received a higher than standard dose ("supradose") of 5 to 12 tablets/day. Despite a twice larger mean maximal dose of Diclectin, women receiving the supradose did not report more prevalent adverse effects of Diclectin. In the supradose group, 32% (31/97) reported sleepiness, tiredness and/or drowsiness compared with 35% (42/122) among the standard dose recipients. There was no association between the dose per kg and rates of reported maternal adverse effects with doses ranging from 0.1 mg/kg to 2.0 mg/kg (1-12 tablets).

Abnormal Hematologic and Clinical Chemistry Findings: None reported.

DRUG INTERACTIONS: Overview: No formal drug-drug interaction studies have been performed with Diclectin.

Drug-Drug Interactions: See Table 1 and Table 2.

Table 1: Diclectin

Theoretical Drug-Drug Interactions for Doxylamine Succinate

Drugs	Effect	Clinical Comment
MAOIs	Enhance	MAOIs may prolong and intensify the effects of doxylamine succinate.
Antimuscarinic Drugs	Additive	There is an increased risk of antimuscarinic side effects when doxylamine is given with other antimuscarinic drugs.
Alcohol and CNS depressants (barbiturates, hypnotics, narcotic analgesics, tranquilizers and sedatives)	Additive	Doxylamine succinate may increase the CNS-depressant effects.

Table 2: Diclectin

Theoretical Drug-Drug Interactions for Pyridoxine Hydrochloride

Drugs	Effect	Clinical Comment
Levodopa	Reduces effectiveness	Pyridoxine enhances peripheral decarboxylation of levodopa reducing the effectiveness of levodopa.

Drug-Food Interactions: Interactions with food have not been established.
Drug-Herb Interactions: Interactions with herbal products have not been established.
Drug-Laboratory Test Interactions: Interactions with laboratory tests have not been established.

DOSAGE AND ADMINISTRATION: Recommended Dose and Dosage Adjustment: Two Diclectin delayed release tablets at bedtime to control nausea and vomiting occurring in the morning; additionally one delayed release tablet in the morning and one delayed release tablet mid-afternoon to control symptoms throughout the day. The dosage schedule may be individualized according to timing, duration, severity and frequency of the symptoms experienced by the patient. Diclectin can be prescribed in any trimester of pregnancy.

Diclectin is a delayed-release formulation that works optimally when given 4 to 6 hours prior to anticipated onset of symptoms. The delay in action may be prolonged when tablets are taken with food.

Diclectin tablets being of a delayed release formulation should not be prescribed on an as needed basis (prn). It is important that Diclectin is taken daily for optimal effect.

A gradual tapering dose of Diclectin is recommended at the time of discontinuation to prevent a sudden onset of symptoms.
Missed Dose: In the event that a dose is missed, it should be taken as soon as possible. However, if it is almost time for the next dose, the missed dose should be skipped. The prescribed dosing schedule should be continued.
Administration: Diclectin is to be taken orally. Diclectin tablets are a delayed release formulation therefore they should not be crushed or split.

OVERDOSAGE:
Diclectin is delayed release therefore signs and symptoms of intoxication may not be apparent immediately.

Signs and symptoms of intoxication may include restlessness, dryness of mouth, dilated pupils, sleepiness, vertigo, mental confusion and tachycardia. If treatment is needed, it consists of gastric lavage or activated charcoal, whole bowel irrigation and a symptomatic treatment.

> For management of a suspected drug overdose, contact your **regional Poison Control Centre**. See the *CPS* Directory section for a list of Poison Control Centres.

ACTION AND CLINICAL PHARMACOLOGY: Mechanism of Action: Diclectin (doxylamine succinate and pyridoxine hydrochloride) provides the action of two unrelated compounds. Doxylamine succinate (an antihistamine) and pyridoxine hydrochloride (vitamin B6) provide anti-nauseant and anti-emetic activity. The delayed action of Diclectin permits the nighttime dose to be effective in the morning hours, when the patient needs it most.
Pharmacokinetics: See Table 3 and Table 4.
Absorption, Distribution, Metabolism and Excretion: Diclectin: A randomized open-label, 2-way crossover relative bioavailability study in 22 healthy adult females compared the pharmacokinetics after a single dose of two (2×[10 mg+10 mg]) Diclectin tablets under fed and fasted conditions. The administration of food delayed the absorption of both doxylamine and pyridoxine by approximately 5 hours. However, this delay did not affect the peak concentration or extent of absorption of doxylamine, as both the C_{max} and AUC were not distinguishable between treatments. In contrast, the peak concentration and extent of absorption of pyridoxine were considerably reduced when administered with food. The effect of food on the pyridoxine component is more complex, in that pyridoxine, pyridoxal and pyridoxal 5'-phosphate, also contribute to the biological activity. Although pyridoxal peak concentrations are somewhat reduced, pyridoxal 5'-phosphate peak concentrations are slightly increased and AUC values for both pyridoxal and pyridoxal 5'-phosphate are not affected by administration under fed conditions. Total pyridoxine mean peak concentrations are slightly reduced but extent of absorption, as measured by AUC, is unaffected by treatment.
Pyridoxine Hydrochloride: Pyridoxine is readily absorbed in the gastrointestinal tract, mainly in the jejunum. Pyridoxine is primarily metabolized in the liver; following phosphorylation, its main active metabolite, pyridoxal 5'-phosphate, is released into the circulation (accounting for at least 60% of circulating vitamin B6) and is highly protein bound; primarily to albumin. The metabolic scheme for pyridoxine is complex, with formation of primary and secondary metabolites along with interconversion back to pyridoxine. These metabolites including pyridoxal, have biologic activity. The major metabolite 4-pyridoxic acid, is inactive and is excreted in urine.
Doxylamine Succinate: Doxylamine is biotransformed in the liver by N-dealkylation to its principle metabolites N-desmethyl and N, N-didesmethyldoxylamine, which are excreted by the kidney.

Doxylamine can cross the blood-brain barrier and has a high affinity for H1 receptors in the brain.

Table 4: Diclectin

Diclectin's Pharmacokinetic Parameters Under Fed and Fasted Conditions in Healthy Female Volunteers for Total Pyridoxine

Value	Total Pyridoxine[a] Mean±SD N=20	
	Fed	Fasted
AUC_{0-t} (pmol·h/mL)	6257.73±3899.06	5224.88± 2983.11
$AUC_{0-\infty}$ (pmol·h/mL)	12 189.53± 7389.52	12 199.21±6764.15
C_{max} (pmol/mL)	533±201	695±183
T_{max} (h)	8.91±1.78	3.45±1.11
Kel (h^{-1})	0.0312±0.0221	0.0313±0.0299
$T_{1/2el}$ (h)	36.67±21.77	49.71±42.52

[a] Total pyridoxine includes pyridoxine, pyridoxal, pyridoxal 5'-phosphate.

Special Populations and Conditions: Race: No data is available on differences in the pharmacokinetics of either doxylamine succinate or pyridoxine hydrochloride in different races.
Hepatic Insufficiency: No data is available on differences in the pharmacokinetics of doxylamine succinate or pyridoxine hydrochloride in patients with hepatic insufficiency.
Renal Insufficiency: No data is available on differences in the pharmacokinetics of doxylamine succinate in renal insufficiency. For pyridoxine hydrochloride some metabolites are excreted renally. There are no data to suggest that this should alter the current dosage recommendation of Diclectin.
Genetic Polymorphism: No data is available.
STORAGE AND STABILITY: Store at room temperature (15 to 30°C).
Protect from light.
Keep out of reach of children.
SPECIAL HANDLING INSTRUCTIONS: No special handling instructions are required.
INFORMATION FOR THE PATIENT: Published in e-CPS, available by subscription at www.e-cps.ca.
DOSAGE FORMS, COMPOSITION AND PACKAGING: Each round, white, film-coated, delayed release tablet, imprinted with the pink image of a pregnant woman, contains: doxylamine succinate 10 mg and pyridoxine HCl 10 mg. Nonmedicinal ingredients: ammonium hydroxide, n-butyl-alcohol, carnauba wax powder, colloidal silicon dioxide, croscarmellose sodium, D&C Red #27, denatured alcohol, FD&C Blue #2, hypromellose, isopropyl alcohol, magnesium stearate, magnesium trisilicate, methacrylic acid copolymer, microcrystalline cellulose 102, PEG 400, PEG 8000, polysorbate 80, propylene glycol, shellac glaze, simethicone, talc and titanium dioxide. Gluten-, lactose-, sulfite- and tartrazine-free. Bottles of 100.

Tablets are imprinted with the pink image of a pregnant woman. The indicia serves as a method to diminish the incidence of erroneous ingestion by pregnant women or erroneous dispensing by pharmacists of therapeutic agents not prescribed or labeled for pregnant women. Noncompliance in the use of prescription medications is common among pregnant women owing to fear over fetal exposure and safety even in the case of drugs with appropriate safety data.

An observational, prospective cross-sectional study was conducted by the manufacturer to determine the teratogenic risk perception of pregnant women when viewing a plain white tablet and a white tablet imprinted with the image of a pregnant woman. The difference in teratogenic risk perception was highly significant (p<0.0001). In the survey group of 132 pregnant women the mean perception of teratogenic risk was decreased by 23.4% when viewing tablets imprinted with the image of a pregnant woman. By reducing the perception of teratogenic risk by pregnant women the pregnancy indicia may increase patient compliance and thus the effectiveness of Diclectin.
Disease Management and Diclectin Surveillance Programs: Since 1996, the Motherisk* Program at the Hospital for Sick Children has maintained a toll-free bilingual (French-English) Nausea and Vomiting of Pregnancy (NVP) Helpline (1-800-436-8477) with the ongoing support of Duchesnay Inc. This service is available to women and healthcare professionals that would like to discuss the impact and management of NVP. Early recognition and treatment can prevent the progression of NVP to hyperemesis gravidarum and maternal and fetal complications.

Further to being a disease management line the NVP Helpline is acting as a surveillance program for Diclectin. This service provides continuous monitoring of adverse events and the safe use of Diclectin during pregnancy while generating valuable research data.

* Motherisk: Hospital for Sick Children, 555 University Ave., Toronto, ON (M5G 1X8). www.motherisk.org. 1-800-436-8477.

Table 3: Diclectin

Diclectin's Pharmacokinetic Parameters Under Fed and Fasted Conditions in Healthy Female Volunteers for Doxylamine/Pyridoxine/Pyridoxal/Pyridoxal 5'-phosphate

Value	Doxylamine Mean±SD N=22		Pyridoxine Mean±SD N=9		Pyridoxal Mean±SD N=16		Pyridoxal 5'-phosphate Mean±SD N=20	
	Fed	Fasted	Fed	Fasted	Fed	Fasted	Fed	Fasted
AUC_{0-t} (ng·h/mL)	1567.23±366.04	1519±428.99	N/A	N/A	118.51±55.09	107.76±62.96	1191.69± 924.39	988.19±685.40
$AUC_{0-\infty}$ (ng·h/mL)	1611.35±372.16	1561.11±429.78	N/A	N/A	N/A	N/A	2462.79±1459.62	2997.77±1793.78
C_{max} (ng/mL)	82.0± 15.5	85.9±17.7	24.0±14.0	55.1±20.3	45.3±16.3	61.4±14.6	40.1±10.4	32.5±7.9
T_{max} (h)	10.6±1.8	5.26±1.55	7.67±1.73	2.81±1.13	9.38±1.76	3.76±0.88	12.7±5.9	12.1±9.1
Kel (h^{-1})	0.0593±0.0098	0.0613±0.0111	N/A	N/A	N/A	N/A	0.0215±0.0090	0.0136±0.0083
$T_{1/2el}$ (h)	11.98±1.91	11.69±2.33	N/A	N/A	N/A	N/A	36.40±12.58	71.90±46.52

Differin® Ⓡ
adapalene
Acne Therapy

Galderma

Differin® XP™ Ⓡ
adapalene
Acne Therapy

Galderma

Date of Preparation: January 13, 1995
Date of Revision: December 19, 2005

SUMMARY PRODUCT INFORMATION:

Route of Administration	Dosage Form/ Strength	Clinically Relevant Nonmedicinal Ingredients
Topical	Cream 0.1%	None For a complete listing see Dosage Forms, Composition and Packaging.
	Gel 0.1%, 0.3%	None For a complete listing see Dosage Forms, Composition and Packaging.

INDICATIONS AND CLINICAL USE: DIFFERIN (adapalene) topical cream and gel and DIFFERIN XP (adapalene) topical gel are indicated for:
- treatment of acne vulgaris

Geriatrics (>65 years of age): Safety and effectiveness in geriatric patients aged 65 years and above have not been established.
Pediatrics (<12 years of age): Safety and effectiveness in children below the age of 12 have not been established.

CONTRAINDICATIONS:
- Patients who are hypersensitive to this drug or to any ingredient in the formulation or component of the container. For a complete listing, see Dosage Forms, Composition and Packaging.
- Patients with eczema or seborrheic dermatitis.

WARNINGS AND PRECAUTIONS: General: For external use only. Avoid contact with the eyes, lips, angles of the nose, mucous membranes and open wounds. Certain cutaneous signs and symptoms such as erythema, dryness, scaling, burning or pruritus are associated with the topical application of retinoids and can also be expected with the use of DIFFERIN (adapalene) topical cream or gel and with DIFFERIN XP (adapalene) topical gel. These treatment-related effects generally occur during the first two to four weeks of therapy and usually resolve as the skin undergoes adjustment with continued use. Depending on the degree of the side effects, patients can be directed to use the medication less frequently or temporarily discontinue use until the symptoms subside (see Dosage and Administration).

Patients should be advised to use non-comedogenic cosmetics. Colour cosmetics such as blushers and powders are acceptable, however, make-up cosmetics should be water based only. Cosmetics must be removed by thorough cleansing before the area is treated.

As with any retinoid, exposure to excessive sunlight, including sunlamps, should be avoided while using the preparation, or a suitably effective sunscreen product and protective clothing over the treated areas is recommended when exposure cannot be avoided. Weather extremes, such as wind or cold, also may be irritating to patients under treatment with adapalene. As with other retinoids, use of "waxing" as a depilatory method should be avoided on skin treated with adapalene.

Special Populations: Pregnant Women: It is recommended that topical adapalene should not be used by pregnant women. Topical adapalene should be used by women of childbearing years only after contraceptive counselling.

There have been rare reports of birth defects among babies born to women exposed to topical retinoids during pregnancy. However, there are no well controlled prospective studies of the use of topical retinoids, including adapalene, in pregnant women. A retrospective study of mothers exposed to topical tretinoin during the first trimester of pregnancy found no increase in the incidence of birth defects.

Adapalene administered orally at doses of ≥25 mg/kg/day (38 times the Maximum Recommended Human Dose [MRHD] based on mg/m² comparisons for rats or 65 times MRHD for rabbits) has been shown to be teratogenic. No teratogenic effects were seen in rats at oral doses of up to 5.0 mg/kg/day adapalene (7.6 times the MRHD). Cutaneous teratology studies in rats and rabbits at doses of 0.6 (0.03 %), 2.0 (0.1 %) and 6.0 (0.3 %) mg/kg/day (17 times the MRHD for rats or 32 times the MRHD for rabbits) exhibited no teratogenicity. At 2 mg/kg/day (0.1% adapalene gel), no adverse events were observed in rabbits and only a marginal increase in the incidence of additional lumbar ribs was observed in rats. However, at 6 mg/kg/day (0.3% adapalene gel), in addition to the recorded increase in foetal rib numbers in the rat and rabbit, there were also other skeletal anomalies in both species. There are no adequate and well-controlled studies in pregnant women.

Nursing Women: It is not known whether this drug is excreted in human milk. Animal pharmacology studies indicate that adapalene is excreted in milk at levels lower than plasma levels. Because many drugs are excreted in human milk, caution should be exercised when DIFFERIN topical cream or gel or DIFFERIN XP topical gel is administered to a nursing mother.
Pediatrics (12-16 years of age): No specific monitoring or hazards are associated with the use of the product in pediatric patients between the ages of 12 and 16 years. Safety and effectiveness in children below the age of 12 have not been established.
Geriatrics (>65 years of age): Safety and effectiveness in geriatric patients age 65 and above have not been established.

ADVERSE REACTIONS: Adverse Drug Reaction Overview: Treatment-related adverse reactions typically associated with use of DIFFERIN and DIFFERIN XP include mild to moderate application site reactions, such as skin irritation characterized by scaling, dryness, erythema, burning and stinging. DIFFERIN XP results in a slightly greater incidence of these events, as would be expected with the higher concentration of adapalene. These reactions usually occur early in the treatment, and tend to resolve after 2 to 4 weeks of therapy (see Warnings and Precautions).

Clinical Trial Adverse Drug Reactions: Because clinical trials are conducted under very specific conditions the adverse reaction rates observed in the clinical trials may not reflect the rates observed in practice and should not be compared to the rates in the clinical trials of another drug. Adverse drug reaction information from clinical trials is useful for identifying drug-related adverse events and for approximating rates.

DIFFERIN (adapalene) Topical Cream or Topical Gel: In clinical trials with DIFFERIN topical gel and cream 0.1%, most of the reactions occurred within two to four weeks of initiation of therapy and were generally observed to resolve with continued use of the product or temporary adjustment of the treatment schedule. Contact allergy to topical adapalene was not reported during clinical trials. To date, all adverse effects of DIFFERIN topical cream or gel 0.1% have been reversible upon discontinuation of therapy.

DIFFERIN XP (adapalene) Topical Gel: In a multi-centre, placebo- and active-controlled Phase III clinical trial, signs and symptoms of local cutaneous irritation were monitored in 258 adult acne patients who used DIFFERIN XP topical gel 0.3% once daily for 12 weeks. Of the patients who experienced cutaneous irritation (erythema, scaling, dryness, and/or burning/stinging), the majority of cases were mild to moderate in severity, occurred in the first week of treatment, and decreased thereafter.

In a one-year, open-label safety study of 551 patients with acne vulgaris who used DIFFERIN XP, the pattern of adverse events was similar to the 12-week controlled study. The percentage of subjects who experienced cutaneous irritation (scaling, erythema, dryness, and/or stinging/burning) greater than baseline was highest after one week of treatment and decreased thereafter, continuing to decrease during the one-year treatment period.

The proportion of subjects with adverse events was generally higher for the DIFFERIN XP group compared to the adapalene gel 0.1% group, as was expected with the higher concentration. Almost all related adverse events were in the Skin and Appendages body system and most were mild to moderate in severity.

Table 1: DIFFERIN/DIFFERIN XP
Related Adverse Events From Open, and Vehicle- and Active-Controlled Studies

	DIFFERIN XP adapalene gel 0.3% n=1087 (%)	DIFFERIN adapalene gel 0.1% n=1463 (%)	DIFFERIN adapalene cream 0.1% n=311 (%)	Gel Vehicle n=134 (%)
Total No. (%) of Subjects with Related[a] Adverse Event(s)	267 (24.6%)	153 (10.5%)	16 (5.1%)	6 (4.5%)
Skin and Appendages	263 (24.2%)	164 (11.2%)	17 (5.5%)	6 (4.5%)
Skin Dry	117 (10.8%)	58 (4.0%)	1 (0.3%)	2 (1.5%)
Erythema	27 (2.5%)	18 (1.2%)	0 (0%)	0 (0%)
Skin Discomfort	70 (6.4%)	40 (2.7%)	1 (0.3%)	0 (0%)
Desquamation	28 (2.6%)	9 (0.6%)	0 (0%)	0 (0%)
Pruritus	18 (1.7%)	13 (0.9%)	0 (0%)	0 (0%)
Sunburn	21 (1.9%)	13 (0.9%)	3 (1.0%)	2 (1.5%)
Irritant Dermatitis	59 (5.4%)	33 (2.3%)	0 (0%)	0 (0%)
Skin Irritation	0 (0%)	4 (0.4%)	5 (1.6%)	0 (0%)

[a] Related=Possibly, probably, or definitely related.

Less Common Clinical Trial Adverse Drug Reactions (<1%): The following less common events have been designated as related (possibly, probably, definitely) to treatment with DIFFERIN and DIFFERIN XP, considering all patients in the clinical trials in acne vulgaris:
Skin and Appendages: eczema, contact dermatitis, atopic dermatitis, skin edema, dermatitis, acne, worsening of treated disease, urticaria, skin discolouration, seborrhea, herpes simplex, vesicular rash, eyelid edema, burning/stinging.
Body as a Whole: pain, facial edema.
Special Senses: eye pain, keratoconjunctivitis.
Abnormal Hematologic and Clinical Chemistry Findings: No significant abnormal values were observed in the short term controlled studies or the long term safety study.
Post-Market Adverse Drug Reactions: The following isolated (one report each) serious, unexpected adverse events have been designated as probably/possibly related to treatment with an adapalene topical formulation: papilloedema, hepatitis/cholectasis, convulsions, foetal disorders.

DRUG INTERACTIONS: Overview: There are no known interactions with other medications which are likely to be used topically and concurrently with DIFFERIN (adapalene) topical cream or gel or with DIFFERIN XP (adapalene) topical gel. Absorption of adapalene through human skin is low, and therefore interaction with systemic medications is unlikely.
Drug-Drug Interactions: As DIFFERIN and DIFFERIN XP have the potential for local irritation, it is possible that concomitant use of abrasive cleansers, strong drying agents, or irritant products may produce additive irritant effects Particular caution should be exercised in using preparations containing sulfur, resorcinol, or salicylic acid in combination with DIFFERIN topical cream or gel or DIFFERIN XP. If these preparations have been used, it is advisable not to start therapy with DIFFERIN until the effects of such preparations have subsided.

Other cutaneous anti-acne treatments (e.g., erythromycin topical solution, clindamycin phosphate topical solution 1% or benzoyl peroxide products in concentrations up to 10%) may be used in the morning when DIFFERIN topical cream or gel or DIFFERIN XP is used at night.
Drug-Herb Interactions: Interactions with herbal products have not been established.
Drug-Laboratory Test Interactions: Interactions with laboratory tests have not been established.

DOSAGE AND ADMINISTRATION: Dosing Considerations: DIFFERIN (adapalene) topical cream and gel or DIFFERIN XP (adapalene) topical gel should be applied to the affected areas of the face, chest and back once a day before retiring and after washing. A small amount should be applied to provide a thin film, avoiding eyes, lips and mucous membranes. This medication should not be applied to cuts, abrasions, eczematous, or sunburned skin.

Discontinue treatment if a severe local inflammatory response is experienced. Reinstitute therapy when the reaction has subsided, initially applying the preparation less frequently. Once daily application may be resumed if it is judged that the patient is able to tolerate the treatment.

Clinical improvement is expected to be clearly evident after four to eight weeks of treatment, with further improvement expected with continued use. Cutaneous safety of DIFFERIN topical gel has been demonstrated over a six-month period of treatment. Cutaneous safety of DIFFERIN XP topical gel has been demonstrated over a 12-month period of treatment.
Missed Dose: Dosing should continue as per usual the following evening, and the usual amount should be applied.

OVERDOSAGE:
DIFFERIN (adapalene) topical cream and gel and DIFFERIN XP (adapalene) topical gel are intended for cutaneous use only. If the medication is applied excessively, no more rapid or better results will be obtained and marked redness, peeling or discomfort may occur.

The acute oral toxicity of adapalene topical gel, 0.1% in mice and rats is greater than 10 mL/kg (10 mg/kg). Inadvertent oral ingestion of adapalene may lead to the same adverse effects as those associated with excessive oral intake of Vitamin A including teratogenesis in women of childbearing years. Therefore, in such cases, pregnancy testing should be carried out in women of childbearing years. In the event of accidental ingestion of the product, an appropriate method of gastric emptying might be considered.

For management of a suspected drug overdose, CPhA recommends that you contact your **regional Poison Control Centre**. See the *CPS* Directory section for a list of Poison Control Centres.

ACTION AND CLINICAL PHARMACOLOGY: Mechanism of Action: Adapalene is a chemically stable, retinoid-like compound. Biochemical and pharmacological profile studies have demonstrated that adapalene is a potent modulator of cellular differentiation, keratinization and inflammatory processes all of which represent important features in the pathology of acne vulgaris. Mechanistically, adapalene binds to specific retinoic acid nuclear receptors but, unlike tretinoin, does not bind to the cytosolic receptor protein. Although the exact mode of action of adapalene is unknown, current evidence suggests that topical adapalene normalizes the differentiation of follicular epithelial cells resulting in decreased microcomedone formation.
Pharmacodynamics: Studies in acne patients provide clinical evidence that topical adapalene is effective in reducing the non-inflammatory acne lesions (open and closed comedones). Adapalene inhibits the chemotactic (directional) and chemokinetic (random) responses of human polymorphonuclear leucocytes in in vitro assay models; it also inhibits the metabolism of arachidonic acid, by lipoxidation, to inflammatory mediators. This profile suggests that the cell mediated inflammatory component of acne is modified by adapalene. Studies in human patients provide clinical evidence that topical adapalene is effective in reducing the inflammatory components of acne (i.e., papules and pustules).
Pharmacokinetics: See Table 2.
Absorption: Absorption of adapalene through human skin is low. No quantifiable levels of parent substance have been found in the plasma of patients following chronic adapalene gel 0.1% application in controlled clinical trials (limit of quantification=0.25 ng/mL). In adult patients with acne vulgaris who received daily applications of 0.3% gel for 10 days, the mean $AUC_{(0\text{-}24h)}$ on Day 10 was 8.94 ng·h/mL (SD:8.99) and the mean C_{max} was 0.553 ng/mL (SD:0.466). The C_{max} ranged from <0.1 to 2 ng/mL and the maximum $AUC_{(0\text{-}24h)}$ value obtained was 36.1 ng·h/mL. The terminal apparent half-life ranged from 13 to 16 hours, thereby indicating that a pharmacokinetic steady-state was reached before Day 10.

Table 2: DIFFERIN XP

Summary of Adapalene's Pharmacokinetic Parameters in Adult Patients with Acne Vulgaris Following Application of 0.3% Gel

	C_{max}	$t_{½}$ (h)	AUC_{0-24}	Clearance
Repeated Dose Mean	0.553±0.466 ng/mL[a]	13–16[b]	8.94±8.99 ng·h/mL[c]	Within 72 hours

[a] Derived from 15/16 subjects.
[b] Derived from 7/16 subjects.
[c] Derived from 14/16 subjects.

Distribution: Classical plasma protein binding techniques were not feasible for adapalene due to the physiochemical properties of the molecule. However, an alternative method was adopted which measures the partitioning of the drug between plasma or protein solutions and erythrocytes. When ^{3}H-adapalene was incubated with human whole blood, 26% was bound to erythrocytes and total binding of adapalene in blood was >99%. Adapalene bound primarily to lipoproteins and human serum albumin.
Metabolism: Following 24-hour incubation with human hepatocytes, more than 90% of adapalene has been metabolized. Both metabolites and adapalene showed a possibility for conjugation—predominantly glucuronidation and sulfatation.
Excretion: Excretion appears to be primarily by the biliary route. The majority of an administered dose of 0.3% gel was excreted by 144 hours post dose and no drug was detected after the 6th day following last application. Under maximized conditions, the mean total unchanged drug substance excreted in the faeces was 0.07%±0.06% of the total dose applied (range, 0.02% to 0.19%).

STORAGE AND STABILITY: DIFFERIN (adapalene) topical cream and gel and DIFFERIN XP (adapalene) topical gel should be stored at room temperature (15 to 30°C). Keep from freezing. Keep container tightly closed. Keep in a safe place out of the reach of children.

INFORMATION FOR THE PATIENT: Published in e-CPS, available by subscription at www.e-cps.ca.

DOSAGE FORMS, COMPOSITION AND PACKAGING: DIFFERIN: Cream: Each g of topical cream contains: adapalene 0.1% (1 mg). Nonmedicinal ingredients: carbomer 934P, cyclomethicone, edetate disodium, glycerin, methyl gluceth-20 sesquistearate, methyl glucose sesquistearate, methylparaben, phenoxyethanol, propylparaben, purified water, squalane and trolamine. Tubes of 60 g.
Gel: Each g of topical gel contains: adapalene 0.1% (1 mg). Nonmedicinal ingredients: carbomer 940, edetate disodium, methylparaben, poloxamer 182, propylene glycol, purified water and sodium hydroxide and/or hydrochloric acid for pH adjustment. Tubes of 60 g.
DIFFERIN XP: Each g of topical gel contains: adapalene 0.3% (3 mg). Nonmedicinal ingredients: carbomer 940, edetate disodium, methylparaben, poloxamer 124, propylene glycol, purified water and sodium hydroxide and/or hydrochloric acid for pH adjustment. Tubes of 60 g.

Diflucan™ Ⓟ

fluconazole

Antifungal

Pfizer

PHARMACOLOGY: Fluconazole is a highly selective inhibitor of fungal cytochrome P450 sterol C-14-α-demethylation. Mammalian cell demethylation is much less sensitive to fluconazole inhibition. The subsequent loss of normal sterols correlates with the accumulation of 14-α-methyl sterols in fungi and may be responsible for the fungistatic activity of fluconazole.

Fluconazole is a polar bis-triazole antifungal drug. Studies have shown that fluconazole exhibits specificity as an inhibitor of the fungal as opposed to mammalian cytochrome P450 mediated reactions, including those involved in steroid biosynthesis and drug metabolism. Many of the clinical advantages of fluconazole are a result of its unique pharmacokinetic properties.
Pharmacokinetics: Adults: Absorption: The pharmacokinetic properties of fluconazole are similar following administration by the i.v. or oral routes and do not appear to be affected by gastric pH. In normal volunteers, the bioavailability of orally administered fluconazole is over 90% compared with i.v. administration. Essentially all of the administered drug reaches systemic circulation; thus, there is no evidence of first-pass metabolism of the drug. In addition, no adjustment in dosage is necessary when changing from p.o. to i.v. or vice versa.

Peak plasma concentrations (C_{max}) in fasted normal volunteers occur rapidly following oral administration, usually between 1 and 2 hours of dosing with a terminal plasma elimination half-life of approximately 30 hours (range 20 to 50 hours) after oral administration. The long plasma elimination half-life provides the basis for once daily dosing with fluconazole in the treatment of fungal infections.

In fasted normal volunteers, administration of a single oral 400 mg dose of fluconazole leads to a mean C_{max} of 6.72 μg/mL (range: 4.12 to 8.08 μg/mL) and after single oral doses of 50 to 400 mg, fluconazole plasma concentrations and AUC (area under the plasma concentration-time curve) are dose proportional.

In normal volunteers, oral bioavailability as measured by C_{max} and AUC was not affected by food when fluconazole was administered as a single 50 mg capsule; however T_{max} was doubled.

Steady-state concentrations are reached within 5 to 10 days following oral doses of 50 to 400 mg given once daily. Administration of a loading dose on the first day of treatment consisting of twice the usual daily dose results in plasma concentrations close to steady state by the second day.
Pharmacokinetics in Children: In children, the following pharmacokinetic data {mean (% cv)} have been reported (see Table 1).

Table 1: Diflucan

Pharmacokinetics in Children

Age Studied	Dose (mg/kg)	Clearance (mL/min/kg)	Half-life (hours)	C_{max} (μg/mL)	V_{dss} (L/kg)
9 months–13 years	Single—Oral 2 mg/kg	0.40 (38%) n=14	25.0	2.9 (22%) n=16	—
9 months–13 years	Single—Oral 8 mg/kg	0.51 (60%) n=15	19.5	9.8 (20%) n=15	—
5–15 years	Multiple i.v. 2 mg/kg	0.49 (40%) n=4	17.4	5.5 (25%) n=5	0.722 (36%) n=4
5-15 years	Multiple i.v. 4 mg/kg	0.59 (64%) n=5	15.2	11.4 (44%) n=6	0.729 (33%) n=5
5-15 years	Multiple i.v. 8 mg/kg	0.66 (31%) n=7	17.6	14.1 (22%) n=8	1.069 (37%) n=7

Clearance corrected for body weight was not affected by age in these studies. Mean body clearance in adults is reported to be 0.23 mL/min/kg (17%).

In premature newborns (gestation age 26 to 29 weeks), the mean (% cv) clearance within 36 hours of birth was 0.180 (35%, n=7) mL/min/kg, which increased with time to a mean of 0.218 (31%, n=9) mL/min/kg 6 days later and 0.333 (56%, n=4) mL/min/kg 12 days later. Similarly, the half-life was 73.6 hours, which decreased with time to a mean of 53.2 hours 6 days later and 46.6 hours 12 days later.

The dose equivalency scheme (see Table 2) should generally provide equivalent exposure in pediatric and adult patients.

Table 2: Diflucan

Dose Equivalency

Pediatric Patients	Adults
3 mg/kg	100 mg
6 mg/kg	200 mg
12 mg/kg[a]	400 mg

[a] Some older children may have clearances similar to that of adults. Absolute doses exceeding 600 mg/day are not recommended.

Distribution: The apparent volume of distribution of fluconazole approximates that of total body water. Plasma protein binding is low (11 to 12%) and is constant over the concentration range tested (0.1 to 10 mg/L). This degree of protein binding is not clinically meaningful. Following either single- or multiple-oral doses for up to 14 days, fluconazole penetrates into all body tissues and fluids studied (see Table 3). In normal volunteers, saliva concentrations of fluconazole were equal to or slightly greater than plasma concentrations regardless of dose, route, or duration of dosing. In patients with bronchiectasis, sputum concentrations of fluconazole following a single 150 mg oral dose were equal to plasma concentrations at both 4 and 24 hours post dose. In patients with fungal meningitis, fluconazole concentrations in the CSF are approximately 80% of the corresponding plasma concentrations. Whole blood concentrations of fluconazole indicated that the drug freely enters erythrocytes and maintains a concentration equivalent to that of plasma.

Table 3: Diflucan

Distribution of Fluconazole

Tissue or Fluid	Ratio of Fluconazole Tissue (Fluid)/Plasma Concentration[a]
Cerebrospinal fluid[b]	0.5–0.9
Saliva	1
Sputum	1
Blister fluid	1
Urine	10
Normal skin	10
Nails	1
Blister skin	2

[a] Relative to concurrent concentrations in plasma in subjects with normal renal function.
[b] Independent of degree of meningeal inflammation.

Metabolism and Excretion: Fluconazole is cleared primarily by renal excretion, with approximately 80% of the administered dose appearing in the urine as unchanged drug. Following administration of radiolabeled fluconazole, greater than 90% of the radioactivity is excreted in the urine. Approximately 11% of the radioactivity in urine is due to metabolites. An additional 2% of the total radioactivity is excreted in feces.

The pharmacokinetics of fluconazole do not appear to be affected by age alone but are markedly affected by reduction in renal function. There is an inverse relationship between the elimination half-life and creatinine clearance. The dose of fluconazole may need to be reduced in patients with impaired renal function (see Dosage). A 3-hour hemodialysis session decreases plasma concentrations by approximately 50%.
Pharmacodynamics: The effects of fluconazole on the metabolism of carbohydrates, lipids, adrenal and gonadal hormones were assessed. In normal volunteers, fluconazole administration (doses ranging from 200 to 400 mg once daily for up to 14 days) was associated with small and inconsistent effects on testosterone concentrations, endogenous corticosteroid concentrations, and the ACTH-stimulated cortisol response. In addition, fluconazole appears to have no clinically significant effects on carbohydrate or lipid metabolism in man.

INDICATIONS: For the treatment of oropharyngeal and esophageal candidiasis. Fluconazole is also effective for the treatment of serious systemic candidal infections, including urinary tract infection, peritonitis and pneumonia.

Cryptococcal meningitis.

Prevention of the recurrence of cryptococcal meningitis in patients with acquired immunodeficiency syndrome (AIDS).

Specimens for fungal culture and other relevant laboratory studies (serology, histopathology) should be obtained prior to therapy to isolate and identify causative organisms. Therapy may be instituted before the results of the cultures and other laboratory studies are known; however, once these results become available, anti-infective therapy should be adjusted accordingly.
Prophylaxis: Fluconazole is also indicated to decrease the incidence of candidiasis in patients undergoing bone marrow transplantation who receive cytotoxic chemotherapy and/or radiation therapy.

CONTRAINDICATIONS: In patients who have shown hypersensitivity to fluconazole or to any of its excipients. There is no information regarding cross hypersensitivity between fluconazole and other azole antifungal agents. Caution should be used in prescribing fluconazole to patients with hypersensitivity to other azoles.

Coadministration of terfenadine is contraindicated in patients receiving fluconazole at multiple doses of 400 mg or higher based upon results of a multiple dose interaction study (see Precautions).

Coadministration of cisapride is contraindicated in patients receiving fluconazole (see Precautions).

WARNINGS: Hepatic injury: Fluconazole has been associated with rare cases of serious hepatic toxicity, including fatalities, primarily in patients with serious underlying medical conditions. In cases of fluconazole associated hepatotoxicity, no obvious relationship to total daily dose, duration of therapy, sex or age of the patient has been observed. Fluconazole hepatotoxicity has usually, but not always been reversible on discontinuation of therapy. Patients who develop abnormal liver function tests during fluconazole therapy should be monitored for the development of more severe hepatic injury. Fluconazole should be discontinued if clinical signs and symptoms consistent with liver disease develop that may be attributable to fluconazole.
Anaphylaxis: In rare cases, anaphylaxis has been reported.
Dermatologic: Patients have rarely developed exfoliative skin disorders during treatment with fluconazole. In patients with serious underlying diseases (predominantly AIDS and malignancy) those have rarely resulted in a fatal outcome. Patients who develop rashes during treatment with fluconazole should be monitored closely and the drug discontinued if lesions progress.

PRECAUTIONS: QT Prolongation: Some azoles, including fluconazole, have been associated with prolongation of the QT interval on the electrocardiogram. During post-marketing surveillance, there have been very rare cases of QT prolongation and torsade de pointes in patients taking fluconazole. These reports included seriously ill patients with multiple confounding risk factors, such as structural heart disease, electrolyte abnormalities and concomitant medications that may have been contributory. Fluconazole should be administered with caution to patients with these potentially proarrhythmic conditions (see Precautions, Drug Interactions and Adverse Effects).
Pregnancy: There are no adequate and well-controlled studies in pregnant women. There have been reports of multiple congenital abnormalities in infants whose mothers were treated with high dose (400 to 800 mg/day) fluconazole therapy for coccidioidomycosis (an unapproved indication). Exposure to fluconazole began during the first trimester in all cases and continued for 3 months or longer. Fluconazole is not recommended in pregnant women unless the potential benefit outweighs the potential risk to mother and fetus.

Fluconazole was administered orally to pregnant rabbits during organogenesis in 2 studies: at 5, 10 and 20 mg/kg, and at 5, 25 and 75 mg/kg respectively. Maternal weight gain was impaired at all dose levels, and abortions occurred at 75 mg/kg (approximately 9.4×the maximum recommended human dose); no adverse fetal effects were detected. In several studies in which pregnant rats were treated orally with fluconazole during organogenesis, maternal weight gain was impaired and placental weights were increased at the 25 mg/kg dose. There were no fetal effects at 5 or 10 mg/kg; increases in fetal anatomical variants (supernumerary ribs, renal pelvis dilation) and delays in ossification were observed at 25 and 50 mg/kg and higher doses. At doses ranging from 80 to 320 mg/kg (approximately 10 to 40×the maximum recommended human dose), embryolethality in rats was increased and fetal abnormalities included wavy ribs, cleft palate and abnormal cranio-facial ossification. These effects are consistent with the inhibition of estrogen synthesis in rats and may be a result of known effects of lowered estrogen on pregnancy, organogenesis and parturition.

Women of Childbearing Potential: Since the teratologic effects of fluconazole in humans are unknown, women taking fluconazole should consider using adequate contraception (see Pregnancy).

There have been reports of multiple congenital abnormalities in infants whose mothers were treated with high dose (400 to 800 mg/day) fluconazole therapy for coccidioidomycosis (an unapproved indication). Exposure to fluconazole began during the first trimester in all cases and continued for 3 months or longer. Since there are no adequate studies in pregnant women to assess the potential for fetal risk, fluconazole should not be used in pregnant women unless the potential benefit outweighs the potential risk to the fetus.

Lactation: Fluconazole is secreted in human breast milk at concentrations similar to plasma, hence its use in nursing mothers is not recommended.

Children: An open-label, randomized, controlled trial has shown fluconazole to be effective in the treatment of oropharyngeal candidiasis in children 6 months to 13 years of age.

In a noncomparative study of children with serious systemic fungal infections, fluconazole was effective in the treatment of candidemia (10 of 11 patients cured) and disseminated candidiasis (5 of 6 patients cured or improved).

Fluconazole was effective for the suppression of cryptococcal meningitis and/or disseminated cryptococcal infection in a group of 6 children treated in a compassionate study of fluconazole for the treatment of life-threatening or serious mycosis. There is no information regarding the efficacy of fluconazole for primary treatment of cryptococcal meningitis in children.

In addition, the use of fluconazole in children with cryptococcal meningitis, candida esophagitis or systemic candida infections is consistent with the approved use of fluconazole in similar indications for adults and, is supported by pharmacokinetic studies in children (see Pharmacology) establishing dose proportionality between children and adults (see Dosage).

The safety of fluconazole in children has been established in 577 children ages 1 day to 17 years who received doses ranging from 1 to 15 mg/kg/day for 1 to 1616 days (see Adverse Effects).

Efficacy of fluconazole has not been established in infants less than 6 months of age. A small number of patients (29) ranging in age from 1 day to 6 months have been treated safely with fluconazole.

Geriatrics: Fluconazole was well tolerated by patients aged 65 years and over.

In a small number of elderly patients with bone marrow transplant (BMT) in which fluconazole was administered prophylactically there was a greater incidence of drug discontinuation due to adverse reactions (4.3%) than in younger patients (1.7%).

Superinfections: Development of resistance to fluconazole has not been studied; however, there have been reports of cases of superinfection with Candida species other than *C. albicans*, which are often inherently not susceptible to fluconazole (e.g., *Candida krusei*). Such cases may require alternative antifungal therapy.

As for other anti-infectives used prophylactically, prudent medical practice dictates that fluconazole be used judiciously in prophylaxis, in view of the theoretical risk of emergence of resistant strains.

Drug Interactions: Clinically or potentially significant drug interactions between fluconazole and the following agents/classes have been observed.

Benzodiazepines (Short Acting): Following oral or i.v. administration of midazolam, fluconazole resulted in substantial increases in midazolam concentrations and psychomotor effects. This effect on midazolam appears to be more pronounced following oral administration of fluconazole than with fluconazole administered i.v. If concomitant benzodiazepine therapy, such as midazolam or triazolam, is necessary in patients being treated with fluconazole, consideration should be given to decreasing the benzodiazepine dosage, and the patients should be appropriately monitored.

Cimetidine: Absorption of orally administered fluconazole does not appear to be affected by gastric pH. Fluconazole 100 mg was administered as a single oral dose alone and 2 hours after a single dose of cimetidine 400 mg to 6 healthy male volunteers. After the administration of cimetidine, there was a significant decrease in fluconazole AUC (area under the plasma concentration-time curve) and C_{max}. There was a mean±SD decrease in fluconazole AUC of 13%±11% (range −3.4 to −31%) and C_{max} decreased 19%±14% (range: −5 to −40%). However, the administration of cimetidine 600 to 900 mg i.v. over a 4-hour period (from 1 hour before to 3 hours after a single oral dose of fluconazole 200 mg) did not affect the bioavailability or pharmacokinetics of fluconazole in 24 healthy male volunteers.

Coumarin-Type Anticoagulants: In a clinical trial, there was a significant increase in prothrombin time response (area under the prothrombin time-time curve) following a single dose of warfarin (15 mg) administered to 13 normal male volunteers following oral fluconazole 200 mg administered daily for 14 days as compared to the administration of warfarin alone. There was a mean ±SD increase in the prothrombin time response (area under the prothrombin time-time curve) of 7%±4% (range: −2 to 13%). Mean is based on data from 12 subjects as one of 13 subjects experienced a 2-fold increase in his prothrombin time response.

During the postmarketing experience, as with some azole antifungals, bleeding events (bruising, epistaxis, gastrointestinal bleeding, hematuria, and melena) have been reported, in association with increases in prothrombin time in patients receiving fluconazole concurrently with warfarin.

Prothrombin time may be increased in patients receiving concomitant fluconazole and coumarin-type anticoagulants. Careful monitoring of prothrombin time in patients receiving fluconazole and coumarin-type anticoagulants is recommended.

Cyclosporine: Cyclosporine AUC and C_{max} were determined before and after the administration of fluconazole 200 mg daily for 14 days in 8 renal transplant patients who had been on cyclosporine therapy for at least 6 months and on a stable cyclosporine dose for at least 6 weeks. There was a significant increase in cyclosporine AUC, C_{max}, C_{min} (24-hour concentration), and a significant reduction in apparent oral clearance following the administration of fluconazole. The mean±SD increase in AUC was 92%±43% (range: 18 to 147%). The C_{max} increased 60%±48% range (range: −5 to 133%). The C_{min} increased 157%±96% (range: 33 to 360%). The apparent oral clearance decreased 45%±15% (range: −15 to −60%). Fluconazole administered at 100 mg daily dose does not affect cyclosporine pharmacokinetic levels in patients with bone marrow transplants. Fluconazole may significantly increase cyclosporine levels in renal transplant patients with or without renal impairment. Careful monitoring of cyclosporine concentrations and serum creatinine is recommended in patients receiving fluconazole and cyclosporine.

Drugs Prolonging the QTc Interval: The use of fluconazole in patients concurrently taking drugs metabolized by the Cytochrome P450 system may be associated with elevations in the serum levels of these drugs. In the absence of definitive information caution should be used when coadministering fluconazole and such agents (see Precautions—QT Prolongation). Patients should be carefully monitored.

Astemizole: Definitive interaction studies with fluconazole have not been conducted. The use of fluconazole may be associated with elevations in serum levels of astemizole. Caution should be used when coadministering fluconazole with astemizole. Patients should be carefully monitored.

Cisapride: There have been reports of cardiac events including torsades de pointes in patients to whom fluconazole and cisapride were coadministered. A controlled study found that concomitant fluconazole 200 mg once daily and cisapride 20 mg four times a day yielded a significant increase in cisapride plasma levels and prolongation of QTc interval. Coadministration of cisapride is contraindicated in patients receiving fluconazole (see Contraindications).

Terfenadine: Because of the occurrence of serious cardiac dysrhythmias secondary to prolongation of the QTc interval in patients receiving azole antifungals in conjunction with terfenadine, interaction studies have been performed. In one study, 6 healthy volunteers received terfenadine 60 mg b.i.d. for 15 days. Fluconazole 200 mg was administered daily from days 9 through 15. Fluconazole did not affect terfenadine plasma concentrations. Terfenadine acid metabolite AUC increased 36%±36% (range: 7 to 102%) from day 8 to day 15 with the concomitant administration of fluconazole. There was no change in cardiac repolarization as measured by Holter QTc intervals. However, another study at a 400 mg and 800 mg daily dose of fluconazole demonstrated that fluconazole taken in doses of 400 mg/day or greater significantly increases plasma levels of terfenadine when taken concomitantly. Therefore the combined use of fluconazole at doses of 400 mg or higher with terfenadine is contraindicated (see Contraindications). Patients should be carefully monitored if they are being concurrently prescribed fluconazole at multiple doses lower than 400 mg/day with terfenadine.

Hydrochlorothiazide: Concomitant oral administration of 100 mg fluconazole and 50 mg hydrochlorothiazide for 10 days in 13 normal volunteers resulted in a significant increase in fluconazole AUC and C_{max} compared to fluconazole given alone. There was a mean±SD increase in fluconazole AUC and C_{max} of 45%±31% (range: 19 to 114%) and 43%±31% (range: 19 to 122%), respectively. These changes are attributed to a mean±SD reduction in renal clearance of 30%±12% (range −10 to −50%).

Oral Contraceptives: In pharmacodynamic studies, single and multiple 50 mg oral doses of fluconazole produced an overall mean increase in ethinyl estradiol or levonorgestrel pharmacokinetics in healthy women taking oral contraceptives. At 200 mg of fluconazole daily, the AUCs of ethinyl estradiol and levonorgestrel were increased, 40% and 24%, respectively.

Twenty-five normal females received daily doses of both 200 mg of fluconazole tablets or placebo for 2, 10-day periods. The treatment cycles were 1 month apart with all subjects receiving fluconazole during one cycle and placebo during the other. The order of study treatment was random. Single doses of an oral contraceptive tablet containing levonorgestrel and ethinyl estradiol were administered on the final treatment day (day 10) of both cycles. Following administration of 200 mg of fluconazole, the mean percentage increase of AUC for levonorgestrel compared to placebo was 25% (range: −12 to 82%) and the mean percentage increase for ethinyl estradiol compared to placebo was 38% (range: −11 to 101%). Both of these increases were statistically significantly different from placebo.

Oral Hypoglycemics: The effects of fluconazole on the pharmacokinetics of the sulfonylurea oral hypoglycemic agents tolbutamide, glipizide, and glyburide were evaluated in 3 placebo-controlled studies in normal volunteers. All subjects received the sulfonylurea alone as a single dose and again as a single dose following the administration of fluconazole 100 mg daily for 7 days. In these 3 studies, 22/46 (47.8%) of fluconazole-treated patients and 9/22 (40.1%) of placebo-treated patients experienced symptoms consistent with hypoglycemia.

Tolbutamide: In 13 normal male volunteers, there was a significant increase in tolbutamide (500 mg single dose) AUC and C_{max} following the administration of fluconazole. There was a mean±SD increase in tolbutamide AUC of 26%±9% (range: 12 to 39%). Tolbutamide C_{max} increased 11%±9% (range −6 to 27%).

Glipizide: The AUC and C_{max} of glipizide (2.5 mg single dose) were significantly increased following the administration of fluconazole in 13 normal male volunteers. There was a mean±SD increase in AUC of 49%±13% (range: 27 to 73%) and an increase in C_{max} of 19%±23% (range: −11 to 79%).

Glyburide: The AUC and C_{max} of glyburide (5 mg single dose) were significantly increased following the administration of fluconazole in 20 normal male volunteers. There was a mean±SD increase in AUC of 44%±29% (range: −13 to 115%) and C_{max} increased 19%±19% (range: −23 to 62%). Five subjects required oral glucose following the ingestion of glyburide after 7 days of fluconazole administration.

Clinically significant hypoglycemia may be precipitated by the use of fluconazole with oral hypoglycemic agents; 1 fatality has been reported from hypoglycemia in association with combined fluconazole and glyburide use. Fluconazole reduces the metabolism of tolbutamide, glyburide, and glipizide and increases the plasma concentration of these agents. When fluconazole is used concomitantly with these or other sulfonylurea oral hypoglycemic agents, blood glucose concentrations should be carefully monitored and the dose of the sulfonylurea should be adjusted as necessary.

Phenytoin: Phenytoin AUC was determined after 4 days of phenytoin dosing (200 mg daily, orally for 3 days, followed by 250 mg i.v. for 1 dose) both with and without the administration of fluconazole (oral fluconazole 200 mg daily for 16 days) in 10 normal male volunteers. There was a significant increase in phenytoin AUC. The mean±SD increase in phenytoin AUC was 88%±68% (range: 16 to 247%). The absolute magnitude of this interaction is unknown because of the intrinsically nonlinear disposition of phenytoin.

Fluconazole increases the plasma concentrations of phenytoin. Careful monitoring of phenytoin concentrations in patients receiving fluconazole and phenytoin is recommended.

Rifabutin: There have been reports that an interaction exists when fluconazole is administered concomitantly with rifabutin, leading to increased serum levels of rifabutin. There have been reports of uveitis in patients to whom fluconazole and rifabutin were coadministered. Patients receiving rifabutin and fluconazole concomitantly should be carefully monitored.

Rifampin: Administration of a single oral 200 mg dose of fluconazole after 15 days of rifampin administered as 600 mg daily in 8 healthy male volunteers resulted in a significant decrease in fluconazole AUC and a significant increase in apparent oral clearance of fluconazole. There was a mean±SD reduction in fluconazole AUC of 23%±9% (range: −13 to −42%). Apparent oral clearance of fluconazole increased 32%±17% (range: 16 to 72%). Fluconazole half-life decreased from 33.4±4.4 hours to 26.8±3.9 hours.

Rifampin enhances the metabolism of concurrently administered fluconazole. Depending on clinical circumstances, consideration should be given to increasing the dose of fluconazole when it is administered with rifampin.

Tacrolimus: There have been reports that an interaction exists when fluconazole is administered concomitantly with tacrolimus, leading to increased serum levels of tacrolimus. There have been reports of nephrotoxicity in patients to whom fluconazole and tacrolimus were coadministered. Patients receiving tacrolimus and fluconazole concomitantly should be carefully monitored.

Theophylline: The pharmacokinetics of theophylline were determined from a single i.v. dose of aminophylline (6 mg/kg) before and after the oral administration of fluconazole 200 mg daily for 14 days in 16 normal male volunteers. There were significant increases in theophylline AUC, C_{max}, and half-life with a corresponding decrease in clearance. The mean±SD theophylline AUC increased 21%±16% (range: −5 to 48%). The C_{max} increased 13%±17% (range: −13 to 40%). Theophylline clearance decreased 16%±11% (range: −32 to 5%). The half-life of theophylline increased from 6.6±1.7 hours to 7.9±1.5 hours. Patients who are receiving high doses theophylline or who are otherwise at increased risk for theophylline toxicity should be observed for signs of theophylline toxicity while receiving fluconazole, and therapy modified appropriately if signs of toxicity develop.

Zidovudine: Plasma zidovudine concentrations were determined on 2 occasions (before and following fluconazole 200 mg daily for 15 days) in 13 volunteers with AIDS or ARC who were on a stable zidovudine dose for at least 2 weeks. There was a significant increase in zidovudine AUC following the administration of fluconazole. The mean±SD increase in AUC was 20%±32% (range: −27 to 104%). The metabolite, GZDV, to parent drug ratio significantly decreased after the administration of fluconazole, from 7.6±3.6 to 5.7±2.2. Patients receiving this combination should be monitored for the development of zidovudine-related adverse reactions.

Drugs exhibiting no significant pharmacokinetic interactions with fluconazole: Antacid: Administration of Maalox (20 mL) to 14 normal male volunteers immediately prior to a single dose of fluconazole 100 mg had no effect on the absorption or elimination of fluconazole.

Interaction studies with other medications have not been conducted, but such interactions may occur.

Drug/Laboratory Test Interactions: None known.

ADVERSE EFFECTS: Adults: Sixteen percent of over 4000 patients treated with fluconazole in clinical trials of 7 days or more experienced adverse events.

Treatment was discontinued in 1.5% of patients due to adverse clinical events and in 1.3% of patients due to laboratory test abnormalities.

Adverse clinical events were reported more frequently in HIV infected patients (21%) than in non-HIV infected patients (13%). However, the patterns of adverse events in HIV infected and non-HIV infected patients were similar. The proportions of patients discontinuing therapy due to clinical adverse events were similar in the 2 groups (1.5%).

The 2 most serious adverse clinical events noted during clinical trials were exfoliative skin disorders and hepatic necrosis.

Because most of these patients had serious underlying disease (predominantly AIDS or malignancy) and were receiving multiple concomitant medications, including many known to be hepatotoxic or associated with exfoliative skin disorders, the causal association of these reactions with fluconazole is uncertain. Two cases of hepatic necrosis and one exfoliative skin disorder (Stevens-Johnson syndrome) were associated with a fatal outcome (see Warnings).

The following treatment-related clinical adverse events occurred at an incidence of 1% or greater in 4048 patients receiving fluconazole for 7 or more days in clinical trials:

Central and Peripheral Nervous System: headache (1.9%).

Dermatologic: skin rash (1.8%).

Gastrointestinal: abdominal pain (1.7%), diarrhea (1.5%), nausea (3.7%) and vomiting (1.7%).

Other treatment-related clinical adverse events which occurred less commonly (0.2 to <1%) are presented by organ system below:

Skin and Appendages: pruritus.

Musculoskeletal: myalgia.

Central and Peripheral Nervous Systems: convulsions, dizziness, paresthesia, tremor, vertigo.

Autonomic Nervous System: dry mouth, increased sweating.

Psychiatric: insomnia, somnolence.

Gastrointestinal: anorexia, constipation, dyspepsia, flatulence.

Liver and Biliary System: cholestasis, hepatocellular damage, jaundice.

Special Senses: taste perversion.

Hematopoietic: anemia.

General: fatigue, malaise, asthenia, fever.

Immunologic: In rare cases, anaphylaxis has been reported.

In addition, the following adverse events have occurred under conditions where a causal association is uncertain (e.g., open trials, during postmarketing experience):

Cardiovascular: QT prolongation, torsade de pointes (see Precautions—QT Prolongation).

Central and Peripheral Nervous System: seizures.

Dermatologic: alopecia, exfoliative skin disorders including Stevens-Johnson syndrome and toxic epidermal necrolysis (see Warnings).

Hematopoietic and Lymphatic: leukopenia, including neutropenia and agranulocytosis, thrombocytopenia.

Body as a Whole: anaphylaxis including angioedema, face edema, pruritus, and urticaria.

Liver/Biliary: hepatic failure, hepatitis.

Metabolic: hypercholesterolemia, hypertriglyceridemia, hypokalemia.

Laboratory Test Abnormalities: Liver Function: Clinically significant increases were observed in the following proportions of patients: AST 1%, ALT 1.2%, alkaline phosphatase 1.2%, total bilirubin 0.3%. The incidence of elevated serum transaminases was independent of age or route (oral or i.v) of administration but was greater in patients taking fluconazole concomitantly with one or more of the following medications: rifampin, phenytoin, isoniazid, valproic acid or oral hypoglycemic agents. Clinically significant increases also were more frequent in patients who: 1) had AST or ALT elevations greater than 3 times the upper limit of normal (>3×ULN) at the time of entering the study (baseline), 2) had a diagnosis of hepatitis at any time during the study and, 3) were identified as alcohol abusers. The overall rate of serum transaminase elevations of more than 8 times the upper limit of normal was approximately 1% in patients treated with fluconazole during clinical trials (see Table 4).

Table 4: Diflucan

Laboratory Test Abnormalities—Liver Enzymes

Lab Parameter	Number[a] of Patients	% Abnormal	% Drug-related	Number of Patients	% Abnormal	% Drug-related
	Baseline >3×ULN			Baseline <3×ULN		
AST	53	9.4	3.8	3007	4.2	0.8
ALT	65	3.1	0.0	2874	4.8	1.0
	Hepatitis Patients			Non-hepatitis Patients		
AST	160	10.6	1.9	2900	3.9	0.8
ALT	140	11.4	2.1	2799	4.4	1.0
	Alcohol Abuse			Non-alcohol Abuse		
AST	42	9.5	2.4	3018	4.2	0.9
ALT	40	10.0	2.5	2899	4.7	1.0
	Received I.V. Fluconazole			Never Received I.V. Fluconazole		
AST	144	5.6	1.4	2916	4.2	0.9
ALT	139	5.0	0.7	2800	4.7	1.0
	≥65 Years Old			<65 Years Old		
AST	277	4.3	1.1	2783	4.3	0.9
ALT	258	3.9	1.2	2681	4.8	1.0

[a] Note: Only patients who had measurements at baseline and during therapy were included.
Legend:
ULN=Upper Limit of Normal.

Renal Function: Clinically significant increases were observed in the following proportions of patients: BUN (0.4%) and creatinine (0.3%).

Hematological Function: Clinically meaningful deviations from baseline in hematologic values which were possibly related to fluconazole were observed in the following proportions of patients: hemoglobin (0.5%), white blood cell count (0.5%) and total platelet count (0.6%).

Children: In Phase II/III clinical trials conducted in the U.S. and in Europe, 577 pediatric patients, ages 1 day to 17 years were treated with fluconazole at doses ranging up to 15 mg/kg/day for up to 1616 days. Thirteen percent of children experienced treatment related adverse events. The most commonly reported events were vomiting (5.4%), abdominal pain (2.8%), nausea (2.3%) and diarrhea (2.1%). Treatment was discontinued in 2.6% of patients due to adverse clinical events and in 1% of patients due to laboratory test abnormalities.

OVERDOSE:

Symptoms: There have been reports of overdosage with fluconazole and in one case, a 42-year-old patient infected with human immunodeficiency virus developed hallucinations and exhibited paranoid behavior after reportedly ingesting 8200 mg of fluconazole. The patient was admitted to the hospital, and his condition resolved within 48 hours.

Treatment: In the event of overdose, symptomatic treatment (with supportive measures and gastric lavage if necessary) may be adequate. Fluconazole is largely excreted in urine. A 3-hour hemodialysis session decreases plasma levels by approximately 50%.

Mice and rats receiving very high doses of fluconazole, whether orally or i.v., displayed a variety of nonspecific, agonal signs such as decreased activity, ataxia, shallow respiration, ptosis, lacrimation, salivation, urinary incontinence and cyanosis. Death was sometimes preceded by clonic convulsions.

> For management of a suspected drug overdose, CPhA recommends that you contact your **regional Poison Control Centre**. See the *CPS* Directory section for a list of Poison Control Centres.

DOSAGE: Oral (Tablets and Oral Suspension) and I.V. Administration: Fluconazole is well absorbed and excreted predominantly unchanged in urine following oral administration in man. The oral bioavailability is essentially complete (greater than 90%), and is independent of dose. Peak plasma concentrations after oral administration are attained rapidly, usually within 2 hours of dosing. **Since oral absorption is rapid and almost complete, the daily dose of fluconazole is the same for oral tablets and suspension and i.v. administration.** The terminal plasma elimination half-life is approximately 30 hours (range 20 to 50 hours).

The daily dose of fluconazole and the route of administration should be based on the infecting organism, the patient's condition and the response to therapy. Treatment should be continued until clinical parameters and laboratory tests indicate that an active fungal infection has been cured or has subsided. An inadequate period of treatment may lead to recurrence of active infection. Patients with AIDS and cryptococcal meningitis or recurrent oropharyngeal candidiasis usually require maintenance therapy to prevent relapse.

Recommended Dosages in Adults and Children (see also Pharmacology): Treatment: Loading Dose: **Administration of a loading dose on the first day of treatment, consisting of twice the usual daily dose, results in plasma concentrations close to steady state by the second day. Patients with acute infections should be given a loading dose equal to twice the daily dose, not to exceed a maximum single dose of 400 mg in adults or 12 mg/kg in children, on the first day of treatment.**

Dosage Equivalency Scheme: See Table 5.

Table 5: Diflucan

Dosage Equivalency Scheme

Pediatric Patients	Adults
3 mg/kg	100 mg
6 mg/kg	200 mg
12 mg/kg[a]	400 mg

[a] Some older children may have clearances similar to that of adults. Absolute doses exceeding 600 mg/day are not recommended.

Recommended Treatment Guidelines: See Table 6.

Table 6: Diflucan

Recommended Treatment Guidelines

Indication	Adults	Children
Oropharyngeal Candidiasis	100 mg once daily for at least 2 weeks to decrease the likelihood of relapse	3 mg/kg once daily for at least 2 weeks to decrease the likelihood of relapse
Esophageal Candidiasis	100 to 200 mg once daily for a minimum of 3 weeks, and for at least 2 weeks following resolution of symptoms	3 to 6 mg/kg once daily for a minimum of 3 weeks, and for at least 2 weeks following resolution of symptoms
Systemic Candidiasis (Candidemia and Disseminated Candidal Infections)	200 to 400 mg once daily for a minimum of 4 weeks, and for at least 2 weeks following resolution of symptoms	6 to 12 mg/kg/day have been used in an open, noncomparative study of a small number of patients
Cryptococcal Meningitis	200 to 400 mg once daily. The duration of therapy for cryptococcal meningitis is unknown, it is recommended that the initial therapy should last a minimum of 10 weeks	6 to 12 mg/kg once daily. The recommended duration for initial therapy is 10-12 weeks after the cerebrospinal fluid becomes culture-negative
Prevention of Recurrence of Cryptococcal Meningitis in Patients with AIDS	200 mg once daily	6 mg/kg once daily

Premature Neonates: Experience with fluconazole in neonates is limited to pharmacokinetic studies in premature newborns (see Pharmacology). Based upon the prolonged half-life seen in premature newborns (gestational age 26 to 29 weeks), these children in the first 2 weeks of life, should receive the same dosage (mg/kg) as in older children, but administered every 72 hours. After the first 2 weeks, these children should be dosed once daily.

Neonates: No information regarding fluconazole pharmacokinetics in full-term newborns is available.

Prophylaxis in Adult Patients: The recommended fluconazole daily dosage for the prevention of candidiasis in adult patients undergoing bone marrow transplantation is 400 mg once daily. Patients who are anticipated to have severe granulocytopenia (less than 500 neutrophils/mm^3) should start fluconazole prophylaxis several days before the anticipated onset of neutropenia and continue for 7 days after the neutrophil count rises above 1000 cells/mm^3.

Fluconazole may be administered either orally or by i.v. infusion. The i.v. infusion of fluconazole should be administered at a maximum rate of approximately 200 mg/hour given as a continuous infusion (see Directions for Use).

Impaired Renal Function: Adults: Fluconazole is cleared primarily by renal excretion as unchanged drug. In patients with impaired renal function, an initial loading dose of 50 to 400 mg should be given (for children, see below). After the loading dose, the daily dose (according to indication) should be based on Table 7.

Table 7: Diflucan

Dosage in Adult Patients with Impaired Renal Function

Creatinine Clearance (mL/min)	Creatinine Clearance (mL/s)	Percent Recommended Dose
>50	>0.83	100%
21–50 (no dialysis)	0.35–0.83 (no dialysis)	50%
11–20 (no dialysis)	0.18–0.34 (no dialysis)	25%
Regular hemodialysis	Regular hemodialysis	100% after each dialysis

When serum creatinine is the only measure of renal function available, the following formula (based on sex, weight and age of the patient) should be used to estimate the creatinine clearance:

mL/min:

$$\text{Males: } \frac{\text{weight (kg)} \times (140\text{–age})}{72 \times \text{serum creatinine (mg/100 mL)}}$$

Females: 0.85 × the above value.

mL/s:

$$\text{Males: } \frac{\text{weight (kg)} \times (140\text{–age})}{50 \times \text{serum creatinine } (\mu\text{mol/L})}$$

Females: 0.85 × the above value.

Children: Although the pharmacokinetics of fluconazole has not been studied in children with renal insufficiency, dosage reduction in children with renal insufficiency should parallel that recommended for adults. The following formula may be used to estimate creatinine clearance in children:

$$K \times \frac{\text{linear length or height (cm)}}{\text{serum creatinine (mg/100 mL)}}$$

(Where K=0.55 for children older than 1 year and 0.45 for infants.)

Directions for Use: Mixing Directions: Powder for Oral Suspension: Prepare a suspension at time of dispensing as follows: Tap bottle until all powder flows freely. Add 24 mL of water and shake vigorously to suspend powder and produce 35 mL suspension. Each 5 mL contains 50 mg fluconazole at a concentration of 10 mg/mL, for a total fluconazole content of 350 mg per bottle. Shake oral suspension well before using.

Directions for Use: Injection: Inspect visually for particulate matter or discoloration prior to administration. Do not use if cloudiness or precipitation is evident.

Reject the contents as unsterile if the metal seal is broken. **Not intended for multidose use:** discard any portion not used when the seal is first broken.

Connect an i.v. giving set to the bottle of fluconazole i.v. solution and also insert a venting set through the bung. **Infuse the i.v. solution at a maximum rate of 200 mg/hour.** Flush fluconazole i.v. solution remaining in the giving set with sterile normal saline. Because fluconazole is available as a dilute saline solution, consideration should be given to the rate of fluid administration in patients requiring sodium or fluid restriction.

Incompatibility: It is recommended that fluconazole i.v. be infused separately.

Compatibility: Administration Sets (Giving Sets): The i.v. infusion is compatible with (i.e., not susceptible to absorption) sets constructed of a delivery tube (PVC) luer lock (modified phenylene oxide), flash ball (latex) drip chamber (polypropylene) and piercing spike (polypropylene).

SUPPLIED: I.V.: Each mL of sterile aqueous solution for direct infusion contains: fluconazole 2 mg and sodium chloride 9 mg. Clear glass bottles of 100 mL (2×100 mL), affording doses of 200 mg fluconazole, sealed with a rubber bung. Store at 15 to 30°C. Do not freeze.

Powder for Oral Suspension: On reconstitution with water (24 mL) each mL of the orange-flavored suspension contains: fluconazole 10 mg (i.e., equivalent to fluconazole 50 mg/5 mL). Nonmedicinal ingredients: citric acid, colloidal silicon dioxide, natural orange flavor, sodium benzoate, sodium citrate, sucrose, titanium dioxide and xanthan gum. Bottles of 350 mg in HDPE bottles of 35 mL.

Before reconstitution (i.e., dry powder): Store at 15 to 30°C. **After reconstitution:** The reconstituted suspension is stable for 14 days at 5 to 30°C. Protect from freezing. Shake well before each use. Discard unused portion after 2 weeks (14 days).

Tablets: 50 mg: Each pink tablet, marked with "Pfizer" on one side and "Diflucan 50" on the other side, contains: fluconazole 50 mg. Nonmedicinal ingredients: croscarmellose sodium, dibasic calcium phosphate anhydrous, FD&C Red No. 40 aluminum lake dye, magnesium stearate, microcrystalline cellulose and povidone. Opaque polyethylene bottles of 50. Store at 15 to 30°C. **100 mg:** Each pink tablet, marked with "Pfizer" on one side and "Diflucan 100" on the other side, contains: fluconazole 100 mg. Nonmedicinal ingredients: croscarmellose sodium, dibasic calcium phosphate anhydrous, FD&C Red No. 40 aluminum lake dye, magnesium stearate, microcrystalline cellulose and povidone. Opaque polyethylene bottles of 50 and 100. Store at 15 to 30°C.

(Shown in Product Identification Section)

Diflucan 150™

fluconazole

Antifungal

Pfizer

Date of Preparation: November 7, 1994
Date of Revision: May 7, 2010

SUMMARY PRODUCT INFORMATION:

Route of Administration	Dosage Form/ Strength	Clinically Relevant Nonmedicinal Ingredients
Oral	Capsule, 150 mg	Lactose, maize starch, colloidal silicon dioxide, magnesium stearate and sodium lauryl sulphate For a complete listing of nonmedicinal ingredients see Dosage Forms, Composition and Packaging.

INDICATIONS AND CLINICAL USE: DIFLUCAN 150 (fluconazole) is indicated for the single-dose treatment of vaginal candidiasis (yeast infections due to Candida) and is clinically proven to cure most vaginal yeast infections.

CONTRAINDICATIONS: DIFLUCAN 150 (fluconazole) is contraindicated in patients who have shown hypersensitivity to fluconazole or to any of the excipients used. See Dosage Forms, Composition and Packaging of the product monograph for a complete listing of excipients. There is no information regarding cross hypersensitivity between fluconazole and other azole antifungal agents. Caution should be used by individuals having hypersensitivity to other azoles when using fluconazole.

Co-administration of terfenadine* is contraindicated in patients receiving fluconazole at multiple doses of 400 mg or higher based upon results of a multiple dose interaction study (see Warnings and Precautions).

Co-administration of cisapride* is contraindicated in patients receiving fluconazole (see Warnings and Precautions).

WARNINGS AND PRECAUTIONS: DIFLUCAN 150 (fluconazole) is indicated for single dose only. Some (not all) adverse experiences have been reported in patients following exposure to multiple doses of fluconazole.

Clinically significant warnings and precautions for DIFLUCAN 150 (fluconazole) are listed below.

General: The convenience of the single oral dose fluconazole regimen for the treatment of vaginal yeast infections **should be weighed against the acceptability of a higher incidence of drug related adverse events** with oral fluconazole (26%) versus intravaginal agents (16%) in comparative clinical studies where no difference in efficacy was demonstrated (see Adverse Reactions).

Fluconazole administered in combination with ethinyl estradiol- and levonorgestrel-containing oral contraceptives produced an overall mean increase in ethinyl estradiol and levonorgestrel levels; however, in some patients there were decreases up to 47% and 33% of ethinyl estradiol and levonorgestrel levels, respectively (see Drug Interactions). The data presently available indicate that the decreases in some individual ethinyl estradiol and levonorgestrel AUC values with fluconazole treatment may be the result of random variation. While there is evidence that fluconazole can inhibit the metabolism of ethinyl estradiol and levonorgestrel, there is no evidence that fluconazole is a net inducer of ethinyl estradiol or levonorgestrel metabolism. The clinical significance of these effects is presently unknown.

Cardiovascular: QT Prolongation: Some azoles, including fluconazole, have been associated with prolongation of the QT interval on the electrocardiogram. During post-marketing surveillance, there have been very rare cases of QT prolongation and torsades de pointes in patients taking fluconazole. These reports included seriously ill patients with multiple confounding risk factors, such as structural heart disease, electrolyte abnormalities and concomitant medications that may have been contributory. Fluconazole should be administered with caution to patients with these potentially proarrhythmic conditions (see Drug Interactions and Adverse Reactions).

Dermatologic: In very rare cases, during the treatment of systemic and vaginal infections, patients have developed exfoliative skin disorders (Stevens-Johnson Syndrome, Toxic Epidermal Necrolysis) during treatment with fluconazole.

Hepatic/Biliary/Pancreatic: In the treatment of systemic infections, multiple doses of fluconazole have been associated with rare cases of serious hepatic toxicity, including fatalities primarily in patients with serious underlying medical conditions. In cases of fluconazole-associated hepatotoxicity, no obvious relationship to total daily dose, duration of therapy, sex or age of the patient has been observed. Fluconazole hepatotoxicity has usually, but not always, been reversible on discontinuation of therapy.

Hypersensitivity: In rare cases, anaphylaxis and angioedema have been reported in patients using fluconazole.

Special Populations: Pregnant Women: There are no adequate and well-controlled studies in pregnant women. Single-dose oral fluconazole 150 mg does not appear to increase the risk of congenital anomalies. There have been reports of multiple congenital abnormalities in infants whose mothers were treated with high dose (400-800 mg/day) fluconazole therapy for coccidioidomycosis (an unapproved indication). Exposure to fluconazole began during the first trimester in all cases and continued for three months or longer. Fluconazole should not be used in pregnant women unless the potential benefit outweighs the potential risk to the fetus. Women of child-bearing potential taking fluconazole for vaginal candidiasis should consider using adequate contraception.

Fluconazole was administered orally to pregnant rabbits during organogenesis in two studies, at 5, 10 and 20 mg/kg and at 5, 25 and 75 mg/kg respectively. Maternal weight gain was impaired at all dose levels, and abortions occurred at 75 mg/kg (approximately 9.4× the maximum recommended human dose); no adverse fetal effects were detected. In several studies in which pregnant rats were treated orally with fluconazole during organogenesis, maternal weight gain was impaired and placental weights were increased at the 25 mg/kg dose. There were no fetal effects at 5 or 10 mg/kg; increases in fetal anatomical variants (supernumerary ribs, renal pelvis dilation) and delays in ossification were observed at 25 and 50 mg/kg and higher doses. At doses ranging from 80 mg/kg to 320 mg/kg (approximately 10-40× the maximum recommended human dose) embryolethality in rats was increased and fetal abnormalities included wavy ribs, cleft palate and abnormal cranio-facial ossification. These effects are consistent with the inhibition of estrogen synthesis in rats and may be a result of known effects of lowered estrogen on pregnancy, organogenesis and parturition.

Nursing Women: DIFLUCAN 150 is secreted in human breast milk at concentrations similar to plasma, hence its use in nursing mothers is not recommended.

Pediatrics: DIFLUCAN 150 should not be used by girls less than 12 years of age unless advised by a physician.

ADVERSE REACTIONS: Adverse Drug Reaction Overview: Clinical Trial Adverse Drug Reactions: In patients with vaginal candidiasis treated with fluconazole (150 mg) as a single oral dose, the adverse events documented in two controlled North American trials were as follows: See Table 1.

* Not marketed in Canada.

Table 1: DIFLUCAN 150
Adverse Events Documented in Two Controlled North American Trials

	Percent of Patients with Side Effects	
	Fluconazole (n=448)	**Intravaginal Products (n=422)**
Drug Related Side Effects	26.1	15.9
Nausea	6.7	0.7
Abdominal Pain	5.6	1.7
Diarrhea	2.7	0.5
Dyspepsia	1.3	0.2
Headache	12.9	6.6
Application Site Reactions	0.0	4.5
Dizziness	1.3	0.0
Taste Perversion	1.3	0.0
Most of the reported side effects were mild to moderate in severity.		

Less Common Clinical Trial Adverse Drug Reactions: Occasional allergic reactions including pruritus and urticaria were reported.

Post-Market Adverse Drug Reactions: In marketing experience of single dose fluconazole, rare cases of anaphylactic reaction and angioedema have been reported.

In addition, the following adverse experiences have been reported in patients under conditions (e.g. open trials, marketing experience fluconazole) where a causal relationship is uncertain or in patients treated with multiple doses of fluconazole:

Cardiovascular: QT prolongation, torsades de pointes (see Warnings and Precautions, QT Prolongation).
Central and Peripheral Nervous Systems: seizures.
Dermatologic: alopecia, exfoliative skin disorders including Stevens-Johnson syndrome and toxic epidermal necrolysis (see Warnings and Precautions).
Gastrointestinal: vomiting.
Hematopoietic and Lymphatic: leukopenia including neutropenia and agranulocytosis, thrombocytopenia.
Immunologic: face edema.
Body as a Whole: urticaria.
Liver/Biliary: hepatic failure, hepatitis, hepatocellular necrosis, jaundice.
Metabolic/Nutritional: hypercholesterolemia, hypertriglyceridemia, hypokalemia.

DRUG INTERACTIONS: Overview: Drug-Drug Interactions: Clinically or potentially significant drug interactions between fluconazole and the following agents/classes have been observed.

Benzodiazepines (short acting): Following oral or intravenous administration of midazolam, fluconazole resulted in substantial increases in midazolam concentrations and psychomotor effects. This effect on midazolam appears to be more pronounced following oral administration of fluconazole than with fluconazole administered intravenously. If concomitant benzodiazepine therapy, such as midazolam or triazolam, is necessary in patients being treated with fluconazole, consideration should be given to decreasing the benzodiazepine dosage.

Cimetidine: Absorption of orally administered fluconazole does not appear to be affected by gastric pH. Fluconazole 100 mg was administered as a single oral dose alone and two hours after a single dose of cimetidine 400 mg to six healthy male volunteers. After the administration of cimetidine, there was a significant decrease in fluconazole AUC (area under the plasma concentration-time curve) and C_{max}. There was a mean ± SD decrease in fluconazole AUC of 13%±11% (range: -3.4 to -31%) and C_{max} decreased 19%±14% (range: -5 to -40%). However, the administration of cimetidine 600 mg to 900 mg intravenously over a 4-hour period (from 1 hour before to 3 hours after a single oral dose of fluconazole 200 mg) did not affect the bioavailability or pharmacokinetics of fluconazole in 24 healthy male volunteers.

Coumarin-Type Anticoagulants: In a clinical trial, there was a significant increase in prothrombin time response (area under the prothrombin time-time curve) following a single dose of warfarin (15 mg) administered to 13 normal male volunteers following oral fluconazole 200 mg administered daily for 14 days as compared to the administration of warfarin alone. There was a mean ± SD increase in the prothrombin time response (area under the prothrombin time-time curve) of 7%±4% (range: -2 to 13%). Mean is based on data from 12 subjects as one of 13 subjects experienced a 2-fold increase in his prothrombin time response.

During the post-marketing experience, as with some azole antifungals, bleeding events (bruising, epistaxis, gastrointestinal bleeding, hematuria, and melena) have been reported, in association with increases in prothrombin time in patients receiving fluconazole concurrently with warfarin.

Prothrombin time may be increased in patients receiving concomitant fluconazole and coumarin-type anticoagulants.

Cyclosporine: Cyclosporine AUC and C_{max} were determined before and after the administration of fluconazole 200 mg daily for 14 days in eight renal transplant patients who had been on cyclosporine therapy for at least 6 months and on a stable cyclosporine dose for at least 6 weeks. There was a significant increase in cyclosporine AUC, C_{max}, C_{min} (24-hour concentration), and a significant reduction in apparent oral clearance following the administration of fluconazole. The mean ± SD increase in AUC was 92% ± 43% (range: 18 to 147%). The C_{max} increased 60%±48% range (range: -5 to 133%). The C_{min} increased 157%±96% (range: 33 to 360%). The apparent oral clearance decreased 45%±15% (range: -15 to -60%). Fluconazole administered at 100 mg daily dose does not affect cyclosporine pharmacokinetic levels in patients with bone marrow transplants. Fluconazole may significantly increase cyclosporine levels in renal transplant patients with or without renal impairment.

Drugs Prolonging the QTc Interval: The use of fluconazole in patients concurrently taking drugs metabolized by the Cytochrome P-450 system may be associated with elevations in the serum levels of these drugs.

Astemizole*: Definitive interaction studies with fluconazole have not been conducted. The use of fluconazole may be associated with elevations in the serum levels of astemizole. Caution should be used when coadministering fluconazole with astemizole. Patients should be carefully monitored.

Cisapride*: There have been reports of cardiac events including torsade de pointes in patients to whom fluconazole and cisapride were coadministered. A controlled study found that concomitant fluconazole 200 mg once daily and cisapride 20 mg four times a day yielded a significant increase in cisapride plasma levels and prolongation of QTc interval. Co-administration of cisapride is contraindicated in patients receiving fluconazole (see Contraindications).

Terfenadine*: Because of the occurrence of serious cardiac dysrhythmias secondary to prolongation of the QTc interval in patients receiving azole antifungals in conjunction with terfenadine, interaction studies have been performed. In one study, 6 healthy volunteers received terfenadine 60 mg BID for 15 days. Fluconazole 200 mg was administered daily from days 9 through 15. Fluconazole did not affect terfenadine plasma concentrations. Terfenadine acid metabolite AUC increased 36%±36% (range: 7 to 102%) from day 8 to day 15 with the concomitant administration of fluconazole. There was no change in cardiac repolarization as measured by Holter QTc intervals. However, another study at a 400 mg and 800 mg daily dose of fluconazole demonstrated that fluconazole taken in doses of 400 mg per day or greater significantly increases plasma levels of terfenadine when taken concomitantly. Therefore the combined use of fluconazole at doses of 400 mg or higher with terfenadine is contraindicated (see Contraindications). Patients should be carefully monitored if they are being concurrently prescribed fluconazole at multiple doses lower than 400 mg/day with terfenadine.

Hydrochlorothiazide: Concomitant oral administration of 100 mg fluconazole and 50 mg hydrochlorothiazide for 10 days in 13 normal volunteers resulted in a significant increase in fluconazole AUC and C_{max} compared to fluconazole given alone. There was a mean ± SD increase in fluconazole AUC and C_{max} of 45%±31% (range: 19 to 114%) and 43%±31% (range: 19 to 122%), respectively. These changes are attributed to a mean ± SD reduction in renal clearance of 30%±12% (range -10 to -50%).

Oral Contraceptives: Oral contraceptives were administered as a single dose both before and after the oral administration of fluconazole 50 mg once daily for 10 days in 10 healthy women. There was no significant difference in ethinyl estradiol or levonorgestrel AUC after the administration of fluconazole. The mean increase in ethinyl estradiol AUC was 6% (range: −47 to 108%) and levonorgestrel AUC increased 17% (range: −33 to 141%).

Twenty-five normal females received daily doses of both 200 mg fluconazole or placebo for two, ten-day periods. The treatment cycles were one month apart with all subjects receiving fluconazole during one cycle and placebo during the other. The order of study treatment was random. Single doses of an oral contraceptive tablet containing levonorgestrel and ethinyl estradiol were administered on the final treatment day (day 10) of both cycles. Following administration of 200 mg of fluconazole, the mean percentage increase of AUC for levonorgestrel compared to placebo was 25% (range: −12 to 82%) and the mean percentage increase for ethinyl estradiol compared to placebo was 38% (range: −11 to 101%). Both of these increases were statistically significantly different from placebo.

Oral Hypoglycemics: The effects of fluconazole on the pharmacokinetics of the sulfonylurea oral hypoglycemic agents tolbutamide, glipizide, and glyburide were evaluated in three placebo-controlled studies in normal volunteers. All subjects received the sulfonylurea alone as a single dose and again as a single dose following the administration of fluconazole 100 mg daily for 7 days. In these three studies, 22/46 (47.8%) of fluconazole-treated patients and 9/22 (40.1%) of placebo-treated patients experienced symptoms consistent with hypoglycemia.

Tolbutamide: In 13 normal male volunteers, there was a significant increase in tolbutamide (500 mg single dose) AUC and C_{max} following the administration of fluconazole. There was a mean ± SD increase in tolbutamide AUC of 26%±9% (range: 12 to 39%). Tolbutamide C_{max} increased 11%±9% (range: −6 to 27%).

Glipizide: The AUC and C_{max} of glipizide (2.5 mg single dose) were significantly increased following the administration of fluconazole in 13 normal male volunteers. There was a mean ± SD increase in AUC of 49%±13% (range: 27 to 73%) and an increase in C_{max} of 19%±23% (range: −11 to 79%).

Glyburide: The AUC and C_{max} of glyburide (5 mg single dose) were significantly increased following the administration of fluconazole in 20 normal male volunteers. There was a mean ± SD increase in AUC of 44%±29% (range: −13 to 115%) and C_{max} increased 19%±19% (range: −23 to 62%). Five subjects required oral glucose following the ingestion of glyburide after 7 days of fluconazole administration.

Clinically significant hypoglycemia may be precipitated by the use of fluconazole with oral hypoglycemic agents; one fatality has been reported from hypoglycemia in association with combined fluconazole and glyburide use. Fluconazole reduces the metabolism of tolbutamide, glyburide, and glipizide and increases the plasma concentration of these agents.

Phenytoin: Fluconazole increases the plasma concentrations of phenytoin. Phenytoin AUC was determined after 4 days of phenytoin dosing (200 mg daily, orally for 3 days, followed by 250 mg intravenously for one dose) both with and without the administration of fluconazole (oral fluconazole 200 mg daily for 16 days) in 10 normal male volunteers. The mean ± SD increase in phenytoin AUC was 88%±68% (range: 16 to 247%). The absolute magnitude of this interaction is unknown because of the intrinsically non-linear disposition of phenytoin.

Rifabutin: There have been reports that an interaction exists when fluconazole is administered concomitantly with rifabutin, leading to increased serum levels of rifabutin. There have been reports of uveitis in patients to whom fluconazole and rifabutin were coadministered.

Rifampin: Administration of a single oral 200 mg dose of fluconazole after 15 days of rifampin administered as 600 mg daily in 8 healthy male volunteers resulted in a significant decrease in fluconazole AUC and a significant increase in apparent oral clearance of fluconazole. There was a mean ± SD reduction in fluconazole AUC of 23%±9% (range: −13 to −42%). Apparent oral clearance of fluconazole increased 32%±17% (range: 16 to 72%). Fluconazole half-life decreased from 33.4±4.4 hours to 26.8±3.9 hours.

Rifampin enhances the metabolism of concurrently administered fluconazole.

Tacrolimus: There have been reports that an interaction exists when fluconazole is administered concomitantly with tacrolimus, leading to increased serum levels of tacrolimus. There have been reports of nephrotoxicity in patients to whom fluconazole and tacrolimus were coadministered.

Theophylline: The pharmacokinetics of theophylline were determined from a single intravenous dose of aminophylline (6 mg/kg) before and after the oral administration of fluconazole 200 mg daily for 14 days in 16 normal male volunteers. There were significant increases in theophylline AUC, C_{max} and half-life with a corresponding decrease in clearance. The mean ± SD theophylline AUC increased 21%±16% (range: −5 to 48%). The C_{max} increased 13%±17% (range: −13 to 40%). Theophylline clearance decreased 16%±11% (range: −32 to 5%). The half-life of theophylline increased from 6.6±1.7 hours to 7.9±1.5 hours.

Zidovudine: Plasma zidovudine concentrations were determined on two occasions (before and following fluconazole 200 mg daily for 15 days) in 13 volunteers with AIDS or ARC who were on a stable zidovudine dose for at least two weeks. There was a significant increase in zidovudine AUC following the administration of fluconazole. The mean ± SD increase in AUC was 20%±32% (range: −27 to 104%). The metabolite, GZDV, to parent drug ratio significantly decreased after the administration of fluconazole, from 7.6±3.6 to 5.7±2.2.

Drugs Exhibiting No Significant Pharmacokinetic Interactions with Fluconazole: Antacids: Administration of Maalox (20 mL) to 14 normal male volunteers immediately prior to a single dose of fluconazole 100 mg had no effect on the absorption or elimination of fluconazole.

Interaction studies with other medications have not been conducted, but such interactions may occur.

Drug-Food Interactions: Interactions with foods have not been established.

Drug-Herb Interactions: Interactions with herbal products have not been established.

DOSAGE AND ADMINISTRATION: **Dosing Considerations:** The recommended dosage of DIFLUCAN 150 for vaginal candidiasis is 150 mg as a single oral dose.

Recommended Dose and Dosage Adjustment: There is no need to adjust single dose therapy for vaginal candidiasis because of impaired renal function.

OVERDOSAGE:

Symptoms: There have been reports of overdosage with fluconazole and in one reported case, a 42-year-old patient infected with human immunodeficiency virus developed hallucinations and exhibited paranoid behaviour after reportedly ingesting 8200 mg of fluconazole. The patient was admitted to the hospital, and his condition resolved within 48 hours.

Treatment: In the event of overdose, symptomatic treatment (with supportive measures and gastric lavage if necessary) may be adequate. Fluconazole is largely excreted in urine. A three hour hemodialysis session decreases plasma levels by approximately 50%.

Mice and rats receiving very high doses of fluconazole, whether orally or intravenously, displayed a variety of nonspecific, agonal signs such as decreased activity, ataxia, shallow respiration, ptosis, lacrimation, salivation, urinary incontinence and cyanosis. Death was sometimes preceded by clonic convulsions.

> For management of a suspected drug overdose, CPhA recommends that you contact your **regional Poison Control Centre**. See the *CPS* Directory section for a list of Poison Control Centres.

ACTION AND CLINICAL PHARMACOLOGY: Mechanism of Action: Fluconazole is a highly selective inhibitor of fungal cytochrome P-450 sterol C-14-α-demethylation. Mammalian cell demethylation is much less sensitive to fluconazole inhibition. The subsequent loss of normal sterols correlates with the accumulation of 14-α-methyl sterols in fungi and may be responsible for the fungistatic activity of fluconazole.

Pharmacodynamics: The effects of fluconazole on the metabolism of carbohydrates, lipids, adrenal and gonadal hormones were assessed. In normal volunteers, fluconazole administration at doses ranging from 200 to 400 mg once daily for up to 14 days was associated with small and inconsistent effects on testosterone concentrations, endogenous corticosteroid concentrations, and the ACTH-stimulated cortisol response. In addition, fluconazole appears to have no clinically significant effects on carbohydrate or lipid metabolism in man.

Pharmacokinetics: Fluconazole is a polar bis-triazole antifungal drug. Studies have shown that fluconazole exhibits specificity as an inhibitor of the fungal as opposed to mammalian cytochrome P-450 mediated reactions, including those involved in steroid biosynthesis and drug metabolism. Many of the clinical advantages of fluconazole are a result of its unique pharmacokinetic properties.

Absorption: The pharmacokinetic properties of fluconazole are similar following administration by the intravenous or oral routes and do not appear to be affected by gastric pH. In normal volunteers, the bioavailability of orally administered fluconazole is over 90% compared with intravenous administration. Essentially all of the administered drug reaches systemic circulation; thus, there is no evidence of first-pass metabolism of the drug. In addition, no adjustment in dosage is necessary when changing from p.o. to i.v. or vice versa.

Peak plasma concentrations (C_{max}) in fasted normal volunteers occur rapidly following oral administration, usually between 1 and 2 hours of dosing with a terminal plasma elimination half-life of approximately 30 hours (range 20-50 hours) after oral administration. The long plasma elimination half-life provides the basis for once daily dosing with fluconazole in the treatment of fungal infections.

In fasted normal volunteers, administration of a single oral 150 mg dose of fluconazole produced a mean C_{max} of 2.70 μg/mL (range: 1.91 to 3.70 μg/mL).

In normal volunteers, oral bioavailability as measured by C_{max} and AUC was not affected by food when fluconazole was administered as a single 50 mg capsule; however, T_{max} was doubled.

Distribution: The apparent volume of distribution of fluconazole approximates that of total body water. Plasma protein binding is low (11-12%) and is constant over the concentration range tested (0.1 mg/L to 10 mg/L). This degree of protein binding is not clinically meaningful.

A single oral 150 mg dose of fluconazole administered to 27 patients penetrated into vaginal tissue, resulting in tissue: plasma ratios ranging from 0.94 to 1.14 over the first 48 hours following dosing.

A single oral 150 mg dose of fluconazole administered to 14 patients penetrated into vaginal fluid, resulting in fluid: plasma ratios ranging from 0.36 to 0.71 over the first 72 hours following dosing.

Metabolism and Excretion: Fluconazole is cleared primarily by renal excretion, with approximately 80% of the administered dose appearing in the urine as unchanged drug. Following administration of radiolabelled fluconazole, greater than 90% of the radioactivity is excreted in the urine. Approximately 11% of the radioactivity in urine is due to metabolites. An additional 2% of the total radioactivity is excreted in feces.

The pharmacokinetics of fluconazole do not appear to be affected by age alone but are markedly affected by reduction in renal function. There is an inverse relationship between the elimination half-life and creatinine clearance. There is no need to adjust single dose therapy for vaginal candidiasis because of impaired renal function.

STORAGE AND STABILITY: DIFLUCAN 150 Capsules (fluconazole) 150 mg: Store between 15-30°C.

INFORMATION FOR THE PATIENT: Published in e-CPS, available by subscription at www.e-cps.ca.

DOSAGE FORMS, COMPOSITION AND PACKAGING: Each hard white gelatin capsule, marked with Pfizer logo, contains: fluconazole 150 mg. Nonmedicinal ingredients: colloidal silicon dioxide, lactose, magnesium stearate, maize starch and sodium lauryl sulfate; capsule shell: gelatin and titanium dioxide. Unit dose blister packs of 1.

(Shown in Product Identification Section)

Diflucortolone ℞

CPhA Monograph

see *Corticosteroids: Topical*

Diflunisal ℞

Nonsteroidal Anti-inflammatory Agent

CPhA Monograph

Date of Preparation: November 2004
Date of Revision: October 2010

> This monograph has been compiled by CPhA and reviewed by experts. It may contain information different from that found in Health Canada-approved Product Monographs. The reader is referred to the *CPS* Editorial Policy for more information.

SUMMARY PRODUCT INFORMATION:

Route of Administration	Dosage Form	Strength
Oral	Tablet	250 mg, 500 mg

INDICATIONS AND CLINICAL USE: Health Canada approved indications include:

- Relief of mild to moderate pain accompanied by inflammation in conditions such as musculoskeletal trauma, post-dental extraction or post-episiotomy. Single doses of diflunisal provide analgesia similar to that of other nonsteroidal anti-inflammatory drugs (NSAIDs) for a duration of about 12 hours.
- Symptomatic relief of osteoarthritis and rheumatoid arthritis.

NSAIDs do not prevent disease progression and will only decrease inflammation (and thus relieve symptoms) for as long as the patient continues to take the drug.

Geriatrics: Diflunisal should be used with caution in individuals 65 years of age or older since increasing age may be associated with increased risk of adverse reactions. See Warnings and Precautions.

Pediatrics: Safety and efficacy of diflunisal in children have not been established. Use of the drug in children younger than 12 years of age is not recommended. Because diflunisal is a derivative of salicylic acid, the possibility that diflunisal may be associated with an increased risk of developing Reye's syndrome in children with varicella infections or influenza-type illnesses cannot be excluded.

CONTRAINDICATIONS: Active peptic ulcer, a history of recurrent ulceration, or active inflammatory disease of the GI system. Known or suspected hypersensitivity to the drug or other nonsteroidal anti-inflammatory drugs. The potential for cross-reactivity between different NSAIDs must be kept in mind.

Diflunisal should not be used in patients with the complete or partial syndrome of ASA-intolerance (rhinosinusitis, urticaria/angioedema, nasal polyps, asthma) in whom asthma, anaphylaxis, urticaria/angioedema, rhinitis or other allergic manifestations are precipitated by ASA or other nonsteroidal anti-inflammatory agents. Fatal anaphylactoid reactions have occurred in such individuals. As well, individuals with the above medical problems are at risk of a severe reaction even if they have taken NSAIDs in the past without any adverse effects.

Significant hepatic impairment or active liver disease.

Severely impaired or deteriorating renal function (creatinine clearance <30 mL/min). Individuals with lesser degrees of renal impairment are at risk of deterioration of their renal function when prescribed NSAIDs and must be monitored.

Diflunisal should not be used in the presence of known hyperkalemia (also see Warnings and Precautions, Fluid and Electrolyte Balance).

Perioperatively in coronary artery bypass graft (CABG) surgery; other NSAIDs studied in this setting showed an increased incidence of cardiovascular thromboembolic events, deep surgical infections and sternal wound complications.

Diflunisal is not recommended for use with other NSAIDs because of the absence of evidence demonstrating synergistic benefits and the potential for additive side effects.

WARNINGS AND PRECAUTIONS: General: Aseptic Meningitis: In occasional cases, with some NSAIDs, the symptoms of aseptic meningitis (stiff neck, severe headaches, nausea and vomiting, fever or clouding of consciousness) have been observed. Patients with autoimmune disorders (systemic lupus erythematosus, mixed connective tissues diseases, etc.) seem to be predisposed. Therefore, in such patients, the health provider must be vigilant to the development of this complication.

Infection: In common with other anti-inflammatory drugs, diflunisal may suppress fever.

Reye's Syndrome: ASA has been associated with Reye's syndrome. Because diflunisal is a derivative of salicylic acid, the possibility of its association with Reye's syndrome cannot be excluded.

Cardiovascular: Some patients may develop new-onset hypertension, and those with pre-existing hypertension may develop worsening of blood pressure control when placed on an NSAID. Regular monitoring of blood pressure should be performed under such circumstances. NSAIDs may exacerbate heart failure.

The risk of cardiovascular complications in patients receiving NSAIDs is not clearly defined. Use of some NSAIDs has been associated with an increased risk of serious cardiovascular adverse effects (myocardial infarction, stroke, thrombotic events). Patients with pre-existing cardiovascular disease or cardiovascular risk factors and those with a longer duration of therapy may be at higher risk. Short-term use of NSAIDs, especially at low doses, does not appear to be associated with an increased risk of serious cardiovascular events except immediately following coronary artery bypass graft (CABG) surgery.

Fluid and Electrolyte Balance: Fluid retention and edema have been observed in patients treated with diflunisal. Therefore, as with many other NSAIDs, the possibility of precipitating heart failure in elderly patients or those with compromised cardiac function should be borne in mind. Diflunisal should be used with caution in patients with heart failure, hypertension or other conditions predisposing to fluid retention. Ask patients who are at risk for fluid retention to weigh themselves at regular intervals to assist in monitoring for fluid accumulation. With nonsteroidal anti-inflammatory treatment there is a potential risk of hyperkalemia, particularly in patients with conditions such as diabetes mellitus or renal failure; elderly patients; or in patients receiving concomitant therapy with angiotensin-II receptor antagonists, adrenergic blockers, angiotensin-converting enzyme inhibitors or potassium-sparing diuretics. Patients at risk should be monitored periodically during long-term therapy.

Dependence/Tolerance/Withdrawal: Habituation, tolerance and addiction have not been reported.

Gastrointestinal: Serious GI toxicity, such as ulceration, perforation, obstruction and gastrointestinal bleeding, sometimes severe and occasionally fatal, can occur at any time, with or without symptoms in patients treated with NSAIDs including diflunisal. While upper GI events are more common, NSAIDs may cause toxicity throughout the gastrointestinal tract.

GI symptoms, such as dyspepsia, are common, usually developing early in therapy. Health providers should remain alert for ulceration and bleeding in patients treated with NSAIDs, even in the absence of previous GI tract symptoms.

In patients observed in clinical trials of NSAIDs, symptomatic upper GI ulcers, gross bleeding, or perforation appear to occur in approximately 1% of patients treated for 3 to 6 months and in about 2% to 4% of patients treated for 1 year. The risk continues beyond 1 year. The incidence of these complications is related to dose, past history of known ulcer disease, and advanced age (see Special Populations).

Diflunisal should be given under close medical supervision to patients with a history of ulcer of the upper gastrointestinal tract or inflammatory disease of the gastrointestinal tract such as ulcerative colitis and Crohn's disease. In these cases the health provider must weigh the benefits of treatment against the possible hazards.

Health providers should inform patients about the signs and symptoms of serious GI toxicity and instruct them to contact a health provider immediately if they experience persistent dyspepsia or other symptoms or signs suggestive of gastrointestinal ulceration or bleeding. Because serious GI tract ulceration and bleeding can occur without warning symptoms, health providers should follow chronically treated patients and watch for the signs and symptoms of ulceration and bleeding and should inform the patients of the importance of this follow-up. If ulceration is suspected or confirmed, or if GI bleeding occurs, diflunisal should be discontinued immediately, appropriate treatment instituted and the patient monitored closely.

No studies, to date, have identified any group of patients not at risk of developing ulceration and bleeding. The major risk factors are a prior history of serious GI events and increasing age. Possible risks factors include *H. pylori* infection, long-term NSAID use, excess alcohol intake, smoking, and concomitant use of oral corticosteroids, anticoagulants, antiplatelet agents (including ASA), or selective serotonin reuptake inhibitors (SSRIs).

Genitourinary: Some NSAIDs are associated with persistent urinary symptoms (bladder pain, dysuria, urinary frequency), hematuria or cystitis. The onset of these symptoms may occur at any time after the initiation of therapy with an NSAID. Should urinary symptoms occur, in the absence of an alternate explanation, treatment with diflunisal should be stopped to ascertain if symptoms disappear. This should be done before urological investigations or treatments are considered.

Hematologic: Drugs inhibiting prostaglandin biosynthesis interfere with platelet function to varying degrees; therefore, patients who may be adversely affected by such an action, such as those on anticoagulants or suffering from hemophilia or platelet disorders should be carefully observed when diflunisal is administered.

Antiplatelet agents are used for the prevention of thrombosis or to reduce the risk of nonfatal myocardial infarction (MI), nonfatal cerebral thrombosis or embolism, and death in the following clinical situations: acute MI, secondary prevention following MI, patients with a history of transient ischemic attack(s), ischemic stroke, chronic stable angina, unstable angina or coronary artery disease. Whether antiplatelet agents confer significant benefit as primary prevention in low-risk patient populations remains unclear.

Antiplatelet agents are used to prevent thrombotic complications in patients undergoing procedures such as coronary angioplasty, coronary artery bypass or carotid endarterectomy. They are used to prevent thrombosis in patients with atrial fibrillation who cannot take warfarin. Diflunisal and other NSAIDs have no proven efficacy as antiplatelet agents and cannot be used as a substitute for acetylsalicylic acid (ASA) or other antiplatelet agents under these conditions.

Concomitant administration of diflunisal with low-dose ASA increases the risk of GI ulceration and associated complications. If the two drugs must be used together, extra caution is warranted.

Blood dyscrasias (such as neutropenia, leukopenia, thrombocytopenia, aplastic anemia and agranulocytosis) associated with the use of NSAIDs are rare, but could occur with severe consequences.

Hepatic/Biliary/Pancreatic: As with other NSAIDs, borderline elevations of one or more liver enzyme tests (AST, ALT, ALP) may occur in up to 15% of patients. These abnormalities may progress, may remain essentially unchanged, or may be transient with continued therapy.

A patient with symptoms and/or signs suggesting liver dysfunction, or in whom an abnormal liver test has occurred, should be evaluated for evidence of the development of a more severe hepatic reaction while on therapy with this drug. Severe hepatic reactions including jaundice and cases of fatal hepatitis have been reported with NSAIDs.

Although such reactions are rare, if abnormal liver tests persist or worsen, if clinical signs and symptoms consistent with liver disease develop (e.g., jaundice), or if systemic manifestations occur (e.g., eosinophilia, associated with rash, etc.), the drug should be discontinued.

If there is a need to prescribe this drug in the presence of impaired liver function, it must be done under strict observation.

Immune: Cross-sensitivity: Patients sensitive to any one of the NSAIDs may be sensitive to any of the other NSAIDs also.

ASA-Intolerance: As with NSAIDs in general, some patients may experience urticaria and angioedema upon exposure to diflunisal. Diflunisal should not be given to patients with the complete or partial syndrome of ASA-intolerance (see Contraindications).

Serious Skin Reactions: In rare cases, serious skin reactions such as Stevens-Johnson syndrome, toxic epidermal necrolysis, exfoliative dermatitis and erythema multiforme have been associated with the use of some NSAIDs. Because the incidence of these reactions is low, they have usually been noted during post-marketing surveillance in patients taking other medications also associated with the potential development of these serious skin reactions. Thus, causality is not clear. These reactions are potentially life threatening but may be reversible if the causative agent is discontinued and appropriate treatment instituted. Patients should be advised that if they experience a skin rash they should discontinue the NSAID and contact their physician for assessment and advice, including which additional therapies to discontinue.

Ophthalmologic: Blurred and/or diminished vision has been reported with the use of diflunisal and other NSAIDs. If such symptoms develop, the drug should be discontinued and an ophthalmologic examination performed; ophthalmic examination should be carried out at periodic intervals in any patient receiving this drug for an extended period of time.

Renal: Long-term administration of NSAIDs to animals has resulted in renal papillary necrosis and other abnormal renal pathology. In humans, there have been reports of acute interstitial nephritis with hematuria, proteinuria, and occasionally nephrotic syndrome.

A second form of renal toxicity has been seen in patients with pre-renal conditions leading to the reduction in renal blood flow or blood volume, where the renal prostaglandins have a supportive role in the maintenance of renal perfusion. In these patients, administration of an NSAID may cause a dose-dependent reduction in prostaglandin formation and may precipitate overt renal decompensation. Patients at greatest risk of this reaction are those with impaired renal function (GFR <60 mL/min or 1 mL/s), patients on salt-restricted diets, those with heart failure, cirrhosis or liver dysfunction, those taking diuretics, angiotensin-converting enzyme inhibitors, angiotensin-II receptor blockers, cyclosporine or ASA and the elderly. Serious or life-threatening renal failure has been reported in patients with normal or impaired renal function after short-term therapy with NSAIDs. Even patients at risk who demonstrate the ability to tolerate an NSAID under stable conditions may decompensate during periods of added stress, for example during states of fluid restriction as can occur during gastroenteritis. Discontinuation of NSAID therapy is usually followed by recovery to the pretreatment state.

NSAIDs can increase the risk of hyperkalemia (see Fluid and Electrolyte Balance). In patients on dialysis, NSAIDs should be used with caution.

Respiratory: ASA-induced asthma is an uncommon but very important indication of ASA and NSAID sensitivity. It occurs more frequently in patients with asthma who have nasal polyps.

Special Populations: Pregnant Women: Until more is known about the safety of diflunisal, it should not be used during pregnancy. A positive association has been reported between NSAIDs and spontaneous abortions. It is suggested that diflunisal not be used in women attempting to conceive as it blocks blastocyte implantation in animals.

In the latter half of pregnancy, due to the diverse recorded and potential effects of NSAIDs such as premature closure of the ductus arteriosus and pulmonary hypertension or oligohydramnios, the use of these agents should be avoided. If therapeutic use in pregnancy is required, the pregnancy should be managed by obstetricians or other health providers with particular expertise in high-risk pregnancies.

Nursing Women: Diflunisal is excreted in human milk in concentrations of 2% to 7% of those in plasma. Experience with the use of diflunisal in lactating women is not available. Shorter-acting agents with more available published information (e.g., ibuprofen) may be preferable, especially while nursing a newborn or preterm infant.

Pediatrics: Safety and efficacy of diflunisal in children have not been established. Use of the drug in children younger than 12 years of age is not recommended. Because diflunisal is a derivative of salicylic acid, the possibility that diflunisal may be associated with an increased risk of developing Reye's syndrome in children with varicella infections or influenza-type illnesses cannot be excluded.

Geriatrics: Patients older than 65 years and frail or debilitated patients are most susceptible to a variety of adverse reactions from NSAIDs; the incidence of these adverse reactions increases with dose and duration of treatment. In addition, these patients are less tolerant of ulceration and bleeding. Most reports of fatal GI events are in this population, especially those with cardiovascular disease. Older patients are also at risk of lower esophageal ulceration and bleeding.

For such patients, consider a starting dose lower than the one usually recommended, with individual adjustment when necessary and under close supervision.

Monitoring and Laboratory Tests: Diflunisal may cause falsely elevated values of serum salicylate when measured by various laboratory assays; therefore, serum salicylate concentrations should be interpreted with caution in patients receiving diflunisal.

Occupational Hazards: Some patients may experience drowsiness, dizziness, blurred vision, vertigo, tinnitus or hearing loss with the use of diflunisal. If patients experience these side effects, they should exercise caution in carrying out activities that require alertness.

ACTION AND CLINICAL PHARMACOLOGY: Diflunisal is a nonsteroidal drug with analgesic, anti-inflammatory and antipyretic properties. The exact mechanisms have not been clearly established, but many of the actions appear to be associated principally with inhibition of prostaglandin synthesis. Diflunisal is a nonselective inhibitor of cyclooxygenase-1 (COX-1) and cyclooxygenase-2 (COX-2), which catalyze the formation of prostaglandins in the arachidonic acid pathway. Diflunisal appears to exert analgesic, anti-inflammatory and antipyretic activity principally through inhibition of the COX-2 isoenzyme; COX-1 inhibition may be responsible for the gastrointestinal adverse effects of the drug and platelet aggregation.

As is the case with salicylic acid, concentration-dependent pharmacokinetics prevail when diflunisal is administered; a doubling of dosage produces a greater than doubling of drug accumulation. The effect becomes more apparent with repetitive doses. Following single doses, peak plasma concentrations of 41±11 µg/mL (mean±S.D.) were observed following 250 mg doses, 87±17 µg/mL were observed following 500 mg and 124±11 µg/mL following single 1000 mg doses. However, following administration of 250 mg twice a day, a mean peak level of 56±14 µg/mL was observed on day 8, while the mean peak level after 500 mg twice a day for 11 days was 190±33 µg/mL. The plasma half-life of diflunisal is 8 to 12 hours. Because of its long half-life and nonlinear pharmacokinetics, several days are required for diflunisal plasma levels to reach steady state following multiple doses. For this reason, an initial loading dose is necessary to shorten the time to reach steady state levels, and 2 to 3 days of observation are necessary for evaluating changes in treatment regimens if a loading dose is not used.

Pharmacokinetics: Absorption: Diflunisal is rapidly and completely absorbed following oral administration, with peak plasma concentrations occurring between 2 to 3 hours.

Distribution: At least 98% to 99% of diflunisal in plasma is bound to proteins. In healthy individuals, diflunisal has an apparent volume of distribution of 7.53 L.

Metabolism: Diflunisal is metabolized in the liver to glucuronide conjugates. The drug is not metabolized to salicylic acid.

Excretion: In healthy adults, the plasma half-life of diflunisal ranges from 8 to 12 hours. Diflunisal is excreted in the urine as 2 soluble glucuronide conjugates accounting for about 90% of the administered dose. Little or no diflunisal is excreted in the feces.

Special Populations: Renal Insufficiency: The volume of distribution reportedly has increased to 16.2 L in patients with impaired renal function.

ADVERSE REACTIONS: Adverse Drug Reaction Overview: The most common adverse reactions encountered with NSAIDs are gastrointestinal, of which gastric or duodenal ulcer, with or without bleeding, is the most severe. Fatalities have occurred, particularly in the elderly.

Table 1: Diflunisal
Adverse Reactions

3–9%	1–3%	<1%
Gastrointestinal		
Nausea, dyspepsia, GI pain, diarrhea	Vomiting, constipation, flatulence	Peptic ulcer, GI bleeding, anorexia, GI perforation, gastritis
CNS/Psychiatric		
Headache	Dizziness, somnolence, insomnia	Disorientation, vertigo, lightheadedness, paresthesia, nervousness, depression, hallucinations, confusion
Dermatologic		
Rash		Erythema multiforme, Stevens-Johnson syndrome, toxic epidermal necrolysis, exfoliative dermatitis, pruritus, sweating, dry mucous membranes, stomatitis, photosensitivity, urticaria
Special Senses		
	Tinnitus	Transient visual disturbance (including blurred vision)
Hematologic		
		Thrombocytopenia, leukopenia, pancytopenia, agranulocytosis (rarely), hemolytic anemia (rarely)
Renal		
		Cystitis, dysuria, renal impairment (including renal failure), interstitial nephritis, hematuria, proteinuria
Hepatic		
		Jaundice, cholestasis, liver function abnormalities, hepatitis
Miscellaneous		
	Fatigue	Asthenia, edema
Hypersensitivity		
		Acute anaphylactic reaction with bronchospasm, angioedema, hypersensitivity vasculitis, hypersensitivity syndrome

Respiratory: dyspnea.

Cardiovascular: peripheral edema, palpitation, syncope, hypertension, hypotension, heart failure, chest pain, myocardial infarction, arrhythmias.

Miscellaneous: fever, fulminant necrotizing fasciitis, hearing loss, muscle cramps.

Renal: nephrotic syndrome.

DRUG INTERACTIONS: Overview: Diflunisal is highly protein-bound and may displace other highly protein-bound drugs from binding sites. Diflunisal shares some of the drug-drug interactions of other NSAIDs (see Table 2).

Table 2: Diflunisal
Drug-Drug Interactions

Interacting Drug	Effect	Clinical Comment
ACE inhibitors	NSAIDs may diminish the antihypertensive effect of angiotensin-converting enzyme (ACE) inhibitors. Combinations of ACE inhibitors, diuretics and NSAIDs might have an increased risk for acute renal failure and hyperkalemia.	Blood pressure and kidney function should be monitored more closely in this situation, as occasionally there can be a substantial increase in blood pressure.
Acetaminophen	Concomitant administration of diflunisal and acetaminophen to normal volunteers resulted in significantly increased (50%) plasma levels of acetaminophen. Acetaminophen had no effect on plasma levels of diflunisal.	Since acetaminophen in high doses has been associated with hepatotoxicity, concomitant administration of diflunisal and acetaminophen should be used cautiously, with careful monitoring of patients.
Alcohol	There may be an increased risk of GI side effects (including ulceration or GI bleeding) if alcohol is ingested with NSAIDs.	Avoid.
Antacids	Regular administration of aluminum- and/or magnesium hydroxide-containing antacids may reduce plasma levels of diflunisal.	Not likely to be clinically significant with occasional doses of antacids.
Anticoagulants, oral	Numerous studies have shown that the concomitant use of NSAIDs and anticoagulants increases the risk of GI adverse events, such as ulceration and bleeding. The combination may result in prolonged prothrombin times.	Concurrent therapy of diflunisal and warfarin requires close monitoring of INR. Even with therapeutic INR monitoring, increased bleeding may occur.
Antiplatelet agents (e.g., ASA, clopidogrel)	Use of diflunisal with antiplatelet agents may increase bleeding risk (see Warnings and Precautions, Hematologic). Concomitant administration of diflunisal and antiplatelet agents increases the risk for serious GI events.	Some NSAIDs may interfere with the antiplatelet effects of low dose ASA, possibly by competing with ASA for access to the active site of cyclooxygenase-1.
ASA	See Antiplatelet Agents, NSAIDs	
Clopidogrel	See Antiplatelet Agents	
Cyclosporine	Concomitant administration of an NSAID and cyclosporine may increase the nephrotoxic effects of cyclosporine.	This interaction may be related to inhibition of the synthesis of a renal prostaglandin (e.g., prostacyclin). Use concomitantly with caution and monitor renal function closely.
Diuretics	Clinical studies as well as postmarketing observations have shown that NSAIDs can reduce the clinical effects of diuretics.	In normal volunteers, the concomitant administration of diflunisal and furosemide had no effect on the diuretic activity of furosemide. Diflunisal decreased the hyperuricemic effect of furosemide. In normal volunteers, concomitant administration of diflunisal and hydrochlorothiazide resulted in significantly increased plasma levels of hydrochlorothiazide. Diflunisal decreased the hyperuricemic effect of hydrochlorothiazide.
Glucocorticoids	Some studies have shown that the concomitant use of NSAIDs and oral glucocorticoids increases the risk of GI side effects such as ulceration and bleeding.	This is especially the case in older individuals (>65 years of age). Consider cytoprotection with a proton pump inhibitor or misoprostol [*Am J Gastroenterol* 2009;104(3):728-38] to reduce the risk of upper GI tract toxicity.
Lithium	Increased lithium concentrations can occur.	Monitoring of plasma lithium concentrations is advised when stopping or starting an NSAID.
Methotrexate	NSAIDs have been reported to decrease the tubular secretion of methotrexate and potentiate the toxicity.	Avoid the concomitant use of high dose methotrexate; with low dose weekly methotrexate for treatment of inflammatory arthritis, use the combination with caution and monitor for signs and symptoms of toxicity.
NSAIDs	Potential for additive adverse effects.	The use of diflunisal in addition to any other NSAID, including nonprescription agents (e.g., ASA, ibuprofen, naproxen) is not recommended because of the absence of evidence demonstrating synergistic benefits and the potential for additive side effects. In normal volunteers, a small decrease in diflunisal levels was observed when multiple doses of diflunisal and ASA were administered concomitantly. Indomethacin: The administration of diflunisal to normal volunteers receiving indomethacin decreased the renal clearance and significantly increased the plasma levels of indomethacin. Further, the combined use of indomethacin and diflunisal has been associated with fatal GI hemorrhage. Therefore, indomethacin and diflunisal should not be used concomitantly. Ketorolac: Concomitant administration is contraindicated due to the additive risk of serious NSAID toxicities. Naproxen: The concomitant administration of diflunisal and naproxen in normal volunteers had no effect on the plasma levels of naproxen, but significantly decreased the urinary excretion of naproxen and its glucuronide metabolite. Naproxen had no effect on plasma levels of diflunisal. Sulindac: The concomitant administration of diflunisal and sulindac in normal volunteers resulted in lowering of the plasma levels of the active sulfide metabolite by approximately one-third.
Probenecid	Drug clearance and protein binding of diflunisal are decreased.	Monitor for increased diflunisal toxicity.

Drug-Herb Interactions: Use caution with concomitant use of diflunisal and natural health products with anticoagulant or antiplatelet properties including evening primrose oil, feverfew, garlic, ginger, gingko, ginseng, willow bark and others. Monitor for signs of bleeding. Concomitant use may predispose patients to more adverse effects of NSAIDs (gastropathy, increased risk of bleeding).

Drug-Laboratory Test Interactions: Although diflunisal is not metabolized to salicylate, it may cause falsely elevated serum salicylate levels with some assays.

DOSAGE AND ADMINISTRATION:

Dosing Considerations: Diflunisal has slow onset and long duration of action. Diflunisal produces significant analgesia in 1 hour and maximum analgesia in 2 to 4 hours. Analgesic effect lasts 8 to 12 hours. These characteristics should be considered when prescribing the drug.

Recommended Dose and Dosage Adjustment:

Table 3: Diflunisal
Dose in Adult Patients

Indication	Usual Dose	Maximum Dose	Comment
Mild to moderate pain	500 mg every 12 hours		A lower dosage may be appropriate depending on such factors as pain severity, patient response, weight, or advanced age; for example, 500 mg initially, followed by 250 mg every 12 hours.
Osteoarthritis and rheumatoid arthritis	500 mg to 1000 mg daily in 2 divided doses according to patient response.	1000 mg daily	

Dose in Adult Patients with Renal Impairment: In patients with creatinine clearance <50 mL/min, administer 50% of the normal dose.

Administration: Oral: Tablets should be swallowed whole, not crushed or chewed. Diflunisal may be administered with water, milk or meals.

OVERDOSAGE: Ingestion of 15 g has caused death but the usual lethal dose is not known. Signs and symptoms of acute diflunisal overdose may include drowsiness, vomiting, diarrhea, hyperventilation, tachycardia, diaphoresis, tinnitus, stupor, coma, diminished urine output and cardiopulmonary arrest.

For management of a suspected drug overdose, CPhA recommends that you contact your **regional Poison Control Centre**. See the *CPS* Directory section for a list of Poison Control Centres.

Digibind® Ⓟ

digoxin immune Fab (ovine)

Specific Antibody for Digoxin

GlaxoSmithKline

Date of Revision: May 25, 2009

SUMMARY PRODUCT INFORMATION:

Route of Administration	Dosage Form/ Strength	Clinically Relevant Nonmedicinal Ingredients
Intravenous	Sterile lyophilized powder/38 mg of digoxin-specific Fab fragments	Sorbitol and sodium chloride.

INDICATIONS AND CLINICAL USE: DIGIBIND, Digoxin Immune Fab (Ovine) is indicated for:

- treatment of potentially life-threatening digoxin toxicity. Although designed specifically to treat life-threatening digoxin toxicity, it has also been used successfully to treat life-threatening toxicity due to digitoxin. Since human experience is limited the consequences of repeated exposures are unknown, DIGIBIND is not indicated for milder cases of digitalis toxicity.

Manifestations of life-threatening toxicity include severe ventricular arrhythmias such as ventricular tachycardia or ventricular fibrillation, or progressive bradyarrhythmias such as severe sinus bradycardia, or second- or third-degree heart block not responsive to atropine.

Ingestion of more than 10 mg of digoxin in previously healthy adults or 4 mg of digoxin in previously healthy children, or ingestion causing steady-state serum concentrations greater than 10 ng/mL, often results in cardiac arrest. Digitalis-induced progressive elevation of the serum potassium concentration also suggests imminent cardiac arrest. If the potassium concentration exceeds 5 mEq/L in the setting of severe digitalis intoxication, DIGIBIND therapy is indicated.

CONTRAINDICATIONS: There are no known contraindications to the use of DIGIBIND, Digoxin Immune Fab (Ovine).

WARNINGS AND PRECAUTIONS: General: Suicidal ingestion often involves more than one drug; thus, toxicity from other drugs should not be overlooked.

One should consider the possibility of anaphylactic, hypersensitivity or febrile reactions to DIGIBIND, Digoxin Immune Fab (Ovine). If an anaphylactoid reaction occurs, the drug infusion should be discontinued and appropriate therapy initiated using aminophylline, oxygen, volume expansion, diphenhydramine, corticosteroids and airway management as indicated. The need for epinephrine should be balanced against its potential risk in the setting of digitalis toxicity.

Since the Fab fragment of the antibody lacks the antigenic determinants of the Fc fragment, it should pose less of an immunogenic threat to patients than does an intact immunoglobulin molecule. Patients with known allergies would be particularly at risk, as would individuals who have previously received antibodies or Fab fragments raised in sheep.

Papain is used to cleave the whole antibody into Fab and Fc fragments, and traces of papain or inactivated papain residues may be present in DIGIBIND. Patients with allergies to papain, chymopapain, or other papaya extracts also may be particularly at risk.

Skin testing for allergy was performed during the clinical investigation of DIGIBIND. Only one patient developed erythema at the site of skin testing, with no accompanying wheal reaction; this individual had no adverse reaction to systemic treatment with DIGIBIND. Since allergy testing can delay urgently needed therapy, it is not routinely required before treatment of life-threatening digitalis toxicity with DIGIBIND.

Skin Testing: Skin testing may be appropriate for high risk individuals, especially patients with known allergies or those previously treated with DIGIBIND. The intradermal skin test can be performed by:

1. Diluting 0.1 mL of reconstituted DIGIBIND (9.5 mg/mL) in 9.9 mL sterile isotonic saline (1:100 dilution, 95 µg/mL).
2. Injecting 0.1 mL of the 1:100 dilution (9.5 µg) intradermally and observing for an urticarial wheal surrounded by a zone of erythema. The test should be read at 20 minutes.

The scratch test procedure is performed by placing one drop of a 1:100 dilution of DIGIBIND on the skin and then making a ¼ inch scratch through the drop with a sterile needle. The scratch site is inspected at 20 minutes for an urticarial wheal surrounded by erythema. If skin testing causes a systemic reaction, a tourniquet should be applied above the site of testing and measures to treat anaphylaxis should be instituted. Further administration of DIGIBIND should be avoided unless its use is absolutely essential, in which case the patient should be pretreated with corticosteroids and diphenhydramine. The physician should be prepared to treat anaphylaxis.

Standard therapy for digitalis intoxication includes withdrawal of the drug and correction of factors that may contribute to toxicity, such as electrolyte disturbances, hypoxia, acid-base disturbances and agents such as catecholamines. Also, treatment of arrhythmias may include judicious potassium supplements, lidocaine, phenytoin, procainamide and/or propranolol; treatment of sinus bradycardia or atrioventricular block may involve atropine or pacemaker insertion.

Carcinogenesis and Mutagenesis: There have been no long-term studies performed in animals to evaluate carcinogenic potential.

Reproductive Toxicology: Treatment of 5 pregnant baboons with digoxin-specific antibody Fab fragments by intravenous infusion daily for 60 days from approximate Gestation Day 113, which is equivalent to the third trimester in humans (duration of pregnancy in the baboon is approximately 180 days), resulted in no treatment-related adverse effects on tolerability, gestation, parturition or infant viability. Transient antibodies to digoxin-specific antibody Fab fragments were observed in 1 of 5 pregnant animals on Days 15 and 30 of the dosing period, but not later in gestation. Daily exposure to digoxin-specific antibody Fab fragments was at least 3 times higher than average human exposure, based on dose.

Cardiovascular: Patients with intrinsically poor cardiac function may deteriorate from withdrawal of the inotropic action of digoxin. Studies in animals have shown that the reversal of inotropic effect is relatively gradual, occurring over hours. When needed, additional support can be provided by use of intravenous inotropes, such as dopamine or dobutamine, or vasodilators. One must be careful in using catecholamines not to aggravate digitalis toxic rhythm disturbances. Clearly, other types of digitalis glycosides should not be used in this setting. Redigitalization should be postponed, if possible, until the Fab fragments have been eliminated from the body, which may require several days. Patients with impaired renal function may require a week or longer.

Endocrine and Metabolism: Massive digitalis intoxication can cause hyperkalemia; administration of potassium supplements in the setting of massive intoxication may be hazardous (see Warnings and Precautions, Monitoring and Laboratory Tests). After treatment with DIGIBIND Digoxin Immune Fab (Ovine), the serum potassium concentration may drop rapidly and must be monitored frequently, especially over the first several hours after DIGIBIND is given (see Warnings and Precautions, Monitoring and Laboratory Tests).

Renal: The elimination half-life in the setting of renal failure has not been clearly defined. Patients with renal dysfunction have been successfully treated with DIGIBIND. There is no evidence to suggest the time-course of therapeutic effect is any different in these patients than in patients with normal renal function, but excretion of the Fab fragment-digoxin complex from the body is probably delayed. In patients who are functionally anephric, one would anticipate failure to clear the Fab fragment-digoxin complex from the blood by glomerular filtration and renal excretion. Whether failure to eliminate the Fab fragment-digoxin complex in severe renal failure can lead to reintoxication following release of newly unbound digoxin into the blood is uncertain. Such patients should be monitored for a prolonged period for possible recurrence of digitalis toxicity.

Special Populations: Pregnant Women: Treatment of pregnant baboons with digoxin-specific antibody Fab fragments during a period equivalent to the third trimester in humans showed no adverse effects on pregnancy or viability of offspring (see Non-clinical Information). There are no animal data to support use in the first and second trimester.

In the absence of adequate experience of administration of digoxin-specific antibody Fab fragments to pregnant women, the potential benefit to the mother must be weighed against the unknown risks to the fetus.

Nursing Women: It is not known whether this drug is excreted in human milk. Because many drugs are excreted in human milk, caution should be exercised when DIGIBIND is administered to a nursing woman.

Pediatrics: DIGIBIND has been successfully used in infants with no apparent adverse sequelae. As in all other circumstances, use of this drug in infants should be based on careful consideration of the benefits of the drug balanced against the potential risks involved.

Monitoring and Laboratory Tests: DIGIBIND will interfere with digitalis immunoassay measurements. Thus, the standard serum digoxin concentration measurement can be clinically misleading until the Fab fragment is eliminated from the body.

Serum digoxin or digitoxin concentration should be obtained before DIGIBIND administration, if at all possible. These measurements may be difficult to interpret if drawn soon after the last digitalis dose, since at least 6 to 8 hours are required for equilibration of digoxin between serum and tissue. Patients should be closely monitored, including temperature, blood pressure, electrocardiogram and potassium concentration, during and after administration of DIGIBIND. The total serum digoxin concentration may rise precipitously following administration of DIGIBIND, but this will be almost entirely bound to the Fab fragment and therefore not able to react with receptors in the body.

Potassium concentrations should be followed carefully. Severe digitalis intoxication can cause life-threatening elevation in serum potassium concentration by shifting potassium from inside to outside the cell. The elevation in serum potassium concentration can lead to increased renal excretion of potassium. Thus, these patients may have hyperkalemia with total body deficit of potassium. When the effect of digitalis is reversed by DIGIBIND, potassium shifts back inside the cell, with a resulting decline in serum potassium concentration. Hypokalemia may thus develop rapidly. For these reasons, serum potassium concentration should be monitored repeatedly, especially over the first several hours after DIGIBIND is given, and cautiously treated when necessary.

ADVERSE REACTIONS: In general, the adverse reactions of DIGIBIND Digoxin Immune Fab (Ovine) are dose-dependent and occur at doses higher than those needed to achieve a therapeutic effect.

Hence, adverse reactions are less common when DIGIBIND is used within the recommended dose range or therapeutic serum concentration range and when there is careful attention to concurrent medications and conditions.

Allergic reactions to DIGIBIND have been reported rarely. Patients with a history of allergy, especially to antibiotics, appear to be at particular risk (see Warnings and Precautions). In a few instances, low cardiac output states and congestive heart failure could have been exacerbated by withdrawal of the inotropic effects of digitalis. Hypokalemia may occur from reactivation of (sodium, potassium) ATPase (see Warnings and Precautions, Monitoring and Laboratory Tests). Patients with atrial fibrillation may develop a rapid ventricular response from withdrawal of the effects of digitalis on the atrioventricular node.

Very rarely, DIGIBIND can cause thrombocytopenia.

DRUG INTERACTIONS: There are no known drug interactions to the use of DIGIBIND, Digoxin Immune Fab (Ovine).

DOSAGE AND ADMINISTRATION: Dosing Considerations: General Guidelines: The dosage of DIGIBIND, Digoxin Immune Fab (Ovine), varies according to the amount of digitalis (digoxin) to be neutralized. The average dose used during clinical testing was 10 vials.

Recommended Dose and Dosage Adjustment: Dosage for Acute Ingestion of Unknown Amount: 20 vials (760 mg) of DIGIBIND is adequate to treat most life-threatening ingestion in both adults and children. However, in children it is important to monitor for volume overload. The physician may consider administering 10 vials, observing the patient's response, and following with an additional 10 vials if indicated.

Dosage for Toxicity During Chronic Therapy: For **adults**, 6 vials (228 mg) usually is adequate to reverse most cases of toxicity. This dose can be used in patients who are in acute distress or for whom a serum digoxin or digitoxin concentration is not available. In **infants and small children** (≤20 kg) a single vial usually should suffice.

Methods for calculating the dose of DIGIBIND required to neutralize the known or estimated amount of digoxin or digitoxin in the body are given below (see Dosage Calculation).

When determining the dose for DIGIBIND, the following guidelines should be considered:

- Erroneous calculations may result from inaccurate estimates of the amount of digitalis ingested or absorbed, or from non-steady-state serum digitalis concentrations. Inaccurate serum digitalis concentration measurements are a possible source of error. Most serum digoxin assay kits are designed to measure values less than 5 ng/mL. Dilution of samples is required to obtain accurate measures above 5 ng/mL.
- Dosage calculations are based on a steady-state volume of distribution of approximately 5 L/kg for digoxin (0.5 L/kg for digitoxin) to convert serum digitalis concentration to the amount of digitalis in the body. The conversion is based on the principle that body load equals drug steady-state serum concentration multiplied by volume of distribution. These volumes are population averages and vary widely among individuals. Many patients may require higher doses for complete neutralization. Doses should ordinarily be rounded up to the next whole vial.
- If toxicity has not adequately reversed after several hours or appears to recur, readministration of DIGIBIND at a dose guided by clinical judgment may be required.
- Failure to respond to DIGIBIND raises the possibility that the clinical problem is not caused by digitalis intoxication. If there is no response to an adequate dose of DIGIBIND, the diagnosis of digitalis toxicity should be questioned.

Dosage Calculation: Acute Ingestion of Known Amount: Each vial of DIGIBIND contains 38 mg of purified digoxin-specific Fab fragments which will bind approximately 0.5 mg of digoxin (or digitoxin). Thus, one can calculate the total number of vials required by dividing the total digitalis body load in mg by 0.5 mg/vial (see Formula 1).

For toxicity from an acute ingestion, total body load in milligrams will be approximately equal to the amount ingested in milligrams multiplied by 0.80 (to account for incomplete absorption) for digoxin tablets. For digitoxin, the total body load will be approximately equal to the amount ingested in milligrams.

Table 1 gives dosage estimates in number of vials for **adults and children** who have ingested a single large dose of digoxin and for whom the approximate number of tablets is known. The DIGIBIND dose (in number of vials) represented in Table 1 can be approximated using the following formula:

Formula 1:

$$\text{Dose (in \# of vials)} = \frac{\text{Total digitalis body load in mg}}{\text{0.5 mg of digitalis bound/vial}}$$

Table 1: DIGIBIND

Approximate DIGIBIND Dose for Reversal of a Single Large Digoxin Overdose

Number of Digoxin Tablets[a]	DIGIBIND Dose # of Vials
25	10
50	20
75	30
100	40
150	60
200	80

[a] 0.25 mg tablets with 80% bioavailability.

Calculations Based on Steady-State Serum Digoxin Concentrations: Table 2 gives dosage estimates in number of vials for **adult patients** for whom a steady-state serum digoxin concentration is known. The DIGIBIND dose (in number of vials) represented in Table 2 can be approximated using the following formula:

Formula 2: Calculation with digoxin in ng/mL:

$$\text{Dose (in \# of vials)} = \frac{(\text{Serum digoxin concentration in } \textbf{ng/mL}) \times (\text{weight in kg})}{100}$$

Calculation with digoxin in nmol/L (SI units):

$$\text{Dose (in \# of vials)} = \frac{(\text{Serum digoxin concentration in } \textbf{nmol/L}) \times 0.781 \times (\text{weight in kg})}{100}$$

Table 2: DIGIBIND

Adult Dose Estimate of DIGIBIND (in # of Vials) from Steady-state Serum Digoxin Concentration

Patient Weight (kg)	Serum Digoxin Concentration (nmol/L)							
	1	2	4	8	12	16	20	25
40	0.5 v	1 v	2 v	3 v	4 v	5 v	7 v	8 v
60	0.5 v	1 v	2 v	4 v	6 v	8 v	10 v	12 v
70	1 v	2 v	3 v	5 v	7 v	9 v	11 v	14 v
80	1 v	2 v	3 v	5 v	8 v	10 v	13 v	16 v
100	1 v	2 v	4 v	7 v	10 v	13 v	16 v	20 v

Legend: v=vials.

Table 3 gives dosage estimates in milligrams of DIGIBIND for **infants and small children** based on the steady-state serum digoxin concentration. The DIGIBIND dose represented in Table 3 can be estimated by multiplying the dose (in number of vials) calculated from Formula 2 by the amount of DIGIBIND contained in a vial (38 mg/vial) (see Formula 3). Since infants and small children can have much smaller dosage requirements, it is recommended that the 38 mg vial be reconstituted as directed and administered with a tuberculin syringe. For very small doses, a reconstituted vial can be diluted with 34 mL of sterile isotonic saline to achieve a concentration of 1 mg/mL.

Formula 3:

Dose (in mg) = [Dose (in # of vials)]×[38 mg/vial]

Table 3: DIGIBIND

Infants and Small Children Dose Estimates of DIGIBIND (in mg) from Steady-state Serum Digoxin Concentration

Patient Weight (kg)	Serum Digoxin Concentration (nmol/L)							
	1	2	4	8	12	16	20	25
1	0.3[a] mg	0.6[a] mg	1.2[a] mg	2.5[a] mg	4 mg	5 mg	6 mg	8 mg
3	1[a] mg	2[a] mg	4 mg	8 mg	11mg	15 mg	18 mg	23 mg
5	1.5[a] mg	3[a] mg	6 mg	12 mg	18 mg	24 mg	30 mg	38 mg
10	3[a] mg	6 mg	12 mg	24 mg	36 mg	48 mg	60 mg	75 mg
20	6 mg	12 mg	24 mg	48 mg	72 mg	95 mg	119 mg	149 mg

[a] Dilution of reconstituted vial to 1 mg/mL may be desirable.

Calculation Based on Steady-State Digitoxin Concentration: The DIGIBIND dose for digitoxin toxicity can be approximated using the following formula:

Formula 4: Calculation with digitoxin in ng/mL:

$$\text{Dose (in \# of vials)} = \frac{\text{(Serum digitoxin concentration in } \mathbf{ng/mL})\times\text{(weight in kg)}}{1000}$$

Calculation with digitoxin in nmol/L (SI units):

$$\text{Dose (in \# of vials)} = \frac{\text{(Serum digitoxin concentration in } \mathbf{nmol/L})\times 0.765\times\text{(weight in kg)}}{1000}$$

If the dose based on ingested amount differs substantially from that calculated from the serum digoxin or digitoxin concentration, it may be preferable to use the higher dose.

Administration: DIGIBIND is administered by intravenous route over 30 minutes. It is recommended that it be infused through a 0.22 micron membrane filter to ensure no undissolved particulate matter is administered. If cardiac arrest is imminent, it can be given as a bolus injection.

ACTION AND CLINICAL PHARMACOLOGY: Mechanism of Action: DIGIBIND, Digoxin Immune Fab (Ovine), is a sterile lyophilized powder of antigen binding fragments (Fab) derived from specific antidigoxin antibodies raised in sheep. DIGIBIND binds molecules of digoxin, making them unavailable for binding at their site of action on cells in the body. The Fab fragment-digoxin complex accumulates in the blood, from which it is excreted by the kidney. The net effect is to shift the equilibrium away from binding of digoxin to its receptors in the body, thereby, reversing its effects.

The affinity of digoxin for DIGIBIND is in the range of 10^9 to 10^{11} M^{-1}, which is greater than the affinity of digoxin for (sodium, potassium) ATPase, the presumed receptor for its toxic effects. The affinity of DIGIBIND for digitoxin is about ten times less than for digoxin (10^8 to 10^9 M^{-1}).

Pharmacokinetics: After intravenous injection of DIGIBIND in the baboon, digoxin-specific Fab fragments are excreted in the urine with a biological half-life of about 9 to 13 hours. In humans with normal renal function the half-life appears to be 15 to 20 hours. Experimental studies in animals indicate that these antibody fragments have a large volume of distribution in the extracellular space, unlike whole antibody which distributes in a space only about twice that of the plasma volume. Ordinarily, following administration of DIGIBIND, improvement in signs and symptoms of digitalis intoxication begins within one-half hour or less.

STORAGE AND STABILITY: Store under refrigeration (2 to 8°C). Unreconstituted vials can be stored at up to 30°C for a total of 30 days.

Reconstituted Solutions: The contents in each vial should be dissolved with 4 mL of Sterile Water for Injection, by gentle mixing, to give a clear, colourless, approximately isosmotic solution with a protein concentration of 9.5 mg/mL. Reconstituted product should be used promptly. If it is not used immediately, it may be stored under refrigeration at 2 to 8°C for up to 4 hours. The reconstituted product may be diluted with sterile isotonic saline to a convenient volume. Parenteral drug products should be inspected visually for particulate matter and discolouration prior to administration, whenever solution and container permit.

SPECIAL HANDLING INSTRUCTIONS: Not applicable.

INFORMATION FOR THE PATIENT: Published in e-CPS, available by subscription at www.e-cps.ca.

DOSAGE FORMS, COMPOSITION AND PACKAGING: Each vial of sterile, lyophilized powder for injection contains: digoxin-specific Fab fragments 38 mg, sorbitol 75 mg as a stabilizer and sodium chloride 28 mg. Preservative-free. Each vial will bind approximately 0.5 mg digoxin (or digitoxin). Boxes of 1.

Digoxin Injection C.S.D. ℞
digoxin
Cardiotonic Glycoside

Sandoz

Digoxin Pediatric Injection C.S.D. ℞
digoxin
Cardiotonic Glycoside

Sandoz

SUPPLIED: Digoxin Injection: Each mL contains: digoxin 0.25 mg. Nonmedicinal ingredients: citric acid, ethyl alcohol (10%), propylene glycol, sodium phosphate and water for injection. Ampuls of 2 mL, boxes of 10.

Digoxin Pediatric Injection: Each mL contains: digoxin 0.05 mg. Nonmedicinal ingredients: citric acid, ethyl alcohol (10%), propylene glycol, sodium phosphate and water for injection. Ampuls of 1 mL, boxes of 3.

Store between 15 and 30°C. Protect from light. Protect from freezing. Avoid exposure to excessive heat.

Dihydroergotamine (DHE) ℞
dihydroergotamine mesylate
Vascular Headache Therapy

SteriMax

SUPPLIED: Each mL of injectable solution contains: dihydroergotamine mesylate 1 mg. Also contains ethanol 47 mg/mL and glycerol 150 mg. Ampuls of 1 mL, boxes of 5. Protect from light. Store below 25°C. If the solution becomes discolored, do not use.

Dihydroergotamine Mesylate Injection USP ℞
dihydroergotamine mesylate
Vascular Headache Therapy

Sandoz

SUPPLIED: Each mL of sterile injectable solution contains: dihydroergotamine mesylate 1 mg. Also contains anhydrous ethyl alcohol 47 mg, glycerol, methanesulfonic acid to adjust pH and water for injection. Ampoules of 1 mL, boxes of 3. Store between 15 and 30°C. If the solution becomes discoloured, do not use. Protect from light.

Dilantin® Capsules ℞
phenytoin sodium
Anticonvulsant

Pfizer

Date of Revision: January 26, 2010

PHARMACOLOGY: Dilantin (extended phenytoin sodium capsules) is an anticonvulsant drug which can be useful in the treatment of epilepsy. The primary site of action appears to be the motor cortex where spread of seizure activity is inhibited. Possibly by promoting sodium efflux from neurons, phenytoin tends to stabilize the threshold against hyperexcitability caused by excessive stimulation or environmental changes capable of reducing membrane sodium gradient. This includes the reduction of post-tetanic potentiation at synapses. Loss of post-tetanic potentiation prevents cortical seizure foci from detonating adjacent cortical areas. Phenytoin reduces the maximal activity of brain stem centers responsible for the tonic phase of tonic-clonic (grand mal) seizures.

The plasma half-life in man after oral administration of phenytoin averages 22 hours, with a range of 7 to 42 hours. Steady-state therapeutic levels are achieved at least 7 to 10 days after initiation of therapy with recommended doses of 300 mg/day.

When serum level determinations are necessary, they should be obtained at least 7-10 days after treatment initiation, dosage change, or addition or subtraction of another drug to the regimen so that equilibrium or steady-state will have been achieved. Trough levels obtained just prior to the patient's next scheduled dose provide information about clinically effective serum level range and confirm patient compliance. Peak drug levels, obtained at the time of expected peak concentration, indicate an individual's threshold for emergence of dose-related side effects. For Dilantin (extended phenytoin sodium capsules), peak serum levels occur 4-12 hours after administration.

In most patients maintained at a steady dosage, stable phenytoin serum levels are achieved. There may be wide interpatient variability in phenytoin serum levels with equivalent dosages. Patients with unusually low levels may be noncompliant or hypermetabolizers of phenytoin. Unusually high levels result from liver disease, congenital enzyme deficiency or drug interactions which result in metabolic interference. The patient with large variations in phenytoin plasma levels, despite standard doses, presents a difficult clinical problem. Serum level determinations in such patients may be particularly helpful. As phenytoin is highly protein bound, free phenytoin levels may be altered in patients whose protein binding characteristics differ from normal.

Most of the drug is excreted in the bile as inactive metabolites which are then reabsorbed from the intestinal tract and excreted in the urine. Urinary excretion of phenytoin and its metabolites occurs partly with glomerular filtration but more importantly by tubular secretion. Because phenytoin is hydroxylated in the liver by an enzyme system which is saturable at high plasma levels, small incremental doses may increase the half-life and produce very substantial increases in serum levels, when these are in or above the upper therapeutic range. The steady-state level may be disproportionately increased, with resultant intoxication, from an increase in dosage of 10% or more.

INDICATIONS: Dilantin (extended phenytoin sodium capsules) is indicated for the control of generalized tonic-clonic and psychomotor (grand mal and temporal lobe) seizures and prevention and treatment of seizures occurring during or following neurosurgery. Phenytoin serum level determinations may be necessary for optimal dosage adjustments (see Dosage).

CONTRAINDICATIONS: Dilantin (extended phenytoin sodium capsules) is contraindicated in those patients who are hypersensitive to phenytoin or other hydantoins.

WARNINGS: General: Abrupt withdrawal of Dilantin (extended phenytoin sodium capsules) in epileptic patients may precipitate status epilepticus. When, in the judgement of the clinician, the need for dosage reduction, discontinuation, or substitution of alternative antiepileptic medication arises, this should be done gradually. However, in the event of an allergic or hypersensitivity reaction, rapid substitution of alternative therapy may be necessary. In this case, alternative therapy should be an antiepileptic drug not belonging to the hydantoin chemical class.

Anticonvulsant Hypersensitivity Syndrome (AHS) is a rare drug induced, multiorgan syndrome which is potentially fatal and occurs in some patients taking anticonvulsant medication. It is characterized by fever, rash, lymphadenopathy, and other multiorgan pathologies, often hepatic. The mechanism is unknown. The interval between first drug exposure and symptoms is usually 2-4 weeks but has been reported in individuals receiving anticonvulsants for 3 or more months. Patients at higher risk for developing AHS include black patients, patients who have a family history of or who have experienced this syndrome in the past, and immuno-suppressed patients. The syndrome is more severe in previously sensitized individuals. If a patient is diagnosed with AHS, discontinue the phenytoin and provide appropriate supportive measures.

Acute alcoholic intake may increase phenytoin serum levels while chronic alcoholic use may decrease serum levels.

Serious Dermatological Reactions: Steven's-Johnson Syndrome and Toxic Epidermal Necrolysis: Serious and sometimes fatal dermatologic reactions, including Toxic Epidermal Necrolysis (TEN) and Stevens-Johnson Syndrome (SJS), have been reported with phenytoin. In countries with mainly Caucasian populations, these reactions are estimated to occur in 1 to 6 per 10 000 new users, but in some Asian countries (e.g., Taiwan, Malaysia and the Philippines) the risk is estimated to be much higher.

HLA-B*1502: In studies that included small samples of patients of Asian ancestry a strong association was found between the risk of developing SJS/TEN and the presence of HLA-B*1502, an inherited allelic variant of the HLA-B gene. The HLA-B*1502 allele is found almost exclusively in individuals with ancestry across broad areas of Asia*. Results of these studies suggest that the presence of the HLA-B *1502 allele may be one of the risk factors for phenytoin-associated SJS/TEN in patients with Asian ancestry. Therefore, physicians should consider HLA-B *1502 genotyping as a screening tool in these patients. Until further information is available, the use of phenytoin and other anti-epileptic drugs associated with SJS/TEN should also be avoided in patients who test positive for the HLA-B*1502 allele (see Warnings, Asian Ancestry and Allelic Variation in the HLA-B Genotyping and Warnings, Important Limitations of HLA-B Genotyping).

Treatment Recommendations for Dermatological Reactions: Phenytoin should be discontinued at the first sign of a rash, unless the rash is clearly not drug-related. If signs or symptoms suggest SJS/TEN, use of this drug should not be resumed and alternative therapy should be considered. The use of other anti-epileptic drugs associated with SJS/TEN should be avoided in patients who have shown severe dermatological reactions during phenytoin treatment.

Asian Ancestry and Allelic Variation in the HLA-B Genotyping: In studies that included small samples of patients of Asian ancestry a strong association was found between the risk of developing SJS/TEN and the presence of HLA-B*1502, an inherited allelic variant of the HLA-B gene. The HLA-B*1502 allele is found almost exclusively in individuals with ancestry across broad areas of Asia. Results of these studies suggest that the presence of the HLA-B *1502 allele may be one of the risk factors for phenytoin-associated SJS/TEN in patients with Asian ancestry. Therefore, physicians should consider HLA-B *1502 genotyping as a screening tool in these patients. Until further information is available, the use of phenytoin and other anti-epileptic drugs associated with SJS/TEN should also be avoided in patients who test positive for the HLA-B*1502 allele.

Important Limitations of HLA-B Genotyping: HLA-B*1502 genotyping as a screening tool has important limitations and must never substitute for appropriate clinical vigilance and patient management. Many HLA-B*1502-positive Asian patients treated with phenytoin will not develop SJS/TEN, and these reactions can still occur infrequently in HLA-B*1502-negative patients of any ethnicity. The role of other possible factors in the development of, and morbidity from, SJS/TEN, such as antiepileptic drug (AED) dose, compliance, concomitant medications, co-morbidities, and the level of dermatologic monitoring have not been studied.

* The following rates provide a rough estimate of the prevalence of HLA-B*1502 in various populations. Greater than 15% of the population is reported positive in Hong Kong, Thailand, Malaysia, and parts of the Philippines, compared to about 10% in Taiwan and 4% in North China. South Asians, including Indians, appear to have intermediate prevalence of HLA-B*1502, averaging 2 to 4%, but this may be higher in some groups. HLA-B*1502 is present in <1% of the population in Japan and Korea. HLA-B*1502 is largely absent in individuals not of Asian origin (e.g., Caucasians, African-Americans, Hispanics, and Native Americans). The estimated prevalence rates have limitations due to the wide variability in rates that exist within ethnic groups, the difficulties in ascertaining ethnic ancestry and the likelihood of mixed ancestry.

In addition, it should be kept in mind that the majority of phenytoin treated patients who will experience SJS/TEN have this reaction within the first few months of treatment. This information may be taken into consideration when deciding whether to screen genetically at-risk patients currently on phenytoin.

Should signs and symptoms suggest a severe skin reaction such as SJS or TEN, phenytoin should be withdrawn at once.

Literature reports suggest that the combination of phenytoin, cranial irradiation and the gradual reduction of corticosteroids may be associated with the development of erythema multiforme, and/or Stevens-Johnson syndrome, and/or toxic epidermal necrolysis. In any of the above instances, caution should be exercised if using structurally similar compounds (eg, barbiturates, succinimides, oxazolidinediones and other related compounds) in these same patients (see Precautions).

Hepatic/Immunologic: Cases of acute hepatoxicity, including infrequent cases of acute hepatic failure, have been reported with phenytoin. These incidents have been associated with a hypersensitivity syndrome characterized by fever, skin eruptions, and lymphadenopathy, and usually occur with the first 2 months of treatment. Other common manifestations include jaundice, hepatomegaly, elevated serum transaminase levels, leukocytosis, and eosinophilia. The clinical course of acute phenytoin hepatotoxicity ranges from prompt recovery to fatal outcomes. In these patients with acute hepatotoxicity, phenytoin should be immediately discontinued and not re-administered.

Hematopoietic: There have been a number of reports suggesting a relationship between phenytoin and the development of lymphadenopathy (local or generalized) including benign lymph node hyperplasia, pseudolymphoma, lymphoma, and Hodgkin's Disease. Although a cause and effect relationship has not been established, the occurrence of lymphadenopathy indicates the need to differentiate such a condition from other types of lymph node pathology. Lymph node involvement may occur with or without symptoms and signs resembling serum sickness, e.g. fever, rash and liver involvement. In all cases of lymphadenopathy, follow-up observation for an extended period is indicated and every effort should be made to achieve seizure control using alternative antiepileptic drugs.

Metabolic: In view of isolated reports associating phenytoin with exacerbation of porphyria, caution should be exercised in using this medication in patients suffering from this disease.

Psychiatric: Suicidal Ideation and Behaviour: Suicidal ideation and behaviour have been reported in patients treated with antiepileptic agents in several indications.

All patients treated with antiepileptic drugs, irrespective of indication, should be monitored for signs of suicidal ideation and behaviour and appropriate treatment should be considered. Patients (and caregivers of patients) should be advised to seek medical advice should signs of suicidal ideation or behaviour emerge.

An FDA meta-analysis of randomized placebo controlled trials, in which antiepileptic drugs were used for various indications, has shown a small increased risk of suicidal ideation and behaviour in patients treated with these drugs. The mechanism of this risk is not known.

There were 43 892 patients treated in the placebo controlled clinical trials that were included in the meta-analysis. Approximately 75% of patients in these clinical trials were treated for indications other than epilepsy and, for the majority of non-epilepsy indications the treatment (antiepileptic drug or placebo) was administered as monotherapy. Patients with epilepsy represented approximately 25% of the total number of patients treated in the placebo controlled clinical trials and, for the majority of epilepsy patients, treatment (antiepileptic drug or placebo) was administered as adjunct to other antiepileptic agents (i.e., patients in both treatment arms were being treated with one or more antiepileptic drug). Therefore, the small increased risk of suicidal ideation and behaviour reported from the meta-analysis (0.43% for patients on antiepileptic drugs compared to 0.24% for patients on placebo) is based largely on patients that received monotherapy treatment (antiepileptic drug or placebo) for non-epilepsy indications. The study design does not allow an estimation of the risk of suicidal ideation and behaviour for patients with epilepsy that are taking antiepileptic drugs, due both to this population being the minority in the study, and the drug-placebo comparison in this population being confounded by the presence of adjunct antiepileptic drug treatment in both arms.

Pregnancy: A number of reports suggest an association between the use of anticonvulsant drugs by women with epilepsy and a higher incidence of birth defects in children born to these women. Data are more extensive with respect to phenytoin and phenobarbital, but these are also the most commonly prescribed anticonvulsant drugs; less systematic or anecdotal reports suggest a possible similar association with the use of all known anticonvulsant drugs.

The reports suggesting a higher incidence of birth defects in children of drug-treated epileptic women cannot be regarded as adequate to prove a definite cause and effect relationship. There are intrinsic methodologic problems in obtaining adequate data on drug teratogenicity in humans. Genetic factors or the epileptic condition itself may be more important than drug therapy in leading to birth defects. The great majority of mothers on anticonvulsant medication deliver normal infants. It is important to note that anticonvulsant drugs should not be discontinued in patients in whom the drug is administered to prevent major seizures because of the strong possibility of precipitating status epilepticus with attendant hypoxia and threat to life. In individual cases where the severity and frequency of the seizure disorder are such that the removal of medication does not pose a serious threat to the patient, discontinuation of the drug may be considered prior to and during pregnancy, although it cannot be said with any confidence that even minor seizures do not pose some hazard to the developing embryo or fetus. The prescribing physician will wish to weigh these considerations in treating or counseling epileptic women of childbearing potential.

In addition to the reports of the increased incidence of congenital malformations, such as cleft lip/palate and heart malformations in children of women receiving phenytoin and other antiepileptic drugs, there have more recently been reports of a fetal hydantoin syndrome. This consists of prenatal growth deficiency, microcephaly and mental deficiency in children born to mothers who have received phenytoin, barbiturates, alcohol, or trimethadione. However, these features are all interrelated and are frequently associated with intrauterine growth retardation from other causes.

There have been isolated reports of malignancies, including neuroblastoma, in children whose mothers received phenytoin during pregnancy.

An increase in seizure frequency during pregnancy occurs in a high proportion of patients, because of altered phenytoin absorption or metabolism. Periodic measurement of serum phenytoin levels is particularly valuable in the management of a pregnant epileptic patient as a guide to an appropriate adjustment of dosage. However, postpartum restoration of the original dosage will probably be indicated.

Neonatal coagulation defects have been reported within the first 24 hours in babies born to epileptic mothers receiving phenobarbital and/or phenytoin. Vitamin K has been shown to prevent or correct this defect and has been recommended to be given to the mother before delivery and to the neonate after birth.

PRECAUTIONS: General: Phenytoin is not indicated for seizures due to hypoglycemic or other metabolic causes. Appropriate diagnostic procedures should be performed as indicated.

Phenytoin is not effective for absence (petit mal) seizures. If tonic-clonic (grand mal) and absence (petit mal) seizures are present, combined drug therapy is needed.

A small percentage of individuals who have been treated with phenytoin have been shown to metabolize the drug slowly. Slow metabolism may be due to limited enzyme availability and lack of induction; it appears to be genetically determined.

Hepatic/Immunologic: The liver is the chief site of biotransformation of Dilantin (extended phenytoin sodium capsules). Patients with impaired liver function, elderly patients, or those who are gravely ill may show early signs of toxicity.

Toxic hepatitis, liver damage, and hypersensitivity syndrome have been reported and may, in rare cases, be fatal (see Adverse Effects).

Serious Dermatological Reactions: Phenytoin should be discontinued if a skin rash appears (see Warnings regarding drug discontinuation). If the rash is exfoliative, purpuric, or bullous or if lupus erythematosus or Stevens-Johnson syndrome or toxic epidermal necrolysis is suspected, use of this drug should not be resumed and alternative therapy should be considered (see Adverse Effects). If the rash is of a milder type (measles-like or scarlatiniform), therapy may be resumed after the rash has completely disappeared. If the rash recurs upon reinstitution of therapy, further phenytoin medication is contraindicated.

Literature reports suggest that the combination of phenytoin, cranial irradiation and the gradual reduction of corticosteroids may be associated with the development of erythema multiforme, and/or Stevens-Johnson syndrome, and/or toxic epidermal necrolysis. In any of the above instances, caution should be exercised if using structurally similar compounds (e.g. barbiturate, succinimides, oxazolidinediones and other related compounds) in these same patients (see Warnings).

Published literature has suggested that there may be an increased, although still rare, risk of hypersensitivity reactions, including skin rash, SJS, TEN, hepatotoxicity, and Anticonvulsant Hypersensitivity Syndrome in black patients.

† Coadministration with topiramate reduces serum topiramate levels by 59%, and has the potential to increase phenytoin levels by 25% in some patients. The addition of topiramate therapy to phenytoin should be guided by clinical outcome.

‡ Coadministration with Vigabatrin reduces serum phenytoin levels by 20 to 30%. This may be clinically significant in some patients and may require dosage adjustment.

¶ Coadministration with lamotrigine doubles the plasma clearance and reduces the elimination half life of lamotrigine by 50%. This clinically important interaction requires dosage adjustment.

§ Coadministration with topiramate reduces serum topiramate levels by 59%, and has the potential to increase phenytoin levels by 25% in some patients. The addition of topiramate therapy to phenytoin should be guided by clinical outcome.

Hematopoietic : While macrocytosis and megaloblastic anemia have occurred, these conditions usually respond to folic acid therapy. If folic acid is added to phenytoin therapy, a decrease in seizure control may occur.

Metabolic: Hyperglycemia, resulting from the drug's inhibitory effects on insulin release, has been reported. Phenytoin may also raise the serum glucose level in diabetic patients.

Musculoskeletal: Phenytoin and other anticonvulsants that have been shown to induce the CYP450 enzyme are thought to affect bone mineral metabolism indirectly by increasing the metabolism of Vitamin D3. This may lead to Vitamin D deficiency and heightened risk of osteomalacia, bone fractures, osteoporosis, hypocalcemia, and hypophosphatemia in chronically treated epileptic patients (see Adverse Effects, Post-marketing Experience).

Central Nervous System : Serum levels of phenytoin sustained above the optimal range may produce confusional states referred to as "delirium", "psychosis", or "encephalopathy", or rarely, irreversible cerebellar dysfunction. Accordingly, at the first sign of acute toxicity, plasma level determinations are recommended. Dose reduction of phenytoin therapy is indicated if plasma levels are excessive; if symptoms persist, termination is recommended (see Warnings).

Information to Be Provided to the Patient: Patients taking phenytoin should be advised of the importance of adhering strictly to the prescribed dosage regimen, and of informing the physician of any clinical condition in which it is not possible to take the drug orally as prescribed, e.g. surgery, etc.

Patients should also be cautioned on the use of other drugs or alcoholic beverages without first seeking the physician's advice.

Patients should be instructed to call their physician if skin rash develops.

The importance of good dental hygiene should be stressed in order to minimize the development of gingival hyperplasia and its complications.

Do not use capsules which are discoloured.

Laboratory Tests: Phenytoin serum level determinations may be necessary to achieve optimal dosage adjustments.

Drug Interactions: There are many drugs which may increase or decrease phenytoin levels or which phenytoin may affect. Determinations of serum phenytoin concentrations are especially helpful when possible drug interactions are suspected. The **most commonly occurring** drug interactions are listed below:

1. Drugs which may increase phenytoin serum levels include: acute alcohol intake, cimetidine, dicumarol, disulfiram, ethosuximide, methylphenidate, omeprazole, phenothiazines, ticlopidine and topiratmate†. The following drug classes are also included: See Table 1.

Table 1: Dilantin Capsules

Drugs Which May Increase Phenytoin Serum Levels

Drug Classes	Drugs in Each Class (such as)
Analgesic/anti-inflammatory agents	phenylbutazone salicylates
Anesthetics	halothane
Antibacterial agents	chloramphenicol erythromycin isoniazid sulfonamides
Anticonvulsants	felbamate succinimides
Antifungal agents	amphotericin B fluconazole ketoconazole miconazole itraconazole
Benzodiazepines/psychotropic agents	chlordiazepoxide diazepam trazodone
Calcium channel blockers/cardiovascular agents	amiodarone diltiazem nifefipine
H_2-antagonists	cimetidine
Hormones	estrogens
Oral hypoglycemic agents	tolbutamide
Serotonin re-uptake inhibitors	fluoxetine

2. Drugs which may decrease phenytoin levels include: antibacterial agents/fluoroquinolones (such as ciprofloxacin and rifampin), carbamazepine, chronic alcohol abuse, diazoxide, reserpine, sucralfate, theophylline and vigabatrin‡. Molindone Hydrochloride contains calcium ions which interfere with the absorption of phenytoin. Ingestion times of phenytoin and antacid preparations, including antacid preparations containing calcium should be staggered to prevent absorption problems.

3. Drugs which may either increase or decrease phenytoin serum levels include the following: See Table 2.

Table 2: Dilantin Capsules

Drugs Which May Either Increase or Decrease Phenytoin Serum Levels

Drug Classes	Drugs in Each Class (such as)
Anticonvulsants	carbamazepine phenobarbital sodium valproate valproic acid
Antineoplastic agents	
Benzodiazepines	chlordiazepoxide
Phenothiazines	
Psychotropic agents	diazepam

Similarly, the effect of phenytoin on carbamazepine, phenobarbital, valproic acid and sodium valproate serum levels is unpredictable.

4. Although not a true drug interaction, tricyclic antidepressants may precipitate seizures in susceptible patients and phenytoin dosage may need to be adjusted.

5. Drugs whose blood levels and/or effects may be altered by phenytoin include: clozapine, corticosteroids, coumarin anticoagulants, cyclosporine, diazoxide, furosemide, lamotrigine¶, paroxetine, theophylline, topiramate§ and vitamin D. The following drug classes are also included: See Table 3.

Table 3: Dilantin Capsules

Drugs Whose Blood Levels and/or Effects May Be Altered by Phenytoin

Drug Classes	Drugs in Each Class (such as)
Antibacterial agents	doxycycline praziquantel rifampin tetracycline
Antifungal agents	
Antineoplastic agents	
Calcium channel blockers/cardiovascular agents	digitoxin nicardipine nimodipine quinidine verapamil
Hormones	estrogens oral contraceptives
Neuromuscular blocking agents	pancuronium vecuronium
Opioid analgesics	methadone
Oral hypoglycemic agents	chlorpropamide glyburide tolbutamide

Drug-Enteral Feeding/Nutritional Preparations Interaction: Literature reports suggest that patients who have received enteral feeding preparations and/or related nutritional supplements have lower than expected phenytoin plasma levels. It is therefore suggested that phenytoin not be administered concomitantly with an enteral feeding preparation.

More frequent serum phenytoin level monitoring may be necessary in these patients.

Drug/Laboratory Test Interactions: Phenytoin may cause decreased serum levels of protein-bound iodine (PBI). It may also produce lower than normal values for dexamethasone or metyrapone tests. Phenytoin may cause increased serum levels of glucose, alkaline phosphatase, and gamma glutamyl transpeptidase (GGT). Phenytoin may affect blood calcium and blood sugar metabolism tests.

Carcinogenesis: See Warnings.

Pregnancy: See Warnings.

Lactation: Infant breast-feeding is not recommended for women taking this drug because phenytoin appears to be secreted in low concentrations in human milk.

Children: See Dosage.

ADVERSE EFFECTS: Central Nervous System: The most common manifestations encountered with Dilantin (extended phenytoin sodium capsules) therapy are referable to this system and are usually dose-related. These include nystagmus, ataxia, slurred speech, decreased coordination and mental confusion. Dizziness, insomnia, transient nervousness, motor twitchings, and headaches have also been observed. There have also been rare reports of phenytoin induced dyskinesias, including chorea, dystonia, tremor and asterixis, similar to those induced by phenothiazine and other neuroleptic drugs.

A predominantly sensory peripheral polyneuropathy has been observed in patients receiving long-term phenytoin therapy.

Gastrointestinal System: nausea, vomiting, and constipation, toxic hepatitis, and liver damage (see Precautions).

Integumentary System: Dermatological manifestations sometimes accompanied by fever have included scarlatiniform or morbilliform rashes. A morbilliform rash (measles-like) is the most common; other types of dermatitis are seen more rarely. Other more serious forms which may be fatal have included bullous, exfoliative or purpuric dermatitis, lupus erythematosus, and Stevens-Johnson syndrome and toxic epidermal necrolysis (see Warnings).

Hemopoietic System: Hemopoietic complications, some fatal, have occasionally been reported in association with administration of phenytoin. These have included thrombocytopenia, leukopenia, granulocytopenia, agranulocytosis, and pancytopenia with or without bone marrow suppression. While macrocytosis and megaloblastic anemia have occurred, these conditions usually respond to folic acid therapy. Lymphadenopathy including benign lymph node hyperplasia, pseudolymphoma, lymphoma, and Hodgkin's Disease have been reported (see Warnings).

Connective Tissue System: coarsening of the facial features, enlargement of the lips, gingival hyperplasia, hypertrichosis and Peyronie's Disease.

Immunologic: Hypersensitivity syndrome (which may include, but is not limited to symptoms such as arthralgias, eosinophilia, fever, liver dysfunction, lymphadenopathy or rash), systemic lupus erythematosus, periarteritis nodosa, and immunoglobulin abnormalities. Several individual case reports have suggested that there may be an increased, although still rare, incidence of hypersensitivity reactions, including skin rash and hepatoxicity, in black patients (see Warnings and Precautions).

Post-marketing Experience: Musculoskeletal System: Bone fractures and osteomalacia have been associated with long-term (>10 years) use of phenytoin by patients with chronic epilepsy. Osteoporosis and other disorders of bone metabolism such as hypocalcemia, hypophophatemia and decreased levels of Vitamin D metabolites have also been reported (see Precautions, Musculoskeletal).

OVERDOSE:

Symptoms: The lethal dose of Dilantin (extended phenytoin sodium capsules) in pediatric patient is not known. The lethal dose in adults is estimated to be 2 to 5 grams. The initial symptoms are nystagmus, ataxia, and dysarthria. Other signs are tremor, hyperflexia, lethargy, slurred speech, nausea, vomiting. The patient may become comatose and hypotensive. Death is due to respiratory and circulatory depression.

There are marked variations among individuals with respect to phenytoin plasma levels where toxicity may occur. Nystagmus on lateral gaze, usually appears at 80 µmol/L (20 µg/mL), ataxia at 119 µmol/L (30 µg/mL). Dysarthria and lethargy appear when serum concentration is >159 µmol/L (40 µg/mL), but a concentration as high as 198 µmol/L (50 µg/mL) has been reported without evidence of toxicity. As much as 25 times the therapeutic dose has been taken to result in a serum concentration over >396 µmol/L (100 µg/mL) with complete recovery.

Treatment: Treatment is nonspecific since there is no known antidote.

The adequacy of the respiratory and circulatory systems should be carefully observed and appropriate supportive measures employed. Hemodialysis can be considered since phenytoin is not completely bound to plasma proteins. Total exchange transfusion has been used in the treatment of severe intoxication in pediatric patients.

In acute overdosage the possibility of the presence of other CNS depressants, including alcohol, should be borne in mind.

> For management of a suspected drug overdose, contact your **regional Poison Control Centre**. See the *CPS* Directory section for a list of Poison Control Centres.

DOSAGE: Serum concentrations should be monitored and care should be taken when switching a patient from the sodium salt to the free acid form.

Dilantin capsules are formulated with the sodium salt of phenytoin. The free acid form of phenytoin is used in Dilantin-30 Pediatric and Dilantin-125 Suspensions and Dilantin Infatabs. Because there is approximately an 8% increase in drug content with the free acid form over that of the sodium salt, dosage adjustments and serum level monitoring may be necessary when switching from a product formulated with the free acid to a product formulated with the sodium salt and vice versa.

General: Dosage should be individualized to provide maximum benefit. In some cases, serum blood level determinations may be necessary for optimal dosage adjustments; the clinically effective serum level is usually 40-80 µmol/L (10-20 µg/mL). Serum blood level determinations are especially helpful when possible drug interactions are suspected. With recommended dosage, a period of seven to ten days may be required to achieve therapeutic blood levels with Dilantin and changes in dosage (increase or decrease) should not be carried out at intervals shorter than 7 to 10 days.

Adults: Patients who have received no previous treatment may be started on one 100 mg extended phenytoin sodium capsule three times daily, and the dose then adjusted to suit individual requirements. For most adults, the satisfactory maintenance dosage will be three to four capsules (300-400 mg) daily. An increase to six capsules daily may be made, if necessary.

Children: Initially, 5 mg/kg/day in two or three equally divided doses, with subsequent dosage individualized to a maximum of 300 mg daily. A recommended daily maintenance dosage is usually 4 to 8 mg/kg. Children over 6 years old may require the minimum adult dose (300 mg/day). Pediatric dosage forms available include a 30 mg extended phenytoin sodium capsule, a 50 mg palatably flavoured Infatab, or an oral suspension form containing 30 mg of phenytoin in each 5 mL.

Alternative Dose: Once-a-day dosage for adults with 300 mg of extended phenytoin sodium capsules may be considered if seizure control is established with divided doses of three 100 mg capsules daily. Studies comparing divided doses of 300 mg with a single daily dose of this quantity indicated that absorption, peak plasma levels, biologic half-life, difference between peak and minimum values, and urinary recovery were equivalent. Once-a-day dosage offers a convenience to the individual patient or to nursing personnel for institutionalized patients, and is intended only to be used for patients requiring this amount of drug daily. A major problem in motivating noncompliant patients may also be lessened when the patient can take all of his medication once-a-day. However, patients should be cautioned not to inadvertently miss a dose. Only extended phenytoin sodium capsules are recommended for once-a-day dosing.

INFORMATION FOR THE PATIENT: Published in e-CPS, available by subscription at www.e-cps.ca.

SUPPLIED: 30 mg: Each extended, Manufacturer Standard, size 4 hemispherical Coni Snap capsule with a white opaque body and pale pink opaque cap containing a white powder, imprinted with black rectified radial print, "PD" on cap and "Dilantin 30 mg" on body, contains: phenytoin sodium 30 mg. Nonmedicinal ingredients: lactose, magnesium stearate, sugar and talc; capsule shell: D&C Yellow No. 10, FD&C Red No. 3, gelatin and titanium dioxide. Energy: 3.0 kJ (0.7 kcal). Sodium: <1 mmol (2.52 mg). Bottles of 100. Store at controlled room temperature 15-30°C. Protect from light and moisture.

100 mg: Each extended, hard, filled No. 3 capsule USP containing a white powder, with the medium orange cap having the Parke-Davis logo printed in black ink and the white, opaque body having "DILANTIN" over "100 mg" printed in black ink, contains: phenytoin sodium 100 mg. Nonmedicinal ingredients: lactose, magnesium stearate, sugar and talc; capsule shell: D&C Red No. 28, FD&C Yellow No. 6, gelatin and titanium dioxide. Energy: 2.6 kJ (0.6 kcal). Sodium: <1 mmol (8.39 mg). Bottles of 100 and 1000. Store at controlled room temperature 15-30°C. Protect from light and moisture.

(Shown in Product Identification Section)

Dilantin® Infatabs Ⓟ
phenytoin
Anticonvulsant

Pfizer

Dilantin®-30 Suspension Ⓟ
phenytoin
Anticonvulsant

Pfizer

Dilantin®-125 Suspension Ⓟ
phenytoin
Anticonvulsant

Pfizer

Date of Preparation: February 12, 2001
Date of Revision: October 15, 2009

PHARMACOLOGY: DILANTIN Infatabs (phenytoin tablets USP) and DILANTIN-30 Suspension/DILANTIN-125 Suspension (phenytoin oral suspension) are anticonvulsant drugs which can be useful in the treatment of epilepsy. The primary site of action appears to be the motor cortex where spread of seizure activity is inhibited. Possibly by promoting sodium efflux from neurons, phenytoin tends to stabilize the threshold against hyperexcitability caused by excessive stimulation or environmental changes capable of reducing membrane sodium gradient. This includes the reduction of post-tetanic potentiation at synapses. Loss of post-tetanic potentiation prevents cortical seizure foci from detonating adjacent cortical areas. Phenytoin reduces the maximal activity of brain stem centers responsible for the tonic phase of tonic-clonic (grand mal) seizures.

Clinical studies using DILANTIN Infatabs have shown an average plasma half-life of 14 hours with a range of 7 to 29 hours. The plasma half-life of phenytoin in man after oral administration of phenytoin oral suspension averages 22 hours, with a range of 7 to 42 hours. Steady-state therapeutic levels are achieved at least 7 to 10 days after initiation of therapy with recommended doses of 300 mg/day.

When serum level determinations are necessary, they should be obtained at least 7-10 days after treatment initiation, dosage change, or addition or subtraction of another drug to the regimen so that equilibrium or steady-state will have been achieved. Trough levels obtained just prior to the patient's next scheduled dose provide information about clinically effective serum level range and confirm patient compliance. Peak drug levels, obtained at the time of expected peak concentration, indicate an individual's threshold for emergence of dose-related side effects. For DILANTIN Infatabs, DILANTIN-30 Suspension and DILANTIN-125 Suspension, peak serum levels occur 1½-3 hours after administration.

In most patients maintained at a steady dosage, stable phenytoin serum levels are achieved. There may be wide interpatient variability in phenytoin serum levels with equivalent dosages. Patients with unusually low levels may be noncompliant or hypermetabolizers of phenytoin. Unusually high levels result from liver disease, congenital enzyme deficiency or drug interactions which result in metabolic interference. The patient with large variations in phenytoin serum levels, despite standard doses, presents a difficult clinical problem. Serum level determinations in such patients may be particularly helpful. As phenytoin is highly protein bound, free phenytoin levels may be altered in patients whose protein binding characteristics differ from normal.

Most of the drug is excreted in the bile as inactive metabolites which are then reabsorbed from the intestinal tract and excreted in the urine. Urinary excretion of phenytoin and its metabolites occurs partly with glomerular filtration but more importantly by tubular secretion. Because phenytoin is hydroxylated in the liver by an enzyme system which is saturable at high serum levels, small incremental doses may increase the half-life and produce very substantial increases in serum levels when these are in or above the upper therapeutic range. The steady-state level may be disproportionately increased, with resultant intoxication, from an increase in dosage of 10% or more.

Clinical studies show that chewed and unchewed DILANTIN Infatabs are bioequivalent, yield approximately equivalent plasma levels, and are more rapidly absorbed than DILANTIN 100 mg capsules (extended phenytoin capsules, USP).

INDICATIONS: DILANTIN Infatabs (phenytoin tablets USP) and DILANTIN-30 Suspension/DILANTIN-125 Suspension (phenytoin oral suspension USP) are indicated for the control of generalized tonic-clonic (grand mal) and complex partial (psychomotor, temporal lobe) seizures. Phenytoin serum level determinations may be necessary for optimal dosage adjustments (see Pharmacology and Dosage).

CONTRAINDICATIONS: DILANTIN Infatabs (phenytoin tablets USP) and DILANTIN-30 Suspension/DILANTIN-125 Suspension (phenytoin oral suspension USP) are contraindicated in those patients who are hypersensitive to phenytoin or other hydantoins.

WARNINGS: General: Abrupt withdrawal of DILANTIN Infatabs (phenytoin tablets USP) or DILANTIN 30 Suspension/DILANTIN-125 Suspension (phenytoin oral suspension USP) in epileptic patients may precipitate status epilepticus. When, in the judgment of the clinician, the need for dosage reduction, discontinuation, or substitution of alternative anticonvulsant medication arises, this should be done gradually. However, in the event of an allergic hypersensitivity reaction, rapid substitution of alternative therapy may be necessary. In this case, alternative therapy should be an anticonvulsant drug which does not belong to the hydantoin chemical class.

Anticonvulsant Hypersensitivity Syndrome (AHS) is a rare drug induced, multiorgan syndrome which is potentially fatal and occurs in some patients taking anticonvulsant medication. It is characterized by fever, rash, lymphadenopathy, and other multiorgan pathologies, often hepatic. The mechanism is unknown. The interval between first drug exposure and symptoms is usually 2-4 weeks but has been reported in individuals receiving anticonvulsants for 3 or more months. Patients at higher risk for developing AHS include black patients, patients who have a family history of or who have experienced this syndrome in the past, and immuno-suppressed patients. The syndrome is more severe in previously sensitized individuals. If a patient is diagnosed with AHS, discontinue the phenytoin and provide appropriate supportive measures.

Acute alcoholic intake may increase phenytoin serum levels while chronic alcoholic use may decrease serum levels.

Serious Dermatological Reactions: Steven's-Johnson Syndrome and Toxic Epidermal Necrolysis: Serious and sometimes fatal dermatologic reactions, including Toxic Epidermal Necrolysis (TEN) and Stevens-Johnson Syndrome (SJS), have been reported with phenytoin. In countries with mainly Caucasian populations, these reactions are estimated to occur in 1 to 6 per 10 000 new users, but in some Asian countries (e.g., Taiwan, Malaysia and the Philippines) the risk is estimated to be much higher.

HLA-B*1502: In studies that included small samples of patients of Asian ancestry a strong association was found between the risk of developing SJS/TEN and the presence of HLA-B*1502, an inherited allelic variant of the HLA-B gene. The HLA-B*1502 allele is found almost exclusively in individuals with ancestry across broad areas of Asia*. Results of these studies suggest that the presence of the HLA-B *1502 allele may be one of the risk factors for phenytoin-associated SJS/TEN in patients with Asian ancestry. Therefore, physicians should consider HLA-B *1502 genotyping as a screening tool in these patients. Until further information is available, the use of phenytoin and other anti-epileptic drugs associated with SJS/TEN should also be avoided in patients who test positive for the HLA-B*1502 allele (see Warnings, Asian Ancestry and Allelic Variation in the HLA-B Genotyping and Warnings, Important Limitations of HLA-B Genotyping).

Treatment Recommendations for Dermatological Reactions: Phenytoin should be discontinued at the first sign of a rash, unless the rash is clearly not drug-related. If signs or symptoms suggest SJS/TEN, use of this drug should not be resumed and alternative therapy should be considered. The use of other anti-epileptic drugs associated with SJS/TEN should be avoided in patients who have shown severe dermatological reactions during phenytoin treatment.

Literature reports suggest that the combination of phenytoin, cranial irradiation and the gradual reduction of corticosteroids may be associated with the development of erythema multiforme, and/or Stevens-Johnson syndrome, and/or toxic epidermal necrolysis. In any of the above instances, caution should be exercised if using structurally similar compounds (eg, barbiturates, succinimides, oxazolidinediones and other related compounds) in these same patients (see Precautions).

Asian Ancestry and Allelic Variation in the HLA-B Genotyping: In studies that included small samples of patients of Asian ancestry a strong association was found between the risk of developing SJS/TEN and the presence of HLA-B*1502, an inherited allelic variant of the HLA-B gene. The HLA-B*1502 allele is found almost exclusively in individuals with ancestry across broad areas of Asia. Results of these studies suggest that the presence of the HLA-B *1502 allele may be one of the risk factors for phenytoin-associated SJS/TEN in patients with Asian ancestry. Therefore, physicians should consider HLA-B *1502 genotyping as a screening tool in these patients. Until further information is available, the use of phenytoin and other anti-epileptic drugs associated with SJS/TEN should also be avoided in patients who test positive for the HLA-B*1502 allele.

Important Limitations of HLA-B Genotyping: HLA-B*1502 genotyping as a screening tool has important limitations and must never substitute for appropriate clinical vigilance and patient management. Many HLA-B*1502-positive Asian patients treated with phenytoin will not develop SJS/TEN, and these reactions can still occur infrequently in HLA-B*1502-negative patients of any ethnicity. The role of other possible factors in the development of, and morbidity from, SJS/TEN, such as antiepileptic drug (AED) dose, compliance, concomitant medications, co-morbidities, and the level of dermatologic monitoring have not been studied.

In addition, it should be kept in mind that the majority of phenytoin treated patients who will experience SJS/TEN have this reaction within the first few months of treatment. This information may be taken into consideration when deciding whether to screen genetically at-risk patients currently on phenytoin.

Should signs and symptoms suggest a severe skin reaction such as SJS or TEN, phenytoin should be withdrawn at once.

Hepatic/Immunologic: Cases of acute hepatoxicity, including infrequent cases of acute hepatic failure, have been reported with phenytoin. These incidents have been associated with a hypersensitivity syndrome characterized by fever, skin eruptions, and lymphadenopathy, and usually occur within the first 2 months of treatment. Other common manifestations include jaundice, hepatomegaly, elevated serum transaminase levels, leukocytosis, and eosinophilia. The clinical course of acute phenytoin hepatotoxicity ranges from prompt recovery to fatal outcomes. In these patients with acute hepatotoxicity, phenytoin should be immediately discontinued and not re-administered.

Hematopoietic: There have been a number of reports suggesting a relationship between phenytoin and the development of lymphadenopathy (local or generalized) including benign lymph node hyperplasia, pseudolymphoma, lymphoma, and Hodgkin's Disease. Although a cause and effect relationship has not been established, the occurrence of lymphadenopathy indicates the need to differentiate such a condition from other types of lymph node pathology. Lymph node involvement may occur with or without symptoms and signs resembling serum sickness, eg, fever, rash and liver involvement. In all cases of lymphadenopathy, follow-up observation for an extended period is indicated and every effort should be made to achieve seizure control using alternative anticonvulsant drugs.

Metabolic: In view of isolated reports associating phenytoin with exacerbation of porphyria, caution should be exercised in using this medication in patients suffering from this disease.

Psychiatric: Suicidal Ideation and Behaviour: Suicidal ideation and behaviour have been reported in patients treated with antiepileptic agents in several indications.

All patients treated with antiepileptic drugs, irrespective of indication, should be monitored for signs of suicidal ideation and behaviour and appropriate treatment should be considered. Patients (and caregivers of patients) should be advised to seek medical advice should signs of suicidal ideation or behaviour emerge.

An FDA meta-analysis of randomized placebo controlled trials, in which antiepileptic drugs were used for various indications, has shown a small increased risk of suicidal ideation and behaviour in patients treated with these drugs. The mechanism of this risk is not known.

There were 43 892 patients treated in the placebo controlled clinical trials that were included in the meta-analysis. Approximately 75% of patients in these clinical trials were treated for indications other than epilepsy and, for the majority of non-epilepsy indications the treatment (antiepileptic drug or placebo) was administered as monotherapy. Patients with epilepsy represented approximately 25% of the total number of patients treated in the placebo controlled clinical trials and, for the majority of epilepsy patients, treatment (antiepileptic drug or placebo) was administered as adjunct to other antiepileptic agents (i.e., patients in both treatment arms were being treated with one or more antiepileptic drug). Therefore, the small increased risk of suicidal ideation and behaviour reported from the meta-analysis (0.43% for patients on antiepileptic drugs compared to 0.24% for patients on placebo) is based largely on patients that received monotherapy treatment (antiepileptic drug or placebo) for non-epilepsy indications. The study design does not allow an estimation of the risk of suicidal ideation and behaviour for patients with epilepsy that are taking antiepileptic drugs, due both to this population being the minority in the study, and the drug-placebo comparison in this population being confounded by the presence of adjunct antiepileptic drug treatment in both arms.

Pregnancy: A number of reports suggest an association between the use of anticonvulsant drugs by women with epilepsy and a higher incidence of birth defects in children born to these women. Data are more extensive with respect to phenytoin and phenobarbital, but these are also the most commonly prescribed anticonvulsant drugs; fewer systematic or anecdotal reports suggest a possible similar association with the use of all known anticonvulsant drugs.

The reports suggesting a higher incidence of birth defects in children of drug-treated epileptic women cannot be regarded as adequate to prove a definite cause and effect relationship. There are intrinsic methodologic problems in obtaining adequate data on drug teratogenicity in humans. Genetic factors or the epileptic condition itself may be more important than drug therapy in leading to birth defects. The great majority of mothers on anticonvulsant medication deliver normal infants. It is important to note that anticonvulsant drugs should not be discontinued in patients in whom the drug is administered to prevent major seizures because of the strong possibility of precipitating status epilepticus with attendant hypoxia and threat to life. In individual cases where the severity and frequency of the seizure disorder are such that the removal of medication does not pose a serious threat to the patient, discontinuation of the drug may be considered prior to and during pregnancy although it cannot be said with any confidence that even minor seizures do not pose some hazard to the developing embryo or fetus. The prescribing physician will wish to weigh these considerations in treating and counseling epileptic women of childbearing potential.

* The following rates provide a rough estimate of the prevalence of HLA-B*1502 in various populations. Greater than 15% of the population is reported positive in Hong Kong, Thailand, Malaysia, and parts of the Philippines, compared to about 10% in Taiwan and 4% in North China. South Asians, including Indians, appear to have intermediate prevalence of HLA-B*1502, averaging 2 to 4%, but this may be higher in some groups. HLA-B*1502 is present in <1% of the population in Japan and Korea. HLA-B*1502 is largely absent in individuals not of Asian origin (e.g., Caucasians, African-Americans, Hispanics, and Native Americans). The estimated prevalence rates have limitations due to the wide variability in rates that exist within ethnic groups, the difficulties in ascertaining ethnic ancestry and the likelihood of mixed ancestry.

† Coadministration with topiramate reduces serum topiramate levels by 59%, and has the potential to increase phenytoin levels by 25% in some patients. The addition of topiramate therapy to phenytoin should be guided by clinical outcome.

In addition to the reports of increased incidence of congenital malformations, such as cleft lip/palate and heart malformations in children of women receiving phenytoin and other anticonvulsant drugs, there have more recently been reports of a fetal hydantoin syndrome. This consists of prenatal growth deficiency, microcephaly and mental deficiency in children born to mothers who have received phenytoin, barbiturates, alcohol, or trimethadione. However, these features are all interrelated and are frequently associated with intrauterine growth retardation from other causes.

There have been isolated reports of malignancies, including neuroblastoma, in children whose mothers received phenytoin during pregnancy.

An increase in seizure frequency during pregnancy occurs in a high proportion of patients, because of altered phenytoin absorption or metabolism. Periodic measurement of serum phenytoin levels is particularly valuable in the management of a pregnant epileptic patient as a guide to an appropriate adjustment of dosage. However, postpartum restoration of the original dosage will probably be indicated.

Neonatal coagulation defects have been reported within the first 24 hours in babies born to epileptic mothers receiving phenobarbital and/or phenytoin. Vitamin K has been shown to prevent or correct this defect and has been recommended to be given to the mother before delivery and the neonate after birth.

PRECAUTIONS: General: Phenytoin is not indicated for seizures due to hypoglycemic or other metabolic causes. Appropriate diagnostic procedures should be performed as indicated.

Phenytoin is not effective for absence (petit mal) seizures. If tonic-clonic (grand mal) and absence (petit mal) seizures are present, combined drug therapy is needed.

A small percentage of individuals who have been treated with phenytoin have been shown to metabolize the drug slowly. Slow metabolism may be due to limited enzyme availability and lack of induction; it appears to be genetically determined.

Hepatic/Immunologic: The liver is the chief site of biotransformation of DILANTIN Infatabs (phenytoin tablets USP) and DILANTIN-30 Suspension/DILANTIN-125 Suspension (phenytoin oral suspension USP). Patients with impaired liver function, elderly patients, or those who are gravely ill may show early signs of toxicity.

Toxic hepatitis, liver damage, and hypersensitivity syndrome have been reported and may, in rare cases be fatal (see Adverse Effects).

Serious Dermatological Reactions: Phenytoin should be discontinued if a skin rash appears (see "Warnings" regarding drug discontinuation). If the rash is exfoliative, purpuric, or bullous or if lupus erythematosus or Stevens-Johnson syndrome or toxic epidermal necrolysis is suspected, use of this drug should not be resumed and alternative therapy should be considered (see Adverse Effects). If the rash is of a milder type (measles-like or scarlatiniform), therapy may be resumed after the rash has completely disappeared. If the rash recurs upon reinstitution of therapy, further phenytoin medication is contraindicated.

Literature reports suggest that the combination of phenytoin, cranial irradiation and the gradual reduction of corticosteroids may be associated with the development of erythema multiforme, and/or Stevens-Johnson syndrome, and/or toxic epidermal necrolysis. In any of the above instances, caution should be exercised if using structurally similar compounds (eg, barbiturates, succinimides, oxazolidinediones and other related compounds) in these same patients (see Warnings).

Published literature has suggested that there may be an increased, although still rare, risk of hypersensitivity reactions, including skin rash, SJS, TEN, hepatotoxicity, and Anticonvulsant Hypersensitivity Syndrome in black patients.

Hematopoietic: While macrocytosis and megaloblastic anemia have occurred, these conditions usually respond to folic acid therapy. If folic acid is added to phenytoin therapy, a decrease in seizure control may occur.

Metabolic: Hyperglycemia, resulting from the drug's inhibitory effects on insulin release, has been reported. Phenytoin may also raise the serum glucose level in diabetic patients.

Musculoskeletal: Phenytoin and other anticonvulsants that have been shown to induce the CYP450 enzyme are thought to affect bone mineral metabolism indirectly by increasing the metabolism of Vitamin D3. This may lead to Vitamin D deficiency and heightened risk of osteomalacia, bone fractures, osteoporosis, hypocalcemia, and hypophosphatemia in chronically treated epileptic patients (see Adverse Effets, Post-marketing Experience).

Central Nervous System: Serum levels of phenytoin sustained above the optimal range may produce confusional states referred to as "delirium", "psychosis" or "encephalopathy", or rarely irreversible cerebellar dysfunction. Accordingly, at the first sign of acute toxicity, serum drug level determinations are recommended. Dose reduction of phenytoin therapy is indicated if serum levels are excessive; if symptoms persist, termination of phenytoin therapy is recommended (see Warnings).

Information to Be Provided to the Patient: Patients taking phenytoin should be advised of the importance of adhering strictly to the prescribed dosage regimen, and of informing their physician of any clinical condition in which it is not possible to take the drug orally as prescribed, eg, surgery, etc.

Patients should also be cautioned on the use of other drugs or alcoholic beverages without first seeking the physician's advice.

Patients should be instructed to call their physician if skin rash develops.

The importance of good dental hygiene should be stressed in order to minimize the development of gingival hyperplasia and its complications.

Laboratory Tests: Phenytoin serum level determinations may be necessary to achieve optimal dosage adjustments.

Drug Interactions: There are many drugs which may increase or decrease serum phenytoin levels or which phenytoin may affect. Determinations of serum phenytoin concentrations are especially helpful when possible drug interactions are suspected. The **most commonly occurring** drug interactions are listed below:

1. Drugs which may increase phenytoin serum levels include: acute alcohol intake, cimetidine, dicumarol, disulfiram, ethosuximide, methylphenidate, omeprazole, phenothiazines, ticlopidine and topiramate†. The following drug classes are also included: See Table 1.

Table 1: Dilantin Infatabs/Dilantin-30/Dilantin-125

Drugs Which May Increase Phenytoin Serum Levels

Drug Classes	Drugs in Each Class (such as)
Analgesic/anti-inflammatory agents	azapropazone phenylbutazone salicylates
Anesthetics	halothane
Antibacterial agents	chloramphenicol erythromycin isoniazid sulfonamides
Anticonvulsants	felbamate succinimides
Antifungal agents	amphotericin B fluconazole ketoconazole miconazole itraconazole
Benzodiazepines/psychotropic agents	chlordiazepoxide diazepam trazodone
Calcium channel blockers/cardiovascular agents	amiodarone diltiazem nifedipine
H_2-antagonists	cimetidine
Hormones	estrogens

(cont'd)

Table 1: Dilantin Infatabs/Dilantin-30/Dilantin-125 *(cont'd)*

Drugs Which May Increase Phenytoin Serum Levels

Drug Classes	Drugs in Each Class (such as)
Oral hypoglycemic agents	tolbutamide
Serotonin re-uptake inhibitors	fluoxetine paroxetine

2. Drugs which may decrease phenytoin serum levels include: antibacterial agents/fluoroquinolones (such as ciprofloxacin and rifampin), carbamazepine, chronic alcohol abuse, diazoxide, reserpine, sucralfate, theophylline and vigabatrin‡. Molindone Hydrochloride contains calcium ions which interfere with the absorption of phenytoin. Ingestion times of phenytoin and calcium preparations, including antacid preparations containing calcium should be staggered to prevent absorption problems.
3. Drugs which may either increase or decrease phenytoin serum levels include the following: See Table 2.

Table 2: Dilantin Infatabs/Dilantin-30/Dilantin-125

Drugs Which May Either Increase or Decrease Phenytoin Serum Levels

Drug Classes	Drugs in Each Class (such as)
Anticonvulsants	carbamazepine phenobarbital sodium valproate valproic acid
Antineoplastic agents	
Benzodiazepines	chlordiazepoxide
Phenothiazines	
Psychotropic agents	diazepam

Similarly, the effect of phenytoin on carbamazepine, phenobarbital, valproic acid and sodium valproate serum levels is unpredictable.
4. Although not a true drug interaction, tricyclic antidepressants may precipitate seizures in susceptible patients and phenytoin dosage may need to be adjusted.
5. Drugs whose blood levels and/or effects may be altered by phenytoin include: clozapine, corticosteroids, coumarin anticoagulants, cyclosporine, diazoxide, furosemide, lamotrigine¶, paroxetine, theophylline, topiramate§ and vitamin D. The following drug classes are also included: See Table 3.

Table 3: Dilantin Infatabs/Dilantin-30/Dilantin-125

Drugs Whose Blood Levels and/or Effects May Be Altered by Phenytoin

Drug Classes	Drugs in Each Class (such as)
Antibacterial agents	doxycycline praziquantel rifampin tetracycline
Antifungal agents	
Antineoplastic agents	
Calcium channel blockers/cardiovascular agents	digitoxin nicardipine nimodipine quinidine verapamil
Hormones	estrogens oral contraceptives
Neuromuscular blocking agents	alcuronium pancuronium vecuronium
Opioid analgesics	methadone
Oral hypoglycemic agents	chlorpropamide glyburide tolbutamide

Drug-Enteral Feeding/Nutritional Preparations Interaction: Literature reports suggest that patients who have received enteral feeding preparations and/or related nutritional supplements have lower than expected phenytoin plasma levels. It is therefore suggested that phenytoin not be administered concomitantly with an enteral feeding preparation.

More frequent serum phenytoin level monitoring may be necessary in these patients.

Drug/Laboratory Test Interactions: Phenytoin may cause decreased serum levels of protein-bound iodine (PBI). It may also produce lower than normal values for dexamethasone or metyrapone tests. Phenytoin may cause increased serum levels of glucose, alkaline phosphatase, and gamma glutamyl transpeptidase (GGT). Phenytoin may affect blood calcium and blood sugar metabolism tests.

Carcinogenesis: See Warnings.

Pregnancy: See Warnings.

Lactation: Infant breast feeding is not recommended for women taking this drug because phenytoin appears to be secreted in low concentrations in human milk.

Children: See Dosage.

‡ Coadministration with Vigabatrin reduces serum phenytoin levels by 20% to 30%. This may be clinically significant in some patients and may require dosage adjustment.

¶ Coadministration with lamotrigine doubles the plasma clearance and reduces the elimination half life of lamotrigine by 50%. This clinically important interaction requires dosage adjustment.

§ Coadministration with topiramate reduces serum topiramate levels by 59%, and has the potential to increase phenytoin levels by 25% in some patients. The addition of topiramate therapy to phenytoin should be guided by clinical outcome.

ADVERSE EFFECTS: Central Nervous System: The most common manifestations encountered with DILANTIN Infatabs (phenytoin tablets USP) and DILANTIN-30 Suspension/DILANTIN-125 Suspension (phenytoin oral suspension USP) therapy are referable to this system and are usually dose-related. These include nystagmus, ataxia, slurred speech, decreased coordination, and mental confusion. Dizziness, insomnia, transient nervousness, motor twitchings, and headaches have also been observed. There have also been rare reports of phenytoin induced dyskinesias, including chorea, dystonia, tremor and asterixis, similar to those induced by phenothiazine and other neuroleptic drugs.

A predominantly sensory peripheral polyneuropathy has been observed in patients receiving long-term phenytoin therapy.

Gastrointestinal System: nausea, vomiting, constipation, toxic hepatitis, and liver damage (see Precautions).

Integumentary System: Dermatological manifestations sometimes accompanied by fever have included scarlatiniform or morbilliform rashes. A morbilliform rash (measles-like) is the most common; other types of dermatitis are seen more rarely. Other more serious forms which may be fatal have included bullous, exfoliative or purpuric dermatitis, lupus erythematosus, and Stevens-Johnson syndrome and toxic epidermal necrolysis (see Warnings).

Hemopoietic System: Hemopoietic complications, some fatal, have occasionally been reported in association with administration of phenytoin. These have included thrombocytopenia, leukopenia, granulocytopenia, agranulocytosis, and pancytopenia with or without bone marrow suppression. While macrocytosis and megaloblastic anemia have occurred, these conditions usually respond to folic acid therapy. Lymphadenopathy, including benign lymph node hyperplasia, pseudolymphoma, lymphoma, and Hodgkin's Disease has been reported (see Warnings).

Connective Tissue System: coarsening of the facial features, enlargement of the lips, gingival hyperplasia, hypertrichosis and Peyronie's Disease.

Immunologic: Hypersensitivity syndrome (which may include, but is not limited to symptoms such as arthralgias, eosinophilia, fever, liver dysfunction, lymphadenopathy or rash), systemic lupus erythematosus, periarteritis nodosa, and immunoglobulin abnormalities. Several individual case reports have suggested that there may be an increased, although still rare, incidence of hypersensitivity reactions, including skin rash and hepatotoxicity, in black patients (see Warnings and Precautions).

Post-marketing Experience: Musculoskeletal System: Bone fractures and osteomalacia have been associated with long-term (>10 years) use of phenytoin by patients with chronic epilepsy. Osteoporosis and other disorders of bone metabolism such as hypocalcemia, hypophosphatemia and decreased levels of Vitamin D metabolites have also been reported (see Precautions, Musculoskeletal).

OVERDOSE:

Symptoms: The lethal dose of DILANTIN Infatabs (phenytoin tablets USP) and DILANTIN 30 Suspension/DILANTIN 125 Suspension (phenytoin oral suspension USP) in pediatric patients is not known. The lethal dose of phenytoin in adults is estimated to be 2 to 5 grams. The initial symptoms are nystagmus, ataxia, and dysarthria. Other signs are tremor, hyperreflexia, somnolence, drowsiness, lethargy, slurred speech, blurred vision, nausea, vomiting. The patient may become comatose and hypotensive. Death is due to respiratory and circulatory depression.

There are marked variations among individuals with respect to phenytoin plasma levels where toxicity may occur. Nystagmus on lateral gaze, usually appears at 80 µmol/L (20 µg/mL), ataxia at 119 µmol/L (30 µg/mL). Dysarthria and lethargy appear when the serum concentration is >159 µmol/L (40 µg/mL), but a concentration as high as 198 µmol/L (50 µg/mL) has been reported without evidence of toxicity. As much as 25 times the therapeutic dose has been taken to result in a serum concentration over >396 µmol/L (100 µg/mL) with complete recovery.

Treatment: Treatment is nonspecific since there is no known antidote.

The adequacy of the respiratory and circulatory systems should be carefully observed and appropriate supportive measures employed. Hemodialysis can be considered since phenytoin is not completely bound to plasma proteins. Total exchange transfusion has been used in the treatment of severe intoxication in pediatric patients.

In acute overdosage the possibility of the pressure of other CNS depressants, including alcohol, should be borne in mind.

For management of a suspected drug overdose, contact your **regional Poison Control Centre**. See the *CPS* Directory section for a list of Poison Control Centres.

DOSAGE: DILANTIN suspensions are not for parenteral use.

Serum phenytoin concentrations should be monitored and care should be taken when switching a patient from the sodium salt to the free acid form.

DILANTIN extended release capsules are formulated with the sodium salt of phenytoin. The free acid form of phenytoin is used in DILANTIN-30 Suspension and DILANTIN-125 Suspension and DILANTIN Infatabs. Because there is approximately an 8% increase in drug content with the free acid form over that of the sodium salt, dosage adjustments and serum level monitoring may be necessary when switching from a product formulated with the free acid to a product formulated with the sodium salt and vice versa.

General: DILANTIN Infatabs (phenytoin tablets, USP) and DILANTIN-30 Suspension/DILANTIN-125 Suspension (phenytoin oral suspension, USP) are not for once-a-day dosing.

Dosage should be individualized to provide maximum benefit. In some cases, serum blood level determinations may be necessary for optimal dosage adjustments. The clinically effective serum level is usually 40-80 µmol/L (10-20 µg/mL). Serum blood level determinations are especially helpful when possible drug interactions are suspected. With recommended dosage, a period of 7 to 10 days may be required to achieve therapeutic blood levels with DILANTIN and changes in dosage (increase or decrease) should not be carried out at intervals shorter than 7 to 10 days.

Adults: Patients who have received no previous treatment may be started on 2 **DILANTIN Infatabs** 3 times daily or on 1 teaspoonful (5 mL) of **DILANTIN-125 Suspension** 3 times daily, and the dose then adjusted to suit individual requirements. For some adults, the satisfactory maintenance dosage will be 8 **DILANTIN Infatabs** daily; an increase to 12 **DILANTIN Infatabs** may be made, if necessary. With DILANTIN-125 Suspension, an increase to 5 teaspoonfuls (25 mL) daily may be made if necessary.

Children: Initially, 5 mg/kg/day of DILANTIN Infatabs, DILANTIN-30 Suspension or DILANTIN-125 Suspension may be given in 2 or 3 equally divided doses, with subsequent dosage individualized to a maximum of 300 mg daily. A recommended daily maintenance dosage is usually 4 to 8 mg/kg. Children over 6 years may require the minimum adult dose (300 mg/day). If the daily dosage cannot be divided equally, the larger dose should be given at bedtime.

INFORMATION FOR THE PATIENT: Published in e-CPS, available by subscription at www.e-cps.ca.

SUPPLIED: Dilantin Infatabs: Each flavored, triangular shaped, grooved tablet contains: phenytoin (free acid form) 50 mg. Nonmedicinal ingredients: alcohol, magnesium stearate, spearmint oil, sugar and talc. Bottles of 100. Store at controlled room temperature 15 to 30°C. Protect from light and moisture.

Dilantin-30 Suspension: Each 5 mL of flavored, colored suspension contains: phenytoin (free acid form) 30 mg. Nonmedicinal ingredients: alcohol, banana oil, citric acid, glycerin, magnesium aluminum silicate, orange oil, polysorbate 40, Red #2 FD&C, sodium benzoate, sodium carboxymethylcellulose, sugar, vanillin and yellow #6 FD&C. Bottles of 250 mL. Store at controlled room temperature 15 to 30°C and protect from freezing and light.

Dilantin-125 Suspension: Each 5 mL of flavored, colored suspension contains: phenytoin (free acid form) 125 mg. Nonmedicinal ingredients: alcohol, banana oil, citric acid, glycerin, magnesium aluminum silicate, orange oil, polysorbate 40, sodium benzoate, sodium carboxymethyl- cellulose, sugar, vanillin and yellow #6 FD&C. Bottles of 250 mL. Store at controlled room temperature 15 to 30°C and protect from freezing and light.

(Shown in Product Identification Section)

Dilaudid® Ⓝ

hydromorphone HCl

Opioid Analgesic

Purdue Pharma

Date of Preparation: August 8, 2008

PHARMACOLOGY: DILAUDID (hydromorphone hydrochloride) has strong analgesic and antitussive activity. Small doses of hydromorphone produce effective and prompt relief of pain, usually with minimal nausea and vomiting. When given parenterally, hydromorphone's analgesic action is generally apparent within five minutes. The onset of action of oral hydromorphone hydrochloride is somewhat slower, with measurable analgesia occurring within 30 minutes. When sleep follows the administration of hydromorphone, it is usually due to relief of pain, not to hypnosis.

Hydromorphone is approximately 8 times more potent on a milligram basis than morphine. In addition, hydromorphone is better absorbed orally than is morphine, the former approximately 20 to 25% as active orally as i.m. Hydromorphone has greater antitussive potency than codeine on a weight basis; however, its dependence liability is also greater than that of codeine.

After absorption, hydromorphone is metabolized by the liver to the glucuronide conjugate which is then excreted in the urine.

INDICATIONS: DILAUDID (hydromorphone hydrochloride) is indicated for the relief of moderate to severe pain. For post-operative relief of pain.

CONTRAINDICATIONS: DILAUDID (hydromorphone hydrochloride) is contraindicated in patients with known hypersensitivity to the drug; patients with respiratory depression in the absence of resuscitative equipment; in patients with severe CNS depression; patients with intracranial lesions associated with increased intracranial pressure; patients with status asthmaticus; patients with pulmonary edema.

WARNINGS: Drug Dependence: All opioids, like morphine and DILAUDID (hydromorphone hydrochloride), can produce drug dependence and therefore have the potential for being abused. As with other opioid drugs, psychic dependence, physical dependence and tolerance are likely to develop upon repeated administration of hydromorphone, and it should be prescribed and administered with the same degree of caution appropriate for the use of morphine. Abrupt discontinuation of the administration of hydromorphone is likely to result in a withdrawal syndrome (see Precautions, Dependence Liability).

Infants born to mothers physically dependent on hydromorphone will also be physically dependent and may exhibit respiratory difficulties and withdrawal symptoms (see Precautions, Dependence Liability).

Impaired Respiration: Respiratory depression is the chief hazard of hydromorphone. It occurs most frequently in overdose, the elderly, in the debilitated, and in those suffering from conditions accompanied by hypoxia or hypercapnia, when even moderate therapeutic doses may dangerously decrease pulmonary ventilation. This effect may be lessened by careful dose titration as severe pain can antagonize the respiratory depressant action of hydromorphone.

Hydromorphone should be used with extreme caution in patients with chronic obstructive pulmonary disease or cor pulmonale, patients having a substantially decreased respiratory reserve, hypoxia, hypercapnia, or pre-existing respiratory depression. In such patients, even the usual therapeutic doses of opioid analgesics may decrease respiratory drive while simultaneously increasing airway resistance, to the point of apnea.

As mentioned above, severe pain antagonizes the subjective and respiratory depressant actions of hydromorphone. However, should pain suddenly subside, these effects may rapidly become manifest. Patients who are scheduled for cordotomy or other interruptions of pain transmission pathways should not receive hydromorphone within 24 hours of the procedure.

Hypotensive Effect: Opioid analgesics, including hydromorphone, may cause severe hypotension in individuals whose ability to maintain normal blood pressure has already been compromised by depleted blood volume, or the concurrent administration of drugs such as phenothiazines and other tranquilizers, sedative/hypnotics, tricyclic antidepressants or general anesthetics (see also Precautions, Drug Interactions). Hydromorphone may produce orthostatic hypotension in ambulatory patients.

Hydromorphone should be administered with caution to patients in circulatory shock, since vasodilation produced by the drug may further reduce cardiac output and blood pressure.

Rapid intravenous injection of opioid analgesics increases the possibility of hypotension and respiratory depression and should be avoided (see Dosage).

Pregnancy: (see Warnings, Drug Dependence).

Animals: Adequate animal studies on reproduction have not been performed to determine whether hydromorphone affects fertility in males or females. However, animal studies with both morphine and hydromorphone have indicated the possibility of teratogenic effects.

Humans: There are no well-controlled studies in women. Reports based on marketing experience do not identify any specific teratogenic risks following routine (short-term) clinical use. Although there is no clearly defined risk, such reports do not exclude the possibility of infrequent or subtle damage to the human fetus. Hydromorphone should be used in pregnant women only when clearly needed (see Precautions, Dependence Liability).

PRECAUTIONS: General: In diseases, such as malignant cancers, where pain control is the primary focus opioid administration at very high doses is associated with seizures and myoclonus.

If necessary, hydromorphone may be given i.v. but the injection should be given very slowly. Rapid i.v. injection of narcotic analgesic agents, including hydromorphone, increases the possibility of adverse effects, such as hypotension and respiratory depression.

Special Risk Groups: In general, opioids should be given with caution and the initial dose should be reduced for the elderly or debilitated, and those with severe impairment of hepatic, pulmonary or renal function; myxedema or hypothyroidism; adrenocortical insufficiency (i.e. Addison's disease); CNS depression or coma; elevated intracranial pressure; toxic psychosis; prostatic hypertrophy or urethral stricture; gallbladder disease; acute alcoholism; delirium tremens; or kyphoscoliosis.

The administration of opioid analgesics including hydromorphone may obscure the diagnosis or clinical course in patients with acute abdominal conditions.

Opioid analgesics including hydromorphone should also be used with caution in patients about to undergo surgery of the biliary tract, since they may cause spasm of the sphincter of Oddi.

Dependence Liability: Opioid analgesics may cause psychological and physical dependence (see Warnings). Physical dependence results in withdrawal symptoms in patients who abruptly discontinue the drug. Withdrawal symptoms may also be precipitated in the patient with physical dependency by the administration of a drug with opioid antagonist activity, i.e. naloxone or mixed agonist antagonists i.e. pentazocine (see also Overdose, Symptoms and Treatment). Physical dependence usually does not occur to a clinically significant degree until after several weeks of continued opioid usage. Tolerance, in which increasingly large doses are required in order to produce the same degree of analgesia, is initially manifested by a shortened duration of analgesic effect and subsequently, by decreases in the intensity of analgesia. The dose required to produce analgesia is, therefore, related to the degree of tolerance.

In chronic pain patients in whom opioid analgesics are abruptly discontinued, a severe abstinence syndrome should be anticipated. This may be similar to the abstinence syndrome noted in patients withdrawing from heroin.

The latter abstinence syndrome may be characterized by restlessness, lacrimation, rhinorrhea, yawning, perspiration, gooseflesh, restless sleep or "yen", and a mydriasis during the first 24 hours. Those symptoms may increase in severity and over the next 72 hours may be accompanied by increasing irritability, anxiety, weakness, twitching and spasms of muscles, kicking movements, severe backache, abdominal and leg pains, abdominal and muscle cramps, hot and cold flashes, insomnia, nausea, anorexia, vomiting, intestinal spasm, diarrhea, coryza and repetitive sneezing, increase in body temperature, blood pressure, respiratory rate and heart rate.

Because of the excessive loss of fluids through sweating, or vomiting and diarrhea, there is usually marked weight loss, dehydration, ketosis, and disturbances in acid-base balance. Cardiovascular collapse can occur. Without treatment, most observable symptoms disappear in 5 to 14 days; however, there appears to be a phase of secondary or chronic abstinence which may last for 2 to 6 months and is characterized by insomnia, irritability, muscular aches, and autonomic instability.

In the treatment of physical dependence on hydromorphone, the patient may be detoxified by gradual reduction of the dosage, although this is unlikely to be necessary in the terminal cancer patient. If abstinence symptoms become severe, the patient may be given methadone. Temporary administration of tranquilizers and sedatives may aid in reducing patient anxiety. Gastrointestinal disturbances or dehydration should be treated accordingly.

Hydromorphone hydrochloride should be used with caution in patients with alcoholism and other drug dependencies due to increased frequency of opioid tolerance and psychological dependence observed in these patient populations.

Drug Interactions: The concomitant use of other central nervous system depressants including sedatives or hypnotics, general anesthetics, phenothiazines, tranquilizers and alcohol may produce additive depressant effects. Respiratory depression, hypotension and profound sedation or coma may occur. When such combined therapy is contemplated, the dose of one or both agents should be reduced. Opioid analgesics, including hydromorphone may enhance the action of neuromuscular blocking agents and produce an increased degree of respiratory depression.

Pregnancy: During pregnancy, hydromorphone hydrochloride should be administered with caution and after the need of the mother has been considered against the risk for the child. In long-term treatment during pregnancy, the risk of neonatal withdrawal should be considered.

Lactation: Low levels of opioid analgesics have been detected in human milk. As a general rule, nursing should not be undertaken while a patient is receiving hydromorphone since it and other drugs in this class may be excreted in the milk.

Children: Safety and effectiveness in children have not been established. Hydromorphone suppositories are not recommended for use in children.

Geriatrics: In general, dose selection for elderly patients should be cautious and the initial dose should be reduced due to the greater frequency of decreased hepatic, renal or cardiac functions and of concomitant disease or other drug therapy in these patients.

Cough Reflex: Hydromorphone hydrochloride suppresses the cough reflex; as with all opioid analgesics, caution should be exercised when hydromorphone hydrochloride is used post-operatively in patients with pulmonary disease.

Occupational Hazards: Ability to Drive and Use Machines: Hydromorphone hydrochloride may impair mental and/or physical ability required for the performance of potentially hazardous tasks such as driving and operating machinery.

ADVERSE EFFECTS: The adverse effects of DILAUDID (hydromorphone hydrochloride) are similar to those of other opioid analgesics and represent an extension of pharmacological effects of the drug class. The major hazards include respiratory depression and apnea. To a lesser degree, circulatory depression, respiratory arrest, shock and cardiac arrest have occurred.

The most frequently observed adverse effects are constipation, lightheadedness, dizziness, sedation, nausea, vomiting, and sweating. All of these effects, except constipation seem to be more prominent in ambulatory patients and in those not experiencing severe pain. Some adverse reactions in ambulatory patients may be alleviated if the patient lies down. When instituting prolonged therapy with an opioid for chronic pain, the prescription of antiemetics for nausea and vomiting and an appropriate regimen of bowel management for constipation (stool softeners, laxatives etc.) should be considered.

Pain at injection site, local tissue irritation and induration following s.c. injection, particularly when repeated in the same area have occurred.

Sedation: Some degree of sedation is experienced by most patients upon initiation of therapy. This may be at least partly because patients often recuperate from prolonged fatigue after the relief of persistent pain. Most patients develop tolerance to the sedative effects of opioids within three to five days and, if the sedation is not severe, will not require any treatment except reassurance. If excessive sedation persists beyond a few days, the dose of the opioid should be reduced and alternate causes investigated. Some of these are: concurrent CNS depressant medication, hepatic or renal dysfunction, brain metastases, hypercalcemia and respiratory failure. If it is necessary to reduce the dose, it can be carefully increased again after three or four days if it is obvious that the pain is not being well controlled. Dizziness and unsteadiness may be caused by postural hypotension particularly in elderly or debilitated patients and may be alleviated if the patient lies down.

Nausea and Vomiting: Nausea is a common side effect on initiation of therapy with opioid analgesics and is thought to occur by activation of the chemoreceptor trigger zone, stimulation of the vestibular apparatus and through delayed gastric emptying. The prevalence of nausea declines following continued treatment with opioid analgesics. When instituting prolonged therapy with an opioid for chronic pain, the routine prescription of an antiemetic should be considered. In the cancer patient, investigation of nausea should include such causes as constipation, bowel obstruction, uremia, hypercalcemia, hepatomegaly, tumor invasion of celiac plexus and concurrent use of drugs with emetogenic properties. Persistent nausea which does not respond to dosage reduction may be caused by opioid-induced gastric stasis and may be accompanied by other symptoms including anorexia, early satiety, vomiting and abdominal fullness. These symptoms respond to chronic treatment with gastrointestinal prokinetic agents.

Constipation: Practically all patients become constipated while taking opioids on a persistent basis. In some patients, particularly the elderly or bedridden, fecal impaction may result. It is essential to caution the patients in this regard and to institute an appropriate regimen of bowel management at the start of prolonged opioid analgesic therapy. Stool softeners, stimulant laxatives and other appropriate measures should be used as required.

Less Frequently Observed with Opioid Analgesics:

General and CNS: dysphoria, euphoria, weakness, headache, agitation, tremor, uncoordinated muscle movements, alterations of mood (nervousness, apprehension, depression, floating feelings, dreams), muscle rigidity, paresthesia, muscle tremor, blurred vision, nystagmus, diplopia and miosis, hallucinations and disorientation, visual disturbances, insomnia and increased intracranial pressure may occur.

Cardiovascular: flushing of the face, chills, tachycardia, bradycardia, palpitation, faintness, syncope, hypotension and hypertension have been reported.

Respiratory: bronchospasm and laryngospasm have been known to occur.

Gastrointestinal: dry mouth, constipation, biliary tract spasm, anorexia, diarrhea, cramps, ileus and taste alterations have been reported.

Genitourinary: urinary retention or hesitancy, and antidiuretic effects have been reported.

Dermatologic: pruritus, urticaria, other skin rashes, wheal and flare over the vein with intravenous injection, and diaphoresis have been reported with opioid analgesics.

OVERDOSE:

Symptoms: Serious overdosage with DILAUDID (hydromorphone hydrochloride) is characterized by respiratory depression (a decrease in respiratory rate and/or tidal volume, Cheyne-Stokes respiration, cyanosis), extreme somnolence progressing to stupor or coma, skeletal muscle flaccidity, cold and clammy skin, and sometimes bradycardia and hypotension. In severe overdosage, particularly following intravenous injection, apnea, circulatory collapse, cardiac arrest and death may occur.

Treatment: In the treatment of overdosage, primary attention should be given to the re-establishment of adequate respiratory exchange through provision of a patent airway and institution of assisted or controlled ventilation. It should be borne in mind that for individuals who are physically dependent on opioids and are receiving large doses of these drugs, the administration of the usual dose of opioid antagonist will precipitate an acute withdrawal syndrome. The severity will depend on the degree of physical dependence and the dose of the antagonist administered. Use of an opioid antagonist in such persons should be avoided. If necessary to treat serious respiratory depression in the physically dependent patient, the antagonist should be administered with extreme care and by titration, commencing with 10 to 20% of the usual recommended initial dose.

Respiratory depression which may result from overdosage, or unusual sensitivity to hydromorphone in a non-opioid-tolerant patient, can be managed with the opioid antagonist naloxone. A dose of naloxone (usually 0.4 to 2.0 mg) should be administered intravenously, if possible, simultaneously with respiratory resuscitation. The dose can be repeated in 3 minutes. Naloxone should not be administered in the absence of clinically significant respiratory or circulatory depression. Naloxone should be administered cautiously to persons who are known or suspected to be physically dependent on hydromorphone. In such cases, an abrupt or complete reversal of opioid effects may precipitate an acute abstinence syndrome.

Since the duration of action of hydromorphone may exceed that of the antagonist, the patient should be kept under continued surveillance; repeated doses of the antagonist may be required to maintain adequate respiration. Other supportive measures should be applied when indicated.

Supportive measures, including oxygen and vasopressors, should be employed in the management of circulatory shock and pulmonary edema accompanying overdose, as indicated. Cardiac arrest or arrhythmias may require cardiac massage or defibrillation.

For management of a suspected drug overdose, CPhA recommends that you contact your **regional Poison Control Centre**. See the *CPS* Directory section for a list of Poison Control Centres.

DOSAGE: Oral: Orally for adults, 2 to 4 mg every 4 to 6 hours as required.

The oral liquid may be diluted in fruit juice or other beverage, if desired.

Parenteral: The usual adult parenteral dose for pain relief is 2 mg by s.c. or i.m. route every 4 to 6 hours as necessary. If necessary, hydromorphone may be given i.v., but the injection should be given very slowly. Rapid intravenous injection of opioid analgesics increases the possibility of hypotension and respiratory depression. Severe pain can be controlled with 3 to 4 mg every 4 to 6 hours as necessary.

DILAUDID injection has been reported to be physically or chemically incompatible with solutions containing sodium bicarbonate and thiopental sodium.

SUPPLIED: Ampuls: Each mL of sterile solution contains: hydromorphone HCl 2 mg. Nonmedicinal ingredients: citric acid and sodium citrate. Preservative-free. Ampuls of 1 mL, boxes of 25. Store at 15 to 25°C. Protect from light.

Oral Liquid: Each mL of clear, unflavored, syrupy liquid contains: hydromorphone HCl 1 mg. Nonmedicinal ingredients: glycerin, methylparaben, propylparaben and sucrose. Sucrose: 0.5 g/mL. Energy: 8.4 kJ (2 kcal)/mL. Alcohol-free. Amber glass bottles of 450 mL. Store at 15 to 25°C.

Tablets: Each tablet contains: hydromorphone HCl 1 mg (green), 2 mg (orange), 4 mg (yellow) or 8 mg (white, scored). Nonmedicinal ingredients: lactose anhydrous and magnesium stearate. Also contains: D&C Yellow #10 Lake and FD&C Blue #1 Lake (for 1 mg), D&C Red #30 Lake and D&C Yellow #10 Lake (for 2 mg), D&C Yellow #10 Lake (for 4 mg). Tartrazine-free. Bottles of 100. Hospital Control Packs of 4×25. Store at 15 to 25°C.

Dilaudid-HP® Ⓝ
hydromorphone HCl
Opioid Analgesic

Purdue Pharma

Dilaudid-HP-Plus® Ⓝ
hydromorphone HCl
Opioid Analgesic

Purdue Pharma

Dilaudid-XP® Ⓝ
hydromorphone HCl
Opioid Analgesic

Purdue Pharma

Dilaudid® Sterile Powder Ⓝ
hydromorphone HCl
Opioid Analgesic

Purdue Pharma

Date of Preparation: August 8, 2008

> Dilaudid-HP, Dilaudid-HP-Plus, Dilaudid-XP, and reconstituted Dilaudid Sterile Powder are highly concentrated solutions of hydromorphone hydrochloride. They should be used only in opioid tolerant patients requiring high doses or high concentrations of opioid agonists. Do not confuse Dilaudid-HP, Dilaudid-HP-Plus, Dilaudid-XP, and reconstituted Dilaudid Sterile Powder with the lower concentration of the Dilaudid 2 mg/mL ampoules since overdosage and death could result.

PHARMACOLOGY: Hydromorphone is a hydrogenated ketone of morphine. It is an opioid analgesic with many of the effects common to the class of drugs.

Opioid analgesics have multiple actions but exert their primary effects on the CNS and organs containing smooth muscle. The principal actions of therapeutic value are analgesia and sedation. Opioid analgesics also suppress the cough reflex and cause respiratory depression, mood changes, mental clouding, euphoria, dysphoria, nausea, vomiting, increased cerebrospinal fluid pressure, pinpoint constriction of the pupils, increased biliary tract pressure, increased parasympathetic activity and transient hyperglycemia.

The precise mode of analgesic action of opioid analgesics is unknown. However, specific CNS opiate receptors have been identified. Opioids are believed to express their pharmacological effects by combining with these receptors.

The relationship between plasma concentration of hydromorphone and analgesic effect has not been well established. In patients with chronic pain, hydromorphone should be titrated to the dose required to adequately relieve pain without unmanageable side effects. There is no intrinsic limit to the analgesic effect of hydromorphone; adequate doses will relieve even the most severe pain. Clinically, however, dosage limitations are imposed by the adverse effects, primarily respiratory depression; nausea and vomiting which can result from high doses.

Pharmacokinetics: In normal human volunteers hydromorphone is metabolized primarily in the liver. It is excreted predominantly as the glucuronidated conjugate, with small amounts of parent drug and minor amounts of 6-hydroxy reduction metabolites.

Following i.v. administration of hydromorphone to normal volunteers, the mean half-life of elimination was 2.65 ± 0.88 hours. The mean volume of distribution was 91.5 L, suggesting extensive tissue uptake. Hydromorphone is rapidly removed from the bloodstream and distributed to skeletal muscle, kidneys, liver, intestinal tract, lungs, spleen and brain. It also crosses the placental membranes.

Hydromorphone is approximately 5 to 7 times more potent than morphine (i.e., 1.5 to 2 mg of hydromorphone produces analgesia equal to that produced by 10 mg of morphine). After i.m. administration, hydromorphone has a slightly more rapid onset and slightly shorter duration of action than morphine. The duration of analgesia in the non-tolerant patient with usual doses may be up to 4 to 5 hours. However, in opioid tolerant subjects, duration of analgesia will vary substantially depending on tolerance and dose. Dose should be adjusted so that 3 to 4 hours of pain relief may be achieved.

INDICATIONS: Indicated exclusively for the relief of severe pain in patients who require s.c., i.v. or i.m. administered opioids in doses or concentrations higher than those usually needed. Because hydromorphone is highly soluble, a smaller injection volume can be used and discomfort associated with the i.m. or s.c. injection of larger volumes of solution can be minimized.

CONTRAINDICATIONS: Patients who are not already receiving high doses or high concentrations of opioids; patients with known hypersensitivity to the drug; patients with respiratory depression in the absence of resuscitative equipment; in patients with severe CNS depression; and in patients with status asthmaticus. High concentrations of hydromorphone preparations are also contraindicated for use in obstetrical analgesia and are not intended for use except in patients with severe pain.

WARNINGS: Drug Dependence: All opioids, like morphine and hydromorphone, can produce drug dependence and therefore have the potential for being abused. As with other opioid drugs, psychic dependence, physical dependence and tolerance are likely to develop upon repeated administration of hydromorphone, and it should be prescribed and administered with the same degree of caution appropriate for the use of morphine. Abrupt discontinuation of the administration of hydromorphone is likely to result in a withdrawal syndrome (see Precautions, Dependence Liability).

Infants born to mothers physically dependent on hydromorphone will also be physically dependent and may exhibit respiratory difficulties and withdrawal symptoms (see Precautions, Dependence Liability).

Impaired Respiration: Respiratory depression is the chief hazard of hydromorphone. It occurs most frequently in overdose, in the elderly, in the debilitated, and in those suffering from conditions accompanied by hypoxia or hypercapnia, when even moderate therapeutic doses may dangerously decrease pulmonary ventilation. This effect may be lessened by careful dose titration as severe pain can antagonize the respiratory depressant action of hydromorphone.

Hydromorphone should be used with extreme caution in patients with chronic obstructive pulmonary disease or cor pulmonale, patients having a substantially decreased respiratory reserve, hypoxia, hypercapnia, or pre-existing respiratory depression. In such patients, even the usual therapeutic doses of opioid analgesics may decrease respiratory drive while simultaneously increasing airway resistance, to the point of apnea.

As mentioned above, severe pain antagonizes the subjective and respiratory depressant actions of hydromorphone. However, should pain suddenly subside, these effects may rapidly become manifest. Patients who are scheduled for cordotomy or other interruptions of pain transmission pathways should not receive hydromorphone within 24 hours of the procedure.

Head Injury and Increased Intracranial Pressure: The respiratory depressant effects of hydromorphone with carbon dioxide retention and secondary elevation of cerebrospinal fluid pressure may be markedly exaggerated in the presence of head injury, other intracranial lesions, or pre-existing increase in intracranial pressure. Opioid analgesics, including hydromorphone, may produce effects which can obscure the clinical course and neurologic signs of further increase in intracranial pressure in patients with head injuries.

Hypotensive Effect: Opioid analgesics, including hydromorphone, may cause severe hypotension in individuals whose ability to maintain normal blood pressure has already been compromised by depleted blood volume, or the concurrent administration of drugs such as phenothiazines and other tranquilizers, sedative/hypnotics, tricyclic antidepressants or general anesthetics (see Precautions, Drug Interactions). Hydromorphone may produce orthostatic hypotension in ambulatory patients.

Hydromorphone should be administered with caution to patients in circulatory shock, since vasodilation produced by the drug may further reduce cardiac output and blood pressure.

Rapid intravenous injection of opioid analgesics increases the possibility of hypotension and respiratory depression and should be avoided (see Dosage)

Pregnancy: (see Warnings, Drug Dependence): Animals: Adequate animal studies on reproduction have not been performed to determine whether hydromorphone affects fertility in males or females. However, animal studies with both morphine and hydromorphone have indicated the possibility of teratogenic effects.

Humans: There are no well-controlled studies in women. Reports based on marketing experience do not identify any specific teratogenic risks following routine (short-term) clinical use. Although there is no clearly defined risk, such reports do not exclude the possibility of infrequent or subtle damage to the human fetus. Hydromorphone should be used in pregnant women only when clearly needed (see Labor and Delivery and Precautions, Dependence Liability).

Labor and Delivery: High concentration hydromorphone preparations are contraindicated in labor and delivery (see Contraindications).

PRECAUTIONS: General:

> When used at high concentrations, the delivery of precise lower doses of hydromorphone may be difficult. Therefore, high concentration hydromorphone preparations should be used only if the amount of hydromorphone required can be delivered accurately.

Where high concentration hydromorphone preparations are indicated, the patient is presumed to be receiving an opioid to which tolerance has developed and the initial dose of hydromorphone selected, should therefore be estimated on the basis of the relative potency of hydromorphone and the opioid previously used by the patient (see Dosage).

In diseases, such as malignant cancers, where pain control is the primary focus opioid administration at very high doses is associated with seizures and myoclonus.

Special Risks Groups: In general, opioids should be given with caution and the initial dose should be reduced for the elderly or debilitated, and those with severe impairment of hepatic, pulmonary or renal function; myxedema or hypothyroidism; adrenocortical insufficiency (i.e. Addison's disease); CNS depression or coma; elevated intracranial pressure; toxic psychosis; prostatic hypertrophy or urethral stricture; gallbladder disease; acute alcoholism; delirium tremens; or kyphoscoliosis.

The administration of opioid analgesics including hydromorphone may obscure the diagnosis or clinical course in patients with acute abdominal conditions.

Opioid analgesics including hydromorphone should also be used with caution in patients about to undergo surgery of the biliary tract, since they may cause spasm of the sphincter of Oddi.

Dependence Liability: Opioid analgesics may cause psychological and physical dependence (see Warnings). Physical dependence results in withdrawal symptoms in patients who abruptly discontinue the drug. Withdrawal symptoms may also be precipitated in the patient with physical dependency by the administration of a drug with opioid antagonist activity, i.e. naloxone or mixed agonist antagonists i.e. pentazocine (see Overdose: Symptoms and Treatment). Physical dependence usually does not occur to a clinically significant degree until after several weeks of continued opioid usage. Tolerance, in which increasingly large doses are required in order to produce the same degree of analgesia, is initially manifested by a shortened duration of analgesic effect and subsequently, by decreases in the intensity of analgesia. The dose required to produce analgesia is, therefore, related to the degree of tolerance.

In chronic pain patients in whom opioid analgesics are abruptly discontinued, a severe abstinence syndrome should be anticipated. This may be similar to the abstinence syndrome noted in patients withdrawing from heroin.

The latter abstinence syndrome may be characterized by restlessness, lacrimation, rhinorrhea, yawning, perspiration, gooseflesh, restless sleep or "yen", and a mydriasis during the first 24 hours. Those symptoms may increase in severity and over the next 72 hours may be accompanied by increasing irritability, anxiety, weakness, twitching and spasms of muscles, kicking movements, severe backache, abdominal and leg pains, abdominal and muscle cramps, hot and cold flashes, insomnia, nausea, anorexia, vomiting, intestinal spasm, diarrhea, coryza and repetitive sneezing, increase in body temperature, blood pressure, respiratory rate and heart rate.

Because of the excessive loss of fluids through sweating, or vomiting and diarrhea, there is usually marked weight loss, dehydration, ketosis, and disturbances in acid-base balance. Cardiovascular collapse can occur. Without treatment, most observable symptoms disappear in 5 to 14 days; however, there appears to be a phase of secondary or chronic abstinence which may last for 2 to 6 months and is characterized by insomnia, irritability, muscular aches, and autonomic instability.

In the treatment of physical dependence on hydromorphone, the patient may be detoxified by gradual reduction of the dosage, although this is unlikely to be necessary in the terminal cancer patient. If abstinence symptoms become severe, the patient may be given methadone. Temporary administration of tranquilizers and sedatives may aid in reducing patient anxiety. Gastrointestinal disturbances or dehydration should be treated accordingly.

Hydromorphone should be used with caution in patients with alcoholism and other drug dependencies due to increased frequency of opioid tolerance and psychological dependence observed in these patient populations.

Drug Interactions: The concomitant use of other CNS depressants including sedatives or hypnotics, general anesthetics, phenothiazines, tranquilizers and alcohol may produce additive depressant effects. Respiratory depression, hypotension and profound sedation or coma may occur. When such combined therapy is contemplated, the dose of one or both agents should be reduced. Opioid analgesics, including hydromorphone, may enhance the action of neuromuscular blocking agents and produce an increased degree of respiratory depression.

Pregnancy: During pregnancy, hydromorphone should be administered with caution and after the need of the mother has been considered against the risk for the child. In long-term treatment during pregnancy, the risk of neonatal withdrawal should be considered.

Lactation: Low levels of opioid analgesics have been detected in human milk. As a general rule, nursing should not be undertaken while a patient is receiving hydromorphone since it and other drugs in this class may be excreted in the milk.

Children: Safety and effectiveness in children have not been established.

Geriatrics: In general, dose selection for elderly patients should be cautious and the initial dose should be reduced due to the greater frequency of decreased hepatic, renal or cardiac functions and of concomitant disease or other drug therapy in these patients.

Cough Reflex: Hydromorphone suppresses the cough reflex; as with all opioid analgesics, caution should be exercised when hydromorphone is used post-operatively in patients with pulmonary disease.

Occupational Hazards: Ability to Drive and Use Machines: Hydromorphone may impair mental and/or physical ability required for the performance of potentially hazardous tasks such as driving and operating machinery.

ADVERSE EFFECTS: The adverse effects of hydromorphone are similar to those of other opioid analgesics and represent an extension of pharmacological effects of the drug class. The major hazards include respiratory depression and apnea. To a lesser degree, circulatory depression, respiratory arrest, shock and cardiac arrest have occurred.

The most frequently observed adverse effects are constipation, lightheadedness, dizziness, sedation, nausea, vomiting, and sweating. All of these effects, except constipation, seem to be more prominent in ambulatory patients and in those not experiencing severe pain. Some adverse reactions in ambulatory patients may be alleviated if the patient lies down. When instituting prolonged therapy with an opioid for chronic pain, the prescription of antiemetics for nausea and vomiting and an appropriate regimen of bowel management for constipation (stool softeners, laxatives, etc.) should be considered.

Sedation: Some degree of sedation is experienced by most patients upon initiation of therapy. This may be at least partly because patients often recuperate from prolonged fatigue after the relief of persistent pain. Most patients develop tolerance to the sedative effects of opioids within 3 to 5 days and, if the sedation is not severe, will not require any treatment except reassurance. If excessive sedation persists beyond a few days, the dose of the opioid should be reduced and alternate causes investigated. Some of these are: concurrent CNS depressant medication, hepatic or renal dysfunction, brain metastases, hypercalcemia and respiratory failure. If it is necessary to reduce the dose, it can be carefully increased again after 3 or 4 days if it is obvious that the pain is not being well controlled. Dizziness and unsteadiness may be caused by postural hypotension particularly in elderly or debilitated patients and may be alleviated if the patient lies down.

Nausea and Vomiting: Nausea is a common side effect on initiation of therapy with opioid analgesics and is thought to occur by activation of the chemoreceptor trigger zone, stimulation of the vestibular apparatus and through delayed gastric emptying. The prevalence of nausea declines following continued treatment with opioid analgesics. When instituting prolonged therapy with an opioid for chronic pain, the routine prescription of an antiemetic should be considered. In the cancer patient, investigation of nausea should include such causes as constipation, bowel obstruction, uremia, hypercalcemia, hepatomegaly, tumor invasion of celiac plexus and concurrent use of drugs with emetogenic properties. Persistent nausea which does not respond to dosage reduction may be caused by opioid-induced gastric stasis and may be accompanied by other symptoms including anorexia, early satiety, vomiting and abdominal fullness. These symptoms respond to chronic treatment with gastrointestinal prokinetic agents.

Constipation: Practically all patients become constipated while taking opioids on a persistent basis. In some patients, particularly the elderly or bedridden, fecal impaction may result. It is essential to caution the patients in this regard and to institute an appropriate regimen of bowel management at the start of prolonged opioid analgesic therapy. Stool softeners, stimulant laxatives and other appropriate measures should be used as required.

Less Frequently Observed with Opioid Analgesics:

General and CNS: dysphoria, euphoria, weakness, headache, agitation, tremor, uncoordinated muscle movements, alterations of mood (nervousness, apprehension, depression, floating feelings, dreams), muscle rigidity, paresthesia, muscle tremor, blurred vision, nystagmus, diplopia and miosis, hallucinations and disorientation, visual disturbances, insomnia and increased intracranial pressure may occur.
Cardiovascular: flushing of the face, chills, tachycardia, bradycardia, palpitation, faintness, syncope, hypotension and hypertension have been reported.
Respiratory: bronchospasm and laryngospasm have been known to occur.
Gastrointestinal: dry mouth, constipation, biliary tract spasm, anorexia, diarrhea, cramps, ileus and taste alterations have been reported.
Genitourinary: urinary retention or hesitancy, and antidiuretic effects have been reported.
Dermatologic: pruritus, urticaria, other skin rashes, wheal and flare over the vein with i.v. injection, and diaphoresis have been reported with opioid analgesics.

OVERDOSE:

Symptoms: Serious overdosage with hydromorphone is characterized by respiratory depression, somnolence progressing to stupor or coma, skeletal muscle flaccidity, cold and clammy skin, constricted pupils and sometimes bradycardia and hypotension. In serious overdosage, particularly following i.v. injection, apnea, circulatory collapse, cardiac arrest and death may occur.

Treatment: In the treatment of overdosage, primary attention should be given to the re-establishment of adequate respiratory exchange through provision of a patent airway and institution of assisted or controlled ventilation. It should be borne in mind that for individuals who are physically dependent on opioids and are receiving large doses of these drugs, the administration of the usual dose of an opioid antagonist will precipitate an acute withdrawal syndrome. The severity will depend on the degree of physical dependence and the dose of the antagonist administered. Use of an opioid antagonist in such persons should be avoided. If necessary to treat serious respiratory depression in the physically dependent patient, the antagonist should be administered with extreme care and by titration, commencing with 10 to 20% of the usual recommended initial dose.

Respiratory depression which may result from overdosage, or unusual sensitivity to hydromorphone, in a nonopioid-tolerant patient, can be managed with the opioid antagonist naloxone. A dose of naloxone (usually 0.4 to 2 mg) should be administered i.v., if possible, simultaneously with respiratory resuscitation. The dose can be repeated in 3 minutes. Naloxone should not be administered in the absence of clinically significant respiratory or circulatory depression. Naloxone should be administered cautiously to persons who are known or suspected to be physically dependent on hydromorphone. In such cases, an abrupt or complete reversal of opioid effects may precipitate an acute abstinence syndrome.

Since the duration of action of hydromorphone may exceed that of the antagonist, the patient should be kept under continued surveillance; repeated doses of the antagonist may be required to maintain adequate respiration. Other supportive measures should be applied when indicated.

Supportive measures, including oxygen and vasopressors, should be employed in the management of circulatory shock and pulmonary edema accompanying overdose, as indicated. Cardiac arrest or arrhythmias may require cardiac massage or defibrillation.

For management of a suspected drug overdose, CPhA recommends that you contact your **regional Poison Control Centre**. See the *CPS* Directory section for a list of Poison Control Centres.

DOSAGE:

Dilaudid-HP, Dilaudid-HP-Plus, Dilaudid-XP and Reconstituted Dilaudid Sterile Powder are highly concentrated solutions of hydromorphone HCl. They should be used only in opioid-tolerant patients requiring high doses or high concentrations of opioid agonists. Do not confuse Dilaudid-HP, Dilaudid-HP-Plus, Dilaudid-XP and Reconstituted Dilaudid Sterile Powder with the lower concentration of the Dilaudid 2 mg/mL ampuls since overdosage and death could result.

High concentration hydromorphone preparations are indicated for relief of severe pain in opioid-tolerant patients. Thus, these patients will already have received opioid analgesics. If the patient is being changed from one injectable form of hydromorphone to higher concentration hydromorphone preparations, similar doses should be used, depending on the patient's clinical response to the drug. If high concentration hydromorphone preparations are substituted for a different opioid analgesic, Table 1 is provided as a guide to determine the approximate equivalent dose of hydromorphone.

Table 1: Dilaudid-HP, Dilaudid-HP-Plus, Dilaudid-XP, Dilaudid Sterile Powder

Opioid Analgesics: Approximate Analgesic Equivalences[a]

Drug	Equivalent Dose (mg)[b] (compared to morphine 10 mg i.m.) Parenteral	Oral	Duration of Action (hours)
Strong Opioid Agonists			
Morphine (single dose)	10	60	3–4
(chronic dose)	10	20–30[c]	3–4
Hydromorphone	1.5–2	6–7.5	2–4
Anileridine	25	75	2–3
Levorphanol	2	4	4–8
Meperidine[d]	75	300	1–3
Oxymorphone	1.5	5 (rectal)	3-4
Methadone[e]			
Heroin	5–8	10–15	3–4
Weak Opioid Agonists			
Codeine	120	200	3–4
Oxycodone	5–10	10–15	2–4
Propoxyphene	50	100	2–4
Mixed Agonist-Antagonists[f]			
Pentazocine[d]	60	180	3–4
Nalbuphine	10		3–6
Butorphanol	2		3–4

[a] References: Cancer Pain: A Monograph on the Management of Cancer Pain, Health and Welfare Canada, 1984. Foley, K.M., New Engl. J. Med. 313: 84-95, 1985. Aronoff, G.M. and Evans, W.O., In: Evaluation and Treatment of Chronic Pain, 2nd Ed., G.M. Aronoff (Ed.), Williams and Wilkins, Baltimore, pp. 359-368, 1992. Cherny, N.I. and Portenoy, R.K., In: Textbook of Pain, 3rd Ed., P.H. Wall and R. Melzack (Eds.), Churchill Livingstone, London, pp. 1437-1467, 1994.
[b] Most of these data were derived from single-dose, acute pain studies and should be considered an approximation for selection of doses when treating chronic pain.
[c] For acute pain, the oral dose of morphine is 6 times the injectable dose. However, for chronic dosing this ratio becomes 2 or 3:1, possibly due to the accumulation of active metabolites.
[d] These drugs are not recommended for the management of chronic pain.
[e] Extremely variable equianalgesic dose. Patients should undergo personalized titration starting at an equivalent to 1/10 of the morphine dose.
[f] Mixed agonist-antagonists can precipitate withdrawal in patients on pure opioid agonists.

In open clinical trials with hydromorphone in patients with terminal cancer, both s.c. and i.m. injections of hydromorphone were well-tolerated, with minimal pain and/or burning at the injection site. Mild erythema was rarely noted after i.m. injection. S.C. injections of hydromorphone were particularly well tolerated when administered with a short, 30 gauge needle. In addition, continuous s.c. infusions of hydromorphone have been shown to be well tolerated. The most common adverse reaction is local tissue redness which can be relieved with more frequent site changes. Experience with administration of hydromorphone by the i.v. route is limited. Should i.v. administration be necessary, the injection should be given slowly, over at least 2 to 3 minutes. Rapid i.v. injection of opioid analgesics increases the possibility of hypotension and respiratory depression. The i.v. route is usually painless.

A gradual increase in dose may be required if analgesia is inadequate, tolerance occurs, or if pain severity increases. The first sign of tolerance is usually a reduced duration of effect.

Reconstitution for Parenteral Products: Dilaudid Sterile Powder is provided sterile as 250 mg of hydromorphone HCl in a 30 mL vial. It can be reconstituted to desired concentration with sterile water for injection, 0.9% sodium chloride or 5% dextrose. Table 2 provides information on the amount of diluent to be added in order to prepare a variety of concentrations.

Table 2: Dilaudid Sterile Powder

Amount of Diluent to be Added to Vial Resulting in a Desired Concentration

Volume of Diluent to be added to Vial	Resulting Volume	Nominal Concentration per mL
24.8 mL	25.0 mL	10 mg/mL
12.4 mL	12.5 mL	20 mg/mL
4.9 mL	5.0 mL	50 mg/mL
2.4 mL	2.5 mL	100 mg/mL
1.6 mL	1.67 mL	150 mg/mL
1.1 mL	1.25 mL	200 mg/mL
0.9 mL	1.0 mL	250 mg/mL

The information provided in Table 3 is only for physical compatibility and chemical stability of the reconstituted solutions. Continued sterility of the reconstituted solution is dependent on the procedures and equipment used during the preparation of the solution. Each pharmacist must address these factors in determining the duration of use of the solution prepared. The usual recommendation for reconstituted solutions is 24 hours at room temperature or 72 hours under refrigeration.

Dilaudid Sterile Powder for injection is physically compatible and chemically stable in the diluents and containers shown in Table 3.

Table 3: Dilaudid Sterile Powder

Physical Compatibility and Chemical Stability of the Reconstituted Solutions

Diluent	Final Concentration (mg) Hydromorphone HCl/mL	Storage Condition	Type of Container	[a]Physical and Chemical Stability (In Days)
Sterile Water for Injection	10, 100, 250	Room Temperature	Amber Glass	42
		Refrigerated (Fridge)	Amber Glass	42
Sterile Water for Injection	10, 100, 250	Room Temperature	Pharmacia Cassettes	42
		Refrigerated (Fridge)	Pharmacia Cassettes	42
Sterile Water for Injection	10, 100, 250	37°C dry heat incubator (after storage in fridge)	Pharmacia Cassettes	10 days after 42 days storage in fridge
0.9% Sodium Chloride Solution	10, 100	Room Temperature	Amber Glass	28
5% Dextrose Solution	10, 100	Room Temperature	Amber Glass	28

[a] This information does not address sterility. Please see the previous paragraph for further comments.

Solutions made from Dilaudid Sterile Powder (as well as Dilaudid-HP, -HP-Plus and -XP) can be administered by i.v., i.m. or s.c. routes including i.v. and s.c. continuous infusion.

Note: Parenteral drug products should be inspected visually for particulate matter and discoloration prior to administration, whenever solution and container permit. A slight yellowish discoloration may develop in Dilaudid solutions. This yellowish coloration is proportional to hydromorphone concentration and has a tendency to increase over time. The coloration is of an aesthetic nature and not a result of chemical degradation. No loss of potency has been demonstrated. Also note that Dilaudid does not contain any preservatives; therefore, unused portions of the remaining drug in the vial should be discarded.

SUPPLIED: Dilaudid-HP: Each mL of sterile solution contains: hydromorphone HCl 10 mg, citric acid 2 mg and sodium citrate 2 mg, in Water for Injection. No added preservatives. Amber ampuls of 1 and 5 mL, boxes of 10. Single use amber vials with white flip-off caps of 50 mL, boxes of 2.
Dilaudid-HP-Plus: Each mL of sterile solution contains: hydromorphone HCl 20 mg, citric acid 2 mg and sodium citrate 2 mg, in Water for Injection. No added preservatives. Single use amber vials with brown flip-off caps of 50 mL, boxes of 2.
Dilaudid-XP: Each mL of sterile solution contains: hydromorphone HCl 50 mg, citric acid 2 mg and sodium citrate 2 mg, in Water for Injection. No added preservatives. Single use amber vials with yellow flip-off caps of 50 mL, boxes of 2.
Dilaudid Sterile Powder: Each vial contains: sterile lyophilized hydromorphone HCl 250 mg. No added preservatives. Amber vials of 30 mL with black flip-off caps, boxes of 4.
Store between 15 and 25°C. Protect from light. Do not use beyond the expiry date indicated on the label.

Diltiazem [Pr]

CPhA Monograph

see *Calcium Channel Blockers*

Diltiazem Hydrochloride Injection [Pr]

diltiazem HCl
Antiarrhythmic

Sandoz

SUPPLIED: Each mL of solution contains: diltiazem hydrochloride 5 mg. Nonmedicinal ingredients: citric acid, sodium citrate dihydrate, sodium hydroxide and/or hydrochloric acid to adjust pH, sorbitol solution 70% and water for injection. Single use vials of 5 and 10 mL, boxes of 5. Discard unused portion. Store between 2 and 8°C. Protect from light. Do not freeze. If product is stored at room temperature, discard after 1 month.

Dimenhydrinate

dimenhydrinate
Antiemetic

Sandoz

SUPPLIED: Dimenhydrinate Injection USP IM: Ampuls: Each mL contains: dimenhydrinate 50 mg. Nonmedicinal ingredients: propylene glycol and water for injection. Preservative-free. Ampuls of 1 mL, boxes of 10.
Multidose Vials: Each mL contains: dimenhydrinate 50 mg. Nonmedicinal ingredients: benzyl alcohol, propylene glycol and water for injection. Vials of 5 mL, boxes of 3 and 10.
Dimenhydrinate IV Injection: Each mL contains dimenhydrinate 10 mg. Nonmedicinal ingredients: ethyl alcohol and water for injection. Single use vials of 5 mL, boxes of 10. Discard unused portion.
Store between 15 and 30°C.
Sandoz Dimenhydrinate Suppository: 50 mg: Each suppository contains: dimenhydrinate 50 mg. Boxes of 10 and 100.
100 mg: Each suppository contains: dimenhydrinate 100 mg. Boxes of 10 and 100.

Dimetane® Expectorant-C Ⓝ

brompheniramine maleate—phenylephrine HCl—guaifenesin—codeine phosphate
Antihistamine—Decongestant—Expectorant—Antitussive

Pfizer Consumer Healthcare

Dimetane® Expectorant-DC Ⓝ

brompheniramine maleate—phenylephrine HCl—guaifenesin—hydrocodone bitartrate
Antihistamine—Decongestant—Expectorant—Antitussive

Pfizer Consumer Healthcare

INDICATIONS: The temporary relief of coughing and the complications of allergic states including manifestations such as perennial and seasonal allergic rhinitis. The symptomatic relief of cough, nasal stuffiness and rhinitis accompanying the common cold and other upper respiratory tract infections.

CONTRAINDICATIONS: Hypersensitivity to any of the ingredients and patients receiving MAO inhibitors. Should not be used to treat lower respiratory tract symptoms including asthma.

Patients allergic to codeine or other opioids, have suffered head injury, are at risk of blocked intestines or suffer from seizures.

WARNINGS: No data supplied by the manufacturer.

PRECAUTIONS: Keep out of reach of children.

Product may cause drowsiness or excitability, especially in children.

Do not exceed recommended dosage.

Stop use and consult a physician if symptoms or cough worsen or persist for more than 7 days, or if high fever, rash or persistent headache is present, as these could be signs of a serious condition.

Patients should be advised to use under the direction of a physician if medication has been taken in the last 14 days for high blood pressure or depression, including monoamine oxidase inhibitors (MAOIs), or if taking other antihistamines, decongestants, tranquilizers or sedating drugs.

Before prescribing medication to suppress or modify cough, it is important to ascertain that the underlying cause of the cough is identified, that modification of the cough does not increase the risk of clinical or physiologic complications, and that appropriate therapy for the primary disease is provided.

Administer with caution to patients with cardiac or peripheral vascular disease, glaucoma, hyperthyroidism, diabetes mellitus or hypertension, persistent chronic cough (as occurs with smoking), breathing problems or shortness of breath, chronic lung disease (e.g., chronic bronchitis, asthma or emphysema), prostate enlargement and bladder neck obstruction and in pregnancy or lactation.

Occupational Hazards: Patients should be cautioned not to operate vehicles or hazardous machinery until their response to the drug has been determined. Since the depressant effects of antihistamines are additive to those of other drugs affecting the CNS, patients should be cautioned against drinking alcoholic beverages or taking hypnotics, sedatives, psychotherapeutic agents or other drugs with CNS depressant effects during antihistaminic therapy.

Guaifenesin has been shown to produce a color interference with certain clinical laboratory determinations of 5-hydroxyindoleacetic acid (5-HIAA) and vanillylmandelic acid (VMA).

Dimetane Expectorant-DC: In young children the respiratory centre is especially susceptible to the depressant action of narcotic cough suppressants. Benefit-to-risk ratio should be carefully considered especially in children with respiratory embarrassment, e.g., croup. Estimation of dosage relative to the child's age and weight is of great importance.

Pregnancy: Since hydrocodone crosses the placental barrier, its use in pregnancy is not recommended.

As hydrocodone may inhibit peristalsis, patients with chronic constipation should be given Dimetane Expectorant-DC only after weighing the potential therapeutic benefit against the hazards involved.

Dimetane Expectorant-C contains codeine—may produce drug dependence.

Dimetane Expectorant-DC contains hydrocodone—may be habit forming.

ADVERSE EFFECTS: Hypersensitivity reactions to brompheniramine maleate, including skin rashes, urticaria, hypotension and thrombocytopenia may occur rarely. Drowsiness, lassitude, nausea, giddiness, dryness of the mouth, mydriasis, increased irritability or excitement may be encountered.

OVERDOSE:

Symptoms: May vary from CNS depression to stimulation. Stimulation is particularly likely in children as a result of antihistamine overdosage. Atropine-like signs and symptoms such as dry mouth, fixed, dilated pupils, flushing and gastrointestinal symptoms may also occur.

Treatment: If vomiting has not occurred spontaneously, the patient should be induced to vomit. This is best done by administering syrup of ipecac. Precautions against aspiration must be taken, especially in infants and children. If vomiting is unsuccessful, gastric lavage is indicated within 3 hours after ingestion and even later if large amounts of milk or cream were given beforehand. Emesis or lavage should be followed by the administration of activated charcoal. Stimulants should not be used. Vasopressors may be used to treat hypotension. Naloxone may be used to treat codeine or hydrocodone toxicity.

> For management of a suspected drug overdose, CPhA recommends that you contact your **regional Poison Control Centre**. See the *CPS* Directory section for a list of Poison Control Centres.

DOSAGE: Dimetane Expectorant-C and Dimetane Expectorant-DC: Adults and children over 12 years: 10 mL (2 tsps) every 6 hours. Maximum 4 doses (8 tsp) per day. Children under 12 years: Do not use.

SUPPLIED: Dimetane Expectorant-C: Each 5 mL of palatable, cherry-red liquid, menthol and raspberry taste and odor, contains: brompheniramine maleate 2 mg, phenylephrine HCl 5 mg, guaifenesin 100 mg and codeine phosphate 10 mg. Nonmedicinal ingredients: alcohol, citric acid, D&C Red No. 33, edetate disodium, FD&C Red No. 40, flavors, glycerin, propylene glycol, sodium benzoate, sodium carboxymethylcellulose, sodium saccharin and water. Energy: 43.5 kJ (10.39 kcal)/5 mL. Sodium: <1 mmol (0.8 mg). Bottles of 1 L.
Dimetane Expectorant-DC: Each 5 mL of cherry-red liquid, menthol and raspberry taste and odor, contains: hydrocodone bitartrate 1.8 mg, brompheniramine maleate 2 mg, phenylephrine HCl 5 mg and guaifenesin 100 mg. Nonmedicinal ingredients: alcohol, citric acid, D&C Red No. 33, FD&C Red No. 40, flavors, glycerin, invert sugar, sodium benzoate and water. Energy: 48 kJ (11.48 kcal)/5 mL. Sodium: <1 mmol (0.8 mg). Bottles of 1 L.

Dimetapp® Chewables for Kids

brompheniramine maleate—phenylephrine HCl
Antihistamine—Decongestant

Pfizer Consumer Healthcare

Dimetapp® DM Cough & Cold Liquid

brompheniramine maleate—dextromethorphan HBr—phenylephrine HCl
Antihistamine—Antitussive—Decongestant

Pfizer Consumer Healthcare

Dimetapp® Extra Strength DM Cough & Cold Liquid

brompheniramine maleate—dextromethorphan HBr—phenylephrine HCl
Antihistamine—Cough Suppressant—Decongestant

Pfizer Consumer Healthcare

Dimetapp® Extra Strength Liquid

brompheniramine maleate—phenylephrine HCl
Antihistamine—Decongestant

Pfizer Consumer Healthcare

Dimetapp® Liquid

brompheniramine maleate—phenylephrine HCl
Antihistamine—Decongestant

Pfizer Consumer Healthcare

INDICATIONS: Liquid and Extra Strength Liquid: Symptomatic, temporary relief of the allergic manifestations of respiratory illnesses such as the common cold, seasonal allergies, etc.
DM Cough and Cold Liquid and Extra Strength DM Cough & Cold Liquid: Symptomatic, temporary relief of the allergic manifestations of cough, nasal congestion, runny nose accompanying colds and other respiratory infections.
Chewables for Kids: For the symptomatic, temporary relief of the allergic manifestations of seasonal allergies and the common cold.

CONTRAINDICATIONS: Hypersensitivity to any of the ingredients, marked hypertension and in patients receiving MAO inhibitors (MAOIs) or for 2 weeks after stopping the MAOI drug.

PRECAUTIONS: Keep out of reach of children.

Product may cause drowsiness or excitability.

Do not exceed recommended dosage.

Do not use longer than 7 days. Do not give with other antihistamines, nasal decongestants or any other cough and cold, medications since harm may occur.

Stop use and consult a physician if symptoms or cough worsen or persist for more than 7 days, or are accompanied by high fever (>38°C) or the production of thick yellow/green phlegm, as these could be signs of a serious condition.

Do not use when child is engaged in activities requiring mental alertness. Do not give with sedatives and tranquilizers as this may increase drowsiness.

Administer with caution to patients with cardiac or peripheral vascular diseases, glaucoma, hyperthyroidism, chronic lung disease (chronic bronchitis, asthma or emphysema), breathing problems or shortness of breath, diabetes mellitus, hypertension, prostate enlargement and bladder neck obstruction and in pregnancy and lactation.

Occupational Hazards: Patients should be cautioned not to operate vehicles or hazardous machinery until their response to the drug has been determined. Since the depressant effects of antihistamines are additive to those of other drugs affecting the CNS, patients should be cautioned against drinking alcoholic beverages or taking hypnotics, sedatives, psychotherapeutic agents or other drugs with CNS depressant effects during antihistaminic therapy.

Pregnancy: Safe use during pregnancy has not been established.

ADVERSE EFFECTS: Side effects may include: allergic reaction, breathing difficulties, convulsions, drowsiness, hallucinations and rapid heart rate.

Liquid and Extra Strength Liquid: Hypersensitivity reactions including skin rashes, urticaria, hypotension and thrombocytopenia have been reported on rare occasions. Drowsiness, lassitude, nausea, giddiness, mydriasis, dryness of the mouth, increased irritability or excitement may occur.

DM Cough and Cold Liquid and Extra Strength DM Cough & Cold Liquid: Hypersensitivity reactions including skin rashes, urticaria, hypotension and thrombocytopenia have been reported as adverse effects to brompheniramine maleate. Drowsiness, lassitude, nausea, giddiness, mydriasis, dryness of the mouth, increased irritability or excitement may be encountered. These occur rarely, however, and are reversible upon reduction of dosage or withdrawal of the drug.

Chewables for Kids: Hypersensitivity reactions including skin rashes, urticaria have been reported on rare occasions. Dryness of the mouth and increased irritability or excitement may be encountered. See Liquid and Extra Strength Liquid.

OVERDOSE:
In case of accidental overdose, contact a physician or poison control centre immediately, even if there are no symptoms.

For management of a suspected drug overdose, CPhA recommends that you contact your **regional Poison Control Centre**. See the *CPS* Directory section for a list of Poison Control Centres.

DOSAGE: Liquid Products: Use only the measuring device provided.
Chewables for Kids: Administer every 4 to 6 hours. Children 6 to 12 years: 2 chewable tablets. Maximum 12 tablets in 24 hours. Children under 6 years: **Do not use.**
Cold Liquid & DM Cough and Liquid: Administer every 4 to 6 hours. Maximum 6 doses in 24 hours. Adults and children 12 years and over: 2 teaspoonfuls (10 mL). Children 6 to under 12 years: 1 teaspoonful (5 mL). Children under 6 years: **Do not use.**
Extra Strength Liquid and Extra Strength DM Cough & Cold Liquid: Administer every 4 to 6 hours as follows: Maximum 6 doses in 24 hours. Adults and children 12 years and over: 1 teaspoonful (5 mL). Children 6 to under 12 years: ½ teaspoonful (2.5 mL). Children under 6 years: **Do not use.**

SUPPLIED: Chewables for Kids: Each chewable tablet contains: brompheniramine maleate 1 mg and phenylephrine HCl 2.5 mg. Nonmedicinal ingredients: carmine, carrageenan, croscarmellose sodium, flavors, fumaric acid, glycine, magnesium stearate, maltodextrin, mannitol, microcrystalline cellulose, polyethylene oxide, silicon dioxide and sucralose. Blisters of 20.
DM Cough & Cold Liquid: Each 5 mL of red, cherry-vanilla flavored liquid contains: brompheniramine maleate 2 mg, phenylephrine HCl 5 mg, and dextromethorphan HBr 10 mg. Nonmedicinal ingredients: citric acid, D&C Red No. 33, FD&C Red No. 40, flavors, propylene glycol, sodium benzoate, sodium cyclamate, sorbitol and water. Energy: 43.12 kJ (10.3 kcal)/5 mL. Sodium: <1 mmol (3.65 mg)/5 mL. Alcohol- and sucrose-free. Bottles of 100 and 250 mL.
DM Cough & Cold Liquid: Dye-Free: Each 5 mL of clear, cherry-vanilla flavored liquid contains: brompheniramine maleate 2 mg and phenylephrine HCl 5 mg and dextromethorphan HBr 10 mg. Nonmedicinal ingredients: citric acid, flavors, propylene glycol, sodium benzoate, sodium cyclamate, sorbitol and water. Energy: 43.12 kJ (7.71 kcal)/5 mL. Sodium <1 mmol (3.65 mg)/5 mL. Alcohol- and sucrose-free. Bottles of 100 mL.
Extra Strength DM Cough and Cold Liquid: Each 5 mL of red, cherry-vanilla flavored liquid contains: brompheniramine maleate 4 mg, phenylephrine HCl 10 mg and dextromethorphan HBr 20 mg. Nonmedicinal ingredients: citric acid, D&C Red No. 33, FD&C Red No. 40, flavors, maltol, propylene glycol, sodium benzoate, sodium cyclamate, sorbitol and water. Energy: 43.12 kJ (10.3 kcal)/5 mL. Sodium: <1 mmol (3.35 mg)/5 mL. Alcohol- and sucrose-free. Bottles of 100 and 250 mL.
Extra Strength Liquid: Each 5 mL of purple-colored, grape-flavored liquid contains: brompheniramine maleate 4 mg and phenylephrine HCl 10 mg. Nonmedicinal ingredients: citric acid, D&C Red No. 33, FD&C Blue No. 1, FD&C Red No. 40, flavors, propylene glycol, sodium benzoate, sorbitol and water. Energy: 32.32 kJ (7.72 kcal)/5 mL. Sodium: <1 mmol (0.8 mg)/5 mL. Alcohol- and sucrose-free. Bottles of 100 and 250 mL.
Liquid: Each 5 mL of purple-colored, grape-flavored liquid contains: brompheniramine maleate 2 mg and phenylephrine HCl 5 mg. Nonmedicinal ingredients: citric acid, D&C Red No. 33, FD&C Blue No. 1, FD&C Red No. 40, flavors, propylene glycol, sodium benzoate, sorbitol and water. Energy: 32.28 kJ (7.71 kcal)/5 mL. Sodium: <1 mmol (0.8 mg)/5 mL. Alcohol- and sucrose-free. Bottles of 100 and 250 mL.
Liquid: Dye-Free: Each 5 mL of clear, grape-flavored liquid contains: brompheniramine maleate 2 mg and phenylephrine HCl 5 mg. Nonmedicinal ingredients: citric acid, flavor, propylene glycol, sodium benzoate, sorbitol and water. Energy: 32.28 kJ (7.71 kcal)/5 mL. Sodium: <1 mmol (0.8 mg)/5 mL. Alcohol- and sucrose-free. Bottles of 100 mL.

Dimetapp®-C Syrup Ⓝ
brompheniramine maleate—codeine phosphate—phenylephrine HCl
Antihistamine—Cough Suppressant—Decongestant

Pfizer Consumer Healthcare

INDICATIONS: For the symptomatic, temporary relief of coughing, nasal congestion, runny nose, sneezing and lacrimation accompanying the common cold and other upper respiratory infections.
CONTRAINDICATIONS: Hypersensitivity to any of the ingredients, marked hypertension and in patients receiving MAO inhibitors.
Patients allergic to codeine or other opioids, have suffered head injury, are at risk of blocked intestines or suffer from seizures.
PRECAUTIONS: Keep out of reach of children.
Product may cause drowsiness or excitability, especially in children.
Do not exceed recommended dosage.
Patients should be advised to stop use and consult a physician if symptoms or cough worsen or persist for more than 7 days, or if high fever is present, as these could be signs of a serious condition.
Administer with caution to patients with cardiac or peripheral vascular disease, glaucoma, hypertension, persistent chronic cough (as occurs with smoking), breathing problems or shortness of breath, hyperthyroidism, bladder neck obstruction, diabetes, chronic lung disease (e.g., chronic bronchitis, asthma or emphysema), and in pregnancy or lactation.
Patients should be advised to use under the direction of a physician if medication has been taken in the last 14 days, for high blood pressure or depression, including monoamine oxidase inhibitors (MAOIs), or if taking other antihistamines, decongestants, tranquilizers or sedating drugs.
Consult your doctor if you feel sedated or drowsy, confused, have shallow breathing or have severe constipation.
Sedatives and tranquilizers may increase drowsiness.
Avoid alcoholic beverages, (alcohol may increase drowsiness), driving a motor vehicle or operating machinery.
Codeine may cause harm to a breast fed baby. Contact your physician immediately if you are breastfeeding and your baby is having difficulty breathing or feeding, or is very sleepy or limp.
Occupational Hazards: Until the drowsiness potential has been determined, the patient should be cautioned against engaging in operations requiring alertness.
ADVERSE EFFECTS: Drowsiness, lassitude, nausea, giddiness, dryness of the mouth, mydriasis, increased irritability or excitement may be encountered rarely. Codeine may produce drug dependence and therefore has the potential for being abused.
OVERDOSE:
In case of accidental overdose, contact a physician or poison control centre immediately, even if there are no symptoms.

For management of a suspected drug overdose, CPhA recommends that you contact your **regional Poison Control Centre**. See the *CPS* Directory section for a list of Poison Control Centres.

DOSAGE: Administer every 4 hours, not to exceed 6 doses in a 24-hour period. Adults: 10 mL (2 tsps). Children under 12 years: **Do not use.**

SUPPLIED: Each 5 mL of light blue-colored, grape-flavored syrup contains: brompheniramine maleate 2 mg, phenylephrine HCl 5 mg and codeine phosphate 10 mg. Nonmedicinal ingredients: citric acid, flavors, FD&C Blue No. 1, FD&C Red No. 40, propylene glycol, sodium benzoate, sodium saccharin, sorbitol and water. Energy: 34.75 kJ (8.3 kcal)/5 mL. Sodium: <1 mmol (1.06 mg)/5 mL. Alcohol- and sucrose-free. Bottles of 1 L.

Dimethyl Sulfoxide Irrigation USP Ⓟ
dimethyl sulfoxide
Intravesical Instillation for the Treatment of Interstitial Cystitis

Sandoz

SUPPLIED: Each mL of sterile solution contains: dimethyl sulfoxide 50% w/w in water for injection. Pyrogen free. Discard unused portion. Clear single use vials of 50 mL, boxes of 1. Store between 15 and 30°C. Protect from light. Do not autoclave. Not for injection.

Diodoquin® Ⓟ
iodoquinol
Amebicide

Glenwood

PHARMACOLOGY: Iodoquinol is amebicidal against *E. histolytica*, *D. fragilis* and *G. lamblia* and is considered effective against the trophozoite and cyst forms.
INDICATIONS: In the treatment of intestinal amebiasis.
CONTRAINDICATIONS: Hypersensitivity to any 8-hydroxy-quinoline or iodine-containing preparations, hepatic damage and pre-existing optic neuropathy.
WARNINGS: Optic neuritis, optic atrophy, and peripheral neuropathy have been reported following prolonged high dosage therapy with halogenated 8-hydroxyquinolines. Long-term use of this drug should be avoided.
Pregnancy: Safety for use in pregnancy has not been established.
Lactation: Safety for use during lactation has not been established.
PRECAUTIONS: Iodoquinol should be used with caution in patients with thyroid disease.
Protein-bound serum iodine levels may be increased during treatment with iodoquinol and therefore interfere with certain thyroid function tests. These effects may persist for as long as 6 months after discontinuation of therapy. Discontinue the drug if hypersensitivity reactions occur.
ADVERSE EFFECTS: Skin: various forms of skin eruptions (acneiform papular and pustular; bullae; vegetating or tuberots iododerma), urticaria and pruritus.
Gastrointestinal: nausea, vomiting, abdominal cramps, diarrhea, and pruritus ani.
Fever, chills, headache, vertigo, and enlargement of thyroid have been reported. Optic neuritis, optic atrophy and peripheral neuropathy have been reported in association with prolonged high-dosage 8-hydroxyquinoline therapy.
OVERDOSE:
No data supplied by the manufacturer.

For management of a suspected drug overdose, CPhA recommends that you contact your **regional Poison Control Centre**. See the *CPS* Directory section for a list of Poison Control Centres.

DOSAGE: 210 mg: Usual adult dose: 3 tablets 3 times daily, after meals for 20 days. Children 6 to 12 years: 2 tablets t.i.d. Children under 6: 1 tablet/6.8 kg of body weight, divided into 3 daily doses for 20 days.
650 mg: Usual adult dose: 1 tablet 3 times a day for 20 days, to be taken after meals. Children: For 20 days, 40 mg/kg of body weight daily divided into 3 doses, not to exceed 1.95 g in 24 hours, for 20 days.

SUPPLIED: Each tablet contains: iodoquinol USP 210 or 650 mg. Nonmedicinal ingredients: colloidal silicon dioxide NF, croscarmellose sodium NF, lactose anhydrous NF, magnesium stearate NF, microcrystalline cellulose NF and povidone USP. Bottles of 100. Store at controlled room temperature 15 to 30°C.

Diophenyl-T® Ⓟ
phenylephrine HCl—tropicamide
Mydriatic—Cycloplegic

Sandoz

SUPPLIED: Each mL of ophthalmic solution contains: phenylephrine HCl 5% and tropicamide 0.8%. Nonmedicinal ingredients: benzalkonium chloride as preservative, disodium edetate, purified water and sodium metabisulfite. Plastic dropper bottles of 15 mL. Store between 15 and 30°C. Keep container tightly closed; do not use if solution is discoloured.

Diopred® Ⓟ
prednisolone acetate
Corticosteroid

Sandoz

SUPPLIED: Each mL of sterile ophthalmic suspension contains: prednisolone acetate 1 %. Nonmedicinal ingredients: benzalkonium chloride 0.01% as preservative, boric acid, disodium edetate, hydroxypropyl methylcellulose, polysorbate 80, sodium bisulphite, sodium chloride, sodium citrate and purified water. Plastic dropper bottles of 5 and 10 mL. Store between 15 and 30°C.

Diovan® Ⓟ
valsartan
Angiotensin II AT1 Receptor Blocker

Novartis Pharmaceuticals

Date of Revision: January 23, 2009

SUMMARY PRODUCT INFORMATION:

Route of Administration	Dosage Form/ Strength	Clinically Relevant Nonmedicinal Ingredients
Oral	40 mg, 80 mg, 160 mg and 320 mg tablets	Colloidal silicon dioxide, crospovidone, magnesium stearate, and microcrystalline cellulose For a complete listing see Dosage Forms, Composition and Packaging.

INDICATIONS AND CLINICAL USE: DIOVAN (valsartan) is indicated for:
- **Hypertension:**
  - For the treatment of mild to moderate essential hypertension.
  - DIOVAN may be administered alone, or concomitantly with thiazide diuretics.
  - The safety and efficacy of concurrent treatment with DIOVAN and angiotensin converting enzyme inhibitors have not been established.
- **Following Myocardial Infarction:**
  - To reduce cardiovascular mortality in clinically stable patients with signs or symptoms of left ventricular dysfunction in conjunction with acute myocardial infarction when the use of an angiotensin-converting enzyme inhibitor (ACEI) is not appropriate.
  - The combination of valsartan and an angiotensin-converting enzyme inhibitor (ACEI) has not been shown to result in clinically relevant improvement in cardiovascular outcome over valsartan use alone. Accordingly, such combined use is not recommended.
- **Chronic Heart Failure:**
  - Diovan can be used in patients with chronic heart failure who have been shown to be intolerant to an angiotensin converting enzyme inhibitor. There is no evidence that Diovan provides added benefits when it is used with ACE inhibitors.

Geriatrics (>65 years of age): No overall difference in efficacy or safety observed versus younger patients, but greater sensitivity of some older individuals cannot be ruled out.
Pediatrics (<18 years of age): The safety and effectiveness of DIOVAN in children and adolescents (below the age of 18 years) have not been established.

CONTRAINDICATIONS:
- DIOVAN is contraindicated in patients who are hypersensitive to this drug or to any ingredient in the formulation or component of the container (see Dosage Forms, Composition and Packaging).

WARNINGS AND PRECAUTIONS:

Serious Warnings and Precautions
When used in pregnancy **angiotensin receptor (AT_1) blockers (ARB)** can cause injury to or even death of the developing fetus. When pregnancy is detected, DIOVAN should be discontinued as soon as possible (see Warnings and Precautions, Special Populations).

Cardiovascular: Hypotension: Occasionally, symptomatic hypotension has occurred after administration of valsartan, in some cases after the first dose. It is more likely to occur in patients who are volume-depleted by diuretic therapy, dietary salt restriction, dialysis, diarrhea, or vomiting. In these patients, because of the potential fall in blood pressure, therapy should be started under close medical supervision. Similar considerations apply to patients with ischemic heart or cerebrovascular disease, in whom an excessive fall in blood pressure could result in myocardial infarction or cerebrovascular accident.

Caution should be exercised when initiating therapy after acute myocardial infarction. Patients with heart failure or those in the early post-myocardial infarction period that are given DIOVAN commonly have some reduction in blood pressure, but discontinuation of therapy is usually not necessary if patients are well screened prior to instituting treatment and found to be clinically stable. If symptomatic hypotension does occur, consideration should be given to dosage reduction (see Dosage and Administration, Following Myocardial Infarction). In patients treated following myocardial infarction, the recommended regimen of valsartan has been observed to result in a greater incidence of hypotension as a serious adverse event than the conventional dosage regimen of captopril in this indication (see Adverse Reactions, Following Myocardial Infarction).

In patients with heart failure, a greater incidence of hypotension has been reported. Monitoring and dose adjustment should be considered.

Valvular Stenosis: There is concern on theoretical grounds that patients with aortic stenosis might be at a particular risk of decreased coronary perfusion, because they do not develop as much afterload reduction.

Hepatic/Biliary/Pancreatic: On average, patients with mild to moderate chronic liver disease have twice the exposure to valsartan of healthy volunteers as measured by AUC and C_{max}. Care should be exercised in administering DIOVAN to these patients (see Action and Clinical Pharmacology, Pharmacokinetics).

Renal: As a consequence of inhibiting the renin-angiotensin-aldosterone system, changes in renal function have been seen in susceptible individuals. In patients whose renal function may depend on the activity of the renin-angiotensin-aldosterone system, such as patients with bilateral renal artery stenosis, unilateral renal artery stenosis to a solitary kidney, or severe congestive heart failure, treatment with agents that inhibit this system has been associated with oliguria, progressive azotemia, and rarely, acute renal failure and/or death. In susceptible patients, concomitant diuretic use may further increase risk.

Following myocardial infarction, major renal dysfunction was observed to occur more frequently with valsartan than with captopril monotherapy (see Adverse Reactions, Following Myocardial Infarction). The role of modestly lower blood pressure that may occur with valsartan compared to captopril monotherapy is not known.

The incidence of clinically relevant hyperkalemia has also been observed to be increased with valsartan (see Adverse Reactions, Laboratory Findings). Patients exposed to potassium-sparing diuretics and/or potassium supplements were more likely to develop hyperkalemia. Accordingly, their use should be carefully monitored or avoided (see Drug Interactions, Agents Increasing Serum Potassium).

Some patients with heart failure have developed increases in blood urea nitrogen, serum creatinine, and potassium. These effects are more likely to occur in patients with pre-existing renal impairment. Dosage reduction and/or discontinuation of DIOVAN may be required. In the Valsartan Heart Failure Trial, in which 93% of patients were on concomitant ACE inhibitors, treatment was discontinued for elevations in creatinine or potassium in a total of 1.0% on valsartan vs. 0.2% on placebo.

Use of valsartan should include appropriate assessment of renal function.

Special Populations: Pregnant Women: Drugs that act directly on the renin-angiotensin-aldosterone-system (RAAS) can cause fetal and neonatal morbidity and death when administered to pregnant women. When pregnancy is detected, DIOVAN should be discontinued as soon as possible.

The use of ARB is not recommended during pregnancy. Epidemiological evidence regarding the risk of teratogenicity following exposure to angiotensin converting enzyme inhibitors (another class of therapeutic products interfering with the RAAS) during the first trimester of pregnancy has not been conclusive; however a small increase in risk cannot be excluded. Given the current evidence available on the risk with ARB, similar risks may exist for this class of drugs. Patients planning pregnancy should be changed to alternative anti-hypertensive treatments which have an established safety profile for use in pregnancy. When pregnancy is diagnosed, treatment with angiotensin II antagonists should be stopped immediately, and, if appropriate, alternative therapy should be started.

The use of ARBS during the second and third trimesters is known to induce human fetotoxicity (decreased renal function, oligohydramnios, skull ossification retardation) and neonatal toxicity (renal failure, hypotension, hyperkalaemia).

There have been reports of spontaneous abortion, oligohydramnios and newborn renal dysfunction, when pregnant women have inadvertently taken valsartan.

Infants with histories of in utero exposure to an angiotensin II AT_1 receptor blocker should be closely observed for hypotension, oliguria, and hyperkalemia. If oliguria occurs, attention should be directed toward support of blood pressure and renal perfusion. Exchange transfusion may be required as a means of reversing hypotension and/or substituting for impaired renal function; however, limited experience with those procedures has not been associated with significant clinical benefit. Valsartan is not removed from plasma by dialysis.

Animal Data: No teratogenic effects were observed when valsartan was administered orally to pregnant mice and rats at doses up to 600 mg/kg/day and to pregnant rabbits at oral doses up to 10 mg/kg/day. However, significant decreases in fetal weight, pup birth weight, pup survival rate and slight delays in developmental milestones were observed in studies in which parental rats were treated orally with valsartan at maternally toxic (reduction in body weight gain and food consumption) doses of 600 mg/kg/day during organogenesis or late gestation and lactation. In rabbits, fetotoxicity associated with maternal toxicity (mortality) was observed at doses of 5 and 10 mg/kg/day.

Nursing Women: It is not known whether valsartan is excreted in human milk but significant levels have been found in the milk of lactating rats. Because many drugs are excreted in human milk and because of their potential for affecting the nursing infant adversely, a decision should be made whether to discontinue nursing or discontinue the drug, taking into account the importance of the drug to the mother.

Pediatrics: The safety and effectiveness of DIOVAN in children and adolescents (below the age of 18 years) have not been established.

Geriatrics (>65 years of age): In controlled clinical trials no overall age-related differences were seen in the adverse effect profile but greater sensitivity in some older individuals cannot be ruled out.

ADVERSE REACTIONS: Clinical Trial Adverse Drug Reactions: Because clinical trials are conducted under very specific conditions the adverse reaction rates observed in the clinical trials may not reflect the rates observed in practice and should not be compared to the rates in the clinical trials of another drug. Adverse drug reaction information from clinical trials is useful for identifying drug-related adverse events and for approximating rates.

Hypertension: DIOVAN has been evaluated for safety in over 4300 patients treated for hypertension, including more than 600 treated for over 6 months and more than 330 for over 1 year. Of these, 3634 were treated with valsartan monotherapy in controlled clinical trials.

In controlled clinical trials, discontinuation due to AEs occurred in 3.1% and 4.0% of patients treated with DIOVAN monotherapy and placebo, respectively.

The following potentially serious adverse reactions have been reported rarely with valsartan in controlled clinical trials: syncope, hypotension.

Table 1 is based on double-blind controlled trials in patients treated with DIOVAN monotherapy at doses of 80 to 160 mg/day. The table includes all AEs with an incidence of 1% or greater in the DIOVAN treatment group, irrespective of causal relationship to study drug. No AE appeared to have an incidence related to dose. Therefore, AEs are grouped irrespective of dose.

Table 1: DIOVAN

Hypertension: Occurrence of Adverse Events During Double-blind Controlled Trials in Patients Treated with DIOVAN Monotherapy at Doses of 80 to 160 mg/day

	DIOVAN N=2827 (%)	Placebo N=1007 (%)
Central Nervous System		
Headache	8.5	13.6
Dizziness	2.8	3.9
Respiratory System		
Upper Respiratory Tract Infection	2.9	2.3
Coughing	2.7	1.3
Rhinitis	1.8	2.0
Sinusitis	1.5	1.7
Pharyngitis	1.3	0.7
Bronchitis	1.1	1.3
Digestive System		
Diarrhea	2.5	1.6
Abdominal Pain	1.3	0.9
Nausea	1.5	2.2
Dyspepsia	1.1	1.8
Musculoskeletal System		
Arthralgia	1.3	0.9
Back Pain	2.2	1.5
Body as a Whole		
Fatigue	1.9	1.3
Other		
Viral Infection	3.1	2.6

In a study conducted with patients taking DIOVAN at starting doses of 20 mg to 320 mg, an increased incidence of dizziness was observed with DIOVAN 320 mg (9%) compared to DIOVAN 20 to 160 mg (2 to 4%). In another study where patients were up-titrated to the 320 mg dose of DIOVAN, the incidence of dizziness was comparable to the 160 mg dose (1%).

In double-blind controlled trials, the following adverse events were reported with DIOVAN at an occurrence rate of less than 1% regardless of drug relationship: orthostatic effects, chest pain, palpitations, myalgia, asthenia, somnolence, vertigo, impotence, epistaxis, fibrosing alveolitis (one case), allergic reactions, urticaria, pruritus and rash.

Following Myocardial Infarction: Table 2 shows the frequency of selected serious adverse events (≥0.4% in any treatment group) for the valsartan, valsartan + captopril, and captopril treatment groups in a large, randomized double-blind trial. Serious adverse events related to the disease under study have not been included in this table.

Table 2: DIOVAN

Following Myocardial Infarction: Selected Serious Adverse Events by Treatment (Safety Population)

	Valsartan n=4885 (%)	Valsartan+Captopril n=4862 (%)	Captopril n=4879 (%)
Hypotension[a]	2.8	3.3	2.0
Syncope	0.7	0.6	0.6
Dizziness	0.4	0.4	0.3
Renal causes[b]	3.1	3.0	2.0
Hyperkalemia	0.4	0.6	0.4
Atrial fibrillation	1.0	0.7	0.8
Cough	0.3	0.5	0.4
Taste disturbances[c]	0.1	0.4	0.3

[a] This term includes SAEs related to hypotension, orthostatic hypotension.
[b] This term includes SAEs related to acute renal failure, chronic renal failure, blood creatinine increased.
[c] This term includes ageusia, dysgeusia, hypogeusia.

Major renal dysfunction was observed in 3.8%, 3.7%, and 2.6% of patients in the valsartan, valsartan + captopril, and captopril treatment groups, respectively. Major renal dysfunction was defined as death from a renal cause, a serious adverse event suggestive of renal failure, and temporary or permanent discontinuation of study drug for a renal cause.

Heart Failure: The adverse experience profile of valsartan in heart failure patients was consistent with the pharmacology of the drug and the health status of the patients for the doses of valsartan used in the Valsartan Heart Failure Trial.

Abnormal Hematologic and Clinical Chemistry Findings: Laboratory Findings: These laboratory findings pertain to trials in hypertension, except as otherwise indicated.

Hyperkalemia: In hypertensive patients, greater than 20% increases in serum potassium were observed in 5.0% of valsartan-treated patients compared to 3.0% of placebo-treated patients. Hyperkalemia as an adverse event occurred in 2.3%, 2.4%, and 1.5% of post-myocardial infarction patients treated with valsartan, valsartan + captopril, and captopril, respectively. In heart failure patients, greater than 20% increases in serum potassium were observed in 10.0% of valsartan-treated patients compared to 5.1% of placebo-treated patients.

Creatinine: Minor elevations in creatinine occurred in 1.1% of patients treated with valsartan and 0.8% of patients given placebo in controlled clinical trials in hypertensive patients. In post-myocardial infarction patients, doubling of serum creatinine was observed in 4.2% of valsartan-treated patients, 4.8% of valsartan + captopril-treated patients, and 3.4% of captopril-treated patients. In heart failure patients, increases in serum creatinine greater than 50% were observed in 3.9% of valsartan-treated patients compared to 0.9% of placebo-treated patients.

Blood Urea Nitrogen (BUN): In heart failure trials, increases in blood urea nitrogen (BUN) greater than 50% were observed in 16.6% of patients treated with valsartan as compared to 6.3% of patients treated with placebo.

Hemoglobin and Hematocrit: In controlled clinical trials, greater than 20% decreases in hemoglobin and hematocrit were observed in 0.4% and 0.8%, respectively, of patients treated with valsartan compared with 0.1% and 0.1% of patients given placebo. One valsartan patient discontinued treatment for microcytic anemia.

Uric Acid: In placebo-controlled trials, elevations of uric acid levels (baseline versus terminal lab) occurred in 2.6% of patients receiving valsartan monotherapy, 8.2% receiving valsartan and hydrochlorothiazide, 6.0% receiving hydrochlorothiazide alone and 2.3% receiving placebo.

Neutropenia: Neutropenia was observed in 1.9% of patients treated with valsartan and 0.8% of patients treated with placebo.

In controlled clinical trials, thrombocytopenia was observed in 0.1% of patients.

Post-Market Adverse Drug Reactions: Other adverse reactions reported rarely in post-marketing use include: anaphylaxis (very rarely), angioedema (involving swelling of the face, lips and/or tongue), renal impairment (very rare), photosensitivity, increase in blood pressure and taste disorders.

Cases of muscle pain, muscle weakness, myositis and rhabdomyolysis have been reported in patients receiving angiotensin II receptor blockers.

DRUG INTERACTIONS: Drug-Drug Interactions: Diuretics: Patients on diuretics, and especially those in whom diuretic therapy was recently instituted, may occasionally experience an excessive reduction in blood pressure after initiation of therapy with DIOVAN. The possibility of symptomatic hypotension with the use of DIOVAN can be minimized by discontinuing the diuretic prior to initiation of treatment (see Warnings and Precautions, Cardiovascular, Hypotension). No drug interaction of clinical significance has been identified with thiazide diuretics.

Agents Increasing Serum Potassium: Since DIOVAN decreases the production of aldosterone, potassium-sparing diuretics or potassium supplements should be given only for documented hypokalemia and with frequent monitoring of serum potassium. Potassium-containing salt substitutes should also be used with caution.

Lithium Salts: As with other drugs which eliminate sodium, lithium clearance may be reduced. Therefore, serum lithium levels should be monitored carefully if lithium salts are to be administered.

Warfarin: Co-administration of valsartan and warfarin over 3 days did not affect the bioavailability of valsartan. Co-administration had no effect on activated partial thromboplastin time (APTT) and resulted in a 12% increase in prothrombin time (PT).

Digoxin: A single dose of digoxin administered with a single dose of valsartan did not result in a clinically significant interaction. No steady state data are available.

Drug-Food Interactions: See Action and Clinical Pharmacology, Pharmacokinetics, Absorption.

DOSAGE AND ADMINISTRATION: Dosing Considerations: Hepatic Impairment: No initial dosage adjustment is required in patients with mild to moderate liver disease. Care should be exercised in patients with liver disease (see Action and Clinical Pharmacology, Pharmacokinetics, and Warnings and Precautions, Hepatic/Biliary/Pancreatic).

Renal Impairment: No initial dosage adjustment is required for patients with renal impairment including those patients requiring hemodialysis. Appropriate monitoring of these patients is however recommended (see Action and Clinical Pharmacology, Pharmacokinetics, and Warnings and Precautions, Renal).

Elderly: No dosage adjustment is usually necessary (see Warnings and Precautions, Special Populations, Geriatrics).

Concomitant Diuretic Therapy: In patients receiving diuretics, DIOVAN therapy should be initiated with caution, since these patients may be volume-depleted and thus more likely to experience hypotension following initiation of additional anti-hypertensive therapy. Whenever possible, all diuretics should be discontinued two to three days prior to the administration of DIOVAN to reduce the likelihood of hypotension (see Warnings and Precautions, Hypotension, and Drug Interactions, Diuretics). If this is not possible because of the patient's condition, DIOVAN should be administered with caution and the blood pressure monitored closely. Thereafter, the dosage should be adjusted according to the individual response of the patient.

Recommended Dose and Dosage Adjustment: Hypertension: Initiation of therapy requires consideration of recent antihypertensive drug treatment, the extent of blood pressure elevation, salt restriction, and other pertinent clinical factors (see Warnings and Precautions, Hypotension). The dosage of antihypertensive agents used with DIOVAN may need to be adjusted.

The recommended initial dose of DIOVAN is 80 mg once daily. The antihypertensive effect is present within 2 weeks and maximal reduction is usually attained within 4 weeks following initiation of therapy. In patients whose blood pressure is not adequately controlled, the daily dose may be increased to a maximum of 320 mg or a thiazide diuretic added.

It is not recommended to prescribe the maximum dose of 320 mg without prior up-titration.

DIOVAN should be administered consistently with or without food (see Action and Clinical Pharmacology, Pharmacokinetics).

Following Myocardial Infarction: DIOVAN may be initiated as early as 12 hours after a myocardial infarction in clinically stable patients. In order to diminish the risk of hypotension, the recommended starting dose is 20 mg twice daily. Thereafter, patients may be uptitrated within 7 days to 40 mg twice daily, with subsequent titrations to a target maintenance dose of 160 mg twice daily, as tolerated. If symptomatic hypotension or renal dysfunction occurs, consideration should be given to dosage reduction. DIOVAN should be given with other standard post-myocardial infarction treatment, including thrombolytics, aspirin and statins, as indicated.

Concomitant use of beta-blockers is to be encouraged with DIOVAN in this clinical setting, if indicated, since further substantial relative risk reduction may be expected with such use over that of valsartan alone.

Heart Failure: The recommended starting dose of DIOVAN is 40 mg twice daily. Titration every two weeks to 80 mg and 160 mg twice daily should be done to the highest dose tolerated by the patient. Consideration should be given to reduce the dose of concomitant diuretics. The maximum recommended dose is 160 mg twice daily.

Missed Dose: Patients should try to take their dose at the same time each day, preferably in the morning. However, if they have forgotten to take the dose during the day, they should carry on with the next dose at the usual time. They should not double doses.

OVERDOSAGE:

Limited data are available in regard to overdosage with DIOVAN (valsartan) in humans. The most likely manifestations of overdosage would be hypotension and tachycardia; bradycardia could occur from parasympathetic (vagal) stimulation. Depressed level of consciousness, circulatory collapse and shock have been reported. If symptomatic hypotension should occur, supportive treatment should be instituted.

Valsartan is not removed from the plasma by dialysis.

For the management of a suspected drug overdose, contact your regional Poison Control Centre.

> For management of a suspected drug overdose, CPhA recommends that you contact your **regional Poison Control Centre**. See the *CPS* Directory section for a list of Poison Control Centres.

ACTION AND CLINICAL PHARMACOLOGY: Mechanism of Action: DIOVAN (valsartan) is an orally active angiotensin II AT_1 receptor blocker.

Valsartan acts selectively on AT_1, the receptor subtype that mediates the known cardiovascular actions of angiotensin II, the primary vaso-active hormone of the renin-angiotensin-system. The AT_2 receptor subtype, found in tissues such as brain, endometrium, myometrium and fetal kidney and adrenals, plays no known role in cardiovascular homeostasis to date. Valsartan does not exhibit any partial AT_1 receptor agonist activity and has essentially no activity at the AT_2 receptor. Valsartan does not bind to or block other hormone receptors or ion channels known to be important in cardiovascular regulation. The primary metabolite, valeryl 4-hydroxy valsartan, is essentially inactive.

Angiotensin II has a wide variety of physiological effects; many are either directly or indirectly involved in blood pressure regulation. A potent vasoconstrictor, angiotensin II exerts a direct pressor response. In addition, it promotes sodium retention and aldosterone secretion.

Blockade of angiotensin II AT_1 receptors results in two- to three-fold increase in plasma renin and angiotensin II plasma concentrations in hypertensive patients. Long-term effects of increased AT_2 receptor stimulation by angiotensin II are unknown.

Valsartan does not inhibit angiotensin converting enzyme (ACE), also known as kininase II, the enzyme that converts angiotensin I to angiotensin II and degrades bradykinin.

Administration of valsartan to patients with type II diabetes and microalbuminuria has resulted in significant reduction of urinary albumin excretion.

Pharmacodynamics: Valsartan inhibits the pressor effect of an angiotensin II infusion. An oral dose of 80 mg inhibits the pressor effect by about 80% at peak with approximately 30% inhibition persisting for 24 hours.

After a single oral dose, the antihypertensive activity of valsartan has an onset within approximately 2 hours and peaks within 4-6 hours in most patients.

The anti-hypertensive effect of valsartan persists for 24 hours after dosing. Trough/peak ratio ranges from 0.54 to 0.76. DIOVAN reduces blood pressure in hypertensive patients without affecting pulse rate.

During repeated dosing, the maximum blood pressure reduction with any dose is generally attained within 4 weeks, and is sustained during long-term therapy. Combinations with hydrochlorothiazide produce additional reduction in blood pressure.

There is no apparent rebound effect after abrupt withdrawal of valsartan therapy.

Although data available to date indicate a similar pharmacodynamic effect of valsartan in black and white hypertensive patients, this should be viewed with caution since antihypertensive drugs that affect the renin-angiotensin system, such as ACE inhibitors and angiotensin II AT_1 receptor blockers, have generally been found to be less effective in low-renin hypertensives (frequently blacks).

Pharmacokinetics: Since its pharmacokinetics are linear in the 80 to 320 mg dose range, valsartan does not accumulate appreciably in plasma following repeated administration.

The DIOVAN tablet and capsule dosage forms were found to be bioequivalent in a two-treatment, three period, repeated measure, randomized cross-over study conducted in 40 healthy volunteers and comparing the 320 mg tablet formulation to 2×160 mg capsule. The median T_{max} values were similar and the mean C_{max} values were nearly identical (2.75 h versus 3.00 h and 6.162 mg/dL versus 6.164 mg/dL, respectively for the tablet and capsule). The $AUC_{0-\infty}$ was of 42.68 h·mg/L for the tablet and 39.829 h·mg/L for the capsule.

Absorption: The mean absolute bioavailability of valsartan is about 23%, but with high variability. Peak plasma concentration is reached 2 to 4 hours after dosing. Giving DIOVAN with food reduces the area under the valsartan plasma concentration curve (AUC) by 48%. After about 8 hours however, plasma valsartan concentrations are similar in the fed and fasted state.

Distribution: Valsartan is 94-97% bound to serum protein, mainly serum albumin. Steady-state volume of distribution is about 17 L, indicating that valsartan does not distribute into tissues extensively.

Metabolism: Following intravenous administration, valsartan shows bi-exponential decay kinetics ($t_{1/2}\alpha$ <1 hour and $t_{1/2}\beta$ between 5-9 hours). Plasma clearance is relatively slow (about 2 L/h) when compared with hepatic blood flow (about 30 L/h). Valsartan biotransformation does not seem to involve the cytochrome P-450 system. The enzyme(s) responsible for valsartan metabolism have not been identified.

Excretion: Following administration of an oral solution of ^{14}C labelled valsartan, 83% of absorbed valsartan is excreted in the feces and 13% in the urine, mainly as unchanged compound.

Special Populations and Conditions: Pediatrics: The safety and effectiveness of DIOVAN in children and adolescents (below the age of 18 years) have not been established.

Geriatrics: Exposure to valsartan is about 50% higher as measured by AUC and C_{max} and the half life is longer in elderly subjects than in young subjects. However, this difference has not been shown to have any clinical significance.

Gender: Plasma concentrations are similar in males and females.

Hepatic Insufficiency: On average, patients with mild to moderate chronic liver disease have twice the exposure to valsartan of healthy volunteers as measured by AUC and C_{max} (see Warnings and Precautions, and Dosage and Administration).

Renal Insufficiency: Renal clearance accounts for only 30% of total plasma clearance. There is no apparent correlation between renal function and exposure to valsartan, as measured by AUC and C_{max}, in patients with different degrees of renal impairment. In patients with renal failure undergoing hemodialysis, limited information showed that exposure to valsartan is comparable to that in patients with creatinine clearance >10 mL/min.

STORAGE AND STABILITY: Protect from moisture and heat (store at 15-30°C).

SPECIAL HANDLING INSTRUCTIONS: Not applicable.

INFORMATION FOR THE PATIENT: Published in e-CPS, available by subscription at www.e-cps.ca.

DOSAGE FORMS, COMPOSITION AND PACKAGING: 40 mg: Each yellow, ovaloid, scored on one side, slightly convex tablet with bevelled edges, debossed on one side with DO and with NVR on the other side, contains: valsartan 40 mg. Nonmedicinal ingredients: colloidal silicon dioxide, crospovidone, magnesium stearate and microcrystalline cellulose; coating: black iron oxide, hydroxypropyl methylcellulose, polyethylene glycol, red iron oxide, titanium dioxide and yellow iron oxide. Cartons containing 2 blister strips of 14 tablets. Since the 40 mg tablets are scored on one side, these may be used to initiate therapy following myocardial infarction (see Dosage and Administration, Following Myocardial Infarction).

80 mg: Each pale red, round shaped tablet with bevelled edges, debossed with DV on one side and NVR on the other, contains: valsartan 80 mg. Nonmedicinal ingredients: colloidal silicon dioxide, crospovidone, magnesium stearate and microcrystalline cellulose; coating: black iron oxide, hydroxypropyl methylcellulose, polyethylene glycol, red iron oxide and titanium dioxide. Cartons containing 2 blister strips of 14 tablets.

160 mg: Each grey orange, ovaloid shaped tablet with bevelled edges, debossed with DX on one side and NVR on the other, contains: valsartan 160 mg. Nonmedicinal ingredients: colloidal silicon dioxide, crospovidone, magnesium stearate and microcrystalline cellulose; coating: black iron oxide, hydroxypropyl methylcellulose, polyethylene glycol, red iron oxide, titanium dioxide and yellow iron oxide. Cartons containing 2 blister strips of 14 tablets.

320 mg: Each dark grey-violet, ovaloid tablet with bevelled edges, slightly convex, debossed with DXL on one side and NVR on the other, contains: valsartan 320 mg. Nonmedicinal ingredients: colloidal silicon dioxide, crospovidone, magnesium stearate and microcrystalline cellulose; coating: black iron oxide, hydroxypropyl methylcellulose, polyethylene glycol, red iron oxide, titanium dioxide and yellow iron oxide. Cartons containing 2 blister strips of 14 tablets.

(Shown in Product Identification Section)

Diovan®-HCT ℞

valsartan—hydrochlorothiazide

Angiotensin II AT1 Receptor Blocker—Diuretic

Novartis Pharmaceuticals

Date of Revision: June 29, 2009

SUMMARY PRODUCT INFORMATION:

Route of Administration	Dosage Form/ Strength	Clinically Relevant Nonmedicinal Ingredients
Oral	Tablets: 80 mg/12.5 mg, 160 mg/12.5 mg, 160 mg/25 mg, 320 mg/12.5 mg, 320 mg/25 mg	Colloidal silicon dioxide, crospovidone, magnesium stearate and microcrystalline cellulose For a complete listing see Dosage Forms, Composition and Packaging.

INDICATIONS AND CLINICAL USE: DIOVAN-HCT (valsartan and hydrochlorothiazide) is indicated for the treatment of mild to moderate essential hypertension in patients for whom combination therapy is appropriate.

DIOVAN-HCT is not indicated for initial therapy (see Dosage and Administration).

Patients should be titrated on individual drugs. If the fixed combination represents the dose and dosing frequency determined by this titration, the use of DIOVAN-HCT may be more convenient in the management of patients. If during maintenance therapy dosage adjustment is necessary it is advisable to use the individual drugs.

Geriatrics (>65 years of age): No overall age-related differences were seen in the adverse effect profile but greater sensitivity in some older individuals cannot be ruled out and appropriate caution is recommended.

Pediatrics (<18 years of age): The safety and efficacy of DIOVAN-HCT in children and adolescents (below the age of 18 years) have not been established and use in this age group is not recommended.

CONTRAINDICATIONS:

- DIOVAN-HCT (valsartan and hydrochlorothiazide) is contraindicated in patients who are hypersensitive to this drug or to any ingredient in the formulation or component of the container (see Dosage Forms, Composition and Packaging).
- Because of the hydrochlorothiazide component, it is also contraindicated in patients with anuria, and in patients who are hypersensitive to other sulfonamide-derived drugs.
- DIOVAN-HCT is also contraindicated in pregnant women.

WARNINGS AND PRECAUTIONS:

Serious Warnings and Precautions

When used in pregnancy, **angiotensin receptor (AT$_1$) blockers (ARB)** can cause injury to or even death of the developing fetus. When pregnancy is detected, DIOVAN-HCT should be discontinued as soon as possible (see Contraindications and Warnings and Precautions, Special Populations).

Cardiovascular: Hypotension: Occasionally, symptomatic hypotension has occurred after administration of valsartan, in some cases after the first dose. It is more likely to occur in patients who are volume-depleted by diuretic therapy, dietary salt restriction, dialysis, diarrhea, or vomiting. In these patients, because of the potential fall in blood pressure, therapy should be started under close medical supervision. Similar considerations apply to patients with ischemic heart or cerebrovascular disease, in whom an excessive fall in blood pressure could result in myocardial infarction or cerebrovascular accident.

Valvular Stenosis: There is concern on theoretical grounds that patients with aortic stenosis might be at a particular risk of decreased coronary perfusion when treated with vasodilators, because they do not develop as much after load reduction.

Endocrine and Metabolism: Treatment with thiazide diuretics, including hydrochlorothiazide, has been associated with hyponatremia and hypochloremic alkalosis. Patients receiving thiazides should be carefully observed for clinical signs of fluid and electrolyte imbalance (hyponatremia, hypochloremic alkalosis and hypokalemia). Periodic determinations of serum electrolytes to detect possible electrolyte disturbance should be performed at appropriate intervals. Warning signs or symptoms of fluid and electrolyte imbalance include dryness of the mouth, thirst, weakness, lethargy, drowsiness, restlessness, muscle pains or cramps, muscular fatigue, hypotension, oliguria, tachycardia, and gastrointestinal disturbances such as nausea and vomiting.

Hypokalemia may develop, especially with brisk diuresis, when severe cirrhosis is present, or after prolonged therapy.

Interference with adequate oral electrolyte intake will also contribute to hypokalemia. Hypokalemia can sensitize or exaggerate the response of the heart to the toxic effects of digitalis (e.g. increased ventricular irritability).

Any chloride deficit during thiazide therapy is generally mild and usually does not require specific treatment except under extraordinary circumstances (as in liver disease or renal disease). Dilutional hyponatremia may occur in edematous patients in hot weather; appropriate therapy is water restriction rather than administration of salt, except in rare instances, when the hyponatremia is life threatening. In actual salt depletion, appropriate replacement is the therapy of choice.

Hyperuricemia may occur or acute gout may be precipitated in certain patients receiving thiazide therapy.

Thiazides may decrease serum PBI levels without signs of thyroid disturbance.

Thiazides have been shown to increase excretion of magnesium; this may result in hypomagnesia.

Thiazides may decrease urinary calcium excretion. Thiazides may cause intermittent and slight elevation of serum calcium in the absence of known disorders of calcium metabolism. Marked hypercalcemia may be evidence of hidden hyperparathyroidism. Thiazides should be discontinued before carrying out tests for parathyroid function.

Increases in cholesterol, triglyceride and glucose levels may be associated with thiazide diuretic therapy, including hydrochlorothiazide.

Hepatic/Biliary/Pancreatic: In general, no dosage adjustment is needed in patients with mild to moderate liver disease. However, care should be exercised in patients with liver disease, especially in those patients with biliary obstructive disorders, as the major portion of valsartan is eliminated in the bile. No information is available in patients with severe liver disease (see Action and Clinical Pharmacology, Pharmacokinetics).

Thiazides should be used with caution in patients with impaired hepatic function or progressive liver disease, since minor alterations of fluid and electrolyte balance may precipitate hepatic coma.

Renal: Renal Impairment: As a consequence of inhibiting the renin-angiotensin-aldosterone system, changes in renal function have been seen in susceptible individuals. In patients whose renal function may depend on the activity of the renin-angiotensin-aldosterone system, such as patients with bilateral renal artery stenosis, unilateral renal artery stenosis to a solitary kidney, or severe congestive heart failure, treatment with agents that inhibit this system has been associated with oliguria, progressive azotemia, and rarely, acute renal failure and/or death. In susceptible patients, concomitant diuretic use may further increase risk.

Use of valsartan should include appropriate assessment of renal function.

Thiazides should be used with caution.

Because of the hydrochlorothiazide component, DIOVAN-HCT (valsartan and hydrochlorothiazide) is not recommended in patients with severe renal impairment (creatinine clearance ≤30 mL/min).

Azotemia: Azotemia may be precipitated or increased by hydrochlorothiazide. Cumulative effects of the drug may develop in patients with impaired renal function. If increasing azotemia and oliguria occur during treatment of severe progressive renal disease the diuretic should be discontinued.

Sensitivity/Resistance: Sensitivity reactions to hydrochlorothiazide may occur in patients with or without a history of allergy or bronchial asthma.

The possibility of exacerbation or activation of systemic lupus erythematosus has been reported in patients treated with hydrochlorothiazide.

Special Populations: Pregnant Women: Drugs that act directly on the renin-angiotensin-aldosterone-system (RAAS) can cause fetal and neonatal morbidity and death when administered to pregnant women. When pregnancy is detected, DIOVAN-HCT (valsartan and hydrochlorothiazide) should be discontinued as soon as possible.

The use of ARB is not recommended during pregnancy. Epidemiological evidence regarding the risk of teratogenicity following exposure to angiotensin converting enzyme inhibitors (another class of therapeutic products interfering with the RAAS) during the first trimester of pregnancy has not been conclusive; however a small increase in risk cannot be excluded. Given the current evidence available on the risk with ARB, similar risks may exist for this class of drugs. Patients planning pregnancy should be changed to alternative anti-hypertensive treatments which have an established safety profile for use in pregnancy. When pregnancy is diagnosed, treatment with angiotensin II antagonists should be stopped immediately, and, if appropriate, alternative therapy should be started.

The use of ARBS during the second and third trimesters is known to induce human fetotoxicity (decreased renal function, oligohydramnios, skull ossification retardation) and neonatal toxicity (renal failure, hypotension, hyperkalaemia).

There have been reports of spontaneous abortion, oligohydramnios and newborn renal dysfunction, when pregnant women have inadvertently taken valsartan.

Infants with histories of in utero exposure ARBs should be closely observed for hypotension, oliguria, and hyperkalemia. If oliguria occurs, attention should be directed toward support of blood pressure and renal perfusion. Exchange transfusion may be required as a means of reversing hypotension and/or substituting for impaired renal function; however, limited experience with those procedures has not been associated with significant clinical benefit. Valsartan is not removed from plasma by dialysis.

Thiazides cross the placental barrier and appear in cord blood. The routine use of diuretics, including hydrochlorothiazide in otherwise healthy pregnant women is not recommended and exposes mother and fetus to unnecessary hazard including fetal or neonatal jaundice, thrombocytopenia and possibly other adverse experiences which have occurred in the adult. Diuretics do not prevent development of toxemia of pregnancy and there is no satisfactory evidence that they are useful in the treatment of toxemia.

Animal Data: No teratogenic effects were observed when valsartan was administered orally to pregnant mice and rats at doses up to 600 mg/kg/day and to pregnant rabbits at oral doses up to 10 mg/kg/day. However, significant decreases in fetal weight, pup birth weight, pup survival rate and slight delays in developmental milestones were observed in studies in which parental rats were treated orally with valsartan at maternally toxic (reduction in body weight gain and food consumption) doses of 600 mg/kg/day during organogenesis or late gestation and lactation. In rabbits, fetotoxicity associated with maternal toxicity (mortality) was observed at doses of 5 and 10 mg/kg/day.

Nursing Women: It is not known whether valsartan is excreted in human milk but significant levels have been found in the milk of lactating rats. Thiazides appear in human milk. Because many drugs are excreted in human milk and because of their potential for affecting the nursing infant adversely, a decision should be made whether to discontinue nursing or discontinue the drug, taking into account the importance of the drug to the mother.

Pediatrics (<18 years of age): The safety and efficacy of DIOVAN-HCT in children and adolescents (below the age of 18 years) have not been established and use in this age group is not recommended.

Geriatrics (>65 years of age): No overall age-related differences were seen in the adverse effect profile but greater sensitivity in some older individuals cannot be ruled out and appropriate caution is recommended.

ADVERSE REACTIONS: Clinical Trial Adverse Drug Reactions: Because clinical trials are conducted under very specific conditions the adverse reaction rates observed in the clinical trials may not reflect the rates observed in practice and should not be compared to the rates in the clinical trials of another drug. Adverse drug reaction information from clinical trials is useful for identifying drug-related adverse events and for approximating rates.

DIOVAN-HCT (valsartan and hydrochlorothiazide) has been evaluated for safety in more than 7616 patients treated for essential hypertension. Of these, 4372 were treated with DIOVAN-HCT in controlled clinical trials with a mean exposure of 8 weeks.

In controlled clinical trials, discontinuation due to Adverse Experiences (AEs) occurred in 2.3 % and 3.1 % of patients treated with DIOVAN-HCT and placebo, respectively. The most common AEs resulting in discontinuation of therapy with Diovan-HCT were dizziness and headache.

The most common serious AEs with DIOVAN-HCT were myocardial infarction and chest pain.

Table 1 is based on double-blind, active or placebo-controlled trials in patients treated with DIOVAN-HCT at doses of 80 mg/12.5 mg, 80 mg/25 mg, 160 mg/12.5 mg, 160 mg/25 mg, 320 mg/12.5 mg and 320 mg/25 mg, DIOVAN at doses of 80 mg, 160 mg, and 320 mg, and HCT at doses of 12.5 mg and 25 mg. The table includes all AEs with an incidence of 1% or greater in either the DIOVAN-HCT, DIOVAN monotherapy, HCT monotherapy, or placebo group, irrespective of causal relationship to study drug.

Table 1: DIOVAN-HCT

Occurrence of Adverse Events During Double-blind Controlled Trials in Patients Treated with DIOVAN-HCT at Doses of 80 mg/12.5 mg, 80 mg/25 mg, 160 mg/12.5 mg, 160 mg/25 mg, 320 mg/12.5 mg and 320 mg/25 mg

	Vaslartan/HCTZ N=4372	Valsartan N=2447	Hydrochlorothiazide N=535	Placebo N=262
	n (%)	n (%)	n (%)	n (%)
Ear and Labyrinth Disorders				
Vertigo	35 (0.8)	10 (0.4)	6 (1.1)	1 (0.4)
Gastrointestinal Disorders				
Diarrhoea	48 (1.1)	41 (1.7)	10 (1.9)	3 (1.1)
Nausea	37 (0.8)	21 (0.9)	10 (1.9)	4 (1.5)
Dyspepsia	25 (0.6)	18 (0.7)	6 (1.1)	1 (0.4)
Vomiting	13 (0.3)	11 (0.4)	1 (0.2)	4 (1.5)
Toothache	9 (0.2)	4 (0.2)	1 (0.2)	3 (1.1)
Constipation	6 (0.1)	3 (0.1)	12 (2.2)	2 (0.8)
General Disorders				
Fatigue	72 (1.6)	26 (1.1)	22 (4.1)	4 (1.5)
Oedema peripheral	25 (0.6)	27 (1.1)	10 (1.9)	3 (1.1)
Infections				
Nasopharyngitis	103 (2.4)	67 (2.7)	15 (2.8)	5 (1.9)
Upper respiratory tract infection	53 (1.2)	49 (2.0)	23 (4.3)	9 (3.4)
Influenza	37 (0.8)	22 (0.9)	8 (1.5)	3 (1.1)
Bronchitis	33 (0.8)	15 (0.6)	6 (1.1)	3 (1.1)
Sinusitis	29 (0.7)	23 (0.9)	7 (1.3)	6 (2.3)
Urinary tract infection	26 (0.6)	12 (0.5)	7 (1.3)	1 (0.4)
Metabolic and Nutrition Disorders				
Hypokalaemia	7 (0.2)	2 (0.1)	13 (2.4)	2 (0.8)
Musculoskeletal and Connective Tissue Disorders				
Back pain	52 (1.2)	37 (1.5)	11 (2.1)	7 (2.7)
Arthralgia	44 (1.0)	25 (1.0)	8 (1.5)	3 (1.1)
Myalgia	25 (0.6)	15 (0.6)	6 (1.1)	1 (0.4)
Pain in extremity	21 (0.5)	10 (0.4)	11 (2.1)	0 (0.0)
Muscle cramp	18 (0.4)	3 (0.1)	10 (1.9)	3 (1.1)
Nervous System Disorders				
Headache	161 (3.7)	126 (5.1)	54 (10.1)	38 (14.5)
Dizziness	153 (3.5)	49 (2.0)	27 (5.0)	10 (3.8)
Somnolence	11 (0.3)	8 (0.3)	1 (0.2)	3 (1.1)
Hypoaesthesia	10 (0.2)	5 (0.2)	2 (0.4)	4 (1.5)
Sinus headache	4 (0.1)	7 (0.3)	3 (0.6)	3 (1.1)
Migraine	2 (0.0)	7 (0.3)	0 (0.0)	4 (1.5)
Psychiatric Disorders				
Insomnia	16 (0.4)	12 (0.5)	3 (0.6)	3 (1.1)
Renal and Urinary Disorders				
Pollakiuria	30 (0.7)	11 (0.4)	8 (1.5)	2 (0.8)
Respiratory, Thoracic and Mediastinal Disorders				
Cough	52 (1.2)	37 (1.5)	11 (2.1)	2 (0.8)
Pharyngolaryngeal pain	30 (0.7)	12 (0.5)	6 (1.1)	1 (0.4)

(cont'd)

Table 1: DIOVAN-HCT *(cont'd)*

Occurrence of Adverse Events During Double-blind Controlled Trials in Patients Treated with DIOVAN-HCT at Doses of 80 mg/12.5 mg, 80 mg/25 mg, 160 mg/12.5 mg, 160 mg/25 mg, 320 mg/12.5 mg and 320 mg/25 mg

	Vaslartan/HCTZ N=4372	Valsartan N=2447	Hydrochlorothiazide N=535	Placebo N=262
	n (%)	n (%)	n (%)	n (%)
Sinus congestion	19 (0.4)	7 (0.3)	12 (2.2)	3 (1.1)
Nasal congestion	16 (0.4)	14 (0.6)	7 (1.3)	0 (0.0)
Skin and Subcutaneous Tissue Disorders				
Rash	11 (0.3)	10 (0.4)	6 (1.1)	1 (0.4)

Evaluation of the AEs in the total active-, or placebo-controlled safety population, showed that the most common events, regardless of relationship to treatment in patients treated with valsartan 320 mg/HCTZ were, dizziness, nasopharyngitis, headache and fatigue. The incidence of hypotension was 0.7% in patients treated with valsartan 320 mg/HCTZ.

Less Common Clinical Trial Adverse Drug Reactions (<1%): Body as a Whole: arthritis, asthenia, hypersensitivity, influenza, contusion, insomnia, peripheral oedema, pyrexia, sprains and strains.

Cardiovascular: angina pectoris, hypotension, myocardial infarction, palpitations, tachycardia, ventricular systoles.

Digestive: motion sickness, stomach discomfort.

Ear and Labyrinth: ear pain.

Gastrointestinal: abdominal pain, dry mouth, dyspepsia, flatulence, gastritis, toothache, vomiting.

Muscoskeletal and Connective Tissue: arthralgia, myalgia, muscle strain.

Metabolic and Nutritional: diabetes mellitus, gout, hypokalaemia, hyperuricaemia.

Nervous System/Psychiatric: anxiety, somnolence.

Renal and Urinary System: micturition frequency, urinary tract infection, pollakiuria.

Respiratory, Thoracic, Mediastinal: bronchitis, chest discomfort/pain, dyspnea pharyngolaryngeal pain, sinus congestion, sinusitis.

Reproductive: erectile dysfunction.

Skin and Subcutaneous Tissue: rash.

Special Senses: blurred vision, conjunctivitis, vertigo, tinnitus, visual disturbance.

Other: viral infection.

Abnormal Hematologic and Clinical Chemistry Findings: Laboratory Findings: Potassium: In the double-blind, active or placebo-controlled trials potassium decrease of >20% was observed most frequently with HCTZ 25 mg (9.7%), followed by HCTZ 12.5 mg (6.3%), valsartan/HCTZ 320/25 mg (4.5%), valsartan 320/12.5 mg (3.8%), and valsartan 320 mg (2.0%) compared to placebo (3.1%). Also some patients showed serum potassium increase >20 % but no dose relationship could be demonstrated.

Liver Function Tests: Occasional elevations of liver enzymes occurred in DIOVAN-HCT treated patients.

Creatinine/Blood Urea Nitrogen (BUN)/Uric Acid: Minor elevations in creatinine and BUN occurred in 1.9% and 14.7%, respectively, of patients treated with DIOVAN-HCT and 0.4% and 6.3%, respectively, of patients given placebo in controlled clinical trials. Uric acid increase of >50% was observed most frequently with valsartan/HCTZ 320/25 mg (5.5%), followed by valsartan/HCTZ 320/12.5 mg (2.8%), HCTZ 25 mg (2.0%), valsartan 320 mg (1.7%), and HCTZ 12.5 mg (0.8%) compared to placebo (1.6%).

Hemoglobin and Hematocrit: Greater than 20% decreases in hemoglobin and hematocrit were observed in less than 0.1% of patients treated with DIOVAN-HCT compared with 0.0% of patients given placebo.

Neutropenia: Neutropenia was observed in 0.1% of patients treated with DIOVAN-HCT and 0.4% of patients treated with placebo.

Post-Market Adverse Drug Reactions: Other adverse reactions reported rarely in post-marketing use of DIOVAN alone include: anaphylaxis (very rarely), angioedema (involving swelling of the face, lips and/or tongue), photosensitivity, increase in blood pressure and taste disorders. Very rare cases of impaired renal function have also been reported.

Cases of muscle pain, muscle weakness, myositis and rhabdomyolysis have been reported in patients receiving angiotensin II receptor blockers.

Cases of syncope were reported with DIOVAN-HCT. It is unknown whether this effect was causally related to the therapy.

DRUG INTERACTIONS: Drug-Drug Interactions: Diuretics: Patients on diuretics, and especially those in whom diuretic therapy was recently instituted, may occasionally experience an excessive reduction in blood pressure after initiation of therapy with valsartan. The possibility of symptomatic hypotension with the use of valsartan can be minimized by discontinuing the diuretic prior to initiation of treatment (see Warnings and Precautions, Cardiovascular, Hypotension, and Dosage and Administration). No drug interaction of clinical significance has been identified with thiazide diuretics.

Agents Increasing Serum Potassium: Since valsartan decreases the production of aldosterone, potassium-sparing diuretics or potassium supplements should be given only for documented hypokalemia and with frequent monitoring of serum potassium when valsartan therapy is instituted. Potassium-containing salt substitutes should also be used with caution. Concomitant thiazide diuretic use may attenuate any effect that valsartan may have on serum potassium.

Lithium Salts : As with other drugs which eliminate sodium, lithium clearance may be reduced in the presence of valsartan. Therefore, serum lithium levels should be monitored carefully if lithium salts are to be administered with valsartan. Lithium generally should not be given with diuretics. Diuretic agents reduce the renal clearance of lithium and add a high risk of lithium toxicity.

Warfarin: Co-administration of valsartan and warfarin over 3 days did not affect the bioavailability of valsartan. Co-administration of valsartan and warfarin resulted in a 12% increase in prothrombin time (PT) but had no effect on activated partial thromboplastin time (APTT).

Digoxin: A single dose of digoxin administered with a single dose of valsartan did not result in a clinically significant interaction. No steady state data are available. Thiazide-induced electrolyte disturbances may predispose to digitalis-induced arrhythmias.

Curare Derivatives: Thiazide drugs, including hydrochlorothiazide, may increase the responsiveness to curare derivatives such as d-tubocurarine.

Insulin: Insulin requirements in diabetic patients treated with diuretics may be increased, decreased or unchanged. Diabetes mellitus which has been latent may become manifest during thiazide administration.

Alcohol, Barbiturates, or Narcotics: Diuretic potentiation of orthostatic hypotension may occur.

Corticosteroids, ACTH: Intensified electrolyte depletion, particularly hypokalemia, may occur when steroids are given concomitantly with diuretics.

Pressor Amines (e.g. norepinephrine): In the presence of diuretics possible decreased response to pressor amines may be seen but not sufficient to preclude use.

Non-Steroidal Anti-Inflammatory Drugs: In some patients, the administration of a non-steroidal anti-inflammatory agent can reduce the diuretic, natriuretic, and antihypertensive effects of loop, potassium-sparing and thiazide diuretics. Therefore, when DIOVAN-HCT and non-steroidal anti-inflammatory agents are used concomitantly, the patient should be observed closely to determine if the desired effect of the diuretic is obtained.

Others: Co-administration of thiazide diuretics, including hydrochlorothiazide, may increase the incidence of hypersensitivity reactions to allopurinol, may increase the risk of adverse effects caused by amantadine, may enhance the hyperglycemic effect of diazoxide, and may reduce the renal excretion of cytotoxic drugs (e.g. cyclophosphamide, methotrexate) and potentiate their myelosuppresive effects.

The bioavailability of thiazide-type diuretics may be increased by anticholinergic agents (e.g. atropine, biperiden), apparently due to a decrease in gastrointestinal motility and the stomach emptying rate.

There have been reports in the literature of hemolytic anemia occurring with concomitant use of hydrochlorothiazide and methyldopa.

Absorption of thiazide diuretics, including hydrochlorothiazide, is decreased by cholestyramine.

Administration of thiazide diuretics, including hydrochlorothiazide, with vitamin D or with calcium salts may potentiate the rise in serum calcium.

Concomitant treatment with cyclosporin may increase the risk of hyperuricemia and gout-type complications.

Patients receiving hydrochlorothiazide concomitantly with carbamazepine may develop hyponatremia. Such patients should therefore be advised about the possibility of hyponatremic reactions, and should be monitored accordingly.

Drug-Food Interactions: DIOVAN-HCT may be administered with our without food, however it should be taken consistently with respect to food intake (see Dosage and Administration).

DOSAGE AND ADMINISTRATION: Dosing Considerations: Dosage must be individualized. The fixed combination is not for initial therapy. The dose of DIOVAN-HCT (valsartan and hydrochlorothiazide) should be determined by the titration of the individual components.

Hepatic Impairment: No initial dosage adjustment in valsartan is required in patients with mild to moderate liver disease. However, because thiazide diuretics may precipitate hepatic coma, care should be exercised when administering a fixed combination product containing hydrochlorothiazide (see Warnings and Precautions).

Renal Impairment : No initial dosage adjustment is required for patients with renal impairment including those patients requiring hemodialysis. Appropriate monitoring of these patients is however recommended.

The usual regimens of therapy with DIOVAN-HCT may be followed as long as the patient's creatinine clearance is >30 mL/min. In patients with more severe renal impairment, loop diuretics are preferred to thiazides, so DIOVAN-HCT is not recommended.

Elderly: No dosage adjustment is usually necessary however see Warnings and Precautions.

Recommended Dose and Dosage Adjustment: Once the patient has been stabilized on the individual components as described below, DIOVAN-HCT tablet, 80 mg/12.5 mg, 160 mg/12.5 mg, 160 mg/25 mg, 320 mg/12.5 mg, or 320 mg/25 mg once daily may be substituted if the doses on which the patient was stabilized are the same as those in the fixed combination (see Indications and Clinical Use and Warnings and Precautions).

The maximum recommended dose is 320 mg valsartan and 25 mg hydrochlorothiazide and the titration will be based on physician's judgment according to severity of hypertension and other associated risk factors.

DIOVAN-HCT may be administered with our without food, however it should be taken consistently with respect to food intake.

Valsartan Monotherapy: The recommended starting dose of DIOVAN is 80 mg once daily. The antihypertensive effect is present within 2 weeks and maximal reduction is usually attained within 4 weeks following initiation of therapy. In patients whose blood pressure is not adequately controlled, the daily dose may be increased to a maximum of 320 mg or a thiazide diuretic added.

Diuretic-Treated Patients: In patients receiving diuretics, valsartan therapy should be initiated with caution, since these patients may be volume-depleted and thus more likely to experience hypotension following initiation of additional anti-hypertensive therapy. Whenever possible, all diuretics should be discontinued two to three days prior to the administration of DIOVAN-HCT to reduce the likelihood of hypotension (see Warnings and Precautions and Drug Interactions). If this is not possible because of the patient's condition, DIOVAN-HCT should be administered with caution and the blood pressure monitored closely. Thereafter, the dosage should be adjusted according to the individual response of the patient.

Missed Dose: Patients should try to take their dose at the same time each day, preferably in the morning. However, if they have forgotten to take the dose during the day, they should carry on with the next dose at the usual time. They should not double doses.

OVERDOSAGE:

No specific information is available on the treatment of overdosage with DIOVAN-HCT (valsartan and hydrochlorothiazide). Treatment is symptomatic and supportive.

Valsartan: Limited data are available in regard to overdosage with DIOVAN (valsartan) in humans. The most likely manifestations of overdosage would be hypotension, which could lead to depressed level of consciousness, circulatory collapse and/or shock, and/or tachycardia. If symptomatic hypotension should occur, supportive treatment should be instituted.

Valsartan is not removed from the plasma by dialysis.

Hydrochlorothiazide: The most common signs and symptoms observed are those caused by electrolyte depletion (hypokalemia, hypochloremia, hyponatremia) and dehydration resulting from excessive diuresis. If digitalis has also been administered, hypokalemia may accentuate cardiac arrhythmias.

The degree to which hydrochlorothiazide is removed by hemodialysis has not been established.

For management of a suspected drug overdose, contact your **regional Poison Control Centre**. See the *CPS* Directory section for a list of Poison Control Centres.

ACTION AND CLINICAL PHARMACOLOGY: DIOVAN-HCT (valsartan and hydrochlorothiazide) combines the actions of valsartan, an orally active angiotensin II AT_1 receptor blocker, and that of a diuretic, hydrochlorothiazide.

Mechanism of Action: Valsartan: Valsartan acts selectively on AT_1, the receptor subtype that mediates the known cardiovascular actions of angiotensin II, the primary vaso-active hormone of the renin-angiotensin-system. The AT_2 receptor subtype, found in tissues such as brain, endometrium, myometrium and fetal kidney and adrenals, plays no known role in cardiovascular homeostasis to date. Valsartan does not exhibit any partial AT_1 receptor agonist activity and has essentially no activity at the AT_2 receptor. Valsartan does not bind to or block other hormone receptors or ion channels known to be important in cardiovascular regulation. The primary metabolite, valeryl 4-hydroxy valsartan, is essentially inactive.

Angiotensin II has a wide variety of physiological effects; many are either directly or indirectly involved in blood pressure regulation. A potent vasoconstrictor, angiotensin II exerts a direct pressor response. In addition it promotes sodium retention and aldosterone secretion.

Blockade of angiotensin II AT_1 receptors results in two- to three-fold increase in plasma renin and angiotensin II plasma concentrations in hypertensive patients. Long-term effects of increased AT_2 receptor stimulation by angiotensin II are unknown.

Valsartan does not inhibit angiotensin converting enzyme (ACE), also known as kininase II, the enzyme that converts angiotensin I to angiotensin II and degrades bradykinin.

Hydrochlorothiazide: Hydrochlorothiazide is a thiazide diuretic. Thiazides affect the renal tubular mechanism of electrolyte reabsorption, directly increasing excretion of sodium and chloride in approximately equivalent amounts. Indirectly, the diuretic action of hydrochlorothiazide reduces plasma volume with consequent increases in plasma renin activity, increases in aldosterone secretion, increases in urinary potassium loss, and decreases in serum potassium. The renin-aldosterone link is mediated by angiotensin II, therefore co-administration of an angiotensin II AT_1 Receptor Blocker tends to reverse the potassium loss associated with thiazide diuretics.

Hydrochlorothiazide is useful in the treatment of hypertension. It may be used alone or as an adjunct to other antihypertensive drugs. Hydrochlorothiazide does not affect normal blood pressure.

Pharmacodynamics: Valsartan: Valsartan inhibits the pressor effect of an angiotensin II infusion. An oral dose of 80 mg inhibits the pressor effect by about 80% at peak with approximately 30% inhibition persisting for 24 hours.

After a single oral dose, the antihypertensive activity of valsartan has an onset within approximately 2 hours and peaks within 4-6 hours in most patients.

The anti-hypertensive effect of valsartan persists for 24 hours after dosing. Trough/peak ratio ranges from 0.54 to 0.76. Valsartan reduces blood pressure in hypertensive patients without affecting heart rate.

During repeated dosing, the maximum blood pressure reduction with any dose is generally attained within 4 weeks, and is sustained during long-term therapy. Combinations with hydrochlorothiazide produce additional reduction in blood pressure.

There is no apparent rebound effect after abrupt withdrawal of valsartan therapy.

Although data available to date indicate a similar pharmacodynamic effect of valsartan in black and white hypertensive patients, this should be viewed with caution since antihypertensive drugs that affect the renin-angiotensin system, such as ACE inhibitors and angiotensin II AT_1 receptor blockers, have generally been found to be less effective in low-renin hypertensives (frequently blacks).

Hydrochlorothiazide: Onset of the diuretic action following oral administration occurs in 2 hours and the peak action in about 4 hours. Diuretic activity lasts about 6-12 hours.

Valsartan-Hydrochlorothiazide: The components of DIOVAN-HCT have been shown to have additive effect on blood pressure reduction, reducing blood pressure to a greater degree than either component used alone.

The antihypertensive effect of DIOVAN-HCT is sustained for a 24-hour period. In clinical studies of at least one year duration, the antihypertensive effect was maintained with continued therapy. Despite the significant decrease in blood pressure, administration of DIOVAN-HCT had no clinically significant effect on heart rate.

Pharmacokinetics: Valsartan: Since its pharmacokinetics are linear in the 80 to 320 mg dose range, valsartan does not accumulate appreciably in plasma following repeated administration. Plasma concentrations are similar in males and females.

Absorption: The mean absolute bioavailability of valsartan is about 23%, but with high variability. Peak plasma concentration is reached 2 to 4 hours after dosing.

Distribution: Valsartan is 94-97% bound to serum protein, mainly serum albumin. Steady-state volume of distribution is about 17 L, indicating that valsartan does not distribute into tissues extensively.

Metabolism: Following intravenous administration, valsartan shows bi-exponential decay kinetics ($t_{½}\alpha$ <1 hour and $t_{½}\beta$ between 5-9 hours). Plasma clearance is relatively slow (about 2 L/hr) when compared with hepatic blood flow (about 30 L/hr).

Valsartan biotransformation does not seem to involve the cytochrome P450 system. The enzyme(s) responsible for valsartan metabolism have not been identified.

Excretion: Following administration of an oral solution of ^{14}C labeled valsartan, 83% of absorbed valsartan is excreted in the feces and 13% in the urine, mainly as unchanged compound.

Hydrochlorothiazide: The absorption of hydrochlorothiazide following an oral dose is rapid with a t_{max} of approximately 2 hours. The distribution and elimination kinetics have generally been described by a bi-exponential decay function, with a terminal half-life of 6-15 hours.

Absolute bioavailability of hydrochlorothiazide is 60-80% after oral administration, with >95% of the absorbed dose being excreted unchanged in the urine.

Hydrochlorothiazide crosses the placental but not the blood-brain barrier and is excreted in breast milk.

Valsartan-Hydrochlorothiazide: The systemic availability of hydrochlorothiazide is reduced by about 30% when co-administered with valsartan. The kinetics of valsartan are not markedly affected by the co-administration of hydrochlorothiazide. This observed interaction has no impact on the combined used of valsartan and hydrochlorothiazide.

Special Populations and Conditions: Pediatrics: The pharmacokinetics of valsartan have not been investigated in patients <18 years of age.

Geriatrics: Exposure to valsartan is about 50% higher as measured by AUC and C_{max} and the half-life is longer in elderly subjects than in young subjects. However, this difference has not been shown to have any clinical significance.

Gender: Plasma concentrations are similar in males and females.

Hepatic Insufficiency: On average, patients with mild to moderate chronic liver disease have twice the exposure to valsartan of healthy volunteers as measured by AUC and C_{max} (see Warnings and Precautions, and Dosage and Administration).

Renal Insufficiency: Renal clearance accounts for only 30% of total plasma clearance. There is no apparent correlation between renal function and exposure to valsartan, as measured by AUC and C_{max}, in patients with different degrees of renal impairment. In patients with renal failure undergoing hemodialysis, limited information showed that exposure to valsartan is comparable to that in patients with creatinine clearance >10 mL/min.

Valsartan is not removed from plasma by dialysis.

STORAGE AND STABILITY: Protect from moisture. Store at 15-30°C.

SPECIAL HANDLING INSTRUCTIONS: Not applicable.

INFORMATION FOR THE PATIENT: Published in e-CPS, available by subscription at www.e-cps.ca.

DOSAGE FORMS, COMPOSITION AND PACKAGING: 80 mg/12.5 mg: Each light orange, ovaloid, film-coated tablet, imprinted with "HGH" on one side and "CG" on the other, contains: valsartan 80 mg and hydrochlorothiazide 12.5 mg. Nonmedicinal ingredients: colloidal silicon dioxide, crospovidone, magnesium stearate and microcrystalline cellulose; coating: hydroxypropyl methylcellulose, polyethylene glycol, red iron oxide, talc, titanium dioxide and yellow iron oxide. Blister strips of 14, cartons of 2.

160 mg/12.5 mg: Each dark red, ovaloid, film-coated tablet, imprinted with "HHH" on one side and "CG" on the other, contains: valsartan 160 mg and hydrochlorothiazide 12.5 mg. Nonmedicinal ingredients: colloidal silicon dioxide, crospovidone, magnesium stearate and microcrystalline cellulose; coating: hydroxypropyl methylcellulose, polyethylene glycol, red iron oxide, talc and titanium dioxide. Blister strips of 14, cartons of 2.

160 mg/25 mg: Each brown, ovaloid, film-coated tablet, imprinted with "HXH" on one side and "NVR" on the other, contains: valsartan 160 mg and hydrochlorothiazide 25 mg. Nonmedicinal ingredients: colloidal silicon dioxide, crospovidone, magnesium stearate and microcrystalline cellulose; coating: black iron oxide, hydroxypropyl methylcellulose, polyethylene glycol, red iron oxide, talc, titanium dioxide and yellow iron oxide. Blister strips of 14, cartons of 2.

320 mg/12.5 mg: Each pink, ovaloid, film-coated tablet, imprinted with "NVR" on one side and "HIL" on the other, contains: valsartan 320 mg and hydrochlorothiazide12.5 mg. Nonmedicinal ingredients: colloidal silicon dioxide, crospovidone, magnesium stearate and microcrystalline cellulose; coating: black iron oxide, hydroxypropyl methylcellulose, polyethylene glycol, red iron oxide, talc and titanium dioxide. Blister strips of 14, cartons of 2.

320 mg/25 mg: Each yellow, ovaloid, film-coated tablet, imprinted with "NVR" on one side and "CTI" on the other, contains: valsartan 320 mg and hydrochlorothiazide 25 mg. Nonmedicinal ingredients: colloidal silicon dioxide, crospovidone, magnesium stearate and microcrystalline cellulose; coating: hydroxypropyl methylcellulose, polyethylene glycol, talc, titanium dioxide and yellow iron oxide. Blister strips of 14, cartons of 2.

(Shown in Product Identification Section)

Diovol®

magnesium hydroxide—aluminum hydroxide

Antacid

Church & Dwight

SUPPLIED: Caplets: Each light blue, oval, convex, beveled edged, opaque, film-coated, mint-flavored caplet, plain on one side, intagliated DIOVOL on the other, contains: dried aluminum hydroxide gel 200 mg and magnesium hydroxide 200 mg. Nonmedicinal ingredients: alumina, cellulose, cornstarch, FD&C Blue No. 2, FD&C Red No. 3, flavor, gelatin, glycerin, magnesium stearate, propylene glycol and titanium dioxide. Energy: 0.83 kJ (<0.2 kcal). Gluten-, sucrose- and tartrazine-free. Boxes of 10 and 50 in push-through format.

Suspension: Each 5 mL of opaque, white suspension with a mint flavor (pH: 7.3 to 8.5) contains: aluminum hydroxide 165 mg (as aluminum hydroxide compressed gel) and magnesium hydroxide 200 mg. Nonmedicinal ingredients: benzyl alcohol, calcium disodium EDTA, cetylpyridinium chloride, glycerin, guar gum, peppermint flavour, purified water, saccharin sodium, sodium cyclamate and sorbitol. Energy: 7.0 kJ (1.7 kcal). Sodium: less than 1 mg/5mL. Sucrose- and tartrazine-free. Bottles of 350 mL. Protect from freezing.

Tablets: Each round, flat, white tablet with beveled edges, intagliated DIOVOL on one side, contains: aluminum hydroxide and magnesium carbonate co-dried gel 300 mg (equivalent to aluminum hyroxide 184 mg) and magnesium hydroxide 100 mg. Nonmedicinal ingredients: calcium cyclamate, cellulose, flavor, gelatin, magnesium stearate, mannitol, sorbitol, starch (corn) and talc. Energy: 7.5 kJ (1.8 kcal). Sodium: <1 mmol (1 mg). Sucrose- and tartrazine-free. Cartons of 50 in push-through format.

Diovol Plus®

aluminum hydroxide—magnesium hydroxide—simethicone

Antacid—Antiflatulent

Church & Dwight

Diovol Plus® AF

calcium carbonate—magnesium hydroxide—simethicone

Antacid—Antiflatulent

Church & Dwight

INDICATIONS: Provides fast relief of heartburn, acid indigestion, and gas.

CONTRAINDICATIONS: Alkalosis; hypermagnesemia; where distention may be due to partial or complete intestinal obstruction. Not recommended for severely debilitated patients or those with impaired renal function.

WARNINGS: Do not take more than 16 tablets or 80 mL during a 24-hour period. Do not take for more than 2 weeks or if symptoms recur, unless directed by a physician. Do not take if you suffer from kidney disease, except on your physician's advice. Do not take within 2 hours of another medicine, because the effectiveness of the medicine may be altered. Antacids can interfere with the absorption of iron preparations and/or tetracyclines.

PRECAUTIONS: Magnesium salts, in the presence of renal insufficiency, may cause CNS depression. Aluminum hydroxide, in the presence of low phosphorus diets, may cause phosphorus deficiency. Aluminum salts tend to cause constipation. Do not administer concomitantly with tetracycline antibiotics or iron preparations.

ADVERSE EFFECTS: No data supplied by the manufacturer.

OVERDOSE:

Treatment: Symptomatic.

> For management of a suspected drug overdose, CPhA recommends that you contact your **regional Poison Control Centre**. See the *CPS* Directory section for a list of Poison Control Centres.

DOSAGE: Adults: 10 to 20 mL of suspension, or 2 to 4 tablets taken 4 times a day 20 to 60 minutes after meals and at bedtime or as directed by the physician. Suspension may be taken undiluted or with water. Tablets may be chewed or sucked.

SUPPLIED: Diovol Plus: Suspension: Each 5 mL of white to off-white, peppermint or tropical-fruit-flavored suspension with a milky appearance contains: aluminum hydroxide (as aluminum hydroxide compressed gel) 165 mg, magnesium hydroxide 200 mg and simethicone 25 mg. Nonmedicinal ingredients: benzyl alcohol, calcium disodium EDTA, cetylpyridinium chloride, D&C yellow #10 (fruit-flavored suspension), flavor, glycerin, guar gum, purified water, saccharin sodium, sodium cyclamate and sorbitol. Energy: 7.0 kJ (1.7 kcal). Sodium: <1 mg/5 mL. Sucrose- and tartrazine-free. pH: 7.5 to 8.5. Bottles of 350 mL. Protect from freezing.

Tablets: Each round, flat, beveled edge tablet, monogrammed DIOVOL PLUS on one side, fruit-flavored (yellow, single layer) or peppermint (⅔ white, ⅓ yellow), contains: aluminum hydroxide and magnesium carbonate co-dried gel 300 mg (equivalent to aluminum hydroxide 184 mg), magnesium hydroxide 100 mg and simethicone 25 mg. Nonmedicinal ingredients: calcium cyclamate, cellulose, D&C Yellow 10, FD&C Yellow 6 (mint tablets), flavors, gelatin, magnesium stearate, mannitol, sorbitol, starch (corn) and talc. Energy: 8.4 kJ (2 kcal). Sodium: <1 mmol (1 mg). Gluten-, sucrose- and tartrazine-free. Boxes of 50 and 100 in push through format. Boxes of 50 in push through format (Diovol Plus fruit-flavored).

Diovol Plus AF: Liquid: Each 5 mL of white to off-white peppermint flavored suspension with a milky appearance contains: calcium carbonate, magnesium hydroxide 200 mg and simethicone 25 mg. Nonmedicinal ingredients: benzyl alcohol, calcium disodium EDTA, cetylpyridinium chloride, flavor, glycerin, guar gum, purified water, saccharin sodium, sodium cyclamate and sorbitol. Energy: 7.0 kJ (1.7 kcal). Sodium: <1 mg/5 mL. Sucrose- and tartrazine-free. Bottles of 350 mL. Protect from freezing.

Tablets: Each round, flat, beveled-edge white tablet, mint flavored, monogrammed DIOVOL PLUS on one side and AF on the other side contains: calcium carbonate, magnesium hydroxide 200 mg and simethicone 25 mg. Nonmedicinal ingredients: calcium cyclamate, flavor, gelatin, magnesium stearate and mannitol. Energy: 10.5 kJ (2.5 kcal). Sodium: <1 mmol (1 mg). Boxes of 50.

Dipentum® 🄿

olsalazine sodium

Lower Gastrointestinal Anti-inflammatory

UCB

SUPPLIED: Each opaque, beige, hard gelatin capsule contains: olsalazine sodium 250 mg. Nonmedicinal ingredients: magnesium stearate; shell: black iron oxide, caramel, gelatin and titanium dioxide. Bottles of 100. Store in a well closed container at room temperature (15 to 30°C).

Diphenhydramine Hydrochloride Injection USP

diphenhydramine HCl

Antihistaminic

Sandoz

SUPPLIED: Each mL contains: diphenhydramine HCl 50 mg, sodium hydroxide and/or hydrochloric acid to adjust pH and water for injection. Preservative-free. Single use vials of 1 mL, boxes of 10. Store between 15 and 30°C. Discard unused portion.

Diphenylhydantoin 🄿

CPhA Monograph

see *Phenytoin*

Diprivan® 🄿

propofol

I.V. Emulsion—Anesthetic—Sedative

AstraZeneca

Date of Preparation: April 12, 2000
Date of Revision: July 21, 2004

PHARMACOLOGY: Propofol is an i.v. hypnotic agent for use in the induction and maintenance of general anesthesia or sedation. The drug, an alkylphenol formulated in an oil-in-water emulsion, is chemically distinct from currently available i.v. anesthetic agents. I.V. injection of a therapeutic dose of propofol produces hypnosis rapidly and smoothly, usually within 40 seconds from the start of an injection (one arm-brain circulation time), although induction times >60 seconds have been observed.

Pharmacokinetics: Adults: The pharmacokinetic profile of propofol can be described by a 3-compartment open model. After a single bolus dose, there is fast distribution from blood into tissues ($t_{1/2}\alpha$: 1.8 to 8.3 min), high metabolic clearance ($t_{1/2}\beta$: 34 to 66 min) and a terminal slow elimination from poorly perfused tissues ($t_{1/2}\gamma$: 184 to 480 min). With 12- and 24-hour samplings, $t_{1/2}\gamma$ values of 502 and 674 min, respectively, were observed.

Propofol has large volumes of distribution as would be expected with a highly lipophilic anesthetic agent. The volume of central compartment (V_c) is between 21 and 56 L (0.35 to 0.93 L/kg based on a 60 kg patient), and the volume of distribution at steady state (V_{ss}) is between 171 and 364 L (2.85 to 6.07 L/kg). Values for volume of distribution during the terminal phase (V_d) are 2 to 3 times the corresponding V_{ss} values.

The termination of the anesthetic or sedative effects of propofol after a single i.v. bolus or a maintenance infusion is due to extensive redistribution from the CNS to other tissues and high metabolic clearance, both of which will decrease blood concentrations. The mean propofol concentration at time of awakening is 1 µg/mL (range: 0.74 to 2.2 µg/mL). Recovery from anesthesia or sedation is rapid. When propofol is used for both induction (2.0 to 2.5 mg/kg) and maintenance (0.1 to 0.2 mg/kg/min) of anesthesia, the majority of patients are generally awake, responsive to verbal command and oriented in approximately 7 to 8 minutes. Recovery from the effects of propofol occurs due to rapid metabolism and is not dependent on the terminal elimination half-life since the blood levels achieved in this phase are not clinically significant.

A study in 6 subjects showed that 72 and 88% of the administered radio-labeled dose was recovered in the urine within 24 hours and 5 days, respectively. Less than 2% was excreted in the feces. Unchanged drug was less than 0.3%. Propofol is chiefly metabolized by conjugation in the liver to inactive metabolites which are excreted by the kidney. Propofol glucuronide accounts for about 50% of the administered dose. The remainder consists of the 1- and 4-glucuronide and 4-sulfate conjugates of 2,6-diisopropyl-1,4-quinol.

The total body clearance (Cl) of propofol ranges from 1.6 L/min to 2.3 L/min (0.026 to 0.038 L/min/kg based on a 60 kg patient). This clearance exceeds estimates of hepatic blood flow, suggesting possible extrahepatic metabolism.

The pharmacokinetics of propofol do not appear to be altered by gender or chronic hepatic cirrhosis. The effects of acute hepatic failure on the pharmacokinetics of propofol have not been studied. In renal failure, the data is based on very limited findings. There was a trend towards longer half-lives, although the differences versus control patients did not reach statistical significance. With increasing age, the dose of propofol needed to achieve a defined anesthetic endpoint (dose-requirement) decreases. Elderly patients had higher propofol blood concentrations at 2 minutes than young ones (6.07 vs 4.15 µg/mL), probably due to a significantly lower initial distribution volume (20 vs 26 L). The relatively high blood concentrations during the first few minutes can predispose elderly patients to cardiorespiratory effects including hypotension, apnea, airway obstruction and/or oxygen desaturation. The clearance of propofol also decreased from a mean±S.D. of 1.8±0.4 L/min in young patients (18 to

35 years) to 1.4±0.4 L/min in elderly patients (65 to 80 years). The reduced clearance could decrease maintenance propofol requirements and prolong recovery if inappropriate infusions are used. Obesity is associated with significantly larger volumes of distribution (399 L vs 153 L) and clearance rates (2.8 L/min vs 1.8 L/min) but there is no change in the elimination half-life.

When given by an infusion for up to 2 hours, the pharmacokinetics of propofol appear to be independent of dose (0.05 to 0.15 mg/kg/min; 3 to 9 mg/kg/hour) and similar to i.v. bolus pharmacokinetics. Pharmacokinetics are linear over recommended infusion rates.

Propofol is highly protein-bound (97 to 99%); the degree of binding seems to be unrelated to either sex or age.

In the presence of propofol, alfentanil concentrations were higher than expected based upon the rate of infusion. However, alfentanil did not affect the pharmacokinetics of propofol (see Dosage, Compatibility and Stability, Premixing with alfentanil).

Pharmacokinetics in Adult Patients in Intensive Care Unit (ICU): Regarding most parameters, the pharmacokinetics of propofol in these patients are similar to those of patients undergoing anesthesia/sedation for short surgical procedures. However, the terminal half-life ($t_{1/2}\gamma$) is substantially prolonged after long-term infusion, reflecting extensive tissue distribution.

Pharmacokinetics in Children: The results were obtained in ASA I children, ranging in age from 3 to 10 years, who received a single bolus dose of propofol, 2.5 mg/kg. Propofol was rapidly distributed from blood into tissue ($t_{1/2}\alpha$: 1.5 to 4.1 min), metabolic clearance was high ($t_{1/2}\beta$: 9.3 to 56.1 min) and terminal elimination slow ($t_{1/2}\gamma$: 209 to 735 min). The volume of central compartment (V_c) ranged between 0.53 to 0.72 L/kg, the volume of distribution at steady state (V_{ss}) was between 2.1 to 10.9 L/kg and clearance (Cl) ranged between 0.032 to 0.040 L/min/kg. The mean plasma concentration of propofol at awakening was 2.3 µg/mL.

Clinical Pharmacology: Propofol induces anesthesia in a dose-dependent manner. In unpremedicated, ASA I or II patients, propofol induced anesthesia in 87% and 95% of patients at doses of 2.0 and 2.5 mg/kg, respectively. Elderly patients require lower doses; for unpremedicated patients older than 55 years of age, the mean dose requirement was 1.66 mg/kg. Premedication profoundly alters dose requirements; at 1.75 mg/kg, propofol induced anesthesia in 65% of patients who had no premedication and in 85% and 100% of patients who received diazepam or papaveretum-hyoscine premedication, respectively.

During induction of anesthesia, the hemodynamic effects of propofol vary. If spontaneous ventilation is maintained, the major cardiovascular effects are arterial hypotension (sometimes greater than a 30% decrease) with little or no change in heart rate and no appreciable decrease in cardiac output. If ventilation is assisted or controlled (positive pressure ventilation), the degree and incidence of decrease in cardiac output are accentuated. Maximal fall in blood pressure occurs within the first few minutes of the administration of a bolus dose. The fall in arterial pressure is greater under propofol anesthesia than under anesthesia induced by thiopental or methohexital. Increases in heart rate with propofol are generally less pronounced or absent after an induction dose, than after equivalent doses of these other 2 agents.

During maintenance of anesthesia with propofol, systolic and diastolic blood pressures generally remain below pre-anesthetic levels, although the depth of anesthesia, the rate of maintenance infusion as well as stimulation from tracheal intubation and/or surgery may increase or decrease blood pressure. Heart rate may also vary as a function of these factors but will generally remain below preanesthetic levels.

In the presence of a potent opioid (e.g., fentanyl), the blood pressure lowering effect of propofol is substantially increased. Fentanyl also decreases heart rate and this might lead to a significant decrease in cardiac output.

Age is highly correlated with the fall in blood pressure. In elderly subjects, both the incidence and degree of hypotension are greater than in younger subjects. Thus, a lower induction dose and a slower maintenance rate of administration should be used in the elderly (see Dosage). Particular caution should be exercised in elderly patients with severe coronary and/or cerebral arteriosclerosis; reduction in perfusion pressure may impair adequate blood supply to these organs.

Insufficient data are available regarding the cardiovascular effects of propofol when used for induction and/or maintenance of anesthesia or sedation in elderly, hypotensive, debilitated or other ASA III and IV patients. However, limited information suggests that these patients may have more profound cardiovascular responses. It is recommended that if propofol is used in these patients, a lower induction dose and a slower maintenance rate of administration of the drug be used (see Warnings and Dosage).

The first respiratory disturbance after a bolus dose of propofol is a profound fall in tidal volume leading to apnea in many patients. There has been no accompanying cough or hiccough and otherwise anesthesia is smooth. However, there might be some difficulty in uptake of volatile agents if respiration is not assisted.

In unpremedicated, healthy patients, there is a steep dose-response relationship regarding apnea; 0% and 44% of patients had apnea after receiving 2.0 and 2.5 mg/kg of propofol, respectively. Fentanyl enhanced both the incidence and the onset of apnea and the episode lasted for >60 seconds in the majority of patients.

Opioid premedication—in the presence of hyoscine—affected respiratory function (rate of respiration and minute volume) substantially more than atropine premedication. Respiratory function was more depressed when these premedicants were combined with propofol than when they were combined with thiopental. Enhanced respiratory depression with propofol and an opioid have been observed in the postoperative period.

During maintenance, propofol (0.1 to 0.2 mg/kg/min; 6 to 12 mg/kg/hour) caused a decrease in ventilation usually associated with an increase in carbon dioxide tension which may be marked depending upon the rate of administration and other concurrent medication (e.g., narcotics, sedatives, etc.). **Propofol was not evaluated in patients with any respiratory dysfunction.**

During sedation, attention must be given to the cardiorespiratory effects of propofol. Hypotension, apnea, airway obstruction, and/or oxygen desaturation can occur, especially with a rapid bolus injection. During initiation of sedation, slow infusion or slow injection techniques are preferable over rapid bolus administration, and during maintenance of sedation, a variable rate infusion is preferable over intermittent bolus administration in order to minimize undesirable cardiorespiratory effects. In the elderly, debilitated and ASA III or IV patients, rapid (single or repeated) bolus dose administration should not be used for sedation (see Warnings).

Clinical and preclinical studies suggest that propofol is rarely associated with elevation of plasma histamine levels and does not cause signs of histamine release.

Clinical and preclinical studies show that propofol does not suppress the adrenal response to ACTH.

Preliminary findings in patients with normal intraocular pressure indicate that propofol anesthesia produces a decrease in intraocular pressure which may be associated with a concomitant decrease in systemic vascular resistance.

Propofol is devoid of analgesic or antanalgesic activity.

INDICATIONS: Induction and Maintenance of General Anesthesia: Propofol is a short-acting i.v. general anesthetic agent that can be used for both induction and maintenance of anesthesia as part of a balanced anesthesia technique, including total i.v. anesthesia (TIVA), for inpatient and outpatient surgery.

Propofol is also indicated for pediatric anesthesia in children 3 years of age and older.

Conscious Sedation for Surgical and Diagnostic Procedures: Adults: Propofol, when administered i.v. as directed, can be used to initiate and maintain sedation in conjunction with local/regional anesthesia in patients undergoing surgical procedures. Propofol may also be used for sedation during diagnostic procedures (see Warnings and Precautions).

Pediatrics: Propofol is not recommended for sedation in children under the age of 18, during surgical/diagnostic procedures, as safety and efficacy have not been established.

Sedation During Intensive Care: Adults: Propofol should only be administered to intubated, mechanically ventilated, adult patients in the Intensive Care Unit (ICU) to provide continuous sedation and control of stress responses. In this setting, propofol should be administered only by or under the supervision of persons trained in general anesthesia or critical care medicine.

Pediatrics: See Contraindications.

CONTRAINDICATIONS: When general anesthesia or sedation are contraindicated. In patients with a known allergy and/or hypersensitivity to propofol or to lipid emulsions. For the sedation of children 18 years or younger receiving intensive care.

WARNINGS: For general anesthesia or sedation for surgical/diagnostic procedures, propofol should be administered only by persons trained in the administration of general anesthesia and not involved in the conduct of surgical/diagnostic procedures. Patients should be continuously monitored and facilities for maintenance of a patent airway, artificial ventilation, and oxygen enrichment and circulatory resuscitation must be immediately available.

For sedation of intubated, mechanically ventilated, adult patients in the Intensive Care Unit (ICU), propofol should be administered only by persons trained in general anesthesia or critical care medicine.

In the elderly, debilitated and ASA III or IV patients, rapid (single or repeated) bolus administration should not be used during general anesthesia or sedation in order to minimize undesirable cardiorespiratory depression including hypotension, apnea, airway obstruction and/or oxygen desaturation.

Propofol should not be coadministered through the same i.v. catheter with blood or plasma because compatibility has not been established. In vitro tests have shown that aggregates of the globular component of the emulsion vehicle have occurred with blood/plasma/serum from humans and animals. The clinical significance is not known.

The neuromuscular blocking agents, atracurium and mivacurium should not be given through the same i.v. line as propofol without prior flushing.

Propofol should not be used in obstetrics including Cesarean section deliveries, because propofol crosses the placenta and may be associated with neonatal depression.

Propofol should not be used for Intensive Care Unit (ICU) sedation in patients who have severely disordered fat metabolism because the vehicle of propofol is similar to that of Intralipid 10%. The restrictions that apply to Intralipid 10% should also be considered when using propofol in the ICU.

Extreme care should be used in administering propofol in patients with impaired left ventricular function because propofol may produce a negative inotropic effect.

Extreme care should be used in administering propofol in patients who are hypotensive, hypovolemic or in shock because propofol may cause excessive arterial hypotension.

Extreme care should be used in administering propofol in elderly, debilitated or other ASA III or IV patients.

Strict aseptic techniques must always be maintained during handling as propofol is a single-use parenteral product, for use in an individual patient, and contains no antimicrobial preservatives. The vehicle is capable of supporting rapid growth of microorganism (see Precautions and Dosage). Failure to follow aseptic handling procedures may result in microbial contamination causing fever/infection/sepsis which could lead to life-threatening illness.

Propofol lacks vagolytic activity and has been associated with reports of bradycardia (occasionally profound) and also asystole. The i.v. administration of an anticholinergic agent before induction, or during maintenance of anesthesia should be considered, especially in situations where vagal tone is likely to predominate or when propofol is used in conjunction with other agents likely to cause a bradycardia.

Since various manifestations of seizures have been reported during propofol anesthesia, special care should be taken when giving the drug to epileptic patients.

Occupational Hazards: Patients receiving propofol on an outpatient basis should not engage in hazardous activities requiring complete mental alertness such as driving a motor vehicle or operating machinery until the effects of propofol have completely subsided.

PRECAUTIONS: General: In adults and children, attention should be paid to minimize pain on administration of propofol. Transient local pain during i.v. injection may be reduced by prior injection of i.v. lidocaine (1 mL of a 1% solution.)

Patients should be continuously monitored for early signs of significant hypotension and/or bradycardia. Treatment may include increasing the rate of i.v. fluid, elevation of lower extremities, use of pressor agents or administration of anticholinergic agents (e.g., atropine) or use of plasma volume expanders. Apnea often occurs during induction and may persist for more than 60 seconds. Ventilatory support may be required. Because propofol is a lipid emulsion, caution should be exercised in patients with disorders of lipid metabolism such as primary hyperlipoproteinemia, diabetic hyperlipemia and pancreatitis.

When propofol is administered as a sedative for surgical or diagnostic procedures, patients should be continuously monitored by persons not involved in the conduct of the surgical/diagnostic procedure. Oxygen supplementation should be immediately available and provided where clinically indicated; and oxygen saturation should be monitored in all patients. Patients should be continuously monitored for early signs of hypotension, apnea, airway obstruction and/or oxygen desaturation. These cardiorespiratory effects are more likely to occur following rapid initiation (loading) boluses or during supplemental maintenance boluses, especially in the elderly, debilitated and ASA III or IV patients.

As with other sedative agents, when propofol is used for sedation during operative procedures, involuntary patient movements may occur. During procedures requiring immobility these movements may be hazardous to the operative site.

Since propofol is rarely used alone, an adequate period of evaluation of the awakened patient is indicated to ensure satisfactory recovery from general anesthesia or sedation prior to discharge of the patient from the recovery room or to home. Very rarely the use of propofol may be associated with the development of a period of postoperative unconsciousness, which may be accompanied by an increase in muscle tone. This may or may not be preceded by a period of wakefulness. Although recovery is spontaneous, appropriate care of an unconscious patient should be administered.

Intensive Care Unit (ICU) Sedation–Adults: **Strict aseptic techniques must be followed when handling propofol as the vehicle is capable of supporting rapid growth of microorganisms** (see Warnings and Dosage).

Very rarely reports of metabolic acidosis, rhabdomyolysis, hyperkalemia, and/or cardiac failure, in some cases with a fatal outcome, have been received concerning seriously ill patients receiving propofol for ICU sedation (see Adverse Effects; Spontaneous Reports and Publications). These reports demonstrated that a failure of oxygen delivery to the tissues was likely to have occurred. A causal relationship between these reported events and propofol has not been established. All sedatives and therapeutic agents used in the ICU (including propofol) should be titrated to maintain optimal oxygen delivery and hemodynamic parameters.

The administration of propofol should be initiated as a continuous infusion and changes in the rate of administration made slowly (>5 min) in order to minimize hypotension and avoid acute overdosage.

Patients should be monitored for early signs of significant hypotension and/or cardiovascular depression, which may be profound. These effects are responsive to discontinuation of propofol, i.v. fluid administration, and/or vasopressor therapy.

As with other sedative medications, there is wide interpatient variability in propofol dosage requirements, and these requirements may change with time.

Patients who receive large doses of narcotics during surgery may require very small doses of propofol for appropriate sedation.

Abrupt discontinuation of propofol infusion prior to weaning should be avoided since, due to the rapid clearance of propofol, it may result in rapid awakening with associated anxiety, agitation and resistance to mechanical ventilation. Infusions of propofol should be adjusted to maintain a light level of sedation throughout the weaning process.

Since propofol is formulated in an oil-water emulsion, patients should be monitored for lipemia. Administration of propofol should be adjusted if fat is being inadequately cleared from the body. A reduction in the quantity of concurrently administered lipids is indicated to compensate for the amount of lipid infused as part of the propofol formulation; 1 mL of propofol contains approximately 0.1 g of fat (1.1 kcal).

The long-term administration of propofol to patients with renal failure and/or hepatic insufficiency has not been evaluated.

EDTA is a chelator of metal ions, including zinc. The need for supplemental zinc should be considered during prolonged administration of propofol, particularly in patients who are predisposed to zinc deficiency, such as those with burns, diarrhea and/or major sepsis.

Intensive Care Unit (ICU) Sedation– Children under 18 years of age: See Contraindications.

Sedation during Surgical/Diagnostic Procedures in Children Under 18 years of Age: Propofol is not recommended for sedation during surgical/diagnostic procedures in children under the age of 18, as safety and efficacy have not been established.

Pediatric Use for General Anaesthesia: In the absence of sufficient clinical experience, propofol is not recommended for anesthesia in children less than 3 years of age (see Indications and Dosage).

Pregnancy: Propofol should not be used in pregnancy. Propofol has been used during termination of pregnancy in the first trimester. Teratology studies in rats and rabbits show some evidence of delayed ossification or abnormal cranial ossification; however, such developmental delays are not considered indicative of a teratogenic effect. Reproductive studies in rats suggest that administration of propofol to the dam adversely affects perinatal survival of the offspring.

Lactation: Propofol is not recommended for use in nursing mothers because preliminary findings indicate that it is excreted in human milk and the effects of oral absorption of small amounts of propofol are not known.

Geriatrics: Elderly patients may be more sensitive to the effects of propofol; therefore, the dosage of propofol should be reduced in these patients according to their condition and clinical response (see Pharmacology, Pharmacokinetics and Dosage).

Cardiac Anesthesia: Propofol was evaluated in 328 patients undergoing coronary artery bypass graft (CABG). Of these patients 85% were males (mean age 61, range 32 to 83) and 15% were females (mean age 65, range 42 to 86).

The majority of patients undergoing CABG had good left ventricular function. Experience in patients with poor left ventricular function, as well as, in patients with hemodynamically significant valvular or congenital heart disease is limited.

Slower rates of administration should be utilized in premedicated patients, geriatric patients, patients with recent fluid shift, or patients who are hemodynamically unstable. Any fluid deficits should be corrected prior to administration of propofol. In those patients where additional fluid therapy may be contraindicated, other measures, e.g., elevation of lower extremities, or use of pressor agents, may be useful to offset the hypotension which is associated with the induction of anesthesia with propofol.

Neurosurgical Anesthesia: When using propofol in patients with increased intracranial pressure (ICP) or impaired cerebral circulation, significant decreases in mean arterial pressure should be avoided because of the resultant decreases in cerebral perfusion pressure. When increased ICP is suspected, hyperventilation and hypocarbia should accompany the administration of propofol (see Dosage).

Drug Interactions: Propofol has been used in association with spinal and epidural anesthesia and with a range of premedicants, muscle relaxants, inhalational agents, analgesic agents and with local anesthetic agents; no significant adverse interactions have been observed.

ADVERSE EFFECTS: Anesthesia and Sedation for Surgical/Diagnostic Procedures: During induction of anesthesia in clinical trials, hypotension and apnea occurred in the majority of patients. The incidence of apnea varied considerably, occurring in between 30 and 100% of patients depending upon premedication, speed of administration and dose (see Pharmacology). Decreases in systolic and diastolic pressures ranged between 10 and 28%, but were more profound in the elderly and in ASA III and IV patients. Excitatory phenomena occurred in up to 14% of adult patients and in 33 to 90% of pediatric patients; they consisted most frequently of spontaneous musculoskeletal movements and twitching and jerking of the hands, arms, feet or legs. Epileptiform movements including convulsions and opisthotonus have occurred rarely, but a causal relationship with propofol has not been established. Flushing and rash have occurred in 10 to 25% of pediatric patients. Local pain occurred during i.v. injection of propofol at an incidence of 28% when veins of the dorsum of the hand were used and 5% when the larger veins of the forearm and the antecubital fossa were used. Propofol increased plasma glucose concentrations significantly, but no other significant changes in hematological or biochemical values were observed.

In the sedation clinical trials, the adverse reaction profile of propofol was similar to that seen during anesthesia. The most common adverse reactions included hypotension, nausea, pain and/or hotness at injection site and headache. Respiratory events included upper airway obstruction, apnea, hypoventilation, dyspnea and cough.

Rarely, clinical features of anaphylaxis, which may include angioedema, bronchospasm, erythema and hypotension, occur following propofol administration.

Very rarely the use of propofol may be associated with the development of a period of postoperative unconsciousness, which may be accompanied by an increase in muscle tone. This may or may not be preceded by a period of wakefulness.

There have been reports of postoperative fever.

Pulmonary edema may be a potential side effect associated with the use of propofol.

As with other anesthetics, sexual disinhibition may occur during recovery.

Intensive Care Unit (ICU) Sedation–Adults: The most frequent adverse reactions during Intensive Care Unit (ICU) sedation were hypotension (31.5%), hypoxia (6.3%), and hyperlipemia (5.5%). In some patients, hypotension was severe. Other reactions considered severe were observed in single patients and included ventricular tachycardia, decreased cardiac output, decrease in vital capacity and negative inspiratory force, increase in triglycerides, and agitation. Two patients with head injury suffered renal failure with severe increases in BUN accompanied in one patient by an increase in creatinine.

There have been very rare reports of rhabdomyolysis when propofol has been administered at doses greater than 4 mg/kg/h for ICU sedation.

Very rarely pancreatitis has been observed following the use of propofol for induction and maintenance of anesthesia, and for intensive care sedation. A causal relationship has not been clearly established.

Table 1 compares the overall occurrence rates of adverse reactions in propofol patients from non-ICU and ICU clinical trials where the rate of occurrence was greater than 1%. Major differences include lack of metabolic/nutritional (hyperlipemia) and respiratory events in the non-ICU group and lack of nausea, vomiting, headache, movement and injection site events in the ICU group.

Table 1: Diprivan

Non-ICU vs ICU Adverse Events Occurring in Greater Than 1% of Propofol Patients

Body System	Event	Non-ICU	ICU
Number of patients		2588	127
Cardiovascular	Hypotension	7.38%	31.50%
	Bradycardia	2.82%	3.94%
	Hypertension	2.82%	1.57%
	Arrhythmia	1.24%	0.79%
	Tachycardia	0.81%	3.15%
	Cardiovascular Disorder	0.23%	2.36%
	Hemorrhage	0.23%	1.57%
	Atrial Fibrillation	0.15%	1.57%
	Cardiac Arrest	0.12%	3.15%
	Ventricular Tachycardia	0.08%	1.57%
Digestive	Nausea	14.57%	0%
	Vomiting	8.31%	0%
	Abdominal Cramping	1.24%	0%
Nervous	Movement	4.44%	0%
	Headache	1.78%	0%
	Dizziness	1.70%	0%
	Twitching	1.47%	0%
	Agitation	0.19%	2.36%
	Intracranial Hypertension	0%	3.94%
Metabolic/Nutritional	Hyperlipemia	0.08%	5.51%
	Acidosis	0.04%	1.57%
	Creatinine Increased	0%	2.36%
	BUN Increased	0%	1.57%
	Hyperglycemia	0%	1.57%
	Hypernatremia	0%	1.57%
	Hypokalemia	0%	1.57%
Respiratory	Dyspnea	0.43%	1.57%
	Hypoxia	0.08%	6.30%
	Acidosis	0%	1.57%
	Pneumothorax	0%	1.57%
Other	Injection Site:		
	Pain	8.11%	0%
	Burning/Stinging	7.77%	0%
	Fever	1.89%	2.36%
	Hiccough	1.78%	0%
	Cough	1.55%	0%
	Rash	1.20%	1.57%
	Anemia	0.35%	1.57%
	Kidney Failure	0%	1.57%

(cont'd)

Table 1: Diprivan *(cont'd)*

Non-ICU vs ICU Adverse Events Occurring in Greater Than 1% of Propofol Patients

Adverse reactions reported at an incidence of 1% or less during anesthesia and sedation for surgical/diagnostic procedures:

Cardiovascular: significant hypotension, premature atrial contractions, premature ventricular contractions, tachycardia, syncope, abnormal ECG, bigeminy, edema.

Respiratory: burning in throat, tachypnea, dyspnea, upper airway obstruction, wheezing, bronchospasm, laryngospasm, hypoventilation, hyperventilation, sneezing.

Excitatory: hypertonia, dystonia, rigidity, tremor.

Central Nervous System: confusion, dizziness, paresthesia, somnolence, shivering, abnormal dreams, agitation, delirium, euphoria, fatigue.

Injection Site: phlebitis, thrombosis, hives/itching, redness/discoloration.

Digestive: hypersalivation, dry mouth.

Skin and Appendages: flushing/rash (for incidence in children, see above), urticaria, pruritus.

Special Senses: diplopia, amblyopia, tinnitus.

Musculoskeletal: myalgia.

Urogenital: urine retention, discoloration of urine.

Adverse reactions reported at an incidence of 1% or less during ICU sedation:

Cardiovascular: arrhythmia, extrasystole, heart block, right heart failure, bigeminy, ventricular fibrillation, heart failure, myocardial infarction.

Respiratory: lung function decreased, respiratory arrest.

Central Nervous System: seizure, thinking abnormal, akathisia, chills, anxiety, confusion, hallucinations.

Digestive: ileus, hepatomegaly.

Metabolic/Nutritional: osmolality increased.

Urogenital: green urine, urination disorder, oliguria.

Body as a Whole: sepsis, trunk pain, whole body weakness.

Post Marketing Experience: Clinical Trial: A randomised, controlled, clinical trial that evaluated the safety and effectiveness of propofol versus standard sedative agents (SSA) in paediatric ICU patients has been conducted. In that study, a total of 327 paediatric patients were randomized to receive either propofol 2% (113 patients), propofol 1% (109 patients), or an SSA (e.g. lorazepam, chloral hydrate, fentanyl, ketamine, morphine, or phenobarbital).

Propofol therapy was initiated at an infusion rate of 5.5 mg/kg/hr and titrated as needed to maintain sedation at a standardized level. The results of the study showed an increase in the number of deaths in patients treated with propofol as compared to SSAs. A total of 25 patients died during the trial or within the 28-day follow-up period: 12 (11%) in the propofol 2% treatment group, 9 (8%) in the propofol 1% treatment group, and 4 (4%) in the SSA treatment group.

Spontaneous Reports and Publications: There are several publications identifying an association in adults between high infusion rates (greater than 5 mg/kg/h) of propofol for more than 48 hours in ICUs and a potentially fatal constellation of adverse events characterized by metabolic acidosis, rhabdomyolysis, hyperkalemia and cardiovascular collapse (see Precautions).

The majority of the above-reported cases occurred in adults with head injury. These patients were treated with propofol at infusion rates greater than 5 mg/kg/h in an attempt to control intracranial hypertension It is unclear at this time whether propofol at these high infusion rates can provide enhanced intracranial pressure reduction. A causal relationship between these adverse events and propofol and/or the lipid carrier cannot yet be established.

Similar findings were first reported in the literature in 1992 in children who received high doses of propofol in the ICU. Since the 1992 publication, several similar reports have been published, including an article that summarized 18 cases of children who received propofol infusions and suffered serious adverse events, including death.

Drug Abuse and Dependence: Rare cases of self-administration of propofol by health care professionals have been reported, including some fatalities.

OVERDOSE:

Symptoms: To date, there is no known case of acute overdosage, and no specific information on emergency treatment of overdosage is available. If accidental overdosage occurs, propofol administration should be discontinued immediately. Overdosage is likely to cause cardiorespiratory depression. Respiratory depression should be treated by artificial ventilation with oxygen. Cardiovascular depression may require repositioning of the patient by raising the patient's legs, increasing the flow rate of i.v. fluids and if severe may require the administration of plasma volume expanders and/or pressor agents.

Treatment: See Symptoms.

For management of a suspected drug overdose, CPhA recommends that you contact your **regional Poison Control Centre**. See the *CPS* Directory section for a list of Poison Control Centres.

DOSAGE: Strict aseptic techniques must always be maintained during handling as propofol is a single-use parenteral product, for use in an individual patient, and contains no antimicrobial preservatives. The vehicle is capable of supporting rapid growth of microorganisms. Failure to follow aseptic handling procedures may result in microbial contamination causing fever/infection/sepsis which could lead to life-threatening illness.

Propofol should be shaken well before use.

General: Dosage and rate of administration should be individualized and titrated to the desired effect according to clinically relevant factors including preinduction and concomitant medications, age, ASA status and level of debilitation of the patient. In heavily premedicated patients, both the induction and maintenance doses should be reduced.

Induction of General Anesthesia: Most **adult patients** under 55 years of age and classified ASA I and II are likely to require 2 to 2.5 mg/kg of propofol for induction when unpremedicated or when premedicated with oral benzodiazepines or i.m. narcotics. For induction, it is recommended that propofol should be titrated (approximately 40 mg every 10 seconds by bolus injection or infusion) against the response of the patient until the clinical signs show the onset of general anesthesia.

It is important to be familiar and experienced with the appropriate i.v. use of propofol before treating **elderly, debilitated and/or adult patients in ASA Physical Status Classes III and IV**. These patients may be more sensitive to the effects of propofol; therefore, the dosage of propofol should be reduced in these patients by approximately 50% (20 mg every 10 seconds) according to their condition and clinical response. A rapid bolus should not be used as this will increase the likelihood of undesirable cardiorespiratory depression including hypotension, apnea, airway obstruction and/or oxygen desaturation (see Warnings, Precautions and Table 2).

During **cardiac anesthesia**, a rapid bolus induction should be avoided. A slow rate of approximately 20 mg every 10 seconds until induction onset (0.5 to 1.5 mg/kg) should be used.

Most children over 8 years of age require approximately 2.5 mg/kg of propofol for induction of anesthesia. Children 3 to 8 years of age may require somewhat higher doses, however the dose should be titrated by administering propofol slowly until the clinical signs show the onset of anesthesia. Propofol is not recommended for induction of anesthesia in children less than 3 years of age. Reduced dosage is recommended for children of ASA Classes III and IV.

Additionally, as with most anesthetic agents, the effects of propofol may be potentiated in patients who have received i.v. sedative or narcotic premedications shortly prior to induction.

Maintenance of General Anesthesia: Anesthesia can be maintained by administering propofol by infusion or intermittent i.v. bolus injection. The patient's clinical response will determine the infusion rate or the amount and frequency of incremental injections.

When administering propofol by infusion, drop counters, syringe pumps or volumetric pumps must be used to provide controlled infusion rates.

Continuous Infusion: Propofol 0.1 to 0.2 mg/kg/min (6 to 12 mg/kg/h) administered in a variable rate infusion with 60 to 70% nitrous oxide and oxygen provides anesthesia for patients undergoing general surgery. Maintenance by infusion of propofol should immediately follow the induction dose in order to provide satisfactory or continuous anesthesia during the induction phase. During this initial period following the induction injection higher rates of infusion are generally required (0.15 to 0.20 mg/kg/min; 9 to 12 mg/kg/h) for the first 10 to 15 minutes. Infusion rates should subsequently be decreased by 30 to 50% during the first half-hour of maintenance. Changes in vital signs (increases in pulse rate, blood pressure, sweating and/or tearing) that indicate a response to surgical stimulation or lightening of anesthesia may be controlled by the administration of propofol 25 mg (2.5 mL) to 50 mg (5.0 mL) incremental boluses and/or by increasing the infusion rate. If vital sign changes are not controlled after a 5-minute period, other means such as a narcotic, barbiturate, vasodilator or inhalation agent therapy should be initiated to control these responses.

For minor surgical procedures (i.e., body surface) 60 to 70% nitrous oxide can be combined with a variable rate propofol infusion to provide satisfactory anesthesia. With more stimulating surgical procedures (i.e., intra-abdominal) supplementation with i.v. analgesic agents should be considered to provide a satisfactory anesthetic and recovery profile. When supplementation with nitrous oxide is not provided, administration rate(s) of propofol and/or opioids should be increased in order to provide adequate anesthesia.

Infusion rates should always be titrated downward in the absence of clinical signs of light anesthesia until a mild response to surgical stimulation is obtained in order to avoid administration of propofol at rates higher than are clinically necessary. Generally, rates of 0.05 to 0.1 mg/kg/min should be achieved during maintenance in order to optimize recovery times.

During **cardiac anesthesia**, when propofol is used as the primary agent, maintenance infusion rates should not be less than 0.10 mg/kg/min and should be supplemented with analgesic levels of continuous opioid administration. When an opioid is used as the primary agent, propofol maintenance rates should not be less than 0.05 mg/kg/min. Higher doses of propofol will reduce the opioid requirements.

For **children**, the average rate of administration varies considerably, but rates between 0.10 to 0.25 mg/kg/min (6 to 15 mg/kg/h) should achieve satisfactory anesthesia. These infusion rates may be subsequently reduced depending on patient response and concurrent medication.

Intermittent Bolus: Increments of propofol 25 mg (2.5 mL) to 50 mg (5.0 mL) may be administered with nitrous oxide in patients undergoing general surgery. The incremental boluses should be administered when changes in vital signs indicate a response to surgical stimulation or light anesthesia.

Propofol has been used in conjunction with a wide variety of agents commonly used in anesthesia such as atropine, scopolamine, glycopyrrolate, diazepam, depolarizing and nondepolarizing muscle relaxants, and narcotic analgesics, as well as with inhalational and regional anesthetic agents. No pharmacological incompatibilities have been encountered.

Lower doses of propofol may be required when used as an adjunct to regional anesthesia.

Sedation During Surgical or Diagnostic Procedures–Adults: When propofol is administered for sedation, rates of administration should be individualized and titrated to clinical response. In most patients, the rates of propofol administration will be approximately 25 to 30% of those used for maintenance of general anesthesia.

During initiation of sedation, slow injection or slow infusion techniques are preferable over rapid bolus administration. During maintenance of sedation, a variable rate infusion is preferable over intermittent bolus dose administration.

Initiation of Sedation: Slow Injection: Most adult patients will generally require 0.5 to 1 mg/kg administered over 3 to 5 minutes and titrated to clinical response.

In the elderly, debilitated, hypovolemic and ASA III or IV patients, the dosage of propofol should be reduced to approximately 70 to 80% of the adult dosage and administered over 3 to 5 minutes.

Infusion: Sedation may be initiated by infusing propofol at 0.066 to 0.100 mg/kg/min (4 to 6 mg/kg/h) and titrating to the desired level of sedation while closely monitoring respiratory function.

Maintenance of Sedation: Patients will generally require maintenance rates of 0.025 to 0.075 mg/kg/min (1.5 to 4.5 mg/kg/h) during the first 10 to 15 minutes of sedation maintenance.

Infusion rates should always be titrated downward in the absence of clinical signs of light sedation until mild responses to stimulation are obtained in order to avoid sedative administration of propofol at rates higher than are clinically necessary.

In addition to the infusion, bolus administration of 10 to 15 mg may be necessary if a rapid increase in sedation depth is required.

In the elderly, debilitated, hypovolemic and ASA III or IV patients, the rate of administration and the dosage of propofol should be reduced to approximately 70 to 80% of the adult dosage according to their condition, responses, and changes in vital signs. Rapid (single or repeated) bolus dose administration should not be used for sedation in these patients (see Warnings).

Intensive Care Unit (ICU) Sedation: Propofol should be individualized according to the patient's condition and response, blood lipid profile, and vital signs.

Table 2: Diprivan

Dosage Guide

Indication	Dosage and Administration
Induction of General Anesthesia	
	Dosage should be individualized. **Adult Patients less than 55 Years of Age:** Are likely to require 2 to 2.5 mg/kg (approximately 40 mg every 10 seconds until induction onset). **Elderly, Debilitated and/or Adult ASA III or IV Patients:** Are likely to require 1 to 1.5 mg/kg (approximately 20 mg every 10 seconds until induction onset) but dose should be carefully titrated to effect. **Cardiac Anesthesia:** Patients are likely to require 0.5 to 1.5 mg/kg (approximately 20 mg every 10 seconds until induction onset). **Neurosurgical Patients:** Are likely to require 1 to 2 mg/kg (approximately 20 mg every 10 seconds until induction onset). **Pediatric Patients:** Children over 8 years of age require approximately 2.5 mg/kg. Children 3 to 8 years of age may require somewhat higher doses but doses should be titrated slowly to the desired effect. In the absence of sufficient clinical experience, propofol is not recommended for anesthesia in children less than 3 years of age (see Indications and Precautions). Reduced dosage is recommended for children of ASA Classes III and IV.
Maintenance of General Anesthesia	
Infusion	**Variable rate infusion titrated to the desired clinical effect.** **Adult Patients less than 55 Years of Age:** Generally, 0.1 to 0.2 mg/kg/min (6 to 12 mg/kg/h). **Elderly, Debilitated and/or Adult ASA III or IV Patients:** Generally, 0.05 to 0.1 mg/kg/min (3 to 6 mg/kg/h). **Cardiac Anesthesia:** Most patients require: primary propofol with secondary opioid: 0.1 to 0.15 mg/kg/min (6 to 9 mg/kg/h); low dose propofol with primary opioid: 0.05 to 0.1 mg/kg/min (3 to 6 mg/kg/h). **Neurosurgical Patients:** Generally, 0.1 to 0.2 mg/kg/min (6 to 12 mg/kg/h). **Pediatric Patients:** Generally, 0.10 to 0.25 mg/kg/min (6 to 15 mg/kg/h).
Intermittent Bolus	Increments of 25 to 50 mg, as needed.
Surgical/Diagnostic Sedation	
	Dosage and rate should be individualized and titrated to the desired clinical effect. **Adult Patients less than 55 Years of Age:** Are likely to require 0.5 to 1 mg/kg over 3 to 5 min to initiate sedation, followed by 0.025 to 0.075 mg/kg/min (1.5 to 4.5 mg/kg/h) for continued sedation. **Elderly, debilitated, hypovolemic and/or ASA III or IV patients:** The dosage and rate of administration may need to be reduced in these patients by approximately 20 to 30% (see previous section for details). **Pediatric Patients:** Propofol is not recommended for sedation during surgical/diagnostic procedures in children under the age of 18, as safety and efficacy have not been established (see Indications).
Initiation and Maintenance of ICU Sedation in Intubated, Mechanically Ventilated, Adult Patients	
	Dosage and rate of infusion should be individualized. **Adult Patients:** For initiation, most patients require an infusion of 0.005 mg/kg/min (0.3 mg/kg/h) for at least 5 minutes. Subsequent increments of 0.005 to 0.010 mg/kg/min (0.3 to 0.6 mg/kg/h) over 5 to 10 minutes may be used until desired level of sedation is achieved. For maintenance, most patients require 0.005 to 0.050 mg/kg/min (0.3 to 3 mg/kg/h). The long-term administration of propofol to patients with renal failure and/or hepatic insufficiency has not been evaluated. **Pediatric Patients:** See Contraindications.

Adults: For intubated, mechanically ventilated, adult patients, Intensive Care Unit (ICU) sedation should be initiated slowly with a continuous infusion in order to titrate to desired clinical effect and minimize hypotension. When indicated, initiation of sedation should begin at 0.005 mg/kg/min (0.3 mg/kg/h). The infusion rate should be increased by increments of 0.005 to 0.010 mg/kg/min (0.3 to 0.6 mg/kg/h) until the desired level of sedation is achieved. A minimum period of 5 minutes between adjustments should be allowed for onset of peak drug effect.

Most adult patients require maintenance rates of 0.005 to 0.050 mg/kg/min (0.3 to 3 mg/kg/h). Dosages of propofol should be reduced in patients who have received large dosages of narcotics. As with other sedative medications, there is interpatient variability in dosage requirements and these requirements may change with time (see Table 2).

Bolus administration of 10 to 20 mg should only be used to rapidly increase sedation depth in patients where hypotension is not likely to occur. A rapid bolus should not be used as this will increase the likelihood of hypotension. Patients with compromised myocardial function, intravascular volume depletion or abnormally low vascular tone (e.g., sepsis) may be more susceptible to hypotension.

Children under 18 years of age: Propofol is contraindicated for the sedation of children 18 years or younger receiving intensive care.

Compatibility and Stability: Propofol can be premixed with alfentanil. Propofol should not be mixed with other therapeutic agents prior to administration.

The neuromuscular blocking agents, atracurium and mivacurium should not be given through the same i.v. line as propofol without prior flushing.

Dilution Prior to Administration: When propofol is diluted prior to administration, it should only be diluted with 5% Dextrose Injection, USP, and it should not be diluted to a concentration less than 2 mg/mL because it is an emulsion. Dilutions should be prepared aseptically immediately before administration and should not be used beyond 6 hours of preparation. In diluted form it has been shown to be more stable when in contact with glass than with plastic (95% potency after 2 hours of running infusion in plastic).

Premixing with Alfentanil: propofol may be premixed with alfentanil injection containing 500 µg/mL alfentanil in the ratio of 20:1 to 50:1 v/v. Mixtures should be prepared using sterile technique and used within 6 hours of preparation.

Administration into a Running I.V. Catheter: Compatibility of propofol with the coadministration of blood/serum/plasma has not been established (see Warnings). Propofol has been shown to be compatible with the following i.v. fluids when administered into a running i.v. catheter: 5% Dextrose Injection, USP; Lactated Ringers Injection, USP; Lactated Ringers and 5% Dextrose Injection; 5% Dextrose and 0.45% Sodium Chloride Injection, USP; 5% Dextrose and 0.2% Sodium Chloride Injection, USP.

Handling Procedures: Parenteral drug products should be inspected visually for particulate matter and discoloration prior to administration whenever solution and container permit. Do not freeze.

Do not use if there is evidence of separation of the phases of the emulsion.

Aseptic techniques must be applied to the handling of the drug. Propofol contains no antimicrobial preservatives and the vehicle supports growth of microorganisms. When propofol is to be aspirated it should be drawn aseptically into a sterile syringe or i.v. administration set immediately after breaking the vial seal. Administration should commence without delay. Asepsis must be maintained for both propofol and the infusion equipment throughout the infusion period. Any drugs or fluids added to the infusion line must be administered close to the cannula site. Propofol must not be administered via a microbiological filter.

Propofol is for single use in an individual patient only. If a vial is utilized for infusion, both the reservoir of propofol and the infusion line must be discarded and replaced as appropriate at the end of the procedure or at 12 hours, whichever is sooner (when using **diluted** propofol see Dilution Prior to Administration).

Since propofol contains no preservative or bacteriostatic agents, any unused portions of propofol or solutions containing propofol should be discarded at the end of the surgical procedure.

Dilution for i.v. Infusion: Propofol 1% w/v may be pre-mixed with alfentanil injection containing 500 µg/mL alfentanil in the ratio of 20:1 to 50:1 v/v. Mixtures should be prepared using sterile technique and used within 6 hours of preparation.

SUPPLIED: Each mL of white, oil in water emulsion contains: propofol 10 mg for i.v. administration. Nonmedicinal ingredients: disodium edetate, egg phosphatide, glycerol, soybean oil and water for injection with sodium hydroxide to adjust pH. It is isotonic with a pH of 6.5 to 8.5. Glass vials of 20, 50 and 100 mL for single infusion only. Store between 2 and 25°C; do not freeze. The emulsion should be visually inspected for particulate matter, emulsion separation and discoloration prior to use. Any unused portions of propofol or solutions containing propofol should be discarded at the end of the surgical procedure.

Diprolene® Glycol Ⓟ

betamethasone dipropionate

Topical Corticosteroid

Schering-Plough

PHARMACOLOGY: Provides anti-inflammatory, antipruritic and vasoconstrictive effects. The propylene glycol components of the vehicle increase penetration and enhance the local effectiveness of betamethasone.

INDICATIONS: For the relief of the inflammatory manifestations of resistant or severe psoriasis and corticosteroid-responsive dermatoses.

CONTRAINDICATIONS: In viral diseases including vaccinia, varicella, herpes simplex, and fungal infections; also, tuberculosis of the skin. Diprolene products are contraindicated in those patients with a history of sensitivity reactions to betamethasone dipropionate, other corticosteroids or to any of the components of Diprolene products.

WARNINGS: Do not use in or near the eyes since Diprolene Glycol is not formulated for ophthalmic use.

This product should not be used under occlusive dressing.

The lotion contains isopropyl alcohol and may cause stinging or burning upon application to abraded or sun-burned skin.

Pregnancy: Since safety of topical corticosteroid use in pregnant women has not been established, drugs of this class should be used during pregnancy only if the potential benefit justifies the potential risk to the fetus. Drugs of this class should not be used extensively in large amounts or for prolonged periods of time in pregnant patients.
Lactation: Since it is not known whether topical administration of corticosteroids can result in sufficient systemic absorption to produce detectable quantities in breast milk, a decision should be made to discontinue nursing or to discontinue the drug, taking into account the importance of the drug to the mother.
Children: This product is not recommended for use in children under 12 years of age.

Pediatric patients may demonstrate greater susceptibility to topical corticosteroid-induced HPA axis suppression and to exogenous corticosteroid effects because of greater absorption due to a larger skin surface area to body weight ratio.

HPA axis suppression, Cushing's syndrome, linear growth retardation, delayed weight gain, and intracranial hypertension have been reported in children receiving topical corticosteroids. Manifestations of adrenal suppression in children include low plasma cortisol levels and absence of response to ACTH stimulation. Manifestations of intracranial hypertension include a bulging fontanelle, headaches and bilateral papilledema.

PRECAUTIONS: Suitable precautions should be taken in using topical glucocorticoids in patients with stasis dermatitis and other skin diseases with impaired circulation; hypersensitive subjects and in patients with glaucoma.

Patients should be advised to inform subsequent physicians of the prior use of glucocorticoids.

If irritation, sensitization, excessive dryness develop with its use, treatment should be discontinued.

During the use of topical corticosteroids, infections may occur.

If an overt infection is present, appropriate antimicrobial treatment is indicated.

If symptomatic response is not noted within a few days to a week, the local application of corticosteroids should be discontinued and the patient re-evaluated.

Prolonged use of corticosteroid preparations may produce striae or atrophy of the skin or s.c. tissues. It this occurs, treatment should be discontinued.

Diprolene lotion and cream have been shown to suppress the hypothalamic-pituitary adrenal (HPA) axis with repeated application of 7 mL/day and 7 g/day, respectively.

Application of corticosteroids over extensive lesions, or failure to follow dosage schedule may result in significant systemic absorption producing hypercortisolism manifesting itself by adrenal suppression, moon facies, striae and suppression of growth.

Systemic absorption of topical corticosteroids will be increased with the use of more potent corticosteroid formulations, with prolonged usage or if extensive body surface areas are treated. Therefore, patients receiving large doses of potent topical corticosteroids, applied to a large surface area should be evaluated periodically for evidence of HPA axis suppression. If HPA axis suppression occurs, an attempt should be made to withdraw the drug, to reduce the frequency of application, or to substitute with a less potent corticosteroid agent.

Recovery of HPA axis function is generally prompt and complete upon discontinuation of the drug. Infrequently, signs and symptoms of corticosteroid withdrawal may occur, requiring supplemental systemic corticosteroid therapy.

ADVERSE EFFECTS: The following adverse reactions were reported with this product: mild to moderate transient folliculitis, increased erythema, itching and vesiculation, perilesional scaling, telangiectasia, dryness, stinging, burning, skin atrophy, local irritation, urticaria. Rarely reported adverse effects include: tingling, prickly skin, tightening or cracking of skin, warm feeling, laminar scaling, follicular rash, hyperesthesia and pruritus. Subnormal plasma cortisol levels were also reported.

The following local adverse skin reactions have been reported with the use of topical steroids: itching, folliculitis, striae, hypertrichosis, change in pigmentation, secondary infection, perioral dermatitis, allergic contact dermatitis, maceration of the skin, acneiform eruptions and miliaria.

Adrenal suppression has also been reported following topical corticosteroid therapy. Posterior subcapsular cataracts have been reported following systemic use of corticosteroids.

OVERDOSE:

Symptoms: Excessive or prolonged use of topical corticosteroids can suppress pituitary-adrenal function, resulting in secondary-adrenal insufficiency and produce manifestations of hypercorticism, including Cushing's disease.

Treatment: Appropriate symptomatic treatment is indicated. Acute hypercorticoid symptoms are virtually reversible. Treat electrolyte imbalance if necessary. In case of chronic toxicity, slow withdrawal of corticosteroids is advised.

> For management of a suspected drug overdose, CPhA recommends that you contact your **regional Poison Control Centre**. See the *CPS* Directory section for a list of Poison Control Centres.

DOSAGE: Cream and Ointment: A thin film of cream or ointment should be applied to cover completely the affected area once daily, in the morning. It may also be applied twice daily, in the morning and at night or as directed by the physician. Treatment should be discontinued when the dermatologic disorder is controlled. According to clinical response, duration of therapy may vary from a few days to a longer period of time. However, treatment should not be continued for more than 4 weeks without patient re-evaluation.
Lotion: A few drops of lotion should be applied to cover completely the affected area and a gentle massage should be effected until the lotion disappears. Once a day for 3 weeks, is the usual frequency of application.

The cream, lotion and ointment should not be used under an occlusive dressing.

SUPPLIED: Cream: Each g of cream contains: betamethasone dipropionate USP, micronized, equivalent to 0.5 mg (0.05%) betamethasone USP. Nonmedicinal ingredients: carbomer 940, propylene glycol, sodium hydroxide, titanium dioxide and purified water. Aluminum tubes of 15 and 50 g.
Lotion: Each g of lotion contains: betamethasone dipropionate USP, micronized, equivalent to 0.5 mg (0.05%) betamethasone USP. Nonmedicinal ingredients: carbomer 940, isopropyl alcohol, propylene glycol, sodium hydroxide and purified water. Plastic squeeze bottles of 30 and 60 mL.
Ointment: Each g of ointment contains: betamethasone dipropionate USP, micronized, equivalent to 0.5 mg (0.05%) betamethasone USP. Nonmedicinal ingredients: propylene glycol monostearate, propylene glycol, white wax and white petrolatum. Aluminum tubes of 15 and 50 g.

Store at 2 to 25°C.

Diprosalic® 🅿

betamethasone dipropionate—salicylic acid
Topical Corticosteroid—Keratolytic

Schering-Plough

PHARMACOLOGY: Betamethasone dipropionate with salicylic acid combines the anti-inflammatory, antipruritic and vasoconstrictive activity of betamethasone dipropionate with the keratolytic effects of salicylic acid.

INDICATIONS: Diprosalic lotion and/or ointment provide anti-inflammatory, antipruritic and keratolytic activity in the topical management of subacute and chronic hyperkeratotic and dry dermatoses responsive to corticosteroid therapy.

CONTRAINDICATIONS: In viral diseases including vaccinia, varicella, herpes simplex, and fungal infections; also, tuberculosis of the skin. Hypersensitivity to any one of the components of Diprosalic is a contraindication to its use.

WARNINGS: These drugs should not be used in or near the eyes since Diprosalic is not formulated for ophthalmic use. Avoid contact with mucous membranes. As well, keep Diprosalic Lotion away from the genital area and other orifices.
Children: Any of the side effects that have been reported following systemic use of corticosteroids, including adrenal suppression, may also occur with topical corticosteroids, especially in infants and children.

Systemic absorption of topical corticosteroids or salicylic acid will be increased if extensive body surface areas are treated or if the occlusive technique is used. Suitable precautions should be taken under these conditions or when long-term use is anticipated, particularly in infants and children.

Pediatric patients may demonstrate greater susceptibility to topical corticosteroid-induced HPA axis suppression and to exogenous corticosteroid effects than mature patients because of a greater absorption due to a larger skin surface area to body weight ratio. Use of topical corticosteroids in children should be limited to the least amount compatible with an effective therapeutic regimen. Chronic corticosteroid therapy may interfere with growth and development of children.

HPA axis suppression, Cushing's syndrome, linear growth retardation, delayed weight gain, and intracranial hypertension have been reported in children receiving topical corticosteroids. Manifestations of adrenal suppression in children include low plasma cortisol levels and absence of response to ACTH stimulation. Manifestations of intracranial hypertension include a bulging fontanelle, headaches, and bilateral papilledema.
Pregnancy: Since safety of topical corticosteroid use in pregnant women has not been established, drugs of this class should be used during pregnancy only if the potential benefit justifies the potential risk to the fetus. Drugs of this class should not be used extensively in large amounts or for prolonged periods of time in pregnant patients.
Lactation: Since it is not known whether topical administration of corticosteroids can result in sufficient systemic absorption to produce detectable quantities in breast milk, a decision should be made to discontinue nursing or to discontinue the drug, taking into account the importance of the drug to the mother.
PRECAUTIONS: Suitable precautions should be taken in using topical corticosteroids in patients with stasis dermatitis and other skin diseases with impaired circulation.

Prolonged use of corticosteroid preparations may produce striae or atrophy of the skin or subcutaneous tissue. If this occurs, treatment should be discontinued.

Patients should be advised to inform subsequent physicians of the prior use of corticosteroids.

If irritation, sensitization, excessive dryness, or unwanted scaling develops with the use of the product, treatment should be discontinued.

Application over extensive lesions may result in significant systemic absorption producing hypercorticism manifesting itself by adrenal suppression, moon facies, striae and suppression of growth.

If an overt infection is present, appropriate antimicrobial treatment is indicated.

If symptomatic response is not noted within a few days to a week, the local application of corticosteroids should be discontinued and the patient re-evaluated.

Occlusive dressings should not be used.

ADVERSE EFFECTS: The following local adverse skin reactions have been reported with the use of topical steroids; burning, itching, irritation, dryness, folliculitis, hypertrichosis, acneiform eruptions, hypopigmentation, perioral dermatitis, allergic contact dermatitis. The following may occur more frequently with the use of occlusive dressings: maceration of the skin, secondary infection, skin atrophy, striae, miliaria. In addition, the salicylic acid component may cause local reddening of the skin, desquamation, pruritus and smarting. Continuous application of salicylic acid preparations to the skin may cause dermatitis. Hypersensitivity to salicylic acid may occur.

OVERDOSE:

Symptoms: Excessive or prolonged use of topical corticosteroids can suppress pituitary-adrenal function, resulting in secondary adrenal insufficiency, and produce manifestations of hypercorticism, including Cushing's disease.

Excessive or prolonged use of topical preparations containing salicylic acid may cause symptoms of salicylism. Overdosage of salicylates may cause temporary hearing or visual disturbances, drowsiness and nausea. If this occurs, discontinue use until symptoms disappear.

Treatment: Appropriate symptomatic treatment is indicated. Acute hypercorticoid symptoms are usually reversible. Treat electrolyte imbalance, if necessary. In case of chronic toxicity, slow withdrawal of corticosteroids is advised.

Treatment of salicylism is symptomatic. Measures should be taken to rid the body rapidly of salicylate. Administer oral sodium bicarbonate to alkalinize the urine and force diuresis.

> For management of a suspected drug overdose, CPhA recommends that you contact your **regional Poison Control Centre**. See the *CPS* Directory section for a list of Poison Control Centres.

DOSAGE: Lotion: A thin film should be applied to cover completely the affected areas of the scalp. The usual frequency of application is twice daily.
Ointment: A thin film should be applied to cover completely the affected area. The ointment should be massaged gently and thoroughly into the skin. The usual frequency of application is twice daily, in the morning and at night.

For some patients, adequate maintenance may be achieved with less frequent application.

Diprosalic should not be used under occlusive dressing.

SUPPLIED: Lotion: Each g contains: 0.64 mg of betamethasone dipropionate USP, equivalent to 0.5 mg of betamethasone USP and 20 mg of salicylic acid. Nonmedicinal ingredients: edetate disodium, hydroxypropyl methylcellulose, isopropyl alcohol, water and sodium hydroxide to adjust pH to approximately 5. Plastic squeeze bottles of 30 mL and 60 mL.
Ointment: Each g contains: 0.64 mg of betamethasone dipropionate USP, equivalent to 0.5 mg of betamethasone USP and 30 mg of salicylic acid in a paraben-free ointment base of white petrolatum and mineral oil. Tubes of 15 and 50 g.

Store between 2 and 25°C. Protect from light.

Diprosone® 🅿

betamethasone dipropionate
Topical Corticosteroid

Schering-Plough

PHARMACOLOGY: Many clinical studies have established the efficacy and relative safety of betamethasone dipropionate in a variety of steroid responsive dermatological conditions.

In the course of clinical investigations, special emphasis was placed on the more troublesome conditions such as psoriasis and/or atopic dermatitis.

INDICATIONS: Betamethasone dipropionate cream and/or ointment provides anti-inflammatory, antipruritic and antiallergic activity in the topical management of corticosteroid-responsive dermatoses. Such disorders include: psoriasis, contact dermatitis (dermatitis venenata), atopic dermatitis (infantile eczema, allergic dermatitis), neurodermatitis (lichen simplex chronicus, lichen planus, eczema, eczematous dermatitis), intertrigo, dyshidroses (pompholyx), seborrheic dermatitis, exfoliative dermatitis, solar dermatitis, stasis dermatitis, anogenital and senile pruritus. The lotion is formulated to spread easily without adherence to hairy areas to facilitate treatment of dermatoses, such as psoriasis, and seborrheic dermatitis of the scalp.

CONTRAINDICATIONS: Topical steroids are contraindicated in:

1. Untreated bacterial, tubercular and fungal infections involving the skin, and in certain viral diseases such as herpes simplex, chickenpox, and vaccinia.
2. Hypersensitivity to any of the components.

WARNINGS: *Pregnancy:* Since safety of topical corticosteroid use in pregnant women has not been established, drugs of this class should be used during pregnancy only if the potential benefit justifies the potential risk to the fetus. Drugs of this class should not be used extensively in large amounts or for prolonged periods of time in pregnant patients.
Lactation: Since it is not known whether topical administration of corticosteroids can result in sufficient systemic absorption to produce detectable quantities in breast milk, a decision should be made to discontinue nursing or to discontinue the drug, taking into account the importance of the drug to the mother.
Children: Any of the side effects that have been reported following systemic use of corticosteroids, including adrenal suppression, may also occur with topical corticosteroids, especially in infants and children.

Systemic absorption of topical corticosteroids will be increased if extensive body surface areas are treated or if the occlusive technique is used. Suitable precautions should be taken under these conditions or when long-term use is anticipated, particularly in infants and children. Pediatric patients may demonstrate greater susceptibility than mature patients to topical corticosteroid-induced HPA axis suppression and to exogenous corticosteroid effects because of greater absorption due to a larger skin surface area to body weight ratio. Use of topical corticosteroids in children should be limited to the least amount compatible with an effective therapeutic regimen. Chronic corticosteroid therapy may interfere with growth and development of children.

HPA axis suppression, Cushing's syndrome, linear growth retardation, delayed weight gain, and intracranial hypertension have been reported in children receiving topical corticosteroids. Manifestations of adrenal suppression in children include low plasma cortisol levels and absence of response to ACTH stimulation. Manifestations of intracranial hypertension include a bulging fontanelle, headaches and bilateral papilledema.

The lotion contains isopropyl alcohol, and may cause stinging upon application to abraded or sun-burned skin. Do not use in or near the eyes.

PRECAUTIONS: Topical corticosteroids should be used with caution on lesions close to the eye.

Although hypersensitivity reactions have been rare with topically applied steroids, the drug should be discontinued and appropriate therapy initiated if there are signs of sensitivity or irritation.

In cases of bacterial or fungal infections of the skin, appropriate antimicrobial agents should be used as primary therapy. If it is considered necessary, betamethasone dipropionate may be used as an adjunct to control inflammation, erythema, and itching.

If a symptomatic response is not noted within a few days to a week, the local applications of betamethasone dipropionate should be discontinued until the infection is brought under control.

Significant systemic absorption may occur when steroids are applied over large areas of the body, especially under occlusive dressings. To minimize this possibility, when long-term therapy is anticipated, interrupt treatment periodically or treat one area of the body at a time.

Patients should be advised to inform subsequent physicians of the prior use of corticosteroids.

Occlusive dressings should not be applied if there is an elevation of body temperature.

ADVERSE EFFECTS: The following local adverse reactions have been reported rarely with the use of topical corticosteroids: burning, itching, irritation, dryness, folliculitis, hypertrichosis, acneiform eruptions, hypopigmentation, perioral dermatitis, allergic contact dermatitis. The following may occur more frequently with occlusive dressings: maceration of the skin, secondary infection, skin atrophy, striae, miliaria.

OVERDOSE:

Symptoms: Excessive or prolonged use of topical corticosteroids can suppress pituitary-adrenal function, resulting in secondary adrenal insufficiency, and produce manifestations of hypercorticism, including Cushing's disease.

Treatment: Appropriate symptomatic treatment is indicated. Acute hypercorticoid symptoms are usually reversible. Treat electrolyte imbalance, if necessary. In case of chronic toxicity, slow withdrawal of corticosteroids is advised.

> For management of a suspected drug overdose, CPhA recommends that you contact your **regional Poison Control Centre**. See the *CPS* Directory section for a list of Poison Control Centres.

DOSAGE: A thin film should be applied to completely cover the affected area. Massage gently and thoroughly into the skin. The usual frequency of application is twice daily. For some patients adequate maintenance therapy may be achieved with less frequent application.

SUPPLIED: Cream: Each g of cream contains: betamethasone dipropionate USP equivalent to 0.5 mg (0.05%) betamethasone USP, in a water miscible base. Nonmedicinal ingredients: cetostearyl alcohol, chlorocresol, mineral oil, monobasic sodium phosphate, phosphoric acid, polyethylene glycol 1000 monocetyl ether, sodium hydroxide, water and white petrolatum. Tubes of 15 and 50 g.

Lotion: Each g of lotion contains: betamethasone dipropionate USP equivalent to 0.5 mg (0.05%) betamethasone USP. Nonmedicinal ingredients: carbomer 934P, isopropyl alcohol, sodium hydroxide to adjust pH and water. Plastic squeeze bottles of 30 and 75 mL.

Ointment: Each g of ointment contains: betamethasone dipropionate USP equivalent to 0.5 mg (0.05%) betamethasone USP, in a lanolin free base. Nonmedicinal ingredients: white petrolatum USP. Tubes of 15 and 50 g.

Store between 2 and 30°C.

Ditropan XL® Ⓟ

oxybutynin chloride

Anticholinergic—Antispasmodic

Janssen-Ortho

Date of Preparation: January 30, 2002
Date of Revision: March 3, 2009

SUMMARY PRODUCT INFORMATION:

Route of Administration	Dosage Form/ Strength	Clinically Relevant Nonmedicinal Ingredients
Oral	Extended-release tablet, 5 mg and 10 mg	Lactose For a complete listing of nonmedicinal ingredients, see Dosage Forms, Composition and Packaging.

INDICATIONS AND CLINICAL USE: DITROPAN XL (oxybutynin chloride) is indicated for the relief of the symptoms of urge incontinence, urgency and frequency in patients with overactive bladder (U-UI).

Geriatrics (>65 years of age): The efficacy of DITROPAN XL is similar in patients younger or older than 65 years.

Pediatrics (<18 years of age): The safety and efficacy of DITROPAN XL in children have not been established.

CONTRAINDICATIONS: DITROPAN XL is contraindicated in patients with urinary retention, gastric retention, and other severe decreased gastrointestinal motility conditions, uncontrolled narrow-angle glaucoma and in patients who are at risk for these conditions.

DITROPAN XL is contraindicated in patients who have demonstrated hypersensitivity to the drug substance or other components of the product. For a complete listing of the nonmedicinal ingredients, see Dosage Forms, Composition and Packaging.

WARNINGS AND PRECAUTIONS: General: As with any other nondeformable material, caution should be used when administering DITROPAN XL (oxybutynin chloride) to patients with pre-existing severe gastrointestinal narrowing (pathologic or iatrogenic). There have been rare reports of obstructive symptoms in patients with known strictures in association with the ingestion of other drugs in nondeformable controlled-release formulations.

Patients should be informed that DITROPAN XL should be swallowed whole with the aid of liquids. Patients should not chew, divide, or crush tablets. The medication is contained within a nonabsorbable shell designed to release the drug at a controlled rate. The tablet shell is eliminated from the body; patients should not be concerned if they occasionally notice in their stool something that looks like a tablet.

Patients should be informed that, when administered in the presence of high environmental temperature, anticholinergics such as DITROPAN XL can cause heat prostration (fever and heat stroke due to decreased sweating).

Because anticholinergic agents such as DITROPAN XL may produce drowsiness (somnolence) or blurred vision, patients should be advised to exercise caution.

Alcohol or other sedative drugs may enhance the drowsiness caused by anticholinergic agents such as DITROPAN XL.

Cardiovascular: Although there are no clinical trial or post-marketing data to confirm the potential for DITROPAN XL to aggravate certain pre-existing cardiac conditions, this product is in the class of anticholinergic medications which are known to have cardiac effects. Prescribers should therefore use caution when prescribing DITROPAN XL to patients with coronary heart disease, congestive heart failure, cardiac arrhythmias, tachycardia or hypertension.

Although no formal QT studies have been conducted for oxybutynin formulations, there have been very rare reports of QT interval prolongation with oxybutynin use. Newer antimuscarinic agents used in the treatment of urinary incontinence have been reported to prolong the QT/QTc interval of the electrocardiogram. Some drugs that cause QT/QTc prolongation may increase the risk of the rare, but serious ventricular arrhythmia—torsades de pointes. Patients at risk for QT/QTc prolongation, such as those with clinically relevant heart failure, long QT syndrome, recent significant hypokalemia, or receiving other drugs known to prolong QT/QTc, should be appropriately monitored when receiving oxybutynin. Patients who develop prolonged QT/QTc or symptoms of possible arrhythmia such as dizziness, palpitations, or fainting should be evaluated electrocardiographically and for electrolyte disturbances.

Gastrointestinal: DITROPAN XL should be administered with caution to patients with gastrointestinal obstructive disorders because of the risk of gastric retention (see Contraindications).

Administration of DITROPAN XL to patients with severe ulcerative colitis may precipitate toxic megacolon.

DITROPAN XL, like other anticholinergic drugs, may decrease gastrointestinal motility and should be used with caution in patients with conditions such as ulcerative colitis, and intestinal atony (see Contraindications).

DITROPAN XL should be used with caution in patients who have gastroesophageal reflux and/or who are concurrently taking drugs (such as bisphosphonates) that can cause or exacerbate esophagitis.

Genitourinary: DITROPAN XL should be administered with caution to patients with clinically significant bladder obstruction because of the risk of urinary retention (see Contraindications).

Hepatic: DITROPAN XL should be used with caution in patients with hepatic disease.

Neurologic: DITROPAN XL is associated with anticholinergic central nervous system (CNS) effects (see Adverse Reactions, Post-Market Adverse Drug Reactions). Patients should be monitored for signs of anticholinergic CNS effects (e.g. confusion, sedation, anxiety, nervousness, hallucinations, psychotic disorder, agitation and memory impairment), particularly in the first few months after beginning treatment or increasing the dose. If a patient experiences anticholinergic CNS effects, drug discontinuation or dose reduction should be considered.

DITROPAN XL, like other anticholinergic drugs, should be administered with caution to patients with pre-existing dementia treated with cholinesterase inhibitors due to the risk of aggravation of symptoms.

DITROPAN XL should be used with caution in patients with myasthenia gravis.

Renal: DITROPAN XL should be used with caution in patients with renal disease.

Special Populations: Pregnant Women: The safety of DITROPAN XL administration to women who are or who may become pregnant has not been established. Therefore, DITROPAN XL should not be given to pregnant women, unless, in the judgment of the physician, the probable clinical benefits outweigh the possible hazards.

Nursing Women: It is not known whether this drug is excreted in human milk. Because many drugs are excreted in human milk, caution should be exercised when DITROPAN XL is administered to a nursing woman.

Pediatrics (<18 years of age): The safety and efficacy of DITROPAN XL in children have not been established.

Geriatrics (>65 years of age): The pharmacokinetics of DITROPAN XL are similar in patients younger or older than 65 years.

ADVERSE REACTIONS: Adverse Drug Reaction Overview: The most common adverse events reported were the expected side effects of anticholinergic agents which include, but are not limited to, dry mouth, constipation and blurred vision. The incidence of dry mouth was dose related.

Clinical Trial Adverse Drug Reactions: Because clinical trials are conducted under very specific conditions, the adverse reaction rates observed in the clinical trials may not reflect the rates observed in practice and should not be compared to the rates in the clinical trials of another drug. Adverse drug reaction information from clinical trials is useful for identifying drug-related adverse events and for approximating rates.

The safety and efficacy of DITROPAN XL were evaluated in a total of 580 participants who received DITROPAN XL in four clinical trials (429 patients), and four pharmacokinetic studies (151 healthy volunteers). The 429 patients were treated with 5-30 mg/day for up to 4.5 months.

Three of the four clinical trials allowed dose adjustments based on efficacy and adverse events and one was a fixed-dose escalation design.

Adverse events from the three controlled clinical studies and one open-label study in which 429 patients were treated with 5-30 mg/day of DITROPAN XL are provided in the first column of Table 1. Adverse events from two additional fixed-dose, active-controlled clinical trials in which 576 patients were treated with a fixed dose of DITROPAN XL 10 mg/day for a 12-week duration are provided in the second column of Table 1. The adverse events are reported regardless of causality.

For patients receiving 5-30 mg/day DITROPAN XL, the discontinuation rate for all adverse events was 6.8%. The most frequent adverse event causing early discontinuation of study medication was nausea (1.9%). The rate and severity of anticholinergic effects reported by patients less than 65 years old and those 65 years and older were similar.

The most common adverse events reported by the 429 patients receiving 5-30 mg/day DITROPAN XL were the expected side effects of anticholinergic agents, including dry mouth, constipation, and somnolence. The incidence of all dry mouth events at doses up to 30 mg was 60.8%; 1.2% of patients treated with DITROPAN XL discontinued due to dry mouth. At the fixed dose of 10 mg/day, the incidence of all dry mouth events was 29.3% of which 20.8% were mild.

Table 1: DITROPAN XL

Incidence (%) of Adverse Events Reported by ≥5% of Patients Using DITROPAN XL (5-30 mg/day) and % of Corresponding Adverse Events in Two Fixed Dose (10 mg/day) Studies

Body System	Adverse Event	DITROPAN XL 5–30 mg/day (n=429)	DITROPAN XL 10 mg/day (n=576)
General	Headache	9.8	6.4
	Asthenia	6.8	3.0
	Pain	6.8	3.8
Digestive	Dry Mouth	60.8	29.3
	Constipation	13.1	6.6
	Diarrhea	9.1	7.8
	Nausea	8.9	2.4
	Dyspepsia	6.8	4.9
Nervous	Somnolence	11.9	2.1
	Dizziness	6.3	4.2
Respiratory	Rhinitis	5.6	1.7
Special Senses	Blurred Vision	7.7	1.6
	Dry Eyes	6.1	3.1
Urogenital	Urinary Tract Infection	5.1	5.2

A complete list of pooled adverse events reported by patients participating in the 4 adjustable-dose and 2 fixed-dose studies are presented in Table 2. A total of 1006 subjects were treated with DITROPAN XL (5-30 mg/day) from 3 to up to 23 weeks in these trials. Table 2 includes adverse events, regardless of investigator assessment of causality, reported by ≥1% of subjects in either treatment group. A dash represents an incidence of less than 1%. The adverse events for DITROPAN immediate-release (IR) formulation, which was the comparator in three of the trials, are also presented.

Post-Market Adverse Drug Reactions: Additional rare adverse drug reactions reported from worldwide post-marketing experience with DITROPAN XL include:

Psychiatric Disorders: hallucinations; psychotic disorder, agitation and memory impairment (very rare).

Nervous System Disorders: convulsions.

Cardiac Disorders: arrhythmia, tachycardia.

Vascular Disorders: flushing.

Skin and Subcutaneous Tissue Disorders: rash.

Renal and Urinary Disorders: impotence.

Injury, Poisoning and Procedural Complications: fall.

Other Oxybutynin Chloride Formulations: Other adverse events have been reported with other oxybutynin chloride formulations: cycloplegia, mydriasis, suppression of lactation and QT interval prolongation.

Table 2: DITROPAN XL

Adverse Events Reported by ≥1% of Subjects in Either Treatment Group in Clinical Trials of DITROPAN XL

System/ Organ Class Preferred Term	% DITROPAN XL subjects reporting event (n=1006)	% DITROPAN IR subjects reporting event (n=199)
Infections and Infestations		
Urinary Tract Infection	5.2	6.5
Nasopharyngitis	2.5	1.5
Upper Respiratory Tract Infection	2.2	2.5
Sinusitis	1.7	—
Bronchitis	1.2	2.0
Cystitis	1.0	1.0
Fungal infection	—	1.0
Metabolism and Nutrition Disorders		
Fluid Retention	—	1.0
Psychiatric Disorders		
Insomnia	2.8	5.5
Depression	1.7	—
Nervousness	1.5	6.5
Confusional State	1.0	2.5
Nervous System Disorders		
Headache	7.8	7.5
Somnolence	5.7	14.0
Dizziness	4.9	16.6
Dysgeusia	1.1	1.5
Sinus Headache	—	2.0
Eye Disorders		
Keratoconjunctivitis Sicca	4.2	2.5
Vision Blurred	4.2	9.6
Eye Irritation	—	1.0
Cardiac Disorders		
Palpitations	1.5	4.5
Sinus Arrhythmia	—	1.0
Vascular Disorders		
Hypertension	1.3	—
Flushing	—	1.0
Respiratory, Thoracic and Mediastinal Disorders		
Nasal Dryness	2.8	4.5
Cough	2.4	3.0
Pharyngolaryngeal Pain	1.9	1.5
Dry throat	1.6	2.5
Sinus Congestion	—	2.0
Hoarseness	—	1.0
Asthma	—	1.0
Nasal Congestion	—	2.0
Gastrointestinal Disorders		
Dry mouth	41.6	71.4
Constipation	9.1	15.1
Diarrhea	6.8	3.5
Nausea	5.2	11.6
Dyspepsia	4.7	6.0
Gastroesophageal Reflux Disease	1.6	—

(cont'd)

Table 2: DITROPAN XL *(cont'd)*

Adverse Events Reported by ≥1% of Subjects in Either Treatment Group in Clinical Trials of DITROPAN XL

System/ Organ Class Preferred Term	% DITROPAN XL subjects reporting event (n=1006)	% DITROPAN IR subjects reporting event (n=199)
Abdominal Pain	1.5	2.5
Loose Stools	1.4	3.0
Flatulence	1.2	2.5
Vomiting	1.2	1.5
Abdominal Pain Upper	—	3.0
Dysphagia	—	1.5
Aptyalism	—	1.0
Eructation	—	1.0
Tongue Coated	—	1.0
Skin and Subcutaneous Tissue Disorders		
Dry Skin	2.6	3.0
Pruritus	1.3	1.5
Musculoskeletal and Connective Tissue Disorders		
Back pain	2.4	2.0
Arthralgia	1.5	2.0
Pain in extremity	1.3	1.0
Flank pain	—	1.0
Renal and Urinary Disorders		
Urinary Retention	4.7	6.0
Urinary Hesitation	2.3	8.5
Dysuria	1.7	2.5
Pollakiuria	—	1.0
General Disorders and Administration Site Conditions		
Fatigue	3.1	3.0
Edema Peripheral	2.5	4.0
Asthenia	1.7	2.5
Chest Pain	1.3	—
Pain	—	1.0
Thirst	—	1.0
Edema	—	1.0
Investigations		
Blood Pressure Increased	1.0	1.5
Blood Glucose Increased	—	1.5
Blood pressure decreased	—	1.0
Injury, Poisoning and Procedural Complications		
Fall	—	1.0

Note: Includes adverse events, regardless of investigator assessment of causality, reported by ≥1% of the subjects in either treatment group.

DRUG INTERACTIONS: Overview: The concomitant use of oxybutynin with other anticholinergic drugs or with other agents which produce dry mouth, constipation, somnolence (drowsiness), and/or other anticholinergic-like effects may increase the frequency and/or severity of such effects.

Anticholinergic agents may potentially alter the absorption of some concomitantly administered drugs due to anticholinergic effects on gastrointestinal motility. This may be of concern for drugs with a narrow therapeutic index.

Drug-Drug Interactions: Mean oxybutynin plasma concentrations were approximately two-fold higher when DITROPAN XL was administered with ketoconazole, a potent CYP3A4 inhibitor.

Other inhibitors of the cytochrome P450 3A4 enzyme system, such as antimycotic agents (e.g., itraconazole and miconazole) or macrolide antibiotics (e.g., erythromycin and clarithromycin), may alter oxybutynin mean pharmacokinetic parameters (i.e., C_{max} and AUC). The clinical relevance of such potential interactions is not known. Caution should be used when such drugs are co-administered.

Concurrent ingestion of an antacid (20 mL of an antacid containing aluminum hydroxide, magnesium hydroxide, and simethicone) with DITROPAN XL did not significantly affect the exposure of oxybutynin or desethyloxybutynin.

Concurrent ingestion of a proton pump inhibitor (20 mg omeprazole) with DITROPAN XL did not significantly affect the exposure of oxybutynin or desethyloxybutynin.

Drug-Food Interactions: The rate and extent of absorption and metabolism of oxybutynin are similar under fed and fasted conditions.

Drug-Herb Interactions: Interactions with herbal products have not been established.

Drug-Lifestyle Interactions: Patients should be informed that alcohol may enhance the drowsiness caused by anticholinergic agents such as oxybutynin.

DOSAGE AND ADMINISTRATION: **Dosing Considerations:** DITROPAN XL (oxybutynin chloride) must be swallowed whole with the aid of liquids, and must not be chewed, divided, or crushed.

DITROPAN XL may be administered with or without food.

DITROPAN XL should be taken at a consistent time each day.

Recommended Dose and Dosage Adjustment: Initiating Therapy: In adults, the usual starting dose of DITROPAN XL is 5 or 10 mg once daily at a consistent time each day. Dosage may be adjusted in 5 mg increments to achieve a balance of efficacy and tolerability (up to a maximum of 30 mg/day). In general, dosage adjustment may proceed at approximately weekly intervals.

Converting from Immediate-Release Formulations to DITROPAN XL: Patients already taking immediate-release oxybutynin chloride tablets may be switched to the nearest equivalent total daily dose of DITROPAN XL. Patients who are not fully continent on immediate-release oxybutynin may tolerate higher doses of DITROPAN XL, administered in 5 mg increments, and may achieve a greater improvement in their incontinence symptoms. Subsequent adjustment to higher or lower doses should be initiated as clinically warranted.

Missed Dose: The missed dose should be taken as soon as possible. If it is almost time for the next dose, the missed dose should not be taken. Instead, the next scheduled dose should be taken. Doses should not be doubled.

OVERDOSAGE:

The continuous release of oxybutynin from DITROPAN XL (oxybutynin chloride) should be considered in the treatment of overdosage. Patients should be monitored for at least 24 hours. Treatment should be symptomatic and supportive. Activated charcoal as well as a cathartic may be administered.

Overdosage with oxybutynin has been associated with anticholinergic effects including CNS excitation, flushing, fever, dehydration, cardiac arrhythmia, vomiting, and urinary retention.

Ingestion of 100 mg oxybutynin chloride in association with alcohol has been reported in a 13-year-old boy who experienced memory loss, and a 34-year-old woman who developed stupor, followed by disorientation and agitation on awakening, dilated pupils, dry skin, cardiac arrhythmia, and retention of urine. Both patients fully recovered with symptomatic treatment.

> For management of a suspected drug overdose, CPhA recommends that you contact your **regional Poison Control Centre**. See the *CPS* Directory section for a list of Poison Control Centres.

ACTION AND CLINICAL PHARMACOLOGY: Mechanism of Action: DITROPAN XL (oxybutynin chloride) is a tertiary amine anticholinergic agent which exerts antimuscarinic as well as direct antispasmodic action on smooth muscle. In addition to its smooth muscle relaxing effects, oxybutynin chloride exerts an analgesic and a local anesthetic effect.

Oxybutynin chloride relaxes bladder smooth muscle. In patients with uninhibited neurogenic and reflex neurogenic bladder, cystometric studies have demonstrated that oxybutynin chloride increases bladder (vesical) capacity, diminishes the frequency of uninhibited contractions of the detrusor muscle, and delays the initial desire to void. DITROPAN XL thus decreases urgency and frequency of both incontinent episodes and voluntary urination.

Pharmacodynamics: Several studies have assessed oxybutynin's urodynamic effect (increase in bladder capacity) as measured by cystometry. The onset of action was rapid (within 1 h) following 5 mg oral oxybutynin chloride. The effect was seen up to 10 hours post-drug administration. Intravesical administration of oxybutynin chloride has also shown increase in bladder capacity within 1-1.5 h after drug instillation.

Pharmacokinetics: Absorption: Oxybutynin chloride is readily absorbed from the gastrointestinal tract. Following the first dose of DITROPAN XL, oxybutynin plasma concentrations rise for 4 to 6 hours; thereafter, steady concentrations are maintained for up to 24 hours.

The relative bioavailabilities of R- and S-oxybutynin from DITROPAN XL are 156% and 187%, respectively, compared with immediate-release oxybutynin chloride tablets. The mean pharmacokinetic parameters for R- and S-oxybutynin are summarized in Table 3. The plasma concentration-time profiles for R- and S-oxybutynin are similar in shape; Figure 1 shows the profile for R-oxybutynin.

Table 3: DITROPAN XL

Following a Single Dose of DITROPAN XL 10 mg (n=43) Mean (SD) R- and S-Oxybutynin Pharmacokinetic Parameters

Parameters (units)	R-Oxybutynin	S-Oxybutynin
C_{max} (ng/mL)	1.0 (0.6)	1.8 (1.0)
T_{max} (h)	12.7 (5.4)	11.8 (5.3)
$t_{1/2}$ (h)	13.2 (6.2)	12.4 (6.1)
$AUC_{(0-48)}$ (ng·h/mL)	18.4 (10.3)	34.2 (16.9)
AUC_{inf} (ng·h/mL)	21.3 (12.2)	39.5 (21.2)

Figure 1: DITROPAN XL

Mean R-oxybutynin Plasma Concentrations Following a Single Dose of DITROPAN XL 10 mg and Immediate-release (IR) Oxybutynin 5 mg Administered Every 8 hours (n=23 for each treatment)

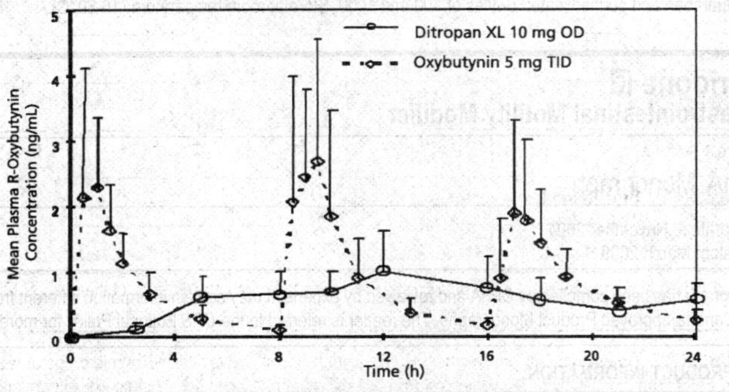

Steady-state oxybutynin plasma concentrations are achieved by Day 3 of repeated DITROPAN XL dosing, with no drug accumulation or change in oxybutynin and desethyloxybutynin pharmacokinetic parameters. The rate and extent of absorption and metabolism of oxybutynin are similar under fed and fasted conditions.

Distribution: Plasma concentrations of oxybutynin decline biexponentially following intravenous or oral administration. The volume of distribution is 193 L after intravenous administration of 5 mg oxybutynin chloride.

Metabolism: Oxybutynin is metabolized primarily by the cytochrome P450 enzyme systems, particularly CYP3A4 found mostly in the liver and gut wall. Its metabolic products include phenylcyclohexylglycolic acid, which is pharmacologically inactive, and desethyloxybutynin, which is pharmacologically active. Following DITROPAN XL administration, plasma concentrations of R- and S-desethyloxybutynin are 73% and 92%, respectively, of concentrations observed with immediate-release oxybutynin chloride tablets.

Excretion: Oxybutynin is extensively metabolized by the liver, with less than 0.1% of the administered dose excreted unchanged in the urine.

Dose Proportionality: Pharmacokinetic parameters of oxybutynin and desethyloxybutynin (C_{max} and AUC) following administration of DITROPAN XL are dose proportional.

Special Populations and Conditions: Pediatrics: The pharmacokinetics of DITROPAN XL were not evaluated in individuals younger than 18 years of age. The pharmacokinetics of immediate-release oxybutynin chloride in children (5-13 years) are similar to those in adults.

Geriatrics: The pharmacokinetics of DITROPAN XL are similar in patients younger or older than 65 years. In frail elderly patients treated with immediate-release oxybutynin chloride, C_{max} and AUC values were approximately twice those in elderly patients or young adult volunteers.

Gender: There are no significant differences in the pharmacokinetics of oxybutynin in healthy male and female volunteers following administration of DITROPAN XL.

Race: Available data suggest that there are no significant differences in the pharmacokinetics of oxybutynin based on race in healthy volunteers following administration of DITROPAN XL.

Hepatic Insufficiency: There is no experience with the use of DITROPAN XL in patients with hepatic insufficiency.

Renal Insufficiency: There is no experience with the use of DITROPAN XL in patients with renal insufficiency.

STORAGE AND STABILITY: Store between 15 and 30°C. Protect from moisture and humidity.

INFORMATION FOR THE PATIENT: Published in e-CPS, available by subscription at www.e-cps.ca.

DOSAGE FORMS, COMPOSITION AND PACKAGING: 5 mg: Each round, pale yellow, extended-release tablet, imprinted with "5 XL", contains: oxybutynin chloride USP 5 mg. Nonmedicinal ingredients: butylated hydroxytoluene, cellulose acetate, hydroxypropyl methylcellulose, lactose, magnesium stearate, polyethylene glycol, polyethylene oxide, polysorbate 80, sodium chloride, synthetic iron oxides and titanium dioxide. Bottles of 100 and 500.

10 mg: Each round, pink, extended-release tablet, imprinted with "10 XL", contains: oxybutynin chloride USP 10 mg. Nonmedicinal ingredients: butylated hydroxytoluene, cellulose acetate, hydroxypropyl methylcellulose, lactose, magnesium stearate, polyethylene glycol, polyethylene oxide, polysorbate 80, sodium chloride, synthetic iron oxides and titanium dioxide. Bottles of 100 and 500.

System Components and Performance: DITROPAN XL uses osmotic pressure to deliver oxybutynin chloride at a controlled rate over approximately 24 hours. The system, which resembles a conventional tablet in appearance, comprises an osmotically active bilayer core surrounded by a semipermeable membrane. The bilayer core is composed of a drug layer containing the drug and excipients, and a push layer containing osmotically active components. There is a precision-laser drilled orifice in the semipermeable membrane on the drug-layer side of the tablet. In an aqueous environment, such as the gastrointestinal tract, water permeates through the membrane into the tablet core, causing the drug to go into suspension and the push layer to expand. This expansion pushes the suspended drug out through the orifice. The semipermeable membrane controls the rate at which water permeates into the tablet core, which in turn controls the rate of drug delivery. The controlled rate of drug delivery into the gastrointestinal lumen is thus independent of pH or gastrointestinal motility. The function of DITROPAN XL depends on the existence of an osmotic gradient between the contents of the bilayer core and the fluid in the gastrointestinal tract. Since the osmotic gradient remains constant, drug delivery remains essentially constant. The biologically inert components of the tablet remain intact during gastrointestinal transit and are eliminated in the feces as an insoluble shell.

(Shown in Product Identification Section)

Dixarit® ℞

clonidine HCl

Vascular Stabilizer for the Treatment of Menopausal Flushing

Boehringer Ingelheim

Date of Revision: January 20, 2007

SUMMARY PRODUCT INFORMATION:

Route of Administration	Dosage Form/ Strength	Clinically Relevant Nonmedicinal Ingredients
Oral	Tablet/0.025 mg	Lactose For a complete listing see Dosage Forms, Composition and Packaging.

INDICATIONS AND CLINICAL USE: DIXARIT (clonidine hydrochloride) is indicated for the relief of menopausal flushing in patients for whom hormonal replacement therapy is either unnecessary or not desirable.

Pediatrics (<18 years of age): Safety and effectiveness in children has not been established.

CONTRAINDICATIONS: DIXARIT (clonidine hydrochloride) is contraindicated in patients with known hypersensitivity to the active substance or to any of the ingredients of the product. For a complete listing, see Dosage Forms, Composition and Packaging.

DIXARIT is contraindicated in patients with severe bradyarrhythmia resulting from either sick sinus syndrome or atrioventricular block of 2nd or 3rd degree; patients with sinus node function impairment.

WARNINGS AND PRECAUTIONS: General: DIXARIT (clonidine hydrochloride) can have a hypotensive effect especially in high doses. In patients whose blood pressure decreases to an intolerable extent when taking DIXARIT, treatment should be discontinued.

It has been demonstrated that an excessive rise in blood pressure, should it occur on discontinuation of DIXARIT, can be reversed by resumption of clonidine hydrochloride therapy or by intravenous phentolamine.

An abrupt withdrawal of higher doses of clonidine hydrochloride is followed in some cases by an excess of circulating catecholamines. Therefore, caution should be exercised in concomitant use of drugs which affect the metabolism, tissue uptake or pressor effects of these amines (monoamine oxidase inhibitors, tricyclic antidepressants and beta-blocking agents).

DIXARIT (clonidine hydrochloride 0.025 mg) should not be confused with Catapres (clonidine hydrochloride 0.1 mg, 0.2 mg). Catapres is a higher dosage form of the same active ingredient, clonidine hydrochloride, and is used for treating hypertension. Catapres is available as white tablets of 0.1 mg and orange tablets containing 0.2 mg of clonidine. Caution should however be exercised in patients receiving antihypertensive therapy because of the possibility of an additive effect.

Patients who engage in potentially hazardous activities such as operating machinery or driving should be warned of the possible sedative effect of clonidine hydrochloride. Caution should be exercised in the concomitant administration of sedatives, tranquilizing drugs or alcohol.

Patients should be instructed not to discontinue therapy without consulting their physician. Following sudden discontinuation of DIXARIT after prolonged treatment with high doses, restlessness, palpitations, rapid rise in blood pressure, nervousness, tremor, headache or nausea have been reported. When discontinuing therapy with DIXARIT, the physician should reduce the dose gradually over 2-4 days.

A few instances of a condition resembling Raynaud's phenomenon have been reported with the higher doses of clonidine as used in the therapy of hypertension. Caution should be observed if patients with Raynaud's disease or thromboangiitis obliterans are to be treated with DIXARIT.

Cardiovascular: Because it can lower blood pressure at high doses, DIXARIT (clonidine hydrochloride) should be used with caution in patients with severe coronary insufficiency, recent myocardial infarction, cerebral vascular disease, or chronic renal failure. DIXARIT should be used with caution in patients with mild to moderate bradyarrhythmia such as low sinus rhythm, with disorders of cerebral or peripheral perfusion, polyneuropathy, and constipation, patients with heart failure or severe coronary heart disease.

Depending on the dose given, DIXARIT can lower the heart and pulse rate. In patients with diseases affecting the rhythmic and atrioventricular conduction system of the heart, arrhythmias have been observed after high doses.

DIXARIT should be monitored particularly carefully in patients with heart failure or severe coronary disease.

Ophthalmologic: In several studies clonidine hydrochloride produced a dose-dependent increase in the incidence and severity of spontaneously occurring retinal degeneration in albino rats treated for six months or longer. In view of this retinal degeneration, eye examinations were performed in 908 hypertensive patients prior to the start of clonidine hydrochloride therapy, who were then examined periodically thereafter. In 353 of these 908 patients, examinations were performed for periods of 24 months or longer. Except for the dryness of the eyes, no drug-related abnormal ophthalmologic findings were recorded and clonidine hydrochloride did not alter retinal function as shown by specialized tests such as the electroretinogram and macular dazzle.

Psychiatric: Patients with a known history of depression should be carefully supervised while under treatment with clonidine as there have been occasional reports of further depressive episodes occurring in such patients.

Renal: Clonidine and its metabolites are extensively excreted with urine. As a result, DIXARIT should be used with caution in patients with renal insufficiency. As with any drug excreted primarily in the urine, smaller doses of the drug are often effective in treating patients with a degree of renal failure. In patients exhibiting renal failure or insufficiency, periodic determination of the BUN is indicated. If, in the physician's opinion, a rising BUN is significant, the drug should be stopped.

Special Populations: Pregnant Women: When rats were given clonidine hydrochloride alone in doses as low as one-third the maximum recommended daily human dose, some embryotoxicity was evident. There are, however, no adequate and well-controlled studies in pregnant women. Thus, use of clonidine hydrochloride in pregnancy is not recommended.
Nursing Women: The use of DIXARIT during lactation is not recommended due to a lack of supporting information.
Pediatrics (<18 years of age): Safety and effectiveness in children has not been established.

ADVERSE REACTIONS: Adverse Drug Reaction Overview: Most adverse reactions associated with the use of DIXARIT (clonidine hydrochloride) are mild and diminish with continued therapy.

Accumulated clinical and postmarketing data indicate that the most frequently occurring adverse reactions are dryness of mouth, sedation and reduction of blood pressure.

Occasionally, constipation, nausea and vomiting, headache, malaise, impotence, decreased libido, gynaecomastia, orthostatic symptoms, paresthesia of the extremities, Raynauds's phenomenon, pain in the parotid gland, dryness of the nasal mucosa and reduced lacrymal flow (caution: contact lens wearers) as well as skin reactions with symptoms such as rash, urticaria, pruritus, and alopecia have been observed.

In rare instances, sleep disturbances, nightmares, depression, perceptual disorders, hallucinations, confusion, disturbances of accommodation and transient elevations of blood sugar have been reported.

In very rare cases, pseudo-obstruction of the large bowel has been observed in predisposed patients.

Clonidine may cause or potentiate bradyarrhythmic conditions such as sinus bradycardia or atrioventricular-block.

Adverse events reported during treatment with DIXARIT include, fatigue, muscle or joint pain and cramps, drowsiness and dizziness. In addition, there have been isolated reports of accelerated rate of dental caries due to continual dry mouth, in patients receiving higher doses of clonidine hydrochloride.

DRUG INTERACTIONS: Overview: The doses of DIXARIT used during clinical trials in menopausal flushing, 0.05 mg b.i.d., did not produce significant changes in blood pressure. Caution should, however, be exercised in patients receiving antihypertensive therapy because of the possibility of an additive effect. The reduction in blood pressure induced by clonidine can be further potentiated by concurrent administration of agents such as diuretics, vasodilators, beta-receptor blockers, calcium antagonists and ACE-inhibitors.

Concomitant use of β-receptor blockers and/or cardiac glycosides can further lower heart rate (bradycardia) or cause dysrhythmia (atrioventricular block) in isolated cases.

It cannot be ruled out that concomitant administration of a beta-receptor blocker will cause or potentiate peripheral vascular disorders.

Orthostatic regulation disturbances may be provoked or aggravated by concomitant administration of tricyclic antidepressants or neuroleptics with alpha-receptor blocking properties.

Withdrawal of higher doses of clonidine hydrochloride may result in an excess of circulating catecholamines (see Warnings and Precautions). Therefore, caution should be exercised in concomitant use of drugs which affect the metabolism, tissue uptake or pressor effects of these amines (monoamine oxidase inhibitors, tricyclic antidepressants and beta blocking agents, respectively).

If combined treatment with a β-blocker necessitates the interim interruption of antihypertensive therapy or even total discontinuation, the β-blocker must always be discontinued slowly first, reducing the dose gradually to avoid sympathetic hyperactivity. DIXARIT must then be reduced gradually over several days if previously given in high dosages.

If clonidine hydrochloride and tricyclic antidepressants are administered as concurrent therapy, the effect of clonidine hydrochloride may be reduced, thus necessitating an increase in the dosage of DIXARIT. Amitriptyline in combination with clonidine hydrochloride enhances the manifestation of corneal lesions in rats.

Clonidine hydrochloride may enhance the CNS-depressive effects of alcohol, barbiturates or other sedatives.

Substances with alpha$_2$-receptor blocking properties such as phenolamine or tolazoline may abolish the alpha$_2$-receptor mediated effects of clonidine in a dose-dependent manner. Therefore, depending upon the dose administered, tolazoline is suitable as an antidote.

DOSAGE AND ADMINISTRATION: Recommended Dose and Dosage Adjustment: The recommended dose for the treatment of menopausal flushing is 0.05 mg of DIXARIT (clonidine hydrochloride) twice daily. If after two to four weeks there has been no remission, the treatment should be discontinued and the patient reassessed.

Attempts should be made to discontinue treatment at three to six month intervals for patient re-evaluation of menopausal symptoms.

Missed Dose: If a dose of DIXARIT is missed, patients should take the dose as soon as possible and then return to their normal schedule.

Administration: The tablets should be swallowed whole with water.

OVERDOSAGE:
The signs and symptoms of clonidine hydrochloride overdosage are due to generalised sympathetic depression and include pupillary constriction, hypotension, hypothermia, bradycardia, lethargy, irritability, weakness, somnolence, diminished or absent reflexes, vomiting and hypoventilation. With large overdoses, reversible cardiac conduction defects or arrhythmias, coma, apnea, seizures and transient hypertension have been reported.

In a patient who ingested 100 mg clonidine hydrochloride, plasma clonidine levels were 60 ng/mL (one hour), 190 ng/mL (1.5 hours), 370 ng/mL (two hours) and 120 ng/mL (5.5 and 6.5 hours). This patient developed hypertension followed by hypotension, bradycardia, apnea, hallucinations, semicoma, and premature ventricular contractions. The patient fully recovered after intensive treatment.

Clonidine overdosage usually responds to symptomatic treatment, volume expansion for hypotension and careful cardiovascular monitoring. Gastric lavage, followed by administration of activated charcoal if a large dose has been taken, can be initiated within two hours of ingestion if the airway can be protected. Routine hemodialysis is of limited benefit since a maximum of 5% of circulating clonidine is removed.

Intravenous naloxone has been used as antidote to clonidine poisoning, with inconsistent results. If other efforts fail, these agents may provide some benefit in reversing the effects of clonidine.

> For management of a suspected drug overdose, CPhA recommends that you contact your **regional Poison Control Centre**. See the *CPS* Directory section for a list of Poison Control Centres.

ACTION AND CLINICAL PHARMACOLOGY: Mechanism of Action: DIXARIT (clonidine hydrochloride) reduces the response of peripheral vessels to either vasoconstrictor or vasodilator stimuli. Clonidine hydrochloride, the active ingredient, is an α-adrenergic agonist which also has some α-adrenergic antagonist effects.

DIXARIT therapy has been shown to reduce the frequency, severity, and duration of flushing attacks associated with the menopausal syndrome. There is a gradual onset of therapeutic response, and a gradual return of symptoms on interruption of treatment.

DIXARIT will not correct or relieve other menopausal changes that are due to hormonal deficiencies.

Clonidine stimulates alpha-adrenoreceptors in the brain stem, resulting in reduced sympathetic outflow from the central nervous system and a decrease in peripheral resistance, renal vascular resistance, heart rate, and blood pressure. Renal blood flow and glomerular filtration rate remain essentially unchanged.

Clonidine hydrochloride acts relatively rapidly. The patient's blood pressure declines within 30 to 60 minutes after an oral dose, the maximum decrease occurring within 2 to 4 hours. The plasma level of clonidine peaks in approximately 3 to 5 hours and the plasma half-life from 12-16 hours. The half-life increases up to 41 hours in patients with severe impairment of renal function. Following oral administration about 40-60% of the absorbed dose is recovered in the urine as unchanged drug in 24 hours. About 50% of the absorbed dose is metabolized in the liver.

Acute studies with clonidine hydrochloride in humans have demonstrated a moderate reduction (15%-20%) of cardiac output in the supine position with no change in the peripheral resistance, at a 45° tilt there is a smaller reduction in cardiac output and a decrease in peripheral resistance. During long-term therapy, cardiac output tends to return to controlled values, while peripheral resistance remains decreased.

Slowing of the pulse rate has been observed in most patients given clonidine, but the drug does not alter normal hemodynamic response to exercise.

Other studies in patients have provided evidence of a reduction in plasma renin activity and in the excretion of aldosterone and catecholamines, but the exact relationship of these pharmacologic actions to the antihypertensive effect has not been fully elucidated.

Clonidine acutely stimulates growth hormone release in both children and adults, but does not produce a chronic elevation of growth hormone with long-term use.

Pharmacodynamics: In man, a significant plasma level (0.20 µg% of clonidine) can be detected one hour after oral administration of a single dose of 390 µg. Since clonidine is approximately 50% bound, this reflects an actual free plasma level.

Sixty-five percent (65%) of the orally administered drug is excreted in the urine and an estimated 22% in the feces. Fifty-eight percent of the activity in human urine at 24 hours, and 44% at 48 hours is unchanged clonidine. Four different metabolites have been detected in man.

The blood pressure reduction due to higher doses of clonidine does not cause significant alterations in renal blood flow in the supine position. In the erect position, a consistent decrease in renal vascular resistance is seen.

STORAGE AND STABILITY: The DIXARIT tablets should be stored at room temperature (15-30°C).

INFORMATION FOR THE PATIENT: Published in e-CPS, available by subscription at www.e-cps.ca.

DOSAGE FORMS, COMPOSITION AND PACKAGING: Each blue, sugar-coated, round, biconvex tablet contains: 0.025 mg of clonidine HCl. Nonmedicinal ingredients: Tablet core: $CaHPO_4$, colloidal silica, FD&C Blue #2, lactose (fine), magnesium stearate, maize starch, polyvinylpyrrolidone and soluble starch. Sugar coating: carnauba wax, FD&C Blue #2, gum arabic, polyethylene glycol 6000, polyvinylpyrrolidone, sucrose, talc, titanium dioxide and white wax. Bottles of 100.

Doak™ Oil
mineral oil—tar distillate—isopropyl palmitate
Antipruritic Bath Oil

Stiefel, a GSK company

Doak™ Oil Forte
mineral oil—tar distillate—isopropyl palmitate
Antipruritic Bath Oil

Stiefel, a GSK company

SUPPLIED: Each bottle contains: mineral oil, isopropyl palmitate and "Doak" tar distillate 2% (Doak Oil) or 10% (Doak Oil Forte). Nonmedicinal ingredients: acetulan, amerchol L-101, fragrance A-833, isopropyl palmitate, light mineral oil and nonoxinol-4. Bottles of 250 mL.

Dobutamine Injection Pr
dobutamine HCl
Sympathomimetic

Hospira

SUPPLIED: Each mL of clear, practically colorless sterile, nonpyrogenic solution, contains: dobutamine HCl 12.5 mg. Nonmedicinal ingredients: sodium metabisulfite and water for injection. Hydrochloric acid and/or sodium hydroxide to adjust pH. Must be diluted prior to i.v. use as directed. Single dose vials of 20 mL, boxes of 5. Store between 15 to 25°C.

Dobutamine Injection USP Pr
dobutamine HCl
Sympathomimetic

Sandoz

SUPPLIED: Each mL contains: dobutamine 12.5 mg (as hydrochloride), sodium metabisulfite 0.24 mg, hydrochloric acid and/or sodium hydroxide to adjust pH and water for injection. Single use vials of 20 mL, boxes of 10. Store between 15 and 30°C. Protect from light. Discard unused portion.

Docusate Sodium
docusate sodium
Stool Softener

Taro

SUPPLIED: Each orange, oval-shaped soft gelatin capsule contains: docusate sodium USP 100 mg. Nonmedicinal ingredients: ethyl vanillin, FD&C Red No. 40, FD&C Yellow No. 6, gelatin, glycerin, methylparaben, polyethylene glycol (PEG 400), propylene glycol, propylparaben and purified water. Bottles of 100 and 1000. Store at room temperature (15-30°C).

Domperidone Pr
Upper Gastrointestinal Motility Modifier

CPhA Monograph

Date of Preparation: November 2004
Date of Revision: March 2009

> This monograph has been compiled by CPhA and reviewed by experts. It may contain information different from that found in Health Canada-approved Product Monographs. The reader is referred to the CPS Editorial Policy for more information.

SUMMARY PRODUCT INFORMATION:

Route of Administration	Dosage Form	Strength
Oral	Tablet	10 mg

INDICATIONS AND CLINICAL USE: Health Canada-approved indications include:

- symptomatic management of upper gastrointestinal motility disorders associated with chronic and subacute gastritis and diabetic gastroparesis. Symptoms that can be improved by use of domperidone include nausea, vomiting, bloating, early satiety and gastric distention. Domperidone is an alternative to metoclopramide for acute and recurrent diabetic gastroparesis. Limited data from randomized trials exist to guide management, however, expert opinion as reflected in the American Gastroenterological Association [*Gastroenterology* 2004;127(5):1592-622] and the American Motility Association [*Neurogastroenterol Motil* 2006;18(4):263-83] guidelines for management of gastroparesis, recommend domperidone as one of the treatment modalities. Symptom improvement may be because of its antiemetic effect rather than its motor stimulatory actions with respect to gastric and upper GI motility. Long-term efficacy of domperidone in diabetic gastroparesis has not been established though there is no evidence that symptomatic improvement diminishes.
- prevention of gastrointestinal symptoms, such as nausea and vomiting, associated with the use of dopamine agonists used in Parkinson's disease. In patients with Parkinson's disease, domperidone improves gastric emptying without blocking the central dopaminergic actions of levodopa and dopamine agonists. Because domperidone reduces the incidence of nausea and vomiting, it may allow patients to tolerate higher doses of dopamine agonists.

Uses Not Approved in Canada:

- Domperidone has a limited role in the management of gastroesophageal reflux disease (GERD) as antisecretory agents (proton pump inhibitors and histamine H_2-receptor antagonists) are the mainstay of therapy. Domperidone may be of benefit as an adjunct to PPIs in patients with gas-bloat syndrome or gastroparesis after fundoplication [*Am J Gastroenterol* 2007;102(9):2036-45].
- Although not studied in well-designed clinical trials, domperidone may improve symptoms in a subset of patients with functional dyspepsia who have delayed gastric emptying and patients who have gastric dysrhythmias [*Am J Gastroenterol* 2001;96(3):689-96; *Am J Gastroenterol* 1989;84(9):1069-75].
- Domperidone may be used in the treatment of nausea and vomiting associated with moderately emetogenic cytotoxic drugs and it compares favorably with metoclopramide [*Biomedicine* 1978;29(7):242-4; *Cancer Chemother Pharmacol* 1978;1(4):215-8].
- Domperidone may be used as primary or adjunctive therapy in headache disorders accompanied by nausea and vomiting. Because of its antiemetic effects, domperidone may improve oral absorption of other drugs used to manage the headache.
- Patients with anorexia nervosa or bulimia nervosa may have reduced gut motility [*Scand J Gastroenterol* 2003;38(6):573-87], thus, domperidone may be used to relieve symptoms of bloating and constipation [*Ann Intern Med* 2001;134(11):1048-59].
- Domperidone has been used in nursing mothers to improve lactation. Prior to initiating domperidone, any modifiable factors such as frequency and thoroughness of breast emptying have to be evaluated and addressed. Further, women who are unresponsive to counselling, relaxation techniques and mechanical expression may consider taking domperidone. Close follow-up on baby and mother is essential [*CMAJ* 2004;171(7):725-6].

Pediatrics: In children with chronic vomiting or regurgitation, domperidone resulted in either resolution or marked improvement of symptoms. [*Postgrad Med J* 1979;55(Suppl 1):40-2]. It has also been used to prevent pediatric nausea and vomiting induced by cytotoxic drugs. Current evidence, however, does not support domperidone as a first-line antiemetic in children. Children with symptomatic reflux disease with upper GI motility abnormalities may benefit from domperidone [*J Pediatr* 1985;106(2):311-6].

CONTRAINDICATIONS:

- Patients who are hypersensitive to domperidone or to any ingredient in the formulation.
- Patients in whom gastrointestinal stimulation could prove dangerous, such as those with preexisting gastrointestinal hemorrhage, mechanical perforation or obstruction.
- Patients taking ketoconazole concomitantly.

WARNINGS AND PRECAUTIONS: Cardiovascular: QT interval prolongation and ventricular tachyarrhythmias have occurred after administration of high doses of domperidone by the intravenous route. QT interval prolongation has also been documented in adults receiving the combination of orally administered domperidone and ketoconazole, therefore, avoid the combination.

In adults, hypokalemia has been associated as a risk factor for QT interval prolongation. A baseline electrocardiogram and serum potassium measurement may be useful prior to initiation of domperidone.

Endocrine and Metabolism: Caution is advised when administering domperidone to patients with a history of breast cancer, as certain breast cancers are thought to be prolactin-dependant. Serum prolactin levels increase during chronic administration of domperidone and return to baseline after discontinuation. Gynecomastia with long term domperidone use has been reported in men. Galactorrhea and breast tenderness have been reported in women. Galactorrhea usually occurs within the first 14 days of therapy but can take as long as 3 months to appear. Upon discontinuation, galactorrhea usually resolves within a week but may resolve gradually over a period of 2 months.

Gastrointestinal: See Contraindications.

Hepatic/Biliary/Pancreatic: Domperidone is metabolized primarily by the liver (see Dosage and Administration, Hepatic Impairment).

Neurologic: Domperidone does not readily cross the blood-brain barrier, therefore, CNS effects occur rarely. Extrapyramidal symptoms are more likely to occur in infants and in patients given more than the maximum recommended dosage.

Renal: Domperidone does not interact with renal or peripheral dopamine D_1 receptors and has no appreciable effect on plasma renin or aldosterone levels.

Special Populations: Pregnant Women: Pregnancy Category C. Conclusive evidence is not available as to whether domperidone is safe to use in pregnancy. A small percentage of the maternal dose crosses the placenta in animals though this is not known for humans. Given the low molecular weight, availability of unbound drug and prolonged elimination half-life, theoretically, domperidone may cross the placenta. It is not known what risk, if any, this poses for the fetus.

Nursing Women: Domperidone appears in the breast milk where the concentration is approximately 25% of the maternal serum concentration. The drug has been used to increase daily milk production in women who are nursing and have insufficient milk production. The American Academy of Pediatrics considers domperidone to be compatible with breastfeeding.

Pediatrics (birth to 16 years old): Although still rare, a higher incidence of CNS adverse effects has been noted in infants, possibly because of the incompletely developed blood-brain barrier of very young children. QT interval prolongation occurred in a 4-month-old infant treated with domperidone 0.6 mg/kg three times daily and resolved upon discontinuation of the drug. Hyperprolactinemia, galactorrhea, breast enlargement and neuroleptic syndrome occurred in a 3-month-old infant on maintenance hemodialysis who was treated with domperidone 0.25 mg/kg tid. The symptoms resolved and prolactin levels decreased after withdrawal of domperidone. Significant association between oral domperidone therapy (mean daily dose 1.3±0.7 mg/kg daily) and QT interval prolongation in neonates and infants has been demonstrated [*J Pediatr* 2008;153(5):663-6]. In this study, advanced gestational age and serum potassium at the upper limit of normal, were significantly and independently associated with significant QT interval prolongation.

Monitoring and Laboratory Tests: Patients may exhibit elevated serum prolactin levels. Elevations of serum AST, ALT and cholesterol have also been noted (<1%).

ADVERSE REACTIONS:

Table 1: Domperidone

Adverse Drug Reactions

Body System	Effect (%)
Cardiovascular	edema, palpitations (0.5%)
CNS	headache (1.2%) insomnia, dizziness, thirst, lethargy, irritability, nervousness (<1%) acute dystonic reactions (rare in adults)
Dermatologic	skin rash, itching, urticaria (<1%)
Endocrine and Metabolism	breast enlargement, galactorrhea, menstrual irregularities, hot flushes, mastalgia, elevated serum prolactin (1.3%)
Gastrointestinal	dry mouth (1.9%) abdominal cramps, diarrhea, regurgitation, appetite changes, nausea, heartburn, constipation (<1%)
Miscellaneous	stomatitis, conjunctivitis, urinary frequency, dysuria, leg cramps, asthenia, drug intolerance; elevation of AST, ALT, cholesterol (<1%)

DRUG INTERACTIONS: Overview: Domperidone decreases gastric emptying times; thus, it has the potential to alter the absorption of concomitantly administered medications. CYP3A4 is the major hepatic enzyme involved in the metabolism of domperidone. The potential exists for interactions between domperidone and drugs that induce or inhibit CYP3A4, such as phenobarbital, phenytoin, and the azole antifungals. Ketoconazole significantly inhibits CYP3A4-mediated metabolism of domperidone in vitro. Plasma levels of domperidone (C_{max} and AUC) increased threefold when coadministered with domperidone in healthy volunteers. QTc prolongation (10 to 20 msec) occurred in individuals receiving the combination of domperidone 10 mg four times daily plus ketoconazole 200 mg twice daily, but not domperidone alone.

Drug-Drug Interactions: See Table 2.

Drug-Food Interactions: See Action and Clinical Pharmacology, Pharmacokinetics.

Table 2: Domperidone

Drug-Drug Interactions

Interacting Drug	Effect	Clinical Comment
Ketoconazole	Approximately threefold increase in domperidone plasma levels resulting in QT interval prolongation.	Avoid use of this combination
Anticholinergics	May decrease effectiveness of domperidone.	Preliminary studies suggest that anticholinergics may antagonize the prokinetic effects of domperidone.
Monoamine oxidase inhibitors (MAOIs)	Possible hypertensive crisis.	This is a theoretical caution based on increased dopamine levels in sympathetic nerve terminals when MAOIs are given with domperidone.

DOSAGE AND ADMINISTRATION: Dosing Considerations: Can be crushed and dissolved for administration through nasogastric, gastrotomy or jejunostomy tubes [*Am J Gastroenterol* 2007;102(9):2036-45].

Duration of Therapy: The recommended maximum duration of therapy is 12 weeks, although longer courses of therapy are sometimes prescribed, especially in gastroparesis, which is a chronic problem.

Recommended Dose and Dosage Adjustment: Adults: For symptoms of upper gastrointestinal dysmotility; acute nausea and vomiting; to manage side effects of dopamine agonists in the treatment of Parkinson's disease: Start at 10 mg, 15 to 30 minutes before meals and at bedtime if needed, increasing to 20 mg three or four times daily if the desired response is not achieved. The maximum recommended total daily dose is 80 mg.

As a galactagogue, domperidone is usually given at an oral dose of 60 to 80 mg daily though 30 mg daily has been used [*CMAJ* 2001;164(1):17-21].

Although not an approved indication, domperidone has been used in children. Pediatrics (>1 month old): For gastroesophageal reflux disease; acute nausea and vomiting: 1.2 to 2.4 mg/kg daily divided in 3 to 4 doses, 15 to 30 minutes before meals and at bedtime, not to exceed a total daily dose of 80 mg. See Warnings and Precautions, Special Populations, Pediatrics (birth to 16 years old).

Renal Impairment: As the kidneys are a minor route of elimination, it is not anticipated that domperidone would accumulate in patients with renal insufficiency. Older literature state renal excretion of domperidone as 1.7 to 2.4%. Limited pharmacokinetics data suggest that in patients with severe renal insufficiency, the dose interval may need to be extended. May require twice daily dosing instead of four times a day [*Am J Gastroenterol* 2007;102(9):2036-45].

Hepatic Impairment: As domperidone is mainly metabolized by the liver, it is likely that hepatic insufficiency would lead to decreased metabolism of domperidone in proportion to the degree of hepatic impairment. No specific dose adjustment guidelines are available; however, caution is advised when prescribing domperidone for patients with severe hepatic dysfunction. Such patients should be monitored for increased side effects and response to domperidone.

Administration: Patients taking domperidone for dysmotility should take it 15-30 minutes before eating.

OVERDOSAGE:

For management of a suspected drug overdose, CPhA recommends that you contact your **regional Poison Control Centre**. See the *CPS* Directory section for a list of Poison Control Centres.

ACTION AND CLINICAL PHARMACOLOGY: Mechanism of Action: Domperidone is a peripheral dopamine antagonist that selectively blocks the effect of dopamine at D_2 receptors in myenteric motor neurons and the chemoreceptor trigger zone (CTZ). Through this action it stimulates peristalsis and helps coordinate antral and duodenal contractions, improving gastric motility. The antiemetic effects of domperidone are largely due to blockade of dopamine receptors in the CTZ, although there is indirect evidence to suggest that some of the antiemetic effect stems from its prokinetic properties. Domperidone does not readily cross the blood-brain barrier and has no appreciable effect on dopamine receptors in the brain. Domperidone does not have significant effects at renal or peripheral D_1 receptors.

Pharmacodynamics: In patients with symptoms of upper gastrointestinal tract dysmotility such as those resulting from gastroparesis, for example, domperidone has been shown to significantly improve gastric emptying rates. Domperidone normalizes gastric slow-wave activity that can contribute to symptoms of nausea in patients with upper gastrointestinal motility disorders. It helps synchronize peristaltic contractions, thus improving the movement of both solids and liquids through the stomach and duodenum. Domperidone has no effect on esophageal or colonic motility. Domperidone stimulates release of prolactin from the pituitary gland. In in vitro and ex vivo experiments conducted with clinically relevant concentrations of the drug, domperidone exhibited cardiac electrophysiologic effects similar to those of cisapride and class III antiarrhythmic drugs.

Pharmacokinetics: Absorption: Domperidone is rapidly absorbed when administered orally under fasting conditions. The peak serum concentration occurs approximately 30 minutes after oral ingestion under fasting conditions. Oral bioavailability is low (13 to 17%) due to a high degree of both hepatic first-pass and gut wall metabolism. Bioavailability increases significantly when the drug is administered after a meal, although the time to achieve peak serum concentrations is increased. Patients taking the drug for dysmotility should take it 15 to 30 minutes before eating.

Distribution: Domperidone is rapidly and extensively distributed into tissues with an apparent volume of distribution of 5.7 L/kg. Domperidone has a high affinity for GI tissue and a high concentration of the drug is found in the esophagus, stomach and small intestine. Plasma protein binding is approximately 92%. Domperidone does not readily cross the blood-brain barrier.

Metabolism: Domperidone is subject to extensive first-pass metabolism both in the gut wall and liver. Domperidone is metabolized to several inactive metabolites by CYP3A4-mediated hydroxylation and oxidative N-dealkylation.

Excretion: A small amount of domperidone (<1%) is excreted unchanged in urine and approximately 6% in the feces. The elimination half-life after oral administration is 7.5 hours in healthy subjects.

Dopamine HCl and 5% Dextrose Injection ℞

dopamine HCl—dextrose

Sympathomimetic

Baxter

SUPPLIED: Each mL of sterile, nonpyrogenic solution contains: dopamine HCl USP in 5% dextrose injection USP in Viaflex Plus plastic (polyvinyl chloride) containers in the following sizes and concentrations: see Table 1.

Table 1: Dopamine HCl and 5% Dextrose Injection

Supplied

Total Volume (mL)	Total Dopamine HCl Content (mg)	Dopamine HCl Concentration (μg/mL)
250	200	800
250	400	1600
250	800	3200
500	800	1600

Store below 25°C. Protect from light and freezing.

Dopamine HCl and Dextrose Injection Pr

dopamine HCl—dextrose

Sympathomimetic

Hospira

SUPPLIED: Dopamine HCl and Dextrose Injection is a sterile, nonpyrogenic solution in a single-dose flexible (polyester) container. Each mL contains: dopamine HCl 800 µg, 1600 µg or 3200 µg, dextrose monohydrate 50 mg, sodium metabisulfite 0.5 mg as a stabilizer, hydrochloric acid (may also contain sodium hydroxide) for pH adjustment. pH approximately 3.8 (2.5 to 4.5) and the osmolarity approximately 261 mOsm/L (800 µg/mL), 269 mOsm/L (1600 µg/mL) or 286 mOsm/L (3200 µg/mL). Flexible (polyester) single-dose containers of 250 mL (800 µg/mL or 3200 µg/mL) and 250 and 500 mL (1600 µg/mL).

Store at room temperature (25°C). Protect from light, freezing and extreme heat.

Note: Dopamine HCl and dextrose as well as other dextrose solutions without electrolytes, should **not** be administered simultaneously with blood through the same infusion set, because of the possibility that pseudoagglutination of red cells may occur.

Parenteral drugs should be visually inspected for particulate matter and discoloration prior to administration, whenever solution and container permit; do not use the solution if it is darker than slightly yellow or discolored in any other way.

Do not use in series connections.

Do not administer unless solution is clear and container undamaged. Discard unused portion.

Doribax™ Pr

doripenem

Antibacterial

Janssen-Ortho

Date of Preparation: September 1, 2009
Date of Revision: April 13, 2010

SUMMARY PRODUCT INFORMATION:

Route of Administration	Dosage Form/ Strength	Clinically Relevant Nonmedicinal Ingredients
Intravenous infusion	Sterile powder/500 mg/vial doripenem (as doripenem monohydrate)	None

INDICATIONS AND CLINICAL USE: DORIBAX (doripenem for injection) is a carbapenem antibiotic indicated for the treatment of adults (18 years and older) with the following infections when caused by susceptible strains of the designated microorganisms:

Nosocomial Pneumonia, Including Ventilator-Associated Pneumonia caused by *S. aureus* (methicillin-susceptible strains only), *S. pneumoniae*, *E. cloacae*, *E. coli*, *K. pneumoniae*, *H. influenzae* and *P. aeruginosa*.

Note: Adjunctive use of an aminoglycoside was permitted in the nosocomial pneumonia clinical studies.

Complicated Intra-Abdominal Infections caused by *E. coli*, *K. pneumoniae*, *P. aeruginosa*, *B. fragilis*, *B. thetaiotaomicron*, *B. caccae*, *B. uniformis*, *B. vulgatus*, *S. intermedius*, *S. constellatus* and *P. micros*.

Complicated Urinary Tract Infections, Including Pyelonephritis caused by *E. coli*, *K. pneumoniae*, *P. aeruginosa*, *P. mirabilis*, and *A. baumannii*.

Appropriate specimens for bacteriological examination should be obtained in order to isolate and identify causative organisms and to determine their susceptibility to doripenem. Once these results are available, antimicrobial therapy should be adjusted accordingly. In the absence of such data, local epidemiology and susceptibility patterns may contribute to the empiric selection of therapy. Empiric therapy with DORIBAX may be initiated before the results of these tests are known.

Geriatrics (≥65 years of age): Evidence from clinical studies suggests that use in the geriatric population is not associated with significant differences in safety or effectiveness (see Warnings and Precautions, Special Populations, Geriatrics (>65 years of age)). Population pharmacokinetic data showed there is no independent effect of age on the pharmacokinetics of doripenem. Dosage adjustment is not required in elderly patients with normal renal function (see Dosage and Administration, Patients with Renal Impairment).

Pediatrics (<18 years of age): No data available (see Warnings and Precautions, Special Populations, Pediatrics (<18 years of age)).

CONTRAINDICATIONS: DORIBAX is contraindicated in patients with known hypersensitivity to doripenem monohydrate or to other drugs in the same class or in patients who have demonstrated anaphylactic reactions to beta-lactams.

WARNINGS AND PRECAUTIONS:

> **Serious Warnings and Precautions**
> **Serious and occasionally fatal hypersensitivity (anaphylactic) reactions have been reported in patients receiving beta-lactams. Anaphylactic and anaphylactoid reactions have been observed with DORIBAX (see Warnings and Precautions, Immune, Hypersensitivity Reactions).**

General: Prescribing DORIBAX in the absence of a proven or strongly suspected bacterial infection is unlikely to provide benefit to the patient and may increase the risk of the development of drug-resistant bacteria.

Experience in patients who are severely immunocompromised, receiving immunosuppressive therapy, and patients with severe neutropenia is limited since this population was excluded from clinical trials.

Seizures have been infrequently reported during treatment with carbapenems.

DORIBAX should not be used to treat infections caused by methicillin resistant staphylococci.

Doripenem reduced serum valproic acid concentrations to sub-therapeutic levels in healthy subjects. Therapeutic monitoring of valproic acid and use of alternative therapies should be considered in patients (see Drug Interactions).

Gastrointestinal: *C. difficile*-Associated Disease: *C. difficile*-associated disease (CDAD) has been reported with use of many antibacterial agents, including DORIBAX. CDAD may range in severity from mild diarrhea to fatal colitis. It is important to consider this diagnosis in patients who present with diarrhea, or symptoms of colitis, pseudomembranous colitis, toxic megacolon, or perforation of colon subsequent to the administration of any antibacterial agent. CDAD has been reported to occur over 2 months after the administration of antibacterial agents.

Treatment with antibacterial agents may alter the normal flora of the colon and may permit overgrowth of *C. difficile*. *C. difficile* produces toxins A and B, which contribute to the development of CDAD. CDAD may cause significant morbidity and mortality. CDAD can be refractory to antimicrobial therapy.

If the diagnosis of CDAD is suspected or confirmed, appropriate therapeutic measures should be initiated. Mild cases of CDAD usually respond to discontinuation of antibacterial agents not directed against *C. difficile*. In moderate to severe cases, consideration should be given to management with fluids and electrolytes, protein supplementation, and treatment with an antibacterial agent clinically effective against *C. difficile*. Surgical evaluation should be instituted as clinically indicated, as surgical intervention may be required in certain severe cases (see Adverse Reactions).

Hepatic/Biliary/Pancreatic: The safety, efficacy and pharmacokinetics of DORIBAX in patients with known hepatic impairment have not been established.

Immune: Hypersensitivity Reactions: Serious and occasionally fatal hypersensitivity (anaphylactic) and serious skin reactions have been reported in patients receiving beta-lactam antibiotics (see Contraindications). Anaphylactic and anaphylactoid reactions have been observed with DORIBAX. These reactions are more likely to occur in individuals with a history of sensitivity to multiple allergens. Before therapy with DORIBAX is instituted, careful inquiry should be made to determine whether the patient has had a previous hypersensitivity reaction to other carbapenems, cephalosporins, penicillins or other allergens. If this product is to be given to a penicillin- or other beta lactam-allergic patient, caution should be exercised because cross-hyperreactivity among beta-lactam antibiotics has been clearly documented. If an allergic reaction to DORIBAX occurs, discontinue the drug. Serious acute hypersensitivity (anaphylactic) reactions require emergency treatment with epinephrine and other emergency measures, including oxygen, IV fluids, IV antihistamines, corticosteroids, pressor amines and airway management, as clinically indicated.

Renal: In patients with moderately or severely impaired renal function (CrCl >10 to ≤50 mL/min), dosage adjustment is required (see Dosage and Administration, Patients with Renal Impairment). In such patients, renal function should be monitored.

Evidence from clinical studies suggests more adverse events occurred in patients with moderately or severely impaired renal function than patients with CrCl >50 mL/min. Most adverse events that occurred at a higher rate in patients with moderately or severely impaired renal function also occurred at a higher rate in patients ≥65 years of age, as would be expected since renal function declines with age. Clinical response rates were also lower for these patients as compared to patients with normal renal function. There is limited clinical experience with this population, and in addition there are no clinical data for patients with severe renal impairment using the four-hour DORIBAX infusion. PK/PD modeling indicates a potential for reduced efficacy of DORIBAX against pathogens with MICs ≥4 µg/mL in certain situations, even when using the extended duration of infusion of four hours (see Dosage and Administration and Action and Clinical Pharmacology, Pharmacodynamics).

No data on the safety and efficacy in patients with end-stage renal disease (CrCl ≤10 mL/min) or those on dialysis compared to non-renally impaired patients are available.

Due to limited clinical data and an expected increased exposure of doripenem and its metabolite, DORIBAX should be used with caution in patients with severe renal impairment (see Action and Clinical Pharmacology, Special Populations and Conditions, Renal Insufficiency).

DORIBAX can be removed by hemodialysis. In subjects with end-stage renal disease requiring dialysis administered DORIBAX 500 mg, the mean total recovery of doripenem and doripenem M-1 in the dialysate following a 4-hour dialysis session was 259 mg (52% of the dose). However, there is insufficient information to make dose adjustment recommendations in patients with end-stage renal disease (CrCl ≤10 mL/min) or in patients on dialysis. Therefore, DORIBAX is not recommended for patients with CrCl ≤10 mL/min or in patients on any type of dialysis.

Respiratory: Pneumonitis with Inhalation Use: When used investigationally in clinical trials via inhalation, pneumonitis has occurred. DORIBAX should not be administered by this route.

Special Populations: Pregnant Women: There are no adequate and well-controlled studies in pregnant women. DORIBAX should be used during pregnancy only if the potential benefit justifies the potential risk to the mother and fetus.

Doripenem was not teratogenic and did not produce effects on ossification, developmental delays or fetal weight in preclinical studies. Because animal reproduction studies are not always predictive of a human response, this drug should be used during pregnancy only if clearly needed.

Nursing Women: It is not known whether DORIBAX is excreted in human milk. A study in rats has shown that doripenem and its metabolite are transferred to milk. Because many drugs are excreted in human milk, DORIBAX should be administered to nursing mothers only when the potential benefit justifies the potential risk to the baby.

Pediatrics (<18 years of age): Safety and effectiveness in pediatric patients below the age of 18 have not been established. Therefore, use in patients under 18 years of age is not recommended.

Geriatrics (>65 years of age): Of the total number of subjects in clinical studies treated with DORIBAX, 31% were 65 years and over, while 14% were 75 years and over. No differences were seen in clinical cure rates in elderly patients versus younger patients with nosocomial pneumonia. Clinical cure rates in complicated intra-abdominal and complicated urinary tract infections were slightly lower in patients ≥65 years of age and also in the subgroup of patients ≥75 years of age versus patients <65. Cure rates were similar between DORIBAX and comparator treatment groups.

Population pharmacokinetic data showed there is no independent effect of age (18 years or older) on the pharmacokinetics of doripenem. Dose adjustment is not required in elderly patients with normal renal function.

DORIBAX is known to be excreted substantially by the kidney, and the risk of adverse reactions to this drug may be greater in patients with impaired renal function. Because elderly patients are more likely to have decreased renal function, care should be taken in dose selection, and it may be useful to monitor renal function (see Renal).

ADVERSE REACTIONS: Adverse Drug Reaction Overview: The overall rate of adverse drug reactions assigned by clinical investigators as being possibly or probably related to DORIBAX in Phase 3 clinical trials was 24%. The most common adverse drug reactions (≥1%) assigned by clinical investigators as being possibly or probably related to DORIBAX in clinical trials were diarrhoea (3.4%), headache (3.2%), phlebitis (3.2%), nausea (2.7%), vomiting (1.6%), hepatic enzymes increased (1.2%), gamma-glutamyltransferase increased (1.1%), and rash (1.0%). The majority (97%) of related adverse drug reactions were reported as mild or moderate in severity. Serious adverse drug reactions were atrial fibrillation, atrial flutter, renal failure, renal impairment, cholestasis, liver function test abnormal, convulsion, and hypotension; each was reported once (<0.1%). During clinical trials, the most common related adverse drug reaction (≥0.2%) that led to DORIBAX discontinuation was hepatic enzyme increased (0.2%). DORIBAX was discontinued due to a related adverse drug reaction in 1.2% of patients.

Clinical Trial Adverse Drug Reactions: Because clinical trials are conducted under very specific conditions the adverse drug reaction rates observed in the clinical trials may not reflect the rates observed in practice and should not be compared to the rates in the clinical trials of another drug. Adverse drug reaction information from clinical trials is useful for identifying drug-related adverse events and for approximating rates.

The safety of DORIBAX in patients with nosocomial pneumonia (NP), complicated intra-abdominal infection (cIAI), and complicated urinary tract infection (cUTI) was evaluated in five Phase 3 double-blind, controlled trials and 1 Phase 3 non-comparative study (cUTI) involving 3086 adult patients (1761 of whom received DORIBAX). Adverse drug reactions due to DORIBAX that occurred at a rate ≥1% (as judged by the investigator to be possibly or probably related to DORIBAX) are listed in Table 1. Adverse drug reactions with an incidence of <1.0% and ≥0.1% (as judged by the investigator to be possibly or probably related to DORIBAX) are listed in Table 2.

Table 1: DORIBAX

Adverse Drug Reactions (%) Observed in Six Phase 3 Clinical Trials Occurring at a Rate ≥1%

Body System or Organ Class Dictionary-Derived Term	DORIBAX (N=1761) %	COMPARATOR (N=1325) %
Gastrointestinal Disorders	8.3	7.8
Diarrhoea	3.4	4.3
Nausea	2.7	1.7
Vomiting	1.6	1.1
Investigations	4.2	4.9
Hepatic enzyme increased	1.2	1.4
Gamma-glutamyltransferase increased	1.1	1.4
Nervous System Disorders	4.1	2.0
Headache	3.2	1.1
Vascular Disorders	3.6	2.0
Phlebitis	3.2	1.7
Skin and Subcutaneous Tissue Disorders	2.4	1.8
Rash	1.0	0.2

The following significant but non-serious adverse drug reactions (as judged by the investigator as probably/possibly related to DORIBAX) occurred at a rate of <0.1% arrhythmia, delirium, rhabdomyolysis, vasculitis, coagulopathy, encephalopathy, bronchospasm, generalized edema, urticaria localized and swelling face.

Table 2: DORIBAX

Less Common Clinical Trial Adverse Drug Reactions Observed in Six Phase 3 Clinical Trials Occurring at a Rate of <1.0% and ≥0.1%

Body System or Organ Class	Dictionary-Derived Term
Gastrointestinal Disorders	Dyspepsia, abdominal pain, constipation, abdominal distension, abdominal pain upper, flatulence, gastritis, stomatitis
Investigations	Blood alkaline phosphatase increased, alanine aminotransferase increased, aspartate aminotransferase increased, blood creatinine increased, platelet count increased, blood creatine phosphokinase increased, blood lactate dehydrogenase increased, eosinophil count increased, blood pressure decreased, liver function test abnormal
Nervous System Disorders	Dizziness, dysgeusia, tremor
Vascular Disorders	Hypertension, hypotension
Infections and Infestations	Fungal infection, oral candidiasis, vulvovaginal mycotic infection, vulvovaginitis, vaginal infection, vaginal candidiasis, wound infection, candidiasis, fungal skin infection, urinary tract infection fungal, *C. difficile* colitis (see Warnings and Precautions, Gastrointestinal)
Skin and Subcutaneous Tissue Disorders	Pruritus, hyperhidrosis, rash papular, pruritus generalised
General Disorders and Administration Site Conditions	Pyrexia, asthenia, injection site pain, infusion site pain, injection site phlebitis
Metabolism and Nutrition Disorders	Hypokalaemia, hypoglycaemia, anorexia, decreased appetite, hypercholesterolaemia, hypomagnesaemia
Blood and Lymphatic System Disorders	Anaemia, thrombocythaemia, eosinophilia
Reproductive System and Breast Disorders	Genital pruritus female, polymenorrhoea
Hepatobiliary Disorders	Cholestasis, hepatitis, hepatitis cholestatic, hepatitis toxic
Respiratory, Thoracic and Mediastinal Disorders	Hiccups, pleural effusion
Psychiatric Disorders	Anxiety, insomnia
Renal and Urinary Disorders	Dysuria, renal failure acute
Immune System Disorders	Hypersensitivity
Ear and Labyrinth Disorders	Vertigo

Abnormal Hematologic and Clinical Chemistry Findings: Table 3 shows the most frequently observed drug-related laboratory abnormalities reported as an adverse experience during treatment with DORIBAX.

Table 3: DORIBAX

Incidence (%) of Specific Drug-Related Chemical and Hematologic Laboratory Adverse Experiences Reported in 6 Phase 3 Clinical Trials Occurring at a Rate ≥0.1%

Laboratory Adverse Experiences	Incidence (%)
Chemistry	
Gamma-glutamyltransferase ↑	1.1
Blood alkaline phosphatase ↑	0.6
Alanine aminotransferase ↑	0.5
Aspartate aminotransferase ↑	0.3
Blood creatinine ↑	0.3
Blood creatine phosphokinase ↑	0.2
Blood lactate dehydrogenase ↑	0.2
Hematology	
Platelet count ↑	0.3
Eosinophil count ↑	0.2

Post-Market Adverse Drug Reactions: The following adverse reactions have been identified during post-approval use of DORIBAX. Because these reactions were reported voluntarily from a population of uncertain size, it is not possible to reliably estimate their frequency:
Blood and the Lymphatic System Disorders: thrombocytopenia, neutropenia.
Immune System Disorders: anaphylaxis.
Skin and Subcutaneous Tissue Disorders: toxic epidermal necrolysis, Stevens-Johnson syndrome.

The following treatment-emergent adverse events (known to occur with beta-lactams including carbapenems) have been reported voluntarily during post-approval use of DORIBAX. They are included due to their seriousness, although it is not possible to estimate their frequency and causality has not been established: interstitial pneumonia, seizure, agranulocytosis, leukopenia.

Hemolytic anemia and pancytopenia have been reported during treatment with carbapenems.

DRUG INTERACTIONS: Overview: In vitro studies in human liver microsomes and hepatocytes indicate that doripenem does not inhibit the major cytochrome P450 isoenzymes. Therefore, DORIBAX is not expected to inhibit clearance of drugs that are metabolized by these metabolic pathways in a clinically relevant manner.

DORIBAX also is not expected to have enzyme-inducing properties based on in vitro studies in cultured human hepatocytes.
Drug-Drug Interactions: Probenecid: Probenecid competes with doripenem for active tubular secretion and thus reduces the renal clearance of doripenem. Probenecid increased doripenem AUC by 75% and plasma half-life by 53%. Coadministration of probenecid with DORIBAX is not recommended.

Valproic Acid: Reduction in serum valproic acid concentrations to below the therapeutic concentration range (50 to 100 μg/mL) was observed by 12 hours after initiation of doripenem in healthy subjects co-administered both drugs. Patients with seizure disorders controlled with valproic acid or sodium valproate may be at an increased risk for breakthrough seizures when treated with DORIBAX concomitantly. Alternative antibacterial and anticonvulsant therapies or supplemental anti-convulsant therapy should be considered. A similar drug interaction involving other carbapenem antibacterials and valproic acid or sodium valproate has been described in published case reports. Therefore, valproic acid concentrations in the blood should be monitored if DORIBAX is administered concomitantly with valproic acid or sodium valproate. The pharmacokinetics of doripenem were unaffected by the co-administration of valproic acid.
Drug-Food Interactions: Interactions with food have not been established.
Drug-Herb Interactions: Interactions with herbal products have not been established.
Drug-Laboratory Test Interactions: Interactions with laboratory tests have not been established.

DOSAGE AND ADMINISTRATION: Dosing Considerations: On the basis of pharmacokinetic data in patients with moderate to severe renal impairment, the dose of DORIBAX should be adjusted (see Recommended Dose and Dosage Adjustment, Patients with Renal Impairment).
Recommended Dose and Dosage Adjustment: The recommended dose of DORIBAX for patients aged 18 years and older is 500 mg administered every 8 hours by intravenous infusion. The recommended dosage and infusion time by indication are described in Table 4.

Table 4: DORIBAX

Dosage of DORIBAX by Indication

Indication	Dosage	Frequency	Infusion Time (hours)	Duration
Nosocomial Pneumonia including ventilator-associated pneumonia	500 mg	Every 8 hours	1 or 4[a]	7–14 days[b]
Complicated Intra-Abdominal Infection	500 mg	Every 8 hours	1	5–14 days[b]
Complicated UTI, including pyelonephritis	500 mg	Every 8 hours	1	10 days[b,c]

[a] One-hour infusions are recommended for treatment of patients with nosocomial pneumonia. For patients with late onset VAP (>5 days ventilation) who are at risk for infection with less susceptible pathogens, four-hour infusions are recommended (based primarily on pharmacokinetic/pharmacodynamic modeling). [See Action and Clinical Pharmacology, Pharmacodynamics. See also Dosage and Administration, Reconstitution and Dilution.]
[b] Duration includes a possible switch to an appropriate oral therapy, after at least 3 days of parenteral therapy, once clinical improvement has been demonstrated.
[c] Duration can be extended up to 14 days for patients with concurrent bacteremia; data for this regimen is limited to *E. coli* infections only).

DORIBAX was given for up to 14 days in clinical studies and the safety of longer durations of therapy has not been established.
Patients with Renal Impairment: Following a single 500 mg dose of DORIBAX, the mean AUC of doripenem in subjects with mild (CrCl >50 mL/min), moderate (CrCl 31-50 mL/min), and severe (CrCl ≤30 mL/min) renal impairment was 1.6-, 2.8-, and 5.1-times that of age-matched healthy subjects with normal renal function (CrCl >80 mL/min), respectively.

In patients whose creatinine clearance (CrCl) is >50 mL/min, no dosage adjustment is necessary. In patients with moderate renal impairment (CrCl ≥30 to ≤50 mL/min), the dosage of DORIBAX should be 250 mg administered every 8 hours as a 1-hour i.v. infusion. In patients with severe renal impairment (CrCl >10 to <30 mL/min), the dosage of DORIBAX should be 250 mg administered every 12 hours as a 1-hour i.v. infusion. For patients with late onset VAP (>5 days ventilation) who are at risk for infection with less susceptible pathogens, 4-hour infusions are recommended, with dose adjustments made for CrCl as described above; this recommendation is based on PK/PD modeling and target attainment is not always reached for less susceptible pathogens (see Warnings and Precautions, Renal and Action and Clinical Pharmacology, Pharmacodynamics, PK/PD Index).

The following formula may be used to estimate CrCl. The serum creatinine used in the formula should represent a steady state of renal function.

Males:

$$\text{Creatinine clearance (mL/min)} = \frac{\text{Weight (kg)} \times (140-\text{age in years})}{72 \times \text{serum creatinine (mg/dL)}}$$

Females:

$$\text{Creatinine clearance (mL/min)} = 0.85 \times \text{value calculated for males}$$

DORIBAX is hemodialyzable; however, there is insufficient information to make dose adjustment recommendations in patients with CrCl ≤10 mL/min or those on hemodialysis. Therefore, DORIBAX is not recommended for patients with CrCl ≤10 mL/min or on any type of dialysis (see Warnings and Precautions, Renal and Action and Clinical Pharmacology, Special Populations and Conditions, Renal Insufficiency).
Patients with Hepatic Impairment: The safety, efficacy and pharmacokinetics of DORIBAX in patients with known hepatic impairment have not been established. As doripenem does not appear to undergo hepatic metabolism, the pharmacokinetics of DORIBAX are not expected to be affected by hepatic impairment.
Other: No dosage adjustment is recommended based on age (18 years of age and older), gender or race (see Action and Clinical Pharmacology, Special Populations and Conditions, Pediatrics, Gender and Race).
Administration: DORIBAX is to be reconstituted and then further diluted prior to administration by intravenous infusion. Each vial contains 500 mg doripenem and is for single use only.
Reconstitution and Dilution: Aseptic technique must be followed in preparation of the infusion solution.

5% Dextrose should not be used for infusion durations lasting longer than one hour.
Preparation of 500 mg Dose:

1. Add 10 mL of sterile water for injection or 0.9% sodium chloride injection (normal saline) and gently shake to form a suspension.
2. Inspect the suspension visually for foreign material. Note: the suspension is not for direct infusion.
3. Withdraw the suspension using a syringe and needle and add it to an infusion bag containing 100 mL of normal saline or 5% dextrose.
4. To ensure complete transfer of the vial contents, repeat steps 1 to 2, and withdraw the second 10 mL suspension using a syringe and needle and add it to the same infusion bag. Infuse all of this solution to administer a 500 mg dose of doripenem.

Preparation of a 250 mg Dose for Patients with Moderate or Severe Renal Impairment (see Recommended Dose and Dosage Adjustment, Patients with Renal Impairment):

1. Add 10 mL of sterile water for injection or 0.9% sodium chloride injection (normal saline) and gently shake to form a suspension.
2. Inspect the suspension visually for foreign material. Note: the suspension is not for direct infusion.
3. Withdraw the suspension using a syringe and needle and add it to an infusion bag containing 100 mL of normal saline or 5% dextrose.
4. To ensure complete transfer of the contents of the vial to the infusion solution, repeat steps 1 to 2, and withdraw the second 10 mL suspension using a syringe and needle and add it to the same infusion bag.
5. Remove 60 mL of this solution from the bag and discard. Infuse all of the remaining solution to administer a 250 mg dose of doripenem.

DORIBAX infusions range from clear, colourless solutions to solutions that are clear and slightly yellow. Variations in colour within this range do not affect the potency of the product.

Parenteral drug products should be inspected visually for particulate matter and discolouration prior to use, whenever solution and container permit.

Compatibility and Stability: The compatibility of DORIBAX with other drugs has not been established. DORIBAX should not be mixed with or physically added to solutions containing other drugs.

Storage of Reconstituted Suspension: Upon reconstitution with sterile water for injection or 0.9% sodium chloride (normal saline) injection, DORIBAX suspension in the vial may be held for 1 hour prior to transfer and dilution in the infusion bag.

Storage of the Infusion Solution: Following dilution with normal saline or 5% dextrose, DORIBAX infusions stored at room temperature or under refrigeration should be completed according to the times in Table 5.

Table 5: DORIBAX

Storage of Infusion Solutions Prepared in Normal Saline or 5% Dextrose

Diluent	Stability Time (hours) Room Temp.	Stability Time (hours) 2–8°C (Refrigeration)
Normal saline	12	72[a]
5% Dextrose[b]	4	24[b,a]

[a] Once removed from the refrigerator, infusions should be completed within the room temperature stability time, provided the total refrigeration time, time to reach room temperature and infusion time does not exceed refrigeration stability time.
[b] 5% Dextrose should not be used for infusion durations longer than 1 hour.

Constituted DORIBAX suspension or DORIBAX infusion should not be frozen.

OVERDOSAGE:

Information on overdosage with DORIBAX in humans is not available. The highest total daily dose administered in Phase I clinical trials was 3 g (1 g every 8 hours) and no new safety concerns were identified. In the event of overdose, DORIBAX should be discontinued and general supportive treatment given until renal elimination takes place.

DORIBAX can be removed by hemodialysis. In subjects with end-stage renal disease administered DORIBAX 500 mg, the mean total recovery of doripenem and doripenem M-1 in the dialysate following a 4-hour hemodialysis session was 259 mg (52% of the dose). However, no information is available on the use of hemodialysis to treat overdosage.

For management of a suspected drug overdose, contact your regional Poison Control Centre. See the *CPS Directory* section for a list of Poison Control Centres.

ACTION AND CLINICAL PHARMACOLOGY: Doripenem is a synthetic broad spectrum beta-lactam carbapenem antibacterial agent with in vitro antibacterial activity against aerobic and anaerobic gram-positive and gram-negative bacteria.

Mechanism of Action: Doripenem exerts its bactericidal activity by inhibiting bacterial cell wall biosynthesis.

Interaction with Other Antimicrobials: In vitro, doripenem showed little potential to antagonize or be antagonized by other antibiotics.

Mechanisms of Resistance: Bacterial resistance mechanisms that affect doripenem include drug inactivation by carbapenem-hydrolyzing enzymes, mutant or acquired PBPs, decreased outer membrane permeability and active efflux. Doripenem is stable to hydrolysis by most beta-lactamases, including penicillinases and cephalosporinases produced by gram-positive and gram-negative bacteria, with the exception of carbapenem hydrolyzing beta-lactamases.

Pharmacodynamics: PK/PD Index: Similar to other beta-lactam antimicrobial agents, the time (% of the dosing interval) that the plasma concentration of free doripenem exceeds the MIC (%fT>MIC) of the infecting organism has been shown to best correlate with efficacy in nonclinical pharmacokinetic/pharmacodynamic studies. %fT>MIC (±SD) required to achieve a bacteriostatic effect, 1 $\log_{10}$ reduction and 2 $\log_{10}$ reduction in a neutropenic murine thigh infection model were 29% (±5.3), 36% (±7.4), and 43% (±7.1) respectively. Based on human pharmacokinetic modeling and simulations, extending the infusion time to 4 hours generally increases the %fT>MIC for the recommended dose Estimates of PK/PD target attainment rates are summarized in Table 6.

Table 6: DORIBAX

Estimated Target Attainment Rates (%) for DORIBAX PK/PD Target of 35% fT>MIC

Renal Function/ Dosing Regimen	MIC (µg/mL)	Infusion Time Creatinine Clearance (CrCl, mL/min) 1-hour infusion		4-hour infusion	
		CrCl=51 to 215 mL/min		CrCl=51 to 215 mL/min	
Normal Renal Function and Mild Renal Impairment/ 500 mg every 8 hours	1	91.8		100	
	2	68.4		100	
	4	25.3		90.0	
		CrCl=50	CrCl=30	CrCl=50	CrCl=30
Moderate Renal Impairment/250 mg every 8 hours	1	99.8	100	100	100
	2	91	99.8	99.9	100
	4	16.2	71.4	49.5	85.5
		CrCl=29	CrCl=10	CrCl=29	CrCl=10
Severe Renal Impairment/250 mg every 12 hours	1	99.4	100	100	100
	2	87.0	100	99.9	100
	4	14.8	97.5	40.8	98.7

PK/PD target of 35% fT>MIC corresponds to exposure required to achieve approximately 1 $\log_{10}$ reduction in a neutropenic murine thigh infection model.
PK data were obtained from 303 subjects, including 176 healthy volunteers, 109 patients with cUTI and pyelonephritis, and 18 patients with nosocomial pneumonia. A two-compartment model with zero- order input and first-order elimination best described the PK of doripenem following i.v. administration. 5000 subjects were simulated per Monte Carlo simulation scenario.

QT Study: In a randomized, positive- and placebo-controlled crossover QT study, 60 healthy subjects were administered DORIBAX 500 mg i.v. every 8 hours infused over 1 hour × 4 doses and DORIBAX 1g i.v. every 8 hours infused over 1 hour × 4 doses, placebo, and a single oral dose of positive control. At both the 500 mg and 1g doripenem doses, no significant effect on QTc interval was detected at peak plasma concentration or at any other time.

Pharmacokinetics: Plasma Concentrations: Average plasma concentrations (µg/mL) of doripenem following single 1-hour and 4-hour intravenous infusions of a 500 mg dose administered to healthy adult subjects with normal renal function (CrCL ≥80 mL/min) are presented in Table 7.

Table 7: DORIBAX

Plasma Concentrations of Doripenem After Single-Dose Administration

Dose and Infusion Duration	Time Relative to Start of Infusion (hour) / Average Plasma Concentration (µg/mL) 0.5	1	2	3	4	6	7	8	9
500 mg over 1 hour	20.2	20.9	6.13	2.69	1.41	0.45	—	0.13	—
500 mg over 4 hours	4.01	5.70	7.26	8.12	8.53	1.43	0.78	—	0.28

The pharmacokinetics of doripenem (C_{max} and AUC) are linear over a dose range of 500 mg to 1 g when intravenously infused over either 1 or 4 hours. There is no accumulation of doripenem following multiple intravenous infusions of either 500 mg or 1 g administered every 8 hours for 7 to 10 days in patients with normal renal function.

Plasma Pharmacokinetic Parameters: Mean (SD) plasma pharmacokinetic parameters of doripenem following multiple intravenous infusions of 500 mg administered every 8 hours over 30 minutes to healthy adult subjects with normal renal function (CrCL ≥80 mL/min) are presented in Table 8.

Table 8: DORIBAX

Plasma Pharmacokinetic Parameters of Doripenem After Multiple-Dose Administration

Parameter	500 mg Over 30 Minutes q8h
N	5
T_{max}[a] (h)	0.50 (0.50–0.50)
C_{max} (µg/mL)	31.4 (3.61)
AUC_τ (µg·h/mL)	35.5 (4.42)
$t_{1/2}$ (h)	0.872 (0.0723)
Accumulation Ratio[b]	0.926 (0.0808)

[a] Expressed as median (minimum-maximum).
[b] Calculated as AUC_τ (multiple-dose) divided by AUC_τ (single-dose).

Absorption: DORIBAX is administered intravenously and therefore has 100% bioavailability.

Distribution: The average binding of doripenem to plasma proteins is approximately 8.1% and is independent of plasma drug concentrations. The volume of distribution at steady state of doripenem is approximately 16.8 L, similar to extracellular fluid volume (18.2 L) in man. Doripenem penetrates well into several body fluids and tissues, achieving concentrations either matching or exceeding those required to inhibit most susceptible bacteria. Concentrations achieved in selected tissues and fluids following administration of DORIBAX are shown in Table 9.

Table 9: DORIBAX

Doripenem Concentrations in Selected Tissues and Fluids

Tissue or Fluid	Dose (mg)	Infusion Duration (h)	Number of Samples or Subjects[a]	Sampling Period	Concentration Range (µg/mL or µg/g)	Tissue- or Fluid-To-Plasma Concentration Ratio (%) Mean (Range)
Myometrium	250	0.5	20	40–360 min	BQL-9.04[b]	39.2 (0.00–85.9)
Cervix uteri	250	0.5	20	40–360 min	BQL-8.94[b]	37.5 (0.00–96.9)
Portio Vaginalis	250	0.5	20	40–360 min	BQL-9.89[b]	39.5 (0.00–123)
Endometrium	250	0.5	16	40–360 min	BQL-6.66[c]	37.8 (0.00–86.0)
Oviduct	250	0.5	20	40–360 min	BQL-10.6[d]	35.1 (0.00–106)
Ovary	250	0.5	12	40–360 min	BQL-4.83[e]	33.0 (0.00–108)
Retroperitoneal Fluid	250	0.5	9[f]	30–90 min[g]	3.15–52.4	80.8 (22.5–409)
	500	0.5	4[f]	240–240 min[g]	9.53–13.9	31.7 (25.4–44.7)
Prostate	250	0.5 or 1	8	60–160 min	0.760–10.3	81.3 (15.0–426)
	500	0.5 or 1	5	90–130 min	1.04–4.51	33.5 (18.7–49.9)
Peritoneal Exudates	250	0.5	5[f]	30–150 min[g]	2.36–5.17	25.1 (14.4–47.3)
Gallbladder	250	0.5	10	20–215 min	BQL-1.87[h]	8.02 (0.00–44.4)
Bile	250	0.5	10	20–215 min	BQL-15.4[d]	117 (0.00–611)
	500	0.5, 1 or 4	118	0–4 h	623 (BQL[e]-3360)[i]	—

(cont'd)

Table 9: DORIBAX *(cont'd)*

Doripenem Concentrations in Selected Tissues and Fluids

Tissue or Fluid	Dose (mg)	Infusion Duration (h)	Number of Samples or Subjects[a]	Sampling Period	Concentration Range (μg/mL or μg/g)	Tissue- or Fluid-To-Plasma Concentration Ratio (%) Mean (Range)
Urine	500	0.5, 1 or 4	118	4–8 h	47.1 (BQL[e]-635)[i]	—

[a] Unless stated otherwise, only one sample was collected per subject.
[b] Below quantitation limit (BQL) in 3 subjects.
[c] BQL in 2 subjects.
[d] BQL in 4 subjects.
[e] BQL in 1 subject.
[f] Serial samples were collected and maximal concentration is reported for each subject.
[g] t_{max} range.
[h] BQL in 6 subjects.
[i] Median (range) of average concentrations over the collection interval.

In addition, although clinical relevance is uncertain, concentrations approximating 3 μg/mL or μg/g or higher have been achieved in joint fluid, synovial membrane, bony tissue and skin tissue following a 250 mg dose of DORIBAX.

Metabolism: Metabolism of doripenem to a microbiologically inactive ring-opened metabolite occurs primarily via dehydropeptidase-I. No CYP450-mediated in vitro metabolism of doripenem could be detected in the presence or absence of NADPH.

Doripenem degraded less than 20% after a 90-minute incubation with recombinant human renal DHP-I similar to the rate for meropenem, whereas imipenem underwent extensive hydrolysis.

Excretion: Doripenem is primarily eliminated unchanged by the kidneys. Mean plasma terminal elimination half-life of doripenem in healthy young adults is approximately 1 hour and plasma clearance is approximately 15.9 L/hour. Mean renal clearance is 10.3 L/hour. The magnitude of this value, coupled with the significant decrease in the elimination of doripenem seen with concomitant probenecid administration, suggests that doripenem undergoes both glomerular filtration and tubular secretion. In healthy young adults given a single 500 mg dose of DORIBAX, 71% and 15% of the dose was recovered in urine as unchanged drug and ring-opened metabolite, respectively. Following the administration of a single 500 mg dose of radiolabeled doripenem to healthy young adults, less than 1 % of the total radioactivity was recovered in feces.

Special Populations and Conditions: Pediatrics: The pharmacokinetics of doripenem have not been established in patients under 18 years of age.

Geriatrics: The impact of age on the pharmacokinetics of doripenem was evaluated in healthy male and female subjects ≥66 years of age. Doripenem AUC increased 49% in elderly adults relative to young adults. These changes were mainly attributed to age-related changes in creatinine clearance. No dosage adjustment is recommended for elderly patients with normal renal function (see Dosage and Administration, Other).

Gender: The effect of gender on the pharmacokinetics of doripenem was evaluated in healthy male and female subjects. Doripenem AUC was 15% higher in females compared to males. No dose adjustment is recommended based on gender (see Dosage and Administration, Other).

Race: The effect of race on doripenem pharmacokinetics was examined through a population pharmacokinetic analysis. No significant difference in mean doripenem clearance was observed across race groups and therefore no dosage adjustment is recommended based on race (see Dosage and Administration, Other).

Hepatic Insufficiency: The pharmacokinetics of doripenem in patients with hepatic impairment have not been established. As doripenem does not appear to undergo hepatic metabolism, the pharmacokinetics of DORIBAX are not expected to be affected by hepatic impairment (see Dosage and Administration, Patients with Hepatic Impairment).

Renal Insufficiency: Following a single 500 mg dose of DORIBAX, AUC increased 1.6 fold, 2.8-fold, and 5.1 fold in subjects with mild (CrCl 51-79 mL/min), moderate (CrCl 31-50 mL/min), and severe renal impairment (CrCl ≤30 mL/min), respectively, compared to age-matched healthy subjects with normal renal function (CrCl ≥80 mL/min). Dosage adjustment is recommended in patients with moderate to severe renal impairment (see Dosage and Administration, Patients with Renal Impairment).

Plasma Pharmacokinetic Parameters in Subjects with Renal Impairment: Mean (SD) plasma pharmacokinetic parameters of doripenem following a single infusion of 500 mg doripenem administered over 1-hour in healthy volunteers with and without renal impairment are presented in Table 10.

Table 10: DORIBAX

Plasma Pharmacokinetic Parameters of Doripenem After Single-Dose (500 mg over 1 hour) Administration in Healthy Volunteers with and without Renal Impairment

PK Parameter	Normal Renal Function (CrCl ≥80 mL/min)	Mild Renal Impairment (CrCl 51–79 mL/min)	Moderate Renal Impairment (CrCl 31–50 mL/min)	Severe Renal Impairment (CrCl 10–30 mL/min)
Number of subjects	8	6	6	6
C_{max} (μg/mL)	31.7 (9.20)	41.3 (9.42)	38.5 (5.95)	36.4 (6.28)
t_{max} (h)[a]	0.5 (0.50–0.50)	0.5 (0.50–0.50)	0.5 (0.25–0.50)	0.5 (0.25–0.75)
AUC_{∞} (μg·h/mL)	37.3 (5.35)	61.4 (18.0)	106 (18.6)	190 (26.4)
$t_{1/2}$ (h)	1.11 (0.192)	1.31 (0.377)	2.67 (0.638)	4.62 (0.496)
CL (L/h)	13.7 (1.98)	8.64 (2.05)	4.84 (0.750)	2.68 (0.389)
V_{ss} (L)	16.5 (3.57)	13.3 (5.07)	15.7 (3.33)	16.8 (2.77)

[a] Expressed as median (minimum-maximum).

STORAGE AND STABILITY: DORIBAX vials should be stored at 15-30°C.

For infusion solution storage conditions, see Dosage and Administration, Compatibility and Stability, Storage of the Infusion Solution.

DORIBAX must be reconstituted and then further diluted prior to infusion (see Dosage and Administration, Administration).

INFORMATION FOR THE PATIENT: Published in e-CPS, available by subscription at www.e-cps.ca.

DOSAGE FORMS, COMPOSITION AND PACKAGING: Each vial of sterile powder contains: doripenem 500 mg (on an anhydrous basis). Sterile single use clear glass vials of 20 mL.

Dostinex™ Pr

cabergoline

Dopamine Receptor Agonist

Paladin

Date of Revision: May 15, 2009

SUMMARY PRODUCT INFORMATION:

Route of Administration	Dosage Form/ Strength	Clinically Relevant Nonmedicinal Ingredients
Oral	Tablet/0.5 mg	Leucine USP and Lactose anhydrous For a complete listing see Dosage Forms, Composition and Packaging.

INDICATIONS AND CLINICAL USE: DOSTINEX is indicated for:

- **Treatment of hyperprolactinemic disorders:** DOSTINEX (cabergoline) is indicated for the treatment of hyperprolactinemic disorders, either idiopathic or due to pituitary adenomas.
- **Inhibition of physiological lactation:** DOSTINEX (cabergoline) is indicated for the prevention of the onset of physiological lactation in the puerperium for clearly defined medical reasons.

These medical reasons may include birth of a still born baby, neonatal death, conditions interfering with suckling (cleft lip or palate of the baby), severe acute or chronic mental illness or medical conditions, maternal disease which may be transmitted to the baby that require medications which are excreted in the milk.

DOSTINEX is not indicated for the purpose of suppression of already established post partum lactation.

Geriatrics (>65 years of age): Very limited data concerning experience of treatment of hyperprolactinemia in the elderly are available. However, available data do not indicate a special risk for this population.

Pediatrics (<16 years of age): Safety and effectiveness of DOSTINEX in pediatric patients have not been established.

CONTRAINDICATIONS: DOSTINEX (cabergoline) is contraindicated in patients with:

- uncontrolled hypertension,
- a history of pulmonary, pericardial and retroperitoneal fibrotic disorders (see Warnings and Precautions),
- anatomical evidence of cardiac valvulopathy of any valve (eg, echocardiogram showing valve leaflet thickening, valve restriction, valve mixed restriction-stenosis). Echocardiogram is required at pretreatment in patients being treated for hyperprolactinemic disorders (see Warnings and Precautions),
- a known hypersensitivity to this drug or any ergot derivatives and to any ingredient in the formulation. For a complete listing, see Dosage Forms, Composition and Packaging.

WARNINGS AND PRECAUTIONS: General: Dopamine agonists in general should not be used in patients with pregnancy-induced hypertension, for example, preeclampsia and eclampsia, unless the potential benefit is judged to outweigh the possible risk.

Initial doses higher than 1 mg may produce orthostatic hypotension. Care should be exercised when administering DOSTINEX (cabergoline) with other medications known to lower blood pressure.

The effects of alcohol on overall tolerability of DOSTINEX are currently unknown.

Before DOSTINEX administration, pregnancy should be excluded and after treatment pregnancy should be prevented for at least one month.

Cardiovascular: DOSTINEX should be given with caution to subjects with cardiovascular disease and Raynaud's syndrome. Symptomatic hypotension can occur with DOSTINEX administration. Care should be exercised when administering DOSTINEX concomitantly with other drugs known to lower blood pressure.

Fibrosis: As with other ergot derivatives, pleural effusion/pulmonary fibrosis has been reported following long-term administration of cabergoline. Therefore, DOSTINEX should not be used in patients with a history of, or current signs and/or symptoms of respiratory or cardiac disorders linked to fibrotic tissue (see Contraindications). Erythrocyte sedimentation rate (ESR) has been found to be abnormally increased in association with pleural effusion/fibrosis. Chest x-ray examination is recommended in cases of unexplained ESR increases to abnormal values. Serum creatinine measurements can also be used to help in the diagnosis of fibrotic disorder. Following diagnosis of pleural effusion/pulmonary fibrosis, the discontinuance of cabergoline has been reported to result in improvement of signs and symptoms.

Treatment for Hyperprolactinemia: Before Initiating Treatment: All patients must undergo a cardiovascular evaluation, including echocardiogram to assess the potential presence of asymptomatic valvular disease. It is also appropriate to perform baseline investigations of erythrocyte sedimentation rate or other inflammatory markers, lung function/chest X-ray and renal function prior to initiation of therapy.

During Treatment: Fibrotic disorders can have an insidious onset and patients should be regularly monitored for possible manifestations of progressive fibrosis. Therefore, during treatment, attention should be paid to the signs and symptoms of:

- Pleuro-pulmonary disease such as dyspnoea, shortness of breath, persistent cough or chest pain.
- Renal insufficiency or ureteral/abdominal vascular obstruction that may occur with pain in the loin/flank and lower limb oedema as well as any possible abdominal masses or tenderness that may indicate retroperitoneal fibrosis.
- Cardiac failure: cases of valvular and pericardial fibrosis have often manifested as cardiac failure. Therefore, valvular fibrosis (and constrictive pericarditis) should be excluded if such symptoms occur.

Clinical diagnostic monitoring for development of fibrotic disorders, as appropriate, is essential.

Additional appropriate investigations such as erythrocyte sedimentation rate, and serum creatinine measurements should be performed if necessary to support a diagnosis of a fibrotic disorder.

The need for other clinical monitoring (e.g., physical examination including cardiac auscultation, X-ray, CT scan) should be determined on an individual basis.

Cardiac Valvulopathy: There have been post-marketing reports of cardiac valvulopathy involving one or more valves in patients taking DOSTINEX. The incidence of treatment emergent cardiac valvulopathy has not yet been determined, although some studies have suggested that the risk is cumulative, and asymptomatic cases of valvulopathy have been identified using echocardiography.

Valvulopathy has been reported with substantially greater frequency during treatment with ergot derivatives with 5-HT2B agonist activity, including cabergoline, compared to non-ergot dopamine agonists.

DOSTINEX is contraindicated in patients with a history of cardiac valvulopathy (see Contraindications). Physicians should inform patients/caregivers of the risk of cardiac valvulopathy.

Treatment of Hyperprolactinemia: Before Initiating Treatment: All patients must undergo a cardiovascular evaluation, including echocardiogram to assess the potential presence of asymptomatic valvular disease. In patients with valvular regurgitation, it is not known whether cabergoline treatment might worsen the underlying disease. If fibrotic valvular disease is detected, the patient should not be treated with cabergoline (see Contraindications).

During Treatment: Fibrotic disorders can have an insidious onset and patients should be regularly monitored for possible manifestations of progressive fibrosis. Therefore, during treatment, attention should be paid to the signs and symptoms of:

- Cardiac failure: cases of valvular and pericardial fibrosis have often manifested as cardiac failure. Therefore, valvular fibrosis (and constrictive pericarditis) should be excluded if such symptoms occur.

Following treatment initiation, the first echocardiogram must occur within 3-6 months; thereafter, the frequency of echocardiographic monitoring should be determined by appropriate individual clinical assessment with particular emphasis on the above-mentioned signs and symptoms, but must occur at least every 6 to 12 months.

Cabergoline should be discontinued if an echocardiogram reveals new or worsened valvular regurgitation, valvular restriction or valve leaflet thickening (see Contraindications).

The need for other clinical monitoring (e.g., physical examination including cardiac auscultation, X-ray, CT scan) should be determined on an individual basis.

Gastrointestinal: DOSTINEX should be given with caution to subjects with peptic ulcer and gastrointestinal bleeding.

Hepatic/Biliary/Pancreatic: Since cabergoline is extensively metabolised by the liver, caution should be used, and careful monitoring exercised, when administering DOSTINEX to patients with hepatic impairment.

Neurologic: Cabergoline has been associated with somnolence. Sudden sleep onset episodes that can be associated with dopamine agonists usually occur in patients with Parkinson's disease. A reduction of dosage or termination of therapy may be considered.

Patients being treated with cabergoline should be warned of the potential for experiencing somnolence. Patients should be cautioned about engaging in activities where impaired alertness may put themselves or others at risk of serious injury or death (e.g. operating machines) in case somnolence does occur.

Psychiatric: DOSTINEX should be given with caution to subjects with a history of mental disease. Particular care should be taken when patients are taking concomitant psychoactive medication (see Drug Interactions).

Pathological gambling, aggression, psychotic behavior, increased libido, and hypersexuality have been reported in patients treated with dopamine agonists including cabergoline. This has been generally reversible upon reduction of the dose or treatment discontinuation.

Renal: DOSTINEX should be given with caution to subjects with renal insufficiency.

Special Populations: Pregnant Women: Reproduction studies have been performed with cabergoline in mice, rats, and rabbits administered by gavage. There are, however, no adequate and well-controlled studies in pregnant women. Because animal reproduction studies are not always predictive of human response, this drug should be used during pregnancy only if clearly needed. Before DOSTINEX administration, pregnancy should be excluded and after treatment pregnancy should be prevented for at least one month.

Nursing Women: Based on information from animal studies, excretion in human milk is very likely. Because many drugs are excreted in human milk and because of the potential for serious adverse reactions in nursing infants from cabergoline, a decision should be made whether to discontinue nursing or to discontinue the drug, taking into account the importance of the drug to the mother.

Due to this interference with lactation, DOSTINEX should not be given to women postpartum who are breastfeeding or who are planning to breastfeed.

Pediatrics: Safety and effectiveness of DOSTINEX in pediatric patients have not been established.

Geriatrics: Very limited data concerning experience of treatment of hyperprolactinemia in the elderly are available. However, available data do not indicate a special risk for this population.

Monitoring and Laboratory Tests: Erythrocyte sedimentation rate (ESR) has been found to be abnormally increased in association with pleural effusion/fibrosis. Chest x-ray examination is recommended in cases of unexplained ESR increases to abnormal values. Serum creatinine measurements can also be used to help in the diagnosis of fibrotic disorder.

Treatment of Hyperprolactinemia: Before Initiating Treatment: All patients must undergo a cardiovascular evaluation, including echocardiogram to assess the potential presence of asymptomatic valvular disease. It is also appropriate to perform baseline investigations of erythrocyte sedimentation rate or other inflammatory markers, lung function/chest X-ray and renal function prior to initiation of therapy. In patients with valvular regurgitation, it is not known whether cabergoline treatment might worsen the underlying disease. If fibrotic valvular disease is detected, the patient should not be treated with cabergoline (see Contraindications).

During Treatment: Fibrotic disorders can have an insidious onset and patients should be regularly monitored for possible manifestations of progressive fibrosis. Therefore, during treatment, attention should be paid to the signs and symptoms of:

- Pleuro-pulmonary disease such as dyspnoea, shortness of breath, persistent cough or chest pain.
- Renal insufficiency or ureteral/abdominal vascular obstruction that may occur with pain in the loin/flank and lower limb oedema as well as any possible abdominal masses or tenderness that may indicate retroperitoneal fibrosis.
- Cardiac failure: cases of valvular and pericardial fibrosis have often manifested as cardiac failure. Therefore, valvular fibrosis (and constrictive pericarditis) should be excluded if such symptoms occur.

Clinical diagnostic monitoring for development of fibrotic disorders, as appropriate, is essential. Following treatment initiation, the first echocardiogram must occur within 3-6 months; thereafter, the frequency of echocardiographic monitoring should be determined by appropriate individual clinical assessment with particular emphasis on the above-mentioned signs and symptoms, but must occur at least every 6 to 12 months.

Cabergoline should be discontinued if an echocardiogram reveals new or worsened valvular regurgitation, valvular restriction or valve leaflet thickening (see Contraindications).

The need for other clinical monitoring (e.g., physical examination including cardiac auscultation, X-ray, CT scan) should be determined on an individual basis.

Additional appropriate investigations such as erythrocyte sedimentation rate, and serum creatinine measurements should be performed if necessary to support a diagnosis of a fibrotic disorder.

Information to Be Provided to the Patient: A patient should be instructed to notify her physician if she suspects she is pregnant, becomes pregnant, or intends to become pregnant during therapy. A pregnancy test should be done if there is any suspicion of pregnancy and continuation of treatment should be discussed with her physician.

ADVERSE REACTIONS: Adverse Drug Reaction Overview: Hyperprolactinemic Disorders: The safety of DOSTINEX (cabergoline) has been evaluated in more than 900 patients with hyperprolactinemic disorders. Most adverse events were mild or moderate in severity (see Table 1 and Table 2 for the incidence of most common adverse events during the placebo-controlled studies). The most common adverse events were nausea, headache and dizziness and the most common reason for discontinuation was dizziness.

Inhibition of Physiological Lactation: Most side effects were transient and mild to moderate in severity. In women treated for **inhibition** of physiologic lactation the most frequently occurring adverse events were asymptomatic decreases in blood pressure, dizziness/vertigo, headache, nausea, and abdominal pain. In addition, on rare occasions, palpitations, epigastric pain, somnolence, epistaxis, and transient hemianopia have been reported (see Warnings and Precautions).

Clinical Trial Adverse Drug Reactions: Because clinical trials are conducted under very specific conditions the adverse reaction rates observed in the clinical trials may not reflect the rates observed in practice and should not be compared to the rates in the clinical trials of another drug. Adverse drug reaction information from clinical trials is useful for identifying drug-related adverse events and for approximating rates.

Hyperprolactinemic Disorders: In a 4 week, double-blind, placebo-controlled study, treatment consisted of placebo or cabergoline at fixed doses of 0.125, 0.5, 0.75, or 1 mg twice weekly. Doses were halved during the first week. Since a possible dose-related effect was observed for nausea only, the four cabergoline treatment groups have been combined. The incidence of the most common adverse events during the placebo-controlled study is presented in Table 1.

Table 1: DOSTINEX

Incidence of Reported Adverse Events During the 4-Week, Double-Blind, Placebo-Controlled Trial

Adverse Event[a]	Cabergoline (n=168) 0.125 to 1 mg 2 times a week	Placebo (n=20)
	Number (%)	
Gastrointestinal		
Nausea	45 (27)	4 (20)
Constipation	15 (10)	0
Abdominal pain	9 (5)	1 (5)
Dyspepsia	4 (2)	0
Vomiting	4 (2)	0
Central and Peripheral Nervous Systems		
Headache	43 (26)	5 (25)
Dizziness	25 (15)	1 (5)
Paresthesia	2 (1)	0
Vertigo	2 (1)	0
Body as a Whole		
Asthenia	15 (9)	2 (10)
Fatigue	12 (7)	0
Hot flashes	2 (1)	1 (5)
Psychiatric		
Somnolence	9 (5)	1 (5)
Depression	5 (3)	1 (5)
Nervousness	4 (2)	0
Autonomic Nervous System		
Postural hypotension	6 (4)	0
Reproductive—Female		
Breast pain	2 (1)	0
Dysmenorrhea	2 (1)	0
Vision		
Abnormal vision	2 (1)	0

[a] Reported at ≥1% for cabergoline.

In the 8-week, double-blind period of the comparative trial with bromocriptine, DOSTINEX (at a dose of 0.5 mg twice weekly) was discontinued due to an adverse event in 4 of 221 patients (2%) while bromocriptine (at a dose of 2.5 mg two times a day) was discontinued due to an adverse event in 14 of 231 patients (6%). The most common reasons for discontinuation from DOSTINEX were headache, nausea and vomiting (3, 2 and 2 patients respectively); the most common reasons for discontinuation from bromocriptine were nausea, vomiting, headache, and dizziness or vertigo (10, 3, 3, and 3 patients respectively). The incidence of the most common adverse events during the double-blind portion of the comparative trial with bromocriptine is presented in Table 2.

Table 2: DOSTINEX

Incidence of Reported Adverse Events During the 8-Week, Double-Blind Period of the Comparative Trial with Bromocriptine

Adverse Event[a]	Cabergoline (n=221)	Bromocriptine (n=231)
	Number (%)	
Gastrointestinal		
Nausea	63 (29)	100 (43)
Constipation	15 (7)	21 (9)
Abdominal pain	12 (5)	19 (8)
Dyspepsia	11 (5)	16 (7)
Vomiting	9 (4)	16 (7)
Dry mouth	5 (2)	2 (1)
Diarrhea	4 (2)	7 (3)
Flatulence	4 (2)	3 (1)
Throat irritation	2 (1)	0
Toothache	2 (1)	0
Central and Peripheral Nervous Systems		
Headache	58 (26)	62 (27)
Dizziness	38 (17)	42 (18)
Vertigo	9 (4)	10 (4)
Paresthesia	5 (2)	6 (3)
Body as a Whole		
Asthenia	13 (6)	15 (6)
Fatigue	10 (5)	18 (8)
Syncope	3 (1)	3 (1)
Influenza-like symptoms	2 (1)	0
Malaise	2 (1)	0
Periorbital edema	2 (1)	2 (1)
Peripheral edema	2 (1)	1
Psychiatric		

(cont'd)

Table 2: DOSTINEX *(cont'd)*

Incidence of Reported Adverse Events During the 8-Week, Double-Blind Period of the Comparative Trial with Bromocriptine

	Cabergoline (n=221)	Bromocriptine (n=231)
Adverse Event[a]	**Number (%)**	
Depression	7 (3)	5 (2)
Somnolence	5 (2)	5 (2)
Anorexia	3 (1)	3 (1)
Anxiety	3 (1)	3 (1)
Insomnia	3 (1)	2 (1)
Impaired concentration	2 (1)	1
Nervousness	2 (1)	5 (2)
Cardiovascular		
Hot flashes	6 (3)	3 (1)
Hypotension	3 (1)	4 (2)
Dependent edema	2 (1)	1
Palpitation	2 (1)	5 (2)
Reproductive—Female		
Breast pain	5 (2)	8 (3)
Dysmenorrhea	2 (1)	1
Skin and Appendages		
Acne	3 (1)	0
Pruritus	2 (1)	1
Musculoskeletal		
Pain	4 (2)	6 (3)
Arthralgia	2 (1)	0
Respiratory		
Rhinitis	2 (1)	9 (4)
Vision		
Abnormal vision	2 (1)	2 (1)

[a] Reported at ≥1% for cabergoline.

Less Common Clinical Trial Adverse Drug Reactions (<1%): Hyperprolactinemic Disorders: Body as a Whole: facial edema, influenza-like symptoms, malaise.
Cardiovascular System: hypotension, syncope, palpitations.
Digestive System: dry mouth, flatulence, diarrhea, anorexia.
Metabolic and Nutritional Systems: weight loss, weight gain.
Nervous System: somnolence, nervousness, paresthesia, insomnia, anxiety.
Respiratory System: nasal stuffiness, epistaxis.
Skin and Appendages: acne, pruritus.
Special Senses: abnormal vision.
Urogenital System: dysmenorrhea, increased libido.
Other Conditions: The safety of cabergoline has been evaluated in approximately 1200 patients with Parkinson's disease in controlled and uncontrolled studies at dosages of up to 11.5 mg/day which greatly exceeds the maximum recommended dosage of cabergoline for hyperprolactinemic disorders. In addition to the adverse events that occurred in the patients with hyperprolactinemic disorders, the most common adverse events in patients with Parkinson's disease were dyskinesia, hallucinations, confusion, peripheral edema and sudden onset sleep. Heart failure, pleural effusion, pulmonary fibrosis, and gastric or duodenal ulcer occurred rarely. One case of constrictive pericarditis has been reported.
Post-Market Adverse Drug Reactions: The following events have been reported in patients who have received cabergoline: aggression, alopecia, blood creatinine phosphokinase increased, delusions, dyspnea, edema, congenital abnormalities, fibrosis, hepatic function abnormal, hypersensitivity reaction, hypersexuality, increased libido, liver function tests abnormal, pathological gambling, psychotic disorder, rash, respiratory disorder, respiratory failure, sudden sleep onset, valvulopathy. It should be noted that the uncontrolled nature of post-marketing surveillance makes it difficult to determine definitively if a reported event was actually caused by cabergoline, or to reliably assess causation in individual cases (see Warnings and Precautions).

The prevalence of asymptomatic valvular regurgitation is significantly greater than that of non-ergot dopamine agonists (see Contraindications and Warnings and Precautions).

DRUG INTERACTIONS: Overview: Ergot-alkaloids: Although there is no conclusive evidence of an interaction between DOSTINEX (cabergoline) and other ergot alkaloids, the concomitant use of these medications during long-term treatment with DOSTINEX is not recommended.
Dopamine Antagonists: Since DOSTINEX exerts its therapeutic effect by direct stimulation of dopamine receptors, it should not be concurrently administered with drugs that have dopamine-antagonist activity (such as phenothiazines, butyrophenones, thioxanthenes, metoclopramide) since these might reduce the prolactin-lowering effect of DOSTINEX.
Macrolide Antibiotics: By analogy with ergot derivatives, DOSTINEX should not be used in association with macrolide antibiotics (e.g., erythromycin) since systemic bioavailability and also adverse effects could increase.
Drug-Food Interactions: Food is not noted to affect the absorption of DOSTINEX (see Dosage and Administration, Dosing Considerations and Action and Clinical Pharmacology, Pharmacokinetics).

DOSAGE AND ADMINISTRATION: Dosing Considerations: Since the tolerability of this class of compounds is improved when administered with food, it is recommended, that DOSTINEX (cabergoline) be taken with meals, for all the therapeutic indications. Food is not noted to affect the absorption of DOSTINEX (see Drug Interactions, Drug-Food Interactions, Action and Clinical Pharmacology, Pharmacokinetics).

Recommended Dose and Dosage Adjustment: Adults: Treatment of Hyperprolactinaemia: The recommended initial dosage of DOSTINEX is 0.5 mg per week given in one or two (one-half of one 0.5 mg tablet) doses (e.g. on Monday and Thursday) per week. The weekly dose should be increased gradually, preferably by adding 0.5 mg per week at monthly intervals until an optimal therapeutic response is achieved. The therapeutic dosage is usually 1 mg per week and ranges from 0.25 mg to 2 mg per week.

The weekly dose may be given as a single administration or divided into two or more doses per week according to patient tolerability. Division of the weekly dose into multiple administrations is advised when doses higher than 1 mg per week are to be given, since the tolerability of doses greater than 1 mg taken as a single weekly dose has been evaluated only in a few patients.

Patients should be evaluated during dose escalation to determine the lowest dosage that produces the therapeutic response. Monitoring of serum prolactin levels at monthly intervals is advised since, once the effective therapeutic dosage regimen has been reached, serum prolactin normalisation is usually observed within 2 to 4 weeks.

After a normal serum prolactin level has been maintained for 6 months, DOSTINEX may be discontinued, with periodic monitoring of the serum prolactin level to determine whether or when treatment with DOSTINEX should be reinstituted.
Missed Dose: If a dose of this medication has been missed, it should be taken as soon as possible. However, if it is almost time (e.g. 1 day) before the next dose, skip the missed dose and go back to the regular dosing schedule. Do not double doses.
Inhibition of Physiological Lactation: For **inhibition of physiological lactation** the recommended therapeutic dosage is 1 mg (two 0.5 mg tablets) given as a single dose. DOSTINEX should be administered during the first day post-partum.
Administration: DOSTINEX is to be administered by the oral route.

OVERDOSAGE:
There is no experience with DOSTINEX (cabergoline) in humans of overdosage when used in the proposed indications. Doses of DOSTINEX up to 4.5 mg per week have been used in hyperprolactinemic patients. Symptoms of overdose would likely be those of over-stimulation of dopamine receptors. These might include nausea, vomiting, gastric complaints, hypotension, or thought/perception disturbances (hallucinations), nasal congestion and syncope.

General supportive measures should be undertaken to remove any unabsorbed drug and maintain blood pressure if necessary. In addition, the administration of dopamine antagonist drug may be advisable. Measures to support blood pressure should be taken if necessary.

For management of a suspected drug overdose, contact your **regional Poison Control Centre**. See the *CPS* Directory section for a list of Poison Control Centres.

ACTION AND CLINICAL PHARMACOLOGY: Mechanism of Action: Cabergoline, the active ingredient in DOSTINEX (cabergoline), is a dopaminergic ergoline derivative endowed with a potent and long-lasting prolactin-lowering activity. It acts by direct stimulation of the D_2-dopamine receptors on pituitary lactotrophs, thus inhibiting prolactin secretion. In rats the compound decreases prolactin secretion at oral doses of 3 to 25 μg/kg, and in vitro at a concentration of 45 pg/mL. In addition, cabergoline exerts a central dopaminergic effect via D_2 receptor stimulation at oral doses higher than those effective in lowering serum prolactin levels.
Pharmacodynamics: The long-lasting prolactin-lowering effect of cabergoline is probably due to its long persistence in the target organ as suggested by the slow elimination of total radioactivity from the pituitary after a single oral dose in rats ($t_{½}$ of approximately 60 hours).

The pharmacodynamic effects of cabergoline have been studied in healthy volunteers, puerperal women and hyperprolactinemic patients. After a single oral administration of cabergoline (0.3 to 1.5 mg), a significant decrease in serum prolactin levels was observed in each of the populations studied. The effect is prompt (within 3 hours from administration) and persistent (up to 7 to 28 days in healthy volunteers and hyperprolactinemic patients, and up to 14 to 21 days in puerperal women). The prolactin lowering effect is dose-related both in terms of degree of effect and duration of action.

With regard to the endocrine effects of cabergoline not related to the antiprolactinemic effect, available data from humans confirm the experimental findings in animals indicating that the test compound is endowed with a selective action with no effect on basal secretion of other pituitary hormones or cortisol. The pharmacodynamic actions of cabergoline not correlated with the therapeutic effect relate only to blood pressure decrease. The maximal hypotensive effect of a single dose usually occurs during the first 6 hours after drug intake and is dose-dependent both in terms of maximal decrease and frequency.
Pharmacokinetics: The pharmacokinetic and metabolic profiles of cabergoline have been studied in healthy volunteers of both sexes and in female hyperprolactinemic patients.
Absorption: After oral administration of the labeled compound, radioactivity was rapidly absorbed from the gastrointestinal tract as the peak of radioactivity in plasma was between 0.5 and 4 hours. Ten days after administration, about 18% and 72% of the radioactive dose of ^{14}C cabergoline was recovered in the urine and feces, respectively. Unchanged drug in urine accounted for 2% to 3% of the dose. Food does not appear to affect absorption and disposition of cabergoline.
Distribution: In vitro experiments showed that the drug at concentrations of 0.1 to 10 ng/mL is 41% to 42% bound to plasma proteins.
Metabolism: In urine, the main metabolite identified was 6-allyl-8b-carboxy-ergoline, which accounted for 4% to 6% of the dose. Three additional metabolites were identified in urine, which accounted overall for less than 3% of the dose. The metabolites have been found to be much less potent than cabergoline in inhibiting prolactin secretion in vitro.

The pharmacokinetics of cabergoline were found to be dose independent in healthy volunteers at doses of 0.5 to 1.5 mg. On the basis of the elimination half-life, steady state conditions should be achieved after 4 weeks, as confirmed by the mean peak plasma levels of cabergoline obtained after a single dose (37±8 pg/mL) and after a 4-week multiple-dose regimen (101±43 pg/mL). While renal insufficiency has been shown not to modify cabergoline kinetics, hepatic insufficiency of severe degree (>10 Child Pugh score, maximum score 12) has been shown to be associated with an increase of AUC.
Excretion: The low urinary excretion of unchanged cabergoline has been confirmed also in studies with non radioactive product. The elimination half-life of cabergoline, estimated from urinary excretion rates, is long (63 to 68 hours in healthy volunteers and 79 to 115 hours in hyperprolactinemic patients as assessed by radioimmunoassay).
Special Populations and Conditions: Renal Insufficiency: The pharmacokinetics of cabergoline were not altered in patients with moderate-to-severe renal insufficiency as assessed by creatinine clearance.
Hepatic Insufficiency: Hepatic insufficiency of severe degree (>10 Child Pugh score, maximum score 12) has been shown to be associated with an increase of AUC (about six-fold).

STORAGE AND STABILITY: Store at controlled room temperature 15 to 25°C.

SPECIAL HANDLING INSTRUCTIONS: Not applicable.

INFORMATION FOR THE PATIENT: Published in e-CPS, available by subscription at www.e-cps.ca.

DOSAGE FORMS, COMPOSITION AND PACKAGING: Each white, scored, capsule-shaped tablet, scored on one side, with the letter P and the letter U on either side of the breakline and the number 700 engraved on the other side of the tablet, contains: cabergoline 0.5 mg. Nonmedicinal ingredients: lactose anhydrous and leucine. Bottles of 8.

(Shown in Product Identification Section)

Dovobet®

calcipotriol—betamethasone dipropionate

Topical Antipsoriatic Agent—Vitamin D Analogue—Corticosteroid

LEO Pharma

Date of Preparation: June 26, 2001
Date of Revision: November 5, 2008

SUMMARY PRODUCT INFORMATION:

Route of Administration	Dosage Form/Strength	Clinically Relevant Nonmedicinal Ingredients
Topical	Ointment, 50 μg/g calcipotriol and 0.5 mg/g betamethasone (as dipropionate)	None For a complete listing see Dosage Forms, Composition and Packaging.

INDICATIONS AND CLINICAL USE: DOVOBET (calcipotriol and betamethasone dipropionate) ointment is indicated for:

- The topical treatment of psoriasis vulgaris for up to 4 weeks.
- DOVOBET should not be used on the face.

CONTRAINDICATIONS:
- Patients who are hypersensitive to DOVOBET (calcipotriol and betamethasone dipropionate), to any ingredient in the formulation or to components of the tube. For a complete listing, see Dosage Forms, Composition and Packaging.
- Ophthalmic use
- treatment of viral, fungal or bacterial skin infections, tuberculosis of the skin, syphilitic skin infections, chicken pox, eruptions following vaccinations, and in viral diseases such as herpes simplex, varicella and vaccinia.

WARNINGS AND PRECAUTIONS: General: If DOVOBET (calcipotriol and betamethasone dipropionate) is used in excess of the maximum recommended weekly amount of 100 g, it is important to monitor the serum calcium levels at regular intervals due to the risk of hypercalcemia secondary to excessive absorption of calcipotriol. If the serum calcium level becomes elevated, therapy should be discontinued and the serum calcium level monitored until it returns to normal.

Carcinogenesis and Mutagenesis: Calcipotriol when used in combination with ultraviolet radiation (UVR) may enhance the known skin carcinogenic effect of UVR.

Endocrine and Metabolism: Application on large areas of damaged skin, under occlusive dressings, or in skin folds should be avoided since it increases systemic absorption of corticosteroids and the risk of adverse effects such as adrenal suppression with the potential for glucocorticosteroid insufficiency after withdrawal of treatment. Manifestations of Cushing's syndrome, hyperglycaemia and glucosuria can also be produced in some patients by systemic absorption of topical corticosteroids. Occlusive dressings should not be applied if body temperature is elevated.

All of the adverse effects associated with systemic use of corticosteroids, including adrenal suppression, may also occur following topical administration of corticosteroid containing products such as DOVOBET, especially in children.

Skin: DOVOBET should not be used on the face since this may give rise to itching and erythema of the facial skin. Patients should be instructed to wash their hands after each application of DOVOBET in order to avoid inadvertent transfer to the face. Should facial dermatitis develop in spite of these precautions, DOVOBET therapy should be discontinued.

Prolonged use of corticosteroid-containing preparations may produce striae or atrophy of the skin or subcutaneous tissues. Therefore, it is recommended that corticosteroid treatment be interrupted periodically, and that one area of the body be treated at a time. Topical corticosteroids should be used with caution on lesions of the face, groin and axillae as these areas are more prone to atrophic changes than other areas of the body. If skin atrophy occurs, discontinue treatment. There may be a risk of rebound psoriasis when discontinuing corticosteroids after prolonged periods of use (see Adverse Reactions).

Special Populations: Pregnant Women: The safety of calcipotriol and/or topical corticosteroids for use during pregnancy has not been established. Although studies in experimental animals have not shown teratogenic effects with calcipotriol, studies with corticosteroids have shown teratogenic effects. The use of DOVOBET is not recommended in pregnant women.

Nursing Women: The safety of calcipotriol and/or topical corticosteroids for use in nursing women has not been established. It is not known whether calcipotriol can be excreted in breast milk or if topical application of corticosteroids can lead to sufficient systemic absorption to produce detectable quantities in breast milk. The use of DOVOBET is not recommended in nursing women.

Pediatrics (<18 years of age): There is no clinical trial experience with the use of DOVOBET in children. Children may demonstrate greater susceptibility to systemic steroid related adverse effects due to a larger skin surface area to body weight ratio as compared to adults.

Monitoring and Laboratory Tests: Treatment with DOVOBET (calcipotriol and betamethasone dipropionate) in the recommended amounts (see Dosage and Administration) does not generally result in changes in laboratory values. However, in patients at risk for hypercalcaemia it is recommended that baseline serum calcium levels be obtained before starting treatment with subsequent monitoring of serum calcium levels at suitable intervals. If serum calcium becomes elevated, DOVOBET administration should be discontinued and serum calcium levels should be measured once weekly until they return to normal. Patients with marginally elevated serum calcium may be treated with DOVOBET, provided that serum calcium is monitored at suitable intervals.

ADVERSE REACTIONS: In clinical trials, the most common adverse reaction associated with DOVOBET (calcipotriol and betamethasone dipropionate) was pruritus. Pruritus was usually mild and no patients were withdrawn from treatment.

Calcipotriol is associated with local reactions such as transient lesional and perilesional irritation. Rare cases of hypersensitivity reaction have been reported. Hypercalcemia can develop but is usually related to excessive administration (i.e. greater than the recommended weekly amount of 100 g ointment or 5 mg calcipotriol—see Dosage and Administration).

Topical corticosteroids can cause the same spectrum of adverse effects associated with systemic steroid administration, including adrenal suppression. Adverse effects associated with topical corticosteroids are generally local and include dryness, itching, burning, local irritation, striae, atrophy of the skin or subcutaneous tissues, telangiectasia, hypertrichosis, folliculitis, skin hypopigmentation, allergic contact dermatitis, maceration of the skin, miliaria, or secondary infection. If applied to the face, acne rosacea or perioral dermatitis can occur. In addition, there are reports of the development of pustular psoriasis from chronic plaque psoriasis following reduction or discontinuation of potent topical corticosteroid products.

In a randomized, double-blind, parallel group, safety study of psoriasis patients with at least moderate disease severity, DOVOBET ointment was used intermittently on an 'as needed' basis under medical supervision (N=207). Patients were followed for up to 52 weeks. The median amount of study drug used was 15.4 g/week. The effects of DOVOBET ointment on calcium metabolism were not studied and the effects on adrenal suppression were not adequately studied. The following adverse drug reactions were reported in 1% or more of patients: pruritus (5.8%), psoriasis (5.3%), skin atrophy (based on a dermatologist's visual assessment) (1.9%), folliculitis (1.9%), burning sensation (1.4%), skin depigmentation (1.4%), and erythema (1.0%). One case of serious flare-up of psoriasis was reported.

DRUG INTERACTIONS: There is no experience of concomitant therapy with other antipsoriatic drugs.

DOSAGE AND ADMINISTRATION: Dosing Considerations:
- DOVOBET (calcipotriol and betamethasone dipropionate) is **for topical use only** and not for ophthalmic use.
- There is no clinical trial experience with the use of DOVOBET in children.

Recommended Dose and Dosage Adjustment: DOVOBET should be applied topically to the affected areas once daily for up to 4 weeks. After satisfactory improvement has occurred, the drug can be discontinued. If recurrence takes place after discontinuation, treatment may be reinstituted.

The maximum recommended adult dose of DOVOBET ointment is 100 g per week.

Missed Dose: If a dose is missed, the patient should apply DOVOBET as soon as he/she remembers and then continue on as usual.

OVERDOSAGE:

Due to the calcipotriol component of DOVOBET (calcipotriol and betamethasone dipropionate), excessive administration (i.e. more than the recommended weekly amount of 100 g) may cause elevated serum calcium, which rapidly subsides when treatment is discontinued. In such cases, it is recommended to monitor serum calcium levels once weekly until they return to normal.

Excessive or prolonged use of topical corticosteroids can suppress pituitary-adrenal function, resulting in secondary adrenal insufficiency and manifestations of hypercorticoidism, including Cushing's disease. Recovery is usually prompt and complete upon steroid discontinuation. In cases of chronic toxicity, slow withdrawal of corticosteroids is recommended.

> For management of a suspected drug overdose, CPhA recommends that you contact your **regional Poison Control Centre**. See the *CPS* Directory section for a list of Poison Control Centres.

ACTION AND CLINICAL PHARMACOLOGY: Mechanism of Action: DOVOBET is a combination of the vitamin D analogue calcipotriol and the corticosteroid betamethasone dipropionate.

Calcipotriol is a non-steroidal antipsoriatic agent, derived from the naturally occurring vitamin D. Calcipotriol exhibits a vitamin D-like effect by competing for the $1,25(OH)_2D_3$ receptor. Calcipotriol is as potent as $1,25(OH)_2D_3$, the naturally occurring active form of vitamin D, in regulating cell proliferation and cell differentiation, but much less active than $1,25(OH)_2D_3$ in its effect on calcium metabolism. Calcipotriol induces differentiation and suppresses proliferation of keratinocytes (without any evidence of a cytotoxic effect), thus reversing the abnormal keratinocyte changes in psoriasis. The therapeutic goal envisaged with calcipotriol is thus a normalization of epidermal growth.

Topical corticosteroids such as betamethasone dipropionate have anti-inflammatory, anti-pruritic, and vasoconstrictive properties. The mechanism of the anti-inflammatory activity is generally unclear. However, corticosteroids are thought to induce phospholipase A_2 inhibitor proteins, preventing arachidonic acid release and the biosynthesis of potent mediators of inflammation.

Clinical Pharmacology : A large multicentre, randomized, double-blind clinical trial has shown DOVOBET ointment (50 µg/g calcipotriol plus 0.5 mg/g betamethasone (as dipropionate)) administered twice daily to be more efficacious and to provide faster onset of action than either of the individual components alone (calcipotriol or betamethasone dipropionate) for the treatment of plaque psoriasis. These findings were supported by a second large, multicentre, randomised, double-blind trial comparing DOVOBET twice daily to calcipotriol and betamethasone dipropionate, each in their currently marketed formulations. A third large, multicentre, randomised, double-blind trial found DOVOBET once daily to be more efficacious than vehicle alone and calcipotriol twice daily (betamethasone alone was not evaluated). It was also demonstrated that once daily DOVOBET was similar to twice daily DOVOBET for most of the efficacy measures. In all three studies, DOVOBET was effective in terms of reducing PASI (Psoriasis Area and Severity Index) score and thickness of target lesions. Furthermore, a significant proportion of patients on DOVOBET achieved marked improvement or clearance at the end of 4 weeks of treatment. Clinical improvement occurred rapidly and a significant improvement was evident within 1 week of treatment. DOVOBET was well tolerated with the most common adverse reaction being mild pruritus. In one additional study, patients were treated with DOVOBET once daily for 8 weeks. Optimal population results in this study were seen between 4 and 5 weeks of treatment. The therapeutic goal envisioned with DOVOBET is to provide an effective, rapid acting topical agent for initial treatment of psoriasis and/or for treatment of flare-ups of psoriasis.

Pharmacokinetics: A pharmacokinetic study of calcipotriol ointment demonstrated that the apparent systemic absorption over 12 hours is approximately 5.5% of the dose in normal subjects and in psoriatic patients. Topical application of corticosteroids to normal skin results in minimal absorption. Only small amounts of drug reach the dermis and are then absorbed into the systemic circulation. However, absorption may be greater when corticosteroids are applied to certain areas of the body (such as the axilla and scrotum) or if the epidermis is damaged by disease or inflammation. Continued absorption of corticosteroids may occur, even after washing, due to retention of the drug in the stratum corneum. The individual pharmacokinetics of calcipotriol and betamethasone dipropionate, are not affected by their combined presence in DOVOBET ointment. Under normal conditions of use, systemic absorption of calcipotriol and/or betamethasone from DOVOBET is not expected to have any effects.

STORAGE AND STABILITY: Store at 5 to 25°C. Use within 12 months of first opening the tube. For easy application do not refrigerate, this is to prevent pulling of delicate skin.

INFORMATION FOR THE PATIENT: Published in e-CPS, available by subscription at www.e-cps.ca.

DOSAGE FORMS, COMPOSITION AND PACKAGING: Each g of faintly translucent white to yellowish ointment contains: calcipotriol 50 µg plus betamethasone (as dipropionate) 0.5 mg. Nonmedicinal ingredients: alpha-tocopherol, liquid paraffin, polyoxypropylene-15-stearyl ether and white soft paraffin. Lacquered aluminium tubes of 60 and 120 g (equipped with an aluminium membrane).

Dovonex® Ⓟ
calcipotriol
Topical Nonsteroidal Antipsoriatic

LEO Pharma

Date of Preparation: October 27, 1992
Date of Revision: April 29, 2010

SUMMARY PRODUCT INFORMATION:

Route of Administration	Dosage Form/ Strength	Clinically Relevant Nonmedicinal Ingredients
Topical	Ointment and Cream, 50 µg/g calcipotriol Scalp solution, 50 µg/mL calcipotriol	None For a complete listing see Dosage Forms, Composition and Packaging.

INDICATIONS AND CLINICAL USE: DOVONEX (calcipotriol) cream and ointment is indicated for:
- the topical treatment of psoriasis
- combination use with a moderate to very potent topical corticosteroid, cyclosporin A or acitretin.

DOVONEX scalp solution is indicated for:
- the topical treatment of scalp psoriasis.

DOVONEX cream, ointment and scalp solution are not generally recommended for severe extensive psoriasis.
DOVONEX is not recommended for use on the face.

CONTRAINDICATIONS:
- Patients who are hypersensitive to DOVONEX (calcipotriol) cream, ointment or scalp solution, to any ingredient in the formulations or components of the containers. For a complete listing, see Dosage Forms, Composition and Packaging.
- **Not for ophthalmic use.**
- When DOVONEX is used in combination with other antipsoriatic therapies, all available information on "Contraindications" for the other antipsoriatic therapy/therapies apply and should be considered.

WARNINGS AND PRECAUTIONS: General: When DOVONEX (calcipotriol) is used in combination with other antipsoriatic therapies, all available information on "Warnings and Precautions" for the other antipsoriatic therapy/therapies apply and should be considered.

DOVONEX cream, ointment and scalp solution are not generally recommended for severe extensive psoriasis. If calcipotriol is used for severe extensive psoriasis, it is important to monitor the serum calcium levels at regular intervals due to the risk of hypercalcemia secondary to excessive absorption of calcipotriol when there is extensive skin involvement. If the serum calcium level becomes elevated, calcipotriol therapy should be discontinued and the serum calcium level monitored in these patients until it returns to normal.

Carcinogenesis and Mutagenesis: Calcipotriol when used in combination with ultra-violet radiation (UVR) may enhance the known skin carcinogenic effect of UVR. This potential risk is based on the preclinical finding in mice of a reduced time to tumor formation from long term exposure to UVR and topically applied calcipotriol.

Skin: DOVONEX is not recommended for use on the face since this may give rise to itching and erythema of the facial skin. Patients should be instructed to wash their hands after using calcipotriol to avoid inadvertent transfer to the face from other body parts. Should facial dermatitis develop in spite of these precautions, calcipotriol therapy should be discontinued.

DOVONEX should be used cautiously in skin folds, where the natural occlusion may give rise to an increase of the irritant effect of calcipotriol.

Special Populations: Pregnant Women: Safety for use during pregnancy has not yet been established, although studies in experimental animals have not shown teratogenic effects. Calcipotriol should be used in women during pregnancy only if the anticipated benefit clearly outweighs the potential risk.

Nursing Women: It is not known whether calcipotriol could be excreted in breast milk. Calcipotriol should be used in women during breast feeding only if the anticipated benefit clearly outweighs the potential risk.

Infants (<2 yrs of age): There is inadequate experience with the use of calcipotriol in infants under 2 years of age to recommend use in this age group. Use beneath diapers has not been investigated and should be avoided as diapers may be occlusive.

Pediatrics (2-14 years of age): Administration to children should be supervised by a responsible individual to ensure proper administration and dosage. There is no experience in children with the use of DOVONEX in combination with other antipsoriatic therapies.

Monitoring and Laboratory Tests: Treatment with DOVONEX in the recommended amounts (see Dosage and Administration) does not generally result in changes in laboratory values. However, it is recommended that baseline serum calcium levels be obtained in all patients before starting treatment with calcipotriol, with subsequent monitoring of these serum calcium levels at suitable intervals. The monitoring of serum calcium levels is particularly important if the total dose of calcipotriol exceeds the recommended amount or if calcipotriol is used for severe psoriasis with extensive skin involvement. If serum calcium becomes elevated, calcipotriol treatment should be discontinued and the levels of serum calcium should be measured once weekly until the serum calcium levels return to normal values. Patients with marginally elevated serum calcium may be treated with calcipotriol, provided that serum calcium is monitored at suitable intervals.

ADVERSE REACTIONS: In clinical trials reported to-date, the most common adverse reactions have been related to lesional and perilesional irritation. Some patients develop face and scalp irritation which is likely related to the inadvertent transfer of DOVONEX (calcipotriol) cream or ointment from other body parts. Facial irritation may also occur with the use of DOVONEX scalp solution from inadvertent transfer of the scalp solution to the face. One unconfirmed case of Koebner phenomenon and three unconfirmed cases of hypersensitivity reaction to calcipotriol have been reported. Occasionally hypercalcemia has been reported usually related to excessive (greater than the recommended weekly amount, see Dosage and Administration) use of topical calcipotriol or when excessive absorption of calcipotriol has occurred when used for severe psoriasis with extensive skin involvement (see Warnings and Precautions).

Clinical studies have shown that combination of DOVONEX once daily plus a **moderately potent to very potent** topical corticosteroid once daily reduces skin irritation due to calcipotriol. Combination of DOVONEX plus cyclosporin A (2 mg/kg/day) or DOVONEX plus acitretin (20-70 mg/day) did not affect the incidence of short term adverse effects compared to cyclosporin A or acitretin plus placebo ointment. The combination of DOVONEX plus PUVA or UVB phototherapy did not affect the incidence of short term adverse effects compared to PUVA or UVB plus placebo ointment/cream.

DRUG INTERACTIONS: With the exception of topical corticosteroids, (see Dosage and Administration), there is no experience of concomitant therapy with other topical antipsoriatic drugs applied to the same skin area.

DOSAGE AND ADMINISTRATION: Dosing Considerations:

- DOVONEX (calcipotriol) is **for topical use only** and not for ophthalmic use.
- There is no clinical trial experience with use of DOVONEX scalp solution in children.
- There is no experience in children with the use of DOVONEX in combination with other antipsoriatic therapies.

Recommended Dose and Dosage Adjustment: The maximum recommended weekly dose of DOVONEX cream and/or ointment is:

Age (years)	DOVONEX Cream or Ointment, g/week	Total Calcipotriol mg/week
2–5	25	1.25
6–10	50	2.5
11–14	75	3.75
Adults (over 14)	100	5

The maximum weekly dose of DOVONEX cream and/or ointment for children is based on the adult dose of 100 g/week adjusted for body surface area (maximum 50 g/week/m^2). The dosage regimen is based on the following expected body surface area: age 2-5 years, 0.5 m^2 (25% of adult); age 6-10 years, 1.0 m^2 (50% of adult); age 11-14 years, 1.5 m^2 (75% of adult).

The maximum recommended adult weekly dose of DOVONEX scalp solution is 60 mL (3 mg calcipotriol). There is no clinical trial experience with use of DOVONEX scalp solution in children.

When the cream, ointment, or scalp solution are used together, the total dose of calcipotriol should not exceed the recommended weekly amount for each age group (i.e. 2-5 years, 1.25 mg; 6-10 years, 2.5 mg; 11-14 years, 3.75 mg; Adults, 5 mg in any week).

Missed Dose: If an application of DOVONEX is missed, it should be used as soon as the patient remembers and further dosing resumed as usual.

Administration: DOVONEX 50 µg/g ointment or cream is available for use on the body and; a 50 µg/mL scalp solution is available for hairy areas.

DOVONEX Used as Monotherapy: DOVONEX should be applied topically to the affected areas twice daily (i.e. in the morning and in the evening). Application can be reduced to once daily (i.e. in the morning or in the evening) for maintenance treatment when appropriate. After satisfactory improvement has occurred, the drug can be discontinued. If recurrence takes place after discontinuation, the treatment may be reinstituted.

DOVONEX Used as Combination Therapy: DOVONEX can be used in combination with a moderately potent to very potent topical corticosteroid (see Action and Clinical Pharmacology). DOVONEX and the steroid should be applied once daily at alternate times (i.e. morning versus evening application).

DOVONEX can be used twice daily in combination with low dose cyclosporin A (i.e. 2 mg/kg/ day) or in combination with acitretin (20-70 mg/day) (see Action and Clinical Pharmacology).

The use of DOVONEX in combination with other treatments (i.e. topical steroids, cyclosporin A or acitretin) improves efficacy allowing for dosage reduction of the other treatments. There is no experience in children with the use of DOVONEX in combination with other antipsoriatic therapies.

OVERDOSAGE:

Hypercalcemia does not occur at the usual dose of DOVONEX (calcipotriol) (see Dosage and Administration). Excessive use (i.e. more than the recommended weekly amount) may cause elevated serum calcium, which rapidly subsides when treatment is discontinued. In such cases, the monitoring of serum calcium levels once weekly until the serum calcium returns to normal levels is recommended.

For management of a suspected drug overdose, CPhA recommends that you contact your **regional Poison Control Centre**. See the *CPS* Directory section for a list of Poison Control Centres.

ACTION AND CLINICAL PHARMACOLOGY: Mechanism of Action: Calcipotriol is a non-steroidal antipsoriatic agent, derived from naturally occurring vitamin D. Calcipotriol exhibits a vitamin D-like effect by competing for the 1,25$(OH)_2D_3$ receptor. Calcipotriol is as potent as 1,25$(OH)_2D_3$, the naturally occurring active form of vitamin D, in regulating cell proliferation and cell differentiation, but much less active than 1,25$(OH)_2D_3$ in its effect on calcium metabolism. Calcipotriol induces differentiation and suppresses proliferation (without any evidence of a cytotoxic effect) of keratinocytes, thus reversing the abnormal keratinocyte changes in psoriasis. The therapeutic goal envisaged with calcipotriol is thus a normalization of epidermal growth.

Clinical Pharmacology: Clinical trials have shown DOVONEX cream and ointment (calcipotriol 50 µg/g) and DOVONEX scalp solution (calcipotriol 50 µg/mL) to be efficacious and well-tolerated in the topical treatment of psoriasis vulgaris (plaque psoriasis). Clinical improvement usually occurred rapidly and was evident within 2 weeks of treatment. The symptoms of thickness, erythema and scaling, as well as extent of psoriasis, were all markedly improved. The efficacy and safety of DOVONEX ointment and cream are similar with best results obtained at the end of up to 6 to 8 weeks of treatment. Long-term control of psoriasis lasting up to 12 months has been demonstrated in clinical trials with DOVONEX ointment.

Clinical trials have demonstrated the efficacy and safety of once daily DOVONEX administration in combination with once daily administration of a moderately potent to very potent topical corticosteroid. Twice daily application of DOVONEX is safe and effective when combined with systemic drug therapy (cyclosporin A or acitretin). In clinical studies, DOVONEX ointment was combined with either cyclosporin A (2 mg/kg/day) for up to 6 weeks or with acitretin (20-70 mg/day) for up to 12 weeks. Improved efficacy achieved through combination therapy allowed once daily steroid administration or reductions in the required dose of cyclosporin A or acitretin, thereby reducing the potential for dose related adverse effects associated with these agents. Combination of DOVONEX plus a moderately potent to very potent corticosteroid was also shown to reduce skin irritation due to calcipotriol. Combination of DOVONEX with systemic drug therapy did not affect the incidence of short term adverse events compared to systemic drug therapy alone.

Three pivotal trials to evaluate the safety and efficacy of DOVONEX scalp solution were conducted in patients with scalp psoriasis. There was a statistically significant improvement in the scalp psoriasis with a positive effect on total sign score, redness, thickness, scaliness and extent of scalp psoriasis.

Pharmacokinetics: A pharmacokinetic study of DOVONEX ointment has demonstrated that the apparent systemic absorption of the applied dose of calcipotriol over 12 hours is approximately 5.5% of the dose in normal subjects and in psoriatic patients.

Special Populations and Conditions: Pediatrics: The safety, efficacy and tolerability of DOVONEX ointment in children (ages 2 to 14 years) has been demonstrated by an 8 week open-label trial as well as an 8 week double-blind vehicle controlled trial. DOVONEX was significantly more effective than vehicle in reducing the symptoms of redness, thickness and scaliness, and in the overall assessment of efficacy. No significant effects on haematology, serum and urine biochemistry parameters (including calcium levels) and parameters of bone formation or resorption were observed after 8 weeks of treatment (maximum dose 50 g/week/m^2 body surface area).

STORAGE AND STABILITY: Cream: Store at room temperature (15-25°C).

Ointment: Do not store above 25°C. Use within 6 months of first opening of tube.

May be refrigerated. For easy application use at room temperature (this is to prevent pulling of delicate skin).

Scalp Solution: Store below 25°C. Use within 3 months of first opening of bottle.

INFORMATION FOR THE PATIENT: Published in e-CPS, available by subscription at www.e-cps.ca.

DOSAGE FORMS, COMPOSITION AND PACKAGING: Cream: Each g of white cream contains: calcipotriol 50 µg. Nonmedicinal ingredients: cetostearyl alcohol, chloroallylhexaminium (dowicil 200), disodium edetate, disodium phosphate dihydrate, glycerol 85%, liquid paraffin, macrogol cetostearyl ether, purified water and white soft paraffin. Lacquered aluminum tubes of 120 g.

Ointment: Each g of faintly translucent white to yellowish ointment contains: calcipotriol 50 µg. Nonmedicinal ingredients: disodium edetate, disodium phosphate dihydrate, DL-α-tocopherol, liquid paraffin, polyoxyethylene-(2)-stearyl ether, propylene glycol, purified water and white soft paraffin. Lacquered aluminum tubes of 60 g.

Scalp Solution: Each mL of colorless, slightly viscous solution contains: calcipotriol 50 µg. Nonmedicinal ingredients: hydroxypropyl cellulose, isopropanol, levomenthol, propylene glycol, purified water and sodium citrate. Polyethylene bottles of 60 and 120 mL.

Doxercalciferol Pr

CPhA Monograph

see *Vitamin D*

Doxorubicin HCl for Injection USP Pr

doxorubicin HCl

Antineoplastic

Hospira

SUPPLIED: Each vial of sterile lyophilized red powder contains: doxorubicin HCl 10, 50 or 150 mg. Nonmedicinal ingredients: lactose (52.6 mg, 263.1 mg and 789.4 mg respectively). Contains no preservative. Single use vials, cartons of 1. Store between 15 and 25°C. Protect from light. Discard unused portion.

Doxycin Pr

doxycycline hyclate

Antibiotic

Riva

SUPPLIED: Capsules: Each aqua capsule, imprinted H539 contains: doxycycline hyclate USP equivalent to doxycycline 100 mg. Nonmedicinal ingredients: cellulose, colloidal silicon, lactose, magnesium stearate and stearic acid. Alcohol-, gluten-, paraben-, sucrose- and sulfite-free. Bottles of 100 and 300.

Tablets: Each orange, film-coated tablet, scored on one side and embossed DOXYCIN 100 on the other side, contains: doxycycline hyclate USP equivalent to doxycycline 100 mg. Nonmedicinal ingredients: carnauba wax, cellulose, colloidal silicon, D&C Yellow, FD&C Blue, FD&C Red, FD&C Yellow, hydroxypropyl methylcellulose, magnesium stearate, polyethylene glycol, polysorbate 80, sodium starch glycolate, starch, stearic acid and titanium dioxide. Alcohol-, gluten-, paraben-, sucrose- and sulfite-free. Bottles of 100 and 300. Boxes of 10 and 20 (peel off unit dose blister).

Doxycycline Pr

CPhA Monograph

see *Tetracyclines*

Drisdol®

ergocalciferol

Vitamin D Deficiency Prevention

sanofi-aventis

SUPPLIED: Each mL of solution contains: vitamin D_2 (ergocalciferol solution USP) 8288 IU in propylene glycol. Approximately, 207.2 IU per drop, (40 drops=approximately 1 mL). Nonmedicinal ingredients: propylene glycol. Alcohol-, lactose-, parabens-, starch-, sucrose- and tartrazine-free. Bottles of 60 mL with 1 mL calibrated dropper. Store at 15-30°C.

Dristan®

phenylephrine HCl—chlorpheniramine maleate—acetaminophen

Decongestant—Antihistamine—Analgesic

Pfizer Consumer Healthcare

Dristan® Extra Strength

phenylephrine HCl—chlorpheniramine maleate—acetaminophen

Decongestant—Antihistamine—Analgesic

Pfizer Consumer Healthcare

INDICATIONS: Dristan/Dristan Extra Strength: For the symptomatic, temporary relief of colds, sinusitis, hay fever or other upper respiratory allergies, nasal congestion, sneezing, runny nose, fever, headache, minor aches and pains.

CONTRAINDICATIONS: Hypersensitivity to any of the components. Patients receiving MAO inhibitors.

PRECAUTIONS: Dristan/Dristan Extra Strength: Keep out of reach of children.

Stop use and ask a doctor or healthcare professional if symptoms worsen on persist for more than 5 days unless directed by a doctor.

Do not exceed recommended dosage.

Use with caution on elderly patients or patients with allergy to acetaminophen, chronic alcoholism, serious liver or kidney disease, diabetes, heart or thyroid disease, high blood pressure, chronic lung disease, glaucoma, difficulty in urination due to enlarged prostate, or pregnant or nursing, or taking antidepressants, other antihistamines, tranquilizers, or sedating drugs.

This package contains enough medication to seriously harm a child.

Do not use if you have an allergy to acetaminophen or any of the listed ingredients.

Do not use without consulting your physician if you suffer from chronic alcoholism, serious liver or kidney disease, diabetes, heart or thyroid disease, high blood pressure, breathing problems or chronic lung disease, (e.g. chronic bronchitis, asthma or emphysema), glaucoma, difficulty urinating due to an enlarged prostate, or if you are pregnant, nursing or under a physician's care.

Individuals who have taken medication for high blood pressure or depression in the last 14 days, including monoamine oxidase inhibitors (MAOIs), other antihistamines, or other nasal decongestants, should use only as directed by a physician.

Do not use with other products containing acetaminophen.

Taking more than the recommended daily dose may cause severe and possibly fatal liver damage. Stop use and consult a doctor if you develop allergic reactions such as wheezing, rash or itching, if symptoms last more than 5 days or fever lasts more than 3 days.

Consult a doctor before use prior to combining with sedatives, tranquilizers, medication for high blood pressure or depression or any other medication including prescription drugs, salicylates, nasal decongestants or pain and fever medications.

May cause drowsiness or excitability.

Avoid alcoholic beverages, driving a motor vehicle or operating machinery.

Occupational Hazards: Patients should be cautioned not to operate vehicles or hazardous machinery until their response to the drug has been determined. Since the depressant effects of antihistamines are additive to those of other drugs affecting the CNS, patients should be cautioned against drinking alcoholic beverages or taking hypnotics, sedatives, psychotherapeutic agents or other drugs with CNS depressant effects during antihistamine therapy.

Pregnancy: Caution should be exercised before giving to women who are pregnant.

Lactation: Caution should be exercised before giving to women who are nursing a baby.

ADVERSE EFFECTS: Slight to moderate drowsiness may occur. Other possible adverse reactions may include restlessness, dry mouth, nervousness, visual disturbances, dermatitis, weakness and nausea, vomiting, stomach pain and loss of appetite.

Pseudoephedrine may cause mild stimulation, particularly in patients sensitive to sympathomimetic drugs.

In therapeutic doses, acetaminophen is relatively nontoxic. Chronic use of large doses of acetaminophen may produce more significant toxicity.

Renal: Nephropathy, including papillary renal failure has been reported following consumption of large amounts of acetaminophen. Renal tubular necrosis has been associated occasionally with hepatic injury produced by acetaminophen overdose.

Hematologic: Neutropenia and thrombocytopenia purpura have been reported and rarely agranulocytosis.

Immune: Laryngeal edema, angioedema and anaphylactoid reactions may occur rarely.

Hepatic: Hepatic toxicity has been associated with acetaminophen in overdose. Chronic use of high doses, e.g., ≥5 g daily for several weeks in adults or 150 mg/kg/day for 2 to 4 days in children, has also been associated with hepatotoxicity. Alcoholics, patients with liver disease, the malnourished and patients taking drugs that induce hepatic microsomal enzymes, may be at increased risk for hepatic toxicity.

Respiratory: May aggravate bronchospasm in patients sensitive to ASA or other analgesics.

OVERDOSE:

For management of a suspected drug overdose, CPhA recommends that you contact your **regional Poison Control Centre**. See the *CPS* Directory section for a list of Poison Control Centres.

DOSAGE: Dristan: Adults 12 years and over: 2 tablets every 4-6 hours not to exceed 8 tablets daily. Children under 12 years: **Do not use.**

Dristan Extra Strength: Adults 12 years and over: 2 caplets every 4-6 hours not to exceed 8 caplets daily. Children under 12 years: **Do not use.** Use only on the advice of a physician.

SUPPLIED: Dristan: Each yellow and white layered regular strength tablet contains: phenylephrine HCl 5 mg, chlorpheniramine maleate 2 mg and acetaminophen 325 mg. Nonmedicinal ingredients: calcium stearate, celluloses, croscarmellose sodium, crospovidone, D&C Yellow No. 10, FD&C Yellow No. 6, povidone, pregelatinized starch and stearic acid. Energy: 0.19 kJ (0.05 kcal). Blister packages of 24, 48 and 72. Store at room temperature (15 to 30°C).

Dristan Extra Strength: Each yellow and white layered extra strength caplet contains: phenylephrine HCl 5 mg, chlorpheniramine maleate 2 mg and acetaminophen 500 mg. Nonmedicinal ingredients: calcium stearate, croscarmellose sodium, crospovidone, D&C Yellow No. 10, FD&C Yellow No. 6, hypromellose, microcrystalline cellulose, polyethylene glycol, povidone, pregelatinized starch and stearic acid. Energy: 0.80 kJ (0.19 kcal). Blister packages of 24. Store at room temperature (15 to 30°C).

Dristan® Long Lasting Nasal Mist/Spray

oxymetazoline HCl

Nasal Decongestant

Pfizer Consumer Healthcare

PHARMACOLOGY: The sympathomimetic action of oxymetazoline constricts the smaller arterioles of the nasal passages, producing a prolonged (up to 12 hours), gentle and decongesting effect.

INDICATIONS: For prompt temporary relief of nasal congestion due to the common cold, sinusitis, hay fever or other upper respiratory allergies for up to 12 hours.

CONTRAINDICATIONS: Narrow angle glaucoma, rhinitis sicca. Concurrent therapy with MAO inhibitors. Hypersensitivity to any component. Sensitivity to even small doses of adrenergic substances as manifested by sleeplessness, dizziness, lightheadedness, weakness, tremulousness, or cardiac arrhythmias. Do not use for irrigation or displacement after sinus operations in which the dura may have been entered.

PRECAUTIONS: For adults only. Do not exceed the recommended dose. Do not use for more than 7 days.

Stop use and ask your doctor if symptoms persist for more than 7 days.

Systemic effects from the use of topical decongestants can occur due to rapid absorption from the nasal mucous membrane, especially when it is inflamed, and from gastrointestinal absorption if given in excess so that the nasally applied solution is swallowed. Such reactions are most likely to occur in infants, young children and the elderly.

Because of the possibility of generalized vasoconstriction and tachycardia, use sympathomimetic amines very cautiously in patients with hypertension, heart disease, including angina, hyperthyroidism, diabetes mellitus, advanced arteriosclerotic conditions and those patients receiving tricyclic antidepressants.

To help prevent contamination from nasal secretions, rinse spray tips in hot water after each use. Use of this dispenser by more than one person may spread infection.

Caution: **May cause temporary stinging or burning sensations.**

Do not use if you have an allergy to any of the listed ingredients.

Prolonged or excessive use may cause an increase in nasal congestion. Keep all medicine safely away from children.

Do not use without consulting your physician if you have high blood pressure, heart disease, diabetes, thyroid disease or difficulty urinating due to prostate enlargement, or if you are pregnant or nursing, or taking other nasal decongestants.

Do not use if you have taken medication for high blood pressure or depression including monoamine oxidase inhibitors (MAOIs) in the last 14 days.

Children: Overdosage in children may produce profound CNS depression, possibly requiring intensive supportive treatment.

Pregnancy: Clinical data are inadequate to establish conditions for safe use in pregnancy or in women of childbearing potential.

ADVERSE EFFECTS: The following adverse effects may occur with topical nasal decongestants: burning, stinging, dryness of the nasal mucosa, sneezing, palpitations, tachycardia, cardiac arrhythmias, increase in blood pressure, headache, lightheadedness, nervousness, insomnia, blurred vision, drowsiness, CNS depression. Prolonged or excessive use may cause an increase in nasal congestion.

OVERDOSE:

In case of accidental overdose, call a physician or poison control center immediately, even if there are no symptoms.

For management of a suspected drug overdose, CPhA recommends that you contact your **regional Poison Control Centre**. See the *CPS* Directory section for a list of Poison Control Centres.

DOSAGE: Tilt head slightly forward. Place nozzle loosely to nostril. Spray firmly. Breathe deeply. Repeat 2 to 3 times for each nostril. Use every 10 to 12 hours as required. Maximum 2 doses in 24 hours. Adult use only. Children under 12: **Do not use.**

SUPPLIED: Dristan Long Lasting Nasal Mist: Each bottle contains: oxymetazoline HCl 0.05%. Nonmedicinal ingredients: benzalkonium chloride, benzyl alcohol, disodium edetate, hypromellose, phosphoric acid, sodium chloride, sodium phosphate and water. Plastic squeeze bottles of 15 and 30 mL.

Dristan Long Lasting Mentholated Nasal Spray: Each bottle contains: oxymetazoline HCl 0.05%. Nonmedicinal ingredients: benzalkonium chloride, benzyl alcohol, camphor, disodium edetate, ethyl alcohol, eucalyptol, hypromellose, menthol, phosphoric acid, sodium chloride, sodium phosphate and water. Plastic squeeze bottles of 15 and 30 mL.

Dristan® Nasal Mist

phenylephrine HCl—pheniramine maleate

Nasal Decongestant—Antihistamine

Pfizer Consumer Healthcare

PHARMACOLOGY: Phenylephrine is a sympathomimetic agent that constricts the smaller arterioles of the nasal passages producing a gentle and predictable decongesting effect. Pheniramine is an antihistamine that controls rhinorrhea, sneezing and lacrimation associated with elevated histamine levels in disorders of the respiratory tract.

INDICATIONS: Prompt temporary relief of nasal congestion due to colds, sinusitis, hay fever or other upper respiratory allergies.

CONTRAINDICATIONS: Hypersensitivity to any of the ingredients and patients receiving MAO inhibitors.

PRECAUTIONS: Do not exceed recommended dosage because symptoms may occur such as burning, stinging, sneezing or increase of nasal discharge. Do not use this product for more than 3 days. If symptoms persist, consult a physician. To help prevent contamination from nasal secretions, rinse spray tip in hot water after each use. Use of this dispenser by more than one person may spread infection. For adult use only. Do not give this product to children under 12 years except under the advice and supervision of a physician. Keep these and all medicines out of children's reach. In case of accidental ingestion, seek professional assistance or contact a Poison Control Centre immediately.

Prolonged or excessive use may cause an increase in nasal congestion.

Do not use without consulting your physician if you have high blood pressure, heart disease, diabetes, thyroid disease or difficulty urinating due to prostate enlargement, or if you are pregnant or nursing.

Do not use if you have taken medication for high blood pressure or depression in the last 14 days, including monoamine oxidase inhibitors (MAOIs), tranquilizers, sedating drugs or other nasal decongestants.

Caution: **May cause temporary stinging or burning sensations.**

OVERDOSE:

In case of accidental overdose, contact a physician or poison control centre immediately, even if there are no symptoms.

For management of a suspected drug overdose, CPhA recommends that you contact your **regional Poison Control Centre**. See the *CPS* Directory section for a list of Poison Control Centres.

DOSAGE: Tilt head slightly forward. Place nozzle loosely to nostril. Spray firmly. Breathe deeply. Repeat 2 to 3 times for each nostril. Use every 4 hours as required. Do not use in children under 12 years of age.

SUPPLIED: Each bottle contains: phenylephrine HCl 0.5% and pheniramine maleate 0.2%. Nonmedicinal ingredients: benzalkonium chloride, benzyl alcohol, disodium edetate, hypromellose, phosphoric acid, sodium chloride, sodium phosphate and water. Plastic squeeze bottles of 15 and 30 mL.

Droperidol Injection USP Ⓟ

droperidol

Neuroleptic—Antiemetic

Sandoz

SUPPLIED: Each mL of colourless, sterile, aqueous solution contains: droperidol 2.5 mg, lactic acid and/or sodium hydroxide to adjust pH and water for injection. Single use amber vials of 2 mL, boxes of 10. Store between 15 and 30°C. Protect from light.

Dukoral®

oral, inactivated travellers' diarrhea and cholera vaccine

Active Immunizing Agent

sanofi pasteur

Date of Revision: November 2007

SUMMARY PRODUCT INFORMATION:

Route of Administration	Dosage Form/ Strength	Vaccine	Clinically Relevant Nonmedicinal Ingredients
Oral	Oral Suspension	*V. cholerae* O1 Inaba classic strain, heat inactivated: ca. 2.5×10^{10} vibrios *V. cholerae* O1 Inaba El Tor strain, formalin inactivated: ca. 2.5×10^{10} vibrios *V. cholerae* O1 Ogawa classic strain, heat inactivated: ca. 2.5×10^{10} vibrios *V. cholerae* O1 Ogawa classic strain, formalin inactivated: ca. 2.5×10^{10} vibrios **Total:** ca. 1×10^{11} vibrios Recombinant cholera toxin B subunit (rCTB): 1 mg	**Sodium Hydrogen Carbonate**, one sachet (5.6 g) contains: sodium hydrogen carbonate saccharin sodium For a complete listing see Dosage Forms, Composition and Packaging.

DESCRIPTION: DUKORAL [Oral, Inactivated Travellers' Diarrhea and Cholera Vaccine] contains killed whole *V. cholerae* O1 bacteria and the recombinant non-toxic B-subunit of the cholera toxin (CTB). Bacterial strains of both Inaba and Ogawa serotypes and of El Tor and Classical biotypes are included in the vaccine. The vaccine is a whitish suspension in a single-dose glass vial. The sodium hydrogen carbonate is supplied as white effervescent granules with a raspberry flavour, which should be dissolved in a glass of water. Each dose of vaccine is supplied with one sachet of sodium hydrogen carbonate.

INDICATIONS AND CLINICAL USE: DUKORAL [Oral, Inactivated Travellers' Diarrhea and Cholera Vaccine] is indicated for the prevention of and protection against travellers' diarrhea (TD) and/or cholera in adults and children 2 years of age and older who will be visiting areas where there is a risk of contracting TD caused by enterotoxigenic *E. coli* (ETEC) or cholera caused by *V. cholerae.*

Protection against ETEC diarrhea and cholera can be expected about one week after the primary immunization series is completed.

CONTRAINDICATIONS: Allergy to any component of DUKORAL [Oral, Inactivated Travellers' Diarrhea and Cholera Vaccine] (see components listed in Dosage Forms, Composition and Packaging), or its container, or an anaphylactic or other allergic reaction to a previous dose of DUKORAL is a contraindication to vaccination.

Immunization with DUKORAL should be deferred in the presence of any acute illness, including acute gastrointestinal illness or acute febrile illness to avoid superimposing adverse effects from the vaccine on the underlying illness or mistakenly identifying a manifestation of the underlying illness as a complication of vaccine use. A minor illness such as mild upper respiratory infection is not reason to defer immunization.

WARNINGS AND PRECAUTIONS: General: Do not administer this vaccine parenterally. This vaccine must be taken orally (by mouth).

Before administration, take all appropriate precautions to prevent adverse reactions. This includes a review of the patient's history concerning possible hypersensitivity to the vaccine or similar vaccine, previous immunization history, the presence of any contraindications to immunization and current health status.

Before administration of any vaccine, health-care providers should inform the patient, parent or guardian of the benefits and risks of immunization, inquire about the recent health status of the patient and comply with any local requirements regarding information to be provided to the patient before immunization and the importance of completing the immunization series.

Gastrointestinal: As with any vaccine, immunization with DUKORAL [Oral, Inactivated Travellers' Diarrhea and Cholera Vaccine] may not protect 100% of susceptible persons.

Travellers should use care in the choice of food and water supply and use good hygienic measures.

Immune: Immunocompromised persons (whether from disease or treatment) may not obtain the expected immune response. If possible, consideration should be given to delaying vaccination until after the completion of any immunosuppressive treatment.

DUKORAL can be given to HIV-infected persons. Clinical trials have shown no vaccine-associated adverse events and no change in disease clinical progression. Limited data are available on immunogenicity and safety of the vaccine. Vaccine protective efficacy has not been studied among HIV-infected persons. However, in a field study in Mozambique the protective efficacy was 84% in a population with approximately 25% HIV prevalence.

Formaldehyde is used during the manufacturing process and trace amounts may be present in the final product. Caution should be taken in subjects with known hypersensitivity to formaldehyde.

As with all products, the possibility of allergic reactions in persons sensitive to components of the vaccine should be evaluated.

DUKORAL confers protection specific to *V. cholerae* serogroup O1. DUKORAL has not been demonstrated to protect against cholera caused by *V. cholerae* serogroup O139 or other species of Vibrio.

Special Populations: Pregnant Women: The effect of DUKORAL [Oral, Inactivated Travellers' Diarrhea and Cholera Vaccine] on embryo-fetal development has not been assessed and animal studies on reproductive toxicity have not been conducted. No specific clinical studies have been performed to address this issue. The vaccine is therefore not recommended for use in pregnancy. However, DUKORAL is an inactivated vaccine that does not replicate. DUKORAL is also given orally and acts locally in the intestine. Therefore, in theory, DUKORAL should not pose any risk to the human fetus. Administration of DUKORAL to pregnant women may be considered after careful evaluation of the benefits and risks.

Nursing Women: DUKORAL may be given to lactating women.

Pediatrics: DUKORAL has been given to children between 1 and 2 years of age in safety and immunogenicity studies, but the protective efficacy has not been studied in this age group. Therefore, DUKORAL is not recommended for children less than 2 years of age.

Geriatrics: DUKORAL has been given to persons over the age of 65 in clinical trials, but there are only very limited data on protective efficacy of the vaccine in this age group. However, this group can be expected to be at risk of more severe complications of disease if infected by ETEC or cholera and therefore may obtain greater benefit from vaccination.

ADVERSE REACTIONS: Adverse Drug Reaction Overview: In clinical trials conducted in Bangladesh, Peru and Sweden, gastrointestinal symptoms were reported with similar frequency in vaccine and placebo groups. No serious adverse reactions were reported.

Clinical Trial Adverse Drug Reactions: The safety of DUKORAL [Oral, Inactivated Travellers' Diarrhea and Cholera Vaccine] was assessed in clinical trials, including both adults and children, conducted in endemic and non-endemic countries for cholera and ETEC producing heat-labile enterotoxin (LT). Over 94 000 doses of DUKORAL were administered during the clinical trials. Evaluation of safety varied between trials with respect to mode of surveillance, definition of symptoms and time of follow-up. In the majority of studies adverse events were assessed by passive surveillance. The most frequently reported adverse reactions occurred at similar frequencies in vaccine and placebo groups. These included gastrointestinal symptoms including abdominal pain, diarrhea, loose stools, nausea and vomiting.

Frequency Classification: Very common: ≥1/10 (≥10%). Common (frequent): ≥1/100 and <1/10 (≥1% and <10%). Uncommon (infrequent): ≥1/1000 and <1/100 (≥0.1% and <1%). Rare: ≥1/10 000 and <1/1000 (≥0.01% and <0.1%). Very rare: <1/10 000 (<0.01%), including isolated reports.

Metabolism and Nutrition Disorders: Rare: loss of or poor appetite. Very rare: dehydration.

Nervous System Disorders: Uncommon: headache. Rare: dizziness. Very rare: drowsiness, insomnia, fainting, reduced sense of taste.

Respiratory, Thoracic and Mediastinal Disorders: Rare: respiratory symptoms (including rhinitis and cough).

Gastrointestinal Disorders: Uncommon: diarrhea, abdominal pain, abdominal cramps, stomach/abdominal gurgling (gas), abdominal discomfort. Rare: nausea, vomiting. Very rare: dyspepsia, sore throat.

Skin and Subcutaneous Tissue Disorders: Very rare: sweating, rash.

Musculoskeletal and Connective Tissue Disorders: Very rare: joint pain.

General Disorders and Administration Site Conditions: Rare: fever, malaise. Very rare: fatigue, shivers.

Post-Market Adverse Drug Reactions: Additional adverse reactions reported (very rare <1/10 000) during post-marketing surveillance, following distribution of approximately 7 000 000 vaccine doses, are listed below:

Blood and Lymphatic System Disorders: lymphadenitis.

Gastrointestinal Disorders: flatulence.

General Disorders and Administration Site Conditions: pain, flu-syndrome, asthenia, chills.

Infections and Infestations: gastroenteritis.

Nervous System Disorders: paraesthesia.

Respiratory Thoracic and Mediastinal Disorders: dyspnoea, increased sputum.

Skin and Subcutaneous Tissue Disorders: urticaria, angioedema, pruritus.

Vascular Disorders: hypertension.

Physicians, nurses and pharmacists should report any adverse occurrences temporally related to the administration of the product in accordance with local requirements and to the Global Pharmacovigilance Department, Sanofi Pasteur Limited, 1755 Steeles Avenue West, Toronto, ON, M2R 3T4, Canada. 1-888-621-1146 (phone) or 416-667-2435 (fax).

DRUG INTERACTIONS: Overview: There are obvious practical advantages to giving more than one vaccine at the same time, especially in preparation for foreign travel or when there is doubt that the patient will return for further doses of vaccine. Most of the commonly used antigens can safely be given simultaneously. No increase in the frequency or severity of clinically significant side effects has been observed. The immune response to each antigen is generally adequate and comparable to that found in patients receiving these vaccines at separate times.

Drug-Drug Interactions: The administration of an encapsulated oral typhoid vaccine and DUKORAL [Oral, Inactivated Travellers' Diarrhea and Cholera Vaccine] should be separated by at least 8 hours.

Oral administration of other vaccines and medicinal products should be avoided 1 hour before and 1 hour after vaccination.

DUKORAL has been administered concomitantly with yellow fever vaccine to 55 subjects. The yellow fever antibody response was similar to that seen in the 58 subjects who received the yellow fever vaccine alone. However, no results are available to evaluate the safety of concomitant administration of the two vaccines or to evaluate the immune response to DUKORAL when administered with yellow fever vaccine.

Drug-Food Interactions: Food and drink should be avoided 1 hour before and 1 hour after vaccination as the vaccine is acid labile. Food and/or drink may increase acid production in the stomach and the effect of the vaccine may be impaired.

DUKORAL should only be mixed with the supplied effervescent granules dissolved in water.

DOSAGE AND ADMINISTRATION: To Prevent Travellers' Diarrhea Caused by ETEC: Primary Immunization for Adults and Children 2 Years and Older:

- 2 doses orally at least 1 week apart.
- 1st dose at least 2 weeks before departure.
- 2nd dose 1 week after the 1st dose and at least 1 week before departure.
- Protection against traveller's diarrhea caused by ETEC starts 1 week after the second dose and will last for 3 months.
- If more than 6 weeks elapse between the 1st and 2nd dose, the primary immunization should be re-started.

Booster for Adults and Children 2 Years and Older:

- If the patient received the last dose between 3 months and 5 years before, one booster dose will renew the protection.
- If more than 5 years has passed since the last dose, complete primary immunization (2 doses) is recommended.

To Prevent Cholera: Primary Immunization for Adults and Children 6 Years and Older:

- 2 doses orally at least 1 week apart.
- 1st dose at least 2 weeks before departure.
- 2nd dose 1 week after the 1st dose at least 1 week before departure.
- Protection against cholera starts 1 week after the second dose and will last for 2 years.
- If more than 6 weeks elapse between the 1st and 2nd dose, the primary immunization should be re-started.

Booster for Adults and Children 6 Years and Older:

- If the patient received the last dose between 2 and 5 years before, one booster dose will renew the protection.
- If more than 5 years has passed since the last dose, complete primary immunization (2 doses) is recommended.

Primary Immunization for Children 2 to 6 Years: 3 doses orally at least 1 week apart and finishing at least 1 week before departure.

- 1st dose at least 3 weeks before departure; 2nd dose 1 week later; 3rd dose 1 week later and at least one week before departure.
- Protection against cholera starts after 1 week and will last for 6 months for children 2 to 6 years.
- If more than 6 weeks elapse between the 1st and 2nd dose, the primary immunization should be re-started.

Booster for Children 2 to 6 Years:

- If the patient received the last dose between 6 months and 5 years before, one booster dose will renew the protection.
- If more than 5 years has passed since the last dose, complete primary immunization (3 doses) is recommended.

Important Information About Taking DUKORAL: Do not eat or drink for 1 hour before and 1 hour after taking the vaccine.

Do not take any other medicine for 1 hour before and 1 hour after taking the vaccine.

Use only cool water to mix the vaccine. (See How to Prepare DUKORAL.) **Do not use any other liquid.**

How to Prepare DUKORAL: Mix the vaccine according to the directions below:

Step 1: Dissolve the powder from the sachet in 5 oz. (150 mL) of cool water.

For adults and children 6 years and older—proceed to Step 2.

For children 2 to 6 years—discard half the mixture and proceed to Step 2.

Step 2: Shake the small glass vial that contains the vaccine to mix it well.

Step 3: Open the vial and add the vaccine to the liquid in the glass. Stir well and drink immediately.

If the mixture is not drunk immediately, it should be consumed within 2 hours of mixing. Keep it at room temperature.

Missed Dose: If the second dose is missed, it can be taken at any time within six weeks. Food and drink are to be avoided for 1 hour before and 1 hour after.

OVERDOSAGE:

Data on overdose are extremely limited. Adverse reactions reported are consistent with those seen after the recommended dosing.

For management of a suspected drug overdose, CPhA recommends that you contact your **regional Poison Control Centre**. See the *CPS* Directory section for a list of Poison Control Centres.

ACTION AND CLINICAL PHARMACOLOGY: Mechanism of Action: DUKORAL [Oral, Inactivated Travellers' Diarrhea and Cholera Vaccine] consists of killed *V. cholerae* and the non-toxic recombinant cholera toxin B subunit. The vaccine acts locally in the gastrointestinal tract to induce an IgA antitoxic and antibacterial response (including memory) comparable to that induced by cholera disease itself. The protection against cholera is specific for both biotype and serotype. O-antigens as well as toxin B subunit will induce immunity. Most ETEC strains produce an enterotoxin which is structurally, pathophysiologically and immunologically similar to cholera toxin. This enterotoxin is neutralized by antibodies against cholera toxin B subunit. Hence, the vaccine confers protection against ETEC, as well as cholera.

Pharmacodynamics: In clinical trials DUKORAL has been shown to prevent TD caused by enterotoxigenic *E. coli* and cholera caused by *V. cholerae* O1 (classical and El Tor biotypes). Protection against ETEC diarrhea and cholera can be expected about one week after the primary immunization series is completed.

Duration of Effect: Effect on Cholera: Clinical results have revealed a protective efficacy against cholera of 80-85% for the first six months in all age categories. In adults and children over the age of 6, protective efficacy over a 3-year follow-up period averaged about 63% (without a booster dose). Children under the age of 2 were not examined, but protective efficacy in the 2-6 year age range was satisfactory for the first six months.

Effect on ETEC: Protective efficacy with reference to all TD will vary depending on the prevalence of ETEC. There are considerable variations between different seasons and geographic areas. Protective efficacy against ETEC lasts about 3 months.

STORAGE AND STABILITY: Store at 2 to 8°C. **Do not freeze.**

The vaccine can be stored at room temperature (<27°C) for up to two weeks on one occasion only. After reconstitution the vaccine should be consumed within 2 hours.

The sodium hydrogen carbonate sachet may be stored separately at room temperature (<27°C).

Do not use after expiration date.

INFORMATION FOR THE PATIENT: Published in e-CPS, available by subscription at www.e-cps.ca.

DOSAGE FORMS, COMPOSITION AND PACKAGING: Vaccine: One dose contains: *V. cholerae* O1 Inaba classic strain, heat inactivated: ca. 2.5×10^{10} vibrios; *V. cholerae* O1 Inaba El Tor strain, formalin inactivated: ca. 2.5×10^{10} vibrios; *V. cholerae* O1 Ogawa classic strain, heat inactivated: ca. 2.5×10^{10} vibrios; *V. cholerae* O1 Ogawa classic strain, formalin inactivated: ca. 2.5×10^{10} vibrios; Total: ca. 1×10^{11} vibrios; recombinant cholera toxin B subunit (rCTB): 1 mg; sodium dihydrogen phosphate; disodium hydrogen phosphate; sodium chloride; water for injection to 3 mL.

Sodium hydrogen carbonate: one sachet (5.6 g) contains: sodium hydrogen carbonate, citric acid, sodium carbonate, saccharin sodium, sodium citrate, raspberry flavour.

The stopper of the vial for this product does not contain natural rubber latex. DUKORAL [Oral, Inactivated Travellers' Diarrhea and Cholera Vaccine] is supplied in a package containing: Package of 1 dose vial of vaccine and 1 sachet (5.6 g) sodium hydrogen carbonate. Package of 2×1 dose vial of vaccine and 2 sachets (5.6 g) sodium hydrogen carbonate. Package of 20×1 dose vial of vaccine and 20 sachets (5.6 g) sodium hydrogen carbonate.

Dulcolax®

bisacodyl

Laxative

Boehringer Ingelheim

Date of Revision: December 18, 2008

SUMMARY PRODUCT INFORMATION:

Route of Administration	Dosage Form/ Strength	Clinically Relevant Nonmedicinal Ingredients
Oral	Tablet 5 mg	Lactose, sucrose, and tartrazine (yellow). Please refer to the complete listing of ingredients in Dosage Forms, Composition and Packaging.
Rectal	Suppositories 5 mg, 10 mg	Hard fat

INDICATIONS AND CLINICAL USE: DULCOLAX is indicated for:

- relief of occasional constipation
- Under medical supervision, for the preparation of diagnostic procedures, in pre- and postoperative treatment, and in conditions which require defecation to be facilitated.

CONTRAINDICATIONS: DULCOLAX is contraindicated in:

- Patients who are hypersensitive to this drug or to any ingredient in the formulation or component of the container. For a complete listing, see Dosage Forms, Composition and Packaging.
- Patients with ileus, intestinal obstruction, acute abdominal conditions like acute appendicitis, acute inflammatory bowel diseases, severe abdominal pain associated with nausea and vomiting which may be indicative of more severe conditions.
- Severe dehydration.
- In case of rare hereditary conditions that may be incompatible with an excipient of the product (lactose or sucrose) see Warnings and Precautions.

WARNINGS AND PRECAUTIONS: General: As with all laxatives, DULCOLAX should not be taken on a continuous daily basis or for extended periods without investigating the cause of constipation. Prolonged excessive use may lead to fluid and electrolyte imbalance and hypokalaemia.

Do not use DULCOLAX in the presence of abdominal pain, nausea, fever or vomiting, or within two hours of another medicine since the desired effect of the other medicine may be reduced.

Dizziness and/or syncope have been reported in patients who have taken DULCOLAX. The details available for these cases suggest that the events would be consistent with defecation syncope (or syncope attributable to straining at stool), or with a vasovagal response to abdominal pain which may be related to the constipation that prompted the patients in question to resort to the use of laxatives and not necessarily to the administration of DULCOLAX itself.

The use of suppositories may lead to painful sensations and local irritation, especially in anal fissures and ulcerative proctitis and should be used in these conditions under medical advice or as directed by a physician.

DULCOLAX coated tablets contain lactose and sucrose. One coated tablet contains 33.2 mg lactose and 23.4 mg sucrose (saccharose), resulting in 66.4 mg lactose and 46.8 mg sucrose per maximum recommended daily dose for treatment of constipation. For preparation of diagnostic procedure this will result in 132.8 mg of lactose and 93.6 mg sucrose per maximum recommended daily dose in adults. Patients with the rare hereditary conditions of galactose intolerance, e.g. galactosaemia, or fructose intolerance should not take DULCOLAX tablets.

The tablet formulation contains tartrazine as a colouring agent; this agent may cause allergic reactions. Patients with tartrazine allergy should not take Dulcolax tablets.

Dependence/Tolerance: Since extended use of any laxative can cause dependence for bowel function, do not take for more than one week unless directed by a health professional. If the use of DULCOLAX every day for a week does not result in a bowel movement, a doctor should be consulted immediately.

Special Populations: Pregnant Women: There are no adequate and well-controlled studies in pregnant women. For use during pregnancy, it is recommended that medical advice from a physician first be obtained. As with all medications, DULCOLAX should only be taken during pregnancy on medical advice.

Nursing Women: Whether DULCOLAX passes into breast milk has not been characterized in detail, but detection of trace amounts of milk has been reported. As with all medications, DULCOLAX should only be taken by nursing women on medical advice.

Pediatrics: Children should not be given DULCOLAX without medical advice.

ADVERSE REACTIONS: Post-Market Adverse Drug Reactions: Immune System Disorders: anaphylactic reactions, angioneurotic oedema and other hypersensitivity.

Gastrointestinal Disorders: colitis, abdominal cramps, abdominal pain, diarrhoea, vomiting, nausea, abdominal discomfort.

DRUG INTERACTIONS: The concomitant use of diuretics or adreno-corticosteroids may increase the risk of electrolyte imbalance if excessive doses of DULCOLAX are taken.

Electrolyte imbalance may lead to increased sensitivity to cardiac glycosides.

DULCOLAX tablets have an enteric coating and should not be taken together with products reducing the acidity of the upper gastrointestinal tract, such as milk, antacids or certain proton pump inhibitors.

DOSAGE AND ADMINISTRATION: Dosing Considerations: DULCOLAX should be used under medical supervision for the preparation of diagnostic procedures, in pre- and postoperative treatment and in medical conditions which require defecation to be facilitated.

Recommended Dose and Dosage Adjustment: Unless prescribed by the physician otherwise, the following dosages are recommended:

- **For constipation:**
  - **Adults and children over 12 years:** Take one to two coated tablets (5-10 mg) orally or one adult suppository (10 mg) rectally.
  - **Children 6-12 years:** Give one coated tablet (5 mg) orally or one paediatric suppository (5 mg) rectally.
  - **Children under 6 years:** Use only as directed by your doctor.
- **For diagnostic procedures or pre-operatively to achieve complete evacuation of the intestine:**
  - **Adults:** Two to four coated tablets (10-20 mg) orally the night before the procedure, followed by one suppository (10 mg) in the morning of the procedure.
  - **Children 6 years and over:** One coated tablet (5 mg) orally at bedtime, and one paediatric suppository (5 mg) inserted rectally the following morning.

Administration: It is recommended to take DULCOLAX coated tablet(s) at night to have a bowel movement the following morning.

Tablets have a special coating and therefore should not be taken together with products reducing the acidity of the upper gastrointestinal tract, such as milk, antacids or certain proton pump inhibitors in order not to prematurely dissolve the enteric coating.

Tablets should be swallowed whole with an adequate amount of fluid.

Suppositories should take from about 15 minutes to 1 hour to stimulate a bowel movement. They should be unwrapped and inserted into the rectum pointed end first.

OVERDOSAGE:

Symptoms: If high doses are taken, watery stools (diarrhoea), abdominal cramps, and a clinically significant loss of potassium and other electrolytes can occur.

DULCOLAX, as with other laxatives, when taken in chronic overdose may cause chronic diarrhoea, abdominal pain, hypokalaemia, secondary hyperaldosteronism and renal calculi. Renal tubular damage, metabolic alkalosis and muscle weakness secondary to hypokalaemia have also been described in association with chronic laxative abuse.

Treatment: Within a short time after ingestion of oral forms of DULCOLAX, absorption can be minimized or prevented by inducing vomiting or gastric lavage. Replacement of fluids and correction of electrolyte imbalance may be required. This is especially important in the elderly and the young.

Administration of antispasmodics may be of value.

> For management of a suspected drug overdose, contact your **regional Poison Control Centre**. See the *CPS* Directory section for a list of Poison Control Centres.

STORAGE AND STABILITY: Store out of the reach of children.
Tablets: Store at room temperature (15-30°C).
Suppositories: Store at room temperature (15-25°C).

INFORMATION FOR THE PATIENT: Published in e-CPS, available by subscription at www.e-cps.ca.

DOSAGE FORMS, COMPOSITION AND PACKAGING: Suppositories: Each rectal suppository contains: bisacodyl 5 mg (children formula) or 10 mg (adult formula). Nonmedicinal ingredient: hard fat. Boxes of 3 (5 mg); boxes of 3, 6 and 100 (10 mg).
Tablets: Each yellow, enteric-coated tablet contains: bisacodyl 5 mg. Nonmedicinal ingredients: acacia, beeswax, carnauba wax, corn starch, dibutyl phthalate, eudragit, glycerine, lactose, magnesium stearate, polyethylene glycol, sucrose, talc, tartrazine (yellow) and titanium dioxide. Packages of 10, 30, 60 and 100.

(Shown in Product Identification Section)

Duofilm® Liquid
salicylic acid—lactic acid
Verrucae Therapy

Stiefel, a GSK company

SUPPLIED: Each mL contains: salicylic acid USP 16.7% and lactic acid USP 16.7% in flexible collodion. Bottles of 15 mL with brush applicator.

Duofilm® Patch
salicylic acid
Verrucae Therapy

Stiefel, a GSK company

SUPPLIED: Each medicated patch contains: salicylic acid 40% w/w. Nonmedicinal ingredients: plaster-base vehicle. Boxes of 12 medicated patches and 12 adhesive cover-up discs.

Duofilm® Plantar Patch
salicylic acid
Plantar Wart Treatment

Stiefel, a GSK company

SUPPLIED: Each medicated plantar patch contains: salicylic acid 40% w/w in a plaster base. Nonmedicinal ingredient: plaster-base vehicle. Boxes of 24 medicated patches and 24 protective pads.

Duoforte® 27
salicylic acid
Verrucae Therapy

Stiefel, a GSK company

INDICATIONS: For common, plantar and mosaic warts.

CONTRAINDICATIONS: Diabetics or patients with impaired blood circulation should not use this product without the advice of a health professional. Do not use on moles, birthmarks or unusual warts with hair growing from them. Do not use near eyes or mucous membranes.

WARNINGS: Do not use on inflamed and/or infected skin.

PRECAUTIONS: For external use only. Duoforte 27 gel is highly flammable and should be kept away from fire or flame. Keep tube tightly capped when not in use. Store at controlled room temperature.

If spilled on mucous membranes or in eyes, flush with water, remove precipitated collodion and flush with water for an additional 15 minutes. Contact physician. Keep this and all medication out of reach of children.

OVERDOSE:

> For management of a suspected drug overdose, CPhA recommends that you contact your **regional Poison Control Centre**. See the *CPS* Directory section for a list of Poison Control Centres.

DOSAGE: Thoroughly wash the affected area and soak the wart in warm water for at least 5 minutes. Dry completely with a clean towel. Warts can be contagious, so be sure no one else uses the towel. Remove the soft portion of the wart by gently rubbing with an emery board, pumice stone or coarse washcloth. Apply a thin layer directly to the wart using the pointed applicator tip. Take care to keep away from the skin surrounding the wart.

The gel will dry and form an acrylic barrier, protecting the wart and aiding in the penetration of the medication.

Apply Duoforte 27 gel once each day and continue treatment as directed by physician. If skin irritation develops or if there appears to be no improvement within 10 days or if the condition persists after 14 days of the treatment, contact physician.

SUPPLIED: Each g contains: salicylic acid 27% w/w in a nonmedicinal polyacrylic collodion gel. Nonmedicinal ingredients: polybutylene, ethyl lactate, polymethylmethacrylate, alcohol absolute, flexible collodion and hydroxypropylcellulose. Tubes of 15 g with applicator tips.

Duoplant®
salicylic acid—lactic acid—formalin
Plantar Wart Remover

Stiefel, a GSK company

SUPPLIED: Each g contains: salicylic acid USP 25%, lactic acid USP 10%, formalin 5% in a specially formulated base. Nonmedicinal ingredients: lanolin anhydrous, mineral oil light 90, paraffin wax and white soft petrolatum. Plastic tubes of 30 g. Store between 15 and 30°C.

PLANTAR WART REMOVAL KIT: Each kit contains: 1 tube of Duoplant 30 g, 1 emery file, 20 self-adhesive bandages, 2 cushion pads and detailed instructions for use.

DuoTrav® Pr
travoprost—timolol maleate
Elevated Intraocular Pressure Therapy—Prostaglandin F2α Analogue and Beta-adrenergic Receptor Blocker

Alcon

Date of Preparation: March 15, 2006
Date of Revision: October 23, 2008

PHARMACOLOGY: Mechanism of Action: DUOTRAV (travoprost/timolol) Ophthalmic Solution contains two active components, travoprost and timolol maleate, which lower intraocular pressure by complementary mechanisms of action.

Travoprost free acid is a highly selective FP prostanoid receptor agonist that has been shown to reduce intraocular pressure by increasing uveoscleral and conventional outflow. Reduction of intraocular pressure starts within approximately two hours after administration, and the maximum effect is reached after 12 hours. Significant lowering of intraocular pressure can be maintained for periods exceeding 24 hours with a single dose. Repeated observations over a period of one year indicate that the intraocular pressure lowering effect of travoprost is well maintained.

Timolol maleate is a $beta_1$ and $beta_2$ (non-selective) adrenergic receptor blocking agent that does not have significant intrinsic sympathomimetic, direct myocardial depressant, or local anesthetic (membrane-stabilizing) activity. The precise mechanism of the ocular hypotensive action of timolol is not definitively established. Tonography and fluorophotometry studies in man suggest that its predominant action is related to reduced aqueous humor formation. However, in some studies a slight increase in outflow facility was also observed. The onset of reduction of intraocular pressure following administration of timolol can usually be detected within one-half hour after a single dose. The maximum effect usually occurs in one to two hours and significant lowering of intraocular pressure can be maintained for periods as long as 24 hours with a single dose. Repeated observations over a period of one year indicate that the intraocular pressure-lowering effect of timolol is well maintained.

Pharmacokinetics/Pharmacodynamics: DUOTRAV (travoprost/timolol) Ophthalmic Solution, when applied topically to the eye, has the action of reducing elevated as well as normal intraocular pressure, whether or not accompanied by glaucoma. Elevated intraocular pressure is a major risk factor in the pathogenesis of glaucomatous visual field loss. The higher the level of intraocular pressure, the greater the likelihood of glaucomatous visual field loss and optic nerve damage. The Advanced Glaucoma Intervention Study (AGIS) established elevated intraocular pressure as a positive risk factor for glaucomatous visual field loss. Eyes with intraocular pressures below 18 mmHg at all visits were found to have little to no visual field loss during the six-year monitoring period.

Absorption: Travoprost and timolol are absorbed through the cornea. Travoprost undergoes rapid ester hydrolysis in the cornea to the active free acid. In travoprost studies, peak plasma concentrations of the free acid were observed within 30 minutes after dosing. Following topical ocular administration of DUOTRAV solution once-daily in healthy subjects (N=15) for 3 days, the travoprost free acid was not quantifiable in plasma samples from the majority of subjects (80%, N=12/15) and was not detectable in any samples one hour after dosing. In those subjects in whom travoprost free acid was measurable (≥0.01 ng/mL, the assay limit of quantitation), plasma concentration ranged from 0.010 to 0.020 ng/mL. The mean peak timolol steady-state concentration was 0.692 ng/mL±0.384 ng/mL after once-daily administration of DUOTRAV solution. Timolol T_{max} was observed within one hour after dosing.

Distribution: Travoprost free acid can be measured in the aqueous humor during the first few hours in animals and in human plasma only during the first hour after topical ocular administration of DUOTRAV solution. Timolol can be measured in human aqueous humor after topical ocular administration of timolol and in plasma for up to 12 hours after topical ocular administration of DUOTRAV solution.
Metabolism: Travoprost, an isopropyl ester prodrug, is hydrolyzed by esterases in the cornea to its pharmacologically active free acid. Systemically, travoprost free acid is metabolized to inactive metabolites via beta-oxidation of the α (carboxylic acid) chain to give the 1,2-dinor and 1,2,3,4-tetranor analogs, via oxidation of the 15-hydroxyl moiety, as well as via reduction of the 13,14 double bond in primates. The plasma elimination of the free acid was rapid with a mean apparent $t_{½}$ of approximately 45 minutes. There was no difference in plasma concentrations between Days 1 and 3, indicating steady-state was reached early and there was no accumulation.

In humans, timolol is primarily metabolized by two pathways involving ring-opening oxidation of the morpholine ring. One route yields an ethanolamine side chain on the thiadiazole ring and the other giving an ethanolic side chain on the morpholine nitrogen and a second similar side chain with a carbonyl group adjacent to the nitrogen. The apparent terminal elimination $t_{½}$ of timolol in plasma is approximately 4 hours after topical ocular administration of DUOTRAV solution.
Excretion: Travoprost free acid and its metabolites are mainly excreted by the kidneys. In humans, less than 2% of a topical ocular dose of travoprost was recovered in urine as free acid. Timolol and its metabolites are primarily excreted by the kidneys. Approximately 20% of a timolol dose is excreted in the urine unchanged and the remainder excreted in urine as metabolites.

INDICATIONS: DUOTRAV (travoprost/timolol) Ophthalmic Solution is indicated for the reduction of elevated intraocular pressure (IOP) in patients with open-angle glaucoma or ocular hypertension who are insufficiently responsive to beta-blockers, prostaglandins, or other IOP lowering agents AND when the use of DUOTRAV solution (the fixed combination drug) is considered appropriate.

DUOTRAV solution should not be used to initiate therapy.

The use of DUOTRAV solution is not recommended for paediatric patients.

For details of information obtained from Clinical Trials with DUOTRAV solution, see Dosage.

CONTRAINDICATIONS: Note: DUOTRAV solution is a combination of travoprost 0.004% and timolol 0.5% as timolol maleate. When DUOTRAV solution is prescribed, the relevant Product Monographs for travoprost and/or timolol maleate should be consulted.

DUOTRAV (travoprost/timolol) Ophthalmic Solution is contraindicated in patients who:

- are hypersensitive to this drug or to any ingredient in the formulation (see Supplied) or component of the container.
- have bronchial asthma
- have a history of bronchial asthma
- have severe chronic obstructive pulmonary disease (see Warnings)
- have sinus bradycardia
- have second or third degree atrioventricular block
- have overt cardiac failure (see Warnings)
- have cardiogenic shock

WARNINGS: For topical ophthalmic use only.
Note: DUOTRAV solution is a combination of travoprost 0.004% and timolol 0.5% as timolol maleate. When DUOTRAV solution is prescribed, the relevant Product Monographs for travoprost and/or timolol maleate should be consulted.

If signs of serious reactions or hypersensitivity occur, discontinue use of this preparation.
Ocular Effects: Travoprost and other prostaglandin analogues have been reported to cause changes to pigmented tissues. The most frequently reported changes have been increased pigmentation of the iris and periorbital tissue (eyelid) and increased pigmentation and growth of eyelashes. These changes may be permanent.

DUOTRAV (travoprost/timolol) Ophthalmic Solution may gradually change eye colour, increasing the amount of brown pigmentation in the iris. The colour change is due to increased melanin content in stromal melanocytes on the iris rather than to an increase in the number of melanocytes, although the exact mechanism of action is unknown at this time. Typically the brown pigmentation around the pupil spreads concentrically towards the periphery in affected eyes, but the entire iris or parts of it may become more brown. Iris pigmentation changes may be more noticeable in patients with mixed coloured irides, i.e., blue-brown, grey-brown, yellow-brown, and green-brown, however, it has also been observed in patients with brown eyes. The change in iris colour occurs slowly and may not be noticeable for several months to years. The long-term effects on the melanocytes and the consequences of potential injury to the melanocytes and/or deposition of pigment granules to other areas of the eye are currently unknown. Patients should be informed of the possibility of iris colour change since the increased pigmentation is permanent. Patients should be examined regularly and, depending on the clinical situation, treatment may be stopped if increased pigmentation ensues.

Eyelid skin darkening has been reported in association with the use of DUOTRAV solution. DUOTRAV solution may gradually change eyelashes in the treated eye; these changes include increased length, thickness, pigmentation, and/or number of lashes.

Patients who are expected to receive treatment in only one eye should be informed about the potential for increased brown pigmentation of the iris, periorbital and/or eyelid tissue, and eyelashes in the treated eye and thus heterochromia between the eyes. They should also be advised of the potential for a disparity between the eyes in length, thickness, and/or number of eyelashes.
Systemic Effects: The same adverse reactions found with systemic administration of beta-adrenergic blocking agents may occur with topical administration of DUOTRAV solution due to the beta-adrenergic component, timolol. For example, severe respiratory reactions and cardiac reactions, including death due to bronchospasm in patients with asthma, and rarely death in association with cardiac failure, have been reported following systemic or ophthalmic administration of timolol maleate (see Contraindications).
Cardiac Failure: Because of the timolol maleate component, cardiac failure should be adequately controlled before beginning treatment with DUOTRAV solution. Patients with a history of severe cardiac disease should be watched for signs of cardiac failure and have their pulse rates checked.

Caution should be exercised in treating patients with severe cardiovascular disease.
Anaphylaxis: While taking beta-blockers, patients with a history of atopy or a history of severe anaphylactic reactions to a variety of allergens may be more reactive to repeated accidental, diagnostic, or therapeutic challenge with such allergens. Such patients may be unresponsive to the usual doses of epinephrine used to treat anaphylactic reactions.
Obstructive Pulmonary Disease: Patients with chronic obstructive pulmonary disease (e.g., chronic bronchitis, emphysema) of mild or moderate severity, bronchospastic disease, or a history of bronchospastic disease (other than bronchial asthma or a history of bronchial asthma, in which DUOTRAV solution is contraindicated [see Contraindications]) should, in general, not receive beta-blockers or products containing them, including DUOTRAV.
Diabetes Mellitus: Beta-adrenergic blocking agents should be administered with caution in patients subject to spontaneous hypoglycemia or to diabetic patients (especially those with labile diabetes) who are receiving insulin or oral hypoglycemic agents. Beta-adrenergic receptor blocking agents may mask the signs and symptoms of acute hypoglycemia.
Angle-closure Glaucoma: DUOTRAV solution should not be used alone in the treatment of acute angle-closure glaucoma.
Concomitant Therapy: Timolol may interact with other drugs (see also information under Precautions, Drug Interactions). The effect on intraocular pressure or the known effects of systemic beta-blockers may be exaggerated when DUOTRAV solution is given to patients already receiving an oral beta-blocking agent. The use of two local beta-blockers or two local prostaglandins is not recommended.
Pregnancy: No adequate and well-controlled studies have been performed in pregnant women. DUOTRAV solution should be used during pregnancy only if the potential benefit justifies the potential risk to the fetus.
Teratogenic Effects: Travoprost was teratogenic in rats. Travoprost administered intravenously to pregnant rats from gestation Days 6-17 at a dose of 10 µg/kg/day, induced a slight increase in the incidence of skeletal malformations such as fused sternebrae, domed head and hydrocephaly. No effect was observed at 3 µg/kg/day (75 times the maximum recommended human dose (MRHOD) of 0.04 µg/kg/day). The no effect level for fetal external, visceral or skeletal malformation was observed after 1.0 µg/kg/day subcutaneous administration during gestation days 6-16 to pregnant mice, though postimplantation loss was increased at that dose, but not at 0.3 µg/kg/day.

Teratogenicity studies with timolol in mice, rats, and rabbits at oral doses up to 50 mg/kg/day (7000 times the MRHOD demonstrated no evidence of fetal malformations. Although delayed fetal ossification was observed at this dose in rats, there were no adverse effects on postnatal development of offspring. Doses of 1000 mg/kg/day (142 000 times the MRHOD) were maternotoxic in mice and resulted in an increased number of fetal resorptions. Increased fetal resorptions were also seen in rabbits at doses of 14 000 times the MRHOD, in this case without apparent maternotoxicity.
Children: The use of DUOTRAV solution in paediatric patients is currently not recommended. The safety and efficacy of the use of DUOTRAV solution in children has not been established.

PRECAUTIONS: Note: DUOTRAV solution is a combination of travoprost 0.004% and timolol 0.5% as timolol maleate. When DUOTRAV solution is prescribed, the relevant Product Monographs for travoprost and/or timolol maleate should be consulted.
General: Patients prescribed IOP-lowering medication should be routinely monitored for IOP status.

Patients may slowly develop increased brown pigmentation of the iris. This change is permanent and may not be noticeable for months to years (see Warnings).

DUOTRAV solution should be used with caution in patients with active intraocular inflammation (iritis/uveitis).

Macular edema, including cystoid macular edema, has been reported during treatment with prostaglandin $F_{2\alpha}$ analogues such as travoprost. These reports have mainly occurred in aphakic patients, pseudophakic patients with a torn posterior lens capsule, or in patients with known risk factors for macular edema. DUOTRAV solution should be used with caution in these patients.
Contact Lenses: DUOTRAV solution contains the preservative benzalkonium chloride, which may be deposited in soft contact lenses; therefore, DUOTRAV solution should not be administered while wearing these lenses. The lenses should be removed before application of the drops and not be reinserted earlier than 15 minutes after use.
Choroidal Detachment: Choroidal detachment after filtration procedures has been reported with administration of aqueous suppressant therapy (e.g., timolol maleate, acetazolamide). Management of eyes with chronic or recurrent choroidal detachment should include stopping all forms of aqueous suppressant therapy and treating endogenous inflammation vigorously.
Major Surgery: The necessity or desirability of withdrawal of beta-adrenergic blocking agents prior to major surgery is controversial. If necessary during surgery, the effects of beta-adrenergic blocking agents may be reversed by sufficient doses of such agonists as isoproterenol, dopamine, dobutamine or levarterenol.
Thyrotoxicosis: Beta-adrenergic blocking agents may mask certain clinical signs of hyperthyroidism (e.g., tachycardia). Patients suspected of developing thyrotoxicosis should be managed carefully to avoid abrupt withdrawal of beta-adrenergic blocking agents that might precipitate a thyroid storm.
Muscle Weakness: Beta-adrenergic blockade has been reported to increase muscle weakness consistent with certain myasthenic symptoms (e.g., diplopia, ptosis and generalized weakness). Timolol maleate has been reported rarely to increase muscle weakness in some patients with myasthenia gravis or myasthenic symptoms.
Cerebrovascular Insufficiency: Because of potential effects of beta-adrenergic blocking agents on blood pressure and pulse, these agents should be used with caution in patients with cerebrovascular insufficiency. If signs or symptoms suggesting reduced cerebral blood flow develop following initiation of therapy with DUOTRAV solution, alternative therapy should be considered.
Renal/Hepatic Impairment: DUOTRAV solution has not been studied in patients with renal impairment; caution should be exercised in treating such patients.
Pregnancy: There are no adequate and well-controlled studies of DUOTRAV solution in pregnant women. Because animal reproduction studies are not always predictive of human response, DUOTRAV solution should be used during pregnancy only if the potential benefit to the mother justifies potential risk to the fetus. See Warnings.
Lactation: Timolol maleate has been detected in human milk following oral and ophthalmic drug administration. It is not known whether travoprost and/or its metabolites are excreted in human milk, although in animal studies, travoprost has been shown to be excreted in milk. Because of the potential for serious adverse reactions from timolol maleate or travoprost in nursing infants, a decision should be made whether to discontinue nursing or to discontinue the drug, taking into account the importance of the drug to the mother.
Children: The use of DUOTRAV solution in paediatric patients is currently not recommended. The safety and efficacy of the use of DUOTRAV solution in children has not been established (see Warnings).
Geriatrics: No overall differences in safety or effectiveness have been observed between elderly and other adult patients.
Occupational Hazards: DUOTRAV solution, as with other similar medications, can potentially cause fatigue and/or drowsiness in some patients. Patients who engage in hazardous activities should be cautioned of the potential for a decrease in mental alertness.
Drug Interactions: No specific interaction studies have been performed with DUOTRAV solution.
Beta-adrenergic Blocking Agents: Patients who are receiving a beta-adrenergic blocking agent orally and DUOTRAV solution should be observed for potential additive effects of beta-blockade, both systemic and on intraocular pressure. The concomitant use of two topical beta-adrenergic blocking agents is not recommended.
Calcium Antagonists: Caution should be used in the coadministration of beta-adrenergic blocking agents, such as the timolol found in DUOTRAV, and oral or intravenous calcium antagonists because of possible atrioventricular conduction disturbances, left ventricular failure, and hypotension. In patients with impaired cardiac function, coadministration should be avoided.
Catecholamine-depleting Drugs: Close observation of the patient is recommended when a beta blocker is administered to patients receiving catecholamine-depleting drugs such as reserpine, because of possible additive effects and the production of hypotension and/or marked bradycardia, which may result in vertigo, syncope, or postural hypotension.
Digitalis and Calcium Antagonists: The concomitant use of beta-adrenergic blocking agents with digitalis and calcium antagonists may have additive effects in prolonging atrioventricular conduction time.
Quinidine: Potentiated systemic beta-blockade (e.g., decreased heart rate) has been reported during combined treatment with quinidine and timolol, possibly because quinidine inhibits the metabolism of timolol via the P-450 enzyme, CYP2D6.
Clonidine: Oral beta-adrenergic blocking agents may exacerbate the rebound hypertension which can follow the withdrawal of clonidine. There have been no reports of exacerbation of rebound hypertension with ophthalmic timolol maleate.
Injectable Epinephrine: (See Warnings, Anaphylaxis.)
CNS Depressants: Although specific drug interaction studies have not been conducted with DUOTRAV solution, the possibility of an additive or potentiating effect with CNS depressants (alcohol, barbiturates, opiates, sedatives, or anesthetics) should be considered.
Tricyclic Antidepressants: Tricyclic antidepressants have been reported to blunt the hypotensive effect of systemic clonidine. It is not known whether the concurrent use of these agents with DUOTRAV solution can lead to an interference in IOP lowering effect.

No data are available on the level of circulating catecholamines after DUOTRAV solution is instilled. Caution, however, is advised in patients taking tricyclic antidepressants which can affect the metabolism and uptake of circulating amines.
Epinephrine: Mydriasis resulting from concomitant use of timolol maleate and epinephrine has been reported occasionally.
Information to Be Provided to the Patient by the Physician: Patients should be advised to carefully take note of the proper use of the medication and other precautions contained in the package insert.

Patients with bronchial asthma, a history of bronchial asthma, severe chronic obstructive pulmonary disease, sinus bradycardia, second- or third-degree atrioventricular block, cardiac failure, or patients receiving monoamine oxidase (MAO) inhibitor therapy should be advised not to take this product (see Contraindications).

Patients should be instructed to avoid allowing the tip of the dispensing container to contact the eye or surrounding structures. If handled improperly, ocular solutions can become contaminated by common bacteria known to cause ocular infections. Serious damage to the eye and subsequent loss of vision may result from using contaminated solutions.

There have been reports of bacterial keratitis associated with the use of multiple dose containers of topical ophthalmic products. These containers had been inadvertently contaminated by patients who, in most cases, had a concurrent corneal disease or a disruption of the ocular epithelial surface.

Patients should also be advised that if they have ocular surgery or develop an intercurrent ocular condition (e.g., trauma or infection), they should immediately seek their physician's advice concerning the continued use of the present multidose container.

If more than one topical ophthalmic drug is being utilized, the drugs should be administered at least ten minutes apart.
Patient wearing Contact Lenses: The preservative in DUOTRAV solution, benzalkonium chloride, may be absorbed by soft (hydrophilic) contact lenses. Patients wearing soft contact lenses should be instructed to wait at least 15 minutes after instilling DUOTRAV solution to insert soft contact lenses.

ADVERSE EFFECTS: Clinical Trial Adverse Drug Reactions: Adverse Drug Reaction Overview: In clinical trials 721 subjects/patients were exposed to DUOTRAV (travoprost/timolol) Ophthalmic Solution administered once-daily for up to 12 months. This included 15 subjects with short-term exposure in a single pharmacokinetic study and 706 patients with open-angle glaucoma or ocular hypertension in long-term studies. No serious ophthalmic or systemic adverse reactions specifically related to DUOTRAV solution were reported in any study. The adverse drug reactions are limited to those reported previously with travoprost and/or timolol maleate. In the clinical trials 4.6% of patients discontinued therapy with DUOTRAV solution due to adverse drug reactions.
Clinical Trial Adverse Drug Reactions: Because clinical trials are conducted under very specific conditions the adverse drug reaction rates observed in the clinical trials may not reflect the rates observed in practice and should not be compared to the rates in the clinical trials of another drug. Adverse reaction information from clinical trials is useful for identifying drug-related adverse events and for approximating rates.
Adverse Drug Reactions in Clinical Trials Providing Short-Term Exposure: In a single pharmacokinetic trial of crossover design (C-02-35), 15 subjects had short-term exposure (3 days) to DUOTRAV solution. The most frequently reported adverse drug reaction was ocular hyperaemia. No subject discontinued therapy as a result of any adverse drug reaction in this study and no subject experienced a serious adverse drug reaction. See Table 1.

Table 1: DUOTRAV

All Adverse Drug Reactions Occurring in Subjects with Exposure to DUOTRAV Solution—Short-Term Study (C-02-35)

	DUOTRAV Solution N=15 %	Travatan Solution N=15 %	Timolol 0.5% N=14 %
Eye Disorders			
Ocular hyperaemia	86.7	46.7	28.6
Eye irritation	13.3	13.3	
Eye pruritus	6.7		
Eyelids pruritus	6.7		
Abnormal sensation in eye	6.7	6.7	
Blurred vision	6.7		7.1
Respiratory, Thoracic and Mediastinal Disorder			
Postnasal drip	6.7	6.7	7.1
General Disorders and Administration Site Conditions			
Thirst	6.7		
Investigations			
Intraocular pressure decreased	6.7		

Adverse drug reactions coded using MedDRA version 8.0.
This table includes all reported ocular and non-ocular adverse drug reactions.

Less Common Clinical Trial Adverse Drug Reactions (<1%) in Subjects with Short-Term Exposure to DUOTRAV Solution: Due to the small sample size in this trial, a single reported adverse drug reaction in the DUOTRAV solution or TRAVATAN solution treatment group resulted in an incidence of 6.7%, while in the Timolol treatment group a single adverse drug reaction resulted in an incidence of 7.1%.

Adverse Drug Reactions in Clinical Trials Providing Long-Term Exposure: In 5 clinical trials (C-01-69, C-01-70, C-02-03, C-02-28, and C-02-41), 706 patients with open-angle glaucoma or ocular hypertension had long-term exposure (6 weeks to 1 year) to DUOTRAV solution. No serious ophthalmic or systemic adverse drug reactions related to DUOTRAV solution were reported in any trial providing long-term exposure. The most frequently reported adverse drug reaction was ocular hyperaemia (13.9%). Almost all patients (98%) who experienced ocular hyperaemia did not discontinue therapy as a result of this reaction. Additional adverse drug reactions that occurred at an incidence of ≥1.0% in patients with long-term exposure to DUOTRAV solution included the following: See Table 2.

Table 2: DUOTRAV

Adverse Drug Reactions Occurring at an Incidence of ≥1% in Patients with Exposure to DUOTRAV Solution—Long-Term Studies (C-01-69, C-01-70, C-02-03, C-02-28, C-02-41)

	DUOTRAV N=706 %	Latanoprost 0.005%/ Timolol 0.5% N=200 %	TRAVATAN+Timolol 0.5% N=313 %	TRAVATAN Solution N=86 %	Timolol 0.5% N=176 %
Eye Disorders					
Ocular hyperaemia	13.9	2.5	18.8	11.6	1.7
Eye irritation	6.1	3.0	10.9	5.8	5.7
Eye pruritus	4.5	2.0	4.8	2.3	0.5
Dry eye	2.5	1.0	2.9	2.3	1.7
Abnormal sensation in eye	2.3	3.5	2.9	2.3	1.7
Growth of eyelashes	1.6	—	2.2	1.2	—
Eye pain	1.3	0.5	—	—	—
Photophobia	1.3	—	1.6	1.2	—
Blurred vision	1.1	—	1.6	—	2.8
Punctate keratitis	1.0	0.5	1.9	1.2	—

Adverse drug reactions coded using MedDRA version 8.0.
No non-ocular adverse drug reactions occurred at an incidence ≥1%.

In a twelve month study with DUOTRAV solution ocular photographs were taken of the iris using a standardized procedure and evaluated by a centralized reading center masked to study treatment in order to assess effects on iris pigmentation. Following an initial latent period the incidence of iris pigmentation changes increased in both treatment groups from Month 6 to Month 12 as shown in Table 3.

Table 3: DUOTRAV

Patients with Iris Pigmentation Changes[a] (C-02-28)

DUOTRAV			Latanoprost 0.005%/Timolol 0.5%		
	N[c]	%		N[c]	%
Month 6 (N=169)[b]	1	0.6	Month 6 (N=161)[b]	1	0.6
Month 12 (N=166)[b]	4	2.4	Month 12 (N=163)[b]	2	1.2

[a] Changes based upon review of ocular photographs by a centralized reading center.
[b] N values represent number of patients with ocular photographs.
[c] N values represent number of patients with iris pigmentation changes.

Less Common Clinical Trial Adverse Drug Reactions (<1%) in Patients with Long-Term Exposure to DUOTRAV Solution: Adverse drug reactions that occurred at an incidence of <1.0% in patients with long-term exposure to DUOTRAV solution included the following: See Table 4.

Table 4: DUOTRAV

Adverse Drug Reactions Occurring at an Incidence of <1% in Patients with Exposure to DUOTRAV Solution—Long-Term Studies (C-01-69, C-01-70, C-02-03, C-02-28, C-02-41)

MedDRA SOC	MedDRA PT
Psychiatric Disorders	nervousness
Nervous System Disorders	dizziness, headache
Eye Disorders	anterior chamber cells, anterior chamber flare, dermatitis eyelid, erythema of eyelid, ocular discomfort, periorbital disorder, asthenopia, eyelids pruritus, visual acuity reduced, conjunctival haemorrhage, conjunctivitis allergic, eye swelling, eyelid irritation, eyelid oedema, eyelid pain, lacrimation increased, visual disturbance, corneal staining, blepharitis, conjunctival oedema, eye allergy, xerophthalmia
Vascular Disorders	hypertension
Respiratory, Thoracic and Mediastinal Disorders	postnasal drip, bronchospasm, cough, dyspnoea, throat irritation
Skin and Subcutaneous Tissue Disorders	skin hyperpigmentation, dermatitis contact, distichiasis, hypertrichosis, urticaria
Musculoskeletal and Connective Tissue Disorders	pain in extremity
Renal and Urinary Disorders	chromaturia
General Disorders and Administration Site Conditions	thirst
Investigations	alanine aminotransferase increased[a], aspartate aminotransferase increased[a], blood pressure diastolic decreased, blood pressure diastolic increased, blood pressure increased, heart rate decreased, heart rate irregular, intraocular pressure decreased

[a] No clinical laboratory evaluations were performed. These adverse drug reactions were based upon patient reports. Adverse drug reactions are presented in order of decreasing incidence; when reactions occurred at the same incidence they are presented alphabetically.
Adverse drug reactions coded using MedDRA version 8.0.
Legend: SOC=System Organ Class; PT=Preferred term.

Additional Adverse Drug Reactions Observed with the Individual Components of DUOTRAV Solution: The following additional adverse drug reactions have been seen with one of the individual components of DUOTRAV solution (TRAVATAN solution or Timolol), have not been presented in the preceding tables or text, and may potentially occur with DUOTRAV solution. For further detailed information, please consult the individual Product Monographs for TRAVATAN solution or Timolol. See Table 5.

Table 5: DUOTRAV

Additional Adverse Drug Reactions Previously Observed in One of the Individual Components and That May Potentially Occur with DUOTRAV Solution

	TRAVATAN	Timolol
MedDRA SOC	MedDRA PT	MedDRA PT
Metabolism and Nutrition Disorders	—	hypoglycemia
Psychiatric Disorders	—	depression
Nervous System Disorders	—	cerebrovascular accident, cerebral ischaemia, myasthenia gravis, syncope, paresthesia
Eye Disorders	asthenopia, conjunctivitis, conjunctival follicles, conjunctival disorder, eyelid margin crusting, eyelid oedema, iris hyperpigmentation, iritis, macular oedema, uveitis	conjunctivitis, corneal disorder, diplopia, eyelid ptosis
Cardiac Disorders	—	arrhythmia, atrioventricular block, cardiac arrest, cardiac failure, palpations
Vascular Disorders	hypotension	hypotension
Respiratory, Thoracic and Mediastinal Disorders	asthma	nasal congestion, respiratory failure
Gastrointestinal Disorders	—	diarrhoea, nausea
Skin and Subcutaneous Tissue Disorders	hair growth abnormal, skin discolouration	alopecia, rash
General Disorders and Administration Site Conditions	—	asthenia, chest pain

Adverse drug reactions coded using MedDRA version 8.0.
Legend: SOC=System Organ Class; PT=Preferred term.

Abnormal Hematologic and Clinical Chemistry Findings: No clinical laboratory evaluations for the analysis of safety were performed during the clinical development of DUOTRAV solution. The clinical laboratory adverse drug reactions presented in Table 4 were based upon patient reports. For further information, please consult the individual Product Monographs for TRAVATAN solution or Timolol.

Post-Market Adverse Drug Reactions: The individual components TRAVATAN (travoprost ophthalmic solution, 0.004%) and Timolol (timolol maleate ophthalmic solution, 0.1%, 0.25%, and 0.5%) are registered in numerous countries. Based upon a review of spontaneous post-marketing reports of adverse events to date, TRAVATAN solution and Timolol are well-tolerated and safe for use as indicated.

In post-market, a few reports of iritis/uveitis associated with the use of travoprost have been published. These cases occurred a few days after travoprost use in patients without a history of iritis/uveitis. All of these cases resolved after stopping travoprost with or without corticosteroid treatment. As spontaneous event reports frequently provide incomplete data, report of a spontaneous event does not necessarily constitute an admission that TRAVATAN solution or Timolol caused or contributed to the event.

The following additional adverse drug reactions (presented in alphabetical order), not presented in the preceding tables or text, have been reported via postmarketing surveillance with one of the individual components of DUOTRAV solution (TRAVATAN solution or Timolol) and may potentially occur with DUOTRAV solution. See Table 6.

Table 6: DUOTRAV

Additional Adverse Drug Reactions Reported Via Postmarketing Surveillance for One of the Individual Components and That May Potentially Occur with DUOTRAV Solution

	TRAVATAN Solution	Timolol
MedDRA SOC	**MedDRA PT**	**MedDRA PT**
Infections and Infestations	herpes simplex ophthalmic, influenza, urinary tract infection NOS	conjunctivitis ineffective, eye infection
Neoplasms Benign, Malignant and Unspecified (Incl Cysts And Polyps)	gastrointestinal carcinoma	
Blood and Lymphatic System Disorders	thrombocytopenia	
Immune System Disorders	anaphylactic shock, hypersensitivity NOS	hypersensitivity
Endocrine Disorders	hirsutism	
Metabolism and Nutrition Disorders	hyperglycaemia NOS, hypoglycaemia NOS, weight fluctuation	
Psychiatric Disorders	aggression, anxiety, anxiety aggravated, depression aggravated, insomnia, sleep disorder NOS	
Nervous System Disorders	amnesia, aphonia, cerebrovascular accident, dysgeusia, epilepsy NOS, facial neuralgia NOS, hypertonia, hypoaesthesia, hypokinesia, loss of consciousness, memory impairment, migraine NOS, motor dysfunction NOS, paraesthesia, paresis, somnolence, syncope, tremor, vasovagal attack	dysgeusia, somnolence
Eye Disorders	accommodation disorder, angle closure glaucoma, anterior chamber disorder NOS, anterior chamber pigmentation, blepharospasm, blindness, blindness transient, blindness unilateral, chalazion, choroiditis, colour blindness NOS, conjunctival cyst, corneal disorder NOS, corneal oedema, cyanopsia, cycloplegia, extraocular muscle paresis, eye disorder NOS, eye haemorrhage NOS, eye inflammation NOS, eyelid disorder NOS, glaucoma NOS, iridocyclitis, iris adhesions, iris cyst, keratitis, macular hole, madarosis, miosis, myopia aggravated, photopsia, pupillary light reflex tests abnormal, retinal detachment, retinal disorder, retinal haemorrhage, retinal vein occlusion, rubeosis iridis, vitreous haemorrhage	dacryostenosis acquired, eye discharge, eye inflammation, eyelid disorder, eyelid margin crusting, keratoconjunctivitis sicca, keratopathy, lid margin discharge, optic nerve disorder, scleral discolouration
Ear and Labyrinth Disorders	ear pain, hypoacusis, tinnitus, vertigo	vertigo
Cardiac Disorders	angina pectoris, arrhythmia, atrioventricular block NOS, bradycardia NOS, cardiac arrest, cardiac disorder NOS, cardiac failure NOS, cyanosis, extrasystoles NOS, myocardial infarction, palpitations, palpitations, tachycardia NOS, ventricular tachycardia	bradycardia, cardiac failure
Vascular Disorders	arterial pressure NOS decreased, circulatory collapse, flushing, hypertensive crisis	flushing, hot flush
Respiratory, Thoracic and Mediastinal Disorders	asthma aggravated, chronic obstructive airways disease exacerbated, dry throat, dyspnoea exacerbated, epistaxis, expectoration, nasal congestion, nasal dryness, oropharyngeal swelling, pharyngolaryngeal pain	apnoea, increased upper airway secretion, respiratory disorder
Gastrointestinal Disorders	abdominal pain, chapped lips, diarrhoea NOS, dyspepsia, gastric function disorder NOS, gastrointestinal disorder, gastrointestinal upset, mouth haemorrhage, nausea, vomiting	
Hepatobiliary Disorders	autoimmune hepatitis	
Skin and Subcutaneous Tissue Disorders	alopecia, angioneurotic oedema, cold sweat, dry skin, eczema NOS, eczema weeping, erythema, hair colour changes, hyperhidrosis, localised skin reaction, photosensitivity reaction, prurigo, pruritus, pruritus generalized, rash NOS, skin depigmentation, skin disorder, skin reaction, skin tightness, sweating increased, trichiasis, urticaria NOS	dermatitis, dermatitis exfoliative, dry skin, eczema, erythema, lichenification, periorbital oedema, pruritus, psoriasis, rash macular, scab, skin disorder, skin irritation
Musculoskeletal and Connective Tissue Disorders	arthralgia, back pain, limb discomfort NOS, neck pain, pain in jaw, tendon disorder NOS	
Renal and Urinary Disorders	anuria, haematuria, incontinence NOS, micturition frequency decreased, pollakiuria, urine flow decreased	
Reproductive System and Breast Disorders	benign prostatic hyperplasia, breast mass NOS, erectile dysfunction NOS, peyronie's disease, priapism	menorrhagia
Congenital, Familial and Genetic Disorders	coloboma , epidermal naevus	

(cont'd)

Table 6: DUOTRAV *(cont'd)*

Additional Adverse Drug Reactions Reported Via Postmarketing Surveillance for One of the Individual Components and That May Potentially Occur with DUOTRAV Solution

	TRAVATAN Solution	Timolol
MedDRA SOC	**MedDRA PT**	**MedDRA PT**
General Disorders and Administration Site Conditions	asthenia, chest discomfort, chest pain, chest pressure sensation, condition aggravated, drug ineffective, facial pain, fall, fatigue, feeling abnormal, feeling hot, influenza like illness, lethargy, malaise, no adverse drug effect, oedema peripheral, pain	chest discomfort, drug ineffective, fatigue, unevaluable event
Investigations	arterial pressure NOS increased, blood bilirubin increased, blood cholesterol increased, heart rate abnormal, heart rate increased, intraocular pressure increased, liver function test abnormal, prostatic specific antigen increased, retinogram abnormal, serum ferritin increased, transferrin increased, weight decreased	heart rate increased, intraocular pressure increased
Injury, Poisoning and Procedural Complications	accident NOS, accidental overdose, corneal injury NOS, face injury, head injury, injury	Excoriation
Surgical and Medical Procedures	cardiac pacemaker insertion	

Adverse drug reactions coded using MedDRA version 8.0.
Legend: SOC=System Organ Class; PT=Preferred term.

OVERDOSE:

Symptoms: There are no human data available on overdosage with DUOTRAV (travoprost/timolol) Ophthalmic Solution or TRAVATAN (travoprost ophthalmic solution).

Symptoms of systemic timolol overdosage are: bradycardia, hypotension, bronchospasm, and cardiac arrest. If such symptoms occur, treatment should be symptomatic and supportive.

Treatment: Specific therapeutic measures for the treatment of overdosage with timolol maleate are reproduced below for ease of reference.

Gastric Lavage: If ingested.

Symptomatic bradycardia: Use atropine sulfate intravenously in a dosage of 0.25 to 2 mg to induce vagal blockade. If bradycardia persists, intravenous isoproterenol hydrochloride should be administered cautiously. In refractory cases the use of transvenous cardiac pacemaker may be considered.

Hypotension: Use sympathomimetic pressor drug therapy, such as dopamine, dobutamine or levarterenol. In refractory cases the use of glucagons hydrochloride has been reported to be useful.

Bronchospasm: Use isoproterenol hydrochloride. Additional therapy with aminophylline may be considered.

Acute cardiac failure: Conventional therapy with digitalis, diuretics and oxygen should be instituted immediately. In refractory cases the use of intravenous aminophylline is suggested. This may be followed if necessary by glucagon hydrochloride which as been reported to be useful.

Heart block (second or third degree): Use isoproterenol hydrochloride or a transvenous cardiac pacemaker.

> For management of a suspected drug overdose, CPhA recommends that you contact your **regional Poison Control Centre**. See the *CPS* Directory section for a list of Poison Control Centres.

DOSAGE: The recommended dosage is one drop in the affected eye(s) once-daily in the morning. The dosage of DUOTRAV (travoprost/timolol) Ophthalmic Solution should not exceed once-daily since it has been shown that more frequent administration of prostaglandin analogues may decrease the intraocular pressure lowering effect. If one dose is missed treatment should continue with the next dose as normal.

The use of DUOTRAV solution may be considered in patients who require both timolol and travoprost. If more than one topical ophthalmic drug is being used, the drugs should be administered at least five minutes apart.

INFORMATION FOR THE PATIENT: Published in e-CPS, available by subscription at www.e-cps.ca.

SUPPLIED: Each mL of sterile, isotonic, buffered, preserved, aqueous solution contains: travoprost 0.04 mg and timolol maleate 6.8 mg (equivalent to 5 mg timolol base). Nonmedicinal ingredients: benzalkonium chloride, boric acid, edetate disodium, hydrochloric acid, mannitol, polyoxyl 40 hydrogenated castor oil, purified water and tromethamine. Alcon DROP-TAINER package system comprises a white, opaque, polypropylene dispenser bottle with a natural polypropylene dropper tip and a dark blue polypropylene closure. Tamper evidence is provided with a neck-band which shrinks to conform around the closure and neck area of the package. Bottles of 4 mL containing 2.5 mL solution. Bottles of 7.5 mL containing 5 mL solution. A 2.5 mL bottle of DUOTRAV solution contains at least 94 drops of solution. Store at 2-25°C. No refrigeration required.

Duovent® UDV Ⓟ

ipratropium bromide—fenoterol HBr

Bronchodilator

Boehringer Ingelheim

Date of Revision: August 14, 2009

SUMMARY PRODUCT INFORMATION:

Route of Administration	Dosage Form/ Strength	All Nonmedicinal Ingredients
Inhalation	Solution/0.5 mg of ipratropium bromide and 1.25 mg fenoterol hydrobromide in 4 mL of isotonic saline	Sodium chloride, hydrochloric acid

INDICATIONS AND CLINICAL USE: DUOVENT UDV (ipratropium bromide/fenoterol hydrobromide) is indicated for:

- treatment of bronchospasm associated with acute severe exacerbations of bronchial asthma or chronic obstructive pulmonary disease (COPD).

DUOVENT UDV inhalation solution must be administered by means of nebulizer using gas flow (oxygen or compressed air).

Concomitant use of DUOVENT UDV (ipratropium bromide/fenoterol hydrobromide) with other sympathomimetic agents is not recommended since the combined use may lead to deleterious cardiovascular effects. If concomitant use is necessary, this should take place only under strict medical supervision.

Pediatrics (<12 years of age): DUOVENT UDV is not currently indicated for use in children under 12 years of age as the dosing regimen and evidence concerning its safety in this age group have not been established.

CONTRAINDICATIONS:

- Patients with a known hypersensitivity to the component drugs, sympathomimetic amines, atropinics or to any of the product components. For a complete listing, see Dosage Forms, Composition and Packaging.
- DUOVENT UDV (ipratropium bromide/fenoterol hydrobromide) is also contraindicated in patients with tachyarrhythmias and hypertrophic obstructive cardiomyopathy.

WARNINGS AND PRECAUTIONS: General: Like other inhalation solutions that contain β_2 agonists, DUOVENT UDV (ipratropium bromide/fenoterol hydrobromide) should not be used on a regular basis without appropriate concomitant anti-inflammatory therapy (see Dosage and Administration).

Care should be taken in patients suffering from myocardial insufficiency, cardiac arrhythmias, recent myocardial infarction, severe organic heart and/or other vascular disorders, hypertension, hyperthyroidism, insufficiently controlled diabetes mellitus, or pheochromocytoma.

If therapy does not produce a significant improvement or if the patient's condition gets worse, medical advice must be sought in order to determine a new plan of treatment. In the case of acute or rapidly worsening dyspnea, a doctor should be consulted immediately.

Increasing use of β_2 agonists to control symptoms of bronchial obstruction, especially administration on a regular basis or in high amounts, indicates deterioration of asthma control. Under these conditions, the patient's therapy plan has to be revised. It is inadequate simply to increase the use of bronchodilators under these circumstances, in particular over extended periods of time (see Dosage and Administration).

Concomitant use of DUOVENT UDV (ipratropium bromide/fenoterol hydrobromide) with other sympathomimetic agents is not recommended since the combined use may lead to deleterious cardiovascular effects. If concomitant use is necessary, this should take place only under strict medical supervision.

The bronchodilating action of sympathomimetic drugs may be antagonized by β adrenergic blocking agents with the result that the respiratory status of patients may worsen when the two drugs are used concomitantly. In patients requiring concomitant treatment with DUOVENT UDV and a β adrenergic blocking agent, the use of a relatively cardioselective β blocker (e.g. metoprolol, atenolol, acebutolol) must be considered. During the concomitant treatment, patients should be monitored carefully for possible deterioration in pulmonary function or for the need to adjust the dosage of either drug.

Caution is advised against accidental release of the solution into the eyes.

DUOVENT UDV should be used with caution in patients with glaucoma, prostatic hyperplasia, urinary retention or bladder neck obstruction and in asthmatic or emphysematous patients who also have acute and recurring congestive heart failure or in patients sensitive to sympathomimetic amines.

To ensure the proper dosage administration, the patient should be instructed by the physician or other health professional on the proper use and maintenance of the nebulizer.

Failure to respond to a **previously effective dose** usually indicates a significant deterioration in the patient's asthmatic condition. The patient should be instructed to contact his/her physician immediately in these circumstances and warned on no account to exceed the recommended dose.

Three retrospective case-control studies, from one group in New Zealand, have suggested that there may be an increased risk of death in those patients using Berotec (fenoterol hydrobromide) whom the studies classified as 'severe' asthmatics. These conclusions have not been confirmed by other studies and are subject to considerable debate and ongoing studies.

Cardiovascular: Cardiovascular effects may be seen with sympathicomimetic drugs, including DUOVENT. There is some evidence from post-marketing data and published literature of rare occurrences of myocardial ischaemia associated with beta-agonists. Patients with underlying severe heart disease (e.g. ischaemic heart disease, arrhythmia or severe heart failure) who are receiving DUOVENT, should be warned to seek medical advice if they experience chest pain or other symptoms of worsening heart disease. Attention should be paid to assessment of symptoms such as dyspnoea and chest pain, as they may be of either respiratory or cardiac origin.

Fatalities, the exact cause of which is unknown, have been reported following excessive use of sympathomimetic amines by inhalation. Cardiac arrest was noticed in several instances.

Endocrine and Metabolism: In common with other β adrenergic agents, fenoterol hydrobromide can induce reversible metabolic changes. These are most pronounced during **infusions** of the drug and include hyperglycemia and hypokalemia.

Potentially serious hypokalemia may result from β_2 agonist therapy, mainly from parenteral and nebulized administration. Particular caution is advised in acute severe asthma, as hypokalemia may be potentiated by concomitant treatment with xanthine derivatives, steroids and diuretics; the adverse effects of hypokalemia may be exacerbated by hypoxia. It is recommended that serum potassium levels be monitored in such situations.

Hypokalemia will increase the susceptibility of digitalis-treated patients to cardiac arrhythmias.

Gastrointestinal: Patients with cystic fibrosis may be more prone to gastro-intestinal motility disturbances.

Immune: Immediate hypersensitivity reactions may occur after administration of DUOVENT, as demonstrated by rare cases of urticaria, angio-edema, bronchospasm, oropharyngeal oedema and anaphylaxis.

Ophthalmologic: Glaucoma, Angle-Closure: Care should be taken to ensure that the nebulizer mask fits the patient's face properly and that nebulized solution does not escape into the eyes (ie, use swimming goggles with the mask, or use a mouth piece). In patients with glaucoma or narrow anterior chambers, the administration by nebulizer of DUOVENT UDV should be avoided unless measures (e.g., use of swimming goggles or mouthpiece) are taken to ensure that nebulized solution does not reach the eye. Exposure of the eyes of such patients to a nebulized combination of ipratropium bromide and a β_2 agonist solution (i.e., DUOVENT UDV) has been reported to result in increased intraocular pressure and/or acute angle closure. There have been isolated reports of ocular complications (i.e., mydriasis, increased intraocular pressure, angle closure glaucoma, eye pain) when nebulized ipratropium bromide either alone or in combination with an adrenergic β_2 agonist solution has escaped into the eyes. In the event that glaucoma is precipitated or worsened, treatment should include standard measures for this condition.

Eye pain or discomfort, blurred vision, visual halos, or colored images in association with red eyes from conjunctival congestion and corneal oedema may be signs of acute narrow angle glaucoma. Should any combination of these symptoms develop, treatment with miotic drops should be initiated and specialist advice sought immediately.

Respiratory: Paradoxic Bronchospasm: Some patients receiving inhaled β adrenergic agonists have developed severe paradoxical bronchospasm, which has been life-threatening. The cause of this refractory state is unknown. If it occurs, the preparation should be discontinued immediately and alternative therapy instituted.

Use of DUOVENT UDV in Conjunction with IPPV: It has been reported in several cases that the use of intermittent positive-pressure ventilation in acute asthma attacks was related to lethal episodes of hypoxia and pneumothorax. This method of drug administration may be ineffective in patients with severe obstruction and greatly increased airway resistance, and it may induce severe hypercapnia and hypoxia. During intermittent positive-pressure ventilation therapy, the monitoring of arterial blood gases is highly desirable.

In patients with bronchial asthma and mild COPD, on-demand (symptom-oriented) treatment may be preferable to regular use.

Special Populations: Pregnant Women: The safety of DUOVENT UDV in pregnancy and lactation has not been established. It should be used with caution before childbirth in view of the inhibiting effect of fenoterol on uterine contractions.

Autoradiographic studies in gravid rats showed no detectable amounts of fenoterol in the fetus. Direct blood and tissue studies in several animal species and in man showed that the levels of fenoterol and its conjugates were 10 to 20 times lower in the fetus than in the maternal tissues.

Nursing Women: It is unknown whether ipratropium is excreted into breast milk. But it is unlikely that ipratropium would reach the infant to an important extent especially when administered to the mother by inhalation. However, because many drugs are excreted in breast milk, caution should be exercised when DUOVENT is administered to a nursing woman.

Pediatrics (<12 years of age): DUOVENT UDV is not currently indicated for use in children under 12 years of age as the dosing regimen and evidence concerning its safety in this age group have not been established.

ADVERSE REACTIONS: Adverse Drug Reaction Overview: Frequent undesirable effects of DUOVENT UDV (ipratropium bromide/fenoterol hydrobromide) are fine tremor of skeletal muscles and nervousness, less frequent are tachycardia, increased heart rate, dizziness, palpitations or headache, especially in hypersensitive patients.

Potentially serious hypokalemia may result from $beta_2$ agonist therapy.

In isolated cases there may be local reactions such as dryness of the mouth, throat irritation, pharyngitis or allergic reactions. As with use of other inhalation therapy, cough, local irritation (such as phyaryngitis, throat irritation) and inhalation induced bronchospasm have been reported.

As with other β agonist containing products, nausea, vomiting, sweating, weakness and myalgia/muscle cramps may occur.

In rare cases, decrease in diastolic blood pressure, increase in systolic blood pressure, arrythmias, particularly after higher doses, atrial fibrillation and supraventricular tachycardia and myocardial ischaemia may occur.

In individual cases, psychological alterations have been reported under inhalational therapy with β agonist containing products.

Because of the low systemic absorption of ipratropium bromide, ocular accommodation disturbances, gastrointestinal motility disturbances (vomiting, constipation, and diarrhea) and urinary retention are rare and reversible.

Ocular side effects (including accommodation disturbances and glaucoma) may occur (see Warnings and Precautions).

Skin reactions or allergic-type reactions such as skin rash, angioedema of the tongue, lips and face, urticaria, laryngospasm and anaphylactic reactions have been reported.

Clinical Trial Adverse Drug Reactions: Because clinical trials are conducted under very specific conditions the adverse reaction rates observed in the clinical trials may not reflect the rates observed in practice and should not be compared to the rates in the clinical trials of another drug. Adverse drug reaction information from clinical trials is useful for identifying drug-related adverse events and for approximating rates.

The adverse reactions noted for the individual components of DUOVENT UDV inhalation solution are as follows:
Ipratropium Bromide: The frequency of adverse reactions recorded in 214 patients receiving Atrovent (ipratropium bromide) solution was as follows (given by adverse effect : % of patients): dry mouth or throat (9.3); bad taste (5.1); tremor (4.2); exacerbation of symptoms (4.2); burning eyes (0.9); nausea (0.9); sweating (0.9); cough (0.9); headache (0.5); palpitations (0.5).

The adverse effect judged to be most severe was exacerbation of symptoms. This occurred in 8 patients treated with Atrovent solution alone, 6 of whom withdrew from the clinical studies.

Bronchospasm occurred in 3 patients with acute severe asthma who received Atrovent solution alone. In two patients, this was reversed after therapy with a β_2 sympathomimetic solution. The third patient received no other therapy.

Table 1 compares the incidence of adverse effects of the combination of Atrovent and a β_2 agonist solution with that of the β_2 agonist alone.

Table 1: DUOVENT UDV

Comparison of Adverse Effects

Adverse Effect	Atrovent-β_2 Agonist (% of 94 patients)	β_2 Agonist (% of 96 patients)
Tremor	31.9	26.0
Dry Mouth	16.0	28.1
Bad Taste	16.0	13.5
Vomiting	2.1	2.1
Palpitations	2.1	1.0
Headache	1.1	2.1
Cough	1.1	0.0
Flushing	1.1	0.0
Dizziness	0.0	1.0
Numbness in Leg	0.0	1.0

There have been isolated reports of ocular effects such as mydriasis, increased intraocular pressure, and acute glaucoma associated with the escape of nebulized ipratropium bromide (alone or in combination with a β_2 agonist) solution into the eyes.

Fenoterol Hydrobromide: At the most frequently used dosage of Berotec (fenoterol hydrobromide) solution of 0.5 to 1.0 mg, tremor occurred in 12% of patients. At higher doses of Berotec solution (up to 2.5 mg), given for the treatment of severe asthma in a hospital emergency room, mild to moderate tremor occurred in 32% of patients. Other adverse reactions in decreasing order of frequency included nervousness, dizziness, headache, lightheadedness, and palpitations.

In 104 patients who received the highest recommended dosage of 2.5 mg of Berotec solution, increases in heart rate of 10% or greater within 4 hours after drug administration were observed in 21% of the patients. However, at least an equal number of patients had decreased heart rate of a similar magnitude in the same time period. The remainder showed no significant pulse rate changes.

Local irritation or allergic reactions have been reported rarely. As with other bronchodilators, cough and, very rarely, paradoxical bronchospasm have been observed (see Warnings and Precautions).

Potentially serious hypokalemia may result from β_2 agonist therapy.

DRUG INTERACTIONS: Overview: Other β adrenergic agents, anticholinergics, xanthine derivatives (such as theophylline) and corticosteroids may enhance the effect of DUOVENT UDV inhalation solution. The concurrent administration of other beta mimetics, systemically available anticholinergics and xanthine derivatives (e.g. theophylline) may increase the adverse reactions.

A potentially serious reduction in bronchodilation may occur during concurrent administration of beta receptor blocking agents and fenoterol hydrobromide as these two agents inhibit the effects of one another (see Warnings and Precautions).

Beta agonist induced hypokalemia may be increased by concomitant treatment with xanthine derivatives, corticosteroids, and diuretics. This should be taken into account particularly in patients with severe airway obstruction.

Hypokalemia may result in an increased susceptibility to arrhythmias in patients receiving digoxin. Additionally, hypoxia may aggravate the effects of hypokalemia on cardiac rhythm. It is recommended that serum potassium levels are monitored in such situations.

Avoid concomitant use of $beta_2$-agonist containing medicinal products with monoamine oxidase inhibitors, tricyclic antidepressants or with other sympathomimetic agents since their combined effect on the cardiovascular system may be deleterious to the patient.

Inhalation of halogenated hydrocarbon anesthetics such as halothane, trichloroethylene and enflurane may increase the susceptibility of the cardiovascular effects of beta agonists.

Labour and Delivery: Beta adrenergic agents have been shown to delay preterm labour in some reports. There are no well-controlled studies which demonstrate that such agents will stop preterm labour or prevent labour at term. Cautious use of β adrenergics for the relief of bronchospasm is therefore required in pregnant patients to avoid interference with uterine contractility.

Lactation: The safety of DUOVENT during lactation has not been established.

DOSAGE AND ADMINISTRATION: Dosing Considerations: COPD: Chronic Bronchitis and Emphysema: DUOVENT UDV (ipratropium bromide/fenoterol hydrobromide) Inhalation Solution dosage should be individualized, and patient response should be monitored to determine the requirement for more than a single bronchodilator by the prescribing physician on an ongoing basis. Concomitant anti-inflammatory therapy should be considered for patients with steroid-responsive chronic obstructive pulmonary disease (COPD).

Counselling on smoking cessation should be the first step in treating patients with chronic obstructive pulmonary disease (COPD) who smoke, independent of the clinical presentation i.e. chronic bronchitis (with or without airflow limitation) or emphysema.

Smoking cessation produces symptomatic benefits and has been shown to confer a survival advantage by slowing or stopping the progression of chronic bronchitis and emphysema.

Asthma: DUOVENT UDV (ipratropium bromide/fenoterol hydrobromide) Inhalation Solution should be used only under medical supervision in patients with severe acute exacerbations of asthma who require more than a single bronchodilator.

In accordance with the present practice for asthma treatment, concomitant anti-inflammatory therapy should be part of the regimen if DUOVENT UDV is needed on a regular daily basis.

If a previously effective dosage regimen fails to provide the usual relief, or if the effects of a dose last for less than 3 hours, medical advice should be sought immediately; this is a sign of seriously worsening asthma that requires reassessment of therapy.

Recommended Dose and Dosage Adjustment: Adults and Children 12 years of Age or Over: The usual dose is 4 mL of DUOVENT UDV inhalation solution (each plastic unit dose vial contains a total of 0.5 mg of ipratropium bromide and 1.25 mg fenoterol hydrobromide in 4 mL of isotonic saline). Treatment with DUOVENT UDV inhalation solution may be repeated after 6 hours when necessary.

Not recommended for children under 12 years of age.

Patients should follow the instructions provided by the manufacturer of the nebulising device for proper care, maintenance and cleaning of the equipment.

Missed Dose: If a dose is missed, the next scheduled dose should be taken. An extra dose must not be taken.

Administration: DUOVENT UDV inhalation solution must be administered by means of nebulizer using gas flow (oxygen or compressed air).

Dilution Instructions: If the full content of DUOVENT UDV is to be nebulized, squeeze the plastic vial to empty its contents into the nebulizer chamber. If instructions were given to use a dose less than one complete vial, use a syringe to transfer the necessary amount to the nebulizer chamber. Where wall oxygen is available, the solution is best administered at a flow rate of 6-8 L/min. **Any solution left in the plastic vial must be discarded because DUOVENT UDV does not contain preservatives.** In most cases, dilution of the dose with sterile preservative-free saline is not necessary. However, volumes of DUOVENT solution less than 2 mL are not appropriate for nebulization and must be diluted with sterile preservative-free saline or another suitable nebulizer solution to make-up a total fill volume of 2-5 mL.

OVERDOSAGE:
Symptoms and Treatment: The effects of overdosage are expected to be primarily related to fenoterol. Overdosage resulting in excessive β adrenergic stimulation may cause tachycardia, palpitations, tremor, hypotension, widening of the pulse pressure, anginal pain, flushing, arrhythmia, hypertension and in extreme cases, sudden death. Expected symptoms of overdosage with ipratropium bromide (such as dry mouth, visual accommodation disturbances) are mild because the systemic availability of inhaled ipratropium is very low. If DUOVENT UDV (ipratropium bromide/fenoterol hydrobromide) overdosage occurs, cardiac and respiratory support should be provided as required.

Administration of sedatives, tranquilizers, or in severe cases, intensive therapy may be appropriate for the treatment of overdosage. Beta receptor blockers, preferably β1 selective, are suitable as specific antidotes; however, a possible increase in bronchial obstruction must be taken into account and the dose should be adjusted carefully in patients suffering from bronchial asthma or COPD because of the risk of precipitating severe bronchospasm, which may be fatal.

Furthermore, an increase in mucocilliary clearance has been demonstrated after administration of higher doses of fenoterol.

For management of a suspected drug overdose, contact your **regional Poison Control Centre**. See the *CPS* Directory section for a list of Poison Control Centres.

ACTION AND CLINICAL PHARMACOLOGY: Mechanism of Action: DUOVENT UDV Inhalation solution is a combination of the anticholinergic bronchodilator ipratropium bromide and the β_2 adrenergic bronchodilator fenoterol hydrobromide. Ipratropium bromide is a quaternary ammonium derivative of atropine and is an anticholinergic drug which has bronchodilator properties. Each unit dose vial contains a total of 0.5 mg ipratropium bromide and 1.25 mg fenoterol hydrobromide in 4 mL of normal saline. On inhalation of ipratropium bromide the onset of action is noted within 5 to 15 minutes with a peak response between 1 and 2 hours, lasting about 2 additional hours with subsequent decline from the peak. Bronchodilation is still evident 8 hours after inhalation. Preclinical and clinical evidence suggest no deleterious effect of ipratropium bromide on airway mucous secretion, mucocilliary clearance or gas exchange.

The bronchodilating effect of fenoterol hydrobromide is produced primarily by stimulation of β_2 receptors in the bronchial smooth muscles. When administered by inhalation, fenoterol exerts a significant increase in pulmonary function 5 minutes after administration with a maximal effect in 30 to 60 minutes. This effect remains at the same level for 2-3 hours before gradually declining. A significant degree of bronchodilation has been reported in some studies for 6-8 hours.

The concurrent administration of ipratropium bromide and fenoterol hydrobromide results in dilatation of the bronchi by affecting different pharmacologic sites of action.

Pharmacodynamics: Large single inhaled doses of ipratropium bromide have been given to man without any signs of toxicity. After administration of 400 µg by inhaler (10 times the recommended single dose) to 10 normal subjects, no changes were detected in pulse rate, blood pressure, intraocular pressure, salivary secretion, visual accommodation or electrocardiograms. Likewise, in another study, no changes in pulse rate or salivary secretion were seen when cumulative doses up to 1.2 mg were administered by inhalation to 12 normal volunteers.

Beta-adrenergic effects on the heart such as increase in heart rate and contractility, are caused by the vascular effects of fenoterol, cardiac beta$_2$-receptor stimulation, and at supratherapeutic doses by beta$_1$-receptor stimulation. QTc prolongations, ventricular and supraventricular arrhythmias and myocardia ischemia have been reported following treatment with nebulized fenoterol at a dose of 1 mg. The clinical significance has not been established.

Special studies utilizing therapeutic doses in asthmatic and chronic bronchitic patients, again did not reveal any systemic anticholinergic effects. In one study, 14 patients were treated for 45 days with either Atrovent inhaler 40 µg qid or Atrovent inhaler 40 µg plus oral Berotec 5 mg qid. No changes in visual acuity, intraocular pressure, pupil size or accommodation of vision occurred. Micturition function studies in 20 male patients showed no differences in urinary flow, total flow time and time until maximum flow between placebo and ipratropium bromide inhaler 40 µg tid administered for 3 days.

Deterioration in pulmonary function in patients treated in all clinical trials with therapeutic doses of Atrovent solution was examined. Table 2 shows the number of patients who showed a 15% or greater fall in FEV$_1$ at any time within 2 hours following the administration of the drug. Also shown are the figures for comparative agents used.

Table 2: DUOVENT UDV
Deterioration in Pulmonary Function

Treatment	Incidence
Normal Saline	15/90 (16.7%)
Atrovent Solution	14/214 (6.5%)
Atrovent Inhaler	4/78 (5.1%)
Berotec Solution	4/83 (4.8%)
Atrovent Solution + Berotec Solution	1/81 (1.2%)

Dose titration studies in stable asthmatic patients with Atrovent solution have indicated that maximal improvement in pulmonary function occurs at approximately 250 µg for adults and 125 µg for children over 5 years.

A clinical pharmacology study comparing single doses of Atrovent inhaler (80 µg) and Atrovent solution (250 µg) in 16 stable adult asthmatics was performed. No difference between the regimens was found, based on an improvement in pulmonary function over a 2 hour period.

A wide variety of challenge studies have been conducted using ipratropium bromide as a protective agent. In pharmacologically induced bronchospasm, ipratropium bromide, in clinical doses, was very effective against metacholine and acetylcholine, moderately effective against propranolol but had little or no effect against histamine or serotonin. Studies in exercise induced bronchospasm have yielded variable results. Some investigations have indicated that ipratropium bromide has little or no effect but other studies have shown that some patients are protected against bronchospasm induced by exercise. Likewise, the protective effects of ipratropium bromide against cold air induced bronchospasm have been variable.

Antigen challenge studies have demonstrated that Atrovent offers some protection against the "early" allergic asthma response, but has no effect on the "late" response.

Pharmacokinetics: The pharmacokinetics of ipratropium bromide and fenoterol are not altered when the two drugs are administered concurrently.

Ipratropium Bromide: Absorption: Ipratropium bromide is absorbed quickly after oral inhalation of a nominal dose of 40 µg administered from a pressurized metered dose inhaler. The peak plasma concentration (mean C_{max}=32 pg/mL) is reached within 5 minutes after inhalation. The therapeutic effect of ipratropium bromide is produced by a local action in the airways. Therefore time courses of bronchodilation and systemic pharmacokinetics do not run in parallel. The time to reach peak plasma concentration was similar to that seen after oral administration, likely reflecting the large fraction of inhaled dose which is deposited in the pharyngeal mucosa and swallowed. The absolute bioavailability after oral administration is approximately 2%.

Distribution: Intravenous administration of 1.0 mg in man showed a rapid distribution into tissues (half-life of alpha phase approximately 5 minutes), and a terminal half-life (beta phase) of 3-4 hours. Plasma concentrations after inhaled ipratropium bromide were 1000 times lower than equipotent oral or intravenous doses (15 and 0.15 mg, respectively).

The half-life of the terminal elimination phase is about 1.6 hours. The total clearance of the active ingredient is 2.3 L/min. Approximately 40% of the clearance is renal (0.9 L/min) and 60% non-renal i.e. mainly hepato-metabolic.

Radio-labelled technetium was administered with Atrovent (ipratropium bromide) solution in an adult dose finding study. Table 3 outlines the doses reaching the patient. The figures for Atrovent inhaler are published estimates.

Table 3: DUOVENT UDV
Doses Reaching the Patient

Dose Available (µg)	Amount Reaching Patient (µg)	Lung Dose (µg)
500	53	17.0
250	27	8.5
125	13	4.3
40 (Atrovent Inhaler)	40	4.4

The drug is minimally (less than 20%) bound to plasma proteins. The ipratropium ion does not cross the blood-brain barrier, consistent with the quaternary amine structure of the molecule. It is not known if the placental barrier is crossed.

Metabolism: Up to eight metabolites of ipratropium have been detected in man, rat and dog. However, the main metabolites bind poorly to the muscarinic receptor.

Excretion: In man, about 70% of the ^{14}C labelled drug is excreted unchanged after i.v. administration and only one metabolite exceeds 10% of the total radioactivity. The elimination of ipratropium and its metabolites occurs primarily via the kidneys with less than 10% of the total intravenous dose excreted via the biliary or fecal route. After oral or inhaled doses, however, up to 90% of the radiolabelled dose is detectable in the feces, suggesting relatively low lung deposition and poor absorption of the swallowed portion.

Thirty-nine percent of the active ingredient is excreted renally after intravenous administration, 4.4%-13.1% after inhalation from a metered dose inhaler is excreted as unchanged compound in urine.

Fenoterol: Absorption: In man, fenoterol is rapidly absorbed from the gastrointestinal tract, with an absorption level of 60%. After administration of tritium labelled fenoterol, peak plasma levels (2.5% of the oral dose) are reached in two hours, the half-life of radioactivity being 6 to 7 hours. When given from a pressured container, absorption proceeds in two phases: the first one is essentially independent of the dose and apparently takes place between the first and fourth subdivisions of the bronchial tree. The second phase appears to be identical to oral absorption. After inhalation, blood levels remain almost unchanged for 7 hours (0.3-0.4 ng/mL fenoterol).

Following intravenous administration, three phases were observed, whereby the half-life of the terminal phase was approximately 3 hours.

Distribution: Fenoterol is very rapidly taken up by the tissues, where it conjugated to the extent of 99% (as sulfates).

Metabolism: Unlike isoproterenol, fenoterol is not metabolized by catechol-O-methyl transferase.

Excretion: The resulting metabolites are excreted via the kidneys (40% within the first 48 hours after oral administration) and the bile (fecal excretion: 40% of the oral dose).

STORAGE AND STABILITY: Unopened unit dose vials of DUOVENT UDV should be stored at room temperature (15-25°C) and protected from heat and light. If necessary, the solution may be diluted with preservative-free sterile sodium chloride solution 0.9% and used immediately. Any solution remaining in the vial must be discarded.

INFORMATION FOR THE PATIENT: Published in e-CPS, available by subscription at www.e-cps.ca.

DOSAGE FORMS, COMPOSITION AND PACKAGING: Each mL of clear, colorless solution contains: ipratropium bromide 0.125 mg and fenoterol hydrobromide 0.3125 mg. Nonmedicinal ingredients: hydrochloric acid to adjust the pH and sodium chloride. Plastic single dose units, strips of 10. Cartons containing 2 strips of 10x4 mL UDVs. Each UDV strip is packaged in an aluminum/Low Density Polyethylene (LDPE) pouch.

Duragesic® MAT Ⓝ

fentanyl transdermal system
Opioid Analgesic

Janssen-Ortho

Date of Preparation: December 20, 1991
Date of Revision: July 26, 2010

SUMMARY PRODUCT INFORMATION:

Route of Administration	Dosage Form/Strength	Nonmedicinal Ingredients
Transdermal	Patch Five strengths with 2.1, 4.2, 8.4, 12.6, and 16.8 mg fentanyl per patch, delivering 12, 25, 50, 75, 100 µg/h fentanyl respectively for 72 hours	Polyester/EVA backing film, polacrylate adhesive, orange ink

INDICATIONS AND CLINICAL USE: Adults: DURAGESIC MAT (fentanyl transdermal system) is indicated in the management of persistent, moderate to severe chronic pain that cannot be managed by other means such as opioid combination products or immediate-release opioids, and only in patients:

- who require continuous around-the-clock opioid analgesia for an extended period of time and
- who are already receiving opioid therapy at a total daily dose of at least 60 mg/day Morphine Equivalents.

The initial dose of DURAGESIC MAT should be obtained or calculated from the conversion tables (see Dosage and Administration), and must **not** be higher than that dose which is equivalent to the total dose of opioids the patient is receiving at the time of the switch to the patch.

Because serious or life-threatening hypoventilation could occur, DURAGESIC MAT should not be used in:

- non-opioid-tolerant patients
- the management of postoperative pain

Special Populations: Pediatrics: The use of DURAGESIC MAT in children under 18 years of age is not recommended, as dosage requirements for the safe and efficacious use of fentanyl transdermal system have not been established for this patient population. Life-threatening hypoventilation has been reported in some pediatric patients receiving fentanyl transdermal system.

Geriatrics and Debilitated Patients: In elderly, cachectic, or debilitated patients, DURAGESIC MAT may have altered pharmacokinetics due to poor fat stores, muscle wasting or altered clearance (see Dosage and Administration). Therefore, it may be appropriate, according to clinical judgment, to initiate these patients on a lower DURAGESIC MAT dose than that which the conversion tables recommend, including the use of the 12 µg/h dose by itself or in combination with another dose, provided the patient is not opioid-naive (see Contraindications). The 12 µg/h strength may also be used for dose titration up or down, as using small increments for dose adjustment is recommended to enhance tolerability of opioid therapy (see Dosage and Administration).

CONTRAINDICATIONS: Because serious or life-threatening hypoventilation could occur, DURAGESIC MAT is contraindicated in:

1. patients with acute or perioperative pain, especially use in out-patient or day surgeries (see Warnings and Precautions, Peri-Operative Considerations);
2. patients with mild, intermittent or short duration pain that can otherwise be managed;
3. opioid-naive patients, at any dose;
4. situations of significant respiratory depression, especially in unmonitored settings where there is a lack of resuscitative equipment; and
5. patients who have acute or severe bronchial asthma.

Because serious or life-threatening hypoventilation could occur, the maximum initiation dose of DURAGESIC MAT should not be higher than that equivalent to the total dose of opioids the patient is receiving at the time of the switch (see conversion tables in Dosage and Administration).

DURAGESIC MAT is contraindicated in patients who have or are suspected of having paralytic ileus.

DURAGESIC MAT is contraindicated in patients with known hypersensitivity to fentanyl or to the adhesives present in the system.

WARNINGS AND PRECAUTIONS: General: Use in non-opioid-tolerant patients, or use of an initiating dose which is higher than the opioid equivalent to which the patient is tolerant at the time of the switch, may lead to fatal respiratory depression.

The following contraindications reduce the potential risk of serious or life-threatening hypoventilation: DURAGESIC MAT should not be used in the management of acute or postoperative pain since there is no opportunity for dose titration during short-term use and serious or life-threatening hypoventilation could result. Similarly, DURAGESIC MAT should not be administered to patients who do not have some degree of tolerance to opioid-induced side effects. DURAGESIC MAT should ONLY be prescribed to patients who require continuous opioids for pain management, and who are tolerant to at least the morphine equivalent of the lowest initiating DURAGESIC MAT dose.

The initial dose of DURAGESIC MAT should be obtained from the conversion tables in Dosage and Administration, and must not be higher than that dose which is equivalent to the total dose of opioids the patient is receiving at the time of the switch to the patch. It may be appropriate, according to clinical judgment, to initiate some patients on a lower DURAGESIC MAT dose than that which the conversion tables recommend, which may include use of the 12 µg/h dose. Opioid-naive patients should not be given DURAGESIC MAT at any dose, inclusive of 12 µg/h (see Contraindications). In general, the 12 µg/h dose, which allows for smaller dose increases than does the 25 µg/h patch, is to be used for titration/adjustments of dosage (see Dosage and Administration).

The use of DURAGESIC MAT in children under 18 years of age is not recommended as dosage requirements for the safe and efficacious use of DURAGESIC MAT have not been established for this patient population. Life-threatening hypoventilation has been reported in some pediatric patients receiving fentanyl transdermal system.

DURAGESIC MAT should only be prescribed by persons knowledgeable in the continuous administration of potent opioids, in the management of patients receiving potent opioids for treatment of pain and in the detection and management of respiratory depression including the use of opioid antagonists.

Since serum fentanyl concentrations decline gradually after system removal, patients who have experienced serious adverse events should be monitored for at least 24 hours after DURAGESIC MAT removal or until the adverse reaction has subsided.

As with other CNS depressants, patients who have received DURAGESIC MAT should be closely monitored especially for signs of respiratory depression until a stable maintenance dose is reached.

Due to the formation of a subcutaneous depot of fentanyl, not only does continued exposure occur after system removal but, in the case of removal prior to attainment of peak fentanyl exposure, fentanyl plasma levels may in fact continue to increase after removal of DURAGESIC MAT patches.

DURAGESIC MAT patches are intended for transdermal use on intact skin only; use on compromised skin can lead to increased exposure to fentanyl.

Placing DURAGESIC MAT in the mouth, chewing it, swallowing it, or using it in any ways other than indicated may cause choking or overdose that could result in death.

Risk of Unintentional Increase in Drug Exposure: Patients with Fever: Serum fentanyl concentrations could theoretically increase by approximately one-third for patients with a body temperature of 40°C due to temperature-dependent increases in fentanyl release from the system and increased skin permeability. Patients who develop fever should be monitored for opioid side effects and have their DURAGESIC MAT dose adjusted if necessary.

External Heat Sources: There is a potential for temperature-dependent increases in fentanyl released from the system resulting in possible overdose and death. A clinical pharmacology trial conducted in healthy adult subjects has shown that the application of heat over the DURAGESIC MAT system increased mean fentanyl AUC values by 120% and mean C_{max} values by 61%. All patients should be advised to avoid exposing the DURAGESIC MAT application site to direct external heat sources, such as heating pads, electric blankets, heated water beds, heat lamps, hot water bottles, saunas and hot whirlpool spa baths, intensive sunbathing, etc.

Accidental Exposure to DURAGESIC MAT: Serious medical consequences, including death, have occurred when people were accidentally exposed to fentanyl transdermal system. Examples of accidental exposure include transfer of a fentanyl transdermal system patch while hugging, sharing a bed, or moving a patient.

Disposal of DURAGESIC MAT: DURAGESIC MAT should be kept out of the reach of children before and after use.

Used systems should be folded so that the adhesive side of the system adheres to itself, then flushed down the toilet immediately upon removal. If the drug adhesive layer accidentally contacts the skin, the area should be washed with clear water. Patients should dispose of any systems remaining from a prescription as soon as they are no longer needed. Unused systems should be removed from their pouch, folded so that the adhesive side of the system adheres to itself, then flushed down the toilet (see Dosage and Administration and Special Handling Instructions).

Cardiovascular: Intravenous fentanyl may produce bradycardia. Fentanyl should be administered with caution to patients with bradyarrhythmias.

Concomitant Use of Central Nervous System Depressants: When patients are receiving DURAGESIC MAT, the dose of additional opioids or other CNS- depressant drugs (including alcohol beverages, benzodiazepines, general anesthetics, muscle relaxants and sedating over-the-counter antihistamines) should be reduced by at least 50%. The concomitant use of CNS depressants may result in hypotension, respiratory depression and profound sedation, coma or death (see Drug Interactions).

Concomitant Use of CYP3A4 Inhibitors: The concomitant use of DURAGESIC MAT with potent cytochrome P450 3A4 inhibitors (ritonavir, ketoconazole, itraconazole, troleandomycin, clarithromycin, nelfinavir, nefazodone, verapamil, diltiazem, amiodarone, amprenavir, fosamprenavir, aprepitant, fluconazole, erythromycin and grapefruit juice) may result in an increase in fentanyl plasma concentrations, which could increase or prolong adverse drug effects and may cause potentially fatal respiratory depression. In this situation special patient care and observation are appropriate. Therefore, the concomitant use of transdermal fentanyl and CYP 3A4 inhibitors is not recommended unless the patient is closely monitored, for an extended period of time, for signs of respiratory depression, with dosage adjustments made as warranted (see Drug Interactions).

Potential for Abuse and Diversion: DURAGESIC MAT contains a high concentration of a potent opioid, fentanyl, which along with other opioids of the morphine type has high potential for abuse and associated risk of fatal overdose due to respiratory depression. The high fentanyl content in DURAGESIC MAT patches may be a particular target for abuse and diversion, with alternative routes of administration potentially resulting in overdose from uncontrolled delivery of the opioid.

This risk should be considered when administering, prescribing, or dispensing DURAGESIC MAT in situations where the healthcare professional is concerned about increased risk of misuse, abuse or diversion.

Concerns about abuse, addiction and diversion should not prevent the proper management of pain. Patients should be assessed for their clinical risks for opioid abuse or addiction prior to being prescribed opioids. All patients receiving opioids should be routinely monitored for signs of misuse and abuse.

Since DURAGESIC MAT may be diverted for non-medical use, careful record keeping of prescribing information, including quantity, frequency, and renewal requests is strongly advised. Proper assessment of the patient, proper prescribing practices, periodic re-evaluation of therapy, and proper dispensing and storage are appropriate measures that help to limit abuse of opioid drugs (see Dependence/Tolerance).

Dependence/Tolerance: Drug Dependence vs. Abuse: Fentanyl is an opioid substance and can produce drug dependence similar to that produced by morphine. DURAGESIC MAT, therefore, has the potential for abuse. However, tolerance as well as both physical and psychological dependence may develop upon repeated administration of opioids, and are not by themselves evidence of an addictive disorder or abuse. Iatrogenic addiction following appropriate opioid administration for relief of severe pain is relatively rare. Physicians should not let concerns of physical dependence deter them from using adequate amounts of opioids in the management of severe pain when such use is indicated. Patients at increased risk of opioid abuse may still be appropriately treated with modified-release opioid formulations; however, these patients will require monitoring for signs of misuse, abuse or addiction.

Drug or Alcohol Dependence: Use of DURAGESIC MAT in combination with CNS depressants, including alcohol, can result in increased risk to the patient (see Drug Interactions).

DURAGESIC MAT should be used with caution in individuals who have a history of drug or alcohol abuse, especially those outside a medically controlled environment. While the management of severe pain in patients with a history of addiction requires special consideration, the use of opioids is not necessarily contraindicated in these patients. There may also be an increased risk of diversion in this population; this risk may be decreased by attention to patterns of prescription requests, and by prescribing opioids only as part of an ongoing relationship between a patient and a healthcare provider.

"Drug seeking" behaviour includes emergency calls or visits near the end of office hours; refusal to undergo appropriate examination, testing or referral; repeated "loss" of prescriptions; tampering with prescriptions; "doctor shopping" to obtain additional prescriptions; and reluctance to provide prior medical records or contact information for other treating physician(s).

Head Injuries and Increased Intracranial Pressure: DURAGESIC MAT should not be used in patients who may be particularly susceptible to the intracranial effects of CO_2 retention such as those with evidence of increased intracranial pressure, impaired consciousness, or coma. Opioids may obscure the clinical course of patients with head injury. DURAGESIC MAT should be used with caution in patients with brain tumours.

Peri-Operative Considerations: DURAGESIC MAT is contraindicated for perioperative pain relief, especially in the elective surgical setting. In the case of planned chordotomy, or other pain-relieving operations, patients should not be treated with DURAGESIC MAT within 72 hours before the operation and should not be used in the immediate post-operative period. Thereafter, if DURAGESIC MAT is to be continued after the patient recovers from the post-operative period, a new dosage should be administered in accordance with the changed need for pain relief, if needed, and to reduce the risk of withdrawal in highly opioid-tolerant patients.

The administration of analgesics in the perioperative period should be managed by health care providers with adequate training and experience (e.g., an anesthesiologist) (see Contraindications).

Hepatic/Biliary/Pancreatic: Because of the hepatic metabolism of fentanyl, DURAGESIC MAT should be used with caution in patients with liver dysfunction.

DURAGESIC MAT may cause spasm of the sphincter of Oddi and should be used with caution in patients with biliary tract disease, including acute pancreatitis. Opioids like DURAGESIC MAT may cause increases in the serum amylase concentration.

If patients with hepatic impairment receive DURAGESIC MAT, they should be observed carefully for signs of fentanyl toxicity and the dose of DURAGESIC MAT reduced if necessary.

Psychomotor Impairment: DURAGESIC MAT may impair mental and/or physical ability required for the performance of potentially hazardous tasks such as driving a car or operating machinery. Patients using DURAGESIC MAT should not drive or operate dangerous machinery unless they are tolerant to the effects of the drug.

Renal: Because of the renal excretion of fentanyl, DURAGESIC MAT should be used with caution in patients with kidney dysfunction.

If patients with renal impairment receive DURAGESIC MAT, they should be observed carefully for signs of fentanyl toxicity and the dose reduced if necessary.

Respiratory: Respiratory Depression: As with all potent opioids, some patients may experience significant respiratory depression (including respiratory distress, apnea, bradypnea, hypoventilation, dyspnea) with DURAGESIC MAT; caution must be exercised and patients carefully observed for untoward reactions. While most patients using DURAGESIC MAT chronically develop tolerance to fentanyl-induced hypoventilation, episodes of slowed respiration may occur at any time during therapy. A small number of patients have experienced clinically significant hypoventilation with fentanyl transdermal system; medical intervention generally was not required in these instances. The incidence of respiratory depression increases as the fentanyl transdermal system dose is increased.

Hypoventilation can occur throughout the therapeutic range of fentanyl serum concentrations. However, the risk of hypoventilation increases at serum fentanyl concentrations greater than 2 ng/mL in non-opioid-tolerant patients, especially for patients who have an underlying pulmonary condition or who receive usual doses of opioids or other CNS drugs associated with hypoventilation in addition to DURAGESIC MAT (see Drug Interactions regarding the use of concomitant CNS active drugs). The use of DURAGESIC MAT should be monitored by clinical evaluation. As with other drug-level measurements, serum fentanyl concentrations may be useful clinically, although they do not reflect patients' sensitivity to fentanyl and should not be used by physicians as a sole indicator of effectiveness or toxicity.

The duration of the respiratory depressant effect of DURAGESIC MAT may extend beyond the removal of the system (see also Overdosage concerning respiratory depression).

Use in Patients with Chronic Pulmonary Disease: Fentanyl should be used with caution in patients with chronic pulmonary disease, patients with decreased respiratory reserve and others with potentially compromised respiration. Normal analgesic doses of opioids may further decrease respiratory drive in these patients to the point of respiratory failure.

Information to Be Provided to the Patient: Consumer Information is included in the package of DURAGESIC MAT patches dispensed to the patient.

Patients receiving DURAGESIC MAT patches should be given the following instructions by the physician:

1. Patients should be informed that accidental ingestion or use by individuals (including children) other than the patient for whom it was originally prescribed, may lead to severe, even fatal, consequences.
2. Patients should be advised that DURAGESIC MAT patches contain fentanyl, an opioid pain medicine similar to morphine, hydromorphone, methadone, oxycodone, and oxymorphone.
3. Patients should be advised that each DURAGESIC MAT patch may be worn continuously for 72 hours, and that each patch should be applied to a different skin site after removal of the previous transdermal patch.
4. Patients should be advised that DURAGESIC MAT patches should be applied to intact, non-irritated, and non-irradiated skin on a flat surface such as the chest, back, flank, or upper arm. Additionally, patients should be advised of the following:
   - In young children or persons with cognitive impairment, the patch should be put on the upper back to lower the chances that the patch will be removed and placed in the mouth.
   - Hair at the application site should be clipped (not shaved) prior to patch application.
   - If the site of DURAGESIC MAT application must be cleansed prior to application of the patch, do so with clear water.
   - Do not use soaps, oils, lotions, alcohol, or any other agents that may irritate the skin or alter its characteristics.
   - Allow the skin to dry completely prior to patch application.
5. Patients should be advised that DURAGESIC MAT should be applied immediately upon removal from the sealed package and after removal of the protective liner. Additionally the patient should be advised of the following:
   - The DURAGESIC MAT patch should not be used if the seal is broken, or if it is altered, cut, or damaged in any way prior to application. The transdermal patch should be pressed firmly in place with the palm of the hand for 30 seconds, making sure the contact is complete, especially around the edges.
   - The patch should not be folded so that only part of the patch is exposed.
6. Patients should be advised that, while wearing the patch, they should avoid exposing the DURAGESIC MAT application site to direct external heat sources, such as:
   - heating pads,
   - electric blankets,
   - heat lamps,
   - saunas,
   - hot tubs, and
   - heated water beds, etc.
7. Patients should be advised that there is a potential for temperature-dependent increase in fentanyl release from the patch that could result in an overdose of fentanyl; therefore, if patients develop a high fever while wearing the patch they should contact their physician.
8. Patients should be advised that if they experience problems with adhesion of the DURAGESIC MAT patch, they may tape the edges of the patch with first aid tape. If problems with adhesion persist, patients may overlay the patch with a transparent adhesive film dressing.
9. Patients should be advised that if the patch falls off before 72 hours a new patch may be applied to a different skin site.
10. Patients should be advised to fold (so that the adhesive side adheres to itself) and immediately flush down the toilet used DURAGESIC MAT patches after removal from the skin.
11. Patients should be instructed that, if the drug adhesive layer accidentally contacts the skin, the area should be washed clean with clear water and not soap, alcohol, or other chemicals, because these products may increase the ability of fentanyl to go through the skin.
12. Patients should be advised that the dose of DURAGESIC MAT should **never** be adjusted without the prescribing health care professional's instruction.
13. Patients should be advised that DURAGESIC MAT may impair mental and/or physical ability required for the performance of potentially hazardous tasks (e.g., driving, operating machinery).
14. Patients should be advised to refrain from any potentially dangerous activity when starting on DURAGESIC MAT or when their dose is being adjusted, until it is established that they have not been adversely affected.
15. Patients should be advised that DURAGESIC MAT should not be combined with alcohol or other CNS depressants (e.g. sleep medications, tranquilizers) because dangerous additive effects may occur, resulting in serious injury or death.
16. Patients should be advised to consult their physician or pharmacist if other medications are being or will be used with DURAGESIC MAT.
17. Patients should be advised of the potential for severe constipation.
18. Patients should be advised that if they have been receiving treatment with DURAGESIC MAT and cessation of therapy is indicated, it may be appropriate to taper the DURAGESIC MAT dose, rather than abruptly discontinue it, due to the risk of precipitating withdrawal symptoms.
19. Patients should be advised that DURAGESIC MAT contains fentanyl, a drug with high potential for abuse.
20. Patients, family members and caregivers should be advised to protect DURAGESIC MAT from theft or misuse in the work or home environment.
21. Patients should be advised that DURAGESIC MAT should never be given to anyone other than the individual for whom it was prescribed because of the risk of death or other serious medical problems to that person for whom it was not intended.

22. Patients should be instructed to keep DURAGESIC MAT in a secure place out of the reach of children due to the high risk of **fatal respiratory depression**.
23. When DURAGESIC MAT is no longer needed, the unused patches should be removed from their pouches, folded so that the adhesive side of the patch adheres to itself, and flushed down the toilet.
24. Women of childbearing potential who become or are planning to become pregnant should be advised to consult a physician prior to initiating or continuing therapy with DURAGESIC MAT.
25. Patients should be informed that accidental exposure or misuse may lead to death or other serious medical problems.
26. Patients should be informed that, if the patch dislodges and accidentally sticks to the skin of another person, they should immediately take the patch off, wash the exposed area with water and seek immediate medical attention for the accidentally exposed individual.

Special Populations: Pregnant Women: Fentanyl has been shown to impair fertility and to have an embryocidal effect in rats when given in intravenous doses 0.3 times the human dose for a period of 12 days. No evidence of teratogenic effects has been observed after the administration of fentanyl to rats. The safe use of fentanyl has not been established with respect to possible adverse effects upon human fetal development. Neonatal withdrawal syndrome has been reported in newborn infants with chronic maternal use of fentanyl transdermal system during pregnancy. Therefore, DURAGESIC MAT should not be used in women of childbearing potential unless, in the judgment of the physician, the potential benefits outweigh the possible hazards.

Use of DURAGESIC MAT during childbirth is not recommended because fentanyl passes through the placenta and may cause respiratory depression in the newborn child.

Nursing Women: Fentanyl is excreted in human milk; therefore, DURAGESIC MAT is not recommended for use in nursing women because of the possibility of effects in their infants.

Pediatrics (<18 years of age): The use of DURAGESIC MAT in children under 18 years of age is not recommended, as dosage requirements for the safe and efficacious use of fentanyl transdermal system have not been established for this patient population. Life-threatening hypoventilation has been reported in some pediatric patients receiving fentanyl transdermal system.

Geriatrics and Debilitated Patients: In elderly, cachectic, or debilitated patients, DURAGESIC MAT may have altered pharmacokinetics due to poor fat stores, muscle wasting or altered clearance (see Dosage and Administration). Therefore, it may be appropriate, according to clinical judgment, to initiate these patients on a lower DURAGESIC MAT dose than that which the conversion tables recommend, including the use of the 12 µg/h dose by itself or in combination with another dose, provided the patient is not opioid-naive (see Contraindications). The 12 µg/h strength may also be used for dose titration up or down, as using small increments for dose adjustment is recommended to enhance tolerability of opioid therapy (see Dosage and Administration). As with all DURAGESIC MAT patients, they should be carefully monitored for pain levels and adverse events, particularly hypoventilation.

ADVERSE REACTIONS: Clinical Trial Adverse Drug Reactions: Cancer Trials—Adults: Open-Label and Active-Control Double-Blind Studies: The safety of fentanyl transdermal system has been evaluated in 153 cancer patients and 357 postoperative patients. The duration of fentanyl transdermal system use varied in cancer patients, 56% of patients used fentanyl transdermal system for over 30 days, 28% continued treatment for more than 4 months, and 10% used fentanyl transdermal system for more than 1 year. In cancer patients, fentanyl transdermal system was administered in doses of 25 µg/h to 600 µg/h. Patients with acute pain used fentanyl transdermal system for 1 to 3 days.

Respiratory depression, the most serious adverse reaction, was observed in 3 (2%) of the cancer patients and 13 (4%) of postoperative patients. Hypotension and hypertension were observed in 11 (3%) and 4 (1%) of the opioid-naive patients.

Placebo-Controlled Study: Adverse events occurring at a greater frequency than placebo were identified in a placebo-controlled clinical trial of fentanyl transdermal system (25 µg/h to 100 µg/h) in cancer patients. Patients were stabilized on morphine for 7 days, and those who achieved adequate pain relief (n=131) were then switched to fentanyl transdermal system. During the initial open-label dose-titration and stabilization period of 15 days, a total of 43 patients dropped out; four experienced dyspnea, 3 nausea and 1 severe hallucinations.

Following this stabilization period, the nine-day double-blind period began, with patients randomized to either continue the dose of fentanyl transdermal system achieved during stabilization (n=47) or to switch to placebo (n=48). Rescue morphine was available. The median dose of fentanyl transdermal system was 50 µg/h. Adverse events during this period, as reported by at least 1 fentanyl transdermal system patient (2.1%), and with a higher frequency of occurrence versus placebo include: vomiting (4.3% vs 0%), and the following events at 2.1% vs. 0%: abscess, vertigo, hemorrhage, abdominal pain and jaundice.

Chronic Non-Cancer Pain Trials—Adults: The safety findings from the two primary trials (FEN-INT-12, n=248 patients, and FEN-INT-13, n=532 patients) are described below.

Safety Findings: Adverse events related to respiratory depression (reported as either bradypnea or hypoventilation) have been reported in 3/780 (0.4%) of the CNCP patients, leading to discontinuation in all three cases.

There were nine deaths (all in the one-year trial): four were due to cardiac events, three to pneumonia, one to a cerebrovascular event, and one to cancer.

The discontinuation rates were 16% for the one-month crossover trial (FEN-INT-12) and 43% for the one-year trial (FEN-INT-13).

Of the 780 patients, 149 (19%) received less than one month fentanyl transdermal system treatment, 272 (35%) used fentanyl transdermal system for one to six months, 137 (18%) for six months to one year, and 222 patients (28%) continued treatment for more than one year.

Among patients who completed the one-year trial (n=301 of 530 ITT patients), the mean dose at the 12-month endpoint was 90.4 µg/h, with the most common dose being 75 µg/h.

Most Common Adverse Events: A causal relationship of adverse events to fentanyl transdermal system was not always determined. The most commonly observed adverse events in the non-cancer chronic pain clinical trials, regardless of causal relationship, are: nausea or vomiting, somnolence, constipation, sweating, headache, dizziness, pruritus and depression.

Other reported adverse reactions occurring in >1% of patients that are probably or likely related to fentanyl transdermal system treatment are:

Application Site: application site reaction.
Body as a Whole: fatigue, pain, malaise, asthenia, hot flushes, withdrawal syndrome, back pain, rigors, temperature changed sensation.
Central & Peripheral Nervous System: tremor, vertigo, hypertonia.
Gastrointestinal System: dry mouth, diarrhea, abdominal pain, dyspepsia.
Heart Rate and Rhythm: palpitation.
Liver and Biliary System: hepatic enzymes increased, gamma-GT increased.
Metabolic and Nutritional: weight decreased, LDH increased.
Psychiatric: anorexia, anxiety, confusion, insomnia, nervousness, agitation, hallucination, concentration impaired, emotional lability, amnesia.
Respiratory System: dyspnea.
Skin and Appendages: rash erythematous, skin disorder.

Chronic Pain Trials—Pediatrics: The safety of fentanyl transdermal system has been evaluated in 293 opioid-tolerant pediatric patients (age 18 years or less) with chronic pain, with n=63 receiving fentanyl transdermal system for at least 2 months. Approximately 60% of the patients had underlying pain due to malignancy. The number of patients in the lower age ranges were as follows: n=2 patients <2 years old; n=65 patients 2 to <6 years old; n=100 patients 6 to <12 years old. The most commonly reported adverse events regardless of causality include: vomiting (14.3%), nausea (11.6%), constipation (9.2%), pruritus (8.2%), and somnolence (5.8%). Three patients experienced respiratory depression within 96 hours of beginning fentanyl transdermal system; two of these patients died. The underlying condition of the patients contributed to the deaths. The third patient's decreased respiratory rate was resolved after temporary discontinuation of fentanyl transdermal system.

Dosing recommendations for the safe and effective use of DURAGESIC MAT in this patient population have not been established, in view of the combination of: i) the variety of factors which could lead to overexposure from DURAGESIC MAT in children as compared to adults (including smaller body weight and significantly different body surface area; differential skin characteristics; potential for magnification, compared to adults, of the impact of amount of body fat stores, muscle wasting, fever, external heat), and ii) the limitations in both formal PK data (see Action and Clinical Pharmacology, Pharmacokinetics, Special Populations and Conditions) and exposure data (as above).

Post-Market Adverse Drug Reactions: In post-marketing experience, deaths from hypoventilation have been reported in cases of inappropriate use of fentanyl transdermal system.

Other opioid-related adverse reactions include: nausea, vomiting, constipation, hypotension, bradycardia, somnolence, headache, confusion, hallucination, euphoria, pruritus, sweating, tachycardia, paresthesia, sexual dysfunction, and urinary retention.

Skin reactions such as rash, erythema and itching have occasionally been reported. These reactions usually resolve within 24 hours or upon removal of the patch.

There have been very rare reports of anaphylactic and anaphylactoid reaction, including Stevens-Johnson syndrome, airway constriction, swelling, anaphylactic shock, and two deaths that occurred within 24 hours of the anaphylactic reaction. In one case, it was the care-giver of the patient who experienced dyspnea, urticaria and swelling, within ten minutes of applying the patch to the patient.

There have also been rare reports of convulsions, including clonic convulsions and grand mal convulsions. In two cases, vegetative state or coma was reported to immediately follow the convulsions.

Opioid withdrawal symptoms, such as nausea, vomiting, diarrhea, anxiety and shivering are possible in some patients after conversion from their previous opioid analgesic to DURAGESIC MAT or if therapy is stopped suddenly. There have been very rare reports of newborn infants experiencing neonatal withdrawal syndrome when mothers chronically used fentanyl transdermal system during pregnancy (see Warnings and Precautions, Special Populations, Pregnant Women).

DRUG INTERACTIONS: Overview: Additive Effects of Other CNS Depressants: Hypoventilation, hypotension and profound sedation or coma may occur with the concomitant use of other central nervous system depressants (including other opioids, sedatives or hypnotics, general anesthetics, phenothiazines, tranquilizers); skeletal muscle relaxants, sedating antihistamines, and alcoholic beverages may produce additive depressant effects. When combined therapy is contemplated, the dose of each agent should be reduced by at least 50%.

Drug-Drug Interactions: CYP 3A4 Inhibitors: Fentanyl, a high clearance drug, is rapidly and extensively metabolized mainly by the human cytochrome P450 3A4 isoenzyme system (CYP3A4); therefore, potential interactions may occur when DURAGESIC MAT is given concurrently with agents that affect CYP3A4 activity. Coadministration with agents that induce 3A4 activity may reduce the efficacy of DURAGESIC MAT. The concomitant use of transdermal fentanyl with ritonavir or other potent 3A4 inhibitors such as ketoconazole, itraconazole, troleandomycin, clarithromycin, nelfinavir, nefazodone, verapamil, diltiazem, amiodarone, amprenavir, fosamprenavir, aprepitant, fluconazole, erythomycin and grapefruit juice may result in an increase in fentanyl plasma concentrations which could increase or prolong adverse drug effects and may cause serious respiratory depression (see also Warnings and Precautions, Concomitant Use of CYP3A4 Inhibitors). In this situation, special patient care and observation are appropriate. The concomitant use of CYP3A4 inhibitors and DURAGESIC MAT is not recommended, unless the patient is closely monitored.

MAO Inhibitors: Severe and unpredictable potentiation by MAO inhibitors has been reported with opioid analgesics. Since the safety of fentanyl in this regard has not been established, the use of fentanyl in patients who have received MAO inhibitors during the previous 14-day period is not recommended. Conversely, the use of MAO inhibitors in patients who have received fentanyl in the previous 14-day period is not recommended.

DOSAGE AND ADMINISTRATION: General: DURAGESIC MAT should only be prescribed by persons knowledgeable in the continuous administration of potent opioids, in the management of patients receiving potent opioids for treatment of pain, and in the detection and management of respiratory depression including the use of opioid antagonists.

At the time of the switch to DURAGESIC MAT from other opioids, patients must be tolerant to opioid therapy of comparable potency to that of the intended initiating dose. Use of DURAGESIC MAT in patients who are non-opioid-tolerant, or insufficiently tolerant, may lead to fatal respiratory depression.

Dosing Considerations: DURAGESIC MAT doses must be individualized based upon the status of each patient and should be assessed at regular intervals after application. Proper optimization of doses scaled to the relief of the individual's pain should aim at the regular administration of the lowest dose of DURAGESIC MAT which will achieve the overall treatment goal of satisfactory pain relief with acceptable side effects. Dosage of the drug must be individualized according to the response and tolerance of the patient. The most important factor to be considered in determining the appropriate dose is the extent of pre-existing opioid tolerance. Reduced doses of DURAGESIC MAT are suggested for the elderly and other groups discussed in Warnings and Precautions.

There has been no systematic evaluation of DURAGESIC MAT as an initial opioid analgesic in the management of chronic pain. Most patients in the clinical trials were converted to fentanyl transdermal system from other opioid therapies on which inadequate to moderate pain control had been experienced prior to conversion.

Initiation of DURAGESIC MAT in patients who are opioid-naïve is contraindicated at any dose (see Contraindications). The initial dose of DURAGESIC MAT should be obtained from the conversion tables in Dosage and Administration, and must not be higher than that dose which is equivalent to the total dose of opioids the patient is receiving at the time of the switch to the patch. It may be appropriate, according to clinical judgment, to initiate some patients on a lower DURAGESIC MAT dose than that which the conversion tables recommend, including the use of the 12 µg/h dose by itself or in combination with another dose, provided the patient is not opioid-naive (see Contraindications).

In general the 12 µg/h dose, which allows for smaller dose increases than does the 25 µg/h patch, is to be used for titration/adjustments of dosage (For oral morphine equivalency in dose adjustment, see Recommended Dose and Dosage Adjustment, Dose Adjustment, Titration Dose Increment). The 12 µg/h dose is not included in the conversion tables (Table 1 and Table 2) because it is generally not to be used as the initiating dose.

Opioid analgesics may be only partially effective in relieving dysesthetic pain, postherpetic neuralgia, stabbing pains, activity-related pain and some forms of headache. That is not to say that patients with these types of pain should not be given an adequate trial of opioid analgesics, but it may be necessary to refer such patients at an early time to other forms of pain therapy.

DURAGESIC MAT has a high potential for abuse and diversion (see Warnings and Precautions).

Concomitant Use of CYP3A4 Inhibitors: The concomitant use of DURAGESIC MAT with potent cytochrome P450 3A4 inhibitors (ritonavir, ketoconazole, itraconazole, troleandomycin, clarithromycin, nelfinavir, nefazodone, verapamil, diltiazem, amiodarone, amprenavir, fosamprenavir, aprepitant, fluconazole, erythromycin and grapefruit juice) may result in an increase in fentanyl plasma concentrations, which could increase or prolong adverse drug effects and may cause potentially fatal respiratory depression. Patients concomitantly exposed to DURAGESIC MAT and potent CYP3A4 inhibitors should be carefully monitored for an extended period of time and dosage adjustments should be made if warranted (see Drug Interactions).

Recommended Dose and Dosage Adjustment: Pediatrics: The use of DURAGESIC MAT in children under 18 years of age is not recommended as dosage requirements for the safe and efficacious use of fentanyl transdermal system have not been established for this patient population. Life-threatening hypoventilation has been reported in some pediatric patients receiving fentanyl transdermal system.

Adults: Initial Dose Selection: In selecting an initial DURAGESIC MAT dose, attention should be given to 1) the daily dose, potency, and characteristics of the opioid the patient has been taking previously (e.g. whether it is a pure agonist or mixed agonist-antagonist), 2) the reliability of the relative potency estimates used to calculate the DURAGESIC MAT dose needed (potency estimates may vary with the route of administration), 3) the degree of opioid tolerance, and 4) the general condition and medical status of the patient.

At the time of the switch to DURAGESIC MAT, patients must be tolerant to opioid therapy of comparable potency to that of the intended initiating dose. It may be appropriate, according to clinical judgment, to initiate some patients on a lower DURAGESIC MAT dose than that which the conversion tables recommend, which may include use of the 12 µg/h dose. The 12 µg/h dose is not included in the conversion tables (Table 1 and Table 2), because it is generally to be used for dose adjustment rather than as the initiation dose, except in the case of patients who, because of their clinical status, are to be initiated on a lower dose than that which the conversion tables recommend. Overestimating the DURAGESIC MAT dose when converting patients from another opioid medication can result in fatal overdose with the first dose. Due to the mean elimination half-life of 17 hours of DURAGESIC MAT, patients who are thought to have had a serious adverse event, including overdose, will require monitoring and treatment for at least 24 hours or until the adverse event has subsided.

Parenteral/Oral/Equianalgesic Potency Conversion: To convert adult patients from oral or parenteral opioids to DURAGESIC MAT, use Table 1.

Alternatively, for adult patients taking opioids or doses not listed in Table 1, use the following methodology:

1. Calculate the previous 24-hour analgesic requirement expressed in morphine equivalents.
2. Use Table 2 to convert this equianalgesic morphine dose to the recommended initial DURAGESIC MAT dose. **This conversion recommendation is intentionally conservative to minimize the potential for DURAGESIC MAT overdosage.**

For delivery rates in excess of 100 µg/h, multiple systems may be applied.

Because of the gradual increase in serum fentanyl concentration over the first 24 hours following initial system application, the initial evaluation of the maximum analgesic effect of DURAGESIC MAT cannot be made before 24 hours of wearing. Patients should use short-acting analgesics after the initial dose application as needed until analgesic efficacy with DURAGESIC MAT is attained.

Initial Dose Selection in Elderly, Cachectic, or Debilitated Patients: In patients from these populations, DURAGESIC MAT may have altered pharmacokinetics due to poor fat stores, muscle wasting or altered clearance. Therefore, it may be appropriate, according to clinical judgment, to initiate these patients on DURAGESIC MAT at a dose level lower than that which the conversion tables recommend, including the use of the 12 µg/h dose by itself or in combination with another dose, provided the patient is not opioid-naive (see Contraindications). As with all DURAGESIC MAT patients, they should be carefully monitored for pain levels and adverse events, particularly hypoventilation.

Dose Adjustment: Dose titration is the key to success with opioid analgesic therapy. The recommended initial DURAGESIC MAT dose based upon the daily morphine dose is conservative, and 50% of patients are likely to require a dose increase after initial application of DURAGESIC MAT. If analgesia is insufficient after the initial application, the first dosage increase should occur three days after application, while all subsequent dosage increases should occur six days following the previous application.

Initial Dosage Increase: The initial DURAGESIC MAT dosage may be increased after 3 days based on the daily dose of supplemental analgesics required by the patients in the second or third day of the initial application.

All Other Dosage Increases: Physicians are advised that it may take up to 6 days after increasing the dose of DURAGESIC MAT for the patient to reach equilibrium on the new dose. Therefore, patients should wear a higher dose through two applications before any further increase in dosage is made on the basis of the average daily use of a supplemental analgesic.

Titration Dose Increment: Dosage of DURAGESIC MAT must be individualized according to the pain relief and tolerance of the patient. Appropriate dose increments should be based on the daily dose of supplementary opioids, using the ratio of 45-59 mg/24 hours of oral morphine to a 12 µg/h increase in DURAGESIC MAT dose. For example, if at the end of the required 6-day duration with a new patch strength, a patient is consuming an average daily dose of 150 mg of oral morphine, then the recommended DURAGESIC MAT dose increase would be 3×12 µg/h, which can be achieved by three 12 µg/h patches, or one of 25 µg/h and one of 12 µg/h. The use of 12 µg/h in the ratio for calculation of DURAGESIC MAT dose increases allows for achieving smaller increments when needed, i.e. increments that are as close as possible to the actual average amount of supplementary oral morphine. Some patients may continue to require periodic supplemental doses of short-acting analgesic for 'breakthrough' pain.

Maintenance: The majority of patients are adequately maintained with DURAGESIC MAT administered every 72 hours. A small number of patients may not achieve adequate analgesia using this dosing interval and may require systems to be applied every 48 hours rather than every 72 hours. If breakthrough pain repeatedly occurs at the end of the dosing interval, it is generally an indication for a dosage increase rather than more frequent administration. An increase in the DURAGESIC MAT dose should be considered before changing dosing intervals in order to maintain patients on a 72-hour regimen.

Some patients may require additional or alternative methods of opioid administration when the DURAGESIC MAT dose exceeds 300 µg/h.

Decreased Dosing or Discontinuation of DURAGESIC MAT: Following the successful relief of severe pain, periodic attempts should be made to reduce the opioid dose. Lower doses or complete discontinuation of the opioid analgesic may become feasible due to physiological change or improved mental state of the patient.

Opioid withdrawal symptoms, such as nausea, vomiting, diarrhea, anxiety and shivering are possible in some patients after conversion or dose decrease.

For patients requiring discontinuation of opioids, a gradual downward titration is recommended since it is not known at what dose level the opioid may be discontinued without producing the signs and symptoms of abrupt withdrawal (see Dose Adjustment, Titration Dose Increment).

For all downward titration, it is important to note that it takes 17 hours or more for the fentanyl serum concentration to fall by 50% after system removal.

Safe Use of Table 1 and Table 2: To convert patients to another opioid, remove DURAGESIC MAT and titrate the dose of the new analgesic, based upon the patient's report of pain, until adequate analgesia has been attained.

Table 1 and Table 2 should not be used to convert from DURAGESIC MAT to other opioid therapies. Because the conversion to DURAGESIC MAT is conservative, use of Table 1 and Table 2 for conversion to other analgesic therapies can overestimate the dose of the new agent. Overdosage of the new analgesic agent is possible.

Table 1: DURAGESIC MAT[a]

Dose Conversion Guidelines

Dose Conversion Guidelines are Unidirectional and for Chronic Use.
Use this table to convert patients from the Current Analgesic ONLY to DURAGESIC MAT.
Do NOT use this table to convert patients from DURAGESIC MAT to other opioids; doing so may result in overdose and toxicity

Current Analgesic	**Daily Dosage (mg/d)**						
Oral morphine	60–134	135–179	180–224	225–269	270–314	315–359	360–404
IM/IV morphine (based on a 1:3 IM:PO ratio)	20–44	45–60	61–75	76–90	NA[b]	NA[b]	NA[b]
Oral oxycodone	30–66	67–90	91–112	113–134	135–157	158–179	180–202
Oral codeine	150–447	448–597	598–747	748–897	898–1047	1048–1197	1198–1347
Oral hydromorphone	8–16	17–22	23–28	29–33	34–39	40–45	46–51
IV hydromorphone[c]	4.0–8.4	8.5–11.4	11.5–14.4	14.5–16.5	16.6–19.5	19.6–22.5	22.6–25.5
	↓	↓	↓	↓	↓	↓	↓
DURAGESIC MAT Dose	**25 µg/h**	**37 µg/h**	**50 µg/h**	**62 µg/h**	**75 µg/h**	**87 µg/h**	**100 µg/h**

[a] **Table 1 should not be used to convert from DURAGESIC MAT to other therapies because this conversion to DURAGESIC MAT is conservative. Use of Table 1 for conversion to other analgesic therapies can overestimate the dose of the new agent. Overdosage of the new analgesic agent is possible (see Dosage and Administration, Safe Use of Table 1 and Table 2).**

[b] NA reflects insufficient data available for guidance. Prescribers should make these conversions very carefully and conservatively.

[c] The conversion ratio of parenteral hydromorphone to oral hydromorphone of 1:2 is based on clinical experience in patients with chronic pain. Reference: Parenteral Drug Therapy Manual, Vancouver General Hospital, Pharmaceutical Clinical Services.

Table 2: DURAGESIC MAT[b]

Recommended Initial DURAGESIC MAT Dose Based upon Daily Oral Morphine Dose[a]

	Oral 24-hour morphine (mg/day)	**DURAGESIC MAT Dose (µg/h)**
Dose Adjustment	45–59	12
Initiation Dose	60–134	25
	135–179	25+12
	180–224	50
	225–269	50+12
	270–314	75
	315–359	75+12

(cont'd)

Table 2: DURAGESIC MAT[b] *(cont'd)*

Recommended Initial DURAGESIC MAT Dose Based upon Daily Oral Morphine Dose[a]

Oral 24-hour morphine (mg/day)	**DURAGESIC MAT Dose (µg/h)**
360–404	100
405–494	125
495–584	150
585–674	175
675–764	200
765–854	225
855–944	250
945–1034	275
1035–1124	300

[a] In clinical trials these ranges of chronic daily oral morphine doses were used as a basis for conversion to fentanyl transdermal system. See Recommended Dose and Dosage Adjustment, Dose Adjustment.

[b] 12 µg/h dose is included in this table for dose adjustment. 12 µg/h dose generally should not be used as the initiating dose, except in the case of patients for whom clinical judgment deems it appropriate to start DURAGESIC MAT at less than 25 µg/h; DURAGESIC MAT at any dose is contraindicated in opioid-naive patients (see Contraindications).

Administration: Application of DURAGESIC MAT Patch: DURAGESIC MAT should be applied to non-irritated and non-irradiated skin on a flat surface such as the chest, back, flank, or upper arm. Hair at the application site should be clipped (not shaved) prior to application. If the site of DURAGESIC MAT application must be cleansed prior to application of the system, do so with clear water. Do not use soaps, oils, lotions, alcohol, or any other agents that may irritate the skin or alter its characteristics. Allow the skin to dry completely prior to system application.

DURAGESIC MAT should be applied immediately upon removal from the sealed package. The system should not be altered, e.g., cut, in any way prior to its application. The transdermal system should be pressed firmly in place with the palm of the hand for 30 seconds, making sure the contact is complete, especially around the edges.

Each DURAGESIC MAT system may be worn continuously for 72 hours. A new system should be applied on a different skin site after removal of the previous transdermal system.

Disposal of DURAGESIC MAT Patch: Used systems should be folded so that the adhesive side of the system adheres to itself, then flushed down the toilet immediately upon removal (see Special Handling Instructions).

OVERDOSAGE:

Symptoms: The manifestations of fentanyl overdosage are an extension of its pharmacologic actions with the most serious effect being respiratory depression.

Treatment: For management of respiratory depression, immediate countermeasures include removing the DURAGESIC MAT and physically or verbally stimulating the patient. These actions can be followed by administration of a specific opioid antagonist such as naloxone. The duration of respiratory depression following an overdose may be longer than the effects of the opioid antagonist's action (the half-life of naloxone ranges from 30 to 81 minutes). The interval between IV antagonist doses should be carefully chosen because of the possibility of re-narcotization after system removal; repeated administration of naloxone may be necessary. Reversal of the opioid effect may result in acute onset of pain and release of catecholamines.

If the clinical situation warrants, establish and maintain a patent airway, administer oxygen and assist or control respiration as indicated, and use an oropharyngeal airway or endotracheal tube if necessary. If depressed respiration is associated with muscular rigidity, an intravenous neuromuscular blocking agent may be required to facilitate assisted or controlled respiration. Adequate body temperature and fluid intake should be maintained.

If severe or persistent hypotension occurs, the possibility of hypovolemia should be considered, and managed with appropriate parenteral fluid therapy.

> For management of a suspected drug overdose, contact your regional Poison Control Centre. See the *CPS* Directory section for a list of Poison Control Centres.

ACTION AND CLINICAL PHARMACOLOGY: Pharmacodynamics: Fentanyl is an opioid analgesic which interacts predominantly with the µ-opioid receptor. Fentanyl produces analgesia, sedation, respiratory depression, constipation, and physical dependence but appears to have less emetic activity than other opioid analgesics. Fentanyl may produce muscle rigidity, miosis, cough reflex suppression, alterations in mood, bradycardia and bronchoconstriction.

Analgesic blood levels of fentanyl may cause nausea and vomiting directly by stimulating the chemoreceptor trigger zone, but nausea and vomiting are significantly more common in ambulatory than in recumbent patients, as is postural syncope.

Opioids increase the tone and decrease the propulsive contractions of the smooth muscle of the gastrointestinal tract. The resultant prolongation in gastrointestinal transit time may be responsible for the constipating effect of fentanyl. Because opioids may increase biliary tract pressure, some patients with biliary colic may experience worsening rather than relief of pain.

While opioids generally increase the tone of urinary tract smooth muscle, the net effect tends to be variable, in some cases producing urinary urgency, in others, difficulty in urination.

At therapeutic dosages, fentanyl usually does not exert major effects on the cardiovascular system. However, some patients may exhibit orthostatic hypotension and fainting.

Histamine assays and skin wheal testing in man indicate that histamine release rarely occurs with fentanyl. Assays in man show no clinically significant histamine release in dosages up to 50 µg/kg.

Both the minimum effective concentration and the concentration at which toxicity occurs rise with increasing tolerance. The rate of development of tolerance varies widely among individuals.

Pharmacokinetics: DURAGESIC MAT provides continuous systemic delivery of fentanyl for up to 72 hours. Fentanyl is released along the concentration gradient existing between the drug adhesive layer of the system and the lower concentration in the skin.

Adults : Fentanyl Transdermal System: Absorption: Fentanyl is released at a relatively constant rate. The concentration gradient existing between the matrix and the lower concentration in the skin drives drug release. Following initial fentanyl transdermal system administration, serum fentanyl concentrations increase gradually, generally leveling off between 12 and 24 hours and remaining relatively constant for the remainder of the 72-hour application period. Peak serum levels of fentanyl generally occur between 24 and 72 hours after the first application.

Serum fentanyl concentrations achieved are proportional to the fentanyl transdermal system delivery rate (see Table 3). With continuous use, serum fentanyl concentrations continue to rise for the first few system applications. After several sequential 72-hour applications, patients reach and maintain a steady-state serum concentration that is determined by individual variation in skin permeability and body clearance of fentanyl.

After fentanyl transdermal system removal, serum fentanyl concentrations decline gradually, falling about 50% in approximately 17 (range 13-22) hours. Continued absorption of fentanyl from the skin accounts for a slower disappearance of the drug from the serum than is seen after an IV infusion, where the apparent half-life ranges from 3-12 hours.

Distribution: The average volume of distribution for fentanyl is 6 L/kg (range 3-8, n=8). The average clearance in patients undergoing various surgical procedures is 46 L/h (range 27-75, n=8). The plasma protein binding for fentanyl is about 84%.

Metabolism: Skin does not appear to metabolize fentanyl delivered transdermally. Fentanyl is metabolized primarily in the liver. This was determined in a human keratinocyte cell assay and in clinical studies in which 92% of the dose delivered from the system was accounted for as unchanged fentanyl that appeared in the systemic circulation. In humans, the drug is metabolized primarily by N-dealkylation to norfentanyl and other inactive metabolites.

Table 3: DURAGESIC MAT

Pharmacokinetic Parameters of TTS (fentanyl) in Adults

	Mean (SD) Maximal Concentration C_{max} (ng/mL)	Mean (SD) Time to Maximal Concentration T_{max} (h)
Fentanyl transdermal system 12 µg/h	0.3 (0.2)	27.5 (9.6)
Fentanyl transdermal system 25 µg/h	0.6 (0.3)	38.1 (18.0)
Fentanyl transdermal system 50 µg/h	1.4 (0.5)	34.8 (15.4)
Fentanyl transdermal system 75 µg/h	1.7 (0.7)	33.5 (14.5)
Fentanyl transdermal system 100 µg/h	2.5 (1.2)	36.8 (15.7)

Excretion: Within 72 hours of IV fentanyl administration, approximately 75% of the fentanyl dose is excreted in urine, mostly as metabolites, with less than 10% representing unchanged drug. Approximately 9% of the dose is recovered in the feces, primarily as metabolites.

DURAGESIC MAT: Bioequivalence and Dose Proportionality: Bioequivalence between fentanyl transdermal system and DURAGESIC MAT has been evaluated in single-application, and multi-application studies. To block the opioid effects of fentanyl during study treatment, each subject received oral naltrexone 50 mg as an opioid antagonist in each treatment period starting 14 hours before the first system application, then twice daily through 24 hours after removal of the fourth system.

Study C-2002-046 was a pharmacokinetic study to evaluate the bioequivalency of DURAGESIC MAT 100 µg/h to fentanyl transdermal system 100 µg/h after single application in healthy subjects (n=38). The study was an open-label, two-treatment, two-sequence, four-period, replicate, crossover study. Each subject received each treatment twice in an alternate fashion in separate treatment periods. In each period, 25 blood samples were taken at specific times for fentanyl pharmacokinetic analysis. Table 4 summarizes the pharmacokinetic parameters for serum fentanyl, and results from statistical analysis of the log-transformed pharmacokinetic parameters for the study.

Table 4: DURAGESIC MAT

Fentanyl 100 µg/h. Geometric Mean. Arithmetic Mean (CV %)

Parameter	DURAGESIC MAT	Fentanyl Transdermal System	% Ratio of Geometric Means	90% Confidence Interval (%)
AUC_T (ng· h/mL)	190 196.6 (26.2)	166 170.2 (23.2)	114.46%	109.52, 119.78
AUC_I (ng· h/mL)	202.9 211.2 (29.5)	176 181.3 (25.2)	115.28%	110.32, 120.46
C_{max} (ng/mL)	3.329 3.483 (31.17)	3.066 3.174 (26.96)	108.58%	102.29, 115.25
T_{max} (h)	31.777 (47.58)	38.216 (35.62)		
$T_{½}$ (h)	21.8 (33.1)	20.5 (31.6)		

Note: T_{max} and $T_{½}$ for C-2002-046 are expressed as arithmetic mean (CV%) only.

C-2002-049 was a randomized, open-label, 2-treatment, 2-sequence, 2-period crossover study in which the bioequivalence of DURAGESIC MAT 100 µg/h with fentanyl transdermal system 100 µg/h after repeated application was evaluated in 37 healthy subjects. In each treatment period, subjects wore 4 systems consecutively, each for a duration of 72 hours. Assessment of predose concentrations before the second, third, and fourth applications suggest that steady state was achieved by the fourth application. The ratio of least square mean values for log-transformed $AUC_{216-288}$, C_{max}, and C_{min} for the DURAGESIC MAT relative to the fentanyl transdermal system treatment were 109%, 106%, and 107%, respectively. The results that indicate DURAGESIC MAT 100 µg/h is bioequivalent to fentanyl transdermal system 100 µg/h at steady state are summarized in Table 5.

Table 5: DURAGESIC MAT

Fentanyl 100 µg/h. Geometric Mean. Arithmetic Mean (CV %)

Parameter	DURAGESIC MAT	Fentanyl Transdermal System	% Ratio of Geometric Means	90% Confidence Interval
AUC_{tau} (ng· h/mL)	200.6 216.2 (37.6)	182.2 190.1 (30.1)	110.10%	102.49, 116.48
C_{max} (ng/mL)	4.319 4.798 (46.22)	4.0 4.572 (73.84)	107.98%	95.56, 118.09
C_{min} (ng/mL)	1.561 1.681 (38.48)	1.453 1.504 (26.53)	107.43%	98.96, 114.85
T_{max} (h)	28.4063 (49.51)	26.4631 (47.65)		

Note: T_{max} for C-2002-049 are expressed as arithmetic mean (CV%) only.

Study C-2002-048: The dose relationship of DURAGESIC MAT 25, 50, 75, and 100 µg/h was evaluated in a single dose 4-treatment, 4-sequence, 4-period, crossover study with 36 subjects. Data for linearity of pharmacokinetics and dose proportionality of DURAGESIC MAT are summarized in Table 6.

Table 6: DURAGESIC MAT

Data for Linearity of Pharmacokinetics and Dose Proportionality of DURAGESIC MAT

Serum Fentanyl Pharmacokinetic Parameters: Mean (SD)				
DURAGESIC MAT	25 µg/h	50 µg/h	75 µg/h	100 µg/h
C_{max} (ng/mL)	0.85 (0.26)	1.72 (0.53)	2.32 (0.86)	3.36 (1.28)
AUC_t (ng·h/mL)	51.4 (14.9)	100.4 (26.7)	146.6 (46.2)	196.4 (59.3)
AUC_{inf} (ng·h/mL)	55.0 (16.3)	108 (30.9)	159.4 (50.1)	210.7 (63.7)

(cont'd)

Table 6: DURAGESIC MAT *(cont'd)*

Data for Linearity of Pharmacokinetics and Dose Proportionality of DURAGESIC MAT

Statistical Analysis of Log-transformed Parameters, Normalized to 25 µg/h

DURAGESIC MAT	50 µg/h		75 µg/h		100 µg/h	
	Ratio (%)	90% CI	Ratio (%)	90% CI	Ratio (%)	90% CI
ln C_{max}	100.36	(93.30, 107.95)	89.76	(83.46, 96.53)	97.33	(90.48, 104.69)
ln AUC_t	97.59	(91.67, 103.89)	94.49	(88.77, 100.58)	95.50	(89.71, 101.67)
ln AUC_{inf}	98.32	(92.46, 104.54)	96.02	(90.32, 102.09)	95.68	(89.98, 101.74)

Special Populations and Conditions: Pediatrics Under 18 Years of Age: In a pharmacokinetic study with non-opioid-tolerant patients, 8 children aged 1.5 to 5 years old on **25 µg/h** patches were compared to 8 adults on **50 µg/h** patches. The comparative "dose per mean body weight" i.e. µg/h/kg was 1.67 for children vs 0.67 for adults. Mean C_{max} was 50% higher in the children and mean AUC ~25% higher, with both mean T_{max} and mean half-life shorter (approx. 50% and 75% of the adult values, respectively). For 6 of the 8 children, there was no apparent plateau in plasma concentrations. Adjusting for either body weight or body surface area, clearance in pediatric subjects was found to be about 20%-40% higher than in adults.

Analyses of population pharmacokinetics data in pediatrics indicate that the variability in fentanyl AUC and C_{max} values at steady state (C_{ss}) correlated with changes in body surface area (BSA) values observed in subjects. An increase in BSA of 0.1 m^2 is predicted to result in a 4.8% increase in clearance and 4.6% decrease in C_{ss}.

Dosing recommendations for the safe and effective use of DURAGESIC MAT in this patient population have not been established, in view of the combination of:

i. the variety of factors which could lead to overexposure from DURAGESIC MAT in children as compared to adults (including smaller body weight and significantly different body surface area; differential skin characteristics; potential for magnification, compared to adults, of the impact of amount of body fat stores, muscle wasting, fever, external heat), and
ii. the limitations in both formal PK data (as above) and exposure data (see Adverse Reactions, Clinical Trial Adverse Drug Reactions, Chronic Pain Trials—Pediatrics)

Geriatrics or Debilitated Patients: In elderly, cachectic, or debilitated patients, DURAGESIC MAT may have altered pharmacokinetics due to poor fat stores, muscle wasting or altered clearance. The clearance of fentanyl may be reduced, and the terminal half-life prolonged (see Dosage and Administration).

Data from intravenous studies with fentanyl suggest that elderly patients may have reduced clearance, a prolonged half-life, and they may be more sensitive to the drug than younger patients. In a study conducted with DURAGESIC MAT healthy elderly subjects had fentanyl pharmacokinetics which did not differ significantly from healthy young subjects although peak serum concentrations tended to be lower and mean half-life values were prolonged to approximately 34 hours. Elderly patients should be observed carefully for signs of fentanyl toxicity and the dose reduced if necessary (see Dosage and Administration).

Hepatic Insufficiency: In a study conducted with patients with hepatic cirrhosis, the pharmacokinetics of a single 50 µg/hr application of fentanyl transdermal system were assessed. Although t_{max} and $t_{1/2}$ were not altered, the mean plasma C_{max} and AUC values increased by approximately 35% and 73%, respectively, in these patients. Patients with hepatic impairment should be observed carefully for signs of fentanyl toxicity and the dose of DURAGESIC MAT reduced if necessary.

Renal Insufficiency: Data obtained from a study administering IV fentanyl in patients undergoing renal transplantation suggest that the clearance of fentanyl may be reduced in this patient population. If patients with renal impairment receive DURAGESIC MAT, they should be observed carefully for signs of fentanyl toxicity and the dose reduced if necessary.

STORAGE AND STABILITY: DURAGESIC MAT is stable for 2 years from date of manufacturing when stored in sealed pouch between 15 and 30°C.

SPECIAL HANDLING INSTRUCTIONS: DURAGESIC MAT should be kept out of the reach of children before and after use.

Do not cut DURAGESIC MAT patches.

Used systems should be folded so that the adhesive side of the system adheres to itself, then flushed down the toilet immediately upon removal. If the drug adhesive layer accidentally contacts the skin, the area should be washed with clear water. Do not use soap, alcohol or other solvents as these may enhance the drug's ability to penetrate the skin. Patients should dispose of any systems remaining from a prescription as soon as they are no longer needed. Unused systems should be removed from their protective pouch, folded so that the adhesive side of the patch adheres to itself, and flushed down the toilet.

Wash hands with water only, after applying or removing the patch.

INFORMATION FOR THE PATIENT: Published in e-CPS, available by subscription at www.e-cps.ca.

DOSAGE FORMS, COMPOSITION AND PACKAGING: DURAGESIC MAT is a transdermal patch providing continuous systemic delivery of fentanyl, a potent opioid analgesic, for 72 hours.

DURAGESIC MAT fentanyl matrix system is a multilaminated product comprised of a siliconized polyethylene terephthalate (PET) protective liner and two functional layers: (1) a backing layer of polyethylene terephthalate/ethyl vinyl acetate (PET/EVA) film, (2) a drug in adhesive layer containing polyacrylate adhesive and fentanyl. The peelable protective liner covering the adhesive layer must be removed before the system can be applied. The composition per unit area of all system sizes is identical.

DURAGESIC MAT is available in five different strengths. Each system is labelled with a nominal flux that represents the average amount of drug delivered to the systemic circulation per hour across average skin. The active component of the system is fentanyl. The amount of fentanyl released from each system per hour is proportional to the surface area (25 µg/h per 10.5 cm^2). The 5.25, 10.5, 21, 31.5 and 42 cm^2 systems are designed to deliver 12, 25, 50, 75 or 100 µg/h fentanyl to the systemic circulation, representing approximately 0.3, 0.6, 1.2, 1.8 or 2.4 mg per day, respectively. The remaining components are pharmacologically inactive.

Total fentanyl contents and system sizes for the five strengths are summarized in Table 7.

Table 7: DURAGESIC MAT

Total Fentanyl Contents and System Sizes for the Five Strengths

System	Nominal Fentanyl Delivery Rate (µg/h)	Total Fentanyl Content (mg)	System Size (cm^2)
DURAGESIC MAT 12[a]	12	2.1	5.25
DURAGESIC MAT 25	25	4.2	10.5
DURAGESIC MAT 50	50	8.4	21.0
DURAGESIC MAT 75	75	12.6	31.5
DURAGESIC MAT 100	100	16.8	42.0

[a] Nominal delivery rate 12.5 µg/hr.

Each carton contains 5 individually packaged systems.

(Shown in Product Identification Section)

Duratocin™ ℞
carbetocin
Uterotonic Agent

Ferring

PHARMACOLOGY: Carbetocin is a long-acting synthetic octapeptide analogue of oxytocin with agonist properties. It can be administered i.v. as a single dose immediately following cesarean delivery under epidural or spinal anesthesia, to prevent uterine atony and postpartum hemorrhage.

The clinical and pharmacological properties of carbetocin are similar to those of naturally occurring oxytocin, another posterior pituitary hormone. Like oxytocin, carbetocin binds to oxytocin receptors present on the smooth musculature of the uterus, resulting in rhythmic contractions of the uterus, increased frequency of existing contractions, and increased uterine tone. The oxytocin receptor content of the uterus is very low in the nonpregnant state, and increases during pregnancy, reaching a peak at the time of delivery. Therefore carbetocin has no effect on the nonpregnant uterus, and has a potent uterotonic effect on the pregnant and immediate postpartum uterus.

The onset of uterine contraction following carbetocin administration by either the i.v. or i.m. route is rapid, with a firm contraction being obtained within 2 minutes. The total duration of action of a single i.v. injection of carbetocin on uterine activity is about 1 hour suggesting that carbetocin may act long enough to prevent postpartum hemorrhage in the immediate postpartum period. In comparison to oxytocin, carbetocin induces a prolonged uterine response when administered postpartum, in terms of both amplitude and frequency of contractions.

When administered immediately postpartum as a single i.v. bolus injection of 100 µg to women delivered by cesarean section under epidural or spinal anesthesia, carbetocin was found to be significantly more effective than placebo in preventing uterine atony and minimizing uterine bleeding.

Carbetocin administration also appears to enhance uterine involution in the early postpartum period.

INDICATIONS: For the prevention of uterine atony and postpartum hemorrhage following elective cesarean section under epidural or spinal anesthesia.

Carbetocin has not been studied in cases involving emergency cesarean section, classical cesarean section, anesthesia other than epidural or spinal, or in patients presenting significant heart disease, history of hypertension, known coagulopathy or evidence of liver, renal or endocrine disease (excluding gestational diabetes). Appropriate studies have not been undertaken and doses have not been established in women following labor or vaginal delivery.

CONTRAINDICATIONS: Because of its long duration of action relative to oxytocin, uterine contractions produced by carbetocin cannot be stopped by simply discontinuing the medication. Therefore carbetocin should not be administered prior to delivery of the infant for any reason, including elective or medical induction of labor. Inappropriate use of carbetocin during pregnancy could theoretically mimic the symptoms of oxytocin overdosage, including hyperstimulation of the uterus with strong (hypertonic) or prolonged (tetanic) contractions, tumultuous labor, uterine rupture, cervical and vaginal lacerations, postpartum hemorrhage, utero-placental hypoperfusion and variable deceleration of fetal heart, fetal hypoxia, hypercapnia, or death.

Carbetocin should not be used in patients with a history of hypersensitivity to oxytocin or carbetocin.

Carbetocin should not be used in patients with vascular disease, especially coronary artery disease, except with extreme caution.

Children: Carbetocin is not intended for use in children.

WARNINGS: Some patients may not have an adequate uterine contraction after a single injection of carbetocin. In these patients, administration of carbetocin should not be repeated and more aggressive treatment with ergometrine or higher doses of oxytocin is warranted. In cases of persistent bleeding, the presence of retained placental fragments, coagulopathy, or trauma to the genital tract should be ruled out.

Although no cases of partial retention or trapping of the placenta have been reported, this remains a theoretical possibility if the drug is administered before delivery of the placenta.

PRECAUTIONS: General: Carbetocin injection use during pregnancy, prior to the delivery of the infant, is contraindicated (see Contraindications).

See Warnings section regarding potential requirement for further oxytocin therapy.

Geriatrics: Carbetocin is not recommended for use in elderly patients.

Lactation: Small amounts of carbetocin have been shown to cross over from plasma into the breast milk of nursing women who were given a 70 µg dose i.m., between 7 and 14 weeks postpartum. The mean peak concentration in breast milk was approximately 50 times lower than in plasma, and the ratio of the milk to plasma area under the concentration vs time curves (M/P_{AUC}) was only 2 to 3%. The small amount of carbetocin transferred into breast milk or colostrum after a single injection, and subsequently ingested by a breast-feeding infant, would not be expected to present a significant safety concern. This is due to the fact that carbetocin would be rapidly degraded by peptidases in the infant gastrointestinal tract.

Oxytocin is known to cause contraction of the myoepithelial cells surrounding the mammary alveoli, thereby stimulating milk let-down. There is no sufficient evidence to determine whether carbetocin can also stimulate milk let-down. However, milk let-down was found to occur normally in 5 nursing women after receiving a 70 µg carbetocin dose by the i.m. route.

Drug Interactions: No specific drug interactions have been reported with carbetocin. However, since carbetocin is closely related in structure to oxytocin, it is possible that some of the same drug interactions could occur.

Severe hypertension has been reported when oxytocin was given 3 to 4 hours following prophylactic administration of a vasoconstrictor in conjunction with caudal block anesthesia. Cyclopropane anesthesia may modify oxytocin's cardiovascular effects, so as to produce unexpected results such as hypotension. Maternal sinus bradycardia with abnormal atrioventricular rhythms has also been noted when oxytocin was used concomitantly with cyclopropane anesthesia.

ADVERSE EFFECTS: The adverse events observed with carbetocin during the clinical trials were of the same type and frequency as the adverse events observed with oxytocin when administered after cesarean section under epidural or spinal anesthesia.

I.V. carbetocin was frequently (10 to 40% of patients) associated with nausea, abdominal pain, pruritus, flushing, vomiting, feeling of warmth, hypotension, headache and tremor.

Infrequent adverse events (1 to 5% of patients) included back pain, dizziness, metallic taste, anemia, sweating, chest pain, pain, dyspnea, chills, tachycardia and anxiety.

OVERDOSE:

Symptoms: Overdosage of carbetocin can be expected to produce enhanced pharmacological effects. Therefore, when carbetocin is administered postpartum, overdosage may be associated with uterine hyperactivity and pain.

Treatment: Treatment consists of symptomatic and supportive management.

> For management of a suspected drug overdose, CPhA recommends that you contact your **regional Poison Control Centre**. See the *CPS* Directory section for a list of Poison Control Centres.

DOSAGE: A single i.v. dose of 100 µg (1 mL) is administered by bolus injection, slowly over 1 minute, only when delivery of the infant has been completed by cesarean section under epidural or spinal anaesthetic. Carbetocin can be administered either before or after delivery of the placenta (see Warnings).

Instructions for Opening Ampuls: 1) Hold ampul with blue dot pointing upwards. Shake or tap ampul to empty the tip. 2) With blue dot pointing upwards, snap off tip by forcing it downwards.

SUPPLIED: Each ampul contains: carbetocin 100 µg (0.1 mg). Nonmedicinal ingredients: glacial acetic acid, sodium chloride and water for injection. Clear glass ampuls of 1 mL, with a white identification ring and a blue dot indicating the cut area. Store at refrigerator temperature (2 to 8°C). Should not be frozen. Once the ampul has been opened, the product should be used immediately.

Duvoid® ℞
bethanechol chloride
Parasympathomimetic Agent

Paladin

SUPPLIED: 10 mg: Each pale orange, flat, beveled, round tablet, bisected and "10" debossed on one side, contains: bethanechol chloride 10 mg. Bisulfite-, gluten-, lactose-, paraben-, sodium-, and tartrazine-free. Bottles of 100. Store below 40°C. Keep container tightly closed.

25 mg: Each white, flat, beveled, round tablet, bisected and "25" debossed on one side, contains: bethanechol chloride 25 mg. Bisulfite-, gluten-, lactose-, paraben-, sodium-, and tartrazine-free. Bottles of 100. Store below 40°C. Keep container tightly closed.

50 mg: Each tan, flat, beveled, round tablet, bisected and "50" debossed on one side, contains: bethanechol chloride 50 mg. Bisulfite-, gluten-, lactose-, paraben-, sodium-, and tartrazine-free. Bottles of 100. Store below 40°C. Keep container tightly closed.

(Shown in Product Identification Section)

D-Vi-Sol®
cholecalciferol
Dietary Supplement Essential for Breastfed Infants

Mead Johnson Nutrition

INDICATIONS: Provides breastfed infants vitamin D which is a factor in the normal development and maintenance of bones and teeth. Helps to prevent vitamin D deficiency.

Supplementation should begin at birth and continue until the infant's diet includes at least 400 IU per day of vitamin D from other dietary sources or until the breastfed infant reaches one year of age. Babies in northern communities (north of 55°, which is about the level of Edmonton) or who have other risk factors (such as dark skin) should get 800 IU per day between October and April, when there is less sunlight.

OVERDOSE:

> For management of a suspected drug overdose, CPhA recommends that you contact your **regional Poison Control Centre**. See the *CPS* Directory section for a list of Poison Control Centres.

DOSAGE: Daily dosage for all full term breast fed infants: 1.0 mL (fill provided dropper to top line). Dispense directly into mouth.

SUPPLIED: Each 1.0 mL contains: vitamin D_3 (cholecalciferol) 400 IU (10 µg). Nonmedicinal ingredients: artificial flavour and colour, citric acid, glycerin, polysorbate 80, purified water, sodium citrate and sodium hydroxide. Bottles of 7.5 and 50 mL; dropper included. All bottles are safety sealed.

E

Ebixa®

memantine HCl

N-methyl-D-aspartate (NMDA) Receptor Antagonist

Lundbeck

Date of Revision: March 22, 2010

Ebixa, indicated for the symptomatic treatment of patients with moderate to severe dementia of the Alzheimer's type, has been issued marketing authorization with conditions, to reflect the promising nature of the clinical evidence and the need for a confirmatory study to verify the clinical benefit. Patients should be advised of the nature of the authorization assessment.

PHARMACOLOGY: Persistent activation of the central nervous system N-methyl-D-aspartate (NMDA) receptors by the excitatory amino acid glutamate has been hypothesized to contribute to the symptomatology of Alzheimer's disease. Memantine is postulated to exert its therapeutic effect through its action as a low to moderate affinity uncompetitive (open channel) NMDA receptor antagonist, which binds preferentially to the NMDA receptor-operated cation channels. It blocks the effects of pathologically elevated sustained levels of glutamate that may lead to neuronal dysfunction. There is no clinical evidence that memantine prevents or slows neurodegeneration or alters the course of the underlying dementing process in patients with Alzheimer's disease. Memantine exhibits low to negligible affinity for other receptors (GABA, benzodiazepine, dopamine, adrenergic, noradrenergic, histamine and glycine) or voltage-dependent Ca^{2+}, Na^+ or K^+ channels. In addition, it does not directly affect the acetylcholine receptor or cholinergic transmission, which have been implicated in the cholinomimetic side effects (e.g., increased gastric acid secretion, nausea and vomiting) seen with acetylcholinesterase inhibitors. Memantine showed antagonist effects at the $5HT_3$ receptor with a potency similar to that for the NMDA receptor.

In vitro studies have shown that memantine does not affect the reversible inhibition of acetylcholinesterase by donepezil or galantamine.

Pharmacokinetics: Absorption: Orally administered memantine is completely absorbed. Oral bioavailability is almost 100%. Time to maximum plasma concentration (t_{max}) following single oral doses of 10 to 40 mg memantine ranged between 3 to 8 hours. It has a terminal elimination half-life of about 60-80 hours, with the majority of the dose excreted unchanged in urine. There is no indication that food influences the absorption of memantine.

Studies in volunteers have demonstrated linear pharmacokinetics in the dose range of 10 to 40 mg. Daily doses of 20 mg lead to steady-state plasma concentrations of memantine ranging from 70 to 150 ng/mL (0.5-1 µM) with large inter-individual variations.

Distribution: The apparent volume of distribution of memantine is approximately 9-11 L/kg and the plasma protein binding is approximately 45%. Memantine rapidly crosses the blood-brain barrier with a CSF/serum ratio of about 0.5.

Metabolism and Elimination: In a study using orally administered ^{14}C-memantine, a mean of 84% of the dose was recovered within 20 days, more than 99% being excreted renally. Memantine undergoes little metabolism being in majority excreted unchanged in urine (75-90%). The remaining dose is converted primarily to three polar metabolites: the N-gludantan conjugate, 6-hydroxy memantine and 1-nitroso-deaminated memantine. These metabolites possess minimal NMDA receptor antagonist activity. The hepatic microsome CYP450 enzyme system does not play a significant role in the metabolism of memantine.

In volunteers with normal kidney function, total clearance (Cl_{tot}) amounts to 170 mL/min/1.73 m^2 and part of total renal clearance is achieved by tubular secretion. Renal handling also involves tubular reabsorption, probably mediated by cation transport proteins. The renal elimination rate of memantine under alkaline urine conditions may be reduced by a factor of 7 to 9 resulting in increased plasma levels of memantine (see Warnings, Genitourinary Conditions). Alkalisation of urine may result from drastic changes in diet, e.g. from a carnivore to a vegetarian diet, or from the massive ingestion of alkalizing gastric buffers.

Special Populations: Elderly Patients: The pharmacokinetics of memantine in young and elderly subjects is similar. No adjustment of dosage on the basis of age is recommended.

Reduced Hepatic Function: Memantine is metabolized to a minor extent into metabolites with no NMDA-antagonistic activity, and is excreted primarily in an unchanged form by the kidneys. In a study comparing the pharmacokinetics of memantine in subjects with normal hepatic function and moderate hepatic impairment (Child-Pugh B), moderate hepatic impairment did not significantly alter the pharmacokinetics of memantine following administration of a single 20 mg oral dose of memantine (see Precautions and Dosage).

Reduced Renal Function: In elderly volunteers with normal and reduced renal function (creatinine clearance of 50 to ≤80 mL/min/1.73 m^2), a significant correlation was observed between creatinine clearance and total renal clearance of memantine. Following a single 20 mg oral dose of memantine, systemic exposure in geriatric subjects with mild and moderate renal impairment was 14% and 39% greater, respectively, compared to geriatric subjects with normal renal function (see Precautions and Dosage).

Clinical Trials: The potential efficacy of Ebixa (memantine hydrochloride) as a treatment for the symptomatic management of moderate to severe Alzheimer's disease was demonstrated by the results of 2 randomized, double-blind, placebo-controlled 6-month clinical studies. Both studies were conducted in patients with Alzheimer's disease. The mean age of patients participating in the Ebixa trials was 76 with a range of 50 to 93 years. Approximately 66% of patients were women. Female patients participating in the clinical trials were required to be at least 50 years of age and at least 2 years postmenopausal or surgically sterile. The racial distribution was approximately 91% Caucasian.

Study Outcome Measures: In each study, the efficacy of Ebixa was evaluated using a dual outcome strategy that included assessment of activities of daily living (modified Alzheimer's Disease Cooperative Study–Activities of Daily Living inventory) (both studies), and a clinician's global assessment of change (Clinician's Interview Based Impression of Change with caregiver input [Study 1]) or a measure of cognition (Severe Impairment Battery [Study 2]).

The Alzheimer's Disease Cooperative Study–Activities of Daily Living inventory ($ADCS\text{-}ADL_{sev}$) consists of a comprehensive battery of ADL questions used to measure the functional capabilities of patients. The inventory is performed by interviewing a caregiver familiar with the behaviour of the patient. The modified $ADCS\text{-}ADL_{sev}$ consists of a subset of 19 items including ratings of the patients' ability to eat, dress, bathe, telephone, travel, shop, and perform other household chores, and has been validated for the assessment of patients with moderate to severe dementia. Each ADL item is rated from the highest level of independent performance to complete loss. The modified $ADCS\text{-}ADL_{sev}$ scoring range is from 0 to 54, with lower scores indicating greater functional impairment.

The Severe Impairment Battery (SIB) is a validated and reliable, multi-item instrument that is sensitive to longitudinal changes in cognitive function in patients with moderate to severe dementia. The SIB assesses selected aspects of cognitive performance including elements of attention, orientation, language, memory, visuospatial ability, construction, praxis, and social interaction. The SIB scoring range is from 0 to 100, with lower scores indicating greater cognitive impairment.

The ability of Ebixa to produce an overall clinical effect was assessed using a Clinician's Interview Based Impression of Change that required the use of caregiver information (CIBIC-Plus). The CIBIC-Plus is a structured instrument that evaluates four domains: general (overall clinical status), functional (including activities of daily living), cognitive, and behavioural. It represents the assessment of a skilled clinician using validated scales based on his/her observation at an interview with the patient, in combination with information supplied by a caregiver familiar with the behaviour of the patient over the interval rated. The CIBIC-Plus is scored as a seven point categorical rating, ranging from a score of 1, indicating "markedly improved" to a score of 4, indicating "unchanged" to a score of 7, indicating "markedly worse."

Study 1 (Twenty-Eight-Week Study): In a study of 28 weeks duration, 252 patients with moderate to severe Alzheimer's disease (diagnosed by DSM-IV and NINCDS-ADRDA criteria, with Mini-Mental State Examination scores ≥3 and ≥14 and Global Deterioration Scale Stages 5-6) were randomized to Ebixa or placebo. For patients randomized to Ebixa, treatment was initiated at 5 mg/day and increased weekly by 5 mg/day to a dose of 20 mg/day (10 mg twice a day). The percentages of randomized patients who completed the study were: placebo 67% and Ebixa 77%. Results are presented for analyses based on all patients (ITT, Intent-to treat population) and carrying their last study observation forward (LOCF analysis). The two primary efficacy endpoints were the mean change from baseline to endpoint (Week 28 LOCF) on the $ADCS\text{-}ADL_{sev}$ and CIBIC-Plus rating at endpoint (Week 28 LOCF).

Effects on the $ADCS\text{-}ADL_{sev}$: Figure 1 illustrates the time course for the change from baseline in the $ADCS\text{-}ADL_{sev}$ score for the two treatment groups over the 28 weeks of the study. At endpoint, the mean difference in the $ADCS\text{-}ADL_{sev}$ change scores for the Ebixa-treated patients compared to the patients on placebo was 2.1 units (p=0.022). Ebixa treatment was statistically significantly superior to placebo.

Figure 1: Ebixa

Time Course of the Change From Baseline in $ADCS\text{-}ADL_{sev}$ Score at Week 28-LOCF (ITT Population)

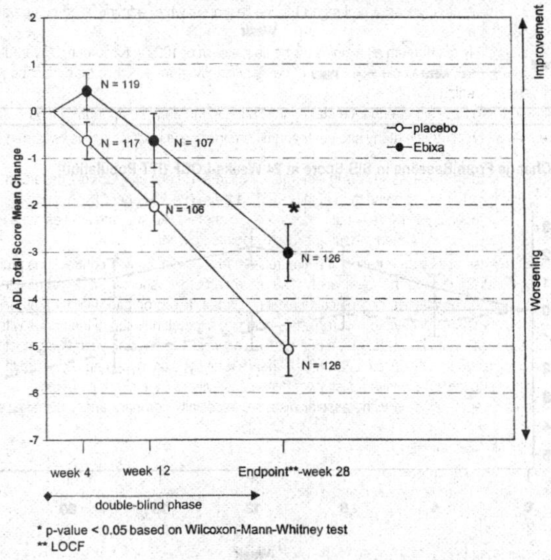

Effects on the CIBIC-Plus: Figure 2 is a histogram of the percentage distribution of CIBIC-Plus scores attained by patients assigned to each of the treatment groups. The Ebixa-placebo difference for these groups of patients in the mean rating was 0.25 units (p=0.06). Ebixa treatment was numerically superior but not statistically significantly superior to placebo.

Figure 2: Ebixa

Distribution of CIBIC-Plus Ratings at Week 28 -LOCF (ITT Population)

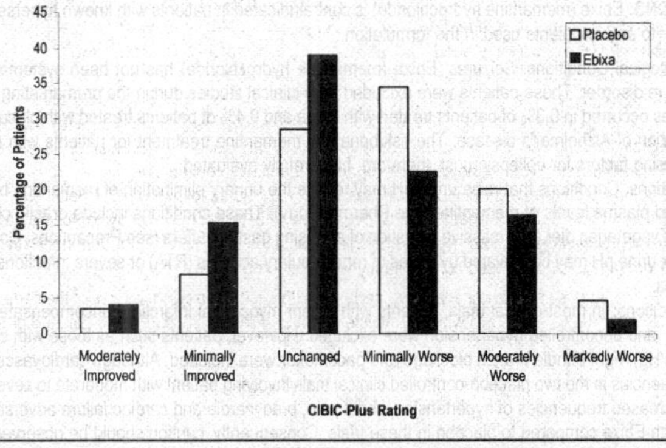

Effects on the SIB: The Severe Impairment Battery was used as a secondary efficacy measure. At study endpoint, the mean difference in the SIB change scores from baseline for the Ebixa-treated patients compared to the patients on placebo was 5.9 units (p<0.001). Ebixa treatment was statistically significantly superior to placebo.

Study 2 (Twenty-Four-Week Study): This 24 week study evaluated the efficacy of memantine as adjunctive therapy with donepezil in 404 patients with moderate to severe Alzheimer's disease (diagnosed by NINCDS-ADRDA criteria, with Mini-Mental State Examination scores ≥5 and ≤14). Patients had been treated with donepezil for at least 6 months and were on a stable dose of donepezil for 3 months prior to randomization to treatment with Ebixa or placebo. All patients continued to receive donepezil while being treated with placebo or memantine. For patients randomized to Ebixa, treatment was initiated at 5 mg/day and increased weekly by 5 mg/day to a dose of 20 mg/day (10 mg twice a day). The percentages of randomized patients who completed the study were: placebo/donepezil 75% and Ebixa/donepezil 85%. The two primary endpoints were the mean changes from baseline to endpoint (Week 24 LOCF) on the $ADCS\text{-}ADL_{sev}$ and SIB.

Effects on the $ADCS\text{-}ADL_{sev}$: Figure 3 illustrates the time course for the change from baseline in the $ADCS\text{-}ADL_{sev}$ score for the two treatment groups over the 24 weeks of the study. The mean difference in the $ADCS\text{-}ADL_{sev}$ change scores for the Ebixa/donepezil treated patients compared to the patients on placebo/donepezil was 1.4 units (p=0.028). Ebixa/donepezil treatment was statistically significantly superior to placebo/donepezil.

Effects on the SIB: Figure 4 illustrates the time course for the change from baseline in SIB score for the two treatment groups over the 24 weeks of the study. The mean difference in the SIB change scores for the Ebixa/donepezil treated patients compared to the patients on placebo/donepezil was 3.4 units (p<0.001). Ebixa/donepezil treatment was statistically significantly superior to placebo/donepezil.

Effects on the CIBIC-Plus: The CIBIC-Plus was used as a secondary efficacy measure. The Ebixa-placebo difference of CIBIC-Plus mean rating was 0.25 units (p=0.027). Ebixa/donepezil treatment was statistically significantly superior to placebo/donepezil.

INDICATIONS: Ebixa (memantine hydrochloride) may be useful as monotherapy or as adjunctive therapy with cholinesterase inhibitors* for the symptomatic treatment of patients with moderate to severe dementia of the Alzheimer's type.

Ebixa tablets should only be prescribed by (or following consultation with) clinicians who are experienced in the diagnosis and management of Alzheimer's disease.

In a 28-week placebo controlled monotherapy trial, patients with moderate to severe Alzheimer's disease showed stabilization or less worsening of functional and cognitive symptoms and of global assessment when treated with Ebixa compared to placebo.

* Cholinesterase inhibitors refers to only those which are approved in Canada for the symptomatic treatment of Alzheimer's disease.

Figure 3: Ebixa

Time Course of the Change From Baseline in ADCS-ADL$_{sev}$ Score at 24 Weeks-LOCF (ITT Population)

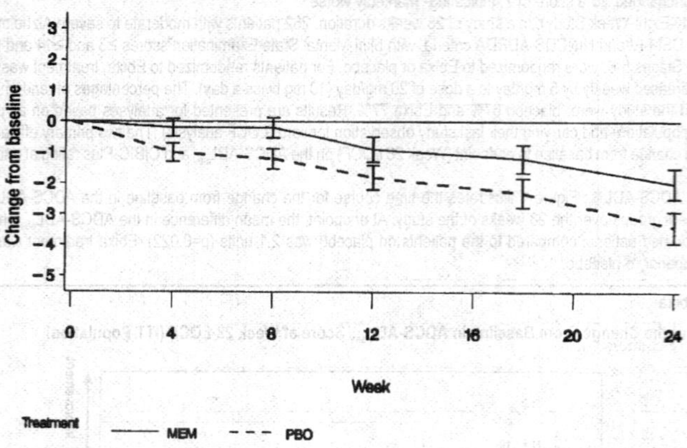

Figure 4: Ebixa

Time Course of the Change From Baseline in SIB Score at 24 Weeks-LOCF (ITT Population)

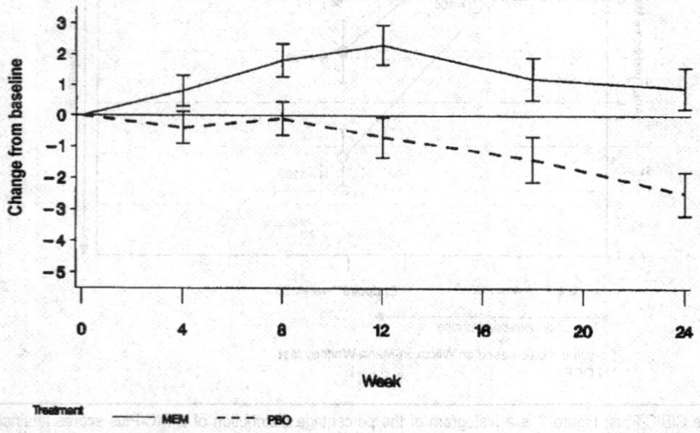

In a 24 week "add-on" placebo controlled trial in which patients were treated with either Ebixa or placebo as add-on to ongoing donepezil therapy, stabilization or less worsening of functional and cognitive symptoms and of global assessment was observed in patients with moderate to severe Alzheimer's disease when treated with Ebixa compared to placebo.

Ebixa has not been studied in controlled clinical trials for the symptomatic treatment of moderate to severe Alzheimer's disease for more than 6 months.

CONTRAINDICATIONS: Ebixa (memantine hydrochloride) is contraindicated in patients with known hypersensitivity to memantine hydrochloride or to any excipients used in the formulation.

WARNINGS: Neurological Conditions: Seizures: Ebixa (memantine hydrochloride) has not been systematically evaluated in patients with a seizure disorder. These patients were excluded from clinical studies during the premarketing testing of Ebixa. In clinical trials, seizures occurred in 0.3% of patients treated with Ebixa and 0.4% of patients treated with placebo. Seizure activity may be a manifestation of Alzheimer's disease. The risk/benefit of memantine treatment for patients with a history of seizure disorder or predisposing factors for epilepsy must, therefore, be carefully evaluated.

Genitourinary Conditions: Conditions that raise urine pH may reduce the urinary elimination of memantine by a factor of 7 to 9, resulting in increased plasma levels of memantine (see Pharmacology). These conditions include drastic changes in diet, e.g. from a carnivore to a vegetarian diet, or a massive ingestion of alkalising gastric buffers (see Precautions, Conditions That Make Urine Alkaline). Also, urine pH may be elevated by states of renal tubulary acidosis (RTA) or severe infections of the urinary tract with Proteus bacteria.

Cardiovascular Conditions: In most clinical trials, patients with recent myocardial infarction, uncompensated congestive heart failure (NYHA III-IV), and uncontrolled hypertension were excluded. However, patients such as those with controlled hypertension (DBP <105 mm/Hg), right bundle branch blockage and pacemaker were included. Although cardiovascular adverse events occurred at low frequencies in the two placebo-controlled clinical trials involving patient with moderate to severe Alzheimer's disease, there were increased frequencies of hypertension, chest pain, bradycardia and cardiac failure adverse events in patients who were treated with Ebixa compared to placebo in these trials. Consequently, caution should be observed when memantine is initiated in patients with cardiovascular conditions.

PRECAUTIONS: Ophthalmic Conditions: In an open label study where Ebixa was administered to 10 elderly patients at a dose of 20 mg per day for approximately 48 months, memantine concentrations in lacrimal fluid were about 3 fold higher than in plasma and did not show ophthalmologic effects. In another 6-month placebo-controlled trial, no major treatment differences were reported for ocular effects but worsening of the corneal condition was reported for slightly more patients treated with Ebixa than placebo (5.4% memantine vs. 3.3% placebo). Repeat-dose toxicology studies demonstrated corneal and lens histopathological changes in rodents treated with Ebixa. Therefore, periodic monitoring of the patient's ophthalmic condition is recommended.

Concomitant Use with Other Drugs: Use with compounds chemically related to N-methyl-D-aspartate (NMDA) antagonists: As these compounds act at the same receptor system as memantine, adverse drug reactions (mainly CNS-related) may be more frequent or pronounced. Pharmacotoxic psychosis has been reported in the literature in two Parkinson's disease patients who were treated concomitantly with memantine, amantadine, L-dopa and terguride (see Precautions, Drug Interactions, Other Agents). The combined use of Ebixa with other compounds chemically related to NMDA antagonists such as amantadine, ketamine or dextromethorphan has not been systematically evaluated and is therefore not recommended.

Conditions That Make Urine Alkaline: The clearance of memantine was reduced by about 80% under alkaline urine conditions at pH 8. Therefore, alterations of urine pH towards the alkaline condition may lead to an accumulation of the drug with a possible increase in adverse effects. Urine pH is altered by diet, drugs (e.g. carbonic anhydrase inhibitors, sodium bicarbonate) and clinical state of the patient (e.g. renal tubular acidosis or severe infections of the urinary tract). Hence, memantine should be used with caution under these conditions (see Pharmacokinetics and Warnings).

Special Populations: Hepatic Impairment: Ebixa undergoes minimal hepatic metabolism and is excreted primarily in its unchanged form by the kidneys. The pharmacokinetics of memantine have been studied in subjects with moderate hepatic impairment (see Pharmacology, Pharmacokinetics). In patients with mild or moderate hepatic impaired function (Child-Pugh A and Child-Pugh B) no dose adjustment is needed. There are no data available for use of memantine in patients with severe hepatic impairment. Therefore, administration of Ebixa is not recommended in patients with severe hepatic impairment.

Renal Impairment: In patients with mildly impaired renal function (creatinine clearance 50-80 mL/min) no dosage adjustment is required. In patients with moderate renal impairment (creatinine clearance 30-49 mL/min) the daily dose should be 10 mg per day. If well tolerated after at least 7 days of treatment, and based on clinical response, the dose may be increased up to 20 mg/day according to the standard titration scheme. In patients with severe renal impairment (creatinine clearance 15-29 mL/min) the daily dosage should be 10 mg per day (see Pharmacology, Pharmacokinetics and Dosage).

Use in Patients ≥85 Years Old: In placebo-controlled clinical studies, the number of patients aged 85 years or older who received memantine at the therapeutic dose of 20 mg/day was 40. There is limited safety information for Ebixa in this patient population.

Use in Patients with Serious Co-morbid Conditions: There is limited information on the safety of memantine treatment in patients with moderate to severe Alzheimer's disease with serious co-morbidities, as these patients were excluded from clinical trials. The use of Ebixa in Alzheimer's disease patients with chronic illnesses common among the geriatric population should be considered only after a proper risk/benefit assessment. Dose escalation in this patient population should proceed with caution.

Pregnancy: Oral treatment of female rats with memantine once daily during organogenesis produced mild maternal toxicity at doses of 6-18 mg/kg/day (3-9 times the Maximum Recommended Human Dose [MRHD] on a mg/m² basis); however, memantine was not teratogenic at doses up to 18 mg/kg/day (9 times the MRHD on a mg/m² basis), the highest dose tested. In a rat reproduction and fertility study, reduced growth and a developmental delay were observed at 18 mg/kg/day (9 times the MRHD on a mg/m² basis).

Memantine doses of 0, 3, 10 and 30 mg/kg/day were orally administered to pregnant rabbits during the period of organogenesis. At 30 mg/kg/day (30 times the MRHD on a mg/m² basis) maternal toxicity and a slight increase in post-implantation loss were observed. No teratogenic effects were observed in rabbits administered memantine 30 mg/kg/day (30 times the MRHD on a mg/m² basis). The maternal and fetal no observed effect level (NOEL) was 10 mg/kg/day (10 times the MRHD on a mg/m² basis).

In a peri and postnatal study, memantine was orally administered to rats at up to 18 mg/kg/day (9 times the MRHD on a mg/m² basis). At 18 mg/kg/day pups showed reduced mean body weights but there was no effect on their development or behaviour. Animal studies showed no indication of an adverse effect of memantine on labour and delivery.

There are no adequate and well-controlled studies of memantine in pregnant women to establish the safe use of Ebixa for this population. Therefore, Ebixa should not be used in women of childbearing potential, unless, in the opinion of the physician, the expected benefits to the patient markedly outweigh the possible hazards to the fetus.

Lactation: It is not known whether memantine is excreted in human breast milk. Therefore Ebixa should not be used in nursing mothers.

Children: The safety and effectiveness of Ebixa in any illness occurring in pediatric patients have not been established. Therefore, Ebixa is not recommended for use in children.

Drug Interactions: Compounds Chemically Related to N-methyl-D-aspartate (NMDA) Antagonists: The combined use of Ebixa with other compounds chemically related to NMDA antagonists such as amantadine, ketamine or dextromethorphan has not been systematically evaluated and is therefore not recommended (see Precautions, Concomitant Use with Other Drugs).

Effects of Ebixa on Substrates of Microsomal Enzymes: In vitro studies conducted with marker substrates of CYP450 enzymes (CYP1A2, -2A6, -2C9, -2D6, -2E1, -3A4) revealed minimal inhibition of these enzymes by memantine. No pharmacokinetic interactions with drugs metabolized by these enzymes are expected.

Effects of Inhibitors and/or Substrates of Microsomal Enzymes on Ebixa: Memantine is predominantly renally eliminated, and drugs that are substrates and/or inhibitors of the CYP450 system are not expected to alter the metabolism of memantine.

Acetylcholinesterase (AChE) Inhibitors: In vitro studies have shown that memantine does not affect the reversible inhibition of acetylcholinesterase by donepezil or galantamine. In young healthy adult subjects (n=19, age range 18-35 years) under steady-state conditions of the AChE inhibitor donepezil HCl (10 mg/day), co-administration of a single 10 mg oral dose of memantine did not affect the pharmacokinetics of either drug and did not affect donepezil-mediated AChE inhibition. In a 24-week study of patients with moderate to severe Alzheimer's disease the adverse event profiles were similar for patients treated with a combination of memantine and donepezil or placebo and donepezil.

In a pharmacokinetic study in healthy adult subjects (n=15, age range 21-55 years), co-administration of memantine (10 mg b.i.d.) did not significantly affect the steady state pharmacokinetics of galantamine (16 mg/day). The effect of galantamine on memantine pharmacokinetics was not evaluated. The safety of co-administering memantine and galantamine in patients with Alzheimer's disease has not been evaluated in clinical trials.

Drugs Eliminated Via Renal Mechanisms: Co-administration of drugs that use the same renal cationic transport system as memantine, such as cimetidine, ranitidine, quinidine, hydrochlorothiazide (HCTZ), triamterene (TA), and nicotine could potentially alter the plasma levels of both agents. Co-administration of Ebixa and hydrochlorothiazide/triamterene (HCTZ/TA) did not affect the bioavailability of either memantine or triamterene, and the bioavailability of HCTZ decreased by 20%. The pharmacokinetics of memantine is similar in smokers and non-smokers, suggesting that nicotine may not affect the disposition of memantine. The potential for compromised renal function in elderly patients should be considered when memantine will be used concomitantly with other drugs eliminated via renal mechanisms (see Precautions and Dosage).

Drugs Highly Bound to Plasma Proteins: Because the plasma protein binding of memantine is low (45%), an interaction with drugs that are highly bound to plasma proteins, such as warfarin and digoxin, is unlikely.

Oral Anticoagulants: In post-marketing experience isolated cases of international normalized ratio (INR) increases have been reported in patients treated concomitantly with memantine and warfarin. Although no causal relationship has been established, close monitoring of prothrombin time or INR is advised for patients treated concomitantly with memantine and oral anticoagulants.

Antihyperglycemic Drugs: In young healthy adult subjects (n=21, age range 19-35 years), co administration of a single 20 mg oral dose of memantine under steady state conditions of glyburide/metformin (1.25 mg glyburide/250 mg metformin) did not affect the pharmacokinetics of memantine, glyburide or metformin. The renal excretion of metformin and memantine, and potential for compromised renal function in elderly patients should be considered when memantine and metformin will be used concomitantly (see Precautions and Dosage).

Other Agents: Since the effects of L-dopa, dopaminergic agonists, and anticholinergics may be enhanced by concomitant treatment with Ebixa, dosage adjustment of these other agents may be necessary.

Carcinogenesis, Mutagenesis and Impairment of Fertility: There was no evidence of carcinogenicity in a 113-week oral study in mice for either sex at doses up to 40 mg/kg/day (10 times the maximum recommended human dose [MRHD] on a mg/m² basis). There was also no evidence of carcinogenicity in rats orally dosed at up to 40 mg/kg/day for 71 weeks followed by 20 mg/kg/day (19 and 10 times the MRHD on a mg/m² basis, respectively) through 128 weeks.

Memantine did not show any genotoxic potential in assays for gene mutation (bacterial and mammalian cells in vitro) or in clastogenicity assays (human lymphocytes in vitro and mouse bone marrow in vivo).

No impairment of fertility or reproductive performance was seen in rats administered up to 18 mg/kg/day (9 times the MRHD on a mg/m² basis) orally from 14 days prior to mating through gestation and lactation in females, or for 60 days prior to mating in males.

ADVERSE EFFECTS: A total of 738 patients were treated with memantine in double-blind, placebo-controlled dementia studies. Of these patients, 592 (80%) completed the studies. Patients were treated with memantine for a mean of 150.3 days. Approximately 60% of patients received memantine for at least 24 weeks.

Adverse Events Leading to Discontinuation of Treatment: In placebo-controlled trials in which dementia patients received doses of Ebixa up to 20 mg/day, 10.8 % (80/738) of the Ebixa-treated patients discontinued treatment due to an adverse event. The discontinuation rate in the placebo-treated patients was 11.2% (81/721). The most frequent adverse event leading to discontinuation was agitation with an observed frequency among patients who discontinued treatment of 1.2% in patients receiving memantine vs. 2.1% in patients administered placebo. None of the other adverse events leading to discontinuation met the criteria for most common adverse events, defined as those occurring at a frequency of at least 2% and at twice the incidence seen in placebo patients.

Adverse Events Reported in Placebo-controlled Dementia Trials: Table 1 lists treatment emergent signs and symptoms that were reported in at least 2% of patients in placebo-controlled dementia trials and for which the rate of occurrence was greater for patients treated with Ebixa than for those treated with placebo. The prescriber should be aware that these figures cannot be used to predict the incidence of adverse events in the course of usual medical practice where patient characteristics and other factors differ from those that prevailed in the clinical trials. Similarly, the cited frequencies cannot be compared with figures obtained from other clinical investigations involving different treatments, uses, and investigators. The cited figures, however, do provide the prescribing physician with some basis for estimating the relative contribution of drug and non-drug factors to the adverse event incidence rate in the population studied.

Other adverse events occurring with an incidence of at least 2% in Ebixa-treated patients but at an equal or lower rate than placebo were agitation, arthralgia, bronchitis, cataract, coughing, depression, diarrhea, fall, gait abnormal, inflicted injury, influenza-like symptoms, insomnia, urinary incontinence and urinary tract infection.

Vital Sign Changes: Ebixa and placebo groups were compared with respect to (1) mean change from baseline in vital signs (pulse, systolic blood pressure, and diastolic blood pressure) and (2) the incidence of patients meeting criteria for potentially clinically significant changes from baseline in these variables. These analyses did not reveal any clinically important changes in vital signs associated with Ebixa treatment.

Laboratory Changes: Ebixa and placebo groups were compared with respect to (1) mean change from baseline in various serum chemistry, hematology, and urinalysis variables and (2) the incidence of patients meeting criteria for potentially clinically significant changes from baseline in these variables. These analyses revealed no clinically important changes in laboratory test parameters associated with Ebixa treatment.

Table 1: Ebixa

Adverse Events Reported in Controlled Clinical Trials in at Least 2% of Patients Receiving Ebixa and at a Higher Frequency than Placebo-treated Patients

Body System Adverse Event	Placebo (N=721) %	Ebixa (N=738) %
Body as a Whole		
Fatigue	0.7	2.3
Pain	1.0	2.4
Cardiovascular System		
Hypertension	2.4	3.3
Central and Peripheral Nervous System		
Dizziness	4.6	6.9
Headache	3.6	5.6
Gastrointestinal System		
Constipation	3.5	6.1
Nausea	2.4	2.8
Vomiting	2.1	3.0
Musculoskeletal System		
Back pain	2.5	2.7
Psychiatric Disorders		
Anorexia	1.2	2.2
Anxiety	0.8	2.6
Confusion	5.5	5.7
Hallucinations	1.2	2.6
Somnolence	2.2	2.8
Respiratory System		
Dyspnea	1.2	2.3

ECG Changes: Ebixa and placebo groups were compared with respect to (1) mean change from baseline in various ECG parameters and (2) the incidence of patients meeting criteria for potentially clinically significant changes from baseline in these variables. These analyses revealed no clinically important changes in ECG parameters associated with Ebixa treatment.

Adverse Events Observed in Placebo-controlled Trial in Patients Previously Treated with Donepezil: In an additional double-blind, placebo-controlled study, 202 patients who had been treated with donepezil for at least 6 months and who had been on stable doses of donepezil for 3 months prior to randomization were treated with memantine for a period of 24 weeks while still receiving donepezil. Of these patients, 172 (85%) completed the study. In this clinical trial, a total of 14.9% (30/202) of the memantine/donepezil patients discontinued the study compared to 25.4% (51/201) of the placebo/donepezil patients. The most frequent reason for discontinuation was adverse events and included 12% of placebo/donepezil patients and 7% of memantine/donepezil patients.

Overall, the safety profile of the memantine/donepezil treated patients was similar to the one observed for the placebo-controlled dementia trials. The adverse events leading to discontinuation of the treatment, and for which the incidence was greater in the memantine/donepezil than in the placebo/donepezil group were: asthenia (memantine 1.0%; placebo 0%) dehydration (memantine 1.5%; placebo 0%) and confusion (memantine 2.0 %; placebo 1.5%).

Table 2 lists treatment emergent signs and symptoms that were reported in at least 2% of patients in placebo-controlled dementia trials and for which the rate of occurrence was greater for patients treated with Ebixa/donepezil than for those treated with placebo/donepezil.

Table 2: Ebixa

Adverse Events Reported in Controlled Clinical Trials in at Least 2% of Patients Receiving Ebixa/donepezil and at a Higher Frequency than Placebo/donepezil-treated Patients

Body System Adverse Event	Placebo/donepezil (N=201) %	Ebixa/donepezil (N=202) %
Body as a Whole		
Chest Pain	0.0	2.5
Fall	7.0	7.4
Fever	0.5	2.0
Oedema Peripheral	4.0	5.0
Pain	0.5	3.0
Cardiovascular System		
Hypertension	1.5	4.5
Central and Peripheral Nervous System		
Gait Abnormal	1.0	3.0
Headache	2.5	6.4
Gastrointestinal System		
Constipation	1.5	3.0
Vomiting	3.0	3.5
Metabolic and Nutritional Disorders		
Weight Increase	0.0	2.5
Musculoskeletal System		
Arthralgia	1.5	2.5
Psychiatric Disorders		
Confusion	2.0	7.9
Depression	3.0	4.0
Red Blood Cell Disorder		
Anemia	0.5	2.0
Reproductive Disorders, Male		
Prostatic Disorder	0.0	4.1
Respiratory System		
Coughing	1.0	3.0
Influenza-like Symptoms	6.5	7.4
Skin and Appendages Disorders		
Rash	1.5	2.5
Urinary System Disorders		
Urinary Tract Infection	5.0	5.9
Urinary Incontinence	3.0	5.4
Micturition Frequency	0.5	2.0

Treatment emergent signs and symptoms that were reported in at least 2% of Ebixa/donepezil treated patients (but less than 9%) and at an equal or lower rate than placebo/donepezil treated patients were abdominal pain, agitation, anorexy, anxiety, asthenia, back pain, bronchitis, dehydration, diarrhea, dizziness, fatigue, fecal incontinence, hallucinations, inflicted injury, insomnia, personality disorder, somnolence, syncope, tremor, upper respiratory tract infection.

Other Adverse Events Observed During Clinical Trials: Ebixa has been administered to approximately 1150 patients with dementia, of whom more than 1000 received the maximum recommended dose of 20 mg/day. Approximately 739 patients received Ebixa for at least 6 months of treatment and 387 patients were treated for approximately a year or more.

All adverse events occurring in at least two patients are included, except for those already listed in Table 1 and Table 2, WHO terms too general to be informative, or events unlikely to be caused by the drug. Also included are the adverse events observed in the placebo-controlled trial in patients who had been previously treated with donepezil prior to Ebixa treatment. Events are classified by body system and listed using the following definitions: frequent—those occurring on one or more occasions in at least 1/100 patients; infrequent—those occurring in less than 1/100 patients but at least in 1/1000 patients. These adverse events are not necessarily related to Ebixa treatment and in most cases were observed at a similar frequency in placebo-treated patients in the controlled studies.

Autonomic Nervous System: Infrequent: sweating increased, mouth dry.

Body as a Whole: Frequent: asthenia, oedema, leg pain, malaise, sepsis, syncope. Infrequent: abscess, allergic reaction, allergy, chest pain precordial, choking, condition aggravated, ESR increased, flushing, hernia NOS, hot flushes, hypothermia, infection, infection fungal, infection viral, moniliasis, edema peripheral, pallor, rigors, sudden death.

Cardiovascular: Frequent: angina pectoris, bradycardia, cardiac failure, cardiac failure left, heart murmur, oedema dependent. Infrequent: aneurysm, arrhythmia, cardiac arrest, embolism pulmonary, fibrillation atrial, heart block, heart disorder, hypertension aggravated, hypotension, hypotension postural, myocardial infarction, palpitation, phlebitis, pulmonary oedema, tachycardia, thrombophlebitis, thrombophlebitis deep, vascular disorder.

Central and Peripheral Nervous System: Frequent: aphasia, ataxia, cerebrovascular disorder, hypokinesia, transient ischemic attack, vertigo. Infrequent: absences, cerebral hemorrhage, coma, convulsions, coordination abnormal, extrapyramidal disorder, hemiparesis, hemiplegia, hyperkinesia, hypertonia, hypoesthesia, muscle contractions involuntary, neuralgia, neuropathy, paralysis, paresthesia, ptosis, speech disorder, stupor, tremor.

Gastrointestinal System: Frequent: abdominal pain, dyspepsia, fecal incontinence, hemorrhoids, tooth disorder. Infrequent: diverticulitis, dysphagia, esophageal ulceration, esophagitis, flatulence, gastroenteritis, gastroesophageal reflux, gastrointestinal disorder NOS, GI hemorrhage, gingivitis, hemorrhage rectum, melena, mucositis NOS, oesophagitis, saliva altered, saliva increased, stomatitis ulcerative, tooth ache, tooth caries.

Hemic and Lymphatic Disorders: Frequent: purpura. Infrequent: epistaxis, hematoma, leukocytosis, leukopenia, polycythemia.

Metabolic and Nutritional Disorders: Frequent: hyperglycemia, hypernatremia, hypokalemia, phosphatase alkaline increased, weight decrease. Infrequent: bilirubinemia, BUN increased, dehydration, diabetes mellitus, diabetes mellitus aggravated, gamma-GT increased, gout, hepatic enzymes increased, hepatic function abnormal, hypercholesterolemia, hyperkalemia, hyperuricemia, hyponatremia, NPN increased, polydipsia, AST increased, ALT increased, thirst.

Musculoskeletal System: Frequent: arthritis, arthrosis, muscle weakness, myalgia. Infrequent: arthritis aggravated, arthritis rheumatoid, bursitis, skeletal pain.

Neoplasms: Infrequent: basal cell carcinoma, breast neoplasm benign (female), breast neoplasm malignant (female), carcinoma, neoplasm NOS, skin neoplasm malignant.

Psychiatric Disorders: Frequent: aggressive reaction, apathy, cognitive disorder, delusion, nervousness. Infrequent: amnesia, appetite increased, concentration impaired, crying abnormal, delirium, depersonalization, emotional lability, libido increased, neurosis, paranoid reaction, paroniria, personality disorder, psychosis, sleep disorder, suicide attempt, thinking abnormal.

Reproductive Disorders: Female: Infrequent: vaginal hemorrhage, moniliasis; Male: Frequent: moniliasis.

Respiratory System: Frequent: pharyngitis, pneumonia, upper respiratory tract infection, rhinitis. Infrequent: apnea, asthma, bronchospasm, hemoptysis, respiratory disorder, sinusitis.

Skin and Appendages: Frequent: bullous eruption, herpes zoster, skin disorder, skin ulceration. Infrequent: alopecia, cellulitis, dermatitis, eczema, pruritus, rash erythematous, seborrhea, skin dry, skin reaction localized, urticaria.

Special Senses: Frequent: cataract, conjunctivitis, eye abnormality, macula lutea degeneration, vision abnormal. Infrequent: blepharitis, blurred vision, conjunctival hemorrhage, corneal opacity, decreased visual acuity, diplopia, ear ache, ear disorder NOS, eye infection, eye pain, glaucoma, hearing decreased, lacrimation abnormal, myopia, xerophthalmia, retinal detachment, retinal disorder, retinal hemorrhage, tinnitus.
Urinary System: Frequent: cystitis, dysuria. Infrequent: hematuria, micturition disorder, polyuria, pyuria, renal function abnormal, urinary retention.
Vascular Disorders: Infrequent: venous thrombosis/thromboembolism.
Post-Market Adverse Drug Reactions: The following adverse events of possible importance, for which there are inadequate data to determine the causal relationship to memantine treatment have been reported to be temporally associated with memantine treatment and are not described elsewhere in labeling: acne, atrioventricular block, bone fracture, carpal tunnel syndrome, cerebral infarction, cholelithiasis, claudication, colitis, depressed level of consciousness (including loss of consciousness and coma), dyskinesia, encephalopathy, gastritis, grand mal convulsions, hepatic failure, hepatitis (including increased ALT and AST), hyperlipidemia, hypoglycemia, ileus, impotence, increased INR, intracranial hemorrhage, lethargy, myoclonus, neuroleptic malignant syndrome, acute pancreatitis, aspiration pneumonia, acute renal failure, otitis media, prolonged QT interval, psychotic reactions, restlessness, sepsis, Stevens-Johnson syndrome, supraventricular tachycardia, tardive dyskinesia, thrombocytopenia.

Alzheimer's disease has been associated with depression, suicidal ideation and suicide. In post-marketing experience these events have been reported in patients treated with Ebixa.

OVERDOSE:

Symptoms: Cases of accidental and intentional overdose have been reported with memantine. The highest ingested dose that has been reported in an overdose is 2000 mg. Reported signs and symptoms in this case were agitation, diplopia and coma followed by full recovery. Fatal overdoses have only been reported when memantine was taken with several other drugs by patients on polytherapy that included memantine. No fatal cases of overdose have been reported in which memantine was taken alone.

Treatment: Because strategies for the management of overdose are continually evolving, it is advisable to contact a regional Poison Control Center for the latest recommendations for the management of a suspected overdose of any drug.

Establish and maintain an airway to ensure adequate ventilation and oxygenation. Gastric lavage and use of activated charcoal should be considered. Cardiac and vital sign monitoring are recommended, along with general symptomatic and supportive measures. There are no specific antidotes for Ebixa. Elimination of memantine can be enhanced by acidification of urine.

> For management of a suspected drug overdose, contact your regional Poison Control Centre. See the *CPS* Directory section for a list of Poison Control Centres.

DOSAGE: Ebixa (memantine hydrochloride) should only be prescribed by (or following consultation with) clinicians who are experienced in the diagnosis and management of Alzheimer's disease. Therapy should only be started if a caregiver is available who will regularly monitor drug intake by the patient. Diagnosis should be made according to current guidelines.
Adults: The recommended maintenance dose for memantine is 20 mg/day. In order to reduce the risk of side effects the maintenance dose is achieved by upward titration as follows: the usual starting dose is 5 mg/day. The dose should then be increased in 5 mg increments to 10 mg/day (5 mg twice a day), 15 mg/day (10 mg and 5 mg as separate doses), and 20 mg/day (10 mg twice a day), depending on the patient's response and tolerability. The minimum recommended interval between dose increases is one week. The recommended dose titration is summarized in the following table.

	10 mg Tablets	
	AM	PM
Week 1	½ tablet	none
Week 2	½ tablet	½ tablet
Week 3	1 tablet	½ tablet
Week 4 and beyond	1 tablet	1 tablet

The tablets can be taken with or without food.
Special Populations: Elderly: On the basis of the clinical studies the recommended dose for patients over the age of 65 years is 20 mg per day (10 mg twice a day) as described above (see Pharmacology, Pharmacokinetics).
Renal Impairment: In patients with mildly impaired renal function (creatinine clearance 50-80 mL/min) no dosage adjustment is required. In patients with moderate renal impairment (creatinine clearance 30-49 mL/min) the daily dose should be 10 mg per day. If well tolerated after at least 7 days of treatment, and based on clinical response, the dose may be increased up to 20 mg/day according to the standard titration scheme. In patients with severe renal impairment (creatinine clearance 15-29 mL/min) the daily dosage should be 10 mg per day (see Pharmacology, Pharmacokinetics and Precautions).
Hepatic Impairment: In patients with mild or moderate hepatic impaired function (Child-Pugh A and Child-Pugh B) no dose adjustment is needed (see Pharmacology, Pharmacokinetics). There are no data available for use of memantine in patients with severe hepatic impairment. Therefore, administration of Ebixa is not recommended in patients with severe hepatic impairment.

INFORMATION FOR THE PATIENT: Published in e-CPS, available by subscription at www.e-cps.ca.

SUPPLIED: Each white to off-white, centrally tapered oblong, biconvex, film-coated tablet with a single break line on both sides, contains: memantine hydrochloride 10 mg. Nonmedicinal ingredients: colloidal anhydrous silica, lactose monohydrate, magnesium stearate, methacrylic acid-ethyl acrylate copolymer, microcrystalline cellulose, polysorbate 80, simethicone emulsion, sodium lauryl sulfate, talc and triacetin. Blister packages of 30. Store in a dry place at room temperature between 15 and 30°C.

(Shown in Product Identification Section)

Edecrin® ℞
ethacrynic acid
Diuretic—Saluretic

Aton Pharma

Sodium Edecrin® ℞
ethacrynate sodium
Diuretic—Saluretic

Aton Pharma

Date of Revision: July 27, 2009

PHARMACOLOGY: EDECRIN (ethacrynic acid) is a saluretic-diuretic agent with marked potency and rapid onset of action. It is chemically unrelated to other diuretics. Patients with congestive heart failure (including acute pulmonary edema), renal edema, hepatic cirrhosis with ascites, and other conditions involving fluid retention have responded well to ethacrynic acid.

EDECRIN has the following major characteristics:

1. Water and electrolyte excretion may be increased several times over that observed with thiazide diuretics. The urinary output is usually dose-dependent and related to the magnitude of fluid accumulation.
2. Electrolyte excretion pattern differs from that of thiazides. Initially, sodium and chloride excretion is usually substantial, and chloride loss exceeds that of sodium. With prolonged therapy, chloride excretion declines, and potassium and hydrogen ion excretion may increase. In patients with increased diuresis excessive amounts of potassium may be excreted. Ethacrynic acid is effective whether or not there is clinical acidosis or alkalosis.
3. Rapid onset of action usually is observed within 30 minutes after an oral dose or within 5 minutes after an intravenous injection.
4. Duration of action is moderate following oral administration (6 to 8 hours). The peak diuretic-saluretic activity occurs in about 2 hours.
5. Sulfhydryl binding propensity differs in certain respects from that of the organomercurials. Its mode of action is not by carbonic anhydrase inhibition.
6. Multiple sites of action. Ethacrynic acid acts on the proximal and distal portions of the tubule, and also on the ascending limb of the loop of Henle.

INDICATIONS: EDECRIN (ethacrynic acid) is especially useful in patients unresponsive to the commonly used diuretics.

It has been found useful in the following conditions: **Congestive Heart Failure, Acute Pulmonary Edema, Renal Edema (Nephrotic syndrome), Hepatic Cirrhosis with Ascites.**

The majority of patients studied to date have been resistant in some degree to other diuretic agents; the remaining patients received ethacrynic acid as their first diuretic in the treatment of edema or were placed on the drug for comparative evaluations.

Experience to date with the use of EDECRIN (ethacrynic acid tablets, USP) for oral maintenance therapy has been limited. The duration of studies has varied from short term investigations to continuous therapy of one year or longer.

Patients with chronic **congestive heart failure** many of whom were unresponsive to other diuretics, have responded successfully to short or long term therapy. These include patients with arteriosclerotic heart disease, rheumatic heart disease, hypertensive cardiovascular disease, pulmonary heart disease, and congenital heart disease. Long term studies in patients who have received ethacrynic acid for over six months have been in patients with cardiac edema secondary to arteriosclerotic or valvular heart disease. The average duration of these studies has been about nine months.

Patients with **acute pulmonary edema** have responded rapidly to the intravenous use of Sodium EDECRIN (ethacrynate sodium for injection, USP). Clinical improvement is coincidental with the large increases in water and electrolyte excretion usually observed to begin within 5 minutes after injection. Ethacrynate sodium offers advantages over other diuretics because of its rapid action and effectiveness.

EDECRIN is indicated for patients with the nephrotic syndrome. The greatest experience with this agent in **renal edema** has been in patients with the nephrotic syndrome. Use of the drug in these patients usually has been of short duration, ranging from one to three months, with treatment usually being initiated in the hospital.

Saluresis and diuresis may be achieved in patients unresponsive to other diuretics. Patients whose response to other diuretics has been suboptimal may obtain a greater effect from ethacrynic acid.

As with other diuretics, hypoproteinemia may reduce responsiveness to ethacrynic acid and the use of salt-poor albumin should be considered. In some patients, larger doses may be necessary to produce effective diuresis in renal than in cardiac edema. Ethacrynic acid is effective in many patients who have significant degrees of renal insufficiency. It has little or no effect on renal blood flow except following pronounced reduction in plasma volume when associated with rapid diuresis. The extreme sensitivity of patients with chronic renal failure to alterations in fluid or electrolyte balance dictates careful clinical and laboratory observation when diuretics are used, and these agents must be discontinued immediately if further deterioration in renal function occurs.

For reasons given below, initiation of diuretic therapy with EDECRIN in the cirrhotic patient with ascites is best carried out in the hospital. When maintenance therapy has been established, the individual can be satisfactorily followed as an outpatient.

Ethacrynic acid is usually effective in patients with cirrhosis who have ascites. Most studies have been of three months' duration, or less. Diuresis and saluresis have occurred in previously unresponsive patients. However, cirrhotic patients tolerate poorly acute shifts in electrolyte balance, and potassium excretion is often augmented as a result of associated aldosteronism. Therefore, careful clinical and laboratory observation is essential to avoid serious loss of potassium and chloride ions and the development of metabolic alkalosis, with resultant hepatic encephalopathy. These effects may be minimized by appropriate adjustment of dosage and by the use of supplemental potassium as the chloride with or without a potassium sparing agent (see Dosage).

A variety of other edematous states have been successfully treated with ethacrynic acid; most of the experience has been of short duration. These include ascites due to malignancy, idiopathic edema, and lymphedema.

Pediatrics: EDECRIN has been found useful in patients of the pediatric age group with the nephrotic syndrome. This experience has been mostly of short duration, in hospitalized patients resistant to other therapy. Pediatric patients with congenital heart disease also have responded to this agent. Information in infants is insufficient to recommend therapy with ethacrynic acid.

CONTRAINDICATIONS: All diuretics, including ethacrynic acid, are contraindicated in anuria. If increasing azotemia and/or oliguria occur during treatment of severe, progressive renal disease, the diuretic should be discontinued.

Until further experience in infants is accumulated, therapy with oral and parenteral ethacrynic acid is contraindicated. (See also Warnings, Pregnant Women and Nursing Women.)

Hypersensitivity to any component of this product.

WARNINGS: EDECRIN (ethacrynic acid) is a potent and rapidly-acting diuretic that may lead to excessive diuresis and natriuresis with water depletion and electrolyte imbalance, which may result in hypokalemia or hypochloremic alkalosis with potassium depletion, hydrogen ion loss and extracellular fluid space contraction. This may occur in patients with marked fluid accumulation or when excessive doses are used but these adverse effects may also be encountered in patients with moderate degrees of edema. The safe use of potent diuretics requires careful understanding of their pharmacologic actions and in particular of their mechanism of development of electrolyte imbalance. Close attention should be given to the directions of use and to identification of the individual patient response to the drug.

Frequent serum electrolyte, CO_2 and BUN determinations should be performed early in therapy and periodically thereafter during active diuresis. Baseline determination of electrolytes and renal function before therapy is recommended when preexisting derangements are suspected. Any electrolyte abnormalities should be corrected or the drug temporarily withdrawn.

Ethacrynic acid should be given with caution to patients with advanced cirrhosis of the liver, particularly those with a history of previous episodes of electrolyte imbalance or hepatic encephalopathy. Like other diuretics it may precipitate hepatic coma and death.

Too vigorous a diuresis, as evidenced by rapid and excessive weight loss, may induce an acute hypotensive episode. In elderly cardiac patients, rapid contraction of plasma volume and the resultant hemoconcentration should be avoided to prevent the development of thromboembolic episodes, such as cerebral vascular thromboses and pulmonary emboli which may be fatal. In patients receiving digitalis glycosides, excessive loss of potassium may precipitate digitalis toxicity. Care should also be exercised in patients receiving potassium-depleting steroids.

The effects of ethacrynic acid on electrolytes are related to its renal pharmacologic activity and are dose-dependent. The possibility of profound electrolyte and water loss may be avoided by weighing the patient throughout the treatment period, by monitoring electrolyte changes, by careful adjustment of dosage, by initiating treatment with small doses, and by using the drug on an intermittent schedule when possible. When excessive diuresis occurs, the drug should be withdrawn until homeostasis is restored. When excessive electrolyte loss occurs, the dosage should be reduced or the drug temporarily withdrawn, and if necessary judicious repletion of losses should be considered.

Avoidance of potassium depletion may be possible by adequate dietary supplementation, intermittent therapy, and when possible by careful liberalization of salt intake. Supplementary potassium chloride may however be required, particularly in cirrhosis or patients with a preexisting degree of aldosteronism.

While potassium supplements may be indicated there have been numerous reports, published and unpublished, concerning non-specific small bowel lesions, consisting of stenosis with or without ulceration, associated with administration of enteric-coated potassium salts alone or with oral diuretics. Surgery was frequently required and deaths have occurred.

Pregnant Women: EDECRIN is not recommended for use in pregnant patients. Use of the drug in women of the child-bearing age requires that its potential benefits be weighed against the possible hazards to the fetus. The safety and efficacy of the drug in toxemia of pregnancy have not been established.

Nursing Women: EDECRIN is contraindicated in nursing mothers. If use of the drug is deemed essential, the patient should stop nursing.

PRECAUTIONS: General: Weakness, muscle cramps, paresthesias, thirst, anorexia, and signs of hyponatremia, hypokalemia, and/or hypochloremic alkalosis may occur following vigorous or excessive diuresis and these may be accentuated by rigid salt restriction. Rarely tetany has been reported following vigorous diuresis. **During therapy with ethacrynic acid, liberalization of salt intake and supplementary potassium chloride are often necessary.**

When metabolic alkalosis may be anticipated, e.g., in cirrhosis with ascites, the use of potassium chloride with or without a potassium sparing agent before and continuously during therapy with ethacrynic acid may mitigate or prevent the hypokalemia. If a potassium sparing agent is used, continued monitoring of electrolytes is still required because of the possible occurrence in this case of hyperkalemia.

In a few patients this diuretic has produced severe, watery diarrhea. If this occurs, it should be discontinued and not readministered.

EDECRIN (ethacrynic acid) has little or no effect on glomerular filtration or on renal blood flow, except following pronounced reductions in plasma volume when associated with rapid diuresis. A transient increase in serum urea nitrogen may occur. This is usually reversible when the drug is discontinued.

Deafness, tinnitus and vertigo with a sense of fullness in the ears have occurred, most frequently in patients with severe impairment of renal function. These symptoms have been associated most often with intravenous administration and with doses in excess of those recommended. The deafness has usually been reversible and of short duration (one to 24 hours). However, in some critically ill patients the hearing loss has been permanent. A number of these patients were also receiving drugs known to be ototoxic.

DRUG INTERACTIONS: Anti-hypertensive Agents : The safety and efficacy of ethacrynic acid in hypertension have not been established. However, the dosage of coadministered antihypertensive agents may require adjustment.

Orthostatic hypotension may occur in patients receiving antihypertensive agents when given ethacrynic acid.

Antibiotics: EDECRIN may increase the ototoxic potential of other drugs such as aminoglycoside antibiotics. Their concurrent use should be avoided.

Warfarin: A number of drugs, including ethacrynic acid, have been shown to displace warfarin from plasma protein; a reduction in the usual anticoagulant dosage may be required in patients receiving both drugs.

Lithium: Lithium should generally not be given to patients receiving diuretics, since diuretics reduce renal clearance of lithium making the risk of lithium toxicity very high in such patients.

Corticosteroid: EDECRIN may increase the risk of gastric hemorrhage associated with corticosteroid treatment.

Patients with Special Diseases and Conditions: Patients with refractory edema or having preexisting degrees of aldosteronism and those receiving potassium depleting steroids are more likely to develop hypokalemia. This may be responsible for increased digitalis toxicity or result in hepatic coma in patients with advanced liver disease. These patients may therefore require potassium supplementation.

ADVERSE REACTIONS: Gastrointestinal: anorexia, malaise, abdominal discomfort or pain, dysphagia, nausea, vomiting, and diarrhea. In a few patients, watery, profuse diarrhea, gastrointestinal bleeding, and acute pancreatitis have been reported.

Metabolic: Reversible hyperuricemia, decreased urinary urate excretion, and hyperglycemia have been reported. Acute gout has been precipitated. Rarely acute symptomatic hypoglycemia with convulsions, jaundice and abnormal tests of hepatocellular function have been reported.

Hematologic: Agranulocytosis, severe neutropenia, thrombocytopenia, and Henoch-Schönlein purpura have been reported rarely.

Special Senses: Vertigo, deafness, and tinnitus, with a sense of fullness in the ears and blurred vision have occurred (see Precautions).

Central Nervous System: fatigue, apprehension, and confusion.

Other: skin rash, headache, fever, chills and hematuria.

Ethacrynate sodium occasionally has caused local irritation and pain, and a rare instance of local thrombophlebitis has been reported after its use.

A number of possibly drug-related deaths have occurred in critically ill patients refractory to other diuretics. These generally have fallen into two categories: (1) patients with severe myocardial disease who have been receiving digitalis and presumably developed acute hypokalemia with fatal arrhythmia; (2) patients with severely decompensated hepatic cirrhosis with ascites, with or without accompanying encephalopathy, who were in electrolyte imbalance and died because of intensification of the electrolyte defect.

OVERDOSAGE:

For management of a suspected drug overdose, CPhA recommends that you contact your **regional Poison Control Centre**. See the *CPS* Directory section for a list of Poison Control Centres.

DOSAGE: Dosage must be regulated carefully to prevent a more rapid or substantial loss of fluid or electrolyte than is indicated or necessary. The magnitude of diuresis and natriuresis is largely dependent on the degree of fluid accumulation present in the patient. Similarly, the extent of potassium excretion is determined in large measure by the presence and magnitude of aldosteronism.

Oral Use: The splitting of EDECRIN 25 mg tablets is not advised.

To Initiate Diuresis: Adults: The smallest dose required to produce gradual weight loss (about 0.5 to 1 kg per day) is recommended.

Onset of diuresis usually occurs at 50 to 100 mg for adults. After diuresis has been achieved, the minimally effective dose (usually from 50 to 200 mg daily) may be given on a continuous or intermittent dosage schedule. Dosage adjustments are usually in 25 to 50 mg increments to avoid derangement of water and electrolyte excretion.

The patient should be weighed under standard conditions before and during the institution of diuretic therapy with this compound. Small alterations in dose might prevent a massive diuretic response.

The following schedule may be helpful in determining the smallest effective dose:

Day 1 - 50 mg (single dose) after a meal.

Day 2 - 50 mg twice daily after meals, if necessary.

Day 3 - 100 mg in the morning and 50 to 100 mg following the afternoon or evening meal, depending upon response to the morning dose.

A few patients may require initial and maintenance doses as high as 200 mg twice daily. These higher doses, which should be achieved gradually, are most often required in patients with severe, refractory edema.

Children: The initial dose should be 25 mg. Careful stepwise increments in dosage of 25 mg should be made to achieve effective maintenance. A dosage for infants has not been established.

Maintenance Therapy: It is usually possible to reduce the dosage and frequency of administration once dry weight has been achieved.

EDECRIN (ethacrynic acid tablets, USP) may be given intermittently after an effective diuresis is obtained with the regimen outlined above. Dosage may be on an alternate daily schedule or more prolonged periods of diuretic therapy may be interspersed with rest periods. Such an intermittent dosage schedule allows time for correction of any electrolyte imbalance and may provide a more efficient diuretic response.

The chloruretic effect of this agent may give rise to retention of bicarbonate and metabolic alkalosis. This may be corrected by giving chloride (ammonium chloride or arginine chloride). Ammonium chloride should not be given to cirrhotic patients.

Ethacrynic acid has additive effects when used with other diuretics. Small doses of ethacrynic acid may be added to existing diuretic regimens to maintain basal weight. This drug may potentiate the action of carbonic anhydrase inhibitors, with augmentation of natriuresis and kaliuresis. Therefore, when adding ethacrynic acid, the initial dose and changes of dose should be in 25 mg increments to avoid electrolyte depletion. Rarely, patients who failed to respond to ethacrynic acid have responded to older established agents.

While many patients do not require supplemental potassium, the use of potassium chloride or potassium sparing agents, or both, during treatment with ethacrynic acid is advisable, especially in cirrhotic or nephrotic patients and in patients receiving digitalis.

Salt liberalization usually prevents the development of hyponatremia and hypochloremia. During treatment with ethacrynic acid, salt may be liberalized to a greater extent than with other diuretics. Cirrhotic patients however, usually require at least moderate salt restriction concomitant with diuretic therapy.

Intravenous Use: Sodium EDECRIN (ethacrynate sodium for injection, USP) is for intravenous use when oral intake is impractical or in urgent conditions, such as acute pulmonary edema.

Adults: The usual intravenous dose for the average sized adult is 50 mg, or 0.5 to 1 mg per kg of body weight. Usually only one dose has been necessary; occasionally a second dose at a new injection site, to avoid possible thrombophlebitis, may be required. A single intravenous dose not exceeding 100 mg has been used in critical situations.

Children: Insufficient pediatric experience precludes recommendation for this age group.

The solution may be given slowly through the tubing of a running infusion or by direct intravenous injection over a period of several minutes.

Ethacrynate sodium should not be given subcutaneously or intramuscularly because of local pain and irritation.

Reconstituted solutions: To reconstitute the dry material, add 50 mL of 5 percent Dextrose Injection or Sodium Chloride Injection to the vial. Occasionally, some 5 percent Dextrose Injection solutions may have a low pH (below 5). The resulting solution with such a diluent may be hazy or opalescent. Intravenous use of such a solution is not recommended.

Parenteral Products: Do not mix this solution with whole blood or its derivatives. Because there is no preservative contained in the vial, a fresh solution should be prepared just prior to each administration. Any unused solution should be discarded.

SUPPLIED: Edecrin: Each white, scored tablet, with ATON 205 on one side and EDECRIN on the other, contains: ethacrynic acid, USP 25 mg. Nonmedicinal ingredients: colloidal silicon dioxide, cornstarch, lactose, magnesium stearate and talc. High density polyethylene bottles of 100. The splitting of EDECRIN 25 mg tablets is not advised. Store in the tightly closed container at room temperature (15-30°C).

Sodium Edecrin: Each vial of dry white material either in a plug form or as a powder, contains: ethacrynate sodium, USP equivalent to ethacrynic acid 50 mg. Nonmedicinal ingredients: mannitol 62.5 mg.

Effexor® XR ℞

venlafaxine HCl

Antidepressant—Anxiolytic

Pfizer

Date of Revision: October 20, 2009

SUMMARY PRODUCT INFORMATION:

Route of Administration	Dosage Form/ Strength	Nonmedicinal Ingredients
Oral	EFFEXOR XR Capsules: hard gelatin capsule (37.5, 75, 150 mg)	Ethylcellulose, gelatin, hydroxypropyl-methyl cellulose, iron oxide, microcrystalline cellulose, talc, titanium dioxide, White Tek SB-0007 and/or Opacode Red S-1-15034 ink

INDICATIONS AND CLINICAL USE: Adults: EFFEXOR XR Venlafaxine Hydrochloride Extended Release Capsules is indicated for:

- Depression: EFFEXOR XR Capsules (extended release) are indicated for the symptomatic relief of major depressive disorder.

  The short-term efficacy of EFFEXOR XR Capsules (extended release) has been demonstrated in placebo-controlled trials of up to 12 weeks.

  The efficacy of EFFEXOR XR Capsules (extended release) in maintaining an antidepressant response for up to 26 weeks following response to 8 weeks of acute treatment was demonstrated in a placebo-controlled trial.
- Generalized Anxiety Disorder (GAD): EFFEXOR XR Capsules are indicated for the symptomatic relief of anxiety causing clinically significant distress in patients with GAD. Anxiety or tension associated with the stress of everyday life usually does not require treatment with an anxiolytic. The effectiveness of EFFEXOR XR in long-term use has been evaluated for up to 6 months in controlled clinical trials.
- Social Anxiety Disorder (Social Phobia): EFFEXOR XR is indicated for the symptomatic relief of Social Anxiety Disorder, also known as Social Phobia.

  Social Anxiety Disorder is characterized by a marked and persistent fear of one or more social or performance situations, in which the person is exposed to unfamiliar people or to possible scrutiny by others. Exposure to the feared situation almost invariably provokes anxiety, which may approach the intensity of a panic attack. The feared situations are avoided or endured with intense anxiety or distress. Fear, anxious anticipation, distress in the feared situation(s) or avoidance of social and/or performance situations that does not interfere significantly with the person's normal routine, occupational or academic functioning, or social life usually does not require treatment with an anxiolytic.

  The efficacy of EFFEXOR XR capsules as a treatment for Social Anxiety Disorder (also known as Social Phobia) was demonstrated in four 12-week, multicenter, placebo-controlled, flexible-dose studies and one 6-month, fixed/flexible-dose study in adult outpatients meeting DSM-IV criteria for Social Anxiety Disorder. These studies evaluating EFFEXOR XR doses in a range of 75-225 mg/day demonstrated that EFFEXOR XR was significantly more effective than placebo for the Liebowitz Social Anxiety Scale Total score, Clinical Global Impressions of Severity of Illness rating, and Social Phobia Inventory.
- Panic Disorder: EFFEXOR XR is indicated for the symptomatic relief of Panic Disorder, with or without agoraphobia, as defined in DSM-IV. Panic Disorder is characterized by the occurrence of unexpected panic attacks and associated concern about having additional attacks, worry about the implications or consequences of the attacks, and/or a significant change in behaviour related to the attacks.

  Panic Disorder (DSM-IV) is characterized by recurrent, unexpected panic attacks, i.e., a discrete period of intense fear or discomfort, in which four (or more) of the following symptoms develop abruptly and reach a peak within 10 minutes: 1) palpitations, pounding heart, or accelerated heart rate; 2) sweating; 3) trembling or shaking; 4) sensations of shortness of breath or smothering; 5) feeling of choking; 6) chest pain or discomfort; 7) nausea or abdominal distress; 8) feeling dizzy, unsteady, light-headed, or faint; 9) derealization (feelings of unreality) or depersonalization (being detached from oneself); 10) fear of losing control; 11) fear of dying; 12) paresthesias (numbness or tingling sensations); 13) chills or hot flushes.

  The efficacy of EFFEXOR XR in the treatment of Panic Disorder was established in two 12-week placebo-controlled trials in adult outpatients with Panic Disorder (DSM-IV). The efficacy of EFFEXOR XR in prolonging time to relapse in Panic Disorder for up to 6 months in responders of a 12-week acute treatment was demonstrated in a placebo-controlled trial.

Long-term Use of EFFEXOR XR: The physician who elects to use EFFEXOR XR for extended periods in the treatment of depression, GAD, Social Anxiety Disorder, or Panic Disorder should periodically re-evaluate the long-term usefulness of the drug for the individual patient (see Dosage and Administration).

Geriatrics (>65 years of age): Caution should be exercised in treating the elderly. In Phase II and III clinical trials, no overall differences in effectiveness and safety were observed between these geriatric patients and younger patients, and other reported clinical experience has not identified differences in response between the elderly and younger patients. However, greater sensitivity of some older individuals cannot be ruled out.

Pediatrics (<18 years of age): EFFEXOR XR (venlafaxine) is not indicated for use in children under 18 years of age (see Warnings and Precautions, Potential Association with Behavioral and Emotional Changes, Including Self-harm).

CONTRAINDICATIONS:

- Hypersensitivity: Patients who are hypersensitive to this drug or to any ingredient in the formulation or component of the container.
- Monoamine Oxidase Inhibitors (MAOIs): EFFEXOR XR should not be used in combination with MAOIs or within two weeks of terminating treatment with MAOIs. Treatment with MAOIs should not be started until 2 weeks after discontinuation of EFFEXOR XR therapy.

  Adverse reactions, some serious, have been reported when EFFEXOR XR therapy is initiated soon after discontinuing an MAOI and when an MAOI is initiated soon after discontinuation of EFFEXOR XR. These reactions have included tremor, myoclonus, diaphoresis, nausea, vomiting, flushing, dizziness, hyperthermia with features resembling neuroleptic malignant syndrome, seizures and death. In patients receiving antidepressants with pharmacological properties similar to venlafaxine in combination with an MAOI, there have also been reports of serious, sometimes fatal, reactions. For a selective serotonin reuptake inhibitor, these reactions have included hyperthermia, rigidity, myoclonus, autonomic instability with possible rapid fluctuations of vital signs, and mental status changes that include extreme agitation progressing to delirium and coma. Some cases presented with features resembling neuroleptic malignant syndrome. Severe hypothermia and seizures, sometimes fatal, have been reported in association with the combined use of tricyclic antidepressants and MAOIs. These reactions have also been reported in patients who have recently discontinued these drugs and have been started on an MAOI.

WARNINGS AND PRECAUTIONS: Potential Association with Behavioral and Emotional Changes, Including Self-harm: Pediatrics: Placebo-controlled Clinical Trial Data:

- **Recent analyses of placebo-controlled clinical trial safety databases from SSRIs and other newer antidepressants suggest that use of these drugs in patients under the age of 18 may be associated with behavioral and emotional changes, including an increased risk of suicidal ideation and behaviour over that of placebo.**
- **The small denominators in the clinical trial database, as well as the variability in placebo rates, preclude reliable conclusions on the relative safety profiles among the drugs in the class.**

Adults and Pediatrics: Additional Data:

- **There are clinical trial and post-marketing reports with SSRIs and other newer antidepressants, in both pediatrics and adults, of severe agitation-type adverse events coupled with self-harm or harm to others. The agitation-type events include: akathisia/psychomotor restlessness, agitation, disinhibition, emotional lability, hostility, aggression, depersonalization. In some cases, the events occurred within several weeks of starting treatment.**

  Rigorous clinical monitoring for suicidal ideation or other indicators of potential for suicidal behaviour is advised in patients of all ages. This includes monitoring for agitation-type emotional and behavioral changes.

  Patients, their families, and their caregivers should be encouraged to be alert to the emergence of anxiety, agitation, panic attacks, insomnia, irritability, hostility, aggressiveness, impulsivity, akathisia (psychomotor restlessness), hypomania, mania, other unusual changes in behaviour, worsening of depression, and suicidal ideation, especially when initiating therapy or during any change in dose or dosage regimen. The risk of suicide attempt must be considered, especially in depressed patients (see Overdosage).

Discontinuation Symptoms: Patients currently taking EFFEXOR XR should not be discontinued abruptly, due to risk of discontinuation symptoms (see Warnings and Precautions, Discontinuation Symptoms). At the time that a medical decision is made to discontinue an SSRI or other newer antidepressant drug, a gradual reduction in the dose wherever possible, rather than an abrupt cessation, is recommended.

General: Allergic Reactions: Patients should be advised to notify their physician if they develop a rash, hives or a related allergic phenomenon.

Hypertension: General: Dose-related increases in blood pressure have been reported in some patients treated with venlafaxine. Also, rare cases of hypertensive crisis and malignant hypertension have been reported in normotensive and treated-hypertensive patients in post-marketing experience (see Acute Severe Hypertension).

Caution should be exercised in patients whose underlying conditions might be compromised by increases in blood pressure.

Acute Severe Hypertension: Cases of severe elevated blood pressure requiring immediate treatment have been reported in postmarketing experience, including reports of hypertensive crisis and malignant hypertension. The reports included normotensives and treated-hypertensive patients as well. Pre-existing hypertension should be controlled before treatment with venlafaxine. All patients should have their blood pressure evaluated before starting venlafaxine and monitored regularly during treatment. Patients should be told to consult their doctors if they have symptoms associated with acute severe hypertension, such as headache (particularly in the back of head/neck when waking up), stronger heart beat and possibly more rapid, palpitations, dizziness, easy fatigability, blurred vision, chest pain.

Sustained Hypertension: Venlafaxine treatment has been associated with sustained hypertension (see Table 1). Sustained increases in blood pressure could have adverse consequences. Therefore, it is recommended that patients have their blood pressure monitored before starting venlafaxine and then regularly during treatment. For patients who experience a sustained increase in blood pressure while receiving venlafaxine, either dose reduction or discontinuation should be considered after a benefit-risk assessment is made.

Venlafaxine Immediate Release Tablets: Treatment with immediate release venlafaxine HCl tablets was associated with modest but sustained increases in blood pressure during premarketing studies. Sustained hypertension, defined as treatment-emergent supine diastolic blood pressure (SDBP) ≥90 mm Hg and ≥10 mm Hg above baseline for 3 consecutive visits, showed the following incidence and dose-relationship: (see Table 1).

Table 1: EFFEXOR XR

Probability of Sustained Elevation in SDBP

Probability of Sustained Elevation in SDBP (Pool of Premarketing Depression Studies with Venlafaxine HCl)		
Treatment Group	**(%) Incidence of Sustained Elevation in SDBP**	
Venlafaxine	**Immediate Release Tablets**	**Extended Release EFFEXOR XR**
<100 mg/day	2	3
101–200 mg/day	5	2
201–300 mg/day	6	4
>300 mg/day	13	NE[a]
Placebo	2	0

a Not evaluable.

An analysis of the blood pressure increases in patients with sustained hypertension and in the 19 patients who were discontinued from treatment because of hypertension (<1% of total venlafaxine-treated group) showed that most of the blood pressure increases were in the range of 10 to 15 mm Hg, SDBP.

EFFEXOR XR Capsules: Depression: In placebo-controlled premarketing depression studies with EFFEXOR XR, a final on-therapy mean increase in supine diastolic pressure (SDBP) of <1.2 mm Hg was observed for EFFEXOR XR-treated patients compared with a mean decrease of 0.2 mm Hg for placebo-treated patients. Less than 3% of EFFEXOR XR patients treated with doses of 75 to 300 mg/day had sustained elevations in blood pressure (defined as treatment-emergent SDBP ≥90 mm Hg and ≥10 mm Hg above baseline for 3 consecutive on-therapy visits). An insufficient number of patients received doses of EFFEXOR XR >300 mg/day to evaluate systematically sustained blood pressure increases. Less than 1% of EFFEXOR XR-treated patients in double-blind, placebo-controlled premarketing depression studies discontinued treatment because of elevated blood pressure compared with 0.4% of placebo-treated patients.

Generalized Anxiety Disorder (GAD): In placebo-controlled premarketing anxiety studies with EFFEXOR XR 37.5-225 mg/day, a final on-drug mean increase in SDBP of 0.4 mm Hg was observed for EFFEXOR XR-treated patients compared with a mean decrease of 0.8 mm Hg for placebo treated patients.

Social Anxiety Disorder (Social Phobia): In 4 placebo-controlled premarketing Social Anxiety Disorder studies with EFFEXOR XR 75-225 mg/day up to 12 weeks, a final on-drug mean increase in SDBP of 0.9 mm Hg was observed for EFFEXOR XR-treated patients compared with a mean decrease of 1.6 mm Hg for placebo-treated patients. In one placebo-controlled premarketing Social Anxiety Disorder study with EFFEXOR XR up to 6 months, a final on-drug mean decrease in SDBP of 0.2 mm Hg was observed for EFFEXOR XR-treated patients who received fixed doses of 75 mg/day and a mean increase of 1.5 mm Hg was observed for EFFEXOR XR-treated patients who received flexible doses of 150 to 225 mg/day, compared with a mean decrease of 0.6 mm Hg for placebo-treated patients.

Among patients treated with 75-225 mg per day of EFFEXOR XR in all premarketing Social Anxiety Disorder studies, 0.6% (5/771) experienced sustained hypertension.

In all premarketing Social Anxiety Disorder studies with patients treated with 75-225 mg per day, 0.6% (5/771) of the EFFEXOR XR-treated patients discontinued treatment because of elevated blood pressure.

Panic Disorder: In placebo-controlled premarketing Panic Disorder studies with EFFEXOR XR 75-225 mg/day up to 12 weeks, a final on-drug mean increase in SDBP of 0.3 mm Hg was observed for EFFEXOR XR-treated patients compared with a mean decrease of 1.1 mm Hg for placebo-treated patients.

Among patients treated with 75 to 225 mg/day of EFFEXOR XR in premarketing Panic Disorder studies up to 12 weeks, 0.9% (9/973) experienced sustained hypertension.

In premarketing Panic Disorder studies up to 12 weeks, 0.5% (5/1001) of the EFFEXOR XR-treated patients discontinued treatment because of elevated blood pressure.

Serotonin Syndrome: As with other serotonergic agents, serotonin syndrome, a potentially life threatening condition, may occur with venlafaxine treatment, particularly with concomitant use of other agents that may affect the serotonergic neurotransmitter systems (please see Serotonin Syndrome/Neuroleptic Malignant Syndrome, and Drug Interactions, Drug-Drug Interactions, Serotonergic Drugs).

Discontinuation Symptoms: Discontinuation symptoms have been assessed both in patients with depression and those with anxiety. Abrupt discontinuation, dose reduction, or tapering of venlafaxine at various doses has been found to be associated with the appearance of new symptoms, the frequency of which increased with increased dose level and with longer duration of treatment. If venlafaxine is used until or shortly before birth, discontinuation effects in the newborn should be considered.

Reported symptoms include aggression, agitation, anorexia, anxiety, asthenia, confusion, convulsions, coordination impaired, diarrhoea, dizziness, dry mouth, dysphoric mood, fasciculation, fatigue, flu-like symptoms, headache, hypomania, impaired coordination and balance, insomnia, nausea, nightmares, nervousness, paresthesia, electric shock sensations, sensory disturbances (including shock like electrical sensations), sleep disturbances, somnolence, sweating, tinnitus, tremor, vertigo, and vomiting. Where such symptoms occurred they were usually self-limiting but in a few patients continued for several weeks. In premarketing studies, the majority of discontinuation reactions were mild and resolved without treatment.

Discontinuation effects are well known to occur with antidepressants, and, therefore, it is recommended that the dosage be tapered gradually whenever possible and the patient monitored. Time to event onset after dose reduction or discontinuation can vary in individual patients and range from the same day to several weeks. (See also Adverse Reactions, Discontinuation Symptoms; Dosage and Administration, Discontinuing Venlafaxine.)

Venlafaxine Treatment During Pregnancy—Effects on Newborns: Post-marketing reports indicate that some neonates exposed to venlafaxine, SSRIs (Selective Serotonin Reuptake Inhibitors), or other newer antidepressants late in the third trimester have developed complications requiring prolonged hospitalization, respiratory support, and tube feeding. Such complications can arise immediately upon delivery. When treating a pregnant woman with EFFEXOR XR during the third trimester, the physician should carefully consider the potential risks and benefits of treatment (see Warnings and Precautions, Special Populations, Pregnant Women; Dosage and Administration, Special Patients Populations, Treatment of Pregnant Women During the Third Trimester.

Psychomotor Impairment: In healthy volunteers receiving an immediate release venlafaxine formulation at a stable regimen of 150 mg/day, some impairment of psychomotor performance was observed. Patients should be cautioned about operating hazardous machinery, including automobiles, or engaging in tasks requiring alertness until they have been able to assess the drug's effect on their own psychomotor performance.

The following additional precautions are listed alphabetically.

Cardiovascular: Hypertension: See Warnings and Precautions, General, Hypertension.

Cardiac Disease: Venlafaxine has not been evaluated or used to any appreciable extent in patients with a recent history of myocardial infarction or unstable heart disease. Patients with these diagnoses were systematically excluded from many clinical studies during the product's clinical trials. Therefore it should be used with caution in these patients.

Evaluation of the electrocardiograms for 769 patients who received venlafaxine immediate release tablets in 4- to 6-week double-blind trials showed that the incidence of trial-emergent conduction abnormalities did not differ from that with placebo.

The electrocardiograms for 357 patients who received EFFEXOR XR and 285 patients who received placebo in 8 to 12 week double-blind, placebo-controlled trials in depression were analyzed. The mean change from baseline in corrected QT interval (QTc) for EFFEXOR XR-treated patients in depression studies was increased relative to that for placebo-treated patients (increase of 4.7 msec for EFFEXOR XR and decrease of 1.9 msec for placebo). The clinical significance of this change is unknown. Three of 705 EFFEXOR XR-treated patients in phase III studies experienced QTc prolongation to 500 msec during treatment. Baseline QTc was >450 msec for all 3 patients.

Electrocardiograms are available for 815 patients who received EFFEXOR XR and 379 patients who received placebo in up to 6-month, double-blind, placebo-controlled trials in Generalized Anxiety Disorder. The mean change from baseline in the corrected QT interval (QTc) for EFFEXOR XR-treated patients in the GAD studies did not differ significantly from that with placebo. One of the 815 EFFEXOR XR-treated patients experienced QTc prolongation to 593 msec. Baseline QTc was 460 msec for this one patient.

Electrocardiograms were evaluated for 401 patients who received EFFEXOR XR and 444 patients who received placebo in four 12-week double-blind, placebo-controlled trials in Social Anxiety Disorder. The mean change from baseline in QTc for EFFEXOR XR-treated patients in the 12-week Social Anxiety Disorder studies was increased relative to that for placebo-treated patients (increase of 4.1 msec for EFFEXOR XR and decrease of 1.4 msec for placebo). Electrocardiograms were evaluated for 101 patients who received EFFEXOR XR 75 mg/day, 96 patients who received 150-225 mg/day, and 90 patients who received placebo in one 6-month double-blind, placebo-controlled trial in Social Anxiety Disorder. A mean decrease from baseline in QTc of 0.05 ms was observed for patients treated with EFFEXOR XR 75 mg/day, a mean increase from baseline in QTc of 3.4 ms was observed for patients treated with EFFEXOR XR 150-225 mg/day, and a mean increase from baseline in QTc of 0.5 ms was observed for patients treated with placebo in the 6-month Social Anxiety Disorder study.

Electrocardiograms were evaluated for 661 patients who received EFFEXOR XR and 395 patients who received placebo in three 10- to 12-week double-blind, placebo-controlled trials in Panic Disorder. The mean change from baseline in QTc for EFFEXOR XR-treated patients in the Panic Disorder studies was increased relative to that for placebo-treated patients (increase of 1.5 msec for EFFEXOR XR and decrease of 0.7 msec for placebo).

No case of sudden unexplained death or serious ventricular arrhythmia, which are possible clinical sequelae of QTc prolongation, was reported in EFFEXOR XR pre-marketing studies.

The mean heart rate was increased by about 3-4 beats per minute during treatment with venlafaxine in clinical trials of depression and GAD. The mean change from baseline in heart rate for EFFEXOR XR-treated patients in the Social Anxiety Disorder studies was significantly higher than that for placebo (a mean increase of 5 beats per minute for EFFEXOR XR and no change for placebo).

The mean change from baseline in heart rate for EFFEXOR XR-treated patients in the Panic Disorder studies was significantly higher than that for placebo (a mean increase of 3 beats per minute for EFFEXOR XR and a mean decrease of less than 1 beat per minute for placebo).

Increases in heart rate can occur, particularly with higher doses. Caution should be exercised in patients whose underlying conditions might be compromised by increases in heart rate.

Concomitant Illness: Clinical experience with venlafaxine in patients with concomitant systemic illness is limited. Caution is advised in administering venlafaxine to patients with diseases or conditions that could affect hemodynamic responses or metabolism (see also Warnings and Precautions, General, Hypertension. Patients should be questioned about any prescription or "over the counter drugs, herbal or natural products or dietary supplements" that they are taking, or planning to take, since there is a potential for interactions.

Dependence/Tolerance: In vitro studies revealed that venlafaxine has virtually no affinity for opiate, benzodiazepine, phencyclidine (PCP), or N-methyl-D-aspartic acid (NMDA) receptors. It has no significant CNS stimulant activity in rodents. In primate drug discrimination studies, venlafaxine showed no significant stimulant or depressant abuse liability.

While venlafaxine has not been systematically studied in clinical trials for its potential for abuse, there was no indication of drug-seeking behaviour in the clinical trials. However, it is not possible to predict on the basis of premarketing experience the extent to which a CNS active drug will be misused, diverted, and/or abused once marketed. Consequently, physicians should carefully evaluate patients for history of drug abuse and follow such patients closely, observing them for signs of misuse or abuse of venlafaxine (e.g., development of tolerance, incrementation of dose, drug-seeking behaviour).

Endocrine and Metabolism: Serum Cholesterol Elevation: Clinically relevant increases in total serum cholesterol were recorded in 5.3% of venlafaxine-treated patients and 0.0% of placebo-treated patients treated for at least 3 months in placebo-controlled trials in Major Depressive Disorders. (See Monitoring Laboratory Changes, Serum Cholesterol Elevation.)

Consistent with the above findings, elevations of High Density Lipoprotein Cholesterol (HDL), Low Density Lipoprotein Cholesterol (LDL) and the overall ratio of Total Cholesterol/HDL have been observed in placebo controlled clinical trials for Social Anxiety Disorder (SAD) and Panic Disorder.

Measurement of serum cholesterol levels (including a complete lipid profile/fractionation and an assessment of the patient's individual risk factors) should be considered especially during long-term treatment.

Changes in Appetite and Weight: Treatment-emergent anorexia and weight loss were more commonly reported for venlafaxine-treated patients than for placebo-treated patients in depression and GAD, Social Anxiety Disorder and Panic Disorder trials. Significant weight loss, especially in underweight depressed/GAD patients, may be an undesirable result of treatment. Venlafaxine is not recommended for weight loss alone or in combination with other products such as phentermine or sibutramine. Based on the known mechanisms of action, the potential harm of coadministration includes the possibility of serotonin syndrome. (See Drug Interactions, Drug-Drug Interactions, Serotonergic Drugs.)

Gastrointestinal: Results of testing in healthy volunteers demonstrated differences in the gastrointestinal tolerability of different formulations of venlafaxine. Data from healthy volunteers showed reduced incidence and severity of nausea with EFFEXOR XR capsules, compared with immediate release tablets.

In a 12-week study comparing immediate release tablets with EFFEXOR XR capsules, once daily, EFFEXOR XR was significantly more effective at weeks 8 and 12, compared with immediate release tablets given twice daily for treating major depression. Analysis of safety data from this trial showed that the incidence of treatment-emergent nausea and nausea severity over time were lower with EFFEXOR XR than with immediate release tablets. Additionally, the incidence of vomiting was lower with EFFEXOR XR than with immediate release tablets.

Genitourinary: Hyponatremia: Cases of hyponatremia may occur with venlafaxine, usually in volume-depleted or dehydrated patients. Elderly patients, patients taking diuretics, and patients who are otherwise volume depleted, may be at greater risk for this event.

The hyponatremia appeared to be reversible when venlafaxine was discontinued.

Inappropriate Antidiuretic Hormone Secretion: Cases of Syndrome of Inappropriate Antidiuretic Hormone (SIADH) secretion may occur with venlafaxine, usually in volume-depleted or dehydrated patients. Elderly patients, and patients taking diuretics, and patients who are otherwise volume depleted, may be at greater risk for this event.

Hematologic: Abnormal Bleeding: There have been reports of abnormal bleeding (most commonly ecchymosis) associated with venlafaxine treatment. While a causal relationship to venlafaxine is unclear, impaired platelet aggregation may result from platelet serotonin depletion and contribute to such occurrences.

Skin and other mucous membrane bleedings have been reported following treatment with venlafaxine. Venlafaxine should therefore be used with caution in patients concomitantly treated with drugs that give an increased risk for bleeding (e.g. anticoagulants, nonsteroidal anti-inflammatories and ASA) and in patients with a known tendency for bleeding or those with predisposing conditions. The risk of skin and mucous membrane bleeding, including gastrointestinal hemorrhage, may be increased in patients taking venlafaxine.

Hepatic/Biliary/Pancreatic: In patients with hepatic impairment, the pharmacokinetic disposition of both venlafaxine and ODV are significantly altered. Dosage adjustment is necessary in these patients (see Dosage and Administration, Recommended Dose and Dosage Adjustment, Patients with Hepatic Impairment and Patients with Renal Impairment).

Immune: Venlafaxine and O-desmethylvenlafaxine produced only limited effects in immunological studies which were generally at doses greater than those required to produce antidepressant effects in animals.

Neurologic: Seizures: EFFEXOR XR should be used cautiously in patients with a history of seizures, and should be promptly discontinued in any patient who develops seizures. Seizures have also been reported as a discontinuation symptom (see also Warnings and Precautions, Discontinuation Symptoms; Adverse Reactions, Discontinuation Symptoms; Dosage and Administration, Discontinuing Venlafaxine).

During premarketing testing, seizures were reported in 8 out of 3082 immediate release tablet-treated patients (0.3%). In 5 of the 8 cases with immediate release tablets, patients were receiving doses of 150 mg/day or less. During premarketing depression studies no seizures were seen in 705 EFFEXOR XR Capsule-treated patients. Premarketing, no seizures occurred among 1381 EFFEXOR XR-treated patients in Generalized Anxiety Disorder studies or among 277 EFFEXOR XR-treated patients in Social Anxiety Disorder Studies. In Panic Disorder studies, 1 seizure occurred among 1001 EFFEXOR XR-treated patients (0.1%). However, patients with a history of convulsive disorders were excluded from most of these studies. EFFEXOR XR should be used cautiously in patients with a history of seizures, and should be promptly discontinued in any patient who develops seizures.

Serotonin Syndrome/Neuroleptic Malignant Syndrome: On rare occasions serotonin syndrome or neuroleptic malignant syndrome-like events have occurred in association with treatment with SSRIs, including venlafaxine, particularly when given in combination with other serotonergic and/or neuroleptic/antipsychotic drugs. As these syndromes may result in potentially life-threatening conditions, treatment with venlafaxine should be discontinued if patients develop a combination of symptoms possibly including hyperthermia, rigidity, myoclonus, autonomic instability with possible rapid fluctuations of vital signs, mental status changes including confusion, irritability, extreme agitation progressing to delirium and coma and supportive symptomatic treatment should be initiated. Due to the risk of serotonergic syndrome or neuroleptic malignant syndrome venlafaxine should not be used in combination with MAO inhibitors or serotonin-precursors (such as L-tryptophan, oxitriptan) and should be used with caution in patients receiving other serotonergic drugs (triptans, lithium, tramadol, St. John's Wort, most tricyclic antidepressants) or neuroleptics/antipsychotics (see Contraindications and Drug Interactions, Drug-Drug Interactions, Serotonergic Drugs).

Ophthalmologic: Mydriasis: Mydriasis may occur in association with venlafaxine. It is recommended that patients with raised intra-ocular pressure or patients at risk for acute narrow-angle glaucoma (angle closure glaucoma) be closely monitored.

Psychiatric: Suicide: The possibility of a suicide attempt in seriously depressed patients is inherent to the illness and may persist until significant remission occurs. Close supervision of patients should accompany initial drug therapy, and consideration should be given to the need for hospitalization of high risk patients.

Patients, their families, and their caregivers should be encouraged to be alert to the emergence of anxiety, agitation, panic attacks, insomnia, irritability, hostility, aggressiveness, impulsivity, akathisia (psychomotor restlessness), hypomania, mania, other unusual changes in behaviour, worsening of depression, and suicidal ideation, especially when initiating therapy or during any change in dose or dosage regimen.

The risk of suicide attempt must be considered, especially in depressed patients, and the smallest quantity of drug, consistent with good patient management, should be provided to reduce the risk of overdose with this drug.

The same precautions observed when treating patients with depression should be observed when treating patients with GAD or Social Anxiety Disorder. (See Warnings and Precautions, Potential Association with Behavioral and Emotional Changes, Including Self-harm.)

Insomnia and Nervousness: Treatment-emergent insomnia and nervousness were more commonly reported for patients treated with venlafaxine than with placebo (see Adverse Reactions) in depression, GAD, Social Anxiety Disorder and Panic Disorder studies, as shown in Table 2.

Table 2: EFFEXOR XR

Incidence of Insomnia and Nervousness in Placebo-controlled Depression, GAD, Social Anxiety Disorder, and Panic Disorder Trials

	Depression		GAD		Social Anxiety Disorder		Panic Disorder	
Symptom	**EFFEXOR XR n=357**	**Placebo n=285**	**EFFEXOR XR n=1381**	**Placebo n=555**	**EFFEXOR XR n=819**	**Placebo n=695**	**EFFEXOR XR n=1001**	**Placebo n=662**
Insomnia	17%	11%	15%	10%	24%	8%	17%	9%
Nervousness	10%	5%	6%	4%	10%	5%	4%	6%

Insomnia and nervousness each led to drug discontinuation in 0.9% of the patients treated with EFFEXOR XR in depression studies.

In GAD trials, insomnia and nervousness led to drug discontinuation in 3% and 2%, respectively, of the patients treated with EFFEXOR XR up to 8 weeks and 2% and 0.7%, respectively, of the patients treated with EFFEXOR XR up to 6 months. In Social Anxiety Disorder trials, insomnia and nervousness led to drug discontinuation in 2% and 1%, respectively, of the patients treated with EFFEXOR XR up to 12 weeks and 2% and 3%, respectively, of the patients treated with EFFEXOR XR up to 6 months. In Panic Disorder trials, insomnia and nervousness led to drug discontinuation in 1% and 0.1%, respectively, of the patients treated with EFFEXOR XR up to 12 weeks.

Activation of Mania/Hypomania: During Phase II and III trials, mania or hypomania occurred in 0.5% of venlafaxine immediate release tablet-treated patients and in 0.3% and 0% of EFFEXOR XR Capsule-treated patients in depression and anxiety studies respectively. In premarketing Social Anxiety Disorder studies, 0.2% of EFFEXOR XR-treated patients and no placebo-treated patients experienced mania or hypomania. In premarketing Panic Disorder studies, 0.1% of EFFEXOR XR-treated patients and 0.0% placebo-treated patients experienced mania or hypomania. Mania or hypomania occurred in 0.4% of all venlafaxine-treated patients. Mania/hypomania has also been reported in a small proportion of patients with major affective disorder who were treated with other marketed antidepressants. As with all antidepressants, EFFEXOR XR should be used cautiously in patients with a history or family history of bipolar disorder.

A major depressive episode may be the initial presentation of bipolar disorder. Patients with bipolar disorder may be at an increased risk of experiencing manic episodes when treated with antidepressants alone. Therefore, the decision to initiate symptomatic treatment of depression should only be made after patients have been adequately assessed to determine if they are at risk for bipolar disorder.

Renal: In patients with renal impairment (GFR=10-70 mL/min), the pharmacokinetic disposition of both venlafaxine and ODV are significantly altered. **Dosage adjustment is necessary in these patients** (see Dosage and Administration, General, Patients with Hepatic or Renal Impairment and Recommended Dose and Dosage Adjustment, Patients with Renal Impairment).

Sexual Function/Reproduction: See Adverse Reactions.

Special Populations: Pregnant Women: There are no adequate and well controlled studies with venlafaxine in pregnant women. Therefore, venlafaxine should only be used during pregnancy if clearly needed. Patients should be advised to notify their physician if they become pregnant or intend to become pregnant during therapy.

Post-marketing reports indicate that some neonates exposed to venlafaxine, SSRIs (Selective Serotonin Reuptake Inhibitors), or other newer antidepressants late in the third trimester have developed complications requiring prolonged hospitalization, respiratory support, and tube feeding. Such complications can arise immediately upon delivery. Reported clinical findings have included respiratory distress, cyanosis, apnea, seizures, temperature instability, feeding difficulty, vomiting, hypoglycemia, hypotonia, hypertonia, hyperreflexia, tremor, jitteriness, irritability, and constant crying. These features are consistent with either a direct toxic effect of SSRIs and other newer antidepressants, or, possibly a drug discontinuation syndrome. It should be noted that, in some cases, the clinical picture is consistent with serotonin syndrome (see Warnings and Precautions, Serotonin Syndrome/Neuroleptic Malignant Syndrome). When treating a pregnant woman with EFFEXOR XR during the third trimester, the physician should carefully consider the potential risks and benefits of treatment. (See Dosage and Administration, Treatment of Pregnant Women During the Third Trimester.)

Nursing Women: Because venlafaxine and its active metabolite, O-desmethylvenlafaxine, have been reported to be excreted in human milk, lactating women should not nurse their infants while receiving venlafaxine. If the mother is taking EFFEXOR XR while nursing, the potential for discontinuation effects in the infant upon cessation of nursing should be considered.

Pediatrics (<18 years of age): EFFEXOR XR (venlafaxine) is not indicated for use in children under 18 years of age (see Warnings and Precautions, Potential Association with Behavioral and Emotional Changes, Including Self-harm).

Geriatrics (>65 years of age): Of the 2897 patients in Phase II and III trials with venlafaxine immediate release tablets, 357 (12%) were 65 years of age or older. Forty three (4%) of the patients in premarketing depression and 77 (6%) in GAD trials respectively, with EFFEXOR XR Capsules, were 65 years of age or older. Ten (1%) patients in placebo-controlled Social Anxiety Disorder studies were 65 years or older. Sixteen (2%) patients in placebo-controlled Panic Disorder studies were 65 years or older. No overall differences in effectiveness and safety were observed between these geriatric patients and younger patients, and other reported clinical experience has not identified differences in response between the elderly and younger patients. However, greater sensitivity of some older individuals cannot be ruled out.

Monitoring and Laboratory Tests: Self-harm: Rigorous clinical monitoring for suicidal ideation or other indicators of potential for suicidal behaviour is advised in patients of all ages. This includes monitoring for agitation-type emotional and behavioral changes (see Warnings and Precautions, Potential Association with Behavioral and Emotional Changes, Including Self-harm).

Sustained Hypertension and Acute Severe Hypertension: Venlafaxine treatment has been associated with sustained hypertension. Also, cases of severe elevated blood pressure requiring immediate treatment have been reported in postmarketing experience, including hypertensive crisis and malignant hypertension. The reports included normotensives and treated-hypertensive patients as well. It is recommended that patients receiving venlafaxine have their blood pressure evaluated before starting venlafaxine and monitored regularly during treatment.

For patients who experience a sustained increase in blood pressure while receiving venlafaxine, either dose reduction or discontinuation should be considered after a benefit-risk assessment is made. Patients should be told to consult their doctors if they have symptoms associated with acute severe hypertension such as headache (particularly in the back of head/neck when waking up), stronger heart beat and possibly more rapid, palpitations, dizziness, easy fatigability, blurred vision, chest pain. (See also Warnings and Precautions, General, Hypertension.)

Serum Cholesterol Elevation: Clinically relevant increases in total serum cholesterol were recorded in 5.3% of venlafaxine-treated patients and 0.0% of placebo-treated patients treated for at least 3 months in placebo-controlled trials in Major Depressive Disorder. (See Adverse Reactions, Laboratory Changes—Cholesterol.)

Consistent with the above findings, elevations of High Density Lipoprotein Cholesterol (HDL), Low Density Lipoprotein Cholesterol (LDL) and the overall ratio of Total Cholesterol/HDL have been observed in placebo controlled clinical trials for Social Anxiety Disorder (SAD) and Panic Disorder.

Measurement of serum cholesterol levels (including a complete lipid profile/fractionation and an assessment of the patient's individual risk factors) should be considered especially during long-term treatment.

ADVERSE REACTIONS: Clinical Trial Adverse Drug Reactions: Because clinical trials are conducted under very specific conditions the adverse reaction rates observed in the clinical trials may not reflect the rates observed in practice and should not be compared to the rates in the clinical trials of another drug. Adverse drug reaction information from clinical trials is useful for identifying drug-related adverse events and for approximating rates.

Commonly Observed Adverse Reactions: During depression trials, the most commonly observed adverse events associated with the use of venlafaxine immediate release tablets and EFFEXOR XR (incidence of 5% or greater) and not seen at an equivalent incidence among placebo-treated patients (i.e., incidence for immediate release formulation/EFFEXOR XR at least twice that for placebo), derived from the 2% incidence Table 4, were:

Venlafaxine Immediate Release: asthenia, sweating, nausea, constipation, anorexia, vomiting, somnolence, dry mouth, dizziness, nervousness, anxiety, tremor, blurred vision, and abnormal ejaculation/orgasm and impotence in men.

EFFEXOR XR: abnormal dreams, anorexia, dizziness, dry mouth, nausea, nervousness, somnolence, sweating, and tremor as well as abnormal ejaculation/orgasm in men.

During GAD trials, the most commonly observed adverse events associated with the use of EFFEXOR XR, derived from the 2% incidence Table 6 were: nausea, dry mouth, anorexia, abnormal ejaculation, constipation, sweating, abnormal vision, impotence in men, vasodilatation, dizziness, somnolence, libido decreased, abnormal dreams, yawn and tremor.

During Social Anxiety Disorder trials, the following adverse events occurred in at least 5% of the EFFEXOR XR patients and at a rate at least twice that of the placebo group for the four 12-week placebo-controlled trials for the Social Anxiety Disorder indication (Table 8): asthenia, nausea, anorexia, constipation, insomnia, dry mouth, somnolence, nervousness, libido decreased, tremor, yawn, sweating, abnormal vision, as well as abnormal ejaculation, impotence, and anorgasmia in men. In a 6-month Social Anxiety Disorder trial, the following adverse events occurred in at least 5% of the patients who received either dose of EFFEXOR XR and at a rate at least twice that of the placebo group (Table 9): asthenia, vasodilatation, anorexia, constipation, nausea, dizziness, dry mouth, libido decreased, nervousness, paresthesia, somnolence, tremor, twitching pharyngitis, yawn, sweating, abnormal vision, as well as abnormal ejaculation and impotence in men, and dysmenorrhea in women.

During Panic Disorder trials, the following adverse events occurred in at least 5% of the EFFEXOR XR patients and at a rate at least twice that of the placebo group for the placebo-controlled trials for the Panic Disorder indication (Table 10): anorexia, constipation, dry mouth, somnolence, tremor, abnormal ejaculation in men, and sweating.

Adverse Reactions that Led to Discontinuation of Treatment in Clinical Trials: Nineteen percent (537/2897) of venlafaxine immediate release and 12% (88/705) of EFFEXOR XR-treated patients in Phase II and III depression studies discontinued treatment due to an adverse reaction. Approximately 18% of the 1381 patients who received EFFEXOR XR capsules for up to 8 weeks in placebo-controlled clinical trials for GAD discontinued treatment due to an adverse experience, compared with 12% of the 555 placebo-treated patients in those studies. Approximately 14% of the 562 patients who received EFFEXOR XR capsules for up to 12 weeks in 4 placebo-controlled clinical trials for social anxiety disorder discontinued treatment due to an adverse experience, compared with 5% of the 566 placebo-treated patients in those studies. Approximately 20% of the 257 patients who received EFFEXOR XR capsules in a 6-month placebo-controlled clinical trial for social anxiety disorder discontinued treatment due to an adverse experience, compared with 7% of the 129 placebo-treated patients in that study. The more common events (≥1%) associated with discontinuation of treatment in all 5 trials and considered to be drug-related (i.e., those events associated with dropout at a rate approximately twice or greater for venlafaxine compared to placebo) are shown in Table 3.

Table 3: EFFEXOR XR

Adverse Reactions (%) Leading to Discontinuation of Treatment

	Immediate Release Venlafaxine Depression Indication (n=2897)	**Placebo Depression Indication (n=609)**	**EFFEXOR XR Depression Indication (n=705)**	**Placebo Depression Indication (n=285)**	**EFFEXOR XR GAD Indication (n=1381)**	**Placebo GAD Indication (n=555)**	**EFFEXOR XR Social Anxiety Indication (n=819)**	**Placebo Social Anxiety Indication (n=695)**
CNS								
Somnolence	3	1	2	<1	3	<1	2	<1
Insomnia	3	1	<1	<1	3	<1	2	<1

(cont'd)

Table 3: EFFEXOR XR *(cont'd)*

Adverse Reactions (%) Leading to Discontinuation of Treatment

	Immediate Release Venlafaxine Depression Indication (n=2897)	Placebo Depression Indication (n=609)	EFFEXOR XR Depression Indication (n=705)	Placebo Depression Indication (n=285)	EFFEXOR XR GAD Indication (n=1381)	Placebo GAD Indication (n=555)	EFFEXOR XR Social Anxiety Indication (n=819)	Placebo Social Anxiety Indication (n=695)
Dizziness	3	<1	2	1	4	2	2	<1
Nervousness	2	<1	<1	1	2	<1	<1	0
Anxiety	2	1	<1	<1	1[b]	1	<1	<1
Tremor	<1	<1	<1	<1	1	0	<1	<1
Gastrointestinal								
Dry Mouth	2	<1	<1	0	2	<1	<1	<1
Anorexia	1	<1	<1	<1	<1	<1	<1	<1
Nausea	6	1	4	<1	8	<1	3	<1
Vomiting	<1	<1	1	0	1	<1	<1	0
Urogenital								
Abnormal Ejaculation[a]	3	0	<1	<1	<1	0	<1	0
Impotence[a]	<1	<1	0	0	<1	0	2	0
Other								
Headache	3	1	2[b]	1	3	<1	1	<1
Asthenia	2	<1	<1	1	3	<1	2	<1
Sweating	2	<1	<1	0	2	<1	<1	<1

[a] Percentages based on the number of males.
[b] Greater than 1% but active drug rate not twice rate for placebo.

Incidence in Controlled Trials: Table 4 enumerates adverse events that occurred at an incidence of 2% or more, and were more frequent than in the placebo group, among venlafaxine-treated depressed patients.

Venlafaxine Immediate Release: Patients participated in 4- to 8- week placebo-controlled trials in which doses in the range of 75 to 375 mg/day were administered.

EFFEXOR XR: Patients participated in 8- to 12-week placebo-controlled trials in which doses in the range of 75 to 225 mg/day were administered.

Reported adverse events were classified using a standard COSTART-based Dictionary terminology.

The prescriber should be aware that the cited frequencies for EFFEXOR XR cannot be compared with figures obtained from other clinical investigations of venlafaxine tablets which involved different treatments, uses and investigators. The cited figures for EFFEXOR XR, however, do provide the prescribing physician with some basis for estimating the relative contribution of drug and non-drug factors to the side effect incidence rate in the population studied.

Table 4: EFFEXOR XR

Treatment-emergent Adverse Experience Incidence in Placebo-controlled Clinical Trials (%)[a] in Depressed Patients

Body System/ Preferred Term	Venlafaxine Immediate Release (n=1033)	Placebo (n=609)	EFFEXOR XR (n=357)	Placebo (n=285)
Body as a Whole				
Headache	25	24	26[b]	33
Asthenia	12	6	8	7
Infection	6	5	6[b]	9
Chills	3	<1	<1	1
Cardiovascular				
Vasodilatation	4	3	4	2
Increased Blood Pressure/ Hypertension	2	<1	4	1
Tachycardia	2	<1	<1	<1
Dermatological				
Sweating	12	3	14	3
Rash	3	2	1	1
Gastrointestinal				
Nausea	37	11	31	12
Constipation	15	7	8	5
Anorexia	11	2	8	4
Diarrhea	8	7	8[b]	9
Vomiting	6	2	4	2

(cont'd)

Table 4: EFFEXOR XR *(cont'd)*

Treatment-emergent Adverse Experience Incidence in Placebo-controlled Clinical Trials (%)[a] in Depressed Patients

Body System/ Preferred Term	Venlafaxine Immediate Release (n=1033)	Placebo (n=609)	EFFEXOR XR (n=357)	Placebo (n=285)
Dyspepsia	5	4	7[b]	9
Flatulence	3	2	4	3
Metabolic				
Weight Loss	1	<1	3	0
Nervous				
Somnolence	23	9	17	8
Dry Mouth	22	11	12	6
Dizziness	19	7	20	9
Insomnia	18	10	17	11
Nervousness	13	6	10	5
Anxiety	6	3	2[b]	5
Tremor	5	1	5	2
Abnormal Dreams	4	3	7	2
Hypertonia	3	2	1	0
Paresthesia	3	2	3	1
Libido Decreased	2	<1	3	<1
Agitation	2	<1	3	1
Depression	1	1	3	<1
Thinking Abnormal	2	<1	<1	1
Respiration				
Pharyngitis	4	4	7	6
Yawn	3	0	3	0
Special Senses				
Abnormal Vision	6	2	4	<1
Taste Perversion	2	<1	1	<1

(cont'd)

Table 4: EFFEXOR XR *(cont'd)*

Treatment-emergent Adverse Experience Incidence in Placebo-controlled Clinical Trials (%)[a] in Depressed Patients

Body System/ Preferred Term	Venlafaxine Immediate Release (n=1033)	Placebo (n=609)	EFFEXOR XR (n=357)	Placebo (n=285)
Urogenital System				
Abnormal Ejaculation/Orgasm	12[c]	<1[c]	16[c]	<1[c]
Impotence	6[c]	<1[c]	4[c]	<1[c]
Anorgasmia	<1[d]	<1[d]	3[d]	<1[d]
Urinary Frequency	3	2	1	1
Urination Impaired	2	<1	<1	0

[a] Events reported by at least 2% of patients treated with venlafaxine immediate release/EFFEXOR XR are included, and are rounded to the nearest %. Events for which the venlafaxine immediate release/EFFEXOR XR incidence was equal to or less than placebo included the following: abdominal pain, accidental injury, anxiety, back pain, bronchitis, diarrhea, dysmenorrhoea, dyspepsia, flu syndrome, headache, infection, pain, palpitation, rhinitis and sinusitis.

[b] Incidence greater than 2%, but active drug incidence less than incidence for placebo.

[c] Incidence based on number of male patients (for venlafaxine immediate release: n=439, Placebo: n=245; for EFFEXOR XR: n=126, Placebo: n=108).

[d] Incidence based on number of female patients (for venlafaxine immediate release: n=594, Placebo: n=364; for EFFEXOR XR: n=231, Placebo: n=177).

Dose Dependency of Adverse Events: A comparison of adverse event rates in a fixed-dose study comparing venlafaxine immediate release tablets 75, 225, and 375 mg/day with placebo in depressed patients revealed a dose dependency for some of the more common adverse events associated with venlafaxine use, as shown in the table that follows (Table 5). The rule for including events was to enumerate those that occurred at an incidence of 5% or more for at least one of the venlafaxine groups and for which the incidence was at least twice the placebo incidence for at least one venlafaxine group. Tests for potential dose relationships for these events (Cochran-Armitage Test, with a criterion of exact 2-sided p-value ≤0.05) suggested a dose-dependency for several adverse events in this list, including chills, hypertension, anorexia, nausea, agitation, dizziness, somnolence, tremor, yawning, sweating, and abnormal ejaculation.

Table 5: EFFEXOR XR

Treatment-emergent Adverse Experience Incidence (%) in a Dose Comparison Trial in Depressed Patients

Body System/ Preferred Term	Placebo (n=92)	Venlafaxine Immediate Release Tablets (mg/day)		
		75 (n=89)	225 (n=89)	375 (n=88)
Body as a Whole				
Abdominal Pain	3.3	3.4	2.2	8
Asthenia	3.3	16.9	14.6	14.8
Chills	1.1	2.2	5.6	6.8
Infection	2.2	2.2	5.6	2.3
Cardiovascular				
Hypertension	1.1	1.1	2.2	4.5
Vasodilatation	0	4.5	5.6	2.3
Digestive System				
Anorexia	2.2	14.6	13.5	17
Dyspepsia	2.2	6.7	6.7	4.5
Nausea	14.1	32.6	38.2	58
Vomiting	1.1	7.9	3.4	6.8
Nervous				
Agitation	0	1.1	2.2	4.5
Anxiety	4.3	11.2	4.5	2.3
Dizziness	4.3	19.1	22.5	23.9
Insomnia	9.8	22.5	20.2	13.6
Libido Decreased	1.1	2.2	1.1	5.7
Nervousness	4.3	21.3	13.5	12.5
Somnolence	4.3	16.9	18	26.1
Tremor	0	1.1	2.2	10.2
Respiratory				
Yawn	0	4.5	5.6	8
Skin and Appendages				
Sweating	5.4	6.7	12.4	19.3
Special Senses				

(cont'd)

Table 5: EFFEXOR XR *(cont'd)*

Treatment-emergent Adverse Experience Incidence (%) in a Dose Comparison Trial in Depressed Patients

Body System/ Preferred Term	Placebo (n=92)	Venlafaxine Immediate Release Tablets (mg/day)		
		75 (n=89)	225 (n=89)	375 (n=88)
Abnormality of Accommodation	0	9.1	7.9	5.6
Urogenital System				
Abnormal Ejaculation/Orgasm	0	4.5	2.2	12.5
Impotence	0	5.8	2.1	3.6
(Number of men)	(n=63)	(n=52)	(n=48)	(n=56)

Table 6 and Table 7 enumerate adverse events that occurred at an incidence of 2% or more, and at a higher rate than the placebo group, among EFFEXOR XR-treated anxious patients.

Table 6: EFFEXOR XR

Treatment-emergent Adverse Event Incidence (%) in Placebo-controlled EFFEXOR XR North American Clinical Trials (210 US, 214 US and 218 US) in GAD Patients[a,b] (8-28 Weeks, Dosage Range 75-225 mg)

Body System/ Preferred Term	EFFEXOR XR (n=600)	Placebo (n=328)
Body as a Whole		
Asthenia	16	10
Accidental Injury	5	4
Fever	3	2
Chills	3	<1
Cardiovascular System		
Vasodilatation	8	3
Hypertension	4	3
Tachycardia	3	2
Digestive System		
Nausea	46	18
Dry Mouth	24	9
Diarrhea	16	13
Anorexia	13	3
Constipation	12	6
Vomiting	7	4
Flatulence	3	2
Nervous System		
Dizziness	27	13
Somnolence	24	11
Insomnia	24	15
Nervousness	13	8
Libido Decreased	6	3
Abnormal Dreams	6	3
Tremor	5	2
Hypertonia	4	3
Paresthesia	3	2
Thinking Abnormal	3	2
Twitching	3	<1
Trismus	2	<1
Confusion	2	<1
Respiratory System		
Yawn	5	<1
Cough Increased	4	3
Skin and Appendages		

(cont'd)

Table 6: EFFEXOR XR *(cont'd)*

Treatment-emergent Adverse Event Incidence (%) in Placebo-controlled EFFEXOR XR North American Clinical Trials (210 US, 214 US and 218 US) in GAD Patients[a,b] (8-28 Weeks, Dosage Range 75-225 mg)

Body System/ Preferred Term	EFFEXOR XR (n=600)	Placebo (n=328)
Sweating	12	2
Special Senses		
Abnormal Vision	8	1
Urogenital System		
Abnormal Ejaculation/Orgasm (male)[c]	15	0
Anorgasmia	4	<1
(male)[c]	5	<1
(female)[d]	3	0
Urinary Frequency	4	2
Impotence (male)[c]	6	<1
Urination Impaired	2	0
Menstrual Disorder (female)[d]	3	2

[a] Incidence rounded to the nearest %, for events reported by at least 2% of patients treated with EFFEXOR XR, except the following events which had an incidence equal to or less than placebo: abdominal pain, agitation, anxiety, arthralgia, back pain, chest pain, depression, dyspepsia, flu syndrome, headache, infection, migraine, myalgia, neck pain, pain, palpitation, pharyngitis, rash, rhinitis, sinusitis, and tinnitus.
[b] <1% indicates an incidence greater than zero but less than 1%.
[c] Incidence is based on number of male patients (for EFFEXOR XR: n=242, Placebo: n=131).
[d] Incidence is based on number of female patients (for EFFEXOR XR: n=358, Placebo: n=197).

Table 7: EFFEXOR XR

Treatment-emergent Adverse Event Incidence (%) in a Dose Comparison Trial (378 EU, 24 Weeks) with GAD Patients[a,c]

Body System/ Preferred Term	Placebo (n=130)	EFFEXOR XR 37.5 mg (n=140)	EFFEXOR XR 75 mg (n=134)	EFFEXOR XR 150 mg (n=137)
Body as a Whole				
Accidental Injury	4	5	5	7
Asthenia	9	11	13	12
Back Pain	5	7	5	5
Chest Pain	2	5	2	2[b]
Cyst	0	1	2	0
Flu Syndrome	6	6	5	7
Headache	26	28	24	25
Infection	4	9	5	12
Withdrawal Syndrome	0	0	0	2
Cardiovascular System				
Hypertension	2	1	2	5
Migraine	<1	4	2[b]	2[b]
Tachycardia	0	0	2[b]	2
Vasodilation	2[b]	4	2[b]	4
Digestive System				
Anorexia	2[b]	4	2[b]	3
Constipation	5	8	13	15
Diarrhea	8	8	7	10
Dry Mouth	4	6	13	17
Dyspepsia	5	4	6	3
Nausea	14	22	34	42
Vomiting	6	5	8	7
Musculoskeletal System				
Arthralgia	4	4	5	2[b]
Myalgia	2[b]	1	<1	3
Tenosynovitis	<1	2	0	0

(cont'd)

Table 7: EFFEXOR XR *(cont'd)*

Treatment-emergent Adverse Event Incidence (%) in a Dose Comparison Trial (378 EU, 24 Weeks) with GAD Patients[a,c]

Body System/ Preferred Term	Placebo (n=130)	EFFEXOR XR 37.5 mg (n=140)	EFFEXOR XR 75 mg (n=134)	EFFEXOR XR 150 mg (n=137)
Nervous System				
Abnormal Dreams	2[b]	4	6	3
Anxiety	6	5	2[b]	7
Depersonalization	<1	<1	<1	2
Depression	2[b]	4	2	<1
Dizziness	14	15	22	31
Hypertonia	<1	3	2[b]	3
Insomnia	10	7	12	15
Libido Decreased	<1	3	2[b]	4
Nervousness	2[b]	4	3	3
Paresthesia	2	1	2	10
Somnolence	4	1	6	7
Thinking Abnormal	0	2	0	0
Tremor	0	2	4	4
Vertigo	<1	2	2	0
Respiratory System				
Bronchitis	<1	3	2[b]	4
Cough Increased	2[b]	3	3	2
Dyspnea	2[b]	1	2	0
Rhinitis	2[b]	4	4	4
Sinusitis	<1	4	5	4
Yawn	0	0	2	5
Skin and Appendages				
Eczema	<1	2	2[b]	2[b]
Rash	2[b]	<1	3	2
Sweating	5	9	11	18
Special Senses				
Abnormal Vision	2[b]	<1	8	4
Conjunctivitis	0	4	2[b]	2[b]
Mydriasis	0	<1	<1	2
Tinnitus	<1	4	4	3
Urogenital System				
Abnormal Ejaculation/Orgasm (male)[d]	0	1	0	2
Anorgasmia (male)[d]	0	2	0	8
(female)[e]	0	0	0	2
Dysmenorrhea (female)[e]	3	4	1	1
Dysuria	0	<1	2	2[b]
Impotence (male)[d]	0	2	2	3
Menorrhagia (female)[e]	0	3	1	2
Urinary Frequency	2[b]	2	<1	2[b]

[a] Incidence rounded to the nearest %, for events reported by at least 2% of patients in any EFFEXOR XR treatment group and at an incidence greater than the respective placebo incidence.
[b] Incidence is less than 2% but rounds to 2%.
[c] <1% indicates an incidence greater than zero but less than 1%.
[d] Incidence is based on number of male patients (for EFFEXOR XR: n=60 (37.5 mg), 51 (75 mg), 48 (150 mg); Placebo: n=54).
[e] Incidence is based on number of female patients (for EFFEXOR XR: n=80 (37.5 mg), 83 (75 mg), 89 (150 mg); Placebo: n=76).

Table 8 and Table 9 enumerate adverse events that occurred at an incidence of 2% or more, and were more frequent than in the placebo group, among venlafaxine-treated patients with Social Anxiety Disorder in 12-week and 6-month studies, respectively.

Table 8: EFFEXOR XR

Treatment-emergent Adverse Event Incidence (%) in Short-term, Placebo-controlled EFFEXOR XR Clinical Trials (387 EU/CA, 388 EU, 392-US, and 393 US) in Social Anxiety Disorder Patients[a,c] (12 Weeks, Dosage Range 75-225 mg)

Body System/ Preferred Term	EFFEXOR XR (n=562)	Placebo (n=566)
Body as a Whole		
Asthenia	19	8
Abdominal Pain	6	4
Accidental Injury	4	3
Cardiovascular System		
Hypertension	5	3
Palpitation	3	2[b]
Vasodilatation	2	1
Digestive System		
Nausea	30	9
Anorexia	15	2
Constipation	9	3
Diarrhea	7	5
Dyspepsia	6	5
Vomiting	4	2
Metabolic and Nutritional		
Weight Loss	3	<1
Nervous System		
Insomnia	23	8
Somnolence	18	7
Dry Mouth	15	4
Dizziness	15	8
Libido Decreased	9	2
Nervousness	9	4
Tremor	6	2[b]
Anxiety	6	4
Agitation	3	1
Abnormal Dreams	3	1
Thinking Abnormal	2	<1
Twitching	2	0
Sleep Disorder	2[b]	<1
Trismus	2[b]	0
Respiratory System		
Yawn	7	<1
Sinusitis	2[b]	1
Skin		
Sweating	15	4
Special Senses		
Abnormal Vision	5	1
Tinnitus	2[b]	<1
Urogenital System		
Abnormal Ejaculation/Orgasm (men)[d]	12	<1
(women)[e]	2[b]	<1
Impotence[d]	7	2[b]
Anorgasmia (men)[d]	7	<1
(women)[e]	4	0

(cont'd)

Table 8: EFFEXOR XR *(cont'd)*

Treatment-emergent Adverse Event Incidence (%) in Short-term, Placebo-controlled EFFEXOR XR Clinical Trials (387 EU/CA, 388 EU, 392-US, and 393 US) in Social Anxiety Disorder Patients[a,c] (12 Weeks, Dosage Range 75-225 mg)

Body System/ Preferred Term	EFFEXOR XR (n=562)	Placebo (n=566)
Menstrual Disorder[e]	2[b]	1
Urinary Frequency	2[b]	<1

[a] Incidence rounded to the nearest %, for events reported by at least 2% of patients in any EFFEXOR XR treatment group, and at an incidence greater than the respective placebo incidence.
[b] Incidence is less than 2% but rounds to 2%.
[c] <1% means greater than zero but less than 1%.
[d] Percentage based on the number of males (EFFEXOR XR=308, Placebo=284).
[e] Percentage based on the number of females (EFFEXOR XR=254, Placebo=282).

Table 9: EFFEXOR XR

Treatment-emergent Adverse Event Incidence (%) in a Long-term, Placebo-controlled EFFEXOR XR Clinical Trial (390 US) in Social Anxiety Disorder Patients[a,c] (6 Months, Dosage Range 75-225 mg)

Body System/ Preferred Term	EFFEXOR XR 75 mg (n=128)	EFFEXOR XR 150–225 mg (n=129)	Placebo (n=129)
Body as a Whole			
Allergic Reaction	<1	2[b]	<1
Asthenia	25	19	11
Back Pain	9	5	8
Chest Pain	3	2	0
Fever	3	0	2
Flu Syndrome	9	4	6
Headache	57	45	43
Pain	9	5	7
Cardiovascular System			
Hypertension	3	7	4
Palpitation	3	4	<1
Postural Hypotension	2[b]	<1	0
Vasodilatation	2	5	2
Digestive System			
Anorexia	19	22	3
Constipation	8	9	2
Diarrhea	13	9	10
Dyspepsia	11	12	11
Dysphagia	0	2	0
Flatulence	3	4	2[b]
Nausea	37	34	10
Vomiting	5	4	3
Hemic and Lymphatic			
Ecchymosis	<1	2	0
Metabolic and Nutritional			
Hyperlipemia	2[b]	0	0
Weight Gain	2	<1	<1
Musculoskeletal System			
Leg Cramps	2[b]	<1	0
Nervous System			
Abnormal Dreams	3	4	<1
Agitation	3	2[b]	2[b]
Amnesia	2[b]	<1	0
Apathy	<1	2[b]	0
Depersonalization	2	<1	0
Dizziness	24	19	12

(cont'd)

Table 9: EFFEXOR XR *(cont'd)*

Treatment-emergent Adverse Event Incidence (%) in a Long-term, Placebo-controlled EFFEXOR XR Clinical Trial (390 US) in Social Anxiety Disorder Patients[a,c] (6 Months, Dosage Range 75-225 mg)

Body System/ Preferred Term	EFFEXOR XR 75 mg (n=128)	EFFEXOR XR 150–225 mg (n=129)	Placebo (n=129)
Dry Mouth	23	19	6
Insomnia	26	30	16
Libido Decreased	5	10	2
Libido Increased	2[b]	0	<1
Nervousness	10	14	6
Paresthesia	4	6	2[b]
Sleep Disorder	0	2[b]	<1
Somnolence	24	29	14
Tremor	2	7	2[b]
Twitching	2	5	<1
Vertigo	<1	2[b]	0
Respiratory System			
Asthma	2[b]	2	0
Dyspnea	2[b]	<1	0
Pharyngitis	11	9	5
Rhinitis	13	6	7
Upper Respiratory Infection	8	5	7
Yawn	5	12	0
Skin			
Contact Dermatitis	0	2	0
Rash	5	<1	3
Sweating	10	12	2
Urticaria	<1	2	0
Special Senses			
Abnormal Vision	3	7	3
Conjunctivitis	<1	2	0
Mydriasis	2[b]	4	0
Taste Perversion	0	2[b]	<1
Tinnitus	0	2	<1
Urogenital System			
Urinary Frequency	0	2[b]	<1
Urination Impaired	2[b]	2[b]	0
Urine Abnormality	0	2[b]	0
Abnormal Ejaculation/Orgasm (men)[d]	12	18	1
(women)[e]	0	2	0
Amenorrhea[e]	0	4	0
Anorgasmia (men)[d]	0	3	0
(women)	0	4	0
Dysmenorrhea[e]	13	12	5
Impotence[d]	3	8	0
Menstrual Disorder[e]	0	2	0
Metrorrhagia[e]	3	0	0
Unintended Pregnancy[e]	2[b]	0	0
Uterine Spasm[e]	2[b]	0	0

[a] Incidence rounded to the nearest %, for events reported by at least 2% of patients in any EFFEXOR XR treatment group, and at an incidence greater than the respective placebo incidence.
[b] Incidence is less than 2% but rounds to 2%.
[c] <1% means greater than zero but less than 1%.
[d] Percentage based on the number of males (EFFEXOR XR 75 mg=67, EFFEXOR XR 150-225 mg=79, Placebo=73).
[e] Percentage based on the number of females (EFFEXOR XR 75 mg=61, EFFEXOR XR 150-225 mg=50, Placebo=56).

Table 10 enumerates adverse events that occurred at an incidence of 2% or more, and were more frequent than in the placebo group, among venlafaxine-treated patients with Panic Disorder.

Table 10: EFFEXOR XR

Treatment-emergent Adverse Event Incidence (%) in Short-term, Placebo-controlled EFFEXOR XR Clinical Trials (391-CA/EU, 353-US/CA, 398-EU and 399-AC) in Panic Disorder Patients[a,b] (10-12 Weeks, Dosage Range 37.5-225 mg)

Body System/ Preferred Term	EFFEXOR XR (n=1001)	Placebo (n=662)
Body as a Whole		
Asthenia	10	8
Cardiovascular System		
Hypertension	4	3
Vasodilatation	3	2
Tachycardia[d]	2	<1
Digestive System		
Nausea	21	14
Dry Mouth	12	6
Constipation	9	3
Anorexia	8	3
Nervous System		
Insomnia	17	9
Somnolence	12	6
Dizziness	11	10
Tremor	5	2
Libido Decreased	4	2
Vertigo[d]	2	1
Skin		
Sweating	10	2
Urogenital System		
Abnormal Ejaculation (men)[c]	7	<1
Impotence (men)[c]	4	<1
Anorgasmia (men)[c]	2	0

[a] Adverse events for which the EFFEXOR XR reporting rate was less than or equal to the placebo rate are not included. These events are: abdominal pain, abnormal vision, accidental injury, anxiety, back pain, diarrhea, dysmenorrhea, dyspepsia, flu syndrome, headache, infection, nervousness, pain, paresthesia, pharyngitis, rash, rhinitis, and vomiting.
[b] <1% means greater than zero but less than 1%.
[c] Percentage based on the number of males (EFFEXOR XR=335, Placebo=238).
[d] Occurred at less than 2% but frequency rounded up to 2%.

Adaptation to Certain Adverse Events: In premarketing experience with venlafaxine immediate release Tablets over a 6-week period, and EFFEXOR XR capsules over a 12 week period, there was evidence of adaptation to some adverse events with continued therapy (e.g., dizziness and nausea), but less to other effects (e.g., abnormal ejaculation and dry mouth). The incidence of nausea in the GAD studies, during weeks 1 and 2 were 28% and 14% for EFFEXOR XR-treated patients and 6% and 4% for placebo-treated patients, respectively. The incidence of dizziness during weeks 1 and 2 were 12% and 6% for EFFEXOR XR-treated patients and 4% and 4% for placebo-treated patients, respectively.

Discontinuation Symptoms: Abrupt discontinuation, dose reduction, or tapering of venlafaxine at various doses has been found to be associated with the appearance of new symptoms, the frequency of which increased with increased dose level and with longer duration of treatment. Symptoms associated with discontinuation include but are not limited to: aggression, agitation, anorexia, anxiety, asthenia, confusion, convulsions, coordination impaired, diarrhoea, dizziness, dry mouth, dysphoric mood, fasciculation, fatigue, flu-like symptoms, headache, hypomania, impaired coordination and balance, insomnia, nausea, nightmares, nervousness, paresthesia, electric shock sensations, sensory disturbances (including shock like electrical sensations), sleep disturbances, somnolence, sweating, tinnitus, tremor, vertigo, and vomiting. Where such symptoms occurred they were usually self-limiting but in a few patients continued for several weeks. In premarketing studies, the majority of discontinuation reactions were mild and resolved without treatment.

Patients should be monitored for these or any other symptoms when discontinuing treatment, regardless of the indication for which EFFEXOR XR is being prescribed. If intolerable symptoms occur following a decrease in the dose or upon discontinuation of treatment, dose titration should be managed on the basis of the patient's clinical response (see Warnings and Precautions, Discontinuation Symptoms and Dosage and Administration, General, Discontinuing Venlafaxine for details).

Vital Sign Changes: Treatment with venlafaxine immediate release tablets (averaged over all dose groups) in clinical trials was associated with a mean increase in pulse rate of approximately 3 beats per minute, compared to no change for placebo. It was associated with mean increases in diastolic blood pressure ranging from 0.7 to 2.5 mm Hg averaged over all dose groups, compared to mean decreases ranging from 0.9 to 3.8 mm Hg for placebo. However, there is a dose dependency for blood pressure increase (see Warnings and Precautions, Sustained Hypertension for effects on blood pressure).

Treatment with EFFEXOR XR Capsules for up to 12 weeks in premarketing depression trials was associated with a mean increase in pulse rate of approximately 2 beats per minute, compared with 1 beat per minute for placebo. It was associated with mean increases in diastolic blood pressure ranging from 0.7 to 0.9 mm Hg, compared with mean decreases ranging from 0.5 to 1.4 mm Hg for placebo. EFFEXOR XR treatment for up to 6 months in premarketing placebo-controlled Generalized Anxiety Disorder trials was associated with a mean final on-therapy increase in pulse rate of approximately 2 beats per minute, compared with less than 1 beat per minute for placebo.

EFFEXOR XR treatment for up to 12 weeks in 4 premarketing placebo-controlled Social Anxiety Disorder trials was associated with mean final on-therapy increase in pulse rate of approximately 3 beats per minute, compared with an increase of approximately 1 beat per minute for placebo. EFFEXOR XR treatment for up to 6 months in a premarketing placebo-controlled Social Anxiety Disorder trial was associated with mean final on-therapy increase of approximately 2 beats per minute in the 75 mg/day group and an increase of approximately 4 beats per minute in the 150 to 225 mg/day group, compared with an increase of approximately 2 beats per minute for placebo.

Mean changes in supine diastolic blood pressure were also associated with venlafaxine treatment in the Social Anxiety Disorder trials (see Warnings and Precautions, Sustained Hypertension).

EFFEXOR XR treatment for up to 12 weeks in premarketing placebo-controlled Panic Disorder trials was associated with mean final on-therapy increase in pulse rate of approximately 1 beat per minute, compared with a decrease of less than 1 beat per minute for placebo. A dose-dependence effect was noted in the 2 fixed-dose studies. In one study, no change in mean pulse rate was observed in the placebo and EFFEXOR XR 75 mg dosage groups, and a mean increase of 1 beat/min was observed in the EFFEXOR XR 150 group. In another study, there was a mean increase of less than 1 beat/min in both placebo and EFFEXOR XR 75 mg groups, and a mean increase of 3 beats/min in the EFFEXOR XR 225 mg group.

Mean changes in supine diastolic blood pressure and sustained hypertension were also associated with EFFEXOR XR treatment in the Panic Disorder trials (see Warnings and Precautions, Sustained Hypertension).

Laboratory Changes—Cholesterol: Clinically and statistically relevant increases in cholesterol levels have been noted in studies using venlafaxine immediate release tablets and EFFEXOR XR Capsules (see Warnings and Precautions, Serum Cholesterol Elevation).

Venlafaxine Immediate Release Tablets: Patients treated with venlafaxine immediate release tablets for at least 3 months in placebo-controlled 12-month extension trials for Major Depressive Disorders had a mean final on-therapy increase in total cholesterol of 9.1 mg/dL (0.2364 mmol/L) compared with a decrease of 7.1 mg/dL (0.1835 mmol/L) among placebo-treated patients. This increase was duration dependent over the study period and tended to be greater with higher doses. Clinically relevant increases in serum cholesterol, defined as 1) a final on-therapy increase in serum cholesterol ≥50 mg/dL (1.2930 mmol/L) from baseline and to a value ≥261 mg/dL (6.7495 mmol/L) or 2) an average on-therapy increase in serum cholesterol ≥50 mg/dL (1.2930 mmol/L) from baseline and to a value ≥261 mg/dL (6.7495 mmol/L), were recorded in 5.3% of venlafaxine-treated patients and 0.0% of placebo-treated patients.

EFFEXOR XR Capsules: EFFEXOR XR (venlafaxine hydrochloride) extended-release capsules treatment for up to 12 weeks in premarketing placebo-controlled trials for major depressive disorder was associated with a mean final on-therapy increase in serum cholesterol concentration of approximately 1.5 mg/dL (0.0381 mmol/L) compared with a mean final decrease of 7.4 mg/dL (0.1919 mmol/L) for placebo.

EFFEXOR XR treatment for up to 8 weeks and up to 6 months in premarketing placebo-controlled GAD trials was associated with mean final on-therapy increases in serum cholesterol concentration of approximately 1.0 mg/dL (0.0247 mmol/L) and 2.3 mg/dL (0.0606 mmol/L), respectively while placebo subjects experienced mean final decreases of 4.9 mg/dL (0.1278 mmol/L) and 7.7 (0.1990 mmol/L) mg/dL, respectively.

Elevations of total serum cholesterol, High Density Lipoprotein Cholesterol (HDL), Low Density Lipoprotein Cholesterol (LDL) and the overall ratio of Total Cholesterol/HDL have been observed in placebo controlled clinical trials for Social Anxiety Disorder and Panic Disorder.

Measurement of serum cholesterol levels (including a complete lipid profile/fractionation and an assessment of the patient's individual risk factors) should be considered especially during long-term treatment.

Patients treated with EFFEXOR XR for up to 12 weeks in 4 premarketing placebo-controlled Social Anxiety Disorder trials had a mean final on-therapy increases in total serum cholesterol concentration of approximately 8.8 mg/dL (0.227 mmol/L), increases in HDL cholesterol of 2.3 mg/dL (0.059 mmol/L), and increases in LDL cholesterol of 5.4 mg/dL (0.139 mmol/L). Patients treated with EFFEXOR XR 75 mg/day for up to 6 months in a premarketing placebo-controlled Social Anxiety Disorder trial had a mean final on-therapy decrease in total serum cholesterol concentration of approximately 0.5 mg/dL (0.013 mmol/L), decrease in HDL cholesterol of 1.0 mg/dL (0.025 mmol/L), and increase in LDL cholesterol of 0.2 mg/dL (0.006 mmol/L). Patients treated with EFFEXOR XR 150-225 mg/day for up to 6 months in the same premarketing placebo-controlled Social Anxiety Disorder trial had a mean final on-therapy increase in total serum cholesterol concentration of approximately 12.5 mg/dL (0.322 mmol/L), increase in HDL cholesterol of 1.0 mg/dL (0.026 mmol/L), and increase in LDL cholesterol of 8.2 mg/dL (0.213 mmol/L).

Patients treated with EFFEXOR XR for up to 12 weeks in premarketing placebo-controlled Panic Disorder trials had a mean final on-therapy increases in total serum cholesterol concentration of approximately 5.8 mg/dL (0.149 mmol/L), increases in HDL cholesterol of 1.9 mg/dL (0.050 mmol/L), and increases in LDL cholesterol of 2.9 mg/dL (0.076 mmol/L). A dose-dependence effect in serum cholesterol concentration was noted in the 2 fixed-dose studies. In one study, a mean decrease of 2.9 mg/dL (0.07 mmol/L) was observed in the placebo group, and mean increases of 2.1 mg/dL (0.05 mmol/L) and 5.1 mg/dL (0.13 mmol/L) were observed in the EFFEXOR XR 75 mg and 150 mg dosage groups, respectively. In another study, a mean decrease of 4.8 mg/dL (0.12 mmol/L) was observed in the placebo group, and mean increases of 2.3 mg/dL (0.06 mmol/L) and 11.5 mg/dL (0.30 mmol/L) were observed in the EFFEXOR XR 75 mg and 225 mg dosage groups, respectively.

ECG Changes: In an analysis of ECGs obtained in 769 patients treated with venlafaxine immediate release tablets and 450 patients treated with placebo in controlled clinical trials in depression, the only statistically significant difference observed was for heart rate, i.e., a mean increase from baseline of 4 beats per minute for venlafaxine immediate release tablets.

An analysis of ECGs was obtained in 357 patients treated with EFFEXOR XR and 285 patients treated with placebo in controlled clinical trials in depression, in 815 patients who received EFFEXOR XR and 379 patients who received placebo for up to 6 months in double-blind, placebo-controlled trials in GAD, 593 patients who received EFFEXOR XR and 534 patients who received placebo for up to 12 weeks in double-blind, placebo-controlled trials in Social Anxiety Disorder, and in 661 patients who received EFFEXOR XR and 395 patients who received placebo for up to 12 weeks in double-blind, placebo-controlled trials in Panic Disorder were analyzed. The mean change from baseline in corrected QT interval (QTc) for EFFEXOR XR-treated patients was increased relative to that for placebo-treated patients in the clinical trials for depression, Social Anxiety Disorder and Panic Disorder (see Warnings and Precautions, Cardiac Disease).

In North American clinical trials for Generalized Anxiety Disorder, mean reductions in PR interval (3-6 msec decrease) were reported during EFFEXOR XR treatment which represented statistically significant differences from the corresponding placebo groups (1-3 msec increase). The clinical significance of these changes is not definitively known.

Other Events Observed During the Premarketing Evaluation of Venlafaxine: During the premarketing assessment of venlafaxine immediate release tablets, multiple doses were administered to 2897 patients in phase II-III depression studies. Multiple doses of EFFEXOR XR were administered to 705 patients in phase III depression studies (as well as 96 patients on venlafaxine immediate release tablets), to 1381 patients in phase III GAD studies, 819 patients in phase III Social Anxiety Disorder studies and 1314 patients in phase III Panic Disorder studies. The conditions and duration of exposure to venlafaxine in both development programs varied greatly, and included (in overlapping categories) open and double-blind studies, uncontrolled and controlled studies, inpatient (venlafaxine immediate release tablets only) and outpatient studies, fixed-dose and titration studies. Untoward events associated with this exposure were recorded by clinical investigators using terminology of their own choosing. Consequently, it is not possible to provide a meaningful estimate of the proportion of individuals experiencing adverse events without first grouping similar types of untoward events into a smaller number of standardized event categories.

In the tabulations that follow, reported adverse events were classified using a standard COSTART-based Dictionary terminology. The frequencies presented, therefore, represent the proportion of the 7212 patients exposed to multiple doses of either formulation of venlafaxine who experienced an event of the type cited on at least one occasion while receiving venlafaxine. All reported events are included except those already listed in Table 4 (MDD), Table 5 (MDD dose related), Table 6 (GAD NA), Table 7 (GAD 378), Table 8 (SAD ST), Table 9 (SAD LT), and Table 10 (PD), and those events for which a drug cause was remote. If the COSTART term for an event was so general as to be uninformative, it was replaced with a more informative term. **It is important to emphasize that, although the events reported occurred during treatment with venlafaxine, they were not necessarily caused by it.**

* Based on the number of men and women, as appropriate.

Events are further categorized by body system and listed in order of decreasing frequency according to the following definitions: frequent adverse events are those occurring on one or more occasions in at least 1/100 patients; infrequent adverse events are those occurring in 1/100 to 1/1000 patients; rare adverse events are those occurring in fewer than 1/1000 patients.

Body as a Whole: Frequent: chest pain substernal. Infrequent: angioedema, face edema, intentional injury, malaise, moniliasis, neck rigidity, overdose, pelvic pain, photosensitivity reaction, suicide attempt. Rare: anaphylaxis, appendicitis, bacteremia, body odour, carcinoma, cellulitis, granuloma, halitosis.

Cardiovascular System: Common: palpitations. Infrequent: angina pectoris, arrhythmia, bradycardia, extrasystoles, hypotension, peripheral vascular disorder (mainly cold feet and/or cold hands), syncope. Rare: aortic aneurysm, arteritis, first degree atrioventricular block, bigeminy, bundle branch block, capillary fragility, cardiovascular disorder (includes mitral valve and circulatory disturbances), cerebral ischemia, coronary artery disease, heart arrest, congestive heart failure, hematoma, mucocutaneous hemorrhage, myocardial infarct, pallor, QT and QTc interval prolonged, sinus arrhythmia, thrombophlebitis varicose vein, venous insufficiency.

Digestive System: Frequent: increased appetite. Infrequent: bruxism, colitis, dysphagia, tongue edema, eructation, esophagitis, gastritis, gastroenteritis, gastrointestinal ulcer, gingivitis, glossitis, rectal hemorrhage, hemorrhoids, melena, oral moniliasis, stomatitis, mouth ulceration. Rare: abdominal distension, biliary pain, cheilitis, cholecystitis, cholelithiasis, duodenitis, esophageal spasms, hematemesis, gastroesophageal reflux disease, gum hemorrhage, hepatitis, ileitis, jaundice, intestinal obstruction, liver tenderness, parotitis, periodontitis, proctitis, rectal disorder, increased salivation, salivary gland enlargement, soft stools, tongue discoloration.

Endocrine System: Rare: galactorrhea, goiter, hyperthyroidism, hypothyroidism, thyroid nodule, thyroiditis.

Hemic and Lymphatic System: Infrequent: anemia, gastrointestinal hemorrhage, leukocytosis, leukopenia, lymphadenopathy, thrombocythemia, mucous membrane bleeding. Rare: basophilia, bleeding time increased, cyanosis, eosinophilia, lymphocytosis, multiple myeloma, purpura, thrombocytopenia.

Metabolic and Nutritional: Frequent: edema, serum cholesterol increase. Infrequent: alkaline phosphatase increased, dehydration, hypercholesterolemia, hyperglycemia, hypokalemia, AST increased, ALT increased, thirst, SIADH. Rare: alcohol intolerance, bilirubinemia, BUN increased, creatinine increased, diabetes mellitus, glycosuria, gout, healing abnormal, hemochromatosis, hypercalcinuria, hyperkalemia, hyperphosphatemia, hyperuricemia, hypocholesterolemia, hypoglycemia, hyponatremia, hypophosphatemia, hypoproteinemia, uremia.

Musculoskeletal System: Infrequent: arthritis, arthrosis, bone spurs, bursitis, myasthenia. Rare: bone pain, muscle cramp, muscle spasm, musculoskeletal stiffness, pathological fracture, myopathy, osteoporosis, osteosclerosis, plantar fasciitis, rheumatoid arthritis, tendon rupture.

Nervous System: Frequent: hypesthesia. Infrequent: akathisia/psychomotor restlessness, ataxia, circumoral paresthesia, CNS stimulation, emotional lability, euphoria, hallucinations, hostility, hyperesthesia, hyperkinesias, hypotonia, impaired coordination and balance, manic reaction, myoclonus, neuralgia, neuropathy, psychosis, serotonergic syndrome, seizure, abnormal speech, stupor, suicidal ideation. Rare: abnormal/changed behaviour, adjustment disorder, akinesia, alcohol abuse, aphasia, bradykinesia, buccoglossal syndrome, cerebrovascular accident, convulsion, feeling drunk, loss of consciousness, delusions, dementia, dystonia, energy increased, facial paralysis, abnormal gait, Guillain-Barré Syndrome, homicidal ideation, hyperchlorhydria, hysteria, impulse control difficulties, hypokinesia, motion sickness, neuritis, nystagmus, paranoid reaction, paresis, psychotic depression, reflexes decreased, reflexes increased, torticollis.

Respiratory System: Infrequent: chest congestion, epistaxis, hyperventilation, laryngismus, laryngitis, pneumonia, voice alteration. Rare: atelectasis, hemoptysis, hiccup, hypoventilation, hypoxia, larynx edema, pleurisy, pulmonary embolus, sleep apnea, sputum increased.

Skin and Appendages: Frequent: pruritus. Infrequent: acne, alopecia, dry skin, maculopapular rash, psoriasis. Rare: brittle nails, erythema nodosum, exfoliative dermatitis, lichenoid dermatitis, hair discoloration, skin discoloration, furunculosis, hirsutism, leukoderma, miliaria, petechial rash, pruritic rash, pustular rash, vesiculobullous rash, seborrhea, skin atrophy, skin hypertrophy, skin striae, sweating decreased.

Special Senses: Infrequent: diplopia, dry eyes, eye pain, otitis media, parosmia, photophobia, taste loss. Rare: blepharitis, cataract, chromatopsia, conjunctival edema, corneal lesion, deafness, exophthalmos, eye hemorrhage, glaucoma, hyperacusis, retinal hemorrhage, subconjunctival hemorrhage, keratitis, labyrinthitis, miosis, papilledema, decreased pupillary reflex, otitis externa, scleritis, uveitis, visual field defect, vitreous disorder.

Urogenital System: Frequent: erectile dysfunction*. Infrequent: albuminuria, cystitis, hematuria, leukorrhea*, kidney calculus, kidney pain, kidney function abnormal, nocturia, breast pain, prostatic disorder (includes prostatitis, enlarged prostate, and prostate irritability)*, polyuria, pyuria, urinary incontinence, urinary retention, urinary urgency, vaginal hemorrhage*, vaginitis*. Rare: abortion*, anuria, balanitis*, bladder pain, breast discharge, breast engorgement, breast enlargement, endometriosis*, fibrocystic breast, calcium crystalluria, cervicitis*, ovarian cyst*, prolonged erection*, female lactation*, gynecomastia*, hypomenorrhea*, mastitis*, menopause*, oliguria, orchitis, pyelonephritis, salpingitis*, urolithiasis, uterine hemorrhage*, vaginal dryness*.

Post-Market Adverse Drug Reactions Not Listed as Clinical Trial Adverse Event: Voluntary reports of adverse events other than those above, temporally associated with the use of venlafaxine, that have been received since market introduction and that may have no causal relationship with the use of venlafaxine include the following:

Body as a Whole: anaphylaxis, congenital anomalies, neuroleptic malignant syndrome-like events (including the case of a 10-year old boy who may have been taking methylphenidate, was treated and recovered), serotonin syndrome.

Cardiovascular System: congestive heart failure, deep vein thrombosis, heart arrest, hemorrhage, myocardial infarction, ECG abnormalities (such as atrial fibrillation, bigeminy, supraventricular tachycardia, ventricular extrasystole, ventricular fibrillation and ventricular tachycardia, including torsades de pointes).

Digestive System: bruxism, diarrhoea, gastrointestinal bleeding, hepatic events (including GGT elevation; abnormalities of unspecified liver function tests; fatty liver, liver damage, necrosis or failure, fulminant hepatitis, including rare fatalities), pancreatitis, diarrhoea.

Endocrine System: prolactin increased.

Hemic and Lymphatic Systems: agranulocytosis, aplastic anemia, neutropenia, pancytopenia.

Metabolic and Nutritional: CPK increased, dehydration, hepatitis, LDH increased, syndrome of inappropriate antidiuretic hormone secretion, weight loss.

Musculoskeletal: rhabdomyolysis.

Nervous System: abnormal gait, agitation, catatonia, delirium, extrapyramidal symptoms (including dyskinesia, dystonia, tardive dyskinesia), grand mal seizures, increased muscle tonus, involuntary movements, panic, paresthesia, neuroleptic malignant syndrome, sedation, shock-like electrical sensations (in some cases, subsequent to the discontinuation of venlafaxine or tapering of dose), aggressive ideation and acts, including harm to others.

Respiratory System: interstitial lung disease (including pulmonary eosinophilia).

Skin and Appendages: toxic epidermal necrolysis/Stevens-Johnson syndrome, erythema multiforme, sweating including night sweats.

Special Senses: angle closure glaucoma, eye hemorrhage, tinnitus.

Urogenital System: renal failure.

DRUG INTERACTIONS:

> **Serious Drug Interactions**
> - **Monoamine Oxidase Inhibitors: See Contraindications.**

Overview: Venlafaxine is not highly bound to plasma proteins; therefore, administration of venlafaxine to a patient taking another drug that is highly protein bound should not cause increased free concentrations of the other drug.

The risk of using venlafaxine in combination with other CNS-active drugs has not been systematically evaluated. Consequently, caution is advised if the concomitant administration of venlafaxine and such drugs is required.

As with all drugs, the potential for interaction by a variety of mechanisms is a possibility.

Drug-Drug Interactions:

- **Monoamine Oxidase Inhibitors: See Contraindications and Dosage and Administration, Switching Patients to or from a Monoamine Oxidase Inhibitor.**
- Other CNS-Active Drugs: The risk of using venlafaxine in combination with other CNS-Active drugs has not been systematically evaluated. Consequently, caution is advised if the concomitant administration of venlafaxine and such drugs is required.
- Serotonergic Drugs: Based on the known mechanism of action of venlafaxine and the potential for serotonin syndrome, a potentially life threatening condition, caution is advised when venlafaxine is co-administered with other drugs that may affect the serotonergic neurotransmitter systems (such as triptans, selective serotonin reuptake inhibitors, other SNRIs, linezolid (an antibiotic which is a reversible non-selective MAOI; see Contraindications), lithium, sibutramine or tramadol, or with serotonin precursors, such as tryptophan supplements). Rare postmarketing reports describe patients with symptoms suggestive of, or diagnostic of, serotonin syndrome, following the combined use of a selective serotonin reuptake inhibitor (SSRI) with

5HT1-agonists (triptans) or lithium. If concomitant treatment with EFFEXOR XR and a triptan (e.g., almotriptan, sumatriptan, rizatriptan, naratriptan, zolmitriptan), tricyclic antidepressants, or other drugs or agents with serotonergic activity (including but not limited to fenfluramine, tryptophan and silbutramine; the antibiotic linezolid; St. John's Wort) is clinically warranted, appropriate observation of the patient for acute and long-term adverse events is advised. (See also Warnings and Precautions, Endocrine and Metabolism, Changes in Appetite and Weight and Warnings and Precautions, Neurologic, Serotonin Syndrome/Neuroleptic Malignant Syndrome.)

Serotonin syndrome symptoms may include mental status changes, autonomic instability, neuromuscular aberrations and/or gastrointestinal symptoms.

- Alcohol: The possibility of additive psychomotor impairment should be considered if venlafaxine is used in combination with alcohol. Patients should be advised to avoid alcohol while taking venlafaxine.
- Lithium: The steady-state pharmacokinetics of venlafaxine 150 mg administered as 50 mg every 8 hours was not affected when a single 600 mg oral dose of lithium was administered to 12 healthy male subjects. ODV was also unaffected. Venlafaxine had no effect on the pharmacokinetics of lithium. (Also see Other CNS-Active Drugs.)
- Diazepam: The steady-state pharmacokinetics of venlafaxine 150 mg administered as 50 mg every 8 hours was not affected when a single 10 mg oral dose of diazepam was administered to 18 healthy male subjects. ODV was also unaffected. Venlafaxine had no effect on the pharmacokinetics of diazepam or its active metabolite, desmethyldiazepam. Additionally, venlafaxine administration did not affect the psychomotor and psychometric effects induced by diazepam.
- Cimetidine: Concomitant administration of cimetidine and venlafaxine in a steady-state study for both drugs in 18 healthy male subjects resulted in inhibition of first-pass metabolism of venlafaxine. The oral clearance of venlafaxine was reduced by about 43%, and the exposure (AUC) and maximum concentration (C_{max}) of the drug were increased by about 60%. However, there was no effect on the pharmacokinetics of ODV. The overall pharmacological activity of venlafaxine plus ODV is expected to increase only slightly, and no dosage adjustment should be necessary for most normal adults. However, for patients with pre-existing hypertension, for elderly patients and for patients with hepatic or renal dysfunction, the interaction associated with the concomitant use of cimetidine and venlafaxine is not known and potentially could be more pronounced. Therefore, caution is advised with such patients.
- Haloperidol: Venlafaxine administered under steady-state conditions at 150 mg/day in 24 healthy subjects decreased total oral-dose clearance (Cl/F) of a single 2 mg dose of haloperidol by 42%, which resulted in a 70% increase in haloperidol AUC. In addition, the haloperidol C_{max} increased 88% when coadministered with venlafaxine, but the haloperidol elimination half-life ($t_{½}$) was unchanged. The mechanism explaining this finding is unknown.
- Imipramine: Venlafaxine did not affect the pharmacokinetics of imipramine and 2-OH-imipramine. However, AUC, C_{max} and C_{min} of desipramine (the active metabolite of imipramine) increased by approximately 35% in the presence of venlafaxine. The 2-OH-desipramine AUCs increased by at least 2.5 fold (with venlafaxine 37.5 mg q12h) and by 4.5 fold (with venlafaxine 75 mg q12h). The clinical significance of elevated 2-OH-desipramine levels is unknown.

  Imipramine partially inhibited the CYP2D6-mediated formation of ODV. However, the total concentration of active compounds (venlafaxine plus ODV) was not affected by coadministration with imipramine, and no dosage adjustment is required.
- Metoprolol: Concomitant administration of venlafaxine (50 mg every 8 hours for 5 days) and metoprolol (100 mg every 24 hours for 5 days) to healthy volunteers in a pharmacokinetic interaction study for both drugs resulted in an increase of plasma concentrations of metoprolol by approximately 30-40% without altering the plasma concentrations of its active metabolite, α-hydroxymetoprolol. The clinical relevance of this finding is unknown. Metoprolol did not alter the pharmacokinetic profile of venlafaxine or its active metabolite, O-desmethyl venlafaxine. (See also Warnings and Precautions, General, Hypertension.)
- Risperidone: Venlafaxine administered under steady-state conditions at 150 mg/day slightly inhibited the CYP2D6-mediated metabolism of risperidone (administered as a single 1 mg oral dose) to its active metabolite, 9-hydroxyrisperidone, resulting in an approximate 32% increase in risperidone AUC. However, venlafaxine co-administration did not significantly alter the pharmacokinetic profile of the total active moiety (risperidone plus 9-hydroxyrisperidone).
- Indinavir: In a study of 9 healthy volunteers, venlafaxine administered under steady-state conditions at 150 mg/day resulted in a 28% decrease in the AUC of a single 800 mg oral dose of indinavir and a 36% decrease in indinavir C_{max}. Indinavir did not affect the pharmacokinetics of venlafaxine and ODV. The clinical significance of this finding is unknown.
- Ketoconazole: A pharmacokinetic study with ketoconazole in extensive (EM) and poor metabolizers (PM) of CYP2D6 resulted in higher plasma concentrations of both venlafaxine and ODV in subjects following administration of ketoconazole. Venlafaxine C_{max} increased by 26% in EM subjects and 48% in PM subjects. C_{max} values for ODV increased by 14% and 29% in EM and PM subjects, respectively. Venlafaxine AUC increased by 21% in EM subjects and 70% in PM subjects. AUC values for ODV increased by 23% and 33% in EM and PM subjects, respectively.
- Drugs Highly Bound to Plasma Proteins: Venlafaxine is not highly bound to plasma proteins; therefore, administration of venlafaxine to a patient taking another drug that is highly protein bound should not cause increased free concentrations of the other drug.
- Drugs Metabolized by Cytochrome P450 Isoenzymes: The metabolic pathways for venlafaxine include CYP2D6 and CYP3A4. Venlafaxine is primarily metabolized to its active metabolite, ODV, by the cytochrome P450 enzyme CYP2D6. CYP3A4 is a minor pathway relative to CYP2D6 in the metabolism of venlafaxine.

  In vitro studies indicate that venlafaxine is a relatively weak inhibitor of CYP2D6. These findings have been confirmed in vivo by a clinical drug interaction study comparing the effect of venlafaxine with that of fluoxetine on the CYP2D6-mediated metabolism of dextromethorphan to dextrorphan.
- Drugs that Inhibit Cytochrome P450 Isoenzymes—CYP2D6-Inhibitors: In vitro and in vivo studies indicate that venlafaxine is metabolized to its active metabolite, ODV, by CYP2D6, the isoenzyme that is responsible for the genetic polymorphism seen in the metabolism of many antidepressants. Therefore, the potential exists for a drug interaction between drugs that inhibit CYP2D6 mediated metabolism and venlafaxine.

  Drug interactions that reduce the metabolism of venlafaxine to ODV (see Imipramine above) potentially increase the plasma concentrations of venlafaxine and lower the concentrations of the active metabolite. Concomitant use of CYP2D6 inhibitors and venlafaxine may reduce the metabolism of venlafaxine to ODV, resulting in increased plasma concentrations of venlafaxine and decreased concentrations of ODV. As venlafaxine and ODV are both pharmacologically active, no dosage adjustment is required when venlafaxine is coadministered with a CYP2D6 inhibitor.
- CYP3A3/4 Inhibitors: In vitro studies indicate that venlafaxine is likely metabolized to a minor, less active metabolite, N-desmethylvenlafaxine, by CYP3A3/4. Concomitant use of CYP3A4 inhibitors and venlafaxine may increase levels of venlafaxine and ODV (see Ketoconazole above). Therefore, caution is advised when combining venlafaxine with a CYP3A4 inhibitor.
- CYP2D6 and 3A4 Inhibitors: Interactions between concomitant intake of inhibitors of both CYP2D6 and CYP3A3/4 with venlafaxine have not been studied. However, this concomitant use would be expected to increase venlafaxine plasma concentrations. Because the two primary metabolic pathways for venlafaxine are through CYP2D6 and, to a lesser extent, CYP3A3/4, concomitant intake of inhibitors of both of these isoenzymes is not recommended during treatment with venlafaxine.
- CYP3A4: Venlafaxine did not inhibit CYP3A4 in vitro. This finding was confirmed in vivo by clinical drug interaction studies in which venlafaxine did not inhibit the metabolism of several CYP3A4 substrates, including alprazolam, diazepam, and terfenadine.
- CYP1A2: Venlafaxine did not inhibit CYP1A2 in vitro. This finding was confirmed in vivo by a clinical drug interaction study in which venlafaxine did not inhibit the metabolism of caffeine, a CYP1A2 substrate.
- CYP2C9: Venlafaxine did not inhibit CYP2C9 in vitro. This finding was confirmed in vivo by a clinical drug interaction study in which venlafaxine did not inhibit the metabolism of tolbutamide, a CYP2C9 substrate.
- CYP2C19: Venlafaxine did not inhibit the metabolism of diazepam, which is partially metabolized by CYP2C19 (see Diazepam above).

Post-Marketing Reports of Drug-Drug Interactions: There have been reports of elevated clozapine levels that were temporally associated with adverse events including seizures, following the addition of venlafaxine. There have been reports of increases in prothrombin time, partial thromboplastin time, or INR when venlafaxine was given to patients receiving warfarin therapy.

Electroconvulsive Therapy: There are no clinical data on the use of electroconvulsive therapy combined with EFFEXOR XR treatment.

Drug-Food Interactions: Food has no significant effect on the absorption of venlafaxine or on the subsequent formation of ODV.

Drug-Herb Interactions: St. John's Wort: In common with SSRIs, pharmacodynamic interactions between EFFEXOR XR and the herbal remedy St. John's Wort may occur and may result in an increase in undesirable effects.

Drug-Lifestyle Interactions: Interference with Cognitive and Motor Performance: In healthy volunteers receiving an immediate release venlafaxine formulation at a stable regimen of 150 mg/day, some impairment of psychomotor performance was observed. Patients should be cautioned about operating hazardous machinery, including automobiles, or engaging in tasks requiring alertness until they have been able to assess the drug's effect on their own psychomotor performance.

Drug Abuse and Dependence: Physical and Psychological Dependence: In vitro studies revealed that venlafaxine has virtually no affinity for opiate, benzodiazepine, phencyclidine (PCP), or N-methyl-D-aspartic acid (NMDA) receptors. It has no significant CNS stimulant activity in rodents. In primate drug discrimination studies, venlafaxine showed no significant stimulant or depressant abuse liability. While venlafaxine has not been systematically studied in clinical trials for their potential for abuse, there was no indication of drug-seeking behaviour in the clinical trials. However, it is not possible to predict on the basis of premarketing experience the extent to which a CNS active drug will be misused, diverted, and/or abused once marketed. Consequently, physicians should carefully evaluate patients for history of drug abuse and follow such patients closely, observing them for signs of misuse or abuse of venlafaxine (e.g., development of tolerance, incrementation of dose, drug-seeking behaviour).

DOSAGE AND ADMINISTRATION: Dosing Considerations: General: EFFEXOR XR is not indicated for use in children under 18 years of age (see Warnings and Precautions, Potential Association with Behavioral and Emotional Changes, Including Self-harm).

Discontinuing Venlafaxine: When discontinuing venlafaxine after more than 1 week of therapy, it is generally recommended that the dose be tapered gradually to minimize the risk of discontinuation symptoms. Discontinuation symptoms have been assessed both in patients with depression and in those with GAD. Abrupt discontinuation, dose reduction, or tapering of venlafaxine at various doses has been found to be associated with the appearance of new symptoms, the frequency of which increased with higher dose levels and with longer duration of treatment. Reported symptoms include but are not limited to the following: aggression, agitation, anorexia, anxiety, asthenia, confusion, convulsions, impaired coordination and balance, diarrhoea, dizziness, dry mouth, dysphoric mood, fasciculation, fatigue, flu-like symptoms, headache, hypomania, insomnia, nausea, nightmares, nervousness, paresthesia, electric shock sensations, sensory disturbances (including shock like electrical sensations), sleep disturbances, somnolence, sweating, tinnitus, vertigo, and vomiting. Where such symptoms occurred they were usually self-limiting but in a few patients continued for several weeks. It is therefore recommended that the dosage of EFFEXOR XR be tapered gradually whenever possible and the patient monitored. The period required for tapering may depend on the dose, duration of therapy and the individual patient. If venlafaxine has been used for more than 6 weeks, tapering over at least a two week period is recommended (see Warnings and Precautions, Potential Association with Behavioral and Emotional Changes, Including Self-harm) and also Discontinuation Symptoms; Adverse Reactions, Discontinuation Symptoms).

Patients with Hepatic or Renal Impairment: Dosage adjustments are required (see Dosage and Administration, Special Patients Populations).

Switching Patients to or from a Monoamine Oxidase Inhibitor: At least 14 days should elapse between discontinuation of an MAOI and initiation of therapy with EFFEXOR XR. In addition, at least 14 days should be allowed after stopping EFFEXOR XR before starting an MAOI (see Contraindications).

Switching Patients from Immediate Release Tablets: Depressed patients who are currently being treated at a therapeutic dose with immediate release tablets may be switched to EFFEXOR XR at the nearest equivalent dose (mg/day), e.g., 37.5 mg immediate release two-times-a-day to 75 mg EFFEXOR XR once daily. However, individual dosage adjustments may be necessary.

Recommended Dose and Dosage Adjustment: Adults: Patients with Major Depressive Disorder: The recommended dose for EFFEXOR XR is 75 mg/day, administered once daily with food, either in the morning or in the evening. For some patients, it may be desirable to start at 37.5 mg/day for 4-7 days to allow new patients to adjust to the medication before increasing to 75 mg/day. Each capsule should be swallowed whole with water. It should not be divided, crushed, chewed, or placed in water. While the relationship between dose and antidepressant response for EFFEXOR XR has not been adequately explored patients not responding to the initial 75 mg may benefit from dose increases. Depending on tolerability and the need for further clinical effect, the dose should be increased by up to 75 mg/day up to a maximum of 225 mg/day as a single dose for moderately depressed outpatients. Dose increments should be made at intervals of approximately 2 weeks or more, but not less than 4 days. There is very limited experience with EFFEXOR XR at doses higher than 225 mg/day, or in severely depressed inpatients.

Patients with Generalized Anxiety Disorder (GAD): The recommended starting dose of EFFEXOR XR is 37.5 mg/day administered as a single dose, taken with food, for 4-7 days. The usual dose is 75 mg/day administered as a single dose. Subsequent dosage increments of up to 75 mg/day may be considered, if clinically warranted. Dose increments should be made as needed at intervals of not less than 4 days. The maximum recommended daily dose is 225 mg/day as a single dose.

Patients with Social Anxiety Disorder (Social Phobia): For most patients, the recommended dose for EFFEXOR XR is 75 mg/day, administered in a single dose. For some patients, it may be desirable to start at 37.5 mg/day for 4 to 7 days, to allow new patients to adjust to the medication before increasing to 75 mg/day. Depending on tolerability and if clinically warranted, dose increases should be in increments of up to 75 mg/day, as needed, up to a maximum of 225 mg/day. Dose increments should be made at intervals of not less than 4 days.

Panic Disorder: It is recommended that initial single doses of 37.5 mg/day of EFFEXOR XR be used for 7 days. The recommended treatment dose is 75 mg/day, administered in a single dose. Although a dose response relationship for effectiveness in patients with Panic Disorder was not clearly established in fixed-dose studies, certain patients not responding to 75 mg/day may benefit from dose increases to a maximum of 225 mg/day. Dose increases should be in increments of up to 75 mg/day, as needed, and should be made at intervals of at least 7 days.

Maintenance/Continuation/Extended Treatment: There is no body of evidence available to answer the question of how long a patient should continue to be treated with EFFEXOR XR for depression, GAD, Social Anxiety Disorder or Panic Disorder.

During long-term therapy for any indication, the EFFEXOR XR dosage should be maintained at the lowest effective dose and the need for continuing treatment should be periodically reassessed.

Depression: It is generally agreed that acute episodes of major depression require several months or longer of sustained pharmacotherapy beyond response to the acute episode. Whether the dose needed to induce remission is identical to the dose needed for maintenance is unknown.

Maintenance of efficacy of EFFEXOR XR has been shown in a placebo controlled study in which patients responding during 8 weeks of acute treatment with EFFEXOR XR were assigned randomly to placebo or to the same dose of EFFEXOR XR [75, 150, or 225 mg/day, in the morning (i.e. qAM)] during 26 weeks of maintenance treatment.

It is not known whether or not the dose of EFFEXOR XR needed for maintenance treatment is identical to the dose needed to achieve an initial response. Patients should be periodically reassessed to determine the need for maintenance treatment and the appropriate dose for such treatment.

Social Anxiety Disorder: In patients with Social Anxiety Disorder, there are no efficacy data beyond 6 months of treatment with EFFEXOR XR. The need for continuing medication in patients with Social Anxiety Disorder who improve with EFFEXOR XR treatment should be periodically reassessed.

Panic Disorder: In one study in Panic Disorder, in which patients who were responders in the final 2 weeks of a 12-week acute treatment with EFFEXOR XR were assigned randomly to placebo or to the same dose of EFFEXOR XR (75, 150, or 225 mg/day) during 6 months of maintenance treatment, patients continuing EFFEXOR XR treatment showed a significant longer time to relapse than patients switched to placebo.

Special Patients Populations: Treatment of Pregnant Women During the Third Trimester: Post-marketing reports indicate that some neonates exposed to immediate release venlafaxine or EFFEXOR XR, SSRIs (Selective Serotonin Reuptake Inhibitors), or other newer antidepressants late in the third trimester have developed complications requiring prolonged hospitalization, respiratory support, and tube feeding. (See Warnings and Precautions, Special Populations, Pregnant Women). When treating a pregnant woman with EFFEXOR XR during the third trimester, the physician should carefully consider the potential risks and benefits of treatment.

Due to the potential for discontinuation symptoms, if a decision is taken to discontinue EFFEXOR XR treatment, a gradual reduction in the dose rather than an abrupt cessation is recommended (see Warnings and Precautions, Discontinuation Symptoms).

Elderly Patients: No dose adjustment is recommended for elderly patients solely on the basis of their age. As with any antidepressant or anxiolytic, drug for treatment of Social Anxiety Disorder, or Panic Disorder, however, caution should be exercised in treating the elderly. When individualizing the dosage, extra care should be taken when increasing the dose.

Pediatrics: EFFEXOR XR is not indicated for use in children under 18 years of age (see Warnings and Precautions, Potential Association with Behavioral and Emotional Changes, Including Self-harm).

Patients with Hepatic Impairment: Given the decrease in clearance and increase in elimination half-life for both venlafaxine and ODV that is observed in patients with hepatic cirrhosis compared with normal subjects (see Action and Clinical Pharmacology, Hepatic Insufficiency), the total daily dose should be reduced by about 50% in patients with mild to moderate hepatic impairment. For such patients, it may be desirable to start at 37.5 mg/day. Because of individual variability in clearance in these patients, individualization of dosage may be desirable. Since there was much individual variability in clearance between patients with cirrhosis, it may be necessary to reduce the dose by even more than 50%, and individualization of dosing may be desirable in some patients.

Patients with Renal Impairment: Given the decrease in clearance for venlafaxine and increase in elimination half-life for both venlafaxine and ODV that is observed in patients with renal impairment (GFR=10-70 mL/min) compared to normal subjects (see Action and Clinical Pharmacology, Renal Insufficiency) the total daily dose should be decreased by 25%-50%. In patients undergoing hemodialysis, the total daily dose must be reduced by 50% and the dose be withheld until the dialysis treatment is completed (4 hrs). For such patients, it may be desirable to start at 37.5 mg/day. Since there is so much individual variability in clearance among patients with renal impairment, individualization of dosing may be desirable.

Missed Dose: If a dose is missed, it should not be made up for it by doubling up on the dose next time. The next dose should be taken as scheduled.
Administration: Administer once daily with food, either in the morning or in the evening.

OVERDOSAGE:
Venlafaxine Immediate Release Tablets: There were 14 reports of acute overdose with immediate release tablets (venlafaxine HCl), either alone or in combination with other drugs and/or alcohol, among the patients included in the premarketing evaluation. The majority of the reports involved ingestions in which the total dose of venlafaxine taken was estimated to be no more than several-fold higher than the usual therapeutic dose. The 3 patients who took the highest doses were estimated to have ingested approximately 6.75 g, 2.75 g and 2.5 g. The resultant peak plasma levels of venlafaxine for the latter 2 patients were 6.24 and 2.35 μg/mL, respectively, and the peak plasma levels of O-desmethylvenlafaxine were 3.37 and 1.30 μg/mL, respectively. Plasma venlafaxine levels were not obtained for the patient who ingested 6.75 g of venlafaxine. All 14 patients recovered without sequelae. Most patients reported no symptoms. Among the remaining patients, somnolence was the most commonly reported symptom. The patient who ingested 2.75 g of venlafaxine was observed to have 2 generalized convulsions and a prolongation of QTc to 500 msec, compared with 405 msec at baseline. Mild sinus tachycardia was reported in 2 of the other patients.
EFFEXOR XR Capsules: Among the patients included in the premarketing evaluation of venlafaxine extended release capsules, there were 2 reports of acute overdosage with EFFEXOR XR in depression trials, either alone or in combination with other drugs. One patient took a combination of 6 g of EFFEXOR XR and 2.5 mg of lorazepam. This patient was hospitalized, treated symptomatically, and recovered without any untoward effects. The other patient took 2.85 g of EFFEXOR XR. This patient reported paresthesia of all four limbs but recovered without sequelae. There were 2 reports of acute overdose with EFFEXOR XR in anxiety trials. One patient took a combination of 0.75 g EFFEXOR XR and 200 mg of paroxetine and 50 mg of zolpidem. This patient was described as being alert, able to communicate, and a little sleepy. This patient was hospitalized, treated with activated charcoal, and recovered without any untoward effects. The other patient took 1.2 g of EFFEXOR XR. This patient recovered and no other specific problems were found. The patient had moderate dizziness, nausea, numb hands and feet, and hot-cold spells 5 days after the overdose. There were no reports of acute overdose with EFFEXOR XR in Social Anxiety Disorder trials. There were 2 reports of acute overdose with EFFEXOR XR in Panic Disorder trials. One patient took 0.675 g of EFFEXOR XR once and the other patient took 0.45 g of EFFEXOR XR for 2 days. No signs or symptoms were associated with either overdose and no actions were taken to treat them.
Post-Marketing Experience with EFFEXOR (Dosage Form Unknown): In postmarketing experience, overdose with venlafaxine was reported predominantly in combination with alcohol and/or other drugs. The most commonly reported events in overdose include tachycardia, changes in level of consciousness (ranging from somnolence to coma), mydriasis, convulsion, and vomiting. Other events reported include electrocardiographic changes (e.g., prolongation of QT interval, bundle branch block, QRS prolongation), ventricular tachycardia, bradycardia, hypotension, delayed rise in plasma creatine kinase levels, rhabdomyolysis, liver necrosis, serotonin syndrome, vertigo, and death. Muscle enzymes should be monitored in patients with venlafaxine overdose to detect development of rhabdomyolysis at an early stage and to initiate appropriate treatment. According to postmarketing overdose reports with venlafaxine (where overdose amounts were provided) fatal acute overdoses have been reported with venlafaxine alone at doses as low as approximately 1 gram.

Published retrospective studies report that venlafaxine overdosage may be associated with an increased risk of fatal outcomes compared to that observed with SSRI antidepressant products, but lower than that for tricyclic antidepressants. Epidemiological studies have shown that venlafaxine-treated patients have a higher burden of suicide risk factors than SSRI patients. The extent to which the finding of an increased risk of fatal outcomes can be attributed to the toxicity of venlafaxine in overdosage as opposed to some characteristics of venlafaxine-treated patients is not clear. Prescriptions for venlafaxine should be written for the smallest quantity of drug consistent with good patient management, in order to reduce the risk of overdose.
Overdosage Management: Treatment should consist of those general measures employed in the management of overdosage with any antidepressant. Ensure an adequate airway, oxygenation, and ventilation. Monitor cardiac rhythm and vital signs. General supportive and symptomatic measures are also recommended. Induction of emesis is not recommended. Gastric lavage with a large bore orogastric tube with appropriate airway protection, if needed, may be indicated if performed soon after ingestion or in symptomatic patients. Activated charcoal should be administered. Due to the large volume of distribution of this drug, forced diuresis, dialysis, hemoperfusion and exchange transfusion are unlikely to be of benefit. No specific antidotes for venlafaxine are known.

In managing overdosage, consider the possibility of multiple drug involvement. The physician should consider contacting a poison control centre for current information on the treatment of any overdose.

> For management of a suspected drug overdose, CPhA recommends that you contact your **regional Poison Control Centre**. See the *CPS* Directory section for a list of Poison Control Centres.

ACTION AND CLINICAL PHARMACOLOGY: Mechanism of Action: Venlafaxine is a phenethylamine bicyclic derivative, chemically unrelated to tricyclic, tetracyclic or other available antidepressant or anxiolytic agents.

The mechanism of venlafaxine's antidepressant action in humans is believed to be associated with its potentiation of neurotransmitter activity in the CNS. Preclinical studies have shown that venlafaxine and its active metabolite, O-desmethylvenlafaxine (ODV), are potent inhibitors of neuronal serotonin and norepinephrine reuptake and weak inhibitors of dopamine reuptake.
Pharmacodynamics: Venlafaxine and ODV have no significant affinity for muscarinic, histaminergic, or α_1-adrenergic receptors in vitro. Pharmacologic activity at these receptors is hypothesized to be associated with the various anticholinergic, sedative, and cardiovascular effects seen with other psychotropic drugs. Venlafaxine and ODV do not possess monoamine oxidase (MAO) inhibitory activity.
Pharmacokinetics: Venlafaxine Immediate Release Formulation: Venlafaxine is well absorbed, with peak plasma concentrations occurring approximately 2 hours after dosing. Venlafaxine is extensively metabolized, with O-desmethylvenlafaxine, (ODV, the only major active metabolite) peak plasma levels occurring approximately 4 hours after dosing. Following single doses of 25 to 75 mg, mean (±SD) peak plasma concentrations of venlafaxine range from 37±14 to 102±41 ng/mL, respectively, and are reached in 2±1 hours, and mean peak ODV plasma concentrations range from 61±13 to 168±37 ng/mL and are reached in 4±2 hours. Approximately 87% of a single dose of venlafaxine is recovered in the urine within 48 hours as either unchanged venlafaxine (5%), unconjugated ODV (29%), conjugated ODV (26%), or other minor inactive metabolites (27%), and 92% of the radioactive dose is recovered within 72 hours. Therefore, renal elimination of venlafaxine and its metabolites is the primary route of excretion.
EFFEXOR XR Capsules: After administration of EFFEXOR XR (venlafaxine hydrochloride, extended release capsules, the peak plasma concentrations of venlafaxine and ODV are attained within 6.0±1.5 and 8.8±2.2 hours, respectively. The rate of absorption of venlafaxine from the EFFEXOR XR capsule is slower than its rate of elimination. Therefore, the apparent elimination half-life of venlafaxine following administration of EFFEXOR XR (15±6 hours) is actually the absorption half-life instead of the true disposition half-life (5±2) hours observed following administration of a venlafaxine hydrochloride immediate release tablet.
Multiple-dose Pharmacokinetic Profile (Immediate Release Tablets and Extended Release Capsules): Steady-state concentrations of both venlafaxine and ODV in plasma are attained within 3 days of oral multiple dose therapy. The clearance of venlafaxine is slightly (15%) lower following multiple doses than following a single dose.

Venlafaxine and ODV exhibited approximately linear kinetics over the dose range of 75 to 450 mg/day.

The mean±SD steady-state plasma clearances of venlafaxine and ODV are 1.3±0.6 and 0.4±0.2 L/h/kg, respectively; apparent elimination half-life is 5±2 and 11±2 hours, respectively; and apparent (steady-state) volume of distribution is 7.5±3.7 and 5.7±1.8 L/kg, respectively.

Venlafaxine and ODV renal clearances are 49±27 and 94±56 mL/h/kg, respectively, which correspond to 5±3.0% and 25±13% of an administered venlafaxine dose recovered in urine as venlafaxine and ODV, respectively.

When equal daily doses of venlafaxine were administered as either an immediate release tablet or the extended release capsule, the exposure (AUC, area under the concentration curve) to both venlafaxine and ODV was similar for the two treatments, and the fluctuation in plasma concentrations was slightly lower following treatment with the extended release capsule. Therefore, the EFFEXOR XR capsules provide a slower rate of absorption, but the same extent of absorption (i.e., AUC), as the venlafaxine immediate release tablet.

Results of testing in healthy volunteers demonstrated differences in the gastrointestinal tolerability of different formulations of venlafaxine. Data from healthy volunteers showed reduced incidence and severity of nausea with EFFEXOR XR capsules, compared with immediate release tablets.

Venlafaxine and ODV are 27 and 30% bound to human plasma proteins, respectively. Therefore, administration of venlafaxine to a patient taking another drug that is highly protein-bound should not cause increased free concentrations of the other drug. Following intravenous administration, the steady-state volume of distribution of venlafaxine is 4.4±1.9 L/kg, indicating that venlafaxine distributes well beyond the total body water.

Absorption: Venlafaxine is well absorbed; after administration of EFFEXOR XR (venlafaxine hydrochloride, extended release capsules), the peak plasma concentrations of venlafaxine and ODV are attained within 6.0±1.5 and 8.8±2.2 hours, respectively. The rate of absorption of venlafaxine from the EFFEXOR XR capsule is slower than its rate of elimination. Therefore, the apparent elimination half-life of venlafaxine following administration of EFFEXOR XR (15±6 hours) is actually the absorption half-life instead of the true disposition half-life (5±2) hours observed following administration of a venlafaxine hydrochloride immediate release tablet. On the basis of mass balance studies, at least 92% of a single dose of venlafaxine is absorbed.

Food has no significant effect on the absorption of venlafaxine or on the subsequent formation of ODV.
Distribution: Following intravenous administration, the steady-state volume of distribution of venlafaxine is 4.4±1.9 L/kg, indicating that venlafaxine distributes well beyond the total body water. Venlafaxine and ODV are 27 and 30% bound to human plasma proteins, respectively. Therefore, administration of venlafaxine to a patient taking another drug that is highly protein-bound should not cause increased free concentrations of the other drug.
Metabolism: Following absorption, venlafaxine undergoes extensive presystemic metabolism in the liver. The absolute bioavailability of venlafaxine is approximately 45%. The primary metabolite of venlafaxine is ODV, which is an active metabolite. Venlafaxine is also metabolized to N-desmethylvenlafaxine, N,O-didesmethylvenlafaxine, and other minor metabolites. In vitro studies indicate that the formation of ODV is catalysed by CYP2D6 and that the formation of N-desmethylvenlafaxine is catalysed by CYP3A3/4. The results of the in vitro studies have been confirmed in a clinical study with subjects who are CYP2D6 poor and extensive metabolizers. However, despite the metabolic differences between the CYP2D6 poor and extensive metabolizers, the total exposure to the sum of the two active species (venlafaxine and ODV, which have comparable activity) was similar in the two metabolizer groups.
Excretion: Approximately 87% of a single dose of venlafaxine is recovered in the urine within 48 hours as either unchanged venlafaxine (5%), unconjugated ODV (29%), conjugated ODV (26%), or other minor inactive metabolites (27%), and 92% of the radioactive dose is recovered within 72 hours. Therefore, renal elimination of venlafaxine and its metabolites is the primary route of excretion.
Special Populations and Conditions: Pediatrics: Safety and efficacy in children below the age of 18 have not been established. EFFEXOR XR (venlafaxine) is not indicated for use in children under 18 years of age.
Geriatrics: Population pharmacokinetic analyses of 547 venlafaxine-treated patients from three studies involving both venlafaxine immediate release tablets and venlafaxine extended release capsules showed that age does not significantly affect the pharmacokinetics of venlafaxine. A 20% reduction in clearance was noted for ODV in subjects over 60 years old; this was possibly caused by the decrease in renal function that typically occurs with aging. Dosage adjustment based upon age is generally not necessary.
Gender: Population pharmacokinetic analyses of 547 venlafaxine-treated patients from three studies involving both venlafaxine immediate release tablets and venlafaxine extended release capsules showed that sex does not significantly affect the pharmacokinetics of venlafaxine. Dosage adjustment based upon gender is generally not necessary.
Hepatic Insufficiency: In 9 patients with hepatic cirrhosis, the pharmacokinetic disposition of both venlafaxine and ODV was significantly altered. Venlafaxine elimination half-life was prolonged by about 30%, and clearance was decreased by about 50% in cirrhotic patients compared to normal subjects. ODV elimination half-life was prolonged by about 60% and clearance decreased by about 30% in cirrhotic patients compared to normal subjects.

A large degree of inter-subject variability was noted. Three patients with more severe cirrhosis had a more substantial decrease in venlafaxine clearance (about 90%) compared to normal subjects. **Dosage adjustment is necessary in patients with hepatic impairment** (see Dosage and Administration, Special Patients Populations).
Renal Insufficiency: In patients with moderate to severe impairment of renal function (GFR=10-70 mL/min), venlafaxine elimination half-life was prolonged by 50%, and clearance was decreased by about 24% compared to normal subjects. ODV elimination half-life was prolonged by about 40%, but clearance was unchanged.

In dialysis patients, venlafaxine elimination half-life was prolonged by about 180% and clearance was decreased by about 57%. In dialysis patients, ODV elimination half-life was prolonged by about 142%, and clearance was reduced by about 56% compared to normal subjects.

A large degree of inter-subject variability was noted.

Dosage adjustment is necessary in patients with renal impairment (see Dosage and Administration, Special Patients Populations).
Genetic Polymorphism: Plasma concentrations of venlafaxine were higher in CYP2D6 poor metabolizers than extensive metabolizers. Because the total exposure (AUC) of venlafaxine and ODV was similar in poor and extensive metabolizer groups, there is no need for different venlafaxine dosing regimens for these two groups.
STORAGE AND STABILITY: Store at room temperature (15-30°C), in a dry place.
SPECIAL HANDLING INSTRUCTIONS: None.
INFORMATION FOR THE PATIENT: Published in e-CPS, available by subscription at www.e-cps.ca.
DOSAGE FORMS, COMPOSITION AND PACKAGING: 37.5 mg: Each extended release, hard gelatin capsule, with gray cap and peach body, with "W" and "Effexor XR" on the cap and "37.5" on the body, in red ink, contains: venlafaxine HCl equivalent to venlafaxine base 37.5 mg. Nonmedicinal ingredients: ethylcellulose, gelatin, hydroxypropyl methylcellulose, iron oxide, microcrystalline cellulose, Opacode Red S-1-15034 ink, talc and titanium dioxide. Gluten-free. Bottles of 15, 90 and 100.
75 mg: Each extended release, hard gelatin capsule, with peach cap and body, with "W" and "Effexor XR" on the cap and "75" on the body, in red ink, contains: venlafaxine HCl equivalent to venlafaxine base 75 mg. Nonmedicinal ingredients: ethylcellulose, gelatin, hydroxypropyl methylcellulose, iron oxide, microcrystalline cellulose, Opacode Red S-1-15034 ink, talc and titanium dioxide. Gluten-free. Bottles of 15, 90 and 100.
150 mg: Each extended release, hard gelatin capsule, with dark orange cap and body, with "W" and "Effexor XR" on the cap and "150" on the body, in white ink, contains: venlafaxine HCl equivalent to venlafaxine base 150 mg. Nonmedicinal ingredients: ethylcellulose, gelatin, hydroxypropyl methylcellulose, iron oxide, microcrystalline cellulose, talc, titanium dioxide and White Tek SB-0007. Gluten-free. Bottles of 15, 90 and 100.

(Shown in Product Identification Section)

Effient™ Ⓟ
prasugrel HCl
Platelet Aggregation Inhibitor

Lilly

Date of Preparation: April 16, 2010

SUMMARY PRODUCT INFORMATION:

Route of Administration	Dosage Form/Strength	All Nonmedicinal Ingredients
Oral	Tablet, 10 mg	Lactose, iron oxide yellow, iron oxide red, croscarmellose sodium, hypromellose, mannitol, microcrystalline cellulose, vegetable magnesium stearate, titanium dioxide, and triacetin

INDICATIONS AND CLINICAL USE: EFFIENT (prasugrel hydrochloride), coadministered with acetylsalicylic acid (ASA), is indicated for the early and long-term secondary prevention of atherothrombotic events in patients with acute coronary syndrome (ACS) who are to be managed with percutaneous coronary intervention (PCI) as follows:

- unstable angina (UA) or non-ST-segment elevation myocardial infarction (NSTEMI) managed with PCI
- ST-segment elevation myocardial infarction (STEMI) managed with primary or delayed PCI.

Geriatrics (≥75 years of age): EFFIENT is not recommended in patients ≥75 years of age because of the increased risk of fatal and intracranial bleeding (see Warnings and Precautions, Adverse Reactions and Action and Clinical Pharmacology).
Pediatrics (<18 years of age): No data is available on the safety and efficacy of EFFIENT in children below the age of 18. Use in this population is not recommended (see Warnings and Precautions and Action and Clinical Pharmacology).
CONTRAINDICATIONS: EFFIENT (prasugrel hydrochloride) is contraindicated in:

- patients with a known history of transient ischemic attack (TIA) or stroke (see Adverse Reactions).
- patients with active pathological bleeding, such as peptic ulcer or intracranial hemorrhage.
- patients with severe hepatic impairment (Child-Pugh Class C) (see Dosage and Administration and Action and Clinical Pharmacology).

- patients who are hypersensitive to this drug or to any ingredient in the formulation or component of the container (see Dosage Forms, Composition and Packaging).

WARNINGS AND PRECAUTIONS:

> **Risk of Bleeding**
> EFFIENT increases the risk of bleeding.
> - In patients ≥75 years of age, EFFIENT is not recommended because of the increased risk of fatal and intracranial bleeding (see Warnings and Precautions, Special Populations, Adverse Reactions and Action and Clinical Pharmacology).
> - In patients with body weight <60 kg, EFFIENT is not recommended because of increased risk of major bleeding. This is due to an increase in exposure to the active metabolite of prasugrel (see Warnings and Precautions, Special Populations, Adverse Reactions and Action and Clinical Pharmacology).

In addition, use EFFIENT cautiously in patients:

- with a propensity to bleed (e.g. due to recent trauma, recent surgery, recent or recurrent gastrointestinal (GI) bleeding, active peptic ulcer disease, or severe hepatic impairment) (see Adverse Reactions and Action and Clinical Pharmacology).
- with concomitant administration of medications that may increase the risk of bleeding, including oral anticoagulants, non steroidal anti-inflammatory drugs (NSAIDs), and fibrinolytics (see Action and Clinical Pharmacology).

If a patient is to undergo elective surgery and an antiplatelet effect is not desired, EFFIENT should be discontinued at least 7 days prior to surgery (see Action and Clinical Pharmacology).

For patients with active bleeding for whom reversal of the pharmacological effects of EFFIENT is required, platelet transfusion may be appropriate.

Discontinuation of EFFIENT: In patients with ACS who are managed with PCI, premature discontinuation of any antiplatelet medication, including EFFIENT, could result in an increased risk of thrombosis, myocardial infarction, or death due to the patient's underlying disease. Patients who require premature discontinuation of EFFIENT (e.g. secondary to active bleeding) should be monitored for atherothrombotic events. Once the patient is stabilized, at the discretion of the patient's treating physician, EFFIENT should be restarted as soon as possible.

Gastrointestinal: EFFIENT should be used with caution in patients with recent or recurrent gastrointestinal bleeding.

Hematologic: Thrombotic Thrombocytopenic Purpura (TTP) has been reported with the use of other thienopyridines. TTP is a serious condition and requires prompt treatment. EFFIENT administration was not associated with TTP in clinical trials supporting registration, which included over 7500 EFFIENT-treated patients.

Hepatic: No dosage adjustment is necessary in subjects with mild to moderate hepatic impairment (Child-Pugh Class A and B). The pharmacokinetics and pharmacodynamics of EFFIENT in patients with severe hepatic disease (Child-Pugh Class C) have not been studied. EFFIENT should not be used in this population due to the potential risk of bleeding (see Contraindications and Action and Clinical Pharmacology).

Neoplasms: During TRITON-TIMI 38, newly diagnosed malignancies were reported in 1.6% and 1.2% of patients treated with prasugrel and clopidogrel, respectively. The sites contributing to the differences were primarily colon and lung. These observations are yet to be confirmed as either causally-related or random occurrences. The non-clinical studies were negative for carcinogenicity and tumour stimulation. Bleeding in patients taking antiplatelet therapy warrants diagnostic investigation since it may unmask a previously unsuspected lesion (e.g. tumour, ulcer).

Peri-Operative Considerations: If a patient is to undergo elective surgery and an antiplatelet effect is not desired, EFFIENT should be discontinued at least 7 days prior to surgery (see Action and Clinical Pharmacology).

Renal: No dosage adjustment is necessary for patients with renal impairment, including patients with end-stage renal disease (see Action and Clinical Pharmacology).

Special Populations: Pregnant Women: There are no adequate and well-controlled studies in pregnant women.

Because animal reproduction studies are not always predictive of a human response, EFFIENT should be used during pregnancy only if the potential benefit to the mother justifies the potential risk to the fetus.

In embryo fetal developmental toxicology studies in rats and rabbits at doses up to 300 mg/kg/day (>240 times the recommended daily human maintenance dose on a mg/m² basis), there was no evidence of malformations.

Non Teratogenic Effects: At doses causing effects on maternal body weight and/or food consumption in rats and rabbits (300 mg/kg/day), a slight decrease in offspring body weight (relative to controls) was observed.

In prenatal and postnatal rat studies, maternal treatment with EFFIENT had no effect on fertility of male and female offspring at oral doses up to 300 mg/kg per day.

Nursing Women: There are no clinical studies in lactating women. A study in rats has shown that prasugrel metabolites are excreted in the animals' milk. It is not known whether this drug is excreted in human milk. Because many drugs are excreted in human milk and because of the potential for serious adverse reactions in nursing infants, EFFIENT should not be used by lactating women.

Pediatrics (<18 of age): Safety and effectiveness in pediatric patients have not been established.

Geriatrics (≥75 years of age): Of the total number of EFFIENT-treated patients in TRITON, 13.2% were ≥75 years of age. Individuals ≥75 years of age had an increased risk of bleeding (including fatal and intracranial bleeding). Due to an increase in exposure to the active metabolite of prasugrel and possibly a greater sensitivity to bleeding in patients ≥75 years of age compared to patients <75 years of age, the use of EFFIENT in this population is not recommended (see Adverse Reactions and Action and Clinical Pharmacology).

Body weight: Of the total number of EFFIENT patients in the TRITON study, 4.6% had body weight <60 kg. Individuals with body weight <60 kg had an increased risk of bleeding and an increased exposure to the active metabolite of prasugrel. For patients <60 kg, EFFIENT is not recommended (see Adverse Reactions and Action and Clinical Pharmacology).

Ethnicity: No dose adjustment is necessary based on ethnicity alone (see Action and Clinical Pharmacology).

ADVERSE REACTIONS: Adverse Drug Reaction Overview: In the All ACS population of Study TAAL, the percent of Treatment Emergent Adverse Events (TEAEs) (80.34% versus 80.02%), Serious Adverse Events (SAEs) (24.70% versus 24.26%), and prespecified clinically significant TEAEs (13.40% versus 12.25%) were similar for the prasugrel- and clopidogrel-treated groups, respectively. Similar results were seen between the UA/NSTEMI and the STEMI populations for both treatment groups.

The 3 most frequently reported common (occurring at an incidence of ≥1%) hemorrhagic TEAEs (preferred terms) in both treatment groups were contusion, hematoma, and epistaxis. Similar results were seen in the UA/NSTEMI and STEMI populations.

A total of 5213 (77.33%) prasugrel- and 5229 (77.86%) clopidogrel-treated subjects in TAAL experienced ≥1 non-hemorrhagic TEAE. In the All ACS population, the common non-hemorrhagic TEAEs of pyrexia and a greater tendency to bruise (preferred terms), coronary revascularization, fatigue, MI, musculoskeletal pain, constipation, and cardiac failure (preferred terms) were reported. The majority of non-hemorrhagic TEAEs were mild to moderate in severity, and the incidence was comparable between subjects treated with prasugrel and those treated with clopidogrel.

Gastrointestinal hemorrhage (preferred term) was the only commonly reported hemorrhagic SAE for either prasugrel- or clopidogrel-treated subjects in the All ACS UA/NSTEMI, and STEMI populations.

The non-hemorrhagic SAE of non-cardiac chest pain, coronary artery restenosis, chest pain, and angina pectoris were commonly reported by both prasugrel- and clopidogrel-treated subjects in the All ACS population.

Drug Discontinuation: The rate of study drug discontinuation due to adverse events was 7.2% for EFFIENT and 6.3% for clopidogrel. Of these, bleeding was the most common adverse reaction for both drugs leading to study drug discontinuation (2.5% for EFFIENT and 1.4% for clopidogrel).

Clinical Trial Adverse Drug Reactions: Because clinical trials are conducted under very specific conditions the adverse reaction rates observed in the clinical trials may not reflect the rates observed in practice and should not be compared to the rates in the clinical trials of another drug. Adverse drug reaction information from clinical trials is useful for identifying drug-related adverse events and for approximating rates.

TRITON (TAAL/TIMI 38 Trial): During clinical development, 7681 patients with atherosclerosis with or without ACS who did or did not undergo PCI were exposed to EFFIENT in 5 studies using clopidogrel as the comparator.

Safety in patients with ACS undergoing PCI was evaluated in a clopidogrel-controlled study, TRITON, in which 6741 patients were treated with EFFIENT (60 mg loading dose and 10 mg once daily maintenance dose) for a median of 14.5 months (5802 patients were treated for over 6 months; 4136 patients were treated for more than 1 year). The population was 27 to 96 years of age, 25% female, and 92% Caucasian. The TRITON protocol provided for all patients to receive aspirin. The dose of clopidogrel in this study was 300 mg loading dose and 75 mg once daily maintenance dose.

Bleeding: Non-Coronary Artery Bypass Graft (CABG) Related Bleeding: In TRITON, the frequency of patients experiencing a non-CABG-related bleeding event is shown in Table 1. The most common site of spontaneous non-CABG-related Thrombolysis in Myocardial Infarction (TIMI) Major or Minor bleeding was the GI tract (1.7% rate with EFFIENT and 1.3% rate with clopidogrel); the most frequent site of provoked bleeding was the arterial puncture site (1.3% rate with EFFIENT and 1.2% with clopidogrel).

Table 1: EFFIENT

TRITON Incidence of Non-CABG Related Bleeding[a] (% Patients) for All ACS, UA/NSTEMI and STEMI

	All ACS		UA/NSTEMI		STEMI	
Event	**EFFIENT[b] +ASA (N=6741)**	**Clopidogrel[b] +ASA (N=6716)**	**EFFIENT[b] +ASA (N=5001)**	**Clopidogrel[b] +ASA (N=4980)**	**EFFIENT[b] +ASA (N=1740)**	**Clopidogrel[b] +ASA (N=1736)**
TIMI Major bleeding[c]	2.2	1.7	2.2	1.6	2.2	2.0
Life-threatening[d]	1.3	0.8	1.3	0.8	1.2	1.0
Fatal	0.3	0.1	0.3	0.1	0.4	0.1
Symptomatic ICH[e]	0.3	0.3	0.3	0.3	0.2	0.2
Requiring inotropes	0.3	0.1	0.3	0.1	0.3	0.2
Requiring surgical intervention	0.3	0.3	0.3	0.3	0.1	0.2
Requiring transfusion (≥4 units)	0.7	0.5	0.6	0.3	0.8	0.8
TIMI Minor bleeding[f]	2.4	1.9	2.3	1.6	2.7	2.6

[a] Centrally adjudicated events defined by the TIMI Study Group criteria.
[b] Other standard therapies were used as appropriate. The TRITON protocol provided for all patients to receive aspirin.
[c] Any intracranial hemorrhage or any clinically overt bleeding associated with a fall in hemoglobin ≥5 g/dL.
[d] Life-threatening is a subset of TIMI Major bleeding and includes the types indented below. Patients may be counted in more than one row.
[e] ICH=intracranial hemorrhage.
[f] Clinically overt bleeding associated with a fall in hemoglobin of ≥3 g/dL but <5 g/dL.

Patients <60 kg: In TRITON, non-CABG-related TIMI Major or Minor bleeding rates for patients in two weight groups were as follows (see Dosage and Administration and Warnings and Precautions):

Weight	EFFIENT	Clopidogrel
<60 kg (N=664)	10.1% (0% fatal)	6.5% (0.3% fatal)
≥60 kg (N=12 672)	4.2% (0.3% fatal)	3.3% (0.1% fatal)

Geriatrics (≥75 years): In TRITON, non-CABG-related TIMI Major or Minor bleeding rates for patients in two age groups were as follows (see Dosage and Administration and Warnings and Precautions):

Age	EFFIENT	Clopidogrel
≥75 years (N=1785)	9.0% (1.0% fatal)	6.9% (0.1% fatal)
<75 years (N=11 672)	3.8% (0.2% fatal)	2.9% (0.1% fatal)

CABG-Related Bleeding: In TRITON, 437 patients underwent CABG during the course of the study. Of those patients, the rate of CABG-related TIMI Major or Minor bleeding was 14.1% for the EFFIENT group and 4.5% in the clopidogrel group. The higher risk for bleeding events in subjects treated with EFFIENT persisted up to 7 days from the most recent dose of study drug.

Bleeding Reported as Adverse Reactions: Table 2 shows the incidence of hemorrhagic adverse reactions.

Table 2: EFFIENT

Hemorrhagic Adverse Reactions with an Incidence in the EFFIENT Group of ≥1% in TRITON

MedDRA Preferred Term	EFFIENT	Clopidogrel
Contusion	6.9	3.9
Hematoma	6.5	5.6
Epistaxis	6.2	3.3
Ecchymosis	2.2	1.7
Vessel Puncture Site Hematoma	2.0	1.6
Puncture Site Hemorrhage	1.8	1.3
Hematuria	1.5	1.3
Gastrointestinal Hemorrhage[a]	1.5	1.0

[a] Approximately 50% of patients experiencing GI bleeding had GI pathology.

Other Adverse Reactions: In TRITON, non-hemorrhagic adverse drug reactions for EFFIENT and clopidogrel, respectively, are as follows: rash (2.8%, 2.4%) and anemia (2.2%, 2.0%).

In TRITON, in patients with or without a history of TIA or stroke, the incidence of stroke was as follows:

History of TIA or stroke	EFFIENT	Clopidogrel
Yes (N=518)	6.5% (2.3% ICH[a])	1.2% (0% ICH[a])
No (N=13 090)	0.9% (0.2% ICH[a])	1.0% (0.3% ICH[a])

[a] ICH=Intracranial hemorrhage.

EFFIENT-treated patients with a history of TIA or a history of ischemic stroke more than 3 months prior to randomization had a higher rate of ischemic or hemorrhagic stroke compared to clopidogrel-treated patients. Patients with a history of ischemic stroke within 3 months of randomization or hemorrhagic stroke were excluded from TRITON. EFFIENT has not been studied without aspirin (ASA) in patients with prior history of TIA or stroke.

Neoplasms: During TRITON-TIMI 38, newly diagnosed malignancies were reported in 1.6% and 1.2% of patients treated with prasugrel and clopidogrel, respectively. The sites contributing to the differences were primarily colon and lung. These observations are yet to be confirmed as either causally-related or random occurrences. The non-clinical studies were negative for carcinogenicity and tumour stimulation. Bleeding in patients taking antiplatelet therapy warrants diagnostic investigation since it may unmask a previously unsuspected lesion (e.g. tumour, ulcer).

Less Common Clinical Trial Adverse Drug Reactions (<1%): Additional important hemorrhagic reactions in TRITON for EFFIENT and clopidogrel, respectively, are as follows: rectal hemorrhage (0.6%, 0.3%), hemoptysis (0.6%, 0.5%), gingival bleeding (0.5%, 0.6%), hematochezia (0.5%, 0.4%), subcutaneous hematoma (0.5%, 0.2%), postprocedural hemorrhage (0.5%, 0.2%), retroperitoneal hemorrhage (0.3%, 0.2%), and eye hemorrhage (0.2%, 0.1%).

DRUG INTERACTIONS: Warfarin: Because of the potential for increased risk of bleeding, warfarin and EFFIENT should be coadministered with caution (see Action and Clinical Pharmacology).

Nonsteroidal Anti-Inflammatory Drugs (NSAIDs): Concomitant administration with chronic NSAIDs has not been studied. Because of the potential for increased risk of bleeding, chronic NSAIDs and EFFIENT should be coadministered with caution (see Action and Clinical Pharmacology).

Other Concomitant Medications: EFFIENT can be concomitantly administered with drugs metabolized by cytochrome P450 enzymes (including statins) or with drugs that are inducers or inhibitors of cytochrome P450 enzymes (see Action and Clinical Pharmacology).

EFFIENT can also be concomitantly administered with aspirin, heparin, digoxin, and drugs that elevate gastric pH, including proton pump inhibitors and H_2 blockers (see Action and Clinical Pharmacology).

Potential for Other Drugs to Affect EFFIENT: Acetylsalicylic Acid: ASA (150 mg daily with an additional single 900 mg) did not alter EFFIENT-mediated inhibition of platelet aggregation.

Heparin: A single intravenous dose of unfractionated heparin (100 U/kg) did not significantly alter the EFFIENT-mediated inhibition of platelet aggregation. Likewise, EFFIENT did not significantly alter the effect of heparin on measures of coagulation.

Statins: Atorvastatin (80 mg daily) did not alter the pharmacokinetics of EFFIENT and its inhibition of platelet aggregation. Therefore, statins that are substrates of CYP3A are not anticipated to have an effect on the pharmacokinetics of EFFIENT or its inhibition of platelet aggregation.

Drugs that Elevate Gastric pH: Daily coadministration of ranitidine (an H_2 blocker) or lansoprazole (a proton pump inhibitor) did not change the metabolite's AUC and T_{max}, but decreased the C_{max} by 14% and 29%, respectively. In TRITON, EFFIENT was administered without regard to coadministration of a proton pump inhibitor (PPI) or H_2 blocker with no significant effect on efficacy in prasugrel patients.

Nonsteroidal Anti-Inflammatory Drugs (NSAIDs): Concomitant administration with chronic NSAIDs has not been studied. Because of the potential for increased risk of bleeding, chronic NSAIDs and EFFIENT should be coadministered with caution (see Warnings and Precautions).

Inhibitors of CYP3A: Ketoconazole (400 mg daily), a selective and potent inhibitor of CYP3A4, did not affect EFFIENT-mediated inhibition of platelet aggregation or the active metabolite's AUC and T_{max}, but decreased the C_{max} by 34 to 46%. Therefore, CYP3A inhibitors such as verapamil, diltiazem, indinavir, ciprofloxacin, clarithromycin, and grapefruit juice are not anticipated to have a significant effect on the pharmacokinetics of the active metabolite.

Inducers of Cytochromes P450: Rifampicin (600 mg daily), a potent inducer of CYP3A and CYP2B6, and an inducer of CYP2C9, CYP2C19, and CYP2C8, did not significantly change the pharmacokinetics of EFFIENT and its inhibition of platelet aggregation. Therefore, known CYP3A inducers such as rifampicin, carbamazepine, and other inducers of cytochromes P450 are not anticipated to have significant effect on the pharmacokinetics of the active metabolite.

Clopidogrel: Following administration of 75 mg PLAVIX daily for 10 days, healthy subjects were placed on 10 mg daily of EFFIENT, with or without a 60 mg loading dose. Throughout the study, all subjects were concurrently taking 81 mg of aspirin once daily. Higher inhibition of platelet aggregation (p<0.001) was observed with EFFIENT with no increase in adverse reactions. Mean inhibition of platelet aggregation increased from 52 to 94% 1 hour after switching to the 60 mg loading dose of EFFIENT. After switching to 10 mg daily of EFFIENT without a loading dose, platelet aggregation increased gradually to the higher prasugrel-mediated steady state inhibition (about 70%) in 4 to 5 days.

Potential for EFFIENT to Affect Other Drugs: In vitro metabolism studies demonstrate that EFFIENT's main circulating metabolites are not likely to cause clinically significant inhibition of CYP1A2, CYP2C9, CYP2C19, CYP2D6, or CYP3A, or induction of CYP1A2 or CYP3A.

Drugs Metabolized by CYP2C9 and 2C19: EFFIENT did not inhibit CYP2C9 or CYP2C19, as it did not affect the pharmacokinetics of S-warfarin or R-warfarin. Because of the potential for increased risk of bleeding, warfarin and EFFIENT should be coadministered with caution (see Warnings and Precautions).

Drugs Metabolized by CYP2B6: EFFIENT is a weak inhibitor of CYP2B6. In healthy subjects, EFFIENT decreased exposure to hydroxybupropion, a CYP2B6-mediated metabolite of bupropion, by 23%, which is not considered to be clinically significant. EFFIENT is not anticipated to have significant effect on the pharmacokinetics of drugs that are primarily metabolized by CYP2B6, such as halothane, cyclophosphamide, propofol, and nevirapine.

Effect on Digoxin: EFFIENT has no clinically significant effect on the pharmacokinetics of digoxin. When EFFIENT was coadministered with digoxin, a substrate of P-glycoprotein transporter, the AUC of digoxin was not altered, while C_{max} decreased by 17%.

Drug-Food Interactions: EFFIENT can be administered without regard to food (see Action and Clinical Pharmacology).

Drug-Herb Interactions: Interactions with herbal products have not been established.

Drug-Laboratory Test Interactions: Interactions with laboratory tests have not been established.

DOSAGE AND ADMINISTRATION: Recommended Dose and Dosage Adjustment: EFFIENT should be initiated with a single 60 mg loading dose and then continued at a 10 mg once daily dose for long-term treatment. Patients taking EFFIENT should also take ASA (75 mg to 325 mg) daily.

Clinical trial data demonstrate the benefit of long-term treatment with EFFIENT coadministered with ASA, compared with clopidogrel coadministered with ASA.

EFFIENT may be administered with or without food (see Action and Clinical Pharmacology).

It is generally recommended that antiplatelet therapy be administered promptly in the management of ACS because many cardiovascular events occur within hours of initial presentation. In the clinical trial that established the efficacy of EFFIENT, EFFIENT and the control drug were not administered to UA/NSTEMI patients until coronary anatomy was established. For the small fraction of patients that required urgent CABG after treatment with EFFIENT, the risk of significant bleeding was substantial (see Warnings and Precautions). Because the large majority of patients are managed without CABG, however, treatment can be considered before determining coronary anatomy if need for CABG is considered unlikely. The advantages of earlier treatment with EFFIENT must then be balanced against the increased rate of bleeding in patients who do need to undergo urgent CABG.

Missed Dose: If a scheduled daily dose of EFFIENT is missed, it should be taken as soon as possible. If the doses for an entire day are forgotten, resume taking EFFIENT at its usual dose the next day. Do not take two doses at the same time.

Discontinuation of EFFIENT: In patients with ACS who are managed with PCI, premature discontinuation of any antiplatelet medication, including EFFIENT, could result in an increased risk of thrombosis, myocardial infarction, or death due to the patient's underlying disease. Patients who require premature discontinuation of EFFIENT (e.g. secondary to active bleeding) should be monitored for atherothrombotic events. Once the patient is stabilized, at the discretion of the patient's treating physician, EFFIENT should be restarted as soon as possible.

If a patient is to undergo elective surgery and an antiplatelet effect is not desired, EFFIENT should be discontinued at least 7 days prior to surgery (see Action and Clinical Pharmacology).

OVERDOSAGE:

Signs and Symptoms: Overdose following EFFIENT administration may lead to prolonged bleeding time and subsequent bleeding complications. In rats, lethality was observed only after administration of the very high dose of 2000 mg/kg. Symptoms of acute toxicity in dogs included emesis, increased serum alkaline phosphatase, and hepatocellular atrophy. Symptoms of acute toxicity in rats included mydriasis, irregular respiration, decreased locomotor activity, ptosis, staggering gait, and lacrimation. Platelet inhibition by prasugrel is rapid and irreversible, lasting for the life of the platelet, and is unlikely to be increased in the event of an overdose.

Treatment: No data are available on the reversal of the pharmacological effect of EFFIENT; however, based on biological plausibility, platelet transfusion and/or other blood products may be considered.

For management of a suspected drug overdose, contact your regional Poison Control Centre. See the *CPS* Directory section for a list of Poison Control Centres.

ACTION AND CLINICAL PHARMACOLOGY: Mechanism of Action: EFFIENT is an inhibitor of platelet activation and aggregation through the irreversible binding of its active metabolite to the $P2Y_{12}$ class of ADP receptors on platelets. A variety of drugs that inhibit platelet function have been shown to decrease morbid events in people with established atherosclerotic disease. Since platelets participate in the initiation and/or evolution of thrombotic complications of atherosclerotic disease, inhibition of platelet function can result in the reduction of the rate of cardiovascular events such as death, myocardial infarction, or stroke.

Pharmacodynamics: Inhibition of ADP-induced platelet aggregation to 20 μM or 5 μM ADP (termed "platelet inhibition" in the following section) measured by light transmission aggregometry has been assessed in clinical pharmacology studies in healthy subjects and patients with stable atherosclerosis for both EFFIENT and clopidogrel used as active comparator with or without aspirin. Following a 60 mg loading dose of EFFIENT, platelet inhibition occurred as early as 30 minutes and 15 minutes, respectively for 20 μM and 5 μM ADP (see Figure 1). This rapid onset of action is a result of the rapid biotransformation of EFFIENT to its active metabolite which is responsible for the inhibition of platelet aggregation.

Mean maximum platelet inhibition after a 60 mg loading dose of EFFIENT was 79% and 83%, respectively for 20 μM and 5 μM ADP, with ≥89% of all subjects achieving at least 50% inhibition of platelet aggregation by 1 hour for both ADP concentrations.

Mean steady state inhibition of platelet aggregation (IPA) was 69% and 74%, respectively for 20 μM and 5 μM ADP, and was achieved following 3 to 5 days of 10 mg maintenance dosing with a preceding loading dose of EFFIENT. Greater than 98% of subjects had ≥20% inhibition of platelet aggregation during maintenance dosing. The extent of inhibition of platelet aggregation is dependent on the dose of EFFIENT and exposure of the active metabolite.

EFFIENT-mediated inhibition of platelet aggregation exhibited low between-subject (9%) and within-subject (12%) variability (standard deviation) in both 20 μM and 5 μM ADP. Platelet aggregation gradually returned to baseline values after treatment in 7 to 9 days following a single 60 mg loading dose of EFFIENT and in 5 days following discontinuation of maintenance dosing at steady state.

Figure 1: EFFIENT

Least Square Mean (±95% CI) Inhibition of 20 μM and 5 μM ADP-induced Platelet Aggregation (IPA) Measured by Light Transmission Aggregometry after EFFIENT 60 mg/10 mg (o) Loading Dose and Maintenance Dose and Clopidogrel 300 mg/75 mg (•), respectively. Arrows (↓) Indicate Day of Dose Administration

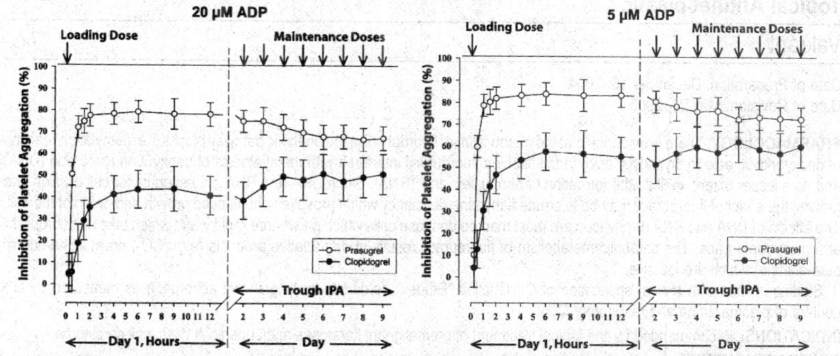

The IPA achieved in response to prasugrel was significantly higher than that observed for clopidogrel responders. Among clopidogrel responders, the onset of IPA was still slower than that achieved following administration of prasugrel (Study TAAJ). Prasugrel 10 mg MD produced significantly greater IPA (p<.01) than the approved 75 mg clopidogrel MD. The prasugrel 60 mg LD also achieved significantly more rapid onset and greater levels of IPA (p<.001) (20 μM ADP) than the clopidogrel 300 mg LD (Studies TAAA and TAAE). A 60/10 mg LD/MD of prasugrel provided more rapid onset (beginning 30 minutes following LD) of higher and less variable IPA than was achieved with 600/75 mg or 600/150 mg LD/MD of clopidogrel in patients undergoing PCI (Studies TABR and TABL). The 60 mg LD doubled the level of IPA compared to the 300 mg LD of clopidogrel. In addition, there were ≤3% PD poor responders with the prasugrel 60 mg LD compared to approximately 52% PD poor responders for the clopidogrel 300 mg LD. During maintenance dosing there were 0% PD poor responders with prasugrel 10 mg MD compared to 45% in the clopidogrel 75 mg MD group (Study TAAD). Based on the results of these studies, a prasugrel 60 mg LD and a daily 10 mg MD were selected for Study TAAL (Study TAAH). In a Phase 2 study (Study TABN), subjects with ACS received a 900 mg loading dose of clopidogrel. They were then randomly assigned to prasugrel 10 mg or clopidogrel 150 mg as a daily maintenance dose (MD) for 14±2 days. Subjects were then switched directly (without a washout period) to the alternative MD treatment for an additional 14±2 days. The prasugrel 10 mg MD regimen resulted in significantly greater platelet inhibition than clopidogrel 150 mg MD or a 900 mg LD.

Pharmacokinetics: EFFIENT is a prodrug and is rapidly metabolized to a pharmacologically active metabolite and inactive metabolites. The active metabolite's exposure (AUC) has moderate to low between-subject (27%) and within-subject (19%) variability. EFFIENT's pharmacokinetics are similar in healthy subjects, patients with stable atherosclerosis, and patients undergoing percutaneous coronary intervention.

Absorption: Following oral administration, ≥79% of the dose is absorbed. The absorption and metabolism are rapid, with peak plasma concentrations (C_{max}) of the active metabolite occurring approximately 30 minutes after dosing. The active metabolite's exposure (AUC) increases proportionally over the therapeutic dose range. In a study of healthy subjects, AUC of the active metabolite was unaffected by a high fat, high calorie meal, but C_{max} was decreased by 49% and the time to reach C_{max} (T_{max}) was increased from 0.5 to 1.5 hours. EFFIENT was administered without regard to food in TRITON. Therefore, EFFIENT can be administered without regard to food.

Distribution: The active metabolite binding to human serum albumin (4% buffered solution) was 98%.

Metabolism: EFFIENT is not detected in plasma following oral administration. It is rapidly hydrolyzed in the intestine to a thiolactone, which is then converted to the active metabolite by a single step of cytochrome P450 metabolism, primarily by CYP3A4 and CYP2B6 and to a lesser extent by CYP2C9 and CYP2C19. The active metabolite is further metabolized to two inactive compounds by S-methylation or conjugation with cysteine.

In healthy subjects, patients with stable atherosclerosis, and patients with ACS receiving EFFIENT, there was no relevant effect of genetic variation in CYP3A5, CYP2B6, CYP2C9, or CYP2C19 on the pharmacokinetics of EFFIENT or its inhibition of platelet aggregation.

Excretion: Approximately 68% of the EFFIENT dose is excreted in the urine and 27% in the feces, as inactive metabolites. The active metabolite has an elimination half-life of about 7.4 hours (range 2 to 15 hours).

Pharmacogenomics: Both prasugrel and clopidogrel are pro-drugs that must be metabolized to their active moieties. Whereas the pharmacokinetics of prasugrel's active metabolite are not known to be affected by genetic variations in CYP2B6, CYP2C9, CYP2C19, or CYP3A5, the pharmacokinetics of clopidogrel's active metabolite are affected by CYP2C19 genotype, and approximately 30% of Caucasians, 40% of African descent, and 60% of Asians are reduced-metabolizers.

Special Populations and Conditions: Pediatrics (<18 of age): Pharmacokinetics and pharmacodynamics of EFFIENT have not been evaluated in a pediatric population.

Geriatrics (≥75 years of age): In a study of 32 healthy subjects between the ages of 20 and 80 years, age had no significant effect on pharmacokinetics of EFFIENT or its inhibition of platelet aggregation. In TRITON, the mean exposure (AUC) of the active metabolite was 19% higher in patients ≥75 years of age compared to patients <75 years of age. Due to an increase in exposure to the active metabolite of prasugrel and possibly a greater sensitivity to bleeding in patients ≥75 years of age compared to patients <75 years of age, EFFIENT is not recommended in this patient population (see Warnings and Precautions and Adverse Reactions).

Gender: Pharmacokinetics of EFFIENT are similar in men and women.

Race: In clinical pharmacology studies, after adjusting for body weight, the AUC of the active metabolite was approximately 19% higher in Chinese, Japanese, and Korean subjects compared to Caucasian subjects. Within the Chinese, Japanese, and Korean subjects there was no difference in exposure amongst these groups. Exposure in subjects of African and Hispanic descent is comparable to that of Caucasians.

Hepatic Insufficiency: Pharmacokinetics of EFFIENT and its inhibition of platelet aggregation were similar in subjects with mild to moderate hepatic impairment compared to healthy subjects.

Pharmacokinetics and pharmacodynamics of EFFIENT in patients with severe hepatic disease (Child-Pugh Class C) have not been studied. EFFIENT should not be used due to the potential risk of bleeding in this population (see Contraindications and Warnings and Precautions).

Renal Insufficiency: Pharmacokinetics of EFFIENT and its inhibition of platelet aggregation are similar in patients with moderate renal impairment (CrCL=30 to 50 mL/min) and healthy subjects. EFFIENT-mediated inhibition of platelet aggregation was also similar in patients with end-stage renal disease (ESRD) who required hemodialysis compared to healthy subjects, although C_{max} and AUC of the active metabolite decreased 51% and 42%, respectively, in ESRD patients (see Warnings and Precautions).

Body Weight: The mean exposure (AUC) of the active metabolite is approximately 30 to 40% higher in healthy subjects with a body weight of <60 kg compared to those weighing ≥60 kg. Individuals with body weight <60 kg had an increased risk of bleeding and an increased exposure to the active metabolite of prasugrel. EFFIENT is not recommended in this patient population (see Warnings and Precautions and Adverse Reactions).

Smoking: Pharmacokinetics of EFFIENT are similar in smokers and non-smokers.

STORAGE AND STABILITY: Store at 25°C; excursions permitted to 15 to 30°C. Dispense product in original packaging. Keep product in package and do not remove until ready to use. Do not break the tablet.

SPECIAL HANDLING INSTRUCTIONS: Store product in original blister packaging.

INFORMATION FOR THE PATIENT: Published in e-CPS, available by subscription at www.e-cps.ca.

DOSAGE FORMS, COMPOSITION AND PACKAGING: Each beige, double-arrow-shaped, film-coated, not scored tablet, debossed with "10 MG" on one side and "4759" on the other side contains: prasugrel hydrochloride10.98 mg equivalent to prasugrel 10 mg. During manufacture and storage prasugrel hydrochloride undergoes partial conversion to prasugrel free base to within controlled limits. Nonmedicinal ingredients: croscarmellose sodium, hypromellose, mannitol, microcrystalline cellulose and vegetable magnesium stearate; color coatings: hypromellose, iron oxide red, iron oxide yellow, lactose, titanium dioxide and triacetin. Blister packages of 28 (2×14) and 30 (5×6).

(Shown in Product Identification Section)

Efudex® Ⓟ

fluorouracil

Topical Antineoplastic

Valeant

Date of Preparation: December 15, 2004
Date of Revision: May 24, 2005

PHARMACOLOGY: There is evidence that the metabolism of fluorouracil in the anabolic pathway blocks the methylation reaction of deoxyuridylic acid to thymidylic acid. In this fashion fluorouracil interferes with the synthesis of deoxyribonucleic acid (DNA) and, to a lesser extent, inhibits the formation of ribonucleic acid (RNA). Since DNA and RNA are essential for cell division and growth, the effect of fluorouracil may be to create a thymine deficiency which provokes unbalanced growth and death of the cell. The effects of DNA and RNA deprivation are most marked on those cells which grow more rapidly and which take up fluorouracil at a more rapid pace. The catabolic metabolism of fluorouracil results in degradative products (e.g., CO_2, urea, alpha-fluoro-beta-alanine) which are inactive.

Studies in man with topical application of C^{14}-labelled "Efudex" demonstrate insignificant absorption as measured by C^{14} content of plasma, urine and respiratory CO_2.

INDICATIONS: Recommended for the topical treatment of premalignant keratoses and superficial basal cell carcinoma.

CONTRAINDICATIONS: In patients with known hypersensitivity to any of its components.

WARNINGS: If an occlusive dressing is used, there may be an increase in the incidence of inflammatory reactions in the adjacent normal skin.

Prolonged exposure to ultraviolet light should be avoided while under treatment with fluorouracil because the intensity of the reaction may be increased.

Pregnancy: Since fluorouracil is known to have teratogenic properties, the potential value of its use in women of child-bearing potential should be weighed against the risks involved.

Appropriate therapy for pre-existing concomitant inflammatory dermatoses should be instituted before using the drug.

PRECAUTIONS: The cream is preferably applied with a nonmetal applicator or suitable glove; if it is applied with the fingertips, the hands should be washed immediately afterward. Fluorouracil should be applied with care near the eyes, nostrils and mouth. To rule out the presence of a frank neoplasm, a biopsy should be made of those lesions failing to respond to treatment or recurring after treatment.

ADVERSE EFFECTS: The most frequently encountered local reactions are pain, pruritus, hyperpigmentation and burning at the site of application. Other local reactions include dermatitis, scarring, soreness and tenderness. Insomnia, stomatitis, suppuration, scaling, swelling, irritability, medicinal taste, photosensitivity and lacrimation have also been reported.

Laboratory abnormalities reported include leukocytosis, thrombocytopenia, toxic granulation and eosinophilia.

OVERDOSE:

Symptoms: Since fluorouracil is applied topically, it is highly unlikely that an overdosage would occur. In the event that this preparation is accidentally ingested, signs of toxicity may include diarrhea, stomatitis, thrombocytopenia (platelets <100 000) and leukopenia (WBC <3500).

Treatment: These symptoms may be ameliorated by leucovorin.

> For management of a suspected drug overdose, CPhA recommends that you contact your **regional Poison Control Centre**. See the *CPS* Directory section for a list of Poison Control Centres.

DOSAGE: The cream should be applied twice daily with a nonmetal applicator or suitable glove in an amount of the cream sufficient to cover the lesion. When applied to a lesion, a response occurs with the following sequence: erythema, usually followed by vesiculation, erosion, ulceration, necrosis and epithelization. The lower frequency and intensity of activity in adjacent normal skin indicate a selective cytotoxic property. Medication should be continued until the inflammatory reaction reaches the erosion, ulceration, and necrosis stage, at which time use of the drug should be terminated. The usual duration of therapy is from 2 to 4 weeks. Complete healing of the lesion may not be evident for 1 to 2 months following cessation of fluorouracil therapy.

While the patient is undergoing topical fluorouracil therapy, consideration can be given to curettage, wound excision and removal of pathological tissue.

INFORMATION FOR THE PATIENT: Published in e-CPS, available by subscription at www.e-cps.ca.

SUPPLIED: Each g of cream contains: fluorouracil 5% (50 mg/g) in a vanishing cream base. Nonmedicinal ingredients: methylparaben, polysorbate 60, propylene glycol, propylparaben, stearyl alcohol and white petrolatum. Sulfite-free. Tubes of 40 g. Store at 15 to 30°C. For external use only.

Elaprase™ Ⓟ

idursulfase

Enzyme Replacement Therapy

Paladin

Date of Preparation: June 13, 2007

SUMMARY PRODUCT INFORMATION:

Route of Administration	Dosage Form/ Strength	Clinically Relevant Nonmedicinal Ingredients
Intravenous (IV)	2 mg/mL concentrate for solution for infusion	None

INDICATIONS AND CLINICAL USE: ELAPRASE (idursulfase) is indicated for:

- enzyme replacement therapy in patients with Hunter syndrome (Mucopolysaccharidosis II, MPS II). ELAPRASE has been shown to improve walking capacity in these patients.

CONTRAINDICATIONS:

- Patients who are hypersensitive to this drug or to any ingredient in the formulation or component of the container. For a complete listing, see Dosage Forms, Composition and Packaging.

WARNINGS AND PRECAUTIONS:

> **Serious Warnings and Precautions**
> **Risk of hypersensitivity reactions.**
> **Anaphylactoid reactions, which have the potential to be life threatening, have been observed in some patients treated with ELAPRASE.**
> **Patients with compromised respiratory function or acute respiratory disease may be at risk of serious exacerbation of their respiratory dysfunction due to infusion related reactions. These patients require additional monitoring. Late-emergent anaphylactoid reactions have been observed after ELAPRASE administration. Patients who have experienced severe and refractory anaphylactoid reactions may require prolonged observation times.**
> **Due to the potential for severe infusion reactions appropriate medical support measures should be readily available when ELAPRASE is administered.**

General: ELAPRASE is not expected to affect the ability to drive or use machines.

A registry for patients with Hunter syndrome (the Hunter Outcome Survey) has been established in order to better understand the variability and progression of the disease and monitoring and evaluation of treatments. Patients should be encouraged to participate in the process and advised that their participation may involve a long-term follow-up. Information on the registry program may be obtained by calling 1-888-550-6060.

Hepatic: No studies have been performed in patients with hepatic impairment.

Immune: In clinical trials with ELAPRASE, 11 of 108 patients (10%) experienced anaphylactoid reactions during 19 of 8274 infusions (0.2%). Reactions have included respiratory distress, hypoxia, decreased blood pressure, angioedema, or seizure. If severe allergic or anaphylactoid reactions occur, it is recommended that the administration of ELAPRASE be discontinued immediately and appropriate treatment initiated. The current medical standards for emergency treatment are to be observed.

The most common infusion-related reactions included cutaneous reactions (rash, pruritus, and urticaria), pyrexia, headache, hypertension, and flushing. Infusion-related reactions were treated or ameliorated by slowing the infusion rate, interrupting the infusion, or by administration of medicines, such as antihistamines, antipyretics, low-dose corticosteroids (prednisone and methylprednisolone), or beta-agonist nebulization. Reactions were more severe in patients with compromised respiratory function or respiratory illnesses. No patient discontinued treatment with ELAPRASE due to an infusion reaction during clinical studies.

Special care should be taken when administering an infusion in patients with severe underlying airway disease. These patients should be closely monitored and infused with ELAPRASE in an appropriate clinical setting. Caution must be exercised in the management and treatment of such patients by limitation or careful monitoring of antihistamine and other sedative medication use.

Consider delaying ELAPRASE infusion in patients who present with an acute febrile respiratory illness.

Patients using supplemental oxygen should have this treatment readily available during infusion in the event of an infusion-related reaction.

Across clinical studies, 53/106 patients (50%) developed anti-idursulfase IgG antibodies at some point. Six (6) of the IgG positive patients also tested positive for IgM antibodies, and 2 patients tested positive for IgA antibodies. No patient developed IgE antibodies during any study. Fourteen (14) of the IgG positive patients had antibodies that demonstrated neutralizing activity in an in vitro assay. In the 53-week placebo-controlled study, rates of seropositivity peaked by Weeks 18 to 27 and steadily declined thereafter for the remainder of the study.

In general, patients who tested positive for IgG antibodies were more likely to have infusion-related adverse events than those who did not test positive. However, overall rates of infusion-related adverse events declined over time, regardless of antibody status.

Renal: No studies have been conducted in patients with renal impairment.

Special Populations: Pregnant Women: There is no experience with ELAPRASE treatment in pregnant women. Reproduction studies in pregnant female animals have not been conducted with ELAPRASE. It is not known whether idursulfase crosses the placenta.

Nursing Women: It is not known whether ELAPRASE is excreted in human milk.

Pediatrics and Geriatrics: Children, adolescents, and adults responded similarly to treatment with ELAPRASE. Studies in patients under the age of 5 and over the age of 65 have not been performed.

Monitoring and Laboratory Tests: No special laboratory tests are required for patients receiving ELAPRASE, other than the usual tests that are required for monitoring patients with Hunter syndrome.

ADVERSE REACTIONS: Adverse Drug Reaction Overview: Adverse reactions were commonly reported in association with infusions. The most common infusion-related reactions were headache, fever, cutaneous reactions (rash, pruritus, erythema, and urticaria), and hypertension. The frequency of infusion-related reactions decreased over time with continued ELAPRASE treatment. Adverse drug reactions (ADRs) that were reported during the 53-week placebo-controlled study were almost all mild to moderate in severity.

Clinical Trial Adverse Drug Reactions: Because clinical trials are conducted under very specific conditions the adverse reaction rates observed in the clinical trials may not reflect the rates observed in practice and should not be compared to the rates in the clinical trials of another drug. Adverse drug reaction information from clinical trials is useful for identifying drug-related adverse events and for approximating rates.

Table 1 lists those adverse drug reactions observed during the 53-week placebo-controlled study in the patients treated with 0.5 mg/kg weekly ELAPRASE compared to patients receiving placebo. Information is presented by system organ class and frequency. Frequency is given as very common (>1/10) or common (>1/100, <1/10). The occurrence of an event in a single patient is defined as common in view of the small number of patients treated in the trial.

Adverse drug reactions were defined in Table 1 as treatment-emergent events with suspected causality and excluded non-serious events that were reported only once in a single patient; treatment emergent events with an excess incidence of at least 9% compared with placebo were also considered as adverse drug reactions. Adverse reactions occurring only in placebo-treated patients are excluded. Note: All types of rash and all types of urticaria have been combined.

Table 1: ELAPRASE
Adverse Drug Reactions in the 53-week Placebo-controlled Clinical Trial (n (%))

System Organ Class	Adverse Drug Reaction (Preferred Term)	ELAPRASE 0.5 mg/kg Weekly (n=32)	Placebo (n=32)
Nervous System Disorders			
Very Common:	Headache	9 (28.1)	8 (25.0)
Common:	Dizziness	2 (6.3)	2 (6.3)
	Tremor	2 (6.3)	0
Eye Disorders			
Common:	Lacrimation increased	2 (6.3)	0
Cardiac Disorders			
Common:	Arrhythmia[a]	1 (3.1)	0
	Cyanosis	1 (3.1)	0
Vascular Disorders			

(cont'd)

Table 1: ELAPRASE *(cont'd)*

Adverse Drug Reactions in the 53-week Placebo-controlled Clinical Trial (n (%))

System Organ Class	Adverse Drug Reaction (Preferred Term)	ELAPRASE 0.5 mg/kg Weekly (n=32)	Placebo (n=32)
Very Common:	Hypertension	6 (18.8)	6 (18.8)
Common:	Flushing	3 (9.4)	3 (9.4)
	Hypotension	2 (6.3)	3 (9.4)
Respiratory, Thoracic and Mediastinal Disorders			
Common:	Cough	3 (9.4)	1 (3.1)
	Wheezing	2 (6.3)	0
	Tachypnoea	2 (6.3)	1 (3.1)
	Dyspnoea	1 (3.1)	1 (3.1)
	Bronchospasm	1 (3.1)	0
	Pulmonary embolism[a]	1 (3.1)	0
Gastrointestinal Disorders			
Very Common:	Dyspepsia	4 (12.5)	0
Common:	Nausea	3 (9.4)	3 (9.4)
	Abdominal pain	2 (6.3)	2 (6.3)
	Diarrhoea	2 (6.3)	1 (3.1)
	Swollen tongue	2 (6.3)	0
Skin and Subcutaneous Tissue Disorders			
Very Common:	Rash	8 (25.0)	6 (18.8)
	Pruritus	7 (21.9)	3 (9.4)
	Urticaria	5 (15.6)	0
Common:	Erythema	2 (6.3)	0
	Eczema	1 (3.1)	0
	Face oedema	1 (3.1)	0
Musculoskeletal and Connective Tissue Disorders			
Very Common:	Chest pain	7 (21.9)	0
Common:	Arthralgia	1 (3.1)	1 (3.1)
General Disorders and Administration Site Conditions			
Very Common:	Pyrexia	7 (21.9)	8 (25.0)
	Infusion site swelling	4 (12.5)	1 (3.1)
Common:	Oedema peripheral	2 (6.3)	0

[a] See serious adverse reactions below.

In clinical studies, serious adverse reactions were reported in a total of 5 patients who received 0.5 mg/kg of ELAPRASE weekly or every other week. Four patients experienced a hypoxic episode during one or several infusions, which necessitated oxygen therapy in 3 patients with severe underlying obstructive airway disease (2 with a tracheostomy). The most severe episode, which was associated with a short seizure, occurred in a patient who received his infusion while he had a febrile respiratory exacerbation. In this patient, who had less severe underlying disease, spontaneous resolution occurred shortly after the infusion was interrupted. These events did not recur with subsequent infusions using a slower infusion rate and administration of pre-infusion medication, usually with low-dose steroids, antihistamine, and beta-agonist nebulization. The fifth patient, who had pre-existing cardiopathy, was diagnosed with ventricular premature complexes and pulmonary embolism during the study.

Adverse drug reactions that occurred in the 0.5 mg/kg weekly ELAPRASE group with a frequency less than those included in Table 1 (single event reported) are listed here by MedDRA System Organ Class and preferred term:

Blood and Lymphatic System Disorders: anemia, lymphadenitis, thrombocytopenia.
Psychiatric Disorders: anxiety.
Nervous System Disorders: depressed level of consciousness, hyperaesthesia.
Eye Disorders: conjunctivitis allergic, vision blurred.
Ear and Labyrinth Disorders: vertigo.
Cardiac Disorders: palpitations.
Respiratory, Thoracic and Mediastinal Disorders: nasal congestion, pharyngitis, rhinorrhoea
Gastrointestinal Disorders: abdominal pain upper, gastroenteritis, loose stools.
Musculoskeletal and Connective Tissue Disorders: back pain, bone pain, muscle cramp, myalgia, neck pain.
Renal and Urinary Disorders: enuresis, nocturia.
General Disorders and Administration Site Conditions: feeling cold, inflammation localized, injection site joint swelling, malaise, pain, rigors, sensation of foreign body.
Investigations: blood alkaline phosphatase increased, blood bilirubin increased, blood lactate dehydrogenase increased, blood uric acid increased, haemoglobin decreased, heart rate decreased, heart rate increased.

Table 2 enumerates treatment emergent adverse events (regardless of investigator causality assessment) that occurred in the 53-week placebo-controlled clinical trial with a difference of more than 2 patients between the 0.5 mg/kg weekly ELAPRASE and placebo treatment groups. Reported frequencies of adverse events have been classified by MedDRA terms.

Across studies, 53/106 patients (50%) developed anti-idursulfase IgG antibodies at some point. Six (6) of the IgG positive patients also tested positive for IgM antibodies, and 2 patients tested positive for IgA antibodies. No patient developed IgE antibodies during any study. Fourteen (14) of the IgG positive patients had antibodies that demonstrated neutralizing activity in an in vitro assay. In the 53-week study, rates of seropositivity peaked by Weeks 18 to 27 and steadily declined thereafter for the remainder of this study.

Patients who tested positive for IgG antibodies at any time during the clinical trials had an increased incidence rate of infusion-related reactions, including hypersensitivity reactions. However, overall rates of infusion-related adverse events declined over time, regardless of antibody status. The reduction of urinary GAG excretion was somewhat less in patients for whom circulating anti-idursulfase antibodies were detected.

Table 2: ELAPRASE

Treatment Emergent Adverse Events with a Difference of More Than 2 Patients Between 0.5 mg/kg ELAPRASE Weekly and Placebo Treatment Groups (n (%))

System Organ Class	Adverse Event (Preferred Term)	ELAPRASE 0.5 mg/kg Weekly (n=32)	Placebo (n=32)
Infections and Infestations	Hordeolum	0	3 (9.4)
Psychiatric Disorders	Depression	3 (9.4)	0
Nervous System Disorders	Headache	19 (59.4)	14 (43.8)
	Dizziness	4 (12.5)	8 (25.0)
Ear and Labyrinth Disorders	Ear disorder	3 (9.4)	0
	Hypoacusis	1 (3.1)	4 (12.5)
Respiratory, Thoracic, and Mediastinal Disorders	Cough	16 (50.0)	19 (59.4)
	Pharyngitis	13 (40.6)	10 (31.3)
	Dyspnoea	4 (12.5)	9 (28.1)
	Epistaxis	2 (6.3)	5 (15.6)
Gastrointestinal Disorders	Diarrhoea	11 (34.4)	15 (46.9)
	Vomiting	8 (25.0)	16 (50.0)
	Abdominal pain upper	5 (15.6)	2 (6.3)
	Dyspepsia	4 (12.5)	0
Skin and Subcutaneous Tissue Disorders	Rash	14 (43.8)	11 (34.4)
	Pruritus	10 (31.3)	5 (15.6)
	Urticaria	5 (15.6)	0
	Acne	3 (9.4)	0
Musculoskeletal and Connective Tissue Disorders	Chest pain	7 (21.9)	0
General Disorders and Administration Site Conditions	Infusion site swelling	4 (12.5)	1 (3.1)
	Asthenia	3 (9.4)	0
	Fall	0	4 (12.5)
	Catheter site pain	0	3 (9.4)
Investigations	Alanine aminotransferase increased	0	4 (12.5)
	Aspartate aminotransferase increased	0	3 (9.4)
Injury, Poisoning, and Procedural Complications	Arthropod bite	3 (9.4)	0
	Abrasion	0	3 (9.4)

Post-Market Adverse Drug Reactions: In post-marketing experience, 2 patients have had symptoms and signs suggestive of late-emergent anaphylactoid reactions approximately 24 hours after treatment and recovery from an initial anaphylactoid reaction. These symptoms required treatment with inhaled beta-adrenergic agonists, epinephrine, anti-histamines, corticosteroids and hospitalization in 1 patient, and with corticosteroids in the second patient. With appropriate pre-treatment and monitoring, both patients continued weekly ELAPRASE treatments. Because of the potential for late-emergent anaphylactoid reactions, patients who experience initial severe or refractory reactions may require prolonged observation dependant on the clinical needs.

DRUG INTERACTIONS: No serious drug interactions have been reported.

Overview: Based on its metabolism in cellular lysosomes, idursulfase would not be a candidate for cytochrome P450 mediated drug-drug interactions.

Drug-Drug Interactions: No formal drug interaction studies have been conducted with ELAPRASE.

Drug-Food Interactions: Interactions with food have not been established.

Drug-Herb Interactions: Interactions with herbal products have not been established.

Drug-Laboratory Test Interactions: Interactions with laboratory tests have not been established.

DOSAGE AND ADMINISTRATION: Dosing Considerations:

- ELAPRASE (idursulfase) is intended for use under the supervision of a physician or other experienced health care provider.
- The infusion rate may be slowed and/or temporarily stopped, based on clinical judgment, when infusion-related reactions occur (see Administration).

Recommended Dose and Dosage Adjustment: ELAPRASE is administered at a dose of 0.5 mg/kg body weight every week by intravenous infusion.

Administration: The total volume of infusion may be administered over a period of 1 to 3 hours. Patients may require longer infusion times due to infusion reactions; however, infusion times should not exceed 8 hours. The initial infusion rate should be 8 mL/hr for the first 15 minutes. If the infusion is well tolerated, the rate may be increased by 8 mL/hr increments at 15 minute intervals in order to administer the full volume within the desired period of time. However, at no time should the infusion rate exceed 100 mL/hr. The infusion rate may be slowed and/or temporarily stopped, based on clinical judgment, when infusion-related reactions occur.

See Special Handling Instructions for method of dilution.

OVERDOSAGE:
There is no experience with overdosage of ELAPRASE in humans. Single intravenous doses of idursulfase up to 20 mg/kg were not lethal in male rats or cynomolgus monkeys (approximately 40 times the recommended human dose based on body weight) and there were no signs of toxicity.

> For management of a suspected drug overdose, CPhA recommends that you contact your **regional Poison Control Centre**. See the *CPS* Directory section for a list of Poison Control Centres.

ACTION AND CLINICAL PHARMACOLOGY: Mechanism of Action: Hunter syndrome (Mucopolysaccharidosis II, MPS II) is an X-linked recessive disease caused by insufficient levels of the lysosomal enzyme iduronate-2-sulfatase. This enzyme cleaves the terminal 2-O-sulfate moieties from the glycosaminoglycans (GAG) dermatan sulfate and heparan sulfate. Due to the missing or defective iduronate-2-sulfatase enzyme in patients with Hunter syndrome, GAG progressively accumulate in the lysosomes of a variety of cells, leading to cellular engorgement, organomegaly, tissue destruction, and organ system dysfunction.

ELAPRASE is a formulation of idursulfase, a purified form of human iduronate-2-sulfatase, a lysosomal enzyme. Idursulfase is produced by recombinant DNA technology in a human cell line. Idursulfase is an enzyme that hydrolyzes the 2-sulfate esters of terminal iduronate sulfate residues from the glycosaminoglycans dermatan sulfate and heparan sulfate in the lysosomes of various cell types.

Pharmacodynamics: Idursulfase is a 525-amino acid glycoprotein with a molecular weight of approximately 76 kilodaltons. The enzyme contains eight asparagine-linked glycosylation sites occupied by complex oligosaccharide structures. ELAPRASE is a formulation of idursulfase, a purified form of human iduronate-2-sulfatase, a lysosomal enzyme. Idursulfase is produced by recombinant DNA technology in a human cell line. Idursulfase is an enzyme that hydrolyzes the 2-sulfate esters of terminal iduronate sulfate residues from the glycosaminoglycans dermatan sulfate and heparan sulfate in the lysosomes of various cell types.

Treatment of Hunter syndrome patients with ELAPRASE provides exogenous enzyme for uptake into cellular lysosomes. Mannose-6-phosphate (M6P) residues on the oligosaccharide chains allow specific binding of the enzyme to the M6P receptors on the cell surface, leading to cellular internalization of the enzyme, targeting to intracellular lysosomes and subsequent catabolism of accumulated GAG.

Pharmacokinetics: Idursulfase is taken up by selective receptor-mediated mechanisms involving binding to mannose-6-phosphate receptors. Upon internalization by cells, it is localized within cellular lysosomes, thereby limiting distribution of the protein. Degradation of idursulfase is achieved by generally well understood protein hydrolysis mechanisms to produce small peptides and amino acids. Since metabolic degradation of this product is expected to occur in cells via normal proteolytic mechanisms, no metabolism studies were conducted in humans.

The pharmacokinetic characteristics of idursulfase were evaluated in several studies in patients with Hunter syndrome (see Table 3). The serum concentration of idursulfase was quantified using an antigen-specific ELISA assay. The area under the concentration-time curve (AUC) increased in a greater than dose proportional manner as the dose increased from 0.15 mg/kg to 1.5 mg/kg following a single 1-hour infusion of ELAPRASE.

Table 3: ELAPRASE

Comparison of Initial and Repeat-Dose PK Parameters for All Evaluable Patient Samples—Based on Idursulfase Concentration Data (Mean (SD))

	PK Parameter				
Week	**C_{max} (µg/mL)**	**AUC (min· µg/mL)**	**$T_{½}$ (min)**	**Cl (mL/min/kg)**	**V_{ss} (% BW)**
TKT024 Week 1 (n=28)	1.64 (0.55)	234 (82)	50 (36)	2.55 (0.97)	19.2% (7.50%)
TKT024 Week 27 (n=30)	1.17 (0.41)	165 (48)	39 (17)	3.45 (1.03)	23.30% (10.8%)
TKT024EXT Week 1 (n=44)	1.20 (0.65)	192 (70)	60 (16)	2.95 (0.93)	24.30% (12.3%)

STORAGE AND STABILITY: Store at 2 to 8°C (in a refrigerator).

Do not use ELAPRASE after the expiration date on the vial.

This product contains no preservatives. The product should be diluted in an infusion bag using strict aseptic technique. The diluted solution should be used immediately. If immediate use is not possible, the diluted solution can be stored refrigerated at 2 to 8°C for up to 24 hours, or must be administered within 8 hours if held at room temperature.

SPECIAL HANDLING INSTRUCTIONS: ELAPRASE should be prepared and administered by a healthcare professional.

1. Determine the total volume of ELAPRASE to be administered and the number of vials needed based on the patient's weight and the recommended dose of 0.5 mg/kg.

$$\text{Patient's weight (kg)} \times 0.5 \text{ mg per kg of ELAPRASE} \div 2 \text{ mg per mL} = \text{Total \# mL of ELAPRASE}$$

$$\text{Total \# mL of ELAPRASE} \div 3 \text{ mL per vial} = \text{Total \# of vials}$$

   Round up to determine the number of whole vials needed from which to withdraw the calculated volume of ELAPRASE to be administered.
2. Perform a visual inspection of each vial. ELAPRASE is a clear to slightly opalescent, colorless solution. Do not use if the solution in the vials is discolored or particulate matter is present. ELAPRASE should not be shaken.
3. Withdraw the calculated volume of ELAPRASE from the appropriate number of vials.
4. Using strict aseptic technique, dilute the total calculated volume of ELAPRASE in 100 mL of 0.9% Sodium Chloride Injection, USP. Once diluted into normal saline, the solution in the infusion bag should be mixed gently, but not shaken. Diluted solution stored at room temperature should be discarded if not administered within 8 hours of preparation. Diluted solution may be stored refrigerated for up to 24 hours.
5. Use of an infusion set equipped with a 0.2 micrometer (µm) filter is recommended. ELAPRASE should not be infused with other products in the infusion tubing.
6. ELAPRASE is supplied in single-use vials. Remaining ELAPRASE left in a vial after withdrawing the patient's calculated dose should be disposed of in accordance with local requirements.

INFORMATION FOR THE PATIENT: Published in e-CPS, available by subscription at www.e-cps.ca.

DOSAGE FORMS, COMPOSITION AND PACKAGING: Each single use vial of sterile, aqueous, clear to slightly opalescent, colorless solution contains: a 2 mg/mL solution of idursulfase protein (6 mg) in an extractable volume of 3 mL. The concentrate must be further diluted; see Special Handling Instructions. Nonmedicinal ingredients: polysorbate 20, sodium chloride, sodium phosphate dibasic, heptahydrate, sodium phosphate monobasic, monohydrate and Water for Injection. Type I glass vials of 5 mL. The vials are closed with a butyl rubber stopper with fluororesin coating and an aluminum overseal with a blue flip-off plastic cap. Cartons of 1 vial.

Elidel® Ⓟ
pimecrolimus
Topical Calcineurin Inhibitor

Novartis Pharmaceuticals

Date of Preparation: March 10, 2003
Date of Revision: August 6, 2008

SUMMARY PRODUCT INFORMATION:

Route of Administration	Dosage Form/Strength	Clinically Relevant Nonmedicinal Ingredients
Topic	Cream 1%	Benzyl alcohol For a complete listing see Dosage Forms, Composition and Packaging.

INDICATIONS AND CLINICAL USE: ELIDEL (pimecrolimus) Cream 1% is indicated as a second-line therapy for short-term and intermittent long-term therapy of mild to moderate atopic dermatitis in non-immunocompromised patients 2 years of age and older, in whom the use of alternative, conventional therapies is deemed inadvisable because of potential risks, or in the treatment of patients who are not adequately responsive to or intolerant of alternative, conventional therapies. For additional safety information, please refer to Warnings and Precautions.

CONTRAINDICATIONS: ELIDEL (pimecrolimus) Cream, 1% is contraindicated in individuals who have known or suspected hypersensitivity to pimecrolimus or any of the components of the cream.

WARNINGS AND PRECAUTIONS:

> Long-term safety of topical calcineurin inhibitors has not been established. Although a causal relationship has not been established, rare cases of skin malignancy and lymphoma have been reported in patients treated with topical calcineurin inhibitors, including ELIDEL Cream 1%.
> Therefore:
> - Continuous long-term use of ELIDEL Cream 1% should be avoided, and application limited to areas of involvement with atopic dermatitis.
> - ELIDEL Cream 1% is not indicated in children less than 2 years of age.

General: ELIDEL (pimecrolimus) Cream, 1% should not be applied to areas of active cutaneous viral infections.

ELIDEL has not been evaluated for its efficacy and safety in the treatment of clinically infected atopic dermatitis. Before commencing treatment with ELIDEL, clinical infections at treatment sites should be cleared.

While patients with atopic dermatitis are predisposed to surface infections including eczema herpeticum (Kaposi's varicelliform eruption) treatment with ELIDEL may be associated with an increased risk of varicella zoster virus infection (chickenpox or shingles), herpes simplex virus infection, or eczema herpeticum. In presence of these skin infections, ELIDEL treatment at the site of infection should be discontinued until the viral infection is cleared.

Although patients treated with ELIDEL experienced overall a lower incidence of bacterial skin infections as compared to patients treated with the vehicle, patients with severe atopic dermatitis may have an increased risk of skin bacterial infections (impetigo) during treatment with ELIDEL.

Cases of lymphadenopathy (0.9%) were reported in patients treated with ELIDEL. These cases of lymphadenopathy were usually related to infections and noted to resolve upon appropriate antibiotic therapy. However, in the absence of clear etiology for the lymphadenopathy, or in the presence of acute infectious mononucleosis, discontinuation of ELIDEL should be considered. Patients who developed lymphadenopathy should be monitored to ensure that the lymphadenopathy resolves.

Carcinogenesis and Mutagenesis: In clinical studies, cases of skin papilloma or warts (1%) were observed in pediatric patients treated with ELIDEL. In cases where patients have worsening of skin papillomas or do not respond to conventional therapy, discontinuation of ELIDEL should be considered until complete resolution of the warts is achieved.

Animal photocarcinogenicity study: Despite the absence of observed phototoxicity in humans, ELIDEL Cream and its vehicle shortened the time to skin papilloma formation. It is prudent for patients to minimize or avoid exposure to natural or artificial sunlight. The enhancement of ultraviolet carcinogenicity is not necessarily dependent on phototoxic mechanisms.

Animal studies of monkey and mice using pimecrolimus administered at high and sustained doses were associated with lymphoma formation. Chronic topical dosing of ELIDEL Cream 1% or vehicle alone in hairless mice with concurrent exposure to UV radiation decreased the median time to onset of skin tumor formation.

Immune: There are no data to support use of ELIDEL in immunocompromised patients.

Ophthalmologic: ELIDEL (pimecrolimus) Cream, 1% is not for ophthalmic use.

Skin: ELIDEL Cream should not be used in patients with Netherton's syndrome due to the potential for increased systemic absorption of pimecrolimus.

The use of ELIDEL may cause local symptoms such as skin burning, which are mostly mild and transient. If the application site reaction is severe, the risk-benefit of treatment with ELIDEL should be considered.

Special Populations: Pregnant Women: There are no adequate and well-controlled studies in pregnant women. Studies in rats and rabbits, by dermal and oral administration gave no evidence of a teratogenic potential of pimecrolimus. Because animal reproduction studies are not always predictive of human response, this drug should be used only if clearly needed during pregnancy.

Nursing Women: It is not known whether this drug is excreted in human milk. Because of the potential for serious adverse reactions in nursing infants from pimecrolimus, a decision should be made whether to discontinue nursing or to discontinue the drug, taking into account the importance of the drug to the mother.

Pediatrics (>2 years of age): ELIDEL may be used in pediatric patients 2 years of age and older. ELIDEL is not recommended for use in pediatric patients below the age of 2 years. Studies have been conducted in pediatric patients below 2 years of age (3 months to 23 months). Certain adverse event incidences, including pyrexia, URI, cough, rhinitis, viral rash, and wheezing, were found to be higher in patients treated with ELIDEL in comparison with patients treated with vehicle.

The effects of ELIDEL on the developing immune system in infants are unknown.

Geriatrics (>65 years of age): Clinical studies of ELIDEL did not include sufficient numbers of subjects aged 65 and older to establish efficacy and safety of the drug in geriatric patients.

Information to Be Provided to the Patient/Guardian: Patients using ELIDEL should receive the following information and instructions:

Patients should use ELIDEL as directed by the physician. ELIDEL is for external use only. Patients should wash their hands after application if hands are not an area for treatment. Care should be taken to avoid contact with nose, eyes and mouth. If accidentally applied to these areas, the cream should be thoroughly wiped off and rinsed off with water.

- Patients should minimize or avoid exposure to natural or artificial sunlight (tanning beds or UVA/B treatment) while using ELIDEL.
- Patients should not use this medication for any disorder other than that for which it was prescribed.
- Patients should report any signs of adverse reactions to their physician.
- Before applying ELIDEL after a bath or shower, be sure your skin is completely dry.
- Therapy should be discontinued after signs and symptoms of atopic dermatitis have resolved. If no improvement is seen following 3 weeks of treatment, or in case of disease exacerbation, ELIDEL therapy should be discontinued and patients should consult their physicians.

ADVERSE REACTIONS: Adverse Drug Reaction Overview: In human dermal safety studies, ELIDEL did not induce contact sensitization, phototoxicity, or photoallergy, nor did it show any cumulative irritation. ELIDEL did not elicit skin atrophy compared to topical corticosteroid use.

In a one year safety study in pediatric patients age 2-17 years old involving sequential use of ELIDEL Cream and a topical corticosteroid, 43% of ELIDEL patients and 68% of vehicle patients used corticosteroids during the study. Corticosteroids were used for more than 7 days by 34% of ELIDEL patients and 54% of vehicle patients. An increased incidence of impetigo, skin infection, superinfection (infected atopic dermatitis), rhinitis, and urticaria were found in the patients that had used ELIDEL Cream and topical corticosteroid sequentially as compared to ELIDEL Cream alone.

In 3 randomized, double-blind vehicle-controlled pediatric studies and one active controlled adult study, 843 and 328 patients respectively, were treated with ELIDEL Cream 1%. In these clinical trials, 48 (4%) of the 1171 ELIDEL patients and 13 (3%) of 408 vehicle-treated patients discontinued therapy due to adverse events. Discontinuations for AEs were primarily due to application site reactions, and cutaneous infections. The most common application site reaction was application site burning, which occurred in 8-26% of patients treated with ELIDEL Cream.

Clinical Trial Adverse Drug Reactions: Because clinical trials are conducted under very specific conditions the adverse reaction rates observed in the clinical trials may not reflect the rates observed in practice and should not be compared to the rates in the clinical trials of another drug. Adverse drug reaction information from clinical trials is useful for identifying drug-related adverse events and for approximating rates.

Table 1 depicts the incidence of adverse events pooled across the 2 identically designed 6 week studies with their open label extensions and the 1 year safety study for pediatric patients ages 2-17. Data from the adult active control study is also included in this table. Adverse events are listed regardless of relationship to study drug.

A clinical study showed that the incidence of overall viral skin infections were significantly increased in the ELIDEL treated group compared to the vehicle control group (12.4% vs. 6.3%, p=0.038).

In clinical trials, there were two cases of cancer (squamous cell carcinoma of the skin and colon carcinoma) out of 19 000 patients on ELIDEL, and 5 cases of cancer (gastric cancer, melanoma, malignant histiocytosis, leukemia, and thyroid cancer) out of 4000 patients given the control, 4 out of 5 of which were on topical corticosteroids. Clinical studies show no evidence of an increased risk of cancer.

Table 1: ELIDEL

Treatment Emergent Adverse Events (1%) in ELIDEL Treatment Groups

	Pediatric Patients[a] Vehicle-Controlled (6 weeks)		Pediatric Patients Open Label (20 weeks)	Pediatric Patients[a] Vehicle-Controlled (1 year)		Adult Active Comparator (1 year)
	ELIDEL Cream (N=267) N (%)	Vehicle (N=136) N (%)	ELIDEL Cream (N=335) N (%)	ELIDEL Cream (N=272) N (%)	Vehicle (N=75) N (%)	ELIDEL Cream (N=328) N (%)
At least 1 AE	182 (68.2%)	97 (71.3%)	240 (72.0%)	230 (84.6%)	56 (74.7%)	256 (78.0%)
Infections and Infestations						
Upper Respiratory Tract Infection NOS	38 (14.2%)	18 (13.2%)	65 (19.4%)	13 (4.8%)	6 (8.0%)	14 (4.3%)
Nasopharyngitis	27 (10.1%)	10 (7.4%)	32 (19.6%)	72 (26.5%)	16 (21.3%)	25 (7.6%)
Skin Infection NOS	8 (3.0%)	9 (5.1%)	18 (5.4%)	6 (2.2%)	3 (4.0%)	21 (6.4%)
Influenza	8 (3.0%)	1 (0.7%)	22 (6.6%)	36 (13.2%)	3 (4.0%)	32 (9.8%)
Ear Infection NOS	6 (2.2%)	2 (1.5%)	19 (5.7%)	9 (3.3%)	1 (1.3%)	2 (0.6%)
Otitis Media	6 (2.2%)	1 (0.7%)	10 (3.0%)	8 (2.9%)	4 (5.3%)	2 (0.6%)
Impetigo	5 (1.9%)	3 (2.2%)	12 (3.6%)	11 (4.0%)	4 (5.3%)	8 (2.4%)
Bacterial Infection	4 (1.5%)	3 (2.2%)	4 (1.2%)	3 (1.1%)	0	6 (1.8%)
Folliculitis	3 (1.1%)	1 (0.7%)	3 (0.9%)	6 (2.2%)	3 (4.0%)	20 (6.1%)
Sinusitis	3 (1.1%)	1 (0.7%)	11 (3.3%)	6 (2.2%)	1 (1.3%)	2 (0.6%)
Pneumonia NOS	3 (1.1%)	1 (0.7%)	5 (1.5%)	0	1 (1.3%)	1 (0.3%)
Pharyngitis NOS	2 (0.7%)	2 (1.5%)	3 (0.9%)	22 (8.1%)	2 (2.7%)	3 (0.9%)
Pharyngitis Streptococcal	2 (0.7%)	2 (1.5%)	10 (3.0%)	0	<1%	0
Molluscum Contagiosum	2 (0.7%)	0	4 (1.2%)	5 (1.8%)	0	0
Staphylococcal Infection	1 (0.4%)	5 (3.7%)	7 (2.1%)	0	<1%	3 (0.9%)
Bronchitis NOS	1 (0.4%)	3 (2.2%)	4 (1.2%)	29 (10.7%)	6 (8.0%)	8 (2.4%)
Herpes Simplex	1 (0.4%)	0	4 (1.2%)	9 (3.3%)	2 (2.7%)	13 (4.0%)
Tonsillitis NOS	1 (0.4%)	0	3 (0.9%)	17 (6.3%)	0	2 (0.6%)
Viral Infection NOS	2 (0.7%)	1 (0.7%)	1 (0.3%)	18 (6.6%)	1 (1.3%)	0
Gastroenteritis NOS	0	3 (2.2%)	2 (0.6%)	20 (7.4%)	2 (2.7%)	6 (1.8%)
Chickenpox	2 (0.7%)	0	3 (0.9%)	8 (2.9%)	3 (4.0%)	1 (0.3%)
Skin Papilloma	1 (0.4%)	0	2 (0.6%)	9 (3.3%)	<1%	0
Tonsillitis Acute NOS	0	0	0	7 (2.6%)	0	0
Upper Respiratory Tract Infection Viral NOS	1 (0.4%)	0	3 (0.9%)	4 (1.5%)	0	1 (0.3%)
Herpes Simplex Dermatitis	0	0	1 (0.3%)	4 (1.5%)	0	2 (0.6%)
Bronchitis Acute NOS	0	0	0	4 (1.5%)	0	0
Eye Infection NOS	0	0	0	3 (1.1%)	<1%	1 (0.3%)
General Disorders and Administration Site Conditions						
Application Site Burning	28 (10.4%)	17 (12.5%)	5 (1.5%)	23 (8.5%)	5 (6.7%)	85 (25.9%)
Pyrexia	20 (7.5%)	12 (8.8%)	41 (12.2%)	34 (12.5%)	4 (5.3%)	4 (1.2%)
Application Site Irritation NOS	8 (3.0%)	7 (5.1%)	7 (2.1%)	9 (3.3%)	2 (2.7%)	48 (14.6%)
Application Site Irritation	8 (3.0%)	8 (5.9%)	3 (0.9%)	1 (0.4%)	3 (4.0%)	21 (6.4%)
Influenza Like Illness	1 (0.4%)	0	2 (0.6%)	5 (1.8%)	2 (2.7%)	6 (1.8%)
Application Site Erythema	1 (0.4%)	0	0	6 (2.2%)	0	7 (2.1%)
Application Site Pruritus	3 (1.1%)	2 (1.5%)	2 (0.6%)	5 (1.8%)	0	18 (5.5%)
Respiratory, Thoracic and Mediastinal Disorders						
Cough	31 (11.6%)	11 (8.1%)	31 (9.3%)	43 (15.8%)	8 (10.7%)	8 (2.4%)
Nasal Congestion	7 (2.6%)	2 (1.5%)	6 (1.8%)	4 (1.5%)	1 (1.3%)	2 (0.6%)

(cont'd)

Table 1: ELIDEL *(cont'd)*
Treatment Emergent Adverse Events (1%) in ELIDEL Treatment Groups

	Pediatric Patients[a] Vehicle-Controlled (6 weeks)		Pediatric Patients Open Label (20 weeks)	Pediatric Patients[a] Vehicle-Controlled (1 year)		Adult Active Comparator (1 year)
	ELIDEL Cream (N=267) N (%)	Vehicle (N=136) N (%)	ELIDEL Cream (N=335) N (%)	ELIDEL Cream (N=272) N (%)	Vehicle (N=75) N (%)	ELIDEL Cream (N=328) N (%)
Rhinorrhea	5 (1.9%)	1 (0.7%)	3 (0.9%)	1 (0.4%)	1 (1.3%)	0
Asthma Aggravated	4 (1.5%)	3 (2.2%)	13 (3.9%)	3 (1.1%)	1 (1.3%)	0
Sinus Congestion	3 (1.1%)	1 (0.7%)	2 (0.6%)	<1%	<1%	3 (0.9%)
Rhinitis	1 (0.4%)	0	5 (1.5%)	12 (4.4%)	5 (6.7%)	7 (2.1%)
Wheezing	1 (0.4%)	1 (0.7%)	4 (1.2%)	2 (0.7%)	<1%	0
Asthma NOS	2 (0.7%)	1 (0.7%)	11 (3.3%)	10 (3.7%)	2 (2.7%)	8 (2.4%)
Epistaxis	0	1 (0.7%)	0	9 (3.3%)	1 (1.3%)	1 (0.3%)
Dyspnea NOS	0	0	0	5 (1.8%)	1 (1.3%)	2 (0.6%)
Gastrointestinal Disorders						
Abdominal Pain Upper	11 (4.1%)	6 (4.4%)	10 (3.0%)	15 (5.5%)	5 (6.7%)	1 (0.3%)
Sore Throat	9 (3.4%)	5 (3.7%)	15 (5.4%)	22 (8.1%)	4 (5.3%)	12 (3.7%)
Vomiting NOS	8 (3.0%)	6 (4.4%)	14 (4.2%)	18 (6.6%)	6 (8.0%)	2 (0.6%)
Diarrhea NOS	3 (1.1%)	1 (0.7%)	2 (0.6%)	21 (7.7%)	4 (5.3%)	7 (2.1%)
Nausea	1 (0.4%)	3 (2.2%)	4 (1.2%)	11 (4.0%)	5 (6.7%)	6 (1.8%)
Abdominal Pain NOS	1 (0.4%)	1 (0.7%)	5 (1.5%)	12 (4.4%)	3 (4.0%)	1 (0.3%)
Toothache	1 (0.4%)	1 (0.7%)	2 (0.6%)	7 (2.6%)	1 (1.3%)	2 (0.6%)
Constipation	1 (0.4%)	0	2 (0.6%)	10 (3.7%)	<1%	0
Loose Stools	0	1 (0.7%)	4 (1.2%)	<1%	<1%	0
Reproductive System and Breast Disorders						
Dysmenorrhea	3 (1.1%)	0	5 (1.5%)	3 (1.1%)	1 (1.3%)	4 (1.2%)
Eye Disorders						
Conjunctivitis NEC	2 (0.7%)	1 (0.7%)	7 (2.1%)	6 (2.2%)	3 (4.0%)	10 (3.0%)
Skin and Subcutaneous Tissue Disorders						
Urticaria	3 (1.1%)	0	1 (0.3%)	1 (0.4%)	<1%	3 (0.9%)
Acne NOS	0	1 (0.7%)	1 (0.3%)	4 (1.5%)	<1%	6 (1.8%)
Immune System Disorders						
Hypersensitivity NOS	11 (4.1%)	6 (4.4%)	16 (4.8%)	14 (5.1%)	1 (1.3%)	11 (3.4%)
Injury and Poisoning						
Accident NOS	3 (1.1%)	1 (0.7%)	1 (0.3%)	<1%	1 (1.3%)	0
Laceration	2 (0.7%)	1 (0.7%)	5 (1.5%)	<1%	<1%	0
Musculoskeletal, Connective Tissue and Bone Disorders						
Back Pain	1 (0.4%)	2 (1.5%)	1 (0.3%)	<1%	0	6 (1.8%)
Arthralgias	0	0	1 (0.3%)	3 (1.1%)	1 (1.3%)	5 (1.5%)
Ear and Labyrinth Disorders						
Earache	2 (0.7%)	1 (0.7%)	0	8 (2.9%)	2 (2.7%)	0
Nervous System Disorders						
Headache	37 (13.9%)	12 (8.8%)	38 (11.3%)	69 (25.4%)	12 (16.0%)	23 (7.0%)

[a] Ages 2-17 years.
Legend: NOS=not otherwise specified.

Post-Market Adverse Drug Reactions: The following adverse reactions have been reported in patients also having used ELIDEL Cream. Because these reactions are reported voluntarily from a population of uncertain size, it is not always possible to reliably estimate their frequency or establish a causal relationship to drug exposure.

General: Alcohol intolerance has been rarely (<1 out of 1000) reported in patients treated with ELIDEL 1% Cream. In most cases, flushing, rash, burning, itching or swelling occurred shortly after the intake of alcohol.

Allergic reactions (e.g. rash, urticaria, angioedema) and skin discoloration (e.g. hypopigmentation, hyperpigmentation) have been rarely reported in patients treated with ELIDEL. Very rarely, anaphylactic reactions, including erythroderma and anaphylactic shock have been reported.

Hematology/Oncology: Isolated cases of malignant neoplasms were reported from post-marketing surveillance for patients also having used ELIDEL Cream 1%. The malignancies included T- and B-cell type lymphomas, skin neoplasms (basal cell carcinoma, squamous cell carcinoma, melanoma), and malignancies of various organs. A causal relationship between the use of ELIDEL Cream 1% and the reported cases has not been established. Because these reactions are reported voluntarily from a population of uncertain size, it is not possible to reliably estimate their frequency or establish a causal relationship to drug exposure.

DRUG INTERACTIONS: Overview: Potential interactions between ELIDEL and other drugs, including immunizations, have not been systematically evaluated. Although very low blood levels of pimecrolimus are detected in a minority of patients after topical application, the concomitant administration of known CYP3A inhibitors in patients with wide spread and/or erythrodermic diseases should be done with caution.

Some examples of these drugs are: erythromycin, itraconazole, ketoconazole, fluconazole, calcium channel blocker and cimetidine.

DOSAGE AND ADMINISTRATION: Recommended Dose and Dosage Adjustment: Apply a thin layer of ELIDEL (pimecrolimus) Cream, 1% to sufficiently cover the affected skin area twice daily. ELIDEL may be used on all skin surfaces, including the head, neck, and intertriginous areas.

ELIDEL Cream should be used for short or long intermittent periods of treatment. Therapy should be stopped upon clearance of the signs and symptoms of atopic dermatitis (e.g. pruritus, inflammation and erythema). Treatment should be discontinued if resolution of disease occurs. If no improvement occurs after 3 weeks of treatment, or in case of disease exacerbation, ELIDEL therapy should be discontinued and patients should consult their physicians.

The use of ELIDEL under occlusion has not been studied, therefore occlusive dressings are not recommended.

OVERDOSAGE:
There has been no experience of overdose with ELIDEL (pimecrolimus) Cream, 1%. No incidents of accidental ingestion have been reported.

For management of a suspected drug overdose, CPhA recommends that you contact your **regional Poison Control Centre**. See the *CPS* Directory section for a list of Poison Control Centres.

ACTION AND CLINICAL PHARMACOLOGY: Mechanism of Action: The exact mechanism of action of pimecrolimus in atopic dermatitis is not known. However, it has been demonstrated that pimecrolimus binds with high affinity to macrophilin-12 and inhibits the calcium-dependent phosphatase, calcineurin. As a consequence, it inhibits T cell activation by blocking the transcription of early cytokines. In particular, pimecrolimus inhibits at nanomolar concentrations Interleukin-2 and interferon gamma (Th1-type) and Interleukin-4 and Interleukin-10 (Th2-type) cytokine synthesis in human T cells. In addition, pimecrolimus prevents the release of cytokines and pro-inflammatory mediators from mast cells in vitro after stimulation by antigen/IgE. Pimecrolimus does not affect the growth of, or IL-8 release from, keratinocyte, fibroblast, and endothelial cell lines.

Pharmacokinetics: Pediatrics: Systemic exposure to pimecrolimus was investigated in 58 pediatric patients aged 3 months to 4 years and 8 to 14 years. For these patients, atopic dermatitis (AD) lesions involving 10-92% of the total body surface area were treated with ELIDEL (pimecrolimus) Cream, 1% twice daily for 3 weeks.

Blood concentrations measured in the youngest patients aged 3 to 23 months were consistently low, ranging from below the assay limit of quantitation (LoQ: 0.1 ng/mL) to 2.6 ng/mL. In earlier studies, blood concentrations in pediatric patients 8 months to 14 years of age were also low, ranging from below the LoQ (0.5 ng/mL) to 2.0 ng/mL. Overall, the majority of concentrations measured was below the limit of quantitation and there was no evidence of higher blood concentrations in patients even with a high proportion of their total body surface area (%TBSA) under treatment (>70% TBSA).

Adults: The range of blood concentrations measured in adult AD patients (≥18 years of age) was similar to that in pediatric patients. The highest blood level of pimecrolimus measured in adults was 1.4 ng/mL. In 8 adult AD patients the $AUC_{(0\text{-}12h)}$ values ranged from 2.5 to 11.4 ng·h/mL.

In 40 adult patients treated for up to 1 year with ELIDEL, blood concentrations of pimecrolimus were low. A maximum blood concentration of 0.8 ng/mL was observed in only 2 patients in week 6 of treatment. There was no increase of blood concentration over time in any patient during the 12 months of treatment. In 13 adult patients with hand dermatitis treated with ELIDEL twice daily for 3 weeks (palmar and dorsal surfaces of hands treated, overnight occlusion), the maximum blood concentration of pimecrolimus was 0.91 ng/mL.

Absorption, Distribution, Metabolism, and Excretion: In man, the fate of pimecrolimus in the body following topical application could not be determined due to low systemic absorption and low resultant blood concentrations of pimecrolimus. No drug metabolism was observed in human skin in vitro.

After single oral administration in healthy subjects, unchanged pimecrolimus was the major drug-related component in blood and there were numerous minor metabolites of moderate polarity that appeared to be products of O-demethylations and oxygenation.

Drug related radioactivity was excreted principally via the feces (78.4%) and only a small fraction (2.5%) was recovered in urine. Total mean recovery of radioactivity was 80.9%. Parent compound was not detected in urine and less than 1% of radioactivity in feces was accounted for by unchanged pimecrolimus.

STORAGE AND STABILITY: Store at room temperature (15-30°C). Do not freeze. The in-use (consumption) period of the tube, following piercing of the aluminum membrane, is 12 months.

INFORMATION FOR THE PATIENT: Published in e-CPS, available by subscription at www.e-cps.ca.

DOSAGE FORMS, COMPOSITION AND PACKAGING: Each g of cream contains: pimecrolimus 10 mg (1%). Nonmedicinal ingredients: benzyl alcohol, cetyl alcohol, citric acid, mono- and di-glycerides, oleyl alcohol, propylene glycol, sodium cetostearyl sulfate, sodium hydroxide, stearyl alcohol, triglycerides and water. Tubes of 30 and 60 g.

(Shown in Product Identification Section)

Eligard® Pr

leuprolide acetate

Luteinizing Hormone-Releasing Hormone (LHRH) Analog

sanofi-aventis

Date of Revision: August 11, 2010

SUMMARY PRODUCT INFORMATION:

Route of Administration	Dosage Form/ Strength	Clinically Relevant Nonmedicinal Ingredients
Subcutaneous Injection	Injectable solutions of: 7.5 mg (10.2 mg leuprolide acetate/syringe) [1-Month] 22.5 mg (28.2 mg leuprolide acetate/syringe) [3-Month] 30 mg (35.8 mg leuprolide acetate/syringe) [4-Month] Injectable suspension of: 45 mg (58.2 mg leuprolide acetate/syringe) [6-Month]	N-methyl-2-pyrrolidone Poly (DL-lactide-co-glycolide)

INDICATIONS AND CLINICAL USE: ELIGARD (leuprolide acetate) are indicated for the palliative treatment of advanced prostate cancer (stage D2).

ELIGARD should be administered by a health care professional.

Geriatrics (>70 years of age): The majority (>70%) of the patients studied in the clinical trials for ELIGARD were 70 years and older.

Pediatrics (<12 years of age): The safety and effectiveness of ELIGARD in pediatric patients have not been established (see Warnings and Precautions).

CONTRAINDICATIONS: ELIGARD is contraindicated in patients with hypersensitivity to Luteinizing Hormone-Releasing Hormone (LH-RH), LH-RH analogs or any of the components of ELIGARD. Anaphylactic reactions to synthetic LH-RH or LH-RH analogs have been reported in literature. For a complete listing, see Dosage Forms, Composition and Packaging.

ELIGARD is contraindicated in women who are, or may become, pregnant while receiving the drug. There are possibilities that fetal harm and spontaneous abortions may occur. The use of ELIGARD in nursing mothers is not recommended.

WARNINGS AND PRECAUTIONS: General: ELIGARD, like other LH-RH analogs, causes a transient increase in serum concentration of testosterone during the first week of treatment. Patients may experience worsening of symptoms or onset of new symptoms, including bone pain, neuropathy, hematuria, or ureteral or bladder outlet obstruction. Cases of spinal cord compression, which may contribute to paralysis with or without fatal complications, have been reported with LH-RH analogs. If spinal cord compression or renal impairment due to ureteral obstruction develops, standard treatment of these complications should be instituted.

Patients with metastatic vertebral lesions and/or with urinary tract obstruction should begin leuprolide therapy under close supervision.

Carcinogenesis and Mutagenesis: Two-year carcinogenicity studies were conducted with leuprolide acetate in rats and mice. In rats, a dose-related increase of benign pituitary hyperplasia and benign pituitary adenomas were noted at 24 months when the drug was administered subcutaneously at high daily doses (0.6 to 4 mg/kg). There was a significant but not dose-related increase of pancreatic islet-cell adenomas in females and testicular interstitial cell adenomas in males (highest incidence in the low dose group). In mice, no leuprolide acetate-induced tumors or pituitary abnormalities were observed at a dose as high as 60 mg/kg for two years. Patients have been treated with leuprolide acetate for up to two years with doses as high as 20 mg/day without demonstrable pituitary abnormalities. No carcinogenicity studies have been conducted with ELIGARD.

Mutagenicity studies have been performed with leuprolide acetate using bacterial and mammalian systems and with ELIGARD 7.5 mg in bacterial systems. These studies provided no evidence of a mutagenic potential.

Dependence/Tolerance: No drug dependence has been reported with the use of leuprolide.

Endocrine and Metabolism: Changes in Bone Density: Bone loss can be expected as part of natural aging and can also be anticipated during the hypoandrogenic state caused by long-term use of leuprolide acetate. In patients with significant risk factors for decreased bone mineral content and/or bone mass such as family history of osteoporosis, chronic use of corticosteroids or anticonvulsants or chronic abuse of alcohol or tobacco, leuprolide acetate may pose additional risk. In these patients, risk versus benefit must be weighed carefully before initiation of leuprolide acetate therapy.

Long-term administration of leuprolide will cause suppression of pituitary gonadotropins and gonadal hormone production with clinical symptoms of hypogonadism. These changes have been observed to reverse on discontinuation of therapy. However, whether the clinical symptoms of induced hypogonadism will reverse in all patients has not yet been established.

Renal and Hepatic: All clinical studies and kinetic evaluations have been conducted in patients with adequate hepatic and renal function.

Special Populations: Pregnant Women: ELIGARD is contraindicated in women who are, or may become pregnant while receiving the drug and in women who are nursing, as safety and effectiveness have not been established in this group of patients.

Nursing Women: ELIGARD is not indicated for use in nursing women as safety and effectiveness have not been established in this group of patients.

Pediatrics (<12 years of age): ELIGARD is not indicated for use in children as safety and effectiveness have not been established in this group of patients.

Geriatrics (>70 years of age): The majority (>70%) of the patients studied in the clinical trials for ELIGARD were 70 years and older.

Race: In clinical pharmacokinetic studies, mean serum leuprolide concentration profiles were similar among subjects after administration of ELIGARD 7.5 mg (26 White, 2 Black), ELIGARD 22.5 mg (19 White, 4 Black, 2 Hispanic), ELIGARD 30 mg (18 White, 4 Black, 2 Hispanic), and ELIGARD 45 mg (17 White, 7 Black, 3 Hispanic).

Monitoring and Laboratory Tests: Renal function tests, blood urea nitrogen (BUN) and creatinine may rarely be elevated during the first few days of therapy in prostate cancer patients before returning to normal. In clinical trials with ELIGARD however, no significant difference was observed from baseline to 7 days following injection in terms of the number of patients who demonstrated an elevation from normal to above normal levels of creatinine and BUN.

Response to ELIGARD may be monitored by periodically measuring serum concentrations of testosterone and prostate specific antigen. Results of testosterone determinations are dependent on assay methodology. It is advisable to be aware of the type and precision of the assay methodology to make appropriate clinical and therapeutic decisions.

The effects of leuprolide on bone lesions may be monitored by bone scans, while its effects on prostatic lesions may be monitored by ultrasonography, and/or CT scan in addition to digital rectal examination. Intravenous pyelogram, ultrasonography, or CT scan may also be utilized to diagnose or assess the status of obstructive uropathy.

ADVERSE REACTIONS: Adverse Drug Reaction Overview: ELIGARD, like other LH-RH analogs, caused a transient increase in serum testosterone concentrations during the first 2 weeks of treatment (first week of treatment for 4-Month and 6-Month). Therefore, potential exacerbations of signs and symptoms of the disease during the first few weeks of treatment are of concern in patients with vertebral metastases and/or urinary obstruction or hematuria. If these conditions are aggravated, it may lead to neurological problems such as weakness and/or paresthesia of the lower limbs or worsening of urinary symptoms (see Warnings and Precautions).

In clinical trials of non-orchiectomized prostate cancer patients treated with ELIGARD 7.5 mg, 22.5 mg, 30 mg and 45 mg, none of the 1338 injections and subsequent transient increases in testosterone were associated with an exacerbation of disease symptoms.

Some adverse effects reported with ELIGARD are due primarily to its pharmacological action of sex hormone suppression. The safety of ELIGARD 7.5 mg (1-Month) and ELIGARD 22.5 mg (3-Month) was evaluated in orchiectomized and non-orchiectomized patients with advanced prostate cancer in three clinical trials. The safety of ELIGARD 30 mg (4-Month) and ELIGARD 45 mg (6-Month) was evaluated in 50 and 63 patients with advanced prostate cancer, respectively.

Local adverse events reported after injection of ELIGARD 7.5 mg (1-Month), ELIGARD 22.5 mg (3-Month), ELIGARD 30 mg (4-Month) and ELIGARD 45 mg (6-Month) were typical of those frequently associated with similar subcutaneously injected products and included transient burning and stinging (27.5 % of injections) and pain at the site of injection (3.9 % of injections), which were typically mild in intensity, brief in duration (one minute or less) and non-recurrent over time.

The majority of study injections were not associated with reports of injection site adverse events.

Other local adverse events that were reported rarely (<2.6%) following the administration of ELIGARD 7.5 mg, 22.5 mg, 30 mg and 45 mg included erythema (1.7%), bruising (2.0%), pruritus (0.8%), induration and ulceration (0.3%). These events were mostly reported as mild and generally resolved within a few days post injection.

Clinical Trial Adverse Drug Reactions: ELIGARD 7.5 mg (1-Month), 22.5 mg (3-Month), 30 mg (4-Month) and 45 mg (6-Month): The following possibly or probably related systemic adverse events were reported by ≥2% of the patients using ELIGARD 7.5 mg, 22.5 mg, 30 mg and 45 mg in clinical studies (see Table 1).

Table 1: ELIGARD

Incidence (%) of Possibly or Probably Related Systemic Adverse Events Reported by ≥2% of Patients Treated with ELIGARD 7.5 mg [1 injection every month for up to 6 months], ELIGARD 22.5 mg [1 injection every 3 months for up to 6 months], ELIGARD 30 mg [1 injection every 4 months for up to 8 months] and ELIGARD 45 mg [1 injection every 6 months for up to 12 months]

Body System	Adverse Events	7.5 mg (n=128) %	22.5 mg (n=117) %	30 mg (n=90) %	45 mg (n=111) %
Body as a Whole	Malaise and Fatigue	21 (16.4)	—	—	—
	Dizziness	4 (3.1)	—	4 (4.4)	—
Cardiovascular	Vasodilation/Hot flashes/flushing[a]	70 (54.7)	66 (56.4)	66 (73.3)	64 (57.7)
General disorders	Fatigue	See Body as a Whole	7 (6.0)	12 (13.3)	13 (11.7)
	Weakness	—	—	—	4 (3.6)
Genitourinary	Atrophy of Testes[a]	6 (4.7)	—	4 (4.4)	8 (7.2)
	Testicular Pain	—	—	2 (2.2)	—
	Gynecomastia[a]	—	—	2 (2.2)	4 (3.6)
Digestive	Gastroenteritis/Colitis	3 (2.2)	—	—	—
Gastrointestinal	Nausea	—	4 (3.4)	2 (2.2)	—
Musculoskeletal	Arthralgia	—	4 (3.4)	—	—
	Myalgia	—	—	2 (2.2)	5 (4.5)
	Pain in Limb	—	—	—	3 (2.7)
Renal and Urinary	Urinary Frequency	—	3 (2.6)	2 (2.2)	—
	Nocturia	—	—	2 (2.2)	—

(cont'd)

Table 1: ELIGARD *(cont'd)*

Incidence (%) of Possibly or Probably Related Systemic Adverse Events Reported by ≥2% of Patients Treated with ELIGARD 7.5 mg [1 injection every month for up to 6 months], ELIGARD 22.5 mg [1 injection every 3 months for up to 6 months], ELIGARD 30 mg [1 injection every 4 months for up to 8 months] and ELIGARD 45 mg [1 injection every 6 months for up to 12 months]

Body System	Adverse Events	7.5 mg (n=128) %	22.5 mg (n=117) %	30 mg (n=90) %	45 mg (n=111) %
Skin	Pruritus (not otherwise specified)	—	3 (2.6)	—	—
	Alopecia	—	—	2 (2.2)	—
	Clamminess[a]	—	—	4 (4.4)	—
	Night Sweats[a]	—	—	3 (3.3)	3 (2.7)
Psychiatric	Decreased Libido[a]	—	—	3 (3.3)	—

[a] Expected pharmacological consequences of testosterone suppression.

In the ELIGARD 7.5 mg clinical trial, hot flashes were reported as mild in 80% of patients, moderate in 18.6 % patients and severe in 1.4 % of patients. A total of 84 hot flashes/flushing events were reported in the ELIGARD 22.5 mg clinical trial; of these, 73 of 84 (87%) were described as mild and 11 of 84 (11%) as moderate. No severe events were reported in the ELIGARD 22.5 mg study. In the patient population studied for ELIGARD 30 mg, a total of 75 hot flashes were reported in 66 patients. Of these, 57 events (76%) were described as mild; 16 (21%) as moderate; 2 (3%) as severe. A total of 89 hot flash events were reported in the ELIGARD 45 mg study. Of these, 62 events (70%) were described as mild and 27 events (30%) as moderate.

Less Common Clinical Trial Adverse Drug Reactions (<2%): The following possibly or probably related systemic adverse events were reported by <2% of the patients using ELIGARD 7.5 mg (1-Month), 22.5 mg (3-Month), 30 mg (4-Month) and 45 mg (6-Month) in clinical studies.

ELIGARD 7.5 mg (1-Month): General: sweating, insomnia, syncope.
Gastrointestinal: flatulence, constipation.
Hematologic: decreased red blood cell count, hematocrit and hemoglobin (anemia).
Metabolic: weight gain.
Musculoskeletal: tremor, backache, joint pain.
Nervous: disturbance of smell and taste, depression, vertigo.
Skin: alopecia.
Urogenital: testicular soreness, impotence, decreased libido, gynecomastia, breast soreness.
ELIGARD 22.5 mg (3-Month): Cardiovascular: hypertension, hypotension.
General: rigors, weakness, lethargy, pain (not otherwise specified), fever.
Urinary: difficulties with urination, pain on urination, scanty urination, bladder spasm, blood in urine and urinary retention.
Reproductive and Breast: breast tenderness, testicular atrophy and pain, enlarged breasts, impotence.
Gastrointestinal: stomach upset, constipation, dry mouth.
ELIGARD 30 mg (4-Month): General: lethargy.
Reproductive: breast enlargement*, erectile dysfunction*, reduced penis size*.
Renal/Urinary: urinary urgency, incontinence.
Musculoskeletal: muscle atrophy, limb pain.
Psychiatric: insomnia, depression, loss of libido*.
ELIGARD 45 mg (6-Month): In addition, the following possibly or probably related systemic adverse events were reported by 1% of the patients (2/111) using ELIGARD 45 mg in the clinical study:
General: lethargy.
Reproductive: penile disorder*.
Renal/Urinary: nocturia, nocturia aggravated.
Psychiatric: loss of libido*.

Abnormal Hematologic and Clinical Chemistry Findings: Abnormalities of certain parameters were observed, but are difficult to assess in this population. For both ELIGARD 7.5 mg and ELIGARD 22.5 mg abnormal values were observed in ≥5% of the study population for the following analyses at any time during the study: increased eosinophils, neutrophils, BUN, total cholesterol, triglycerides, alanine aminotransferase (ALT), alkaline phosphatase (ALP) and creatine kinase (CK). Decreased red blood cell count, hematocrit, and hemoglobin were observed.

In addition, for ELIGARD 7.5 mg, decreased white blood cells, as well as increased sodium, lactate dehydrogenase (LDH) and International Normalized Ratio (INR) were observed for ≥5% of the study population. For ELIGARD 22.5 mg, increased creatinine and aspartate aminotransferase (AST) were observed in ≥5% of the study population.

Post-Market Adverse Drug Reactions: Post-market studies have not been conducted with ELIGARD.

DRUG INTERACTIONS: Overview: No formal drug interaction studies have been conducted with ELIGARD. No data is available on the interaction with alcohol.
Drug-Drug Interactions: Interactions with drugs have not been established.
Drug-Food Interactions: Interactions with food have not been established.
Drug-Herb Interactions: Interactions with herbal products have not been established.
Drug-Laboratory Interactions: Therapy with leuprolide results in suppression of the pituitary-gonadal system. Results of diagnostic tests of pituitary gonadotropic and gonadal functions conducted during and after leuprolide therapy may be affected.

DOSAGE AND ADMINISTRATION:

Dosing Considerations: ELIGARD should be administered by a health care professional.

ELIGARD 7.5, 22.5, 30 and 45 mg administered subcutaneously is designed to provide continuous sustained release of leuprolide for 1, 3, 4 and 6 months, respectively.

Recommended Dose and Dosage Adjustment: ELIGARD 7.5 mg (1-Month): The recommended dose of ELIGARD (1-Month) is 7.5 mg administered monthly as a single subcutaneous injection after mixing with a special polymer formulation (see Administration). The total deliverable injection weight per dose is 250 mg including 7.5 mg leuprolide acetate. The total volume administered per dose is approximately 0.25 mL.

ELIGARD 22.5 mg (3-Month): The recommended dose of ELIGARD (3-Month) is 22.5 mg administered every three months as a single subcutaneous injection after mixing with a special polymer formulation (see Administration). The total deliverable injection weight per dose is 375 mg including 22.5 mg of leuprolide acetate. The total volume administered per dose is approximately 0.37 mL.

ELIGARD 30 mg (4-Month): The recommended dose of ELIGARD 30 mg (4-Month) is 30 mg administered every four months as a single subcutaneous injection after mixing with a special polymer formulation (see Administration). The total deliverable injection weight per dose is 500 mg including 30 mg of leuprolide acetate. The total volume administered per dose is approximately 0.50 mL.

ELIGARD 45 mg (6-Month): The recommended dose of ELIGARD 45 mg (6-Month) is 45 mg administered every six months as a single subcutaneous injection after mixing with a special polymer formulation (see Administration). The total deliverable injection weight per dose is 375 mg including 45 mg of leuprolide acetate. The total volume administered per dose is approximately 0.375 mL.

Missed Dose: Maintaining testosterone suppression is important in treating the symptoms of hormone-dependent prostate cancer. Missing an appointment by a few days should not disrupt the benefits of treatment, but keeping a consistent schedule of ELIGARD injections is an important part of treatment.

Administration: As with other drugs administered by subcutaneous injection, the injection site should be varied periodically. The specific injection location chosen should be an area with sufficient soft or loose subcutaneous tissue. In clinical trials, the injection was administered in the upper- or mid-abdominal area. Avoid areas with brawny or fibrous subcutaneous tissue or locations that could be rubbed or compressed (i.e., with a belt or clothing waistband).

As with all parenteral drug products, syringes as well as reconstituted drug solutions, should be inspected visually for particulate matter, precipitate, discoloration and leakage prior to administration. Solutions showing particulate matter, precipitate, discoloration or leakage should not be used.

Prior to administration, the syringes are removed from the trays, the syringe tip caps are removed, and the syringes are coupled. The product is prepared by passing the formulation from syringe to syringe until a homogenous solution (homogenous suspension for ELIGARD 45 mg product) is achieved. The syringes are decoupled and the sterile needle is affixed to the male syringe. The Domrex Needle Guard device must be affixed on the syringe prior to the injection to help prevent accidental needle stick injuries following the injection. The health care professional should carefully read the leaflet provided with the device before use.

Mixing and Administration Procedure: ELIGARD 7.5 mg (1-Month), 22.5 mg (3-Month), 30 mg (4-Month) and 45 mg (6-Month).

Important: Allow the product to reach room temperature before using. Once mixed, the product must be administered within 30 minutes.

Follow the instructions as directed to ensure proper preparation of ELIGARD prior to administration:

ELIGARD is packaged in tray packaging.

The tray packaging contains two thermoformed trays. One tray contains the sterile Syringe A pre-filled with the ATRIGEL polymer system, a long white replacement plunger rod and a desiccant pouch. The other tray contains the sterile Syringe B pre-filled with leuprolide acetate powder, a sterile needle and a desiccant pouch. The two trays are placed into a paperboard carton.

1. On a clean field, open the trays and remove the contents. Discard the desiccant pack(s).
2. Pull out the blue-tipped short plunger rod and attached stopper from Syringe B and discard. Gently insert the long, white replacement plunger rod into the gray primary stopper remaining in Syringe B by twisting it in place.
3. Unscrew the clear cap from Syringe A. Remove the gray rubber cap from Syringe B.
4. Join the two syringes together by pushing in and twisting until secure.
5. Inject the liquid contents of Syringe A into Syringe B containing the leuprolide acetate. Thoroughly mix the product by pushing the contents of both syringes back and forth between syringes (approximately 45 seconds) to obtain a uniform solution (suspension for ELIGARD 45 mg product). When thoroughly mixed, the solution (suspension for ELIGARD 45 mg product) will appear a colourless to tan color. Please note: Product must be mixed as described; shaking will not provide adequate mixing of the product.
6. Hold the syringes vertically with Syringe B on the bottom. The syringes should remain securely coupled. Draw the entire mixed product into Syringe B (short, wide syringe) by depressing the Syringe A plunger and slightly withdrawing the Syringe B plunger. Uncouple Syringe A while continuing to push down on the Syringe A plunger. Please note: Small air bubbles will remain in the formulation—this is acceptable.
7. Hold Syringe B upright. Remove the cap on the bottom of the sterile needle cartridge by twisting it. Attach the needle cartridge to the end of Syringe B by pushing in and turning the needle until it is firmly seated. Do not twist the needle onto the syringe until it is stripped.
8. Affix the Domrex Needle Guard device on the syringe. The health care professional should carefully follow the detailed instructions provided by the manufacturer (Domrex Pharma Inc.) with the device.
9. Choose an injection site on the abdomen, upper buttocks, or anywhere with adequate amounts of subcutaneous tissue that does not have excessive pigment, nodules, lesions, or hair. Since you can vary the injection site with a subcutaneous injection, choose an area that hasn't recently been used.
10. Cleanse the injection-site area with an alcohol swab.
11. Pull off the clear needle cartridge cover prior to administration.
12. Using the thumb and forefinger of your nondominant hand, grab and bunch the area of skin around the injection site.
13. Using your dominant hand, insert the needle quickly. The approximate angle you use will depend on the amount and fullness of the subcutaneous tissue and the length of the needle.
14. After the needle is inserted, release the skin with your nondominant hand.
15. Inject the drug using a slow, steady push. Press down on the plunger until the syringe is empty.
16. Withdraw the needle quickly at the same angle used for insertion. Activate the Domrex Needle Guard device. The health care professional should carefully follow the detailed instructions provided by the manufacturer (Domrex Pharma Inc.) with the device.
17. Gently massage the injection area with a cotton ball or gauze pad.
18. Discard all components safely in an appropriate biohazard container.
19. Remove your gloves and wash your hands. Document both the procedure and the patient's response to the injection.

OVERDOSAGE: There is no clinical experience with the effects of an acute overdose. Because the acute animal toxicity of the drug is low, adverse effects are not expected. No difference in adverse reactions was observed in patients who subcutaneously received either 1 or 10 mg/day leuprolide for up to three years or 20 mg/day for up to two years.

> For management of a suspected drug overdose, contact your regional Poison Control Centre. See the *CPS Directory* section for a list of Poison Control Centres.

ACTION AND CLINICAL PHARMACOLOGY: Mechanism of Action: Leuprolide acetate is a synthetic nonapeptide analog of naturally occurring luteinizing hormone-releasing hormone (LH-RH) that, when given continuously, inhibits pituitary gonadotropin secretion and suppresses testicular and ovarian steroidogenesis. The analog possesses greater potency than the natural hormone. Leuprolide acetate is chemically unrelated to steroids.

Unlike steroid hormones, leuprolide exerts specific action on the pituitary gonadotrophs and the human reproductive tract. This specificity reduces the likelihood of secondary adverse effects such as gynecomastia, thromboembolism, edema, liver and gallbladder involvement.

In humans, administration of leuprolide acetate results in an initial increase in circulating levels of luteinizing hormone (LH) and follicle stimulating hormone (FSH), leading to a transient increase in levels of gonadal steroids. However, continuous administration of leuprolide acetate results in decreased levels of LH and FSH. As a result, testosterone is reduced in males to levels associated with castration (≤50 ng/dL in serum), and estrogen in females is reduced to postmenopausal levels. These decreases are observed within two to four weeks after the start of treatment and are maintained as long as treatment continues. Castrate levels of testosterone in prostate cancer patients have been demonstrated for periods of up to seven years. The effect is reversible upon discontinuation of drug therapy.

ELIGARD is an injectable polymer-based, extended-release formulation of leuprolide acetate. Subcutaneous (SC) injections of 7.5 mg (1-Month), 22.5 mg (3-Month), 30 mg (4-Month) and 45 mg (6-Month) of ELIGARD provide sustained levels of leuprolide acetate over the respective dosing intervals, resulting in continuous suppression of gonadal testosterone synthesis.

In the majority of prostate cancer patients administered monthly SC injections of ELIGARD, 7.5 mg (1-Month) and repeated injections of ELIGARD 22.5 mg (3-Month), ELIGARD 30 mg (4-Month), or ELIGARD 45 mg (6-Month) testosterone levels increased above baseline during the first week, declining thereafter at or below baseline levels by the end of the second and third week, respectively. Castrate levels of testosterone were generally reached within two to four weeks of administration and were maintained for the duration of the treatment.

Pharmacodynamics: After each injection of ELIGARD 7.5 mg, mean serum leuprolide levels peaked during the first day, then fell rapidly to sustained levels between 0.2-2 ng/mL. In response to this pattern of leuprolide exposure, serum testosterone levels rose initially, from 408±60 ng/dL at baseline to 600±74 ng/dL on Day 3, then fell to below castrate levels (≤50 ng/dL) within three weeks after the first dose (38±9 ng/dL on Day 21). Mean serum testosterone remained relatively constant (7.1-17.9 ng/dL) for the rest of the 84-day study.

For ELIGARD 22.5 mg, in response to leuprolide exposure, serum testosterone levels rose initially, to 610±246 ng/dL on Day 2, then fell to below castrate levels (≤50 ng/dL) within three weeks after the first dose (28±18 ng/dL on Day 21). Mean serum testosterone remained relatively constant (7-13 ng/dL) for the rest of the six-month (168-day) study, and did not increase following administration of the second dose at month three (Day 84).

After each injection of ELIGARD 30 mg, mean serum leuprolide levels peaked during the first day, then fell rapidly to sustained levels of 0.1-1.0 ng/mL. In response to this pattern of leuprolide exposure, mean serum testosterone levels rose initially, from 385.5 (±18.04) ng/dL at baseline, to 588±40 ng/dL on Day 3, then fell to below castrate levels (≤50 ng/dL) within 3 weeks after the first dose (31.7±4.2 ng/dL on Day 21). Levels of testosterone remained between 6-12 ng/dL for the remainder of the 224 day study.

* Expected pharmacological consequence of testosterone suppression.

The pharmacodynamic response following repeated administration of ELIGARD 45 mg (6-Month) in 28 patients with advanced prostate cancer is shown in Figure 1. After each injection, mean serum leuprolide levels peaked during the first day, then fell rapidly to sustained levels of 0.2-2.0 ng/mL. In response to this pattern of leuprolide exposure, mean serum testosterone levels rose initially, from 585±49 ng/dL on Day 3, then fell to below castrate levels (≤50 ng/dL) within 3 weeks after the first dose (30.4±3.0 ng/dL on Day 21). Levels of testosterone remained between 6-12 ng/dL for the remainder of the 12-month study.

Figure 1: ELIGARD 45 mg (6-Month)

Pharmacodynamic response to ELIGARD 45 mg (6-Month) showing serum levels of leuprolide (open circles, N=27) and testosterone (closed circles, N=28) after two consecutive SC injections at six-month intervals in advanced prostate cancer patients. Doses administrated on Day 0 and Month 6 (Day 168)

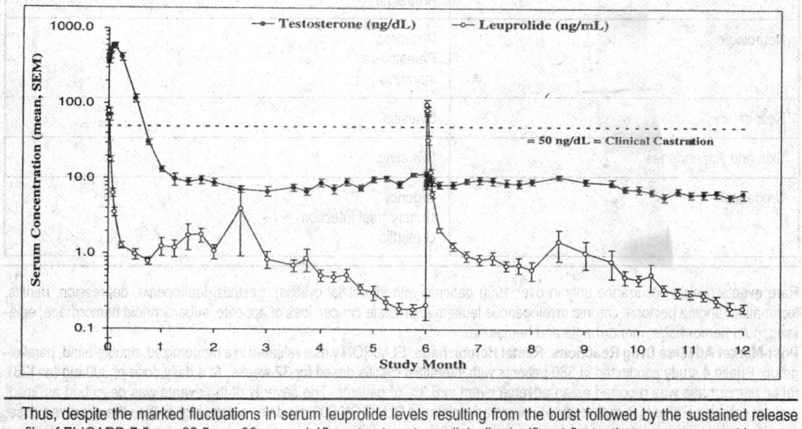

Thus, despite the marked fluctuations in serum leuprolide levels resulting from the burst followed by the sustained release profile of ELIGARD 7.5 mg, 22.5 mg, 30 mg and 45 mg treatment, no clinically significant fluctuations were observed in serum testosterone levels, which remained continuously suppressed once they had fallen to castrate levels. The initial rise and fall in testosterone levels produced by ELIGARD 7.5 mg, 22.5 mg, 30 mg and 45 mg were of a magnitude and timecourse similar to those observed with other leuprolide formulations, and are related to the mechanism by which continuous exposure to LH-RH analogs suppresses gonadal steroidogenesis via hypophyseal desensitization. No acute-on-chronic or breakthrough responses were seen in testosterone concentrations after the second and third dose of ELIGARD.

There were no acute-on-chronic or breakthrough testosterone responses during the burst phase after the second dose of ELIGARD 22.5 (3-Month).

No acute-on-chronic responses were seen in testosterone concentrations after the first and second dose of ELIGARD 30 mg (4-Month) and only one patient had a breakthrough response with a single serum testosterone value of 53 ng/dL after the second dose (Day 113). The patient resuppressed at Day 115 and remained suppressed throughout the remainder of the study.

No acute-on-chronic responses were seen in testosterone concentrations after the first and second dose of ELIGARD 45 mg (6-Month) and none of the patients exhibited a breakthrough response during the study.

Pharmacokinetics: Absorption: The pharmacokinetics of ELIGARD in patients with advanced prostate cancer were determined over two dosing intervals for ELIGARD 22.5 mg (3-Month), ELIGARD 30 mg (4-Month) and ELIGARD 45 mg (6-Month) and over three dosing intervals for ELIGARD 7.5 mg (1-Month). Repeated treatment of advanced prostate cancer patients with ELIGARD products at their intended dosing interval produced serum leuprolide profiles similar to those of other effective leuprolide depot formulations. After the subcutaneous administration of each ELIGARD depot formulation, an initial burst phase characterized by high serum leuprolide concentrations was followed by a plateau phase during which serum leuprolide concentrations remained relatively constant over the remainder of each dosing interval. There was no evidence of accumulation after repeated administration, with similar serum profiles observed after the first, and each subsequent dose of ELIGARD. Serum leuprolide concentrations during the plateau phase were occasionally below detection, with no effect on testosterone suppression. The sustained-release pharmacokinetic profile of each ELIGARD formulation was associated with continuous testosterone suppression in close to 100% of patients over the intended 1-month, 3-month, 4-month or 6-month dosing interval. See Table 2 for clinical pharmacokinetic parameters of ELIGARD.

Table 2: ELIGARD

Clinical Pharmacokinetic Parameters of ELIGARD

Subcutaneous Administration in Patients with Advanced Prostate Cancer								
	Burst Phase (Day 0–3)			Plateau Phase (Day 3–end of interval)			Total Dosing Interval	
	C_{max} (ng/mL)	T_{max} (h)	AUC (ng·h/mL)	C_{max} (ng/mL)	C_{min} (ng/mL)	AUC (ng·h/mL)	C last (ng/mL)	AUC (ng·h/mL)
ELIGARD 45 mg (6-Month), N=27								
Dose 1	82.0	4.43	1558	6.7	0.12	4362	0.21	5922
Dose 2	102.4	4.75	2357	3.4	0.12	3216	0.20	5573
ELIGARD 30 mg (4-Month), N=24								
Dose 1	150	3.3	2080	2.6	0.07	1471	0.08	3551
Dose 2	192	3.0	2659	1.9	0.06	1083	0.07	3743
ELIGARD 22.5 mg (3-Month), N=25								
Dose 1	127	4.6	2227	2.4	0.15	1419	0.34	3646
Dose 2	107	4.5	1955	2.7	0.25	1925	0.30	3880
ELIGARD 7.5 mg (1-Month), N=8 (single dose study)								
Dose 1	26.3	4.1	350.6	2.69	0.175	514.9	0.36	865.6
ELIGARD 7.5 mg (1-Month), N=20								
Dose 1	25.3	4.6	435.3	2.68	0.169	438.1	0.42	873.4
Dose 2	ND	ND	ND	2.02	0.360	499.6	0.45	ND
Dose 3	ND	ND	ND	1.78	0.328	475.7	0.45	ND

Distribution: The mean steady-state volume of distribution of leuprolide following intravenous bolus administration to healthy male volunteers was 27 L. In vitro binding to human plasma proteins ranged from 43% to 49%.

Metabolism: In healthy male volunteers, a 1 mg bolus of leuprolide administered intravenously revealed that the mean systemic clearance was 8.34 L/h, with a terminal elimination half-life of approximately 3 hours based on a two compartment model. The major metabolite of leuprolide is a pentapeptide (M-1) metabolite. No metabolism study was conducted with ELIGARD.

Excretion: No excretion study was conducted with ELIGARD.

Special Populations and Conditions: Pediatrics: The safety and effectiveness of ELIGARD in pediatric patients have not been established (see Warnings and Precautions).

Geriatrics: The majority (>70%) of the patients studied in the clinical trials for ELIGARD were 70 years and older.

Gender: Only male patients were included in studies with ELIGARD.

Race: In the patients studied, mean serum leuprolide concentrations were similar. See Table 3 for race distribution of all subjects in ELIGARD studies.

Table 3: ELIGARD

Race Distribution of All Subjects in ELIGARD Studies

	AGL0205 ELIGARD 45 mg Study (%)	AGL0001 ELIGARD 30 mg Study (%)	AGL9909 ELIGARD 22.5 mg Study (%)	AGL9904 ELIGARD 7.5 mg Study (%)
White	84 (75.7)	71 (78.9)	93 (79.5)	92 (76.7)
Black	19 (17.1)	10 (11.1)	13 (11.1)	15 (12.5)
Hispanic	6 (5.4)	8 (8.9)	7 (6.0)	13 (10.8)
Asian	1 (0.9)	0	3 (2.6)	0
Other	1 (0.9)	1 (1.1)	1 (0.9)	0

Hepatic and Renal Insufficiency: The pharmacokinetics of the drug in hepatically (renally) -impaired patients have not been determined.

Genetic Polymorphism: The effect of genetic polymorphism on the pharmacokinetics of ELIGARD was not studied.

STORAGE AND STABILITY: ELIGARD should be kept refrigerated between 2-8°C.

ELIGARD can be stored at room temperature (15-30°C) in original packaging for a period of 8 weeks prior to administration. Once mixed, ELIGARD should be discarded if not used within 30 minutes.

SPECIAL HANDLING INSTRUCTIONS: Allow the product to reach room temperature before using.

INFORMATION FOR THE PATIENT: Published in e-CPS, available by subscription at www.e-cps.ca.

DOSAGE FORMS, COMPOSITION AND PACKAGING: ELIGARD 7.5 mg (1-Month) (10.2 mg leuprolide acetate per syringe): ELIGARD 7.5 mg (1-Month) is supplied in two separate prefilled, sterile syringes whose contents are mixed immediately prior to administration. The two syringes are joined and the single dose product is mixed until it is homogenous. One syringe contains the ATRIGEL Delivery System, and the other contains leuprolide acetate. The ATRIGEL Delivery System is a polymeric (non gelatin containing) delivery system consisting of a biodegradable, 34% poly (DL-Lactide-co-glycolide)(PLGH) polymer formulation dissolved in a biocompatible solvent, 66% N-methyl-2-pyrrolidone (NMP). PLGH is a co-polymer with a 50:50 molar ratio of DL-lactide to glycolide containing carboxyl end groups. The second syringe contains 10.2 mg lyophilized leuprolide acetate and is designed to deliver 7.5 mg of leuprolide acetate at the time of subcutaneous injection.

ELIGARD 7.5 mg (1-Month) is available in a single use tray packaging. The tray packaging contains the two-syringe mixing system, a 20-gauge half-inch needle, and two silicone desiccant pouches to control moisture uptake. A needle safety device, the Domrex Needle Guard (manufactured by Domrex Pharma Inc.), is also included to help prevent accidental needle stick injuries. An instructions leaflet is provided with the device.

ELIGARD 22.5 mg (3-Month) (28.2 mg leuprolide acetate per syringe): ELIGARD 22.5 mg (3-Month) is supplied in two separate prefilled, sterile syringes whose contents are mixed immediately prior to administration. The two syringes are joined and the single dose product is mixed until it is homogenous. One syringe contains the ATRIGEL Delivery System, and the other contains leuprolide acetate. The ATRIGEL Delivery System is a polymeric (non gelatin containing) delivery system consisting of a biodegradable, 45% poly (DL-Lactide-co-glycolide)(PLG) polymer formulation dissolved in a biocompatible solvent, 55% N-methyl-2-pyrrolidone (NMP). PLG is a co-polymer with a 75:25 molar ratio of DL-lactide to glycolide with hexanediol. The second syringe contains 28.2 mg lyophilized leuprolide acetate and is designed to deliver 22.5 mg of leuprolide acetate at the time of SC injection.

ELIGARD 22.5 mg (3-Month) is available in a single use tray packaging. The tray packaging contains the two-syringe mixing system, a 20-gauge half-inch needle, and two desiccant pouches to control moisture uptake. A needle safety device, the Domrex Needle Guard (manufactured by Domrex Pharma Inc.), is also included to help prevent accidental needle stick injuries. An instructions leaflet is provided with the device.

ELIGARD 30 mg (4-Month) (35.8 mg leuprolide acetate per syringe): ELIGARD 30 mg (4-Month) is supplied in two separate prefilled, sterile syringes whose contents are mixed immediately prior to administration. The two syringes are joined and the single dose product is mixed until it is homogenous. One syringe contains the ATRIGEL Delivery System, and the other contains leuprolide acetate. The ATRIGEL Delivery System is a polymeric (non gelatin containing) delivery system consisting of a biodegradable, 45% poly (DL-Lactide-co-glycolide) (PLG) polymer formulation dissolved in a biocompatible solvent, 55% N-methyl-2-pyrrolidone (NMP). PLG is a co-polymer with a 75:25 molar ratio of DL-lactide to glycolide with hexanediol. The second syringe contains 35.8 mg lyophilized leuprolide acetate and is designed to deliver 30 mg of leuprolide acetate at the time of subcutaneous injection.

ELIGARD 30 mg (4-Month) is available in a single use tray packaging. The tray packaging contains the two-syringe mixing system, a 20-gauge 5/8-inch needle, and two silicone desiccant pouches to control moisture uptake. A needle safety device, the Domrex Needle Guard (manufactured by Domrex Pharma Inc.), is also included to help prevent accidental needle stick injuries. An instructions leaflet is provided with the device.

ELIGARD 45 mg (6-Month) (58.2 mg leuprolide acetate per syringe): ELIGARD 45 mg (6-Month) is supplied in two separate prefilled, sterile syringes whose contents are mixed immediately prior to administration. The two syringes are joined and the single dose product is mixed until it is homogenous. One syringe contains the ATRIGEL Delivery System, and the other contains leuprolide acetate. The ATRIGEL Delivery System is a polymeric (non gelatin containing) delivery system consisting of a biodegradable, 50% poly (DL-Lactide-co-glycolide) (PLG) polymer formulation dissolved in a biocompatible solvent, 50% N-methyl-2-pyrrolidone (NMP). PLG is a co-polymer with a 85:15 molar ratio of DL-lactide to glycolide with hexanediol. The second syringe contains 58.2 mg lyophilized leuprolide acetate and is designed to deliver 45 mg of leuprolide acetate at the time of subcutaneous injection.

ELIGARD 45 mg (6-Month) is available in a single use tray packaging. The tray packaging contains the two-syringe mixing system, a 18-gauge 5/8-inch needle, and two silicone desiccant pouches to control moisture uptake. A needle safety device, the Domrex Needle Guard (manufactured by Domrex Pharma Inc.), is also included to help prevent accidental needle stick injuries. An instructions leaflet is provided with the device.

Can't find information on a particular drug? Consult the CPhA Monograph Index in the front pages of the *CPS*. The CPhA monographs are compiled by the editorial staff of the Canadian Pharmacists Association and reviewed by expert Canadian physicians and pharmacists.

Elmiron® Ⓟ

pentosan polysulfate sodium

Glycosaminoglycan Substitute

Janssen-Ortho

Date of Preparation: September 28, 1998
Date of Revision: July 11, 2008

SUMMARY PRODUCT INFORMATION:

Route of Administration	Dosage Form/ Strength	Clinically Relevant Nonmedicinal Ingredients
Oral	Capsules 100 mg	For a complete listing, see Dosage Forms, Composition and Packaging.

INDICATIONS AND CLINICAL USE: ELMIRON (pentosan polysulfate sodium) is indicated for the initial and maintenance treatment of interstitial cystitis.
Pediatrics (<18 years of age): Safety and effectiveness in children and adolescents below the age of 18 years have not been established.

CONTRAINDICATIONS: Patients who are hypersensitive to this drug or to any ingredient in the formulation or component of the container. For a complete listing, see Dosage Forms, Composition and Packaging.

WARNINGS AND PRECAUTIONS: General: ELMIRON is a weak anticoagulant (only 1/15 the activity of heparin) and has been used in prevention of thrombotic disease.
Carcinogenesis and Mutagenesis: Long-term carcinogenicity studies in rats showed no evidence of carcinogenic potential at exposures up to 60 times the maximum recommended human dose (MRHD) on a mg/kg basis. In a 2-year carcinogenicity study in mice, there was an increase in hemangiosarcomas in male mice and hepatocellular neoplasms in male and female mice at a dose approximately 117 times the MRHD on a mg/kg basis. No mutagenic activity has been observed.
Hematologic: A small number of bleeding complications of ecchymosis, epistaxis, and gum hemorrhage have been reported (see Adverse Reactions). At a daily dose of 300 mg (n=128), rectal hemorrhage was reported as an adverse event in 6.3% of patients.

Patients at increased hemorrhagic risk due to diseases such as ulcerative GI lesions, aneurysms, internal or external hemorrhoids, thrombocytopenia, hemophilia, polyps or diverticulae should also be evaluated carefully if they are to receive ELMIRON.
Hepatic: Pentosan polysulfate sodium is desulfated by both the liver and the spleen. The extent to which hepatic insufficiency or splenic disorders may increase the bioavailability of the parent or active metabolites of pentosan polysulfate sodium is not known. Caution should be exercised when using ELMIRON in these patients.

Mildly (<2.5×normal) elevated transaminase, alkaline phosphatase, γ-glutamyl transpeptidase, and lactic dehydrogenase occurred in 1.2% of patients. The increases usually appeared 3 to 12 months after the start of ELMIRON therapy, and were not associated with jaundice or other clinical signs or symptoms. These abnormalities are usually transient, may remain essentially unchanged, or may rarely progress with continued use.
Peri-Operative Considerations: Patients undergoing invasive procedures, having signs or symptoms of underlying coagulopathy or who are otherwise at increased risk of bleeding (due to other therapies such as coumarin anticoagulants e.g. warfarin, heparin, tPA, streptokinase, high-dose aspirin, or nonsteroidal anti-inflammatories) should be evaluated for hemorrhagic risk.
Reproduction: Reproductive studies performed in the rat had no effect on fertility. The effect of pentosan polysulfate sodium on spermatogenesis has not been investigated.
Special Populations: Pregnant Women: There are no adequate and well-controlled studies in pregnant women. Therefore, this drug should be used during pregnancy only if the potential benefit clearly exceeds the potential risk.
Nursing Women: It is not known if ELMIRON is excreted in human milk. Many drugs are excreted in human milk; therefore, caution should be exercised when ELMIRON is administered to a nursing mother.
Pediatrics (<18 years of age): Safety and effectiveness in children and adolescents below the age of 18 years have not been established. This drug should be kept out of the reach of children.

ADVERSE REACTIONS: Adverse Drug Reaction Overview: ELMIRON is usually well tolerated. Reported adverse reactions are infrequent and usually do not require discontinuation of treatment. The most common reactions are gastrointestinal, hematologic or dermatologic (see Warnings and Precautions). Adverse events reported are summarized in Table 1 and Table 2.

Table 1: ELMIRON

Low Frequency (≤3%) Adverse Events Reported in Patients Treated with ELMIRON

Body System	Adverse Event
Body as a Whole	Headache
Digestive	GI discomfort Diarrhea Nausea
Skin and Appendages	Alopecia Rash

Table 2: ELMIRON

Uncommon (≤1%) Adverse Events Reported in Patients Treated with ELMIRON

Body System	Adverse Event
Body as a Whole	Malaise Pelvic pain
Digestive	Liver function abnormalities Vomiting Mouth ulcer Colitis Esophagitis Gastritis
Hematologic	Anemia Ecchymosis Prothrombin decrease Thrombocytopenia Retinal hemorrhage
Hypersensitive Reactions	Allergic reaction Photosensitivity

(cont'd)

Table 2: ELMIRON *(cont'd)*

Uncommon (≤1%) Adverse Events Reported in Patients Treated with ELMIRON

Body System	Adverse Event
Metabolic	Weight gain Weight loss Edema
Musculoskeletal	Myalgia Arthralgia
Neurologic	Dizziness Paresthesia Insomnia
Respiratory	Sinusitis
Skin and Appendages	Sweating
Urogenital	Urgency Urinary tract infection Urethritis

Rare events (single occurrence only in over 1000 patients with interstitial cystitis): gastritis, leukopenia, depression, rhinitis, lacrimation, angina pectoris, chronic myelogenous leukemia, prostate cancer, loss of appetite, subarachnoid hemorrhage, epistaxis, gum hemorrhage, menorrhagia and hematuria.
Post-Market Adverse Drug Reactions: Rectal Hemorrhage: ELMIRON was evaluated in a randomized, double-blind, parallel-group, Phase 4 study conducted in 380 patients with interstitial cystitis dosed for 32 weeks. At a daily dose of 300 mg (n=128), rectal hemorrhage was reported as an adverse event in 6.3% of patients. The severity of the events was described as "mild" in most patients. Patients in that study who were administered ELMIRON 900 mg daily, a dose higher than the approved dose, experienced a higher incidence of rectal hemorrhage, 15%.
Liver Function Abnormality: A randomized, double-blind, parallel-group, Phase 2 study was conducted in 100 men (51 ELMIRON and 49 placebo) dosed for 16 weeks. At a daily dose of 900 mg, a dose higher than the approved dose, elevated liver function tests were reported as an adverse event in 11.8% (n=6) of ELMIRON treated patients and 2% (n=1) of placebo-treated patients.

DRUG INTERACTIONS: Drug-Drug Interactions: In a study in which healthy subjects (24 completed) received pentosan polysulfate sodium 100 mg or placebo every 8 hours for 7 days, and were titrated with warfarin to an INR of 1.4 to 1.8, the pharmacokinetic parameters of R-warfarin and S-warfarin were similar in the absence or presence of pentosan polysulfate sodium. Prothrombin time, partial thromboplastin time and INR for warfarin + placebo and warfarin + pentosan polysulfate sodium were comparable. See also Warnings and Precautions, Peri-Operative Considerations.

Drug interactions with other anticoagulant drugs have not been studies.

Care should be taken when administering ELMIRON to patients receiving anticoagulant drugs such as warfarin, heparin, tPA, streptokinase, high-dose aspirin, and nonsteroidal anti-inflammatory drugs.

DOSAGE AND ADMINISTRATION: Dosing Considerations: The capsules should be taken with water at least 1 hour before meals or 2 hours after meals.
Recommended Dose: The recommended dose of ELMIRON is 300 mg/day taken as one 100 mg capsule orally three times daily.

Some patients with interstitial cystitis may require 6 to 8 weeks of therapy with ELMIRON to achieve relief of symptoms. Long-term continuation of ELMIRON therapy is necessary for persistent therapeutic effect.

OVERDOSAGE:
Overdose has not been reported. Based upon the pharmacodynamics of the drug, toxicity is likely to be reflected as anticoagulation, bleeding, thrombocytopenia, liver function abnormalities, and gastric distress. (See Action and Clinical Pharmacology and Warnings and Precautions.) At a daily dose of 900 mg for 32 weeks (n=127) in a clinical trial, rectal hemorrhage was reported as an adverse event in 15% of patients. At a daily dose of ELMIRON 900 mg for 16 weeks in a clinical trial that enrolled 51 patients in the ELMIRON group and 49 in the placebo group, elevated liver function tests were reported as an adverse event in 11.8% of patients in the ELMIRON group and 2% of patients in the placebo group. In the event of acute overdosage, the patient should be given gastric lavage if possible, carefully observed and given symptomatic and supportive treatment.

> For management of a suspected drug overdose, CPhA recommends that you contact your **regional Poison Control Centre.** See the *CPS* Directory section for a list of Poison Control Centres.

ACTION AND CLINICAL PHARMACOLOGY: Mechanism of Action: ELMIRON is orally bioavailable pentosan polysulfate sodium. Its mechanism of action is thought to be adherence to the bladder surface supplementing the defective natural glycosaminoglycan layer. It is hypothesized that this action ameliorates the symptoms of interstitial cystitis.
Pharmacodynamics: ELMIRON is intended for the treatment of interstitial cystitis. In interstitial cystitis patients, a deficient or defective bladder protective glycosaminoglycan layer allows diffusion of irritating components in urine through to the underlying bladder wall. The resultant inflammatory response in the bladder wall produces the symptoms of interstitial cystitis. Definitive proof for this is not available.

In addition to its action as a glycosaminoglycan replacement in the bladder, pentosan polysulfate sodium has weak anticoagulant effect, fibrinolytic effect, a lipolytic effect and anti-inflammatory actions.
Pharmacokinetics: Absorption: In a clinical pharmacology study in which healthy female volunteers received a single oral 300 mg or 450 mg dose of pentosan polysulfate sodium containing radiolabeled drug under fasted conditions, mean maximal levels of plasma radioactivity were seen approximately 2 hours after dosing. Based on urinary excretion of radioactivity, a mean of approximately 6% of a radiolabeled oral dose of pentosan polysulfate sodium is absorbed and reaches the systemic circulation. In clinical trials, ELMIRON, was administered with water 1 hour before or 2 hours after meals; the effect of food on absorption of pentosan polysulfate sodium is not known.
Distribution: Parenteral radiolabelled studies in animals indicate significant distribution to the uroepithelium of the genitourinary tract with lesser amounts found in the liver, spleen, lung, skin, periosteum and bone marrow. Erythrocyte penetration is very low.
Metabolism: The absorbed fraction of a dose of pentosan polysulfate sodium is metabolized by partial desulfation in the liver and spleen, and by partial depolymerization in the kidney to a large number of metabolites. Both the desulfation and depolymerization can be saturated with continued dosing.
Excretion: Following oral administration of a 300 or 450 mg dose of pentosan polysulfate sodium containing radiolabeled drug to groups of healthy subjects, plasma radioactivity declined with mean half-lives of 27 and 20 hours, respectively. Most of an orally administered dose of pentosan polysulfate sodium (mean 84%) is excreted in feces as unchanged drug. A mean of 6% of an oral dose is excreted in the urine, mostly as desulfated and depolymerized metabolites. Only a small fraction of the administered dose (mean 0.14%) is recovered as intact drug.
Special Populations: No data are available in geriatric patients or in patients with hepatic or renal impairment. See also Warnings and Precautions, Hepatic.
STORAGE AND STABILITY: Store at controlled room temperature (15 to 30° C).
INFORMATION FOR THE PATIENT: Published in e-CPS, available by subscription at www.e-cps.ca.
DOSAGE FORMS, COMPOSITION AND PACKAGING: Each white, opaque, hard gelatin capsule, imprinted with "BNP7600", contains: pentosan polysulfate sodium 100 mg. Nonmedicinal ingredients: gelatin, magnesium stearate, microcrystalline cellulose and titanium dioxide. Bottles of 100.

(Shown in Product Identification Section)

The reader is invited to consult CPhA's monograph **Corticosteroids: Topical**.

Elocom®

mometasone furoate

Corticosteroid

Schering-Plough

PHARMACOLOGY: Mometasone furoate has anti-inflammatory, antipruritic and vasoconstrictive actions. The exact mechanism, however, of corticosteroids in each disease is uncertain. Mometasone furoate has been shown to have topical (dermatologic) and systemic pharmacologic and metabolic effects characteristic of this class of drugs.

INDICATIONS: For the relief of inflammatory and pruritic manifestations of corticosteroid-responsive dermatoses such as psoriasis and atopic dermatitis. The lotion formulation may be applied to scalp lesions.

CONTRAINDICATIONS: Hypersensitivity to any one of the components or to other corticosteroids is a contraindication to its use. Topical steroids are contraindicated in untreated fungal, bacterial and viral (i.e. herpes simplex, chickenpox and vaccinia) infections involving the skin.

WARNINGS: Any of the side effects that have been reported following systemic use of corticosteroids, including adrenal suppression, may also occur with topical corticosteroids, especially in infants and children.

Systemic absorption of topical corticosteroids will be increased if extensive body surface areas are treated or if the occlusive technique is used. Suitable precautions should be taken under these conditions or when long-term use is anticipated, particularly in infants and children. Pediatric patients may demonstrate greater susceptibility to topical corticosteroid-induced HPA axis suppression and Cushing's syndrome than mature patients because of a larger skin surface area to body weight ratio. Use of topical corticosteroids in children should be limited to the least amount compatible with an effective therapeutic regimen. Chronic corticosteroid therapy may interfere with growth and development of children.

The lotion contains isopropyl alcohol and may cause stinging or burning upon application to abraded or sun-burned skin. Do not use in or near the eyes.

PRECAUTIONS: Geriatrics: Suitable precautions should be taken in using topical glucocorticoids in patients with impaired circulation suffering from stasis dermatitis and other skin diseases.

Pregnancy: Since safety of topical corticosteroid use in pregnant women has not been established, drugs of this class should be used during pregnancy only if the potential benefit justifies the potential risk to the fetus. Drugs of this class should not be used extensively in large amounts or for prolonged periods of time in pregnant patients.

Lactation: Since it is not known whether topical administration of corticosteroids can result in sufficient systemic absorption to produce detectable quantities in breast milk, a decision should be made whether to discontinue nursing or to discontinue the drug, taking into account the importance of the drug to the mother.

General: Patients should be advised to inform subsequent physicians of the prior use of glucocorticoids.

If irritation, sensitization, excessive dryness develop with the use of mometasone furoate, treatment should be discontinued and appropriate therapy instituted.

Although mometasone furoate is poorly absorbed, nevertheless, application of corticosteroids over extensive lesions, or exceeding the dosage schedule may result in significant systemic absorption producing hypercorticism manifesting itself by adrenal suppression, moon facies, striae and suppression of growth.

During the use of topical corticosteroids, infections may occur. If an overt infection is present, appropriate antimicrobial treatment is indicated. If symptomatic response is not noted within a few days to a week, the local application of corticosteroids should be discontinued and the patient re-evaluated.

Prolonged use of corticosteroid preparations may produce striae or atrophy of the skin or s.c. tissues. If this occurs, treatment should be discontinued.

Mometasone furoate is not formulated for ophthalmic use and should not be used in or near the eyes.

ADVERSE EFFECTS: The following local adverse reactions have been reported:

Cream: During clinical studies in 319 patients: burning (1), pruritus (1), skin atrophy (3).

Ointment: During clinical studies in 812 patients: burning (13), pruritus (8), skin atrophy (8), tingling/stinging (7), and furunculosis (3).

Lotion: During clinical studies in 457 patients: burning (9 or 2%), pruritus (4 or 1%), skin atrophy (6 or 2%) (shininess, thinness, striae, telangiectasia), acneiform reactions (3 or <1%).

The following local adverse reactions have been reported infrequently when other topical dermatologic corticosteroids have been used as recommended. These reactions are listed in an approximate decreasing order of occurrence: burning, itching, irritation, dryness, folliculitis, hypertrichosis, acneiform eruptions, hypopigmentation, perioral dermatitis, allergic contact dermatitis, maceration of the skin, secondary infection, skin atrophy, striae, miliaria.

Adrenal suppression has also been reported following topical corticosteroid therapy. Posterior subcapsular cataracts have been reported following systemic use of corticosteroids.

Cream: The overall incidence of side effects was 1.6%, i.e. 5 of 319 subjects and patients reported treatment-related adverse experiences.

Ointment: The overall incidence of side effects was 4.9%, i.e. 40 of 812 subjects reported treatment-related adverse experiences.

Lotion: The overall incidence of side effects was 5.1%, i.e. 31 of 613 subjects and patients reported treatment-related adverse experiences.

Side effects were mild to moderate and were those typically associated with topical corticosteroid formulations after 7 days of treatment.

No systemic treatment-related adverse experiences were seen.

OVERDOSE:

Symptoms: No specific antidote is available and treatment should be symptomatic.

Excessive, prolonged use of topical corticosteroids can suppress pituitary-adrenal function resulting in secondary adrenal insufficiency.

Percutaneous absorption of corticosteroids can occur when large amounts of corticosteroids are applied. Toxic effects may include ecchymosis of skin, peptic ulceration, hypertension, aggravation of infection, hirsutism, acne, edema and muscle weakness due to protein depletion.

Treatment: Appropriate symptomatic treatment is indicated. Acute hypercorticoid symptoms are virtually reversible. Treat electrolyte imbalance, if necessary. In cases of chronic toxicity, slow withdrawal of corticosteroids is advised.

Treatment of a patient with systemic toxic manifestations consists of assuring and maintaining a patent airway and supporting ventilation using oxygen and assisted or controlled respiration as required. This will be sufficient in the management of most reactions. Should circulatory depression occur, vasopressors such as ephedrine or metaraminol and i.v. fluids may be used. Should a convulsion persist despite oxygen therapy, small increments of an ultra-short acting barbiturate (pentobarbital or secobarbital) may be given i.v. Allergic reactions are characterized by cutaneous lesions, urticaria, edema or anaphylactoid reactions.

For management of a suspected drug overdose, CPhA recommends that you contact your **regional Poison Control Centre**. See the *CPS* Directory section for a list of Poison Control Centres.

DOSAGE: Cream/Ointment: Apply a thin film to the affected skin areas once daily.

Lotion: Apply a few drops of the lotion to affected skin areas including scalp sites once daily; massage gently and thoroughly until medication disappears.

Do not use occlusive dressings.

SUPPLIED: Cream: Each g of white to off-white uniform cream contains: mometasone furoate 1 mg. Nonmedicinal ingredients: aluminum starch octenylsuccinate, ceteareth-20, hexylene glycol, phosphoric acid to adjust the pH, propylene glycol stearate, purified water, stearyl alcohol, titanium dioxide, white petrolatum and white wax. Tubes of 15 and 50 g. Store between 2 and 30°C.

Lotion: Each g of lotion contains: mometasone furoate 1 mg. Nonmedicinal ingredients: hydroxypropylcellulose, isopropyl alcohol, phosphoric acid to adjust the pH, propylene glycol, purified water and sodium phosphate monobasic monohydrate. Plastic bottles of 30 and 75 mL. Store between 2 and 30°C.

Ointment: Each g of ointment contains: mometasone furoate 1 mg. Nonmedicinal ingredients: hexylene glycol, phosphoric acid to adjust the pH, propylene glycol stearate, purified water, white petrolatum and white wax. Tubes of 15 and 50 g. Store between 2 and 30°C.

Eloxatin®

oxaliplatin

Antineoplastic Agent

sanofi-aventis

Date of Revision: January 13, 2009

SUMMARY PRODUCT INFORMATION:

Route of Administration	Dosage Form/ Strength	Clinically Relevant Nonmedicinal Ingredients
Intravenous infusion	Lyophilized powder 50 mg and 100 mg	Lactose monohydrate
	Aqueous solution 50 mg/10 mL, 100 mg/20 mL and 200 mg/40 mL	Water for injection

(See Dosage and Administration.)

INDICATIONS AND CLINICAL USE: ELOXATIN (oxaliplatin for injection) in combination with infusional 5-fluorouracil/leucovorin (5-FU/LV) is indicated for:

- Adjuvant treatment of patients with stage III (Dukes' C) colon cancer after complete resection of primary tumor. The indication is based on a demonstrated improvement in disease-free survival. Survival data at 6 years show a numerical improvement in overall survival.
- Treatment of patients with metastatic colorectal cancer.

Geriatrics (≥65 years of age): In patients previously untreated for metastatic colorectal cancer, patients ≥65 years (99 of 279 patients) receiving ELOXATIN in combination with 5-FU/LV experienced more fatigue, dehydration, diarrhea, leukopenia, and syncope than patients <65 years, although the difference was not statistically significant. Starting doses were the same in both age groups. In the adjuvant trial, patients ≥65 years receiving the ELOXATIN combination therapy (393 of 1108 patients) experienced more grade 3-4 granulocytopenia and diarrhea than patients <65 years, although the difference was not statistically significant. The efficacy of ELOXATIN on disease free survival benefit in patients ≥65 years of age was not conclusive in the adjuvant trial (see Dosage and Administration).

Pediatrics (≤22 years of age): There is no indication for use of oxaliplatin in children. The effectiveness of oxaliplatin single agent in the pediatric populations with solid tumors has not been established (see Warnings and Precautions).

CONTRAINDICATIONS: ELOXATIN should not be administered to patients:

- with a history of known allergy to ELOXATIN or other platinum compounds or to any ingredient in the formulation or component of the container. For a complete listing, see Dosage Forms, Composition and Packaging.
- who are breast-feeding.
- who are pregnant.
- with severe renal impairment (creatinine clearance Cl_{Cr} <30 mL/min).

WARNINGS AND PRECAUTIONS:

Serious Warnings and Precautions

- **ELOXATIN should be administered under the supervision of a qualified physician experienced in the use of cancer chemotherapeutic agents.**
- **Anaphylactic Reactions**—See Warnings and Precautions, Immune; Cardiovascular.
- **Hepatotoxicity**—See Warnings and Precautions, Hepatic/Biliary/Pancreatic.
- **Myelosuppression—Neutropenia and Thrombocytopenia**—See Warnings and Precautions, Hematologic.
- **Neuropathy—Sensory and Motor**—See Warnings and Precautions, Neurologic; Adverse Reactions, Adverse Drug Reaction Overview, Other Clinical Trial Adverse Drug Reactions and Post-Market Adverse Drug Reactions, Nervous System Disorders.
- **Respiratory—Interstitial lung disease (including fatalities)** has been reported with ELOXATIN use. See Warnings and Precautions, Respiratory; Adverse Reactions, Other Clinical Trial Adverse Drug Reactions, Respiratory, Thoracic and Mediastinal Disorders.

General: No studies on the effects on the ability to drive and operate machinery have been performed. However ELOXATIN treatment resulting in an increased risk of dizziness, nausea and vomiting, and neurologic gait and balance disorders may have influence on the ability to drive and operate machinery.

Vision abnormalities, in particular transient vision loss (reversible following therapy discontinuation) were reported with Eloxatin administration (see Other Clinical Trial Adverse Drug Reactions and Post-Market Adverse Drugs Reactions, Eye Disorders). Transient blindness episodes lasting for periods of seconds or minutes may recur repeatedly during the event duration (usually hours to days). Therefore, patients should be warned of the potential effect of these events on the ability to drive or operate machinery.

Carcinogenesis and Mutagenesis: ELOXATIN was shown to be mutagenic and clastogenic in mammalian test systems in vitro and in vivo. The teratogenic potential of ELOXATIN was manifested by the embryonic mortality, decreased fetal weight and delayed ossifications in rats at doses up to 12 mg/m²/day. This daily dose is approximately one-sixth of the recommended human dose. Related compounds with similar mechanism of action and genotoxicity profiles have been reported to be teratogenic. ELOXATIN may increase the risk of genetic defects or fetal malformations. ELOXATIN is contraindicated in pregnancy, and males are advised not to father a child during treatment and up to 6 months thereafter. Because ELOXATIN may cause irreversible infertility, men are advised to seek counseling on sperm storage before starting treatment.

Carcinogenicity studies have not been performed with ELOXATIN. However given that ELOXATIN is genotoxic, it should be considered a human carcinogen, which should be taken into consideration for the overall risk/benefit in the adjuvant setting.

Cardiovascular: No formal clinical cardiac safety studies have been carried out. Preclinical data are limited. No standard hERG or Purkinje fibre tests have been done. Cardiotoxicity was observed in dogs. No formal clinical QT studies with ELOXATIN were done. The effect of ELOXATIN in combination with 5-HT_3 blocker antiemetics (given as pre-medication in clinical studies) on QTc has not been formally studied. In case of grade 3 or grade 4 hypersensitivity reaction associated with hemodynamic instability (e.g., bradycardia, tachycardia, hypotension, hypertension) ECG monitoring should be done.

Gastrointestinal: Gastrointestinal toxicity, which manifests as nausea and vomiting, warrants prophylactic and/or therapeutic antiemetic therapy (see Adverse Reactions).

Dehydration, ileus, intestinal obstruction, hypokalemia, metabolic acidosis, and even renal disorders, may be associated with severe diarrhea/emesis, particularly when combining ELOXATIN with 5-FU. In rare cases, colitis, including *C. difficile* diarrhea, have occurred (see Adverse Reactions, Other Clinical Trial Adverse Drug Reactions).

Patients must be adequately informed of the risk of diarrhea/emesis after ELOXATIN/5-FU administration in order to contact urgently their treating physician for appropriate management (see Monitoring and Laboratory Tests).

Hematologic: Patients must be adequately informed of the risk of neutropenia after ELOXATIN/5-FU administration in order to contact urgently their treating physician for appropriate management (see Monitoring and Laboratory Tests). Thrombocytopenia is commonly seen with ELOXATIN combination therapy, although the risk of grade 3 or 4 bleeding is low (see Adverse Reactions, Clinical Trial Adverse Drug Reactions). Anemia (rarely presenting as Hemolytic Uremic Syndrome) can also occur.

Hepatic/Biliary/Pancreatic: Routine monitoring of liver function should be performed on all patients receiving ELOXATIN. Hepatotoxicity with the use of ELOXATIN plus 5-FU/LV has been noted in clinical studies (see Adverse Reactions, Clinical Trial Adverse Drug Reactions, "Hepatic Adverse Events" Table 4, Table 6 and Table 9). Hepatic vascular disorders should be considered, and if appropriate, should be investigated in cases of abnormal liver function test results or portal hypertension, which cannot be explained by liver metastases. There is evidence that ELOXATIN causes liver sinusoidal obstruction syndrome, also known as veno-occlusive disease of the liver, which, on liver biopsy is manifested as peliosis, nodular regenerative hyperplasia, and perisinusoidal fibrosis. In the literature, there is a case report of fatal hepatic failure following liver metastasis resection in a patient treated pre-operatively with ELOXATIN. Very rare cases of hepatic failure, hepatitis and rare cases of pancreatitis have been reported in the post-market setting (see Adverse Reactions, Other Clinical Trial Adverse Drug Reactions).

Immune: Hypersensitivity, anaphylactic reactions, and/or allergic reactions are reported with the use of ELOXATIN. The incidence of Grade 3 or 4 events was 2-3% across clinical studies. In the post-marketing experience, some cases of anaphylaxis have been fatal. These allergic reactions can occur within minutes of ELOXATIN administration, and can include rash, urticaria, erythema, pruritus, and, rarely, bronchospasm and hypotension. Patients with a history of allergic reaction to platinum compounds should be monitored for allergic symptoms. In case of an anaphylactic-like reaction to ELOXATIN, the infusion should be immediately discontinued and appropriate symptomatic treatment initiated. These reactions are usually managed with epinephrine, corticosteroid, and antihistamine therapy. ELOXATIN rechallenge is contraindicated (see Boxed Serious Warnings and Precautions).

Neurologic: ELOXATIN is consistently associated with two types of sensory neuropathy:

1. **An acute, reversible, sensory peripheral neuropathy can develop (reported in 85 to 95% of patients) at the end of the 2-hour ELOXATIN infusion, or within 1 to 2 days of dosing. It usually resolves between cycles, but frequently recurs with further cycles.** Symptoms may be precipitated or exacerbated by exposure to cold temperatures or objects. The symptoms usually present as transient paresthesias, dysesthesias and hypoesthesias in the hands, feet, perioral area, or throat. Other symptoms occasionally observed include, abnormal tongue sensation, dysarthria, eye pain, and throat or chest tightness. In addition, acute motor symptoms, including jaw spasms, muscle spasms, involuntary muscle contractions, ptosis, vocal cord paralysis and cranial nerve dysfunction have been reported. Acute neuropathy (all grades) occurred in 58% of patients with metastatic colorectal cancer receiving ELOXATIN plus 5-FU/LV but grade 3/4 events occurred in only 4% of patients. In any individual cycle, acute neurotoxicity was observed in about one third of patients.

   An acute syndrome of pharyngolaryngeal dysesthesia occurs in 1-2% of patients, and is characterized by subjective sensations of dysphagia or dyspnea, feeling of suffocation, without any evidence of respiratory distress (no cyanosis or hypoxia) or of laryngospasm or bronchospasm (no stridor or wheezing). Because cold temperatures can precipitate or exacerbate acute neurological symptoms, ice (mucositis prophylaxis) should be avoided during ELOXATIN infusion (see Dosage and Administration, Recommended Dose and Dosage Adjustment).

2. **A persistent peripheral sensory neuropathy can develop. It is characterised by paresthesias, dysesthesias and/or hypoesthesias, and may include deficits in proprioception, thus resulting in difficulties performing activities of daily living (ADLs). This can result in difficulty with delicate movements such as writing or buttoning, as well as difficulty walking due to impaired proprioception.**

   In adjuvant patients, sensory neuropathy was reported in 92% (all Grades) and 13% (Grade 3) of patients. The median cycle of onset for grade 3 neuropathy was cycle 9. At the 28-day follow-up after the last treatment cycle, 60% of all patients had neuropathy of any grade (Grade 1-40%; Grade 2-16%; Grade 3-5%) decreasing to 21% at 18 months (Grade 1-17%; Grade 2-3%; Grade 3-1%). At the 48-month follow-up, neuropathy status was as follows: Grade 0-62%; Grade 1-9%; Grade 2-2%; Grade 3-0.5%; not evaluable-26.5%. This suggests that there can be partial or complete recovery of sensory neuropathy over time after cessation of therapy. However, in some cases, an increase in severity of the sensory neuropathy was reported years after completion of adjuvant therapy.

   The long term impact of the neuropathy is difficult to measure, and needs to be considered carefully in the overall risk/benefit ratio during therapy with ELOXATIN.

   In patients previously untreated for metastatic colorectal cancer, neuropathy was reported in 82% (all Grades) and 19% (Grade 3/4), and in the previously treated patients in 79% (all Grades) and 11% (Grade 3/4). The probability of developing peripheral sensory neuropathy is dependent upon the cumulative dose of oxaliplatin administered. These symptoms may improve in some patients upon discontinuation of ELOXATIN.

   NCI CTC grading definitions are as follows:

Grade	Definition
Grade 0	No change or none
Grade 1	Mild paresthesias, loss of deep tendon reflexes
Grade 2	Mild or moderate objective sensory loss, moderate paresthesias
Grade 3	Severe objective sensory loss or paresthesias that interfere with function

Sensory peripheral neurotoxicity of ELOXATIN should be carefully monitored, especially if coadministered with other medications with specific neurological toxicity (see Boxed Serious Warnings and Precautions; Adverse Reactions; Monitoring and Laboratory Tests). The risk factors that make a patient more likely to develop neuropathy have not been identified.

One case of posterior reversible encephalopathy syndrome (PRES) has been reported in the literature in a patient treated with oxaliplatin and 5-FU/LV, although the cause/effect relationship cannot be established with certainty.

Respiratory: ELOXATIN has been uncommonly associated with pulmonary fibrosis/interstitial lung disease (<1% of study patients). In the adjuvant trial, the combined incidence of cough and dyspnea in patients receiving ELOXATIN plus 5-FU/LV compared to patients receiving infusional 5-FU/LV alone was 7% vs 5% (all grades) and 0.8% vs 0.1% (Grade 3-4), respectively. In previously untreated patients with metastatic colorectal cancer, the combined incidence of cough, dyspnea and hypoxia in patients receiving ELOXATIN plus 5-FU/LV vs irinotecan plus 5-FU/LV was 43% vs 32% (all grades) and 7% vs 5% (Grade 3-4). In previously treated patients, the combined incidence of cough, dyspnea and hypoxia in patients receiving ELOXATIN plus 5-FU/LV vs 5-FU/LV alone was 30% vs 21% (all grades) and 5% vs 2% (Grade 3-4). One fatal case of eosinophilic pneumonia was reported in a patient receiving combination ELOXATIN therapy on study.

In case of unexplained respiratory symptoms such as non-productive cough, dyspnea, crackles, or radiological pulmonary infiltrates, ELOXATIN should be discontinued until further pulmonary investigation excludes interstitial lung disease (see Boxed Serious Warnings and Precautions and Adverse Reactions). Fatal cases of interstitial lung disease have been reported in the post-market setting.

Skin: In case of ELOXATIN extravasation, the infusion must be stopped immediately and usual local symptomatic treatment initiated. Extravasation of ELOXATIN may result in local pain and inflammation that may be severe and lead to complications, including necrosis and injection site reaction, including redness, swelling, and pain. In the literature, tissue necrosis has been reported with ELOXATIN extravasation.

Special Populations: Pregnant Women: To date, there is no available information on safety of use in pregnant women. Based on preclinical findings, ELOXATIN is likely to be lethal and/or teratogenic to the human foetus at the recommended therapeutic doses. Therefore, ELOXATIN is contraindicated in pregnancy.

As with other cytotoxic agents, effective contraceptive measures should be taken in potentially fertile patients (male and female) prior to initiating chemotherapy with ELOXATIN (see Contraindications).

Nursing Women: Excretion in breast milk has not been studied. Breast-feeding is contraindicated during ELOXATIN therapy (see Contraindications).

Geriatrics (≥65 years of age): In patients previously untreated for metastatic colorectal cancer, patients ≥65 years (99 of 279 patients) receiving ELOXATIN in combination with 5-FU/LV experienced more fatigue, dehydration, diarrhea, leukopenia, and syncope than patients <65 years, although the difference was not statistically significant. Starting doses were the same in both age groups. In the adjuvant trial, patients ≥65 years receiving the ELOXATIN combination therapy (393 of 1108) experienced more grade 3-4 granulocytopenia and diarrhea than patients <65 years although the difference was not statistically significant.

Pediatrics (≤22 years of age): Oxaliplatin single agent has been evaluated in pediatric population in 2 Phase I (69 patients) and 2 Phase II (90 patients) studies. A total of 159 pediatric patients (7 months-22 years of age) with solid tumors have been treated. The effectiveness of oxaliplatin single agent in the pediatric populations treated has not been established. Accrual in both Phase II studies was stopped for lack of tumor response (see Indications and Clinical Use).

Hepatic Insufficiency: No increase in ELOXATIN acute toxicities was observed in the subset of patients with abnormal liver function tests at baseline. No specific dose adjustment for patients with abnormal liver function tests was performed during clinical development.

Renal Insufficiency: The primary route of platinum elimination is renal. Clearance of ultrafilterable platinum is decreased in patients with mild, moderate and severe renal impairment. A pharmacodynamic relationship between platinum ultrafiltrate levels and clinical safety and effectiveness has not been established (see Action and Clinical Pharmacology).

ELOXATIN has not been studied in patients with severe renal impairment (see Contraindications).

Due to limited information on safety in patients with moderately impaired renal function, administration should be considered after suitable appraisal of the benefit/risk for the patient. In this situation, treatment may be initiated at the normally recommended dose and renal function should be closely monitored and dose adjusted according to toxicity.

Monitoring and Laboratory Tests: Complete blood count with differential, hemoglobin, platelets, and blood chemistries, including ALT, AST, bilirubin, creatinine, magnesium and electrolytes should be performed prior to the start of therapy and before each subsequent course (see Dosage and Administration, Recommended Dose and Dosage Adjustment).

There have been reports while on study and from post-marketing surveillance of prolonged prothrombin time and INR occasionally associated with hemorrhage in patients who received ELOXATIN plus 5-FU/LV while on anticoagulants. Patients receiving ELOXATIN plus 5-FU/LV and requiring oral anticoagulants may require closer monitoring (see Drug Interactions).

Patients receiving ELOXATIN combination therapy should be monitored for diarrhea, vomiting, and mucositis, which can lead to severe/life-threatening dehydration. If this occurs, discontinue ELOXATIN until improvement or resolution (see Dosage and Administration, Recommended Dose and Dosage Adjustment).

A neurological examination should be performed before each administration and periodically thereafter. See Dosage and Administration, Recommended Dose and Dosage Adjustment for guidance if neurological symptoms occur.

ADVERSE REACTIONS: Adverse Drug Reaction Overview: Both 5-FU and ELOXATIN are associated with gastrointestinal and hematologic adverse events. When ELOXATIN is administered in combination with 5-FU, the incidence of these events is increased.

The most common adverse reactions in patients treated with ELOXATIN in combination with 5-FU in the adjuvant colon and metastatic colorectal cancer trials were peripheral sensory neuropathies, fatigue, thrombocytopenia, anemia, neutropenia, nausea, vomiting, diarrhea, stomatitis and increase in hepatic enzymes and alkaline phosphatase (see Warnings and Precautions).

Blood and Lymphatic System Disorders: Anemia, neutropenia and thrombocytopenia were reported with the combination of ELOXATIN and infusional 5-FU/LV (see Adverse Reactions, Clinical Trial Adverse Drug Reactions).

In adjuvant patients the incidence of febrile neutropenia was 0.1% in the 5-FU/LV infusion arm and 0.7% in the ELOXATIN plus 5-FU/LV arm. The incidence of febrile neutropenia in the patients previously untreated for metastatic colorectal cancer was 15% (3% of cycles) in the irinotecan plus 5-FU/LV arm and 4% (less than 1% of cycles) in the ELOXATIN plus 5-FU/LV arm. The incidence of febrile neutropenia in the previously treated patients was 1% in the 5-FU/LV arm and 5% (less than 1% of cycles) in the ELOXATIN plus 5-FU/LV combination arm.

In adjuvant patients the incidence of thrombocytopenia (all grades) was 77% vs 19% (ELOXATIN plus 5-FU/LV vs 5-FU/LV) while grade 3-4 thrombocytopenia incidence was 1.7% vs 0.4%. There were more bleeding events in the ELOXATIN plus 5-FU/LV arm (gastrointestinal hemorrhage 0.5%; hematemesis 0.3%; rectal hemorrhage 1.3%). The incidence of thrombocytopenia in patients previously untreated for metastatic colorectal cancer was higher in the ELOXATIN plus 5-FU/LV arm vs irinotecan plus 5-FU/LV arm (all grade thrombocytopenia: 70% vs 26%; grade 3 and 4: 5% vs 2%). However, bleeding events in the ELOXATIN plus 5-FU/LV arm were infrequent and included: epistaxis, rectal bleeding, melena, vaginal bleeding, hematuria, and hemoptysis. The incidence of thrombocytopenia in patients previously treated for metastatic colorectal cancer was higher in the ELOXATIN plus 5-FU/LV arm vs the 5-FU/LV arm (all grade thrombocytopenia: 67% vs 21%; grade 3 and 4: 6% vs 0%).

Hemolytic Uremic Syndrome has been rarely reported with the use of ELOXATIN.

Gastrointestinal Disorders: Anorexia, nausea, vomiting, diarrhea, stomatitis/mucositis and abdominal pain were commonly reported in the adjuvant treatment of patients with colon cancer and the previously untreated and treated patients for metastatic colorectal cancer (see Adverse Reactions, Clinical Trial Adverse Drug Reactions).

Dehydration, hypokalemia, metabolic acidosis, ileus, intestinal obstruction and renal disorders may be associated with severe diarrhea or vomiting, particularly when ELOXATIN is combined with 5-FU (see Warnings and Precautions and Adverse Reactions, Post-Market Adverse Drug Reactions).

General Disorders and Administration Site Conditions: Fever and rigors (tremors) either from infection (with or without febrile neutropenia) or possibly from immunological mechanism were reported in the adjuvant treatment of patients with colon cancer and in the previously untreated and treated patients for metastatic colorectal cancer (see Adverse Reactions, Clinical Trial Adverse Drug Reactions).

Injection Site: Injection site reactions, including local pain, redness, swelling and thrombosis have been reported (see Adverse Reactions, Clinical Trial Adverse Drug Reactions). In the literature, tissue necrosis has been reported with ELOXATIN extravasation.

Immune System Disorders: Allergic reactions such as: skin rash (particularly urticaria), conjunctivitis, rhinitis and anaphylactic reactions were reported (see Warnings and Precautions and Adverse Reactions, Clinical Trial Adverse Drug Reactions).

Musculoskeletal and Connective Tissue Disorders: Back pain was reported in patients receiving ELOXATIN plus 5-FU/LV as adjuvant therapy and in the previously treated patients for metastatic colorectal cancer. In case of such adverse reaction, hemolysis (as part of Hemolytic Uremic Syndrome) which has been rarely reported should be investigated (see Adverse Reactions, Clinical Trial Adverse Drug Reactions).

Nervous System Disorders: ELOXATIN is frequently associated with acute and chronic sensory peripheral neuropathy. There have been very rare reports of symptoms compatible with a diagnosis of Guillain-Barre Syndrome, for which a causal relationship has not been established (see Adverse Reactions, Other Clinical Trial Adverse Drug Reactions).

Peripheral sensory neuropathy was reported in adjuvant patients treated with the ELOXATIN combination with a frequency of 92% (all Grades) and 13% (Grade 3). In patients previously untreated for metastatic colorectal cancer, neuropathy was reported in 82% (all Grades) and 19% (Grade 3/4), and in the previously treated patients in 79% (all Grades) and 11% (Grade 3/4) events.

Peripheral Sensory Neuropathy: Acute Sensory Neuropathy: These symptoms usually develop at the end of the 2-hour ELOXATIN infusion or within a few hours, abate spontaneously within the next hours or days, and frequently recur with further cycles. They may be precipitated or exacerbated by exposure to cold temperatures or objects. They usually present as transient paresthesia, dysesthesia and hypoesthesia. An acute syndrome of pharyngolaryngeal dysesthesia occurs in 1-2% of patients and is characterized by subjective sensations of dysphagia or dyspnea, feeling of suffocation, without any evidence of respiratory distress (no cyanosis or hypoxia) or of laryngospasm or bronchospasm (no stridor or wheezing).

Dysesthesia/Paresthesia of Extremities and Peripheral Neuropathy: The dose limiting toxicity of ELOXATIN is neurological. It involves a sensory peripheral neuropathy characterised by peripheral dysesthesia and/or paresthesia with or without cramps, often triggered by the cold (85 to 95% of patients).

The duration of these symptoms, which usually recede between the cycles of treatment, increases with the number of treatment cycles. The onset of pain and/or a functional disorder and their duration are indications for dose adjustment, or even treatment discontinuation (see Warnings and Precautions and Dosage and Administration). This functional disorder, including difficulties in executing delicate movements, is a possible consequence of sensory impairment. The risk of occurrence of a functional disorder for a cumulative dose of approximately 800 mg/m² (i.e. 10 cycles) is 15% or less. The neurological signs and symptoms improve when treatment is discontinued in the majority of cases.

Other Neurologic Manifestations: Other symptoms occasionally observed include cranial nerve dysfunction which may occur as a single, isolated event or several events may occur in combination. These include: ptosis, diplopia, aphonia, dysphonia, hoarseness, sometimes described as vocal cord paralysis, abnormal tongue sensation or dysarthria, sometimes described as aphasia, trigeminal neuralgia, facial pain, fasciculations, eye pain, decrease of visual acuity, visual field disorders, transient blindness (reversible following therapy discontinuation), amaurosis and amaurosis fugax. In addition, the following have been observed: jaw spasm, muscle spasms, involuntary muscle contractions, muscle twitching, myoclonus, abnormal coordination, abnormal gait, ataxia, balance disorders and throat or chest tightness/pressure/discomfort/pain (see Warnings and Precautions, General).

Skin and Subcutaneous Tissue Disorders: Alopecia in patients receiving ELOXATIN has been reported across clinical studies with an incidence of approximately one third (all grades), most cases being mild hair loss only.

Clinical Trial Adverse Drug Reactions: Patients Treated in the Adjuvant Setting for Colon Cancer: One thousand one hundred and eight (1108) patients with colon cancer were treated adjuvantly in a clinical study with ELOXATIN in combination with infusional 5-FU/LV.

Treatment was discontinued due to an adverse event in 15% of patients on the ELOXATIN plus infusional 5-FU/LV arm compared to 6% of patients on the 5-FU/LV only arm.

The incidence of death within 28 days of last treatment, regardless of causality, was 0.5% (n=6) in both the ELOXATIN combination (primarily septic deaths) and infusional 5-FU/LV arms, respectively.

Deaths within 60 days from initiation of therapy were 0.3% (n=3) in both the ELOXATIN combination and infusional 5-FU/LV arms, respectively.

Although specific events can vary, the overall frequency of adverse events was similar in men and women and in patients <65 and ≥65 years. However, the following grade 3/4 events were more common in females regardless of treatment arm: diarrhea, fatigue, granulocytopenia, nausea and vomiting. In patients ≥65 years old, the incidence of grade 3/4 granulocytopenia and diarrhea was higher than in younger patients, although the difference was not statistically significant.

Table 1 provides adverse events reported in the adjuvant treatment of patients with colon cancer pivotal study for events with overall incidences ≥5% in the arm combining ELOXATIN and 5-FU/LV.

Table 1: ELOXATIN

Adverse Events Reported in the Adjuvant Treatment of Patients with Colon Cancer Pivotal Clinical Trial (≥5% of all Patients in the ELOXATIN+5-FU/LV arm)—by Body System

Adverse Event (WHO/Pref)	ELOXATIN+5-FU/LV N=1108 All Grades (%)	ELOXATIN+5-FU/LV N=1108 Grade 3/4 (%)	5-FU/LV N=1111 All Grades (%)	5-FU/LV N=1111 Grade 3/4 (%)
Any Event	100	70	99	31
Application Site Disorders				
Injection Site Reaction	11	3	10	3
Body as a Whole—General Disorders				
Allergic Reaction	10	3	2	<1
Fatigue	44	4	38	1
Fever	27	1	12	1
Pain	5	<1	5	<1
Weight Increase	10	<1	10	<1
Central and Peripheral Nervous System Disorders				
Headache	7	<1	5	<1
Overall Peripheral Sensory Neuropathy[b]	92	12	16	<1
Sensory Disturbance	8	<1	1	0
Gastrointestinal System Disorders				
Abdominal Pain	18	1	17	2
Anorexia	13	1	8	<1
Constipation	22	1	19	<1
Diarrhea	56	11	48	7
Dyspepsia	8	<1	5	0
Nausea	74	5	61	2
Stomatitis	42	3	40	2
Vomiting	47	6	24	1
Liver and Biliary System Disorders				
Bilirubinemia	20	4	20	5
Hepatic Enzyme Increased	57	2	34	1
Metabolic and Nutritional Disorders				
Phosphatase Alkaline Increased	42	<1	20	<1
Platelet, Bleeding and Clotting Disorders				
Epistaxis	16	<1	12	0
Thrombocytopenia	77	2	19	<1
Red Blood Cell Disorders				
Anemia	76	1	67	<1
Resistance Mechanism Disorders				
Infection	25	4	25	3
Respiratory System Disorders				
Dyspnea	5	1	3	<1
Rhinitis	6	0	8	<1
Skin and Appendage Disorders				
Alopecia[a]	30	0	28	0
Skin Disorders	32	2	36	2
Special Senses Disorders				
Taste Perversion	12	<1	8	0
Vision Disorders				
Conjunctivitis	9	1	15	1

(cont'd)

Table 1: ELOXATIN *(cont'd)*

Adverse Events Reported in the Adjuvant Treatment of Patients with Colon Cancer Pivotal Clinical Trial (≥5% of all Patients in the ELOXATIN+5-FU/LV arm)—by Body System

Adverse Event (WHO/Pref)	ELOXATIN+5-FU/LV N=1108 All Grades (%)	ELOXATIN+5-FU/LV N=1108 Grade 3/4 (%)	5-FU/LV N=1111 All Grades (%)	5-FU/LV N=1111 Grade 3/4 (%)
White Cell and RES Disorders				
Granulocytopenia	79	41	40	5

[a] Alopecia: only grades 1 and 2 according to the NCI grading scale used.
[b] Overall Peripheral Sensory Neuropathy: only grades 1, 2 and 3 according to the NCI grading scale used.
RES: reticulo-endothelial system.

The following additional most common and potentially important adverse events regardless of treatment causality were reported in less than 5% of the patients in the ELOXATIN combined with 5-FU/LV arm in the pivotal study in the adjuvant treatment of patients with colon cancer.
Body as a Whole—General Disorders: chest pain.
Central & Peripheral Nervous System Disorders: dizziness.
Metabolic/Laboratory: Magnesium levels were not prospectively tested.
Psychiatric Disorders: insomnia.
Respiratory System Disorders: coughing.
Vision Disorders: abnormal lacrimation.
White Cell and Reticulo-endothelial System Disorders: leukopenia.
Patients Previously Untreated for Metastatic Colorectal Cancer: Two hundred and fifty-nine (259) patients were treated in the ELOXATIN plus 5-FU/LV combination arm of the randomized trial in patients previously untreated for metastatic colorectal cancer.

Twenty-six percent (26%) of patients in the ELOXATIN plus 5-FU/LV combination arm and 8% in the irinotecan plus 5-FU/LV arm had to discontinue treatment because of adverse effects related most commonly to gastrointestinal, hematologic or neurologic adverse events.

The incidence of death within 30 days of treatment in the previously untreated for metastatic colorectal cancer study, regardless of causality, was 3% with the ELOXATIN plus 5 FU/LV, 5% with irinotecan plus 5-FU/LV and 3% with ELOXATIN plus irinotecan. Deaths within 60 days from initiation of therapy were 2% with ELOXATIN plus 5-FU/LV, 5% with irinotecan plus 5-FU/LV and 3% with ELOXATIN plus irinotecan. Deaths within 60 days from initiation of therapy on the ELOXATIN plus 5-FU/LV arm were attributed to disease progression, sepsis, dehydration/electrolyte imbalance, and liver failure.

The following adverse events were reported more frequently in patients ≥65 years old on the ELOXATIN and 5-FU/LV combination arm: constitutional symptoms, fatigue, anorexia, dehydration, leukopenia, musculoskeletal events, syncope and pulmonary events.

For any class of adverse event (all inclusive), the overall reported cases were similar across arms and populations. When Grade 3 or 4 events were evaluated, the female patient population reported a higher number of events independent of treatment arm.

Table 2 provides adverse events reported in the previously untreated for metastatic colorectal cancer pivotal study for events with overall incidences ≥5% in the ELOXATIN and 5-FU/LV combination arm.

Table 2: ELOXATIN

Adverse Events Reported in Patients Previously Untreated for Metastatic Colorectal Cancer Clinical Trial (≥5% of all Patients in the ELOXATIN+5-FU/LV Arm)—by Body System

Adverse Event (WHO/Pref)	ELOXATIN+5-FU/LV N=259 All Grades (%)	ELOXATIN+5-FU/LV N=259 Grade 3/4 (%)	Irinotecan+5-FU/LV N=256 All Grades (%)	Irinotecan+5-FU/LV N=256 Grade 3/4 (%)	ELOXATIN+irinotecan N=258 All Grades (%)	ELOXATIN+irinotecan N=258 Grade 3/4 (%)
Any Event	99	82	98	70	99	76
Allergy/Immunology						
Allergic Rhinitis	10	0	6	0	6	0
Hypersensitivity	12	2	5	0	6	1
Cardiovascular						
Oedema	15	0	13	<1	10	1
Thrombosis	6	5	6	6	3	3
Constitutional Symptoms						
Fatigue	70	7	58	11	66	16
Fever—No ANC[a]	16	1	9	<1	9	0
Rigors	8	<1	2	0	7	0
Sweating	5	0	6	0	12	0
Weight Loss	11	0	9	<1	11	<1
Dermatology/Skin						
Alopecia	38	0	44	0	67	0
Dermatology NOS[a]	6	0	1	0	2	0
Dry Skin	6	0	2	0	5	0
Flushing	7	0	2	0	5	0
Injection Site Reaction	6	0	1	0	4	1
Pruritus	6	0	4	0	2	0
Rash	11	<1	4	0	7	1

(cont'd)

Table 2: ELOXATIN *(cont'd)*

Adverse Events Reported in Patients Previously Untreated for Metastatic Colorectal Cancer Clinical Trial (≥5% of all Patients in the ELOXATIN+5-FU/LV Arm)—by Body System

	ELOXATIN+5-FU/LV N=259		Irinotecan+5-FU/LV N=256		ELOXATIN+irinotecan N=258	
Adverse Event (WHO/Pref)	**All Grades (%)**	**Grade 3/4 (%)**	**All Grades (%)**	**Grade 3/4 (%)**	**All Grades (%)**	**Grade 3/4 (%)**
Skin Reaction—Hand/foot Syndrome	7	1	2	<1	1	0
Gastrointestinal						
Anorexia	35	2	25	4	27	5
Constipation	32	4	27	2	21	2
Dehydration	9	5	16	11	14	7
Diarrhea—Colostomy	13	2	16	7	16	3
Diarrhea—No Colostomy	56	12	65	29	76	25
Dyspepsia	12	0	7	0	5	<1
Dysphagia	5	0	3	0	3	<1
Flatulence	9	0	6	0	5	<1
Mouth Dryness	5	0	2	0	3	0
Nausea	71	6	67	15	83	19
Stomatitis	38	0	25	1	19	<1
Taste	14	0	6	0	8	<1
Vomiting	41	4	43	13	64	23
Hemorrhage						
Epistaxis	10	0	2	0	2	<1
Infection/Febrile Neutropenia						
Infection—ANC[a]	8	8	12	11	9	8
Infection—No ANC[a]	10	4	5	1	7	2
Neurology						
Anxiety	5	0	2	0	6	<1
Depression	9	1	5	<1	7	1
Dizziness	8	<1	6	0	10	1
Insomnia	13	0	9	0	11	0
Neuro-sensory	12	1	2	0	9	1
Paresthesias	77	18	16	2	62	7
Pharyngo-laryngeal Dysesthesias	38	2	1	0	28	1
Ocular/Visual						
Abnormal Vision	5	0	2	<1	6	1
Tearing	9	0	1	0	2	<1
Pain						
Abdominal Pain	29	8	31	7	39	10
Arthralgia	5	<1	5	0	8	<1
Headache	13	<1	6	<1	9	<1
Myalgia	14	2	6	0	9	2
Pain	7	1	5	1	6	1
Pulmonary						
Cough	35	1	25	2	17	<1
Dyspnea	18	7	14	3	11	2
Renal/Genitourinary						
Urinary Frequency	5	1	2	<1	3	1

[a] ANC: absolute neutrophil count; NOS: Not otherwise specified.

The following additional most common and potentially important adverse events regardless of treatment causality were reported in less than 5% of the patients in the ELOXATIN and 5-FU/LV combination arm in the previously untreated for metastatic colorectal cancer pivotal study.

Cardiovascular: hypertension, hypotension, prothrombin time.
Dermatology/Skin: nail changes, pigmentation changes, urticaria.
Gastrointestinal: gastrointestinal not otherwise specified (NOS).
Hemorrhage: rectal bleeding.
Infection/Febrile Neutropenia: catheter infection, febrile neutropenia, unknown infection.
Metabolic/Laboratory: magnesium levels were not prospectively tested.
Neurology: syncope, vertigo.
Pain: bone pain, chest pain, neuralgia, rectal pain.
Pulmonary: hiccups, hypoxia, pneumonitis, pulmonary NOS.
Renal/Genitourinary: creatinine, dysuria.

Patients Previously Treated for Metastatic Colorectal Cancer: Seven hundred and ninety one (791) patients were studied in a randomized trial in patients with refractory and relapsed colorectal cancer in which 268 patients received the combination of ELOXATIN and 5-FU/LV.

Fourteen percent (14%) of patients in the ELOXATIN and 5-FU/LV combination arm and 7% in the 5-FU/LV arm of the previously treated study had to discontinue treatment because of adverse effects related to allergy, fatigue, gastrointestinal events, hematological events or neuropathies.

The incidence of death within 30 days of treatment in the previously treated study, regardless of causality, was 6% with the ELOXATIN and 5-FU/LV combination, 6% with ELOXATIN alone and 5% with 5-FU/LV.

The following adverse events were reported more frequently in patients ≥65 years old on the ELOXATIN and 5-FU/LV combination arm: cellulitis, general cardiovascular disorders, anorexia, dehydration, platelet, bleeding and clotting disorders and secondary terms.

For any class of adverse event (all inclusive), the proportion of patients reporting adverse events (all grade) was similar across arms and patient populations (male, female). When Grade 3 or 4 events were evaluated, the female patient population reported a higher number of events independent of treatment arm.

Table 3 provides adverse events reported in the previously treated pivotal study for events with overall incidences ≥5% in the ELOXATIN and 5-FU/LV combination arm.

Table 3: ELOXATIN

Adverse Events Reported in Patients Previously Treated for Metastatic Colorectal Cancer Clinical Trial (≥5% of all Patients in the ELOXATIN and 5-FU/LV Arm)—by Body System

	ELOXATIN+5-FU/LV (N=268)		ELOXATIN (N=266)		5-FU/LV (N=257)	
Adverse Event (WHO/Pref)	**All Grades (%)**	**Grade 3/4 (%)**	**All Grades (%)**	**Grade 3/4 (%)**	**All Grades (%)**	**Grade 3/4 (%)**
Any Event	100	81	100	46	98	44
Application Site Disorders						
Injection Site Reaction	13	3	7	0	7	1
Autonomic Nervous System Disorders						
Flushing	10	0	3	0	2	0
Body as a Whole						
Accidental Injury	7	0	2	0	4	0
Allergic Reaction	8	1	3	1	2	1
Chest Pain	8	1	4	<1	5	1
Fatigue	75	10	59	10	57	6
Fever	31	0	20	1	19	1
Pain	16	2	13	3	12	3
Rigors	11	0	7	0	5	0
Weight Decrease	9	<1	8	0	6	0
Cardiovascular Disorders, General						
Oedema Legs	8	<1	5	1	6	1
Peripheral Oedema	6	0	3	<1	5	1
Central & Peripheral Nervous System Disorders						
Dizziness	15	1	7	<1	9	<1
Headache	16	<1	14	0	10	1
Neuropathy	6	<1	9	0	2	<1
Paresthesia	54	7	49	2	13	0
Sensory Disturbance	58	4	58	4	2	0
Gastrointestinal System Disorders						
Abdominal Pain	35	4	32	6	33	5
Anorexia	33	3	25	2	22	2
Constipation	33	1	32	2	24	1
Diarrhea	65	11	40	3	42	2
Dyspepsia	13	0	7	0	9	0
Flatulence	9	0	5	<1	8	0

(cont'd)

Table 3: ELOXATIN *(cont'd)*

Adverse Events Reported in Patients Previously Treated for Metastatic Colorectal Cancer Clinical Trial (≥5% of all Patients in the ELOXATIN and 5-FU/LV Arm)—by Body System

Adverse Event (WHO/Pref)	ELOXATIN+5-FU/LV (N=268) All Grades (%)	ELOXATIN+5-FU/LV (N=268) Grade 3/4 (%)	ELOXATIN (N=266) All Grades (%)	ELOXATIN (N=266) Grade 3/4 (%)	5-FU/LV (N=257) All Grades (%)	5-FU/LV (N=257) Grade 3/4 (%)
Hiccup	5	<1	2	0	1	<1
Intestinal Obstruction	5	5	4	3	2	2
Mucositis NOS[a]	8	1	2	0	9	1
Nausea	68	10	58	4	53	2
Stomatitis	28	2	8	0	22	1
Vomiting	44	9	38	5	27	2
Metabolic and Nutritional Disorders						
Dehydration	9	4	5	3	4	2
Musculoskeletal System Disorders						
Arthralgia	10	1	8	<1	11	3
Back Pain	16	2	11	<1	17	4
Myalgia	6	<1	4	0	2	0
Neoplasms						
Aggravated Neoplasm Malignant	13	12	10	9	13	13
Platelet, Bleeding & Clotting Disorders						
Epistaxis	11	0	3	0	3	0
Hematuria	6	2	1	0	3	1
Thrombocytopenia	15	5	5	1	0	0
Psychiatric Disorders						
Anxiety	7	<1	6	0	5	0
Depression	7	<1	5	0	5	<1
Insomnia	16	0	9	<1	5	0
Red Blood Cell Disorders						
Anemia	20	5	7	1	11	2
Respiratory System Disorders						
Coughing	19	2	10	<1	13	0
Dyspnea	20	3	13	4	13	2
Pharyngitis	10	0	2	0	7	0
Rhinitis	13	0	6	0	7	0
Sinusitis	6	0	3	0	4	0
Upper Resp. Tract Infection	12	1	7	0	9	0
Skin and Appendage Disorders						
Alopecia	8	0	3	<1	4	0
Rash	14	0	4	0	5	0
Skin Exfoliation	9	1	2	0	11	1
Sweating Increased	7	0	8	0	4	0
Special Senses Other, Disorders						
Taste Perversion	12	0	3	0	4	0
Urinary System Disorders						
Dysuria	6	<1	1	0	2	<1
Urinary Tract Infection	5	<1	5	2	4	1
Vision Disorders						
Abnormal Lacrimation	8	0	1	0	8	0

(cont'd)

Table 3: ELOXATIN *(cont'd)*

Adverse Events Reported in Patients Previously Treated for Metastatic Colorectal Cancer Clinical Trial (≥5% of all Patients in the ELOXATIN and 5-FU/LV Arm)—by Body System

Adverse Event (WHO/Pref)	ELOXATIN+5-FU/LV (N=268) All Grades (%)	ELOXATIN+5-FU/LV (N=268) Grade 3/4 (%)	ELOXATIN (N=266) All Grades (%)	ELOXATIN (N=266) Grade 3/4 (%)	5-FU/LV (N=257) All Grades (%)	5-FU/LV (N=257) Grade 3/4 (%)
White cell and RES Disorders[a]						
Decreased Neutrophils	5	2	0	0	<1	<1
Granulocytopenia	52	41	1	0	9	3
Leukopenia	9	4	0	0	1	<1

[a] NOS: Not otherwise specified; RES: Reticulo-Endothelial System.

The following additional most common and potentially important adverse events regardless of treatment causality were reported in less than 5% of the patients in the ELOXATIN and 5-FU/LV combination arm in the previously treated for metastatic colorectal cancer pivotal study.
Body as a Whole—General Disorders: ascites.
Cardiovascular Disorders, General: oedema.
Central and Peripheral Nervous System Disorders: ataxia.
Gastrointestinal System Disorders: dry mouth, gastroesophageal reflux, tenesmus.
Heart Rate and Rhythm Disorders: tachycardia.
Metabolic/Laboratory: magnesium levels were not prospectively tested.
Musculoskeletal System Disorders: bone pain.
Platelet, Bleeding and Clotting Disorders: bruise, deep thrombophlebitis, melena, rectal hemorrhage.
Respiratory System Disorders: pneumonia.
Skin and Appendage Disorders: dry skin, erythematous rash, pruritus, skin disorder.
Vision Disorders: abnormal vision, conjunctivitis.
White Cell and Recticulo-Endothelial System Disorders: febrile neutropenia.
Abnormal Hematologic and Clinical Chemistry Findings: Patients Treated in the Adjuvant Setting for Colon Cancer: See Table 4 and Table 5.

Table 4: ELOXATIN

Hepatic Adverse Events in Patients with Colon Cancer Receiving Adjuvant Therapy (≥5% of Patients)

Hepatic Parameter	ELOXATIN+5-FU/LV (N=1108) All Grades (%)	ELOXATIN+5-FU/LV (N=1108) Grade 3/4 (%)	5-FU/LV (N=1111) All Grades (%)	5-FU/LV (N=1111) Grade 3/4 (%)
Hepatic Enzymes Elevation	57	2	34	1
Phosphatase Alkaline Increased	42	<1	20	<1
Bilirubinemia	20	4	20	5

Table 5: ELOXATIN

Hematologic Adverse Events in Patients with Colon Cancer Receiving Adjuvant Therapy (≥5% of Patients)

Adverse Event[a] (WHO/Pref)	ELOXATIN+5-FU/LV (N=1108) All Grades (%)	ELOXATIN+5-FU/LV (N=1108) Grade 3/4 (%)	5-FU/LV (N=1111) All Grades (%)	5-FU/LV (N=1111) Grade 3/4 (%)
Anemia	76	1	67	0.3
Neutropenia	79	41	40	5
Thrombocytopenia	77	2	19	<1

[a] The hematology data were collected by NCI grade; no laboratory values were collected. The worst grade observed during each cycle period was reported.

Patients Previously Untreated for Metastatic Colorectal Cancer: See Table 6, Table 7 and Table 8.

Table 6: ELOXATIN

Hepatic Adverse Events in Patients Previously Untreated for Metastatic Colorectal Cancer (≥5% of Patients)

Adverse Event (WHO/Pref)	ELOXATIN+5-FU/LV N=259 All Grades (%)	ELOXATIN+5-FU/LV N=259 Grade 3/4 (%)	Irinotecan+5-FU/LV N=256 All Grades (%)	Irinotecan+5-FU/LV N=256 Grade 3/4 (%)	ELOXATIN+irinotecan N=258 All Grades (%)	ELOXATIN+irinotecan N=258 Grade 3/4 (%)
Alkaline Phosphatase	16	0	7	0	16	2
ALT[a]	6	1	2	0	5	2
AST[a]	17	1	2	<1	11	1
Bilirubin Total	6	<1	3	1	3	2
Hypoalbuminemia	8	0	5	2	9	<1

[a] AST: aspartate aminotransferase; ALT: alanine aminotransferase.

Table 7: ELOXATIN

Hematologic Adverse Events in Patients Previously Untreated for Metastatic Colorectal Cancer (≥5% of Patients)

Adverse Event (WHO/Pref)	ELOXATIN+5-FU/LV N=259 All Grades (%)	ELOXATIN+5-FU/LV N=259 Grade 3/4 (%)	Irinotecan+5-FU/LV N=256 All Grades (%)	Irinotecan+5-FU/LV N=256 Grade 3/4 (%)	ELOXATIN+irinotecan N=258 All Grades (%)	ELOXATIN+irinotecan N=258 Grade 3/4 (%)
Anemia	27	3	28	4	25	3
Leukopenia	87	20	84	23	78	25
Lymphopenia	6	2	4	1	5	2
Neutropenia	81	54	77	46	73	39
Thrombocytopenia	71	5	26	3	45	4

Table 8: ELOXATIN

Metabolic Adverse Events in Patients Previously Untreated for Metastatic Colorectal Cancer (≥5% of Patients)

Adverse Event (WHO/Pref)	ELOXATIN+5-FU/LV N=259 All Grades (%)	ELOXATIN+5-FU/LV N=259 Grade 3/4 (%)	Irinotecan+5-FU/LV N=256 All Grades (%)	Irinotecan+5-FU/LV N=256 Grade 3/4 (%)	ELOXATIN+irinotecan N=258 All Grades (%)	ELOXATIN+irinotecan N=258 Grade 3/4 (%)
Hyperglycemia	14	2	11	3	12	3
Hypocalcemia	7	0	5	1	4	0
Hypokalemia	11	3	7	4	6	2
Hyponatremia	8	2	7	4	4	1

Patients Previously Treated For Metastatic Colorectal Cancer: See Table 9, Table 10 and Table 11.

Table 9: ELOXATIN

Hepatic Clinical Chemistry Abnormalities in Patients Previously Treated for Metastatic Colorectal Cancer (≥5% of Patients)

Clinical Chemistry	ELOXATIN+5-FU/LV (N=268) All Grades (%)	ELOXATIN+5-FU/LV (N=268) Grade 3/4 (%)	ELOXATIN (N=266) All Grades (%)	ELOXATIN (N=266) Grade 3/4 (%)	5-FU/LV (N=257) All Grades (%)	5-FU/LV (N=257) Grade 3/4 (%)
Alkaline Phosphatase	60	4	60	7	50	5
ALT[a]	36	0	39	1	27	1
AST[a]	53	0	57	4	42	2
Bilirubin Total	13	1	15	4	20	6
Lactate Dehydrogenase	53	22	53	23	46	24

[a] AST: aspartate aminotransferase; ALT: alanine aminotransferase.

Table 10: ELOXATIN

Clinically Significant Hematologic Abnormalities by Preferred Term and Body System in Patients Previously Treated for Metastatic Colorectal Cancer (≥5% of Patients)

Adverse Event (WHO/Pref)	ELOXATIN+5-FU/LV (N=268) All Grades (%)	ELOXATIN+5-FU/LV (N=268) Grade 3/4 (%)	ELOXATIN (N=266) All Grades (%)	ELOXATIN (N=266) Grade 3/4 (%)	5-FU/LV (N=257) All Grades (%)	5-FU/LV (N=257) Grade 3/4 (%)
Anemia	84	5	61	2	67	2
Leukopenia	81	27	13	<1	35	2
Neutropenia	77	52	7	0	25	6
Thrombocytopenia	67	6	28	2	21	0

Table 11: ELOXATIN

Metabolic Adverse Event by Preferred Term and Body System in Patients Previously Treated for Metastatic Colorectal Cancer (≥5% of Patients)

Adverse Event (WHO/Pref)	ELOXATIN+5-FU/LV (N=268) All Grades (%)	ELOXATIN+5-FU/LV (N=268) Grade 3/4 (%)	ELOXATIN (N=266) All Grades (%)	ELOXATIN (N=266) Grade 3/4 (%)	5-FU/LV (N=257) All Grades (%)	5-FU/LV (N=257) Grade 3/4 (%)
Hypokalemia	9	6	3	2	3	1

Other Clinical Trial Adverse Drug Reactions: Frequencies are defined using the following convention: very common (≥10%); common (≥1%, <10%); uncommon (≥0.1%, <1%); rare (≥0.01%, <0.1%): very rare (<0.01%), not known (cannot be estimated from the available data).

Blood and Lymphatic System Disorders: Rare: hemolysis.

Ear and Labyrinth Disorders: Rare: deafness.

Eye Disorders: Rare: visual acuity reduced transiently, optic neuritis, transient vision loss reversible following therapy discontinuation, visual field disturbances. Several cases of positive rechallenge associated with subsequent cycles of chemotherapy were reported indicating probable causal relationship to ELOXATIN.

Gastrointestinal Disorders: Very common: Dehydration, hypokalemia, metabolic acidosis, ileus, intestinal obstruction, renal disorders may be associated with severe diarrhea/vomiting, particularly when ELOXATIN is combined with 5-FU. Common: gastrointestinal hemorrhage. Rare: colitis, including *C. difficile* diarrhea.

General Disorders and Administration Site Conditions: Very common: asthenia.

Extravasation may also result in local pain and inflammation, which may be severe and lead to complications including necrosis, especially when ELOXATIN is infused through a peripheral vein.

Hepatobiliary Disorders: Rare: pancreatitis. Very rare: hepatic failure, hepatitis, liver sinusoidal obstruction syndrome, also known as veno-occlusive disease of liver, or pathological manifestations related to such liver disorder, including nodular regenerative hyperplasia, peliosis hepatis, perisinusoidal fibrosis. Clinical manifestations of this syndrome may be portal hypertension and/or increased transaminases.

Immune System Disorders: Common: anaphylactic reactions including bronchospasm, sensation of chest pain, angioedema, hypotension, anaphylactic shock. Rare: immuno-allergic hemolytic anemia, immuno-allergic thrombocytopenia.

Nervous System Disorders: Very common: acute neuro-sensory manifestations, dysesthesia, paresthesia of extremities and peripheral neuropathy. Rare: dysarthria, Lhermitte's sign, loss of deep tendon reflexes. Very rare: Reports of symptoms compatible with a diagnosis of Guillain-Barre Syndrome. Causal relationship has not been established.

Renal and Urinary Disorders: Very rare: acute tubular necrosis, acute interstitial nephritis and acute renal failure were reported.

Respiratory, Thoracic and Mediastinal Disorders: Rare: acute interstitial lung diseases (including fatalities), pulmonary fibrosis (see Warnings and Precautions).

Vascular Disorders: Common: hypertension, thromboembolic events, including deep vein thrombosis.

Post-Market Adverse Drug Reactions: The following events have been reported from worldwide post-marketing experience.

Blood and Lymphatic System Disorders: hemolytic uremic syndrome.

Eye Disorders: amaurosis, amaurosis fugax. Cases of positive rechallenge associated with subsequent cycles of chemotherapy were reported indicating probable causal relationship to ELOXATIN.

Few cases of optic ischemic neuropathy were reported without established causal relationship.

Metabolism and Nutrition Disorders: hypomagnesemia.

Musculoskeletal and Connective Tissue Disorders: rhabdomyolysis.

Nervous System Disorders: convulsion.

Posterior reversible encephalopathy syndrome (PRES) has been reported in the literature in a patient treated with oxaliplatin and 5-FU/LV, although the cause/effect relationship cannot be established with certainty.

DRUG INTERACTIONS: Overview: No specific cytochrome P-450-based drug interaction studies have been conducted.

In vitro, ELOXATIN is not metabolized by, nor does it inhibit, human cytochrome P450 isoenzymes. No P450-mediated drug-drug interactions are therefore anticipated in patients.

Since platinum-containing species are eliminated primarily through the kidney, clearance of these products may be decreased by coadministration of potentially nephrotoxic compounds; although, this has not been specifically studied (see Action and Clinical Pharmacology).

Drug-Drug Interactions: In patients who have received a single dose of 85 mg/m² of ELOXATIN immediately before administration of 5-FU, no change in the level of exposure to 5-FU has been observed. No pharmacokinetic interaction between 85 mg/m² ELOXATIN and 5-FU/LV has been observed in patients treated every 2 weeks. Increases of 5-FU plasma concentrations by approximately 20% have been observed with doses of 130 mg/m² ELOXATIN administered every 3 weeks. The approved dose of ELOXATIN is 85 mg/m² every 2 weeks in combination with 5-FU/LV (see Dosage and Administration).

In vitro, platinum was not displaced from plasma proteins by the following medications: erythromycin, salicylate, sodium valproate, granisetron and paclitaxel.

There have been reports while on study and from post-marketing surveillance of prolonged prothrombin time and INR occasionally associated with hemorrhage in patients who received ELOXATIN plus 5-FU/LV while on anticoagulants. Patients receiving ELOXATIN plus 5-FU/LV and requiring oral anticoagulants may require closer monitoring.

Drug-Food Interactions: Interactions with food have not been established.

Drug-Herb Interactions: Interactions with herbal products have not been established.

Drug-Laboratory Test Interactions: Interactions with laboratory tests have not been established.

DOSAGE AND ADMINISTRATION: Dosing Considerations:

- Dosage given should be adjusted according to tolerability.
- If severe/life-threatening diarrhea, neurotoxicity or hematological toxicity occurs, a dose adjustment may be required (see Warnings and Precautions and Dosage and Administration, Recommended Dose and Dosage Adjustment).

Recommended Dose and Dosage Adjustment: Administer ELOXATIN in combination with 5-FU/LV every 2 weeks. For metastatic disease, treatment is recommended until disease progression or unacceptable toxicity. For adjuvant use, treatment is recommended for a total of 12 cycles (6 months). The recommended dose schedule given every 2 weeks is as follows:

Day 1: ELOXATIN 85 mg/m² IV infusion in 250 to 500 mL of 5% (50 mg/mL) glucose solution (D5W) is given at the same time as leucovorin 200 mg/m² IV infusion in 5% glucose solution (D5W), over 2 to 6 hours in separate bags using a Y-line.

Followed by 5-FU 400 mg/m² IV bolus given over 2-4 minutes, followed by 5-FU 600 mg/m² IV infusion in 500 mL of 5% glucose solution (D5W) (recommended) as a 22-hour continuous infusion.

Day 2: Leucovorin 200 mg/m² IV infusion over 2 hours.

Followed by 5-FU 400 mg/m² IV bolus given over 2-4 minutes, followed by 5-FU 600 mg/m² IV infusion in 500 mL of 5% glucose solution (D5W) (recommended) as a 22-hour continuous infusion. See Figure 1.

Figure 1: ELOXATIN

Recommended Dose Schedule

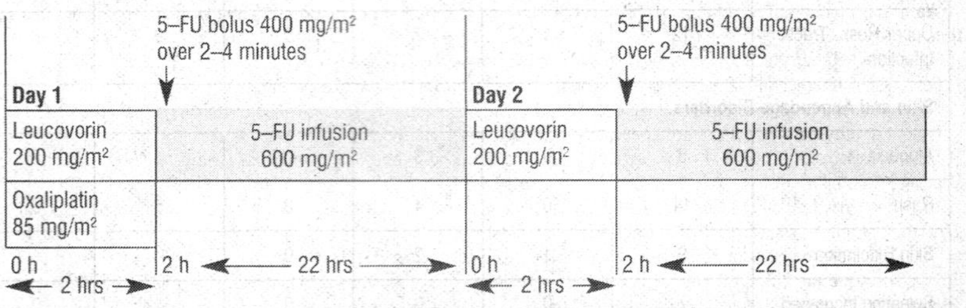

Geriatrics (≥65 years of age): Starting dose in this age group is the same. In studies of patients with metastatic colorectal cancer, patients ≥65 years receiving ELOXATIN in combination with 5-FU/LV experienced more fatigue, dehydration, diarrhea, leukopenia, and syncope than patients <65 years, although the difference was not statistically significant. In the adjuvant trial, patients ≥65 years receiving the ELOXATIN combination therapy experienced more grade 3/4 granulocytopenia and diarrhea than patients <65 years, although the difference was not statistically significant.

Gastrointestinal: Adjuvant Stage III Colon Cancer: If severe/life-threatening gastrointestinal toxicity (NCI CTC grade 3-4) occurs despite prophylactic treatment, ELOXATIN must be discontinued until resolution. A dose reduction of ELOXATIN to 75 mg/m² and bolus 5-FU to 300 mg/m² and infusional 5-FU to 500 mg/m² over 22 hours is recommended at subsequent cycles.

Metastatic Colorectal Cancer: After recovery from grade 3 or 4 gastrointestinal toxicity (despite prophylactic treatment), a dose reduction of ELOXATIN to 65 mg/m² and 5-FU by 20% (300 mg/m² bolus and 500 mg/m² 22-hour infusion) is recommended.

Hematologic: Adjuvant Stage III Colon Cancer: After recovery from grade 3-4 neutropenia (ANC <1.0×10⁹/L) or grade 3-4 thrombocytopenia (platelets <50×10⁹/L), a dose reduction of ELOXATIN to 75 mg/m² and bolus 5-FU to 300 mg/m² and infusional 5-FU to 500 mg/m² over 22 hours is recommended. The next dose should be delayed until neutrophils ≥1.5×10⁹/L and platelets ≥75×10⁹/L.

Metastatic Colorectal Cancer: After recovery from grade 3/4 neutropenia (ANC <1.0×10⁹/L) or grade 3/4 thrombocytopenia (platelets <50×10⁹/L), a dose reduction of ELOXATIN to 65 mg/m² and 5-FU by 20% (300 mg/m² bolus and 500 mg/m² 22-hour infusion) is recommended. The next dose should be delayed until: neutrophils ≥1.5×10⁹/L and platelets ≥75×10⁹/L.

Neurologic: For patients (any indication) who develop acute laryngo-pharyngeal dysesthesia (see Adverse Reactions), during or within the hours following the 2-hour infusion, the next ELOXATIN infusion should be administered over 6 hours. To prevent such dysesthesia, inform the patient to avoid exposure to cold and to avoid ingesting fresh/cold food or/and beverages during or within the hours following ELOXATIN administration.

No dose adjustment is required to the 5-FU/LV regimen for neurotoxicity.

Adjuvant Stage III Colon Cancer: Neurotoxicity was graded using the NCI CTC grading system (see Warnings and Precautions). For patients who experience persistent grade 2 neurotoxicity (mild or moderate objective sensory loss, moderate paresthesias), the ELOXATIN dose should be reduced to 75 mg/m². For patients with persistent grade 3 neurotoxicity, therapy should be discontinued.

Metastatic Colorectal Cancer: In the metastatic colorectal cancer trials, neurotoxicity was graded using a study-specific neurotoxicity scale, and dose adjustments for ELOXATIN were recommended, as follows: See Table 12.

Table 12: ELOXATIN

Neurologic Toxicity Scale for Oxaliplatin Dose Adjustments

Toxicity (Grade)	Duration of Toxicity		Persistent[a] Between Cycles
	1–7 Days	>7 Days	
Paresthesias/dysesthesias[b] that do not interfere with function (Grade 1)	No change	No change	No change
Paresthesias/dysesthesias[b] interfering with function, but not activities of daily living (ADL) (Grade 2)	No change	No change	65 mg/m²
Paresthesias/dysesthesias[b] with pain or with functional impairment that also interfere with ADL (Grade 3)	No change	65 mg/m²	Stop
Persistent paresthesias/dysesthesias that are disabling or life-threatening (Grade 4)	Stop	Stop	Stop
Acute (during or after the 2 hour infusion) laryngopharyngeal dysesthesias[b]	↑ duration of next infusion to 6 hours[c]	↑ duration of next infusion to 6 hours[c]	↑ duration of next infusion to 6 hours[c]

[a] Not resolved by the beginning of the next cycle.
[b] May have been cold-induced.
[c] May also have been pre-treated with benzodiazepines.

Renal Insufficiency: ELOXATIN has not been studied in patients with severe renal impairment. In patients with moderate renal impairment, treatment may be initiated at the normally recommended dose and renal function should be closely monitored. Dose should be adjusted according to toxicity (see Contraindications and Warnings and Precautions, Special Populations).

Hepatic Insufficiency: No increase in ELOXATIN acute toxicities was observed in the subset of patients with abnormal liver function tests at baseline. No specific dose adjustment for patients with abnormal liver function tests was performed during clinical development.

Administration: ELOXATIN is considered moderately emetogenic. Premedication with antiemetics, including 5-HT_3 blockers with or without dexamethasone, is recommended.

The administration of ELOXATIN does not require prehydration.

ELOXATIN is administered by intravenous infusion.

ELOXATIN lyophilized powder must be reconstituted and further diluted before use (see Reconstitution and Dilution Before Infusion).

ELOXATIN aqueous solution must be diluted before use (see Dilution Before Infusion).

ELOXATIN diluted in 250 to 500 mL of 5% glucose solution to give a concentration not less than 0.2 mg/mL must be infused via a central venous line or peripheral vein over 2 to 6 hours.

In the event of extravasation, administration must be discontinued immediately.

Instruction for Use with Leucovorin (as calcium folinate or disodium folinate): ELOXATIN 85 mg/m² IV infusion in 250 to 500 mL of 5% glucose solution is given at the same time as leucovorin IV infusion in 5% glucose solution, over 2 to 6 hours, using a Y-line placed immediately before infusion.

These two drugs should not be combined in the same infusion bag.

Leucovorin must not contain trometamol as an excipient and must only be diluted using isotonic 5% glucose solution, never in alkaline solutions or sodium chloride or chloride containing solutions.

For information on leucovorin, see the Product Monograph and package insert.

Instruction for Use with 5-FU: ELOXATIN should always be administered before fluoropyrimidines—i.e. 5-FU.

After ELOXATIN administration, flush the line and then administer 5-FU.

For information on 5-FU, see the Product Monograph and package insert.

Reconstitution: ELOXATIN Lyophilized Powder: ELOXATIN lyophilized powder must be reconstituted and further diluted before use.

Only the recommended diluents should be used to reconstitute and then dilute the freeze-dried product.

Water for injection or 5% glucose solution should be used as solvent to reconstitute the lyophilized powder in solution.

- For a vial of 50 mg: add 10 mL of solvent to obtain a concentration of 5 mg oxaliplatin/mL
- For a vial of 100 mg: add 20 mL of solvent to obtain a concentration of 5 mg oxaliplatin/mL

Reconstitution must **never** be performed with a sodium chloride solution or other chloride-containing solutions.

Do not administer the reconstituted solution without further dilution.

From a microbiological point of view, the reconstituted solution should be diluted immediately with 5 % glucose solution (see Dilution Before Infusion).

Inspect visually for clarity, particulate matter, precipitate, discoloration and leakage prior to use. Only clear solutions without particles, precipitate, discoloration or leakage should be used.

The medicinal product is for single-use only. Any unused solution should be discarded.

ELOXATIN Aqueous Solution: ELOXATIN aqueous solution does not need to be reconstituted. The aqueous solution **must be diluted** with 5% glucose solution before use (see Dilution Before Infusion).

Dilution Before Infusion: Only 5% glucose infusion solution is to be used to dilute the product.

Never use sodium chloride or chloride containing solutions for dilution.

Inspect visually for clarity, particulate matter, precipitate, discoloration and leakage prior to use. Only clear solutions without particles, precipitate, discoloration or leakage should be used.

The medicinal product is for single-use only. Any unused solution should be discarded.

Needles or intravenous administration sets containing aluminum parts that may come in contact with ELOXATIN **should not** be used for the preparation or mixing of the drug. Aluminum has been reported to cause degradation of platinum compounds.

The compatibility of ELOXATIN solution for infusion has been tested with representative, PVC-based, administration sets.

ELOXATIN Lyophilized Powder: Withdraw the required amount of reconstituted solution from the vial(s) and then dilute with 250 mL to 500 mL of a 5% glucose solution to give an ELOXATIN concentration between not less than 0.2 mg/mL and 0.7 mg/mL (0.70 mg/mL is the highest concentration in clinical practice for an oxaliplatin dose of 85 mg/m²).

The concentration range over which the physico-chemical stability of ELOXATIN has been demonstrated is 0.2 mg/mL to 2.0 mg/mL. After dilution in 5% glucose solution, chemical and physical in-use stability has been demonstrated for 24 hours at 2°C to 8°C. From a microbiological point of view, this infusion preparation should be used immediately. If not used immediately, in-use storage times and conditions prior to use are the responsibility of the user and would normally not be longer than 24 hours at 2°C to 8°C unless dilution has taken place in controlled and validated aseptic conditions.

ELOXATIN Aqueous Solution: Withdraw the required amount of concentrate from the vial(s) and then dilute with 250 mL to 500 mL of a 5% glucose solution to give an ELOXATIN concentration between not less than 0.2 mg/mL and 0.7 mg/mL (0.70 mg/mL is the highest concentration in clinical practice for an oxaliplatin dose of 85 mg/m²).

The concentration range over which the physico-chemical stability of ELOXATIN has been demonstrated is 0.2 mg/mL to 2.0 mg/mL. After dilution in 5% glucose solution, chemical and physical in-use stability has been demonstrated for 24 hours at 25°C and 48 hours at 2°C to 8°C. From a microbiological point of view, this infusion preparation should be used immediately. If not used immediately, in-use storage times and conditions prior to use are the responsibility of the user and would normally not be longer than 24 hours at 2°C to 8°C unless dilution has taken place in controlled and validated aseptic conditions.

Incompatibilities:

- **Do not** administer undiluted.
- Only 5% glucose infusion solution is to be used to dilute the product.
- **Do not** reconstitute or dilute ELOXATIN with saline or other solutions containing chloride ions (including calcium, potassium or sodium chloride).
- The diluted medicinal product should not be mixed with other medicinal products in the same infusion bag or infusion line. ELOXATIN can be coadministered with leucovorin via a Y-line (see Dosage and Administration, Administration, Instruction for Use with Leucovorin (as calcium folinate or disodium folinate)).
- **Do not** mix with alkaline medicinal products or solutions, in particular 5-FU, leucovorin preparations containing trometamol as an excipient and trometamol salts of others active substances. Alkaline medicinal products or solutions will adversely affect the stability of ELOXATIN.
- **Do not** use injection equipment containing aluminium.

Disposal: Remnants of the medicinal product as well as all materials that have been used for reconstitution, for dilution and administration must be destroyed according to hospital standard procedures applicable to cytotoxic agents in accordance with local requirements related to the disposal of hazardous waste.

OVERDOSAGE:

The approved dose of ELOXATIN is 85 mg/m² every 2 weeks in combination with 5-FU/LV (see Dosage and Administration). In cases of overdose, exacerbation of adverse events can be expected.

In addition to thrombocytopenia, the anticipated complications of an ELOXATIN overdose include hypersensitivity reaction, myelosuppression, nausea and vomiting, diarrhea, neurotoxicity and cardiotoxicity.

Several cases of overdoses have been reported with ELOXATIN. Adverse events observed were grade 4 thrombocytopenia (<25 000/mm³) without any bleeding, anemia, blood creatinine increased, sensory neuropathy such as paresthesia, dysesthesia, laryngospasm and facial muscle spasms, asthenia, fatigue, anxiety, dizziness, gastrointestinal disorders such as diarrhea, nausea, vomiting, stomatitis, flatulence, abdomen enlarged and grade 4 intestinal obstruction, grade 4 dehydration, dyspnea, wheezing, hypotension, chest pain, respiratory failure and severe bradycardia.

Among overdose cases, one patient was mistakenly administered ELOXATIN instead of carboplatin. The patient received a total ELOXATIN dose of 500 mg and experienced dyspnea, wheezing, paresthesia, profuse vomiting and chest pain on the day of administration. The patient developed respiratory failure and severe bradycardia, and subsequent resuscitation efforts failed. Another patient who was mistakenly administered a 700 mg dose experienced rapid onset of dysesthesia. Inpatient supportive care was given, including hydration, electrolyte support and platelet transfusion. Recovery occurred 15 days after the overdose. The maximum dose of ELOXATIN that has been administered in a single infusion is 825 mg. The patient who received this ELOXATIN dose experienced intestinal obstruction, dehydration, nausea, flatulence and an enlarged abdomen. The treatment was discontinued and the patient recovered.

There is no known antidote for ELOXATIN overdose. Patients suspected of receiving an overdose should be monitored and supportive treatment should be administered.

For management of a suspected drug overdose, CPhA recommends that you contact your **regional Poison Control Centre**. See the *CPS* Directory section for a list of Poison Control Centres.

ACTION AND CLINICAL PHARMACOLOGY: Mechanism of Action: ELOXATIN is a platinum-type alkylating agent. It undergoes nonenzymatic conversion in physiologic solutions to active derivatives via displacement of the labile oxalate ligand. Several transient reactive species are formed, including monoaquo and diaquo 1,2-diaminocyclohexane (DACH) platinum, which covalently bind with macromolecules. Both inter- and intrastrand Pt-DNA crosslinks are formed. Crosslinks are formed between the N7 positions of two adjacent guanines (GG), adjacent adenine-guanines (AG), and guanines separated by an intervening nucleotide (GNG). These crosslinks inhibit DNA replication and transcription leading to cytotoxic and antitumor effects.

Pharmacodynamics: The antitumor activity of oxaliplatin relevant to the proposed indication is confirmed both in vitro and in vivo in human colorectal cancer models. Oxaliplatin demonstrates in vitro cytotoxicity against HT-29, CaCo2 and HEC59 colon cancer cells. Oxaliplatin as a single agent displays only modest in vivo antitumor activity in HT-29 and DLD2 human colon cancer xenografts. Oxaliplatin is additively effective with 5-FU against human colonic tumor xenograft in vivo.

Pharmacokinetics: Absorption: Maximum platinum concentrations in blood, plasma and plasma ultrafiltrate were reached at the end of 2-hour infusion of oxaliplatin at 85 mg/m². Low interpatient variability in C_{max} values was observed in plasma and whole blood (CV 19% and 16%, respectively). Variability in C_{max} in ultrafiltrate was higher (CV 45%). Following biotransformation in vivo, the reactive products from oxaliplatin bind plasma proteins, cellular proteins and DNA. The reactive oxaliplatin derivatives are present as a fraction of the unbound platinum in plasma ultrafiltrate.

The C_{max} obtained after a single 2-hour IV infusion of ELOXATIN at a dose of 85 mg/m² expressed as ultrafilterable platinum was 0.814 μg/mL.

Interpatient and intrapatient variability in ultrafilterable platinum exposure (AUC_{0-48}) assessed over 3 cycles was moderate to low (23% and 6%, respectively). A pharmacodynamic relationship between platinum ultrafiltrate levels and clinical safety and effectiveness has not been established. See Table 13.

Table 13: ELOXATIN

Summary of Pharmacokinetic Parameters in Patients Following Single Dosing of ELOXATIN at 85 mg/m² q2w (every two weeks)

	C_{max} (μg/mL)	$t_{½α}$ (h)	$t_{½β}$ (h)	$t_{½γ}$ (h)	AUC_{0-inf} (μg·h/mL)	Clearance (L/h)	Volume of distribution (L)
Mean	0.814	0.43	16.8	391	4.68	17.4	440
SD	0.193	0.35	5.74	406	1.4	6.35	199

Distribution: The volume of distribution obtained after a single 2-hour IV infusion of ELOXATIN at a dose of 85 mg/m² expressed as ultrafilterable platinum was 440 L.

At the end of a 2-hour infusion of ELOXATIN, approximately 15% of the administered platinum is present in the systemic circulation. The remaining 85% is rapidly distributed into tissues or eliminated in the urine. The relative distribution ratio of platinum between blood cells, plasma, and plasma ultrafiltrate is approximately 3.1: 3.7: 1.0.

In patients, plasma protein binding of platinum is irreversible and is greater than 90%. The main binding proteins are albumin and gamma-globulins. Platinum also binds irreversibly and accumulates (approximately 2-fold) in erythrocytes. Based on AUC values, statistically significant accumulation of platinum was observed in blood cells with a mean terminal-phase half-life of 589±89.8 hrs.

No platinum accumulation was observed in plasma ultrafiltrate following 85 mg/m² every two weeks.

Metabolism: Oxaliplatin undergoes extensive nonenzymatic biotransformation in patients and no intact drug was detectable in plasma ultrafiltrate at the end of a 2-hour infusion. There is no evidence of cytochrome P450-mediated metabolism in vitro.

Up to 17 platinum-containing derivatives have been observed in plasma ultrafiltrate samples from patients, including several cytotoxic species (monochloro DACH platinum, dichloro DACH platinum, and monoaquo and diaquo DACH platinum) and a number of noncytotoxic, conjugated species.

Excretion: The decline of ultrafilterable platinum levels following oxaliplatin administration is triphasic, characterized by two relatively short distribution phases ($t_{½α}$: 0.43 hours and $t_{½β}$: 16.8 hours) and a long terminal elimination phase ($t_{½γ}$: 391 hours).

The major route of platinum elimination is renal excretion. At five days after a single 2-hour infusion of ELOXATIN, urinary elimination accounted for about 54% of the platinum eliminated, with fecal excretion accounting for only about 2%. Platinum was cleared from plasma at a rate (9-19 L/h) that was similar to or exceeded the average human glomerular filtration rate (GFR: 7.5 L/h). The volume of distribution was high with interpatient variability of 33-45%. A significant decrease in clearance of ultrafilterable platinum from 17.6±2.18 L/h to 9.95±1.91 L/h in renal impairment (creatinine clearance 12-57 mL/min) was observed together with a statistically significant decrease in distribution volume from 330±40.9 to 241±36.1 L. The renal clearance of ultrafilterable platinum is significantly correlated with GFR (see Adverse Reactions).

Special Populations and Conditions: Pediatrics: See Indications and Clinical Use and Warnings and Precautions, Special Populations, Pediatrics (≤22 years of age).

Geriatrics: There was no significant effect of age (26-72 years) on the clearance of ultrafilterable platinum.

Gender: There was no significant effect of gender on the clearance of ultrafilterable platinum.

Hepatic Insufficiency: Mild to moderate hepatic impairment did not affect the clearance of platinum in a clinically significant manner. No increase in ELOXATIN acute toxicities was observed in the subset of patients with abnormal liver function tests at baseline. No specific dose adjustment for patients with abnormal liver function tests was performed during clinical development (see Warnings and Precautions and Dosage and Administration).

Renal Insufficiency: The primary route of platinum elimination is renal. The AUC_{0-48} of platinum in the plasma ultrafiltrate increases as renal function decreases. The AUC_{0-48} of platinum in patients with mild (creatinine clearance, CL_{cr} 50 to 80 mL/min), moderate (CL_{cr} 30 to <50 mL/min) and severe (CL_{cr} <30 mL/min) renal impairment is increased by about 60, 140 and 190%, respectively, compared to patients with normal renal function (CL_{cr} >80 mL/min) (see Warnings and Precautions and Dosage and Administration).

STORAGE AND STABILITY: ELOXATIN Lyophilized Powder: The product should be stored between 15°C to 30°C. Do not freeze. For long-term storage, protect product from light.

ELOXATIN Aqueous Solution: The product should be stored between 15°C to 30°C. Do not freeze. For long-term storage, protect product from light.

SPECIAL HANDLING INSTRUCTIONS: As with other potentially toxic compounds, care should be exercised in the handling and preparation of ELOXATIN solutions.

The handling of this cytotoxic agent by healthcare personnel requires every precaution to guarantee the protection of the handler and his surroundings. If ELOXATIN powder, reconstituted solution, concentrate or solution for infusion contacts the skin or the mucous membranes, wash immediately and thoroughly with water.

Procedures for the handling and disposal of anticancer drugs should be considered. Several guidelines on this subject have been published. There is no general agreement that all of the procedures recommended in the guidelines are necessary or appropriate.

INFORMATION FOR THE PATIENT: Published in e-CPS, available by subscription at www.e-cps.ca.

DOSAGE FORMS, COMPOSITION AND PACKAGING: ELOXATIN Aqueous Solution: Each clear, glass, single-use vial with a gray stopper and crimping seal with flip-off cap contains: 50 mg, 100 mg or 200 mg of oxaliplatin as a sterile, preservative-free, aqueous solution at a concentration of 5 mg/mL. Nonmedicinal ingredients: water for injection, USP.

ELOXATIN Lyophilized Powder: Each clear, single-use, glass vial with a gray stopper and crimping seal with flip-off cap contains: 50 mg or 100 mg of oxaliplatin as a sterile, preservative-free lyophilized powder for reconstitution. Nonmedicinal ingredients: lactose monohydrate at 450 mg and 900 mg in the 50 mg and 100 mg dosage strengths, respectively.

Eltor® 120

pseudoephedrine HCl

Nasal Decongestant—Sympathomimetic—Bronchodilator

sanofi-aventis

SUPPLIED: Each white caplet, engraved "ELTOR" on one side contains: pseudoephedrine HCl 120 mg in specially formulated pellets designed to provide a continuous release of the active therapeutic agent over a 12-hour period. Nonmedicinal ingredients: hypromellose, magnesium stearate, methylcellulose, silicon dioxide and sucrose. Blister packs of 12 and 24.

(Shown in Product Identification Section)

Eltroxin® Ⓟ

levothyroxine sodium

Thyroid Hormone

Triton Pharma

Date of Revision: November 3, 2009

SUMMARY PRODUCT INFORMATION:

Route of Administration	Dosage Form/ Strength	Clinically Relevant Nonmedicinal Ingredients
Oral	Tablet—50, 100, 150, 200 and 300 µg	Lactose For a complete listing see Dosage Forms, Composition and Packaging.

INDICATIONS AND CLINICAL USE: ELTROXIN (levothyroxine sodium) is indicated as:

- replacement or supplemental therapy in patients of any age or state (including pregnancy) with hypothyroidism of any etiology except transient hypothyroidism during the recovery phase of subacute thyroiditis.
- Specific indications are: primary hypothyroidism resulting from thyroid dysfunction, primary atrophy, or partial or total absence of thyroid gland, or from the effects of surgery, radiation or drugs, with or without the presence of goiter, including subclinical hypothyroidism; secondary (pituitary) hypothyroidism; and tertiary (hypothalamic) hypothyroidism
- a pituitary TSH suppressant in the treatment or prevention of various types of euthyroid goiters, including thyroid nodules, subacute or chronic lymphocytic thyroiditis (Hashimoto's), multinodular goiter, and in conjunction with surgery and radioactive iodine therapy in the management of thyrotropin-dependent well-differentiated papillary or follicular carcinoma of the thyroid.

CONTRAINDICATIONS: ELTROXIN (levothyroxine sodium) is contraindicated in:

- Patients with an apparent hypersensitivity to thyroid hormones or any of the inactive product constituents.
- Patients with untreated subclinical (suppressed serum TSH with normal T_3 and T_4 levels) or overt thyrotoxicosis of any etiology.
- Patients with acute myocardial infarction.
- Patients with uncorrected adrenal insufficiency, as thyroid hormones increase tissue demands for adrenocortical hormones and may thereby precipitate acute adrenal crisis (see Warnings and Precautions).

WARNINGS AND PRECAUTIONS:

Serious Warnings and Precautions
Thyroid hormones, including ELTROXIN, either alone or with other therapeutic agents, should not be used for the treatment of obesity or for weight loss. In euthyroid patients, doses within the range of daily hormonal requirements are ineffective for weight reduction. Larger doses may produce serious or even life threatening manifestations of toxicity, particularly when given in association with sympathomimetic amines such as those used for their anorectic effects.

General: ELTROXIN (levothyroxine sodium) has a narrow therapeutic index. Regardless of the indication for use, careful dosage titration is necessary to avoid the consequences of over- or under- treatment. These consequences include, among others, effects on growth and development, cardiovascular function, bone metabolism, reproductive function, cognitive function, emotional state, gastrointestinal function, and on glucose and lipid metabolism. Many drugs interact with levothyroxine sodium necessitating adjustments in dosing to maintain therapeutic response (see Drug Interactions).

The bioavailability of levothyroxine may differ to some extent among marketed brands. Once the patient is stabilized on a particular brand of levothyroxine sodium caution should be exercised when a change in drug product brand is implemented.

It has been shown that differences in formulations of levothyroxine, despite an identical content of active ingredient, may be associated with differences in fractional gastrointestinal absorption. These differences may not be observed through measurement of total T_3 and T_4 serum levels. It is therefore, recommended that patients who are switched from one levothyroxine formulation to another be retitrated to the desired thyroid function. Accuracy in retitration can best be achieved by using sensitive thyrotropin assays.

Seizures have been reported rarely in association with the initiation of levothyroxine sodium therapy, and may be related to the effect of thyroid hormone on seizure threshold.

Lithium blocks the TSH-mediated release of T_4 and T_3. Thyroid function should therefore be carefully monitored during lithium initiation, stabilization, and maintenance. If hypothyroidism occurs during lithium treatment, a higher than usual levothyroxine sodium dose may be required.

Cardiovascular: Levothyroxine sodium should be used with caution in patients with cardiovascular disorders, including angina, coronary artery disease, and hypertension, and in the elderly who have a greater likelihood of occult cardiac disease. In these patients, levothyroxine sodium therapy should be initiated at lower doses than those recommended in younger individuals or in patients without cardiac diseases (see Warnings and Precautions, Special Populations, Geriatrics (>50 years of age) and Dosage and Administration). If cardiac symptoms develop or worsen, the levothyroxine sodium dose should be reduced or withheld for one week and then cautiously restarted at a lower dose. Over-treatment with levothyroxine sodium may have adverse cardiovascular effects such as an increase in heart rate, cardiac wall thickness, and cardiac contractility and may precipitate angina or arrhythmias. Patients with coronary artery disease who are receiving levothyroxine sodium therapy should be monitored closely during surgical procedures, since the possibility of precipitating cardiac arrhythmias may be greater in those treated with levothyroxine. Concomitant administration of thyroid hormone and sympathomimetic agents to patients with coronary artery disease may increase the risk of coronary insufficiency.

Endocrine and Metabolism: Thyroid hormones, either alone or together with other therapeutic agents, should not be used for the treatment of obesity or for weight loss. In euthyroid patients, doses within the range of daily hormonal requirements are ineffective for weight reduction. Larger doses may produce serious or even life-threatening manifestations of toxicity, particularly when given in association with sympathomimetic amines such as those used for their anorectic effects.

Effects on Bone Mineral Density: In women, long-term levothyroxine therapy has been associated with increased bone resorption, thereby decreasing bone mineral density, especially in postmenopausal women on greater replacement doses or in women who are receiving suppressive doses of levothyroxine sodium. The increased bone resorption may be associated with increased serum levels and urinary excretion of calcium and phosphorous, elevations in bone alkaline phosphatase and suppressed serum parathyroid hormone levels. Therefore, it is recommended that patients receiving levothyroxine sodium be given the minimum dose necessary to achieve the desired clinical and biochemical response.

Patients with Nontoxic Diffuse Goiter or Nodular Thyroid Disease: In patients with non-toxic diffuse goiter or nodular thyroid disease, particularly the elderly or those with underlying cardiovascular disease, levothyroxine therapy is contraindicated if the serum TSH level is already suppressed due to the risk of precipitating overt thyrotoxicosis (see Contraindications). If the serum TSH level is not suppressed, levothyroxine sodium should be used with caution in conjunction with careful monitoring of thyroid function for evidence of hyperthyroidism and clinical monitoring for potential associated adverse cardiovascular signs and symptoms of hyperthyroidism.

Associated Endocrine Disorders: Hypothalamic/pituitary Hormone Deficiencies: In patients with secondary or tertiary hypothyroidism, additional hypothalamic/pituitary hormone deficiencies should be considered, and, if diagnosed, treated for adrenal insufficiency.

Autoimmune Polyglandular Syndrome: Use of levothyroxine sodium in patients with concomitant diabetes mellitus, diabetes insipidus or adrenal cortical insufficiency may aggravate the intensity of their symptoms. Appropriate adjustments of the various therapeutic measures directed at these concomitant endocrine diseases may therefore be required. Treatment of myxedema coma may require simultaneous administration of glucocorticoids (see Dosage and Administration).

Hematologic: T_4 enhances the response to anticoagulant therapy. Prothrombin time should be closely monitored in patients taking both levothyroxine sodium and oral anticoagulants, and the dosage of anticoagulant adjusted accordingly.

Sexual Function/Reproduction: The use of levothyroxine sodium is also unjustified in the treatment of male or female infertility unless this condition is associated with hypothyroidism.

Special Populations: Pregnant Women: Studies in pregnant women have not shown that levothyroxine sodium increases the risk of fetal abnormalities if administered during pregnancy. If levothyroxine sodium is used during pregnancy, the possibility of fetal harm appears remote.

Thyroid hormones cross the placental barrier to some extent. T_4 levels in the cord blood of athyroid fetuses have been shown to be about one-third of maternal levels. Nevertheless, maternal-fetal transfer of T_4 may not prevent in utero hypothyroidism.

Hypothyroidism during pregnancy is associated with a higher rate of complications, including spontaneous abortion, preeclampsia, stillbirth and premature delivery. Maternal hypothyroidism may have an adverse effect on fetal and childhood growth and development. On the basis of current knowledge, levothyroxine sodium should therefore not be discontinued during pregnancy, and hypothyroidism diagnosed during pregnancy should be treated. Studies have shown that during pregnancy T_4 concentrations may decrease and TSH concentrations may increase to values outside normal ranges. Postpartum values are similar to preconception values. Elevations in TSH may occur as early as the fourth week of gestation.

Pregnant women who are maintained on levothyroxine sodium should have their TSH measured periodically. An elevated TSH should be corrected by an increase in levothyroxine sodium dose. After pregnancy, the dose can be decreased to the optimal preconception dose. A serum TSH level should be obtained six to eight weeks postpartum.

Nursing Women: Minimal amounts of thyroid hormones are excreted in human milk. Thyroid hormones are not associated with serious adverse reactions and do not have known tumorigenic potential. While caution should be exercised when levothyroxine sodium is administered to a nursing woman, adequate replacement doses of levothyroxine sodium are generally needed to maintain normal lactation.

Pediatrics (All ages including neonates): Congenital Hypothyroidism: Infants with congenital hypothyroidism appear to be at increased risk for other congenital anomalies, with cardiovascular anomalies (pulmonary stenosis, atrial septal defect, and ventricular septal defect) being the most common association.

Rapid restoration of normal serum T_4 concentrations is essential to prevent deleterious neonatal thyroid hormone deficiency effects on intelligence, overall growth, and development. Treatment should be initiated immediately upon diagnosis and generally maintained for life. The therapeutic goal is to maintain serum total T_4 or FT_4 in the upper half of the normal range and serum TSH in the normal range.

An initial starting dose of 10 to 15 µg/kg/day (ages 0 to 3 months) will generally increase serum T_4 concentrations to the upper half of the normal range in less than 3 weeks. Clinical assessment of growth, development, and thyroid status should be monitored frequently. In most cases, the levothyroxine sodium dose per body weight will decrease as the patient grows through infancy and childhood (see Dosage and Administration, Recommended Dose and Dosage Adjustment, Pediatric Dosage, Table 2). Prolonged use of large doses in infants may be associated with temperament problems, which appear to be transient.

Thyroid function tests (serum total T_4 or FT_4, and TSH) should be monitored closely and used to determine the adequacy of levothyroxine sodium therapy. Serum T_4 normalization is usually followed by a rapid decline in TSH. Nevertheless, TSH normalization may lag behind T_4 normalization by 2 to 3 months or longer. The relative serum TSH elevation is more marked in the early months, but can persist to some degree throughout life. In rare patients TSH remains relatively elevated despite clinical euthyroidism and age-specific normal total T_4 or FT_4 levels. Increasing the levothyroxine sodium dosage to suppress TSH into the normal range may produce overtreatment, with an elevated serum T_4 and clinical features of hyperthyroidism including: irritability, increased appetite with diarrhea, and sleeplessness. Another risk of prolonged overtreatment in infants is premature cranial synostosis.

Acquired Hypothyroidism: The initial levothyroxine sodium dose varies with age and body weight, and should be adjusted to maintain serum total T_4 or free T_4 levels in the upper half of the normal range. In general, unless there are overriding clinical concerns, children should be started on a full replacement dose. Children with underlying heart disease should be started at lower dosages, with careful upward titration. Children with severe, longstanding hypothyroidism may also be started on a lower initial dose followed by an upward titration, attempting to avoid premature epiphyseal closure. The recommended dose per body weight decreases with age (see Dosage and Administration, Recommended Dose and Dosage Adjustment, Pediatric Dosage, Table 2).

Treated children may resume growth at a greater than normal rate (period of transient catch-up growth). In some cases the catch-up may be adequate to normalize growth. However, severe and prolonged hypothyroidism may reduce adult height. Excessive thyroxine replacement may initiate accelerated bone maturation, producing disproportionate skeletal age advancement and shortened adult stature.

If transient hypothyroidism is suspected hypothyroidism permanence may be assessed after the child reaches 3 years of age. Levothyroxine therapy may be interrupted for 30 days and serum T_4 and TSH measured. Low T_4 and elevated TSH confirm permanent hypothyroidism; therapy should be re-instituted. If T_4 and TSH remain in the normal range, a presumptive diagnosis of transient hypothyroidism can be made. In this instance, continued clinical monitoring and periodic thyroid function test reevaluation may be warranted.

Since some more severely affected children may become clinically hypothyroid when treatment is discontinued for 30 days, an alternate approach is to reduce the replacement dose of levothyroxine sodium by half during the 30-day trial period. If, after 30 days, the serum TSH is elevated above 20 mU/L, the diagnosis of permanent hypothyroidism is confirmed, and full replacement therapy should be resumed. However, if the serum TSH has not risen to greater than 20 mU/L, levothyroxine sodium treatment should be discontinued for another 30-day trial period followed by repeat serum T_4 and TSH testing.

Geriatrics (>50 years of age): Because of the increased prevalence of cardiovascular disease among the elderly, levothyroxine therapy should not be initiated at the full replacement dose (see Warnings and Precautions and Dosage and Administration).

Monitoring and Laboratory Tests: Treatment of patients with levothyroxine sodium requires periodic assessment of thyroid status by appropriate laboratory tests and clinical evaluation. Selection of appropriate tests for the diagnosis and management of thyroid disorders depends on patient variables such as presenting signs and symptoms, pregnancy, and concomitant medications. A measurement of free T_4 and TSH levels, using a sensitive TSH assay, are recommended to confirm a diagnosis of thyroid disease. Normal ranges for these parameters are age-specific in newborns and younger children.

TSH alone or initially may be useful for thyroid disease screening and for monitoring therapy for primary hypothyroidism as a linear inverse correlation exists between serum TSH and free T_4. Measurement of total serum T_4 and T_3, resin T_3 uptake, and free T_3 concentrations may also be useful. Antithyroid microsomal antibodies are an indicator of autoimmune thyroid disease. Positive microsomal antibody presence in an euthyroid patient is a major risk factor for the development of hypothyroidism. An elevated serum TSH in the presence of a normal T_4 may indicate subclinical hypothyroidism. Intracellular resistance to thyroid hormone is quite rare, and is suggested by clinical signs and symptoms of hypothyroidism in the presence of high serum T_4 levels. Adequacy of levothyroxine sodium therapy for hypothyroidism of pituitary or hypothalamic origin should be assessed by measuring free T_4, which should be maintained in the upper half of the normal range. Measurement of TSH is not a reliable indicator of response to therapy for this condition. Adequacy of levothyroxine sodium therapy for congenital and acquired pediatric hypothyroidism should be assessed by measuring serum total T_4 or free T_4; these should be maintained in the upper half of the normal range. In congenital hypothyroidism, serum TSH normalization may lag behind serum T_4 normalization by 2 to 3 months or longer. In rare patients, serum TSH remains relatively elevated despite clinical euthyroidism and age-specific normal T_4 or free T_4 levels (see Warnings and Precautions, Special Populations, Pediatrics (All ages including neonates)).

Carcinogenesis and Mutagenesis: Although animal studies to determine the mutagenic or carcinogenic potential of thyroid hormones have not been performed, synthetic T_4 is identical to that produced by the human thyroid gland. A reported association between prolonged thyroid hormone therapy and breast cancer has not been confirmed and patients receiving levothyroxine sodium for established indications should not discontinue therapy.

ADVERSE REACTIONS: Adverse Drug Reaction Overview: Adverse reactions other than those indicative of thyrotoxicosis as a result of therapeutic overdosage, either initially or during the maintenance periods, are rare (see Overdosage). Seizures have been reported rarely with the institution of levothyroxine sodium therapy. Pseudotumor cerebri and slipped capital femoral epiphysis have also been reported in children receiving levothyroxine therapy. Over treatment in children may result in craniosynostosis and premature closure of the epiphyses with resultant compromised adult height.

Inadequate doses of ELTROXIN (levothyroxine sodium) may produce or fail to resolve symptoms of hypothyroidism. Hair loss may occur during the initial months of therapy, but is generally transient. The incidence of continued hair loss is unknown.

Adverse reactions associated with levothyroxine sodium are primarily those of hyperthyroidism due to therapeutic overdosage (see Warnings and Precautions and Overdosage). They include the following:

General: fatigue, increased appetite, weight loss, heat intolerance, fever, and excessive sweating.
Cardiovascular System: palpitations, tachycardia, arrhythmias, increased pulse and blood pressure, heart failure, angina, myocardial infarction and cardiac arrest.
Central Nervous System: headache, hyperactivity, nervousness, anxiety, irritability, emotional lability, and insomnia.
Dermatologic: hair loss, flushing.
Endocrine System: decreased bone mineral density.
Gastrointestinal System: diarrhea, vomiting, abdominal cramps, and elevations in liver function tests.
Musculoskeletal System: tremors, muscle weakness.
Reproductive System: menstrual irregularities, impaired fertility.
Respiratory System: dyspnea.

Hypersensitivity reactions to inactive ingredients have occurred in patients treated with thyroid hormone products. These include urticaria, pruritus, skin rash, flushing, angioedema, various GI symptoms (abdominal pain, nausea, vomiting and diarrhea), fever, arthralgia, serum sickness and wheezing. Hypersensitivity to levothyroxine itself is not known to occur.

DRUG INTERACTIONS: Overview: The magnitude and relative clinical importance of the effects noted below are likely to be patient-specific and may vary by such factors as age, gender, race, intercurrent illnesses, dose of either agents, additional concomitant medications, and timing of drug administration. Any agent that alters thyroid hormone synthesis, secretion, distribution, effect on target tissues, metabolism, or elimination may alter the optimal therapeutic dose of ELTROXIN (levothyroxine sodium).

Drug-Drug Interactions: Many drugs affect thyroid hormone pharmacokinetics and metabolism (e.g., absorption, synthesis, secretion, catabolism, protein binding, and target tissue response) and may alter the therapeutic response to levothyroxine sodium. In addition, thyroid hormones and thyroid status have varied effects on the pharmacokinetics and actions of other drugs. A listing of drug-thyroidal axis interactions is contained in Table 1.

The list of drug-thyroidal axis interactions in Table 1 may not be comprehensive due to the introduction of new drugs that interact with the thyroidal axis or the discovery or previously unknown interactions. The prescriber should be aware of this fact and should consult appropriate reference sources (e.g., package inserts of newly approved drugs, medical literature) for additional information if a drug-drug interaction with levothyroxine is suspected.

Anticoagulants: Levothyroxine levels increase the response to oral anticoagulant therapy. Therefore, a decrease in the dose of anticoagulant may be warranted with correction of the hypothyroid state or when the levothyroxine sodium dose is increased. Prothrombin time should be closely monitored to permit appropriate and timely dosage adjustments (see Table 1).

Table 1: ELTROXIN

Drug-Thyroidal Axis Interactions

Drug or Drug Class	Effect
Drug-Thyroidal Axis Interactions — Drugs that may reduce TSH secretion—the reduction is not sustained; therefore, hypothyroidism does not occur	
Dopamine/Dopamine Agonists Glucocorticoids Octreotide	Use of these agents may result in a transient reduction in TSH secretion when administered at the following doses: Dopamine (greater than or equal to 1 µg/kg/min); Glucocorticoids (hydrocortisone greater than or equal to 100 mg/day or equivalent); Octreotide (greater than 100 µg/day).
Drugs That Alter Thyroid Hormone Secretion — Drugs that may decrease thyroid hormone secretion, which may result in hypothyroidism	
Aminoglutethimide Amiodarone Iodide (including iodine-containing radiographic contrast agents) Lithium Thioamides • Methimazole • Propylthiouracil (PTU) • Carbimazole Sulfonamides Tolbutamide	Long-term lithium therapy can result in goiter in up to 50% of patients, and either subclinical or overt hypothyroidism, each in up to 20% of patients. The fetus, neonate, elderly and euthyroid patients with underlying thyroid disease (e.g., Hashimoto's thyroiditis or with Grave's disease previously treated with radioiodine or surgery) are among those individuals who are particularly susceptible to iodine-induced hypothyroidism. Oral cholecystographic agents and amiodarone are slowly excreted, producing more prolonged hypothyroidism than parenterally administered iodinated contrast agents. Long-term aminoglutethimide therapy may minimally decrease T_4 and T_3 levels and increase TSH, although all values remain within normal limits in most patients.
Drugs That May Increase Thyroid Hormone Secretion, Which May Result in Hyperthyroidism	
Amiodarone Iodide (including iodine-containing radiographic contrast agents)	Iodide and drugs that contain pharmacologic amounts of iodide may cause hyperthyroidism in euthyroid patients with Grave's disease previously treated with antithyroid drugs or in euthyroid patients with thyroid autonomy (e.g., multinodular goiter or hyperfunctioning thyroid adenoma). Hyperthyroidism may develop over several weeks and may persist for several months after therapy discontinuation. Amiodarone may induce hyperthyroidism by causing thyroiditis.

(cont'd)

Table 1: ELTROXIN *(cont'd)*

Drug-Thyroidal Axis Interactions

Drug or Drug Class	Effect
Drugs That May Decrease T_4 Absorption, Which May Result in Hypothyroidism	
Antacids • Aluminum & Magnesium Hydroxides • Simethicone Bile Acid Sequestrants • Cholestyramine • Colestipol Calcium Carbonate Cation Exchange Resins • Kayexalate Ferrous Sulfate Sucralfate	Concurrent use may reduce the efficacy of levothyroxine by binding and delaying or preventing absorption, potentially resulting in hypothyroidism. Calcium carbonate may form an insoluble chelate with levothyroxine, and ferrous sulfate likely forms a ferric-thyroxine complex. Administer levothyroxine at least four (4) hours apart from these agents.
Drugs That May Alter T_4 and T_3 Serum Transport—but FT_4 Concentration Remains Normal; and Therefore, the Patient Remains Euthyroid	
Drugs that may increase serum TBG Concentration Clofibrate Estrogen-containing Oral Contraceptives Estrogens (oral) Heroin/Methadone 5-Fluorouracil Mitotane Tamoxifen	Drugs that may decrease serum TBG Concentration Androgens/Anabolic Steroids Asparaginase Glucocorticoids Slow-Release Nicotinic Acid
Drugs That May Cause Protein-Binding Site Replacement	
Furosemide (greater than 80 mg IV) Heparin Hydantoins Non Steroidal Anti-Inflammatory Drugs • Fenamates • Phenylbutazone Salicylates (greater than 2 g/day)	Administration of these agents with levothyroxine results in an initial transient increase in FT_4. Continued administration results in a decrease in Serum T_4 and normal FT_4 and TSH concentrations and, therefore, patients are clinically euthyroid. Salicylates inhibit binding of T_4 and T_3 to TBG and transthyretin. An initial increase in serum FT_4 is followed by return of FT_4 to normal levels with sustained therapeutic serum saliyclate concentrations, although total-T_4 levels may decrease by as much as 30%.
Drugs That May Alter T_4 and T_3 Metabolism — Drugs that may increase hepatic metabolism, which may result in hypothyroidism	
Carbamazepine Hydantoins Phenobarbital Rifampin	Stimulation of hepatic microsomal drug-metabolizing enzyme activity may cause increased hepatic degradation of levothyroxine, resulting in increased levothyroxine requirements. Phenytoin and carbamazepine reduce serum protein binding of levothyroxine, and total- and free-T_4 may be reduced by 20% to 40%, but most patients have normal serum TSH levels and are clinically euthyroid.
Drugs That May Decrease T_4 5'-Deiodinase Activity	
Amiodarone Beta-adrenergic antagonists • (e.g., Propranolol greater than 160 mg/day) Glucocorticoids • (e.g., Dexamethasone greater than or equal to 4 mg/day) Propylthiouracil (PTU)	Administration of these enzyme inhibitors decreases the peripheral conversion of T_4 to T_3, leading to decreased T_3 levels. However, serum T_4 levels are usually normal but may occasionally be slightly increased. In patients treated with large doses of propranolol (greater than 160 mg/day), T_3 and T_4 levels change slightly, TSH levels remain normal, and patients are clinically euthyroid. It should be noted that actions of particular beta-adrenergic antagonists may be impaired when the hypothyroid patient is converted to the euthyroid state. Short-term administration of large doses of glucocorticoids may decrease serum T_3 concentrations by 30% with minimal change in serum T_4 levels. However, long-term glucocorticoid therapy may result in slightly decreased T_3 and T_4 levels due to decreased TBG production (see above).
Miscellaneous	
Anticoagulants (oral) • Coumarin Derivatives • Indandione Derivatives	Thyroid hormones appear to increase the catabolism of vitamin K-dependent clotting factors, thereby increasing the anticoagulant activity of oral anticoagulants. Concomitant use of these agents impairs the compensatory increases in clotting factor synthesis. Prothrombin time should be carefully monitored in patients taking levothyroxine and oral anticoagulants and the dose of anticoagulant therapy adjusted accordingly.
Antidepressants • Tricyclics (e.g., Amitriptyline) • Tetracyclics (e.g., Maprotiline) • Selective Serotonin Reuptake Inhibitors (SSRIs; e.g., Sertraline)	Concurrent use of tri/tetracyclic antidepressants and levothyroxine may increase the therapeutic and toxic effects of both drugs, possibly due to increased receptor sensitivity to catecholamines. Toxic effects may include increased risk of cardiac arrhythmias and CNS stimulation; onset of action of tricyclics may be accelerated. Administration of sertraline in patients stabilized on levothyroxine may result in increased levothyroxine requirements.
Antidiabetic Agents • Biguanides • Meglitinides • Sulfonylureas • Thiazolidinediones • Insulin	Addition of levothyroxine to antidiabetic or insulin therapy may result in increased antidiabetic agent or insulin requirements. Careful monitoring of diabetic control is recommended, especially when thyroid therapy is started, changed, or discontinued.
Cardiac glycosides	Serum digitalis glycoside levels may be reduced in hyperthyroidism or when the hypothyroid patient is converted to the euthyroid state. Therapeutic effect of digitalis glycosides may be reduced.

(cont'd)

Table 1: ELTROXIN *(cont'd)*

Drug-Thyroidal Axis Interactions

Drug or Drug Class	Effect
Cytokines • Interferon-alpha • Interleukin-2	Therapy with interferon-alpha has been associated with the development of antithyroid microsomal antibodies in 20% of patients and some have transient hypothyroidism, hyperthyroidism, or both. Patients who have antithyroid antibodies before treatment are at higher risk for thyroid dysfunction during treatment. Interleukin-2 has been associated with transient painless thyroiditis in 20% of patients. Interferon-beta and-gamma have not been reported to cause thyroid dysfunction.
Growth Hormones • Somatrem • Somatropin	Excessive use of thyroid hormones with growth hormones may accelerate epiphyseal closure. However, untreated hypothyroidism may interfere with growth response to growth hormone.
HMG-CoA reductase inhibitors (statins) • Lovastatin • Simvastatin	Some statins may increase thyroid hormone requirements. It is unknown if this occurs with all statins. Close monitoring of thyroid function and appropriate thyroxine dose adjustments may be necessary when thyroxine and statins are co-prescribed.
Ketamine	Concurrent use may produce marked hypertension and tachycardia; cautious administration to patients receiving thyroid hormone therapy is recommended.
Methylxanthine Bronchodilators • (e.g., Theophylline)	Decreased theophylline clearance may occur in hypothyroid patients; clearance returns to normal when the euthyroid state is achieved.
Radiographic agents	Thyroid hormones may reduce the uptake of ^{123}I, ^{131}I, and ^{99m}Tc.
Sympathomimetics	Concurrent use may increase the effects of sympathomimetics or thyroid hormone. Thyroid hormones may increase the risk of coronary insufficiency when sympathomimetic agents are administered to patients with coronary artery disease.
Chloral Hydrate Diazepam Ethionamide Metoclopramide 6-Mercaptopurine Nitroprusside Para-aminosalicylate sodium Perphenazine Resorcinol (excessive topical use) Thiazide Diuretics	These agents have been associated with thyroid hormone and/or TSH level alterations by various mechanisms.

Digitalis Glycosides: The therapeutic effects of digitalis glycosides may be reduced by levothyroxine sodium. Serum digitalis glycoside levels may be decreased when a hypothyroid patient becomes euthyroid, necessitating an increase in the dose of digitalis glycosides (see Table 1).

Drug-Food Interactions: Consumption of certain foods may affect levothyroxine absorption thereby necessitating adjustments in dosing. Soybean flour (infant formula), cotton seed meal, walnuts, calcium and calcium-fortified orange juice, and dietary fibre may bind and decrease the absorption of levothyroxine sodium from the gastrointestinal tract.

Drug-Laboratory Test Interactions: A number of drugs or moieties are known to alter serum levels of TSH, T_4 and T_3 and may thereby influence the interpretation of laboratory tests of thyroid function (see Drug Interactions).

1. Changes in TBG concentration should be taken into consideration when interpreting T_4 and T_3 values. Drugs such as estrogens and estrogen-containing oral contraceptives increase serum TBG concentrations. TBG concentrations may also be increased during pregnancy, in infectious hepatitis and acute intermittent porphyria. Decreases in TBG concentrations are observed in nephrosis, severe hypoproteinemia, severe liver disease, acromegaly, and after androgen or corticosteroid therapy. Familial hyper- or hypo-thyroxine-binding- globulinemias have been described. The incidence of TBG deficiency is approximately 1 in 9000. Certain drugs such as salicylates inhibit the protein-binding of T_4. In such cases, the unbound (free) hormone should be measured.
2. Persistent clinical and laboratory evidence of hypothyroidism despite an adequate replacement dose suggests either poor patient compliance, impaired absorption, drug interactions, or decreased potency of the preparation due to improper storage.

DOSAGE AND ADMINISTRATION:

Dosing Considerations: The dosage and rate of administration of ELTROXIN (levothyroxine sodium) is determined by the indication, and must in every case be individualized according to patient response and laboratory findings.

Adult Dosage: Hypothyroidism: The goal of therapy for primary hypothyroidism is to achieve and maintain a clinical and biochemical euthyroid state with consequent resolution of hypothyroid signs and symptoms. The starting dose of levothyroxine sodium the frequency of dose titration, and the optimal full replacement dose must be individualized for every patient, and will be influenced by such factors as age, weight, cardiovascular status, presence of other illness, and the severity and duration of hypothyroid symptoms.

In patients with hypothyroidism resulting from pituitary or hypothalamic disease, the possibility of secondary adrenal insufficiency should be considered, and if present, treated with glucocorticoids prior to initiation of levothyroxine sodium. The adequacy of levothyroxine sodium therapy should be assessed in these patients by measuring FT_4, which should be maintained in the upper half of the normal range, in addition to clinical assessment. Measurement of TSH is not a reliable indicator of response to therapy for this condition.

TSH Suppression in Thyroid Cancer and Thyroid Nodules: The rationale for TSH suppression therapy is that a reduction in TSH secretion may decrease the growth and function of abnormal thyroid tissue. Exogenous thyroid hormone may inhibit recurrence of tumour growth and may produce regression of metastases from well-differentiated (follicular and papillary) carcinoma of the thyroid. It is used as ancillary therapy of these conditions following surgery or radioactive iodine therapy. Medullary and anaplastic carcinoma of the thyroid is unresponsive to TSH suppression therapy. TSH suppression is also used in treating nontoxic solitary nodules and multinodular goiters.

No controlled studies have compared the various degrees of TSH suppression in the treatment of either benign or malignant thyroid nodular disease. Further, the effectiveness of TSH suppression for benign nodular disease is controversial. The dose of levothyroxine sodium used for TSH suppression should therefore be individualized by the nature of the disease, the patient being treated, and the desired clinical response, weighing the potential benefits of therapy against the risks of iatrogenic thyrotoxicosis. In general, levothyroxine sodium should be given in the smallest dose that will achieve the desired clinical response.

Pediatric Dosage: Congenital or Acquired Hypothyroidism: The levothyroxine sodium pediatric dosage varies with age and body weight. Levothyroxine sodium should be given at a dose that maintains T_4 or free T_4 in the upper half of the normal range and serum TSH in the normal range (see Warnings and Precautions, Special Populations, Pediatrics (All ages including neonates)). Normalization of TSH may lag significantly behind T_4 in some infants. In general, despite the smaller body size of children, the dosage (on a weight basis) required to sustain full development and general thriving is higher than in adults (see Table 2).

Recommended Dose and Dosage Adjustment: Adult Dosage: Hypothyroidism: The usual full replacement dose of levothyroxine sodium for younger, healthy adults is approximately 1.7 µg/kg/day administered once daily. In the elderly, the full replacement dose may be altered by decreases in T_4 metabolism and levothyroxine sodium absorption. Older patients may require less than 1 µg/kg/day. Children generally require higher doses (see Pediatric Dosage). Women who are maintained on levothyroxine sodium during pregnancy may require increased doses (see Warnings and Precautions, Special Populations, Pregnant Women).

Therapy is usually initiated in younger, healthy adults at the anticipated full replacement dose. Clinical and laboratory evaluations should be performed at 6 to 8 week intervals (2 to 3 weeks in severely hypothyroid patients), and the dosage adjusted until the serum TSH concentration is normalized and signs and symptoms resolve. In older patients or in younger patients with a history of cardiovascular disease, the starting dose should be lowered and gradually increased every 3 to 6 weeks until TSH is normalized and signs and symptoms resolve. If cardiac symptoms develop or worsen, the cardiac disease should be evaluated and the dose of levothyroxine sodium reduced. Rarely, worsening angina or other signs of cardiac ischemia may prevent achieving a TSH in the normal range.

Treatment of subclinical hypothyroidism may require lower than usual replacement doses, e.g. 1 µg/kg/day. Patients for whom treatment is not initiated should be monitored yearly for changes in clinical status, TSH, and thyroid antibodies.

Few patients require doses greater than 200 µg/day. An inadequate response to daily doses of 300 to 400 µg/day is rare, and may suggest malabsorption, poor patient compliance, and/or drug interactions.

Once optimal replacement is achieved, clinical and laboratory evaluations should be conducted at least annually or whenever warranted by a change in patient status. Levothyroxine sodium products from different manufacturers should not be used interchangeably unless retesting of the patient and retitration of the dosage, as necessary, accompanies the product switch.

Myxedema Coma: Myxedema coma represents the extreme expression of severe hypothyroidism and is considered a medical emergency. It is characterized by hypothermia, hypotension, hypoventilation, hyponatremia, and bradycardia. In addition to restoration of normal thyroid hormone levels, therapy should be directed at the correction of electrolyte disturbances and possible infection. Because the mortality rate of patients with untreated myxedema coma is high, treatment must be started immediately, and should include appropriate supportive therapy and corticosteroids to prevent adrenal insufficiency. Possible precipitating factors should also be identified and treated.

Myxedema coma is a life-threatening emergency characterized by poor circulation and hypometabolism, and may result in unpredictable absorption of levothyroxine sodium from the gastrointestinal tract. Therefore, oral thyroid hormone drug products, such as levothyroxine sodium are not recommended to treat this condition. Thyroid hormone products formulated for intravenous administration should be administered.

TSH Suppression in Thyroid Cancer and Thyroid Nodules: For well-differentiated thyroid cancer, TSH is generally suppressed to less than 0.1 mU/L. Doses of levothyroxine sodium greater than 2 µg/kg/day are usually required. The efficacy of TSH suppression in reducing the size of benign thyroid nodules and in preventing nodule regrowth after surgery is controversial. Nevertheless, when treatment with levothyroxine sodium is warranted, TSH is generally suppressed to a higher target range (e.g. 0.1 to 0.3 mU/L) than that employed for the treatment of thyroid cancer. Levothyroxine sodium therapy may also be considered for patients with nontoxic multinodular goiter who have a TSH in the normal range, to moderately suppress TSH (e.g. 0.1 to 0.3 mU/L).

Levothyroxine sodium should be administered with caution to patients in whom there is a suspicion of thyroid gland autonomy, in view of the fact that the effects of exogenous hormone administration will be additive to endogenous thyroid hormone production.

Pediatric Dosage: Congenital or Acquired Hypothyroidism: Therapy is usually initiated at the full replacement dose (see Table 2). Infants and neonates with very low (<5 µg/dL) or undetectable serum T_4 levels should be started at higher end of the dosage range (e.g. 50 µg daily). A lower dose (e.g. 25 µg daily) should be considered for neonates at risk of cardiac failure, increasing every few days until a full maintenance dose is reached. In children with severe, longstanding hypothyroidism, levothyroxine sodium should be initiated gradually, with an initial 25 µg dose for two weeks, then increasing by 25 µg every 2 to 4 weeks until the desired dose, based on serum T_4 and TSH levels, is achieved.

Table 2: ELTROXIN

Levothyroxine Sodium Dosing Guidelines for Pediatric Hypothyroidism

Age	Daily Dose Per Kg Body Weight[a]
0–3 months	10–15 µg/kg/day
3–6 months	8–10 µg/kg/day
6–12 months	6–8 µg/kg/day
1–5 years	5–6 µg/kg/day
6–12 years	4–5 µg/kg/day
>12 years but growth and puberty incomplete	2–3 µg/kg/day
Growth and puberty complete	1.6–1.7 µg/kg/day

[a] The dose should be adjusted based on clinical response and laboratory parameters (see Warnings and Precautions, Monitoring and Laboratory Tests, Pediatrics (All ages including neonates)).

Serum T_4 and TSH measurements should be evaluated at the following intervals, with subsequent dosage adjustments to normalize serum total T_4 or FT_4 and TSH: 2 and 4 weeks after therapy initiation, every 1 to 2 months during the first year of life, every 2 to 3 months between 1 and 3 years of age, every 3 to 12 months thereafter until growth is completed.

Evaluation at more frequent intervals is indicated when compliance is questioned or abnormal laboratory values are obtained. Patient evaluation is also advisable approximately 6 to 8 weeks after any change in levothyroxine sodium dose.

Missed Dose: If a scheduled daily dose is missed, the dose should be taken as soon as the patient remembers, unless it is almost time for the patient's next dose. Two doses should not be taken together. If more than two doses are missed, the patient should consult with their doctor.

Administration: Pediatrics: Levothyroxine sodium tablets may be given to infants and children who cannot swallow intact tablets by crushing the tablet and suspending the freshly crushed tablet in a small amount of water (5 to 10 mL), breast milk or non-soybean based formula. The suspension can be given by spoon or dropper. **Do not store the suspension for any period of time.** The crushed tablet may also be sprinkled over a small amount of food, such as apple sauce. Foods or formula containing large amounts of soybean, fibre, or iron should not be used for administering levothyroxine sodium.

OVERDOSAGE:

Signs and Symptoms: Excessive doses of ELTROXIN (levothyroxine sodium) result in a hypermetabolic state indistinguishable from thyrotoxicosis of endogenous origin. Signs and symptoms of thyrotoxicosis include exophthalmic goiter, weight loss, increased appetite, palpitations, nervousness, diarrhea, abdominal cramps, sweating, tachycardia, increased pulse and blood pressure, cardiac arrhythmias, angina pectoris, tremors, insomnia, heat intolerance, fever, and menstrual irregularities. In addition, confusion and disorientation may occur. Cerebral embolism, shock, coma, and death have been reported. Seizures have occurred in a child ingesting 18 mg of levothyroxine. Symptoms are not always evident or may not appear until several days after ingestion of levothyroxine sodium.

Treatment of Overdosage: Levothyroxine sodium should be reduced in dose or temporarily discontinued if signs and symptoms of overdosage appear.

In the treatment of acute massive levothyroxine sodium overdosage, symptomatic and supportive therapy should be instituted immediately. Treatment is aimed at reducing gastrointestinal absorption and counteracting central and peripheral effects, mainly those of increased sympathetic activity. Cholestyramine and activated charcoal have also been used to decrease levothyroxine sodium absorption. Beta-receptor antagonists, particularly propranolol, are useful in counteracting many of the effects of increased central and peripheral sympathetic activity, especially when no contraindications exist for its use. Provide respiratory support as needed; control congestive heart failure and arrhythmia, control fever, hypoglycemia, and fluid loss as necessary. Large doses of antithyroid drugs (e.g. methimazole, carbimazole, or propylthiouracil) followed in one to two hours by large doses of iodine may be given to inhibit synthesis and release of thyroid hormones. Cardiac glycosides may be administered if congestive heart failure develops. Glucocorticoids may be administered to inhibit the conversion of T_4 to T_3. Plasmapheresis, charcoal hemoperfusion and exchange transfusion have been reserved for cases in which continued clinical deterioration occurs despite conventional therapy. Since T_4 is extensively protein bound, very little drug will be removed by dialysis.

For management of a suspected drug overdose, contact your regional Poison Control Centre. See the *CPS Directory* section for a list of Poison Control Centres.

ACTION AND CLINICAL PHARMACOLOGY: Mechanism of Action: The synthesis and secretion of the major thyroid hormones, L-thyroxine (T_4) and L-triiodothyronine (T_3), from the normally functioning thyroid gland are regulated by complex feedback mechanisms of the hypothalamic-pituitary-thyroid axis. The thyroid gland is stimulated to secrete thyroid hormones by the action of thyrotropin (thyroid stimulating hormone, TSH), which is produced in the anterior pituitary gland. TSH secretion is in turn controlled by thyrotropin-releasing hormone (TRH) produced in the hypothalamus, circulating thyroid hormones, and possibly other mechanisms. Thyroid hormones circulating in the blood act as feedback inhibitors of both TSH and TRH secretion. Thus, when serum concentrations of T_3 and T_4 are increased, secretion of TSH and TRH decreases. Conversely, when serum thyroid hormone concentrations are decreased, secretion of TSH and TRH is increased. Administration of exogenous thyroid hormones to euthyroid individuals results in suppression of endogenous thyroid hormone secretion.

The mechanisms by which thyroid hormones exert their physiologic actions have not been completely elucidated, but it is thought that their principal effects are exerted through control of DNA transcription and protein synthesis. T_4 and T_3 are transported into cells by passive and active mechanisms. T_3 in cell cytoplasm and T_3 generated from T_4 within the cell diffuse into the nucleus and bind to thyroid receptor proteins, which appear to be primarily attached to DNA. Receptor binding leads to activation or repression of DNA transcription, thereby altering the amounts of mRNA and resultant proteins. Changes in protein concentrations are responsible for the metabolic changes observed in organs and tissues.

Thyroid hormones enhance oxygen consumption of most body tissues and increase the basal metabolic rate and metabolism of carbohydrates, lipids, and proteins. Thus, they exert a profound influence on every organ system and are of particular importance in the development of the central nervous system. Thyroid hormones also appear to have direct effects on tissues, such as increased myocardial contractility and decreased systemic vascular resistance.

The physiologic effects of thyroid hormones are produced primarily by T_3, a large portion of which (approximately 80%) is derived from the deiodination of T_4 in peripheral tissues. About 70 to 90 percent of peripheral T_3 is produced by monodeiodination of T_4 at the 5 position (outer ring). Peripheral monodeiodination of T_4 at the 5 position (inner ring) results in the formation of reverse triiodothyronine (rT_3), which is calorigenically inactive.

Levothyroxine, at doses individualized according to patient response, is effective as replacement or supplemental therapy in hypothyroidism of any etiology, except transient hypothyroidism during the recovery phase of subacute thyroiditis.

Levothyroxine is also effective in the suppression of pituitary TSH secretion in the treatment or prevention of various types of euthyroid goiters, including thyroid nodules, Hashimoto's thyroiditis, multinodular goiter and, as adjunctive therapy in the management of thyrotropin-dependent well-differentiated thyroid cancer (see Indications and Clinical Use, Warnings and Precautions and Dosage and Administration).

Pharmacokinetics: Absorption: Few clinical studies have evaluated the kinetics of orally administered thyroid hormone. In animals, the most active sites of absorption appear to be the proximal and mid-jejunum. T_4 is not absorbed from the stomach and little, if any, drug is absorbed from the duodenum. There seems to be no absorption of T_4 from the distal colon in animals. A number of human studies have confirmed the importance of an intact jejunum and ileum for T_4 absorption and have shown some absorption from the duodenum. Studies involving radioiodinated T_4 fecal tracer excretion methods, equilibration, and AUC methods have shown that absorption varies from 48 to 80 percent of the administered dose. The extent of absorption is increased in the fasting state and decreased in malabsorption syndromes, such as sprue. Absorption may also decrease with age. The degree of T_4 absorption is dependent on the product formulation as well as on the character of the intestinal contents, the intestinal flora, including plasma protein and soluble dietary factors, which bind thyroid hormone, making it unavailable for diffusion. Decreased absorption may result from administration of infant soybean formula, ferrous sulfate, sodium polystyrene sulfonate, aluminum hydroxide, sucralfate, or bile acid sequestrants. T_4 absorption following intramuscular administration is variable. The relative bioavailability of levothyroxine sodium tablets, compared to an equal nominal dose of oral levothyroxine sodium solution, is approximately 93%.

Distribution: Distribution of thyroid hormones in human body tissues and fluids has not been fully elucidated. More than 99% of circulating hormones is bound to serum proteins, including thyroxine-binding globulin (TBG), thyroxine-binding prealbumin (TBPA), and albumin (TBA). T_4 is more extensively and firmly bound to serum proteins than is T_3. Only unbound thyroid hormone is metabolically active. The higher affinity of TBG and TBPA for T_4 partly explains the higher serum levels, slower metabolic clearance, and longer serum elimination half-life of this hormone.

Certain drugs and physiologic conditions can alter the binding of thyroid hormones to serum proteins and/or the concentrations of the serum proteins available for thyroid hormone binding. These effects must be considered when interpreting the results of thyroid function tests. (See Warnings and Precautions, Monitoring and Laboratory Tests and Drug Interactions.)

Metabolism: The liver is the major site of degradation for both hormones. T_4 and T_3 are conjugated with glucuronic and sulfuric acids and excreted in the bile. There is an enterohepatic circulation of thyroid hormones, as they are liberated by hydrolysis in the intestine and reabsorbed. A portion of the conjugated material reaches the colon unchanged, is hydrolyzed there, and is eliminated as free compounds in the feces. In man, approximately 20 to 40 percent of T_4 is eliminated in the stool. About 70 percent of the T_4 secreted daily is deiodinated to yield equal amounts of T_3 and rT_3. Subsequent deiodination of T_3 and rT_3 yields multiple forms of diiodothyronine. A number of other minor T_4 metabolites have also been identified. Although some of these metabolites have biologic activity, their overall contribution to the therapeutic effect of T_4 is minimal.

Excretion: Thyroid hormones are primarily eliminated by the kidneys. T_4 is eliminated slowly from the body (see Table 3), with a half-life of 6 to 7 days. T_3 has a half-life of 1 to 2 days.

Table 3: ELTROXIN

Pharmacokinetic Parameters of Thyroid Hormones in Euthyroid Patients

Hormone	Ratio in Thyroglobulin	Biologic Potency	$t_{½}$ (days)	Protein Binding (%)[b]
Levothyroxine, T_4	10 to 20	14	6 to 7[a]	99.96
Liothyronine T_3	1		<2	99.5

[a] Three to four days in hyperthyroidism, nine to ten days in hypothyroidism.
[b] Includes TBG, TBPA, and TBA.

STORAGE AND STABILITY: Store between 15 and 25°C. Protect from light.

INFORMATION FOR THE PATIENT: Published in e-CPS, available by subscription at www.e-cps.ca.

DOSAGE FORMS, COMPOSITION AND PACKAGING: 50 µg: Each white, scored, round tablet, engraved with "50", contains: levothyroxine sodium, USP 50 µg. Nonmedicinal ingredients: acacia powder, cornstarch, lactose and magnesium stearate. Gluten- and tartrazine-free. Bottles of 500.

100 µg: Each yellow, scored, round tablet, engraved with "100", contains: levothyroxine sodium, USP 100 µg. Nonmedicinal ingredients: acacia powder, colorcon yellow, cornstarch, lactose and magnesium stearate. Gluten- and tartrazine-free. Bottles of 500.

150 µg: Each blue, scored, round tablet, engraved with "150", contains: levothyroxine sodium, USP 150 µg. Nonmedicinal ingredients: acacia powder, colorcon blue, cornstarch, lactose and magnesium stearate. Gluten- and tartrazine-free. Bottles of 500.

200 µg: Each pink, scored, round tablet, engraved with "200", contains: levothyroxine sodium, USP 200 µg. Nonmedicinal ingredients: acacia powder, cornstarch, erythrosine, lactose and magnesium stearate. Gluten- and tartrazine-free. Bottles of 500.

300 µg: Each green, scored, round tablet, engraved with "300", contains: levothyroxine sodium, USP 300 µg. Nonmedicinal ingredients: acacia powder, colorcon green, cornstarch, lactose and magnesium stearate. Gluten- and tartrazine-free. Bottles of 100 and 500.

(Shown in Product Identification Section)

Emadine® Ⓟ

emedastine difumarate

Antiallergic

Alcon

SUPPLIED: Each mL of sterile ophthalmic solution contains: emedastine difumarate equivalent to emedastine 0.5 mg (0.05%) and benzalkonium chloride 0.01% as preservative. Nonmedicinal ingredients: hydrochloric acid and/or sodium hydroxide, hydroxypropyl methylcellulose, purified water, sodium chloride and tromethamine. Drop-Tainer dispensers of 5 mL. Store at 4 to 30°C. Protect from light.

Emcyt® Ⓟ

estramustine sodium phosphate

Antineoplastic

Pfizer

Date of Revision: July 14, 2008

Caution: Estramustine is a potent drug and should be prescribed only by physicians experienced with cancer chemotherapeutic drugs (see Warnings and Precautions). Blood counts, as well as renal and hepatic function tests, should be performed regularly. Discontinue the drug if abnormal renal or hepatic function is seen. Capsules should not be opened.

PHARMACOLOGY: Estramustine has a dual mode of action. The intact molecule acts as an antimitotic agent and after hydrolysis of the carbamate ester bridge the released estrogens exert an antigonadotrophic effect. The low level of clinically manifested side effects may be due to the fact that estramustine binds to a protein present in the tumor tissue, which results in an accumulation of the drug at the target site.

INDICATIONS: The treatment of metastatic prostatic carcinoma (stage D) in patients whose disease is refractory to hormonal therapy. Estramustine may produce either a stabilization or regression of the disease process and improvement in ability to function.

CONTRAINDICATIONS: In patients with any of the following conditions: known hypersensitivity to either estradiol or to nitrogen mustard, severe hepatic or cardiac disease or active thrombophlebitis or thromboembolic disorders.

WARNINGS: Estramustine should be used with caution in patients with a history of thrombophlebitis, thrombosis or thromboembolic disorders, especially if associated with estrogen therapy. Caution should also be used in patients with cerebral vascular or coronary artery disease.

Angioneurotic edema has been reported in few cases during estramustine therapy, with or without concomitant medication.

Glucose Tolerance: Because glucose tolerance may be decreased, diabetic patients should be carefully observed while receiving estramustine.

Elevated Blood Pressure: Because hypertension may occur, blood pressure should be monitored periodically.

PRECAUTIONS: Estramustine should be administered by individuals experienced in the use of antineoplastic therapy. Professional staff administering estramustine should exercise particular care to prevent spillage and contact with the drug. Should skin contact occur, the area should be vigorously washed with soap and cold water and material used for cleansing disposed of by incineration.

Fluid Retention: Exacerbation of pre-existing or incipient peripheral edema or congestive heart disease has been seen in some patients receiving estramustine therapy. Other conditions which might be influenced by fluid retention, such as epilepsy, migraine, or renal dysfunction, require careful observation.

Estramustine may be poorly metabolized in patients with impaired liver function and should be administered with caution in such patients. Liver function tests should be performed at regular intervals.

Calcium/Phosphorous Metabolism: Because estramustine may influence the metabolism of calcium and phosphorus, it should be used with caution in patients with metabolic bone diseases that are associated with hypercalcemia or in patients with renal insufficiency. Patients with prostate cancer and osteoblastic metastases are at risk for hypocalcemia and should have calcium levels closely monitored.

Mutagenesis, Carcinogenesis: Although testing by the Ames method failed to demonstrate mutagenicity for estramustine, it is known that both estradiol and nitrogen mustard are mutagenic. Patients should therefore be advised to use contraceptive measures during therapy with estramustine.

Immunosuppressant Effects/Increased Susceptibility to Infections: Administration of live or live-attenuated vaccines in patients immunocompromised by chemotherapeutic agents including estramustine, may result in serious or fatal infections. Vaccination with a live vaccine should be avoided in patients receiving estramustine. Killed or inactivated vaccines may be administered; however, the response to such vaccines may be diminished.

Laboratory Tests: Certain endocrine and liver function tests may be affected by estrogen-containing drugs. Abnormalities of hepatic enzymes and of bilirubin have occurred in patients receiving estramustine, but have seldom been severe enough to require cessation of therapy. Such tests should be done at appropriate intervals during therapy and repeated 2 months after the drug has been withdrawn.

Sexual Function and Reproduction: It is known that both estradiol and nitrogen mustard are mutagenic, and therefore males undergoing treatment with estramustine should employ contraceptive measures.

Food/Drug Interactions: Estrogens have been reported to increase both therapeutic activity and toxicity of tricyclic antidepressants, probably via inhibition of their metabolism.

Food like milk, milk products or drugs which contain calcium or other polyvalent ions may impair the absorption of estramustine and must not be taken simultaneously with estramustine.

Angioneurotic edema has been reported in few cases when estramustine was administered concomitantly with ACE-inhibitors.

Effects on Ability to Drive and Use Machines: The effect of estramustine on the ability to drive or use machinery has not been systematically evaluated.

ADVERSE EFFECTS: Gastrointestinal disturbances (most commonly transient nausea, but occasionally vomiting, and rarely diarrhea) sometimes occur during the first two weeks of therapy. In a few cases thrombocytopenia, leukopenia and elevated transaminases/bilirubin have been noted but were completely reversible on reduction of dosage or temporary (1 to 2 weeks) withdrawal of the drug. Other cases of anemia, muscular weakness, depression, headache, confusion and lethargy may rarely occur. A few cases of allergic skin rashes, edema and anginal complaints have been reported. Cardiovascular adverse reactions such as fluid retention/edema, thromboembolism, ischemic heart disease, congestive heart failure, myocardial infarction and hypertension may occur during treatment. A few cases of angioneurotic edema have been reported during estramustine therapy, with or without concomitant medication. Therapy with estramustine is to be immediately discontinued, should angioneurotic edema occur. As with conventional estradiol therapy, thromboembolic disorders, gynecomastia, reduced libido and potency may occur.

OVERDOSE:

Symptoms: Although, there has been no experience with overdoses of Emcyt (estramustine sodium phosphate) to date, it is reasonable to expect that such episodes may produce pronounced manifestations of the known adverse reactions associated with estramustine, particularly gastrointestinal symptoms.

Treatment: In the event of overdosage, treatment should be symptomatic and supportive. Gastric lavage should be performed and measures taken to encourage diuresis. Hematologic and hepatic parameters should be monitored for at least 6 weeks after overdosage of estramustine.

For management of a suspected drug overdose, CPhA recommends that you contact your **regional Poison Control Centre**. See the *CPS* Directory section for a list of Poison Control Centres.

DOSAGE: The recommended dose of estramustine is 14 mg/kg of body weight/day (i.e., one 140 mg capsule for each 10 kg), given in 3 or 4 divided doses. Most patients have been treated at a dose range of 10 to 16 mg/kg/day.

Treatment for at least 30 days is recommended before assessing the benefits of therapy and may be continued as long as a favorable response lasts. If no response is observed after 4-6 weeks, treatment should be discontinued. Some patients have been maintained on therapy for more than 2 years at doses ranging from 10 to 16 mg/kg of body weight/day.

The capsules should be taken at not less than 1 hour before or 2 hours after meals.

The capsules should be swallowed with a glass of water. Milk, milk products or calcium containing drugs (such as calcium-containing antacids) must not be used simultaneously with estramustine capsules.

INFORMATION FOR THE PATIENT: Published in e-CPS, available by subscription at www.e-cps.ca.

SUPPLIED: Each white, opaque, hard gelatin capsule contains: estramustine sodium phosphate 140 mg. Nonmedicinal ingredients: gelatin capsule, isopropanol, magnesium stearate, silica and sodium laurylsulfate. Bisulfite-, gluten-, lactose- and tartrazine-free. Bottles of 100. Store at 2 to 25°C.

(Shown in Product Identification Section)

Emend® Ⓟ

aprepitant

Neurokinin 1 (NK1) Receptor Antagonist

Merck Frosst

Date of Revision: March 4, 2010

SUMMARY PRODUCT INFORMATION:

Route of Administration	Dosage Form/ Strength	Clinically Relevant Nonmedicinal Ingredients
Oral	Capsule/80 mg, 125 mg	For a complete listing see Dosage Forms, Composition and Packaging.

INDICATIONS AND CLINICAL USE: EMEND (aprepitant), in combination with a $5\text{-}HT_3$ antagonist class of antiemetics and dexamethasone, is indicated for the:

- prevention of acute and delayed nausea and vomiting due to highly emetogenic cancer chemotherapy
- prevention of nausea and vomiting in women due to treatment with moderately emetogenic cancer chemotherapy.

Geriatrics (≥65 years of age): In clinical studies, the efficacy and safety of EMEND in the elderly (≥65 years) were comparable to those seen in younger patients (<65 years). No dosage adjustment is necessary in elderly patients.

Pediatrics (<18 years of age): No data available.

CONTRAINDICATIONS:

- Patients who are hypersensitive to this drug or to any ingredient in the formulation. For a complete listing, see Dosage Forms, Composition and Packaging.
- EMEND should not be used concurrently with pimozide, terfenadine, astemizole, or cisapride. Inhibition of cytochrome P450 isoenzyme 3A4 (CYP3A4) by aprepitant could result in elevated plasma concentrations of these drugs, potentially causing serious or life-threatening reactions (see Drug Interactions).

WARNINGS AND PRECAUTIONS:

Serious Warnings and Precautions

Drug interactions with:

- Medicinal product that are metabolized through CYP3A4 (see Drug Interactions).
- Warfarin (see Drug Interactions).
- Hormonal contraception (see Drug Interactions).

Special Populations: Pregnant Women: Reproductive studies have been performed in rats and rabbits at doses up to 1.5 times the systemic exposure at the adult human dose and have revealed no evidence of impaired fertility or harm to the fetus due to aprepitant. However, there are no adequate and well-controlled studies in pregnant women; therefore, EMEND is not recommended for use during pregnancy unless clearly necessary.

Nursing Women: Aprepitant is excreted in the milk of lactating rats. It is not known whether this drug is excreted in human milk; therefore, breastfeeding is not recommended during treatment with EMEND.

Pediatrics (<18 years of age): Safety and effectiveness of EMEND in pediatric patients have not been established.

Geriatrics (≥65 years of age): In 2 well-controlled clinical studies, of the total number of patients (N=544) treated with EMEND, 31% were 65 and over, while 5% were 75 and over. No overall differences in safety or effectiveness were observed between these subjects and younger subjects. Greater sensitivity of some older individuals cannot be ruled out. Dosage adjustment in the elderly is not necessary.

ADVERSE REACTIONS: Clinical Trial Adverse Drug Reactions: The overall safety of aprepitant was evaluated in approximately 4300 individuals.

Highly Emetogenic Chemotherapy: In 2 well-controlled clinical trials in patients receiving cisplatin-based chemotherapy, 544 patients were treated with aprepitant during Cycle 1 of chemotherapy and 413 of these patients continued into the Multiple-Cycle extension for up to 6 cycles of chemotherapy. EMEND was given in combination with ondansetron and dexamethasone and was generally well tolerated. Most adverse experiences reported in these clinical studies were described as mild to moderate in intensity.

In Cycle 1, clinical adverse experiences were reported in approximately 69% of patients treated with the aprepitant regimen compared with approximately 68% of patients treated with standard therapy. Table 1 shows the percent of patients with clinical adverse experiences reported at an incidence ≥3%.

Table 1: EMEND

All Adverse Experiences, Regardless of Causality, (incidence ≥3%) Occurring in Patients Receiving Highly Emetogenic Chemotherapy Who Were Treated with the Aprepitant Regimen for Chemotherapy Induced Nausea and Vomiting (CINV) in Clinical Studies (Cycle 1)

	Aprepitant Regimen N=544 %	Standard Therapy N=550 %
Body As a Whole/Site Unspecified		
Abdominal Pain	(4.6)	(3.3)
Asthenia/Fatigue	(17.8)	(11.8)
Dehydration	(5.9)	(5.1)
Dizziness	(6.6)	(4.4)
Fever	(2.9)	(3.5)
Mucous Membrane Disorder	(2.6)	(3.1)
Digestive System		
Constipation	(10.3)	(12.2)
Diarrhea	(10.3)	(7.5)
Epigastric Discomfort	(4.0)	(3.1)
Gastritis	(4.2)	(3.1)
Heartburn	(5.3)	(4.9)
Nausea	(12.7)	(11.8)
Vomiting	(7.5)	(7.6)
Eyes, Ears, Nose, and Throat		
Tinnitus	(3.7)	(3.8)
Hemic and Lymphatic System		
Neutropenia	(3.1)	(2.9)
Metabolism and Nutrition		
Anorexia	(10.1)	(9.5)
Nervous System		
Headache	(8.5)	(8.7)
Insomnia	(2.9)	(3.1)
Respiratory System		
Hiccups	(10.8)	(5.6)

(cont'd)

Table 1: EMEND (cont'd)

In addition, isolated cases of serious adverse experiences, regardless of causality, of bradycardia, disorientation, and perforating duodenal ulcer were reported in highly emetogenic CINV clinical studies.

Moderately Emetogenic Chemotherapy: During Cycle 1 of 2 moderately emetogenic chemotherapy studies, 868 patients were treated with the aprepitant regimen and 686 of these patients continued into extensions for up to 4 cycles of chemotherapy. In the combined analysis of Cycle 1 data for these 2 studies, adverse experiences were reported in approximately 69% of patients treated with the aprepitant regimen compared with approximately 72% of patients treated with standard therapy.

In the combined analysis of Cycle 1 data for these 2 studies, the adverse experience profile in both moderately emetogenic chemotherapy studies was generally comparable to the highly emetogenic chemotherapy studies. Table 2 shows the percent of patients with clinical adverse experiences reported at an incidence ≥3%.

Table 2: EMEND

All Adverse Experiences, Regardless of Causality, (incidence ≥3%) Occurring in Patients Receiving Moderately Emetogenic Chemotherapy Who Were Treated with the Aprepitant Regimen for CINV in Clinical Studies (Cycle 1)

	Aprepitant Regimen N=868 %	Standard Therapy N=846 %
Blood and Lymphatic System Disorders		
Neutropenia	(5.8)	(5.6)
Metabolism and Nutrition Disorders		
Anorexia	(6.2)	(7.2)
Psychiatric Disorders		
Insomnia	(2.6)	(3.7)
Nervous System Disorders		
Dizziness	(2.8)	(3.4)
Headache	(13.2)	(14.3)
Gastrointestinal Disorders		
Constipation	(10.3)	(15.5)
Diarrhea	(7.6)	(8.7)
Dyspepsia	(5.8)	(3.8)
Nausea	(5.8)	(5.1)
Stomatitis	(3.1)	(2.7)
Skin and Subcutaneous Tissue Disorders		
Alopecia	(12.4)	(11.9)
General Disorders and General Administration Site Conditions		
Asthenia	(4.7)	(4.6)
Fatigue	(15.4)	(15.6)

In a combined analysis of these two studies, isolated cases of serious adverse experiences were similar in the two treatment groups.

Additional Clinical Trial Adverse Experiences (>0.5% and greater than standard therapy), Regardless of Causality, Occurring in Patients Receiving Highly and Moderately Emetogenic Chemotherapy: Blood and Lymphatic System Disorders: anemia, febrile neutropenia, thrombocytopenia.

Cardiac Disorders: myocardial infarction, palpitations, tachycardia.

Eye Disorders: conjunctivitis.

Gastrointestinal Disorders: abdominal pain upper, acid reflux, deglutition disorder, dry mouth, dysgeusia, dysphagia, eructation, flatulence, obstipation, salivation increased.
General Disorders and Administrative Site Conditions: edema, malaise, pain, rigors.
Infections and Infestations: candidiasis, herpes simplex, lower respiratory infection, oral candidiasis, pharyngitis, septic shock, upper respiratory infection, urinary tract infection.
Investigations: weight loss.
Metabolism and Nutrition Disorders: appetite decreased, diabetes mellitus, hypokalemia.
Musculoskeletal and Connective Tissue Disorders: arthralgia, back pain, muscular weakness, musculoskeletal pain, myalgia.
Neoplasms Benign, Malignant and Unspecified (Including Cysts and Polyps): malignant neoplasm, non-small cell lung carcinoma.
Nervous System: peripheral neuropathy, sensory neuropathy, taste disturbance, tremor.
Psychiatric Disorders: anxiety disorder, confusion, depression.
Renal and Urinary Disorders: dysuria, renal insufficiency.
Reproductive System and Breast Disorders: pelvic pain.
Respiratory, Thoracic and Mediastinal Disorders: cough, dyspnea, nasal secretion, pharyngolaryngeal pain, pneumonitis, pulmonary embolism, respiratory insufficiency, vocal disturbance.
Skin and Subcutaneous Tissue Disorders: acne, diaphoresis, pruritus, rash.
Vascular Disorders: deep venous thrombosis, flushing, hot flush, hypertension, hypotension.

Stevens-Johnson syndrome was reported as a serious adverse experience in a patient receiving aprepitant with cancer chemotherapy in another CINV study.

Abnormal Hematologic and Clinical Chemistry Findings: Table 3 shows the percent of patients with laboratory adverse experiences reported at an incidence ≥3% in patients receiving highly emetogenic chemotherapy.

Table 3: EMEND

All Laboratory Abnormalities, Regardless of Causality, (incidence ≥3%) Occurring in Patients Receiving Highly Emetogenic Chemotherapy Who Were Treated with the Aprepitant Regimen for CINV in Clinical Studies (Cycle 1)

	Aprepitant Regimen N=544 %	Standard Therapy N=550 %
ALT increased	(6.0)	(4.3)
AST increased	(3.0)	(1.3)
Blood urea nitrogen increased	(4.7)	(3.5)
Serum creatinine increased	(3.7)	(4.3)
Proteinuria	(6.8)	(5.3)

Table 4 shows the percent of patients with laboratory adverse experiences reported at an incidence ≥3% in patients receiving moderately emetogenic chemotherapy.

Table 4: EMEND

Percent of Patients Receiving Moderately Emetogenic Chemotherapy with Laboratory Adverse Experiences (Incidence ≥3%)—Cycle 1

	Aprepitant Regimen (N=868)	Standard Therapy (N=846)
Neutrophil Count Decreased	4.6	4.6
White Blood Cell Count Decreased	5.1	4.7

The following additional laboratory adverse experiences (incidence >0.5% and greater than standard therapy), regardless of causality, were reported in patients treated with aprepitant regimen: alkaline phosphatase increased, hyperglycemia, hyponatremia, leukocytes increased, erythrocyturia, leukocyturia. The adverse experiences of increased AST and ALT were generally mild and transient.

The adverse experience profiles in the Multiple-Cycle extensions of Highly and Moderately Emetogenic Chemotherapy studies for up to 6 cycles of chemotherapy were generally similar to those observed in Cycle 1.

Post-Market Adverse Drug Reactions: Regardless of causality with EMEND, the following adverse events have been reported rarely or very rarely and occur with multiple confounding factors: loss of consciousness, depressed level of consciousness, convulsion, somnolence, paresthesia, syndrome of inappropriate antidiuretic hormone, hallucination, pruritus, rash, urticaria, and hypersensitivity reactions including anaphylactic reactions.

DRUG INTERACTIONS:

Serious Drug Interactions

- EMEND should be used with caution in patients receiving concomitant medicinal products that are primarily metabolized through CYP3A4 and CYP2C9, including chemotherapy agents. Inhibition of CYP3A4 by aprepitant could result in elevated plasma concentrations of these concomitant medicinal products. Induction of CYP2C9 by aprepitant could result in decreased plasma concentrations of these concomitant medicinal products (see Contraindications and Drug Interactions).
- The effect of EMEND on the pharmacokinetics of orally administered CYP3A4 substrates is greater than the effect of EMEND on the pharmacokinetics of intravenously administered CYP3A4 substrates.
- Coadministration of EMEND with warfarin results in decreased prothrombin time, reported as International Normalized Ratio (INR). In patients on chronic warfarin therapy, the prothrombin time (INR) should be closely monitored in the 2-week period, particularly at 7 to 10 days, following initiation of the 3-day regimen of EMEND with each chemotherapy cycle (see Drug Interactions).
- The efficacy of hormonal contraceptives during and for 28 days after administration of EMEND may be reduced. Alternative or back-up methods of contraception should be used during treatment with EMEND and for 1 month following the last dose of EMEND (see Drug Interactions).

Overview: Aprepitant is a substrate, a moderate inhibitor, and an inducer of CYP3A4. Aprepitant is also an inducer of CYP2C9.

Chronic continuous use of EMEND is not recommended because it has not been studied and because the drug interaction profile may change during chronic dosing.

Effect of aprepitant on the Pharmacokinetics of Other Agents: As a moderate inhibitor of CYP3A4, aprepitant can increase plasma concentrations of coadministered medicinal products that are metabolized through CYP3A4. EMEND may increase the plasma concentration of orally administered CYP3A4 substrates to a greater extent than if the substrate was administered intravenously.

Aprepitant has been shown to induce the metabolism of S(-) warfarin and tolbutamide, which are metabolized through CYP2C9. Coadministration of EMEND with these drugs or other drugs that are known to be metabolized by CYP2C9, such as phenytoin, may result in lower plasma concentrations of these drugs.

Effect of Other Agents on the Pharmacokinetics of Aprepitant: Aprepitant is a substrate for CYP3A4; therefore, coadministration of EMEND with drugs that inhibit CYP3A4 activity may result in increased plasma concentrations of aprepitant. Consequently, concomitant administration of EMEND with strong CYP3A4 inhibitors (e.g., ketoconazole, itraconazole, nefazodone, troleandomycin, clarithromycin, ritonavir, nelfinavir) should be approached cautiously. Moderate CYP3A4 inhibitors (e.g., diltiazem) resulted in a 2-fold increase in plasma concentrations of aprepitant; therefore, concomitant administration should also be approached with caution.

Aprepitant is a substrate for CYP3A4; therefore, coadministration of EMEND with drugs that strongly induce CYP3A4 activity (e.g., rifampin, carbamazepine, phenytoin) may result in reduced plasma concentrations of aprepitant that may result in decreased efficacy of EMEND.

Drug-Drug Interactions: See Table 5.

Table 5: EMEND

Established or Potential Drug-drug Interactions

Proper Name	Ref	Effect	Clinical Comment
Pimozide	T	↑ pimozide concentration	Potentially causing serious or life-threatening reactions.
Terfenadine	T	↑ terfenadine concentration	Potentially causing serious or life-threatening reactions.
Astemizole	T	↑ astemizole concentration	Potentially causing serious or life-threatening reactions.
Cisapride	T	↑ cisapride concentration	Potentially causing serious or life-threatening reactions.
Warfarin	CT	↓ Warfarin concentration ↓ INR	In patients on chronic warfarin therapy, the INR should be closely monitored in the 2-week period, particularly at 7 to 10 days, following initiation of the 3-day regimen of EMEND with each chemotherapy cycle (see Warnings and Precautions).
Tolbutamide	CT	↓ tolbutamide concentration	Aprepitant induces the metabolism of drug metabolized by CYP2C9.
Phenytoin	T	↓ phenytoin concentration	Aprepitant induces the metabolism of drug metabolized by CYP2C9.
Dexamethasone	CT	↑ dexamethasone concentration	The usual oral dexamethasone doses should be reduced by approximately 50% when coadministered with EMEND, to achieve exposures of dexamethasone similar to those obtained when it is given without EMEND.
Methylprednisolone	CT	↑ methylprednisolone concentration	The usual IV methylprednisolone dose should be reduced by approximately 25%, and the usual oral methylprednisolone dose should be reduced by approximately 50% when coadministered with EMEND, to achieve exposures of methylprednisolone similar to those obtained when it is given without EMEND.
Hormone contraceptives with all routes of administration	CT	↓ hormone concentration	The efficacy of hormonal contraceptives during and for 28 days after administration of EMEND may be reduced. Alternative or back-up methods of contraception should be used during treatment with EMEND and for 1 month following the last dose of EMEND (see Warnings and Precautions).
Midazolam oral and IV	CT	↑ midazolam concentration	The potential effects of increased plasma concentrations of midazolam or other benzodiazepines metabolized via CYP3A4 (alprazolam, triazolam) should be considered when coadministering these agents with EMEND.
Ketoconazole	CT	↑ aprepitant concentration	Concomitant administration of EMEND with strong CYP3A4 inhibitors should be approached cautiously.
Rifampin	CT	↓ aprepitant concentration	Coadministration of EMEND with drugs that induce CYP3A4 activity may result in reduced plasma concentrations and decreased efficacy of EMEND.
Diltiazem	CT	↑ aprepitant and diltiazem concentration	No clinically meaningful changes in ECG, heart rate, or blood pressure beyond those changes induced by diltiazem alone.
Paroxetine	CT	↓ aprepitant and paroxetine concentration	

Legend: CT=clinical trial; T=theoretical.

EMEND is unlikely to interact with drugs that are substrates for the P-glycoprotein transporter, as demonstrated by the lack of interaction of EMEND with digoxin in a clinical drug interaction study.

5-HT$_3$ Antagonists: In clinical drug interaction studies, aprepitant did not have clinically important effects on the pharmacokinetics of ondansetron administered intravenously, granisetron administered orally, or hydrodolasetron (the active metabolite of dolasetron) following oral administration of dolasetron.

Chemotherapeutic Agents: Chemotherapy agents that are known to be metabolized by CYP3A4 include docetaxel, paclitaxel, etoposide, irinotecan, ifosfamide, imatinib, vinorelbine, vinblastine and vincristine. In clinical studies, EMEND was administered with the following chemotherapeutic agents metabolized primarily or in part by CYP3A4: etoposide, vinorelbine, docetaxel, and paclitaxel. The doses of these agents were not adjusted to account for potential drug interactions. However, caution is advised and additional monitoring may be appropriate in patients receiving chemotherapy agents known to be metabolized by CYP3A4, especially those not studied in the clinical trials, including vinblastine, vincristine and ifosfamide (see Warnings and Precautions).

Docetaxel: In a clinical study, EMEND did not influence the pharmacokinetics of docetaxel.

Etoposide, Paclitaxel: No pharmakinetic studies to determine the effect of EMEND on the concentration of etoposide or paclitaxel were performed.

Vinorelbine: In a separate pharmacokinetic study, EMEND (125 mg/80 mg regimen) did not influence the pharmacokinetics of vinorelbine.

Drug-Food Interactions: EMEND may be administered with or without food.

Drug-Herb Interactions: Interactions with herbal products have not been established.

Drug-Laboratory Test Interactions: Interactions with laboratory tests have not been established.

DOSAGE AND ADMINISTRATION: **Dosing Considerations:** EMEND is indicated for use for a maximum of 3 consecutive days per chemotherapy cycle.

EMEND has not been demonstrated to be effective as a single anti-emetic agent and must be administered with other anti-emetic agents.

Recommended Dose and Dosage Adjustment: The recommended dose of EMEND is 125 mg orally 1 hour prior to chemotherapy treatment (Day 1) and 80 mg once daily in the morning on Days 2 and 3.

In clinical studies with EMEND, the following regimen was used for the prevention of nausea and vomiting associated with cisplatin-based highly emetogenic cancer chemotherapy:

	Day 1	Day 2	Day 3	Day 4
EMEND[a]	125 mg orally	80 mg orally	80 mg orally	none
Dexamethasone[b]	12 mg orally	8 mg orally	8 mg orally	8 mg orally
Ondansetron[c]	32 mg IV	none	none	none

[a] EMEND was administered orally 1 hour prior to chemotherapy treatment on Day 1 and in the morning on Days 2 and 3.
[b] Dexamethasone was administered 30 minutes prior to chemotherapy treatment on Day 1 and in the morning on Days 2 through 4. **The dose of dexamethasone was chosen to account for drug interactions. Increasing the dose of dexamethasone is not recommended (see Drug Interactions).**
[c] Ondansetron was administered 30 minutes prior to chemotherapy treatment on Day 1.

For highly emetic chemotherapy, there is only limited efficacy data with EMEND in combination with oral ondansetron or other 5-HT_3 antagonist class of antiemetics and dexamethasone.

In a clinical study with EMEND, the following regimen was used for the prevention of nausea and vomiting associated with moderately emetogenic cancer chemotherapy:

	Day 1	Day 2	Day 3
EMEND[a]	125 mg orally	80 mg orally	80 mg orally
Dexamethasone[b]	12 mg orally	none	none
Ondansetron[c]	2×8 mg orally	none	none

[a] EMEND was administered orally 1 hour prior to chemotherapy treatment on Day 1 and in the morning on Days 2 and 3.
[b] Dexamethasone was administered 30 minutes prior to chemotherapy treatment on Day 1. **The dose of dexamethasone was chosen to account for drug interactions. Increasing the dose of dexamethasone is not recommended (see Drug Interactions).**
[c] Ondansetron 8-mg capsule was administered 30 to 60 minutes prior to chemotherapy treatment and one 8-mg capsule was administered 8 hours after the first dose on Day 1.

For moderately emetogenic chemotherapy, there is only limited efficacy data with EMEND in combination with other 5-HT_3 antagonist class of antiemetics and dexamethasone.

See Drug Interactions for additional information on the administration of EMEND with corticosteroids.

Refer to each product's respective Product Monograph for additional information on coadministered antiemetic agents.

EMEND may be taken with or without food.

No dosage adjustment is necessary for the elderly.

No dosage adjustment is necessary based on gender or race.

No dosage adjustment is necessary for patients with severe renal insufficiency (creatinine clearance <30 mL/min) or for patients with end stage renal disease undergoing hemodialysis.

No dosage adjustment is necessary for patients with mild to moderate hepatic insufficiency (Child-Pugh score 5 to 9). There are no clinical data in patients with severe hepatic insufficiency (Child-Pugh score >9).

OVERDOSAGE:
No specific information is available on the treatment of overdosage with EMEND. Single doses up to 600 mg of aprepitant were generally well tolerated in healthy subjects. Aprepitant was generally well tolerated when administered as 375 mg once daily for up to 42 days to patients in non-CINV studies. In 33 cancer patients, administration of a single 375-mg dose of aprepitant on Day 1 and 250 mg once daily on Days 2 to 5 was generally well tolerated.

Drowsiness and headache were reported in one patient who ingested 1440 mg of aprepitant.

In the event of overdose, EMEND should be discontinued and general supportive treatment and monitoring should be provided. Because of the antiemetic activity of aprepitant, drug-induced emesis may not be effective.

Aprepitant cannot be removed by hemodialysis.

> For management of a suspected drug overdose, contact your regional Poison Control Centre. See the *CPS* Directory section for a list of Poison Control Centres.

ACTION AND CLINICAL PHARMACOLOGY: **Mechanism of Action:** Aprepitant has a unique mode of action; it is a selective high affinity antagonist at human substance P neurokinin 1 (NK_1) receptors. Counter-screening assays showed that aprepitant was at least 3000-fold selective for the NK_1 receptor over other enzyme, transporter, ion channel and receptor sites including the dopamine and serotonin receptors that are targets for existing chemotherapy induced nausea and vomiting (CINV) therapies.

NK_1-receptor antagonists have been shown pre-clinically to inhibit emesis induced by cytotoxic chemotherapeutic agents, such as cisplatin, via central actions. Preclinical and human Positron Emission Tomography (PET) studies with aprepitant have shown that it is brain penetrant and occupies brain NK_1 receptors. Preclinical studies show that aprepitant has a long duration of central activity, inhibits both the acute and delayed phases of cisplatin-induced emesis, and augments the antiemetic activity of the 5-HT_3-receptor antagonist ondansetron and the corticosteroid dexamethasone against cisplatin-induced emesis.

Pharmacokinetics: See Table 6.

Table 6: EMEND
Summary of Pharmacokinetic Parameters of EMEND in Healthy Subjects

	C_{max} (µg/mL)	$AUC_{0\text{-}24hr}$ (µg·hr/mL)
Day 1 oral dose aprepitant 125 mg	1.5	19.5
Day 3 oral dose aprepitant 80 mg	1.4	20.1

Absorption: The mean absolute oral bioavailability of aprepitant is approximately 60 to 65% and the mean peak plasma concentration (C_{max}) of aprepitant occurred at approximately 4 hours (T_{max}). Oral administration of the capsule with a standard breakfast had no clinically meaningful effect on the bioavailability of aprepitant.

The pharmacokinetics of aprepitant are non-linear across the clinical dose range. In healthy young adults, the increase in $AUC_{0\text{-}\infty}$ was 26% greater than dose proportional between 80-mg and 125-mg single doses administered in the fed state.

Following oral administration of a single 125-mg dose of EMEND on Day 1 and 80 mg once daily on Days 2 and 3, the $AUC_{0\text{-}24hr}$ was approximately 19.5 µg·hr/mL and 20.1 µg·hr/mL on Day 1 and Day 3, respectively. The C_{max} of 1.5 µg/mL and 1.4 µg/mL were reached in approximately 4 hours (T_{max}) on Day 1 and Day 3, respectively.

Distribution: Aprepitant is greater than 95% bound to plasma proteins. The geometric mean apparent volume of distribution at steady state (Vd_{ss}) is approximately 66 L in humans.

Aprepitant crosses the placenta in rats, and crosses the blood brain barrier in rats and ferrets. PET studies in humans indicate that aprepitant crosses the blood brain barrier (see Action and Clinical Pharmacology).

Metabolism: Aprepitant undergoes extensive metabolism. In healthy young adults, aprepitant accounts for approximately 24% of the radioactivity in plasma over 72 hours following a single oral 300-mg dose of [^{14}C]-aprepitant, indicating a substantial presence of metabolites in the plasma. Seven metabolites of aprepitant, which are only weakly active, have been identified in human plasma. The metabolism of aprepitant occurs largely via oxidation at the morpholine ring and its side chains. In vitro studies using human liver microsomes indicate that aprepitant is metabolized primarily by CYP3A4 with minor metabolism by CYP1A2 and CYP2C19, and no metabolism by CYP2D6, CYP2C9, or CYP2E1.

Excretion: Aprepitant is eliminated primarily by metabolism; aprepitant is not renally excreted. Following administration of a single oral 300-mg dose of [^{14}C]-aprepitant to healthy subjects, 5% of the radioactivity was recovered in urine and 86% in feces.

The apparent plasma clearance of aprepitant ranged from approximately 60 to 84 mL/min. The apparent terminal half-life ranged from approximately 9 to 13 hours.

Special Populations and Conditions: Pediatrics: The pharmacokinetics of EMEND have not been evaluated in patients below 18 years of age.

Geriatrics: Following oral administration of a single 125-mg dose of EMEND on Day 1 and 80 mg once daily on Days 2 through 5, the $AUC_{0\text{-}24hr}$ of aprepitant was 21% higher on Day 1 and 36% higher on Day 5 in elderly (≥65 years) relative to younger adults. The C_{max} was 10% higher on Day 1 and 24% higher on Day 5 in elderly relative to younger adults. These differences are not considered clinically meaningful. No dosage adjustment for EMEND is necessary in elderly patients.

Gender: Following oral administration of a single 125-mg dose of EMEND, the C_{max} for aprepitant is 16% higher in females as compared with males. The half-life of aprepitant is 25% lower in females as compared with males and its T_{max} occurs at approximately the same time. No dosage adjustment for EMEND is necessary based on gender.

Race: Following oral administration of a single 125-mg dose of EMEND, the $AUC_{0\text{-}24hr}$ is approximately 25% and 29% higher in Hispanics as compared with Caucasians and Blacks, respectively. The C_{max} is 22% and 31% higher in Hispanics as compared with Caucasians and Blacks, respectively. These differences are not considered clinically meaningful. No dosage adjustment for EMEND is necessary based on race.

Hepatic Insufficiency: EMEND was well tolerated in patients with mild to moderate hepatic insufficiency. Following administration of a single 125-mg dose of EMEND on Day 1 and 80 mg once daily on Days 2 and 3 to patients with mild hepatic insufficiency (Child-Pugh score 5 to 6), the $AUC_{0\text{-}24hr}$ of aprepitant was 11% lower on Day 1 and 36% lower on Day 3, as compared with healthy subjects given the same regimen. In patients with moderate hepatic insufficiency (Child-Pugh score 7 to 9), the $AUC_{0\text{-}24hr}$ of aprepitant was 10% higher on Day 1 and 18% higher on Day 3, as compared with healthy subjects given the same regimen. These differences in $AUC_{0\text{-}24hr}$ are not considered clinically meaningful; therefore, no dosage adjustment for EMEND is necessary in patients with mild to moderate hepatic insufficiency.

There are no clinical or pharmacokinetic data in patients with severe hepatic insufficiency (Child-Pugh score >9).

Renal Insufficiency: A single 240-mg dose of EMEND was administered to patients with severe renal insufficiency (CrCl <30 mL/min) and to patients with end stage renal disease (ESRD) requiring hemodialysis.

In patients with severe renal insufficiency, the $AUC_{0\text{-}\infty}$ of total aprepitant (unbound and protein bound) decreased by 21% and C_{max} decreased by 32%, relative to healthy subjects. In patients with ESRD undergoing hemodialysis, the $AUC_{0\text{-}\infty}$ of total aprepitant decreased by 42% and C_{max} decreased by 32%. Due to modest decreases in protein binding of aprepitant in patients with renal disease, the AUC of pharmacologically active unbound drug was not significantly affected in patients with renal insufficiency compared with healthy subjects. Hemodialysis conducted 4 or 48 hours after dosing had no significant effect on the pharmacokinetics of aprepitant; less than 0.2% of the dose was recovered in the dialysate.

No dosage adjustment for EMEND is necessary for patients with severe renal insufficiency or for patients with ESRD undergoing hemodialysis.

STORAGE AND STABILITY: Blisters: Store at room temperature (15-30°C) in the original package.

INFORMATION FOR THE PATIENT: Published in e-CPS, available by subscription at www.e-cps.ca.

DOSAGE FORMS, COMPOSITION AND PACKAGING: 80 mg: Each white, opaque hard gelatin capsule with 461 and 80 mg printed radially in black ink, contains: aprepitant 80 mg. Nonmedicinal ingredients: hydroxypropyl cellulose, microcrystalline cellulose, sodium lauryl sulfate and sucrose; capsule shell: gelatin and titanium dioxide. Blister packages of 2 and 6. Tri-Pack contains 2 capsules of 80 mg and 1 capsule of 125 mg.

125 mg: Each opaque, hard gelatin capsule with white body and pink cap with 462 and 125 mg printed radially in black ink, contains: aprepitant 125 mg. Nonmedicinal ingredients: hydroxypropyl cellulose, microcrystalline cellulose, sodium lauryl sulfate and sucrose; capsule shell: gelatin, red ferric oxide, titanium dioxide and yellow ferric oxide. Blister packages of 6. Tri-Pack contains 2 capsules of 80 mg and 1 capsule of 125 mg.

(Shown in Product Identification Section)

Emend® IV Pr

fosaprepitant dimeglumine

Neurokinin 1 (NK1) Receptor Antagonist

Merck Frosst

Date of Revision: March 23, 2010

SUMMARY PRODUCT INFORMATION:

Route of Administration	Dosage Form/ Strength	Clinically Relevant Nonmedicinal Ingredients
Intravenous	Lyophilized powder/115 mg/vial	For a complete listing see Dosage Forms, Composition and Packaging.

INDICATIONS AND CLINICAL USE: EMEND IV (fosaprepitant dimeglumine), in combination with a 5-HT_3 antagonist class of antiemetics and dexamethasone, is indicated for the:

1. prevention of acute and delayed nausea and vomiting due to highly emetogenic cancer chemotherapy.
2. prevention of nausea and vomiting in women due to treatment with moderately emetogenic cancer chemotherapy.

Approval of EMEND IV is based on the bioequivalence study indicating that 115 mg of the pro-drug, fosaprepitant, is equivalent to 125 mg oral aprepitant in regard to aprepitant exposure. No clinical trials that involved the use of fosaprepitant and both dexamethasone and a 5-HT_3 antagonist class of antiemetics have been submitted. (See also Drug Interactions and Dosage and Administration.)

Geriatrics (≥65 years of age): In clinical studies, the efficacy and safety of aprepitant in the elderly (≥65 years) were comparable to those seen in younger patients (<65 years). No dosage adjustment is necessary in elderly patients.

Pediatrics (<18 years of age): No data available.

CONTRAINDICATIONS:

- Patients who are hypersensitive to EMEND IV, aprepitant, polysorbate 80, or to any ingredient in the formulation. For a complete listing, see Dosage Forms, Composition and Packaging.
- EMEND IV should not be used concurrently with pimozide, terfenadine, astemizole, or cisapride. Inhibition of cytochrome P450 isoenzyme 3A4 (CYP3A4) by aprepitant could result in elevated plasma concentrations of these drugs, potentially causing serious or life-threatening reactions (see Drug Interactions).

WARNINGS AND PRECAUTIONS:

> **Serious Warnings and Precautions**
> Drug interactions with:
> - Medicinal products that are metabolized through CYP3A4 (see Drug Interactions)
> - Warfarin (see Drug Interactions)
> - Hormonal contraception (see Drug Interactions)

Isolated reports of immediate hypersensitivity reactions including flushing, erythema, and dyspnea have occurred during infusion of fosaprepitant. These hypersensitivity reactions have generally responded to discontinuation of the infusion and administration of appropriate therapy. The infusion should not be reinitiated in patients who experience hypersensitivity reactions (see Contraindications).

Special Populations: Pregnant Women:
There are no adequate and well-controlled studies in pregnant women; therefore, EMEND IV are not recommended for use during pregnancy unless clearly necessary.

Nursing Women: EMEND IV, when administered intravenously, is rapidly converted to aprepitant. Aprepitant is excreted in the milk of lactating rats. It is not known whether this drug is excreted in human milk; therefore, breastfeeding is not recommended during treatment with EMEND IV.

Pediatrics (<18 years of age): Safety and effectiveness of EMEND IV in pediatric patients have not been established.

Geriatrics (≥65 years of age): In 2 well-controlled clinical studies, of the total number of patients (N=544) treated with aprepitant, 31% were 65 and over, while 5% were 75 and over. No overall differences in safety or effectiveness were observed between these subjects and younger subjects. Greater sensitivity of some older individuals cannot be ruled out. Dosage adjustment in the elderly is not necessary.

ADVERSE REACTIONS: Clinical Trial Adverse Drug Reactions: No clinical trials that involved the use of fosaprepitant and both dexamethasone and a 5-HT_3 antagonist class of antiemetics have been submitted. Since EMEND IV is converted to aprepitant, those adverse reactions associated with aprepitant are to be expected to occur with EMEND IV. The overall safety of aprepitant was evaluated in approximately 4300 individuals. Injection site adverse reaction can also be expected.

Fosaprepitant (intravenous formulation): In a randomized, open-label crossover, bioequivalence study, 66 subjects were dosed with 115 mg of EMEND IV intravenously and 125 mg of aprepitant orally. Systemic exposure of 115 mg of intravenous EMEND IV is equivalent to 125 mg oral aprepitant. The following drug related clinical adverse experiences were reported in subjects dosed with EMEND IV: infusion site pain, 5 (7.6%); infusion site induration, 1 (1.5%); headache, 2 (3%).

Oral Aprepitant: Highly Emetogenic Chemotherapy: In 2 well-controlled clinical trials in patients receiving cisplatin-based chemotherapy, 544 patients were treated with aprepitant during Cycle 1 of chemotherapy and 413 of these patients continued into the Multiple-Cycle extension for up to 6 cycles of chemotherapy. Oral aprepitant was given in combination with ondansetron and dexamethasone and was generally well tolerated. Most adverse experiences reported in these clinical studies were described as mild to moderate in intensity.

In Cycle 1, clinical adverse experiences were reported in approximately 69% of patients treated with the aprepitant regimen compared with approximately 68% of patients treated with standard therapy.

Table 1 shows the percent of patients with clinical adverse experiences reported at an incidence ≥3%.

Table 1: EMEND IV

All Adverse Experiences, Regardless of Causality, (incidence ≥3%) Occurring in Patients Receiving Highly Emetogenic Chemotherapy Who Were Treated with the Aprepitant Regimen for Chemotherapy Induced Nausea and Vomiting (CINV) in Clinical Studies (cycle 1)

	Aprepitant Regimen N=544 %	Standard Therapy N=550 %
Body as a Whole/Site Unspecified		
Abdominal pain	(4.6)	(3.3)
Asthenia/fatigue	(17.8)	(11.8)
Dehydration	(5.9)	(5.1)
Dizziness	(6.6)	(4.4)
Fever	(2.9)	(3.5)
Mucous Membrane Disorder	(2.6)	(3.1)
Digestive System		
Constipation	(10.3)	(12.2)
Diarrhea	(10.3)	(7.5)
Epigastric Discomfort	(4.0)	(3.1)
Gastritis	(4.2)	(3.1)
Heartburn	(5.3)	(4.9)
Nausea	(12.7)	(11.8)
Vomiting	(7.5)	(7.6)
Eyes, Ears, Nose, and Throat		
Tinnitus	(3.7)	(3.8)
Hemic and Lymphatic System		
Neutropenia	(3.1)	(2.9)
Metabolism and Nutrition		
Anorexia	(10.1)	(9.5)
Nervous System		
Headache	(8.5)	(8.7)
Insomnia	(2.9)	(3.1)
Respiratory System		
Hiccups	(10.8)	(5.6)

In addition, isolated cases of serious adverse experiences, regardless of causality, of bradycardia, disorientation, and perforating duodenal ulcer were reported in highly emetogenic CINV clinical studies.

Moderately Emetogenic Chemotherapy: During Cycle 1 of 2 moderately emetogenic chemotherapy studies, 868 patients were treated with the aprepitant regimen and 686 of these patients continued into extensions for up to 4 cycles of chemotherapy. In the combined analysis of Cycle 1 data for these 2 studies, adverse experiences were reported in approximately 69% of patients treated with the aprepitant regimen compared with approximately 72% of patients treated with standard therapy.

In the combined analysis of Cycle 1 data for these 2 studies, the adverse experience profile in the moderately emetogenic chemotherapy studies was generally comparable to the highly emetogenic chemotherapy studies. Table 2 shows the percent of patients with clinical adverse experiences reported at an incidence ≥3%.

In a combined analysis of these two studies, isolated cases of serious adverse experiences were similar in the two treatment groups.

Additional Clinical Trial Adverse Experiences (>0.5% and greater than standard therapy), Regardless of Causality, Occurring in Patients Receiving Highly and Moderately Emetogenic Chemotherapy with Aprepitant Regimen: Blood and Lymphatic System Disorders: anemia, febrile neutropenia, thrombocytopenia.

Cardiac Disorders: myocardial infarction, palpitations, tachycardia.

Eye Disorders: conjunctivitis.

Gastrointestinal Disorders: abdominal pain upper, acid reflux, deglutition disorder, dry mouth, dysgeusia, dysphagia, eructation, flatulence, obstipation, salivation increased.

General Disorders and Administrative Site Conditions: edema, malaise, pain, rigors.

Infections and Infestations: candidiasis, herpes simplex, lower respiratory infection, oral candidiasis, pharyngitis, septic shock, upper respiratory infection, urinary tract infection.

Investigations: weight loss.

Metabolism and Nutrition Disorders: appetite decreased, diabetes mellitus, hypokalemia.

Musculoskeletal and Connective Tissue Disorders: arthralgia, back pain, muscular weakness, musculoskeletal pain, myalgia.

Neoplasms Benign, Malignant and Unspecified (including cysts and polyps): malignant neoplasm, non-small cell lung carcinoma.

Nervous System: peripheral neuropathy, sensory neuropathy, taste disturbance, tremor.

Psychiatric Disorders: anxiety disorder, confusion, depression.

Renal and Urinary Disorders: dysuria, renal insufficiency.

Reproductive System and Breast Disorders: pelvic pain.

Respiratory, Thoracic and Mediastinal Disorders: cough, dyspnea, nasal secretion, pharyngolaryngeal pain, pneumonitis, pulmonary embolism, respiratory insufficiency, vocal disturbance.

Skin and Subcutaneous Tissue Disorders: acne, diaphoresis, pruritus, rash. Fosaprepitant injections may result in injection site erythema, induration and pain.

Vascular Disorders: deep venous thrombosis, flushing, hot flush, hypertension, hypotension.

Stevens-Johnson syndrome was reported as a serious adverse experience in a patient receiving aprepitant with cancer chemotherapy in another CINV study.

Table 2: EMEND IV

All Adverse Experiences, Regardless of Causality, (incidence ≥3%) Occurring in Patients Receiving Moderately Emetogenic Chemotherapy Who Were Treated with the Aprepitant Regimen for CINV in Clinical Studies (cycle 1)

	Aprepitant Regimen N=868 %	Standard Therapy N=846 %
Blood and Lymphatic System Disorders		
Neutropenia	(5.8)	(5.6)
Metabolism and Nutrition Disorders		
Anorexia	(6.2)	(7.2)
Psychiatric Disorders		
Insomnia	(2.6)	(3.7)
Nervous System Disorders		
Dizziness	(2.8)	(3.4)
Headache	(13.2)	(14.3)
Gastrointestinal Disorders		
Constipation	(10.3)	(15.5)
Diarrhea	(7.6)	(8.7)
Dyspepsia	(5.8)	(3.8)
Nausea	(5.8)	(5.1)
Stomatitis	(3.1)	(2.7)
Skin and Subcutaneous Tissue Disorders		
Alopecia	(12.4)	(11.9)
General Disorders and General Administration Site Conditions		
Asthenia	(4.7)	(4.6)
Fatigue	(15.4)	(15.6)

Abnormal Hematologic and Clinical Chemistry Findings: Table 3 shows the percent of patients with laboratory adverse experiences reported at an incidence ≥3% in patients receiving highly emetogenic chemotherapy.

Table 3: EMEND IV

All Laboratory Abnormalities, Regardless of Causality, (incidence ≥3%) Occurring in Patients Receiving Highly Emetogenic Chemotherapy Who Were Treated with the Aprepitant Regimen for CINV in Clinical Studies (cycle 1)

	Aprepitant Regimen N=544 %	Standard Therapy N=550 %
ALT increased	(6.0)	(4.3)
AST increased	(3.0)	(1.3)
Blood urea nitrogen increased	(4.7)	(3.5)
Serum creatinine increased	(3.7)	(4.3)
Proteinuria	(6.8)	(5.3)

Table 4 shows the percent of patients with laboratory adverse experiences reported at an incidence ≥3% in patients receiving moderately emetogenic chemotherapy.

The following additional laboratory adverse experiences (incidence >0.5% and greater than standard therapy), regardless of causality, were reported in patients treated with aprepitant regimen: alkaline phosphatase increased, hyperglycemia, hyponatremia, leukocytes increased, erythrocyturia, leukocyturia. The adverse experiences of increased AST and ALT were generally mild and transient.

Table 4: EMEND IV

Percent of Patients Receiving Moderately Emetogenic Chemotherapy with Laboratory Adverse Experiences (Incidence ≥3%)—Cycle 1

	Aprepitant Regimen (N=868)	Standard Therapy (N=846)
Neutrophil Count Decreased	4.6	4.6
White Blood Cell Count Decreased	5.1	4.7

The adverse experience profiles in the Multiple-Cycle extensions of Highly and Moderately Emetogenic Chemotherapy studies for up to 6 cycles of chemotherapy were generally similar to those observed in Cycle 1.

Post-Market Adverse Drug Reactions: Regardless of causality with aprepitant the following adverse events have been reported rarely or very rarely and occur with multiple confounding factors: loss of consciousness, depressed level of consciousness, convulsion, somnolence, paresthesia, syndrome of inappropriate antidiuretic hormone, hallucination, pruritus, rash, urticaria, and hypersensitivity reactions including anaphylactic reactions.

Immediate hypersensitivity reactions have been observed during the infusion of fosaprepitant which may include the following: flushing, erythema, dyspnea (see Warnings and Precautions).

DRUG INTERACTIONS: Following the infusion of fosaprepitant 115 mg, a higher aprepitant C_{max} (~2-fold) was observed compared to oral aprepitant (125 mg). A theoretical risk for increased adverse experiences due to a higher peak aprepitant exposure cannot be ruled out.

Serious Drug Interactions
- Fosaprepitant is rapidly converted to aprepitant, which is a moderate inhibitor of CYP3A4 when administered as a 3-day antiemetic dosing regimen for CINV. Fosaprepitant should be used with caution in patients receiving concomitant medicinal products that are primarily metabolized through CYP3A4 and CYP2C9, including chemotherapy agents. Inhibition of CYP3A4 by aprepitant could result in elevated plasma concentrations of these concomitant medicinal products. Induction of CYP2C9 by aprepitant could result in decreased plasma concentrations of these concomitant medicinal products (see Contraindications and Drug Interactions).
- The effect of oral aprepitant on the pharmacokinetics of orally administered CYP3A4 substrates is greater than the effect of oral aprepitant on the pharmacokinetics of intravenously administered CYP3A4 substrates.
- Coadministration of aprepitant with warfarin results in decreased prothrombin time, reported as International Normalized Ratio (INR). In patients on chronic warfarin therapy, the prothrombin time (INR) should be closely monitored in the 2-week period, particularly at 7 to 10 days, following initiation of the 3-day regimen of fosaprepitant followed by oral aprepitant with each chemotherapy cycle (see Drug Interactions).
- The efficacy of hormonal contraceptives during and for 28 days after administration of fosaprepitant or aprepitant may be reduced. Alternative or back-up methods of contraception should be used during treatment with fosaprepitant or aprepitant and for 1 month following the last dose (see Drug Interactions).

Overview: Drug interactions following administration of fosaprepitant are likely to occur with drugs that interact with oral aprepitant. The following information was derived from data with oral aprepitant and one study conducted with fosaprepitant and oral midazolam.

Aprepitant is a substrate, a moderate inhibitor, and an inducer of CYP3A4. Aprepitant is also an inducer of CYP2C9.

Chronic continuous use of EMEND IV is not recommended because it has not been studied and because the drug interaction profile may change during chronic dosing.

Effect of Aprepitant on the Pharmacokinetics of Other Agents: As a moderate inhibitor of CYP3A4, aprepitant can increase plasma concentrations of orally coadministered medicinal products that are metabolized through CYP3A4. Aprepitant may increase the plasma concentration of orally administered CYP3A4 substrates to a greater extent than if the substrate was administered intravenously.

Aprepitant has been shown to induce the metabolism of S(-) warfarin and tolbutamide, which are metabolized through CYP2C9. Coadministration of fosaprepitant or oral aprepitant with these drugs or other drugs that are known to be metabolized by CYP2C9, such as phenytoin, may result in lower plasma concentrations of these drugs.

Effect of Other Agents on the Pharmacokinetics of Aprepitant: Aprepitant is a substrate for CYP3A4; therefore, coadministration of fosaprepitant or aprepitant with drugs that inhibit CYP3A4 activity may result in increased plasma concentrations of aprepitant. Consequently, concomitant administration of fosaprepitant or aprepitant with strong CYP3A4 inhibitors (e.g., ketoconazole, itraconazole, nefazodone, troleandomycin, clarithromycin, ritonavir, nelfinavir) should be approached cautiously. Moderate CYP3A4 inhibitors (e.g., diltiazem) resulted in a 2-fold increase in plasma concentrations of aprepitant; therefore, concomitant administration should also be approached with caution.

Aprepitant is a substrate for CYP3A4; therefore, coadministration of fosaprepitant or aprepitant with drugs that strongly induce CYP3A4 activity (e.g., rifampin, carbamazepine, phenytoin) may result in reduced plasma concentrations and decreased efficacy.

Drug-Drug Interactions: See Table 5.

Table 5: EMEND IV

Established or Potential Drug-Drug Interactions

Proper name	Ref	Effect	Clinical Comment
Pimozide	T	↑ pimozide concentration	Potentially causing serious or life-threatening reactions.
Terfenadine	T	↑ terfenadine concentration	Potentially causing serious or life-threatening reactions.
Astemizole	T	↑ astemizole concentration	Potentially causing serious or life-threatening reactions.
Cisapride	T	↑ cisapride concentration	Potentially causing serious or life-threatening reactions.
Warfarin	CT	↓ Warfarin concentration ↓ INR	In patients on chronic warfarin therapy, the INR should be closely monitored in the 2-week period, particularly at 7 to 10 days, following initiation of the 3-day regimen of fosaprepitant followed by aprepitant with each chemotherapy cycle (see Warnings and Precautions).
Tolbutamide	CT	↓ tolbutamide concentration	Aprepitant induces the metabolism of drug metabolized by CYP2C9.
Phenytoin	T	↓ phenytoin concentration	Aprepitant induces the metabolism of drug metabolized by CYP2C9.
Dexamethasone	CT	↑ dexamethasone concentration	The usual oral dexamethasone doses should be reduced by approximately 50% when coadministered with a regimen of fosaprepitant followed by aprepitant, to achieve exposures of dexamethasone similar to those obtained when it is given without EMEND.
Methylprednisolone	CT	↑ methylprednisolone concentration	The usual IV methylprednisolone dose should be reduced by approximately 25%, and the usual oral methylprednisolone dose should be reduced by approximately 50% when coadministered with a regimen of fosaprepitant followed by aprepitant, to achieve exposures of methylprednisolone similar to those obtained when it is given without aprepitant.
Hormone contraceptives with all routes of administration	CT	↓ hormone concentration	The efficacy of hormonal contraceptives during and for 28 days after administration fosaprepitant or aprepitant may be reduced. Alternative or back-up methods of contraception should be used during treatment with fosaprepitant or aprepitant and for 1 month following the last dose (see Warnings and Precautions).
Midazolam oral and IV	CT	↑ midazolam concentration	The potential effects of increased plasma concentrations of midazolam or other benzodiazepines metabolized via CYP3A4 (alprazolam, triazolam) should be considered when coadministering these agents with a 3-day regimen of EMEND IV followed by EMEND.
Ketoconazole	CT	↑ aprepitant concentration	Concomitant administration of fosaprepitant and aprepitant with strong CYP3A4 inhibitors should be approached cautiously.
Rifampin	CT	↓ aprepitant concentration	Coadministration of fosaprepitant and aprepitant with drugs that induce CYP3A4 activity may result in reduced plasma concentrations and decreased efficacy of EMEND.
Diltiazem	CT	↑ aprepitant and diltiazem concentration	No clinically meaningful changes in ECG, heart rate, PR interval or blood pressure beyond those changes induced by diltiazem alone.
Paroxetine	CT	↓ aprepitant and paroxetine concentration	

Legend: CT=clinical trial; T=theoretical.

Fosaprepitant or aprepitant are unlikely to interact with drugs that are substrates for the P-glycoprotein transporter, as demonstrated by the lack of interaction of oral aprepitant with digoxin in a clinical drug interaction study.

5-HT$_3$ Antagonists: In clinical drug interaction studies, aprepitant did not have clinically important effects on the pharmacokinetics of ondansetron administered intravenously, granisetron administered orally, or hydrodolasetron (the active metabolite of dolasetron) following oral administration of dolasetron.

Chemotherapeutic Agents: Chemotherapy agents that are known to be metabolized by CYP3A4 include docetaxel, paclitaxel, etoposide, irinotecan, ifosfamide, imatinib, vinorelbine, vinblastine and vincristine. In clinical studies, the oral aprepitant regimen was administered with the following chemotherapeutic agents metabolized primarily or in part by CYP3A4: etoposide, vinorelbine, docetaxel, and paclitaxel. The doses of these agents were not adjusted to account for potential drug interactions. However, caution is advised and additional monitoring may be appropriate in patients receiving chemotherapy agents known to be metabolized by CYP3A4, especially those not studied in the clinical trials, including vinblastine, vincristine and ifosfamide (see Warnings and Precautions).

Docetaxel: In a separate pharmacokinetic study, oral aprepitant did not influence the pharmacokinetics of docetaxel.

Etoposide, Paclitaxel: No pharmacokinetic studies to determine the effect of oral aprepitant on the concentration of etoposide or paclitaxel were performed.

Vinorelbine: In a separate pharmacokinetic study, oral aprepitant (125 mg/80 mg regimen) did not influence the pharmacokinetics of vinorelbine.

Drug-Food Interactions: EMEND IV may be administered with or without food.

Drug-Herb Interactions: Interactions with herbal products have not been established.

Drug-Laboratory Test Interactions: Interactions with laboratory tests have not been established.

DOSAGE AND ADMINISTRATION: Dosing Considerations: EMEND IV (115 mg) may be substituted for EMEND (125 mg) prior to chemotherapy, on Day 1 only of the CINV regimen as an infusion administered over 15 minutes.

EMEND IV has not been demonstrated to be effective as a single anti-emetic agent and must be administered with other anti-emetic agents.

Recommended Dose and Dosage Adjustment: The 3-day CINV regimen includes EMEND IV (115 mg) 30 minutes prior to chemotherapy or EMEND (125 mg orally) 1 hour prior to chemotherapy on Day 1; EMEND (80 mg orally) on Days 2 and 3; in addition to a corticosteroid and a 5-HT$_3$ antagonist.

In clinical studies with EMEND, the following regimen was used for the prevention of nausea and vomiting associated with cisplatin-based highly emetogenic cancer chemotherapy:

	Day 1	Day 2	Day 3	Day 4
EMEND[a]	125 mg orally	80 mg orally	80 mg orally	none
Dexamethasone[b]	12 mg orally	8 mg orally	8 mg orally	8 mg orally
Ondansetron[c]	32 mg IV	none	none	none

a EMEND was administered orally 1 hour prior to chemotherapy treatment on Day 1 and in the morning on Days 2 and 3.

b Dexamethasone was administered 30 minutes prior to chemotherapy treatment on Day 1 and in the morning on Days 2 through 4. **The dose of dexamethasone was chosen to account for drug interactions. Increasing the dose of dexamethasone is not recommended (see Drug Interactions).**

c Ondansetron was administered 30 minutes prior to chemotherapy treatment on Day 1.

For highly emetic chemotherapy, there is only limited efficacy data with EMEND in combination with oral ondansetron or other 5-HT$_3$ antagonist class of antiemetics and dexamethasone.

In a clinical study with EMEND, the following regimen was used for the prevention of nausea and vomiting associated with moderately emetogenic cancer chemotherapy:

	Day 1	Day 2	Day 3
EMEND[a]	125 mg orally	80 mg orally	80 mg orally
Dexamethasone[b]	12 mg orally	none	none
Ondansetron[c]	2×8 mg orally	none	none

[a] EMEND was administered orally 1 hour prior to chemotherapy treatment on Day 1 and in the morning on Days 2 and 3.
[b] Dexamethasone was administered 30 minutes prior to chemotherapy treatment on Day 1. **The dose of dexamethasone was chosen to account for drug interactions. Increasing the dose of dexamethasone is not recommended (see Drug Interactions).**
[c] Ondansetron 8 mg capsule was administered 30 to 60 minutes prior to chemotherapy treatment and one 8 mg capsule was administered 8 hours after the first dose on Day 1.

For moderately emetogenic chemotherapy, there is only limited efficacy data with EMEND in combination with other 5-HT_3 antagonist class of antiemetics and dexamethasone.

See Drug Interactions for additional information on the administration of fosaprepitant or aprepitant with corticosteroids.

Refer to each product's respective Product Monograph for additional information on coadministered antiemetic agents.

No dosage adjustment is necessary for the elderly.

No dosage adjustment is necessary based on gender or race.

No dosage adjustment is necessary for patients with severe renal insufficiency (creatinine clearance <30 mL/min) or for patients with end stage renal disease undergoing hemodialysis.

No dosage adjustment is necessary for patients with mild to moderate hepatic insufficiency (Child-Pugh score 5 to 9). There are no clinical data in patients with severe hepatic insufficiency (Child-Pugh score >9).

Administration: EMEND IV is for IV infusion only, upon reconstitution and dilution and for single use only.

Instructions for Reconstitution and Dilution: Preparation of EMEND IV for Injection:

1. Aseptically inject 5 mL 0.9% Sodium Chloride for injection (saline) into the vial. Assure that saline is added to the vial along the vial wall in order to prevent foaming. Swirl the vial gently. Avoid shaking and jetting saline into the vial.
2. Aseptically prepare an infusion bag filled with 110 ml 0.9% NaCl for injection
3. Aseptically withdraw the entire volume from the vial and transfer it into an infusion bag containing 110 mL of saline to yield a total volume of 115 mL and a final concentration of approximately 1 mg fosaprepitant/mL. Gently invert the bag 2-3 times.

The reconstituted and diluted solutions should be used immediately; however, after reconstitution and dilution the final drug solution is stable for 24 hours at ambient room temperature (at or below 25°C).

Reconstituted and diluted solutions should be inspected for discoloration, cloudiness and particulate matter before administration whenever solution and container permit. Discard unused portion.

EMEND IV is incompatible with any solutions containing divalent cations (e.g., Ca^{2+}, Mg^{2+}), including Hartman's and Lactated Ringer's Solution. EMEND IV must not be reconstituted or mixed with solutions for which physical and chemical compatibility have not been established.

OVERDOSAGE:

No specific information is available on the treatment of overdosage. Single doses up to 200 mg of fosaprepitant IV and 600 mg of aprepitant were generally well tolerated in healthy subjects. Three out of 33 subjects receiving 200 mg of fosaprepitant experienced mild injection site thrombosis. Aprepitant was generally well tolerated when administered as 375 mg once daily for up to 42 days to patients in non-CINV studies. In 33 cancer patients, administration of a single 375 mg dose of aprepitant on Day 1 and 250 mg once daily on Days 2 to 5 was generally well tolerated.

Drowsiness and headache were reported in one patient who ingested 1440 mg of aprepitant.

In the event of overdose, EMEND IV should be discontinued and general supportive treatment and monitoring should be provided. Because of the antiemetic activity of aprepitant, drug-induced emesis may not be effective.

Aprepitant cannot be removed by hemodialysis.

For management of a suspected drug overdose, contact your regional Poison Control Centre. See the *CPS* Directory section for a list of Poison Control Centres.

ACTION AND CLINICAL PHARMACOLOGY: Mechanism of Action: Fosaprepitant is a prodrug of aprepitant and accordingly, its antiemetic effects are attributable to aprepitant.

Aprepitant has a unique mode of action; it is a selective high affinity antagonist at human substance P neurokinin 1 (NK_1) receptors. Counter-screening assays showed that aprepitant was at least 3000-fold selective for the NK_1 receptor over other enzyme, transporter, ion channel and receptor sites including the dopamine and serotonin receptors that are targets for existing chemotherapy induced nausea and vomiting (CINV) therapies.

NK_1-receptor antagonists have been shown pre-clinically to inhibit emesis induced by cytotoxic chemotherapeutic agents, such as cisplatin, via central actions. Preclinical and human Positron Emission Tomography (PET) studies with aprepitant have shown that it is brain penetrant and occupies brain NK_1 receptors. Preclinical studies show that aprepitant has a long duration of central activity, inhibits both the acute and delayed phases of cisplatin-induced emesis, and augments the antiemetic activity of the 5-HT_3-receptor antagonist ondansetron and the corticosteroid dexamethasone against cisplatin-induced emesis.

Pharmacokinetics: See Table 6.

Table 6: EMEND IV

Summary of Pharmacokinetic Parameters of EMEND in Healthy Subjects

	C_{max} (µg/mL)	AUC_{0-24hr} (µg· hr/mL)
Day 1 oral dose aprepitant 125 mg	1.5	19.5
Day 3 oral dose aprepitant 80 mg	1.4	20.1

Absorption: Following a single intravenous dose of fosaprepitant administered as a 15-minute infusion to healthy volunteers the mean $AUC_{0-\infty}$ of aprepitant was 31.7 (±14.3) µg·hr/mL and the mean maximal aprepitant concentration (C_{max}) was 3.27 (±1.16) µg/mL. The mean aprepitant plasma concentration at 24 hours postdose was similar between the 125 mg oral aprepitant dose and the 115 mg intravenous fosaprepitant dose.

Aprepitant after Fosaprepitant Administration: The AUC of aprepitant which is formed following administration of 115 mg of the IV prodrug fosaprepitant was equivalent to the AUC of 125 mg of orally administered aprepitant. Mean plasma concentrations following single doses are depicted in Figure 1.

The mean absolute oral bioavailability of aprepitant is approximately 60 to 65% and the mean peak plasma concentration (C_{max}) of aprepitant occurred at approximately 4 hours (T_{max}). Oral administration of the capsule with a standard breakfast had no clinically meaningful effect on the bioavailability of aprepitant.

The pharmacokinetics of aprepitant are non-linear across the clinical dose range. In healthy young adults, the increase in $AUC_{0-\infty}$ was 26% greater than dose proportional between 80 mg and 125 mg single doses administered in the fed state.

Following oral administration of a single 125 mg dose of EMEND on Day 1 and 80 mg once daily on Days 2 and 3, the AUC_{0-24hr} was approximately 19.5 µg·hr/mL and 20.1 µg·hr/mL on Day 1 and Day 3, respectively. The C_{max} of 1.5 µg/mL and 1.4 µg/mL were reached in approximately 4 hours (T_{max}) on Day 1 and Day 3, respectively.

Distribution: Fosaprepitant is rapidly converted to aprepitant.

Aprepitant is greater than 95% bound to plasma proteins. The geometric mean apparent volume of distribution at steady state (Vd_{ss}) is approximately 66 L in humans.

Aprepitant crosses the placenta in rats, and crosses the blood brain barrier in rats and ferrets. PET studies in humans indicate that aprepitant crosses the blood brain barrier (see Action and Clinical Pharmacology).

Metabolism: Fosaprepitant was rapidly converted to aprepitant in in vitro incubations with liver preparations from nonclinical species (rat and dog) and humans. Furthermore, fosaprepitant underwent rapid and nearly complete conversion to aprepitant in S9 preparations from multiple other human tissues including kidney, lung and ileum. Thus, it appears that the conversion of fosaprepitant to aprepitant can occur in multiple extrahepatic tissues in addition to the liver. In humans, fosaprepitant administered intravenously was rapidly converted to aprepitant within 30 minutes following the end of infusion.

Aprepitant undergoes extensive metabolism. In healthy young adults, aprepitant accounts for approximately 24% of the radioactivity in plasma over 72 hours following a single oral 300 mg dose of [^{14}C]-aprepitant, indicating a substantial presence of metabolites in the plasma. Seven metabolites of aprepitant, which are only weakly active, have been identified in human plasma. The metabolism of aprepitant occurs largely via oxidation at the morpholine ring and its side chains. In vitro studies using human liver microsomes indicate that aprepitant is metabolized primarily by CYP3A4 with minor metabolism by CYP1A2 and CYP2C19, and no metabolism by CYP2D6, CYP2C9, or CYP2E1.

All metabolites observed in urine, feces and plasma following an intravenous 100 mg [^{14}C]-fosaprepitant dose were also observed following an oral dose of [^{14}C]-aprepitant. Upon conversion of 115 mg of fosaprepitant to aprepitant, 18.3 mg of phosphate is liberated from fosaprepitant.

Figure 1: EMEND IV

Mean Plasma Concentration of Aprepitant Following 125 mg Oral Aprepitant and 115 mg IV Fosaprepitant

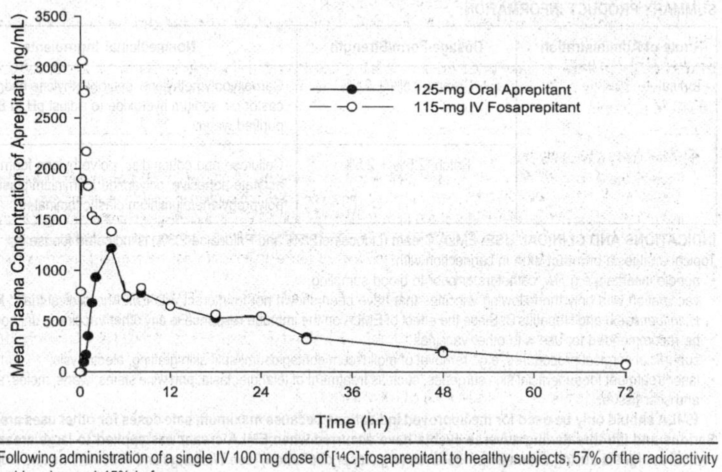

Excretion: Following administration of a single IV 100 mg dose of [^{14}C]-fosaprepitant to healthy subjects, 57% of the radioactivity was recovered in urine and 45% in feces.

Aprepitant is eliminated primarily by metabolism; aprepitant is not renally excreted. Following administration of a single oral 300 mg dose of [^{14}C]-aprepitant to healthy subjects, 5% of the radioactivity was recovered in urine and 86% in feces.

The apparent plasma clearance of aprepitant ranged from approximately 60 to 84 mL/min. The apparent terminal half-life ranged from approximately 9 to 13 hours.

Special Populations and Conditions: Pediatrics: The pharmacokinetics of EMEND and EMEND IV have not been evaluated in patients below 18 years of age.

Geriatrics: Following oral administration of a single 125 mg dose of EMEND on Day 1 and 80 mg once daily on Days 2 through 5, the AUC_{0-24hr} of aprepitant was 21% higher on Day 1 and 36% higher on Day 5 in elderly (≥65 years) relative to younger adults. The C_{max} was 10% higher on Day 1 and 24% higher on Day 5 in elderly relative to younger adults. These differences are not considered clinically meaningful. No dosage adjustment for EMEND is necessary in elderly patients.

Gender: Following oral administration of a single 125 mg dose of aprepitant, the C_{max} for aprepitant is 16% higher in females as compared with males. The half-life of aprepitant is 25% lower in females as compared with males and its T_{max} occurs at approximately the same time. No dosage adjustment is necessary based on gender.

Race: Following oral administration of a single 125 mg dose of aprepitant, the AUC_{0-24hr} is approximately 25% and 29% higher in Hispanics as compared with Caucasians and Blacks, respectively. The C_{max} is 22% and 31% higher in Hispanics as compared with Caucasians and Blacks, respectively. These differences are not considered clinically meaningful. No dosage adjustment is necessary based on race.

Hepatic Insufficiency: Fosaprepitant is metabolized in various extrahepatic tissues; therefore hepatic insufficiency is not expected to alter the conversion of fosaprepitant to aprepitant.

Oral aprepitant was well tolerated in patients with mild to moderate hepatic insufficiency. Following administration of a single 125 mg dose of oral aprepitant on Day 1 and 80 mg once daily on Days 2 and 3 to patients with mild hepatic insufficiency (Child-Pugh score 5 to 6), the AUC_{0-24hr} of aprepitant was 11% lower on Day 1 and 36% lower on Day 3, as compared with healthy subjects given the same regimen. In patients with moderate hepatic insufficiency (Child-Pugh score 7 to 9), the AUC_{0-24hr} of aprepitant was 10% higher on Day 1 and 18% higher on Day 3, as compared with healthy subjects given the same regimen. These differences in AUC_{0-24hr} are not considered clinically meaningful; therefore, no dosage adjustment is necessary in patients with mild to moderate hepatic insufficiency.

There are no clinical or pharmacokinetic data in patients with severe hepatic insufficiency (Child-Pugh score >9).

Renal Insufficiency: A single 240 mg dose of aprepitant was administered to patients with severe renal insufficiency (CrCl<30 mL/min) and to patients with end stage renal disease (ESRD) requiring hemodialysis.

In patients with severe renal insufficiency, the $AUC_{0-\infty}$ of total aprepitant (unbound and protein bound) decreased by 21% and C_{max} decreased by 32%, relative to healthy subjects. In patients with ESRD undergoing hemodialysis, the $AUC_{0-\infty}$ of total aprepitant decreased by 42% and C_{max} decreased by 32%. Due to modest decreases in protein binding of aprepitant in patients with renal disease, the AUC of pharmacologically active unbound drug was not significantly affected in patients with renal insufficiency compared with healthy subjects. Hemodialysis conducted 4 or 48 hours after dosing had no significant effect on the pharmacokinetics of aprepitant; less than 0.2% of the dose was recovered in the dialysate.

No dosage adjustment is necessary for patients with severe renal insufficiency or for patients with ESRD undergoing hemodialysis.

STORAGE AND STABILITY: Vials: Store at 2-8°C.

INFORMATION FOR THE PATIENT: Published in e-CPS, available by subscription at www.e-cps.ca.

DOSAGE FORMS, COMPOSITION AND PACKAGING: Each vial of white to off-white lyophilized solid contains: fosaprepitant dimeglumine 188 mg equivalent to fosaprepitant 115 mg. Nonmedicinal ingredients: edetate disodium, lactose anhydrous, polysorbate 80 and sodium hydroxide and/or hydrochloric acid (for pH adjustment). Glass vials of 10 mL, cartons of 1.

EMLA® Cream
lidocaine—prilocaine
Topical Anesthetic for Dermal Analgesia

AstraZeneca

EMLA® Patch
lidocaine—prilocaine
Topical Anesthetic for Dermal Analgesia

AstraZeneca

Date of Preparation: May 2, 2000
Date of Revision: May 25, 2010

SUMMARY PRODUCT INFORMATION:

Route of Administration	Dosage Form/Strength	Nonmedicinal Ingredients
Topical	Cream, 2.5% + 2.5%	Carboxypolymethylene, polyoxyethylene hydrogenated castor oil, sodium hydroxide to adjust pH to 8.7-9.7, purified water.
	Patch, 2.5% + 2.5%	Cellulose and cotton disc, polyethylene foam with acrylate adhesive, polyamide/aluminium/plastic and polypropylene/aluminium/plastic laminates.

INDICATIONS AND CLINICAL USE: EMLA Cream (Lidocaine 2.5% and Prilocaine 2.5%) is indicated for use in:
Topical analgesia of **intact skin** in connection with:
- needle insertion, e.g., i.v. catheters or prior to blood sampling;
- vaccination with only the following vaccines that have been shown not to interact with EMLA in clinical trials: MMR, DPTP, *H. influenzae* b and Hepatitis B. Since the effect of EMLA on the immune response to any other vaccine is unknown, it cannot be recommended for use with other vaccines;
- superficial surgical procedures, e.g., removal of molluscum contagiosum, split skin grafting, electrolysis;
- laser treatment for superficial skin surgeries, such as treatment of telangiectasia, port wine stains, warts, moles, skin nodules, and scar tissue.

EMLA should only be used for the approved indications because maximum safe doses for other uses are not known. Serious and life-threatening adverse events have occurred when EMLA cream was applied to large areas of skin for topical analgesia during cosmetic procedures (e.g., laser depilation) (see Warnings and Precautions and Adverse Reactions).

Topical analgesia of **genital mucosa** in connection with:
- local infiltration anesthesia;
- surgical procedures lasting not longer than 10 minutes on small superficial localized lesions, e.g., removal of condylomata by laser or cautery, and biopsies.

Topical analgesia of **leg ulcers** in connection with:
- mechanical/sharp cleansing/debridement, e.g., the removal of necrotic tissue and debris by curettes, scissors, tweezers, etc.

EMLA Patch (Lidocaine 2.5% and Prilocaine 2.5%) is indicated for use in:
Topical analgesia of **intact skin** in connection with:
- needle insertion, e.g., i.v. catheters or prior to blood sampling;
- vaccination with only the following vaccines that have been shown not to interact with EMLA in clinical trials: MMR, DPTP, *H. influenzae* b and Hepatitis B. Since the effect of EMLA on the immune response to any other vaccine is unknown, it cannot be recommended for use with other vaccines.

CONTRAINDICATIONS: EMLA (lidocaine and prilocaine) is contraindicated in:
- patients who are hypersensitive to local anesthetics of the amide type or to any ingredients in the formulation (see Dosage Forms, Composition and Packaging);
- patients with congenital or idiopathic methemoglobinemia;
- procedures requiring large amounts of EMLA over a large body area that are not conducted in a facility where the healthcare professionals are trained in the diagnosis and management of dose-related toxicity and other acute emergencies that may arise and, the appropriate resuscitative treatments and equipment required for management of toxic reactions and related emergencies are available;
- infants who require treatment with methemoglobin-inducing agents, e.g., sulfonamides, and are 12 months of age or younger (see Drug Interactions);
- preterm infants (defined as gestational age less than 37 weeks).

WARNINGS AND PRECAUTIONS: General: Serious and life-threatening systemic adverse events, including methemoglobinemia, central nervous system toxicity and cardiovascular collapse have occurred when EMLA cream was applied to large areas of skin for topical analgesia during cosmetic procedures (e.g., laser depilation) (see Adverse Reactions and Overdosage). EMLA should only be used for the approved indications because maximum safe doses for other uses are not known.

Patients should be instructed to strictly adhere to dosing recommendations and to limit the dose and area of application (see Dosage and Administration).

When using EMLA in younger children, especially infants under the age of 3 months, care must be taken to ensure that the caregiver understands the need to limit the dose and area of application and to prevent accidental ingestion (see Dosage and Administration). Children should be closely observed during and after use of topical anesthetics, as they are at greater risk than adults for serious adverse events (e.g., methemoglobinemia).

Repeated doses of EMLA (lidocaine and prilocaine) may increase blood levels of lidocaine and prilocaine. EMLA should be used with caution in patients who may be more sensitive to the systemic effects of lidocaine and prilocaine including acutely ill, debilitated, or elderly patients, and patients with severe hepatic impairment (see Dosage and Administration).

Due to insufficient data on absorption, EMLA should not be applied to open wounds as a result of trauma. Note: Leg ulcers often follow a slight trauma but are not classified as traumatic wounds.

Special care should also be employed to ensure the occlusive bandage or patch is secure. This will avoid accidental dislocation and exposure of EMLA, especially in young children.

EMLA is not recommended in any clinical situation where it can penetrate or migrate into the middle ear. Tests on laboratory animals (guinea pigs) have shown that EMLA has an ototoxic effect when instilled into the middle ear. When the same animals were exposed to EMLA in the external auditory canal, no abnormalities were seen. EMLA causes minor structural damage to the tympanic membrane in rats when applied directly to the membrane.

Carcinogenesis and Mutagenesis: The active substances in EMLA, lidocaine and prilocaine, have not been evaluated for carcinogenicity in animal studies following topical application; neither has EMLA the eutectic mixture of lidocaine and prilocaine bases. Metabolites of prilocaine have been shown to be carcinogenic after life-time, once-daily oral exposure in laboratory animals.

Chronic oral toxicity studies of o-toluidine, a metabolite of prilocaine, in mice (150-2400 mg/kg) and rats (150-800 mg/kg) have shown that o-toluidine is a carcinogen in both species at all doses tested. A non-carcinogenic dose in rats or mice has not been established. The lowest tumor-inducing dose tested in animals (150 mg/kg) corresponds to approximately 30 times the amount of o-toluidine to which a 50 kg subject would be exposed following the application of 60 g of EMLA Cream for 24 hours on the intact skin, assuming an extent of absorption of 30%, and 100% conversion to o-toluidine. Based on a yearly exposure (once daily dosing with o-toluidine in animals and 5 treatment sessions with 60 g EMLA Cream in humans), the safety margins would be approximately 2200 times when comparing the exposure in animals to man.

Genotoxicity tests with lidocaine showed no evidence of mutagenic potential. A metabolite of lidocaine, 2,6-xylidine, showed weak evidence of activity in some genotoxicity tests. A chronic oral toxicity study of the metabolite 2,6-xylidine (0, 14, 45, 135 mg/kg) administered in feed to rats showed that there was a significantly greater incidence of nasal cavity tumors in male and female animals that had daily oral exposure to the highest dose of 2,6-xylidine for 2 years. The lowest tumor-inducing dose tested in animals (135 mg/kg) corresponds to approximately 60 times the amount of 2,6-xylidine to which a 50 kg subject would be exposed following the application of 60 g of EMLA Cream for 24 hours on the intact skin, assuming an extent of absorption of 15%, and 80% conversion to 2,6-xylidine. Based on a yearly exposure (once daily dosing with 2,6-xylidine in animals and 5 treatment sessions with 60 g EMLA Cream in humans), the safety margins would be approximately 4700 times when comparing the exposure in animals to man.

Hepatic: Because amide-type local anesthetics are metabolized by the liver, these drugs, especially repeated doses, should be used cautiously in patients with hepatic disease. For patients with severe hepatic disease, a reduced capacity to metabolize local anesthetics may increase the risk of developing toxic plasma concentrations (see Dosage and Administration).

Ophthalmologic: EMLA should not be applied to, or near to, the eyes as it causes corneal irritation if it comes into contact with the cornea. This reaction may be reversible. In addition, the loss of protective reflexes may allow corneal irritation and potential abrasion. Take care to avoid accidental contact of EMLA with the eyes (e.g., rubbing the eyes after using fingers to apply EMLA elsewhere), as the analgesic effect may result in damage from undetected foreign bodies. If eye contact does occur, immediately rinse the eye in water or sodium chloride solution and protect the eye until sensation returns.

Renal: In individuals with normal renal function, the extent of systemic absorption of lidocaine and prilocaine is low, 5-14% after cutaneous application, higher on genital mucosa and leg ulcer. Only a small fraction of lidocaine and prilocaine (2-5%) is excreted unchanged in the urine, as the primary metabolism occurs in the liver (see Action and Clinical Pharmacology). The pharmacokinetics of lidocaine and its main metabolite were not altered significantly in haemodialysis patients (n=4) who received an intravenous dose of lidocaine. Therefore, renal impairment is not expected to significantly affect the pharmacokinetics of lidocaine and prilocaine when EMLA is used according to dosage instructions (see Dosage and Administration).

Skin: Care should be taken when applying EMLA to patients with atopic dermatitis. A more rapid and greater absorption through the skin is observed in these patients. A shorter application time should be used (see Action and Clinical Pharmacology). There have been two reports of purpura at the application site after 60 minutes. After a repeated application of 30 minutes in one of these patients, no reaction was seen. There are not sufficient data available to characterize absorption or local reactions, nor to permit dosing recommendations.

Vaccination: Lidocaine and prilocaine have been shown to inhibit viral and bacterial growth. The effect of EMLA on intradermal injections of live vaccines has not been determined.

Special Populations: EMLA is contraindicated for patients with congenital or idiopathic methemoglobinemia and for infants 12 months of age or younger who require treatment with methemoglobin-inducing drugs (see also Contraindications). Patients with glucose-6-phosphate dehydrogenase deficiency are more susceptible to drug-induced methemoglobinemia.

Patients who are acutely ill, debilitated or elderly, and patients with severe hepatic impairment may require dosing adjustments commensurate with age, weight and physical condition, because they may be more sensitive to systemic effects due to increased blood levels of lidocaine and prilocaine following repeated doses of EMLA (see also Dosage and Administration).

Pregnant Women: The safety of EMLA during pregnancy has not been established in humans. Lidocaine and prilocaine cross the placental barrier and may be absorbed by the fetal tissues. It is reasonable to assume that lidocaine and prilocaine have been used in a large number of pregnant women and women of child-bearing age. No specific disturbances to the reproductive process have so far been reported, e.g., an increased incidence of malformations or other directly or indirectly harmful effects on the fetus. However, care should be given during early pregnancy when maximum organogenesis takes place.

Labor and Delivery: Should EMLA be used concomitantly with other products containing lidocaine and/or priolocaine during labor and delivery, the total dose contributed by all formulations should be considered.

Nursing Women: Lidocaine and, in all probability, prilocaine, are excreted in human milk, but in such small quantities that there is generally no risk of the infant being affected at therapeutic dose levels due to low systemic absorption.

Pediatrics: Children should be closely observed during and after use of topical anesthetics, as they are at greater risk than adults for serious adverse events (e.g., methemoglobinemia).

When using EMLA in younger children, especially infants under the age of 3 months, care must be taken to ensure that the caregiver understands the need tolimit the dose and area of application and to prevent accidental ingestion (see Dosage and Administration).

In neonates (minimum gestation age: 37 weeks) and children weighing less than 20 kg, the area and duration of application should be limited (see Dosage And Administration, Table 3).

EMLA should not be applied to the genital mucosa of children or infants due to insufficient data on absorption.

In infants below the age of 3 months, the capacity of the MetHb reductase is lower than in older children and in adults. A transient, clinically insignificant increase in methemoglobin levels is commonly observed up to 12 hours after an application of EMLA.

EMLA should not be used:
- in patients with congenital or idiopathic methemoglobinemia;
- in infants who require treatment with methemoglobin-inducing agents such as sulfonamides, and are 12 months of age or younger (see also Contraindications, Warnings and Precautions, Drug Interactions, Adverse Reactions);
- in preterm infants (defined as a gestational age less than 37 weeks).

Parents should be reminded of the importance of emotional and psychological support of younger children undergoing medical or surgical procedures.

Geriatrics: Greater sensitivity of some older individuals cannot be ruled out. There are insufficient data to evaluate quantitative differences in systemic plasma levels of lidocaine and prilocaine between geriatric and non-geriatric patients following application of EMLA.

During intravenous studies, the elimination half-life of lidocaine was statistically significantly longer in elderly patients (2.5 hours) than in younger patients (1.5 hours).

No studies are available on the intravenous pharmacokinetics of prilocaine in elderly patients (see Action and Clinical Pharmacology).

ADVERSE REACTIONS: The adverse drug reactions included below for EMLA (lidocaine and prilocaine) represent data from both clinical and post-marketing experience (see Table 1).

Table 1: EMLA

Adverse Drug Reactions

	Adverse Reactions
Intact Skin (for all age groups)	
Common Events (>1%)	At the application site: transient local reactions such as paleness, erythema (redness) and edema.
Uncommon Events (>0.1% and <1%)	At the application site: skin sensations, e.g., an initial mild burning or itching sensation; local paresthesia such as tingling.
Rare Events (<0.1%)	In rare cases, local anesthetics have been associated with allergic reactions; in the most severe instances, anaphylactic shock. There have also been rare cases of discrete local lesions at the application site, described as purpuric or petechial, especially after longer application times in children with atopic dermatitis or molluscum contagiosum. Corneal irritation after accidental eye exposure. Prilocaine in high doses may cause an increase in the methemoglobin level particularly in conjunction with methemoglobin-inducing agents (e.g., sulfonamides) (see Overdosage).
Very Rare Events (<0.01%)	In very rare cases, central nervous system toxicity (e.g. convulsion, dizziness, loss of consciousness, somnolence) and cardiovascular collapse (e.g. cardiac arrest, hypoxia, respiratory arrest) have occurred after very high doses of EMLA[a].
Genital Mucosa	

(cont'd)

Table 1: EMLA *(cont'd)*

Adverse Drug Reactions

	Adverse Reactions
Common Events (>1%)	Application site: transient local reactions such as erythema (redness), edema and paleness; local sensations, e.g., an initial, usually mild, burning sensation, itch or warmth.
Uncommon Events (>0.1% and <1%)	Application site: local paresthesia such as tingling.
Rare Events (<0.1%)	In rare cases, local anesthetics have been associated with allergic reactions; in the most severe instances, anaphylactic shock.
Leg Ulcer	
Common Events (>1%)	Transient local reactions at the application site such as paleness, erythema (redness) and edema. Skin sensations, e.g., an initial usually mild burning, itch or warmth at the application site.
Uncommon Events (>0.1% and <1%)	Skin irritation at the application site.
Rare Events (<0.1%)	In rare cases, local anesthetics have been associated with allergic reactions; in the most severe instances, anaphylactic shock.

[a] During post-marketing experience serious and life threatening systemic adverse events, including methemoglobinemia, central nervous system toxicity and cardiovascular collapse, have occurred when EMLA cream was applied to large areas of skin for topical analgesia during cosmetic procedures (e.g., laser depilation).

DRUG INTERACTIONS: Overview: Lidocaine is mainly metabolized in the liver to its two major pharmacologically active metabolites, monoethylglycinexylidine (MEGX) and glycinexylidine (GX), by CYP1A2 and CYP3A4 and has a high hepatic extraction ratio. Prilocaine is mainly metabolized to o-toluidine in the liver, by unestablished mechanisms. Only a small proportion (2-5%) of lidocaine and prilocaine is excreted unchanged in the urine. The hepatic clearance of lidocaine, and probably prilocaine, is expected to depend largely on blood flow.

With the low systemic exposure to lidocaine and prilocaine and short duration of topical application of EMLA (lidocaine and prilocaine), metabolic drug-drug interactions of clinical significance with lidocaine or prilocaine are unlikely.

Clinically relevant pharmacodynamic drug interactions may occur with EMLA and other local anesthetics or structurally related drugs, and Class I and Class III antiarrhythmic drugs due to additive effects.

Metabolism of prilocaine can accentuate the formation of methemoglobin. Co-administration of EMLA and other methemoglobin-inducing agents to patients 12 months of age or younger may result in clinical signs of methemoglobinemia (see Contraindications, Warnings and Precautions, Drug Interactions, Adverse Reactions).

Drug-Drug Interactions: Local Anesthetics and Agents Structurally Related to Amide-type Local Anesthetic: Large doses of EMLA Cream and EMLA Patch should be used with caution in patients receiving other local anesthetics or agents structurally related to amide-type local anesthetics (e.g. antiarrhythmics such as mexiletine), as the toxic effects are additive.

Antiarrhythmic Drugs: Class 1 Antiarrhythmic Drugs: Class 1 antiarrhythmic drugs (such as mexiletine) should be used with caution since toxic effects are additive and potentially synergistic (see Contraindications regarding infants, Adverse Reactions, and Overdosage).

Class III Antiarrhythmic Drugs: Caution is advised when using Class III antiarrhythmic drugs concomitantly with EMLA due to potential pharmacodynamic or pharmacokinetic interactions, or both. A drug interaction study has shown that the plasma concentration of lidocaine may be increased following administration of a therapeutic dose of intravenous lidocaine to patients treated with amiodarone (n=6). Case reports have described symptoms of lidocaine toxicity in patients treated concomitantly with lidocaine and amiodarone. Patients treated with Class III antiarrhythmic drugs (e.g. amiodarone) should be kept under close surveillance and ECG monitoring should be considered, since cardiac effects of these drugs and EMLA Cream may be additive.

Drugs that Reduce the Clearance of Lidocaine: Drugs that reduce the clearance of lidocaine (eg, cimetidine or beta-blockers) may cause potentially toxic plasma concentrations when lidocaine is given in repeated high doses over a long time period. Such interactions are not expected to be clinically relevant when lidocaine (eg, EMLA cream) is used for short term treatment at recommended doses.

Methemoglobinemia: Prilocaine, a component of EMLA, accentuates the formation of methemoglobin (MetHb) by a mechanism involving metabolism of prilocaine to o-toluidine and subsequent oxidation of hemoglobin to MetHb. The in vivo reduction of MetHb back to O_2Hb is dependent on the presence of MetHb reductase.

In patients treated concomitantly with EMLA and other methemoglobin-inducing agents including but not limited to sulfonamides, acetanilid, aniline dyes, benzocaine, chloroquine, dapsone, naphthalene, nitrates and nitrites, nitrofurantoin, nitroglycerin, nitroprusside, pamaquine, para-aminosalicylic acid, phenacetin, phenobarbital, phenytoin, primaquine and quinine, EMLA may induce the formation of methemoglobin and result in overt clinical signs of methemoglobinemia (see Contraindications and Overdosage).

Acetaminophen has been shown to induce methemoglobin formation in vitro and in animals. In humans, methemoglobin formation is very rare at therapeutic doses and overdoses of acetaminophen.

Drug-Food Interactions: Interactions of lidocaine and prilocaine with food have not been established.

Drug-Herb Interactions: Interactions of lidocaine and prilocaine with herbs have not been established.

Drug-Laboratory Tests Interactions: Interactions of lidocaine and prilocaine with laboratory tests have not been established.

DOSAGE AND ADMINISTRATION: Dosing Considerations: Conditions where dosing may require adjustment:

- in acutely ill, debilitated or elderly patients, and patients with severe hepatic impairment who are more sensitive to systemic effects due to increased blood levels of lidocaine and prilocaine from repeated doses of EMLA (lidocaine and prilocaine)
- in patients who are administered other local anesthetics or amide type local anesthetics (see Drug Interactions)
- in debilitated patients, or those with impaired elimination, smaller application areas are recommended to avoid toxicity. Decreased duration of application is not recommended as this may decrease the analgesic effect

Children should be closely observed during and after use of topical anesthetics, as they are at greater risk than adults for serious adverse events (e.g., methemoglobinemia).

Recommended Dose and Dosage Adjustment: EMLA should only be used for approved indications because maximum safe doses for other uses are not known.

Serious and life threatening adverse events have occurred when EMLA cream was applied to large areas of skin for topical analgesia during cosmetic procedures (e.g., laser depilation) (see Contraindications, Adverse Reactions and Overdosage).

Do not exceed dosages outlined in the tables below.

At each recommended dose (g cream/cm² skin area), the depth and effectiveness of analgesia are dependent upon the total time elapsed between application and procedure (i.e., total time is a combination of the period of cream application and the period following the removal of the cream up until the procedure is performed).

Table 2 and Table 3 detail dosing recommendations for EMLA Cream, for adults and pediatrics, respectively, while Table 4 provides common references for the size of each specific recommended maximum skin area.

Table 5 and Table 6 detail dosing recommendations for EMLA patch, for adults and pediatrics respectively.

1 g of EMLA Cream administered from the 30 g aluminium tube is equivalent to a ribbon of cream of approximately 3.5 cm (approximately 1.5 inches).

Administration: See Information for the Patient—Instructions for Application.

OVERDOSAGE:

A few fatal cases have been reported with limited information and doses unknown, therefore a causal relationship to EMLA (lidocaine and prilocaine) could not be established.

Table 2: EMLA Cream

Adults: Recommended Dosage of EMLA Cream According to Body Surface, and Procedure

Surface	Procedure	Cream Application
Intact Skin	Minor procedures, e.g., needle insertion, surgical treatment of localized lesions, and laser treatment.[a,b]	Apply a thick layer of cream under an occlusive dressing to selected area(s). Remove the dressing and clean the area of any excess cream thoroughly prior to the procedure. In general, approx. 1.5 g/10 cm². Approx. 2 g (½ of 5 g tube) for a minimum of 1 hour. Maximum 5-hour application[c].
	Dermal procedures performed on larger areas, in a hospital setting, e.g., split-skin grafting.[d]	1.5–2 g/10 cm², up to a total of 60 g. Maximum recommended treated area: 400 cm²[d]. Minimum application time: 2 hours. Maximum application time: 5 hours[c].
Genital Mucosa	Surgical procedures lasting not longer than 10 minutes on localized lesions, e.g., removal of genital warts, and prior to local infiltration anesthesia.	Approx. 2 g (½ of 5 g tube) per lesion for 5–10 minutes. Maximum 10 g[e]. Occlusion is not necessary. Commence procedure immediately after removal of cream.
Leg Ulcers	Mechanical cleansing/debridement of leg ulcers[f]	Approx. 1–2 g/10 cm² area, up to a total of 10 g. Minimum 30 minutes application time, with up to 60 minutes for necrotic tissue with a thicker penetration barrier. Cleansing should start immediately after removal of the cream.

[a] EMLA should only be used for approved indications because maximum safe doses for other uses are not known. Serious and life threatening adverse events have occurred when EMLA cream was applied to large areas of skin for topical analgesia during cosmetic procedures (e.g. laser depilation).

[b] Topical analgesia with EMLA has been evaluated in clinical trials in which laser treatments were for superficial skin surgeries, such as treatment of telangiectasia, port wine stains, warts, moles, skin nodules, and scar tissue.

[c] There is no benefit to application times longer than 5 hours, as the analgesic effectiveness of the cream dissipates over time.

[d] In clinical trials evaluating the analgesic effects of EMLA during split skin grafting, EMLA was well tolerated when applied to treatment areas of approximately 50 to 400 cm² (n=232). A small number of patients in these clinical trials had EMLA applied to treatment areas >400 cm² (n=8).

[e] Pharmacokinetic data for doses larger than 10 g are not available.

[f] In the treatment of leg ulcers, EMLA Cream has been repeatedly applied (up to 15 times within a 1-2 month period, at intervals of 1 to 4 days), with no apparent loss of effect or increase in local reaction.

Table 3: EMLA Cream

Pediatrics: Maximum Recommended Dosage of EMLA Cream According to Age

Age	Cream Application
In general, approx. 1 g/10 cm² area for 1 hour under a dressing to minimize the potential for the child to accidental spread the cream outside of the treatment area. Remove the dressing and clean the area of any excess cream thoroughly prior to the procedure.	
Neonates 0–3 months or <5 kg[a,b] (minimal gestational age is 37 weeks)	0.5 to 1.0 g, and up to 10 cm² area for approximately 1 hour. Standard dose=1.0 g. Maximum 1-hour application[c,d]. No more than one application site at a time. The safety of repeated dosing has not been established.
Infants 3 up to 12 months[b] and >5 kg	Up to 2 g and 20 cm² for approximately 1 hour[e]. Maximum 4-hour application.
Children 1–6 years and >10 kg	Up to 10 g and 100 cm² for a minimum of 1 hour. Maximum 5-hour application[f].
Children 7–12 years and >20 kg	Up to 20 g and 200 cm² for a minimum of 1 hour. Maximum 5-hour application[f].

[a] Infants less than 3 months of age are at higher risk of methemoglobinemia due to immature reductase enzyme pathways.

[b] Until further clinical data is available, EMLA should not be used in infants who require treatment with methemoglobin-inducing agents, i.e., sulfonamides, and are 12 months of age or younger.

[c] The safety of a longer application time has not been established.

[d] Of eight cases of neonates with >5% methemoglobin, misuse was documented in seven (overdose, or concomitant methemoglobin-inducing meds.)

[e] No clinically significant increase in methemoglobin levels has been observed after an application time of up to 4 hours on 16 cm².

[f] There is no benefit to application times longer than 5 hours, as the analgesic effectiveness of the cream dissipates over time.

Please note: If a patient greater than 3 months old does not meet the minimum weight requirement, the maximum total dose of EMLA Cream should be restricted to that which corresponds to the patient's weight.

Table 4: EMLA Cream

Conversion of Maximum Recommended Skin Areas (cm²) to Inches² and to a Reference Object of Comparable Size

cm²	inch²	Area Reference
10	approx. 2	A little larger than the size of a two dollar coin ("toonie").
16	approx. 3	A little larger than the size of a credit card.
100	approx. 4	A little larger than the size of two credit cards.
200	approx. 6	A little larger than the size of a standard postcard.

Symptoms—General: Local anesthetic toxicity is manifested by symptoms of nervous system excitation and in severe cases, central nervous and cardiovascular depression.

In the unlikely event of toxicity following epidermal application of EMLA, signs of systemic toxicity anticipated would be similar in nature to those observed following other routes of administration of local anesthetics.

Methemoglobinemia: Rare cases of methemoglobinemia have been reported.

Mild methemoglobinemia is characterized by tissue cyanosis, a bluish-grey or brownish discoloration of the skin, especially around the lips and nail beds, which is not reversed by breathing 100% oxygen. Clinical signs may also include pallor and marbleization.

Severe methemoglobinemia (MetHb concentrations above approximately 25%) is associated with signs of hypoxemia, ie. dyspnea, tachycardia and depression of consciousness.

Drug-induced methemoglobinemia may occur with the use of drugs including but not limited to sulfonamides, acetanilid, aniline dyes, benzocaine, chloroquine, dapsone, naphthalene, nitrates and nitrites, nitrofurantoin, nitroglycerin, nitroprusside, pamaquine, para-aminosalicylic acid, phenacetin, phenobarbital, phenytoin, primaquine and quinine.

Acetaminophen has been shown to induce methemoglobin formation in vitro and in animals. In humans, methemoglobin formation is very rare at therapeutic doses and overdoses of acetaminophen.

It should be kept in mind that EMLA is contraindicated for patients with congenital or idiopathic methemoglobinemia and for infants 12 months of age or younger who require treatment with methemoglobin-inducing drugs. Patients with glucose-6-phosphate dehydrogenase deficiency are more susceptible to drug-induced methemoglobinemia (see also Contraindications, Warnings and Precautions).

Table 5: EMLA Patch

Adults: Recommended Dosage of EMLA Patch

Surface	Procedure	Patch Application
Intact Skin only	Minor procedures, e.g., needle insertion.	Apply patch(es) only to selected skin area(s) <10 cm^2. One or more patches applied for a minimum of 1 hour. Maximum 5-hour application[a]. Remove patch and clean the area thoroughly prior to procedure.

[a] There is no benefit to application times longer than 5 hours, as the analgesic effectiveness of the cream in the patch dissipates over time.

Table 6: EMLA Patch

Pediatrics: Maximum Recommended Dosage of EMLA Patch by Age Group

Age	Patch Application
	Apply patch(es) only to selected skin area(s) <10 cm^2[a]. Remove patch and clean the area thoroughly prior to procedure.
Neonates 0 up to 3 months or <5 kg[b,c]	1 patch applied for approx. 1 hour. Maximum 1-hour application[d]. No more than 1 patch applied at the same time. The safety of repeated dosing has not been established.
Infants 3 up to 12 months[c] and >5 kg	Patch applied for approx. 1 hour[d]. Maximum 4-hour application. No more than 2 patches applied at the same time[e].
Children 1–6 years and >10 kg	One or more patches applied for a minimum of 1 hour. Maximum 5-hour application[f]. Maximum dose is 10 g (10 patches).
Children 7–12 years and >20 kg	One or more patches applied for a minimum of 1 hour. Maximum 5-hour application[f]. Maximum dose is 20 g (20 patches).

[a] The size of the patch makes it less suitable for use on certain parts of the body in neonates and infants.
[b] Infants less than 3 months of age are at higher risk of methemoglobinemia due to immature reductase enzyme pathways.
[c] Until further clinical data is available, EMLA should not be used in infants who require treatment with methemoglobin-inducing agents, i.e., sulfonamides, and are 12 months of age or younger.
[d] The safety of a longer application time has not been established.
[e] No clinically significant increase in methemoglobin levels has been observed after an application time of up to 4 hours on 16 cm^2.
[f] There is no benefit to application times longer than 5 hours, as the analgesic effectiveness of the cream in the patch dissipates over time.
Please note: If a patient greater than 3 months old does not meet the minimum weight requirement, the maximum total dose of EMLA Patch should be restricted to that which corresponds to the patient's weight.

Class 1 Antiarrhythmic Drugs: Class 1 antiarrhythmic drugs (such as mexiletine) should be used with caution since the toxic effects are additive and potentially synergistic.
Treatment: Severe neurological symptoms (convulsions, CNS depression) must be treated symptomatically by respiratory support and the administration of anticonvulsive drugs.

In neonates, methemoglobin concentrations of up to 5-6% are not considered to be of clinical significance, with treatment of symptomatic methemoglobinemia not typically necessary unless methemoglobin concentrations are above 25-30%. However, the severity of clinical symptoms should be the primary consideration in the decision to initiate treatment, rather than the level of methemoglobin. Most patients recovered spontaneously after removal of the cream. Methemoglobinemia may be treated with a slow intravenous injection of methylene blue. It has been reported in published literature that methylene blue should be used cautiously as a treatment for methemoglobinemia in patients with glucose-6-phosphate dehydrogenase deficiency because it may not be effective for these patients and may cause hemolytic anemia.

There are anecdotal reports of patients consuming EMLA Cream or Patches; all cases resolved without serious injury. Such patients should be monitored for symptoms of systemic toxicity.

> For management of a suspected drug overdose, contact your regional Poison Control Centre. See the *CPS* Directory section for a list of Poison Control Centres.

ACTION AND CLINICAL PHARMACOLOGY: Mechanism of Action and Pharmacodynamics: EMLA (Eutectic Mixture of Local Anesthetics) (lidocaine and prilocaine) is a 1:1 oil/water emulsion of a eutectic mixture of lidocaine and prilocaine bases. Dermal analgesia is a result of the migration of lidocaine and prilocaine into the epidermal and dermal layers of the skin followed by the accumulation of these agents in the vicinity of dermal pain receptors and nerve endings. Lidocaine and prilocaine are both amide-type local anesthetic agents. They stabilize the neuronal membrane preventing the initiation and conduction of nerve impulses, thereby effecting local anesthetic action. EMLA provides dermal analgesia; the depth of which depends upon the application time and the applied dose. Analgesia may be less for deeper structures.

EMLA may produce a transient biphasic vascular response involving initial vasoconstriction followed by vasodilation at the application site (see Adverse Reactions). In patients with atopic dermatitis, a shorter biphasic response involving initial vasoconstriction followed by vasodilation may be seen. Erythema may be observed after 30 to 60 minutes.
General Pharmacokinetics: Absorption: Systemic absorption of lidocaine and prilocaine from EMLA is dependent upon several factors, including: the applied dose, area of application and duration of application. Additional factors include thickness of the skin (which varies in different areas of the body), vascularity of the skin in the area of application, the presence of any condition in which the skin is not healthy and intact (e.g. sunburn, rash), and shaving. Following application to leg ulcers, the characteristics of the ulcers may also affect the absorption.
Atopic Dermatitis: It is well known that patients with atopic dermatitis show abnormal vascular reactions to pharmacological stimuli. In patients with atopic dermatitis, percutaneous absorption of EMLA is more rapid and greater than in normal skin. In two patients, within one hour after application of 4-6 g EMLA to a 25 cm^2 area of the forearm, lidocaine and prilocaine plasma levels were higher than those observed in normal skin. However, in these patients, the systemic plasma levels were 100 times lower than those associated with toxicity. In patients with atopic dermatitis, a shorter application time should be used (see Warnings and Precautions, Skin). It should be noted, however, that dermatological procedures were not performed in the above patients. Clinical data are not available at present to permit dosage recommendations.
Distribution and Metabolism: Prilocaine has a larger distribution volume than lidocaine which results in lower plasma concentrations of prilocaine when equal amounts of prilocaine and lidocaine are administered. At concentrations produced by application of EMLA, lidocaine is approximately 60-80% bound to plasma proteins, primarily alpha-1-acid glycoprotein. At much higher plasma concentrations (1 to 4 μg/mL of free base), the plasma protein binding of lidocaine is concentration dependent. Prilocaine is 55% bound to plasma proteins.

It is not known if lidocaine or prilocaine are metabolized in the skin. Lidocaine is metabolized rapidly by the liver to a number of metabolites including monoethylglycinexylidide (MEGX) and glycinexylidide (GX), both of which have pharmacologic activity similar to, but less potent than that of lidocaine. Prilocaine is metabolized in both the liver and kidneys by amidases to various metabolites including ortho-toluidine and N-n-propylalanine.
Excretion: The half-life of lidocaine elimination from the plasma following IV administration is approximately 65 to 150 minutes (mean 110,±24 SD, n=13). More than 98% of an absorbed dose of lidocaine can be recovered in the urine as metabolites or parent drug. The systemic clearance is 10 to 20 mL/min/kg (mean 13,±3 SD, n=13). The elimination half-life of prilocaine is approximately 10 to 150 minutes (mean 70,±48 SD, n=13). The systemic clearance is 18 to 64 mL/min/kg (mean 38,±15 SD, n=13).

During intravenous studies, the elimination half-life of lidocaine was statistically significantly longer in elderly patients (2.5 hours) than in younger patients (1.5 hours). No studies are available on the intravenous pharmacokinetics of prilocaine in elderly patients (see Warnings and Precautions, Geriatrics).
Specific Pharmacokinetics for Lidocaine and Prilocaine in EMLA Products: There is considerable inter-subject variability in lidocaine and prilocaine plasma levels. In pre-marketing studies, all plasma levels of lidocaine and prilocaine after topical administration of EMLA products have been found to be below 1.2 μg/mL. These are below the levels associated with systemic toxicity (5 μg/mL).

STORAGE AND STABILITY: EMLA Cream (lidocaine and prilocaine) in aluminium tubes should be stored at room temperature (15-30°C). Protect from freezing.

EMLA Patch (lidocaine and prilocaine) should be stored at room temperature (15-30°C). Protect from freezing. Single use. Do not reuse.

INFORMATION FOR THE PATIENT: Published in e-CPS, available by subscription at www.e-cps.ca.

DOSAGE FORMS, COMPOSITION AND PACKAGING: Cream: Each g of cream (5%) contains: lidocaine 25 mg and prilocaine 25 mg as a 1:1 oil/water emulsion. Nonmedicinal ingredients: carboxypolymethylene, polyoxyethylene hydrogenated castor oil, purified water and sodium hydroxide to adjust pH to 8.7 to 9.7. Aluminum tubes of 5 g with 2 occlusive dressings and tubes of 30 g without dressings.
Patch: Each single dose unit patch in the form of an occlusive dressing contains: lidocaine 25 mg and prilocaine 25 mg. It is composed of a laminate backing, an absorbent cellulose disc, and an adhesive tape ring. The disc contains 1 g of the EMLA emulsion, the active contact surface area being approximately 10 cm^2. The surface area of the entire patch is approximately 40 cm^2. Nonmedicinal ingredients: carboxypolymethylene, polyoxyethylene hydrogenated castor oil, purified water and sodium hydroxide to adjust pH to 8.7-9.7; patch components: cellulose and cotton disc, polyethylene foam with acrylate adhesive, polyamide/aluminium/plastic and polypropylene/aluminium/plastic laminates. Boxes of 2 or 20 single-use patches.

(Shown in Product Identification Section)

> The reader is invited to consult CPhA's monograph **Corticosteroids: Topical**.

Emo-Cort® ℞
hydrocortisone
Topical Corticosteroid

Stiefel, a GSK company

SUPPLIED: Cream: Each container of white, odorless, washable cream contains: hydrocortisone USP 1% or 2.5%. Nonmedicinal ingredients: ceteareth-20, cetearyl alcohol, germaben II, mineral oil (heavy), purified water and white petrolatum. Plastic jars of 45 g (1%). Plastic tubes of 45 g (2.5%). Plastic jars of 225 g (2.5%). Protect from excessive heat. Avoid freezing.
Lotion: Each bottle of white, odorless, washable lotion contains: hydrocortisone USP 1% or 2.5%. Nonmedicinal ingredients: ceteareth-20, emulsifying wax, germaben II, isopropyl myristate, purified water and sorbitol solution. Plastic bottles of 60 mL. Protect from excessive heat. Avoid freezing.
Scalp Solution: Each bottle of clear, odorless hydroalcoholic solution contains: hydrocortisone USP 2.5%. Nonmedicinal ingredients: isopropyl alcohol, polyethylene glycol and purified water. Plastic bottles of 60 mL. Store below 30°C.

Enablex® ℞
darifenacin HBr
Muscarinic M3 Selective Receptor Antagonist

Novartis Pharmaceuticals

Date of Preparation: November 8, 2005
Date of Revision: January 5, 2009

SUMMARY PRODUCT INFORMATION:

Route of Administration	Dosage Form/ Strength	Clinically Relevant Nonmedicinal Ingredients
Oral	Extended release tablet, 7.5 mg, 15 mg	Dibasic calcium phosphate anhydrous, hypromellose

INDICATIONS AND CLINICAL USE: ENABLEX (darifenacin) is indicated for the treatment of overactive bladder. Overactive bladder is used to describe a collection of urinary symptoms composed of urgency, with or without urge incontinence, usually with frequency and nocturia, in the absence of proven infection or other obvious pathology.
Geriatrics: >65 Years Of Age: In clinical studies (31.4% of patients were >65 years of age), the safety and efficacy profile of darifenacin 7.5 mg and 15 mg in patients aged over 65 years are comparable to the younger population and were not affected by age.
>75 Years Of Age: In clinical studies, the safety and efficacy profile of darifenacin 7.5 mg and 15 mg in patients aged over 75 years are comparable to the younger population and were not affected by age. This information is based on 75 patients over 75 years of age, that were included in the four pivotal darifenacin phase III studies (see also Warnings and Precautions).
Pediatrics: The safety and effectiveness of ENABLEX in pediatric patients have not been established.

CONTRAINDICATIONS: ENABLEX (darifenacin) extended release tablets are contraindicated in patients with, or at risk of, urinary retention, gastric retention or uncontrolled narrow-angle glaucoma.

ENABLEX is also contraindicated in patients with known hypersensitivity to the drug or its ingredients.

WARNINGS AND PRECAUTIONS: Risk of Urinary Retention and Gastrointestinal Obstructive Disorders: ENABLEX (darifenacin) should be administered with caution to the following:

- Patients with clinically significant bladder outflow obstruction because it may worsen symptoms of urinary retention;
- Patients with gastrointestinal obstructive disorders, such as pyloric stenosis, because of the risk of gastrointestinal obstruction;
- Patients with severe constipation (≤2 bowel movements per week) (see Contraindications) or
- Patients with risk of decreased gastrointestinal motility.

Narrow-Angle Glaucoma: ENABLEX should be used with caution in patients with narrow-angle glaucoma.
Hepatic/Biliary/Pancreatic: There are no special dosing requirements for patients with mild hepatic impairment (Child Pugh A). The daily dose of ENABLEX (darifenacin) should not exceed 7.5 mg for patients with moderate hepatic impairment (Child Pugh B). ENABLEX has not been studied in patients with severe hepatic impairment (Child Pugh C) and therefore is not recommended for use in this patient population (see Action and Clinical Pharmacology and Dosage and Administration).
Renal: There is insufficient evidence to determine whether a dose reduction is necessary in patients with severe renal failure.
Special Populations: Pregnant Women: There are no studies of ENABLEX in pregnant women. ENABLEX should be used during pregnancy only if the benefit to the mother outweighs the potential risk to the fetus.
Nursing Women: ENABLEX is excreted into the milk of rats. It is not known whether ENABLEX is excreted into human milk and therefore caution should be exercised before ENABLEX is administered to a nursing woman.
Pediatrics: The safety and effectiveness of ENABLEX in pediatric patients have not been established.
Geriatrics: The recommended starting dose for the elderly is 7.5 mg daily. After 2 weeks of starting therapy, patients should be reassessed for efficacy and safety. For those patients who have an acceptable tolerability profile but require greater symptom relief, the dose may be increased to 15 mg daily, based on individual response. (See Action and Clinical Pharmacology, Special Populations and Conditions.)

In clinical studies, the safety and efficacy profile of darifenacin 7.5 mg and 15 mg in patients aged over 75 years is comparable to the younger population and were not affected by age. This information is based on 75 patients over 75 years of age that were included in the four pivotal darifenacin phase III studies.

ADVERSE REACTIONS: During the clinical development of ENABLEX (darifenacin), a total of 7271 patients and healthy volunteers have been treated with doses of darifenacin from 3.75 to 60 mg once daily (recommended doses are 7.5 and 15 mg once daily) for up to one year duration of therapy, resulting in more than 2000 patient-years exposure, for overactive bladder and other indications.

Table 1 lists the adverse events (regardless of causality) reported in 3% or more patients treated with 7.5 or 15 mg ENABLEX Extended Release Tablets in fixed-dose, placebo-controlled Phase III studies.

The majority of adverse events in ENABLEX treated subjects were mild or moderate and mostly occurred during the first two weeks of treatment. The incidence of serious adverse events was similar for 7.5 mg, 15 mg and placebo. The profile of adverse events remained consistent across all populations and dose studied. There is a tendency for adverse reactions, particularly those classified as mild to moderate, to increase with increasing dose.

The most frequently reported adverse events in the pivotal trials were dry mouth and constipation. However as seen in Table 2, the patient discontinuation rates due to these events were low.

Consistent with M_3 muscarinic receptor selectivity, the incidence of central nervous system adverse events at all doses was similar to placebo in the population tested. The incidence of cardiovascular adverse events, such as tachycardia, were less than 1% at all doses and did not increase with dose.

No clinically significant changes in QT interval were observed in clinical trials of volunteers and patients (n=964 treated, n=261 placebo) with ENABLEX up to and including doses of 60 mg (4 times the recommended dose).

Table 1: ENABLEX

Incidence of Adverse Events, Regardless of Causality, Reported in ≥2% of Patients Treated with ENABLEX Extended Release Tablets in Fixed-dose, Placebo-controlled Phase III Studies

Adverse Event	Darifenacin 7.5 mg N=337 %	Darifenacin 15 mg N=334 %	Placebo N=388 %
Dry Mouth	68 (20.2)	118 (35.3)	32 (8.2)
Constipation	50 (14.8)	71 (21.3)	24 (6.2)
Dyspepsia	9 (2.7)	28 (8.4)	10 (2.6)
Headache	15 (4.5)	17 (5.1)	21 (5.4)
Respiratory Tract Infection	9 (2.7)	17 (5.1)	26 (6.7)
Urinary Tract Infection	16 (4.7)	15 (4.5)	10 (2.6)
Abdominal Pain	8 (2.4)	13 (3.9)	2 (0.5)
Asthenia	5 (1.5)	9 (2.7)	5 (1.3)
Flu Syndrome	7 (2.1)	7 (2.1)	10 (2.6)
Dizziness	3 (0.9)	7 (2.1)	5 (1.3)
Dry Eyes	5 (1.5)	7 (2.1)	2 (0.5)
Back Pain	8 (2.4)	5 (1.5)	12 (3.1)
Nausea	9 (2.7)	5 (1.5)	6 (1.5)
Pharyngitis	9 (2.7)	4 (1.2)	9 (2.3)
Diarrhea	7 (2.1)	3 (0.9)	7 (1.8)

Discontinuations due to any adverse events occurred in 1.2% and 4.5% of 7.5 mg and 15 mg ENABLEX patients treated in fixed-dose placebo controlled trials, respectively and in 1.3% of placebo subjects. There were no discontinuations due to laboratory test abnormalities.

Table 2: ENABLEX

Frequency of Discontinuations for the Most Common Adverse Events

	Darifenacin 7.5 mg N=337 %	Darifenacin 15 mg N=334 %	Placebo N=388 %
Dry Mouth	0 (0.0)	3 (0.9)	0 (0.0)
Constipation	2 (0.6)	4 (1.2)	1 (0.3)

Acute urinary retention (AUR) requiring treatment was reported in a total of 16 patients in the ENABLEX phase I-III clinical trials. Of these 16 cases, 7 were reported as serious adverse events, including one patient with detrusor hyperreflexia secondary to a stroke, one patient with benign prostatic hypertrophy (BPH), one patient with irritable bowel syndrome (IBS) and four OAB patients taking darifenacin 30 mg daily. Of the remaining nine cases, none were reported as serious adverse events. Three occurred in OAB patients taking the recommended doses, and two of these required bladder catheterization for 1-2 days.

In addition, the following adverse events were reported, regardless of causality, by less than 2% of ENABLEX patients in either the 7.5 mg or 15 mg once daily darifenacin dose groups in the fixed-dose, placebo-controlled Phase III studies:

Body as a Whole: accidental injury; pain; face edema.

Cardiovascular: hypertension.

Digestive: vomiting; flatulence, ulcerative stomatitis.

Metabolic and Nutritional: peripheral edema; weight gain; ALT increased, AST increased; edema

Musculoskeletal: arthralgia.

Nervous: insomnia; somnolence; thinking abnormal.

Respiratory: bronchitis; rhinitis; sinusitis; cough increased.

Skin and Appendages: rash; dry skin; pruritus; sweating.

Special Senses: abnormal vision; taste perversion.

Urogenital: urinary tract disorder; vaginitis; impotence; bladder pain.

In one flexible dose titration study (n=395) evaluating the dosing regimen approved for marketing, the overall ADR profile was comparable to that observed in the pooled analysis of three pivotal fixed-dose studies, with the most relevant difference in the very common ADRs. Dry mouth was reported in 18.7% of patients treated with darifenacin and in 8.7% of those treated with placebo. Constipation was reported in 20.9% and 7.9% of patients treated with darifenacin and placebo, respectively. The discontinuation rates due to these ADRs in patients treated with darifenacin were low (dry mouth: 0.7%; constipation: 2.2%).

The incidence of adverse events with the doses of ENABLEX 7.5 mg and 15 mg decreased during the treatment period up to 6 months. A similar trend is also seen for the discontinuation rates.

Abnormal Hematologic and Clinical Chemistry Findings: There was no indication of an increased incidence of laboratory test abnormalities in subjects treated with darifenacin in long term studies.

DRUG INTERACTIONS: Drug-Drug Interactions: Effects of Other Drugs on Darifenacin: Darifenacin metabolism is primarily mediated by the cytochrome P450 enzymes CYP2D6 and CYP3A4. Therefore, inducers of CYP3A4 or inhibitors of either of these enzymes may alter darifenacin pharmacokinetics.

CYP 2D6 Inhibitors: No special dosing requirements are necessary in the presence of CYP 2D6 inhibitors. Darifenacin exposure following 30 mg once daily dosing (twice the maximum recommended therapeutic dose) was 33% higher in the presence of the potent CYP 2D6 inhibitor paroxetine 20 mg.

CYP 3A4 Inhibitors: The daily dose of darifenacin should not exceed 7.5 mg when co-administered with potent CYP3A4 inhibitors (e.g. ketoconazole, itraconazole, miconazole, troleandomycin, clarithromycin, nefazodone and ritonavir) (see Dosage and Administration). When the 7.5 mg once-daily dose of darifenacin was given to steady-state and co-administered with the potent CYP 3A4 inhibitor ketoconazole, mean darifenacin exposure was increased 5.3 fold.

No special dosing requirements are necessary in the presence of moderate CYP 3A4 inhibitors. Darifenacin exposure following 30 mg once daily dosing (twice the maximum recommended therapeutic dose) was 34%, 84% and 95% higher in the presence of cimetidine, fluconazole and erythromycin, respectively.

Effects of Darifenacin on Other Drugs: The potential for clinical doses of darifenacin to act as inhibitors of CYP 2D6 or CYP 3A4 substrates was investigated in specific clinical interaction studies.

CYP 2D6 substrates: Caution should be taken when darifenacin is used concomitantly with medications that are predominantly metabolized by CYP 2D6 and which have a narrow therapeutic window, such as flecainide, thioridazine and tricyclic antidepressants.

The mean exposure of imipramine, a CYP 2D6 substrate, was increased 70% in the presence of steady-state darifenacin 30 mg once daily (twice the maximum recommended therapeutic dose). This was accompanied by a 3.6-fold increase in the exposure of desipramine, the active metabolite of imipramine.

CYP 3A4 Substrates: Darifenacin (30 mg once daily) had no clinically relevant effect on the exposure of the CYP 3A4 substrate midazolam.

Darifenacin (30 mg once daily) had no effect on the pharmacokinetics of the oral contraceptives levonorgestrel or ethinylestradiol.

Other Drugs: Warfarin: The effect of warfarin on prothrombin time was not significantly altered when co-administered with darifenacin 30 mg/day (twice the maximum recommended daily dose).

Digoxin: Routine therapeutic drug monitoring for digoxin should be continued. Darifenacin 30 mg qd (twice the maximum dose) co-administered with digoxin at steady-state resulted in a small but potentially clinically significant, 16%, increase in digoxin exposure.

Therapeutic drug monitoring for digoxin should be performed when initiating and ending darifenacin treatment as well as changing the darifenacin dose.

Antimuscarinic Agents: The concomitant use of ENABLEX with other antimuscarinic agents may increase the frequency and/or severity of antimuscarinic pharmacological effects such as dry mouth, constipation and blurred vision.

In vitro studies: In vitro human microsomal studies have shown that darifenacin does not inhibit CYP 1A2 or CYP 2C9 up to concentrations of 1·10^5 nM. In comparison, the average peak unbound concentration of darifenacin at steady state following 15 mg dosing is 0.24 nM.

Drug-Food Interactions: There is no effect of food on multiple dose pharmacokinetics from extended release tablets.

Drug-Lifestyle Interactions: Effects on ability to drive and use machines: No studies of the effects of ENABLEX on the ability to drive and use machines have been performed. However, antimuscarinics such as ENABLEX may produce dizziness or blurred vision. Patients experiencing these side effects should not drive or use machines.

DOSAGE AND ADMINISTRATION: Dosing Considerations: Use in Children: The safety and effectiveness of ENABLEX in pediatric patients with overactive bladder or any other condition have not been investigated.

Use in Elderly: There are no special dosing requirements for the elderly.

Gender: No special dosing requirements are necessary based on gender.

Renal Insufficiency: There are no special dosing requirements for patients with renal impairment.

Hepatic Impairment: There is a risk of increased exposure in this population, however, no dose adjustment is required in patients with mild hepatic impairment (Child Pugh A). For patients with moderate hepatic impairment (Child Pugh B) or when co-administered with potent CYP3A4 inhibitors (e.g. ketoconazole, itraconazole, miconazole, troleandomycin and nefazodone), the daily dose of ENABLEX should not exceed 7.5 mg. ENABLEX is not recommended for use in patients with severe hepatic impairment (Child Pugh C) (see Action and Clinical Pharmacology, Special Populations and Conditions).

Recommended Dose and Dosage Adjustment: The recommended starting dose of ENABLEX (darifenacin) Extended Release Tablets is 7.5 mg once daily. For those patients starting on 7.5 mg daily and requiring greater symptom relief, the dose may be increased to 15 mg daily as early as two weeks after starting therapy, based on individual response.

ENABLEX Extended Release Tablets should be taken once daily. They may be taken with or without food, and should be swallowed whole and not chewed, divided or crushed.

OVERDOSAGE:

No cases of overdose were recorded in the ENABLEX (darifenacin) clinical development programme that included doses as high as 60 mg daily (4 times the recommended maximum daily dose). Moreover, in a study evaluating the interaction between ketoconazole and daily doses of 30 mg darifenacin, the systemic plasma exposure exceeded the systemic exposure observed after a 60 mg dose by a factor of two, with no reported SAEs. The most commonly reported adverse events were typical of those expected from a drug with anti-muscarinic M_3-receptor antagonist activity.

Overdosage with antimuscarinic agents can potentially result in severe antimuscarinic effects. Treatment should be symptomatic and supportive when necessary. Treatment should be aimed at reversing the antimuscarinic symptoms under careful medical supervision.

For management of a suspected drug overdose, CPhA recommends that you contact your **regional Poison Control Centre**. See the *CPS Directory* section for a list of Poison Control Centres.

ACTION AND CLINICAL PHARMACOLOGY: Mechanism of Action: Darifenacin is a potent muscarinic M_3 selective receptor antagonist that exhibits, in vitro, a nine to 59-fold selectivity for the human M_3 receptor over human M_1, M_2, M_4 and M_5 receptors. The M_3 receptor is the major subtype that modulates urinary bladder muscle contraction.

Darifenacin has a clinically significant effect on bladder function.

Pharmacodynamics: Individuals with full CYP 2D6 activity are referred to as extensive metabolizers (EMs). The estimated mean oral bioavailability of darifenacin in EMs at steady-state is 15% and 19% for 7.5 and 15 mg extended release tablets, respectively.

Pharmacokinetics: Following administration of the extended release tablets maximum plasma levels are reached approximately 7 h after dosing and steady-state plasma levels are achieved by the sixth day of dosing. At steady-state, peak to trough fluctuations in darifenacin concentrations are small (peak to trough fluctuations: 0.87 for 7.5 mg and 0.76 for 15 mg) (Figure 1), thereby maintaining therapeutic plasma levels over the dosing interval. The estimated half-life ($t_{1/2}$) for the extended release tablet is 12.8 to 18.7 hours.

Absorption: In healthy volunteers, darifenacin is rapidly and completely (>98%) absorbed after oral administration, although oral bioavailability is limited by first pass metabolism (see Metabolism).

Distribution: Darifenacin is a lipophilic base and is 98% bound to plasma proteins (primarily to alpha-1-acid- glycoprotein). The steady-state volume of distribution (V_{ss}) is estimated to be 163 L. Based on free drug levels in animal cerebrospinal fluid and plasma, darifenacin shows negligible concentrations in the CSF, suggesting low penetration of the blood brain barrier.

Metabolism: Darifenacin is extensively metabolized by the liver following oral dosing. Metabolism is mediated by cytochrome P450 enzymes CYP 2D6 and CYP 3A4. The three main metabolic routes are as follows: (i) monohydroxylation in the dihydrobenzofuran ring; (ii) dihydrobenzofuran ring opening; (iii) N-dealkylation of the pyrrolidine nitrogen.

The initial products of the hydroxylation and N-dealkylation pathways are major circulating metabolites but none contributes significantly to the overall clinical effect of darifenacin. One of the hydroxylated derivatives has some anti-M_3 muscarinic receptor activity. This metabolite's contribution to overall activity is negligible.

Variability in Metabolism: A subset of individuals are devoid of CYP 2D6 enzyme activity (i.e. approximately 7% of the Caucasian population). Therefore, the metabolism of darifenacin in these poor metabolizers (PMs) will be principally mediated via CYP 3A4. The darifenacin ratios (poor metabolisers: extensive metabolisers) for C_{max} and AUC following darifenacin 15 mg once-daily at steady state were 1.9 and 1.7, respectively.

Population pharmacokinetic analyses of Phase 3 data indicated that on average PMs have 55% higher steady-state exposure than EMs. However, there is considerable overlap between the ranges of exposures seen in EM and PM populations and clinical experience confirms that there are no special dosing requirements for PMs.

Excretion: Following administration of an oral dose of ^{14}C-darifenacin solution to healthy volunteers, approximately 60% of the radioactivity was recovered in the urine and 40% in the feces. Only a small percentage of the excreted dose was unchanged darifenacin (3%). Estimated darifenacin clearance is 40 L/h (11.1 mL/s) for EMs and 32 L/h (8.9 mL/s) for PMs.

Figure 1: ENABLEX

Steady-State Darifenacin Plasma Concentration Profile from Once Daily Dosing with Extended Release Tablets

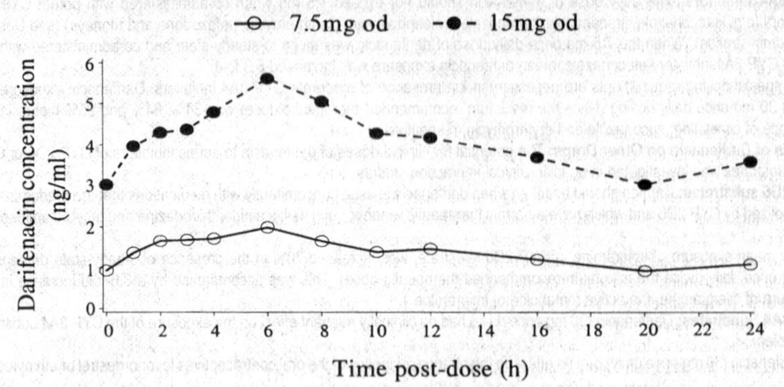

Special Populations and Conditions: Pediatrics: The pharmacokinetics of darifenacin have not been studied in the pediatric population.

Geriatrics: In a population pharmacokinetic study, there was a 23% per decade increase in bioavailability of darifenacin in subjects over the age of 65. However, there was considerable overlap between the ranges of exposure seen in younger and older patients, and, in the pivotal trials, no difference in safety and efficacy was observed in the elderly (>65 years of age) as compared to the overall population.

Gender: A population pharmacokinetic analysis of patient data indicated that darifenacin exposure at steady state was 28% lower in males than in females. In pivotal clinical studies, the safety and efficacy profiles of males and females were not found to be significantly different.

Race: The effect of race on the pharmacokinetics of darifenacin has not been characterized.

Hepatic Insufficiency: The daily dose of darifenacin should not exceed 7.5 mg for patients with moderate hepatic impairment (Child Pugh B) (see Warnings and Precautions, Dosage and Administration). There are no special dosing requirements for patients with mild hepatic impairment (Child Pugh A).

Darifenacin pharmacokinetics were investigated in subjects with mild (Child Pugh A) or moderate (Child Pugh B) impairment of hepatic function given darifenacin 15 mg once daily to steady-state. Mild hepatic impairment had no effect on the pharmacokinetics of darifenacin. However, protein binding of darifenacin was affected by moderate hepatic impairment.

After adjusting for plasma protein binding, unbound darifenacin exposure was estimated to be 4.7-fold higher in subjects with moderate hepatic impairment than subjects with normal hepatic function.

Subjects with severe hepatic impairment (Child Pugh C) have not been studied, and therefore darifenacin is not recommended for use in these patients (see Warnings and Precautions, Dosage and Administration).

Renal Insufficiency: A study of subjects with varying degrees of renal function [creatinine clearance between 10 and 136 mL/min (0.17 and 2.27 mL/s)] given darifenacin 15 mg once daily to steady-state demonstrated no relationship between renal function and darifenacin clearance. There is insufficient evidence to determine whether a dose reduction is necessary in patients with a greater degree of impairment.

STORAGE AND STABILITY: ENABLEX extended release tablets should be stored at 15 to 30°C and protected from light.

INFORMATION FOR THE PATIENT: Published in e-CPS, available by subscription at www.e-cps.ca.

DOSAGE FORMS, COMPOSITION AND PACKAGING: 7.5 mg: Each once-a-day extended release, white, round, shallow, convex film-coated tablet for oral use, debossed with "DF" on one side and "7.5" on the reverse contains darifenacin 7.5 mg as darifenacin hydrobromide. Nonmedicinal ingredients: dibasic calcium phosphate anhydrous, hypromellose, magnesium stearate, PEG 400, talc and titanium dioxide. Blister packs of 28 (7 or 14 tablets per blister).

15 mg: Each once-a-day extended release, light peach, round, shallow, convex film-coated tablet for oral use, debossed with "DF" on one side and "15" on the reverse contains: darifenacin 15 mg as darifenacin hydrobromide. Nonmedicinal ingredients: dibasic calcium phosphate anhydrous, hypromellose, iron oxide red, iron oxide yellow, magnesium stearate, PEG 400, talc and titanium dioxide. Blister packs of 28 (7 or 14 tablets per blister).

(Shown in Product Identification Section)

Enalapril

CPhA Monograph

see ***ACE Inhibitors***

Enalaprilat

CPhA Monograph

see ***ACE Inhibitors***

Enbrel®

etanercept

Biological Response Modifier

Amgen

Date of Revision: August 12, 2010

SUMMARY PRODUCT INFORMATION:

Route of Administration	Dosage Form/ Strength	Clinically Relevant Nonmedicinal Ingredients
Subcutaneous injection (SC)	Sterile solution for injection/50 mg/mL prefilled syringe (0.98 mL per syringe) and 50 mg/mL autoinjector (0.98 mL) Lyophilized powder for reconstitution/25 mg/vial	Not applicable For a complete listing see Dosage Forms, Composition and Packaging.

DESCRIPTION: ENBREL (etanercept) is a dimeric fusion protein consisting of the extracellular ligand-binding portion of the human 75 kilodalton (p75) tumor necrosis factor receptor (TNFR) linked to the Fc portion of human immunoglobulin (IgG1). Etanercept is produced by recombinant DNA technology in a Chinese hamster ovary (CHO) mammalian cell expression system. It consists of 934 amino acids and has an apparent molecular weight of approximately 150 kilodaltons.

INDICATIONS AND CLINICAL USE: ENBREL is indicated for:

- treatment of moderately to severely active rheumatoid arthritis (RA) in adults. Treatment is effective in reducing the signs and symptoms of RA, inducing major clinical response, inhibiting the progression of structural damage, and improving physical function. ENBREL can be initiated in combination with methotrexate (MTX) in adult patients or used alone.
- reducing signs and symptoms of moderately to severely active polyarticular juvenile idiopathic arthritis (JIA) in patients aged 4 to 17 years who have had an inadequate response to one or more disease-modifying antirheumatic drugs (DMARDs). ENBREL has not been studied in children less than 4 years of age.
- reducing signs and symptoms, inhibiting the progression of structural damage of active arthritis, and improving physical function in adult patients with psoriatic arthritis (PsA). ENBREL can be used in combination with methotrexate in adult patients who do not respond adequately to methotrexate alone.
- reducing signs and symptoms of active ankylosing spondylitis (AS).
- treatment of adult patients with chronic moderate to severe plaque psoriasis who are candidates for systemic therapy or phototherapy.

Improvement may be seen as early as 1 week after initial administration of ENBREL in adults, and within 2 weeks in children. Attainment of full effect was usually seen by 3 months in both populations and remained durable thereafter with continued treatment with ENBREL. Some patients see continuing improvement after 3 months of treatment with ENBREL.

After discontinuation of ENBREL, symptoms of arthritis generally returned within a month. Reintroduction of treatment with ENBREL in adults after discontinuation of up to 18 months resulted in the same magnitudes of response as patients who received ENBREL without interruption of therapy based on results of open-label studies. Reintroduction of ENBREL to children after discontinuation up to 4 months also resulted in a subsequent response to therapy.

Geriatrics (>65 years of age): Four hundred and eighty RA patients in clinical studies were age 65 or older. No overall differences in safety or effectiveness were observed between these patients and younger patients.

One hundred thirty-eight patients with plaque psoriasis in clinical studies were age 65 or older. No overall differences in effectiveness were observed between younger and older patients with psoriasis. Because there is greater sensitivity and predisposition of older individuals to infection, caution should be used in treating the elderly (see Warnings and Precautions, Special Populations, Geriatrics (>65 years of age)).

Pediatrics (<4 years of age): ENBREL is indicated for treatment of polyarticular juvenile idiopathic arthritis in patients who have had an inadequate response to one or more DMARDs. ENBREL has not been studied in children <4 years of age.

The safety and efficacy of ENBREL in pediatric patients with plaque psoriasis have not been studied.

CONTRAINDICATIONS:

- Patients who are hypersensitive to ENBREL or to any of its components. For a complete listing of the components, see Dosage Forms, Composition and Packaging.
- Patients with, or at risk of, sepsis syndrome, such as immunocompromised and HIV+ patients.

WARNINGS AND PRECAUTIONS:

Serious Warnings and Precautions

Infections

- **Serious infections leading to hospitalization or death, including sepsis, tuberculosis (TB), invasive fungal and other opportunistic infections, have been observed with the use of TNF blocking agents including ENBREL. Cases of TB may be due to reactivation of latent TB infection or to new infection.**
- **Treatment with ENBREL should not be initiated in patients with active infections including TB, chronic or localized infections. Administration of ENBREL should be discontinued if a patient develops a serious infection or sepsis.**
- **Physicians also should exercise caution when considering the use of ENBREL in patients with a history of recurring or latent infections, including TB, or with underlying conditions, which may predispose patients to infections, such as advanced or poorly controlled diabetes.**
- **Before starting treatment with ENBREL, all patients should be evaluated for both active and inactive ('latent') TB. If inactive ('latent') TB is diagnosed, treatment for latent TB should be started with anti-TB therapy before the initiation of ENBREL.**
- **Patients should be monitored for the development of signs and symptoms of infection during and after treatment with ENBREL, including the possible development of tuberculosis in patients who tested negative for latent tuberculosis infection prior to initiating therapy (see further details in Infections).**

Malignancies

- **Lymphoma and other malignancies, some fatal, have been reported in children and adolescent patients treated with TNF blockers, including ENBREL (see further detail in Malignancies, Pediatric Patients).**

Infections: Serious and sometimes fatal infections due to bacterial, mycobacterial, invasive fungal, viral, or other opportunistic pathogens have been reported in patients receiving TNF-blocking agents. Tuberculosis, histoplasmosis, aspergillosis, candidiasis, coccidioidomycosis, listeriosis, and pneumocystosis have been reported (see Adverse Reactions, Infections). Patients have frequently presented with disseminated rather than localized disease. Many of the serious infections have occurred in patients on concomitant immunosuppressive therapy that, in addition to their underlying disease, could predispose them to infections.

Treatment with ENBREL should not be initiated in patients with an active infection, including clinically important localized infections. The risks and benefits of treatment should be considered prior to initiating therapy in patients:

- **With chronic or recurrent infection**
- **Who have been exposed to tuberculosis**
- **Who have resided or traveled in areas of endemic tuberculosis or mycoses, such as histoplasmosis, coccidioidomycosis, or blastomycosis**
- **With underlying conditions that may predispose them to infection such as advanced or poorly controlled diabetes.**

Cases of reactivation of tuberculosis or new tuberculosis infections have been observed in patients receiving ENBREL, including patients who have previously received treatment for latent or active tuberculosis. Patients should be evaluated according to the Canadian Tuberculosis Standards guidelines for tuberculosis risk factors and tested for latent infection prior to initiating ENBREL and during therapy as appropriate. Prescribers are reminded of the risk of false negative tuberculin skin test results, especially in patients who are severely ill or immuno-compromised.

If active tuberculosis is diagnosed, ENBREL therapy should not be initiated. If inactive ('latent') tuberculosis is diagnosed, treatment for latent TB should be started with anti-tuberculosis therapy before the initiation of ENBREL. In this situation, the benefit/risk balance of ENBREL therapy should be very carefully considered. Anti-tuberculosis therapy should also be considered prior to initiation of ENBREL in patients with a past history of latent or active tuberculosis in whom an adequate course of treatment cannot be confirmed, and for patients with a negative test for latent tuberculosis but having risk factors for tuberculosis infection. Consultation with a physician with expertise in the treatment of tuberculosis is recommended to aid in the decision whether initiating anti-tuberculosis therapy is appropriate for an individual patient.

Patients should be monitored for the development of signs and symptoms of infection during and after treatment with ENBREL, including the possible development of tuberculosis in patients who tested negative for latent tuberculosis infection prior to initiating therapy. Tests for latent tuberculosis infection may be falsely negative while on therapy with ENBREL.

Tuberculosis should be strongly considered in patients who develop a new infection during ENBREL treatment, especially in patients who have previously or recently traveled to countries with a high prevalence of tuberculosis, or who have had close contact with a person with active tuberculosis.

Histoplasmosis and other invasive fungal infections are not consistently recognized in patients taking TNF blockers, including ENBREL. This has resulted in delays in appropriate treatment, sometimes resulting in death. For patients who reside or travel in regions where mycoses are endemic, invasive fungal infection should be suspected if they develop a serious systemic illness. Appropriate empiric antifungal therapy may be initiated while a diagnostic workup is being performed. Antigen and antibody testing for histoplasmosis may be negative in some patients with active infection. When feasible, the decision to administer empiric antifungal therapy in these patients should be made in consultation with a physician with expertise in the diagnosis and treatment of invasive fungal infections and taking into account both the risk for severe fungal infection and the risks of antifungal therapy.

ENBREL should be discontinued if a patient develops a serious infection or sepsis. A patient who develops a new infection during treatment with ENBREL should be closely monitored, undergo a prompt and complete diagnostic workup appropriate for an immunocompromised patient, and antimicrobial therapy should be initiated, as appropriate.

In post-marketing studies of patients with juvenile idiopathic arthritis, serious infections have been reported in approximately 3% of patients. Sepsis has also been reported in the post-market setting (0.8%).

Neurologic: Treatment with TNF blocking agents, including ENBREL, has been associated with rare cases of new onset or exacerbation of central nervous system disorders, including demyelinating disorders, some presenting with mental status changes and some associated with permanent disability, and with peripheral nervous system demyelinating disorders. Rare cases of transverse myelitis, optic neuritis, and new onset or exacerbation of seizure disorders have been observed in association with ENBREL therapy. Guillain-Barré like syndromes have been reported very rarely in postmarketing experience with ENBREL therapy. While no clinical trials have been performed evaluating ENBREL therapy in patients with multiple sclerosis, other TNF antagonists administered to patients with multiple sclerosis have been associated with increases in disease activity. Prescribers should exercise caution in considering the use of ENBREL in patients with pre-existing or recent-onset or peripheral central nervous system demyelinating disorders. Development of new, confirmed central nervous system demyelination in patients on ENBREL warrants consideration of discontinuation of the medication.

Hematologic: Rare cases (less than 1 case out of 1000 patients treated) of neutropenia, leukopenia, thrombocytopenia, anemia and pancytopenia (including aplastic anemia), some with fatal outcomes, have been reported in patients treated with ENBREL. Cases of pancytopenia occurred as early as two weeks after initiating ENBREL therapy. The causal relationship to ENBREL therapy remains unclear. While the majority of patients who developed pancytopenia had recent or concurrent exposure to other anti-rheumatic medications known to be associated with myelosuppression (eg, methotrexate, leflunomide, azathioprine, and cyclophosphamide), some patients had no recent or concurrent exposure to such therapies. Although no high risk group has been identified, caution should be exercised in patients being treated with ENBREL who have a previous history of significant hematologic abnormalities. All patients should be advised to seek immediate medical attention if they develop signs and symptoms suggestive of blood dyscrasias or infection (eg, persistent fever, bruising, bleeding, pallor) while on ENBREL. Discontinuation of ENBREL therapy should be considered in patients with confirmed significant hematologic abnormalities.

Patients treated with anakinra plus etanercept (3/139, 2%) developed neutropenia (ANC <1×10⁹/L). While neutropenic, one of these patients developed cellulitis that resolved with antibiotic therapy.

Malignancies: Lymphomas: In the controlled portions of clinical trials of all the TNF-blocking agents, more cases of lymphoma have been observed among patients receiving the TNF blocker compared to control patients. In the controlled and open-label portions of clinical trials of ENBREL in RA, AS, and PsA patients, the observed rate of lymphoma was 0.10 cases per 100 patient-years. This is 3-fold higher than expected in the general population. Patients with rheumatoid arthritis or psoriasis, particularly those with highly active disease and/or chronic exposure to immunosuppressant therapies, may be at a higher risk (up to several fold) for the development of lymphoma.

Leukemia: Cases of acute and chronic leukemia have been reported in association with post-marketing TNF-blocker use in rheumatoid arthritis and other indications. Even in the absence of TNF-blocker therapy, patients with rheumatoid arthritis may be at higher risk (approximately 2-fold) than the general population for the development of leukemia.

During the controlled portions of ENBREL trials, 2 cases of leukemia were observed among 5445 (0.06 cases per 100 patient-years) ENBREL-treated patients versus 0 among 2890 (0%) control patients (duration of controlled treatment ranged from 3 to 48 months).

Among 15 401 patients treated with ENBREL in controlled and open portions of clinical trials representing approximately 23 325 patient-years of therapy, the observed rate of leukemia was 0.03 cases per 100 patient-years (see Adverse Reactions, Clinical Trial Adverse Drug Reactions, Malignancies).

Other Malignancies: For malignancies other than lymphoma and non-melanoma skin cancer, there was no difference in exposure-adjusted rates between the ENBREL and control arms in the controlled portions of clinical studies for all indications. Analysis of the malignancy rate in combined controlled and uncontrolled portions of studies has demonstrated that types and rates are similar to what is expected in the general population based on the Surveillance, Epidemiology, and End Results (SEER) Database of the National Cancer Institute and suggest no increase in rates over time.

Whether treatment with ENBREL might influence the development and course of malignancies in adults is unknown (see Adverse Reactions, Less Common Clinical Trial Adverse Drug Reactions, Malignancies).

Melanoma and Non-melanoma Skin Cancer (NMSC): Melanoma and non-melanoma skin cancer (NMSC) have been reported in patients treated with TNF-antagonists, including ENBREL. In controlled and open portions of clinical trials among 15 401 patients treated with ENBREL representing approximately 23 325 patient-years of therapy, the observed rate of melanoma was 0.043 cases per 100 patient years. In controlled clinical trials of rheumatology (RA, AS, PsA) patients, the observed rate of NMSC was 0.41 cases per 100 patient-years in the ENBREL-treated patients compared to 0.37 cases per 100 patient-years among control patients. In controlled clinical trials of psoriasis patients, the observed rate of NMSC was 3.54 cases per 100 patient-years in the ENBREL-treated patients compared to 1.28 cases per 100 patient-years among control patients (see Adverse Reactions, Clinical Trial Adverse Drug Reactions, Malignancies). Post-marketing cases of Merkel cell carcinoma have been reported very infrequently in patients treated with ENBREL. Risk factors for melanoma or NMSC include cumulative exposure to ultraviolet light, increasing age, male gender, fair complexion, history of acute sunburn or skin cancer, tobacco use, and immunosuppressive agents. Periodic skin examination should be considered for all patients at increased risk for skin cancers.

Pediatric Patients: Malignancies, some fatal, have been reported among children, adolescents and young adults (≤22 years of age) who initiated treatment with TNF-blocking agents (initiation of therapy at ≤18 years of age), including ENBREL. These cases were reported post-marketing and are derived from a variety of sources including registries and spontaneous post-marketing reports. Approximately half the cases were lymphomas, including Hodgkin's and non-Hodgkin's lymphoma. Of these cases, hepatosplenic T-cell lymphoma was not reported in patients treated with ENBREL. The other cases represented a variety of different malignancies and included rare malignancies usually associated with immunosuppression and malignancies that are not usually observed in children and adolescents. Approximately half of these malignancies occurred in patients being treated for inflammatory bowel disease; approximately one-third of the cases occurred in patients being treated for JIA. The malignancies occurred after a median of 30 months of therapy (range 1 to 84 months). Most of the patients were receiving concomitant immunosuppressants.

In clinical trials of 696 patients treated with ENBREL, representing 1282 patient-years of therapy, no malignancies, including lymphoma or NMSC, have been reported.

Wegener's Granulomatosis: In a randomized placebo controlled study of 180 patients with Wegener's granulomatosis, the addition of ENBREL to standard treatment (including cyclophosphamide, methotrexate, and corticosteroids) was no more efficacious than standard therapy alone. Patients receiving ENBREL experienced more non-cutaneous malignancies than patients receiving placebo. The role of ENBREL in this finding is uncertain due to imbalances between the two arms of the study including age, disease duration, and use of cyclophosphamide. The use of ENBREL in patients with Wegener's granulomatosis receiving immunosuppressive agents is not recommended. The use of ENBREL in any patients receiving concurrent cyclophosphamide therapy is not recommended.

General: Parenteral administration of any biologic product should be attended by appropriate precautions in case an allergic or untoward reaction occurs. Allergic reactions associated with administration of ENBREL during clinical trials have been reported in <2% of patients. If any serious allergic or anaphylactic reaction occurs, administration of ENBREL should be discontinued immediately and appropriate therapy initiated.

Caution: The needle cap on the prefilled syringe and on the SureClick autoinjector contains dry natural rubber (a derivative of latex), which may cause allergic reactions in individuals sensitive to latex.

Concurrent ENBREL and Anakinra Treatment: Serious infections and neutropenia were seen in clinical studies with concurrent use of anakinra and ENBREL with no added clinical benefit compared to ENBREL alone. Because of the nature of the adverse events seen with combination of ENBREL and anakinra therapy, the combination of ENBREL and anakinra is not recommended (see Drug Interactions).

Concurrent ENBREL and Abatacept Treatment: In clinical studies, concurrent administration of abatacept and ENBREL resulted in increased incidences of serious adverse events and did not demonstrate increased clinical benefit. Use of ENBREL with abatacept is not recommended (see Drug-Drug Interactions).

Switching between Biological DMARDS: When switching from one biologic to another, patients should continue to be monitored for signs of infection.

Cardiovascular: There have been post-marketing reports of worsening of congestive heart failure (CHF), with and without identifiable precipitating factors, in patients taking ENBREL. Physicians should exercise caution when using ENBREL in patients who also have CHF.

Two large clinical trials (2048 patients) evaluating the use of ENBREL in the treatment of heart failure were terminated early due to lack of efficacy. There was a suggestion of worse heart failure outcomes in patients with moderate to severe CHF (NYHA Class IIIB) receiving ENBREL treatment compared to patients receiving placebo in one of the two trials.

Immune: Immunosuppression and Immunocompetence: The possibility exists for anti-TNF therapies, including ENBREL, to affect host defenses against infections and malignancies since TNF mediates inflammation and modulates cellular immune responses. In a study of 49 patients with RA treated with ENBREL, there was no evidence of depression of delayed-type hypersensitivity, depression of immunoglobulin levels, or change in enumeration of effector cell populations. The role of ENBREL in the development and course of malignancies as well as active and/or chronic infections is not fully understood. The safety and efficacy of ENBREL in patients with immunosuppression or chronic infections have not been evaluated.

Immunizations: Live vaccines (including yellow fever, BCG, rubella, polio, cholera, typhoid and varicella) should not be given concurrently with ENBREL. No data are available on the secondary transmission of infection by live vaccines in patients receiving ENBREL.

No data are available on the effects of vaccination in RA patients receiving ENBREL. Most psoriatic arthritis patients receiving ENBREL were able to mount effective B-cell immune response to pneumococcal polysaccharide vaccine, but titers in aggregate were moderately lower and fewer patients had two-fold rises in titers compared to patients not receiving ENBREL. The clinical significance of this is unknown. In a study of 205 adult patients with psoriatic arthritis, antibody response to polysaccharide pneumococcal vaccine was similar in patients receiving placebo or ENBREL for the following antigens: 9V, 14, 18C, 19F and 23F.

It is recommended that JIA patients, if possible, be brought up to date with all immunizations in agreement with current immunizations guidelines prior to initiating ENBREL therapy. Two JIA patients developed varicella infection and signs and symptoms of aseptic meningitis, which resolved without sequelae. Patients with a significant exposure to varicella virus should temporarily discontinue ENBREL therapy and be considered for prophylactic treatment with Varicella Zoster Immune Globulin.

Autoimmunity: Treatment with ENBREL may result in the formation of autoantibodies and, rarely, can result in the development of lupus-like syndrome or autoimmune hepatitis, which may resolve following withdrawal of ENBREL. If a patient develops symptoms and findings suggestive of a lupus-like syndrome or autoimmune hepatitis following treatment with ENBREL, treatment should be discontinued and the patient should be carefully evaluated.

Hepatic/Biliary/Pancreatic: Hepatitis B Reactivation: Very rare cases of Hepatitis B virus (HBV) reactivation have been reported in patients treated with TNF antagonists. In the majority of cases, patients were also being treated with other immunosuppressive drugs, including methotrexate, azathioprine, and/or corticosteroids. Reactivation of HBV is not unique to TNF antagonists and has been reported with other immunosuppressive drugs. Therefore, a direct causal relationship to TNF antagonists has not been established. Patients at risk for HBV infection should be evaluated for prior evidence of HBV infection before initiating TNF antagonist therapy. Those identified as chronic HBV carriers (i.e. surface antigen positive) should be monitored for signs and symptoms of active HBV infection throughout the course of therapy and for several months following discontinuation of therapy.

Use in Patients with Moderate to Severe Alcoholic Hepatitis: Physicians should use caution when using ENBREL in patients with moderate to severe alcoholic hepatitis. In a study of 48 hospitalized patients treated with ENBREL or placebo for moderate to severe alcoholic hepatitis, the mortality rate in patients treated with ENBREL was similar to patients treated with placebo at one month but significantly higher after six months. Therefore, the use of ENBREL for the treatment of patients with alcoholic hepatitis is not recommended.

Carcinogenesis, Mutagenesis, and Impairment of Fertility: Long-term animal studies have not been conducted to evaluate the carcinogenic potential of ENBREL or its effect on fertility. Mutagenesis studies were conducted in vitro and in vivo, and no evidence of mutagenic activity was observed.

Special Populations: Pregnant Women: There have been no studies in pregnant women. ENBREL should not be used during pregnancy unless benefits outweigh the risks (see Adverse Reactions and Warnings and Precautions). ENBREL has no established use in labour or delivery.

Developmental toxicity studies have been performed in rats and rabbits at doses ranging from 60- to 100-fold higher than the human dose and have revealed no evidence of harm to the fetus due to ENBREL. Because animal reproduction studies are not always predictive of human response, this drug should be used during pregnancy only if clearly needed.

Pregnancy Registry: To monitor outcomes of pregnant women exposed to ENBREL, a pregnancy registry has been established. Physicians are encouraged to register patients by calling 1-877-311-8972.

Nursing Women: It is not known whether ENBREL is excreted in human milk or absorbed systemically after ingestion. Because many drugs and immunoglobulins are excreted in human milk, and because of the potential of serious adverse reactions in nursing infants from ENBREL, a decision should be made whether to discontinue nursing or to discontinue the drug.

Pediatrics: ENBREL is indicated for treatment of polyarticular juvenile idiopathic arthritis in patients who have had an inadequate response to one or more DMARDs. In post-marketing studies with juvenile idiopathic arthritis, serious infections have been reported in approximately 3% of patients. Sepsis has also been reported in the post-market setting (0.8%). The long-term effects of ENBREL therapy on skeletal, behavioural, cognitive, sexual and immune maturation and development in children are unknown.

A higher rate of adverse events was noted when juvenile idiopathic arthritis patients in an observational registry received ENBREL therapy in combination with methotrexate. As the juvenile idiopathic arthritis patients receiving combination therapy had more severe disease, since they had failed prior therapeutic trials with either ENBREL or methotrexate alone, it remains unclear whether the higher event rate is related to therapy or underlying disease severity.

There have been reports of Inflammatory Bowel Disease (IBD) in juvenile idiopathic arthritis (JIA) patients receiving ENBREL, which is not effective for the treatment of IBD. A causal relationship with ENBREL is unclear because clinical manifestations of bowel inflammation have also been observed in untreated JIA patients.

ENBREL has not been studied in children <2 years of age.

The safety and efficacy of ENBREL in pediatric patients with plaque psoriasis have not been studied.

Geriatrics (>65 years of age): Four hundred and eighty clinical study patients in RA were age 65 or older. No overall differences in safety or effectiveness were observed between these patients and younger patients.

One hundred and thirty-eight plaque psoriasis patients in clinical studies were age 65 or older. No overall differences in effectiveness were observed between younger and older psoriasis patients. In controlled trials of plaque psoriasis, rates of serious adverse events were seen at a frequency of <1.5% among ENBREL- and placebo-treated patients in the first 3 months of treatment. However, in patients greater than 65 years of age treated with ENBREL 50 mg twice weekly, serious adverse events occurred at a higher rate than in younger patients. In long-term open-label trials of plaque psoriasis serious non-infectious adverse events were infrequent and exposure-adjusted event rates generally remained stable throughout ENBREL treatment. Although data for patients aged 65 or greater in the long-term trials are limited, adverse events, including serious adverse events, occurred at a higher frequency for patients treated with 50 mg twice weekly (see Adverse Reactions, Adverse Drug Reaction Overview).

Greater sensitivity of some older individuals cannot be ruled out. Predisposition of older individuals to infection justifies greater caution when treating the elderly.

Use in Diabetics: There have been reports of hypoglycemia following initiation of ENBREL in patients receiving medication for diabetes, necessitating a reduction in anti-diabetic medication in some of these patients.

ADVERSE REACTIONS: Adverse Drug Reaction Overview: Adverse Reactions in Adult Patients with RA, Psoriatic Arthritis, Ankylosing Spondylitis or Plaque Psoriasis: ENBREL has been studied in 1442 patients with RA followed for up to 80 months, in 169 adult patients with psoriatic arthritis for up to 24 months, in 222 patients with ankylosing spondylitis for up to 48 months and in 1864 patients with plaque psoriasis for up to 36 months. ENBREL has over one million patient-years of exposure post-market.

Among patients with RA treated in placebo-controlled studies, serious adverse events occurred at a frequency of 4% in 349 patients treated with ENBREL compared to 5% of 152 placebo-treated patients. In a subsequent study (Study III), serious adverse events occurred at a frequency of 6% in 415 patients treated with ENBREL compared to 8% of 217 methotrexate-treated patients. Among adult patients with psoriatic arthritis, serious adverse events occurred at a frequency of 4% in 101 patients treated with ENBREL compared to 4% of 104 placebo-treated patients.

In controlled trials of plaque psoriasis, rates of serious adverse events were seen at a frequency of <1.5% among ENBREL- and placebo-treated patients in the first 3 months of treatment. However, in patients greater than 65 years of age treated with ENBREL 50 mg twice weekly, serious adverse events occurred at a higher rate than in younger patients.

In long-term open-label trials of plaque psoriasis serious non-infectious adverse events were infrequent and exposure-adjusted event rates generally remained stable throughout ENBREL treatment. Although data for patients aged 65 or greater in the long-term trials are limited, adverse events, including serious adverse events, occurred at a higher frequency for patients treated with 50 mg twice weekly.

Among RA patients in placebo-controlled, active-controlled, and open-label trials of ENBREL, infections and malignancies were the most common serious adverse events observed. Other infrequent serious adverse events observed in RA, psoriatic arthritis, ankylosing spondylitis or plaque psoriasis clinical trials are listed below by body system:

Cardiovascular: cardiomyopathy, fainting, heart failure, hypertension, hypotension, myocardial infarction, myocardial ischemia, deep vein thrombosis, thrombophlebitis.

Digestive: cholecystitis, diarrhea, esophageal ulcer, gastrointestinal hemorrhage, pancreatitis, appendicitis.

General: impaired healing, asthenia.

Hematologic/Lymphatic: lymphadenopathy, myelodysplastic syndrome, necrotizing granulomatous lymphadenitis.

Hepatic: hepatic disorder, hepatic steatosis.

Musculoskeletal: bursitis, fistula, fracture nonunion, polymyositis.

Nervous: anxiety, cerebral ischemia, convulsion, depression, multiple sclerosis.
Respiratory: asthma, dyspnea, pulmonary embolism, sarcoidosis.
Skin: worsening psoriasis.
Urogenital: membranous glomerulonephropathy, kidney calculus.

In a randomized controlled trial in which 51 patients with RA received ENBREL 50 mg twice weekly and 25 patients received ENBREL 25 mg twice weekly, the following serious adverse events were observed in the 50 mg twice weekly arm: gastrointestinal bleeding, normal pressure hydrocephalus, seizure, and stroke. No serious adverse events were observed in the 25 mg arm.

In controlled trials, the proportion of patients who discontinued treatment due to adverse events was approximately 4% in both the ENBREL and placebo treatment groups. The vast majority of these patients were treated with the recommended dose of 25 mg SC twice weekly. In plaque psoriasis studies, ENBREL doses studied were 25 mg SC once or twice a week and 50 mg SC once or twice a week. In three randomized, placebo-controlled studies of plaque psoriasis, the safety profile for patients receiving 50 mg twice a week was similar to those receiving 25 mg once or twice weekly, and all were similar to placebo. No cumulative toxicities were observed in long term studies in plaque psoriasis up to 144 weeks and ankylosing spondylitis up to 192 weeks.

Among patients with rheumatoid arthritis in placebo-controlled studies, deaths occurred in 10 of 2696 (0.37%) ENBREL-treated patients compared to 3 of 1167 (0.26%) placebo-treated patients. In controlled and uncontrolled RA studies there were 58 deaths in 6973 patient treated with at least one dose of ENBREL over an exposure period of 11 765 patient-years (exposure-adjusted rate of 0.49). Among patients with plaque psoriasis in placebo-controlled studies, deaths occurred in 1 of 1245 (0.08%) ENBREL-treated patients compared to 0 of 720 placebo-treated patients. In controlled and uncontrolled psoriasis studies there were 10 deaths in 4361 patient treated with at least one dose of ENBREL over an exposure period of 3966 patient-years (exposure-adjusted rate of 0.25). No deaths were reported in PsA, AS, or JIA studies.

Clinical Trial Adverse Drug Reactions: Because clinical trials are conducted under very specific conditions the adverse reaction rates observed in the clinical trials may not reflect the rates observed in practice and should not be compared to the rates in the clinical trials of another drug. Adverse drug reaction information from clinical trials is useful for identifying drug-related adverse events and for approximating rates.

Adverse reactions reported in at least 1% of all patients who received ENBREL in placebo-controlled RA trials (including the combination methotrexate trial) are outlined in Table 1. Adverse reactions reported in juvenile idiopathic arthritis, adult psoriatic arthritis, ankylosing spondylitis, and plaque psoriasis trials were similar to those reported in RA clinical trials.

Table 1: ENBREL

Percent of RA Patients Reporting Adverse Reactions ≥1% by Body System and Preferred Term in Controlled Clinical Trials[a]

	Placebo-Controlled Percent of patients		Active-Controlled Percent of patients	
Body System Preferred Term	**Placebo (N=152)**	**Etanercept (N=349)**	**Methotrexate (N=217)**	**Etanercept (N=415)**
Injection site reaction	10	37	7	33
Infection[b]	32	35	72	64
Non-upper respiratory infection[c]	31	39	60	51
Upper respiratory infection[c]	16	29	39	31
Other Adverse Events				
Body as a Whole				
Headache	3	3	13	12
Asthenia	0	1	7	5
Abdominal pain	1	1	5	4
Injection site hemorrhage	0	0	2	4
Pain	1	0	1	1
Mucous membrane disorder	0	1	2	0
Chills	0	0	2	0
Face edema	0	0	1	0
Fever	0	0	1	0
Cardiovascular System				
Vasodilation	1	1	1	1
Hypertension	0	0	0	1
Digestive System				
Nausea	3	2	18	9
Diarrhea	1	1	5	7
Dyspepsia	0	0	3	6
Mouth ulcer	0	1	11	4
Constipation	1	0	3	2
Vomiting	0	0	4	1
Anorexia	0	0	2	1
Flatulence	0	0	2	1
Stomatitis aphthous	0	0	2	1
Dry mouth	0	1	0	1
Stomatitis	0	0	3	0
Hemic and Lymphatic System				
Ecchymosis	1	0	2	2
Metabolic and Nutritional Disorders				
Peripheral edema	0	0	1	2
Weight increased	0	0	1	1
Abnormal healing	0	0	1	0
Musculoskeletal System				
Leg cramps	0	1	1	0
Nervous System				
Dizziness	1	3	5	5
Vertigo	0	0	0	1
Respiratory System				
Rhinitis	2	2	5	4
Dyspnea	0	0	1	3
Pharyngitis	0	1	2	2
Cough increased	1	1	2	1
Epistaxis	0	0	3	0
Voice alteration	0	0	1	0
Skin and Appendages				
Rash	2	3	10	6
Alopecia	0	1	11	5
Pruritus	1	2	1	2
Urticaria	1	0	2	1
Sweat	0	0	1	1
Nail disorder	0	0	2	0
Special Senses				
Dry eye	0	0	0	1
Tinnitus	0	0	0	1
Amblyopia	0	0	1	0

(cont'd)

Table 1: ENBREL (cont'd)

[a] Includes data from the double-blinded studies in which patients received concurrent MTX therapy.
[b] Infection (total) includes data from all three placebo-controlled trials. Body system and relationship to study drug was not collected for infections.
[c] Non-URI and URI include data only from two placebo-controlled trials where infections were collected separately from adverse events (placebo N=110, Etanercept N=213).
Legend: N=Number of subjects having received at least 1 dose of study drug; Percent=n/N*100.

Less Common Clinical Trial Adverse Drug Reactions (<1%): The following adverse reactions were reported at an incidence of <1% (occurring in more than 1 patient, with higher frequency than placebo):
Body as a Whole: enlarged abdomen, general edema, hernia, infection, injection site reaction, malaise, overdose, Sjögren's syndrome.
Cardiovascular: cerebrovascular accident, hypotension, myocardial infarction, phlebitis, deep thrombophlebitis.
Gastrointestinal: increased appetite, colitis, dysphagia, glossitis, gum hemorrhage, rectal hemorrhage.
Hemic and Lymphatic System: petechia.
Metabolic and Nutritional Disorders: edema, hypercholesteremia, hyperglycemia.
Musculoskeletal System: arthrosis, bone disorder, fibrosis tendon, bone necrosis.
Nervous System: nervousness, neuropathy.
Respiratory System: bronchitis, lung carcinoma, hemoptysis, laryngitis.
Skin and Appendages: skin carcinoma, dermatitis exfoliative, skin hypertrophy, skin discoloration, skin ulcer.
Special Senses: corneal lesion, ear disorder, eye hemorrhage, otitis media.
Urogenital System: cervix disorder, cystitis, dysuria, gynecomastia, uterine hemorrhage, kidney polycystic, cervix neoplasm, polyuria, urine urgency.
Injection Site Reactions: In controlled trials in rheumatologic indications, approximately 37% of patients treated with ENBREL developed injection site reactions. In controlled trials in patients with plaque psoriasis, approximately 14% of patients treated with ENBREL developed injection site reactions during the first 3 months of treatment. In a long-term plaque psoriasis study the exposure-adjusted rate of injections site reactions was 12.2 per 100 patient-years for patients treated with ENBREL 50 mg twice weekly over 96 weeks compared to 6.1 per 100-patient-years for placebo-treated patients (treated for 12 weeks). All injection site reactions were described as mild to moderate (erythema and/or itching, pain, or swelling). Injection site reactions generally occurred in the first month, if they occurred at all, did not necessitate study drug discontinuation, and subsequently decreased in frequency after the first month. The mean duration was 3 to 5 days. No treatment was given for approximately 90% of injection site reactions, and most of the patients who were given treatment received topical preparations, such as corticosteroids, or oral antihistamines. There have been common occurrences (7%) of redness at a previous injection site when subsequent injections were given; however, no intervention was necessary. In post-marketing experience, there have been reported cases (1.8% of all patients treated) of injection site bleeding and bruising observed in conjunction with ENBREL therapy.
Infections: The percent of patients reporting infections in controlled studies of ENBREL in psoriasis, rheumatoid arthritis, psoriatic arthritis and ankylosing spondylitis is provided in Table 2. The most common type of infection was upper respiratory infection.

Table 2: ENBREL

Percent of Patients Reporting Infections Across Controlled Studies in Psoriasis, Rheumatoid Arthritis, Psoriatic Arthritis and Ankylosing Spondylitis

	Event		
	Total Infections	**Non-URI**	**URI**
Psoriasis			
Placebo (N=271)	26%	17%	9%
ENBREL (N=1244)	30%	21%	10%
Rheumatoid Arthritis (Placebo-Controlled)			
Placebo (N=152)	32%	31%	16%
ENBREL (N=349)	35%	39%	29%[a]
Rheumatoid Arthritis (Active-Controlled)			
MTX (N=217)	72%	60%	39%
ENBREL (N=415)	64%[a]	51%	31%
Psoriatic Arthritis			
Placebo (N=104)	43%	20%	23%
ENBREL (N=101)	40%	19%	21%
Ankylosing Spondylitis			
Placebo (N=139)	30%	20%	12%
ENBREL (N=138)	41%	24%	20%[a]

[a] Fisher's exact p-value <0.05.
Legend: URI=upper respiratory infection.

In placebo-controlled trials in RA, psoriatic arthritis, ankylosing spondylitis, and plaque psoriasis no increase in the incidence of serious infections was observed (approximately 1% in both placebo and ENBREL-treated groups). In all clinical trials in RA, serious infections experienced by patients have included pyelonephritis, bronchitis, septic arthritis, abdominal abscess, cellulitis, osteomyelitis, wound infection, pneumonia, foot abscess, leg ulcer, diarrhea, sinusitis and sepsis. The rate of serious infections has not increased in open-label extension trials and is similar to that observed in controlled trials (Table 3). Serious infections, including sepsis and death, have also been reported during post-marketing use of ENBREL. Some have occurred within a few weeks after initiating treatment with ENBREL. Many of the patients had underlying conditions (e.g., diabetes, congestive heart failure, history of active or chronic infections) in addition to their RA. Data from a sepsis clinical trial not specifically in patients with RA suggest that ENBREL treatment may increase mortality in patients with established sepsis.

Table 3: ENBREL

Serious Infections Over Time

	All ENBREL[a] (n=1341)		
Year	**Number of Subjects**	**Number of Subjects with Events**	**Incidence Rate**
1	1341	46	0.034
2	1088	27	0.025
3	984	29	0.029
4	865	21	0.024
5	740	17	0.023
6	425	7	0.016

[a] Controlled trials and open-label extension studies in RA.

In controlled trials in adult patients with psoriatic arthritis, there were no differences in rates of infection among patients treated for up to 1 year with ENBREL and those treated with placebo, and no serious infections occurred in patients treated with ENBREL.

In a controlled trial in patients with ankylosing spondylitis, rates of infection were also similar to those observed in the controlled studies of patients with RA or psoriatic arthritis. No increase in the incidence of serious infections was observed in patients treated with ENBREL.

In clinical trials in plaque psoriasis, serious infections experienced by ENBREL-treated patients have included cellulitis, gastroenteritis, pneumonia, abscess, osteomyelitis, viral meningitis, myositis, fascial infection and septic shock.

In 2 studies in which patients were receiving both etanercept and anakinra for up to 24 weeks, the incidence of serious infections was 7%. The most common infections consisted of bacterial pneumonia (4 cases) and cellulitis (4 cases). One patient with pulmonary fibrosis and pneumonia died due to respiratory failure.

In post-marketing experience infections have been observed with various pathogens including viral, bacterial, mycobacterial, fungal, and protozoal organisms. Infections, including opportunistic infections (including atypical mycobacterial infection, herpes zoster, aspergillosis, *P. jiroveci* pneumonia, histoplasmosis, candidiasis, coccidioidomycosis, and listeriosis), have been noted and have been reported in patients receiving ENBREL alone or in combination with immunosuppressive agents.

In global ENBREL clinical studies of 20 070 patients (28 308 patient-years of therapy), tuberculosis was observed in approximately 0.01% of patients. In 15 438 patients (23 524 patient-years of therapy) from clinical studies in the US and Canada, tuberculosis was observed in approximately 0.007% of patients. These studies include reports of pulmonary and extra-pulmonary tuberculosis (see Warnings and Precautions, Infections).

In 38 ENBREL clinical trials and 4 cohort studies in all approved indications representing 27 169 patient-years of exposure (17 696 patients) from the United States and Canada, no histoplasmosis infections were reported among patients treated with ENBREL. Data from clinical studies and post-marketing reports suggest that differences may exist in the risk of invasive histoplasmosis infection among TNF blockers. Nonetheless, post-marketing cases of serious and sometimes fatal fungal infections, including histoplasmosis, have been reported with TNF blockers, including ENBREL (see Warnings and Precautions, Infections).

Malignancies: Information is available from 10 953 adult patients with 17 123 patient-years and 696 pediatric patients with 1282 patient-years of experience across 45 ENBREL clinical studies.

Lymphomas: In the controlled portions of clinical trials of TNF-blocking agents, more cases of lymphoma have been observed among patients receiving a TNF blocker compared to control patients. During the controlled portions of ENBREL trials in adult patients with RA, AS, and PsA, 2 lymphomas were observed among 3306 ENBREL-treated patients versus 0 among 1521 control patients (duration of controlled treatment ranged from 3 to 36 months).

Among 6543 adult rheumatology (RA, PsA, AS) patients treated with ENBREL in controlled and uncontrolled portions of clinical trials, representing approximately 12 845 patient-years of therapy, the observed rate of lymphoma was 0.10 cases per 100 patient-years. This was 3-fold higher than the rate of lymphoma expected in the general population based on the SEER Database. An increased rate of lymphoma up to several-fold has been reported in the RA patient population, and may be further increased in patients with more severe disease activity.

Among 4410 adult psoriasis patients treated with ENBREL in clinical trials up to 36 months, representing approximately 4278 patient-years of therapy, the observed rate of lymphoma was 0.05 cases per 100 patient-years, which is comparable to the rate in the general population. No cases were observed in ENBREL- or placebo-treated patients during the controlled portions of these trials.

Leukemia: Cases of acute and chronic leukemia have been reported in association with post-marketing TNF-blocker use in rheumatoid arthritis and other indications. Even in the absence of TNF-blocker therapy, patients with rheumatoid arthritis may be at higher risk (approximately 2-fold) than the general population for the development of leukemia.

During the controlled portions of ENBREL trials, 2 cases of leukemia were observed among 5445 (0.06 cases per 100 patient-years) ENBREL-treated patients versus 0 among 2890 (0%) control patients (duration of controlled treatment ranged from 3 to 48 months).

Among 15 401 patients treated with ENBREL in controlled and open portions of clinical trials representing approximately 23 325 patient-years of therapy, the observed rate of leukemia was 0.03 cases per 100 patient-years.

Other Malignancies: For malignancies other than lymphoma and non-melanoma skin cancer, there was no difference in exposure-adjusted rates between the ENBREL and control arms in the controlled portions of clinical studies for all indications. Analysis of the malignancy rate in combined controlled and uncontrolled portions of studies has demonstrated that types and rates are similar to what is expected in the general population based on the SEER database and suggest no increase in rates over time.

Whether treatment with ENBREL might influence the development and course of malignancies in adults is unknown.

Melanoma and Non-melanoma skin cancer (NMSC): Melanoma and non-melanoma skin cancer (NMSC) have been reported in patients treated with TNF-antagonists, including ENBREL. Among 15 401 patients treated with ENBREL in controlled and open portions of clinical trials representing approximately 23 325 patient-years of therapy, the observed rate of melanoma was 0.043 cases per 100 patient years. Among 3306 adult rheumatology (RA, PsA, AS) patients treated with ENBREL in controlled clinical trials, representing approximately 2669 patient-years of therapy, the observed rate of NMSC was 0.41 cases per 100 patient-years vs. 0.37 cases per 100 patient-years among 1521 control patients representing 1077 patient-years. Among 1245 adult psoriasis patients treated with ENBREL in controlled clinical trials, representing approximately 283 patient-years of therapy, the observed rate of NMSC was 3.54 cases per 100 patient-years vs. 1.28 cases per 100 patient-years among 720 control patients representing 156 patient-years.

Among 89 patients with Wegener's granulomatosis receiving ENBREL in a randomized, placebo-controlled trial, 5 experienced a variety of non-cutaneous solid malignancies compared with none receiving placebo (see Warnings and Precautions, Wegener's Granulomatosis).

Autoantibodies: Patients had serum samples tested for autoantibodies at multiple time points. In RA Studies I and II, the percentage of patients evaluated for antinuclear antibodies (ANA) who developed new positive ANA (1:40) was higher in patients treated with ENBREL (11%) than in placebo-treated patients (5%). The percentage of patients who developed new positive anti-double-stranded DNA antibodies was also higher by radioimmunoassay (15% of patients treated with ENBREL compared to 4% of placebo-treated patients) and by Crithidia luciliae assay (3% of patients treated with ENBREL compared to none of placebo-treated patients). The proportion of patients treated with ENBREL who developed anticardiolipin antibodies was similarly increased compared to placebo-treated patients. In Study III, no pattern of increased autoantibody development was seen in ENBREL patients compared to methotrexate patients.

The impact of long-term treatment with ENBREL on the development of autoimmune diseases is unknown. Rare adverse event reports have described patients with rheumatoid factor positive and/or erosive RA who have developed additional autoantibodies in conjunction with rash and other features suggesting a lupus-like syndrome.

Immunogenicity: Patients with RA, psoriatic arthritis, ankylosing spondylitis or plaque psoriasis were tested at multiple time points for antibodies to ENBREL. Non-neutralizing antibodies to the TNF receptor portion or other protein components of the ENBREL drug product were detected at least once in sera of approximately 6% of adult patients with RA, psoriatic arthritis, ankylosing spondylitis or plaque psoriasis. In long-term plaque psoriasis studies up to 144 weeks, the percentage of patients testing positive at any time point assessed was 3%-10%. Results from JIA patients were similar to those seen in adult RA patients treated with ENBREL. In all clinical studies with ENBREL to date, there has been no apparent correlation of antibody development to clinical response or adverse events. Neutralizing antibodies have not been observed with ENBREL.

The data reflect the percentage of patients whose test results were considered positive for antibodies to ENBREL in an ELISA assay and are highly dependent on the sensitivity and specificity of the assay. Additionally, the observed incidence of any antibody positivity in an assay is highly dependent on several factors including assay sensitivity and specificity, assay methodology, sample handling, timing of sample collection, concomitant medications, and underlying disease. For these reasons, comparison of the incidence of antibodies to ENBREL with incidence of antibodies to other products may be misleading.

Patients with Heart Failure: Two randomized placebo-controlled studies have been performed in patients with CHF. In one study, patients received either ENBREL 25 mg twice weekly, 25 mg three times weekly, or placebo. In a second study, patients received either ENBREL 25 mg once weekly, 25 mg twice weekly, or placebo. Results of the first study suggested higher mortality in patients treated with ENBREL at either schedule compared to placebo. Results of the second study did not corroborate these observations. Analyses did not identify specific factors associated with increased risk of adverse outcomes in heart failure patients treated with ENBREL (see Warnings and Precautions, Cardiovascular).

Adverse Reactions in Pediatric Patients: In general, the adverse events in pediatric patients were similar in frequency and type as those seen in adult patients. Differences from adult and other special considerations are discussed in the following paragraphs.

Severe adverse reactions reported in 69 JIA patients ages 4 to 17 years included varicella, gastroenteritis, depression/personality disorder, cutaneous ulcer, esophagitis/gastritis, group A streptococcal septic shock, type I diabetes mellitus, and soft tissue and post-operative wound infection.

Forty-three of 69 (62%) children with JIA experienced an infection while receiving ENBREL during the 3 months of the study (part 1 open-label), and the frequency and severity of infections was similar in 58 patients completing 12 months of open-label extension therapy. The types of infections reported in JIA patients were generally mild and consistent with those commonly seen in outpatient pediatric populations.

The following adverse events were reported more commonly in 69 JIA patients receiving 3 months of ENBREL compared to the 349 adult RA patients in placebo-controlled trials. These included headache (19% of patients, 1.7 events per patient-year), nausea (9%, 1.0 events per patient-year), abdominal pain (19%, 0.74 events per patient-year), and vomiting (13%, 0.74 events per patient-year).

In clinical studies of children with JIA, adverse events reported in those aged 2 to 4 years were similar to adverse events reported in older children.

In post-marketing experience, the following additional serious adverse events have been reported in pediatric patients: abscess with bacteremia, optic neuritis, pancytopenia, neutropenia, leukopenia, thrombocytopenia, anemia, seizures, tuberculous arthritis, urinary tract infection including urosepsis, coagulopathy, cutaneous vasculitis, bronchitis, gastroenteritis and transaminase elevation. Other significant adverse events have included depression. The frequency of these events and their causal relationship to ENBREL therapy is unknown.

The long-term effects of ENBREL therapy on skeletal, behavioural, cognitive, sexual and immune maturation and development in children are unknown.

A higher rate of adverse events was noted when JIA patients in an observational registry received ENBREL therapy in combination with methotrexate. As the juvenile idiopathic arthritis patients receiving combination therapy had more severe disease, since they had failed prior therapeutic trials with either ENBREL or methotrexate alone, it remains unclear whether the higher event rate is related to therapy or underlying disease severity.

Other: In a study with etanercept manufactured by a modified process major adverse events included the following. Twelve subjects (5.4%) experienced 13 serious adverse events. One subject experienced a benign lung neoplasm. One subject (0.4%) experienced a life-threatening non-infectious event (pulmonary embolism) and 14 subjects (6.3%) experienced severe non-infectious adverse events. One serious event (urinary tract infection) was considered infectious. One adverse event of hepatic neoplasm malignant (serious) and one squamous cell carcinoma (non-serious) were reported. Overall, the safety profile was comparable to the etanercept manufactured using the previous process.

Post-Market Adverse Drug Reactions: Additional adverse events have been identified during post-marketing use of ENBREL. Because these events are reported voluntarily from a population of uncertain size, it is not always possible to reliably estimate their frequency or establish a causal relationship to ENBREL exposure. These adverse events include, but are not limited to, the following (listed by body system):

Body as a Whole: angioedema, fatigue, fever, flu syndrome, generalized pain, weight gain.

Cardiovascular: chest pain, vasodilation (flushing), new-onset congestive heart failure.

Digestive: altered sense of taste, anorexia, diarrhea, dry mouth, intestinal perforation.
Hematologic/Lymphatic: adenopathy, anemia, aplastic anemia, leukopenia, neutropenia, pancytopenia, thrombocytopenia.
Hepatobiliary: autoimmune hepatitis, elevated transaminase.
Immune: macrophage activation syndrome.
Musculoskeletal: joint pain, lupus-like syndrome with manifestations including rash consistent with subacute or discoid lupus.
Neoplasms Benign, Malignant and Unspecified: Merkel cell carcinoma.
Nervous: paresthesias, stroke, seizures and central nervous system events suggestive of multiple sclerosis or isolated demyelinating conditions such as transverse myelitis or optic neuritis.
Ocular: dry eyes, ocular inflammation, uveitis.
Respiratory: dyspnea, interstitial lung disease, pulmonary disease, worsening of prior lung disorder.
Skin: cutaneous vasculitis, including leukocytoclastic vasculitis (with several symptom manifestations), erythema multiforme, Stevens-Johnson syndrome, toxic epidermal necrolysis, pruritus, subcutaneous nodules, urticaria, new or worsening psoriasis (all sub-types including pustular and palmoplantar).

DRUG INTERACTIONS: Overview: Specific drug interaction studies have not been conducted with ENBREL. ENBREL has not been formally evaluated in combination with other DMARDs such as gold, antimalarials, sulfasalazine, penicillamine, azathioprine, cyclophosphamide, or leflunomide and the benefits and risks of such combinations are unknown.

Drug-Drug Interactions: ENBREL can be used in combination with methotrexate in adult patients with rheumatoid arthritis or psoriatic arthritis.

No clinically significant pharmacokinetic drug-drug interactions were observed in studies with digoxin and warfarin.

A higher rate of adverse events was noted when juvenile idiopathic arthritis patients in an observational registry received ENBREL therapy in combination with methotrexate. As the juvenile idiopathic arthritis patients receiving combination therapy had more severe disease, since they had failed prior therapeutic trials with either ENBREL or methotrexate alone, it remains unclear whether the higher event rate is related to therapy or underlying disease severity.

Patients in a clinical study who were on established therapy with sulfasalazine, to which ENBREL was added, experienced a statistically significant decrease in mean white blood cell counts in comparison to groups treated with either ENBREL or sulfasalazine alone. The significance of this observation is unknown.

Concurrent introduction of etanercept and anakinra therapies has not been associated with increased clinical benefit to patients. In a study in which patients with active RA were treated for up to 24 weeks with concurrent ENBREL and anakinra therapy, a 7% rate of serious infections was observed, which was higher than that observed with ENBREL alone (0%). Two percent of patients treated concurrently with ENBREL and anakinra developed neutropenia (ANC $<1\times10^9$/L).

In a study of patients with Wegener's granulomatosis, the addition of ENBREL to standard therapy (including cyclophosphamide) was associated with a higher incidence of non-cutaneous malignancies. Although the role of ENBREL in this finding is uncertain, the use of ENBREL in any patients receiving concurrent cyclophosphamide therapy is not recommended.

In clinical studies, concurrent administration of abatacept and ENBREL resulted in increased incidences of serious adverse events and did not demonstrate increased clinical benefit. Use of ENBREL with abatacept is not recommended.

DOSAGE AND ADMINISTRATION:

Dosing Considerations: ENBREL is intended for use under the guidance and supervision of a physician who has sufficient knowledge of RA, juvenile idiopathic arthritis, psoriatic arthritis, ankylosing spondylitis, or plaque psoriasis and who has fully familiarized himself/herself with the efficacy/safety profile of ENBREL. Patients may self-inject only if their physician determines that it is appropriate and with medical follow-up, as necessary, after proper training in measurement of the correct dose and injection technique.

Recommended Dose and Dosage Adjustment: General: A 50 mg dose should be given as one subcutaneous (SC) injection using either a 50 mg single-use prefilled syringe or single-use prefilled SureClick autoinjector. A 50 mg dose can also be given as two 25 mg SC injections using the 25 mg multiple-use vial.

When administering ENBREL as two 25 mg injections in adults or children, the injections should be given either on the same day once weekly or 3 or 4 days apart.

Adult RA, Psoriatic Arthritis, and Ankylosing Spondylitis Patients: The recommended dose of ENBREL for adult patients with rheumatoid arthritis, psoriatic arthritis, or ankylosing spondylitis is 50 mg per week. Methotrexate, glucocorticoids, salicylates, nonsteroidal anti-inflammatory drugs (NSAIDs), or analgesics may be continued during treatment with ENBREL. Based on a study of 50 mg ENBREL twice weekly in patients with RA that suggested higher incidence of adverse reactions but similar American College of Rheumatology (ACR) response rates, doses higher than 50 mg per week are not recommended.

Adult Plaque Psoriasis Patients: The recommended starting dose of ENBREL for adult patients is a 50 mg dose given twice weekly (administered 3 or 4 days apart) for 3 months followed by a reduction to a maintenance dose of 50 mg per week. A maintenance dose of 50 mg given twice weekly has also been shown to be efficacious.

JIA Patients: The recommended dose of ENBREL for pediatric patients ages 4 to 17 years with active polyarticular JIA is 0.8 mg/kg per week (up to a maximum of 50 mg per week). The 50 mg prefilled syringe or SureClick autoinjector may be used for pediatric patients weighing 63 kg (138 pounds) or more. Glucocorticoids, nonsteroidal anti-inflammatory drugs (NSAIDs), or analgesics may be continued during treatment with ENBREL. Concurrent use with methotrexate and higher doses of ENBREL have not been studied in pediatric patients.

Missed Dose: Patients who miss a dose of ENBREL should be advised to contact their doctor to find out when to take their next dose of ENBREL.

Administration: Preparation of ENBREL Using the Single-use Prefilled Syringe or Single-use Prefilled SureClick Autoinjector: Before injection, ENBREL may be allowed to reach room temperature (approximately 15 to 30 minutes). **Do not** remove the needle cap while allowing the prefilled syringe or SureClick autoinjector to reach room temperature.

Prior to administration, visually inspect the solution for particulate matter and discolouration. There may be small white particles of protein in the solution. This is not unusual for proteinaceous solutions. The solution should not be used if discoloured or cloudy, or if foreign particulate matter is present.

Preparation of ENBREL Using the Multiple-use Vial: ENBREL should be reconstituted aseptically with 1 mL of the supplied Sterile Bacteriostatic Water for Injection (BWFI), USP (0.9% benzyl alcohol), giving a solution of 1.0 mL containing 25 mg of ENBREL.

A vial adapter is supplied for use when reconstituting the lyophilized powder. However, the vial adapter should not be used if multiple doses are going to be withdrawn from the vial. If the vial will be used for multiple doses, a 25-gauge needle should be used for mixing and withdrawing ENBREL and a 27-gauge needle should be used for injecting ENBREL, as the vial adapter is not recommended for multi-use. The needles and syringe should be used only once. The reconstituted solution is clear and colourless and should be used within 14 days.

During reconstitution of ENBREL, if not using the vial adapter, the diluent should be injected very slowly into the vial. Some foaming will occur. This is normal. To avoid excessive foaming, do not shake or vigorously agitate. The contents should be swirled gently during dissolution. Generally, dissolution of ENBREL takes less than 10 minutes. Reconstitution with the supplied BWFI yields a multiple-use preservative solution that expires 14 days after reconstitution. For pediatric patients to be treated with less than a 25 mg dose, write the date in the area marked "Mixing Date:" on the supplied sticker and attach the sticker to the vial immediately after reconstitution. Contents of one vial of ENBREL solution should not be mixed with, or transferred into, the contents of another vial of ENBREL.

Visually inspect the solution for particulate matter and discolouration prior to administration. The solution should not be used if discoloured or cloudy, or if particulate matter remains. Withdraw the solution into the syringe, removing only the dose to be given from the vial. Some foam or bubbles may remain in the vial.

Sites for injection include the thigh, abdomen, or upper arm. Injection sites should be rotated. New injections should be given at least one inch from an old site and never into areas where the skin is tender, bruised, red, or hard.

No other medications should be added to solutions containing ENBREL, and ENBREL should not be reconstituted with other diluents. Do not filter reconstituted solution during preparation or administration.

OVERDOSAGE:
The maximum tolerated dose of ENBREL has not been established in humans. Toxicology studies have been performed in monkeys at doses up to 30 times the human dose with no evidence of dose-limiting toxicities. No dose-limiting toxicities have been observed during clinical trials of ENBREL. Single IV doses up to 60 mg/m² have been administered to 32 healthy volunteers (25 males; 7 females) in an endotoxemia study without evidence of dose-limiting toxicities. The highest dose level evaluated in RA patients has been a single IV loading dose of 32 mg/m² followed by SC doses of 16 mg/m² (~25 mg) administered twice weekly. In one RA trial, one patient mistakenly self-administered 62 mg ENBREL SC twice weekly for 3 weeks without experiencing adverse effects.

> For management of a suspected drug overdose, contact your regional Poison Control Centre. See the *CPS* Directory section for a list of Poison Control Centres.

ACTION AND CLINICAL PHARMACOLOGY: Mechanism of Action: ENBREL (etanercept) is a dimeric fusion protein consisting of the extracellular ligand-binding portion of the human 75 kilodalton (p75) tumor necrosis factor receptor (TNFR) linked to the Fc portion of human IgG1. It consists of 934 amino acids and has an apparent molecular weight of approximately 150 kilodaltons.

Etanercept binds specifically to soluble and cell surface tumour necrosis factor (TNF) and blocks its interaction with cell surface TNF receptors. Etanercept inactivates TNF without causing in vitro lysis of cells involved in the immune response. TNF is a naturally occurring cytokine, or immune system protein, that is implicated in the development and progression of inflammatory, infectious, and autoimmune diseases. TNF plays an important role in the inflammatory processes of rheumatoid arthritis (RA), polyarticular juvenile idiopathic arthritis (JIA), ankylosing spondylitis and the resulting joint pathology. In addition, TNF plays an important role in the inflammatory process of plaque psoriasis and resulting skin pathology. Elevated levels of TNF are found in the synovial fluid of RA patients, in both the synovium and psoriatic plaques of patients with psoriatic arthritis and plaque psoriasis and in serum and synovial tissue of patients with ankylosing spondylitis. In plaque psoriasis, infiltration by inflammatory cells including T-cells leads to increased TNF levels in psoriatic lesions, compared with levels in uninvolved skin.

Two distinct receptors for TNF (TNFRs), a 55 kilodalton protein (p55) and a 75 kilodalton protein (p75), exist naturally as monomeric molecules on cell surfaces and in soluble forms. Biological activity of TNF is dependent upon binding to either cell surface TNFR.

Etanercept is a dimeric soluble form of the p75 TNF receptor that can bind to two TNF molecules. This dimeric binding provides substantially greater competitive inhibition of TNF than monomeric soluble receptors.

Much of the joint pathology in RA is mediated by proinflammatory molecules that are linked in a network controlled by TNF.

Etanercept competitively inhibits binding of both TNF α and TNF β (lymphotoxin α [LT α]) to cell surface TNF receptors, rendering TNF biologically inactive. Etanercept does not cause lysis of TNF-producing cells in vitro, in the presence or absence of complement.

Pharmacodynamics: Etanercept also modulates biological responses that are induced or regulated by TNF, including expression of adhesion molecules responsible for leukocyte migration (ie, E-selectin and to a lesser extent intercellular adhesion molecule-1 [ICAM-1]), serum levels of cytokines (eg, IL-6, IL-1), and serum levels of matrix metalloproteinase-3 (MMP-3 or stromelysin). Etanercept has been shown to affect several animal models of inflammation, including murine collagen-induced arthritis.

Pharmacokinetics: After administration of 25 mg ENBREL by a single subcutaneous (SC) injection to 25 patients with RA, a mean±standard deviation half-life of 102±30 hours was observed with a clearance of 160±80 mL/h. A maximum serum concentration (C_{max}) of 1.1±0.6 µg/mL and time to C_{max} of 69±34 hours was observed in these patients following a single 25 mg dose. After 6 months of twice weekly 25 mg doses in these same RA patients, the mean C_{max} was 2.4±1.0 µg/mL (N=23). Patients exhibited a two- to seven-fold increase in peak serum concentrations and approximately four-fold increase in $AUC_{0\text{-}72\,h}$ (range 1 to 17 fold) with repeated dosing. Serum concentrations in patients with RA have not been measured for periods of dosing that exceed 6 months.

In another study, serum concentration profiles at steady state were comparable among patients with RA treated with 50 mg ENBREL once weekly and those treated with 25 mg ENBREL twice weekly. The mean (±standard deviation) C_{max}, C_{min}, and partial AUC were 2.4±1.5 mg/L, 1.2±0.7 mg/L, and 297±166 mg·h/L, respectively, for patients treated with 50 mg ENBREL once weekly (N=21); and 2.6±1.2 mg/L, 1.4±0.7 mg/L, and 316±135 mg·h/L for patients treated with 25 mg ENBREL twice weekly (N=16). Serum concentrations in patients with plaque psoriasis treated with 50 mg ENBREL twice weekly were approximately twice that of 25 mg ENBREL twice weekly treatment; mean (±SD) of 3.8±1.9 mg/L and 1.9±1.1 mg/L, at 12 weeks respectively.

Special Populations and Conditions: Pediatrics: Pediatric patients with JIA (ages 4 to 17 years) were administered 0.4 mg/kg of ENBREL twice weekly (up to a maximum dose of 50 mg per week) for up to 18 weeks. The average serum concentration after repeated dosing was 2.1 µg/mL, with a range of 0.7 to 4.3 µg/mL compared to a serum concentration of 3.1 µg/mL, with a range of 0.9 to 5.6 µg/mL in adults. Preliminary data suggests that the clearance of ENBREL is reduced slightly in children ages 4 to 8 years. Population pharmacokinetic analyses predict that administration of 0.8 mg/kg of ENBREL once weekly in children will result in Cmax 11% higher, and Cmin 20% lower at steady state as compared to administration of 0.4 mg/kg of ENBREL twice weekly. The predicted pharmacokinetic differences between the regimens in JIA patients are of the same magnitude as the differences observed between twice weekly and weekly regimens in adult RA patients. Serum concentrations of ENBREL in children with JIA aged 2 to 4 years were similar to serum concentrations of ENBREL in older children with JIA.

Concomitant methotrexate does not alter the pharmacokinetics of ENBREL in adults. The pharmacokinetics of concomitant MTX in children with JIA ages 4 to 17 has not been evaluated.

Gender: Pharmacokinetic parameters were not different between men and women and did not vary with age in adult patients.

Hepatic Insufficiency: No formal pharmacokinetic studies have been conducted to examine the effect of hepatic impairment on ENBREL disposition or potential interactions with methotrexate.

Renal Insufficiency: No formal pharmacokinetic studies have been conducted to examine the effect of renal impairment on ENBREL disposition or potential interactions with methotrexate.

STORAGE AND STABILITY: ENBREL **Single-use Prefilled Syringe and ENBREL Single-use Prefilled SureClick Autoinjector:** Do not use ENBREL beyond the expiration date stamped on the carton or syringe label. ENBREL must be refrigerated at 2 to 8°C. **Do not freeze.** Keep the product in the original carton to protect from light until the time of use. Do not shake.

ENBREL **Multiple-use Vial:** Do not use a dose tray beyond the date stamped on the carton, dose tray label, vial label, or diluent syringe label. The dose tray containing ENBREL (sterile powder) must be refrigerated at 2 to 8°C. **Do not freeze.**

Reconstituted solutions of ENBREL prepared with the supplied Sterile Bacteriostatic Water for Injection, USP (0.9% benzyl alcohol) may be stored in the original vial for up to 14 days at 2 to 8°C, with overall room temperature exposure of less than 12 hours during storage and handling/usage. Discard reconstituted solution after 14 days.**Product stability and sterility cannot be assured after 14 days.**

Keep in a safe place out of the reach of children.

SPECIAL HANDLING INSTRUCTIONS: Information to Be Provided to the Patient: ENBREL is provided as a single-use prefilled syringe, a single-use prefilled SureClick autoinjector, or a multiple-use vial. The needle cap on the prefilled syringe and on the SureClick autoinjector contains dry natural rubber (a derivative of latex), which should not be handled by persons sensitive to latex. One ENBREL 50 mg prefilled syringe or ENBREL 50 mg SureClick autoinjector provides a dose equivalent to two 25 mg vials of lyophilized ENBREL.

If a patient or caregiver is to administer ENBREL, he/she should be instructed in injection techniques and how to measure the correct dose to ensure the safe administration of ENBREL. The first injection should be performed under the supervision of a qualified health care professional. The patient or caregiver ability to inject subcutaneously should be assessed. Alcohol swabs and cotton balls or gauze are required for the injections and will need to be obtained separately. A puncture-resistant container for disposal of needles, syringes, and autoinjectors should be used. Patients and caregivers should be instructed in the technique of proper syringe and needle disposal, and be cautioned against reuse of these items. If product is intended for multiple-use, additional syringes, and needles, will be required.

INFORMATION FOR THE PATIENT: Published in e-CPS, available by subscription at www.e-cps.ca.

DOSAGE FORMS, COMPOSITION AND PACKAGING: Multiple-use Vials: Each vial contains a sterile, white, preservative-free lyophilized powder. Reconstitution with 1 mL of the supplied Sterile Bacteriostatic Water for Injection (BWFI), USP (containing 0.9% benzyl alcohol) yields a multiple-use, clear, and colourless solution with a pH of 7.4±0.3 containing 25 mg etanercept. Nonmedicinal ingredients: mannitol, sucrose and tromethamine. Cartons of 4 dose trays. Each dose tray contains: one 25 mg vial of etanercept, one diluent syringe (1 mL Sterile Bacteriostatic Water for Injection, USP, containing 0.9% benzyl alcohol), one 27-gauge ½ inch needle, one vial adapter, and one plunger. Each carton contains four "Mixing Date:" stickers. A single dose replacement tray is available, if needed.

Single-use Prefilled Syringes: Each single-use prefilled syringe contains: 0.98 mL (minimum deliverable volume of 0.94 mL) of a 50 mg/mL clear and colourless, sterile, preservative-free, formulated at pH 6.3±0.2 solution of etanercept. There may be small white particles of protein in the solution. Nonmedicinal ingredients: L-arginine hydrochloride, sodium chloride, sodium phosphate dibasic anhydrous, sodium phosphate monobasic monohydrate and sucrose. Cartons of 4 single-dose prefilled syringes with 27-gauge, ½ inch needles. A single syringe replacement carton is available if needed. Administration of one 50 mg/mL prefilled syringe of ENBREL provides a dose equivalent to two 25 mg multi-use vials of lyophilized ENBREL, when vials are reconstituted and administered as recommended.

Single-use Prefilled SureClick Autoinjector : Each single-use use prefilled SureClick autoinjector contains: 0.98 mL (minimum deliverable volume of 0.94 mL) of a 50 mg/mL clear and colourless, formulated at pH 6.3±0.2 solution of etanercept. There may be small white particles of protein in the solution. Nonmedicinal ingredients: L-arginine hydrochloride, sodium chloride, sodium phosphate dibasic anhydrous, sodium phosphate monobasic monohydrate and sucrose. Preservative-free. Cartons of 4 SureClick autoinjectors. A single autoinjector replacement carton is available if needed. Administration of one 50 mg/mL ENBREL SureClick autoinjector provides a dose equivalent to two 25 mg multi-use vials of lyophilized ENBREL, when vials are reconstituted and administered as recommended.

Endocet® Ⓝ

oxycodone HCl—acetaminophen

Opioid Analgesic

Bristol-Myers Squibb

SUPPLIED: Each white to off-white tablet, scored on one side, embossed with "0636" on the other, contains: oxycodone HCl 5 mg and acetaminophen 325 mg. Nonmedicinal ingredients: cornstarch, microcrystalline cellulose, povidone, pregelatinized starch, silicone dioxide and stearic acid. Lactose-, sodium- and tartrazine-free. Bottles of 100 and 500. Store at room temperature (15 to 30°C).

Endometrin® Ⓟ

progesterone

Progestin

Ferring

Date of Preparation: September 30, 2009

SUMMARY PRODUCT INFORMATION:

Route of Administration	Dosage Form/ Strength	Clinically Relevant Nonmedicinal Ingredients
Vaginal	Effervescent vaginal tablets 100 mg	Lactose monohydrate, polyvinylpyrrolidone, adipic acid, sodium bicarbonate, sodium lauryl sulfate, magnesium stearate, pregelatinized starch, and colloidal silicone dioxide For a complete listing see Dosage Forms, Composition and Packaging.

INDICATIONS AND CLINICAL USE: Endometrin is indicated for progesterone supplementation in women undergoing in vitro fertilization.

Geriatrics: No clinical data have been collected in patients over age 65.

Pediatrics: This drug is not intended for pediatric use and no clinical data have been collected in children.

CONTRAINDICATIONS: Endometrin should not be used in individuals with any of the following conditions:

- Previous allergic reactions to progesterone or any of the ingredients of Endometrin [see Summary Product Information]
- Known missed abortion or ectopic pregnancy
- Liver disease
- Known or suspected breast cancer
- Active arterial or venous thromboembolism or severe thrombophlebitis or cerebro-vascular disease, or a history of these events.
- Acute Porphyria

WARNINGS AND PRECAUTIONS: General:

- A pretreatment physical examination should include special reference to breasts, pelvic organs as well as Papanicolaou smear.
- In all cases of irregular vaginal bleeding adequate diagnostic measures should be undertaken.
- Progesterone may cause fluid retention and conditions which might be influenced by this (e.g., epilepsy, migraine, asthma, cardiac or renal dysfunction) require careful observation.
- The pathologist should be informed of progesterone therapy when relevant specimens are submitted.
- Endometrin should not be recommended for use with other vaginal products (such as antifungal products) as this may alter progesterone release and absorption from the vaginal insert [see Drug Interactions].

Cardiovascular: The physician should be alert to earliest signs of myocardial infraction, cerebrovascular disorders, arterial or venous thromboembolism (venous thromboembolism or pulmonary embolism), thrombophlebitis or retinal thrombosis. Endometrin should be discontinued if any of these are suspected.

Endocrine and Metabolism: Decrease in glucose tolerance has been noted in a few patients when taking oestrogen-progestin combination drugs. The mechanism for this is unknown. Diabetic patients should be carefully monitored while receiving progesterone therapy.

Psychiatric: Patients who have a history of depression should be carefully observed. Endometrin should be discontinued if serious depression recurs.

Special Populations: Pregnant Women: Endometrin has been used to support embryo implantation and maintain clinical pregnancy in one clinical study. The live birth outcomes of these pregnancies were as follows:

- Among the 404 subjects treated with Endometrin twice daily, 143 subjects had livebirths consisting of 85 singletons, 56 twins, and 2 triplets. In this treatment group, 13 subjects had a spontaneous abortion, 1 subject had an ectopic pregnancy, and 7 subjects reported fetal birth defects (3.4% based on 203 live births).
- Among the 404 subjects treated with Endometrin three times daily, 155 subjects had livebirths consisting of 91 singletons, 60 twins, and 4 triplets. In this treatment group, 22 subjects had a spontaneous abortion, 4 subjects had an ectopic pregnancy, and 7 subjects reported fetal birth defects (3.1% based on 223 live births).

Birth defects reported in the Endometrin twice daily group included: one fetus with a cleft palate and intrauterine growth retardation, one fetus with spina bifida, three fetuses with congenital heart defects, one fetus with an umbilical hernia, and one fetus with an intestinal anomaly.

Birth defects reported in the Endometrin three times daily group included: one fetus with an esophageal fistula, one fetus with hypospadias and an underdeveloped right ear, one fetus with Down's and an atrial septal defect, one fetus with congenital heart anomalies, one fetus with DiGeorge's syndrome, one fetus with a hand deformity, and one fetus with cleft palate.

Nursing Women: Detectable amounts of progesterone have been identified in the milk of mothers receiving oral progestins. The effect of this on the nursing infant has not been determined. Endometrin should not be used during lactation.

Pediatrics: This drug is not intended for pediatric use and no clinical data have been collected in children.

Geriatrics: No clinical data have been collected in patients over age 65.

ADVERSE REACTIONS: Adverse Drug Reaction Overview: Endometrin was well tolerated after exposure in more than 860 subjects in clinical trials and in well over 6000 cycles in clinical practice worldwide. No serious adverse events (SAEs) were assessed as being related to the Endometrin treatment. No deaths were reported during any of the trials.

Clinical Trial Adverse Drug Reactions: Because clinical trials are conducted under very specific conditions the adverse reaction rates observed in the clinical trials may not reflect the rates observed in practice and should not be compared to the rates in the clinical trials of another drug. Adverse drug reaction information from clinical trials is useful for identifying drug-related adverse events and for approximating rates.

The safety data reflect exposure to Endometrin in 808 infertile women (74.9% White, 10.3% Hispanic, 5.4% Black, 5 % Asian, and 4.6% Other) in a single In Vitro Fertilization 10 week clinical study. Endometrin was studied at doses of 100 mg twice daily and 100 mg three times daily. The adverse reactions that occurred at a rate greater than or equal to 2% in either Endometrin group are summarized in Table 1.

Other less common reported adverse reactions included genital itching, vaginal burning sensation, and vaginal discomfort. These may, in part, be due to the excipient sodium lauryl sulfate. Urticaria was reported in 0.2% of the subjects in each Endometrin group and peripheral edema in 0.2% in Endometrin 100 mg three times daily group.

Endometrin is also expected to have adverse reactions similar to other drugs containing progesterone that may include breast tenderness, bloating, mood swings, irritability, drowsiness and fluid retention.

DRUG INTERACTIONS: Drug-Drug Interactions: No formal drug-drug interaction studies have been conducted for Endometrin. Drugs known to induce the hepatic cytochrome-P450-3A4 system (such as rifampin, carbamazepine) may increase the elimination of progesterone. The effect of concomitant vaginal products on the exposure of progesterone from Endometrin has not been assessed. Endometrin is not recommended for use with other vaginal products (such as antifungal products) as this may alter progesterone release and absorption from the vaginal insert [see Warnings and Precautions].

Drug-Food Interactions: Food can increase the bioavailability of progesterone administered orally. However, this is not relevant to Endometrin since it is administered vaginally.

Table 1: Endometrin

Number and Frequency of Reported Adverse Reactions in Women Treated with Endometrin in a Study Involving in Vitro Fertilization

Body System Preferred Term	Endometrin 100 mg Twice Daily (N=404)	Endometrin 100 mg Three Times Daily (N=404)
Gastrointestinal Disorders		
Abdominal pain	50 (12%)	50 (12%)
Nausea	32 (8%)	29 (7%)
Abdominal distention	18 (4%)	17 (4%)
Constipation	9 (2%)	14 (3%)
Vomiting	13 (3%)	9 (2%)
General Disorders & Administration Site Conditions		
Fatigue	7 (2%)	12 (3%)
Infections and Infestations		
Urinary tract infection	9 (2%)	4 (1%)
Injury, Poisoning and Procedural Complications		
Post-oocyte retrieval pain	115 (28%)	102 (25%)
Nervous System Disorder		
Headache	15 (4%)	13 (3%)
Reproductive System and Breast Disorders		
Ovarian hyperstimulation syndrome	30 (7%)	27 (7%)
Uterine spasm	15 (4%)	11 (3%)
Vaginal bleeding	13 (3%)	14 (3%)

Table 2: Endometrin

Mean (±Standard Deviation) Serum Progesterone Pharmacokinetic Parameters

Pharmacokinetic Parameter (unit)	Endometrin 100 mg Twice Daily (N=6)	Endometrin 100 mg Three Times Daily (N=6)
Single Dosing		
C_{max} (nmol/L)	54.06±20.67	62.96±22.89
T_{max} (hr)	24.0±0.0	17.3±7.4
$AUC_{0\text{-}24}$ (nmol·hr/L)	690.06±359.18	903.12±454.74
Day 5 of Multiple Dosing		
C_{max} (nmol/L)	58.83±17.49	76.64±17.80
T_{max} (hr)	18.0±9.4	18.0±9.4
C_{min} (nmol/L)	28.30±14.31	34.66±21.30
C_{avg} (nmol/L)	44.52±15.26	50.56±13.64
$AUC_{0\text{-}24}$ (nmol·hr/L)	1039.86±403.86	1386±337.08

Legend: C_{max}=maximum progesterone serum concentration; T_{max}=time to maximum progesterone concentration; C_{avg}=average progesterone serum concentration; $AUC_{0\text{-}24}$=area under the drug concentration versus time curve from 0-24 hours post dose; C_{min}=minimum progesterone serum concentration.

DOSAGE AND ADMINISTRATION: Dosing Considerations: The dose of Endometrin is 100 mg administered vaginally two or three times daily starting at the day after oocyte retrieval and continuing for up to 10 weeks total duration.

Recommended Dose and Dosage Adjustment: Endometrin administered into the vagina twice daily (BID) and three times daily (TID) dosing have both been shown to be efficacious. However specific populations may derive greater benefits from BID or TID dosing regimen and the clinician can tailor treatment to the patient. For women <35 years of age and those patients with adequate ovarian reserve, Endometrin BID would be the appropriate dose. For patients aged 35 and older and those with diminished ovarian reserve, TID dosing would be the preferred regimen. Serum progesterone levels may be measured 7 days post fertilization and used to guide therapy.

Missed Dose: If a patient misses a dose, the patient should be instructed to take the dose as soon as she remembers. The patient should also be instructed **not** to use more than her daily dose and **not** to double dose.

Administration: The patient should also be instructed **not** to use any other vaginal products when using Endometrin and to follow the steps below.

1. Unwrap the applicator.
2. Put one insert in the space provided at the end of the applicator. The insert should fit snugly and not fall out.
3. Whilst you are standing, sitting, or when lying on your back with your knees bent, gently place the thin end of the applicator well into the vagina.
4. Push the plunger to release the insert.
5. Remove the applicator and throw it away in the trash.

OVERDOSAGE:

Treatment of overdosage consists of discontinuation of Endometrin together with institution of appropriate symptomatic and supportive care.

For management of a suspected drug overdose, CPhA recommends that you contact your **regional Poison Control Centre**. See the *CPS* Directory section for a list of Poison Control Centres.

ACTION AND CLINICAL PHARMACOLOGY: Mechanism of Action: Progesterone is a naturally occurring steroid that is secreted by the ovary, placenta, and adrenal gland. In the presence of adequate estrogen, progesterone transforms a proliferative endometrium into a secretory endometrium. Progesterone is necessary to increase endometrial receptivity for implantation of an embryo. Once an embryo is implanted, progesterone acts to maintain a pregnancy.

Pharmacokinetics: A pharmacokinetic study was performed to assess the pharmacokinetics of 2 dose regimen of Endometrin, 100 mg BID and 100 mg TID. A summary of the pharmacokinetic parameters results is presented in Table 2.

Absorption: Progesterone serum concentrations increased following the administration of the Endometrin Vaginal Insert in 12 healthy pre-menopausal females. On single dosing, the mean C_{max} was 54.06±20.67 nmol/L in the Endometrin twice daily group and 62.96±22.89 nmol/L in the Endometrin three times daily group. On multiple dosing, steady-state concentrations were attained within approximately 1 day after initiation of treatment with Endometrin. Both Endometrin regimens provided average serum concentrations of progesterone exceeding 31.45 nmol/L on Day 5.

Distribution: Progesterone is approximately 96 % to 99 % bound to serum proteins, primarily to serum albumin and corticosteroid binding globulin.

Metabolism: Progesterone is metabolized primarily by the liver largely to pregnanediols and pregnanolones. Pregnanediols and pregnanolones are conjugated in the liver to glucuronide and sulfate metabolites. Progesterone metabolites that are excreted in the bile may be deconjugated and may be further metabolized in the gut via reduction, dehydroxylation, and epimerization.

Excretion: Progesterone undergoes renal and biliary elimination. Following injection of labeled progesterone, 50-60% of the excretion of metabolites occurs via the kidney; approximately 10% occurs via the bile and feces. Overall recovery of the labeled material accounts for 70% of an administered dose. Only a small portion of unchanged progesterone is excreted in the bile.

STORAGE AND STABILITY: Endometrin (progesterone) is available as 100 mg effervescent vaginal tablets packed individually in a sealed foil pouch. Store Endometrin at 20-25°C. Excursions permitted to 15-30°C.

INFORMATION FOR THE PATIENT: Published in e-CPS, available by subscription at www.e-cps.ca.

DOSAGE FORMS, COMPOSITION AND PACKAGING: Each white to off-white oblong-shaped effervescent vaginal tablet, debossed with "FPI" on one side and "100" on the other side, contains: micronized progesterone and delivers 100 mg of progesterone in a base. Nonmedicinal ingredients: adipic acid, colloidial silicone dioxide, lactose monohydrate, magnesium stearate, polyvinylpyrrolidone, pregelatinized starch, sodium bicarbonate and sodium lauryl sulfate. Cartons packed with 21 vaginal tablets packed individually in a sealed foil pouch and 21 disposable polyethylene vaginal applicators.

Engerix®-B

hepatitis B vaccine (recombinant)

Injectable Vaccine for Active Immunization Against Infection Caused by All Known Subtypes of Hepatitis B Virus

GlaxoSmithKline

Date of Revision: September 23, 2008

SUMMARY PRODUCT INFORMATION:

Route of Administration	Dosage Form/ Strength	Clinically Relevant Nonmedicinal Ingredients
Intramuscular Injection	Injection 0.5 mL, 1.0 mL, 5 mL, and 10 mL suspensions of 20 µg/mL hepatitis B surface antigen	Aluminum hydroxide, multi-dose presentations (5 mL and 10 mL suspensions) contain 2-phenoxyethanol and trace amounts of thimerosal (<0.5 µg mercury for each 0.5 mL pediatric dose and <1.0 µg mercury for each 1.0 mL adolescent/adult dose). The single dose (0.5 mL and 1 mL) formulation is thimerosal free. For a complete listing see Dosage Forms, Composition and Packaging.

DESCRIPTION: The hepatitis B virus induces a severe form of viral hepatitis. Other causative agents are hepatitis A virus, and the non-A, non-B hepatitis viruses. Hepatitis D virus, a defective virus requiring the "keeper function" of the hepatitis B virus, occurs either as a co-infection or super-infection in a HBsAg carrier.

Transmission of the virus occurs through percutaneous contact with contaminated blood, serum or plasma. Infection may also occur by the exposure of mucous surfaces, or intact or damaged skin to other body fluids such as saliva, mucosal secretions and semen.

There is no specific treatment for hepatitis. The incubation period may be as long as 6 months, followed by a very complex clinical course of an acute or chronic nature, often leading to hospitalization.

Viral hepatitis caused by hepatitis B virus is a major worldwide health problem, though the incidence and epidemiology vary widely among geographical areas and population subgroups.

In Canada, the United States and Northern Europe, 4% to 6% of the population are infected during their lifetime (mostly young adults); between 5% and 10% of infections lead to persistent viremia (carrier state). Certain population subgroups in these areas, however, are at high risk (see Indications and Clinical Use).

In Asia, infection often occurs early in life, leading to a hepatitis B marker prevalence of more than 70% in the general population and a carrier rate of up to 20%.

It is estimated that the reservoir of persistent hepatitis B surface antigen carriers amounts to 350 million people worldwide. Carriers are at a high risk of developing chronic liver disease which may lead to cirrhosis or primary hepatocellular carcinoma. A significant reduction in the incidence of hepatocellular carcinoma has been observed in children aged 6 to14 years following a nationwide hepatitis B vaccination in Taiwan. This resulted from a significant decline in the prevalence of hepatitis B antigen, the persistence of which is an essential factor in the development of hepatocellular carcinoma.

Vaccination against hepatitis B is expected in the long term to reduce the overall incidence of both hepatitis B and the chronic complications such as chronic active hepatitis and cirrhosis.

INDICATIONS AND CLINICAL USE: ENGERIX-B (hepatitis B vaccine (recombinant)) is indicated for:

- active immunization against hepatitis B virus infection.

The vaccine will not protect against infection caused by hepatitis A and non-A non-B hepatitis viruses. As hepatitis D (caused by the delta agent) does not occur in the absence of hepatitis B infection or carrier state, it can be expected that hepatitis D will also be prevented by vaccination with ENGERIX-B.

The vaccine can be administered at any age from birth onwards. It may be used to start a primary course of vaccination or as a booster dose. It may also be used to complete a primary course of vaccination started with plasma-derived or yeast-derived vaccines or as a booster dose in subjects who have previously received a primary course of vaccination with plasma-derived or yeast-derived vaccines.

In areas of low prevalence of hepatitis B, vaccination is strongly recommended in subjects who are at increased risk of infection. These include the following groups:

- **Health Professionals:** physicians and surgeons; oral surgeons and dentists; nurses, dental nurses, dental hygienists, podiatrists; IV teams and operating room personnel; paramedical personnel in close contact with patients; staff in hemodialysis, nephrology, hepatology, hematology and oncology units; laboratory personnel handling blood and other clinical specimens; blood bank and plasma fractionation workers; pathologists and morgue attendants; cleaning staff who handle waste in hospitals; emergency and first aid workers; ambulance staff; dental, medical and nursing students.
- **Patients:** patients receiving frequent blood transfusion or clotting factor concentrates, such as those in oncology units and those with thalassemia, sickle-cell anemia, cirrhosis, hemophilia, etc.; patients on hemodialysis.
- **Personnel and Residents of Institutions:** persons with frequent and/or close contacts with high-risk groups; prisoners and prison staff; residents and staff of institutions for the developmentally challenged (those who are in contact with aggressive biting residents being at highest risk).
- **Persons at increased risk due to their sexual practices:** males having sexual contact with other males; others with multiple sexual partners or with a recent history of sexually transmitted disease.
- **Persons who use injectable drugs illicitly.**
- **Travellers to areas of high endemicity and their close contacts.**
- **Household contacts of any of the above groups and of patients with acute or chronic hepatitis B infection.**
- **Infants born of HBsAg-positive mothers.**
- **Chronic Liver Disease (CLD):** subjects with chronic liver disease; subjects at risk of developing CLD (e.g. Hepatitis C virus carriers, persons who abuse alcohol).
- **Others:** police; fire fighters; armed forces personnel; morticians and embalmers; those who through their work or personal lifestyle may be exposed to the hepatitis B virus.

In areas of both low and high prevalence, vaccination should be offered to all young children and neonates at risk, as well as to adult high risk groups.

CONTRAINDICATIONS: ENGERIX-B (hepatitis B vaccine (recombinant)):

- should not be administered to subjects with known hypersensitivity to any component of the vaccine or having shown signs of hypersensitivity after previous ENGERIX-B administration. For a complete listing of the components, see Dosage Forms, Composition and Packaging.
- should not be administered to subjects with severe febrile infections as for any vaccine. However, the presence of a minor infection does not contraindicate vaccination.

Human immunodeficiency virus (HIV) infection is not considered as a contraindication for hepatitis B vaccination (see Warnings and Precautions).

WARNINGS AND PRECAUTIONS: General: As with all injectable vaccines, appropriate medical treatment and supervision should always be readily available in case of a rare anaphylactic reaction following the administration of the vaccine.

ENGERIX-B (hepatitis B vaccine (recombinant)) should not be administered in the gluteal region or intradermally since these routes of administration may result in a lower immune response. Intradermal administration may also result in severe local reactions.

The vaccine must never be administered intravenously.

A new sterile syringe and a new sterile needle should always be used to prevent the transmission from one subject to another of infectious agents, such as the hepatitis B virus, non-A, non-B hepatitis virus or the human immunodeficiency virus (HIV).

Hepatic: Patients with chronic liver disease or hepatitis C carriers should not be precluded from vaccination against hepatitis B. The vaccine could be advised since hepatitis B virus (HBV) infection can be severe in these patients. The HBV vaccination should be considered on a case by case basis by the physician.

Immune: Because hepatitis B has a long incubation period it is possible that there may be latent infection at the time of vaccination. ENGERIX-B may not prevent hepatitis B in such cases.

Patients who develop symptoms suggestive of hypersensitivity after an injection should not receive further injections of ENGERIX-B (see Contraindications).

The immune response to hepatitis B vaccine is related to a number of factors, including older age, male gender, obesity, smoking habits and route of administration. In subjects who may respond less well to the administration of the hepatitis B vaccine (e.g. more than 40 years of age, etc.), additional doses may be considered.

Patients with HIV infection should not be precluded from vaccination against hepatitis B. The vaccine could be advised since hepatitis B virus (HBV) infection can be severe in these patients. The HBV vaccination should be considered on a case by case basis by the physician.

In HIV infected patients and persons with an impaired immune system, adequate anti-HBs antibody titers may not be obtained after the primary immunization course and such patients may therefore require administration of additional doses of vaccine (see Dosage and Administration).

Renal: In hemodialysis patients, adequate anti-HBs antibody titers may not be obtained after the primary immunization course and such patients may therefore require administration of additional doses of vaccine (see Dosage and Administration).

Special Populations: Pregnant Women: The effect of the antigen (HBsAg) on fetal development is unknown as adequate studies with ENGERIX-B have not been conducted during pregnancy and adequate animal reproduction studies are not available. However, vaccination of a pregnant woman may be considered in order to prevent hepatitis B in high-risk situations.

Nursing Women: Adequate human data on use during lactation and adequate animal reproduction studies are not available. It is not known whether ENGERIX-B is excreted in human milk. Because many drugs are excreted in human milk, caution should be exercised when ENGERIX-B is administered to a nursing woman.

Pediatrics: The potential risk of apnoea and the need for respiratory monitoring for 48-72 hours should be considered when administering the primary immunization series to very premature infants (born ≤28 weeks of gestation) and particularly for those with a previous history of respiratory immaturity. As the benefit of vaccination is high in this group of infants, vaccination should not be withheld or delayed.

ADVERSE REACTIONS: Clinical Trial Adverse Drug Reactions: Because clinical trials are conducted under very specific conditions the adverse reaction rates observed in the clinical trials may not reflect the rates observed in practice and should not be compared to the rates in the clinical trials of another drug. Adverse drug reaction information from clinical trials is useful for identifying drug-related adverse events and for approximating rates.

The safety profile presented in Table 1 is based on data from more than 5300 subjects.

Table 1: ENGERIX-B

Safety Profile

Frequency	Adverse Event	System/Organ Class
Very Common ≥10%	irritability	Psychiatric disorders
	headache (with 10 µg formulation)	Nervous system disorders
	pain and redness at the injection site, fatigue	General disorders and administration site conditions
Common ≥1% and <10%	appetite loss	Metabolism and nutrition disorders
	headache (with 20 µg formulation), drowsiness	Nervous system disorders
	gastrointestinal symptoms (such as nausea, vomiting, diarrhea, abdominal pain)	Gastrointestinal disorders
	swelling at the injection site, malaise, injection site reaction (such as induration), fever (≥37.5°C)	General disorders and administration site conditions
Uncommon ≥0.1% and <1%	dizziness	Nervous system disorders
	myalgia	Musculoskeletal and connective tissue disorders
	Influenza-like illness	General disorders and administration site conditions
Rare ≥0.01% and <0.1%	lymphadenopathy	Blood and lymphatic system disorders
	paraesthesia	Nervous system disorders
	rash, pruritus, urticaria	Skin and subcutaneous tissue disorders
	arthralgia	Musculoskeletal and connective tissue disorders

Post-Market Adverse Drug Reactions: The following adverse reactions have been reported with ENGERIX-B. See Table 2.

Table 2: ENGERIX-B

Post-Market Adverse Reactions

Infections and infestations	Meningitis
Blood and lymphatic system disorder	Thrombocytopenia
Immune system disorders	Anaphylaxis, allergic reactions including anaphylactoid reactions and mimicking serum sickness
Nervous system disorders	Encephalopathy, encephalitis, neuritis, neuropathy, paralysis, convulsions, hypoaesthesia, multiple sclerosis[a], optic neuritis, Guillain-Barre syndrome[a]
Vascular disorders	Hypotension, vasculitis, syncope
Skin and subcutaneous tissue disorders	Angioneurotic oedema, lichen planus, erythema multiforme
Musculoskeletal and connective tissue disorders	Arthritis, muscular weakness
Hepatic system disorders	Abnormal liver function tests
Respiratory system disorders	Bronchospasm

[a] "A number of studies have demonstrated no link between hepatitis B vaccine and multiple sclerosis, Guillain-Barre syndrome (GBS), ..." (Canadian Immunization Guide 7th Edition 2006).

In a comparative trial in subjects from 11 years up to and including 15 years of age, the incidence of local and general solicited symptoms reported after a two-dose regimen of ENGERIX-B (hepatitis B vaccine (recombinant)) 20 μg was similar overall to that reported after the standard three-dose regimen of ENGERIX-B 10 μg.

DRUG INTERACTIONS: Not applicable.

DOSAGE AND ADMINISTRATION: Recommended Dose and Dosage Adjustment: The recommended Standard schedule for ENGERIX-B (hepatitis B vaccine [recombinant]) is three doses administered at 0, 1 and 6 months.

For more Accelerated protection a three dose schedule (0, 1, 2 with a booster dose at month 12) results in the development of protective anti-HBs titres by 3 months. The booster dose (at 12 months) is required to maintain prolonged protective anti-HBs titres.

In circumstances in adults, where a very Rapid induction of protection is required, e.g. persons travelling to areas of high endemicity and who commence a course of vaccination against hepatitis B within one month prior to departure, a schedule of three intramuscular injections given at 0, 7 and 21 days may be used. When this schedule is applied, a booster dose should be administered 12 months after the first dose for longer term protection (see Action and Clinical Pharmacology for seroconversion rates).

Dosage: Adults 20 Years and Over: A dose of 20 μg of antigen protein in 1 mL suspension is recommended for adults.

Neonates, Infants, Children and Adolescents up to 19 Years Inclusive: A dose of 10 μg of antigen protein in 0.5 mL suspension is recommended for neonates, infants, children and adolescents up to 19 years of age inclusive.

When the pediatric presentation is not available, other presentations may be used for withdrawing the appropriate dose.

Alternative Dosing (adolescents 11-15 years): A dose of 20 μg of antigen protein in 1 mL suspension may be administered in subjects from 11 years up to and including 15 years of age according to a 0, 6 months schedule (see Action and Clinical Pharmacology).

Patients with Renal Insufficiency Including Patients Undergoing Hemodialysis 16 Years of Age and Above: The primary immunization schedule for patients with renal insufficiency including patients undergoing hemodialysis is four double doses (2×20 μg) at elected date, 1 month, 2 months and 6 months from the date of the first dose. The immunization schedule should be adapted in order to ensure that the anti-HBs antibody titre remains above the accepted protective level of 10 IU/L.

Patients with Renal Insufficiency Including Patients Undergoing Hemodialysis up to and Including 15 Years of Age: Patients with renal insufficiency including patients undergoing hemodialysis have a reduced immune response to hepatitis B vaccine. Consideration should be given to serological testing following a complete course of ENGERIX-B. Additional doses of vaccine may need to be considered to ensure a protective anti-HBs level >10 IU/L.

Immunocompromised Patients: A 2 mL (2×1 mL) dose of ENGERIX-B 40 μg (2×20 μg) is recommended (see Action and Clinical Pharmacology).

ENGERIX-B can effectively boost anti-HBs responses initially elicited by either plasma-derived or yeast-derived vaccines.

For individuals in whom a primary vaccination schedule has been initiated with a plasma-derived vaccine, dosing may be continued with ENGERIX-B.

Table 3: ENGERIX-B

Dosage and Administration Table

Vaccination Schedule	Age	Dose/Volume (μg/mL)	Dosing Schedule (months)				
			0	1	2	6	12
Standard (3 doses)	≥20 years of age	20/1.0	x	x		x	
Standard	0–19 years of age	10/0.5	x	x		x	
Accelerated	≥20 years of age	20/1.0	x	x	x		x
	0–19 years of age	10/0.5	x	x	x		x
Rapid	≥20 years of age	20/1.0	0,7d, 21d xxx d=days				x
Alternative	11–15 years of age	20/1.0	x			x	

Booster Doses: Routine booster vaccinations in immunocompetent persons are not recommended since protection has been shown to last for at least 15 years. Studies of long term protective efficacy, however, will determine whether booster doses of vaccine are ever needed. It is important to recognize that absence of detectable anti-HBs does not mean lack of protection, because immune memory persists. Booster doses in this situation are not indicated.

Immunocompromised persons often respond suboptimally to the vaccine. Subsequent hepatitis B virus (HBV) exposures in these individuals can result in disease or the carrier state. Therefore, booster doses may be necessary in this population. The optimal timing of booster doses for immunocompromised individuals who are at continued risk of HBV exposure is not known and should be based on the severity of the compromised state and annual monitoring for the presence of anti-HBs.

Administration: Check the expiry date of the vaccine carefully. Do not use vaccine beyond its expiry date.

The vaccine should be inspected visually for any foreign particulate matter and/or coloration prior to administration. Before use of ENGERIX-B, the vaccine should be well shaken to resuspend the sediment of fine white particles of adjuvant (aluminium hydroxide) which settles during storage and to obtain a slightly opaque, white suspension. Discard if the content appears otherwise.

When using a multidose vial, each dose should be taken with a sterile needle and syringe. As with other vaccines, a dose of vaccine should be withdrawn under strict aseptic conditions and precautions taken to avoid contamination of the contents. When using vial, use different needles to pierce the rubber stopper and to inject the vaccine.

Clean the skin at the site of injection with a suitable antiseptic and dry with a piece of dry sterile cotton. Disinfect the rubber stopper with antiseptic; wipe it dry with a dry, sterile cotton swab; then using a sterile needle, withdraw the vaccine from the vial into a sterile syringe.

ENGERIX-B should be injected intramuscularly. In adults the injection should be given in the deltoid region. In neonates and infants it may be preferable to inject ENGERIX-B in the anterolateral thigh because of the small size of their deltoid muscle. In special circumstances the vaccine may be administered subcutaneously in patients with severe bleeding tendencies (e.g., hemophiliacs).

ENGERIX-B must not be given intravenously or intradermally. ENGERIX-B may be administered simultaneously with hepatitis B immunoglobulin (HBIG); however it must be administered at a separate injection site.

OVERDOSAGE:

Cases of overdose have been reported during post-marketing surveillance. Adverse events reported following overdosage were similar to those reported with normal vaccine administration.

For management of a suspected drug overdose, CPhA recommends that you contact your **regional Poison Control Centre**. See the *CPS* Directory section for a list of Poison Control Centres.

ACTION AND CLINICAL PHARMACOLOGY: Mechanism of Action: ENGERIX-B induces specific humoral antibodies against HBsAg (anti-HBs antibodies). It is generally accepted that an anti-HBs titre greater than 10 IU/L correlates with protection against hepatitis B virus infection. More than 90% of healthy adults, children and neonates developed protective anti-HBs titres one month after completing a primary vaccination schedule of ENGERIX-B (hepatitis B vaccine (recombinant)).

STORAGE AND STABILITY: ENGERIX-B (hepatitis B vaccine (recombinant)) should be shipped under refrigeration and stored at 2 to 8°C. **Do not freeze.** Vaccine which has been frozen is no longer potent and should be discarded.

The single dose container does not contain a preservative. The entire contents of a single dose container must be withdrawn and should be used immediately upon withdrawal.

For multidose vaccine, discard unused portion no longer than 24 hours after first puncture.

When stored at 2 to 8°C, ENGERIX-B is stable until the expiry date shown on the label.

INFORMATION FOR THE PATIENT: Published in e-CPS, available by subscription at www.e-cps.ca.

DOSAGE FORMS, COMPOSITION AND PACKAGING: 0.5 mL: Each 0.5 mL single pediatric dose vial contains: hepatitis B surface antigen 10 μg adsorbed onto Al^{+++} 0.25 mg as aluminum hydroxide. Preservative-free. Cartons of 1 with Prescribing Information leaflet.

1 mL: Each 1 mL single adolescent/adult dose vial contains: hepatitis B surface antigen 20 μg adsorbed onto Al^{+++} 0.5 mg as aluminum hydroxide. Preservative-free. Cartons of 1 with Prescribing Information leaflet.

5 mL: Each 5 mL multidose vial for mass immunization programs contains: hepatitis B surface antigen 100 μg adsorbed onto Al^{+++} 5 mg as aluminum hydroxide. Also contains 5.0 mg/mL of 2-phenoxyethanol as preservative. Cartons of 1 with Prescribing Information leaflet.

10 mL: Each 10 mL multidose vial for mass immunization programs contains: hepatitis B surface antigen 200 μg adsorbed onto Al^{+++} 5 mg as aluminum hydroxide. Also contains 5.0 mg/mL of 2-phenoxyethanol as preservative. Cartons of 1 with Prescribing Information leaflet.

The ENGERIX-B multidose (5 mL and 10 mL) formulation contains a trace amount of thimerosal (<0.5 μg mercury for each 0.5 mL pediatric dose and <1.0 μg mercury for each 1.0 mL adolescent/adult dose) from the manufacturing process. The ENGERIX-B single dose (0.5 mL and 1 mL) formulation is thimerosal free.

Enoxaparin

CPhA Monograph

see *Heparins: Low Molecular Weight*

Entex® LA

pseudoephedrine HCl—guaifenesin

Decongestant—Expectorant

Purdue Pharma

Date of Preparation: April 25, 2001
Date of Revision: September 17, 2009

PHARMACOLOGY: Pseudoephedrine is an alpha-adrenergic receptor agonist (sympathomimetic) which produces vasoconstriction by stimulating alpha-receptors within the mucosa of the respiratory tract. Clinically, pseudoephedrine shrinks swollen mucous membranes, reduces tissue hyperemia, edema and nasal congestion, and increases nasal airway patency.

Guaifenesin promotes lower respiratory tract drainage by thinning bronchial secretions, lubricates irritated respiratory tract membranes through increased mucus flow, and facilitates removal of viscous, inspissated mucus. As a result of these combined actions, sinus and bronchial drainage is improved, and dry, nonproductive coughs become more productive.

A study was conducted in 30 healthy subjects to determine the bioavailability and pharmacokinetics of the Entex LA tablet under steady state conditions relative to corresponding immediate release pseudoephedrine hydrochloride and guaifenesin liquids.

One Entex LA tablet was administered every 12 hours for 9 consecutive doses, and the immediate release liquids (300 mg guaifenesin and 60 mg pseudoephedrine HCl) were administered four times daily for 18 consecutive doses.

Plasma levels of guaifenesin and pseudoephedrine for the tablets and for the immediate release liquids were determined at various times over a 12 hour dosing interval.

The extent of absorption of guaifenesin and pseudoephedrine as measured by the AUC (area under the plasma concentration-time curve) were comparable for Entex LA and the immediate release liquids.

INDICATIONS: Entex LA reduces nasal congestion, helps decongest sinus openings and promotes nasal and/or sinus drainage. Entex LA helps bronchial tubes by thinning mucus and loosening phlegm in conjunction with other measures for productive (wet) coughs such as ensuring hydration by drinking water and increasing air humidity, as needed.

CONTRAINDICATIONS: Entex LA is contraindicated in individuals with known hypersensitivity to sympathomimetics, severe hypertension, or in patients receiving MAO inhibitors.

WARNINGS: See Precautions.

PRECAUTIONS: This product should not be taken by persons who have high blood pressure, peripheral vascular disease, prostate disease, glaucoma, heart or thyroid disease, diabetes, persistent/chronic cough; or by pregnant/nursing women, or by persons taking high blood pressure medication or an antidepressant containing a monoamine oxidase inhibitor, except under the advice and supervision of a physician.

Information to Be Provided to the Patient:

- Consult a physician if symptoms worsen, last for more than a week, are accompanied by high fever (>38°C) or the production of thick yellow/green phlegm, or if you have peripheral vascular disease, glaucoma, high blood pressure, heart or thyroid disease, diabetes or prostate disease.
- Do not use if you are allergic to any of the ingredients. Discontinue use if allergic reactions such as wheezing, rash or itching develop.
- Do not give with any other cough and cold medications since harm may occur, unless recommended by a healthcare practitioner.
- Consult a healthcare practitioner prior to combining with any other medications, including natural health products, prescription drugs or nonprescription drugs.
- Do not exceed recommended single and maximum daily dose. Overdose may result in harm.

In Case of Overdose: Call a Regional Poison Control Centre and/or your doctor and/or your local emergency number immediately, or go to your a local hospital emergency, even if you do not notice any signs or symptoms. Keep all medicines out of the reach of children.

Do not crush or chew tablets.

Drug Interactions: Entex LA should not be used in patients taking other sympathomimetics or MAO inhibitors.

Drug/Laboratory Test Interactions: Guaifenesin has been reported to interfere with clinical laboratory determinations of urinary 5-hydroxyindole-acetic acid (5-HIAA) and urinary vanillylmandelic acid (VMA).

Pregnancy: Animal reproduction studies have not been conducted with Entex LA. It is also not known whether Entex LA can cause fetal harm when administered to a pregnant woman or can affect reproduction capacity. Entex LA should not be used in pregnancy unless the potential benefits outweigh the possible risks.

Lactation: It is not known whether the drugs in Entex LA are excreted in human milk. Because many drugs are excreted in human milk and because of the potential for serious adverse reactions in nursing infants, a decision should be made whether to discontinue nursing or to discontinue the product, taking into account the importance of the drug to the mother.

Children: Entex LA is not recommended for children under 12 years of age.

ADVERSE EFFECTS: Possible adverse reactions include nervousness, insomnia, restlessness, dizziness, headache, nausea, or gastric irritation. These reactions rarely, if ever, require discontinuation of therapy. Chest tightness has been reported on occasion. Urinary retention may occur in patients with prostatic hypertrophy.

OVERDOSE:

Treatment: The treatment of overdosage should provide symptomatic and supportive care. If the amount ingested is considered dangerous or excessive, induce vomiting with ipecac syrup unless the patient is convulsing, comatose, or has lost the gag reflex, in which case perform gastric lavage using a large bore tube. If indicated, follow with activated charcoal and saline cathartic. Since the effects of Entex LA may last up to 12 hours, continue treatment for at least that length of time.

For management of a suspected drug overdose, CPhA recommends that you contact your **regional Poison Control Centre**. See the *CPS* Directory section for a list of Poison Control Centres.

DOSAGE: Adults and children 12 years of age and over: one (1) tablet twice daily (every 12 hours), maximum 2 tablets daily. Do not exceed the single and maximum daily dose. Do not use for longer than 7 days.

Entex LA is not recommended for children under 12 years of age.

Tablets **may be broken in half** for ease of administration without affecting release of medication but should not be crushed or chewed prior to swallowing.

SUPPLIED: Each yellow, capsule-shaped, scored tablet, imprinted with "Entex LA" on one side and unmarked on the scored side, contains: pseudoephedrine HCl 120 mg and guaifenesin 600 mg in a special base to provide a prolonged 12-hour therapeutic effect. Nonmedicinal ingredients: compressible sugar, D&C Yellow No. 10, FD&C Yellow No. 6, hydroxypropyl cellulose, hydroxypropyl methylcellulose, magnesium stearate, polyethylene glycol, silicon dioxide, stearic acid and titanium dioxide. Cartons of 16. Store below 30°C protected from moisture.

(Shown in Product Identification Section)

Entocort® Capsules ℞

budesonide

Glucocorticosteroid for the Treatment of Crohn's Disease Affecting the Ileum and/or Ascending Colon

AstraZeneca

Date of Revision: March 2, 2009

PHARMACOLOGY: The active ingredient of ENTOCORT capsules, budesonide, is a potent nonhalogenated synthetic glucocorticosteroid with high topical potency and weak systemic effects.

The exact mechanism of action of glucocorticosteroids in the treatment of Crohn's disease is not fully understood. Anti-inflammatory actions, such as the inhibition of inflammatory mediator release and inhibition of immunological cellular responses, are probably important.

Data from clinical pharmacology studies and controlled clinical trials indicate that ENTOCORT capsules, at least partly, act topically. Budesonide undergoes an extensive degree (approximately 90%) of biotransformation in the liver to metabolites with low glucocorticosteroid activity. The glucocorticosteroid activity of the major metabolites, 6β-hydroxybudesonide and 16α-hydroxyprednisolone, is less than 1% of that of budesonide. The metabolism of budesonide is primarily mediated by CYP3A4, an isozyme of cytochrome P450.

The favorable separation between topical anti-inflammatory and systemic effect is due to strong glucocorticosteroid receptor affinity and an effective first pass metabolism by the liver with a short half-life. A glucocorticosteroid with such a profile is of particular importance for the local treatment of inflammatory bowel diseases such as Crohn's disease. With regard to treatment of this disease with glucocorticosteroids, it is essential to achieve a high local anti-inflammatory activity in the bowel wall with systemic side effects, e.g., on the hypothalamic pituitary adrenal (HPA) axis function, as low as possible.

INDICATIONS: ENTOCORT (budesonide) capsules are indicated for: the treatment of mild to moderate active Crohn's disease involving the ileum and/or the ascending colon and the maintenance of clinical remission of mild to moderate Crohn's disease involving the ileum and/or the ascending colon for up to 3 months.

CONTRAINDICATIONS: ENTOCORT (budesonide) capsules are contraindicated for the following: Systemic or local bacterial, fungal or viral infections. Known hypersensitivity to any of the ingredients. Active tuberculosis.

WARNINGS: Glucocorticosteroids can reduce the response of the HPA-axis to stress. In situations where patients are subject to surgery or other stress situations, supplementation with a conventional glucocorticosteroid is recommended.

Special care is demanded in treatment of patients transferred from conventional systemic steroids to ENTOCORT (budesonide) capsules, as disturbances in the HPA axis could be expected in these patients.

PRECAUTIONS: Glucocorticosteroids may mask some signs of infections and new infections may appear. A decreased resistance to localized infection has been observed during glucocorticosteroid therapy. Viral infections such as chickenpox and measles can have a more serious or fatal course in patients on immunosuppressant glucocorticosteroids. In adults who have not had these diseases, particular care should be taken to avoid exposure. If exposed to chickenpox or measles, therapy with varicella zoster immune globulin (VZIG) or pooled i.v. immunoglobulin (IVIG), as appropriate, may be indicated. If chickenpox develops, treatment with antiviral agents may be considered.

Although treatment with ENTOCORT (budesonide) capsules causes significantly less lowering of plasma cortisol compared to conventional glucocorticosteroids, the knowledge with regard to treatment during the following conditions is limited and therefore cautioned: active peptic ulcer, osteoporosis, acute glomerulonephritis, myasthenia gravis, exanthematous diseases, diverticulitis, thrombophlebitis, psychic disturbances, diabetes (or family history of diabetes), cataracts and glaucoma (or family history of glaucoma) which may cause elevation of intraocular pressure, hypertension, hyperthyroidism, acute coronary disease, limited cardiac reserve and pregnancy. In such cases the benefits of an oral glucocorticosteroid must be weighed against the risks.

With the recommended therapeutic doses of budesonide, the risk/benefit ratio seems to be low for the long-term systemic effects. However, as with any other glucocorticosteroid, patients should be carefully followed up for systemic adverse effects. During long-term therapy, adrenal function and hematological status should be periodically assessed.

Particular care is needed in patients who are transferred from systemic glucocorticosteroid treatment with higher systemic effect to ENTOCORT capsules. When ENTOCORT is used to replace prednisolone in steroid dependent patients, the daily dose should not exceed 6 mg. When treatment with ENTOCORT capsules is initiated, the prednisolone dose should be tapered, as these patients may experience adrenal cortical suppression. Therefore, monitoring of adrenocortical function may be considered in these patients. Some patients feel unwell in a nonspecific way during the withdrawal phase, e.g., pain in muscles and joints. Sometimes this can also unmask allergies e.g. rhinitis and eczema, which were previously controlled by the systemic drug. A general insufficient glucocorticosteroid effect should be suspected if, in rare cases, symptoms such as tiredness, headache, nausea and vomiting should occur. In these cases a temporary increase in the dose of systemic glucocorticosteroids is sometimes necessary.

Patients should be advised to inform subsequent physicians of the prior use of glucocorticosteroids.

Glucocorticosteroids should be used with caution in patients if there is a probability of bowel perforation as well as the probability of obstruction, abscess or other pyogenic infection and fresh intestinal anastomoses. Aggravation of diabetes mellitus or stimulation of manifestations of latent diabetes mellitus may be caused by glucocorticosteroid therapy.

There may be an enhanced systemic effect of budesonide in patients with liver cirrhosis since the metabolism of budesonide may be impaired and, as with other glucocorticosteroids, there may be enhanced effects in those with hypothyroidism. Reduced liver function may affect the elimination of corticosteroids. The i.v. pharmacokinetics of budesonide are, however, similar in cirrhotic patients and in healthy subjects. The pharmacokinetics after oral ingestion of budesonide were affected by compromised liver function as evidenced by increased systemic availability.

In vivo studies in male subjects, have shown that oral administration of ketoconazole (a known inhibitor of CYP3A activity in the liver and in the intestinal mucosa, see Drug Interactions, Ketoconazole) caused a 4- to 7-fold increase of the systemic exposure to oral budesonide. If treatment with ketoconazole (and possibly other azoles such as fluconazole, itraconazole or miconazole) together with budesonide is indicated, reduction of the budesonide dose should be considered if side effects typical of systemic glucocorticosteroids occur.

After extensive intake of grapefruit juice (observed in male subjects taking in 600 mL of concentrated grapefruit juice per day for 4 days), the systemic exposure for oral budesonide increased approximately 2-fold. Grapefruit juice inhibits CYP3A activity predominantly in the intestinal mucosa. As with other drugs primarily being metabolized through CYP3A, regular ingestion of grapefruit or its juice, should be avoided in connection with budesonide administration (other juices such as orange juice or apple juice do not inhibit CYP3A). See Drug Interactions, Grapefruit Juice.

Glucocorticosteroid therapy may cause hyperacidity of peptic ulcer.

ASA should be used cautiously in conjunction with glucocorticosteroids in hypoprothrombinemia.

Pregnancy: Administration of ENTOCORT capsules during pregnancy should be avoided unless there are compelling reasons. In experimental animal studies, budesonide was found to cross the placental barrier. Like other glucocorticosteroids, budesonide is teratogenic to rodent species. High doses of budesonide administered s.c. produced fetal malformations, primarily skeletal defects, in rabbits, rats, and in mice. The relevance of these findings to humans has not yet been established. In the absence of further studies in humans, budesonide should be used during pregnancy only if the potential benefits clearly outweigh the risk to the fetus. Infants born of mothers who have received substantial doses of glucocorticosteroids during pregnancy should be carefully observed for hypoadrenalism.

Lactation: Budesonide is excreted in breast milk. However, based on data from inhaled budesonide, at therapeutic doses of ENTOCORT, exposure to the infant is anticipated to be low. The use of ENTOCORT capsules in nursing mothers requires that the possible benefits of the drug be weighed against the potential hazards to the mother, or infant.

Children: The safety and effectiveness of ENTOCORT capsules in children have not been established, therefore use in this age group is not recommended.

Drug Interactions: To date, budesonide has not been observed to interact with other drugs used for the treatment of inflammatory bowel diseases.

Elevated plasma levels and enhanced effects of corticosteroids have been reported in women also receiving estrogens or oral contraceptives. However, a low-dose combination (ethinylestradiol/desogestrel: 30 μg/150 μg) oral contraceptive that more than doubled the plasma concentration of oral prednisolone, had no significant effect on the plasma concentration of oral budesonide.

The metabolism of budesonide is primarily mediated by CYP3A4, an isozyme of cytochrome P450. Inhibition of this enzyme by e.g. ketoconazole (and possibly other azoles such as fluconazole, itraconazole or miconazole), cyclosporin, troleandomycin, erythromycin or grapefruit juice can therefore increase the systemic exposure to budesonide.

Cimetidine: The kinetics of budesonide were investigated in healthy subjects without and with cimetidine, 1000 mg daily. After a 4 mg oral dose the values of C_{max} (nmol/L) and systemic availability (%) of budesonide without and with cimetidine (3.3 vs 5.1 nmol/L and 10 vs 12%, respectively) indicated a slight inhibitory effect on hepatic metabolism of budesonide, caused by cimetidine. This should be of little clinical importance.

Ketoconazole: Ketoconazole, a potent inhibitor of cytochrome P450 3A, the main metabolic enzyme for corticosteroids, increases plasma levels of orally ingested budesonide.

Omeprazole: At recommended doses, omeprazole has no effect on the pharmacokinetics of oral budesonide.

ADVERSE EFFECTS: In clinical trials, most adverse events experienced by patients or healthy volunteers receiving ENTOCORT (budesonide) capsules were of mild to moderate intensity and were classified as non-serious. A total of 577 patients with Crohn's disease were treated with ENTOCORT capsules for induction and maintenance of remission, in controlled clinical trials.

Adverse events reported in patients during induction of remission (n=399) with ENTOCORT capsules included dyspepsia (9%), muscle cramps (4%), palpitations (2%), blurred vision (3%), skin reactions including rash and urticaria (6%), and menstrual disorders (2%).

A similar adverse event profile was reported in patients during 3 long term (up to 12 months) maintenance treatment studies (n=178) with ENTOCORT capsules. The nature and incidence of adverse events was generally the same or less than observed during treatment for induction of remission.

Other side effects that have been reported include hypokalemia, tremor, and behavioural changes such as nervousness, insomnia, and mood swings.

Side effects typical of systemic glucocorticosteroids (such as Cushingoid features and reduced growth velocity) may occur. The systemic effects of budesonide on the HPA-axis were found to be dose-dependent.

In very rare cases, anaphylactic reactions have been reported during post marketing use.

OVERDOSE:

Symptoms: Reports of acute toxicity and/or death following overdosage with glucocorticosteroids are rare. Thus, acute overdosage with ENTOCORT (budesonide) capsules, even in excessive doses, is not expected to be a clinical problem. In the event of acute overdosage, no specific antidote is available. Treatment consists of immediate gastric lavage or emesis followed by supportive and symptomatic therapy.

Occasional overdosing will not give any obvious symptoms in most cases but it will decrease the plasma cortisol level and increase the number and percentage of circulating neutrophils. The number and percentage of eosinophils will decrease concurrently. Stopping the treatment or decreasing the dose will abolish the induced effects.

Habitual overdosing may cause hypercorticism and HPA suppression. Decreasing the dose or stopping the therapy, with the accepted procedures for discontinuing prolonged oral therapy with systemic steroids, will abolish the effects, although the restitution of the HPA axis may be a slow process and during periods with pronounced physical stress (severe infections, trauma, surgical operations, etc.) it may be advisable to supplement with conventional systemic steroids.

Treatment: See Symptoms.

For management of a suspected drug overdose, contact your **regional Poison Control Centre**. See the *CPS* Directory section for a list of Poison Control Centres.

DOSAGE: Active Disease: The recommended daily dose for induction of remission is 9 mg, administered once daily in the morning, for up to 8 weeks. The dose should be taken before meals. Full effect is usually achieved within 2-4 weeks.

Maintenance of Remission: Following an 8 week course of treatment for the active disease and once the patient's symptoms are controlled (CDAI <150), ENTOCORT 6 mg is recommended, administered daily in the morning before breakfast, for maintenance of clinical remission up to 3 months. If symptom control is still maintained at 3 months, an attempt to taper to complete cessation is recommended. The rate of tapering should be patient-specific and the patient should be monitored by the treating physician during this period. Continued treatment with ENTOCORT 6 mg for more than 3 months has not been shown to provide substantial clinical benefit.

The capsules should be swallowed whole with water, and not chewed, broken or crushed before being swallowed.

INFORMATION FOR THE PATIENT: Published in e-CPS, available by subscription at www.e-cps.ca.

SUPPLIED: Each controlled ileal release, 2-piece hard gelatin capsule, with an opaque light grey body and an opaque pink cap, printed "CIR/3mg" in black radial ink, contains: micronized budesonide 3 mg. Nonmedicinal ingredients: acetyltributyl citrate, dimethicone, ethylcellulose, gelatin, iron oxide, methacrylic acid copolymer, polysorbate 80, sodium lauryl sulfate, sugar spheres (sucrose and maize starch), talc, titanium dioxide and triethylcitrate. High density polyethylene bottles of 100 with a polypropylene screw cap.

There is a desiccant pellet in the cap. The capsules should be dispensed and stored in the original container. The patient should be advised to keep the bottle tightly capped. Store at controlled room temperature (15 to 30°C).

(Shown in Product Identification Section)

Entocort® Enema Ⓟ

budesonide

Glucocorticosteroid

AstraZeneca

Date of Preparation: February 15, 2000

Date of Revision: March 2, 2009

PHARMACOLOGY: Budesonide is a potent nonhalogenated synthetic glucocorticosteroid with strong topical and weak systemic effects.

Budesonide has a high topical anti-inflammatory potency. It undergoes an extensive degree (approximately 90%) of biotransformation in the liver to metabolites with low glucocorticosteroid activity. The glucocorticosteroid activity of the major metabolites, 6β-hydroxybudesonide and 16α-hydroxyprednisolone, is less than 1% of that of budesonide. The metabolism of budesonide is primarily mediated by CYP3A4, an isozyme of cytochrome P450.

The favourable separation between topical anti-inflammatory and systemic effect is due to strong glucocorticosteroid receptor affinity and an effective first-pass metabolism with a short half-life.

A glucocorticosteroid with such a profile is of particular importance for the local treatment of inflammatory bowel diseases (IBD) such as ulcerative colitis (UC). With regard to treatment of these diseases with glucocorticosteroids, it is essential to achieve a high local anti-inflammatory activity in the bowel wall with systemic side effects, for example, on the hypothalamic-pituitary-adrenal (HPA) axis function, as low as possible. At the recommended doses, budesonide enema causes no or small suppression of plasma cortisol.

Pharmacokinetics: Absorption in healthy subjects after rectal dosing of 2 mg budesonide low viscosity enema is rapid and essentially complete within 3 hours. The mean maximal plasma concentration after rectal administration is 3±2 nmol/L, reached within 1.5 hours. Similar results are obtained in patients suffering from distal ulcerative colitis. The mean systemic availability after rectal dosing is 15±12%. The plasma half-life is between 2 and 3 hours in adults.

INDICATIONS: In the management of distal ulcerative colitis (rectum, sigmoid and descending colon).

CONTRAINDICATIONS: Budesonide is contraindicated for the following: Local contraindications to the use of budesonide include imminent bowel perforation as well as the probability of obstruction, abscess or other pyogenic infection, fresh intestinal anastomoses, extensive fistulas and sinus tracts; systemic or local bacterial, fungal or viral infections; known hypersensitivity to any of the ingredients; active tuberculosis; ocular herpes simplex, and acute psychosis.

WARNINGS: Special care is demanded in treatment of patients transferred from systemic steroids to budesonide as disturbances in the hypothalamic-pituitary-adrenal axis could be expected in these patients.

PRECAUTIONS: Glucocorticosteroids may mask some signs of infections and new infections may appear. A decreased resistance to localized infection has been observed during corticosteroid therapy. Viral infections such as chicken pox and measles can have a more serious or fatal course in patients on immunosuppressant corticosteroids. In adults who have not had these diseases, particular care should be taken to avoid exposure. If exposed to chicken pox or measles, therapy with varicella zoster immune globulin (VZIG) or pooled i.v. immunoglobulin (IVIG), as appropriate, may be indicated. If chicken pox develops, treatment with antiviral agents may be considered.

At recommended doses, budesonide enema causes no clinically important changes in basal plasma cortisol levels or in the response to stimulation with ACTH. The effects on morning plasma cortisol and adrenal function are significantly less compared with prednisolone enema 25 mg daily. However, knowledge with regard to treatment of the following conditions is limited and therefore cautioned: active or latent peptic ulcer, osteoporosis, acute glomerulonephritis, myasthenia gravis, exanthematous diseases, diverticulitis, thrombophlebitis, psychic disturbances, diabetes, hypertension, hyperthyroidism, acute coronary disease, limited cardiac reserve and pregnancy. In such cases the benefits of a corticosteroid enema must be weighed against the risks.

There are still insufficient data on the long-term systemic effect of budesonide. With the recommended therapeutic doses, the risk/benefit ratio seems to be very low. However, as with any other glucocorticosteroid, patients should be carefully followed up for systemic adverse effects. During long-term therapy, pituitary-adrenal function and haematological status should be periodically assessed.

Some patients feel unwell in a nonspecific way during the withdrawal phase, e.g., pain in muscles and joints. A general insufficient glucocorticosteroid effect should be suspected if, in rare cases, symptoms such as tiredness, headache, nausea and vomiting should occur. In these cases a temporary increase in the dose of systemic glucocorticosteroids is sometimes necessary.

Glucocorticosteroid enemas should be administered with caution in patients with severe ulcerative colitis because these patients are predisposed to perforations of the bowel wall.

Patients should be advised to inform subsequent physicians of the prior use of glucocorticosteroids.

Aggravation of diabetes mellitus or stimulation of manifestations of latent diabetes mellitus may be caused by corticosteroid therapy.

There may be an enhanced effect of budesonide in patients with liver cirrhosis and, as with other glucocorticosteroids, there may be enhanced effects in those with hypothyroidism. Reduced liver function may affect the elimination of corticosteroids. The i.v. pharmacokinetics of budesonide are, however, similar in cirrhotic patients and in healthy subjects. The pharmacokinetics after oral ingestion of budesonide were affected by compromised liver function as evidenced by increased systemic availability.

In vivo studies in male subjects have shown that oral administration of ketoconazole (a known inhibitor of CYP3A activity in the liver and the intestinal mucosa, caused a 4- to 7-fold increase of the systemic exposure to oral budesonide. Therefore, it cannot be excluded that concomitant administration of budesonide enema and ketoconazole (and possibly other azoles such as fluconazole, itraconazole or miconazole) may result in increased systemic availability of budesonide (see Precautions, Drug Interactions).

Glucocorticosteroid therapy may cause hyperacidity of peptic ulcer.

ASA should be used cautiously in conjunction with corticosteroids in hypoprothrombinemia.

Glucocorticosteroids may cause elevation of intraocular pressure in glaucoma patients.

Pregnancy: Administration of budesonide during pregnancy should be avoided unless there are compelling reasons. In experimental animal studies, budesonide was found to cross the placental barrier. Like other glucocorticosteroids, budesonide is teratogenic to rodent species. High doses of budesonide administered s.c. produced fetal malformations, primarily skeletal defects, in rabbits, rats, and in mice. The relevance of these findings to humans has not yet been established. In the absence of further studies in humans, budesonide should be used during pregnancy only if the potential benefits clearly outweigh the risk to the fetus. Infants born of mothers who have received substantial doses of corticosteroids during pregnancy should be carefully observed for hypoadrenalism.

Lactation: Budesonide is excreted in breast milk. However, based on data from inhaled budesonide, at therapeutic doses of ENTOCORT, exposure to the infant is anticipated to be low. The use of budesonide in nursing mothers requires that the possible benefits of the drug be weighed against the potential hazards to the mother, or infant.

Children: The safety and effectiveness of budesonide in children have not been established; therefore, use in this age group is not recommended.

Drug Interactions: To date, budesonide has not been observed to interact with other drugs used for the treatment of inflammatory bowel diseases.

Elevated plasma levels and enhanced effects of corticosteroids have been reported in women also receiving estrogens or oral contraceptives. However, a low-dose combination (ethinylestradiol/desogestrel: 30 µg/150 µg) oral contraceptive that more than doubled the plasma concentration of oral prednisolone had no significant effect on the plasma concentration of oral budesonide.

The metabolism of budesonide is primarily mediated by CYP3A4, an isozyme of cytochrome P450. Inhibition of this enzyme by e.g. ketoconazole (and possibly other azoles such as fluconazole, itraconazole or miconazole), cyclosporin, troleandomycin or erythromycin can therefore increase the systemic exposure to budesonide.

Cimetidine: The kinetics of budesonide were investigated in healthy subjects without and with cimetidine, 1000 mg daily. After a 4 mg oral dose the values of C_{max} (nmol/L) and systemic availability (%) of budesonide without and with cimetidine (3.3 vs 5.1 nmol/L and 10 vs 12%, respectively) indicated a slight inhibitory effect on hepatic metabolism of budesonide, caused by cimetidine. This should be of little clinical importance.

Omeprazole: At recommended doses, omeprazole has no effect on the pharmacokinetics of oral budesonide.

ADVERSE EFFECTS: No major side effects attributable to the use of budesonide have been reported. During clinical trials, the frequency of subjectively reported side effects in a total of 247 patients and healthy volunteers given 2 mg budesonide, once daily in the morning, was low.

The most common adverse reactions are gastrointestinal disturbances, e.g., flatulence, nausea, diarrhea. These symptoms were reported in 23 of the 247 patients (9%) receiving 2 mg of budesonide. Psychiatric symptoms (insomnia, agitation, anxiety, depression, dysphoria, emotional lability, somnolence) were reported in 7 patients (3%) receiving 2 mg budesonide. Skin reactions (rash, urticaria) occurred in 5 patients (2%).

Systemic effects of budesonide on the HPA-axis function were found to be dose-dependent. In rare cases, signs or symptoms of systemic glucocorticosteroid effects, including hypofunction of the adrenal gland, may occur with rectally administered glucocorticosteroids, probably depending on dose, treatment time, concomitant and previous glucocorticosteroid intake, and individual sensitivity. Rectal administration of high concentrations of budesonide (10 mg/dose) resulted in significant suppression of endogenous cortisol concentrations as measured by plasma and urinary cortisol levels.

In patients in whom systemic steroids are reduced or stopped, withdrawal symptoms due to decreased systemic activity may occur.

In very rare cases, anaphylactic reactions have been reported during post marketing use.

OVERDOSE:

Symptoms: Acute overdosage with budesonide, even in excessive doses, is not expected to be a clinical problem. When used chronically at excessive doses, systemic corticosteroid effects such as hypercorticism and adrenal suppression may appear. If such changes occur, the dosage of budesonide should be discontinued consistent with accepted procedures for discontinuing prolonged oral steroid therapy. However, the dosage form, enema, and the route of administration make any prolonged overdosage unlikely.

Occasional overdosing will not give any obvious symptoms in most cases but it will decrease the plasma cortisol level and increase the number and percentage of circulating neutrophils. The number and percentage of eosinophils will decrease concurrently. Stopping the treatment or decreasing the dose will abolish the induced effects.

Habitual overdosing may cause hypercorticism and hypothalamic-pituitary-adrenal suppression. Decreasing the dose or stopping the therapy will abolish these effects, although the restitution of the HPA-axis may be a slow process and during periods with pronounced physical stress (severe infections, trauma, surgical operations, etc.) it may be advisable to supplement with systemic steroids.

Treatment: See Symptoms.

> For management of a suspected drug overdose, contact your **regional Poison Control Centre**. See the *CPS* Directory section for a list of Poison Control Centres.

DOSAGE: 1 retention enema is given nightly to the patient for 4 weeks. If the patient is not in remission after 4 weeks, the treatment period may be prolonged to 8 weeks.

ENTOCORT Enema is reconstituted by adding 1 dispersible tablet into the enema bottle, whereafter the bottle is vigorously shaken for at least 10 seconds or until the tablet is completely dissolved. The tablet will disintegrate rapidly and the suspension will turn slightly yellowish.

INFORMATION FOR THE PATIENT: Published in e-CPS, available by subscription at www.e-cps.ca.

SUPPLIED: Each retention enema contains: budesonide 0.02 mg/mL and consists of 2 components, a dispersible tablet and a vehicle. The enema is reconstituted before use. The volume of the reconstituted enema is 115 mL. Since the residual volume is about 15 mL, the dose administered to the patient is about 2 mg budesonide. The tablets are provided in an aluminum blister package and the vehicle is in a polyethylene bottle equipped with a rectular nozzle. Each tablet contains: micronized budesonide 2.3 mg. Nonmedicinal ingredients: tablet: colloidal silicon dioxide, cross-linked polyvidone, lactose, lactose anhydrous, magnesium stearate and riboflavin-5-phosphate sodium; vehicle: methylparaben, propylparaben, purified water and sodium chloride. Cartons of 7 dispersible tablets and vehicle solutions. Store at 15 to 30°C. After preparation of the enema, the solution is intended for immediate use.

(Shown in Product Identification Section)

Entrophen

ASA

Nonsteroidal Anti-inflammatory—Analgesic—Antipyretic—Platelet Aggregation Inhibitor

PendoPharm

SUPPLIED: Chewable Tablets: Each chewable, salmon colored, round, biconvex tablet, embossed "81" contains: ASA 81 mg. Nonmedicinal ingredients: cornstarch, D&C Yellow No. 10 Aluminum Lake, FD&C Red No. 40 Lake, mannitol, orange flavor, sodium saccharin and stearic acid. Bottles of 30 and 120. Store at room temperature between 15 and 30°C. Protect from moisture.

Enteric Coated Caplets: 325 mg: Each yellow, capsule shaped, enteric-coated caplet contains: ASA 325 mg. Nonmedicinal ingredients: cornstarch, guar gum, hydrogenated vegetable oil, iron oxide yellow, methacrylic acid copolymer, methylated silica, methylcellulose, microcrystalline cellulose, polydimethylsiloxane, polyethylene glycol, polyvinyl alcohol, silica, sodium bicarbonate, sodium lauryl sulfate, sorbitan tristearate, soy lecithin, talc, titanium dioxide and triethyl citrate. Bottles of 100 and 1000. Store at room temperature between 15 and 30°C. Protect from moisture.

650 mg: Each orange, capsule shaped, enteric-coated caplet contains: ASA 650 mg. Nonmedicinal ingredients: cornstarch, FD&C Yellow No. 6 Aluminum Lake, guar gum, hydrogenated vegetable oil, methacrylic acid colopolymer, methylated silica, methylcellulose, microcrystalline cellulose, polydimethylsiloxane, polyethylene glycol, polyvinyl alcohol, silica, sodium bicarbonate, sodium lauryl sulfate, sorbitan tristearate, soy lecithin, talc, titanium dioxide and triethyl citrate. Bottles of 100. Store at room temperature between 15 and 30°C. Protect from moisture.

Enteric Coated Tablets: 81 mg: Each round, white, enteric-coated tablet contains: ASA 81 mg. Nonmedicinal ingredients: cornstarch, lactose, methacrylic acid copolymer, methylated silica, methylcellulose, polydimethylsiloxane, polyethylene glycol, silica, sodium bicarbonate, sodium lauryl sulfate, sorbitan tristearate, stearic acid, talc, titanium dioxide and trietyl citrate. Bottles of 30, 120 and 180. Store at room temperature between 15 and 30°C. Protect from moisture.

325 mg: Each brown, round, enteric-coated tablet contains: ASA 325 mg. Nonmedicinal ingredients: cornstarch, FD&C Blue No. 1 Aluminum Lake, FD&C Red No. 40 Aluminum Lake, FD&C Yellow No. 6 Aluminum Lake, guar gum, hydrogenated vegetable oil, methacrylic acid copolymer, methylated silica, methylcellulose, microcrystalline cellulose, polydimethylsiloxane, polyethylene glycol, polyvinyl alcohol, silica, sodium bicarbonate, sodium lauryl sulfate, sorbitan tristearate, soy lecithin, talc, titanium dioxide and triethyl citrate. Bottles of 100. Store at room temperature between 15 and 30°C. Protect from moisture.

500 mg: Each pink, enteric-coated tablet contains: ASA 500 mg. Nonmedicinal ingredients: cornstarch, FD&C Red No. 40 Aluminum Lake, guar gum, hydrogenated vegetable oil, methacrylic acid copolymer, methylated silica, methylcellulose, microcrystalline cellulose, polydimethylsiloxane, polyethylene glycol, polyvinyl alcohol, silica, sodium bicarbonate, sodium lauryl sulfate, sorbitan tristearate, soy lecithin, talc, titanium dioxide and triethyl citrate. Bottles of 100. Store at room temperature between 15 and 30°C. Protect from moisture.

650 mg: Each orange, enteric-coated tablet contains: ASA 650 mg. Nonmedicinal ingredients: cornstarch, FD&C Yellow No. 6 aluminum lake, guar gum, hydrogenated vegetable oil, methacrylic acid copolymer, methylated silica, methylcellulose, microcrystalline cellulose, polydimethylsiloxane, polyethylene glycol, polyvinyl alcohol, silica, sodium bicarbonate, sodium lauryl sulfate, sorbitan tristearate, soy lecithin, talc, titanium dioxide and triethyl citrate. Bottles of 100. Store at room temperature between 15 and 30°C. Protect from moisture.

Enuclene™

tyloxapol

Cleaning/Lubricating Solution for Artificial Eyes

Alcon

SUPPLIED: Each mL of sterile, buffered solution contains: tyloxapol 0.25%. Nonmedicinal ingredients: benzalkonium chloride (as preservative), boric acid, dibasic sodium phosphate, hydroxypropyl methylcellulose and purified water. Drop-Tainer dispensers of 15 mL.

Ephedrine Sulfate Injection USP

ephedrine sulfate

Sympathomimetic

Hospira

SUPPLIED: Each mL of sterile, nonpyrogenic solution contains: ephedrine sulfate 50 mg. pH 4.5 to 7.0; the 5% solution has a concentration of 0.35 mOsm/mL (approx.) Nonmedicinal ingredients: water for injection. Single dose ampoules of 1 mL, boxes of 50. Store at room temperature. Protect from light. Discard unused portion.

Ephedrine Sulfate Injection USP

ephedrine sulfate

Alpha and Beta Adrenergic Agonist

Sandoz

SUPPLIED: Each mL of solution contains: ephedrine sulfate 50 mg. Nonmedicinal ingredients: sodium hydroxide or sulfuric acid to adjust pH and water for injection. Ampoules of 1 mL, boxes of 10. Store between 15 and 30°C. Protect from light.

EpiCeram®

ceramides—cholesterol—free fatty acids

Topical Therapeutic Skin Barrier Emulsion

Pediapharm

Date of Preparation: August 31, 2010

SUMMARY PRODUCT INFORMATION: EpiCeram Skin Barrier Emulsion is a steroid-free, fragrance-free, ceramide-dominant formulation.

INDICATIONS AND CLINICAL USE: EpiCeram Skin Barrier Emulsion is to be used to treat dry skin conditions and to manage and relieve the burning and itching associated with various types of dermatoses, including atopic dermatitis. EpiCeram Skin Barrier Emulsion helps to relieve dry, waxy skin by maintaining a moist wound and skin environment, which is beneficial to the healing process.

CONTRAINDICATIONS: EpiCeram Skin Barrier Emulsion is contraindicated in persons with known hypersensitivity to any of the components of the formulation.

WARNINGS AND PRECAUTIONS: EpiCeram Skin Barrier Emulsion does not contain a sunscreen and should always be used in conjunction with a sunscreen in sun exposed areas. In radiation dermatitis and/or in conjunction with ongoing radiation therapy, apply following radiation therapy. Do not apply within 4 hours prior to radiation therapy. Apply twice daily or as indicated by the radiation therapist. After application, a temporary tingling sensation may occur (10 to 15 minutes). Keep this and similar products out of the reach of children. Follow directions for use. If condition does not improve within 10 to 14 days, consult a physician.

Precautions and Observations: For the treatment of any dermal wound, consult a physician.

- Use EpiCeram Skin Barrier Emulsion only as directed.
- EpiCeram Skin Barrier Emulsion is non-toxic; however it is for external use only and should not be ingested or taken internally.
- If clinical signs of infection are present, appropriate treatment should be initiated. If clinically indicated, use of EpiCeram Skin Barrier Emulsion may be continued during the anti-infective therapy.
- If the condition does not improve within 10-14 days, consult a physician.
- EpiCeram Skin Barrier Emulsion does not contain a sunscreen and should always be used in conjunction with a sun screen in sun exposed areas.
- In radiation dermatitis and/or in conjunction with ongoing radiation therapy, apply following radiation therapy.
- Do not apply within 4 hours prior to radiation therapy. Apply twice daily or as indicated by the radiation therapist.
- Following the application of EpiCeram Skin Barrier Emulsion a temporary tingling sensation may occur (10-15 minutes).
- Keep this and other similar products out of the reach of children.

ACTION AND CLINICAL PHARMACOLOGY: The stratum corneum is a multilayered tissue composed of flattened anucleated corneocytes embedded in a lipid-enriched extracellular matrix. This matrix is derived from lipid sheets extruded from the lamellar bodies. Lamellar bodies fuse with the plasma membrane of the granular cell and discharge lipids and enzymes into the extracellular space. Enzymatic processing of the extracellular lipids is required to generate the mature lamellae. The corneocytes with the extracellular lipid surroundings provide the mechanical protection and water regulation of the skin barrier. In patients with atopic dermatitis, this lipid barrier is markedly reduced.

EpiCeram is a ceramide-dominant, physiologic, lipid-based emulsion that provides an optimal **3:1:1 ratio of ceramides, cholesterol and free fatty acids** to replenish the skin barrier in atopic skin.

EpiCeram normalizes the skin barrier through multiple proposed mechanisms:

- Creation of a barrier to prevent transepidermal water loss
- Bulk replenishment of physiologic lipids
- Enrichment of high quality of ceramides
- Delivery of an optimal ratio of ceramides, cholesterol, and free fatty acids
- Formulation is buffered at pH 5.5

In a study designed to assess the efficacy of EpiCeram in correcting the lipid-biochemical abnormalities in atopic dermatitis (AD), EpiCeram reduced clinical disease severity after 14 and 28 days of therapy (Efficacy of a lipid-based barrier repair formulation in moderate-to-severe paediatric atopic dermatitis, Sugarman, JL, J Drugs in Dermatol. 2009;8(12):1106-1111).

Table 1: EpiCeram

Clinical Endpoints Following Treatment with EpiCeram

	Time	Mean	Change (%)[a]	Significance
SCORAD (0 to 72)	Baseline	37.2	—	—
	Day 14	23.6	37	<0.001
	Day 28	18.5	51	<0.001
Pruritus[b]	Baseline	6.1		
	Day 14	3.9	39	<0.001
	Day 28	2.8	52	<0.001
Sleep Habits[b]	Baseline	4.1	—	—
	Day 14	2.2	42	<0.001
	Day 28	1.4	62	<0.001

[a] Reduction from baseline.
[b] Ten-point scale where 0=none.

The study, a five-center, investigator-blinded, randomized trial, compared EpiCeram to fluticasone propionate cream (Cutivate) in 121 patients with moderate-to-severe AD. Primary outcome measures were: 1) Reduction in disease severity, assessed as SCORAD scores; 2) improvement in pruritus; and 3) changes in sleep habits.

Results showed that EpiCeram reduced clinical disease severity, decreased pruritus, and improved sleep habits both 14 and 28 days after initiation of therapy. The EpiCeram-treated group did not differ significantly from the fluticasone-treated group by 28 days in terms of SCORAD, pruritus, and sleep habit scores.

SCORAD scores decreased 37% and 51% from the baseline at 14 and 28 days respectively (Table 1; p <0.001). Subjective pruritus and sleep habits scores decreased in parallel, and to a comparable extent (Table 1). Both the patients/family self-assessment and IGA scores also demonstrated parallel, highly significant improvement at 14 and 28 days.

Based upon changes in SCORAD and IGA scores, there was no statistical difference between the ceramide-dominant, barrier formulation and fluticasone propionate at 28 days (Table 2). Both agents demonstrated significant improvements in pruritus, sleep habits, and patient/family assessment scores at both 14 and 28 days, changes that did not differ significantly from one another. Fluticasone propionate-treated subjects demonstrated significantly faster improvement in SCORAD and IGA scores at 14 days (p<0.05) (Table 2). Thus, with the exception of SCORAD and IGA scores at day 14, the ceramide-dominant barrier formulation and fluticasone propionate cream demonstrated comparable efficacy for moderate-to-severe atopic dermatitis.

Table 2: EpiCeram

Statistical Comparisons of Responses to EpiCeram and Fluticasone

	Mean Reduction from Baseline	
SCORAD (0 to 72)	**EpiCeram (%)**	**Fluticasone (%)**
Day 14	13.6 (36.6)	18.5 (57.6)
Anova p-value: 0.021; Rank sum p-value: 0.081		
Day 28	18.7 (50.7)	22.2 (66.7)
Anova p-value: 0.134; Rank sum p-value: 0.363		

SCORAD: 0=no evidence of disease.

DOSAGE AND ADMINISTRATION: **Instructions for Use:** Apply in a thin layer to the affected skin areas 2 times per day (or as needed) and massage gently into the skin. If the skin is broken, cover EpiCeram Skin Barrier Emulsion with a dressing of choice.

Information to Be Provided to the Patient:

- Patients should use EpiCeram as directed by the physician. EpiCeram is for external topical use only; patients should wash their hands after application.
- Patients should not use EpiCeram for any disorder other than that for which it is prescribed.
- EpiCeram is recommended to be used b.i.d. in atopic dermatitis on targeted area as directed by your physician; it can be used as a prophylactic on areas prone to repeated atopic dermatitis.
- Should EpiCeram be prescribed along with steroids or a topical immunomodulator, it is recommended to apply EpiCeram on affected areas of the skin just a few minutes before to allow proper penetration. To ensure efficacy of EpiCeram in combination therapy, it should never be mixed with any other product.
- EpiCeram should not be mixed on skin with an emollient or moisturizer.

STORAGE AND STABILITY: Store at 15 to 30°C. Do not freeze.

DOSAGE FORMS, COMPOSITION AND PACKAGING: Each tube of emulsion contains: capric acid, cholesterol, citric acid, conjugated linoleic acid, dimethicone, disodium EDTA, E. Cerifera (candelilla) wax, food starch, modified corn syrup solids, glycerin, glyceryl stearate, hydroxypropyl bispalmitamide MEA (ceramide), palmitic acid, PEG-100 stearate, petrolatum, phenoxyethanol, potassium hydroxide, purified water, sorbic acid, squalane and xanthan gum. Tubes of 50 g.

Epinephrine

epinephrine

Sympathomimetic

Hospira

PHARMACOLOGY: The actions of epinephrine resemble the effects of stimulation of adrenergic nerves. It acts on both alpha and beta receptor sites of sympathetic effector cells. Its most prominent actions are on the beta receptors of the heart, vascular and other smooth muscle. When given by rapid i.v. injection, it produces a rapid rise in blood pressure, mainly systolic, by direct stimulation of cardiac muscle which increases the strength of ventricular contraction, increasing the heart rate and constriction of the arterioles in the skin, mucosa and splanchnic areas of the circulation.

When given by slow i.v. injection, epinephrine usually produces only a moderate rise in systolic and a fall in diastolic pressure. Although some increase in pulse pressure occurs, there is usually no great elevation in mean blood pressure. Accordingly, the compensatory reflex mechanisms that come into play with a pronounced increase in blood pressure do not antagonize the direct cardiac actions of epinephrine as much as with catecholamines that have a predominant action on alpha receptors.

Total peripheral resistance decreases by action of epinephrine on beta receptors of the skeletal muscle vasculature and blood flow is thereby enhanced. Usually this vasodilator effect of the drug on the circulation predominates so that the modest rise in systolic pressure which follows slow injection or absorption is mainly the result of direct cardiac stimulation and increase in cardiac output. In some instances, peripheral resistance is not altered or may even rise owing to a greater ratio of alpha to beta activity in different vascular areas.

Epinephrine relaxes the smooth muscles of the bronchi and iris and is a physiologic antagonist of histamine. The drug also produces an increase in blood sugar and glycogenolysis in the liver.

Pharmacokinetics: I.V. injection produces an immediate and intensified response. Following i.v. injection, epinephrine disappears rapidly from the blood stream.

Epinephrine is rapidly inactivated in the body and is degraded by enzymes in the liver and other tissues. The larger portion of injected doses is excreted in the urine as inactivated compounds and the remainder either partly unchanged or conjugated.

The drug becomes fixed in the tissues and is inactivated chiefly by enzymatic transformation to metanephrine or normetanephrine, either of which is subsequently conjugated and excreted in the urine in the form of sulfates and glucuronides. Either sequence results in the formation of 3-methoxy-4 hydroxy-mandelic acid (vanillyl-mandelic acid; VMA) which also is detectable in the urine.

Sodium chloride added to render the solution isotonic for injection of the active ingredient is present in amounts insufficient to affect serum electrolyte balance of sodium (Na^+) and chloride (Cl^-) ions.

INDICATIONS: In general, the most common uses of parenteral epinephrine are to relieve respiratory distress due to bronchospasm, to provide rapid relief of hypersensitivity (anaphylactic or anaphylactoid) reactions to drugs, animal serums and other allergens, and to prolong the action of infiltration anesthetics. Its cardiac effects may be of use in restoring cardiac rhythm in cardiac arrest due to various causes, and attacks of transitory atrioventricular (AV) heart block and syncopal seizures (Stokes-Adams syndrome), but it is not used in cardiac failure or in hemorrhagic, traumatic, or cardiogenic shock.

In acute attacks of ventricular standstill, physical measures should be applied first. When external cardiac compression and attempts to restore the circulation by electrical defibrillation or use of a pacemaker fail, intracardiac puncture and intramyocardial injection of epinephrine may be effective.

Epinephrine is used as a hemostatic agent.

It is also used in treating mucosal congestion of hay fever, rhinitis, and acute sinusitis; to relieve bronchial asthmatic paroxysms; in syncope due to complete heart block or carotid sinus hypersensitivity; for symptomatic relief of serum sickness, urticaria, angioneurotic edema; for resuscitation in cardiac arrest following anesthetic accidents; in simple (open angle) glaucoma; for relaxation of uterine musculature and to inhibit uterine contractions. Epinephrine injection can be utilized to prolong the action of intraspinal and local anesthetics (see Contraindications).

CONTRAINDICATIONS: In patients with known hypersensitivity to sympathomimetic amines, in patients with angle closure glaucoma, and patients in shock (nonanaphylactic). It should not be used in patients anesthetized with agents such as cyclopropane or halothane as these may sensitize the heart to arrhythmic action of sympathomimetic drugs.

Epinephrine should not ordinarily be used in cases where vasopressor drugs may be contraindicated, e.g., in thyrotoxicosis, diabetes, patients receiving MAO inhibitors, in obstetrics when maternal blood pressure is in excess of 130/80 or during labor, and in hypertension and other cardiovascular disorders.

WARNINGS: Inadvertently induced high arterial blood pressure may result in angina pectoris, aortic rupture or cerebral hemorrhage.

Epinephrine may induce potentially serious cardiac arrhythmias in patients not suffering from heart disease and patients with organic heart disease or who are receiving drugs that sensitize the myocardium.

Parenterally administered epinephrine initially may produce constriction of renal blood vessels and decrease urine formation, and large doses may cause complete renal shutdown.

Epinephrine and Beta-blockers: There may be increased difficulty in treating an allergic-type reaction in patients on beta-blockers. In these patients, the reaction may be more severe due to pharmacologic effects of the beta-blockers and problems with fluid changes (see Precautions, Drug Interactions).

Epinephrine is the preferred treatment for serious allergic or other emergency situations even though this product contains sodium metabisulfite, a sulfite that may cause allergic-type reactions including anaphylactic symptoms or life-threatening or less severe asthmatic episodes in certain susceptible persons. The alternatives to using epinephrine in a life-threatening situation may not be satisfactory. The presence of a sulfite in this product should not deter administration of the drug for treatment of serious allergic or other emergency situations.

PRECAUTIONS: Although epinephrine can produce ventricular fibrillation, its actions in restoring electrical activity in asystole and in enhancing defibrillation of the fibrillating ventricle are well documented. The drug, however, should be used with caution in patients with ventricular fibrillation.

In patients with prefibrillatory rhythm, i.v. epinephrine must be used judiciously, with extreme caution, because of its excitatory action on the heart. Since the myocardium is sensitized to this action of the drug by many anesthetic agents, epinephrine may convert asystole to ventricular fibrillation if used in the treatment of anesthetic cardiac accidents.

Epinephrine should be used cautiously in the elderly and in patients with hyperthyroidism, hypertension, diabetes and cardiac diseases/arrhythmias. Patients with long-standing bronchial asthma and emphysema, who have developed degenerative heart disease, should be administered the drug with extreme caution.

Fatalities may also result from pulmonary edema because of the peripheral constriction and cardiac stimulation produced. Rapidly acting vasodilators such as nitrites, or alpha-blocking agents may counteract the marked pressor effects of epinephrine.

Drug Interactions: Beta-blockers: There may be increased difficulty in treating an allergic-type reaction in patients on beta-blockers. In these patients, the reaction may be more severe due to pharmacologic effects of the beta-blockers and problems with fluid changes. Epinephrine should be administered with caution, since it may not have its usual effects in the treatment of anaphylaxis. On the one hand, larger doses of epinephrine may be needed to overcome the bronchospasm, while on the other, these doses can be associated with excessive alpha adrenergic stimulation with consequent hypertension, reflex bradycardia and heart-block and possible potentiation of bronchospasm. Alternatives to the use of large doses of epinephrine include vigorous supportive care such as fluids and the use of beta agonists including parenteral salbutamol or isoproterenol to overcome bronchospasm and norepinephrine to overcome hypotension.

Sympathomimetic Drugs: Epinephrine should not be administered concomitantly with other sympathomimetic drugs (such as isoproterenol) because of possible additive effects and increased toxicity. Combined effects may induce serious cardiac arrhythmias. They may be administered alternately when the preceding effect of another such drug has subsided.

Cyclopropane or Halogenated Hydrocarbons: Administration of epinephrine to patients receiving cyclopropane or halogenated hydrocarbon general anesthetics such as halothane, which sensitize the myocardium, may induce cardiac arrhythmias (see Contraindications). When encountered, such arrhythmias may respond to administration of a beta-adrenergic blocking drug.

Diuretics: Diuretic agents may decrease vascular response to pressor drugs such as epinephrine.

Guanethidine: Epinephrine may antagonize the neuron blockade produced by guanethidine, resulting in decreased antihypertensive effect and requiring increased dosage of the latter.

MAO Inhibitors: All vasopressors should be used cautiously in patients taking MAO inhibitors (see Contraindications).

Others: The effects of epinephrine may be potentiated by tricyclic antidepressants; certain antihistamines, e.g., diphenhydramine, tripelennamine, chlorpheniramine and sodium levothyroxine.

Epinephrine also should be used cautiously with other drugs (e.g., digitalis glycosides) that sensitize the myocardium to the actions of sympathomimetic drugs.

Pregnancy: Epinephrine has been shown to be teratogenic in rats when given in doses about 25 times the human doses. It is not known whether epinephrine can cause fetal harm when administered to a pregnant woman or can affect reproduction capacity. Epinephrine should be given to a pregnant woman only if clearly needed.

Labor and Delivery: Parenteral administration of epinephrine, if used to support blood pressure during low or other spinal anesthesia for delivery, can cause acceleration of fetal heart rate and should not be used in obstetrics when maternal blood pressure exceeds 130/80 (see Contraindications). Epinephrine may delay the second stage of labor.

ADVERSE EFFECTS: Transient and minor side effects of anxiety, headache, fear and palpitations may occur with systemic therapeutic doses, especially in hyperthyroid individuals. Adverse effects, such as cardiac arrhythmias and excessive rise in blood pressure, may also occur with systemic therapeutic doses or inadvertent overdosage. Other adverse reactions include: cerebral hemorrhage, hemiplegia, subarachnoid hemorrhage, anginal pain in patients with angina pectoris, anxiety, restlessness, throbbing headache, tremor, weakness, dizziness, pallor and respiratory difficulty.

OVERDOSE:

Symptoms: Erroneous administration of large doses of epinephrine may lead to precordial distress, vomiting, headache, dyspnea, as well as unusually elevated blood pressure (see Warnings).

Treatment: Toxic effects of overdosage can be counteracted by injection of an alpha-adrenergic blocker and a beta-adrenergic blocker. In the event of a sharp rise in blood pressure, rapid-acting vasodilators such as the nitrites, or alpha-adrenergic blocking agents can be given to counteract the marked pressor effect of large doses of epinephrine.

For management of a suspected drug overdose, CPhA recommends that you contact your **regional Poison Control Centre**. See the *CPS* Directory section for a list of Poison Control Centres.

DOSAGE: Epinephrine injection is administered by the following routes: i.v., intracardiac (left ventricular chamber), s.c. or i.m., and via endotracheal tube in the bronchial tree.

Note: The s.c. is the preferred route of administration. If given i.m., injection into the buttocks should be avoided, due to the possibility of poor absorption.

Hypersensitivity Reaction: Adults: For bronchial asthma and certain allergic manifestations, e.g., angioedema, urticaria, serum sickness, anaphylactic shock, use epinephrine 0.2 to 1 mg (0.2 to 1 mL of a 1 mg/mL solution [1:1000]) s.c. or i.m. S.C. doses may be repeated at 10- to 15-minute intervals in patients with anaphylactic shock. In patients with asthma, s.c. doses may be given at 20-minute to 4-hour intervals, depending on the severity of the condition and the response of the patient. In severe anaphylactic shock, i.v. administration may be necessary since absorption of the drug may be impaired with s.c. or i.m. administration. If necessary, 0.1 to 0.25 mg of epinephrine (1 to 2.5 mL of a 0.1 mg/mL solution [1:10 000]) may be administered i.v. slowly (over 5 to 10 minutes) and repeated every 5 to 15 minutes as necessary. Start with small doses and increase if required.

Children: For bronchial asthma and other allergic manifestations in pediatric patients, administer 0.01 mg/kg (0.01 mL/kg of 1 mg/mL solution [1:1000]) or 0.3 mg/m² (0.3 mL/m² of a 1 mg/mL solution [1:1000]) to a maximum of 0.5 mg (0.5 mL of a 1 mg/mL solution [1:1000]) s.c. Doses may be repeated at 20-minute to 4-hour intervals, depending on the severity of the condition and the response of the patient. In severe anaphylactic shock, i.v. administration may be necessary since absorption of the drug may be impaired with s.c. administration. If necessary, some clinicians recommend an initial i.v. epinephrine dose of 0.1 mg (10 mL of a 1:100 000 dilution prepared by diluting 0.1 mL of a 1 mg/mL solution [1:1000]) with 10 mL of 0.9% sodium chloride injection given over 5 to 10 minutes (the initial dose may have to be reduced in young children), followed by a continuous infusion at an initial rate of 0.1 µg/kg/min (to a maximum of 1.5 µg/kg/min).

Cardiac Resuscitation: Adults: A dose of 0.5 mg i.v. (range 0.1 to 1 mg, usually as 1 to 10 mL of a 0.1 mg/mL solution [1:10 000]). I.V. doses may be repeated every 5 minutes if needed. Adult intracardiac doses of 0.1 to 1 mg (usually as 1 to 10 mL of a 0.1 mg/mL solution [1:10 000]) have been recommended. External cardiac massage should follow intracardiac administration to permit the drug to enter coronary circulation.

Children: The usual **pediatric** i.v. dose is 0.01 mg/kg (0.1 mL/kg of 0.1 mg/mL solution [1:10 000]). I.V. doses may be repeated every 5 minutes if needed.

The usual **neonatal** i.v. dose is 0.01 to 0.03 mg/kg (0.1 to 0.3 mL/kg of a 0.1 mg/mL solution [1:10 000]). I.V. doses may be repeated every 5 minutes if necessary.

Endotracheal Dosage: Alternatively, as a means for advanced cardiac life support, when vascular access is hampered and patients intubated, epinephrine can be administered via the endotracheal tube directly into the bronchial tree. To aid delivery of the drug via an endotracheal tube, the dose may be diluted with 0.9% sodium chloride. Adults: 1 mg (10 mL of a 0.1 mg/mL solution [1:10 000]). Children: 0.01 mg/kg (0.1 mL/kg of a 0.1 mg/mL solution [1:10 000]). Neonates: 0.01 to 0.03 mg/kg (0.1 to 0.3 mL/kg of a 0.1 mg/mL solution [1:10 000]).

Regional Anesthesia: A final concentration of 1:100 000 to 1:200 000 of epinephrine injection is recommended for infiltration injection, nerve block, caudal or other epidural blocks. From 0.2 to 0.4 mg of epinephrine (0.2 to 0.4 mL of a 1 mg/mL solution [1:1000]) may be mixed with spinal anesthetic agents.

SUPPLIED: 1:1000: Each mL of sterile, nonpyrogenic solution contains: epinephrine 1 mg, sodium chloride added to adjust tonicity, sodium metabisulfite 0.9 mg as an antioxidant, hydrochloric acid for pH adjustment and water for injection. Ampuls of 1 mL, boxes of 5×10.

1:10 000: Each mL of sterile, nonpyrogenic solution contains: epinephrine 0.1 mg, sodium chloride 8.16 mg, sodium metabisulfite 0.46 mg as an antioxidant, citric acid, anhydrous, sodium citrate, dihydrate (as buffers) and water for injection. May contain additional citric acid and/or sodium citrate for pH adjustment -pH 3.3 (2.2 to 5.0). Abboject syringes of 10 mL, boxes of 10. Lifeshield syringes of 10 mL, boxes of 10.

The solution contains no bacteriostatic or antimicrobial agent and is intended for use as a single-dose injection. When smaller doses are required, the unused portion should be discarded.

Note: This product contains sodium metabisulfite: use with caution (see Warnings).

Parenteral drug products should be inspected visually for particulate matter and discoloration prior to administration, whenever solution and container permit.

Protect from freezing and extreme heat. Store at controlled room temperature (15 to 30°C).

Protect from light by retaining product in carton until ready for use.

Note: Do not use the injection if its color is pinkish or darker than slightly yellow or if it contains a precipitate. Do not administer unless solution is clear and seal is intact. Discard unused portion.

EpiPen®

epinephrine

Catecholamine—Sympathomimetic

King Pharmaceuticals

EpiPen® Jr

epinephrine

Catecholamine—Sympathomimetic

King Pharmaceuticals

Date of Preparation: July 14, 2006

Date of Revision: October 23, 2009

SUMMARY PRODUCT INFORMATION:

Route of Administration	Dosage Form/ Strength	Nonmedicinal Ingredients
Intramuscular Injection inject into anterolateral aspect of the thigh. Do not inject into the buttock.	EpiPen Syringe, 1:1000 Unidose 0.3 mg epinephrine auto-injector EpiPen Jr Syringe, 1:2000 Unidose 0.15 mg epinephrine auto-injector	Hydrochloric acid, sodium chloride, sodium metabisulfite, water for injection

INDICATIONS AND CLINICAL USE: EpiPen (0.3 mL Epinephrine Injection, USP, 1:1000) and EpiPen Jr (0.3 mL Epinephrine Injection, USP, 1:2000) are indicated for the emergency treatment of anaphylactic reactions in patients who are determined to be at increased risk for anaphylaxis, including individuals with a history of anaphylactic reactions. Selection of the appropriate dosage strength is determined according to patient body weight (see Dosage and Administration).

EpiPen and EpiPen Jr are intended for immediate self-administration for the emergency treatment of severe allergic reactions (Type I), including anaphylaxis associated with:

- foods (e.g., peanuts, tree nuts, shellfish, fish, milk, eggs, and wheat)
- stinging insects (e.g., Order Hymenoptera, including bees, wasps, hornets, yellow jackets, and fire ants) and biting insects (e.g., mosquitoes and black flies)
- medications
- latex
- idiopathic anaphylaxis
- exercise-induced anaphylaxis
- other allergens

Epinephrine is the drug of choice for the emergency treatment of severe allergic reactions. The strong vasoconstrictor action of epinephrine, through its effect on alpha adrenergic receptors, quickly counteracts vasodilation and increased vascular permeability which can lead to loss of intravascular fluid volume and hypotension during anaphylactic reactions.

EpiPen and EpiPen Jr are designed as emergency supportive therapy only and not as a replacement or substitute for subsequent medical or hospital care, nor are they intended to supplant insect venom hyposensitization.

Clinical Signs and Symptoms of Anaphylaxis: Anaphylaxis is a serious, acute, allergic reaction that may cause death. It has a sudden onset and generally lasts less than 24 hours. Because anaphylaxis is a generalized reaction, a wide variety of clinical signs and symptoms may be observed.

One to 2% of the general population are estimated to be at risk for anaphylaxis from food allergies and insect stings, with a lower reported prevalence for drugs and latex. People with asthma are at particular risk.

Symptoms of Anaphylaxis May Include: Oral: pruritus of lips, tongue, and palate, edema of lips and tongue; metallic taste in the mouth.

Cutaneous: flushing, pruritus, urticaria, angioedema, morbilliform rash, and pilor erecti.

Gastrointestinal: nausea, abdominal pain, vomiting, and diarrhea.

Respiratory: Laryngeal: pruritus and "tightness" in the throat, dysphagia, dysphonia, hoarseness, wheezing, and cough: Nasal: nasal pruritus, congestion, rhinorrhea, sneezing, and sensation of itching in the external auditory canals.

Cardiovascular: feeling of faintness, syncope, chest pain, dysrhythmia, hypotension. **Note:** Hypotension is a sign of anaphylaxis. Patients should be treated in the early stages of anaphylaxis to prevent hypotension from developing.

Other: periorbital pruritus, erythema and edema, conjunctival erythema, and tearing; lower back pain and uterine contractions in women; aura of "doom."

The severity of previous anaphylactic reactions does not determine the severity of future reactions, and subsequent reactions could be the same, better, or worse. The severity may depend on the degree of sensitivity, the dose of allergen, and other factors.

Research shows that fatalities from anaphylaxis are often associated with failure to use epinephrine or a delay in the use of epinephrine treatment.

Epinephrine should be administered as early as possible after the onset of symptoms of a severe allergic response. Patients requiring epinephrine will not always have predictable reactions. Adequate warning signs are not always present before serious reactions occur.

It is recommended that epinephrine be given at the start of any reaction associated with a known or suspected allergen contact. In patients with a history of severe cardiovascular collapse on exposure to an allergen, the physician may advise that epinephrine be administered immediately after exposure to that allergen, and before any reaction has begun.

Epinephrine may prove to be life saving when used as directed immediately following exposure to an allergen.

In most patients, epinephrine is effective after 1 injection. However, symptoms may recur and further injections may be required to control the reaction. Epinephrine can be re-injected every 5 to 15 minutes until there is resolution of the anaphylaxis or signs of adrenaline excess (such as palpitations, tremor, uncomfortable apprehension and anxiety).

All individuals receiving emergency epinephrine must be immediately transported to hospital, ideally by ambulance, for evaluation and observation. Repeat attacks have occurred hours later without additional exposure to the offending allergen. Therefore, it is recommended that a patient suffering from an anaphylactic reaction be observed in an emergency facility for an appropriate period because of the possibility of either a "biphasic" reaction (a second reaction) or a prolonged reaction. At least a four hour period of observation is advised, although this time may vary. The attending physician will take into consideration such factors as the severity of the reaction, the patient's response and history and the distance from the hospital to the patient's home.

Anaphylactic reactions typically follow a uniphasic course; however, 20% will be biphasic in nature. The second phase usually occurs after an asymptomatic period of 1 to 8 hours, but may occur up to 38 hours (mean 10 hours) after the initial reaction. About one third of the second-phase reactions are more severe, one third are as severe, and one third are less severe. The second-phase reactions can occur even following administration of corticosteroids.

Following treatment of anaphylaxis, the patient must stay within close proximity to a hospital or where he or she can call 911 for the next 48 hours.

Protracted anaphylaxis, which is frequently associated with profound hypotension and sometimes lasts longer than 24 hours, is minimally responsive to aggressive therapy, and has a poor prognosis.

CONTRAINDICATIONS: There are no absolute contraindications to the use of epinephrine in a life-threatening allergic situation.

WARNINGS AND PRECAUTIONS: General: Patients with a history of anaphylaxis are at risk for subsequent episodes and even death. All patients who have had one or more episodes of anaphylaxis should have injectable epinephrine with them or with their parent or caregiver at all times, and should wear some form of medical identification bracelet or necklace.

Following the resolution of an anaphylactic episode and discharge from hospital, the patient should immediately obtain and fill a new EpiPen or EpiPen Jr auto-injector prescription.

Epinephrine injection (1:1000 and 1:2000) is not intended as a substitute for medical attention or hospital care. In conjunction with the administration of epinephrine, the patient should seek appropriate medical care.

Antihistamines and asthma medications must not be used as first line treatment for an anaphylactic reaction.

Accidental injection into the hands or feet may result in loss of blood flow to the affected areas and should be avoided. If there is an accidental injection into these areas, the patient must go immediately to the nearest emergency room for treatment. Epinephrine should only be injected into the anterolateral aspect of the thigh. Every effort should be made to avoid possible inadvertent intravascular administration through appropriate selection of an injection site such as the thigh. Do not inject into the buttock. Large doses or accidental intravenous injection of epinephrine may result in cerebral hemorrhage due to a sharp rise in blood pressure. Rapidly acting vasodilators can counteract the marked pressor effects of epinephrine.

The presence of a condition listed below is not a contraindication to epinephrine administration in an acute, life-threatening situation. Therefore, patients with these conditions, or any other person who might be in a position to administer epinephrine to a patient with these conditions experiencing anaphylaxis, should be instructed about the circumstances under which epinephrine should be used.

Cardiovascular: Epinephrine use should be avoided in patients with cardiogenic, traumatic, or hemorrhagic shock; cardiac dilation; and/or cerebral arteriosclerosis.

Epinephrine should be used with caution in patients with cardiac arrhythmias, coronary artery or organic heart disease, hypertension, or in patients who are on medications that may sensitize the heart to arrhythmias, e.g., digitalis, diuretics, or anti-arrhythmics. In such patients, epinephrine may precipitate or aggravate angina pectoris as well as produce ventricular arrhythmias.

Patients with hypertension or hyperthyroidism are prone to more severe or persistent effects.

Endocrine and Metabolism: Patients with diabetes may develop increased blood glucose levels following epinephrine administration.

Neurologic: Epinephrine use should be avoided in patients with organic brain damage.

Patients with Parkinson's disease may notice a temporary worsening of symptoms after treatment with epinephrine.

Ophthalmologic: Epinephrine use should be avoided in patients with narrow-angle glaucoma.

Respiratory: There is a significantly increased risk of respiratory symptoms in patients with concomitant asthma, especially if poorly controlled. These patients are at increased risk of death from anaphylaxis.

Fatalities may also occur from pulmonary edema resulting from peripheral constriction and cardiac stimulation.

Sensitivity/Resistance: This product contains sodium metabisulfite, a substance which may cause allergic-type reactions including anaphylactic symptoms or mild to severe asthmatic episodes in certain susceptible persons.

Nevertheless, epinephrine is the drug of choice for serious allergic reactions and the presence of a sulfite in this product should not deter administration of the drug for treatment of serious allergic or other emergency situations, even if the patient is sulfite-sensitive.

Sexual Function/Reproduction: No studies have been conducted to determine epinephrine's potential effect on fertility.

Special Populations: Pregnant Women: Although there are no adequate and well-controlled studies in pregnant women, epinephrine should be used in pregnancy only if the potential benefit justifies the potential risk to the fetus.

Pediatrics (patients 15-30 kg): There are no data to suggest a difference in safety or effectiveness of epinephrine between adults and children in this weight group.

See Dosage and Administration for dosage requirements based on weight.

Geriatrics (>65 years of age): Elderly patients with hypertension, coronary artery disease or cardiac arrythmias are particularly at risk for epinephrine overdose. More careful monitoring and avoidance of epinephrine overdose is recommended for these patients.

ADVERSE REACTIONS: Adverse Drug Reaction Overview: Adverse reactions of epinephrine include transient, moderate anxiety; feelings of over stimulation; apprehensiveness; restlessness; tremor; weakness; shakiness; dizziness; sweating; tachycardia; palpitations; pallor; nausea and vomiting; headache; and/or respiratory difficulties. Ventricular arrhythmias may follow administration of epinephrine. While these symptoms occur in some patients treated with epinephrine, they are likely to be more pronounced in patients with hypertension or hyperthyroidism. These signs and symptoms usually subside rapidly, especially with bed rest.

Some patients may be at greater risk of developing adverse reactions after epinephrine administration. These include elderly individuals, pregnant women, and patients with diabetes.

Patients with coronary artery disease are prone to more severe or persistent effects, and may experience angina.

Excessive doses cause acute hypertension. Rapid rises in blood pressure have produced cerebral hemorrhage, particularly in elderly patients with cardiovascular disease.

Arrhythmias, including fatal ventricular fibrillation, have been reported, particularly in patients with underlying cardiac disease or those receiving certain drugs (see Drug Interactions).

The potential for epinephrine to produce these types of adverse reactions does not contraindicate its use in an acute life-threatening allergic reaction.

DRUG INTERACTIONS: Overview: There are no known contraindications to the use of epinephrine in a life-threatening allergic reaction.

Drug-Drug Interactions: Epinephrine should be used with caution in patients who are on medications that may sensitize the heart to arrhythmias, e.g., digitalis, diuretics, or anti-arrhythmics. In such patients, epinephrine may precipitate or aggravate angina pectoris as well as produce ventricular arrhythmias.

Caution is advised in patients receiving cardiac glycosides or diuretics, since these agents may sensitize the myocardium to beta-adrenergic stimulation and make cardiac arrhythmias more likely.

The effects of epinephrine may be potentiated by tricyclic antidepressants, monoamine oxidase inhibitors, sodium levothyroxine, and certain antihistamines, notably chlorpheniramine, tripelennamine, and diphenhydramine.

The cardiostimulating and bronchodilating effects of epinephrine are antagonized by beta-adrenergic blocking drugs, such as propranolol. Anaphylaxis may be made worse by beta blockers because these drugs decrease the effectiveness of epinephrine.

The vasoconstricting and hypertensive effects of epinephrine are antagonized by alpha-adrenergic blocking drugs, such as phentolamine.

Phenothiazines may also reverse the pressor effects of epinephrine.

Deaths have been reported in asthmatic patients treated with epinephrine following the use of isoproterenol, orciprenaline, salbutamol, and long acting beta agonists.

Drug-Lifestyle Interactions: Cocaine sensitizes the heart to catecholamines (as does uncontrolled hyperthyroidism), and epinephrine use in these patients should be cautious.

DOSAGE AND ADMINISTRATION: Dosing Considerations: Dosage in any specific patient should be based on body weight. A physician who prescribes EpiPen or EpiPen Jr should take appropriate steps to ensure that the patient thoroughly understands the indications and use of the device. The physician should review with the patient, in detail, the Information for the Patient section and operation of the auto-injector.

EpiPen and EpiPen Jr contain 2 mL of solution but deliver a single dose of 0.3 mL **only**, with 1.7 mL remaining in the unit **after use**.

Inject only into the anterolateral aspect of the thigh.

Recommended Dose and Dosage Adjustment: EpiPen: EpiPen delivers a dose of 0.3 mg in 0.3 mL of 1:1000 dilution of epinephrine injection, USP. EpiPen is intended for adults and children who weigh 30 kg or more.

EpiPen Jr: EpiPen Jr delivers a dose of 0.15 mg in 0.3 mL of 1:2000 dilution of epinephrine injection, USP. EpiPen Jr is intended for children who weigh between 15 kg and 30 kg.

Since the dose of epinephrine delivered from EpiPen Jr is fixed at 0.15 mg, the physician can consider other forms of injectable epinephrine if doses lower than 0.15 mg are felt to be necessary (e.g., for children weighing less than 15 kg).

Administration: Patients with a history of severe allergic reactions should be instructed about the circumstances under which epinephrine should be used (see Indications and Clinical Use).

The patient's physician or pharmacist should review the package insert in detail with the patient or caregiver to ensure that he/she understands the indications and use of EpiPen or EpiPen Jr.

Actual demonstration of the injection technique by a physician or a pharmacist is recommended. A training device for patient instruction purposes is also available.

EpiPen and EpiPen Jr are intended for intramuscular use in the anterolateral aspect of the thigh, through clothing if necessary. **Do not inject into the buttock.**

OVERDOSAGE:

Epinephrine is rapidly inactivated in the body, and treatment following overdose with epinephrine is primarily supportive. If necessary, pressor effects may be counteracted by rapidly acting vasodilators or alpha-adrenergic blocking drugs. If prolonged hypotension follows such measures, it may be necessary to administer another pressor drug.

Overdosage of epinephrine may produce extremely elevated arterial pressure, which may result in cerebrovascular hemorrhage, particularly in elderly patients. Overdosage sometimes also results in extreme pallor and coldness of the skin, metabolic acidosis, and kidney failure. Suitable corrective measures must be taken in such situations. Epinephrine overdosage can also cause transient bradycardia followed by tachycardia, and these may be accompanied by potentially fatal cardiac arrhythmias. Treatment of arrhythmias consists of administration of a beta-adrenergic blocking drug such as propranolol.

If an epinephrine overdose induces pulmonary edema that interferes with respiration, treatment consists of a rapidly acting alpha-adrenergic blocking drug and/or intermittent positive-pressure respiration.

Premature ventricular contractions may appear within 1 minute after injection and may be followed by multifocal ventricular tachycardia (prefibrillation rhythm).

Subsidence of the ventricular effects may be followed by atrial tachycardia and occasionally by atrioventricular block.

For management of a suspected drug overdose, CPhA recommends that you contact your **regional Poison Control Centre**. See the *CPS* Directory section for a list of Poison Control Centres.

ACTION AND CLINICAL PHARMACOLOGY: Epinephrine acts on both alpha- and beta-adrenergic receptors. Through its action on alpha-adrenergic receptors, epinephrine counters the vasodilation and high vascular permeability that occurs during an anaphylactic reaction that can lead to loss of intravascular fluid volume and hypotension. Through its action on beta-adrenergic receptors, epinephrine causes bronchial smooth muscle relaxation that helps alleviate bronchospasm, wheezing, and dyspnea that may occur during anaphylaxis.

Epinephrine also helps to alleviate pruritus, urticaria, and angioedema, and may be effective in relieving gastrointestinal and genitourinary symptoms of anaphylaxis because of its relaxant effects on the smooth muscle of the stomach, intestine, and urinary bladder. Epinephrine contracts the smooth muscle of the uterus.

Epinephrine, when given intramuscularly or subcutaneously, has a rapid onset and short duration of action.

STORAGE AND STABILITY: Always store EpiPen or EpiPen Jr in the carrier tube with the blue safety release on until you need to use it. Store at 25°C; **excursions permitted to** 15-30°C. Do not refrigerate. Protect from light. Periodically check to make sure the solution in the auto-injector is not brown in color. Replace if it is discolored or contains a precipitate.

INFORMATION FOR THE PATIENT: Published in e-CPS, available by subscription at www.e-cps.ca.

DOSAGE FORMS, COMPOSITION AND PACKAGING: EpiPen or EpiPen Jr auto-injectors are designed to be compact and easy to carry, and to provide emergency treatment when medical care is not immediately available.

Highly sensitive individuals should have epinephrine injectable products readily available at all times.

EpiPen: Each auto-injector contains: 2 mL epinephrine injection 1:1000 and is designed to deliver a single dose of epinephrine 0.3 mg in 0.3 mL. Nonmedicinal ingredients: sodium chloride 6 mg, sodium metabisulfite 1.67 mg and hydrochloric acid to adjust pH. Latex-free. Packages of 1 auto-injector and packages of 6 units.

EpiPen Jr: Each auto-injector contains: 2 mL epinephrine injection 1:2000 and is designed to deliver a single dose of epinephrine 0.15 mg in 0.3 mL. Nonmedicinal ingredients: sodium chloride 6 mg, sodium metabisulfite 1.67 mg and hydrochloric acid to adjust pH. Latex-free. Packages of 1 auto-injector.

(Shown in Product Identification Section)

Epirubicin Hydrochloride for Injection Ⓟ

epirubicin HCl

Antineoplastic

Hospira

Date of Preparation: November 14, 2007

Caution: Epirubicin Hydrochloride for Injection is a potent drug and should be used only by physicians experienced with cancer chemotherapeutic drugs (see Warnings and Precautions). Blood counts and hepatic function tests should be performed regularly. Irreversible cardiac toxicity may occur as the cumulative dose approaches 1000 mg/m². Cardiac monitoring is advised in those patients who have received mediastinal radiotherapy, other anthracycline or anthracene therapy, with pre-existing cardiac disease, or received prior epirubicin cumulative doses exceeding 650 mg/m².

Secondary acute myeloid leukemia (AML) with or without a preleukemic phase (myelodysplastic syndrome or MDS) has been reported in patients treated with epirubicin-containing regimens. The cumulative risk of developing treatment-related AML/MDS in 7110 patients with early breast cancer who received adjuvant treatment with epirubicin-containing regimens was estimated as 0.27% at 3 years, 0.46% at 5 years, and 0.55% at 8 years.

SUMMARY PRODUCT INFORMATION:

Route of Administration	Dosage Form/ Strength	Clinically Relevant Nonmedicinal Ingredients
Intravenous	Lyophilized powder for injection/ 50 mg vials	Lactose For a complete listing see Dosage Forms, Composition and Packaging.

INDICATIONS AND CLINICAL USE: Epirubicin Hydrochloride for Injection has been used successfully as a single agent and in combination with other chemotherapeutic agents to produce regression in a variety of tumour types such as lymphoma, lung, cancer of the breast, ovary and stomach.

Epirubicin Hydrochloride for Injection is recommended for the treatment of metastatic breast cancer.

Epirubicin Hydrochloride for Injection may also be used as a component in the adjuvant treatment of early stage breast cancer for pre- and peri- menopausal women.

Epirubicin Hydrochloride for Injection is also recommended in small cell lung cancer (both limited and extensive disease) advanced non-small cell lung cancer, non-Hodgkin's lymphoma, Hodgkin's disease, Stage III and IV (FIGO) ovarian carcinoma and metastatic and locally unresectable gastric carcinoma.

In addition, several other solid tumours have shown responsiveness to Epirubicin Hydrochloride for Injection but data are not yet sufficient to justify specific recommendations.

CONTRAINDICATIONS:

- Hypersensitivity to epirubicin or any other component of the product, or other anthracyclines or anthracenediones such as doxorubicin hydrochloride, daunorubicin hydrochloride, mitoxantrone or mitomycin C.
- marked persistent myelosuppression induced by prior treatment with other antitumour agents or by radiotherapy;
- severe hepatic impairment;
- severe myocardial insufficiency;
- recent myocardial infarction;
- severe arrhythmias;
- history of severe cardiac disease;
- previous treatments with maximum cumulative doses of epirubicin and/or other anthracyclines and anthracenediones (see Warnings and Precautions).

WARNINGS AND PRECAUTIONS: Cardiac Function: Cardiotoxicity is a risk of anthracycline treatment that may be manifested by early (i.e., acute) or late (i.e., delayed) events.

Early (i.e., Acute) Events: Early cardiotoxicity of epirubicin consists mainly of sinus tachycardia and/or ECG abnormalities such as non-specific ST-T wave changes. Tachyarrhythmias, including premature ventricular contractions, ventricular tachycardia, and bradycardia, as well as atrioventricular and bundle-branch block have also been reported. These effects do not usually predict subsequent development of delayed cardiotoxicity, are rarely of clinical importance, and are generally not a consideration for the discontinuation of epirubicin treatment.

Late (i.e., Delayed) Events: Delayed cardiotoxicity usually develops late in the course of therapy with epirubicin or within 2 to 3 months after treatment termination, but later events several months to years after completion of treatment have also been reported. Delayed cardiomyopathy is manifested by reduced left ventricular ejection fraction (LVEF) and/or signs and symptoms of congestive heart failure (CHF) such as dyspnea, pulmonary edema, dependent edema, cardiomegaly and hepatomegaly, oliguria, ascites, pleural effusion, and gallop rhythm. Life-threatening CHF is the most severe form of anthracycline-induced cardiomyopathy and represents the cumulative dose-limiting toxicity of the drug.

Cardiac function should be assessed before patients undergo treatment with epirubicin and must be monitored throughout therapy to minimize the risk of incurring severe cardiac impairment. The risk may be decreased through regular monitoring of LVEF during the course of treatment with prompt discontinuation of epirubicin at the first sign of impaired function. The appropriate quantitative method for repeated assessment of cardiac function (evaluation of LVEF) includes multi-gated radionuclide angiography (MUGA) or echocardiography (ECHO). A baseline cardiac evaluation with an ECG and either a MUGA scan or an ECHO is recommended, especially in patients with risk factors for increased cardiotoxicity. Repeated MUGA or ECHO determinations of LVEF should be performed, particularly with higher, cumulative anthracycline doses. The technique used for assessment should be consistent throughout follow-up.

Congestive heart failure and/or cardiomyopathy may be encountered several weeks after discontinuation of Epirubicin Hydrochloride for Injection therapy.

Given the risk of cardiomyopathy, a cumulative dose of 900 to 1000 mg/m² epirubicin should generally not be exceeded. Risk factors for cardiac toxicity include active or dormant cardiovascular disease, prior or concomitant radiotherapy to the mediastinal/pericardial area, previous therapy with other anthracyclines or anthracenediones, and concomitant use of other drugs with the ability to suppress cardiac contractility. Cardiac function monitoring must be particularly strict in patients receiving high cumulative doses and in those with risk factors. While cardiotoxicity with epirubicin may occur at lower cumulative doses whether or not cardiac risk factors are present, it may be more likely to occur at lower cumulative doses in patients with these risk factors.

Available evidence appears to indicate that cardiotoxicity is cumulative across members of the anthracycline and anthracene class of drugs. Patients who have previously received other anthracyclines and anthracenes are at particular risk for possible cardiotoxic effects of Epirubicin Hydrochloride for Injection at a lower total dose than previously untreated patients and, therefore, should be carefully monitored. The total dose of Epirubicin Hydrochloride for Injection administered to a patient should take into account: prior or concomitant therapy with related compounds such as doxorubicin and daunorubicin or anthracene derivatives; and/or radiotherapy to the mediastinal area.

Anthracycline-induced cardiac failure is often resistant to currently available therapeutic and physical measures used for the treatment of cardiac failure. Early clinical diagnosis of drug-induced heart failure is essential. Treatment measures include digitalis, diuretics, peripheral vasodilators, low salt diet, and bed rest. Severe cardiac toxicity may occur precipitously without antecedent EKG changes. An EKG, echocardiogram or radionuclide angiography (MUGA) performed at baseline and prior to each dose or course after a cumulative dose of 650 mg/m² is suggested. Transient EKG changes consisting of T-wave flattening, S-T depression and arrhythmias occurring up to two weeks after a dose or course of Epirubicin Hydrochloride for Injection are presently not considered indications for suspension of Epirubicin Hydrochloride for Injection therapy.

Epirubicin Hydrochloride for Injection cardiomyopathy has been reported to be associated with a reduction of the ejection fraction as determined by radionuclide scan or echocardiography. None of these tests have yet consistently identified those individual patients that are approaching their maximally tolerated cumulative dose of Epirubicin Hydrochloride for Injection. If test results indicate a change in cardiac status associated with Epirubicin Hydrochloride for Injection therapy, the benefit of continued therapy must be carefully weighed against the risk of producing irreversible cardiac damage.

Hematologic Toxicity: Careful haematologic monitoring is required since bone marrow depression, primarily of leukocytes may occur. Haematologic profiles should be assessed before and during each cycle of therapy with epirubicin, including differential white blood cell counts (WBC).

With the recommended dosage schedule (see Dosage and Administration) leukopenia is transient, reaching its nadir 10-14 days after treatment, with recovery usually occurring by the 21st day. White blood cell counts as low as 1000/mm³ are to be expected during treatment with Epirubicin Hydrochloride for Injection.

Red blood cell and platelet levels should be monitored since they may also be depressed. Hematologic toxicity may require dose reduction or delay or suspension of Epirubicin Hydrochloride for Injection therapy. Persistent myelosuppression may result in infection or hemorrhage.

Epirubicin Hydrochloride for Injection may potentiate the toxicity of other anticancer therapies as well as radiation induced toxicity to the myocardium, mucosa and skin. Patients should recover from acute toxicities (such as stomatitis, neutropenia, thrombocytopenia and generalized infections) of prior cytotoxic treatment before beginning treatment with Epirubicin Hydrochloride for Injection.

While treatment with high doses of epirubicin (e.g., ≥90 mg/m² every 3 to 4 weeks) causes adverse events generally similar to those seen at standard doses (<90 mg/m² every 3 to 4 weeks), the severity of the neutropenia and stomatitis/mucositis may be increased. Treatment with high doses of the drug does require special attention for possible clinical complications due to profound myelosuppression.

Hepatic/Biliary/Pancreatic: Epirubicin is extensively metabolized by the liver and its major route of elimination is the hepatobiliary system. Serum total bilirubin and AST levels should be evaluated before and during treatment with epirubicin. Patients with elevated bilirubin or AST may experience slower clearance of drug with an increase in overall toxicity. Lower doses are recommended in these patients (see Dosage and Administration). Patients with severe hepatic impairment should not receive epirubicin (see Contraindications).

Renal: Serum creatinine should be assessed before and during therapy. Dosage adjustment is necessary in patients with serum creatinine >5 mg/dL (see Dosage and Administration).

Secondary Leukemia: The occurrence of secondary acute myeloid leukemia (AML) with or without a preleukemic phase (myelodysplastic syndrome or MDS) has been reported in patients treated with epirubicin-containing regimens. Such cases could have a short (1-3 years) latency period (see below and in Table 2 under Adverse Reactions).

The quantified risk of developing acute myeloid leukemia (AML), including myelodysplastic syndrome (MDS), following epirubicin or epirubicin-containing therapy, has been estimated by analyzing data collected prospectively from 19 randomized trials for the adjuvant treatment of early breast cancer, that were either company-sponsored or conducted by independent institutions (including the National Institute of Canada's MA.5 trial). As of 31 December 2001, 28 (0.39%) of the 7110 evaluable patients treated with epirubicin, had presented with either AML or MDS. An additional 4 patients were diagnosed with other types of leukemia: 3 with acute lymphoblastic leukemia (ALL), and 1 with chronic lymphocytic leukemia (CLL). The time elapsed from the start of adjuvant treatment to the diagnosis of AML/MDS ranged from 8 to 126 months, with a median of 33 months. Of the 23 cases of AML/MDS for whom cytogenetic information was available, in 12 there was evidence of balanced chromosome translocations, and in 7 these translocations involved chromosome 11 or 21. Therapy-induced leukemia secondary to topoisomerase inhibitors generally has a short induction period (6 months to 5 years) and is known to be associated with translocations involving chromosome 11 or 21.

In this most recent analysis, the cumulative risk of developing AML/MDS in the 7110 patients treated with epirubicin was 0.27% (95% confidence interval 0.14%, 0.40%) at 3 years, 0.46% (95% confidence interval 0.28%, 0.65%) at 5 years, and 0.55% (95% confidence interval, 0.33%, 0.78%) at 8 years. AML/MDS rates increased with epirubicin dose per cycle, and cumulative dose. For instance, in the MA.5 trial, in patients that received intensive doses of epirubicin (120 mg/m²), the incidence of AML/MDS was 1.1% at 5 years with no additional cases observed during the second 5 years (years 6-10) of follow-up.

Since the completion of these analyses, in the period up to and including September 2003, further spontaneous, literature and study reports of AML/MDS have been received.

In addition, in 10 trials for the treatment of advanced breast cancer (3061 patients, follow-up until March 1999), two cases of AML occurred. However, due to the small number of cases and the limited follow-up as a result of the natural history of advanced breast cancer in these patients, risk estimates could not be made for this patient population.

General: Epirubicin Hydrochloride for Injection must not be administered by intramuscular or subcutaneous injection.

Severe local tissue necrosis can occur if Epirubicin Hydrochloride for Injection is extravasated during intravenous administration. Extravasation may occur with or without an accompanying stinging or burning sensation even if blood returns well on aspiration of the infusion needle (see Dosage and Administration). If signs or symptoms of extravasation occur the injection or infusion should be terminated immediately and restarted in another vein.

As with other cytotoxic agents, thrombophlebitis and thromboembolic phenomena, including pulmonary embolism (in some cases fatal) have been coincidentally reported with the use of epirubicin.

Epirubicin Hydrochloride for Injection is mutagenic, clastogenic, and carcinogenic in animals and has been associated with an increased risk of secondary leukemia (AML) in clinical trials of adjuvant treatment of breast cancer (see Adverse Reactions). In addition, epirubicin could induce chromosomal damage in human spermatozoa. Men undergoing treatment with epirubicin should use effective contraceptive methods.

Epirubicin may cause amenorrhea or premature menopause in premenopausal women.

Epirubicin Hydrochloride for Injection imparts a red colouration to the urine for 1 or 2 days after administration. Patients should be advised to expect this during active therapy.

Special Populations: Pregnant Women and Nursing Women: There is no conclusive information about epirubicin adversely affecting human fertility, or causing teratogenesis; however, at high doses Epirubicin Hydrochloride for Injection is embryotoxic and teratogenic in rats and embryotoxic and abortifacient in rabbits. There are no studies in pregnant women. Therefore, women of childbearing potential should be advised to avoid pregnancy.

Epirubicin should be used during pregnancy only if the potential benefit justifies the potential risk to the fetus. If Epirubicin Hydrochloride for Injection is to be used during pregnancy, or if the patient becomes pregnant during therapy, the patient should be informed of the potential hazard to the fetus. Mothers should be advised not to breast-feed while undergoing chemotherapy with Epirubicin Hydrochloride for Injection.

Monitoring and Laboratory Tests: Initial treatment with Epirubicin Hydrochloride for Injection requires close observation of the patient and extensive laboratory monitoring. Like other cytotoxic drugs, Epirubicin Hydrochloride for Injection may induce hyperuricemia secondary to rapid lysis of neoplastic cells. The physician should monitor the patient's serum chemistry and blood uric acid level and be prepared to institute appropriate measures that might be necessary to control this problem. Hydration, urine alkalinization, and prophylaxis with allopurinol to prevent hyperuricemia may minimize potential complications of tumor-lysis syndrome.

Epirubicin Hydrochloride for Injection is not an anti-microbial agent.

Information to Be Provided to the Patient: Patients should be counseled about the known adverse effects that they could experience during chemotherapy with Epirubicin Hydrochloride for Injection, including cardiotoxicity, myleosuppression and risk of infection, thrombocytopenia, anemia, nausea, vomiting, and stomatitis.

Physicians should also clearly lay out early on the risks and benefits of the various chemotherapeutic options available, thus enabling the patient to make an informed treatment choice. Patients should be aware that higher dose regimens may have a greater toxicity that includes secondary leukemia. Wherever possible, the physician should discuss the information presented in the Information for the Patient.

ADVERSE REACTIONS: Dose limiting toxicities are myelosuppression and cardiotoxicity (see Warnings and Precautions). Other reactions reported are:

Cutaneous: Reversible partial or complete alopecia occurs in most patients. Alopecia and lack of beard growth in males are usually reversible. Recall of skin reaction associated with prior radiotherapy may occur with Epirubicin Hydrochloride for Injection administration. Local toxicity, rash/itch and skin changes may also occur.

Gastrointestinal: Acute nausea and vomiting occurs frequently in most patients. This may be alleviated by antiemetic therapy. Mucositis (stomatitis and esophagitis) has been reported to occur 5-10 days after administration. This may lead to ulceration and represents a site of origin for severe infections. Diarrhea has been reported. Most patients recover from this adverse event by the third week of therapy.

Local: Severe cellulitis, vesication, local pain and tissue necrosis can occur if Epirubicin Hydrochloride for Injection is extravasated during administration (see Dosage and Administration). Erythematous streaking and/or transient urticaria along the vein proximal to the site of administration may occur. Venous sclerosis may result from injection into small veins or repeated injection into the same vein. Following the recommended administration procedures may minimize the risk of phlebitis/thrombophlebitis at the injection site (see Special Handling Instructions).

Hematological: A dose-dependent, reversible leukopenia and/or granulocytopenia (neutropenia) are the predominant manifestations of epirubicin bone marrow/haematologic toxicity and represents the acute dose-limiting toxicity of this drug. Leukopenia and neutropenia are usually more severe after administration of high-dose regimens; under these conditions appropriate bone marrow support (eg. peripheral blood progenitor cells and/or colony-stimulating factors) may be required. Thrombocytopenia and anemia may also occur. Clinical consequences of severe myelosuppression include fever, infection, sepsis/septicemia, septic shock, hemorrhage, tissue hypoxia, or death.

Secondary Leukemia: See Warnings and Precautions.

Body as a Whole: Phlebitis, fever and malaise/asthenia have been reported following administration of Epirubicin Hydrochloride for Injection.

Drug-related adverse events also occurred in the following systems:

Endocrine: amenorrhea and hot flashes.

Cardiovascular: asymptomatic drops in left ventricular ejection fraction and congestive heart failure.

Ocular: conjunctivitis, keratitis.

Other: infection, acute lymphocytic leukemia, acute myelogenous leukemia.

Adverse Reactions in Early Breast Cancer Adjuvant Treatment: On-Study Events: Integrated safety data are available from two studies (Studies MA.5 and GFEA-05 (FASG-05), evaluating epirubicin-containing combination regimens in patients with early breast cancer. Of the 1260 patients treated in these studies, 620 patients received the higher-dose epirubicin regimen (FEC-100/CEF-120), 280 patients received the lower-dose epirubicin regimen (FEC-50), and 360 patients received CMF. Serotonin-specific anti-emetic therapy and colony-stimulating factors were not used in these trials. Clinically relevant acute adverse events are summarized in Table 1.

Table 1: Epirubicin Hydrochloride for Injection

Clinically Relevant Acute Adverse Events in Patients with Early Breast Cancer

	% of Patients					
	FEC-100/CEF-120 (N=620)		FEC-50 (N=280)		CMF (N=360)	
Event	Grades 1-4	Grades 3/4	Grades 1-4	Grades 3/4	Grades 1-4	Grades 3/4
Haematologic						
Leukopenia	80.3	58.6	49.6	1.5	98.1	60.3
Neutropenia	80.3	67.2	53.9	10.5	95.8	78.1
Anemia	72.2	5.8	12.9	0	70.9	0.9

(cont'd)

Table 1: Epirubicin Hydrochloride for Injection *(cont'd)*
Clinically Relevant Acute Adverse Events in Patients with Early Breast Cancer

	% of Patients					
	FEC-100/CEF-120 (N=620)		FEC-50 (N=280)		CMF (N=360)	
Event	Grades 1-4	Grades 3/4	Grades 1-4	Grades 3/4	Grades 1-4	Grades 3/4
Thrombocytopenia	48.8	5.4	4.6	0	51.4	3.6
Endocrine						
Amenorrhea	71.8	0	69.3	0	67.7	0
Hot flashes	38.9	4.0	5.4	0	69.1	6.4
Body as a Whole						
Lethargy	45.8	1.9	1.1	0	72.7	0.3
Fever	5.2	0	1.4	0	4.5	0
Gastrointestinal						
Nausea/vomiting	92.4	25.0	83.2	22.1	85.0	6.4
Mucositis	58.5	8.9	9.3	0	52.9	1.9
Diarrhea	24.8	0.8	7.1	0	50.7	2.8
Anorexia	2.9	0	1.8	0	5.8	0.3
Infection						
Infection	21.5	1.6	15.0	0	25.9	0.6
Febrile neutropenia	NA	6.1	0	0	NA	1.1
Ocular						
Conjunctivitis/keratitis	14.8	0	1.1	0	38.4	0
Skin						
Alopecia	95.5	56.6	69.6	19.3	84.4	6.7
Local toxicity	19.5	0.3	2.5	0.4	8.1	0
Rash/itch	8.9	0.3	1.4	0	14.2	0
Skin changes	4.7	0	0.7	0	7.2	0

Legend: FEC & CEF=cyclophosphamide+epirubicin+fluorouracil; CMF=cyclophosphamide+methotrexate+flurouracil; NA=not available.
Grade 1 or 2 changes in transaminase levels were observed but were more frequently seen with CMF than with CEF.

Delayed Events: Table 2 describes the incidence of delayed adverse events in patients participating in the MA.5 and GFEA-05 (FASG-05) trials.

Table 2: Epirubicin Hydrochloride for Injection
Long-Term Adverse Events in Patients with Early Breast Cancer (5-year follow-up data)[a]

	% of Patients		
Event	FEC-100/CEF-120 (N=620)	FEC-50 (N=280)	CMF (N=360)
Cardiac Events			
Asymptomatic drops in LVEF	1.8	1.4	0.8
CHF	1.5	0.4	0.3
AML/MDS			
AML	0.8	0	0.3
MDS	0	0	0

[a] In study MA.5 cardiac function was not monitored after 5 years. In study GFEA-05 (FASG-05) monitoring of cardiac function was optional.

Within the first 5 year follow-up period, two cases of acute lymphoid leukemia (ALL) were also observed in patients receiving epirubicin. However, an association between anthracyclines such as epirubicin and ALL has not been clearly established.

Over the 10 year follow-up period for study GFEA-05 (FASG-05), the overall incidence of cardiac events in patients treated with FEC-100 remained similar to that reported in patients receiving FEC-50. There were, however, two new cases of decreased left ventricular ejection fraction reported in FEC-100 treated patients. Therefore, the incidence of decreased left ventricular ejection fraction was 1.1% (3/280) in the FEC-50 group and 3% (8/266) in the FEC-100 group. No new cases of delayed CHF were reported. Thus the frequency of CHF remains at 0.4% (1/280) in the FEC-50 and at 1.1% (3/266) in the FEC-100 group. In a subset of patient from this study who were without disease at median follow up time of 102 months, a subsequent analysis of long term cardiac function identified 2 patients with CHF amongst the 85 FEC-100 patients evaluated. Cardiac function was not monitored after 5 years in MA.5 study.

No new cases of secondary leukemia were reported in the 10 year follow up for both MA.5 and GFEA-05 (FASG-05) trials.

Post-Market Adverse Drug Reactions: Gastrointestinal: pain or burning sensation, erythema, erosions, ulcerations, bleeding, dehydration, hyperpigmentation of the oral mucosa.
Cutaneous: flushes, skin and nail hyperpigmentation, photosensitivity, hypersensitivity to irradiated skin (radiation-recall reaction).
Hypersensitivity Reactions: urticaria, anaphylaxis, fever, chills, shock.
Vascular: phlebitis, thrombophlebitis.
Urological: red colouration of urine for 1 to 2 days after administration.

DRUG INTERACTIONS: Epirubicin is mainly used in combination with other cytotoxic drugs. Additive toxicity may occur especially with regard to bone marrow/haematologic and gastro-intestinal effects (see Warnings and Precautions). The use of epirubicin in combination chemotherapy with other potentially cardiotoxic drugs, as well as the concomitant use of other cardioactive compounds (e.g., calcium channel blockers), requires monitoring of cardiac function throughout treatment.

Cimetidine increased the AUC of epirubicin by 50% when given for seven days, starting five days before chemotherapy. Cimetidine should be stopped prior to treatment with epirubicin.

DOSAGE AND ADMINISTRATION: Refer to Special Handling Instructions.

Recommended Dose and Dosage Adjustment: A variety of dose schedules have been used. The following recommendations are for use as a single agent or in combination with other chemotherapeutic agents.

Dosage is usually calculated on the basis of body surface area. The lower dose should be given to patients with inadequate marrow reserves due to prior therapy or neoplastic marrow infiltration. Standard starting doses and regimens have been used in the elderly.

Hepatic Dysfunction: As Epirubicin Hydrochloride for Injection is extensively metabolized by the liver and excreted primarily by the biliary system, its dosage must be reduced in patients with impaired liver function indicated by elevated bilirubin or serum AST values as follows: Serum bilirubin 21-51 µmol/L or AST 2 to 4 times upper limit of normal—give ½ of recommended starting dose; serum bilirubin >51 µmol/L or AST >4 times upper limit of normal—give ¼ of recommended starting dose. Patients with severe hepatic impairment should not receive epirubicin (see Contraindications).

Renal Dysfunction: While no specific dose recommendation can be made based on the limited available data in patients with renal impairment, lower starting doses are necessary in patients with severe renal impairment (serum creatinine >5 mg/dL).

Other Special Populations: Lower starting doses or longer intervals between cycles may need to be considered for heavily pretreated patients or patients with neoplastic bone marrow infiltration (see Warnings and Precautions). Standard starting doses and regimens have been used in the elderly.

Carcinoma of the Breast: Early Breast Cancer-Adjuvant Treatment: Breast cancer has been managed using epirubicin in combination with various chemotherapeutic agents. The recommended adjuvant treatment of early breast cancer should employ a cyclophosphamide, epirubicin, and 5-fluorouracil combination regimen (CEF 120) in a cycle to be repeated every 4 weeks for 6 cycles as follows:

- cyclophosphamide 75 mg/m² p.o. on days 1 to 14,
- epirubicin 60 mg/m² i.v. on days 1 and 8, and
- 5-fluorouracil 500 mg/m² i.v. days 1 and 8.

Metastatic Breast Cancer: Single Agent: The most commonly used dosage schedule of Epirubicin Hydrochloride for Injection in metastatic breast cancer, when employed as a single agent for adults, is 75-90 mg/m² administered at 21-day intervals. The recommended single dose may be divided over 2 successive days. An alternative weekly dosage schedule of 12.5 to 25 mg/m² has been used and has been reported to produce less clinical toxicity than higher doses given every three weeks.

Combination Therapy: In metastatic breast cancer, epirubicin can be used in combination with cyclophosphamide and 5-fluorouracil (FEC), at a dose of 50 mg/m².

Small Cell Lung Cancer: Single Agent: Epirubicin Hydrochloride for Injection, as a single agent, can be used at 90-120 mg/m² administered every 3 weeks.

Combination Therapy: Epirubicin has been used in several different combinations with other antineoplastic agents at doses ranging from 50-90 mg/m². The following combinations have proven effective: Epirubicin in combination with either cisplatin or ifosfamide; epirubicin with cyclophosphamide and vincristine (CEV); epirubicin with cyclophosphamide and etoposide (CEVP-16) and epirubicin with cisplatin and etoposide.

Non-Small Cell Lung Cancer: Single Agent: Epirubicin Hydrochloride for Injection, as a single agent, can be used at doses of 120-150 mg/m² administered day 1, every 3-4 weeks.

Combination Therapy: Epirubicin, in combination with etoposide, cisplatinum, mitomycin, vindesine and vinblastine, can be used at doses of 90-120 mg/m² administered day 1, every 3-4 weeks.

Non-Hodgkin's Lymphoma: Single Agent: Epirubicin Hydrochloride for Injection, as a single agent, can be used at doses of 75-90 mg/m² at 21-day intervals.

Combination Therapy: Epirubicin at doses of 60-75 mg/m² can be used in combination with cyclophosphamide, vincristine and prednisone with or without bleomycin (replacing doxorubicin in the CHOP, CHOP-Bleo or BACOP regimens) for the treatment of newly diagnosed non-Hodgkin's lymphoma.

Hodgkin's Disease: Combination Therapy: Epirubicin, in combination with bleomycin, vinblastine and dacarbazine, can be used at 35 mg/m² every 2 weeks or 70 mg/m² every 3-4 weeks (replacing doxorubicin in the ABVD regimen).

Ovarian Cancer: Single Agent: In patients with prior therapy, epirubicin can be used as single agent at doses of 50-90 mg/m² at 3-4 week intervals.

Combination Therapy: In patients with prior therapy epirubicin can be used in combination at doses of 50-90 mg/m² at 3-4 week intervals. Epirubicin at doses of 50-90 mg/m² in combination with cisplatin and cyclophosphamide can be used for initial therapy of ovarian cancer repeated at 3-4 week intervals.

Gastric Cancer: Single Agent: Epirubicin, as a single agent, can be used for the treatment of locally unresectable or metastatic gastric carcinoma at doses of 75-100 mg/m².

Combination Therapy: Epirubicin, at a dose of 80 mg/m² can be used in combination with fluorouracil for the treatment of locally unresectable or metastatic gastric carcinoma.

Administration: Care in the administration of Epirubicin Hydrochloride for Injection will reduce the chance of perivenous infiltration. It may also decrease the chance of local reactions such as urticaria and erythematous streaking. On intravenous administration of Epirubicin Hydrochloride for Injection, extravasation may occur with or without an accompanying stinging or burning sensation even if the blood returns well on aspiration of the infusion needle. If any signs or symptoms of extravasation have occurred the injection or infusion should be immediately terminated and restarted in another vein. If it is known or suspected that subcutaneous extravasation has occurred, the following steps are recommended:

1. Attempt aspiration of the infiltrated Epirubicin Hydrochloride for Injection solution.
2. Local intermittent application of ice for up to 3 days.
3. Elevation of the affected limb.
4. Close observation of the lesion.
5. Consultation with a plastic surgeon familiar with drug extravasation if local pain persists or skin changes progress after 3 to 4 days. If ulceration begins, early wide excision of the involved area should be considered.

Epirubicin Hydrochloride for Injection 50 mg vial should be reconstituted with 25 mL of Water for Injection (WFI) to give a final concentration of 2 mg/mL of epirubicin hydrochloride.

Alternatively, Epirubicin Hydrochloride for Injection 50 mg vials can also be reconstituted with 25 mL of Sodium Chloride Solution U.S.P. (0.9%) to give a final concentration of 2 mg/mL of epirubicin hydrochloride. However, it should be noted that **reconstitution in saline will result in a longer reconstitution time.**

Bacteriostatic diluents are not recommended.

After adding the diluent, the vial should be shaken until the contents are dissolved. A slight suspension may form which will completely dissolve on further shaking. The vials are under negative pressure and care should be taken to avoid a pressure build up. The reconstituted solution using WFI is stable for 24 hours at room temperature and 48 hours under refrigeration at 2-8°C. Alternatively, if 0.9% Sodium Chloride was used as the reconstituting diluent, the solution has been shown to be stable for 48 hours at room temperature and 2-8°C. The solution should be protected from exposure to direct light and any unused solution should be discarded.

Epirubicin Hydrochloride for Injection should be slowly administered into the tubing of a freely running intravenous infusion of Sodium Chloride Solution USP (0.9%) or 5% Dextrose Solution USP. The tubing should be attached to a Butterfly needle or other suitable device and inserted preferably into a large vein. If possible, avoid veins over joints or in extremities with compromised venous or lymphatic drainage. To minimize the risk of thrombosis or perivenous extravasation, the usual infusion times range between 3 and 20 minutes depending upon dosage and volume of the infusion solution. The infusion time should be not less than 3 to 5 minutes. A direct push injection is not recommended due to the risk of extravasation, which may occur even in the presence of adequate blood return upon needle aspiration (see Warnings and Precautions). Local erythematous streaking along the vein as well as facial flushing may be indicative of too rapid administration. A burning or stinging may be indicative of perivenous infiltration and the infusion should be immediately terminated and restarted in another vein. Perivenous infiltration may occur painlessly.

Unless specific compatibility data are available, mixing Epirubicin Hydrochloride for Injection with other drugs is not recommended.

Epirubicin Hydrochloride for Injection has been used concurrently with other approved chemotherapeutic agents. Evidence is available that combination chemotherapy is superior to single agents. The benefits and risks of such therapy continue to be elucidated.

For Safe Preparation and Handling of Epirubicin Hydrochloride for Injection refer to Special Handling Instructions.

OVERDOSAGE:
Acute overdosage with Epirubicin Hydrochloride for Injection may cause an acute myocardial dysfunction within 24 hours. Pronounced mucositis, leukopenia and thrombocytopenia could be observed within 7-14 days. Treatment of acute overdosage consists of hospitalization of the severely myelosuppressed patient, platelet and granulocyte transfusions, antibiotics, and symptomatic treatment of mucositis.

For management of a suspected drug overdose, CPhA recommends that you contact your **regional Poison Control Centre**. See the *CPS* Directory section for a list of Poison Control Centres.

ACTION AND CLINICAL PHARMACOLOGY: The mechanism of action of epirubicin, although not completely elucidated, appears to be related to its ability to bind to nucleic acids by intercalation of the planar anthracycline nucleus with the DNA double helix.

Binding to cell membranes as well as to plasma proteins may also be involved. Cell culture studies have demonstrated rapid cell penetration and perinucleolar chromatin binding, rapid inhibition of mitotic activity, mutagenesis and chromosomal aberrations.

Animal studies have shown activity in a wide spectrum of experimental tumours, immunosuppression, mutagenic and carcinogenic properties in rodents, and a variety of toxic effects, including myelosuppression in all species and atrophy of the seminiferous tubules of testes in rats and dogs.

Data from different animal species and in vitro models have shown that epirubicin is less toxic, and in particular less cardiotoxic than doxorubicin.

At equally effective doses, epirubicin produces less severe non-hematologic side effects such as vomiting and mucositis, than doxorubicin.

Early Stage Breast Cancer Studies: Two randomized, open-label, multi center studies evaluated Epirubicin Hydrochloride for Injection 100 to 120 mg/m² in combination with cyclophosphamide and fluorouracil in adjuvant treatment of axillarynode-positive breast cancer with no evidence of distant metastatic disease. (See Adverse Reactions.)

Study MA.5 evaluated 120 mg/m² doses of epirubicin per course in combination with cyclophosphamide and fluorouracil (CEF-120 regimen) versus a CMF (methotrexate) regimen in pre- and peri-menopausal women.

Study GFEA-05 (FASG-05) evaluated 100 mg/m² doses of epirubicin per course in combination with fluorouracil and cyclophosphamide (FEC-100) or lower-dose FEC-50 in pre- and postmenopausal women.

In the pivotal trial MA.5, the Cox proportional model showed that node number is a significant (p=0.0001) outcome predictor overall (conditional risk ratio of 1.7 for ≥4 versus <3 involved nodes). Non-significant trends indicate that the CEF treatment may show superiority over CMF in patients with ≥4 nodes than those with <3. The trial was insufficiently powered to demonstrate a subset difference; it must be borne in mind that the majority of patients (61%) in both treatments had 1-3 positive nodes, yet CEF-120 still produced overall advantages in relapse free survival (RFS) and overall survival (OS) (see below). Nonetheless, CEF versus CMF RFS in the <3 node group was 68 vs. 62%, while in the ≥4 node group the values were 52 vs. 39%.

In the supporting trial GFEA-05 (FASG-05), similar improvements in RFS and OS were observed in both pre- and postmenopausal women treated with FEC-100 compared to FEC-50.

The median follow-up time in the MA.5 study was 8.8 years (range: 0.2 to 12.1 years) and 8.7 years (range: 0.7 to 12.1 years) for the CEF and CMF treatment groups, respectively. In MA.5, the CEF-120 therapy demonstrated superior RFS to CMF, both over the 5- and 10-year followup. The overall reduction in risk of relapse was 24% over 5 years and 22% over 10 years. The 5- and 10-year OS were also greater for the epirubicin-containing CEF-120 regimen than for the CMF regimen. The overall relative reduction in the risk of death was 29% over 5 years and 18% over 10 years.

Pharmacokinetics: Pharmacokinetic studies show an initial rapid elimination of the parent compound from plasma. The terminal half life of elimination of the parent drug from plasma approximates 30-40 hours in humans. Urinary excretion accounts for approximately 9-10% of the administered dose in 48 hours. Biliary excretion represents the major route of elimination, about 40% of the administered dose being recovered in the bile in 72 hours. The major metabolites that have been identified are epirubicinol (13-OH epirubicin) and glucuronides of epirubicin and epirubicinol.

The 4'-O-glucuronidation distinguishes epirubicin from doxorubicin and may account for the faster elimination of epirubicin and its reduced toxicity. Plasma levels of the main metabolite, the 13-OH derivative (epirubicinol) are consistently lower and virtually parallel to those of the unchanged drug.

Impairment of hepatic function results in higher plasma levels.

Distribution studies in the rat have shown that epirubicin does not appear to cross the blood-brain barrier.

STORAGE AND STABILITY: Epirubicin Hydrochloride for Injection should be stored at 15-30°C and protected from light.

Reconstituted Solutions: Recommended Diluents for Reconstitution: Water for Injection (WFI), 0.9% Sodium chloride Injection USP (without bacteriostatic agent).

Table 3: Epirubicin Hydrochloride for Injection

Reconstitution Table

Vial Size	Diluent Added to Vial (mL)	Approximate Available Volume (mL)	Approximate Concentration (mg/mL)
50 mg	25	25	2

See Administration for Instructions.

The solution should be protected from exposure to direct light and any unused solution should be discarded. Please refer to the Table 4 for a summary of the stability of the solutions once it has been reconstituted.

Table 4: Epirubicin Hydrochloride for Injection

Stability of the Solutions After Reconstitution

Reconstituting Diluent	At Room Temperature	At 2-8°C
WFI	24 hours	48 hours
0.9% Sodium Chloride	24 hours	48 hours

Incompatibility: Unless specific compatibility data are available, Epirubicin Hydrochloride for Injection should not be mixed with other drugs.

Contact with any solution of an alkaline pH should be avoided, as it will result in hydrolysis of the drug. Epirubicin should also not be mixed with heparin due to chemical incompatibility that may lead to precipitation.

SPECIAL HANDLING INSTRUCTIONS: Preparation and Handling:

1. Personnel should be trained in good technique for reconstitution and handling. Pregnant staff should be excluded from working with this drug.
2. Preparation of antineoplastic solutions should be done in a vertical laminar flow hood (Biological Safety Cabinet—Class II) and the work surface should be protected by disposable, plastic-backed absorbent paper.
3. Personnel handling epirubicin solutions should wear PVC gloves, safety glasses and protective clothing such as disposable gowns and masks. If epirubicin solutions contact the skin or mucosa, the area should be washed with soap and water or sodium bicarbonate immediately. Do not abrade the skin by using a scrub brush and always wash hands after removing gloves.
4. In case of contact with the eye(s), hold back the eyelid of the affected eye(s) and flush with copious amounts of water for at least 15 minutes, proceed to a physician for medical evaluation.
5. Personnel regularly involved in the preparation and handling of antineoplastics should have blood examinations on a regular basis.

Disposal:

1. Avoid contact with skin and inhalation of airborne particles by use of PVC gloves and disposable gowns and masks.
2. All needles, syringes, vials and other materials which have come in contact with epirubicin should be segregated in plastic bags, sealed, and marked as hazardous waste. Incinerate at 1000°C or higher. Sealed containers may explode if a tight seal exists.
3. If incineration is not available, epirubicin hydrochloride may be detoxified by adding sodium hypochlorite solution (household bleach) to the vial, in sufficient quantity to decolourize the epirubicin, care being taken to vent the vial to avoid a pressure build up of the chlorine gas which is generated. Dispose of detoxified vials in a safe manner.

Needles, Syringes, Disposable and Non-Disposable Equipment: Rinse equipment with an appropriate quantity of sodium hypochlorite solution. Discard the solution in the sewer system with running water and discard disposable equipment in a safe manner. Thoroughly wash non-disposable equipment in soap and water.

Spillage/Contamination: Wear gloves, mask, protective clothing. Treat spilled liquid with sodium hypochlorite solution. Carefully absorb solution with gauze pads or towels, wash area with water and absorb with gauze or towels again and place in a polyethylene bag; seal, double bag and mark as hazardous waste. Disposal of waste by incineration or by other methods approved for hazardous materials. Personnel involved in clean up should wash with soap and water.

INFORMATION FOR THE PATIENT: Published in e-CPS, available by subscription at www.e-cps.ca.

DOSAGE FORMS, COMPOSITION AND PACKAGING: Each vial of sterile red-orange lyophilized powder contains: epirubicin HCl 50.3 mg and lactose monohydrate 251.5 mg. To withdraw exact amount. Glass vials of 50 mg in single vial cartons.

Epirubicin Hydrochloride Injection Ⓟ

epirubicin HCl

Antineoplastic

Hospira

SUPPLIED: Each mL of sterile, clear red solution contains: epirubicin hydrochloride 2 mg, sodium chloride 9 mg and water for injection. Hydrochloric Acid may be used to adjust the pH to 2.5-4.0. Single use clear glass ONCO-TAIN vials of 5, 25, 50, 75 (Pharmacy Bulk Vials) and 100 (Pharmacy Bulk Vials) mL, single vial cartons. Store under refrigeration (2-8°C), protected from light, and retained in original carton until time of use. Do not freeze.

The Epirubicin Hydrochloride Injection vial is for single use only. Unused portions must be discarded. Dispense contents of the Pharmacy Bulk Vial within 8 hours of the initial entry. Discard any unused portion. The contents of the syringes filled from the Pharmacy Bulk Vial should be used within 24 hours at room temperature or 48 hours when refrigerated from the time of the initial entry into the Pharmacy Bulk Vial.

Epival® Ⓟ

divalproex sodium

Anticonvulsant

Abbott

Date of Preparation: November 30, 1983
Date of Revision: May 2, 2008

SUMMARY PRODUCT INFORMATION:

Route of Administration	Dosage Form/ Strength	Clinically Relevant Nonmedicinal Ingredients
Oral	Enteric-Coated Tablet/125 mg, 250 mg, 500 mg	Cellulosic polymers, diacetylated monoglycerides, povidone, pregelatinized starch (contains corn starch), silicon dioxide, talc, titanium dioxide, vanillin and FD&C Red No. 40 (125 mg), FD&C Yellow No. 6 (250 mg), D&C Red No. 30 (500 mg), FD&C Blue No. 2 (500 mg).

INDICATIONS AND CLINICAL USE: EPIVAL (divalproex sodium) enteric-coated tablets are indicated for:

Epilepsy:

- use as sole or adjunctive therapy in the treatment of simple or complex absence seizures, including petit mal, and are useful in primary generalized seizures with tonic-clonic manifestations. Divalproex sodium may also be used adjunctively in patients with multiple seizure types which include either absence or tonic-clonic seizures.

In accordance with the International Classification of Seizures, simple absence is defined as a very brief clouding of the sensorium or loss of consciousness (lasting usually 2 to 15 seconds), accompanied by certain generalized epileptic discharges without other detectable clinical signs. Complex absence is the term used when other signs are also present.

Acute Mania:

- the treatment of the manic episodes associated with bipolar disorder (DSM-III-R).

The safety and effectiveness of EPIVAL for long-term use in mania, that is for more than 3 weeks, has not been evaluated in controlled trials.

EPIVAL is not indicated for use as a mood stabilizer in patients under 18 years of age.

See Contraindications, and Warnings and Precautions for statement regarding serious or fatal hepatic dysfunction.

Geriatrics (≥65 years of age): The safety and efficacy of valproate in elderly patients with epilepsy and mania has not been evaluated in clinical trials. Caution should thus be exercised in dose selection for an elderly patient, recognizing the more frequent hepatic and renal dysfunctions, and limited experience with valproate in this population. For a brief discussion, see Warnings and Precautions, Special Populations, Geriatrics (≥65 years of age); Dosage and Administration and Action and Clinical Pharmacology, Special Populations and Conditions, Geriatrics.

Pediatrics (<18 years of age): When divalproex sodium is used in children under the age of two years, it should be used with extreme caution and as a sole agent. Above the age of two years, experience in epilepsy has indicated that the incidence of fatal hepatotoxicity decreases considerably in progressively older patient groups. For a brief discussion, see Warnings and Precautions, Special Populations, Pediatrics (<18 years of age). The safety and effectiveness of divalproex sodium for the treatment of acute mania has not been studied in individuals below the age of 18 years.

CONTRAINDICATIONS:

- EPIVAL (divalproex sodium) enteric-coated tablets should not be administered to patients with hepatic disease or significant hepatic dysfunction.
- Divalproex sodium is contraindicated in patients with known hypersensitivity to the drug. For a complete listing, see Dosage Forms, Composition and Packaging.
- Divalproex sodium is contraindicated in patients with known urea cycle disorders (see Warnings and Precautions).

WARNINGS AND PRECAUTIONS:

Serious Warnings and Precautions

- **Hepatotoxicity:** Hepatic failure resulting in fatalities has occurred in patients receiving valproic acid and its derivatives. These incidences usually occurred during the first six months of treatment with valproic acid. Caution should be observed when administering valproate products to patients with a prior history of hepatic disease. Patients on multiple anticonvulsants, children, those with congenital metabolic disorders, those with severe seizure disorders accompanied by mental retardation, and those with organic brain disease may be at particular risk. Experience has indicated that children under the age of two years are at a considerably increased risk of developing fatal hepatotoxicity, especially those on multiple anticonvulsants. (See Warnings and Precautions, Hepatic/Biliary/Pancreatic, Serious or Fatal Hepatotoxicity.)
- **Teratogenicity:** Valproate can produce teratogenic effects such as neural tube defects (e.g., spina bifida). Accordingly, the use of the medication in women of childbearing potential requires that the benefits of its use be weighed against the risk of injury to the fetus. (See Warnings and Precautions, Special Populations, Pregnant Women.)
- **Pancreatitis:** Cases of life-threatening pancreatitis have been reported in both children and adults receiving valproate. Some of the cases have been described as hemorrhagic with a rapid progression from initial symptoms to death. Some cases have occurred shortly after initial use as well as after several years of use. (See Warnings and Precautions, Hepatic/Biliary/Pancreatic, Pancreatitis.)

General: Patients with Special Diseases and Conditions: There are in vitro studies that suggest valproate stimulates the replication of the HIV and CMV viruses under certain experimental conditions. The clinical relevance of these in vitro data is unknown.

Carcinogenesis and Mutagenesis: Long-term animal toxicity studies indicate that valproic acid is a weak carcinogen or promoter in rats and mice. The significance of these findings for humans is unknown at present.

Endocrine and Metabolism: Urea Cycle Disorders (UCD): Valproic acid is contraindicated in patients with known urea cycle disorders. Hyperammonemic encephalopathy, sometimes fatal, has been reported following initiation of valproate therapy in patients with urea cycle disorders, a group of uncommon genetic abnormalities, particularly ornithine transcarbamylase deficiency. Prior to initiation of valproate therapy, evaluation for UCD should be considered in the following patients:

1. Those with a history of unexplained encephalopathy or coma, encephalopathy associated with protein load, pregnancy-related or postpartum encephalopathy, unexplained mental retardation, or history of elevated plasma ammonia or glutamine;
2. Those with signs and symptoms of UCD, for example, cyclical vomiting and lethargy, episodic extreme irritability, ataxia, low BUN, protein avoidance;
3. Those with a family history of UCD or a family history of unexplained infant deaths (particularly males);
4. Those with other signs or symptoms of UCD. Patients receiving valproate therapy who develop symptoms of unexplained hyperammonemic encephalopathy should receive prompt treatment (including discontinuation of valproate therapy) and be evaluated for underlying urea cycle disorders (see Contraindications and Warnings and Precautions, Endocrine and Metabolism, Hyperammonemia and Hyperammonemia and Encephalopathy Associated with Concomitant Topiramate Use).

Hyperammonemia: Hyperammonemia has been reported in association with valproate therapy and may be present despite normal liver function tests. In patients who develop unexplained lethargy and vomiting or changes in mental status, hyperammonemic encephalopathy should be considered as a possible cause and serum ammonia level should be measured. If serum ammonia is increased, valproate therapy should be discontinued. Appropriate interventions for treatment of hyperammonemia should be initiated, and such patients should undergo investigation for underlying urea cycle disorders (see Contraindications and Warnings and Precautions, Endocrine and Metabolism, Urea Cycle Disorders (UCD) and Hyperammonemia and Encephalopathy Associated with Concomitant Topiramate Use).

Asymptomatic elevations of serum ammonia are more common and, when present, require close monitoring of serum ammonia levels. If the elevation persists, discontinuation of valproate therapy should be considered.

Hyperammonemia and Encephalopathy Associated with Concomitant Topiramate Use: Concomitant administration of topiramate and valproic acid has been associated with hyperammonemia with or without encephalopathy in patients who have tolerated either drug alone. Clinical symptoms of hyperammonemic encephalopathy often include acute alterations in level of consciousness and/or cognitive function with lethargy or vomiting. In most cases, symptoms and signs abated with discontinuation of either drug. This adverse event is not due to a pharmacokinetic interaction.

It is not known if topiramate monotherapy is associated with hyperammonemia.

Patients with inborn errors of metabolism or reduced hepatic mitochondrial activity may be at an increased risk for hyperammonemia with or without encephalopathy. Although not studied, an interaction of topiramate and valproic acid may exacerbate existing defects or unmask deficiencies in susceptible persons (see Contraindications and Warnings and Precautions, Endocrine and Metabolism, Urea Cycle Disorders (UCD) and Hyperammonemia).

Hematologic: Thrombocytopenia: Because of reports of thrombocytopenia, inhibition of the second phase of platelet aggregation, and abnormal coagulation parameters (e.g., low fibrinogen), platelet counts and coagulation tests are recommended before initiating therapy and at periodic intervals. It is recommended that patients receiving divalproex sodium be monitored for platelet count and coagulation parameters prior to planned surgery. Clinical evidence of hemorrhage, bruising or a disorder of hemostasis/coagulation is an indication for reduction of the dosage or withdrawal of therapy (see also Warnings And Precautions, Hematologic, Dose-related Adverse Reactions: Thrombocytopenia).

Dose-related Adverse Reactions: Thrombocytopenia: The frequency of adverse effects (particularly elevated liver enzymes and thrombocytopenia) may be dose-related. In a clinical trial of divalproex sodium as monotherapy in patients with epilepsy, 34/126 patients (27%) receiving approximately 50 mg/kg/day on average, had at least one value of platelets $\leq 75\times10^9$/L. Approximately half of these patients had treatment discontinued with return of platelet counts to normal. In the remaining patients, platelet counts normalized with continued treatment. In this study, the probability of thrombocytopenia appeared to increase significantly at total valproate concentrations of ≥110 µg/mL (females) or ≥135 µg/mL (males). The therapeutic benefit which may accompany the higher doses should therefore be weighed against the possibility of a greater incidence of adverse events.

In addition, the findings from a crossover clinical trial conducted with EPIVAL ER extended-release tablets, in 44 epilepsy patients, indicate that the frequency of **treatment-emergent** mild thrombocytopenia (platelet count between $100\text{-}150\times10^9$/L) was significantly higher after 12 weeks of treatment with EPIVAL ER than after 12 weeks of treatment with EPIVAL (7 vs 3 low counts, respectively).

Hepatic/Biliary/Pancreatic: Serious or Fatal Hepatotoxicity: Hepatic failure resulting in fatalities has occurred in patients receiving valproic acid and its derivatives. These incidences usually occurred during the first six months of treatment with valproic acid. Caution should be observed when administering valproate products to patients with a prior history of hepatic disease. Patients on multiple anticonvulsants, children, those with congenital metabolic disorders, those with severe seizure disorders accompanied by mental retardation, and those with organic brain disease may be at particular risk.

Experience has indicated that children under the age of two years are at a considerably increased risk of developing fatal hepatotoxicity, especially those on multiple anticonvulsants, those with congenital metabolic disorders, those with severe seizure disorders accompanied by mental retardation, and those with organic brain disease. The risk in this age group decreased considerably in patients receiving valproate as monotherapy. Similarly, patients aged 3 to 10 years were at somewhat greater risk if they received multiple anticonvulsants than those who received only valproate. Above the age of two years, experience in epilepsy has indicated that the incidence of fatal hepatotoxicity decreases considerably in progressively older patients. No deaths have been reported in patients over 10 years of age who received valproate alone.

If valproate products are to be used for the control of seizures in children two years old or younger, it should be used with **extreme caution** and as a sole agent. The benefits of therapy should be weighed against the risks (see Warnings and Precautions, Special Populations, Pediatrics (<18 years of age)).

Serious or fatal hepatotoxicity may be preceded by nonspecific symptoms such as, malaise, weakness, lethargy, facial edema, anorexia, and vomiting. In patients with epilepsy, a loss of seizure control may also occur. Patients should be monitored closely for appearance of these symptoms. Patients and parents should be instructed to report such symptoms. Because of the nonspecific nature of some of the early signs, hepatotoxicity should be suspected in patients who become unwell, other than through obvious cause, while taking valproate products.

Liver function tests should be performed prior to therapy and at frequent intervals thereafter especially during the first 6 months. However, physicians should not rely totally on serum biochemistry since these tests may not be abnormal in all instances, but should also consider the results of careful interim medical history and physical examination.

In high-risk patients, it might also be useful to monitor serum fibrinogen and albumin for decreases in concentration and serum ammonia for increases in concentration. If changes occur, divalproex sodium should be discontinued. Dosage should be titrated to and maintained at the lowest dose consistent with optimal seizure control.

The drug should be discontinued immediately in the presence of significant hepatic dysfunction, suspected or apparent. In some cases, hepatic dysfunction has progressed in spite of discontinuation of drug. The frequency of adverse hepatic effects (particularly elevated liver enzymes may increase with increasing dose. The therapeutic benefit which may accompany the higher doses should therefore be weighed against the possibility of a greater incidence of adverse effects (see Contraindications).

Pancreatitis: Cases of life-threatening pancreatitis have been reported in both children and adults receiving valproate. Some of the cases have been described as hemorrhagic with a rapid progression from initial symptoms to death. Some cases have occurred shortly after initial use as well as after several years of use. The rate based upon the reported cases exceeds that expected in the general population and there have been cases in which pancreatitis recurred after rechallenge with valproate. In clinical trials, there were 2 cases of pancreatitis without alternative etiology in 2416 patients, representing 1044 patient-years experience. Patients and guardians should be warned that abdominal pain, nausea, vomiting, and/or anorexia can be symptoms of pancreatitis that require prompt medical evaluation. If pancreatitis is diagnosed, valproate should ordinarily be discontinued. Alternative treatment for the underlying medical condition should be initiated as clinically indicated.

Neurologic: Driving and Hazardous Occupations: Divalproex sodium may produce CNS depression, especially when combined with another CNS depressant, such as alcohol. Therefore, patients should be advised not to engage in hazardous occupations, such as driving a car or operating dangerous machinery, until it is known that they do not become drowsy from the drug.

Psychiatric: Suicidal ideation may be a manifestation of preexisting psychiatric disorders, and close supervision of high risk patients should accompany initial drug therapy.

Renal: Renal Impairment: Renal impairment is associated with an increase in the unbound fraction of valproate. In several studies, the unbound fraction of valproate in plasma from renally impaired patients was approximately double that for subjects with normal renal function. Accordingly, monitoring of total concentrations in patients with renal impairment may be misleading since free concentrations may be substantially elevated whereas total concentrations may appear to be normal. Hemodialysis in renally impaired patients may remove up to 20% of the circulating valproate.

Sensitivity/Resistance: Multi-organ Hypersensitivity Reaction: Multi-organ hypersensitivity reactions have been rarely reported in close temporal association to the initiation of valproate therapy in adult and pediatric patients (median time to detection 21 days; range 1 to 40). Although there have been a limited number of reports, many of these cases resulted in hospitalization and at least one death has been reported. Signs and symptoms of this disorder were diverse; however, patients typically, although not exclusively, presented with fever and rash associated with other organ system involvement. Other associated manifestations may include lymphadenopathy, hepatitis, liver function test abnormalities, hematological abnormalities (e.g., eosinophilia, thrombocytopenia, neutropenia), pruritus, nephritis, oliguria, hepato-renal syndrome, arthralgia, and asthenia. Because the disorder is variable in its expression, other organ system symptoms and signs, not noted here may occur. If this reaction is suspected, valproate should be discontinued and an alternative treatment started. Although the existence of cross sensitivity with other drugs that produce this syndrome is unclear, the experience amongst drugs associated with multi-organ hypersensitivity would indicate this to be a possibility.

Sexual Function/Reproduction: Fertility: The effect of valproate on testicular development and on sperm production and fertility in humans is unknown.

Skin: Serious Skin Reactions: The dose of lamotrigine should be reduced when co-administered with valproate. Serious skin reactions (such as Stevens-Johnson Syndrome and toxic epidermal necrolysis) have been reported with concomitant lamotrigine and valproate administration (see Lamotrigine Product Monograph for details on lamotrigine dosing with concomitant valproate administration).

Special Populations: Pregnant Women: According to published and unpublished reports in the medical literature, valproic acid may produce teratogenic effects, such as neural tube defects (e.g., spina bifida) in the offspring of human females receiving the drug during pregnancy. There are data that suggest an increased incidence of congenital malformations associated with the use of valproic acid during pregnancy when compared with some other antiepileptic drugs. Therefore, valproic acid should be considered for women of childbearing potential only after the risks have been thoroughly discussed with the patient and weighed against the potential benefits of treatment.

Multiple reports in the clinical literature indicate an association between the use of antiepileptic drugs and an elevated incidence of birth defects in children born to epileptic women taking such medication during pregnancy. The incidence of congenital malformations in the general population is regarded to be approximately 2%; in children of treated epileptic women, this incidence may be increased 2- to 3-fold. The increase is largely due to specific defects such as congenital malformations of the heart, cleft lip and/or palate, craniofacial abnormalities and neural tube defects. Nevertheless, the great majority of mothers receiving antiepileptic medications deliver normal infants.

Neural Tube Defects: The data described below were gained almost exclusively from women who received valproate to treat epilepsy. The incidence of neural tube defects in the fetus is increased in mothers receiving valproic acid during the first trimester of pregnancy. Based upon a single report, it was estimated that the risk of valproic acid-exposed women having children with spina bifida is approximately 1 to 2%.

Other congenital anomalies (e.g., craniofacial defects, cardiovascular malformations and anomalies involving various body systems), compatible and incompatible with life, have been reported. Sufficient data to determine the incidence of these congenital anomalies are not available.

The higher incidence of congenital anomalies in antiepileptic drug-treated women with seizure disorders cannot be regarded as a cause and effect relationship. There are intrinsic methodologic problems in obtaining adequate data on drug teratogenicity in humans; genetic factors or the epileptic condition itself, may be more important than the drug therapy in contributing to congenital anomalies.

There have been reports of developmental delay in the offspring of women who have received valproic acid during pregnancy.

Patients taking valproate may develop clotting abnormalities. A patient who had low fibrinogen when taking multiple anticonvulsants including valproate gave birth to an infant with afibrinogenemia who subsequently died of hemorrhage. If valproic acid is used in pregnancy, the clotting parameters should be monitored carefully.

Hepatic failure, resulting in the death of a newborn and of an infant has been reported following the use of valproate during pregnancy.

Antiepileptic drugs should not be abruptly discontinued in patients to whom the drug is administered to prevent major seizures, because of the strong possibility of precipitating status epilepticus with attendant hypoxia and risks to both the mother and the unborn child. With regard to drugs given for minor seizures, the risks of discontinuing medication prior to or during pregnancy should be weighed against the risk of congenital defects in the particular case and with the particular family history. In individual cases where the severity and frequency of the seizure disorder are such that the removal of medication does not pose a serious threat to the patient, discontinuation of the drug may be considered prior to and during pregnancy, although it cannot be said with any confidence that even minor seizures do not pose some hazard to the developing embryo or fetus.

In summary, current best practice guidelines should be considered in order to provide the optimal counsel to patients regarding the teratogenic risks associated with valproic acid.

Epileptic women of childbearing age should be encouraged to seek the counsel of their physician and should report the onset of pregnancy promptly to him. Where the necessity for continued use of antiepileptic medication is in doubt, appropriate consultation is indicated.

Risk-benefit must be carefully considered when treating or counselling women of childbearing age for bipolar disorder.

If divalproex sodium is used during pregnancy, or if the patient becomes pregnant while taking this drug, the patient should be made aware of the potential hazard to the fetus.

Tests to detect neural tube and other defects using current accepted procedures should be considered a part of routine prenatal care in childbearing women receiving valproate.

Animal studies have demonstrated valproic acid induced teratogenicity, and studies in human females have demonstrated placental transfer of the drug. Increased frequencies of malformations, as well as intrauterine growth retardation and death, have been observed in mice, rats, rabbits, and monkeys following prenatal exposure to valproate. Malformations of the skeletal system are the most common structural abnormalities produced in experimental animals, but neural tube closure defects have been seen in mice exposed to maternal plasma valproate concentrations exceeding 230 µg/mL (2.3 times the upper limit of the human therapeutic range for epilepsy) during susceptible periods of embryonic development.

Administration of an oral dose of 200 mg/kg/day or greater (50% of the maximum human daily dose or greater on a mg/m² basis) to pregnant rats during organogenesis produced malformations (skeletal, cardiac and urogenital) and growth retardation in the offspring. These doses resulted in peak maternal plasma valproate levels of approximately 340 µg/mL or greater (3.4 times the upper limit of the human therapeutic range for epilepsy or greater). Behavioural deficits have been reported in the offspring of rats given a dose of 200 mg/kg/day throughout most of pregnancy.

An oral dose of 350 mg/kg/day (approximately 2 times the maximum human daily dose on a mg/m² basis) produced skeletal and visceral malformations in rabbits exposed during organogenesis. Skeletal malformations, growth retardation, and death were observed in rhesus monkeys following administration of an oral dose of 200 mg/kg/day (equal to the maximum human daily dose on a mg/m² basis) during organogenesis. This dose resulted in peak maternal plasma valproate levels of approximately 280 µg/mL (2.8 times the upper limit of the human therapeutic range for epilepsy).

Nursing Women: Valproic acid is excreted in breast milk. Concentrations in breast milk have been reported to be 1 to 10% of serum concentrations. As a general rule, nursing should not be undertaken while a patient is receiving divalproex sodium. It is not known what effect this may have on a nursing infant.

Pediatrics (<18 years of age): Experience has indicated that children under the age of two years are at a considerably increased risk of developing fatal hepatotoxicity, especially those with the aforementioned conditions (see Warnings and Precautions, Hepatic/Biliary/Pancreatic, Serious or Fatal Hepatotoxicity). When EPIVAL is used in this patient group, it should be used with extreme caution and as a sole agent. The benefits of therapy should be weighed against the risks.

Above the age of 2 years, experience in epilepsy has indicated that the incidence of fatal hepatotoxicity decreases considerably in progressively older patient groups.

Younger children, especially those receiving enzyme-inducing drugs, will require larger maintenance doses to attain targeted total and unbound valproic acid concentrations. The variability in free fraction limits the clinical usefulness of monitoring total serum valproic concentrations. Interpretation of valproic acid concentrations in children should include consideration of factors that affect hepatic metabolism and protein binding.

The safety and effectiveness of divalproex sodium for the treatment of acute mania has not been studied in individuals below the age of 18 years.

Geriatrics (≥65 years of age): Alterations in the kinetics of unbound valproate in the elderly indicate that the initial dosage should be reduced in this population (see Dosage and Administration and Action and Clinical Pharmacology, Special Populations and Conditions, Geriatrics).

The safety and efficacy of valproate in elderly patients with epilepsy and mania has not been evaluated in clinical trials. Caution should thus be exercised in dose selection for an elderly patient, recognizing the more frequent hepatic and renal dysfunctions, and limited experience with valproate in this population.

A study of elderly patients revealed valproate-related somnolence and discontinuation of valproate therapy for this adverse event (see Warnings and Precautions, Special Populations, Geriatrics, Somnolence in the Elderly). The starting dose should be reduced in elderly patients, and dosage reductions or discontinuation should be considered in patients with excessive somnolence (see Dosage and Administration).

Somnolence in the Elderly: In a group of elderly patients (mean age=83 years old, n=172), valproate doses were increased by 125 mg/day to a target dose of 20 mg/kg/day. Compared to placebo a significantly higher number of valproate-treated patients had somnolence, and although not statistically significant, a higher number of valproate-treated patients experienced dehydration. Discontinuations for somnolence were also significantly higher in valproate-treated patients compared to placebo. In approximately one-half of the patients with somnolence, there was also associated reduced nutritional intake and weight loss. In elderly patients, dosage should be increased more slowly and with regular monitoring for fluid intake, dehydration, somnolence, urinary tract infection and other adverse events. Dose reductions or discontinuation of valproate should be considered in patients with decreased food or fluid intake and in patients with excessive somnolence (see Dosage and Administration).

Monitoring and Laboratory Tests: Since valproate may interact with concurrently administered drugs which are capable of enzyme induction, periodic plasma concentration determinations of valproate and concomitant drugs are recommended during the early course of therapy and whenever enzyme-inducing drugs are introduced or withdrawn (see Drug Interactions).

Monitoring Valproate Concentrations: Protein binding of valproate is reduced in the elderly, in patients with renal impairment, and in the presence of other drugs (e.g., acetylsalicylic acid). Accordingly, measurements of plasma levels of valproate may be misleading in these patients, as actual drug exposure may be higher than measured values. See Warnings and Precautions, Hepatic/Biliary/Pancreatic; Endocrine and Metabolism, Hyperammonemia, Hematologic, Thrombocytopenia, and Drug Interactions, Drug-Drug Interactions.

ADVERSE REACTIONS: Epilepsy: The most commonly reported adverse reactions are nausea, vomiting and indigestion. Since divalproex sodium has usually been used with other antiepileptics, it is not possible in most cases to determine whether the adverse reactions mentioned in this section are due to divalproex sodium alone or to the combination of drugs.

Adverse events that have been reported with valproate from epilepsy trials, spontaneous reports, and other sources are listed below by body system.

Gastrointestinal: Nausea, vomiting and indigestion are the most commonly reported side effects at the initiation of therapy. These effects are usually transient and rarely require discontinuation of therapy. Diarrhea, abdominal cramps and constipation have also been reported. Anorexia with some weight loss and increased appetite with some weight gain have also been reported. The administration of delayed-release divalproex sodium may result in reduction of gastrointestinal side effects in some patients. In some patients, many of whom have functional or anatomic (including ileostomy or colostomy) gastrointestinal disorders with shortened gastrointestinal transit times, there have been postmarketing reports of divalproex sodium extended-release tablets in the stool.

CNS Effects: Sedative effects have been noted in patients receiving valproic acid alone but occur most often in patients on combination therapy. Sedation usually disappears upon reduction of other antiepileptic medication.

Hallucination, ataxia, headache, nystagmus, diplopia, asterixis, "spots before the eyes", tremor (may be dose-related), confusion, dysarthria, dizziness, hypesthesia, vertigo, incoordination and parkinsonism have been noted. Rare cases of coma have been reported in patients receiving valproic acid alone or in conjunction with phenobarbital.

Encephalopathy, with or without fever or hyperammonemia, has been reported without evidence of hepatic dysfunction or inappropriate valproate plasma levels. Most patients recovered, with noted improvement of symptoms, upon discontinuation of the drug.

Reversible cerebral atrophy and dementia have been reported in association with valproate therapy.

Dermatologic: Transient increases in hair loss have been observed. Skin rash, photosensitivity, generalized pruritus, erythema multiforme, Stevens-Johnson syndrome (SJS), and petechiae have rarely been noted.

Rare cases of toxic epidermal necrolysis (TEN) have been reported including a fatal case of a six month old infant taking valproate and several other concomitant medications. An additional case of toxic epidermal necrosis resulting in death was reported in a 35 year old patient with AIDS taking several concomitant medications and with a history of multiple cutaneous drug reactions.

Serious skin reactions have been reported with concomitant administration of lamotrigine and valproate (see Drug Interactions).

Endocrine: There have been reports of irregular menses, secondary amenorrhea, breast enlargement, galactorrhea and parotid gland swelling in patients receiving valproic acid.

Abnormal thyroid function tests have been reported (see Drug Interactions, Drug-Laboratory Test Interactions).

There have been rare spontaneous reports of polycystic ovary disease. A cause and effect relationship has not been established.

Psychiatric: Emotional upset, depression, psychosis, aggression, hyperactivity, hostility and behavioural deterioration have been reported.

Musculoskeletal: Weakness has been reported.

Hematopoietic: Thrombocytopenia and inhibition of the secondary phase of platelet aggregation may be reflected in altered bleeding time, petechiae, bruising, hematoma formation, epistaxis, and frank hemorrhage (see Warnings and Precautions, Hematologic, Thrombocytopenia). Relative lymphocytosis, macrocytosis and hypofibrinogenemia have been noted. Leukopenia and eosinophilia have also been reported. Anemia, including macrocytic with or without folate deficiency, aplastic anemia, pancytopenia, bone marrow suppression, agranulocytosis and acute intermittent porphyria have been reported.

Hepatic: Minor elevations of transaminases (e.g., AST and ALT) and LDH are frequent and appear to be dose-related. Occasionally, laboratory tests also show increases in serum bilirubin and abnormal changes in other liver function tests. These results may reflect potentially serious hepatotoxicity (see Warnings and Precautions).

Metabolic: Hyperammonemia (see Warnings and Precautions), hyponatremia and inappropriate ADH secretion. There have been rare reports of Fanconi syndrome occurring primarily in children. Decreased carnitine concentrations have been reported although the clinical relevance is undetermined. Hyperglycinemia (elevated plasma glycine concentration) has been reported and associated with a fatal outcome in a patient with preexisting non-ketotic hyperglycinemia.

Genitourinary: Enuresis and urinary tract infection.

Pancreatic: There have been reports of acute pancreatitis, including rare fatal cases, occurring in patients receiving valproate therapy (see Warnings and Precautions).

Special Senses: Hearing loss, either reversible or irreversible, has been reported; however, a cause and effect relationship has not been established. Ear pain has also been reported.

Other: Allergic reaction, anaphylaxis has been reported. Edema of the extremities has been reported. A lupus erythematosus-like syndrome has been reported rarely. Bone pain, increased cough, pneumonia, otitis media, bradycardia, cutaneous vasculitis, fever, and hypothermia have also been reported.

Clinical Trial Adverse Drug Reactions: Because clinical trials are conducted under very specific conditions the adverse reaction rates observed in the clinical trials may not reflect the rates observed in practice and should not be compared to the rates in the clinical trials of another drug. Adverse drug reaction information from clinical trials is useful for identifying drug-related adverse events and for approximating rates.

EPIVAL versus EPIVAL ER: A 24 week cross-over study compared the safety and efficacy of EPIVAL ER (administered once daily) to that of equal doses of EPIVAL (administered twice daily or three times daily) in the treatment of adolescent and adult epileptic patients with generalized seizures (n=44), two adverse events occurred in significantly more patients on EPIVAL ER than on EPIVAL: asthenia (15.9% vs 6.8% respectively) and treatment-emergent mild thrombocytopenia (16.2% vs 6.8%, respectively).

Bipolar Disorder: The incidence of adverse events has been ascertained based on data from two short-term (21 day) placebo-controlled clinical trials of divalproex sodium in the treatment of acute mania, and from two long-term (up to 3 years) retrospective open trials.

Most Commonly Observed: During the short-term placebo-controlled trials, the six most commonly reported adverse events in patients (N=89) exposed to divalproex sodium were nausea (22%), headache (21%), somnolence (19%), pain (15%), vomiting (12%), and dizziness (12%).

In the long-term retrospective trials (634 patients exposed to divalproex sodium), the six most commonly reported adverse events were somnolence (31%), tremor (29%), headache (24%), asthenia (23%), diarrhea (22%), and nausea (20%).

Associated With Discontinuation of Treatment: In the placebo-controlled trials, adverse events which resulted in valproate discontinuation in at least one percent of patients were nausea (4%), abdominal pain (3%), somnolence (2%), and rash (2%).

In the long-term retrospective trials, adverse events which resulted in valproate discontinuation in at least one percent of patients were alopecia (2.4%), somnolence (1.9%), nausea (1.7%), and tremor (1.4%). The time to onset of these events was generally within the first two months of initial exposure to valproate. A notable exception was alopecia, which was first experienced after 3 to 6 months of exposure by 8 of the 15 patients who discontinued valproate in response to the event.

Controlled Trials: Table 1 summarizes those treatment emergent adverse events reported for patients in the placebo-controlled trials when the incidence rate in the divalproex sodium group was at least 5%. (Maximum treatment duration was 21 days; maximum dose in 83% of patients was between 1000 mg to 2500 mg per day).

Table 1: EPIVAL

Treatment-Emergent Adverse Event Incidence (≥5%) in Short-Term Placebo-Controlled Trials (Oral Administration)

	Percentage of Patients	
Body System/Event	**Divalproex Sodium (N=89)**	**Placebo (N=97)**
Body as a Whole		
Headache	21.3	30.9
Pain	14.6	15.5
Accidental Injury	11.2	5.2
Asthenia	10.1	7.2
Abdominal Pain	9.0	8.2
Back Pain	5.6	6.2
Digestive System		
Nausea	22.5	15.5
Vomiting	12.4[a]	3.1
Diarrhea	10.1	13.4
Dyspepsia	9.0	8.2
Constipation	7.9	8.2
Nervous System		
Somnolence	19.1	12.4
Dizziness	12.4	4.1
Tremor	5.6	6.2
Respiratory System		
Pharyngitis	6.7	9.3
Skin and Appendages		
Rash	5.6	3.1

[a] Statistically significant at $P<0.05$ level.

The following adverse events not listed above were reported by at least 1%, but less than 5%, of the 89 patients from the two placebo-controlled clinical trials of EPIVAL tablets.

Body as a Whole: chest pain, chills, chills and fever, cyst, fever, infection, neck pain, neck rigidity.

Cardiovascular System: hypertension, hypotension, palpitations, postural hypotension, tachycardia, vascular anomaly, vasodilation.

Digestive System: anorexia, fecal incontinence, flatulence, gastroenteritis, glossitis, periodontal abscess.

Hemic and Lymphatic System: ecchymosis.

Metabolic and Nutritional Disorders: edema, peripheral edema.

Musculoskeletal System: arthralgia, arthrosis, leg cramps, twitching.

Nervous System: abnormal dreams, abnormal gait, agitation, ataxia, catatonic reaction, confusion, depression, diplopia, dysarthria, hallucinations, hypertonia, hypokinesia, insomnia, paresthesia, reflexes increased, tardive dyskinesia, thinking abnormalities, vertigo.

Respiratory System: dyspnea, rhinitis.

Skin and Appendages: alopecia, discoid lupus erythematosis, dry skin, furunculosis, maculopapular rash, seborrhea.

Special Senses: abnormal vision, amblyopia, conjunctivitis, deafness, dry eyes, ear disorder, ear pain, eye pain, tinnitus.

Urogenital System: dysmenorrhea, dysuria, urinary incontinence.

Adverse Events in Elderly Patients: In elderly patients (above 65 years of age), there were more frequent reports of accidental injury, infection, pain, and to a lesser degree, somnolence and tremor, when compared to patients 18 to 65 years of age. Somnolence and tremor tended to be associated with the discontinuation of valproate.

DRUG INTERACTIONS:

Serious Drug Interactions

- Rare cases of coma have been reported in patients receiving valproic acid alone or in conjunction with Phenobarbital (see Drug-Drug Interactions).
- Serious skin reactions (such as Stevens-Johnson Syndrome and toxic epidermal necrolysis) have been reported with concomitant lamotrigine and valproate administration (see Drug-Drug Interactions).

Overview: Valproate has been found to be a weak inhibitor of some P450 isozymes, epoxide hydrase, and glucuronyl transferases.

Drugs that affect the level of expression of hepatic enzymes, particularly those that elevate levels of glucuronyl transferases, may increase the clearance of valproate. For example, phenytoin, carbamazepine, and phenobarbital (or primidone) can double the clearance of valproate. Thus, patients on valproate monotherapy will generally have longer half-lives and higher concentrations than patients receiving polytherapy with antiepilepsy drugs.

In contrast, drugs that are inhibitors of cytochrome P450 isozymes, such as antidepressants, may be expected to have little effect on valproate clearance because cytochrome P450 microsomal mediated oxidation is a relatively minor secondary metabolic pathway compared to glucuronidation and beta-oxidation.

The concomitant administration of valproic acid with drugs that exhibit extensive protein binding (e.g., acetylsalicylic acid, carbamazepine, dicumarol, warfarin, tolbutamide, and phenytoin) may result in alteration of serum drug levels.

Since valproate may interact with concurrently administered drugs which are capable of enzyme induction, periodic plasma concentration determinations of valproate and concomitant drugs are recommended during the early course of therapy and whenever enzyme-inducing drugs are introduced or withdrawn.

Drug-Drug Interactions: Table 2 provides information about the potential influence of several commonly prescribed medications on valproate pharmacokinetics as well as the potential influence of valproate on the pharmacokinetics and pharmacodynamics of several commonly prescribed medications. The list is not exhaustive nor could it be, since new interactions are continuously being reported. Please note that drugs may be listed under specific name, family or pharmacologic class. Reading the entire section is recommended.

Drug-Food Interactions: Co-administration of oral valproate products with food should cause no clinical problems in the management of patients with epilepsy.

Drug-Herb Interactions: Interactions with herbal products have not been established.

Drug-Laboratory Test Interactions: Divalproex sodium is partially eliminated in the urine as a ketone-containing metabolite which may lead to a false interpretation of the urine ketone test.

There have been reports of altered thyroid function tests associated with valproic acid; the clinical significance of these is unknown.

Drug-Lifestyle Interactions: Refer to Warnings and Precautions, Neurologic, Driving and Hazardous Occupations for details.

Table 2: EPIVAL

Summary of Drug-Drug Interaction Studies Including Important Interactions, Non-clinically Important Interactions and No Observed Interactions

Concomitant Drug	Ref	Effect	Clinical Comment
Acetaminophen	CT	↔ acetaminophen	Valproate had no effect on any of the pharmacokinetic parameters of acetaminophen when it was concurrently administered to three epileptic patients.
Acetylsalicylic Acid	CT	↑ valproate	A study involving the co-administration of acetylsalicylic acid at antipyretic doses (11 to 16 mg/kg) with valproate to pediatric patients (n=6) revealed a decrease in protein binding and an inhibition of metabolism of valproate. Valproate free fraction was increased 4-fold in the presence of acetylsalicylic acid compared to valproate alone. The beta-oxidation pathway consisting of 2-E-valproic acid, 3-OH-valproic acid, and 3-keto valproic acid was decreased from 25% of total metabolites excreted on valproate alone to 8.3% in the presence of acetylsalicylic acid. Caution should be observed when valproate is administered with drugs affecting coagulation, (e.g., acetylsalicylic acid and warfarin) (see Adverse Reactions).
Alcohol	T	No PK interaction	Valproate may potentiate the CNS depressant action of alcohol.
Amitriptyline/Nortriptyline	CT	In general: ↓ amitriptyline ↓ nortriptyline	Administration of a single oral 50 mg dose of amitriptyline to 15 normal volunteers (10 males and 5 females) who received valproate (500 mg b.i.d.[a]) resulted in a 21% decrease in plasma clearance of amitriptyline and a 34% decrease in the net clearance of nortriptyline.
		Rarely: ↑ amitriptyline ↑ nortriptyline	Rare post-marketing reports of concurrent use of valproate and amitriptyline resulting in an increased amitriptyline and nortriptyline levels have been received. Concurrent use of valproate and amitriptyline has rarely been associated with toxicity. Monitoring of amitriptyline levels should be considered for patients taking valproate concomitantly with amitriptyline. Consideration should be given to lowering the dose of amitriptyline/nortriptyline in the presence of valproate.
Antacids	CT	↔ valproate	A study involving the co-administration of valproate 500 mg with commonly administered antacids (Maalox, Trisogel, and Titralac—160 mEq doses) did not reveal any effect on the extent of absorption of valproate.
Other—Antipsychotics, MAO Inhibitors and Tricyclic Antidepressants			In addition to enhancing central nervous system (CNS) depression when used concurrently with valproic acid, antipsychotics, tricyclic antidepressants and MAO inhibitors may lower the seizure threshold. Dosage adjustments may be necessary to control seizures.
Benzodiazepines			Valproic acid may decrease oxidative liver metabolism of some benzodiazepines, resulting in increased serum concentrations (see Diazepam and Lorazepam).
Carbamazepine/carbamazepine-10,11-epoxide	CT	↓ CBZ ↑ CBZ-E ↓ valproate	Concomitant use of carbamazepine with valproic acid may result in decreased serum concentrations and half-life of valproate due to increased metabolism induced by hepatic microsomal enzyme activity. Monitoring of serum concentrations is recommended when either medication is added to or withdrawn from an existing regimen. Changes in the serum concentration of the 10,11-epoxide metabolite of carbamazepine, however, will not be detected by routine serum carbamazepine assay. Serum levels of carbamazepine (CBZ) decreased 17% while that of carbamazepine-10,11-epoxide (CBZ-E) increased by 45% upon co-administration of valproate and CBZ to epileptic patients.
Chlorpromazine	CT	↑ valproate	A study involving the administration of 100 to 300 mg/day of chlorpromazine to schizophrenic patients already receiving valproate (200 mg b.i.d.[a] revealed a 15% increase in trough plasma levels of valproate. This increase is not considered clinically important.
Cimetidine	T	↑ valproate	Cimetidine may decrease the clearance and increase the half-life of valproic acid by altering its metabolism. In patients receiving valproic acid, serum valproic acid levels should be monitored when treatment with cimetidine is instituted, increased, decreased, or discontinued. The valproic acid dose should be adjusted accordingly.

(cont'd)

Table 2: EPIVAL *(cont'd)*

Summary of Drug-Drug Interaction Studies Including Important Interactions, Non-clinically Important Interactions and No Observed Interactions

Concomitant Drug	Ref	Effect	Clinical Comment
Clonazepam	T	No PK interaction	The concomitant use of valproic acid and clonazepam may induce absence status in patients with a history of absence type seizures.
Clozapine	CT	No interaction	In psychotic patients (n=11), no interaction was observed when valproate was co-administered with clozapine.
Diazepam	CT	↑ diazepam	Valproate displaces diazepam from its plasma albumin binding sites and inhibits its metabolism. Co-administration of valproate (1500 mg daily) increased the free fraction of diazepam (10 mg) by 90% in healthy volunteers (n=6). Plasma clearance and volume of distribution for free diazepam were reduced by 25% and 20%, respectively, in the presence of valproate. The elimination half-life of diazepam remained unchanged upon addition of valproate.
Ethosuximide	CT	↑ ethosuximide	Valproate inhibits the metabolism of ethosuximide. Administration of a single ethosuximide dose of 500 mg with valproate (800 to 1600 mg/day) to healthy volunteers (n=6) was accompanied by a 25% increase in elimination half-life of ethosuximide and a 15% decrease in its total clearance as compared to ethosuximide alone. Patients receiving valproate and ethosuximide, especially along with other anticonvulsants, should be monitored for alterations in serum concentrations of both drugs.
Felbamate	CT	↑ valproate	A study involving the co-administration of 1200 mg/day of felbamate with valproate to patients with epilepsy (n=10) revealed an increase in mean valproate peak concentration by 35% (from 86 to 115 μg/mL) compared to valproate alone. Increasing the felbamate dose to 2400 mg/day increased the mean valproate peak concentration to 133 μg/mL (another 16% increase). A decrease in valproate dosage may be necessary when felbamate therapy is initiated. Lower doses of valproate may be necessary when used concomitantly with felbamate.
Haloperidol	CT	↔ valproate	A study involving the administration of 6 to 10 mg/day of haloperidol to schizophrenic patients already receiving valproate (200 mg b.i.d.[a]) revealed no significant changes in valproate trough plasma levels.
Lamotrigine	CT	↑ lamotrigine ↓ valproate	The effects of sodium valproate on lamotrigine were investigated in six healthy male subjects. Each subject received a single oral dose of lamotrigine alone and with valproic acid 200 mg every 8 hours for six doses starting 1 hour before the lamotrigine dose was given. Valproic acid administration reduced the total clearance of lamotrigine by 21% and increased the plasma elimination half-life from 37.4 hours to 48.3 hours ($p < 0.005$). Renal clearance of lamotrigine was unchanged. In a steady-state study involving 10 healthy volunteers, the elimination half-life of lamotrigine increased from 26 to 70 hours with valproate co-administration (a 165% increase). In a study involving 16 epileptic patients, valproic acid doubled the elimination half-life of lamotrigine. In an open-labelled study, patients receiving enzyme inducing antiepileptic drugs (e.g., carbamazepine, phenytoin, phenobarbital, or primidone) demonstrated a mean lamotrigine plasma elimination half-life of 14 hours while the elimination half-life was 30 hours in patients taking sodium valproate plus an enzyme inducing antiepileptic agent. The latter value is similar to the lamotrigine half-life during monotherapy indicating that valproic acid may counteract the effect of the enzyme inducer. If valproic acid is discontinued in a patient receiving lamotrigine and an enzyme inducing antiepileptic serum lamotrigine concentrations may decrease. Patients receiving combined antiepileptic therapy require careful monitoring when another agent is started, stopped or when the dose is altered. Serious skin reactions (such as Stevens-Johnson Syndrome and toxic epidermal necrolysis) have been reported with concomitant lamotrigine and valproate administration.
Lithium	CT	↔ lithium	In a double-blind placebo-controlled multiple dose crossover study in 16 healthy male volunteers, pharmacokinetic parameters of lithium were not altered by the presence or absence of valproate. The presence of lithium, however, resulted in an 11% to 12% increase in the AUC and C_{max} of valproate. T_{max} was also reduced. Although these changes were statistically significant, they are not likely to have clinical importance. Co-administration of valproate (500 mg b.i.d.[a]) and lithium carbonate (300 mg t.i.d.[a]) to normal male volunteers (n=16) had no effect on the steady-state kinetics of lithium.
Lorazepam	CT	↑ lorazepam	Concomitant administration of valproate (500 mg b.i.d.[a]) and lorazepam (1 mg b.i.d.[a]) in normal male volunteers (n=9) was accompanied by a 17% decrease in the plasma clearance of lorazepam. This decrease is not considered clinically important.

(cont'd)

Table 2: EPIVAL *(cont'd)*

Summary of Drug-Drug Interaction Studies Including Important Interactions, Non-clinically Important Interactions and No Observed Interactions

Concomitant Drug	Ref	Effect	Clinical Comment
Meropenem	C	↓ valproate	Subtherapeutic valproic acid levels have been reported when meropenem was co-administered.
Oral Contraceptive Steroids	CT	No PK interaction	Evidence suggests that there is an association between the use of certain antiepileptic drugs capable of enzyme induction and failure of oral contraceptives. One explanation for this interaction is that enzyme-inducing drugs effectively lower plasma concentrations of the relevant steroid hormones, resulting in unimpaired ovulation. However, other mechanisms, not related to enzyme induction, may contribute to the failure of oral contraceptives. Valproic acid is not a significant enzyme inducer and would not be expected to decrease concentrations of steroid hormones. However, clinical data about the interaction of valproic acid with oral contraceptives are minimal. Administration of a single-dose of ethinyloestradiol (50 µg)/levonorgestrel (250 µg) to 6 women on valproate (200 mg b.i.d.[a]) therapy for 2 months did not reveal any pharmacokinetic interaction.
Phenobarbital	CT	↑ phenobarbital	Valproate was found to inhibit the metabolism of phenobarbital. Co-administration of valproate (250 mg b.i.d.[a] for 14 days) with phenobarbital to normal subjects (n=6) resulted in a 50% increase in half-life and a 30% decrease in plasma clearance of phenobarbital (60 mg single-dose). The fraction of phenobarbital dose excreted unchanged increased by 50% in the presence of valproate. There is evidence for severe CNS depression, with or without significant elevations of barbiturate or valproate serum concentrations. All patients receiving concomitant barbiturate therapy should be closely monitored for neurological toxicity. Serum barbiturate concentrations should be obtained, if possible, and the barbiturate dosage decreased, if appropriate.
Phenytoin	CT	↑ phenytoin	Valproate displaces phenytoin from its plasma albumin binding sites and inhibits its hepatic metabolism. Co-administration of valproate (400 mg t.i.d.[a]) with phenytoin (250 mg) in normal volunteers (n=7) was associated with a 60% increase in the free fraction of phenytoin. Total plasma clearance and apparent volume of distribution of phenytoin increased 30% in the presence of valproate. Both the clearance and apparent volume of distribution of free phenytoin were reduced by 25%. In patients with epilepsy, there have been reports of breakthrough seizures occurring with the combination of valproate and phenytoin. The dosage of phenytoin should be adjusted as required by the clinical situation.
Primidone	T	↑ phenobarbital	Primidone is metabolized into a barbiturate (phenobarbital), and therefore, may also be involved in a similar or identical interaction with valproate as phenobarbital.
Rifampin	CT	↓ valproate	A study involving the administration of a single dose of valproate (7 mg/kg) 36 hours after 5 nights of daily dosing with rifampin (600 mg) revealed a 40% increase in the oral clearance of valproate. Valproate dosage adjustment may be necessary when it is co-administered with rifampin.
Selective Serotonin Re-Uptake Inhibitors (SSRI's)	C	↑ valproate	Some evidence suggests that SSRI's inhibit the metabolism of valproate, resulting in higher than expected levels of valproate.
Tolbutamide	T	↑ tolbutamide	From in vitro experiments, the unbound fraction of tolbutamide was increased from 20% to 50% when added to plasma samples taken from patients treated with valproate. The clinical relevance of this displacement is unknown.
Topiramate	CT	Effect unknown	Concomitant administration of valproic acid and topiramate has been associated with hyperammonemia with and without encephalopathy (see Contraindications and Warnings and Precautions, Endocrine and Metabolism, Urea Cycle Disorders (UCD) and Hyperammonemia and Hyperammonemia and Encephalopathy Associated with Concomitant Topiramate Use).
Warfarin	T	Effect unknown	In an in vitro study, valproate increased the unbound fraction of warfarin by up to 32.6%. The therapeutic relevance of this is unknown, however, coagulation tests should be monitored if valproate therapy is instituted in patients taking anticoagulants. Caution is recommended when valproate is administered with drugs affecting coagulation (see Adverse Reactions).
Zidovudine	CT	↑ zidovudine	In six patients who were seropositive for HIV, the clearance of zidovudine (100 mg q8h) was decreased by 38% after administration of valproate (250 or 500 mg q8h); the half-life of zidovudine was unaffected.

[a] b.i.d.=twice daily; t.i.d.=three times daily
Legend: C=case study; CT=clinical trial; T=theoretical.

DOSAGE AND ADMINISTRATION: Dosing Considerations: Epilepsy: Patients receiving combined antiepileptic therapy require careful monitoring when another agent is started, stopped or when the dose is altered (see Drug Interactions).

As the dosage of divalproex sodium is titrated upward, blood concentrations of phenobarbital, carbamazepine and/or phenytoin may be affected (see Drug Interactions).

Antiepileptic drugs should not be abruptly discontinued in patients in whom the drug is administered to prevent major seizures because of the strong possibility of precipitating status epilepticus with attendant hypoxia and threat to life.

Any changes in dosage and administration, or the addition or discontinuance of concomitant drugs, should ordinarily be accompanied by close monitoring of clinical status and valproate plasma concentrations.

When changing therapy involving drugs known to induce hepatic microsomal enzymes (e.g., carbamazepine) or other drugs with valproate interactions (see Drug Interactions), it is advisable to monitor serum valproate concentrations.

Dosing in Elderly Patients: Due to a decrease in unbound clearance of valproate and possibly a greater sensitivity to somnolence in the elderly, the starting dose should be reduced. Dosage should be increased more slowly and with regular monitoring for fluid and nutritional intake, dehydration, somnolence, urinary tract infection, and other adverse events. Dose reductions or discontinuation of valproate should be considered in patients with decreased food or fluid intake and in patients with excessive somnolence. The ultimate therapeutic dose should be achieved on the basis of clinical response (see Warnings and Precautions).

Dose-Related Adverse Events: The frequency of adverse events (particularly elevated liver enzymes and thrombocytopenia) may be dose related. The probability of thrombocytopenia appears to increase significantly at total valproate concentration of ≥110 µg/mL (females) or ≥135 µg/mL (males) (see Warnings and Precautions). Therefore, the benefit of improved therapeutic effect with higher doses should be weighed against the possibility of a greater incidence of adverse effects.

Recommended Dose and Dosage Adjustment: Epilepsy: EPIVAL (divalproex sodium) enteric-coated tablets are administered orally. The recommended initial dosage is 15 mg/kg/day, increasing at one-week intervals by 5 to 10 mg/kg/day until seizures are controlled or side effects preclude further increases.

The maximal recommended dosage is 60 mg/kg/day. When the total daily dose is 250 mg and over, it should be given in a divided regimen (see Table 3).

Table 3: EPIVAL

Initial Doses by Weight (based on 15 mg/kg/day)

Weight (kg)	Total Daily Dose (mg)	Dosage (mg) Equivalent to Valproic Acid		
		Dose 1	Dose 2	Dose 3
10–24.9	250	125	0	125
25–39.9	500	250	0	250
40–59.9	750	250	250	250
60–74.9	1000	250	250	500
75–89.9	1250	500	250	500

Therapeutic Blood Levels: A good correlation has not been established between daily dose, total serum valproate concentration and therapeutic effect. However, therapeutic valproate serum concentrations for most patients with epilepsy will range from 50 to 100 µg/mL (350 to 700 micromole/L).Some patients may be controlled with lower or higher serum concentrations (see Warnings and Precautions).

Conversion from DEPAKENE to EPIVAL: EPIVAL (divalproex sodium) enteric-coated tablets dissociate to the valproate ion in the gastrointestinal tract. Divalproex sodium tablets are uniformly and reliably absorbed, however, because of the enteric coating, absorption is delayed by an hour when compared to DEPAKENE (valproic acid).

The bioavailability of both types of divalproex sodium tablets (EPIVAL and EPIVAL ER) is equivalent to that of DEPAKENE (valproic acid) capsules.

In patients previously receiving DEPAKENE (valproic acid) therapy, EPIVAL should be initiated at the same daily dosing schedule. After the patient is stabilized on EPIVAL, a dosing schedule of two or three times a day may be elected in selected patients. Changes in dosage administration of valproate or concomitant medications should be accompanied by increased monitoring of plasma concentrations of valproate and other medications, as well as the patient's clinical status.

Acute Mania: EPIVAL is not indicated for the treatment of the symptoms of mania in patients under 18 years of age.

The recommended initial dose is 250 mg three times a day. The dose should be increased as rapidly as possible to achieve the lowest therapeutic dose which produces the desired clinical effect or the desired range of plasma concentrations.

In placebo-controlled trials, 84% of patients received and tolerated maximum daily doses of between 1000 mg/day to 2500 mg/day. The maximum recommended dosage is 60 mg/kg/day.

The relationship of plasma concentration to clinical response has not been established for EPIVAL. In controlled clinical studies, 79% of patients achieved and tolerated serum valproate concentrations between 50 µg/mL and 125 µg/mL.

Missed Dose: The patient should not abruptly stop taking their medication because of the risk of increasing their seizures.

If the patient misses a dose, they should not try to make up for it by doubling up on their next dose. They should take their next regularly scheduled dose and try not to miss any more doses.

Administration: EPIVAL may be taken with or without food.

Patients who experience G.I. irritation may benefit from administration of the drug with food or by a progressive increase of the dose from the initial low level. The tablets should be swallowed without chewing. Co-administration of oral valproate products with food should cause no clinical problems in the management of patients with epilepsy.

OVERDOSAGE:

Overdosage with valproate may result in somnolence, heart block, and deep coma. Fatalities have been reported; however, patients have recovered from valproate levels as high as 2120 µg/mL.

In a reported case of overdosage with valproic acid after ingesting 36 g in combination with phenobarbital and phenytoin, the patient presented in deep coma. An EEG recorded diffuse slowing, compatible with the state of consciousness. The patient made an uneventful recovery.

In overdose situations, the fraction of drug not bound to protein is high and hemodialysis or tandem hemodialysis plus hemoperfusion may result in significant removal of drug. The benefit of gastric lavage or emesis will vary with the time since ingestion. General supportive measures should be applied with particular attention to the prevention of hypovolemia and the maintenance of adequate urinary output.

Naloxone has been reported to reverse the CNS depressant effects of valproic acid overdosage. Because naloxone could theoretically also reverse the antiepileptic effects of valproate, it should be used with caution in patients with epilepsy.

For management of a suspected drug overdose, contact your **regional Poison Control Centre**. See the *CPS* Directory section for a list of Poison Control Centres.

ACTION AND CLINICAL PHARMACOLOGY: Mechanism of Action: EPIVAL (divalproex sodium) has anticonvulsant properties, and is chemically related to valproic acid. Divalproex sodium dissociates to the valproate ion in the gastrointestinal tract. Although its mechanism of action has not yet been established, it has been suggested that its activity in epilepsy is related to increased brain concentrations of gamma-aminobutyric acid (GABA). The effect on the neuronal membrane is unknown.

Pharmacodynamics: A good correlation has not been established between daily dose, serum level and therapeutic effect. In epilepsy, the therapeutic plasma concentration range is believed to be from 50 to 100 µg/mL (350 to 700 micromole/L) of total valproate. Occasional patients may be controlled with serum levels lower or higher than this range (see Dosage and Administration). In placebo-controlled clinical studies in acute mania, 79% of patients were dosed to a plasma concentration between 50 µg/mL and 125 µg/mL. Protein binding of valproate is saturable ranging from 90% at 50 µg/mL to 82% at 125 µg/mL.

Pharmacokinetics: See Table 4.

Table 4: EPIVAL

Summary of the Pharmacokinetic Parameters of EPIVAL in Healthy, Fasting Subjects

Single Dose	Dosage	N	Mean (SD) Pharmacokinetic Parameters C_{max} (mg/L)	T_{max} (h)	$t_{½}$ (h)	AUC_{∞} (mg·h/L)	CL (L/h)	Vd (L)
EPIVAL	2×500 mg QD	28	93.9 (11.7)	4.0 (1.2)	15.2 (5.3)	1818 (345)	—	—

Absorption: Peak serum levels of valproic acid occur in 3 to 4 hours. A slight delay in absorption occurs when the drug is administered with meals but this does not affect the total absorption.

Distribution: Valproic acid is rapidly distributed throughout the body and the drug is strongly bound (90%) to human plasma proteins. Increases in doses may result in decreases in the extent of protein binding and variable changes in valproic acid clearance and elimination.

Protein Binding: The plasma protein binding of valproate is concentration dependent and the free fraction increases from approximately 10% at 40 µg/mL to 18.5% at 130 µg/mL. Protein binding of valproate is reduced in the elderly, in patients with chronic hepatic diseases, in patients with renal impairment, in hyperlipidemic patients, and in the presence of other drugs (e.g., acetylsalicylic acid). Conversely, valproate may displace certain protein-bound drugs (e.g., phenytoin, carbamazepine, warfarin, and tolbutamide) (see Drug Interactions for more detailed information on the pharmacokinetic interactions of valproate with other drugs).

CNS Distribution: Valproate concentrations in cerebrospinal fluid (CSF) approximate unbound concentrations in plasma (ranging from 7 to 25% of total concentration).

Metabolism: Valproate is metabolized almost entirely by the liver. In adult patients on monotherapy, 30-50% of an administered dose appears in urine as a glucuronide conjugate. Mitochondrial (beta)-oxidation is the other major metabolic pathway, typically accounting for over 40% of the dose. Usually, less than 15-20% of the dose is eliminated by other oxidative mechanisms. Less than 3% of an administered dose is excreted unchanged in urine.

Due to the saturable plasma protein binding, the relationship between dose and total valproate concentration is nonlinear; concentration does not increase proportionally with the dose, but rather increases to a lesser extent. The kinetics of unbound drug are linear.

Excretion: Mean plasma clearance and volume of distribution for total valproate are 0.56 L/hr/1.73 m^2 and 11 L/1.73 m^2, respectively. Mean plasma clearance and volume of distribution for free valproate are 4.6 L/hr/1.73 m^2 and 92 L/1.73 m^2, respectively. These estimates cited apply primarily to patients who are not taking drugs that affect hepatic metabolizing enzyme systems. For example, patients taking enzyme-inducing antiepileptic drugs (carbamazepine, phenytoin, and phenobarbital) will clear valproate more rapidly. Because of these changes in valproic acid clearance, monitoring of valproate and concomitant drug concentrations should be intensified whenever enzyme-inducing drugs are introduced or withdrawn.

Elimination of valproic acid and its metabolites occurs principally in the urine, with minor amounts in the feces and expired air. Very little unmetabolized parent drug is excreted in the urine.

The serum half-life ($t_{½}$) of valproic acid is typically in the range of 6 to 16 hours. Half-lives in the lower part of the above range are usually found in patients taking other drugs capable of hepatic enzyme induction.

Special Populations and Conditions: Neonates/Infants: Within the first two months of life, infants have a markedly decreased ability to eliminate valproate compared to children and adults. This is a result of reduced clearance (perhaps due to delay in development of glucuronosyltransferase and other enzyme systems involved in valproate elimination) as well as increased volume of distribution (in part due to decreased plasma protein binding). For example, in one study, the half-life in neonates under 10 days ranged from 10 to 67 hours, compared to a range of 7 to 13 hours in children greater than 2 months.

Pediatrics: Patients between 3 months and 10 years have 50% higher clearances expressed on weight (i.e., mL/min/kg) than do adults. Over the age of 10 years, children have pharmacokinetic parameters that approximate those of adults.

Geriatrics: The capacity of elderly patients (age range: 68 to 89 years) to eliminate valproate has been shown to be reduced compared to younger adults (age range: 22 to 26). Intrinsic clearance is reduced by 39%; the free fraction is increased by 44% (see Dosage and Administration).

Gender: There are no differences in unbound clearance (adjusted for body surface area) between males and females (4.8±0.17 and 4.7±0.07 L/hr per 1.73 m^2, respectively).

Race: The effects of race on the kinetics of valproate have not been studied.

Hepatic Insufficiency: See Contraindications, and Warnings and Precautions for statements regarding hepatic dysfunction and associated fatalities.

Renal Insufficiency: See Warnings and Precautions, Renal, Renal Impairment.

STORAGE AND STABILITY: Store EPIVAL tablets between 15 and 25°C. Tablets should be protected from light.

INFORMATION FOR THE PATIENT: Published in e-CPS, available by subscription at www.e-cps.ca.

DOSAGE FORMS, COMPOSITION AND PACKAGING: 125 mg: Each enteric-coated, salmon-pink tablet contains: divalproex sodium equivalent to valproic acid 125 mg. Nonmedicinal ingredients: cellulosic polymers, diacetylated monoglycerides, FD&C Red No. 40, povidone, pregelatinized starch (contains cornstarch), silicon dioxide, talc, titanium dioxide and vanillin. Alcohol-, gluten-, lactose-, paraben-, sucrose-, sulfite- and tartrazine-free. Bottles of 100.

250 mg: Each enteric-coated, peach-colored tablet contains: divalproex sodium equivalent to valproic acid 250 mg. Nonmedicinal ingredients: cellulosic polymers, diacetylated monoglycerides, FD&C Yellow No. 6, povidone, pregelatinized starch (contains cornstarch), silicon dioxide, talc, titanium dioxide and vanillin. Alcohol-, gluten-, lactose-, paraben-, sucrose-, sulfite- and tartrazine-free. Bottles of 100 and 500.

500 mg: Each enteric-coated, pink-colored tablet contains: divalproex sodium equivalent to valproic acid 500 mg. Nonmedicinal ingredients: cellulosic polymers, D&C Red No. 30, diacetylated monoglycerides, FD&C Blue No. 2, povidone, pregelatinized starch (contains cornstarch), silicon dioxide, talc, titanium dioxide and vanillin. Alcohol-, gluten-, lactose-, paraben-, sucrose-, sulfite- and tartrazine-free. Bottles of 100 and 500.

(Shown in Product Identification Section)

Eprex® Ⓟ

epoetin alfa

Erythropoiesis Regulating Hormone

Janssen-Ortho

Date of Preparation: February 16, 1990
Date of Revision: July 23, 2009

SUMMARY PRODUCT INFORMATION:

Route of Administration	Dosage Form: Sterile Colourless Solution/Strength	Clinically Relevant Nonmedicinal Ingredients
Polysorbate-80 Containing (Human Serum Albumin [HSA]-free formulation) Intravenous/Subcutaneous	**Single-use Pre-filled Syringe with PROTECS needle guard (Polysorbate-80 containing [HSA-free] formulation)** 1000 IU/0.5 mL, 2000 IU/0.5 mL, 3000 IU/0.3 mL, 4000 IU/0.4 mL, 5000 IU/0.5 mL, 6000 IU/0.6 mL, 8000 IU/0.8 mL, 10 000 IU/mL, 20 000 IU/0.5 mL, 30 000 IU/0.75 mL, 40 000 IU/mL	**Single-use Pre-filled Syringe with PROTECS needle guard** Glycine, polysorbate 80, sodium chloride, sodium phosphate monobasic dihydrate, sodium phosphate dibasic dihydrate, in water for injection.
HSA-containing Formulation Intravenous/Subcutaneous	**Multi-use Vial (HSA-containing formulation)** 20 000 IU/mL	**Multi-use Vial** albumin (human) (0.25%), sodium chloride, sodium citrate, citric acid, benzyl alcohol (0.9%) as a preservative, in water for injection.

DESCRIPTION: Erythropoietin is a glycoprotein which stimulates red blood cell production. It is produced in the kidney and stimulates the division and differentiation of committed erythroid progenitors in the bone marrow. EPREX epoetin alfa is a 165 amino acid glycoprotein manufactured by recombinant DNA technology. It has a molecular weight of 30 400 daltons and is produced by mammalian cells into which the human erythropoietin gene has been introduced. The product contains the identical amino acid sequence of isolated natural erythropoietin.

INDICATIONS AND CLINICAL USE: EPREX epoetin alfa is indicated to elevate or maintain the red blood cell level (as manifested by the hematocrit or hemoglobin determinations) and to decrease the need for transfusions. EPREX therapy is not intended for patients who require immediate correction of severe anemia. EPREX epoetin alfa may obviate the need for maintenance transfusions but is not a substitute for emergency transfusion. Blood pressure should be adequately controlled prior to initiation of EPREX therapy and must be closely monitored and controlled during treatment. EPREX therapy is not indicated for other specific causes of anemia with established treatments such as iron or folate deficiencies, hemolysis or gastrointestinal bleeding which should be managed appropriately.

Treatment of Anemia of Chronic Renal Failure: Adults: EPREX therapy is indicated in the treatment of anemia associated with chronic renal failure, including patients on dialysis (end-stage renal disease) and patients not on dialysis (see Dosage and Administration, CRF Patients). Non-dialysis patients with symptomatic anemia considered for therapy should have a hemoglobin less than 100 g/L.

Pediatrics: Epoetin alfa is indicated in infants and children from 1 month old up to 16 years of age for the treatment of anemia associated with CRF requiring dialysis. Safety and effectiveness in pediatric patients less than 1 month old have not been established (see Warnings and Precautions).

Treatment of Anemia in Zidovudine-treated/HIV-infected Patients: EPREX therapy is indicated for the treatment of transfusion-dependent anemia related to therapy with zidovudine in HIV-infected patients. EPREX epoetin alfa is effective in HIV-infected patients treated with zidovudine, when the endogenous serum erythropoietin level is ≤500 mU/mL and when patients are receiving a dose of zidovudine ≤4200 mg/week.

Treatment of Anemia Due to Chemotherapy in Patients with Non-myeloid Malignancies: EPREX is indicated for the treatment of anemia due to the effect of concomitantly administered chemotherapy based on studies that have shown a reduction in the need for RBC transfusions in patients with advanced or metastatic, non-myeloid malignancies receiving chemotherapy for a minimum of 2 months. Studies to determine whether EPREX increases mortality or decreases progression-free/recurrence-free survival are ongoing.

- In patients with a long life expectancy, the decision to administer ESAs should be based on a benefit-risk assessment with the participation of the individual patient. This should take into account the specific clinical context such as (but not limited to) the type of tumor and its stage, the degree of anemia, life expectancy, the environment in which the patient is being treated and known risks of transfusions and ESAs.
- If appropriate, red blood cell transfusion should be the preferred treatment for the management of anemia in patients with a long life expectancy and who are receiving myelosuppressive chemotherapy.
- EPREX is not indicated for use in patients receiving hormonal agents, therapeutic biologic products, or radiotherapy unless receiving concomitant myelosuppressive chemotherapy.

Surgery Patients: EPREX therapy is indicated in the following elective surgery regimens:

Use of EPREX epoetin alfa to Reduce Allogeneic Blood Exposure: EPREX therapy is indicated to treat patients who are undergoing major elective surgery (including patients who do not wish to or are not eligible to participate in an autologous blood donation program) and have a pretreatment hemoglobin of >100 to ≤130 g/L. EPREX therapy is indicated to reduce allogeneic blood transfusions and hasten erythroid recovery in these patients.

Combined Use of EPREX epoetin alfa and ABD: EPREX epoetin alfa is indicated to facilitate autologous blood collection within a predeposit program and may decrease the risk of receiving allogeneic blood transfusions in patients with hemoglobin of 100-130 g/L who are scheduled for major elective surgery and are expected to require more blood than that which can be obtained through autologous blood collection techniques in the absence of epoetin alfa.

Geriatrics (>65 years of age): No data available.

CONTRAINDICATIONS: EPREX epoetin alfa is contraindicated in patients:

- who develop pure red cell aplasia (PRCA) following treatment with any erythropoiesis regulating hormone (see Warnings and Precautions, All Patients, Immune);
- with uncontrolled hypertension;
- with known hypersensitivity to mammalian cell-derived products, albumin (human) or any component of the product (EPREX Sterile Solution is available in some formats, formulated without human serum albumin; see Dosage Forms, Composition and Packaging);
- who for any reason cannot receive adequate antithrombotic treatment.

In addition, the 20 000 IU/mL formulation, preserved with benzyl alcohol, is contraindicated in premature infants and newborns.

The use of EPREX epoetin alfa in patients scheduled for elective surgery and not participating in an autologous blood donation program is contraindicated in patients with severe coronary, peripheral arterial, carotid, or cerebral vascular disease, including patients with recent myocardial infarction or cerebral vascular accident.

Contraindications defined by the guidelines and methods of practice for ABD programs should be respected in patients receiving epoetin alfa.

WARNINGS AND PRECAUTIONS:

Serious Warnings and Precautions

All Patients:

- To minimize the risks for death and serious cardiovascular events, follow the recommended dosage for each indication for EPREX and other erythropoiesis stimulating agents (ESAs) (see Warnings and Precautions, Increased Mortality, Serious Cardiovascular and Thromboembolic Events and Dosage and Administration).
- In surgical patients treated with EPREX for reduction of allogeneic red blood cell transfusions, adequate antithrombotic prophylaxis, as per current standard of care, is recommended in order to reduce the incidence of deep venous thrombosis.
- The multi-use preserved formulation contains benzyl alcohol. Benzyl alcohol has been reported to be associated with an increased incidence of neurological and other complications in premature infants which are sometimes fatal.
- Patients with uncontrolled hypertension should not be treated with EPREX; blood pressure should be controlled adequately before initiation of therapy.
- EPREX should be used with caution in patients with a history of seizures.
- Antibody-mediated pure red cell aplasia (PRCA) has been reported after months to years of treatment with ESAs.

Chronic Renal Failure Patients:

- Patients experienced greater risks for death and serious cardiovascular events when administered ESAs to target higher versus lower hemoglobin levels (135 vs. 113 g/L; 140 vs.100 g/L) in two clinical studies. Individualize dosing to achieve and maintain hemoglobin levels within the range of 100 to 120 g/L.

Cancer Patients:

- ESAs increased the risks for death and serious cardiovascular and thromboembolic events in some controlled clinical trials.
- ESAs shortened overall survival and/or increased the risk of tumour progression or recurrence in some clinical studies in patients with breast, head and neck, lymphoid, cervical and non-small cell lung cancers when dosed to target a hemoglobin of ≥120 g/L.
- To minimize the above risks, use the lowest dose needed to avoid red blood cell (RBC) transfusions.
- Use ESAs only for treatment of anemia due to concomitant myelosuppressive chemotherapy.
- If appropriate, red blood cell transfusion should be the preferred treatment for the management of anemia in patients with a long life expectancy and who are receiving myelosuppressive chemotherapy.
- Discontinue EPREX following completion of a chemotherapy course.

All Patients: General: Creutzfeldt-Jakob Disease (CJD): Some formats of EPREX epoetin alfa contain albumin, a derivative of human blood. Because of careful donor screening and product manufacturing processes, the risk for transmission of viral diseases is extremely remote. The theoretical risk of transmission of Creutzfeldt-Jakob disease also is considered extremely remote. No cases of viral disease transmission or CJD have ever been identified as a result of albumin use.

Carcinogenicity and Mutagenicity: Long-term carcinogenicity studies have not been carried out. Epoetin alfa does not induce bacterial gene mutation (Ames Test), chromosomal aberrations in mammalian cells, micronuclei in mice, or gene mutation at the HGPRT locus.

Cardiovascular: Hypertension: Patients with uncontrolled hypertension should not be treated with EPREX epoetin alfa; blood pressure should be controlled adequately before initiation of therapy. Blood pressure may rise during EPREX therapy, often during the early phase of treatment when the hemoglobin is increasing, especially in CRF patients.

For patients who respond to EPREX therapy with a rapid increase in hemoglobin (e.g., more than 10 g/L in any two-week period), the dose of EPREX epoetin alfa should be reduced because of the possible association of excessive rate of rise of hemoglobin with an exacerbation of hypertension.

All patients on EPREX epoetin alfa should have hematocrit/hemoglobin levels measured at least once a week until a stable level is achieved and periodically thereafter.

In all patients receiving EPREX epoetin alfa, blood pressure should be closely monitored and controlled as necessary. Particular attention should be paid to the development of unusual headaches or an increase in headaches as a possible warning signal.

It may be necessary to initiate or increase antihypertensive treatment during EPREX therapy. If blood pressure cannot be controlled, EPREX epoetin alfa should be discontinued until blood pressure control is re-established. Hypertensive encephalopathy and seizures have been observed in patients with CRF treated with EPREX (see Adverse Reactions, All Patients, Hypertension).

Immune: Pure Red Cell Aplasia: Cases of pure red cell aplasia (PRCA) and of severe anemia, with or without other cytopenias, associated with neutralizing antibodies to erythropoietin have been reported in patients treated with EPREX. This has been reported predominantly in CRF patients receiving EPREX by subcutaneous administration. Any patient who develops a sudden loss of response to EPREX, accompanied by severe anemia and low reticulocyte count should be evaluated for the etiology of loss of effect, including the presence of neutralizing antibodies to erythropoietin. If anti-erythropoietin antibody-associated anemia is suspected, withhold EPREX and other erythropoietic proteins. Contact Janssen-Ortho Inc. at 1-800-567-3331 to perform assays for binding and neutralizing antibodies. EPREX should be permanently discontinued in patients with antibody-mediated anemia. Patients should not be switched to other erythropoietic proteins as antibodies may cross-react (see Adverse Reactions).

Increased Mortality, Serious Cardiovascular and Thromboembolic Events: During hemodialysis, patients treated with EPREX epoetin alfa may require increased anticoagulation with heparin to prevent clotting of the artificial kidney. Clotting of the vascular access (A-V fistula) has occurred at an annualized rate of about 0.25 events per patient-year on EPREX therapy. Overall, for patients with CRF (whether on dialysis or not), other thrombotic events (e.g., myocardial infarction, cerebrovascular accident, transient ischemic attack) have occurred at an annualized rate of less than 0.04 events per patient-year of EPREX therapy. Patients with pre-existing vascular disease should be monitored closely.

Patients with CRF experienced greater risks for death and serious cardiovascular events when administered ESAs to target higher versus lower hemoglobin levels (135 vs. 113 g/L; 140 vs. 100 g/L) in two clinical studies. Patients with CRF and an insufficient hemoglobin response to ESA therapy may be at even greater risk for cardiovascular events and mortality than other patients. EPREX and other ESAs increased the risks for death and for serious cardiovascular and thromboembolic events in controlled clinical trials of patients with cancer. These events included myocardial infarction, stroke, congestive heart failure and an increased risk of serious arterial and venous thromboembolic events including hemodialysis vascular access thrombosis. A rate of hemoglobin rise of >10 g/L over 2 weeks may contribute to these risks.

CRF patients with hypo-responsiveness to ESAs may be at an increased risk for mortality and cardiovascular events. These patients should be evaluated for treatable conditions (see Warnings and Precautions, Lack or Loss of Response and Dosage and Administration, CRF Patients). These risks should be carefully weighed against the benefit to be derived from treatment with ESAs, particularly in cancer patients with increased risk factors of thrombotic vascular events (TVEs), such as patients with a prior history of TVEs (e.g. deep venous thrombosis or pulmonary embolism) (see Dosage and Administration, CRF Patients, Cancer Patients Receiving Chemotherapy).

To minimize the risks for death and serious cardiovascular events, EPREX and other ESAs should follow the recommended dose for each indication. For CRF patients, individualize dosing to achieve and maintain hemoglobin levels within the recommended range of 100-120 g/L. For patients with cancer, use the lowest dose sufficient to avoid blood transfusions. The hemoglobin concentrations should not exceed 120 g/L; the rate of hemoglobin increase should not exceed 10 g/L in any 2-week period (see Dosage and Administration).

Hematologic: The safety and efficacy of EPREX therapy have not been established in patients with underlying hematologic disease (e.g., sickle cell anemia, myelodysplastic syndromes, or hypercoagulable disorders).

Neurologic: Seizures: EPREX epoetin alfa should be used with caution in patients with a history of seizures. Additional close monitoring of all possible risk factors is advisable if the decision is made to use EPREX epoetin alfa to treat patients with a history of seizures.

Given the potential for an increased risk of seizures in CRF patients during the first 90 days of therapy, blood pressure and the presence of premonitory neurologic symptoms should be monitored closely, and CRF patients should be cautioned to avoid potentially hazardous activities such as driving or operating heavy machinery during this period.

It is recommended that the dose of EPREX epoetin alfa be decreased if the hemoglobin increase exceeds 10 g/L in any two-week period.

The safety and efficacy of EPREX therapy have not been established in patients with a known history of a seizure disorder.

Sensitivity/Resistance: The parenteral administration of any biologic product should be attended by appropriate precautions in case allergic or other untoward reactions occur. If an anaphylactoid reaction occurs, EPREX epoetin alfa should be immediately discontinued and appropriate therapy initiated.

Hypersensitivity reactions, including cases of rash, urticaria, anaphylactic reaction, and angioneurotic edema have been reported.

Lack or Loss of Response: Inadequate response to EPREX epoetin alfa should prompt an investigation for causative factors. If the patient fails to respond or to maintain a response, the following etiologies should be considered and evaluated:

1. Iron deficiency: Virtually all patients will eventually require supplemental iron therapy (see Monitoring and Laboratory Tests, Iron Evaluation);
2. Underlying infectious, inflammatory, or malignant processes;
3. Occult blood loss;
4. Underlying hematologic diseases (i.e., thalassemia, refractory anemia, or other myelodysplastic disorders);
5. Vitamin deficiencies: folic acid or vitamin B_{12};
6. Hemolysis;
7. Aluminum intoxication;
8. Osteitis fibrosa cystica;
9. Inflammatory or traumatic episodes;
10. Pure Red Cell Aplasia (PRCA).

Special Populations: Use in Patients with Known Porphyria: Exacerbation of porphyria has been observed rarely in CRF patients treated with EPREX epoetin alfa. However, EPREX epoetin alfa has not caused an increased urinary excretion of porphyrin metabolites in normal volunteers, even in the presence of a rapid erythropoietic response. Nevertheless, EPREX epoetin alfa should be used with caution in patients with known porphyria.

Use in Patients with History of Gout: Increased serum uric acid (and phosphorus) levels have been observed in both normal volunteers and dialysis independent CRF patients treated with EPREX epoetin alfa who experienced a rapid rate of rise of hemoglobin. This effect may be related to an increased rate of nucleic acid synthesis in the bone marrow. Consequently, EPREX epoetin alfa should be administered with caution to patients with a history of gout.

Hepatic Dysfunction: The safety of EPREX epoetin alfa has not been established in patients with hepatic dysfunction.

Pregnant Women: Although epoetin alfa has been shown to have adverse effects in rats when given in doses greater than five times the human dose, it is not known whether it can affect reproduction capacity or cause fetal harm when administered to pregnant women. EPREX epoetin alfa should be given to a pregnant woman only if potential benefit justifies the potential risk to the fetus.

In some female chronic renal failure patients, menses have resumed following EPREX therapy; the possibility of potential pregnancy should be discussed and the need for contraception evaluated.

Nursing Women: It is not known whether EPREX epoetin alfa is excreted in human milk. Because many drugs are excreted in human milk, caution should be exercised when EPREX epoetin alfa is administered to a nursing woman.

Pediatrics: Pediatric Patients on Dialysis: Epoetin alfa is indicated in infants and children from 1 month old up to 16 years of age for the treatment of anemia associated with CRF requiring dialysis. Safety and effectiveness in pediatric patients less than 1 month old have not been established. The safety data from these studies show that there is no increased risk to pediatric CRF patients on dialysis when compared to the safety profile of epoetin alfa in adult CRF patients (see Adverse Reactions). Published literature provides supportive evidence of the safety and effectiveness of epoetin alfa in pediatric patients on dialysis.

Monitoring and Laboratory Tests: Hematology: All patients receiving EPREX epoetin alfa should have hematocrit/hemoglobin levels measured once a week until hematocrit/hemoglobin has been stabilized, and measured periodically thereafter (see Chronic Renal Failure Patients, Monitoring and Laboratory Tests, Hematology for additional laboratory monitoring in CRF patients).

There may be a moderate dose-dependent rise in the platelet count, within the normal range, during treatment with EPREX epoetin alfa. This regresses during the course of continued therapy. In addition, thrombocythemia above the normal range has been reported. The platelet count should be regularly monitored during the first eight weeks of therapy.

Iron Evaluation: In most chronic renal failure, cancer, and HIV-infected patients, the serum ferritin concentrations fall concomitantly with the rise in packed cell volume. Therefore, prior to and during EPREX therapy, the patient's iron stores, including transferrin saturation (serum iron divided by iron binding capacity) and serum ferritin, should be evaluated. Transferrin saturation should be at least 20%, and serum ferritin levels should be at least 100 ng/mL. Supplemental iron, e.g., oral elemental iron or intravenous iron, is recommended to increase and maintain transferrin saturation to levels that will adequately support EPREX epoetin alfa-stimulated erythropoiesis. All surgery patients being treated with EPREX epoetin alfa should receive adequate iron replacement throughout the course of therapy in order to support erythropoiesis and avoid depletion of iron stores (see Dosage and Administration).

Vitamin B_{12} and Folate Evaluation: Prior to starting EPREX therapy, the patient's serum vitamin B_{12} and serum folate should be assessed. A deficiency in vitamin B_{12} and/or folate may blunt the response and should be investigated as per standard clinical practice.

Chronic Renal Failure (CRF) Patients: General: Hemoglobin levels during treatment with ESAs should not exceed 120 g/L in both men and women. The dose of EPREX epoetin alfa should be reduced as the hemoglobin approaches 120 g/L or increases by more than 10 g/L in any 2-week period. Patients with CRF experienced greater risks for death and serious cardiovascular events when administered ESAs to target higher versus lower hemoglobin levels (135 vs. 113 g/L; 140 vs. 100 g/L) in two clinical studies. Individualize dosing to achieve and maintain hemoglobin levels within the range of 100 to 120 g/L (see Dosage and Administration).

Renal: Dialysis Management: Therapy with EPREX epoetin alfa results in an increase in hemoglobin and a decrease in plasma volume, which could potentially affect dialysis efficiency. In studies to date, the resulting increase in hemoglobin did not appear to adversely affect dialyzer function or the efficiency of high flux hemodialysis. During hemodialysis, chronic renal failure patients treated with EPREX epoetin alfa may require increased anticoagulation with heparin to prevent clotting of the artificial kidney.

Chronic renal failure patients who are marginally dialyzed may require adjustments in their dialysis prescription. As with all patients on dialysis, the serum chemistry values [including blood urea nitrogen (BUN), creatinine, phosphorus, and potassium] in patients treated with EPREX epoetin alfa should be monitored regularly to assure the adequacy of the dialysis prescription.

Diet: As the hemoglobin increases and patients experience an improved sense of well-being and quality of life, the importance of compliance with dietary and dialysis prescriptions should be reinforced. In particular, hyperkalemia is not uncommon in patients with CRF.

Predialysis Management: Blood pressure and hemoglobin should be monitored in predialysis patients no less frequently than for ESRD patients maintained on dialysis. Renal function and fluid and electrolyte balance should be closely monitored, as an improved sense of well-being may obscure the need to initiate dialysis in some patients.

Based on information to date, the use of EPREX epoetin alfa in predialysis patients does not accelerate the rate of progression of renal insufficiency.

Monitoring and Laboratory Tests: Hematology: Sufficient time should be allowed to determine a patient's responsiveness to a dosage of EPREX epoetin alfa before adjusting the dose. The hemoglobin should be determined weekly until it has stabilized in the recommended range and the maintenance dose has been established. After any dose adjustment, the hemoglobin should also be measured weekly for at least 2-6 weeks until it has been determined that the hemoglobin has stabilized in response to the dose change. The hemoglobin should then be monitored at regular intervals.

A complete blood count with differential and platelet count should be performed regularly. During clinical trials, modest increases were seen in platelets and white blood cell counts. While these changes were statistically significant, they were not clinically significant and the values remained within normal ranges.

In order to avoid reaching or exceeding the recommended hemoglobin range of 100-120 g/L too rapidly, the guidelines for dose and frequency of dose adjustments (see Dosage and Administration) should be followed.

The elevated bleeding time characteristic of chronic renal failure (CRF) decreases toward normal after correction of anemia in patients treated with EPREX epoetin alfa. Reduction of bleeding time also occurs after correction of anemia by transfusion.

Biochemistry: In patients with CRF, serum chemistry values [including blood urea nitrogen (BUN), uric acid, creatinine, phosphorus, and potassium] should be monitored regularly. During clinical trials in patients on dialysis, modest increases were seen in BUN, creatinine, phosphorus, and potassium. In some CRF patients not on dialysis who were treated with EPREX epoetin alfa, modest increases in serum uric acid and phosphorus were observed. While changes were statistically significant, the values remained within the ranges normally seen in patients with CRF.

In adult patients with CRF not on dialysis, renal function and fluid and electrolyte balance should be closely monitored, as an improved sense of well-being may obscure the need to initiate dialysis in some patients. In patients with CRF not on dialysis, placebo-controlled studies of the progression of renal dysfunction over periods of greater than one year have not been completed. In shorter-term trials in adult patients with CRF not on dialysis, changes in creatinine and creatinine clearance were not significantly different in patients treated with EPREX epoetin alfa, compared with placebo-treated patients. Analysis of the slope of 1/serum creatinine vs. time plots in these patients indicates no significant change in the slope after the initiation of EPREX therapy.

Surgery Patients: General: Combined Use of EPREX epoetin alfa and ABD: Warnings and precautions defined by the guidelines and methods of practice for ABD programs should be respected in patients receiving epoetin alfa.

Use of EPREX epoetin alfa to Reduce Allogeneic Blood Exposure: Thrombotic/Vascular Events: In patients scheduled for major elective orthopedic surgery, thrombotic events can be a risk and this possibility should be carefully weighed against the benefit to be derived from the treatment in this patient group. Patients scheduled for elective surgery should receive adequate antithrombotic prophylaxis as per current standard of care.

An increased incidence of deep vein thrombosis (DVT) was observed in patients receiving epoetin alfa who were undergoing spinal surgery and not receiving prophylactic anticoagulation. Patients should receive adequate antithrombotic prophylaxis in order to reduce the incidence of DVT.

In a randomized, placebo-controlled study of epoetin alfa in adult patients who were undergoing coronary artery bypass surgery and not participating in an autologous blood donation program, increased mortality was observed (7 deaths in 126 patients randomized to epoetin alfa versus no deaths among 56 patients receiving placebo). Among the seven deaths in the epoetin alfa-treated patients, three were related to intercurrent infectious episodes and four of these deaths occurred during the period of study drug administration. All four deaths were associated with thrombotic events and a causative role for epoetin alfa cannot be excluded.

Cardiovascular: Rarely, blood pressure may rise in the perioperative period in patients being treated with EPREX epoetin alfa. Therefore, blood pressure should be monitored.

Thrombotic/Vascular Events: Independent of EPREX treatment, thrombotic and vascular events may occur in surgical patients with underlying cardiovascular disease following repeated phlebotomy. Therefore, routine volume replacement should be performed in such patients in autologous blood donation programs.

Cancer Patients: Increased Mortality and/or Increased Risk of Tumour Progression or Recurrence: ESAs, when administered to target a hemoglobin of >120 g/L, shortened the time to tumour progression in patients with advanced head and neck cancer receiving radiation therapy. ESAs also shortened survival in patients with metastatic breast cancer and in patients with lymphoid malignancy receiving chemotherapy when administered to target a hemoglobin of ≥120 g/L.

In addition, ESAs shortened survival in patients with non-small cell lung cancer and in a study enrolling patients with various malignancies who were not receiving chemotherapy or radiotherapy; in these two studies, ESAs were administered to target a hemoglobin level of ≥120 g/L.

An increased risk of death was observed in a clinical study when ESAs were administered to target hemoglobin of 120 g/L in patients with active malignant disease not being treated with either chemotherapy or radiation therapy. EPREX is not indicated for use in cancer patients who have anemia that is not associated with chemotherapy.

In view of the above, where appropriate red blood cell transfusion should be the preferred treatment for the management of anemia in patients with cancer. The decision to administer ESAs should be based on a benefit-risk assessment with the participation of the individual patient. This should take into account the specific clinical context such as (but not limited to) the type of tumor and its stage, the degree of anemia, life-expectancy, the environment in which the patient is being treated, and known risks of transfusion and ESAs.

Neurologic: Seizures: In a placebo-controlled, double-blind trial utilizing once weekly dosing with epoetin alfa, 1.2% (n=2/168) of safety-evaluable patients treated with epoetin alfa and 0% (n=0/165) of placebo-treated patients had seizures. Seizures in the patients treated with weekly epoetin alfa occurred in the context of a significant increase in hemoglobin from baseline values but significant increases in blood pressure were not seen. Both patients may have had other CNS pathology which may have been related to the seizures.

ADVERSE REACTIONS: All Patients: Hypertension: The most frequent adverse reaction during treatment with EPREX epoetin alfa is a dose-dependent increase in blood pressure or aggravation of existing hypertension. This occurred most commonly in chronic renal failure patients (see Warnings and Precautions).

Hypertensive crises with encephalopathy and seizures have occurred in isolated patients, including previously normotensive patients.

Thrombotic/Vascular Events: Serious adverse drug reactions include venous and arterial thromboses and embolism (including some with fatal outcomes), such as deep venous thrombosis, arterial thrombosis, pulmonary emboli, aneurysms, retinal thrombosis, clotting of vascular access (A-V fistula) and shunt thrombosis (including dialysis equipment). Additionally, cerebrovascular accidents (including cerebral infarction and cerebral hemorrhage) and transient ischemic attacks have been reported in patients receiving epoetin alfa.

In clinical studies conducted in surgery patients with a pretreatment hemoglobin of >100 to ≤130 g/L (the recommended population) and not participating in an ABD program, the rate of deep venous thrombosis (DVT) was similar among patients treated with EPREX epoetin alfa and placebo. However, in patients with a pretreatment hemoglobin of >130 g/L, the rate of DVTs was higher in the group treated with EPREX epoetin alfa than in the placebo-treated group, but within the range of that reported in the literature for orthopedic surgery patients (47-74% without anticoagulant therapy and 3-37% with use of anticoagulant therapy).

In a study examining the use of EPREX epoetin alfa in 182 patients scheduled for coronary artery bypass graft surgery, 23% of patients treated with EPREX epoetin alfa and 29% treated with placebo experienced thrombotic/vascular events. There were four deaths among the patients treated with EPREX epoetin alfa that were associated with a thrombotic/vascular event and a causative role of EPREX epoetin alfa cannot be excluded.

Influenza-like Illness: Influenza-like illness including headaches, joint pains, myalgia and pyrexia may occur, especially at the start of treatment.

Hypersensitivity Reactions: Hypersensitivity reactions, including cases of rash, urticaria, angioneurotic edema and anaphylactic reaction have been reported.

Immune Reactions: In post-marketing reports, very rare cases of pure red cell aplasia (PRCA) have been reported, predominantly in chronic renal failure patients after months to years of treatment with recombinant erythropoietins including EPREX. Most of these reports have been associated with the subcutaneous route of administration. Cases have been rarely reported in patients with hepatitis C treated with interferon and ribavirin, when ESAs are used concomitantly. ESAs are not authorized in the management of anaemia associated with hepatitis C. Neutralizing antibodies to erythropoietins have been reported in most of these patients (see Warnings and Precautions, All Patients, Immune).

Seizures: Seizures have been reported in patients treated with EPREX epoetin alfa.

CRF Patients: Studies analyzed to date indicate that EPREX epoetin alfa is generally well tolerated irrespective of the route of administration. The adverse events reported are frequent sequelae of CRF and are not necessarily attributable to EPREX therapy. In double-blind, placebo-controlled studies involving 335 patients with CRF (both predialysis and treated with dialysis), the events reported in greater than 5% of patients treated with EPREX epoetin alfa (n=200) during the blinded phase were: see Table 1.

Table 1: EPREX

Adverse Events in CRF Patients

Adverse Events	EPREX epoetin alfa (n=200) %	Placebo (n=135) %
Hypertension	24.0	18.5
Headache	16.0	11.9
Arthralgias	11.0	5.9
Nausea	10.5	8.9
Edema	9.0	10.4
Fatigue	9.0	14.1
Diarrhea	8.5	5.9
Vomiting	8.0	5.2
Chest Pain	7.0	8.8
Skin Reaction at Administration Site	7.0	11.9
Asthenia	7.0	11.9
Dizziness	7.0	12.6
Clotted Access	6.8	2.3

Pediatric CRF Patients on Dialysis: Epoetin alfa is generally well tolerated in pediatric dialysis patients. The adverse events reported are typical sequelae for patients on dialysis, and relationship to epoetin alfa therapy has not been established. In double-blind clinical studies involving 123 pediatric dialysis patients, only one event, myalgia, occurred with a statistically significant higher frequency in patients treated with epoetin alfa (20%) than in placebo-treated patients (6%), p=0.03. Adverse events reported in greater than 5% of patients treated with epoetin alfa were: see Table 2.

Table 2: EPREX

Adverse Events Reported at >5% in Pediatric Patients

Adverse Events	Epoetin alfa (n=59) %	Placebo (n=64) %
Hypertension	25.4	17.2
Vomiting	22.0	21.9
Headache	22.0	29.7
Myalgia	20.3	6.3
Abdominal Pain	20.3	25.0
Access Infection	20.3	12.5
Peritonitis	16.9	14.1
Fever	13.6	15.6
Pruritus	11.9	3.1
Upper Respiratory Infection	11.9	14.1
Hyperkalemia	11.9	10.9
Nausea	11.9	12.5
Pharyngitis	10.2	7.8
Cough	10.2	9.4
Constipation	10.2	6.3
Chest Pain	10.2	3.1
Access Complication	10.2	6.3
Dizziness	8.5	10.9
Convulsions	8.5	6.3
Hypotension	8.5	14.1
Influenza-like Symptoms	8.5	6.3
Access Catheter Clotted	8.5	1.6
Thrombosis Vascular Access	6.8	1.6
Pneumonia	6.8	3.1
Increased Nonprotein Nitrogen	5.1	0.0
Arthralgia	5.1	3.1
Hyperphosphatemia	5.1	1.6
Otitis	5.1	1.6
Malaise	5.1	7.8

Adverse events reported at >5% in pediatric patients (see Table 2) that were not previously reported in adult patients include: myalgia, abdominal pain, access infection, peritonitis, fever, pruritus, upper respiratory infection, hyperkalemia, pharyngitis, cough, constipation, access complication, convulsions, hypotension, influenza-like symptoms, thrombosis vascular access, pneumonia, increased nonprotein nitrogen, hyperphosphatemia, otitis, malaise.

The following adverse experiences have been reported at an incidence greater than 1% and less than 5%. No adverse events were reported at an incidence of <1%.

Application Site: injection site reaction.

Body as a Whole: rigors, organ transplant rejection, dialysis complication, syncope, incisional pain, hot flushes, fatigue, edema peripheral, edema periorbital, edema circumoral, access pain, access erythema, access edema, access drainage, access cellulitis.

Cardiovascular: hypertension aggravated, cardiac failure.

CNS/PNS: vertigo, somnolence, paresthesia, migraine, encephalopathy hypertensive.

Endocrine Disorders: glucocorticoids increased.

Gastrointestinal: hemorrhage GI, increased saliva, gastroenteritis, gastrointestinal disorder, gastritis, flatulence, dyspepsia, diarrhea, anorexia.

Hearing/Vestibular: otitis media, earache.

Heart Rate/Rhythm: cardiac arrest.

Hematologic: thrombocythemia, lymphedema, ecchymosis.

Liver and Biliary: infectious hepatitis.

Metabolic/Nutrition: hypokalemia, hypocalcemia, hypercalcemia, ALT increased, hypertriglyceridemia.

Musculoskeletal: limb pain, back pain, skeletal pain, musculo-skeletal disorder, muscle weakness, arthrosis.

Myo/Endo/Pericardial: heart murmur, heart disorder.

Psychiatric Disorder: hallucination.

Reproductive: vaginitis (female), breast mass (male).

Resistance Mechanism: sepsis, infection, viral infection, fungal infection.

Respiratory: wheezing, upper respiratory tract congestion, sinusitis, epistaxis, dyspnea, bronchospasm, atelectasis.

Skin and Appendages: rash, dry skin, maculo-papular rash, folliculitis, erythema, cellulitis, acne.

Urinary Disorders: uremia, urinary tract infection, albuminuria.

Vascular Disorders: superior vena cava syndrome.

Vision Disorders: conjunctivitis, abnormal vision.

Zidovudine-treated/HIV-infected Patients: Adverse experiences reported in clinical trials with EPREX epoetin alfa in zidovudine-treated/HIV-infected patients were consistent with the progression of HIV infection. In double-blind, placebo-controlled studies of 3-month duration involving approximately 300 zidovudine-treated/HIV-infected patients, adverse experiences with an incidence of ≥10% in either patients treated with EPREX epoetin alfa (n=144) or placebo-treated patients were: see Table 3.

Table 3: EPREX

Adverse Events in Zidovudine-treated/HIV-infected Patients

Adverse Events	EPREX epoetin alfa (n=144) %	Placebo (n=153) %
Pyrexia	38	29
Fatigue	25	31

(cont'd)

Table 3: EPREX *(cont'd)*

Adverse Events in Zidovudine-treated/HIV-infected Patients

Adverse Events	EPREX epoetin alfa (n=144) %	Placebo (n=153) %
Headache	19	14
Cough	18	14
Diarrhea	16	18
Rash	16	8
Congestion, Respiratory	15	10
Nausea	15	12
Shortness of Breath	14	13
Asthenia	11	14
Skin Reaction at Administration Site	10	7
Dizziness	9	10

There were no statistically significant differences between treatment groups in the incidence of the above events.

EPREX epoetin alfa does not appear to potentiate progression of HIV disease as measured by: incidence of opportunistic infections; mortality; serum p24 antigen levels; or HIV replication in infected cell lines in vitro.

Cancer Patients: Adverse experiences reported in clinical trials with EPREX epoetin alfa administered thrice weekly in cancer patients were consistent with the underlying disease state. In double-blind, placebo-controlled studies of up to three months duration involving 413 cancer patients, adverse events with an incidence ≥10% in either patients treated with EPREX epoetin alfa or placebo-treated patients were: see Table 4.

Table 4: EPREX

Adverse Events in Cancer Patients

Adverse Events	EPREX epoetin alfa (n=213) %	Placebo (n=200) %
Nausea	23	29
Pyrexia	22	21
Asthenia	17	16
Fatigue	15	20
Vomiting	15	18
Diarrhea	15	9
Edema	14	8
Dizziness	10	9
Skin Reaction at Administration Site	10	10
Constipation	10	9
Shortness of Breath	8	15[a]
Decreased Appetite	8	12
Trunk Pain	8	12
Chills	7	10

[a] Significantly higher incidence for placebo patients (p=0.030).

There were no statistically significant differences in the percentage of patients treated with EPREX epoetin alfa reporting these adverse events compared to the corresponding incidence in placebo-treated patients, except for shortness of breath which occurred at a higher incidence in placebo-treated patients than in patients treated with EPREX epoetin alfa.

Thrombotic vascular events can occur in cancer patients as a consequence of their disease, comorbidities, and treatment. An increased incidence of thromboembolic events has been reported in cancer patients receiving ESAs, including epoetin alfa.

In a placebo-controlled, double-blind trial utilizing once-weekly (QW) dosing with epoetin alfa for up to 4 months involving 333 safety-evaluable cancer patients, adverse events were reported using the NCI Common Toxicity Criteria. Adverse events with an incidence >10% in either patients treated with epoetin alfa or placebo-treated patients were as indicated in Table 5. The safety profile of epoetin alfa administered QW was similar to placebo; adverse events in both groups appeared consistent with events expected in advanced cancer or associated with cancer treatment.

Table 5: EPREX

Percent of Patients in the Weekly Dosing Study Reporting Event

CTC Category Adverse Events (all grades)	Epoetin alfa (n=168) %	Placebo (n=165) %
Fatigue	51	52
Nausea	35	30
Alopecia	25	29
Neurosensory	23	23
Vomiting	20	16
Diarrhea-no colostomy	20	22
Anorexia	18	19
Constipation	18	22
Dyspnea	16	22
Pain	9	11
Anemia	8	13

Based on comparable survival data and on the percentage of patients treated with epoetin alfa QW and placebo-treated patients who discontinued therapy due to death (7% vs 5%), disease progression (7% vs 8%), or adverse experiences (1% vs 1%), the clinical outcome in patients treated with epoetin alfa and placebo-treated patients appeared to be similar.

Surgery Patients: Use of EPREX epoetin alfa to Reduce Allogeneic Blood Exposure: Adverse events were combined for all groups treated with EPREX epoetin alfa and the placebo-treated groups from four orthopedic surgery studies where subjects received EPREX epoetin alfa at a dose of 300 or 100 IU/kg daily, 600 IU/kg weekly, or placebo. Adverse events reported by at least 10% of subjects in any treatment group were: see Table 6.

Table 6: EPREX

Percent of Patients Reporting Event[a]

Adverse Event	300[b] or 100[c] IU/kg EPREX epoetin alfa (daily) (n=546) %	600[d] IU/kg EPREX epoetin alfa (weekly) (n=73) %	Placebo (n=250) %
Pyrexia	45	47	52
Skin Reaction, injection site	42	26	40
Nausea	37	45	34
Constipation	34	51	32
Vomiting	17	21	11
Skin Pain	17	5	19
Insomnia	14	21	11
Headache	13	10	9
Pruritus	12	14	10
Dizziness	10	11	9
Diarrhea	9	10	9
Urinary Tract Infection	8	11	10
Edema	8	11	8
Arthralgia	8	10	6
Urinary Retention	7	11	7
Confusion	5	12	6
Flatulence	4	10	4
Anxiety	3	11	6

[a] All patients participating in orthopedic surgery studies regardless of baseline hemoglobin.
[b] 300 IU/kg daily for either 5 or 10 days prior to surgery, on the day of surgery and either 3 or 4 days following surgery (either 9, 14 or 15 daily doses).
[c] 100 IU/kg daily for 10 days prior to surgery, on the day of surgery and 4 days following surgery (15 daily doses).
[d] 600 IU/kg once a week beginning 3 weeks prior to surgery and on the day of surgery (4 weekly doses).

Similar proportions of patients treated with EPREX epoetin alfa and placebo-treated patients reported each adverse event.

Combined Use of EPREX epoetin alfa and ABD: The incidence of adverse events was calculated across five double-blind, placebo-controlled studies and one single-blind study, combining all patients treated with EPREX epoetin alfa (n=402), regardless of dose administered, and all placebo patients (n=242). Adverse experiences with an incidence of ≥5% in either patients treated with EPREX epoetin alfa or placebo-treated patients were: see Table 7.

Table 7: EPREX

Adverse Events in Surgery Patients

Adverse Event	EPREX epoetin alfa (n=402) %	Placebo (n=242) %
Fatigue	18.41	19.01
Dizziness	12.19	13.64
Nausea	11.44	9.09
Headache	9.20	11.98

(cont'd)

Table 7: EPREX *(cont'd)*

Adverse Events in Surgery Patients

Adverse Event	EPREX epoetin alfa (n=402) %	Placebo (n=242) %
Asthenia	5.47	3.72
Diarrhea	3.48	7.02

In general, there were no notable differences between patients treated with EPREX epoetin alfa and placebo-treated patients in the incidence of any adverse event.

DRUG INTERACTIONS: Overview: No evidence exists that indicates that treatment with EPREX epoetin alfa alters the metabolism of other drugs. However, since cyclosporine is bound by red blood cells, there is potential for a drug interaction. If EPREX epoetin alfa is given concomitantly with cyclosporine, blood levels of cyclosporine should be monitored and the dose of cyclosporine adjusted as necessary.

Drug-Drug Interactions: Interactions with other drugs have not been established.

Drug-Food Interactions: Interactions with food have not been established.

Drug-Herb Interactions: Interactions with herbal products have not been established.

Drug-Laboratory Test Interactions: Interactions with laboratory tests have not been established.

DOSAGE AND ADMINISTRATION: Dosing Considerations: Important: See Warnings and Precautions, Serious Warnings and Precautions Box and Increased Mortality, Serious Cardiovascular and Thromboembolic Events. Follow the recommended dosage for each indication for EPREX.

EPREX may be given either as an IV or SC injection (see Recommended Dose and Dosage Adjustment, CRF Patients).

Self-administration and Information for the Patient: In those situations in which the physician determines that a patient can safely and effectively self-administer EPREX epoetin alfa injection, the patient should be instructed as to the proper dosage and administration. The first few doses should be administered under supervision. Following the initial laboratory and clinical assessment, all patients, including those deemed capable of self-administration, should be monitored for their response to EPREX epoetin alfa, their blood pressure and serum levels as indicated in Warnings and Precautions. Patients should be referred to Information for the Patient. It is not a disclosure of all possible effects. Patients should be informed of the signs and symptoms of allergic drug reaction and advised of appropriate actions.

If home use is prescribed, the patient should be thoroughly instructed in the importance of proper disposal and cautioned against the reuse of needles, syringes, or drug product. A puncture-resistant container for the disposal of used syringes and needles should be available to the patient. The full container should be disposed of according to the directions provided by the physician.

Recommended Dose and Dosage Adjustment: CRF Patients: The recommended dose to initiate therapy of EPREX epoetin alfa is 50 to 100 IU/kg three times per week (TIW) for adult patients. The recommended starting dose for pediatric CRF patients on dialysis is 50 IU/kg three times weekly (TIW). The dose of EPREX epoetin alfa should be reduced as the hemoglobin approaches 120 g/L or increases by more than 10 g/L in any 2-week period.

The dosage of EPREX epoetin alfa should be individualized to achieve and maintain the hemoglobin within the recommended range of 100-120 g/L. If hemoglobin excursions outside the recommended range occur, EPREX dose should be adjusted using the dosing recommendations below.

It should be recognized that subcutaneous administration of recombinant human proteins may increase the risk of immunogenicity. In patients on hemodialysis, the IV route is recommended.

When used intravenously, EPREX Sterile Solution usually has been administered as a slow IV bolus three times per week. While the administration of EPREX epoetin alfa is independent of the dialysis procedure, EPREX solution may be administered into the venous port at the end of the dialysis procedure to obviate the need for additional venous access. Following the change from intravenous to subcutaneous route of administration, the patient should be monitored carefully to ensure that the hemoglobin response is appropriate. Available data suggests that patients with a baseline hemoglobin <60 g/L may require higher maintenance doses than those with a baseline hemoglobin >80 g/L. EPREX therapy is not intended for patients who require immediate correction of severe anemia.

During therapy, hematological parameters should be monitored regularly.

Virtually all patients will eventually require supplemental iron to increase or maintain transferrin saturation to levels that will adequately support EPREX epoetin alfa-stimulated erythropoiesis.

Table 8 provides general therapeutic guidelines.

Table 8: EPREX

General Therapeutic Guidelines

Starting Dose	Reduce Dose When (starting with 25 IU/kg/dose decrement)	Increase Dose If (starting with 25 IU/kg/dose increment)	Maintenance Dose	Recommended Hb Range
Adults: 50-100 IU/kg three times per week IV or SC Pediatric patients: 50 IU/kg three times per week IV or SC	1) Hb approaches 120 g/L or 2) Hb increases >10 g/L in any 2-week period.	Hb does not increase by 10 g/L after 8-12 weeks of therapy, and Hb is below range.	Individually titrate.	100-120 g/L (and not to be exceeded)

In patients with chronic renal failure, maintenance hemoglobin concentration should not exceed 120 g/L.

Dose Adjustment: Following EPREX therapy, a period of time is required for erythroid progenitors to mature and be released into circulation resulting in an eventual increase in hemoglobin. Additionally, red blood cell survival time affects hemoglobin and may vary due to uremia. As a result, the time required to elicit a clinically significant change in hemoglobin (increase or decrease) following any dose adjustment may be 2-6 weeks.

Dose adjustment should not be made more frequently than once a month, unless clinically indicated. After any dose adjustment, the hemoglobin should be determined weekly for at least 2-6 weeks (see Warnings and Precautions, Chronic Renal Failure (CRF) Patients, Monitoring and Laboratory Tests).

- If the hemoglobin is increasing and approaching 120 g/L, the dose should be decreased by approximately 25 IU/kg three times per week. If the reduced dose does not stop the rise in hemoglobin, doses should be temporarily withheld until the hemoglobin begins to decrease, at which point therapy should be re-initiated at a lower dose.
- At any time, if the hemoglobin increases by more than 10 g/L in a two-week period, the dose should be immediately decreased. After the dose reduction, the hemoglobin should be monitored weekly for 2-6 weeks, and further dose adjustments should be made (see Maintenance Dose).
- If a hemoglobin increase of 10 g/L is not achieved after an eight-week period and iron stores are adequate (see Lack or Loss of Response), the dose of EPREX epoetin alfa may be increased in increments of 25 IU/kg three times per week. Further increases of 25 IU/kg three times per week may be added at 4-6 week intervals until the desired response is attained.

Maintenance Dose: The maintenance dose must be individualized for each chronic renal failure patient.

If the hemoglobin remains below, or falls below, the recommended range, iron stores should be re-evaluated. If the transferrin saturation is less than 20%, supplemental iron should be administered. If the transferrin saturation is greater than 20%, the dose of EPREX epoetin alfa may be increased by 25 IU/kg three times per week. Such dose increases should not be made more frequently than once a month, unless clinically indicated, as the response time of the hemoglobin to a dose increase can be 2-6 weeks. Hemoglobin should be measured for 2-6 weeks following dose increases.

Lack or Loss of Response: Over 95% of patients with chronic renal failure responded with clinically significant increases in hemoglobin; virtually all patients were transfusion-independent within approximately two months of initiation of EPREX therapy.

If a patient fails to respond or maintain a response, other etiologies should be considered and evaluated as clinically indicated (see Warnings and Precautions).

For patients whose hemoglobin does not attain a level within the range of 100 to 120 g/L despite the use of appropriate EPREX dose titrations over a 12-week period:

- do not administer higher EPREX doses and use the lowest dose that will maintain a hemoglobin level sufficient to avoid the need for recurrent RBC transfusions,
- evaluate and treat for other causes of anemia (see Warnings and Precautions, Lack or Loss of Response), and
- thereafter, hemoglobin should continue to be monitored and if responsiveness improves, EPREX dose adjustments should be made as described above; discontinue EPREX if responsiveness does not improve and the patient needs recurrent RBC transfusions.

Zidovudine-treated/HIV-infected Patients: Prior to beginning EPREX therapy, it is recommended that the endogenous serum erythropoietin level be determined (prior to transfusion). Available evidence suggests that patients receiving zidovudine with levels >500 mU/mL are unlikely to respond to therapy with EPREX epoetin alfa unless the dose of zidovudine is reduced or temporarily stopped.

Starting Dose: For patients with serum erythropoietin levels ≤500 mU/mL, the recommended starting dose of EPREX epoetin alfa is 100 IU/kg as an intravenous or subcutaneous injection three times weekly for eight weeks.

Increase Dose: During the dose adjustment phase of therapy, the hemoglobin should be monitored weekly. If the response is not satisfactory in terms of reducing transfusion requirements or increasing hemoglobin after eight weeks of therapy, the dose of EPREX epoetin alfa can be increased by 50-100 IU/kg three times per week. Response should be evaluated every 4-8 weeks thereafter and the dose adjusted accordingly by 50-100 IU/kg increments three times per week. If patients have not responded satisfactorily to an EPREX dose of 300 IU/kg three times per week up to month 12 of therapy, further continuation of treatment is not warranted as it is unlikely that they will respond to higher doses of EPREX epoetin alfa.

Maintenance Dose: After attainment of the desired response (i.e., reduced transfusion requirements or increased hemoglobin), the dose of EPREX epoetin alfa should be titrated to maintain the response based on factors such as variations in zidovudine dose and the presence of intercurrent infectious or inflammatory episodes. If the hemoglobin exceeds 120 g/L, the dose should be temporarily withheld until the hemoglobin falls below 120 g/L. Resume dosing at 25% less than the previous dose and titrate the dose to maintain the desired hemoglobin.

Hemoglobin Range: Maximum benefit from EPREX therapy appears to occur when the hemoglobin is maintained in the range of 120-130 g/L; however, the hemoglobin for zidovudine-treated/HIV-infected patients should not exceed 120 g/L.

Cancer Patients Receiving Chemotherapy: EPREX should not be initiated at hemoglobin levels ≥100 g/L. EPREX administration should be discontinued following completion of a chemotherapy course.

Starting Dose: Two EPREX dosing regimens may be used in adults: 150 IU/kg subcutaneously three times per week or 40 000 IU subcutaneously once per week.

Dose Adjustment: Three Times Per Week (TIW):

Starting Dose	150 IU/kg SC (TIW)
Increase dose to 300 IU/kg for four weeks	If the response is not satisfactory i.e., if after four weeks of therapy, no reduction in transfusion requirements or the hemoglobin has not increased by ≥10 g/L
Reduce dose by 25%	If the hemoglobin reaches a level needed to avoid transfusions or increases >10 g/L in any 2 week period
Withhold dose	If hemoglobin exceeds a level needed to avoid transfusions or exceeds 120 g/L. Restart dosing at 25% below the previous dose.
Discontinue	Discontinue EPREX if after 8 weeks of therapy there is no response as measured by increase hemoglobin levels or decrease need for RBC transfusions.

Once Per Week (QW):

Starting Dose	40 000 IU SC (QW)
Increase dose to 60 000 IU/week for four weeks	If the response is not satisfactory i.e., if after four weeks of therapy, no reduction in transfusion requirements or the hemoglobin has not increased by ≥10 g/L
Reduce dose by 25%	If the hemoglobin reaches a level needed to avoid transfusions or increases >10 g/L in any 2 week period
Withhold dose	If hemoglobin exceeds a level needed to avoid transfusions or exceeds 120 g/L. Restart dosing at 25% below the previous dose.
Discontinue	Discontinue EPREX if after 8 weeks of therapy there is no response as measured by increase hemoglobin levels or decrease need for RBC transfusions.

Endogenous Serum Erythropoietin Levels: In patients being treated with cyclic chemotherapy, there does not appear to be a significant relationship between the endogenous serum erythropoietin level and response to EPREX therapy.

Use of EPREX epoetin alfa is not recommended in patients with grossly elevated serum erythropoietin levels (e.g., >200 mU/mL).

Surgery Patients: Use of EPREX epoetin alfa to Reduce Allogeneic Blood Exposure: The recommended dose regimen is 600 IU/kg subcutaneously given once weekly for three weeks (Days -21, -14, and -7) prior to surgery and on the day of surgery.

If the period prior to surgery is less than three weeks, 300 IU/kg subcutaneously may be given as an alternative dosing regimen for 10 consecutive days prior to surgery, on the day of surgery, and for four consecutive days immediately thereafter.

All patients should receive adequate iron replacement. Iron replacement should be initiated no later than the beginning of treatment with EPREX epoetin alfa and should continue throughout the course of therapy.

Combined Use of EPREX epoetin alfa and ABD: EPREX epoetin alfa should be administered twice weekly for three weeks prior to surgery if the presurgical predonation interval permits. At each patient visit, a unit of blood is collected and stored for autologous transfusion if the patient has an acceptable hematocrit or hemoglobin for predonation.

The recommended dosage regimen is 600 IU/kg intravenously twice weekly.

Iron status should be evaluated for all patients prior to treatment with EPREX epoetin alfa. Iron deficiency, if present, should be corrected. To maintain erythropoiesis, adequate iron supplementation is required beginning as soon as possible and should continue throughout the course of therapy. In anemic patients, the cause of anemia should be explored before starting therapy with EPREX epoetin alfa.

Administration: Note: All strengths of EPREX Pre-filled Syringes now contain a "peelable" label on the barrel of the syringe. The peelable portion of the label should be removed from the syringe barrel and affixed to the patient's chart. The peelable label will be used to track Lot numbers and use of EPREX Pre-filled syringes.

1. **Do not shake.** Shaking may denature the glycoprotein, rendering it biologically inactive.
2. Parenteral drug products should be inspected visually for particulate matter and discoloration prior to administration. Do not use any vials or pre-filled syringes exhibiting particulate matter or discoloration.
3. Using aseptic techniques, attach a sterile needle to a sterile syringe. Remove the flip top from the vial containing EPREX Sterile Solution, and wipe the septum with a disinfectant. Insert the needle into the vial, and withdraw into the syringe an appropriate volume of solution.
4. **Intravenous Injection:** EPREX Sterile Solution should be administered over at least one to five minutes, depending on the total dose. While the administration of EPREX is independent of the dialysis procedure, EPREX may be administered into the venous line at the end of the dialysis procedure to obviate the need for additional venous access. A slower injection may be preferable in patients who develop flu-like symptoms.
5. **Subcutaneous Injection:** The maximum volume per injection site should be 1 mL. In case of larger volumes, more than one injection site should be used. The injections should be given in the limbs or the anterior abdominal wall. The patient should always alternate the site for each injection.
6. **Multi-use Vial:** Contains benzyl alcohol as a preservative and can be re-entered. The date of first entry into the vial should be recorded on the inside flap of the box. Discard 30 days after first entry.
7. **Pre-filled Syringe:** Contains no preservative. Discard unused portions.
8. Do not administer by intravenous infusion or mix with other drugs.
9. The multi-use vial contains 0.9% benzyl alcohol which acts as a local anesthetic and may ameliorate subcutaneous injection site discomfort.
10. The phosphate-buffered formulation has been found to mitigate injection site discomfort.

OVERDOSAGE:
The maximum amount of EPREX epoetin alfa that can be safely administered in single or multiple doses has not been determined. Doses of up to 1500 IU/kg three times per week for three to four weeks have been administered to adults without any direct toxic effects of EPREX epoetin alfa itself. Humans have received EPREX epoetin alfa doses as high as 3000 IU/kg in a single day without acute toxic effects.

EPREX therapy can result in polycythemia if the hemoglobin is not carefully monitored and the dose appropriately adjusted. If the recommended range is exceeded, EPREX therapy may be temporarily withheld until the hemoglobin returns to the recommended range; EPREX therapy may then be resumed using a lower dose (see Dosage and Administration). If polycythemia is of concern, phlebotomy may be indicated to decrease the hemoglobin to within acceptable ranges. Supportive care should be provided for hypertensive or convulsive events that may be related to overdosing with EPREX epoetin alfa.

> For management of a suspected drug overdose, CPhA recommends that you contact your **regional Poison Control Centre**. See the *CPS* Directory section for a list of Poison Control Centres.

ACTION AND CLINICAL PHARMACOLOGY: Mechanism of Action: Erythropoietin is a glycoprotein which stimulates red blood cell production. It is produced in the kidney and stimulates the division and differentiation of committed erythroid progenitors in the bone marrow.

Pharmacodynamics: CRF Patients: Erythropoietin is a glycoprotein which stimulates red blood cell production. Endogenous production of erythropoietin is normally regulated by the level of tissue oxygenation. Hypoxia and anemia generally increase the production of erythropoietin, which in turn stimulates erythropoiesis. In normal subjects, plasma erythropoietin levels range from 0.01 to 0.03 U/mL and increase up to 100 to 1000-fold during hypoxia or anemia. In contrast, in patients with chronic renal failure (CRF), production of erythropoietin is impaired, and this erythropoietin deficiency is the primary cause of their anemia.

EPREX epoetin alfa has been shown to stimulate erythropoiesis in anemic patients with CRF, including both patients on dialysis and those who do not require regular dialysis. The first evidence of a response to EPREX epoetin alfa is an increase in the reticulocyte count within 10 days, followed by increases in the red cell count, hemoglobin and hematocrit, usually within 2-6 weeks.

Because several days are required for erythroid progenitors to mature and be released into the circulation, a clinically significant increase in hematocrit is usually not observed in less than 2 weeks and may require up to 6 weeks in some patients. Once the hematocrit reaches the recommended range (30-36%), that level can be sustained by EPREX epoetin alfa in the absence of iron deficiency and concurrent illnesses.

The rate of hematocrit increase varies between patients and is dependent upon the dose of EPREX epoetin alfa, within a therapeutic range of approximately 50-300 IU/kg three times per week. Other factors affecting the rate and extent of response include availability of iron stores, the baseline hematocrit, and the presence of concurrent medical problems.

Intravenously administered EPREX epoetin alfa is eliminated at a rate consistent with first order kinetics with a circulating half-life ranging from approximately 4 to 13 hours in adult and 6.2 to 8.7 hours in pediatric patients with CRF. Within the therapeutic dose range, detectable levels of plasma erythropoietin are maintained for at least 24 hours. After subcutaneous administration of EPREX epoetin alfa to patients with CRF, peak serum levels are achieved within 5-24 hours after administration and decline slowly thereafter. In comparison with intravenous administration, subcutaneously administered EPREX epoetin alfa is more slowly absorbed and results in lower serum levels which are maintained for 48 hours. The estimated AUC_{0-48} for subcutaneous administration is approximately 15% of the AUC_{0-48} for the same dose given intravenously. Despite these differences, EPREX epoetin alfa exhibits a dose-related effect on hematological parameters which is independent of route. There is no apparent difference in half-life between adult patients not on dialysis whose serum creatinine levels were greater than 264 µmol/L (3 mg/dL), and adult patients maintained on dialysis. In normal volunteers, the half-life of intravenously administered EPREX Sterile Solution is approximately 20% shorter than the half-life in CRF patients.

The pharmacokinetic profile of EPREX epoetin alfa in children and adolescents appears to be similar to that of adults. Limited data are available in neonates.

Zidovudine-treated/HIV-infected Patients: Response to EPREX epoetin alfa in zidovudine-treated/HIV-infected patients is manifested by reduced transfusion requirements and increased hematocrit. Responsiveness to EPREX therapy in HIV-infected patients is dependent upon the endogenous serum erythropoietin levels prior to treatment. Zidovudine-treated/HIV-infected patients with endogenous serum erythropoietin levels ≤500 mU/mL respond to EPREX therapy. Patients with endogenous serum erythropoietin levels >500 mU/mL do not appear to respond to EPREX therapy. It appears likely that endogenous serum erythropoietin levels in HIV-infected patients receiving zidovudine are related to the severity of the zidovudine-induced damage to erythroid precursors in the bone marrow.

Cancer Patients: Anemia in cancer patients may be related to the effect of concomitantly administered chemotherapeutic agents. EPREX epoetin alfa administered three times a week (TIW) has been shown to increase hemoglobin and decrease transfusion requirements (after the first month of therapy) in anemic cancer patients. In addition, EPREX epoetin alfa administered once weekly (QW) has been shown to increase hemoglobin and decrease transfusion requirements after the first month of therapy (months 2, 3 and 4) in anemic cancer patients.

In a series of clinical trials enrolling 413 anemic cancer patients who received EPREX epoetin alfa TIW, 289 of whom were receiving cyclic chemotherapy, approximately 75 percent of the patients had endogenous serum erythropoietin levels ≤150 mU/mL, and approximately 5 percent of patients had endogenous serum erythropoietin levels >500 mU/mL. In patients who were being treated with cyclic chemotherapeutic regimens, there was not a statistically significant relationship between response to EPREX therapy and the prestudy endogenous serum erythropoietin level; however, treatment of patients with grossly elevated serum erythropoietin levels (e.g., >200 mU/mL) is not recommended.

In a Phase 1 PK/PD study comparing 150 IU/kg subcutaneous thrice weekly (TIW) dosing to 40 000 IU subcutaneous once weekly (QW) dosing in healthy subjects, the following parameters were estimated using data corrected for predose endogenous erythropoietin concentration during Week 4: mean C_{max} (SD) was 191 (100.1) and 785 (427.3) mIU/mL, respectively; mean (SD) C_{min} was 39 (17.9) and 13 (9.5) mIU/mL, respectively, and mean $t_{½}$ was 31.8 and 39.3 hours, respectively, after the 150 IU/kg TIW dosing (n=24) and 40 000 IU QW (n=22) dosing regimens were administered. Bioavailability of epoetin alfa after the 40 000 IU/week dosing regimen relative to the 150 IU/kg thrice weekly dosing regimen, based on AUC comparison, was 176%.

In another Phase 1 PK/PD study, pharmacokinetic parameters were estimated using data corrected for predose endogenous erythropoietin concentration comparing 150 IU/kg TIW and 40 000 IU QW dosing regimens in healthy subjects (n=6 per arm) and anemic cancer subjects (n=9 per arm). The respective mean (SD) parameters for the 150 IU/kg TIW and 40 000 IU QW regimens in healthy subjects were: C_{max} 163 (53.6) and 1036 (237.9) mIU/mL; C_{min} 29 (10.4) and 9.2 (5.71) mIU/mL; t_{max} 9.0 (3.29) and 21 (7.1) hours; $t_{½}$ 25.2 (6.76) [n=4] and 28.9 (7.98) hours, and CL/F 31.2 (11.48) and 12.6 (3.05) mL/h/kg. The respective mean (SD) parameters for the 150 IU/kg TIW and 40 000 IU QW regimens in the anemic cancer subjects were: C_{max} 263 (179.1) and 931 (596.9) mIU/mL; C_{min} 54 (41.8) and 34 (32.3) mIU/mL; t_{max} 8.3 (8.58) and 43 (16.0) hours; $t_{½}$ 29.9 (2.43) [n=4] and 22.9 (7.55) [n=7] hours and CL/F 45.8 (58.81) and 11.3 (6.45) mL/h/kg. It appeared that the pharmacokinetics of epoetin alfa in anemic cancer subjects were similar to those in healthy subjects.

However, the degree of variability associated with the pharmacokinetic parameters was higher in anemic cancer patients.

Pharmacodynamics: In a PK/PD study comparing the 150 IU/kg thrice weekly and 40 000 IU once weekly dosing regimens in healthy subjects (n=6 per arm) and in anemic cancer subjects (n=9 per arm), the time profiles of changes in percent reticulocytes, hemoglobin, and total red blood cells were similar between the two dosing regimens in both healthy and anemic cancer subjects. The AUCs of the respective pharmacodynamic parameters were similar between the 150 IU/kg TIW and 40 000 IU QW dosing regimens in healthy subjects and also in anemic cancer subjects, although the extent of increase in hemoglobin and RBC count was slightly lower in anemic cancer subjects than in healthy subjects (in terms of AUC of hemoglobin and RBC over the study period).

Surgery Patients: Use of EPREX epoetin alfa to Reduce Allogeneic Blood Exposure: Patients undergoing major elective surgery frequently require transfusion of allogeneic blood, both intraoperatively and postoperatively, resulting from blood loss experienced during and after surgery. In patients with a pretreatment hemoglobin of >100 to ≤130 g/L, EPREX epoetin alfa has been shown to decrease the risk of receiving allogeneic transfusions and hasten erythroid recovery (i.e., increased hemoglobin levels, hematocrit levels, and reticulocyte counts).

Combined Use of EPREX epoetin alfa and Autologous Blood Donation (ABD): EPREX epoetin alfa has been shown to stimulate red blood cell production in order to augment autologous blood collection, and to limit the decline in hematocrit in adult patients scheduled for major elective surgery who are not expected to predeposit their complete perioperative blood needs. The greatest effects are observed in patients with low hematocrit (≤39%).

Pharmacokinetics: Pharmacokinetics and Hematological Responses: Measurement of epoetin alfa following multiple dose intravenous administration revealed a half-life of approximately 4 hours in normal volunteers and a somewhat more prolonged half-life in renal failure patients, approximately 5 hours (ranging to 13 hours). Within the therapeutic dose range, detectable levels of plasma erythropoietin are maintained for at least 24 hours. There is no apparent difference in half-life between patients not on dialysis whose serum creatinine levels were greater than 264 µmol/L (3 mg/dL), and patients maintained on dialysis.

After subcutaneous administration of EPREX epoetin alfa to normal subjects, peak serum levels are achieved within 5-24 hours after administration. In comparison with intravenous administration, subcutaneously administered EPREX epoetin alfa is more slowly absorbed and results in lower serum levels which are maintained for 48 hours. In normal subjects, there was no significant epoetin alfa accumulation when administered under the clinical trial conditions. After multiple doses, similar blood levels were obtained after initial and subsequent injections in normal subjects. In these subjects, the half-life was estimated to be about 24 hours. The bioavailability of subcutaneous epoetin alfa is approximately 20% of that of the intravenously injected epoetin alfa. Despite these differences, EPREX epoetin alfa exhibits an injection-route independent, dose-related effect on hematological parameters.

In normal volunteers, C_{max} values for 40 000 IU once weekly determined in four-week studies were 6 times and $AUC_{(0-168\ h)}$ were 3 times that of the 150 IU/kg thrice weekly dosing regimen. Mean hemoglobin increases are similar with 3.1±0.86 and 3.1±0.84 g/dL for the 150 IU/kg thrice weekly and 40 000 IU once weekly, respectively. The time profiles of changes in hemoglobin and total red blood cells over the one-month study period were similar between the two dosing regimens.

However, statistically significant differences between genders for the AUC_{HEMO} and AUC_{RBC} pharmacodynamic response parameters at 40 000 IU once weekly dosing were noted. Clinical consequences of these differences were not studied as the normal volunteers were not scheduled subject to surgical procedures. When demographic data for the 40 000 IU once weekly and 150 IU/kg t.i.w. regimens were examined separately, or combined and stratified by gender, a significant difference in weight between males and females was detected in each treatment group. Dosing should be individualized on an IU/kg basis (see Dosage and Administration).

Special Populations and Conditions: Pediatrics: No data available.
Geriatrics: No data available.
Gender: No data available.
Race: No data available.
Hepatic Insufficiency: The safety of EPREX epoetin alfa has not been established in patients with hepatic dysfunction.
Renal Insufficiency: Based on information to date, the use of EPREX epoetin alfa in predialysis patients does not accelerate the rate of progression of renal insufficiency.

STORAGE AND STABILITY: Store at 2-8°C. Protect from exposure to light. **Do not freeze. Do not shake.** Multi-use vial should be discarded 30 days after first entry.

When the pre-filled syringe is about to be used, it may be removed from the refrigerator and stored at room temperature (not above 25°C) for one single period of maximum 7 days.

SPECIAL HANDLING INSTRUCTIONS: Store at 2-8°C. Protect from exposure to light. **Do Not Freeze. Do Not Shake.**

INFORMATION FOR THE PATIENT: Published in e-CPS, available by subscription at www.e-cps.ca.

DOSAGE FORMS, COMPOSITION AND PACKAGING: HSA-containing Formulation Multi-use Vials: Each mL of sterile solution contains: epoetin alfa 20 000 IU. Nonmedicinal ingredients: albumin (human) (0.25%) as stabilizer, benzyl alcohol (0.9%) as a preservative, citric acid, sodium chloride, sodium citrate and water for injection. Multi-Use vial (preserved, citrate-buffered) 20 000 IU/mL.

Polysorbate-80 Containing (HSA-free) Formulation Pre-filled Syringes with PROTECS Needle Guard: Each syringe of sterile solution contains: epoetin alfa 1000, 2000, 3000, 4000, 5000, 6000, 8000, 10 000, 20 000, 30 000 or 40 000 IU. Nonmedicinal ingredients: glycine and polysorbate 80 as stabilizers, sodium chloride, sodium phosphate dibasic dihydrate, sodium phosphate monobasic dihydrate and water for injection. Single-use pre-filled syringes (phosphate-buffered) of 1000 IU/0.5 mL, 2000 IU/0.5 mL, 3000 IU/0.3 mL, 4000 IU/0.4 mL, 5000 IU/0.5 mL, 6000 IU/0.6 mL, 8000 IU/0.8 mL, 10 000 IU/mL, 20 000 IU/0.5 mL, 30 000 IU/0.75 mL and 40 000 IU/mL.

To reduce the risk of accidental needle sticks to users, each pre-filled syringe is equipped with the PROTECS needle guard that is automatically activated to cover the needle after complete delivery of the syringe content.

(Shown in Product Identification Section)

Eraxis™ Ⓟ

anidulafungin

Antifungal Agent

Pfizer

Date of Preparation: November 14, 2007
Date of Revision: July 27, 2009

SUMMARY PRODUCT INFORMATION:

Route of Administration	Dosage Form/ Strength	Clinically Relevant Nonmedicinal Ingredients
Intravenous infusion	ERAXIS (anidulafungin powder with solvent): Each active vial contains anidulafungin 100 mg for reconstitution with the companion solvent (30 mL 20% w/w dehydrated alcohol in Water for Injection). The reconstituted solution contains 3.33 mg/mL anidulafungin and the 280 mL infusion solution contains 0.36 mg/mL anidulafungin.	Fructose, ethanol For a complete listing, see Dosage Forms, Composition and Packaging.
	ERAXIS (anidulafungin powder without solvent): Each active vial contains anidulafungin 100 mg for reconstitution with Water for Injection. The reconstituted solution contains 3.33 mg/mL anidulafungin and the 130 mL infusion solution contains 0.77 mg/mL anidulafungin.	Fructose For a complete listing, see Dosage Forms, Composition and Packaging.

INDICATIONS AND CLINICAL USE: ERAXIS (anidulafungin) is indicated for:

- treatment of invasive candidiasis/candidemia in adult non-neutropenic patients.

ERAXIS has not been studied in endocarditis, osteomyelitis, or meningitis due to Candida. Infections caused by *C. krusei* have not been studied. Neutropenic patients have not been studied in sufficient numbers to determine the efficacy of the drug in this group.

CONTRAINDICATIONS: ERAXIS is contraindicated to patients with known hypersensitivity to anidulafungin, any component of ERAXIS, or other echinocandins. For a complete listing see Dosage Forms, Composition and Packaging.

WARNINGS AND PRECAUTIONS: General: The infusion rate should not exceed the recommended infusion rate of 1.1 mg/minute. Infusion associated events are infrequent when the rate of anidulafungin infusion does not exceed 1.1 mg/minute.

Patients with rare hereditary problems of fructose intolerance should not take this medicine.

Carcinogenesis and Mutagenesis: No long-term studies in animals have been performed to evaluate the carcinogenic potential of anidulafungin.

Hepatic/Biliary/Pancreatic: Laboratory abnormalities in liver function tests have been seen in healthy subjects and patients treated with anidulafungin. In some patients with serious underlying medical conditions who were receiving multiple concomitant medications along with anidulafungin, clinically-significant hepatic abnormalities have occurred. Isolated cases of significant hepatic dysfunction, hepatitis, or worsening hepatic failure have been reported in patients; a causal relationship to anidulafungin has not been established. Patients who develop abnormal liver function tests during anidulafungin therapy should be monitored for evidence of worsening hepatic function and evaluated for risk/benefit of continuing anidulafungin therapy.

Special Populations: Pregnant Women: Animal studies have shown no selective reproductive toxicity. There are no adequate and well-controlled studies in pregnant women. Therefore, ERAXIS (anidulafungin) should be used during pregnancy only if the potential benefit justifies the risk to the fetus.

Nursing Women: Animal studies have shown excretion of anidulafungin in breast milk. It is not known whether anidulafungin is excreted in human breast milk. A decision on whether to continue/discontinue breast-feeding or to continue/discontinue therapy with anidulafungin should be made taking into account the benefit of breast-feeding to the child and the benefit of anidulafungin to the woman.

Pediatrics: The experience in children is limited. Use in patients under 18 years of age is not recommended until further data become available, unless the potential benefit justifies the risk (see Dosage and Administration and Action and Clinical Pharmacology, Pharmacokinetics).

ADVERSE REACTIONS: Adverse Drug Reaction Overview: Nine hundred and twenty-nine (929) patients received intravenous anidulafungin in clinical trials (672 in Phase 2/3 studies and 257 in Phase 1 studies). Of the 669 Phase 2/3 patients for whom safety data are available, 505 received anidulafungin for ≥14 days.

Three studies (one comparative vs fluconazole, two non-comparative) assessed the efficacy of anidulafungin (100 mg) in patients with candidemia and other deep tissue Candida infections. In these three studies, a total of 204 patients received anidulafungin, 119 for ≥14 days. Adverse events were typically mild to moderate and seldom led to discontinuation.

Infusion-related adverse events have been reported with anidulafungin, including rash, urticaria, flushing, pruritus, dyspnea, and hypotension. These events can be minimized by infusing anidulafungin at a rate that does not exceed 1.1 mg/minute.

Clinical Trial Adverse Drug Reactions: Because clinical trials are conducted under very specific conditions, the adverse reaction rates observed in the clinical trials may not reflect the rates observed in practice and should not be compared to the rates in the clinical trials of another drug. Adverse drug reaction information from clinical trials is useful for identifying drug-related adverse events and for approximating rates.

Table 1 presents drug-related adverse events (MedDRA) that were reported in ≥2.0% of subjects receiving ERAXIS or fluconazole therapy for candidemia/other Candida infections in the comparative study.

Table 1: ERAXIS

Drug-related[a] Adverse Events Reported in ≥2.0% of Subjects Receiving ERAXIS or Fluconazole Therapy for Candidemia/Other Candida Infections

Preferred Term	ERAXIS 100 mg[b] (N=131) n (%)	Fluconazole 400 mg[b] (N=125) n (%)
Subjects with at Least 1 Treatment-related AE	32 (24.4)	33 (26.4)
Gastrointestinal System		
Diarrhea	4 (3.1)	2 (1.6)
Investigations		
ALT ↑	3 (2.3)	4 (3.2)
AST ↑	1 (0.8)	3 (2.4)
Alkaline phosphatase ↑	2 (1.5)	5 (4.0)
Hepatic enzyme ↑	2 (1.5)	9 (7.2)
Metabolic and Nutritional Systems		
Hypokalemia	4 (3.1)	3 (2.4)
Vascular System		
Deep vein thrombosis	1 (0.8)	3 (2.4)

[a] Treatment-related AEs are defined as those that are possibly or probably related to study treatment, as determined by the investigator.
[b] Maintenance dose.

Less Common Clinical Trial Adverse Drug Reactions: The drug-related adverse events (MedDRA) listed below were reported with frequencies of ≤1.0% in patients receiving ERAXIS therapy for candidemia/other Candida infections in the comparative study (N=131).

Cardiac Disorders: atrial fibrillation, bundle branch block right, sinus arrhythmia, ventricular extrasystoles.
Eye Disorders: vision blurred, eye pain, visual disturbance.
Gastrointestinal Disorders: nausea, abdominal pain upper, fecal incontinence, loose stools.
Hepatobiliary Disorders: cholestasis.
Infections and Infestations: candidiasis, clostridial infection, oral candidiasis.
Investigations: AST ↑, blood amylase ↑, blood creatinine ↑, lipase ↑.
Metabolism and Nutrition Disorders: hyperkalemia, hypercalcemia, hypernatremia.
Nervous System Disorders: headache, convulsion.
Skin and Subcutaneous Tissue Disorders: rash, pruritus generalized, rash papular, urticaria.
Social Circumstances: early adult transition.
Vascular Disorders: deep vein thrombosis, hot flush, hypertension.
Abnormal Hematologic and Clinical Chemistry Findings: The following potentially clinically-significant changes from baseline in hematology values were reported in ≥2.0% of subjects receiving ERAXIS or fluconazole therapy for candidemia/other Candida infections in the comparative study. See Table 2.

Table 2: ERAXIS

Potentially Clinically-significant Changes from Baseline in Hematology Values in ≥2.0% of Subjects Receiving ERAXIS or Fluconazole Therapy for Candidemia/Other Candida Infections

Parameter (Criteria as fold change)	ERAXIS 100 mg[a] (N=131) n (%)			Fluconazole 400 mg[a] (N=125) n (%)		
	On-therapy	EIV	6w FU	On-therapy	EIV	6w FU
Bands	N=55	N=56	N=39	N=49	N=56	N=28
Increase (2.0)	2 (3.6)	2 (3.6)	0	2 (4.1)	3 (5.4)	2 (7.1)
Decrease (0.75)	3 (5.5)	2 (3.6)	3 (7.7)	4 (8.2)	1 (1.8)	1 (3.6)
Basophils	N=90	N=100	N=63	N=79	N=97	N=48
Increase (2.0)	0	0	0	0	0	1 (2.1)
Decrease (0.75)	3 (3.3)	1 (1.0)	0	0	0	0
Eosinophils	N=94	N=103	N=66	N=80	N=98	N=49
Increase (4.0)	3 (3.2)	3 (2.9)	5 (7.6)	7 (8.8)	4 (4.1)	3 (6.1)
Hematocrit	N=105	N=119	N=74	N=84	N=107	N=58
Increase (1.4)	6 (5.7)	2 (1.7)	5 (6.8)	2 (2.4)	4 (3.7)	1 (1.7)
Decrease (0.25)	7 (6.7)	3 (2.5)	5 (6.8)	5 (6.0)	2 (1.9)	2 (3.4)
Hemoglobin	N=105	N=119	N=74	N=85	N=107	N=58
Increase (1.4)	4 (3.8)	3 (2.5)	5 (6.8)	3 (3.5)	4 (3.7)	3 (5.2)
Decrease (0.25)	8 (7.6)	3 (2.5)	5 (6.8)	4 (4.7)	2 (1.9)	2 (3.4)
Lymphocytes	N=99	N=105	N=69	N=82	N=99	N=50
Increase (2.0)	27 (27.3)	22 (21.0)	17 (24.6)	19 (23.2)	20 (20.2)	7 (14.0)
Decrease (0.75)	4 (4.0)	3 (2.9)	0	2 (2.4)	6 (6.1)	0
Monocytes	N=98	N=105	N=67	N=82	N=99	N=50
Increase (2.0)	6 (6.1)	2 (1.9)	3 (4.5)	8 (9.8)	10 (10.1)	1 (2.0)
Decrease (0.75)	4 (4.1)	1 (1.0)	1 (1.5)	1 (1.2)	3 (3.0)	1 (2.0)
Neutrophils	N=99	N=105	N=68	N=82	N=99	N=50
Increase (2.0)	3 (3.0)	1 (1.0)	1 (1.5)	0	2 (2.0)	0
Decrease (0.75)	2 (2.0)	0	0	0	0	0
Platelet Count	N=105	N=119	N=74	N=84	N=107	N=57
Increase (2.0)	12 (11.4)	11 (9.2)	9 (12.2)	6 (7.1)	11 (10.3)	1 (1.8)
Decrease (0.4)	4 (3.8)	4 (3.4)	4 (5.4)	10 (11.9)	5 (4.7)	3 (5.3)
WBC	N=105	N=119	N=74	N=85	N=107	N=58
Increase (2.0)	13 (12.4)	9 (7.6)	2 (2.7)	5 (5.9)	9 (8.4)	4 (6.9)

[a] Maintenance dose.
Legend: EIV=End of IV Therapy; 6w FU=6 week follow-up visit.
Note: Post baseline potentially clinically-significant change values that are within normal range are not included.

The following potentially clinically-significant changes from baseline in chemistry values were reported in ≥2.0% of subjects receiving ERAXIS or fluconazole therapy for candidemia/other Candida infections in the comparative study. See Table 3.

Table 3: ERAXIS

Potentially Clinically-significant Changes from Baseline in Chemistry Values in ≥2.0% of Subjects Receiving ERAXIS or Fluconazole Therapy for Candidemia/Other Candida Infections

Parameter (Criteria as fold change)	ERAXIS 100 mg[a] (N=131) n (%)			Fluconazole 400 mg[a] (N=125) n (%)		
	On-therapy	EIV	6w FU	On-therapy	EIV	6w FU
Alkaline Phosphatase	N=88	N=86	N=61	N=80	N=85	N=48
Increase (2.0)	14 (15.9)	14 (16.3)	5 (8.2)	12 (15.0)	14 (16.5)	10 (20.8)
ALT	N=91	N=86	N=60	N=79	N=84	N=49
Increase (3.0)	5 (5.5)	5 (5.8)	2 (3.3)	2 (2.5)	6 (7.1)	3 (6.1)
AST	N=88	N=86	N=61	N=79	N=86	N=48
Increase (3.0)	4 (4.5)	1 (1.2)	1 (1.6)	2 (2.5)	7 (8.1)	4 (8.3)
BUN	N=98	N=108	N=65	N=83	N=106	N=55
Increase (3.0)	1 (1.0)	3 (2.8)	3 (4.6)	3 (3.6)	2 (1.9)	0
CO_2	N=95	N=108	N=61	N=79	N=98	N=51
Increase (1.3)	6 (6.3)	6 (5.6)	3 (4.9)	7 (8.9)	3 (3.1)	1 (2.0)
Creatinine	N=104	N=114	N=71	N=85	N=108	N=56
Increase (2.0)	3 (2.9)	4 (3.5)	3 (4.2)	2 (2.4)	2 (1.9)	1 (1.8)
Glucose	N=96	N=110	N=62	N=82	N=101	N=54
Increase (3.0)	1 (1.0)	0	2 (3.2)	1 (1.2)	2 (2.0)	2 (3.7)
Decrease (0.4)	6 (6.3)	7 (6.4)	2 (3.2)	6 (7.3)	5 (5.0)	0
Potassium	N=104	N=118	N=70	N=86	N=108	N=56
Increase (1.2)	3 (2.9)	6 (5.1)	1 (1.4)	7 (8.1)	6 (5.6)	2 (3.6)
Decrease (0.15)	14 (13.5)	8 (6.8)	3 (4.3)	12 (14.0)	7 (6.5)	3 (5.4)

(cont'd)

Table 3: ERAXIS *(cont'd)*

Potentially Clinically-significant Changes from Baseline in Chemistry Values in ≥2.0% of Subjects Receiving ERAXIS or Fluconazole Therapy for Candidemia/Other Candida Infections

Parameter (Criteria as fold change)	ERAXIS 100 mg[a] (N=131) n (%)			Fluconazole 400 mg[a] (N=125) n (%)		
	On-therapy	EIV	6w FU	On-therapy	EIV	6w FU
Sodium	**N=103**	**N=118**	**N=70**	**N=86**	**N=109**	**N=56**
Increase (1.1)	3 (2.9)	1 (0.8)	1 (1.4)	3 (3.5)	2 (1.8)	1 (1.8)
Decrease (0.1)	2 (1.9)	2 (1.7)	0	2 (2.3)	1 (0.9)	0
Total Bilirubin	**N=86**	**N=84**	**N=58**	**N=79**	**N=88**	**N=47**
Increase (3.0)	4 (4.7)	1 (1.2)	0	2 (2.5)	6 (6.8)	2 (4.3)

[a] Maintenance dose.
Legend: EIV=End of IV Therapy; 6w FU=6 week follow-up visit.
Note: Post baseline potentially clinically-significant change values that are within normal range are not included.

Post-Market Adverse Drug Reactions: The following adverse events have been reported during the post-approval period of ERAXIS. Because these reactions are reported voluntarily from populations of uncertain size, it is not always possible to reliably estimate their frequency. A causal relationship to ERAXIS could not be excluded for these adverse events. Adverse events were reported in the following SOC (system organ classes):

Metabolism and Nutrition Disorders (dehydration), Hepatobiliary Disorders (bile duct obstruction), General disorders and administration site conditions (injection site reaction). Nervous system disorders (cerebrovascular accident, convulsion), Blood and lymphatic system disorders (leucopenia), Investigations (Blood creatinine increased, blood urea increased, tacrolimus drug level decreased, hepatic enzyme increased, liver function test abnormal, white blood cell count decreased).

DRUG INTERACTIONS: Overview: Preclinical in vitro and in vivo studies and clinical studies have demonstrated that anidulafungin is not a clinically-relevant substrate, inducer or inhibitor of cytochrome P450 isoenzymes. Interaction studies have only been performed in adults. Anidulafungin has negligible renal clearance (<1%). Minimal interactions are expected with concomitant medications (see Action and Clinical Pharmacology, Pharmacokinetics).

In vitro studies showed that anidulafungin is not metabolized by human cytochrome P450 or by isolated human hepatocytes, and anidulafungin does not significantly inhibit the activities of human CYP isoforms (1A2, 2B6, 2C8, 2C9, 2C19, 2D6, 3A4) at clinically-relevant concentrations. Of note, these in vitro studies do not fully exclude possible in vivo interactions.

No clinically-relevant drug-drug interactions were observed with the following drugs likely to be co-administered with anidulafungin.

Drug-Drug Interactions: Drug interaction studies were performed with anidulafungin and other medicinal products likely to be co-administered (Table 4 and Table 5). Co-administration with cyclosporine increased the steady-state AUC of anidulafungin by 22%, and adverse events observed in the study were consistent with adverse events observed from other studies with the administration of anidulafungin alone. A separate in vitro study showed that anidulafungin has no effect on the metabolism of cyclosporine. No dosage adjustment of either drug is recommended when anidulafungin is co-administered with cyclosporine, voriconazole or tacrolimus.

Table 4: ERAXIS

Effect of Other Drugs on the Pharmacokinetic Parameters of Anidulafungin

Co-administered Drug	Dose of Co-administered Drug	Dose of Anidulafungin	N	Mean Ratio (90% CI) of Anidulafungin Pharmacokinetic Parameters with/without Co-administered Drug; No Effect=1.00		Clinical Comment
				C_{max}	AUC	
Cyclosporine	1.25 mg/kg PO BID×4 days	200 mg IV QD×1 day, then 100 mg IV QD×7 days	11	1.08[a]	1.22[a,b]	No dose adjustment required
Voriconazole	400 mg PO BID×1 day, then 200 mg PO BID×3 days	200 mg IV QD×1 day, then 100 mg IV QD×3 days	17	1.01 (0.97 to 1.04)	0.97 (0.95 to 1.00)	No dose adjustment required
Tacrolimus	5 mg PO single dose	200 mg IV QD×1 day, then 100 mg IV QD×9 days	35	1.03 (1.00 to 1.06)	1.07 (1.05 to 1.09)	No dose adjustment required

[a] 90% confidence interval not reported.
[b] Statistically significant (p<0.05).

Table 5: ERAXIS

Effect of Anidulafungin on the Pharmacokinetic Parameters of Other Drugs

Co-administered Drug	Dose of Co-administered Drug	Dose of Anidulafungin	N	Mean Ratio (90% CI) of Co-administered Drug Pharmacokinetic Parameters with/without Anidulafungin; No Effect=1.00		Clinical Comment
				C_{max}	AUC	
Voriconazole	400 mg PO BID ×1 day, then 200 mg PO BID×3 days	200 mg IV QD×1 day, then 100 mg IV QD×3 days	17	0.94 (0.89 to 0.98)	0.97 (0.92 to 1.03)	No dose adjustment required
Tacrolimus	5 mg PO single dose	200 mg IV QD×1 day, then 100 mg IV QD×9 days	35	0.99 (0.90 to 1.09)	1.02 (0.93 to 1.11)	No dose adjustment required

Other Medications: The pharmacokinetics of anidulafungin were examined in 27 patients that were co-administered with liposomal amphotericin B as well as in 27 patients that were co-administered with rifampin (potent CYP450 inducer). The population pharmacokinetic analysis suggested that when compared to data from patients that did not receive amphotericin B or rifampin, the pharmacokinetics of anidulafungin were not significantly altered by co-administration with amphotericin B or rifampin. No dose adjustment for anidulafungin is recommended when coadministered with amphotericin B or rifampin.

Population pharmacokinetic analysis has shown that the pharmacokinetic parameters of anidulafungin were not affected by the presence of concomitant medications which are known metabolic substrates, inhibitors or inducers of **cytochrome P450 isoenzymes.**

Population pharmacokinetic analysis also indicated that overall healthy subjects, HIV positive subjects, and HIV-positive patients with fungal infections appeared to have comparable exposure parameters.

Drug-Food Interactions: Not applicable since ERAXIS (anidulafungin) is a parenterally administered product.

Drug-Herb Interactions: Interactions with herbal products have not been established.

Drug-Laboratory Test Interactions: Interactions with laboratory tests have not been established.

DOSAGE AND ADMINISTRATION: Dosing Considerations: ERAXIS (anidulafungin powder with solvent): ERAXIS (anidulafungin) should be reconstituted with the companion solvent to a concentration of 3.33 mg/mL and subsequently diluted to a concentration of 0.36 mg/mL before use according to the instructions given in Reconstitution.

ERAXIS (anidulafungin powder without solvent): ERAXIS should be reconstituted with Water for Injection to a concentration of 3.33 mg/mL and subsequently diluted to a concentration of 0.77 mg/mL before use according to the instructions given in Reconstitution.

Recommended Dose and Dosage Adjustment: Specimens for fungal culture and other relevant laboratory studies (including histopathology) should be obtained prior to therapy to isolate and identify causative organism(s). Therapy may be instituted before the results of the cultures and other laboratory studies are known. However, once these results become available, antifungal therapy should be adjusted accordingly.

A single 200 mg loading dose should be administered on Day 1, followed by 100 mg daily thereafter. Duration of treatment should be based on the patient's clinical response. In general, antifungal therapy should continue for at least 14 days after the last positive culture.

Renal and Hepatic Impairment: No dosing adjustments are required for patients with mild, moderate or severe hepatic impairment. No dosing adjustments are required for patients with any degree of renal insufficiency, including those on dialysis. Anidulafungin can be given without regard to the timing of hemodialysis (see Action and Clinical Pharmacology, Special Populations and Conditions).

Other Special Populations: No dose adjustments are required for adult patients based on patient gender, ethnicity, HIV positivity, or geriatric status (see Action and Clinical Pharmacology, Special Populations and Conditions).

Children and Adolescents: The experience in children is limited. Use in patients under 18 years of age is not recommended until further data become available, unless the potential benefit justifies the risk (see Warnings and Precautions, Action and Clinical Pharmacology, Pharmacokinetics).

Administration: It is recommended that ERAXIS is administered at a maximum rate of infusion that does not exceed 1.1 mg/minute.

ERAXIS (anidulafungin powder with solvent): Reconstitution: Anidulafungin must be reconstituted with the companion solvent (20% (w/w) dehydrated alcohol in Water for Injection) and subsequently diluted with **only** 5% Dextrose Injection, USP or 0.9% Sodium Chloride Injection, USP (normal saline). The compatibility of reconstituted anidulafungin with intravenous substances, additives, or medications other than 5% Dextrose Injection, USP or 0.9% Sodium Chloride Injection, USP (normal saline) has not been established.

Aseptically reconstitute each vial with the companion diluent (20% (w/w) dehydrated alcohol in Water for Injection) to provide a concentration of 3.33 mg/mL.

The reconstituted solution should be stored at 15-30°C for 3 hours or at 5°C for 2 hours. Do not freeze. The reconstituted solution must be further diluted within an hour and administered within 24 hours.

Dilution and Infusion: Aseptically transfer the contents of the reconstituted vial(s) into an IV bag (or bottle) containing either 5% Dextrose Injection, USP or 0.9% Sodium Chloride Injection, USP (normal saline) obtaining an anidulafungin concentration of 0.36 mg/mL. Table 6 provides the volumes required for each dose.

Table 6: ERAXIS

Dilution Requirements for Anidulafungin Administration

Dose	Number of Kits	Total Reconstituted Volume	Infusion Volume[a]	Total Infusion Volume[b]	Rate of Infusion	Minimum Duration of Infusion
100 mg	1	30 mL (1 kit)	250 mL	280 mL	3.0 mL/min	90 min
200 mg	2	60 mL (2 kits)	500 mL	560 mL	3.0 mL/min	180 min

[a] Either Dextrose Injection, USP or 0.9% Sodium Chloride Injection, USP (normal saline).
[b] Infusion solution concentration is 0.36 mg/mL.

The rate of infusion should not exceed 1.1 mg/minute (equivalent to 3.0 mL/minute).

The infusion solution should be stored at 15-30°C. Do not refrigerate or freeze. For single use only.

ERAXIS (anidulafungin powder without solvent): Reconstitution: Anidulafungin must be reconstituted with Water for Injection and subsequently diluted with **only** 5% Dextrose Injection, USP or 0.9% Sodium Chloride Injection, USP (normal saline). The compatibility of reconstituted anidulafungin with intravenous substances, additives, or medications other than 5% Dextrose Injection, USP or 0.9% Sodium Chloride Injection, USP (normal saline) has not been established.

Aseptically reconstitute each vial with 30 mL Water for Injection to provide a concentration of 3.33 mg/mL.

If not used immediately, the reconstituted solution should be stored at 2-8°C for up to 1 hour. Do not freeze. The reconstituted solution must be further diluted within an hour.

Dilution and Infusion: Aseptically transfer the contents of the reconstituted vial(s) into an IV bag (or bottle) containing either 5% Dextrose Injection, USP or 0.9% Sodium Chloride Injection, USP (normal saline) obtaining an anidulafungin concentration of 0.77 mg/mL. Table 7 provides the volumes required for each dose.

Table 7: ERAXIS

Dilution Requirements for Anidulafungin Administration

Dose	Number of Vials Required	Total Reconstituted Volume	Infusion Volume[a]	Total Infusion Volume[b]	Rate of Infusion	Minimum Duration of Infusion
100 mg	1	30 mL	100 mL	130 mL	1.4 mL/min	90 min
200 mg	2	60 mL	200 mL	260 mL	1.4 mL/min	180 min

[a] Either Dextrose Injection, USP or 0.9% Sodium Chloride Injection, USP (normal saline).
[b] Infusion solution concentration is 0.77 mg/mL.

The rate of infusion should not exceed 1.1 mg/minute (equivalent to 1.4 mL/minute).

If the infusion solution is not used immediately, it should be stored at 2-8°C. The infusion solution must be administered within 24 hours. Do not freeze. For single use only.

Parenteral drug products should be inspected visually for particulate matter and discolouration prior to administration, whenever solution and container permit. If particulate matter or discolouration are identified, discard the solution.

For further information on storage and stability for the infusion and reconstituted solution, see Storage and Stability.

OVERDOSAGE:

As with any overdose, general supportive measures should be utilized as necessary.

During clinical trials a single 400 mg dose of anidulafungin was inadvertently administered as a loading dose. No clinical adverse events were reported. In a study of 10 healthy subjects administered a loading dose of 260 mg followed by 130 mg daily, anidulafungin was well tolerated with no dose limiting toxicity; 3 of the 10 subjects experienced transient, asymptomatic transaminase elevations (≤3×ULN).

Anidulafungin is not dialyzable.

The maximum non-lethal single dose of anidulafungin in rats was 50 mg/kg, a dose which is equivalent to 5 times the recommended daily dose in humans for Candidemia and other Candida infections [100 mg/day], based on the relative body surface area comparison.

> For management of a suspected drug overdose, contact your **regional Poison Control Centre**. See the *CPS* Directory section for a list of Poison Control Centres.

ACTION AND CLINICAL PHARMACOLOGY: Mechanism of Action: ERAXIS (anidulafungin) is a semi-synthetic echinocandin, a lipopeptide synthesized from a fermentation product of *A. nidulans*.

Pharmacodynamics: Anidulafungin selectively inhibits 1,3-β-D glucan synthase, an enzyme present in fungal, but not mammalian cells. This results in inhibition of the formation of 1,3-β-D-glucan, an essential component of the fungal cell wall. Anidulafungin has shown fungicidal activity against Candida species and activity against regions of active cell growth of the hyphae of *A. fumigatus*.

Anidulafungin has in vitro activity against various pathogenic fungi of the Aspergillus and Candida species.

Pharmacokinetics: The pharmacokinetics of anidulafungin following IV administration have been characterized in healthy subjects, special populations and patients. Systemic exposures of anidulafungin are dose-proportional and have low intersubject variability (coefficient of variation <25%) as shown in Table 8. The steady state was achieved on the first day after a loading dose (twice the daily maintenance dose).

Table 8: ERAXIS

Mean (% CV) Steady State Pharmacokinetic Parameters of Anidulafungin Following IV Administration of Anidulafungin Once Daily for 10 Days in Healthy Adult Subjects

	Anidulafungin IV Dosing Regimen (LD/MD, mg)[b]			
PK Parameter[a]	70/35[c,d] (N=6)	150/75 (N=9)	200/100 (N=10)	260/130[d,e] (N=10)
$C_{max,ss}$ [mg/L]	3.5 (13.2)	4.9 (20.3)	8.6 (16.2)	10.9 (11.7)
$C_{min,ss}$ [mg/L]	1.2 (12.6)	1.9 (5.7)	3.2 (21.6)	5.2 (12.6)
AUC_{ss} [mg·h/L]	42.3 (14.5)	65.5 (8.8)	111.8 (24.9)	168.9 (10.8)
CL [L/h]	0.84 (13.5)	1.2 (8.5)	0.94 (24.0)	0.78 (11.3)
$t_{½}$ [h]	43.2 (17.7)	51.2 (6.9)	52.0 (11.7)	50.3 (9.7)

[a] Parameters were obtained from separate studies.
[b] LD/MD: loading dose/maintenance dose once daily.
[c] Data were collected on Day 7.
[d] Safety and efficacy of these doses has not been established.
[e] See Overdosage.

Legend: $C_{max,ss}$=the steady state peak concentration; $C_{min,ss}$=the steady state trough concentration; AUC_{ss}=the steady state area under concentration vs. time curve; CL=clearance; $t_{½}$=the terminal elimination half-life.

The clearance and terminal elimination half-life of anidulafungin are about 1 L/h and 40-50 hours, respectively. Both of these pharmacokinetic parameters have been found to be independent of dosage. The pharmacokinetics of anidulafungin in patients with fungal infections are similar to those observed in healthy subjects (see Special Populations and Conditions, Patients with Fungal Infections).

Distribution: The pharmacokinetics of anidulafungin are characterized by a rapid distribution half-life (0.5-1 hour) and a volume of distribution of 30-50 L that is similar to total body fluid volume. Anidulafungin is extensively bound (>99%) to human plasma proteins.

Metabolism: Hepatic metabolism of anidulafungin has not been observed. Anidulafungin is not a clinically-relevant substrate, inducer, or inhibitor of cytochrome P450 isoenzymes. It is unlikely that anidulafungin will have clinically-relevant effects on the metabolism of drugs metabolized by cytochrome P450 isoenzymes.

Anidulafungin undergoes slow chemical degradation at physiologic temperature and pH to a ring-opened peptide that lacks antifungal activity. The in vitro degradation half-life of anidulafungin under physiologic conditions is approximately 24 hours. In vivo, the ring-opened product is subsequently converted to peptidic degradants and eliminated mainly through biliary excretion.

Excretion: In a single-dose clinical study, radiolabeled (^{14}C) anidulafungin (~88 mg) was administered to healthy subjects. Approximately 30% of the administered radioactive dose was eliminated in the feces over 9 days, of which less than 10% was intact drug. Less than 1% of the administered radioactive dose was excreted in the urine. Anidulafungin concentrations fell below the lower limits of quantitation 6 days post-dose. Negligible amounts of drug-derived radioactivity were recovered in blood, urine, and feces 8 weeks post-dose.

Linearity: Anidulafungin displays linear pharmacokinetics across a wide range of once daily doses (15-130 mg).

Special Populations and Conditions: Patients with Fungal Infections: Population pharmacokinetic analyses from four Phase 2/3 clinical studies including 107 males and 118 female patients with fungal infections showed that the pharmacokinetic parameters of anidulafungin are not affected by age, race, or the presence of concomitant medications which are known metabolic substrates, inhibitors or inducers of **cytochrome P450 isoenzymes**. The pharmacokinetics of anidulafungin in patients with fungal infections are similar to those observed in healthy subjects. The pharmacokinetic parameters of anidulafungin estimated using population pharmacokinetic modeling following IV administration of a maintenance dose of 50 mg/day or 100 mg/day (following a loading dose) are presented in Table 9.

Table 9: ERAXIS

Mean (% CV) Steady State Pharmacokinetic Parameters of Anidulafungin Following IV Administration of Anidulafungin in Patients with Fungal Infections Estimated Using Population Pharmacokinetic Modeling

	Anidulafungin IV Dosing Regimen (LD/MD, mg)[c]	
PK Parameter[a]	100/50	200/100
$C_{max,ss}$ [mg/L]	4.2 (22.4)	7.2 (23.3)
$C_{min,ss}$ [mg/L]	1.6 (42.1)	3.3 (41.8)
AUC_{ss} [mg·h/L]	55.2 (32.5)	110.3 (32.5)
CL [L/h]	1.0 (33.5)	
$t_{½,β}$ [h][b]	26.5 (28.5)	

[a] All the parameters were estimated by population modeling using a two-compartment model with first order elimination; AUC_{ss}, $C_{max,ss}$ and $C_{min,ss}$ (steady state trough plasma concentration) were estimated using individual PK parameters and infusion rate of 1 mg/min to administer recommended doses of 50 or 100 mg/day.
[b] $t_{1/2,β}$ is the predominant elimination half-life that characterizes the majority of the concentration-time profile.
[c] LD/MD: loading dose/maintenance dose.

Pediatrics: The pharmacokinetics of anidulafungin after daily doses were investigated in 24 immunocompromised pediatric (2 to 11 years old) and adolescent (12 to 17 years old) patients with neutropenia. The steady state was achieved on the first day after a loading dose (twice the maintenance dose), and the steady state C_{max} and AUC_{ss} increase in a dose-proportional manner. The systemic exposures following the daily maintenance doses of 0.75 and 1.5 mg/kg/day in patients aged 2 to 17 years old were comparable to those observed in adults following 50 and 100 mg/day, respectively.

Geriatrics: The population pharmacokinetic analysis showed that median clearance differed slightly between the elderly group (patients ≥65, median CL=1.07 L/h) and the non-elderly group (patients <65, median CL=1.22 L/h), however the range of clearance was similar.

Gender: Plasma concentrations of anidulafungin in healthy men and women were similar. In multiple-dose patient studies, drug clearance was slightly faster (approximately 22%) in men.

Ethnicity: Anidulafungin pharmacokinetics were similar among Caucasians, Blacks, Asians, and Hispanics.

HIV Positivity: Dosage adjustments are not required based on HIV status, irrespective of concomitant anti-retroviral therapy.

Hepatic Insufficiency: Anidulafungin is not hepatically metabolized. Anidulafungin pharmacokinetics were examined in subjects with Child-Pugh Class A, B or C hepatic insufficiency. Anidulafungin concentrations were not increased in subjects with any degree of hepatic insufficiency. Although slight decrease in AUC was observed in patients with Child-Pugh C hepatic insufficiency, the decrease was within the range of population estimates noted for healthy subjects.

Renal Insufficiency: Anidulafungin has negligible renal clearance (<1%). In a clinical study of subjects with mild, moderate, severe or end stage (dialysis-dependent) renal insufficiency, anidulafungin pharmacokinetics were similar to those observed in subjects with normal renal function. Anidulafungin is not dialyzable and may be administered without regard to the timing of hemodialysis.

STORAGE AND STABILITY: ERAXIS (anidulafungin powder with solvent): Unreconstituted Vials: Unreconstituted vials should be stored at room temperature 15-30°C.

Reconstituted Solution: The reconstituted solution should be further diluted within an hour. Chemical and physical in-use stability of the reconstituted solution has been demonstrated for 3 hours at 15-30°C and for 2 hours at 5°C. Do not freeze.

Infusion Solution: Chemical and physical in-use stability of the infusion solution has been demonstrated for 24 hours at 25°C. The infusion solution should be stored at 15-30°C. Do not refrigerate or freeze.

ERAXIS (anidulafungin powder without solvent): Unreconstituted Vials: Unreconstituted vials should be **stored at 2-8°C**. Do not freeze.

Reconstituted Solution: Reconstitute with water for injection. If not used immediately, the reconstituted solution should be stored at 2-8°C for up to 1 hour. Do not freeze. Chemical and physical in-use stability of the reconstituted solution has been demonstrated for 1 hour at 5°C.

Infusion Solution: The infusion solution should be stored at 2-8°C, and should be administered within 24 hours. Chemical and physical in-use stability of the infusion solution has been demonstrated for 24 hours at 5°C. Do not freeze.

SPECIAL HANDLING INSTRUCTIONS: Not applicable.

INFORMATION FOR THE PATIENT: Published in e-CPS, available by subscription at www.e-cps.ca.

DOSAGE FORMS, COMPOSITION AND PACKAGING: ERAXIS (anidulafungin powder with solvent): Kits containing 1 vial of 100 mg anidulafungin and 1 vial of 30 mL solvent. Powder: 100 mg anidulafungin lyophile in a 30 mL Type 1 glass vial with an elastomeric stopper and aluminium seal with flip-off cap. Nonmedicinal ingredients: fructose, mannitol, polysorbate 80, tartaric acid and sodium hydroxide and/or hydrochloric acid for pH adjustment. Solvent: 30 mL of 20 % (w/w) dehydrated alcohol in Water for Injection in a Type 1 glass vial with an elastomeric stopper and aluminium seal with flip-off cap.

ERAXIS (anidulafungin powder without solvent): Cartons containing 1 vial of 100 mg anidulafungin. Powder: 100 mg anidulafungin lyophile in a 30 mL Type 1 glass vial with an elastomeric stopper and aluminium seal with flip-off cap. Nonmedicinal ingredients: fructose, mannitol, polysorbate 80, tartaric acid and sodium hydroxide and/or hydrochloric acid for pH adjustment.

Erbitux™ Ⓟ

cetuximab

Antineoplastic

Bristol-Myers Squibb/ImClone LLC

Date of Revision: May 25, 2010

SUMMARY PRODUCT INFORMATION:

Route of Administration	Dosage Form/ Strength	Clinically Relevant Nonmedicinal Ingredients
Intravenous Injection	Injectable liquid Strength: 2 mg/mL, 100 mg cetuximab/50 mL single use vial	For nonmedicinal ingredients see Dosage Forms, Composition and Packaging.

DESCRIPTION: ERBITUX (cetuximab) is a recombinant, human/mouse chimeric monoclonal antibody that binds specifically to the extracellular domain of the human epidermal growth factor receptor (EGFR) with high affinity (Kd=0.2 nM). ERBITUX is genetically engineered by combining the Fv regions of a murine anti-EGFR antibody (M225) with human IgG1 heavy and kappa light chain constant regions. ERBITUX is composed of two identical heavy chains consisting of 449 amino acids each, and two identical light chains consisting of 214 amino acids each, and has an approximate molecular weight of 152 kDa.

INDICATIONS AND CLINICAL USE: Colorectal Cancer: ERBITUX (cetuximab), used in combination with irinotecan, is indicated for the treatment of EGFR-expressing metastatic colorectal carcinoma in patients who are refractory to other irinotecan-based chemotherapy regimens.

ERBITUX administered as a single agent is indicated for the treatment of EGFR-expressing, metastatic colorectal carcinoma in patients who are intolerant to irinotecan-based chemotherapy.

ERBITUX, as a single agent, is also indicated for the treatment of patients with EGFR-expressing metastatic colorectal carcinoma after failure of both irinotecan- and oxaliplatin-based regimens and who have received a fluoropyrimidine, whose tumours have a wild-type (non-mutated) Kirsten rat sarcoma (KRAS) gene. The benefit is based on overall survival in an analysis of patients whose tumours have a wild-type KRAS gene. In the same analysis, there was no treatment benefit with ERBITUX in patients whose tumours have KRAS mutations. Use of ERBITUX is not indicated for the treatment of colorectal cancer in patients with KRAS mutations.

Squamous Cell Carcinoma of the Head and Neck (SCCHN): ERBITUX (cetuximab) is indicated in combination with radiation therapy for the initial treatment of locally or regionally advanced squamous cell carcinoma of the head and neck.

Geriatrics (≥65 years of age): In clinical studies of advanced colorectal cancer, no overall differences in safety or efficacy were observed between patients who were 65 years of age or older and younger patients. Clinical studies of head and neck cancer did not include sufficient number of subjects aged 65 and over to determine whether they respond differently from younger subjects.

Pediatrics: The safety and effectiveness of ERBITUX in pediatric patients have not been established.

CONTRAINDICATIONS: ERBITUX (cetuximab) is contraindicated in patients with known severe hypersensitivity to cetuximab or any component of this product (see Warnings and Precautions).

WARNINGS AND PRECAUTIONS:

> **Serious Warnings and Precautions**
>
> **Infusion Reactions:** Severe infusion reactions occurred with the administration of ERBITUX in approximately 3% of patients in clinical trials, rarely with fatal outcome (<1 in 1000). Approximately 90% of severe infusion reactions were associated with the first infusion of ERBITUX. Severe infusion reactions are characterized by rapid onset of airway obstruction (bronchospasm, stridor, hoarseness), hypotension, shock, loss of consciousness, myocardial infarction and/or cardiac arrest. Fatal anaphylactic reactions may occur despite the use of prophylactic pre-medications. Severe infusion reactions require immediate interruption of the ERBITUX infusion and permanent discontinuation from further treatment (see Warnings and Precautions, Infusion Reactions; Adverse Reactions and Dosage and Administration).
>
> **Cardiopulmonary Arrest:** Cardiopulmonary arrest and/or sudden death occurred in 2% of 208 patients with squamous cell carcinoma of the head and neck treated with radiation therapy and ERBITUX. Carefully consider use of ERBITUX in combination with radiation therapy in head and neck cancer patients with a history of coronary artery disease, congestive heart failure, or arrhythmias, in light of these risks. Closely monitor serum electrolytes, including serum magnesium, potassium and calcium, during and after treatment with ERBITUX (see Warnings and Precautions, Cardiopulmonary Arrest).

Infusion Reactions: Severe, potentially fatal infusion reactions characterized by rapid onset of airway obstruction (bronchospasm, stridor, hoarseness), hypotension, shock, loss of consciousness, myocardial infarction, and/or cardiac arrest have occurred with the administration of ERBITUX (cetuximab).

In clinical studies, severe infusion reactions were observed in 2-5% of patients with fatal outcome in 1 patient (see Dosage and Administration, Dose Modifications).

Approximately 90% of severe infusion reactions were associated with the first infusion of ERBITUX despite the use of prophylactic antihistamines. However, caution must be exercised with every ERBITUX infusion, as there are patients who experienced their first severe infusion reaction during later infusions.

Severe infusion reactions require immediate interruption of the ERBITUX infusion and permanent discontinuation from further treatment. Appropriate physician supervision and supportive medical resources for the treatment of severe infusion reactions, anaphylaxis and cardiac arrest/myocardial infarction must be available. Monitor patients for 1 hour following ERBITUX infusions in a setting with resuscitation equipment and other agents necessary to treat anaphylaxis (e.g., epinephrine, parenteral corticosteroids, intravenous antihistamines, bronchodilators, vasopressors and oxygen). Longer observation periods may be required in patients who experience infusion reactions to confirm resolution of the event. Patients should be observed until all signs and symptoms have completely resolved (see Dosage and Administration, Dose Modifications).

Grade 1 and 2 infusion reactions including chills, fever, and dyspnea usually occurring on the first day of initial dosing, were observed in 13-19% of patients receiving ERBITUX in clinical trials.

In clinical trials, mild to moderate infusion reactions have been managed by slowing the infusion rate of ERBITUX and by employing prophylactic use of antihistamine medications for subsequent doses (see Dosage and Administration).

Cardiopulmonary Arrest: Cardiopulmonary arrest and/or sudden death occurred in 4 (2%) of 208 patients treated with radiation therapy and ERBITUX as compared to none of 212 patients treated with radiation therapy alone in a randomized, controlled ERBITUX trial in patients with SCCHN. Three patients with prior history of coronary artery disease died at home, with myocardial infarction as the presumed cause of death. One of these patients had arrhythmia and one had congestive heart failure. Death occurred 27, 32, and 43 days after the last dose of ERBITUX. One patient with no prior history of coronary artery disease died one day after the last dose of ERBITUX. Carefully consider use of ERBITUX in combination with radiation therapy in head and neck cancer patients with a history of coronary artery disease, congestive heart failure, or arrhythmias in light of these risks. Closely monitor serum electrolytes, including serum magnesium, potassium, and calcium, during and after treatment with ERBITUX (see Warnings and Precautions, Monitoring and Laboratory Tests).

Pulmonary Toxicity: Interstitial lung disease (ILD), including 1 fatality, occurred in 4 (<0.5%) patients receiving ERBITUX in clinical trials. In the events of acute onset or worsening pulmonary symptoms, ERBITUX therapy should be interrupted and a prompt investigation of these symptoms should occur. If ILD is confirmed, ERBITUX should be discontinued and the patient should be treated appropriately.

Carcinogenesis and Mutagenesis, Impairment of Fertility: Long-term animal studies have not been performed to test ERBITUX for the carcinogenic potential or potential to impair fertility. No mutagenic or clastogenic potential of ERBITUX was observed in the Salmonella-*E. coli* (AMES) assay or in the in vivo rat micronucleus test. It is not known if ERBITUX can impair fertility in humans.

Immunogenicity: As with all therapeutic proteins, there is potential for immunogenicity. The incidence of antibodies to ERBITUX was measured by collecting and analysing serum pre-study, prior to selected infusions and during treatment follow-up. Although the data are limited, there does not appear to be any relationship between the appearance of antibodies to ERBITUX and the safety or antitumor activity of the molecule.

The observed incidence of anti-ERBITUX antibody responses may be influenced by the low sensitivity of available assays, sample handling, timing of sample collection, concomitant medications and underlying disease. For these reasons, comparison of the incidence of antibodies to ERBITUX with the incidence of antibodies to other products may be misleading.

Dermatologic Toxicity: Dermatologic toxicities, including acneiform rash, skin drying and fissuring, paronychial inflammation, and infectious sequelae (e.g., *S. aureus* sepsis, abscess formation, blepharitis, conjunctivitis, keratitis, cheillitis, cellulitis) and hypertrichosis, have occurred in patients receiving ERBITUX. Acneiform rash occurred in 76-88% of patients receiving ERBITUX in clinical trials. Severe acneiform rash occurred in 1-17% of patients.

Acneiform rash usually developed within the first two weeks of therapy and resolved in a majority of the patients after cessation of treatment, although in nearly half, the event continued beyond 28 days.

Patients developing dermatologic toxicities while receiving ERBITUX should be monitored for the development of inflammatory or infectious sequelae, and appropriate treatment of these symptoms initiated.

Dose modifications of any future ERBITUX infusions should be instituted in case of severe acneiform rash (see Dosage and Administration, Dose Modifications). Instruct patients to limit sun exposure during treatment with ERBITUX and for 2 months following the last dose of ERBITUX.

Use of ERBITUX in Combination with Radiation and Cisplatin: The safety of ERBITUX in combination with radiation therapy and cisplatin has not been established. Death and serious cardiotoxicity were observed in a single-arm trial with ERBITUX, radiation therapy, and cisplatin (100 mg/m²) in patients with locally advanced SCCHN. Two of 21 patients died, one as a result of pneumonia and one of an unknown cause. Four patients discontinued treatment due to adverse events. Two of these discontinuations were due to cardiac events.

Special Populations: Pregnant Women: Animal data do not suggest a teratogenic effect. However an increased incidence of abortions was observed in monkeys administered doses 1.6 to 4 times greater than human exposure. There are no adequate and well controlled studies of ERBITUX in pregnant women. It is also not known whether ERBITUX can cause foetal harm when administered to a pregnant woman or whether ERBITUX can affect reproduction capacity. IgG molecules are known to cross the placental barrier; therefore ERBITUX may be transmitted from the mother to the developing foetus. Based on animal models, EGFR has been implicated in the control of prenatal development, may be essential for normal organogenesis, and may play a role in proliferation and differentiation in the developing embryo. Therefore, ERBITUX should not be given to a pregnant woman or any woman not employing adequate contraception unless the potential benefit justifies the potential risk to the foetus. If the patient becomes pregnant while receiving this drug, she should be apprised of the potential hazard to the foetus and/or the potential risk for loss of the pregnancy.

Nursing Women: It is not known whether ERBITUX is excreted in human milk. Because human IgG is excreted in human milk, and the potential for absorption and harm to the infant is unknown, women should be advised to discontinue nursing during treatment with ERBITUX and based on the mean half-life, for a minimum of 60 days after the last dose of ERBITUX.

Pediatrics: The safety and effectiveness of ERBITUX in pediatric patients have not been established.

Geriatrics: Of the total number of patients who received ERBITUX with irinotecan or ERBITUX monotherapy in five studies of advanced colorectal cancer, 363 patients were 65 years of age or older. No overall differences in safety or efficacy were observed between these patients and younger patients.

Clinical studies of ERBITUX conducted in patients with head and neck cancer did not include sufficient number of subjects aged 65 and over to determine whether they respond differently from younger subjects. Of the 208 patients with head and neck cancer who received ERBITUX with radiation therapy, 45 patients were 65 years of age or older.

Monitoring and Laboratory Tests: In patients evaluated during clinical trials, hypomagnesemia occurred in 55% of patients receiving ERBITUX and was severe (NCI-CTC Grade 3 and 4) in 6-17%. The onset of hypomagnesemia and accompanying electrolyte abnormalities occurred days to months after initiation of ERBITUX.

Patients should be monitored for hypomagnesemia, and accompanying hypocalcemia and hypokalemia, before and periodically during and following the completion of ERBITUX therapy. Monitoring should continue for a period of time commensurate with the half-life and persistence of the product; i.e. at least 8 weeks following the completion of ERBITUX therapy. Replenish electrolytes as necessary (see Adverse Reactions, Abnormal Hematologic and Clinical Chemistry Findings).

KRAS Testing: Assessment of KRAS mutation status should be performed by an experienced laboratory using a validated test method.

ADVERSE REACTIONS: Adverse Drug Reaction Overview: Across all studies, the most common adverse reactions with ERBITUX (incidence ≥25%) are cutaneous adverse reactions (including rash, pruritus, and nail changes), headache, diarrhea, and infection.

The most serious adverse reactions with ERBITUX are infusion reactions, cardiopulmonary arrest, dermatologic toxicity and radiation dermatitis, sepsis, renal failure, interstitial lung disease, and pulmonary embolus.

Across all studies, ERBITUX was discontinued in 3-10% of patients because of adverse reactions.

Infusion reactions, which included pyrexia, chills, rigors, dyspnea, bronchospasm, angioedema, urticaria, hypertension, and hypotension occurred in 15-21% of patients across studies. Grades 3 and 4 infusion reactions occurred in 2-5% of patients; infusion reactions were fatal in 1 patient.

The incidence of infection was variable across studies, ranging from 13-35%. Sepsis occurred in 1-4% of patients.

Renal failure occurred in 1% of patients with colorectal cancer.

Clinical Trial Adverse Drug Reactions: Because clinical trials are conducted under very specific conditions the adverse reaction rates observed in the clinical trials may not reflect the rates observed in practice and should not be compared to the rates in the clinical trials of another drug. Adverse drug reaction information from clinical trials is useful for identifying drug-related adverse events and for approximating rates.

Infusion Reactions: In clinical trials, severe, potentially fatal infusion reactions were reported. These events include the rapid onset of airway obstruction (bronchospasm, stridor, hoarseness), hypotension, loss of consciousness, and/or cardiac arrest. In clinical studies, severe (NCI CTC Grades 3 and 4) infusion reactions were observed in 2-5% of patients rarely with fatal outcome (<1 in 1000) (see Warnings and Precautions and Dosage and Administration, Dose Modifications). Approximately 90% of severe infusion reactions were associated with the first infusion of ERBITUX despite the use of prophylactic antihistamines. Grade 1 and 2 infusion reactions including chills, fever, and dyspnea usually occurring on the first day of initial dosing, were observed in 13-19% of patients receiving ERBITUX in clinical trials.

Dermatologic Toxicity and Related Disorders: Dermatologic toxicities, including acneiform rash, skin drying and fissuring, paronychial inflammation, and infectious sequelae (e.g., *S. aureus* sepsis, abscess formation, blepharitis, cheilitis, cellulitis) and hypertrichosis have occurred in patients receiving ERBITUX. Acneiform rash occurred in 76-88% of patients receiving ERBITUX in clinical trials. Severe acneiform rash occurred in 1-17% of patients.

Acneiform rash usually developed within the first two weeks of therapy and resolved in a majority of the patients after cessation of treatment, although in nearly half, the event continued beyond 28 days.

Patients developing dermatologic toxicities while receiving ERBITUX should be monitored for the development of inflammatory or infectious sequelae, and appropriate treatment of these symptoms initiated.

Dose modifications of any future ERBITUX infusions should be instituted in case of severe acneiform rash (see Dosage and Administration, Dose Modifications). Instruct patients to limit sun exposure during treatment with ERBITUX.

Squamous Cell Carcinoma of the Head and Neck: Table 1 contains selected adverse events in 420 patients receiving radiation therapy either alone or with ERBITUX for locally or regionally advanced SCCHN. ERBITUX was administered at the recommended dose and schedule (400 mg/m² initial dose, followed by 250 mg/m² weekly). Patients received a median of 8 infusions (range 1-11).

Table 1: ERBITUX

Incidence of Treatment Emergent Adverse Events (≥1%) in Patients with Locoregionally Advanced SCCHN

Worst Grade per Patient	% of Patients			
	Erbitux+Radiation N=208		Radiation Alone N=212	
COSTART Body System COSTART Preferred Term	Grade 1-4	Grade 3/4	Grade 1-4	Grade 3/4
Body as a Whole				
Mucous Membrane Disorder	86	52	86	50
Asthenia	56	4	49	5
Fever	29	1	13	1
Pain	28	6	28	7
Headache	19	<1	8	<1
Chills	16	0	5	0
Infection	13	1	9	1
Moniliasis	8	0	6	<1
Abdominal Pain	7	0	4	1
Chest Pain	5	<1	1	0
Neck Pain	5	<1	7	0
Allergic Reaction	4	2	2	0
Infection Bacterial	4	2	1	<1
Accidental Injury	3	0	1	0
Back Pain	3	<1	1	0
Cellulitis	3	1	1	<1
Face Edema	2	0	4	<1
Injection Site Reaction	2	0	1	0
Abscess	1	1	1	<1
Anaphylactoid Reaction	1	1	0	0
Carcinoma	1	1	1	1
Flu Syndrome	1	0	1	<1
Necrosis	1	1	0	0
Radiation Injury	1	0	2	0
Sepsis	1	<1	2	1
Infection Fungal	0	0	1	<1
Cardiovascular System				
Tachycardia	7	0	3	1
Syncope	5	2	2	1
Hypotension	4	1	4	1
Vasodilatation	4	0	1	0
Hemorrhage	2	0	5	1
Hypertension	2	0	2	1

(cont'd)

Table 1: ERBITUX *(cont'd)*
Incidence of Treatment Emergent Adverse Events (≥1%) in Patients with Locoregionally Advanced SCCHN

Worst Grade per Patient	% of Patients			
	Erbitux+Radiation N=208		Radiation Alone N=212	
COSTART Body System COSTART Preferred Term	**Grade 1-4**	**Grade 3/4**	**Grade 1-4**	**Grade 3/4**
Cardiovascular Disorder	1	0	1	0
Postural Hypotension	1	0	1	0
Arrhythmia	0	0	1	<1
Digestive System				
Dry Mouth	72	5	71	3
Dysphagia	65	26	63	30
Nausea	49	2	37	2
Constipation	35	5	30	5
Vomiting	28	2	23	4
Anorexia	27	2	23	2
Stomatitis	23	5	22	5
Diarrhea	19	2	13	1
Oral Moniliasis	19	0	22	0
Dyspepsia	14	0	9	1
Glossitis	4	<1	4	<1
Flatulence	3	0	1	0
Increased Salivation	3	<1	6	0
Esophagitis	2	1	3	1
Tongue Discoloration	2	0	1	0
Rectal Disorder	1	0	1	0
Rectal Hemorrhage	1	0	1	0
Sialadenitis	1	0	<1	0
Mouth Ulceration	1	0	3	<1
Tongue Disorder	1	0	2	0
Gastroenteritis	<1	0	1	1
Tooth Disorder	<1	0	1	0
Hemic and Lymphatic Systems				
Leukopenia	19	18	20	18
Anemia	3	1	13	6
Thrombocytopenia	2	<1	1	<1
Lymphadenopathy	<1	0	1	<1
Metabolic/Nutritional Disorder				
Weight Loss	84	11	72	7
Dehydration	25	6	19	8
Hyperglycemia	9	6	6	4
Hyponatremia	7	6	9	9
Edema	5	0	6	<1
Hyperkalemia	3	2	2	<1
Hypoproteinemia	3	2	0	0
Cachexia	2	1	4	2
Healing Abnormal	2	0	<1	<1
Hypokalemia	2	1	4	3
Peripheral Edema	2	0	3	0
Weight Gain	2	0	4	0
Alkaline Phosphatase Increased	1	<1	1	0
Bun Increased	1	0	1	<1
Hypercalcemia	1	<1	1	<1
Hyperuricemia	1	0	1	1
Hypocalcemia	1	1	2	1
Hypoglycemia	1	0	2	1
Hypomagnesemia	1	0	2	0
Hypophosphatemia	1	1	2	2
Lactic Dehydrogenase Increased	1	0	<1	<1
ALT Increased	5	2	1	<1
AST Increased	4	2	1	<1
Musculoskeletal System				
Bone Pain	2	0	0	0
Myalgia	2	0	1	0
Arthralgia	1	0	<1	0
Nervous System				
Insomnia	15	0	14	0
Anxiety	11	<1	9	1
Depression	9	1	9	<1
Dizziness	8	<1	7	0
Confusion	6	2	3	1
Paresthesia	4	0	2	0
Trismus	3	0	7	1
Neuropathy	2	0	<1	0
Somnolence	2	0	2	0
Abnormal Gait	1	0	<1	0
Agitation	1	0	1	0
Hallucinations	1	<1	2	1
Speech Disorder	<1	<1	1	0
Respiratory System				
Pharyngitis	26	3	19	4
Cough Increased	20	<1	19	0
Voice Alteration	19	0	22	0
Sputum Increased	13	0	15	1
Dyspnea	9	1	7	4
Larynx Edema	7	0	7	1
Hemoptysis	6	0	4	0
Lung Disorder	6	1	4	1
Respiratory Disorder	5	<1	5	1
Rhinitis	5	0	2	0
Hiccup	4	0	2	0
Pneumonia	4	2	4	3
Asthma	3	0	2	<1
Sinusitis	3	0	1	0
Epistaxis	2	0	1	0
Hypoxia	2	1	<1	<1

(cont'd)

Table 1: ERBITUX *(cont'd)*

Incidence of Treatment Emergent Adverse Events (≥1%) in Patients with Locoregionally Advanced SCCHN

Worst Grade per Patient	% of Patients			
	Erbitux+Radiation N=208		Radiation Alone N=212	
COSTART Body System COSTART Preferred Term	**Grade 1-4**	**Grade 3/4**	**Grade 1-4**	**Grade 3/4**
Laryngitis	2	1	6	<1
Bronchitis	1	<1	2	0
Aspiration Pneumonia	1	1	2	2
Skin and Appendages				
Radiation Dermatitis	86	23	90	18
Acne	62	11	1	0
Rash	28	5	5	1
Dry Skin	22	1	5	0
Application Site Reaction	18	0	12	1
Pruritus	16	0	4	0
Skin Ulcer	6	0	2	0
Skin Discoloration	5	0	7	0
Sweating	5	0	2	0
Maculopapular Rash	4	<1	<1	0
Alopecia	3	0	2	0
Fungal Dermatitis	3	<1	2	0
Nail Disorder	3	0	<1	0
Exfoliative Dermatitis	2	1	<1	0
Skin Disorder	2	0	0	0
Urticaria	2	0	0	0
Herpes Simplex	1	0	1	0
Leukoderma	1	0	1	0
Skin Hypertrophy	<1	0	2	0
Skin Necrosis	0	0	1	1
Special Senses				
Taste Perversion	29	0	28	0
Ear Pain	8	0	9	<1
Otitis Externa	8	1	3	<1
Taste Loss	7	0	7	0
Conjunctivitis	3	0	1	0
Deafness	3	0	2	<1
Ear Disorder	2	0	1	0
Otitis Media	2	0	1	0
Tinnitus	2	0	2	0
Amblyopia	1	0	1	0
Urogenital System				
Urinary Tract Infection	3	1	2	1
Urinary Incontinence	2	0	1	0
Dysuria	1	0	2	0
Urinary Frequency	1	0	1	0
Kidney Function Abnormal	0	0	1	1

Late Radiation Toxicity: The overall incidence of late radiation toxicities (any grade) was higher in ERBITUX in combination with radiation therapy compared with radiation therapy alone. The following sites were affected: salivary glands (65% versus 56%), larynx (52% versus 36%), subcutaneous tissue (49% versus 45%), mucous membrane (48% versus 39%), esophagus (44% versus 35%), skin (42% versus 33%). The incidence of Grade 3 or 4 late radiation toxicities was similar between the radiation therapy alone and the ERBITUX plus radiation treatment groups.

Less Common Clinical Trial Adverse Drug Reactions <1% in Squamous Cell Carcinoma of the Head and Neck—ERBITUX in Combination with Radiotherapy: Body as a Whole: abdomen enlarged, accidental injury, carcinoma, cellulitis, cyst, death, flank pain, flu syndrome, halitosis, infection parasitic, infection superimposed, injection site inflammation, injection site pain, overdose, radiation injury, reaction unevaluable, sepsis, sudden death, viral infection.

Cardiovascular System: arterial anomaly, atrial fibrillation, bradycardia, cardiovascular disorder, heart arrest, migraine, myocardial infarct, myocardial ischemia, pallor, palpitation, peripheral vascular disorder, phlebitis, postural hypotension, thrombosis, vascular anomaly, vasodilatation.

Digestive System: cheilitis, cholelithiasis, duodenal ulcer perforation, fecal impaction, gastritis, gastroenteritis, gastrointestinal disorder, gingivitis, hematemesis, hepatitis, intestinal perforation, liver function tests abnormal, melena, mouth ulceration, pancreatitis, parotid gland enlargement, perforated stomach ulcer, pseudomembranous colitis, salivary gland enlargement, sialadenitis, stomach ulcer, thirst, tongue discoloration, tooth disorder.

Hemic and Lymphatic Systems: ecchymosis, leukocytosis, lymphadenopathy, lymphedema, thromboplastin decreased.

Metabolic/Nutritional Disorders: acidosis, alcohol intolerance, alkaline phosphatase increased, alkalosis, BUN increased, gamma glutamyl transpeptidase increased, glycosuria, healing abnormal, hypercalcemia, hypernatremia, hyperuricemia, hypoglycemia, hypophosphatemia lactic dehydrogenase increased.

Musculoskeletal System: arthralgia, arthritis, bone disorder, generalized spasm, leg cramps, muscle atrophy, myalgia, myasthenia, ptosis.

Nervous System: abnormal gait, aphasia, cerebral ischemia, coma, delirium, emotional lability, hallucinations, hypertonia, manic reaction, movement disorder, myoclonus, nervousness, neuropathy, paralysis sleep disorder, speech disorder, thinking abnormal, tremor, twitching, vertigo.

Respiratory System: aspiration pneumonia, bronchitis, carcinoma of lung, epistaxis, hypoxia, lung fibrosis, pleural effusion, pneumothorax, sinusitis, stridor.

Skin and Appendages: eczema, exfoliative dermatitis, furunculosis, herpes simplex, herpes zoster, hirsutism, leukoderma, lichenoid dermatitis, maculopapular rash, nail disorder, skin carcinoma, skin hypertrophy, skin nodule.

Special Senses: abnormal vision, conjunctivitis, corneal lesion, dry eyes, ear disorder, eye pain, keratoconjunctivitis, lacrimation disorder, otitis media, photophobia, vitreous disorder.

Urogenital System: amenorrhea, hematuria, kidney calculus, menstrual disorder, oliguria, prostatic carcinoma, sexual function abnormal, urinary frequency, urinary incontinence, urination impaired, vaginal hemorrhage, vaginitis.

Colorectal Cancer: 1. Metastatic colorectal carcinoma in patients who are refractory or intolerant to irinotecan-based chemotherapy.

Safety data are presented below for the 774 patients who received ERBITUX (cetuximab) plus irinotecan (n=354) or ERBITUX monotherapy (n=420) in four advanced colorectal cancer studies.

Patients receiving ERBITUX plus irinotecan received a median of 12 doses (with 88/354 [25%] treated for over 6 months), and patients receiving monotherapy received a median of 7 doses (with 36/420 [9%] treated for over 6 months). The range of dosing for patients receiving ERBITUX plus irinotecan was 1-84 infusions, and the range of dosing for patients receiving ERBITUX monotherapy was 1-63 infusions.

The addition of irinotecan to ERBITUX in irinotecan-refractory colorectal cancer patients increased the frequency and severity of a number of adverse events when compared to ERBITUX monotherapy.

These adverse events, typically associated with irinotecan treatment (eg, digestive events and myelosuppression), did not appear to occur at a frequency or severity greater than the reported safety profile of irinotecan in metastatic colorectal cancer. **(Please consult the Product Monograph for irinotecan, Camptosar for full safety information.)** Likewise, the frequency and severity of ERBITUX-associated adverse events did not appear to be exacerbated by the addition of irinotecan.

The most common adverse events (regardless of relationship to study therapy) seen in 354 patients receiving ERBITUX plus irinotecan were acneiform rash (88%), asthenia/malaise (73%), diarrhea (72%), nausea (55%), abdominal pain (45%), and vomiting (41%). The most common grade 3 or 4 adverse events (regardless of relationship to ERBITUX) seen in this group of patients were diarrhea (22%), leukopenia (17%), asthenia/malaise (16%), and acneiform rash (14%).

The most common adverse events (regardless of relationship to study therapy) seen in 420 patients receiving ERBITUX monotherapy were acneiform rash (90%), asthenia/malaise (48%), nausea (29%), fever (27%), constipation (26%), abdominal pain (26%), headache (26%), and diarrhea (25%). The most common grade 3 or 4 adverse events (regardless of relationship to ERBITUX) seen in this group of patients were asthenia/malaise (10%), abdominal pain (9%), acneiform rash (8%), and dyspnea (7%). Thirty-seven (10%) patients receiving ERBITUX plus irinotecan and 17 (4%) patients receiving ERBITUX monotherapy discontinued treatment primarily because of adverse events.

Data in patients with advanced colorectal carcinoma in Table 2 are based on the experience of 354 patients treated with ERBITUX plus irinotecan and 420 patients treated with ERBITUX monotherapy.

Less Common Clinical Trial Adverse Drug Reactions <1%: Information is presented by body system for 354 patients treated with ERBITUX + irinotecan followed by information on 420 patients treated with ERBITUX as monotherapy, in the colorectal cancer trials.

ERBITUX + Irinotecan: Body as a Whole: chills and fever, cholinergic syndrome, injection site edema, lab test abnormal, peritonitis, viral infection, cachexia, death, hypothermia, infection superimposed, injection site hemorrhage, moniliasis, neck rigidity, overdose.

Cardiovascular System: pericardial effusion, heart arrest, migraine, postural hypotension, vascular disorder, arrhythmia, arterial thrombosis, atrial fibrillation, endocarditis, heart failure myocardial infarct, peripheral vascular disorder, pulmonary artery thrombosis, pulmonary embolus, shock, supraventricular extrasystoles, supraventricular tachycardia, thrombophlebitis, vascular headache, ventricular tachycardia.

Table 2: ERBITUX

Incidence of Adverse Events (≥1%) Regardless of Relationship to Study Therapy in Patients with Advanced Colorectal Carcinoma

Body System COSTART Preferred Term[a]	ERBITUX Plus Irinotecan (n=354)		ERBITUX Monotherapy (n=420)	
	Grades 1-4	**Grades 3 and 4**	**Grades 1-4**	**Grades 3 and 4**
	% of Patients			
Body as a Whole				
Asthenia/Malaise[b]	73	16	48	10
Abdominal Pain	45	8	26	9
Fever[c]	34	4	27	
Pain	23	6	17	5
Infusion Reaction[d]	19	3	21	2
Infection	16	1	14	1
Back Pain	16	3	10	2
Headache	14	2	26	2
Chills[c]	11	1	11	
Carcinoma	7	6	1	1
Chest Pain	6		4	

(cont'd)

Table 2: ERBITUX *(cont'd)*

Incidence of Adverse Events (≥1%) Regardless of Relationship to Study Therapy in Patients with Advanced Colorectal Carcinoma

Body System COSTART Preferred Term[a]	ERBITUX Plus Irinotecan (n=354)		ERBITUX Monotherapy (n=420)	
	Grades 1-4	Grades 3 and 4	Grades 1-4	Grades 3 and 4
	% of Patients			
Ascites	5	2	4	2
Flu Syndrome	4		4	
Mucous Membrane Disorder	4		2	
Sepsis	4	4	2	2
Accidental Injury	4		2	
Injection Site Pain	3			
Pelvic Pain	3	1	1	
Infection Bacterial	2	1	1	
Cellulitis	2	1		
Face Edema	2			
Flank Pain	2	1		
Infection Fungal	2		3	
Injection Site Inflammation	2	1		
Injection Site Reaction	2		1	1
Abscess	1	1	1	1
Abdomen Enlarged	1		2	
Cyst	1		2	
Neck Pain	1		1	
Photosensitivity Reaction	1		1	
Cardiovascular				
Hypotension	5	2	1	1
Tachycardia	5		2	
Hypertension	5	1	1	
Vasodilatation	4			
Thrombosis	3	2		
Pallor	2			
Syncope	2	1		
Cardiovascular Disorder	2			
Deep Vein Thrombophlebitis	2	2	1	1
Hemorrhage	2		1	
Palpitation	1		1	
Atrial Fibrillation			1	1
Digestive				
Diarrhea	72	22	25	2
Nausea	55	6	29	2
Vomiting	41	7	25	3
Anorexia	36	4	23	2
Constipation	30	2	26	2
Stomatitis	26	2	10	
Dyspepsia	14		6	
Dry Mouth	6		1	
Flatulence	5		3	
Jaundice	5	3	5	2
Intestinal Obstruction	5	3	6	6
Gastrointestinal Disorder	4	1	3	1
Hepatomegaly	4	1	1	1
Rectal Disorder	4		2	
Rectal Hemorrhage	4		3	
Melena	3		1	
Gastritis	3			
Dysphagia	2		2	1
Gastrointestinal Hemorrhage	2	1	3	1
Oral Moniliasis	2		1	
Mouth Ulceration	2			
Cheilitis	1			
Esophagitis	1	1		
Gingivitis	1			
Glossitis	1		3	
Gum Hemorrhage	1		1	
Tongue Disorder	1		1	
Ulcerative Stomatitis	1		1	
Haematic/Lymphatic				
Leukopenia	25	17		
Anemia	16	5	9	3
Hypochromic Anemia	4			
Thrombocytopenia	2	1	1	
Ecchymosis	2		1	
Prothrombin Decreased	2	2		
Lymphadenopathy	1		1	
Coagulation Disorder	1		1	
Leukocytosis	1		1	
Lymphedema			1	
Metabolic/Nutritional				
Weight Loss	21		7	1
Peripheral Edema	16	1	10	1
Dehydration	15	6	10	3
Hypokalemia	7	4	5	1
Hyperglycemia	6	3	1	
Bilirubinemia	5	4	2	1
Edema	5	1	5	
Alkaline Phosphatase Increased	3	1		
Hypoproteinemia	3	1		
Weight Gain	3			
Hypomagnesemia	3	1	3	
Hyponatremia	3	1		
Hypocalcemia	3	1	1	
AST Increased	3	1		
ALT Increased	2	1		
Cachexia	2	1	1	
Hypovolemia	2	1		

(cont'd)

Table 2: ERBITUX *(cont'd)*

Incidence of Adverse Events (≥1%) Regardless of Relationship to Study Therapy in Patients with Advanced Colorectal Carcinoma

Body System COSTART Preferred Term[a]	ERBITUX Plus Irinotecan (n=354)		ERBITUX Monotherapy (n=420)	
	Grades 1-4	Grades 3 and 4	Grades 1-4	Grades 3 and 4
	% of Patients			
Acidosis	1	1		
Healing Abnormal	1			
Hyperkalemia	1	1		
Hypoglycemia	1			
Hypophosphatemia	1	1	1	
Musculoskeletal				
Myalgia	5		4	
Bone Pain	3		1	
Myasthenia	2		3	
Arthralgia	2		4	
Muscle Atrophy	1		0	
Joint Disorder			1	
Leg Cramps	1		1	
Nervous				
Insomnia	12		10	
Depression	10		7	
Anxiety	9		4	
Dizziness	8	1	5	
Paresthesia	7		4	
Neuropathy	6	1	3	
Somnolence	4	1	3	1
Confusion	3	1	3	1
Tremor	3			
Nervousness	2		1	
Vertigo	2		1	
Neuralgia	1		1	
Twitching	1			
Dry Mouth			2	
Agitation	1		1	
Thinking Abnormal	1	1	1	
Amnesia	1		1	
Convulsion	1	1	1	
Vasodilatation			1	
Respiratory				
Dyspnea[c]	23	2	17	7
Cough Increased	20		11	1
Epistaxis	8		9	
Rhinitis	8		5	
Respiratory Disorder	7		2	
Pharyngitis	5		2	
Pneumonia	5	2	2	2
Lung Disorder	3			
Hiccup	3	1	1	
Asthma	3	1	1	
Pleural Effusion	3	1	4	2

(cont'd)

Table 2: ERBITUX *(cont'd)*

Incidence of Adverse Events (≥1%) Regardless of Relationship to Study Therapy in Patients with Advanced Colorectal Carcinoma

Body System COSTART Preferred Term[a]	ERBITUX Plus Irinotecan (n=354)		ERBITUX Monotherapy (n=420)	
	Grades 1-4	Grades 3 and 4	Grades 1-4	Grades 3 and 4
	% of Patients			
Bronchitis	2	1	1	
Voice Alteration	2		1	
Hemoptysis	1		2	
Sputum Increased	1			
Sinusitis	1		1	
Hypoxia	1	1	1	1
Pulmonary Embolus			1	1
Apnea			1	1
Skin/Appendages				
Acneiform Rash[e]	88	14	90	8
Alopecia	21		4	
Skin Disorder	15	1	4	
Nail Disorder	12		16	
Pruritus	10	1	11	
Sweating	8		4	
Skin Ulcer	4	1	1	
Hirsutism	3		3	
Eczema	2			
Herpes Simplex	1		1	
Skin Discoloration	1			
Hair Disorder	1		4	
Vesiculobullous Rash	1			
Herpes Zoster			1	
Special Senses				
Conjunctivitis	14	1	7	
Taste Perversion	5		1	
Dry Eyes	3		2	
Amblyopia	2		1	
Lacrimation Disorder	2		2	
Abnormal Vision	1			
Blepharitis	1			
Deafness	1		1	
Tinnitus	1			
Ear Disorder	1		1	
Urogenital				
Urinary Tract Infection	8	2	6	1
Hematuria	5	1	3	
Dysuria	3		3	
Kidney Failure	2	2		
Urinary Incontinence	2	1	1	
Urinary Retention	2		1	
Hydronephrosis	1	1	1	
Vaginal Hemorrhage	1		1	
Cystitis	1			
Kidney Function Abnormal	1	1		

(cont'd)

Table 2: ERBITUX *(cont'd)*

Incidence of Adverse Events (≥1%) Regardless of Relationship to Study Therapy in Patients with Advanced Colorectal Carcinoma

Body System COSTART Preferred Term[a]	ERBITUX Plus Irinotecan (n=354)		ERBITUX Monotherapy (n=420)	
	Grades 1-4	Grades 3 and 4	Grades 1-4	Grades 3 and 4
	% of Patients			
Oliguria	1			
Urinary Frequency	1		1	
Urine Abnormality			1	

[a] Adverse events that occurred (toxicity grades 1 through 4) in ≥1% of patients with refractory colorectal carcinoma treated with ERBITUX plus Irinotecan or in ≥1% of patients with refractory colorectal carcinoma treated with ERBITUX monotherapy.
[b] Asthenia/malaise is defined as any events described as "asthenia", "malaise", or "somnolence".
[c] Includes cases reported as infusion reaction.
[d] Infusion reaction is defined as any event described at any time during the clinical study as "allergic reaction" or anaphylactoid reaction", or any events occurring on the first day of dosing described as "allergic reaction", "anaphylactoid reaction", "fever", "chills", "chills and fever", or "dyspnea".
[e] Acneiform rash is defined as any events described as "acne", "rash", "maculopapular rash", "pustular rash", "dry skin", or "exfoliative dermatitis".

Digestive System: cholestatic jaundice, eructation, hepatic failure, tongue disorder, aphthous stomatitis, cholangitis, cholelithiasis, gastroenteritis, ileus, increased salivation, intestinal perforation, pseudomembranous colitis, tenesmus, thirst, tooth caries, abnormal stools, biliary pain, cirrhosis of liver, colitis, duodenal ulcer hemorrhage, enteritis, hematemesis, increased appetite, liver damage, liver function tests abnormal, periodontal abscess, proctitis, stenosis of colon, tooth disorder, ulcerative stomatitis.
Hemic and Lymphatic Systems: thromboplastin decreased, coagulation time increased, disseminated intravascular coagulation, granulocytosis, lymphedema, marrow depression, petechia.
Metabolic and Nutritional System: gamma glutamyl transpeptidase increased, hyperuricemia, lactic dehydrogenase increased, creatinine increased, diabetes mellitus, gout, hypervolemia, BUN increased, cyanosis, hypernatremia, hyperphosphatemia.
Musculoskeletal System: pathological fracture, tetany, bone disorder, bone neoplasm, generalised spasm, joint disorder, myositis.
Nervous System: hypertonia, stupor, aphasia, encephalopathy, hypesthesia, myclonus, peripheral neuritis, speech disorder, akinesia, apathy, ataxia, cerebrovascular accident, coma, emotional lability, foot drop, hallucinations, hemiplegia, hypokinesia, incoordination, meningitis, movement disorder, sleep disorder.
Respiratory System: hyperventilation, lung fibrosis, atelectasis, laryngitis, lung edema, pulmonary embolus.
Skin and Appendages: fungal dermatitis, skin hypertrophy, leukoderma, urticaria, contact dermatitis, erythema nodosum, furunculosis, herpes zoster, psoriasis, purpuric rash, seborrhea, skin carcinoma, subcutaneous nodule.
Special Senses: cataract specified, eye disorder, parosmia photophobia, taste loss, vitreous disorder.
Urogenital System: acute kidney failure, leukorrhea, testis disorder, vaginal moniliasis, albuminuria, hydroureter, kidney pain, urinary tract disorder, urinary urgency, cervix neoplasm, impotence, kidney calculus, nocturia, pyelonephritis, uremia, vaginitis.
ERBITUX Monotherapy: Body as a Whole: lab test abnormal, chills and fever, face edema, hernia, peritonitis, anaphylactoid reaction, cachexia, cellulitis, flank pain, hormone level altered, injection site hemorrhage, injection site inflammation, injection site pain, moniliasis, multiple organ failure, viral infection.
Cardiovascular System: bradycardia, migraine, pallor, thrombosis, arrhythmia, arteriosclerosis, atrial arrhythmia, cardiovascular disorder, heart failure, myocardial infarct, peripheral vascular disorder, postural hypotension, supraventricular tachycardia, syncope, vascular disorder.
Digestive System: gastroenteritis, pancreatitis, tooth disorder, gastritis, hepatic failure, intestinal perforation, large intestine perforation, mouth ulceration, tenesmus, aphthous stomatitis, cheilitis, cholangitis, cholecystitis, cholelithiasis, cholestatic jaundice, eructation, fecal impaction, fecal incontinence, gingivitis, hematemesis, liver damage, liver damage aggravated, liver tenderness, thirst, tongue discoloration.
Hemic and Lymphatic Systems: hypochromic anemia, leukopenia, thromboplastin decreased, coagulation time increased, cyanosis, fibrinogen increased, pancytopenia, purpura.
Metabolic and Nutritional Disorders: creatinine increased, diabetes mellitus, alkaline phosphatase increased, hyperkalemia, hypoglycemia, hypoproteinemia, AST increased, electrolyte depletion, gamma glutamyl transpeptidase increased, generalised edema, hypercalcemia, hypercholesteremia, hyperlipemia, hyponatremia, ALT increased, weight gain.
Musculoskeletal System: generalized spasm, bone disorder.
Nervous System: abnormal gait, hypertonia, peripheral neuritis, ileus, tremor, ataxia, emotional lability, facial paralysis, grand mal convulsion, hallucinations, hyperkinesia, incoordination, libido decreased, neuritis, speech disorder, stupor, vasospasm, withdrawal syndrome.
Respiratory System: lung edema, pneumothorax, atelectasis, laryngismus, lung disorder, sputum increased, aspiration pneumonia, laryngitis, pleural disorder.
Skin and Appendages: fungal dermatitis, cutaneous moniliasis, vesiculobullous rash, application site reaction, eczema, hair discoloration, seborrhoea, skin melanoma, skin nodule, urticaria.
Special Senses: eye disorder, eye pain, abnormal vision, blepharitis, blindness, cataract specified, diplopia, eye hemorrhage, parosmia, photophobia, ptosis, retinal disorder, taste loss.
Urogenital System: acute kidney failure, kidney calculus, leukorrhea, urinary tract disorder, vaginal moniliasis, abnormal ejaculation, balanitis, breast enlargement, epididymitis, impotence, kidney failure, kidney function abnormal, labial edema, metrorrhagia, nocturia, oliguria, polyuria, prostatic disorder, prostatic specific antigen increase, pyuria, urination impaired, urogenital disorder, vaginitis.

2. Metastatic colorectal carcinoma after failure of both irinotecan- and oxaliplatin-based regimens.

ERBITUX was administered at the recommended dose and schedule (400 mg/m² initial dose, followed by 250 mg/m² weekly).

In the prospectively defined, retrospective analysis, 389 out of the 562 patients with pre-treated metastatic CRC receiving ERBITUX plus BSC or BSC alone were evaluated for KRAS status. Of these, 227 patients were determined to have KRAS wild-type tumors. The median duration of ERBITUX treatment for patients with KRAS wild-type was 16 weeks and the median duration of ERBITUX treatment for patients whose tumours have KRAS mutations was 8 weeks. The infusion rate was decreased and/or the infusion temporarily interrupted in 17% of the 117 patients who received ERBITUX and had KRAS wild-type tumours.

Table 3 contains adverse events in the 227 patients with KRAS wild-type, receiving ERBITUX plus BSC or BSC alone.

The safety profile of ERBITUX in patients with KRAS wild-type (n=117) was consistent with the profile of the overall ERBITUX-treated study population (n=288). Patients not eligible for ERBITUX therapy, i.e., those whose tumours express KRAS mutations, may have an increased risk of some adverse events.

Table 3: ERBITUX

Incidence of Adverse Events Occurring in ≥1% of KRAS Wild-Type Patients with Advanced Colorectal Carcinoma Treated with ERBITUX Plus BSC

CTC Category CTC Term	% of Patients			
	ERBITUX Plus BSC (n=117)		BSC Alone (n=110)	
	Any Grades[a]	Grades 3 and 4	Any Grades[a]	Grades 3 and 4
Allergy				
Allergic Rhinitis	8	0	3	0
Auditory				
Inner Ear/Hearing	2	1	1	0
Other—Auditory[c]	2	0	0	0
Blood/Bone Marrow				
Hemoglobin	2	1	3	1
Cardiovascular				
Edema	32	5	31	8
Sinus Tachycardia	5	1	0	0
Hypotension	4	2	3	2
Hypertension	3	0	1	0
Thrombosis/Embolism	3	3	7	7
Supraventricular Arrhythmias	2	2	0	0
Dermatology				
Rash/Desquamation	95	18	19	1
Dry Skin	60	0	16	0
Pruritus	52	3	12	0
Other—Dermatology[c]	34	0	7	2
Nail Changes	28	0	5	0
Alopecia	7	0	5	0
Hand-Foot Skin Reaction	4	0	1	0
Bruising	3	0	2	0
Injection Site Reaction	2	0	0	0
Endocrine				
Hot Flashes/Flushes	4	0	2	0
Flu-Like Symptoms				
Fatigue	91	30	78	25
Fever	25	2	15	0
Rigors, Chills	13	1	3	0
Sweating	8	0	10	0
Other—Flu-Like Symptoms[c]	4	0	2	0
Gastrointestinal				
Anorexia	68	7	64	3
Nausea	61	5	48	6
Constipation	51	3	35	3
Diarrhea	39	2	20	2
Vomiting	37	5	25	4
Stomatitis	31	0	10	0
Other—Gastrointestinal[c]	24	11	15	5
Dyspepsia/Heartburn	15	0	17	0
Mouth Dryness	14	0	7	0
Dehydration	10	3	3	0
Taste Disturbance	10	0	5	0
Dysphagia	7	0	5	0
Ascites	6	3	1	0
Flatulence	4	0	2	0

(cont'd)

Table 3: ERBITUX *(cont'd)*

Incidence of Adverse Events Occurring in ≥1% of KRAS Wild-Type Patients with Advanced Colorectal Carcinoma Treated with ERBITUX Plus BSC

CTC Category CTC Term	% of Patients			
	ERBITUX Plus BSC (n=117)		BSC Alone (n=110)	
	Any Grades[a]	Grades 3 and 4	Any Grades[a]	Grades 3 and 4
Proctitis	3	0	1	0
Hemorrhage				
Epistaxis	9	0	2	0
Melena/GI Bleeding	4	3	5	4
Other—Hemorrhage[c]	4	0	2	2
Rectal Bleeding	4	0	5	0
Hematuria	3	1	1	0
Hemoptysis	3	0	3	0
Vaginal Bleeding	3	0	1	0
Hematemesis	2	2	0	0
Hepatic				
Other—Hepatic[c]	11	6	7	3
Bilirubin	2	2	3	2
Liver Dysfunction	2	2	1	1
Hypersensitivity Reaction				
Infusion Reaction[b]	20	4	—	—
Drug Fever	7	0	—	—
Dyspnea	3	3	—	—
Chills, Rigors	5	0	—	—
Swelling	3	1	—	—
Urticaria	3	1	—	—
Bronchospasm	2	0	—	—
Chest Tightness	2	1	—	—
Flushing	2	0	—	—
Hypertension	2	0	—	—
Hypotension	2	1	—	—
Tachycardia	2	0	—	—
Infection				
Infection Without Neutropenia	40	9	18	5
Lymphatics				
Lymphedema	2	0	2	0
Musculoskeletal				
Other—Musculoskeletal[c]	7	1	0	0
Muscle Weakness	5	3	7	5
Neurology				
Neuropathy—Sensory	49	1	36	2
Insomnia	30	0	13	1
Confusion	17	7	8	1
Depression	15	1	4	0
Anxiety	13	2	3	1
Dizziness	10	1	5	1
Neuropathy—Motor	5	1	5	1
Ataxia	4	0	2	1
Depressed Level of Consciousness	4	1	2	0
Tremor	4	0	2	0

(cont'd)

Table 3: ERBITUX *(cont'd)*

Incidence of Adverse Events Occurring in ≥1% of KRAS Wild-Type Patients with Advanced Colorectal Carcinoma Treated with ERBITUX Plus BSC

CTC Category CTC Term	% of Patients			
	ERBITUX Plus BSC (n=117)		BSC Alone (n=110)	
	Any Grades[a]	Grades 3 and 4	Any Grades[a]	Grades 3 and 4
Extrapyramidal	3	0	1	0
Hallucinations	3	3	3	3
Other—Neurology[c]	3	1	6	1
Speech Impairment	3	2	0	0
Memory Loss	2	0	1	0
Ocular				
Other—Ocular[c]	9	0	0	0
Dry Eye	6	0	0	0
Tearing	4	0	2	0
Conjunctivitis	3	0	0	0
Pain				
Abdominal Pain	59	14	56	13
Pain—Other	57	17	35	6
Headache	38	3	9	0
Arthralgia	14	2	5	0
Bone Pain	14	4	8	1
Chest Pain	11	1	14	1
Myalgia	10	3	8	2
Hepatic Pain	3	1	2	0
Neuropathic Pain	3	0	2	1
Pelvic Pain	3	2	5	0
Pleuritic Pain	3	1	3	0
Rectal/Perirectal Pain	3	0	6	0
Pulmonary				
Dyspnea	48	16	45	14
Cough	26	1	16	2
Hiccoughs	3	0	1	0
Other—Pulmonary[c]	3	1	3	0
Pleural Effusion	2	0	0	0
Voice Changes	2	0	1	0
Renal				
Other—Renal[c]	9	2	5	1
Dysuria	6	0	2	0
Urinary Retention	4	1	2	0
Urine Frequency/Urgency	4	1	10	1
Urine Color Change	3	0	0	0
Incontinence	2	0	5	0
Weight				
Weight Loss	4	0	6	1

[a] Adverse events were graded using the NCI CTC, v 2.0. Excluding AEs reported as cancer death.
[b] Infusion reaction is defined as any event (drug fever, dyspnea, chills rigors, swelling, urticaria, bronchospasm, chest tightness, flushing, hypertension, hypotension, tachycardia, angioedema, nausea, other-hypersensitivity reaction3, pain, pruritus, rash, sweating, or tremors shaking) recorded by the investigator at any time during the clinical study as infusion related.
[c] Events coded using the CTC term "Other" within each category.
BSC=best supportive care; NCI=National Cancer Institute; CTC=common toxicity criteria.

Abnormal Hematologic and Clinical Chemistry Findings: In patients evaluated during clinical trials, hypomagnesemia occurred in 55% of patients receiving ERBITUX and was severe (NCI CTC Grade 3 and 4) in 6-17%. Electrolyte repletion was necessary in some patients and in severe cases, intravenous replacement was required. The onset of hypomagnesemia and electrolyte abnormalities has been reported to occur from days to months after initiation of ERBITUX. Patients should be periodically monitored for hypomagnesemia, and accompanying hypocalcemia and hypokalemia, during and following the completion of ERBITUX therapy. Monitoring should continue for a period of time commensurate with the half-life of the product; i.e. at least 8 weeks following the completion of ERBITUX therapy.

The time to resolution of electrolyte abnormalities is not well known, hence monitoring after ERBITUX treatment is recommended (see Warnings and Precautions, Monitoring and Laboratory Tests).

Post-Market Adverse Drug Reactions: Dermatologic Toxicity and Related Disorders: Very rare cases of skin necrosis have been reported in the post-marketing setting. Dermatologic toxicities with infectious sequelae (for example *S. aureus* sepsis, cellulitis, blepharitis, conjunctivitis, keratitis, cheilitis) have been reported in the post-marketing setting.

Infusion Reactions: Cases of shock and myocardial infarction have been reported in the context of serious infusion reactions.

Hepatobiliary Disorders: Isolated cases of increases in liver enzymes have been reported in the post-marketing setting.

Nervous System Disorders: Cases of aseptic meningitis have been reported in the post-marketing setting.

DRUG INTERACTIONS: Drug-Drug Interactions: A single drug interaction study was performed to investigate the potential for pharmacokinetic interaction between ERBITUX (cetuximab) and irinotecan when given in combination. No pharmacokinetic interaction was observed.

In addition, an integrated population pharmacokinetic analysis across all clinical studies demonstrated that the pharmacokinetics were unaffected by concomitant cisplatin, paclitaxel, doxorubicin, gemcitabine or radiation therapy.

Drug-Herb Interactions: Interactions with herbal products have not been established.

Drug-Laboratory Tests Interactions: Interactions with laboratory tests have not been established.

DOSAGE AND ADMINISTRATION: Recommended Dose and Dosage Adjustment: Colorectal Cancer: Whenever ERBITUX and irinotecan are scheduled to be administered in the same week, irinotecan should be administered after the end of the ERBITUX infusion.

- The recommended initial dose, either as monotherapy or in combination with irinotecan, is 400 mg/m² administered as a 120-minute infusion (maximum infusion rate 10 mg/min).
- The recommended subsequent weekly dose, either as monotherapy or in combination with irinotecan, is 250 mg/m² infused over 60 minutes (maximum infusion rate 10 mg/min) until progression of the underlying disease or unacceptable toxicity.

Squamous Cell Carcinoma of the Head and Neck (SCCHN): ERBITUX is administered in combination with radiation therapy as follows:

- The recommended initial dose is 400 mg/m² administered one week prior to initiation of a course of radiation therapy as a 120-minute intravenous infusion (maximum infusion rate 10 mg/min).
- The recommended subsequent weekly dose (all other infusions) is 250 mg/m² infused over 60 minutes (maximum infusion rate 10 mg/min) for the duration of radiation therapy (6-7 weeks). **Complete ERBITUX administration 1 hour prior to radiation therapy.**

Dose Modifications: Infusion Reactions: (See Warnings and Precautions and Adverse Reactions.)

If the patient experiences a mild or moderate (NCI CTC grade 1 or 2) and non-serious NCI CTC Grade 3-4 infusion reaction, the infusion rate should be reduced by 50%. It is recommended that the ERBITUX infusion rate remain at the lower value for all subsequent infusions.

Occurrences of a severe (grade 3 or 4) infusion reaction require immediate and permanent discontinuation of ERBITUX therapy and may necessitate emergency treatment and/or hospitalisation.

Dermatologic Toxicity: (See Warnings and Precautions and Adverse Reactions.)

If a patient experiences severe acneiform rash (grade 3 or 4), ERBITUX treatment adjustment should be made according to Table 4. If the rash improves and is no longer severe, treatment may be resumed without any change in dose level. The recurrence of severe acneiform rash may require further interruption of therapy with dose reductions at pretreatment after improvement (initially to 200 mg/m² and subsequently to 150 mg/m²) or discontinuation of therapy.

Table 4: ERBITUX

Dose Modifications Guidelines for Rash

Severe Acneiform Rash	ERBITUX	Outcome	ERBITUX Dose Modification
1st Occurrence	Delay infusion 1 to 2 weeks	Improvement No improvement	Continue at 250 mg/m² Discontinue ERBITUX
2nd Occurrence	Delay infusion 1 to 2 weeks	Improvement No improvement	Reduce dose to 200 mg/m² Discontinue ERBITUX
3rd Occurrence	Delay infusion 1 to 2 weeks	Improvement No improvement	Reduce dose to 150 mg/m² Discontinue ERBITUX
4th Occurrence	Discontinue ERBITUX		

Administration: ERBITUX must be administered with the use of a low protein binding 0.22-micron in-line filter. Do not administer ERBITUX as an IV push or bolus.

Do not shake. Do not dilute.

Recommended Premedication: Premedication with an H_1 antagonist (eg, 50 mg of IV diphenhydramine) intravenously 30-60 minutes prior to the first dose should be used. Premedication with an intravenous corticosteroid prior to the first dose may be used. Premedication may be administered for subsequent ERBITUX doses based upon clinical judgment and presence/severity of prior infusion reactions. Anaphylactic reactions may occur despite the use of prophylactic medications. Physicians should always remain vigilant for signs and symptoms of severe infusion reactions (see Warnings and Precautions, Infusion Reactions).

How ERBITUX is Supplied: ERBITUX is supplied as a 50 mL ready-to-use vial that contains 100 mg cetuximab at a concentration of 2 mg/mL in phosphate buffered saline. The solution should be clear and colourless and may contain a small amount of easily visible, white, amorphous cetuximab particulates. The particulates are product-related and do not affect the quality of the product.

Preparation for Administration: Do not shake or dilute.

Prepare infusion using appropriate aseptic technique. ERBITUX should be administered via infusion pump or syringe pump.

To obtain the recommended dose, multiple vials should be pooled aseptically into an infusion container prior to administration. To prevent vacuum formation, a vented needle may be used. **ERBITUX should not be mixed or diluted with other drugs as no studies have been conducted on the physical or biochemical compatibility of ERBITUX mixed with other agents.**

For squamous cell carcinoma of the head and neck complete ERBITUX administration 1 hour prior to radiation therapy.

For colorectal cancer patients receiving ERBITUX in combination with irinotecan, the irinotecan dosage and dose modifications should be performed according to the Product Monograph for Irinotecan (Camptosar). Whenever ERBITUX and irinotecan are scheduled to be administered in the same week, irinotecan should be administered after the end of the ERBITUX infusion.

Saline may be used to clear the infusion set of ERBITUX and to ensure complete dose delivery.

ERBITUX can be administered in an appropriate outpatient setting.

Infusion Pump:

- Draw up the volume of a vial using a sterile syringe attached to an appropriate needle (a vented needle or pin may be used).
- Fill ERBITUX into a sterile evacuated container or bag such as glass containers, polyolefin bags (eg, Baxter Intravia), ethylene vinyl acetate bags (eg, Baxter Clintec), DEHP plasticized PVC bags (eg, Abbott Lifecare), or PVC bags.
- Repeat procedure until the calculated volume has been put into the container. Use a new needle for each vial.
- Administer through a low protein binding 0.22-micrometer in-line filter (placed as proximal to the patient as practical).
- Affix the infusion line and prime it with ERBITUX before starting the infusion.
- Maximum infusion rate should not exceed 10 mg/min.
- Use 0.9% saline solution to flush line at the end of infusion.

Syringe Pump:

- Draw up the volume of a vial using a sterile syringe attached to an appropriate needle (a vented needle or pin may be used).
- Place the syringe into the syringe driver of a syringe pump and set the rate.
- Administer through a low protein binding 0.22-micrometer in-line filter rated for syringe pump use (placed as proximal to the patient as practical).
- Connect up the infusion line and start the infusion after priming the line with ERBITUX.
- Repeat procedure until the calculated volume has been infused.
- Use a new needle and filter for each vial.
- Maximum infusion rate should not exceed 10 mg/min.
- Use 0.9% saline solution to flush line at the end of infusion.

ERBITUX should be piggybacked to the patient's infusion line.

Following the ERBITUX infusion, a 1-hour observation period is recommended. Longer observation periods may be required for patients who experience infusion reactions.

ERBITUX is compatible with:

- polyethylene, ethyl vinyl acetate or polyvinyl chloride bags;
- polyethylene, ethyl vinyl acetate, polyvinyl chloride, polybutadiene or polymethane infusion sets;
- polyethersulfone, polyamide or polysulfone in-line filters.

Care must be taken to ensure aseptic handling when preparing the infusion.

Opened vials should be disposed of as biohazardous waste.

OVERDOSAGE:

There is limited experience with single doses higher than 400 mg/m² body surface area to date or weekly administrations of doses higher than 250 mg/m² body surface area. In clinical studies with doses up to 700 mg/m² given every 2 weeks the safety profile was consistent with that described in Adverse Reactions.

The maximum single dose of ERBITUX administered is 1000 mg/m² in one patient and no adverse events were reported for this patient. There is very limited experience with overdosage in human clinical trials.

> For management of a suspected drug overdose, CPhA recommends that you contact your **regional Poison Control Centre**. See the *CPS* Directory section for a list of Poison Control Centres.

ACTION AND CLINICAL PHARMACOLOGY: EGFR (HER1, c-ErbB-1), a transmembrane glycoprotein, is a member of a structurally-related subfamily of type I receptor tyrosine kinases that includes EGFR (HER1), HER2, HER3, and HER4. The EGFR is expressed in many human cancers including those of the bladder, brain, cervix, colon and rectum, esophagus, head and neck, kidney, lung, ovary, pancreas, and prostate. EGFR is also expressed in normal epithelial tissues, including the skin follicle. ERBITUX (cetuximab) functions as a competitive antagonist that inhibits binding of the ligands, such as epidermal growth factor (EGF) and transforming growth factor-alpha (TGF-α), to the EGFR, and stimulates receptor internalization, leading to a reduction of EGFR expression on the cell surface. This antagonist action inhibits EGFR phosphorylation and activation, resulting in inhibition of cell growth, induction of apoptosis, decreased matrix metalloproteinase (MMP) production, and decreased vascular endothelial growth factor (VEGF) production. In tumours with a wild-type KRAS gene (Kirsten rat sarcoma 2 viral oncogene homolog), activation of KRAS protein by signals from the EGFR contribute to tumour growth, survival, and metastasis. However, in tumours with a mutant KRAS gene, the KRAS protein is continuously active and appears independent of EGFR regulation/activation.

In vitro assays and in vivo animal studies have shown that ERBITUX inhibits the growth and survival of tumour cells that express the EGFR. In vivo animal studies have shown that ERBITUX, in combination with various chemotherapeutic agents: cisplatin, doxorubicin, fluorouracil, gemcitabine, paclitaxel, topotecan and irinotecan, or radiation, enhances the antitumor effects of these agents.

Pharmacokinetics: ERBITUX administered as monotherapy or in combination with concomitant chemotherapy or radiation therapy exhibits nonlinear pharmacokinetics. The area under the concentration time curve (AUC) increased in a greater than dose proportional manner while clearance of cetuximab decreased from 0.08 to 0.02 L/h/m² as the dose increased from 20 to 200 mg/m², it appeared to plateau. The volume of distribution for cetuximab appeared to be independent of dose and approximated 2-3 L/m², a volume approximating the vascular space.

Maximum median serum concentrations (C_{max}) of approximately 181 µg/mL (range: 92-327 µg/mL) were achieved following a 2-hour infusion of 400 mg/m². A 1-hour infusion of 250 mg/m² produced a median C_{max} of approximately 132 µg/mL (range 120-170 µg/mL).

Increases in ERBITUX half-life (Figure 1) and exposure (Figure 2) were approximately dose proportional and predictable across the recommended doses of 400 mg/m² initial dose/250 mg/m² weekly dose.

Figure 1: ERBITUX

ERBITUX Half-life ($t_{½}$) vs Dose

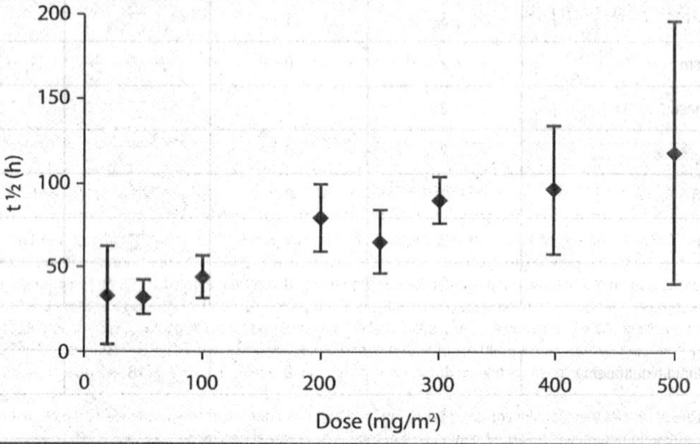

The median half-life of ERBITUX following a weekly dose of 250 mg/m², was 64 hours (range 45 to 104 hours).

Following the recommended dose regimen (400 mg/m² initial dose/250 mg/m² weekly dose), ERBITUX concentrations reached steady state levels by the third weekly infusion with mean peak and trough concentrations across studies ranging from 168 to 235 and 41 to 85 µg/mL respectively. The mean half-life was approximately 112 hours (range 63-230 hours). The pharmacokinetics of cetuximab were similar in patients with SCCHN and those with colorectal cancer.

Figure 2: ERBITUX

ERBITUX Exposure (AUC_{inf}) vs Dose

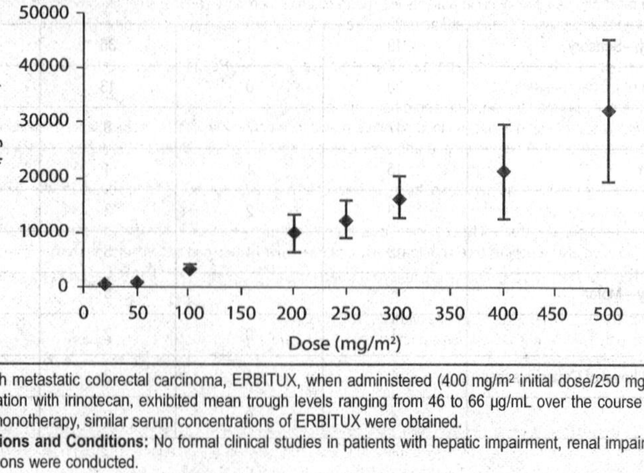

In patients with metastatic colorectal carcinoma, ERBITUX, when administered (400 mg/m² initial dose/250 mg/m² weekly dose) in combination with irinotecan, exhibited mean trough levels ranging from 46 to 66 µg/mL over the course of therapy. When given as monotherapy, similar serum concentrations of ERBITUX were obtained.

Special Populations and Conditions: No formal clinical studies in patients with hepatic impairment, renal impairment, or in pediatric populations were conducted.

A population pharmacokinetic model analysis was used to investigate the potential effects of selected covariates including hepatic and renal function, race, weight, body surface area, and age on ERBITUX pharmacokinetics. None of these covariates appeared to have a statistically significant effect on cetuximab pharmacokinetics suggesting that dose adjustments are not needed for these groups.

Based on a population pharmacokinetic analysis, a small difference in clearance was observed between males and females with CRC however, with females exhibiting a lower maximal clearance. Qualitatively similar, but smaller gender differences in cetuximab clearance were observed in patients with SCCHN. The gender differences do not appear to necessitate any dose modification, because of a similar safety profile.

STORAGE AND STABILITY: Store vials under refrigeration at 2-8°C. Do not freeze. Prepare using appropriate aseptic technique and administer as soon as possible as this product contains no preservatives. ERBITUX (cetuximab) in infusion containers prepared under controlled conditions has been demonstrated to be chemically and physically stable for up to 12 hours at 2-8°C and up to 8 hours at controlled room temperature (20-25°C). It is not recommended to store ERBITUX in the infusion container and any remaining solution should be discarded after 8 hours at controlled room temperature or after 12 hours at 2-8°C.

INFORMATION FOR THE PATIENT: Published in e-CPS, available by subscription at www.e-cps.ca.

DOSAGE FORMS, COMPOSITION AND PACKAGING: Each vial of sterile, preservative-free, injectable liquid contains: cetuximab (2 mg/mL) 100 mg. Nonmedicinal ingredients: hydrochloric acid, NF as 6 M solution, sodium chloride, USP, sodium hydroxide, NF as 10 M solution, sodium phosphate dibasic heptahydrate, USP, sodium phosphate monobasic monohydrate, USP and Water for Injection, USP. Single-use, ready-to-use vials of 50 mL, cartons of 1.

Erdol
ergocalciferol
Vitamin D Supplement

Odan

SUPPLIED: Each mL of solution contains: vitamin D_2 (ergocalciferol solution USP) 8288 IU (207.2 µg) in propylene glycol. Approximately 207 IU (5.17 µg) per drop, (40 drops=approximately 1 mL). Contains no preservatives, artificial flavor, color, lactose, yeast, sodium, sugar, corn, soy, starch, gluten or tartrazine. Bottles of 60 mL with dropper. Store at room temperature (15 to 30°C).

Ergocalciferol
CPhA Monograph

see *Vitamin D*

Ergometrine ℞
CPhA Monograph

see *Ergonovine Maleate*

Ergonovine Maleate ℞
Oxytocic

CPhA Monograph

This monograph has been compiled by CPhA and reviewed by experts. It may contain information different from that found in Health Canada-approved Product Monographs. The reader is referred to the *CPS* Editorial Policy for more information.

PHARMACOLOGY: Ergonovine, also known as ergometrine, directly stimulates contractions of uterine and vascular smooth muscle. The effect on the uterus is more pronounced than that of most other ergot alkaloids, the difference being more marked on the puerperal uterus than on the normal, nonpregnant uterus. Ergonovine is a partial agonist at α-adrenergic, dopaminergic and tryptaminergic receptors. Ergonovine's main effect on the uterus is the production of rhythmic contractions, usually followed by periods of relaxation. Within 6 to 15 minutes after ingestion, oral ergonovine produces a firm tetanic contraction of the postpartum uterus, gradually changing over a period of 90 minutes to a series of clonic contractions that persist for another 90 minutes or more. Parenteral administration causes uterine contractions to begin more rapidly, in 2 or 3 minutes if given i.m., or 1 minute or less if given i.v.

Ergonovine also produces vasoconstriction of coronary arteries and has been used by experienced cardiologists to diagnose coronary artery spasm in patients with variant angina and no major coronary obstruction.

INDICATIONS: Prevention or treatment of postpartum or postabortal hemorrhage due to uterine atony.

CONTRAINDICATIONS: Previous idiosyncrasy or allergic reactions to ergot preparations; pre-eclampsia or eclampsia; hypertension; threatened spontaneous abortion; induction or augmentation of labor.

WARNINGS: See Precautions.

PRECAUTIONS: Ergonovine has been associated with acute attacks of porphyria and should be avoided in patients with porphyria.

Because nausea and vomiting may occur, ergonovine should be administered cautiously to patients under general anesthesia.

Ergonovine must be used cautiously in patients with heart disease; coronary vasoconstriction may occur. Careful monitoring is required if ergonovine is used during cardiac catheterization to diagnose variant angina, as myocardial infarction and death have occurred.

Calcium deficiency can decrease the response of the uterus to ergonovine. Responsiveness can be restored with the cautious administration of i.v. calcium salts.

Prolonged therapy may lead to gangrene and other signs of ergotism.

Drug Interactions: A significant increase in blood pressure may occur, especially when a regional anesthetic containing a vasopressor drug has been used. Avoid prolonged administration or concomitant use of other vasoconstrictors such as sympathomimetics.

Pregnancy: Before ergonovine is administered, the possibility of twin pregnancy should be ruled out and the placenta delivered, to avoid captivation of the placenta.

Lactation: Ergonovine enters breast milk in sufficient quantities to produce ergotism in breast-fed infants during continuous use. However, a single dose of ergonovine, given postpartum to control hemorrhage, need not prevent the mother from breast-feeding.

ADVERSE EFFECTS: Because ergonovine is usually indicated for a short duration, many of the side effects seen with the other ergot alkaloids do not occur.

Central Nervous System: headache, dizziness, vertigo, hallucinations.

Cardiovascular: palpitations, dyspnea, transient chest pain, bradycardia, hypertension that is generally due to an undiluted or too rapid i.v. administration.

Gastrointestinal: nausea and vomiting (usually more common with i.v. administration), diarrhea, abdominal pain.

OVERDOSE:

Symptoms: Acute overdose may cause chest pain, increase or decrease in heart rate or blood pressure, confusion, drowsiness, miosis, peripheral vasoconstriction, respiratory depression, seizures, nausea and vomiting, loss of consciousness, numbness and coldness of the extremities, tingling, hypercoagulability, gangrene of the fingers and toes.

Treatment: Management of acute oral overdose should begin with the administration of activated charcoal and sorbitol, if vomiting is not present. If the patient is vomiting, an antiemetic such as metoclopramide or ondansetron can be used to facilitate the administration of activated charcoal. Seizures should be treated with anticonvulsants. Heparin may be used to manage hypercoagulability. A vasodilator may be required to reverse ischemia in the presence of severe peripheral vasoconstriction, with adjustment of dosage according to heart rate and blood pressure. Hyperbaric oxygen may reverse local tissue hypoxia.

For management of a suspected drug overdose, CPhA recommends that you contact your **regional Poison Control Centre**. See the *CPS* Directory section for a list of Poison Control Centres.

DOSAGE: The immediate postpartum dose of ergonovine, to produce intense uterine contractions and reduce bleeding after delivery of the placenta, is 200 µg (usually administered i.m.). In emergency situations when excessive uterine bleeding has occurred, ergonovine may be administered i.v. over at least 1 minute. It has been recommended that i.v. doses be diluted in 5 mL normal saline. Severe uterine bleeding may require repeated parenteral doses; however, injections will rarely be required more often than every 2 to 4 hours, up to 5 doses. To minimize late postpartum bleeding, 200 or 400 µg may be given orally 2 to 4 times daily, every 6 to 12 hours, until the danger of uterine atony has passed, usually 48 hours.

Eryc™ ℞
erythromycin
Antibiotic

Pfizer

Date of Preparation: September 24, 2003
Date of Revision: January 28, 2009

PHARMACOLOGY: Erythromycin exerts its antibacterial action by binding with the 50S ribosomal subunit of the organism, inhibiting peptide bond formation and protein synthesis within the bacterial cell. The activity is bacteriostatic or bactericidal depending on concentration.

INDICATIONS: ERYC (Erythromycin Capsules) is indicated for the treatment of the following infections caused by susceptible strains of the designated microorganisms.

Upper Respiratory Tract Infections: Those of mild to moderate severity caused by *S. pyogenes* (group A beta-hemolytic streptococci); *S. pneumoniae* (*D. pneumoniae*) and *H. influenzae*. Not all strains of *H. influenzae* are susceptible to erythromycin with usual therapeutic doses.

Lower Respiratory Tract Infections: Those of mild to moderate severity when caused by *S. pyogenes* (group A beta-hemolytic streptococci); *S. pneumoniae* (*D. pneumoniae*) and *M. pneumoniae* (Eaton's agent).

Pertussis (Whooping Cough): Caused by *B. pertussis*. Erythromycin is effective in eliminating the organism from the nasopharynx of infected individuals, rendering them non-infectious. Clinical studies suggest that erythromycin may be helpful in the prophylaxis of pertussis in exposed susceptible individuals.

Diphtheria: As an adjunct to antitoxin in infections due to *C. diphtheriae*, to prevent establishment of carriers and to eradicate the organism in carriers.

Legionnaires' Disease: Caused by *L. pneumophila*. Controlled clinical efficacy studies have not been conducted. In vitro and limited preliminary clinical data suggest that erythromycin can be effective in the treatment of Legionnaires' disease.

Skin and Soft Tissue Infections: Those of mild to moderate severity when caused by *S. pyogenes* and *S. aureus* (resistance of staphylococci may emerge during treatment).

Erythrasma: In the treatment of infections due to *C. minutissimum*.

The treatment of Acne vulgaris.

Sexually Transmitted Diseases: Primary Syphilis: Caused by *T. pallidum*. Erythromycin is an alternative choice for treatment for primary syphilis in patients allergic to the penicillins. Spinal fluid should be examined before treatment and as part of the follow-up after therapy.

Chlamydia Trachomatis Infection: Erythromycin is an alternate choice in the treatment of the following infections when caused by *C. trachomatis*:

a. In infants and children (9 years and older) for conjunctivitis. **Note:** Topical therapy alone for conjunctivitis is **not** adequate.
b. In pregnant women and nursing mothers for urethral, endocervical or rectal infections.
c. In youths and adults, for urethral, endocervical or rectal infections.

Specimens for bacteriologic culture should be obtained prior to therapy in order to isolate and identify the causative organisms and to determine their susceptibility to erythromycin. Therapy may be instituted before results of susceptibility studies are known; however, antibiotic treatment should be re-evaluated when the results become available or if the clinical response is not adequate.

CONTRAINDICATIONS: ERYC (Erythromycin Capsules) should not be used in patients with known hypersensitivity to erythromycin or the product's components, or with infections caused by microorganisms that are resistant to the drug.

ERYC (Erythromycin Capsules) is contraindicated in patients taking terfenadine, astemizole, pimozide, ergotamine, dihydroergotamine or cisapride. There have been post-marketing reports of drug interactions when erythromycin is coadministered with cisapride, astemizole, pimozide or terfenadine resulting in cardiac arrhythmias (QT prolongation, ventricular tachycardia, ventricular fibrillation, and torsades de pointes) most likely due to inhibition of hepatic metabolism of these drugs by erythromycin. Fatalities have been reported (see Precautions, Drug Interactions).

WARNINGS: QT prolongation, ventricular tachycardia, and torsades de pointes have been reported with macrolides, including erythromycin (see Adverse Effects, Contraindications and Precautions, Drug Interactions).

Erythromycin should be administered with caution to any patient who has demonstrated some form of allergy to drugs. If an allergic reaction to erythromycin occurs, administration of the drug should be discontinued. Serious hypersensitivity reactions may require epinephrine, antihistamines or corticosteroids.

Infants born to women treated during pregnancy with oral erythromycin for early syphilis should be treated with an appropriate penicillin regimen since erythromycin does not reach the fetus in adequate concentration.

There have been reports of hepatic dysfunction, with or without jaundice, occurring in patients receiving erythromycin products, particularly erythromycin estolate. If findings suggestive of significant hepatic dysfunction occur, therapy with ERYC (Erythromycin Capsules) should be discontinued.

C. difficile-associated disease (CDAD): *C. difficile*-associated disease (CDAD) has been reported with use of many antibacterial agents, including ERYC (erythromycin). CDAD may range in severity from mild diarrhoea to fatal colitis. It is important to consider this diagnosis in patients who present with diarrhoea, or symptoms of colitis, pseudomembranous colitis, toxic megacolon, or perforation of colon subsequent to the administration of any antibacterial agent. CDAD has been reported to occur over 2 months after the administration of antibacterial agents.

Treatment with antibacterial agents may alter the normal flora of the colon and may permit overgrowth of *C. difficile*. *C. difficile* produces toxins A and B, which contribute to the development of CDAD. CDAD may cause significant morbidity and mortality. CDAD can be refractory to antimicrobial therapy.

If the diagnosis of CDAD is suspected or confirmed, appropriate therapeutic measures should be initiated. Mild cases of CDAD usually respond to discontinuation of antibacterial agents not directed against *C. difficile*. In moderate to severe cases, consideration should be given to management with fluids and electrolytes, protein supplementation, and treatment with an antibacterial agent clinically effective against *C. difficile*. Surgical evaluation should be instituted as clinically indicated, as surgical intervention may be required in certain severe cases (see Adverse Effects).

The risk of myopathy during treatment with certain HMG-CoA reductase inhibitors is increased with concomitant administration of erythromycin. Physicians considering combined therapy should carefully weigh the potential benefits and risks and monitor patients for any signs and symptoms of muscle pain, tenderness, or weakness. (see Precautions, Drug Interactions).

PRECAUTIONS: General: Prolonged or repeated use of ERYC (Erythromycin Capsules) may result in an overgrowth of nonsusceptible bacteria or fungi and organisms initially sensitive to erythromycin. If superinfection occurs, ERYC should be discontinued and appropriate therapy instituted.

Exacerbation of symptoms of myasthenia gravis and new onset of symptoms of myasthenic syndrome has been reported in patients receiving erythromycin therapy.

Since erythromycin is principally excreted by the liver, caution should be exercised when ERYC is administered to patients with impaired hepatic function.

Laboratory Tests: Erythromycin interferes with the fluorometric determination of urinary catecholamines.

Drug Interactions: Terfenadine: Terfenadine undergoes metabolism in the liver by a specific cytochrome P450 isoenzyme. This metabolic pathway may be impaired in patients who are taking erythromycin, an inhibitor of this isoenzyme. Interference with this enzyme can lead to elevated terfenadine plasma levels which may be associated with QT prolongation, and increased risk of ventricular tachyarrhythmias (such as torsades de pointes, ventricular tachycardia, and ventricular fibrillation) (see Contraindications).

Astemizole: Concomitant administration of astemizole with erythromycin is contraindicated because erythromycin is known to impair the Cytochrome P450 enzyme system which also influences astemizole metabolism. There have been two reports to date of syncope with torsades de pointes requiring hospitalization in patients taking astemizole with erythromycin. In each case the QT intervals were prolonged beyond 650 milliseconds at the time of the event; one patient also received ketoconazole and the other patient also had hypokalemia (see Contraindications).

Rare cases of serious cardiovascular adverse events, including death, cardiac arrest and other ventricular arrhythmias have been observed.

Theophylline: The concomitant administration of erythromycin and high doses of theophylline may be associated with increased serum theophylline levels and possible theophylline toxicity. The dose of theophylline may require reduction while patients are receiving ERYC.

Carbamazepine: Erythromycin administration in patients receiving carbamazepine has been reported to cause increased serum levels of carbamazepine with subsequent development of signs of carbamazepine toxicity.

Digoxin/Phenytoin: Concomitant administration of erythromycin and digoxin or phenytoin has been reported to result in elevated serum levels of these agents, leading to toxicity in some patients.

Oral Anticoagulants: There have been reports of increased prothrombin time when erythromycin and oral anticoagulants were used concomitantly. Increased anticoagulation effects due to this drug may be more pronounced in the elderly (see Precautions, Geriatrics).

Ergotamine/Dihydroergotamine: There are reports that ischemic reactions may occur when erythromycin is given concurrently with ergotamine-containing drugs.

Cyclosporin: A rise in plasma cyclosporin levels has been reported during concomitant administration of erythromycin.

Lincomycin/Clindamycin/Chloramphenicol: Erythromycin should be used with caution if administered concomitantly with lincomycin, clindamycin, or chloramphenicol. In vitro experiments have demonstrated that binding sites for erythromycin, lincomycin, clindamycin and chloramphenicol overlap and competitive inhibition may occur.

Triazolam/Midazolam: Erythromycin has been reported to decrease the clearance of triazolam and midazolam and thus may increase the pharmacologic effect of these drugs.

Alfentanil: The concomitant use of erythromycin with alfentanil can significantly inhibit the clearance of alfentanil and may increase the risk of prolonged or delayed respiratory depression.

Lovastatin: Patients receiving concomitant lovastatin and erythromycin should be carefully monitored; cases of rhabdomyolysis have been reported in seriously ill patients.

Cisapride/Pimozide: Rare cases of serious cardiovascular adverse events, including death, cardiac arrest, torsades de pointes, and other ventricular arrhythmias, have been observed in patients taking cisapride concomitantly with macrolide antibiotics including erythromycin.

Atorvastatin: In healthy individuals, coadministration of erythromycin (500 mg qid) was associated with higher plasma concentrations of atorvastatin.

Quinidine: Drug interaction occurring with the concomitant administration of erythromycin and quinidine in their usual oral forms, resulting in QT prolongation, torsades de pointes and cardiac arrest has been reported. Caution and close monitoring is recommended when the drugs are administered concomitantly.

The use of erythromycin in patients taking concurrent drugs which are metabolized by cytochrome P450 (3A4) system may be associated with elevations in serum levels of these other drugs (e.g. pimozide, ergotamine, dihydroergotamine) (see Contraindications). There have been reports of interactions of erythromycin with cyclosporine, tacrolimus, hexobarbital and phenytoin. Serum concentrations of drugs metabolized by the cytochrome P450 system should be monitored closely in patients concurrently receiving erythromycin.

Pregnancy: The safety of ERYC for use during pregnancy has not been established. Erythromycin crosses the placental barrier.

Lactation: The safety of ERYC for use during breast-feeding has not been established. Erythromycin is excreted in breast milk.

Neonates: The safety of ERYC for use in neonates has not been established.

Geriatrics: Clinical studies with ERYC did not include sufficient numbers of subjects aged 65 and over to determine whether they respond differently from younger subjects. In general, dose selection for an elderly patient should be cautious, usually starting at the low end of the dosing range, reflecting the greater frequency of the decreased hepatic, renal, or cardiac function, and of concomitant disease or other drug therapy.

There have been reports of prolonged QT syndrome in geriatric patients receiving erythromycin products.

Elderly patients may experience increased effects of oral anticoagulant therapy while undergoing treatment with erythromycin (see Precautions, Drug Interactions).

ADVERSE EFFECTS: Cardiovascular: QT prolongation, ventricular tachycardia, and torsades de pointes have been reported with macrolides, including erythromycin (see Contraindications, Warnings and Precautions, Drug Interactions).

Gastrointestinal: Abdominal cramping and discomfort have been observed. Nausea, vomiting and diarrhea are also observed, but less frequently. *C. difficile*-associated disease has been observed (see Warnings).

Pancreatitis: There has been a report of a case of erythromycin-induced pancreatitis following erythromycin overdose.

Allergic Reactions: Urticaria, mild skin eruptions and anaphylaxis have been reported.

Hepatotoxicity: There have been reports of hepatic dysfunction, with or without jaundice, occurring in patients receiving erythromycin products.

Miscellaneous: During prolonged or repeated therapy, there is a possibility of overgrowth of nonsusceptible bacteria or fungi and organisms initially sensitive to erythromycin (e.g., *S. aureus, H. influenzae*). If such infections occur, erythromycin should be discontinued and appropriate therapy instituted.

Occasionally there have been reports of reversible hearing loss occurring chiefly in patients with renal insufficiency and in patients receiving high doses of erythromycin.

There have been isolated reports of transient central nervous system side effects including confusion, hallucinations, seizures and vertigo; however, a cause and effect relationship has not been established.

OVERDOSE:

Symptoms: With oral doses of over 2 g per day, abdominal discomfort, nausea or diarrhea may occur. There has been a report of a case of erythromycin-induced pancreatitis following erythromycin overdose.

Treatment: There is no specific treatment for accidental overdosage. ERYC should be discontinued and prompt elimination of unabsorbed drug and all other appropriate measures should be considered which may include use of activated charcoal; otherwise, treatment should be symptomatic. Erythromycin is not removed by peritoneal dialysis or hemodialysis.

For management of a suspected drug overdose, contact your **regional Poison Control Centre**. See the *CPS* Directory section for a list of Poison Control Centres.

DOSAGE: Administration: Blood levels obtained upon administration of ERYC (enteric-coated erythromycin pellets) in the presence of food are above minimum inhibitory concentrations (MICs) of most organisms for which erythromycin is indicated. However, maximum blood levels are obtained in the fasting state (at least 30 minutes and preferably 2 hours before or after a meal).

Adults: The usual dose is 250 mg every 6 hours or 333 mg every 8 hours. If twice-a-day dosage is desired, the recommended dose is 500 mg every 12 hours. Dosage may be increased up to 4 g per day, depending on the severity of infection. Twice-a-day dosing is not recommended when doses larger than 1 g daily are administered.

Children: Age, weight, and severity of the infection are important factors in determining the proper dosage. The usual dosage is 30-50 mg/kg/day in equally divided doses. For the treatment of more severe infections, this dosage may be doubled.

Dosage: Upper and Lower Respiratory Tract and Skin and Soft Tissue Infections: A therapeutic dosage of oral erythromycin should be administered for at least 10 days. The recommended dosage is 1 g per day given in divided doses (2, 3 or 4 times a day), depending on the erythromycin preparation chosen. Depending on the severity of infection doses up to 4 g may be considered; however, a single dose should not exceed 1 g.

Pertussis: Although optimum dosage and duration of therapy have not been established, doses of erythromycin utilized in reported clinical studies were 40 to 50 mg/kg/day, given in divided doses for 5 to 14 days.

Legionnaires' Disease: Large doses of up to 4 g daily in divided doses are necessary for the treatment of known or suspected Legionella infections.

Acne Vulgaris: Initially, up to 1 g per day in divided doses. Depending on clinical response this may then be reduced to 333 to 500 mg per day as a maintenance dose. Extended administration of erythromycin requires regular evaluation, particularly of liver function.

C. Trachomatis Infections:

1. Conjunctivitis in infants: Infants >2000 g: 30 mg/kg/day orally in divided doses for at least 14 days. Infants >1 week to 1 month: 40 mg/kg/day orally in divided doses for at least 14 days. Children 9 years or older as alternative treatment: 40 mg/kg/day orally in divided doses (max. 500 mg qid for 7 days or 250 mg qid for 14 days). **Note:** Topical therapy alone for conjunctivitis is **not** adequate.
2. Urethral, endocervical, rectal infection in pregnant women and nursing mothers: 2 g/day orally in divided doses for 7 days.
3. Youth and adults: urethral, endocervical, rectal infection: 2 g/day orally in divided doses for 7 days.

Note: Erythromycin dosages refer to the use of erythromycin base. Equivalent dosages of other formulations (**except** the estolate which is contraindicated in pregnancy) may be substituted. If erythromycin has been used for treatment, repeat testing after completion of therapy is advisable.

As with all sexually transmitted diseases, follow-up cultures after termination of therapy are recommended in order to assess the microbiological response.

Primary Syphilis: 2-4 g per day given in divided doses either 2, 3 or 4 times-a-day depending on the erythromycin preparation chosen, over a period of 10 to 15 days.

Prophylaxis: For continuous prophylaxis against recurrence of streptococcal infections in adults with a history of rheumatic heart disease, the recommended dose is 250 mg twice-a-day.

See Precautions regarding Alfentanil.

Information to Be Provided to the Patient: ERYC 250 and ERYC 333 mg capsules are not recommended for sprinkling, since the capsules are very full and some of the medication may be lost through spillage. If, however, the capsule is to be opened, care must be taken to open the capsule over food so as not to lose any of the pellets.

1. Hold the capsule with the clear end down. Gently twist off the orange cap to open.
2. Sprinkle the **entire** contents of the capsule on a spoonful of applesauce, fruit jellies, ice cream, etc. The pellets should not be chewed or crushed.
3. Have your child swallow the spoonful of applesauce, fruit jellies or ice cream. Your child should drink some water to make sure all the pellets are swallowed.
4. If the pellets are accidentally spilled, start over with a new capsule.

SUPPLIED: Eryc 250: Each two-tone clear and opaque orange capsule, imprinted "Eryc" and "P-D 696", contains: erythromycin base 250 mg as enteric-coated pellets. Nonmedicinal ingredients: cellulose acetate phthalate, diethyl phthalate, FD&C Yellow No. 6, lactose, methanol, methylene chloride, potassium phosphate monobasic and povidone; capsule shell: FD&C Yellow No. 6, gelatin and titanium dioxide. Gluten-, paraben-, sodium-, sulfite- and tartrazine-free. Bottles of 100 and 500.

Eryc 333: Each two-tone clear and opaque yellow capsule, imprinted "ERYC 333 mg" and "Parke-Davis", contains: erythromycin base 333 mg as enteric-coated pellets. Nonmedicinal ingredients: cellulose acetate phthalate, diethyl phthalate, FD&C Yellow No. 6, lactose, methanol, methylene chloride, potassium phosphate monobasic and povidone; capsule shell: D&C Yellow No. 10, D&C Red No. 33, gelatin and titanium dioxide. Gluten-, paraben-, sulfite- and tartrazine-free. Bottles of 100 and 500.

Store at room temperature below 30°C. Protect from moisture and light.

(Shown in Product Identification Section)

Erysol® Ⓟ

butyl methoxydibenzoylmethane—erythromycin—ethyl alcohol —octyl methoxycinnamate

Topical Acne Therapy

Stiefel, a GSK company

PHARMACOLOGY: Erythromycin exerts its antibacterial action by binding to the 50s ribosomal subunit of susceptible bacteria and suppressing protein synthesis. Erythromycin is usually bacteriostatic but may be bactericidal in high concentrations or against highly susceptible organisms. The precise mechanism of action of erythromycin in the treatment of acne has not been established.

Ethyl alcohol is a drying and peeling agent.

INDICATIONS: In the treatment of inflammatory papular and pustular lesions of acne vulgaris.

Erysol is not indicated for the treatment of cysts or nodules. It is not indicated for use in Grade IV acne.

CONTRAINDICATIONS: In persons who have shown hypersensitivity to erythromycin or any of the other ingredients.

WARNINGS: Erysol is intended for external use only and should be kept away from the eyes, nostrils, mouth and other mucous membranes because of its irritant effects. Concomitant topical anti-acne therapy should be used with caution because a cumulative irritancy effect may occur, especially with preparations having peeling, desquamating or abrasive properties.

PRECAUTIONS: The use of preparations containing antibiotics such as Erysol may be associated with overgrowth of antibiotic resistant organisms, including those initially sensitive to the drug. Cross-resistance between erythromycin and macrolide antibiotics can occur. If this should occur, therapy should be discontinued and appropriate measures taken. A cross-resistance between erythromycin and clindamycin has rarely been reported.

Pregnancy: The safety of Erysol during pregnancy has not been established. Erythromycin crosses the placental barrier.

Lactation: Erythromycin is excreted in human milk. Caution should be exercised whenever Erysol is given to a nursing mother.

ADVERSE EFFECTS: Adverse reactions reported with topical erythromycin preparations such as Erysol include mild to severe skin irritation symptoms including dryness, tenderness, pruritus, desquamation, scaling, coriaceousness, fissuring around the mouth, erythema, urticaria, oiliness and burning sensation.

OVERDOSE:

Symptoms: Accidental ingestion of Erysol (erythromycin and ethyl alcohol) could cause alcoholic intoxication and/or intestinal tract irritation (manifested by abdominal discomfort, cramping, diarrhea or vomiting). Treat with a demulcent.

If Erysol comes into contact with the eye, irrigate with copious amounts of water or irrigation solutions for at least 5 minutes. If discomfort persists, consult a physician.

Excessive frequency of application may result in excessive dryness and scaling, pruritus, tenderness, erythema, desquamation and burning sensation. Discontinue use until condition subsides. Appropriate anti-inflammatory measures may be employed.

Treatment: See Symptoms.

For management of a suspected drug overdose, CPhA recommends that you contact your **regional Poison Control Centre**. See the *CPS* Directory section for a list of Poison Control Centres.

DOSAGE: Apply twice a day to areas affected by acne. These areas should be washed first with a mild soap, rinsed well, and patted dry, followed by application of the gel in a gentle rubbing motion, using fingertips to apply the medication. Wash hands thoroughly after application. Care should be taken to avoid eyes, nostrils, mouth and other mucous membranes.

Ethyl alcohol contributes significantly to the efficacy of Erysol due to its drying and peeling properties. Because ethyl alcohol is potentially irritating, the frequency of application may require adjustment to once a day.

INFORMATION FOR THE PATIENT: Published in e-CPS, available by subscription at www.e-cps.ca.

SUPPLIED: Each g of clear, colorless gel with characteristic odor contains: erythromycin USP 2% (20 mg/g), ethyl alcohol (75%), Parsol MCX 7.5% and Parsol 1789 2%. Sunscreens: SPF15. Nonmedicinal ingredients: cyclomethicone, dioctyl maleate, hydroxypropyl cellulose and isoarachidyl neopentanoate. Tubes of 25 g. Store at 15 to 30°C.

Erythromycin Pr

erythromycin
erythromycin estolate
erythromycin ethylsuccinate
erythromycin lactobionate
erythromycin stearate

Antibiotic

CPhA Monograph

Date of Revision: May 2009

This monograph has been compiled by CPhA and reviewed by experts. It may contain information different from that found in Health Canada-approved Product Monographs. The reader is referred to the *CPS* Editorial Policy for more information.

SUMMARY PRODUCT INFORMATION:

Drug	Route of Administration	Dosage Form	Strength
Single Entity			
Erythromycin	Oral	Tablet	250 mg
	Oral	Capsule, enteric-coated pellets	250 mg, 333 mg
	Topical	Ophthalmic Ointment	5 mg/g
Erythromycin estolate[a]	Oral	Powder for suspension	125 mg/5 mL, 250 mg/5 mL
Erythromycin ethylsuccinate[a]	Oral	Tablet	600 mg
	Oral	Granules for suspension	200 mg/5 mL, 400 mg/5 mL
Erythromycin lactobionate	IV	Powder	500 mg/vial, 1 g/vial
Erythromycin stearate[a]	Oral	Tablet	250 mg, 500 mg
Combinations			
Erythromycin/benzoyl peroxide	Topical	Gel	erythromycin 3% plus benzoyl peroxide 5% per gram (46.6 g)
Erythromycin/ethyl alcohol/ Parsol MCX/Parsol 1789	Topical	Gel	erythromycin 2% plus ethyl alcohol plus Parsol MCX 7.5% plus Parsol 1789 2%
Erythromycin/tretinoin	Topical	Gel	erythromycin 4% plus tretinoin 0.05% erythromycin 4% plus tretinoin 0.01% erythromycin 4% plus tretinoin 0.025%

[a] Erythromycin ethylsuccinate 400 mg is considered equivalent to 250 mg of the base, stearate or estolate.

PHARMACOLOGY: Erythromycin, a macrolide antibiotic produced by *Streptomyces erythreus*, inhibits protein synthesis by binding reversibly to the 50S ribosomal subunits of susceptible microorganisms. Its action may be either bacteriostatic or bactericidal depending on the sensitivity of the microorganism and the concentration of the drug. Erythromycin is generally active against gram-positive cocci, although resistant organisms are increasingly isolated worldwide. Most gram-positive bacilli are also sensitive, including *B. anthracis*, Clostridium, Corynebacterium, Erysipelothrix, *L. monocytogenes* and some Mycobacterium species. Erythromycin is also active in vitro against some gram-negative cocci such as Neisseria, some gram-negative bacilli including Legionella, Pasteurella and Brucella, and gram-negative coccobacilli such as *C. jejuni* and *B. pertussis*.

Erythromycin inhibits some Chlamydia, Actinomyces, *M. pneumoniae*, *U. urealyticum*, Rickettsia, *E. histolytica* and spirochetes (*T. pallidum* and *B. burgdorferi*). Enterobacteriaceae and Pseudomonas are resistant to erythromycin.

Erythromycin binds to motilin receptors in the gut, acting as an agonist. This prokinetic effect results in accelerated gastric emptying, an effect which is utilized therapeutically in the treatment of gastroparesis.

Pharmacokinetics: Absorption of orally administered erythromycin occurs mainly in the duodenum. The bioavailability of the drug is variable and depends on several factors including the formulation of the dosage form administered, acid-stability of the derivative, presence of food in the gastrointestinal tract and gastric emptying time. Peak levels are generally reached within 1 to 4 hours following oral administration.

Erythromycin is widely distributed into most body tissues and fluids including the middle ear exudate in patients with otitis media, and prostatic fluid and semen. It is distributed into breast milk, reaching concentrations approximately 50% of maternal serum concentrations. Erythromycin crosses the placenta; fetal serum concentrations are approximately 5 to 20% of maternal serum concentrations. It does not cross the blood brain barrier.

The extent of binding to plasma proteins varies among the different forms, ranging from 75 to 95%. The half-life ranges from 0.8 to 3 hours. Erythromycin is partly metabolized in the liver and mainly excreted unchanged in the bile; small amounts are also excreted in urine.

Only small amounts of erythromycin are removed by hemodialysis.

INDICATIONS: Erythromycin is usually the drug of choice for the treatment of infections caused by Bartonella spp, *B. pertussis*, Campylobacter spp and *C. minutissimum* (erythasma) as well as for genital ulcers caused by *H. ducreyi* (chancroid).

Erythromycin is also indicated for the treatment of the following infections when caused by susceptible organisms although in many cases newer macrolides (azithromycin and clarithromycin) may be preferred mainly due to better tolerability:

- Respiratory tract infections: pneumonia caused by *M. pneumoniae*, *C. pneumoniae* or *S. pneumoniae*; diphtheria (prophylaxis and treatment); Legionnaires' disease; streptococcal pharyngitis in patients allergic to penicillin; sinusitis (alternative)
- Skin and soft tissue infections: mild-moderate infections
- Urogenital infections: endocervical/urethral/rectal infections caused by *C. trachomatis* (alternative); lymphogranuloma venereum (preferred treatment in pregnancy); granuloma inguinale (Donovanosis); *U. urealyticum* urethritis
- Acne vulgaris
- Chlamydial ophthalmia neonatorum
- Alternative treatment for actinomycosis; anthrax; relapsing fever (Borrelia spp); early Lyme disease (less effective than amoxicillin or doxycycline)

Erythromycin is used in the long-term prophylaxis of rheumatic fever as an alternative to penicillin. Other macrolides (clarithromycin and azithromycin) are recommended in place of erythromycin for use in penicillin-allergic patients in the 2007 American Heart Association recommendations for prevention of bacterial endocarditis mainly due to better tolerability.

Erythromycin is used in the treatment of gastroparesis (iv more effective than oral).

Ophthalmic Ointment: For the treatment of superficial ocular infections involving the conjunctiva and/or cornea caused by organisms susceptible to erythromycin. For prophylaxis of ophthalmia neonatorum due to *N. gonorrhoeae* or *C. trachomatis*.

Topical Gel: Topical treatment of acne vulgaris, primarily in the treatment of the inflammatory papular lesions; superficial infections of the skin.

CONTRAINDICATIONS: Patients who are hypersensitive to erythromycin, its derivatives or to any ingredient in the formulation or component of the container. Erythromycin estolate is contraindicated in persons with pre-existing liver disease or dysfunction and during pregnancy.

The manufacturer states that erythromycin is contraindicated in patients taking cisapride or pimozide (see Precautions).

PRECAUTIONS: The possibility of superinfection caused by overgrowth of nonsusceptible bacteria or fungi should be considered during prolonged or repeated therapy, especially when other antibacterial agents are given concurrently. In such instances the drug should be withdrawn and appropriate treatment instituted.

Use with caution in patients with impaired hepatic function or impaired biliary excretion.

Use high doses of erythromycin with caution, particularly when given parenterally, in patients with a history of cardiac arrhythmias or QT prolongation.

Concomitant use of erythromycin and cisapride or pimozide has been associated with elevated cisapride or pimozide levels resulting in QT prolongation and serious cardiac arrhythmias.

Pseudomembranous colitis associated with erythromycin therapy has been reported.

Erythromycin, particularly the estolate, may cause a reversible cholestatic hepatitis. A prodromal syndrome consisting of abdominal cramps, nausea and vomiting may precede the onset of biliary colic, fever, anorexia and hepatic enlargement with or without jaundice. Leukocytosis and eosinophilia may occur, as well as changes in hepatic enzymes, bilirubin and hepatic function tests.

Hepatotoxicity is most likely to occur in adults who have received erythromycin estolate for longer than 10 days, or with repeated courses. Although the hepatotoxic effects are reversible, symptoms may take several weeks to subside after discontinuation of the drug.

Caution is advised in patients with myasthenia gravis as erythromycin and other macrolides have been associated with aggravation of this condition.

Erythromycin has been associated with infantile hypertrophic pyloric stenosis when used in neonates. As erythromycin may be used for infections associated with significant morbidity and mortality in this population (e.g., pertussis) its use should be preceded by careful consideration to risk and benefit. Caregivers should be advised to contact their physician if the infant develops vomiting or irritability while feeding.

An increased risk of cerebral palsy in children born to mothers given erythromycin for preterm labour (PTL) with intact membranes has been documented [*Lancet* 2008;372(9646):1319-27]. The routine use of antibiotics in PTL is not warranted without obvious infection where a clear benefit is evident. The same risk was not seen in women given erythromycin for preterm premature rupture of the membranes [*Lancet* 2008;372(9646):1310-8].

Topical Gel: For external use only. Avoid contact with the eyes, nostrils, mouth and other mucous membranes. As it contains drying and peeling agents that are potential irritants, reduction in frequency of application may be necessary to avoid excessive irritation. The use of preparations containing antibiotics may be associated with overgrowth of nonsusceptible organisms. If this should occur, therapy should be discontinued and appropriate measures taken. Concomitant topical antiacne therapy should be avoided because a cumulative irritancy effect may occur, particularly with those preparations containing peeling, desquamating or abrasive agents.

Drug Interactions: Erythromycin is an inhibitor of the cytochrome P450 isoenzymes CYP1A2 and CYP3A4. Concomitant use of erythromycin with substrates of these isoenzymes (e.g., alfentanil, alprazolam, atorvastatin, carbamazepine, cisapride, clozapine, colchicine, cyclosporine, felodipine, lovastatin, midazolam, pimozide, quinidine, ritonavir, sertraline, sildenafil, simvastatin, theophylline and verapamil) can result in higher serum concentrations and increased risk of toxicity of these agents, due to inhibition of their metabolism by erythromycin. Close monitoring, dosage adjustment or withholding doses when clinically appropriate (e.g., atorvastatin) may be necessary when erythromycin is used in patients taking these drugs.

Concomitant use of erythromycin and drugs that inhibit CYP3A4 (e.g., ketoconazole, itraconazole, diltiazem, verapamil) was associated with an increased incidence of cardiac-related sudden death according to a population-based study. It appears likely that concomitant use of these drugs may increase plasma erythromycin concentrations resulting in an increased risk of QT prolongation and serious ventricular arrhythmias. Avoid combination with disopyramide. Since erythromycin is a CYP3A4 inhibitor it may also increase plasma diltiazem and verapamil concentrations. It has been suggested that erythromycin not be used concomitantly with these drugs. Because of the high number of potential interactions associated with erythromycin it is recommended to consult a reputable drug interaction reference for more information.

Chloramphenicol: Antagonism with erythromycin. Avoid combination.

Colchicine: Colchicine is a substrate for both CYP3A4 and p-glycoprotein. Because erythromycin inhibits CYP3A4 and p-glycoprotein, colchicine levels may rise. Colchicine toxicity includes abdominal pain, myalgia, vomiting or pancytopenia. Avoid combination.

Dabigatran: Increased systemic exposure and subsequent risk of bleeding may be expected due to inhibition of p-glycoprotein. Concomitant use is not recommended.

Digoxin: In a small proportion of patients (<10%) in which digoxin is metabolized by gastrointestinal bacteria, the concomitant administration of erythromycin may cause increased serum digoxin levels by altering the gastrointestinal flora. Increase in serum digoxin concentration may occur up to several weeks after the discontinuation of erythromycin. With concomitant use, monitor patients for potential increases in the response to digoxin; a lower dose of digoxin may be needed in certain patients.

Ergot Derivatives: Ergot toxicity has been reported with concomitant use of erythromycin. Inhibition of CYP3A4 by erythromycin is the likely mechanism. Select a non-interacting macrolide if possible.

Lincosamide Antibiotics (clindamycin, lincomycin): Antagonism with these agents. Avoid combination.

QT Prolonging Drugs (e.g., amiodarone, amitriptyline, cisapride, disopyramide, mefloquine, quetiapine, quinidine, risperidone, thioridazine): Additive effects may lead to life-threatening ventricular arrythmias. Avoid or monitor as appropriate.

Theophylline Derivatives: Erythromycin inhibits metabolism of theophylline, increasing serum levels and subsequent risk of theophylline toxicity. A decrease in erythromycin levels has been observed with concomitant theophylline and oral erythromycin use.

Warfarin: There have been reports of increased anticoagulant effects when erythromycin is used concurrently with warfarin. Closely monitor INR or prothrombin time when erythromycin is added to or deleted from a drug regimen which includes warfarin. Adjust warfarin dosage as necessary.

Drug-Food Interactions: See Dosage, Oral.

Grapefruit Juice: As an intestinal inhibitor of CYP3A4, grapefruit juice may inhibit metabolism of erythromycin, increasing adverse effects. Grapefruit juice should be avoided during erythromycin therapy.

Pregnant Women: Erythromycin crosses the placenta, reaching fetal serum concentrations of 5 to 20% of maternal serum levels. Erythromycin is used for the treatment of chlamydial infections during pregnancy and has not been associated with an increased risk of fetal malformations. Erythromycin estolate is contraindicated during pregnancy because it has been associated with an increased risk of reversible, subclinical hepatotoxicity in 10% of pregnant women taking the drug. A different formulation should be selected.

Nursing Women: Erythromycin is excreted into breast milk, reaching concentrations of about 50% of the maternal plasma concentration. The use of erythromycin in breast-feeding mothers has not been reported to pose any significant risk to the infant. According to the American Academy of Pediatrics, erythromycin is considered compatible with breast-feeding.

ADVERSE EFFECTS: Cardiovascular: QT_c prolongation, ventricular arrhythmias, torsades de pointes (rare). These effects have been seen more frequently with iv administration.

Gastrointestinal: The most frequent adverse effects are gastrointestinal (such as abdominal pain and cramping) and are dose related. Nausea, vomiting and diarrhea also occur, especially after large doses. Pancreatitis has been reported. Infantile hypertrophic pyloric stenosis (see Precautions).

Hepatic: Elevated transaminase levels (AST, ALT), cholestatic jaundice, cholestatic hepatitis (2 to 4%). Risk of hepatotoxicity is thought to be greater with the estolate and ethylsuccinate salts and with increased duration and dose of therapy.

Hypersensitivity: Serious allergic reactions to erythromycin have been extremely infrequent. Mild allergic reactions, such as urticaria and morbilliform skin rashes have occurred. Should a patient demonstrate signs of anaphylaxis, administer appropriate measures such as epinephrine, corticosteroid and antihistamines, and withdraw the antibiotic.

Local: IV administration may cause venous irritation and thrombophlebitis. These effects may be minimized by using a more dilute solution and infusing slowly.

Neurological: CNS side effects including seizures, hallucinations, confusion and vertigo have been reported occasionally; however, a cause and effect relationship has not been established.

Otic: Reversible ototoxicity, tinnitus and vertigo have been reported rarely. Ototoxicity is more likely in the elderly, in patients receiving large doses or those who have impaired renal or hepatic function.

Topical Gel: Symptoms of irritation: erythema, desquamation, tenderness and excessive dryness.

OVERDOSE:

Symptoms: Nausea, vomiting, diarrhea and abdominal pain are common. Rarely, hypotension, hypothermia and pancreatitis have occurred.

Topical Solution: Accidental ingestion could result in alcoholic intoxication and/or intestinal tract irritation manifested by vomiting, cramping, diarrhea.

Treatment: Milk, food or antacids can be given to minimize gastric discomfort. Activated charcoal should be given for large ingestions.

Topical Solution: Treat with a demulcent. If eye contact with erythromycin topical solution occurs, wash with copious amounts of water for at least 5 minutes. If discomfort persists, a physician should be contacted.

Excessive frequency of application can cause erythema, excessive scaling and sensations of burning and tenderness. Appropriate anti-inflammatory measures (e.g., compresses or topical corticosteroids) may be employed.

> For management of a suspected drug overdose, CPhA recommends that you contact your **regional Poison Control Centre**. See the *CPS* Directory section for a list of Poison Control Centres.

DOSAGE: Oral erythromycin is available as the base or as the estolate, ethylsuccinate or stearate salt. Erythromycin lactobionate is available as a parenteral formulation. Erythromycin base is also available as an ophthalmic ointment and as a topical solution.

Oral: When given orally, erythromycin and its derivatives, with the exception of erythromycin estolate, are variably susceptible to inactivation by acid in the stomach. This can be reduced by administering film-coated erythromycin stearate or base preparations at least 1 hour before meals. Enteric-coated erythromycin base and erythromycin estolate may be taken without regard to meals, although taking the estolate with food lessens gastrointestinal side effects. Erythromycin ethylsuccinate is optimally absorbed when taken immediately following meals.

The following dosages are expressed in terms of erythromycin base. Erythromycin ethylsuccinate 400 mg is considered equivalent to 250 mg of the base, stearate or estolate. Individual product monographs should be consulted for specific information on dosage and administration of the available erythromycin formulations. Unless otherwise specified, the adult dose is given.

Antibacterial: 250 mg every 6 hours; 333 mg every 8 hours; 500 mg every 12 hours (maximum 4 g daily depending on infection severity). Children: 7.5 to 12.5 mg/kg every 6 hours; 15 to 25 mg/kg every 12 hours (maximum 4 g daily depending on infection severity).

Acne: 250 mg every 6 hours; 333 mg every 8 hours; 500 mg every 12 hours. After 4 weeks, maintenance of 333 to 500 mg once daily.

Bartonellosis: 500 mg 4 times daily for at least 3 months.

Chlamydial Infections of Endocervix, Urethra, Rectum or Conjunctiva: The 2008 Canadian STI guidelines recommends, as alternative therapy, an adult dose of 500 mg every 6 hours for 7 days or 250 mg every 6 hours for 14 days. Can substitute with other erythromycin salts. The estolate salt is contraindicated in pregnancy. Erythromycin is the recommended treatment in pregnant and nursing women for chlamydial infections of endocervical, urethral and rectal infection. Perform test of cure in all pregnant and nursing women 3 to 4 weeks after treatment completion.

Children, First Week of Life: <2 kg: 20 mg/kg/day po in divided doses for 14 days; >2 kg: 30 mg/kg/day in divided doses for 14 days. Children, >1 week to 1 month: 40 mg/kg/day in divided doses for 14 days. Children >1 month to 18 years: Alternative choice of therapy: 40 mg/kg/day in divided doses, maximum dose 500 mg four times daily for 7 days or 250 mg four times daily for 14 days. Can substitute with other erythromycin salts. Perform test of cure in all prepubertal children 3 to 4 weeks after treatment completion.

Chancroid: 500 mg every 6–8 hours for 7 days.

Chlamydial Pneumonia of Infancy: 12.5 mg/kg every 6 hours for 14 days.

Diphtheria: As an adjunct with diphtheria antitoxin 500 mg every 6 hours for 14 days. Infants and Children: 10 to 12.5 mg/kg every 6 hours for 14 days (maximum 2 g daily).

Enteritis, Campylobacter (*C. jejuni*): 500 mg 2 times daily for 5 days. Children: 20 mg/kg every 12 hours for 5 days.

Erythasma (*C. minutissimum*): 250 mg 4 times daily for 14 days.

Gastroparesis: 200 mg iv initially then 250 mg 3 times daily, 30 minutes before meals.

Granuloma Inguinale and Lymphogranuloma Venereum: The Canadian STI guidelines recommends, as an alternative choice of therapy, an adult dose of 500 mg every 6 hours for 21 days.

Lyme Disease (Erythema migrans): 500 mg 4 times daily for 14 to 21 days. Children: 12.5 mg/kg every 6 hours for 14 to 21 days. Use recommended only if unable to take amoxicillin, doxycycline and cefuroxime axetil.

Pertussis: 500 mg every 6 hours for 14 days. Infants and Children: 10 to 12.5 mg/kg every 6 hours for 14 days (maximum 2 g daily).

Streptococcal Pharyngitis: 500 mg every 12 hours. Children: 5 to 7.5 mg/kg every 6 hours or 10 to 15 mg/kg every 12 hours for at least 10 days.

Streptococcus Prophylaxis: 250 mg every 12 hours.

Urethritis, Nongonococcal, *U. urealyticum*: 500 mg every 6 hours for 7 days.

Renal Failure: No dosage adjustment is necessary for patients with mild to moderate renal failure. Patients with severe renal failure (ClCr <0.17 mL/s) may receive half of the usual dosage.

Parenteral (IV): For use when large doses of erythromycin are needed but not tolerated orally. Oral therapy should replace iv administration as soon as possible.

Erythromycin must be adequately and properly diluted and administered slowly to avoid local venous irritation.

Adults: Usual dose is 250 to 500 mg every 6 hours. Up to 4 g daily in more severe infections.

Children: 15 to 20 mg/kg daily divided into 4 doses.

Topical: Ophthalmic Ointment: In the treatment of external ocular infections, apply the ointment directly to the infected structure 1 or more times daily, depending on the severity of the infection.

For prophylaxis of neonatal gonococcal or chlamydial conjunctivitis, a ribbon of ointment approximately 0.5 to 1 cm in length should be instilled into each conjunctival sac. The ointment should not be flushed from the eye following instillation. A new tube should be used for each infant. Infants born by cesarean section as well as those delivered by the vaginal route should receive prophylaxis. For treatment of established infection oral therapy is necessary.

Topical Gel: Apply each morning and evening to the areas affected by acne. Before applying, areas should be washed with mild soap, rinsed well and patted dry. Use fingertips to apply medication. Wash hands after use. Because the drying and peeling agents in erythromycin gel are potentially irritating, the frequency of application may require adjustment.

Escitalopram

CPhA Monograph

see *Selective Serotonin Reuptake Inhibitors*

Estalis®

norethindrone acetate—estradiol-17β

Progestin—Estrogen

Novartis Pharmaceuticals

Date of Revision: May 31, 2010

SUMMARY PRODUCT INFORMATION:

Route of Administration	Dosage Form/ Strength	Clinically Relevant Nonmedicinal Ingredients
Transdermal	Patch 140/50 µg/day and 250/50 µg/day	The other substances are silicone (BIO PSA X7-4603), acrylic (Gelva 737)-based multipolymeric adhesive, povidone USP, oleic acid NF, and dipropylene glycol.

INDICATIONS AND CLINICAL USE: ESTALIS (NETA/estradiol-17β) is indicated for:

- the relief of menopausal and postmenopausal symptoms occurring in naturally or surgically induced estrogen deficiency states e.g. hot flushes, sleep disturbances and vulvar and vaginal atrophy.

The above indication is only for women with intact uteri since the regimen includes a progestin whose role is to prevent endometrial hyperplasia/carcinoma.

Geriatrics (>65 years of age): No clinical studies were conducted to evaluate the effect of ESTALIS on women more than 65 years old.

Pediatrics: ESTALIS should not be used in children.

CONTRAINDICATIONS:

- Known or suspected hypersensitivity to this drug or to any ingredient in the formulation or to any component of the patch. For a complete listing, see Dosage Forms, Composition and Packaging.
- Known or suspected estrogen-dependent or progestin-dependent malignant neoplasia such as endometrial cancer
- Endometrial hyperplasia
- Known, suspected or past history of breast cancer
- Known or suspected pregnancy
- Active or past history of confirmed venous thromboembolism (such as deep venous thrombosis or pulmonary embolism) or active thrombophlebitis
- Known thrombophilic disorders
- Liver dysfunction or disease as long as liver function tests have failed to return to normal
- Undiagnosed abnormal genital bleeding
- Active or past history of arterial thromboembolic disease (e.g. stroke, myocardial infarction, coronary heart disease)
- Porphyria
- Partial or complete loss of vision from ophthalmic vascular disease
- Classical migraine
- Breast feeding

WARNINGS AND PRECAUTIONS:

> **Serious Warnings and Precautions**
>
> The Women's Health Initiative (WHI) trial examined the health benefits and risks of oral combined estrogen plus progestin therapy (n=16 608) and oral estrogen-alone therapy (n=10 739) in postmenopausal women aged 50 to 79 years.
>
> The estrogen plus progestin arm of the WHI trial (mean age 63.3 years) indicated an increased risk of myocardial infarction (MI), stroke, invasive breast cancer, pulmonary emboli and deep vein thrombosis in postmenopausal women receiving treatment with combined conjugated equine estrogens (CEE, 0.625 mg/day) and medroxyprogesterone acetate (MPA, 2.5 mg/day) for 5.2 years compared to those receiving placebo.
>
> The estrogen-alone arm of the WHI trial (mean age 63.6 years) indicated an increased risk of stroke and deep vein thrombosis in hysterectomized women treated with CEE-alone (0.625 mg/day) for 6.8 years compared to those receiving placebo.
>
> Therefore, the following should be given serious consideration at the time of prescribing:
>
> - Estrogens with or without progestins **should not** be prescribed for primary or secondary prevention of cardiovascular diseases.
> - Estrogens with or without progestins should be prescribed at **the lowest effective dose** for the approved indication.
> - Estrogens with or without progestins should be prescribed for **the shortest period** possible for the approved indication.

Carcinogenesis and Mutagenesis: Breast Cancer: Available epidemiological data indicate that the use of combined estrogen plus progestin by postmenopausal women is associated with an increased risk of invasive breast cancer. In the estrogen plus progestin arm of the WHI trial, among 10 000 women over a one-year period, there were:

- 8 more cases of invasive breast cancer (38 on combined HRT versus 30 on placebo).

The WHI study also reported that the invasive breast cancers diagnosed in the estrogen plus progestin group were similar in histology but were larger (mean (SD), 1.7 cm (1.1) vs. 1.5 cm (0.9), respectively; P=0.04) and were at a more advanced stage compared with those diagnosed in the placebo group. The percentage of women with abnormal mammograms (recommendations for short-interval follow-up, a suspicious abnormality, or highly suggestive of malignancy) was significantly higher in the estrogen plus progestin group versus the placebo group. This difference appeared at year one and persisted in each year thereafter.

In the estrogen-alone arm of the WHI trial, there was no statistically significant difference in the rate of invasive breast cancer in hysterectomized women treated with conjugated equine estrogens versus women treated with placebo.

It is recommended that estrogens with or without progestins not be given to women with existing breast cancer or those with a previous history of the disease (see Contraindications).

There is a need for caution in prescribing estrogens with or without progestins for women with known risk factors associated with the development of breast cancer, such as strong family history of breast cancer (first degree relative) or who present a breast condition with an increased risk (breast nodules, fibrocystic disease of the breast, abnormal mammograms and/or atypical hyperplasia at breast biopsy).

Other known risk factors for the development of breast cancer such as nulliparity, obesity, early menarche, late age at first full term pregnancy and at menopause should also be evaluated.

It is recommended that women undergo mammography prior to the start of HRT treatment and at regular intervals during treatment, as deemed appropriate by the treating physician and according to the perceived risks for each patient.

The overall benefits and possible risks of hormone replacement therapy should be fully considered and discussed with patients. It is important that the modest increased risk of being diagnosed with breast cancer after 4 years of treatment with combined estrogen plus progestin HRT (as reported in the results of WHI-trial) be discussed with the patient and weighed against its known benefits.

Instructions for regular self-examination of the breasts should be included in this counselling.

Endometrial Hyperplasia & Endometrial Carcinoma: Estrogen should be prescribed with an appropriate dosage of a progestin for women with intact uteri in order to prevent endometrial hyperplasia/carcinoma.

The risk of endometrial hyperplasia/carcinoma in users of unopposed estrogens who have intact uteri is greater than in non-users and appears to depend on the duration of treatment and the estrogen dose. The greatest risk appears to be associated with prolonged use. It has been shown that adequate concomitant progestogen therapy lowers the incidence of endometrial hyperplasia and therefore the potential risk of endometrial carcinoma associated with prolonged use of estrogen therapy (see Action and Clinical Pharmacology, Coadministration of Progestins).

Ovarian Cancer: Some recent epidemiologic studies have found that the use of hormone replacement therapy (estrogen-alone and estrogen plus progestin therapies), in particular for five or more years, has been associated with an increased risk of ovarian cancer.

Hepatocellular Carcinomas: Hepatocellular carcinoma has also been reported in women taking estrogen containing oral contraceptives. The causal relationship of this malignancy to these drugs is not known.

Cardiovascular: The results of the Heart and Estrogen/progestin Replacement Studies (HERS and HERS II) and the Women's Health Initiative (WHI) trial indicate that the use of estrogen plus progestin is associated with an increased risk of coronary heart disease (CHD) in postmenopausal women. The results of the WHI trial indicate that the use of estrogen-alone and estrogen plus progestin is associated with an increased risk of stroke in postmenopausal women.

WHI Trial Findings: In the combined estrogen plus progestin arm of the WHI trial, among 10 000 women over a one-year period, there were:

- 8 more cases of stroke (29 on combined HRT versus 21 on placebo)
- 7 more cases of CHD (37 on combined HRT versus 30 on placebo).

In the estrogen-alone arm of the WHI trial of women with prior hysterectomy, among 10 000 women over a one-year period, there were/was:

• 12 more cases of stroke (44 on estrogen-alone therapy versus 32 on placebo)
• no statistically significant difference in the rate of CHD.

HERS and HERS II Findings: In the Heart and Estrogen/progestin Replacement Study (HERS) of postmenopausal women with documented heart disease (n=2763, average age 66.7 years), a randomized placebo-controlled clinical trial of secondary prevention of coronary heart disease (CHD), treatment with 0.625 mg/day oral conjugated equine estrogen (CEE) plus 2.5 mg medroxyprogesterone acetate (MPA) demonstrated no cardiovascular benefit. Specifically, during an average follow-up of 4.1 years, treatment with CEE plus MPA did not reduce the overall rate of CHD events in postmenopausal women with established coronary heart disease. There were more CHD events in the hormone-treated group than in the placebo group in year 1, but not during the subsequent years.

From the original HERS trial, 2321 women consented to participate in an open label extension of HERS, known as HERS II. Average follow-up in HERS II was an additional 2.7 years, for a total of 6.8 years overall. After 6.8 years, hormone therapy did not reduce the risk of cardiovascular events in women with CHD.

Blood Pressure: Women using hormone replacement therapy sometimes experience increased blood pressure. Blood pressure should be monitored with HRT use. Elevation of blood pressure in previously normotensive or hypertensive patients should be investigated and HRT may have to be discontinued.

Ear/Nose/Throat: Otosclerosis: Estrogens should be used with caution in patients with otosclerosis.

Endocrine and Metabolism: Glucose and Lipid Metabolism: A worsening of glucose tolerance and lipid metabolism have been observed in a significant percentage of peri- and post-menopausal patients. Therefore, diabetic patients or those with a predisposition to diabetes should be observed closely to detect any alterations in carbohydrate or lipid metabolism, especially in triglyceride blood levels.

Women with familial hypertriglyceridemia need special surveillance. Lipid-lowering measures are recommended additionally, before treatment is started.

Calcium and Phosphorus Metabolism: Because the prolonged use of estrogens with or without progestins influences the metabolism of calcium and phosphorus, estrogens with or without progestins should be used with caution in patients with metabolic and malignant bone diseases associated with hypercalcemia, and in patients with renal insufficiency.

Hypothyroidism: Patients who require thyroid hormone replacement therapy and who are also taking estrogen should have their thyroid function monitored regularly to assure that thyroid hormone levels remain in an acceptable range (see Drug Interactions, Drug-Laboratory Test Interactions).

Genitourinary: Vaginal Bleeding: Abnormal vaginal bleeding, due to its prolongation, irregularity or heaviness, occurring during therapy should prompt appropriate diagnostic measures to rule out the possibility of uterine malignancy and the treatment should be re-evaluated.

Uterine Leiomyomata: Pre-existing uterine leiomyomata may increase in size during estrogen use. Growth, pain or tenderness of uterine leiomyomata requires discontinuation of medication and appropriate investigation.

Endometriosis: Symptoms and physical findings associated with a previous diagnosis of endometriosis may reappear or become aggravated with estrogen use.

Hematologic: Venous Thromboembolism: Available epidemiological data indicate that the use of estrogen with or without progestin by postmenopausal women is associated with an increased risk of developing venous thromboembolism (VTE).

In the estrogen plus progestin arm of the WHI trial, among 10 000 women on combined HRT over a one-year period, there were 18 more cases of venous thromboembolism, including 8 more cases of pulmonary embolism.

In the estrogen-alone arm of the WHI trial, among 10 000 women on estrogen therapy over a one-year period, there were 7 more cases of venous thromboembolism, although there was no statistically significant difference in the rate of pulmonary embolism.

Generally recognized risk factors for VTE include a personal history, a family history (the occurrence of VTE in a direct relative at a relatively early age may indicate genetic predisposition), severe obesity (body mass index >30 kg/m^2) and systemic lupus erythematosus. The risk of VTE also increases with age and smoking.

A history of recurrent spontaneous abortions should be investigated to exclude thrombophilic predisposition. In patients in whom thrombophilia is confirmed, the use of ESTALIS is viewed as contraindicated.

The risk of VTE may be temporarily increased with prolonged immobilization, major surgery, or trauma In women on HRT, attention should be given to prophylactic measures to prevent VTE following surgery. Also, patients with varicose veins should be closely supervised. The physician should be alert to the earliest manifestations of thrombotic disorders (thrombophlebitis, retinal thrombosis, cerebral embolism and pulmonary embolism). If these occur or are suspected, hormone therapy should be discontinued immediately given the risks of long-term disability or fatality.

If feasible, estrogens with or without progestins should be discontinued at least 4 weeks before major surgery which may be associated with an increased risk of thromboembolism, or during periods of prolonged immobilization. The treatment should not be restarted until the woman is completely mobile.

Hepatic/Biliary/Pancreatic: Benign Hepatic Adenomas: Benign hepatic adenomas have been associated with the use of combined estrogen and progestin oral contraceptives. Although benign and rare, these tumours may rupture and cause death from intra-abdominal hemorrhage. Such lesions have not yet been reported in association with other estrogen or progestin preparations, but they should be considered if abdominal pain and tenderness, abdominal mass, or hypovolemic shock occurs in patients receiving estrogen.

Gallbladder Diseases: A 2- to 4-fold increase in the risk of gallbladder disease requiring surgery in women receiving postmenopausal estrogens has been reported.

Hepatic Hemangiomas: Particular caution is indicated in women with hepatic hemangiomas, as estrogen may cause an exacerbation of this condition.

Jaundice: Caution is advised in patients with a history of liver and/or biliary disorders. If cholestatic jaundice develops during treatment, the treatment should be discontinued and appropriate investigations carried out.

Liver Function Tests: Liver function tests should be done periodically in subjects who are suspected of having hepatic disease. For information on endocrine and liver function tests, see Monitoring and Laboratory Tests.

Immune: Angioedema: Estrogens may induce or exacerbate symptoms of angioedema, in particular in women with hereditary angioedema.

Systemic Lupus Erythematosus: Particular caution is indicated in women with systemic lupus erythematosus.

Neurologic: Cerebrovascular Insufficiency: Patients who develop visual disturbances, classical migraine, transient aphasia, paralysis or loss of consciousness should discontinue medication.

Dementia: Available epidemiological data indicate that the use of combined estrogen plus progestin in women age 65 and over may increase the risk of developing probable dementia.

The Women's Health Initiative Memory Study (WHIMS), a clinical sub-study of the WHI, was designed to assess whether postmenopausal hormone replacement therapy (oral estrogen plus progestin or oral estrogen-alone) reduces the risk of dementia in women aged 65 and over (age range 65-79 years) and free of dementia at baseline.

In the estrogen plus progestin arm of the WHIMS (n=4532), women with intact uteri were treated with daily 0.625 mg conjugated equine estrogens (CEE) plus 2.5 mg medroxyprogesterone acetate (MPA) or placebo for an average of 4.05 years. The results, when extrapolated to 10 000 women treated over a one-year period showed:

• 23 more cases of probable dementia (45 on combined HRT versus 22 on placebo).

In the estrogen-alone arm of the WHIMS (n=2947), women with prior hysterectomy were treated with daily 0.625 mg CEE or placebo for an average of 5.21 years. The results, when extrapolated to 10 000 women treated over a one-year period showed:

• 12 more cases of probable dementia (37 on estrogen-alone versus 25 on placebo), although this difference did not reach statistical significance.

When data from the estrogen plus progestin arm of the WHIMS and the estrogen alone arm of the WHIMS were combined, as per the original WHIMS protocol, in 10 000 women over a one-year period, there were:

• 18 more cases of probable dementia (41 on estrogen plus progestin or estrogen-alone versus 23 on placebo).

For transdermal estrogen-only or estrogen-progestogen combined products, no large randomized clinical trials have assessed the HRT-associated risk of probable dementia to date. Therefore there are no data to support the conclusion that the frequency of probable dementia is different with ESTALIS.

Epilepsy: Particular caution is indicated in women with epilepsy, as estrogen, with or without progestins, may cause an exacerbation of this condition.

Renal: Fluid Retention: Estrogens with or without progestins may cause fluid retention. Therefore, particular caution is indicated in cardiac or renal dysfunction or asthma. If, in any of the above-mentioned conditions, a worsening of the underlying disease is diagnosed or suspected during treatment, the benefits and risks of treatment should be reassessed based on the individual case.

Skin: Contact Sensitization: Contact sensitization is known to occur with topical applications. Although it is extremely rare, patients who develop contact sensitization to any component of the patch should be warned that a severe hypersensitivity reaction may occur with continuing exposure to the causative agent.

Special Populations: Pregnant Women: ESTALIS must not be used during pregnancy. Both estrogens and progestogens may cause foetal harm when administered to a pregnant woman.

Nursing Women: ESTALIS must not be used while breastfeeding.

Pediatrics: ESTALIS should not be used in children.

Geriatrics (>65 years of age): No clinical studies were conducted to evaluate the effect of estradiol on women more than 65 years old.

Monitoring and Laboratory Tests: Before ESTALIS (norethindrone acetate (NETA)/estradiol-17β) is administered, the patient should have a complete physical examination including a blood pressure determination. Breasts and pelvic organs should be appropriately examined and a Papanicolaou smear should be performed. Endometrial biopsy should be done only when indicated. Baseline tests should include mammography, measurements of blood glucose, calcium, triglycerides and cholesterol, and liver function tests.

The first follow-up examination should be done within 3-6 months after initiation of treatment to assess response to treatment. Thereafter, examinations should be made at intervals at least once a year. Appropriate investigations should be arranged at regular intervals as determined by the physician.

The importance of regular self-examination of the breasts should be discussed with the patient.

Women should be advised that changes in their breasts should be reported to their doctor or nurse.

ADVERSE REACTIONS: Adverse Drug Reaction Overview: See Warnings and Precautions regarding potential induction of malignant neoplasms and adverse effects similar to those of oral contraceptives.

The following adverse reactions have been reported with estrogen/progestin combinations in general.

Blood and Lymphatic System Disorders: altered coagulation tests (see Drug Interactions, Drug-Laboratory Test Interactions).

Cardiac Disorders: palpitations; increase in blood pressure (see Warnings and Precautions). Coronary thrombosis.

Endocrine Disorders: increased blood sugar levels; decreased glucose tolerance.

Eye Disorders: neuro-ocular lesions (e.g., retinal thrombosis, optic neuritis), visual disturbances; steepening of the corneal curvature; intolerance to contact lenses (dry eyes, tear film composition changes).

Gastrointestinal Disorders: nausea; vomiting; abdominal discomfort (cramps, pressure, pain, bloating).

General Disorders and Administration Site Conditions: fatigue; changes in appetite; changes in body weight; change in libido.

Hepatobiliary Disorders: gallbladder disorder; asymptomatic impaired liver function; cholestatic jaundice.

Musculoskeletal and Connective Tissue Disorders: musculoskeletal pain including leg pain not related to thromboembolic disease (usually transient, lasting 3-6 weeks) may occur.

Nervous System Disorders: aggravation of migraine episodes; headaches; dizziness; neuritis.

Psychiatric Disorders: mental depression; nervousness; irritability.

Renal and Urinary Disorders: cystitis; dysuria; sodium retention; edema.

Reproductive System and Breast Disorders: breakthrough bleeding; spotting; change in menstrual flow; dysmenorrhea; vaginal itching/discharge; dyspareunia, endometrial hyperplasia; pre-menstrual-like syndrome; reactivation of endometriosis; changes in cervical erosion and amount of cervical secretion; breast swelling and tenderness.

Skin and Subcutaneous Tissue Disorders: loss of scalp hair; chloasma or melasma, which may persist when drug is discontinued; erythema nodosum; erythema multiforme; hemorrhagic skin eruptions; hirsutism, acne.

Vascular Disorders: isolated cases of thrombophlebitis; thromboembolic disorders.

Overview of Adverse Drug Reactions with ESTALIS: This section summarizes adverse drug reaction data pooled from clinical trials, published investigations and post-marketing experience.

The most commonly reported adverse reaction to ESTALIS (NETA/estradiol-17β) in clinical trials was erythema at the application site. Less than 1% of patients treated sequentially and about 5% of patients treated continuously discontinued therapy due to an application site reaction.

The data on adverse events from 5 pooled clinical trials are included. 3 clinical trials had a 2 years duration and 2 had a 1 year duration. A total safety population of 941 patients on HRT and 207 patients on placebo was identified.

Frequency estimate: very common ≥10%, common ≥1% to <10%; uncommon ≥ 0.1% to <1%; rare ≥0.01% to <0.1%; very rare <0.01%; with unknown frequency.

Most Common Adverse Drug Reactions (≥1%): Psychiatric Disorders: Common: depression, affect lability, insomnia, nervousness.

Nervous System Disorders: Very common: headache. Common: dizziness.

Gastrointestinal Disorders: Common: nausea, abdominal distension, abdominal pain, diarrhoea, dyspepsia.

Skin and Subcutaneous Tissue Disorders: Common: acne, dry skin, pruritus, rash.

Reproductive System and Breast Disorders: Very common: breast pain, breast tenderness, dysmenorrhoea, menstrual disorder. Common: breast enlargement, endometrial hyperplasia, genital discharge, menorrhagia, uterine spasm, vaginal haemorrhage, vaginal infection.

Musculoskeletal and Connective Tissue Disorders: Common: back pain, pain in extremity, pain.

General Disorders and Administration Site Disorders: Common: weight increased. Very common: application site reaction, asthenia. Common: oedema peripheral.

Less Common Clinical Trial Adverse Drug Reactions (<1%): Gastrointestinal Disorders: Uncommon: vomiting.

Hepatobiliary Disorders: Rare: gallbladder disorder, cholelithiasis. Very rare: jaundice cholestatic.

Immune System Disorders: Rare: hypersensitivity.

Investigations: Uncommon: transaminases increased, blood pressure increased.

Neoplasms Benign, Malignant and Unspecified (including cysts and polyps): Uncommon: breast cancer. Rare: cervical polyps, uterine leiomyoma, Fallopian tube cysts.

Nervous System Disorders: Uncommon: migraine. Rare: paraesthesia.

Psychiatric Disorders: Rare: libido increase or decrease.

Skin and Subcutaneous Tissue Disorders: Uncommon: skin discolouration.

Vascular Disorders: Rare: embolism venous.

Adverse Drug Reactions with Unknown Frequency: Skin and Subcutaneous Tissue Disorders: Not known: erythema nodosum, erythema multiforme. Not known: hypersensitivity, including allergic contact dermatitis and isolated cases of anaphylactoid reactions (some of the patients had a history of previous allergy or allergic disorders). Not known: reversible post-inflammatory pigmentation and precipitation or aggravation of porphyria cutanea tarda in predisposed individuals. Not known*: alopecia, chloasma.

Vascular Disorders: Not known: varicose veins.

Abnormal Hematologic and Clinical Chemistry Findings: See Table 1.

Table 1: ESTALIS

Abnormal Hematologic and Clinical Chemistry

Laboratory Parameters	Effect
Antithrombin III	↓
Coagulation factors VII, VIII, IX, X	↑
Corticosteroid binding globulin (CBG)	CBG ↑ in serum → increased circulating sex steroids. Free or biologically active hormone concentrations are unchanged.
Fibrinogen and fibrinogen activity	↑ levels
Folate	↓ serum concentration
T_3	↓ resin uptake, reflecting the elevated TBG
Free T_4	Concentration unaltered
Glucose	Impaired glucose tolerance

* Reported in post-marketing experience.

(cont'd)

Table 1: ESTALIS *(cont'd)*

Abnormal Hematologic and Clinical Chemistry

Laboratory Parameters	Effect
METOPIRONE test	Reduced response
Norepinephrine-induced platelet aggregability	↑
Prothrombin time and partial tromboplastin time	↑
Sex-hormone binding globulin (SHBG)	SHBG↑ in serum → increased circulating sex steroids. Free or biologically active hormone concentrations are unchanged.
Sulfobromophthalein	↑ retention
Triglyceride and phospholipid	↑ serum concentration
Thyroxin-binding globulin (TBG)	↑ → increased circulating total thyroid hormone (T_4) as measured by column or radioimmunoassay

If adverse symptoms persist, the prescription of HRT should be re-considered.

DRUG INTERACTIONS: Overview:

- Estrogens may diminish the efficiency of anticoagulant, antidiabetic and antihypertensive agents.
- Preparations inducing liver enzymes (e.g. barbiturates, hydantoins, carbamazepine, meprobamates, phenylbutazone or rifampicin) may interfere with the activity of orally administered estrogens.

Drug-Drug Interactions: The following section contains information on drug interactions with ethinyl estradiol-containing products (specifically, oral contraceptives) that have been reported in the public literature. It is unknown whether such interactions occur with drug products containing other types of estrogens.

Table 2: ESTALIS

Established or Potential Drug-Drug Interactions

Drug	Ref	Effect	Clinical Comment
Anticonvulsants (phenobarbital, phenytoin, carbamazepine)	T	↑ metabolism of ethinyl estradiol	↓ plasma concentration of estradiol
Acetaminophen	T	↑ AUC and/or plasma concentration of ethinyl estradiol ↓ plasma concentration of acetaminophen	Therapeutic monitoring is recommended
Acid ascorbic	T	↑ AUC and/or plasma concentration of ethinyl estradiol	Therapeutic monitoring is recommended
Aminoglutethimide with medroxyprogesterone acetate (MPA)	T	↓ bioavailability of MPA	Therapeutic monitoring is recommended
Atorvastatin	T	↑ AUC values for ethinyl estradiol by 20%	Therapeutic monitoring is recommended
Clofibric acid	T	↑ clearance of clofibric acid	Therapeutic monitoring is recommended
Cyclosporin	T	↑ plasma concentration of cyclosporine	Therapeutic monitoring is recommended
Morphine	T	↑ clearance of morphine	Therapeutic monitoring is recommended
Prednisolone	T	↑ plasma concentration of prednisolone	Therapeutic monitoring is recommended
Rifampicin[a]	T	↑ metabolism of ethinyl estradiol	↓ plasma concentration of estradiol
Salicylic acid	T	↑ clearance of salicylic acid	Therapeutic monitoring is recommended
Temazepam	T	↑ clearance of temazepam	Therapeutic monitoring is recommended
Theophylline	T	↑ plasma concentration of theophylline	Therapeutic monitoring is recommended
Troglitazone	T	↓ plasma concentrations of ethinyl estradiol by 30%	Therapeutic monitoring is recommended

[a] Clinical pharmacokinetics studies have not demonstrated any consistent effect of antibiotics (other than rifampicin) on plasma concentrations of synthetic steroids.

Legend: C=Case Study; CT=Clinical Trial; T=Theoretical.

Drug-Food Interactions: The interaction of ESTALIS with food has not been studied.

Drug-Herb Interactions: It was found that some herbal products (e.g., St. John's wort) which are available as over-the-counter (OTC) products might interfere with steroid metabolism, and therefore, alter the efficacy and safety of estrogen/progestin products.

Physicians and other health care providers should be made aware of other non-prescription products concomitantly used by the patient, including herbal and natural products obtained from the widely spread health stores.

Drug-Laboratory Test Interactions: The results of certain endocrine and liver function tests may be affected by estrogen-containing products:

- increased prothrombin time and partial thromboplastin time; increased levels of fibrinogen and fibrinogen activity; increased coagulation factors VII, VIII, IX, X; increased norepinephrine-induced platelet aggregability; decreased antithrombin III;
- increased thyroxine-binding globulin (TBG), leading to increased circulating total thyroid hormone (T_4) as measured by column or radioimmunoassay; T_3 resin uptake is decreased, reflecting the elevated TBG; free T_4 concentration is unaltered;
- other binding proteins may be elevated in serum i.e., corticosteroid binding globulin (CBG), sex-hormone binding globulin (SHBG), leading to increased circulating corticosteroids and sex steroids respectively; free or biologically active hormone concentrations are unchanged;
- impaired glucose tolerance;
- increased serum triglyceride and phospholipid concentration.

(See also Table 1 in Abnormal Hematologic and Clinical Chemistry Findings.)

With ESTALIS, no effect on fibrinogen, antithrombin III, TBG, CBG or SHBG and decreases in serum triglycerides have been observed.

The results of the above laboratory tests should not be considered reliable unless therapy has been discontinued for two to four weeks. The pathologist should be informed that the patient is receiving hormone replacement therapy (HRT) when relevant specimens are submitted.

Drug-Lifestyle Interactions: Specific drug-lifestyle interaction studies have not been conducted with ESTALIS. Acute alcohol ingestion during HRT may lead to elevations in circulating estradiol levels.

DOSAGE AND ADMINISTRATION: Dosing Considerations:

- For initiation and maintenance of treatment, the lowest effective dose should always be used.
- Hormone replacement therapy (HRT) involving either estrogen alone or estrogen-progestogen combined therapy should only be continued as long as the benefits outweigh the risks for the individual.
- ESTALIS is used as a continuous treatment (uninterrupted application twice weekly).
- In women who are not currently taking oral estrogens, treatment with ESTALIS (NETA/estradiol-17β) can be initiated at once. In women who are currently taking oral estrogen, treatment with ESTALIS can be initiated on reappearance of menopausal symptoms, following discontinuation of oral therapy.

Therapeutic Regimens: Combination progestin/estrogen regimens are indicated for women with intact uteri. Two ESTALIS (NETA/estradiol-17β) patches are available: 140 µg norethindrone acetate with 50 µg estradiol per day (9 cm²) and 250 µg norethindrone acetate with 50 µg estradiol per day (16 cm²). For all regimens, the requirement for hormone replacement therapy for menopausal symptoms should be reassessed periodically. Attempts to taper or discontinue the medication should be made at 3- to 6-month intervals.

Recommended Dose and Dosage Adjustment: Continuous Combined Regimen: ESTALIS 140/50 or ESTALIS 250/50 µg per day (16 cm²) is worn continuously on the abdomen or buttocks. A new patch should be applied twice weekly during a 28-day cycle. Irregular uterine bleeding may occur particularly in the first 6 months, but generally decreases with time, and often to an amenorrheic state.

If irregular uterine bleeding persists and uterine pathology has been ruled out by appropriate diagnostic measures, it may be more appropriate instead to prescribe ESTALIS using a sequential regimen.

Missed Dose: Patients who miss applying a patch of ESTALIS should apply a new patch as soon as possible. The subsequent patch should be applied according to the original treatment schedule. The interruption of treatment might increase the likelihood of recurrence of symptoms and breakthrough bleeding and spotting.

Administration: Patch Application: The physician should discuss the most appropriate placement of the patch with the patient. Immediately after removal of a patch from the pouch and removal of one-half of the protective liner, the adhesive side of the ESTALIS patch should be placed on a clean, dry area of intact skin and peel off the remaining one-half of the protective liner. The area selected should not be oily, damaged or irritated, and not exposed to the sun. The site selected should also be one at which little wrinkling of the skin occurs during movement of the body (buttocks and lower abdomen). The waistline should be avoided, since tight clothing may dislodge the patch. The patch should be pressed firmly in place with the palm of the hand for at least 10 seconds, making sure there is good contact, especially around the edges. In the event that a patch should fall off, it can be reapplied. If it fails to adhere then a new patch may be applied. In either case, the original treatment schedule should be continued. Patches should not be applied to the same skin site for at least one week.

ESTALIS must not be applied to the breasts to avoid potentially harmful effects on the breast tissue.

OVERDOSAGE:

Symptoms of Overdose: Numerous reports of ingestion of large doses of estrogen products and estrogen-containing oral contraceptives by young children have not revealed acute serious ill effects. Overdosage with estrogen may cause nausea, breast discomfort, fluid retention, bloating or vaginal bleeding in women.

Progestin (norethindrone acetate) overdosage has been characterized by depressed mood, tiredness, acne and hirsutism.

Treatment of Overdose: Owing to the mode of administration (transdermal), plasma levels of estradiol-17β or norethindrone acetate can be rapidly reduced by removal of the patch. Symptomatic treatment should be given.

> For management of a suspected drug overdose, contact your regional Poison Control Centre. See the *CPS* Directory section for a list of Poison Control Centres.

ACTION AND CLINICAL PHARMACOLOGY: Mechanism of Action: ESTALIS (norethindrone acetate (NETA)/estradiol-17ß) is designed to provide continuous estrogen and progestin therapy, in a 28-day treatment cycle, for women with intact uteri.

Transdermally delivered estradiol is metabolized only to a small extent by the skin and by-passes the first pass effect seen with orally administered estrogen products. Therapeutic estradiol serum levels with lower circulating levels of estrone and estrone conjugates are achieved with smaller transdermal doses (daily and total) as compared to oral therapy and more closely approximate premenopausal concentrations.

In a pharmacokinetic study, it was shown that ESTALIS matrix transdermal delivery system achieves estradiol serum levels and estrone to estradiol ratios in the range of those observed in premenopausal women at the early (estradiol >147 pM/L (40 pg/mL)) to mid-follicular phase. These features are maintained for an entire 84 to 96 hour wear period. Multiple applications of ESTALIS (250/50 µg/day, 140/50 µg/day) matrix transdermal delivery system resulted in average estradiol serum concentrations at steady-state of 184 and 165 pM/L (50 and 45 pg/mL), respectively. At the end of the application periods, the average estradiol serum concentrations were 136 and 99 pM/L (37 and 27 pg/mL), respectively. Estradiol has a short elimination half-life of approximately 2 to 3 hours. Therefore, a rapid decline in serum levels is observed after the matrix transdermal delivery system is removed. After removal of the matrix transdermal delivery system, serum concentrations of estradiol return to untreated post-menopausal levels (<73 pM/L (20 pg/mL)) within 4-8 hours.

In a pharmacokinetic study it was shown that multiple applications of ESTALIS (250/50 µg/day, 140/50 µg/day) matrix transdermal delivery systems resulted in average norethindrone serum concentrations at steady-state of 2815 and 1639 pM/L (840 and 489 pg/mL), respectively. At the end of the application period, the average serum concentrations of norethindrone were 2299 and 1293 pM/L (686 and 386 pg/mL), respectively. Serum norethindrone concentrations of ESTALIS increased linearly with increasing doses of NETA. The elimination half-life of norethindrone is reported to be 6 to 8 hours. After removal of the ESTALIS matrix transdermal delivery system, norethindrone serum concentrations diminish rapidly and are less than 168 pM/L (50 pg/mL) within 48 hours.

Minimal fluctuations in serum estradiol and norethindrone concentrations demonstrate consistent deliveries over the application interval. There is no accumulation of estradiol or norethindrone in the circulation following multiple applications.

Pharmacodynamics: Hormone Replacement Therapy: ESTALIS (NETA/estradiol-17β) provides continuous, controlled transdermal delivery of estradiol-17β such that estradiol-17β levels as well as the E2/E1 ratio in postmenopausal women are restored to those seen in the early follicular phase of the premenopausal range (see Pharmacokinetics). ESTALIS thus alleviates the symptoms of estradiol-17β deficiency in postmenopausal women.

Coadministration of Progestins: Estrogen replacement therapy should be supplemented by sequential progestin therapy only in women with intact uteri.

It is not possible to give accurate values for the relative clinical effectiveness of different progestins because careful comparisons are limited in number, and different responses have been used in the published studies. In various tests in women, the relative potencies of the progestins are not the same. Furthermore, some progestins possess more or less estrogenic and androgenic activities than do others.

In general, progestins have been administered sequentially for 10 to 14 days during each estrogen cycle. Published data suggest that 12 to 14 days of sequential progestin treatment during estrogen replacement therapy virtually eliminates the occurrence of endometrial hyperplasia, and thereby irregular bleeding and endometrial carcinoma, compared to estrogen treatment alone. The progestin requirements may vary amongst patients.

Pharmacokinetics: Estradiol-17β: Absorption and Distribution: Metabolism and plasma levels of estradiol-17β delivered transdermally are similar to those in premenopausal women. Estradiol-17β circulates in the blood largely bound to sex hormone binding globulin (SHBG) and albumin.

Administration of ESTALIS every 3 to 4 days in postmenopausal women produces average steady-state estradiol serum concentrations of 165 to 184 pM/L (45 to 50 pg/mL), which are equivalent to the normal ranges observed at early follicular phase in premenopausal women. These concentrations are achieved within 12 to 24 hours following ESTALIS application and are sustained for the entire patch wear period. Minimal fluctuations in serum estradiol concentrations are observed following ESTALIS application, indicating consistent hormone delivery over the application interval. Additionally, transdermal administration of estradiol is reported to produce mean serum concentrations of estradiol comparable to those produced by daily oral administration (oral dose about 20 times the daily transdermal dose).

Concentration data from Phase II and III studies indicate that the pharmacokinetics of estradiol did not change over time, suggesting no evidence of the accumulation of estradiol following extended patch wear period (up to 1 year).

Metabolism: Transdermally delivered estradiol is metabolized only to a small extent by the skin and by-passes the first pass effect seen with orally administered estrogen products. Therapeutic estradiol serum levels with lower circulating levels of estrone and estrone conjugates are achieved with smaller transdermal doses (daily and total) as compared to oral therapy and more closely approximate premenopausal concentrations.

Transdermally applied oestradiol is metabolised in the same way as the endogenous hormone. Oestradiol is metabolised to oestrone, then later–primarily in the liver–to oestriol, epioestriol and catechol oestrogens, which are then conjugated to sulphates and glucuronides.

Excretion: Estradiol has a short elimination half-life of approximately 2 to 3 hours. Therefore, a rapid decline in serum levels is observed after the ESTALIS system is removed. Within 4 to 8 hours following ESTALIS removal, serum estradiol concentrations return to untreated, postmenopausal levels (<73 pM/L (20 pg/mL)).

Norethindrone Acetate: Absorption and Distribution: Progestins used in therapy are well-absorbed through the skin, mucous membranes, and gastrointestinal tract.

Norethindrone steady concentrations are attained within 24 hours of application of the ESTALIS transdermal delivery systems. Minimal fluctuations in serum norethindrone concentrations are observed following ESTALIS treatment, indicating consistent hormone delivery over the application interval. Steady-state norethindrone concentrations are maintained throughout the application interval and are within a therapeutic range sufficient to prevent endometrial hyperstimulation. Serum concentrations of norethindrone increase linearly with increasing doses of norethindrone acetate.

Concentration data from Phase II and III studies indicate that the pharmacokinetics of norethindrone did not change over time, suggesting no evidence of the accumulation of norethindrone following extended patch wear period (up to 1 year).

Metabolism: In plasma, norethindrone is bound approximately 90% to SHBG and albumin.

Norethindrone acetate is hydrolyzed to the active moiety, norethindrone, in most tissues including skin and blood. Norethindrone is primarily metabolized in the liver, however, transdermal administration significantly decreases metabolism because hepatic first-pass uptake is avoided.

Norethindrone undergoes extensive ring A reduction, forming dihydro- and tetrahydro-norethindrone metabolites, which undergo conjugation.

Excretion: The elimination half-life of norethindrone is reported to be 6 to 8 hours. Norethindrone serum concentrations diminish rapidly and are less than <168 pM/L (50 pg/mL) within 48 hours after removal of the ESTALIS transdermal delivery system.

Special Populations and Conditions: Pediatrics: ESTALIS should not be used in children.

Geriatrics (>65 years of age): No clinical studies were conducted to evaluate the effect of estradiol on women more than 65 years old.

Gender: ESTALIS should be used in women only.

Estrogen Pharmacology: Estradiol-17β is the major estrogenic hormone secreted by the human ovary. Among numerous effects, estradiol-17β is largely responsible for the development and maintenance of the female reproductive system and of secondary sexual characteristics. It promotes growth and development of the vagina, uterus, fallopian tubes, and breasts. Estradiol-17β contributes to the shaping of the skeleton, to the maintenance of tone and elasticity of urogenital structures, to changes in the epiphyses of the long bones that allow for the pubertal growth spurt and its termination, to the growth of axillary and pubic hair, and to the pigmentation of the nipples and genitals. Estradiol-17β also affects the release of pituitary gonadotropins.

After menopause, when the ovaries have ceased to function, only small amounts of estradiol-17β are still produced, i.e., from the aromatization of androstenedione to estrone and to a lesser extent, testosterone to estradiol-17ß. Estrone is transformed to estradiol-17β by the enzyme 17β-hydroxysteroid-dehydrogenase. Both enzymes prevail in fat, liver and muscle tissue.

In premenopausal women, the ratio of estradiol-17β (E_2) to estrone (E_1) (i.e., E_2/E_1 ratio) in the plasma is in the range of 0.5 to 2, depending on the phase of the menstrual cycle. The E_2/E_1 ratio for untreated postmenopausal women is below 0.5.

Loss of the ovarian estradiol-17β production after menopause can result in the following: instability of thermoregulation causing hot flushes associated with sleep disturbance and excessive sweating; accelerated loss of bone matrix and mineral, resulting in osteoporosis; alterations in lipid metabolism; urogenital atrophy, causing dyspareunia and urinary incontinence.

The protection against endometrial hyperplasia in women with intact uteri is necessary during long-term therapy. Published data suggest that 12 to 14 days of sequential progestin treatment during estrogen replacement therapy reduces the occurrence of endometrial hyperplasia, and thereby irregular bleeding and endometrial carcinoma, compared to estrogen treatment alone.

Progestin Pharmacology: Norethindrone acetate (NETA) is a potent progestin that essentially mimics the biological effects of progesterone. Tissue effects of NETA are dependent on prior estrogen stimulation, and NETA receptors have been identified in all tissues containing estrogen receptors (see Estradiol-17β).

NETA induces protein synthesis and also reduces the number of estrogen and progestin receptors, thereby limiting excessive growth stimulation of target tissues by estrogen. 17-hydroxysteroid-dehydrogenase, which locally oxidizes estradiol-17β to its weaker estrogenic metabolite estrone, is also induced by NETA.

One of the major targets of NETA is the uterus, where it induces secretory transformation of the estrogen-primed endometrium. Once transformation of the endometrium is completed, the estrogen-primed endometrium is shed resulting in a regular cyclical bleeding.

Progestin is combined to estrogen for protection against endometrial hyperplasia during long-term therapy of women with intact uteri.

STORAGE AND STABILITY: ESTALIS: Store between 2 and 8°C prior to dispensing. Do not freeze.

After dispensing, the patches may be stored unrefrigerated at 20 to 25°C, in which case they should be used within 6 months or before the expiry date, whichever comes first. If the patches are stored in the refrigerator, in this case, they should be used before the expiry date and should be allowed to reach room temperature before application in order to ensure proper adhesion.

Do not store the patches in areas where extreme temperatures can occur. Each patch is individually sealed in a separate pouch. Do not store out of the pouch. Apply immediately upon removal from the protective pouch. Apply whole patches.

Keep out of the reach and sight of children and pets both before use and when disposing of used patches.

Do not use any ESTALIS pack that is damaged or shows signs of tampering.

SPECIAL HANDLING INSTRUCTIONS: See Dosage and Administration, Patch Application.

INFORMATION FOR THE PATIENT: Published in e-CPS, available by subscription at www.e-cps.ca.

DOSAGE FORMS, COMPOSITION AND PACKAGING: ESTALIS is an alcohol-free, adhesive-based matrix transdermal patch comprising three layers. Proceeding from the visible surface toward the surface attached to the skin, these layers are: a backing, an adhesive layer, and a protective liner. The adhesive matrix containing 17ß-estradiol and norethindrone acetate is applied to a polyester/ethylene vinyl acetate laminate film on one side and is protected on the other side by a transparent fluoropolymer coated release liner. The transparent release liner must be removed before the system can be used. Each patch is enclosed in a heat-sealed pouch.

ESTALIS 140/50 and 250/50 contain a fixed combination of norethindrone acetate (NETA) and estradiol-17β. ESTALIS patches release controlled amounts of NETA and estradiol-17ß simultaneously through the skin for up to 4 days.

The active components of the system are estradiol USP and norethindrone acetate USP. The remaining components of the system are pharmacologically inactive; they are: a silicone (BIO PSA X7-4603) and acrylic (Gelva 737)-based multipolymeric adhesive, povidone USP, oleic acid NF, and dipropylene glycol.

The ESTALIS (NETA/estradiol-17β) package consists of the following systems: see Table 3.

Table 3: ESTALIS

ESTALIS Package Composition

	ESTALIS 140/50	ESTALIS 250/50
Estradiol-17β Dosage Nominal in vivo Delivery	50 µg/day	50 µg/day
NETA Dosage Nominal in vivo Delivery	140 µg/day	250 µg/day
Total Estradiol-17β Content	0.62 mg	0.51 mg
Total NETA Content	2.7 mg	4.8 mg
Drug-Releasing Area	9 cm²	16 cm²
Shape of patch	Round	Round
Presentation	Cartons of 8 patches	Cartons of 8 patches

(Shown in Product Identification Section)

Estrace®
estradiol-17β (micronized)
Estrogen

Shire

Date of Preparation: July 24, 2003
Date of Revision: October 15, 2007

SUMMARY PRODUCT INFORMATION:

Route of Administration	Dosage Form/ Strength	Clinically Relevant Nonmedicinal Ingredients
Oral	Tablet 0.5 mg, 1 mg, 2 mg	Lactose, tartrazine (2 mg tablets only) For a complete listing see Dosage Forms, Composition and Packaging.

INDICATIONS AND CLINICAL USE: ESTRACE (17β-estradiol Tablets) tablets are indicated for:

- the symptomatic relief of menopausal symptoms.
- ESTRACE may also contribute to the prevention of osteoporosis in naturally occurring or surgically induced estrogen-deficiency states when combined with other important therapeutics such as diet, calcium and vitamin D intake, smoking cessation and regular physical weight bearing exercises.

The use of ESTRACE in the prevention of osteoporosis is to be considered in light of other available therapies.

In patients with an intact uterus, ESTRACE should always be supplemented by sequential administration of a progestogen in order to prevent endometrial hyperplasia or carcinoma.

CONTRAINDICATIONS: Estrogen including ESTRACE should not be administered to patients with any of the following conditions:

- Liver dysfunction or disease as long as liver function tests have failed to return to normal.
- Known or suspected estrogen-dependent malignant neoplasia (e.g. endometrial cancer).
- Endometrial hyperplasia.
- Known, suspected, or past history of breast cancer.
- Undiagnosed abnormal genital bleeding.
- Known or suspected pregnancy.
- Lactation
- Active or past history of arterial thromboembolic disease (eg. stroke, myocardial infarction, coronary heart disease).
- Classical migraine.
- Active or past history of confirmed venous thromboembolism (such as deep vein thrombosis or pulmonary embolism) or active thrombophlebitis.
- Partial or complete loss of vision or diplopia, from ophthalmic vascular disease.
- Hypersensitivity to this drug or to any ingredient in the formulation or component of the container. For a complete listing, see the Dosage Forms, Composition and Packaging.

WARNINGS AND PRECAUTIONS:

Serious Warnings and Precautions

The Women's Health Initiative (WHI) trial examined the health benefits and risks of combined estrogen plus progestin therapy (n=16 608) and estrogen-alone therapy (n=10 739) in postmenopausal women aged 50 to 79 years.

The estrogen plus progestin arm of the WHI trial indicated increased risk of myocardial infarction (MI), stroke, invasive breast cancer, pulmonary emboli and deep vein thrombosis in postmenopausal women receiving treatment with combined conjugated equine estrogens (CEE, 0.625 mg/day) and medroxyprogesterone acetate (MPA, 2.5 mg/day) for 5.2 years compared to those receiving placebo.

The estrogen-alone arm of the WHI trial indicated an increased risk of stroke and deep vein thrombosis in hysterectomized women treated with CEE-alone (0.625 mg/day) for 6.8 years compared to those receiving placebo.

Therefore, the following should be given serious consideration at the time of prescribing:

1. Estrogens with or without progestins **should not** be prescribed for primary or secondary prevention of cardiovascular diseases.
2. Estrogens with or without progestins should be prescribed at **the lowest effective dose** for the approved indication.
3. Estrogens with or without progestins should be prescribed for **the shortest period** possible for the approved indication.
4. The use of ESTRACE for the prevention of osteoporosis should be considered in light of other available therapies.

Carcinogenesis and Mutagenesis: Breast Cancer: Available epidemiological data indicate that the use of combined estrogen plus progestin by postmenopausal women is associated with an increased risk of invasive breast cancer.

In the estrogen plus progestin arm of the WHI trial, among 10 000 women over a one-year period, there were:

- 8 more cases of invasive breast cancer (38 on combined HRT versus 30 on placebo).

The WHI study also reported that the invasive breast cancers diagnosed in the estrogen plus progestin group were similar in histology but were larger (mean [SD], 1.7 cm [1.1] vs 1.5 cm [0.9], respectively; P=0.04) and were at a more advanced stage compared with those diagnosed in the placebo group. The percentage of women with abnormal mammograms (recommendations for short-interval follow-up, a suspicious abnormality, or highly suggestive of malignancy) was significantly higher in the estrogen plus progestin group versus the placebo group. This difference appeared at year one and persisted in each year thereafter.

In the estrogen-alone arm of the WHI trial, there was no statistically significant difference in the rate of invasive breast cancer in hysterectomized women treated with conjugated equine estrogens versus women treated with placebo.

In a pivotal clinical study with ESTRACE (n=64) on the prevention of early post-menopausal bone loss, three (3) abnormal mammograms were reported post-treatment, however, none showed evidence of malignancy.

It is recommended that estrogens not be given to women with existing breast cancer or those with a previous history of the disease. There is a need for caution in prescribing estrogens for women with known risk factors associated with the development of breast cancer, such as strong family history of breast cancer (first degree relative) or who present a breast condition with an increased risk (abnormal mammograms and/or atypical hyperplasia at breast biopsy). Other known risk factors for the development of breast cancer such as nulliparity, obesity, early menarche, late age at first full term pregnancy and at menopause should also be evaluated.

It is recommended that women undergo mammography prior to the start of HRT treatment and at regular intervals during treatment, as deemed appropriate by the treating physician and according to the perceived risks for each patient.

The overall benefits and possible risks of hormone replacement therapy should be fully considered and discussed with patients. It is important that the modest increased risk of being diagnosed with breast cancer after 4 years of treatment with combined estrogen plus progestin HRT (as reported in the results of WHI-trial) be discussed with the patient and weighed against its known benefits.

Instructions for regular self-examination of the breasts should be included in this counseling.

Endometrial Hyperplasia and Endometrial Carcinoma: The use of unopposed estrogen by women with intact uteri increases the risk of endometrial hyperplasia and endometrial carcinoma. Estrogen should be prescribed with an appropriate dosage of a progestin in women with intact uteri in order to prevent endometrial hyperplasia/carcinoma.

During the conduct of a pivotal clinical study in an open-labeled study of 369 women (mean age=49) with endogenous estrogen deficiency associated with menopausal symptoms, endometrial biopsies were conducted in a subset of 32 subjects prior to and after therapy. Prior to therapy eleven (11) samples were considered abnormal: cystic hyperplasia (4), adenomatous hyperplasia (6) and mixed-inactive hyperplasia (1). One (1) sample biopsy remained abnormal after 11 months of treatment with ESTRACE, changing from cystic hyperplasia to benign cystic hyperplasia.

In a second pivotal clinical study on the prevention of early post-menopausal bone loss, exit endometrial biopsy specimens were obtained for 21 subjects. Abnormalities consistent with estrogen stimulation of the endometrium were found in 27% of these subjects. Two (2) subjects had progression to the point of adenomatous hyperplasia and one (1) subject had atypical nuclear changes. No subjects, however, developed adenocarcinoma of the endometrium.

Ovarian Cancer: Recent epidemiologic studies have found that the use of hormone replacement therapy (estrogen-alone and estrogen plus progestin therapies), in particular for five or more years, has been associated with an increased risk of ovarian cancer.

Cardiovascular: The results of the Heart and Estrogen/progestin Replacement Studies (HERS and HERS II and the Women's Health Initiative (WHI) trial indicate that the use of estrogen plus progestin is associated with an increased risk of coronary heart disease (CHD) in postmenopausal women. The results of the WHI trial indicate that the use of estrogen-alone and estrogen plus progestin is associated with an increased risk of stroke in postmenopausal women.

WHI Trial Findings: In the combined estrogen plus progestin arm of the WHI trial, among 10 000 women over a one-year period, there were:

- 8 more cases of stroke (29 on combined HRT versus 21 on placebo)
- 7 more cases of CHD (37 on combined HRT versus 30 on placebo).

In the estrogen-alone arm of the WHI trial of women with prior hysterectomy, among 10 000 women over a one-year period, there were/was:

- 12 more cases of stroke (44 on estrogen-alone therapy versus 32 on placebo)
- No statistically significant difference in the rate of CHD.

HERS and HERS II Findings: In the Heart and Estrogen/progestin Replacement Study (HERS) of postmenopausal women with documented heart disease (n=2763, average age 66.7 years), a randomized placebo-controlled clinical trial of secondary prevention of coronary heart disease (CHD), treatment with 0.625 mg/day oral conjugated equine estrogen (CEE) plus 2.5 mg medroxyprogesterone acetate (MPA) demonstrated no cardiovascular benefit. Specifically, during an average follow-up of 4.1 years, treatment with CEE plus MPA did not reduce the overall rate of CHD events in postmenopausal women with established coronary heart disease. There were more CHD events in the hormone-treated group than in the placebo group in year 1, but not during the subsequent years.

From the original HERS trial, 2321 women consented to participate in an open label extension of HERS known as HERS II. Average follow-up in HERS II was an additional 2.7 years, for a total of 6.8 years overall. After 6.8 years, hormone therapy did not reduce the risk of cardiovascular events in women with CHD.

Blood Pressure: Women using hormone replacement therapy sometimes experience increased blood pressure. Blood pressure should be monitored with HRT use. Elevation of blood pressure in previously normotensive or hypertensive patients should be investigated and HRT may have to be discontinued.

Endocrine and Metabolism: Glucose and Lipid Metabolism: A worsening of glucose tolerance and lipid metabolism have been observed in a significant percentage of peri- and post-menopausal patients. Therefore, diabetic patients or those with a predisposition to diabetes should be observed closely to detect any alterations in carbohydrate or lipid metabolism, especially in triglyceride blood levels.

Women with familial hyperlipidemias need special surveillance. Lipid-lowering measures are recommended additionally, before treatment is started.

Women with porphyria need special surveillance.

Calcium and Phosphorus Metabolism: Because the prolonged use of estrogens influences the metabolism of calcium and phosphorus, estrogens should be used with caution in patients with metabolic and malignant bone diseases associated with hypercalcemia and in patients with renal insufficiency.

Hypothyroidism: Patients who require thyroid hormone replacement therapy and who are also taking estrogen should have their thyroid function monitored regularly to assure that thyroid hormone levels remain in an acceptable range (see Drug-Laboratory Test Interactions).

Genitourinary: Vaginal Bleeding: Abnormal vaginal bleeding, due to its prolongation, irregularity or heaviness, occurring during therapy should prompt appropriate diagnostic measures to rule out the possibility of uterine malignancy and the treatment should be re-evaluated.

Uterine Leiomyomata: Pre-existing uterine leiomyomata may increase in size during estrogen use. Growth, pain or tenderness of uterine leiomyomata requires discontinuation of medication and appropriate investigation.

Endometriosis: Symptoms and physical findings associated with a previous diagnosis of endometriosis may reappear or become aggravated with estrogen use.

Hematologic: Venous Thromboembolism: Available epidemiological data indicate that use of estrogen with or without progestin by postmenopausal women is associated with an increased risk of developing venous thromboembolism (VTE).

In the estrogen plus progestin arm of the WHI trial, among 10 000 women on combined HRT over a one-year period, there were 18 more cases of venous thromboembolism, including 8 more cases of pulmonary embolism.

In the estrogen-alone arm of the WHI trial, among 10 000 women on estrogen therapy over a one-year period, there were 7 more cases of venous thromboembolism, although there was no statistically significant difference in the rate of pulmonary embolism.

Generally recognized risk factors for VTE include a personal history, a family history (the occurrence of VTE in a direct relative at a relatively early age may indicate genetic predisposition), severe obesity (body mass index >30 kg/m^2) and systemic lupus erythematosus. The risk of VTE also increases with age and smoking.

The risk of VTE may be temporarily increased with prolonged immobilization, major surgery or trauma. In women on HRT, attention should be given to prophylactic measures to prevent VTE following surgery. Also, patients with varicose veins should be closely supervised. The physician should be alert to the earliest manifestations of thrombotic disorders (thrombophlebitis, retinal thrombosis, cerebral embolism and pulmonary embolism). If these occur or are suspected, hormone therapy should be discontinued immediately, given the risks of long-term disability or fatality.

If feasible, estrogens should be discontinued at least 4 weeks before major surgery which may be associated with an increased risk of thromboembolism, or during periods of prolonged immobilization.

Hepatic/Biliary/Pancreatic: Gallbladder Diseases: A 2- to 4-fold increase in the risk of gallbladder disease requiring surgery in women receiving postmenopausal estrogens has been reported.

Jaundice: Caution is advised in patients with a history of liver and/or biliary disorders. If cholestatic jaundice develops during treatment, the treatment should be discontinued and appropriate investigations carried out.

Liver Function Tests: Liver function tests should be done periodically in subjects who are suspected of having hepatic disease. For information on endocrine and liver function tests, see Monitoring and Laboratory Tests.

Neurologic: Cerebrovascular Insufficiency: Patients who develop visual disturbances, classical migraine, transient aphasia, paralysis or loss of consciousness should discontinue medication.

Patients with a previous history of classical migraine and who develop a recurrence or worsening of migraine symptoms should be reevaluated.

Dementia: Available epidemiological data indicate that the use of combined estrogen plus progestin in women age 65 and over may increase the risk of developing probable dementia. The Women's Health Initiative Memory Study (WHIMS), a clinical substudy of the WHI, was designed to assess whether postmenopausal hormone replacement therapy (oral estrogen plus progestin or oral estrogen-alone) reduces the risk of dementia in women aged 65 and over and free of dementia at baseline.

In the estrogen plus progestin arm of the WHIMS (n=4532), women with intact uteri were treated with daily 0.625 mg conjugated equine estrogens (CEE) plus 2.5 mg medroxyprogesterone acetate (MPA) or placebo for an average of 4.05 years. The results, when extrapolated to 10 000 women treated over a one-year period showed:

- 23 more cases of probable dementia (45 on combined HRT versus 22 on placebo).

In the estrogen-alone arm of the WHIMS (n=2947), women with prior hysterectomy were treated with daily 0.625 mg CEE or placebo for an average of 5.21 years. The results, when extrapolated to 10 000 women treated over a one-year period showed:

- 12 more cases of probable dementia (37 on estrogen-alone versus 25 on placebo), although this difference did not reach statistical significance.

When data from the estrogen plus progestin arm of the WHIMS and the estrogen-alone arm of the WHIMS were combined, as per the original WHIMS protocol, in 10 000 women over a one-year period, there were:

- 18 more cases of probable dementia (41 on estrogen plus progestin or estrogen-alone versus 23 on placebo).

Epilepsy: Particular caution is indicated in women with epilepsy, as HRT may cause an exacerbation of this condition.

Renal: Fluid Retention: Estrogens may cause fluid retention. Therefore, particular caution is indicated in cardiac or renal dysfunction, epilepsy or asthma. If, in any of the above-mentioned conditions, a worsening of the underlying disease is diagnosed or suspected during treatment, the benefits and risks of treatment should be reassessed based on the individual case.

Special Populations: Geriatrics (>65 years of age): The use of combined estrogen plus progestin in women aged 65 and over may increase the risk of developing probable dementia (see Warnings and Precautions, Neurologic).

Monitoring and Laboratory Tests: Before ESTRACE is administered, the patient should have a complete physical examination including a blood pressure determination. Breasts and pelvic organs should be appropriately examined and a Papanicolaou smear should be performed. Endometrial biopsy should be done only when indicated. Baseline tests should include mammography, measurements of blood glucose, calcium, triglycerides and cholesterol, and liver function tests.

The first follow-up examination should be done within 3-6 months after initiation of treatment to assess response to treatment. Thereafter, examinations should be made at intervals at least once a year. Appropriate investigations should be arranged at regular intervals as determined by the physician.

The importance of regular self-examination of the breasts should be discussed with the patient.

ADVERSE REACTIONS: Adverse Drug Reaction Overview: See Warnings and Precautions regarding potential induction of malignant neoplasms and adverse effects similar to those of oral contraceptives.

The following adverse reactions have been reported with estrogen/progestin combination in general:

Blood and Lymphatic System Disorders: Altered coagulation tests (see Drug Interactions, Drug-Laboratory Test Interactions).

Cardiac Disorders: palpitations; increase in blood pressure (see Warnings and Precautions); coronary thrombosis.

Congenital, Familial and Genetic disorders: Precipitation or aggravation of porphyria cutanea tarda in predisposed individuals.

Endocrine Disorders: increased blood sugar levels; decreased glucose tolerance.

Eye Disorders: neuro-ocular lesions (e.g., retinal thrombosis, optic neuritis); visual disturbances; steepening of the corneal curvature; intolerance to contact lenses.

Gastrointestinal Disorders: nausea; vomiting; abdominal discomfort (cramps, pressure, pain, bloating).

General Disorders and Administration Site Conditions: fatigue; changes in appetite; anorexia; changes in body weight; change in libido.

Hepatobiliary Disorders: gallbladder disorder; asymptomatic impaired liver function; cholestatic jaundice.

Musculoskeletal and Connective Tissue Disorders: Musculoskeletal pain including leg pain not related to thromboembolic disease (usually transient, lasting 3-6 weeks) may occur.

Nervous System Disorders: aggravation of migraine episodes; headaches; dizziness; neuritis.

Psychiatric Disorders: mental depression; nervousness; irritability.

Renal and Urinary Disorders: cystitis; dysuria; sodium retention; edema.

Reproductive System and Breast Disorders: breakthrough bleeding; spotting; change in menstrual flow; dysmenorrhea; vaginal itching/discharge; dyspareunia; endometrial hyperplasia; increase in size of uterine leiomyomata; vaginal candidiasis; pre-menstrual-like syndrome; reactivation of endometriosis; changes in cervical erosion and amount of cervical secretion; increased cervical mucous; breast swelling, tenderness and secretion.

Skin and Subcutaneous Tissue Disorders: chloasma or melasma, which may persist when drug is discontinued; pigmentation of skin; erythema multiforme; erythema nodosum; haemorrhagic eruption; itching, allergic reactions and rashes; loss of scalp hair; hirsutism and acne.

Vascular Disorders: Isolated cases of: thrombophlebitis; thromboembolic disorders.

Clinical Trial Adverse Drug Reactions: Because clinical trials are conducted under very specific conditions, the adverse drug reaction rates observed in the clinical trials may not reflect the rates observed in practice and should not be compared to the rates in the clinical trials of another drug. Adverse drug reaction information from clinical trials is useful for identifying drug-related adverse events and for approximating rates.

Table 1 summarizes the adverse events reported in a controlled, randomized, double-blind study with ESTRACE for the treatment of osteoporosis in 64 post-menopausal women. ESTRACE was administered in a cyclic manner for up to 18 months with an option to continue for an additional 6 months.

If adverse symptoms persist, the prescription of HRT should be reconsidered.

DRUG INTERACTIONS: Overview: Estrogens may diminish the effectiveness of anticoagulants, antidiabetic and antihypertensive agents.

In vitro and in vivo studies have shown that estrogens are metabolized partially by cytochrome P450 3A4 (CYP 3A4). Therefore, inducers or inhibitors of CYP 3A4 may affect estrogen drug metabolism. Inducers of CYP 3A4 such as St. John's Wort (Hypericum perforatum) preparations, phenobarbital, carbamazepine and rifampin may reduce plasma concentrations of estrogens, possibly resulting in a decrease in therapeutic effects and/or changes in uterine bleeding profile. Inhibitors of CYP 3A4 such as erythromycin, clarithromycin, ketoconazole, itraconazole, ritonavir and grapefruit juice may increase plasma concentrations of estrogens and may result in side effects.

Table 1: ESTRACE

Reported Adverse Events for More Than One Patient Per Dose Group: Symptoms by Treatment Assignment

	0.5 mg ESTRACE n=15 (%)	1.0 mg ESTRACE n=16 (%)	2.0 mg ESTRACE n=16 (%)	Placebo n=16 (%)
Gastrointestinal Disorders				
Nausea	0	0	0	2 (13%)
Constipation	2 (13%)	1 (6%)	0	1 (6%)
General Disorders & Administration Site Conditions				
Asthenia	0	0	2 (13%)	1 (6%)
Investigations				
Weight increased	3 (20%)	3 (19%)	2 (13%)	1 (6%)
Nervous System Disorders				
Headache	0	0	1 (6%)	2 (13%)
Psychiatric Disorders				
Nervousness	1 (7%)	2 (13%)	5 (31%)	2 (13%)
Insomnia	0	1 (6%)	2 (13%)	2 (13%)
Depression	2 (13%)	0	3 (19%)	3 (19%)
Libido decreased	0	0	0	2 (13%)
Renal & Urinary Disorders				
Oedema	2 (13%)	1 (6%)	2 (13%)	1 (6%)
Reproductive System & Breast Disorders				
Menopausal systems[b]	10 (67%)	11 (69%)	11 (69%)	13 (81%)

(cont'd)

Table 1: ESTRACE *(cont'd)*

Reported Adverse Events for More Than One Patient Per Dose Group: Symptoms by Treatment Assignment

	0.5 mg ESTRACE n=15 (%)	1.0 mg ESTRACE n=16 (%)	2.0 mg ESTRACE n=16 (%)	Placebo n=16 (%)
Vaginal haemorrhage	2 (13%)[a]	7 (44%)[a]	9 (56%)[a]	1 (6%)
Vaginitis	1 (7%)	2 (13%)	0	0
Uterine spasm	0	0	2 (13%)	0

[a] Statistically significant at 5% level (Fisher's exact test).
[b] According to MEDRA dictionary, including symptoms such as vasomotor symptoms or hot flushes and vaginal dryness.

Other preparations inducing liver enzymes, (e.g. barbiturates, hydantoins, meprobamate or phenylbutazone) may interfere with the activity of orally administered estrogens.

One in vitro study has shown Cytochrome 1A2 (CYP 1A2) to be partially involved in the metabolism of 17β-estradiol through hydroxylation. The clinical significance of CYP 1A2 metabolism is unknown.

Clinical pharmacokinetic studies have not demonstrated any consistent effect of antibiotics (other than rifampin) on plasma concentrations of synthetic steroids.

Drug-Drug Interactions: Possible drug-drug interactions with ESTRACE specifically have not been established.

Drug-Food Interactions: Inhibitors of CYP 3A4 such as grapefruit juice may increase plasma concentrations of estrogens and may result in side effects.

Drug-Herb Interactions: It was found that some herbal products (e.g. St. John's wort) which are available as over-the-counter (OTC) products might interfere with steroid metabolism and therefore alter the efficacy and safety of estrogen/progestin products.

Physicians and other health care providers should be made aware of other non-prescription products concomitantly used by the patient, including herbal and natural products obtained from the widely spread health stores.

Drug-Laboratory Test Interactions: The results of certain endocrine and liver function tests may be affected by estrogen-containing products.

- increased prothrombin time and partial thromboplastin time; increased levels of fibrinogen and fibrinogen activity; increased coagulation factors VII, VIII, IX, X;
- decreased antithrombin III (although following administration of ESTRACE for 28 days no effect on antithrombin III levels was seen); increased norepinephrine-induced platelet aggregability;
- increased thyroxine-binding globulin (TBG) (although TBG was not affected in clinical trials with ESTRACE), leading to increased circulating total thyroid hormone (T_4) as measured by column or radioimmunoassay; T_3 resin uptake is decreased, reflecting the elevated TBG, free T_4 concentration is unaltered.
- other binding proteins may be elevated in serum i.e. corticosteroid binding globulin (CBG), sex-hormone binding globulin (SHBG), leading to increased circulating corticosteroids and sex steroids respectively; free or biologically active hormone concentrations are unchanged;
- reduced serum folate concentration;
- increased serum triglyceride and phospholipid concentrations;
- impaired glucose tolerance.

The results of the above laboratory tests should not be considered reliable unless therapy has been discontinued for two to four weeks. The pathologist should be informed that the patient is receiving HRT when relevant specimens are submitted.

Drug-Lifestyle Interactions: The effect of lifestyle choices (e.g. smoking) on the use of ESTRACE has not been established.

DOSAGE AND ADMINISTRATION: **Dosing Considerations:** The lowest dose of estrogen required to prevent menopausal symptoms and to prevent development of osteoporosis should be used. ESTRACE should be taken at the same time each day.

ESTRACE should be taken as soon as possible after missing a dose. However the missed dose should be skipped if it is almost time to take the next dose. Patients should be advised not to double the dose.

Recommended Dose and Dosage Adjustment: In general, estrogen is usually administered cyclically for the first 21 to 25 days of each month. In patients with intact uteri a progestin should be sequentially administered for the last 12 to 14 days of estrogen administration in order to prevent development of endometrial hyperplasia/carcinoma as a result of estrogen stimulation.

In hysterectomized patients, estrogen alone should be given continuously.

Menopausal Symptoms: Treatment of menopausal symptoms is usually initiated with 1 mg ESTRACE tablet per day. Thereafter, the dosage should be adjusted to the needs of the individual. Attempts to taper or discontinue the medication should be made at 3 to 6 month intervals.

For Prevention of Osteoporosis: Prophylactic therapy with ESTRACE to prevent postmenopausal bone loss should be initiated with 0.5 mg ESTRACE tablet per day as soon as possible after menopause. The dose may be titrated upward and downward based on the patient's clinical status and plasma estradiol levels. Ideally, plasma estradiol levels should be maintained around 50 pg/mL.

OVERDOSAGE:

Symptoms: Numerous reports of ingestion of large doses of estrogen products and estrogen-containing oral contraceptives by young children have not revealed acute serious ill effects. Over dosage with estrogen may cause nausea, breast discomfort, fluid retention, bloating or vaginal bleeding in women.

Treatment: Remove ingested drug by gastric lavage and give symptomatic treatment.

> For management of a suspected drug overdose, CPhA recommends that you contact your **regional Poison Control Centre**. See the *CPS* Directory section for a list of Poison Control Centres.

ACTION AND CLINICAL PHARMACOLOGY: Mechanism of Action: Estradiol is the most potent physiologic estrogen and, in fact, is the major estrogenic hormone secreted in humans. Estradiol controls the development and maintenance of the female sex organs, the secondary sex characteristics and the mammary glands as well as certain functions of the human uterus and accessory organs, particularly the proliferation of the endometrium, the development of the decidua, and the cyclic changes in the cervix and vagina. The production of estradiol by the ovaries is under the control of pituitary gonadotropins, follicle stimulating hormone (FSH) and luteinizing hormone (LH). In menopausal women, the depletion of ovarian follicles leads to lower plasma estradiol and elevated plasma FSH and LH.

Pharmacodynamics: The active ingredient in ESTRACE tablets is derived from soy beans and it contains only one estrogen, 17β-estradiol, which is structurally identical to the estradiol produced by the human ovary. Estrogens are secreted mainly by the gonads and in a very small amount by the adrenals. In addition, they are formed, to an important degree, from peripheral conversion of adrenal and gonadal androgens to estrogens.

Estradiol is the most potent of the known naturally occurring estrogens in stimulating the growth of the reproductive tissues. Estradiol promotes uterine growth in the rat without undergoing chemical transformation and responsive tissues, such as the uterus and vagina, show a characteristic affinity for estradiol.

Estrogen deficiency is manifested by hot flushes, sweating, insomnia, paresthesia, irritability, and urogenital atrophy. As replacement therapy in estrogen deficiency states (such as menopause), low doses of estradiol in cyclic regimens have been found to relieve such deficiency.

Estrogen deficiency is the main cause of postmenopausal bone loss and contributes to age-associated losses leading to osteoporosis. Numerous clinical studies have demonstrated that estrogen therapy prevents bone loss and reduces the incidence of vertebral, hip, and Colles' fractures.

Although the mechanism of action of estrogen on bone metabolism is still not completely elucidated, estrogens have been shown to have several effects: increase in renal tubular absorption of calcium, thus reducing urinary calcium; decrease in the sensitivity of bone to the parathyroid hormone (PTH); increase in the intestinal absorption of calcium and increase in circulating levels of active 1-25-dihydroxyvitamin D. Recent research has shown that osteoblasts also possess receptors for estrogens.

Pharmacokinetics: A number of steroids with 3 oxygen functions have been identified such as 16-epiestriol, 16-ketoestradiol, 16-hydroxyestrone and 2-methoxyestrone with estradiol being a precursor to these compounds.

Absorption: Micronized 17 β-estradiol is efficiently absorbed by the gastrointestinal tract. The drug passes through the gastrointestinal mucosa and directly into the liver via the portal circulation before its access by the systemic circulation.

Distribution: Estrogens circulate in both unconjugated and conjugated forms in the blood, with the unconjugated estrogens, either free or bound to proteins, mainly albumin, or to the specific sex-hormone binding globulin (SHBG) which shows a great affinity for estradiol.

Metabolism: Estrogens are metabolized mainly in the liver, with the metabolites being conjugated with glucuronic acid or sulfuric acid and even double conjugates such as estriol-3-sulfate-16α-glucuronide are formed. About 1/3 to 1/2 of the circulating estrogens are secreted in the bile and of this fraction 20% is reabsorbed after hydrolysis in the intestinal tract. The exact site of the hydrolysis is not known, but it probably takes place in the intestinal lumen and is catalyzed by enzymes secreted into the intestinal tract or present in the microflora.

Excretion: When administered to humans, about 65% of the dose is excreted in the urine, almost entirely in the water-soluble form as β-glucuronides or sulfate esters. Estrone, estradiol and estriol account for about 1/2 of the excreted products.

STORAGE AND STABILITY: Store at room temperature (15-30°C). Keep container tightly closed and protect from light.

INFORMATION FOR THE PATIENT: Published in e-CPS, available by subscription at www.e-cps.ca.

DOSAGE FORMS, COMPOSITION AND PACKAGING: 0.5 mg: Each white, round, flat-faced, bevel-edged compressed tablet, with MJ logo and "021" on one side and scored on the reverse, contains: estradiol-17β (micronized) 0.5 mg. Nonmedicinal ingredients: acacia, dibasic calcium phosphate, cornstarch, lactose, magnesium stearate, silicon dioxide and talc. Bottles of 100.

1 mg: Each lavender, round, flat-faced, bevel-edged compressed tablet, with MJ logo and "755" on one side and scored on the reverse, contains: estradiol-17β (micronized) 1 mg. Nonmedicinal ingredients: acacia, dibasic calcium phosphate, cornstarch, D&C Red No. 27 aluminum lake, FD&C Blue No. 1, lactose, magnesium stearate, silicon dioxide and talc. Bottles of 100.

2 mg: Each turquoise, round, flat-faced, bevel-edged compressed tablet, with MJ logo and "756" on one side and scored on the reverse, contains: estradiol-17β (micronized) 2 mg. Nonmedicinal ingredients: acacia, dibasic calcium phosphate, cornstarch, FD&C Blue No. 1, FD&C Yellow No. 5 aluminum lake (tartrazine), lactose, magnesium stearate, silicon dioxide and talc. Bottles of 100.

(Shown in Product Identification Section)

Estraderm® ℞
estradiol-17β
Estrogen

Novartis Pharmaceuticals

Date of Preparation: July 21, 1987
Date of Revision: January 23, 2009

SUMMARY PRODUCT INFORMATION:

Route of Administration	Dosage Form/ Strength	Clinically Relevant Nonmedicinal Ingredients
Transdermal	Patch 25, 50 and 100 µg	Cellulose compounds, ethanol, ethylene-vinyl acetate copolymer, light mineral oil, polyester and polyisobutylene

INDICATIONS AND CLINICAL USE: ESTRADERM (estradiol-17β) is indicated for:

- the relief of menopausal and postmenopausal symptoms occurring in naturally or surgically induced estrogen deficiency states.
- the prevention of osteoporosis in naturally occurring or surgically induced estrogen-deficiency states in addition to other important therapeutic measures such as adequate diet, calcium and vitamin D intake, cessation of smoking and regular weight-bearing exercise. In postmenopausal women already diagnosed as having osteoporosis and vertebral fractures, treatment with ESTRADERM may retard further bone loss. ESTRADERM is to be considered in the light of other available therapies for osteoporosis prevention and therapy should only be continued as long as the benefits outweigh the risks for the individual (see Boxed Warnings).

In women with an intact uteri, ESTRADERM should always be supplemented by sequential administration of a progestin whose role is to prevent endometrial hyperplasia/carcinoma.

Geriatrics (>65 years of age): No clinical studies were conducted to evaluate the effect of ESTRADERM on women more than 65 years old.

Pediatrics: ESTRADERM should not be used in children.

CONTRAINDICATIONS:

- Known or suspected hypersensitivity to this drug or to any ingredient in the formulation or to any component of the patch. For a complete listing, see Dosage Forms, Composition and Packaging.
- Liver dysfunction or disease as long as liver function tests have failed to return to normal
- Known or suspected estrogen-dependent malignant neoplasia such as endometrial cancer
- Endometrial hyperplasia
- Known, suspected or past history of breast cancer
- Undiagnosed abnormal genital bleeding
- Known or suspected pregnancy
- Active or past history of arterial thromboembolic disease (e.g. stroke, myocardial infarction, coronary heart disease)
- Active or past history of confirmed venous thromboembolism (such as deep venous thrombosis or pulmonary embolism) or active thrombophlebitis
- Partial or complete loss of vision from ophthalmic vascular disease
- Known thrombophilic disorders
- Porphyria
- Classical migraine
- Breast feeding

WARNINGS AND PRECAUTIONS:

> **Serious Warnings and Precautions**
> The Women's Health Initiative (WHI) trial examined the health benefits and risks of oral combined estrogen plus progestin therapy (n=16 608) and oral estrogen-alone therapy (n=10 739) in postmenopausal women aged 50 to 79 years.
> The estrogen plus progestin arm of the WHI trial (mean age 63.3 years) indicated an increased risk of myocardial infarction (MI), stroke, invasive breast cancer, pulmonary emboli and deep vein thrombosis in postmenopausal women receiving treatment with combined conjugated equine estrogens (CEE, 0.625 mg/day) and medroxyprogesterone acetate (MPA, 2.5 mg/day) for 5.2 years compared to those receiving placebo.
> The estrogen-alone arm of the WHI trial (mean age 63.6 years) indicated an increased risk of stroke and deep vein thrombosis in hysterectomized women treated with CEE-alone (0.625 mg/day) for 6.8 years compared to those receiving placebo.
> Therefore, the following should be given serious consideration at the time of prescribing:
> - Estrogens with or without progestins **should not** be prescribed for primary or secondary prevention of cardiovascular diseases.
> - Estrogens with or without progestins should be prescribed at **the lowest effective dose** for the approved indication.
> - For the prevention of osteoporosis, ESTRADERM treatment should be considered in light of other available therapies.
> - Estrogens with or without progestins should be prescribed for **the shortest period** possible for the approved indication.

Carcinogenesis and Mutagenesis: Breast Cancer: Available epidemiological data indicate that the use of combined estrogen plus progestin HRT by postmenopausal women is associated with an increased risk of invasive breast cancer.

In the estrogen plus progestin arm of the WHI trial, among 10 000 women over a one-year period, there were:

- 8 more cases of invasive breast cancer (38 on combined HRT versus 30 on placebo).

The WHI study also reported that the invasive breast cancers diagnosed in the estrogen plus progestin group were similar in histology but were larger (mean (SD), 1.7 cm (1.1) vs. 1.5 cm (0.9), respectively; P=0.04) and were at a more advanced stage compared with those diagnosed in the placebo group. The percentage of women with abnormal mammograms (recommendations for short-interval follow-up, a suspicious abnormality, or highly suggestive of malignancy) was significantly higher in the estrogen plus progestin group versus the placebo group. This difference appeared at year one and persisted in each year thereafter.

In the estrogen-alone arm of the WHI trial, there was no statistically significant difference in the rate of invasive breast cancer in hysterectomized women treated with conjugated equine estrogens versus women treated with placebo.

It is recommended that estrogens not be given to women with existing breast cancer or those with a previous history of the disease (see Contraindications).

There is a need for caution in prescribing estrogens for women with known risk factors associated with the development of breast cancer, such as strong family history of breast cancer (first degree relative) or who present a breast condition with an increased risk (breast nodules, fibrocystic disease of the breast, abnormal mammograms and/or atypical hyperplasia at breast biopsy).

Other known risk factors for the development of breast cancer such as nulliparity, obesity, early menarche, late age at first full term pregnancy and at menopause should also be evaluated.

It is recommended that women undergo mammography prior to the start of HRT treatment and at regular intervals during treatment, as deemed appropriate by the treating physician and according to the perceived risks for each patient.

The overall benefits and possible risks of hormone replacement therapy should be fully considered and discussed with patients. It is important that the modest increased risk of being diagnosed with breast cancer after 4 years of treatment with combined estrogen plus progestin HRT (as reported in the results of WHI-trial) be discussed with the patient and weighed against its known benefits.

Instructions for regular self-examination of the breasts should be included in this counselling.

Endometrial Hyperplasia & Endometrial Carcinoma: Estrogen should be prescribed with an appropriate dosage of a progestin for women with intact uteri in order to prevent endometrial hyperplasia/carcinoma.

Estrogen-only hormonal therapy in postmenopause is recommended for women without uteri only to avoid unnecessary exposure to progestins. The focus of the clinical program with VIVELLE/ESTRADOT was the demonstration of efficacy in the treatment of postmenopausal symptoms and in the prevention of postmenopausal osteoporosis. Some clinical trials included non-hysterectomized patients who were treated with concomitant progestogen therapy according to the best medical practice at the time, with different dosages, regimens and types of progestin. In addition, endometrial sampling after treatment was not consistently performed and in most cases no baseline data were available to assess the relationship and the effects of the progestogen treatment on the endometrium.

The risk of endometrial hyperplasia/carcinoma in users of unopposed estrogens who have intact uteri is greater than in non-users and appears to depend on the duration of treatment and the estrogen dose. The greatest risk appears to be associated with prolonged use. It has been shown that adequate concomitant progestogen therapy lowers the incidence of endometrial hyperplasia and therefore the potential risk of endometrial carcinoma associated with prolonged use of estrogen therapy (see Dosage and Administration, Coadministration of Progestins).

Ovarian Cancer: Some recent epidemiologic studies have found that the use of hormone replacement therapy (estrogen-alone and estrogen plus progestin therapies), in particular for five or more years, has been associated with an increased risk of ovarian cancer.

Hepatocellular Carcinomas: Hepatocellular carcinoma has also been reported in women taking estrogen-containing oral contraceptives. The causal relationship of this malignancy to these drugs is not known.

Cardiovascular: The results of the Heart and Estrogen/progestin Replacement Studies (HERS and HERS II) and the Women's Health Initiative (WHI) trial indicate that the use of estrogen plus progestin is associated with an increased risk of coronary heart disease (CHD) in postmenopausal women. The results of the WHI trial indicate that the use of estrogen-alone and estrogen plus progestin is associated with an increased risk of stroke in postmenopausal women.

WHI Trial Findings: In the combined estrogen plus progestin arm of the WHI trial, among 10 000 women over a one-year period, there were:

- 8 more cases of stroke (29 on combined HRT versus 21 on placebo)
- 7 more cases of CHD (37 on combined HRT versus 30 on placebo).

In the estrogen-alone arm of the WHI trial of women with prior hysterectomy, among 10 000 women over a one-year period, there were/was:

- 12 more cases of stroke (44 on estrogen-alone therapy versus 32 on placebo)
- no statistically significant difference in the rate of CHD.

HERS and HERS II Findings: In the Heart and Estrogen/progestin Replacement Study (HERS) of postmenopausal women with documented heart disease (n=2763, average age 66.7 years), a randomized placebo-controlled clinical trial of secondary prevention of coronary heart disease (CHD), treatment with 0.625 mg/day oral conjugated equine estrogen (CEE) plus 2.5 mg medroxyprogesterone acetate (MPA) demonstrated no cardiovascular benefit. Specifically, during an average follow-up of 4.1 years, treatment with CEE plus MPA did not reduce the overall rate of CHD events in postmenopausal women with established coronary heart disease. There were more CHD events in the hormone-treated group than in the placebo group in year 1, but not during the subsequent years.

From the original HERS trial, 2321 women consented to participate in an open label extension of HERS, known as HERS II. Average follow-up in HERS II was an additional 2.7 years, for a total of 6.8 years overall. After 6.8 years, hormone therapy did not reduce the risk of cardiovascular events in women with CHD.

Blood Pressure: Women using hormone replacement therapy sometimes experience increased blood pressure. Blood pressure should be monitored with HRT use. Elevation of blood pressure in previously normotensive or hypertensive patients should be investigated and HRT may have to be discontinued.

Ear/Nose/Throat: Otosclerosis: Estrogens should be used with caution in patients with otosclerosis.

Endocrine and Metabolism: Glucose and Lipid Metabolism: A worsening of glucose tolerance and lipid metabolism has been observed in a significant percentage of peri- and post-menopausal patients. Therefore, diabetic patients or those with a predisposition to diabetes should be observed closely to detect any alterations in carbohydrate or lipid metabolism, especially in triglyceride blood levels.

Women with familial hyperlipidemias need special surveillance. Lipid-lowering measures are recommended additionally, before treatment is started.

Calcium and Phosphorus Metabolism: Because the prolonged use of estrogens influences the metabolism of calcium and phosphorus, estrogens should be used with caution in patients with metabolic and malignant bone diseases associated with hypercalcemia and in patients with renal insufficiency.

Hypothyroidism: Patients who require thyroid hormone replacement therapy and who are also taking estrogen should have their thyroid function monitored regularly to assure that thyroid hormone levels remain in an acceptable range (see Drug Interactions, Drug-Laboratory Test Interactions).

Genitourinary: Vaginal Bleeding: Abnormal vaginal bleeding, due to its prolongation, irregularity or heaviness, occurring during therapy should prompt appropriate diagnostic measures, to rule out the possibility of uterine malignancy and the treatment should be re-evaluated.

Uterine Leiomyomata: Pre-existing uterine leiomyomata may increase in size during estrogen use. Growth, pain or tenderness of uterine leiomyomata requires discontinuation of medication and appropriate investigation.

Endometriosis: Symptoms and physical findings associated with a previous diagnosis of endometriosis may reappear or become aggravated with estrogen use.

Hematologic: Venous Thromboembolism: Available epidemiological data indicate that the use of estrogen with or without progestin by postmenopausal women is associated with an increased risk of developing venous thromboembolism (VTE).

In the estrogen plus progestin arm of the WHI trial, among 10 000 women on combined HRT over a one-year period, there were 18 more cases of venous thromboembolism, including 8 more cases of pulmonary embolism.

In the estrogen-alone arm of the WHI trial, among 10 000 women on estrogen therapy over a one-year period, there were 7 more cases of venous thromboembolism, although there was no statistically significant difference in the rate of pulmonary embolism.

Generally recognized risk factors for VTE include a personal history, a family history (the occurrence of VTE in a direct relative at a relatively early age may indicate genetic predisposition), severe obesity (body mass index >30 kg/m²) and systemic lupus erythematosus. The risk of VTE also increases with age and smoking.

A history of recurrent spontaneous abortions should be investigated to exclude thrombophilic predisposition. In patients in whom thrombophilia is confirmed, the use of ESTRADERM is viewed as contraindicated.

The risk of VTE may be temporarily increased with prolonged immobilization, major surgery or trauma. In women on HRT, attention should be given to prophylactic measures to prevent VTE following surgery. Also, patients with varicose veins should be closely supervised. The physician should be alert to the earliest manifestations of thrombotic disorders (thrombophlebitis, retinal thrombosis, cerebral embolism and pulmonary embolism). If these occur or are suspected, hormone therapy should be discontinued immediately given the risks of long-term disability or fatality.

If feasible, estrogens should be discontinued at least 4 weeks before major surgery which may be associated with an increased risk of thromboembolism, or during periods of prolonged immobilization. The treatment should not be restarted until the woman is completely mobile.

Hepatic/Biliary/Pancreatic: Benign Hepatic Adenomas: Benign hepatic adenomas have been associated with the use of combined estrogen and progestin oral contraceptives. Although benign and rare, these tumours may rupture and cause death from intra-abdominal hemorrhage. Such lesions have not yet been reported in association with other estrogen or progestin preparations, but they should be considered if abdominal pain and tenderness, abdominal mass, or hypovolemic shock occurs in patients receiving estrogen.

Gallbladder Diseases: A 2- to 4-fold increase in the risk of gallbladder disease requiring surgery in women receiving postmenopausal estrogens has been reported.

Hepatic Hemangiomas: Particular caution is indicated in women with hepatic hemangiomas, as estrogen may cause an exacerbation of this condition.

Jaundice: Caution is advised in patients with a history of liver and/or biliary disorders. If cholestatic jaundice develops during treatment, the treatment should be discontinued and appropriate investigations carried out.

Liver Function Tests: Liver function tests should be done periodically in subjects who are suspected of having hepatic disease. For information on endocrine and liver function tests, see the section under Monitoring and Laboratory Tests.

Immune: Angioedema: Estrogens may induce or exacerbate symptoms of angioedema, in particular in women with hereditary angioedema.

Systemic Lupus Erythematosus: Particular caution is indicated in women with systemic lupus erythematosus.

Neurologic: Cerebrovascular Insufficiency: Patients who develop visual disturbances, classical migraine, transient aphasia, paralysis or loss of consciousness should discontinue medication.

Dementia: Available epidemiological data indicate that the use of combined estrogen plus progestin in women age 65 and over may increase the risk of developing probable dementia.

The Women's Health Initiative Memory Study (WHIMS), a clinical sub-study of the WHI, was designed to assess whether postmenopausal hormone replacement therapy (oral estrogen plus progestin or oral estrogen-alone) reduces the risk of dementia in women aged 65 and over (age range 65-79 years) and free of dementia at baseline.

In the estrogen plus progestin arm of the WHIMS (n=4532), women with intact uteri were treated with daily 0.625 mg conjugated equine estrogens (CEE) plus 2.5 mg medroxyprogesterone acetate (MPA) or placebo for an average of 4.05 years. The results, when extrapolated to 10 000 women treated over a one-year period showed:

- 23 more cases of probable dementia (45 on combined HRT versus 22 on placebo).

In the estrogen-alone arm of the WHIMS (n=2947), women with prior hysterectomy were treated with daily 0.625 mg CEE or placebo for an average of 5.21 years. The results, when extrapolated to 10 000 women treated over a one-year period showed:

- 12 more cases of probable dementia (37 on estrogen-alone versus 25 on placebo), although this difference did not reach statistical significance.

When data from the estrogen plus progestin arm of the WHIMS and the estrogen alone arm of the WHIMS were combined, as per the original WHIMS protocol, in 10 000 women over a one-year period, there were:

- 18 more cases of probable dementia (41 on estrogen plus progestin or estrogen-alone versus 23 on placebo).

For transdermal estrogen-only or estrogen-progestogen combined products, no large randomized clinical trials have assessed the HRT-associated risk of probable dementia to date. Therefore there are no data to support the conclusion that the frequency of probable dementia is different with ESTRADERM.

Epilepsy: Particular caution is indicated in women with epilepsy, as estrogen, with or without progestins, may cause an exacerbation of this condition.

Renal: Fluid Retention: Estrogens may cause fluid retention. Therefore, particular caution is indicated in cardiac or renal dysfunction, or asthma. If, in any of the above-mentioned conditions, a worsening of the underlying disease is diagnosed or suspected during treatment, the benefits and risks of treatment should be reassessed based on the individual case.

Skin: Contact Sensitization: Contact sensitization is known to occur with topical applications. Although it is extremely rare, patients who develop contact sensitization to any component of the patch should be warned that a severe hypersensitivity reaction may occur with continuing exposure to the causative agent.

Special Populations: Pregnant Women: ESTRADERM must not be used during pregnancy. Both estrogens and progestogens may cause foetal harm when administered to a pregnant woman.

Nursing Women: ESTRADERM must not be used while breastfeeding.

Pediatrics: ESTRADERM should not be used in children.

Geriatrics (>65 years of age): No clinical studies were conducted to evaluate the effect of ESTRADERM on women more than 65 years old.

Monitoring and Laboratory Tests: Before ESTRADERM (estradiol-17β) is administered, the patient should have a complete physical examination including a blood pressure determination. Breasts and pelvic organs should be appropriately examined and a Papanicolaou smear should be performed. Endometrial biopsy should be done only when indicated. Baseline tests should include mammography, measurements of blood glucose, calcium, triglycerides and cholesterol, and liver function tests.

The first follow-up examination should be done within 3-6 months after initiation of treatment to assess response to treatment. Thereafter, examinations should be made at intervals at least once a year. Appropriate investigations should be arranged at regular intervals as determined by the physician.

The importance of regular self-examination of the breasts should be discussed with the patient.

Women should be advised that changes in their breasts should be reported to their doctor or nurse.

ADVERSE REACTIONS: Adverse Drug Reaction Overview: See Warnings and Precautions regarding potential induction of malignant neoplasms and adverse effects similar to those of oral contraceptives.

The following adverse reactions have been reported with estrogen/progestin combinations in general.

Blood and Lymphatic System Disorders: altered coagulation tests (see Drug Interactions, Monitoring and Laboratory Tests).

Cardiac Disorders: palpitations; increase in blood pressure (see Warnings and Precautions); coronary thrombosis.

Endocrine Disorders: increased blood sugar levels; decreased glucose tolerance.

Eye Disorders: neuro-ocular lesions (e.g., retinal thrombosis, optic neuritis), visual disturbances; steepening of the corneal curvature; intolerance to contact lenses.

Gastrointestinal Disorders: nausea; vomiting; abdominal discomfort (cramps, pressure, pain; bloating).

General Disorders and Administration Site Conditions: fatigue; changes in appetite; changes in body weight; change in libido.

Hepatobiliary Disorders: gallbladder disorder; asymptomatic impaired liver function; cholestatic jaundice.

Musculoskeletal and Connective Tissue Disorders: musculoskeletal pain including leg pain not related to thromboembolic disease (usually transient, lasting 3-6 weeks) may occur.

Nervous System Disorders: aggravation of migraine episodes; headaches; dizziness; neuritis.

Psychiatric Disorders: mental depression; nervousness; irritability.

Renal and Urinary Disorders: cystitis; dysuria; sodium retention; edema.

Reproductive System and Breast Disorders: breakthrough bleeding; spotting; change in menstrual flow; dysmenorrhea; vaginal itching/discharge; dyspareunia; endometrial hyperplasia; pre-menstrual-like syndrome; reactivation of endometriosis; changes in cervical erosion and amount of cervical secretion; breast swelling and tenderness.

Skin and Subcutaneous Tissue Disorders: loss of scalp hair; chloasma or melasma, which may persist when drug is discontinued; erythema nodosum; erythema multiforme; hemorrhagic skin eruptions; hirsutism, acne.

Vascular Disorders: isolated cases of thrombophlebitis; thromboembolic disorders.

Clinical Trial Adverse Drug Reactions: This section summarizes adverse drug reaction data pooled from clinical trials, published investigations and post-marketing experience.

The most commonly reported adverse reaction to ESTRADERM (estradiol-17β) in clinical trials was redness and irritation at the application site. This occurred in about 17% of the women treated and caused approximately 2% to discontinue therapy.

The data on adverse events from 5 pooled clinical trials are included. 3 clinical trials had a 2 years duration and 2 had a 1 year duration. A total safety population of 941 patients on HRT and 207 patients on placebo was identified.

Frequency estimate: very common ≥10%, common ≥1% to <10%; uncommon ≥0.1% to <1%; rare ≥0.01% to <0.1%; very rare <0.01%; with unknown frequency. See Table 1.

Table 1: ESTRADERM
Most Common Adverse Drug Reactions (≥1%)

Vascular Disorders	
Common	Varicose veins
Nervous System Disorders	
Common	Dizziness, headache
Gastrointestinal Disorders	
Common	Nausea, abdominal pain, abdominal distension
Skin and Subcutaneous Tissue Disorders	
Common	Rash
Reproductive System and Breast Disorders	
Very common	Breast discomfort
Common	Menstrual disorder
Investigations	
Common	Weight fluctuation
General Disorders and Administration Site Disorders	
Very common	Application site reaction
Common	Oedema

Less Common Clinical Trial Adverse Drug Reactions (<1%): Cardiovascular Disorders: Rare: embolism. Very rare: hypertension.
Hepatobiliary Disorders: Very rare: jaundice cholestatic, liver function test abnormal.
Immune System Disorders: Very rare: anaphylactoid reactions.
Musculoskeletal and Connective Tissue Disorders: Rare: pain in extremity.
Neoplasms Benign, Malignant and Unspecified (including cysts and polyps): Rare: breast cancer.
Skin and Subcutaneous Tissue Disorders: Very rare: generalised pruritus, pigmentation disorders.
Adverse Drug Reactions with Unknown Frequency: Immune System Disorders: Not Known: hypersensitivity.
Skin and Subcutaneous Tissue Disorders: Not Known: erythema nodosum, erythema multiforme.
Abnormal Hematologic and Clinical Chemistry Findings: See Table 2.

Table 2: ESTRADERM
Abnormal Hematologic and Clinical Chemistry

Laboratory Parameters	Effect
Antithrombin III	↓
Coagulation factors VII, VIII, IX, X	↑
Corticosteroid binding globulin (CBG)	CBG ↑ in serum → increased circulating corticosteroids free or biologically active hormone concentrations are unchanged
Fibrinogen and fibrinogen activity	↑ levels
Folate	↓ serum concentration
T_3	↓ resin uptake, reflecting the elevated TBG
Free T_4	concentration unaltered
Glucose	impaired glucose tolerance
METOPIRONE test	reduced response
Norepinephrine-induced platelet aggregability	↑
Prothrombin time and partial tromboplastin time	↑
Sex-hormone binding globulin (SHBG)	SHBG ↑ in serum → increased circulating corticosteroids free or biologically active hormone concentrations are unchanged
Sulfobromophthalein	↑ retention
Triglyceride and Phospholipid	↑ serum concentration
Thyroxin-binding globulin (TBG)	↑ → increased circulating total thyroid hormone (T_4) as measured by column or radioimmunoassay

If adverse symptoms persist, the prescription of HRT should be re-considered.

DRUG INTERACTIONS: Overview:
- Estrogens may diminish the effectiveness of anticoagulant, antidiabetic and antihypertensive agents.
- Preparations inducing liver enzymes (e.g. barbiturates, hydantoins, carbamazepine, meprobamates, phenylbutazone or rifampicin) may interfere with the activity of orally administered estrogens.

Drug-Drug Interactions: The following section contains information on drug interactions with ethinyl estradiol-containing products (specifically, oral contraceptives) that have been reported in the public literature. It is unknown whether such interactions occur with drug products containing other types of estrogens. See Table 3.
Drug-Food Interactions: The interaction of ESTRADERM with food has not been studied.
Drug-Herb Interactions: It was found that some herbal products (e.g., St. John's wort) which are available as over-the-counter (OTC) products might interfere with steroid metabolism, and therefore, alter the efficacy and safety of estrogen/progestin products.
Physicians and other health care providers should be made aware of other non-prescription products concomitantly used by the patient, including herbal and natural products obtained from the widely spread health stores.

Table 3: ESTRADERM
Established or Potential Drug-Drug Interactions

Drug	Ref	Effect	Clinical Comment
Anticonvulsants (phenobarbital, phenytoin, carbamazepin)	T	↑ metabolism of ethinyl estradiol	↓ plasma concentration of estradiol
Acetaminophen	T	↑ AUC and/or plasma concentration of ethinyl estradiol ↓ plasma concentration of acetaminophen	Therapeutic monitoring is recommended
Acid ascorbic	T	↑ AUC and/or plasma concentration of ethinyl estradiol	Therapeutic monitoring is recommended
Aminoglutethimide with medroxyprogesterone acetate (MPA)	T	↓ bioavailability of MPA	Therapeutic monitoring is recommended
Atorvastatin	T	↑ AUC values for ethinyl estradiol by 20%	Therapeutic monitoring is recommended
Clofibric acid	T	↑ clearance of clofibric acid	Therapeutic monitoring is recommended
Cyclosporine	T	↑ plasma concentration of cyclosporine.	Therapeutic monitoring is recommended
Morphine	T	↑ clearance of morphine	Therapeutic monitoring is recommended
Prednisolone	T	↑ plasma concentration of prednisolone	Therapeutic monitoring is recommended
Rifampicin[a]	T	↑ metabolism of ethinyl estradiol	↓ plasma concentration of estradiol
Salicylic acid	T	↑ clearance of salicylic acid	Therapeutic monitoring is recommended
Temazepam	T	↑ clearance of temazepam	Therapeutic monitoring is recommended
Theophylline	T	↑ plasma concentration of theophylline	Therapeutic monitoring is recommended
Troglitazone	T	↓ plasma concentrations of ethinyl estradiol by 30%	Therapeutic monitoring is recommended
Temazepam	T	↑ clearance of temazepam	Therapeutic monitoring is recommended

[a] Clinical pharmacokinetics studies have not demonstrated any consistent effect of antibiotics (other than rifampicin) on plasma concentrations of synthetic steroids.
Legend: C=case study; CT=clinical trial; T=theoretical.

Drug-Laboratory Test Interactions: The results of certain endocrine and liver function tests may be affected by estrogen-containing products:
- increased prothrombin time and partial thromboplastin time; increased levels of fibrinogen and fibrinogen activity; increased coagulation factors VII, VIII, IX, X; increased norepinephrine induced platelet aggregability; decreased antithrombin III;
- increased thyroxine-binding globulin (TBG), leading to increased circulating total thyroid hormone (T_4) as measured by column or radioimmunoassay; T_3 resin uptake is decreased, reflecting the elevated TBG; free T_4 concentration is unaltered;
- other binding proteins may be elevated in serum i.e., corticosteroid binding globulin (CBG), sex-hormone binding globulin (SHBG), leading to increased circulating corticosteroids and sex steroids respectively; free or biologically active hormone concentrations are unchanged;
- impaired glucose tolerance;
- increased serum triglyceride and phospholipid concentration.

(See also Table 2 in Abnormal Hematologic and Clinical Chemistry Findings)
In clinical trials with ESTRADERM, no effect on fibrinogen, antithrombin III, TBG, CBG or SHBG and decreases in serum triglycerides was seen.
The results of the above laboratory tests should not be considered reliable unless therapy has been discontinued for two to four weeks. The pathologist should be informed that the patient is receiving estrogen therapy when relevant specimens are submitted.
Drug-Lifestyle Interactions: Specific drug-lifestyle interaction studies have not been conducted with ESTRADERM.
Acute alcohol ingestion during HRT may lead to elevations in circulating estradiol levels.

DOSAGE AND ADMINISTRATION: Dosing Considerations:
- For all therapeutic indications, the lowest effective dose should be used for maintenance therapy (see Coadministration of Progestins).
- Hormone replacement therapy (HRT) involving either estrogen alone or estrogen-progestogen combined therapy should only be continued as long as the benefits outweigh the risks for the individual.
- In women who are not currently taking oral estrogens, treatment with ESTRADERM (estradiol-17β) can be initiated at once. In women who are currently taking oral estrogens, treatment with ESTRADERM can be initiated on reappearance of menopausal symptoms, following discontinuation of oral therapy.
- ESTRADERM is administered as continuous therapy (uninterrupted application). ESTRADERM should be applied twice weekly i.e., the patch should be changed once every 3-4 days.
- In women with intact uteri, a progestin should be sequentially coadministered for 12 to 14 days per cycle to avoid overstimulation of the endometrium. The addition of sufficient progestin to induce secretory transformation of the endometrium during estrogen replacement therapy is mandatory.
- Abnormal vaginal bleeding, due to its prolongation, irregularity or heaviness, in any patient receiving hormone replacement therapy requires institution of prompt diagnostic measures like endometrial biopsy or curettage to rule out the possibility of uterine malignancy.
- The short term effects of progestin coadministration may include vaginal bleeding during or after progestin treatment, breast tenderness, and mood and weight changes. The long-term effects generally depend on the dosage and type of progestin used. The lowest effective dose of estrogen and progestin should be prescribed (see Coadministration of Progestins).
- ESTRADERM should be prescribed with an appropriate dosage of a progestin for women with intact uteri in order to prevent endometrial hyperplasia/carcinoma. Progestin therapy is not required as part of hormone replacement therapy in women who have had a previous hysterectomy.

See Warnings and Precautions section on the examination of the patient before ESTRADERM administration.

Recommended Dose and Dosage Adjustment:
1. **Menopausal Symptoms**
Treatment of menopausal symptoms is usually initiated with a patch that releases 50 µg estradiol-17β per day i.e. ESTRADERM 50. Thereafter the dosage should be adapted to the needs of the individual.
Breast discomfort, breakthrough or heavy vaginal bleeding, water retention, bloating or nausea (if persisting for more than six weeks), are generally signs that the estrogen dose is too high and needs to be lowered. If on the other hand, the selected dose fails to eliminate the signs and symptoms of estrogen deficiency, a higher dose may be considered.

For maintenance therapy one should always use the lowest dose that still proves effective. The requirement for hormone replacement therapy for menopausal symptoms should be reassessed periodically. Attempts to taper or discontinue the medication should be made at 3 to 6 month intervals.

The doses of ESTRADERM and conjugated estrogens which have been shown to produce the same clinical effect on postmenopausal symptomatology are: ESTRADERM 25: conjugated estrogens 0.3 mg; ESTRADERM 50: conjugated estrogens 0.625 mg, ESTRADERM 100: conjugated estrogens 1.25 mg.

2. **Prevention of Osteoporosis**

For optimal prevention of postmenopausal bone loss in women for whom the drug is indicated, therapy should be initiated as soon as possible after diagnosis of menopause. The dosage of estradiol-17β may require adjustment according to the patient's clinical status, the plasma estradiol-17β levels and the results of bone mineral density studies. Ideally, plasma estradiol-17β levels should be maintained at 184 pM/L (50 pg/mL). To treat patients with established osteoporosis, therapy should be initiated with ESTRADERM 100.

Discontinuation of hormone replacement therapy may reestablish the natural rate of bone loss.

Missed Dose: Patients who miss applying a patch of ESTRADERM, should apply a new patch as soon as possible. The subsequent patch should be applied according to the original treatment schedule. The interruption of treatment might increase the likelihood of recurrence of symptoms.

Administration: Patch Application: The physician should discuss the most appropriate placement of the patch with the patient. Immediately after removal of a patch from the pouch and removal of the protective liner, the adhesive side of the ESTRADERM patch should be placed on a clean, dry area of intact skin. The area selected should not be oily, damaged or irritated, and not exposed to the sun. The site selected should also be one at which little wrinkling of the skin occurs during movement of the body, preferably the buttocks, lower abdomen or hip. The patch may also be placed on the side or lower back. Experience to date has shown that less irritation of the skin occurs on the buttocks than on other sites of application. Therefore, it is advisable to apply ESTRADERM to the buttocks. The waistline should be avoided, since tight clothing may dislodge the patch. The patch should be pressed firmly in place with the palm of the hand, making sure there is good contact, especially around the edges. In the event that a patch should fall off, it can be reapplied. If it fails to adhere then a new patch may be applied. In either case, the original treatment schedule should be continued. Patches should not be applied to the same skin site twice in succession.

ESTRADERM must not be applied to the breasts to avoid potentially harmful effects on the breast tissue.

Coadministration of Progestins: Studies have reported that the addition of a progestin for 10 or more days of a cycle of estrogen administration greatly lowers the incidence of endometrial hyperplasia, and thereby irregular bleeding and endometrial carcinoma, compared to estrogen treatment alone. This applies to women with intact uteri and not to those who have had hysterectomies.

OVERDOSAGE:

Symptoms of Overdose: Numerous reports of ingestion of large doses of estrogen products and estrogen-containing oral contraceptives by young children have not revealed acute serious ill effects. Overdosage with estrogen may cause nausea, breast discomfort, fluid retention, bloating or vaginal bleeding in women.

Treatment of Overdose: Owing to the mode of administration (transdermal), plasma levels of estradiol-17β can be rapidly reduced by removal of the patch. Symptomatic treatment should be given.

For management of a suspected drug overdose, contact your regional Poison Control Centre. See the *CPS* Directory section for a list of Poison Control Centres.

ACTION AND CLINICAL PHARMACOLOGY: Mechanism of Action: ESTRADERM is designed to deliver daily estradiol-17β, a physiologic hormone, transdermally into the systemic circulation. Due to the transdermal route of administration, the estradiol-17β does not undergo first pass liver metabolism. Resultant estradiol-17β plasma levels are comparable to those seen in premenopausal women in the early follicular phase of the menstrual cycle. Estradiol-17β stimulates target tissues such as the uterus, breast and vagina.

ESTRADERM delivers estradiol-17β via skin, which metabolizes estradiol only to a small extent. In comparison, orally administered estrogens are rapidly metabolized by the liver to estrone and its conjugates, giving rise to higher circulating levels of estrogens than estradiol. Therefore, transdermal administration of estradiol produces therapeutic plasma levels with lower circulating levels of estrone conjugates and requires smaller total doses than does oral therapy.

Estrogen replacement therapy decreases the rate of bone loss in menopausal women; evidence of estrogen receptors on bone cells suggests there is a direct effect of estrogen on bone.

Pharmacodynamics: Estradiol: Like all steroid hormones, estrogens exert their metabolic effects intracellularly. In the cells of the target organs, estrogens interact with a specific receptor to form a complex which modulates gene transcription and subsequent protein synthesis. Such receptors have been identified in various organs, e.g. hypothalamus, pituitary, vagina, urethra, uterus, breast and liver, and in osteoblasts.

Estradiol, which from the menarche to the menopause is produced mainly by the ovarian follicles, is the most active estrogen. It is largely responsible for the development and maintenance of the female urogenital system and of secondary sexual characteristics. After the menopause, when the ovaries have ceased to function, only small amounts of estradiol are still produced, from aromatisation of androstenedione and to a lesser extent testosterone, by the aromatase enzyme, yielding estrone and estradiol, respectively. Estrone is further transformed to estradiol by the enzyme 17beta-hydroxysteroid-dehydrogenase. Both enzymes occur in fat, liver, and muscle tissue.

In many women, the cessation of ovarian estradiol production results in vasomotor symptoms (hot flushes), sleep disturbances, and progressive atrophy of the urogenital system.

Hormone Replacement Therapy: ESTRADERM (estradiol-17β) provide continuous, controlled transdermal delivery of estradiol-17β such that estradiol-17β levels as well as the E_2/E_1 ratio in postmenopausal women are restored to those seen in the earlier follicular phase of the premenopausal range (see Pharmacokinetics). ESTRADERM thus alleviate the symptoms of estradiol-17β deficiency in menopausal women.

Placebo-controlled clinical studies have demonstrated that treatment with ESTRADERM 50 or 100 (50 μg or 100 μg per day, respectively) prevents bone loss in postmenopausal women. In recently post-menopausal women, prophylactic treatment with ESTRADERM 100 for 2 years led to a significant increase (3.7% above baseline), in vertebral bone density. Treatment with ESTRADERM 50 showed maintenance of bone density. Initiating treatment with ESTRADERM 100/medroxyprogesterone acetate (MPA) 10-15 years after menopause, prevented further loss of bone density in osteoporotic women with vertebral fractures. Vertebral bone density increased by 7.5% after 1 year.

Pharmacokinetics: Absorption: Studies in postmenopausal women using ESTRADERM patches which provide 25, 50, and 100 μg of exogenous estradiol-17β per day, showed increased blood levels within 4 hours. These levels were linearly proportional to the size of the dose and maintained respective mean serum estradiol-17β levels of 59, 117 and 246 pM/L (16, 32, and 67 pg/mL) above baseline (typically 37 pM/L (10 pg/mL)). At the same time, increases in estrone serum concentration averaged only 1.1, 33, and 100 pM/L (0.3, 9, and 27 pg/mL) above baseline, respectively, providing an average E_2/E_1 ratio between 0.9-1.4, well within the pre-menopausal range. Serum concentrations of estradiol-17β and estrone returned to pre-application levels within 24 hours after removal of the patch.

Distribution: Mean plasma clearance rates of estradiol-17β and estrone in women have been estimated to be 735 L/day per m^2 and 1213 L/day per m^2, respectively. Hence, based on studies with ESTRADERM, for women with a body surface area of 1.4-1.9 m^2, (weight, 48-86 kg; average height 157 cm) ESTRADERM patches which provide 25, 50 and 100 μg/day should maintain mean steady state serum concentrations as follows: see Table 4.

Table 4: ESTRADERM

Mean Steady State Serum Concentrations

Patch	Estradiol Dosage (μg per day)	Expected Increase in Serum Levels of Estradiol (pg/mL) Above Baseline (typically 10 pg/mL)
ESTRADERM 25	25	12–18
ESTRADERM 50	50	24–40
ESTRADERM 100	100	48–85

Estradiol-17β delivered by the transdermal route results in an E_2/E_1 ratio of approximately 1. By comparison, typical E_2/E_1 ratios following oral estrogen therapy are 0.1 to 0.3 because estrone levels increase to a greater extent than estradiol-17β levels. The extensive first-pass liver metabolism leads to supraphysiological plasma concentrations of estrone and, in patients on prolonged treatment, to accumulation of estrone and estrone sulphate.

Metabolism: Metabolism and plasma levels of estradiol-17β delivered transdermally are similar to those in premenopausal women.

Estradiol-17β is rapidly metabolized, primarily in the liver and gut. Its most important metabolites are estriol and estrone and their conjugates (glucuronides, sulphates); these are far less active than estradiol-17β. The bulk of the metabolites is excreted in the urine as glucuronides and sulphates. Estrogen metabolites are also subject to enterohepatic circulation. The skin metabolizes estradiol-17β only to a small extent.

Excretion: The daily urinary output of estradiol-17β conjugates increased 3 to 10 times the baseline values and returned to near baseline values within 2 days after removal of the patch. Multiple-application studies yielded similar results, with urinary output of estradiol-17β conjugates returning to baseline within 3 days of patch removal.

The plasma elimination half-life of estradiol-17β is approximately 1 hour. The short half-life and rapid clearance of estradiol-17β permit a rapid cessation of estrogen therapy when cycling is desirable.

Special Populations and Conditions: Pediatrics: ESTRADERM should not be used in children.

Geriatrics (>65 years of age): No clinical studies were conducted to evaluate the effect of estradiol on women more than 65 years old.

Gender: ESTRADERM should be used in women only.

Estrogen Pharmacology : Estradiol-17β is the major estrogenic hormone secreted by the human ovary. Among numerous effects, estradiol-17β is largely responsible for the development and maintenance of the female reproductive system and of secondary sexual characteristics. It promotes growth and development of the vagina, uterus, fallopian tubes, and breasts. Estradiol-17β contributes to the shaping of the skeleton, to the maintenance of tone and elasticity of urogenital structures, to changes in the epiphyses of the long bones that allow for the pubertal growth spurt and its termination, to the growth of axillary and pubic hair, and to the pigmentation of the nipples and genitals. Estradiol-17β also affects the release of pituitary gonadotropins.

After menopause, when the ovaries have ceased to function, only small amounts of estradiol-17β are still produced, i.e., from the aromatization of androstenedione to estrone and to a lesser extent, testosterone to estradiol-17β. Estrone is transformed to estradiol-17β by the enzyme 17β-hydroxysteroid-dehydrogenase. Both enzymes prevail in fat, liver and muscle tissue.

In premenopausal women, the ratio of estradiol-17β (E_2) to estrone (E_1) (i.e., E_2/E_1 ratio) in the plasma is in the range of 0.5 to 2, depending on the phase of the menstrual cycle. The E_2/E_1 ratio for untreated postmenopausal women is below 0.5.

Loss of the ovarian estradiol-17β production after menopause can result in the following: instability of thermoregulation causing hot flushes associated with sleep disturbance and excessive sweating; accelerated loss of bone matrix and mineral, resulting in osteoporosis; alterations in lipid metabolism; urogenital atrophy, causing dyspareunia and urinary incontinence.

The protection against endometrial hyperplasia in women with intact uteri is necessary during long-term therapy. Published data suggest that 12 to 14 days of sequential progestin treatment during estrogen replacement therapy reduces the occurrence of endometrial hyperplasia, and thereby irregular bleeding and endometrial carcinoma, compared to estrogen treatment alone.

STORAGE AND STABILITY: Store patches below 25°C. Do not freeze.

Each patch is individually sealed in a separate pouch. Do not store out of the pouch. Apply immediately upon removal from the protective pouch. Patches should be applied in whole.

Keep ESTRADERM out of the reach and sight of children and pets both before use and when disposing of used patches.

Do not use any ESTRADERM patch that is damaged or shows signs of tampering.

SPECIAL HANDLING INSTRUCTIONS: See Dosage and Administration, Administration, Patch Application.

INFORMATION FOR THE PATIENT: Published in e-CPS, available by subscription at www.e-cps.ca.

DOSAGE FORMS, COMPOSITION AND PACKAGING: ESTRADERM (estradiol-17β) is a thin, round, multilayer, transparent transdermal therapeutic system, i.e., an adhesive patch, containing estradiol-17β that is designed for application to an area of intact skin.

The ESTRADERM patch comprises five layers. Proceeding from the visible surface toward the surface attached to the skin, these layers are:

- a transparent polyester **backing film**
- a drug **reservoir** of estradiol-17β and ethanol gelled with hydroxypropyl cellulose
- an ethylene vinyl acetate copolymer **release-controlling membrane**
- an **adhesive** formulation of light mineral oil and polyisobutylene
- a **protective liner** of siliconized polyethylene terephthalate film that is attached to the adhesive surface and must be removed before the patch can be used.

The active component of the patch is estradiol-17β. Nonmedicinal ingredients: cellulose compounds, ethanol, ethylene-vinyl acetate copolymer, light mineral oil, polyester and polyisobutylene.

The drug reservoir provides a source for continuous delivery of drug for up to 4 days. ESTRADERM is available in 3 strengths; the composition per unit area is identical.

ESTRADERM (estradiol-17β) is available in the following strengths in patient packs containing 8 patches: See Table 5.

Table 5: ESTRADERM

ESTRADERM Composition

	ESTRADERM 25	ESTRADERM 50	ESTRADERM 100
Estradiol-17β Dosage nominal in vivo delivery	25 μg/day	50 μg/day	100 μg/day
Total Estradiol-17β content	2 mg	4 mg	8 mg
Drug-Releasing Area	5 cm²	10 cm²	20 cm²
Shape of Patch	Round	Round	Oblong
Printed (backing side)	CG DND	—	—

(Shown in Product Identification Section)

Estradot®

estradiol-17β

Estrogen

Novartis Pharmaceuticals

Date of Preparation: December 21, 1995
Date of Revision: June 10, 2004

Warning: As the Women's Health Initiative (WHI) study results indicated increased risk of myocardial infarction (MI), stroke, invasive breast cancer, pulmonary emboli and deep venous thrombosis in postmenopausal women receiving treatment with combined oral conjugated equine estrogens (CE 0.625 mg) and medroxyprogesterone acetate (MPA 2.5 mg) compared to those receiving placebo tablets, the following should be highly considered:

- Estrogens with or without progestins **should not** be prescribed for primary or secondary prevention of cardiovascular diseases.
- Estrogens with or without progestins should be prescribed at **the lowest effective dose** for the approved indications.
- For the prevention of osteoporosis, estrogen treatment should be considered in light of other available therapies.
- Estrogens with or without progestins should be prescribed for **the shortest period** possible for the recognized indications.

PHARMACOLOGY: ESTRADOT is designed to deliver daily estradiol-17β, a physiologic hormone, transdermally into the systemic circulation. Due to the transdermal route of administration, the estradiol-17β does not undergo first-pass liver metabolism. Resultant estradiol-17β plasma levels are comparable to those seen in premenopausal women in the early follicular phase of the menstrual cycle. Estradiol-17β stimulates target tissues such as the uterus, breast and vagina.

ESTRADOT delivers estradiol-17β via the skin, which metabolizes estradiol only to a small extent. In comparison, orally administered estrogens are rapidly metabolized by the liver to estrone and its conjugates, giving rise to higher circulating levels of estrogens than transdermal estradiol. Therefore, transdermal administration of estradiol produces therapeutic plasma levels with lower circulating levels of estrone conjugates and requires smaller total doses than does oral therapy.

Clinical Studies: Relief of menopausal symptoms: Efficacy and safety of another estradiol-17β matrix patch (VIVELLE) in the relief of menopausal and postmenopausal symptoms have been studied in two multicenter, double-blind, placebo-controlled pivotal studies. A total of 356 healthy menopausal women aged 30-65 years (mean 50.5 years) with moderate to severe vasomotor symptoms, a minimum of 6 hot flushes/day, plasma estradiol levels ≤20 pg/mL and plasma FSH levels ≥50 mU/mL were enrolled in the studies. A total of 266 women were randomized to VIVELLE patches (37.5, 50, 75 or 100 µg/day) and 90 were randomized to placebo patches. Over 3 months (3 cycles), the patches were applied to a clear, non-oily area of the abdomen below the waist and were changed twice a week. The evaluable groups consisted of 239 active and 80 placebo patients.

The primary efficacy variable for both studies was the change in the number of hot flushes at the end of the third treatment cycle compared to baseline values. VIVELLE was found to be statistically and clinically superior to placebo at all four doses (Table 1). In addition, VIVELLE significantly reduced the severity of hot flushes, sweating and insomnia compared to placebo.

Table 1: ESTRADOT

Mean Reduction in Number of Hot Flushes—Studies 1003-A and 1003-B Combined

Treatment	N	Baseline	N	Cycle 3
37.5 µg/day	79	10.3	77	−7.1[a]
50 µg/day	44	12.5	43	−7.6[a]
75 µg/day	40	13.0	37	−9.1[a]
100 µg/day	76	11.2	68	−9.0[a]
Placebo	80	10.8	72	−3.0

[a] $p<0.0001$.

Prevention of Osteoporosis: Efficacy and safety of another estradiol-17β matrix patch (VIVELLE) in the prevention of postmenopausal osteoporosis have been studied in a 2-year double-blind, randomized, placebo-controlled, parallel group study. A total of 261 hysterectomized (161) and non-hysterectomized (100), surgically or naturally menopausal women (within 5 years of menopause), with no evidence of osteoporosis (lumbar spine bone mineral density within 2 standard deviation of average peak bone mass, i.e., ≥0.827 g/cm²) were enrolled in this study; 194 patients were randomized to one of the four doses of VIVELLE (100, 50, 37.5 or 25 µg/day) and 67 patients to placebo. Over 2 years, study systems were applied to the buttock or the abdomen twice a week. Nonhysterectomized women received oral medroxy progesterone acetate (2.5 mg/day) throughout the study.

The study population comprised naturally (82%) or surgically (18%) menopausal, hysterectomized (61%) or nonhysterectomized (39%) women with a mean age of 52.0 years (range 27 to 62 years; the mean duration of menopause was 31.7 months (range 2 to 72 months). Two hundred thirty nine (92%) of randomized subjects (178 on active drug, 61 on placebo) contributed data to the analysis of percent change from baseline in bone mineral density (BMD) of the AP lumbar spine, the primary efficacy variable. There was an increase in BMD of the AP lumbar spine in all VIVELLE dose groups; in contrast to this a decrease in AP lumbar spine BMD was observed in placebo patients. All VIVELLE doses were significantly superior to placebo ($p<0.05$) at all time points with the exception of VIVELLE 50 µg/day at 6 months, implying bone preservation for all treatment groups, as opposed to bone loss for placebo.

Analysis of percent change from baseline in femoral neck BMD also showed similar results; all doses of VIVELLE were significantly superior to placebo ($p<0.05$) at 24 months.

Serum osteocalcin (a marker of bone formation) and urinary excretion of cross-link N-telopeptides of type 1 collagen (a marker of bone resorption) generally decreased in active treatment groups, suggesting a decrease in bone turnover. However, the differences were not statistically significant.

Bioequivalence Study: A comparative, multiple dose, cross-over pharmacokinetic study in 30 healthy postmenopausal women demonstrated that the ESTRADOT 5 cm² (50 µg/day) and the VIVELLE 14.5 cm² (50 µg/day) patches produced comparable serum concentrations of estradiol at steady state. Each patch was administered for four 84-hour dosing periods with a 7-day washout period between treatments. Statistical analyses also demonstrated equivalence between the two patches for estradiol pharmacokinetic parameters (Table 2).

Table 2: ESTRADOT

Mean Observed Pharmacokinetic Parameters for Estradiol (E2) Obtained After Treatments with Two Different Transdermal Estradiol Systems (n=30)

Parameter	ESTRADOT 5.0 cm² patch Mean (SD)	VIVELLE 14.5 cm² patch Mean (SD)
C_{max} (pg/mL)	56.7 (30.7)	52.7 (20.0)
T_{max} (h)	30.7 (15.6)	22.0 (13.5)
C_{trough} (pg/mL)	28.1 (19.5)	29.4 (12.3)
% Fluctuation	158.0 (190.8)	89.2 (59.4)
AUC_{0-84} (pg·h/mL)	3088 (1721)	2886 (1147)
AUC_{0-96} (pg·h/mL)	3268 (1865)	3051 (1191)
k_e (h-1)	0.138 (0.079)	0.132 (0.056)
$t_{½}$ (h)	7.7 (7.1)	6.3 (2.7)

INDICATIONS: ESTRADOT (estradiol-17β) is indicated for the relief of menopausal and postmenopausal symptoms occurring in naturally or surgically induced estrogen deficiency states.

ESTRADOT is also indicated for the prevention of osteoporosis in naturally occurring or surgically induced estrogen-deficiency states in addition to other important therapeutic measures such as adequate diet, calcium and vitamin D intake, cessation of smoking and regular weight-bearing exercise. In postmenopausal women already diagnosed as having osteoporosis and vertebral fractures, treatment with ESTRADOT may retard further bone loss. ESTRADOT is to be considered in the light of other available therapies for osteoporosis prevention and therapy should only be continued as long as the benefits outweigh the risks for the individual.

In patients with an intact uterus, estradiol-17β should always be supplemented by sequential administration of a progestin whose role is to prevent endometrial hyperplasia.

CONTRAINDICATIONS: ESTRADOT (estradiol-17β) should not be administered to patients with any of the following conditions:

- Personal history of known or suspected estrogen-dependent neoplasia such as breast or endometrial cancer
- Known or suspected breast cancer
- Active hepatic dysfunction or disease, especially of the obstructive type
- Severe hepatic disease
- Endometrial hyperplasia
- Undiagnosed abnormal vaginal bleeding
- Active or past history of arterial thromboembolic disease (e.g. cerebrovascular accident, myocardial infarction, coronary heart disease)
- Active or past history of confirmed venous thromboembolism (such as deep venous thrombosis or pulmonary embolism) or active thrombophlebitis
- Porphyria
- Partial or complete loss of vision from ophthalmic vascular disease
- Classical Migraine
- Known or suspected pregnancy
- Breast feeding
- Known or suspected hypersensitivity to any component of the patch

WARNINGS: See **Boxed Warning**.

Cardiovascular Disorders: Available epidemiological data indicate that use of estrogen with or without progestin is associated with an increased risk of stroke and coronary heart disease. WHI-trial's results concluded that there are more risks than benefits among women using combined oral Hormone Replacement Therapy (HRT), compared to the group using placebo. In 10 000 women on combined HRT (conjugated equine estrogens/medroxyprogesterone acetate) over one year period, there were seven more cases of coronary heart disease (37 on combined HRT versus 30 on placebo) and eight more cases of strokes (29 versus 21).

In the Heart and Estrogen/progestin Replacement Study (HERS) of postmenopausal women with documented heart disease (n=2763, average age 66.7 years), a randomized placebo-controlled clinical trial of secondary prevention of coronary heart disease (CHD), treatment with 0.625 mg/day oral conjugated equine estrogen (CEE) plus 2.5 mg medroxyprogesterone acetate (MPA) demonstrated no cardiovascular benefit.

Specifically, during an average follow-up of 4.1 years, treatment with CEE plus MPA did not reduce the overall rate of CHD events in postmenopausal women with established coronary heart disease. There were more CHD events in the hormone-treated group than in the placebo group in year 1, but not during the subsequent years.

From the original HERS trial, 2321 women consented to participate in an open label extension of HERS, HERS II. Average follow-up in HERS II was an additional 2.7 years, for a total of 6.8 years overall. After 6.8 years, hormone therapy did not reduce the risk of cardiovascular events in women with CHD.

Breast Cancer: Current epidemiological data indicate that the use of combined HRT is associated with an increased risk of invasive breast cancer. WHI-trial's results suggest that risks exceed benefits among women using combined HRT (conjugated equine estrogens/medroxyprogesterone acetate), compared to the group using placebo. In 10 000 women on combined HRT over one year period, there were eight more cases of invasive breast cancer (38 on combined HRT versus 30 on placebo).

The WHI study reported that the invasive breast cancers diagnosed in the estrogen plus progestin group were similar in histology but were larger (mean (SD), 1.7 cm (1.1) vs. 1.5 cm (0.9), respectively; P=0.04) and were at a more advanced stage compared with those diagnosed in the placebo group.

The WHI trial also reported that the percentage of women with abnormal mammograms (recommendations for short-interval follow-up, a suspicious abnormality, or highly suggestive of malignancy) was significantly higher in the estrogen plus progestin group versus the placebo group. This difference appeared at year one and persisted in each year thereafter.

It is recommended that estrogens not be given to women with existing breast cancer or those with a previous history of the disease. There is a need for caution in prescribing estrogens for women with known risk factors associated with the development of breast cancer, such as strong family history of breast cancer (first degree relative) or who present a breast condition with an increased risk (breast nodules, fibrocystic disease of the breast, abnormal mammograms and/or atypical hyperplasia at breast biopsy). Other known risk factors for the development of breast cancer such as nulliparity, obesity, early menarche, late age at first full term pregnancy and at menopause should also be evaluated.

It is recommended that women undergo mammography prior to the start of HRT treatment and at regular intervals during treatment, as deemed appropriate by the treating physician and according to the perceived risks for each patient.

The overall benefits and possible risks of hormone replacement therapy should be fully considered and discussed with patients. It is important that the increased risk of being diagnosed with breast cancer after 4 years of treatment with HRT (as reported in the results of WHI-trial) be discussed with the patient and weighed against its known benefits.

Instructions for self-examination of the breasts should be included in this counseling.

Venous Thromboembolism: Recent epidemiological data indicate that the use of estrogen with or without progestin is associated with an increased risk of developing venous thromboembolism (VTE). WHI-trial's results suggest that risks exceed benefits among women using combined HRT (conjugated equine estrogens/medroxyprogesterone acetate), compared to the group using placebo. In 10 000 women on combined HRT over a period of one year, there were eighteen more cases of total blood clots in the lungs and legs (34 on combined HRT versus 16 on placebo).

Generally recognized risk factors for VTE include a personal history, a family history (the occurrence of VTE in a direct relative at a relatively early age may indicate genetic predisposition) and severe obesity (body mass index >30 kg/m²). The risk of VTE also increases with age and smoking.

A history of recurrent spontaneous abortions should be investigated to exclude thrombophilic predisposition. In patients in whom this diagnosis is confirmed, the use of HRT is viewed as contraindicated.

The risk of VTE may be temporarily increased with prolonged immobilization, major elective surgery or posttraumatic surgery, or major trauma (if feasible, estrogens should be discontinued at least 4 weeks before major surgery which may be associated with an increased risk of thromboembolism, or during periods of prolonged immobilization). The treatment should not be restarted until the woman is completely mobile. In women on HRT, attention should be given to prophylactic measures to prevent VTE following surgery. Also, patients with varicose veins should be closely supervised although there is no consensus about the possible role of varicose veins in VTE. The physician should be alert to the earliest manifestations of thrombotic disorders (thrombophlebitis, retinal thrombosis, cerebral embolism and pulmonary embolism). If these occur or are suspected, hormone therapy should be discontinued immediately.

Endometrial Hyperplasia and Endometrial Carcinoma: Estrogen-only HRT increases the risk of endometrial hyperplasia (if taken by women with intact uteri). Estrogen-only hormonal therapy in postmenopause is recommended for women without uterus only to avoid unnecessary exposure to progestins. The focus of the clinical program with VIVELLE/ESTRADOT was the demonstration of efficacy in the treatment of postmenopausal symptoms and in the prevention of postmenopausal osteoporosis. Some clinical trials included non-hysterectomized patients who were treated with concomitant progestogen therapy according to the best medical practice at the time, with different dosages, regimens and types of progestin. In addition, endometrial sampling after treatment was not consistently performed and in most cases no baseline data was available to assess the relationship and the effects of the progestogen treatment on the endometrium.

The risk of endometrial cancer in users of unopposed estrogens who have an intact uterus is greater than in non-users and appears to depend on the duration of treatment and the estrogen dose. The greatest risk appears to be associated with prolonged use. It has been shown that adequate concomitant progestogen therapy lowers the incidence of endometrial hyperplasia and therefore the potential risk of endometrial carcinoma associated with prolonged use of estrogen therapy (see Dosage, Coadministration of Progestins).

Ovarian Cancer: In some epidemiological studies, the long-term use of unopposed estrogens in hysterectomised women has been associated with an increased risk of ovarian cancer. It is uncertain whether long-term use of combined HRT (estrogens and progestogens) confers a different risk than estrogen-only HRT products.

Gallbladder Diseases: A 2- to 4-fold increase in the risk of gallbladder disease requiring surgery in women receiving postmenopausal estrogens has been reported with combined oral CE and MPA treatment.

Contact Sensitization: Contact sensitization is known to occur with topical applications. Although it is extremely rare, patients who develop contact sensitization to any component of the patch should be warned that a severe hypersensitivity reaction may occur with continuing exposure to the causative agent.

Benign Hepatic Adenomas and Hepatocellular Carcinomas: Benign hepatic adenomas have been associated with the use of combined estrogen and progestin oral contraceptives. Although benign and rare, these tumors may rupture and cause death from intra-abdominal hemorrhage. Such lesions have not yet been reported in association with other estrogen or progestin preparations, but they should be considered if abdominal pain and tenderness, abdominal mass, or hypovolemic shock occurs in patients receiving estrogen. Hepatocellular carcinoma has also been reported in women taking estrogen-containing oral contraceptives.The causal relationship of this malignancy to these drugs is not known.

Dementia: In a randomized placebo controlled ancillary study of the WHI, the Women's Health Initiative Memory Study (WHIMS), women aged 65 and older (average age 71) treated with oral CEE and MPA for an average follow-up of 4 years were reported to have a two-fold increase in the risk of developing probable dementia. The absolute excess risk of probable dementia was 23 additional cases per 10 000 person-years (45 versus 22) in CEE/MPA treated women and the relative risk was 2.05.

Since only women aged 65 and older were included in this study, it is unknown whether these findings apply to younger postmenopausal women.

The estrogen-only sub-study of the WHIMS is currently on-going and no data are available yet. It is therefore unknown whether these findings apply to estrogen-only therapy.

For transdermal estrogen-only or estrogen-progestogen combined products, no large randomized clinical trials have assessed the HRT-associated risk of probable dementia to date. Therefore there are no data to support the conclusion that the frequency of probable dementia is different with ESTRADOT.

PRECAUTIONS: Before estradiol-17β is administered, the patient should have a complete physical examination including a blood pressure determination. Breasts and pelvic organs should be appropriately examined and a Papanicolaou smear should be performed. Endometrial biopsy should be done when indicated. Baseline tests should include mammography, measurements of blood glucose, calcium, triglycerides and cholesterol, and liver function tests.

The first follow-up examination should be done within 3 to 6 months after initiation of treatment to assess response to treatment. Thereafter, examinations should be made once a year and should include at least those procedures outlined above.

Women should be advised that changes in their breasts should be reported to their doctor or nurse. Investigations, including mammography, should be carried out in accordance with currently accepted screening practices and adapted to the clinical needs of the individual woman.

It is important that patients are encouraged to practice frequent self-examination of the breasts.

If feasible, estrogens should be discontinued at least 4 weeks before major surgery which may be associated with an increased risk of thromboembolism, or during periods of prolonged immobilization.

Women using hormonal replacement therapy (HRT) sometimes experience increased blood pressure. Blood pressure should be monitored with HRT use. Elevation of blood pressure in previously normotensive or hypertensive patients should be evaluated and HRT therapy may have to be discontinued.

Abnormal vaginal bleeding due to its prolongation, irregularity or heaviness occurring during therapy should prompt diagnostic measures like hysteroscopy, endometrial biopsy or curettage to rule out the possibility of uterine malignancy and the treatment should be re-evaluated.

Pre-existing uterine leiomyoma may increase in size during estrogen use. Growth, pain or tenderness of uterine leiomyoma requires discontinuation of medication.

Symptoms and physical findings associated with a previous diagnosis of endometriosis may reappear or become aggravated with estrogen use.

Patients who develop visual disturbances, classical migraine, transient aphasia, paralysis, or loss of consciousness should discontinue medication.

Estrogens may cause fluid retention. Therefore, particular caution is indicated in cardiac or renal dysfunction, epilepsy or asthma. Treatment should be stopped if there is an increase in epileptic seizures. If, in any of the above-mentioned conditions, a worsening of the underlying disease is diagnosed or suspected during treatment, the benefits and risks of treatment should be reassessed based on the individual case.

Because the prolonged use of estrogens influences the metabolism of calcium and phosphorus, estrogens should be used with caution in patients with metabolic and malignant bone diseases associated with hypercalcemia, in patients with renal insufficiency and in patients with otosclerosis.

A worsening of glucose tolerance and lipid metabolism have been observed in a significant percentage of peri- and postmenopausal patients on oral estrogen treatment. Therefore, diabetic patients or those with a predisposition to diabetes should be observed closely to detect any alterations in carbohydrate or lipid metabolism, especially in triglyceride blood levels.

Women with familial hypertriglyceridemia need special surveillance. Lipid-lowering measures are recommended additionally, before treatment is started.

Liver function tests should be done periodically in subjects who are suspected of having hepatic disease. For information on endocrine and liver function tests, see Laboratory Tests.

Caution is advised in patients with a history of estrogen-related jaundice and pruritus. If cholestatic jaundice develops during treatment, the treatment should be discontinued and appropriate investigations carried out.

Drug Interactions: Estrogens may diminish the effectiveness of anticoagulants, antidiabetic and antihypertensive agents.

Preparations inducing liver enzymes (e.g., barbiturates, hydantoins, carbamazepine, meprobamate, phenylbutazone or rifampin) may interfere with the activity of orally administered estrogens.

The following section contains information on drug interactions with ethinyl estradiol-containing products (specifically, oral contraceptives) that have been reported in the public literature. It is unknown whether such interactions occur with drug products containing other types of estrogens.

1. The metabolism of ethinyl estradiol is increased by rifampicin and anticonvulsants such as phenobarbital, phenytoin and carbamazepine. Coadministration of troglitazone and certain ethinyl estradiol containing drug products (e.g., oral contraceptives containing ethinyl estradiol) reduces the plasma concentrations of ethinyl estradiol by 30 percent.

   Ascorbic acid and acetaminophen may increase AUC and/or plasma concentrations of ethinyl estradiol. Coadministration of atorvastatin and certain ethinyl estradiol containing drug products (e.g., oral contraceptives containing ethinyl estradiol) increases AUC values for ethinyl estradiol by 20 percent.

   Clinical pharmacokinetics studies have not demonstrated any consistent effect of antibiotics (other than rifampicin) on plasma concentrations of synthetic steroids.

2. Drug products containing ethinyl estradiol may inhibit the metabolism of other compounds. Increased plasma concentrations of cyclosporin, prednisolone, and theophylline have been reported with concomitant administration of certain drugs containing ethinyl estradiol (e.g., oral contraceptives containing ethinyl estradiol). In addition, these drugs containing ethinyl estradiol may induce the conjugation of other compounds.

   Decreased plasma concentrations of acetaminophen and increased clearance of temazepam, salicylic acid, morphine and clofibric acid have been noted when these drugs were administered with certain ethinyl estradiol containing drug products (e.g., oral contraceptives containing ethinyl estradiol).

   Concomitant administration of aminoglutethimide with medroxyprogesterone acetate (MPA) may significantly reduce the bioavailability of MPA.

   It was found that some herbal products (e.g., St. John's wort) which are available as OTC products might affect metabolism, and therefore, efficacy and safety of estrogen/progestin products.

   Physicians and other health care providers should be aware of other non-prescription products concomitantly used by the patients, including herbal and natural products obtained from the widely spread Health Stores.

Laboratory Tests: The results of certain endocrine and liver function tests may be affected by estrogen-containing products: increased sulfobromophthalein retention; increased prothrombin time and partial thromboplastin time; increased levels of fibrinogen and fibrinogen activity; increased coagulation factors VII, VIII, IX, X; increased norepinephrine-induced platelet aggregability; decreased antithrombin III; increased thyroxine-binding globulin (TBG), leading to increased circulating total thyroid hormone (T_4) as measured by column or radioimmunoassay; free T_3 resin uptake is decreased, reflecting the elevated TBG; free T_4 concentration is unaltered; other binding proteins may be elevated in serum i.e., corticosteroid binding globulin (CBG), sex-hormone binding globulin (SHBG), leading to increased circulating corticosteroids and sex steroids respectively; free or biologically active hormone concentrations are unchanged; reduced response to the Metopirone test; impaired glucose tolerance; reduced serum folate concentration; increased serum triglyceride and phospholipid concentration.

With transdermally administered estradiol-17β, no effect on fibrinogen, antithrombin III, TBG, CBG or SHBG and decreases in serum triglycerides have been observed.

The results of the above laboratory tests should not be considered reliable unless therapy has been discontinued for 2 to 4 months. The pathologist should be informed that the patient is receiving estrogen therapy when relevant specimens are submitted.

Information to Be Provided to the Patient: See Information for the Patient.

ADVERSE EFFECTS: See Warnings and Precautions regarding potential induction of malignant neoplasms and adverse effects similar to those of oral contraceptives.

The most commonly reported adverse reaction to VIVELLE (estradiol-17β), another matrix patch, in clinical trials in patients treated for postmenopausal symptoms was redness and irritation at the application site. This caused approximately 0.8% of patients to discontinue therapy. In a comparative clinical trial, ESTRADOT was found to be less irritating than VIVELLE.

In a 2-year controlled trial in patients with postmenopausal osteoporosis, back pain was reported in 13% of patients treated with the VIVELLE patch and 4.5% of patients treated with placebo. Local application site reactions (patch site erythema, itching, rash, burning, irritation) were reported in approximately 9% of patients treated with active patch and 10% of patients treated with placebo. In most cases the local application site reactions were considered mild; none was considered severe. Two patients out of 259 were discontinued from the trial due to local application site reactions.

The following adverse reactions have been reported with estrogens in general.

Gastrointestinal: nausea, vomiting, abdominal discomfort (cramps, pressure, pain), bloating, gallbladder disorder, asymptomatic impaired liver function, cholestatic jaundice.

Genitourinary: breakthrough bleeding, spotting and vaginal bleeding, change in menstrual flow, dysmenorrhea, vaginal itching/discharge, dyspareunia, dysuria, endometrial hyperplasia, premenstrual-like syndrome, reactivation of endometriosis, cystitis, changes in cervical erosion and amount of cervical secretion.

Skin: allergic contact dermatitis, reversible postinflammatory pigmentation, general pruritus and exanthema, loss of scalp hair, chloasma or melasma, which may persist when drug is discontinued, pigmentation of the skin, erythema nodosum, erythema multiforme, hemorrhagic skin eruptions, precipitation or aggravation of porphyria cutanea tarda in predisposed individuals.

Isolated cases of anaphylactoid reactions (some of the patients had a history of previous allergy or allergic disorders).

Endocrine: breast swelling and tenderness, increased blood sugar levels, decreased glucose tolerance, sodium retention.

Cardiovascular/Hematologic: palpitations, isolated cases of: thrombophlebitis, thromboembolic disorders, exacerbations of varicose veins, increase in blood pressure (see Warnings and Precautions), coronary thrombosis, altered coagulation tests (see Precautions, Laboratory Tests).

Central Nervous System: aggravation of migraine episodes, headaches, mental depression, nervousness, dizziness, fatigue, irritability, neuro-ocular lesions (e.g., retinal thrombosis, optic neuritis).

Dementia has been reported in association with some estrogen-progesterone treatments.

Ophthalmic: visual disturbances, steepening of the corneal curvature, intolerance to contact lenses, neuro-ocular lesions (see Central Nervous System).

Miscellaneous: changes in appetite, changes in body weight, edema, neuritis, change in libido, musculoskeletal pain (including leg pain not related to thromboembolic disease [usually transient, lasting 3 to 6 weeks]. If symptoms persist, the dose of estrogen should be reduced.)

If adverse symptoms persist, the prescription of HRT should be re-considered.

OVERDOSE:

Symptoms: Numerous reports of ingestion of large doses of estrogen products and estrogen-containing oral contraceptives by young children have not revealed acute serious ill effects. Overdosage with estrogen may cause nausea, breast discomfort, fluid retention, bloating or vaginal bleeding in women.

Treatment: Owing to the mode of administration (transdermal), plasma levels of estradiol-17β can be rapidly reduced by removal of the patch.

Symptomatic treatment should be given.

> For management of a suspected drug overdose, CPhA recommends that you contact your **regional Poison Control Centre**. See the *CPS* Directory section for a list of Poison Control Centres.

DOSAGE: For all therapeutic indications, the lowest effective dose should be used for maintenance therapy (see Coadministration of Progestins).

Hormone replacement therapy (HRT) involving either estrogen alone or estrogen-progestogen combined therapy should only be continued as long as the benefits outweigh the risks for the individual.

In women who are not currently taking oral estrogens, treatment with estradiol-17β can be initiated at once. In women who are currently taking oral estrogens, treatment with estradiol-17β can be initiated on reappearance of menopausal symptoms, following discontinuation of oral therapy.

ESTRADOT is administered as continuous therapy (uninterrupted application). ESTRADOT should be applied twice weekly i.e., the patch should be changed once every 3 to 4 days.

In women with an intact uterus, a progestin should be sequentially coadministered for 12 to 14 days per cycle to avoid overstimulation of the endometrium. The addition of sufficient progestin to induce secretory transformation of the endometrium during estrogen replacement therapy is mandatory.

Abnormal vaginal bleeding, due to its prolongation, irregularity or heaviness, in any patient receiving hormone replacement therapy requires institution of prompt diagnostic measures like endometrial biopsy or curettage to rule out the possibility of uterine malignancy.

The short term effects of progestin coadministration may include vaginal bleeding during or after progestin treatment, breast tenderness, and mood and weight changes. The long-term effects generally depend on the dosage and type of progestin used. The lowest effective dose of estrogen and progestin should be prescribed (see Coadministration of Progestins).

See the Precautions section on the examination of the patient before estradiol-17β administration.

Dose Adjustment: Menopausal Symptoms: Treatment of menopausal symptoms is usually initiated with a patch that releases 50 µg estradiol-17β/day i.e., ESTRADOT 50. Thereafter the dosage should be adapted to the needs of the individual.

Breast discomfort, breakthrough or heavy vaginal bleeding, water retention, bloating or nausea (if persisting for more than 6 weeks), are generally signs that the estrogen dose is too high and needs to be lowered. If, on the other hand, the selected dose fails to eliminate the signs and symptoms of estrogen deficiency, a higher dose may be considered.

For maintenance therapy one should always use the lowest dose that still proves effective. The requirement for hormone replacement therapy for menopausal symptoms should be reassessed periodically. Attempts to taper or discontinue the medication should be made at 3- to 6-month intervals.

Prevention of Postmenopausal Osteoporosis: For optimal prevention of postmenopausal bone loss in women for whom the drug is indicated, therapy should be initiated as soon as possible after diagnosis of menopause. The dosage of estradiol-17β may require adjustment according to the patient's clinical status, the plasma estradiol-17β levels and the results of bone mineral density studies. Ideally, plasma estradiol-17β levels should be maintained at 183 pM/L (50 pg/mL).

Discontinuation of hormone replacement therapy may re-establish the natural rate of bone loss.

Patch Application: The physician should discuss the most appropriate placement of the patch with the patient. Immediately after removal of a patch from the pouch and removal of the protective liner, the adhesive side of the ESTRADOT patch should be placed on a clean, dry area of intact skin. The area selected should not be oily, damaged or irritated, and not exposed to the sun. The site selected should also be one at which little wrinkling of the skin occurs during movement of the body, preferably the buttocks, lower abdomen or hip. The patch may also be placed on the side or lower back. The patch should be placed consistently on the same area of the body with each application (i.e., either the buttocks, lower abdomen, hip, side or lower back). Experience to date has shown that less irritation of the skin occurs on the buttocks than on other sites of application. Therefore, it is advisable to apply ESTRADOT to the buttocks. The waistline should be avoided, since tight clothing may dislodge the patch. The patch should be pressed firmly in place with the palm of the hand, making sure there is good contact, especially around the edges. In the event that a patch should fall off, it can be reapplied. If it fails to adhere then a new patch may be applied. In either case, the original treatment schedule should be continued. Patches should not be applied to the same skin site twice in succession.

ESTRADOT must not be applied to the breasts to avoid potentially harmful effects on the breast tissue.

If a woman has forgotten to apply a patch, she should apply a new patch as soon as possible. The subsequent patch should be applied according to the original treatment schedule. The interruption of treatment might increase the likelihood of recurrence of symptoms.

Coadministration of Progestins: Studies have reported that the addition of a progestin for 10 or more days of a cycle of estrogen administration greatly lowers the incidence of endometrial hyperplasia, and thereby irregular bleeding and endometrial carcinoma, compared to estrogen treatment alone.

Wide interpatient variation in absorption occurs with progestins.

The following regimens have been shown, in general, to produce histological and biochemical changes consistent with a uniform secretory pattern in the endometrium: norethindrone 0.7 mg/day orally administered sequentially for 12 days each cycle; medroxyprogesterone acetate (MPA) 10 mg/day (orally) administered sequentially for 12 days each cycle.

There are possible additional risks that may be associated with the inclusion of a progestin in estrogen replacement regimens. The potential risks include adverse effects on carbohydrate and lipid metabolism, mood changes and edema. The choice and dose of progestin may be important in minimizing these adverse effects and may differ among women.

Children: ESTRADOT should not be used in children.

INFORMATION FOR THE PATIENT: Published in e-CPS, available by subscription at www.e-cps.ca.

SUPPLIED: ESTRADOT is available in the 4 following strengths: See Table 3. The matrix provides a source for continuous delivery of drug for up to 4 days. The composition per unit area in each strength is identical. Nonmedicinal ingredients: translucent film: polyolefin; adhesive formulation containing estradiol: acrylic, dipropylene glycol, oleyl alcohol, povidone and silicone; release liner which is attached to the adhesive surface: polyester.

Table 3: ESTRADOT

ESTRADOT Composition

	ESTRADOT 25	ESTRADOT 37.5	ESTRADOT 50	ESTRADOT 75	ESTRADOT 100
Estradiol-17β Dosage nominal in vivo delivery	25 μg/day	37.5 μg/day	50 μg/day	75 μg/day	100 μg/day
Total estradiol-17β content	0.390 mg	0.585 mg	0.78 mg	1.17 mg	1.56 mg
Drug-releasing area	2.5 cm^2	3.75 cm^2	5 cm^2	7.5 cm^2	10 cm^2
Shape of patch	Rounded rectangle	Rounded rectangle	Rounded rectangle	Rounded rectangle	Rounded rectangle

Patient packs of 8. Each patch is individually sealed in a separate pouch. Do not store out of the pouch. Apply immediately upon removal from the protective pouch. Patches should be applied in whole. Store between 2 and 30°C. Do not freeze. Keep ESTRADOT out of reach and sight of children and pets both before use and when disposing of used patches.

(Shown in Product Identification Section)

Estring® Ⓟ

estradiol-17β

Estrogen

Paladin

Date of Preparation: September 22, 2003
Date of Revision: June 29, 2009

SUMMARY PRODUCT INFORMATION:

Route of Administration	Dosage Form/ Strength	Clinically Relevant Nonmedicinal Ingredients
Vaginal	Vaginal Ring, 2 mg	Silicone elastomer, barium sulphate, silicone fluid

INDICATIONS AND CLINICAL USE: ESTRING (17 β-estradiol) is indicated for postmenopausal urogenital complaints due to estrogen deficiency such as feeling of dryness in the vagina (atrophic vaginitis) with or without pruritus vulvae, dyspareunia, dysuria and urinary urgency (atrophic mucosa in the urethra and trigonum).

ESTRING should be prescribed with an appropriate dosage of a progestin for women with intact uteri, in order to prevent endometrial hyperplasia/carcinoma.

The maximum recommended duration of continuous therapy is 2 years.

CONTRAINDICATIONS:

- Known or suspected estrogen-dependent malignant neoplasia (e.g. endometrial cancer).
- Known, suspected, or past history of breast cancer.
- Undiagnosed abnormal genital bleeding.
- Known or suspected pregnancy.
- Known or suspected hypersensitivity to any component of the product. For a complete listing, see Dosage Forms, Composition and Packaging.
- Endometrial hyperplasia.
- Lactation.
- Liver dysfunction or disease as long as liver function tests have failed to return to normal.
- Active or past history of arterial thromboembolic disease (e.g. stroke, myocardial infarction, coronary heart disease).
- Active or past history of confirmed venous thromboembolism (such as deep vein thrombosis or pulmonary embolism) or active thrombophlebitis.
- Partial or complete loss of vision due to ophthalmic vascular disease.

WARNINGS AND PRECAUTIONS:

Serious Warnings and Precautions

The Women's Health Initiative (WHI) trial examined the health benefits and risks of oral combined estrogen plus progestin therapy (n= 16 608) and oral estrogen-alone therapy (n=10 739) in postmenopausal women aged 50 to 79 years.

The estrogen plus progestin arm of the WHI trial (mean age 63.3 years) indicated an increased risk of myocardial infarction (MI), stroke, invasive breast cancer, pulmonary emboli and deep vein thrombosis in postmenopausal women receiving treatment with combined conjugated equine estrogens (CEE, 0.625 mg/day) and medroxyprogesterone acetate (MPA, 2.5 mg/day) for 5.2 years compared to those receiving placebo.

The estrogen-alone arm of the WHI trial (mean age 63.6 years) indicated an increased risk of stroke and deep vein thrombosis in hysterectomized women treated with CEE-alone (0.625 mg/day) for 6.8 years compared to those receiving placebo.

Therefore, the following should be given serious consideration at the time of prescribing:

- Estrogens with or without progestins **should not** be prescribed for primary or secondary prevention of cardiovascular diseases.
- Estrogens with or without progestins should be prescribed at the **lowest effective dose** for the approved indication.
- Estrogens with or without progestins should be prescribed for the **shortest period possible** for the approved indication.

General: Risks and benefits of treatment with ESTRING should be re-assessed at least annually. ESTRING should only be continued as long as the benefits outweigh the risks.

ESTRING is a vaginal administered estrogen product with low systemic absorption following continuous use for 3 months (see Action and Clinical Pharmacology, Pharmacokinetics, Absorption). It is expected that low systemic exposure to estradiol and estrone resulting from ESTRING use should elicit lower estrogen-dependent side effects. However, the following warnings and precautions associated with oral estrogen therapy should be considered in the absence of comparable data with other dosage forms of estrogens.

Carcinogenesis and Mutagenesis: Breast Cancer: Available epidemiological data indicate that the use of combined estrogen plus progestin by postmenopausal women is associated with an increased risk of invasive breast cancer.

In the estrogen plus progestin arm of the WHI trial, among 10 000 women over a one-year period, there were:

- 8 more cases of invasive breast cancer (38 on combined HRT versus 30 on placebo).

The WHI study also reported that the invasive breast cancers diagnosed in the estrogen plus progestin group were similar in histology but were larger (mean [SD], 1.7 cm [1.1] vs 1.5 cm [0.9], respectively; P=0.04) and were at a more advanced stage compared with those diagnosed in the placebo group. The percentage of women with abnormal mammograms (recommendations for short-interval follow-up, a suspicious abnormality, or highly suggestive of malignancy) was significantly higher in the estrogen plus progestin group versus the placebo group. This difference appeared at year one and persisted in each year thereafter.

In the oral estrogen-alone arm of the Women's Health Initiative (WHI) trial, there was no statistically significant difference in the rate of invasive breast cancer in hysterectomized women treated with conjugated equine estrogens versus women treated with placebo.

It is recommended that estrogens not be given to women with existing breast cancer or those with a previous history of the disease (see Contraindications). There is a need for caution in prescribing estrogens of any kind to women with a strong family history (first degree relative) of breast cancer or women who have nodules, fibrocystic disease or abnormal mammograms and/or atypical hyperplasia at breast biopsy.

Other known risk factors for the development of breast cancer such as nulliparity, obesity, early menarche, late age at first full term pregnancy and at menopause should also be evaluated.

It is recommended that women undergo mammography prior to the start of HRT treatment and at regular intervals during treatment, as deemed appropriate by the treating physician and according to the perceived risks for each patient.

The overall benefits and possible risks of hormone replacement therapy should be fully considered and discussed with patients. It is important that the modest increased risk of being diagnosed with breast cancer after 4 years of treatment with HRT (as reported in the results of WHI-trial) be discussed with the patient and weighed against its known benefits.

Instructions for regular self-examination of the breasts should be included in this counselling.

Endometrial Hyperplasia and Endometrial Carcinoma: An increased risk of endometrial cancer has been reported with the use of unopposed estrogen therapy in women with a uterus. The reported endometrial cancer risk among unopposed estrogen users is about 2 to 12-times greater than in nonusers, and appears dependent on duration of treatment and on estrogen dose. Most studies show no significant increased risk associated with use of estrogens for less than 1 year. The greatest risk appears associated with prolonged use, with increased risks of 15 to 24 fold for 5 to 10 years or more. This risk has been shown to persist for at least 8 to 15 years after estrogen therapy is discontinued. There is no evidence that the use of natural estrogens result in a different endometrial risk profile than synthetic estrogens of equivalent estrogen dose. The endometrial safety of long-term or repeated intra-vaginal estrogen administration is uncertain. Adding a progestin to systemic estrogen therapy has been shown to reduce the risk of endometrial hyperplasia, which may be a precursor to endometrial cancer. Therefore, estrogen should be prescribed with an appropriate dosage of a progestin for women with intact uteri in order to prevent endometrial hyperplasia/carcinoma.

Clinical surveillance of all women taking estrogen plus progestin therapy is important. Adequate diagnostic measures, including endometrial sampling when indicated, should be undertaken to rule out malignancy in all cases of undiagnosed persistent or recurring abnormal vaginal bleeding.

Ovarian Cancer: Observational studies have found the use of hormone replacement therapy (estrogen-alone and estrogen plus progestin therapies), in particular for five or more years, has been associated with a small increase in the risk of ovarian cancer.

Cardiovascular: The results of the Heart and Estrogen/progestin Replacement Studies (HERS and HERS II) and the Women's Health Initiative (WHI) trial indicate that the use of continuous combined oral conjugated estrogens (CEE) and medroxyprogesterone acetate (MPA) is associated with an increased risk of coronary heart disease (CHD) in postmenopausal women. The results of the WHI trial indicate that the use of oral estrogen-alone and oral estrogen plus progestin is associated with an increased risk of stroke in postmenopausal women.

Blood Pressure: Women using hormonal replacement therapy (HRT) sometimes experience increased blood pressure. Blood pressure should be monitored with HRT use. Elevation of blood pressure in previously normotensive or hypertensive patients should be investigated and HRT therapy may have to be discontinued.

Endocrine and Metabolism: Estrogen Effects: Although uncommon with ESTRING, certain patients may develop undesirable manifestations of estrogenic stimulation, such as mastodynia.

Glucose and Lipid Metabolism: A worsening of glucose tolerance and lipid metabolism has been observed in a significant percentage of peri- and post-menopausal patients. Therefore, diabetic patients or those with a predisposition to diabetes should be observed closely to detect any alterations in carbohydrate or lipid metabolism, especially in triglyceride blood levels.

Women with familial hyperlipidemias need special surveillance. Lipid-lowering measures are recommended additionally, before treatment is started.

Heme Metabolism: Women with porphyria need special surveillance.

Calcium and Phosphorus Metabolism: Because the prolonged use of estrogens influences the metabolism of calcium and phosphorus, estrogens should be used with caution in patients with metabolic and malignant bone diseases associated with hypercalcemia and in patients with renal insufficiency.

Hypothyroidism: Patients who require thyroid hormone replacement therapy and who are also taking estrogen should have their thyroid function monitored regularly to assure that thyroid hormone levels remain in an acceptable range (see Drug-Drug Interactions, Drug-Laboratory Test Interactions).

Hypocalcemia: Estrogens should be used with caution in individuals with severe hypocalcemia.

Genitourinary: Some women may be unsuitable for treatment with ESTRING, in particular those with short narrow vaginas due to previous surgery or the effect of atrophy, or those with a degree of uterovaginal prolapse severe enough to prevent retention of the ring.

A potential problem related to the vaginal ring is a tendency in a limited number of patients for the ring to slide down, move or fall out. This was noticed primarily during the first 3 weeks of treatment and was the reason for withdrawal from treatment for 3% of the patients on their first ring.

Vaginal Bleeding: Abnormal vaginal bleeding, due to its prolongation, irregularity or heaviness, occurring during therapy should prompt appropriate diagnostic measures to rule out the possibility of uterine malignancy and the treatment should be re-evaluated.

Women should be advised to inform their physician if irritation, pain, discharge, unusual or unexpected bleeding occur during treatment.

Although uncommon with ESTRING, certain patients may develop undesirable manifestations of estrogenic stimulation, such as abnormal uterine bleeding.

Location of ESTRING: Some women have experienced moving or gliding of ESTRING within the vagina. Instances of ESTRING being expelled from the vagina in connection with moving the bowels, strain, or constipation have been reported. If this occurs, ESTRING can be rinsed in lukewarm water and reinserted into the vagina by the patient.

Vaginal Irritation: ESTRING may not be suitable for women with narrow, short, or stenosed vaginas. Narrow vagina, vaginal stenosis, prolapse, and vaginal infections are conditions that make the vagina more susceptible to ESTRING-caused irritation or ulceration. Women with signs or symptoms of vaginal irritation should alert their physician.

In any woman experiencing persistent or severe discomfort due to the presence of the ring or excessive movement of the ring, treatment should be discontinued. Treatment should be discontinued in patients with signs of ulceration or severe inflammation due to unresponsive atrophic vaginitis.

Uterine Leiomyomata: Pre-existing uterine leiomyomata may increase in size during estrogen use. Growth, pain or tenderness of uterine leiomyomata requires discontinuation of medication and appropriate investigation.

Endometriosis: Symptoms and physical findings associated with a previous diagnosis of endometriosis may reappear or become aggravated with estrogen use.

Vaginal Infection: Vaginal infection is generally more common in postmenopausal women due to the lack of the normal flora of fertile women, especially lactobacillus, and the subsequent higher pH. Vaginal infections should be treated with appropriate antimicrobial therapy before initiation of ESTRING. If a vaginal infection develops during use of ESTRING, then ESTRING should be removed and reinserted only after the infection has been appropriately treated.

Toxic Shock Syndrome: A few cases of toxic shock syndrome (TSS) have been reported in women using vaginal rings. TSS is a rare, but serious disease that may cause death. Warning signs of TSS include fever, nausea, vomiting, diarrhea, muscle pain, dizziness, faintness, or a sunburn-rash on face and body.

Hematologic: Venous Thromboembolism: Available epidemiological data indicate that use of oral estrogen with or without progestin by postmenopausal women is associated with an increased risk of developing venous thromboembolism (VTE).

Generally recognized risk factors for VTE include a personal history, a family history (the occurrence of VTE in a direct relative at a relatively early age may indicate genetic predisposition), severe obesity (body mass index >30 kg/m^2) and systemic lupus erythematosus. The risk of VTE also increases with age and smoking.

The risk of VTE may be temporarily increased with prolonged immobilization, major surgery or trauma. In women on HRT, attention should be given to prophylactic measures to prevent VTE following surgery. Also, patients with varicose veins should be closely supervised. The physician should be alert to the earliest manifestations of thrombotic disorders (thrombophlebitis, retinal thrombosis, cerebral embolism and pulmonary embolism). If these occur or are suspected, hormone therapy should be discontinued immediately, given the risks of long-term disability or fatality.

If feasible, estrogens should be discontinued at least 4 weeks before major surgery which may be associated with an increased risk of thromboembolism, or during periods of prolonged immobilization.

Hepatic/Biliary/Pancreatic: Gallbladder Disease: A 2- to 4-fold increase in the risk of gallbladder disease requiring surgery in women receiving postmenopausal estrogens has been reported.

Jaundice: Caution is advised in patients with a history of liver and/or biliary disorders. If cholestatic jaundice develops during treatment, the treatment should be discontinued and appropriate investigations carried out.

Liver Function Tests: Liver function tests should be done periodically in subjects who are suspected of having hepatic disease. For information on endocrine and liver function tests (see Monitoring and Laboratory Tests).

Neurologic: Cerebrovascular Insufficiency: Patients who develop visual disturbances, classical migraine, transient aphasia, paralysis, or loss of consciousness should discontinue medication.

Patients with a previous history of classical migraine and who develop a recurrence or worsening of migraine symptoms should be reevaluated.

Dementia: Available epidemiological evidence indicates that the use of combined oral estrogen plus progestin in women age 65 and over may increase the risk of developing probable dementia.
Epilepsy: HRT may cause an exacerbation of epilepsy.
Renal: Fluid Retention: Estrogens may cause fluid retention. Therefore, particular caution is indicated in cardiac or renal dysfunction, epilepsy or asthma. If, in any of the above-mentioned conditions, a worsening of the underlying disease is diagnosed or suspected during treatment, the benefits and risks of treatment should be reassessed based on the individual case.
Special Populations: Pregnant Women: Estrogens should not be used during pregnancy. Any possibility of pregnancy must be ruled out before prescribing ESTRING. If pregnancy occurs during ESTRING treatment, ESTRING should be discontinued immediately.
Congenital Lesions with Malignant Potential: Estrogen therapy during pregnancy is associated with an increased risk of fetal congenital reproductive tract disorders, and possibly other birth defects. Studies of women who received diethylstilbestrol (DES) during pregnancy have shown that female offspring have an increased risk of vaginal adenosis, squamous cell dysplasia of the uterine cervix and clear cell vaginal cancer later in life; male offspring have an increased risk of urogenital abnormalities and possibly testicular cancer later in life. Although some of these changes are benign, other are precursors of malignancy.
Nursing Women: Estrogens should not be used during lactation. ESTRING should not be prescribed to nursing mothers. Estrogens have been detected in the breast-milk of mothers receiving these drugs, and the effect on breast-fed infants has not been determined. Suppression of lactation may occur.
Pediatrics (<18 years of age): ESTRING is not indicated for use in the pediatric population.
Geriatrics (>65 years of age): Clinical studies of ESTRING did not include sufficient number of subjects aged 65 and over to determine if they responded differently from younger subjects.
Conditions Which Need Supervision: If any of the following conditions are present, have occurred previously, and/or have been aggravated during pregnancy or previous hormone treatment, the patient should be closely supervised. It should be taken into account that these conditions may recur or be aggravated during treatment with vaginal ring, in particular:

- Risk factors for estrogen dependent tumours, e.g. first degree heredity for breast cancer (see above)
- Diabetes mellitus with or without vascular involvement
- Migraine or (severe) headache
- Epilepsy
- A history of, or risk of factors for, thromboembolic disorders (see above)
- Systemic lupus erythematosus
- Liver disorders (e.g. liver adenoma)
- Otosclerosis
- Cholelithiasis
- Leiomyoma (uterine fibroids)
- Endometriosis
- A history of endometrial hyperplasia (see above)
- Hypertension
- Asthma

Reasons for Immediate Withdrawal for Therapy: Therapy should be discontinued in case a contra-indication is discovered and in the following situations :

- Jaundice or deterioration in liver function
- Significant increase in blood pressure
- New onset of migraine-type headache
- Pregnancy

Monitoring and Laboratory Tests: Before ESTRING (estradiol) is administered, the patient should have a complete physical examination including a blood pressure determination. Breasts and pelvic organs should be appropriately examined and a Papanicolaou smear should be performed. Endometrial biopsy should be done when indicated. Baseline tests should include mammography, measurements of blood glucose, calcium, triglycerides and cholesterol, and liver function tests.

The first follow-up examination should be done within 3-6 months after initiation of treatment to assess response to treatment. Thereafter, examinations should be made at intervals at least once a year. Appropriate investigations should be arranged at regular intervals as determined by the physician.

The importance of regular self-examination of the breasts should be discussed with the patient.

Women treated with ESTRING should be advised to keep their regular medical checkups to assess the need for continuing therapy.
X-Ray Procedures: If any x-ray procedures of the lower abdominal tract take place, ESTRING should be removed since the barium sulphate containing core is visible on x-ray and could disturb the procedure or evaluation of x-rays.

ADVERSE REACTIONS: Adverse Drug Reaction Overview: See Warnings and Precautions regarding potential induction of malignant neoplasms and adverse effects similar to those of oral contraceptives.

The following adverse reactions have been reported with estrogen/progestin combination in general:
Reproductive System and Breast Disorders: Breakthrough bleeding; spotting; change in menstrual flow; dysmenorrhea; vaginal itching/discharge; dyspareunia; endometrial hyperplasia; pre-menstrual-like syndrome: reactivation of endometriosis; changes in cervical erosion and amount of cervical secretion, breast swelling and tenderness.
Clinical Trial Adverse Drug Reactions: Because clinical trials are conducted under very specific conditions the adverse drug reaction rates observed in the clinical trials may not reflect the rates observed in practice and should not be compared to the rates in the clinical trials of another drug. Adverse drug reaction information from clinical trials is useful for identifying drug-related adverse events and for approximating rates.

The biological safety of the silicone elastomer has been studied in various in vitro and in vivo test models. The results show that the silicone elastomer is non-toxic, non-pyrogenic, non-irritating, and non-sensitizing. Long-term implantation induced encapsulation equal to or less than the negative control (polyethylene) used in the USP test. No toxic reaction or tumor formation was observed with the silicone elastomer.

In general, ESTRING (estradiol vaginal ring) was well tolerated. In the two pivotal controlled studies, discontinuation of treatment due to an adverse event was required by 5.4% of patients receiving ESTRING and 3.9% of patients receiving conjugated estrogens vaginal cream. The most common reason for withdrawal from ESTRING treatment due to an adverse event were vaginal discomfort and gastrointestinal symptoms.

The adverse events reported with a frequency of 3% or greater in the two pivotal controlled studies by patients receiving ESTRING or conjugated estrogens vaginal cream are listed in Table 1.

Table 1: ESTRING

Adverse Events Reported by 3% or More of Patients Receiving Either ESTRING or Conjugated Estrogens Vaginal Cream in Two Pivotal Controlled Studies

Adverse Events	ESTRING (n=257) %	Conjugated Estrogens Vaginal Cream (n=129) %
Musculoskeletal		
Back Pain	6	8
Arthritis	4	2
Arthralgia	3	5
Skeletal Pain	2	4
CNS/Peripheral Nervous System		
Headache	13	16
Psychiatric		
Insomnia	4	0
Gastrointestinal		
Abdominal Pain	4	2
Nausea	3	2
Respiratory		
Upper Respiratory Tract Infection	5	6
Sinusitis	4	3
Pharyngitis	1	3
Urinary		
Urinary Tract Infection	2	7
Female Reproductive		
Leukorrhea	7	3
Vaginitis	5	2
Vaginal Discomfort/Pain	5	5
Vaginal Hemorrhage	4	5
Asymptomatic Genital Bacterial Growth	4	6
Breast Pain	1	7
Resistance Mechanisms		
Genital Moniliasis	6	7
Body as a Whole		
Flu-like Symptoms	3	2
Hot Flushes	2	3
Allergy	1	4
Miscellaneous		
Family Stress	2	3

Other adverse events (listed alphabetically) occurring at a frequency of 1 to 3% in the two pivotal controlled studies by patients receiving ESTRING include: anxiety, bronchitis, chest pain, cystitis, dermatitis, diarrhea, dyspepsia, dysuria, flatulence, gastritis, genital eruption, genital pruritus, hemorrhoids, leg edema, migraine, otitis media, skin hypertrophy, syncope, toothache, tooth disorder, urinary incontinence.
Less Common Clinical Trial Adverse Drug Reactions: The following additional adverse events were reported at least once by patients receiving ESTRING in the worldwide clinical program, which includes controlled and uncontrolled studies. A causal relationship with ESTRING has not been established.
Body as a Whole: allergic reaction.
CNS/Peripheral Nervous System: dizziness.
Gastrointestinal: enlarged abdomen, vomiting.
Metabolic/Nutritional Disorders: weight decrease or increase.
Psychiatric: depression, decreased libido, nervousness.
Reproductive: breast engorgement, breast enlargement, intermenstrual bleeding, genital edema, vulval disorder.
Skin/Appendages: pruritus, pruritus ani.
Urinary: micturition frequency, urethral disorder.
Vascular: thrombophlebitis.
Vision: abnormal vision.

The following additional adverse reactions have been reported with estrogens:
Genitourinary System: abnormal uterine bleeding/spotting; dysmenorrhea/pelvic pain; increase in size of uterine leiomyomata; vaginitis, including vaginal candidiasis; change in amount of cervical secretion; changes in cervical ectropion; ovarian cancer; endometrial hyperplasia; endometrial cancer.
Breasts: tenderness, enlargement, pain, nipple discharge, galactorrhea; fibrocystic breast changes; breast cancer.
Cardiovascular: deep and superficial venous thrombosis; pulmonary embolism; thrombophlebitis; myocardial infarction; stroke; increase in blood pressure.
Gastrointestinal: nausea, vomiting; abdominal cramps, bloating; cholestatic jaundice; increased incidence of gallbladder disease; pancreatitis, enlargement of hepatic hemangiomas.
Skin: chloasma or melasma that may persist when drug is discontinued; erythema multiforme; erythema nodosum; hemorrhagic eruption; loss of scalp hair; hirsutism, rash.
Eyes: retinal vascular thrombosis; intolerance to contact lenses.
Central Nervous System: headache; migraine; dizziness; mental depression; exacerbation of chorea; nervousness; mood disturbances; irritability; exacerbation of epilepsy, dementia.
Miscellaneous: increase or decrease in weight; glucose intolerance; aggravation of porphyria; edema; arthralgias; leg cramps; changes in libido; angioedema; anaphylactoid/anaphylactic reactions; hypocalcemia (preexisting condition); exacerbation of asthma; increased triglycerides.

If adverse symptoms persist, the prescription of HRT should be re-considered.
Post-Market Adverse Drug Reactions: A few cases of ring adherence to the vaginal wall, making ring removal difficult, have been reported. Vaginal wall ulceration or erosion should be carefully evaluated. If an ulceration or erosion has occurred, consideration should be given to leaving the ring out and not replacing it until healing is complete in order to prevent the ring from adhering to the healing tissue.

A few cases of bowel obstruction and vaginal ring use have been reported. Persistent abdominal complaints consistent with obstruction should be carefully evaluated.

A few cases of toxic shock syndrome have been reported in women using vaginal rings (see Warnings and Precautions, Genitourinary, Toxic Shock Syndrome).

DRUG INTERACTIONS: Overview: ESTRING is a local vaginal estrogen therapy product. The following drug interactions are based on the experience of systemic estrogen treatment.

Estrogens may diminish the effectiveness of anticoagulant, antidiabetic and antihypertensive agents.

Preparations inducing liver enzymes (e.g., barbiturates, hydantoins, carbamazepine, meprobamates, or rifampicin) can enhance estrogen metabolism, resulting in breakthrough bleeding or vaginal spotting.

Drug-Drug Interactions: No formal Drug-Drug Interaction studies with ESTRING have been conducted.

In vitro and in vivo studies have shown that systemic estrogens are metabolized partially by cytochrome P450 3A4 (CYP3A4). Therefore, inducers or inhibitors of CYP3A4 may affect estrogen metabolism.

Inducers of CYP3A4 such as phenobarbital, carbamazepine, and rifampin may reduce plasma concentrations of estrogens, possibly resulting in a decrease in systemic effects and/or changes in the uterine bleeding profile.

Inhibitors of CYP3A4 such as erythromycin, clarithromycin, ketoconazole, itraconazole, ritonavir may increase plasma concentrations of estrogens and may result in side effects.

Use of ESTRING should be discontinued during treatment with vaginal antimicrobial therapy (see Warnings and Precautions, Genitourinary, Vaginal Infection).

Drug-Food Interactions: Inhibitors of CYP3A4 such as grapefruit juice may increase plasma concentrations of estrogens and may result in side effects.

Drug-Herb Interactions: Inducers of CYP3A4 such as St. John's Wort preparations (Hypericum perforatum) may reduce plasma concentrations of estrogens, possibly resulting in a decrease in systemic effects and/or changes in the uterine bleeding profile.

Physicians and other health care providers should be aware of other non-prescription products concomitantly used by the patient, including herbal and natural products from health stores.

Drug-Laboratory Test Interactions: The results of certain endocrine and liver function tests may be affected by estrogen-containing products:

- increased prothrombin time, partial thromboplastin time, and platelet aggregation time; increased platelet count; increased factors II, VII antigen, VIII antigen, VIII coagulant activity, IX, X, XII, VII-X complex, II-VII-X complex, and beta-thromboglobulin; decreased levels of anti-factor Xa and antithrombin III, decreased antithrombin III activity; increased levels of fibrinogen and fibrinogen activity; increased plasminogen antigen and activity.
- Increased thyroid-binding globulin (TBG) levels leading to increased circulating total thyroid hormone levels, as measured by protein-bound iodine (PBI), T4 levels (by column or by radioimmunoassay) or T3 levels by radioimmunoassay. T3 resin uptake is decreased, reflecting the elevated TBG. Free T4 and free T3 concentrations are unaltered. Patients on thyroid replacement therapy may require higher doses of thyroid hormone.
- Other binding proteins may be elevated in serum, (i.e., corticosteroid binding globulin [CBG], sex hormone-binding globulin [SHBG]), leading to increased circulating corticosteroid and sex steroids, respectively. Free hormone concentrations may be decreased. Other plasma proteins may be increased (angiotensinogen/renin substrate, alpha-1-antitrypsin, ceruloplasmin).
- Increased plasma HDL and HDL2 cholesterol subfraction concentrations, reduced LDL cholesterol concentration, increased triglycerides levels.
- Impaired glucose tolerance.

The pathologist should be informed that the patient is receiving hormone replacement therapy (HRT) when relevant specimens are submitted.

DOSAGE AND ADMINISTRATION: Dosing Considerations: Some women may be unsuitable for treatment with ESTRING, in particular those with short narrow vaginas due to previous surgery or the effect of atrophy, or those with a degree of uterovaginal prolapse severe enough to prevent retention of the ring.

ESTRING should be prescribed with an appropriate dosage of a progestin for women with intact uteri in order to prevent endometrial hyperplasia/carcinoma. Progestin therapy is not required as part of hormone replacement therapy in women who have had a previous hysterectomy.

The maximum recommended duration of continuous therapy is 2 years.

Recommended Dose and Dosage Adjustment: One ESTRING (estradiol vaginal ring) is to be inserted as deeply as possible into the upper one-third of the vaginal vault. The ring is to remain in place continuously for three months, after which it is to be removed and, if continuation of therapy is deemed appropriate, replaced by a new ring. The need to continue treatment should be assessed at 3 or 6 month intervals.

Missed Dose: As ESTRING is a symptomatic treatment indicated for the postmenopausal urogenital complaints due to estrogen deficiency, ESTRING may be reintroduce at any time following a period without treatment (missed dose), as long as the patient is still an appropriate candidate for this product. The need to continue treatment should be assessed at 3- to 6-month intervals.

Administration: Instructions for Insertion: ESTRING (estradiol vaginal ring) Insertion: The ring should be pressed into an oval and inserted into the upper third of the vaginal vault. The exact position is not critical. When ESTRING is in place, the patient should not feel anything. If the patient feels discomfort, ESTRING is probably not far enough inside. Gently push ESTRING further into the vagina.

ESTRING Use: ESTRING should be left in place continuously for 90 days and then, if continuation of therapy is deemed appropriate, replaced by a new ESTRING. The patient should not feel ESTRING when it is in place and it should not interfere with sexual intercourse. Straining at defecation may make ESTRING move down in the lower part of the vagina. If so, it may be pushed up again with a finger. If ESTRING is expelled totally from the vagina, it should be rinsed in lukewarm water and reinserted by the patient (or doctor/nurse if necessary).

ESTRING Removal: ESTRING may be removed by hooking a finger through the ring and pulling it out. For patient instructions, see Information for the Patient.

Retention of the ring for greater than 90-days does not represent overdosage but will result in progressively greater underdosage with the attendant risk of loss of efficacy and increasing risk of vaginal infections and/or erosions.

OVERDOSAGE:

Symptoms of Overdose: Numerous reports of ingestion of large doses of estrogen products and estrogen- containing oral contraceptives by young children have not revealed acute serious ill effects. Over dosage with estrogen may cause nausea, breast discomfort, fluid retention, bloating or vaginal bleeding in women.

Treatment of Overdose: Treatment should be discontinued and symptomatic treatment administered.

It is highly unlikely that overdosage would occur with ESTRING (estradiol), as the principle of its release mechanism prevents overdose.

> For management of a suspected drug overdose, CPhA recommends that you contact your **regional Poison Control Centre**. See the *CPS* Directory section for a list of Poison Control Centres.

ACTION AND CLINICAL PHARMACOLOGY: Mechanism of Action: ESTRING (estradiol vaginal ring) is a slightly opaque ring with a whitish core containing a drug reservoir of 2 mg estradiol. Estradiol, silicone polymers and barium sulfate are combined to form the ring. When placed in the vagina, ESTRING releases estradiol, approximately 7.5 µg/24 hours, in a consistent stable manner over 90 days. ESTRING has the following dimensions: outer diameter 55 mm; cross-sectional diameter 9 mm; core diameter 2 mm. One ESTRING should be inserted into the upper third of the vaginal vault, to be worn continuously for three months.

At menopause the ovaries cease to secrete estradiol (E_2), leading to symptoms of estrogen deficiency such as sweating, hot flushes and sleep disturbance. A couple of years after the actual menopause, increasing numbers of women also report symptoms of urogenital estrogen deficiency such as vaginal dryness, genital pruritus, dyspareunia, dysuria and urinary urgency. These latter symptoms respond well to vaginal estrogen replacement therapy.

Pharmacodynamics: The estradiol from ESTRING (estradiol vaginal ring) replaces the missing or decreasing endogenous estrogen production in the post menopausal woman, and eliminates or reduces urogenital estrogen deficiency signs and symptoms. Substitution therapy with estradiol vaginal ring restores vaginal pH to pre-menopausal values and restores the histology and physiology of the vaginal and urethral epithelium to the pre-menopausal state.

In-vivo, estrogens diffuse through cell membranes, distribute throughout the cell, bind to and activate the estrogen receptors, thereby eliciting their biological effects. Estrogen receptors have been identified in tissues of the reproductive tract, breast, pituitary, hypothalamus, liver and bone of women. ESTRING delivers estradiol constantly at a mean rate of 7.5 µg/24 hours for a period of up to 90 days. Its use in post-menopausal patients in Phase I and II studies showed no apparent effects on systemic levels of hepatic protein SHBG, or FSH. Lowering of the pretreatment vaginal pH from a mean of 6.0 to a mean of 4.6 (as found in fertile women) over the 12 to 48 week treatment period, and improvements evident in the vaginal mucosal epithelium seen in all studies attest to the local dynamic effects of estrogens.

Pharmacokinetics: Absorption: Estrogens used in therapeutics are well absorbed through the skin, mucous membranes, and the gastrointestinal (GI) tract. The vaginal delivery of estrogens circumvents first-pass metabolism possibly reducing the induction of several other hepatic proteins.

In a Phase I study of 14 postmenopausal women, the insertion of ESTRING (estradiol vaginal ring) rapidly increased serum estradiol (E_2) levels attesting to the rapid absorption of estradiol via the vaginal mucosa. The time to attain peak serum estradiol levels (T_{max}) was 0.5 to 1 hour. Peak serum estradiol concentrations post-initial burst declined rapidly over the next 24 hours and were virtually indistinguishable from the baseline mean (range: 5 to 22 pg/mL). Serum levels of estradiol and estrone (E_1) over the following 12 weeks during which the ring was maintained in the vaginal vault remained relatively unchanged (see Table 2). The initial estradiol peak post-application of the second ring in the same women resulted in 38% lower C_{max}, apparently due to reduced systemic absorption via the revitalized vaginal epithelium. The relative systemic exposure from the initial peak of ESTRING accounted for approximately 4% of the total estradiol exposure over the 12 week period.

The constant and stable release of estradiol from ESTRING was demonstrated in a Phase II study of 166-222 post-menopausal women who inserted up to four rings consecutively at three month intervals. Low dose systemic delivery of estradiol from ESTRING resulted in mean steady state serum estradiol estimates of 7.8, 7.0, 7.0,8.1 pg/mL at weeks 12, 24, 36, and 48, respectively. Similar reproducibility is also seen in levels of estrone. Lower systemic exposure to estradiol and estrone is further supported by serum levels measured during a pivotal Phase III study.

In post-menopausal women, the mean dose of estradiol systemically absorbed unchanged from ESTRING is 8% [95% CI: 2.8-12.8%] of the daily amount released locally. Low systemic exposure to estradiol and estrone resulting from ESTRING should elicit lower estrogen-dependent effects.

After a brief initial peak (~50 µg), estradiol vaginal ring releases a low and consistent amount of estradiol, approximately 7.5 µg/24 hours, during 90 days. Average in vitro release rates over 7 batches were:

Day 1	Day 9	Day 16	Day 45	Day 90
47.6±6.4 (in µg/24 h)	7.3±0.4	7.7±0.4	7.3±0.2	7.3±0.5

The average in vivo release rate over an 88.4 day period was 9.0±0.06 µg/24 h (n=215), calculated by subtracting the amount of estradiol in the ring at the end of the treatment period from the amount of estradiol measured in the ring before treatment, and averaging the amount over the treatment period. This gives a slightly higher value than is actually released, since it does not take the initial burst of estradiol into account.

Distribution: Circulating, unbound estrogens are known to modulate pharmacological response. Estrogens circulate in blood bound to sex-hormone binding globulin (SHBG) and albumin. A dynamic equilibrium exists between the conjugated and the unconjugated forms of estradiol and estrone, which undergo rapid interconversion.

Metabolism: Exogenously delivered or endogenously derived estrogens are primarily metabolized in the liver to estrone and estriol, which are also found in the systemic circulation. Estrogen metabolites are primarily excreted in the urine as glucuronides and sulphates. Of the several estrogen metabolites, urinary estrone and estrone sulphate (E_1S), post-ESTRING use, are in the normal post-menopausal range.

Excretion: Mean percent dose excreted in the 24-hour urine as estradiol, 4 and 12 weeks post-application of ESTRING in a Phase I study was 5 and 8%, respectively, of the daily released amount.

Table 2: ESTRING

Pharmacokinetic Means Estimates Following ESTRING Application

Estrogen	C_{max} (pg/mL)	$C_{ss\text{-}48\,h}$ (pg/mL)	$C_{ss\text{-}4\,w}$ (pg/mL)	$C_{ss\text{-}12\,w}$ (pg/mL)
Estradiol (E_2)	63.2[a]	11.2	9.5	8.0
Baseline-adjusted E_2[b]	55.6	3.6	2.0	0.4
Estrone (E_1)	66.3	52.5	43.8	47.0
Baseline-adjusted E_1	20.0	6.2	−2.4	0.8

[a] n=14.
[b] Based on means.

STORAGE AND STABILITY: Store at room temperature (15-30°C). Keep in a safe place out of the reach of children and pets.

SPECIAL HANDLING INSTRUCTIONS: Not applicable.

INFORMATION FOR THE PATIENT: Published in e-CPS, available by subscription at www.e-cps.ca.

DOSAGE FORMS, COMPOSITION AND PACKAGING: Each slightly opaque ring, made of a silicone elastomer sheath surrounding a whitish silicone elastomer core, containing a drug reservoir of 2 mg estradiol, barium sulphate as a marker and silicone fluid as a dispersing agent. Each ring contains 2 mg estradiol which is released slowly, 7.5 µg/24 hours. One ring is individually packed in a heat-sealed rectangular pouch consisting of, from outside to inside: polyester/aluminum foil/low density polyethylene. The pouch is provided with a tear-off notch on one side. Each pouch is packed into a cardboard carton containing a Patient Information Leaflet.

(Shown in Product Identification Section)

Estrogel® Ⓟ

estradiol-17β hemihydrate

Estrogen

Schering-Plough

Date of Preparation: September 15, 1998
Date of Revision: February 18, 2009

SUMMARY PRODUCT INFORMATION:

Route of Administration	Dosage Form/ Strength	Clinically Relevant Nonmedicinal Ingredients
Transdermal	Gel 0.06%	Carbopol 980, triethanolamine, ethanol and purified water.

INDICATIONS AND CLINICAL USE: ESTROGEL (17β-estradiol) is indicated for:

- replacement therapy in naturally occurring or surgically induced estrogen deficiency states associated with menopausal and postmenopausal symptoms, e.g. hot flushes, sleep disturbances and atrophic vaginitis.

ESTROGEL should be prescribed with an appropriate dosage of progestin for women with intact uteri in order to prevent endometrial hyperplasia/carcinoma.

Geriatrics: No clinical studies were conducted to evaluate the effect of ESTROGEL on women more than 65 years old.

Pediatrics: ESTROGEL should not be used in children.

CONTRAINDICATIONS: Estrogen and Estrogen/Progestin combinations are contraindicated in patients with any of the following disorders.

- Hypersensitivity to this drug or to any ingredient in the formulation or component of the container. For a complete listing, see Dosage Forms, Composition and Packaging.
- Liver dysfunction or disease as long as liver function tests have failed to return to normal.
- Known or suspected estrogen-dependent or progestin-dependent malignant neoplasia (e.g. endometrial cancer).
- Endometrial hyperplasia.
- Known, suspected, or past history of breast cancer.
- Undiagnosed abnormal genital bleeding.
- Known or suspected pregnancy.
- Active or past history of arterial thromboembolic disease (e.g. stroke, myocardial infarction, coronary heart disease (CHD)).

- Active or past history of confirmed venous thromboembolism (such as deep venous thrombosis or pulmonary embolism) or active thrombophlebitis.
- Partial or complete loss of vision due to ophthalmic vascular disease.
- Breast-feeding.
- Classical migraine.

WARNINGS AND PRECAUTIONS:

Serious Warnings and Precautions

The Women's Health Initiative (WHI) trial examined the health benefits and risks of oral combined estrogen plus progestin therapy (n=16 608) and oral estrogen-alone therapy (n=10 739) in postmenopausal women aged 50 to 79 years.

The estrogen plus progestin arm of the WHI trial (mean age 63.3 years) indicated an increased risk of myocardial infarction (MI), stroke, invasive breast cancer, pulmonary emboli and deep vein thrombosis in postmenopausal women receiving treatment with combined conjugated equine estrogens (CEE, 0.625 mg/day) and medroxyprogesterone acetate (MPA, 2.5 mg/day) for 5.2 years compared to those receiving placebo.

The estrogen-alone arm of the WHI trial (mean age 63.6 years) indicated an increased risk of stroke and deep vein thrombosis in hysterectomized women treated with CEE-alone (0.625 mg/day) for 6.8 years compared to those receiving placebo.

Therefore, the following should be given serious consideration at the time of prescribing:

- Estrogens with or without progestins **should not** be prescribed for primary or secondary prevention of cardiovascular diseases.
- Estrogens with or without progestins should be prescribed at **the lowest effective dose** for the approved indication.
- Estrogens with or without progestins should be prescribed for **the shortest period** possible for the recognized indication.

Carcinogenesis and Mutagenesis: Breast Cancer: Available epidemiological data indicate that the use of combined estrogen plus progestin by postmenopausal women is associated with an increased risk of invasive breast cancer.

In the estrogen plus progestin arm of the WHI trial, among 10 000 women over a one-year period, there were:

- 8 more cases of invasive breast cancer (38 on combined HRT versus 30 on placebo).

The WHI study also reported that the invasive breast cancers diagnosed in the estrogen plus progestin group were similar in histology but were larger (mean [SD], 1.7 cm [1.1] vs 1.5 cm [0.9], respectively; p=0.04) and were at a more advanced stage compared with those diagnosed in the placebo group. The percentage of women with abnormal mammograms (recommendations for short-interval follow-up, a suspicious abnormality, or highly suggestive of malignancy) was significantly higher in the estrogen plus progestin group versus the placebo group. This difference appeared at year one and persisted in each year thereafter.

In the estrogen-alone arm of the WHI trial, there was no statistically significant difference in the rate of invasive breast cancer in hysterectomized women treated with conjugated equine estrogens versus women treated with placebo.

It is recommended that estrogens not be given to women with existing breast cancer or those with a previous history of the disease. (See Contraindications.)

There is a need for caution in prescribing estrogens for women with known risk factors associated with the development of breast cancer, such as strong family history of breast cancer (first degree relative) or who present a breast condition with an increased risk (abnormal mammograms and/or atypical hyperplasia at breast biopsy).

Other known risk factors for the development of breast cancer such as nulliparity, obesity, early menarche, late age at first full term pregnancy and at menopause should also be evaluated.

It is recommended that women undergo mammography prior to the start of hormone replacement therapy (HRT) and at regular intervals during treatment, as deemed appropriate by the treating physician and according to the perceived risks for each patient.

The overall benefits and possible risks of HRT should be fully considered and discussed with patients. It is important that the modest increased risk of being diagnosed with breast cancer after 4 years of treatment with combined estrogen plus progestin HRT (as reported in the results of WHI-trial) be discussed with the patient and weighed against its known benefits.

Other doses of conjugated estrogens and medroxyprogesterone acetate and other combinations of estrogens and progestins were not studied in the WHI trial. In the absence of comparable data, these risks should be assumed to be similar.

Instructions for regular self-examination of the breasts should be included in this counselling.

Endometrial Hyperplasia and Endometrial Carcinoma: Estrogen-only HRT increases the risk of endometrial hyperplasia/carcinoma (if taken by women with intact uteri).

There is evidence from several studies that estrogens, unopposed by progestins, increase the risk of carcinoma of the endometrium in humans. However, administration of a progestin for at least the last 12 to 14 days of an estrogen treatment cycle protects the endometrium from hyperplasia and reduces the risk of endometrial hyperplasia/carcinoma cancer to that of untreated women.

Morphological and biochemical studies have shown that 12-14 days of progestin treatment provides maximal control of endometrial mitotic activity. There are possible additional risks, which may be associated with the inclusion of a progestin in estrogen replacement regimens; therefore the manufacturers' labelling should be consulted. The long-term effects generally depend on the dosage and type of progestin used.

Estrogens should be prescribed with an appropriate dosage of a progestin for women with intact uteri in order to prevent endometrial hyperplasia/carcinoma.

Ovarian Cancer: Some recent epidemiological studies have found that the use of hormone replacement therapy (estrogen-alone and estrogen plus progestin therapies), in particular for five or more years, has been associated with an increased risk of ovarian cancer.

Cardiovascular: The results of the Heart and Estrogen/progestin Replacement Studies (HERS and HERS II) and the Women's Health Initiative (WHI) trial indicate that the use of estrogen plus progestin is associated with an increased risk of CHD in postmenopausal women. The results of the WHI trial indicate that the use of estrogen-alone and estrogen plus progestin is associated with an increased risk of stroke in postmenopausal women.

WHI Trial Findings: In the combined estrogen plus progestin arm of the WHI trial, among 10 000 women over a one-year period, there were:

- 8 more cases of stroke (29 on combined HRT versus 21 on placebo)
- 7 more cases of CHD (37 on combined HRT versus 30 on placebo).

In the estrogen-alone arm of the WHI trial of women with prior hysterectomy, among 10 000 women over a one-year period, there were/was:

- 12 more cases of stroke (44 on estrogen-alone therapy versus 32 on placebo)
- no statistically significant difference in the rate of CHD.

HERS and HERS II Findings: In the Heart and Estrogen/progestin Replacement Study (HERS) of postmenopausal woman with documented heart disease (n=2763, average age 66.7 years), a randomized placebo-controlled clinical trial of secondary prevention of CHD, treatment with 0.625 mg/day oral conjugated equine estrogen (CEE) plus 2.5 mg oral medroxyprogesterone acetate (MPA) demonstrated no cardiovascular benefit. Specifically, during an average follow-up of 4.1 years, treatment with CEE plus MPA did not reduce the overall rate of CHD events in postmenopausal women with established CHD. There were more CHD events in the hormone-treated group than in the placebo group in year 1, but not during the subsequent years. From the original HERS trial, 2321 women consented to participate in an open label extension of HERS known as HERS II. Average follow-up in HERS II was an additional 2.7 years, for a total of 6.8 years overall. After 6.8 years, hormone therapy did not reduce the risk of cardiovascular events in women with CHD.

Blood Pressure: Women using hormonal replacement therapy (HRT) sometimes experience increased blood pressure. Blood pressure should be monitored with HRT use. Elevation of blood pressure in previously normotensive or hypertensive patients should be investigated and HRT therapy may have to be discontinued.

Ear/Nose/Throat: Otosclerosis: Estrogens should be used with caution in patients with otosclerosis.

Endocrine and Metabolism: Glucose and Lipid Metabolism: A worsening of glucose tolerance and lipid metabolism has been observed in a significant percentage of peri- and post-menopausal patients. Therefore, diabetic patients or those with a predisposition to diabetes should be observed closely to detect any alterations in carbohydrate or lipid metabolism, especially in triglyceride blood levels.

Women with familial hyperlipidemias need special surveillance. Lipid lowering measures are recommended additionally, before treatment is started.

Heme Metabolism: Women with porphyria need special surveillance.

Calcium and Phosphorus Metabolism: Because the prolonged use of estrogens influences the metabolism of calcium and phosphorus, estrogens should be used with caution in patients with metabolic and malignant bone diseases associated with hypercalcemia and in patients with renal insufficiency.

Hypothyroidism: Patients who require thyroid hormone replacement therapy and who are also taking estrogen should have their thyroid function monitored regularly to assure that thyroid hormone levels remain in an acceptable range (see Drug Interactions, Drug-Laboratory Test Interactions).

Genitourinary: Vaginal Bleeding: Abnormal vaginal bleeding, due to its prolongation, irregularity or heaviness, occurring during therapy should prompt diagnostic measures to rule out the possibility of uterine malignancy and the treatment should be re-evaluated.

Uterine Leiomyomata: Pre-existing uterine leiomyomata may increase in size during estrogen use. Growth, pain or tenderness of uterine leiomyomata requires discontinuation of medication and appropriate investigation.

Endometriosis: Symptoms and physical findings associated with a previous diagnosis of endometriosis may reappear or become aggravated with estrogen use.

Hematologic: Venous Thromboembolism: Available epidemiological data indicate that use of estrogen with or without progestin by postmenopausal women is associated with an increased risk of developing venous thromboembolism (VTE).

In the estrogen plus progestin arm of the WHI trial, among 10 000 women on combined HRT over a one-year period, there were 18 more cases of venous thromboembolism, including 8 more cases of pulmonary embolism.

In the estrogen-alone arm of the WHI trial, among 10 000 women on estrogen therapy over a one-year period, there were 7 more cases of venous thromboembolism, although there was no statistically significant difference in the rate of pulmonary embolism.

Generally recognized risk factors for VTE include a personal history, a family history (the occurrence of VTE in a direct relative at a relatively early age may indicate genetic predisposition), severe obesity (body mass index >30 kg/m^2) and systemic lupus erythematosus. The risk of VTE also increases with age and smoking.

The risk of VTE may be temporarily increased with prolonged immobilization, major surgery or trauma. In women on HRT, attention should be given to prophylactic measures to prevent VTE following surgery. Also, patients with varicose veins should be closely supervised. The physician should be alert to the earliest manifestations of thrombotic disorders (thrombophlebitis, retinal thrombosis, cerebral embolism and pulmonary embolism). If these occur or are suspected, hormone therapy should be discontinued immediately, given the risk of long-term disability or fatality.

If feasible, estrogens should be discontinued at least 4 weeks before major surgery which may be associated with an increased risk of thromboembolism, or during periods of prolonged immobilization.

Hepatic/Biliary/Pancreatic: Gallbladder Diseases: A 2- to 4-fold increase in the risk of gallbladder disease requiring surgery in women receiving postmenopausal estrogens has been reported.

Hepatic Hemangiomas: Particular caution is indicated in women with hepatic hemangiomas, as estrogen may cause an exacerbation of this condition.

Jaundice: Caution is advised in patients with a history of liver and/or biliary disorders. If cholestatic jaundice develops during treatment, the treatment should be discontinued and appropriate investigations carried out.

Liver Function Tests: Liver function tests should be done periodically in subjects who are suspected of having hepatic disease. For information on endocrine and liver function tests, see Monitoring and Laboratory Tests.

Immune: Angioedema: Estrogens may induce or exacerbate symptoms of angioedema, in particular in women with hereditary angioedema.

Systemic Lupus Erythematosus: Particular caution is indicated in women with systemic lupus erythematosus.

Neurologic: Cerebrovascular Insufficiency: Patients who develop visual disturbances, classical migraine, transient aphasia, paralysis, or loss of consciousness should discontinue medication.

Dementia: Available epidemiological data indicate that the use of combined estrogen plus progestin in women age 65 and over may increase the risk of developing probable dementia.

The Women's Health Initiative Memory Study (WHIMS), a clinical substudy of the WHI, was designed to assess whether postmenopausal hormone replacement therapy (oral estrogen plus progestin or oral estrogen-alone) reduces the risk of dementia in women aged 65 and over (age range 65-79 years) and free of dementia at baseline.

In the estrogen plus progestin arm of the WHIMS (n=4532), women with intact uteri were treated with daily 0.625 mg conjugated equine estrogens (CEE) plus 2.5 mg medroxyprogesterone acetate (MPA) or placebo for an average of 4.05 years. The results, when extrapolated to 10 000 women treated over a one-year period showed:

- 23 more cases of probable dementia (45 on combined HRT versus 22 on placebo).

In the estrogen-alone arm of the WHIMS (n=2947), women with prior hysterectomy were treated with daily 0.625 mg CEE or placebo for an average of 5.21 years. The results, when extrapolated to 10 000 women treated over a one-year period showed:

- 12 more cases of probable dementia (37 on estrogen-alone versus 25 on placebo), although this difference did not reach statistical significance.

When data from the estrogen plus progestin arm of the WHIMS and the estrogen alone arm of the WHIMS were combined, as per the original WHIMS protocol, in 10 000 women over a one-year period, there were:

- 18 more cases of probable dementia (41 on estrogen plus progestin or estrogen-alone versus 23 on placebo).

Epilepsy: Particular caution is indicated in women with epilepsy, as estrogen, with or without progestins, may cause an exacerbation of this condition.

Renal: Fluid Retention: Estrogens may cause fluid retention. Therefore, particular caution is indicated in cardiac or renal dysfunction or asthma. If, in any of the above-mentioned conditions, a worsening of the underlying disease is diagnosed or suspected during treatment, the benefits and risks of treatment should be reassessed based on the individual case.

Skin: Contact Sensitization: Contact sensitization is known to occur with topical applications. Although it is extremely rare, patients who develop contact sensitization to any component of the gel should be warned that a severe hypersensitivity reaction may occur with continuing exposure to the causative agent.

Special Populations: Pregnant Women: ESTROGEL must not be used during pregnancy. Both estrogens and progestins may cause fetal harm when administered to a pregnant woman (see Contraindications).

Nursing Women: ESTROGEL must not be used while breastfeeding (see Contraindications).

Pediatrics: ESTROGEL should not be used in children.

Geriatrics (>65 years of age): No clinical studies were conducted to evaluate the effect of ESTROGEL on women more than 65 years old.

Monitoring and Laboratory Tests: Physical Examination: Before ESTROGEL is administered, the patient should have a complete physical examination including a blood pressure determination. Breasts and pelvic organs should be appropriately examined and a Papanicolaou smear should be performed. Endometrial biopsy should be done only when indicated. Baseline tests should include mammography, measurements of blood glucose, calcium, triglycerides, cholesterol, and liver function tests.

The first follow-up examination should be done within 3-6 months after initiation of treatment to assess response to treatment. Thereafter, examinations should be made at intervals at least once a year. Appropriate investigations should be arranged at regular intervals as determined by the physician.

The importance of regular self-examination of the breasts should be discussed with the patient.

ADVERSE REACTIONS: Adverse Drug Reaction Overview: See Warnings and Precautions regarding potential induction of malignant neoplasms and adverse effects similar to those of oral contraceptives.

The following adverse reactions have been reported with estrogens/progestin combination in general:

Blood and Lymphatic System Disorders: altered coagulation tests (see Warnings and Precautions, Drug Interactions, Drug-Laboratory Test Interactions).

Cardiac Disorders: palpitations; increase in blood pressure (see Warnings and Precautions); coronary thrombosis.

Endocrine Disorders: increased blood sugar levels; decreased glucose tolerance.

Eye Disorders: neuro-ocular lesions (e.g. retinal thrombosis, optic neuritis); visual disturbances; steepening of the corneal curvature; intolerance to contact lenses.

Gastrointestinal Disorders: nausea; vomiting; abdominal discomfort (cramps, pressure, pain, bloating).

General Disorders and Administration Site Conditions: fatigue; changes in appetite; changes in body weight; change in libido.

Hepatobiliary Disorders: gallbladder disorder; asymptomatic impaired liver function; cholestatic jaundice.

Musculoskeletal and Connective Tissue Disorders: Musculoskeletal pain including leg pain not related to thromboembolic disease (usually transient, lasting 3-6 weeks) may occur.

Nervous System Disorders: aggravation of migraine episodes; headaches; dizziness; neuritis.

Psychiatric Disorders: mental depression; nervousness; irritability.

Renal and Urinary Disorders: cystitis; dysuria; sodium retention; edema.

Reproductive System and Breast Disorders: breakthrough bleeding; spotting; change in menstrual flow; dysmenorrhea; vaginal itching/discharge; dyspareunia; endometrial hyperplasia; pre-menstrual-like syndrome; reactivation of endometriosis; changes in cervical erosion and amount of cervical secretion; breast swelling and tenderness.

Skin and Subcutaneous Tissue Disorders: chloasma or melasma, which may persist when drug is discontinued; erythema multiforme; erythema nodosum; hemorrhagic eruptions; loss of scalp hair; hirsutism and acne.

Vascular Disorders: isolated cases of: thrombophlebitis; thromboembolic disorders.

Clinical Trial Adverse Drug Reactions: Because clinical trials are conducted under very specific conditions the adverse drug reaction rates observed in the clinical trials may not reflect the rates observed in practice and should not be compared to the rates in the clinical trials of another drug. Adverse drug reaction information from clinical trials is useful for identifying drug-related adverse events and for approximating rates.

Table 1 summarizes the adverse events reported in a single-centre, double-blind, randomized, parallel group, 2 year study (titled "Percutaneous Oestradiol as prophylaxis in early postmenopausal women) designed to examine the efficacy and safety of ESTROGEL alone or in combination with either micronized progesterone or calcium in the treatment of postmenopausal symptoms as compared to placebo. Fifty-seven (57) patients were randomly divided into four groups and received the following treatment: (1) ESTROGEL 5 g (3 mg E_2) + placebo tablet daily (n=15), (2) ESTROGEL 5 g (3 mg E_2) + 1000 mg oral calcium tablet daily (n=14), (3) placebo (percutaneous) + 1000 mg oral calcium tablet daily (n=15), (4) placebo (percutaneous and oral) (n=13). After 1 year, patients who were receiving ESTROGEL were also administered micronized progesterone from day 13 to 24 of each month.

Table 1: ESTROGEL

Reported Adverse Events in at Least One Patient per Dose Group: Symptoms by Treatment Assignment

Reported Adverse Event	ESTROGEL n (%)	ESTROGEL+ Calcium n (%)	Calcium n (%)	Placebo n (%)
Gastrointestinal disorders	1 (6.7%)	2 (14.3%)	5 (33.3%)	2 (15.4%)
Dysfunctional uterine bleeding with vaginal erosion	2 (13.3%)	2 (14.3%)	1 (6.7%)	0
Vulvovaginal dryness	0	0	2 (13.3%)	1 (7.7%)
Hot flushes	0	0	0	1 (7.7%)
Arthralgia	1 (6.7%)	0	0	0
Benign breast neoplasm	0	0	0	1 (7.7%)
Malignant melanoma in the eye	0	0	1 (6.7%)	0
Duodenal ulcer	0	0	0	1 (7.7%)
Anemia	0	0	0	1 (7.7%)
Application site pruritus with erythema	1 (6.7%)	0	1 (6.7%)	0

Twenty one (21) patients reported adverse events summarized in Table 1. Gastrointestinal (GI) discomfort was reported by 10 patients, 2 in the placebo group, 5 in the calcium only group, 1 in the ESTROGEL only group and 2 in the ESTROGEL + calcium group. The GI effects were attributed to the calcium supplementation. Two incidents of application site pruritus with erythema were reported: 1 in the ESTROGEL group (dropped out of the study before 1 month of treatment) and 1 in the calcium group, who reported application site pruritus with erythema for the first 3 to 6 months. Dysfunctional uterine bleeding with vaginal erosion was reported by 4 patients treated with ESTROGEL or ESTROGEL + calcium. There were no significant changes in any laboratory parameters.

If adverse symptoms persist, the prescription of HRT should be reconsidered.

DRUG INTERACTIONS: Overview: Estrogens may diminish the effectiveness of anticoagulant, antidiabetic and antihypertensive agents.

Preparations inducing liver enzymes (e.g., barbiturates, hydantoins, carbamazepine, meprobamate, phenylbutazone or rifampin) may interfere with the activity of orally administered estrogens.

Drug-Drug Interactions: The following section contains information on drug interactions with ethinyl estradiol-containing products (specifically, oral contraceptives) that have been reported in the public literature (Table 2 and Table 3). It is unknown whether such interactions occur with drug products containing other types of estrogens.

Therapeutic monitoring is recommended.

Table 2: ESTROGEL

Drugs Which May Affect the Concentrations of Ethinyl Estradiol

Drug	Ref	Proposed Mechanism	Effect
Acetaminophen	Literature		Increased AUC and/or plasma concentrations of ethinyl estradiol
Anticonvulsants: Phenobarbital Phenytoin Carbamazepine	Literature	Increased metabolism of ethinyl estradiol	Decreased plasma concentrations of estradiol
Ascorbic acid	Literature		Increased AUC and/or plasma concentrations of ethinyl estradiol
Atorvastatin	Literature		When co-administered with certain ethinyl estradiol containing drug products (e.g. oral contraceptives containing ethinyl estradiol), the AUC values of ethinyl estradiol increase by 20 percent.
Rifampin	Literature	Increased metabolism of ethinyl estradiol	Decreased plasma concentrations of estradiol. Clinical pharmacokinetic studies have not demonstrated any consistent effect of antibiotics (other than rifampin) on plasma concentrations of synthetic steroids.
Troglitazone	Literature		When co-administered with certain ethinyl estradiol containing drug products (e.g. oral contraceptives containing ethinyl estradiol), the plasma concentrations of ethinyl estradiol reduce by 30 percent.

Drug products containing ethinyl estradiol may inhibit the metabolism of other compounds or induce the conjugation of other compounds.

Drug-Food Interactions: Interaction of ESTROGEL with food has not been established.

Drug-Herb Interactions: It was found that some herbal products (e.g. St. John's wort) which are available as over-the-counter (OTC) products might interfere with steroid metabolism and therefore alter the efficacy and safety of estrogen/progestin.

Physicians and other health care providers should be made aware of other non-prescription products concomitantly used by the patient, including herbal and natural products obtained from the widely spread health stores.

Table 3: ESTROGEL

Modification of Other Drug Action by Co-administration with Certain Drugs Containing Ethinyl Estradiol (e.g. oral contraceptives containing ethinyl estradiol)

Drug	Ref	Effect
Acetaminophen	Literature	Decreased plasma concentrations of acetaminophen
Clofibric Acid	Literature	Increased clearance of clofibric acid
Cyclosporin	Literature	Increased plasma concentrations of cyclosporine
Morphine	Literature	Increased clearance of morphine
Prednisolone	Literature	Increased plasma concentrations of prednisolone
Salicylic Acid	Literature	Increased clearance of salicylic acid
Temazepam	Literature	Increased clearance of temazepam
Theophylline	Literature	Increased plasma concentrations of theophylline

Drug-Laboratory Test Interactions: The results of certain endocrine and liver function tests may be affected by estrogen-containing products:

- increased prothrombin time and partial thromboplastin time; increased levels of fibrinogen and fibrinogen activity; increased coagulation factors VII, VIII, IX, X; increased norepinephrine-induced platelet aggregability; decreased antithrombin III;
- increased thyroxine-binding globulin (TBG), leading to increased circulating total thyroid hormone (T4) as measured by column or radioimmunoassay; T3 resin uptake is decreased, reflecting the elevated TBG; free T4 concentration is unaltered;
- other binding proteins may be elevated in serum i.e., corticosteroid binding globulin (CBG), sex-hormone binding globulin (SHBG), leading to increased circulating corticosteroids and sex steroids respectively; free or biologically active hormone concentrations are unchanged;
- impaired glucose tolerance;
- increased serum triglycerides and phospholipids concentration.

Administration of ESTROGEL, alone or in combination with oral micronized progesterone has no effect on antithrombin III. Postmenopausal women treated with ESTROGEL and oral micronized progesterone for three months showed no significant variations in platelet count, thromboelastinogram, factors II, VII, IX, X, prothrombin time, fibrinogen, antithrombin III and plasminogen. No shift towards hypercoagulability was observed. A moderate decrease in platelet aggregation was observed without any related clinical symptoms. In combination with oral micronized progesterone, ESTROGEL does not negatively affect the balance between the vasoactive prostanoids PGI2 and TxA2.

A study has shown that transdermal estradiol improves the anticoagulant response to activated protein C (APC-sensitivity), probably as a result of a decreased factor VIII.

Clinical trials demonstrated no increase of SHBG with percutaneous estradiol or increase to a lesser extent compared to oral conjugated estrogens.

Based on a study, transdermal estradiol did not significantly increase circulating levels of TBG and CBG.

The results of the above laboratory tests should not be considered reliable unless therapy has been discontinued for two to four weeks. The pathologist should be informed that the patient is receiving HRT therapy when relevant specimens are submitted.

Drug-Lifestyle Interactions: Acute alcohol ingestion during HRT may lead to elevations in circulating estradiol levels.

DOSAGE AND ADMINISTRATION:

Dosing Considerations: Because of the variable absorption of ESTROGEL between individuals due to the technique of self administration on the skin, it is recommended to obtain measurement of serum estradiol level after initiation of treatment. This measurement should be done when the patient has developed her technique for ESTROGEL application when she comes for her regular follow-up visit. This measurement should be similar to the serum estradiol level normally produced by the ovary before menopause during the middle part of the follicular phase of the menstrual cycle (150-400 pmol/L).

In women who are not currently taking oral estrogens, treatment with ESTROGEL can be initiated at once. In women who are currently taking oral estrogen, treatment with ESTROGEL can be initiated 1 week after withdrawal of oral therapy or sooner if symptoms reappear before the week's end.

In women with intact uteri, a progestin should be sequentially co-administered for a minimum of 12-14 days each cycle to prevent endometrial hyperplasia.

Continuous, non-cyclic therapy may be indicated in hysterectomized women or in cases where the signs and symptoms of estrogen deficiency become problematic during the treatment-free interval.

There have been no reported cases of biologically significant estradiol transfer from a patient using ESTROGEL to their male partner.

Recommended Dose and Dosage Adjustment: Treatment is usually initiated with 2.5 g ESTROGEL, daily. ESTROGEL is usually administered on a cyclic schedule from day 1 to day 25 of each calendar month or from day 1 to day 21 of a 28-day cycle.

The dose of ESTROGEL should be adjusted as necessary to control symptoms. Attempts to adjust the necessary dosage should be made after two months of treatment. Breast discomfort and/or breakthrough bleeding are generally signs that the dose is too high and needs to be lowered. However, if the selected dose fails to eliminate the signs and symptoms of estrogen deficiency, a higher dose may be prescribed. For maintenance therapy, the lowest effective dose should be used.

Missed Dose: If a dose of ESTROGEL has been missed, the missed dose should be taken as soon as possible. However, if it is almost time for the next dose, the missed dose should be skipped and the regular dosing schedule should be continued. The dose of ESTROGEL should not be doubled.

Administration: ESTROGEL Metered-Dose Pump: Two metered-actuations will deliver 2.5 g of gel (1.5 mg E_2). All of the gel should be applied with the hands over a large area of skin (>2000 cm^2) in a thin, uniform layer.

To measure a 2.5 g dose of ESTROGEL (1.5 mg E_2), press firmly on the pump once and apply the gel to one arm. Repeat applying the gel to the opposite arm. It is recommended to apply ESTROGEL to both arms. Alternate sites of application are the abdomen or the inner thighs. It is not necessary to rotate the site of administration. **ESTROGEL must not be applied to the breasts.** ESTROGEL must not be applied to the face or to irritated or damaged skin. Allow the gel to dry approximately 2 minutes before covering with clothing. ESTROGEL does not stain or smell.

When a new metered-dose pump is opened, it may be necessary to prime the pump by pressing the pump once or twice. The first metered-actuation may not be accurate and should therefore be discarded. The pump contains enough gel for approximately a month's use (i.e. 64 metered-actuations). After that, the amount of gel delivered may be lower and thus, it is recommended to change the pump.

ESTROGEL should be prescribed with an appropriate dosage of a progestin for women with intact uteri in order to prevent endometrial hyperplasia/carcinoma. Progestin therapy is not required as part of hormone replacement therapy in women who have had a previous hysterectomy.

OVERDOSAGE:

Symptoms: Numerous reports of the ingestion of large doses of estrogen products and estrogen-containing oral contraceptives by young children have not revealed acute serious ill effects. Overdosage with estrogen may cause nausea, breast discomfort, fluid retention, abdominal cramps, headache, dizziness, bloating or vaginal bleeding in women.

ESTROGEL does not contain progestins. However, in the case where a progestin is co-administered, progestin (norethindrone acetate) overdosage has been characterized by depressed mood, tiredness, acne and hirsutism.

Treatment: Symptomatic treatment should be given.

For management of a suspected drug overdose, contact your **regional Poison Control Centre**. See the *CPS* Directory section for a list of Poison Control Centres.

ACTION AND CLINICAL PHARMACOLOGY: Mechanism of Action: ESTROGEL is a transdermal preparation which is comprised of a hydro-alcoholic gel containing 0.06% of the physiological hormone, 17β-estradiol (E_2).

Pharmacodynamics: Treatment of postmenopausal women with ESTROGEL provides swift and effective relief from climacteric symptoms such as hot flushes, vaginal atrophy and insomnia. Co-administration of a progestin does not affect the efficacy of ESTROGEL to relieve climacteric symptoms and has been shown to be an effective method to prevent estrogen-induced endometrial hyperplasia.

In general, administration of ESTROGEL, in combination with a progesterone substitute, does not lead to significant changes in systolic and diastolic blood pressure or heart rate in normotensive women. In only one open study, examining normotensive and hypertensive women, was a slight but significant reduction in blood pressure (remaining within the normal range) observed after 3 years of treatment. Administration of ESTROGEL does not lead to any significant change in rennin substrate, even when administered to diabetic patients.

Administration of ESTROGEL has no significant effect on carbohydrate metabolism, even when administered to non-insulin dependent diabetics.

Pharmacokinetics: Percutaneous administration of ESTROGEL produces plasma concentrations of estradiol and estrone that are similar to those observed in the follicular phase of the ovulary cycle.

Absorption: Following application to human skin, ESTROGEL rapidly penetrates the stratum corneum and then diffuses more slowly into the epidermis, dermis and vascular system over several hours. When ESTROGEL is applied on skin, it dries in 2 to 5 minutes.

ESTROGEL 2.5 g was administered to 17 postmenopausal women once daily on the posterior surface of one arm from wrist to shoulder for 14 consecutive days.

Maximal serum concentrations of estradiol and estrone on day 12 were 117 pg/mL and 128 pg/mL, respectively. The time-averaged serum estradiol and estrone concentration over the 24-hour dose interval after administration of 2.5 g ESTROGEL on Day 12 are 76.8 pg/mL and 95.7 pg/mL, respectively.

Table 4: ESTROGEL

Pharmacokinetics

Day	Parameter	Estradiol	Estrone	Estradiol/ Estrone ratio
11	C_{max}	114 pg/mL (44) (417 pmoles/L)	128 pg/mL (57) (473 pmoles/L)	1.02 (42) —
	T_{max}	9.50 (102)	7.83 (106)	0.85 (42)
	AUC $_{(0-24hr)}$	1745 (40)	2343 (56)	—
	C_{avg}	72.2 pg/mL (39) (264 pmoles/L)	92.8 pg/mL (57) (343 pmoles/L)	
12	C_{max}	117 pg/mL (42) (428 pmoles /L)	128 pg/mL (57) (473 pmoles /L)	1.09 (55)
	T_{max}	6.75 (126)	12.7 (70)	0.81 (38)
	AUC $_{(0-24hr)}$	1684 (37)	2326 (54)	
	C_{avg}	76.8 pg/mL (30) (281 pmoles/L)	95.7 pg/mL (53) (354 pmoles /L)	
13	C_{max}	117 pg/mL (51) (428 pmoles /L)	123 pg/mL (63) (455 pmoles/L)	1.08 (35) —
	T_{max}	7.92 (124)	6.50 (111)	0.81 (33)
	AUC $_{(0-24hr)}$	1624 (55)	2142 (62)	
	C_{avg}	70.7 pg/mL (50) (259 pmoles/L)	88.3 pg/mL (60) (326 pmoles/L)	

Legend: C_{max}=maximum serum concentration (pg/mL); T_{max}=time of maximum serum concentration (hr); AUC$_{(0-24hr)}$=area under the serum concentration-time curve from time zero to 24 hr; C_{avg}=average serum concentration (pg/mL).

Mean concentrations-time profiles for estradiol and estrone are shown in Figure 1 and Figure 2.

Figure 1: ESTROGEL

Serum Concentration Time Curves of Estradiol And Estrone on Days 11-13 Following Multiple Administration of ESTROGEL 2.5 g to Postmenopausal Women

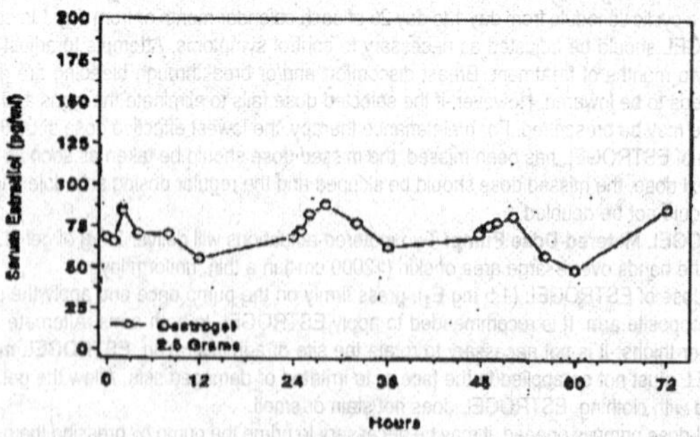

Daily percutaneous administration of ESTROGEL results in increasing plasma estradiol levels, which plateau after 4-5 days of treatment, remaining relatively stable thereafter.

Distribution: The distribution of exogenous estrogens is similar to that of endogenous estrogens. Estrogens are widely distributed in the body and are generally found in higher concentrations in the sex hormone target organs. Estrogens circulate in blood largely bound to sex hormone binding globulin (SHBG) and albumin.

Metabolism: Exogenous estrogens are metabolized in the same manner as endogenous estrogens. Circulating estrogens exist in a dynamic equilibrium of metabolic interconversions. These transformations take place mainly in the liver. Estradiol is converted reversibly to estrone, and both can be converted to estriol, which is the major urinary metabolite. Estrogens also undergo enterohepatic recirculation via sulfate and glucuronide conjugation in the liver, biliary secretion of conjugates into the intestine, and hydrolysis in the gut followed by reabsorption. In postmenopausal women, a significant proportion of the circulating estrogens exist as sulfate conjugates, especially estrone sulfate, which serves as a circulating reservoir for the formation of more active estrogens. Although the clinical significance has not been determined, estradiol from ESTROGEL does not go through the first pass liver metabolism.

Excretion: Estradiol, estrone and estriol are excreted in the urine along with glucuronide and sulfate conjugates.

Special Populations and Conditions: Pediatrics: ESTROGEL should not be used in children.

Geriatrics (>65 years of age): No clinical studies were conducted to evaluate the effect of ESTROGEL® on women more than 65 years old.

Figure 2: ESTROGEL

Serum Concentration Time Curves of Estradiol And Estrone on Days 11-13 Following Multiple Administration of ESTROGEL 2.5 g to Postmenopausal Women

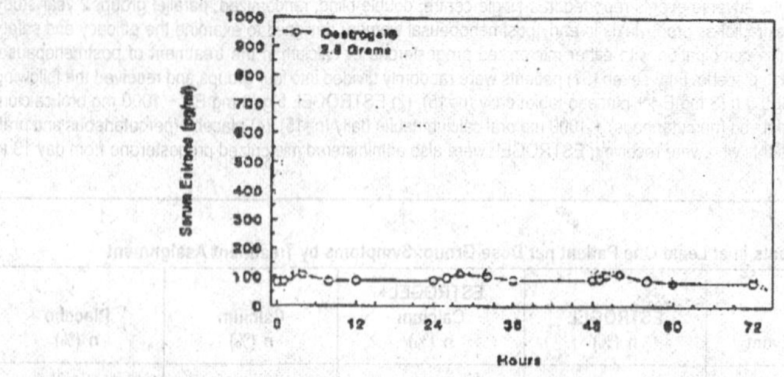

Gender: ESTROGEL should be used in women only.

Estrogen Pharmacology: With daily administration of 2.5 g or 5 g ESTROGEL (corresponding to 1.5 mg or 3 mg estradiol, respectively), mean serum estradiol concentrations of approximately 80 pg/mL (294 pmol/L) and 150 pg/mL (551 pmol/L), respectively, are maintained. Administration of ESTROGEL also results in increased serum estrone concentrations, producing a physiological estradiol/estrone ratio of approximately one. Therefore, serum concentrations of both estradiol and estrone and the serum estradiol/estrone ratio provided by ESTROGEL are consistent with physiological levels observed during the follicular phase of the normal menstrual cycle.

Estrogen exerts a dose-dependent stimulating effect on mitosis (proliferation) of the endometrium. Unopposed estrogen increases the risk of endometrial hyperplasia/carcinoma. Therefore, ESTROGEL should be prescribed with an appropriate dosage of progestin for women with intact uteri.

STORAGE AND STABILITY: Store at controlled room temperature; 15-30°C.

Keep in a safe place out of reach of children.

SPECIAL HANDLING INSTRUCTIONS: See Dosage and Administration, Administration.

INFORMATION FOR THE PATIENT: Published in e-CPS, available by subscription at www.e-cps.ca.

DOSAGE FORMS, COMPOSITION AND PACKAGING: The transdermal gel contains: 17β-estradiol 0.06% as hemihydrate in a specially formulated hydro-alcoholic gel to provide a sustained absorption of the active ingredient. Nonmedicinal ingredients: carbopol 980, ethanol, purified water and triethanolamine. Metered-dose pumps of 80 g. Each metered-actuation delivers 1.25 g of gel (0.75 mg of 17β-estradiol).

Ethambutol ℞

ethambutol HCl

Antimycobacterial

CPhA Monograph

Date of Revision: March 2008

This monograph has been compiled by CPhA and reviewed by experts. It may contain information different from that found in Health Canada-approved Product Monographs. The reader is referred to the *CPS* Editorial Policy for more information.

SUMMARY PRODUCT INFORMATION:

Route of Administration	Dosage Form	Strength
Oral	Tablet	100 mg, 400 mg

INDICATIONS AND CLINICAL USE: Ethambutol is used in the following clinical settings to treat infections caused by susceptible organisms:

- Adjunctive treatment of tuberculosis. Used with isoniazid, rifampin and pyrazinamide, while awaiting susceptibility data. Discontinue ethambutol if the organism is susceptible to isoniazid, rifampin and pyrazinamide. In treatment failure or relapse cases, mycobacterial resistance to other drugs used in initial therapy is frequent. Ethambutol monoresistance is rare; however, this does not change the duration and effectiveness of standard regimens [*Canadian tuberculosis standards.* 6th ed. http://www.phac-aspc.gc.ca/tbpc-latb/pubs/pdf/tbstand07_e.pdf].
- Adjunctive treatment of infections caused by nontuberculous mycobacteria such as *M. avium* complex (*M. avium, M. intracellulare*) and *M. kansasii* [An official ATS/IDSA statement: diagnosis, treatment, and prevention of nontuberculous mycobacterial diseases. *Am J Resp Crit Care Med* 2007;175(4):367-416].

CONTRAINDICATIONS:

- Patients who develop severe hypersensitivity reactions to ethambutol.
- Patients with known optic neuritis unless considerations of risk versus benefit (clinical judgement) determine that it may be used.

WARNINGS AND PRECAUTIONS: Ethambutol may cause optic neuritis with decreased visual acuity, visual field constriction, loss of red-green color vision or scotomata. Ocular toxicity appears to be related to dose and duration of treatment; however, it has occurred rarely after only a few days of therapy. Approximately 6% of patients receiving the drug have exhibited decreases in visual acuity. The effects are generally reversible when detected early and the drug discontinued promptly. Recovery of visual acuity generally occurs over a period of weeks to months after the drug has been discontinued. Some patients have then received ethambutol again, without recurrent loss of visual acuity. In rare cases, recovery may be delayed for up to 1 year or more, or the effects may be irreversible.

The changes in visual acuity may be unilateral or bilateral; hence, each eye must be tested separately and both eyes tested together. Ophthalmoscopy and tests for visual acuity (Snellen eye charts), visual fields (finger perimetry) and color discrimination (Ishihara tests) should be performed before beginning treatment with ethambutol and periodically during drug therapy. Monthly examination is recommended for patients receiving doses greater than 15 mg/kg and in patients with renal insufficiency.

Ophthalmoscopy, finger perimetry and color discrimination should also be included in the baseline evaluation. If corrective lenses are used prior to treatment, they must be worn during visual acuity testing. During 1 to 2 years of ethambutol therapy, a refractive error may develop which must be corrected (by testing visual acuity through a pinhole) in order to obtain accurate results.

In patients with pre-existing visual defects such as cataracts, recurrent inflammatory conditions of the eye, optic neuritis or diabetic retinopathy, the evaluation of changes in visual acuity is more difficult, and care should be taken to ensure that the variations in vision are not due to the underlying disease condition. In such patients, consideration should be given to the expected benefits of ethambutol therapy and the possibility of visual deterioration.

Patients developing ocular toxicities during treatment may show subjective symptoms before, or at the same time as, decreases in visual acuity. All patients receiving ethambutol should be questioned periodically about blurred vision and other subjective eye symptoms. Progressive decreases in visual acuity during therapy must be considered to be due to ethambutol.

Advise patients to promptly report any changes in visual acuity to their physician.

Special Populations: Pregnant Women: There have been no reports linking ethambutol with a higher incidence of congenital birth defects. The American Thoracic Society (ATS), the US Centers for Disease Control and Prevention (CDC) and the Infectious Diseases Society of America (IDSA) consider ethambutol to be safe for use in pregnancy [*MMWR* 2003;52:24].

Nursing Women: Ethambutol is excreted in breast milk. According to the American Academy of Pediatrics, ethambutol is generally considered to be compatible with breast-feeding.
Pediatrics: Ethambutol is often a component of a 4-drug empiric regimen used to treat active tuberculosis in children. Use ethambutol with caution in children who are too young for ophthalmologic monitoring. Ethambutol is not routinely used if visual acuity cannot be monitored. Monitor weight and adjust dose accordingly.
Geriatrics: Use with caution in patients with decreased renal function, especially in the elderly, due to the risk of drug accumulation. Extend ethambutol dosing interval according to the degree of renal impairment (see Table 1: Dose in Adult Patients with Renal Impairment).

ADVERSE REACTIONS: Central Nervous System: headache, dizziness, mental confusion, possible hallucinations, peripheral neuritis (infrequent), mania, psychosis.
Dermatologic: dermatitis, pruritus.
Gastrointestinal: anorexia, nausea, vomiting, abdominal pain, metallic taste.
Hematologic: rare case reports of thrombocytopenia and neutropenia.
Hepatic: jaundice (rare), hepatitis.
Since ethambutol is recommended for therapy in conjunction with one or more other antituberculosis drugs, these changes may be related to concurrent therapy.
Hypersensitivity: anaphylactoid reactions, fever, malaise, Stevens-Johnson syndrome (rare), toxic epidermal necrolysis (rare).
Ophthalmologic: Retrobulbar optic neuritis is dose-dependent, renal function-dependent and is associated with prolonged duration of ethambutol treatment. Patients with retrobulbar optic neuritis complain of bilateral blurry vision, visual acuity impairment and color vision defects (especially red-green color discrimination). Advise patients to report symptoms of blurry vision and to discontinue ethambutol until further testing on visual acuity is performed (see Warnings and Precautions).
Renal: rarely, interstitial nephritis, nephrotoxicity (may be related to other antituberculosis therapy).
Respiratory: pneumonitis, pulmonary infiltrates.
Other: Elevated serum uric acid levels and precipitation of gout have been reported. Joint pain has also been reported.
Monitor for signs and symptoms of immune reconstitution inflammatory syndrome (fever, malaise, local reactions in organs) during tuberculosis therapy after initiation of antiretroviral therapy in patients co-infected with HIV [*Canadian tuberculosis standards*. 6th ed. http://www.phac-aspc.gc.ca/tbpc-latb/pubs/pdf/tbstand07_e.pdf].

DOSAGE AND ADMINISTRATION: Ethambutol can be taken with or without food. If taken concomitantly with aluminum hydroxide, the absorption of ethambutol is reduced. Separate the administration of aluminum hydroxide and ethambutol by at least 4 hours.
For treatment of tuberculosis in HIV-positive patients, once or twice weekly has been associated with higher failure and relapse rates. Daily and three times a week administration is recommended in this population.
Treatment of Active *M. tuberculosis*Disease: Ethambutol should not be used alone in initial treatment or in retreatment. The drug should be administered not more than once every 24 hours (i.e., daily doses should not be divided) or tissue concentrations may not reach therapeutic levels.
Adults: Initial Treatment: As part of a multi-drug regimen in adult patients who have not received previous antituberculosis therapy, administer ethambutol 18 to 26 mg/kg as a single oral dose (up to 1.6 g) every 24 hours [*Canadian tuberculosis standards*. 6th ed. http://www.phac-aspc.gc.ca/tbpc-latb/pubs/pdf/tbstand07_e.pdf]. With directly observed therapy (DOT) the dose is 50 mg/kg twice weekly (up to 4.0 g) or 25 to 30 mg/kg three times weekly (up to 2.4 g). Discontinue ethambutol if organism if susceptible to isoniazid, rifampin and pyrazinamide. Duration of therapy is generally 2 months; however, a longer duration of therapy may be required if organism is resistant to rifampin.
Adults: Retreatment: In adult patients who have received previous antituberculosis therapy, administer ethambutol 25 mg/kg as a single oral dose once every 24 hours, as part of a multi-drug treatment regimen. After 60 days of therapy, or when bacteriologic cultures become negative, decrease the dose to 15 mg/kg once every 24 hours. During the period when a patient is on a daily dose of 25 mg/kg, monthly eye examinations are advised.
Children: The dose for children is 15 to 20 mg/kg (maximum 1 g) daily or 50 mg/kg (maximum 2.5 g) twice weekly [*Canadian tuberculosis standards*. 6th ed. http://www.phac-aspc.gc.ca/tbpc-latb/pubs/pdf/tbstand07_e.pdf]. Intermittent therapy should include directly observed drug administration.
***M. avium* Complex (*M. avium* and *M. intracellulare*) Pulmonary Disease:** For patients with nodular/bronchiectatic disease, the dose of ethambutol is 25 mg/kg three times weekly in combination with clarithromycin 1000 mg or azithromycin 500 mg and rifampin 600 mg, which are also given three times weekly. For patients with fibrocavitary MAC lung disease or severe nodular/bronchiectatic disease, the dose is 15 mg/kg daily in combination with clarithromycin 500 to 1000 mg daily or azithromycin 250 mg daily and rifampin 600 mg daily or rifabutin 150 to 300 mg daily. Consider amikacin or streptomycin three times weekly early in therapy. Treat patients until culture-negative for 1 year [An official ATS/IDSA statement: diagnosis, treatment, and prevention of nontuberculous mycobacterial diseases. *Am J Respir Crit Care Med* 2007;175(4):367-416].
Disseminated *M. avium* Complex Disease: In combination with clarithromycin 1000 mg daily or azithromycin 500 mg daily with or without rifabutin 300 mg daily, the adult dose of ethambutol is 15 mg/kg daily. Discontinue therapy after symptoms have resolved and cell-mediated immune function has been restored [An official ATS/IDSA statement: diagnosis, treatment, and prevention of nontuberculous mycobacterial diseases. *Am J Respir Crit Care Med* 2007;175(4):367-416].
***M. kansasii*:** In combination with rifampin 600 mg daily plus isoniazid 300 mg daily, the adult dose is 15 mg/kg daily for a minimum of 12 months. Treat patients until culture-negative for 1 year.
***M. marinum*:** In combination with rifampin, the adult dose is 15 to 25 mg/kg/day for a minimum of 3 months.
Ethambutol may be used in a dosage of 15 mg/kg/day in combination with other antimycobacterial agents for the treatment of other nontuberculous mycobacterial infections such as those caused by *M. xenopi*.

Table 1: Ethambutol
Dose in Adult Patients with Renal Impairment

Creatinine Clearance	Interval Adjustment
>50 mL/min	Q24H
10–50 mL/min	Q24–36H
<10 mL/min	Q48H

For patients on hemodialysis, 15-25 mg/kg per dose 3 times a week is recommended [The effect of hemodialysis on isoniazid, rifampin, pyrazinamide, and ethambutol. *Am J Resp Crit Care Med* 1999;159(5 Pt 1):1580-4].

OVERDOSAGE:

For management of a suspected drug overdose, CPhA recommends that you contact your **regional Poison Control Centre**. See the *CPS* Directory section for a list of Poison Control Centres.

ACTION AND CLINICAL PHARMACOLOGY: Low-dose ethambutol (15-20 mg/kg daily) is bacteriostatic. High-dose ethambutol (25 mg/kg daily) is bactericidal [*Canadian tuberculosis standards*. 6th ed. http://www.phac-aspc.gc.ca/tbpc-latb/pubs/pdf/tbstand07_e.pdf]. Ethambutol diffuses into actively growing mycobacterium cells, where it inhibits the synthesis of one or more essential metabolites, causing impairment of cell metabolism, arrest of multiplication, and cell death.
Ethambutol is active in vitro and in vivo against strains of *M. tuberculosis, M. bovis, M. avium, M. kansasii, M. marinum, M. xenopi* and *M. intracellulare*. Ethambutol is not active against other bacteria, fungi or viruses.
Resistance develops rapidly if ethambutol is used alone in the treatment of active tuberculosis. Resistance develops in a step-wise manner and may be delayed or prevented by using ethambutol in combination with other antituberculosis agents. Cross-resistance with other antituberculosis drugs has not been reported.
Pharmacokinetics: Ethambutol is about 75 to 80% absorbed after an oral dose. Absorption is rapid and not affected by food.
Two to four hours following a single oral dose of 25 mg/kg of body weight, ethambutol attains a peak serum level of 2 to 5 μg/mL. No drug accumulation has been observed with consecutive single daily doses of 25 mg/kg in patients with normal kidney function, although marked accumulation has been demonstrated in patients with renal insufficiency. Serum concentrations are undetectable 24 hours after the last dose except in some patients with abnormal kidney function.
Ethambutol distributes widely into body fluids and tissues. Concentrations in erythrocytes may reach 2 to 3 times the plasma concentrations. It also appears in the lungs, kidneys and saliva, and to a lesser extent in pleural and ascitic fluids. CSF concentrations reaching 10 to 50% of serum concentrations may occur with inflamed meninges. Ethambutol is not highly bound to plasma proteins. Its volume of distribution is about 1.6-3.2 L/kg. Ethambutol crosses the placenta. Ethambutol distributes into milk in concentrations similar to its plasma concentration. It also distributes into cord blood and amniotic fluid.
The half-life of ethambutol is about 3 to 4 hours in patients with normal kidney function; it may be as long as ≥7 hours in patients with renal insufficiency and 18 to 20 hours in the anephric patient.
Within 24 hours after oral administration, approximately 50% of the initial dose is excreted unchanged in the urine, while an additional 8 to 15% appears as inactive metabolites. The main metabolic path appears to be an initial oxidation of the alcohol to an aldehyde intermediate, followed by conversion to a decarboxylic acid. From 20 to 22% of the initial dose is excreted in the feces as unchanged drug. Ethambutol is removed by peritoneal dialysis and to a lesser extent by hemodialysis.

Etibi® Ⓟ
ethambutol HCl
Antituberculosis Agent

Valeant

SUPPLIED: 100 mg: Each blue, film-coated tablet, single-scored on one side, contains: ethambutol HCl, USP 100 mg. Nonmedicinal ingredients: alcohol, cornstarch, hydroxypropyl cellulose, lactose and magnesium stearate. Bottles of 100.
400 mg: Each blue, film-coated tablet, single-scored on one side and engraved ICN E12 on the other, contains: ethambutol HCl, USP 400 mg. Nonmedicinal ingredients: alcohol, cornstarch, hydroxypropyl cellulose, lactose and magnesium stearate. Bottles of 100.
Protect from light, moisture and excessive heat and store in well-closed containers at controlled room temperature (15 to 30°C).

Etidronate Ⓟ
CPhA Monograph

see *Bisphosphonates: Oral*

Euflex® Ⓟ
flutamide
Nonsteroidal Antiandrogen

Schering-Plough

PHARMACOLOGY: Flutamide demonstrates potent antiandrogenic effects by inhibiting androgen uptake and/or inhibiting nuclear binding of androgen in target tissues. In adult male rats, ventral prostate weights and seminal vesicle weights were markedly reduced by daily administration of flutamide.
Pharmacokinetics: Analysis of plasma, urine, and feces following a single oral 200 mg dose of tritium-labelled flutamide to human volunteers showed that the drug is rapidly and completely absorbed. It is excreted mainly in the urine with 4.2% of the dose excreted in the feces over 72 hours. The composition of plasma radioactivity showed that flutamide is rapidly and extensively metabolized, with flutamide comprising 2.5% of plasma radioactivity 1 hour after administration. At least 6 metabolites have been identified in plasma. The major plasma metabolite is a biologically active alpha-hydroxylated derivative which accounts for 23% of the plasma tritium 1 hour after drug administration. The major urinary metabolite is 2-amino-5-nitro-4-(trifluoromethyl)phenol.
Following a single 250 mg oral dose to normal adult volunteers, low plasma levels of varying amounts of flutamide were detected. The biologically active alpha-hydroxylated metabolite reaches maximum plasma levels in about 2 hours, indicating that it is rapidly formed from flutamide. The plasma half-life for this metabolite is about 6 hours.
Following multiple oral dosing of 250 mg t.i.d. in normal geriatric volunteers, flutamide and its active metabolite approached steady-state plasma levels (based on pharmacokinetic simulations) after the fourth flutamide dose. The half-life of the active metabolite in geriatric volunteers after a single flutamide dose is about 8 hours and at steady-state is 9.6 hours.
Flutamide, in vivo, at steady-state plasma concentrations of 24 to 78 ng/mL is 94 to 96% bound to plasma proteins. The active metabolite of flutamide, in vivo, at steady-state plasma concentrations of 1556 to 2284 ng/mL, is 92 to 94% bound to plasma proteins.
In male rats neither flutamide nor any of its metabolites are preferentially accumulated in any tissue except the prostate after an oral 5 mg/kg dose of ^{14}C-flutamide. Total drug levels were highest 6 hours after drug administration in all tissues. Levels declined at roughly similar rates to low levels at 18 hours. The major metabolite was present at higher concentrations than flutamide in all tissues studied.
Elevations of plasma testosterone and estradiol levels have been noted following flutamide administration.

INDICATIONS: For use in combination with LHRH agonistic analogues (such as leuprolide acetate) for the treatment of metastatic prostatic carcinoma (Stage D_2). To achieve the benefit of the adjunctive therapy with flutamide, treatment must be started simultaneously using both drugs. Also as an adjunctive therapy to orchiectomy, in order to achieve complete androgen blockade.
Flutamide in combination with LHRH agonists are also indicated prior to and during definitive external beam radiotherapy for patients with bulky locally advanced Stage B_2 and Stage C prostatic carcinoma (see Dosage).

CONTRAINDICATIONS: In patients who have shown hypersensitivity to flutamide or any component of this preparation.
In patients with severe hepatic impairment.
Flutamide has not been studied in women and is not indicated for this population, particularly for nonserious or nonthreatening conditions.

WARNINGS: General:
- Gynecomastia occurred in 9% of patients receiving flutamide together with medical castration.
- Physicians must familiarize themselves with the proper use of LHRH before combination medication is contemplated.

Hepatic Injury: There have been postmarketing reports of hospitalization and rarely death due to liver failure in patients taking flutamide. Evidence of hepatic injury included elevated serum transaminase levels, jaundice, hepatic encephalopathy, and death related to acute hepatic failure. The hepatic injury was reversible after prompt discontinuation of therapy in some patients. Approximately half of the reported cases occurred within the initial 3 months of treatment with flutamide.
Serum transaminase levels should be measured prior to starting treatment with flutamide. Flutamide is not recommended in patients whose ALT values exceed twice the upper limit of normal. Serum transaminase levels should then be measured monthly for the first 4 months of therapy, and periodically thereafter. Liver function tests also should be obtained at the first signs and symptoms suggestive of liver dysfunction, e.g., nausea, vomiting, abdominal pain, fatigue, anorexia, "flu-like" symptoms, hyperbilirubinuria, jaundice, or right upper quadrant tenderness. If at any time a patient has jaundice, or their ALT rises above 2 times the upper limit of normal, flutamide should be immediately discontinued with close follow-up of liver function tests until resolution.
Antiandrogen Withdrawal Syndrome: In some patients with metastatic prostate cancer, antiandrogens (steroidal or non-steroidal); may promote, rather than inhibit, the growth of prostate cancer. A decrease in PSA and/or clinical improvement following the discontinuation of antiandrogens have been reported. It is recommended that patients prescribed an antiandrogen, who have PSA progression, should have the antiandrogen discontinued immediately and be monitored for 6-8 weeks for a withdrawal response prior to any decision to proceed with other prostate cancer therapy.
Pregnancy: No studies have been conducted in pregnant or lactating women. Therefore, the possibility that flutamide may cause fetal harm if administered to a pregnant woman, or may be present in the breast milk of lactating women must be considered.
There was decreased 24-hour survival in the offspring of rats treated with flutamide at doses of 30, 100, or 200 mg/kg/day (approximately 3, 9, and 19 times the human dose) during pregnancy. A slight increase in minor variations in the development of the sternebra and vertebra was seen in fetuses of rats at the two higher doses. Feminization of the males also occurred at the two higher dose levels. There was a decreased survival rate in the offspring of rabbits receiving the highest dose (15 mg/kg/day; equal to 1.4 times the human dose).

Lactation: See Pregnancy.

PRECAUTIONS: Periodic liver function tests and sperm count determinations must be performed in patients on long-term treatment with flutamide.

After long-term administration in rats, flutamide produced testicular interstitial cell adenomas and dose-related increases in mammary gland adenomas or carcinomas. The relevance of these findings to humans is unknown. It should be noted that few cases of malignant breast neoplasms have been reported in male patients receiving flutamide; causality has not been established.

Since flutamide tends to elevate plasma testosterone and estradiol levels, fluid retention may occur. Accordingly, flutamide should be used with caution in those patients with cardiac disease.

Hepatic Injury: Treatment with flutamide should not be initiated in patients with serum transaminase levels exceeding 2 to 3 times the upper limit of normal.

Since transaminase abnormalities, cholestatic jaundice, hepatic necrosis and hepatic encephalopathy have been reported with the use of flutamide, periodic liver function tests must be performed in all patients.

Appropriate laboratory testing should be done monthly for the first 4 months, and periodically thereafter, and at the first symptom/sign of liver dysfunction (e.g., pruritus, dark urine, persistent anorexia, jaundice, right upper quadrant tenderness or unexplained "flu-like" symptoms).

If the patient has laboratory evidence of liver injury or jaundice, in the absence of biopsy-confirmed liver metastases, flutamide therapy should be discontinued if the patient develops jaundice or if serum transaminase levels rise to 2 to 3 times the upper limit of normal, even in clinically asymptomatic patients.

The hepatic injury is usually reversible after discontinuation of therapy and in some patients, after dosage reduction. However, there have been reports of death following severe hepatic injury associated with the use of flutamide.

Drug Interactions: Interactions between flutamide and leuprolide have not occurred. In patients receiving long-term oral anticoagulant therapy, increases in prothrombin time have been reported after flutamide monotherapy was initiated. Therefore, close monitoring of prothrombin time is recommended and adjustment of the anticoagulant dose may be necessary when flutamide is administered concomitantly. Cases of increased theophylline plasma concentrations have been reported in patients receiving concomitant theophylline and flutamide tablets. Theophylline is primarily metabolized by CYP 1A2, which is the primary enzyme responsible for the conversion of flutamide to its active agent 2-hydroxyflutamide.

Information to Be Provided to the Patient: Patients should be informed prior to initiating this medication, of the possibility of its causing hepatic dysfunction. Instruct the patient to consult the doctor immediately if symptoms of hepatic dysfunction appear. These include itching of the skin, dark urine (amber or yellow-green urine is not a cause of concern), nausea, vomiting, persistent lack of appetite, yellow eyes or skin, tenderness in the right upper abdomen, or "flu-like" symptoms.

Flutamide is indicated only for use in male patients.

Patients should be informed that flutamide and the drug used for medical castration should be administered concomitantly, and that they should not interrupt their dosing or stop taking these medications without consulting their physician.

ADVERSE EFFECTS: The most frequently reported adverse reactions to flutamide **monotherapy** are gynecomastia and/or breast tenderness, sometimes accompanied by galactorrhea. These reactions disappear upon discontinuation of treatment or reduction in dosage. The incidence of gynecomastia is reduced greatly when flutamide is administered concomitantly with an LHRH agonist.

The most frequently reported (greater than 5%) adverse experiences during treatment with flutamide in combination with an LHRH agonist are listed in Table 1. For comparison, adverse experiences seen with a LHRH agonist and placebo are also listed in Table 1.

Table 1: Euflex

Adverse Effects

	(n=294) Flutamide+LHRH-agonist % All	(n=285) Placebo+LHRH-agonist % All
Hot Flashes	61	57
Loss of Libido	36	31
Impotence	33	29
Diarrhea	12	4
Nausea/Vomiting	11	10
Gynecomastia	9	11
Other	7	9
Other GI	6	4

As shown in Table 1, for both treatment groups, the most frequently occurring adverse experiences (hot flashes, loss of libido, impotence) were those known to be associated with low serum androgen levels and known to occur with LHRH-agonists alone.

The only notable difference between these treatment groups was the higher incidence of diarrhea in the flutamide+LHRH-agonist group (12%; severe in 5%) as compared to the placebo+LHRH-agonist group (4%; severe in less than 1%).

In addition, the following adverse reactions were reported during treatment with flutamide+LHRH-agonist. No causal relatedness of these reactions to drug treatment has been made, and some of the adverse experiences reported are those that commonly occur in elderly patients.

Cardiovascular: hypertension in 1% of patients. Rarely thrombophlebitis, pulmonary embolism, myocardial infarction.

CNS: CNS (drowsiness/confusion/depression/anxiety/nervousness) reactions occurred in 1% of patients. Rarely insomnia, tiredness, headache, dizziness, weakness, malaise, blurred vision and decreased libido have been reported.

Endocrine: gynecomastia in 9% of patients. Rarely breast tenderness sometimes accompanied by galactorrhea.

Gastrointestinal: Nausea/vomiting occurred in 11%; diarrhea 12%, anorexia 4%, and other GI disorders occurred in 6% of patients. Increased appetite, indigestion and constipation have also been reported.

Hematopoietic: Anemia occurred in 6% of patients, leukopenia 3%, thrombocytopenia 1%.

Liver and Biliary: Clinically evident hepatitis and jaundice occurred in <1% of patients.

Skin: Irritation at the injection site and rash occurred in 3% of patients. Photosensitivity reactions have been reported in 5 patients.

Other: Pruritus, ecchymosis, herpes zoster, thirst, lymphedema, lupus-like syndrome, hematuria, reduced sperm counts have been reported rarely in long-term treatment. Edema occurred in 4% of patients; neuromuscular, genitourinary symptoms occurred in 2% of patients. Pulmonary symptoms occurred in <1% of patients.

Additional Adverse Experiences: In addition, the following adverse experiences have been reported during worldwide marketing of flutamide: hemolytic anemia, macrocytic anemia, methemoglobinemia, sulfhemoglobinemia, photosensitivity reactions—including erythema, ulcerations, bullous eruptions, and epidermal necrolysis—and change in urine color to an amber or yellow-green appearance, which can be attributed to flutamide and/or its metabolites. Also observed were cholestatic jaundice, hepatic encephalopathy and hepatic necrosis. The hepatic conditions were usually reversible after discontinuing therapy; however, there have been reports of death following severe hepatic injury associated with use of flutamide. Hyperglycemia and aggravated diabetes mellitus have been reported very rarely.

Two reports of malignant male breast neoplasms in patients being dosed with flutamide have been reported. One involved aggravation of a preexisting nodule which was first detected 3 to 4 months before initiation of flutamide monotherapy in a patient with benign prostatic hypertrophy. After excision, this was diagnosed as a poorly differentiated ductal carcinoma. The other report involved gynecomastia and a nodule noted 2 and 6 months respectively, after initiation of flutamide monotherapy for treatment of advanced prostatic carcinoma. Nine months after the initiation of therapy, the nodule was excised and diagnosed as a moderately differentiated invasive ductal tumor staged T4N0M0, G3, no metastases had advanced.

Laboratory Values: Reported abnormal laboratory test results include elevated AST, ALT; elevated blood urea nitrogen (BUN) and bilirubin levels; less frequently, elevated serum creatinine levels and elevated gamma-glutamyl transferase levels have been reported.

OVERDOSE:

Symptoms: In animal studies with flutamide alone, signs of overdose included hypoactivity, piloerection, slow respiration, ataxia, and/or lacrimation, anorexia, tranquillization, emesis and methemoglobinemia.

Clinical trials have been conducted with flutamide in doses up to 1500 mg/day for periods up to 36 weeks with no serious adverse effects reported. Those adverse reactions reported included gynecomastia, breast tenderness and some increases in AST. The single dose of flutamide ordinarily associated with symptoms of overdose or considered to be life-threatening has not been established.

Treatment: Since flutamide is highly protein bound, dialysis may not be of any use as treatment for overdose. As in the management of overdosage with any drug, it should be borne in mind that multiple agents may have been taken. Gastric lavage may be considered. General supportive care, including frequent monitoring of the vital signs and close observation of the patient, is indicated.

For management of a suspected drug overdose, CPhA recommends that you contact your **regional Poison Control Centre**. See the *CPS* Directory section for a list of Poison Control Centres.

DOSAGE: The recommended dosage of flutamide in combination with orchiectomy or in combination with an LHRH agonist is one 250 mg tablet 3 times a day at 8-hour intervals. In combination with an LHRH agonist, either the two agents may be initiated simultaneously, or flutamide therapy may be started 24 hours prior to initiation of the LHRH agonist.

In the management of bulky locally advanced Stage B_2 and Stage C prostatic carcinoma, the recommended dosage is one 250 mg tablet, 3 times a day at 8-hour intervals. Flutamide should be started simultaneously or 24 hours prior to initiation of the LHRH agonist. Administration of flutamide should begin 8 weeks prior to external beam radiation therapy and continue through the course of radiation therapy.

INFORMATION FOR THE PATIENT: Published in e-CPS, available by subscription at www.e-cps.ca.

SUPPLIED: Each round, biconvex, pale yellow, compressed tablet, engraved with "EUFLEX" on one face, and a single score on the other with the "SP" logo engraved on each side of the score line, contains: flutamide 250 mg. Nonmedicinal ingredients: cellulose, lactose, magnesium stearate, pregelatinized starch, silicon dioxide and sodium lauryl sulfate. Tartrazine-free. Bottles of 100. Store at 15 to 30°C. Protect from light and excessive moisture.

(Shown in Product Identification Section)

Evista® Pr

raloxifene HCl

Selective Estrogen Receptor Modulator

Lilly

Date of Revision: October 10, 2008

SUMMARY PRODUCT INFORMATION:

Route of Administration	Dosage Form/ Strength	Clinically Relevant Nonmedicinal Ingredients[a]
Oral	Tablet/60 mg	Lactose

[a] For a complete listing see Dosage Forms, Composition and Packaging.

INDICATIONS AND CLINICAL USE: EVISTA (raloxifene hydrochloride) is indicated for:

- The treatment of osteoporosis in postmenopausal women.
- The prevention of osteoporosis in postmenopausal women.

Women with diagnosed postmenopausal osteoporosis should be considered for pharmacologic therapy, in conjunction with education and appropriate lifestyle modifications.

No single clinical finding or test result can quantify risk of postmenopausal osteoporosis with certainty. However, clinical assessment can help to identify women at increased risk. Widely accepted risk factors include Caucasian or Asian descent, slender body build, early estrogen deficiency, smoking, alcohol consumption, low calcium diet, sedentary lifestyle, personal history of any fracture after age 40 and family history of osteoporosis. The greater the number of clinical risk factors, the greater the probability of developing postmenopausal osteoporosis. These risk factors may be considered in the decision to use EVISTA for prevention of postmenopausal osteoporosis.

For either osteoporosis treatment or prevention, supplemental calcium and/or vitamin D should be added to the diet if daily intake is inadequate.

Geriatrics: Safety and efficacy in older and younger postmenopausal women in the osteoporosis treatment trial appeared to be comparable (see Warnings and Precautions).

Pediatrics: The safety and efficacy of EVISTA have not been studied in pediatric populations. EVISTA should not be used in pediatric patients (see Warnings and Precautions).

CONTRAINDICATIONS:

- Patients who are hypersensitive to this drug or to any ingredient in the formulation or component of the container. For a complete listing, see Dosage Forms, Composition and Packaging.
- Women of childbearing potential. EVISTA therapy during pregnancy may be associated with an increased risk of congenital defects in the fetus.
- Women with active or past history of venous thromboembolic events, including deep vein thrombosis, pulmonary embolism, and retinal vein thrombosis.

WARNINGS AND PRECAUTIONS: General: Concurrent Estrogen Therapy: Safety information regarding the concurrent use of EVISTA and systemic hormone therapy (estrogen with or without progestin) is limited and therefore concomitant use of EVISTA with systemic estrogens is not recommended.

Endometrium: Unexplained uterine bleeding should be investigated as clinically indicated.

Breast: Any unexplained breast abnormality occurring during EVISTA therapy should be investigated.

Other Osteoporosis Treatment and Prevention Measures: Patients should be instructed to take supplemental calcium and/or vitamin D, if daily dietary intake is inadequate. Weight-bearing exercise should be considered along with the modification of certain behavioral factors, such as cigarette smoking, and/or alcohol consumption, if these factors exist.

Cardiovascular: Vasodilatation: EVISTA is not effective in reducing vasodilatation (hot flashes or flushes) associated with estrogen deficiency. In some patients, vasodilatation may occur upon beginning EVISTA therapy.

Venous Thromboembolic Events (VTE): The risk-benefit balance should be considered in women at risk of thromboembolic disease for any reason. EVISTA should be discontinued at least 72 hours prior to and during prolonged immobilization (e.g. post-surgical recovery, prolonged bed rest) and EVISTA therapy should be resumed only after the patient is fully ambulatory. In clinical trials, EVISTA-treated women had an increased risk of venous thromboembolism (deep vein thrombosis and pulmonary embolism). VTE events reported in the osteoporosis treatment and prevention trials were infrequent (1.44, 3.32 and 3.63 events per 1,000 person-years for placebo, raloxifene 60 mg/day and raloxifene 120 mg/day, respectively). The incidence rate of VTE reported from the Raloxifene Use for The Heart (RUTH) study was 2.70 and 3.88 events per 1,000 person-years for placebo and raloxifene 60 mg/day, respectively.

Other venous thromboembolic events could also occur. A less serious event, superficial thrombophlebitis, also has been reported more frequently with EVISTA. The greatest risk for deep vein thrombosis and pulmonary embolism occurs during the first 4 months of treatment, and the magnitude of risk is similar to that associated with use of hormone replacement therapy.

Stroke: The risk-benefit balance of EVISTA in postmenopausal women with a history of stroke or other significant stroke risk factors, such as transient ischemic attack or atrial fibrillation, should be considered when prescribing EVISTA. The Raloxifene Use for The Heart (RUTH) trial investigated the effects of EVISTA in postmenopausal women (average age=67 years) with known heart disease or at high risk for a coronary event. The RUTH trial demonstrated an increase in mortality due to stroke for EVISTA compared to placebo. The incidence of stroke mortality was 1.5 per 1000 women per year for placebo versus 2.2 per 1000 women per year for EVISTA (p=0.0499). The incidence of stroke, myocardial infarction, hospitalized acute coronary syndrome, cardiovascular mortality, or overall mortality (all causes combined) was comparable for EVISTA and placebo.

Endocrine and Metabolism: Estrogen-Induced Hypertriglyceridemia: Patients with a history of estrogen-induced hypertriglyceridemia can experience an increase in triglyceride levels during treatment with EVISTA. Therefore, triglyceride levels should be followed in such patients and the risk-benefit balance of EVISTA treatment in such cases should be reassessed.

Hepatic Dysfunction: Raloxifene was studied as a single dose in patients with Child-Pugh Class A cirrhosis with total serum bilirubin ranging from 0.6 to 2.0 mg/dL (10.3 to 34.2 mmol/L). Plasma raloxifene concentrations were approximately 2.5 times higher than in controls and correlated with total bilirubin concentrations. Safety and efficacy have not been established in patients with moderate or severe hepatic insufficiency.

Lipid Metabolism: EVISTA lowers serum total and LDL cholesterol by 6% to 11%, but does not affect serum concentrations of total HDL cholesterol or triglycerides. HDL-2 cholesterol subfraction is increased by EVISTA. These effects should be taken into account in therapeutic decisions for patients who may require therapy for hyperlipidemia. Concurrent use of EVISTA and lipid lowering agents has not been studied.

Peri-Operative Considerations: Patient Immobilization: EVISTA should be discontinued at least 72 hours prior to and during prolonged immobilization (e.g. post surgical recovery, prolonged bed rest) and EVISTA therapy should be resumed only after the patient is fully ambulatory because of the increased risk of venous thromboembolic events.

Psychiatric: Cognition and Affect: Any change in cognition and affect during EVISTA therapy should be investigated as clinically indicated.

Special Populations: Pregnant Women: EVISTA should not be used in women who are or may become pregnant (see Contraindications).

Nursing Women: EVISTA should not be used by lactating women (see Contraindications). It is not known whether raloxifene is excreted in human milk.

Premenopausal Use: Safety of EVISTA in premenopausal women has not been established and its use is not indicated.

Pediatrics (<18 years of age): EVISTA should not be used in pediatric patients.

Geriatrics: In the osteoporosis treatment trial of 7705 postmenopausal women, 4621 women were considered geriatric (greater than 65 years old). Of these, 845 women were greater than 75 years old. Safety and efficacy in older and younger postmenopausal women in the osteoporosis treatment trial appeared to be comparable.

Use in Men: There is no indication for use of EVISTA in men.

MONITORING AND LABORATORY TESTS: If EVISTA is given concomitantly with warfarin or other coumarin derivatives, the prothrombin time should be monitored when starting or stopping therapy with EVISTA (see Drug Interactions).

ADVERSE REACTIONS: The safety of raloxifene has been established in Phase 2 and Phase 3 placebo-controlled, estrogen-controlled, and HRT-controlled studies. Twelve studies comprised the primary safety database for the prevention indication, and the safety of raloxifene in the treatment of osteoporosis was assessed in a large, multinational, placebo-controlled trial. In the osteoporosis prevention trials, the duration of treatment ranged from 2 to 30 months and 2036 women were exposed to raloxifene. In the osteoporosis treatment trial, 5129 women were exposed to raloxifene (2557 received 60 mg/day and 2572 received 120 mg/day) for 36 months. The osteoporosis treatment trial was extended by 12 months to a 4th year during which patients were permitted the concomitant use of bisphosphonates, fluorides and calcitonins.

Adverse Drug Reaction Overview: The most commonly observed treatment-emergent adverse events associated with the use of EVISTA in double-blind, placebo-controlled, osteoporosis treatment and prevention clinical trials were vasodilatation and leg cramps.

Vasodilatation events (hot flashes or flushes) were common in placebo-treated women, and the frequency was modestly increased in EVISTA-treated women. The first occurrence of this event was most commonly reported during the first 6 months of treatment and infrequently was reported de novo after that time.

Venous thromboembolism (VTE) and pulmonary embolism are uncommon but serious adverse events associated with raloxifene therapy. The greatest risk for deep vein thrombosis and pulmonary embolism occurs during the first 4 months of treatment.

An increase in mortality due to stroke for EVISTA compared to placebo was demonstrated in the RUTH trial which investigated the effects of EVISTA in postmenopausal women (average age=67 years) with known heart disease or at high risk for a coronary event, (see Warnings and Precautions).

The majority of adverse events occurring during clinical trials were mild and did not require discontinuation of therapy. Discontinuation of therapy due to any clinical adverse experience occurred in 10.9% of 2557 EVISTA-treated women and 8.8% of 2576 placebo-treated women in the osteoporosis treatment trial, and in 11.4% of 581 EVISTA-treated women and 12.2% of 584 placebo-treated women in the osteoporosis prevention trials.

Clinical Trial Adverse Drug Reactions: Because clinical trials are conducted under very specific conditions the adverse reaction rates observed in the clinical trials may not reflect the rates observed in practice and should not be compared to the rates in the clinical trials of another drug. Adverse drug reaction information from clinical trials is useful for identifying drug-related adverse events and for approximating rates.

Adverse Events in Placebo-Controlled Clinical Trials: Table 1 lists adverse events occurring in either the osteoporosis treatment (up to 3 years) or prevention placebo-controlled clinical trials with EVISTA at a frequency ≥1.0% in EVISTA-treated women and at a significantly greater incidence than in placebo-treated women.

Table 1: EVISTA

Adverse Events Occurring in Placebo-Controlled Osteoporosis Clinical Trials (up to 36 months) at a Frequency ≥1.0% in EVISTA-Treated (60 mg once daily) Women and at a Significantly Greater Incidence Than in Placebo-Treated Women

Body System	Osteoporosis Treatment		Osteoporosis Prevention	
	EVISTA (N=2557) %	Placebo (N=2576) %	EVISTA (N=581) %	Placebo (N=584) %
Body as a Whole				
Flu Syndrome	13.5[a]	11.4	14.6	13.5
Leg Cramps	7.0[a]	3.7	5.9[a]	1.9
Cardiovascular				
Vasodilatation	9.7[a]	6.4	24.6	18.3
Metabolic and Nutritional				
Diabetes Mellitus	1.2[a]	0.5	A	A

[a] Significantly (p<0.05) different from placebo.
Legend: A=Placebo incidence greater than or equal to EVISTA incidence.

Glycemic Control: Diabetes mellitus was reported more frequently as an adverse event among EVISTA-treated patients (1.2%) compared with placebo-treated patients (0.5%) in the osteoporosis treatment trial. However, there were no differences between the raloxifene and placebo groups in either fasting glucose or hemoglobin A_{1c} (objective measures of glycemic control) in the osteoporosis treatment trial.

Peripheral Edema in the Treatment and Prevention Trials: A significant dose trend was observed for peripheral edema in the treatment and prevention studies. Cumulative frequency of the event at the 60 mg/day dose was 5.2% for EVISTA-treated patients versus 4.4% for placebo treated patients in the treatment study, and 3.1% for EVISTA-treated patients versus 1.9% for placebo-treated patients in the prevention studies, which was not a statistically significant difference.

48-Month Osteoporosis Treatment Trial Adverse Events: The osteoporosis treatment trial was extended by 12 months to a 4th year during which patients were permitted the concomitant use of bisphosphonates, fluorides and calcitonins. The incidence trend of treatment-emergent adverse events occurring at a frequency ≥1.0% in EVISTA-treated women, and at a significantly greater incidence than in placebo-treated women after year 4 of the osteoporosis treatment trial, were generally similar to the 1 to 3 year results presented in Table 1.

At 48 months in the osteoporosis treatment trial, vasodilatation was reported in 10.6% of patients on EVISTA versus 7.1% of placebo patients (p<0.001), and leg cramps were reported in 9.2% of patients on EVISTA versus 6.0% of placebo patients (p<0.001).

At 48 months in the same osteoporosis treatment trial, flu syndrome (16.2% of EVISTA treated patients versus 14.0% of placebo patients), uterine disorder (endometrial cavity fluid in 12.7% of EVISTA treated patients versus 9.6% of placebo patients), diabetes mellitus (1.5% of EVISTA treated patients versus 0.7% of placebo patients), and peripheral edema (7.1% of EVISTA treated patients versus 6.1% of placebo patients) were also treatment-emergent adverse events which occurred more frequently with patients receiving EVISTA compared to placebo (p<0.05).

Adverse Reactions in a Placebo-Controlled Trial of Postmenopausal Women at Increased Risk for Major Coronary Events: The safety of EVISTA (60 mg once daily) was assessed in a placebo-controlled multinational trial of 10,101 postmenopausal women (age range 55-92) with documented coronary heart disease (CHD) or multiple CHD risk factors. Median study drug exposure was 5.1 years for both treatment groups (see CLINICAL TRIALS). Therapy was discontinued due to an adverse event in 25% of 5044 EVISTA-treated women and 24% of 5057 placebo-treated women. The incidence per year of all-cause mortality was comparable between the raloxifene (2.07%) and placebo (2.25%) groups.

Adverse reactions reported at a frequency of ≥2.0%, which were considered to be possibly related to EVISTA, and which occurred at a statistically significantly greater rate than placebo, were peripheral edema (14.1% raloxifene versus 11.7% placebo), muscle spasms/leg cramps (12.1% raloxifene versus 8.3% placebo), hot flashes (7.8% raloxifene versus 4.7% placebo), venous thromboembolic events (2.0% raloxifene versus 1.4% placebo), and cholelithiasis (3.3% raloxifene versus 2.6% placebo). Although cholelithiasis was reported more frequently for raloxifene than placebo, reports of cholecystectomy (2.3% raloxifene versus 2.0% placebo) were not significantly different.

Bladder cancer was reported in 0.2% (10/5044) of patients on EVISTA versus 0.1% (4/5057) of placebo patients in the RUTH trial. In an osteoporosis placebo-controlled treatment trial, bladder cancer was reported in 0.1% (3/5129) of patients on EVISTA versus 0.2% (4/2576) of placebo patients.

Comparison of EVISTA and Hormone Replacement Therapy Adverse Events: EVISTA (N=317) was compared with continuous combined (N=96) hormone replacement therapy (HRT) or cyclic estrogen plus progestin HRT in 3 clinical trials for prevention of osteoporosis.

The incidence of breast pain (4.4% for EVISTA-treated patients, 37.5% for continuous combined HRT-treated patients, and 29.7% for cyclic estrogen plus progestin HRT-treated patients), vaginal bleeding (6.2% for EVISTA-treated patients, 64.2% for continuous combined HRT-treated patients and 88.5% for cyclic estrogen plus progestin HRT-treated patients), and abdominal pain (6.6% for EVISTA-treated patients, 10.4% for continuous combined HRT-treated patients, and 18.7% for cyclic estrogen plus progestin HRT-treated patients) were significantly lower in EVISTA-treated patients versus patients treated with either form of HRT (p<0.05).

Conversely, the incidence of vasodilatation (28.7% for EVISTA-treated patients, 3.1% for continuous combined HRT-treated patients, and 5.9% for cyclic estrogen plus progestin HRT-treated patients) was significantly greater in EVISTA-treated patients versus patients treated with either form of HRT (p<0.05).

Laboratory Changes: The following changes in analyte concentrations are commonly observed during EVISTA therapy: increased serum HDL-2 cholesterol subfraction and apolipoprotein A1; and reduced serum total cholesterol, LDL cholesterol, fibrinogen, apolipoprotein B, and lipoprotein (a). EVISTA modestly increases hormone-binding globulin concentrations, including sex steroid binding globulin, thyroxine binding globulin, and corticosteroid binding globulin with corresponding increases in measured total hormone concentrations. There is no evidence that these changes in hormone binding globulin concentrations affect concentrations of the corresponding free hormones.

DRUG INTERACTIONS: Clinically Significant Drug-Drug Interactions: Cholestyramine: Cholestyramine, an anion exchange resin, significantly reduces the absorption and enterohepatic cycling of raloxifene and should not be coadministered with raloxifene. Although not specifically studied, it is anticipated that other anion exchange resins would have a similar effect.

Warfarin: Coadministration of raloxifene and warfarin does not alter the pharmacokinetics of either compound. However, modest decreases in prothrombin time have been observed in single-dose studies. If raloxifene is given concurrently with warfarin or other coumarin derivatives, prothrombin time should be monitored.

Drug-Drug Interactions: Ampicillin and Other Oral Antimicrobials: Peak concentrations of raloxifene are reduced with coadministration of ampicillin. The reduction in peak concentrations is consistent with reduced enterohepatic cycling associated with antibiotic reduction of enteric bacteria. Since the overall extent of absorption and the elimination rate of raloxifene are not affected, raloxifene can be concurrently administered with ampicillin. In the osteoporosis treatment trial, co-administered oral antimicrobial agents (including amoxicillin, cephalexin, ciprofloxacin, macrolide antibiotics, sulfamethoxazole/trimethoprim and tetracycline) had no effect on plasma raloxifene concentrations.

Corticosteroids: The chronic administration of raloxifene in postmenopausal women has no effect on the pharmacokinetics of methylprednisolone given as a single oral dose.

Digoxin: Raloxifene has no effect on the pharmacokinetics of digoxin. In the osteoporosis treatment trial, coadministered digoxin had no effect on plasma raloxifene concentration.

Gastrointestinal Medications: Concurrent administration of calcium carbonate or aluminum and magnesium hydroxide-containing antacids does not affect the systemic exposure of raloxifene. In the osteoporosis treatment trial, coadministered gastrointestinal medications (including bisacodyl, cisapride, docusate, H_2-antagonists, laxatives, loperamide, omeprazole and psyllium) had no effect on plasma raloxifene concentration.

Highly Protein-Bound Drugs: Raloxifene is more than 95% bound to plasma proteins. The influence of co-administered highly protein-bound drugs (including diazepam, gemfibrozil, ibuprofen, naproxen and warfarin) on raloxifene plasma concentrations was evaluated in the osteoporosis treatment trial. No clinically significant effects of these agents on raloxifene plasma concentrations were identified. In vitro, raloxifene did not affect the binding of phenytoin, tamoxifen or warfarin.

Highly Glucuronidated Drugs: Raloxifene undergoes extensive first-pass metabolism to glucuronide conjugates. The influence of co-administered highly glucuronidated drugs (including acetaminophen, ketoprofen, morphine and oxazepam) on raloxifene plasma concentrations was evaluated in the osteoporosis treatment trial. No clinically significant effects of these agents on raloxifene plasma concentrations were identified.

Other Medications: The influence of concomitant medications on raloxifene plasma concentrations was evaluated in the osteoporosis treatment clinical trial. The 152 most commonly co-administered medications were grouped by pharmacological class based on their therapeutic use. Frequently co-administered drugs included: ACE inhibitors and angiotensin antagonists, alpha agonists and antagonists, anticholinergics, antidepressants, antimicrobials, antipsychotics, benzodiazepines, beta blockers and agonists, bisphosphonates, calcium channel blockers, diuretics, estrogen preparations, glucocorticoids, guaifenesin, H_1-antagonists, H_2-antagonists and proton pump inhibitors, hypoglycemics, hypolipidemics, iron preparations, muscle relaxants, nitrates, non-benzodiazepine hypnotics, non-steroidal anti-inflammatory drugs (NSAIDs), opioid analgesics, theophylline and thyroid hormone. No clinically relevant effects of the co-administration of any of these agents on raloxifene plasma concentrations were observed.

Drug-Food Interactions: EVISTA can be administered without regard to meals.

Drug-Laboratory Test Interactions: Interactions with laboratory tests have not been established (see Adverse Reactions for additional laboratory safety information).

DOSAGE AND ADMINISTRATION: Recommended Dose: The recommended dosage is one 60 mg EVISTA tablet daily which may be administered any time of day without regard to meals.

Missed Dose: If a scheduled daily dose of EVISTA is missed, it should be taken as soon as remembered and one tablet once daily resumed. Do not take two doses at the same time.

OVERDOSAGE:

In an 8-week study of 63 postmenopausal women, a dose of raloxifene HCl 600 mg/day was safely tolerated. In clinical trials, no overdose of raloxifene has been reported.

In postmarketing spontaneous reports, overdose has been reported very rarely (less than 1 out of 10 000 [<0.01%] patients treated). The highest overdose has been approximately 1.5 grams. No fatalities associated with overdose have been reported. In adults, symptoms reported in patients who took more than 120 mg as a single ingestion included leg cramps and dizziness. In some cases, no adverse events were reported as a result of the overdose.

In accidental overdose in children under 2 years of age, the maximum reported dose has been 180 mg. In children, symptoms reported included ataxia, dizziness, vomiting, rash, diarrhea, tremor, and flushing, as well as elevation in alkaline phosphatase.

There is no specific antidote for raloxifene.

For management of a suspected drug overdose, contact your **regional Poison Control Centre**. See the *CPS* Directory section for a list of Poison Control Centres.

ACTION AND CLINICAL PHARMACOLOGY: Mechanism of Action: Raloxifene is a selective estrogen receptor modulator (SERM) that belongs to the benzothiophene class of compounds. The SERM profile of raloxifene includes estrogen agonist effects on bone and lipid metabolism, and estrogen antagonist effects in uterine and breast tissues. Raloxifene's biological actions, like those of estrogen, are mediated through high-affinity binding to estrogen receptors and regulation of gene expression. This binding results in differential expression of multiple estrogen-regulated genes in different tissues.

Pharmacodynamics: Effects On the Skeleton: During early to middle adult life, bone undergoes continuous remodeling. In this process, local areas of bone resorption are refilled completely by ensuing bone formation; that is, resorption and formation are in balance. The result is that bone mass remains relatively constant. Ovarian estrogen is important for maintenance of this balance in bone turnover. Marked decreases in estrogen availability, such as after oophorectomy or menopause, lead to marked increases in bone resorption, accelerated bone loss and increased risk of fracture. After menopause, bone is initially lost rapidly because the compensatory increase in bone formation is inadequate to offset resorptive losses.

This imbalance between resorption and formation may be related to loss of estrogen, or to age-related impairment of osteoblasts or their precursors. Estrogen replacement therapy reduces resorption of bone by inhibiting the formation and action of osteoclasts, and decreases overall bone turnover. These effects on bone are manifested as reductions in the serum and urine levels of bone turnover markers, histologic evidence of decreased bone resorption and formation, and increased bone mineral density (BMD). Although EVISTA increases BMD to a lesser extent than estrogen, the effects of EVISTA on bone turnover in postmenopausal women parallel those of estrogen, as shown by studies of bone mineral densitometry, radiocalcium kinetics, bone markers, and bone histomorphometry. EVISTA reduces biochemical markers of bone metabolism into the range seen in premenopausal women.

Pharmacokinetics: The disposition of raloxifene has been evaluated in more than 3000 postmenopausal women in selected raloxifene osteoporosis treatment and prevention clinical trials using a population approach. Pharmacokinetic data were also obtained in conventional clinical pharmacology studies in 292 postmenopausal women. Raloxifene exhibits high within-subject variability (approximately 30%) of most pharmacokinetic parameters. Table 2 summarizes the pharmacokinetic parameters of raloxifene.

Table 2: EVISTA

Summary of Raloxifene Pharmacokinetic Parameters in the Healthy Postmenopausal Woman

	C_{max}[a] (ng/mL)/(mg/kg)	$t_{½}$ (h)	$AUC_{0-\infty}$[a] (ng·h/mL)/(mg/kg)	CL/F (L/kg·h)	V/F (L/kg)
Single Dose					
Mean	0.50	27.7	27.2	44.1	2348
CV (%)	52	10.7 to 273[b]	44	46	52
Multiple Dose					
Mean	1.36	32.5	24.2	47.4	2853
CV (%)	37	15.8 to 86.6[b]	36	41	56

a Data normalized based on dose in mg and body weight in kg.
b Range of observed half-life.
Legend: C_{max}=maximum plasma concentration; $t_{½}$=half-life; AUC=area under the curve; CL=clearance; V=volume of distribution; F=bioavailability; CV=coefficient of variation.

Absorption: Raloxifene is absorbed rapidly after oral administration. Approximately 60% of an oral dose is absorbed, but presystemic glucuronide conjugation is extensive. Absolute bioavailability of raloxifene is 2.0%. The time to reach average maximum plasma concentration and bioavailability are functions of systemic interconversion and enterohepatic cycling of raloxifene and its glucuronide metabolites.

Administration of raloxifene HCl with a standardized, high-fat meal increases the absorption of raloxifene slightly, but does not lead to clinically meaningful changes in systemic exposure. EVISTA can be administered without regard to meals.

Distribution: Following oral administration of single doses ranging from 30 to 150 mg of raloxifene HCl, the apparent volume of distribution is 2348 L/kg and is not dose dependent.

Raloxifene and the monoglucuronide conjugates are highly bound to plasma proteins. Raloxifene binds to both albumin and α1-acid glycoprotein, but not to sex steroid binding globulin.

Metabolism: Biotransformation and disposition of raloxifene in humans have been determined following oral administration of ^{14}C-labeled raloxifene. Raloxifene undergoes extensive firstpass metabolism to the glucuronide conjugates: raloxifene-4'-glucuronide, raloxifene-6-glucuronide, and raloxifene-6, 4'-diglucuronide. No other metabolites have been detected, providing strong evidence that raloxifene is not metabolized by cytochrome P450 pathways. Unconjugated raloxifene comprises less than 1% of the total radiolabeled material in plasma. The terminal log-linear portion of the plasma concentration curve for raloxifene and the glucuronides are generally parallel. This is consistent with interconversion of raloxifene and the glucuronide metabolites.

Following intravenous administration, raloxifene is cleared at a rate approximating hepatic blood flow. Apparent oral clearance is 44.1 L/kg·hr. Raloxifene and its glucuronide conjugates are interconverted by reversible systemic metabolism and enterohepatic cycling, thereby prolonging its plasma elimination half-life to 27.7 hours after oral dosing.

Results from single oral doses of raloxifene predict multiple-dose pharmacokinetics. Following chronic dosing, clearance ranges from 40 to 60 L/kg·hr. Increasing doses of raloxifene HCl (ranging from 30 to 150 mg) result in slightly less than a proportional increase in the area under the plasma time concentration curve (AUC).

Excretion: Raloxifene is primarily excreted in feces, and negligible amounts are excreted unchanged in urine. Less than 6% of the raloxifene dose is eliminated in urine as glucuronide conjugates.

Special Populations and Conditions: Geriatrics: The pharmacokinetics of raloxifene are independent of age (42 to 84 years).

Pediatrics: The pharmacokinetics of raloxifene have not been evaluated in a pediatric population.

Gender: Total extent of exposure and oral clearance, normalized for lean body weight, are not significantly different between age-matched male and female volunteers.

Race: Pharmacokinetic differences due to race have been studied in 1712 women including 97.5% Caucasian, 1.0% Asian, 0.7% Hispanic, and 0.5% Black in the osteoporosis treatment trial and in 1053 women including 93.5% Caucasian, 4.3% Hispanic, 1.2% Asian, and 0.5% Black in the osteoporosis prevention trials. There were no discernible differences in raloxifene plasma concentrations among these groups. The influence of race cannot be conclusively determined because of the small numbers of non-Caucasians.

Renal Insufficiency: Since negligible amounts of raloxifene are eliminated in urine, a study in patients with renal insufficiency was not conducted. In the osteoporosis treatment and prevention trials, raloxifene and metabolite concentrations were not affected by renal function in women having estimated creatinine clearance as low as 21 mL/min (0.35 mL/s). EVISTA should be used with caution in patients with moderate or severe renal impairment, Safety and efficacy have not been established in patients with moderate or severe renal impairment.

Hepatic Insufficiency: Raloxifene was studied as a single dose in patients with Child-Pugh Class A cirrhosis with total serum bilirubin ranging from 0.6 to 2.0 mg/dL (10.3 to 34.2 mmol/L). Plasma raloxifene concentrations were approximately 2.5 times higher than in controls and correlated with bilirubin concentrations. Safety and efficacy have not been evaluated further in patients with hepatic insufficiency (see Warnings and Precautions).

STORAGE AND STABILITY: Store at room temperature, 15 to 30°C.

INFORMATION FOR THE PATIENT: Published in e-CPS, available by subscription at www.e-cps.ca.

DOSAGE FORMS, COMPOSITION AND PACKAGING:
Each white, elliptical, film-coated tablet, imprinted on one side with the tablet code 4165 in blue ink, contains: raloxifene HCl 60 mg. Nonmedicinal ingredients: anhydrous lactose, crospovidone, FD&C Blue No. 2 aluminum lake, hydroxypropyl methylcellulose, lactose monohydrate, macrogol 400, magnesium stearate, polysorbate 80, povidone and titanium dioxide E171. Blister packages of 28. Bottles of 30 and 100.

(Shown in product Identification Section)

Evra™ Ⓟ

norelgestromin—ethinyl estradiol

Hormonal Contraceptive

Janssen-Ortho

Date of Preparation: August 8, 2002
Date of Revision: March 16, 2010

SUMMARY PRODUCT INFORMATION:

Route of Administration	Dosage Form/ Strength	Clinically Relevant Nonmedicinal Ingredients
Transdermal	Each transdermal system contains 6 mg norelgestromin (NGMN) and 0.60 mg ethinyl estradiol (EE) and releases approximately 200 µg norelgestromin and 35 µg ethinyl estradiol from the patch every 24 hours.	None For a complete listing see Dosage Forms, Composition and Packaging.

INDICATIONS AND CLINICAL USE: The EVRA (norelgestromin and ethinyl estradiol) transdermal system is indicated for the prevention of pregnancy.

The pharmacokinetic profile for the EVRA transdermal system is different from that of an oral contraceptive. The clinical relevance of the differences in PK profiles between transdermal and oral delivery is not known. (See Warnings and Precautions, General, Transdermal versus Oral Contraceptives and Action and Clinical Pharmacology, Pharmacokinetics, Transdermal versus Oral Contraceptives.)

CONTRAINDICATIONS: The EVRA (norelgestromin and ethinyl estradiol) transdermal system should not be used in women with:

- a history of or actual thrombophlebitis or thromboembolic disorders;
- known thrombophilic conditions;
- a history of or actual cerebrovascular disorders;
- a history of or actual myocardial infarction or coronary artery disease;
- valvular heart disease with complications;
- active liver disease, or history of or actual benign or malignant liver tumours;
- known or suspected carcinoma of the breast;
- carcinoma of the endometrium or other known or suspected estrogen-dependent neoplasia;
- undiagnosed abnormal vaginal bleeding;
- steroid-dependent jaundice, cholestatic jaundice, history of jaundice of pregnancy;
- any ocular lesion arising from ophthalmic vascular disease, such as partial or complete loss of vision, or defect in visual fields;
- known or suspected pregnancy;
- current or history of migraine with focal aura;
- presence of severe or multiple risk factor(s) for arterial or venous thrombosis such as:
  - persistent blood pressure values of ≥160 mm Hg systolic or ≥100 mm Hg diastolic
  - hereditary or acquired predisposition for venous or arterial thrombosis, such as Factor V Leiden mutation and activated protein C (APC-) resistance, antithrombin-III-deficiency, protein C deficiency, protein S deficiency, hyperhomocysteinaemia (e.g. due to MTHFR C677T, A1298 mutations), prothrombin mutation G20210A, and antiphospholipid-antibodies (anticardiolipin antibodies, lupus anticoagulant)
  - severe dyslipoproteinemia
  - heavy smoking (>15 cigarettes per day) and over age 35
  - diabetes mellitus with vascular involvement
- major surgery associated with an increased risk of post-operative thromboembolism;
- prolonged immobilization;
- hypersensitivity to this drug or to any ingredient in the formulation or component of the container. For a complete listing, see Dosage Forms, Composition and Packaging.

WARNINGS AND PRECAUTIONS:

Serious Warnings and Precautions

The risk of venous thromboembolism (VTE) in users of the ORTHO EVRA patch (the formulation of EVRA marketed in the United States) compared to users of oral contraceptives containing norgestimate and 35 µg of EE was assessed in two epidemiological studies with a nested case-control design conducted in women aged 15 to 44 years. One of these studies found an increased risk of VTE for current users of ORTHO EVRA compared to current users of the oral contraceptives [odds ratio 2.46 (95% CI 1.10-5.52)]. The other study did not find an increase in risk of VTE for current users of ORTHO EVRA [odds ratio 0.9 (95% CI 0.5-1.6)] (see Warnings and Precautions, General, Updated Epidemiologic Data).

Prescribers are advised to carefully assess a patient's baseline and cumulative risk of thromboembolism before prescribing hormonal contraceptives, including EVRA. Obesity (BMI ≥30 kg/m²) has been identified as a risk factor for venous thromboembolism. Particular caution should be exercised when prescribing hormonal contraceptives, including EVRA, to women who are obese (see Contraindications; Warnings and Precautions, General, Cardiovascular, Endocrine and Metabolism, Hematologic; and Adverse Reactions).

Cigarette smoking increases the risk of serious adverse effects on the heart and blood vessels. This risk increases with age and becomes significant in hormonal contraceptive users older than 35 years of age. Women should be counselled not to smoke (see Cardiovascular).

Hormonal contraceptives **do not protect** against sexually transmitted diseases including HIV/AIDS. For protection against STDs, it is advisable to use latex condoms **in combination with** hormonal contraceptives.

General: The risk of venous thromboembolism (VTE) among women aged 15-44 who used ORTHO EVRA compared to women who used oral contraceptives containing 30-35 µg of ethinyl estradiol (EE) and either norgestimate (NGM) or levonorgestrel (LNG) has been estimated in three case control studies using electronic healthcare claims data derived from users in the USA. These studies (see Table 1), which used different study designs, reported odds ratios ranging from 0.9 (indicating no increase in risk) to 2.5 (indicating an approximate doubling of risk). One study (i3 Ingenix) included patient chart review to confirm the VTE occurrence (see Warnings and Precautions, Serious Warnings and Precautions).

Table 1: EVRA

Estimates (Odds Ratios) of Venous Thromboembolism Risk in Current Users of ORTHO EVRA Compared to Oral Contraceptive Users

Epidemiologic Study	Comparator Product	Odds Ratio (95% C.I.)
i3 Ingenix	Norgestimate/35 µg Ethinyl Estradiol	2.5[a] (1.1–5.5) 33 months of data Data Set one
		1.4 (0.5–3.7) 24 months of data[c] Data Set two
		2.2 (1.2–4.0) Cumulative[d]

(cont'd)

Table 1: EVRA *(cont'd)*

Estimates (Odds Ratios) of Venous Thromboembolism Risk in Current Users of ORTHO EVRA Compared to Oral Contraceptive Users

Epidemiologic Study	Comparator Product	Odds Ratio (95% C.I.)
Boston Collaborative Drug Surveillance Program (Norgestimate)	Norgestimate/35 µg Ethinyl Estradiol	0.9 (0.5–1.6) initial 36 months of data
		1.1 (0.6–2.1) 17 Month Extension[b]
		2.4[a] (1.2–5.0) 14 Month Extension[b]
		1.2 (0.9–1.8) [Pooled odds ratio from 3 datasets above]
Boston Collaborative Drug Surveillance Program (Levonorgestrel) Database one	Levonorgestrel/30 µg Ethinyl Estradiol	2.0 (0.9–4.1) 48 Months of data
Boston Collaborative Drug Surveillance Program (Levonorgestrel) Database two	Levonorgestrel/30 µg Ethinyl Estradiol	1.3 (0.8–2.0) 69 Months of data

[a] Increase in risk of VTE is statistically significant.
[b] New cases not included in the previous estimates.
[c] Separate estimate from 24 months of data on new cases not included in the previous estimate.
[d] Cumulative odds ratio from Data set one and Data set two.

Transdermal versus Oral Contraceptives: Prescribers should be aware of the differences in pharmacokinetic (PK) profiles of transdermal and oral combined hormonal contraceptives and should exercise caution when making a direct comparison between these parameters. In general, transdermal patches are designed to maintain steady delivery of EE and NGMN over a seven-day period while oral contraceptives are administered on a daily basis and produce daily peaks and troughs. Inter-subject variability (%CV) for PK parameters following delivery from the patch is higher relative to the variability determined from the oral contraceptive. The clinical relevance of the differences in PK profiles between transdermal and oral delivery is not known. (See Action and Clinical Pharmacology, Pharmacokinetics, Transdermal versus Oral Contraceptives.)

Sex Hormone Binding Globulin (SHBG): Published reports have indicated that the mean percent change in concentration of SHBG, a marker of systemic estrogenic activity, is higher following the application of a combined transdermal patch releasing ethinyl estradiol 20 µg and norelgestromin 150 µg per 24 hours than following administration of a daily oral contraceptive. The clinical significance of this finding is not known.

Discontinue Medication at the Earliest Manifestation of:

A. **Thromboembolic and cardiovascular disorders**, such as thrombophlebitis, pulmonary embolism, cerebrovascular disorders, myocardial ischemia, mesenteric thrombosis and retinal thrombosis;
B. **Conditions that predispose to venous stasis and vascular thrombosis**, such as immobilization after accidents or confinement to bed during long-term illness. Other non-hormonal methods of contraception should be used until regular activities are resumed. For use of hormonal contraceptives when surgery is contemplated, see Peri-Operative Considerations;
C. **Visual defects—partial or complete;**
D. **Papilledema or ophthalmic (retinal) vascular lesions;**
E. **Severe headache of unknown etiology or worsening of pre-existing migraine headache.**

Risk of Unintentional Increase in Drug Exposure: (See Drug Interactions, Drug-Lifestyle Interactions and Action and Clinical Pharmacology, Pharmacokinetics, Absorption.)

Patients with Fever: Serum estradiol concentrations could theoretically increase in patients with fever. Any clinical consequences due to any increase in temperature are unknown at this time.

External Heat Sources: Due to a theoretical risk of increased exposure to ethinyl estradiol, all patients should be advised to avoid exposing the EVRA application site to direct external heat sources, such as heating pads, electric blankets, heated water beds, heat lamps, hot water bottles, saunas and hot whirlpool spa baths, intensive sunbathing, etc.

The following information is provided from studies of combination oral contraceptives. The use of the EVRA (norelgestromin and ethinyl estradiol) transdermal system is expected to be associated with similar risks.

The use of combination hormonal contraceptives is associated with increased risks of several serious conditions including myocardial infarction, thromboembolism, stroke, hepatic neoplasia and gallbladder disease, although the risk of serious morbidity or mortality is small in healthy women without underlying risk factors. The risk of morbidity and mortality increases significantly if associated with the presence of other risk factors such as hypertension, hyperlipidemias, obesity and diabetes. The excess risk of venous thromboembolism (VTE) is highest during the first year a woman ever uses a combined hormonal contraceptive.

The information contained in this section is principally based on studies carried out in women who used combination oral contraceptives with higher formulations of estrogens and progestins than those in common use today. The effect of long-term use of combination hormonal contraceptives with lower doses of both estrogen and progestin administered orally or transdermally remains to be determined.

Carcinogenesis and Mutagenesis: Breast Cancer: Increasing age and a strong family history are the most significant risk factors for the development of breast cancer. Other established risk factors include obesity, nulliparity and late age for first full-term pregnancy. The identified groups of women that may be at increased risk of developing breast cancer before menopause are long-term users of hormonal contraceptives (more than eight years) and starters at early age. In a few women, the use of hormonal contraceptives may accelerate the growth of an existing but undiagnosed breast cancer. Since any potential increased risk related to oral contraceptive use is small, there is no reason to change prescribing habits at present.

Women using hormonal contraceptives should be instructed in breast self-examination. Their healthcare providers should be notified whenever any mass is detected. A yearly clinical breast examination is recommended because, if a breast cancer should develop, drugs that contain estrogen may cause a rapid progression.

Hepatocellular Carcinoma: Hepatocellular carcinoma may be associated with oral contraceptives. The risk appears to increase with duration of hormonal contraceptive use. However, the attributable risk (the excess incidence) of liver cancers in oral contraceptive users is extremely small.

Cardiovascular: See also Contraindications; Warnings and Precautions, Boxed Warning, General, Hematologic; and Adverse Reactions.

In the post-market period there have been cases of myocardial infarction, stroke, deep vein thrombosis and pulmonary embolism associated with use of EVRA, with some cases resulting in fatality.

Prescribers are advised to carefully assess a patient's baseline and cumulative risk of thromboembolism and discuss the risk of thromboembolism with all patients before prescribing EVRA.

Predisposing Factors for Coronary Artery Disease: Cigarette smoking increases the risk of serious cardiovascular side effects and mortality. Hormonal contraceptives increase this risk, especially with increasing age. Convincing data are available to support an upper age limit of 35 years for hormonal contraceptive use by women who smoke.

Other women who are independently at high risk for cardiovascular disease include those who suffer from hypertension (persistent blood pressure values ≥140 mm Hg systolic or ≥90 mm Hg diastolic), systemic lupus erythematosus, an abnormal lipid profile or have a family history of diabetes. Whether hormonal contraceptives accentuate this risk is unclear.

In low-risk, non-smoking women of any age, the benefits of hormonal contraceptive use outweigh the possible cardiovascular risks associated with low-dose formulations. Consequently, hormonal contraceptives may be prescribed for these women up to the age of menopause.

Hypertension: Patients with essential hypertension whose blood pressure is well controlled may be given hormonal contraceptives but only under close supervision. If a significant persistent elevation of blood pressure (≥160 mm Hg systolic or ≥100 mm Hg diastolic) in previously normotensive or hypertensive subjects occurs at any time during the administration of the drug and cannot be adequately controlled, cessation of medication is necessary. In general, women who develop hypertension during hormonal contraceptive therapy should be switched to a non-hormonal contraceptive. If other contraceptive methods are not suitable, hormonal contraceptive therapy may continue combined with anti-hypertensive therapy. Regular monitoring of BP throughout hormonal contraception therapy is recommended.

In three clinical trials of EVRA (n=1530, 819 and 748, respectively), mean changes from baseline in systolic and diastolic blood pressure were less than 1 mm Hg.

Endocrine and Metabolism: Obesity: Obesity (BMI ≥30 kg/m²) is generally considered a risk factor for venous thromboembolism.

There have been a number of post-market cases of thromboembolism reported in overweight (BMI ≥25 kg/m²) and obese (BMI ≥30 kg/m²) women using EVRA. Particular caution should be exercised when prescribing hormonal contraceptives, including EVRA, to women who are obese. (See also Warnings and Precautions, Boxed Warning and Hematologic.)

Body Weight ≥90 kg: Analyses of Phase III data suggest that the EVRA (norelgestromin and ethinyl estradiol) transdermal system may be less effective in women with body weight ≥90 kg than in women with lower body weights. Below 90 kg, there was no apparent association between body weight and pregnancy rate.

Lipid and Other Metabolic Effects: A small proportion of women will have adverse lipid changes while on oral contraceptives. Alternative contraception should be used in women with uncontrolled dyslipidemias. (See also Contraindications.) Elevations of plasma triglycerides may lead to pancreatitis and other complications.

Diabetes: Current low-dose hormonal contraceptives exert minimal impact on glucose metabolism. Diabetic patients, or those with a family history of diabetes, should be observed closely to detect any worsening of carbohydrate metabolism. Patients predisposed to diabetes who can be kept under close supervision may be given hormonal contraceptives. Young diabetic patients whose disease is of recent origin, well controlled and not associated with hypertension or other signs of vascular disease such as ocular fundal changes, should be monitored more frequently while using hormonal contraceptives.

In a 6-cycle clinical trial with EVRA, there were no clinically significant changes in fasting blood glucose from baseline to end of treatment.

Genitourinary: Vaginal Bleeding: Persistent irregular vaginal bleeding requires assessment to exclude underlying pathology.

Fibroids: Patients with fibroids (leiomyomata) should be carefully observed. Sudden enlargement, pain or tenderness requires discontinuation of hormonal contraceptive use.

Hematologic: See also Contraindications; Warnings and Precautions, Boxed Warning, General, Cardiovascular, Peri-Operative Considerations; and Adverse Reactions.

In the clinical trials (n=3330 subjects with 1704 women years of exposure), two cases of non-fatal pulmonary embolism were reported with use of EVRA, one of which was postoperative.

In the post-market period there have been cases of myocardial infarction, stroke, deep vein thrombosis and pulmonary embolism associated with use of EVRA, with some cases resulting in fatality.

Prescribers are advised to carefully assess a patient's baseline and cumulative risk of thromboembolism and discuss the risk of thromboembolism with all patients before prescribing EVRA.

Post-Partum Period: There have been post-market cases of thromboembolism reported in women using EVRA up to two months post-partum. Since the immediate postpartum period is associated with an increased risk of thromboembolism, hormonal contraceptives should be started no earlier than four weeks after delivery in women who elect not to breast-feed. If possible, women should be encouraged to use a non-hormonal form of contraception in the three months following delivery. Women who elect to use EVRA in the immediate post-partum period should be carefully monitored for signs and symptoms of thromboembolism.

Post-Abortion/Post-Miscarriage: After an abortion or miscarriage that occurs at or after 20 weeks gestation, hormonal contraceptives may be started either on Day 21 post-abortion or on the first day of the first spontaneous menstruation, whichever comes first. (See Dosage and Administration.)

Obesity: Obesity (BMI ≥30 kg/m²) is generally considered a risk factor for venous thromboembolism

There have been a number of post-market cases of thromboembolism reported in overweight (BMI ≥25 kg/m²) and obese (BMI ≥30 kg/m²) women using EVRA. Particular caution should be exercised when prescribing hormonal contraceptives, including EVRA, to women who are obese. (See also Warnings and Precautions, Boxed Warning and Endocrine and Metabolism.)

Other Risk Factors for Venous Thromboembolism (VTE): Other generalized risk factors for VTE include but are not limited to a personal history of VTE, a family history (the occurrence of VTE in a direct relative at a relatively early age may indicate genetic predisposition), systemic lupus erythematosus and inflammatory bowel disease such as Crohn's disease or ulcerative colitis. The risk of VTE also increases with age and smoking. The risk of VTE may be temporarily increased with prolonged immobilization, major surgery or trauma. Also, patients with varicose veins and leg cast should be closely supervised.

If a hereditary or acquired predisposition to venous thromboembolism is suspected, the woman should be referred to a specialist for advice before deciding on any hormonal contraception use.

Hepatic/Biliary/Pancreatic: Jaundice: Patients who have had jaundice should be given hormonal contraceptives only with great care and under close observation. Oral contraceptive-related cholestasis has been described in women with a history of pregnancy-related cholestasis. Women with a history of cholestasis may have the condition recur with subsequent hormonal contraceptive use.

The development of severe generalized pruritus or icterus requires that the medication be withdrawn until the problem is resolved.

If a patient develops jaundice that proves to be cholestatic in type, the use of hormonal contraceptives should not be resumed. In patients taking hormonal contraceptives, changes in the composition of the bile may occur and an increased incidence of gallstones has been reported.

Hepatic Nodules: Hepatic nodules (adenoma and focal nodular hyperplasia) have been reported, particularly in long-term users of hormonal contraceptives. Although these lesions are extremely rare, they have caused fatal intra-abdominal hemorrhage and should be considered in women with an abdominal mass, acute abdominal pain, or evidence of intra-abdominal bleeding.

Gallbladder Disease: Users of oral contraceptives have a greater risk of developing gallbladder disease requiring surgery within the first year of use. The risk may double after four or five years of use.

Neurologic: Migraine and Headache: The onset or exacerbation of migraine or the development of headaches with a new pattern that is recurrent, persistent or severe requires discontinuation of hormonal contraceptives and evaluation of the cause. Women with migraine headache who take hormonal contraceptives may be at increased risk of stroke (see Contraindications).

Epilepsy/Seizures: There have been very rare cases of seizure/convulsion reported in patients using EVRA (see Adverse Reactions, Post-Market Adverse Drug Reactions). Patients with epilepsy or other seizure disorders who are being treated with anticonvulsants should be monitored closely while using hormonal contraceptives. In some patients being treated with anticonvulsants, a method of contraception other than hormonal contraceptives may be recommended. If a woman experiences new onset or exacerbation of seizures while using EVRA, the use of EVRA should be re-evaluated.

Ophthalmologic: Ocular Disease: Patients who are pregnant or are taking oral contraceptives may experience corneal edema. This may cause visual disturbances and changes in contact lens tolerance in rigid contact lens users; soft contact lenses do not usually cause disturbances. If visual changes or alterations in lens tolerance occur, temporary or permanent cessation of wear may be advised.

Peri-Operative Considerations: Thromboembolic Complications—Post-surgery: A two- to four-fold increase in relative risk of postoperative thromboembolic complications has been reported with the use of hormonal contraceptives. The relative risk of venous thrombosis in women who have predisposing conditions is twice that of women without such medical conditions.

Hormonal contraceptives should be discontinued and an alternative method substituted at least four weeks prior to elective surgery of a type associated with an increase in risk of thromboembolism and during prolonged immobilization. Hormonal contraceptives should not be resumed until the first menstrual period after hospital discharge following surgery or following prolonged immobilization.

Psychiatric: Emotional Disorders: Patients with a history of emotional disturbances, especially the depressive type, may be more prone to have a recurrence of depression while using hormonal contraceptives. In cases of a serious recurrence, a trial of an alternative method of contraception should be made, which may help to clarify the possible relationship. Women with premenstrual syndrome (PMS) may have a varied response to hormonal contraceptives, ranging from symptomatic improvement to worsening of the condition.

Renal: Fluid Retention: Hormonal contraceptives may cause some degree of fluid retention. They should be prescribed with caution, and only with careful monitoring, in patients with conditions which might be aggravated by fluid retention.

Sexual Function/Reproduction: Return to Fertility: After discontinuing hormonal contraceptive therapy, the patient should delay pregnancy until at least one normal spontaneous cycle has occurred in order to date the pregnancy. An alternative contraceptive method should be used during this time. There may be some delay in the patient becoming pregnant following discontinuation of the contraceptive patch, particularly if the patient had irregular menstrual cycles before using the contraceptive patch.

Amenorrhea: In the event of amenorrhea, pregnancy should be ruled out.

Women with a history of oligomenorrhea, secondary amenorrhea or irregular cycles may remain anovulatory or become amenorrheic following discontinuation of estrogen-progestin combination therapy.

Amenorrhea, especially if associated with breast secretion, that continues for six months or more after withdrawal warrants a careful assessment of hypothalamic-pituitary function.

Special Populations: Pregnant Women: Extensive epidemiological studies have revealed no increased risk of birth defects in women who have used oral contraceptives prior to pregnancy.

Hormonal contraceptives should not be taken by pregnant women. However, if conception accidentally occurs while hormonal contraceptives are being used, there is no conclusive evidence that the hormones contained in the contraceptive will harm the developing child. The majority of recent studies also do not indicate a teratogenic effect, particularly insofar as cardiac anomalies and limb reduction defects are concerned, when taken inadvertently during early pregnancy.

Nursing Women: In breast-feeding women, the use of hormonal contraceptives results in the hormonal components being excreted in breast milk and may reduce its quantity and quality. If the use of oral contraceptives is initiated after the establishment of lactation, there does not appear to be any effect on the quantity and quality of the milk.

A few adverse effects on the child have been reported, including jaundice and breast enlargement. The nursing mother should be advised not to use combination hormonal contraceptives, but to use other forms of contraception until she has completely weaned her child.

Pediatrics (<18 years of age): The safety and efficacy of EVRA have not been established in women younger than 18 years of age. Use of this product before menarche is not indicated.

Geriatrics: EVRA is not indicated for use in post-menopausal women.

Renal Impairment: EVRA has not been studied in women with renal impairment. There is a suggestion in the literature that the unbound fraction of ethinyl estradiol is higher. EVRA should be used with supervision in this population.

Hepatic Impairment: EVRA is contraindicated in this population (see Contraindications).

Monitoring and Laboratory Tests: Physical Examination and Follow-up: Before hormonal contraceptives are used, a thorough history and physical examination should be performed, including a blood pressure determination. Breasts, liver, extremities and pelvic organs should be examined. A Papanicolaou smear should be taken if the patient has been sexually active.

The first follow-up visit should be three months after the initiation of hormonal contraceptive therapy. Thereafter, examinations should be performed at least once a year, or more frequently if indicated. Women with a strong family history of breast cancer or who have breast nodules should be monitored with particular care. At each visit, examination should include those procedures that were done at the initial visit, as outlined above or as per the recommendations of the Canadian Task Force on the Periodic Health Examination.

ADVERSE REACTIONS: Adverse Drug Reaction Overview: Listed below are adverse events that have been associated with the use of combination hormonal contraceptives. These are also likely to apply to combination transdermal hormonal contraceptives such as EVRA.

An increased risk of the following serious adverse reactions has been associated with the use of hormonal contraceptives: thrombophlebitis and venous thrombosis with or without embolism; arterial thromboembolism; pulmonary embolism; mesenteric thrombosis; myocardial infarction; cerebral hemorrhage; cerebral thrombosis; hypertension; gallbladder disease; hepatic adenomas or benign liver tumours; neuro-ocular lesions (e.g. retinal thrombosis); congenital anomalies.

The following adverse reactions have also been reported in patients receiving hormonal contraceptives: nausea; vomiting; gastrointestinal symptoms (such as abdominal cramps and bloating); breakthrough bleeding; spotting; change in menstrual flow; amenorrhea during and after treatment; temporary infertility after discontinuation of treatment; edema; chloasma or melasma that may persist; breast changes (tenderness, enlargement, secretion); change in weight (increase or decrease); change in cervical erosion and secretion; diminution in lactation when given immediately postpartum; cholestatic jaundice; migraine; rash (allergic); depression; reduced tolerance to carbohydrates; vaginal candidiasis; change in corneal curvature (steepening); intolerance to contact lenses; administration-site reaction (transdermal, sub-dermal or intramuscular administration only); premenstrual-like syndrome; cataracts; optic neuritis; retinal thrombosis; chorea; changes in appetite; cystitis-like syndrome; rhinitis; headache; nervousness; dizziness; hirsutism; loss of scalp hair; erythema multiforme; erythema nodosum; hemorrhagic eruption; vaginitis; porphyria; impaired renal function; hemolytic uremic syndrome; Raynaud's phenomenon; auditory disturbances; pancreatitis; dysmenorrhea; increase in size of uterine leiomyomata; endocervical hyperplasia; change in libido.

Clinical Trial Adverse Drug Reactions: Because clinical trials are conducted under very specific conditions the adverse reaction rates observed in the clinical trials may not reflect the rates observed in practice and should not be compared to the rates in the clinical trials of another drug. Adverse drug reaction information from clinical trials is useful for identifying drug-related adverse events and for approximating rates.

Two adequate and well-controlled trials demonstrated that the incidence of breakthrough bleeding and spotting with EVRA is statistically and clinically comparable to that seen with CYCLEN (norgestimate/ethinyl estradiol) and TRIPHASIL (levonorgestrel/ethinyl estradiol) tablets.

Presented in Table 2 are the most common treatment-emergent adverse events reported with the use of EVRA in three clinical studies (n=3330), two comparing EVRA to an oral contraceptive, and a third evaluating EVRA alone, occurring in ≥1% of subjects. Treatment-emergent adverse events are all adverse events reported in three clinical studies in subjects receiving EVRA regardless of whether they were deemed by the Investigator to be causally related to EVRA use.

Table 2: EVRA

Incidence (% of patients) of Treatment-Emergent Adverse Events in Three Studies

Body System	EVRA (n=3330) (%)
Gastrointestinal Disorders	nausea (17%), abdominal pain (9%), vomiting (5%), diarrhea (4%), dyspepsia (2%), flatulence (2%), gastroenteritis (2%), toothache (1%)
General Disorders and Administration Site Conditions	application site reaction (17%), Influenza-like symptoms (7%), fatigue (3%), injury (3%), fever (2%), malaise (1%)
Immune System Disorders	allergy (1%)
Infections and Infestations	monoliasis (3%), otitis media (1%)
Investigations	weight increase (3%), cervical smear test positive (1%)
Musculoskeletal and Connective Tissue Disorders	back pain (5%), myalgia (2%), tendon disorder (1%)
Nervous System Disorders	headache (21%), dizziness (3%), migraine (3%)
Psychiatric Disorders	emotional lability (4%), depression (3%), libido decreased (1%)
Renal and Urinary Disorders	urinary tract infection (2%), cystitis (1%)
Reproductive System and Breast Disorders	breast discomfort, (17%), dysmenorrhea (10%), vaginitis (5%), breast pain female (4%), intermenstrual bleeding (3%), menorrhagia (3%), breast engorgement (2%), breast enlargement (2%), leukorrhea (2%), breast fibroadenosis (1%), menstrual disorder (1%)
Respiratory, Thoracic and Mediastinal Disorders	upper respiratory tract infection (10%), pharyngitis (5%), sinusitis (5%), bronchitis (2%), coughing (1%), rhinitis (1%)
Skin and Subcutaneous Tissue Disorders	pruritus (4%), acne (3%), rash (2%), pruritus genital (1%)

Less Common Clinical Trial Adverse Drug Reactions (<1%): Blood and Lymphatic System Disorders: anemia, granulocytopenia, leucopenia, leukocytosis, lymphadenopathy, monocytosis, platelets abnormal, thrombocytopenia.

Cardiac Disorders: angina pectoris, bradycardia, edema dependent, hypertension, hypotension, palpitation, tachycardia.

Ear and Labyrinth Disorders: ear disorder nos, earache, tinnitus, vestibular disorder.

Endocrine Disorders: goitre, hyperprolactinaemia, hypothyroidism.

Eye Disorders: conjunctival discolouration, conjunctivitis, corneal ulceration, exophthalmos, eye abnormality, eye pain, eyelid retraction, myopia, retinal detachment, vision abnormal, xerophthalmia.

Gastrointestinal Disorders: abdomen enlarged, colitis, constipation, enanthema, enteritis, gastritis, gastrointestinal disorder nos, gastroesophageal reflux, gingival bleeding, gingivitis, glossitis, hemorrhoids, mouth dry, periodontal destruction, rectal disorder, saliva increased, stomatitis ulcerative, taste perversion, tenesmus, tooth caries, tooth disorder.

General Disorders and Administration Site Conditions: asthenia, chest pain, application site cellulitis, face edema, hot flushes, edema, edema generalized, edema peripheral, pain, rigors, syncope, thirst, tolerance decreased.

Hepatobiliary Disorders: cholesystitis, cholelithiasis, hepatic function abnormal.

Immune System Disorders: allergic reaction, vasculitis allergic.

Infections and Infestations: abscess, herpes simplex, herpes zoster, infection, infection bacterial, infection fungal, infection viral.

Investigations: globulins increased, AST increased, ALT increased, weight decrease.

Metabolism and Nutrition Disorders: alcohol intolerance, anorexia, appetite increase, dehydration, diabetes mellitus, fat disorder, hypercholesterolemia, hyperglycemia, hypertriglyceridemia, hypoglycaemia, oedema legs, obesity.

Musculoskeletal and Connective Tissue Disorders: arthralgia, arthritis, arthrosis, bursitis, cramps legs, leg pain, muscle weakness, myositis, osteoma, skeletal pain, tendonitis, torticollis.

Neoplasms Benign, Malignant and Unspecified: breast neoplasm benign female, cervical uterine polyp, cervix carcinoma in situ, lipoma, melanoma malignant, neoplasm nos, neuroma, ovarian cyst, phaeochromocytoma, skin neoplasm malignant, thyroid cyst, uterine fibroid.

Nervous System Disorders: convulsions, coordination abnormal, dysphonia, hemiplegia, hypertonia, hypoesthesia, hypotonia, meningitis, migraine aggravated, neuralgia, paraesthesia, stupor, tremor, vertigo.

Psychiatric Disorders: amnesia, anxiety, apathy, crying abnormal, depersonalization, depression aggravated, dyspareunia, insomnia, libido increased, nervousness, paroniria, psychosis manic-depressive, sleep disorder, somnolence, suicide attempt.

Renal and Urinary Disorders: dysuria, micturition frequency, pyelonephritis, renal calculus, renal pain, strangury, urethral disorder, urinary incontinence, urine abnormal.

Reproductive System and Breast Disorders: breast atrophy, cervical dysplasia, cervicitis, cervix lesion, endometriosis, genital ulceration, lactation nonpuerperal, mastitis, ovarian disorder, pelvic inflammation, perineal pain female, uterine disorder nos, uterine spasm, vaginal hemorrhage, vulva disorder, withdrawal bleeding.

Respiratory, Thoracic and Mediastinal Disorders: asthma, bronchospasm, dyspnoea, laryngitis, pleurisy, pneumonia, stridor.

Skin and Subcutaneous Tissue Disorders: alopecia, bullous eruption, chloasma, dermatitis, dermatitis contact, eczema, folliculitis, furunculosis, hypertrichosis, melanosis, nail disorder, paronychia, photosensitivity allergic reaction, photosensitivity reaction, pigmentation abnormal, psoriasis, purpura, rash erythematous, rash maculo-papular, seborrhoea, skin cold clammy, skin depigmentation, skin discolouration, skin disorder, skin dry, sweat gland disorder, sweating increased, urticaria, vasculitis allergic, verruca.

Social Circumstance: drug abuse.

Vascular Disorders: aneurysm, epistaxis, flushing, hematoma, peripheral ischaemia, phlebitis, pulmonary embolism, purpura allergic, thrombophlebitis, thrombophlebitis superficial, vascular disorder, thrombosis arterial leg, vasculitis, vein disorder, vein distended, vein pain, vein varicose.

Post-Market Adverse Drug Reactions: In addition to the adverse events observed in clinical trials listed above, the following other serious and unexpected adverse events have been reported in users of EVRA in the post-marketing period. These adverse events are compiled from spontaneous reports and are listed regardless of frequency and whether or not a causal relationship with EVRA has been established:

Blood and Lymphatic System Disorders: hemolytic uremic syndrome, idiopathic thrombocytopenic purpura, iron deficiency anemia.

Cardiac Disorders: acute coronary syndrome, arrhythmia, atrial tachycardia, cardiac failure, coronary artery atherosclerosis, coronary artery dissection (with fatal outcome), intracardiac thrombus, myocardial infarction, myocarditis (with fatal outcome), pericardial effusion, sinus tachycardia, supraventricular tachycardia.

Congenital, Familial and Genetic Disorders: atrial septal defect, cleft lip, cleft palate, congenital musculoskeletal anomaly, dermoid cyst of ovary, Fallot's tetralogy, limb malformation, skull malformation, ventricular septal defect.

Ear and Labyrinth Disorders: motion sickness, otosclerosis.

Endocrine Disorders: thyroid disorder.

Eye Disorders: amaurosis fugax, blindness, blindness transient, blindness unilateral, cataract, contact lens intolerance, corneal neovascularisation, diplopia, dry eye, eye disorder, eye irritation, eye haemorrhage, eye swelling, iritis, mydriasis, ocular discomfort, ocular hyperaemia, ocular icterus, optic nerve disorder, papilloedema, photophobia, retinal vascular thrombosis, vision blurred, visual acuity reduced, visual disturbance.

Gastrointestinal Disorders: abdominal discomfort, abdominal distension, ascites, colitis ulcerative, edema mouth, gastric disorder gastrointestinal edema, gastrointestinal hemorrhage, gastrointestinal pain, gastrooesophageal reflux disease, hypoaesthesia oral, intestinal ischemia, intestinal obstruction, irritable bowel syndrome, oral mucosal blistering, pancreatic disorder, pancreatitis, rectal hemorrhage, stomach discomfort, umbilical hernia.

General Disorders and Administration Site Conditions: abasia, application site burn, application site dermatitis, application site discolouration, application site erythema, application site irritation, application site pain, application site photosensitivity reaction, application site pruritus, application site swelling, application site urticaria, chest discomfort, chills, cyst rupture, death, difficulty in walking, disease progression, drug ineffective, drug interaction, drug withdrawal syndrome, dysplasia, feeling abnormal, feeling cold, feeling hot and cold, feeling jittery, feeling of body temperature change, gait disturbance, hernia, hunger, irritability, local swelling, swelling, temperature intolerance, therapeutic response delayed.

Hepatobiliary Disorders: cholestasis, gallbladder disorder, hepatic cirrhosis, hepatic failure, hepatic pain, hepatitis, hepatocellular damage, hepatomegaly, jaundice, liver disorder, portal vein thrombosis.

Immune System Disorders: anaphylactic reaction, anaphylactic shock, anaphylactoid reaction, autoimmune disorder, food allergy, hypersensitivity, sarcoidosis.

Infections and Infestations: alpha haemolytic streptococcal infection, appendicitis, breast abscess, cavernous sinus thrombosis, cellulitis, ear infection, encephalitis viral (with fatal outcome), Escherichia urinary tract infection, gastroenteritis viral, gastrointestinal infection, infectious mononucleosis, influenza, joint abscess, nasopharyngitis, osteomyelitis, pelvic inflammatory disease, pneumonia, respiratory tract infection, septic embolus, septic shock, skin infection, staphylococcal infection, streptococcal infection, tonsillitis, vaginal candidiasis, vaginal infection, vaginitis bacterial, vulvovaginal mycotic infection.

Injury, Poisoning and Procedural Complications: brachial plexus injury, closed head injury, collapse of lung, concussion, contusion, drug administration error, drug exposure during pregnancy, drug exposure via breast milk, fall, inappropriate schedule of drug administration, incision site complication, intentional misuse, joint sprain, limb injury, medication error, overdose, road traffic accident, stress fracture, wrist fracture.

Investigations: alanine aminotransferase increased, antithyroid antibody positive, aspartate aminotransferase increased, blood cholesterol increased, blood creatine phosphokinase increased, blood glucose increased, blood lactate dehydrogenase increased, blood pressure increased, blood test abnormal, blood triglycerides increased, cardiac enzymes increased, electrocardiogram abnormal, electrocardiogram T wave abnormal, fetal heart rate decreased, hemoglobin abnormal, haemoglobin decreased, heart rate decreased, heart rate increased, heart rate irregular, hepatic enzyme increased, intraocular pressure increased, liver function test abnormal, red blood cell sedimentation rate increased, smear cervix abnormal, thyroid function test abnormal.

Metabolism and Nutrition Disorders: anorexia, decreased appetite, diabetes mellitus non-insulin-dependent, fluid retention, food intolerance, gestational diabetes, hypokalemia, iron deficiency.

Musculoskeletal and Connective Tissue Disorders: bone pain, flank pain, groin pain, joint effusion, joint swelling, muscle spasms, muscle tightness, muscle twitching, pain in extremity, rhabdomyolysis, rotator cuff syndrome, sensation of heaviness, shoulder pain.

Neoplasms Benign, Malignant and Unspecified: benign hydatidiform mole, brain neoplasm, cervix carcinoma, colon cancer Stage II, colon neoplasm, fibroadenoma of breast, fibromatosis, focal nodular hyperplasia, gastrointestinal carcinoma, hepatic neoplasm, neoplasm malignant, ovarian cancer, peritoneal neoplasm, renal neoplasm, teratoma benign, thyroid gland cancer.

Nervous System Disorders: amnesia, basilar artery thrombosis, benign intracranial hypertension, burning sensation, carotid artery stenosis, cerebral artery occlusion, cerebral hemorrhage, cerebral infarction, cerebral thrombosis, cerebral venous thrombosis (with fatal outcome), cerebrovascular accident (with fatal outcome), coma, depressed level of consciousness, dysarthria, dysgeusia, dyskinesia, encephalitis, facial palsy, facial paresis, formication, grand mal convulsion, hemiparesis, hemorrhagic stroke, intracranial aneurysm, intracranial venous sinus thrombosis, ischemic stroke, lethargy, loss of consciousness, mental impairment, migraine with aura, monoparesis, multiple sclerosis, multiple sclerosis relapse, nervous system disorder, optic neuritis, petit mal epilepsy, polyneuropathy, sinus headache, somnolence, speech disorder, subarachnoid haemorrhage, superior sagittal sinus thrombosis, syncope, thrombotic stroke, transient ischemic attack, transverse sinus thrombosis, tunnel vision, visual field defect.

Pregnancy, Puerperium and Perinatal Conditions: abnormal product of conception, abortion, abortion incomplete, abortion missed, abortion spontaneous, abortion threatened, antepartum hemorrhage, blighted ovum, ectopic pregnancy, fetal disorder, fetal growth retardation, intra-uterine death, oligohydramnios, placenta previa, placental insufficiency, postpartum haemorrhage, preeclampsia, pregnancy, pregnancy-induced hypertension, premature labour, premature separation of placenta, ruptured ectopic pregnancy, twin pregnancy, unintended pregnancy.

Psychiatric Disorders: abnormal behaviour, acute psychosis, affect lability, aggression, anger, attention deficit/hyperactivity disorder, bipolar disorder, completed suicide, confusional state, decreased interest, depressed mood, expressive language disorder, hallucination (auditory, visual), homicidal ideation, mood altered, mood swings, nightmare, panic attack, personality change, stress, suicidal ideation.

Renal and Urinary Disorders: chromaturia, renal disorder, renal failure, renal failure acute, urethral cyst.

Reproductive System and Breast Disorders: adenomyosis, amenorrhea, breast discharge, breast disorder, breast dysplasia, breast mass, breast swelling, breast tenderness, galactorrhea, genital discharge, genital rash, hypertrophy breast, hypomenorrhea, infertility, menometrorrhagia, oligomenorrhea, ovulation pain, pelvic discomfort, pelvic pain, polymenorrhea, premenstrual syndrome, reproductive tract disorder, uterine cyst, uterine hemorrhage, vaginal disorder, vaginal lesion, withdrawal bleeding irregular.

Respiratory, Thoracic and Mediastinal Disorders: acute respiratory distress syndrome, dyspnea, lung consolidation, neonatal respiratory distress syndrome, pharyngeal edema, pharyngolaryngeal pain, pharynx discomfort, pulmonary alveolar hemorrhage (with fatal outcome), pulmonary congestion, pulmonary edema (with fatal outcome), pulmonary alveolar hemorrhage, pulmonary congestion, pulmonary embolism (with fatal outcome), pulmonary hypertension, pulmonary infarction, pulmonary thrombosis, respiratory disorder, respiratory failure, sinus disorder, sleep apnea syndrome, tonsillar disorder.

Skin and Subcutaneous Tissue Disorders: angioneurotic edema, dermatitis allergic, erythema nodusum, hyperhidrosis, night sweats, pigmentation disorder, pruritus generalized, pyoderma gangrenosum, rash generalized, rash papular, rash pruritic, seborrheic dermatitis, skin irritation, skin reaction, swelling face, urticaria generalized, yellow skin.

Surgical and Medical Procedures: abortion induced, appendectomy, dental operation, foot operation, gallbladder operation, hospitalization, hysterectomy, lipectomy, plastic surgery, renal stone removal, salpingo-oophorectomy, surgery, sympathectomy.

Vascular Disorders: angiopathy, arterial thrombosis, cavernous sinus thrombosis, circulatory collapse, deep vein thrombosis (with fatal outcome), diastolic hypertension, embolism, hemorrhage, iliac artery thrombosis, jugular vein thrombosis, malignant hypertension, orthostatic hypotension, pallor, Raynaud's phenomenon, thrombosis (with fatal outcome), vasculitis necrotizing (with fatal outcome), venous thrombosis, venous thrombosis limb.

DRUG INTERACTIONS: Overview: The concurrent administration of **oral** contraceptives with other drugs may result in an altered response to either agent (see Table 3 and Table 4). Similar drug interactions are likely with the transdermal system. It is important to ascertain all drugs that a patient is taking, both prescription and non-prescription, before hormonal contraceptives are prescribed.

Changes in Contraceptive Effectiveness Associated With Co-administration of Other Drugs:

- If a woman on hormonal contraceptives takes a drug or herbal product that induces enzymes, including CYP3A4, that metabolize contraceptive hormones, she should be counselled to use additional contraception or a different method of contraception. Drugs or herbal products that induce such enzymes may decrease the plasma concentrations of contraceptive hormones, and may decrease the effectiveness of hormonal contraceptives or increase breakthrough bleeding. Some drugs or herbal products that may decrease the effectiveness of hormonal contraceptives include:
- barbiturates
- bosentan
- carbamazepine
- griseofulvin
- modafinil
- oxcarbazepine
- phenytoin
- rifampin
- St. John's Wort
- topiramate

HIV Protease Inhibitors and Non-nucleoside Reverse Transcriptase Inhibitors: Significant changes (increase or decrease) in the plasma levels of the estrogen and progestin have been noted in some cases of co-administration of HIV protease inhibitors and non-nucleoside reverse transcriptase inhibitors.

Antibiotics: There have been reports of pregnancy while taking hormonal contraceptives and antibiotics, but clinical pharmacokinetic studies have not shown consistent effects of antibiotics on plasma concentrations of synthetic steroids. In a pharmacokinetic drug interaction study, oral administration of tetracycline HCl, 500 mg q.i.d. for 3 days prior to and 7 days during wear of ORTHO EVRA (the formulation of EVRA marketed in the United States) did not significantly affect the pharmacokinetics of norelgestromin or EE.

Increase in Plasma Hormone Levels Associated With Co-administered Drugs: Some drugs and grapefruit juice may increase the plasma levels of ethinyl estradiol if co-administered. Examples include:

- acetaminophen
- ascorbic acid
- CYP3A4 inhibitors (including itraconazole, ketoconazole, voriconazole and fluconazole)
- grapefruit juice
- HMG-CoA reductase inhibitors (including atorvastatin and rosuvastatin)

Changes in Plasma Levels of Co-administered Drugs: Data from the literature concerning oral combination hormonal contraceptives indicate that they may also affect the pharmacokinetics of some other drugs if used concomitantly.

Examples of drugs whose plasma levels may increase (due to CYP inhibition) include:

- cyclosporine
- omeprazole
- prednisolone
- theophylline
- voriconazole

Examples of drugs whose plasma levels may be decreased (due to induction of glucuronidation) include:

- acetaminophen
- lamotrigine
- morphine
- salicylic acid
- temazepam

Physicians are advised to consult the labelling of concurrently-used drugs to obtain further information about interactions with hormonal contraceptives or the potential for enzyme alterations.

Refer to Oral Contraceptives 1994 (Chapter 8), Health Canada, for possible drug interactions with hormonal contraceptives.

Table 3: EVRA

Drugs that May Decrease the Efficacy of Oral Contraceptives

Class of Compound	Drug	Proposed Mechanism	Suggested Management
Anticonvulsants	Carbamazepine Oxcarbazepine Ethosuximide Lamotrigine Phenobarbital Phenytoin Primidone Topiramate	Induction of hepatic microsomal enzymes. Rapid metabolism of estrogen and increased binding of progestin and ethinyl estradiol to SHBG.	Use higher dose OCs (50 µg ethinyl estradiol), another drug or another method.

(cont'd)

Table 3: EVRA *(cont'd)*

Drugs that May Decrease the Efficacy of Oral Contraceptives

Class of Compound	Drug	Proposed Mechanism	Suggested Management
Antibiotics	Ampicillin Cotrimoxazole Penicillin	Enterohepatic circulation disturbance, intestinal hurry.	For short course, use additional method or use another drug. For long course, use another method.
	Rifampin	Increased metabolism of progestins. Suspected acceleration of estrogen metabolism.	Use another method.
	Chloramphenicol Metronidazole Neomycin Nitrofurantoin Sulfonamides Tetracyclines	Induction of hepatic microsomal enzymes. Also disturbance of enterohepatic circulation.	For short course, use additional method or use another drug. For long course, use another method.
	Troleandomycin	May retard metabolism of OCs, increasing the risk of cholestatic jaundice.	
Antifungals	Griseofulvin	Stimulation of hepatic metabolism of contraceptive steroids may occur.	Use another method.
Sedatives and Hypnotics	Benzodiazepines Barbiturates Chloral Hydrate Glutethimide Meprobamate	Induction of hepatic microsomal enzymes.	For short course, use additional method or another drug. For long course, use another method or higher dose OCs.
Antacids		Decreased intestinal absorption of progestins.	Dose two hours apart.
Other Drugs	Phenylbutazone Antihistamines Analgesics Antimigraine Preparations Vitamin E Modafinil	Reduced OC efficacy has been reported. Remains to be confirmed.	
	Bosentan	Induction of hepatic microsomal enzymes	Consider switching to a non-hormonal contraceptive method or adding a barrier method to oral contraceptive therapy.

Drug-Food Interactions: Interactions with food have not been established.

Drug-Herb Interactions: A possible interaction has been suggested with hormonal contraceptives and the herbal supplement St. John's Wort based on some reports of oral contraceptive users experiencing breakthrough bleeding shortly after starting St. John's Wort. Pregnancies have been reported by users of combined hormonal contraceptives who also used some form of St. John's Wort.

Table 4: EVRA

Modification of Other Drug Action by Oral Contraceptives

Class of Compound	Drug	Modification of Drug Action	Suggested Management
Alcohol		Possible increased levels of ethanol or acetaldehyde.	Use with caution.
Alpha-II Adrenoreceptor Agents	Clonidine	Sedation effect increased.	Use with caution.
Anticoagulants	All	OCs increase clotting factors, decrease efficacy. However, OCs may potentiate action in some patients.	Use another method.
Anticonvulsants	All	Estrogens may increase risk of seizures.	Use another method.
	Lamotrigine	Significantly decreased lamotrigine levels (due to induction of lamotrigine glucuronidation) may lead to breakthrough seizures.	Adjust dose of drug if necessary.
Antidiabetic Drugs	Oral Hypoglycemics and Insulin	OCs may impair glucose tolerance and increase blood glucose.	Use low-dose estrogen and progestin OC or another method. Monitor blood glucose.
Antihypertensive Agents	Guanethidine and Methyldopa	Estrogen component causes sodium retention, progestin has no effect.	Use low-dose estrogen OC or use another method.
	Beta Blockers	Increased drug effect (decreased metabolism).	Adjust dose of drug if necessary.Monitor cardiovascular status.

(cont'd)

Table 4: EVRA *(cont'd)*

Modification of Other Drug Action by Oral Contraceptives

Class of Compound	Drug	Modification of Drug Action	Suggested Management
Antipyretics	Acetaminophen	Increased metabolism and renal clearance.	Dose of drug may have to be increased.
	Antipyrine	Impaired metabolism.	Decrease dose of drug.
	ASA	Effects of ASA may be decreased by the short-term use of OCs.	Patients on chronic ASA therapy may require an increase in ASA dosage.
Aminocaproic Acid		Theoretically, a hypercoagulable state may occur because OCs augment clotting factors	Avoid concomitant use.
Betamimetic Agents	Isoproterenol	Estrogen causes decreased response to these drugs.	Adjust dose of drug as necessary. Discontinuing OCs can result in excessive drug activity.
Caffeine		The actions of caffeine may be enhanced as OCs may impair the hepatic metabolism of caffeine.	Use with caution.
Corticosteroids	Prednisone Prednisolone	Markedly increased serum levels.	Possible need for decrease in dose.
Cyclosporine		May lead to an increase in cyclosporine levels and hepatotoxicity.	Monitor hepatic function. The cyclosporine dose may have to be decreased.
Folic Acid		OCs have been reported to impair folate metabolism.	May need to increase dietary intake, or supplement.
Meperidine		Possible increased analgesia and CNS depression due to decreased metabolism of meperidine.	Use combination with caution.
Phenothiazine Tranquilizers	All Phenothiazines, Reserpine and similar drugs	Estrogen potentiates the hyperprolactinemia effect of these drugs.	Use other drugs or lower dose OCs. If galactorrhea or hyperprolactinemia occurs, use other method.
Sedatives and Hypnotics	Chlordiazepoxide Lorazepam Oxazepam Diazepam	Increased effect (increased metabolism).	Use with caution.
Theophylline	All	Decreased oxidation, leading to possible toxicity.	Use with caution. Monitor theophylline levels.
Tricyclic Antidepressants	Clomipramine (possibly others)	Increased side effects; i.e. depression.	Use with caution.
Vitamin B_{12}		OCs have been reported to reduce serum levels of Vitamin B_{12}.	May need to increase dietary intake, or supplement.

Drug-Laboratory Test Interactions: Laboratory Test Interactions: Certain endocrine and liver function tests and blood components may be affected by hormonal contraceptives:

Coagulation Tests: Factors II, VII, IX, X, XII and XIII: increased; Factor VIII: mild increase; Platelet aggregation and adhesiveness: mild increase in response to common aggregating agents; Fibrinogen: increased; Plasminogen: mild increase; Antithrombin III: mild decrease; Prothrombin time: increased.

Thyroid Function Tests: Protein-Bound Iodine (PBI): increased; Total serum thyroxine (T_4): increased; Thyroid Stimulating Hormone (TSH): unchanged; Free T_3 resin uptake: decreased, reflecting the elevated TBG; Free T_4 concentration: unchanged.

Miscellaneous Tests: Other binding proteins: may be elevated in serum; Sex Hormone Binding Globulins: increased and resulted in elevated levels of total circulating endogenous sex steroids and corticoids; however, free or biologically active levels either decrease or remain unchanged; High-Density Lipoprotein (HDL-C): may increase; Total Cholesterol (Total-C): may increase; Low-Density Lipoprotein (LDL-C): may increase; Triglycerides: may increase; LDL-C/HDL-C ratio: may remain unchanged; Glucose tolerance: may be decreased; Serum folate levels: may be depressed by hormonal contraceptive therapy, this may be of clinical significance if a woman becomes pregnant shortly after discontinuing hormonal contraceptives; Insulin response: mild to moderate increase; c-Peptide response: mild to moderate increase.

Tissue Specimens: Pathologists should be advised of hormonal contraceptive use when specimens from surgical procedures and/or Pap smears are submitted for examination.

Drug-Lifestyle Interactions: When use of EVRA was studied under conditions encountered in a health club (sauna, whirlpool and treadmill), there were slight increases in both steady state concentration (C_{SS}) and area under the curve (AUC) of ethinyl estradiol; however, the C_{SS} values following these treatments were within the reference range. The clinical significance of this finding is not known. Due to a theoretical risk of increased exposure to ethinyl estradiol, all patients should be advised to avoid exposing the EVRA application site to direct external heat sources, such as heating pads, electric blankets, heated water beds, heat lamps, hot water bottles, saunas and hot whirlpool spa baths, intensive sunbathing, etc. (See Warnings and Precautions, General and Action and Clinical Pharmacology, Pharmacokinetics, Absorption.)

Non-Contraceptive Benefits of Hormonal Contraceptives: Several health advantages other than contraception have been reported:

1. Combination hormonal contraceptives reduce the incidence of cancer of the endometrium and ovaries.
2. Hormonal contraceptives reduce the likelihood of developing benign breast disease and, as a result, decrease the incidence of breast biopsies.
3. Hormonal contraceptives reduce the likelihood of development of functional ovarian cysts.
4. Users of hormonal contraceptives have less menstrual blood loss and have more regular cycles, thereby reducing the chance of developing iron-deficiency anemia.
5. The use of hormonal contraceptives may decrease the severity of dysmenorrhea and premenstrual syndrome, and may improve acne vulgaris, hirsutism, and other androgen-mediated disorders.
6. Hormonal contraceptives decrease the incidence of acute pelvic inflammatory disease and, thereby, reduce as well the incidence of ectopic pregnancy.
7. Hormonal contraceptives have potential beneficial effects on endometriosis.

DOSAGE AND ADMINISTRATION: Dosing Considerations: To achieve maximum contraceptive effectiveness, the EVRA (norelgestromin and ethinyl estradiol) transdermal system must be used exactly as directed. Complete instructions to facilitate patient counselling on proper system usage may be found in Information for the Patient.

Recommended Dose and Dosage Adjustment: Transdermal Contraceptive System Overview: This system uses a 28-day, four-week cycle. A new patch is applied each week for three weeks—21 total days. Week Four is patch-free. Withdrawal bleeding is expected during this time.

This means that every new patch will be applied on the same day of the week. This day is known as the "Patch Change Day." For example, if the first patch is applied on a Monday, all subsequent patches should be applied on a Monday. Only one patch should be worn at a time.

The patch should not be cut, damaged or altered in any way. If the patch is cut, damaged or altered in size, contraceptive efficacy may be impaired.

On the day after Week Four ends, a new four-week cycle is started by applying a new patch. Under no circumstances should there be more than a 7-day patch-free interval between dosing cycles.

Clinical trials demonstrated that subjects randomized to EVRA were able to adhere to the weekly dosing regimen better than with daily dosing of oral contraceptives.

Administration:

1. If the patient is starting EVRA for the **first time**, she should **wait until the day she begins her menstrual period**. Either a First Day start or Sunday start may be utilized (see below). The day she applies her first patch will be Day 1. Her "Patch Change Day" will be on this day every week.
2. for **First Day** start: the patient should apply her first patch during the first 24 hours of her period.
   or
   for **Sunday** start: the patient should apply her first patch on the first Sunday after her period starts. She must use back-up contraception for the first week of her first cycle only. If the menstrual period begins on a Sunday, the first patch should be applied on that day. No back-up contraception is needed.
   For both a **First Day** start and a **Sunday** start: a non-hormonal contraceptive (such as a condom or diaphragm) should be used concurrently for the first 7 consecutive days of the first treatment cycle.
3. **Where to apply the patch.** The patch should be applied to clean, dry, intact healthy skin on the buttock, abdomen, upper outer arm or upper torso, in a place where it won't be rubbed by tight clothing. EVRA should not be placed on skin that is red, irritated or cut, nor should it be placed on the breast.
   To prevent interference with the adhesive properties of EVRA, no make-up, creams, lotions, powders or other topical products should be applied to the skin area where the EVRA patch is currently placed or will be applied shortly.
4. **Application of the EVRA patch:** The foil pouch is opened by tearing it along the edge using the fingers. A corner of the patch is grasped firmly and gently removed from the foil pouch. Sometimes patches can stick to the inside of the pouch—the patient should be careful not to accidentally remove the clear liner as she removes the patch. Then half of the clear protective liner is peeled away. The patient should avoid touching the sticky surface of the patch.
5. The patch is positioned on the skin and the other half of the liner is removed. The patient should press down firmly on the patch with the palm of her hand for 10 seconds, making sure that the edges stick well. She should check her patch every day to make sure it is sticking.
6. The patch is worn for 7 days (one week). On the "Patch Change Day", Day 8, the used patch is removed and a new one is applied immediately. The used patch still contains some active hormones—it should be thrown away by carefully folding it in half so that it sticks to itself.
7. A new patch is applied on Week Two (Day 8) and again on Week Three (Day 15), on the usual "Patch Change Day". Patch changes may occur at any time on the Change Day. Consecutive EVRA patches should be applied to a new spot on the skin to help avoid potential irritation, although they may be kept within the same anatomic site.
8. **Week Four is patch-free (Day 22 through Day 28)**, thus completing the four-week contraceptive cycle. Bleeding is expected during this time.
9. **The next four-week cycle is started** by applying a new patch on the usual "Patch Change Day", the day after Day 28, no matter when the menstrual period begins or ends.
   Under no circumstances should there be more than a 7-day patch free interval between dosing cycles.

Patch adhesion was assessed indirectly by replacement rates for complete and partial patch detachment. Experience with more than 70 000 EVRA patches worn for contraception for 6-13 cycles showed that 4.7% of patches were replaced because they either fell off (1.8%) or were partly detached (2.9%). Similarly, in a small study of patch wear under conditions of physical exertion and variable temperature and humidity, less than 2% of patches were replaced for complete or partial detachment.

If the EVRA patch becomes partially or completely detached and remains detached, insufficient drug delivery occurs.

If the patch remains even partly detached:

- **for less than one day** (up to 24 hours), try to reapply it to the same place or replace with a new patch immediately. No back-up contraception is needed. The woman's "Patch Change Day" will remain the same.
- **for more than one day (>24 hours) or if the patient is not sure how long the patch has been detached, she may not be protected from pregnancy.** She should stop the current contraceptive cycle and start a new cycle immediately by putting on a new patch. There is now a new "Day 1" and a new "Patch Change Day." Back-up contraception must be used for the first week of the new cycle only.

A patch should not be re-applied if it is no longer sticky, if it has become stuck to itself or another surface, if it has other material stuck to it or if it has become loose or fallen off before. If a patch cannot be re-attached, a new patch should be applied immediately. Supplemental adhesives or wraps should not be used to hold the EVRA patch in place.

If the patient forgets to change her patch:

- **at the start of any patch cycle** (Week One/Day 1): **She may not be protected from pregnancy.** She should apply the first patch of her new cycle as soon as she remembers. There is now a new "Patch Change Day" and a new "Day 1." The patient must use back-up contraception for the first week of her new cycle.
- **in the middle of the patch cycle (Week Two/Day 8 or Week Three/Day 15):**
  - for **one or two days** (up to 48 hours), she should apply a new patch immediately. The next patch should be applied on the usual "Patch Change Day." No back-up contraception is needed.
  - for **more than two days** (>48 hours), **she may not be protected from pregnancy**. She should stop the current contraceptive cycle and start a new cycle immediately by putting on a new patch. There is now a new "Patch Change Day" and a new "Day 1". The patient must use back-up contraception for one week.
- **at the end of the patch cycle (Week Four/Day 22):** if the patient forgets to remove her patch, she should take it off as soon as she remembers. The next cycle should be started on the usual "Patch Change Day," which is the day after Day 28. No back-up contraception is needed.

Under no circumstances should there be more than a 7-day patch-free interval between dosing cycles. If there are more than 7 patch-free days, **the patient may not be protected from pregnancy** and back-up contraception must be used concurrently for 7 days. As with combined oral contraceptives, the risk of ovulation increases with each day beyond the recommended contraceptive-free period. If coital exposure has occurred during the patch-free interval, the possibility of fertilization should be considered.

Change Day Adjustment: If the patient wishes to move her "Patch Change Day" she should complete her current cycle, removing the third EVRA patch on the correct day. During the patch-free week, a new "Patch Change Day" may be selected by applying a new EVRA patch on the first occurrence of the desired day. In no case should there be more than 7 consecutive patch-free days.

The shorter the patch-free interval, the higher the risk of breakthrough bleeding and spotting replacing the expected withdrawal bleeding. **This practice is for a one-time only change and should not be used as a standard dosing regimen, as there are no long term safety data available on the continuous use of EVRA.**

Switching from an Oral Contraceptive: Treatment with EVRA should begin on the first day of withdrawal bleeding. If there is no withdrawal bleeding within 5 days of the last active (hormone-containing) tablet, pregnancy must be ruled out prior to start of treatment with EVRA. If therapy starts after the first day of withdrawal bleeding, a non-hormonal contraceptive should be used concurrently for 7 days. If more than 7 days elapse after taking the last active oral contraceptive tablet, the patient may have ovulated. The patient should be instructed to consult her physician before initiating treatment with EVRA.

Use after Childbirth: Women who elect not to breast-feed should start contraceptive therapy with EVRA no sooner than 4 weeks after childbirth (see Warnings and Precautions, Hematologic).

Use after Abortion or Miscarriage: After an abortion or miscarriage that occurs before 20 weeks gestation, EVRA may be started immediately. An additional method of contraception is not needed if EVRA is started immediately. Be advised that ovulation may occur within 10 days of an abortion or miscarriage.

After an abortion or miscarriage that occurs at or after 20 weeks gestation, EVRA may be started either on Day 21 post-abortion or on the first day of the first spontaneous menstruation, whichever comes first. The incidence of ovulation on Day 21 post-abortion (at 20 weeks gestation) is not known.

In Case of Vomiting or Diarrhea: Unlike oral contraceptives, dose delivery by transdermal application should be unaffected by vomiting. Dose delivery is also expected to be unaffected by diarrhea.

In Case of Skin Irritation: If patch use results in uncomfortable irritation, a new patch may be applied to a new location until the next Change Day. Only one patch should be worn at a time.

Additional Instructions for All Dosing Regimens: Breakthrough bleeding, spotting, and amenorrhea are frequent reasons for patients discontinuing hormonal contraceptives.

Breakthrough Bleeding or Spotting: In the event of breakthrough bleeding or spotting (bleeding that occurs during EVRA usage), treatment should be continued. This type of bleeding usually disappears after the first few cycles. Non-functional causes should be considered, however, and in cases of undiagnosed persistent or recurrent abnormal bleeding from the vagina, adequate diagnostic measures are indicated to rule out pregnancy or malignancy. If pathology has been excluded, time or a change to another formulation may solve the problem. Changing to a hormonal contraceptive with a higher estrogen content, while potentially useful in minimizing menstrual irregularity, should be done only if necessary since this may increase the risk of thromboembolic disease.

Amenorrhea: Use of hormonal contraceptives in the event of a missed menstrual period:

1. If the woman has not adhered to the prescribed schedule, the possibility of pregnancy should be ruled out at the time of the first missed period.
2. If EVRA has been used correctly, the absence of withdrawal bleeding (bleeding that should occur during the patch-free week) is not necessarily an indication of pregnancy. If the woman has adhered to the prescribed regimen and misses one period, she should continue using her contraceptive patches on the next scheduled Change Day. If the woman has adhered to the prescribed regimen and misses two consecutive periods, pregnancy should be ruled out before continuing hormonal contraceptive use.

OVERDOSAGE:

Serious ill effects have not been reported following accidental ingestion of large doses of hormonal contraceptives. Overdosage may cause nausea and vomiting. Withdrawal bleeding may occur in females. In case of suspected overdose, all transdermal contraceptive systems should be removed and symptomatic treatment given. Liver function tests should be conducted, particularly transaminase levels, 2 to 3 weeks after overdosage.

For management of a suspected drug overdose, contact your **regional Poison Control Centre**. See the *CPS* Directory section for a list of Poison Control Centres.

ACTION AND CLINICAL PHARMACOLOGY: The EVRA (norelgestromin and ethinyl estradiol) transdermal system, with a contact surface area of 20 cm², is a thin, matrix-type transdermal system consisting of three layers. Each transdermal system contains 6.0 mg norelgestromin and 0.60 mg ethinyl estradiol (EE). Each transdermal system releases an average of approximately 200 µg of NGMN and 35 µg of EE every 24 hours. Drug exposure is more appropriately characterized by the pharmacokinetic profile. Systemic exposures (as measured by area under the curve [AUC] and steady state concentration [C_{SS}]) of NGMN and EE during use of EVRA are comparable to those produced by an oral contraceptive containing norgestimate 250 µg/EE 35 µg, and peak concentrations (C_{max}) are lower than those produced by this oral contraceptive.

Each EVRA transdermal system consists of three layers:

1. The backing layer is composed of a beige flexible film consisting of a low-density pigmented polyethylene outer layer and a polyester inner layer. It provides structural support and protects the middle adhesive layer from the environment.
2. The middle layer contains polyisobutylene/polybutene adhesive, crospovidone, non-woven polyester fabric and lauryl lactate as inactive components. The active components in this layer are the hormones, norelgestromin and EE.
3. The third layer is the release liner, which is a transparent polyethylene terephthalate (PET) film with a polydimethylsiloxane coating on the side that is in contact with the middle adhesive layer. The release liner protects the adhesive layer during storage and is removed just prior to application.

The outside of the backing layer is heat-stamped "EVRA™".

Pharmacodynamics: Norelgestromin is the active progestin largely responsible for the progestational activity that occurs in women following application of EVRA. Norelgestromin is also the primary active metabolite produced following oral administration of norgestimate (NGM), the progestin component of the oral contraceptive products CYCLEN (norgestimate/ethinyl estradiol) and TRI-CYCLEN (norgestimate/ethinyl estradiol).

Combination oral contraceptives act by suppression of gonadotropins. Although the primary mechanism of this action is inhibition of ovulation, other alterations include changes in the cervical mucus (which increase the difficulty of sperm entry into the uterus) and the endometrium (which reduce the likelihood of implantation).

Receptor and human sex hormone-binding globulin (SHBG) binding studies, as well as studies in animals and humans, have shown that both norgestimate and norelgestromin exhibit high progestational activity with minimal intrinsic androgenicity. Transdermally-administered norelgestromin, in combination with ethinyl estradiol, does not counteract the estrogen-induced increases in SHBG, resulting in lower levels of free testosterone in serum compared to baseline.

Pharmacokinetics: Absorption: Following application of EVRA, both norelgestromin and EE rapidly appear in the serum, reach a plateau by approximately 48 hours, and are maintained at an approximate steady-state throughout the wear period. C_{SS} concentrations for norelgestromin and EE during one week of patch wear are approximately 0.8 ng/mL and 50 pg/mL, respectively, and are generally consistent from all studies and application sites. These C_{SS} concentrations are well within the reference ranges for norelgestromin (0.6 to 1.2 ng/mL) and EE (25 to 75 pg/mL) established based upon the C_{ave} concentrations in 90% of the individual subjects taking CYCLEN. This was computed from $AUC_{0\text{-}t}/t$ for these analytes from steady-state data following administration of the NGM/EE oral contraceptives.

The absorption of norelgestromin and EE following application of EVRA to the abdomen, buttock, upper outer arm and upper torso (excluding breast) was evaluated in a crossover design study. The results of this study indicated that C_{SS} and AUC for the buttock, upper arm and torso for each analyte were equivalent. While C_{SS} values for the abdomen were within reference ranges for EE 35 µg/NGM 250 µg oral contraceptive users, strict bioequivalence requirements for AUC were not met in this study for the abdomen. However, in a separate parallel-group multiple-application pharmacokinetic study, C_{SS} and AUC for the buttock and abdomen were not statistically different. In a dose-ranging study, EVRA caused effective ovulation suppression when applied to the abdomen. Therefore, all four sites are therapeutically equivalent.

The absorption of norelgestromin and EE following application of EVRA was studied under conditions encountered in a health club (sauna, whirlpool and treadmill) and in a cold-water bath. The results indicated that for norelgestromin there were no significant treatment effects on C_{SS} or AUC when compared to normal wear. For EE, slight increases were observed due to sauna, whirlpool and treadmill; however, the C_{SS} values following these treatments were within the reference range. There was no significant effect of cold water on these parameters. Serum estradiol concentrations could theoretically increase in patients with fever. Any clinical consequences due to an increase in temperature are unknown at this time. Due to a theoretical risk of increased exposure to ethinyl estradiol, all patients should be advised to avoid exposing the EVRA application site to direct external heat sources, such as heating pads, electric blankets, heated water beds, heat lamps, hot water bottles, saunas and hot whirlpool spa baths, intensive sunbathing, etc. See Warnings and Precautions, General and Drug Interactions, Drug-Lifestyle Interactions.

In multiple dose studies, C_{SS} and AUC for norelgestromin and EE were found to increase slightly over time when compared to Week 1 of Cycle 1. In a three-cycle study, these pharmacokinetic parameters reached steady-state conditions during all three weeks of Cycle 3 (see Table 5, Figure 1 and Figure 2).

Table 5: EVRA

Mean (SD) Pharmacokinetic Parameters of Norelgestromin and EE Following Three Consecutive Cycles of EVRA Wear on the Buttock

Analyte	Parameter	Cycle 1 Week 1	Cycle 3 Week 1	Cycle 3 Week 2	Cycle 3 Week 3
Norelgestromin	C_{SS}[a]	0.70 (0.28)	0.70 (0.29)	0.80 (0.23)	0.70 (0.32)
	$AUC_{0\text{–}168}$[b]	107 (44.2)	105 (45.5)	132 (57.1)	120 (52.8)
	$t_{½}$[c]	nc	nc	nc	32.1 (12.9)
EE	C_{SS}[d]	46.4 (17.9)	47.6 (17.3)	59.0 (25.1)	49.6 (27.0)
	$AUC_{0\text{–}168}$[e]	6796 (2673)	7160 (2893)	10 054 (4205)	8840 (5176)
	$t_{½}$[c]	nc	nc	nc	21.0 (9.07)

[a] ng/mL.
[b] ng·h/mL.
[c] h.
[d] pg/mL.
[e] pg·h/mL.
Legend: nc=not calculated.

Figure 1: EVRA

Mean Norelgestromin (NGMN) Serum Concentrations (ng/mL) in Healthy Female Volunteers Following Application of EVRA on the Buttock for Three Consecutive Cycles (Dotted horizontal lines indicate the reference range. Dotted vertical arrow indicates time of patch removal.)

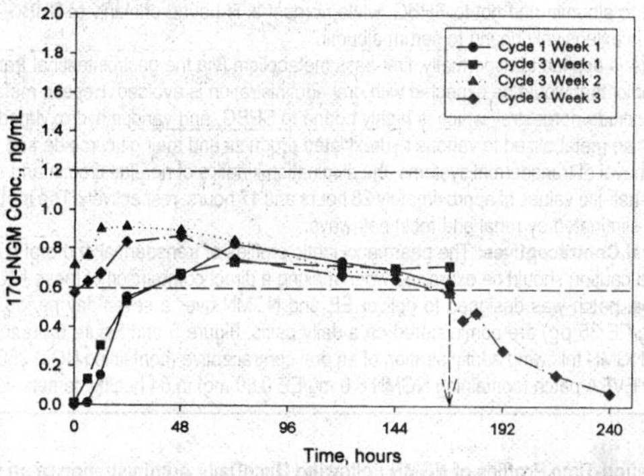

Figure 2: EVRA

Mean Ethinyl Estradiol (EE) Serum Concentrations (pg/mL) in Healthy Female Volunteers Following Application of EVRA on the Buttock for Three Consecutive Cycles (Dotted horizontal lines indicate the reference range. Dotted vertical arrow indicates time of patch removal.)

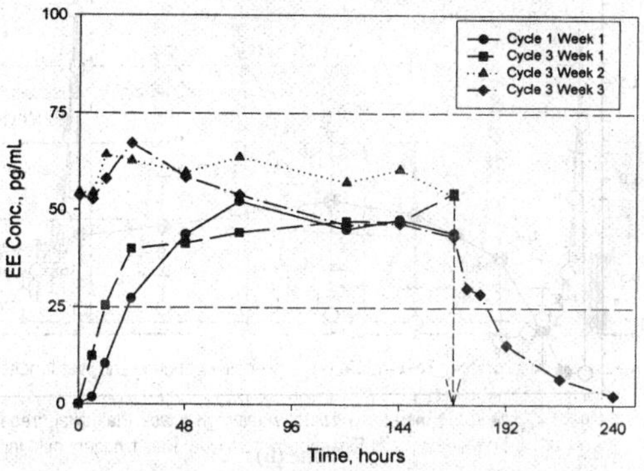

Results from a study of consecutive EVRA wear for 7 days and 10 days indicated that target C_{SS} of norelgestromin and EE were maintained during a 3-day extended wear of EVRA. These findings suggest that clinical efficacy would be maintained even if a scheduled change is missed for as long as 2 full days (see Figure 3 and Figure 4).

Figure 3: EVRA

Mean Norelgestromin (NGMN) Serum Concentrations (ng/mL) Following Application of EVRA to the Abdomen for 7 Days and 10 Days (Dotted horizontal lines indicate the reference range. Solid vertical arrows indicate actual time of patch removal. Dotted vertical arrow indicates theoretical time of patch removal under normal use.)

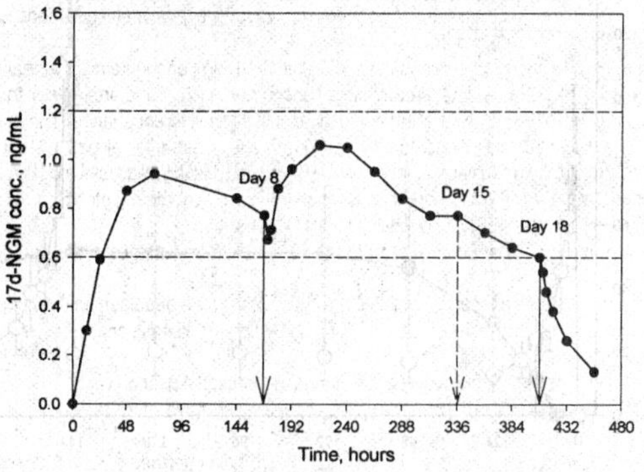

(cont'd)

Figure 4: EVRA

Mean Ethinyl Estradiol (EE) Serum Concentrations (pg/mL) Following Application of EVRA to Abdomen for 7 Days and 10 Days (Dotted horizontal lines indicate reference range. Solid vertical arrows indicate actual time of patch removal. Dotted vertical arrow indicates theoretical time of patch removal under normal use.)

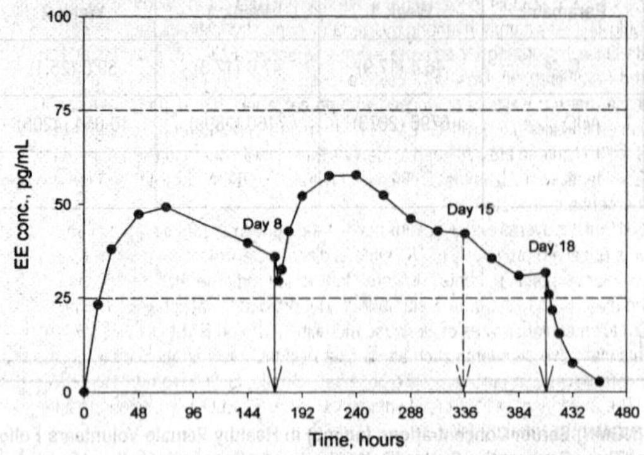

Distribution: Norelgestromin and norgestrel (a serum metabolite of norelgestromin) are highly bound (>97%) to serum proteins. Norelgestromin is bound to albumin and not to SHBG, while norgestrel is bound primarily to SHBG, which limits its biological activity. Ethinyl estradiol is extensively bound to serum albumin.

Metabolism: Since EVRA is applied transdermally, first-pass metabolism (via the gastrointestinal tract and/or liver) of norelgestromin and ethinyl estradiol that would be expected with oral administration is avoided. Hepatic metabolism of norelgestromin occurs and metabolites include norgestrel, which is highly bound to SHBG, and various hydroxylated and conjugated metabolites. Ethinyl estradiol is also metabolized to various hydroxylated products and their glucuronide and sulfate conjugates.

Excretion: Following removal of transdermal systems, the elimination kinetics of norelgestromin and ethinyl estradiol were consistent for all studies with half-life values of approximately 28 hours and 17 hours, respectively. The metabolites of norelgestromin and ethinyl estradiol are eliminated by renal and fecal pathways.

Transdermal versus Oral Contraceptives: The pharmacokinetic profiles of transdermal and oral combined hormonal contraceptives are different and caution should be exercised when making a direct comparison of these PK parameters.

The EVRA transdermal patch was designed to deliver EE and NGMN over a seven-day period while oral contraceptives (containing NGM 250 μg/EE 35 μg) are administered on a daily basis. Figure 5 and Figure 6 present mean pharmacokinetic (PK) profiles for EE and NGMN following administration of an oral contraceptive (containing NGM 250 μg/EE 35 μg) compared to the 7-day transdermal EVRA patch (containing NGMN 6.0 mg/EE 0.60 mg) in 54 healthy female volunteers.

Figure 5: EVRA

Mean Serum Concentration-Time Profiles of NGMN Following OnceDaily Administration of an Oral Contraceptive for 7 days or Application of EVRA to the Buttock in Healthy Female Volunteers

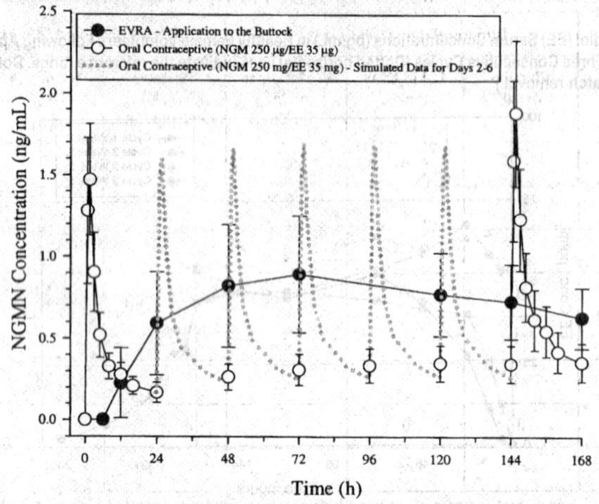

Figure 6: EVRA

Mean Serum Concentration-Time Profiles of EE Following OnceDaily Administration of an Oral Contraceptive for 7 days or Application of EVRA to the Buttock in Healthy Female Volunteers

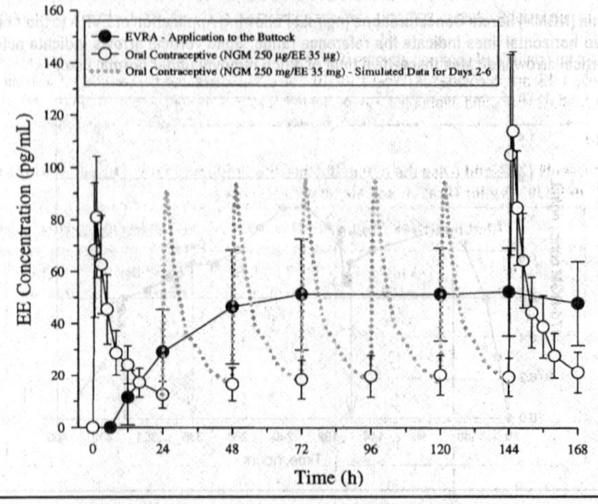

Table 6 provides the mean (%CV) for NGMN and EE pharmacokinetic (PK) parameters.

Table 6: EVRA

Mean (%CV) NGMN and EE Steady State Pharmacokinetic Parameters Following Application of EVRA and Once-daily Administration of an Oral Contraceptive (containing NGM 250 μg/EE 35 μg) in Healthy Female Volunteers

Parameter	EVRA[a]	Oral Contraceptive[b]
NGMN[c]		
C_{max} (ng/mL)	0.934 (37.7)	1.95 (21.3)
$AUC_{0\text{-}168}$ (ng·h/mL)	118 (36.9)	108 (21.5)[d]
C_{ss} (ng/mL)	0.768 (34.0)	0.663 (25.1)[e]
EE		
C_{max} (pg/mL)	58.5 (38.1)	118 (28.7)
$AUC_{0\text{-}168}$ (pg·h/mL)	7289 (35.8)	7226 (28.3)[d]
C_{ss} (ng/mL)	49.9 (34.8)	45.2 (27.8)[e]

[a] Days 1–7.
[b] Week 1.
[c] NGM is rapidly metabolized to NGMN following oral administration.
[d] Average weekly exposure, calculated as AUC_{24}×7.
[e] C_{avg}.

In general, C_{max} values were 2-fold higher for NGMN and EE in subjects administered the oral contraceptive compared to EVRA, while overall exposure (AUC and C_{ss}) was comparable in subjects treated with EVRA. Inter-subject variability (%CV) for the PK parameters following delivery from EVRA was higher relative to the variability determined from the oral contraceptive. The mean pharmacokinetic profiles are different between the two products and caution should be exercised when making a direct comparison of these PK parameters.

The clinical relevance of the difference in PK profile and pharmacodynamic (PD) response between transdermal and oral delivery is not known. (See Warnings and Precautions, General.)

Special Populations and Conditions: Effects of Age, Body Weight, Body Surface Area and Race: The effects of age, body weight, body surface area and race on the pharmacokinetics of norelgestromin and ethinyl estradiol were evaluated in 230 healthy women from nine pharmacokinetic studies of single 7-day applications of EVRA. For both norelgestromin and ethinyl estradiol, increasing age, body weight and body surface area each were associated with slight decreases in C_{ss} and AUC values. However, only a small fraction (10-20%) of the overall variability in the pharmacokinetics of norelgestromin and ethinyl estradiol following application of EVRA may be associated with any or all of the above demographic parameters. There was no significant effect of race with respect to Caucasians, Hispanics and Blacks.

Hepatic Insufficiency: No studies with EVRA have been conducted in women with hepatic impairment. EVRA is contraindicated in patients with hepatic dysfunction (see Contraindications and Warnings and Precautions).

Renal Insufficiency: No studies with EVRA have been conducted in women with renal impairment.

STORAGE AND STABILITY: Store between 15-30°C. Do not refrigerate or freeze. Store patches in their protective pouches inside the original box. Apply patch immediately upon removal from its packaging.

Keep new and used transdermal systems out of the reach of children and pets.

SPECIAL HANDLING INSTRUCTIONS: Disposal of EVRA: Used transdermal systems still contain some active hormones. Used transdermal systems should be carefully folded in half so the adhesive side sticks to itself. The folded patch should be placed in a sturdy container, preferably with a child-resistant cap, and disposed of in the garbage out of the reach of children and pets. Remaining active hormonal ingredients of the patch may have harmful effects if reaching the aquatic environment. Used or unused patches should not be flushed down the toilet or placed in liquid waste disposal systems.

INFORMATION FOR THE PATIENT: Published in e-CPS, available by subscription at www.e-cps.ca.

DOSAGE FORMS, COMPOSITION AND PACKAGING: Each transdermal system sealed within a protective pouch and heat-stamped "EVRA™", contains: norelgestromin 6 mg and ethinyl estradiol 0.60 mg in the middle layer, releasing approximately 200 μg norelgestromin and 35 μg ethinyl estradiol every 24 hours. Backing layer: low-density pigmented polyethylene outer layer and a polyester inner layer; middle layer inactive components: polyisobutylene/polybutene adhesive, crospovidone, non-woven polyester fabric, lauryl lactate; release liner: polyethylene terephthalate film with polydimethylsiloxane coating on one side. The EVRA transdermal system does not contain any metal components. Cartons contain 3 systems each.

(Shown in Product Identification Section)

Exelon® Ⓟ

rivastigmine hydrogen tartrate

Cholinesterase Inhibitor

Novartis Pharmaceuticals

Date of Preparation: April 13, 2000
Date of Revision: May 18, 2010

SUMMARY PRODUCT INFORMATION:

Route of Administration	Dosage Form/Strength	Nonmedicinal Ingredients
Oral	Capsules, 1.5 mg, 3 mg, 4.5 mg, 6 mg	Hydroxypropyl methylcellulose; magnesium stearate; microcrystalline cellulose; silicon dioxide; hard gelatin capsules contain: gelatin, titanium dioxide and red and/or yellow iron oxides
	Oral Solution, 2 mg/mL	Sodium benzoate, citric acid, sodium citrate, quinoline yellow WS dye E104 and purified water

INDICATIONS AND CLINICAL USE: EXELON (rivastigmine hydrogen tartrate) is indicated for the symptomatic treatment of patients with mild to moderate dementia of the Alzheimer's type.

EXELON is indicated for the symptomatic treatment of patients with idiopathic Parkinson's disease, and mild to moderate dementia, with onset at least 2 years after the initial diagnosis of Parkinson's disease, and in whom other causes of dementia have been ruled out.

EXELON has not been studied in controlled clinical trials for longer than 6 months.

EXELON capsules and oral solution should only be prescribed by (or following consultation with) clinicians who are experienced in the diagnosis and management of dementia.

CONTRAINDICATIONS:

- Patients with known hypersensitivity to rivastigmine, other carbamate derivatives or other components of the formulation. For a complete listing, see Dosage Forms, Composition and Packaging.
- Patients with severe liver impairment since it has not been studied in this population.

WARNINGS AND PRECAUTIONS: General: As with other cholinergic substances care must be taken when prescribing EXELON:

- To patients with sick sinus syndrome or conduction defects (sino-atrial block, atrio-ventricular block) (see Cardiovascular).
- To patients with active gastric or duodenal ulcers or patients predisposed to these conditions because gastric acid secretions may be increased (see Gastrointestinal).

- To patients predisposed to urinary obstruction and seizures because cholinomimetics may induce or exacerbate these diseases (see Neurologic).
- To patients with a history of asthma or obstructive pulmonary disease (see Respiratory).

As with other cholinomimetics, adverse effects have been observed shortly after dose increase. They may respond to a dose reduction. In other cases, EXELON has been discontinued (see Dosage and Administration, Dose Interruption).

Anesthesia: EXELON (rivastigmine hydrogen tartrate) as a cholinesterase inhibitor, is likely to exaggerate succinylcholine-type muscle relaxation during anesthesia.

Weight Loss: Cholinesterase inhibitors as well as Alzheimer's disease and dementia associated with Parkinson's disease can be associated with significant weight loss.

In controlled clinical trials of Alzheimer's disease patients, the use of EXELON was associated with weight loss. Women exposed to doses of EXELON at the higher end of the therapeutic range, i.e. usual maintenance dose range of 6-12 mg/day were at greater risk for weight loss. Approximately 24% of women on 6-12 mg/day doses of EXELON had weight loss of equal to or greater than 7% of their baseline weight compared to 6% on placebo. For males, 16% (6-12 mg/day) experienced a similar degree of weight loss compared to 4% on placebo.

In dementia associated with Parkinson's disease, in a single trial of n=541 patients, at a similar dose range as for Alzheimer's disease patients 16.3% of patients had weight loss equal to or greater than 7% of their baseline weight compared to 14% in the placebo group (21.1% drug vs 8.1% placebo for women, and 13.7% drug vs 17.1% placebo for men). The rates in the drug-treated group are similar to those seen in Alzheimer's disease trial (as above), although the relativities with placebo are not.

Where weight loss may be of clinical concern, body weight should be monitored.

Cardiovascular: Because of their pharmacological action, cholinomimetics may have vagotonic effects on heart rate (e.g., bradycardia). The potential for this action may be particularly important to patients with "sick sinus syndrome" or other supraventricular cardiac conduction conditions. In clinical trials patients with serious cardiovascular disease were excluded. Caution should therefore be exercised in treating patients with active coronary artery disease or congestive heart failure. Syncopal episodes have been reported in association with the use of EXELON. It is recommended that EXELON not be used in patients with cardiac conduction abnormalities (except for right bundle branch block) including "sick sinus syndrome" and those with unexplained syncopal episodes.

Gastrointestinal: EXELON is associated with significant gastrointestinal adverse reactions including nausea, vomiting, anorexia and weight loss.

Treatment with EXELON should always be started at a dose of 1.5 mg b.i.d. or 1.5 mg o.d., as clinically indicated, and patients titrated to their maintenance dose. **If treatment with EXELON is interrupted for longer than several days, patients should be instructed to reinitiate treatment with the lowest daily dose and be retitrated (see Dosage and Administration) to reduce the possibility of severe vomiting and its potentially serious sequelae (e.g. very rare post-marketing reports of severe vomiting with esophageal rupture).**

Nausea, vomiting and diarrhea appear more frequently at higher doses (see Adverse Reactions), with nausea and vomiting being more prevalent in women. Females are more sensitive to the cholinergic adverse effects associated with cholinesterase inhibitors and in general are more likely to experience nausea and vomiting than are males. In most cases these effects were of mild to moderate intensity and transient, and they resolved during continued EXELON treatment or upon treatment discontinuation.

Through their primary action, cholinesterase inhibitors may be expected to increase gastric acid secretion due to increased cholinergic activity. Therefore, patients should be monitored for symptoms of active or occult gastrointestinal bleeding, especially those at increased risk for developing ulcers, e.g., those with a history of ulcer disease or those receiving concurrent nonsteroidal anti-inflammatory drugs (NSAIDS). In controlled clinical studies with EXELON in Alzheimer's disease patients, patients with a past history (last 2 years) of peptic ulceration and chronic diseases of the gastrointestinal tract were excluded. In the trial population who received EXELON there was no significant increase, relative to placebo, in the incidence of peptic ulcer disease. The incidence of GI hemorrhage, in controlled clinical trials was <1% (n=6/1923) for EXELON and 0% (n=0/868) for placebo.

Neurologic: Worsening of Tremor and Other Extrapyramidal Symptoms: Like other cholinomimetics, EXELON may exacerbate or induce extrapyramidal symptoms. Worsening of these symptoms (including bradykinesia, dyskinesia, gait abnormality) and an increased incidence of, or severity of, tremor have been observed in patients with dementia associated with Parkinson's disease treated with EXELON. Particularly in the case of tremor, events were observed shortly after dose increase, and may respond to dose reduction (see also Adverse Reactions, Dementia Associated with Parkinson's Disease, Extrapyramidal Symptoms; and Dosage and Administration, Dosing Considerations).

Clinical monitoring is recommended for these adverse events.

Seizures: In placebo controlled clinical trials with EXELON cases of seizures were reported. Cholinomimetics are believed to have some potential to cause generalized convulsions. However, seizure activity also may be a manifestation of Alzheimer's disease. The risk/benefit of EXELON treatment for patients with a history of seizure disorder must therefore be carefully evaluated.

Effects on Ability to Drive and Use Machines: Alzheimer's disease may cause gradual impairment of driving performance or compromise the ability to use machinery. Rivastigmine may induce dizziness and somnolence, mainly when initiating treatment or increasing the dose. Therefore, in patients with dementia treated with rivastigmine, the ability to continue driving or operating complex machines should be routinely evaluated by the treating physician.

EXELON has not been studied in patients with moderately severe or severe Alzheimer's disease, moderately severe or severe dementia associated with Parkinson's disease, or other dementias. The efficacy and safety of EXELON in these patient populations is unknown.

Genetic Polymorphism: The effect of genetic polymorphism of butyrylcholinesterase enzyme on rivastigmine metabolism is unknown.

Genitourinary: Although not reported in clinical trials of EXELON, cholinomimetics may cause bladder spasm.

Hepatic/Biliary/Pancreatic: Pancreatic: In the pivotal clinical trials involving AD patients treated with EXELON, acute pancreatitis was reported as an adverse event in no patient treated with EXELON (0%) and in one patient treated with placebo (<1%). Cases of pancreatitis have been reported during postmarketing experience with EXELON capsules and EXELON PATCH, shortly after initial use as well as after several months or years of use.

Patients experiencing persistent and unexplained upper abdominal pain, that may or may not be accompanied by vomiting and confusion, should promptly seek medical attention.

Laboratory Values: Elevations in Serum Amylase/Lipase levels in Patients with Dementia Associated with Parkinson's Disease: Of patients with normal levels at baseline, 17% receiving EXELON and 10% receiving placebo showed amylase levels beyond the normal range at the second measurement at the end of the Study (Week 24), and 9% and 4% respectively showed lipase levels beyond the normal range. Elevations beyond 2× normal range occurred in 2 of the EXELON patients with respect to amylase levels, 7 with respect to lipase levels, and in 0 placebo patients. Elevations in both amylase and lipase levels occurred in 12 EXELON patients, and in 0 placebo patients; pancreatitis was not recorded as an AE for any patient in the study.

Respiratory: Like other cholinomimetic drugs, EXELON should be used with care in patients with a history of asthma or obstructive pulmonary disease. No experience is available in treating patients with these conditions.

Skin: Skin reactions, including Stevens-Johnson syndrome and blister, have been reported with the use of EXELON. These skin reactions may occur at any time during treatment (see Adverse Reactions, Post-Market Adverse Drug Reactions, Skin and Appendages). During postmarketing experience there have been reports of hypersensitivity type skin reactions with EXELON PATCH that worsened when patients were converted to oral EXELON.

Special Populations: Hepatic Impairment: There is limited information on the pharmacokinetics of EXELON in hepatically impaired patients (see Action and Clinical Pharmacology, Special Populations and Conditions). It is therefore recommended that dose escalation with rivastigmine in hepatically impaired patients be undertaken with caution and under conditions of close monitoring for adverse effects (see Dosage and Administration, Dosing Considerations). EXELON is contraindicated in patients with severe liver impairment since it has not been studied in this population (see Contraindications).

Renal Impairment: There is limited information on the pharmacokinetics of EXELON in renally impaired patients (see Action and Clinical Pharmacology, Special Populations and Conditions). It is therefore recommended that dose escalation with rivastigmine in renally impaired patients be undertaken with caution and under conditions of close monitoring for adverse effects (see Dosage and Administration, Dosing Considerations).

Pregnant Women: The safety of EXELON in pregnant women has not been established. EXELON should not be used in women of childbearing potential unless, in the opinion of the physician, the potential benefit to the patient justifies the potential risk to the fetus.

Nursing Women: It is not known whether EXELON is excreted into human milk, and therefore EXELON should not be used in nursing mothers.

Pediatrics: The safety and effectiveness of EXELON in any illness occurring in pediatric patients have not been established.

Geriatrics: Use in Patients >85 Years Old: In controlled clinical studies in Alzheimer's disease patients, the number of patients over 85 years old who received EXELON in the therapeutic dose range of 6-12 mg/day was 68. Of these patients, 12 received high doses of EXELON (>9-12 mg/day). The safety of EXELON in this patient population has not been adequately characterized.

In Alzheimer's disease patients in controlled clinical trials, nausea, diarrhea, vomiting, dizziness, anorexia, fatigue, dyspepsia and weakness increased with dose. Dose escalation in patients >85 years old should thus proceed with caution (see Dosage and Administration, Dosing Considerations).

Use in Elderly Patients with Serious Comorbid Disease: There is limited information on the safety of EXELON treatment in patients with mild to moderate Alzheimer's disease, or mild to moderate dementia associated with Parkinson's disease, and serious comorbidity. The use of EXELON in Alzheimer's disease patients, or in patient with dementia associated with Parkinson's disease, with chronic illnesses common among the geriatric population, should be considered only after careful risk/benefit assessment and include close monitoring for adverse events. Dose escalation in this patient population should proceed with caution (see Dosage and Administration, Dosing Considerations).

Patients with Vascular Dementia: Patients diagnosed with probable vascular dementia, according to NINDS-AIREN criteria, were randomized to double-blind treatment with EXELON (3-12 mg/day, N=363) or placebo (N=344) for 6 months in a controlled clinical trial. The NINDS-AIREN criteria are designed to identify patients with dementia that appears to be due primarily to vascular causes, and to exclude patients with Alzheimer's disease. Overall, EXELON was not shown to be an effective treatment for patients with vascular dementia in this study.

The study also showed that the overall rate of occurrence of treatment emergent adverse events was lower in vascular dementia patients than what was observed previously in Alzheimer's disease patients. However, rates of serious adverse events were generally greater for vascular dementia patients compared to mild to moderate Alzheimer's disease patients for both EXELON and placebo groups, and may relate to the greater number of co-morbid medical conditions in the vascular dementia population.

In vascular dementia patients, higher rates of all-cause mortality (2.2% on EXELON vs 1.2% on placebo) and certain cardiovascular and cerebrovascular adverse events such as, angina pectoris, myocardial infarction, coronary artery disease, hypertension, dysarthria and cerebrovascular accident were observed in patients who were treated with EXELON compared to those who received placebo. The majority of deaths in patients taking either EXELON or placebo resulted from either cardiovascular or cerebrovascular disorders or respiratory failures.

ADVERSE REACTIONS: Clinical Trial Adverse Drug Reactions: Because clinical trials are conducted under very specific conditions the adverse reaction rates observed in the clinical trials may not reflect the rates observed in practice and should not be compared to the rates in the clinical trials of another drug. Adverse drug reaction information from clinical trials is useful for identifying drug-related adverse events and for approximating rates.

Dementia of the Alzheimer's Type: A total of 1923 patients with mild to moderate Alzheimer's disease were treated in controlled clinical studies with EXELON. Of these patients, 1417 (74%) completed the studies. The mean duration of treatment for all EXELON groups was 154 days (range 1-255 days).

Adverse Events Leading to Discontinuation: Overall, 18% (340/1923) of patients treated with EXELON discontinued from Phase III controlled clinical trials due to adverse events compared to 9% (75/868) in the placebo group. During the titration phases of controlled clinical trials the incidence of discontinuations due to adverse events was 5% for placebo, 5% for EXELON 1-4 mg/day and 21% for EXELON 6-12 mg/day. During the maintenance phases, 3% of patients who received placebo, 3% of patients who received 1-4 mg/day EXELON and 6% of patients who received EXELON 6-12 mg/day withdrew from studies due to adverse events.

Female patients treated with EXELON were approximately twice as likely to discontinue study participation due to adverse events than were male patients [Females: 21%; Males: 12%]. Female patients in clinical studies were found to be more susceptible to gastrointestinal adverse drug reactions and weight loss.

The most common adverse events leading to discontinuation, defined as those occurring in at least 2% of patients and at twice the incidence seen in placebo patients, are shown in Table 1.

Table 1: EXELON

Most Frequent Adverse Events (≥2% and twice the rate in the placebo group) Leading to Withdrawal From Randomized Placebo-controlled Clinical Trials B351, B352, and B303 During Titration and Maintenance Phases[a]

	Titration Phase (Weeks 1–12)			Maintenance Phase (Weeks 13–26)		
	Placebo n=646 (%)	1–4 mg/day n=644 (%)	6–12 mg/day n=824 (%)	Placebo n=588 (%)	1–4 mg/day n=587 (%)	6–12mg/day n=601 (%)
All Events	5	5	21	3	3	6
Nausea	1	1	10	0	<1	1
Vomiting	0	<1	5	0	<1	2
Anorexia	0	<1	3	<1	<1	<1
Dizziness	<1	<1	3	<1	0	1
Abdominal Pain	<1	<1	2	<1	<1	<1
Asthenia	0	0	2	0	0	<1
Fatigue	<1	<1	2	0	0	<1

[a] All patients who received at least one dose of study medication were included in the results for the titration phase. All patients who entered the maintenance phase were represented in the results for the maintenance phase.

Titration and maintenance dosing should remain flexible and be adjusted according to individual needs.

Most Frequent Adverse Clinical Events Seen in Association with the Use of EXELON: The most common adverse events, defined as those occurring at a frequency of at least 5% and twice the placebo rate, are largely predicted by EXELON's cholinomimetic effects. These include nausea, vomiting, dizziness, diarrhea, anorexia, weight loss of >7% of baseline weight, and abdominal pain.

Table 2 presents a comparison of common adverse events (≥5% incidence and twice the placebo rate) by treatment group during titration (Weeks 1-12) and maintenance (Weeks 13-26). The adverse events were generally mild in intensity, more frequent at higher doses, of short duration, and attenuated with continued dosing or discontinuation of drug.

Table 2: EXELON

Common Adverse Events (≥5% and twice the rate in the placebo group) in Randomized Placebo-Controlled Clinical Trials B351, B352, and B303 During Titration and Maintenance Phases[a]

	Titration Phase (Weeks 1–12)			Maintenance Phase (Weeks 13–26)		
Adverse Event	Placebo n=646 (%)	1–4 mg/day n=644 (%)	6–12 mg/day n=824 (%)	Placebo n=588 (%)	1–4 mg/day n=587 (%)	6–12 mg/day n=601 (%)
Nausea	9	15	40	4	8	15
Vomiting	3	5	23	3	5	14
Dizziness	10	10	19	4	6	10
Diarrhea	9	8	16	4	5	9
Anorexia	2	5	13	1	2	4

(cont'd)

Table 2: EXELON *(cont'd)*

Common Adverse Events (≥5% and twice the rate in the placebo group) in Randomized Placebo-Controlled Clinical Trials B351, B352, and B303 During Titration and Maintenance Phases[a]

	Titration Phase (Weeks 1–12)			Maintenance Phase (Weeks 13–26)		
Adverse Event	**Placebo n=646 (%)**	**1–4 mg/day n=644 (%)**	**6–12 mg/day n=824 (%)**	**Placebo n=588 (%)**	**1–4 mg/day n=587 (%)**	**6–12 mg/day n=601 (%)**
Abdominal Pain	4	5	10	3	3	4
Fatigue	4	4	8	1	2	3
Asthenia	2	1	6	1	2	3
Somnolence	2	4	5	1	1	1

[a] All patients who received at least one dose of study medication were included in the results for the titration phase. All patients who entered the maintenance phase were represented in the results for the maintenance phase.

Titration and maintenance dosing should remain flexible and be adjusted according to individual needs.

In an open label study involving 305 patients with Alzheimer's disease the tolerability of a 1.5 mg b.i.d. (3 mg/day) starting dose and dose escalation of 1.5 mg b.i.d. (3 mg/day) at a minimum interval of every two weeks were assessed. A total of 40 of these patients (13%) discontinued the study due to adverse events. The type and incidence of common adverse events reported did not appear to differ substantially from those noted in placebo-controlled studies.

Adverse Events Reported in Controlled Trials: The events cited reflect experience gained under closely monitored condition of clinical trials in a highly selected patient population. In actual clinical practice or in other clinical trials, these frequency estimates may not apply, as the conditions of use, reporting behavior, and the kinds of patients treated may differ. Table 3 lists treatment emergent signs and symptoms that were reported in at least 2% of patients in Phase 3 placebo-controlled trials for which the rate of occurrence was greater for EXELON assigned than placebo assigned patients. There were too few non Caucasian patients enrolled to assess the effect of race on the incidence of adverse events in the Phase III controlled studies. Similarly, there were too few patients aged more than 85 years to systematically assess the effect of advanced age. Female patients were more susceptible to nausea, vomiting, loss of appetite and weight loss.

Table 3: EXELON

Adverse Events Reported in Controlled Clinical Trials in at Least 2% of Patients Receiving EXELON and at a Higher Frequency Than Placebo-Treated Patients

Body System/ Adverse Event	Placebo (n=868)	EXELON (n=1923)
% of Patients with Any Adverse Event	79	87
Autonomic Nervous System		
Sweating Increased	1	3
Body as a Whole		
Fatigue	5	7
Asthenia	2	5
Malaise	2	4
Weight Decrease	<1	2
Cardiovascular Disorders, General		
Hypertension	2	3
Central and Peripheral Nervous Systems		
Dizziness	11	19
Headache	12	15
Somnolence	3	5
Tremor	1	3
Gastrointestinal System		
Nausea	12	37
Vomiting	6	23
Diarrhea	11	16
Anorexia	3	13
Abdominal Pain	6	11
Dyspepsia	4	8
Constipation	4	5
Flatulence	2	4
Eructation	1	2
Psychiatric Disorders		
Insomnia	7	8
Depression	4	5
Anxiety	3	4

(cont'd)

Table 3: EXELON *(cont'd)*

Adverse Events Reported in Controlled Clinical Trials in at Least 2% of Patients Receiving EXELON and at a Higher Frequency Than Placebo-Treated Patients

Body System/ Adverse Event	Placebo (n=868)	EXELON (n=1923)
Hallucination	3	4
Nervousness	3	4
Aggressive Reaction	2	3
Respiratory System		
Rhinitis	3	4
Dyspnea	1	2
Skin and Appendages		
Pruritus	1	2
Urinary System		
Urinary Incontinence	2	3
Micturition Frequency	1	2
Vision Disorders		
Vision Abnormal	1	2

Other Adverse Events Observed During Clinical Trials: EXELON has been administered to over 5297 individuals during clinical trials worldwide. Of these, 4326 patients have been treated for at least 3 months, 3407 patients have been treated for at least 6 months, 2150 patients have been treated for 1 year, 1250 have been treated for 2 years, and 168 have been treated for over 3 years. With regard to exposure to the highest dose, 1679 patients were exposed to mean daily doses of 10-12 mg, 1659 patients treated for 3 months, 1504 patients treated for 6 months, 885 patients treated for 1 year, 629 patients treated for 2 years, and 86 treated for over 3 years.

Treatment emergent signs and symptoms that occurred during 8 controlled clinical trials and 9 open-label trials in North America, Western Europe, Australia, South Africa and Japan were recorded as adverse events by the clinical investigators using terminology of their own choosing. To provide an overall estimate of the proportion of individuals having similar types of events, the events were grouped into a smaller number of standardized categories using a modified WHO dictionary, and event frequencies were calculated across all studies. These categories are used in the listing below. The frequencies represent the proportion of 5297 patients from these trials who experienced that event while receiving EXELON. All adverse events occurring at least 6 times are included, except for those already listed in Table 3, WHO terms too general to be informative, or events less likely to be drug caused. Events are classified by body system and listed using the following definitions: frequent adverse events—those occurring in at least 1/100 patients; infrequent adverse events—those occurring in 1/100 to 1/1000 patients. These adverse events are not necessarily related to EXELON treatment and in most cases were observed at a similar frequency in placebo-treated patients in the controlled studies.

Autonomic Nervous System: Frequent: syncope. Infrequent: cold clammy skin, dry mouth, flushing, increased saliva.

Body as a Whole: Frequent: accidental trauma, allergy, chest pain, edema, fever, hot flushes, influenza-like symptoms, overdose, rigors. Infrequent: allergic reaction, chest pain substernal, edema periorbital, facial edema, feeling cold, halitosis, hypothermia, inflammatory reaction unspecified, pain, pallor, tumor unspecified, unspecified eyelid disorder, weight increase.

Cardiovascular System: Frequent: angina pectoris, cardiac failure, hypotension, myocardial infarction, peripheral edema, postural hypotension. Infrequent: chest pain, coronary artery disorder, ECG abnormal, edema, generalized edema, heart sounds abnormal, myocardial ischemia.

Central and Peripheral Nervous System: Frequent: abnormal gait, ataxia, convulsions, extrapyramidal disorder, paresthesia, vertigo. Infrequent: abnormal coordination, aphasia, apraxia, cerebrovascular accident, coma, dysphonia, hyperkinesia, hyperreflexia, hypertonia, hypoesthesia, hypokinesia, hyporeflexia, involuntary muscle contractions, migraine, neuralgia, neuropathy, nystagmus, paresis, peripheral neuropathy, speech disorder.

Collagen Disorders: Infrequent: rheumatoid arthritis.

Endocrine System: Infrequent: goiter, hypothyroidism.

Gastrointestinal System: Frequent: fecal incontinence, gastritis, tooth disorder. Infrequent: colitis, colorectal polyp, diverticulitis, duodenal ulcer, dysphagia, esophagitis, gastric ulcer, gastroenteritis, gastroesophageal reflux, GI hemorrhage, gingivitis, glossitis, hematemesis, hernia, hiccup, increased appetite, intestinal obstruction, melena, pancreatitis, peptic ulcer, rectal disorder, rectal hemorrhage, tenesmus, tooth caries, ulcerative stomatitis.

Hearing and Vestibular Disorders: Frequent: tinnitus. Infrequent: deafness, earache, ear disorder unspecified, vestibular disorder.

Heart Rate and Rhythm Disorders: Frequent: bradycardia, fibrillation atrial, palpitation. Infrequent: arrhythmia, AV block, bundle branch block, cardiac arrest, extrasystoles, sick sinus syndrome, supraventricular tachycardia, tachycardia.

Injury, Poisoning and Procedural Complications: Infrequent: fall.

Liver and Biliary System Disorders: Infrequent: abnormal hepatic function, cholecystitis, cholelithiasis, increased gamma-glutamyl transferase, increased hepatic enzymes.

Metabolic and Nutritional Disorders: Frequent: dehydration, hypokalemia. Infrequent: cachexia, diabetes mellitus, gout, hypercholesterolemia, hyperglycemia, hyperlipemia, hypoglycemia, hyponatremia, thirst.

Musculoskeletal Disorders: Frequent: arthralgia, arthritis, back pain, bone fracture, leg cramps, leg pain, myalgia, pain. Infrequent: arthropathy, arthrosis, bone disorder, bone pain, bursitis, cramps, hernia, joint malformation, muscle weakness, osteoporosis, spine malformation, stiffness, tendinitis, tendon disorder, vertebral disc disorder.

Neoplasms: Frequent: basal cell carcinoma. Infrequent: bladder carcinoma, carcinoma, colon carcinoma, malignant breast neoplasm (female), malignant skin neoplasm, unspecified adenocarcinoma, unspecified neoplasm.

Platelet, Bleeding, and Clotting Disorders: Frequent: epistaxis. Infrequent: hematoma, purpura, thrombocytopenia, unspecified hemorrhage.

Psychiatric Disorders: Frequent: agitation, behavioral disturbance, confusion, delusion, paranoid reaction, paroniria. Infrequent: abnormal dreaming, amnesia, apathy, decreased libido, delirium, dementia, depersonalization, emotional lability, impaired concentration, increased libido, neurosis, psychosis, sleep disorder, stress reaction, suicidal ideation.

Red Blood Cell Disorders: Frequent: anemia. Infrequent: anemia B_{12} deficiency, hypochromic anemia.

Reproductive Disorders (Female & Male): Frequent: prostatic disorder. Infrequent: atrophic vaginitis, breast pain (female), impotence, intermenstrual bleeding, unspecified uterine disorder, vaginal hemorrhage, vaginitis.

Resistance Mechanism Disorders: Frequent: infection, pneumonia, upper respiratory tract infection, urinary tract infection, viral infection. Infrequent: bacterial infection, cellulitis, cystitis, fungal infection, herpes simplex, herpes zoster, moniliasis, onychomycosis, otitis media, parasitic infection, sepsis.

Respiratory System: Frequent: bronchitis, coughing, pharyngitis, sinusitis. Infrequent: abnormal chest sounds, apnea, bronchospasm, emphysema, hyperventilation, increased sputum, laryngitis, pleural effusion, pulmonary disorder, pulmonary edema, respiratory disorder, respiratory insufficiency.

Skin and Appendages: Frequent: rash, skin disorder, skin ulceration. Infrequent: abscess, acne, alopecia, bullous eruption, contact dermatitis, dermatitis, dry skin, eczema, erythematous rash, furunculosis, genital pruritus, hyperkeratosis, maculo-papular rash, nail disorder, otitis externa, psoriaform rash, seborrhea, skin cyst, skin discoloration, skin exfoliation, skin hypertrophy, sunburn, urticaria, verruca, skin irritation, toxic epidermal necrolysis, erythema, dermatitis allergic.

Special Senses: Infrequent: loss of taste, perversion of taste.

Urinary System Disorders: Frequent: hematuria. Infrequent: acute renal failure, albuminuria, dysuria, micturition disorder, micturition urgency, nocturia, polyuria, pyuria, renal calculus, renal cyst, renal function abnormal, unspecified bladder disorder, urethral disorder, urinary retention.
Vascular (extracardiac) Disorders: Frequent: cerebrovascular disorder. Infrequent: aneurysm, circulatory disorder, hemorrhoids, intracranial hemorrhage, peripheral ischemia, phlebitis, pulmonary embolism, thrombophlebitis deep, thrombosis, varicose vein, vascular disorder.
Vision Disorders: Frequent: cataract, conjunctivitis. Infrequent: abnormal lacrimation, blepharitis, conjunctival hemorrhage, diplopia, eye abnormality, eye pain, glaucoma.
White Cell and Resistance Disorders: Infrequent: leukocytosis, lymphadenopathy.
Dementia Associated with Parkinson's Disease: In the 24 week, double-blind, placebo-controlled trial, n=541 patients were randomized to drug or placebo (2:1 ratio). Of these, 73% of patients in the drug arm completed the study (i.e. did not discontinue from drug treatment), and 82% in the placebo arm. The mean duration of treatment for EXELON-treated patients was 144 days (range 4-197 days).

The overall AE profile of EXELON in this study was consistent with the known profile of patients with Alzheimer's disease, with the exception that frequency of tremor and worsening of Parkinson's disease symptoms in general, is greater compared to placebo. A number of factors beyond that of differing patient populations may affect comparison of AE rates between Alzheimer's disease and Parkinson's disease, including the protocol-specified differences in dosing between the Alzheimer's disease studies, and the sole Parkinson's disease study: a) greater time between dose escalations for the Parkinson's disease patients (4 weeks for Parkinson's disease patients vs 1-2 weeks for Alzheimer's disease patients) and b) lower doses specified for some Alzheimer's disease patients (minimum of 3 mg/day for the Parkinson's disease patients, vs minimum of 1 mg/day for some Alzheimer's disease patients).
Adverse Events Leading to Discontinuation: The rate of discontinuation due to adverse events in the single controlled trial of EXELON was 18.2% for patients receiving 3-12 mg/day compared to 11.2% for patients on placebo during the 24 week study. The most frequent adverse events that led to discontinuation from this study, defined as those occurring in at least 1% of patients receiving EXELON and more frequent than those receiving placebo, were nausea (3.6% EXELON vs 0.6% placebo), vomiting (1.9% EXELON vs 0.6% placebo), and tremor (1.7% EXELON vs 0.0% placebo).
Most Frequent Adverse Clinical Events: The most common adverse events, defined as those occurring at a frequency of at least 5% and twice the placebo rate, are largely predicted by EXELON's cholinergic effects. These include nausea, vomiting, tremor, anorexia, and dizziness.

Table 4 presents a comparison of common adverse events (≥5% incidence and twice the placebo rate) by treatment group during titration (Weeks 1-16) and maintenance (Weeks 17-24).

Table 4: EXELON

Common Adverse Events (≥5% and twice the rate in the placebo group) During the Single Controlled Clinical Trial, Breakdown by Titration and Maintenance Phases[a]

	Titration Phase (Weeks 1–16)		Maintenance Phase (Weeks 17–24)	
Adverse Event	Placebo n=179 %	EXELON n=362 %	Placebo n=158 %	EXELON n=281 %
Nausea	11	27	1	5
Vomiting	2	14	0	4
Tremor	3	9	1	1
Dizziness	1	6	0	<1
Anorexia	2	5	1	2

[a] All patients who received at least one dose of study medication were included in the results for the titration phase. All patients who entered the maintenance phase were represented in the results for the maintenance phase.

Adverse Events Reported in the Controlled Trial: The events cited reflect experience gained under the closely monitored condition of a clinical trial, in a highly selected patient population. In actual clinical practice or in other clinical trials, these frequency estimates may not apply, as the conditions of use, reporting behavior, and the kinds of patients treated may differ. Table 5 lists treatment emergent signs and symptoms that were reported in at least 2% of patients in the EXELON arm (doses of 3-12 mg/day) of placebo-controlled trials and for which the rate of occurrence was greater for patients treated with EXELON than for those treated with placebo. There were too few non-Caucasian patients enrolled to assess the effect of race on the incidence of adverse events in the study. Similarly, there were too few patients aged more than 85 years to systematically assess the effect of advanced age. Female patients were more susceptible to nausea, vomiting, loss of appetite and weight loss.

In general, adverse reactions were less frequent later in the maintenance phase of the treatment.

Table 5: EXELON

Adverse Events Reported in the Single Controlled Clinical Trial in at Least 2% of Patients Receiving EXELON (3–12 mg/day) and at a Higher Frequency than Placebo-Treated Patients

Body System/ Adverse Event	Placebo (n=179)	EXELON (n=362)
Percent of Patients with any Adverse Event	71	84
Gastrointestinal Disorders		
Nausea	11	29
Vomiting	2	17
Diarrhea	4	7
Upper Abdominal Pain	1	4
General Disorders and Administrative Site Conditions		
Fatigue	3	4
Asthenia	1	2
Metabolism and Nutritional Disorders		
Anorexia	3	6
Dehydration	1	2
Nervous System Disorders		
Tremor	4	10

(cont'd)

Table 5: EXELON *(cont'd)*

Adverse Events Reported in the Single Controlled Clinical Trial in at Least 2% of Patients Receiving EXELON (3–12 mg/day) and at a Higher Frequency than Placebo-Treated Patients

Body System/ Adverse Event	Placebo (n=179)	EXELON (n=362)
Dizziness	1	6
Headache	3	4
Somnolence	3	4
Parkinson's Disease (worsening)	1	3
Bradykinesia	2	2
Parkinsonism	1	2
Psychiatric Disorders		
Anxiety	1	4
Insomnia	2	3
Restlessness	2	2
Skin and Subcutaneous Tissue Disorders		
Hyperhidrosis	1	2

Extrapyramidal Symptoms: Like other cholinomimetics, EXELON may exacerbate or induce extrapyramidal symptoms. Worsening of these symptoms (including bradykinesia, dyskinesia, gait abnormality) and an increased incidence of, or severity of, tremor have been observed in patients with dementia associated with Parkinson's disease treated with EXELON. These events led to discontinuation of EXELON in some cases (e.g. discontinuations due to tremor 1.7% on EXELON vs 0% on placebo).

Table 6 lists the number and percentage of patients, from the single controlled study, who experienced pre-defined adverse events that may reflect worsening of Parkinson symptoms. Percentages are listed for those events for which EXELON was numerically higher than placebo; the remaining pre-defined events are listed at the end.

Table 6: EXELON

Pre-Defined Adverse Events That May Reflect Worsening of Parkinsonian Symptoms in Patients with Dementia Associated with Parkinson's Disease[a]

	EXELON n (%)	Placebo n (%)
Total patients studied	362 (100)	179 (100)
Total patients with pre-defined AE(s)	99 (27.3)	28 (15.6)
Tremor	37 (10.2)	7 (3.9)
Worsening of PD/parkinsonism	20 (5.5)	3 (1.7)
Bradykinesia	9 (2.5)	3 (1.7)
Salivary hypersecretion	5 (1.4)	0
Dyskinesia	5 (1.4)	1 (0.6)
Gait abnormality	5 (1.4)	0
Dystonia	3 (0.8)	1 (0.6)
Musculoskeletal stiffness	3 (0.8)	0
Extrapyramidal disorder	1 (0.3)	0
Hypokinesia	1 (0.3)	0
Movement disorder	1 (0.3)	0
Muscle rigidity	1 (0.3)	0
Rigors	1 (0.3)	0
Motor dysfunction	1 (0.3)	0

[a] Pre-defined events that were observed in the EXELON group, but not at a higher rate than for the placebo group, include fall, balance disorders, drooling, on and off phenomena, freezing phenomenon, hypertonia and dysarthria.

Of the reported tremor cases, approx 90% represent one episode, and 47.5% occurred within a week of a dose increase.

Analysis of data on extrapyramidal symptoms utilizing sub-populations of mild (Hoehn and Yahr stage 1.0 to 2.5) vs moderate to severe (Hoehn and Yahr stage 3.0 to 5.0) Parkinson's disease showed no apparent difference between the two sub-groups, except for:

a. From Table 6 above, a greater percentage of EXELON-treated patients in the moderate/severe group experienced the symptoms reflective of worsening of parkinsonian symptoms (32% vs 23%); this was due primarily to the AE "fall" (10% vs 1.6%, respectively) and the AE "worsening of parkinsonian symptoms" (4% vs 0.5%). This pattern was not apparent in the patients who were treated with placebo.
b. The percentage of patients for whom the AE of tremour was resolved during the study was less for the moderate to severe Parkinson's disease group compared to the mild group (47% vs 62%).

Clinical monitoring is recommended for these adverse events (see also Warning and Precautions, Worsening of Tremor and Other Extrapyramidal Symptoms and Dosage And Administration, Dosing Considerations).
Other Adverse Events Observed During Clinical Trials of Dementia Associated with Parkinson's Disease: EXELON has been administered to 485 individuals with dementia associated with Parkinson's disease during clinical trials worldwide. Of these, 413 patients have been treated for at least 3 months, 253 patients have been treated for at least 6 months, and 113 patients have been treated for 1 year.

Additional treatment emergent adverse events in patients with dementia associated with Parkinson's disease, occurring in at least 1 patient (approximately 0.3%) are listed below, excluding events that are already listed above for the dementia of the Alzheimer's type or elsewhere in labeling, WHO terms too general to be informative, relatively minor events, or events unlikely to be drug-caused. Events are classified by body system and listed using the following definitions: frequent adverse events—those occurring in at least 1/100 patients; infrequent adverse events—those occurring in 1/100 to 1/1000 patients. These adverse events are not necessarily related to EXELON treatment and in most cases were observed at a similar frequency in placebo-treated patients in the controlled studies.

Cardiovascular System: Frequent: chest pain. Infrequent: sudden cardiac death.

Central and Peripheral Nervous Systems: Frequent: dyskinesia, transient ischemic attack. Infrequent: dystonia, hemiparesis, epilepsy, restless leg syndrome.

Endocrine System: Infrequent: elevated prolactin level.

Gastrointestinal System: Frequent: dyspepsia. Infrequent: faecaloma, dysphagia, diverticulitis, peritonitis.

Hearing and Vestibular Disorders: Frequent: vertigo. Infrequent: Meniere's disease.

Heart Rate and Rhythm Disorders: Infrequent: Adam-Stokes syndrome.

Liver and Biliary System Disorders: Infrequent: elevated alkaline phosphatase level, elevated gamma-glutamyltransferase level.

Musculoskeletal Disorders: Frequent: back pain Infrequent: muscle stiffness, myoclonus, freezing phenomenon.

Psychiatric Disorders: Frequent: agitation, depression. Infrequent: delusion, insomnia.

Reproductive Disorders (Female & Male): Infrequent: endometrial hypertrophy, mastitis, prostatic adenoma.

Respiratory System: Frequent: dyspnoea. Infrequent: cough

Urinary System Disorders: Infrequent: urinary incontinence, neurogenic bladder.

Vascular (extracardiac) Disorders: Infrequent: vasovagal syncope, vasculitis.

Vision Disorders: Infrequent: blurred vision, blepharospasm, conjunctivitis, retinopathy.

Post-Market Adverse Drug Reactions: EXELON Capsules: Voluntary reports of adverse events temporally associated with EXELON that have been received since market introduction that are not listed above, and that may or may not be causally related to the drug include the following:

Skin and Appendages: Stevens-Johnson syndrome, blister.

Gastrointestinal System: Severe vomiting with esophageal rupture (see Warnings and Precautions, Gastrointestinal).

EXELON PATCH: The following additional adverse events have been identified based on post-marketing spontaneous reports and are not listed above. Because these reactions are reported voluntarily from a population of uncertain size, it is not always possible to reliably estimate their frequency.

Rarely reported: hypertension, application site hypersensitivity, urticaria, blister (including application site and generalized blistering), dermatitis allergic.

Very rarely reported: Worsening of Parkinson's disease in patients with Parkinson's disease who were treated with EXELON PATCH (see Warnings and Precautions); seizure; hepatic failure; Stevens-Johnson syndrome.

Overdose with rivastigmine resulting from medication errors and inappropriate use of EXELON PATCH (e.g. failure to remove the previous day's patch and application of multiple patches at a time) has been reported. As with medication errors and misuse in general, serious medical outcomes, including death, have been reported with EXELON PATCH (see Overdosage for details).

The typical symptoms reported in association with overdose include nausea, vomiting, diarrhea, hypertension, and hallucinations. Bradycardia and/or syncope, that may be associated with malaise or falls, may also occur (see Warnings and Precautions, General; Overdosage).

DRUG INTERACTIONS: Overview: Use with Anticholinergics: Because of their mechanism of action, cholinesterase inhibitors have the potential to interfere with the activity of anticholinergic medications and should not be used with other cholinomimetic drugs.

Use with Cholinomimetics and Other Cholinesterase Inhibitors: In view of its pharmacodynamic effects, rivastigmine should not be given concomitantly with other cholinomimetic drugs. A synergistic effect may be expected when cholinesterase inhibitors are given concurrently with succinylcholine, similar neuromuscular blocking agents or cholinergic agonists such as bethanechol.

Use with Other Psychoactive Drugs: In controlled clinical trials with EXELON few patients received neuroleptics, antidepressants or anticonvulsants, there is thus limited information concerning the interaction of EXELON with these drugs.

Anesthesia: EXELON as a cholinesterase inhibitor, is likely to exaggerate succinylcholine-type muscle relaxation during anesthesia.

Effect of EXELON on the Metabolism of Other Drugs: Rivastigmine is mainly metabolised through hydrolysis by esterases. No in vivo studies have investigated the effects of rivastigmine on the clearance of drugs metabolised by CYP450. Based on in vitro studies, no pharmacokinetic drug interactions with drugs metabolised by the following isoenzyme systems are expected: CYP1A2, CYP2D6, CYP3A4/5, CYP2E1, CYP2C9, CYP2C8, or CYP2C19.

Rivastigmine may inhibit the butyrylcholinesterase mediated metabolism of other drugs (see Actions and Clinical Pharmacology, Pharmacokinetics, Metabolism).

Effect of Other Drugs on the Metabolism of EXELON: Drugs which induce or inhibit CYP450 metabolism are not expected to alter the metabolism of rivastigmine. Formal pharmacokinetic studies to assess the potential for drug interaction with other medications commonly taken by the elderly were not done. Population-pharmacokinetic analyses of a subset (n=359; 6-12 mg/day) of patients with Alzheimer's disease in controlled clinical trials do not suggest that the administration of EXELON with some commonly prescribed medications is associated with an alteration in the kinetics of rivastigmine, or an increased risk of clinically relevant untoward effects. However, the number of patients who received concomitant medications chronically was as follows: anilides (e.g. acetaminophen) (10%), antacids (12%), antianginals (6%), antihistamines (2%), antihypertensives (12%), benzodiazepines (<1%), β-blockers (7%), calcium channel blockers (12%), digitalis glycosides (5%), non-steroidal anti-inflammatory drugs (13%), oral hypoglycemics (3%), and salicylic acid and derivatives (28%).

Drug-Drug Interactions: Studies to assess the potential of EXELON for interaction with digoxin, warfarin, diazepam or fluoxetine were limited to short term, single-dose studies in young healthy volunteers. No significant effects on the pharmacokinetics of these drugs or on the metabolism of rivastigmine were observed. Similar studies in elderly patients were not done.

DOSAGE AND ADMINISTRATION: Dosing Considerations:

- For elderly patients (>85 years old) with low body weight (especially females) or serious comorbid diseases (see Warnings and Precautions), it is recommended to start treatment with less frequent dosing (1.5 mg once a day) and to escalate dosage at a slower rate than for adults.
- For patients with renal or hepatic impairment (see Warnings and Precautions, Special Populations) it is recommended that treatment be started with less frequent dosing (1.5 mg once a day) and that dose escalation be slower than that recommended for adults.
- In a population of cognitively-impaired individuals, safe use of this and all other medications may require supervision.
- Adverse effects (e.g. hypertension and hallucinations in patients with Alzheimer's dementia, and worsening of extrapyramidal symptoms, in particular tremor, in patients with dementia associated with Parkinson's disease) have been observed shortly after dose increase. They may respond to a dose reduction. In other cases, EXELON has been discontinued.

Recommended Dose and Dosage Adjustment: EXELON (rivastigmine hydrogen tartrate) capsules and oral solution should only be prescribed by (or following consultation with) clinicians who are experienced in the diagnosis and management of dementia.

Adults: The usual maintenance dose range for EXELON is 6-12 mg/day. The following dosage escalation recommendations, derived from clinical trial data, are provided as a guide only, as individual tolerance to dose increases will vary. The incidence of cholinergic adverse events associated with EXELON increase with dose and are more prevalent in females (see Adverse Reactions).

Dementia of the Alzheimer's Type: The starting dose of EXELON is 1.5 mg b.i.d. (3 mg/day). If this initial dose is well tolerated, after a minimum of 2 weeks the dose may be increased to 3 mg b.i.d. (6 mg/day). Dose increases above 6 mg/day should proceed cautiously. Increases to 4.5 mg b.i.d. (9 mg/day) and then 6 mg b.i.d. (12 mg/day) should also be based on good tolerability of the current dose and should only be considered after a minimum of two weeks treatment at that dose level. The maximum dose should not exceed 6 mg b.i.d. (12 mg/day).

Dementia Associated with Parkinson's Disease: In dementia associated with Parkinson's disease, the starting dose of EXELON is 1.5 mg b.i.d.; subsequently, the dose may be increased to 3 mg b.i.d.; and further to 4.5 mg b.i.d.; and 6 mg b.i.d.; based on tolerability, with a minimum of 4 weeks at each dose.

Dose Interruption: Following initiation of therapy or any dosage increase, patients should be closely monitored for adverse effects. If adverse effects (e.g. nausea, vomiting, abdominal pain, loss of appetite) are observed during treatment, the patient should be instructed to stop treatment for several doses and then restart at the same dose level, or lower, as clinically indicated. Anytime treatment is interrupted for longer than several days, patients should be instructed to reinitiate treatment with the lowest daily dose (i.e. 1.5 mg b.i.d. or 1.5 mg o.d., as clinically indicated) and be re-titrated to their maintenance dose as described above (see Warnings and Precautions, Gastrointestinal). If side effects persist, the drug should be discontinued.

EXELON oral solution and capsules may be interchanged at equal doses.

EXELON should be taken with food in divided doses in the morning and evening.

Administration: Oral Solution: The prescribed amount of solution should be withdrawn from the container using the oral dosing syringe supplied. EXELON oral solution may be swallowed directly from the syringe or first mixed with a small glass of water, cold fruit juice or soda. Patients should be instructed to stir and drink the mixture.

OVERDOSAGE:

Symptoms: Overdosage with cholinesterase inhibitors can result in cholinergic crisis characterised by severe nausea, vomiting, diarrhoea, hypertension, hallucinations, salivation, sweating, hypotension, respiratory depression, collapse and convulsions. Increasing muscle weakness is a possibility and may result in death if respiratory muscles are involved. Due to the known vagotonic effect of cholinesterase inhibitors on heart rate, bracycardia and/or syncope may also occur.

Treatment: EXELON (rivastigmine hydrogen tartrate) has a short plasma half-life (about 1-2 hours) and a moderate duration of cholinesterase inhibition of 8-12 hours. It is recommended that in cases of asymptomatic overdoses, no further dose of EXELON should be administered for the next 24 hours and that patients be monitored.

As in any case of overdose, general supportive measures should be utilised. Tertiary anticholinergics such as atropine may be used as an antidote for EXELON overdosage. Intravenous atropine sulfate titrated to effect is recommended: an initial dose of 1.0 to 2.0 mg IV with subsequent doses based upon clinical response. Atypical responses in blood pressure and heart rate have been reported with other cholinomimetics when co-administered with quaternary anticholinergics such as glycopyrrolate. Due to the short half-life of EXELON, dialysis (hemodialysis, peritoneal dialysis, or hemofiltration) would not be clinically indicated in the event of an overdose.

In overdoses accompanied by severe nausea and vomiting, the use of antiemetics should be considered. In a documented case of a 46 mg overdose with EXELON, a 69 year old female patient experienced vomiting, incontinence, hypertension, psychomotor retardation and loss of consciousness. The patient was managed conservatively with only supportive measures and fully recovered within 24 hours.

In a documented case of medication error leading to overdose with EXELON PATCH, an 87 year old male patient on a prescribed maintenance dose of one EXELON PATCH 10 (9.5 mg/24 hrs) per day was accidentally administered 6 patches per day on two consecutive days. The patient experienced vomiting, fall and hyperhidrosis and was hospitalized on the second day. At the time of hospitalization he presented with an elevated creatinine level (149 µmol/L; normal range: 70-115 µmol/L) and signs of urinary infection. He was treated by removal of all patches and ciprofloxacin was initiated. Subsequently, the patient developed acute renal failure with anuria and died approximately 14 days after hospitalization. The reporter suspected that overdose contributed to the patient's dehydration and renal failure. Autopsy results were not provided by the reporter.

Dose-related signs of toxicity in animals included lacrimation, excessive salivation, vomiting, decreased locomotor activity, ataxia, twitches/flutters, tremors and clonic convulsions.

> For management of a suspected drug overdose, contact your regional Poison Control Centre. See the *CPS* Directory section for a list of Poison Control Centres.

ACTION AND CLINICAL PHARMACOLOGY: Mechanism of Action: Pathological changes in dementia of the Alzheimer type involve cholinergic neuronal pathways that project from the basal forebrain to the cerebral cortex and hippocampus. A decrease in the function of these cholinergic pathways has been proposed to account for some of the clinical manifestations of dementia. Rivastigmine, a reversible cholinesterase inhibitor of the carbamate-type, is thought to enhance cholinergic neurotransmission by slowing the degradation of acetylcholine released by cholinergic neurons through the inhibition of acetylcholinesterase. If this proposed mechanism of action is correct, rivastigmine's effect may lessen as the disease process advances and fewer cholinergic neurons remain functionally intact.

There is no evidence that rivastigmine alters the course of the underlying dementing process.

Pharmacokinetics: Absorption: Rivastigmine is well absorbed and peak plasma concentrations (C_{max}) are reached in approximately 1 hour. A doubling of the dose within the recommended dose range yields an increase in bioavailability by approximately 3 times the expected increase indicating non-linear pharmacokinetics. The estimated absolute bioavailability for a 3 mg dose in healthy young patients is low (<35%). The elimination half-life ($t_{½}$) of rivastigmine is about 1 to 2 hours in both the young and elderly. Plasma clearance is dose dependent and is approximately 1 L/h/kg at 3 mg in healthy young subjects. In healthy elderly male patients, plasma rivastigmine levels are approximately 30% higher than that noted in young subjects (see Pharmacokinetics, Special Populations and Conditions, Age). When administered with food to healthy young subjects the absorption (T_{max}) of rivastigmine was delayed by 90 min, and C_{max} was lowered while the $AUC_{0-\infty}$ was increased by approximately 25%.

Distribution: Rivastigmine is approximately 40% bound to plasma proteins over a concentration range of 1-to-400 ng/mL. Rivastigmine distributes equally between blood and plasma with a blood-to-plasma partition ratio of 0.9 at concentrations which cover the therapeutic range (1-400 ng/mL). The apparent volume of distribution is 5±3 L/kg. Rivastigmine can be detected in the CSF, reaching peak concentrations in 1-4 hours. Mean AUC_{0-12hr} ratio of CSF/plasma averaged 40±0.5% following 1-6 mg bid doses.

Metabolism: Rivastigmine is subject to first pass clearance and is rapidly and extensively metabolised, primarily via esterase-, including acetylcholinesterase-, mediated hydrolysis to a decarbamylated phenolic metabolite. In vitro preclinical studies suggest that the decarbamylated phenolic metabolite has approximately 10% the activity of the parent compound. The plasma half-life of the decarbamylated phenolic metabolite ranges from 2.5 to 4 hours. Additional metabolites include a sulphate conjugate, a demethylated sulfate conjugate and several unidentified minor metabolites.

Evidence from in vitro studies suggest that the major cytochrome P450 isozymes are minimally involved in rivastigmine metabolism (see Drug Interactions, Overview).

Rivastigmine inhibits acetylcholinesterase (AChE) and butyrylcholinesterase (BuChE) activity. In patients with Alzheimer's disease significant dose-dependent inhibition of AChE and BuChE activity were noted in cerebrospinal fluid, with comparable maximum mean inhibition (62%). In plasma, significant inhibition of BuChE activity is generally observed from 1.5 hours post-dose up to 8 hours post-dose, with a maximum observed inhibition of 51% at 5 mg b.i.d. Rivastigmine may therefore inhibit the butyrylcholinesterase mediated metabolism of other drugs (see Drug Interactions, Overview).

Excretion: Unchanged rivastigmine is not found in the urine; renal excretion is the major route of elimination of the metabolites. Following administration of a single 1 mg or 2.5 mg dose of ^{14}C-labelled rivastigmine, excretion of radioactivity in the urine (expressed as a percent of the administered dose) is over 90% within 24 hours. Approximately 7% of the decarbamylated phenolic metabolite is found in the urine. The sulfate conjugates account for about 40% of the dose. Less than 1% of the administered dose is excreted in the faeces. The accumulation potential of rivastigmine and its decarbamylated phenolic metabolite in patients with Alzheimer's disease has not been systematically studied however, population pharmacokinetic analyses suggest that no accumulation is expected.

Special Populations and Conditions: Age: In a study in which the effect of age on the pharmacokinetics of rivastigmine was assessed, 24 healthy male elderly (age range: 61-71 years) and 24 healthy young patients (age range: 19-40 years) received 1.0 mg or 2.5 mg single oral doses of rivastigmine under fasted conditions. Plasma concentrations of rivastigmine exhibited a wider range of values and tended to be higher in the elderly as compared to young subjects after the 1 mg dose. This difference was more pronounced with the higher dose (2.5 mg) at which rivastigmine plasma concentrations were 30% greater in the elderly than in young subjects. Plasma levels of the decarbamylated phenolic metabolite were not substantially affected by age.

Gender and Race: No specific pharmacokinetic study was conducted to investigate the effect of gender and race on the disposition of rivastigmine. However, retrospective pharmacokinetic analyses suggest that gender and race (Blacks, Oriental, and Caucasians) will not affect the clearance of rivastigmine.

Hepatic Insufficiency: In a single dose study of 10 subjects with biopsy proven liver impairment (Child-Pugh score of 5-12), plasma concentrations of rivastigmine were increased, while that of the decarbamylated phenolic metabolite were decreased by about 60% compared to an age, weight and gender matched control group. The safety and efficacy of rivastigmine in patients with hepatic impairment have not been studied (see Warnings and Precautions, Special Populations).

Renal Insufficiency: In a single-dose study of 8 subjects with moderate renal impairment (GFR=10-50 mL/min) mean peak plasma concentrations of rivastigmine were increased by almost 2.5 fold and overall plasma levels (AUC) of the decarbamylated phenolic metabolite were increased by approximately 50% compared to levels in age, weight, and gender matched control subjects. In this same study, patients with severe renal impairment (GFR <10 mL/min, n=8) showed no difference in rivastigmine blood levels compared to controls. The reason for this discrepancy is unclear. The safety and efficacy of rivastigmine in patients with renal impairment have not been studied (see Warnings and Precautions, Special Populations).

Genetic Polymorphism: The pharmacokinetics of rivastigmine in patients with butyrylcholinesterase enzyme deficiency are unknown (see Warnings and Precautions, Genetic Polymorphism).

Nicotine Use: Population PK analysis showed that nicotine use increases the clearance of oral rivastigmine by 23% (Smokers: n=75; Nonsmokers: n=549).

STORAGE AND STABILITY: Capsules: Store at room temperature (15-30°C).

Oral Solution: Store at room temperature (15-30°C) in original package in an upright position.

INFORMATION FOR THE PATIENT: Published in e-CPS, available by subscription at www.e-cps.ca.

DOSAGE FORMS, COMPOSITION AND PACKAGING: Capsules: 1.5 mg: Each yellow hard gelatin capsule, the strength (1.5 mg) and "Exelon" printed in red on the body of the capsule contains: rivastigmine 1.5 mg (as rivastigmine hydrogen tartrate). Nonmedicinal ingredients: hydroxypropyl methylcellulose, magnesium stearate, microcrystalline cellulose and silicon dioxide; capsule: gelatin, red iron oxide and/or yellow iron oxide and titanium dioxide. Blister strips of 14, cartons of 4.

3 mg: Each orange hard gelatin capsule, the strength (3 mg) and "Exelon" printed in red on the body of the capsule contains: rivastigmine 3 mg (as rivastigmine hydrogen tartrate). Nonmedicinal ingredients: hydroxypropyl methylcellulose, magnesium stearate, microcrystalline cellulose and silicon dioxide; capsule: gelatin, red iron oxide and/or yellow iron oxide and titanium dioxide. Blister strips of 14, cartons of 4.

4.5 mg: Each red hard gelatin capsule, the strength (4.5 mg) and "Exelon" printed in white on the body of the capsule contains: rivastigmine 4.5 mg (as rivastigmine hydrogen tartrate). Nonmedicinal ingredients: hydroxypropyl methylcellulose, magnesium stearate, microcrystalline cellulose and silicon dioxide; capsule: gelatin, red iron oxide and/or yellow iron oxide and titanium dioxide. Blister strips of 14, cartons of 4.

6 mg: Each orange and red hard gelatin capsule, the strength (6 mg) and "Exelon" printed in red on the body of the capsule contains: rivastigmine 6 mg (as rivastigmine hydrogen tartrate). Nonmedicinal ingredients: hydroxypropyl methylcellulose, magnesium stearate, microcrystalline cellulose and silicon dioxide; capsule: gelatin, red iron oxide and/or yellow iron oxide and titanium dioxide. Blister strips of 14, cartons of 4.

Oral Solution: Each mL of clear, yellow solution contains: rivastigmine 2 mg (as rivastigmine hydrogen tartrate). Nonmedicinal ingredients: citric acid, purified water, quinoline yellow WS dye E104, sodium benzoate and sodium citrate. Amber glass bottles of 120 mL with a dip tube and self-aligning plug. The oral solution is packaged with a dispenser set which consists of an assembled oral dosing syringe calibrated in mg that allows dispensing a maximum volume of 3 mL corresponding to a 6 mg dose, with a plastic tube container.

(Shown in Product Identification Section)

Exelon® Patch 5 Pr
rivastigmine
Cholinesterase Inhibitor

Novartis Pharmaceuticals

Exelon® Patch 10 Pr
rivastigmine
Cholinesterase Inhibitor

Novartis Pharmaceuticals

Date of Revision: May 18, 2010

SUMMARY PRODUCT INFORMATION:

Route of Administration	Dosage Form/Strength	Nonmedicinal Ingredients
Transdermal	EXELON PATCH 5, each patch of 5 cm² contains 9 mg rivastigmine base, in vivo release rate of 4.6 mg/24 h EXELON PATCH 10, each patch of 10 cm² contains 18 mg rivastigmine base, in vivo release rate of 9.5 mg/24 h	Acrylic copolymer, poly(butylmethacrylate, methyl-methacrylate), silicone adhesive applied to a flexible polymer backing film, silicone oil, and vitamin E

INDICATIONS AND CLINICAL USE: EXELON PATCH (rivastigmine) is indicated for the symptomatic treatment of patients with mild to moderate dementia of the Alzheimer's type.

EXELON PATCH has not been studied in controlled clinical trials for longer than 6 months.

EXELON PATCH should only be prescribed by (or following consultation with) clinicians who are experienced in the diagnosis and management of Alzheimer's disease.

Geriatrics: Age had no impact on the exposure to rivastigmine in Alzheimer's disease patients treated with EXELON PATCH.

Pediatrics (<18 years of age): No data are available in children. Therefore, the use of EXELON PATCH is not recommended in children under 18 years of age.

CONTRAINDICATIONS:

- Patients with known hypersensitivity to rivastigmine, other carbamate derivatives or other components of the formulation. For a complete listing, see Dosage Forms, Composition and Packaging.
- Patients with severe liver impairment since rivastigmine has not been studied in this population.

WARNINGS AND PRECAUTIONS: General: Overdose with rivastigmine resulting from medication errors and inappropriate use of EXELON PATCH (e.g. failure to remove the previous day's patch before applying a new patch and application of multiple patches at a time) has been reported. As with medication errors and misuse in general, serious medical outcomes, including death, have been reported with EXELON PATCH.

The typical symptoms reported in association with overdose include nausea, vomiting, diarrhea, hypertension, and hallucinations. Bradycardia and/or syncope, that may be associated with malaise or falls, may also occur (see Adverse Reactions, Post-Market Adverse Drug Reactions; Overdosage).

In a population of cognitively-impaired individuals, safe use of this medication may require supervision. Patients and caregivers should be instructed in the proper use of EXELON PATCH (see Warnings and Precautions, Information to Be Provided to the Patient).

The incidence and severity of adverse events generally increases with increasing dose, particularly at dose changes. If treatment is interrupted for more than a few days, it should be reinitiated with EXELON PATCH 5 (rivastigmine).

As with other cholinergic substances care must be taken when prescribing EXELON PATCH:

- To patients with sick sinus syndrome or conduction defects (sino-atrial block, atrio-ventricular block) (see Cardiovascular).
- To patients with active gastric or duodenal ulcers or patients predisposed to these conditions because gastric acid secretions may be increased (see Gastrointestinal).
- To patients predisposed to urinary obstruction and seizures because cholinomimetics may induce or exacerbate these diseases (see Neurologic).
- To patients with a history of asthma or obstructive pulmonary disease (see Respiratory).

EXELON PATCH has not been studied in patients with severe Alzheimer's disease, non Alzheimer dementias or individuals with dementia associated with Parkinson's disease. The efficacy and safety of EXELON PATCH in these patient populations is unknown (see Adverse Reactions, Post-Market Adverse Drug Reactions).

Contact with the eyes should be avoided after handling EXELON PATCH.

Anesthesia: EXELON PATCH (rivastigmine) as a cholinesterase inhibitor, is likely to exaggerate succinylcholine-type muscle relaxation during anesthesia.

Low Body Weight: Patients with body weight below 50 kg may experience more adverse events and may be more likely to discontinue due to adverse events. Particular caution should be exercised when titrating these patients to the maintenance dose.

Cardiovascular: Because of their pharmacological action, cholinomimetics may have vagotonic effects on heart rate (e.g., bradycardia). The potential for this action may be particularly important to patients with "sick sinus syndrome" or other supraventricular cardiac conduction conditions. In clinical trials patients with serious cardiovascular disease were excluded. Caution should therefore be exercised in treating patients with active coronary artery disease or congestive heart failure. Syncopal episodes have been reported in association with the use of EXELON capsules and EXELON PATCH. It is recommended that EXELON PATCH not be used in patients with cardiac conduction abnormalities (except for right bundle branch block) including "sick sinus syndrome" and those with unexplained syncopal episodes.

Gastrointestinal: Treatment with EXELON PATCH at higher than recommended doses is associated with significant gastrointestinal adverse reactions, including nausea, vomiting, diarrhea, anorexia/decreased appetite and weight loss (see Adverse Reactions). Due to the risk of gastrointestinal adverse reactions treatment should always be started with EXELON PATCH 5. A dose increase to EXELON PATCH 10, the maximum recommended maintenance dose, should only occur after a minimum of 4 weeks of treatment with EXELON PATCH 5 and if well tolerated. If treatment is interrupted for longer than a few days, treatment should be reinitiated with EXELON PATCH 5 to reduce the possibility of severe vomiting and its potentially serious sequelae (e.g., there have been very rare postmarketing reports of severe vomiting with esophageal rupture following oral administration) (see Dosage and Administration).

Caregivers should be advised of the high incidence of nausea and vomiting associated with the use of the EXELON PATCH at higher than recommended doses along with the possibility of anorexia and weight loss (see Adverse Reactions). Caregivers should be encouraged to monitor for these adverse events and inform the physician if they occur. It is critical to inform caregivers that if therapy has been interrupted for more than a few days, the next dose should not be administered until they have discussed this with the physician.

Nausea and Vomiting: Gastrointestinal disorders such as nausea and vomiting may occur when initiating treatment and/or increasing the dose. Patients may respond to a dose reduction. In other cases, use of EXELON PATCH has been discontinued.

In the controlled clinical trial, 7% of patients treated with the EXELON PATCH 10 developed nausea, as compared to 23% of patients who received the EXELON capsule at doses up to 6 mg BID and 5% of those who received placebo. In the same clinical trial, 6% of patients treated with EXELON PATCH 10 developed vomiting, as compared with 17% of patients who received the EXELON capsule at doses up to 6 mg BID and 3% of those who received placebo.

The proportion of patients who discontinued treatment due to vomiting was 0% of the patients who received the EXELON PATCH 10 as compared to 2% of patients who received the EXELON capsule at doses up to 6 mg BID and 0% of those who received placebo. Vomiting was severe in 0% of patients who received the EXELON PATCH 10 and 1% of patients who received the EXELON capsule at doses up to 6 mg BID and 0% of those who received placebo. In this study, patients treated with a higher dose of the patch (EXELON PATCH 20) experienced nausea and vomiting at higher frequencies than patients treated with EXELON PATCH 10 (see Adverse Reactions; Dosage and Administration).

Diarrhea: In the controlled clinical trial, 6% of the patients treated with the EXELON PATCH 10 developed diarrhea, as compared with 5% of patients who received the EXELON capsule at doses up to 6 mg BID, and 3% of those who received placebo.

Anorexia/Decreased Appetite: In the controlled clinical trial, 3% of the patients treated with the EXELON PATCH 10 were recorded as developing decreased appetite or anorexia, as compared with 9% of patients who received the EXELON capsule at doses up to 6 mg BID and 2% of those who received placebo.

Weight Loss: Cholinesterase inhibitors as well as Alzheimer's disease can be associated with significant weight loss. Where weight loss may be of clinical concern, body weight should be monitored.

In the controlled clinical trial, 3% of the patients treated with EXELON PATCH 10 had a decreased weight, as compared with 5% of patients who received the EXELON capsule at doses up to 6 mg BID and 1% of those who received placebo. The proportion of patients who had weight loss equal to or greater than 7% of their baseline weight was 8% (5.4% males and 9.6% females) of those treated with EXELON PATCH 10 compared with 11% of patients (9.9% males and 11.4% females) who received the EXELON capsule at doses up to 6 mg BID and 6% (5.0% males and 6.5% females) of those who received placebo.

Peptic Ulcers/Gastrointestinal Bleeding: Through their primary action, cholinesterase inhibitors may be expected to increase gastric acid secretion due to increased cholinergic activity. Therefore, patients should be monitored for symptoms of active or occult gastrointestinal bleeding, especially those at increased risk for developing ulcers, e.g., those with a history of ulcer disease or those receiving concurrent nonsteroidal anti-inflammatory drugs (NSAIDS). Clinical studies of EXELON PATCH have shown no significant increase, relative to placebo, in the incidence of either peptic ulcer disease or gastrointestinal bleeding.

Genetic Polymorphism: The effect of genetic polymorphism of butyrylcholinesterase enzyme on rivastigmine metabolism is unknown.

Genitourinary: Although not reported in clinical trials of EXELON, cholinomimetics may cause bladder spasms.

Neurologic: Seizures: Cholinomimetics are believed to have some potential to cause generalized convulsions. However, seizure activity also may be a manifestation of Alzheimer's disease. The risk/benefit of EXELON PATCH treatment for patients with a history of seizure disorder must therefore be carefully evaluated (see Adverse Reactions, Post-Market Adverse Drug Reactions).

Extrapyramidal symptoms: Like other cholinomimetics, rivastigmine may exacerbate extrapyramidal symptoms. Worsening of parkinsonian symptoms, particularly tremor, has been observed in patients with dementia associated with Parkinson's disease who were treated with EXELON capsules. Such adverse events may also occur with EXELON PATCH. EXELON PATCH is not indicated for the treatment of dementia associated with Parkinson's disease (see Adverse Reactions, Post-Market Adverse Drug Reactions).

In the EXELON PATCH controlled clinical trial 1.4% of patients treated with EXELON PATCH 10 and 0.3% of patients treated with placebo experienced extrapyramidal symptoms including tremor, bradykinesia, dyskinesia and rigidity. Most patients who experienced extrapyramidal symptoms were treated concomitantly with antipsychotics.

Effects on Ability to Drive and Use Machines: Alzheimer's disease may cause gradual impairment of driving performance or compromise the ability to use machinery. Rivastigmine may induce dizziness and somnolence, mainly when initiating treatment or increasing the dose. Therefore, in patients with dementia treated with rivastigmine, the ability to continue driving or operating complex machines should be routinely evaluated by the treating physician.

Pancreatic: In the pivotal clinical trial involving AD patients treated with the EXELON PATCH, acute pancreatitis was reported as an adverse event for one patient treated with EXELON capsule (0.3%) during double-blind treatment and one patient treated with EXELON PATCH (0.2%) during open label treatment. Cases of pancreatitis have also been reported during postmarketing experience with EXELON PATCH and EXELON capsules shortly after initial use as well as after several months or years of use.

Patients experiencing persistent and unexplained upper abdominal pain, that may or may not be accompanied by vomiting and confusion, should promptly seek medical attention.

Respiratory: Like other cholinomimetic drugs, EXELON PATCH should be used with care in patients with a history of asthma or obstructive pulmonary disease. No experience is available in treating patients with these conditions.

Skin: Application site hypersensitivity, urticaria, blister (including application site and generalized blistering), dermatitis allergic have been reported with the use of EXELON PATCH. These skin reactions may occur at any time during treatment. During postmarketing experience there have been reports of hypersensitivity type skin reactions with EXELON PATCH that worsened when patients were converted to oral EXELON (see Adverse Reactions, Skin Irritation, Post-Market Adverse Drug Reactions).

Laboratory Values: Laboratory values were not systematically evaluated during the controlled clinical trial with EXELON PATCH after screening.

Modest elevations in serum amylase and lipase in a clinical trial with EXELON capsules in patients with dementia associated with Parkinson's disease were seen more frequently with EXELON capsule-treatment than in patients receiving placebo. These elevations were not associated with clinical consequences.

Information to Be Provided to the Patient: Consumer Information is included in the package of EXELON PATCH dispensed to the patient.

Patients receiving EXELON PATCH and caregivers should be given the following instructions by the physician:

1. **Importance of Correct Usage**
   Patients or caregivers should be **advised** of the importance of applying the correct dose on the correct part of their body. They should be instructed to **remove any used EXELON PATCH before applying a new one and to apply only one patch per day to one site**. Only one patch should be worn per day to avoid the risk of overdose (see Warnings and Precautions; Adverse Reactions and Overdosage).
   The application site should be rotated in order to minimize skin irritation. The same site should not be used within 14 days. Patches should be replaced every 24 hours and the time of day should be consistent. It may be helpful for this to be part of a daily routine, such as the daily bath or shower.
   Patients or caregivers should be told to avoid exposure of the patch to external heat sources (excess sunlight, saunas, solarium) for long periods of time.
2. **Discarding Used Patches**
   Patients or caregivers should be instructed to fold the patch in half after use and to discard it out of the reach and sight of children and pets. They should also be informed that drug still remains in the patch after 24-hour usage. They should be instructed to avoid eye contact and to wash their hands after handling the patch.
3. **Concomitant Use of Drugs with Cholinergic Action**
   Patients or caregivers should be told that while wearing EXELON PATCH they should not be taking EXELON capsules or other drugs with cholinergic effects.
4. **Gastrointestinal Adverse Events**
   Patients or caregivers should be informed of the potential gastrointestinal adverse events such as nausea, vomiting and diarrhea. Patients and caregivers should be instructed to observe for these adverse reactions at all times, and in particular when treatment is initiated or the dose is increased. Patients and caregivers should be instructed to inform their physician if these adverse events persist as a dose adjustment/reduction may be required.
5. **Monitoring the Patient's Weight**
   Patients or caregivers should be informed that the EXELON PATCH may affect the patient's appetite and/or the patient's weight. Any loss of appetite or weight reduction needs to be monitored.

6. **Missed Doses**
   If the patient has missed a dose, he/she should be instructed to apply a new patch immediately. They may apply the next patch at the usual time the next day, after removing the previous day's patch. Patients should not apply two EXELON patches to make up for one missed. If treatment has been missed for several days, the patient or caregiver should be informed to restart treatment with the starting patch dose of 4.6 mg/24 hours (EXELON PATCH 5). Titration to the next patch dose should proceed after 4 weeks (see Dosage and Administration).

Special Populations: Pregnant Women: The safety of EXELON in pregnant women has not been established. EXELON PATCH should not be used in women of childbearing potential unless, in the opinion of the physician, the potential benefit to the patient justifies the potential risk to the fetus.

Nursing Women: It is not known whether rivastigmine is excreted into human milk, and therefore EXELON PATCH should not be used in nursing mothers. ^{14}CRivastigmine was excreted into the milk of pregnant rats after a single oral dose. In rats given rivastigmine orally, concentrations of rivastigmine plus metabolites were approximately two times higher in milk than in plasma.

Pediatrics: The safety and effectiveness of EXELON in any illness occurring in pediatric patients have not been established.

Geriatrics: Age had no impact on the exposure to rivastigmine in Alzheimer's disease patients treated with EXELON PATCH.

Hepatic Impairment: No study was conducted with the EXELON PATCH in subjects with hepatic impairment (see Action and Clinical Pharmacology, Pharmacokinetics, Special Populations and Conditions). Patients with clinically significant hepatic impairment might experience more adverse events.

Renal Impairment: No study was conducted with the EXELON PATCH in subjects with renal impairment (see Action and Clinical Pharmacology, Pharmacokinetics, Special Populations and Conditions).

Comorbid Disease: Use in elderly patients with serious comorbid disease has not been studied in large phase III-IV clinical studies. The use of EXELON in Alzheimer's disease patients with chronic illnesses common among the geriatric population, should be considered after careful risk/benefit assessment and dose escalation in this patient population should proceed with caution.

Patients with Vascular Dementia: Patients diagnosed with probable vascular dementia, according to NINDS-AIREN criteria, were randomized to double-blind treatment with EXELON capsules (3-12 mg/day, N=363) or placebo (N=344) for 6 months in a controlled clinical trial. The NINDS-AIREN criteria are designed to identify patients with dementia that appears to be due primarily to vascular causes, and to exclude patients with Alzheimer's disease. Overall, EXELON was not shown to be an effective treatment for patients with vascular dementia in this study.

The study also showed that the overall rate of occurrence of treatment emergent adverse events was lower in vascular dementia patients than what was observed previously in Alzheimer's disease patients. However, rates of serious adverse events were generally greater for vascular dementia patients compared to mild to moderate Alzheimer's disease patients for both EXELON and placebo groups, and may relate to the greater number of co-morbid medical conditions in the vascular dementia population.

In vascular dementia patients, higher rates of all-cause mortality (2.2% on EXELON vs 1.2% on placebo) and certain cardiovascular and cerebrovascular adverse events such as, angina pectoris, myocardial infarction, coronary artery disease, hypertension, dysarthria and cerebrovascular accident were observed in patients who were treated with EXELON compared to those who received placebo. The majority of deaths in patients taking either EXELON or placebo resulted from either cardiovascular or cerebrovascular disorders or respiratory failures.

ADVERSE REACTIONS: Clinical Trial Adverse Drug Reactions: Because clinical trials are conducted under very specific conditions the adverse reaction rates observed in the clinical trials may not reflect the rates observed in practice and should not be compared to the rates in the clinical trials of another drug. Adverse drug reaction information from clinical trials is useful for identifying drug-related adverse events and for approximating rates.

In the single controlled clinical trial with the EXELON PATCH, 1190 patients were treated with EXELON PATCH 20, EXELON PATCH 10, EXELON capsule and placebo. The overall incidence of adverse events in patients treated with EXELON PATCH 10 (rivastigmine) was lower than the rate in patients who received EXELON PATCH 20 and EXELON capsule treatment. Nausea and vomiting were the most common adverse events in patients who received active treatment, and occurred at similar rates in both EXELON PATCH 20 and capsule groups. The rates of both these events were substantially lower in the EXELON PATCH 10 group compared to the EXELON PATCH 20 and EXELON capsule groups.

Adverse Events Leading to Discontinuation: Overall, 11% of patients treated with EXELON PATCH 10, 10% of patients treated with EXELON PATCH 20, 9% of patients treated with EXELON capsule, compared to 6% of patients treated with placebo discontinued from the EXELON PATCH controlled clinical trial, due to adverse events. During the titration phase the incidence of discontinuations due to adverse events was 3.6% for placebo, 6.8% for EXELON capsule, 9.6% for EXELON PATCH 10, and 7.3% for EXELON PATCH 20. During the maintenance phase, 2.5% of patients who received placebo, 2.0% of patients who received EXELON capsule, 1.2% of patients who received EXELON PATCH 10, and 3.8% of patients who received EXELON PATCH 20 withdrew due to adverse events.

The most frequent adverse events leading to discontinuation from this study, defined as those occurring in at least 1% of patients receiving EXELON PATCH 20 or EXELON PATCH 10 and more frequent than those receiving placebo, were nausea, vomiting, anorexia, weight decreased, asthenia, application site pruritus, cerebrovascular accident, dizziness, syncope, agitation, anxiety, delirium, erythema and pruritus. Only nausea and vomiting resulted in discontinuation of >1% of patients in an EXELON PATCH treatment group (nausea-EXELON PATCH 20 2% vs placebo 1%; vomiting-EXELON PATCH 20 2% vs placebo <1%). All other adverse events leading to discontinuation occurred in 1% of patients treated with EXELON PATCH and <1% of patients who received placebo.

Most Frequent Adverse Events: The most commonly reported adverse events, defined as those occurring at a frequency of at least 5% in the EXELON PATCH groups and twice the placebo rate, are largely predicted by EXELON's cholinomimetic effects. These are nausea, vomiting and diarrhea. All of these events were more common in the titration phase than during the maintenance phase.

Table 1 presents a comparison of common adverse events (≥5% incidence and twice the placebo rate in the EXELON PATCH groups) by treatment group during titration (weeks 1-16) and maintenance (weeks 17-24) phases.

Table 2 shows the adverse events (≥2% in EXELON PATCH groups) from the 24-week clinical trial conducted with EXELON PATCH in patients with Alzheimer's disease.

Skin Irritation: In clinical trials, skin reactions were measured at each visit using a skin irritation rating scale that rated the degree of erythema, edema, scaling, fissures, pruritus and pain/stinging/burning at the application site. The most commonly observed symptom was erythema which disappeared within 24 hours in the vast majority of patients. During a 24-week double-blind study, symptoms or signs (skin irritation scale) of skin irritation were mainly erythema or pruritus and were mostly slight or mild in severity. Skin irritation rated as severe was observed on at least one occasion in ≤2.2% of EXELON PATCH patients, versus ≤1.0% of placebo patch. Most skin reactions were limited to the application site and resulted in discontinuation in only 2.4% of the patients on EXELON PATCH 10. Among the skin reactions reported as adverse events were the following: application site reactions, application site dermatitis, application site irritation, application site pruritus, application site erythema, application site eczema and peripheral edema. Adverse events reported for more than one patient on any treatment included application site erythema [4 patients (1%) EXELON PATCH 20], application site pruritus [3 patients (1%) EXELON PATCH 20], and application site irritation [2 patients (0.7%) EXELON PATCH 10].

In one crossover trial in 40 healthy volunteers, the application of the patch to the abdomen or outer thigh was more likely to result in skin irritation (mild to moderate erythema), whereas application to the upper arm and chest was less likely to cause skin irritation when compared to application to the upper back (see also Actions and Clinical Pharmacology, Absorption, for effect of application site on plasma concentrations).

Cerebrovascular Accident: In the pivotal clinical trial involving mild to moderate Alzheimer's disease patients treated with EXELON PATCH cerebrovascular accident occurred in 1.0% of patients treated with EXELON PATCH 20, 0.7% of patients treated with EXELON PATCH 10 and 0.3% of patients treated with placebo. The events were fatal in the EXELON PATCH 10 and placebo groups. A lower frequency of cerebrovascular accident was observed in the controlled clinical trials involving patients with mild to moderate Alzheimer's disease who were treated with EXELON capsules.

Other Adverse Events Observed During Clinical Trials: EXELON PATCH has been administered to 1071 patients with Alzheimer's disease during clinical trials worldwide. Of these, 869 patients have been treated for at least 3 months, 706 patients have been treated for at least 6 months, 212 patients have been treated for 1 year.

Treatment-emergent signs and symptoms that occurred during 1 controlled and 4 open-label trials in North America, Europe, Latin America, Asia and Japan were recorded as adverse events by the clinical investigators using terminology of their own choosing.

To provide an overall estimate of the proportion of individuals having similar types of events, the events were grouped into a smaller number of standardized categories using MedDRA dictionary, and event frequencies were calculated across all studies. These categories are used in the listing below. The frequencies represent the proportion of 1071 patients from these trials who experienced that event while receiving EXELON PATCH. All patch doses are pooled. In general, adverse event rates with the patch were dose-related.

All adverse events occurring in at least 1 patient (approximately 0.1%) are included, except for those already listed elsewhere in labeling, too general to be informative, or relatively minor events.

Events are classified by system organ class and listed using the following definitions: Frequent—those occurring in at least 1/100 patients; Infrequent—those occurring in 1/100 to 1/1000 patients. These adverse events are not necessarily related to EXELON PATCH treatment and in most cases were observed at a similar frequency in placebo-treated patients in the controlled studies.

Blood and Lymphatic System Disorders: Frequent: anemia.

Cardiac Disorders: Infrequent: angina pectoris, coronary artery disease, cardiac failure, bradycardia, atrial fibrillation, syncope, electrocardiogram QT prolonged, supraventricular extrasystoles, myocardial infarction, tachycardia, arrhythmia, atrioventricular block.

Ear and Labyrinth Disorders: Infrequent: tinnitus.

Eye Disorders: Infrequent: cataract, glaucoma, vision blurred.

Gastrointestinal System: Frequent: constipation, gastritis, dyspepsia. Infrequent: gastroesophageal reflux disease, hematochezia, peptic ulcer, hematemesis, pancreatitis, salivary hypersecretion.

General Disorders and Administration Site Conditions: Frequent: application site reaction, application site erythema, application site pruritus. Infrequent: application site dermatitis, application site irritation, application site vesicles, peripheral edema, chest pain, application site eczema, hyperpyrexia, malaise.

Hepatobiliary Disorders: Infrequent: cholecystitis.

Infections and Infestations: Frequent: nasopharyngitis, pneumonia. Infrequent: diverticulitis.

Injury, Poisoning and Procedural Complications: Frequent: fall. Infrequent: hip fracture, subdural hematoma.

Metabolic and Nutritional Disorders: Frequent: dehydration. Infrequent: blood amylase increased, blood creatine phosphokinase increased, hyperlipidemia, hypokalemia, hyponatremia, lipase increased.

Musculoskeletal and Connective Tissue Disorders: Infrequent: arthralgia, muscle spasms, myalgia.

Nervous System Disorders: Frequent: tremor. Infrequent: migraine, parkinsonism, extrapyramidal disorder, gait disorder, cerebrovascular accident, cerebral hemorrhage, cerebellar hemorrhage, transient ischemic attack, somnolence.

Psychiatric Disorders: Infrequent: delusion, delirium, hallucinations.

Renal and Urinary Disorders: Frequent: urinary incontinence. Infrequent: pollakiuria, hematuria, nocturia, renal failure.

Reproductive System and Breast Disorders: Infrequent: benign prostatic hyperplasia.

Respiratory, Thoracic, and Mediastinal Disorders: Infrequent: dyspnea, bronchospasm, chronic obstructive pulmonary disease.

Skin and Subcutaneous Tissue Disorders: Frequent: pruritus. Infrequent: erythema, eczema, dermatitis, rash erythematous, skin ulcer, hyperhidrosis.

Vascular Disorders: Infrequent: hypotension.

Additional Adverse Drug Reactions Which Have Been Reported with EXELON Capsules or Oral Solution: The following additional adverse events have been observed in clinical trials with EXELON capsules: confusion (frequent), abnormal liver function tests (infrequent), duodenal ulcers (infrequent).

Post-Market Adverse Drug Reactions: EXELON PATCH: The following additional adverse events have been identified based on post-marketing spontaneous reports and are not listed above. Because these reactions are reported voluntarily from a population of uncertain size, it is not always possible to reliably estimate their frequency.

Rarely reported: hypertension, application site hypersensitivity, urticaria, blister (including application site and generalized blistering), dermatitis allergic.

Very rarely reported: Worsening of Parkinson's disease in patients with Parkinson's disease who were treated with EXELON PATCH (see Warnings and Precautions); seizure; hepatic failure; Stevens-Johnson syndrome.

Overdose with rivastigmine resulting from medication errors and inappropriate use of EXELON PATCH (e.g. failure to remove the previous day's patch and application of multiple patches at a time) has been reported. As with medication errors and misuse in general, serious medical outcomes, including death, have been reported with EXELON PATCH (see Overdosage for details).

The typical symptoms reported in association with overdose include nausea, vomiting, diarrhea, hypertension, and hallucinations. Bradycardia and/or syncope, that may be associated with malaise or falls, may also occur (see Warnings and Precautions, General; Overdosage).

EXELON Capsules: Voluntary reports of adverse events temporally associated with EXELON capsules that have been received since market introduction that may or may not be causally related to the drug include the following:

Skin and Appendages: Stevens-Johnson syndrome, blister.

Gastrointestinal System: Severe vomiting with esophageal rupture, pancreatitis (see Warnings and Precautions, Gastrointestinal, Pancreatic).

Table 1: EXELON PATCH

Common Adverse Events (≥5% and twice the placebo rate in the EXELON PATCH Groups) in the 24-Week Clinical Trial Conducted with EXELON PATCH in Patients with Alzheimer's Disease, During Titration and Maintenance Phases[c]

	Titration Phase (Weeks 1–16)				Maintenance Phase (Weeks 17–24)			
Adverse Event	Placebo n=302 (%)	EXELON Capsules[a] n=294 (%)	EXELON PATCH 10 n=291 (%)	EXELON PATCH 20[b] n=303 (%)	Placebo n=280 (%)	EXELON Capsules 6 mg BID n=250 (%)	EXELON PATCH 10 n=241 (%)	EXELON PATCH 20[b] n=263 (%)
Nausea	5	21	7	17	<1	4	1	6
Vomiting	3	15	6	15	1	3	1	8
Diarrhea	3	5	6	9	<1	<1	1	2
Weight decreased	1	5	2	5	0	1	<1	3
Dizziness	2	6	2	6	0	2	<1	2

a Doses up to 6 mg BID.
b EXELON PATCH 20 did not confer appreciable additional benefit and was associated with significant increases in adverse events.
c All patients who received at least one dose of study medication were included in the results for the titration phase. All patients who entered the maintenance phase were represented in the results for the maintenance phase.

Table 2: EXELON PATCH

Adverse Events (≥2% in EXELON PATCH groups, and occurring with a rate greater than placebo) of the 24-Week Clinical Trial Conducted with EXELON PATCH in Patients with Alzheimer's Disease

	Placebo N=302	EXELON Capsules 6 mg BID N=294	EXELON PATCH 10 Group N=291	EXELON PATCH 20 Group[a] N=303
Percent of patients with AE(s)	46	63	51	66
Ear and Labyrinth Disorders				
Vertigo	1	1	0	2
Gastrointestinal				
Nausea	5	23	7	21
Vomiting	3	17	6	19
Diarrhea	3	5	6	10
Abdominal pain	1	1	2	4
Abdominal pain upper	2	2	1	3
General Disorders and Administrative Site Conditions				
Asthenia	1	6	2	3
Fatigue	1	1	2	2
Infections and Infestations				
Urinary tract infection	1	1	2	2
Investigations				
Weight decreased	1	5	3	8
Metabolism and Nutritional Disorders				
Anorexia	1	5	2	4
Decreased appetite	1	4	1	5
Nervous System Disorders				
Dizziness	2	7	2	7
Headache	2	6	3	4
Psychiatric Disorders				
Depression	1	4	4	4
Insomnia	2	2	1	4
Anxiety	1	2	3	3

a EXELON PATCH 20 did not confer appreciable additional benefit and was associated with significant increases in adverse events.

DRUG INTERACTIONS: Overview: No specific interaction studies have been conducted with EXELON PATCH (rivastigmine).
Use with Anticholinergics: Because of their mechanism of action, cholinesterase inhibitors have the potential to interfere with the activity of anticholinergic medications and should not be given with other cholinomimetic drugs.
Use with Cholinomimetics and Other Cholinesterase Inhibitors: In view of its pharmacodynamic effects, rivastigmine should not be given concomitantly with other cholinomimetic drugs. A synergistic effect may be expected when cholinesterase inhibitors are given concurrently with succinylcholine, similar neuromuscular blocking agents or cholinergic agonists such as bethanechol.
Use with Other Psychoactive Drugs: In controlled clinical trials with EXELON capsules few patients received neuroleptics, antidepressants or anticonvulsants, there is thus limited information concerning the interaction of EXELON with these drugs.
Anesthesia: EXELON as a cholinesterase inhibitor, is likely to exaggerate succinylcholine-type muscle relaxation during anesthesia.
Effect of EXELON on the Metabolism of Other Drugs: Rivastigmine is mainly metabolised through hydrolysis by esterases. No in vivo studies have investigated the effects of EXELON on the clearance of drugs metabolised by CYP450. Based on in vitro studies, no pharmacokinetic drug interactions with drugs metabolised by the following isoenzyme systems are expected: CYP1A2, CYP2D6, CYP3A4/5, CYP2E1, CYP2C9, CYP2C8, or CYP2C19. Thus, no pharmacokinetics interactions are anticipated with other drugs metabolized by these enzymes.

Rivastigmine may inhibit the butyrylcholinesterase mediated metabolism of other drugs (see Actions and Clinical Pharmacology, Pharmacokinetics, Metabolism).
Effect of Other Drugs on the Metabolism of EXELON: Drugs which induce or inhibit CYP450 metabolism are not expected to alter the metabolism of rivastigmine. Formal pharmacokinetic studies to assess the potential for drug interaction with other medications commonly taken by the elderly were not done. Population-pharmacokinetic analyses of a subset (n=359; 6-12 mg/day) of patients with Alzheimer's disease in controlled clinical trials do not suggest that the oral administration of EXELON with some commonly prescribed medications is associated with an alteration in the kinetics of rivastigmine, or an increased risk of clinically relevant untoward effects. However, the number of patients who received concomitant medications chronically was as follows: anilides (e.g. acetaminophen) (10%), antacids (12%), antianginals (6%), antihistamines (2%), antihypertensives (12%), benzodiazepines (<1%), β-blockers (7%), calcium channel blockers (12%), digitalis glycosides (5%), nonsteroidal anti-inflammatory drugs (13%), oral hypoglycemics (3%), and salicylic acid and derivatives (28%).
Drug-Drug Interactions: Studies to assess the potential of EXELON administered orally for interaction with digoxin, warfarin, diazepam or fluoxetine were limited to short term, single-dose studies in young healthy volunteers. No significant effects on the pharmacokinetics of these drugs or on the metabolism of rivastigmine were observed. Similar studies in elderly patients were not done.

DOSAGE AND ADMINISTRATION: Dosing Considerations:

- **Hepatic Impairment:** EXELON PATCH has not been studied in hepatic impairment. Patients with clinically significant hepatic impairment may experience more adverse events. Caution should be used when titrating hepatically impaired patients (see Action and Clinical Pharmacology).
- **Renal Impairment:** EXELON PATCH has not been studied in renal impairment. Dose titration for patients with renal impairment should be undertaken with caution (see Action and Clinical Pharmacology).
- **Low Body Weight:** Patients with body weight below 50 kg may experience more adverse events and may be more likely to discontinue due to adverse events. Particular caution should be exercised when titrating these patients to the maintenance dose.
- Dose escalation for patients with serious comorbid diseases should be undertaken *with particular caution*.
- In a population of cognitively-impaired individuals, safe use of this and all other medications may require supervision (see Warnings and Precautions, Information to Be Provided to the Patient).
- Exposure to sources of heat may increase a drug's ability to penetrate the skin when administered to a patient by transdermal patch and this may result in increased drug exposure. The applied patch area should not be exposed to or have direct contact with external heat sources such as excessive sunlight, heat lamps, heating pads, saunas, hot tubs, etc. This may also occur if the patient has a fever. Patients and caregivers should be advised that the patch area should not be exposed to external heat sources while wearing EXELON PATCH.

Recommended Dose and Dosage Adjustment: EXELON PATCH (rivastigmine) should only be prescribed by (or following consultation with) clinicians who are experienced in the diagnosis and management of Alzheimer's disease. See Table 3.

Table 3: EXELON PATCH

Dosage Form/Strength

Patches	Rivastigmine Base Dose Load[a]	Rivastigmine Base in Vivo Release Rates per 24 h[b]
EXELON PATCH 5	9 mg	4.6 mg
EXELON PATCH 10	18 mg	9.5 mg

a Drug content of the patch.
b Quantity of drug released over a 24-h patch application time interval.

Initial Dose: Treatment is started with EXELON PATCH 5 once a day.

If EXELON PATCH 5 is well tolerated, the dose should be increased to EXELON PATCH 10 after a minimum of four weeks of treatment.
Maintenance Dose: EXELON PATCH 10 is the maximum recommended daily maintenance dose which can be continued for as long as a therapeutic benefit for the patient exists. Higher doses confer no appreciable additional benefit, and are associated with significant increases in the incidence of adverse events (see Adverse Reactions).

Treatment should be temporarily interrupted if gastrointestinal adverse effects are observed, until these adverse effects resolve. Patch treatment can be resumed at the same dose if treatment is not interrupted for more than a few days. Otherwise, treatment should be reinitiated with EXELON PATCH 5.

If adverse effects persist on reinitiation of therapy, the dose should be temporarily reduced to EXELON PATCH 5.
Renal Impairment: No dose adjustment is necessary for patients with renal impairment.
Switching from Capsules or Oral Solution: Patients treated with EXELON capsules or oral solution may be switched to EXELON PATCH as follows:

- A patient who is on a dose of <3 mg BID (<6 mg/day) oral rivastigmine can be switched to EXELON PATCH 5.
- A patient who is on a dose of 3 to 6 mg BID (6 to 12 mg/day) oral rivastigmine may be directly switched to EXELON PATCH 10.

It is recommended to apply the first patch on the day following the last oral dose.
Missed Dose: The missed dose should be taken immediately or at the next scheduled dose. Doses should not be doubled. If therapy has been interrupted for a few days, treatment should be reinitiated with EXELON PATCH 5.
Administration: EXELON PATCH should be applied once a day to clean, dry, hairless, intact healthy skin on the upper or lower back, upper arm, or chest, in a place that will not be rubbed by tight clothing. Application of the patch to other areas, such as the abdomen and thighs, has been shown to decrease the bioavailability of rivastigmine and cause more skin irritation (see Actions and Clinical Pharmacology, Pharmacokinetics and Adverse Reactions, Skin Irritation). The patch should not be applied to skin that is red, irritated, or cut. It is recommended to change the application spot daily to avoid potential irritation, although consecutive patches can be applied to the same anatomic site (e.g., another spot on the same upper arm). The same skin location should not be used within 14 days.

The patch should be pressed down firmly, by applying pressure with the hand over the entire patch for about 10 seconds, making sure that the edges stick well. It can be used in everyday situations, including bathing and during hot weather, however, it should be checked to ensure it has remained well adhered. Showering and washing the EXELON PATCH site is possible without loss of adherence. To ensure proper adherence, the patch should not be applied to wet or damp skin.

The patch should be replaced with a new one after 24 hours. Only one patch should be worn at a time (see Overdosage, Symptoms). Patients and caregivers should be instructed accordingly. (See Warnings and Precautions, Information to Be Provided to the Patient and Information for the Patient.)
Incompatibilities: To prevent interference with the adhesive properties of the patch, the patch should not be applied to a skin area where cream, lotion or powder has recently been applied.

OVERDOSAGE:
Symptoms: Overdosage with cholinesterase inhibitors can result in cholinergic crisis characterised by severe nausea, vomiting, diarrhea, hypertension, hallucinations, salivation, sweating, hypotension, respiratory depression, collapse and convulsions. Increasing muscle weakness is a possibility and may result in death if respiratory muscles are involved. Atypical responses in blood pressure and heart rate have been reported with other cholinomimetics when co-administered with quaternary anticholinergics such as glycopyrrolate.

Due to the known vagotonic effect of cholinesterase inhibitors on heart rate, bradycardia and/or syncope may also occur.

In a documented case of a 46 mg overdose with EXELON capsules, a 69 year old female patient experienced vomiting, incontinence, hypertension, psychomotor retardation and loss of consciousness. The patient was managed conservatively with only supportive measures and fully recovered within 24 hours.

In a documented case of medication error leading to overdose with EXELON PATCH, an 87 year old male patient on a prescribed maintenance dose of one EXELON PATCH 10 (9.5 mg/24 hrs) per day was accidentally administered 6 patches per day on two consecutive days. The patient experienced vomiting, fall and hyperhidrosis and was hospitalized on the second day. At the time of hospitalization he presented with an elevated creatinine level (149 μmol/L; normal range: 70-115 μmol/L) and signs of urinary infection. He was treated by removal of all patches and ciprofloxacin was initiated. Subsequently, the patient developed acute renal failure with anuria and died approximately 14 days after hospitalization. The reporter suspected that overdose contributed to the patient's dehydration and renal failure. Autopsy results were not provided by the reporter.

Dose-related signs of toxicity in animals included lacrimation, excessive salivation, vomiting, decreased locomotor activity, ataxia, twitches/flutters, tremors and clonic convulsions.

Overdose with EXELON PATCH resulting from misuse/medication errors (application of multiple patches at a time) has been reported in the post-marketing setting (see Warnings and Precautions, Adverse Reactions, Post-Market Adverse Drug Reactions). The typical symptoms reported among these cases are similar to those seen with cases of overdose associated with EXELON oral formulations.
Treatment: As rivastigmine has a plasma half-life of about 3.4 hours after patch administration and a duration of acetylcholinesterase inhibition of about 9 hours, it is recommended that in cases of asymptomatic overdose the patch should be immediately removed and no further patch should be applied for the next 24 hours.

In overdoses accompanied by severe nausea and vomiting, the use of antiemetics should be considered.

Symptomatic treatment for other adverse events should also be given as necessary.

Tertiary anticholinergics such as atropine may be used as an antidote for EXELON overdosage. Intravenous atropine sulfate titrated to effect is recommended: an initial dose of 1 to 2 mg IV with subsequent doses based upon clinical response.

Due to the short plasma elimination half-life of rivastigmine after patch administration, dialysis (hemodialysis, peritoneal dialysis, or hemofiltration) would not be clinically indicated in the event of an overdose.

For management of a suspected drug overdose, contact your regional Poison Control Centre. See the *CPS* Directory section for a list of Poison Control Centres.

ACTION AND CLINICAL PHARMACOLOGY: Mechanism of Action: Pathological changes in Dementia of the Alzheimer type involve cholinergic neuronal pathways that project from the basal forebrain to the cerebral cortex and hippocampus. A decrease in the function of these cholinergic pathways has been proposed to account for some of the clinical manifestations of dementia. Rivastigmine, a reversible cholinesterase inhibitor of the carbamate-type, is thought to enhance cholinergic neurotransmission by slowing the degradation of acetylcholine released by cholinergic neurons through the inhibition of acetylcholinesterase. If this proposed mechanism of action is correct, rivastigmine's effect may lessen as the disease process advances and fewer cholinergic neurons remain functionally intact.

There is no evidence that rivastigmine alters the course of the underlying dementing process.

Pharmacodynamics: Rivastigmine inhibits acetylcholinesterase (AChE) and butyrylcholinesterase (BuChE) activity. In patients with Alzheimer's disease significant dose-dependent inhibition of AChE and BuChE activity were noted in cerebrospinal fluid, with comparable maximum mean inhibition (62%). In plasma, significant inhibition of BuChE activity is generally observed from 1.5 hours post-dose up to 8 hours post-dose, with a maximum observed inhibition of 51% at 5 mg b.i.d. Rivastigmine may therefore inhibit the butyrylcholinesterase mediated metabolism of other drugs (see Drug Interactions, Overview).

Pharmacokinetics: Absorption: Absorption of rivastigmine from EXELON PATCH (rivastigmine) transdermal systems is slow. After the first dose, detectable plasma concentrations are observed after a lag time of 0.5-1 hour. Concentrations then rise slowly and typically after 8 hours reach levels close to maximum, although maximum values (C_{max}) are often reached at later times (10-16 hours).

After the peak, plasma concentrations slowly decrease over the remainder of the 24-hour period of application. With multiple dosing (such as at steady state), after the previous patch is replaced with a new one, plasma concentrations initially decrease slowly for about 40 minutes on average, until absorption from the newly applied patch becomes faster than the elimination, and plasma levels begin to rise again to reach a new peak at approximately 8 hours. At steady state, trough levels are approximately 50% of peak levels, in contrast to oral dosing, with which concentrations fall off to virtually zero between doses (see Figure 1 and Figure 2). Although less pronounced than with the oral formulation, the pharmacokinetics of rivastigmine is non-linear, with exposure (C_{max} and AUC) increasing over-proportionally by a factor of 2.6 when escalating from EXELON PATCH 5 to EXELON PATCH 10. The fluctuation index (FI), i.e., a measure of the relative difference between peak and trough concentrations [(C_{max}-C_{min})/C_{avg})], was 0.58 for EXELON PATCH 5 and 0.77 for EXELON PATCH 10, thus demonstrating a much smaller fluctuation between trough and peak concentrations than for the oral formulation (FI=3.96 to 6.24); therefore providing a more continuous delivery of rivastigmine with the patch. As determined by compartmental modeling, EXELON PATCH 10 exhibited exposure approximately the same as that provided by an oral dose of about 6 mg twice daily (i.e., 12 mg/day).

Figure 1: EXELON PATCH

Rivastigmine Plasma Concentrations Following Dermal 24-Hour Patch Application

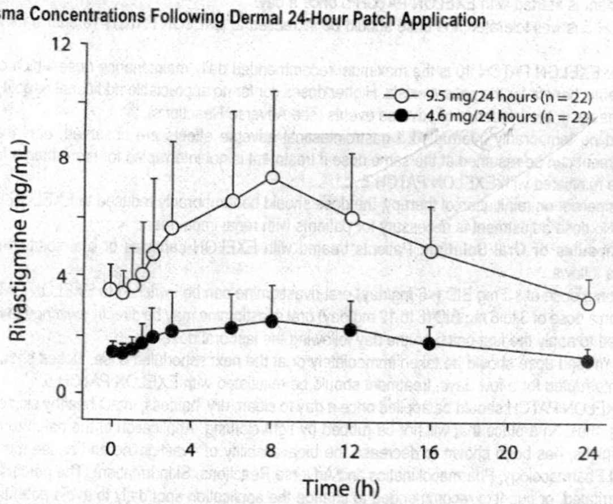

Figure 2: EXELON PATCH

Rivastigmine Plasma Concentrations Following Oral (twice daily) Capsule

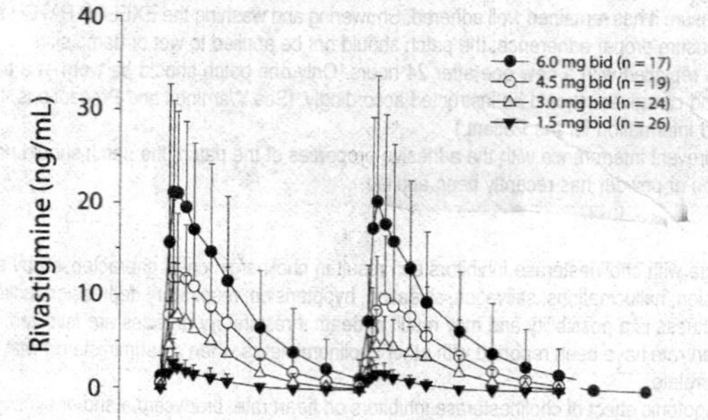

In a single dose study directly comparing the patch (10 cm²) versus oral (3 mg) administration, the inter-subject variability in rivastigmine pharmacokinetic parameters (normalized to dose/kg bodyweight) was 43% (C_{max}) and 49% (AUC_{0-24h}) after the patch versus 74% and 103%, respectively, after the oral capsule. Similarly, inter-subject variability in rivastigmine pharmacokinetic parameters was lower after the patch than after the oral capsule in a steady-state study in Alzheimer's disease patients given repeated doses. The inter-patient variability was at most 45% (C_{max}) and 43% (AUC_{0-24h}) after the patch, while 71% and 73%, respectively, after the oral form.

A relationship between drug exposure at steady state (rivastigmine and metabolite NAP226-90) and bodyweight was observed in Alzheimer's disease patients. Compared to a patient with a body weight of 65 kg, the rivastigmine steady-state concentrations in a patient with a body weight of 35 kg would be approximately doubled, while for a patient with a body weight of 100 kg the concentrations would be approximately halved. The effect of bodyweight on drug exposure suggests special attention to patients with very low body weight during up-titration (see Dosage and Administration).

Rivastigmine was well released from the transdermal system over a 24-hour dermal application with approximately 50% of the drug load released from the system.

Exposure (AUC_∞) to rivastigmine (and metabolite NAP266-90) was highest when the patch was applied to the upper back, chest, or upper arm. Two other sites (abdomen and thigh) could be used if none of the three other sites is available, but the practitioner should keep in mind that the rivastigmine plasma exposure associated with these sites was approximately 20-30% lower (see Adverse Reactions, Skin Irritation, for effect of application site on skin irritation).

There was no relevant accumulation of rivastigmine or the metabolite NAP226-90 in plasma in patients with Alzheimer's disease.

Distribution: Rivastigmine is weakly bound to plasma proteins (approximately 40%). It readily crosses the blood-brain barrier and has an apparent volume of distribution in the range of 1.8-2.7 L/kg.

Metabolism: Rivastigmine is rapidly and extensively metabolized with an apparent elimination half-life in plasma of approximately 3.4 hours after patch removal. Elimination was absorption rate limited (flip-flop kinetics), which explains the longer $t_{½}$ after patch (3.4 hours) versus oral or i.v. administrations (1.4 to 1.7 hours). Metabolism is primarily via cholinesterase-mediated hydrolysis to the decarbamylated metabolite. In vitro, this metabolite shows minimal inhibition of acetylcholinesterase (<10%). Based on evidence from in vitro and animal studies, the major cytochrome P450 isoenzymes are minimally involved in rivastigmine metabolism.

The metabolite-to-parent AUC_∞ ratio was around 0.7 after patch versus 3.5 after oral administration, indicating that much less metabolism occurred after dermal treatment. Less NAP226-90 is formed following patch application, presumably because of the lack of presystemic (hepatic first pass) metabolism.

Excretion: Unchanged rivastigmine is found in trace amounts in the urine; renal excretion of the metabolites is the major route of elimination. Following administration of ^{14}C-rivastigmine, renal elimination was rapid and essentially complete (>90 %) within 24 hours. Less than 1% of the administered dose is excreted in the feces.

Special Populations and Conditions: Pediatrics (<18 years of age): No data are available in children.

Geriatrics: Age had no impact on the exposure to rivastigmine in Alzheimer's disease patients treated with EXELON PATCH.

Hepatic Insufficiency: No study was conducted with EXELON PATCH in subjects with hepatic impairment. After oral administration of EXELON capsules 1-3 mg, the C_{max} of rivastigmine was approximately 60% higher and the AUC of rivastigmine was more than twice as high in subjects with mild to moderate hepatic impairment than in healthy subjects.

Renal Insufficiency: No study was conducted with EXELON PATCH in subjects with renal impairment. After oral administration of EXELON capsules 1-3 mg, C_{max} and AUC of rivastigmine were more than twice as high in Alzheimer's disease patients with moderate renal impairment compared with healthy subjects; however there were no changes in C_{max} and AUC of rivastigmine in Alzheimer's disease patients with severe renal impairment.

STORAGE AND STABILITY: Store at room temperature (15-30°C).

SPECIAL HANDLING INSTRUCTIONS: Keep EXELON PATCH (rivastigmine) in the individual sealed pouch until use.

Used patches should be folded, with the adhesive surfaces pressed together, and discarded safely.

Contact with the eyes should be avoided after handling EXELON PATCH.

INFORMATION FOR THE PATIENT: Published in e-CPS, available by subscription at www.e-cps.ca.

DOSAGE FORMS, COMPOSITION AND PACKAGING: EXELON PATCH (rivastigmine) is a transdermal patch for transdermal administration.

Each patch is a thin, matrix-type transdermal system consisting of three layers when worn by the patient. A fourth layer, the release liner, covers the adhesive layer prior to use and is removed at the time the system is applied to the skin.

EXELON PATCH 5: Each patch of 5 cm² contains: 9 mg rivastigmine base, with in vivo release rate of 4.6 mg/24 hours. The outside of the backing layer is beige and labeled with "PrEXELON* PATCH 5 (rivastigmine) 4.6 mg/24 h" and "AMCX". Nonmedicinal ingredients: acrylic copolymer, poly(butylmethacrylate, methyl-methacrylate), silicone adhesive applied to a flexible polymer backing film, silicone oil and vitamin E. Cartons of 30. Each patch is individually sealed in a separate pouch.

EXELON PATCH 10: Each patch of 10 cm² contains: 18 mg rivastigmine base, with in vivo release rate of 9.5 mg/24 hours. The outside of the backing layer is beige and labeled with "PrEXELON* PATCH 10 (rivastigmine) 9.5 mg/24 h" and "BHDI". Nonmedicinal ingredients: acrylic copolymer, poly(butylmethacrylate, methyl-methacrylate), silicone adhesive applied to a flexible polymer backing film, silicone oil and vitamin E. Cartons of 30. Each patch is individually sealed in a separate pouch.

(Shown in Product Identification Section)

Exjade® Pr

deferasirox

Iron Chelating Agent

Novartis Pharmaceuticals

Date of Preparation: October 18, 2006
Date of Revision: June 18, 2010

Conditional marketing authorization has been issued for EXJADE for the following conditions:
- **the management of chronic iron overload in patients with transfusion-dependent anemias aged six years or older;**
- **the management of chronic iron overload in patients with transfusion-dependent anemias aged two to five who cannot be adequately treated with deferoxamine.**

These marketing authorizations are conditional, pending the results of studies to verify its clinical benefit. Patients should be advised of the nature of the authorization.

Therapy with EXJADE should be initiated and maintained by physicians experienced in the treatment of chronic iron overload due to blood transfusions.

SUMMARY PRODUCT INFORMATION:

Route of Administration	Dosage Form/ Strength	Clinically Relevant Nonmedicinal Ingredients
Oral	Dispersible tablets for oral suspension 125 mg, 250 mg, or 500 mg	Lactose monohydrate For a complete listing see Dosage Forms, Composition and Packaging.

INDICATIONS AND CLINICAL USE: EXJADE (deferasirox) is indicated in the management of chronic iron overload in patients with transfusion-dependent anemias aged 6 years or older.

EXJADE is also indicated in the management of chronic iron overload in patients with transfusion-dependent anemias aged two to five who cannot be adequately treated with deferoxamine.

Therapy with EXJADE should be initiated and maintained by physicians experienced in the treatment of chronic iron overload due to blood transfusions.

Pediatrics (2 to 16 years of age): There are limited data available on the use of EXJADE in children aged 2 to 5 (see Warnings and Precautions, Special Populations, Pediatrics (2 to 16 years of age)). The overall exposure of EXJADE in young children (aged 2 to 5) was about 50% lower than in adults and this age group may require higher maintenance doses than are necessary in adults (see Dosage and Administration).

Geriatrics (≥65 years of age): Four hundred and thirty-one (431) patients ≥65 years of age have been studied in clinical trials of EXJADE (see Warnings and Precautions, Special Populations, Geriatrics (≥65 years of age)). The pharmacokinetics of EXJADE have not been studied in elderly patients. In clinical trials, elderly patients experienced a higher frequency of adverse reactions than younger patients and should be monitored closely for adverse reactions that may require a dose adjustment.

CONTRAINDICATIONS: EXJADE is contraindicated in patients with estimated creatinine clearance <60 mL/min or serum creatinine >2 times the age-appropriate upper limit of normal.

EXJADE is contraindicated in high risk myelodysplastic syndrome (MDS) patients, any other MDS patient with a life expectancy <1 year and patients with other hematological and non-hematological malignancies who are not expected to benefit from chelation therapy due to the rapid progression of their disease.

EXJADE is contraindicated in patients with platelet counts <50 x 10^9/L.

The use of EXJADE (deferasirox) is contraindicated in patients with hypersensitivity to the active substance, deferasirox, or to any of the excipients. For a complete listing of excipients, see Dosage Forms, Composition and Packaging.

WARNINGS AND PRECAUTIONS:

Serious Warnings and Precautions

Therapy with EXJADE should be initiated and maintained by physicians experience in the treatment of chronic iron overload due to blood transfusions.

EXJADE has not been studied in patients with severe renal impairment or severe hepatic impairment.

The following are clinically significant adverse events:

- Acute renal failure
- Hepatic failure
- Gastrointestinal haemorrhage

In some reported cases, these conditions had a fatal outcome. Cases of acute renal failure and hepatic failure (some with a fatal outcome) have been reported following the post-marketing use of EXJADE. Most of these reports are in critically ill patients and in those with significant co-morbidities including liver cirrhosis and multi-organ failure. It is impossible to completely exclude a contributory role for EXJADE in these events. There have been rare reports of gastrointestinal haemorrhages with a fatal outcome, especially in elderly patients who had advanced haematologic malignancies and/or low platelet counts [<50 x 10^9 L]. EXJADE therapy requires laboratory tests of renal and hepatic functions and close patient monitoring.

General: EXJADE should not be combined with other iron chelator therapies as the safety and efficacy of such combinations has not been established.

No studies on the effects of EXJADE on the ability to drive or use machines have been performed. Patients experiencing dizziness should exercise caution when driving or operating machinery.

The decision to remove accumulated iron should be individualized based on anticipated clinical benefits and risks of chelation therapy (see Dosage and Administration).

Cardiovascular: EXJADE has not been studied in patients with acute cardiac failure due to iron overload. Therefore, the use of EXJADE is not recommended in these patients.

Ear/Nose/Throat: Auditory disturbances (high-frequency hearing loss, decreased hearing) have been reported with EXJADE therapy (see Adverse Reactions). Auditory testing is recommended before the start of EXJADE treatment and thereafter at regular intervals.

Gastrointestinal: Gastrointestinal irritation may occur during EXJADE treatment. Upper gastrointestinal ulceration and haemorrhage have been reported uncommonly in patients, including children and adolescents, receiving EXJADE. There have been rare reports of fatal GI haemorrhages, especially in elderly patients who had advanced hematologic malignancies and/or low platelet counts. Multiple ulcers have been observed in some patients (see Adverse Reactions). Physicians and patients should remain alert for signs and symptoms of GI ulceration and haemorrhage during EXJADE therapy and promptly initiate additional evaluation and treatment if a serious GI adverse event is suspected.

Caution should be exercised in patients who are taking EXJADE in combination with drugs that have known ulcerogenic potential, such as NSAIDs, corticosteroids, or oral bisphosphonates, and in patients receiving anticoagulants (see Drug Interactions).

EXJADE contains lactose (1.1 mg lactose for each mg of deferasirox). This medicine is not recommended for patients with rare hereditary problems of galactose intolerance, severe lactase deficiency or glucose-galactose malabsorption.

Hematologic: There have been post-marketing reports (both spontaneous and from clinical trials) of cytopenias in patients treated with EXJADE. Most of these patients had preexisting hematologic disorders that are frequently associated with bone marrow failure (see Adverse Reactions, Post-Market Adverse Drug Reactions). The relationship of these episodes to treatment with EXJADE is unknown. In line with the standard clinical management of such hematological disorders, blood counts should be monitored regularly. Dose interruption of treatment with EXJADE should be considered in patients who develop unexplained cytopenia. Reintroduction of therapy with EXJADE may be considered, once the cause of the cytopenia has been elucidated.

Hepatic/Biliary/Pancreatic: EXJADE has not been studied in patients with hepatic impairment and must be used with caution in hepatic impaired patients. Elevations of serum transaminase levels (greater than 5 times the upper limit of normal) have been observed in 40 patients receiving EXJADE. In these patients, the transaminase levels were already >5 ULN at baseline in 6 of the 40 patients. In 25 of the 40 patients, the transaminase levels at baseline were above the upper limit of normal but less than 5 ULN. There have been postmarketing reports of hepatic failure in patients treated with EXJADE. There are a total of 24 international reports of hepatic failure—21 post-marketing reports and 3 reports from clinical studies. Two of the 24 cases were reported in Canada. Most reports of hepatic failure involved patients with significant comorbidities including liver cirrhosis and multi-organ failure; fatal outcomes were reported in some of these patients. As of the cut-off date above, no patient with normal baseline liver function or without additional life-threatening complications of their underlying disease has developed hepatic failure.

Although uncommon (0.3%), elevations of transaminases greater than 10 times the upper limit of the normal range, suggestive of hepatitis, have been observed in clinical trials. It is recommended that serum transaminases, bilirubin and alkaline phosphatase be monitored before the initiation of treatment, every 2 weeks during the first month and monthly thereafter. If there is an unexplained, persistent and progressive increase in serum transaminase levels, EXJADE treatment should be interrupted.

Ophthalmologic: Ocular disturbances (lens opacities, early cataracts, maculopathies) have been reported with EXJADE therapy (see Adverse Reactions). Ophthalmic testing (including fundoscopy) is recommended before the start of EXJADE treatment and thereafter at regular intervals.

Renal: EXJADE has not been studied in patients with renal impairment. EXJADE treatment has been initiated only in patients with serum creatinine within the age-appropriate normal range and therefore must be used with caution in patients with elevated serum creatinine levels (see Contraindications).

EXJADE-treated patients experienced dose-dependent increases in serum creatinine. Increases in creatinine that were >33% at ≥2 consecutive post baseline visits occurred at a greater frequency in EXJADE-treated patients compared to deferoxamine-treated patients (38% vs. 14%, respectively) in study 0107. In these beta-thalassemia patients, 94% of the creatinine elevations remained within the normal range. Under the dose adjustment instructions, dose reduction was required in one third of patients showing serum creatinine increase. In most patients undergoing dose reductions serum creatinine levels did not return to baseline; in 60% of patients undergoing dose reduction, serum creatinine remained elevated at >33% without progression (see Adverse Reactions, Abnormal Hematologic and Clinical Chemistry Findings).

Cases of acute renal failure (some with fatal outcome) have been reported following the post-marketing use of EXJADE. There have been rare cases of acute renal failure requiring dialysis. For the fatal cases, it is impossible to completely exclude a contributory role of EXJADE to the renal impairment, although the fatalities in these critically ill patients could be attributable to other underlying diseases. The fact that there was an improvement after stopping the treatment in most of the cases with non-fatal acute renal failure is suggestive of a contributory role of EXJADE to these cases (see Adverse Reactions, Post-Market Adverse Drug Reactions).

It is recommended that serum creatinine and/or creatinine clearance be assessed twice before initiating therapy. Weekly monitoring of serum creatinine and/or creatinine clearance is recommended in the first month after initiation or modification of therapy, and monthly thereafter. Patients with pre-existing renal conditions, or patients who are receiving medicinal products that may depress renal function may be more at risk of complications. Care should be taken to maintain adequate hydration in patients (see Dosage and Administration, Dosing Considerations). Dose reduction, interruption, or discontinuations should be considered for elevations in serum creatinine (see Adverse Reactions, Abnormal Hematologic and Clinical Chemistry Findings).

Renal tubulopathy has been reported in patients treated with EXJADE. The majority of these patients were children and adolescents with beta-thalassemia and serum ferritin levels <1500 µg/L.

Tests for proteinuria should be performed monthly. As needed, additional markers of renal tubular function (e.g. glycosuria in non-diabetics and low levels of serum potassium, phosphate, magnesium or urate, phosphaturia, aminoaciduria) may also be monitored. Dose reduction or interruption may be considered if there are abnormalities in levels of tubular markers and/or if clinically indicated.

If there is a progressive increase in serum creatinine beyond the upper limit of normal, EXJADE should be interrupted (see Dosage and Administration).

Skin: Severe skin rashes may occur during EXJADE treatment requiring interruption of treatment.

Rare cases of erythema multiforme have been reported during EXJADE treatment.

Rare cases of serious hypersensitivity reactions (such as anaphylaxis and angioedema) have been reported in patients receiving EXJADE, with the onset of the reaction occurring in the majority of cases within the first month of treatment (see Adverse Reactions, Post-Market Adverse Drug Reactions).

Special Populations: Pregnant Women: There are no adequate and well-controlled studies conducted in pregnant women. No clinical data on exposed pregnancies are available for EXJADE. Studies in animals have shown some reproductive toxicity at maternally toxic doses. The potential risk for humans is unknown. It is therefore recommended that EXJADE should not be used during pregnancy.

Nursing Women: It is not known whether deferasirox is excreted in human milk. In an animal study, deferasirox and its metabolites were present in breast milk of rats following a 10 mg/kg oral dose. The concentration of deferasirox was approximately 20-fold higher in maternal milk than in maternal plasma 4-8 hours post dose. Therefore, women should be advised against breast-feeding while taking EXJADE.

Pediatrics (2 to 16 years of age): There are limited data on the safety and effectiveness of EXJADE in pediatric patients aged 2 to 5. EXJADE has not been associated with growth retardation in children followed for up to 5 years in clinical trials. However, as a precautionary measure, body weight and longitudinal growth in pediatric patients should be monitored at regular intervals (every 12 months).

Geriatrics (≥65 years of age): Four hundred and thirty-one (431) patients ≥65 years of age have been studied in clinical trials of EXJADE. The majority of these patients had myelodysplastic syndrome (MDS, n=393; β-thalassemia, n=2; other anemias, n=36). In general, caution should be used in elderly patients due to the greater frequency of decreased hepatic, renal, or cardiac function, concomitant disease or other drug therapy. In clinical trials, elderly patients experienced a higher frequency of adverse reactions than younger patients and should be monitored closely for adverse reactions that may require a dose adjustment.

Monitoring and Laboratory Tests: Serum ferritin should be measured monthly to assess response to therapy and to evaluate for the possibility of overchelation of iron, although the correlation coefficient between serum ferritin and liver iron content (LIC) was 0.63, and changes in serum ferritin levels may not always reliably reflect changes in LIC. If the serum ferritin falls consistently below 500 µg/L, temporary interruption of EXJADE therapy should be considered (see Dosage and Administration).

As with other iron chelator treatment, the risk of toxicity of EXJADE may be increased when inappropriately given to patients with a low iron burden or with serum ferritin levels that are only slightly elevated.

It is recommended that serum transaminases, bilirubin and alkaline phosphatase be monitored before the initiation of treatment, every 2 weeks during the first month and monthly thereafter. It is recommended that serum creatinine be assessed twice before initiating therapy and monitored weekly for the first month followed by monthly thereafter (see Hepatic/Biliary/Pancreatic and Renal).

Tests for proteinuria should be performed monthly (see Renal).

In line with standard clinical management of hematological disorders, blood counts should be monitored regularly (see Hematologic).

ADVERSE REACTIONS: Adverse Drug Reaction Overview: A total of 652 patients were treated with EXJADE (deferasirox) in therapeutic studies lasting for a median of 366 days in pediatric and adult patients [52 patients between 2 and 5 years of age, 240 patients between 6 and 16 years of age, 330 patients between 17 to 65 years of age and 30 patients ≥65 years]. These 652 patients included 421 with β-thalassemia, 99 with rare anemias, and 132 with sickle cell disease. Of these patients, 302 were male and 456 were Caucasian. In the sickle cell disease population, 89% of patients were black.

The most frequently occurring adverse events (all causalities) in the therapeutic trials of EXJADE were diarrhea, vomiting, nausea, headache, constipation, dyspepsia, abdominal pain, pyrexia, cough, proteinuria, increases in serum creatinine and transaminases, pruritus and skin rash. Gastrointestinal disorders, increases in serum creatinine and skin rash were dose related. Adverse events which most frequently led to dose interruption, dose adjustment, or discontinuation of therapy were skin rash, gastrointestinal disorders, infections, increased creatinine, and increased transaminases.

Clinical Trial Adverse Drug Reactions: Because clinical trials are conducted under very specific conditions the adverse reaction rates observed in the clinical trials may not reflect the rates observed in practice and should not be compared to the rates in the clinical trials of another drug. Adverse drug reaction information from clinical trials is useful for identifying drug-related adverse events and for approximating rates.

The most frequent reactions reported during chronic treatment with EXJADE in adult and pediatric patients include gastrointestinal disturbances in about 26% of patients (mainly nausea, vomiting, diarrhea, or abdominal pain), and skin rash in about 7% of patients. Mild, non-progressive, dose-dependent increases in serum creatinine occurred in 34% of patients (see Abnormal Hematologic and Clinical Chemistry Findings).

Elevations of liver transaminases as suspected drug-related adverse events were reported in about 2% of patients. The increases in liver transaminases were not dose-dependent. Forty percent of these patients had elevated levels (above the upper limit of normal) prior to receiving EXJADE. Elevations of transaminases greater than 10 times the upper limit of the normal range, suggestive of hepatitis, were uncommon (0.3%). High frequency hearing loss and lenticular opacities (early cataracts) have been observed in <1% of patients treated with EXJADE (see Warnings and Precautions, Ear/Nose/Throat and Ophthalmologic).

A total of 652 patients were treated with EXJADE (deferasirox) in therapeutic studies of adult and pediatric patients with β-thalassemia (n=421), rare anemias (n=99) and sickle cell disease (n=132). This population was 46% male, 70% Caucasian and included 292 patients ≤16 years of age. In the sickle cell disease population, 89% of patients were black. A total of 94% of β-thalassemia patients, 70% of patients with rare anemias, and 86% of patients with sickle cell disease patients received therapy for ≥48 weeks.

The data in Table 1 displays the adverse events, regardless of causality, occurring in >5% of patients in either treatment group in the primary efficacy study 0107 in which 296 β-thalassemia patients were treated with EXJADE and 290 patients received deferoxamine as an active comparator. Adverse events which most frequently led to dose interruption, dose adjustment, or discontinuation of therapy were skin rash, gastrointestinal disorders, infections, increased creatinine, and increased transaminases (see Abnormal Hematologic and Clinical Chemistry Findings). Discontinuations due to adverse events with a suspected relationship to EXJADE occurred in 7 patients.

Table 1: EXJADE

Adverse Events Occurring in >5% of β-thalassemia Patients in the Comparative Trial

Preferred Term	EXJADE N=296 n (%)	Deferoxamine N=290 n (%)
Pyrexia	56 (18.9)	69 (23.8)
Headache	47 (15.9)	59 (20.3)
Abdominal Pain	41 (13.9)	28 (9.7)
Cough	41 (13.9)	55 (19.0)
Nasopharyngitis	39 (13.2)	42 (14.5)
Diarrhea	35 (11.8)	21 (7.2)
Creatinine Increased[a]	33 (11.1)	0 (0)
Influenza	32 (10.8)	29 (10.0)
Nausea	31 (10.5)	14 (4.8)
Pharyngolaryngeal Pain	31 (10.5)	43 (14.8)
Vomiting	30 (10.1)	28 (9.7)
Respiratory Tract Infection	28 (9.5)	23 (7.9)
Bronchitis	27 (9.1)	32 (11.0)
Rash	25 (8.4)	9 (3.1)
Abdominal Pain Upper	23 (7.8)	15 (5.2)
Pharyngitis	23 (7.8)	30 (10.3)

(cont'd)

Table 1: EXJADE *(cont'd)*

Adverse Events Occurring in >5% of β-thalassemia Patients in the Comparative Trial

Preferred Term	EXJADE N=296 n (%)	Deferoxamine N=290 n (%)
Arthralgia	22 (7.4)	14 (4.8)
Acute Tonsillitis	19 (6.4)	15 (5.2)
Fatigue	18 (6.1)	14 (4.8)
Rhinitis	18 (6.1)	22 (7.6)
Back Pain	17 (5.7)	32 (11.0)
Ear Infection	16 (5.4)	7 (2.4)
Urticaria	11 (3.7)	17 (5.9)

a >33% increase compared to average baseline values.

The data in Table 2 display the adverse events, regardless of causality, occurring in >1% in the pooled β-thalassemia patients by dose administered. The most frequently reported adverse events were abdominal pain, pyrexia and headache. In the 30 mg/kg dose group, the most frequently reported adverse events were abdominal pain, diarrhea and increased serum creatinine. Skin rash and ALT increase were the only adverse events that resulted in discontinuation.

Table 2: EXJADE

Most Frequently Reported AEs (>1% of all patients)—Pooled β-thalassemia Patients by Dose Administered

Preferred Term	EXJADE 10 mg/kg N=143 Total n (%)	EXJADE 20 mg/kg N=106 Total n (%)	EXJADE 30 mg/kg N=172 Total n (%)	All Patients N=421 Total n (%)
Abdominal Pain	38 (26.6)	21 (19.8)	41 (23.8)	100 (23.8)
Pyrexia	47 (32.9)	31 (29.2)	20 (11.6)	98 (23.3)
Headache	37 (25.9)	20 (18.9)	26 (15.1)	83 (19.7)
Cough	38 (26.6)	17 (16.0)	25 (14.5)	80 (19.0)
Diarrhea	24 (16.8)	9 (8.5)	37 (21.5)	70 (16.6)
Nasopharyngitis	23 (16.1)	16 (15.1)	20 (11.6)	59 (14.0)
Vomiting	28 (19.6)	12 (11.3)	18 (10.5)	58 (13.8)
Rash	12 (8.4)	10 (9.4)	30 (17.4)	52 (12.4)
Nausea	11 (7.7)	11 (10.4)	28 (16.3)	50 (11.9)
Creatinine Increased[a]	2 (1.4)	13 (12.3)	34 (19.8)	49 (11.6)
Laryngeal Pain	20 (14.0)	12 (11.3)	17 (9.9)	49 (11.6)
Pharyngitis	28 (19.6)	9 (8.5)	10 (5.8)	47 (11.2)
Influenza	19 (13.3)	12 (11.3)	13 (7.6)	44 (10.5)
Rhinitis	28 (19.6)	8 (7.5)	6 (3.5)	42 (10.0)
URTI[b]	9 (6.3)	8 (7.5)	24 (14.0)	41 (9.7)
Bronchitis	7 (4.9)	9 (8.5)	20 (11.6)	36 (8.6)
Arthralgia	13 (9.1)	8 (7.5)	13 (7.6)	34 (8.1)
Back Pain	9 (6.3)	16 (15.1)	9 (5.2)	34 (8.1)
Constipation	9 (6.3)	6 (5.7)	12 (7.0)	27 (6.4)
Fatigue	7 (4.9)	6 (5.7)	13 (7.6)	26 (6.2)
Ear Infection	13 (9.1)	7 (6.6)	3 (1.7)	23 (5.5)
Tonsillitis	8 (5.6)	7 (6.6)	6 (3.5)	21 (5.0)
Post Procedural Pain	2 (1.4)	8 (7.5)	10 (5.8)	20 (4.8)
Acute Tonsillitis	2 (1.4)	6 (5.7)	11 (6.4)	19 (4.5)
Asthenia	8 (5.6)	7 (6.6)	4 (2.3)	19 (4.5)
Gastroenteritis	8 (5.6)	6 (5.7)	5 (2.9)	19 (4.5)
Chest Pain	2 (1.4)	8 (7.5)	8 (4.7)	18 (4.3)
Ear Pain	3 (2.1)	5 (4.7)	4 (2.3)	12 (2.9)
Palpitations	1 (0.7)	4 (3.8)	7 (4.1)	12 (2.9)
Tachycardia	5 (3.5)	4 (3.8)	3 (1.7)	12 (2.9)
Transfusion Reaction	7 (4.9)	3 (2.8)	2 (1.2)	12 (2.9)

(cont'd)

Table 2: EXJADE *(cont'd)*

Most Frequently Reported AEs (>1% of all patients)—Pooled β-thalassemia Patients by Dose Administered

Preferred Term	EXJADE 10 mg/kg N=143 Total n (%)	EXJADE 20 mg/kg N=106 Total n (%)	EXJADE 30 mg/kg N=172 Total n (%)	All Patients N=421 Total n (%)
Urticaria	3 (2.1)	4 (3.8)	5 (2.9)	12 (2.9)
Dyspepsia	4 (2.8)	3 (2.8)	4 (2.3)	11 (2.6)
Pain in Extremity	5 (3.5)	3 (2.8)	3 (1.7)	11 (2.6)
Pruritus	3 (2.1)	4 (3.8)	4 (2.3)	11 (2.6)
Rhinorrhoea	1 (0.7)	6 (5.7)	3 (1.7)	10 (2.4)
Sinusitis	0	6 (5.7)	4 (2.3)	10 (2.4)
Transaminases Increased	8 (5.6)	1 (0.9)	1 (0.6)	10 (2.4)
Urinary Tract Infection	2 (1.4)	1 (0.9)	7 (4.1)	10 (2.4)
Herpes Simplex	3 (2.1)	1 (0.9)	5 (2.9)	9 (2.1)
Otitis Media	2 (1.4)	1 (0.9)	6 (3.5)	9 (2.1)
Toothache	2 (1.4)	3 (2.8)	4 (2.3)	9 (2.1)
Anxiety	3 (2.1)	2 (1.9)	3 (1.7)	8 (1.9)
Bone Pain	1 (0.7)	1 (0.9)	6 (3.5)	8 (1.9)
Conjunctivitis	6 (4.2)	1 (0.9)	1 (0.6)	8 (1.9)
Dyspnoea	0	2 (1.9)	6 (3.5)	8 (1.9)
Muscle Cramp	1 (0.7)	0	7 (4.1)	8 (1.9)
Productive Cough	4 (2.8)	3 (2.8)	1 (0.6)	8 (1.9)
Tooth Abscess	2 (1.4)	0	6 (3.5)	8 (1.9)
Abdominal Distension	1 (0.7)	0	6 (3.5)	7 (1.7)
Cholelithiasis	2 (1.4)	1 (0.9)	4 (2.3)	7 (1.7)
Enteritis	5 (3.5)	1 (0.9)	1 (0.6)	7 (1.7)
Epistaxis	4 (2.8)	1 (0.9)	2 (1.2)	7 (1.7)
Erythema	3 (2.1)	2 (1.9)	2 (1.2)	7 (1.7)
Hypoacusis	4 (2.8)	2 (1.9)	1 (0.6)	7 (1.7)
Insomnia	0	3 (2.8)	4 (2.3)	7 (1.7)
Vertigo	2 (1.4)	4 (3.8)	1 (0.6)	7 (1.7)
Alanine Aminotransferase Increased	4 (2.8)	2 (1.9)	0	6 (1.4)
Cardiac Murmur	0	0	6 (3.5)	6 (1.4)
Depression	0	2 (1.9)	4 (2.3)	6 (1.4)
Dizziness	1 (0.7)	2 (1.9)	3 (1.7)	6 (1.4)
Dysmenorrhoea	0	3 (2.8)	3 (1.7)	6 (1.4)
Lymphadenopathy	2 (1.4)	1 (0.9)	3 (1.7)	6 (1.4)
Myalgia	1 (0.7)	1 (0.9)	4 (2.3)	6 (1.4)
Pharyngitis Streptococcal	3 (2.1)	3 (2.8)	0	6 (1.4)
Proteinuria	1 (0.7)	1 (0.9)	4 (2.3)	6 (1.4)
Rash Maculo-papular	0	3 (2.8)	3 (1.7)	6 (1.4)
Seasonal Allergy	0	1 (0.9)	5 (2.9)	6 (1.4)
Abdominal Discomfort	1 (0.7)	0	4 (2.3)	5 (1.2)
Contusion	2 (1.4)	0	3 (1.7)	5 (1.2)
Cystitis	1 (0.7)	1 (0.9)	3 (1.7)	5 (1.2)
Frequent Bowel Movements	1 (0.7)	1 (0.9)	3 (1.7)	5 (1.2)
Oedema Peripheral	0	2 (1.9)	3 (1.7)	5 (1.2)
Respiratory Tract Infection	1 (0.7)	1 (0.9)	3 (1.7)	5 (1.2)
Syncope	2 (1.4)	2 (1.9)	1 (0.6)	5 (1.2)
Viral Infection	1 (0.7)	1 (0.9)	3 (1.7)	5 (1.2)

a >33% increase compared to average baseline values.
b Upper respiratory tract infection.

Less Common Clinical Trial Adverse Drug Reactions (<1%): The less common adverse events which occurred in clinical trials and considered to be related to EXJADE are listed below.
Cardiovascular: QT prolongation*.
General Disorders: pyrexia, oedema, fatigue.
Ear and Labyrinth Disorders: hearing loss.
Eye Disorders: early cataract, maculopathy, optic neuritis.
Gastrointestinal: duodenal ulcer, gastric ulcer (including multiple ulcers), gastritis, gastrointestinal haemorrhage, oesophagitis.
Hepatobiliary: cholelithiasis, hepatitis.
Nervous System: dizziness.
Psychiatric Disorders: anxiety, sleep disorder.
Renal and Urinary Disorders: renal tubulopathy (Fanconi's syndrome).
Respiratory, Thoracic and Mediastinal Disorders: pharyngolaryngeal pain.
Skin and Subcutaneous Tissue Disorders: pigmentation disorder, erythema multiforme.
Abnormal Hematologic and Clinical Chemistry Findings: In the comparative study 0107, 113 patients treated with EXJADE had non-progressive increases in serum creatinine >33% above baseline (see Table 3). Twenty-five (25) patients required dose reductions. Increases in serum creatinine appeared to be dose-related. Of the 17 patients with elevations in ALT levels >5 times the ULN at consecutive visits, one discontinued EXJADE therapy. One patient experienced increases in transaminases to >10×ULN which normalized upon drug discontinuation but then increased sharply upon rechallenge. Increases in transaminases did not appear to be dose-related and most of these patients had elevated transaminases prior to receiving EXJADE therapy.

Table 3: EXJADE

Number (%) of Patients with Increases in ALT or Serum Creatinine in Study 0107

Laboratory Parameter	EXJADE N=296 n (%)	Deferoxamine N=290 n (%)
Serum Creatinine		
No. patients with creatinine >33% and at <ULN ≥2 consecutive post-baseline visits	106 (35.8)	40 (13.8)
No. patients with creatinine increase >33% and >ULN at ≥2 consecutive post-baseline visits	7 (2.4)	1 (0.3)
ALT		
No. patients with ALT >5×ULN at ≥2 post-baseline visits	8 (2.7)	2 (0.7)
No. patients with ALT >5×ULN at ≥2 consecutive post-baseline visits	17 (5.7)	5 (1.7)

A total of 652 patients were treated with EXJADE (deferasirox) in clinical studies 107, 108, and 109. Of these patients, 237 (36%) had an increase in serum creatinine >33% on at least 2 consecutive visits , 68 (11%) of whom underwent dose reduction. The remainder returned to serum creatinine <33% above baseline without dose reduction. Of the 68 patients who underwent dose reduction, 17 (25%) returned to normal, 41 (60%) remained elevated at >33% without progression and the remaining 10 (15%) fluctuated between baseline and 33%.

Based on limited data in patients with sickle cell disease (N=132) and other rare anemias (N=99), the type and frequency of adverse events observed were similar to those observed in patients with β-thalassemia. The adverse event profile in patients <16 years of age was similar to that seen in adults, regardless of disease state.

In 49 adult β-thalassemia patients treated for greater than 1 year and up to 3 years, the type and frequency of adverse events was similar to that seen in patients treated for up to 1 year.

Post-Market Adverse Drug Reactions: Cases of acute renal failure (some with fatal outcome) have been reported following the post-marketing use of EXJADE.

Spontaneously reported adverse reactions, presented below, are reported voluntarily and it is not always possible to reliably establish frequency or a causal relationship to drug exposure.

Post-Market Information: Since the International Birth Date (November 2, 2005), the cumulative exposure to marketed EXJADE is 45 882 patient-years as of April 30, 2009.

Pediatric population : Renal tubulopathy has been reported in patients treated with EXJADE. The majority of these patients were children and adolescents with beta-thalassemia and serum ferritin levels <1500 µg/L.

Renal and Urinary Disorders: acute renal failure (mostly serum creatinine increases ≥2× upper limit of normal, and usually reversible after treatment interruption), hematuria, renal tubular necrosis.
Skin and Subcutaneous Tissue Disorders: leukocytoclastic vasculitis, urticaria, erythema multiforme, alopecia.
Immune System Disorders: hypersensitivity reactions (including anaphylaxis and angioedema).
Gastrointestinal Disorders: duodenal ulcer, gastric ulcer, gastrointestinal bleeding.
Blood and Lymphatic System Disorders: agranulocytosis, neutropenia and thrombocytopenia.
Hepatic/Biliary/Pancreatic: hepatic failure.

DRUG INTERACTIONS: Drug-Drug Interactions: EXJADE should not be combined with other iron chelator therapies as the safety and efficacy of such combinations has not been established.

The concomitant administration of EXJADE and aluminum-containing antacid preparations has not been formally studied. Although deferasirox has a lower affinity for aluminum than for iron, EXJADE should not be taken with aluminum-containing antacid preparations (see Warnings and Precautions).

In a healthy volunteer study, the concomitant administration of EXJADE and midazolam (a CYP3A4 probe substrate) resulted in a decrease of midazolam exposure by 17%. In the clinical setting, this effect may be more pronounced. Therefore, caution should be exercised when deferasirox is combined with substances metabolised through CYP3A4 (e.g. cyclosporin, simvastatin, hormonal contraceptive agents), due to a possible decrease in efficacy.

In a healthy volunteer study, the concomitant administration of EXJADE (single dose of 30 mg/kg) and the potent UDP-glucuronosyltransferase (UGT) inducer rifampicin (repeated dose of 600 mg/day) resulted in a decrease of deferasirox exposure by 44% (90% CI: 37% - 51%). Therefore, the concomitant use of EXJADE with potent UGT inducers (e.g. rifampicin, phenytoin, phenobarbital, ritonavir) may result in a decrease in EXJADE efficacy. If EXJADE and a potent UGT inducer are used concomitantly, increases in the dose of EXJADE should be considered based on clinical response to therapy.

In a healthy volunteer study, the administration of cholestyramine after a single dose of deferasirox resulted in a 45% decrease in deferasirox exposure (AUC).

In a healthy volunteer study, the concomitant administration of EXJADE (repeated dose of 30 mg/kg/day) and the CYP2C8 probe substrate repaglinide (single dose of 0.5 mg) resulted in an increase in repaglinide AUC and C_{max} by 131% and 62%, respectively. If EXJADE and repaglinide are used concomitantly, careful monitoring of glucose levels should be performed. An interaction between EXJADE and other CYP2C8 substrates like paclitaxel cannot be excluded.

In healthy volunteers, EXJADE had no effect on the pharmacokinetics of digoxin. The effect of digoxin on EXJADE pharmacokinetics has not been studied.

The concomitant administration of EXJADE and vitamin C has not been formally studied. Doses of vitamin C up to 200 mg were allowed in clinical studies without negative consequences. High doses of vitamin C should not be used.

Concomitant administration of EXJADE with drugs that have known ulcerogenic potential, such as NSAIDs, corticosteroids, or oral bisphosphonates, and use of EXJADE in patients receiving anticoagulants may increase the risk of gastrointestinal irritation (see Warnings and Precautions).

The interaction of EXJADE with hydroxyurea has not been formally studied. No inhibition of deferasirox metabolism by hydroxyurea is expected based on the results of an in vitro study.

Drug-Food Interactions: EXJADE should be taken on an empty stomach at least 30 minutes before eating the first meal of the day, preferably at the same time each day.

* Three cases of QT interval prolongation were reported in the clinical trials, however, a causal relationship to study drug was not established.

EXJADE tablets for oral suspension can be dispersed in water, orange juice or apple juice. Dispersion of EXJADE in carbonated drinks or milk is not recommended due to foaming and slow dispersion, respectively.

Drug-Herb Interactions: Interactions with herbal products have not been established.

Drug-Laboratory Test Interactions: Interactions between EXJADE and gallium contrast media have not been studied. It is known that the results of gallium-67 imaging may be distorted by the iron chelator deferoxamine due to chelation of gallium-67. It is therefore recommended that EXJADE therapy be interrupted at least five days before gallium-67 scintigraphy.

DOSAGE AND ADMINISTRATION: Recommended Dose and Dosage Adjustment: It is recommended that therapy with EXJADE (deferasirox) be started when a patient has evidence of chronic iron overload, such as the transfusion of approximately 100 mL/kg of packed red blood cells (approximately 20 units for a 40 kg patient) and a serum ferritin consistently >1000 µg/L. Doses should be in mg/kg and must be calculated and rounded to the nearest whole tablet size. EXJADE is available in three strengths (125 mg, 250 mg and 500 mg).

The goals of iron chelation therapy are to remove the amount of iron administered in transfusions and, as required, to reduce the existing iron burden. The decision to remove accumulated iron should be individualized based on anticipated clinical benefit and risks of chelation therapy.

EXJADE should be taken on an empty stomach at least 30 minutes before eating the first meal of the day, preferably at the same time each day.

Starting Dose: The recommended initial daily dose of EXJADE is 10, 20, or 30 mg/kg/day body weight, depending on the patient's transfusion rate and the goal of treatment:

Patients requiring maintenance of an acceptable body iron level:

- An initial daily dose of 10 mg/kg/day is recommended for patients receiving less than 7 mL/kg/month of packed red blood cells (approximately <2 units/month for an adult) and for whom the objective is maintenance of an acceptable body iron level.
- An initial daily dose of 20 mg/kg/day is recommended for patients receiving more than 7 mL/kg/month of packed red blood cells (approximately >2 units/month for an adult) and for whom the objective is maintenance of an acceptable body iron level.

Patients requiring reduction of iron overload:

- An initial daily dose of 20 mg/kg/day is recommended for patients receiving less than 14 mL/kg/month of packed red blood cells (approximately <4 units/month for an adult) and for whom the objective is gradual reduction of iron overload.
- An initial daily dose of 30 mg/kg/day is recommended for patients receiving more than 14 mL/kg/month of packed red blood cells (approximately >4 units/month for an adult) and for whom the objective is gradual reduction of iron overload.

The dose dependent iron excretion (mg/kg/day) was calculated from the change in LIC over one year, the amount of blood transfused and the weight of the patient. Using two example patients of 20 kg and 50 kg, the amount of iron excreted over one year could be calculated in terms of mg/year and transfusion unit-equivalents/year (assuming that one unit of PRBC contains 200 mg iron). Thus in a 50 kg adult, doses of 10, 20 and 30 mg/kg for one year can remove the amount of iron contained in about 20, 36 and 55 units of blood, respectively (i.e. about 1.5, 3 and 4.5 units of blood per month, respectively). In a 20 kg pediatric patient, doses of 10, 20 and 30 mg/kg for one year can remove the amount of iron contained in about 8, 14 and 22 units of blood, respectively (i.e. about 0.6, 1.2 and 1.8 units of blood per month; or 6, 12 and 18 mL/kg/month, respectively). (See Table 4.)

Table 4: EXJADE

Study 0107: Iron Excretion During One Year (PP-2 population, biopsy)

			Iron Excretion (mg/year)		Iron Excretion (transfusion unit equivalents/year)	
Initial Dose (mg/kg)	**n**	**Iron Excretion (mg/kg/day)**	**20 kg patient**	**50 kg patient**	**20 kg patient**	**50 kg patient**
5	8	0.13±0.10	939±726	2349±1816	4.7±3.6	11.7±9.1
10	44	0.22±0.14	1572±1055	3930±2638	7.9±5.3	19.6±13.2
20	64	0.39±0.15	2841±1102	7102±2756	14.2±5.5	35.5±13.8
30	108	0.60±0.23	4378±1712	10945±4280	21.9±8.6	54.7±21.4

Maintenance Dose: It is recommended that serum ferritin be monitored every month and that the dose of EXJADE be adjusted if necessary every 3 to 6 months based on serum ferritin trends. Dose adjustments should be made in steps of 5 or 10 mg/kg and are to be tailored to the individual patient's response and therapeutic goals (maintenance or reduction of body iron burden). In patients with beta-thalassemia not adequately controlled with daily doses of 30 mg/kg, doses of up to 40 mg/kg may be considered. If the serum ferritin falls consistently below 500 µg/L, consideration should be given to temporarily interrupting therapy with EXJADE. As with other iron chelator treatment, the risk of toxicity of EXJADE may be increased when inappropriately high doses are given in patients with a low iron burden or with serum ferritin levels that are only slightly elevated. Doses of EXJADE should not exceed 30 mg/kg per day since, with the exception of beta-thalassemia patients, there is limited experience with doses above this level.

The Liver Iron Concentration (LIC) should be assessed periodically by an appropriate method such as biopsy or MRI in order to verify treatment response.

Dosing Considerations: Geriatrics (≥65 years of age): The pharmacokinetics of EXJADE have not been studied in geriatric patients. The dosing recommendations for elderly patients are the same as described above. In clinical trials, elderly patients experienced a higher frequency of adverse reactions than younger patients and should be monitored closely for adverse reactions that may require a dose adjustment.

Pediatrics (2 to 16 years of age): The dosing recommendations for pediatric patients are the same as for adult patients. In children <6 years of age, exposure was about 50% lower than adults. Since dosing is individually adjusted according to response this difference in exposure is not expected to have clinical consequences. Changes in weight of pediatric patients over time must also be taken into account when calculating the dose.

Patients with Renal Impairment: EXJADE has not been studied in patients with renal impairment (see Contraindications). For adult patients, the daily dose of EXJADE should be reduced by 10 mg/kg if a non-progressive rise in serum creatinine by >33% above the average of the pre-treatment measurements is seen at two consecutive visits, and cannot be attributed to other causes. From those patients who underwent dose reduction, creatinine levels returned to baseline in only 25% of patients and in 60% of them, creatinine levels remained elevated >33% of the average pre-treatment levels. For pediatric patients, the dose should be reduced by 10 mg/kg if serum creatinine levels rise above the age-appropriate upper limit of normal at two consecutive visits. A total of 6 patients <16 years developed creatinine levels >ULN during the core phase of the registration studies. Dose reductions were preformed in 5 patients, in 4 of whom the levels returned to baseline. Creatinine levels fell to <ULN in the fifth patient but remained higher than baseline.

If there is a progressive increase in serum creatinine beyond the upper limit of normal, EXJADE therapy should be interrupted (see Adverse Reactions, Abnormal Hematologic and Clinical Chemistry Findings).

Patients with Hepatic Impairment: EXJADE has not been studied in patients with hepatic impairment and should be used with caution in such patients. EXJADE treatment has been initiated only in patients with baseline liver transaminase levels up to 5 times the upper limit of normal range. The pharmacokinetics of deferasirox were not influenced by such transaminase levels. In patients with severe hepatic impairment (Child-Pugh score 10-15; category C) the starting dose should be reduced. The treating physician should initiate treatment with a dose taking into account general dosing instructions together with the extent of hepatic impairment. Close monitoring of efficacy and safety parameters is recommended. It is recommended that serum transaminase, bilirubin and alkaline phosphatase be monitored before the initiation of treatment, every 2 weeks during the first month and monthly thereafter. If there is an unexplained, persistent, and progressive increase in serum transaminase levels EXJADE treatment should be interrupted.

Patients with Skin Rash: Skin rashes may occur during EXJADE treatment. Severe skin rashes may require interruption of EXJADE treatment.

Gender: Females have a moderately lower apparent clearance (by 17.5%) for deferasirox compared to males. Since dosing is individually adjusted according to response this difference in clearance is not expected to have clinical consequences.

Missed Dose: If a dose is missed it should be taken as soon as remembered on that day, and the next dose should be taken as planned. Doses should not be doubled to make up for a missed dose.

Administration: Reconstitution: EXJADE tablets should be completely dispersed by stirring in water, orange juice, or apple juice until a fine suspension is obtained. Doses of <1 g should be dispersed in 100 mL of liquid and doses of >1 g in 200 mL of liquid. After swallowing the suspension, any residue should be resuspended in a small volume of liquid and swallowed. Tablets must not be chewed, split, crushed or swallowed whole.
Incompatibilities: Dispersion in carbonated drinks or milk is not recommended due to foaming and slow dispersion, respectively.

OVERDOSAGE:
Cases of overdose (2-3 times the prescribed dose for several weeks) have been reported with EXJADE (deferasirox). In one case, this resulted in subclinical hepatitis which resolved without long-term consequences after a dose interruption. Single doses up to 80 mg/kg in iron overloaded β-thalassemic patients have been tolerated with nausea and diarrhea noted. In healthy volunteers, single doses of up to 40 mg/kg were tolerated.

Acute signs of overdose may include nausea, vomiting, headache, and diarrhea. Overdose should be treated by induction of emesis or by gastric gavage, and by symptomatic treatment.

> For management of a suspected drug overdose, contact your regional Poison Control Centre. See the *CPS* Directory section for a list of Poison Control Centres.

ACTION AND CLINICAL PHARMACOLOGY: Mechanism of Action: EXJADE (deferasirox) is an orally active chelator that is highly selective for iron (as Fe^{3+}). It is a tridentate ligand that binds iron with high affinity in a 2:1 ratio. Although its highest affinity is for iron, deferasirox has a significant affinity for aluminium. Deferasirox has very low affinity for zinc and copper, and there are variable decreases in the serum concentration of these trace metals after the administration of deferasirox. The clinical significance of these decreases is uncertain.
Pharmacodynamics: Pharmacodynamic effects tested in an iron balance metabolic study showed that deferasirox (10, 20 and 40 mg/kg/day) was able to induce net iron excretion (0.119, 0.329 and 0.445 mg Fe/kg body weight/day, respectively) within the clinically relevant range (0.1-0.5 mg Fe/kg/day). Iron excretion was predominantly fecal.

Daily treatment with EXJADE at doses of 20 and 30 mg/kg for one year in frequently transfused adult and pediatric patients with beta-thalassemia led to reductions in indicators of total body iron; liver iron concentration was reduced by about 0.4 and 8.9 mg Fe/g liver (biopsy dry weight) on average, respectively, and serum ferritin was reduced by about 36 and 926 μg/L on average, respectively. At these same doses the ratios of iron excretion: iron intake were 1.02 (indicating net iron balance) and 1.67 (indicating net iron removal), respectively. EXJADE induced similar responses in iron-overloaded patients with other anemias. Daily doses of 10 mg/kg for one year could maintain liver iron and serum ferritin levels and induce net iron balance in patients receiving infrequent transfusions or exchange transfusions.

The effect of 20 and 40 mg/kg of deferasirox on QT interval was evaluated in a single-dose, double-blind, randomized, placebo- and active-controlled (moxifloxacin 400 mg), parallel group study in 182 healthy male and female volunteers aged 18-65 years. No evidence of prolongation of the QTc interval was observed in this study; however, the relevance of this study to long-term EXJADE use is unknown.
Pharmacokinetics: Absorption: EXJADE (deferasirox) is absorbed following oral administration with a median time to maximum plasma concentration (t_{max}) of about 1.5 to 4 hours. The C_{max} and AUC of deferasirox increase approximately linearly with dose after both single administration and under steady-state conditions. Exposure to deferasirox increased by an accumulation factor of 1.3 to 2.3 after multiple doses. The absolute bioavailability (AUC) of deferasirox tablets for oral suspension is 70% compared to an intravenous dose.

Total exposure (AUC) was approximately doubled when taken along with a high-fat breakfast (fat content >50% of calories) and increased by about 50% when taken along with a standard breakfast. The bioavailability (AUC) of deferasirox was moderately elevated when taken 30 minutes before meals with normal content (25% elevation) or high fat content (13% elevation). EXJADE must therefore be taken on an empty stomach at least 30 minutes before eating, preferably at the same time each day (see Dosage and Administration).

The total exposure (AUC) to deferasirox when taken after dispersion of tablets in orange juice or apple juice was equivalent to the exposure after dispersion in water (relative AUC ratios of 103% and 90%, respectively).
Distribution: Deferasirox is highly (~99%) protein bound almost exclusively to serum albumin. The percentage of deferasirox confined to the blood cells was 5% in humans. The volume of distribution at steady state (V_{ss}) of deferasirox is 14.37±2.69 L in adults.
Metabolism: Glucuronidation is the main metabolic pathway for deferasirox, with subsequent biliary excretion. Deconjugation of glucuronidates in the intestine and subsequent reabsorption (enterohepatic recycling) is likely to occur. Deferasirox is mainly glucuronidated by UGT1A1 and to a lesser extent UGT1A3. CYP450-catalysed (oxidative) metabolism of deferasirox appears to be minor in humans (about 8%). No evidence for induction or inhibition of CYP450 enzymes (CYP1A1, CYP1A2 and CYP2D6) at therapeutic doses has been observed. No inhibition of deferasirox metabolism by hydroxyurea was observed in an in vitro study. Deferasirox undergoes enterohepatic recycling.
Excretion: Deferasirox and metabolites are primarily (84% of the dose) excreted in the feces. Renal excretion of deferasirox and metabolites is minimal (8% of the dose). The mean elimination half-life ($t_{1/2}$) ranged from 8 to 16 hours.

STORAGE AND STABILITY: Store at room temperature (15-30°C). Protect from moisture.

Keep in the original package. Keep in a safe place out of the reach of children and pets.

INFORMATION FOR THE PATIENT: Published in e-CPS, available by subscription at www.e-cps.ca.

DOSAGE FORMS, COMPOSITION AND PACKAGING: 125 mg: Each off-white, round, flat dispersible tablet with beveled edge and imprinted with "J 125" on one side and "NVR" on the other, contains: deferasirox 125 mg. Nonmedicinal ingredients: colloidal silicon dioxide, crospovidone, lactose monohydrate, magnesium stearate, microcrystalline cellulose, povidone (K30) and sodium lauryl sulfate. Blisters of 28.
250 mg: Each off-white, round, flat dispersible tablet with beveled edge and imprinted with "J 250" on one side and "NVR" on the other, contains: deferasirox 250 mg. Nonmedicinal ingredients: colloidal silicon dioxide, crospovidone, lactose monohydrate, magnesium stearate, microcrystalline cellulose, povidone (K30) and sodium lauryl sulfate. Blisters of 28.
500 mg: Each off-white, round, flat dispersible tablet with beveled edge and imprinted with "J 500" on one side and "NVR" on the other, contains: deferasirox 500 mg. Nonmedicinal ingredients: colloidal silicon dioxide, crospovidone, lactose monohydrate, magnesium stearate, microcrystalline cellulose, povidone (K30) and sodium lauryl sulfate. Blisters of 28.

(Shown in Product Identification Section)

Experience™
senna leaves (Senna angustifolia)
Herbal Medicine

Awareness Corporation/dba AwarenessLife

SUPPLIED: Each capsule contains: senna leaves (Senna angustifolia) 300 mg. Nonmedicinal ingredients: black seed (Nigella sativa), corn silk (Stigmata maydis), fennel seed (Foeniculum vulgare), kelp (Fucus vesiculosus), psyllium seed husk (Plantago ovata) and solomon's seal [rhizome] (Polygonatum multiflorum); capsule: vegetable cellulose. No artificial colors, caffeine, flavors, preservatives, or salt. Bottles of 90. Store in a cool, dry place. Keep out of reach of children.

(Shown in Product Identification Section)

Extavia® Pr
interferon beta-1b
Immunomodulator

Novartis Pharmaceuticals

Date of Revision: November 27, 2009

SUMMARY PRODUCT INFORMATION:

Route of Administration	Dosage Form/ Strength	Clinically Relevant Nonmedicinal Ingredients
Subcutaneous	Lyophilized powder: 0.3 mg of interferon beta-1b/single-use vial Diluent: 1.2 mL of sodium chloride 0.54% solution/single-use syringe	Albumin human, USP For a complete listing see Dosage Forms, Composition and Packaging.

DESCRIPTION: EXTAVIA (interferon beta-1b) is a purified, sterile, lyophilized protein product produced by recombinant DNA techniques and formulated for use by injection.

INDICATIONS AND CLINICAL USE: EXTAVIA (interferon beta-1b) is indicated for:
- the treatment of patients with a single demyelinating event accompanied by at least two clinically silent lesions typical of multiple sclerosis (MS) on magnetic resonance imaging, to delay progression to definite MS. Before initiating treatment with EXTAVIA, alternate diagnoses should first be excluded.
- the reduction of the frequency of clinical exacerbations in ambulatory patients with relapsing-remitting multiple sclerosis. Relapsing-remitting MS is characterized by recurrent attacks of neurologic dysfunction followed by complete or incomplete recovery.
- the slowing of progression in disability and the reduction of the frequency of clinical exacerbations in patients with secondary-progressive multiple sclerosis.

The safety and efficacy of EXTAVIA in primary progressive MS have not been evaluated.
Pediatrics (<18 years of age): Safety and efficacy in children under 18 years of age have not been established.

CONTRAINDICATIONS:
- Patients with a history of hypersensitivity to natural or recombinant interferon beta, albumin human or to any other ingredient in the formulation. For a complete listing, see Dosage Forms, Composition and Packaging.
- Pregnant women.

WARNINGS AND PRECAUTIONS: Cardiovascular: Rare cases of cardiomyopathy have been reported. If this occurs, and a relationship to EXTAVIA (interferon beta-1b) is suspected, treatment should be discontinued.

Symptoms of flu syndrome observed with EXTAVIA therapy may prove stressful to patients with severe cardiac conditions. Patients with cardiac disease such as angina, congestive heart failure, or arrhythmia should be monitored closely for worsening of their clinical conditions.
Dependence/Tolerance: No evidence or experience suggests that abuse or dependence occurs with EXTAVIA therapy; however, the risk of dependence has not been systematically evaluated.
Endocrine and Metabolism: Rare cases of thyroid dysfunction (hyper- as well as hypothyroidism) associated with the use of EXTAVIA have been reported.
Hepatic/Biliary/Pancreatic: Rare post-market cases of serious hepatic injury, including autoimmune hepatitis, hepatitis and hepatic failure, have been reported with interferon beta treatment for multiple sclerosis.

It is recommended that liver function testing occur at baseline, every month for the first 6 months of treatment and at 6-month intervals thereafter. Dose reduction or discontinuation of therapy should be considered if alanine aminotransferase (ALT) levels increase 5 times above the upper limit of normal.

Interferon beta therapy should be initiated with caution in patients with a history of significant liver disease or alcohol abuse and in patients with clinical evidence of acute liver disease.

Caution must be exercised when prescribing drugs with documented hepatotoxicity to patients on interferon beta therapy for multiple sclerosis.

In rare cases, pancreatitis has been observed with EXTAVIA use, often associated with hypertriglyceridemia.
Hypersensitivity: Serious hypersensitivity reactions (rare but severe acute reactions such as bronchospasm, anaphylaxis and urticaria) may occur.
Immune: The administration of cytokines to patients with pre-existing monoclonal gammopathy has been associated with the development of systemic capillary leak syndrome with shock-like symptoms and fatal outcome.
Immunogenicity: As with all therapeutic proteins, there is a potential for immunogenicity. Serum samples in controlled clinical trials were collected every 3 months for monitoring of development of antibodies to EXTAVIA.

In the different controlled clinical trials, between 23% and 41% of the patients developed serum interferon beta-1b neutralizing activity confirmed by at least two consecutive positive titres; of these patients, between 43% and 55% converted to a stable antibody negative status (based on two consecutive negative titres) during the subsequent observational period of the respective study.

The development of neutralizing activity is associated with a reduction in clinical efficacy only with regard to relapse activity. Some analyses suggest that this effect might be larger in patients with higher titre levels of neutralizing activity.

In the study of patients with a single clinical event suggestive of multiple sclerosis, neutralizing activity measured every 6 months was observed at least once in 32% (88) of the patients treated early with EXTAVIA; of these, 47% (41) returned to negative status over a 3 year period. Within this period, the development of neutralizing activity was not associated with a reduction in clinical efficacy (with regard to time to clinically definite multiple sclerosis [CDMS], and time to confirmed EDSS progression).

New adverse events have not been associated with the development of neutralizing activity.

It has been demonstrated in vitro that EXTAVIA cross reacts with natural interferon beta. However, this has not been investigated in vivo and its clinical significance is uncertain.

There are sparse and inconclusive data on patients who have developed neutralizing activity and have completed EXTAVIA therapy.

The decision to continue or discontinue treatment should be based on clinical disease activity rather than on neutralizing activity status.
Neurologic: Rare cases of seizures have been reported with interferon beta therapy. EXTAVIA should be administered with caution to patients with a history of seizure disorders.

This product contains human albumin and hence carries an extremely remote risk for transmission of viral diseases. A theoretical risk for transmission of Creutzfeld-Jakob disease (CJD) is also considered extremely remote.

The effect of EXTAVIA on the ability to drive and use machinery has not been investigated.
Psychiatric: In the RR-MS clinical trial, one suicide and four attempted suicides were observed among 372 study patients during a 3-year period. All five patients received EXTAVIA (three in the 0.05 mg [1.6 MIU] group and two in the 0.25 mg [8.0 MIU] group). There were no attempted suicides in patients on study who did not receive EXTAVIA. In the SP-MS study there were 5 suicide attempts in the placebo group and 3 in the EXTAVIA group including one patient in each group who committed suicide. Depression and suicide have been reported to occur in patients receiving interferon alpha, a related compound. Patients treated with EXTAVIA should be informed that depression and suicidal ideation may be a side effect of the treatment and should report these symptoms immediately to the prescribing physician. Patients exhibiting depression should be monitored closely and cessation of therapy should be considered.
Sexual Function/Reproduction: Studies in female rhesus monkeys with normal menstrual cycles, at doses up to 0.33 mg (10.7 MIU)/kg/day (equivalent to 32 times the recommended human dose based on body surface area comparison) showed no apparent adverse effects on the menstrual cycle or on associated hormonal profiles (progesterone and estradiol) when administered over 3 consecutive menstrual cycles. The extrapolability of animal doses to human doses is not known. Effects of EXTAVIA on women with normal menstrual cycles are not known.
Special Populations: Pregnant Women: EXTAVIA was not teratogenic at doses up to 0.42 mg (13.3 MIU)/kg/day in rhesus monkeys, but demonstrated dose-related abortifacient activity when administered at doses ranging from 0.028 mg (0.89 MIU)/kg/day (2.8 times the recommended human dose based on body surface area comparison) to 0.42 mg (13.3 MIU)/kg/day (40 times the recommended human dose based on body surface area comparison). The extrapolability of animal doses to human doses is not known. Lower doses were not studied in monkeys. Spontaneous abortions while on treatment were reported in 4 patients who participated in the EXTAVIA RR-MS clinical trial, whereas there was one induced abortion in each of the placebo and EXTAVIA groups in the SP-MS trial. EXTAVIA given to rhesus monkeys on gestation days 20 to 70 did not cause teratogenic effects; however, it is not known if teratogenic effects exist in humans. There are no adequate and well-controlled studies in pregnant women.
Women of Childbearing Age: Women of childbearing potential should take reliable contraceptive measures. If the patient becomes pregnant or plans to become pregnant while taking EXTAVIA, the patient should discontinue therapy. It is not known if interferons alter the efficacy of oral contraceptives.
Nursing Women: It is not known whether EXTAVIA is excreted in human milk. Given that many drugs are excreted in human milk, there is a potential for serious adverse reactions in nursing infants, therefore a decision should be made whether to discontinue nursing or discontinue EXTAVIA treatment.

Pediatrics (<18 years of age): Safety and efficacy in children under 18 years of age have not been established.

Information to Be Provided to the Patient: Patients should be informed of the potential risk of liver injury with interferon beta therapy, and of the requirement for frequent laboratory testing for liver function (see Monitoring and Laboratory Tests). Patients should be informed of the symptoms suggesting liver dysfunction, such as jaundice, malaise, fatigue, nausea, vomiting, abdominal pain, dark urine, and pruritus, and advised to consult their physician immediately if such symptoms arise.

Patients should be instructed in injection techniques to assure the safe self-administration of EXTAVIA (see below and Information for the Patient).

Instruction on Self-injection Technique and Procedures: It is recommended that the first injection be administered by, or under the direct supervision of, a physician. Appropriate instructions for reconstitution of EXTAVIA and self-injection, using aseptic techniques, should be given to the patient. A careful review of Information for the Patient is also recommended.

Patients should be cautioned against the re-use of needles or syringes and instructed in safe disposal procedures. Information on how to acquire a puncture-resistant container for disposal of used needles and syringes should be given to the patient along with instructions for safe disposal of full containers.

Overall, 80% of patients in the two controlled clinical trials reported injection site reactions at one or more times during therapy. Post-marketing experience has been consistent with this finding, with infrequent reports of injection site necrosis.

The onset of injection site necrosis usually appears early in therapy with most cases reported to have occurred in the first two to three months of therapy. The number of sites where necrosis has been observed was variable.

Rarely, the area of necrosis has extended to subcutaneous fat or fascia. Response to treatment of injection site necrosis with antibiotics and/or steroids has been variable. In some of these patients elective debridement and, less frequently, skin grafting took place to facilitate healing which could take from three to six months.

Some patients experienced healing of necrotic skin lesions while EXTAVIA therapy continued. In other cases new necrotic lesions developed even after therapy was discontinued.

The nature and severity of all reported reactions should be carefully assessed.

To minimize the risk of injection site necrosis patients should be advised to use an aseptic injection technique and rotate the injection sites with each dose. Patient understanding and use of aseptic self-injection technique and procedures should be periodically re-evaluated.

The incidence of injection site reactions may be reduced by the use of an autoinjector. In the pivotal study of patients with a single clinical event suggestive of MS an autoinjector was used by the majority of patients. Injection site reactions, as well as injection site necrosis, were observed less frequently in this study than in the other pivotal studies.

Flu-like symptoms are not uncommon following initiation of therapy with EXTAVIA. In the controlled MS clinical trials, acetaminophen and non-steroidal anti-inflammatory drugs (NSAIDs) were permitted for relief of fever or myalgia.

Patients should be cautioned not to change the dosage or the schedule of administration without medical consultation.

Awareness of Adverse Reactions: Patients should be advised about the common adverse events associated with the use of EXTAVIA, particularly injection site reactions and the flu-like symptom complex (see Adverse Reactions).

Patients should be cautioned to report depression or suicidal ideation (see Warnings and Precautions, Psychiatric).

Patients should be advised about the abortifacient potential of EXTAVIA (see Warnings and Precautions, Special Populations, Pregnant Women).

Monitoring and Laboratory Tests: The following laboratory tests are recommended prior to initiating EXTAVIA therapy and at periodic intervals thereafter: thyroid function test, hemoglobin, complete and differential white blood cell counts, platelet counts and blood chemistries including liver function tests. It is recommended that liver function testing occur at baseline, every month for the first 6 months of treatment and at 6-month intervals thereafter. Dose reduction or discontinuation of therapy should be considered if alanine aminotransferase (ALT) levels increase 5 times above the upper limit of normal. A pregnancy test, chest roentgenogram and ECG should also be performed prior to initiating EXTAVIA therapy.

In the controlled MS trials, patients were monitored every 3 months. The study protocol stipulated that EXTAVIA therapy be discontinued in the event the absolute neutrophil count fell below 750/mm³. When the absolute neutrophil count had returned to a value greater than 750/mm³, therapy could be restarted at a 50% reduced dose. No patients were withdrawn or dose-reduced for neutropenia or lymphopenia. Similarly, if AST/ALT levels exceeded 10 times the upper limit of normal, or if the serum bilirubin exceeded 5 times the upper limit of normal, therapy was discontinued. In each instance, hepatic enzyme abnormalities returned to normal following discontinuation of therapy. When measurements had decreased to below these levels, therapy could be restarted at a 50% dose reduction, if clinically appropriate. Dose was reduced in two patients due to increased liver enzymes; one continued on treatment and one was ultimately withdrawn.

In the study conducted in patients with a single clinical event suggestive of MS, five EXTAVIA patients (1.7%) were withdrawn due to increased hepatic enzymes (AST/ALT), two of them after a dose reduction.

ADVERSE REACTIONS: Adverse Drug Reaction Overview: The most frequently observed adverse reactions are a flu-like symptom complex (fever, chills, arthralgia, malaise, sweating, headache or myalgia) and injection site reactions. Flu-like symptoms may be reduced by administration of acetaminophen or NSAIDs. Dose titration was used at the start of treatment in the clinically isolated syndrome and secondary-progressive MS studies in order to increase the tolerability of EXTAVIA (see Dosage and Administration).

Clinical Trial Adverse Drug Reactions: The following adverse events were observed in placebo-controlled clinical studies of EXTAVIA (interferon beta-1b), at the recommended dose of 0.25 mg (8 MIU), in patients with relapsing-remitting MS (n=124), secondary-progressive MS (n=360), and in patients with a single clinical event suggestive of MS (n=292). Because clinical trials are conducted under very specific conditions the adverse reaction rates observed in the clinical trials may not reflect the rates observed in practice and should not be compared to the rates in the clinical trials of another drug. Adverse drug reaction information from clinical trials is useful for identifying drug-related adverse events and for approximating rates.

1. Relapsing-remitting MS: Injection site reactions (85%) and injection site necrosis (5%) occurred after administration of EXTAVIA. Inflammation, pain, hypersensitivity, necrosis, and non-specific reactions were significantly associated (P<0.05) with the 0.25 mg (8 MIU) EXTAVIA-treated group, compared to placebo. Only inflammation, pain, and necrosis were reported as severe events. The incidence rate for injection site reactions was calculated over the course of 3 years. This incidence rate decreased over time, with 79% of patients experiencing the event during the first 3 months of treatment compared to 47% during the last 6 months. The median time to the first occurrence of an injection site reaction was 7 days. Patients with injection site reactions reported these events 183.7 days per year. Three patients withdrew from the 0.25 mg (8 MIU) EXTAVIA-treated group for injection site pain.

Flu-like symptom complex was reported in 76% of the patients treated with 0.25 mg (8 MIU) EXTAVIA. A patient was defined as having a flu-like symptom complex if flu-like syndrome or at least two of the following symptoms were concurrently reported: fever, chills, myalgia, malaise or sweating. Only myalgia, fever and chills were reported as severe in more than 5% of the patients. The incidence rate for flu-like symptom complex was also calculated over the course of 3 years. The incidence rate of these events decreased over time, with 60% of patients experiencing the event during the first 3 months of treatment compared to 10% during the last 6 months. The median time to the first occurrence of flu-like symptom complex was 3.5 days and the median duration per patient was 7.5 days per year.

Twenty-one (28%) of the 76 females of childbearing age treated at 0.25 mg (8 MIU) EXTAVIA and 10 (13%) of the 76 females of childbearing age treated with placebo reported menstrual disorders. All reports were of mild to moderate severity and included: intermenstrual bleeding and spotting, early or delayed menses, decreased days of menstrual flow, and clotting and spotting during menstruation.

Mental disorders such as depression, anxiety, emotional lability, depersonalization, suicide attempts, and confusion were observed in this study. Two patients withdrew for confusion. One suicide and four attempted suicides were also reported. It is not known whether these symptoms may be related to the underlying neurological basis of MS, to EXTAVIA treatment, or to a combination of both. Some similar symptoms have been noted in patients receiving interferon alpha and both interferons are thought to act through the same receptor. Patients who experience these symptoms should be monitored closely and cessation of therapy should be considered.

Additional common clinical and laboratory adverse events associated with the use of EXTAVIA are listed in the following paragraphs. These events occurred at an incidence of 5% or more in the 124 MS patients treated with 0.25 mg (8 MIU) EXTAVIA every other day for periods of up to three years in the controlled trial, and at an incidence that was at least twice that observed in the 123 placebo patients. Common adverse clinical and laboratory events associated with the use of EXTAVIA were: injection site reaction (85%); lymphocyte count <1500/mm³ (82%); ALT >5 times baseline value (19%); absolute neutrophil count <1500/mm³ (18%); menstrual disorder (17%); WBC <3000/mm³ (16%); palpitation (8%); dyspnea (8%); cystitis (8%); hypertension (7%); breast pain (7%); tachycardia (6%); gastrointestinal disorders (6%); total bilirubin >2.5 times baseline value (6%); somnolence (6%); laryngitis (6%); pelvic pain (6%); menorrhagia (6%); injection site necrosis (5%); peripheral vascular disorders (5%).

A total of 277 MS patients have been treated with EXTAVIA in doses ranging from 0.025 mg (0.8 MIU) to 0.5 mg (16 MIU). During the first three years of treatment, withdrawals due to clinical adverse events or laboratory abnormalities not mentioned above included: fatigue (2%, 6 patients); cardiac arrhythmia (<1%, 1 patient); allergic urticarial skin reaction to injections (<1%, 1 patient); headache (<1%, 1 patient); unspecified adverse events (<1%, 1 patient); "felt sick" (<1%, 1 patient).

Table 1 enumerates adverse events and laboratory abnormalities that occurred at an incidence of 2% or more among the 124 MS patients treated with 0.25 mg (8 MIU) EXTAVIA every other day for periods of up to three years in the controlled trial and at an incidence that was at least 2% more than that observed in the 123 placebo patients. Reported adverse events have been re-classified using the standard COSTART glossary to reduce the total number of terms employed in Table 1. In the following table, terms so general as to be uninformative, and those events where a drug cause was remote have been excluded.

Table 1: EXTAVIA

Incidence of Adverse Events and Laboratory Abnormalities (Regardless of Causality) ≥2% and >2% Difference (EXTAVIA vs Placebo) in the Relapsing-remitting MS Study

System Organ Class Adverse Event	Placebo n=123	EXTAVIA 0.25 mg (8 MIU) n=124
Infections and Infestations		
Sinusitis	26%	36%
Laryngitis	2%	6%
Neoplasms, Benign, Malignant and Unspecified		
Cyst	2%	4%
Breast neoplasm	0%	2%
Blood and Lymphatic System Disorders		
Lymphadenopathy	11%	14%
Endocrine Disorders		
Goiter	0%	2%
Metabolism and Nutrition Disorders		
Glucose <55 mg/dL	13%	15%
Weight gain	0%	4%
Weight loss	2%	4%
Psychiatric Disorders		
Depression	24%	25%
Anxiety	13%	15%
Nervousness	5%	8%
Suicide attempt	0%	2%
Nervous System Disorders		
Dizziness	28%	35%
Hypertonia	24%	26%
Myasthenia	10%	13%
Migraine	7%	12%
Somnolence	3%	6%
Confusion	2%	4%
Speech disorder	1%	3%
Convulsion	0%	2%
Hyperkinesia	0%	2%
Amnesia	0%	2%
Eye Disorders		
Conjunctivitis	10%	12%
Abnormal vision	4%	7%
Cardiac Disorders		
Palpitation[a]	2%	8%
Tachycardia	3%	6%
Vascular Disorders		
Hypertension	2%	7%
Peripheral vascular disorder	2%	5%
Hemorrhage	1%	3%
Respiratory, Thoracic and Mediastinal Disorders		
Dyspnea[a]	2%	8%
Gastrointestinal Disorders		

(cont'd)

Table 1: EXTAVIA *(cont'd)*

Incidence of Adverse Events and Laboratory Abnormalities (Regardless of Causality) ≥2% and >2% Difference (EXTAVIA vs Placebo) in the Relapsing-remitting MS Study

System Organ Class Adverse Event	Placebo n=123	EXTAVIA 0.25 mg (8 MIU) n=124
Diarrhea	29%	35%
Abdominal pain	24%	32%
Constipation	18%	24%
Vomiting	19%	21%
Gastrointestinal disorder	3%	6%
Skin and Subcutaneous Tissue Disorders		
Sweating[a]	11%	23%
Alopecia	2%	4%
Necrosis	0%	2%
Musculoskeletal and Connective Tissue Disorders		
Myalgia[a]	28%	44%
Pelvic pain	3%	6%
Renal and Urinary Disorders		
Cystitis	4%	8%
Urinary urgency	2%	4%
Reproductive System and Breast Disorders		
Dysmenorrhea	11%	18%
Menstrual disorder[a]	8%	17%
Metrorrhagia	8%	15%
Breast pain	3%	7%
Menorrhagia	3%	6%
Fibrocystic breast	1%	3%
General Disorders and Administration Site Conditions		
Injection site reaction[a]	37%	85%
Headache	77%	84%
Flu-like symptom complex[a]	56%	76%
Fever[a]	41%	59%
Pain	48%	52%
Asthenia[a]	35%	49%
Chills[a]	19%	46%
Malaise[a]	3%	15%
Generalized edema	6%	8%
Injection site necrosis[a]	0%	5%
Investigations		
Lymphocytes <1500/mm^3	67%	82%
ALT >5 times baseline[a]	6%	19%
ANC <1500/mm^3[a]	6%	18%
WBC <3000/mm^3[a]	5%	16%
Total bilirubin >2.5 times baseline	2%	6%
Urine protein >1+	3%	5%
AST >5 times baseline[a]	0%	4%

[a] Significantly associated with EXTAVIA treatment (P<0.05).

It should be noted that the figures cited in Table 1 cannot be used to predict the incidence of side effects in the course of usual medical practice where patient characteristics and other factors differ from those that prevailed in the clinical trials. The cited figures do provide the prescribing physician with some basis for estimating the relative contribution of drug and non-drug factors to the side effect incidence rate in the population studied.

2. Secondary-progressive MS: The incidence of adverse events that occurred in at least 2% of patients treated with 8 MIU EXTAVIA or placebo for up to three years, **or** where an adverse event was reported at a frequency at least 2% higher with EXTAVIA than that observed for placebo-treated patients in the secondary-progressive study, is presented in Table 2. Adverse events significantly associated with EXTAVIA compared to placebo (P<0.05) are also indicated in Table 2.

Table 2: EXTAVIA

Incidence of Adverse Events (Regardless of Causality) ≥2% or >2% Difference (EXTAVIA vs Placebo) in the Secondary-progressive MS Study

System Organ Class Adverse Event	Placebo n=358	EXTAVIA 0.25 mg (8 MIU) n=360
Infections and Infestations		
Rhinitis	32%	28%
Urinary tract infection	25%	22%
Pharyngitis	20%	16%
Infection	11%	13%
Bronchitis	12%	9%
Sinusitis	6%	6%
Pneumonia	5%	5%
Abscess[a]	2%	4%
Upper respiratory tract infection	2%	3%
Herpes simplex	2%	3%
Herpes zoster	2%	1%
Blood and Lymphatic System Disorders		
Leukopenia[a]	5%	10%
Lymphadenopathy	1%	3%
Anemia	5%	2%
Ecchymosis	2%	1%
Immune System Disorders		
Allergic reaction	3%	2%
Metabolism and Nutrition Disorders		
Weight loss	3%	2%
Hypercholesterolemia	2%	1%
Psychiatric Disorders		
Depression	31%	27%
Insomnia	8%	12%
Emotional lability	11%	8%
Anxiety	5%	6%
Nervousness	3%	4%
Nervous System Disorders		
Headache	41%	47%
Hypertonia[a]	31%	41%
Myasthenia	40%	39%
Neuropathy	41%	38%
Paresthesia	39%	35%
Abnormal gait	34%	34%
Ataxia	23%	19%
Dizziness	14%	14%
Incoordination	13%	11%
Vertigo	12%	8%
Paralysis	10%	8%
Somnolence	8%	8%
Tremor	9%	6%
Sleep disorder	5%	6%
Hypesthesia	4%	6%
Neuralgia	7%	5%
Movement disorder	6%	5%

(cont'd)

Table 2: EXTAVIA *(cont'd)*

Incidence of Adverse Events (Regardless of Causality) ≥2% or >2% Difference (EXTAVIA vs Placebo) in the Secondary-progressive MS Study

System Organ Class Adverse Event	Placebo n=358	EXTAVIA 0.25 mg (8 MIU) n=360
Migraine	3%	4%
Spastic paralysis	1%	3%
Speech disorder	5%	2%
Dysarthria	4%	2%
Convulsion	2%	2%
Hyperesthesia	2%	2%
Optic neuritis	2%	2%
Amnesia	3%	1%
Hemiplegia	2%	1%
Thinking abnormal	2%	1%
Myoclonus	2%	0%
Eye Disorders		
Abnormal vision	15%	11%
Amblyopia	10%	7%
Diplopia	9%	7%
Eye pain	5%	4%
Eye disorder	2%	3%
Conjunctivitis	3%	2%
Ear and Labyrinth Disorders		
Otitis media	3%	2%
Deafness	3%	1%
Ear disorder	2%	1%
Tinnitus	2%	1%
Cardiac Disorders		
Palpitation	3%	2%
Syncope	3%	2%
Tachycardia	1%	2%
Vascular Disorders		
Vasodilatation	4%	6%
Peripheral vascular disorder	5%	5%
Hypertension[a]	2%	4%
Hypotension	4%	2%
Hemorrhage	2%	2%
Respiratory, Thoracic and Mediastinal Disorders		
Cough increased	10%	5%
Dyspnea	2%	3%
Sore throat	1%	2%
Asthma	2%	1%
Thorax pain	2%	1%
Voice alteration	2%	1%
Gastrointestinal Disorders		
Nausea	13%	13%
Constipation	12%	12%
Abdominal pain[a]	6%	11%
Diarrhea	10%	7%
Gastroenteritis	5%	6%

(cont'd)

Table 2: EXTAVIA *(cont'd)*

Incidence of Adverse Events (Regardless of Causality) ≥2% or >2% Difference (EXTAVIA vs Placebo) in the Secondary-progressive MS Study

System Organ Class Adverse Event	Placebo n=358	EXTAVIA 0.25 mg (8 MIU) n=360
Vomiting	6%	4%
Dysphagia	5%	4%
Gastrointestinal disorder	5%	4%
Tooth disorder	4%	4%
Dyspepsia	4%	4%
Anorexia	2%	4%
Flatulence	1%	3%
Fecal incontinence	3%	2%
Gastritis	2%	2%
Gastrointestinal pain	0%	2%
Gingivitis	0%	2%
Dry mouth	2%	1%
Colitis	2%	0%
Skin and Subcutaneous Tissue Disorders		
Rash[a]	12%	20%
Sweating increased	6%	6%
Pruritus	6%	6%
Skin disorder	4%	4%
Eczema	4%	2%
Alopecia	2%	2%
Acne	2%	2%
Dry skin	3%	1%
Subcutaneous hematoma	3%	1%
Seborrhea	2%	1%
Musculoskeletal and Connective Tissue Disorders		
Back pain	24%	26%
Myalgia[a]	9%	23%
Arthralgia	20%	20%
Pain in extremity	12%	14%
Neck pain	6%	5%
Chest pain	4%	5%
Bone fracture (not spontaneous)	5%	3%
Muscle cramps	3%	3%
Spontaneous bone fracture	3%	3%
Arthritis	1%	2%
Joint disorder	1%	2%
Renal and Urinary Disorders		
Urinary incontinence	15%	8%
Urinary urgency	7%	8%
Urinary tract disorder	10%	7%
Cystitis	9%	7%
Increased urinary frequency	5%	6%
Urinary retention	6%	4%
Dysuria	2%	2%
Nocturia	1%	2%
Pyelonephritis	0%	2%

(cont'd)

Table 2: EXTAVIA *(cont'd)*

Incidence of Adverse Events (Regardless of Causality) ≥2% or >2% Difference (EXTAVIA vs Placebo) in the Secondary-progressive MS Study

System Organ Class Adverse Event	Placebo n=358	EXTAVIA 0.25 mg (8 MIU) n=360
Kidney pain	2%	0%
Reproductive System and Breast Disorders		
Metrorrhagia	6%	12%
Menstrual disorder	13%	9%
Impotence	4%	7%
Vaginitis	4%	3%
Amenorrhea	4%	3%
Menopause	4%	2%
Menorrhagia	4%	2%
Vaginal moniliasis	2%	2%
Prostatic disorder	1%	2%
Breast pain	2%	1%
General Disorders and Administration Site Conditions		
Asthenia	58%	63%
Flu syndrome[a]	40%	61%
Injection site inflammation[a]	4%	48%
Injection site reaction[a]	10%	46%
Fever[a]	13%	40%
Pain	25%	31%
Chills[a]	7%	23%
Injection site pain	5%	9%
Malaise	5%	8%
Peripheral edema	7%	7%
Injection site necrosis[a]	0%	5%
Chills and fever[a]	0%	3%
Injection site hemorrhage	2%	2%
Investigations		
Laboratory test abnormal	1%	3%
Liver function test abnormal	1%	3%
ALT increased	2%	2%
Injury, Poisoning and Procedural Complications		
Accidental injury	17%	14%

[a] Significantly associated with EXTAVIA treatment (P<0.05).

Seventy-four (74) patients discontinued treatment due to adverse events (23 on placebo and 51 on EXTAVIA). Injection site reactions were significantly associated with early termination of treatment in the EXTAVIA group compared to placebo (P<0.05). The highest frequency of adverse events leading to discontinuation involved the nervous system, of which depression (7 on placebo and 11 on EXTAVIA) was the most common.

3. Single Clinical Event Suggestive of MS: The incidence of all adverse events reported during the two-year study duration that occurred in ≥1% of patients treated with 8 MIU EXTAVIA and with a higher frequency versus the placebo group is presented in Table 3. The most frequent adverse events reported for EXTAVIA were injection site reaction (48.3%), flu syndrome (44.2%), headache (26.7%), and asthenia (21.6%).

The frequency of some adverse events decreased substantially from the first year to the second year of the study. The proportion of EXTAVIA-treated patients experiencing flu syndrome was reduced from 42% in the first year to 13% in the second year. Also, injection site reactions occurred less frequently during the second year (30%) than during the first year (46%).

Table 3: EXTAVIA

Incidence of Adverse Events (Regardless of Causality) ≥1% Occurring More Frequently in EXTAVIA (vs Placebo) Patients With a Single Demyelinating Event Suggestive of MS

System Organ Class Adverse Event (Preferred Term, MedDRA Version 9.0)	Placebo (n=176)	EXTAVIA 0.25 mg (8 MIU) (n=292)
Infections and Infestations		
Infection	3.4%	5.8%
Herpes simplex	1.1%	1.4%
Tooth abscess	0.6%	1.0%
Herpes zoster	0%	1.0%
Blood and Lymphatic System Disorders		
Leukopenia[a]	5.7%	18.2%
Lymphadenopathy	0.6%	1.4%
Thrombocytopenia	0.6%	1.4%
Immune System Disorders		
Hypersensitivity	1.7%	4.5%
Endocrine Disorders		
Hypothyroidism	1.1%	1.4%
Metabolism and Nutrition Disorders		
Hypoglycemia	0%	1.0%
Psychiatric Disorders		
Insomnia	4.0%	8.2%
Affect lability	2.3%	4.1%
Nervousness	1.1%	1.4%
Nervous System Disorders		
Headache[a]	17.0%	26.7%
Optic neuritis	2.3%	2.7%
Migraine	1.7%	2.4%
Hypertonia	1.1%	2.1%
Visual field defect	0%	1.4%
Hemiplegia	0.6%	1.0%
Myoclonus	0%	1.0%
Eye Disorders		
Visual disturbance[a]	0.6%	3.4%
Eye pain	2.8%	3.1%
Vision blurred	0%	1.7%
Conjunctivitis	1.1%	1.4%
Diplopia	0.6%	1.0%
Cardiac Disorders		
Palpitations	0.6%	1.4%
Tachycardia	0%	1.4%
Vascular Disorders		
Hypertension	0%	2.1%
Hypotension	0%	1.4%
Respiratory, Thoracic and Mediastinal Disorders		
Cough	2.3%	2.4%
Epistaxis	0.6%	1.4%
Gastrointestinal Disorders		
Vomiting[a]	1.1%	5.1%
Abdominal pain	2.8%	4.8%
Diarrhea	1.7%	4.1%
Tooth disorder	1.7%	2.4%
Gastritis	0.6%	1.7%
Aphthous stomatitis	0.6%	1.4%

(cont'd)

Table 3: EXTAVIA *(cont'd)*

Incidence of Adverse Events (Regardless of Causality) ≥1% Occurring More Frequently in EXTAVIA (vs Placebo) Patients With a Single Demyelinating Event Suggestive of MS

System Organ Class Adverse Event (Preferred Term, MedDRA Version 9.0)	Placebo (n=176)	EXTAVIA 0.25 mg (8 MIU) (n=292)
Constipation	0.6%	1.0%
Glossodynia	0%	1.0%
Skin and Subcutaneous Tissue Disorders		
Rash[a]	2.8%	11.0%
Hyperhidrosis	1.1%	2.1%
Pruritus	1.1%	2.1%
Urticaria	0.6%	2.1%
Skin disorder	0%	1.4%
Psoriasis	0.6%	1.0%
Eczema	0%	1.0%
Musculoskeletal and Connective Tissue Disorders		
Back pain	6.8%	9.9%
Pain in extremity	3.4%	6.2%
Arthralgia	5.7%	5.8%
Renal and Urinary Disorders		
Proteinuria	1.1%	2.7%
Urinary incontinence	0.6%	1.0%
Micturition urgency	0.6%	1.0%
Nocturia	0%	1.0%
Reproductive System and Breast Disorders		
Dysmenorrhea[b]	0%	2.4%
Ejaculation disorder[c]	0%	2.4%
Metrorraghia[b]	0%	1.9%
Vaginal candidiasis[b]	0%	1.4%
Impotence[c]	0%	1.2%
General Disorders and Administration Site Conditions		
Injection site reaction[a]	8.5%	48.3%
Influenza-like illness[a]	18.2%	44.2%
Asthenia	17.0%	21.6%
Pyrexia[a]	4.5%	13.0%
Injection site pain	2.8%	5.8%
Chills[a]	1.1%	5.5%
Pain	4.0%	4.1%
Gait disturbance	0.6%	2.1%
Malaise	0.6%	1.0%
Chest pain	0%	1.0%
Injection site inflammation	0%	1.0%
Injection site necrosis	0%	1.0%
Investigations		
Alanine aminotransferase increased[a]	4.5%	15.4%
Aspartate aminotransferase increased[a]	2.8%	11.0%
Liver function test abnormal[a]	1.1%	5.5%
Laboratory test abnormal	1.7%	2.1%
Gamma-glutamyltransferase increased	0.6%	1.0%
Injury, Poisoning and Procedural Complications		
Injury	4.0%	5.5%
Subcutaneous hematoma	2.8%	3.4%
Post-procedural complication	0%	1.4%

(cont'd)

[a] Significantly associated with EXTAVIA treatment (P<0.05).
[b] Incidence in females only (n=207).
[c] Incidence in males only (n=85).

Serious adverse events were reported by equal proportions (6.8%) of patients in the two treatment groups. Eight EXTAVIA patients (2.7%) experienced adverse events which led to premature discontinuation of the study.

A 3-year integrated analysis combined safety data from the 2-year placebo-controlled study and the pre-planned follow-up study. The incidence of adverse events reported in ≥10% of overall patients is presented in Table 4.

Table 4: EXTAVIA

Incidence of Adverse Events ≥10% of Overall Patients in Integrated 3-Year Analysis

System Organ Class Adverse event (Preferred term, MedDRA version 11.0)	Delayed Treatment (n=176)	Early Treatment (n=292)
Infections and Infestations		
Upper respiratory tract infection	29.5%	26.0%
Pharyngitis	13.6%	12.7%
Blood and Lymphatic System Disorders		
Leukopenia	12.5%	22.3%
Psychiatric Disorders		
Depression	20.5%	15.4%
Insomnia	10.2%	10.6%
Nervous System Disorders		
Multiple sclerosis relapse	43.2%	30.1%
Headache	27.8%	31.8%
Paresthesia	24.4%	25.0%
Skin and Subcutaneous Tissue Disorders		
Rash	8.5%	14.4%
Musculoskeletal and Connective Tissue Disorders		
Back pain	10.2%	13.0%
General Disorders and Administration Site Conditions		
Injection site reaction (various kinds)[a]	41.5%	57.2%
Flu-like symptom complex[b]	47.7%	51.4%
Asthenia	26.7%	25.7%
Pyrexia	9.7%	15.8%
Investigations		
ALT increased	6.8%	15.8%

[a] "Injection site reaction (various kinds)" comprises all adverse events occurring at the injection site, ie, the terms "injection site edema", "injection site hemorrhage", "injection site hypersensitivity", "injection site inflammation", "injection site mass", "injection site necrosis", "injection site pain", and "injection site reaction".
[b] "Flu-like syndrome complex" denotes the terms "flu syndrome" and/or a combination of at least two adverse events from "fever", "chills", "myalgia", "malaise", or "sweating".
Abbreviations: ALT—alanine aminotransferase.

Flu-like symptoms and injection site reactions were observed less frequently than in the other pivotal trials. To increase tolerability of EXTAVIA, dose titration was performed and NSAIDs were administered at start of therapy. Moreover, an autoinjector was used by the majority of patients throughout the study.

Other events observed during pre-marketing evaluation of various doses of EXTAVIA in 1440 patients are listed in the paragraphs that follow. Given that most of the events were observed in open and uncontrolled studies, the role of EXTAVIA in their causation cannot be reliably determined.

Blood and Lymphatic System Disorders: chronic lymphocytic leukemia, hemoglobin less than 9.4 g/100 mL, petechia, platelets less than 75 000/mm³, and splenomegaly.
Cardiac Disorders: angina pectoris, arrhythmia, atrial fibrillation, cardiomegaly, cardiac arrest, cerebral ischemia, endocarditis, heart failure, myocardial infarct, pericardial effusion, syncope, ventricular extrasystoles, and ventricular fibrillation.
Ear and Labyrinth Disorders: deafness, ear pain, otitis externa, and otitis media.
Endocrine Disorders: Cushing's syndrome, diabetes insipidus, diabetes mellitus, hypothyroidism, and inappropriate ADH.
Eye Disorders: blepharitis, blindness, dry eyes, diplopia, iritis, keratoconjunctivitis, mydriasis, photophobia, retinitis, and visual field defect.

Gastrointestinal Disorders: aphthous stomatitis, ascites, cardiospasm, cheilitis, cholecystitis, cholelithiasis, duodenal ulcer, dry mouth, enteritis, esophagitis, fecal impaction, fecal incontinence, flatulence, gastritis, gingivitis, glossitis, hematemesis, ileus, increased salivation, intestinal obstruction, melena, nausea, oral leukoplakia, oral moniliasis, pancreatitis, proctitis, salivary gland enlargement, stomach ulcer, taste loss, taste perversion, and tenesmus.
General Disorders and Administration Site Conditions: edema, hernia, hypothermia, and photosensitivity.
Hepatobiliary Disorders: alkaline phosphatase greater than 5 times baseline value, hepatitis, and hepatomegaly.
Immune System Disorders: anaphylactoid reaction.
Infections and Infestations: abscess, cellulitis, infection, periodontal abscess, peritonitis, and sepsis.
Metabolism and Nutrition Disorders: alcohol intolerance, calcium greater than 11.5 mg/dL, glucose greater than 160 mg/dL, glycosuria, hypoglycemic reaction, ketosis, and thirst.
Musculoskeletal and Connective Tissue Disorders: arthritis, arthrosis, bursitis, dystonia, leg cramps, muscle atrophy, myopathy, myositis, ptosis, and tenosynovitis.
Neoplasms, Benign, Malignant and Unspecified: adenoma, carcinoma of the lung, hepatic neoplasia, sarcoma, skin benign neoplasm, skin carcinoma, spider angioma, and uterine neoplasm.
Nervous System Disorders: abnormal gait, acute brain syndrome, aphasia, ataxia, brain edema, chronic brain syndrome, coma, delirium, depersonalization, facial paralysis, foot drop, hemiplegia, hydrocephalus, hypalgesia, hyperesthesia, incoordination, libido decreased, meningitis, neuralgia, neuropathy, nystagmus, oculogyric crisis, ophthalmoplegia, papilledema, paralysis, reflexes decreased, shock, subdural hematoma, torticollis, and tremor.
Psychiatric Disorders: agitation, apathy, delusions, dementia, depersonalization, euphoria, hallucinations, manic reaction, neurosis, paranoid reaction, psychosis, and stupor.
Renal and Urinary Disorders: anuria, BUN greater than 40 mg/dL, hematuria, kidney calculus, kidney failure, kidney tubular disorder, nephritis, nocturia, oliguria, polyuria, urethritis, urinary incontinence, and urinary retention.
Reproductive System and Breast Disorders: balanitis, breast engorgement, cervicitis, epididymitis, gynecomastia, impotence, leukorrhea, salpingitis, and uterine fibroids enlarged.
Respiratory, Thoracic and Mediastinal Disorders: apnea, asthma, atelectasis, cyanosis, hemoptysis, hiccup, hyperventilation, hypoventilation, hypoxia, interstitial pneumonia, lung edema, parosmia, pleural effusion, pneumonia, and pneumothorax.
Skin and Subcutaneous Tissue Disorders: contact dermatitis, erythema nodosum, exfoliative dermatitis, furunculosis, hirsutism, leukoderma, lichenoid dermatitis, maculopapular rash, psoriasis, seborrhea, skin hypertrophy, skin necrosis, skin ulcer, urticaria, and vesiculobullous rash.
Vascular Disorders: cerebral hemorrhage, gastrointestinal hemorrhage, hypotension, intracranial hypertension, postural hypotension, pulmonary embolus, rectal hemorrhage, subarachnoid hemorrhage, thrombophlebitis, thrombosis, vaginal hemorrhage, varicose vein, vasospasm, and venous pressure increased.
Abnormal Hematologic and Clinical Chemistry Findings: 1. Relapsing-remitting MS: In the relapsing-remitting MS study, the most common laboratory abnormalities included: lymphocyte count <1500/mm³ (82%); ALT >5 times baseline value (19%); absolute neutrophil count <1500/mm³ (18%) (no patients had absolute neutrophil counts <500/mm³); WBC <3000/mm³ (16%); total bilirubin >2.5 times baseline value (6%).

Three patients were withdrawn from treatment with 0.25 mg (8 MIU) EXTAVIA for abnormal liver enzymes including one following dose reduction (see Warnings and Precautions, Monitoring and Laboratory Tests).
2. Secondary-progressive MS: Significantly more patients on active therapy (14.4% vs 4.7% on placebo) had elevated ALT values (>5 times baseline value). Elevations were also observed in AST and gamma-GT values in the EXTAVIA group throughout the study. In the EXTAVIA group, most ALT abnormalities resolved spontaneously with continued treatment whereas some resolved upon dose reduction or temporary discontinuation of treatment.

Lymphopenia (<1500/mm³) was observed in 90.9% of EXTAVIA patients compared to 74.3% of placebo patients and neutropenia (<1400/mm³) was noted in 18.0% EXTAVIA and 5.1% placebo patients.
3. Single Clinical Event Suggestive of MS: The following laboratory abnormalities were reported at a significantly higher incidence in the EXTAVIA group: lymphocyte count <1500/mm³: EXTAVIA 79.1% vs placebo 45.5%; ALT >5 times baseline value: EXTAVIA 17.8% vs placebo 4.5%; absolute neutrophil count <1500/mm³: EXTAVIA 10.6% vs placebo 2.3%; WBC <3000/mm³: EXTAVIA 10.6% vs placebo 1.7%; AST >5 times baseline value: EXTAVIA 6.2% vs placebo 0.6%.

Bilirubin values of Grade 3 or 4 were reported in five EXTAVIA patients and in one placebo patient.

Five patients discontinued EXTAVIA due to elevated liver function tests (see Warnings and Precautions, Monitoring and Laboratory Tests).

There were no relevant differences between the EXTAVIA and placebo groups for lipid profile, thyroid function parameters, other serum chemistry parameters or urinalysis parameters.
Post-Market Adverse Drug Reactions: Rare post-marketing cases of adverse hepatic reactions have been reported, including autoimmune hepatitis, hepatitis and hepatic failure requiring liver transplantation.

DRUG INTERACTIONS: Drug-Drug Interactions: Interactions between EXTAVIA and other drugs have not been evaluated. Although studies designed to examine drug interactions have not been done, it was noted that EXTAVIA patients (n=180) have received corticosteroid or ACTH treatment of relapses for periods of up to 28 days.

EXTAVIA administered in three cancer patients over a dose range of 0.025 mg (0.8 MIU) to 2.2 mg (71 MIU) led to a dose-dependent inhibition of antipyrine elimination. The effect of alternate-day administration of 0.25 mg (8 MIU) EXTAVIA on drug metabolism in MS patients is unknown.

Interferons have been reported to reduce the activity of hepatic cytochrome P450-dependent enzymes in humans and animals. Caution should be exercised when EXTAVIA is administered in combination with agents that have a narrow therapeutic index and are largely dependent on the hepatic cytochrome P450 system for clearance.
Drug-Food Interactions: Interactions with food have not been established.
Drug-Herb Interactions: Interactions with herbal products have not been established.
Drug-Laboratory Test Interactions: Interactions with laboratory tests have not been established.

DOSAGE AND ADMINISTRATION: Dosing Considerations: For subcutaneous use only.
EXTAVIA (interferon beta-1b) should only be prescribed by (or following consultation with) clinicians who are experienced in the diagnosis and management of multiple sclerosis.
Recommended Dose and Dosage Adjustment: The recommended dose of EXTAVIA for both relapsing-remitting and secondary-progressive MS patients is 0.25 mg (8 MIU) injected subcutaneously every other day. Limited data regarding the activity of a lower dose in relapsing-remitting MS are presented in the Clinical Trials section.

Dose titration was used at the start of treatment in the clinically isolated syndrome and secondary-progressive MS studies in order to increase the tolerability of EXTAVIA.

In the study in patients with a single clinical event suggestive of MS (clinically isolated syndrome), dosage was increased as shown in Table 5.

Table 5: EXTAVIA
Schedule for Dose Titration[a]

Treatment Day	Dose	Volume
1, 3, 5	0.0625 mg (2 MIU)	0.25 mL
7, 9, 11	0.125 mg (4 MIU)	0.5 mL
13, 15, 17	0.1875 mg (6 MIU)	0.75 mL
≥19	0.250 mg (8 MIU)	1.0 mL

a Titration scheme as used in the study in patients with a single clinical event suggestive of multiple sclerosis. The titration period may be adjusted if any significant adverse reaction occurs.

In the secondary-progressive MS study, patients initiated treatment with half the dose (4 MIU s.c. every other day) for a period of 2 weeks prior to escalating to the recommended dose of 8 MIU (s.c. every other day).

Efficacy of treatment for longer than 2 years has not been substantially demonstrated in relapsing-remitting multiple sclerosis. For secondary-progressive multiple sclerosis, safety and efficacy data beyond 3 years are not available.

In patients with a single clinical event suggestive of MS, efficacy has been demonstrated over a period of three years.
Missed Dose: If an injection is missed, it should be given as soon as feasible. The next injection should be given two days later.
Administration: Reconstitution: To reconstitute lyophilized EXTAVIA for injection, use the vial adapter to inject the entire contents of the prefilled diluent syringe containing Sodium Chloride 0.54% Solution into the EXTAVIA vial. Gently swirl the vial of EXTAVIA to dissolve the drug completely; do not shake. Inspect the reconstituted product visually and discard the product before use if it contains particulate matter or is discolored. After reconstitution with diluent, each mL of solution contains 0.25 mg (8 MIU) interferon beta-1b, 13 mg albumin human USP and 13 mg mannitol USP.

Vial Content	Volume of Diluent to be Added to Vial	Approximate Available Volume	Nominal Concentration per mL
0.3 mg interferon beta-1b	1.2 mL	1.2 mL	0.25 mg/mL

Subcutaneous Injection: Withdraw 1 mL of reconstituted solution from the vial back into the syringe, fitted with a ½-inch needle, and inject the solution subcutaneously. Sites for self-injection include arms, abdomen, buttocks and thighs. All components are suitable for single use only; unused portions should be discarded (see Information for the Patient for self-injection procedure).

OVERDOSAGE:

For management of a suspected drug overdose, CPhA recommends that you contact your **regional Poison Control Centre**. See the *CPS* Directory section for a list of Poison Control Centres.

ACTION AND CLINICAL PHARMACOLOGY: Mechanism of Action: Interferons are a family of naturally occurring proteins, which have molecular weights ranging from 15 000 to 21 000 daltons. Three major classes of interferons have been identified: alpha, beta and gamma. Interferon beta-1b, interferon alpha, and interferon gamma have overlapping yet distinct biologic activities. The activities of interferon beta are species-restricted and, therefore, the most pertinent pharmacological information on EXTAVIA (interferon beta-1b) is derived from studies of human cells in culture and in vivo.

Interferon beta-1b has been shown to possess both antiviral and immunomodulatory activities. The mechanisms by which EXTAVIA exerts its actions in multiple sclerosis are not clearly understood. However, it is known that the biologic response-modifying properties of interferon beta-1b are mediated through its interactions with specific cell receptors found on the surface of human cells. The binding of interferon beta-1b to these receptors induces the expression of a number of interferon-induced gene products (eg, 2',5'-oligoadenylate synthetase, protein kinase, and indoleamine 2,3-dioxygenase) that are believed to be the mediators of the biological actions of interferon beta-1b. A number of these interferon-induced products have been readily measured in the serum and cellular fractions of blood collected from patients treated with interferon beta 1b.
Pharmacokinetics: Given that serum concentrations of interferon beta-1b are low or not detectable following subcutaneous administration of 0.25 mg (8 MIU) or less of EXTAVIA (interferon beta-1b), pharmacokinetic information in MS patients receiving the recommended dose of EXTAVIA is not available. Following single and multiple daily subcutaneous administrations of 0.5 mg (16 MIU) EXTAVIA to healthy volunteers (n=12), serum interferon beta-1b concentrations were generally below 100 IU/mL. Peak serum interferon beta-1b concentrations occurred between 1 to 8 hours, with a mean peak serum interferon concentration of 40 IU/mL. Bioavailability, based on a total dose of 0.5 mg (16 MIU) EXTAVIA given as two subcutaneous injections at different sites, was approximately 50%.

After intravenous administration of EXTAVIA (0.006 mg [0.2 MIU] to 2.0 mg [64 MIU]), similar pharmacokinetic profiles were obtained from healthy volunteers (n=12) and from patients with diseases other than MS (n=142). In patients receiving single intravenous doses up to 2.0 mg (64 MIU), increases in serum concentrations were dose proportional. Mean serum clearance values ranged from 9.4 mL/min·kg⁻¹ to 28.9 mL/min·kg⁻¹ and were independent of dose. Mean terminal elimination half-life values ranged from 8.0 minutes to 4.3 hours and mean steady-state volume of distribution values ranged from 0.25 L/kg to 2.88 L/kg. Three-times-a-week intravenous dosing for 2 weeks resulted in no accumulation of interferon beta-1b in the serum of patients. Pharmacokinetic parameters after single and multiple intravenous doses of EXTAVIA were comparable.

STORAGE AND STABILITY: Before reconstitution: Store between 2-25°C. Excursions between 25 and 30°C are permitted as long as they do not exceed a maximum of 30 days. Do not freeze. Do not use beyond the expiration date indicated on the labels of the EXTAVIA vial and the prefilled diluent syringe.
After Reconstitution: The reconstituted product contains no preservative. If not used immediately, store under refrigeration between 2 and 8°C **and use within 3 hours of reconstitution**. Do not freeze.

INFORMATION FOR THE PATIENT: Published in e-CPS, available by subscription at www.e-cps.ca.

DOSAGE FORMS, COMPOSITION AND PACKAGING: Each single-use vial of lyophilized powder contains: 0.3 mg (9.6 MIU) interferon beta-1b, 15 mg albumin human USP and 15 mg mannitol USP. Cartons containing 15 single-use blister packs. Each single-use pack contains the necessary components to prepare and inject a single dose of EXTAVIA: 1 vial of medication, 1 prefilled diluent syringe (containing 1.2 mL of Sodium Chloride 0.54% solution), 1 vial adapter with attached 27 gauge, ½" needle, and 3 alcohol wipes. **The single-use blister pack can only be used with the EXTAVIA Auto-Injector II.**

Ezetrol® Pr

ezetimibe

Cholesterol Absorption Inhibitor

Merck Frosst-Schering Pharma, G.P.

Date of Revision: October 19, 2009

SUMMARY PRODUCT INFORMATION:

Route of Administration	Dosage Form/ Strength	Clinically Relevant Nonmedicinal Ingredients
Oral	Tablet 10 mg	Lactose monohydrate

INDICATIONS AND CLINICAL USE: EZETROL (ezetimibe) is indicated as an adjunct to lifestyle changes, including diet, when the response to diet and other non-pharmacological measures alone has been inadequate.
Primary Hypercholesterolemia: EZETROL, administered alone or with an HMG-CoA reductase inhibitor (statin), is indicated for the reduction of elevated total cholesterol (total-C), low density lipoprotein cholesterol (LDL-C), apolipoprotein B (Apo B), and triglycerides (TG) and to increase high density lipoprotein cholesterol (HDL-C) in patients with primary (heterozygous familial and non-familial) hypercholesterolemia.

EZETROL, administered in combination with fenofibrate, is indicated for the reduction of elevated total-C, LDL-C, Apo B, and non-HDL-C in patients with mixed hyperlipidemia.
Homozygous Familial Hypercholesterolemia (HoFH): EZETROL, administered with a statin, is indicated for the reduction of elevated total-C and LDL-C levels in patients with HoFH as an adjunct to treatments such as LDL apheresis or if such treatments are not possible.
Homozygous Sitosterolemia (Phytosterolemia): EZETROL is indicated for the reduction of elevated sitosterol and campesterol levels in patients with homozygous familial sitosterolemia.

CONTRAINDICATIONS: Hypersensitivity to any component of this medication.

When EZETROL is to be administered with a statin or with fenofibrate, the contraindications to that medication should be reviewed before starting concomitant therapy.

The combination of EZETROL with a statin is contraindicated in patients with active liver disease or unexplained persistent elevations in serum transaminases.

All statins and fenofibrate are contraindicated in pregnant and nursing women. When EZETROL is administered with a statin or with fenofibrate in a woman of childbearing potential, refer to the product labeling for that medication (see Warnings and Precautions, Special Populations, Pregnant Women).

WARNINGS AND PRECAUTIONS:

Serious Warnings and Precautions
- hepatitis
- pancreatitis
- myopathy/rhabdomyolysis
- myalgia
- anaphylaxis (see Adverse Reactions, Post-Market Adverse Drug Reactions)

General: When EZETROL is to be administered with a statin or with fenofibrate, please refer also to the Product Monograph for that medication. Note that all statins and fenofibrate are contraindicated in pregnant women (see the Product Monograph for the medication; see Warnings and Precautions, Special Populations, Pregnant Women).

Hepatic/Biliary/Pancreatic: Concomitant Administration with a Statin or Fenofibrate: When EZETROL is initiated in a patient already taking a statin or fenofibrate, liver function tests should be considered at initiation of EZETROL therapy, and then as indicated (see Adverse Reactions, Abnormal Hematologic and Clinical Chemistry Findings).

When EZETROL is initiated at the same time as a statin or fenofibrate, liver function tests should be performed at initiation of therapy and according to the recommendations of that medication (see Adverse Reactions, Abnormal Hematologic and Clinical Chemistry Findings).

Liver Enzymes: In controlled monotherapy studies, the incidence of consecutive elevations (≥3 times the upper limit of normal [ULN]) in serum transaminases was similar between EZETROL (0.5%) and placebo (0.3%).

In controlled coadministration trials in patients receiving EZETROL with a statin, the incidence of consecutive transaminase elevations (≥3×ULN) was 1.3% compared to 0.4% in patients on a statin alone.

Patients with Liver Impairment: The pharmacokinetics of ezetimibe were examined in patients with impaired liver function as defined by the Child-Pugh scoring system.

- In patients with mild hepatic insufficiency (Child-Pugh score 5 or 6), the mean area under the curve (AUC) for total ezetimibe (after a single 10 mg dose of EZETROL) was increased approximately 1.7-fold compared to healthy subjects. No dosage adjustment is necessary for patients with mild hepatic insufficiency.
- In patients with moderate hepatic insufficiency (Child-Pugh score 7 to 9), the mean AUC for total ezetimibe (after multiple doses of 10 mg daily) was increased approximately 4-fold on Day 1 and Day 14 compared to healthy subjects. Due to the unknown effects of the increased exposure to ezetimibe in patients with moderate (Child-Pugh score 7 to 9) or severe (Child-Pugh score >9) hepatic insufficiency, ezetimibe is not recommended in these patients.
- No pharmacokinetic studies with ezetimibe have been carried out in patients with either active liver disease or unexplained and persistent elevations in serum transaminases. It is recommended that care be exercised in such patients.

The coadministration of EZETROL and a statin is contraindicated in patients with active liver disease or unexplained and persistent elevations in serum transaminases.

Post-marketing reports of adverse events have included rare cases of hepatitis in patients taking EZETROL, although causality has not been proven. If patients develop signs or symptoms of hepatitis, liver function should be evaluated.

Concomitant Administration with Fibrates: The coadministration of ezetimibe with fibrates other than fenofibrate has not been studied. Therefore, coadministration of EZETROL and fibrates (other than fenofibrate) is not recommended (see Drug Interactions).

Fenofibrate: If cholelithiasis is suspected in a patient receiving EZETROL and fenofibrate, gallbladder studies are indicated and alternative lipid-lowering therapy should be considered (see Adverse Reactions and the Product Monograph for fenofibrate).

Pancreatitis: Post-marketing reports of adverse events have included rare cases of acute pancreatitis occurring in patients taking EZETROL, although causality has not been proven. The diagnosis of acute pancreatitis should be considered in patients taking EZETROL who develop sudden acute abdominal pain.

Muscle Effects: Myopathy/Rhabdomyolysis: Myopathy and rhabdomyolysis are known adverse effects of statins and fibrates. Post-marketing reports of adverse events have included rare cases of myopathy/rhabdomyolysis occurring in patients taking EZETROL with or without a statin, regardless of causality. Myopathy/Rhabdomyolysis should be considered in patients presenting with muscle pain during treatment with EZETROL with or without a statin or fenofibrate, and consideration given to discontinuation of the drugs. Most cases of myopathy/rhabdomyolysis resolved when drugs were discontinued.

Myalgia: In controlled clinical trials, the incidence of myalgia was 5.0% for EZETROL vs 4.6% for placebo (see Adverse Reactions, Table 2). Post-marketing reports of adverse events have included myalgia in patients taking EZETROL with or without a statin, regardless of causality. Patients should be instructed to contact their physician if they experience persistent and severe muscle pains with no obvious cause.

A number of patients treated with EZETROL, in whom myalgia occurred had previously experienced myalgia (with or without elevated CK levels) with statin therapy. Patients with a history of statin intolerance (myalgia with or without elevated CK levels) should be closely monitored for adverse muscle events during treatment with EZETROL.

Renal: Renal Insufficiency: After a single 10 mg dose of EZETROL in patients with severe renal disease, the mean AUC for total ezetimibe was increased approximately 1.5-fold compared to healthy subjects. Accordingly, no dosage adjustment is necessary for renal impaired patients.

Special Populations: Pregnant Women: No clinical data on exposed pregnancies are available for EZETROL. The effects of ezetimibe on labour and delivery in pregnant women are unknown. Note that all statins and fenofibrate are **contraindicated** in pregnant women (see the Product Monograph for the medication). Caution should be exercised when prescribing to pregnant women.

Nursing Women: Studies in rats have shown that ezetimibe is excreted in milk. It is not known whether ezetimibe is excreted into human breast milk, therefore, EZETROL should not be used in nursing mothers unless the potential benefit justifies the potential risk to the infant. Note that all statins and fenofibrate are **contraindicated** in nursing women (see the Product Monograph for the medication).

Pediatrics: The pharmacokinetics of EZETROL in adolescents (10 to 18 years) have been shown to be similar to that in adults. Treatment experience with EZETROL in the pediatric population is limited to 4 patients (9 to 17 years) in the sitosterolemia study and 5 patients (11 to 17 years) in the HoFH study. Treatment with EZETROL in children (<10 years) is not recommended.

Geriatrics: Plasma concentrations for total ezetimibe are about 2-fold higher in the elderly (≥65 years) than in the young (18 to 45 years). LDL-C reduction and safety profile are comparable between elderly and young subjects treated with EZETROL. Therefore, no dosage adjustment is necessary in the elderly.

Sex: Plasma concentrations for total ezetimibe are slightly higher (<20%) in women than in men. LDL-C reduction and safety profile are comparable between men and women treated with ezetimibe. Therefore, no dosage adjustment is necessary on the basis of sex.

Race: Based on a meta-analysis of pharmacokinetic studies, there were no pharmacokinetic differences between Blacks and Caucasians.

ADVERSE REACTIONS: Adverse Drug Reaction Overview: The most commonly reported adverse events in clinical studies were upper respiratory tract infection, headache, myalgia and back pain. In post-marketing use, serious adverse events reported rarely or very rarely, regardless of causality, included hepatitis, hypersensitivity reactions, pancreatitis and myopathy/rhabdomyolysis.

When EZETROL is to be administered with a statin or fenofibrate, please refer also to the Product Monograph for that medication.

Clinical Trial Adverse Drug Reactions: EZETROL clinical trial experience involved 2486 patients in placebo-controlled monotherapy trials (1691 treated with EZETROL) and 4547 patients in active controlled trials (449 of whom were treated with EZETROL alone and 1708 treated with EZETROL plus a statin and 185 patients treated with EZETROL and fenofibrate). The studies were of 8 to 14 weeks duration. The overall incidence of adverse events reported with EZETROL was similar to that reported with placebo and the discontinuation rates due to treatment related adverse events was similar between EZETROL (2.3%) and placebo (2.1%).

Monotherapy: Adverse experiences reported in ≥2% of patients treated with EZETROL and at an incidence greater than placebo in placebo-controlled studies of EZETROL, regardless of causality assessment, are shown in Table 1.

The frequency of less common adverse events was comparable between EZETROL and placebo.

Only two patients out of the 1691 patients treated with EZETROL alone reported serious adverse reactions-one with abdominal pain plus panniculitis, and one with arm pain and palpitation.

In monotherapy placebo-controlled clinical trials, 4% of patients treated with EZETROL and 3.8% of patients treated with placebo were withdrawn from therapy due to adverse events.

Table 1: EZETROL[a]

Clinical Adverse Events Occurring in ≥2% of Patients Treated with EZETROL and at an Incidence Greater than Placebo, Regardless of Causality

Body System/Organ Class Adverse Event	Placebo (%) n=795	EZETROL 10 mg (%) n=1691
Body as a Whole—General Disorders		
Fatigue	1.8	2.2
Gastrointestinal System Disorders		
Abdominal pain	2.8	3.0
Diarrhea	3.0	3.7
Infection and Infestations		
Infection viral	1.8	2.2
Pharyngitis	2.1	2.3
Sinusitis	2.8	3.6
Musculoskeletal System Disorders		
Arthralgia	3.4	3.8
Back pain	3.9	4.1
Respiratory System Disorders		
Coughing	2.1	2.3

[a] Includes patients who received placebo or EZETROL alone reported in Table 2.

Combination with a Statin: EZETROL has been evaluated for safety in combination studies in more than 2000 patients. In general, adverse experiences were similar between EZETROL administered with a statin and a statin alone. However, the frequency of increased transaminases was slightly higher in patients receiving EZETROL administered with a statin than in patients treated with a statin alone (see Warnings and Precautions, Hepatic/Biliary/Pancreatic; Patients with Liver Impairment).

Clinical adverse experiences reported in ≥2% of patients and at an incidence greater than placebo in four placebo-controlled trials where EZETROL was administered alone or initiated concurrently with various statins, regardless of causality assessment, are shown in Table 2.

Table 2: EZETROL[a]

Clinical Adverse Events Occurring in ≥2% of Patients and at an Incidence Greater than Placebo, Regardless of Causality, in EZETROL/Statin Combination Studies

Body System/Organ Class Adverse Event	Placebo (%) n=259	EZETROL 10 mg (%) n=262	All Statins[b] (%) n=936	EZETROL + All Statins[b] (%) n=925
Body as a Whole—General Disorders				
Chest pain	1.2	3.4	2.0	1.8
Dizziness	1.2	2.7	1.4	1.8
Fatigue	1.9	1.9	1.4	2.8
Headache	5.4	8.0	7.3	6.3
Gastrointestinal System Disorders				
Abdominal pain	2.3	2.7	3.1	3.5
Diarrhea	1.5	3.4	2.9	2.8
Infection and Infestations				
Pharyngitis	1.9	3.1	2.5	2.3
Sinusitis	1.9	4.6	3.6	3.5
Upper respiratory tract infection	10.8	13.0	13.6	11.8
Musculoskeletal System Disorders				
Arthralgia	2.3	3.8	4.3	3.4
Back pain	3.5	3.4	3.7	4.3
Myalgia	4.6	5.0	4.1	4.5

[a] Includes four placebo-controlled combination studies in which EZETROL was initiated concurrently with a statin.
[b] All statins=all doses of all statins.

In coadministration placebo-controlled clinical trials, 5.7% of patients treated with EZETROL coadministered with a statin, 4.3% of patients treated with statin alone, 5.0% of patients treated with EZETROL alone, and 6.2% of patients treated with placebo were withdrawn from therapy due to adverse events.

Combination with Fenofibrate: In a clinical study involving 625 patients treated for up to 12 weeks and 576 patients treated for up to 1 year, coadministration of EZETROL and fenofibrate was well tolerated. This study was not designed to compare treatment groups for infrequent events. Incidence rates (95% CI) for clinically important elevations (>3×ULN, consecutive) in serum transaminases were 4.5% (1.9, 8.8) and 2.7% (1.2, 5.4) for fenofibrate monotherapy and EZETROL coadministered with fenofibrate, respectively, adjusted for treatment exposure. Corresponding incidence rates for cholecystectomy were 0.6% (0.0, 3.1) and 1.7% (0.6, 4.0) for fenofibrate monotherapy and EZETROL coadministered with fenofibrate, respectively (see Warnings and Precautions, Fenofibrate and Drug Interactions). There were no CPK elevations >10×ULN in either treatment group in this study.

Abnormal Hematologic and Clinical Chemistry Findings: In controlled clinical monotherapy trials, the incidence of clinically important consecutive elevations in serum transaminases (ALT and/or AST ≥3×ULN) was similar between EZETROL (0.5%) and placebo (0.3%). In coadministration trials, the incidence was 1.3% for patients treated with EZETROL coadministered with a statin and 0.4% for patients treated with a statin alone. These elevations were generally asymptomatic, not associated with cholestasis, and returned to baseline levels after discontinuation of therapy or with continued treatment.

In clinical trials there was no excess of myopathy or rhabdomyolysis associated with EZETROL compared with the relevant control arm (placebo or statin alone). However, myopathy and rhabdomyolysis are known adverse reactions to statins and other lipid-lowering drugs. In clinical trials, the incidence of CK >10×ULN was 0.2% for EZETROL vs 0.1% for placebo, and 0.1% for EZETROL coadministered with a statin vs 0.4% for statin alone.

Post-Market Adverse Drug Reactions: The following adverse events have been reported rarely or very rarely, regardless of causality: increased CK (creatine phosphokinase); myalgia (see Warnings and Precautions); myopathy/rhabdomyolysis (see Warnings and Precautions); elevations of liver transaminases; hepatitis (see Warnings and Precautions); hypersensitivity reactions, including anaphylaxis, angioedema, rash and urticaria; erythema multiforme; nausea; pancreatitis (see Warnings and Precautions); thrombocytopenia; arthralgia; dizziness; cholelithiasis; cholecystitis; depression; paresthesia.

DRUG INTERACTIONS:

Serious Drug Interactions
- cyclosporine

Overview: Drug-drug interactions are known or suspected with cholestyramine, cyclosporine and fibrates.

Drug-Drug Interactions: Cytochrome P450 System: No clinically significant pharmacokinetic interactions have been observed between ezetimibe and drugs known to be metabolized via CYP 1A2, 2D6, 2C8, 2C9, and 3A4 isoenzymes, or N-acetyltransferase such as caffeine, dextromethorphan, tolbutamide, and IV midazolam. It has been shown that ezetimibe neither induces, nor inhibits, these cytochrome P450 isoenzymes.

Anticoagulants: Concomitant administration of ezetimibe (10 mg once daily) had no significant effect on bioavailability of warfarin and prothrombin time in a study of twelve healthy adult males. As with the initiation of any medication in patients treated with warfarin or another coumarin anticoagulant, additional International Normalised Ratio (INR) measurements are recommended for patients administered warfarin or another coumarin anticoagulant concomitantly with EZETROL.

Digoxin: Concomitant administration of ezetimibe (10 mg once daily) had no significant effect on the bioavailability of digoxin and the ECG parameters (HR, PR, QT, and QTc intervals) in a study of twelve healthy adult males.

Oral Contraceptives: Coadministration of ezetimibe (10 mg once daily) with oral contraceptives had no significant effect on the bioavailability of ethinyl estradiol or levonorgestrel in a study of eighteen healthy adult females.

Cimetidine: Multiple doses of cimetidine (400 mg twice daily) had no significant effect on the oral bioavailability of ezetimibe and total ezetimibe in a study of twelve healthy adults.

Antacids: Concomitant antacid (aluminum and magnesium hydroxide) administration decreased the rate of absorption of ezetimibe but had no effect on the bioavailability of ezetimibe. This decreased rate of absorption is not considered clinically significant.

Glipizide: In a study of twelve healthy adult males, steady-state levels of ezetimibe (10 mg once daily) had no significant effect on the pharmacokinetics and pharmacodynamics of glipizide. A single dose of glipizide (10 mg) had no significant effect on the exposure to total ezetimibe or ezetimibe.

Cholestyramine: Concomitant cholestyramine administration decreased the mean AUC of total ezetimibe (ezetimibe+ezetimibe-glucuronide) approximately 55%. The incremental LDL-C reduction due to adding ezetimibe to cholestyramine may be lessened by this interaction.

Fibrates: The safety and effectiveness of ezetimibe coadministered with fenofibrate have been evaluated in a clinical study (see Warnings and Precautions and Adverse Reactions); coadministration of ezetimibe with other fibrates has not been studied. Fibrates may increase cholesterol excretion into the bile, leading to cholelithiasis. In a preclinical study in dogs, ezetimibe increased cholesterol in the gallbladder bile. Although the relevance of this preclinical finding to humans is unknown, coadministration of EZETROL with fibrates (other than fenofibrate) is not recommended until use in patients is studied.

Fenofibrate: In a pharmacokinetic study, concomitant fenofibrate administration increased total ezetimibe concentrations approximately 1.5-fold. This increase is not considered clinically significant.

Gemfibrozil: In a pharmacokinetic study, concomitant gemfibrozil administration increased total ezetimibe concentrations approximately 1.7-fold. This increase is not considered clinically significant. No clinical data are available.

Statins: No clinically significant pharmacokinetic interactions were seen when ezetimibe was coadministered with atorvastatin, simvastatin, pravastatin, lovastatin, fluvastatin or rosuvastatin.

Cyclosporine: Caution should be exercised when initiating ezetimibe in the setting of cyclosporine. Cyclosporine concentrations should be monitored in patients receiving EZETROL and cyclosporine.

In a study of eight post-renal transplant patients with creatinine clearance of >50 mL/min on a stable dose of cyclosporine, a single 10 mg dose of ezetimibe resulted in a 3.4-fold (range 2.3- to 7.9-fold) increase in the mean AUC for total ezetimibe compared to a healthy control population from another study (n=17). In a different study, a renal transplant patient with severe renal insufficiency (creatinine clearance of 13.2 mL/min/1.73 m^2) who was receiving multiple medications, including cyclosporine, demonstrated a 12-fold greater exposure to total ezetimibe compared to concurrent controls.

In contrast, in a two-period crossover study in twelve healthy subjects, daily administration of 20 mg ezetimibe for 8 days with a single 100-mg dose of cyclosporine on Day 7 resulted in a mean 15% increase in cyclosporine AUC (range 10% decrease to 51% increase) compared to a single 100-mg dose of cyclosporine alone.

DOSAGE AND ADMINISTRATION: Dosing Considerations:
- Patients should be placed on a standard cholesterol-lowering diet at least equivalent to the NCEP Adult Treatment Panel III (ATP III) TLC diet before receiving EZETROL, and should continue on this diet during treatment with EZETROL. If appropriate, a program of weight control and physical exercise should be implemented.
- Prior to initiating therapy with EZETROL, secondary causes for elevations in plasma lipid levels should be excluded. A lipid profile should also be performed.

Recommended Dose and Dosage Adjustment: The recommended dose of EZETROL is 10 mg once daily orally, alone, with a statin, or with fenofibrate. EZETROL can be taken with or without food at any time of the day but preferably at the same time each day.

Use in the Elderly: No dosage adjustment is required for elderly patients (see Warnings and Precautions, Special Populations, Geriatrics).

Use in Pediatric Patients: Children and adolescents ≥10 years: No dosage adjustment is required (see Warnings and Precautions, Special Populations, Pediatrics).

Use in Patients with Hepatic Impairment: No dosage adjustment is required in patients with mild hepatic insufficiency (Child-Pugh score 5 to 6). Treatment with EZETROL is not recommended in patients with moderate (Child-Pugh score 7 to 9) or severe (Child-Pugh score >9) liver dysfunction (see Warnings and Precautions, Hepatic/Biliary/Pancreatic, Patients with Liver Impairment).

Use in Patients with Renal Impairment: No dosage adjustment is required for patients with renal impairment (see Warnings and Precautions, Renal, Renal Insufficiency).

Coadministration with Bile Acid Sequestrants: EZETROL should be administered either 2 hours or longer before or 4 hours or longer after administration of a bile acid sequestrant (see Drug Interactions, Drug-Drug Interactions, Cholestyramine).

Missed Dose: The recommended dosing regimen is one tablet, once daily. If a dose is missed, the patient should be counselled to resume the usual schedule of one tablet daily.

OVERDOSAGE:

In clinical studies, administration of ezetimibe, 50 mg/day to 15 healthy subjects for up to 14 days, or 40 mg/day to 18 patients with primary hypercholesterolemia for up to 56 days, was generally well tolerated.

A few cases of overdosage with EZETROL have been reported; most have not been associated with adverse experiences. Reported adverse experiences have not been serious. In the event of an overdose, symptomatic and supportive measures should be employed.

For management of a suspected drug overdose, contact your regional Poison Control Centre. See the *CPS* Directory section for a list of Poison Control Centres.

ACTION AND CLINICAL PHARMACOLOGY: Mechanism of Action: EZETROL is in a new class of lipid-lowering compounds that selectively inhibit the intestinal absorption of cholesterol and related plant sterols. EZETROL is orally active, with a unique mechanism of action that differs from other classes of cholesterol-reducing compounds e.g., HMG-CoA reductase inhibitors (statins), bile acid sequestrants (resins), fibric acid derivatives, plant stanols. The molecular target of ezetimibe is the sterol transporter, Niemann-Pick C1-Like 1 (NPC1L1), which is responsible for the intestinal uptake of cholesterol and phytosterols.

Although ezetimibe is rapidly absorbed and is extensively metabolized to an active phenolic glucuronide which reaches the systemic circulation after oral administration (see Action and Clinical Pharmacology, Pharmacokinetics, Absorption), its action is localized at the brush border of the small intestine where it inhibits the absorption of cholesterol, leading to a decrease in the delivery of intestinal cholesterol to the liver. This results in a reduction of hepatic cholesterol stores and an increase in clearance of cholesterol from the blood. Ezetimibe does not increase bile acid excretion in contrast to bile acid sequestrants and does not inhibit cholesterol synthesis in the liver as do statins. EZETROL and statins have distinct mechanisms of action that provide complementary cholesterol reduction. Administration of EZETROL with fenofibrate is effective in improving serum total-C, LDL-C, Apo B, TG, HDL-C, and non-HDL-C in patients with mixed hyperlipidemia.

Clinical studies have demonstrated that elevated levels of total-C, low density lipoprotein cholesterol (LDL-C) and apolipoprotein B (Apo B; the major protein constituent of LDL), promote atherosclerosis in humans. In addition, decreased levels of high density lipoprotein cholesterol (HDL-C) are associated with the development of atherosclerosis. Epidemiologic studies have established that cardiovascular morbidity and mortality vary directly with the level of total-C and LDL-C and inversely with the level of HDL-C. Like LDL, cholesterol-enriched triglyceride-rich lipoproteins, including very low density lipoproteins (VLDL), intermediate density lipoproteins (IDL), and remnants, can also promote atherosclerosis. **The effects of ezetimibe given either alone or in addition to a statin or fenofibrate on cardiovascular morbidity and mortality have not been established.**

Pharmacodynamics: Preclinical studies in animals were performed to determine the selectivity of ezetimibe for inhibiting cholesterol absorption. Ezetimibe inhibited the absorption of [^{14}C]-cholesterol with no effect on the absorption of triglycerides, fatty acids, bile acids, progesterone, ethinyl estradiol, or the fat soluble vitamins A and D.

In a study of hypercholesterolemic patients, EZETROL inhibited intestinal cholesterol absorption by 54%, compared with placebo. EZETROL had no clinically meaningful effect on the plasma concentrations of the fat-soluble vitamins A, D, and E, and did not impair adrenocortical steroid hormone production.

Pharmacokinetics: Absorption: After oral administration, ezetimibe is rapidly absorbed and extensively conjugated to a phenolic glucuronide (ezetimibe-glucuronide) form which is at least as pharmacologically active as the parent drug. Mean ezetimibe peak plasma concentrations (C_{max}) of 3.4 to 5.5 ng/mL were attained within 4 to 12 hours (T_{max}). Ezetimibe-glucuronide mean C_{max} values of 45 to 71 ng/mL were achieved between 1 and 2 hours (T_{max}). The extent of absorption and absolute bioavailability of ezetimibe cannot be determined as the compound is virtually insoluble in aqueous media suitable for injection.

Concomitant food administration (high fat or non-fat meals) had no effect on the extent of absorption of ezetimibe when administered as EZETROL 10 mg tablets. C_{max} of ezetimibe was increased by 38% when taken with high fat meals.

Distribution: Ezetimibe and ezetimibe-glucuronide are bound 99.7% and 88 to 92% to human plasma proteins, respectively.

Metabolism: Ezetimibe is metabolized primarily in the small intestine and liver via glucuronide conjugation (a phase II reaction) with subsequent biliary and renal excretion. Minimal oxidative metabolism (a phase I reaction) has been observed in all species evaluated. Ezetimibe and ezetimibe-glucuronide are the major compounds detected in plasma. The conjugated ezetimibe-glucuronide constitutes 80-90% of plasma drug levels with ezetimibe the remaining 10-20%. Both ezetimibe and ezetimibe-glucuronide are slowly eliminated from plasma with evidence of significant enterohepatic recycling. The half-life for ezetimibe and ezetimibe-glucuronide is approximately 22 hours.

Excretion: Following oral administration of ^{14}C-ezetimibe (20 mg) to human subjects, total ezetimibe (ezetimibe+ezetimibe-glucuronide) accounted for approximately 93% of the total radioactivity in plasma. Approximately 78% and 11% of the administered radioactivity were recovered in the faeces and urine, respectively, over a 10-day collection period. After 48 hours, there were no detectable levels of radioactivity in the plasma. Ezetimibe was the major component in faeces (69% of the administered dose) while ezetimibe-glucuronide was the major component in urine and accounted for 9% of the administered dose.

STORAGE AND STABILITY: Store between 15 and 30°C. Protect from moisture.

INFORMATION FOR THE PATIENT: Published in e-CPS, available by subscription at www.e-cps.ca.

DOSAGE FORMS, COMPOSITION AND PACKAGING: Each white to off-white, capsule-shaped tablet, debossed with "414" on one side, contains: ezetimibe 10 mg. Nonmedicinal ingredients: croscarmellose sodium, lactose monohydrate, magnesium stearate, microcrystalline cellulose, povidone and sodium laurylsulfate. Blisters of 30. HDPE bottles of 100.

(Shown in Product Identification Section)

F

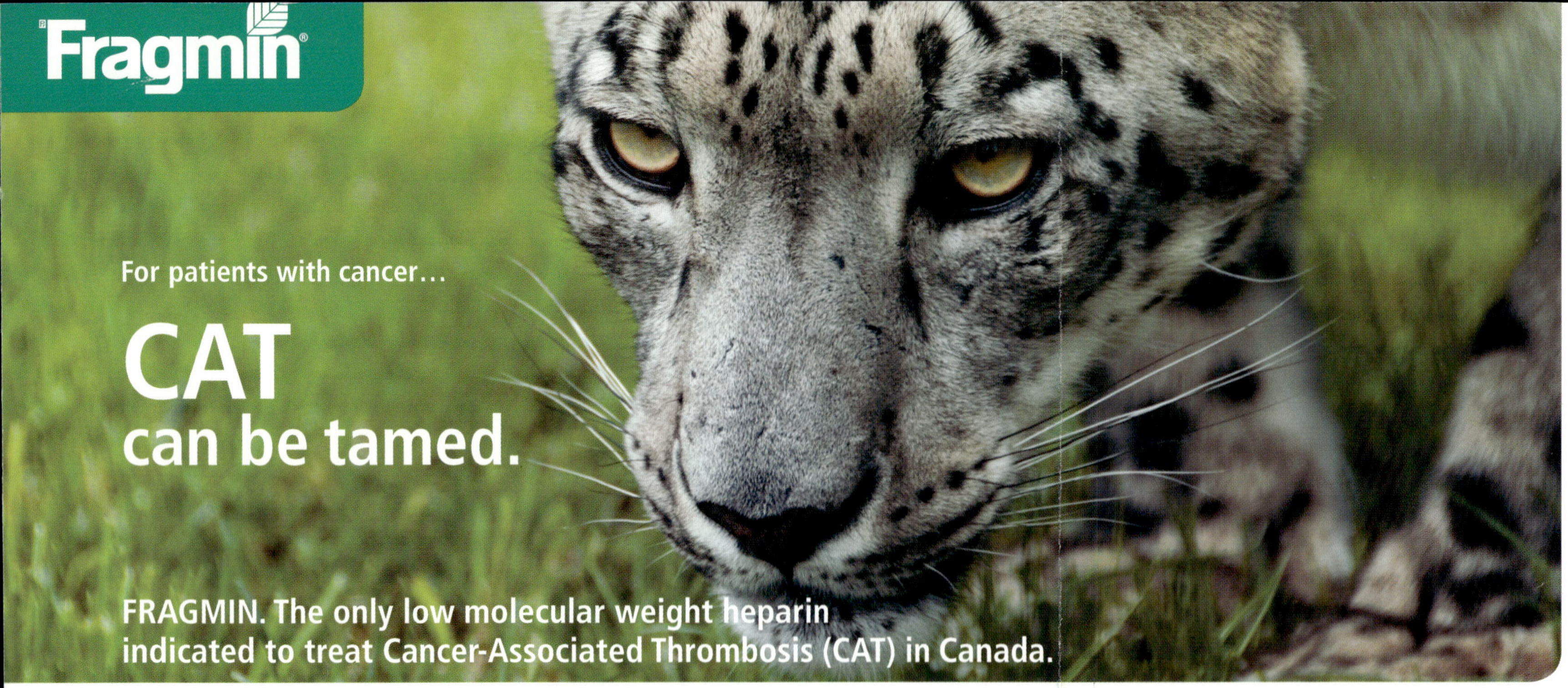

FRAGMIN is indicated for the extended treatment of symptomatic VTE to prevent recurrence of VTE in patients with cancer.

Venous thromboembolism (VTE) is a frequent medical complication in patients with cancer, occurring in 4% to 20% of cases.

FRAGMIN Achieved A Statistically Significant 52% Relative-Risk Reduction In Recurrent VTE vs. Oral Anticoagulant Therapy*,†

(27/336 vs. 53/336; p=0.002)

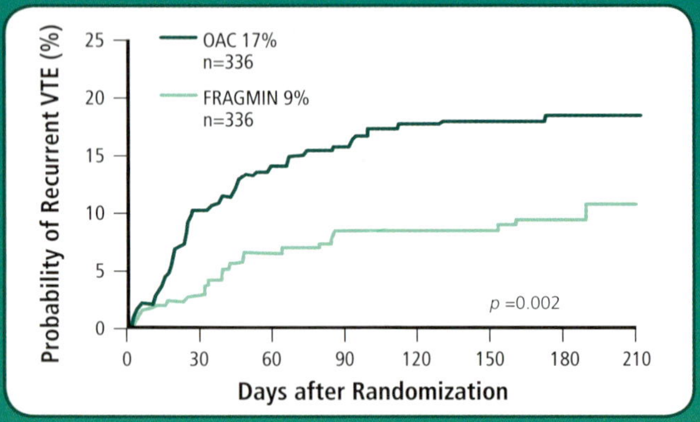

Adapted from Lee *et al*, *N Eng J Med* 2003.
*Absolute risk reduction: 8%, 95% CI: 0.30–0.77.

No Significant Difference In The Incidence Of Bleeding Between FRAGMIN And Oral Anticoagulant Therapy (OAC) Was Demonstrated.†

	FRAGMIN n=336	OAC n=336	*p* value
Minor Bleeding	8%	15%	n/a
Major Bleeding	6%	4%	0.27
All Bleeding	**14%**	**19%**	0.09

Adapted from Lee *et al*, *N Eng J Med* 2003 and FRAGMIN Product Monograph, 2009.

- Evidence-based FRAGMIN dosing: 200 IU/kg sc once daily (maximum 18,000 IU daily) for the first month, followed by a maintenance dose of ~150 IU/kg sc once daily for 2–6 months sc.
- INR or APTT monitoring is not required.§
- FRAGMIN is eligible for reimbursement under many provincial formularies.

F

Adverse Events: Clinically significant adverse reactions with FRAGMIN and other LMWHs include bleeding events and local reactions, with a low incidence of thrombocytopenia and allergic reactions. In clinical trials with hospitalized patients with severely restricted mobility, the incidence of thrombocytopenia was 0.54% at days 14 and 21. Injection site hematomas are a common side effect with FRAGMIN, occurring at a frequency of <5% with lower (prophylaxis) doses and <10% with higher (treatment) doses.
FRAGMIN should be used with care in patients with hepatic insufficiency, renal insufficiency or a history of gastrointestinal ulceration. Please consult the Prescribing Information for complete dosing instructions, warnings and precautions, and adverse events.

The multi-dose vial of FRAGMIN (25,000 IU/mL) contains benzyl alcohol (14 mg/mL) as a preservative. Benzyl alcohol has been associated with a potentially fatal "Gasping Syndrome" in neonates. Because benzyl alcohol may cross the placenta, FRAGMIN preserved with benzyl alcohol should not be used in pregnant women.

FRAGMIN should NOT be administered intra-muscularly.
FRAGMIN CANNOT BE USED INTERCHANGEABLY (UNIT FOR UNIT) WITH UNFRACTIONATED HEPARIN (UFH) OR OTHER LOW MOLECULAR WEIGHT HEPARINS (LMWHs) AS THEY DIFFER IN THEIR MANUFACTURING PROCESS, MOLECULAR WEIGHT DISTRIBUTION, ANTI-Xa AND ANTI-IIa ACTIVITIES, UNITS AND DOSAGES. SPECIAL ATTENTION AND COMPLIANCE WITH INSTRUCTIONS FOR USE OF EACH SPECIFIC PRODUCT ARE REQUIRED DURING ANY CHANGE IN TREATMENT.

Contraindications: FRAGMIN should not be used in patients who have: hypersensitivity to FRAGMIN or any of its constituents, including benzyl alcohol (when using the 25,000 IU multi-dose vial) or to other low molecular weight heparins and/or heparin or pork products; history of confirmed or suspected immunologically mediated heparin-induced thrombocytopenia (delayed-onset severe thrombocytopenia), and/or in patients in whom an *in vitro* platelet-aggregation test in the presence of FRAGMIN is positive; septic endocarditis (endocarditis lenta, subacute endocarditis); uncontrollable active bleeding; major blood-clotting disorders; acute gastroduodenal ulcer; cerebral hemorrhage; severe uncontrolled hypertension; diabetic or hemorrhagic retinopathy; other conditions or diseases involving an increased risk of hemorrhage; injuries to and operations on the central nervous system, eyes and ears; spinal/epidural anesthesia is contraindicated where repeated high doses of FRAGMIN (100–120 IU/kg given twice daily or 200 IU/kg once daily) are required, due to an increased risk of bleeding.

§ Platelet counts should be determined prior to the start of treatment with FRAGMIN and subsequently, twice weekly for the duration of treatment. Caution is recommended when administering FRAGMIN to patients with congenital or drug-induced thrombocytopenia, or platelet defects. Measurement of peak anti-Xa levels at about 4 hours post-dose should be considered in patients at higher risk of bleeding and receiving FRAGMIN, such as the elderly, patients with renal impairment or the extremes of body weight, during pregnancy, or for children.

Fragmin®
dalteparin sodium
ONCE-DAILY antithrombotic efficacy with easy dosing.

FRAGMIN® Pfizer Health AB, owner/
Pfizer Canada Inc., Licensee

Pfizer

PAAB Member R&D

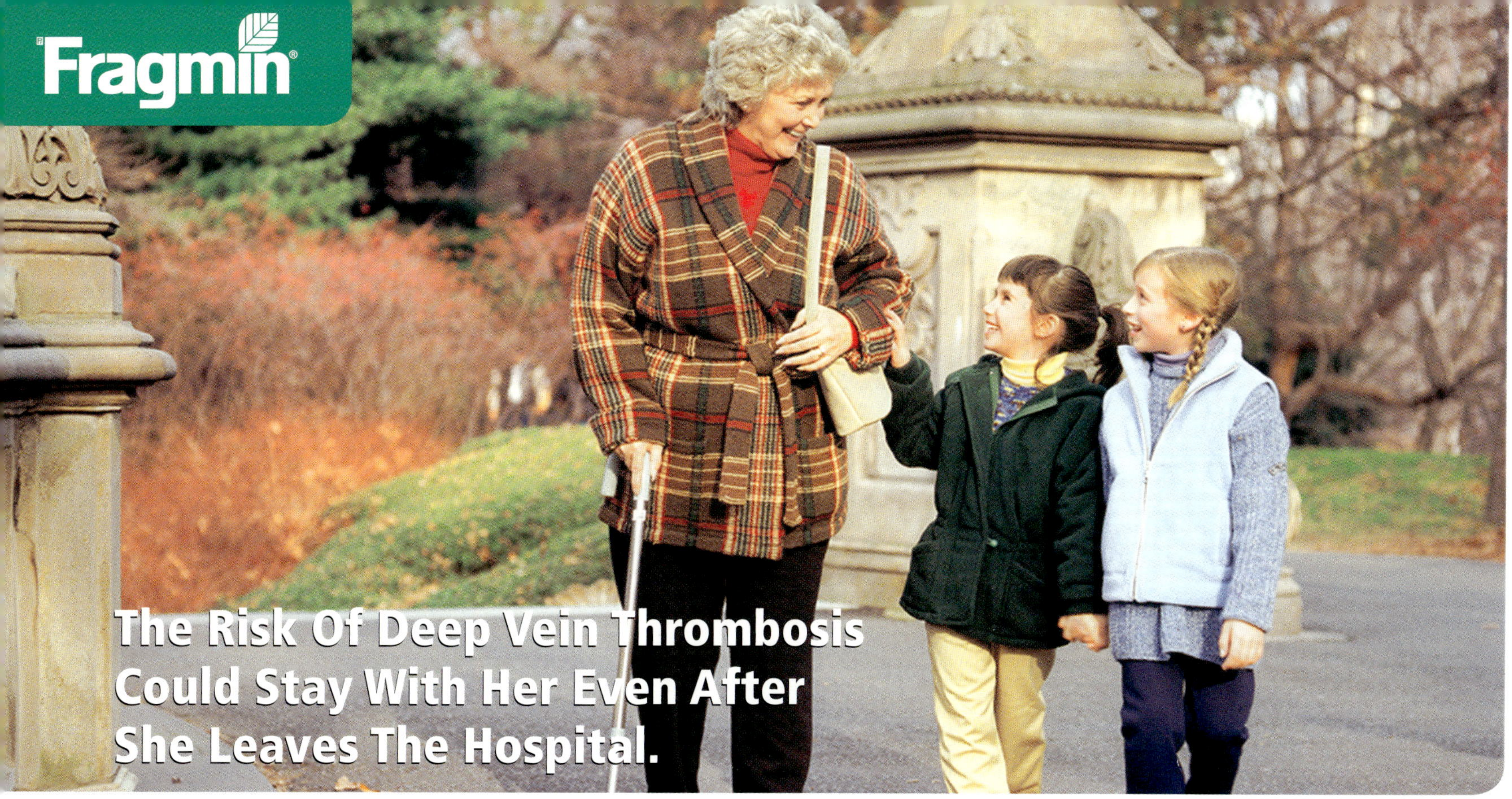

Beyond her hospital stay, [Pr]FRAGMIN® may help manage the risk.[*]

FRAGMIN is indicated for thromboprophylaxis in conjunction with surgery.

Post-operative use of FRAGMIN resulted in a significant reduction in the relative risk of venographically identified DVT compared to warfarin:[†]

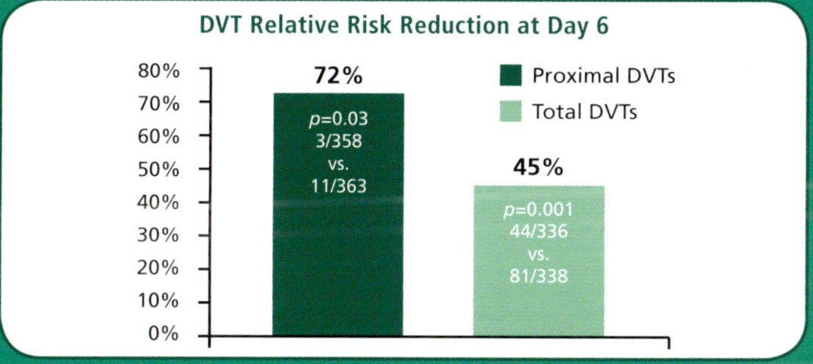

ARR dalteparin – all DVTs: 10.9; proximal DVTs: 2.2; CI: 95%. DVTs assessed on day 6 +/- 2 or at time of discharge from hospital if this occurred earlier.

FRAGMIN showed no significant differences in the incidence of major or minor bleeding risk compared to warfarin.[†,‡]

	Major Bleeding (% pts)		Minor Bleeding (% pts)	
	Day 0–1	Day 2–8	Day 0–1	Day 2–8
Post-Operative FRAGMIN (n=487)	5.7	0.8	0.6	1.6
Warfarin (n=489)	4.1	0.4	0.4	1.6

Adapted from Hull *et al. Arch Intern Med* 2000.

- In elective hip surgery, 5000 IU s.c. is given the evening before the operation and then 5000 IU s.c. the following evenings. Treatment is continued until the patient is mobilized, generally 5–7 days or longer.
- INR or APTT monitoring is not required.[§]
- FRAGMIN is eligible for reimbursement under many provincial formularies.

Adverse Events: Clinically significant adverse reactions with FRAGMIN and other LMWHs include bleeding events and local reactions, with a low incidence of thrombocytopenia and allergic reactions. In clinical trials with hospitalized patients with severely restricted mobility, the incidence of thrombocytopenia was 0.54% at days 14 and 21. Injection site hematomas are a common side effect with FRAGMIN, occurring at a frequency of <5% with lower (prophylaxis) doses and <10% with higher (treatment) doses.

FRAGMIN should be used with care in patients with hepatic insufficiency, renal insufficiency or a history of gastrointestinal ulceration. Please consult the Prescribing Information for complete dosing instructions, warnings and precautions, and adverse events.

The multi-dose vial of FRAGMIN (25,000 IU/mL) contains benzyl alcohol (14 mg/mL) as a preservative. Benzyl alcohol has been associated with a potentially fatal "Gasping Syndrome" in neonates. Because benzyl alcohol may cross the placenta, FRAGMIN preserved with benzyl alcohol should not be used in pregnant women.

FRAGMIN should NOT be administered intra-muscularly.

FRAGMIN CANNOT BE USED INTERCHANGEABLY (UNIT FOR UNIT) WITH UNFRACTIONATED HEPARIN (UFH) OR OTHER LOW MOLECULAR WEIGHT HEPARINS (LMWHs) AS THEY DIFFER IN THEIR MANUFACTURING PROCESS, MOLECULAR WEIGHT DISTRIBUTION, ANTI-Xa AND ANTI-IIa ACTIVITIES, UNITS AND DOSAGES. SPECIAL ATTENTION AND COMPLIANCE WITH INSTRUCTIONS FOR USE OF EACH SPECIFIC PRODUCT ARE REQUIRED DURING ANY CHANGE IN TREATMENT.

Contraindications: FRAGMIN should not be used in patients who have: hypersensitivity to FRAGMIN or any of its constituents, including benzyl alcohol (when using the 25,000 IU multi-dose vial) or to other low molecular weight heparins and/or heparin or pork products; history of confirmed or suspected immunologically mediated heparin-induced thrombocytopenia (delayed-onset severe thrombocytopenia), and/or in patients in whom an *in vitro* platelet-aggregation test in the presence of FRAGMIN is positive; septic endocarditis (endocarditis lenta, subacute endocarditis); uncontrollable active bleeding; major blood-clotting disorders; acute gastroduodenal ulcer; cerebral hemorrhage; severe uncontrolled hypertension; diabetic or hemorrhagic retinopathy; other conditions or diseases involving an increased risk of hemorrhage; injuries to and operations on the central nervous system, eyes and ears; spinal/epidural anesthesia is contraindicated where repeated high doses of FRAGMIN (100–120 IU/kg given twice daily or 200 IU/kg once daily) are required, due to an increased risk of bleeding.

[Pr]Fragmin®
dalteparin sodium
ONCE-DAILY antithrombotic efficacy with easy dosing.

FRAGMIN® Pfizer Health AB, owner/
Pfizer Canada Inc., Licensee

Pfizer

PAAB

Member R&D

For your *NEW* osteoporosis patients

Covered by most Provincial Formularies[1,2,3,4,5,6,7,8,*]

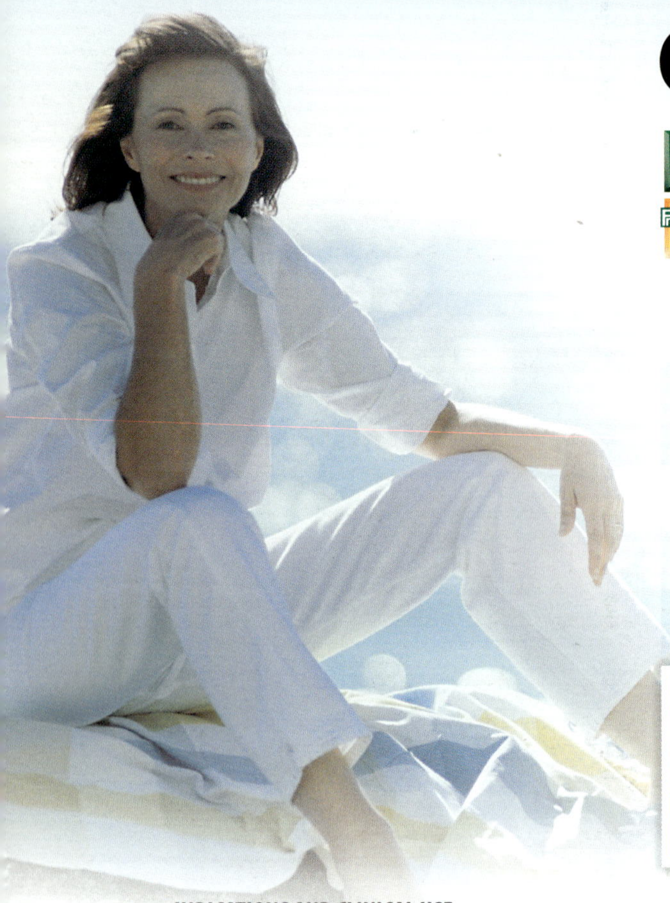

Choose

Pr FOSAVANCE® 70/5600

alendronate sodium/cholecalciferol (Vitamin D_3)

WITH

✓ The demonstrated fracture prevention of alendronate

PLUS

✓ The benefits of a weekly dose of 5600 IU Vitamin D_3[9,**]

70 mg alendronate	5600 IU Vitamin D_3

in a single once-weekly tablet[9,**]

INDICATIONS AND CLINICAL USE

FOSAVANCE® (bone metabolism regulator and Vitamin D), containing alendronate sodium, a bisphosphonate, and cholecalciferol (Vitamin D_3), is indicated for the treatment of osteoporosis in postmenopausal women and men. The alendronate sodium component of FOSAVANCE® increases bone mass and can prevent fractures including those of the hip and spine (vertebral compression fractures). The recommended dosage is one tablet of FOSAVANCE® (70 mg/2800 IU) or FOSAVANCE® (70 mg/5600 IU) once weekly. The appropriate dosage of FOSAVANCE® must be determined by the physician based on the patient's vitamin D requirement.

SELECTED IMPORTANT SAFETY INFORMATION

Like other bisphosphonate containing products, FOSAVANCE® may cause local irritation of the upper gastrointestinal mucosa.

Osteonecrosis of the jaw (ONJ) has been reported in patients with cancer receiving treatment regimens including bisphosphonates. The majority of reports occurred following tooth extractions with delayed healing and involved cancer patients treated with intravenous bisphosphonates. Many of these patients were also receiving chemotherapy and corticosteroids. However, some cases have also occurred in patients receiving oral bisphosphonate treatment for postmenopausal osteoporosis and other diagnoses. The majority of reported cases have been associated with dental procedures such as tooth extraction. Many had signs of local infection, including osteomyelitis. A dental examination with appropriate preventive dentistry should be considered prior to treatment with bisphosphonates in patients with concomitant risk factors. Known risk factors for osteonecrosis of the jaw include a diagnosis of cancer, concomitant therapies (e.g., chemotherapy, radiotherapy, corticosteroids, immunosuppressive drugs), poor oral hygiene, co-morbid disorders (e.g., periodontal and/or other pre-existing dental disease, anemia, coagulopathy, infection, diabetes mellitus), smoking, and heavy alcohol use.

FOSAVANCE® is contraindicated for use in patients with abnormalities of the esophagus which delay esophageal emptying such as stricture or achalasia, inability to stand or sit upright for at least 30 minutes, hypersensitivity to any component of this product, hypocalcemia or renal insufficiency with creatinine clearance <0.58 mL/s (<35 mL/min).

FOSAVANCE® alone should not be used to treat Vitamin D deficiency (commonly defined as 25(OH)D <22.5 nmol/L). Caution should be exercised in patients with diseases associated with unregulated overproduction of 1,25-dihydroxyvitamin D, as Vitamin D_3 supplementation may worsen hypercalcemia and/or hypercalciuria in these patients.

In a study of osteoporotic postmenopausal women and men, the safety profile of FOSAVANCE® (70 mg/2800 IU) was similar to that of PrFOSAMAX® 70 mg once weekly. The safety profile of FOSAVANCE® (70 mg/2800 IU) administered with an additional 2800 IU Vitamin D_3 was similar to that of FOSAVANCE® (70 mg/2800 IU). In a clinical study, the most common drug-related adverse experiences reported in ≥1% of patients taking FOSAMAX® 70 mg tablet Once Weekly were abdominal pain (3.7%), musculoskeletal (bone, muscle, joint) pain (2.9%), dyspepsia (2.7%), acid regurgitation (1.9%), and nausea (1.9%).

* See respective Formularies for details (not covered in MAN and PEI).

** The appropriate dosage of FOSAVANCE® must be determined by the physician based on the patient's vitamin D requirement. All patients must receive supplemental calcium and/or vitamin D, if intake is inadequate. Patients suffering from osteoporosis are at an increased risk for vitamin D insufficiency. FOSAVANCE® alone should not be used to treat vitamin D deficiency (commonly defined as 25-hydroxyvitamin D <22.5 nmol/L or 9 ng/mL). Patients must wait at least 30 minutes after swallowing FOSAVANCE® before taking the first food, beverage, or any oral medicines, including other vitamins and supplements.

MERCK

Merck Frosst Canada Ltd., Kirkland, Quebec

PLEASE CONSULT THE PRODUCT MONOGRAPH FOR INFORMATION ABOUT INDICATIONS, CONTRAINDICATIONS, WARNINGS AND PRECAUTIONS WITH RESPECT TO UPPER GASTROINTESTINAL EVENTS, CLINICAL ADVERSE EVENTS, DRUG INTERACTIONS, AND DOSAGE AND ADMINISTRATION.

BEFORE PRESCRIBING **FOSAVANCE®**, PLEASE CONSULT THE ENCLOSED PRESCRIBING INFORMATION.

Please visit our website at **www.merckfrosst.com**

PAAB

FSD-11-CDN-34491170-JA-CPS

F

Fabrazyme® Ⓟ
agalsidase beta
Enzyme Replacement Therapy

Genzyme

Date of Revision: August 3, 2006

SUMMARY PRODUCT INFORMATION:

Route of Administration	Dosage Form/Strength	Clinically Relevant Nonmedicinal Ingredients
Intravenous infusion	Lyophilized powder for reconstitution and intravenous infusion, 5 mg, 35 mg	There are no clinically relevant nonmedicinal ingredients. For a complete listing of nonmedicinal ingredients, see Dosage Forms, Composition and Packaging.

DESCRIPTION: Fabrazyme (agalsidase beta) is a recombinant enzyme intended for use as replacement for the human enzyme, α galactosidase A, (α-GAL). The characteristics of Fabrazyme were consistent with the limited data (molecular weight, pH optimum and isoelectric focusing (IEF) patterns) available about the enzyme isolated from human sources (plasma, placenta, liver and spleen). α-GAL catalyzes the hydrolysis to ceramide dihexoside and galactose of globotriaosylceramide (GL-3) and other α-galactyl-terminated neutral glycosphingolipids, such as galabiosylceramide and blood group B substances. Accumulation of undegraded forms of these glycosphingolipids is the primary pathological process in Fabry disease.

INDICATIONS AND CLINICAL USE: Fabrazyme (agalsidase beta) is indicated for long-term enzyme replacement therapy in patients with a confirmed diagnosis of Fabry disease. Fabrazyme reduces globotriaosylceramide (GL-3) levels in the vascular endothelium and slows the rate of clinical progression in Fabry disease as manifested by renal, cardiac and cerebrovascular outcomes.

Pediatrics (<16 years of age): No pediatric patients below the age of 16 years were included in the clinical studies. However, since Fabrazyme treats the underlying pathology of Fabry disease by significantly clearing GL-3 from vascular endothelium of the kidney, heart and skin, pediatric patients would be expected to benefit from treatment. (See Warnings and Precautions, Pediatrics (<16 years of age).)

CONTRAINDICATIONS: Treatment with Fabrazyme (agalsidase beta) is contraindicated if there is clinical evidence of anaphylaxis to agalsidase beta or any of the excipients.

WARNINGS AND PRECAUTIONS: Infusion Reactions: As with any intravenously administered protein product, patients may develop antibodies to the protein and immune mediated reactions are possible. In addition, most Fabry patients have no detectable α-GAL protein levels or activity. Therefore, it is expected that the majority of patients will develop IgG antibodies (seroconvert) upon treatment. Patients with antibodies to Fabrazyme (agalsidase beta) have a higher risk of infusion associated reactions (see Adverse Reactions). The mean time to seroconversion was within 3 months of the first infusion with Fabrazyme. The percentage of patients with IARs peaked early in the treatment period and coincided with IgG seroconversion.

In clinical trials, infusion-associated reactions were the most frequently reported related adverse events occurring in patients treated with Fabrazyme. These IARs included events of chills, fever (pyrexia/body temperature increased/hyperthermia), temperature change sensation (feeling cold/feeling hot), hypertension (blood pressure increased) nausea, vomiting, flushing (hot flush), paraesthesia (burning sensation), fatigue (lethargy/malaise/asthenia), pain (pain in extremity), headache, chest pain (chest discomfort), and pruritus (pruritus generalized). The majority of these infusion-associated reactions were assessed as mild or moderate in intensity.

As a preventive measure, it is recommended that patients are treated with antipyretics prior to an infusion. If an infusion-associated reaction occurs, regardless of pretreatment, the adverse events have been successfully managed by decreasing the infusion rate, temporarily stopping the infusion, and/or administering non-steroidal anti-inflammatory drugs, antipyretics, antihistamines and/or corticosteroids to ameliorate the symptoms. Because of the potential for severe IARs, appropriate medical support measures should be readily available when Fabrazyme is administered. IARs have occurred in some patients after receiving pretreatment with antipyretics, antihistamines, and/or oral steroids. IARs declined in frequency with continued use of Fabrazyme. However, IARs may still occur despite extended duration of Fabrazyme treatment.

Patients who experience an infusion-associated reaction during a Fabrazyme infusion should be treated with caution when Fabrazyme is re-administered. If severe allergic or anaphylactoid reactions occur, immediate discontinuation of the administration of Fabrazyme and current medical standards for emergency treatment are to be observed.

The initial IV infusion rate should be no more than 0.25 mg/min (15 mg/hr). The infusion rate may be slowed in the event of infusion-associated reactions. After patient tolerance to the infusion is well established, the infusion rate may be increased gradually in increments of 0.05 to 0.08 mg/min (increments of 3 to 5 mg/hr) with each subsequent infusion.

Special Populations: The Fabry Registry, sponsored by Genzyme Corporation, is an ongoing, observational database that tracks natural history and outcomes of patients with Fabry disease. Participation is open to all physicians managing patients with Fabry disease. Physicians are encouraged to collaborate, share observations, and generate hypotheses for evaluation, as well as assist in the collection of clinical data in an effort to guide and assess future therapeutic interventions.

The primary objectives of the Registry are:

- To enhance the understanding of the variability, progression and natural history of Fabry disease, including heterozygous females with the disease;
- To assist the Fabry medical community with the development of recommendations for monitoring patients and reports on patient outcomes to help optimize patient care;
- To characterize and describe the Fabry population as a whole; and
- To evaluate the long term safety and effectiveness of Fabrazyme.

For a more detailed description of the Fabry Registry, please refer to the Fabry Registry Protocol, or contact The Fabry Registry team at 1-800-745-4447 or refer to the website, www.LSDregistry.net.

Pregnant Women: Reproduction studies have been performed in rats at daily doses up to 30 times the human dose and have revealed no evidence of impaired fertility or harm to the fetus due to Fabrazyme. However, since clinical trials have not been carried out in pregnant women with Fabry disease and there is no other clinical data to indicate safety in pregnancy, caution should be exercised if Fabrazyme is to be used during pregnancy.

Nursing Women: It is not known whether Fabrazyme is secreted in human milk. However, since clinical trials have not been carried out in nursing women with Fabry disease and there is no other clinical data to indicate safety in this clinical situation, caution should be exercised if Fabrazyme is to be administered to nursing women.

Pediatrics (<16 years of age): No pediatric patients below the age of 16 years were included in the clinical studies. However, since Fabrazyme treats the underlying pathology of Fabry disease by significantly clearing GL-3 from vascular endothelium of the kidney, heart and skin, pediatric patients would be expected to benefit from treatment.

Geriatrics: Clinical studies did not include any subjects aged 65 and over.

ADVERSE REACTIONS: Adverse Drug Reaction Overview: The most frequently reported related adverse events in the clinical trials are infusion associated and include: rigors (shaking chills), fever, temperature change sensation (feels cold), headache, nausea, rhinitis (nasal congestion), dyspnea, chest pain, flushing, hypertension, vomiting, and pruritus.

The most common serious adverse drug reactions requiring intervention (interruption or discontinuation of Fabrazyme), hospitalization or medications were also IARs, including urticaria, fever, chills, tachycardia, tightness in chest/throat, or hypertension/hypotension (see Warnings and Precautions: Infusion Reactions). Most patients develop IgG antibodies to Fabrazyme (see Warnings and Precautions: Infusion Reactions). Some patients developed IgE or skin test reactivity specific to Fabrazyme. Physicians should consider testing patients who experienced allergic reactions suspected to be IgE-mediated for IgE antibody development. Physicians should also consider the risks and benefits of continued treatment in patients with anti-Fabrazyme IgE. Skin testing can be considered based on the patient's clinical presentation of symptoms.

Patients who have had a positive skin test or who have tested positive for anti-Fabrazyme IgE may be successfully re-challenged with Fabrazyme. The initial re-challenge administration should be a low dose at a lower infusion rate e.g., 1/2 the therapeutic dose at 1/25 the initial standard recommended rate. Once a patient tolerates the infusion, the dose may be increased to reach the approved dose of 1.0 mg/kg and the infusion rate may be increased by slowly titrating upwards, as tolerated.

There are no marketed tests for antibodies against Fabrazyme. If testing is warranted, contact your local Genzyme representative or Genzyme Corporation at (800) 745-4447.

The adverse events associated with Fabrazyme infusion have been successfully managed using standard medical practices, such as reduction in infusion rate and/or premedication with, or additional administration of non-steroidal, anti inflammatory drugs, antipyretics, antihistamines and/or corticosteroids.

Clinical Trial Adverse Drug Reactions: Because clinical trials are conducted under very specific conditions, the adverse reaction rates observed in the clinical trials may not reflect the rates observed in practice and should not be compared to the rates in the clinical trials of another drug. Adverse drug reaction information from clinical trials is useful for identifying drug-related adverse events and for approximating rates.

In clinical studies Fabrazyme (agalsidase beta) infusions were generally well tolerated.

Adverse events reported to be related to Fabrazyme in a total of 71 patients treated for up to 48 months (Phase 3 Double-Blind/Open Label Extension studies) and up to 5 months (Phase 2 Japan Bridging study) are listed by system organ class in Table 1. The majority of these adverse events were judged to be mild to moderate in severity. Currently available data demonstrate that the total number of patients experiencing any related adverse event on the same day as infusion has decreased over time.

Table 1: Fabrazyme

Incidence of Related[a] Adverse Events from Start of Treatment with Fabrazyme Up to Infusion 96 (42 Months) (Three Studies combined: Phase 3 Double Blind, Phase 3 Extension and Phase 2 Japan)

Body System	(5–10%)	(10–50%)	(>50%)
Body as a Whole — General	Pain, Fatigue, Leg pain, Malaise	Temperature changed sensation, Fever, Chest pain	Rigors
Cardiovascular — General	Edema in extremities	Hypertension	—
Central/Peripheral Nervous System	Dizziness, Paraesthesia	Headache	—
Gastro-Intestinal System	—	Nausea, Abdominal pain, Vomiting	—
Heart Rate and Rhythm	Tachycardia, Bradycardia	—	—
Musculoskeletal System	—	Myalgia	—
Red Blood Cell	—	—	—
Respiratory System	Bronchospasm, Throat tightness	Rhinitis, Dyspnea	—
Secondary Terms	—	Fabry pain (extremity pain)	—
Skin and Appendages	Urticaria	Pruritus	—
Urinary System	—	—	—

[a] Related adverse events is defined as Possible, Probably, Definite, and Unknown. For the Phase 2 Japan study, related adverse events defined as Unlikely/Remote were also included.

A review of individual adverse event terms reported during clinical trials in which a reasonable relationship to the administration of Fabrazyme was not demonstrated include syncope, tremor, somnolence, lacrimation abnormal, and vision abnormal.

The most frequently reported related adverse events are infusion associated and include (in decreasing order of frequency): rigors (shaking chills), fever, temperature change sensation (feels cold), nausea, headache, flushing, rhinitis (nasal congestion), vomiting, chest pain, dyspnoea, pruritus, and hypertension.

The majority of these infusion associated adverse drug reactions (ADRs) can be attributed to the formation of IgG antibodies and/or complement activation and were not IgE mediated. During clinical studies, 52 of 58 (90%) patients in the Phase 3 double-blind and Phase 3 Extension study (with up to 48 months of exposure) developed IgG antibodies to Fabrazyme. Forty-four (85%) of the 52 patients seroconverted within three months of treatment with Fabrazyme. By 42-48 months of therapy, >50% of the seroconverted patients have demonstrated a downward trend in antibody titer based on a 4-fold reduction in titer. Seven patients have tolerized (no detectable antibody by radioimmunoprecipitation (RIP)). There is no evidence that the immune response inhibited or neutralized activity of Fabrazyme.

No patient experienced anaphylaxis. Only a small number of patients have experienced reactions suggestive of immediate (Type 1) hypersensitivity. The adverse events associated with Fabrazyme infusion have been successfully managed using standard medical practices, such as reduction in infusion rate and/or premedication with, or additional administration of nonsteroidal, anti inflammatory drugs, antipyretics, antihistamines and corticosteroids.

Adverse events reported to be related to Fabrazyme in a total of 63 patients who received 1 mg/kg of Fabrazyme in the randomized (2:1), double blind, placebo controlled study is listed by system organ class in Table 2. Fifty-one patients were randomized to Fabrazyme and 31 patients were randomized to placebo and, throughout the course of the study, 12 patients transitioned to open-label therapy after experiencing an event. All patients were treated with acetaminophen prior to the infusions.

Table 2: Fabrazyme

Incidence of Related Adverse Events[a] in the Double Blind Study (AGAL-008-00)

Body System	Very Common (>10%)	Common (5-10%)
Body as a Whole – General	Fever, Rigors	Chest pain, Fatigue, Pain, Temperature changed sensation
Cardiovascular – General	Hypertension	Hypotension
Central/Peripheral Nervous System	—	Dizziness, Paraesthesia, Tremor
Gastro-Intestinal System	—	Nausea, Vomiting
Heart Rate and Rhythm	—	Tachycardia
Musculoskeletal System	—	Myalgia

(cont'd)

Table 2: Fabrazyme *(cont'd)*

Incidence of Related Adverse Events[a] in the Double Blind Study (AGAL-008-00)

Body System	Very Common (>10%)	Common (5-10%)
Secondary Terms	—	Fabry pain
Skin and Appendages	—	Pruritus, Rash, Urticaria
Vascular (Extracardiac)	—	Flushing

[a] Related adverse event is defined as Possible, Probably, Definite or Unknown. AE terminology from WHOART dictionary.

During the AGAL-008-00 study, the following adverse events that were considered to be related by the reporting investigator and occurred within the frequency range of 1-4% were: injection site reaction, back pain, hot flushes, leg pain, malaise, oedema mouth, oedema peripheral, pallor, cardiomegaly, heart disorder, heart valve disorders, oedema dependent, headache, hypoaesthesia, vertigo, abdominal pain, diarrhoea, gastroenteritis, hepatic enzymes increased, oedema legs, phosphatase alkaline increased, thirst, skeletal pain, thrombosis venous arm, agitation, anxiety, somnolence, dysmenorrhoea, antibodies drug specific, bronchospasm, coughing, pharyngitis, pneumonia, rhinitis, throat tightness, angioedema, rash erythematous, rash maculopapular, skin disorder, vasospasm and vision abnormal.

During the AGAL-008-00 trial, one patient was reported to have 2 asymptomatic episodes of QTc prolongation (>450 msec) which could not be attributed to Fabrazyme treatment. The first occurrence was while the patient was receiving placebo and the second was during open-label Fabrazyme treatment. Overall, during the double-blind placebo controlled period of the study, 8 of 29 placebo patients and 23 of 48 Fabrazyme patients had centrally-read QTc prolongations. There was no statistically significant difference between the two groups.

The majority of patients experienced related adverse drug reactions (ADRs) on the day of infusion. These reactions most often consisted of fever and chills. Infusion-associated reactions included additional symptoms such as mild to moderate dyspnoea, throat tightness, chest tightness, flushing, pruritus, urticaria, rhinitis, temperature changed sensation, tremor (3 reports of shaking and one report of generalized tremor), Fabry pain, hypoaesthesia, paraesthesia, fatigue, pallor, vision abnormal bronchial constriction, bronchospasm, coughing, tachypnea and/or wheezing; cardiovascular symptoms including moderate hypertension, tachycardia, chest pain, pain, palpitations; gastrointestinal symptoms including abdominal pain, nausea, vomiting; infusion-related pain including pain at the extremities, myalgia; and headache.

The majority of these infusion-associated ADRs are thought to be due to the formation of IgG antibodies and/or complement activation. Forty-three out of the 63 patients (68%) who received drug at any time during the AGAL-008-00 double-blind, randomized, placebo-controlled study developed IgG antibodies to Fabrazyme. Seventy percent of the patients randomized to Fabrazyme seroconverted within 3 months of their first Fabrazyme infusion. Six Fabrazyme patients demonstrated a downward trend in antibody titer, defined as a ≥ four-fold reduction in titer from the peak measurement to the last measurement, while 4 Fabrazyme patients tolerized. There is no evidence that the immune response inhibited or neutralized the activity of Fabrazyme.

The hypersensitivity reactions were managed by a reduction in the rate of infusion together with the administration of antipyretics, antihistamines and/or corticosteroids.

Among the 10 female patients who received Fabrazyme (2 in the Phase 3 and 8 in the AGAL-008-00 double-blind clinical trials), 4 patients tolerized, 6 patients did not develop IgG antibodies.

DRUG INTERACTIONS: Drug-Drug Interactions: Interactions with other drugs have not been established. No in vitro metabolism studies have been carried out. Because it is a protein, Fabrazyme is an unlikely candidate for cytochrome P450 mediated drug-drug interactions.

Drug-Food Interactions: Interactions with food have not been established.

Drug-Herb Interactions: Interactions with herbal products have not been established.

Drug-Laboratory Test Interactions: Interactions with laboratory tests have not been established.

DOSAGE AND ADMINISTRATION: Dosing Considerations:

- Renal Disease: No changes in dose are necessary for patients with renal insufficiency.
- Liver Disease: Studies in patients with hepatic insufficiency were not performed.

Recommended Dose and Dosage Adjustment: The recommended dosage of Fabrazyme (agalsidase beta) is 1.0 mg/kg body weight infused every 2 weeks as an IV infusion.

The initial IV infusion rate should be no more than 0.25 mg/min (15 mg/hr). The infusion rate may be slowed in the event of infusion-associated reactions. After patient tolerance to the infusion is well established, the infusion rate may be increased gradually in increments of 0.05 to 0.08 mg/min (increments of 3 to 5 mg/hr) with each subsequent infusion.

In clinical trials, pretreatment with an antipyretic and/or an antihistamine was used to manage a single or recurrent mild moderate infusion associated reaction(s). Pretreatment with an antihistamine, antipyretic and/or corticosteroid was used to manage a single severe or recurrent moderate severe infusion associated reaction(s). The selection of pretreatment medication and dose should be based on the patient's age, weight and severity of the reaction. The time of administration should be based on the onset of action of the medication selected. A decrease in infusion rate should also be considered. If the infusion proceeds without incident, consideration may be given to increasing infusion rates in a stepwise manner and to reducing premedication.

Administration: Instructions for Use: Fabrazyme does not contain any preservatives.

Vials are for single use only. Any unused product should be discarded. Pneumatic tube systems should not be used for transport of this product.

Excessive agitation of this product should be avoided. Do not use filter needles during the preparation of the infusion. The diluted solution may be filtered through an in line low protein binding 0.2 µm filter during administration.

Materials Inventory: The following items are suggested for the reconstitution and administration of Fabrazyme: Fabrazyme (vials); sterile water for injection, USP; 0.9% sodium chloride injection, USP (normal saline); tape; two syringes for reconstitution and dilution; two needles; in-line low protein-binding particulate filter (0.2 µm) (Optional); administration set with flow-regulating device or intravenous infusion pump and tubing; i.v. kit; anaphylaxis kit; angiocatheter; gloves; alcohol wipes; arm board; medication label.

Reconstitution and Dilution (using Aseptic Technique):

1. Fabrazyme vials and diluent should be allowed to reach room temperature prior to reconstitution (approximately 30 minutes). The number of vials needed is based on the patient's body weight (kg) and the recommended dose of 1.0 mg/kg. Select the appropriate number of vials so that the total number of mg is equal to or greater than the patient's number of kg of body weight.
2. Reconstitute each 35 mg vial of Fabrazyme by **slowly** injecting 7.2 mL of Sterile Water for Injection, USP down the inside wall of each vial. Roll and tilt each vial gently. Each vial will yield a 5.0 mg/mL clear, colorless solution (total extractable dose per vial is 35 mg, 7.0 mL).
   Reconstitute each 5 mg vial of Fabrazyme by **slowly** injecting 1.1 mL of Sterile Water for Injection, USP down the inside wall of each vial. Roll and tilt each vial gently. Each vial will yield a 5.0 mg/mL clear, colorless solution (total extractable dose per vial is 5 mg, 1.0 mL).
3. Visually inspect the reconstituted vials for particulate matter and discoloration. Do not use vials exhibiting particulate matter or discoloration. Report lot number to hospital pharmacist for vials exhibiting particulate matter or discoloration.
4. Slowly withdraw the reconstituted solution from each vial and further dilute with 0.9 % Sodium Chloride Injection, USP to a **final total volume of 500 mL**. Be sure to inject the reconstituted Fabrazyme solution directly into the sodium chloride solution rather than into the air within the infusion bag. Total infusion volumes as low as 100 mL have been used in a clinical trial.
5. Gently invert infusion bag to mix the solution, avoiding vigorous shaking and agitation. Use immediately.
6. Fabrazyme should not be infused in the same intravenous line with other products.

OVERDOSAGE:

There have been no reports of overdose with Fabrazyme (agalsidase beta). In clinical trials, patients received doses up to 3.0 mg/kg body weight.

For management of a suspected drug overdose, CPhA recommends that you contact your **regional Poison Control Centre**. See the *CPS* Directory section for a list of Poison Control Centres.

ACTION AND CLINICAL PHARMACOLOGY: Mechanism of Action: In Fabry disease, deficiency of the lysosomal enzyme α-GAL leads to progressive accumulation of glycosphingolipids, predominantly GL-3, in most body tissues and fluids. This excessive accumulation of GL-3 is the primary pathological process which, over a period of years or decades, triggers a cascade of events that results in disease expression.

GL-3 buildup in the vascular wall results in narrowing and thrombosis of arteries and arterioles. This derangement of the vascular network often involves capillaries and has been implicated in the development of peripheral neuritis, angiokeratoma corporis diffusum universale, renal failure, myocardial infarction and cerebral infarction. The most significant clinical manifestations of Fabry disease are renal failure, cardiomyopathy, and cerebrovascular accidents resulting in chronic morbidity and premature death.

Fabrazyme is intended as an enzyme replacement therapy to provide an exogenous source of α-GAL in Fabry disease patients. This recombinant human α-GAL (r-hαGAL) will catalyze the hydrolysis of glycosphingolipids including GL-3 in the lysosomes of multiple cell types and tissues.

Pharmacokinetics: Plasma profiles of Fabrazyme were studied at 0.3, 1.0 and 3.0 mg/kg in a Phase 1/2 dose-finding study. The area under the plasma concentration-time curve (AUC_{∞}) and the clearance did not increase proportionately with increasing doses, demonstrating that the enzyme follows non-linear pharmacokinetics. Terminal half-life was dose independent with a range of 45-102 minutes.

Pharmacokinetics of Fabrazyme was evaluated in 11 Fabry patients in Europe participating in a Phase 3 double-blind clinical trial. Following an intravenous infusion of 1 mg/kg of Fabrazyme over a period averaging 280 to 300 minutes, mean maximum plasma concentrations (C_{max}) ranged from 2.09-3.49 µg/mL. The mean AUC_{∞} ranged from 372-784 µg/mL·min. The mean volume of distribution (V_z) was 0.23-0.49 L/kg and the mean volume of distribution at steady state (V_{ss}) was 0.12-0.57 L/kg. Mean plasma clearance ranged from 1.75-4.87 mL/min/kg and the mean elimination half-life ($t_{1/2}$) ranged from 82.3-119 minutes.

Pharmacokinetics of Fabrazyme was also evaluated in 13 Fabry patients in Japan participating in a Phase 2 open-label clinical trial. The results of these evaluations show that Fabrazyme pharmacokinetics are comparable in Caucasian and Japanese Fabry patients.

STORAGE AND STABILITY: Store Fabrazyme (agalsidase beta) under refrigeration between 2-8°C. This product contains no preservatives. Use immediately after reconstitution (within 3 hours).

Do not use Fabrazyme after the expiration date on the vial.

INFORMATION FOR THE PATIENT: Published in e-CPS, available by subscription at www.e-cps.ca.

DOSAGE FORMS, COMPOSITION AND PACKAGING: 5 mg: Each vial of sterile, nonpyrogenic, white to off-white lyophilized cake or powder, contains: agalsidase beta 5.5 mg total amount, which allows for an extractable dose of 5 mg/vial, mannitol 33 mg, sodium phosphate monobasic, monohydrate 3 mg, sodium phosphate dibasic, heptahydrate 8.8 mg. Single-use, clear Type I glass 5 mL vials. The closure consists of a siliconized butyl stopper and an aluminum seal with a plastic grey flip-off cap. 1, 5 and 10 vials per carton. Not all package sizes may be marketed.

35 mg: Each vial of sterile, nonpyrogenic, white to off-white lyophilized cake or powder, contains: agalsidase beta 37 mg total amount, which allows for an extractable dose of 35 mg/vial, mannitol 222 mg, sodium phosphate monobasic, monohydrate 20.4 mg, sodium phosphate dibasic, heptahydrate 59.2 mg. Single-use, clear Type I glass 20 mL vials. The closure consists of a siliconized butyl stopper and an aluminum seal with a plastic purple flip-off cap. 1, 5 and 10 vials per carton. Not all package sizes may be marketed.

Famvir® Ⓟ

famciclovir

Antiviral Agent

Novartis Pharmaceuticals

Date of Preparation: January 18, 2001
Date of Revision: July 20, 2010

SUMMARY PRODUCT INFORMATION:

Route of Administration	Dosage Form/ Strength	Clinically Relevant Nonmedicinal Ingredients
Oral	Tablets/125 mg, 250 mg and 500 mg	Lactose For a complete listing see Dosage Forms, Composition and Packaging.

INDICATIONS AND CLINICAL USE: FAMVIR (famciclovir) tablets are indicated:

- for the treatment of acute herpes zoster (shingles).
- for the treatment or suppression of recurrent episodes of genital herpes in immunocompetent adults.
- for the treatment of recurrent episodes of mucocutaneous herpes simplex infections in HIV-infected patients.

Early treatment of acute herpes zoster (shingles) in immune-competent individuals with oral famciclovir resulted in decreased time to loss of vesicles; decreased time to loss of crusts; and decreased viral shedding.

The results of clinical studies indicate that early treatment of acute herpes zoster with oral famciclovir resulted in decreased duration of post-herpetic neuralgia. Those most likely to benefit are patients who initiate treatment within 48 hours of onset of rash or are greater than 50 years of age or those patients with severe pain at the time of treatment initiation.

In clinical studies of immunocompetent patients with recurrent genital herpes (typically ≥6 episodes in a 12 month period) famciclovir suppressed lesional episodes, slowed the rate to first recurrence and patients were more likely to remain free from recurrences for a 12 month period. Suppressive therapy in patients with fewer than 6 episodes of genital herpes in a 12 month period was not evaluated in these clinical studies.

Initiation of famciclovir treatment of recurrent genital herpes during the prodrome or as soon as possible after the onset of lesions resulted in decreased duration of viral shedding, decreased time to lesion healing and decreased time to resolution of symptoms (including pain, tenderness, itching and burning).

CONTRAINDICATIONS: Patients who have known hypersensitivity to FAMVIR (famciclovir) or to any ingredient in the formulation or component of the container. For a complete listing, see Dosage Forms, Composition and Packaging.

WARNINGS AND PRECAUTIONS: General: The efficacy of FAMVIR (famciclovir) has not been established for first episode genital herpes infections, disseminated zoster, or in immunocompromised patients with herpes zoster (see Action and Clinical Pharmacology). Dosage adjustment is required when administering famciclovir to patients with moderate or severe renal dysfunction (see Dosage and Administration). No special precautions are required for patients with well-compensated hepatic impairment. Famciclovir has not been studied in patients with severe uncompensated hepatic impairment (see Action and Clinical Pharmacology).

Genital herpes is a sexually transmitted disease with an increased risk of transmission during acute episodes. There are no data evaluating whether FAMVIR will prevent transmission of infection to others. Patients should be advised to avoid intercourse when lesions and/or symptoms are present (even if treatment with an anti-viral has been initiated) in order to avoid infecting partners. Genital herpes can also be transmitted in the absence of symptoms through asymptomatic viral shedding.

FAMVIR 125 mg, 250 mg and 500 mg tablets contain lactose (26.9 mg, 53.7 mg and 107.4 mg, respectively). Patients with rare heredity problems of galactose intolerance, a severe case of lactase deficiency or glucose-galactose malabsorption should not take FAMVIR 125 mg, 250 mg and 500 mg tablets.

Special Populations: Pregnant Women: Although animal studies have not shown any embryotoxic or teratogenic effects with famciclovir or penciclovir, the safety of famciclovir in human pregnancy has not been established. Because animal reproductive studies are not always predictive of human response, famciclovir should, therefore, not be used in pregnancy unless the potential benefits are considered to outweigh the potential risks associated with treatment.

Nursing Women: Following oral administration of famciclovir to lactating rats, penciclovir is excreted in milk. It is not known whether it (penciclovir) is excreted in human milk, thus, a decision should be made whether to discontinue nursing or to discontinue the drug, taking into account the importance of the drug to the mother.

Pediatrics: Safety and efficacy in children under the age of 18 years have not been established.

Race: The impact of race on the safety and efficacy of FAMVIR has not been established.

Geriatrics: Of 816 patients with herpes zoster in clinical studies who were treated with famciclovir, 248 (30.4%) were >65 years of age and 103 (13%) were >75 years of age. No overall differences were observed in safety between younger and older patients (see Adverse Reactions).

Impairment of Fertility: As with other drugs of this class, testicular toxicity has been observed in animals receiving both famciclovir and penciclovir. Two placebo-controlled studies in a total of 130 otherwise healthy men with a normal sperm profile over an 8 week baseline period and recurrent genital herpes receiving oral famciclovir (250 mg bid) (n=66) or placebo (n=64) therapy for 18 weeks showed no evidence of significant effects on sperm count, motility or morphology during treatment or during an 8 week follow-up. Preliminary results of another placebo-controlled trial in a total of 117 otherwise healthy men with recurrent genital herpes and a normal sperm profile over an 8 week baseline period receiving famciclovir (250 mg bid, n=59) and placebo (n=58) therapy for 52 weeks showed no evidence of significant effects in sperm concentration, total sperm count, percent motility, percent abnormal morphology and percent dead sperm during treatment or during a 12 week follow-up.

Effects on Ability to Drive and Use Machines: FAMVIR can cause dizziness, drowsiness or confusion in very rare cases. Patients who experience any of these symptoms while taking FAMVIR should take special care when driving or using machines (see Adverse Reactions, Post-Market Adverse Drug Reactions).

ADVERSE REACTIONS: Clinical Trial Adverse Drug Reactions: Because clinical trials are conducted under very specific conditions the adverse reaction rates observed in the clinical trials may not reflect the rates observed in practice and should not be compared to the rates in the clinical trials of another drug. Adverse drug reaction information from clinical trials is useful for identifying drug-related adverse events and for approximating rates.

Adverse Drug Reaction Overview: Immunocompetent Patients: The most frequent adverse reactions reported during herpes zoster clinical trials with oral FAMVIR (famciclovir) three times daily were as shown in Table 1.

Table 1: FAMVIR

Patients (%) Reporting Adverse Events Related[a] to Study Medication by Preferred Term in Famciclovir Zoster Trials within 30 Days of the Last Dose

	Famciclovir	Placebo
Patients Receiving Study Medication	816	146
Event	%	%
Body as a Whole		
Headache	7.1	6.8
Fatigue	1.6	0.7
Fever	1.1	0.0
Rigors	0.6	1.4
Herpes Zoster Symptoms	0.5	1.4
Central Nervous System		
Dizziness	1.5	0.7
Somnolence	1.2	2.7
Gastrointestinal		
Nausea	4.3	8.2
Diarrhea	1.8	2.1
Abdominal Pain	1.5	0.0
Constipation	1.0	0.0
Vomiting	1.2	0.7
Anorexia	0.5	1.4
Dermatologic		
Pruritus	1.2	0.7
Sweating Increased	1.0	0.0
Hepatic		
ALT Increased	0.6	1.4
Gamma GT Increased	0.6	1.4
Hepatic Enzymes Increased	0.2	1.4
Special Senses		
Tinnitus	0.0	1.4

[a] Includes events assessed by the investigator as related, probably related, possibly related and adverse events where the relationship was unassessable or missing.

The most frequent adverse reactions reported within 30 days of the last dose, during genital herpes clinical trials with oral FAMVIR were as shown in Table 2.

Table 2: FAMVIR

Patients (%) Reporting Adverse Events Related[a] to Study Medication by Preferred Term in Famciclovir Genital Herpes Trials

	Famciclovir	Placebo
Patients Receiving Study Medication	1500	255
Event	%	%
Body as a Whole		
Headache	5.5	3.9
Fatigue	1.5	1.6

(cont'd)

Table 2: FAMVIR *(cont'd)*

Patients (%) Reporting Adverse Events Related[a] to Study Medication by Preferred Term in Famciclovir Genital Herpes Trials

	Famciclovir	Placebo
Patients Receiving Study Medication	1500	255
Event	%	%
Central Nervous System		
Dizziness	2.3	3.1
Gastrointestinal		
Nausea	4.9	3.9
Diarrhea	1.8	1.6
Dyspepsia	1.3	1.2
Abdominal Pain	0.9	1.6
Autonomic Nervous System		
Dry Mouth	0.3	1.2

[a] Includes events assessed by the investigator as related, probably related, possibly related or where relationship was unassessable or not given.

The most frequent adverse events (incidence of >1%) are listed in Table 3 for patients receiving double-blind FAMVIR or placebo for at least 10 months in the two 12-month-long trials.

Table 3: FAMVIR

Patients (%) Reporting A/Es Related[a] to Study Medication by Preferred Term in Famciclovir Genital Herpes Suppression Trials

	Famciclovir	Placebo
Patients Receiving Study Medication	458	63
Event	%	%
Body as a Whole		
Headache	8.7	9.5
Central Nervous System		
Dizziness	1.5	0
Gastrointestinal		
Abdominal Pain	2.4	4.8
Dyspepsia	2.0	3.2
Nausea	1.5	3.2
Diarrhea	1.3	0
Flatulence	1.1	0
Enzyme Abnormality[b]	2.2	3.2
Bilirubinemia	1.3	1.6
Leukopenia	1.3	0

[a] Includes events assessed by the investigator as related, probably related, possibly related and AEs where the relationship was unassessable or missing.
[b] Reports of elevated lipase.

HIV-Infected Patients: In a controlled study of HIV-infected patients, the overall percentages of patients reporting adverse events were comparable for famciclovir and acyclovir. The most frequently reported events (≥2% in any group) are listed in Table 4.

Table 4: FAMVIR

Adverse Events[a] Reported by Preferred Term in HIV-Infected Patients

	Famciclovir	Acyclovir
Patients Receiving Study Medication	150	143
Event	%	%
Headache	13.3	9.1
Nausea	8.7	8.4
Diarrhea	4.7	4.9
Vomiting	3.3	2.1
Fatigue	2.0	0.7
Creatine Phosphokinase Increased	2.0	0.7
Abdominal Pain	1.3	3.5

[a] Includes adverse events considered by the investigators to be related, possibly related or of unknown relationship to study medication.

Post-Market Adverse Drug Reactions: Because they are reported spontaneously from a population of unknown size, estimates of frequency of post-marketing adverse events cannot be made. The following events have been chosen for inclusion due to their seriousness, frequency of reporting, potential causal connection to FAMVIR, or a combination of these factors: headache, nausea and confusion (including delirium, disorientation, confusional state, occurring predominantly in the elderly), rash, urticaria, pruritus, serious skin reactions (e.g. erythema multiforme, Steven-Johnson syndrome, toxic epidermal necrolysis), edema, vomiting, dizziness, somnolence (predominantly in the elderly), hallucinations and jaundice and abnormal liver function tests.
Abnormal Hematological and Clinical Chemistry Findings: In post-market experience, thrombocytopenia has been reported.

DRUG INTERACTIONS: Effects of Other Medicinal Products on Famciclovir: No clinically significant alterations in penciclovir (active metabolite of famciclovir) pharmacokinetics were observed following single dose administration of 500 mg famciclovir after pretreatment with multiple doses of cimetidine, allopurinol, theophylline, zidovudine, or promethazine or when given shortly after an antacid (magnesium and aluminium hydroxide), or concomitantly with emtricitabine. Furthermore, no clinically significant effect on penciclovir pharmacokinetics was observed following multiple-dose (t.i.d.) administration of famciclovir (500 mg) with multiple doses of digoxin.

Probenecid and other drugs that affect renal physiology could affect plasma levels of penciclovir.

The conversion of the inactive metabolite 6-deoxy penciclovir (formed by deacetylation of famciclovir) to penciclovir is catalysed by aldehyde oxidase. Interactions with other drugs metabolized by this enzyme and/or inhibiting this enzyme could potentially occur. Clinical interaction studies of famciclovir with cimetidine and promethazine, in vitro inhibitors of aldehyde oxidase, did not show relevant effects on the formation of penciclovir. However raloxifene, the most potent aldehyde oxidase inhibitor observed in vitro, could affect the formation of penciclovir.
Effects of Famciclovir on Other Medicinal Products: The pharmacokinetics of digoxin were not altered by concomitant administration of single or multiple (t.i.d) doses of famciclovir (500 mg). No clinically significant effects on the pharmacokinetics of zidovudine, its metabolite zidovudine glucuronide or emtricitabine were observed following a single oral dose of 500 mg famciclovir coadministered with zidovudine or emtricitabine.

Although famciclovir is only a weak inhibitor of aldehyde oxidase in vitro, interactions with drugs metabolized by aldehyde oxidase could potentially occur. Evidence from preclinical studies has shown no potential for induction of cytochrome P450 enzymes and inhibition of CYP3A4.

DOSAGE AND ADMINISTRATION: Recommended Dose and Dosage Adjustment: Herpes Zoster Infections: The recommended dose is 500 mg 3 times per day for 7 days. Therapy should be initiated within 72 hours of the onset of the rash.
Herpes Simplex Infections: Immunocompetent Patients: Recurrent Genital Herpes Episodes: The recommended dosage is 125 mg twice a day for 5 days. Initiation of treatment is recommended during the prodromal period or as soon as possible after onset of lesions.
Suppression of Recurrent Genital Herpes Episodes: The recommended dosage is 250 mg twice daily for up to 1 year. The safety and efficacy of Famvir therapy beyond one year of treatment has not been established.
HIV-Infected Patients: For recurrent episodes of mucocutaneous herpes simplex infection, the recommended dosage is 500 mg twice a day for 7 days.

FAMVIR (famciclovir) tablets should be swallowed whole and may be taken with or without food.
Dosage in Renally Impaired Patients: In patients with moderately or severely reduced renal function, dosage reduction is recommended (see Table 5).

Table 5: FAMVIR

Dosage in Reduced Renal Function

Indication	Creatinine Clearance (mL/min/1.73 m²)	Dosage
Herpes Zoster	≥60	500 mg every 8 hours
	40–59	500 mg every 12 hours
	20–39	500 mg every 24 hours
	<20	250 mg every 48 hours
Recurrent Genital Herpes	≥40	125 mg every 12 hours
	20–39	125 mg every 24 hours
	<20	125 mg every 48 hours
Suppression of Recurrent Genital Herpes	≥40	250 mg every 12 hours
	20–39	125 mg every 12 hours
	<20	125 mg every 24 hours
Recurrent episodes of mucocutaneous herpes simplex infections in HIV-infected patients	≥40	500 mg every 12 hours
	20–39	500 mg every 24 hours
	<20	250 mg every 24 hours

Hemodialysis Patients: Following each dialysis treatment, the recommended dose of famciclovir is 250 mg (herpes zoster) or 125 mg (genital herpes) in immunocompetent patients and 250 mg (recurrent episodes of mucocutaneous herpes simplex) in HIV-infected patients.
Dosage in Hepatically Impaired Patients: No dosage adjustment is required in patients with well-compensated hepatic impairment. No data are available for patients with severe uncompensated hepatic impairment (see Action and Clinical Pharmacology).
Missed Dose: If a dose of FAMVIR is missed, it should be taken as soon as the patient remembers. The next dose should be taken at the normal time.

The patient should carry on as normal until they have finished all the tablets.

Do not double-dose.

OVERDOSAGE:
No acute overdosage has been reported. Appropriate symptomatic and supportive therapy should be given. Penciclovir is dialyzable; plasma concentrations are reduced by approximately 75% following 4 h hemodialysis.

In patients with underlying renal disease who have received inappropriately high doses of famciclovir for their level of renal function, acute renal failure has been reported frequently.

For management of a suspected drug overdose, contact your regional Poison Control Centre. See the *CPS* Directory section for a list of Poison Control Centres.

ACTION AND CLINICAL PHARMACOLOGY: FAMVIR (famciclovir) is the orally administered pro-drug of the antiviral agent penciclovir. Famciclovir itself has no antiviral activity until it is biotransformed to penciclovir. Studies in volunteers have shown that famciclovir is well absorbed and produces plasma penciclovir concentrations superior to those obtained following oral administration of penciclovir alone.

The mean bioavailability of penciclovir after administration of oral famciclovir is 77%. The mean peak plasma concentration of penciclovir, following a 500 mg oral dose of famciclovir was 3.3 µg/mL and occurred at a mean time of 0.89 hours post-dose. Plasma concentration time curves of penciclovir are similar following single and repeat dosing. The terminal plasma elimination half-life of penciclovir after both single and repeat oral dosing with famciclovir is 2.3 hours. The elimination of famciclovir is by metabolism, principally to penciclovir and its 6-deoxy precursor, which are subsequently excreted in urine (see Pharmacokinetics).

Mechanism of Action: Penciclovir is a substituted guanine analogue with potent and selective antiviral activity against varicella zoster virus and other human herpes viruses. Penciclovir is in the same class of antiviral drugs as acyclovir, and both are phosphorylated by viral thymidine kinase and then by cellular enzymes to the active triphosphate form in virus-infected cells. Penciclovir triphosphate inhibits viral DNA polymerase competitively with deoxyguanosine triphosphate and is incorporated into the extending DNA chain, preventing significant chain elongation. Consequently, viral DNA synthesis and, therefore, viral replication are inhibited. Inhibition of the virus reduces the period of viral shedding, limits the degree of spread and level of pathology, and thereby facilitates healing.

Penciclovir is not readily phosphorylated in uninfected cells and does not inhibit cellular DNA synthesis even at concentrations >20 times those achieved in clinical usage.
Pharmacokinetics: Absorption: Following oral administration, famciclovir is rapidly, extensively and consistently absorbed and converted to the antivirally active compound, penciclovir. The mean (range) bioavailability of penciclovir after oral famciclovir is 77% (69.5-84.5%). The extent of systemic availability (AUC) of penciclovir from oral famciclovir is unaffected by food.

In a healthy male volunteer study using a single oral dose of famciclovir, the pharmacokinetics of penciclovir were linear over the famciclovir dose range 125 to 750 mg. The mean (range) peak plasma concentration of penciclovir, calculated from dose normalised estimates across all single dose healthy male volunteer studies, following a single 500 mg dose of famciclovir was 3.3 µg/mL (range 1.3-6.3 µg/mL) and occurred at a mean time of 0.89 hours post-dose (range 0.5-5.0 hours). The mean terminal half-life of penciclovir was 2.3 hours (range 0.99-5.26 hours).

Pharmacokinetic parameter estimates of penciclovir following oral administration of a single dose of famciclovir to patients with uncomplicated herpes zoster were essentially identical to values reported in healthy volunteers matched for age. Repeated oral dosing of famciclovir every 8 hours for up to 7 days in patients with herpes zoster infections had no significant effect on the pharmacokinetics of penciclovir compared to that described after single doses of famciclovir. The terminal plasma half-life of penciclovir in patients with herpes zoster was 2.8 h and 2.7 h, respectively, after single and repeated doses of famciclovir.
Distribution: Plasma protein binding of penciclovir and its 6-deoxy precursor is low (<20%) and penciclovir distributes freely between plasma and blood cells.
Metabolism: Following oral administration little or no famciclovir is detected in plasma or urine since famciclovir is rapidly converted via deacetylation and oxidation to penciclovir. An in vitro study using human liver microsomes demonstrated that cytochrome P450 does not play an important role in famcyclovir metabolism. The conversion of B-deoxy penciclovir is catalyzed by aldehyde oxidase.
Excretion: Little or no famciclovir is detected in plasma or urine since famciclovir undergoes extensive first-pass metabolism to penciclovir. The major metabolites identified in plasma and urine are penciclovir (67±4% of radioactivity in plasma at 1.5 h following a 500 mg oral dose of [^{14}C] famciclovir and 82±2.2% of radioactivity in 0-24 h urine) and, to a lesser extent, its 6-deoxy precursor, which has no antiviral activity (11±4% in plasma and 7±0.5% in urine at the corresponding time points). Other minor, virally inactive metabolites identified in human urine are monoacetylated penciclovir and 6-deoxy monoacetylated penciclovir (each <0.5% of the dose).

Renal clearance values for penciclovir exceed creatinine clearance indicating that net active tubular secretion and glomerular filtration contribute to renal elimination.
Renal Impaired Patients: The apparent plasma clearance, renal clearance, and plasma elimination rate constant of penciclovir decreased linearly with reductions in renal function, both after single and repeated dosing. Dose adjustment is necessary in patients with renal insufficiency (see Dosage and Administration).
Hepatically Impaired Patients: Following single oral administration of famciclovir to patients with well-compensated hepatic impairment, there was no change in the extent of availability of penciclovir compared with healthy volunteers. There was, however, a decrease in the rate of availability of penciclovir in the hepatically impaired subjects. Mean maximum plasma concentrations of penciclovir were decreased by 43% and the time to maximum plasma concentrations increased by 0.75 hours. However, no dosage adjustment for patients with well-compensated hepatic impairment is recommended. The pharmacokinetics of penciclovir following oral famciclovir in patients with severe uncompensated hepatic impairment has not been studied.
HIV-Infected Patients: Following oral administration of a single dose of 500 mg famciclovir to HIV positive patients, the pharmacokinetic parameters of penciclovir were comparable to those observed in healthy subjects.
Elderly Subjects: Based on cross-study comparisons, the mean penciclovir AUC was about 40 % higher and penciclovir renal clearance about 20% lower after oral administration of famciclovir in elderly volunteers (65-79 years) compared to younger volunteers. Some of this difference may be due to differences in renal function between the two age groups. No dose adjustment based on age is recommended unless renal function is impaired (see Dosage and Administration).
Gender: Small differences in renal clearance of penciclovir between females and males have been reported and were attributed to gender differences in renal function. No dose adjustment based on gender is recommended.

STORAGE AND STABILITY: Store at controlled room temperature (15-30°C).

INFORMATION FOR THE PATIENT: Published in e-CPS, available by subscription at www.e-cps.ca.

DOSAGE FORMS, COMPOSITION AND PACKAGING: 125 mg: Each white, round, biconvex, film-coated tablet, with bevelled edges, debossed with FV on one side and 125 on the other, contains: famciclovir 125 mg. Nonmedicinal ingredients: hydroxypropyl cellulose, hydroxypropyl methylcellulose, lactose, magnesium stearate, polyethylene glycols, sodium starch glycolate and titanium dioxide. Blister packages of 10.
250 mg: Each white, round, biconvex, film-coated tablet, with bevelled edges, debossed with FV on one side and 250 on the other, contains: famciclovir 250 mg. Nonmedicinal ingredients: hydroxypropyl cellulose, hydroxypropyl methylcellulose, lactose, magnesium stearate, polyethylene glycols, sodium starch glycolate and titanium dioxide. Bottles of 30 and 60. Blister packages of 30.
500 mg: Each white, oval, biconvex, film-coated tablet, with bevelled edges, debossed with FAMVIR on one side and 500 on the other, contains: famciclovir 500 mg. Nonmedicinal ingredients: hydroxypropyl cellulose, hydroxypropyl methylcellulose, lactose, magnesium stearate, polyethylene glycols, sodium starch glycolate and titanium dioxide. Bottles of 30 and 60. Blister packages of 21.

(Shown in Product Identification Section)

Faslodex® Ⓟ

fulvestrant

Nonagonist Estrogen Receptor Antagonist

AstraZeneca

Date of Preparation: February 10, 2004
Date of Revision: December 11, 2006

SUMMARY PRODUCT INFORMATION:

Route of Administration	Dosage Form/Strength	Clinically Relevant Nonmedicinal Ingredients
Intramuscular Injection	Pre-filled syringe injection 50 mg/mL	Ethanol 96%, benzyl alcohol, benzyl benzoate, castor oil

INDICATIONS AND CLINICAL USE: FASLODEX (fulvestrant) is indicated for the hormonal treatment of locally advanced or metastatic breast cancer in postmenopausal women, regardless of age, who have disease progression following prior endocrine therapy.
Geriatrics: No changes in dose are necessary for elderly patients.
Pediatrics: FASLODEX is not recommended for use in the pediatric population, as safety and efficacy have not been established in this age group.

CONTRAINDICATIONS:
- Patients with known hypersensitivity to fulvestrant or to any of the excipients. For a complete listing of ingredients, see Dosage Forms, Composition and Packaging.
- Pregnant or lactating women.

WARNINGS AND PRECAUTIONS: Body as a Whole: FASLODEX (fulvestrant) is unlikely to impair the ability of patients to drive or operate machinery. However, during treatment with FASLODEX, asthenia has been reported, and caution should be observed by those patients who experience this symptom when driving or operating machinery.

Hematologic: Due to the route of administration (intramuscular injection), caution should be used before treating patients on anticoagulants or patients with bleeding diatheses or thrombocytopenia.

Hepatic/Biliary/Pancreatic: Fulvestrant is metabolised primarily in the liver. Caution should be used with FASLODEX in patients with hepatic impairment, as clearance may be reduced. Pharmacokinetic data show that the mean clearance is reduced 2.2 fold in subjects with moderate hepatic impairment in comparison to healthy subjects (see Action and Clinical Pharmacology, Special Populations and Conditions, Hepatic Insufficiency). The safety profile in patients with mild hepatic impairment was similar to that seen in patients with no hepatic impairment in clinical trials of advanced breast cancer.

Fulvestrant has not been investigated in subjects with severe hepatic impairment. The potential risk/benefit to such patients should be carefully considered before administration of FASLODEX.

Renal: Caution should be used before treating patients with creatinine clearance less than 30 mL/min.

Special Populations: Pregnant Women: FASLODEX (fulvestrant) is contraindicated in pregnant women.

FASLODEX can cause fetal harm if administered to a pregnant woman. Women of childbearing potential should be advised not to become pregnant while receiving FASLODEX.

If a patient becomes pregnant while receiving FASLODEX she should be apprised of the potential hazard to the fetus, or the potential risk for loss of pregnancy.

Nursing Women: FASLODEX is contraindicated in lactating women.

FASLODEX is found in rats' milk at levels significantly higher than those in rat plasma. It is not known if fulvestrant is excreted in human milk. However, since many drugs are excreted in human milk, and because of the potential for serious adverse reactions from FASLODEX in nursing infants, a decision should be made whether to discontinue nursing or to discontinue the drug.

Pediatrics: FASLODEX is not recommended for use in the pediatric population, as safety and efficacy have not been established in this age group.

ADVERSE REACTIONS: Adverse Drug Reaction Overview: Table 1 summarizes the adverse drug reactions seen in FASLODEX (fulvestrant) clinical trials and post-marketing experience.

Table 1: FASLODEX

Summary of Adverse Drug Reactions Seen in Clinical Trials and Post-Marketing Experience

Very common (>10%)	Cardiovascular	Hot flushes, which are predominately mild in nature.
Common (>1%–≤10%)	Gastrointestinal	Gastrointestinal disturbance including nausea, vomiting, diarrhea, and anorexia, which were usually mild in nature.
	Hepatobiliary	Elevated liver enzymes, the vast majority <2×ULN (upper limit of normal).
	Nervous system	Headache, usually mild.
	Skin	Rash, usually mild in nature.
	Urogenital	Urinary tract infections, usually mild in nature.
	Whole Body	Injection site reactions including mild transient pain and inflammation (frequency based on administration of one 5 mL injection, the recommended administration), and asthenia, usually mild or moderate in nature.
Uncommon (>0.1%–≤1%)	Immune System	Hypersensitivity reactions including angioedema and urticaria. These reactions may occur shortly after injection, or in one reported case of angioedema, several days after injection. Local injection site reactions (e.g. pruritus, urticaria) may occur even after prior uneventful injections, and have been reported to develop with time into a systemic allergic response (e.g. widespread urticaria). FASLODEX therapy may need to be discontinued.

Clinical Trial Adverse Drug Reactions: Because clinical trials are conducted under very specific conditions the adverse reaction rates observed in the clinical trials may not reflect the rates observed in practice and should not be compared to the rates in the clinical trials of another drug. Adverse drug reaction information from clinical trials is useful for identifying drug-related adverse events and for approximating rates.

In patients with locally advanced or metastatic breast cancer treated with FASLODEX, the most commonly reported adverse events (irrespective of causality) were vasodilation (hot flushes), nausea and injection site reactions. Injection site reactions, with mild transient pain and inflammation, occurred in 7% of patients (1% of injections) when given the 5 mL injection in the predominantly European Clinical trial (9238IL/0020). In the North American trial (9238IL/0021), where patients were given a 250 mg dose of fulvestrant as two 2.5 mL injections, injection site reaction occurred in 27% of patients (5% of all administered injections).

Approximately 47% of patients experienced adverse events reported as treatment related; however, only 0.9% of patients stopped therapy because of such events in the clinical trial programme.

Table 2 lists adverse events reported with an incidence of ≥5% in the two controlled trials 9238IL/0020 and 9238IL/0021, regardless of causality, during treatment or the specified safety follow-up period (defined as 8 weeks after the last injection or 30 days after ingestion of the last tablet).

Table 2: FASLODEX

Adverse Events Occurring at an Incidence of ≥5% (irrespective of causality): Combined Results From Trials 9238IL/0020 and 9238IL/0021

Body System and Adverse Event[a]	FASLODEX 250 mg (IM injection/month) N=423 (%)	Anastrozole 1 mg (oral tablet/day) N=423 (%)
Body as a Whole	68.3	67.6
Asthenia	22.7	27.0
Pain	18.9	20.3
Headache	15.4	16.8
Back Pain	14.4	13.2
Abdominal Pain	11.8	11.6
Injection Site Pain[b]	10.9	6.6
Pelvic Pain	9.9	9.0
Chest Pain	7.1	5.0
Flu Syndrome	7.1	6.4
Fever	6.4	6.4
Accidental Injury	4.5	5.7
Cardiovascular System	30.3	27.9
Vasodilation	17.7	17.3
Digestive System	51.5	48.0
Nausea	26.0	25.3
Vomiting	13.0	11.8
Constipation	12.5	10.6
Diarrhea	12.3	12.8
Anorexia	9.0	10.9
Hemic and Lymphatic Systems	13.7	13.5
Anemia	4.5	5.0
Metabolic and Nutritional Disorders	18.2	17.7
Peripheral Edema	9.0	10.2
Musculoskeletal System	25.5	27.9
Bone Pain	15.8	13.7
Arthritis	2.8	6.1
Nervous System	34.3	33.8
Dizziness	6.9	6.6
Insomnia	6.9	8.5
Paresthesia	6.4	7.6
Depression	5.7	6.9
Anxiety	5.0	3.8
Respiratory System	38.5	33.6
Pharyngitis	16.1	11.6
Dyspnea	14.9	12.3
Cough increased	10.4	10.4
Skin and Appendages	22.2	23.4
Rash	7.3	8.0
Sweating	5.0	5.2
Urogenital System	18.2	14.9
Urinary tract infection	6.1	3.5

(cont'd)

Table 2: FASLODEX *(cont'd)*

[a] A patient may have more then one adverse event.

[b] All patients on FASLODEX received injections, but only those anastrozole patients who were in the North American study received placebo injections.

DRUG INTERACTIONS: Overview: FASLODEX (fulvestrant) does not significantly inhibit any of the major cytochrome P450 (CYP) isoenzymes in vitro, and results from a clinical pharmacokinetic trial in 8 healthy males involving co-administration of fulvestrant (36 mg intramuscularly) with midazolam (7.5 mg p.o.) also suggest that therapeutic doses of fulvestrant will have no inhibitory effects on CYP3A4. In addition, although fulvestrant can be metabolised by CYP3A4 in vitro, a clinical study in 8 healthy males with rifampicin (600 mg p.o.), an inducer of CYP3A4, showed no change in the pharmacokinetics of a 10 mg IV dose of fulvestrant as a result of the induction of CYP3A4. Results from a clinical study in 18 healthy subjects (17 male, 1 female) with ketoconazole (400 mg daily), a potent inhibitor of CYP3A4, also indicated that there is no clinically relevant change in the pharmacokinetics of an 8 mg IV dose of fulvestrant. Dosage adjustment is not necessary in patients co-prescribed CYP3A4 inhibitors or inducers.

Drug-Drug Interactions: There are no known drug-drug interactions requiring dose adjustment.

Drug-Food Interactions: Interactions with particular foods have not been established.

Drug-Herb Interactions: Interactions with herbal products have not been established.

Drug-Laboratory Test Interactions: Interactions with laboratory tests have not been established.

DOSAGE AND ADMINISTRATION: Recommended Dose and Dosage Adjustment: Adult Females: The recommended dose of FASLODEX (fulvestrant) is 250 mg, administered intramuscularly into the buttock at intervals of 1 month as a single 5 mL injection. It is recommended that the injection be administered slowly.

Patients with hepatic insufficiency: No dose adjustments are recommended for patients with Child-Pugh category A and B hepatic impairment. However, as the clearance of fulvestrant may be decreased in patients with hepatic impairment, these patients should be monitored for side effects when treated with fulvestrant (see Action and Clinical Pharmacology, Special Populations and Conditions, Hepatic Insufficiency). The use of fulvestrant has not been evaluated in patients or pharmacokinetic study subjects with Child-Pugh C hepatic impairment.

Patients with renal insufficiency: No dose adjustments are recommended for patients with a creatinine clearance greater than 30 mL/min. Safety and efficacy have not been evaluated in patients with creatinine clearance less than 30 mL/min.

Elderly: No dose adjustment is required for elderly patients.

Children: Not recommended for use in children or adolescents, as safety and efficacy have not been established in this age group.

Administration: Instructions for use, handling and disposal:

1. Remove glass syringe barrel from tray and check that it is not damaged.
2. Peel open the safety needle (SafetyGlide) outer packaging. For complete SafetyGlide instructions refer below to the "SafetyGlide Instructions From Becton Dickinson".
3. Break the seal of the white plastic cover on the syringe luer connector to remove the cover with the attached rubber tip cap.
4. Twist to lock the needle to the luer connector.
5. Remove the needle sheath.
6. Remove excess gas from the syringe (a small gas bubble may remain).
7. Administer intramuscularly slowly into the buttock.
8. Immediately activate needle protection device upon withdrawal from patient by pushing lever arm completely forward until needle tip is fully covered.
9. Visually confirm that the lever arm has fully advanced and the needle tip is covered. If unable to activate, discard immediately into an approved sharps collector.

SafetyGlide Instructions From Becton Dickinson: SafetyGlide is a trademark of Becton Dickinson and Company. Reorder number 305917.

Warning: Do not autoclave SafetyGlide needle before use. Hands must remain behind the needle at all times during use and disposal.

Peel apart packaging of the SafetyGlide, break the seal of the white plastic cover on the syringe luer connector and attach the SafetyGlide needle to the Luer Lock of the syringe by twisting.

Transport filled syringe to point of administration.

Pull shield straight off needle to avoid damaging needle point.

Administer injection following package instruction.

For user convenience, the needle "bevel up" position is oriented to the lever arm.

Immediately activate needle protection device upon withdrawal from patient by pushing lever arm completely forward until needle tip is fully covered.

Visually confirm that the lever arm has fully advanced and the needle tip is covered. If unable to activate, discard immediately into an approved sharps collector.

Activation of the protective mechanism may cause minimal splatter of fluid that may remain on the needle after injection.

For greatest safety, use a one-handed technique and activate away from self and others.

After single use, discard in an approved sharps collector in accordance with applicable regulations and institutional policy.

Becton Dickinson guarantees the contents of their unopened or undamaged packages to be sterile, non-toxic and non-pyrogenic.

OVERDOSAGE:

There is no clinical experience of overdosage with FASLODEX (fulvestrant) in humans. Animal studies have shown no adverse effects with intramuscular doses of greater than 400-fold of the clinical dose. Further animal studies, in which fulvestrant was dosed either monthly or twice monthly and achieved plasma levels several-fold higher than those seen in humans, showed no effects other than those related directly or indirectly to antiestrogen activity.

If overdosage occurs, this should be managed symptomatically.

For management of a suspected drug overdose, CPhA recommends that you contact your **regional Poison Control Centre**. See the *CPS* Directory section for a list of Poison Control Centres.

ACTION AND CLINICAL PHARMACOLOGY: Mechanism of Action: FASLODEX (fulvestrant) is an estrogen receptor (ER) antagonist that has a mode of action leading to downregulation of ER protein. Fulvestrant is a nonagonist ER antagonist that blocks the trophic actions of estrogens without itself having any partial agonist (estrogen-like) activity. Fulvestrant binds to estrogen receptors in a competitive manner with an affinity comparable to that of estradiol.

Fulvestrant is a reversible inhibitor of the growth of estrogen-sensitive human breast cancer cells in vitro. Fulvestrant inhibits the growth of estrogen-sensitive xenografts of human breast cancer in nude mice, prevents the establishment of tumours from xenografts of human breast cancer cells, and suppresses the growth of breast tumours. Furthermore, fulvestrant inhibits the growth of tamoxifen-resistant breast cancer cells in vitro and of tamoxifen-resistant breast tumours in vivo. Fulvestrant resistant breast tumours may also be cross-resistant to tamoxifen.

Pharmacodynamics: A clinical trial in postmenopausal women with primary breast cancer has shown that a single 250 mg dose of fulvestrant significantly downregulates ER expression in ER positive tumours, when compared to placebo. This same study also showed for fulvestrant a significant decrease in progesterone receptor (PgR) expression compared to placebo after 15-22 days of treatment. These data are consistent with fulvestrant having no agonist activity.

A trial in healthy postmenopausal volunteers showed that, compared to placebo, pre-treatment with 250 mg fulvestrant resulted in significantly reduced stimulation of the postmenopausal endometrium in volunteers treated with 20 µg per day ethinyl estradiol. Mean endometrial thickness after treatment with 250 mg fulvestrant was 4.2 mm, and with placebo it was 11.22 mm.

In postmenopausal women, the absence of changes in plasma concentrations of FSH and LH in response to fulvestrant treatment (250 mg monthly) suggests no peripheral steroidal effects. The reduction in levels of sex hormone-binding globulin indicates a lack of agonist properties.

Pharmacokinetics: Following intravenous or intramuscular administration, fulvestrant is rapidly cleared at a rate approximating the hepatic blood flow (nominally 10.5 mL plasma/min/kg). FASLODEX long-acting intramuscular injection maintains plasma fulvestrant concentrations within a range of 2- to 3-fold difference between peak and trough concentrations over a period of at least 28±3 days after injection. Administration of 250 mg of fulvestrant intramuscularly every month results in limited accumulation, approaching steady-state levels after approximately 3 to 6 doses, with an approximate 2-fold increase in plasma AUC.

Results from single-dose studies of fulvestrant are predictive of multiple-dose pharmacokinetics (see Table 3).

Table 3: FASLODEX

Summary of Fulvestrant Pharmacokinetic Parameters in Postmenopausal Advanced Breast Cancer Patients After Intramuscular Administration of a 250 mg Dose (Mean±SD)

	C_{max} ng/mL	C_{min} ng/mL	AUC ng·d/mL	$t_{1/2}$ days	CL mL/min
Single dose	8.5±5.4	2.6±1.1	131±62.0	39.8±10.8	690±226
Multiple dose steady state	15.8±2.4	7.4±1.7	328±48	49.9	537±57

Absorption: Fulvestrant is not administered orally.

Distribution: Fulvestrant is subject to extensive and rapid distribution; the apparent volume of distribution at steady state is large (approximately 3 to 5 L/kg), which suggests that the compound distribution is largely extravascular. Fulvestrant is highly (99%) bound to plasma proteins. VLDL, LDL, and HDL lipoprotein fractions appear to be the major binding components. The role of sex hormone-binding globulin, if any, could not be determined. No studies were conducted on drug-drug competitive protein binding interactions, as most reported interactions of this type involved binding to albumin and α-1-acid-glycoproteins.

Metabolism: Biotransformation and disposition of fulvestrant in humans have been determined following intramuscular and intravenous administration of ^{14}C-labelled fulvestrant. Metabolism of fulvestrant appears to involve combinations of a number of possible biotransformation pathways analogous to those of endogenous steroids, including oxidation, aromatic hydroxylation, and conjugation with glucuronic acid and/or sulphate at the 2-, 3-, and 17-positions of the steroid nucleus, and oxidation of the side chain sulphoxide. The metabolism of fulvestrant in humans yields a similar profile of metabolites to that found in other species. Identified metabolites are either less active or exhibit similar activity to fulvestrant in antiestrogen models. Studies using human liver preparations and recombinant human enzymes indicate that CYP3A4 is the only P450 isoenzyme involved in the oxidation of fulvestrant. However, the relative contribution of P450 and non-P450 routes in vivo is unknown.

Excretion: Fulvestrant is rapidly cleared by the hepatobiliary route with the overall rate of elimination being determined by the mode of administration, i.e., with monthly administration of FASLODEX long acting intramuscular formulation, exposure, and hence elimination, is primarily determined by the rate of release from the injection site. Excretion is primarily via the feces (approximately 90%). Renal elimination of drug-related material is negligible (less than 1%).

Special Populations and Conditions: Geriatrics: No difference in the fulvestrant pharmacokinetic profile was detected with regard to age (range 33 to 89 years).

Gender: Following administration of a single intravenous dose, there were no pharmacokinetic differences between men and either premenopausal or postmenopausal women. Similarly, there were no apparent differences between men and postmenopausal women after intramuscular administration.

Race: In the advanced breast cancer treatment trials, the potential for pharmacokinetic differences due to race have been evaluated in 294 women including 87.4% Caucasian, 7.8% Black, and 4.4% Hispanic. No discernible differences in fulvestrant plasma pharmacokinetics were observed among these groups. In a separate trial, pharmacokinetic data from postmenopausal Japanese women living in Japan were comparable to those obtained in non-Japanese patients.

Hepatic Insufficiency: The pharmacokinetics of fulvestrant has been evaluated in a single-dose clinical trial conducted in 21 subjects (4-7 subjects with Child-Pugh category A and 4-7 with category B hepatic impairment due to cirrhosis, 7 healthy subjects), using a high dose (100 mg) of a shorter duration intramuscular injection formulation. There was a 1.3 and 2.2-fold reduction in mean clearance in subjects with Child-Pugh category A and B hepatic impairment respectively compared to healthy subjects. Child-Pugh category C subjects were not evaluated; it is expected that clearance would be further reduced in this group of subjects.

Modelled intramuscular mean steady state plasma concentrations of fulvestrant in subjects with Child-Pugh category A and B hepatic impairment fall within the upper 95% confidence limit of the mean steady state concentrations expected for patients with normal hepatic function given the intramuscular formulation. Given the known safety profile of fulvestrant, no dose adjustment is considered to be necessary in patients with Child-Pugh category A or B hepatic impairment, although they should be monitored for side effects.

STORAGE AND STABILITY: Store refrigerated at 2 to 8°C. Store in original package. Single dose syringe. Discard unused portion.

INFORMATION FOR THE PATIENT: Published in e-CPS, available by subscription at www.e-cps.ca.

DOSAGE FORMS, COMPOSITION AND PACKAGING: Each mL of clear, colorless to yellow, viscous liquid for injection contains: fulvestrant 50 mg. Nonmedicinal ingredients: benzyl alcohol, benzyl benzoate, castor oil and ethanol 96%. Prefilled syringes of 5 mL. The syringe is presented in a tray with polystyrene plunger rod and a safety needle (SafetyGlide) for connection to the barrel.

As with all parenteral drug products, syringes should be inspected visually for clarity, particulate matter, precipitate, discolouration and leakage prior to administration. Solutions showing haziness, particulate matter, precipitate, discoloration or leakage should not be used.

(Shown in Product Identification Section)

Fasturtec® Ⓟ

rasburicase

Uricolytic Agent

sanofi-aventis

Date of Revision: February 9, 2007

Caution: FASTURTEC (rasburicase) should be administered only under the supervision of a physician who is experienced in the use of cancer chemotherapeutic agents.

PHARMACOLOGY: FASTURTEC (rasburicase) is a recombinant urate-oxidase enzyme produced by a genetically modified *S. cerevisiae* strain. The cDNA coding for rasburicase was cloned from a strain of *A. flavus*.

FASTURTEC is a highly potent uricolytic agent that catalyzes enzymatic oxidation of uric acid into an inactive and soluble metabolite (allantoin) which is easily excreted by the kidneys in the urine. In humans, uric acid is the final step in the catabolic pathway of purines. Rasburicase is only active at the end of the purine catabolic pathway.

Pharmacokinetics: Pharmacokinetics of rasburicase were evaluated in two studies that enrolled patients with lymphoid leukemia (B and T cell), non-Hodgkin's lymphoma (including Burkitt's lymphoma) or acute myelogenous leukemia. Rasburicase exposure, as measured by AUC_{0-24} and C_{max}, tended to increase linearly with doses over a limited dose range (0.15 to 0.20 mg/kg). The overall elimination half-life was 18 hours. No accumulation of rasburicase was observed between days 1 and 5 of dosing. Rasburicase mean volume of distribution was 110 to 127 mL/kg.

INDICATIONS: FASTURTEC (rasburicase) is indicated for the treatment and prophylaxis of hyperuricemia in pediatric and adult cancer patients.

CONTRAINDICATIONS: FASTURTEC (rasburicase) should not be administered to patients with a known history of anaphylactic reactions or known history of hypersensitivity reactions to FASTURTEC or any of the excipients. Studies have not been conducted in patients with severe allergies or asthma.

FASTURTEC should not be administered to patients with a known history of glucose-6-phosphate dehydrogenase deficiency (G6PD) or other cellular metabolic disorders known to cause hemolytic anemia.

WARNINGS: Clinical experience with FASTURTEC (rasburicase) demonstrates that FASTURTEC, like other proteins, has the potential to induce allergic responses in humans. Clinical experience with FASTURTEC demonstrates that patients should be closely monitored for the onset of allergic-type adverse events, especially urticaria or bronchospasm. If any serious allergic or anaphylactic reaction occurs, FASTURTEC therapy should be immediately and permanently discontinued, and appropriate therapy initiated.

The safety and efficacy of FASTURTEC has been established for a treatment duration of up to seven days. Because the safety and efficacy of other schedules have not been established, dosing beyond seven days or administration of more than one course of FASTURTEC is not currently recommended pending further clinical studies. Therefore, repeated treatment with interruptions is not recommended.

Hemolysis: Hemolysis has been reported in patients receiving FASTURTEC.

FASTURTEC administration should be immediately and permanently discontinued in any patient developing hemolysis and appropriate measures initiated.

Glucose-6-Phosphate Dehydrogenase (G6PD) Deficiency: FASTURTEC administered to patients with glucose-6-phosphate dehydrogenase (G6PD) deficiency can cause severe hemolysis. Therefore, FASTURTEC is contraindicated in individuals deficient in glucose-6-phosphate dehydrogenase (G6PD), in order to prevent hemolytic anemia in this patient population.

It is recommended that patients at higher risk for G6PD deficiency (e.g. patients of African or Mediterranean ancestry) be screened prior to starting FASTURTEC therapy.

Methemoglobinemia: FASTURTEC use has been associated with methemoglobinemia on rare occasions. FASTURTEC administration should be immediately and permanently discontinued in any patient identified as having developed methemoglobinemia and appropriate measures initiated.

Pregnancy: FASTURTEC has been shown to be teratogenic in rabbits given doses of 10, 50 and 100 times the human dose and in rats given doses 250 times the human dose.

Animal studies with respect to effects on parturition and postnatal development have not been conducted with FASTURTEC. It is also not known whether FASTURTEC can cause fetal harm when administered to a pregnant woman or can affect reproduction capacity. FASTURTEC should be given to a pregnant woman only if the potential benefit to the mother justifies the potential risk to the fetus.

Lactation: It is not known whether this drug is excreted in human milk. Because many drugs are excreted in human milk, FASTURTEC should not be used in breast-feeding women.

Immunogenicity: Antibodies to FASTURTEC have been detected in 24 of 28 (86%) healthy adult volunteers within 6 weeks of a single intravenous infusion. In clinical studies, 24 of 218 patients (11%) who received a single 5-7 day course of intravenous FASTURTEC produced detectable antibody responses within 4 weeks of administration. Clinically significant allergic reactions to FASTURTEC occurred in clinical studies; the relative risk of an allergic reaction in patients who develop anti-FASTURTEC antibodies has not been determined (refer to Table 1).

Pending further clinical trials to assess safety and efficacy in retreated patients, patients should not receive more than one course of FASTURTEC. Any patient with a serious hypersensitivity reaction should have FASTURTEC permanently discontinued.

PRECAUTIONS: General: Age and gender do not significantly affect the pharmacokinetics of FASTURTEC (rasburicase) in healthy subjects and patients as indicated by population pharmacokinetic analysis.

Renal function revealed no clinically meaningful changes in population pharmacokinetic analysis. Therefore no dose adjustment is necessary for renally impaired patients.
Leukapheresis/Exchange Transfusions: Patients who require leukapheresis or exchange transfusion due to hyperleukocytosis within 12 hours of receiving a dose of FASTURTEC (rasburicase), may require repeat dosing since these procedures may remove FASTURTEC from the system.
Drug Interactions: No specific in vivo clinical drug interaction studies have been performed. FASTURTEC does not metabolize allopurinol, methylprednisolone, etoposide, daunorubicin, cyclophosphamide and vincristine, or the following anti-metabolites, 6-mercaptopurine, methotrexate, cytarabine and thioguanine, in vitro. No metabolic-based drug interactions are therefore anticipated with these agents in patients.
FASTURTEC is adjunct therapy administered to cancer chemotherapy patients and has been administered with concomitant medications. Given the efficacy of rasburicase in patients, it is judged that the concomitant administrations of cytotoxic drugs does not significantly modify the uricolytic activity of FASTURTEC.
Rasburicase did not affect the activity of the following isoenzymes: CYP1A, CYP2A, CYP2B, CYP2C, CYP2E, and CYP3A in animal studies, suggesting no induction nor inhibition potential. Clinically relevant P450-mediated drug-drug interactions are therefore not anticipated in patients based on the dosing schedule recommended.
Laboratory Test Interactions: Although use of FASTURTEC does not require any special schedule of uric acid monitoring beyond standard practice, a special handling procedure for plasma samples is required to avoid ex vivo enzymatic degradation of uric acid by the drug at room temperature.
Procedure for Blood Collection: Blood must be collected into pre-chilled tubes containing heparin anticoagulant. Samples must be immediately immersed in an ice water bath. Plasma samples must be prepared by centrifugation in a pre-cooled centrifuge (4°C). Finally, the plasma must be maintained in an ice water bath and analyzed for uric acid within four hours.
FASTURTEC is not known to alter the accuracy of any other laboratory tests.
Carcinogenesis, Mutagenesis, Impairment of Fertility: FASTURTEC was non-genotoxic in the Ames, unscheduled DNA synthesis, chromosome analysis, mouse lymphoma, and micronucleus tests.
FASTURTEC did not affect reproductive performance or fertility in male or female rats.
Children: FASTURTEC has been shown to be safe and effective in children over the age of one month.
Immunogenicity: Caution should be used in patients with a history of atopic allergies.

ADVERSE EFFECTS: Adverse events were reported in pediatric and adult patients in various clinical efficacy and safety studies, as well as in one study, which was specifically designed to collect further safety and tolerability data of FASTURTEC (rasburicase).
In a study of 28 healthy volunteers, only two adverse events (headache of moderate intensity) were reported.
In the clinical studies in patients, the adverse events that were judged to be at least in part related to FASTURTEC include: allergic reactions, including anaphylaxis (with signs and symptoms which include chest pain, dyspnea, hypotension and/or urticaria), rash, rhinitis, bronchospasm, diarrhea, fever, headache, nausea, and vomiting. The incidence of these events are presented in Table 1.

Table 1: FASTURTEC
Incidence of Adverse Events

	Comparator Study				Non-Comparator Studies	
	Allopurinol (N=25)		FASTURTEC (N=27)		FASTURTEC (N=320)	
Adverse Event	All Grades	Grade 3 or 4	All Grades	Grade 3 or 4	All Grades	Grade 3 or 4
Any allergic reaction	12.0%	0	3.7%	0	2.5%	0.6%
Any rash	12.0%	0	14.8%	3.7%	23.4%	0.9%
Diarrhoea	16.0%	4.0%	29.6%	0	19.4%	0.9%
Fever	32.0%	4.0%	40.7%	0	37.5%	6.6%
Headache	12.0%	0	25.9%	0	25.3%	0.9%
Nausea	24.0%	8.0%	33.3%	3.7%	30.9%	1.6%
Vomiting	36.0%	4.0%	55.6%	3.7%	46.6%	1.3%

The following additional adverse events occurred in ≥5% of patients (not considered related to FASTURTEC treatment): abdominal pain, anemia, back pain, constipation, coughing, dyspnea, epistaxis, granulocytopenia, hyperglycemia, hypertension, hypocalcemia, hypotension, injection site pain, injection site reaction, mucositis, pain, pharyngitis, sepsis, skeletal pain, thrombocytopenia.
Uncommon cases of hemolysis which could be related to G6PD deficiency and methemoglobinemia have been reported.

OVERDOSE:
The maximum dose of FASTURTEC that has been administered as a single dose is 0.2 mg/kg; the maximum daily dose that has been administered is 0.4 mg/kg/day. According to the mechanism of action of FASTURTEC, an overdose will lead to low or undetectable plasma uric acid concentrations and increased production of hydrogen peroxide. Patients suspected of receiving an overdose should be monitored for hemolysis and general supportive measures should be initiated as no specific antidote for FASTURTEC has been identified.

For management of a suspected drug overdose, CPhA recommends that you contact your **regional Poison Control Centre**. See the *CPS* Directory section for a list of Poison Control Centres.

DOSAGE: FASTURTEC (rasburicase) should be administered as a single daily dose of 0.2 mg/kg daily for up to 7 days. Administration of FASTURTEC does not require a change in chemotherapy timing or schedule and chemotherapy may be initiated as soon as four hours after the first dose. Age and gender do not significantly affect the pharmacokinetics of FASTURTEC in patients as indicated by population pharmacokinetic analysis.
FASTURTEC must first be reconstituted in the solvent provided. The reconstituted solution must then be diluted in sterile normal saline solution for injection and administered intravenously over 30 minutes (see below).
Reconstitution and Dilution Procedure: Add 1 mL of the provided reconstitution solution (solvent) to each vial containing 1.5 mg of FASTURTEC and mix by swirling very gently. **Do not vortex.** The required quantity of solution (according to the patient's weight and the dose per kilogram) is to be further diluted with 50 mL sterile normal saline solution. This final solution is to be infused over 30 minutes. **No filters should be used for the infusion.** The reconstituted or diluted solution should be used immediately (within 3 hours), as FASTURTEC does not contain any bacteriostatic agents. Although not recommended, they may be stored for up to 24 hours at 2-8°C.
Do not administer as a bolus infusion.
FASTURTEC should be infused through a separate infusion line. If use of a separate line is not possible, the line should be flushed with at least 15 mL of saline solution prior to and after infusion with FASTURTEC.
Parenteral drug products should be inspected visually for particulate matter and discoloration prior to administration, whenever solution and container permit.

Vial Size	Volume of Solvent to be Added to Vial	Nominal Concentration per mL
1.5 mg	1 mL	1.5 mg

Stability and Storage Recommendations: The lyophilized drug product and the solution for reconstitution should be stored at 2-8°C for a maximum of 36 months. **Do not freeze.** Protect from light.
The reconstituted or diluted solution should be used immediately (within 3 hours), as FASTURTEC does not contain any bacteriostatic agents. Although not recommended, they may be stored for up to 24 hours at 2-8°C.
Do not administer as a bolus infusion.

SUPPLIED: Each vial of sterile lyophilized powder contains: rasburicase 1.5 mg, mannitol 10.6 mg, L-alanine 15.9 mg, and between 12.6 and 14.3 mg of dibasic sodium phosphate. Colorless glass vials of 3 mL with a rubber stopper. The accompanying sterile solution for reconstitution is composed of 1 mL sterile water for injection, USP, and 1 mg poloxamer 188 (anti-aggregation agent). Clear, glass ampoules of 2 mL. Packs of 3 vials and 3 ampoules.

Felodipine ℞

CPhA Monograph

see *Calcium Channel Blockers*

Femara® ℞

letrozole

Nonsteroidal Aromatase Inhibitor—Inhibitor of Estrogen Biosynthesis—Antitumor Agent

Novartis Pharmaceuticals

Date of Preparation: May 16, 1997
Date of Revision: September 29, 2008

FEMARA, indicated for:
- The adjuvant treatment of postmenopausal women with hormone receptor-positive early breast cancer;
- The extended adjuvant treatment of hormone receptor-positive early breast cancer in postmenopausal women who have received approximately 5 years of prior standard adjuvant tamoxifen therapy;

has been issued market authorization with conditions, pending the results of studies to verify its clinical benefit. Patients should be advised of the nature of the market authorization granted.
FEMARA, indicated for:
- The first-line therapy in postmenopausal women with advanced breast cancer;
- The hormonal treatment of advanced/metastatic breast cancer in women with natural or artificially-induced postmenopausal status, who have disease progression following antiestrogen therapy;

has been issued market authorisation without conditions.
FEMARA should be administered under the supervision of a qualified physician experienced in the use of anti-cancer agents.

SUMMARY PRODUCT INFORMATION:

Route of Administration	Dosage Form/ Strength	Clinically Relevant Nonmedicinal Ingredients
Oral	Tablets, 2.5 mg	Lactose For a complete listing see Dosage Forms, Composition and Packaging.

INDICATIONS AND CLINICAL USE: FEMARA (letrozole) is indicated for the adjuvant treatment of postmenopausal women with hormone receptor-positive early breast cancer.
Approval is based on superior Disease-Free Survival (DFS) compared to tamoxifen from the overall study population, at a median follow-up of 26 months. However, DFS advantage of FEMARA over tamoxifen was not observed in the subset of patients with node-negative disease.
FEMARA (letrozole) is also indicated for the extended adjuvant treatment of hormone receptor-positive early breast cancer in postmenopausal women who have received approximately 5 years of prior standard adjuvant tamoxifen therapy.
Although the intended duration of extended adjuvant therapy with FEMARA is 5 years, randomized, double-blinded data on efficacy endpoints is limited to a median follow-up of 28 months. After this time, the study was unblinded and patients who had received placebo had the option to switch in a non-randomized fashion to treatment with FEMARA. At a median follow-up of 30 months, a non-significant increase in deaths (P=0.749) occurred in the letrozole arm in node-negative patients (HR 1.1 (CI 0.62, 1.96): 24/1298 in the FEMARA arm versus 22/1301 in the placebo arm). The clinical evidence collected to date demonstrates a statistically significant increase in disease-free survival, but no overall survival advantage has been consistently demonstrated.
FEMARA (letrozole) is indicated as first-line therapy in postmenopausal women with advanced breast cancer.
FEMARA (letrozole) is also indicated for the hormonal treatment of advanced/metastatic breast cancer in women with natural or artificially-induced postmenopausal status, who have disease progression following antiestrogen therapy.

CONTRAINDICATIONS:
- Premenopausal endocrine status, pregnancy, lactation (see Warnings and Precautions).
- Patients who are hypersensitive to letrozole, other aromatase inhibitors, or to any ingredient in the formulation or component of the container. For a complete listing, see Dosage Forms, Composition and Packaging.
- In the absence of clinical experience with the use of FEMARA in children or adolescents (under 18 years of age), FEMARA should not be used in these patients.

WARNINGS AND PRECAUTIONS:

Serious Warnings and Precautions
FEMARA (letrozole) should be administered under supervision of a qualified physician experienced in the use of anti-cancer agents.
- Osteoporosis (see Musculoskeletal).

General: Clinical trial evidence (median follow-up duration of 26 months in the adjuvant setting, 49 months in the extended adjuvant setting) is insufficient to assess adverse effects associated with long term use of letrozole for five years.
Ability to Drive and Use Machines: Since fatigue and dizziness have been observed with the use of FEMARA, and somnolence has been reported uncommonly, caution is advised when driving or using machines.
Cardiovascular: In the adjuvant setting, the use of some aromatase inhibitors, including FEMARA, may increase the risk of cardiovascular events compared to tamoxifen. The overall incidence of cardiovascular events in the BIG 1-98 study for FEMARA and tamoxifen arms was 9.7 vs. 10.5%, respectively. However, a higher incidence of events was seen for FEMARA vs. tamoxifen, including cardiac failure (0.9 vs. 0.4%, respectively), myocardial infarction (0.8 vs. 0.4%, respectively), fatal cardiac events (0.6 vs. 0.3%, respectively) and numerically higher fatal stroke (0.15%, 6 cases vs. 0.03%, 1 case, respectively), and a lower incidence was seen for thromboembolic events (1.4% vs. 3.0%, respectively). Patients with non-malignant systemic diseases (cardiovascular, renal, hepatic, lung embolism etc.) which would prevent prolonged follow-up were ineligible from enrolment in the BIG 1-98 trial (see Adverse Reactions, Clinical Trial Adverse Drug Reactions).
In the extended adjuvant setting, in a 5-year, phase III trial, after a median follow-up of 28 months, the incidence of cardiovascular events any time after randomization was comparable between treatment arms; 6.8% in the FEMARA arm compared to 6.5% in the placebo arm. The most frequent cardiovascular events were: new or worsening angina (1.4% in the FEMARA arm vs. 1.0% in the placebo arm), myocardial infarction (0.6% in the FEMARA arm vs. 0.7% in the placebo arm), and stroke/transient ischemic attack (0.9% in the FEMARA arm vs. 0.9% in the placebo arm). These results were obtained prior to unblinding the study.

The updated results obtained from this Phase III study after study unblinding showed that after a median follow-up of approximately 49 months, the frequency of cardiovascular events any time after randomization was higher in the FEMARA arm than in placebo arm until the switch (11.1% vs. 8.6%, respectively). The most frequent cardiovascular events included arrhythmia (4.0% in the FEMARA arm vs. 3.3% in the placebo arm until switch), new or worsening angina (1.7% on FEMARA vs. 1.2% on placebo until switch), and stroke/transient ischemic attack (1.7% on FEMARA vs. 1.3% on placebo until the switch).

At a median follow-up of approximately 49 months, the number of deaths attributed to a cardiovascular cause during treatment or within 30 days of stopping treatment was slightly higher in the placebo arm [16/2577 (0.6%)] than in the FEMARA arm [10/2566 (0.4%)], but the difference was not statistically significant. Of the 16 deaths attributed to a cardiovascular cause in the placebo arm, 12 occurred in the group of 1129 patients who did not switch to FEMARA after study unblinding, and 4 occurred in the group of 1448 patients who did switch to FEMARA. There was a statistically significant higher incidence of fatal stroke in the FEMARA arm [5/2566 (0.2%)] than in the placebo arm (0/2577) (P<0.0001)). (See also Adverse Reactions, Clinical Trial Adverse Drug Reactions).

Musculoskeletal: Bone Mineral Density: FEMARA reduces circulating estrogen levels. The use of estrogen lowering agents, including FEMARA, may cause a reduction in bone mineral density (BMD) with a possible consequent increased risk of osteoporosis and fracture. Osteoporosis and/or bone fractures have been reported with the use of FEMARA (see also Special Populations, Geriatrics and Adverse Reactions, Clinical Trial Adverse Drug Reactions). Therefore, monitoring of overall bone health is recommended during treatment with FEMARA. Women should have their osteoporosis risk assessed and managed according to local clinical practice and guidelines.

In the 5-year, phase III trial for extended adjuvant therapy, after a median follow-up of 28 months, the incidence of self-reported osteoporosis any time after randomization was higher in patients who received FEMARA (6.9%) than in patients who received placebo (5.5%) (P=0.042). The incidence of clinical fractures any time after randomization was slightly higher in patients who received FEMARA than who received placebo (5.9% vs. 5.5% respectively; P=0.548, not statistically significant). Fracture rates any time after randomization in patients with a history of osteoporosis were 10.6% in the FEMARA arm compared to 7.3% in the placebo arm; the difference is not statistically significant (P=0.161). In patients with a previous history of fractures, fracture rates were 12.2% in the FEMARA arm compared to 8.7% in the placebo arm; the difference is not statistically significant (P=0.177). These results were obtained prior to the study unblinding.

After the study unblinding, patients randomized to the placebo arm were offered to switch to FEMARA or discontinue treatment.

The updated results obtained from this phase III trial after unblinding showed that at a median follow-up of approximately 49 months, the incidence of osteoporosis, any time after randomization, was higher in the FEMARA arm (12.3%) than in the placebo until switch arm (7.4%) and the FEMARA after switch arm (3.6%).

Fracture rates any time after randomization in patients with a history of osteoporosis were 17.7% (55/311) in FEMARA arm compared to 10.9% (33/304) in placebo until switch arm and 5.6% (9/162) in the FEMARA after switch arm. In patients with a previous history of fractures, fracture rates any time after randomization were 18.1% (52/287) in the FEMARA arm compared to 12.2% (37/304) in the placebo arm until switch, and 10.2% (17/167) in the FEMARA after switch arm.

The interpretation of the updated results is confounded by the fact that after study unblinding, 56% of patients randomized placebo opted to switch to FEMARA, resulting in different median exposure to treatment (47 months for FEMARA, 28 months for placebo until switch and 20 months for FEMARA after switch). (See also Adverse Reactions, Clinical Trial Adverse Drug Reactions.) The study is ongoing.

Sexual Function/Reproduction: Reproductive Toxicology: Letrozole was evaluated for maternal toxicity as well as embryotoxic, fetotoxic and teratogenic potential in female rats following oral administration of daily doses of 0.003, 0.01 or 0.03 mg/kg on gestation days 6 through 17. Oral administration of letrozole to pregnant rats resulted in teratogenicity and maternal toxicity at 0.03 mg/kg. Embryotoxicity and fetotoxicity were seen at doses of ≥0.003 mg/kg and there was an increase in the incidence of fetal malformation among the animals treated. However it is not known whether this was an indirect consequence of the pharmacological activity of FEMARA (inhibition of estrogen biosynthesis) or a direct drug effect.

Special Populations: Hepatic Impairment: In a single dose trial with 2.5 mg letrozole in volunteers with hepatic impairment, mean AUC values of the volunteers with moderate hepatic impairment was 37% higher than in normal subjects, but still within the range seen in subjects with normal hepatic function. In a study comparing the pharmacokinetics of letrozole after a single oral dose of 2.5 mg in eight subjects with liver cirrhosis and severe non-metastatic hepatic impairment (Child-Pugh score C) to those in healthy volunteers (N=8), AUC and $t_{½}$ increased by 95 % and 187%, respectively. Breast cancer patients with severe hepatic impairment are thus expected to be exposed to higher levels of letrozole than patients without severe hepatic dysfunction. Long term effects of this increased exposure have not been studied.

These results indicate that no dosage adjustment is necessary for breast cancer patients with mild to moderate hepatic dysfunction. However, since letrozole elimination depends mainly on intrinsic metabolic clearance, caution is recommended. Insufficient data are available to recommend a dose adjustment in breast cancer patients with severe non-metastatic hepatic impairment. Therefore, such patients should be kept under close supervision for adverse events.

Renal Impairment: Pharmacokinetics of a single 2.5 mg letrozole dose were unchanged in a study in postmenopausal women with varying degrees of renal function (24-hour creatinine clearance=9-116 mL/min.). In a study in 364 patients with advanced breast cancer there was no significant association between letrozole plasma levels and calculated CL_{cr} (range 22.9-211.9 mL/min). No dosage adjustment is required in patients with CL_{cr} ≥10 mL/min. No data are available for patients with CL_{cr} ≤9 mL/min. The potential risks and benefits to such patients should be considered carefully before prescribing letrozole.

Pregnant Women: Letrozole should not be given to pregnant women (see Contraindications).

Women of Child-Bearing Potential: There have been post-market reports of spontaneous abortions and congenital anomalies in infants of mothers who have taken FEMARA. Letrozole should not be given to women with premenopausal endocrine status (see Contraindications). Women who are not premenopausal but have the potential to become pregnant, including women who are perimenopausal or who recently became postmenopausal, should use appropriate contraception while being treated with FEMARA (see also Sexual Function/Reproduction, Reproductive Toxicology).

Nursing Women: Letrozole should not be administered to nursing mothers (see Contraindications).

Geriatrics: There have been no age-related effects observed on the pharmacokinetics of letrozole.

In the adjuvant setting, more than 8000 postmenopausal women were enrolled in the clinical study. In total, 36% of patients were aged 65 years or older at enrolment, while 12% were 75 or older. Although more adverse events were generally reported in elderly patients irrespective of study treatment allocation, the differences between the two treatment groups were similar to those of younger patients.

In a 5-year, phase III trial for extended adjuvant therapy, after a median follow-up of 28 months, fracture rates recorded any time after randomization in patients 65 years and older were 7.1% (77/1090) in the FEMARA arm compared to 7.5 % (77/1033) in the placebo arm; the difference is not statistically significant (P=0.738). These results were obtained prior to study unblinding.

After the study unblinding, patients randomized to the placebo arm were offered to switch to FEMARA or discontinue treatment.

The updated results obtained from this phase III trial after unblinding at a median follow-up of approximately 49 months, showed that the fracture rates any time after randomization in patients 65 years and older were 12.2% (133/1090) in FEMARA arm compared to 10.2% (105/1032) in placebo until switch arm and 6.9% (34/495) in FEMARA after switch arm.

The interpretation of the updated results is confounded by the fact that after study unblinding, 56% of patients randomized placebo opted to switch to FEMARA, resulting in different median exposure to treatment (47 months for FEMARA, 28 months for placebo until switch and 20 months for FEMARA after switch). (See also Adverse Reactions, Clinical Trial Adverse Drug Reactions.) The study is ongoing.

Monitoring and Laboratory Tests: Plasma Lipids: In the adjuvant setting, the use of aromatase inhibitors, including FEMARA, may increase lipid levels (see Adverse Reactions, Clinical Trial Adverse Drug Reactions). Women should have their cholesterol levels assessed and managed according to current clinical practice and guidelines.

ADVERSE REACTIONS: Adverse Drug Reaction Overview: Adverse Events in Adjuvant Study BIG 1-98: The Data and Safety Monitoring Committee, after review of the primary analysis results of the BIG 1-98 study, observed a difference in incidence in grade 5 myocardial infarctions (9 vs. 2 in the letrozole and tamoxifen arms, respectively) and recommended that these cardiac events and certain other safety data be reviewed. As a result, a blinded medical review of more than 2000 patients with pre-specified adverse events (cardiovascular events, fractures, arthritis/arthralgia, myalgia, any adverse event leading to discontinuation) or death without a prior cancer event was conducted following the primary analysis of the adjuvant trial BIG 1-98. This medical review resulted in a change in the cause of death for 25 patients, 19 of which were reclassified from a cardiac cause to either "sudden death, cause unknown" (9 cases in letrozole arm, 7 cases in tamoxifen arm) or to "other" (3 cases in letrozole arm). Some adverse events (such as arthritis/arthralgia and edema) reported in the primary analysis did not meet the definition of a treatment-emergent adverse event as they were present at baseline and did not worsen in severity during treatment. The BIG 1-98 study is currently ongoing, and the medical review is being conducted on an ongoing basis; the updated efficacy and safety results from the study will be made available at the 5-year median treatment duration. It is important to note that these updated safety data will not be comparable with those of the primary analysis. Extrapolation of the absolute risk of these pre-specified events as a function of time cannot be reasonably established.

FEMARA was generally well tolerated as adjuvant treatment of early breast cancer. In the adjuvant setting (26 months median follow-up) approximately 91% vs. 86% of the patients allocated to FEMARA or tamoxifen, respectively, experienced adverse events. Generally, the observed adverse events were mainly mild or moderate in nature, and most were associated with estrogen deprivation. The most frequently reported adverse events in the adjuvant setting were hot flushes (letrozole: 33.7%, tamoxifen: 38.0%), arthralgia/arthritis (letrozole: 21.2%, tamoxifen 13.5%), and night sweats (letrozole: 14.1%, tamoxifen: 16.4%).

Adverse Events in Extended Adjuvant Study MA-17: Adverse events discussed below were analyzed irrespective of relationship to study treatment.

FEMARA was generally well tolerated as extended adjuvant treatment in women who have received prior standard adjuvant tamoxifen treatment. In the phase III trial for extended adjuvant therapy, after a median follow-up of 28 months 87.2% vs. 84.5% of the patients on FEMARA or placebo experienced adverse events. The most frequent events were: hot flushes (FEMARA 49.7% vs. placebo 43.3%), fatigue (lethargy, asthenia, malaise) (FEMARA 33.8% vs. placebo 32.2%), arthralgia/arthritis (FEMARA 27.7% vs. placebo 22.2%); and sweating (diaphoresis) (24.3% vs. placebo 22.5%).

After the study unblinding, patients randomized to placebo arm were offered to switch to FEMARA. The placebo results beyond 28 months median follow-up are confounded by the fact that 56% of patients randomised placebo opted to switch to FEMARA and that dates of onset for general adverse events (based on self-report) were not recorded. In most cases, therefore, it cannot be determined if the adverse events in the placebo group occurred before switch to FEMARA or after switch to FEMARA. General adverse event data after unblinding of the study should therefore be interpreted with caution.

In the extended adjuvant study after study unblinding at a median follow-up of approximately 49 months the overall incidence of adverse events reported during study treatment or within 30 days irrespective of causality was 94.2% in FEMARA, 91.1% in placebo not switched and 94.1% in placebo patients switched to FEMARA. The most frequent adverse events were: hot flushes (60.3% in FEMARA vs. 52.6% in placebo not switched), fatigue (lethargy, malaise, asthenia) (45.0% in FEMARA vs. 44.8% in placebo not switched), arthralgia/arthritis (37.9% in FEMARA vs. 26.8% in placebo not switched), sweating (diaphoresis) (34.0% in FEMARA vs. 29.8% in placebo not switched).

Most frequently reported adverse events from the clinical trials in adjuvant and extended adjuvant are summarized in Table 1, Table 2 and Table 3.

Adverse Events in First-Line and Second-Line Treatment of Advanced Breast Cancer: FEMARA (letrozole) was generally well tolerated across all studies as first-line and second-line treatment for advanced breast cancer. Approximately one third of patients treated with FEMARA can be expected to experience adverse reactions. The most frequently reported adverse reactions in the clinical trials were hot flushes, nausea and fatigue. Many adverse reactions can be attributed to the normal physiological consequences of estrogen deprivation (e.g., hot flushes, alopecia and vaginal bleeding). The adverse drug reactions reported from clinical trials are summarized for first-line and second-line treatment with FEMARA.

Clinical Trial Adverse Drug Reactions: Adverse Events in Adjuvant Treatment of Early Breast Cancer in Postmenopausal Women: The median duration of adjuvant treatment was 24 months and the median duration of follow-up for safety was 26 months for patients receiving FEMARA and tamoxifen.

Certain adverse events were prospectively specified for analysis, based on the known pharmacologic properties and side effect profiles of the two drugs.

Most adverse events reported (82%) were grade 1 and grade 2 applying the Common Toxicity Criteria Version 2.0. Serious adverse events that were suspected to be related to study treatment were significantly less frequent with FEMARA (177 patients, 4.5%) than with tamoxifen (276 patients, 6.9%). Table 1 describes the most frequently reported adverse events irrespective of relationship to study treatment in the adjuvant BIG 1-98 trial (safety population, during treatment or within 30 days of stopping treatment).

In the adjuvant setting, total cholesterol levels remained stable over 5 years (median 1-3% decrease) in the FEMARA arm whereas there was an expected slight decrease (median 10-15% decrease) over time observed in the tamoxifen arm. Hypercholesterolemia recorded at least once as a check-listed adverse event was more frequent in patients treated with FEMARA (43%) compared with tamoxifen (19%). Hypercholesterolemia recorded from non-fasting laboratory evaluations was defined as an increase in total serum cholesterol in patients who had baseline values of total serum cholesterol within the normal range, and then subsequently, had an increase in total serum cholesterol of 1.5 ULN at least one time. The incidence of laboratory evaluated hypercholesterolemia was more frequent in patients treated with letrozole (5.6%) compared to tamoxifen (1.3%) (see Table 1).

Overall, the incidence of cardiovascular events was similar in the FEMARA and tamoxifen arms (9.7 vs. 10.5%, respectively), although more patients receiving FEMARA compared to tamoxifen were reported to have cardiac failure (0.9 vs. 0.4%, respectively), myocardial infarction (0.8 vs. 0.4%, respectively), fatal cardiac events (0.6 vs. 0.3%, respectively), and numerically higher fatal stroke (0.15%, 6 cases vs. 0.03%, 1 case, respectively). As expected, thromboembolic events were more frequent in patients on tamoxifen compared to FEMARA (3.0 vs. 1.4%), respectively.

Patients with other non-malignant systemic diseases (cardiovascular, renal, hepatic, lung embolism etc.) which would prevent prolonged follow-up were ineligible from enrolment in the BIG 1-98 trial. Patients with previous DVT (deep vein thrombosis) were only included if medically suitable.

See Adverse Events in Extended Adjuvant Therapy in Early Breast Cancer, Median Treatment Duration of 24 Months for data with respect to placebo.

FEMARA treatment was associated with a significantly higher risk of osteoporosis (2.0 vs. 1.1% with tamoxifen). Bone fractures were significantly higher in the FEMARA arm than the tamoxifen arm (5.7 vs. 4.0%, respectively).

Table 1: FEMARA

Most Frequently Reported Adverse Events Irrespective of Relationship to Study Drug in the Adjuvant Trial BIG 1-98

Preferred Term	Letrozole N=3975 n (%)	Tamoxifen N=3988 n (%)
Hot flashes/flushes	1338 (33.7)	1515 (38.0)
Arthralgia/arthritis	841 (21.2)	537 (13.5)
Night sweats	561 (14.1)	654 (16.4)
Nausea	378 (9.5)	418 (10.5)
Fatigue (lethargy, malaise, asthenia)	333 (8.4)	345 (8.7)
Edema	286 (7.2)	288 (7.2)
Myalgia	256 (6.4)	243 (6.1)
Bone fractures	226 (5.7)	161 (4.0)
Hypercholesterolemia[a, b]	173 (5.6)	40 (1.3)
Vaginal bleeding	177 (4.5)	413 (10.4)
Depression	144 (3.6)	155 (3.9)
Headache	143 (3.6)	126 (3.2)
Vaginal irritation	139 (3.5)	122 (3.1)
Vomiting	109 (2.7)	107 (2.7)
Dizziness/light-headedness	97 (2.4)	112 (2.8)
Osteoporosis	80 (2.0)	44 (1.1)

(cont'd)

Table 1: FEMARA *(cont'd)*

Most Frequently Reported Adverse Events Irrespective of Relationship to Study Drug in the Adjuvant Trial BIG 1-98

Preferred Term	Letrozole N=3975 n (%)	Tamoxifen N=3988 n (%)
Constipation	59 (1.5)	95 (2.4)
Cataract	48 (1.2)	39 (1.0)
Breast pain	40 (1.0)	47 (1.2)
Cardiac failure	36 (0.9)	15 (0.4)
Anorexia	33 (0.8)	31 (0.8)
Myocardial infarction	31 (0.8)	17 (0.4)
Angina pectoris	27 (0.7)	24 (0.6)
Ovarian cyst	17 (0.4)	14 (0.4)
Endometrial proliferation disorders	10 (0.3)	73 (1.8)
Other endometrial disorders	3 (<0.1)	4 (0.1)

[a] Based on number of patients with normal serum cholesterol levels at baseline and developing at least one value greater than 1.5 times the upper limit of normal in the laboratory, measuring total serum cholesterol. Approximately 90% of the measured values were non-fasting measurements.
[b] Denominator is number of patients with baseline measurements of total serum cholesterol—letrozole, n=3105; tamoxifen, n=3129.

Adverse Events in Extended Adjuvant Therapy in Early Breast Cancer, Median Treatment Duration of 24 Months: Table 2 describes the adverse events occurring at a frequency of at least 2% in any treatment group in a well-controlled clinical study in which over 5100 postmenopausal patients with receptor-positive or unknown primary breast cancer patients who had remained disease-free after completion of adjuvant treatment with tamoxifen were randomly assigned either FEMARA or placebo. The median duration of extended adjuvant treatment was 24 months and the median duration of follow-up for safety was 28 months for patients receiving letrozole and placebo. Most adverse events reported were grade 1 or grade 2 based on the Common Toxicity Criteria Version 2.0.

Table 2: FEMARA

Most Frequently Reported Adverse Events Irrespective of Relationship to Study Drug (median treatment duration 24 months) in the Extended Adjuvant Trial MA-17

	Letrozole N=2563 n (%)	Placebo N=2573 n (%)
Any Adverse Event	2234 (87.2)	2174 (84.5)
Cardiac Disorders	90 (3.5)	113 (4.4)
Eye Disorders	91 (3.6)	79 (3.1)
Gastrointestinal	725 (28.3)	731 (28.4)
Constipation	290 (11.3)	304 (11.8)
Nausea	221 (8.6)	212 (8.2)
Diarrhea NOS	128 (5.0)	143 (5.6)
Abdominal pain NOS	74 (2.9)	86 (3.3)
Vomiting	75 (2.9)	83 (3.2)
Dyspepsia	72 (2.8)	82 (3.2)
General Disorders	1155 (45.1)	1090 (42.4)
Asthenia	862 (33.6)	826 (32.1)
Edema NOS	471 (18.4)	416 (16.2)
Chest pain	59 (2.3)	69 (2.7)
Pain NOS	56 (2.2)	47 (1.8)
Infections and Infestations	166 (6.5)	163 (6.3)
Investigation	184 (7.2)	147 (5.7)
Weight increased	55 (2.1)	51 (2.0)
Weight decreased	52 (2.0)	38 (1.5)
Metabolism and Nutrition Disorders	551 (21.5)	537 (20.9)
Hypercholesterolaemia	401 (15.6)	398 (15.5)
Anorexia	119 (4.6)	96 (3.7)
Musculoskeletal Disorders	978 (38.2)	836 (32.5)
Arthralgia	565 (22.0)	465 (18.1)
Arthritis NOS	173 (6.7)	124 (4.8)
Myalgia	171 (6.7)	122 (4.7)

(cont'd)

Table 2: FEMARA *(cont'd)*

Most Frequently Reported Adverse Events Irrespective of Relationship to Study Drug (median treatment duration 24 months) in the Extended Adjuvant Trial MA-17

	Letrozole N=2563 n (%)	Placebo N=2573 n (%)
Fractures	152 (5.9)	142 (5.5)
Back pain	129 (5.0)	112 (4.4)
Bone pain	70 (2.7)	81 (3.1)
Pain in extremity	70 (2.7)	62 (2.4)
Neoplasms Benign, Malignant and Unspecified	51 (2.0)	48 (1.9)
Nervous System Disorders	865 (33.7)	819 (31.8)
Headache	516 (20.1)	508 (19.7)
Dizziness	363 (14.2)	342 (13.3)
Psychiatric Disorders	320 (12.5)	276 (10.7)
Insomnia	149 (5.8)	120 (4.7)
Depression	115 (4.5)	104 (4.0)
Anxiety	78 (3.0)	73 (2.8)
Renal Disorders	130 (5.1)	100 (3.9)
Reproductive Disorders	303 (11.8)	357 (13.9)
Vulvovaginal dryness	137 (5.3)	127 (4.9)
Vaginal haemorrhage	123 (4.8)	171 (6.6)
Respiratory Disorders	280 (10.9)	261 (10.1)
Dyspnoea	140 (5.5)	137 (5.5)
Cough	96 (3.7)	94 (3.7)
Skin Disorders	830 (32.4)	787 (30.6)
Sweating increased	619 (24.2)	577 (22.4)
Alopecia	112 (4.4)	83 (3.2)
Rash NOS	41 (1.6)	53 (2.1)
Vascular Disorders	1376 (53.7)	1230 (47.8)
Flushing[a]	1273 (49.7)	1114 (43.3)
Hypertension NOS	122 (4.8)	110 (4.3)
Lymphoedema NOS	68 (2.7)	79 (3.1)

[a] Includes terms "hot flashes/hot flushes".
Legend: NOS: not otherwise specified.

The incidence of self-reported osteoporosis from the MA-17 core study was significantly higher in patients who received FEMARA 6.9% (176) than in patients who received placebo 5.5% (141) (P=0.042). The incidence of clinical fractures was 5.9% (152) in patients who received FEMARA compared to 5.5% (142) in patients who received placebo, the difference is not statistically significant (P=0.548).

Results (median duration of follow-up was 20 months) from the MA-17 bone sub-study demonstrated that, at 2 years, compared to baseline, patients receiving letrozole had a mean decrease (versus baseline) of 3% versus 0.4% (P=0.048) in placebo for hip bone mineral density. There was no significant difference in terms of lumbar spine bone mineral density.

The incidence of cardiovascular ischemic events from the MA-17 core study was comparable between patients who received FEMARA 6.8% (175) and placebo 6.5% (167) (P=NS).

Results from the MA-17 lipid study (median follow-up 36 months) did not show significant differences between the FEMARA and placebo groups. Subjects did not have a prior history of hyperlipidemia. The study continues to investigate the long term impact of FEMARA on lipid levels. As per normal clinical practice and guidelines for post-menopausal women, physicians should continue their routine monitoring of lipid levels on a regular basis.

Adverse Events in Extended Adjuvant Therapy in Early Breast Cancer, Median Treatment Duration of 47 Months and a Median Follow-up of 49 Months: Adverse events discussed below were analyzed irrespective of relationship to study treatment.

Table 3 compares the self-reported adverse events irrespective of drug relationship experienced in the randomized FEMARA arm at a median treatment duration of 24 months and 47 months. The table describes the adverse events occurring in the safety population at a cut-off frequency of at least 2%. Most of these adverse events were grade 1 or grade 2 based on Common Toxicity Criteria Version 2.0. The placebo comparison after unblinding is not reliable due to the fact that 56% of patients randomized placebo opted to switch to FEMARA and dates of onset for general adverse events (based on self-report) were not recorded. In most cases, therefore, it cannot be determined if the adverse events in the placebo group occurred before switch to FEMARA or after switch to FEMARA. The safety population after study unblinding consists of 2566 patients in the FEMARA arm, 1129 patients in the placebo not switched arm and 1448 patients in the FEMARA after switch from placebo arm. The median 24 months of treatment duration versus the median 47 months of treatment duration comparison is presented to indicate the evolution of adverse events in the FEMARA arm over time.

The most frequent adverse events irrespective of drug relationship (cut-off frequency of at least 2%) reported in the 604/2566 (23.5%) patients randomized to the FEMARA arm who had actually completed 5 years of treatment were: flushing (384, 64%), asthenia (288, 47.4%), increased sweating (241, 40%), headache (221, 37%), arthralgia (220, 36%), hypercholesterolemia (187, 31%), edema NOS (160, 26.5%) and dizziness (145, 24%).

In contrast to general self-reported adverse events presented in Table 3, dates of onset were recorded for serious adverse events (SAE) and for targeted adverse events of fracture, osteoporosis and cardiovascular events. The comparison between the FEMARA randomized arm to placebo until switch is therefore more meaningful for these events.

Table 3: FEMARA

Most Frequently Reported Adverse Events Irrespective of Relationship to Study Drug in the Extended Adjuvant Trial MA-17

	Letrozole (median treatment duration 24 months) N=2563 n (%)	Letrozole (median treatment duration 47 months) N=2566 n (%)
Any Adverse Event	2234 (87.2)	2418 (94.2)
Cardiac Disorders	90 (3.5)	135 (5.3)
Eye Disorders	91 (3.6)	138 (5.4)
Gastrointestinal	725 (28.3)	1030 (40.1)
Constipation	290 (11.3)	432 (16.8)
Nausea	221 (8.6)	355 (13.8)
Diarrhea NOS	128 (5.0)	199 (7.8)
Vomiting NOS	75 (2.9)	116 (4.5)
Abdominal pain NOS	74 (2.9)	112 (4.4)
Dyspepsia	72 (2.8)	122 (4.8)
Flatulence	47 (1.8)	55 (2.1)
General Disorders	1155 (45.1)	1462 (57.0)
Asthenia	862 (33.6)	1139 (44.4)
Edema NOS	471 (18.4)	632 (24.6)
Chest pain	59 (2.3)	83 (3.2)
Pain NOS	56 (2.2)	68 (2.7)
Edema peripheral	41 (1.6)	59 (2.3)
Fatigue	9 (0.4)	51 (2.0)
Infections and Infestations	166 (6.5)	251 (9.8)
Investigation	184 (7.2)	251 (9.8)
Weight increased	55 (2.1)	69 (2.7)
Weight decreased	52 (2.0)	74 (2.9)
Metabolism and Nutrition Disorders	551 (21.5)	811 (31.6)
Hypercholesterolaemia	401 (15.6)	582 (22.7)
Anorexia	119 (4.6)	178 (6.9)
Hyperglycaemia NOS	48 (1.9)	78 (3.0)
Musculoskeletal Disorders	978 (38.2)	1288 (50.2)
Arthralgia	565 (22.0)	806 (31.4)
Arthritis NOS	173 (6.7)	349 (13.6)
Myalgia	171 (6.7)	318 (12.4)
Fractures	152 (5.9)	279 (10.9)
Back pain	129 (5.0)	162 (6.3)
Bone pain	70 (2.7)	157 (6.1)
Pain in extremity	70 (2.7)	90 (3.5)
Muscle cramp	39 (1.5)	52 (2.0)
Neoplasms Benign, Malignant and Unspecified	51 (2.0)	83 (3.2)
Nervous System Disorders	865 (33.7)	1200 (46.8)
Headache	516 (20.1)	792 (30.9)
Dizziness	363 (14.2)	547 (21.3)
Sensory disturbance NOS	41 (1.6)	65 (2.5)
Hypoaesthesia	41 (1.6)	60 (2.3)
Memory impairment	35 (1.4)	52 (2.0)
Psychiatric Disorders	320 (12.5)	425 (16.6)
Insomnia	149 (5.8)	204 (8.0)
Depression	115 (4.5)	158 (6.2)

(cont'd)

Table 3: FEMARA *(cont'd)*

Most Frequently Reported Adverse Events Irrespective of Relationship to Study Drug in the Extended Adjuvant Trial MA-17

	Letrozole (median treatment duration 24 months) N=2563 n (%)	Letrozole (median treatment duration 47 months) N=2566 n (%)
Anxiety	78 (3.0)	103 (4.0)
Renal Disorders	130 (5.1)	172 (6.7)
Pollakiuria	47 (1.8)	65 (2.5)
Incontinence NOS	45 (1.8)	56 (2.2)
Reproductive Disorders	303 (11.8)	412 (16.1)
Vulvovaginal dryness	137 (5.3)	184 (7.2)
Vaginal haemorrhage	123 (4.8)	157 (6.1)
Respiratory Disorders	280 (10.9)	396 (15.4)
Dyspnoea	140 (5.5)	208 (8.1)
Cough	96 (3.7)	141 (5.5)
Skin Disorders	830 (32.4)	1117 (43.5)
Sweating increased	619 (24.2)	867 (33.8)
Alopecia	112 (4.4)	147 (5.7)
Dry skin	42 (1.6)	59 (2.3)
Rash NOS	41 (1.6)	58 (2.3)
Dermatitis exfoliative NOS	34 (1.3)	54 (2.1)
Vascular Disorders	1376 (53.7)	1662 (64.8)
Flushing[a]	1273 (49.7)	1548 (60.3)
Hypertension NOS	122 (4.8)	178 (6.9)
Lymphoedema NOS	68 (2.7)	91 (3.5)

[a] Includes terms "hot flashes/hot flushes".
Legend: NOS: Not Otherwise Specified.

Osteoporosis and Fracture: After the study unblinding, patients randomized to the placebo arm were offered to switch to FEMARA or discontinue treatment.

The updated results from the MA-17 core safety population obtained after unblinding, showed that at a median follow-up of 49 months, the incidence of osteoporosis any time after randomization was higher in patients originally randomized in the FEMARA arm than for patients in the placebo until switch arm [12.3% in FEMARA arm vs. 7.4% in placebo until switch arm (P<0.001)].

The incidence of bone fractures, any time after randomization, was significantly higher in patients who received FEMARA than for placebo until switch (10.9% vs. 7.2%, respectively). In the placebo patients who switched to FEMARA, newly diagnosed osteoporosis, any time after switching, was reported in 3.6% while fractures were reported in 5.1% any time after switching.

In the randomized FEMARA arm, 1.9% of patients experienced more than one fracture, compared with 1.1% in the placebo until switch group and 1.0% in the FEMARA after switch from placebo group. Of the 74/1448 patients who experienced a fracture after switching to FEMARA from placebo, 12 patients had previously experienced a fracture on placebo (and 3 of these patients had experienced more than one fracture on placebo).

The interpretation of the updated results in the core study is confounded by the fact that after study unblinding, 56% of patients randomized placebo opted to switch to FEMARA, resulting in different median exposure to treatment (47 months for FEMARA, 28 months for placebo until switch and 20 months for FEMARA after switch from placebo).

Updated results (median follow-up was 40 months) from the bone mineral density (BMD) sub-study conducted in a subset of 219 patients (117 on FEMARA and 102 on placebo, including 77 placebo/FEMARA switchers), demonstrated that, at 2 years, compared to baseline, patients receiving FEMARA had a median decrease of 3.8% in hip BMD compared to 2.0% in the placebo until switch group (P=0.018). There were no statistically significant differences in median % changes from baseline in hip BMD at any other measured time-points other than at 2 years. There were no statistically significant changes in lumbar spine BMD at any time between FEMARA and placebo until switch groups. In the 77 placebo patients who switched to FEMARA, BMD in the hip and lumbar spine showed a median decrease from baseline of approximately 1-2% at each of the first, second and third annual visits after switching to FEMARA. The treatment duration in each group was median 38 months for FEMARA, 22 months for placebo until switch and 22 months for FEMARA after switch from placebo respectively. (See also Warnings and Precautions, Musculoskeletal and Special Populations, Geriatrics.)

Cardiovascular Events: As reported in Table 4, at a median follow-up of 49 months, the incidence of cardiovascular events any time after randomization was 11.1% for FEMARA versus 8.6% for placebo until switch. This is higher than the incidence reported at 28 months follow-up (6.8% in the FEMARA arm compared with 6.5% in the placebo arm, see also Warnings and Precautions, Cardiovascular).

Table 4: FEMARA

Cardiovascular Disease any Time After Randomization in the MA-17 Study (safety population), Median Follow-up 49 Months

	Letrozole N=2566 n (%)	Placebo Until Switch[a] N=2577 n (%)	Letrozole After Switch[b] N=1448 n (%)
Cardiovascular Disease			
No	2280 (88.9)	2355 (91.4)	1392 (96.1)
Yes	286 (11.1)	222 (8.6)	56 (3.9)
Type of Cardiovascular Disease			

(cont'd)

Table 4: FEMARA *(cont'd)*

Cardiovascular Disease any Time After Randomization in the MA-17 Study (safety population), Median Follow-up 49 Months

	Letrozole	Placebo Until Switch[a]	Letrozole After Switch[b]
	N=2566 n (%)	N=2577 n (%)	N=1448 n (%)
Angina requiring CABG	12 (0.5)	13 (0.5)	2 (0.1)
Myocardial Infarction	34 (1.3)	24 (0.9)	4 (0.3)
New or worsening angina	44 (1.7)	32 (1.2)	6 (0.4)
Angina requiring PTCA	14 (0.5)	11 (0.4)	1 (0.1)
Thromboembolic event	25 (1.0)	16 (0.6)	7 (0.5)
Stroke/transient ischemic attack	43 (1.7)	33 (1.3)	6 (0.4)
Other	179 (7.0)	140 (5.4)	35 (2.4)
Arrhythmia	103 (4.0)	85 (3.3)	16 (1.1)
Cardiac	66 (2.6)	51 (2.0)	11 (0.8)
Vascular	28 (1.1)	21 (0.8)	4 (0.3)
Valvular	9 (0.4)	5 (0.2)	3 (0.2)
CNS/Cerebrovascular	7 (0.3)	3 (0.1)	0
Other	8 (0.3)	11 (0.4)	7 (0.5)

[a] After randomization but until switch to letrozole, if switch occurred; if switch did not occur, then until date of last contact.
[b] After switch until date of last contact.

The most frequent cause of non-cancer death during study treatment or within 30 days of stopping treatment (regardless of treatment arm) was cardiovascular. (See Warnings and Precautions, Cardiovascular.)

The incidence of serious adverse events (all grades 1-5) regardless of study drug relationship was 0.5% in the FEMARA group, 1.3% in the placebo not switched arm and 0.3% in FEMARA after switch arm. Breast cancer related death reported during treatment or within 30 days of stopping treatment occurred in 0.5% of patients in the FEMARA arm, 0.8% in the placebo not switched arm and 0.3% in the FEMARA after switch arm. Non-breast cancer related death reported during treatment or within 30 days of stopping treatment occurred in 1.7% of patients in the FEMARA arm, 2.6% in the placebo not switched arm and 0.5% in the FEMARA after switch arm.

Lipids: Updated results (median follow-up was approximately 50 months) from the lipid sub-study showed no significant differences between the FEMARA and placebo groups at any time.

The MA-17 study is ongoing. The final study results are pending.

Adverse Events in First-Line Therapy: Overall, 455 post-menopausal patients with locally advanced or metastatic breast cancer were treated with FEMARA in a well-controlled clinical trial and the median time of exposure was 11 months. The incidence of adverse experiences was similar for FEMARA and tamoxifen. The most frequently reported adverse experiences were bone pain, hot flushes, back pain, nausea, arthralgia and dyspnea. Discontinuations for adverse experiences other than progression of tumour occurred in 10/455 (2%) of patients on FEMARA and in 15/455 (3%) of patients on tamoxifen.

Table 5 shows the frequency of adverse events considered possibly related to trial drug that have been reported with an incidence of more than 2.0% (whether for FEMARA (letrozole) or for tamoxifen) in a well-controlled clinical study with FEMARA (2.5 mg daily) and tamoxifen (20 mg daily).

Table 5: FEMARA

Frequency of Adverse Events (Experience >2%)

Adverse Event System Organ Class/Preferred Term	FEMARA N=455 (%)	Tamoxifen N=455 (%)
Gastrointestinal Disorders		
Nausea	6.6	6.4
Constipation	2.4	1.3
Vomiting	2.2	1.5
General Disorders and Administration Site Conditions		
Fatigue	2.6	2.4
Metabolism and Nutrition Disorders		
Appetite Decreased	1.6	3.3
Appetite Increased	1.8	2.0
Nervous System Disorders		
Headache	2.2	2.4
Skin and Subcutaneous Tissue Disorders		
Alopecia	5.5	3.3
Sweating Increased	2.0	2.9
Vascular Disorders		
Hot Flushes	16.7	14.3
Thromboembolic Events	1.5	1.9

* Including paresthesia, hypoesthesia.

Adverse Events in Second-Line Therapy: Table 6 shows in decreasing order of frequency the AEs—considered possibly related to trial drug according to the investigator—that have been reported with an incidence of more than 1.0% for FEMARA (letrozole) in a controlled clinical trial with FEMARA (2.5 mg daily) and megestrol acetate (160 mg daily) for up to 33 months.

Table 6: FEMARA

Frequency of Adverse Events (Experience >1%)

Adverse Event	FEMARA % (N=174)	Megestrol Acetate % (N=189)
Headache	6.9	4.8
Nausea	6.3	4.2
Peripheral edema	6.3	3.7
Fatigue	5.2	6.3
Hot flushes	5.2	3.7
Hair thinning	3.4	1.1
Rash[a]	3.4	0.5
Vomiting	2.9	1.6
Dyspepsia	2.9	1.6
Weight increase	2.3	8.5
Musculoskeletal pain[b]	2.3	1.1
Anorexia	2.3	1.1
Vaginal bleeding	1.7	3.2
Leukorrhea	1.7	2.6
Constipation	1.7	2.1
Dizziness	1.1	3.7
Increased appetite	1.1	3.7
Increased sweating	1.1	2.1

[a] Including: erythematous rash, maculopapular rash.
[b] Including: arm pain, back pain, leg pain, skeletal pain.

There were no differences in the incidence and severity of adverse reactions in patients ≤55 years, 55-69 years and ≥70 years.

Post-Market Adverse Drug Reactions: Spontaneously reported adverse drug reactions are presented below. Because these events are reported voluntarily from a population of uncertain size, it is not always possible to reliably estimate their frequency or clearly establish a causal relationship to FEMARA exposure.

Blood and Lymphatic System Disorders: leukopenia.
Cardiac Disorders: palpitations, tachycardia, atrial fibrillation, atrial flutter, cardiac failure.
Eye Disorders: cataract, eye irritation, blurred vision.
Gastrointestinal Disorders: dyspepsia, abdominal pain, stomatitis, dry mouth.
General Disorders and Administration Site Conditions: pyrexia, mucosal dryness, thirst.
Hepato-Biliary Disorders: increased hepatic enzymes, hepatitis.
Immune System Disorders: anaphylactic reaction.
Infections and Infestations: urinary tract infection.
Investigations: weight increase, weight loss, increase in aminotransferases.
Musculoskeletal and Connective Tissue Disorders: myalgia, osteoporosis, bone fractures.
Neoplasms Benign, Malignant and Unspecified (incl. cysts and polyps): tumour pain.
Nervous System Disorders: memory impairment, dysesthesia*, taste disturbance, cerebrovascular accident.
Psychiatric Disorders: anxiety†.
Renal and Urinary Disorders: increased urinary frequency.
Reproductive System and Breast Disorders: vaginal discharge.
Respiratory, Thoracic and Mediastinal Disorders: cough.
Skin and Subcutaneous Tissue Disorders: rash‡, pruritus, dry skin, urticaria, angioedema, erythema multiforme, toxic epidermal necrolysis.
Vascular Disorders: thrombophlebitis¶, hypertension, pulmonary embolism, arterial thrombosis, cerebrovascular infarction, ischemic cardiac events.

DRUG INTERACTIONS: Drug-Drug Interactions: Clinical trials of interaction with FEMARA (letrozole) and cimetidine or warfarin indicate that coadministration does not result in clinically significant drug interactions.

A review of the clinical trial database indicated no evidence of other clinically relevant interactions with other commonly prescribed drugs.

In vitro, letrozole inhibits the cytochrome P450 isoenzymes 2A6 and moderately 2C19. CYP2A6 does not play a major role in drug metabolism. In in vitro experiments letrozole was not able to substantially inhibit the metabolism of diazepam (a substrate of CYP2C19) at concentrations approximately 100-fold higher than those observed in plasma at steady-state. Thus clinically relevant interactions with CYP2C19 are unlikely to occur. However, caution should be used in the concomitant administration of drugs whose disposition is mainly dependent on these isoenzymes and whose therapeutic index is narrow.

Use with Other Anticancer Agents: Co-administration of FEMARA and tamoxifen 20 mg daily resulted in a reduction of letrozole plasma levels by 38% on average. The clinical significance of this finding has not been explored in prospective clinical trials.

There is no clinical experience to date on the use of FEMARA in combination with other anti-cancer agents.

Drug-Food Interactions: Food slightly decreases the rate of absorption (median t_{max} 1 hour fasted vs. 2 hours fed and mean C_{max} 129±20.3 nmol/L fasted vs. 98.7±18.6 nmol/L fed), but the extent of absorption (area under the curve (AUC)) remains unchanged. This minor effect on absorption rate is not considered to be of clinical relevance and therefore letrozole may be taken with or without food.

Drug-Laboratory Test Interactions: No clinically significant changes in the results of clinical laboratory tests have been observed.

DOSAGE AND ADMINISTRATION: Dosing Considerations:

- Insufficient data available to recommend dose adjustment in patients with severe hepatic impairment (see Patients with Hepatic and/or Renal Impairment).

† Including nervousness, irritability.
‡ Including erythematous, maculopapular, psoriaform and vesicular rash.
¶ Including superficial and deep thrombophlebitis.

Recommended Dose and Dosage Adjustment: Adult and Elderly Patients: The recommended dose is one 2.5 mg tablet once daily. No dose adjustment is required for elderly patients.

In the adjuvant setting, the intended duration of treatment is 5 years, although data are limited to a median follow-up of 26 months.

In the extended adjuvant setting, treatment with FEMARA (letrozole) is intended for 5 years, although scientific evidence collected to date covers a median follow-up of 49 months.

In the first- and second-line advanced breast cancer settings, FEMARA (letrozole) treatment should continue until further tumour progression is evident.

Patients with Hepatic and/or Renal Impairment: No dosage adjustment is required for patients with renal impairment (creatinine clearance ≥10 mL/min) or moderate hepatic impairment. Insufficient data are available to recommend a dose adjustment in breast cancer patients with severe non-metastatic hepatic impairment. Therefore, patients with severe hepatic impairment (Child-Pugh score C) should be kept under close supervision for adverse events (see Warnings and Precautions).

Missed Dose: The missed dose should be taken as soon as the patient remembers. However, if it is almost time for the next dose, the missed dose should be skipped, and the patient should go back to her regular dosage schedule. Do not double doses.

OVERDOSAGE:

Isolated cases of FEMARA (letrozole) overdose have been reported. In these instances, the highest single dose ingested was 62.5 mg or 25 tablets. While no serious adverse events were reported in these cases, because of the limited data available, no firm recommendations for treatment can be made. In single dose studies the highest dose used was 30 mg, which was well tolerated; in multiple dose trials, the largest dose of 10 mg was well tolerated.

For management of suspected drug overdose, contact your regional poison control centre. In general, treatment of overdose with letrozole should be supportive and symptomatic. Vital signs should be monitored in all patients. Complete blood count (CBC) and liver function tests should be monitored in symptomatic patients. Fluid and electrolyte status should be monitored in patients with significant vomiting and/or diarrhea. Administration of activated charcoal may be appropriate in some cases.

> For management of a suspected drug overdose, contact your **regional Poison Control Centre**. See the *CPS* Directory section for a list of Poison Control Centres.

ACTION AND CLINICAL PHARMACOLOGY: Mechanism of Action: FEMARA (letrozole) is a potent and highly specific non-steroidal aromatase inhibitor. It inhibits the aromatase enzyme by competitively binding to the heme of the cytochrome P450 subunit of the enzyme, resulting in a reduction of estrogen biosynthesis in all tissues.

Pharmacodynamics: FEMARA exerts its antitumour effect by depriving estrogen-dependent breast cancer cells of one of their growth stimuli. In postmenopausal women, estrogens are derived mainly from the action of the aromatase enzyme, which converts adrenal androgens—primarily androstenedione and testosterone—to estrone (E1) and estradiol (E2). The suppression of estrogen biosynthesis in peripheral tissues and the malignant tissue can be achieved by specifically inhibiting the aromatase enzyme.

In healthy postmenopausal women, single oral doses of 0.1, 0.5 and 2.5 mg letrozole suppressed serum estrone by 75-78% and estradiol by 78% from baseline. Maximum suppression is achieved in 48-78 hours.

In postmenopausal women with advanced breast cancer, daily letrozole doses of 0.1 to 5 mg suppress estradiol, estrone and estrone sulphate plasma levels by 75-95% from baseline in all patients treated. With 0.5 mg doses and higher, many plasma levels of estrone and estrone sulphate are below the limit of detection of the assays, indicating that higher estrogen suppression is achieved with these doses. Estrogen suppression was maintained throughout treatment in all patients.

Letrozole is highly specific in inhibiting aromatase activity. Impairment of adrenal steroidogenesis has not been observed. No clinically relevant changes in the plasma levels of cortisol, aldosterone, 11-deoxycortisol, 17-hydroxy-progesterone, ACTH (adrenocorticotropic hormone) or in plasma renin activity were found in postmenopausal patients treated with 0.1 to 5 mg letrozole daily. The ACTH stimulation test performed after 6 and 12 weeks of treatment with daily doses of 0.1 to 5 mg letrozole did not indicate any attenuation of aldosterone or cortisol production. Thus, glucocorticoid or mineralocorticoid supplementation is not required.

Letrozole had no effect on plasma androgen concentrations (androstenedione and testosterone) among healthy postmenopausal women after single doses of 0.1, 0.5 and 2.5 mg, or on plasma androstenedione concentrations among postmenopausal patients treated with daily doses of 0.1 to 5 mg. These results indicate that accumulation of androgenic precursors does not occur. Plasma levels of LH and FSH are not affected by letrozole in patients, nor is thyroid function as evaluated by TSH, T_4 and T_3 uptake.

Pharmacokinetics: Absorption: Letrozole is rapidly and completely absorbed from the gastrointestinal tract (absolute bioavailability=99.9%). Food slightly decreases the rate of absorption (median t_{max} 1 hour fasted vs. 2 hours fed and mean C_{max} 129±20.3 nmol/L fasted vs. 98.7±18.6 nmol/L fed), but the extent of absorption (area under the curve (AUC)) remains unchanged. This minor effect on absorption rate is not considered to be of clinical relevance and therefore letrozole may be taken with or without food.

Distribution: Letrozole is rapidly and extensively distributed into tissues (Vd_{SS}=1.87±0.47 L/kg). Plasma protein binding is approximately 60%, mainly to albumin. The letrozole concentration in erythrocytes is about 80% of that in plasma. After administration of 2.5 mg ^{14}C-labelled letrozole, approximately 82% of the radioactivity in plasma was unchanged compound. Systemic exposure to metabolites is therefore low.

Metabolism: Metabolic clearance to a pharmacologically inactive carbinol metabolite, CGP 44645, is the major elimination pathway of letrozole (Cl_m=2.1 L/h), but it is relatively slow when compared to hepatic blood flow (about 90 L/h). The cytochrome P450 isoenzymes 3A4 and 2A6 were found to be capable of converting letrozole to this metabolite. Formation of minor unidentified metabolites and direct renal and fecal excretion play only a minor role in the overall elimination of letrozole. Within 2 weeks after administration of 2.5 mg ^{14}C-labelled letrozole to healthy postmenopausal volunteers, 88.2±7.6% of the radioactivity was recovered in urine and 3.8±0.9% in feces. At least 75% of the radioactivity recovered in urine up to 216 hours (84.7±7.8% of the dose) was attributed to the glucuronide of the carbinol metabolite, about 9% to two unidentified metabolites, and 6% to unchanged letrozole.

Excretion: The apparent terminal elimination half-life in plasma is about 2 days. After daily administration of 2.5 mg steady-state levels are reached within 2 to 6 weeks. Plasma concentrations at steady-state are approximately 7 times higher than concentrations measured after a single dose of 2.5 mg, while they are 1.5 to 2 times higher than steady-state values predicted from the concentrations measured after a single dose, indicating a slight non-linearity in the pharmacokinetics of letrozole upon daily administration of 2.5 mg. Since steady state levels are maintained over time, it can be concluded that no continuous accumulation of letrozole occurs.

STORAGE AND STABILITY: Protect from heat (store at room temperature 15 to 30°C). Protect from moisture.

Keep out of reach and sight of children and pets.

INFORMATION FOR THE PATIENT: Published in e-CPS, available by subscription at www.e-cps.ca.

DOSAGE FORMS, COMPOSITION AND PACKAGING:

Each dark yellow, round, slightly biconvex tablet with beveled edges bearing the imprint "FV" on one side and "CG" on the other, contains: letrozole 2.5 mg. Nonmedicinal ingredients: cellulose compounds (microcrystalline cellulose and methylhydroxypropylcellulose), corn starch, iron oxide, lactose, magnesium stearate, polyethylene glycol, sodium starch glycolate, silicon dioxide, talc and titanium dioxide. Blister packages of 30.

(Shown in Product Identification Section)

femHRT® Ⓟ

norethindrone acetate—ethinyl estradiol

Estrogen-Progestin Combination

Warner Chilcott

Date of Preparation: August 12, 2010

INDICATIONS AND CLINICAL USE: femHRT tablets are a combination of ethinyl estradiol (estrogen) and norethindrone acetate (progestin) intended for continuous administration as hormone replacement therapy.

femHRT is indicated for:

- Relief of menopausal and postmenopausal symptoms occurring in naturally or surgically induced estrogen deficiency states;
- Symptomatic treatment of vulvar and vaginal atrophy associated with menopause;
- Prevention of osteoporosis in naturally occurring or surgically induced estrogen-deficiency states in addition to other important therapeutic measures such as sufficient calcium and vitamin D intake, cessation of smoking and regular physical weight bearing exercise. When prescribing solely for the prevention of postmenopausal osteoporosis, therapy should only be considered for women at significant risk of osteoporosis, and non-estrogen medications should be carefully considered.

femHRT is recommended for use only in patients with an intact uterus, since the regimen includes a progestin whose role is to prevent endometrial hyperplasia.

Estrogen replacement therapy reduces bone resorption and retards or halts postmenopausal loss. When estrogen therapy is discontinued, bone mass declines at a rate comparable to that in the immediate postmenopausal period. There is no evidence that estrogen replacement therapy restores bone mass to premenopausal levels.

At skeletal maturity there are sex and race differences in both the total amount of bone present and its density, in favour of men. Thus, women are at higher risk than men because they start with less bone mass and, for several years following natural or induced menopause, the rate of bone mass decline is accelerated. White and Asian women are also at higher risk than black women.

Early menopause is one of the strongest predictors for development of osteoporosis. In addition, other factors affecting the skeleton, which are associated with osteoporosis, include genetic factors (small build, family history), endocrine factors (nulliparity, thyrotoxicosis, hyperparathyroidism, Cushing's syndrome, hyperprolactinemia, type I diabetes), lifestyle (cigarette smoking, alcohol abuse, sedentary lifestyles), and nutrition (below average body weight, low dietary calcium intake).

The mainstays for decreasing the risk of osteoporosis are an adequate calcium and vitamin D intake, weight bearing exercise, smoking cessation and when indicated, pharmacologic measures. Postmenopausal women absorb dietary calcium less efficiently than premenopausal women and require an average of 1500 mg/day of elemental calcium to remain in neutral calcium balance. By comparison, premenopausal women require about 1000 mg/day, and the average calcium intake in North America is 400-600 mg/day. Therefore, when not contraindicated, calcium supplementation may be helpful. Vitamin D supplementation of 400-800 IU/day may also be required to ensure adequate daily intake in postmenopausal women.

Weight bearing exercise and nutrition are important in the prevention and management of osteoporosis. Immobilization and prolonged bed rest produce rapid bone loss, while weigh-bearing exercise has been shown to reduce bone loss and increase bone mass. The optimal types and amount of physical activity that would prevent osteoporosis have not been established; however, in two studies, an hour of walking and running exercises two or three times weekly significantly increased lumbar spine bone mass.

CONTRAINDICATIONS: femHRT (norethindrone acetate and ethinyl estradiol) is contraindicated in patients with any of the following disorders:

- Active hepatic dysfunction or disease, especially of the obstructive type
- Personal history of known or suspected estrogen/progestin-dependent neoplasia, such as breast or endometrial cancer
- Endometrial hyperplasia
- Undiagnosed abnormal genital bleeding
- Known or suspected pregnancy
- Lactation
- Active or past history of arterial thromboembolic disease (e.g., stroke, myocardial infarction, coronary heart disease)
- Classical migraine
- Active or past history of confirmed venous thromboembolism (such as deep venous thrombosis or pulmonary embolism) or active thrombophlebitis
- Partial or complete loss of vision due to ophthalmic disease
- Known or suspected hypersensitivity to any components of the medication

WARNINGS AND PRECAUTIONS:

> **Serious Warnings and Precautions**
> As the Women's Health Initiative (WHI) study results indicated increased risk of myocardial infarction (MI), stroke, invasive breast cancer, pulmonary emboli, and deep vein thrombosis in postmenopausal women during 5 years of treatment with combined 0.625 mg conjugated equine estrogens and 2.5 mg medroxyprogesterone acetate compared to those receiving placebo tablets, the following should be highly considered:
> - Estrogens with or without progestins **should not** be prescribed for primary or secondary prevention of cardiovascular diseases.
> - Other combinations of estrogens and progestins were not studied in the WHI and, in the absence of comparable data, these risks should be assumed to be similar. Because of these risks, estrogens with or without progestins should be prescribed at the **lowest effective doses and for the shortest duration** possible for the recognized indication.
> - When prescribing solely for the prevention of postmenopausal osteoporosis, therapy should only be considered for women at significant risk of osteoporosis, and non-estrogen medications should be carefully considered.

General: Before femHRT (norethindrone acetate and ethinyl estradiol) is administered, the patient should have a complete physical examination including a blood pressure determination. Breasts and pelvic organs should be appropriately examined and a Papanicolaou smear should be performed. Endometrial thickness should be evaluated by ultrasound and/or by endometrial biopsy, when indicated. Baseline tests should include mammography, measurements of blood glucose, calcium, triglycerides and cholesterol, and liver function tests.

The first follow-up examination should be done within 3-6 months after initiation of treatment to assess response to treatment. Thereafter, examinations should be made every 6-12 months and should include at least those procedures outlined above.

It is important that patients are encouraged to practice frequent self-examination of the breasts.

Carcinogenesis and Mutagenesis: Breast Cancer: Current epidemiological data indicate that the use of combined HRT is associated with an increased risk of invasive breast cancer. The WHI trial results concluded that there are more risks than benefits among women using combined HRT (0.625 mg conjugated equine estrogens/2.5 mg medroxyprogesterone acetate) compared to the group using placebo. In 10 000 women on combined HRT over one year period, there were eight more cases of invasive breast cancer (38 on combined HRT versus 30 on placebo per 10 000 person-years).

The WHI study reported that the invasive breast cancers diagnosed in the estrogen plus progestin group were similar in histology but were larger (mean [SD], 1.7 cm [1.1] vs. 1.5 cm [0.9], respectively; P=0.04) and were at a more advanced stage compared with those diagnosed in the placebo group.

The WHI trial also reported that the percentage of women with abnormal mammograms (recommendations for short-interval follow-up, a suspicious abnormality, or highly suggestive of malignancy) was significantly higher in the estrogen plus progestin group versus the placebo group. This difference appeared at year one and persisted in each year thereafter.

Two breast neoplastic events occurred across the four pivotal femHRT trials described in the Clinical Trials section. Both events occurred in Study 376-359: One breast cancer occurred on Day 164 in a subject randomized to 0.5/2.5 (n=136) dose. Tumor marker studies were negative for estrogen and progesterone receptors. A recurrence of cancer was reported on follow-up. One breast cancer occurred at an unknown onset date in a subject randomized to the 1/5 dose (n=146). Drug was permanently discontinued. On follow-up, drug-related causality could not be ruled out.

It is recommended that estrogens not be given to women with existing breast cancer or those with a previous history of the disease. There is a need for caution in prescribing estrogens for women with known risk factors associated with the development of breast cancer, such as strong family history of breast cancer (first degree relative) or who present a breast condition with an increased risk (abnormal mammograms and/or atypical hyperplasia at breast biopsy). Other known risk factors for the development of breast cancer such as nulliparity, obesity, early menarche, late age at first full term pregnancy and at menopause should also be evaluated.

It is recommended that women undergo mammography before starting HRT, and at regular intervals during treatment, as deemed appropriate by the treating physician and according to the perceived risks for each patient.

The overall benefits and possible risks of hormone replacement therapy should be fully considered and discussed with patients. It is important that the modest increase in risk of being diagnosed with breast cancer after 4 years of treatment with HRT (as reported in the results of the WHI trial) be discussed with the patient and weighed against its known benefits.

Instructions for regular self-examination should be included in this counselling.

Endometrial Hyperplasia and Endometrial Carcinoma: There is evidence from several studies that estrogens unopposed by progestins increase the risk of carcinoma of the endometrium in humans. femHRT (norethindrone acetate and ethinyl estradiol) provides plasma norethindrone levels within the appropriate range to counteract the effects of ethinyl estradiol on the endometrium.

In the CHART Study (376-359), it has been demonstrated that when norethindrone acetate is administered with ethinyl estradiol, the incidence of endometrial hyperplasia (a possible precursor of endometrial cancer) is reduced to the level observed in placebo users. No cases of endometrial hyperplasia were detected with femHRT 0.5/2.5 and 1/5 doses administered for 2 years. femHRT 0.5/2.5 and 1/5 treatment groups did not differ from placebo with regard to the degree of endometrial proliferation.

Study 376-401 assessed the safety and endometrial protective effect of femHRT 1/5 in healthy, postmenopausal women. At the end of 1 year, there were no cases of endometrial hyperplasia reported with femHRT 1/5.

Clinical surveillance of all women taking estrogen/progestin combinations is important. Adequate diagnostic measures, including endometrial sampling when indicated, should be undertaken to rule out malignancy in all cases of undiagnosed persistent or recurring abnormal vaginal bleeding.

Cardiovascular: Available epidemiological data indicate that use of estrogen with or without progestin is associated with an increased risk of stroke and coronary heart disease. The WHI trial results concluded that there are more risks than benefits among women using combined Hormone Replacement Therapy (HRT), consisting of 0.625 mg conjugated equine estrogens plus 2.5 mg medroxyprogesterone acetate, compared to the group using placebo. In 10 000 women on this combined HRT over one year period, there were seven more cases of coronary heart disease (37 on combined HRT versus 30 on placebo per 10 000 person years) and eight more cases of strokes (29 versus 21 per 10 000 person years).

No cardiovascular event occurred in the femHRT clinical trials described in the Clinical Trials section using the recommended therapeutic doses of femHRT.

In the Heart and Estrogen/Progestin Replacement Study (HERS) of postmenopausal women with documented heart disease (n=2763, average age 66.7 years), a randomized placebo-controlled clinical trial of secondary prevention of coronary heart disease (CHD), treatment with 0.625 mg/day oral conjugated equine estrogen (CEE) plus 2.5 mg medroxyprogesterone acetate (MPA) demonstrated no cardiovascular benefit. Specifically, during an average follow-up of 4.1 years, treatment with CEE plus MPA did not reduce the overall rate of CHD in postmenopausal women with established coronary heart disease. There were more CHD events in the hormone-treated group than in the placebo group in year 1, but not during the subsequent years.

From the original HERS trial, 2321 women consented to participate in an open label extension of HERS, HERS II. Average follow-up in HERS II was an additional 2.7 years, for a total of 6.8 years overall. After 6.8 years, hormone therapy did not reduce the risk of cardiovascular events in women with CHD.

In Study 376-359, one transient ischemic attack was reported on Day 611 in a subject randomized to the femHRT 0.5/2.5 dose (n=136). The patient recovered from the upper extremity numbness, and medication was discontinued at study completion on Day 730.

Venous Thromboembolism: Recent epidemiological data indicate that the use of estrogen with or without progestin is associated with an increased risk of developing venous thromboembolism (VTE). The WHI trial results concluded that there are more risks than benefits among women using combined HRT (0.625 mg conjugated equine estrogens/2.5 mg medroxyprogesterone acetate), compared to the group using placebo. In 10 000 women on combined HRT over a period of one year, there were eighteen more cases of total blood clots in the lungs and legs (34 on combined HRT versus 16 on placebo per 10 000 person-years).

One venous thromboembolic event occurred across the four pivotal femHRT trials described in the Clinical Trials section. One deep venous thrombosis was reported on Day 588 of Study 376-359 in a subject randomized to the femHRT 1/5 dose (n=146). Study medication was discontinued, and the subject was hospitalized for anticoagulant therapy. Diagnosis upon hospital discharge was resolving deep vein thrombosis.

Generally recognized risk factors for VTE include a personal history, a family history (the occurrence of VTE in a direct relative at a relatively early age may indicate genetic predisposition) and severe obesity (body mass index >30 kg/m^2). The risk of VTE also increases with age and smoking.

The risk of VTE may be temporarily increased with prolonged immobilization, major elective surgery or post-traumatic surgery, or major trauma. If feasible, hormone replacement therapy should be discontinued at least 4 weeks before major surgery or during periods of prolonged immobilization, since these events may be associated with an increased risk of thromboembolism. In women on HRT, attention should be given to prophylactic measures to prevent VTE following surgery. Also, patients with varicose veins should be closely supervised.

The physician should be alert to the earliest manifestations of thrombotic disorders (thrombophlebitis, retinal thrombosis, cerebral embolism and pulmonary embolism). If these occur or are suspected, femHRT therapy should be discontinued immediately.

Blood Pressure: Women using hormone replacement therapy sometimes experience increased blood pressure, which, in most cases, returns to normal upon discontinuing the drug. Blood pressure should be monitored with HRT use. Elevation of blood pressure in previously normotensive or hypertensive patients should be evaluated, and femHRT therapy may have to be discontinued.

Endocrine and Metabolism: Because the prolonged use of estrogens influences the metabolism of calcium and phosphorus, estrogens should be used with caution in patients with metabolic and malignant bone diseases associated with hypercalcemia and in patients with renal insufficiency.

A worsening of glucose tolerance and lipid metabolism has been observed in a significant percentage of peri- and postmenopausal patients. Therefore, diabetic patients or those with a predisposition to diabetes should be observed closely to detect any alterations in carbohydrate or lipid metabolism, especially in triglyceride blood levels.

Women with familial hypertriglyceridemia or porphyria need special surveillance. Lipid lowering measures are recommended before starting treatment in these women.

Genitourinary: Abnormal vaginal bleeding that is prolonged, irregular or heavy, occurring during therapy should prompt diagnostic measures like endometrial biopsy or dilation and curettage (D&C) to rule out the possibility of uterine malignancy, and the treatment should be re-evaluated.

Pre-existing uterine leiomyoma may increase in size during estrogen use. This is usually minimal, especially in patients who are well past the menopause. Growth, pain or tenderness of uterine leiomyoma requires prompt attention and, if necessary, discontinuation of medication.

Symptoms and physical findings associated with a previous diagnosis of endometriosis may reappear or become aggravated with estrogen use.

Hematologic: If feasible, hormone replacement therapy should be discontinued at least 4 weeks before major surgery or during periods of prolonged immobilization, since these events may be associated with an increased risk of thromboembolism.

Hepatic/Biliary/Pancreatic: A 2 to 4 fold increase in the risk of gallbladder disease requiring surgery in women receiving postmenopausal estrogens has been reported. Caution is advised in patients with a history of estrogen-related jaundice and pruritus. If cholestatic jaundice develops during treatment with femHRT, the drug should be discontinued and appropriate investigations carried out.

Liver function tests should be done periodically in subjects who are suspected of having hepatic disease. For information on endocrine and liver function tests, see the section under Monitoring and Laboratory Tests.

The effect of hepatic disease on the disposition of femHRT has not been evaluated. However, ethinyl estradiol and norethindrone may be poorly metabolized in patients with impaired liver function (see Contraindications).

Neurologic: Patients who develop visual disturbances, classical migraine, transient aphasia, paralysis, or loss of consciousness should discontinue medication.

Renal: Estrogens may cause fluid retention. Therefore, particular attention is indicated in cardiac or renal dysfunction, epilepsy or asthma. Treatment should be stopped if there is an increase in epileptic seizures. If, in any of the above-mentioned conditions, a worsening of the underlying disease is diagnosed or suspected during treatment, the benefits and risks of treatment should be reassessed based on the individual case.

The effect of renal disease on the disposition of femHRT has not been evaluated. In premenopausal women with chronic renal failure undergoing peritoneal dialysis who received multiple doses of an oral contraceptive containing ethinyl estradiol and norethindrone, plasma ethinyl estradiol concentrations were higher and norethindrone concentrations were unchanged compared to concentrations in premenopausal women with normal renal function.

Special Populations: Pregnant Women: Estrogens/progestins should not be used during pregnancy (see Contraindications).

Geriatrics (≥65 years of age): Current epidemiological evidence suggests that the use of combined HRT is associated with an increased risk of developing dementia. The Women's Health Initiative Memory Study, a clinical sub study of the WHI, followed 4532 post-menopausal women age 65 and over and free of dementia at baseline. There was a reported two-fold increase in the relative risk of developing probable dementia after an average follow-up of 4.05 years in the group treated with daily 0.625 mg conjugated equine estrogen plus 2.5 mg medroxyprogesterone versus those treated with placebo (hazard ratio [HR] 2.05, 95% confidence interval [CI], 1.21-3.480. This increased risk would result in an additional 23 cases of dementia per 10 000 women per year (45 vs. 22 per 10 000 person-years; P=0.01).

The pharmacokinetics of norethindrone acetate and ethinyl estradiol was not affected by age (age range 40-62), in the postmenopausal population studied.

Monitoring and Laboratory Tests: The results of certain endocrine and liver function tests may be affected by estrogen-containing products:

- Increased sulfobromophthalein retention
- Increased prothrombin time and partial thromboplastin time; increased levels of fibrinogen and fibrinogen activity; increased coagulation factors VII, VIII, IX, and X; increased norepinephrine-induced platelet aggregability; decreased antithrombin III
- Increased thyroxin-binding globulin (TBG), leading to increased circulating total thyroid hormone (T4) as measured by column or radioimmunoassay; free T3 resin uptake is decreased, reflecting the elevated TBG; free T4 concentration is unaltered
- Other binding proteins may be elevated in serum, i.e., corticosteroid binding globulin (CBG), sex-hormone binding globulin (SHBG), leading to increased circulating corticosteroids and sex steroids respectively; free or biologically active hormone concentrations are unchanged
- Impaired glucose tolerance
- Reduced response to the METOPIRONE test
- Reduced serum folate concentration
- Increased serum triglyceride and phospholipid concentration

The results of the above laboratory tests should not be considered reliable unless therapy has been discontinued for 2 to 4 weeks. The pathologist should be informed that the patient is receiving estrogen-progestin therapy when relevant specimens are submitted.

ADVERSE REACTIONS: Adverse events reported in placebo controlled clinical studies of femHRT at a frequency of ≥5% are shown in Table 1.

Table 1: femHRT

All Treatment-Emergent Adverse Events Reported at a Frequency of ≥5% of Patients with femHRT

	Percent of Patients (%)		
Body System/Adverse Event	**Placebo N=247**	**femHRT 0.5/2.5 N=244**	**femHRT 1/5 N=258**
Body as a Whole	40.1	38.5	39.5
Headache	14.6	15.2	18.2
Back Pain	5.3	5.3	4.7
Viral Infection	7.7	8.6	7.0
Digestive System	24.4	30.5	33.0
Nausea and/or Vomiting	5.3	5.3	7.4
Abdominal Pain	4.5	10.2	8.1
Dyspepsia	2.0	5.3	3.1
Diarrhea	3.6	5.7	3.9
Musculoskeletal System	21.7	20.3	20.4
Arthralgia	6.9	2.9	5.8
Myalgia	8.5	8.6	7.8
Psychobiologic Function	8.3	7.9	14.1
Nervousness	1.6	1.6	5.4
Depression	3.6	3.7	5.8
Respiratory System	37.2	33.9	35.6
Rhinitis	15.4	12.7	15.1
Sinusitis	9.7	9.4	8.1
Urogenital System	25.0	31.6	40.8
Breast Pain	5.3	9.0	8.1
Urinary Tract Infection	3.2	3.7	6.2
Vaginitis	4.9	4.5	5.4

Post-Market Adverse Drug Reactions: The following adverse reactions have been reported with estrogens/progestin combinations in general:

Gastrointestinal: nausea, vomiting, abdominal discomfort (cramps, pressure, pain), bloating, gallbladder disorder, asymptomatic impaired liver function, cholestatic jaundice.

Genitourinary: breakthrough bleeding, spotting, change in menstrual flow, dysmenorrhea, vaginal itching/discharge, dyspareunia, endometrial hyperplasia, premenstrual-like syndrome, reactivation of endometriosis, cystitis, changes in cervical erosion and amount of cervical secretion.

Skin: chloasma or melasma, which may persist when drug is discontinued, erythema multiforme, erythema nodosum, hemorrhagic eruption, loss of scalp hair, hirsutism, acne.

Endocrine: breast swelling and tenderness, increased blood sugar levels, decreased glucose tolerance, sodium retention.

Cardiovascular/Hematologic: palpitations, isolated cases of thromobophlebitis, thromboembolic disorder, exacerbation of varicose veins, increase in blood pressure (see Warnings and Precautions), coronary thrombosis, altered coagulation tests, (see Monitoring and Laboratory Tests under Warnings and Precautions).

Central Nervous System: aggravation of migraine episodes, headaches, mental depression, nervousness, dizziness, fatigue, irritability, neuro-ocular lesions (e.g., retinal thrombosis, optic neuritis).

Ophthalmic: visual disturbances, steepening of the corneal curvature, intolerance to contact lenses, neuro-ocular lesions (see Central Nervous System).

Miscellaneous: changes in appetite, changes in body weight, edema, neuritis, change in libido; musculoskeletal pain, including leg pain not related to thromboembolic disease (usually transient, lasting 3-6 weeks), may occur.

If adverse symptoms persist, the prescription of hormone replacement therapy should be re-evaluated.

DRUG INTERACTIONS: Overview: No drug-drug interaction studies have been conducted with femHRT. The following section contains information on drug interactions with ethinyl estradiol-containing products (specifically, oral contraceptives) that have been reported in the published literature. It is unknown whether such interactions occur with femHRT or drug products containing other types of estrogens.

Drug-Drug Interactions: Estrogens may diminish the effectiveness of anticoagulants, antidiabetic and antihypertensive agents.

Preparations inducing liver enzymes (e.g., barbiturates, hydantoins, carbamazepine, meprobamates, phenylbutazone, rifampin) may interfere with the activity of orally administered estrogens.

- The metabolism of ethinyl estradiol is increased by rifampin and anticonvulsants such as phenobarbital, phenytoin and carbamazepine. Coadministration of troglitazone and certain ethinyl estradiol-containing drug products (e.g., oral contraceptives containing ethinyl estradiol) reduce the plasma concentration of ethinyl estradiol by 30 percent.

Ascorbic acid and acetaminophen (gram doses) may increase AUC and/or plasma concentration of ethinyl estradiol. Coadministration of atorvastatin and ethinyl estradiol-containing oral contraceptives increased AUC values for ethinyl estradiol by 20%.

Clinical pharmacokinetic studies have not demonstrated any consistent effect of antibiotics (other than rifampin) on plasma concentrations of synthetic steroids.

- Drug products containing ethinyl estradiol may inhibit the metabolism of other compounds. Increased plasma concentrations of cyclosporine, prednisolone and theophylline have been reported with concomitant administration of oral contraceptives containing ethinyl estradiol. In addition, these drugs containing ethinyl estradiol may induce the conjugation of other compounds.

  Decreased plasma concentrations of acetaminophen and increased clearance of temazepam, salicylic acid, morphine and clofibric acid have been noted when these drugs were administered with certain ethinyl estradiol-containing drug products (e.g., oral contraceptive containing ethinyl estradiol).

Drug-Food Interactions: femHRT may be taken without regard to meals.

Drug-Herb Interactions: It was found that some herbal products (e.g., St. John's Wort), which are available as OTC products might affect metabolism, and therefore, efficacy and safety of estrogen/progestin combination products.

Physicians and other healthcare providers should be aware of other non-prescription products concomitantly used by the patient, including "herbal" and "natural" products made widely available through Health Food and pharmacy outlets.

DOSAGE AND ADMINISTRATION:

Dosing Considerations: Treated patients with an intact uterus should be monitored closely for signs of endometrial cancer, and appropriate diagnostic measures should be taken to rule out malignancy in the event of persistent or recurring vaginal bleeding. Patients should be evaluated at least annually for breast abnormalities and more often, if there are any symptoms.

Recommended Dose and Dosage Adjustment: femHRT (norethindrone acetate and ethinyl estradiol) therapy consists of a single tablet to be taken once daily, without regard for meals.

1. **Treatment of Vasomotor Symptoms**
   femHRT 0.5/2.5 or 1/5 should be given once daily for the treatment of moderate to severe vasomotor symptoms associated with the menopause. Patients should be re-evaluated within 3-6 months after initiation of treatment, to assess response to treatment.
2. **Symptomatic Treatment of Vulvar and Vaginal Atrophy Associated with Menopause**
   femHRT 0.5/2.5 or 1/5 should be given once daily for the treatment of vulvar and vaginal atrophy associated with the menopause. Patients should be re-evaluated within 3-6 months after initiation of treatment, to assess response to treatment.
3. **Prevention of Osteoporosis**
   femHRT 0.5/2.5 or 1/5 should be given once daily to prevent postmenopausal osteoporosis. Response to therapy can be assessed by measurement of bone mineral density.

Missed Dose: If the patient forgets to take the pill at the usual time, it should be taken as soon as she remembers. If it is almost time for the next pill, the missed dose should be skipped and the next pill in the pack should be taken. Two pills should not be taken at once.

OVERDOSE:

Symptoms: Numerous reports of ingestion of large doses of estrogen products and estrogen-containing oral contraceptives by young children have not revealed acute serious ill effects. Overdosage with estrogen may cause nausea, breast discomfort, fluid retention, bloating or vaginal bleeding in women.

Progestin (norethindrone acetate) overdosage has been characterized by depressed mood, tiredness, acne and hirsutism.

Treatment: In case of overdose or accidental ingestion by children, the physician should observe the patient closely and provide symptomatic treatment. Gastric lavage should be given if considered necessary.

For management of a suspected drug overdose, contact your regional Poison Control Centre. See the *CPS* Directory section for a list of Poison Control Centres.

ACTION AND CLINICAL PHARMACOLOGY:

Mechanism of Action: femHRT (norethindrone acetate and ethinyl estradiol, NA/EE) is a continuous dosage regimen of an estrogen-progestin combination for oral administration as hormone replacement therapy (HRT). femHRT manages hypoestrogenic states, especially those associated with menopause, and following oophrectomy.

Estrogen drug products, including ethinyl estradiol, act by regulating the transcription of a limited number of genes. Estrogens diffuse through cell membranes, distribute themselves throughout the cell, and bind to and activate the nuclear estrogen receptor, a DNA-binding protein, which is found in estrogen-responsive tissues. The activated estrogen receptor binds to specific DNA sequences, or hormone-response elements, which enhance the transcription of adjacent genes and in turn lead to the observed effects. Estrogen receptors have been identified in tissues of the reproductive tract, breast, pituitary, hypothalamus, liver, arterial wall and bone of women.

Progestins, including norethindrone, exert their effects in target cells by binding to specific progesterone receptors that interact with progesterone response elements in target genes. Progesterone receptors have been identified in the female reproductive tract, breast, pituitary, hypothalamus, bone, skeletal tissue and central nervous system. Norethindrone produces similar endometrial changes to those of naturally occurring hormone progesterone.

Pharmacodynamics: Estrogens: Estrogens are largely responsible for the development and maintenance of the female reproductive system and secondary sexual characteristics. Although circulating estrogens exist in a dynamic equilibrium of metabolic interconversion, estradiol is the principal intracellular human estrogen and is substantially more potent than its metabolites, estrone and estriol, at the receptor level. The primary source of estrogen in normally cycling adult women is the ovarian follicle, which secretes 70 to 500 µg of estradiol daily, depending on the phase of the menstrual cycle. After menopause, most endogenous estrogen is produced by conversion of androstenedione, secreted by the adrenal cortex, to estrone by peripheral tissues. Thus, estrone and the sulfate-conjugated form, estrone sulfate, are the most abundant circulating estrogens in postmenopausal women. The pharmacologic effects of ethinyl estradiol are similar to those of endogenous estrogens.

Circulating estrogens modulate the pituitary secretion of the gonadotropins, luteinizing hormone (LH) and follicle stimulating hormone (FSH) through a negative feedback mechanism. Estrogen replacement therapy acts to reduce the elevated levels of these hormones seen in postmenopausal women.

Estrogen replacement therapy decreases the rate of bone loss in menopausal women; evidence of estrogen receptors on bone cells suggests there is a direct effect of estrogen on bone. Estrogens also have direct effects on arterial walls through genomic and non-genomic effects.

Progestin: It has been established that the inclusion of either cyclic or continuous progestin, including norethindrone acetate, in hormone replacement therapy inhibits endometrial proliferation induced by estrogen. The inhibition of endometrial proliferation is associated with a reduction in risk of endometrial hyperplasia and the attendant risk of carcinoma in women with intact uteri.

Progestin compounds enhance cellular differentiation and generally oppose the actions of estrogens by decreasing estrogen receptor levels, increasing local metabolism of estrogens to less active metabolites, or inducing gene products that blunt cellular responses to estrogen.

Pharmacokinetics: Absorption: Norethindrone acetate (NA) and ethinyl estradiol (EE) are rapidly absorbed from femHRT tablets, with maximum plasma concentrations of norethindrone and ethinyl estradiol generally occurring 1 to 2 hours postdose. Both are subject to first-pass metabolism after oral dosing, resulting in a bioavailability of approximately 64% for norethindrone and 55% for ethinyl estradiol. Bioavailability of femHRT tablets is similar to that from solution for norethindrone and slightly less for ethinyl estradiol absorption. Administration of femHRT with a high fat meal decreases rate but not extent of ethinyl estradiol absorption. The extent of norethindrone absorption is increased by 27% following administration with food.

The full pharmacokinetic profile of femHRT (0.5 mg NA/2.5 µg EE and 1 mg NA/5 µg EE) was not characterized due to assay sensitivity limitations. Multiple-dose pharmacokinetics of 1 mg NA/10 µg EE tablets were studied in 18 postmenopausal women. Mean plasma concentrations of norethindrone and ethinyl estradiol are shown in Figure 1 and pharmacokinetic parameters are found in Table 2. Based on a population pharmacokinetic analysis, mean steady-state concentrations of norethindrone for the 1 mg NA/5 µg EE (1/5) and 1 mg NA/10 µg EE (1/10) tablets are slightly more than proportional to dose when compared to the 0.5 mg NA/ 2.5 µg EE (0.5/2.5) tablet, which is largely explained by higher sex hormone binding globulin (SHBG) concentrations. Mean steady-state plasma concentrations of ethinyl estradiol for the femHRT 0.5/2.5 and femHRT 1/5 tablets are proportional to dose, but there is a less than proportional increase in steady state concentration for the NA/EE 1/10 tablet.

Based on a population pharmacokinetic analysis, average estimates of steady-state concentrations (Css) of norethindrone and ethinyl estradiol in femHRT (NA/EE) tablets are shown in Table 3.

Distribution: Volume of distribution of norethindrone and ethinyl estradiol ranges from 2 to 4 L/kg. Plasma protein binding of both steroids is extensive (>95%); norethindrone binds to both albumin and sex hormone binding globulin (SHBG), whereas ethinyl estradiol binds only to albumin. Although ethinyl estradiol does not bind to SHBG, it induces SHBG synthesis. femHRT increases serum SHBG concentrations approximately 2.6-fold over pretreatment values.

Figure 1: femHRT

Mean Steady-state (Day 87) Plasma Norethindrone and Ethinyl Estradiol Concentrations Following Chronic Administration of NA 1 mg/EE 10 µg Tablets

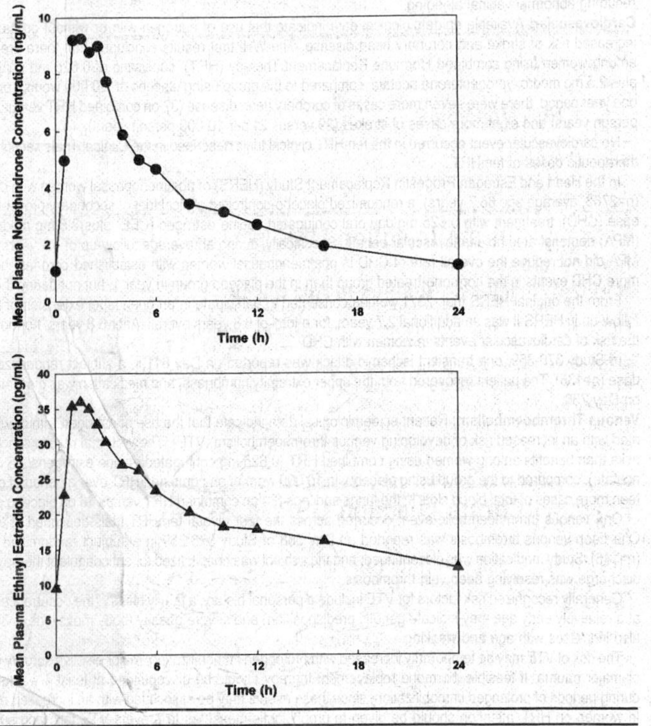

Table 2: femHRT

Mean (SD) Single-Dose (Day 1) and Steady-State (Day 87) Pharmacokinetic Parameters[a] Following Administration of 1 mg NA/10 µg EE Tablets

	C_{max}	t_{max}	$AUC_{(0-24)}$	CL/F	$t_{1/2}$
Norethindrone	ng/mL	hr	ng· hr/mL	mL/min	hr
Day 1	6.0 (3.3)	1.8 (0.8)	29.7 (16.5)	588 (416)	10.3 (3.7)
Day 87	10.7 (3.6)	1.8 (0.8)	81.8 (36.7)	226 (139)	13.3 (4.5)
Ethinyl Estradiol	pg/mL	hr	pg· hr/mL	mL/min	hr
Day 1	33.5 (13.7)	2.2 (1.0)	339 (113)	ND[b]	ND[b]
Day 87	38.3 (11.9)	1.8 (0.7)	471 (132)	383 (119)	23.9 (7.1)

[a] C_{max}=maximum plasma concentration; t_{max}=time of C_{max}; $AUC_{(0-24)}$=area under the plasma concentration-time curve over the dosing interval; and CL/F=apparent oral clearance; $t_{1/2}$=elimination half-life.
[b] ND=not determined.

Table 3: femHRT

Average Steady-State Concentrations (Css) of Norethindrone and Ethinyl Estradiol in NA/EE Tablets

	mg NA/µg EE		
	0.5/2.5	**1/5**	**1/10**
Norethindrone (ng/mL)	1.1	2.6	2.9
Ethinyl Estradiol (pg/mL)	5.4	11.4	17.2

Metabolism: Norethindrone acetate is rapidly deacetylated to norethindrone after oral administration, and the disposition of norethindrone acetate is indistinguishable from that of orally administered norethindrone. Norethindrone undergoes extensive biotransformation, primarily via reduction, followed by sulfate and glucuronide conjugation. The majority of metabolites in the circulation are sulfates, with glucuronides accounting for most of the urinary metabolites. A small amount of norethindrone acetate is metabolically converted to ethinyl estradiol, such that exposure to ethinyl estradiol following administration of 1 mg of norethindrone acetate is equivalent to oral administration of 2.8 mcg ethinyl estradiol. Ethinyl estradiol is also extensively metabolized, by both oxidation and by conjugation with sulfate and glucuronide. Sulfates are the major circulating conjugates of ethinyl estradiol and glucuronides predominate in the urine. The primary oxidative metabolite is 2-hydroxy ethinyl estradiol, formed by the CYP3A4 isoform of cytochrome P450. Part of the first-pass metabolism of ethinyl estradiol is believed to occur in gastrointestinal mucosa. Ethinyl estradiol may undergo enterohepatic circulation.

Excretion: Norethindrone and ethinyl estradiol are excreted in both urine and feces, primarily as metabolites. Plasma clearance values for norethindrone and ethinyl estradiol are similar (approximately 0.4 L/hr/kg). Steady-state elimination half-lives of norethindrone and ethinyl estradiol following administration of NA 1 mg/EE 10 µg tablets are approximately 13 hours and 24 hours, respectively.

Special Populations and Conditions: Geriatrics: The pharmacokinetics of norethindrone acetate and ethinyl estradiol was not affected by age (age range 40-62), in the postmenopausal population studied.

Hepatic Insufficiency: The effect of hepatic disease on the disposition of femHRT has not been evaluated. However, ethinyl estradiol and norethindrone may be poorly metabolized in patients with impaired liver function (see Contraindications).

Renal Insufficiency: The effect of renal disease on the disposition of femHRT has not been evaluated. In premenopausal women with chronic renal failure undergoing peritoneal dialysis who received multiple doses of an oral contraceptive containing ethinyl estradiol and norethindrone, plasma ethinyl estradiol concentrations were higher and norethindrone concentrations were unchanged compared to concentrations in premenopausal women with normal renal function.

STORAGE AND STABILITY: Store at controlled room temperature, 15-25°C.

INFORMATION FOR THE PATIENT: Published in e-CPS, available by subscription at www.e-cps.ca.

DOSAGE FORMS, COMPOSITION AND PACKAGING: 0.5/2.5: Each white, oval tablet, debossed with "PD" on one side and "145" on the other side, contains: norethindrone acetate 0.5 mg and ethinyl estradiol 2.5 µg. Nonmedicinal ingredients: calcium stearate, cornstarch, lactose monohydrate and microcrystalline cellulose. Blister cards of 28. Bottles of 90.

1/5: Each white, D-shaped tablet, debossed with "WC" on one side and "144" on the other side, contains: norethindrone acetate 1 mg and ethinyl estradiol 5 µg. Nonmedicinal ingredients: calcium stearate, cornstarch, lactose monohydrate and microcrystalline cellulose. Blister cards of 28. Bottles of 90.

(Shown in Product Identification Section)

Fentanyl Ⓝ

CPhA Monograph

see *Opioids*

Fentanyl Citrate Injection USP Ⓝ

fentanyl citrate

Narcotic Analgesic—Adjunct to Anesthesia

Hospira

SUPPLIED: Each mL of sterile, nonpyrogenic solution contains: fentanyl 50 µg as the citrate in water for injection. The solution may contain sodium hydroxide or hydrochloric acid for pH adjustment. The solution contains no bacteriostat, antimicrobial agent or added buffer and is intended only for use as a single dose injection. Ampoules of 2, 5, 10 and 20 mL and flip-top vials of 10 and 20 mL. Protect from light. Avoid excessive heat. Protect from freezing. Store at room temperature (25°C); however, brief exposure up to 40°C does not adversely affect the product.

Fentanyl Citrate Injection USP Ⓝ

fentanyl citrate

Opioid Analgesic—Adjunct to Anesthesia

Sandoz

SUPPLIED: Each mL of sterile aqueous solution contains: fentanyl 50 µg as citrate. Nonmedicinal ingredients: citric acid and/or sodium hydroxide to adjust pH and water for injection. Preservative-free. Ampuls of 2 mL, boxes of 10. Single-use vials of 5, 10 and 20 mL, boxes of 5. Pharmacy bulk vials of 50 mL, boxes of 1. Discard unused portion. Store between 15 and 30°C. Protect from light.

Fer-In-Sol®

ferrous sulfate

Hematinic

Mead Johnson Nutrition

INDICATIONS: Helps to prevent iron deficiency.

CONTRAINDICATIONS: Hemosiderosis, hemochromatosis, hemolytic anemia.

PRECAUTIONS: Oral iron preparations may aggravate existing peptic ulcer, regional enteritis and ulcerative colitis.

Iron compounds taken orally can impair the absorption of tetracycline antibiotics. Antacids given concomitantly with iron compounds decrease iron absorption. When iron drops or syrup are given to babies some darkening of the teeth may occur. This is not serious and may be removed by rubbing the teeth with baking soda.

It is very important that the appropriate dose is given as there is enough iron in the entire bottle of Fer-in-Sol to seriously harm a child. Dose should be recommended and monitored by the physician depending on iron requirements. If a child has ingested enough iron to cause toxicity, nausea, vomiting and diarrhea will usually result.

ADVERSE EFFECTS: Mild gastrointestinal upsets may rarely occur in iron-sensitive patients.

OVERDOSE:

> For management of a suspected drug overdose, CPhA recommends that you contact your **regional Poison Control Centre**. See the *CPS* Directory section for a list of Poison Control Centres.

DOSAGE: Drops: Children 0 to 2 years: Supplementation Dose: 0.5 to 1 mL daily or as directed. Therapeutic Dose: 5 mL daily or as directed by your physician. Divide into 3 doses and must take with food.

Syrup: For prevention of iron deficiency (administer once daily), or as directed by physician. Children 0 to 6 yrs: 1.25 mL; 6 to 12 yrs: 2.5 mL; adults: 5 mL. For treatment of iron deficiency, divide into 3 doses and administer between meals, mixed with water or fruit juice, or as directed by physician. Children 0 to 2 years: 2.5 to 5 mL; 2 to 6 years: 5 mL; 6 to 12 years: 5 to 12 mL; adults: 10 to 15 mL.

SUPPLIED: Drops: Each 1.0 mL of liquid contains: ferrous sulfate 75 mg (equivalent to 15 mg elemental iron). Nonmedicinal ingredients: artificial flavouring, citric acid anhydrous, ethyl alcohol, purified water, sodium bisulfite, sorbitol solution and sugar. Alcohol: 0.16%. Bottles of 50 mL with calibrated dropper.

Syrup: Each 5 mL of syrup contains: ferrous sulfate 150 mg (equivalent to 30 mg elemental iron). Each teaspoonful contains 5 mL. Nonmedicinal ingredients: artificial flavouring, citric acid anhydrous, purified water, sodium bisulfite, sodium chloride, sorbitol solution, sugar and sulfuric acid. Alcohol-free. Bottles of 250 mL.

All bottles have child-resistant closures and are safety sealed.

Fermentol®

pepsin

Digestant

Church & Dwight

SUPPLIED: Each 30 mL of green-colored, transparent liquid contains: pepsin 100 mg. Nonmedicinal ingredients: alcohol, D&C Green No. 5 and Yellow No. 10, FD&C Yellow No. 6, flavor, glycerin, polysorbate, sodium benzoate, sodium cyclamate and sugar. Hydrochloric acid and sodium hydroxide to adjust pH. Energy: 133 kJ (32 kcal.). Sodium <1mmol (10 mg). Gluten- and tartrazine-free. pH: 4.4 to 4.6. Bottles of 500 mL.

Ferodan™ Infant Drops

ferrous sulfate

Hematinic

Odan

Ferodan™ Syrup

ferrous sulfate

Hematinic

Odan

Ferodan™ Tablets

ferrous sulfate

Hematinic

Odan

SUPPLIED: Infant Drops: Each mL of light amber to green/gold solution with an aromatic fruity flavor contains: ferrous sulfate $7H_2O$ USP 75 mg (equivalent to elemental iron 15 mg). Nonmedicinal ingredients: citric acid, flavors (lemon, pineapple and strawberry), glycerin, purified water, sodium bisulfite, sorbitol and sucrose. Gluten-, lactose- and tartrazine-free. Plastic amber bottles of 50 mL with child resistant closures and calibrated dropper.

Syrup: Each 5 mL of light amber solution with an aromatic fruity flavor contains: ferrous sulfate $7H_2O$ USP 150 mg (equivalent to elemental iron 30 mg). Nonmedicinal ingredients: citric acid, flavors (lemon, pineapple and strawberry), glycerin, purified water, sodium benzoate, sodium bisulfite, sorbitol and sucrose. Gluten-, lactose- and tartrazine-free. Plastic amber unidose vials of 10 mL. Plastic amber bottles of 250 and 500 mL with child-resistant closures and safety seals.

Tablets: Each red, round odorless tablet contains: 300 mg of ferrous sulfate $7H_2O$ (equivalent to 60.27 mg of elemental iron). Nonmedicinal ingredients: carnauba wax, crospovidone, FD&C Blue # 2, FD&C Red # 40, FD&C Yellow # 6, hypromellose, magnesium stearate, microcrystalline cellulose, polyethylene glycol, povidone, titanium dioxide and triacetin. Gluten-, lactose- and tartrazine-free. White plastic bottles of 1000.

Ferrous Fumarate

CPhA Monograph

see *Iron Salts: Oral*

Ferrous Gluconate

CPhA Monograph

see *Iron Salts: Oral*

Ferrous Sulfate

CPhA Monograph

see *Iron Salts: Oral*

Finacea® Ⓟ

azelaic acid

Antirosacea Agent

Bayer

Date of Revision: February 22, 2010

SUMMARY PRODUCT INFORMATION:

Route of Administration	Dosage Form/ Strength	Clinically Relevant Nonmedicinal Ingredients
Topical	Gel/15%	Benzoic acid, disodium edetate, lecithin, medium-chain triglycerides, polyacrylic acid, polysorbate 80, propylene glycol, sodium hydroxide For a complete listing see Dosage Forms, Composition and Packaging.

INDICATIONS AND CLINICAL USE: FINACEA (azelaic acid gel) is indicated for:

- Topical treatment of inflammatory papules and pustules and erythema of mild to moderate rosacea.

CONTRAINDICATIONS:

- FINACEA (azelaic acid gel) is contraindicated in individuals with a history of hypersensitivity to azelaic acid, propylene glycol or to any other component of the formulation. For a complete listing, see Dosage Forms, Composition and Packaging.

WARNINGS AND PRECAUTIONS: General: FINACEA (azelaic acid gel) should be used only as directed by a physician.

FINACEA is for dermatological use only, and not for ophthalmic, oral, rectal or intravaginal use.

Carcinogenesis and Mutagenesis: Long-term animal studies have not been performed to evaluate the carcinogenic potential of FINACEA Gel. Azelaic acid was not mutagenic or clastogenic in a battery of in vitro [Ames assay, HGPRT in V79 cells (Chinese hamster lung cells), and chromosomal aberration assay in human lymphocytes] and in vivo [dominant lethal assay in mice and mouse micronucleus assay] genotoxicity tests.

Oral administration of azelaic acid at dose levels up to 2500 mg/kg/day [162 times the maximum recommended human dose based on body surface area] did not affect fertility or reproductive performance in male or female rats.

Skin: FINACEA contains benzoic acid and propylene glycol which may cause mild irritant cutaneous and mucocutaneous reactions. Care should be taken to avoid contact with the eyes, mouth and other mucous membranes, and patients should be instructed accordingly. In the event of accidental contact, the eyes, mouth and/or affected mucous membranes should be washed with large amounts of water. If eye irritation persists, patients should consult a physician.

If pronounced local irritation occurs, patients should be directed to temporarily use the medication less frequently or to discontinue use for a few days. In case of sensitization, or if severe irritation persists, FINACEA should be discontinued and appropriate therapy instituted.

There have been isolated reports of hypopigmentation after use of azelaic acid. Since azelaic acid has not been well studied in patients with a dark complexion, these patients should be monitored for early signs of hypopigmentation.

Special Populations: Pregnant Women: Experience with the use of FINACEA by pregnant women is very limited and does not permit assessment of the product safety during pregnancy.

Reproduction toxicology studies were conducted with systemically administered (oral) azelaic acid in rats, rabbits and cynomolgus monkeys. Embryotoxicity was observed in rats, rabbits and monkeys given maternally toxic oral doses of azelaic acid during organogenesis. This effect was observed in rats given 2500 mg/kg/day (125 times the maximum recommended human dose based on body surface area), rabbits given 150 or 500 mg/kg/day (15 or 49 times the maximum recommended human dose based on body surface area) and cynomolgus monkeys given 500 mg/kg/day (50 times the maximum recommended human dose based on body surface area). No teratogenic effects were observed.

Because animal reproduction studies are not always predictive of human response, this drug should be used during pregnancy only if clearly needed.

Nursing Women: Equilibrium dialysis was used to assess human milk partitioning in vitro. At an azelaic acid concentration of 25 µg/mL, the milk/plasma distribution coefficient was 0.7 and the milk/buffer distribution was 1.0, indicating that passage of the drug into the maternal milk may occur. Since less than 4% of a topically applied dose is systemically absorbed, the uptake of azelaic acid into maternal milk is not expected to cause a significant change from baseline azelaic acid levels in the milk. However, caution should be exercised when FINACEA is administered to a nursing mother.
Pediatrics (<18 years of age): The safety and effectiveness of FINACEA in pediatric patients has not been established.
Geriatrics (>65 years of age): Clinical studies of FINACEA did not include sufficient numbers of subjects aged 65 and over to determine whether they respond differently than younger subjects.

ADVERSE REACTIONS: Adverse Drug Reaction Overview: Local skin irritation (mostly burning or itching sensations, occasionally reddening and scaling) may occur, usually at the start of treatment with FINACEA (azelaic acid gel). In the majority of cases, the irritation symptoms are mild and generally regress during the course of treatment. In very rare cases, allergic skin reactions (e.g., rash) may occur (see Contraindications).
Clinical Trial Adverse Drug Reactions: Because clinical trials are conducted under very specific conditions, the adverse reaction rates observed in the clinical trials may not reflect the rates observed in practice and should not be compared to the rates in the clinical trials of another drug. Adverse drug reaction information from clinical trials is useful for identifying drug-related adverse events and for approximating rates.

In pivotal studies (two 12-week, vehicle-controlled clinical trials; n=664), safety was monitored in the 333 patients who used FINACEA and the 331 patients who used the gel vehicle.

Table 1: FINACEA

Cutaneous Adverse Events Occurring in 1% or More of Subjects in Two Clinical Trials in Rosacea Patients, by Treatment Group and Maximum Intensity[a]

	FINACEA n=333 (100%)			Vehicle n=331 (100%)		
	Mild n=86 (26%)	Moderate n=44 (13%)	Severe n=20 (6%)	Mild n=49 (15%)	Moderate n=27 (8%)	Severe n=5 (2%)
Cutaneous						
Burning/stinging/tingling	66 (20%)	30 (9%)	12 (4%)	8 (2%)	6 (2%)	2 (1%)
Pruritus	24 (7%)	14 (4%)	3 (1%)	9 (3%)	6 (2%)	0 (0%)
Scaling/dry skin/xerosis	21 (6%)	8 (2%)	4 (1%)	33 (10%)	12 (4%)	1 (0%)
Erythema/irritation	6 (2%)	6 (2%)	1 (0%)	8 (2%)	4 (1%)	2 (1%)
Edema	3 (1%)	2 (1%)	1 (0%)	3 (1%)	0 (0%)	0 (0%)
Contact dermatitis	2 (1%)	2 (1%)	0 (0%)	1 (0%)	0 (0%)	0 (0%)
Acne	2 (1%)	1 (0%)	0 (0%)	1 (0%)	0 (0%)	0 (0%)
Seborrhea	2 (1%)	0 (0%)	0 (0%)	0 (0%)	0 (0%)	0 (0%)
Photosensitivity	1 (0%)	0 (0%)	0 (0%)	3 (1%)	1 (0%)	1 (0%)
Skin disease	1 (0%)	0 (0%)	0 (0%)	1 (0%)	2 (1%)	0 (0%)

[a] Subjects may have >1 cutaneous adverse event; thus, the sum of the frequencies of the preferred terms may exceed the number of subjects with at least 1 cutaneous adverse event.

No phototoxicity or photoallergenicity was reported in the controlled clinical studies and in human dermal safety studies.
Less Common Clinical Trial Adverse Drug Reactions (<1%): Cardiovascular: vasodilatation.
Genitourinary: exacerbation of recurrent herpes labialis, herpes simplex and herpes zoster infections.
Respiratory: worsening of asthma.
Skin: acne flare, nevi, hirsutism, vitiligo depigmentation, small depigmented spots, hypertrichosis, reddening (signs of keratosis pilaris), mycosis.
Post-Market Adverse Drug Reactions: Adverse events occurring post-market with FINACEA are consistent with those reported during clinical trials.

DRUG INTERACTIONS: Overview: There have been no formal studies evaluating the interaction of FINACEA (azelaic acid gel) with other drugs.

The pivotal clinical trials excluded concomitant use of medications that affect rosacea.

DOSAGE AND ADMINISTRATION: Recommended Dose and Dosage Adjustment: FINACEA (azelaic acid gel) is intended for topical use only.

Before application, the skin should be thoroughly washed and patted dry with a soft towel. Only very mild soaps or mild soapless cleansing lotions should be used.

A thin layer of FINACEA (0.5 g or approximately 2.5 cm of gel) should be applied twice daily, in the morning and evening, to the entire affected areas and gently massaged into the skin. The use of occlusive dressings or wrappings should be avoided, and the hands should be washed following application. During application, contact with the eyes should be avoided. In case of accidental exposure, the eyes should be rinsed with plenty of water.

It is important to use FINACEA continuously over the entire period of treatment.

In the event of skin irritation, the amount of gel per application should be reduced or the frequency of use of FINACEA should be decreased to once a day until the irritation ceases. If required, the treatment should be interrupted for a few days.

Avoid contact with the mouth, eyes and other mucous membranes. If FINACEA comes in contact with the eyes, wash with large amounts of water and consult a physician if eye irritation persists.

The hands should be washed after application of FINACEA.

The duration of use of FINACEA can vary from person to person and also depends on the severity of rosacea. Significant initial therapeutic effects have been observed after four to eight weeks of treatment.

Non-medicated cosmetics or cosmetics free of substances causing acniforme eruptions or irritations may be applied after the application of FINACEA has dried.

Patients should be instructed to avoid spicy foods, hot foods and drinks, and alcoholic beverages.

OVERDOSAGE:
FINACEA (azelaic acid gel) is intended for cutaneous use only. If pronounced local irritation occurs due to excessive application, patients should be directed to temporarily use the medication less frequently or to discontinue use until symptoms and signs subside (see Warnings and Precautions).

Acute toxicology studies in laboratory animals do not indicate that acute intoxication is to be expected following oral ingestion of large amounts of the drug.

> For management of a suspected drug overdose, CPhA recommends that you contact your **regional Poison Control Centre**. See the *CPS* Directory section for a list of Poison Control Centres.

ACTION AND CLINICAL PHARMACOLOGY: Pharmacodynamics: Azelaic acid has been characterized as anti-keratinizing and anti-bacterial. The mechanisms by which azelaic acid interferes with the pathogenic events in rosacea are unknown, but appear to include an anti-inflammatory effect. In vitro findings indicate that azelaic acid inhibits the production and/or release of reactive pro-inflammatory oxygen species from neutrophils. The clinical relevance of this in vitro effect is unknown.

Pharmacokinetics: Absorption: Endogenous plasma concentration (20 to 80 ng/mL) and daily urinary excretion (4 to 28 mg) of azelaic acid are highly dependent on dietary intake. The percutaneous absorption of azelaic acid after topical application of azelaic acid 15% gel is unknown. After topical application of an azelaic acid 20% cream, approximately 4% of azelaic acid is systemically absorbed. There was no difference between azelaic acid 15% gel and azelaic acid 20% cream in the urinary excretion of azelaic acid in patients with facial acne treated over a period of 8 weeks. Additionally, plasma azelaic acid concentrations in rosacea patients treated with FINACEA gel twice daily for at least 8 weeks are within the range of endogenous plasma azelaic acid concentrations. This indicates that FINACEA does not increase plasma azelaic acid concentration beyond the range derived from nutrition and endogenous metabolism.
Metabolism: Azelaic acid is a dietary constituent (found in whole-grain cereals and animal products), and can be formed endogenously from longer-chain dicarboxylic acids, metabolism of oleic acid, and β-oxidation of monocarboxylic acids. Negligible cutaneous metabolism occurs after topical application.
Excretion: Azelaic acid is mainly excreted unchanged in the urine, but undergoes some β-oxidation to shorter-chain dicarboxylic acids. The observed half-lives in healthy subjects are approximately 45 minutes after oral dosing and 12 hours after topical dosing of the cream, indicating percutaneous absorption rate-limited kinetics.

STORAGE AND STABILITY: Store at room temperature (between 15 and 30°C).

SPECIAL HANDLING INSTRUCTIONS: Keep out of the reach of children before and after use.

INFORMATION FOR THE PATIENT: Published in e-CPS, available by subscription at www.e-cps.ca.

DOSAGE FORMS, COMPOSITION AND PACKAGING: Each g contains: azelaic acid 0.15 g (15% w/w) in an aqueous gel base. Nonmedicinal ingredients: benzoic acid (as a preservative), disodium edetate, lecithin, medium-chain triglycerides, polyacrylic acid, polysorbate 80, propylene glycol, purified water and sodium hydroxide to adjust pH. Tubes of 5 and 50 g. Each tube is made of aluminum, with a membrane closure, an internal epoxide resin coating, a white exterior and a screw cap made of high-density polyethylene.

Fiorinal® Ⓒ

ASA—caffeine—butalbital

Analgesic—Sedative

Novartis Pharmaceuticals

Date of Revision: July 19, 2004

INDICATIONS: For tension (or muscle contraction) headache and conditions where a simultaneous sedative and analgesic action is required, such as mixed migraine headaches, menstrual and postpartum tension and pain.

CONTRAINDICATIONS: FIORINAL is contraindicated under the following conditions:

1. Hypersensitivity or intolerance to ASA, caffeine, or butalbital or to any of the components.
2. Patients with a hemorrhagic diathesis (e.g., hemophilia, hypoprothrombinemia, von Willebrand's disease, the thrombocytopenias, thrombasthenia and other ill-defined hereditary platelet dysfunctions, severe vitamin K deficiency and severe liver damage).
3. Patients with the syndrome of nasal polyps, angioedema and bronchospastic reactivity to ASA or other nonsteroidal anti-inflammatory drugs. Anaphylactoid reactions have occurred in such patients.
4. Peptic ulcer or other serious gastrointestinal lesions.
5. Patients with porphyria.
6. In patients with overdosage of, or intoxication due to alcohol, hypnotics, analgesics and psychotropic drugs.

WARNINGS: Therapeutic doses of ASA can cause anaphylactic shock and other severe allergic reactions. It should be ascertained if the patient is allergic to ASA, although a specific history of allergy may be lacking.

Significant bleeding can result from ASA therapy in patients with peptic ulcer or other gastrointestinal lesions, and in patients with bleeding disorders.

ASA administered pre-operatively may prolong the bleeding time.

Butalbital is habit-forming and potentially abusable. Consequently, the extended use of FIORINAL is not recommended.

A possible association between Reye's syndrome and the use of salicylates has been suggested but not established. Reye's syndrome has also occurred in many patients not exposed to salicylates. However, caution is advised when prescribing salicylate-containing medications for children, teenagers and young adults with influenza or chickenpox.

PRECAUTIONS: Because of its ASA content, FIORINAL should be used with caution in patients with a history of bleeding tendencies or peptic ulceration, in patients on anticoagulant therapy and in patients with underlying hemostatic defects.

Precautions should be taken when administering salicylates to persons with known allergies. Hypersensitivity to ASA is particularly likely in patients with nasal polyps and relatively common in those with asthma.

Long-term use of preparations containing barbiturates may lead to habituation and physical dependence. FIORINAL, because of its butalbital content, should be avoided in patients with head injury, in whom a depressed CNS is suspected. Similarly, it should not be used in patients with actual or a predisposition towards respiratory depression.

FIORINAL should be prescribed with caution for certain special-risk patients, such as the elderly or debilitated, and those with severe impairment of renal or hepatic function, coagulation disorders, head injuries, elevated intracranial pressure, acute abdominal conditions, hypothyroidism, urethral stricture, Addison's disease, prostatic hypertrophy, or in osteomalacia and osteoporosis.

Occupational Hazards: Barbiturate containing preparations may impair the mental and/or physical alertness required for the efficient performance of hazardous tasks such as driving a vehicle or operating machinery.

Pregnancy: It is not known whether FIORINAL can cause fetal harm when administered to a pregnant woman or can affect reproduction capacity.

Ingestion of ASA prior to delivery may prolong delivery or lead to bleeding in the mother or neonate.

Lactation: ASA, caffeine and barbiturates are excreted in breast milk in small amounts, but the significance of their effects on nursing infants is not known. Because of potential for serious adverse reactions in nursing infants from FIORINAL, a decision should be made whether to discontinue nursing or to discontinue the drug, taking into account the importance of the drug to the mother.

During pregnancy and lactation, FIORINAL should be taken only as prescribed.

Drug Interactions: The concomitant use of alcohol or other CNS depressants may have an additive effect, and patients should be warned accordingly.

The CNS effects of butalbital may be enhanced by monoamine oxidase (MAO) inhibitors.

In patients receiving concomitant corticosteroids and chronic use of ASA, withdrawal of corticosteroids may result in salicylism because corticosteroids enhance renal clearance of salicylates and their withdrawal is followed by return to normal rates of renal clearance.

FIORINAL may enhance the effects of:

1. Oral antidiabetic agents and insulin, causing hypoglycemia by contributing an additive effect if dosage of FIORINAL exceeds maximum recommended dosage.
2. Oral anticoagulants, causing bleeding by inhibiting prothrombin formation in the liver and displacing anticoagulants from plasma protein binding sites.
3. 6-mercaptopurine and methotrexate, causing bone marrow toxicity and blood dyscrasias by displacing these drugs from secondary binding sites, and, in the case of methotrexate, also reducing its excretion.
4. Nonsteroidal anti-inflammatory agents, increasing the risk of peptic ulceration and bleeding by contributing additive effects.
5. Other narcotic analgesics, alcohol, general anesthetics, tranquilizers such as chlordiazepoxide, sedative-hypnotics, or other CNS depressants, causing increased CNS depression.

FIORINAL may diminish the effects of: uricosuric agents such as probenecid and sulfinpyrazone, reducing their effectiveness in the treatment of gout. ASA competes with these agents for protein binding sites.

The prolonged ingestion of barbiturates gives rise to enzyme induction. This increases the rate of metabolism of certain drugs, including oral anticoagulants and oral contraceptives, thus reducing their effectiveness.

Drug/Laboratory Test Interactions: ASA: ASA may interfere with the following laboratory determinations in blood: serum amylase, fasting blood glucose, cholesterol, protein, aspartate aminotransferase (AST), uric acid, prothrombin time and bleeding time. ASA may interfere with the following laboratory determinations in urine: glucose, 5-hydroxyindoleacetic acid, Gerhardt ketone, vanillylmandelic acid (VMA), uric acid, diacetic acid, and spectrophotometric detection of barbiturates.

Dependance: FIORINAL products have the potential for being abused and should be avoided in chronic pain states leading to continuous daily use.

ADVERSE EFFECTS: The most frequent adverse reactions are drowsiness and dizziness. Less frequent adverse reactions are constipation, rash, miosis, lightheadedness and gastrointestinal disturbances including nausea, vomiting and flatulence. A single incidence of bone marrow suppression has been reported with the use of FIORINAL. Several cases of dermatological reactions including toxic epidermal necrolysis and erythema multiforme have been reported.

OVERDOSE:

Symptoms: 1) Acute barbiturate poisoning: drowsiness, confusion and coma, with reduced or absent reflexes; prominent, persistent respiratory depression; hypotension, followed by circulatory collapse and a typical shock like state in severe intoxication; respiratory complications, renal failure, and, possibly, death. 2) Acute ASA poisoning: principal toxic effects include hyperpnea; hypercapnia; acid-base disturbances with the development of metabolic acidosis, especially in children; and gastrointestinal irritation with vomiting and abdominal pain. Also, acetone odour in breath, tinnitus, sweating, hyperthermia, dehydration, hypoprothrombinemia with spontaneous bleeding, restlessness, delirium, convulsions and coma may occur. 3) Acute caffeine poisoning: insomnia, restlessness, tinnitus and flashes of light; tachycardia and extrasystoles; tremor, delirium and coma, following high doses in the region of 10 g. Death has not been reported with caffeine overdosage.

Note: Because large doses of barbiturates alone may cause marked respiratory and CNS depression, an even more profound depressant effect may be expected after an overdosage of FIORINAL.

The dangers of FIORINAL overdosage are increased when the drug is ingested in the presence of alcohol, phenothiazines, minor tranquilizers and/or narcotics.

Treatment: The management of acute FIORINAL overdosage may involve the treatment of the toxic effects of all its constituents, with the possible exception of caffeine, which is toxic in very high doses only. Generally, it is the management of the barbiturate intoxication and the correction of the acid-base imbalance due to salicylism which demand most attention. The therapeutic procedures most commonly employed are:

Elimination of the offending drug: 1) Emesis: if the patient is conscious, induce vomiting with syrup of ipecac (15 to 30 mL). 2) Perform gastric lavage followed by the administration of activated charcoal if the pharyngeal and laryngeal reflexes are present and if less than 4 hours have elapsed since ingestion. Do not attempt gastric lavage on the unconscious patient unless cuffed endotracheal intubation has been performed to prevent aspiration and pulmonary complications. 3) Catharsis: Following gastric lavage, a saline cathartic (sodium or magnesium sulfate 30 g in 250 mL of water) may be introduced and left in the stomach. 4) Encourage diuresis by administration of i.v. fluids assisted, if necessary, by 100 to 150 mL 25% mannitol solution given slowly i.v. Note: Mannitol should not be mixed with blood in a transfusion set, as red cell crenation and agglutination may occur. 5) Alkalinization of the urine (see caution): i.v. isotonic sodium bicarbonate solution accelerates urinary excretion of barbiturates. Maximum alkalinization may be more successfully attained if the sodium bicarbonate infusion is accompanied by acetazolamide 250 mg given as a single i.v. injection every 6 hours. (Caution: perform urinary alkalinization with care in children). 6) peritoneal dialysis and hemodialysis have been used with success in acute barbiturate intoxication and may be life saving. However, before embarking on either method, weigh the risks inherent to these procedures against the risk of not using them at all.

Maintenance of adequate pulmonary ventilation: Respiratory depression is an early and often profound manifestation of acute barbiturate poisoning. Meticulous attention to this aspect of treatment is essential. Perform pharyngeal and tracheal suction diligently to remove excess mucous secretions. Judicious administration of oxygen is also indicated. However, oxygen without assisted respiration must be used with caution, as its use in hypoventilation hypoxia may result in further respiratory depression and hypercapnia. In more critical cases, endotracheal intubation or tracheotomy, with or without assisted respiration, may be necessary.

Correction of hypotension: Vigorous treatment is essential, as circulatory collapse and renal failure are frequent causes of death. 1) Mild cases: the usual head down position and other supportive measures may be adequate. 2) Severe cases: Vasopressors (dopamine, levarterenol) may be given i.v. with the usual precautions and serial blood pressure monitoring.

Special features due to salicylate overdosage: 1) The prominent features of salicylate intoxication are metabolic acidosis and electrolyte disturbance, and these require evaluation and correction. Sodium bicarbonate 400 mg (5 mEq)/kg as a 1% solution in 5% dextrose water is not only effective in correcting acidosis, but effectively and rapidly accelerates salicylate excretion by the kidneys. The administration of sodium bicarbonate must be carefully monitored with frequent blood pH and plasma CO_2 content determinations, as large amounts of sodium bicarbonate may result in severe alkalosis, particularly in children. THAM, an osmotic alkalinizing diuretic, also greatly increases the excretion of salicylate. This is given as a 0.3 molar solution at a rate not exceeding 5 mL/kg/hour. Potassium deficiency may occur and should be corrected. 2) Treat hyperthermia and dehydration with ice packs and i.v. fluids. 3) Treat hypoprothrombinemia with vitamin K_1 50 mg given daily i.v. 4) Hemodialysis, peritoneal dialysis or exchange transfusion are indicated in very severe salicylate intoxication. However, in FIORINAL overdosage, these measures are indicated mainly for barbiturate intoxication but would be effective for both.

General supportive measures: 1) Good nursing care is of prime importance, particularly in the comatose patient, and should include regular observation and accurate recording of the vital signs and depth of coma, maintenance of a free airway, frequent turning, and other routine measures usually adopted with unconscious patients. 2) Careful supervision and recording of fluid intake and output is essential. 3) Take blood samples to determine barbiturate blood concentrations and for electrolyte and other pertinent blood studies.

> For management of a suspected drug overdose, CPhA recommends that you contact your **regional Poison Control Centre**. See the *CPS* Directory section for a list of Poison Control Centres.

DOSAGE: Adults: 2 capsules at once, followed if necessary, by 1 capsule every 3 to 4 hours; up to 6 capsules daily, or as prescribed.

Children: 1 to 3 capsules a day, according to age.

SUPPLIED: Each hard gelatin, oblong capsule, purple opaque with blue opaque cap, printed with "FIORINAL" and "⚠" in white ink contains: butalbital, USP 50 mg, caffeine, USP 40 mg and ASA, USP 330 mg. Nonmedicinal ingredients: cornstarch, microcrystalline cellulose, stearic acid and talc. Bottles of 100.

Fiorinal®-C ¼, ½ Ⓝ

ASA—caffeine—codeine phosphate—butalbital

Analgesic—Sedative

Novartis Pharmaceuticals

Date of Revision: July 20, 2004

INDICATIONS: The relief of acute and chronic pain of mild, moderate, or severe degree, which is accompanied by tension or anxiety and in all indications where a simultaneous sedative and analgesic action is required, such as: tension headache, musculoskeletal pain, including low back pain, postoperative, post-partum pain, dysmenorrhea, pain associated with dental procedures, neoplastic disease or trauma.

CONTRAINDICATIONS: FIORINAL-C is contraindicated under the following conditions:

1. Hypersensitivity or intolerance to ASA, caffeine, or butalbital or to any of the components.
2. Patients with a hemorrhagic diathesis (e.g., hemophilia, hypoprothrombinemia, von Willebrand's disease, the thrombocytopenias, thrombasthenia and other ill-defined hereditary platelet dysfunctions, severe vitamin K deficiency and severe liver damage).
3. Patients with the syndrome of nasal polyps, angioedema and bronchospastic reactivity to ASA or other nonsteroidal anti-inflammatory drugs. Anaphylactoid reactions have occurred in such patients.
4. Peptic ulcer or other serious gastrointestinal lesions.
5. Patients with porphyria.
6. In patients with overdosage of, or intoxication due to alcohol, hypnotics, analgesics and psychotropic drugs.

WARNINGS: Therapeutic doses of ASA can cause anaphylactic shock and other severe allergic reactions. It should be ascertained if the patient is allergic to ASA, although a specific history of allergy may be lacking.

Significant bleeding can result from ASA therapy in patients with peptic ulcer or other gastrointestinal lesions, and in patients with bleeding disorders.

ASA administered pre-operatively may prolong the bleeding time.

In the presence of head injury or other intracranial lesions, the respiratory depressant effects of codeine and other narcotics may be markedly enhanced, as well as their capacity for elevating cerebrospinal fluid pressure. Narcotics also produce other CNS depressant effects, such as drowsiness, that may further obscure the clinical course of patients with head injuries.

Codeine or other narcotics may obscure signs on which to judge the diagnosis or clinical course of patients with acute abdominal conditions.

Butalbital and codeine are both habit-forming and potentially abusable. Consequently, the extended use of FIORINAL-C is not recommended.

A possible association between Reye's syndrome and the use of salicylates has been suggested but not established. Reye's syndrome has also occurred in many patients not exposed to salicylates. However, caution is advised when prescribing salicylate-containing medications for children, teenagers and young adults with influenza or chickenpox.

PRECAUTIONS: Because of its ASA content, FIORINAL-C should be used with caution in patients with a history of bleeding tendencies or peptic ulceration, in patients on anticoagulant therapy and in patients with underlying hemostatic defects.

Precautions should be taken when administering salicylates to persons with known allergies. Hypersensitivity to ASA is particularly likely in patients with nasal polyps and relatively common in those with asthma.

Long-term use of preparations containing barbiturates and/or codeine may lead to habituation and physical dependence. FIORINAL-C, because of its codeine and butalbital content, should be avoided in patients with head injury, in whom a depressed CNS is suspected. Similarly, it should not be used in patients with actual or a predisposition towards respiratory depression.

FIORINAL-C should be prescribed with caution for certain special-risk patients, such as the elderly or debilitated, and those with severe impairment of renal or hepatic function, coagulation disorders, head injuries, elevated intracranial pressure, acute abdominal conditions, hypothyroidism, urethral stricture, Addison's disease, prostatic hypertrophy, or in osteomalacia and osteoporosis.

Occupational Hazards: Barbiturate containing preparations may impair the mental and/or physical alertness required for the efficient performance of hazardous tasks such as driving a vehicle or operating machinery.

Pregnancy: It is not known whether FIORINAL-C can cause fetal harm when administered to a pregnant woman or can affect reproduction capacity.

Ingestion of ASA prior to delivery may prolong delivery or lead to bleeding in the mother or neonate. Use of codeine during labour may lead to respiratory depression in the neonate.

Lactation: ASA, caffeine, barbiturates and codeine are excreted in breast milk in small amounts, but the significance of their effects on nursing infants is not known. Because of potential for serious adverse reactions in nursing infants from FIORINAL-C, a decision should be made whether to discontinue nursing or to discontinue the drug, taking into account the importance of the drug to the mother.

During pregnancy and lactation, FIORINAL-C should be taken only as prescribed.

Drug Interactions: The concomitant use of alcohol or other CNS depressants may have an additive effect, and patients should be warned accordingly.

The CNS effects of butalbital may be enhanced by monoamine oxidase (MAO) inhibitors.

In patients receiving concomitant corticosteroids and chronic use of ASA, withdrawal of corticosteroids may results in salicylism because corticosteroids enhance renal clearance of salicylates and their withdrawal is followed by return to normal rates of renal clearance.

The prolonged ingestion of barbiturates gives rise to enzyme induction. This increases the rate of metabolism of certain drugs, including oral anticoagulants and oral contraceptives, thus reducing their effectiveness.

FIORINAL-C may enhance the effects of:

1. Oral antidiabetic agents and insulin, causing hypoglycemia by contributing an additive effect if dosage of FIORINAL-C exceeds maximum recommended daily dosage.
2. Oral anticoagulants, causing bleeding by inhibiting prothrombin formation in the liver and displacing anticoagulants from plasma protein binding sites.
3. 6-mercaptopurine and methotrexate, causing bone marrow toxicity and blood dyscrasias by displacing these drugs from secondary binding sites, and, in the case of methotrexate, also reducing its excretion.
4. Nonsteroidal anti-inflammatory agents, increasing the risk of peptic ulceration and bleeding by contributing additive effects.
5. Other narcotic analgesics, alcohol, general anesthetics, tranquilizers such as chlordiazepoxide, sedative-hypnotics, or other CNS depressants, causing increased CNS depression.

FIORINAL-C may diminish the effects of: uricosuric agents such as probenecid and sulfinpyrazone, reducing their effectiveness in the treatment of gout. ASA competes with these agents for protein binding sites.

Drug/Laboratory Test Interactions: ASA: ASA may interfere with the following laboratory determinations in blood: serum amylase, fasting blood glucose, cholesterol, protein, aspartate aminotransferase (AST), uric acid, prothrombin time and bleeding time. ASA may interfere with the following laboratory determinations in urine: glucose, 5-hydroxyindoleactic acid, Gerhardt ketone, vanillylmandelic acid (VMA), uric acid, diacetic acid, and spectrophotometric detection of barbiturates.

Codeine: Codeine may increase serum amylase levels.

Children: Safety and effectiveness in pediatric patients have not been established.

Dependance: FIORINAL-C products have the potential for being abused and should be avoided in chronic pain states leading to continuous daily use.

ADVERSE EFFECTS: Commonly Observed: The most commonly reported adverse events associated with the use of FIORINAL-C and not reported at an equivalent incidence by placebo-treated patients were nausea and/or abdominal pain, drowsiness and dizziness. Vomiting, constipation, skin rash and miosis are possible adverse effects.

Incidence in Controlled Clinical Trials: Table 1 summarizes the incidence rates of the adverse events reported by at least 1% of the FIORINAL-C treated patients in controlled clinical trials comparing FIORINAL-C to placebo, and provides a comparison to the incidence rates reported by the placebo-treated patients.

The prescriber should be aware that these figures cannot be used to predict the incidence of side effects in the course of usual medical practice where patient characteristics and other factors differ from those that prevailed in the clinical trials. Similarly, the cited frequencies cannot be compared with figures obtained from other clinical investigations involving different treatments, uses, and investigators.

Other Adverse Events Reported During Controlled Clinical Trials: The listing that follows represents the proportion of the 382 patients exposed to FIORINAL-C while participating in the controlled clinical trials who reported, on at least one occasion, an adverse event of the type cited. All reported adverse events, except those already presented in Table 1, are included. It is important to emphasize that, although the adverse events reported did occur while the patient was receiving FIORINAL-C, the adverse events were not necessarily caused by FIORINAL-C.

Adverse events are classified by body system and frequency. "Frequent" is defined as an adverse event which occurred in at least 1/100 (1%) of the patients; all adverse events listed in Table 1 are frequent. "Infrequent" is defined as an adverse event that occurred in less than 1/100 patients but at least 1/1000 patients. All adverse events tabulated below are classified as infrequent.

Central nervous: headache, shaky feeling, tingling, agitation, fainting, fatigue, heavy eyelids, high energy, hot spells, numbness, and sluggishness.

Autonomic nervous: dry mouth and hyperhidrosis.

Gastrointestinal: vomiting, difficulty swallowing, and heartburn.

Cardiovascular: tachycardia.

Musculoskeletal: leg pain and muscle fatigue.

Genitourinary: diuresis.

Miscellaneous: pruritus, fever, earache, nasal congestion, and tinnitus.

Post-Marketing Reported Adverse Events: Voluntary reports of adverse drug events, temporally associated with FIORINAL-C, that have been received since market introduction and that were not reported in clinical trials by the patients treated with FIORINAL-C, are listed below. Many or most of these events may have no causal relationship with the drug and are listed according to body system.

Central nervous: abuse, addiction, anxiety, depression, disorientation, hallucination, hyperactivity, insomnia, libido decrease, nervousness, neuropathy, psychosis, sedation, sexual activity increase, slurred speech, twitching, unconsciousness, vertigo.

Autonomic nervous: epistaxis, flushing, miosis, salivation.

Gastrointestinal: anorexia, appetite increased, constipation, diarrhea, esophagitis, gastroenteritis, gastrointestinal spasm, hiccup, mouth burning, pyloric ulcer.

Cardiovascular: chest pain, hypotensive reaction, palpitations, syncope.

Skin: erythema, erythema multiforme, exfoliative dermatitis, hives, rash, toxic epidermal necrolysis.

Urinary: kidney impairment, urinary difficulty.

Miscellaneous: allergic reaction, anaphylactic shock, cholangiocarcinoma, drug interaction with erythromycin (stomach upset), edema.

The following adverse drug events may be borne in mind as potential effects of the components of FIORINAL-C. Potential effects of high dosage are listed in the Overdose section.

ASA: occult blood loss, hemolytic anemia, iron deficiency anemia, gastric distress, heartburn, nausea, peptic ulcer, prolonged bleeding time, acute airway obstruction, renal toxicity when taken in high doses for prolonged periods, impaired urate excretion, hepatitis.

Caffeine: cardiac stimulation, irritability, tremor, dependence, nephrotoxicity, hyperglycemia.
Codeine: nausea, vomiting, drowsiness, lightheadedness, constipation, pruritus.

Table 1: FIORINAL-C

Adverse Events Reported by at Least 1% of FIORINAL-C Treated Patients During Placebo Controlled Clinical Trials

	Incidence Rate of Adverse Events	
Body System/Adverse Event	**FIORINAL-C (N=382) %**	**Placebo (N=377) %**
Central Nervous		
Drowsiness	2.4	0.5
Dizziness/Lightheadedness	2.6	0.5
Intoxicated Feeling	1.0	0.0
Gastrointestinal		
Nausea/Abdominal Pain	3.7	0.8

OVERDOSE:

Symptoms: 1) Acute barbiturate poisoning: drowsiness, confusion and coma, with reduced or absent reflexes; prominent, persistent respiratory depression; hypotension, followed by circulatory collapse and a typical shock like state in severe intoxication; respiratory complications, renal failure, and, possibly, death. 2) Acute ASA poisoning: principal toxic effects include hyperpnea; hypercapnia; acid-base disturbances with the development of metabolic acidosis, especially in children; and gastrointestinal irritation with vomiting and abdominal pain. Also, acetone odour in breath, tinnitus, sweating, hyperthermia, dehydration, hypoprothrombinemia with spontaneous bleeding, restlessness, delirium, convulsions and coma may occur. 3) Acute caffeine poisoning: insomnia, restlessness, tinnitus and flashes of light; tachycardia and extrasystoles; tremor, delirium and coma, following high doses in the region of 10 g. Death has not been reported with caffeine overdosage. 4) Acute codeine poisoning: symptoms will be more pronounced with the capsules containing the higher doses. These include the triad of: pinpoint pupils, marked depression of respiration, and loss of consciousness. Convulsions may occur.

Note: Because large doses of barbiturate alone may cause marked respiratory and CNS depression, an even more profound depressant effect may be expected after an overdosage of FIORINAL-C.

The dangers of Fiorinal-C overdosage are increased when the drug is ingested in the presence of alcohol, phenothiazines, minor tranquilizers and/or narcotics.

Treatment: The management of acute FIORINAL-C overdosage may involve the treatment of the toxic effects of all its constituents, with the possible exception of caffeine, which is toxic in very high doses only. Generally, it is the management of the barbiturate intoxication, the correction of the acid-base imbalance due to salicylism and the reversal of the effects of codeine which demand most attention. The therapeutic procedures most commonly employed are:

Elimination of the offending drug: 1) Emesis: if the patient is conscious, induce vomiting with syrup of ipecac (15 to 30 mL). 2) Perform gastric lavage followed by the administration of activated charcoal if the pharyngeal and laryngeal reflexes are present and if less than 4 hours have elapsed since ingestion. Do not attempt gastric lavage on the unconscious patient unless cuffed endotracheal intubation has been performed to prevent aspiration and pulmonary complications. 3) Catharsis: Following gastric lavage, a saline cathartic (sodium or magnesium sulfate 30 g in 250 mL of water) may be introduced and left in the stomach. 4) Encourage diuresis by administration of i.v. fluids assisted, if necessary, by 100 to 150 mL 25% mannitol solution given slowly i.v. Note: Mannitol should not be mixed with blood in a transfusion set, as red cell crenation and agglutination may occur. 5) Alkalinization of the urine (see caution): i.v. isotonic sodium bicarbonate solution accelerates urinary excretion of barbiturates. Maximum alkalinization may be more successfully attained if the sodium bicarbonate infusion is accompanied by acetazolamide 250 mg given as a single i.v. injection every 6 hours. (Caution: perform urinary alkalinization with care in children). 6) peritoneal dialysis and hemodialysis have been used with success in acute barbiturate intoxication and may be life saving. However, before embarking on either method, weigh the risks inherent to these procedures against the risk of not using them at all.

Maintenance of adequate pulmonary ventilation: Respiratory depression is an early and often profound manifestation of acute barbiturate poisoning. Meticulous attention to this aspect of treatment is essential. Perform pharyngeal and tracheal suction diligently to remove excess mucous secretions. Judicious administration of oxygen is also indicated. However, oxygen without assisted respiration must be used with caution, as its use in hypoventilation hypoxia may result in further respiratory depression and hypercapnia. In more critical cases, endotracheal intubation or tracheotomy, with or without assisted respiration, may be necessary.

Correction of hypotension: Vigorous treatment is essential, as circulatory collapse and renal failure are frequent causes of death. 1) Mild cases: the usual head down position and other supportive measures may be adequate. 2) Severe cases: Vasopressors (dopamine, levarterenol) may be given i.v. with the usual precautions and serial blood pressure monitoring.

Narcotic antagonism: Naloxone injection may reverse the respiratory depression caused by codeine and should be used until respiration improves.

Note: Respiratory depression caused by barbiturates will not respond to narcotic antagonists. Unwitting overdosage with narcotic antagonists may occur in an attempt to reverse respiratory depression caused by mixed barbiturate-codeine intoxication.

Special features due to salicylate overdosage: 1) The prominent features of salicylate intoxication are metabolic acidosis and electrolyte disturbance, and these require evaluation and correction. Sodium bicarbonate 400 mg (5 mEq)/kg as a 1% solution in 5% dextrose water is not only effective in correcting acidosis, but effectively and rapidly accelerates salicylate excretion by the kidneys. The administration of sodium bicarbonate must be carefully monitored with frequent blood pH and plasma CO_2 content determinations, as large amounts of sodium bicarbonate may result in severe alkalosis, particularly in children. THAM, an osmotic alkalinizing diuretic, also greatly increases the excretion of salicylate. This is given as a 0.3 molar solution at a rate not exceeding 5 mL/kg/hour. Potassium deficiency may occur and should be corrected. 2) Treat hyperthermia and dehydration with ice packs and i.v. fluids. 3) Treat hypoprothrombinemia with vitamin K_1 50 mg given daily i.v. 4) Hemodialysis, peritoneal dialysis or exchange transfusion are indicated in very severe salicylate intoxication. However, in FIORINAL-C overdosage, these measures are indicated mainly for barbiturate intoxication but would be effective for both.

General supportive measures: 1) Good nursing care is of prime importance, particularly in the comatose patient, and should include regular observation and accurate recording of the vital signs and depth of coma, maintenance of a free airway, frequent turning, and other routine measures usually adopted with unconscious patients. 2) Careful supervision and recording of fluid intake and output is essential. 3) Take blood samples to determine barbiturate blood concentrations and for electrolyte and other pertinent blood studies.

> For management of a suspected drug overdose, CPhA recommends that you contact your **regional Poison Control Centre**. See the *CPS* Directory section for a list of Poison Control Centres.

DOSAGE: Adults: 1 or 2 capsules at once, followed if necessary, by 1 capsule every 3 to 4 hours, up to 6 capsules daily, or as prescribed.

SUPPLIED: Fiorinal-C ¼ Capsules: Each hard gelatin oblong capsule, white opaque body with blue opaque cap, printed with FIORINAL-C 1/4 and △ in black ink contains: butalbital, USP 50 mg, caffeine, USP 40 mg, ASA, USP 330 mg, codeine phosphate, USP 15 mg. Nonmedicinal ingredients: cornstarch, microcrystalline cellulose, stearic acid and talc. Bottles of 100 and 500.
Fiorinal-C ½ Capsules: Each hard gelatin oblong capsule, light blue opaque with blue opaque cap, printed with FIORINAL-C 1/2 and △ in black ink contains: butalbital, USP 50 mg, caffeine, USP 40 mg, ASA, USP 330 mg and codeine phosphate, USP 30 mg. Nonmedicinal ingredients: cornstarch, microcrystalline cellulose, stearic acid and talc. Bottles of 100 and 500.

(Shown in Product Identification Section)

Firmagon® Pr

degarelix acetate

Gonadotropin-Releasing Hormone Receptor Antagonist

Ferring

Date of Preparation: November 6, 2009

SUMMARY PRODUCT INFORMATION:

Route of Administration	Dosage Form/ Strength	Clinically Relevant Nonmedicinal Ingredients
Subcutaneous Injection	Powder for injection: 120 mg/vial Powder for injection: 80 mg/vial	Mannitol For a complete listing see Dosage Forms, Composition and Packaging.

INDICATIONS AND CLINICAL USE: FIRMAGON (degarelix) is a gonadotropin-releasing hormone (GnRH) receptor antagonist (blocker) indicated for testosterone suppression in patients with advanced hormone-dependent prostate cancer in whom androgen deprivation is warranted.

Approval of FIRMAGON for prostate cancer is based on testosterone suppression to castrate levels. Evidence of palliation or prolongation of survival has not been established for FIRMAGON in prostate cancer.

Geriatrics (>65 years of age): The patient population tested in the clinical program was typical of the intended target population of patients with prostate cancer. The mean age was 74 years (range 47 to 98 years), with 82% age 65 and over and 42% age 75 and over.

Pediatrics (<18 years of age): FIRMAGON is not indicated in pediatric patients.

Women (>18 years of age): FIRMAGON is not indicated for use in women.

CONTRAINDICATIONS: Hypersensitivity to degarelix or to any of the excipients.

FIRMAGON is not indicated for use in women and is contraindicated in women who are or who may become pregnant.

WARNINGS AND PRECAUTIONS:

> **Serious Warnings and Precautions**
> FIRMAGON (degarelix) should be prescribed by a qualified health professional that is experienced in the use of hormonal therapy in prostate cancer. FIRMAGON should be administered under the supervision of a physician (see Dosage and Administration).
> FIRMAGON has not been studied in patients with severe hepatic or severe renal impairment (see Hepatic/Biliary/Pancreatic and Renal below).
> The following are clinically significant adverse events:
> - QT prolongation (see Cardiovascular below and Drug Interactions, Drug-Drug Interactions).
> - Osteoporosis (see Musculoskeletal below and Adverse Reactions, Other Clinical Trial Adverse Drug Reactions).

General: The data available on efficacy and safety experience with degarelix is limited to a one year treatment.

Route of Administration: FIRMAGON is for **subcutaneous administration only** and is **not** to be administered intravenously. Gently pull back the plunger to check if blood is aspirated. If blood appears in the syringe, the reconstituted product can no longer be used. Discontinue the procedure and discard the syringe and the needle (reconstitute a new dose for the patient). (See Dosage and Administration.)

FIRMAGON is administered as a subcutaneous injection in the abdominal region. As with other drugs administered by subcutaneous injection, the injection site should vary periodically. Injections should be given in areas of the abdomen that will not be exposed to pressure, e.g. not close to waistband or belt nor close to the ribs.

Cardiovascular: An increased risk of heart disease has been observed in men who have had orchiectomy or who have been treated with a GnRH agonist or antiandrogen monotherapy. In the randomized, active-controlled trial comparing degarelix to leuprolide, mild/moderate hypertension occurred in 26 (6%) patients in the pooled degarelix group and 8 (4%) patients in the leuprolide 7.5 mg group; myocardial infarction occurred in 5 (1%) patients in the pooled degarelix group and 4 (2%) patients in the leuprolide 7.5 mg group. Screening for and intervention to prevent/treat cardiovascular disease is warranted.

Effect on QT/QTc Interval: Long-term androgen deprivation therapy prolongs the QT interval. Physicians should consider whether the benefits of androgen deprivation therapy outweigh the potential risk in patients with congenital long QT syndrome, electrolyte abnormalities, or congestive heart failure and in patients taking Class IA (e.g. quinidine, procainamide), Class III (e.g. amiodarone, sotalol, dofetilide, ibutilide)), or Class IC (e.g. flecainide, propafenone) antiarrhythmic medications.

In the randomized, active-controlled trial comparing degarelix to leuprolide, periodic electrocardiograms were performed. Both therapies showed QT/QTc intervals exceeding 450 msec in approximately 20% of the patients. Seven patients, three (<1%) in the pooled degarelix group and four (2%) patients in the leuprolide 7.5 mg group, had a QTcF ≥500 msec. From baseline to end of study the median change for degarelix was 12.3 msec and for leuprolide was 16.7 msec.

Endocrine and Metabolism: Changes in Glucose Tolerance: A reduction in glucose tolerance has been observed in men who have had orchiectomy or who have been treated with a GnRH agonist. Development or aggravation of diabetes may occur; therefore diabetic patients may require more frequent monitoring of blood glucose when receiving androgen deprivation therapy. The effect of degarelix on insulin and glucose levels has not been studied.

Hematologic: Anemia is a known physiological consequence of testosterone suppression. In the randomized, active-controlled trial comparing degarelix to leuprolide, anemia occurred in fourteen (3%) patients in the pooled degarelix group and ten (5%) patients in the leuprolide 7.5 mg group.

Hepatic/Biliary/Pancreatic: Patients with known or suspected hepatic disorder have not been included in long-term clinical trials with degarelix. Mild, transient increases in ALT and AST have been seen, these were not accompanied by a rise in bilirubin or clinical symptoms. Monitoring of liver function in patients with known or suspected hepatic disorder is advised during treatment.

A single dose of 1 mg degarelix administered as an intravenous infusion over 1 hour has been studied in a pharmacokinetic study in 16 non-prostate cancer patients with mild to moderate hepatic impairment. Compared to non-prostate cancer patients with normal liver function, the exposure of degarelix decreased by 10% and 18% in patients with mild and moderate hepatic impairment, respectively. Therefore, dose adjustment is not necessary in patients with mild or moderate hepatic impairment. However, since hepatic impairment can lower degarelix exposure, it is recommended that in patients with hepatic impairment testosterone concentrations should be monitored on a monthly basis until medical castration is achieved. Once medical castration is achieved, an every-other-month testosterone monitoring approach could be considered.

Patients with severe hepatic dysfunction have not been studied and caution is therefore warranted in this group.

Immune: Hypersensitivity: Degarelix has not been studied in patients with a history of severe untreated asthma, anaphylactic reactions, severe urticaria or angioedema. No immediate onset of generalized hypersensitivity was seen in the development program.

Musculoskeletal: Changes in Bone Density: Decreased bone density has been reported in the medical literature in men who have had orchiectomy or who have been treated with a GnRH agonist. It can be anticipated that long periods of medical castration in men will have effects on bone density. Bone density has not been measured during treatment with degarelix.

Neurologic: No studies on the effects of degarelix on the ability to drive and use machines have been performed. However, fatigue and dizziness are common adverse reactions that might influence the ability to drive and use machines.

Renal: No pharmacokinetic studies in renally impaired patients have been conducted. Approximately 20-30% of a given dose of degarelix is excreted unchanged in the urine. A population pharmacokinetics analysis of the data from the confirmatory Phase III study has demonstrated that the clearance of degarelix in patients with moderate CrCL <50 mL/min, renal impairment is reduced by 23%: therefore dose adjustment in patients with mild or moderate renal impairment is not recommended. Data on patients with severe renal impairment are scarce and caution is therefore warranted in this patient category.

Special Populations: Pregnant Women: FIRMAGON is contraindicated in women who are or who may become pregnant. Fetal harm can occur when administered to pregnant women based on nonclinical reproductive studies (see Contraindications).

Nursing Women: FIRMAGON is not indicated for use in women and is contraindicated in women who are or who may become pregnant. It is not known whether this drug is excreted in human milk. Because many drugs are excreted in human milk and because of the potential for serious adverse reactions in nursing infants from degarelix, a decision should be made whether to discontinue nursing or discontinue the drug taking into account the importance of the drug to the mother.

Pediatrics (<18 years of age): Safety and effectiveness in pediatric patients have not been established.

Geriatrics (>65 years of age): Of the total number of subjects in clinical studies of FIRMAGON, 82% were age 65 and over, while 42% were age 75 and over. No overall differences in safety or effectiveness were observed between these subjects and younger subjects, but greater sensitivity of some older individuals cannot be ruled out.

Monitoring and Laboratory Tests:

- Therapy with FIRMAGON results in suppression of the pituitary gonadal axis. Results of diagnostic tests of pituitary gonadotropic and gonadal functions conducted during and after FIRMAGON therapy may be affected.
- The therapeutic effect of FIRMAGON should be monitored by measuring serum concentrations of prostate-specific antigen (PSA) periodically. If PSA increases, serum concentrations of testosterone should be measured.
- A screening electrocardiogram (ECG) is recommended prior to initiation of treatment with FIRMAGON.
- Baseline measurements of serum potassium, calcium, and magnesium levels are recommended. Monitoring of serum electrolyte levels during treatment is recommended in those patients at risk for an electrolyte abnormality. Electrolyte abnormalities may prolong the QT interval.

ADVERSE REACTIONS: Adverse Drug Reaction Overview: In total, 1839 patients with prostate cancer have been exposed to degarelix, including 1567 exposed for at least 6 months and 1178 exposed for more than one year. Degarelix was studied primarily in an active-controlled trial (N=610) and in uncontrolled trials, including long-term extension studies evaluating safety and tolerability.

The population was male patients with prostate cancer; the median age was 74 years and the age range was 47 to 98 years of age. Patients were given degarelix at monthly (N=1259) or 3-monthly (N=580) intervals. Most patients have received mean monthly doses of 60-120 mg, given as subcutaneous injections at 28-days intervals (N=875). The most commonly observed adverse reactions during degarelix therapy included injection site reactions (e.g. pain, erythema, swelling, nodule or induration), hot flashes, increased weight, fatigue, dizziness, anemia and increases in serum levels of transaminases and gamma-glutamyl-transferase (GGT). The majority of the adverse reactions were Grade 1 or 2, with Grade 3/4 adverse reaction incidences of 1% or less. Adverse reactions reported as uncommon were cardiac arrhythmia (incl. atrial fibrillation, QT-prolongation), hypertension, hyperglycemia/diabetes mellitus, hypersensitivity (including urticaria, rash and pruritus), osteoporosis/osteopenia and renal impairment.

The most commonly observed adverse reactions during degarelix therapy in the confirmatory Phase III trial (N=409) were due to the expected physiological effects of testosterone suppression, including hot flashes and weight increase (reported in 25% and 7%, of patients receiving treatment for one year) and injection site reactions. Transient chills, fever or influenza like illness were reported to occur hours after dosing (in 3%, 2% and 1% of patients, respectively).

Clinical Trial Adverse Drug Reactions: Degarelix was studied in an active-controlled trial (N=610) in which patients with prostate cancer were randomized to receive degarelix (subcutaneous) or leuprolide (intramuscular) monthly for 12 months. Adverse events reported in 5% of patients or more regardless of causality are shown in Table 1.

Table 1: FIRMAGON

Adverse Events Reported in ≥5% of Patients in an Active Controlled Study

	Degarelix 240/160 mg (subcutaneous) N=202 %	Degarelix 240/80 mg (subcutaneous) N=207 %	Leuprolide 7.5 mg (intramuscular) N=201 %
Percentage of subjects with adverse events	83	79	78
Body as a Whole			
Injection site adverse events	44	35	<1
Weight increase	11	9	12
Fatigue	6	3	6
Chills	3	5	0
Cardiovascular System			
Hot flash	26	26	21
Hypertension	7	6	4
Musculoskeletal System			
Back pain	6	6	8
Arthralgia	3	5	9
Urogenital System			
Urinary tract infection	1	5	9
Digestive System			
Increases in transaminases and GOT	10	10	5
Constipation	3	5	5
Nausea	5	4	4
Hypercholesterolemia	6	3	2

The most frequently reported adverse reactions at the injection sites were pain (28%), erythema (17%), swelling (6%), induration (4%) and nodule (3%) with the FIRMAGON 240/80 mg dosing regimen. These adverse reactions were mostly transient, of mild to moderate intensity, occurred primarily with the starting dose and led to few discontinuations (<1%). Grade 3 injection site reactions occurred in 2% or less of patients receiving degarelix.

Hepatic laboratory abnormalities were primarily Grade 1 or 2 and were generally reversible. Grade 3 hepatic laboratory abnormalities occurred in less than 1% of patients. Changes in hepatic laboratory values were similar for degarelix and the comparator.

In 1-5% of patients in the active controlled trial the following adverse reactions, not already listed, were considered related to degarelix by the investigator:

Body as a Whole: asthenia, fever, night sweats.

Digestive System: nausea.

Nervous System: dizziness, headache, insomnia.

In uncontrolled trials the following adverse reactions, not already listed, were reported to be drug-related by the investigator in ≥1% of patients: erectile dysfunction, gynecomastia, hyperhidrosis, testicular atrophy, and diarrhea.

Abnormal Hematologic and Clinical Chemistry Findings: Changes in Laboratory Parameters: Changes in laboratory values seen during one year of treatment were in the same range for degarelix and a GnRH-agonist (leuprolide) used as comparator. Markedly abnormal (>3*ULN) liver transaminase values (ALT, AST and GGT) were seen in 2-6% of patients with normal values prior to treatment, following treatment with both medicinal products. Marked decrease in hematological values, hematocrit (<0.37) and hemoglobin (<115 g/L) were seen in 40% and 13-15%, respectively, of patients with normal values prior to treatment, following treatment with both medicinal products. It is unknown to what extent this decrease in hematological values was caused by the underlying prostate cancer and to what extent it was a consequence of androgen deprivation therapy. Markedly abnormal values of potassium (>5.8 mmol/L), creatinine (>177 mmol/L) and BUN (>10.7 mmol/L) in patients with normal values prior to treatment, were seen in 6%, 2% and 15% of degarelix treated patients and 3%, 2% and 14% of leuprolide treated patients, respectively.

Other Clinical Trial Adverse Drug Reactions: The following less common adverse reactions were reported in the active-controlled trial.

- Cardiovascular: atrio-ventricular first degree block, hypertension, vaso-vagal reaction
- Haematologic: anemia
- Immune: hypersensitivity, urticaria
- Musculoskeletal: musculoskeletal pain, muscular weakness
- Renal: renal impairment, pollakiuria, micturition urgency

Anti-Degarelix Antibody Development: Anti-degarelix antibody development has been observed in 10% of patients after treatment with degarelix for 1 year. There is no indication that the efficacy or safety of degarelix treatment is affected by antibody formation. Efficacy and safety data in relation to antibody development beyond one year is not available.

Changes in Bone Density: Decreased bone density has been reported in the medical literature in men who have had orchiectomy or who have been treated with a GnRH agonist. It can be anticipated that long periods of medical castration in men will have effects on bone density. Bone density has not been measured during treatment with degarelix.

During the one year treatment in CS21, 0.7% of degarelix and 2.5% of leuprolide patients reported fractures and/or osteoporosis or osteopenia. See Table 2.

Table 2: FIRMAGON

Patient Reported Incidences of Fractures, Osteoporosis and Osteopenia

	CS21	
	Degarelix (N=409)	Leuprolide (N=201)
Any fracture, osteoporosis or osteopenia	3 (0.7 %)	5 (2.48%)
Osteoporosis	1 (0.24%)	1 (0.49%)
Osteopenia	0 (0.0%)	0 (0.0%)
Any fracture	2 (0.49)	4 (1.99%)
Fracture of long tubular bone, spine or pelvis[a]	2 (0.49%)	4 (1.99%)

[a] Excluding fractures of minor bones (i.e. face, rib, clavicular bone, patella, hands and feet).

In the pooled degarelix safety database, where the median duration of follow-up has been 1.2 years (mean 1.7 years), 3.3% of prostate cancer patients have reported bone mineral density/osteoporosis-related adverse events.

DRUG INTERACTIONS: Drug-Drug Interactions: No drug-drug interaction studies have been performed.

Since androgen deprivation treatment may prolong the QTc interval, the concomitant use of degarelix with medicinal products known to prolong the QTc interval or medicinal products able to induce torsades de pointes should be carefully evaluated. Such medicinal products include but are not limited to the examples that follow: Class IA (e.g. quinidine, disopyramide), Class III (e.g. amiodarone, sotalol, dofetilide, ibutilide), or Class IC (e.g. flecainide, propafenone) antiarrhythmic medicinal products, antipsychotics (e.g. chlorpromazine), antidepressants (e.g. amitriptyline, nortriptyline), opioids (e.g. methadone), macrolide antibiotics and analogues (e.g. erythromycin, clarithromycin, azithromycin), quinolone antibiotics (e.g. moxifloxacin), pentamidine, antimalarials (e.g. quinine), azole antifungals, cisapride, 5-hydroxytryptamine (5-HT_3) receptor antagonists (e.g. ondansetron), and beta-2 adrenoceptor agonists (e.g. salbutamol).

Degarelix is not a substrate for the human CYP450 system (as demonstrated in vitro) and has not been shown to induce or inhibit CYP1A2, CYP2B6, CYP2C8, CYP2C9, CYP2C19, CYP2D6, CYP2E1, or CYP3A4/5 to any great extent in vitro. Therefore, clinically significant pharmacokinetic drug-drug interactions are unlikely.

Drug-Food Interactions: Interactions with food have not been established.

Drug-Herb Interactions: Interactions with herbal products have not been established.

Drug-Laboratory Test Interactions: Therapy with FIRMAGON results in suppression of the pituitary gonadal axis. Results of diagnostic tests of pituitary gonadotropic and gonadal functions conducted during and after FIRMAGON therapy may be affected.

The therapeutic effect of FIRMAGON should be monitored by measuring serum concentrations of prostate-specific antigen (PSA) periodically. If PSA increases, serum concentrations of testosterone should be measured.

DOSAGE AND ADMINISTRATION: Dosing Considerations: FIRMAGON should be administered by a health professional.

The therapeutic effect of FIRMAGON should be monitored by clinical parameters and by measuring prostate specific antigen (PSA) serum levels. Clinical studies have shown that testosterone (T) suppression occurs immediately after administration of the starting dose with 96% of the patients having plasma testosterone at medical castration levels (T≤0.5 ng/mL) after three days and 100% after one month. Long term treatment with the maintenance dose up to 1 year shows that 97% of the patients have sustained suppressed testosterone levels (T≤0.5 ng/mL).

In case the patient's clinical response appears to be sub-optimal, it should be confirmed that serum testosterone levels are remaining sufficiently suppressed.

Since FIRMAGON does not induce a testosterone surge it is not necessary to add an anti-androgen as surge protection at initiation of therapy.

FIRMAGON is supplied as a powder to be reconstituted with Sterile Water for Injection, USP. The reconstitution procedure needs to be carefully followed. Administration of other concentrations is not recommended. The reconstituted solution should be a clear liquid, free of undissolved matter. See Instructions for Reconstitution and Administration below.

FIRMAGON is administered as a subcutaneous injection in the abdominal region. As with other drugs administered by subcutaneous injection, the injection site should vary periodically. Injections should be given in areas of the abdomen that will not be exposed to pressure, e.g. not close to waistband or belt nor close to the ribs.

The first maintenance dose should be given one month after the starting dose.

The patient should be instructed to return every month after the starting dose and thereafter for their next injections.

Method of Administration: FIRMAGON must be reconstituted prior to administration. FIRMAGON is administered by **subcutaneous injection only**. FIRMAGON should **not** be administered intravenously. Voir Table 3.

Table 3: FIRMAGON

Dosage for Adult Males

Starting Dose	Maintenance Dose—Monthly Administration
240 mg given as two subcutaneous injections of 120 mg at a concentration of 40 mg/mL	80 mg given as one subcutaneous injection at a concentration of 20 mg/mL

The first maintenance dose should be given one month after the starting dose.

Starting Dose: 240 mg given as two subcutaneous injections of 120 mg at concentration of 40 mg/mL: One vial of FIRMAGON 120 mg contains 120 mg degarelix as degarelix acetate. Each vial is to be reconstituted with 3 mL of sterile water for injection. 3 mL is withdrawn to deliver 120 mg degarelix at a concentration of 40 mg/mL. One starting dose comprises 240 mg given as two 3 mL subcutaneous injections of 120 mg each.

Maintenance Dose: Monthly administration of 80 mg administered as one subcutaneous Injection: One vial of FIRMAGON 80 mg contains 80 mg degarelix as degarelix acetate. Each vial is to be reconstituted with 4.2 mL of sterile water for injection. 4 mL is withdrawn to deliver 80 mg degarelix at a concentration of 20 mg/mL. One maintenance dose comprises 80 mg given as one 4 mL injection.

Recommended Dose and Dosage Adjustment: Dose Adjustment in Specific Patient Populations: Elderly, Hepatically or Renally impaired: There is no need to adjust the dose for the elderly or in patients with mild or moderate liver or kidney function impairment. Patients with severe liver or kidney dysfunction have not been studied and caution is therefore warranted.

There is no relevant indication for FIRMAGON in women and children.

Missed Dose: Maintaining testosterone suppression is important in treating the symptoms of hormone-dependent prostate cancer. Missing an appointment by a few days should not disrupt the benefits of treatment, but keeping a consistent schedule of FIRMAGON injections is an important part of treatment.

Administration: FIRMAGON is for **subcutaneous administration only** and is **not** to be administered intravenously.

FIRMAGON is administered as a subcutaneous injection in the abdominal region. As with other drugs administered by subcutaneous injection, the injection site should vary periodically. Injections should be given in areas where the patient will not be exposed to pressure, e.g., not close to waistband or belt and not close to the ribs.

FIRMAGON is supplied as a powder to be reconstituted with water for injection. The reconstitution procedure needs to be carefully followed. Administration of other concentrations is not recommended. The reconstituted solution should be a clear liquid, free of undissolved matter.

Starting Dose: One starting dose comprises of two vials of degarelix for injection 120 mg and two vials of solvent 6 mL (3.0 mL should be withdrawn for each vial). After reconstitution the concentration is 40 mg/mL.

Maintenance Dose: One maintenance dose comprises one vial of powder for injection 80 mg and one vial of solvent 6 mL (4.2 mL should be withdrawn). After reconstitution the concentration is 20 mg/mL.

Instructions for Reconstitution and Administration: FIRMAGON has a unique reconstitution process. It is important to read the instructions carefully. Remember to keep the vials vertical at all times, keep the syringe in the vial at all times and **not** to shake the vial.

After reconstitution, the product should be injected immediately. Chemical and physical in-use stability of the reconstituted solution has been demonstrated for 2 hours after solvent addition. From a microbiological point of view, once reconstituted, the product should be administered immediately.

Note:
- Gloves should be worn during preparation and administration
- Reconstituted drug must be administered within 2 hours after addition of Sterile Water for Injection, USP (WFI)
- Keep the vial vertical at all times
- Do not shake the vials
- Follow aseptic technique

FIRMAGON 120 mg: The Treatment Starter pack contains 2 vials of FIRMAGON 120 mg degarelix as degarelix acetate that must be prepared for 2 subcutaneous injections. Hence, the instructions here below need to be repeated a second time.

Prepare FIRMAGON 120 mg for reconstitution by gathering the following:
- 2 vials of FIRMAGON 120 mg powder
- 2 vials of 6 mL of Sterile Water for Injection, USP (WFI); Do not use Bacteriostatic Water for Injection
- 2 reconstitution needles—21G/0.8×50 mm
- 2 administration needles for subcutaneous injection—27G/0.4×25 mm
- 2 injection syringes (5 mL)

1. Draw up 3 mL WFI with a reconstitution needle (21G/0.8×50 mm).
2. Inject the WFI slowly into the FIRMAGON 120 mg vial. To keep the product and syringe sterile, do not remove the syringe and the needle.
3. Keeping the vial in an upright position, swirl it very gently until the liquid looks clear and without undissolved powder or particles. If the powder adheres to the vial over the liquid surface, the vial can be tilted slightly to dissolve powder. Avoid shaking to prevent foam formation. A ring of small air bubbles on the surface of the liquid is acceptable. The reconstitution procedure may take up to 15 minutes.
4. Tilt the vial slightly and keep the needle in the lowest part of the vial. Withdraw 3 mL of FIRMAGON 120 mg without turning the vial upside down.
5. Exchange the reconstitution needle with the administration needle for deep subcutaneous injection (27G /0.4×25 mm). Remove any air bubbles.
6. Inject 3 mL of FIRMAGON 120 mg subcutaneously immediately after reconstitution.
   - Grasp the skin of the abdomen, elevate the subcutaneous tissue. Insert the needle deeply at an angle of not less than 45 degrees.
   - Gently pull back the plunger to check if blood is aspirated. If blood appears in the syringe, the reconstituted product can no longer be used. Discontinue the procedure and discard the syringe and the needle (reconstitute a new dose for the patient).
7. Repeat reconstitution procedure for the second dose. Choose a different injection site and inject 3 mL.

FIRMAGON 80 mg: The Treatment Maintenance pack contains 1 vial of FIRMAGON 80 mg degarelix as degarelix acetate that must be prepared for subcutaneous injection.

Prepare FIRMAGON 80 mg for reconstitution by gathering the following;
- 1 vial of FIRMAGON 80 mg powder
- 1 vial of 6.0 mL of Sterile Water for Injection, USP (WFI); Do not use Bacteriostatic Water for Injection
- 1 reconstitution needle—21G/0.8×50 mm
- 1 administration needle for sc injection—27G/0.4×25 mm
- 1 injection syringe (5 mL)

1. Draw up 4.2 mL WFI with the reconstitution needle (21G/0.8×50 mm).
2. Inject the WFI slowly into the FIRMAGON 80 mg vial. To keep the product and syringe sterile, do not remove the syringe and the needle.
3. Keeping the vial in an upright position, swirl it very gently until the liquid looks clear and without undissolved powder or particles. If the powder adheres to the vial over the liquid surface, the vial can be tilted slightly to dissolve powder. Avoid shaking to prevent foam formation. A ring of small air bubbles on the surface of the liquid is acceptable. The reconstitution procedure may take up to 15 minutes.
4. Tilt the vial slightly and keep the needle in the lowest part of the vial. Withdraw 4 mL of FIRMAGON 80 mg without turning the vial upside down.
5. Exchange the reconstitution needle with the administration needle for deep subcutaneous injection (27G/0.4×25 mm). Remove any air bubbles.
6. Inject 4 mL of FIRMAGON 80 mg subcutaneously immediately after reconstitution.
   - Grasp the skin of the abdomen, elevate the subcutaneous tissue. Insert the needle deeply at an angle of not less than 45 degrees.
   - Gently pull back the plunger to check if blood is aspirated. If blood appears in the syringe, the reconstituted product can no longer be used. Discontinue the procedure and discard the syringe and the needle (reconstitute a new dose for the patient).

OVERDOSAGE:

There have been no reports of overdose with FIRMAGON. In case of overdose, discontinue FIRMAGON, treat the patient symptomatically, and institute supportive measures.

> For management of a suspected drug overdose, CPhA recommends that you contact your **regional Poison Control Centre**. See the *CPS* Directory section for a list of Poison Control Centres.

ACTION AND CLINICAL PHARMACOLOGY: Mechanism of Action: Degarelix is a selective GnRH receptor antagonist (blocker) that competitively and reversibly binds to the pituitary GnRH receptors, thereby rapidly reducing the release of gonadotropins luteinizing hormone (LH) and follicle stimulating hormone (FSH), and thereby reducing the secretion of testosterone by the testes. Prostatic carcinoma is known to be androgen sensitive and responds to androgen deprivation therapy. Unlike GnRH agonists, GnRH antagonists do not induce an LH surge with subsequent testosterone surge and potential symptomatic flare after the initiation of treatment.

Pharmacodynamics: A single dose of FIRMAGON 240 mg followed by a monthly maintenance dose of 80 mg rapidly causes a decrease in the concentrations of luteinizing hormone (LH), follicle stimulating hormone (FSH), and subsequently testosterone. The plasma concentration of dihydrotestosterone (DHT) decreases in a similar manner to testosterone.

FIRMAGON is effective in achieving and maintaining testosterone suppression well below the medical castration level of 0.5 ng/mL. See Figure 1.

Figure 1: FIRMAGON

Plasma Testosterone from Day 0 to 364 for Degarelix 240 mg/80 mg (median with interquartile ranges)

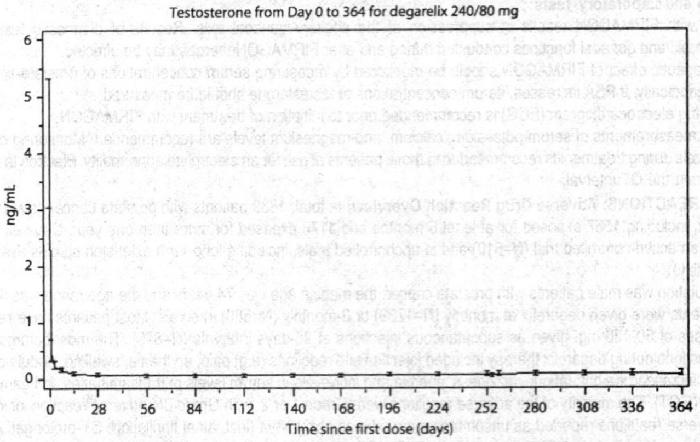

Maintenance monthly dosing of degarelix 80 mg resulted in sustained testosterone suppression in 97% of patients for at least one year. Median testosterone levels after one year of treatment were 0.087 ng/mL [interquartile range 0.06-0.15] N=167.

Prostate specific antigen (PSA) levels were lowered by 64% two weeks after administration of degarelix, by 85% after one month, 95% after three months, and remained suppressed throughout the one year of treatment. These PSA results should be interpreted with caution because of the heterogeneity of the patient population studied. No evidence has shown that the rapidity of PSA decline is related to a clinical benefit.

The effect of degarelix on QT has not been investigated in a thorough QT/QTc study.

Pharmacokinetics: Absorption: FIRMAGON forms a depot upon subcutaneous administration, from which degarelix is released to the circulation.

Following subcutaneous administration of degarelix 240 mg at a concentration of 40 mg/mL to prostate cancer patients in the pivotal study CS21, AUC 0-28 days was 635 (602-668) day*ng/mL, Cmax was 66.0 (61.0-71.0) ng/mL and occurred at tmax 40 (37-42) hours. Mean trough values were approximately 11-12 ng/mL after the starting dose and 11-16 ng/mL after maintenance dosing of 80 mg at a concentration of 20 mg/mL. Degarelix decreases in a biphasic fashion, with a median terminal half-life (t½) of approximately 43 days for the starting dose or 28 days for the maintenance dose, as estimated based on population pharmacokinetics modeling. The long half-life after subcutaneous administration is a consequence of a very slow release of degarelix from the FIRMAGON depot formed at the injection site(s). The pharmacokinetic behavior of the drug is strongly influenced by its concentration in the injection solution. Thus, Cmax and bioavailability tend to decrease with increasing dose concentration while the t½ is increased. Therefore, no other dose concentrations than the recommended should be used.

Distribution: The distribution volume of degarelix after intravenous administration is approximately 1 L/kg in healthy elderly men. This indicates that degarelix is distributed throughout total body water. In vitro plasma protein binding of degarelix is estimated to be approximately 90%.

Metabolism: Degarelix is subject to common peptidic degradation during passage through the hepato-biliary system and is mainly excreted as peptide fragments in the feces. No quantitatively significant metabolites were detected in plasma samples after subcutaneous administration. In vitro studies have shown that degarelix is not a substrate, inducer nor inhibitor of CYP450 or P-glycoprotein transporter systems.

Excretion: In healthy men, approximately 20-30% of a given dose of degarelix was renally excreted, suggesting that approximately 70-80% is excreted via the hepato-biliary system in humans. The clearance after an intravenous administration is approximately 35-50 mL/h/kg in healthy elderly men.

Special Populations and Conditions: Renal Insufficiency: No pharmacokinetic studies in renally impaired patients have been conducted. Only about 20-30% of a given dose of degarelix is excreted unchanged by the kidneys. A population pharmacokinetics analysis of the data from the confirmatory Phase III trial has demonstrated that the clearance of degarelix in patients with moderate renal impairment is reduced by 23%; therefore dose adjustment in patients with mild or moderate renal impairment is not recommended. Data on patients with severe renal impairment are scarce and caution is therefore warranted in this patient population.

Hepatic Insufficiency: Degarelix has been studied in a pharmacokinetic study in patients with mild to moderate hepatic impairment. No signs of increased exposure in the hepatically impaired were observed compared to healthy subjects. Dose adjustment is not necessary in patients with mild or moderate hepatic impairment. Patients with severe hepatic dysfunction have not been studied and caution is therefore warranted in this group.

Geriatrics: The patient population tested in the clinical program was typical of the intended target population of patients with prostate cancer. The mean age was 74 years (range 47 to 98 years).

Effect of Age, Weight and Race: Population pharmacokinetic analysis shows only a small change in clearance of degarelix related to age and weight. Therefore, dose adjustment is not warranted.

STORAGE AND STABILITY: Degarelix Powder for Injection: Store at 25°C (excursions permitted to15-30°C).

Sterile Water for Injection: Store at 25°C (excursions permitted to 15-30°C).

SPECIAL HANDLING INSTRUCTIONS: The instruction for reconstitution must be followed carefully. After reconstitution, the product should be injected immediately. Chemical and physical in-use stability of the reconstituted solution has been demonstrated for two hours after solvent addition. From a microbiological point of view, once reconstituted, the product should be administered immediately.

INFORMATION FOR THE PATIENT: Published in e-CPS, available by subscription at www.e-cps.ca.

DOSAGE FORMS, COMPOSITION AND PACKAGING: Starting dose (240 mg, 40 mg/mL): 1 pack contains: 2 single use vials of FIRMAGON containing degarelix 120 mg powder as degarelix acetate for injection with mannitol, 2 single use vials for reconstitution containing 6 mL sterile water for injection, USP (3.0 mL has to be withdrawn from each 6 mL vial); 2 syringes (5 mL), 2 reconstitution needles (21G/0.8×50 mm) and 2 injection needles (27G/0.4×25 mm).

Maintenance dose (80 mg, 20 mg/mL): 1 pack contains: 1 single use vial of FIRMAGON containing degarelix 80 mg powder as degarelix acetate for injection with mannitol, 1 single use vial for reconstitution containing 6 mL sterile water for injection, USP (4.2 mL has to be withdrawn from each 6 mL vial); 1 syringe (5 mL), 1 reconstitution needle (21G/0.8×50 mm) and 1 injection needle (27G/0.4×25 mm).

Flagyl® Ⓟ

metronidazole

Antibacterial—Antiprotozoal

sanofi-aventis

Date of Revision: November 6, 2009

PHARMACOLOGY: Metronidazole is bactericidal against anaerobic bacteria, it exerts trichomonacidal activity and is also active against *G. lamblia* and *E. histolytica*. Its exact mechanism of action has not been entirely determined as yet. It has been proposed that an intermediate in the reduction of metronidazole, produced only in anaerobic bacteria and protozoa is bound to deoxyribonucleic acid and electron-transport proteins, inhibits subsequent nucleic acid synthesis.

At present, the mechanism by which topical metronidazole reduces the lesions and erythema associated with acne rosacea is not precisely known. Despite the established antimicrobial effects of metronidazole, there is no evidence that the suppression of bacteria or parasitic mites harbored in the skin is directly responsible for its beneficial effects in rosacea. In vitro and in vivo studies indicate that metronidazole has direct antiinflammatory activity and affects neutrophil chemotaxis and cell-mediated immunity.

An antioxidant action via inhibition of neutrophil-generated reactive oxygen species has also been demonstrated; this action is believed to underlie its anti-inflammatory effect. It has been proposed that the reduction in rosacea lesions and erythema is the result of anti-inflammatory or immunosuppressive actions of metronidazole.

Pharmacokinetics: Following oral administration, metronidazole is completely absorbed with plasma concentration usually reaching a peak within 1 to 2 hours. After single oral 500 mg doses, peak plasma levels of approximately 13 mg/L were obtained. On a regimen of 500 mg t.i.d. administered by the i.v. route, a steady state was achieved after approximately 3 days. The mean peak and trough concentrations measured at that time were 26 and 12 mg/L respectively, and the elimination half-life was approximately 7 to 8 hours. Comparison of the pharmacokinetics of oral and i.v. metronidazole revealed that the area under the plasma metronidazole concentration against time curves were essentially identical.

There is negligible percutaneous absorption following topical application of metronidazole 1% cream. In healthy volunteers who applied a single 100 mg dose of ^{14}C-labelled metronidazole 2% cream to intact skin, no metronidazole could be detected in plasma after 12 hours. Only about 1% and 0.1% of the applied dose could be found in urine and feces, respectively. After once-daily application of the 1% cream for 1 month, only traces (about 1% of the C_{max} of a 200 mg oral dose) could be detected in 25% of patients. In the rest of the patients, no detectable plasma levels were found.

In two kinetic studies in which a single metronidazole 1.5 g dose was infused intravenously over a 50-60 minutes period in volunteers, a peak level of 30-40 mg/L was obtained 1 hour after the start of infusion and fell to 10 mg/L at 12 h and 4 mg/L at 24 hour.

Excretion and Metabolism: The major route of elimination of metronidazole and its metabolites is via the urine (60-80% of the dose) with fecal excretion accounting for 6 to 15% of the dose. The metabolites that appear in the urine result primarily from side chain oxidation (i.e., 1-(β hydroxyethyl)-2-hydroxymethyl 5-nitroimidazole and 2-methyl-5 nitroimidazole-1-yl-acetic acid) and glucuronide conjugation, with unchanged metronidazole accounting for approximately 20% of the total.

Metronidazole is the major component appearing in the plasma with lesser quantities of the 2-hydroxymethyl metabolite also being present. The ratio of these components varies with time but the maximum concentration of the metabolite (C_{max}) is approximately 20% of the C_{max} of metronidazole for the oral route of administration.

Protein Binding: Less than 20% of the circulating metronidazole is bound to plasma proteins.

Tissue Distribution: The concentrations of metronidazole found in various tissues and body fluids are given in Table 1.

Table 1: Flagyl

Concentrations of Metronidazole in Various Tissues and Body Fluids

Tissue or Fluid	Dose Administered	Tissue or Fluid Level	Plasma Level
Bile	500 mg q.i.d. p.o.×10 days	26 mg/L (on day 5) 20 mg/L (on day 15)	N/A[a] N/A
Saliva	500 mg p.o. single dose	7 mg/L (at 2–3 hour)	N/A
Placenta	250 mg p.o. single dose	0–1.4 mg/kg (at 4–5 hour)	3–6.9 mg/L (maternal)
Embryo	250 mg p.o. single dose	0–1 mg/kg	3–6.9 mg/L (maternal)
Breast milk	200 mg p.o.	1.3–3.4 mg/L	1.8–3.9 mg/L
Cerebrospinal fluid	500 mg p.o. b.i.d.	11–13.9 mg/L	8.3–15.4 mg/L
Pus (brain abscess)	400 mg p.o. t.i.d.	35 mg/L inflamed meninges	N/A
	600 mg i.v. t.i.d.	43 mg/L	N/A
Pus (pulmonary empyema)	400 mg, p.o. q.i.d.	24.2 mg/L	N/A

[a] Not available.

Decreased Renal Function: Decreased renal function does not appear to alter the single dose pharmacokinetics of metronidazole, although the elimination half-life of the metabolites is prolonged.

Hemodialysis: During hemodialysis, the hydroxy metabolite is removed from the plasma about 3 times more rapidly than in normal subjects. Comparison of the elimination half-lives of metronidazole and two metabolites are given in Table 2.

Therefore, no accumulation should occur in anuric patients undergoing regular dialysis.

Continuous Ambulatory Peritoneal Dialysis: Metronidazole was given I.V. at 750 mg to five patients undergoing continuous ambulatory peritoneal dialysis (CAPD). Insignificant changes were noted in the pharmacokinetic parameters of metronidazole (apparent volume of distribution, elimination half-life, total body clearance). Peritoneal dialysis does not appear to reduce the serum levels of metronidazole metabolites.

Impaired Liver Function: In patients with impaired liver function, the plasma clearance of metronidazole is decreased and accumulation can therefore result.

Table 2: Flagyl

Metronidazole Elimination in Normal Subjects and in Patients with Renal Insufficiency Following a Single Intravenous Dose of Metronidazole (500 mg)

	Elimination Half-Life (hours)		
		Patients	
Compound	Normal Subjects	On Dialysis	Between Dialysis
Metronidazole	7.3±1	2.6±0.7	7.2±2.4
1-(β-hydroxyethyl) 2-hydroxymethyl-5 nitroimidazole	9.8±1.3	7.8±4.1	34±43
2-methyl-5-nitroimidazole-1-yl-acetic acid	—	7.9±4.1	138±82

INDICATIONS: Protozoal Infections:

- Trichomonal infections in men as well as in women.
- Hepatic and intestinal amebiasis.
- Giardiasis.

Bacterial Vaginosis: The 1988 Canadian Guidelines for the Treatment of Sexually Transmitted Diseases in Neonates, Children, Adolescents and Adults recommends metronidazole for the treatment of this condition.

Bacterial Infections: Treatment: Metronidazole is indicated in the treatment of serious anaerobic intra-abdominal infections due to susceptible anaerobic bacteria, such as *B. fragilis* (and other species of Bacteroides), Clostridium, Fusobacterium, Peptococcus, and Peptostreptococcus species. In the treatment of most serious anaerobic infections, intravenous metronidazole is usually administered initially. This may be followed by oral therapy with Flagyl capsules at the discretion of the physician.

Culture and susceptibility studies should be performed to determine the causative organisms and their susceptibility to metronidazole. Based on clinical judgment and anticipated bacteriological findings, therapy may be started while awaiting the results of these tests. However, modification of the treatment may be necessary once these results become available.

In mixed aerobic and anaerobic infections, consideration should be given to the concomitant administration of an antibiotic appropriate for the treatment of the aerobic component of the infection (see Warnings).

Flagyl (metronidazole) has also been used in the treatment of a small number of cases of brain or lung infections (some with abscesses) caused by anaerobic bacteria.

CONTRAINDICATIONS: Flagyl (metronidazole) is contraindicated in patients with a prior history of hypersensitivity to metronidazole or other nitroimidazole derivatives.

Flagyl should not be administered to patients with active neurological disorders or a history of blood dyscrasia, hypothyroidism or hypoadrenalism.

WARNINGS: Metronidazole has been shown to be carcinogenic in mice and rats (see Precautions). Unnecessary use of the drug should be avoided. Its use should be reserved for the conditions described in Indications.

Flagyl (metronidazole) has no direct activity against aerobic or facultative anaerobic bacteria. In patients with mixed aerobic-anaerobic infections appropriate concomitant antibiotics active against the aerobic component should be considered.

Known or previously unrecognized moniliasis may present more prominent symptoms after treatment with Flagyl.

Severe neurological disturbances (i.e. convulsive seizures and peripheral neuropathy) have been reported in patients treated with Flagyl. These have been observed very infrequently.

Occupational Hazards: Patients should be warned about the potential for confusion, dizziness, hallucinations, convulsions or transient visual disorders, and advised not to drive or operate machinery if these symptoms occur.

Flagyl should be used with caution in patients with active or chronic severe peripheral and central nervous system diseases due to the risk of neurological aggravation.

Patients should be advised not to take alcohol or alcohol-containing medicines during Flagyl therapy and for at least one day afterwards because of the possibility of a disulfiram-like (Antabuse effect) reaction.

PRECAUTIONS: General: Where there is clinical evidence of a trichomonal infection in the sexual partner, he should be treated concomitantly to avoid reinfection.

A rare case of reversible but profound neurological deterioration has been reported following a single oral dose of Flagyl (metronidazole); it is therefore advisable that a patient taking Flagyl for the first time not be left unattended for a period of two hours. The appearance of abnormal neurologic signs demands prompt discontinuation of Flagyl therapy and, when severe, immediate medical attention. Gastric lavage may be considered if no more than two or three hours have elapsed since administration of the drug.

If for compelling reasons, Flagyl must be administered longer than the usually recommended duration, it is recommended that patients should be monitored for adverse reactions such as peripheral or central neuropathy (such as paresthesia, ataxia, dizziness, convulsive seizures).

Treatment with Flagyl should be discontinued if ataxia or any other symptom of central nervous system (CNS) involvement occurs.

Patients with severe hepatic disease (including hepatic encephalopathy) metabolize metronidazole slowly with resultant accumulation of metronidazole and its metabolites in the plasma. Accordingly, for such patients, doses of Flagyl below those usually recommended should be administered and with caution.

Treatment with Flagyl should be discontinued should pancreatitis occur once other causes of this disease are excluded.

Administration of solutions containing sodium ions may result in sodium retention. Care should be taken when administering metronidazole injection to patients receiving corticosteroids or to those predisposed to edema.

Patients should be warned that Flagyl may darken urine. This is probably due to a metabolite of metronidazole and seems to have no clinical significance (see Adverse Effects).

Hematologic: Transient eosinophilia and leukopenia have been observed during treatment with Flagyl. Haematological tests, especially regular total and differential leukocyte counts are advised if administration for more than 10 days or a second course of therapy is considered to be necessary.

Carcinogenesis, Mutagenesis, Impairment of Fertility: **Metronidazole has been shown to be carcinogenic in the mouse and in the rat.** However similar studies in the hamster have given negative results. Metronidazole has been shown to be mutagenic in bacteria in vitro. In studies conducted in mammalian cells in vitro as well as in rodent in vivo, there was inadequate evidence of mutagenic effect of metronidazole.

Prominent among the effects in the mouse was the promotion of pulmonary tumorigenesis. This has been observed in all six reported studies in that species, including one study in which the animals were dosed on an intermittent schedule (administration during every fourth week only). At very high dose levels (approximately 1500 mg/m^2 which is approximately 3 times the most frequently recommended human dose for a 50 kg adult based on mg/m^2), there was a statistically significant increase in the incidence of malignant liver tumors in males. Also, the published results of one of the mouse studies indicate an increase in the incidence of malignant lymphomas as well as pulmonary neoplasms associated with lifetime feeding of the drug. All these effects are statistically significant.

Several long-term oral dosing studies in the rat have been completed. There were statistically significant increases in the incidence of various neoplasms, particularly in mammary and hepatic tumors, among female rats administered metronidazole over those noted in the concurrent female control groups. Two lifetime tumorigenicity studies in hamsters have been performed and reported to be negative.

The use of Flagyl for longer treatment than usually required should be carefully weighed since it has been shown to be carcinogenic in mice and rats (see Warnings).

Fertility studies have been performed in mice at doses up to six times the maximum recommended human oral dose (based on mg/m^2) and have revealed no evidence of impaired fertility.

Pregnancy: Metronidazole crosses the placental barrier and enters the fetal circulation rapidly. Although Flagyl has been given to pregnant women without apparent complication, its effects on human fetal organogenesis are not known; it is advisable that administration of Flagyl be avoided in pregnant patients and be withheld during the first trimester of pregnancy. In serious anaerobic infections, if the administration of Flagyl to pregnant patients is considered to be necessary, its use requires that the potential benefits to the mother be weighed against the possible risks to the fetus.

Lactation: Metronidazole is secreted in breast milk in concentrations similar to those found in plasma. Administration of Flagyl should be avoided in the nursing mother.

Children: Clinical experience in children is very limited. The monitoring of this group of patients is particularly important. The safety and effectiveness of intravenous metronidazole in children has not been established.

Laboratory Test Interferences: Flagyl interferes with serum AST, ALT, LDH, triglycerides and hexokinase glucose determinations which are based on the decrease in ultraviolet absorbance which occurs when NADH is oxidized to NAD. Metronidazole causes an increase in absorbance at the peak of NADH (340 nm) resulting in falsely decreased values.

Drug Interactions: Patients taking Flagyl should be warned against consuming alcoholic beverages and drugs containing alcohol during therapy and for at least one day afterwards, because of the possibility of a disulfiram-like (antabuse effect) reaction (flushing, vomiting, tachycardia). This reaction appears to be due to the inhibition of the oxidation of acetaldehyde, the primary metabolite of alcohol.

Administration of disulfiram and Flagyl has been associated with acute psychoses and confusion in some patients; therefore, these drugs should not be used concomitantly.

Metronidazole has been reported to potentiate the anticoagulant effect of warfarin resulting in a prolongation of prothrombin time and increased hemorrhagic risk caused by decreased hepatic catabolism. This possible drug interaction should be considered when Flagyl is prescribed for patients on this type of anticoagulant therapy. In case of coadministration, prothrombin time should be more frequently monitored and anticoagulant therapy adjusted during treatment with Flagyl.

In single dose studies, metronidazole injection did not interfere with the biotransformation of diazepam, antipyrine or phenytoin in man. However, patients maintained on phenytoin were found to have toxic blood levels after oral metronidazole administration. Phenytoin concentration returned to therapeutic blood level after discontinuance of metronidazole.

The metabolism of metronidazole has been reported to be increased by concurrent administration of phenobarbital or phenytoin. It is recommended that increased doses of metronidazole Injection be considered in such cases.

Cyclosporin: Risk of elevation of cyclosporin serum levels. Serum cyclosporin and serum creatinine should be closely monitored when coadministration is necessary.

A slight potentiation of the neuromuscular blocking activity of vecuronium has been reported in patients administered metronidazole at a dose of 15 mg/kg.

Concomitant use of lithium and Flagyl may result in lithium intoxication due to decreased renal clearance of lithium. Persistent renal damage may develop. When Flagyl must be administered to patients on lithium therapy, it may be prudent to consider tapering or discontinuing lithium temporarily when feasible. Otherwise frequent monitoring of lithium, creatinine and electrolyte levels and urine osmolality should be done.

Flagyl has been reported to reduce the clearance of 5-fluorouracil resulting in increased toxicity of 5-fluorouracil.

Busulfan: Plasma levels of busulfan may be increased by metronidazole, which may lead to severe busulfan toxicity.

ADVERSE EFFECTS: Gastrointestinal Disorders: diarrhea, nausea, vomiting, epigastric distress, epigastric pain, dyspepsia, constipation, coated tongue, dry mouth, taste disorders including metallic taste, oral mucositis. Reversible cases of pancreatitis have been reported infrequently.

Infections and Infestations: Rare cases of pseudomembranous colitis have been reported.

Hepatobiliary Disorders: Very rare cases of reversible abnormal function tests and cholestatic hepatitis sometimes with jaundice have been reported.
Blood and Lymphatic System Disorders: Transient eosinophilia, neutropenia, very rare cases of agranulocytosis and thrombocytopenia have been reported.
Skin and Subcutaneous Tissue Disorders: rash and pruritus.
Immune System Disorders: hypersensitivity reactions including flushing, urticaria, fever, angioedema, exceptional anaphylactic shocks, very rare pustular eruptions.
Cardiovascular Disorders: palpitation and chest pain.
Nervous System Disorders: convulsive seizures, peripheral sensory neuropathy, transient ataxia, dizziness, drowsiness, insomnia and headache.

Very rare reports of encephalopathy (e.g. confusion) and subacute cerebellar syndrome (e.g. ataxia, dysarthria, gait impairment, nystagmus, and tremor) have been reported, which may resolve with discontinuation of the drug.

Peripheral neuropathies have been reported in a few patients on moderately high to high-dose prolonged oral treatment with metronidazole. It would appear that the occurrence is not directly related to the daily dosage and that an important predisposing factor is the continuation of oral and/or i.v. medication for several weeks or months.

Profound neurological deterioration, within 2 hours after Flagyl administration has been reported. The occurrence is not directly related to the dosage level.
Psychiatric Disorders: confusion, hallucinations, and depressed mood.
Eye Disorders: transient vision disorders such as diplopia, myopia.
Metabolism and Nutrition Disorders: An antithyroid effect has been reported by some investigators but three different clinical studies failed to confirm this. Anorexia has been reported.
General Disorders and Administration Site Conditions: Thrombophlebitis has occurred with I.V. administration. Fever has been reported.
Other: Proliferation of *C. albicans* in the vagina, vaginal dryness and burning; dysuria; occasional flushing and headaches, especially with concomitant ingestion of alcohol; altered taste of alcoholic beverages.

Darkening of the urine has been reported. This is probably due to a metabolite of metronidazole and seems to have no clinical significance (see Precautions). Reversible lowering of serum lipids has been reported.
Reproductive System and Breast Disorders: A single case of gynecomastia has been reported which resolved on discontinuing metronidazole administration.

OVERDOSE:

Symptoms: Single oral doses of metronidazole, up to 12 g have been reported in suicide attempts and accidental overdoses. Symptoms were limited to vomiting, ataxia and slight disorientation. Neurotoxic effects, including seizures and peripheral neuropathy have been reported after 5 to 7 days of oral doses of 6 to 10.4 g every other day.

Treatment: There is no specific antidote. Early gastric lavage may remove a large amount of the drug; otherwise, symptomatic and supportive treatment should be instituted.

For management of a suspected drug overdose, CPhA recommends that you contact your **regional Poison Control Centre**. See the *CPS* Directory section for a list of Poison Control Centres.

DOSAGE: Treatment of Trichomoniasis: Consideration should be given to use Flagyl therapy (oral or vaginal) in female patients, only when trichomonal infection has been confirmed by appropriate diagnostic techniques. In the male patient, oral Flagyl is recommended in those who are evidently the source of reinfection in female consorts and those with demonstrated urogenital trichomoniasis (see Warnings).
Oral Administration: Single-Dose Treatment: For both women and men, 2 g administered as a single dose after a meal.
Standard Ten-Day Treatment: Women: One 250 mg tablet twice a day, morning and night for 10 consecutive days.
Men: One 250 mg tablet twice a day for 10 consecutive days.

For both men and women, it may be occasionally necessary to give a second ten-day course after 4 to 6 weeks.
Vaginal Treatment: Cream: One applicator full of Flagyl Cream once or twice a day into the vagina for 10 or 20 consecutive days even during menstruation. The applicator should not be used after the 7th month of pregnancy.
Treatment of Amebiasis: Adults: Intestinal Amebiasis: Three 250 mg tablets three times daily for 5 to 7 days.
Amebic Abscesses of the Liver: Two to three 250 mg tablets three times daily for 5 to 7 days.
Children: Administer 35 to 50 mg/kg/day in three divided doses for 5 to 7 days.
Treatment of Giardiasis: Adults: One 250 mg tablet twice daily for 5 to 7 days.
Children: Administer 25 to 35 mg/kg/day in two divided doses for 5 to 7 days.
Note: The efficacy of the recommended dosages for the treatment of amebiasis and giardiasis has been demonstrated. However, the optimal dose, the duration of treatment and the risk of recurrence have not been completely established.
Treatment of Bacterial Vaginosis: Adults: 500 mg orally twice a day for 7 days. Concurrent treatment of sexual partners is not usually indicated.
Anaerobic Infections: Adults: Treatment: In the treatment of most serious anaerobic infections, i.v. metronidazole is usually administered initially. This may be followed by oral therapy with Flagyl capsules at the discretion of the physician.

Duration of therapy depends upon clinical and bacteriological assessment. Treatment for seven days should be satisfactory for most patients. However, in cases where infection sites cannot be drained or which are liable to endogenous recontamination by anaerobic pathogens, a longer treatment may be required.
Oral Administration: 500 mg every 8 hours.
Severe Hepatic Disease: Patients with severe hepatic disease metabolize metronidazole slowly, with resultant accumulation of metronidazole and its metabolites. Accordingly, doses below those usually recommended should be administered and with caution. However, due to a lack of pharmacokinetic information, specific dosage recommendations cannot be given for these patients. Therefore, close monitoring of blood metronidazole levels and of the patients for signs of toxicity are recommended (see Warnings and Precautions).
Severe Impairment of Renal Function and Anuria: The elimination half-life of metronidazole in anuric patients is not significantly altered. However, the elimination half-lives of the metabolites of metronidazole are significantly increased (3- to 13-fold). Consequently, although metronidazole would not be expected to accumulate in these patients, accumulation of the metabolites would be expected. The potential for toxicity of these metabolites is not known.
Patients on Hemodialysis: The dose of Flagyl need not be specifically reduced since accumulated metabolites may be rapidly removed by hemodialysis.
Patients on Peritoneal Dialysis: Peritoneal dialysis does not appear to reduce serum levels of metronidazole metabolites.

Patients with severe impairment of renal function who are not undergoing hemodialysis should be monitored closely for signs of toxicity.
Children: The safety and effectiveness of Flagyl in children is not known. Due to lack of pharmacokinetic data, no dosage recommendations can be made (see Precautions).

SUPPLIED: Oral Capsules: Each pale green and light gray capsule, printed ⊛ and 500, contains: metronidazole 500 mg. Nonmedicinal ingredients: black ink, D&C Red No. 33, D&C Yellow No. 10, FD&C Blue No. 1, FD&C Green No. 3, gelatin, lactose monohydrate, magnesium stearate, polacrilin potassium, silicon dioxide, sodium lauryl sulfate and titanium dioxide. Sodium: <1 mmol (5.47 mg). Tartrazine-free. Bottles of 100. Store between 15 to 30°C.
Vaginal Cream: Each tube contains: metronidazole 10% w/w in a cream base. Nonmedicinal ingredients: glycerin, glyceryl monostearate, methylparaben, propylparaben, purified water, stearic acid and trolamine. Tartrazine-free. Tubes of 60 g with applicator. Store between 15 to 30°C.

(Shown in Product Identification Section)

Flagystatin® Ⓟ
metronidazole—nystatin
Trichomonacide—Moniliacide

sanofi-aventis

Date of Revision: May 1, 2006

PHARMACOLOGY: Flagyl shows little or no effect on the cardiovascular, respiratory or autonomic nervous systems of dogs, rats and mice.

In vitro, activity was studied using decreasing concentrations of metronidazole which were added to a series of *T. vaginalis* cultures maintained at 37°C. A 1:400 000 dilution of metronidazole kills up to 99% of the trichomonads in 24 hours.

In vivo, 0.5 mL of a 48-hour culture of *T. vaginalis* injected under the dorsal skin in a control and a test group of mice revealed, seven days later, extensive abscess-like lesions swarming with trichomonads in the control group and normal subcutaneous tissue free of trichomonads in the animals which had received oral metronidazole in a daily dosage of 12.5 mg/kg of body weight.

Nystatin is not absorbed from mucous membranes; therefore, no systemic manifestations are observed after local application of the product.

In vitro, Nystatin is fungistatic against *C. albicans* at a concentration of 3.12 µg/mL (4.4-6.2 U/mL) in liquid medium. A fungicidal activity is observed after a 5-hour contact with 1000 µg/mL (1400-2000 U/mL) or after 24 hours with 100 µg/mL (140-200 U/mL).

In vivo, rabbits were infested by the oral route with 2.5 x 108 cells of *C. albicans*. The administration of 50 mg/kg (100 000 U/kg) per os for 3 days reduced the number of organisms found in the feces from a few millions to less than 20 yeast cells per g.

Mortality in rabbits infested with *C. albicans* by the I.V. route is usually 100%. It is reduced to 62.5% when 20 mg (40 000 IU) is administered twice daily by the S.C. route for 4 days.

Metronidazole and Nystatin do not show antagonism in vitro. It was demonstrated that, when used in combination, (in the proportion of 5 µg of metronidazole to 1 unit of Nystatin as in Flagystatin vaginal inserts) Nystatin does not alter the antitrichomonal activity of Flagyl and that Flagyl does not affect the anticandidal activity of Nystatin. Furthermore, the presence of excessive amounts of either product failed to alter the specific effectiveness of the other.

It was also shown that both Flagystatin vaginal inserts and ovules and Flagystatin cream exert antitrichomonal and anticandidal activities comparable to those of the individual components.

INDICATIONS: Mixed vaginal infection due to *T. vaginalis* and *C. albicans*.

CONTRAINDICATIONS: Hypersensitivity to either of the components. Combined treatment with oral Flagyl should be avoided in cases of active neurological disorders or a history of blood dyscrasia, hypothyroidism or hypoadrenalism unless in the opinion of the physician the benefits outweigh the possible hazard to the patient. See also Flagyl monograph.

WARNINGS: Nystatin possesses little or no antibacterial activity while metronidazole is selective against certain anaerobic bacteria; therefore, Flagystatin may not be effective in bacterial vaginal infections and should not be prescribed unless there is direct evidence of trichomonal infestation.

PRECAUTIONS: Where there is evidence of trichomonal infestation in the sexual partner, he should be treated concomitantly with oral Flagyl to avoid reinfestation.

It is possible that adverse effects normally associated with oral administration of metronidazole may occur following the vaginal administration of Flagystatin.

When administering oral Flagyl (see Flagyl Product Monograph) the following precautions must be borne in mind.

Patients should be warned against consuming alcohol, because of a possible disulfiram-like reaction. Although no persistent hematologic abnormalities have been observed in clinical studies, total and differential leukocyte counts should be made before and after treatment, especially if a second course of oral Flagyl therapy is needed.

Metronidazole passes the placental barrier. Although it has been given to pregnant women without apparent complication, it is advisable that oral use be avoided in pregnant patients and the drug be withheld during the first trimester of pregnancy.

Oral treatment should be discontinued if ataxia or any other symptom of CNS involvement occurs.

ADVERSE EFFECTS: Infrequent and minor adverse reactions reported to date include: vaginal burning and granular sensation; bitter taste, nausea and vomiting, already known to occur with metronidazole were mainly seen when oral metronidazole was administered concomitantly with Flagystatin local treatment.

In the course of clinical trials, reactions, not necessarily related to the product, were observed: spots on the skin around the knees, welts all over the body, aching and swelling of wrists and ankles, pruritus, headache, coated tongue and fatigue.

OVERDOSE:

Symptoms: No case of accidental massive ingestion of Flagystatin has been reported yet. However, should this occur, symptoms such as nausea, vomiting, diarrhea and slight disorientation may be observed.

Treatment: No specific antidote. Treatment should be symptomatic after gastric lavage.

For management of a suspected drug overdose, CPhA recommends that you contact your **regional Poison Control Centre**. See the *CPS* Directory section for a list of Poison Control Centres.

DOSAGE: One vaginal ovule, or one applicatorful of Flagystatin cream daily, inserted deep into the vagina, for 10 consecutive days. If after 10 days of treatment a cure has not been achieved a second 10-day course of treatment should be given. If Trichomonas vaginalis has not been completely eliminated, oral Flagyl 250 mg b.i.d. should be administered for 10 days.

SUPPLIED: Vaginal Cream: Each applicatorful of cream delivers: metronidazole 500 mg and nystatin 100 000 units. Nonmedicinal ingredients: methylparaben 0.12%, propylparaben 0.04%. Tartrazine-free. Tubes of 55 g with applicator.
Vaginal Ovules: Each ovule contains: metronidazole 500 mg and nystatin 100 000 units. Boxes of 10 with applicator.

Flarex® Ⓟ
fluorometholone acetate
Corticosteroid

Alcon

SUPPLIED: Each mL of sterile ophthalmic suspension contains: fluorometholone acetate 0.1%. Nonmedicinal ingredients: benzalkonium chloride 0.01% (as preservative), edetate disodium, hydrochloric acid and/or sodium hydroxide (to adjust pH), hydroxyethyl cellulose, monobasic sodium phosphate, purified water, sodium chloride and tyloxapol. Plastic Drop-Tainer dispensers of 5 mL. Protect from freezing. Store upright at room temperature.

Fleet Enema®
sodium phosphates
Laxative

Johnson & Johnson • Merck

Fleet Enema® Mineral Oil
mineral oil
Laxative

Johnson & Johnson • Merck

PHARMACOLOGY: Fleet Enema: Useful as a laxative in the relief of constipation, and as a bowel evacuant for a variety of diagnostic, surgical and therapeutic indications. Dibasic sodium phosphate and monobasic sodium phosphate are poorly absorbed from the gastrointestinal tract and retain water in the lumen of the intestine. When administered rectally as an enema, they produce a watery evacuation of the bowel. Fleet Enema provides cleansing action and induces complete emptying of the left colon usually in 2 to 5 minutes.
Fleet Enema Mineral Oil: Serves to soften and lubricate the contents of the intestinal tract, easing their passage without irritating the mucosa. Results approximate a normal bowel movement in that only the rectum, sigmoid and part or all of the descending colon are evacuated. Results are usually obtained in 2 to 15 minutes.

INDICATIONS: Fleet Enema: Useful as a laxative in the relief of constipation. As a routine enema, when bowel evacuation is needed for proctoscopy and sigmoidoscopy, preoperative cleansing and general postoperative care, to help relieve fecal or barium impaction, collecting stool specimens, during pregnancy and pre- and postnatally.

Fleet Enema Mineral Oil: Lubricant laxative. For the relief of occasional constipation. Especially suitable for bowel cleansing when straining might be dangerous, painful, or unproductive, as in: hypertension, cardiovascular syndromes, pelvic hernia, hemorrhoids, care of many postoperative conditions, gastrointestinal irritations, atonic colon, impaction in the paralyzed patient, chronic pelvic inflammatory disease and abdominal aneurysm; to obtain the laxative benefits of mineral oil when oral cathartics are contraindicated.

CONTRAINDICATIONS: Fleet Enema: Should **not** be used when the following medical problems exist: appendicitis (or symptoms of), intestinal blockage, ulcerative colitis, ileitis, heart disease, rectal bleeding, high blood pressure, kidney disease.
Fleet Enema: Children: Not recommended for infants under 6 months of age.
Fleet Enema Mineral Oil: Should **not** be used when the following medical problems exist: appendicitis (or symptoms of), intestinal blockage, ulcerative colitis, ileitis, rectal bleeding, kidney disease.

WARNINGS: Fleet Enema: Do **not** use in the presence of abdominal pain, nausea, fever or vomiting, (this could refer to signs of appendicitis or inflamed bowel), cardiac disease, severe dehydration or debility.

Frequent or prolonged use of enemas may result in dependence for bowel function. Use only when needed or when prescribed by a physician.
Children and Geriatrics: Children and elderly persons are more sensitive to the effects of enemas.
Fleet Enema Mineral Oil: Do **not** use in the presence of abdominal pain, nausea, fever or vomiting (this could refer to signs of appendicitis or inflamed bowel).

Frequent or prolonged use of enemas may result in dependence for bowel function.
Children and Geriatrics: Give to children only on the advice of, and as directed by a physician. Children and elderly persons are more sensitive to the effects of enemas.

PRECAUTIONS: Fleet Enema: **Do not administer to children under 2 years of age except on the advice of a physician.** In dehydrated or debilitated patients, volume of solution administered must be carefully determined since the solution is hypertonic and may cause further dehydration. Care should be taken to ensure that the contents of the bowel are expelled after administration. Repeated usage at short intervals should be avoided. Laxative products should not be used longer than 1 week unless directed by a physician.
Fleet Enema Mineral Oil: **Do not administer to children under 2 years of age except on the advice of a physician.** Care should be taken to ensure that the contents of the bowel are expelled after administration. Laxative products should not be used longer than 1 week unless directed by a physician.

ADVERSE EFFECTS: No data supplied by the manufacturer.

OVERDOSE:
No data supplied by the manufacturer.

For management of a suspected drug overdose, CPhA recommends that you contact your **regional Poison Control Centre**. See the *CPS* Directory section for a list of Poison Control Centres.

DOSAGE: For rectal use only.
Fleet Enema: Adults: 120 mL. Children 2 to 12 years: 60 mL as a single dose or as directed by a physician. Children under 2 years: consult a physician.

The enema does not require warming. May be used at room temperature.
Preferred Position: Lying on left side with knees flexed, or in the knee-chest position. Remove protective cap from the prelubricated rectal tube before using. Insert tube gently, pointing it in the direction of the navel. Slowly squeeze bottle to empty contents into rectum. Rubber diaphragm at base of tube prevents accidental leakage and assures controlled flow of the enema solution. Withdraw the tube from rectum. (An extra amount of solution is provided to allow for the quantity normally remaining in bottle after squeezing.) Maintain position until defecation impulse is felt, usually within 2 to 5 minutes.
Fleet Enema Mineral Oil: Adults and children 12 years and older: 120 mL as a single dose. Children 2 to 12 years: 60 mL as a single dose. Children under 2 years: Consult a physician.

The enema should first be warmed by placing bottle in water at body temperature.
Preferred Position: Lying on left side with knees flexed, or in the knee-chest position. Remove protective cap from the prelubricated rectal tube before using. Insert the tube gently pointing it in the direction of the navel and squeeze bottle to empty contents into rectum. Rubber diaphragm at base of tube prevents accidental leakage and assures controlled flow of the enema solution. Withdraw the tube from rectum. (An extra amount of oil solution is provided to allow for the quantity normally remaining in bottle after squeezing.) The body position should be maintained until a strong urge to have a bowel movement is felt or the enema should be retained for length of time indicated by physician. Results are usually felt within 2 to 15 minutes. Contents of the bowel should then be expelled.

SUPPLIED: Fleet Enema: Each 100 mL of solution contains: monobasic sodium phosphate 16 g and dibasic sodium phosphate 6 g in single dose disposable unit. Nonmedicinal ingredients: sodium methylhydroxybenzoate. Ready-to-use, hand size plastic squeeze bottles of 130 mL, with a 5 cm prelubricated rectal tube and protective cap. Also available: Fleet Enema Pediatric (sodium phosphates enema) (65 mL).
Fleet Enema Mineral Oil: Each single dose disposable unit of solution contains: mineral oil USP 130 mL. Ready-to-use hand-size plastic squeeze bottle, with a 5 cm prelubricated rectal tube and protective cap.

Flintstones®
multiple vitamins and minerals
Vitamin—Mineral Supplement

Bayer Consumer Care

SUPPLIED: Multiple Vitamins: Each flavoured, chewable, shaped tablet contains: vitamin A (as acetate) 480 µg (1600 IU), thiamine (vitamin B_1) (thiamine mononitrate) 1.5 mg, riboflavin (vitamin B_2) (riboflavin) 1.5 mg, vitamin B_6 (pyridoxine hydrochloride) 1 mg, vitamin B_{12} (cyanocobalamin) 3 µg, vitamin C (sodium ascorbate) 50 mg, vitamin D (cholecalciferol) 10 µg (400 IU), folate (folic acid) 0.1 mg and niacinamide (niacinamide) 8 mg. Nonmedicinal ingredients: butylated hydroxytoluene, citric acid, dl-alpha tocopherol, FD&C Blue #2, FD&C Red #3, FD&C Red #40, FD&C Yellow #6, flavours (grape, orange, strawberry and tangerine), gelatin, glycerides of stearic and palmytic acids, invert sugar, magnesium stearate, malic acid, maltodextrin, microcrystalline cellulose, pectin, silica gel, sodium aluminosilicate, sodium benzoate, sodium citrate, sorbic acid, soybean oil, starch, stearic acid, sucrose and triglycerides. Bottles of 60.
Multiple Vitamins Complete: Each flavored, chewable, shaped tablet contains: vitamin A (as acetate) 480 µg (1600 IU), thiamine (vitamin B_1) (thiamine mononitrate) 1.5 mg, riboflavin (vitamin B_2) (riboflavin) 1.5 mg, vitamin B_6 (pyridoxine hydrochloride) 1 mg, vitamin B_{12} (cyanocobalamin) 3 µg, biotin (biotin) 30 µg, vitamin C (sodium ascorbate) 50 mg, vitamin D (cholecalciferol) 10 µg (400 IU), vitamin E (dl-alpha tocopheryl acetate) 4.5 mg (10 IU), folate (folic acid) 0.1 mg, niacinamide (niacinamide) 8 mg, pantothenic acid (calcium d-pantothenate) 10 mg, calcium (calcium phosphate dibasic) 160 mg, copper (cupric oxide) 1 mg, iron (ferrous fumarate) 4 mg and phosphorus (calcium phosphate dibasic) 125 mg. Nonmedicinal ingredients: aspartame, butylated hydroxytoluene, carrageenan, citric acid, FD&C Blue #2, FD&C Red #3, FD&C Red #40, FD&C Yellow #6, flavours (cherry, grape, lemon, orange, raspberry and tutti-fruitti), gelatin, glycerides of stearic and palmytic acids, hydrogenated vegetable oil, magnesium stearate, malic acid, monoammonium glycyrrhizinate, pectin, silica gel, sodium aluminosilicate, sodium benzoate, sodium citrate, sorbic acid, sorbitol, soybean oil, starch, stearic acid, sucrose and triglycerides. Bottles of 60 and 150.
Multiple Vitamins Plus Iron: Each flavoured, chewable, shaped tablet contains: vitamin A (as acetate) 480 µg (1600 IU), thiamine (vitamin B_1) (thiamine mononitrate) 1.5 mg, riboflavin (vitamin B_2) (riboflavin) 1.5 mg, vitamin B_6 (pyridoxine hydrochloride) 1 mg, vitamin B_{12} (cyanocobalamin) 3 µg, vitamin C (sodium ascorbate) 50 mg, vitamin D (cholecalciferol) 10 µg (400 IU), folate (folic acid) 0.1 mg, niacinamide (niacinamide) 8 mg and iron (ferrous fumarate) 4 mg. Nonmedicinal ingredients: butylated hydroxytoluene, citric acid, dl-alpha tocopherol, FD&C Blue #2, FD&C Red #3, FD&C Red #40, FD&C Yellow #6, flavours (grape, orange, strawberry and tangerine), gelatin, glycerides of stearic and palmytic acids, invert sugar, magnesium stearate, malic acid, maltodextrin, microcrystalline cellulose, pectin, silica gel, sodium aluminosilicate, sodium benzoate, sodium citrate, sorbic acid, soybean oil, starch, stearic acid, sucrose and triglycerides. Bottles of 60.
Multiple Vitamins with Extra C: Each flavoured, chewable, shaped tablet contains: vitamin A (as acetate) 480 µg (1600 IU), thiamine (vitamin B_1) (thiamine mononitrate) 1.5 mg, riboflavin (vitamin B_2) (riboflavin) 1.5 mg, vitamin B_6 (pyridoxine hydrochloride) 1 mg, vitamin B_{12} (cyanocobalamin) 3 µg, vitamin C (sodium ascorbate and ascorbic acid) 250 mg, vitamin D (cholecalciferol) 10 µg (400 IU), folate (folic acid) 0.1 mg and niacinamide (niacinamide) 8 mg. Nonmedicinal ingredients: butylated hydroxytoluene, citric acid, dl-alpha tocopherol, FD&C Blue #2, FD&C Red #3, FD&C Red #40, FD&C Yellow #6, flavours (grape, orange, strawberry and tangerine), fructose, gelatin, glycerides of stearic and palmytic acids, hypromellose, invert sugar, magnesium stearate, malic acid, maltodextrin, microcrystalline cellulose, pectin, silica gel, sodium aluminosilicate, sodium benzoate, sodium citrate, sorbic acid, soybean oil, starch, stearic acid, sucrose and triglycerides. Bottles of 60.
Sour Gummies: Each gummy contains: vitamin A (as acetate) 480 µg (1600 IU), vitamin B_6 (pyridoxine hydrochloride) 2 mg, vitamin B_{12} (cyanocobalamin) 6 µg, vitamin C (ascorbic acid) 20 mg, vitamin D (cholecalciferol) 5 µg (200 IU), vitamin E (dl-alpha tocopheryl acetate) 4.5 mg (10 IU) and folate (folic acid) 100 µg. Nonmedicinal ingredients: acacia gum, calcium citrate, calcium lactate, citric acid, corn starch, dl-alpha tocopherol, FD&C Blue #1, FD&C Red #40, FD&C Yellow #5, FD&C Yellow #6, flavours (apple, cherry and orange), gelatin, glucose syrup, lactic acid, malic acid, maltodextrin, silicon dioxide, starch sodium octenylsuccinate, sucrose and water. Bottles of 50.
Gummies: Each gummy contains: vitamin A (as acetate) 480 µg (1600 IU), vitamin B_6 (pyridoxine hydrochloride) 2 mg, vitamin B_{12} (cyanocobalamin) 6 µg, vitamin C (ascorbic acid) 20 mg, vitamin D (cholecalciferol) 5 µg (200 IU), vitamin E (dl-alpha tocopheryl acetate) 4.5 mg and folate (folic acid) 100 µg. Nonmedicinal ingredients: acacia gum, beeswax, carnauba wax, citric acid, corn starch, dl-alpha tocopherol, FD&C Blue #1, FD&C Red #40, FD&C Yellow #6, flavours (cherry, fruit punch and orange), gelatin, glucose syrup, maltodextrin, silicon dioxide, starch sodium octenylsuccinate, sucrose, vegetable oil and water. Bottles of 50.

Flolan® for Injection Ⓟ
epoprostenol sodium
Vasodilator

GlaxoSmithKline

Date of Revision: March 11, 2008

PHARMACOLOGY: FLOLAN (epoprostenol sodium), also known as prostacyclin, PGI_2 or PGX, a metabolite of arachidonic acid, is a naturally occurring prostaglandin. Epoprostenol has 2 major pharmacological actions: (1) direct vasodilation of pulmonary and systemic arterial vascular beds, and (2) inhibition of platelet aggregation. In animals, the vasodilatory effects of epoprostenol reduce right and left ventricular afterload and increase cardiac output and stroke volume. The effect of epoprostenol on heart rate in animals varies with dose. At low doses, there is vagally mediated bradycardia, but at higher doses, epoprostenol causes reflex tachycardia in response to direct vasodilation and hypotension. No major effects on cardiac conduction have been observed. Additional pharmacologic effects of epoprostenol in animals include bronchodilation, inhibition of gastric acid secretion and decreased gastric emptying.
Pharmacokinetics: Epoprostenol is rapidly hydrolyzed at neutral blood pH and is also subject to enzymatic degradation. Animal studies using tritium-labelled epoprostenol have indicated a high clearance (93 mL/min/kg), small volume of distribution (357 mL/kg) and a short half-life (2.7 minutes). During infusions in animals, steady-state plasma concentrations of tritium-labelled epoprostenol were reached within 15 minutes and were proportional to infusion rates.

No available chemical assay is sufficiently sensitive and specific to assess the in vivo human pharmacokinetics of epoprostenol. The in vitro half-life of epoprostenol in human blood at 37°C and pH 7.4 is approximately 6 minutes; the in vivo half-life of epoprostenol in man is therefore expected to be no greater than 6 minutes. The in vitro pharmacologic half-life of epoprostenol in human plasma, based on inhibition of platelet aggregation, is 10.6 minutes in males (n=954) and 10.8 minutes in females (n=1024).

Tritium-labelled epoprostenol has been administered to humans in order to identify the metabolic products of epoprostenol. Epoprostenol is metabolized to 6-keto-$PGF_{1\alpha}$ (formed by spontaneous degradation) and 6,15-diketo-13,14-dihydro-$PGF_{1\alpha}$ (enzymatically formed), both of which have pharmacological activity at orders of magnitude less than epoprostenol in animal test systems. The recovery of radioactivity in urine and feces over a 1-week period was 82% and 4% of the administered dose, respectively. Fourteen additional minor metabolites have been isolated from urine, indicating that epoprostenol is extensively metabolized in man.
Pharmacodynamics: Acute Hemodynamic Effects of FLOLAN in Pulmonary Hypertension: Acute i.v. infusions of FLOLAN for up to 15 minutes in patients with primary pulmonary hypertension and secondary pulmonary hypertension due to Scleroderma Spectrum of Diseases (SSD) produced dose-related increases in cardiac index (CI) and stroke volume (SV), and dose-related decreases in pulmonary vascular resistance (PVR), total pulmonary resistance (TPR), and mean systemic arterial pressure (SAPm). The effects of FLOLAN on mean pulmonary artery pressure (PAPm) were variable and minor.
Chronic Hemodynamic Effects of FLOLAN in Primary Pulmonary Hypertension (PPH): Chronic hemodynamic effects were generally similar to acute effects. CI, SV, and arterial oxygen saturation were increased, and PAPm, right atrial pressure (RAP), TPR, and systemic vascular resistance (SVR) were decreased in patients who received FLOLAN chronically, compared to those who did not.

Survival was improved in NYHA functional Class III and Class IV PPH patients treated with FLOLAN for 12 weeks in a multicentre, open, randomized, parallel, controlled study. At the end of the treatment period, 8 of 40 patients receiving standard therapy alone had died, whereas none of the 41 patients receiving FLOLAN had died (p=0.003).

Table 1 illustrates the treatment-related hemodynamic changes in these patients after 8 or 12 weeks of treatment.

Table 1: FLOLAN for Injection

Hemodynamics During Chronic Administration of FLOLAN in Patients with PPH

Hemodynamic Parameter	Baseline		Mean Change from Baseline at End of Treatment Period[a]	
	FLOLAN (n=52)	Conventional Therapy (n=54)	FLOLAN (n=48)	Conventional Therapy (n=41)
CI (L/min/m²)	2.0	2.0	0.3[b]	−0.1
PAPm (mm Hg)	60	60	−5[b]	1
PVR (Wood U)	16	17	−4[b]	1
SAPm (mm Hg)	89	91	−4	−3
SV (mL/beat)	44	43	6[b]	−1
TPR (Wood U)	20	21	−5[b]	1

[a] At 8 weeks: FLOLAN n=10; Conventional Therapy n=11 (n is the number of patients with hemodynamic data).
At 12 weeks: FLOLAN n=38; Conventional Therapy n=30 (n is the number of patients with hemodynamic data).
[b] Denotes statistically significant difference between FLOLAN and Conventional Therapy groups.
Legend: CI=cardiac index; PAPm=mean pulmonary arterial pressure; PVR=pulmonary vascular resistance; SAPm=mean systemic arterial pressure; SV=stroke volume; TPR=total pulmonary resistance.

Chronic Infusion in Secondary Pulmonary Hypertension (SPH) due to SSD: Hemodynamic Effects: Chronic continuous infusions of FLOLAN in patients with SPH due to scleroderma spectrum of diseases (SSD) were studied in a prospective, open, randomized trial of 12 weeks duration comparing FLOLAN plus conventional therapy to conventional therapy alone. Except for the 5 New York Heart Association (NYHA) functional Class II patients, all patients were either functional Class III or Class IV. The patients principally had pulmonary vascular manifestations of the collagen-vascular disease, with minimal evidence of interstitial lung disease and with total lung capacities greater than 60% of the predicted normal. Dosage of FLOLAN was determined as described in Dosage and averaged 11.2 ng/kg/min at study end. Conventional therapy varied among patients and included oxygen and diuretics in two-thirds of the patients, oral vasodilators in 40% of the patients, and digoxin in a third of the patients. A statistically significant increase in CI, and statistically significant decreases in PAPm, RAP, PVR, and SAPm were observed in patients who received FLOLAN chronically compared to those who did not. Table 2 illustrates the treatment-related hemodynamic changes in these patients after 12 weeks of treatment.

Table 2: FLOLAN for Injection

Hemodynamics During Chronic Administration of FLOLAN in Patients with SPH due to SSD

Hemodynamic Parameter	Baseline		Mean Change from Baseline at 12 Weeks	
	FLOLAN (n=56)	Conventional Therapy (n=55)	FLOLAN (n=50)	Conventional Therapy (n=48)
PAPm (mm Hg)	51	49	−5[a]	1
RAP (mm Hg)	13	11	−1[a]	1
PVR (Wood U)	14	11	−5[a]	1
SAPm (mm Hg)	93	89	−8[a]	−1

[a] Denotes statistically significant difference between FLOLAN and Conventional Therapy groups (n is the number of patients with hemodynamic data).

Legend: CI=cardiac index; PAPm=mean pulmonary arterial pressure; RAP=right atrial pressure; PVR=pulmonary vascular resistance; SAPm=mean systemic arterial pressure.

Clinical Effects: Statistically significant improvement was observed in exercise capacity, as measured by the 6-minute walk, in patients receiving continuous i.v. FLOLAN plus conventional therapy for 12 weeks, compared to those receiving conventional therapy alone. Improvements were apparent as early as the first week of therapy. Increases in exercise capacity were accompanied by statistically significant improvements in dyspnea and fatigue, as measured by the Borg Dyspnea Index and Dyspnea Fatigue Index. By week 12, NYHA Functional Class improved in 21 of 51 (41%) patients treated with FLOLAN compared to none of the 48 patients treated with conventional therapy alone.

No statistical difference in survival over 12 weeks was observed in SPH patients treated with FLOLAN. At the end of the treatment period, 4 of 56 (7%) patients receiving FLOLAN died, whereas 5 of 55 (9%) patients receiving conventional therapy died.

INDICATIONS: FLOLAN (epoprostenol sodium) is indicated for the long-term i.v. treatment of primary pulmonary hypertension (PPH) and secondary pulmonary hypertension (SPH) due to scleroderma spectrum of diseases (SSD) in NYHA functional Class III and Class IV patients who did not respond adequately to conventional therapy.

Prior to initiation of therapy, the potential benefit of FLOLAN should be weighed against the risks associated with use of the drug and the presence of an indwelling central venous catheter.

FLOLAN should be used only by clinicians experienced in the diagnosis and treatment of pulmonary hypertension. The diagnosis of PPH or SPH due to SSD should be carefully established by standard clinical tests.

CONTRAINDICATIONS: The chronic use of FLOLAN (epoprostenol sodium) in patients with congestive heart failure (CHF) due to severe left ventricular systolic dysfunction is contraindicated. A large study evaluating the effect of FLOLAN on survival in NYHA Class III and IV patients with CHF due to severe left ventricular systolic dysfunction was terminated after an interim analysis of 471 patients revealed a higher mortality in patients receiving FLOLAN plus conventional therapy than in those receiving conventional therapy alone.

FLOLAN is also contraindicated in patients with known or suspected hypersensitivity to the drug or any of its excipients, or to structurally related compounds.

FLOLAN should not be used chronically in patients who develop pulmonary edema during dose initiation.

WARNINGS: FLOLAN (epoprostenol sodium) must be reconstituted only as directed using specific Sterile Diluent for FLOLAN. FLOLAN must not be reconstituted or mixed with any other parenteral medications or solutions prior to or during administration.

FLOLAN is not to be used for bolus administration (see Adverse Effects, Adverse Events During Acute Dose Escalation).

Abrupt Withdrawal: Abrupt withdrawal (including interruptions in drug delivery) or sudden large reductions in dosage of FLOLAN may result in symptoms associated with rebound pulmonary hypertension, including dyspnea, dizziness, and asthenia. In clinical trials, there were rare reports of deaths considered attributable to the interruption of FLOLAN. Abrupt withdrawal should be avoided.

Pulmonary Edema: A minority of patients have pulmonary hypertension associated with pulmonary veno-occlusive disease. Some of these patients develop pulmonary edema during dose initiation. Where pulmonary edema arises within hours to days of starting FLOLAN infusion, a diagnosis of veno-occlusive disease should be considered. In such cases, consideration should be given to discontinuation of FLOLAN. The FLOLAN should be discontinued after dose tapering.

FLOLAN should not be used chronically in patients who develop pulmonary edema during dose initiation.

Sepsis: Sepsis is a known risk associated with the presence of an indwelling central venous catheter and requires immediate access to expert medical care (see Adverse Effects, Adverse Events Attributable to the Drug Delivery System).

PRECAUTIONS: FLOLAN (epoprostenol sodium) is a potent pulmonary and systemic vasodilator. The cardiovascular effects during infusion disappear within 30 minutes of the end of administration. Acute dose initiation with FLOLAN must be performed in a hospital setting with adequate personnel and equipment for physiologic monitoring and emergency care.

Epoprostenol is a potent inhibitor of platelet aggregation, therefore, an increased risk for hemorrhagic complications should be considered, particularly for patients with other risk factors for bleeding (see Risk of Bleeding and Drug Interactions).

Because of the high pH of the final infusion solutions, care should be taken to avoid extravasation during their administration and consequent risk of tissue damage.

During the early phase of chronic administration, intense patient education is required.

Due to the potential for problems associated with the drug delivery system, immediate access to medical care should be available during chronic treatment.

FLOLAN is infused continuously through a permanent indwelling central venous catheter via a small, portable infusion pump. Thus, therapy with FLOLAN requires commitment by the patient to drug reconstitution, drug administration, care of the permanent central venous catheter, and access to intense and ongoing patient education. Sterile technique must be adhered to in preparing the drug and in the care of the catheter, and even brief interruptions in the delivery of FLOLAN may result in rapid symptomatic deterioration. The decision to receive FLOLAN for pulmonary hypertension should be based upon the understanding that there is a high likelihood that therapy with FLOLAN will be needed for prolonged periods, possibly years, and the patient's ability to accept and care for a permanent i.v. catheter and infusion pump should be carefully considered.

Based on clinical trials, the acute hemodynamic response to FLOLAN did not correlate well with survival during chronic use of FLOLAN. Dosage of FLOLAN during chronic use should be adjusted at the first sign of recurrence or worsening of symptoms attributable to pulmonary hypertension or the occurrence of adverse events associated with FLOLAN (see Dosage). Following dosage adjustments, standing and supine blood pressure and heart rate should be monitored closely for several hours.

During ongoing treatment, patients should avoid situations which promote vasodilation such as saunas, hot baths and sunbathing. Severe hypotension has been seen in patients treated with chronic FLOLAN infusions under such circumstances.

FLOLAN use has been associated with an increased incidence of bradycardia in patients with pulmonary hypertension and with episodes of severe hypotension, including fatalities.

Elevated serum glucose levels have been reported during infusion of FLOLAN in man but these are not inevitable.

Hypotension may be profound in overdose and may result in loss of consciousness (see Overdose).

Risk of Bleeding: Prothrombin times should be monitored because anticoagulant therapy is generally recommended in these patients. Platelet counts should also be monitored.

Drug Interactions: Additional reductions in blood pressure may occur when FLOLAN is administered with diuretics, antihypertensive agents or other vasodilators. When NSAIDs or other drugs affecting platelet aggregation are used concomitantly, there is the potential for FLOLAN to increase the risk of bleeding. In clinical trials, FLOLAN was used with digoxin, diuretics, anticoagulants, oral vasodilators and supplemental oxygen.

The vasodilator effects of FLOLAN may augment or be augmented by concomitant use of other vasodilators.

In a pharmacokinetic substudy in patients with congestive heart failure receiving furosemide or digoxin in whom FLOLAN therapy was initiated, apparent oral clearance values for furosemide (n=23) and digoxin (n=30) were decreased by 13% and 15%, respectively, on the second day of therapy and returned to baseline values by day 87. The change in furosemide clearance value is not likely to be clinically significant. However, patients on digoxin may show elevations of digoxin concentrations after initiation of therapy with FLOLAN, which may be clinically significant in patients prone to digoxin toxicity.

Pregnancy: There are no adequate and well-controlled studies in pregnant women.

Labor and Delivery: The use of FLOLAN during labor, vaginal delivery, or caesarean section has not been studied in humans.

Lactation: It is not known whether this drug is excreted in human milk. Because many drugs are excreted in human milk, consideration should be given to discontinuation of breast-feeding when FLOLAN is to be administered to a nursing woman.

Children: The safety and effectiveness of FLOLAN in children have not been established.

Geriatrics: Clinical studies of FLOLAN did not include sufficient numbers of patients aged 65 and over to determine whether they respond differently from younger patients. In general, dose selection for an elderly patient should be made carefully, reflecting the greater frequency of decreased hepatic, renal, or cardiac function and of concomitant disease or other drug therapy.

Occupational Hazards: Ability to perform tasks that require judgement, motor or cognitive skills: Pulmonary hypertension and its therapeutic management may affect the ability to drive and operate machinery.

ADVERSE EFFECTS: During clinical trials, adverse events were classified as follows: (1) adverse events during dose escalation, (2) adverse events during chronic dosing, and (3) adverse events associated with the drug delivery system.

Adverse Events During Dose Escalation: In early clinical trials, FLOLAN was increased in 2 ng/kg/min increments until such times as the patients developed symptomatic intolerance. The most common adverse events and those that limited further increases in dose were generally related to the major pharmacologic effect of FLOLAN, i.e., vasodilation. Table 3 lists the adverse events reported during dose escalation in decreasing order of frequency as well as the % of cases where the event was dose-limiting. Age-related differences (<16 vs ≥16 years) in the incidence of adverse events are shown in Table 4.

Adverse Events During Chronic Administration: Interpretation of adverse events is complicated by the clinical features of pulmonary hypertension, which may be similar to some of the pharmacologic effects of FLOLAN (e.g., dizziness, syncope). Adverse events probably related to the underlying disease include dyspnea, fatigue, chest pain, edema, hypoxia, right ventricular failure and pallor. Several adverse events, on the other hand, can clearly be attributed to FLOLAN. These include jaw pain, flushing, headache, diarrhea, nausea and vomiting, flu-like symptoms and anxiety/nervousness.

Adverse Events During Chronic Administration for PPH: In an effort to separate the adverse effects of the drug from the adverse effects of the underlying disease, Table 5 lists adverse events that occurred at a rate at least 10% different in the 2 groups in controlled trials for PPH.

Table 3: FLOLAN for Injection

Adverse Events During Dose Escalation

Adverse Events Occurring in ≥1% of Patients	FLOLAN (n=391) % of Patients Where Event was Reported	FLOLAN (n=391) % of Patients Where Event was Dose-limiting
Flushing	58	14
Headache	49	18
Nausea/Vomiting	32	19
Hypotension	16	15
Anxiety, nervousness, agitation	11	7
Chest pain	11	7
Dizziness	8	4
Bradycardia	5	4
Abdominal pain	5	2
Musculoskeletal pain	3	2
Dyspnea	2	2
Back pain	2	—
Sweating	1	≤1
Dyspepsia	1	≤1
Hypesthesia/Paresthesia	1	≤1
Tachycardia	1	≤1

Table 4: FLOLAN for Injection

Age-related Adverse Events During Dose Escalation

Adverse Events	<16 Years (n=63) % of Patients Reporting Event	≥16 Years (n=328) % of Patients Reporting Event
Flushing	14	66
Headache	8	57
Nausea/Vomiting	40	30
Hypotension	14	16
Anxiety, nervousness, agitation	21	9
Chest pain	0	13
Dizziness	2	9
Bradycardia	6	5

(cont'd)

Table 4: FLOLAN for Injection *(cont'd)*

Age-related Adverse Events During Dose Escalation

Adverse Events	<16 Years (n=63) % of Patients Reporting Event	≥16 Years (n=328) % of Patients Reporting Event
Abdominal pain	6	5

Table 5: FLOLAN for Injection

Adverse Events Regardless of Attribution Occurring in Patients with PPH During Chronic Administration in Controlled Trials with ≥10% Difference Between FLOLAN and Conventional Therapy Alone

Adverse Event	FLOLAN (n=52) % of Patients	Conventional Therapy (n=54) % of Patients
Occurrence More Common with FLOLAN		
General		
Chills/Fever/Sepsis/Flu-like symptoms	25	11
Cardiovascular		
Tachycardia	35	24
Flushing	42	2
Gastrointestinal		
Diarrhea	37	6
Nausea/Vomiting	67	48
Musculoskeletal		
Jaw pain	54	0
Myalgia	44	31
Non-specific musculoskeletal pain	35	15
Neurological		
Anxiety/Nervousness/Tremor	21	9
Dizziness	83	70
Headache	83	33
Hypesthesia, hyperesthesia, paresthesia	12	2
Occurrence More Common with Conventional Therapy		
Cardiovascular		
Heart failure	31	52
Syncope	13	24
Shock	0	13
Respiratory		
Hypoxia	25	37

Thrombocytopenia, dry mouth, lassitude, chest tightness, reddening over the infusion site, occlusion of the long i.v. catheter and bleeding at various sites have been reported during uncontrolled clinical trials and post marketing clinical use in patients receiving FLOLAN.

Table 6 lists those additional adverse events reported in PPH patients receiving FLOLAN plus conventional therapy versus conventional therapy alone during controlled clinical trials where the difference in incidence of the event between treatment groups was <10%.

Table 6: FLOLAN for Injection

Adverse Events Regardless of Attribution Occurring During Chronic Administration in Controlled Trials with <10% Difference between FLOLAN and Conventional Therapy Alone

Adverse Event	FLOLAN (n=52) % of Patients	Conventional Therapy (n=54) % of Patients
General		
Asthenia	87	81
Cardiovascular		
Angina pectoris	19	20
Arrhythmia	27	20
Bradycardia	15	9
Supraventricular tachycardia	8	0

(cont'd)

Table 6: FLOLAN for Injection *(cont'd)*

Adverse Events Regardless of Attribution Occurring During Chronic Administration in Controlled Trials with <10% Difference between FLOLAN and Conventional Therapy Alone

Adverse Event	FLOLAN (n=52) % of Patients	Conventional Therapy (n=54) % of Patients
Pallor	21	30
Cyanosis	31	39
Palpitation	63	61
Cerebrovascular accident	4	0
Hypotension	27	31
Myocardial ischemia	2	6
Gastrointestinal		
Abdominal pain	27	31
Anorexia	25	30
Ascites	12	17
Constipation	6	2
Metabolic		
Edema	60	63
Hypokalemia	6	4
Weight reduction	27	24
Weight gain	6	4
Musculoskeletal		
Arthralgia	6	0
Bone pain	0	4
Chest pain	67	65
Neurological		
Confusion	6	11
Convulsion	4	0
Depression	37	44
Insomnia	4	4
Respiratory		
Cough increase	38	46
Dyspnea	90	85
Epistaxis	4	2
Pleural effusion	4	2
Skin and Appendages		
Pruritus	4	0
Rash	10	13
Sweating	15	20
Special Senses		
Amblyopia	8	4
Vision abnormality	4	0
Other		
Hemorrhage	19	11

Although the number of patients was small, in controlled trials there was a trend towards increased incidence of bradycardia associated with chronic treatment in patients <16 vs those ≥16 years of age.

Adverse Events During Chronic Administration for SPH due to SSD: In an effort to separate the adverse effects of the drug from the adverse effects of the underlying disease, Table 7 lists adverse events that occurred at a rate at least 10% difference between the 2 groups in the controlled trial for patients with SPH.

Table 7: FLOLAN for Injection

Adverse Events Regardless of Attribution Occurring in Patients with SPH due to SSD with ≥10% Difference Between FLOLAN and Conventional Therapy Alone

Adverse Event	FLOLAN % n=56	Conventional Therapy % n=55
Occurrence More Common with FLOLAN		
Cardiovascular		
Flushing	23	0
Hypotension	13	0
Gastrointestinal		
Anorexia	66	47
Nausea/Vomiting	41	16
Diarrhea	50	5
Musculoskeletal		
Jaw pain	75	0
Pain/Neck pain/Arthralgia	84	65
Neurological		
Headache	46	5
Skin and Appendages		
Skin ulcer	39	24
Eczema/Rash/Urticaria	25	4
Occurrence More Common with Conventional Therapy		
Cardiovascular		
Cyanosis	54	80
Pallor	32	53
Syncope	7	20
Gastrointestinal		
Ascites	23	33
Esophageal reflux/Gastritis	61	73
Metabolic		
Weight decrease	45	56
Neurological		
Dizziness	59	76
Respiratory		
Hypoxia	55	65

Table 8 lists additional adverse events reported in SPH due to SSD patients receiving FLOLAN plus conventional therapy or conventional therapy alone during controlled clinical trials.

Adverse Events Attributable to the Drug Delivery System: Chronic infusions of FLOLAN are delivered using a small, portable infusion pump through an indwelling central venous catheter. During controlled PPH trials of up to 12 weeks duration, up to 21% of patients reported a local infection and up to13% of patients reported pain at the venous catheter insertion site. During a 12-week controlled trial of SPH due to SSD, 14% of patients reported a local infection and 9% of patients reported pain at the venous catheter insertion site. During subsequent long-term follow-up in clinical trials of PPH, sepsis was reported at least once in 14% of patients and occurred at a rate of 0.32 infections per patient per year in patients treated with FLOLAN. When suspected, sepsis should be diagnosed and treated quickly. It is therefore important that these patients have immediate access to expert medical care. Malfunctions in the delivery system resulting in an inadvertent bolus of, or a reduction in, FLOLAN were associated with symptoms related to excess or insufficient FLOLAN, respectively, that may lead to serious consequences including death (see Warnings, Adverse Effects, Adverse Events During Chronic Administration and Overdose).

Table 8: FLOLAN for Injection *(cont'd)*

Adverse Events Regardless of Attribution Occurring in Patients with SPH due to SSD with <10% Difference Between FLOLAN and Conventional Therapy Alone

Adverse Event[a]	FLOLAN % n=56	Conventional Therapy % n=55
General		
Asthenia	100	98
Hemorrhage/Hemorrhage injection site/Hemorrhage rectal	11	2
Infection/Rhinitis	21	20
Chills/Fever/Sepsis/Flu-like symptoms	13	11
Cardiovascular		
Heart failure/Heart failure right	11	13
Myocardial infarction	4	0
Palpitation	63	71
Shock	5	5
Tachycardia	43	42
Thrombocytopenia	4	0
Vascular disorder peripheral	96	100
Vascular disorder	95	89
Gastrointestinal		
Abdominal enlargement	4	0
Abdominal pain	14	7
Constipation	4	2
Flatulence	5	4
Metabolic		
Edema/Edema peripheral/Edema genital	79	87
Hypercalcemia	48	51
Hyperkalemia	4	0
Thirst	0	4
Musculoskeletal		
Arthritis	52	45
Back pain	13	5
Chest pain	52	45
Cramps leg	5	7
Respiratory		
Cough increase	82	82
Dyspnea	100	100
Epistaxis	9	7
Pharyngitis	5	2
Pleural effusion	7	0
Pneumonia	5	0
Pneumothorax	4	0
Pulmonary edema	4	2
Respiratory disorder	7	4
Sinusitis	4	4
Neurological		
Anxiety/Hyperkinesia/Nervousness/Tremor	7	5
Depression/Depression psychotic	13	4
Hyperesthesia/Hypesthesia/Paresthesia	5	0
Insomnia	9	0
Somnolence	4	2
Skin and Appendages		
Collagen disease	82	84

(cont'd)

Table 8: FLOLAN for Injection *(cont'd)*

Adverse Events Regardless of Attribution Occurring in Patients with SPH due to SSD with <10% Difference Between FLOLAN and Conventional Therapy Alone

Adverse Event[a]	FLOLAN % n=56	Conventional Therapy % n=55
Pruritus	4	2
Sweat	41	36
Urogenital		
Hematuria	5	0
Urinary tract infection	7	0

a Table lists adverse events which occurred in at least 2 patients in either group.

OVERDOSE:

Symptoms: Signs and symptoms of excessive doses of FLOLAN are the expected dose-limiting pharmacologic effects of FLOLAN including flushing, headache, hypotension, tachycardia, nausea, vomiting and diarrhea. Treatment will ordinarily require dose reduction of FLOLAN.

One patient with secondary pulmonary hypertension accidentally received 50 mL of an unspecified concentration of FLOLAN. The patient vomited and became unconscious with an initially unobtainable blood pressure. FLOLAN was discontinued, and the patient regained consciousness within seconds.

Treatment: See Symptoms.

For management of a suspected drug overdose, CPhA recommends that you contact your **regional Poison Control Centre**. See the *CPS* Directory section for a list of Poison Control Centres.

DOSAGE: FLOLAN (epoprostenol sodium) must be reconstituted only with specific Sterile Diluent for FLOLAN. Reconstituted solutions of FLOLAN must not be diluted or administered with other parenteral solutions or medications (see Warnings).

FLOLAN is not to be used for bolus administration.

During acute dose-ranging, asymptomatic increases in pulmonary artery pressure coincident with increases in cardiac output occurred rarely. In such cases, dose reduction should be considered, but such an increase does not imply that chronic treatment is contraindicated. However, in the rare occurrence of pulmonary edema, chronic treatment is contraindicated.

During chronic use, FLOLAN is delivered continuously on an ambulatory basis through a permanent indwelling central venous catheter. Unless contraindicated, anticoagulant therapy should be administered to PPH patients receiving FLOLAN to reduce the risk of pulmonary thromboembolism or systemic embolism through a patent foramen ovale. In order to reduce the risk of infection, aseptic technique must be used in the reconstitution and administration of FLOLAN as well as in routine catheter care. Because FLOLAN is metabolized rapidly, even brief interruptions in the delivery of FLOLAN may result in symptoms associated with rebound pulmonary hypertension including dyspnea, dizziness, and asthenia. The decision to initiate therapy with FLOLAN should be based upon the understanding that there is a high likelihood that i.v. therapy with FLOLAN will be needed for prolonged periods, possibly years, and the patient's ability to accept and care for a permanent i.v. catheter and infusion pump should be carefully considered.

Dosage: FLOLAN can be used in acute vasoreactivity studies, to assess pulmonary vasodilator capacity.

Continuous chronic infusion of FLOLAN should be administered through a central venous catheter. Temporary peripheral i.v. infusion may be used until central access is established. Chronic infusion of FLOLAN should be initiated at 2 ng/kg/min and increased until dose-limiting pharmacological effects are elicited or until a tolerance limit to the drug is established and further increases in the infusion rate are not clinically warranted (see Dosage Adjustments). If dose-limiting pharmacologic effects occur, then the infusion rate should be decreased to an appropriate chronic infusion rate whereby the pharmacologic effects of FLOLAN are tolerated. In clinical trials, the most common dose-limiting adverse events were nausea, vomiting, hypotension, sepsis, headache, abdominal pain, or respiratory disorder (most treatment-limiting adverse events were not serious). If the initial infusion rate of 2 ng/kg/min is not tolerated, a lower dose which is tolerated by the patient should be identified.

In the controlled 12-week trial in SPH due to SSD, for example, the dose increased from a mean starting dose of 2.2 ng/kg/min. During the first 7 days of treatment, the dose was increased daily to a mean dose of 4.1 ng/kg/min on Day 7 of treatment. At the end of week 12, the mean dose was 11.2 ng/kg/min. The mean incremental increase was 2 to 3 ng/kg/min every 3 weeks.

Dosage Adjustments: Changes in the chronic infusion rate should be based on persistence, recurrence or worsening of the patient's symptoms of pulmonary hypertension and the occurrence of adverse events due to excessive doses of FLOLAN. In general, the need for increases in dose from the initial chronic dose should be expected over time.

Increments in dose should be considered if symptoms of pulmonary hypertension persist or recur after improving. The infusion should be increased by 1 to 2 ng/kg/min increments at intervals sufficient to allow assessment of clinical response and tolerability; these intervals should be of at least 15 minutes. Following establishment of a new chronic infusion rate, the patient should be observed, and standing and supine blood pressure and heart rate monitored for several hours to ensure that the new dose is tolerated.

During chronic infusion, the occurrence of dose-limiting pharmacologic events may necessitate a decrease in infusion rate, but the adverse event may occasionally resolve without dosage adjustment. Dosage decreases should generally be made gradually in 2 ng/kg/min decrements every 15 minutes or longer until the dose-limiting effects resolve. Abrupt withdrawal of FLOLAN or sudden large reductions in infusion rates should be avoided. Except in life-threatening situations (e.g., unconsciousness, collapse, etc.), infusion rates of FLOLAN should be adjusted only under the direction of a physician.

In patients receiving lung transplants, doses of FLOLAN were tapered after the initiation of cardiopulmonary bypass.

Administration: FLOLAN is administered by continuous i.v. infusion via a central venous catheter using an ambulatory infusion pump as recommended by the physician. During initiation of treatment, FLOLAN may be administered peripherally.

The ambulatory infusion pump used to administer FLOLAN should: (1) be small and lightweight, (2) be able to adjust infusion rates in 2 ng/kg/min increments, (3) have occlusion, end of infusion, and low battery alarms, (4) be accurate to ±6% of the programmed rate, (5) be positive pressure driven (continuous or pulsatile) with intervals between pulses not exceeding 3 minutes at infusion rates used to deliver FLOLAN, and (6) have design characteristics that minimize the likelihood of accidental bolus administration. The reservoir should be made of polyvinyl chloride, polypropylene, or glass. The infusion pump used in the most recent clinical trials was the CADD-1 HFX 5100 (SIMS Deltec). A 152 cm microbore non-DEHP extension set with proximal antisyphon valve, low priming volume (0.9 mL), and in-line 0.22 micron filter was used during clinical trials.

To avoid potential interruptions in drug delivery, the patient should have access to a back-up infusion pump and additional i.v. infusion sets. A multi-lumen catheter should be considered if other i.v. therapies are routinely administered.

Preliminary data suggest that peristaltic pumps may have advantages over syringe pumps.

Prior to use, reconstituted solutions of FLOLAN must be protected from light and must be refrigerated at 2 to 8°C if not used immediately. Under these conditions, reconstituted FLOLAN solution may be stored for up to 24 hours before being transferred to the infusion pump. Reconstituted FLOLAN solution that has not been transferred to the infusion pump within 24 hours (i.e., that has been stored for more than 24 hours) is to be discarded. Do not freeze reconstituted solutions of FLOLAN.

Once placed in the pump, a single reservoir of reconstituted FLOLAN solution can be administered for up to 24 hours by maintaining the temperature between 2 to 8°C with the use of 2 frozen 170 mL gel packs in a cold pouch. The gel packs should be changed every 12 hours, or every 8 hours if the ambient temperature approaches 30°C. **When stored or in use, reconstituted FLOLAN must not be exposed to direct sunlight.**

Reconstitution: Parenteral drug products should be inspected visually for particulate matter and discoloration prior to administration whenever solution and container permit.

FLOLAN is only stable when reconstituted with specific Sterile Diluent for FLOLAN. FLOLAN must not be reconstituted or mixed with any other parenteral medications or solutions prior to or during administration.

A concentration for the solution of FLOLAN should be selected that is compatible with the infusion pump being used with respect to minimum and maximum flow rates, reservoir capacity, and the infusion pump criteria listed above. FLOLAN, when administered chronically, should be prepared in a drug delivery reservoir appropriate for the infusion pump with a total reservoir volume of at least 100 mL. FLOLAN should be prepared using 2 vials of the specific **Sterile Diluent** for FLOLAN for use during a 24-hour period.

Infusion Rates During Acute Dose Escalation: Generally, 3000 and 10 000 ng/mL are satisfactory concentrations to deliver between 2 to 16 ng/kg/min in adults. Infusion rates may be calculated using the following formula:

$$\text{Infusion Rate (mL/h)} = \frac{[\text{Dose (ng/kg/min)} \times \text{Weight (kg)} \times 60\ \text{min/h}]}{\text{Final Concentration (ng/mL)}}$$

Table 9, Table 10, Table 11 and Table 12 provide infusion rates for doses up to 16 ng/kg/min based upon patient weight, drug delivery rate, and concentration of the solution of FLOLAN to be used. These tables may be used to select the most appropriate concentration of FLOLAN that will result in an infusion rate between the minimum and maximum flow rates of the infusion pump and which will allow the desired duration of infusion from a given reservoir volume.

Table 9: FLOLAN for Injection

Infusion Rates for FLOLAN at a Concentration of 3000 ng/mL

Patient Weight (kg)	Dose or Drug Delivery Rate (ng/kg/min)							
	2	4	6	8	10	12	14	16
	Infusion Delivery Rate (mL/hr)							
10	—	—	1.2	1.6	2.0	2.4	2.8	3.2
20	—	1.6	2.4	3.2	4.0	4.8	5.6	6.4
30	1.2	2.4	3.6	4.8	6.0	7.2	8.4	9.6
40	1.6	3.2	4.8	6.4	8.0	9.6	11.2	12.8
50	2.0	4.0	6.0	8.0	10.0	12.0	14.0	16.0
60	2.4	4.8	7.2	9.6	12.0	14.4	16.8	19.2
70	2.8	5.6	8.4	11.2	14.0	16.8	19.6	22.4
80	3.2	6.4	9.6	12.8	16.0	19.2	22.4	25.6
90	3.6	7.2	10.8	14.4	18.0	21.6	25.2	28.8
100	4.0	8.0	12.0	16.0	20.0	24.0	28.0	32.0

Table 10: FLOLAN for Injection

Infusion Rates for FLOLAN at a Concentration of 5000 ng/mL

Patient Weight (kg)	Dose or Drug Delivery Rate (ng/kg/min)							
	2	4	6	8	10	12	14	16
	Infusion Delivery Rate (mL/hr)							
10	—	—	—	1.0	1.2	1.4	1.7	1.9
20	—	1.0	1.4	1.9	2.4	2.9	3.4	3.8
30	—	1.4	2.2	2.9	3.6	4.3	5.0	5.8
40	1.0	1.9	2.9	3.8	4.8	5.8	6.7	7.7
50	1.2	2.4	3.6	4.8	6.0	7.2	8.4	9.6
60	1.4	2.9	4.3	5.8	7.2	8.6	10.1	11.5
70	1.7	3.4	5.0	6.7	8.4	10.1	11.8	13.4
80	1.9	3.8	5.8	7.7	9.6	11.5	13.4	15.4
90	2.2	4.3	6.5	8.6	10.8	13.0	15.1	17.3
100	2.4	4.8	7.2	9.6	12.0	14.4	16.8	19.2

Table 11: FLOLAN for Injection

Infusion Rates for FLOLAN at a Concentration of 10 000 ng/mL

Patient Weight (kg)	Dose or Drug Delivery Rate (ng/kg/min)						
	4	6	8	10	12	14	16
	Infusion Delivery Rate (mL/hr)						
20	—	—	1.0	1.2	1.4	1.7	1.9
30	—	1.1	1.4	1.8	2.2	2.5	2.9
40	1.0	1.4	1.9	2.4	2.9	3.4	3.8
50	1.2	1.8	2.4	3.0	3.6	4.2	4.8
60	1.4	2.2	2.9	3.6	4.3	5.0	5.8
70	1.7	2.5	3.4	4.2	5.0	5.9	6.7
80	1.9	2.9	3.8	4.8	5.8	6.7	7.7

(cont'd)

Table 11: FLOLAN for Injection *(cont'd)*

Infusion Rates for FLOLAN at a Concentration of 10 000 ng/mL

Patient Weight (kg)	Dose or Drug Delivery Rate (ng/kg/min)						
	4	6	8	10	12	14	16
	Infusion Delivery Rate (mL/hr)						
90	2.2	3.2	4.3	5.4	6.5	7.6	8.6
100	2.4	3.6	4.8	6.0	7.2	8.4	9.6

Table 12: FLOLAN for Injection

Infusion Rates for FLOLAN at a Concentration of 15 000 ng/mL

Patient Weight (kg)	Dose or Drug Delivery Rate (ng/kg/min)						
	4	6	8	10	12	14	16
	Infusion Delivery Rate (mL/hr)						
30	—	—	1.0	1.2	1.4	1.7	1.9
40	—	1.0	1.3	1.6	1.9	2.2	2.6
50	—	1.2	1.6	2.0	2.4	2.8	3.2
60	1.0	1.4	1.9	2.4	2.9	3.4	3.8
70	1.1	1.7	2.2	2.8	3.4	3.9	4.5
80	1.3	1.9	2.6	3.2	3.8	4.5	5.1
90	1.4	2.2	2.9	3.6	4.3	5.0	5.8
100	1.6	2.4	3.2	4.0	4.8	5.6	6.4

Infusion Rates During Chronic Infusion: More concentrated solutions than those described in Table 9 through Table 10, Table 11 and Table 12 may be necessary in some cases where higher drug delivery rates are indicated. Generally, over time, the daily dose of FLOLAN requires up-titration.

INFORMATION FOR THE PATIENT: Published in e-CPS, available by subscription at www.e-cps.ca.

SUPPLIED: Each vial of sterile, freeze-dried powder contains: epoprostenol sodium equivalent to epoprostenol 0.5 mg (500 000 ng) or 1.5 mg (1 500 000 ng). Nonmedicinal ingredients: glycine, mannitol, sodium chloride and sodium hydroxide (added to adjust pH). Flint glass vials, individually packaged in a carton. Store at 15 to 25°C. Protect from light.

Each vial of sterile diluent contains: glycine 94 mg, sodium chloride 73.3 mg, sodium hydroxide (added to adjust pH) and water for injection USP q.s. to 50 mL. Glass vials of 50 mL, trays of 2. Store at 15 to 25°C. **Do not freeze.**

Flomax® CR ℞

tamsulosin HCl

Selective Antagonist of Alpha1A/1D Adrenoreceptor Subtypes in the Prostate and Bladder

Boehringer Ingelheim

Date of Preparation: May 28, 1998
Date of Revision: January 21, 2008

SUMMARY PRODUCT INFORMATION:

Route of Administration	Dosage Form/ Strength	Clinically Relevant Nonmedicinal Ingredients
Oral	Controlled release tablet 0.4 mg	none For a complete listing see Dosage Forms, Composition and Packaging.

INDICATIONS AND CLINICAL USE: FLOMAX CR (tamsulosin hydrochloride) is indicated for the treatment of Lower Urinary Tract Symptoms (LUTS) associated with benign prostatic hyperplasia (BPH).

Geriatrics (>65 years of age): Tamsulosin hydrochloride has been found to be a safe and effective alpha$_1$ adrenoceptor antagonist when administered at therapeutic doses (0.4 mg once daily) to patients over the age of 65 years.

Pediatrics: FLOMAX CR is not indicated for use in children.

CONTRAINDICATIONS: FLOMAX CR (tamsulosin hydrochloride) is contraindicated in patients known to have hypersensitivity including drug induced angioedema to tamsulosin or any component of the FLOMAX CR controlled release formulation. For a complete listing, see Dosage Forms, Composition and Packaging.

WARNINGS AND PRECAUTIONS: As with all α_1-adrenoceptor antagonists, a reduction in blood pressure can occur in individual cases during treatment with FLOMAX CR, as a result of which, rarely, syncope can occur. At the first signs of orthostatic hypotension (dizziness, weakness), the patient should sit or lie down until the symptoms have disappeared.

Patients beginning treatment with FLOMAX CR should be cautioned to avoid situations where injury could result should syncope occur (see Adverse Reactions).

General: FLOMAX CR (tamsulosin hydrochloride) is not indicated for the treatment of hypertension.

Carcinoma of the Prostate: Carcinoma of the prostate and BPH cause many of the same symptoms. These two diseases frequently co-exist. Patients should be evaluated to rule out the presence of carcinoma of the prostate.

Orthostatic Hypotension: While syncope is the most severe orthostatic symptom of α_1-adrenoceptor antagonists, other symptoms can occur (dizziness and postural hypotension). In a phase III, randomized, double-blind, placebo-controlled trial involving male patients treated once daily with either 0.4 mg FLOMAX CR (n=350) or placebo (n=356), both supine and standing blood pressure were monitored over the course of the 12 week treatment period. There was a small, clinically insignificant decrease from baseline in mean supine and standing systolic/diastolic BP in both treatment groups; the decrease in BP from baseline in the FLOMAX CR group (<2 mmHg) was comparable to the placebo group (<1.5 mmHg). There were no cases of orthostatic hypotension or syncope reported in either treatment group.

Patients in occupations in which orthostatic hypotension could be dangerous should be treated with caution.

If hypotension occurs, the patient should be placed in the supine position and if this measure is inadequate, volume expansion with intravenous fluids or vasopressor therapy may be used. A transient hypotensive response is not a contraindication to further therapy with FLOMAX CR.

Hepatic/Biliary/Pancreatic: The treatment of patients with severe hepatic impairment should be approached with caution as no studies have been conducted in this patient population. No dose adjustment is warranted in hepatic insufficiency.

Renal: The treatment of patients with severe renal impairment (creatinine clearance of <10 mL/min) should be approached with caution, as these patients have not been studied.

Intraoperative Floppy Iris Syndrome: During cataract surgery, a variant of small pupil syndrome known as Intraoperative Floppy Iris Syndrome (IFIS) has been reported during post-marketing surveillance in association with alpha-$_1$ blocker therapy, including FLOMAX. Most reports to date were in patients taking FLOMAX when IFIS occurred, but in some cases, FLOMAX had been stopped prior to surgery. In most of these cases, the FLOMAX had been stopped recently prior to surgery (2 to 14 days), but in a few cases, IFIS was reported after the patient had been off FLOMAX for a longer period. This variant of small pupil syndrome is characterized by the combination of a flaccid iris that billows in response to intraoperative irrigation currents, progressive intraoperative miosis despite preoperative dilation with standard mydriatic drugs and potential prolapse of the iris toward the phacoemulsification incisions. The patient's ophthalmologist should be prepared for possible modifications to their surgical technique, such as the utilization of iris hooks, iris dilator rings, or viscoelastic substances. The benefit of stopping alpha-$_1$ blocker therapy, including FLOMAX prior to cataract surgery has not been established.

Special Populations: Pregnant Women: FLOMAX CR is not indicated for use in women. Studies in pregnant rats and rabbits at daily doses of 300 and 50 mg/kg, respectively (30 000 and 5000 times the anticipated human dose), revealed no evidence of harm to the fetus. There are no adequate data on the use of tamsulosin in pregnant women; therefore the potential risk from the use of tamsulosin during pregnancy in humans is unknown.

Nursing Women: FLOMAX CR is not indicated for use in women.

Pediatrics: FLOMAX CR is not indicated for use in children.

Geriatrics (>65 years of age): There were no pharmacokinetic studies conducted in geriatric patients with FLOMAX CR. Cross-study comparisons of overall exposure (AUC) and half-life of FLOMAX capsules indicate that the pharmacokinetic disposition of tamsulosin may be slightly prolonged in geriatric males compared to young healthy male volunteers. However, FLOMAX capsules have been found to be a safe and effective alpha$_1$ adrenoreceptor antagonist when administered at therapeutic doses to patients over the age of 65 years.

Gender Effects: FLOMAX CR is not indicated for use in women. Safety, effectiveness, and pharmacokinetics have not been evaluated in women.

Monitoring and Laboratory Tests: No laboratory test interactions with FLOMAX CR are known. Treatment with FLOMAX CR for up to 3 months had no significant effect on prostate specific antigen (PSA).

Information to Be Provided to the Patient: Patients should be advised not to crush or chew FLOMAX CR tablets. These tablets are specially formulated to control the delivery of tamsulosin HCl to the blood stream.

There are no specific studies conducted with FLOMAX CR and the ability to drive vehicles or use machinery. However patients should be advised that dizziness can occur with FLOMAX CR, requiring caution in people who must drive, operate machinery, or perform hazardous tasks.

Patients should be advised about the possibility of priapism as a result of treatment with FLOMAX CR and other similar medications. Patients should be informed that this reaction is extremely rare, but if not brought to immediate medical attention, can lead to permanent erectile dysfunction (impotence).

ADVERSE REACTIONS: Adverse Drug Reaction Overview: Information on the safety profile of FLOMAX CR was derived from two, 3-month placebo-controlled clinical trials involving 1840 male subjects. Of these, 563 were treated with FLOMAX CR 0.4 mg, 709 with FLOMAX capsules 0.4 mg and 568 with placebo. The results suggest that FLOMAX CR 0.4 mg and FLOMAX capsules 0.4 mg were very well tolerated with the AE profile of FLOMAX CR 0.4 mg tending to be more favourable than that of FLOMAX capsules.

In these studies, 3.6% of patients taking FLOMAX CR (0.4 mg) discontinued from the study due to adverse events compared with 1.2% in the placebo group. The most frequently reported Treatment Emergent Adverse Events (TEAE) in the FLOMAX CR 0.4 mg group were dizziness and those related to abnormal ejaculation, although the incidence of both were comparable to placebo.

Impotence and other events related to sexual function are commonly associated with other alpha$_1$-blockers, however in the 3-month studies with FLOMAX CR there were minimal effects on sexual function and ejaculatory disorders/abnormalities with no reports of priapism. The difference in incidence of ejaculatory disorders/abnormalities between FLOMAX CR and placebo was not statistically significant. No patient discontinued treatment with FLOMAX CR 0.4 mg due to ejaculatory disorders/abnormalities.

Clinical Trial Adverse Drug Reactions: Because clinical trials are conducted under very specific conditions the adverse reaction rates observed in the clinical trials may not reflect the rates observed in practice and should not be compared to the rates in the clinical trials of another drug. Adverse drug reaction information from clinical trials is useful for identifying drug-related adverse events and for approximating rates. (See Table 1 and Table 2).

Table 1: FLOMAX CR

Treatment-Emergent Adverse Events in ≥2% of Patients Receiving Either Tamsulosin or Placebo During the 3 Month Placebo and Active-Controlled Study

SOC/Preferred term	Placebo N=356	FLOMAX CR Tablets 0.4 mg N=360	Tamsulosin Capsules 0.4 mg N=709
Any TEAE	71 (19.9%)	93 (25.8%)	168 (23.7%)
Cardiac disorders	8 (2.2%)	8 (2.2%)	16 (2.3%)
Gastrointestinal disorders	7 (2.0%)	14 (3.9%)	34 (4.8%)
General Disorders and administration site conditions	2 (0.6%)	8 (2.2%)	11 (1.6%)
Infections and infestations	16 (4.5%)	20 (5.6%)	32 (4.5%)
Investigations	10 (2.8%)	6 (1.7%)	10 (1.4%)
Musculoskeletal and connective tissue disorders	7 (2.0%)	9 (2.5%)	12[a] (1.7%)
Nervous system disorders	9 (2.5%)	11 (3.1%)	29 (4.1%)
Reproductive system and breast disorders	2 (0.6%)	12 (3.3%)	28 (3.9%)
Respiratory, thoracic and mediastinal disorders	3 (0.8%)	10 (2.8%)	20 (2.8%)
Vascular disorders	8 (2.2%)	6[b] (1.7%)	15 (2.1%)

[a] Post database lock: deletion of 1 AE.
[b] Post database lock: addition of 1 AE.
Number (%) of patients
A patient may experience an AE more than once or may experience more than one AE within the same SOC.

Table 2: FLOMAX CR

Number (%) of Patients With TEAES Commonly Associated With $_{A1}$–AR Antagonists During the 3 Month Placebo and Active-Controlled Study

SOC/Preferred term	Placebo N=356	FLOMAX CR tablets 0.4 mg N=360	Tamsulosin Capsules 0.4 mg N=709
Non-cardiovascular class effects			
Retrograde ejaculation	1 (0.3%)	6 (1.7%)	10 (1.4%)

(cont'd)

Table 2: FLOMAX CR *(cont'd)*

Number (%) of Patients With TEAES Commonly Associated With $_{A1}$–AR Antagonists During the 3 Month Placebo and Active-Controlled Study

SOC/Preferred term	Placebo N=356	FLOMAX CR tablets 0.4 mg N=360	Tamsulosin Capsules 0.4 mg N=709
Ejaculation Failure	0 (0.0%)	0 (0.0%)	2 (0.3%)
Semen volume reduced	0 (0.0%)	1 (0.3%)	2 (0.3%)
Ejaculation delayed	0 (0.0%)	1 (0.3%)	2 (0.3%)
Ejaculation disorder NOS	0 (0.0%)	0 (0.0%)	6 (0.8%)
Abnormal Ejaculation Pooled	1 (0.3%)	7 (1.9%)	22 (3.1%)
Headache NOS	4 (1.1%)	3 (0.8%)	10 (1.4%)
Asthenia	1 (0.3%)	1 (0.3%)	1 (0.1%)
Fatigue	1 (0.3%)	3 (0.8%)	2 (0.3%)
Somnolence	0 (0.0%)	0 (0.0%)	2 (0.3%)
Rhinitis NOS	0 (0.0%)	1 (0.3%)	2 (0.3%)
Nasal congestion	0 (0.0%)	1 (0.3%)	1 (0.1%)
Nasal obstruction	0 (0.0%)	0 (0.0%)	0 (0.0%)
Sub-Total	7 (2.0%)	16 (4.4%)	36 (5.1%)
Cardiovascular class effects			
Dizziness	5 (1.4%)	5 (1.4%)	9 (1.3%)
Dizziness aggravated	0 (0.0%)	0 (0.0%)	2 (0.3%)
Dizzy spell	0 (0.0%)	0 (0.0%)	1 (0.1%)
Dizziness Pooled	5 (1.4%)	5 (1.4%)	12 (1.7%)
Palpitations	2 (0.6%)	2 (0.6%)	1 (0.1%)
Tachycardia NOS	0 (0.0%)	1 (0.3%)	2 (0.3%)
Hypotension NOS	1 (0.3%)	0 (0.0%)	2 (0.3%)
Orthostatic hypotension	0 (0.0%)	0 (0.0%)	3 (0.4%)
Dizziness postural	0 (0.0%)	0 (0.0%)	2 (0.3%)
Syncope	0 (0.0%)	0 (0.0%)	1 (0.1%)
Orthostatic/circulatory collapse	0 (0.0%)	0 (0.0%)	0 (0.0%)
Depressed level of/loss of consciousness	0 (0.0%)	1 (0.3%)	1 (0.1%)
Sub-Total	8 (2.2%)	9 (2.5%)	23 (3.2%)
Total	13 (3.7%)	25 (6.9%)	55 (7.8%)

A patient may experience an AE more than once or may experience more than one AE within the same SOC.

Angioedema or priapism were not reported in the phase 2 or 3 studies.

Post-Market Adverse Drug Reactions: The following adverse reactions have been reported during the use of tamsulosin hydrochloride at a frequency of:

>1% and <10%: Nervous System Disorders: dizziness.
>0.1% and <1%: Cardiac Disorders: palpitations.
Gastrointestinal Disorders: constipation, diarrhea, nausea, and vomiting.
General Disorders and Administration Site Conditions: asthenia.
Nervous Systems Disorders: headache.
Reproductive System and Breast Disorders: abnormal ejaculation.
Respiratory, Thoracic and Mediastinal Disorders: rhinitis.
Skin and Subcutaneous Tissue Disorders: rash, pruritus, urticaria.
Vascular Disorders: postural hypotension.
>0.01% and <0.1%: syncope, angioedema.
<0.01%: priapism.

During cataract surgery, a variant of small pupil syndrome known as Intraoperative Floppy Iris Syndrome (IFIS) has been reported during post-marketing surveillance in association with alpha-$_1$ blocker therapy, including FLOMAX (see Warnings and Precautions).

An open label extension study involving 609 male patients with lower urinary tract symptoms (LUTS) associated with BPH demonstrated sustained efficacy, safety and long-term tolerability of tamsulosin for up to 6 years.

DRUG INTERACTIONS: Overview: There were no drug interaction studies conducted specifically with FLOMAX CR tablets and it is expected that the interaction profile would not be any different than that of FLOMAX capsules. As with FLOMAX capsules, caution should be exercised with concomitant administration of FLOMAX CR and other alpha-adrenergic blocking agents.

No clinically significant drug-drug interactions were observed when FLOMAX capsules 0.4 mg or 0.8 mg were administered with one of the following therapeutic agents: nifedipine, atenolol, enalapril, digoxin, furosemide or theophylline.

Drug-Drug Interactions: Nifedipine, Atenolol, Enalapril: No dosage adjustments are necessary when FLOMAX CR is administered concomitantly with Procardia XL (nifedipine), atenolol, or enalapril. In three studies in hypertensive subjects (age range 47-79 years) whose blood pressure was controlled with stable doses of Procardia XL (nifedipine), atenolol or enalapril for at least three months, FLOMAX 0.4 mg capsules for seven days followed by FLOMAX 0.8 mg capsules for another seven days (n=8 per study) resulted in no clinically significant effects on blood pressure and pulse rate compared to placebo (n=4 per study).

Warfarin: A definitive drug-drug interaction study between tamsulosin and warfarin was not conducted. Results from limited in-vitro and in-vivo studies are inconclusive. Therefore, caution should be exercised with concomitant administration of warfarin and FLOMAX CR.

Digoxin and Theophylline: No dosage adjustments are necessary when FLOMAX CR is administered concomitantly with digoxin or theophylline. In two studies in healthy volunteers (n=10 per study; age range 19-39 years), receiving FLOMAX capsules 0.4 mg/day for two days, followed by FLOMAX capsules 0.8 mg/day for five to eight days, single intravenous doses of digoxin 0.5 mg or theophylline 5 mg/kg resulted in no change in the pharmacokinetics of digoxin or theophylline.

Furosemide: No dosage adjustments are necessary when FLOMAX CR is administered concomitantly with furosemide. The pharmacokinetic and pharmacodynamic interaction between FLOMAX capsules 0.8 mg/day (steady-state) and furosemide 20 mg intravenously (single dose) was evaluated in ten healthy volunteers (age range 21-40 years). FLOMAX capsules had no effect on the pharmacodynamics (excretion of electrolytes) of furosemide. While furosemide produced a 11% to 12% reduction in tamsulosin C_{max} and AUC, these changes are expected to be clinically insignificant and do not require adjustment of the FLOMAX CR dosage.

Cimetidine: The effects of cimetidine at the highest recommended dose (400 mg every six hours for six days) on the pharmacokinetics of a single FLOMAX 0.4 mg capsules dose was investigated in ten healthy volunteers (age range 21-38 years). Treatment with cimetidine resulted in a moderate increase in tamsulosin AUC (44%) due to a significant decrease (26%) in the clearance of tamsulosin. Therefore, FLOMAX CR should be used with caution in combination with cimetidine.

Drug-Laboratory Test Interactions: No laboratory test interactions with FLOMAX CR are known. Treatment with FLOMAX CR for up to 3 months had no significant effect on prostate specific antigen (PSA).

DOSAGE AND ADMINISTRATION: Dosing Considerations: FLOMAX CR (tamsulosin hydrochloride) 0.4 mg once daily is recommended as the dose for the treatment of lower urinary tract symptoms (LUTS) associated with Benign Prostatic Hyperplasia (BPH).

Missed Dose: If a dose of FLOMAX CR is missed, the missed dose can be taken later the same day. If a day is missed, the missed dose should be skipped and the regular dosing schedule should be resumed. Doses must not be doubled.

Administration: FLOMAX CR should be taken at the same time each day with or without food. FLOMAX CR tablets must be swallowed whole, as crushing or chewing will interfere with the controlled release of the active ingredient.

OVERDOSAGE:

Should overdosage of FLOMAX CR (tamsulosin hydrochloride) lead to hypotension, (see Warnings and Precautions), support of the cardiovascular system is of first importance. Restoration of blood pressure and normalization of heart rate may be accomplished by keeping the patient in the supine position. If this measure is inadequate, then administration of intravenous fluids should be considered. If necessary, vasopressors should then be used and renal function should be monitored and supported as needed. Laboratory data indicate that tamsulosin is 94% to 99% protein bound: therefore dialysis is unlikely to be of benefit.

Measures such as emesis, can be taken to impede absorption. When large quantities are involved, gastric lavage can be applied and activated charcoal and an osmotic laxative, such as sodium sulphate can be administered.

Acute overdose with 5 mg tamsulosin hydrochloride has been reported. Acute hypotension (systolic blood pressure 70 mmHg), vomiting and diarrhoea were observed, which were treated with fluid replacement and the patient was discharged the same day. One patient reported an overdose of 30×0.4 mg FLOMAX capsules. Following the ingestion of the capsules, the patient reported a headache judged to be severe and probably drug-related that resolved the same day.

> For management of a suspected drug overdose, CPhA recommends that you contact your **regional Poison Control Centre**. See the *CPS* Directory section for a list of Poison Control Centres.

ACTION AND CLINICAL PHARMACOLOGY: Mechanism of Action: FLOMAX CR (tamsulosin hydrochloride) is an alpha$_1$ adrenoreceptor (AR) blocking agent used for the treatment of lower urinary tract symptoms (LUTS) associated with benign prostatic hyperplasia (BPH). It exhibits selectivity for both alpha$_{1A}$ and alpha$_{1D}$ receptors over the alpha$_{1B}$ AR subtype. These three AR subtypes have a distinct distribution pattern in human tissue. Whereas approximately 70% of the alpha$_1$-receptors in human prostate are of the alpha$_{1A}$ subtype, the human bladder contains predominantly the alpha$_{1D}$ subtype while blood vessels express predominantly alpha$_{1B}$ subtype.

Stimulation/antagonism of each of the receptor subtypes gives rise to a distinct pharmacological effect.

Lower Urinary Tract Symptoms (LUTS) suggestive of benign prostatic obstruction (BPO) formerly referred to as symptomatic benign prostatic hyperplasia (BPH) are very common in men >50 years old; the prevalence increases with age. The symptoms associated with LUTS/BPH are comprised of two underlying components: the static and dynamic. The static component is related to an increase in prostate size caused, in part, by a proliferation of smooth muscle cells in the prostatic stroma. However, the severity of BPH symptoms and the degree of urethral obstruction do not correlate well with the size of the prostate. The dynamic component is a function of an increase in smooth muscle tone in the prostate and bladder neck leading to constriction of the bladder outlet. Smooth muscle tone is mediated by the sympathetic nervous stimulation of alpha$_1$ adrenoreceptors, which are abundant in the prostate, prostatic capsule, prostatic urethra, and bladder neck. Blockade of these adrenoreceptors can cause smooth muscles in the bladder neck and prostate to relax, resulting in an improvement in urine flow rate and a reduction in symptoms of BPH.

It is further believed that blockade of alpha$_{1D}$ subtypes in the human obstructed bladder may be responsible for reducing detrusor overactivity and subsequent relief of storage symptoms.

FLOMAX CR (tamsulosin hydrochloride) is not intended for use as an antihypertensive drug.

Pharmacodynamics: The FLOMAX CR (tamsulosin hydrochloride) tablet is a novel formulation based on the Oral-Controlled Absorption System (OCAS), a patented gel matrix controlled-release technology designed to provide a consistent slow release of tamsulosin which is maintained throughout the gastro-intestinal tract, resulting in an adequate exposure, with little fluctuation, over 24 hours.

The pharmacokinetics of tamsulosin from the OCAS have been evaluated in adult healthy volunteers with doses ranging from 0.4 mg to 1.6 mg.

Pharmacokinetics: Absorption: After a single oral dose of 0.4 mg FLOMAX CR in the fasted state, the plasma concentration of tamsulosin gradually increased reaching C_{max} at a median time of 6 hours. At steady state, which is reached by day 4 of multiple dosing, plasma concentrations of tamsulosin peak at 4-6 hours in the fasted and fed state. Peak plasma concentrations increase from approximately 6 ng/mL after the first dose to 11 ng/mL in steady state. After C_{max} is reached, the plasma concentration decreases, but at approximately 16-24 hours post-dose, a small increase or second plateau is observed. The absolute bioavailability of tamsulosin from FLOMAX CR was estimated to be 55-59%.

A study conducted at steady state with 0.4 mg FLOMAX CR demonstrated that the plasma concentration-time profile in the fed state was bioequivalent to the fasted state, indicating the absence of a food effect (Table 3).

Table 3: FLOMAX CR

Mean Pharmacokinetic Parameters of Tamsulosin at Steady Stage Following Administration of Once Daily Doses of 0.4 mg FLOMAX CR in Both the Fed and Fasted State

Parameter	FLOMAX CR 0.4 mg (Fed) (n=24)	FLOMAX CR 0.4 mg (Fasted) (n=24)
$AUC_{0\text{-}inf}$ (ng·h/mL)	291.1	278.7
C_{max} (ng/mL)	11.1	10.7
C_{24} (ng/mL)	4.8	4.6
T_{max} (h)	4.16	4.75
$T_{1/2}$ (h)	14.6	15.6

The 0.4 mg FLOMAX CR Controlled-Release tablet is not bioequivalent to the 0.4 mg FLOMAX capsule, as the test/reference ratio for C_{max} and AUC did not fall within the predefined limits of 80-125%. The plasma concentration-time profile presented in Figure 1 shows the lack of a pronounced spike in C_{max} with FLOMAX CR tablets compared with capsules which may be consistent with a more favourable safety profile.

Distribution: The mean steady-state apparent volume of distribution of tamsulosin after intravenous administration to ten healthy male adults was 16 litres, which is suggestive of distribution into extracellular fluids in the body. Additionally, whole body autoradiographic studies in mice, rats and dogs indicate that tamsulosin is widely distributed to most tissues including kidney, prostate, liver, gall bladder, heart, aorta, and brown fat, and minimally distributed to the brain, spinal cord, and testes.

Figure 1: FLOMAX CR
Mean Tamsulosin Plasma vs. Time Profiles of FLOMAX CR 0.4 mg and Tamsulosin Capsules, 0.4 mg (N=12)

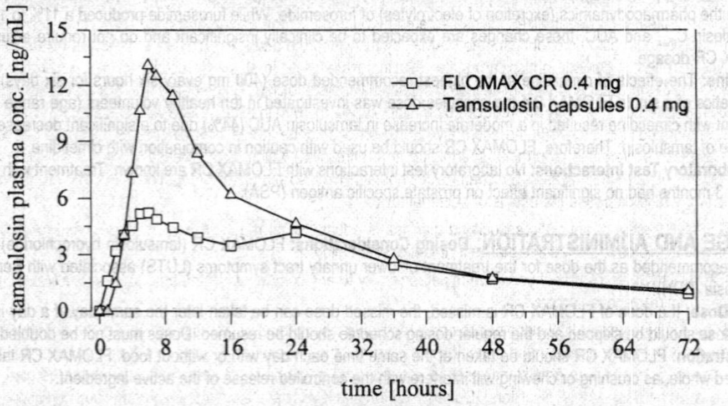

Tamsulosin is extensively bound to human plasma proteins (94% to 99%), primarily alpha-1-acid glycoprotein (AAG) in humans, with linear binding over a wide concentration range (20 to 600 ng/mL). The results of two-way in vitro studies indicate that the binding of tamsulosin to human plasma proteins is not affected by amitriptyline, diclofenac, glyburide, simvastatin plus simvastatin-hydroxy acid metabolite, warfarin, diazepam, propranolol, trichlormethiazide, or chlormadinone. Likewise, tamsulosin had no effect on the extent of binding of these drugs.

Metabolism: Tamsulosin is extensively metabolized by cytochrome P450 enzymes (CYP3A) in the liver, followed by extensive glucuronide or sulfate conjugation of metabolites. On administration of a dose of radiolabelled tamsulosin to four healthy volunteers, 97% of the administered radioactivity was recovered, with urine (76%) representing the primary route of excretion compared to feces (21%) over 168 hours. Less than 10% of the dose was recovered as unchanged (parent) compound in the urine.

Metabolites of tamsulosin do not contribute significantly to tamsulosin adrenoreceptor antagonist activity. Furthermore, there is no enantiomeric bioconversion from tamsulosin [R(−) isomer] to the S(+) isomer in studies with mice, rats, dogs, and humans.

Incubations with human liver microsomes showed no evidence of clinically significant interactions between tamsulosin and drugs which are known to interact or be metabolized by hepatic enzymes, such as amitriptyline, diclofenac, albuterol (beta agonist), glyburide (glibenclamide), finasteride (5 alpha-reductase inhibitor for treatment of BPH), and warfarin. No dose adjustment is warranted in hepatic insufficiency.

Excretion: Tamsulosin undergoes restrictive clearance in humans, with a relatively low systemic clearance (2.88 L/h). Tamsulosin exhibits linear pharmacokinetics following single or multiple dosing of FLOMAX CR resulting in a proportional increase in C_{max} and AUC with increasing doses. Intrinsic clearance is independent of tamsulosin binding to AAG, but diminishes with age, resulting in a 40% overall higher exposure (AUC) in subjects of age 55 to 75 years compared to subjects of age 20 to 32 years.

Following intravenous or oral administration of an immediate-release formulation, the elimination half-life of tamsulosin in plasma ranged from five to seven hours. Because of absorption rate-controlled pharmacokinetics with the FLOMAX CR formulation, the apparent half-life of tamsulosin increases to approximately 12 to 15 hours in healthy volunteers.

Special Populations and Conditions: Pediatrics: FLOMAX CR is not indicated for use in children. Pharmacokinetics have not been evaluated in pediatrics.

Geriatrics: There were no pharmacokinetic studies conducted in geriatric patients with FLOMAX CR. Cross-study comparisons of overall exposure (AUC) and half-life of FLOMAX capsules indicate that the pharmacokinetic disposition of tamsulosin may be slightly prolonged in geriatric males compared to young healthy male volunteers. However, FLOMAX capsules have been found to be a safe and effective alpha1 adrenoreceptor antagonist when administered at therapeutic doses to patients over the age of 65 years.

Gender: FLOMAX CR is not indicated for use in women. Pharmacokinetics have not been evaluated in women.

Hepatic Insufficiency: The pharmacokinetics of tamsulosin have been compared in subjects with hepatic dysfunction (n=8) and in normal subjects (n=8). While a change in the overall plasma concentration of tamsulosin was observed as the result of altered binding to AAG, the unbound (active) concentration of tamsulosin does not change significantly with only a modest (32%) change in intrinsic clearance of unbound tamsulosin. Therefore, patients with mild to moderate hepatic dysfunction do not require an adjustment in FLOMAX dosage.

Renal Insufficiency: The pharmacokinetics of tamsulosin have been compared in subjects with moderate (n=6) or severe (n=6) renal impairment and in normal subjects (n=6). While a change in the overall plasma concentration of tamsulosin was observed as the result of altered binding to AAG, the unbound (active) concentration of tamsulosin, as well as the intrinsic clearance, remained relatively constant. Therefore, patients with such renal impairment do not require an adjustment in FLOMAX dosing. Patients with end stage renal disease (Cl_{cr} <10mL/min) have not been studied.

STORAGE AND STABILITY: Store at room temperature (15-30°C).

INFORMATION FOR THE PATIENT: Published in e-CPS, available by subscription at www.e-cps.ca.

DOSAGE FORMS, COMPOSITION AND PACKAGING: Each controlled-release tablet for oral administration contains: tamsulosin HCl 0.4 mg. Nonmedicinal ingredients: hypromellose, iron oxide yellow E172, macrogol 7 000 000, macrogol 8000 and magnesium stearate. Aluminum foil blister packs of 10 and 30.

(Shown in Product Identification Section)

Flonase®

fluticasone propionate

Corticosteroid for Nasal Use

GlaxoSmithKline

Date of Preparation: June 14, 2001
Date of Revision: November 25, 2004

PHARMACOLOGY: Fluticasone is a potent anti-inflammatory steroid. When administered intranasally in therapeutic doses, it has a direct anti-inflammatory action on the nasal mucosa, the mechanism of which is not yet completely defined.

The onset of action is not immediate, and 2 to 3 days treatment may be required before maximum relief is obtained. This is because the anti-inflammatory activities of glucocorticoids are related to specific steroid effects, which involve several biochemical events, including protein synthesis.

Following intranasal dosing of fluticasone (200 µg/day), steady-state maximum plasma concentrations were not quantifiable in most subjects (<0.01 ng/mL). The highest C_{max} observed was 0.017 ng/mL. Direct absorption in the nose is negligible due to the low aqueous solubility with the majority of the dose being eventually swallowed. When administered orally the systemic exposure is <1% due to poor absorption and pre-systemic metabolism. The total systemic absorption arising from both nasal and oral absorption of the swallowed dose is therefore negligible.

In clinical trials, no hypothalamic-pituitary-adrenal (HPA) axis effects have been observed. Following intranasal dosing of fluticasone (200 µg/day), no significant change in 24-hour serum cortisol AUC was found compared to placebo (ratio 1.01; 90% CI: 0.9 to 1.14).

INDICATIONS: For the treatment of seasonal allergic rhinitis including hay fever, and perennial rhinitis poorly responsive to conventional treatment. In patients with allergic rhinitis, fluticasone is also indicated for the management of associated sinus pain and pressure.

Regular usage is essential for full therapeutic benefit, since maximum relief may not be obtained until after 2 to 3 days of treatment.

CONTRAINDICATIONS: In patients with a history of hypersensitivity to any of its ingredients, and in patients with untreated fungal, bacterial, or tuberculosis infections of the respiratory tract.

WARNINGS: In patients previously on systemic steroids, either over prolonged periods or in high doses, the replacement with a topical corticosteroid can be accompanied by symptoms of withdrawal, e.g., joint and/or muscular pain, lassitude, and depression and, in severe cases, adrenal insufficiency may occur, necessitating the temporary resumption of systemic steroid therapy.

Careful attention must be given to patients with asthma or other clinical conditions in whom a rapid decrease in systemic steroids may cause a severe exacerbation of their symptoms.

A drug interaction study of intranasal fluticasone propionate in healthy subjects has shown that ritonavir (a highly potent cytochrome P450 3A4 inhibitor) can greatly increase fluticasone propionate plasma concentrations, resulting in markedly reduced serum cortisol concentrations. During post-marketing use, there have been reports of clinically significant drug interactions in patients receiving intranasal or inhaled fluticasone propionate and ritonavir, resulting in systemic corticosteroid effects including Cushing's syndrome and adrenal suppression. Therefore, concomitant use of fluticasone propionate and ritonavir should be avoided, unless the potential benefit to the patient outweighs the risk of systemic corticosteroid side-effects.

PRECAUTIONS: General: Patients should be informed that the full effect of fluticasone therapy is not achieved until 2 to 3 days of treatment have been completed. Treatment of seasonal rhinitis should, if possible, start before the exposure to allergens.

Although fluticasone will control seasonal allergic rhinitis in most cases, an abnormally heavy challenge of summer allergens may in certain instances necessitate appropriate additional therapy.

Under most circumstances, treatment with corticosteroids should not be stopped abruptly but tapered off gradually. Patients should be advised to inform subsequent physicians of prior use of corticosteroids.

Steroid Replacement by Fluticasone: The replacement of a systemic steroid with fluticasone must be gradual and carefully supervised by the physician. The guidelines under Dosage should be followed in all such cases.

Effect on Infection: Corticosteroids may mask some signs of infection and new infections may appear. A decreased resistance to localized infections has been observed during corticosteroid therapy; this may require treatment with appropriate therapy or stopping the administration of fluticasone.

Patients who are on drugs that suppress the immune system are more susceptible to infections than healthy individuals. Chickenpox and measles, for example, can have a more serious or even fatal course in nonimmune children or adults on corticosteroids. In such children or adults who have not had these diseases, particular care should be taken to avoid exposure. How the dose, route, and duration of corticosteroid administration affect the risk of developing a disseminated infection is not known. The contribution of the underlying disease and/or prior corticosteroid treatment to the risk is also not known. If exposed to chickenpox, prophylaxis with varicella zoster immune globulin (VZIG) may be indicated. If exposed to measles, prophylaxis with pooled i.m. immunoglobulin (IG), as appropriate, may be indicated. If chickenpox develops, treatment with antiviral agents may be considered.

Systemic Effects: Use of excessive doses of corticosteroids may lead to signs or symptoms of hypercorticism, suppression of HPA function, and/or reduction of growth velocity in children or teenagers. Physicians should closely follow the growth of children and adolescents taking corticosteroids, by any route, and weigh the benefits of corticosteroid therapy against the possibility of growth suppression if growth appears slowed.

Although systemic effects have been minimal with recommended doses of fluticasone aqueous nasal spray, potential risk increases with larger doses. Therefore, larger than recommended doses of fluticasone aqueous nasal spray should be avoided.

Drug Interactions: Under normal circumstances, very low plasma concentrations of fluticasone propionate are achieved after intranasal dosing, due to extensive first pass metabolism and high systemic clearance mediated by cytochrome P450 3A4 in the gut and liver. Hence, clinically significant drug interactions involving fluticasone propionate are unlikely.

A drug interaction study of intranasal fluticasone propionate in healthy subjects has shown that ritonavir (a highly potent cytochrome P450 3A4 inhibitor) can greatly increase fluticasone propionate plasma concentrations, resulting in markedly reduced serum cortisol concentrations. During post-marketing use, there have been reports of clinically significant drug interactions in patients receiving intranasal or inhaled fluticasone propionate and ritonavir, resulting in systemic corticosteroid effects including Cushing's syndrome and adrenal suppression. Therefore, concomitant use of fluticasone propionate and ritonavir should be avoided, unless the potential benefit to the patient outweighs the risk of systemic corticosteroid side-effects.

This study has shown that other inhibitors of cytochrome P450 3A4 produce negligible (erythromycin) and minor (ketoconazole) increases in systemic exposure to fluticasone propionate without notable reductions in serum cortisol concentrations. However, there have been a few case reports during world-wide post-market use of adrenal cortisol suppression associated with concomitant use of azole anti-fungals and inhaled fluticasone propionate. Therefore, care is advised when co-administering potent cytochrome P450 3A4 inhibitors (e.g. ketoconazole) as there is potential for increased systemic exposure to fluticasone propionate.

Long-term Effects: During long-term therapy, HPA axis function and hematological status should be assessed.

The long-term effects of fluticasone in humans are still unknown, in particular, its local effects; the possibility of atrophic rhinitis and/or pharyngeal candidiasis should be kept in mind.

Hypothyroidism and Cirrhosis: There is an enhanced effect of corticosteroids on patients with hypothyroidism and in those with cirrhosis.

Use of Corticosteroids and ASA: ASA should be used cautiously in conjunction with corticosteroids in hypothrombinemia.

Effect of Corticosteroids on Wound Healing: In patients who have had recent nasal surgery or trauma, a nasal corticosteroid should be used with caution until healing has occurred, because of the inhibitory effect of corticosteroids on wound healing.

Proper Use of Drug: To ensure proper dosage and administration of the drug, the patient should be instructed by a physician or other health professional in the use of fluticasone (see Information for the Patient).

Pregnancy: The safety of fluticasone in pregnancy has not been established. If used, the expected benefits should be weighed against the potential hazard to the fetus, particularly during the first trimester of pregnancy.

Like other glucocorticosteroids, fluticasone is teratogenic to rodent species. Adverse effects typical of potent corticosteroids are only seen at high systemic exposure levels; direct intranasal application ensures minimal systemic exposure. The relevance of these findings to humans has not yet been established. Infants born of mothers who have received substantial doses of glucocorticosteroids during pregnancy should be carefully observed for hypoadrenalism.

Lactation: Glucocorticosteroids are excreted in human milk. It is not known whether fluticasone is excreted in human milk.

When measurable plasma levels were obtained in lactating laboratory rats following s.c. administration, there was evidence of fluticasone in the breast milk. However, following intranasal administration to primates, no drug was detected in the plasma, and it is therefore unlikely that the drug would be detectable in milk. The use of fluticasone in nursing mothers requires that the possible benefits of the drug be weighed against the potential hazards to the infant.

Children: Fluticasone is not presently recommended for children younger than 4 years of age due to limited clinical data in this age group.

Until greater clinical experience has been gained, the continuous, long-term treatment of children under age 12 is not recommended.

ADVERSE EFFECTS: Adverse reactions in controlled clinical studies with fluticasone have been primarily associated with irritation of the nasal mucous membranes, and are consistent with those expected from application of a topical medication to an already inflamed membrane. The adverse reactions reported by patients treated with fluticasone were similar to those reported by patients receiving placebo.

The most frequently reported adverse reactions (≥1% in any treatment group) considered by the investigator to be potentially related to fluticasone or placebo in trials of seasonal allergic rhinitis are listed in Table 1. These studies, conducted in 948 adults and in 499 children, evaluated 14 to 28 days of treatment with recommended doses of fluticasone compared with placebo.

Table 1: Flonase
Adverse Reactions Reported Most Frequently in Clinical Trials of Seasonal Allergic Rhinitis

	Adults (age ≥12 years)			Children (age 4-11 years)		
	Flonase 100 µg b.i.d. (n=312) %	Flonase 200 µg o.d. (n=322) %	Placebo (n=314) %	Flonase 100 µg o.d. (n=167) %	Flonase 200 µg o.d. (n=164) %	Placebo (n=168) %
Nasal Burning	2.2	3.4	2.5	1.8	2.4	1.2
Pharyngitis	1.3	1.6	<1	<1	0	0
Runny Nose	<1	1.6	<1	<1	<1	<1

(cont'd)

Table 1: Flonase *(cont'd)*

Adverse Reactions Reported Most Frequently in Clinical Trials of Seasonal Allergic Rhinitis

	Adults (age ≥12 years)			Children (age 4-11 years)		
	Flonase 100 µg b.i.d. (n=312) %	Flonase 200 µg o.d. (n=322) %	Placebo (n=314) %	Flonase 100 µg o.d. (n=167) %	Flonase 200 µg o.d. (n=164) %	Placebo (n=168) %
Blood in Nasal Mucous	0	1.6	<1	0	<1	0
Epistaxis	1.6	2.8	2.2	3.0	3.7	3.6
Sneezing	<1	1.2	2.2	0	<1	0
Crusting in Nostrils	0	0	0	1.2	0	0
Nasal Congestion	0	0	0	0	1.2	0
Nasal Ulcer	<1	0	0	1.2	1.2	1.2
Headache	1.3	2.5	1.9	1.2	1.2	1.2

In two 6-month trials involving 831 patients aged 12 to 75 years with perennial allergic rhinitis, the adverse reactions reported by patients treated with fluticasone were similar in type and incidence to those reported in seasonal trials, with the exception of epistaxis (≤13.3%) and blood in nasal mucous (≤8.3%). In addition to the events reported most frequently in the seasonal trials, patients receiving fluticasone in the 6-month trials reported nasal soreness (≤2.5%), nasal excoriation (≤2.0%), sinusitis (≤1.6%), and nasal dryness (≤1.3%).

Infrequent adverse reactions (incidence of 0.1% to 1% and greater than placebo) reported by patients receiving fluticasone at the recommended daily dose of 200 µg (or 100 µg/day for children 4 to 11 years of age) in the aforementioned clinical trials included pharyngeal irritation, nasal stinging, nausea and vomiting, unpleasant smell and taste, and sinus headache (0.3%); lacrimation, eye irritation, xerostomia, cough, urticaria, and rash (0.2%); and nasal septum perforation (0.1%).

Postmarketing Surveillance: The following events have been identified during postapproval use of fluticasone in clinical practice.

General: headache and hypersensitivity reactions including angioedema, skin rash, edema of the face or tongue, pruritus, urticaria, bronchospasm, wheezing, dyspnea and anaphylaxis/anaphylactic reactions have been reported.

Ear, Nose and Throat: alteration or loss in sense of taste and/or smell and, rarely, nasal septal perforation, nasal ulcer, sore throat, throat irritation and dryness, cough, hoarseness, and voice changes.

Eye: dryness and irritation of the eyes, conjunctivitis, blurred vision, and very rarely, glaucoma, increased intraocular pressure, and cataracts.

OVERDOSE:

Symptoms: Like any other nasally administered corticosteroid, acute overdosing is unlikely in view of the total amount of active ingredient present. However, when used chronically in excessive doses or in conjunction with other corticosteroid formulations, systemic corticosteroid effects such as hypercorticism and adrenal suppression may appear. If such changes occur, the dosage of fluticasone should be discontinued slowly, consistent with accepted procedures for discontinuation of chronic steroid therapy (see Dosage).

The restoration of HPA axis function may be slow. During periods of pronounced physical stress (i.e., severe infections, trauma, surgery) a supplement with systemic steroids may be advisable.

Treatment: See Symptoms.

For management of a suspected drug overdose, CPhA recommends that you contact your **regional Poison Control Centre**. See the *CPS* Directory section for a list of Poison Control Centres.

DOSAGE: See Warnings.

The therapeutic effects of corticosteroids, unlike those of decongestants, are not immediate. Since the effect of fluticasone depends on its regular use, patients must be instructed to take the nasal inhalation at regular intervals and not, as with other nasal sprays, as they feel necessary.

Adults and Children 12 years of age and older: The usual dosage is 2 sprays (50 µg each) in each nostril once a day (total daily dosage, 200 µg). Some patients with severe rhinitis may benefit from 2 sprays in each nostril every 12 hours. The recommended maximum daily dose is 400 µg (4 sprays in each nostril).

Children 4 to 11 years of age: The usual dosage is 1 or 2 (50 µg/actuation) sprays in each nostril in the morning (100 or 200 µg/day). The recommended maximum daily dose is 200 µg (2 sprays in each nostril).

The safety and efficacy of fluticasone in children below 4 years of age have not been established and, therefore, fluticasone is not recommended in this patient population.

Until greater clinical experience has been gained, the continuous, long-term treatment of children under age 12 is not recommended.

An improvement of symptoms usually becomes apparent within a few days after the start of therapy. However, symptomatic relief may not occur in some patients for as long as 2 weeks. Fluticasone should not be continued beyond three weeks in the absence of significant symptomatic improvement.

In the presence of excessive nasal mucous secretion or edema of the nasal mucosa, the drug may fail to reach the site of action. In such cases it is advisable to use a nasal vasoconstrictor for 2 to 3 days prior to starting treatment with fluticasone. Patients should be instructed on the correct method of use, which is to blow the nose, then insert the nozzle carefully into the nostril, compress the opposite nostril and actuate the spray while inspiring through the nose, with the mouth closed (see Information for the Patient).

Careful attention must be given to patients previously treated for prolonged periods with systemic corticosteroids when transferred to fluticasone. Initially, fluticasone and the systemic corticosteroid must be given concomitantly, while the dose of the latter is gradually decreased. The usual rate of withdrawal of the systemic steroid is the equivalent of 1 mg of prednisone every 4 days if the patient is under close supervision. If continuous supervision is not feasible, the withdrawal of the systemic steroid should be slower, approximately 1 mg of prednisone (or equivalent) every 10 days. If withdrawal symptoms appear, the previous dose of the systemic steroid should be resumed for a week before further decrease is attempted.

INFORMATION FOR THE PATIENT: Published in e-CPS, available by subscription at www.e-cps.ca.

SUPPLIED: Each 100 mg of spray delivered by the metered nasal adaptor (1 actuation), contains: micronised fluticasone propionate 50 µg. Nonmedicinal ingredients: benzalkonium chloride, dextrose, microcrystalline cellulose and carboxymethylcellulose sodium, phenylethyl alcohol, polysorbate 80 and purified water. Amber glass bottles containing sufficient formulation for 120 metered sprays (16 g net weight). Store between 4 and 30°C. Shake gently before use.

(Shown in Product Identification Section)

Florastor®

Saccharomyces boulardii lyo

Natural Health Product

Medical Futures

PHARMACOLOGY: Saccharomyces boulardii lyo is ingested and reaches the small and large intestine in a viable state. Under normal conditions the cells do not enter into the circulatory system. Saccharomyces boulardii lyo does not permanently colonize the human intestinal tract. Bacteria exert their pathogenicity via toxins in the intestines. Saccharomyces boulardii lyo secretes a 54 kDa protein protease that neutralizes toxins secreted by bacteria. Some bacteria produce toxins that increase the intracellular level of cyclic adenosine monophosphate (cAMP) by activating the adenylate cyclase in intestinal epithelial cells. This triggers active secretion of chloride and bicarbonate resulting in diarrhea. In studies, Saccharomyces boulardii lyo inhibited approximately 50% of the water and sodium secretion caused by cholera toxin (CT) compared with loops treated with CT alone. Toxins A and B secreted by *C. difficile* are reduced by a factor of 100 to 1000 in mice treated with Saccharomyces boulardii lyo. Saccharomyces boulardii lyo increases the absorptive transport of chloride in intestinal electrolyte transport. Saccharomyces boulardii lyo releases polyamines (spermine, spermidine and putrescine) which help increase the activity of dissaccharidase enzymes (lactase, sucrase and maltase). Saccharomyces boulardii lyo also stimulates production of IgA and IgG in the intestinal mucosa which may help decrease the effects of bacterial toxins.

INDICATIONS: Helps prevent antibiotic associated diarrhea in adults. Helps reduce the symptoms related to acute diarrhea (infectious) in adults. Helps to treat acute diarrhea (infectious) in children.

CONTRAINDICATIONS: Do not use if you have hypersensitivity to any component of the product (especially allergy to yeast) or if you have a central venous catheter.

WARNINGS: Discontinue use and consult a health care practitioner if symptoms of digestive upset (e.g., diarrhea) occur, worsen or persist beyond 3 days. Do not open the capsules in the surrounding of patients having a central venous catheter. Lactose intolerance. Consult a health care practitioner prior to use this drug if you have an abnormal condition of the gastrointestinal tract lining (i.e. ulcer or other GI tract disorders). Do not use Florastor if you have an immune-compromised condition (e.g. AIDS, lymphoma, long-term corticosteroid treatment). Consult a health care practitioner prior to use if you have an abnormal condition of the gastrointestinal tract lining (i.e. ulcer or other GI tract disorders). Do not use if you are experiencing nausea, fever, vomiting, bloody diarrhea or severe abdominal pain. Treatment does not replace rehydration when this is necessary.

PRECAUTIONS: *Pregnancy:* There are no adequate and well-controlled studies in pregnant women. It is classified as Pregnancy category B.

Lactation: Saccharomyces boulardii lyo is not excreted in human milk. However, caution should be exercised when Saccharomyces boulardii lyo is given to nursing women.

ADVERSE EFFECTS: Rarely: flatulence, pruritus, rash, angioedema. Very rarely: anaphylactic reaction.

OVERDOSE:

Treatment: No overdoses have been reported with Saccharomyces boulardii lyo. In the event of overdose, patients should be carefully observed and given supportive treatment.

For management of a suspected drug overdose, CPhA recommends that you contact your **regional Poison Control Centre**. See the *CPS* Directory section for a list of Poison Control Centres.

DOSAGE: Duration of use: 1 week.

Adults: 2 capsules daily (1 capsule in the morning and 1 capsule in the evening). May be recommended up to 6 capsules per day by health care practitioners.

Children (age 1 to 12): 1 capsule in the morning and 1 capsule in the evening.

SUPPLIED: Each capsule contains 5×10^9 CFU of Saccharomyces boulardii. (Equivalent to 250 mg). Nonmedicinal ingredients: hydroxypropylmethylcellulose, lactose monohydrate, magnesium stearate and titanium dioxide (E171). Gluten- and wheat- free. **Do not use if seal is broken. Store at 15-30°C in a dry area. No need to refrigerate.**

Florazole® ER ℞

metronidazole

Antibacterial—Antiprotozoal

Ferring

PHARMACOLOGY: Metronidazole has activity against most obligately anaerobic bacteria and many protozoa. It is inactive against fungi, viruses and most aerobic or facultatively anaerobic bacteria.

Metronidazole exerts an antimicrobial effect in an anaerobic environment by the following possible mechanism: Once metronidazole enters the organism, the drug is reduced by intracellular electron transport proteins. Because of this alteration to the metronidazole molecule, a concentration gradient is maintained which promotes the drug's intracellular transport. Presumably, free radicals are formed which, in turn, react with cellular components resulting in death of the microorganism.

INDICATIONS: For the treatment of symptomatic women with bacterial vaginosis.

CONTRAINDICATIONS: In patients with a prior history of hypersensitivity to metronidazole or other nitroimidazole derivatives.

Pregnancy: Metronidazole is contraindicated in the first trimester of pregnancy.

WARNINGS: Convulsive Seizures and Peripheral Neuropathy: Convulsive seizures and peripheral neuropathy, the latter characterized mainly by numbness or paresthesia of an extremity, have been reported in patients treated with metronidazole. The appearance of abnormal neurologic signs demands the prompt discontinuation of metronidazole therapy. Metronidazole should be administered with caution to patients with CNS diseases.

Studies in rats and mice have provided some evidence that metronidazole may cause tumors in these species, when administered orally for long periods, at high doses.

The relevance of these findings in humans is not known.

Occupational Hazards: Patients should be warned about potential for confusion, dizziness, hallucination, or convulsion and advised not to drive or operate machinery if these symptoms occur.

PRECAUTIONS: General: Patients with severe hepatic disease metabolize metronidazole slowly, with resultant accumulation of metronidazole and its metabolites in the plasma. Accordingly, for such patients, doses below those usually recommended should be administered, cautiously.

Known or previously unrecognized candidiasis may present more prominent symptoms during therapy with metronidazole and requires treatment with a candidacidal agent.

Treatment with metronidazole should be discontinued should pancreatitis occur, once other causes of this disease have been excluded.

A rare case of reversible but profound neurological deterioration has been reported following a single oral dose of metronidazole. It is therefore advised that a patient taking metronidazole for the first time should not be left unattended for a period of 2 hours. The appearance of abnormal neurological symptoms demands prompt discontinuation of metronidazole therapy and, when severe, immediate medical attention. Gastric lavage may be considered, if no more than 2 or 3 hours have elapsed since administration of the drug.

Treatment with metronidazole should be discontinued if ataxia or any other symptoms of CNS involvement occur.

Hematologic Effects: Metronidazole is a nitroimidazole and should be used with caution in patients with evidence of or history of blood dyscrasia. A mild leukopenia has been observed during its administration; however, no persistent hematologic abnormalities attributable to metronidazole have been observed in clinical studies. Total and differential leukocyte counts should be made before and after retreatments.

Pregnancy: Metronidazole crosses the placental barrier and enters the fetal circulation rapidly. No fetotoxicity was observed when metronidazole was administered orally to pregnant mice at 60 mg/m²/day, which is approximately 10% of the human dose when expressed as mg/m². However, in a single small study where the drug was administered intraperitoneally, some intrauterine deaths were observed. The relationship of these findings to the drug is unknown. There are, however, no adequate and well-controlled studies in pregnant women. Because animal reproduction studies are not always predictive of human response, this drug should be used during pregnancy only if clearly needed.

Lactation: Metronidazole is secreted in human milk in concentrations similar to those found in plasma. If a nursing mother is treated with metronidazole, the breast milk should be expressed and discarded during treatment. Breast-feeding can be resumed 24 to 48 hours after treatment.

Drug/Laboratory Test Interactions: Metronidazole may interfere with certain types of determinations of serum chemistry values, such as AST, ALT, LDH, triglycerides, and glucose hexokinase. Values of zero may be observed. All of the assays in which interference has been reported involve enzymatic coupling of the assay to oxidation reduction of nicotinamide adenine dinucleotide ($NAD^+ \leftrightarrow NADH$). Interference is due to the similarity in absorbance peaks of NADH (340 nm) and metronidazole (322 nm) at pH 7.

Geriatrics: Decreased renal function does not alter the single-dose pharmacokinetics of metronidazole. However, plasma clearance of metronidazole is decreased in patients with decreased liver function. Therefore, in elderly patients, monitoring of serum levels may be necessary to adjust the metronidazole dosage accordingly.

Children: Safety and effectiveness in pediatric patients have not been established.

Drug Interactions: Alcohol: Alcoholic beverages should not be consumed during metronidazole therapy and for at least 2 days afterward because abdominal cramps, nausea, vomiting, headaches, and flushing may occur.

Disulfiram: Psychotic reactions have been reported in alcoholic patients who are using metronidazole and disulfiram concurrently. Metronidazole should not be given to patients who have taken disulfiram within the last 2 weeks.

5-fluorouracil: Metronidazole has been reported to reduce the clearance of 5-fluorouracil resulting in increased toxicity of 5-fluorouracil.

Vecuronium: A slight potentiation of the neuromuscular blocking activity of vecuronium has been reported in patients administered metronidazole at a dose of 15 mg/kg.

Anticoagulants: Metronidazole has been reported to potentiate the anticoagulant effect of warfarin and other oral coumarin anticoagulants, resulting in a prolongation of prothrombin time. This possible drug interaction should be considered when metronidazole is prescribed for patients on this type of anticoagulant therapy.

Liver Enzyme-Inducing Drugs: The simultaneous administration of drugs that induce microsomal liver enzymes, such as phenytoin or phenobarbital, may accelerate the elimination of metronidazole, resulting in reduced plasma levels; impaired clearance of phenytoin has been reported.

Liver Enzyme-Reducing Drugs: The simultaneous administration of drugs that decrease microsomal liver enzyme activity, such as cimetidine, may prolong the half life and decrease plasma clearance of metronidazole.

Lithium: In patients stabilized on relatively high doses of lithium, short-term metronidazole therapy has been associated with elevation of serum lithium and, in a few cases, signs of lithium toxicity. Serum lithium and serum creatinine levels should be obtained several days after beginning metronidazole to detect any increase that may precede clinical symptoms of lithium intoxication.

ADVERSE EFFECTS: In 2 multicentre clinical trials, a total of 418 patients received metronidazole extended release tablets orally once daily for 5 or 7 days.

In these 2 multicentre trials, the following adverse events occurred with an incidence of 2% or greater (see Table 1).

Table 1: Florazole ER

Adverse Events with Incidence ≥2%

Adverse Event	Florazole ER 750 mg × 5 days (N=151)	Florazole ER 750 mg × 7 days (N=267)
Abdominal Pain	7 (5%)	10 (4%)
Allergy	3 (2%)	1 (0%)
Anorexia	3 (2%)	1 (0%)
Cervicitis	3 (2%)	0 (0%)
Coughing	3 (2%)	4 (1%)
Diarrhea	6 (4%)	11 (4%)
Dizziness	2 (1%)	11 (4%)
Dysmenorrhea	6 (4%)	9 (3%)
Dyspepsia	3 (2%)	5 (2%)
Dysuria	3 (2%)	2 (1%)
Flatulence	2 (1%)	5 (2%)
Headache	22 (15%)	48 (18%)
Infection Bacterial	12 (8%)	19 (7%)
Influenza-like Symptoms	10 (7%)	17 (6%)
Intermenstrual Bleeding	1 (1%)	6 (2%)
Leukorrhea	3 (2%)	2 (1%)
Moniliasis	9 (6%)	9 (3%)
Mouth Dry	4 (3%)	5 (2%)
Nausea	23 (15%)	28 (10%)
Nervousness	2 (1%)	5 (2%)
Pain	7 (5%)	4 (1%)
Perineal Pain Female	0 (0%)	6 (2%)
Pharyngitis	4 (3%)	8 (3%)
Pruritus Genital	5 (3%)	14 (5%)
Rash	4 (3%)	1 (0%)
Rhinitis	6 (4%)	12 (4%)
Sinusitis	4 (3%)	7 (3%)
Taste Perversion	10 (7%)	23 (9%)
Upper Respiratory Tract Infection	8 (5%)	11 (4%)
Urinary Tract Infection	4 (3%)	6 (2%)
Urine Abnormal	6 (4%)	7 (3%)
Vaginitis	16 (11%)	39 (15%)
Vomiting	1 (1%)	6 (2%)

The following reactions have also been reported during treatment with metronidazole:

CNS: Two serious adverse reactions reported in patients treated with metronidazole have been convulsive seizures and peripheral neuropathy, the latter characterized mainly by numbness or paresthesia of an extremity. Since persistent peripheral neuropathy has been reported in some patients receiving prolonged administration of metronidazole, patients should be specifically warned about these reactions and should be told to stop the drug and report immediately to their physicians if any neurologic symptoms occur. In addition, patients have reported dizziness, vertigo, incoordination, ataxia, confusion, irritability, depression, weakness, and insomnia (see Warnings).

Gastrointestinal: The most common adverse reactions reported have been referable to the GI tract, particularly nausea reported by about 12% of patients, sometimes accompanied by headache, anorexia, and occasionally vomiting, diarrhea, epigastric distress, and abdominal cramping. Constipation has also been reported.

A sharp, unpleasant metallic taste is not unusual. Furry tongue, glossitis, and stomatitis have occurred; these may be associated with a sudden overgrowth of Candida which may occur during therapy. Rare cases of pancreatitis, which generally abated on withdrawal of the drug, have been reported.

Hematopoetic: reversible neutropenia (leukopenia); rarely, reversible thrombocytopenia.

Cardiovascular: Flattening of the T-wave may be seen in electrocardiographic tracings.

Hypersensitivity: urticaria, erythematous rash, flushing, nasal congestion, dryness of the mouth (or vagina or vulva), and fever.

Renal: dysuria, cystitis, polyuria, incontinence, and a sense of pelvic pressure. Instances of darkened urine have been reported by approximately 1 patient in 100 000. Although the pigment which is probably responsible for this phenomenon has not been positively identified, it is almost certainly a metabolite of metronidazole and seems to have no clinical significance.

Other: Proliferation of Candida in the vagina, dyspareunia, decrease of libido, proctitis, and fleeting joint pains sometimes resembling "serum sickness". If patients receiving metronidazole drink alcoholic beverages, they may experience abdominal distress, nausea, vomiting, flushing, or headache. A modification of the taste of alcoholic beverages has also been reported.

OVERDOSE:

Symptoms: Single oral doses of metronidazole, up to 15 g, have been reported in suicide attempts and accidental overdoses. Symptoms reported include nausea, vomiting and ataxia.

Oral metronidazole has been studied as a radiation sensitizer in the treatment of malignant tumors. Neurotoxic effects, including seizures and peripheral neuropathy, have been reported after 5 to 7 days of doses of 6 to 10.4 g every other day.

Treatment: There is no specific treatment for metronidazole overdose; therefore, management of the patient should consist of symptomatic and supportive therapy.

> For management of a suspected drug overdose, CPhA recommends that you contact your **regional Poison Control Centre**. See the *CPS* Directory section for a list of Poison Control Centres.

DOSAGE: The recommended oral dose for the treatment of bacterial vaginosis is one 750 mg tablet daily for 7 consecutive days.

When metronidazole extended release tablets are taken with food there is an increase in the rate and extent of absorption; therefore, it is recommended that metronidazole extended release be taken under fasting conditions, at least 1 hour before or 2 hours after meals.

When repeat courses of the drug are required, it is recommended that an interval of 4 to 6 weeks elapse between courses. Total and differential leukocyte counts should be made before and after retreatments.

Patients with severe hepatic disease metabolize metronidazole slowly, with resultant accumulation of metronidazole and its metabolites in the plasma. Accordingly, for such patients, doses below those usually recommended should be administered, cautiously. Close monitoring of plasma metronidazole levels and toxicity is recommended.

Severe Impairment of Renal Function and Anuria: The elimination half-life of metronidazole in anuric patients is not significantly altered. However, the elimination half-lives of metabolites of metronidazole are slightly increased. Consequently, although metronidazole would not be expected to accumulate, accumulation of the metabolites would be expected.

Patients with severe impairment of renal function who are not undergoing hemodialysis should be monitored closely for signs of toxicity.

Patients on Hemodialysis: The dose of metronidazole need not be specifically reduced since accumulated metabolites may be rapidly removed by hemodialysis.

Patients on Peritoneal Dialysis: Peritoneal dialysis does not appear to reduce serum levels of metronidazole metabolites.

INFORMATION FOR THE PATIENT: Published in e-CPS, available by subscription at www.e-cps.ca.

SUPPLIED: Each oval, blue, film-coated, extended-release tablet, with FLORAZOLE ER on one side and 750 mg on the other, contains: metronidazole 750 mg. Nonmedicinal ingredients: FD&C Blue No. 2 Aluminium Lake, hydroxypropyl methylcellulose, lactose, magnesium stearate, poly (meth) acrylic acid ester copolymers, polyethylene glycol, polysorbate 80, silicon dioxide, simethicone emulsion, talc and titanium dioxide. Bottles of 30. Store in a dry place under controlled room temperature at 15 to 25°C. Dispense in a well-closed container with a child-resistant closure.

Florinef® ℞

fludrocortisone acetate

Mineralocorticoid for Renal Insufficiency

Paladin

Date of Revision: May 1, 2009

PHARMACOLOGY: The physiologic action of fludrocortisone is similar to that of hydrocortisone. However, the effects of fludrocortisone, particularly on electrolyte balance, but also on carbohydrate metabolism, are considerably heightened and prolonged. In small oral doses, fludrocortisone produces marked sodium retention and increased urinary potassium excretion. It also causes a rise in blood pressure, apparently because of these effects on electrolyte levels. In larger doses, fludrocortisone inhibits endogenous adrenal cortical secretion, thymic activity, and pituitary corticotropin excretion: promotes the deposition of liver glycogen; and, unless protein intake is adequate, induces negative nitrogen balance.

INDICATIONS: Partial replacement therapy for primary and secondary adrenocortical insufficiency in Addison's disease and for the treatment of salt losing adrenogenital syndrome.

CONTRAINDICATIONS: Corticosteroids are contraindicated in patients with systemic fungal infections.

PRECAUTIONS: Because of its marked effect on sodium retention, the use of fludrocortisone in the treatment of conditions other than those indicated herein is not advised.

Corticosteroids may mask some signs of infection, and new infections may appear during their use. There may be decreased resistance and inability to localize infection when corticosteroids are used. If an infection occurs during fludrocortisone therapy, it should be promptly controlled by suitable antimicrobial therapy.

Prolonged use of corticosteroids may produce posterior subcapsular cataracts, glaucoma with possible damage to the optic nerves, and may enhance the establishment of secondary ocular infections due to fungi or viruses.

Average and large doses of hydrocortisone or cortisone can cause elevation of blood pressure, salt and water retention, and increased excretion of potassium. These effects are less likely to occur with the synthetic derivatives except when used in large doses. However, since fludrocortisone is a potent mineralocorticoid, both the dosage and salt intake should be carefully monitored in order to avoid the development of hypertension, edema, or weight gain. Periodic checking of serum electrolyte levels is advisable during prolonged therapy; dietary salt restriction and potassium supplementation may be necessary. All corticosteroids increase calcium excretion.

Patients should not be vaccinated against smallpox while on corticosteroid therapy. Other immunization procedures should not be undertaken in patients who are on corticosteroids, especially on high dose, because of possible hazards of neurological complications and a lack of antibody response.

The use of fludrocortisone in patients with active tuberculosis should be restricted to those cases of fulminating or disseminated tuberculosis in which the corticosteroid is used for the management of the disease in conjunction with an appropriate antituberculous regimen. If corticosteroids are indicated in patients with latent tuberculosis or tuberculin reactivity, close observation is necessary since reactivation of the disease may occur. During prolonged corticosteroid therapy these patients should receive chemoprophylaxis.

Pregnancy: Since adequate human reproduction studies have not been done with corticosteroids, the use of these drugs in pregnancy, nursing mothers, or women of childbearing potential requires that the possible benefits of the drug be weighed against the potential hazards to the mother, embryo, fetus or nursing infant. Infants born of mothers who have received substantial doses of corticosteroids during pregnancy should be carefully observed for signs of hypoadrenalism.

Lactation: See Pregnancy.

Adverse reactions to corticosteroids may be produced by too rapid withdrawal or by continued use of large doses.

To avoid drug induced adrenal insufficiency, supportive dosage may be required in times of stress (such as trauma, surgery, or severe illness) both during treatment with fludrocortisone and for a year afterwards.

There is an enhanced corticosteroid effect in patients with hypothyroidism and in those with cirrhosis.

Corticosteroids should be used cautiously in patients with ocular herpes simplex because of possible corneal perforation.

The lowest possible dose of corticosteroid should be used to control the condition being treated. A gradual reduction in dosage should be made when possible.

Psychic derangements may appear when corticosteroids are used. These may range from euphoria, insomnia, mood swings, personality changes, and severe depression, to frank psychotic manifestations. Existing emotional instability or psychotic tendencies may also be aggravated by corticosteroids.

ASA should be used cautiously in conjunction with corticosteroids in patients with hypoprothrombinemia.

Corticosteroids should be used with caution in patients with nonspecific ulcerative colitis if there is a probability of impending perforation, abscess, or other pyogenic infection.

Corticosteroids should also be used cautiously in patients with diverticulitis, fresh intestinal anastomoses, active or latent peptic ulcer, renal insufficiency, hypertension, osteoporosis, acute glomerulonephritis, vaccinia, varicella, exanthema, Cushing's syndrome, antibiotic resistant infections, diabetes mellitus, congestive heart failure, chronic nephritis, thromboembolitic tendencies, thrombophlebitis, convulsive disorders, metastatic carcinoma, and myasthenia gravis.

Growth and development of infants and children on prolonged corticosteroid therapy should be carefully observed.

ADVERSE EFFECTS: In the recommended small dosages, the side effects seen with cortisone and its derivatives are not usually a problem with fludrocortisone. However, the following untoward effects should be kept in mind, particularly when this agent is used over a prolonged period of time or in conjunction with cortisone or a similar glucocorticoid:

Fluid and Electrolyte Disturbances: sodium retention, fluid retention, congestive heart failure in susceptible patients, potassium loss, hypokalemic alkalosis, and hypertension.

Musculoskeletal: muscle weakness, steroid myopathy, loss of muscle mass, osteoporosis, vertebral compression fractures, aseptic necrosis of femoral and humeral heads, pathologic fracture of long bones, and spontaneous fractures.

Gastrointestinal: peptic ulcer with possible perforation and hemorrhage, pancreatitis, abdominal distention, and ulcerative esophagitis.

Dermatologic: impaired wound healing, thin fragile skin, bruising, petechiae and ecchymoses, facial erythema, increased sweating, subcutaneous fat atrophy, purpura, striae, hyperpigmentation of the skin and nails, hirsutism, and acneiform eruptions; reactions to skin tests may be suppressed.

Neurological: convulsions, increased intracranial pressure with papilledema (pseudotumor cerebri) usually after treatment, vertigo, headache, and severe mental disturbances.

Endocrine: menstrual irregularities; development of the Cushingoid state; suppression of growth in children; secondary adrenocortical and pituitary unresponsiveness, particularly in times of stress (e.g. trauma, surgery, or illness); decreased carbohydrate tolerance; manifestations of latent diabetes mellitus; and increased requirements for insulin or oral hypoglycemic agents in diabetics.

Ophthalmic: posterior subcapsular cataracts, increased intraocular pressure, glaucoma, and exophthalmos.

Metabolic: hyperglycemia, glycosuria, and negative nitrogen balance due to protein catabolism.

Others: Other adverse reactions that may occur following the administration of a corticosteroid are necrotizing angiitis, thrombophlebitis, aggravation or masking of infections, insomnia, syncopal episodes, and anaphylactoid reactions.

OVERDOSE:

For management of a suspected drug overdose, CPhA recommends that you contact your **regional Poison Control Centre**. See the *CPS* Directory section for a list of Poison Control Centres.

DOSAGE: Addison's disease: Usual dose is 0.1 mg daily, although dosage ranging from 0.1 mg 3 times a week to 0.2 mg daily has been employed. In the event transient hypertension develops as a consequence of therapy, the dose should be reduced to 0.05 mg daily. Fludrocortisone is preferably administered in conjunction with cortisone (10 to 37.5 mg daily in divided doses) or hydrocortisone (10 to 20 mg daily in divided doses).

Salt losing adrenogenital syndrome: 0.1 to 0.2 mg daily.

SUPPLIED: Each white, scored tablet, imprinted with "RPC" and "059" contains: fludrocortisone acetate 0.1 mg. Bottles of 100. Store between 2 and 8°C.

(Shown in Product Identification Section)

Flovent® HFA Ⓟ
fluticasone propionate
Corticosteroid for Oral Inhalation

GlaxoSmithKline

Flovent® Diskus® Ⓟ
fluticasone propionate
Corticosteroid for Oral Inhalation

GlaxoSmithKline

Date of Revision: March 31, 2010

SUMMARY PRODUCT INFORMATION:

Route of Administration	Dosage Form/Strength	Nonmedicinal Ingredients
Oral Inhalation	Powder for Inhalation/50, 100, 250, and 500 μg/blister	Lactose and milk protein. For a complete listing see Dosage Forms, Composition and Packaging.
Oral Inhalation	Inhalation Aerosol/50, 125, and 250 μg/metered dose	1,1,1,2-tetrafluoroethane (HFA-134a). For a complete listing see Dosage Forms, Composition and Packaging.

INDICATIONS AND CLINICAL USE: FLOVENT (fluticasone propionate) is indicated for:

- the prophylactic management of steroid-responsive bronchial asthma in adults and children. For children, this includes patients not controlled on currently available prophylactic medication.

Geriatrics: There is no need to adjust the dose in elderly patients.

Adults and Adolescents 16 years of age and older: Mild Asthma: PEF values greater than 80% of predicted at baseline with less than 20% variability. Patients requiring intermittent symptomatic bronchodilator asthma medication on more than an occasional basis.

Moderate Asthma: PEF values 60-80% of predicted at baseline with 20-30% variability. Patients requiring regular asthma medication and patients with unstable or worsening asthma on currently available prophylactic therapy or bronchodilator alone.

Severe Asthma: PEF values less than 60% of predicted at baseline with greater than 30% variability. Patients with severe, chronic asthma. On introduction of inhaled fluticasone propionate, many patients who are dependent on systemic corticosteroids for adequate control of symptoms may be able to reduce significantly or to eliminate their requirements for oral corticosteroids.

Severe asthma requires regular medical assessment as death may occur. Patients with severe asthma have constant symptoms and frequent exacerbations, with limited physical capacity. These patients will require high dose inhaled (see Dosage and Administration) or oral corticosteroid therapy. Sudden worsening of symptoms may require increased corticosteroid dosage which should be administered under urgent medical supervision.

Pediatrics (12 months of age and older): FLOVENT DISKUS is indicated for any child 4 years of age and older, and FLOVENT HFA inhalation aerosol is indicated for children 12 months of age and above who require prophylactic medication, including patients not controlled on currently available prophylactic medication.

At present there are insufficient clinical data to recommend the use of FLOVENT DISKUS in children younger than 4 years and the use of FLOVENT HFA inhalation aerosol in children younger than 12 months.

CONTRAINDICATIONS:

- Patients with a history of hypersensitivity to any of its ingredients (see Dosage Forms, Composition and Packaging) and in patients with untreated fungal, bacterial or tuberculous infections of the respiratory tract.
- Patients with IgE mediated allergic reactions to lactose or milk (see Dosage Forms, Composition and Packaging).
- In the primary treatment of status asthmaticus or other acute episodes of asthma, or in patients with moderate to severe bronchiectasis.

WARNINGS AND PRECAUTIONS: General: It is essential that the patients be instructed that FLOVENT (fluticasone propionate) is a preventative agent which must be taken daily at the intervals recommended by their doctors and is not to be used as acute treatment for an asthmatic attack.

Patients should be advised to inform subsequent physicians of the prior use of corticosteroids.

Discontinuance: Treatment with FLOVENT should not be stopped abruptly, but tapered off gradually.

Ear/Nose/Throat: See Immune, Candidiasis.

Endocrine and Metabolism: Systemic Steroid Replacement by Inhaled Steroid: Particular care is needed in asthmatic patients who are transferred from systemically active corticosteroids to inhaled corticosteroids because deaths due to adrenal insufficiency have occurred during and after transfer. For the transfer of patients being treated with oral corticosteroids, FLOVENT should first be added to the existing oral steroid therapy, which is then gradually withdrawn.

Patients with adrenocortical suppression should be monitored regularly and the oral steroid reduced cautiously. Some patients transferred from other inhaled steroids or oral steroids remain at risk of impaired adrenal reserve for a considerable time after transferring to inhaled fluticasone propionate.

After withdrawal from systemic corticosteroids, a number of months are required for recovery of hypothalamic-pituitary-adrenal (HPA) function. During this period of HPA suppression, patients may exhibit signs and symptoms of adrenal insufficiency when exposed to trauma, surgery or infections, particularly gastroenteritis. Although FLOVENT may provide control of asthmatic symptoms during these episodes, it does not provide the systemic steroid which is necessary for coping with these emergencies. The physician may consider supplying oral steroids for use in times of stress (e.g. worsening asthma attacks, chest infections, surgery) (see Overdosage).

During periods of stress or a severe asthmatic attack, patients who have been withdrawn from systemic corticosteroids should be instructed to resume systemic steroids immediately and to contact their physician for further instruction. These patients should also be instructed to carry a warning card indicating that they may need supplementary systemic steroids during periods of stress or a severe asthma attack. To assess the risk of adrenal insufficiency in emergency situations, routine tests of adrenal cortical function, including measurement of early morning and evening cortisol levels, should be performed periodically in all patients. An early morning resting cortisol level may be accepted as normal only if it falls at or near the normal mean level.

Transfer of patients from systemic steroid therapy to FLOVENT may unmask allergic conditions outside the pulmonary tract that were previously suppressed by the systemic steroid therapy (e.g. rhinitis, conjunctivitis and eczema). These allergies should be symptomatically treated with anti-histamine and/or topical preparations, including topical steroids.

The replacement of a systemic steroid with inhaled steroid must be gradual and carefully supervised by the physician since upon withdrawal systemic symptoms (e.g. joint and/or muscular pain, lassitude, and depression) may occur despite maintenance or improvement of respiratory function. The guidelines under Dosage and Administration should be followed in all such cases.

Systemic Effects: Systemic effects may occur with any inhaled corticosteroid, particularly at high doses prescribed for long periods; these effects are much less likely to occur than with oral corticosteroids (see Overdosage). Possible systemic effects include Cushing's syndrome, Cushingoid features, adrenal suppression, growth retardation in children and adolescents, decrease in bone mineral density, cataract and glaucoma. It is important, therefore, that the dose of inhaled corticosteroid is titrated to the lowest dose at which effective control is maintained (see Adverse Reactions).

The long-term effects of fluticasone propionate in human subjects are still unknown. The local effects of the drug on developmental or immunologic processes in the mouth, pharynx, trachea, and lungs are unknown. There is also no information about the possible long-term systemic effects of the agent (see Monitoring and Laboratory Tests).

During post-marketing use, there have been reports of clinically significant drug interactions in patients receiving intranasal or inhaled fluticasone propionate and ritonavir, resulting in systemic corticosteroid effects including Cushing's syndrome and adrenal suppression. Therefore, concomitant use of fluticasone propionate and ritonavir should be avoided, unless the potential benefit to the patient outweighs the risk of systemic corticosteroid side effects (see Drug Interactions).

Metabolic Effects: Certain individuals can show greater susceptibility to the effects of inhaled corticosteroid than do patients.

There is an enhanced effect of corticosteroids on patients with hypothyroidism.

There have been very rare reports of increases in blood glucose levels (see Adverse Reactions) and this should be considered when prescribing to patients with a history of diabetes mellitus.

Hematologic: Eosinophilic Conditions: In rare cases, patients on inhaled fluticasone propionate may present with systemic eosinophilic conditions, with some patients presenting with clinical features of vasculitis consistent with Churg-Strauss syndrome, a condition that is often treated with systemic corticosteroid therapy. These events usually, but not always, have been associated with the reduction and/or withdrawal of oral corticosteroid therapy following the introduction of fluticasone propionate. Cases of serious eosinophilic conditions have also been reported with other inhaled corticosteroids in this clinical setting. Physicians should be alert to eosinophilia, vasculitic rash, worsening pulmonary symptoms, cardiac complications, and/or neuropathy presenting in their patients. A causal relationship between fluticasone propionate and these underlying conditions has not been established.

Hepatic/Biliary/Pancreatic: There is an enhanced effect of corticosteroids on patients with cirrhosis.

Immune: Candidiasis: Therapeutic dosages frequently cause the appearance of *C. albicans* (thrush) in the mouth and throat. The development of pharyngeal and laryngeal candidiasis is a cause for concern because the extent of its penetration into the respiratory tract is unknown. Patients may find it helpful to rinse and gargle with water after using fluticasone propionate. Symptomatic candidiasis can be treated with topical anti-fungal therapy while still continuing to use FLOVENT.

Infection: Corticosteroids may mask some signs of infections and new infections may appear. Patients who are on drugs that suppress the immune system are more susceptible to infections than healthy individuals. Chickenpox and measles, for example, can have a more serious or even fatal course in susceptible children or adults on corticosteroids. In such children or adults who have not had these diseases, particular care should be taken to avoid exposure. How the dose, route, and duration of corticosteroid administration affect the risk of developing a disseminated infection is not known. The contribution of the underlying disease and/or prior corticosteroid treatment to the risk is also not known. If exposed to chickenpox, prophylaxis with varicella zoster immune globulin (VZIG) may be indicated. If exposed to measles, prophylaxis with intramuscular pooled immunoglobulin (IG) may be indicated. If chickenpox develops, treatment with antiviral agents may be considered.

Respiratory: As with other inhalation therapy, paradoxical bronchospasm may occur characterized by an immediate increase in wheezing after dosing. This should be treated immediately with a fast-acting inhaled bronchodilator (e.g. salbutamol) to relieve acute asthmatic symptoms. FLOVENT should be discontinued immediately, the patient assessed, and if necessary, alternative therapy instituted.

Special Populations: Pregnant Women: The safety of fluticasone propionate in pregnancy has not been established. If used, the expected benefits should be weighed against the potential risk to the fetus, particularly during the first trimester of pregnancy.

Like other glucocorticoids, fluticasone propionate is teratogenic to rodent species. Adverse effects typical of potent corticosteroids are only seen at high systemic exposure levels; administration by inhalation ensures minimal systemic exposure. The relevance of these findings to humans has not yet been established since well-controlled trials relating to fetal risk in humans are not available. Infants born of mothers who have received substantial doses of glucocorticoids during pregnancy should be carefully observed for hypoadrenalism.

Nursing Women: Glucocorticoids are excreted in human milk. The excretion of fluticasone propionate into human breast milk has not been investigated. When measurable plasma levels were obtained in lactating laboratory rats following subcutaneous administration there was evidence of fluticasone propionate in the breast milk. However, plasma levels in patients following inhaled fluticasone propionate at recommended doses are likely to be low. The use of fluticasone propionate in nursing mothers requires that the possible benefits of the drug be weighted against the potential risk to the infant.

Pediatrics (12 months of age and older): Fluticasone propionate is not presently recommended for children younger than 12 months of age due to limited clinical data in this age group.

Spacer Devices: Spacer devices may be used in patients, such as young children, who have difficulty coordinating inhalation with the actuation of a metered dose inhaler (MDI). The dosage of FLOVENT HFA should be adjusted according to individual response. For patients whose asthma has been stabilized without the use of a spacer device, continuation of therapy with a spacer may require a dosage adjustment. The use of different spacer devices may result in variable effects on drug delivery.

Monitoring and Laboratory Tests: Increasing use of fast-acting inhaled bronchodilators to control symptoms indicates deterioration of asthma control. Sudden and progressive deterioration in asthma control is potentially life-threatening and consideration should be given to increasing corticosteroid dosage. Patients should be instructed to contact their physicians if they find that relief with short-acting bronchodilator treatment becomes less effective or they need more inhalations than usual. During such episodes, patients may require therapy with systemic corticosteroids.

FLOVENT is not indicated for rapid relief of bronchospasm but for regular daily treatment of the underlying inflammation. Patients will require a fast and short acting inhaled bronchodilator (e.g. salbutamol) to relieve acute asthmatic symptoms. There is no evidence that control of bronchial asthma can be achieved by the administration of FLOVENT in amounts greater than the recommended dosages.

Lack of response or severe exacerbations of asthma should be treated by increasing the dose of FLOVENT and, if necessary, by giving a systemic steroid and/or an antibiotic if there is an infection.

During long-term therapy, HPA axis function and haematological status should be assessed periodically.

It is recommended that the height of children receiving prolonged treatment with inhaled corticosteroids is regularly monitored (see Adverse Reactions).

ADVERSE REACTIONS: Adverse Drug Reaction Overview: In general, inhaled corticosteroid therapy may be associated with dose dependent increases in the incidence of ocular complications, reduced bone density, suppression of HPA axis responsiveness to stress, and inhibition of growth velocity in children. Such events have been reported rarely in clinical trials with FLOVENT (fluticasone propionate).

Glaucoma may be exacerbated by inhaled corticosteroid treatment for asthma or rhinitis. In patients with established glaucoma who require long-term inhaled corticosteroid treatment, it is prudent to measure intraocular pressure before commencing the inhaled corticosteroid and to monitor it subsequently. In patients without established glaucoma, but with a potential for developing intraocular hypertension (e.g. the elderly), intraocular pressure should be monitored at appropriate intervals.

In elderly patients treated with inhaled corticosteroids, the prevalence of posterior subcapsular and nuclear cataracts is probably low but increases in relation to the daily and cumulative lifetime dose. Cofactors such as smoking, ultraviolet B exposure, or diabetes may increase the risk. Children may be less susceptible.

A reduction of growth velocity in children or teenagers may occur as a result of inadequate control of chronic diseases such as asthma or from use of corticosteroids for treatment. Physicians should closely follow the growth of all children taking corticosteroids by any route and weigh the benefits of corticosteroid therapy and asthma control against the possibility of growth suppression if any child's or adolescent's growth appears slowed.

Osteoporosis and fracture are the major complications of long-term asthma treatment with parenteral or oral steroids. Inhaled corticosteroid therapy is also associated with dose-dependent bone loss although the degree of risk is very much less than with oral steroid. This risk may be offset by estrogen replacement in post-menopausal women, and by titrating the daily dose of inhaled steroid to the minimum required to maintain optimal asthma control. It is not yet known whether the peak bone density achieved during youth is adversely affected if substantial amounts of inhaled corticosteroid are administered prior to 30 years of age. Failure to achieve maximal bone density during youth could increase the risk of osteoporotic fracture when those individuals reach 60 years of age and older.

No major side effects attributable to the use of FLOVENT have been reported. Adverse reactions in controlled clinical studies with FLOVENT have been primarily those normally associated with asthma. Apart from asthma and related events and pharmacologically predicted events (candidiasis and hoarseness), there were no dose-related trends. The adverse reactions reported by patients treated with FLOVENT were similar to those reported by patients treated with beclomethasone dipropionate.

There have been very rare reports of anxiety, sleep disorders and behavioural changes, including hyperactivity and irritability (predominantly in children and adolescents).

Clinical Trial Adverse Drug Reactions: Because clinical trials are conducted under very specific conditions the adverse reaction rates observed in the clinical trials may not reflect the rates observed in practice and should not be compared to the rates in the clinical trials of another drug. Adverse drug reaction information from clinical trials is useful for identifying drug-related adverse events and for approximating rates.

Use in adolescents and adults: Table 1 lists adverse events considered by the investigator to be potentially drug-related that occurred at a rate of 3% or greater in any treatment group during clinical trials comparing FLOVENT HFA inhalation aerosol and FLOVENT inhalation aerosol (CFC formulation) at a dosage of 500 µg twice daily for one year. The FLOVENT DISKUS adverse events profile is similar in incidence and nature at 500 µg bid for 4 weeks.

Table 1: FLOVENT

Adverse Experience Incidence (percentage of patients) in Clinical Trials in Adolescent and Adult Patients

Adverse Event	FLOVENT HFA 500 µg bid (n=366) (%)	FLOVENT[a] 500 µg bid (n=371) (%)	FLOVENT DISKUS 500 µg bid (n=443) (%)
Hoarseness/Dysphonia	7	7	1.5
Oral Candidiasis	6	7	<1
Asthma & related events	6	5	1
Sore Throat	4	2	<1

[a] FLOVENT (fluticasone propionate) inhalation aerosol formulated with CFC propellants.

There have been very rare reports of anxiety, sleep disorders and behavioural changes, including hyperactivity and irritability (predominantly in children and adolescents).

There have been common reports of contusions (skin bruising).

Use in Children: In children 4-17 years of age, receiving FLOVENT DISKUS, the incidence of drug-related adverse events were similar in incidence and nature to that seen in adults.

In children 4 to 16 years of age, receiving FLOVENT HFA inhalation aerosol versus FLOVENT inhalation aerosol (CFC formulation), the incidence and nature of adverse events whether considered by the investigator to be drug-related or not, were similar in each treatment group. The most commonly reported events were upper respiratory tract infection, headache, viral infections, throat irritation and rhinitis.

In children 12 months to 4 years of age, receiving FLOVENT HFA inhalation aerosol the nature of adverse events were as expected for this subject population. The majority of the adverse events reported were primarily from the ear, nose and throat and lower respiratory body systems. The most commonly reported adverse events whether considered by the investigator to be drug-related or not, were upper respiratory tract infection, cough, fever, asthma and rhinitis.

Overall, the incidence and nature of the adverse events reported for FLOVENT HFA and FLOVENT inhalation aerosol CFC formulation were similar.

There have been very rare reports of anxiety, sleep disorders and behavioural changes, including hyperactivity and irritability (predominantly in children and adolescents).

Post-Market Adverse Drug Reactions: There have been uncommon reports of cutaneous hypersensitivity reactions. There have also been rare reports of hypersensitivity reactions manifesting as angioedema (mainly facial and oropharyngeal edema), respiratory symptoms (dyspnea and/or bronchospasm) and very rarely, anaphylactic reactions.

Very rare occurrences of Cushing's syndrome, Cushingoid features, anxiety, sleep disorders and behavioural changes, including hyperactivity and irritability (predominantly in children and adolescents) have been reported.

Very rarely, hyperglycemia has been reported.

DRUG INTERACTIONS: Overview: Under normal circumstances, low plasma concentrations of fluticasone propionate are achieved after inhaled dosing, due to extensive first pass metabolism and high systemic clearance mediated by cytochrome P450 3A4 in the gut and liver. Hence, clinically significant drug interactions involving fluticasone propionate are unlikely.

A drug interaction study of intranasal fluticasone propionate in healthy subjects has shown that ritonavir (a highly potent cytochrome P450 3A4 inhibitor) can greatly increase fluticasone propionate plasma concentrations, resulting in markedly reduced serum cortisol concentrations. During post-marketing use, there have been reports of clinically significant drug interactions in patients receiving intranasal or inhaled fluticasone propionate and ritonavir, resulting in systemic corticosteroid effects including Cushing's syndrome and adrenal suppression. Therefore, concomitant use of fluticasone propionate and ritonavir should be avoided, unless the potential benefit to the patient outweighs the risk of systemic corticosteroid side effects.

This study has shown that other inhibitors of cytochrome P450 3A4 produce negligible (erythromycin) and minor (ketoconazole) increases in systemic exposure to fluticasone propionate without notable reductions in serum cortisol concentrations. However, there have been a few case reports during worldwide post-market use of adrenal cortisol suppression associated with concomitant use of azole anti-fungals and inhaled fluticasone propionate. Therefore, care is advised when co-administering potent cytochrome P450 3A4 inhibitors (e.g. ketoconazole) as there is potential for increased systemic exposure to fluticasone propionate.

Drug-Drug Interactions: See Table 2.

Table 2: FLOVENT

Established or Potential Drug-Drug Interactions

Proper name	Ref	Effect	Clinical comment
Ritonavir	CT, PM	Systemic effects including Cushing's syndrome and adrenal suppression.	Concomitant use of fluticasone propionate and ritonavir should be avoided. (See Drug Interactions, Overview.)
Other inhibitors of cytochrome P450 3A4	CT	Increased systemic exposure to fluticasone propionate.	Care is advised when co-administering potent cytochrome P450 3A4 inhibitors. (See Drug Interactions, Overview.)
Acetylsalicylic acid	T		Use with caution in conjunction with corticosteroids in hypoprothrombinemia.

Legend: CT=Clinical Trial; PM=Post-marketing; T=Theoretical.

DOSAGE AND ADMINISTRATION: Dosing Considerations: The lowest dose of FLOVENT (fluticasone propionate) required to maintain good asthma control should be used. When the patient's asthma is well controlled, a reduction in the dose of FLOVENT should be attempted in order to identify the lowest possible dose required to maintain control. Such an attempt at dose reduction should be carried out on a regular basis.

Patients using inhaled bronchodilators should be advised to use the bronchodilator before the FLOVENT in order to enhance the penetration of FLOVENT into the bronchial tree. Several minutes should lapse between the use of the two inhalers to allow for some bronchodilation to occur.

In the presence of excessive mucous secretion, the drug may fail to reach the bronchioles. Therefore, if an obvious response is not obtained after ten days, a short course of systemic corticosteroid treatment might be in order. Continuation of treatment with inhaled fluticasone propionate usually maintains the improvement achieved, the systemic steroid being gradually withdrawn.

Treatment with FLOVENT should not be stopped abruptly, but tapered off gradually.

Physicians should be aware that, due to the improved potency of FLOVENT, the dose may be different than that required with some other inhaled steroids.

It is intended that each prescribed dose of FLOVENT HFA be given by a minimum of two inhalations twice daily. However, the prescribed dose of FLOVENT DISKUS may be given by a single inhalation twice daily.

Recommended Dosage: Adults and adolescents 16 years of age and older: Usual dosage is 100 to 500 µg twice daily. Patients should be given a starting dose of FLOVENT which is appropriate for the severity of their disease (see Indications and Clinical Use) as follows:

Asthma Severity	FLOVENT Dose
Mild	100 to 250 µg twice daily
Moderate	250 to 500 µg twice daily
Severe	500 µg twice daily. Very severe patients requiring higher doses of corticosteroids such as those patients currently requiring oral steroids may use doses up to 1000 µg twice daily.

The dose may then be adjusted until control is achieved or reduced to the minimum effective dose according to the individual response.

Alternatively, the starting dose of FLOVENT may be gauged at half the total daily dose of beclomethasone dipropionate or equivalent as administered by metered-dose inhaler.

Onset of effect occurs within 4-7 days, although some benefit may be apparent as soon as 24 hours of the start of treatment with FLOVENT for patients who have not previously received inhaled steroids. If no improvement is noted in this time frame, an increase in dose should be considered.

Children 4-16 years of age: The usual starting dose is 50 or 100 µg twice daily and many children's asthma will be well controlled with this regimen. For those patients whose asthma is not sufficiently controlled, additional benefit may be obtained by increasing the FLOVENT DISKUS dose up to 200 µg twice daily. Children should be given a starting dose of inhaled fluticasone propionate which is appropriate for the severity of their disease. The recommended dosing is as follows:

FLOVENT Dose	Recommended Administration
50 µg twice daily	One inhalation of FLOVENT DISKUS 50 µg twice daily
100 µg twice daily	Two inhalations of FLOVENT HFA 50 µg twice daily or One inhalation of FLOVENT DISKUS 100 µg twice daily
200 µg twice daily	Two inhalations of FLOVENT DISKUS 100 µg twice daily

FLOVENT HFA inhalation aerosol is only available in 50, 125 and 250 µg/metered dose. It is intended that each prescribed dose of FLOVENT HFA be given by a minimum of two inhalations twice daily. For children 4-16 years of age, it therefore does not permit 50 µg b.i.d. to be administered by a minimum of two inhalations twice daily, nor does it offer the pediatric dose of 200 µg b.i.d. In these cases, FLOVENT DISKUS 50 µg/blister or 100 µg/blister should be considered.

The dose should be adjusted until control is achieved or reduced to the minimum effective dose according to the individual response. This is particularly important in the younger children with severe symptoms who are receiving the larger daily dose.

Children 12 months to 4 years of age: Younger children should be given 100 µg of FLOVENT HFA twice daily administered via a pediatric spacer device with a face mask such as a BABYHALER spacer device.

Clinical trials in 12 month to 4 year old children have shown that the optimal control of asthma symptoms is achieved with 100 µg twice daily. Higher doses of inhaled drug are required in younger children compared to older children because of reduced efficiency of drug delivery due to smaller airways and increased nasal breathing.

The diagnosis and treatment of asthma should be kept under regular review.

Dosage Adjustment: The dosage of FLOVENT should be adjusted according to individual response. For patients whose asthma has been stabilized without the use of a spacer device, continuation of therapy with a spacer may require a dosage adjustment. The use of different spacer devices may result in variable effects on drug delivery.
Special patient groups: There is no need to adjust the dose in elderly patients or those with hepatic or renal impairment.
Patients receiving systemic steroids: The transfer of steroid-dependent patients to FLOVENT, and their subsequent management, needs special care mainly because recovery from impaired adrenocortical function, caused by prolonged systemic therapy, is slow. Patients' bronchial asthma should be stable before being given FLOVENT in addition to the usual maintenance dose of systemic steroid. After about a week, gradual withdrawal of the systemic steroid is started by reducing the daily dose by 1 mg of prednisone, or its equivalent of other corticosteroid, at not less than weekly intervals, if the patient is under close observation. In children, the usual rate of withdrawal is 1 mg of the daily dose of prednisone every eight days when under close supervision. **If continuous supervision is not feasible, the withdrawal of the systemic steroid should be slower**, approximately 1 mg of the daily dose of prednisone (or equivalent) every ten and every twenty days in adults and in children, respectively. A slow rate of withdrawal cannot be over-emphasized.

If withdrawal symptoms appear, the previous dose of the systemic drug should be resumed for a week before any further decrease is attempted. Patients who have been treated with systemic steroids for long periods of time or at a high dose may have adrenocortical suppression. In these patients adrenocortical function should be monitored regularly and their dose of systemic steroid reduced cautiously.

Some patients feel unwell during the withdrawal phase experiencing symptoms such as joint and/or muscular pain, lassitude, and depression, despite maintenance or even improvement of respiratory function. Such patients should be encouraged to persevere with FLOVENT but should be watched carefully for objective signs of adrenal insufficiency such as hypotension and weight loss. If evidence of adrenal insufficiency occurs, the systemic steroid dosage should be boosted temporarily and thereafter further withdrawal should be continued more slowly.

Transferred patients whose adrenocortical function is impaired should carry a warning card indicating that they need supplementary treatment with systemic steroids during periods of stress, e.g. surgery, chest infection, or severe asthma attack. Consideration should be given to supplying such patients with oral steroids to use in an emergency. The dose of inhaled fluticasone propionate should be increased at this time and then reduced to the maintenance level after the systemic steroid has been discontinued.

Exacerbations of bronchial asthma which occur during the course of treatment with FLOVENT should be treated with a short course of systemic steroid which is gradually tapered as these symptoms subside. Under stressful conditions or when the patient has a severe exacerbation of bronchial asthma, after complete withdrawal of the systemic steroid, use of the latter must be resumed in order to avoid relative adrenocortical insufficiency.

There are some patients who cannot completely discontinue the oral corticosteroid. In these cases, a minimum maintenance dosage should be given in addition to FLOVENT.
Missed Dose: If a single dose is missed, instruct the patient to take the next dose when it is due.
Administration: FLOVENT HFA inhalation aerosol and DISKUS are to be administered by oral inhalation only.

Patients must be instructed, as described in Information for the Patient, in the correct method of using FLOVENT HFA inhalation aerosol or DISKUS to ensure that the drug reaches the target areas within the lungs.

Since the effect of FLOVENT depends on its regular use and on the proper technique of inhalation, the patient should be made aware of the prophylactic nature of therapy with inhaled fluticasone propionate, and that for optimum benefit FLOVENT should be taken regularly even when the patient is asymptomatic.

As a general rule, rinsing the mouth and gargling with water after each inhalation can help in preventing the occurrence of candidiasis. Cleansing dentures has the same effect.
Inhalation Aerosol: Before the first use of FLOVENT HFA inhalation aerosol and after periods of greater than seven days without use, the inhaler should be primed before treatment by actuating the inhaler once.

Inhalation aerosol actuation should be synchronised with inspiration to ensure optimum delivery of drug to the lungs.

The use of the open-mouth technique to administer FLOVENT HFA inhalation aerosol has not been investigated in clinical trials.
Diskus: FLOVENT DISKUS is a device for delivering the dry powder formulation of fluticasone propionate. When using FLOVENT DISKUS, the usual prescribed dose is one blister (inhalation) twice a day.

OVERDOSAGE:
Acute inhalation of FLOVENT (fluticasone propionate) doses in excess of those approved may lead to temporary suppression of the hypothalamic-pituitary-adrenal axis. This does not usually require emergency action, as normal adrenal function typically recovers within a few days.

If higher than approved doses are continued over prolonged periods, significant adrenocortical suppression is possible. There have been very rare reports of acute adrenal crisis occurring in children exposed to higher than approved dosages (typically 1000 µg daily and above), over prolonged periods (several months or years); observed features included hypoglycemia and sequelae of decreased consciousness and/or convulsions. Situations which could potentially trigger acute adrenal crisis include exposure to trauma, surgery or infection or any rapid reduction in dosage. Patients receiving higher than approved dosages should be managed closely and the dose reduced gradually.

Chronic use of inhaled fluticasone propionate in daily doses in excess of the recommended dosage may lead to some degree of adrenal suppression. Monitoring of adrenal reserve may be indicated. Gradual reduction of the inhaled dose may be required. Treatment with inhaled FLOVENT should be continued at a dose sufficient to control asthma.

> For management of a suspected drug overdose, contact your regional Poison Control Centre. See the *CPS* Directory section for a list of Poison Control Centres.

ACTION AND CLINICAL PHARMACOLOGY: Mechanism of Action: FLOVENT (fluticasone propionate) is a highly potent glucocorticoid anti-inflammatory steroid. When administered by inhalation at therapeutic dosages it has direct potent anti-inflammatory action within the lungs, resulting is reduced symptoms and exacerbations of asthma and less adverse effects than systemically administered corticosteroids.

In comparison with beclomethasone dipropionate, fluticasone propionate has demonstrated greater topical potency.
Pharmacodynamics: Fluticasone propionate has many pharmacokinetic and pharmacodynamic features similar to those of other inhaled glucocorticoids used for the treatment of asthma. However, in contrast to these other steroids, a combination of incomplete gastrointestinal absorption and high first pass metabolic extraction ensures that virtually no fluticasone propionate swallowed after oral inhalation reaches the systemic circulation.
Pharmacokinetics: Following intravenous administration, the pharmacokinetics of fluticasone propionate are proportional to dose. Fluticasone propionate is extensively distributed within the body. The volume of distribution at steady state is approximately 300 L and had a very high clearance which is estimated to be 1.1 L/min indicating extensive hepatic extraction. Peak plasma fluticasone propionate concentrations are reduced by approximately 98% within 3-4 hours and only low plasma concentrations are associated with the terminal half-life, which is approximately 8 hours.

Following oral administration of fluticasone propionate, 87-100% of the dose is excreted in the faeces. Following doses of either 1 or 16 mg, up to 20% and 75% respectively, is excreted in the faeces as the parent compound. There is a non-active major metabolite. Absolute oral bioavailability is negligible (<1%) due to a combination of incomplete absorption from the gastrointestinal tract and extensive first-pass metabolism. Following inhaled dosing in healthy volunteers, absolute systemic bioavailability of fluticasone propionate varies between approximately 10-30% of the nominal dose depending on the inhalation device used. Systemic absorption of fluticasone propionate occurs mainly through the lungs, and is initially rapid then prolonged.

The plasma protein binding of fluticasone propionate is 91%. Fluticasone propionate is extensively metabolised by the CYP3A4 enzyme to an inactive carboxylic acid derivative.
STORAGE AND STABILITY: Inhalation Aerosol: Replace the mouthpiece cover firmly and snap it into position. Store at room temperature (15 to 30°C). Protect from frost and direct sunlight.
DISKUS: Store between 2 and 25°C in a dry place. Protect from frost and direct sunlight. FLOVENT DISKUS is sealed in a foil overwrap which should only be opened when it is to be used for the first time. Once opened the foil overwrap should be discarded.
SPECIAL HANDLING INSTRUCTIONS: Inhalation Aerosol: Contents under pressure. Container may explode if heated. Do not place in hot water or near radiators, stoves, or other sources of heat. Even when apparently empty, do not puncture or incinerate container or store at temperatures over 30°C.

As with most inhaled medications in pressurised canisters, the therapeutic effect of this medication may decrease when the canister is cold.
INFORMATION FOR THE PATIENT: Published in e-CPS, available by subscription at www.e-cps.ca.

DOSAGE FORMS, COMPOSITION AND PACKAGING: Inhalation Aerosol: Each actuation of the pressurized metered-dose inhaler delivers: 50, 125, or 250 µg of fluticasone propionate suspended in propellant HFA-134a (1,1,1,2-tetrafluoroethane). This product does not contain chlorofluorocarbons (CFCs) as the propellant. The 50 µg strength of FLOVENT HFA inhalation aerosol is available in 120 dose containers. The 125 µg and 250 µg strengths of FLOVENT HFA inhalation aerosol are available in 60 and 120 dose containers. FLOVENT HFA inhalation aerosol is a pressurized metered-dose inhaler (MDI) consisting of an aluminum canister fitted with a metering valve. The 50 µg canister is fitted into the supplied peach actuator/adaptor. The 125 µg canister is fitted into the supplied orange actuator/adaptor. The 250 µg canister is fitted into the supplied red/brown actuator/adaptor. A dust cap is fitted over the actuator's mouthpiece when not in use.
Diskus: Each inhalation of the dry powder inhalation device delivers: 50, 100, 250, or 500 µg of fluticasone propionate. It also contains lactose (milk sugar), including milk protein, which acts as the "carrier". FLOVENT DISKUS is a plastic inhaler device containing a foil strip with 60 blisters. Each blister contains 50, 100, 250, or 500 µg of the active ingredient fluticasone propionate.

(Shown in Product Identification Section)

Fluanxol® Ⓟ
flupenthixol dihydrochloride
Antipsychotic

Lundbeck

Fluanxol® Depot Ⓟ
flupenthixol decanoate
Antipsychotic

Lundbeck

Date of Preparation: February 17, 1995
Date of Revision: September 10, 2004

PHARMACOLOGY: Flupenthixol decanoate is the decanoate ester of a thioxanthene derivative with antipsychotic properties. The esterification of flupenthixol results in the slow release of the drug from the injection site with consequent prolongation of duration of action. The onset of action usually occurs in the range of 24 to 72 hours after injection and the improvement of symptoms continues for 2 to 4 weeks. However, there is considerable variation in the individual response of patients to flupenthixol and its use for maintenance therapy requires careful supervision.

Flupenthixol dihydrochloride is a thioxanthene derivative with antipsychotic properties.

The exact mechanism of action of flupenthixol has not been established. Its effects resemble those of the phenothiazine, fluphenazine, in that it belongs among the antipsychotic drugs which are less likely to cause sedation and hypotension, but have greater propensity for producing extrapyramidal reactions.
Pharmacokinetics: In pharmacokinetic studies measuring flupenthixol blood levels, peak concentrations of the drug were found between days 4 and 7, following i.m. injections of 40 mg of flupenthixol 2% or 10%. It could still be detected in the blood 3 weeks after injection. The metabolites of flupenthixol appear to be inactive.

Flupenthixol dihydrochloride is well absorbed from the gastrointestinal tract. Based upon radioisotope monitoring in man, the drug reaches maximum serum concentrations within 3 to 8 hours. It has not yet been possible to accurately define the metabolic pathways in man; however, the metabolites of flupenthixol appear to be inactive. Flupenthixol is excreted mainly in the feces, with some excretion also occurring in the urine.

INDICATIONS: The maintenance therapy of chronic schizophrenic patients whose main manifestations do not include excitement, agitation or hyperactivity.

CONTRAINDICATIONS: In patients with known hypersensitivity to the thioxanthenes. The possibility of cross-sensitivity between the thioxanthenes and phenothiazine derivatives should be considered.

Flupenthixol is also contraindicated in the presence of CNS depression due to any cause, comatose states, suspected or established subcortical brain damage, blood dyscrasias, pheochromocytoma, liver damage, cerebrovascular or renal insufficiency, and severe cardiovascular disorders. It is not indicated for the management of severely agitated psychotic patients, psychoneurotic patients or geriatric patients with confusion and/or agitation. As with phenothiazines, flupenthixol should not be used concomitantly with large doses of hypnotics due to the possibility of potentiation.

WARNINGS: Tardive Dyskinesia: Tardive dyskinesia is a syndrome consisting of potentially irreversible, involuntary, dyskinetic movement that may develop in patients receiving treatment with antipsychotic drugs (see Adverse Effects). Although the syndrome appears to be most prevalent in the elderly, especially elderly female patients, it is impossible to predict at the onset of treatment which patients are likely to develop tardive dyskinesia.

Both the risk of developing tardive dyskinesia and the likelihood that it will become irreversible increase with the total cumulative dose of the antipsychotic agent and the duration of treatment. However, less commonly, the syndrome can develop after relatively brief periods of treatment at low doses. Although there is no established treatment of tardive dyskinesia, the syndrome may remit, partially or completely, following withdrawal of the antipsychotic drug. Antipsychotic treatment may itself suppress the signs and symptoms of tardive dyskinesia, possibly masking the underlying process. However, the effects of symptomatic suppression on the long-term course of the syndrome are not known.

In view of these considerations, flupenthixol should be prescribed in a manner that is most likely to minimize the risk of tardive dyskinesia. As with any antipsychotic drug, flupenthixol should be administered at the smallest dose and for the shortest duration of treatment that is consistent with a satisfactory clinical response. Chronic use should be reserved for patients who appear to be obtaining a substantial benefit from the drug. The need for continued treatment should be reassessed at periodic intervals.

If the signs and symptoms of tardive dyskinesia develop during treatment with flupenthixol, withdrawal of the drug should be considered. However, some patients may require continued antipsychotic treatment despite the presence of this syndrome.
Neuroleptic Malignant Syndrome: Neuroleptic malignant syndrome is a potentially fatal symptom complex that has been reported in association with neuroleptic drugs (see Adverse Effects). The clinical manifestations of neuroleptic malignant syndrome are hyperpyrexia, muscle rigidity, altered mental status (including catatonic signs), and evidence of autonomic instability (irregularity of pulse or blood pressure, tachycardia, diaphoresis, and cardiac arrhythmias). Additional signs may include elevated creatine phosphokinase, myoblobinuria (rhabdomyolysis), and acute renal failure.

The diagnostic evaluation of patients with this syndrome is complicated. Cases in which the clinical presentation includes both serious medical illness (e.g., pneumonia, systemic infection, etc.) and untreated or inadequately treated extrapyramidal signs and symptoms should be identified. Other important considerations in the differential diagnosis include central anticholinergic toxicity, heat stroke, drug fever and primary central nervous system pathology.

The management of neuroleptic malignant syndrome should include the immediate discontinuation of antipsychotic drugs and nonessential concurrent therapies. Intensive symptomatic treatment and medical monitoring is required. Concomitant serious medical problems for which specific treatments are available should be dealt with appropriately. No general agreement exists regarding specific pharmacological treatment regimens for uncomplicated neuroleptic malignant syndrome.

If a patient requires antipsychotic drug treatment following recovery from neuroleptic malignant syndrome, the potential reintroduction of drug therapy should be carefully considered. As recurrences of neuroleptic malignant syndrome have been reported, careful patient monitoring is necessary.
Pregnancy: Safety in pregnancy has not been established. Therefore, it should not be administered to women of childbearing potential or during lactation, unless, in the opinion of the physician, the expected benefit to the patient outweighs the potential risk to the fetus or child.
Lactation: See Pregnancy.
Children: Safety and efficacy in children have not been established, and its use is not recommended in the pediatric age group.

Severe adverse reactions requiring immediate medical attention may occur and are difficult to predict. Therefore, the evaluation of tolerance and response, and establishment of adequate maintenance therapy require careful stabilization of each patient under continuous, close medical observation and supervision.

Flupenthixol is not recommended for excitable, overactive or manic patients, and the relative lack of sedating effect may cause restlessness and insomnia. The drug should be used with caution in patients with parkinsonism or severe arteriosclerosis.
Occupational Hazards: Although flupenthixol is a relatively non-sedating drug, sedation may occur in some patients. Therefore, ambulatory patients should be warned about engaging in activities such as driving a car or operating machinery and about the concomitant use of alcohol and other CNS depressant drugs, since potentiation of their effects may occur.

Flupenthixol should be used with caution in patients with a history of convulsive disorders since it may lower the convulsive threshold.

The possibility of the development of irreversible dyskinesia should be borne in mind when patients are on prolonged therapy.

The antiemetic effect observed with flupenthixol in animal studies may also occur in man; therefore, the drug may mask signs of toxicity due to overdosage of other drugs, or it may mask the symptoms of disease, such as brain tumor or intestinal obstruction.

Although its anticholinergic properties are relatively weak, flupenthixol should be used with caution in patients who are known or are suspected to have glaucoma, and in those patients who might be exposed to extreme heat, or organophosphorus insecticides or who are receiving atropine or related drugs. Paralytic ileus has occasionally been reported, particularly in the elderly, when several drugs with anticholinergic effects have been used simultaneously.

Blood dyscrasias and liver damage have been reported with this class of drugs, but only eosinophilia has been reported to date with flupenthixol. Therefore, routine blood counts and hepatic function tests are advisable, particularly during the first months of therapy. Should either of these disorders occur, supportive treatment should be instituted and the drug discontinued.

Photosensitivity reactions, pigmentary retinopathy, and lenticular and corneal deposits, although not reported to date with flupenthixol, have been reported with related drugs.

Caution should be observed when using a drug of this category in patients who may have a propensity for development of defects in cardiac conduction.

Patients on large doses of flupenthixol who are undergoing surgery should be watched carefully for possible hypotensive phenomena, and anesthetic or CNS depressant drug dosages may have to be reduced.

To lessen the likelihood of adverse reactions related to drug accumulation, patients on long-term therapy, particularly on high doses, should be evaluated periodically to decide whether the maintenance dosage can be lowered or drug therapy discontinued.

Neuroleptic drugs elevate prolactin levels; the elevation persists during chronic administration. Tissue culture experiments indicate that approximately one-third of human breast cancers are prolactin-dependent in vitro, a factor of potential importance if the prescription of these drugs is contemplated in a patient with a previously detected breast cancer. Although disturbances such as galactorrhea, amenorrhea, gynecomastia and impotence have been reported, the clinical significance of elevated serum prolactin levels is unknown for most patients. An increase in mammary neoplasms has been found in rodents after chronic administration of neuroleptic drugs. Neither clinical studies, nor epidemiologic studies conducted to date, however, have shown an association between chronic administration of these drugs and mammary tumorogenesis; the available evidence is considered too limited to be conclusive at this time.

Withdrawal Emergent Neurological Signs: Abrupt withdrawal after short-term administration of antipsychotic drugs does not generally pose problems. However, transient dyskinetic signs are experienced by some patients on maintenance therapy after abrupt withdrawal. The signs are very similar to those described under Tardive Dyskinesia, (see Warnings and Adverse Effects), except for duration. Although it is not known whether gradual withdrawal of antipsychotic drugs will decrease the incidence of withdrawal emergent neurological signs, gradual withdrawal would appear to be advisable.

PRECAUTIONS: See Warnings.

ADVERSE EFFECTS: The most common adverse reactions reported with flupenthixol have been extrapyramidal symptoms, occurring in up to 30% of patients.

Flupenthixol shares many of the pharmacologic properties of other thioxanthenes and phenothiazines. Therefore, the known adverse reactions of these drugs should be borne in mind when flupenthixol is used.

Central Nervous System: Extrapyramidal symptoms, including hypo- and hyperkinetic states, tremors, pseudoparkinsonism, dystonia, hypertonia, akathisia, oculogyric crises, opisthotonos, hyperreflexia and tardive dyskinesia (see Warnings and below). The symptoms, if they are to occur, usually appear within the first few days of drug administration and can usually be controlled or totally curtailed by reduction in dosage and/or standard anticholinergic antiparkinsonian medication. The incidence of extrapyramidal symptoms appears to be more frequent with the first few injections of flupenthixol, and diminishes thereafter. The routine prophylactic use of antiparkinsonian medication is not recommended. Extrapyramidal reactions may be alarming, and patients should be forewarned and reassured.

Other CNS effects reported with flupenthixol include restlessness, insomnia, overactivity, psychomotor agitation, hypomania, epileptiform convulsions, headache, drowsiness, somnolence, depression, fatigue, and anergia.

Persistent Tardive Dyskinesia: As with all antipsychotic agents, tardive dyskinesia may appear in some patients on long-term therapy or may occur after drug therapy has been discontinued. The risk seems to be greater in elderly patients on high dose therapy, especially females. The symptoms are persistent and in some patients appear to be irreversible. The syndrome is characterized by rhythmical involuntary movements of the tongue, face, mouth, or jaw (e.g. protrusion of tongue, puffing of cheeks, puckering of mouth, chewing movements). Sometimes these may be accompanied by involuntary movements of the extremities.

There is no known effective treatment for tardive dyskinesia; antiparkinsonian agents usually do not alleviate the symptoms of this syndrome. It is suggested that all antipsychotic agents be discontinued if these symptoms appear. Should it be necessary to reinstitute treatment, or increase the dosage of the agent, or switch to a different antipsychotic agent, the syndrome may be masked. The physician may be able to reduce the risk of this syndrome by minimizing the unnecessary use of neuroleptic drugs and reducing the dose or discontinuing the drug, if possible, when manifestations of this syndrome are recognized, particularly in patients over the age of fifty. It has been reported that fine vermicular movements of the tongue may be an early sign of the syndrome and if the medication is stopped at that time, the syndrome may not develop. See Warnings.

Autonomic Nervous System: Dry mouth, blurred vision, constipation, excessive salivation, excessive perspiration, nausea, difficulty in micturition, dizziness, palpitations and fainting have been observed with flupenthixol but are uncommon. Miosis, mydriasis, paralytic ileus, polyuria, nasal congestion, glaucoma, tachycardia, hypotension, hypertension, fluctuations in blood pressure, non specific ECG changes and cardiac arrhythmias have been reported with related drugs. If hypotension occurs, **epinephrine should not be used** as a pressor agent since a paradoxical further lowering of blood pressure may result.

Metabolic and Endocrine: Weight change, galactorrhea, elevation in serum prolactin levels, impotence, loss of libido, and sexual excitement have been reported with flupenthixol. Related drugs have been also associated with breast enlargement, menstrual irregularities, false positive pregnancy tests, peripheral edema, gynecomastia, hypo- and hyperglycemia and glycosuria.

Toxic and Allergic: Eosinophilia, jaundice and increased levels of AST, ALT and alkaline phosphatase have been reported with flupenthixol. Other antipsychotic drugs have been associated with leukopenia, agranulocytosis, thrombocytopenic or nonthrombocytopenic purpura, hemolytic anemia and pancytopenia. If any soreness of the mouth, gums or throat or any symptoms of upper respiratory infection occur and confirmatory leukocyte count indicates cellular depression, therapy should be discontinued and other appropriate measures instituted immediately.

Skin reactions, such as pruritus, rash, urticaria, erythema, seborrhea, eczema, exfoliative dermatitis, and contact dermatitis have been reported with flupenthixol or related drugs. The possibility of anaphylactoid reactions occurring in some patients should be borne in mind.

Miscellaneous: Sudden, unexpected and unexplained deaths have occasionally been reported in patients who have received certain phenothiazine derivatives. Previous brain damage or seizures may be predisposing factors; high doses should be avoided in known seizure patients. Several patients have shown flare ups of psychotic behavior patterns shortly before death. Autopsy findings have usually revealed acute fulminating pneumonia or pneumonitis, aspiration of gastric contents or intramyocardial lesions.

The following adverse reactions have also occurred with phenothiazine derivatives: photosensitivity, systemic lupus erythematosus-like syndrome, hypotension severe enough to cause fatal cardiac arrest, altered ECG and EEG tracings, altered CSF proteins, cerebral edema, asthma, laryngeal edema, and angioneurotic edema. Skin pigmentation, and lenticular and corneal opacities have been seen with long-term use of phenothiazines.

OVERDOSE:

Symptoms: Sedation, frequently preceded by extreme agitation, excitement and confusion. Extrapyramidal symptoms may develop, and respiratory and circulatory collapse may occur.

Treatment: Symptomatic. In cases of oral overdosing, gastric lavage should be carried out immediately and measures aimed at supporting the respiratory and cardiovascular systems instituted. If overdosing with parenteral flupenthixol occurs, no further injections should be given until the patient shows signs of relapse and the dosage should then be decreased. An airway should be maintained. Severe hypotension calls for the immediate use of an i.v. vasopressor drug, such as levarterenol. Epinephrine should **not** be used, as a further lowering of blood pressure may result. Antiparkinsonian medication should be administered only if extrapyramidal symptoms develop.

For management of a suspected drug overdose, CPhA recommends that you contact your **regional Poison Control Centre**. See the *CPS* Directory section for a list of Poison Control Centres.

DOSAGE: Injection: Flupenthixol is administered by deep i.m. injection, preferably in the gluteus maximus. Flupenthixol is **not** for i.v. use.

As a long acting depot preparation, flupenthixol has been found useful in the maintenance treatment of non agitated chronic schizophrenic patients who have been stabilized with short acting neuroleptics and might benefit from transfer to a longer acting injectable medication. The changeover of medication should aim at maintaining a clinical outcome similar to or better than that obtained with the previous therapy. To achieve and maintain the optimum dose, the changeover from other neuroleptic medication should proceed gradually and constant supervision is required during the period of dosage adjustment in order to minimize the risk of overdosage or insufficient suppression of psychotic symptoms before the next injection.

Patients not previously treated with long acting depot neuroleptics should be given an initial test dose of 5 mg (0.25 mL) to 20 mg (1.0 mL) of flupenthixol 2%. An initial dose of 20 mg (1.0 mL) of flupenthixol 2% is usually well tolerated; however, a 5 mg (0.25 mL) test dose of flupenthixol 2% is recommended in elderly, frail and cachectic patients, and in patients whose individual or family history suggests a predisposition to extrapyramidal reactions. In the subsequent 5 to 10 days, the therapeutic response and the appearance of extrapyramidal symptoms should be carefully monitored. Oral neuroleptic drugs may be continued, but in diminishing dosage, during this period.

In patients previously treated with long acting depot neuroleptics who displayed good tolerance to these drugs, an initial dose of 20 to 40 mg (1.0 to 2.0 mL) of flupenthixol 2% may be adequate.

Subsequent doses and the frequency of administration must be determined for each patient. There is no reliable dosage comparability between a shorter acting neuroleptic and depot flupenthixol, and, therefore, the dosage of the long acting drug must be individualized.

Except in particularly sensitive patients, a second dose of 20 (1.0 mL) to 40 mg (2.0 mL) of flupenthixol 2% can be given 4 to 10 days after the initial injection. Subsequent dosage adjustments are made in accordance with the response of the patient, but the majority of patients can be adequately controlled by 20 to 40 mg (1.0 to 2.0 mL) of flupenthixol 2% every 2 to 3 weeks. The optimal amount of the drug has been found to vary with the clinical circumstances and individual response. Doses greater than 80 mg (4.0 mL) of flupenthixol 2% are usually not deemed necessary, although higher doses have been used occasionally in some patients.

Although the response to a single injection usually lasts for 2 to 3 weeks, it may last for 4 weeks or more, particularly when higher doses are used. Since higher doses increase the incidence of extrapyramidal reactions and other adverse effects, the amount of drug used should not be increased merely in order to prolong the intervals between injections. With higher doses there may also be more variability in the action of flupenthixol and, therefore, unit dose increments should not exceed 20 mg (1.0 mL) of flupenthixol 2%. After an appropriate dosage adjustment is achieved, regular and continuous supervision and reassessment is considered essential in order to permit any further dosage adjustments that might be required to ensure use of the lowest effective individual dose and avoid troublesome side effects.

Patients who require higher doses of flupenthixol to control symptoms of schizophrenia and/or those who complain of discomfort with a large injection volume may be administered flupenthixol 10% (100 mg/mL) in preference to flupenthixol 2% (20 mg/mL).

As with all oily injections it is important to ensure, by aspiration before injection, that inadvertent intravascular injection does not occur.

Instruction for use: As with all parenteral drug products, the injection should be inspected visually for clarity, particulate matter, precipitate, discoloration and leakage prior to administration, whenever solution and container permit. Solution showing haziness, particulate matter, precipitate, discoloration or leakage should not be used. Discard unused portion.

Tablets: The dosage should be individualized and adjusted according to the severity of symptoms and tolerance to the drug. The initial recommended dose is 1 mg, 3 times daily. This may be increased, if necessary by 1 mg every 2 to 3 days until there is effective control of psychotic symptoms. The usual maintenance dosage is 3 to 6 mg daily in divided doses, although doses of up to 12 mg daily or more have been used in some patients.

During the initial therapeutic period, disturbance of sleep may occur, especially in those patients who have previously received neuroleptics possessing a marked sedative effect. In this event, the evening dose may be reduced.

Until further clinical evidence is available, it is not recommended for use in children.

Following stabilization on flupenthixol dihydrochloride tablets, patients may be treated with flupenthixol decanoate administered by the i.m. route.

INFORMATION FOR THE PATIENT: Published in e-CPS, available by subscription at www.e-cps.ca.

SUPPLIED: Fluanxol: 0.5 mg: Each ochre-yellow, sugar-coated, round, biconvex tablet contains: flupenthixol dihydrochloride 0.5 mg. Also contains sucrose. Bottles of 100.

3 mg: Each ochre-yellow, sugar-coated, round, biconvex tablet contains: flupenthixol dihydrochloride 3 mg. Also contains sucrose. Bottles of 100.

Fluanxol Depot: 2% Solution: Each mL contains: flupenthixol decanoate 20 mg. Ampoules of 2 mL, packages of 5. Vials of 10 mL.

10% Solution: Each mL contains: flupenthixol decanoate 100 mg. Vials of 2 mL.

Solutions are yellowish and consist of flupenthixol decanoate 2% or 10% in medium-chain triglycerides. Store between 15 and 25°C. Protect from light.

(Shown in Product Identification Section)

Fluconazole Injection Ⓟ

fluconazole

Antifungal

Baxter

Date of Preparation: December 3, 2004

SUMMARY PRODUCT INFORMATION:

Route of Administration	Dosage Form/ Strength	Clinically Relevant Nonmedicinal Ingredients
Intravenous Infusion	200 mg/100 mL, 400 mg/200 mL	Sodium chloride

INDICATIONS AND CLINICAL USE: Fluconazole is indicated for:

- Treatment of oropharyngeal and esophageal candidiasis, and cryptococcal meningitis. Fluconazole is also effective for the treatment of serious systemic candidal infections, including urinary tract infection, peritonitis, and pneumonia.
- Prevention of the recurrence of cryptococcal meningitis in patients with acquired immunodeficiency syndrome (AIDS).

Specimens for fungal culture and other relevant laboratory studies (serology, histopathology) should be obtained prior to therapy to isolate and identify causative organisms. Therapy may be instituted before the results of the cultures and other laboratory studies are known; however, once these results become available, anti-infective therapy should be adjusted accordingly.

Prophylaxis: Fluconazole is also indicated to decrease the incidence of candidiasis in patients undergoing bone marrow transplantation who receive cytotoxic chemotherapy and/or radiation therapy.

Geriatrics: Fluconazole was well tolerated by patients aged 65 years and over. In a small number of elderly patients with bone marrow transplant (BMT) in which fluconazole was administered prophylactically there was a greater incidence of drug discontinuation due to adverse reactions (4.3%) than in younger patients (1.7%).

Pediatrics: An open-label, randomized, controlled trial has shown fluconazole to be effective in the treatment of oropharyngeal candidiasis in children 6 months to 13 years of age.

In a non-comparative study of children with serious systemic fungal infections, fluconazole was effective in the treatment of candidemia (10 of 11 patients cured) and disseminated candidiasis (5 of 6 patients cured or improved).

Fluconazole was effective for the suppression of cryptococcal meningitis and/or disseminated cryptococcal infection in a group of 6 children treated in a compassionate study of fluconazole for the treatment of life-threatening or serious mycosis. There is no information regarding the efficacy of fluconazole for primary treatment of cryptococcal meningitis in children.

In addition, the use of fluconazole in children with cryptococcal meningitis, candidal esophagitis or systemic candidal infections is consistent with the approved use of fluconazole in similar indications for adults, and is supported by pharmacokinetic studies in children (see Action and Clinical Pharmacology) establishing dose proportionality between children and adults (see Dosage and Administration).

The safety of fluconazole in children has been established in 577 children ages 1 day to 17 years who received doses ranging from 1 to 15 mg/kg/day for 1 to 1616 days (see Adverse Reactions).

Efficacy of fluconazole has not been established in infants less than 6 months of age. A small number of patients (29) ranging in age from 1 day to 6 months have been treated safely with fluconazole.

CONTRAINDICATIONS: Fluconazole is contraindicated in patients who have shown hypersensitivity to fluconazole or to any of its excipients. There is no information regarding cross hypersensitivity between fluconazole and other azole antifungal agents. Caution should be used in prescribing fluconazole to patients with hypersensitivity to other azoles.

Coadministration of terfenadine is contraindicated in patients receiving fluconazole at multiple doses of 400 mg or higher based upon results of a multiple dose interaction study (see Warnings and Precautions).

Co-administration of cisapride is contraindicated in patients receiving fluconazole (see Warnings and Precautions).

QT Prolongation: Some azoles, including fluconazole, have been associated with prolongation of the QT interval on the electrocardiogram. During post-marketing surveillance, there have been very rare cases of QT prolongation and torsade de pointes in patients taking fluconazole. These reports included seriously ill patients with multiple confounding risk factors, such as structural heart disease, electrolyte abnormalities and concomitant medications that may have been contributory. Fluconazole should be administered with caution to patients with these potentially proarrhythmic conditions. (See Warnings and Precautions, Drug Interactions, Drugs Prolonging the QTc Interval and Adverse Reactions.)

WARNINGS AND PRECAUTIONS:

Serious Warnings and Precautions

- Hepatic injury: Fluconazole has been associated with rare cases of serious hepatic toxicity, including fatalities, primarily in patients with serious underlying medical conditions. In cases of fluconazole-associated hepatotoxicity, no obvious relationship to total daily dose, duration of therapy, sex or age of the patient has been observed. Fluconazole hepatotoxicity has usually, but not always been reversible on discontinuation of therapy. Patients who develop abnormal liver function tests during fluconazole therapy should be monitored for the development of more severe hepatic injury. Fluconazole should be discontinued if clinical signs and symptoms consistent with liver disease develop that may be attributable to fluconazole.
- Anaphylaxis: In rare cases, anaphylaxis has been reported.
- Dermatologic: Patients have rarely developed exfoliative skin disorders during treatment with fluconazole. In patients with serious underlying diseases (predominantly AIDS and malignancy) those have rarely resulted in a fatal outcome. Patients who develop rashes during treatment with fluconazole should be monitored closely and the drug discontinued if lesions progress.

Please also see Drug Interactions (Serious Drug Interactions).

Sensitivity/Resistance: Development of resistance to fluconazole has not been studied; however, there have been reports of cases of superinfection with Candida species other than *C. albicans*, which are often inherently not susceptible to fluconazole (e.g., *C. krusei*). Such cases may require alternative antifungal therapy.

As for other anti-infectives used prophylactically, prudent medical practice dictates that fluconazole be used judiciously in prophylaxis, in view of the theoretical risk of emergence of resistant strains.

Special Populations: Pregnant Women: There are no adequate and well-controlled studies in pregnant women. There have been reports of multiple congenital abnormalities in infants whose mothers were treated with high dose (400-800 mg/day) fluconazole therapy for coccidioidomycosis (an unapproved indication). Exposure to fluconazole began during the first trimester in all cases and continued for three months or longer. Fluconazole is not recommended in pregnant women unless the potential benefit outweighs the potential risk to mother and fetus.

Fluconazole was administered orally to pregnant rabbits during organogenesis in two studies: at 5, 10 and 20 mg/kg, and at 5, 25 and 75 mg/kg respectively. Maternal weight gain was impaired at all dose levels, and abortions occurred at 75 mg/kg (approximately 9.4× the maximum recommended human dose); no adverse fetal effects were detected. In several studies in which pregnant rats were treated orally with fluconazole during organogenesis, maternal weight gain was impaired and placental weights were increased at the 25 mg/kg dose. There were no fetal effects at 5 or 10 mg/kg; increases in fetal anatomical variants (supernumerary ribs, renal pelvis dilation) and delays in ossification were observed at 25 and 50 mg/kg and higher doses. At doses ranging from 80 mg/kg to 320 mg/kg (approximately 10-40× the maximum recommended human dose), embryolethality in rats was increased and fetal abnormalities included wavy ribs, cleft palate and abnormal cranio-facial ossification. These effects are consistent with the inhibition of estrogen synthesis in rats and may be a result of known effects of lowered estrogen on pregnancy, organogenesis and parturition.

Nursing Women: Fluconazole is secreted in human breast milk at concentrations similar to plasma, hence its use in nursing mothers is not recommended.

Women of Child-bearing Potential: Since the teratologic effects of fluconazole in humans are unknown, women taking fluconazole should consider using adequate contraception (see Pregnant Women).

There have been reports of multiple congenital abnormalities in infants whose mothers were treated with high dose (400-800 mg/day) fluconazole therapy for coccidioidomycosis (an unapproved indication). Exposure to fluconazole began during the first trimester in all cases and continued for three months or longer. Since there are no adequate studies in pregnant women to assess the potential for fetal risk, fluconazole should not be used in pregnant women unless the potential benefit outweighs the potential risk to the fetus.

Pediatrics (birth to 16 years old): Fluconazole was effective for the suppression of cryptococcal meningitis and/or disseminated cryptococcal infection in a group of 6 children treated in a compassionate study of fluconazole for the treatment of life-threatening or serious mycosis. There is no information regarding the efficacy of fluconazole for primary treatment of cryptococcal meningitis in children.

Efficacy of fluconazole has not been established in infants less than 6 months of age.

ADVERSE REACTIONS: Adverse Drug Reaction Overview: Sixteen percent of over 4000 patients treated with fluconazole in clinical trials of 7 days or more experienced adverse events.

Treatment was discontinued in 1.5% of patients due to adverse clinical events and in 1.3% of patients due to laboratory test abnormalities.

Adverse clinical events were reported more frequently in HIV infected patients (21%) than in non-HIV infected patients (13%). However, the patterns of adverse events in HIV infected and non-HIV infected patients were similar. The proportions of patients discontinuing therapy due to clinical adverse events were similar in the two groups (1.5%).

The two most serious adverse clinical events noted during clinical trials with fluconazole were:

1. Exfoliative skin disorders
2. Hepatic necrosis

Because most of these patients had serious underlying disease (predominantly AIDS or malignancy) and were receiving multiple concomitant medications, including many known to be hepatotoxic or associated with exfoliative skin disorders, the causal association of these reactions with fluconazole is uncertain. Two cases of hepatic necrosis and one exfoliative skin disorder (Stevens-Johnson syndrome) were associated with a fatal outcome (see Warnings and Precautions).

Clinical Trial Adverse Drug Reactions: The following treatment-related clinical adverse events occurred at an incidence of 1% or greater in 4,048 patients receiving fluconazole for 7 or more days in clinical trials:

Central and Peripheral Nervous System: headache (1.9%).

Dermatologic: skin rash (1.8%).

Gastrointestinal: abdominal pain (1.7%), diarrhea (1.5%), nausea (3.7%) and vomiting (1.7%).

Children: In Phase II/III clinical trials conducted in the United States and in Europe, 577 pediatric patients, ages 1 day to 17 years were treated with fluconazole at doses ranging up to 15 mg/kg/day for up to 1616 days. Thirteen percent of children experienced treatment-related adverse events. The most commonly reported events were vomiting (5.4%), abdominal pain (2.8%), nausea (2.3%), and diarrhea (2.1%). Treatment was discontinued in 2.6% of patients due to adverse clinical events and in 1.0% of patients due to laboratory test abnormalities.

Less Common Clinical Trial Adverse Drug Reactions: Other treatment-related clinical adverse events which occurred less commonly (0.2 to <1%) are presented by organ system below:

Skin and Appendages: pruritus.

Musculoskeletal: myalgia.

Central and Peripheral Nervous System: convulsions, dizziness, paresthesia, tremor, vertigo.

Autonomic Nervous System: dry mouth, increased sweating.

Psychiatric: insomnia, somnolence.

Gastrointestinal: anorexia, constipation, dyspepsia, flatulence.

Liver and Biliary System: cholestasis, hepatocellular damage, jaundice.

Special Senses: taste perversion.

Hematopoietic: anemia.

General: fatigue, malaise, asthenia, fever.

Immunologic: In rare cases, anaphylaxis has been reported.

Abnormal Hematologic and Clinical Chemistry Findings: Liver Function: Clinically significant increases were observed in the following proportions of patients: AST 1%, ALT 1.2%, alkaline phosphatase 1.2%, total bilirubin 0.3%. The incidence of elevated serum aminotransferases was independent of age or route (p.o. or i.v.) of administration but was greater in patients taking fluconazole concomitantly with one or more of the following medications: rifampin, phenytoin, isoniazid, valproic acid, or oral hypoglycemic agents. Clinically significant increases also were more frequent in patients who: 1) had AST or ALT elevations greater than three times the upper limit of normal (>3×ULN) at the time of entering the study (baseline), 2) had a diagnosis of hepatitis at any time during the study and, 3) were identified as alcohol abusers. The overall rate of serum aminotransferase elevations of more than 8 times the upper limit of normal was approximately 1% in patients treated with fluconazole during clinical trials (see Table 1).

Table 1: Fluconazole Injection

Laboratory Test Abnormalities—Liver Enzymes

Lab Parameter	#[a] of Patients	% Abnormal	% Drug-related	# of Patients	% Abnormal	% Drug-related
		Baseline >3×ULN			Baseline <3×ULN	
AST	53	9.4	3.8	3007	4.2	0.8
ALT	65	3.1	0.0	2874	4.8	1.0
		Hepatitis Patients			Non-hepatitis Patients	
AST	160	10.6	1.9	2900	3.9	0.8
ALT	140	11.4	2.1	2799	4.4	1.0
		Alcohol Abuse			Non-alcohol Abuse	
AST	42	9.5	2.4	3018	4.2	0.9
ALT	40	10.0	2.5	2899	4.7	1.0
		Received IV Fluconazole			Never Received IV Fluconazole	
AST	144	5.6	1.4	2916	4.2	0.9
ALT	139	5.0	0.7	2800	4.7	1.0
		≥65 Years Old			<65 Years Old	
AST	277	4.3	1.1	2783	4.3	0.9
ALT	258	3.9	1.2	2681	4.8	1.0

[a] Note: Only patients who had measurements at baseline and during therapy were included.

Renal Function: Clinically significant increases were observed in the following proportions of patients: blood urea nitrogen (0.4%) and creatinine (0.3%).

Hematological Function: Clinically meaningful deviations from baseline in hematologic values which were possibly related to fluconazole were observed in the following proportions of patients: hemoglobin (0.5%), white blood cell count (0.5%), and total platelet count (0.6%).

Post-Market Adverse Drug Reactions: In addition, the following adverse events have occurred under conditions where a causal association is uncertain (e.g. open trials, during post-marketing experience):

Cardiovascular: QT Prolongation, torsade de pointes (see Contraindications, QT Prolongation).

Central and Peripheral Nervous System: seizures.

Dermatologic: alopecia, exfoliative skin disorders including Stevens-Johnson syndrome and toxic epidermal necrolysis (see Warnings and Precautions).

Hematopoietic and Lymphatic: leucopoenia, including neutropenia and agranulocytosis, thrombocytopenia.

Immunologic: anaphylaxis including angioedema, face edema, pruritus and urticaria.

Liver/Biliary: hepatic failure, hepatitis (see Warnings and Precautions).

Metabolic: hypercholesterolemia, hypertriglyceridemia, hypokalemia.

DRUG INTERACTIONS:

Serious Drug Interactions

- Drugs prolonging the QTc interval: The use of fluconazole in patients concurrently taking drugs metabolized by the Cytochrome P-450 system may be associated with elevations in the serum levels of these drugs. In the absence of definitive information caution should be used when coadministering fluconazole and such agents. Patients should be carefully monitored.
- Oral Hypoglycemics: Clinically significant hypoglycemia may be precipitated by the use of fluconazole with oral hypoglycemic agents; one fatality has been reported from hypoglycemia in association with combined fluconazole and glyburide use. Fluconazole reduces the metabolism of tolbutamide, glyburide, and glipizide and increases the plasma concentration of these agents. When fluconazole is used concomitantly with these or other sulfonylurea oral hypoglycemic agents, blood glucose concentrations should be carefully monitored and the dose of the sulfonylurea should be adjusted as necessary. (See Oral Hypoglycemics.)

Overview: Clinically or potentially significant drug interactions between fluconazole and the following agents/classes have been observed:

Benzodiazepines (Short Acting): Following oral or intravenous administration of midazolam, fluconazole resulted in substantial increases in midazolam concentrations and psychomotor effects. This effect on midazolam appears to be more pronounced following oral administration of fluconazole than with fluconazole administered intravenously. If concomitant benzodiazepine therapy, such as midazolam or triazolam, is necessary in patients being treated with fluconazole, consideration should be given to decreasing the benzodiazepine dosage, and the patients should be appropriately monitored.

Cimetidine: Absorption of orally administered fluconazole does not appear to be affected by gastric pH. Fluconazole 100 mg was administered as a single oral dose alone and two hours after a single dose of cimetidine 400 mg to six healthy male volunteers. After the administration of cimetidine, there was a significant decrease in fluconazole AUC (area under the plasma concentration-time curve) and C_{max}. There was a mean ±SD decrease in fluconazole AUC of 13%±11% (range −3.4 to −31%) and C_{max} decreased 19%±14% (range: −5 to −40%). However, the administration of cimetidine 600 mg to 900 mg intravenously over a 4-hour period (from 1 hour before to 3 hours after a single oral dose of fluconazole 200 mg) did not affect the bioavailability or pharmacokinetics of fluconazole in 24 healthy male volunteers.

Coumarin-Type Anticoagulants: In a clinical trial, there was a significant increase in prothrombin time response (area under the prothrombin time-time curve) following a single dose of warfarin (15 mg) administered to 13 normal male volunteers following oral fluconazole 200 mg administered daily for 14 days as compared to the administration of warfarin alone. There was a mean ±SD increase in the prothrombin time response (area under the prothrombin time-time curve) of 7%±4% (range: −2 to 13%). Mean is based on data from 12 subjects as one of 13 subjects experienced a 2-fold increase in his prothrombin time response.

During the post-marketing experience, as with some azole antifungals, bleeding events (bruising, epistaxis, gastrointestinal bleeding, hematuria, and melena) have been reported, in association with increases in prothrombin time in patients receiving fluconazole concurrently with warfarin.

Prothrombin time may be increased in patients receiving concomitant fluconazole and coumarin-type anticoagulants. Careful monitoring of prothrombin time in patients receiving fluconazole and coumarin-type anticoagulants is recommended.

Cyclosporine: Cyclosporine AUC and C_{max} were determined before and after the administration of fluconazole 200 mg daily for 14 days in eight renal transplant patients who had been on cyclosporine therapy for at least 6 months and on a stable cyclosporine dose for at least 6 weeks. There was a significant increase in cyclosporine AUC, C_{max}, C_{min} (24-hour concentration), and a significant reduction in apparent oral clearance following the administration of fluconazole. The mean ±SD increase in AUC was 92%±43% (range: 18 to 147%). The C_{max} increased 60%±48% (range: −5 to 133%). The C_{min} increased 157%±96% (range: 33 to 360%). The apparent oral clearance decreased 45%±15% (range: −15 to −60%). Fluconazole administered at 100 mg daily dose does not affect cyclosporine pharmacokinetic levels in patients with bone marrow transplants. Fluconazole may significantly increase cyclosporine levels in renal transplant patients with or without renal impairment. Careful monitoring of cyclosporine concentrations and serum creatinine is recommended in patients receiving fluconazole and cyclosporine.

Drugs Prolonging the QTc Interval: Astemizole: Definitive interaction studies with fluconazole have not been conducted. The use of fluconazole may be associated with elevations in serum levels of astemizole. Caution should be used when coadministering fluconazole with astemizole. Patients should be carefully monitored.

Cisapride: There have been reports of cardiac events including torsade de pointes in patients to whom fluconazole and cisapride were coadministered. A controlled study found that concomitant fluconazole 200 mg once daily and cisapride 20 mg four times a day yielded a significant increase in cisapride plasma levels and prolongation of QTc interval. Co-administration of cisapride is contraindicated in patients receiving fluconazole (see Contraindications).

Terfenadine: Because of the occurrence of serious cardiac dysrhythmias secondary to prolongation of the QTc interval in patients receiving azole antifungals in conjunction with terfenadine, interaction studies have been performed. In one study, 6 healthy volunteers received terfenadine 60 mg BID for 15 days. Fluconazole 200 mg was administered daily from days 9 through 15. Fluconazole did not affect terfenadine plasma concentrations. Terfenadine acid metabolite AUC increased 36%±36% (range: 7 to 102%) from day 8 to day 15 with the concomitant administration of fluconazole. There was no change in cardiac repolarization as measured by Holter QTc intervals. However, another study at a 400 mg and 800 mg daily dose of fluconazole demonstrated that fluconazole taken in doses of 400 mg per day or greater significantly increases plasma levels of terfenadine when taken concomitantly. Therefore the combined use of fluconazole at doses of 400 mg or higher with terfenadine is contraindicated (see Contraindications). Patients should be carefully monitored if they are being concurrently prescribed fluconazole at multiple doses lower than 400 mg/day with terfenadine.

Hydrochlorothiazide: Concomitant oral administration of 100 mg fluconazole and 50 mg hydrochlorothiazide for 10 days in 13 normal volunteers resulted in a significant increase in fluconazole AUC and C_{max} compared to fluconazole given alone. There was a mean ±SD increase in fluconazole AUC and C_{max} of 45%±31% (range: 19 to 114%) and 43%±31% (range: 19 to 122%), respectively. These changes are attributed to a mean ±SD reduction in renal clearance of 30%±12% (range −10 to −50%).

Oral Contraceptives: In pharmacodynamic studies, single and multiple 50 mg oral doses of fluconazole produced an overall mean increase in ethinyl estradiol or levonorgestrel pharmacokinetics in healthy women taking oral contraceptives. At 200 mg of fluconazole daily, the AUCs of ethinyl estradiol and levonorgestrel were increased, 40% and 24%, respectively.

Twenty-five normal females received daily doses of both 200 mg fluconazole tablets or placebo for two, 10-day periods. The treatment cycles were one month apart with all subjects receiving fluconazole during one cycle and placebo during the other. The order of study treatment was random. Single doses of an oral contraceptive tablet containing levonorgestrel and ethinyl estradiol were administered on the final treatment day (day 10) of both cycles. Following administration of 200 mg of fluconazole, the mean percentage increase of AUC for levonorgestrel compared to placebo was 25% (range: −12 to 82%) and the mean percentage increase for ethinyl estradiol compared to placebo was 38% (range: −11 to 101%). Both of these increases were statistically significantly different from placebo.

Oral Hypoglycemics: The effects of fluconazole on the pharmacokinetics of the sulfonylurea oral hypoglycemic agents tolbutamide, glipizide, and glyburide were evaluated in three placebo-controlled studies in normal volunteers. All subjects received the sulfonylurea alone as a single dose and again as a single dose following the administration of fluconazole 100 mg daily for 7 days. In these three studies, 22/46 (47.8%) of fluconazole-treated patients and 9/22 (40.1%) of placebo-treated patients experienced symptoms consistent with hypoglycemia.

Tolbutamide: In 13 normal male volunteers, there was a significant increase in tolbutamide (500 mg single dose) AUC and C_{max} following the administration of fluconazole. There was a mean ±SD increase in tolbutamide AUC of 26%±9% (range: 12 to 39%). Tolbutamide C_{max} increased 11%±9% (range −6 to 27%).

Glipizide: The AUC and C_{max} of glipizide (2.5 mg single dose) were significantly increased following the administration of fluconazole in 13 normal male volunteers. There was a mean ±SD increase in AUC of 49%±13% (range: 27 to 73%) and an increase in C_{max} of 19%±23% (range: −11 to 79%).

Glyburide: The AUC and C_{max} of glyburide (5 mg single dose) were significantly increased following the administration of fluconazole in 20 normal male volunteers. There was a mean ±SD increase in AUC of 44%±29% (range: −13 to 115%) and C_{max} increased 19%±19% (range: −23 to 62%). Five subjects required oral glucose following the ingestion of glyburide after 7 days of fluconazole administration.

Phenytoin: Phenytoin AUC was determined after 4 days of phenytoin dosing (200 mg daily, orally for 3 days, followed by 250 mg intravenously for one dose) both with and without the administration of fluconazole (oral fluconazole 200 mg daily for 16 days) in 10 normal male volunteers. There was a significant increase in phenytoin AUC. The mean ±SD increase in phenytoin AUC was 88%±68% (range: 16 to 247%). The absolute magnitude of this interaction is unknown because of the intrinsically non-linear disposition of phenytoin.

Fluconazole increases the plasma concentrations of phenytoin. Careful monitoring of phenytoin concentrations in patients receiving fluconazole and phenytoin is recommended.

Rifabutin: There have been reports that an interaction exists when fluconazole is administered concomitantly with rifabutin, leading to increased serum levels of rifabutin. There have been reports of uveitis in patients to whom fluconazole and rifabutin were coadministered. Patients receiving rifabutin and fluconazole concomitantly should be carefully monitored.

Rifampin: Administration of a single oral 200 mg dose of fluconazole after 15 days of rifampin administered as 600 mg daily in 8 healthy male volunteers resulted in a significant decrease in fluconazole AUC and a significant increase in apparent oral clearance of fluconazole. There was a mean ±SD reduction in fluconazole AUC of 23%±9% (range: −13 to −42%). Apparent oral clearance of fluconazole increased 32%±17% (range: 16 to 72%). Fluconazole half-life decreased from 33.4±4.4 hours to 26.8±3.9 hours.

Rifampin enhances the metabolism of concurrently administered fluconazole. Depending on clinical circumstances, consideration should be given to increasing the dose of fluconazole when it is administered with rifampin.

Tacrolimus: There have been reports that an interaction exists when fluconazole is administered concomitantly with tacrolimus, leading to increased serum levels of tacrolimus. There have been reports of nephrotoxicity in patients to whom fluconazole and tacrolimus were coadministered. Patients receiving tacrolimus and fluconazole concomitantly should be carefully monitored.

Theophylline: The pharmacokinetics of theophylline were determined from a single intravenous dose of aminophylline (6 mg/kg) before and after the oral administration of fluconazole 200 mg daily for 14 days in 16 normal male volunteers. There were significant increases in theophylline AUC, C_{max}, and half-life with a corresponding decrease in clearance. The mean ±SD theophylline AUC increased 21%±16% (range: −5 to 48%). The C_{max} increased 13%±17% (range: −13 to 40%). Theophylline clearance decreased 16%±11% (range: −32 to 5%). The half-life of theophylline increased from 6.6±1.7 hours to 7.9±1.5 hours. Patients who are receiving high doses of theophylline or who are otherwise at increased risk for theophylline toxicity should be observed for signs of theophylline toxicity while receiving fluconazole, and therapy modified appropriately if signs of toxicity develop.

Zidovudine: Plasma zidovudine concentrations were determined on two occasions (before and following fluconazole 200 mg daily for 15 days) in 13 volunteers with AIDS or ARC who were on a stable zidovudine dose for at least two weeks. There was a significant increase in zidovudine AUC following the administration of fluconazole. The mean ±SD increase in AUC was 20%±32% (range: −27 to 104%). The metabolite, GZDV, to parent drug ratio significantly decreased after the administration of fluconazole, from 7.6±3.6 to 5.7±2.2. Patients receiving this combination should be monitored for the development of zidovudine-related adverse reactions.

Drugs exhibiting no significant pharmacokinetic interactions with fluconazole:

Antacid: Administration of Maalox (20 mL) to 14 normal male volunteers immediately prior to a single dose of fluconazole 100 mg had no effect on the absorption or elimination of fluconazole.

Interaction studies with other medications have not been conducted, but such interactions may occur.

Drug-Drug Interactions: The drugs listed in Table 2 are based on either drug interaction case reports or studies, or potential interactions due to the expected magnitude and seriousness of the interaction (i.e. those identified as contraindicated).

Drug-Food Interactions: None known.

Drug-Herb Interactions: None known.

Drug-Laboratory Test Interactions: None known.

Table 2: Fluconazole Injection
Established or Potential Drug-Drug Interactions

Name	Reference	Effect	Clinical Comment
Benzodiazepines (short acting)	NA	Substantial increases in benzodiazepines concentration and psychomotor effects	If concomitant benzodiazepine therapy, such as midazolam or triazolam, is necessary in patients being treated with fluconazole, consideration should be given to decreasing the benzodiazepine dosage, and the patients should be appropriately monitored.
Cimetidine	CT	Significant decrease in fluconazole AUC and C_{max}	The administration of cimetidine 600 mg to 900 mg intravenously over a 4-hour period (from 1 hour before to 3 hours after a single oral dose of fluconazole 200 mg) did not affect the bioavailability or pharmacokinetics of fluconazole in 24 healthy male volunteers.
Coumarin-Type Anticoagulants	CT and PM	Significant increase in prothrombin time, bleeding events	Careful monitoring of prothrombin time in patients receiving fluconazole and coumarin-type anticoagulants is recommended.
Cyclosporine	CT	Significant increase in cyclosporine AUC, C_{max} and C_{min}	Fluconazole may significantly increase cyclosporine levels in renal transplant patients with or without renal impairment. Careful monitoring of cyclosporine concentrations and serum creatinine is recommended in patients receiving fluconazole and cyclosporine.
Astemizole	T	Possible increase in serum levels of Astemizole	Caution should be used when coadministering fluconazole with astemizole. Patients should be carefully monitored.
Cisapride	C	Cardiac events including torsade de pointes	Co-administration of cisapride is contraindicated in patients receiving fluconazole (see Contraindications).
Terfenadine	CT	Serious cardiac dysrhythmias	The combined use of fluconazole at doses of 400 mg or higher with terfenadine is contraindicated (see Contraindications). Patients should be carefully monitored if they are being concurrently prescribed fluconazole at multiple doses lower than 400 mg/day with terfenadine.
Hydrochlorothiazide	CT	Significant increase in fluconazole AUC and C_{max}	These changes are attributed to a mean ±SD reduction in renal clearance of 30%±12% (range −10 to −50%).
Oral Contraceptives	CT	Overall increase in AUCs of ethinyl estradiol and levonorgestrel	NA
Tolbutamide	CT	Significant increase in tolbutamide AUC and C_{max}	When fluconazole is used concomitantly with these or other sulfonylurea oral hypoglycemic agents, blood glucose concentrations should be carefully monitored and the dose of the sulfonylurea should be adjusted as necessary.
Glipizide	CT	Significant increase in glipizide AUC and C_{max}	When fluconazole is used concomitantly with these or other sulfonylurea oral hypoglycemic agents, blood glucose concentrations should be carefully monitored and the dose of the sulfonylurea should be adjusted as necessary.
Glyburide	CT	Significant increase in glyburide AUC and C_{max}	When fluconazole is used concomitantly with these or other sulfonylurea oral hypoglycemic agents, blood glucose concentrations should be carefully monitored and the dose of the sulfonylurea should be adjusted as necessary.
Phenytoin	CT	Significant increase in phenytoin AUC	The absolute magnitude of this interaction is unknown because of the intrinsically non-linear disposition of phenytoin. Fluconazole increases the plasma concentrations of phenytoin. Careful monitoring of phenytoin concentrations in patients receiving fluconazole and phenytoin is recommended.
Rifabutin	C	Increase serum levels of rifabutin, uveitis	Patients receiving rifabutin and fluconazole concomitantly should be carefully monitored.
Rifampin	CT	Significant decrease in fluconazole AUC, and decrease in fluconazole half-life	Rifampin enhances the metabolism of concurrently administered fluconazole. Depending on clinical circumstances, consideration should be given to increasing the dose of fluconazole when it is administered with rifampin.
Tacrolimus	C	Increase serum levels of tacrolimus, nephrotoxicity	Patients receiving tacrolimus and fluconazole concomitantly should be carefully monitored.
Theophylline	CT	Significant increases in theophylline AUC, C_{max} and half-life with a corresponding decrease in clearance	Patients who are receiving high doses of theophylline or who are otherwise at increased risk for theophylline toxicity should be observed for signs of theophylline toxicity while receiving fluconazole, and therapy modified appropriately if signs of toxicity develop.

(cont'd)

Table 2: Fluconazole Injection *(cont'd)*

Established or Potential Drug-Drug Interactions

Name	Reference	Effect	Clinical Comment
Zidovudine	CT	Significant increase in zidovudine AUC	Patients receiving this combination should be monitored for the development of zidovudine-related adverse reactions.

Legend:
C=case study.
CT=clinical trial.
T=theoretical.
PM=post-marketing.

DOSAGE AND ADMINISTRATION:

Dosing Considerations: The most suitable product format with intended route of administration and daily dosage of fluconazole should be based on the infecting organism, the patient's condition and the response to therapy. Treatment should be continued until clinical parameters and laboratory tests indicate that an active fungal infection has been cured or has subsided. An inadequate period of treatment may lead to recurrence of active infection. Patients with AIDS and cryptococcal meningitis or recurrent oropharyngeal candidiasis usually require maintenance therapy to prevent relapse.

Recommended Dose and Dosage Adjustment: Adults and Children (see also Action and Clinical Pharmacology): Loading Dose: Administration of a loading dose on the first day of treatment, consisting of twice the usual daily dose, results in plasma concentrations close to steady state by the second day. Patients with acute infections should be given a loading dose equal to twice the daily dose, not to exceed a maximum single dose of 400 mg in adults or 12 mg/kg in children, on the first day of treatment. See Table 3 and Table 4.

Table 3: Fluconazole Injection

Dosage Equivalency Scheme

Pediatric Patients		Adults
3 mg/kg		100 mg
6 mg/kg		200 mg
12 mg/kg[a]		400 mg

[a] Some older children may have clearances similar to that of adults. Absolute doses exceeding 600 mg/day are not recommended.

Table 4: Fluconazole Injection

Recommended Treatment Guidelines

Indication	Adults	Children
Oropharyngeal Candidiasis	100 mg once daily for at least 2 weeks to decrease the likelihood of relapse.	3 mg/kg once daily for at least 2 weeks to decrease the likelihood of relapse.
Esophageal Candidiasis	100 mg to 200 mg once daily for a minimum of 3 weeks, and for at least 2 weeks following resolution of symptoms.	3 mg/kg to 6 mg/kg once daily for a minimum of 3 weeks, and for at least 2 weeks following resolution of symptoms.
Systemic Candidiasis (Candidemia and Disseminated Candidal Infections)	200 mg to 400 mg once daily for a minimum of 4 weeks, and for at least 2 weeks following resolution of symptoms.	6 mg/kg to 12 mg/kg per day have been used in an open, non-comparative study of a small number of patients.
Cryptococcal Meningitis	200 mg to 400 mg once daily. The duration of therapy for cryptococcal meningitis is unknown, it is recommended that the initial therapy should last a minimum of 10 weeks.	6 mg/kg to 12 mg/kg once daily. The recommended duration for initial therapy is 10–12 weeks after the cerebrospinal fluid becomes culture-negative.
Prevention of Recurrence of Cryptococcal Meningitis in Patients with AIDS	200 mg once daily.	6 mg/kg once daily.

Premature Neonates: Experience with fluconazole in neonates is limited to pharmacokinetic studies in premature newborns (see Action and Clinical Pharmacology). Based upon the prolonged half-life seen in premature newborns (gestation age 26 to 29 weeks), these children, in the first two weeks of life, should receive the same dosage (mg/kg) as in older children, but administered every 72 hours. After the first two weeks, these children should be dosed once daily.

Neonates: No information regarding fluconazole pharmacokinetics in full-term newborns is available.

Prophylaxis in Adult Patients: The recommended fluconazole daily dosage for the prevention of candidiasis in adult patients undergoing bone marrow transplantation is 400 mg once daily. Patients who are anticipated to have severe granulocytopenia (less than 500 neutrophils per mm^3) should start fluconazole prophylaxis several days before the anticipated onset of neutropenia and continue for 7 days after the neutrophil count rises above 1000 cells per mm^3.

The intravenous infusion of fluconazole should be administered at a maximum rate of approximately 200 mg/hour given as a continuous infusion.

Dosage in Patients with Impaired Renal Function: Adults: Fluconazole is cleared primarily by renal excretion as unchanged drug. In patients with impaired renal function, an initial loading dose of 50 to 400 mg should be given (for children, see below). After the loading dose, the daily dose (according to indication) should be based on Table 5.

Table 5: Fluconazole Injection

Dosage in Adult Patients with Impaired Renal Function

Creatinine Clearance (mL/min)	Creatinine Clearance (mL/sec)	Percent Recommended Dose
>50	>0.83	100%
21–50 (no dialysis)	0.35–0.83 (no dialysis)	50%
11–20 (no dialysis)	0.18–0.34 (no dialysis)	25%
Regular hemodialysis	Regular hemodialysis	100% after each dialysis

When serum creatinine is the only measure of renal function available, the following formula (based on sex, weight, and age of the patient) should be used to estimate the creatinine clearance.

Creatinine Clearance Calculations:

Males:

$$\text{mL/min} = \frac{\text{Weight (kg)} \times (140\text{–age})}{72 \times \text{serum creatinine (mg/100 mL)}}$$

or

$$\text{mL/sec} = \frac{\text{Weight (kg)} \times (140\text{–age})}{50 \times \text{serum creatinine } (\mu\text{mol/L})}$$

Females: 0.85×above value

Children: Although the pharmacokinetics of fluconazole have not been studied in children with renal insufficiency, dosage reduction in children with renal insufficiency should parallel that recommended for adults. The following formula may be used to estimate creatinine clearance in children:

$$K \times \frac{\text{linear length or height (cm)}}{\text{serum creatinine (mg/100 mL)}}$$

(Where K=0.55 for children older than 1 year and 0.45 for infants.)

Administration: Fluconazole Injection in INTRAVIA plastic containers is available in two different container sizes providing different total doses; 200 mg/100 mL and 400 mg/200 mL (see Dosage Forms, Composition and Packaging). Please ensure the appropriate dosage is administered based on the physician's order. In the event the inappropriate container size is administered, please see Overdosage.

Fluconazole Injection in INTRAVIA plastic containers is intended only for intravenous infusion using sterile equipment. The intravenous infusion of fluconazole should be administered at a maximum rate of approximately 200 mg/hour given as a continuous infusion.

Do not remove unit from overwrap until ready to use. The overwrap is a moisture barrier. The inner bag maintains the sterility of the product.

Inspect visually for particulate matter or discoloration prior to administration. Do not use if cloudiness or precipitation is evident or if the seal is not intact.

Not intended for multidose use: Single use. Discard any unused portion.

Connect an intravenous giving set to the container of fluconazole injection solution. **Infuse fluconazole injection solution at a maximum rate of 200 mg/hour.** Flush fluconazole intravenous solution remaining in the giving set with sterile normal saline. Because fluconazole is available as a dilute saline solution, consideration should be given to the rate of fluid administration in patients requiring sodium or fluid restriction.

Caution: Do not use plastic containers in series connections. Such use could result in air embolism due to residual air being drawn from the primary container before administration of the fluid from the secondary container is completed. Do not add supplemental medication.

Incompatibility: It is recommended that fluconazole injection for intravenous infusion be infused separately.

Compatibility : Administration sets ("giving" sets): Fluconazole injection for intravenous infusion is compatible with (i.e. not susceptible to absorption) sets constructed of a delivery tube (PVC) luer lock (modified phenylene oxide), flash ball (latex) drip chamber (polypropylene) and piercing spike (polypropylene).

Reconstitution: Not applicable.

OVERDOSAGE:

Symptoms: There have been reports of overdosage with fluconazole and in one case, a 42-year old patient infected with human immunodeficiency virus developed hallucinations and exhibited paranoid behavior after reportedly ingesting 8200 mg of fluconazole. The patient was admitted to the hospital, and his condition resolved within 48 hours.

Treatment: In the event of overdose, symptomatic treatment (with supportive measures and gastric lavage if necessary) may be adequate. Fluconazole is largely excreted in urine. A three hour hemodialysis session decreases plasma levels by approximately 50%.

Mice and rats receiving very high doses of fluconazole, whether orally or intravenously, displayed a variety of nonspecific, agonal signs such as decreased activity, ataxia, shallow respiration, ptosis, lacrimation, salivation, urinary incontinence and cyanosis. Death was sometimes preceded by clonic convulsions.

> For management of a suspected drug overdose, CPhA recommends that you contact your **regional Poison Control Centre**. See the *CPS* Directory section for a list of Poison Control Centres.

ACTION AND CLINICAL PHARMACOLOGY:

Mechanism of Action: Fluconazole is a highly selective inhibitor of fungal cytochrome P-450 sterol C-14-α-demethylation. Mammalian cell demethylation is much less sensitive to fluconazole inhibition. The subsequent loss of normal sterols correlates with the accumulation of 14-α-methyl sterols in fungi and may be responsible for the fungistatic activity of fluconazole.

Pharmacodynamics: The effects of fluconazole on the metabolism of carbohydrates, lipids, adrenal and gonadal hormones were assessed. In normal volunteers, fluconazole administration (doses ranging from 200 to 400 mg once daily for up to 14 days) was associated with small and inconsistent effects on testosterone concentrations, endogenous corticosteroid concentrations, and the ACTH-stimulated cortisol response. In addition, fluconazole appears to have no clinically significant effects on carbohydrate or lipid metabolism in man.

Pharmacokinetics: Absorption: Human Adults: The pharmacokinetic properties of fluconazole are similar following administration by the intravenous or oral routes and do not appear to be affected by gastric pH. In normal volunteers, the bioavailability of orally administered fluconazole is over 90% compared with intravenous administration. Essentially all of the administered drug reaches systemic circulation; thus, there is no evidence of first-pass metabolism of the drug. In addition, no adjustment in dosage is necessary when changing from p.o. to i.v. or vice versa.

Peak plasma concentrations (C_{max}) in fasted normal volunteers occur rapidly following oral administration, usually between 1 and 2 hours of dosing with a terminal plasma elimination half-life of approximately 30 hours (range 20-50 hours) after oral administration. The long plasma elimination half-life provides the basis for once daily dosing with fluconazole in the treatment of fungal infections.

In fasted normal volunteers, administration of a single oral 400 mg dose of fluconazole leads to a mean C_{max} of 6.72 µg/mL (range: 4.12 to 8.08 µg/mL) and after single oral doses of 50-400 mg, fluconazole plasma concentrations and AUC (area under the plasma concentration-time curve) are dose proportional.

In normal volunteers, oral bioavailability as measured by C_{max} and AUC was not affected by food when fluconazole was administered as a single 50 mg capsule; however T_{max} was doubled.

Steady-state concentrations are reached within 5-10 days following oral doses of 50-400 mg given once daily. Administration of a loading dose on the first day of treatment of twice the usual daily dose results in plasma concentrations close to steady-state by the second day.

Distribution: The apparent volume of distribution of fluconazole approximates that of total body water. Plasma protein binding is low (11-12%) and is constant over the concentration range tested (0.1 mg/L to 10 mg/L). This degree of protein binding is not clinically meaningful. Following either single- or multiple-oral doses for up to 14 days, fluconazole penetrates into all body tissues and fluids studied (see Table 6). In normal volunteers, saliva concentrations of fluconazole were equal to or slightly greater than plasma concentrations regardless of dose, route, or duration of dosing. In patients with bronchiectasis, sputum concentrations of fluconazole following a single 150 mg oral dose were equal to plasma concentrations at both 4 and 24 hours post dose. In patients with fungal meningitis, fluconazole concentrations in the CSF (cerebrospinal fluid) are approximately 80% of the corresponding plasma concentrations. Whole blood concentrations of fluconazole indicated that the drug freely enters erythrocytes and maintains a concentration equivalent to that of plasma.

Table 6: Fluconazole Injection
Distribution of Fluconazole

Tissue or Fluid	Ratio of Fluconazole Tissue (Fluid)/Plasma Concentration[a]
Cerebrospinal fluid[b]	0.5–0.9
Saliva	1
Sputum	1
Blister fluid	1
Urine	10
Normal skin	10
Nails	1
Blister skin	2

[a] Relative to concurrent concentrations in plasma in subjects with normal renal function.
[b] Independent of degree of meningeal inflammation.

Metabolism and Excretion: Fluconazole is cleared primarily by renal excretion, with approximately 80% of the administered dose appearing in the urine as unchanged drug. Following administration of radiolabeled fluconazole, greater than 90% of the radioactivity is excreted in the urine. Approximately 11% of the radioactivity in urine is due to metabolites. An additional 2% of the total radioactivity is excreted in feces.

The pharmacokinetics of fluconazole do not appear to be affected by age alone but are markedly affected by reduction in renal function. There is an inverse relationship between the elimination half-life and creatinine clearance. The dose of fluconazole may need to be reduced in patients with impaired renal function (see Dosage and Administration). A 3-hour hemodialysis session decreases plasma concentrations by approximately 50%.

Special Populations and Conditions: Pediatrics: In children, the following pharmacokinetic data {MEAN (% cv)} have been reported: See Table 7.

Table 7: Fluconazole Injection
Pharmacokinetics in Children

Age Studied	Dose (mg/kg)	Clearance (mL/min/kg)	Half-life (Hours)	C_{max} (µg/mL)	Vdss (L/kg)
9 Months-13 years	Single-Oral 2 mg/kg	0.40 (38%) N=14	25.0	2.9 (22%) N=16	—
9 Months-13 years	Single-Oral 8 mg/kg	0.51 (60%) N=15	19.5	9.8 (20%) N=15	—
5–15 years	Multiple i.v. 2 mg/kg	0.49 (40%) N=4	17.4	5.5 (25%) N=5	0.722 (36%) N=4
5–15 years	Multiple i.v. 4 mg/kg	0.59 (64%) N=5	15.2	11.4 (44%) N=6	0.729 (33%) N=5
5–15 years	Multiple i.v. 8 mg/kg	0.66 (31%) N=7	17.6	14.1 (22%) N=8	1.069 (37%) N=7

Clearance corrected for body weight was not affected by age in these studies. Mean body clearance in adults is reported to be 0.23 mL/min/kg (17%).

In premature newborns (gestation age 26 to 29 weeks), the mean (% cv) clearance within 36 hours of birth was 0.180 mL/min/kg (35%, N=7), which increased with time to a mean of 0.218 mL/min/kg (31%, N=9) six days later and 0.333 mL/min/kg (56%, N=4) 12 days later. Similarly, the half-life was 73.6 hours, which decreased with time to a mean of 53.2 hours six days later and 46.6 hours 12 days later.

The following dose equivalency scheme should generally provide equivalent exposure in pediatric and adult patients: See Table 8.

Table 8: Fluconazole Injection
Dosage Equivalency Scheme

Pediatric Patients	Adults
3 mg/kg	100 mg
6 mg/kg	200 mg
12 mg/kg[a]	400 mg

[a] Some older children may have clearances similar to that of adults. Absolute doses exceeding 600 mg/day are not recommended.

Animals: Table 9 illustrates key parameters of fluconazole in the mouse, rat, and dog as compared to man.

Table 9: Fluconazole Injection
Pharmacokinetics in Animals Compared to Man

Parameter	Mouse	Rat	Dog	Man
Elimination Half-life (hr)	5.0 (2.6)	4.0	15 (13)	20–50
Plasma Clearance (mL/min/kg)	2.0 (6.2)	2.2	0.62 (0.65)	— (0.28)
Renal Clearance (mL/min/kg)	1.4 (5.0)	1.8	0.30 (0.46)	0.27 (0.26)
Urinary Excretion (% of unchanged drug)	70 (68)	82	63 (72)	80 (75)
Total Urinary Recovery[a] (% of dose)	79 (78)	—	72 (80)	91

[a] Total radioactivity.
Values in parentheses are from i.v. administration; all others are from oral administration.

In all species and man: (1) C_{max} levels are similar after normalization for different body mass, (2) volume of distribution is about 0.8 L/kg, (3) plasma protein binding is in the range of 11-12% and (4) bioavailability is greater than 80%.

Plasma concentrations of fluconazole generally declined in a monophasic manner with first order kinetics. The elimination half-life ranges from about 2 to 5 hours in the mouse to approximately 30 hours in man (range 20-50 hours). The longer elimination half-life in man is a consequence of low plasma clearance (0.28 mL/min/kg) relative to the normal glomerular filtration rate (1.8 mL/min/kg).

STORAGE AND STABILITY: Store at 5-25°C. Do not freeze. Avoid excessive heat.

SPECIAL HANDLING INSTRUCTIONS: Not applicable.

DOSAGE FORMS, COMPOSITION AND PACKAGING: Each mL of sterile aqueous solution for direct intravenous infusion contains: fluconazole 2 mg, sodium chloride solution 9 mg and Water for Injection. Osmolarity: 315 mOsmol/L (calc). pH: 5.5 (4.0 to 6.5). INTRAVIA plastic containers of 100 mL (10×100 mL) and 200 mL (10×200 mL), affording doses of 200 mg and 400 mg fluconazole, respectively.

The flexible container is manufactured from a specially designed multilayer plastic (PL2408). Solutions in contact with the plastic container leach out certain chemical components from the plastic in very small amounts; however, biological testing was supportive of the safety of the plastic container materials. The flexible container has a foil overwrap. Water can permeate the plastic into the overwrap, but the amount is insufficient to significantly affect the premixed solution.

Fluconazole Injection 🅿
fluconazole
Antifungal

Sandoz

SUPPLIED: Each mL of sterile aqueous solution for direct infusion contains: fluconazole 2 mg, sodium chloride for isotonicity, hydrochloric acid and/or sodium hydroxide to adjust pH and water for injection. Single use vials of 100 mL, boxes of 1. Store between 15 and 30°C. Protect from freezing. Protect from light. Discard unused portion.

Fludrocortisone 🅿
CPhA Monograph

see *Corticosteroids: Systemic*

Flumazenil Injection
flumazenil
Benzodiazepine Antagonist

Sandoz

SUPPLIED: Each mL contains: flumazenil 0.1 mg. Nonmedicinal ingredients: acetic acid, edetate disodium, hydrochloric acid and/or sodium hydroxide, methylparaben, propylparaben, sodium chloride and water for injection. Multidose vials of 5 mL, boxes of 10. Store at 15-30°C. Protect from light. Discard unused portion 28 days after the initial puncture.

Flumethasone 🅿
CPhA Monograph

see *Corticosteroids: Eye Ear Nose*

see *Corticosteroids: Topical*

FluMist®
influenza vaccine (live, attenuated)
Intranasal Spray

AstraZeneca

Date of Preparation: July 20, 2010

SUMMARY PRODUCT INFORMATION:

Route of Administration	Dosage Form/ Strength	Clinically Relevant Nonmedicinal Ingredients
Intranasal	Spray, 0.2 mL	Gelatin hydrolysate (porcine Type A), sucrose, arginine, gentamicin For a complete listing see Dosage Forms, Composition and Packaging.

DESCRIPTION: FLUMIST [influenza vaccine (live, attenuated)] is a live, trivalent vaccine for administration by intranasal spray. Each 0.2 mL dose contains $10^{6.5\text{-}7.5}$ FFU (fluorescent focus units) of live attenuated influenza virus reassortants of each of three strains propagated in specific pathogen-free (SPF) eggs from SPF chicken flocks. The three strains used for the 2010-2011 season are: A/California/7/2009 (H1N1), A/Perth/16/2009 (H3N2), and B/Brisbane/60/2008. This influenza vaccine complies with the WHO recommendation (northern hemisphere) for the 2010-2011 influenza season.

The influenza virus strains in FLUMIST are (a) cold-adapted (ca) (i.e., they replicate efficiently at 25°C, a temperature that is restrictive for replication of many wild-type influenza viruses); (b) temperature-sensitive (ts) (i.e., they are restricted in replication at 37°C (Type B strains) or 39°C (Type A strains), temperatures at which many wild-type influenza viruses grow efficiently); and (c) attenuated (att) (they do not produce classic influenza-like illness in the ferret model of human influenza infection). The cumulative effect of the antigenic properties and the ca, ts, and att phenotypes is that the attenuated vaccine viruses replicate in the nasopharynx and induce protective immunity.

INDICATIONS AND CLINICAL USE: FLUMIST [influenza vaccine (live, attenuated)] is indicated for the active immunization of individuals 2-59 years of age against influenza caused by virus subtypes A and type B contained in the vaccine.

CONTRAINDICATIONS: FLUMIST is contraindicated in individuals with a history of hypersensitivity, especially anaphylactic reactions, to eggs, egg proteins, gentamicin, gelatin, or arginine or to any other ingredient in the formulation. For a complete listing, see Dosage Forms, Composition and Packaging.

FLUMIST is contraindicated in individuals with a history of hypersensitivity to previous influenza vaccination.

WARNINGS AND PRECAUTIONS: General: As with most vaccines, supervision and treatment by an appropriately trained healthcare professional should always be readily available in case of an anaphylactic event following the administration of the vaccine.

Administration of FLUMIST, a live attenuated virus vaccine, to immunosuppressed persons should be based on careful consideration of potential benefits and risks. Data supporting the safety and efficacy of FLUMIST in immunocompromised individuals are limited. FLUMIST has been administered to approximately 170 children and adults with mild to moderate immunosuppression due to HIV infections and 10 children with mild to moderate immunosuppression due to cancer.

Vaccine recipients should be informed that FLUMIST is an attenuated live virus vaccine and has the potential for transmission to immunocompromised contacts. Vaccine recipients should attempt to avoid, whenever possible, close association with severely immunocompromised individuals (e.g., bone marrow transplant recipients requiring isolation) for at least 2 weeks following vaccination. Peak incidence of vaccine virus recovery occurred 2-3 days post-vaccination in clinical studies. In circumstances where contact with severely immunocompromised individuals is unavoidable, the potential risk of transmission of the influenza vaccine virus should be weighed against the risk of acquiring and transmitting wild-type influenza virus.

Those under the age of 18 years receiving aspirin therapy or aspirin-containing therapy should avoid vaccination with FLUMIST due to the association of Reye's syndrome with aspirin and wild-type influenza infection.

Neurologic: If Guillain-Barré syndrome has occurred within 6 weeks of any prior influenza vaccination, the decision to give FLUMIST should be based on careful consideration of the potential benefits and potential risks (see Adverse Reactions).

Respiratory: FLUMIST should not be administered to individuals with severe asthma (e.g. currently requiring therapy with oral glucocorticosteroids or high dose inhaled glucocorticosteroids) or active wheezing (medically attended wheezing in the seven days prior to vaccination) because these individuals have not been adequately studied in clinical trials.

Special Populations: Pregnant Women: Animal reproduction studies and studies in pregnant or lactating women have not been conducted with FLUMIST.

The effect of the vaccine on embryo-fetal and pre-weaning development was evaluated in developmental toxicity studies of pregnant rats and pregnant ferrets. No adverse effects on pregnancy, parturition, lactation or embryo-fetal development were observed in either study. No adverse effects on pre-weaning development were observed in the rat study. No fetal malformations or other evidence of teratogenesis were observed.

FLUMIST should be given to pregnant women only if clearly needed.

Nursing Women: Animal reproduction studies and studies in pregnant or lactating women have not been conducted with FLUMIST.

It is not known whether FLUMIST is excreted in human milk. Therefore, as some viruses are excreted in human milk caution should be exercised if FLUMIST is administered to nursing mothers.

Pediatrics (<24 months): Do not administer FLUMIST to children <24 months of age due to increased risk of wheezing (see Adverse Reactions).

ADVERSE REACTIONS: Adverse Drug Reaction Overview: In clinical studies, the safety of FLUMIST was evaluated in over 28 500 children and adolescents 2 to 17 years of age and over 4350 adults 18-59 years of age. The most common adverse reaction observed in clinical studies in all ages was nasal congestion/rhinorrhea.

Clinical Trial Adverse Drug Reactions: Because clinical trials are conducted under very specific conditions the adverse reaction rates observed in the clinical trials may not reflect the rates observed in practice and should not be compared to the rates in the clinical trials of another drug. Adverse drug reaction information from clinical trials is useful for identifying drug-related adverse events and for approximating rates.

Adverse Reactions in Children and Adolescents: Seven placebo controlled studies and four active controlled studies were pooled to evaluate solicited events occurring in children and adolescents 2-17 years of age. Table 1 presents an analysis of solicited events post dose 1 occurring in at least 1% of FLUMIST recipients and includes rates for these solicited events from active controlled studies. A total of 7336 children and adolescents 2 to 17 years of age received at least 1 dose of FLUMIST in Year 1 of dosing in controlled studies and provided data for the pooled safety analysis.

Solicited events were those about which parents/guardians were specifically queried after vaccination with FLUMIST. In these studies, solicited events were documented within 10 days post vaccination. Solicited events post dose 2 for FLUMIST were similar to those post dose 1, and were generally observed at a lower frequency.

Table 1: FLUMIST

Summary of Solicited Events Observed During Days 0 to 10 after Dose 1 for FLUMIST and either Placebo or Active Control Recipients; Children and Adolescents 2-17 Years of Age

	Placebo Controlled Studies[a]		Active Controlled Studies[b]	
Solicited Event	**FluMist N=258–3245[c] (%)**	**Placebo N=191–1994[c] (%)**	**FluMist N=3931–4108[c] (%)**	**Injectable Influenza Vaccine N=3982–4118[c] (%)**
Any solicited event	74.2	69.5	70.4	64.8
Runny/stuffy nose	63.7	56.9	56.7	45.0
Cough	39.9	41.6	33.6	35.6
Decreased appetite	24.1	21.7	15.9	15.2
Irritability	21.2	19.7	13.8	12.5
Abdominal pain	14.1	12.3	12.3	11.5
Decreased activity[d]	13.8	11.7	13.1	11.8
Headache	13.4	6.5	13.8	12.3
Vomiting	12.3	13.7	6.8	6.9
Sore throat	10.1	8.2	11.6	11.2
Muscle ache	8.1	5.2	5.7	6.9
Chills	6.2	7.8	5.8	5.1
Fever				
≥38.0°C	11.2	9.7	9.3	8.6
≥38.5°C	6.0	5.6	5.1	5.1
≥39.0°C	2.5	2.5	2.3	2.4
≥39.5°C	1.1	1.0	0.8	0.9

a Includes Studies D153-P002, D153-P501 Year 1, D153-P502 Year 1, D153-P504 Year 1, D153-P511, D153 P513, and D153-P526. Follow-up time for Study D153-P526 was Days 0-6 post dose.
b Includes Studies MI-CP111, D153-P002, D153-P514, and D153-P515.
c Number of subjects evaluated for the specific solicited event. Range reflects differences in data collection between pooled studies.
d Collected as decreased activity/tiredness/weakness/malaise.

In MI-CP111, an active-controlled study, an increased rate of wheezing through 42 days was observed in children 6-23 months of age (5.9% FLUMIST versus 3.8% injectable influenza vaccine) (see Warnings and Precautions). The rate of wheezing was not increased in FLUMIST recipients 24 months and older (2.1% FLUMIST versus 2.5% injectable influenza vaccine).

In the same study, an increased rate of hospitalizations (for any cause) through 180 days after final vaccination dose was observed in children 6-11 months of age (6.1% FLUMIST versus 2.6% injectable influenza vaccine). The rate of hospitalizations was not increased in FLUMIST recipients 12 months and older (2.5% FLUMIST versus 2.9% injectable influenza vaccine).

Adverse Reactions in Adults: Twelve placebo controlled studies and three active controlled studies were pooled to evaluate solicited events in adults 18-59 years of age. Table 2 presents an analysis of solicited events occurring in at least 1% of FLUMIST recipients and includes rates for these solicited events from active controlled studies. A total of 3301 adults 18-59 years of age received FLUMIST dosing and provided data for the pooled safety analysis in controlled studies. In these studies, solicited events were documented for 6 days post vaccination.

Table 2: FLUMIST

Summary of Solicited Events Observed During Days 0 to 6 Post Dose in FLUMIST and either Placebo or Active Control Recipients; Adults 18-59 years of age

	Placebo Controlled Studies[a]		Active Controlled Studies[b]	
Solicited Event	**FluMist N=64–3265[c] (%)**	**Placebo N=65–1711[c] (%)**	**FluMist N=10–80[c] (%)**	**Injectable Influenza Vaccine N=11–77[c] (%)**
Any solicited event	69.1	58.9	62.5	58.4
Runny/stuffy nose	43.6	26.2	40.0	33.8
Headache	37.5	34.5	25.0	36.4
Sore throat	24.7	15.2	15.0	11.7
Malaise[d]	23.8	19.3	11.4	20.5
Muscle ache	15.4	13.7	16.3	18.2
Cough	13.1	10.2	18.8	14.3
Chills	7.7	5.6	6.3	6.5
Decreased appetite	5.8	8.9	2.3	9.1
Abdominalpain/stomach ache	4.7	6.2	0.0	9.1
Vomiting	3.5	3.8	2.3	2.3
Fever				
≥38.0°C	0.9	1.2	2.5	0.0
≥38.5°C	0.2	0.4	1.3	0.0
≥39.0°C	0.1	0.0	1.3	0.0

a Includes Studies AV001, AV003, AV004, AV005, AV009, D145-P501, D153-P001, D153-P003, D153-P004, D153-P507, D153-P510 and DMID 98-005.
b Includes Studies AV003, D153-P003, and D153-P004.
c Number of subjects evaluated for the specific solicited event. Range reflects differences in data collection between pooled studies.
d Collected as decreased activity/tiredness/weakness/malaise.

Serious Adverse Events: In the pooled safety analysis for subjects 2 to 17 years of age, 0.45% (129/28,873) of subjects exposed to FLUMIST reported at least 1 serious adverse event (SAE) during Days 0 to 42 post dose in the first year of dosing. The majority of these were either infectious (0.23%) or respiratory (0.05%) events, including gastroenteritis, pneumonia, otitis media, and asthma. Of the 2.22% (182/8,202) subjects who reported at least 1 SAE during Days 0 to 180 post dose in the first year of dosing, the majority reported infectious (1.52%), respiratory (0.28%) or gastrointestinal (0.23%) events, including pneumonia, gastroenteritis, asthma, and otitis media. During Days 0 to 42 post dosing, in studies with an active control, 0.75% (32/4245) of subjects who received FLUMIST and 1.01% (43/4278) subjects who received injectable influenza vaccine reported at least 1 SAE, and in placebo controlled studies, 0.49% (52/10 693) of subjects who received FLUMIST and 0.55% (31/5677) of subjects who received placebo reported at least 1 SAE. During Days 0 to 180 post dosing, in studies with an active control, 2.28% (94/4130) of subjects who received FLUMIST and 2.45% (102/4163) of subjects who received injectable influenza vaccine reported at least 1 SAE, and in placebo controlled studies, 2.91% (70/2408) of subjects who received FLUMIST and 2.72% (42/1546) subjects who received placebo reported at least 1 SAE.

In the pooled safety analysis for subjects 18 to 59 years of age, 0.18% (8/4376) of subjects exposed to FLUMIST reported at least 1 SAE during Days 0 to 28 post dose. Two gastroenteritis events were reported; all other events occurred in 1 subject each. In placebo controlled studies, 0.18% (6/3315) of subjects who received FLUMIST and 0.29% (5/1740) of subjects who received placebo reported at least 1 SAE during Days 0 to 28 post dose.

Death: Among the over 40 000 children and adolescents less than 18 years of age who received FLUMIST in clinical studies, there were eight deaths reported within 180 days of FLUMIST dosing. Of the 8 deaths, 4 occurred within 42 days after the last dose of FLUMIST due to septicemia escherichial and malnutrition protein-calorie, bronchopneumonia, accidental drowning, and accident at home and 4 occurred between 43 and 180 days after FLUMIST dosing due to diarrhea and sepsis, encephalopathy, suffocation, and posterior fossa tumor and malignant hyperthermia.

Among the over 4350 adults 18-59 years of age who received FLUMIST in clinical studies, there were 2 deaths reported within 180 days of FLUMIST dosing: one due to homicide and one due to drowning. In addition, 4 subjects died within 180 days of receipt of concurrent FLUMIST and injectable influenza vaccine in a study that enrolled subjects with stable chronic obstructive pulmonary disease (COPD): two due to COPD; one due to a gastrointestinal hemorrhage; and one due to an acute myocardial infarction.

None of the deaths described in children, adolescents, and adults were considered by the medical monitor or investigator to be related to FLUMIST.

Post-Market Adverse Drug Reactions: The following adverse reactions have been identified during post-approval use of FLUMIST. Because these reactions are reported voluntarily from a population of uncertain size, it is not always possible to reliably estimate their frequency or establish a causal relationship to vaccine exposure.

Congenital, Familial and Genetic: exacerbation of symptoms of mitochondrial encephalomyopathy (Leigh syndrome).
Immune System: hypersensitivity reactions (including anaphylactic reaction, facial edema and urticaria).
Nervous System: Guillain-Barré syndrome, Bell's Palsy.
Respiratory, Thoracic and Mediastinal: epistaxis.
Skin and Subcutaneous Tissue: rash.
DRUG INTERACTIONS: See Table 3.

DOSAGE AND ADMINISTRATION: Recommended Dose and Dosage Adjustment: FLUMIST [influenza vaccine (live, attenuated)] is a spray for intranasal administration by a health care professional. The recommended dose for previously vaccinated and unvaccinated children and adults is:

Age Group	Vaccination Status	Dosage Schedule
Children (2–8 years)	Not previously vaccinated with seasonal influenza vaccine	2 doses (0.2 mL[a] each, at least 4 weeks apart)
	Previously vaccinated with seasonal influenza vaccine	1 dose (0.2 mL[a])
Children, adolescents and adults 9–59 years	Not applicable	1 dose (0.2 mL[a])

a Administer as 0.1 mL per nostril.

For children 2-8 years of age not previously vaccinated with seasonal influenza vaccine, 2 doses of FLUMIST, 4 weeks apart, is recommended.

Annual revaccination with influenza vaccine is recommended because immunity declines over time, and because circulating strains of influenza virus can change from year to year.

Table 3: FLUMIST

Established or Potential Drug-Drug Interactions

FLUMIST	Effect	Clinical comment
Antiviral agents that are active against influenza A and/or B viruses	Not evaluated	Based upon the potential for influenza antiviral agents to reduce the effectiveness of FLUMIST, it is recommended not to administer FLUMIST until 48 hours after the cessation of influenza antiviral therapy. It is recommended not to administer influenza antiviral agents until two weeks after administration of FLUMIST unless medically indicated. If influenza antiviral agents and FLUMIST are administered concomitantly, revaccination should be considered when appropriate.
Aspirin therapy and aspirin-containing therapy	Association of Reye's syndrome with aspirin and wild-type influenza infection.	Those under the age of 18 years receiving aspirin therapy or aspirin-containing therapy should avoid vaccination with FLUMIST. Do not use aspirin-containing therapy for 4 weeks after vaccination with FLUMIST.
Concomitant vaccines	No interaction: measles, mumps, rubella, varicella vaccines	Concurrent administration of FLUMIST has been studied with: • measles, mumps and rubella vaccine (819 children 11 to 23 months of age) • measles, mumps and rubella vaccine and the varicella vaccine (430 children 12 to15 months of age) Adverse events were similar to those seen in other clinical studies with FLUMIST. No evidence of interference with immune responses to measles, mumps, rubella, varicella, or FLUMIST was observed.

Administration: Each sprayer contains a single dose of FLUMIST; approximately one-half of the contents should be administered into each nostril. Once FLUMIST has been administered, the sprayer should be disposed of according to the standard procedures for medical waste (e.g., sharps container or biohazard container).

1. **Check expiration date.** Product must be used before the date on sprayer label.
2. Remove rubber tip protector. Do not remove dose-divider clip at the other end of the sprayer.
3. With the patient in an upright position, place the tip just inside the nostril to ensure FluMist is delivered into the nose.
4. With a single motion, depress plunger **as rapidly as possible** until the dose-divider clip prevents you from going further.
5. Pinch and remove the dose-divider clip from plunger.
6. Place the tip just inside the other nostril and with a single motion, depress plunger **as rapidly as possible** to deliver remaining vaccine.

DO NOT INJECT. DO NOT USE A NEEDLE.

Note: Active inhalation (i.e., sniffing) is not required by the patient during FluMist administration

OVERDOSAGE:

No data are available relevant to overdose with FLUMIST vaccine.

> For management of a suspected drug overdose, contact your regional Poison Control Centre. See the *CPS* Directory section for a list of Poison Control Centres.

ACTION AND CLINICAL PHARMACOLOGY: Mechanism of Action: Immune mechanisms conferring protection against influenza following receipt of FLUMIST vaccine are not fully understood. Likewise, naturally acquired immunity to wild-type influenza has not been completely elucidated. Serum antibodies, mucosal antibodies and influenza-specific T cells may play a role in prevention and recovery from infection.

Influenza illness and its complications follow infection with influenza viruses. Global surveillance of influenza identifies yearly antigenic variants. Antibody against one influenza virus type or subtype confers limited or no protection against another. Furthermore, antibody to one antigenic variant of influenza virus might not protect against a new antigenic variant of the same type or subtype. Frequent development of antigenic variants through antigenic drift is the virologic basis for seasonal epidemics and the reason for the usual change of one or more new strains in each year's influenza vaccine. Therefore, influenza vaccines are standardized to the WHO recommendation (northern hemisphere) to contain the strains (i.e., typically two subtype A and one type B) representing the influenza viruses likely to be circulating in North America in the upcoming winter.

STORAGE AND STABILITY: Store in a refrigerator (2-8°C) upon receipt and until use. **Do not freeze.**

Use the product as indicated by the expiration date on the sprayer label.

INFORMATION FOR THE PATIENT: Published in e-CPS, available by subscription at www.e-cps.ca.

DOSAGE FORMS, COMPOSITION AND PACKAGING: FLUMIST is a spray for intranasal delivery. Each 0.2 mL pre-filled, single-use glass sprayer contains: $10^{6.5\text{-}7.5}$ FFU (fluorescent focus units) of live attenuated influenza virus reassortants of each of the three strains for the specific season. Nonmedicinal ingredients: arginine hydrochloride, dibasic potassium phosphate, gelatin hydrolysate (porcine Type A), gentamicin (a trace residual), monobasic potassium phosphate, monosodium glutamate and sucrose. Preservative-free (e.g., no thimerosal). The intranasal sprayer contains no latex. Packages of 5.

Flunarizine

CPhA Monograph

see *Calcium Channel Blockers*

Flunisolide

CPhA Monograph

see *Corticosteroids: Eye Ear Nose*

Fluocinolone

CPhA Monograph

see *Corticosteroids: Topical*

Fluocinonide

CPhA Monograph

see *Corticosteroids: Topical*

Fluor-A-Day®

sodium fluoride

Dental Caries Prophylaxis

PendoPharm

SUPPLIED: Drops: Each mL of clear, colorless and odorless liquid contains: sodium fluoride USP 5.56 mg (equivalent to 1 mg fluoride ion per 8 drops). Nonmedicinal ingredients: methylparaben and purified water. Bottles of 60 mL.

Tablets: 0.25 mg: Each chewable, train-shaped, white, raspberry-flavored, compressed tablet contains: sodium fluoride USP 0.55 mg (equivalent to 0.25 mg fluoride ion) in a specially formulated anticaries vehicle containing xylitol. Bottles of 120.

0.5 mg: Each chewable, car-shaped, white, raspberry-flavored, compressed tablet contains: sodium fluoride USP 1.10 mg (equivalent to 0.5 mg fluoride ion) in a specially formulated anticaries vehicle containing xylitol. Bottles of 120.

1 mg: Each chewable, airplane-shaped, white, raspberry-flavored, compressed tablet contains: sodium fluoride USP 2.21 mg (equivalent to 1 mg fluoride ion) in a specially formulated anticaries vehicle containing xylitol. Bottles of 120.

Fluorescite®

fluorescein sodium

Ophthalmic Diagnostic Aid

Alcon

SUPPLIED: Each ampul contains: a sterile aqueous solution of fluorescein sodium (equivalent to fluorescein) 10% (5 mL ampuls), or 25% (2 mL ampuls). Sodium hydroxide and/or hydrochloric acid to adjust pH, and water for injection. Store at 8 to 27°C; do not freeze.

Fluorometholone

CPhA Monograph

see *Corticosteroids: Eye Ear Nose*

Fluoroquinolones

besifloxacin
ciprofloxacin
ciprofloxacin HCl
gatifloxacin
levofloxacin
moxifloxacin HCl
norfloxacin
ofloxacin

Anti-infective

CPhA Monograph

Date of Revision: October 2010

> This monograph has been compiled by CPhA and reviewed by experts. It may contain information different from that found in Health Canada-approved Product Monographs. The reader is referred to the *CPS* Editorial Policy for more information.

SUMMARY PRODUCT INFORMATION:

Drug	Route of Administration	Dosage Form	Strength
Besifloxacin	Ophthalmic	Suspension	6 mg/mL
Ciprofloxacin	IV	Solution	2 mg/mL, 10 mg/mL
	Oral	Suspension	10 g/100 mL
		Immediate-release tablet	250 mg, 500 mg, 750 mg
		Extended-release tablet	500 mg, 1000 mg
Ciprofloxacin HCl	Ophthalmic	Ointment	3 mg/g
		Solution	3 mg/mL
Ciprofloxacin HCl/ dexamethasone	Otic	Suspension	ciprofloxacin 3 mg/mL plus dexamethasone 1 mg/mL
Gatifloxacin	Ophthalmic	Solution	3 mg/mL
Levofloxacin	IV	Solution	5 mg/mL
	Oral	Tablet	250 mg, 500 mg, 750 mg
Moxifloxacin HCl	IV	Solution	400 mg/250 mL
	Oral	Tablet	400 mg
	Ophthalmic	Solution	5 mg/mL
Norfloxacin	Oral	Tablet	400 mg
Ofloxacin	Oral	Tablet	200 mg, 300 mg, 400 mg
	Ophthalmic	Solution	0.3%

PHARMACOLOGY: The original quinolone anti-infective agent was nalidixic acid, a 1,8-naphthyridine compound that was identified among the by-products of quinine synthesis. The addition of a fluorine atom at position 6 distinguishes fluoroquinolones from the basic quinolone structure. Other structural modifications have led to the development of agents with improved antibacterial spectra and varying pharmacokinetic properties and toxicities.

The mechanism of action of fluoroquinolones is believed to be inhibition of bacterial DNA synthesis, specifically targeting types II and IV topoisomerases. These enzymes prevent excessive positive supercoiling of cellular DNA that tends to occur during and after replication. This ultimately leads to arrested DNA replication and cell death. Generally, inhibition of topoisomerase type IV is associated with activity versus gram-positive bacteria, while inhibition of topoisomerase type II (DNA gyrase) correlates with activity against gram-negative organisms.

Fluoroquinolones exhibit concentration-dependent bacterial killing, with a post-antibiotic effect (the time period after which surviving bacteria resume growth following exposure to an antibacterial agent) of about 1 to 2 hours. Bacterial killing against gram-negative infections is reported to be optimal when the ratio of the peak serum drug concentration to the minimum inhibitory concentration is approximately 10:1 to 12:1 in immunocompetent patients and higher in immunocompromised patients.

Quinolones have been classified into four generations based mainly on their spectra of activity, although third- and fourth-generation agents are not classified consistently by different authors. Generally, ciprofloxacin, norfloxacin and ofloxacin have expanded gram-negative coverage over first-generation quinolones (nalidixic acid), as well as activity against some atypical pathogens. Levofloxacin (the L-isomer of ofloxacin) and moxifloxacin, often termed the "respiratory quinolones," add gram-positive coverage, including penicillin-resistant *S. pneumoniae*. Moxifloxacin has some activity versus anaerobes, including the *B. fragilis* group. Ciprofloxacin possesses the highest antipseudomonal potency of the quinolones although resistance is not uncommon. The spectra of activity of the fluoroquinolones are presented in Table 1. Gatifloxacin, oral and iv, was voluntarily withdrawn from the Canadian market as of June 2006; an ophthalmic preparation is still available.

Proposed mechanisms of resistance to fluoroquinolones include chromosomal mutations that lead to modification of the target sites (DNA gyrase and topoisomerase IV), changes in the diffusion channels of the outer bacterial membrane and multidrug-resistance efflux pumps that actively extrude drug from the cytoplasm. Resistance can develop rapidly, even during a single course of therapy, particularly with Pseudomonas species.

Pharmacokinetics: Absorption: The fluoroquinolones are well absorbed following oral administration. Peak serum drug concentrations occur within 1 to 3 hours.

Distribution: With the exception of norfloxacin, which does not distribute well into tissues with its lower bioavailability, fluoroquinolones penetrate well into tissues, achieving concentrations comparable to and sometimes higher than those in plasma, in tissues such as the bronchial mucosa, lung, gallbladder, prostate and genital tract. They also reach high concentrations in neutrophils and macrophages, which contributes to their activity against intracellular pathogens such as *C. pneumoniae*, *M. pneumoniae* and *L. pneumophila*. CSF levels are much lower than serum concentrations, even in the presence of inflamed meninges. Those fluoroquinolones whose primary route of elimination is renal reach high concentrations in kidney tissue and in the urine.

Elimination: Some quinolones are eliminated primarily by the kidney; others are metabolized in the liver to varying degrees, and then excreted via the kidneys or gut.

Levofloxacin, norfloxacin and ofloxacin are eliminated through the kidney with minimal hepatic metabolism. Dosage adjustment is required in patients with reduced renal function.

Ciprofloxacin is eliminated mostly unchanged in the urine (about 60%) and feces (about 40%). Dosage adjustment may be necessary in patients with significant renal impairment.

Moxifloxacin is metabolized in the liver, mainly via conjugation, rather than through cytochrome P450 oxidative metabolism. The resulting inactive conjugates are excreted in the urine and feces. Dosage adjustment is usually not required in patients with mild to moderate hepatic insufficiency. The manufacturer recommends this agent not be used in patients with severe hepatic impairment.

The half-lives of the fluoroquinolones range from 4 to 14 hours. Ciprofloxacin and norfloxacin are administered every 12 hours. Levofloxacin (for most indications), moxifloxacin and ofloxacin are administered every 24 hours. The iv and oral doses of levofloxacin and moxifloxacin are equivalent.

Pharmacokinetic parameters of individual fluoroquinolones are presented in Table 2.

INDICATIONS: The specific clinical role of individual fluoroquinolone agents is the subject of debate, primarily concerned with the risk of emerging bacterial resistance. Because of this, recommendations and policies on the use of fluoroquinolones vary among health care institutions and organizations and may not reflect the approved indications for each agent.

Health Canada-approved Indications: Besifloxacin, ciprofloxacin, gatifloxacin, moxifloxacin and ofloxacin ophthalmic solutions, suspensions or ointments are used in the treatment of acute superficial infections of the eye, such as bacterial conjunctivitis, when caused by susceptible bacteria. Ciprofloxacin is used topically in combination with dexamethasone in the management of otitis externa when caused by susceptible bacteria.

Table 3 summarizes the indications approved by Health Canada for systemic use of fluoroquinolones.

Systemic ciprofloxacin can be used in treatment of the following infections when caused by susceptible bacteria: respiratory infections including acute exacerbations of chronic bronchitis, acute sinusitis and pneumonia, although not first-line therapy if *S. pneumoniae* is a suspected pathogen; uncomplicated or complicated urinary tract infections; prostatitis; bone and joint infections; skin and soft tissue infections; infectious diarrhea; typhoid fever; eradication of meningococci in carriers (not indicated for treatment of meningococcal meningitis); intra-abdominal infections, in combination with other agents; and febrile neutropenia, in combination with other agents. Ciprofloxacin extended release tablets are only indicated for urinary tract infections, when caused by susceptible bacteria.

In general, norfloxacin is used only in the treatment of infections of the urinary tract, when caused by susceptible bacteria.

Levofloxacin and moxifloxacin, also termed "respiratory quinolones", are principally for the treatment of community-acquired pneumonia (CAP). According to the Infectious Disease Society of America/American Thoracic Society Consensus Guidelines on the Management of Community-Acquired Pneumonia in Adults [*Clin Infect Dis* 2007;44(Suppl 2):S27-72], respiratory quinolones are suggested as first-line initial therapy in the outpatient management of CAP in patients with medical comorbidities (e.g., chronic lung, heart, liver or renal disease, diabetes, alcoholism, malignancies, asplenia or immunosuppression) or risk factors for drug-resistant *S. pneumoniae* such as use of antimicrobials within the past 3 months. They are also first-line agents for CAP in patients admitted to hospital (non-ICU). Selection of empiric therapy should also be based on local epidemiology and resistance patterns. Respiratory quinolones are also used for the treatment of acute bacterial sinusitis and acute bacterial exacerbations of COPD.

Moxifloxacin is indicated for the treatment of complicated intra-abdominal infections due to polymicrobial or monomicrobial infections caused by *B. fragilis*, *B. thetaiotaomicron*, *C. perfringens*, *E. faecalis* (vancomycin-sensitive strains only), *E. coli*, *P. mirabilis* and *S. anginosus*. Moxifloxacin is also indicated for the treatment of complicated skin and skin structure infections in hospitalized patients, when caused by susceptible strains of *E. cloacae*, *E. coli*, *K. pneumoniae* or *S. aureus*.

Uses Without Health Canada Approval: Table 4 summarizes uses of fluoroquinolones without Health Canada approval.

Anthrax: Ciprofloxacin is recommended for post-exposure prophylaxis and treatment of cutaneous and inhalational anthrax [*JAMA* 2002;287(17):2236-52].

Bone and Joint Infections: Fluoroquinolones may be used in the treatment of osteomyelitis caused by susceptible organisms [*Semin Plast Surg* 2009;23(2):90-9].

Table 1: Fluoroquinolones

Spectra of Activity[a]

Quinolone	Gram-negative Coverage	Gram-positive Coverage	Atypical Pathogens	Other
Besifloxacin[b]	*H. influenzae*[c]	*S. aureus* (methicillin-sensitive) *S. epidermidis* *S. pneumoniae* *S. mitis* *S. oralis*	—	—
Ciprofloxacin	Enterobacteriaceae[d] Acinetobacter Aeromonas *H. influenzae*[c] *M. catarrhalis* *N. gonorrhoeae*[e] *N. meningitidis* *P. aeruginosa* *P. multocida*	*S. aureus* (methicillin-sensitive)	*L. pneumophila* *M. pneumoniae* *C. pneumoniae*	*B. anthracis* some Mycobacterium spp.
Gatifloxacin[b]	*H. influenzae*[c]	*S. aureus* (methicillin-sensitive) *S. epidermidis* *S. pneumoniae*	—	—
Levofloxacin	Enterobacteriaceae[d] Acinetobacter Aeromonas *H. influenzae*[c] *M. catarrhalis* *N. gonorrhoeae*[e] *N. meningitidis* *P. multocida*	*S. aureus* (methicillin-sensitive) Streptococci, Groups A, B, C and G *S. pneumoniae*	*L. pneumophila* *M. pneumoniae* *C. pneumoniae*	*B. anthracis* *C. trachomatis* Mycobacterium spp.
Moxifloxacin	Enterobacteriaceae[d] Acinetobacter Aeromonas *H. influenzae*[c] *M. catarrhalis* *N. gonorrhoeae*[e] *N. meningitidis* *P. multocida*	*S. aureus* (methicillin-sensitive) Streptococci, Groups A, B, C and G *S. pneumoniae*	*L. pneumophila* *M. pneumoniae* *C. pneumoniae*	*B. anthracis* Mycobacterium spp.
Norfloxacin[f]	Enterobacteriaceae[d] Acinetobacter Aeromonas	—		
Ofloxacin	Enterobacteriaceae[d] Acinetobacter Aeromonas *H. influenzae*[c] *M. catarrhalis* *N. gonorrhoeae*[e] *N. meningitidis* *P. multocida*	*S. aureus* (methicillin-sensitive)	*L. pneumophila* *M. pneumoniae* *C. pneumoniae*	*C. trachomatis* some Mycobacterium spp.

[a] Organisms are included if they are usually sensitive to the agent in question. Differences in sensitivity exist among various regions and health care institutions.
[b] Spectrum of activity of ophthalmic preparation only.
[c] Includes beta-lactamase-producing strains.
[d] Includes most clinically important species, such as Citrobacter, Enterobacter, Klebsiella, Morganella, Providencia, Salmonella, Serratia and Shigella spp as well as *P. mirabilis*, *P. vulgaris*, *Y. enterocolitica* and *E. coli*.
[e] Quinolone resistance among *N. gonorrhoeae* has increased in the last several years with a 28% incidence reported in Ontario in 2006 [*CMAJ* 2009;180(3):287-90].
[f] Urinary tract pathogens only.

Crohn's Disease: While the exact role of antibiotics in the treatment of Crohn's disease is under debate, ciprofloxacin (+/- metronidazole) has been used as an alternative treatment in mild-moderate colonic Crohn's disease. It is also used in the treatment of pouchitis and perianal fistulae. It is not generally used to treat ulcerative colitis [*Inflamm Bowel Dis* 2006;12(7):651-64].

Endocarditis: Ciprofloxacin, levofloxacin or moxifloxacin are alternative agents in the treatment of endocarditis caused by HACEK organisms (*Haemophilus parainfluenzae*, *H. aphrophilus*, *Actinobacillus actinomycetemcomitans*, *Cardiobacterium hominis*, *Eikenella corrodens* and *Kingella kingae*) [*Circulation* 2005;111:3167-84].

Mycobacterial Infections: Levofloxacin and moxifloxacin are considered alternative agents as part of a multi-drug regimen for the treatment of drug-resistant *M. tuberculosis* [*Am J Respir Crit Care Med* 2003;167(4):603-62; *Canadian Tuberculosis Standards 2007*, 6th ed.].

In cases of treatment failure with first-line agents, ciprofloxacin, levofloxacin or moxifloxacin may be considered in a multi-drug regimen for the treatment of *Mycobacterium avium* complex infections although evidence of efficacy is minimal [*MMWR Recomm Rep* 2009;58(RR-4):1-207].

Table 2: Fluoroquinolones

Pharmacokinetic Parameters (Oral Administration)

Fluoroquinolone	Absorption (%)	Bioavailability (%)	Time to Peak Concentration (hours)	Volume of Distribution (L/kg)	Protein Binding (%)	Elimination Half-life (hours)	Principal Route of Elimination
Ciprofloxacin	Rapid, 50–85	70–80	Immediate release: 0.5–2 Extended release: 1–2.5	2–3	20–30	Children: 2.5 Adults (normal renal function): 3–5	Renal
Levofloxacin	Rapid and complete	>99	1–2	0.92–1.36	24–38	6–8	Renal
Moxifloxacin	Well absorbed	~90	0.75–3.5	1.7–2.7	~50	Oral: 12 IV: 15	Hepatic
Norfloxacin	<40	Not available	1–1.5	3.2±1.4	~15	3	Renal
Ofloxacin	Rapid and complete	98	1.2–2.4	2.4–3.5	~20	9	Renal

Table 3: Fluoroquinolones:

Health Canada-approved Indications of Systemic Fluoroquinolones

Indications	Ciprofloxacin[a]	Levofloxacin	Moxifloxacin	Norfloxacin	Ofloxacin
Acute sinusitis	•[b]	•	•		
Acute exacerbation of chronic bronchitis	•	•	•		•
Pneumonia	•	•	•		•
Bone and joint infections	•				
Infectious diarrhea	•				
Complicated intra-abdominal infections	•[c]		•		
Febrile neutropenia	•[d]				
Pelvic inflammatory disease[e]					•[f]
Urethritis or cervicitis[e]	•[f]			•[g]	•[f]
Prostatitis	•	•			•
Urinary tract infections (uncomplicated/complicated UTIs, pyelonephritis)	•	•		•	•
Septicemia	•				
Skin and soft tissue infections	•	•	•		•
Typhoid fever	•				
Elimination of *N. meningitidis* nasopharyngeal colonization[h]	•				

[a] Extended-release ciprofloxacin tablets are only approved for urinary tract infections.
[b] Ciprofloxacin is no longer recommended for acute sinusitis because of poor coverage of *S. pneumoniae*. Fluoroquinolones should be reserved for (severe situations) due to the concern of resistance associated with overuse [Anti-infective Review Panel. *Anti-infective Guidelines for Community-acquired Infections*. Toronto: MUMS Guideline Clearinghouse; 2010].
[c] Used IV in combination with metronidazole.
[d] Used empirically in combination with piperacillin.
[e] According to the Canadian Sexually Transmitted Infections guidelines update 2008, due to the rapid increase in quinolone resistant *N. gonorrhoeae*, quinolones may be considered as an alternative treatment option only if quinolone susceptibility is demonstrated.
[f] Due to *N. gonorrhoeae* or *C. trachomatis*.
[g] Due to *N. gonorrhoeae*.
[h] Not indicated for the treatment of meningococcal meningitis.

Sexually Transmitted Infections: According to the Canadian Sexually Transmitted Infections guidelines update 2008, quinolones are no longer preferred drugs for the treatment of gonococcal infections. However, uncomplicated gonorrhea involving the urethra, cervix, rectum or pharynx can be treated with ciprofloxacin (or ofloxacin—approved use) but only if antimicrobial susceptibility demonstrates sensitivity to quinolones. Levofloxacin (or ofloxacin—approved use) in combination with metronidazole (optional) are alternative regimens as outpatient therapy for pelvic inflammatory disease (PID). Alternative parenteral therapies for PID in an inpatient setting include either ciprofloxacin plus doxycycline or levofloxacin; the addition of metronidazole should be considered for anaerobic coverage. Ciprofloxacin is a first-line option for the treatment of chancroid and is considered an alternative treatment of granuloma inguinale [*Canadian Guidelines on Sexually Transmitted Infections*, 2008 ed.].

Traveller's Diarrhea: Levofloxacin, norfloxacin and ofloxacin have also been used for the prevention and treatment of traveller's diarrhea where appropriate [*Can Commun Dis Rep* 2001;27:1-12].

Typhoid Fever: Ciprofloxacin (approved use) or ofloxacin are preferred treatment options for typhoid fever when susceptibility is demonstrated. Nalidixic acid resistance is commonly used as an indicator of reduced susceptibility to fluoroquinolones and a predictor of poor clinical response. Ideally, minimum inhibitory concentrations for specific fluoroquinolones should be obtained if nalidixic acid-resistant *S. typhi* is detected [*JAMA* 2009;302(8):859-65].

Fluoroquinolones are used in other bacterial infections where susceptibility is demonstrated, e.g., osteomyelitis, septicemia. The results of culture and sensitivity testing should guide the completion of therapy.

Table 4: Fluoroquinolones

Uses Without Health Canada Approval

Indication	Ciprofloxacin	Levofloxacin	Moxifloxacin	Norfloxacin	Ofloxacin
Anthrax	•				
Bone and joint infections		•	•		•
Crohn's disease	•				
Infectious diarrhea		•		•	•
Infective endocarditis	•	•	•		
Pelvic inflammatory disease	•	•			
Septicemia		•	•		
Drug-resistant tuberculosis		•	•		
Typhoid fever					•

CONTRAINDICATIONS: Patients who are hypersensitive to a fluoroquinolone or to any ingredient in the formulation or component of the container.

According to the manufacturer of ciprofloxacin, the concurrent administration of ciprofloxacin and tizanidine is contraindicated due to a significant increase in serum tizanidine and subsequent clinically significant side effects (see Drug Interactions).

WARNINGS: See Precautions.

PRECAUTIONS: Cardiovascular: Dose-related prolongation of the QT interval has been reported with several fluoroquinolones. Torsades de pointes has occurred rarely. The incidence of QT prolongation has varied among the fluoroquinolones in post-marketing studies and whether it is a class effect is controversial. It appears to be only rarely (<1 per million) associated with ciprofloxacin use.

QT prolongation is associated with a risk of developing potentially life-threatening ventricular arrhythmias such as torsades de pointes, particularly in the presence of hypokalemia or hypomagnesemia. Because of this, some fluoroquinolone product monographs include recommendations to either avoid the drug in question or use it with caution in patients known to have risk factors such as pre-existing QT prolongation or concurrent drug therapy that also can prolong the QT interval (e.g., azole antifungals, erythromycin, clarithromycin, methadone and antiarrhythmic agents such as amiodarone, procainamide, quinidine and sotalol). Further experience with fluoroquinolones will shed more light on the risk associated with individual agents.

Central Nervous System: Seizures, increased intracranial pressure, toxic psychosis, CNS stimulation including hallucinations, agitation, tremors and other symptoms have been reported in patients taking fluoroquinolones, sometimes following the first dose. Fluoroquinolones should be used with caution in patients with a history of CNS disorders such as epilepsy or those predisposed to seizures, e.g., patients on drug therapy that lowers the seizure threshold. Fluoroquinolones should be discontinued if serious CNS side effects occur.

Dermatologic: Moderate to severe phototoxicity reactions have occurred in patients taking certain fluoroquinolones, particularly agents that are halogenated at position 8 (in addition to the fluorine atom at position 6). Such agents (e.g., lomefloxacin, sparfloxacin) are not available in Canada. Phototoxic reactions develop within just a few hours after administration of the drug and may occur in virtually any patient who has received sufficient drug dosage and sufficient intensity and duration of ultraviolet exposure. Patients should avoid direct sun or other ultraviolet light exposure while taking fluoroquinolones and discontinue their use if a phototoxic reaction occurs.

Skin rashes have occurred in patients taking fluoroquinolones (see Precautions, Hypersensitivity).

Endocrine: Hypoglycemia has occurred in patients taking fluoroquinolones, particularly when combined with oral hypoglycemic agents. Close monitoring of blood glucose is important when fluoroquinolones are used in patients taking oral hypoglycemic agents. Hyperglycemia has also been reported in patients receiving fluoroquinolones. Hypo- and hyperglycemia appear to be reported more often in gatifloxacin-treated patients. Gatifloxacin, oral and iv, is no longer available in Canada as of June 2006.

Gastrointestinal: Pseudomembranous colitis has been reported with every class of antibacterial agents, including fluoroquinolones. This possibility should be considered when patients present with diarrhea subsequent to taking fluoroquinolones.

Hepatic: Elevations in ALT, AST, ALP and total bilirubin levels have been reported; liver enzyme abnormalities are mild and reversible upon fluoroquinolone discontinuation. There have been reports of more serious hepatic disorders including hepatitis and hepatic failure with levofloxacin and moxifloxacin.

Hemodynamic: Intravenous doses of fluoroquinolones should be given by slow infusion over 60 minutes to avoid causing hypotension or other adverse effects such as seizures.

Hypersensitivity: Serious hypersensitivity reactions, including anaphylaxis and death, have occurred during fluoroquinolone therapy, sometimes following the first dose. Fluoroquinolones should be discontinued if a hypersensitivity reaction is suspected.

Musculoskeletal: Tendinopathy, including tendinitis or tendon rupture requiring surgical repair, has occurred with the use of fluoroquinolones, primarily involving the shoulder joint, hand or Achilles tendon. It appears to occur more often in men, the elderly or in patients who have recently taken corticosteroids. If tendinitis occurs, fluoroquinolone therapy should be discontinued, physical exercise should be avoided and a physician consulted. Arthropathy has also been reported with fluoroquinolone use. Joint pain, stiffness and swelling of weight-bearing joints are common clinical manifestations. It appears to occur in younger patients. If arthropathy occurs, fluoroquinolone therapy should be discontinued and a physician consulted.

Ophthalmic: Ophthalmic solutions of besifloxacin, ciprofloxacin, gatifloxacin, moxifloxacin or ofloxacin must **not** be injected into the eye.

Otic: Ciprofloxacin otic drops are not for injection and not to be used in the eye.

Renal: Crystalluria has been reported rarely with the use of fluoroquinolones. Adequate hydration should be maintained to avoid this occurrence.

Resistance: The development of resistance to fluoroquinolones is of concern. Since their introduction, fluoroquinolone resistance has increased substantially among strains of *C. jejuni* and *N. gonorrhoeae* as well as some other gram-negative species. The prevalence of fluoroquinolone-resistant strains of *S. pneumoniae* has been shown to correlate with the frequency of fluoroquinolone use. Prudent use of these agents is encouraged to curb growing resistance.

Pregnant Women: While not every fluoroquinolone has been studied, ciprofloxacin and ofloxacin have been shown to cross the placenta, and the other agents are expected to as well, based on their structure and molecular weight. Fluoroquinolones have not been proven to be associated with a specific or increased risk of malformations in the developing fetus. However, it is generally recommended that these agents not be used during pregnancy, especially during the 1st trimester, as safer alternatives are usually available.

Nursing Women: Fluoroquinolones are excreted in breast milk. When first marketed, their use during lactation was not recommended because of the potential for arthropathy or other toxicity in exposed infants; however, there is little clinical evidence of harmful effects of fluoroquinolone exposure through lactation. Based on the limited data available, the American Academy of Pediatrics considers ciprofloxacin and ofloxacin to be compatible with breast-feeding.

Pediatrics: Mainly because of concerns about cartilage toxicity in studies of juvenile animals and because fluoroquinolones have not been extensively studied in children, their use has been discouraged in children under 18 years. Further, except for ciprofloxacin, little is known about their pharmacokinetics in the pediatric population. However, they have been used in children and some expert groups recommend that they be formally studied because of their potential usefulness in the treatment of serious infections such as acute pulmonary exacerbations of cystic fibrosis, febrile neutropenia or infections involving resistant *S. pneumoniae*, Pseudomonas, multidrug-resistant gram-negative bacilli or severe enteric infections caused by *Salmonella* and *Shigella* spp. Further evidence will clarify whether fluoroquinolones have the same safety profile in children as in adults or whether there is an additional risk specific to the pediatric population.

Drug Interactions: General: Ciprofloxacin, norfloxacin and ofloxacin are inhibitors of the cytochrome P450 isoenzyme, CYP1A2, and can decrease the clearance of substrates of this isoenzyme.

Agents that Prolong the QT Interval: Because some fluoroquinolones may prolong the QT interval, caution is advised when administering with other agents associated with QT interval prolongation. See Precautions, Cardiovascular.

Antacids, Metallic Cations: The extent of absorption and consequently the bioavailability of fluoroquinolones can be substantially reduced in the presence of sucralfate (up to 98% when given within 2 hours of fluoroquinolone administration) or metallic cations, e.g., aluminum, calcium, iron, magnesium or zinc. In general, it is recommended that doses of fluoroquinolones be separated by several hours (up to 8) from doses of sucralfate or metallic cations; however, it is uncertain whether this will completely eliminate the risk of subtherapeutic fluoroquinolone levels. Ideally, these agents should be avoided or alternatives used during the course of fluoroquinolone therapy.

Anticoagulants, Oral: There have been case reports of an enhanced hypoprothrombinemic response to warfarin in patients taking these agents concomitantly. The clinical significance of this interaction is controversial. Consider increased monitoring of INR when fluoroquinolones are initiated or discontinued in patients taking warfarin.

Caffeine: As inhibitors of CYP1A2, ciprofloxacin, norfloxacin and ofloxacin can significantly reduce the metabolism of caffeine and enhance its side effects. Advise patients to minimize their caffeine intake during therapy.

Hypoglycemic Agents, Oral: Hypoglycemia has occurred in patients taking oral glyburide who were prescribed ciprofloxacin or gatifloxacin, possibly because of decreased metabolism of the glyburide. Monitor patients taking oral hypoglycemic agents for enhanced hypoglycemic effect during therapy with a fluoroquinolone. Gatifloxacin, oral and iv, was voluntarily withdrawn from the Canadian market as of June 2006.

Methadone: The use of fluoroquinolones may increase the toxicity of methadone via two independent mechanisms. Methadone is metabolized by CYP 1A2 and therefore its use with ciprofloxacin, norfloxacin and ofloxacin can result in elevated serum levels. Since methadone is also associated with dose-dependent QT prolongation concomitant use with some fluoroquinolones may enhance this effect. If a fluoroquinolone is deemed necessary monitor for side effects, including cardiovascular parameters, of methadone carefully.

NSAIDs: A few case reports and animal studies suggest there may be an increased risk of seizures when NSAIDs and fluoroquinolones are used concomitantly. Although the risk appears low, caution is advised in individuals at risk of seizures, e.g., impaired renal function, seizure disorder.

Probenecid: By blocking their tubular secretion, probenecid may prolong the half-life and increase serum levels of renally excreted fluoroquinolones. The clinical significance of this interaction is not known but should be considered when the drugs are used concomitantly. Monitor for adverse effects.

Theophylline: Because it is a major substrate of CYP1A2, theophylline's clearance can be significantly reduced by ciprofloxacin, norfloxacin and ofloxacin, which are inhibitors of the isoenzyme. Theophylline toxicity can result. Monitor patients for signs of toxicity if theophylline is used concomitantly with ciprofloxacin, norfloxacin or ofloxacin. Consider monitoring theophylline levels.

Tizanidine: Ciprofloxacin is contraindicated in combination with tizanidine. Ciprofloxacin decreases the metabolism of tizanidine, likely through inhibition of CYP 1A2, thereby increasing its toxicity (decreased blood pressure and heart rate, dizziness and drowsiness). Although not reported, this interaction may theoretically occur with norfloxacin and ofloxacin as they are strong inhibitors of CYP 1A2.

ADVERSE EFFECTS: (See also Precautions): Although fluoroquinolones are generally well tolerated, certain adverse effects are relatively common (approximately 2% to 20%) with all agents in the class, including gastrointestinal symptoms such as nausea, vomiting, diarrhea and abdominal pain, and CNS effects such as headache, dizziness, drowsiness, insomnia, restlessness and tremor.

Less common adverse effects (<1%) include manic reactions (reported most often with ciprofloxacin) and taste perversion. Many other adverse effects have been included in fluoroquinolone product monographs; however, a causal relationship with the fluoroquinolone was not necessarily established.

OVERDOSAGE:

Symptoms: Serious toxicity resulting from acute fluoroquinolone overdose is uncommon. Rarely, seizures or renal failure have occurred. Seizures may be due to inhibition of GABA, possibly due to chelation of synaptic magnesium. Some fluoroquinolones may prolong the QT interval.

Treatment: Management of fluoroquinolone overdose is mainly supportive. In patients with very large ingestions, the administration of activated charcoal within 1 hour of ingestion may limit systemic exposure. Adequate hydration is important. ECG monitoring may be recommended due to possible QT-prolongation. Seizures can be treated with benzodiazepines. Barbiturates can be added if necessary, to increase GABA activity. With the exception of moxifloxacin, fluoroquinolones are not readily removed by dialysis.

For management of a suspected drug overdose, CPhA recommends that you contact your **regional Poison Control Centre**. See the *CPS* Directory section for a list of Poison Control Centres.

DOSAGE: General adult dosing information is presented in Table 5. While fluoroquinolones have been used in children, their use is generally restricted to very specific indications and is, ideally, monitored by infectious disease specialists (see also Precautions, Pediatrics). Ciprofloxacin has been given to children in doses of 20 to 30 mg/kg/day po or iv divided every 12 hours with maximum doses of 1.5 g/day orally and 800 mg/day iv. Children with cystic fibrosis have received up to 40 mg/kg/day divided every 12 hours with a maximum of 2 g/day orally.

Dose and duration of therapy in adults often depend on the susceptibility and severity of the infection and response to the fluoroquinolone. Some patients whose initial therapy is iv may be switched to oral therapy to complete the course, if deemed appropriate by the clinician. Consult individual product monographs and specialized references for further information.

Table 5: Fluoroquinolones

Adult Dosage[a]

Drug	Oral[b]	IV	Ophthalmic[c] or Otic	Comments
Besifloxacin	N/A	N/A	1 drop 3 times daily for 7 days.	Ophthalmic Drops: Not for injection into the eye.
Ciprofloxacin	500–1500 mg per day, usually in 2 divided doses (Q12H) for 7–14 days. *N. meningitidis* nasopharyngeal colonization: 750 mg as a single dose. Traveller's diarrhea treatment: 500 mg Q12H for 3 days. Uncomplicated UTI: 500 mg once daily (extended release) or 250 mg Q12H (immediate-release) for 3 days. Complicated UTI or pyelonephritis: increase dose to 1000 mg daily for 7–14 days.	400–1200 mg per day, in 2 to 3 divided doses.[d]	Ophthalmic Drops (usual dose): 1–2 drops of 0.3% solution every 2 h while awake for 2 days then 2 drops every 4 h while awake for 5 days. Ophthalmic Ointment (usual dose): Apply a 1.25 cm ribbon of 0.3% ointment 3 times daily for 2 days then twice daily for 5 days. Otic Drops (ciprofloxacin 0.3% in combination with dexamethasone 0.1%): Shake suspension well and instill 4 drops twice daily for 7 days.	Oral: Absorbed faster on an empty stomach. Oral suspension must be mixed properly with the provided diluent and shaken vigorously for 15 seconds prior to each dose. Suspension is stable at room temperature and under refrigeration for 14 days. Ophthalmic Drops: Not for injection into the eye. Otic Drops: Not for injection; not to be used in the eye.
Gatifloxacin	N/A	N/A	1 drop every 2 h (max 8 times/day) for 2 days then 1 drop 4 times daily for days 3–7.	Ophthalmic Drops: Not for injection into the eye.
Levofloxacin	Usual dose is 250–750 mg once daily. Duration ranges from 3 days to 10–14 days. Chronic bacterial prostatitis is treated for 28 days.	Same as oral dose.[d]	N/A	Oral: May be taken with or without food.
Moxifloxacin	400 mg once daily for all indications, for 5–21 days.	Same as oral dose.[d]	1 drop 3 times daily for a total of 7 days.	Oral: May be taken with or without food. Ophthalmic Drops: Not for injection into the eye.
Norfloxacin	400 mg Q12H for 7–10 days.	N/A	N/A	Oral: Take on an empty stomach.
Ofloxacin	300–400 mg Q12H for 7–14 days. Prostatitis due to *E.coli* is treated for 6 weeks.	N/A	1–2 drops every 2–4 h for 2 days then 1–2 drops 4 times daily for 8 days.	Oral: May be taken with or without food. Ophthalmic Drops: Not for injection into the eye.

[a] All patients taking fluoroquinolones should be advised to drink plenty of fluids to prevent crystalluria, to consult their physician or pharmacist about discontinuing products that contain aluminum, calcium, magnesium, iron or zinc during therapy, separating the doses by several hours or using alternate therapy while taking the fluoroquinolone and to avoid exposure to direct sunlight or other sources of ultraviolet light.

[b] Indicated duration of therapy is for majority of infections. Exceptions exist, however not all exceptions are listed, e.g., single dose therapy for gonorrhea, longer term therapy for osteomyelitis (up to 3 months). See individual monographs.

[c] The use of contact lenses should be avoided during therapy. Patients should be instructed on how to avoid contaminating the tip of the eye dropper bottle.

[d] Fluoroquinolones should be properly diluted and given by slow iv infusion, over 60 minutes.

Table 6: Ciprofloxacin

Dose in Adult Patients with Renal Impairment

Creatinine Clearance	Dosage Adjustment
>50 mL/min	Usual dose
10–50 mL/min	50–75%
<10 mL/min	50%

Renal Impairment: Dosage in renal impairment for ciprofloxacin, levofloxacin, norfloxacin and ofloxacin appears in Table 6, Table 7, Table 8 and Table 9, respectively. No dosage adjustment is required for moxifloxacin in renal impairment.

Table 7: Levofloxacin

Dose in Adult Patients with Renal Impairment

Creatinine Clearance	Dosage and Interval Adjustment
>50 mL/min	Usual dose
10–50 mL/min	Initial dose 500–750 mg, then 250–750 mg Q24–48H
<10 mL/min	Initial dose 500 mg, then 250–500 mg Q48H

Table 8: Norfloxacin

Dose in Adult Patients with Renal Impairment

Creatinine Clearance	Interval Adjustment
>50 mL/min	Q12H
10–50 mL/min	Q12–24H
<10 mL/min	Q24H

Table 9: Ofloxacin

Dose in Adult Patients with Renal Impairment

Creatinine Clearance	Dosage and Interval Adjustment
>50 mL/min	Usual dose
10–50 mL/min	200–400 mg Q24H
<10 mL/min	200 mg Q24H

Fluorouracil Injection

5-fluorouracil

Antineoplastic

Sandoz

SUPPLIED: Each mL of solution contains: 5-fluorouracil USP 50 mg, water for injection; sodium hydroxide is added to solubilize the compound and as a pH adjuster. Pharmacy bulk vials of 100 mL containing 5000 mg fluorouracil USP, packs of 1. Latex-free stoppers: stoppers contain no dry natural rubber. Although Fluorouracil Injection (5-fluorouracil) solution may discolour slightly during storage, the potency, and safety are not adversely affected, and are maintained until the expiry date. Store between 15 and 30°C. Protect from light. Do not freeze.

Fluorouracil Injection USP

5-fluorouracil

Antineoplastic

Hospira

SUPPLIED: Each mL of sterile aqueous solution contains: 5-fluorouracil (5-FU) 50 mg. Nonmedicinal ingredients: none. May contain sodium hydroxide as pH adjusters. Contains no preservative. Pharmacy bulk ONCO-TAIN clear glass vials of 100 mL, cartons of 1. Store between 15 and 25°C. Protect from light and heat. Discard unused portion.

Fluoxetine

CPhA Monograph

see *Selective Serotonin Reuptake Inhibitors*

Fluphenazine

fluphenazine decanoate—fluphenazine HCl

Antipsychotic

CPhA Monograph

Date of Revision: October 2010

This monograph has been compiled by CPhA and reviewed by experts. It may contain information different from that found in Health Canada-approved Product Monographs. The reader is referred to the *CPS* Editorial Policy for more information.

SUMMARY PRODUCT INFORMATION:

Fluphenazine Salt	Route of Administration	Dosage Form	Strength
Fluphenazine HCl	Oral	Tablet	1 mg, 2 mg, 2.5 mg, 5 mg
Fluphenazine decanoate	IM	Long-acting injection	25 mg/mL, 100 mg/mL

PHARMACOLOGY: Fluphenazine is a high-potency, short-acting piperazine phenothiazine antipsychotic. The ability of phenothiazines to ameliorate the positive symptoms of psychotic disorders (hallucinations, delusions) is believed to be mediated by antagonism of postsynaptic dopamine D_2 receptors in the mesolimbic tract. Extrapyramidal side effects and hyperprolactinemia have been attributed to antagonism of postsynaptic D_2 receptors in the nigrostriatal and tuberoinfundibular dopaminergic tracts, respectively.

Fluphenazine also weakly antagonizes histamine H_1 receptors (associated with sedation and weight gain), alpha$_1$ adrenergic receptors (orthostatic hypotension, reflex tachycardia) and muscarinic M_1 receptors (anticholinergic effects such as dry mouth, dry eyes, blurred vision, constipation and urinary retention). Because fluphenazine has a higher affinity for D_2 receptors than for H_1, M_1 or alpha$_1$ adrenergic receptors, it has a higher propensity to cause EPS than side effects associated with other receptors.

Pharmacokinetics: Rapid absorption occurs following oral administration. Fluphenazine is distributed into most body tissues. It is highly bound to plasma proteins. Onset of action for oral doses is ≤1 hour. The reported half-life ranges from 13 to 33 hours or more.

Fluphenazine is a substrate and inhibitor of the cytochrome P450 isoenzymes, CYP1A2 and CYP2D6.

Fluphenazine decanoate, a fluphenazine ester, is available in an injectable, sesame oil–based formulation. Both esterification and the oil-based vehicle slow the release of fluphenazine from tissues after im or sc injection, resulting in a longer duration of action. The onset of action of fluphenazine decanoate is 24 to 72 hours and the average duration of action is 3 to 4 weeks.

INDICATIONS: Health Canada-approved indications include:

- management of psychotic disorders including schizophrenia.

CONTRAINDICATIONS:

- Patients who are hypersensitive to fluphenazine or to any ingredient in the formulation or component of the container.
- Patients with:
  - severe CNS depression or coma
  - bone marrow suppression
  - blood dyscrasias
  - severe hepatic disease

WARNINGS:

Serious Warnings and Precautions

- The use of phenothiazines such as fluphenazine has been associated with acute and chronic extrapyramidal reactions including dystonias, akathisia, parkinsonian symptoms, neuroleptic malignant syndrome (NMS) and tardive dyskinesia (TD). NMS can be life-threatening, especially when not recognized and addressed early, and TD may not resolve after drug discontinuation. See Adverse Effects.
- The use of antipsychotic agents in elderly patients has been associated with a dose-related increase in all-cause mortality, with an inverse relationship to duration of use. The risk may be higher with first-generation or "conventional" antipsychotics compared to second-generation or "atypical" agents in this population [*N Engl J Med* 2005;353(22):2335-41; *CMAJ* 2007;176 (5):627-32. doi:10.1503/cmaj.061250]. The use of antipsychotic agents in older patients should be carefully considered, and first-generation agents should be avoided when possible.

PRECAUTIONS: Abrupt Withdrawal: Sudden discontinuation of antipsychotics can result in symptoms such as nausea, vomiting, diarrhea, sweating, insomnia and confusion. Psychosis and movement disorders can also be precipitated. Antipsychotics should be discontinued gradually.

Cardiovascular: Fluphenazine may cause hypotension. It should be used with caution in the elderly (see Serious Warnings and Precautions), patients with alcohol dependency or cardiovascular disease, or in patients undergoing surgery. The dosage of anesthetics and CNS depressants may have to be reduced in the perioperative period. ECG changes have been associated with the administration of phenothiazines. These changes appear to be reversible and related to a disturbance in repolarization. Use fluphenazine with caution in patients with cardiovascular disease.

CNS: Fluphenazine may lower the seizure threshold. Use the drug cautiously in patients with a history of seizures.

Phenothiazines affect thermoregulation. Use fluphenazine with caution in patients who may be exposed to extreme heat or cold.

Dermatologic: Photosensitivity may occur. Patients should apply a broad spectrum sunscreen prior to sunlight exposure.

Endocrine: Patients with hypocalcemia may be more susceptible to dystonic reactions (see Adverse Effects). Fluphenazine can elevate prolactin levels and can lead to galactorrhea, amenorrhea, gynecomastia, and sexual dysfunction (in both men and women). The correlation with prolactin levels and these adverse effects is low.

Hematologic: Blood dyscrasias including agranulocytosis have occurred in patients taking antipsychotics. These reactions are rare with phenothiazines, and most have occurred between the fourth and tenth week of treatment. Monitor patients during that time for the appearance of sore throat, fever and weakness. If these symptoms occur, discontinue the drug if STAT white blood cell and differential counts confirm a suspected hematologic reaction.

Hepatic: Fluphenazine should be used with caution in patients who have impaired liver function or alcohol-related liver disease. CNS depression may be potentiated. If bilirubinemia or icterus occurs, discontinue the drug and perform liver function tests.

Respiratory: Use cautiously in patients with respiratory difficulties as CNS depression may cause respiratory failure in these patients.

Occupational Hazards: Warn patients that fluphenazine may impair their ability to safely perform activities requiring full mental alertness, such as driving or operating machinery. Potentiation of the effects of alcohol may also occur.

Drug Interactions: Drug-Drug Interactions: See Table 1.

Table 1: Fluphenazine

Drug-Drug Interactions

Interacting Drug	Effect	Comment
Anticholinergic agents (e.g., antihistamines, antiparkinsonian drugs, atropine, tricyclic antidepressants)	Additive anticholinergic side effects (e.g., constipation, urinary retention, blurred vision, dry eyes, dry mouth, cognitive impairment)	Monitor for increased anticholinergic effects.
CNS depressants	Fluphenazine may enhance the CNS depressant effects of drugs including alcohol, anticonvulsants, antidepressants antihistamines, barbiturates, benzodiazepines	Monitor therapy to prevent and/or manage excessive sedation.
CYP2D6 inhibitors, strong (e.g., fluoxetine, paroxetine, quinidine, ritonavir)	May result in decreased clearance of fluphenazine	Consider a therapeutic alternative for one of the interacting drugs, or monitor and adjust fluphenazine dose.
Dopaminergic agents (e.g., bromocriptine, cabergoline, levodopa, pramipexole, ropinirole)	Fluphenazine may antagonize the dopaminergic effects of these drugs resulting in decreased efficacy	Avoid combination.
Lithium	Lithium may enhance the neurotoxic effects of phenothiazines. Rare cases of severe neurotoxicity have been reported.	If lithium and fluphenazine are used concurrently, monitor closely for signs of adverse neurologic effects, especially if serum concentrations of lithium are in the upper range. Avoid combining these agents at high doses.

Drug-Herb Interactions: Avoid concurrent use of phenothiazines with kava kava, gotu kala, valerian and St. John's wort because these herbs may increase CNS depression. Kava kava may also provide additive dopamine antagonism. Avoid dong quai because of a possible increased risk of photosensitization.

Pregnancy: Phenothiazines readily cross the placenta but have not been associated with an increased risk of congenital abnormalities and are considered relatively safe during pregnancy when used in low doses. They should be used in the lowest effective dose for the shortest possible time and avoided near term if possible, to prevent adverse effects on the fetus.

Lactation: Phenothiazines are distributed into breast milk but are likely safe due to a low milk:plasma concentration ratio. Use the lowest effective dose and monitor infant for signs of adverse effects such as drowsiness, lethargy or extrapyramidal symptoms.

Children: Safety and efficacy of fluphenazine in children under 12 years of age has not been established.

Geriatrics: See Serious Warnings and Precautions.

Use reduced dosages. Older patients may be at greater risk for developing extrapyramidal or parkinsonian symptoms, and may be more susceptible to sedation or to the anticholinergic effects of phenothiazines (e.g., constipation, blurred vision, urinary retention, cognitive impairment).

ADVERSE EFFECTS: Adverse effects with different phenothiazines vary in type, frequency and mechanism, i.e., some are dose-related, while others involve individual patient sensitivity.

In general, members of the piperazine group of phenothiazines have more marked stimulating effects, are more likely to cause motor disorders associated with extrapyramidal reactions, particularly in children, but are less likely to cause blood dyscrasias, hypotension, tachycardia and drowsiness, compared to other phenothiazine groups. More common adverse effects (incidence ≥2%) are described in Table 2.

Table 2: Fluphenazine

More Common Adverse Effects (≥2%)

Body System	Effect	Comment
Autonomic Nervous System	Anticholinergic effects such as dry mouth, dry eyes, blurred vision, constipation, urinary retention (particularly problematic for men with benign prostatic hyperplasia)	Anticholinergic effects may improve spontaneously with continued therapy. Treatment options include reducing dose of fluphenazine or switching to an antipsychotic with less propensity to cause anticholinergic effects.
	Impaired temperature regulation	Inform patients about hazards associated with exposure to extreme heat or cold.
Central Nervous System	Sedation	Dose-related; older patients more susceptible.
	Paradoxical agitation, insomnia	
	Acute onset extrapyramidal effects such as parkinsonism, akathisia, dystonic reactions	More common with high-potency antipsychotics such as fluphenazine; use lowest effective dose for shortest possible time and regularly re-evaluate need for continued therapy. Management options include dosage reduction, switching to a 2nd generation antipsychotic, use of medications such as benzodiazepines (akathisia), anticholinergic agents (dystonia, parkinsonism) or beta-blockers (akathisia).
	Late onset extrapyramidal effects such as tardive dyskinesia (TD), typically characterized by rhythmical involuntary movements of the tongue, face, mouth or jaw (e.g., protrusion of the tongue, puffing of the cheeks, puckering of the mouth and chewing movements)	There is no evidence-based drug treatment for this syndrome. Management includes discontinuing the antipsychotic, switching to a 2nd generation agent if necessary. Fine vermicular movements of the tongue may be an early sign of TD and discontinuing the drug when this occurs might prevent full onset of the syndrome.
Cardiovascular	Hypotension, tachycardia, ECG changes (e.g., QTc prolongation)	Hypotension less common with high-potency agents.
Dermatologic	Photosensitivity, photoallergic reactions	Recommend use of sunscreen.
Endocrine	Polydipsia; weight gain, dysglycemia, hyperlipidemia, hyperprolactinemia (manifestations include gynecomastia, mastalgia, galactorrhea, menstrual changes, sexual dysfunction)	Encourage healthy diet and lifestyle to minimize cardiovascular risk factors; hyperprolactinemic symptoms may respond to dosage reduction.
Genitourinary	Sexual dysfunction including anorgasmia, ejaculatory dysfunction, erectile dysfunction	May remit with continued therapy; dosage reduction may be helpful.

Less Common Adverse Effects (<2%): CNS: Neuroleptic Malignant Syndrome (NMS): This rare but potentially fatal syndrome characterized by muscle rigidity, fever/hyperthermia, labile blood pressure and fluctuating levels of consciousness, can occur in patients taking fluphenazine or other antipsychotics. NMS appears to occur more commonly in young males. Dehydration is an additional risk factor. Patients need to be aware of the importance of adequate hydration, particularly in situations involving environmental exposure to extreme heat.

Hematologic: agranulocytosis, leukopenia, granulocytopenia, eosinophilia, thrombocytopenia, anemia, aplastic anemia, pancytopenia.

Hepatic: cholestatic jaundice; symptoms generally subside following discontinuation of the drug, but cholestasis may be prolonged.

OVERDOSAGE:

Symptoms: Symptoms of fluphenazine overdose are an extension of its pharmacologic actions. The primary symptoms observed are extrapyramidal reactions, hypotension and sedation. Mild or early intoxication may appear as restlessness and confusion, which may progress to coma. Altered temperature regulation can occur; both hypothermia and hyperthermia have been reported. Neuroleptic malignant syndrome can occur in overdose, though it most often occurs with therapeutic doses (see Adverse Effects). Other symptoms may include tachycardia, cardiac arrhythmias, seizures, miosis, and respiratory and/or vasomotor collapse. Anticholinergic symptoms tend to be less prominent with fluphenazine compared to less potent phenothiazines.

Treatment: Patients who have ingested fluphenazine in overdose occasionally require respiratory and hemodynamic support. This may include intubation, ventilation, boluses of isotonic iv fluids, and inotropic support. Once the patient's airway is adequately protected, 1 dose of activated charcoal (1 g/kg body weight) can be administered up to 120 minutes following oral overdose to minimize absorption of fluphenazine. The utility of this intervention decreases with time, and it may not influence clinical outcome. Patients with seizures should be treated with benzodiazepines, or if necessary, barbiturates. Ventricular arrhythmias are uncommon, and may be treated with boluses of sodium bicarbonate (typically 1-2 mEq/kg) as well as antiarrhythmics such as lidocaine. In the rare patient with torsades de pointes, iv magnesium sulfate and/or an overdrive pacemaker should be used. Acute dystonic reactions may be treated with iv benztropine or diphenhydramine.

For management of a suspected drug overdose, CPhA recommends that you contact your **regional Poison Control Centre**. See the *CPS* Directory section for a list of Poison Control Centres.

DOSAGE: **Dosing Considerations:** Dosage should be initiated at a low level and increased gradually, carefully noting the clinical response. Patients on long-term therapy should be evaluated periodically to evaluate the need for continued therapy. Avoid using first-generation antipsychotic agents in elderly patients when possible (see Warnings, Serious Warnings and Precautions).

Oral:
Initial Dose for Adults: 2.5 to 10 mg daily in divided doses every 6 to 8 hours. Doses greater than 20 mg should be used with caution.
Maintenance: When satisfactory improvement has been achieved, dosage should be gradually reduced to the lowest dose that will maintain relief of symptoms. The usual maintenance dose is 1 to 5 mg daily as a single dose.
Geriatrics: If chlorpromazine is used in elderly patients, lower dosages are recommended: 1 to 2.5 mg as an initial dose.
Parenteral Depot Injection: For maintenance therapy, in patients who have been stabilized on oral fluphenazine therapy and may benefit from switching to long-acting injections because of poor adherence or for other reasons. A precise formula for converting patients from oral to depot therapy has not been established. It has been proposed that fluphenazine decanoate 12.5 mg every 3 weeks is approximately equivalent to an oral fluphenazine HCl dosage of 10 mg daily.

The usual adult dose of fluphenazine decanoate in the management of chronic schizophrenia is 12.5 to 25 mg im or sc every 2 to 3 weeks. The duration of effect may be longer in some patients.

Flurazepam

CPhA Monograph

see *Benzodiazepines*

Fluticasone

CPhA Monograph

see *Corticosteroids: Eye Ear Nose*

see *Corticosteroids: Inhaled*

see *Corticosteroids: Topical*

Fluvastatin

CPhA Monograph

see *HMG-CoA Reductase Inhibitors*

Fluviral® (2010-2011)

split-virion influenza virus vaccine trivalent, inactivated

Active Immunizing Agent

ID Biomedical

Date of Revision: April 30, 2010

SUMMARY PRODUCT INFORMATION:

Route of Administration	Dosage Form/ Strength	Clinically Relevant Nonmedicinal Ingredients
IM	Suspension for Injection 15 µg influenza virus Hemagglutinin/strain/0.5 mL dose	Thimerosal, trace amounts of egg proteins, formaldehyde, sodium deoxycholate and sucrose For a complete listing see Dosage Forms, Composition and Packaging.

DESCRIPTION: FLUVIRAL is a trivalent, split-virion influenza vaccine prepared from virus grown in the allantoic cavity of embryonated hens' eggs. The virus is inactivated with ultraviolet light treatment followed by formaldehyde treatment, purified by centrifugation and disrupted with sodium deoxycholate. FLUVIRAL is used for active immunization against influenza disease caused by the influenza subtypes A and type B contained in the vaccine.

FLUVIRAL conforms to the current requirements of the World Health Organization (WHO). The influenza virus strains for the 2010-2011 season are A/California/7/2009 (H1N1)-like strain (A/California/7/2009 NYMC X-179A), A/Perth/16/2009 (H3N2)-like strain (A/Victoria/210/2009 NYMC X-187) and B/Brisbane/60/2008-like strain (B/Brisbane/60/2008).

INDICATIONS AND CLINICAL USE: FLUVIRAL, split-virion influenza vaccine, is indicated for the active immunization against influenza caused by the specific strains of influenza virus contained in the vaccine in adults and children 6 months of age or older. The National Advisory Committee on Immunization (CCDR, October 2009) recommends administration of influenza vaccines to the following groups:

1. **People at high risk of influenza-related complications or those more likely to require hospitalization:**
   - Adults (including pregnant women) and children with the following chronic health conditions:
     - cardiac or pulmonary disorders (including bronchopulmonary dysplasia, cystic fibrosis, and asthma)
     - diabetes mellitus and other metabolic diseases
     - cancer, immunodeficiency, immunosuppression (due to underlying disease and/or therapy)
     - renal disease
     - anemia or hemoglobinopathy
     - conditions that compromise the management of respiratory secretions and are associated with an increased risk of aspiration
     - children and adolescents with conditions treated for long periods with acetylsalicylic acid
   - People of any age who are residents of nursing homes and other chronic care facilities
   - People ≥65 years of age
   - Healthy children aged 6 to 23 months of age
   - Healthy pregnant women (the risk of influenza-related hospitalization increases with length of gestation; e.g. it is higher in the third than the second trimester).
2. **People capable of transmitting influenza to those at high risk:**
   - Health care and other care providers in facilities and community settings who, through their activities, are capable of transmitting influenza to those at high risk of influenza complications.
   - Household contacts (adults and children) of individuals at high risk of influenza-related complications (whether or not the individual at high risk has been immunized):
     - Household contacts of individuals at high risk, as listed in the section above
     - Household contacts of infants <6 months of age who are at high risk of complications from influenza but for whom influenza vaccine is not approved, and
     - Members of a household expecting a newborn during the influenza season
   - Those providing regular child care to children ≤24 months of age, whether in or out of the home.
   - Those who provide services within closed or relatively closed settings to persons at high risk (e.g. crew on ships).
3. **Others:**
   - People who provide essential community services
   - People in direct contact during culling operations with poultry infected with avian influenza

Note: Healthy persons aged 2 to 64 years without contraindication are also encouraged to receive influenza vaccine even if they are not in one of the aforementioned priority groups.
Pediatrics: Healthy children aged 6 to 23 months are at increased risk of influenza-associated hospitalization compared with healthy older children and young adults. Children and adolescents (aged 6 months to 18 years) treated for long periods with ASA may be at increased risk of Reye Syndrome after influenza infection.
Geriatrics (≥65 years of age): The risk of severe morbidity and mortality related to influenza is moderately increased in healthy persons over 65 years of age but is not nearly as great as in persons with chronic underlying disease.
HIV-Infected Persons: Limited information exists regarding the frequency and severity of influenza illness among HIV-infected persons, but reports suggest that symptoms may be prolonged and the risk for complications increased for some HIV-infected persons. Because influenza can result in serious illness and complications, vaccination is a prudent precaution and will result in protective antibody levels in many recipients. However, the antibody response to vaccine may be low in persons with advanced HIV-related illnesses; giving a second dose of vaccine 4 or more weeks after the first does not improve the immune response for these persons. Further studies are also required to determine whether influenza immunization can adversely affect patients infected with HIV. To date, some studies indicate that influenza immunization can be associated with transient increases in plasma HIV concentration, but no study has demonstrated an adverse effect of this temporary change on HIV disease progression.
Pregnant Women: Vaccination is recommended for pregnant women in high-risk groups (see above section). Vaccine is considered safe for pregnant women—regardless of their stage of pregnancy. Although excess morbidity and mortality were observed among pregnant women during the pandemic outbreaks in 1918-19 and 1957-58, further studies are needed to determine whether pregnancy per se is a risk factor that warrants routine influenza immunization. Pregnant women should be immunized in their third trimester if they are expected to deliver during influenza season, as they will become household contacts of their newborn (children <6 months of age are at increased risk of complications from influenza).
Breast-Feeding Mothers: Influenza immunization does not adversely affect the health of breast-feeding mothers or their infants. Breast-feeding is not a contraindication for influenza immunization.

People at high risk of influenza complications embarking on foreign travel to destinations where influenza is likely to be circulating should be vaccinated with the most current available vaccine. In the tropics, influenza can occur throughout the year. In the southern hemisphere, peak activity occurs from April through September. In the northern hemisphere, peak activity occurs from November through March.

Employers and their employees should consider yearly influenza immunization for healthy working adults as this has been shown to decrease work absenteeism because of respiratory and other illnesses.

Concern has been raised regarding the possibility that a pandemic influenza strain may emerge through human-avian gene reassortment within workers directly involved in poultry culling operations, who may become simultaneously infected with a human influenza virus strain and an avian influenza virus strain. This is a theoretical concern, given that this gene reassortment has not been documented to date. FLUVIRAL protects against human but not avian influenza strains. Immunization is recommended for those directly involved in the destruction (culling) of avian influenza-infected poultry before the culling operation. Direct involvement may be defined as sufficient contact with infected poultry to allow transmission of avian virus to the exposed person. The relevant individuals include those performing the cull as well as others (such as supervising veterinarians and inspectors) who may be directly exposed to the avian virus. Those persons who would be expected by reason of their employment to come into direct contact with infected poultry during culling operations in the event of potential avian influenza outbreaks should be immunized with trivalent influenza vaccine on a yearly basis prior to the human influenza season (CCDR, October 2009).

CONTRAINDICATIONS:

- Known or suspected hypersensitivity to FLUVIRAL, to thimerosal, or to any other ingredient in the formulation or component of the container. For a complete listing, see Dosage Forms, Composition and Packaging.
- Vaccination is not recommended for subjects who develop anaphylactic type reactions when they eat eggs (urticaria (hives), oedema of the mouth and throat, difficulty in breathing, hypotension and shock). Allergic reactions are extremely rare and usually attributable to extreme sensitivity to certain components of the vaccine, probably to trace amounts of residual egg protein. Subjects whose allergy to eggs is not of the anaphylactic type, as well as those who are allergic to chicken and to feathers may be vaccinated.
- Subjects with an acute respiratory infection or with any other active infection or serious febrile illness. On the other hand, a minor indisposition such as a mild infection of the upper respiratory tract is not necessarily a contraindication to vaccination.

WARNINGS AND PRECAUTIONS:

Serious Warnings and Precautions
- Sterile epinephrine hydrochloride solution 1:1000 should always be readily available in case of an acute anaphylactic reaction following administration of the vaccine.

General: Influenza vaccine can inhibit the clearance of warfarin and theophylline. However, clinical studies have not shown any adverse effects attributable to these drugs in people receiving influenza vaccine.
Hematologic: As with other vaccines administered intramuscularly, FLUVIRAL should be given with caution in individuals with bleeding disorders such as hemophilia or on anticoagulant therapy to avoid the risk of hematoma following the injection.
Immune: It is possible that the protective immune response following influenza vaccination may not develop in subjects undergoing immunosuppressive therapy.

Corticosteroid therapy can result in immunosuppression although the exact dose and duration of therapy required to suppress the immune system is not well defined. Persons treated with high doses of systemic steroids, e.g., ≥2 mg/kg/day of prednisone orally for more than 2 weeks, or ≥60 mg prednisone/day in an adult, should be considered to have a compromised immune system.
Local Skin Reactions at Vaccination Sites: Soreness and redness at the injection site may occur and may last for up to two days. Prophylactic acetaminophen may decrease the frequency of pain at the injection site.
Neurologic: If Guillain-Barré syndrome has occurred within 6 weeks of receipt of prior influenza vaccine, the decision to give FLUVIRAL should be based on the careful consideration of the potential benefits and risks.

Immunization should be delayed in a patient with an active neurologic disorder, but should be considered when the disease process has been stabilized.
Respiratory: Revaccination of individuals who have previously experienced oculo-respiratory symptoms is safe. Previously affected individuals should be encouraged to be revaccinated. The risk of recurrence of oculo-respiratory symptoms after revaccination is minimal compared to the serious threat posed by influenza. Please refer to most current NACI recommendations regarding revaccination of subjects who experienced more severe oculo-respiratory syndrome.
Special Populations: Pregnant Women: The National Advisory Committee on Immunization considers influenza vaccine safe in pregnancy.
Pediatrics: In infants <6 months of age, influenza vaccine is less immunogenic than in infants and children aged 6 to 18 months. Therefore, immunization with currently available influenza vaccine is not recommended for infants <6 months.

Since the likelihood of febrile convulsions is greater in children aged 6 to 35 months, special care should be taken in weighing relative risks and benefits in this group.
Monitoring and Laboratory Tests: False positive ELISA serologic tests for HIV-1, Hepatitis C, and especially HTLV-1 may occur following influenza vaccination. These transient false-positive results may be due to cross-reactive IgM elicited by the vaccine. For this reason, a definitive diagnosis of HIV-1, Hepatitis C, or HTLV-1 infection requires a positive result from a virus-specific confirmatory test (e.g, Western Blot or immunoblot).

ADVERSE REACTIONS: Adverse Drug Reaction Overview: The most commonly reported adverse drug reactions with FLUVIRAL are pain and redness at the injection site, fatigue, headache and myalgia. Common reactions are red eyes, sore throat, cough, arthralgia, swelling at the injection site, fever, chills, malaise and chest tightness. Reactions are generally mild and of limited duration. Prophylactic acetaminophen may decrease the frequency of some side effects in adults.

Immediate, allergic-type responses, such as hives, angioedema, allergic asthma, or systemic anaphylaxis occur extremely rarely. These reactions probably result from sensitivity to some vaccine component—most likely residual egg proteins (see Contraindications).
Clinical Trial Adverse Drug Reactions: Because clinical trials are conducted under very specific conditions the adverse reaction rates observed in the clinical trials may not reflect the rates observed in practice and should not be compared to the rates in the clinical trials of another drug. Adverse drug reaction information from clinical trials is useful for identifying drug-related adverse events and for approximating rates.

FLUVIRAL was administered to 2220 adult and elderly subjects in six clinical trials. General symptoms were solicited by a diary aid used by the subjects for 3 days post-vaccination.

Adverse reactions considered possibly related to vaccination have been categorised by frequency as follows: very common (≥1/10), common (≥1/100 to <1/10), uncommon (≥1/1000 to <1/100), rare (≥1/10 000 to <1/1000), very rare (<1/10 000).
Infections and Infestations: Uncommon: upper respiratory tract infection.

Nervous System Disorders: Very common: headache. Uncommon: dizziness.
Eye Disorders: Common: red eyes*.
Respiratory, Thoracic and Mediastinal Disorders: Common: sore throat*, cough*.
Gastrointestinal Disorders: Uncommon: nausea.
Skin and Subcutaneous Tissue Disorders: Uncommon: swelling of the face*.
Musculoskeletal and Connective Tissue Disorders: Very common: myalgia. Common: arthralgia.
General Disorders and Administration Site Conditions: Very common: pain and redness at the injection site, fatigue. Common: swelling at the injection site, fever, chills, malaise, chest tightness*.

A study was conducted in 130 children aged 3-12 years. The data in the Table 1 show the percentage of reported symptoms to FLUVIRAL split-virion vaccine versus a competitor subvirion vaccine. The most frequently reported local reaction was soreness at the injection site and usually resolved in 1-2 days. The most common systemic reactions were headache, loss of appetite and muscle aches. There were no significant differences between the two groups.

Table 1: FLUVIRAL

Percentage of Subjects Reporting Symptoms

Subjects Aged 3–12 Years	Fluviral (n=65)	Competitor (n=65)
Local Reactions (%)		
Soreness	57	58
Redness	12	14
Swelling	15	22
Limitation of movement	12	14
Systemic Reactions (%)		
Headache	15	17
Loss of appetite	12	8
Muscle aches	14	11
Chills	3	6
Nausea	3	3
Vomiting	1	0
Diarrhea	6	6
Redness/rash	3	3

Post-Market Adverse Drug Reactions: Oculo-respiratory Syndrome (ORS) has been reported in Canada, US and Europe following administration of influenza vaccines. The symptoms associated with the ORS are red eyes, respiratory symptoms and facial oedema. Most cases are mild in severity and resolve spontaneously regardless of the influenza vaccine administered.

Revaccination of subjects with history of ocular or respiratory symptoms is considered to be safe regardless of the influenza vaccine used for the initial vaccination or the revaccination. Since the 2000-2001 influenza season when the symptom was first identified, the incidence of ORS has slowly declined and reporting rates are returning to background levels reported prior to 2000.

There have been reports of other neurological illnesses, including facial paralysis, encephalitis, encephalopathy, demyelinating disease and labyrinthitis, associated with other influenza vaccines. Any relationship, other than temporal, to the vaccine has not been established.

Unlike the 1976-77 swine influenza vaccine, subsequent vaccines prepared from other virus strains have not been clearly associated with an increased frequency of Guillain-Barré syndrome. Influenza vaccine is not known to predispose to Reye's syndrome.

Notification of Reactions: It is desirable that all unusual reactions, arising from any vaccination whatsoever, or following shortly thereafter, be reported to the manufacturer of the product and to the provincial epidemiologist.

DRUG INTERACTIONS: Drug-Drug Interactions: Influenza vaccine can inhibit the clearance of warfarin and theophylline. However, clinical studies have not shown any adverse effects attributable to these drugs in people receiving influenza vaccine.

The target groups for influenza and pneumococcal vaccination overlap considerably. Health care providers should take the opportunity to vaccinate eligible persons against pneumococcal disease during the same visit at which influenza vaccine is given. The concurrent administration of the two vaccines at different sites does not increase the risk of side effects. Pneumococcal vaccine, however, is not administered annually, as in the case of influenza vaccine.

Children at high risk may receive influenza vaccine at the same time but at a different site from that used for routine pediatric vaccines.

DOSAGE AND ADMINISTRATION: Recommended Dose and Dosage Adjustment: See Table 2.

Table 2: FLUVIRAL

Influenza Vaccine Dosage, by Age Group

Age Group	Dosage	Route
6–35 months	1×0.25 mL or 2×0.25 mL[a]	IM
3–8 years	1×0.50 mL or 2×0.50 mL[a]	IM
9 years and older	1×0.50 mL	IM

[a] Two doses administered at least one month apart are recommended for children younger than 9 years of age receiving influenza vaccine for the first time.

The recommended site of vaccination is the deltoid muscle for adults and older children. The preferred site for infants and young children is the anterolateral aspect of the thigh.

Check the expiry date of the vaccine carefully. Any vaccine beyond its expiry date should not be used.

Administration: FLUVIRAL vaccine must not be administered intravenously.

FLUVIRAL is an opalescent translucent to off-white liquid suspension. Inspect FLUVIRAL visually for particulate matter and/or discoloration prior to administration. If either of these conditions exist, the vaccine should not be administered.

Shake the multidose vial vigorously each time before withdrawing a dose of vaccine.

Proper aseptic technique should be used for withdrawal of each dose from the multidose vial. Once entered, return the multidose vial to the recommended storage conditions, between 2 and 8°C. Once entered, the multidose vial should be discarded after 28 days.

* These symptoms can be associated to the oculo-respiratory syndrome (ORS). ORS consists of the following signs and symptoms: bilateral red eyes and/or respiratory symptoms (cough, wheeze, chest tightness, difficulty breathing, difficulty swallowing, hoarseness or sore throat) and/or facial swelling. Although not explicitly identified as ORS during the clinical trials, these symptoms were solicited to detect possible cases of that syndrome.

A separate sterile 1-cc syringe and needle or a sterile disposable 1-cc unit should be used for each injection to prevent transmission of hepatitis B, HIV, or other infectious agents from one person to another.

Disinfect the skin at the site of injection with a suitable antiseptic and wipe dry with sterile cotton wool. The injection of FLUVIRAL **should be given intramuscularly**, usually into the deltoid muscle. **Do not inject influenza vaccine intravenously.** No data are available on subcutaneous administration of FLUVIRAL.

All vaccinees should be observed for about 15 minutes after vaccination. If an anaphylactic reaction develops, sterile epinephrine hydrochloride (1:1000) should be administered.

OVERDOSAGE:
In a study by Matzkin and Nili (1984), following administration of a dose of flu vaccine 10 times greater than the recommended dose of 0.5 mL, adverse events were not significantly different between study and control subjects.

There have been reports of patients who received higher than recommended doses of FLUVIRAL. The adverse events noted in these patients were similar to those reported from patients who had received the recommended dose.

For management of a suspected drug overdose, contact your regional Poison Control Centre. See the *CPS* Directory section for a list of Poison Control Centres.

ACTION AND CLINICAL PHARMACOLOGY: Mechanism of Action: FLUVIRAL, split-virion inactivated influenza vaccine, promotes an active immunization against influenza strains A (H1N1 and H3N2) and B. Within seven days after injection of the vaccine there is an increase in circulating antibody to the viral hemagglutinin and peripheral blood lymphocytes are primed to respond to in vitro stimulation by vaccine antigens. As with other inactivated influenza vaccines, immunization is based on the humoral component of the specific immunological defense system, namely immunoglobulin G (IgG) antibodies against viral hemagglutinin (HA) and neuraminidase antigens. The effectiveness of inactivated influenza vaccines correlates with the age and immunocompetence of the vaccine recipient and the degree of similarity between the virus strains used in the preparation of the vaccines and those prevailing in the population.

Cytotoxic T lymphocyte response occurs after administrations of either killed or live virus vaccines and is detectable in the absence of demonstrable antibody response.

Pharmacodynamics/Pharmacokinetics: No pharmacodynamics studies and no pharmacokinetics studies have been conducted with FLUVIRAL in accordance with its status as a vaccine.

Duration of Effect: Both humoral and cell-mediated responses are thought to play a role in immunity to influenza. Immunity declines over the year following vaccination. The production and persistence of antibody after vaccination depends on numerous factors, including age, prior and subsequent exposure to antigens, presence of immunodeficiency states, and polymorphisms in HLA class II molecules. Humoral antibody levels, which correlate with vaccine protection, are generally achieved by 2 weeks after immunization. It is postulated that immunity after administration of the inactivated vaccine lasts <1 year. However, in the elderly, antibody levels may fall below protective levels within 4 months. Data are not available to support a recommendation for the administration of a second dose of influenza vaccine in elderly individuals in order to boost immunity.

STORAGE AND STABILITY: FLUVIRAL must be stored between 2 and 8°C. **Do not freeze.** Freezing destroys activity. Do not use vaccine that has been frozen.

Store in the original package in order to protect from light.

Do not use vaccine after the expiration date.

Once entered, the multidose vial should be discarded after 28 days.

SPECIAL HANDLING INSTRUCTIONS: FLUVIRAL and materials used during vaccination should be disposed of in the same way as other drugs administered by injection. Since split-virion influenza vaccine is an inactivated vaccine, it presents no risk of contaminating the work area during manipulation.

INFORMATION FOR THE PATIENT: Published in e-CPS, available by subscription at www.e-cps.ca.

DOSAGE FORMS, COMPOSITION AND PACKAGING: The composition of FLUVIRAL is established in agreement with the recommendations of the Canadian National Advisory Committee on Immunization (NACI) and the World Health Organization (WHO). For the 2010-2011 season, each dose of 0.5 mL of FLUVIRAL contains: 15 µg HA-A/California/7/2009 (H1N1)-like strain (A/California/7/2009 NYMC X-179A), 15 µg HA-A/Perth/16/2009 (H3N2)-like strain (A/Victoria/210/2009 NYMC X-187), 15 µg HA-B/Brisbane/60/2008-like strain (B/Brisbane/60/2008). The vaccine is formulated with phosphate buffered saline composed of: sodium chloride, potassium chloride, sodium phosphate dibasic heptahydrate, potassium phosphate monobasic and water for injection. Thimerosal (100 µg/mL) is added as a preservative. The vaccine also contains trace residual amounts of egg proteins, formaldehyde, sodium deoxycholate and sucrose. Antibiotics are not used in the manufacture of this vaccine. Vials of 5 mL (10 doses). FLUVIRAL packaging does not contain latex.

Fluvoxamine ℞

CPhA Monograph

see *Selective Serotonin Reuptake Inhibitors*

FML® ℞

fluorometholone

Corticosteroid

Allergan

SUPPLIED: Each mL of sterile ophthalmic suspension contains: fluorometholone 0.1%. Nonmedicinal ingredients: benzalkonium chloride 0.004% (as preservative), edetate disodium, Liquifilm (polyvinyl alcohol), polysorbate 80, sodium chloride, sodium phosphate dibasic and sodium phosphate monobasic. Plastic dropper bottles of 5 and 10 mL.

FML Forte® ℞

fluorometholone

Corticosteroid—Anti-inflammatory

Allergan

SUPPLIED: Each mL of sterile ophthalmic suspension contains: fluorometholone 0.25%. Nonmedicinal ingredients: benzalkonium chloride 0.005% (as preservative), edetate disodium, polysorbate 80, polyvinyl alcohol, sodium biphosphate, sodium chloride and sodium phosphate. Plastic dropper bottles of 5 and 10 mL. Protect from freezing. Shake well before using.

Folic Acid ℞

Anemia Therapy

CPhA Monograph

Date of Revision: October 2007

This monograph has been compiled by CPhA and reviewed by experts. It may contain information different from that found in Health Canada-approved Product Monographs. The reader is referred to the *CPS* Editorial Policy for more information.

SUMMARY PRODUCT INFORMATION:

Route of Administration[a]	Dosage Form[a]	Strength[a]
Oral	Capsule	0.8 mg
	Tablet	0.4 mg, 1 mg, 5 mg, 25 mg
Parenteral	Injectable solution	5 mg/mL

[a] Table includes single-entity folic acid products only. For specific product information consult Health Canada's Drug Product Database http://www.hc-sc.gc.ca/dhp-mps/prodpharma/databasdon/index_e.html

PHARMACOLOGY: Folic acid, also known as folate, pteroylglutamic acid or vitamin B_9, is a water-soluble B complex vitamin. After absorption from the gastrointestinal tract, folic acid is converted in the liver to tetrahydrofolic acid which is a cofactor in the biosynthesis of purines and thymidylates of nucleic acids. An exogenous source of folic acid is necessary for the synthesis of nucleoproteins and maintenance of normal erythropoiesis.

Folic acid deficiency can lead to megaloblastic and macrocytic anemias, as a result of impairment of thymidylate synthesis. Within 48 hours of beginning treatment with folic acid, the bone marrow of patients with megaloblastic anemia due to folate deficiency begins to become normoblastic. Reticulocytosis begins within 2 to 5 days.

Folic acid occurs in a variety of foods in the form of polyglutamate conjugates. Folic acid found in oral or injectable pharmaceutical preparations is synthetically derived.

Studies have provided strong scientific support for periconceptual prophylaxis with folic acid in reducing the risk of fetal neural tube defects.

Folic acid has been shown to reduce elevated fasting plasma homocysteine levels. A causal relationship between elevated homocysteine levels and cardiovascular disease has been postulated but has not been proven. Although epidemiologic studies using folic acid looked promising, prospective clinical trials in the prevention of cardiovascular disease have largely been disappointing.

Although folic acid is not effective in the treatment of methotrexate overdose, it is used during long-term, low-dose methotrexate therapy to prevent or treat associated folate deficiency, prevent methotrexate toxicity and to prevent hyperhomocysteinemia.

Pharmacokinetics: Folic acid polyglutamates from food sources are enzymatically hydrolyzed in the gastrointestinal tract to monoglutamates prior to absorption, which occurs mainly in the proximal small intestine. In the presence of malabsorption syndrome, folic acid from oral supplements will still be absorbed, whereas absorption of folic acid from food sources may be impaired.

Following absorption of 1 mg or less, folic acid is converted in the liver and plasma to its metabolically active form tetrahydrofolic acid, which is then distributed into all body tissues. Normal serum folate concentrations range from 11 to 34 nmol/mL. The liver contains about 50% of total body folate stores. Larger doses of folic acid may escape metabolism by the liver and appear in the blood mainly as folic acid.

Following oral administration of single 0.1 to 0.2 mg doses of folic acid in healthy adults, only a trace amount of the drug appears in urine. Following administration of large doses, the renal tubular reabsorption maximum is exceeded and excess folate is excreted unchanged in urine. After doses of about 2.5 to 5 mg, about 50% of a dose is excreted in urine and after a 15 mg dose, up to 90% may be recovered in urine. Small amounts of orally administered folic acid have been recovered from feces.

INDICATIONS: Folic acid is used in the treatment of megaloblastic and macrocytic anemias caused by folate deficiency. It is also used in the treatment of megaloblastic anemias of pregnancy, infancy and childhood, as well as megaloblastic anemias associated with primary liver disease, alcoholic cirrhosis, intestinal strictures, anastomoses or sprue. In large doses, folic acid is used in the treatment of tropical sprue.

There is strong evidence that prophylactic therapy with folic acid, prior to and during pregnancy, can reduce the risk of fetal neural tube defects. Health Canada recommends that all women of child bearing potential, whether planning pregnancy or not, should maintain an adequate daily intake of folic acid (see Dosage).

Folic acid is not effective in reversing the effects of folic acid reductase inhibitors such as methotrexate, for which leucovorin calcium (folinic acid) must be used. However, folic acid is used during long-term, low-dose methotrexate therapy to prevent methotrexate toxicity, particularly oral ulceration and gastrointestinal irritation, to treat or prevent folate deficiency and to prevent hyperhomocysteinemia.

CONTRAINDICATIONS: Folic acid is contraindicated in patients with hypersensitivity to folic acid products.

WARNINGS: See Precautions.

PRECAUTIONS: Use only as an adjunct to treatment with vitamin B_{12} whenever pernicious anemia is present or suspected. The use of folic acid in pernicious anemia without adequate vitamin B_{12} therapy may result in hematologic improvement, while neurologic manifestations continue to progress. Signs or symptoms of vitamin B_{12} deficiency (e.g., chronic malaise, sore tongue, numbness of the fingers) should be investigated before starting supplementation with folic acid.

Folic acid is not effective as an antidote or in the rescue treatment of overdosage of folic acid antagonists such as methotrexate.

Drug Interactions: Folic acid therapy in folate deficient individuals may decrease serum levels of phenytoin.

Drugs that can cause folate deficiency include phenytoin, isoniazid, primidone, barbiturates, oral contraceptives, ethanol, sulfasalazine, cycloserine, glutethimide, methotrexate, pyrimethamine, trimethoprim and triamterene.

When cholestyramine and folic acid are administered together, there may be a reduction or delay in folic acid absorption. If concomitant therapy is required, folic acid should be administered at least 1 hour before or 4 to 6 hours after cholestyramine.

Pregnancy: Pregnant women are more prone to develop folate deficiency which can lead to complications and fetal abnormalities (see Pharmacology).

Lactation: Folic acid is actively excreted in human breast milk. Adverse effects in breast-fed infants have not been documented with intake of normal daily requirements of folic acid during lactation.

ADVERSE EFFECTS: Folic acid is relatively nontoxic but has rarely caused allergic reactions including erythema, pruritus and/or urticaria. High doses (e.g., 15 mg/day) have rarely been associated with various gastrointestinal symptoms and CNS effects such as altered sleep patterns, difficulty concentrating, irritability, overactivity, excitement, mental depression, confusion and impaired judgement.

OVERDOSE:

For management of a suspected drug overdose, CPhA recommends that you contact your **regional Poison Control Centre**. See the *CPS* Directory section for a list of Poison Control Centres.

DOSAGE: To prevent deficiency, adequate dietary intake of folic acid is preferred over supplementation whenever possible. Food sources include asparagus, spinach, legumes (e.g., beans, lentils), avocados, cantaloupe, fortified cereal and grain products, and liver.

Treatment of Deficiency: Oral: The usual therapeutic dose of folic acid for adults and children is 0.25 to 1 mg daily; however, some patients may require higher doses. Within the first 48 hours of treatment, the bone marrow begins to become normoblastic. Reticulocytosis begins within 2 to 5 days. To maintain a normoblastic marrow, lower daily maintenance doses of folic acid are used: adults and children 4 years and over, 0.4 mg; children up to 4 years, 0.3 mg; infants, 0.1 mg. Higher maintenance doses may be required in certain patients such as alcoholics, patients with hemolytic anemia or chronic infections, or pregnant women taking certain anticonvulsants (e.g., valproic acid or carbamazepine).

Higher doses have been recommended for the treatment of tropical sprue: 3 to 15 mg daily.

Prophylaxis of Neural Tube Defects (NTD): Health Canada recommends that all women who could become pregnant should take a multivitamin containing 0.4 mg of folic acid every day starting at least 3 months before pregnancy and throughout the first 3 months of pregnancy.

Women with a history of pregnancy complicated by NTD are considered at high risk for recurrence and are advised to consider taking 4 mg folic acid daily when not using reliable birth control (or at least 2 to 4 weeks prior to conception), continuing until 10 to 12 weeks after last menstrual period.

Women with no previous history of NTD-affected pregnancy but who may be at increased risk due to 1st degree relative (child, sibling or parent) with NTD, or for medical reasons such as type I diabetes or therapy with valproic acid or carbamazepine, are advised to consider taking 1 to 5 mg folic acid daily while not using reliable birth control, continuing for 10 to 12 weeks after last menstrual period. Higher doses (4 to 5 mg daily) should not be taken as a multivitamin because of the risk of intake of harmful amounts of other components such as vitamins A and D.

Prevention of Methotrexate Toxicity (see Indications): 0.4 to 1 mg daily.

Parenteral: When the oral route is not feasible, an equivalent dose of folic acid may be given by iv, sc or deep im injection. However, most patients with malabsorption syndrome are still able to absorb oral folic acid supplements.

Products with strengths less than 1 mg are available without a prescription.

Foradil® Ⓟ

formoterol fumarate

Bronchodilator

Novartis Pharmaceuticals

Date of Preparation: March 6, 1997
Date of Revision: October 16, 2008

PHARMACOLOGY: FORADIL (formoterol fumarate) is a potent selective long-acting (12 hours) β_2-adrenergic stimulant. It exerts a bronchodilator effect in patients with reversible airways obstruction. The effect is seen within 1 to 3 minutes and is still significant 12 hours after inhalation.

Single-dose studies have shown that FORADIL is effective in preventing bronchospasm induced by allergen, exercise, cold air, histamine or methacholine challenge. The bronchoprotective effect of FORADIL against methacholine provocation has been shown to persist for 12 hours.

In vitro, FORADIL inhibits the release of histamine and leukotrienes from passively sensitized human lung. In humans, formoterol was more effective than salbutamol at suppressing late phase airway obstruction and increased airway responsiveness to allergen. The clinical significance of these findings is unclear because the long duration of action of formoterol may produce an apparent effect on late phase reactions due to functional antagonism.

Pharmacokinetics: As for other inhaled drugs, it is likely that 90% of formoterol administered from an inhaler is swallowed and absorbed from the gastrointestinal tract (see Pharmacology). Formoterol fumarate acts locally in the lung; plasma levels therefore do not predict therapeutic effect. Systemic levels of formoterol are low or undetectable after inhalation of recommended doses.

INDICATIONS: Asthma: FORADIL (formoterol fumarate) is indicated as long-term, twice-daily administration in the maintenance treatment of asthma in patients 6 years of age and older with reversible obstructive airways disease, including patients with symptoms of nocturnal asthma, who are using optimal corticosteroid treatment and experiencing regular or frequent breakthrough symptoms requiring use of a short-acting bronchodilator. FORADIL should not be used in patients whose asthma can be managed by occasional use of short-acting inhaled β_2-agonists.

Corticosteroids should not be stopped because formoterol is prescribed.

Long-acting β_2-adrenergic agonists may increase the risk of asthma exacerbation and possibly asthma-related death (see Warnings). When treating asthma patients, FORADIL should be used only as additional therapy for patients whose conditions are not adequately controlled using low-to medium-dose inhaled corticosteroids or the severity of whose disease clearly warrants the initiation of treatment with two maintenance therapies, including FORADIL. It is not indicated for patients whose asthma can be managed by occasional use of inhaled short-acting β_2-agonists or for patients whose asthma can be successfully managed by inhaled corticosteroids along with occasional use of inhaled short-acting inhaled β_2-agonists.

Formoterol is a long-acting β_2-agonist and should not be used as a rescue medication. To relieve acute asthmatic symptoms a short-acting inhaled bronchodilator (e.g., salbutamol) should be used.

Chronic Obstructive Pulmonary Disease (COPD): FORADIL (formoterol fumarate) is indicated as long-term, twice-daily administration in the treatment of adults with chronic obstructive pulmonary disease (COPD) including chronic bronchitis and emphysema.

CONTRAINDICATIONS: FORADIL (formoterol fumarate) is contraindicated patients with cardiac tachyarrhythmias. FORADIL contains lactose (see Supplied) and is contraindicated in patients with an allergy to lactose, milk or in those who have ever had any unusual or allergic reaction to formoterol fumarate.

WARNINGS: Use in Asthma (see also General Warnings for Asthma and COPD):

Warning: Long-acting β_2-adrenergic agonists may increase the risk of asthma exacerbation and possibly asthma-related death. When treating asthma patients FORADIL should be used only as additional therapy for patients whose conditions are not adequately controlled using low- to medium-dose inhaled corticosteroids or the severity of whose disease clearly warrants the initiation of treatment with two maintenance therapies, including FORADIL. Data from a large placebo-controlled US study (Salmeterol Multi-center Asthma Research Trial, also known as "SMART") comparing the safety of another long-acting β_2-adrenergic agonist (salmeterol) to that of a placebo added to the original asthma therapy showed an increase in asthma-related deaths in patients receiving salmeterol. This finding with salmeterol may also apply to formoterol (a long-acting β_2-adrenergic agonist), the active ingredient in FORADIL.

Important Information:

FORADIL (formoterol fumarate) should not be initiated in patients with significantly worsening or acutely deteriorating asthma (see Precautions).

FORADIL should not be used to treat acute symptoms. It is crucial to advise patients accordingly and prescribe a short-acting, inhaled bronchodilator for this purpose. Medical attention should be sought if patients find that short-acting relief bronchodilator treatment becomes less effective or that they need more inhalations than usual (see Precautions).

FORADIL is not a substitute for inhaled or oral corticosteroids. Its use is complementary to them. Corticosteroids should not be stopped when FORADIL is initiated. Patients must be warned not to stop or reduce corticosteroid therapy without medical advice (see Precautions).

FORADIL and the Management of Asthma: The management of asthma should normally follow a stepwise program, with patient response closely monitored and lung function tests regularly conducted. The following recommendations are stated in the current Canadian Consensus Guidelines for the long-acting β_2-adrenergic agonists:

- Oral or inhaled corticosteroids should not be stopped.
- Long-acting β_2-agonists should not be used as monotherapy.
- Long-acting β_2-agonists should be used as add-on therapy to low- to medium-dose inhaled corticosteroids.
- Adequate education should be provided to the patient regarding the use of long-acting β_2-agonists and the acute treatment of asthma, with close follow-up to ensure compliance.
- Long-acting β_2-agonists should not be introduced in patients with significantly worsening or acutely deteriorating asthma.

Increasing use of short-acting inhaled β_2-agonists to control symptoms indicates deterioration of asthma control and the need to reassess the patient's therapy.

Sudden or progressive deterioration in asthma control is potentially life-threatening; the treatment plan must be re-evaluated, and consideration given to increasing corticosteroid therapy. In patients at risk, daily peak flow monitoring with precise instructions for acceptable variation limits should be considered.

Beta-adrenergic Blockers: Beta-adrenergic blockers, especially noncardioselective agents, should not be administered to asthmatic patients (see Precautions, Drug Interactions) since these antagonize the action of β_2-agonists including FORADIL and may produce severe, resistant bronchospasm.

Do not Exceed Recommended Dosage: Fatalities, the exact cause of which is unknown, have been reported following excessive use of inhaler preparations containing sympathomimetic amines. The exact cause of death is unknown but cardiac arrest following an unexpected development of a severe acute asthmatic crisis and subsequent hypoxia is suspected. In individual patients, any β_2-agonist may have a clinically adverse cardiac effect. The incidence of mortality in patients receiving FORADIL is consistent with that typically seen in the asthmatic population. In an open-label, uncontrolled study conducted in Europe an overall crude mortality rate of approximately 14 per 1000 person years (8 of 1393 patients followed for 4.8±2.6 months) was reported.

General Warnings for Asthma and COPD: Cardiovascular and Other Non-pulmonary Effects: Potentially serious ECG changes (such as increased QT_c interval) and hypokalemia may result from β_2-agonist therapy. Although clinically not significant, a small increase in QT_c interval and/or decrease in serum potassium has been reported at therapeutic doses of formoterol. The effects of single doses of formoterol at 12 to 96 µg were studied in 22 adult asthmatics, all of whom were receiving inhaled corticosteroids and an inhaled short-acting β_2-agonist prior to entering the trial. The number of patients whose longest measured QT_c in this trial was >440 msec was greater for placebo (3 patients) than it was for formoterol 12 µg (no patient), 24 µg (2 patients), and 48 µg (2 patients). Five patients treated with formoterol 96 µg showed QT_c prolongations >440 msec. Six patients had clinically meaningful (K^+ <3.2 mmol/L) hypokalemia at 96 µg, compared with one each at 12 and 48 µg. It is not known if these effects become clinically significant when concomitant medications causing similar effects are prescribed and/or in the presence of heart diseases, hypokalemia, or hypoxia. Particular caution is advised in severe asthma as these effects may be potentiated by hypoxia and concomitant treatment with xanthine derivatives, steroids and diuretics. Hypokalemia will increase the susceptibility of digitalis patients to cardiac arrhythmias (see Precautions). It is recommended that serum potassium levels be monitored in such situations.

Paradoxical Bronchospasm: As with other inhaled medication, paradoxical bronchospasm (which can be life-threatening) has been reported following the use of FORADIL. If it occurs, treatment with FORADIL should be discontinued immediately and alternative therapy instituted.

Labor and Delivery: There are no well-controlled human studies that have investigated the effects of formoterol on preterm labor or labor at term. Because of the potential for β-agonist interference with uterine contractility, use of β_2-agonists, such as FORADIL, during labor should be restricted to those patients in whom the benefits clearly outweigh the risks.

PRECAUTIONS: Use in Asthma (see also General Precautions for Asthma and COPD): Do not introduce FORADIL as a treatment for acutely deteriorating asthma. FORADIL (formoterol fumarate) is intended for the maintenance treatment of asthma (see Indications) and should not be introduced in acutely deteriorating asthma, which is a potentially life-threatening condition. There are no data demonstrating that long-acting β_2-agonists provide greater efficacy than or additional efficacy to short-acting, inhaled β_2-agonists in patients with worsening asthma. As with other long-acting β_2-agonists, serious acute respiratory events, including fatalities, have been reported in patients receiving FORADIL, some of which have occurred in patients with severe asthma and/or patients in whom asthma has been acutely deteriorating. Although it is not possible from these reports to determine the causal relationship between long-acting β_2-agonists and these adverse events, the use of a long-acting β_2-agonist in patients with acutely deteriorating asthma is inappropriate (see Warnings, Postmarketing Experience).

Do not use FORADIL to treat acute symptoms. FORADIL should not be used to relieve acute asthma symptoms. When prescribing FORADIL, the physician must also provide the patient with a short-acting, inhaled β_2-agonist (e.g., salbutamol) for treatment of symptoms that occur acutely, despite regular twice-daily use of FORADIL.

When beginning treatment with FORADIL, patients who have been taking short-acting, inhaled β_2-agonists on a regular basis (e.g., q.i.d.) should be instructed to discontinue the regular use of these drugs and use them only for symptomatic relief if they develop acute asthma symptoms while using FORADIL (see Information for the Patient or Guardian). Although formoterol has a rapid onset of action (1 to 3 minutes), current asthma management guidelines recommend that long-acting inhaled bronchodilators should be used only as twice-daily maintenance bronchodilator therapy.

Watch for increased need for short-acting, inhaled β_2-agonists. Asthma may deteriorate acutely over a period of hours or chronically over several days or longer. If the patient's short-acting inhaled β_2-agonist becomes less effective or a patient needs more inhalation than usual, this may be a marker of destabilization of asthma. In this setting, the patient requires reassessment of the treatment regimen. Those patients who require increasing doses or inhalations of short-acting β_2-agonists for relief of symptoms should consult a physician for re-evaluation. **Increasing the daily dosage of FORADIL in this situation is not appropriate. FORADIL should not be used more frequently than twice daily or at higher doses than recommended.**

Do not use FORADIL as a substitute for oral or inhaled corticosteroids. Patients must be warned not to stop or reduce corticosteroid therapy without medical advice, even if they feel better as a result of FORADIL treatment.

Use in Children 6 Years of Age or Older and Asthma Severity Reassessment: In children 6 years of age or older the severity of asthma may be variable with age and periodic reassessment should be considered to determine if continued maintenance therapy with FORADIL is still indicated. Compliance, especially neglect of anti-inflammatory therapy and overuse of short-acting β_2-agonists, should be carefully followed in children 6 years of age or older receiving long-acting β_2-agonists.

General Precautions for Asthma and COPD: Do not exceed recommended dosage. As with other inhaled β_2-agonist drugs, FORADIL should not be used more often or at higher doses than recommended. Fatalities have been reported in association with excessive use of inhaled sympathomimetic drugs (see below).

Cardiovascular and Other Medical Conditions: Usually no effect on the cardiovascular or CNS is seen after the administration of formoterol at recommended doses, but the cardiovascular and CNS effects seen with all sympathomimetic drugs (e.g., increased heart rate, cardiac contractility, tremor) can occur while using formoterol. Potentially serious ECG changes and hypokalemia were seen at increased doses (96 µg or 4 times the recommended maximum dose) of inhaled formoterol. Therefore, special care and supervision, with particular emphasis on dosage limits, is required in patients receiving FORADIL when the following conditions may exist: ischemic heart disease, cardiac arrhythmias, especially third degree AV block, severe cardiac decompensation, idiopathic subvalvular aortic stenosis, hypertrophic obstructive cardiomyopathy, thyrotoxicosis, known or suspected prolongation of the QT-interval (QT_c >0.44 seconds). Formoterol itself may induce prolongation of the QTc interval.

Use with caution in patients with idiopathic hypertrophic subvalvular aortic stenosis, in whom an increase in the pressure gradient between the left ventricle and the aorta may occur, causing increased strain on the left ventricle.

Hypokalemia: Potentially serious Hypokalemia may occur as a result of $beta_2$-agonist therapy, including FORADIL. Hypokalemia may increase susceptibility to cardiac arrhythmias. Particular caution is advised in patients with severe asthma as Hypokalemia may be potentiated by hypoxia and concomitant treatment. It is recommended that serum potassium levels be monitored in such situations.

Immediate Hypersensitivity Reactions: Immediate hypersensitivity reactions may occur after administration of FORADIL. FORADIL contains lactose and is contraindicated in patients with allergy to lactose, milk or in those who have ever had any unusual or allergic reaction to formoterol (see Contraindications).

Metabolic Effects: Due to the hyperglycemic effect of β_2-stimulants including FORADIL, additional blood glucose controls are recommended in diabetic patients.

Pregnancy: The safety of FORADIL during pregnancy has not yet been established (see Warnings, Labor and Delivery).

Lactation: FORADIL was found to be excreted in the milk of lactating rats after oral administration. It is not known whether inhaled FORADIL passes into the breast milk in humans. Therefore, mothers nursing their infants should refrain from taking FORADIL.

Labor and Delivery: See Warnings.

Geriatrics: No special considerations are required in elderly patients.

Children: FORADIL is not recommended for use in children younger than 6 years of age.

Occupational Hazards: Effect on Ability to Drive and Use Machines: Patients experiencing dizziness or other similar side effects should be advised to refrain from driving or using machines.

Drug Interactions: Short-acting β_2-agonists: Aerosol bronchodilators of the short-acting adrenergic stimulant type may be used for relief of breakthrough symptoms while using formoterol. However, increasing use of such preparations to control symptoms indicates deterioration of asthma control and the need to reassess the patient's therapy.

Concomitant administration of other sympathomimetic agents may potentiate the undesirable effects of FORADIL.

MAO Inhibitors and Tricyclic Antidepressants: FORADIL should be administered with extreme caution in patients being treated with monoamine oxidase inhibitors, tricyclic antidepressants, or drugs known to prolong the QTc interval because the action of formoterol on the cardiovascular system may be potentiated by these agents. Drugs that are known to prolong the QT interval have an increased risk of ventricular arrhythmias.

Corticosteroids, Methylxanthines and Diuretics: Concomitant treatment with xanthine derivatives, steroids, or diuretics may potentiate a possible hypokalemic effect of β_2-agonists. See General Precautions for Asthma and COPD. Hypokalemia may increase susceptibility to cardiac arrhythmias in patients treated with digitalis.

β-adrenergic Blockers: β-adrenergic blockers may weaken or antagonize the effect of FORADIL. Therefore FORADIL should not be given together with β-adrenergic blockers (including eye drops) unless there are compelling reasons for their use.

Other Drugs: Drugs such as quinidine, disopyramide, procainamide, phenothiazines, antihistamines, and tricyclic antidepressants may be associated with QT-interval prolongation and an increased risk of ventricular arrhythmia (see Warnings).

Information to Be Provided to the Patient or Guardian: See Information for the Patient or Guardian and package insert for illustrations. It is important that patients understand how to use FORADIL capsules with the supplied Aerolizer inhalation device and how it should be used in relation to other asthma or COPD medications they are taking. Patients/Guardians should be given the following information:

i. The recommended dosage (1 or 2 capsules twice daily, morning and evening) should not be exceeded.
ii. FORADIL is not meant to relieve acute asthma or COPD symptoms and extra doses should not be used for that purpose. Acute symptoms should be treated with a short-acting, inhaled β_2-agonist such as salbutamol (the physician should provide the patient with such medication and instruct the patient in how it should be used).
iii. The physician should be notified immediately if any of the following situations occur, which may be a sign of seriously worsening asthma: decreased effectiveness of short-acting, inhaled β_2-agonists; need for more inhalations than usual of short-acting, inhaled β_2-agonists.
iv. FORADIL should not be used as monotherapy or as a substitute for oral or inhaled corticosteroids. FORADIL should be used only as an add-on therapy to low- to medium-dose inhaled corticosteroids. The dosage of these medications should not be changed and treatment should not be stopped without consulting the prescribing physician, even if the patient feels better after initiating treatment with FORADIL.
v. Patients should be cautioned regarding potential adverse cardiovascular effects, such as palpitations or chest pain.
vi. In patients receiving FORADIL, other inhaled medications should be used only as directed by the physician.
vii. Guardians of children who have been prescribed FORADIL should be alerted to the general concern regarding asthma therapy compliance, especially neglect of anti-inflammatory therapy and overuse of short-acting β_2-agonists.

ADVERSE EFFECTS: The adverse reactions observed with FORADIL (formoterol fumarate) in controlled, comparative and non-comparative clinical studies were dose-dependent and corresponded to those known to occur with other β_2-adrenergic agonists.

Asthma: The most common adverse reactions (<10%) were tremor, palpitations, headache, dizziness, and oropharyngeal irritation. Rarely (<1%) muscle cramps, myalgia, tachycardia, agitation, anxiety, nervousness, insomnia, and, very rarely (<0.01%) aggravated bronchospasm.

The clinical trial program conducted with FORADIL has involved over 6000 patients. The profile of adverse events considered to be causally related to treatment from 3 controlled multidose trials of 3 months duration with FORADIL dry powder inhaler is presented in Table 1.

Table 1: FORADIL
Adverse Event Profile in Three 3-Month Controlled Trials (≥1%)

	Total Number of Patients Reporting (%)				
	Formoterol			Salbutamol	
	I: 12 µg b.i.d.	II: 24 µg b.i.d.	I+II	400 µg q.i.d.	Placebo
Total Number of Patients	**292**	**197**	**489**	**294**	**101**
Cardiovascular System					
Palpitations	2 (0.7)	5 (2.5)	7 (1.4)	10 (3.4)	1 (1.0)
Nervous System					
Tremor	6 (2.1)	10 (5.1)	16 (3.3)	6 (2.0)	1 (1.0)
Headache	9 (3.1)	4 (2.0)	13 (2.7)	10 (3.4)	2 (2.0)
Dizziness	5 (1.7)	2 (1.0)	7 (1.4)	3 (1.0)	0

The adverse event profile in 3 controlled clinical trials of up to 12 months' duration in children 5 to 15 years of age was similar to that reported in adults.

Based on its worldwide use involving over 6 million of patient-treatment-months since first introduction onto the market in 1990, the adverse events profile of FORADIL is in keeping with those observed in controlled clinical trials.

Isolated cases of the following adverse events have been reported through spontaneous reporting from those countries where the product is already marketed: hypersensitivity reactions such as severe hypotension, urticaria, angioedema, pruritus, exanthema. Peripheral edema, taste perversion, nausea.

COPD: FORADIL has been evaluated for safety in patients with COPD in 2 multi-centre, controlled studies with ipratropium or theophylline as reference therapy. In these studies, the maximum exposure to ipratropium was 3 months compared with 12 months for the other groups (formoterol, placebo and theophylline).

Table 2: FORADIL
Adverse Event Profile in 2 Controlled Studies

	Total Number of Patients Reporting (%)					
	Formoterol					
	I: 12 µg b.i.d.	II: 24 µg b.i.d.	I + II	Placebo	Ipratropium 40 µg q.i.d.	Theophylline 200-400[a] mg b.i.d.
Total Number of Patients	**405**	**406**	**811**	**420**	**194**	**209**
Digestive System						
Dry Mouth	4 (1.0)	3 (0.7)	7 (0.86)	2 (0.48)	2 (1.0)	0
Musculoskeletal System						
Cramps Muscle	4 (1.0)	9 (2.2)	13 (1.6)	0	2 (1.0)	0
Nervous System						
Headache	8 (2.0)	8 (2.0)	16 (2.0)	7 (1.7)	5 (2.6)	15 (7.1)
Tremor	4 (1.0)	10 (2.5)	14 (1.7)	1 (0.24)	0	10 (4.8)
Anxiety	4 (1.0)	1 (0.2)	5 (0.6)	0	0	2 (1.0)
Insomnia	4 (1.0)	0	4 (0.5)	2 (0.5)	2 (1.0)	7 (3.4)
Dysphonia	1 (0.2)	4 (1.0)	5 (0.61)	0	2 (1.0)	0
Respiratory System						
Coughing	2 (0.5)	5 (1.2)	7 (0.9)	5 (1.2)	2(1.0)	0
Dyspnea	0	5 (1.2)	5 (0.6)	2 (0.5)	5 (2.6)	0
Skin and Appendages						
Pruritus	4 (1.0)	0	4 (0.5)	1 (0.2)	0	1 (0.5)

[a] Open-label theophylline arm (doses had to be adjusted according to serum levels).

The type and most frequent adverse events that were considered treatment-related and occurred at an incidence of ≥1% in the FORADIL treated groups are presented in Table 2.

Postmarketing Experience: The following post-marketing events have been reported in patients treated with FORADIL:

Metabolism and Nutrition Disorders: hypokalemia, hyperglycaemia.

Cardiovascular and Other Medical Conditions: electrocardiogram QT prolonged, cardiac arrhythmias, syncope.

Rare reports of anaphylactic reactions, including severe hypotension and angioedema, have also been received in association with the use of FORADIL.

OVERDOSE:

Symptoms: An overdosage of FORADIL (formoterol fumarate) is likely to lead to effects that are typical of β_2-adrenergic stimulants: nausea, vomiting, headache, tremor, somnolence, palpitations, tachycardia, ventricular arrhythmias, metabolic acidosis, hypokalemia, hyperglycemia.

Treatment: Supportive and symptomatic treatment is indicated. Serious cases should be hospitalized.

Use of cardioselective β-adrenergic blockers may be considered, but only subject to extreme caution since the use of β-adrenergic blocker medication may provoke bronchospasm.

For management of a suspected drug overdose, contact your **regional Poison Control Centre**. See the *CPS* Directory section for a list of Poison Control Centres.

DOSAGE: **Asthma: Long-acting β_2-adrenergic agonists may increase the risk of asthma exacerbation and possibly asthma-related death (see Warnings). When treating asthma patients, FORADIL should be used only as additional therapy for patients whose conditions are not adequately controlled using low-to medium-dose inhaled corticosteroids or the severity of whose disease clearly warrants the initiation of treatment with two maintenance therapies, including FORADIL. It is not indicated for patients whose asthma can be managed by occasional use of inhaled short-acting β_2-agonists or for patients whose asthma can be successfully managed by inhaled corticosteroids along with occasional use of inhaled short-acting inhaled β_2-agonists.**

FORADIL (formoterol fumarate) should not be initiated in patients with significantly worsening or acutely deteriorating asthma, which may be a life-threatening condition (see Precautions).

FORADIL is not a replacement for inhaled or oral corticosteroid therapy; its use is complementary to it. Patients must be warned not to stop or reduce anti-inflammatory therapy without medical advice, even if they feel better on FORADIL.

FORADIL should not be used to treat acute symptoms. It is crucial to inform patients of this and prescribe a short-acting, inhaled β_2-agonist for this purpose. The need for additional symptomatic bronchodilator therapy is usually reduced with FORADIL. Medical attention should be sought if patients find that short-acting relief bronchodilator treatment becomes less effective or if they need more inhalations than usual.

Bronchodilators should not be the only or main treatment in patients with moderate to severe asthma. Patients with severe asthma require regular medical assessment since death may occur. These patients will require high-dose inhaled or oral corticosteroid therapy. Sudden worsening of symptoms may require increased corticosteroid dosage which should be administered under medical supervision (see Precautions).

Long-term Maintenance Therapy: Adults: 1 capsule (12 µg) is inhaled using the Aerolizer inhaler twice daily, in the morning and evening. In severe cases, adults may require 2 capsules (2×12 µg) twice daily, in the morning and evening. In adults, the maximum recommended daily dose of FORADIL is 48 µg.

Children (6 to 16 years): One capsule (12 µg) is inhaled using the Aerolizer inhaler twice daily, in the morning and evening. In severe cases, children may require 2 capsules (2×12 µg) twice daily, in the morning and evening. A daily dose of 48 µg should not be exceeded. In children the severity of asthma may be variable with age and periodic reassessment should be considered to determine if continued maintenance therapy with FORADIL is still indicated (see Precautions).

If a previously effective dosage fails to provide the usual relief, medical advice should be sought immediately; this is a sign of seriously worsening asthma that requires reassessment of therapy.

COPD: Adults: 1 or 2 capsules (12 µg or 24 µg) is inhaled using the Aerolizer inhaler twice daily, in the morning and evening.

General Considerations for Asthma and COPD: FORADIL should not be used more than twice daily with a 12-hour interval between doses.

Special Instructions for Asthma and COPD: Only use FORADIL capsules with the Aerolizer inhaler that is provided with each prescription refill. Do not use another type of inhaler with the capsules. Do not use other capsules in the Aerolizer inhaler.

Always use the new Aerolizer inhaler that is supplied with each prescription refill. To ensure proper administration of the drug, the physician or other health professional should show the patient how to operate the Aerolizer inhaler.

It is important for the patient to understand that the gelatin capsule might fragment and small pieces of gelatin might reach the mouth or throat during inhalation. The tendency for this to happen is minimized by not piercing the capsule more than once.

Remove the capsules from the blister pack **only immediately** before use.

The emitted dose from 1 capsule when inhaled by the Aerolizer inhaler is 9.6 µg.

INFORMATION FOR THE PATIENT: Published in e-CPS, available by subscription at www.e-cps.ca.

SUPPLIED: Each clear, hard gelatin capsule of white free flowing powder for inhalation only, contains: formoterol fumarate 12 µg. Use capsules only with the supplied Aerolizer inhalation device. Nonmedicinal ingredients: lactose. Cartons of 60 along with 1 Aerolizer inhalation device. Protect from heat (i.e., store between 15 to 25°C) and humidity.

(Shown in Product Identification Section)

Fortaz® ℞
ceftazidime pentahydrate
Antibiotic

GlaxoSmithKline

Date of Revision: September 4, 2007

PHARMACOLOGY: In vitro studies indicate that the bactericidal action of ceftazidime, a semisynthetic cephalosporin antibiotic, results from inhibition of bacterial cell wall synthesis.

Ceftazidime has a high affinity for the Penicillin-Binding Protein-3 (PBP-3) and moderate affinity for the PBP-1a of certain gram-negative organisms such as *E. coli* and *P. aeruginosa*. The affinity for PBP-1b is much less than that for either PBP-3 or PBP-1a. PBP-3 is involved in the process of cross-wall formation (septation). Binding to this protein results in formation of filaments and eventual death of the bacterium. PBP-1a and PBP-1b are involved in longitudinal wall synthesis (elongation) prior to septation. Binding to these proteins results in spheroplast formation followed by rapid lysis.

Ceftazidime has high affinity for PBP-1 and PBP-2 of *S. aureus*. However, the drug's affinity for PBP-3 is very much less in this organism.

Ceftazidime is poorly absorbed when given orally (e.g. following a 250 mg dose the average urinary recovery was less than 1% of the dose). Doses of 250, 500 and 1000 mg administered as a single bolus injection over 1 minute resulted in peak serum concentrations within 20 minutes. Mean urinary recovery of unchanged drug over 24 hours ranged from 77.4 to 85.5% with over 50% being excreted in the first 2 to 4 hours. Single i.v. infusions of 500, 1000 and 2000 mg administered over 20 to 30 minutes to normal adult volunteers resulted in peak serum concentrations within 30 minutes. Mean urinary recovery of unchanged drug over 24 hours ranged from 83.7 to 87.1% with over 50% being excreted in the first 2 to 4 hours. In both routes, serum concentration-time curves follow a biexponential decay.

Peak serum concentrations following i.m. injections of 500 or 1000 mg occurred at 1 hour. Mean urinary recovery of ceftazidime over 24 hours ranged from 78.9 to 84.6%.

No accumulation of drug was noted during repeated i.m. doses of ceftazidime (1 g, t.i.d., 10 days).

In vitro studies with human serum revealed that 5 to 23% of ceftazidime is protein bound and is independent of drug concentration.

Ceftazidime is not metabolized. Metabolites were not detected either in the serum by HPLC or in the urine by chromatography or bioautography.

Hepatic clearance (i.e. biliary excretion) accounts for less than 1% of the total clearance of ceftazidime in the presence of normally functioning kidneys.

The mean renal clearance of ceftazidime was 97.6 mL/min (range 76 to 110 mL/min). The calculated plasma clearance of 116.4 mL/min (range 97 to 139 mL/min) indicated nearly complete elimination of ceftazidime by the renal route. Administration of probenecid prior to dosing had no effect on the elimination kinetics of ceftazidime. This suggested that ceftazidime is eliminated by glomerular filtration and is not actively secreted by renal tubular mechanisms.

INDICATIONS: For the treatment of patients with infections caused by susceptible strains of the designated organisms in the following diseases:

Lower Respiratory Tract Infections: Pneumonia caused by *P. aeruginosa*; *H. influenzae* including ampicillin-resistant strains; Klebsiella species; Enterobacter species; *P. mirabilis*; *E. coli*; Serratia species; *S. pneumoniae*; and *S. aureus* including ampicillin-resistant (but not methicillin-resistant) strains.

Urinary Tract Infections: caused by *P. aeruginosa*; Enterobacter species; Proteus species (indole positive and negative); Klebsiella species; and *E. coli*.

Due to the nature of the underlying conditions which usually predispose patients to Pseudomonas infections of the lower respiratory and urinary tracts, a good clinical response accompanied by bacterial eradication may not be achieved despite evidence of in vitro sensitivity.

Skin Structure Infections: caused by *P. aeruginosa*; Klebsiella species; *E. coli*; *P. mirabilis*; Enterobacter species; *S. aureus*, including ampicillin-resistant (but not methicillin-resistant) strains; and *S. pyogenes*.

Bacteremia/Septicemia: caused by *P. aeruginosa*; Klebsiella species; *E. coli*; Serratia species; *S. pneumoniae*; *S. aureus*, including ampicillin-resistant (but not methicillin-resistant) strains; and *S. epidermidis*.

Bone Infections: caused by *P. aeruginosa*; *P. mirabilis*; Enterobacter species; and *S. aureus*, including ampicillin-resistant (but not methicillin-resistant) strains.

Peritonitis: caused by *E. coli*; Klebsiella species; and Peptostreptococcus species. Patients infected with Bacteroides species have also responded.

Meningitis: caused by *H. influenzae* and *N. meningitidis*. Ceftazidime has also been used successfully in a limited number of cases of meningitis due to *P. aeruginosa*.

Specimens for bacteriologic culture should be obtained prior to therapy in order to identify the causative organisms and to determine their susceptibilities to ceftazidime. Therapy may be instituted before results of susceptibility testing are known. However, modification of the treatment may be required once these results become available.

CONTRAINDICATIONS: Patients who have shown hypersensitivity to ceftazidime or the cephalosporin group of antibiotics.

WARNINGS: Before therapy with ceftazidime is instituted, careful enquiry should be made to determine whether the patient has had previous hypersensitivity reactions to ceftazidime, cephalosporins, penicillins, or other drugs. Ceftazidime should be administered with caution to any patient who has demonstrated some form of allergy, particularly to drugs. Special care is indicated in patients who have experienced an allergic reaction to penicillins or other beta-lactams. If an allergic reaction to ceftazidime occurs, treatment should be discontinued and standard agents (e.g. epinephrine, antihistamines, corticosteroids) administered as necessary.

Pseudomembranous colitis has been reported to be associated with treatment with ceftazidime (and other broad-spectrum antibiotics). Therefore, it is important to consider its diagnosis in patients administered ceftazidime who develop diarrhea. Treatment with broad-spectrum antibiotics, including ceftazidime, alters the normal flora of the colon and may permit overgrowth of Clostridia. Studies indicate that a toxin produced by *C. difficile* is one primary cause of antibiotic-associated colitis. Mild cases of colitis may respond to drug discontinuance alone. Moderate to severe cases should be managed with fluid, electrolyte, and protein supplementation as indicated. When the colitis is not relieved by discontinuance of ceftazidime administration or when it is severe, consideration should be given to the administration of vancomycin or other suitable therapy. Other possible causes of colitis should also be considered.

PRECAUTIONS: Ceftazidime should be administered with caution to individuals with a history of gastrointestinal disease, particularly colitis.

Patients with impaired renal function (i.e. creatinine clearance of 50 mL/min/1.73 m² or less) should be placed on the special dosage schedule for ceftazidime (see Dosage). Normal dosages in these individuals are likely to produce excessive serum concentrations of ceftazidime. Elevated levels of ceftazidime in these patients could lead to convulsions.

The concomitant administration of aminoglycosides and some cephalosporins has caused nephrotoxicity. Although transient elevations of BUN and serum creatinine have been observed in clinical studies, there is no evidence that ceftazidime, when administered alone, is significantly nephrotoxic. However, the effect of administering it concomitantly with aminoglycosides is not known. Studies suggest that the concomitant use of potent diuretics, such as furosemide and ethacrynic acid, may increase the risk of renal toxicity with cephalosporins.

Ceftazidime is eliminated via the kidneys, therefore the dosage should be reduced according to the degree of renal impairment. Neurological sequelae have occasionally been reported when the dose has not been reduced appropriately (see Dosage, Adults with Impaired Renal Function and Adverse Effects).

Prolonged treatment may result in the overgrowth of nonsusceptible organisms, including species originally sensitive to the drug. Repeated evaluation of the patient's condition is essential. If superinfection occurs during therapy, appropriate measures should be taken.

Development of resistance during the administration of ceftazidime has been observed for *S. aureus*, members of the Enterobacteriaceae family, Acinetobacter species, Pseudomonas species, and Serratia species.

Chloramphenicol is antagonistic in vitro with ceftazidime and other cephalosporins. The clinical relevance of this finding is unknown, but if concurrent administration of ceftazidime with chloramphenicol is proposed, the possibility of antagonism should be considered.

In common with other antibiotics, ceftazidime may affect the gut flora, leading to lower estrogen reabsorption and reduced efficacy of combined oral contraceptives.

Pregnancy: Safety in pregnancy has not been established. The use of ceftazidime in pregnant women requires that the likely benefit from the drug be weighed against the possible risk to the mother and fetus.

Reproduction studies have been performed in mice and rats employing ceftazidime doses of up to 25 times those usually administered to humans. These studies have revealed no evidence of impaired fertility or harm to the fetus caused by ceftazidime. Animal reproduction studies, however, are not always predictive of human response.

Lactation: Ceftazidime is excreted in human milk in low concentrations (3.8 to 5.2 mg/L). The clinical significance of this is unknown, therefore, caution should be exercised when ceftazidime is administered to a nursing mother.

Geriatrics: The elimination of ceftazidime may be reduced due to impairment of renal function.

Drug-laboratory Test Interactions: Ceftazidime may cause a false-positive reaction for glucose in the urine with copper reduction tests (Benedict's or Fehling's solution). As a false-negative result may occur in the ferricyanide test, it is recommended that either glucose oxidase or hexokinase method be used to determine blood plasma glucose levels in patients receiving ceftazidime.

Ceftazidime does not interfere in the alkaline picrate assay for creatinine.

A positive Coombs' test has been reported during treatment with cephalosporins. This phenomenon can interfere with cross-matching of blood.

ADVERSE EFFECTS: The most common adverse effects have been local reactions following i.v. injection, allergic reactions, and gastrointestinal reactions. Other adverse effects have been encountered less frequently.

Local (2.8% of patients): thrombophlebitis or phlebitis and pain with i.v. administration. Pain after i.m. injection.

Hypersensitivity (2.7% of patients): pruritus, urticaria, allergic exanthema, and fever. There have been rare reports of toxic epidermal necrolysis. Angioderma and anaphylaxis (including bronchospasm and/or hypotension) have been reported very rarely.

Gastrointestinal (<4% of patients): diarrhea, nausea, vomiting, colitis and abdominal pain. Pseudomembranous colitis has been reported (see Warnings). Oral thrush has been reported very rarely.

CNS (<1% of patients): headache, dizziness, hallucinations, and lethargy. There have been reports of neurological sequelae including tremor, myoclonia, convulsions and coma occurring in patients with renal impairment in whom the dose of ceftazidime has not been appropriately reduced.

Renal (<1% of patients): transient elevations of blood urea, BUN and serum creatinine.

Hepatic (<4% of patients): transient elevations of serum bilirubin, alkaline phosphatase, LDH, AST, ALT and GGT.

Hematopoietic: eosinophilia (3.4%), positive direct Coombs' test (5.1%), and with an incidence of <1%: thrombocytosis, transient leukopenia, neutropenia, agranulocytosis, thrombocytopenia, lymphocytosis and, very rarely, hemolytic anemia.

Hepatobiliary Tract and Pancreas: very rarely, jaundice.

Miscellaneous (<1% of patients): paresthesia, blurred vision, bad taste, flushing, candidiasis, and vaginitis.

OVERDOSE:

Symptoms: Overdosage of cephalosporins can lead to neurological sequelae, including encephalopathy, convulsions and coma.

Treatment: Excessive serum levels of ceftazidime can be reduced by hemodialysis or peritoneal dialysis.

For management of a suspected drug overdose, CPhA recommends that you contact your **regional Poison Control Centre**. See the *CPS* Directory section for a list of Poison Control Centres.

DOSAGE: Ceftazidime may be administered either i.v. or i.m. after reconstitution.

Dosage and route of administration should be determined by severity of infection, susceptibility of the causative organism(s), and condition of the patient. The i.v. route is preferable for patients with septicemia, peritonitis or other severe or life-threatening infections, or for patients who may be poor risks because of lowered resistance resulting from such debilitating conditions as malnutrition, trauma, surgery, diabetes, heart failure, or malignancy, particularly if shock is present or pending.

The usual duration of treatment is 7 to 14 days. For Streptococcal infections, therapy should be continued for at least 10 days.

Adults: 0.5 to 6 g daily administered in equally divided doses every 8 to 12 hours (see Table 1).

Table 1: Fortaz

Dosage in Adults

Type of Infection	Daily Dose (g)	Frequency and Route
Uncomplicated pneumonia or skin structure infection	1.5–3	0.5–1 g i.m. or i.v. q8h
Uncomplicated urinary tract infections	0.5	250 mg i.m. or i.v. q12h
Complicated urinary tract infections	1–1.5	500 mg i.m. or i.v. q8h or q12h
Bone infections	4	2 g i.v. q12h
Peritonitis or septicemia	6	2 g i.v. q8h
Meningitis	6	2 g i.v. q8h

For the treatment of infections caused by Staphylococcus species, a dosage of 1 or 2 g administered every 8 hours is recommended. For the treatment of infections (except those confined to the urinary tract) caused by Enterobacter species, a dosage of at least 1 g administered every 8 hours is recommended.

Children: (see Table 2).

Table 2: Fortaz

Dosage in Children

Type of Infection	Age Group[a] Dosage	Dosage
Infections other than meningitis	1 month–2 months	25–50 mg/kg i.v. q12h to a maximum of 6 g/day
	2 months–12 years	30–50 mg/kg i.v. q8h to a maximum of 6 g/day
Meningitis	1 month–12 years	50 mg/kg i.v. q8h to a maximum of 6 g/day

[a] The maximum daily dose in children is 6 g.

Neonates (aged 0 to 28 days): In children aged 1 month or less the recommended dose is 25 to 50 mg/kg given twice daily.

Data indicate that the half-life of ceftazidime in neonates increases with decreasing gestational age and can be 3 to 4 times that in adults. An adjustment in dosing interval may be necessary with an increasing degree of prematurity. Additionally, clearance may increase rapidly in the first 2 to 3 weeks of life, necessitating a readjustment of dose and/or dosing interval.

Geriatrics: In acutely ill elderly patients with reduced renal clearance of ceftazidime, the daily dosage should not exceed 3 g.

Impaired Hepatic Function: No adjustment in dosage is required for patients with hepatic dysfunction, provided renal function is not impaired.

Adults with Impaired Renal Function: Ceftazidime is excreted almost exclusively by glomerular filtration. In patients in whom the glomerular filtration rate (GFR) is less than or equal to 50 mL/min (0.83 mL/s), the dosage must be reduced to compensate for its slower excretion. After an initial loading dose of 1 g, a maintenance dosage schedule should be followed (see Table 3).

Table 3: Fortaz

Recommended Maintenance Doses in Renal Insufficiency

Creatinine Clearance		Recommended Unit Dose		
mL/min/1.73 m²	mL/s/1.73 m²	Moderate Infections	Severe Infections	Frequency[a] of Dosing
31–50	0.51–0.83	1 g	1.5 g	q12h
16–30	0.26–0.50	1 g	1.5 g	q24h
6–15	0 .10–0.25	500 mg	750 mg	q24h
≤5	≤0.09	500 mg	750 mg	q48h

[a] If the severity of the infection necessitates an increase in the dosing frequency, serum concentrations of ceftazidime should be used as guidelines.

When only serum creatinine levels are known, the following formulas may be used to estimate creatinine clearance. The serum creatinine must represent a steady state of renal function.

Males:

$$\text{Creatinine clearance (mL/s)} = \frac{\text{Weight (kg)} \times (140-\text{age})}{49 \times \text{serum creatinine } (\mu\text{mol/L})}$$

or

$$\text{Creatinine clearance (mL/min)} = \frac{\text{Weight (kg)} \times (140-\text{age})}{72 \times \text{serum creatinine (mg/dL)}}$$

Females: 0.85 × above value.

Mean serum half-life of ceftazidime in patients with no kidney function was reduced, from a range of 24.0 to 35.4 hours between dialysis sessions, to a range of 2.8 to 4.6 hours during hemodialysis. Therefore, a loading dose of 1 g is recommended, followed by 0.5 to 1 g after each hemodialysis period. Serum concentrations of ceftazidime should be carefully monitored and used as a basis to adjust the dosage.

Ceftazidime can also be used in patients undergoing peritoneal dialysis and continuous ambulatory peritoneal dialysis. In such patients, a loading dose of 1 g is suggested, followed by 500 mg every 24 hours. Serum concentrations of ceftazidime should be carefully monitored and used as a basis to adjust the dosage.

Administration: I.M.: Ceftazidime may be administered by deep i.m. injection into a large muscle mass such as the upper outer quadrant of the gluteus maximus or vastus lateralis. The maximum dose should be 1 g for a single i.m. injection.

I.V.: Intermittent I.V. Administration: The reconstituted solution may be slowly injected into the vein over a period of 3 to 5 minutes or given through the tubing of an administration set. During the infusion of the solution containing ceftazidime, the administration of other solutions should be discontinued temporarily.

Continuous I.V. Infusion: Ceftazidime may also be administered over a longer period of time.

Note: If therapy is carried out in combination with an aminoglycoside antibiotic, each should be administered at different sites because of a physical incompatibility. An aminoglycoside should not be mixed with this product in the same container.

Reconstitution: Caution: Ensure adequate venting. Addition of diluent generates a positive pressure.

I.M.: Solutions for reconstitution are sterile water for injection or, if required, Bacteriostatic Water for Injection with benzyl alcohol or parabens (not for use in neonates) and 0.5 to 1.0% Lignocaine Hydrochloride Injection. See Table 4.

Table 4: Fortaz

Reconstitution Table: I.M. Use

Vial Size	Diluent to be added to Vial	Approximate Available Volume	Approximate Average Concentration
1 g	3 mL	3.9 mL	280 mg/mL

Shake well until dissolved.

I.V.: Solutions for reconstitution are Sterile Water for Injection. See Table 5.

Table 5: Fortaz

Reconstitution Table: I.V. Use

Vial Size	Diluent to be added to Vial	Approximate Available Volume	Approximate Average Concentration
1 g	10 mL	10.9 mL	100 mg/mL
2 g	10 mL	11.7 mL	175 mg/mL

Shake well until dissolved. The prepared solution may be further diluted to the desired volume with any of the solutions listed under Solutions for I.V. Infusion.

Direct I.V. Injection: Reconstitute as directed above.

Intermittent I.V. Infusion: Reconstitute as directed above for 1 g or 2 g vials.

Continuous I.V. Infusion: Vials: Reconstitute 1 g or 2 g vials with 10 mL Sterile Water for Injection. The appropriate quantity of the reconstituted solution may be added to an i.v. bottle containing any of the solutions listed under Solutions for I.V. Infusion.

Pharmacy Bulk Vial 6 g: **The availability of the pharmacy bulk vial is restricted to hospitals with a recognized i.v. admixture program.**

This product does not contain any preservatives. The Pharmacy Bulk Vial is intended for multiple dispensing for i.v. use only, employing a single puncture. Reconstitute with 26 mL Sterile Water for Injection. See Table 6.

Table 6: Fortaz

Reconstitution Table: Pharmacy Bulk Vial

Vial Size	Diluent to be added to Vial	Approximate Available Volume	Approximate Average Concentration
6 g	26 mL	30 mL	200 mg/mL

Shake well until dissolved. Following reconstitution with Sterile Water for Injection, the solution should be dispensed and diluted for use within 8 hours at room temperature (not exceeding 25°C). Any unused reconstituted solution should be discarded after 8 hours. The appropriate quantity of the reconstituted solution may be added to an i.v. bottle containing any of the solutions listed below.

Solutions for I.V. Infusion: 0.9 % Sodium Chloride Injection, M/6 Sodium Lactate Injection, Ringers Injection USP, Lactated Ringers Injection USP, 5% Dextrose Injection, 5% Dextrose and 0.225% Sodium Chloride Injection, 5% Dextrose and 0.45% Sodium Chloride Injection, 5% Dextrose and 0.9% Sodium Chloride Injection, 10% Dextrose Injection, 10% Invert Sugar in Water for Injection and Normosol-M in 5% Dextrose Injection, Sterile Water for Injection.

Stability: Reconstituted solutions should be administered within 12 hours when stored at room temperature (not exceeding 25°C), and within 48 hours when refrigerated, from the time of reconstitution, both when prepared as bolus injections, i.m. or i.v., and as infusion admixtures with the recommended i.v. diluents.

Incompatibility: Ceftazidime should not be added to blood products, protein hydrolysates or amino acids. It should not be mixed together with an aminoglycoside. Ceftazidime is less stable in Sodium Bicarbonate Injection than in other i.v. fluids; therefore it is not recommended as a diluent.

Precipitation has been reported when vancomycin has been added to ceftazidime in solution. Therefore, it would be prudent to flush giving sets and the i.v. lines between administration of these two agents.

SUPPLIED: I.M. or Direct I.V. Injection: Each vial contains: the equivalent of 1 g ceftazidime. Packs of 10.

I.V. injection or infusion: Each vial contains: the equivalent of 1 g and 2 g ceftazidime. Packs of 10.

Each pharmacy bulk vial contains: the equivalent of 6 g ceftazidime. Packs of 6.

Vials contain a mixture of ceftazidime pentahydrate and sodium carbonate. Sodium carbonate at a concentration of 118 mg/g of ceftazidime activity has been admixed to facilitate dissolution. Total sodium content of the mixture is approximately 2.3 mEq/g (54 mg of ceftazidime activity). Gluten- and tartrazine-free.

Ceftazidime pentahydrate is a white to cream-colored powder. Solutions range in color from light yellow to amber, depending upon the diluent and volume used. The pH of freshly reconstituted solutions ranges from 5.0 to 7.5.

Store the dry powder below 25°C. Protect from light.

Forteo® Ⓟ

teriparatide (rDNA origin)

Bone Formation Agent

Lilly

Date of Revision: February 9, 2010

SUMMARY PRODUCT INFORMATION:

Route of Administration	Dosage Form/Strength	Clinically Relevant Nonmedicinal Ingredients
Subcutaneous Injection	Sterile Solution for Subcutaneous Injection, 250 µg/mL in 3 mL prefilled pen, 250 µg/mL in 2.4 mL prefilled pen	None For a complete listing see Dosage Forms, Composition and Packaging.

DESCRIPTION: FORTEO [teriparatide (rDNA origin) injection] contains recombinant human parathyroid hormone (1-34), [rhPTH(1-34)], which has an identical sequence to the 34 N-terminal amino acids (the biologically active region) of the 84-amino acid human parathyroid hormone. Teriparatide (rDNA origin) is manufactured using a strain of *E. coli* modified by recombinant DNA technology.

INDICATIONS AND CLINICAL USE: FORTEO [teriparatide (rDNA origin) injection] is indicated:

- For the treatment of postmenopausal women with severe osteoporosis who are at high risk of fracture or who have failed or are intolerant to previous osteoporosis therapy.
- To increase bone mass in men with primary or hypogonadal severe osteoporosis who have failed or are intolerant to previous osteoporosis therapy. The effects of FORTEO on risk for fracture in men have not been demonstrated.

- For the treatment of osteoporosis associated with sustained systemic glucocorticoid therapy in men and women who are at increased risk for fracture.

The diagnosis of severe osteoporosis may be confirmed by the finding of low bone mass or the presence or history of osteoporotic fracture. While non-vertebral fractures are usually clinically apparent, vertebral fractures also may be manifested by back pain, height loss, or kyphosis.

Geriatrics: Of the patients receiving FORTEO in the osteoporosis treatment trial of 1637 postmenopausal women, 75% were 65 and over and 23% were 75 and over. No significant differences in bone response and no new safety findings were seen in geriatric patients receiving FORTEO as compared with younger patients.

Of the patients receiving FORTEO in the osteoporosis treatment trial of 437 men, 39% were 65 and over and 13% were 75 and over. Fracture efficacy endpoints have not been evaluated in these patients. No significant differences in bone response and no new safety findings were seen in geriatric patients receiving FORTEO as compared with younger patients.

Of the 214 patients that received FORTEO in an active comparator trial of glucocorticoid-induced osteoporosis, 28% were 65 and over and 9% were 75 and over. No significant differences in bone response and no new safety findings were seen in geriatric patients (≥65) receiving FORTEO as compared with younger patients.

Pediatrics: The safety and efficacy of FORTEO have not been studied in pediatric populations. FORTEO is not indicated for use in pediatric patients or young adults with open epiphysis (see Warnings and Precautions, Special Populations, Pediatrics).

CONTRAINDICATIONS: FORTEO [teriparatide (rDNA origin) injection] is contraindicated for:

- Hypersensitivity to teriparatide or any of its excipients.
- Pre-existing hypercalcemia.
- Severe renal impairment.
- Metabolic bone diseases other than primary osteoporosis (including hyperparathyroidism and Paget's disease of the bone).
- Unexplained elevations of alkaline phosphatase.
- Prior external beam or implant radiation therapy involving the skeleton.
- Bone metastases or a history of skeletal malignancies.
- Pregnancy and nursing mothers (see Warnings and Precautions, Special Populations).
- Pediatric patients or young adults with open epiphysis (see Warnings and Precautions, Special Populations).

WARNINGS AND PRECAUTIONS:

Serious Warnings and Precautions

Physicians should become familiar with the full content of the Product Monograph prior to prescribing FORTEO [teriparatide (rDNA origin) injection]. FORTEO should be prescribed only to patients for whom the potential benefits outweigh the potential risk. In rats, teriparatide caused an increase in the incidence of osteosarcoma that was dose and treatment duration dependent at systemic exposures ranging from 3 to 60 times the exposure in humans given a 20 µg dose. FORTEO should not be prescribed to patients who are at increased baseline risk for osteosarcoma (see Contraindications and Warnings and Precautions, Carcinogenicity).

Carcinogenicity: Two carcinogenicity bioassays were conducted in Fischer 344 rats. In these studies, rats were given daily subcutaneous teriparatide injections at doses that resulted in systemic exposures between 3 and 60 times higher than the systemic exposure observed in humans following a subcutaneous dose of 20 µg (based on AUC comparison). Teriparatide treatment resulted in increases in the incidence of bone tumours, including osteosarcoma, that occurred in association with dose-dependant exaggerated increases in bone mass. The studies showed that the occurrence of bone tumours was dependent upon dose and duration of exposure. The clinical significance of the observations in rats has not been established. Osteosarcoma has not been observed in teriparatide clinical trials.

FORTEO should not be prescribed to patients who are at increased baseline risk for osteosarcoma (e.g. Paget's disease, pediatric and young adult with open epiphyses, history of radiation therapy involving the skeleton, etc.)

General: The safety and efficacy of FORTEO [teriparatide (rDNA origin) injection] have been evaluated up to 2 years in studies GHAC, GHAJ, GHBJ and GHCA (median 19 months in women in study GHAC and 10 months in men in study GHAJ). An additional clinical study (GHBZ) evaluated the safety and efficacy of FORTEO for up to 3 years. The maximum lifetime exposure to FORTEO for an individual patient is 24 months.

In clinical trials, the frequency of urolithiasis was similar in patients treated with FORTEO and placebo. However, FORTEO has not been studied in patients with active urolithiasis. If active urolithiasis or pre-existing hypercalciuria are suspected, measurement of urinary calcium excretion should be considered. FORTEO should be used with caution in patients with active or recent urolithiasis because of the potential to exacerbate this condition.

Hypotension: In short-term clinical studies with teriparatide, isolated episodes of transient orthostatic hypotension were observed. Typically, an event began within 4 hours of dosing and spontaneously resolved within a few minutes to a few hours. When transient orthostatic hypotension occurred, it happened within the first several doses, was relieved by placing subjects in a reclining position, and did not preclude continued treatment. Patients experiencing symptoms associated with hypotension should not drive or operate machinery until they become asymptomatic.

Information to Be Provided to the Patient: For safe and effective use of FORTEO, the physician should inform patients about the following:

General: Physicians should instruct their patients to read the Information for the Patient Leaflet and Pen User Manual before starting therapy with FORTEO and re-read them each time the prescription is renewed.

Osteosarcomas in Rats: Patients should be made aware that FORTEO caused osteosarcomas in rats and that the clinical relevance of these findings is unknown.

Orthostatic Hypotension: Patients should be instructed that if they feel lightheaded after injection, they should sit or lie down until the symptoms resolve. If symptoms persist or worsen, patients should be instructed to consult a physician before continuing treatment. Patients experiencing symptoms associated with hypotension should not drive or operate machinery until they become asymptomatic (see Warnings and Precautions, Hypotension).

Hypercalcemia: Although symptomatic hypercalcemia was not observed in clinical trials, physicians should instruct patients to contact a health care provider if they develop persistent symptoms of hypercalcemia (i.e., nausea, vomiting, constipation, lethargy, muscle weakness).

Use of the Pen: Patients should be instructed on how to properly use the prefilled delivery device (refer to Pen User Manual) and properly dispose of needles, and be advised not to share their pens with other patients.

Other Osteoporosis Treatment and Prevention Measures: Patients should be informed regarding the roles of supplemental calcium and/or vitamin D, weight-bearing exercise, and modification of certain behavioral factors such as cigarette smoking and/or alcohol/coffee consumption.

Special Populations: Pregnant Women and Women of Childbearing Potential: FORTEO should not be administered to women who are pregnant. The effect of teriparatide treatment on human fetal development has not been studied. Women of childbearing potential should use effective methods of contraception during use of FORTEO. Should pregnancy occur, FORTEO should be discontinued (see Contraindications).

Nursing Women: There have been no clinical studies to determine if teriparatide is secreted into breast milk. FORTEO should not be administered to nursing mothers (see Contraindications).

Pediatrics: FORTEO has not been studied in pediatric populations. FORTEO should not be used in children or young adults with open epiphyses (see Contraindications).

Premenopausal Women: Before initiating therapy with FORTEO in premenopausal women with glucocorticoid-induced osteoporosis, risk factors such as low BMD, length and dosage of glucocorticoid therapy, previous fractures, family history, high bone turnover, level of underlying disease activity, low sex steroid level or low body mass index, should be considered.

Geriatrics: Of the patients receiving FORTEO in the osteoporosis treatment trial of 1637 postmenopausal women, 75% were 65 and over and 23% were 75 and over. No significant differences in bone response and no new safety findings were seen in geriatric patients receiving FORTEO as compared with younger patients.

Of the patients receiving FORTEO in the osteoporosis treatment trial of 437 men, 39% were 65 and over and 13% were 75 and over. Fracture efficacy endpoints have not been evaluated in these patients. No significant differences in bone response and no new safety findings were seen in geriatric patients receiving FORTEO as compared with younger patients.

Of the 214 patients that received FORTEO in an active comparator trial of glucocorticoid-induced osteoporosis, 28% were 65 and over and 9% were 75 and over. No significant differences in bone response and no new safety findings were seen in geriatric patients (≥65) receiving FORTEO as compared with younger patients.

Monitoring and Laboratory Tests: Serum Calcium: FORTEO transiently increases serum calcium, with the maximal effect observed at approximately 4 to 6 hours post-dose. By 16 hours post-dose, serum calcium generally has returned to or near baseline. These effects should be kept in mind because serum calcium concentrations observed within 16 hours after a dose may reflect the pharmacologic effect of teriparatide. Persistent hypercalcemia was not observed in clinical trials with FORTEO. If persistent hypercalcemia is detected, treatment with FORTEO should be discontinued pending further evaluation of the cause of hypercalcemia.

Patients known to have an underlying hypercalcemic disorder, such as primary hyperparathyroidism, should not be treated with FORTEO (see Contraindications).

Urinary Calcium: FORTEO increases urinary calcium excretion, but the frequency of hypercalciuria in clinical trials was similar for patients treated with FORTEO and placebo (see Action and Clinical Pharmacology, Pharmacodynamics, Urinary Calcium Excretion).

Renal Function: No clinically important adverse renal effects were observed in clinical studies. Assessments included creatinine clearance; measurements of blood urea nitrogen (BUN), creatinine, and electrolytes in serum; urine specific gravity and pH; and examination of urine sediment. Long-term evaluation of patients with severe renal insufficiency, patients undergoing acute or chronic dialysis, or patients who have functioning renal transplants has not been performed. Caution should be exercised in patients with moderate and severe renal impairment.

Serum Uric Acid: FORTEO increases serum uric acid concentrations. In clinical trials, 2.8% of FORTEO patients had serum uric acid concentrations above the upper limit of normal compared with 0.7% of placebo patients. However, the hyperuricemia did not result in an increase in gout, arthralgia, or urolithiasis.

ADVERSE REACTIONS: Adverse Drug Reaction Overview: The safety of teriparatide has been evaluated in 24 clinical trials that enrolled over 2800 women and men. Four long-term, Phase 3 clinical trials included one large placebo-controlled, double-blind multicentre trial with 1637 postmenopausal women, one placebo-controlled, double-blind multicentre trial with 437 men, and two active-controlled trials including 393 postmenopausal women. Teriparatide doses ranged from 5 to 100 µg/day in short-term trials and 20 to 40 µg/day in the long-term trials. A total of 1943 of the patients studied received teriparatide, including 815 patients at 20 µg/day and 1107 patients at 40 µg/day. In the long-term clinical trials, 1137 patients were exposed to teriparatide for greater than 1 year (500 at 20 µg/day and 637 at 40 µg/day). The maximum exposure duration to teriparatide was 2 years. Adverse events associated with FORTEO [teriparatide (rDNA origin) injection] usually were mild and generally did not require discontinuation of therapy.

The safety of teriparatide has also been evaluated in a Phase 3 randomized, double blind, doubledummy, active controlled clinical trial that enrolled 428 men and women with glucocorticoidinduced osteoporosis. Patients received either FORTEO 20 µg/day plus oral placebo (n=214) or alendronate 10 mg/day plus injectable placebo (n=214) for up to 3 years.

An additional Phase 3, randomized, multinational, multicenter, open-label study that enrolled 868 patients evaluated safety and efficacy of up to 24 months continuous treatment with 20 µg/day of FORTEO.

Clinical Trial Adverse Drug Reactions: In the two Phase 3, placebo-controlled clinical trials in men and postmenopausal women, early discontinuation due to an adverse event occurred in 5.6% of patients assigned to placebo and 7.1% of patients assigned to FORTEO.

Table 1 lists adverse events occurring in the Phase 3, placebo-controlled clinical trials in postmenopausal women and in men at a frequency ≥2.0% in the FORTEO groups and in more FORTEO-treated patients than in placebo-treated patients. Adverse events are shown without attribution of causality.

Table 1: FORTEO

Adverse Events in Placebo-controlled Clinical Trials (Irrespective of Causality)[a]

	% Patients	
Body System	**FORTEO (N=691)**	**Placebo (N=691)**
Body as a Whole		
Pain	21.3	20.5
Headache	7.5	7.4
Asthenia	8.7	6.8
Neck Pain	3.0	2.7
Cardiovascular		
Hypertension	7.1	6.8
Angina Pectoris	2.5	1.6
Syncope	2.6	1.4
Digestive System		
Nausea	8.5	6.7
Constipation	5.4	4.5
Diarrhea	5.1	4.6
Dyspepsia	5.2	4.1
Vomiting	3.0	2.3
Gastrointestinal Disorder	2.3	2.0
Tooth Disorder	2.0	1.3
Metabolic		
Hyperuricemia	2.8	0.7
Musculoskeletal		
Arthralgia	10.1	8.4
Leg Cramps	2.6	1.3
Nervous System		
Dizziness	8.0	5.4
Depression	4.1	2.7
Insomnia	4.3	3.6
Vertigo	3.8	2.7
Respiratory System		

(cont'd)

Table 1: FORTEO *(cont'd)*

Adverse Events in Placebo-controlled Clinical Trials (Irrespective of Causality)[a]

	% Patients	
Body System	**FORTEO (N=691)**	**Placebo (N=691)**
Rhinitis	9.6	8.8
Cough Increased	6.4	5.5
Pharyngitis	5.5	4.8
Dyspnea	3.6	2.6
Pneumonia	3.9	3.3
Skin and Appendages		
Rash	4.9	4.5
Sweating	2.2	1.7

[a] Treatment emergent adverse events that occurred at a frequency ≥2% in patients treated with FORTEO at 20 µg/day irrespective of causality assessment by Clinical Study Investigators.
COSTART terminology.

Treatment emergent adverse events considered by Clinical Study Investigators to be causally related to FORTEO, reported by at least 1% of FORTEO-treated patients and reported in more FORTEO-treated patients than placebo-treated patients are: dizziness, nausea, arthralgia, asthenia and headache. Leg cramps is an adverse event that may also be causally related to FORTEO.

Note: The incidence of hypertension, syncope, dyspepsia, rhinitis, and pharyngitis in patients treated with teriparatide 40 µg/day (twice the recommended dose) was lower than the incidence in placebo treated-patients.

During the 18-month primary phase of a double-blind, double-dummy, active comparatorcontrolled study in men and women with glucocorticoid-induced osteoporosis, early discontinuation due to treatment-emergent adverse events (TEAEs) occurred in 31 (15%) patients assigned to FORTEO (N=214) and in 25 (12%) patients assigned to alendronate (N=214). Over 24 months, the early discontinuation due to TEAEs occurred in 35 (16.4%) patients assigned to FORTEO (N=214) and in 27 (12.6%) patients assigned to alendronate (N=214).

Table 2 lists drug-related adverse events reported in ≥1% of patients treated with FORTEO or Alendronate 10 mg/day in a clinical trial of men and women with Glucocorticoid-induced Osteoporosis up to 24 months.

Table 2: FORTEO

Drug-Related[a] Adverse Events Reported in ≥1% of Patients Treated with FORTEO 20 µg/day or Alendronate 10 mg/day in a Principle Clinical Trial in Men and Women with Glucocorticoid-induced Osteoporosis. Study B3D-US-GHBZ, 24 Month Data

	FORTEO (N=214) (%)	**Alendronate (N=214) (%)**
Gastrointestinal Disorders		
Nausea	7.0	2.3
Abdominal pain upper	3.3	3.3
Vomiting	2.8	3.3
Abdominal pain	1.4	0.9
Dyspepsia	1.4	0.9
Gastric ulcer	0	1.4
Nervous System Disorders		
Dizziness	3.3	0.9
Headache	3.3	0.9
Musculoskeletal and Connective Tissue Disorders		
Muscle spasms	0.9	1.9

[a] Considered to be possibly related by Clinical Study Investigators.
MedDRA (version 10.0) terminology.

The 24-month study, B3D-EW-GHCA (EUROFORS), was a multinational, multicenter, prospective, open-label Phase 3/4 trial in postmenopausal women with osteoporosis. Study GHCA had 2 substudies in which all patients received FORTEO 20 µg/day plus calcium and vitamin D during the first 12 months. In substudy 1, patients were randomized to receive an additional one year of therapy with either FORTEO 20 µg/day or raloxifene 60 mg/day, or no treatment. In substudy 2, all patients received 24 months of FORTEO 20 µg/day. All patients received supplemental calcium and Vitamin D.

Table 3 lists drug-related adverse events reported in ≥1% of patients. Most reports of possibly drug related TEAEs occurred in the first 6-month interval of the study.

Table 3: FORTEO

Drug-Related[a] Adverse Events Reported in ≥1% of Patients Treated with FORTEO 20 µg/day in a Clinical Trial in Women with Osteoporosis. Study B3D-EW-GHCA (EUROFORS), 24 Month Data

	FORTEO (N=866) (%)
Gastrointestinal Disorders	
Nausea	8.0
Vomiting	1.3
Diarrhea	1.2
Nervous System Disorders	
Headache	4.4
Dizziness	2.9
Vertigo	1.5
Muscloskeletal and Connective Tissue Disorders	
Muscle cramp	4.3
Pain in extremity	1.3
Arthralgia	1.7
Back pain	1.0
Other	
Hypercalcemia	3.1
Injection site erythema	1.3

(cont'd)

Table 3: FORTEO *(cont'd)*

[a] Considered to be possibly related by Clinical Study Investigators.
MedDRA (version 7.0) terminology.

Serum Calcium: FORTEO transiently increases serum calcium, with the maximal effect observed at approximately 4 to 6 hours post-dose. Serum calcium measured at least 16 hours post-dose was not different from pretreatment levels. In clinical trials, the frequency of at least 1 episode of transient hypercalcemia in the 4 to 6 hours after FORTEO administration was increased from 1.5% of women and none of the men treated with placebo to 11.1% of women and 6.0% of men treated with FORTEO. The number of patients treated with FORTEO whose transient hypercalcemia was verified on consecutive measurements was 3.0% of women and 1.3% of men.

Immunogenicity: In a large clinical trial, antibodies that cross reacted with teriparatide were detected in 2.8% of female patients receiving FORTEO. Generally, antibodies were first detected following 12 months of treatment and diminished after withdrawal of therapy. There were no effects of the antibodies on serum calcium or bone mineral density (BMD) response.

Post-Market Adverse Drug Reactions: Since global market introduction, adverse events reported have included:

- Possible allergic events soon after injection: acute dyspnea, oro/facial edema, generalized urticaria, chest pain (less than 1 in 1000 patients treated).
- Since first marketing in 2002, spontaneous reports of anaphylaxis (irrespective of causality assessment) have been reported very rarely (<1 in 25 000 patients treated). In these very rare case reports, patients typically had alternative diagnoses explaining the events or subsequent negative rechallenge.
- Cases of bone tumor and osteosarcoma have been reported rarely in the postmarketing period. The causality to FORTEO use is unclear. Long term osteosarcoma surveillance studies are ongoing.
- In the post-marketing data analysis of benign, malignant and unspecified neoplasms, the ratio of cases reported for both men and women is equivalent.
- Hypercalcemia greater than 2.76 mmol/L (less than 1 in 100 patients treated).
- Hypercalcemia greater than 3.25 mmol/L (less than 1 in 1000 patients treated).
- Muscle spasms, such as of the leg or back, are reported commonly (≥1 in 100 and <1 in 10 patients treated), sometimes shortly after the first dose.
- Serious back spasms have been reported very rarely (less than 1 in 10 000 patients treated).

DRUG INTERACTIONS: Drug-Drug Interactions: Hydrochlorothiazide: In a study of 20 healthy subjects, the co-administration of 25-mg hydrochlorothiazide with teriparatide did not affect the serum calcium response to teriparatide 40 µg. The 24-hour urine excretion of calcium was reduced by a clinically insignificant amount (15%). The effect of co-administration of a higher dose of hydrochlorothiazide with teriparatide on serum calcium levels has not been studied.

Furosemide: In a study of 9 healthy subjects and 17 patients with mild, moderate, and severe renal insufficiency (creatinine clearance 13 to 72 mL/min), co-administration of intravenous furosemide (20 to 100 mg) with teriparatide 40 µg resulted in small increases in the serum calcium (2%) and 24-hour urine calcium (37%) responses to teriparatide that did not appear to be clinically important.

Digoxin: In a study of 15 healthy people administered digoxin daily to steady state, a single FORTEO 20 µg dose did not alter the effect of digoxin on the systolic time interval (from electrocardiographic Q-wave onset to aortic valve closure, a measure of digoxin's calcium-mediated cardiac effect). However, sporadic case reports have suggested that hypercalcemia may predispose patients to digitalis toxicity. Because FORTEO [teriparatide (rDNA origin) injection] transiently increases serum calcium, FORTEO should be used with caution in patients taking digoxin.

DOSAGE AND ADMINISTRATION: FORTEO [teriparatide (rDNA origin) injection] should be administered as a subcutaneous injection into the thigh or abdominal wall. The recommended dosage is 20 µg once a day.

The safety and efficacy of FORTEO have been evaluated up to 2 years in studies GHAC, GHAJ, GHBJ and GHCA (median 19 months in women in study GHAC and 10 months in men in study GHAJ). An additional clinical study (GHBZ) evaluated the safety and efficacy of FORTEO for up to 3 years. The maximum lifetime exposure to FORTEO for an individual patient is 24 months.

FORTEO should be administered initially under circumstances in which the patient can sit or lie down if symptoms of orthostatic hypotension occur (see Warnings and Precautions, Information to Be Provided to the Patient).

Patients should receive supplemental calcium and vitamin D if dietary intake is inadequate.

FORTEO should not be used in patients with severe renal impairment (see Contraindications).

FORTEO is a clear and colourless solution. Do not use if solid particles appear or if the solution is cloudy or coloured. The FORTEO pen should not be used past the stated expiration date.

No data are available on the safety or efficacy of intravenous or intramuscular injection of FORTEO.

OVERDOSAGE:
No cases of overdose were reported during clinical trials with FORTEO [teriparatide (rDNA origin) injection]. Teriparatide has been administered in single doses of up to 100 µg and in repeated doses of up to 60 µg/day for 6 weeks. The effects of overdose that might be expected include a delayed hypercalcemic effect and risk of orthostatic hypotension. Nausea, vomiting, dizziness, and headache might also occur.

In post-marketing spontaneous reports, there have been cases of medication error in which the entire contents (up to 800 µg) of the FORTEO pen have been administered as a single dose. Transient events reported have included nausea, weakness/lethargy and hypotension. In some cases, no adverse events occurred as a result of the overdose. No fatalities associated with overdose have been reported.

Overdose Management: There is no specific antidote for teriparatide. Treatment of suspected overdose should include discontinuation of FORTEO, monitoring of serum calcium and phosphorus, and implementation of appropriate supportive measures, such as hydration.

For management of a suspected drug overdose, CPhA recommends that you contact your **regional Poison Control Centre**. See the *CPS* Directory section for a list of Poison Control Centres.

ACTION AND CLINICAL PHARMACOLOGY: Mechanism of Action: Endogenous 84-amino-acid parathyroid hormone (PTH) is the primary regulator of calcium and phosphate metabolism in bone and kidney. Physiological actions of PTH include regulation of bone metabolism, renal tubular reabsorption of calcium and phosphate, and intestinal calcium absorption. The biological actions of PTH and teriparatide are mediated through binding to specific high-affinity cell-surface receptors. Teriparatide and the 34 N-terminal amino acids of PTH bind to these receptors with the same affinity and have the same physiological actions on bone and kidney. Teriparatide is not expected to accumulate in bone or other tissues.

The skeletal effects of teriparatide depend upon the pattern of systemic exposure. Once-daily administration of teriparatide stimulates new bone formation on trabecular and cortical (periosteal and/or endosteal) bone surfaces by preferential stimulation of osteoblastic activity over osteoclastic activity. In monkey studies, teriparatide improved trabecular microarchitecture and increased bone mass and strength by stimulating new bone formation in both cancellous and cortical bone. In humans, the anabolic effects of teriparatide manifest as an increase in skeletal mass, an increase in markers of bone formation and resorption, and an increase in bone strength. By contrast, continuous excess of endogenous PTH, as occurs in hyperparathyroidism, may be detrimental to the skeleton because bone resorption may be stimulated more than bone formation.

Pharmacodynamics: Effects on Mineral Metabolism: Teriparatide affects calcium and phosphorus metabolism in a pattern consistent with the known actions of endogenous PTH (e.g., increases serum calcium and decreases serum phosphorus).

Serum Calcium Concentrations: When FORTEO 20 µg is administered once daily, the serum calcium concentration increases transiently, beginning approximately 2 hours after dosing and reaching a maximum concentration between 4 and 6 hours (median increase, 0.1 mmol/L). The serum calcium concentration begins to decline approximately 6 hours after dosing and returns to baseline by 16 to 24 hours after each dose.

In a clinical study of postmenopausal women with osteoporosis, the median peak serum calcium concentration measured 4 to 6 hours after dosing with FORTEO [teriparatide (rDNA origin) injection] was 2.42 mmol/L at 12 months. The peak serum calcium remained below 2.76 mmol/L in >99% of women at each visit. Sustained hypercalcemia was not observed.

In this study, 11.1% of women treated with FORTEO had at least 1 serum calcium value above the upper limit of normal (2.64 mmol/L) at the 4- to 6-hour post-dose peak measurement compared with 1.5% of women treated with placebo. The 24-hour post-dose trough serum calcium measurement was unchanged from baseline in both groups. The percentage of women treated with FORTEO whose serum calcium was above the upper limit of normal on consecutive 4- to 6-hour post-dose measurements was 3.0% compared with 0.2% of women treated with placebo. In these women, calcium supplements and/or FORTEO doses were reduced. The timing of these dose reductions was at the discretion of the investigator. FORTEO dose adjustments were made at varying intervals after the first observation of increased serum calcium (median 21 weeks). During these intervals, there was no evidence of progressive increases in serum calcium.

In a clinical study of men with either primary or hypogonadal osteoporosis, the effects on serum calcium were similar to those observed in postmenopausal women. The median peak serum calcium concentration measured 4 to 6 hours after dosing with FORTEO was 2.35 mmol/L at 12 months. The peak serum calcium remained below 2.76 mmol/L in 98% of men at each visit. Sustained hypercalcemia was not observed.

In this study, 6.0% of men treated with FORTEO daily had at least 1 serum calcium value above the upper limit of normal (2.64 mmol/L) at the 4- to 6-hour post-dose peak measurement compared with none of the men treated with placebo. The 24-hour post-dose trough serum calcium measurement was unchanged from baseline in both groups. The percentage of men treated with FORTEO whose serum calcium was above the upper limit of normal on consecutive measurements was 1.3% (2 men) compared with none of the men treated with placebo. Although calcium supplements and/or FORTEO doses could have been reduced in these men, only calcium supplementation was reduced (see Warnings and Precautions and Adverse Reactions).

FORTEO has not been studied in patients with pre-existing hypercalcemia. These patients should be excluded from treatment with FORTEO because of the possibility of exacerbating hypercalcemia (see Contraindications).

Urinary Calcium Excretion: In a long-term (median of 19 months) study of postmenopausal women with osteoporosis, who received 1000 mg of supplemental calcium and at least 400 IU of vitamin D, FORTEO slightly increased urinary calcium excretion. The median values at 6 and 12 months were 0.76 mmol/day (30 mg/day) and 0.30 mmol/day (12 mg/day) higher, respectively, than those of placebo-treated patients. The median urinary excretion of calcium was 4.8 mmol/day (190 mg/day) at 6 months and 4.2 mmol/day (170 mg/day) at 12 months. The incidence of hypercalciuria (>7.5 mmol calcium/day or 300 mg/day) was not different from that in placebo-treated subjects.

In a long-term (median of 10 months) study of men with osteoporosis, who received 1000 mg of supplemental calcium and at least 400 IU of vitamin D, FORTEO had inconsistent effects on urinary calcium excretion. The median values at 1 and 6 months were 0.50 mmol/day (20 mg/day) higher and 0.20 mmol/day (8.0 mg/day) lower, respectively, than those of placebo-treated patients. The median urinary excretion of calcium was 5.6 mmol/day (220 mg/day) at 1 month and 5.3 mmol/day (210 mg/day) at 6 months. The incidence of hypercalciuria (>7.5 mmol Ca/day or 300 mg/day) was not different from that in placebo-treated subjects.

Phosphorus and Vitamin D: In single-dose studies, teriparatide produced transient phosphaturia and mild transient reductions in serum phosphorus concentration. However, hypophosphatemia (<0.74 mmol/L or 2.4 mg/dL) was not observed in long term (median of 10 and 19 months) clinical trials with FORTEO.

In clinical studies of daily FORTEO, the median serum concentration of 1,25-dihydroxyvitamin D at 12 months was increased by 19% in women and 14% in men, compared to baseline. In the placebo group, this concentration decreased by 2% in women and increased by 5% in men. The median serum 25-hydroxyvitamin D concentration at 12 months was decreased by 19% in women and 10% in men compared to baseline. In the placebo group, this concentration was unchanged in women and increased by 1% in men.

Effects on Markers of Bone Turnover: Daily administration of FORTEO to men and postmenopausal women with osteoporosis stimulated bone formation, as shown by rapid increases in the formation markers: serum bone-specific alkaline phosphatase (BSAP) and procollagen I carboxy-terminal propeptide (PICP). Peak concentrations of PICP approximately 41% above baseline were observed at 1 month of treatment, followed by a decline to near-baseline values by 12 months. BSAP concentrations had increased by 1 month of treatment and continued to rise more slowly from 6 through 12 months. Maximum increases of BSAP achieved were 45% above baseline in women and 23% in men. After discontinuation of therapy, BSAP concentrations returned toward baseline. The increases in formation markers were accompanied by secondary increases in the markers of bone resorption: urinary N-telopeptide (NTX) and urinary deoxypyridinoline (DPD), consistent with the physiological coupling of bone formation and resorption in skeletal remodelling. Changes in BSAP, NTX, and DPD were somewhat lower in men than in women, possibly because of lower systemic exposure to teriparatide in men.

Pharmacodynamics in Men and Women with Glucocorticoid-Induced Osteoporosis: Glucocorticoid-Induced Osteoporosis: The primary effect of glucocorticoids on bone is to inhibit osteoblastic bone-forming activity. Glucocorticoids also increase bone resorption.

Effects on Markers of Bone Turnover: During 18 months (the primary phase) of therapy in a 36-month double-blind, double-dummy, active comparator-controlled study of patients with glucocorticoid-induced osteoporosis who received either FORTEO 20 µg/day or alendronate 10 mg/day, daily administration of FORTEO stimulated new bone formation as shown by increases from baseline in the serum concentration of biochemical markers of bone formation including BSAP, PICP, and aminoterminal propeptide of type I collagen (PINP) (see Table 4). FORTEO also stimulated bone resorption as shown by increases from baseline in serum concentrations of C-terminal telopeptide of type I collagen (CTX). Alendronate 10 mg/day induced decreases from baseline in the serum concentration of BSAP, PICP, PINP and CTX (see Table 4). The effects of FORTEO on bone turnover markers in patients with glucocorticoid-induced osteoporosis were qualitatively similar to the effects in postmenopausal women with osteoporosis not taking glucocorticoids.

Table 4: FORTEO

Median Percent Changes[a,b] from Baseline in Bone Biomarkers in Patients with Glucocorticoid-Induced Osteoporosis

Treatment Duration	PINP (µg/L)		BSAP (µg/L)		PICP (µg/L)		CTX (pmol/L)	
	FORTEO	ALN	FORTEO	ALN	FORTEO	ALN	FORTEO	ALN
1 month	64	−17	19	−5	36	−12	11	−46
6 month	70	−50	31	−20	0	−27	45	−56
18 month	35	−48	16	−21	−11	−28	9	−64

a The median percent changes in FORTEO-treated patients were significantly different (p<0.01) compared with alendronate-treated (ALN) patients for each biomarker at all time points.

b Values represent median percent changes with n=54 to 99 among the 4 biomarkers at the different time points.

Calcium and Phosphorus Concentrations: In the study of patients with glucocorticoid-induced osteoporosis, the effects of FORTEO on serum calcium and phosphorus were similar to those observed in postmenopausal women with osteoporosis not taking glucocorticoids.

Pharmacokinetics: Absorption: Teriparatide is extensively absorbed after subcutaneous injection; the absolute bioavailability is approximately 95% based on pooled data from 20-, 40-, and 80-µg doses administered into the abdominal wall. The rates of absorption and elimination are rapid. The peptide reaches peak serum concentrations about 30 minutes after subcutaneous injection of a 20-µg dose and declines to non-quantifiable concentrations within 3 hours. Peak molar concentrations of teriparatide briefly exceed the upper limit of normal for endogenous PTH by 4- to 5-fold.

Metabolism: No metabolism or excretion studies have been performed with teriparatide. However, the mechanisms of metabolism and elimination of PTH(1-34) and intact endogenous PTH have been extensively described in published literature. Peripheral metabolism of PTH is believed to occur by non-specific enzymatic mechanisms in the liver followed by excretion via the kidneys.

Distribution and Elimination: Systemic clearance of teriparatide (approximately 62 L/hr in women and 94 L/hr in men) exceeds the rate of normal liver plasma flow, consistent with both hepatic and extra-hepatic clearance. Volume of distribution, following intravenous injection, is approximately 0.12 L/kg. Inter-subject variability in systemic clearance and volume of distribution is 25% to 50%. The half-life of teriparatide in serum is 5 minutes when administered by intravenous injection and approximately 1 hour when administered by subcutaneous injection. The longer half-life following subcutaneous administration reflects the time required for absorption from the injection site.

Special Populations and Conditions: Pediatrics: The pharmacokinetics of teriparatide have not been evaluated in pediatric populations (see Warnings and Precautions, Special Populations, Pediatrics).

Geriatrics: No differences in teriparatide pharmacokinetics were detected with regard to age (range 31 to 85 years).

Gender: Although systemic exposure to teriparatide is approximately 20% to 30% lower in men than in women, the recommended dose for both genders is 20 µg/day.

Race: The populations included in the pharmacokinetic analyses were predominantly Caucasian (98.5%) with less than 1.5% representing Hispanic, Asian, and other origins. The influence of race on serum teriparatide concentrations has not been determined.

Hepatic Insufficiency: Non-specific proteolytic enzymes in the liver (possibly Kupffer cells) cleave PTH(1-34) and PTH(1-84) into fragments that are cleared from the circulation mainly by the kidney. No studies have been performed in patients with hepatic impairment.

Renal Insufficiency: No pharmacokinetic differences were identified in 11 patients with mild or moderate renal insufficiency [creatinine clearance (CrCl) 30 to 72 mL/min] administered a single dose of teriparatide. In 5 patients with severe renal insufficiency (CrCl<30 mL/min), the AUC and $T_{1/2}$ of teriparatide were increased by 73% and 77%, respectively. Maximum serum concentration of teriparatide was not increased. No studies have been performed in patients undergoing dialysis for chronic renal failure (see Contraindications).

Heart Failure: No clinically relevant pharmacokinetic, blood pressure, pulse rate, or other safety differences were identified in 13 patients with stable heart failure (New York Heart Association Class I to III and additional evidence of cardiac dysfunction) after administration of two 20 µg doses of FORTEO. There are no data from patients with severe heart failure.

STORAGE AND STABILITY: The FORTEO [teriparatide (rDNA origin) injection] pen should be stored under refrigeration at 2-8°C at all times. During the use period, time out of the refrigerator should be minimized; the dose may be delivered immediately following removal from the refrigerator. When stored under refrigerated conditions, FORTEO is stable until date of expiry. Do not freeze. Do not use FORTEO if it has been frozen.

Instructions for Pen Use: Patients and caregivers who administer FORTEO [teriparatide (rDNA origin) injection] should receive appropriate training and instruction on the proper use of the FORTEO pen from a qualified health professional. It is important to read, understand, and follow the instructions for using the pen in the FORTEO Pen User Manual. Failure to do so may result in inaccurate dosing. The 3 mL prefilled pen must be primed before each dose. The 2.4 mL prefilled pen is not primed before each dose. Each FORTEO pen can be used for up to 28 days including the first injection. After the 28 day use period, discard the FORTEO pen, even if it still contains some unused solution. Never share a FORTEO pen.

INFORMATION FOR THE PATIENT: Published in e-CPS, available by subscription at www.e-cps.ca.

DOSAGE FORMS, COMPOSITION AND PACKAGING: Supplied as a sterile, colorless, clear, solution for injection in a 3 mL cartridge contained in a prefilled delivery device (pen). Each mL of solution for injection contains: teriparatide 250 µg (corrected for acetate, chloride, and water content) and 3 mg metacresol (preservative) in addition to glacial acetic acid, sodium acetate (anhydrous), mannitol, and water for injection. Hydrochloric acid solution and/or sodium hydroxide solution may have been added to adjust the product to pH 4. Each 3 mL or 2.4 mL prefilled injection pen delivers 20 µg of teriparatide per dose.

(Shown in Product Identification Section)

The reader is invited to consult CPhA's monograph **Bisphosphonates: Oral**.

Fosamax® Ⓟ

alendronate sodium

Bone Metabolism Regulator

Merck Frosst

Date of Revision: October 8, 2009

SUMMARY PRODUCT INFORMATION:

Route of Administration	Dosage Form/ Strength	Clinically Relevant Nonmedicinal Ingredients
Oral	Tablets 5 mg, 10 mg, 40 mg, 70 mg	Lactose anhydrous For a complete listing see Dosage Forms, Composition and Packaging.
Oral	Oral Solution 70 mg/75 mL	For a complete listing see Dosage Forms, Composition and Packaging.

INDICATIONS AND CLINICAL USE: FOSAMAX (alendronate sodium) is indicated for:

- The treatment and prevention of osteoporosis in postmenopausal women.
  - For the treatment of osteoporosis, FOSAMAX increases bone mass and prevents fractures, including those of the hip and spine (vertebral compression fractures).

    Osteoporosis may be confirmed by the finding of low bone mass (for example, at least 2.0 standard deviations below the premenopausal mean) or by the presence or history of osteoporotic fracture.
  - For the prevention of osteoporosis, FOSAMAX may be considered in postmenopausal women who are at risk of developing osteoporosis and for whom the desired clinical outcome is to maintain bone mass and to reduce the risk of future fracture.

    Bone loss is particularly rapid in postmenopausal women younger than age 60. Risk factors often associated with the development of postmenopausal osteoporosis include early menopause; moderately low bone mass; thin body build; Caucasian or Asian race; and family history of osteoporosis. The presence of such risk factors may be important when considering the use of FOSAMAX for prevention of osteoporosis.
- The treatment of osteoporosis in men to reduce the incidence of fractures.
- The treatment and prevention of glucocorticoid-induced osteoporosis in men and women.
- The treatment of Paget's disease of bone in men and women.
  - Treatment is indicated in patients with Paget's disease of bone having serum alkaline phosphatase at least two times the upper limit of normal, or those who are symptomatic, or those at risk for future complications from their disease.

CONTRAINDICATIONS:

- Patients who are hypersensitive to this drug or to any ingredient in the formulation. For a complete listing, see Dosage Forms, Composition and Packaging.
- Abnormalities of the esophagus which delay esophageal emptying such as stricture or achalasia.
- Inability to stand or sit upright for at least 30 minutes.

- Patients at increased risk of aspiration should not receive FOSAMAX oral solution.
- Hypocalcemia (see Warnings and Precautions).
- Renal insufficiency with creatinine clearance <0.58 mL/s [<35 mL/min] (see Dosage and Administration).

WARNINGS AND PRECAUTIONS: General: To facilitate delivery to the stomach and thus reduce the potential for esophageal irritation, patients should be instructed to swallow each tablet of FOSAMAX with a **full** glass of water. To facilitate gastric emptying, patients should drink at least 60 mL (a quarter of a cup) of water after taking FOSAMAX oral solution. Patients should be instructed not to lie down for at least 30 minutes **and** until after their first food of the day. Patients should not chew or suck on the tablet because of a potential for oropharyngeal ulceration. Patients should be specifically instructed not to take FOSAMAX at bedtime or before arising for the day. Patients should be informed that failure to follow these instructions may increase their risk of esophageal problems. Patients should be instructed that if they develop symptoms of esophageal disease (such as difficulty or pain upon swallowing, retrosternal pain or new or worsening heartburn) they should stop taking FOSAMAX immediately and consult their physician.

Causes of osteoporosis other than estrogen deficiency, aging and glucocorticoid use should be considered.

Osteonecrosis of the Jaw: Osteonecrosis of the jaw (ONJ) has been reported in patients with cancer receiving treatment regimens including bisphosphonates. The majority of reports occurred following tooth extractions with delayed healing and involved cancer patients treated with intravenous bisphosphonates. Many of these patients were also receiving chemotherapy and corticosteroids. However, some cases have also occurred in patients receiving oral bisphosphonate treatment for postmenopausal osteoporosis and other diagnoses. The majority of reported cases have been associated with dental procedures such as tooth extraction. Many had signs of local infection, including osteomyelitis.

A dental examination with appropriate preventive dentistry should be considered prior to treatment with bisphosphonates in patients with concomitant risk factors. Known risk factors for osteonecrosis of the jaw include a diagnosis of cancer, concomitant therapies (e.g., chemotherapy, radiotherapy, corticosteroids, immunosuppressive drugs), poor oral hygiene, co-morbid disorders (e.g., periodontal and/or other pre-existing dental disease, anemia, coagulopathy, infection, diabetes mellitus), smoking, and heavy alcohol use.

Patients who develop osteonecrosis of the jaw should receive appropriate antibiotic therapy and/or oral surgery and discontinuation of bisphosphonate therapy should be considered based on individual benefit/risk assessment. Dental surgery may exacerbate the condition. For patients requiring dental procedures (e.g. tooth extraction, dental implants), there are no definitive data available to establish whether discontinuation of bisphosphonate treatment reduces the risk of ONJ.

Clinical judgment of the treating physician and/or oral surgeon should guide the management plan, including bisphosphonate treatment, of each patient based on individual benefit/risk assessment.

Musculoskeletal: In post marketing experience, severe and occasionally incapacitating bone, joint, and/or muscle pain has been reported in patients taking bisphosphonates that are approved for the prevention and treatment of osteoporosis (see Adverse Reactions). However, such reports have been infrequent. This category of drugs includes FOSAMAX. Most of the patients were postmenopausal women. The time to onset of symptoms varied from one day to several months after starting the drug. Most patients had relief of symptoms after stopping the medication. A subset had recurrence of symptoms when rechallenged with the same drug or another bisphosphonate.

In placebo-controlled clinical studies of FOSAMAX, the percentages of patients with these symptoms were similar in the FOSAMAX and placebo groups.

Low-energy fractures of the subtrochanteric and proximal femoral shaft have been reported in some alendronate-treated patients. Some were stress fractures (also known as insufficiency fractures) occurring in the absence of trauma. Some patients experienced prodromal pain in the affected area, often associated with imaging features of stress fracture, weeks to months before a complete fracture occurred. Patients with suspected stress fractures should be evaluated, including evaluation for causes of stress fractures (e.g., vitamin D deficiency, malabsorption, glucocorticoid use, lower extremity arthritis or fracture, extreme or increased exercise, diabetes mellitus, chronic alcohol abuse), and receive appropriate orthopedic care. Interruption of alendronate therapy in patients with stress fractures should be considered based on individual benefit/risk assessment.

Endocrine and Metabolism: Hypocalcemia must be corrected before initiating therapy with FOSAMAX (see Contraindications). Other disorders affecting mineral metabolism (such as Vitamin D deficiency) should be treated. In patients with these conditions, serum calcium and symptoms of hypocalcemia should be monitored during therapy with FOSAMAX. Symptomatic hypocalcemia has been reported rarely, both in patients with predisposing conditions and patients without known predisposing conditions. Patients should be advised to report to their physicians any symptoms of hypocalcemia, such as paresthesias or muscle spasms. Physicians should carefully evaluate patients who develop hypocalcemia during therapy with FOSAMAX for predisposing conditions.

Due to the positive effects of FOSAMAX in increasing bone mineral, small, asymptomatic decreases in serum calcium and phosphate may occur, especially in patients with Paget's disease, in whom the pretreatment rate of bone turnover may be greatly elevated, and in patients receiving glucocorticoids, in whom calcium absorption may be decreased.

Ensuring adequate calcium and Vitamin D intake is especially important in patients with Paget's disease of bone and in patients receiving glucocorticoids.

Gastrointestinal: FOSAMAX, like other bisphosphonates, may cause local irritation of the upper gastrointestinal mucosa.

Esophageal adverse experiences, such as esophagitis, esophageal ulcers and esophageal erosions, rarely followed by esophageal stricture or perforation, have been reported in patients receiving treatment with FOSAMAX. In some cases these have been severe and required hospitalization. Physicians should therefore be alert to any signs or symptoms signaling a possible esophageal reaction and patients should be instructed to discontinue FOSAMAX immediately and seek medical attention if they develop dysphagia, odynophagia, retrosternal pain or new or worsening heartburn.

The risk of severe esophageal adverse experiences appears to be greater in patients who lie down after taking FOSAMAX and/or who fail to swallow it with the recommended amount of water, and/or who continue to take FOSAMAX after developing symptoms suggestive of esophageal irritation. Therefore, it is very important that the full dosing instructions are provided to, and understood by, the patient (see Dosage and Administration).

Because of possible irritant effects of FOSAMAX on the upper gastrointestinal mucosa and a potential for worsening of the underlying disease, caution should be used when FOSAMAX is given to patients with active upper gastrointestinal problems, such as dysphagia, esophageal diseases (including known Barrett's esophagus), gastritis, duodenitis, or ulcers.

While no increased risk was observed in extensive clinical trials, there have been rare (post-marketing) reports of gastric and duodenal ulcers, some severe and with complications.

Special Populations: Pregnant Women: FOSAMAX has not been studied in pregnant women and should not be given to them.

Nursing Women: FOSAMAX has not been studied in nursing mothers and should not be given to them.

Pediatrics (<18 years of age): FOSAMAX is not indicated for use in children.

Geriatrics: In clinical studies, there was no age-related difference in the efficacy or safety profiles of FOSAMAX.

Monitoring and Laboratory Tests: Not applicable.

ADVERSE REACTIONS: Clinical Trial Adverse Drug Reactions: Because clinical trials are conducted under very specific conditions the adverse drug reaction rates observed in the clinical trials may not reflect the rates observed in practice and should not be compared to the rates in the clinical trials of another drug. Adverse drug reaction information from clinical trials is useful for identifying drug-related adverse events and for approximating rates.

In clinical studies, FOSAMAX was generally well tolerated. In studies of up to five years in duration, side effects, which usually were mild, generally did not require discontinuation of therapy.

FOSAMAX has been evaluated for safety in clinical studies in approximately 7200 postmenopausal women.

Treatment of Osteoporosis: Postmenopausal Women: In two, three-year, placebo-controlled, double-blind, multicenter studies (United States and Multinational) of virtually identical design, with a total of 994 postmenopausal women, the overall safety profiles of FOSAMAX 10 mg/day and placebo were similar. Discontinuation of therapy due to any clinical adverse experience occurred in 4.1% of 196 patients treated with FOSAMAX 10 mg/day and 6.0% of 397 patients treated with placebo.

Adverse experiences considered by the investigators as possibly, probably, or definitely drug-related in ≥1% of patients treated with either FOSAMAX 10 mg/day or placebo are presented in Table 1.

One patient treated with FOSAMAX (10 mg/day), who had a history of peptic ulcer disease and gastrectomy and who was taking concomitant acetylsalicylic acid (ASA) developed an anastomotic ulcer with mild hemorrhage, which was considered drug-related. ASA and FOSAMAX were discontinued and the patient recovered.

In the two-year extension (treatment years 4 and 5) of the above studies, the overall safety profile of FOSAMAX 10 mg/day was similar to that observed during the three-year placebo-controlled period. Additionally, the proportion of patients who discontinued FOSAMAX 10 mg/day due to any clinical adverse experience was similar to that during the first three years of the study.

In the Fracture Intervention Trial, discontinuation of therapy due to any clinical adverse experience occurred in 9.1% of 3236 patients treated with FOSAMAX 5 mg/day for two years and 10 mg/day for either one or two additional years and 10.1% of 3223 patients treated with placebo. Discontinuations due to upper gastrointestinal adverse experiences were: FOSAMAX, 3.2%; placebo, 2.7%. The overall adverse experience profile was similar to that seen in other studies with FOSAMAX 5 or 10 mg/day.

In a one-year, double-blind multicenter study, the overall safety and tolerability profiles of FOSAMAX 70 mg once weekly and FOSAMAX 10 mg daily were similar. The adverse experiences considered by the investigators as possibly, probably, or definitely drug-related in ≥1% of patients in either treatment group are presented in Table 2.

Table 1: FOSAMAX

Drug-Related[a] Adverse Experiences Reported in ≥1% of Patients Treated for Osteoporosis

	FOSAMAX 10 mg/day % (n=196)	Placebo % (n=397)
Gastrointestinal		
Abdominal Pain	6.6	4.8
Nausea	3.6	4.0
Dyspepsia	3.6	3.5
Constipation	3.1	1.8
Diarrhea	3.1	1.8
Flatulence	2.6	0.5
Acid Regurgitation	2.0	4.3
Esophageal Ulcer	1.5	0.0
Vomiting	1.0	1.5
Dysphagia	1.0	0.0
Abdominal Distention	1.0	0.8
Gastritis	0.5	1.3
Musculoskeletal		
Musculoskeletal (bone, muscle or joint) pain	4.1	2.5
Muscle Cramp	0.0	1.0
Nervous System/Psychiatric		
Headache	2.6	1.5
Dizziness	0.0	1.0
Special Senses		
Taste Perversion	0.5	1.0

[a] Considered possibly, probably or definitely drug-related as assessed by the investigators.

Table 2: FOSAMAX

Drug-Related[a] Adverse Experiences Reported in ≥1% of Patients Treated for Osteoporosis

	FOSAMAX 70 mg Once Weekly % (n=519)	FOSAMAX 10 mg/day % (n=370)
Gastrointestinal		
Abdominal Pain	3.7	3.0
Dyspepsia	2.7	2.2
Acid Regurgitation	1.9	2.4
Nausea	1.9	2.4
Abdominal Distention	1.0	1.4
Constipation	0.8	1.6
Flatulence	0.4	1.6
Gastritis	0.2	1.1
Gastric Ulcer	0.0	1.1
Musculoskeletal		
Musculoskeletal Pain (bone, muscle, joint)	2.9	3.2
Muscle Cramp	0.2	1.1

[a] Considered possibly, probably, or definitely drug-related as assessed by the investigators.

Men: In two placebo-controlled, double-blind, multicenter studies in men (a two-year study of FOSAMAX 10 mg/day [n=146] and a one-year study of FOSAMAX 70 mg once weekly [n=109]), the safety profile of FOSAMAX was generally similar to that seen in postmenopausal women. The rates of discontinuation of therapy due to any clinical adverse experience were 2.7% for FOSAMAX 10 mg/day vs. 10.5% for placebo, and 6.4% for FOSAMAX 70 mg once weekly vs. 8.6% for placebo.

Other Studies in Men and Women: In a ten-week endoscopy study in men and women (n=277; mean age: 55) no difference was seen in upper gastrointestinal tract lesions between FOSAMAX 70 mg once weekly and placebo.

In an additional one-year study in men and women (n=335; mean age: 50) the overall safety and tolerability profiles of FOSAMAX 70 mg once weekly were similar to that of placebo and no difference was seen between men and women.

Prevention of Osteoporosis in Postmenopausal Women: The safety of FOSAMAX 5 mg/day in postmenopausal women 40-60 years of age has been evaluated in three double-blind, placebo-controlled studies involving over 1400 patients randomized to receive FOSAMAX for either two or three years. In these studies the overall safety profiles of FOSAMAX 5 mg/day and placebo were similar. Discontinuation of therapy due to any clinical adverse experience occurred in 7.5% of 642 patients treated with

FOSAMAX 5 mg/day and 5.7% of 648 patients treated with placebo. Adverse experiences reported by the investigators as possibly, probably or definitely drug-related in ≥1% of patients treated with either FOSAMAX 5 mg/day or placebo are presented in Table 3.

Table 3: FOSAMAX

Drug-Related[a] Adverse Experiences Reported in ≥1% of Patients—Prevention of Osteoporosis

	FOSAMAX 5 mg/day % (n=642)	Placebo % (n=648)
Gastrointestinal		
Abdominal Pain	1.7	3.4
Acid Regurgitation	1.4	2.5
Diarrhea	1.1	1.7
Dyspepsia	1.9	1.7
Nausea	1.4	1.4

[a] Considered possibly, probably, or definitely drug-related as assessed by the investigators.

Concomitant Use with Estrogen/Hormone Replacement Therapy: In two studies (of one and two years' duration) of postmenopausal osteoporotic women (total: n=853), the safety and tolerability profile of combined treatment with FOSAMAX 10 mg once daily and estrogen±progestin (n=354) was consistent with those of the individual treatments.

Treatment and Prevention of Glucocorticoid-Induced Osteoporosis: In two, one-year, placebo-controlled, double-blind, multicenter studies in patients receiving glucocorticoid treatment, the overall safety and tolerability profiles of FOSAMAX 5 or 10 mg/day were generally similar to that of placebo. Adverse experiences reported by the investigators as possibly, probably or definitely drug-related in ≥1% of patients treated with either FOSAMAX 5 or 10 mg/day or placebo are presented in Table 4.

Table 4: FOSAMAX

Drug-Related[a] Adverse Experiences Reported in ≥1% of Patients—Treatment and Prevention of Glucocorticoid-induced Osteoporosis

	FOSAMAX 10 mg/day % (n=157)	FOSAMAX 5 mg/day % (n=161)	Placebo % (n=159)
Gastrointestinal			
Abdominal Pain	3.2	1.9	0.0
Acid Regurgitation	2.5	1.9	1.3
Constipation	1.3	0.6	0.0
Melena	1.3	0.0	0.0
Nausea	0.6	1.2	0.6
Diarrhea	0.0	0.0	1.3
Nervous System/Psychiatric			
Headache	0.6	0.0	1.3

[a] Considered possibly, probably, or definitely drug-related as assessed by the investigators.

The overall safety and tolerability profile in the glucocorticoid-induced osteoporosis population that continued therapy for the second year of the studies was consistent with that observed in the first year.

Paget's Disease of Bone: In clinical studies (Paget's disease and osteoporosis), adverse experiences reported in 175 patients taking FOSAMAX 40 mg/day for 3-12 months were similar to those in postmenopausal women treated with FOSAMAX 10 mg/day. However, there was an apparent increased incidence of upper gastrointestinal adverse experiences in patients taking FOSAMAX 40 mg/day (17.7% FOSAMAX vs 10.2% placebo). Isolated cases of esophagitis and gastritis resulted in discontinuation of treatment.

Additionally, musculoskeletal pain (bone, muscle or joint), which has been described in patients with Paget's disease treated with other bisphosphonates, was reported by the investigators as possibly, probably, or definitely drug-related in approximately 6% of patients treated with FOSAMAX 40 mg/day versus approximately 1% of patients treated with placebo, but rarely resulted in discontinuation of therapy. Discontinuation of therapy due to any clinical adverse experience occurred in 6.4% of patients with Paget's disease treated with FOSAMAX 40 mg/day and 2.4% of patients treated with placebo.

Less Common Clinical Trial Adverse Drug Reactions (<1%): Skin: Rarely, rash and erythema have occurred.

Abnormal Hematologic and Clinical Chemistry Findings: Laboratory Tests: In double-blind, multicenter, controlled studies, asymptomatic, mild, and transient decreases in serum calcium and phosphate were observed in approximately 18 and 10%, respectively, of patients taking FOSAMAX versus approximately 12 and 3% of those taking placebo. However, the incidences of decreases in serum calcium to <8.0 mg/dL (2.0 mM) and serum phosphate to ≤2.0 mg P*/dL (0.65 mM) were similar in both treatment groups.

In a small, open-label study, at higher doses (80 mg/day) some patients had elevated transaminases. However, this was not observed at 40 mg/day. No clinically significant toxicity was associated with these laboratory abnormalities.

Rare cases of leukemia have been reported following therapy with other bisphosphonates. Any causal relationship to either the treatment or to the patients' underlying disease has not been established.

Post-Market Adverse Drug Reactions: Post-Marketing Experience: The following adverse reactions have been reported in post-marketing use:

Body as a Whole: hypersensitivity reactions including urticaria and rarely angioedema. As with other bisphosphonates, transient symptoms as in an acute-phase response (myalgia, malaise, asthenia and rarely, fever) have been reported with FOSAMAX, typically in association with initiation of treatment. Rarely, symptomatic hypocalcemia has occurred, both in association with predisposing conditions and in patients without known predisposing conditions. Rarely, peripheral edema.

Dental: Localized osteonecrosis of the jaw (ONJ) has been reported rarely with oral bisphosphonate treatment. ONJ is generally associated with local infection (including osteomyelitis), tooth extraction with delayed healing (see Warnings and Precautions, General).

Gastrointestinal: esophagitis, esophageal erosions, esophageal ulcers, rarely esophageal stricture or perforation, and oropharyngeal ulceration. Some of these have been serious and required hospitalization. Rarely, gastric or duodenal ulcers, some severe and with complications (see Warnings and Precautions and Dosage and Administration).

Musculoskeletal: bone, joint, and/or muscle pain, rarely severe and/or incapacitating (see Warnings and Precautions); joint swelling; low-energy femoral shaft fracture (see Warnings and Precautions).

Nervous System: dizziness, vertigo, dysgeusia.

Skin: rash (occasionally with photosensitivity), pruritus, alopecia, rarely severe skin reactions, including Stevens-Johnson syndrome and toxic epidermal necrolysis.

Special Senses: rarely uveitis, scleritis or episcleritis.

* P=elemental phosphorus.

DRUG INTERACTIONS: Overview: Animal studies have demonstrated that FOSAMAX is highly concentrated in bone and is retained only minimally in soft tissue. No metabolites have been detected. Although alendronate is bound approximately 78% to plasma protein in humans, its plasma concentration is so low after oral dosing that only a small fraction of plasma-binding sites is occupied, resulting in a minimal potential for interference with the binding of other drugs. Alendronate is not excreted through the acidic or basic transport systems of the kidney in rats, and thus it is not anticipated to interfere with the excretion of other drugs by those systems in humans. In summary, FOSAMAX is not expected to interact with other drugs based on effects on protein binding, renal excretion, or metabolism of other drugs.

Drug-Drug Interactions: If taken at the same time it is likely that calcium supplements, antacids, other multivalent cations and other oral medications will interfere with absorption of FOSAMAX. Therefore, patients must wait at least one-half hour after taking FOSAMAX before taking any other oral medication.

Intravenous ranitidine was shown to double the bioavailability of oral alendronate. The clinical significance of this increased bioavailability and whether similar increases will occur in patients given oral H_2-antagonists is unknown; no other specific drug interaction studies were performed.

Concomitant use of hormone replacement therapy (HRT [estrogen±progestin]) and FOSAMAX was assessed in two clinical studies of one or two years' duration in postmenopausal osteoporotic women. Combined use of FOSAMAX and HRT resulted in greater increases in bone mass, together with greater decreases in bone turnover, than seen with either treatment alone. In these studies, the safety and tolerability profile of the combination was consistent with those of the individual treatments (see Adverse Reactions, Clinical Trial Adverse Drug Reactions, Concomitant Use with Estrogen/Hormone Replacement Therapy). The studies were too small to detect antifracture efficacy, and no significant differences in fracture incidence among the treatment groups were found.

Specific interaction studies were not performed. FOSAMAX was used in osteoporosis studies in men, postmenopausal women, and glucocorticoid users, with a wide range of commonly prescribed drugs without evidence of clinical adverse interactions.

In clinical studies, the incidence of upper gastrointestinal adverse events was increased in patients receiving daily therapy with dosages of FOSAMAX greater than 10 mg and acetylsalicylic acid-containing products. This was not observed in a study with FOSAMAX 70 mg once weekly.

FOSAMAX may be administered to patients taking nonsteroidal anti-inflammatory drugs (NSAIDs). In a three-year, controlled, clinical study (n=2027) during which a majority of patients received concomitant NSAIDs, the incidence of upper gastrointestinal adverse events was similar in patients taking FOSAMAX 5 or 10 mg/day compared to those taking placebo. However, since NSAID use is associated with gastrointestinal irritation, caution should be used during concomitant use with FOSAMAX.

Drug-Food Interactions: Food and beverages other than **plain water** may markedly reduce the absorption and effectiveness of alendronate. FOSAMAX must be taken at least one-half hour before the first food, beverage, or medication of the day with plain water only (see Dosage and Administration, Administration).

Drug-Herb Interactions: Herbal products may interfere with the absorption of alendronate. FOSAMAX must be taken at least one-half hour before any herbal products.

Drug-Laboratory Interactions: Interactions with laboratory tests have not been established.

Drug-Lifestyle Interactions: No studies on the effects on the ability to drive and use machines have been performed. However, certain adverse reactions that have been reported with FOSAMAX (e.g., dizziness, vertigo, visual disturbances, and severe bone, muscle or joint pain) may affect some patients' ability to drive or operate machinery. Individual responses to FOSAMAX may vary.

DOSAGE AND ADMINISTRATION: Recommended Dose: Treatment of Osteoporosis in Postmenopausal Women and in Men: The recommended dosage is:

- one 70 mg tablet once weekly

  or
- one bottle of 70 mg oral solution once weekly

  or
- one 10 mg tablet once daily.

Prevention of Osteoporosis in Postmenopausal Women: The recommended dosage is 5 mg once a day.

Treatment and Prevention of Glucocorticoid-Induced Osteoporosis in Men and Women: The recommended dosage is 5 mg once a day, except for postmenopausal women not receiving estrogen, for whom the recommended dosage is 10 mg once a day.

Paget's Disease of Bone in Men and Women: The recommended treatment regimen is 40 mg once a day for six months.

Retreatment of Paget's Disease: In clinical studies in which patients were followed every six months, relapses during the 12 months following therapy occurred in 9% (3 out of 32) of patients who responded to treatment with FOSAMAX. Specific retreatment data are not available, although responses to FOSAMAX were similar in patients who had received prior bisphosphonate therapy and those who had not. Retreatment with FOSAMAX may be considered, following a six-month post-treatment evaluation period, in patients who have relapsed based on increases in serum alkaline phosphatase (which should be measured periodically). Retreatment may also be considered in those who failed to normalize their serum alkaline phosphatase.

Dosage Adjustment: No dosage adjustment is necessary for the elderly or for patients with mild-to-moderate renal insufficiency (creatinine clearance 0.58 to 1 mL/s [35 to 60 mL/min]). FOSAMAX is not recommended for patients with more severe renal insufficiency (creatinine clearance <0.58 mL/s [<35 mL/min]) due to lack of experience.

Missed Dose: Patients should be instructed that if they miss a dose of FOSAMAX 70 mg once weekly, they should take one dose on the morning after they remember. They should not take two doses on the same day but should return to taking one dose once a week, as originally scheduled on their chosen day.

Administration: FOSAMAX must be taken at least one-half hour before the first food, beverage, or medication of the day with plain water only. Other beverages (including mineral water), food, and some medications are known to reduce the absorption of FOSAMAX (see Drug Interactions). Waiting less than 30 minutes will lessen the effect of FOSAMAX by decreasing its absorption into the body.

FOSAMAX should only be taken upon arising for the day. To facilitate delivery to the stomach and thus reduce the potential for esophageal irritation, a FOSAMAX tablet should be swallowed with a **full** glass of water (200-250 mL). To facilitate gastric emptying, FOSAMAX oral solution should be followed by at least 60 mL (a quarter of a cup) of water. Patients should not lie down for at least 30 minutes **and** until after their first food of the day. FOSAMAX should not be taken at bedtime or before arising for the day. Failure to follow these instructions may increase the risk of esophageal adverse experiences (see Warnings and Precautions).

All patients must receive supplemental calcium and Vitamin D, if dietary intake is inadequate.

Although no specific studies have been conducted on the effects of switching patients on another therapy for osteoporosis or Paget's disease to FOSAMAX, there are no known or theoretical safety concerns related to FOSAMAX in patients who previously received any other antiosteoporotic or antipagetic therapy.

OVERDOSAGE:

No specific information is available on the treatment of overdosage with FOSAMAX. Hypocalcemia, hypophosphatemia, and upper gastrointestinal adverse events, such as upset stomach, heartburn, esophagitis, gastritis, or ulcer, may result from oral overdosage. Milk or antacids should be given to bind alendronate. Due to the risk of esophageal irritation, vomiting should not be induced and the patient should remain fully upright.

Dialysis would not be beneficial.

For management of a suspected drug overdose, contact your regional Poison Control Centre. See the *CPS* Directory section for a list of Poison Control Centres.

ACTION AND CLINICAL PHARMACOLOGY: Mechanism of Action: FOSAMAX is a bisphosphonate that acts as a potent, specific inhibitor of osteoclast-mediated bone resorption. Bisphosphonates are synthetic analogs of pyrophosphate that bind to the hydroxyapatite found in bone.

Pharmacodynamics: Alendronate is a bisphosphonate that binds to bone hydroxyapatite and specifically inhibits the activity of osteoclasts, the bone-resorbing cells. Alendronate reduces bone resorption with no direct effect on bone formation, although the latter process is ultimately reduced because bone resorption and formation are coupled during bone turnover.

Osteoporosis in Postmenopausal Women: Osteoporosis is characterized by low bone mass that leads to an increased risk of fracture. The diagnosis can be confirmed by the finding of low bone mass, evidence of fracture on x-ray, a history of osteoporotic fracture, or height loss or kyphosis, indicative of vertebral fracture. Osteoporosis occurs in both males and females but is most common among women following the menopause, when bone turnover increases and the rate of bone resorption exceeds that of bone formation. These changes result in progressive bone loss and lead to osteoporosis in a significant proportion of women over age 50. Fractures, usually of the spine, hip, and wrist, are the common consequences. From age 50 to age 90, the risk of hip fracture in white women increases 50-fold and the risk of vertebral fracture 15- to 30-fold. It is estimated that approximately 40% of 50-year-old women will sustain one or more osteoporosis-related fractures of the spine, hip, or wrist during their remaining lifetimes. Hip fractures, in particular, are associated with substantial morbidity, disability, and mortality.

Daily oral doses of alendronate (5, 20, and 40 mg for six weeks) in postmenopausal women produced biochemical changes indicative of dose-dependent inhibition of bone resorption, including decreases in urinary calcium and urinary markers of bone collagen degradation (such as deoxypyridinoline and cross-linked N-telopeptides of type I collagen). These biochemical changes tended to return toward baseline values as early as 3 weeks following the discontinuation of therapy with alendronate and did not differ from placebo after 7 months.

Long-term treatment of osteoporosis with FOSAMAX 10 mg/day (for up to five years) reduced urinary excretion of markers of bone resorption, deoxypyridinoline and cross-linked N-telopeptides of type I collagen, by approximately 50% and 70%, respectively, to reach levels similar to those seen in healthy premenopausal women. Similar decreases were seen in patients in osteoporosis prevention studies who received FOSAMAX 5 mg/day. The decrease in the rate of bone resorption indicated by these markers was evident as early as one month and at three to six months reached a plateau that was maintained for the entire duration of treatment with FOSAMAX. In osteoporosis treatment studies, FOSAMAX 10 mg/day decreased the markers of bone formation, osteocalcin and bone specific alkaline phosphatase by approximately 50%, and total serum alkaline phosphatase, by approximately 25 to 30%, to reach a plateau after 6 to 12 months. In osteoporosis prevention studies, FOSAMAX 5 mg/day decreased osteocalcin and total serum alkaline phosphatase by approximately 40% and 15%, respectively. Similar reductions in the rate of bone turnover were observed in postmenopausal women during a one-year study with FOSAMAX 70 mg once weekly for the treatment of osteoporosis. These data indicate that the rate of bone turnover reached a new steady-state, despite the progressive increase in the total amount of alendronate deposited within bone.

As a result of inhibition of bone resorption, asymptomatic reductions in serum calcium and phosphate concentrations were also observed following treatment with FOSAMAX. In the long-term studies, reductions from baseline in serum calcium (approximately 2%) and phosphate (approximately 4 to 6%) were evident the first month after the initiation of FOSAMAX 10 mg. No further decreases in serum calcium were observed for the five-year duration of treatment, however, serum phosphate returned toward prestudy levels during years three through five. Similar reductions were observed with FOSAMAX 5 mg/day. In a one-year study with FOSAMAX 70 mg once weekly, similar reductions were observed at 6 and 12 months. The reduction in serum phosphate may reflect not only the positive bone mineral balance due to FOSAMAX but also a decrease in renal phosphate reabsorption.

Osteoporosis in Men: Even though osteoporosis is less prevalent in men than in postmenopausal women, a significant proportion of osteoporotic fractures occur in men. The prevalence of vertebral deformities appears to be similar in men and women. Treatment of men with osteoporosis with FOSAMAX 10 mg/day for two years reduced urinary excretion of cross-linked N-telopeptides of type I collagen by approximately 60% and bone-specific alkaline phosphatase by approximately 40%. Similar reductions were observed in a one-year study in men with osteoporosis receiving FOSAMAX 70 mg once weekly.

Glucocorticoid-Induced Osteoporosis: Sustained use of glucocorticoids is commonly associated with development of osteoporosis and resulting fractures (especially vertebral, hip, and rib). It occurs both in males and females of all ages. Osteoporosis occurs as a result of inhibited bone formation and increased bone resorption resulting in net bone loss. Alendronate decreases bone resorption without directly inhibiting bone formation.

In clinical studies of up to two years' duration, FOSAMAX 5 and 10 mg/day reduced cross-linked N-telopeptides of type 1 collagen (a marker of bone resorption) by approximately 60% and reduced bone-specific alkaline phosphatase and total serum alkaline phosphatase (markers of bone formation) by approximately 15 to 30% and 8 to 18%, respectively. As a result of inhibition of bone resorption, FOSAMAX 5 and 10 mg/day induced asymptomatic decreases in serum calcium (approximately 1 to 2%) and serum phosphate (approximately 1 to 8%).

Paget's Disease of Bone: Paget's disease of bone is a chronic, focal skeletal disorder characterized by greatly increased and disorderly bone remodeling. Excessive osteoclastic bone resorption is followed by osteoblastic new bone formation, leading to the replacement of the normal bone architecture by disorganized, enlarged, and weakened bone structure.

Clinical manifestations of Paget's disease range from no symptoms to severe morbidity due to bone pain, bone deformity, pathological fractures, and neurological and other complications. Serum alkaline phosphatase, the most frequently used biochemical index of disease activity, provides an objective measure of disease severity and response to therapy.

FOSAMAX decreases the rate of bone resorption directly, which leads to an indirect decrease in bone formation. In clinical trials, FOSAMAX 40 mg once daily for six months produced significant decreases in serum alkaline phosphatase as well as in urinary markers of bone collagen degradation. As a result of the inhibition of bone resorption, FOSAMAX induced generally mild, transient, and asymptomatic decreases in serum calcium and phosphate.

Pharmacokinetics:

Table 5: FOSAMAX

Summary of Pharmacokinetic Parameters in the Normal Population

	Mean	90% Confidence Interval
Absolute bioavailability of 5 mg tablet, taken 2 hours before first meal of the day	0.63% (females)	(0.48, 0.83)
Absolute bioavailability of 10 mg tablet, taken 2 hours before first meal of the day	0.78% (females)	(0.61, 1.04)
	0.59% (males)	(0.43, 0.81)
Absolute bioavailability of 40 mg tablet, taken 2 hours before first meal of the day	0.60% (females)	(0.46, 0.78)
Absolute bioavailability of 70 mg tablet, taken 2 hours before first meal of the day	0.57% (females)	(0.44, 0.73)
Renal clearance mL/s (mL/min) (n=6)	1.18 (71)	(1.07, 1.3) (64,78)

Absorption: Relative to an intravenous (IV) reference dose, the mean oral bioavailability of alendronate in women was 0.64% for doses ranging from 5 to 70 mg when administered after an overnight fast and two hours before a standardized breakfast. Oral bioavailability of the 10 mg tablet in men was 0.59% (see Table 5).

A study examining the effect of timing of a meal on the bioavailability of alendronate was performed in 49 postmenopausal women. Bioavailability was decreased (by approximately 40%) when 10 mg alendronate was administered either 0.5 or 1 hour before a standardized breakfast, when compared to dosing 2 hours before eating. In studies of treatment and prevention of osteoporosis, alendronate was effective when administered at least 30 minutes before breakfast.

Bioavailability was negligible whether alendronate was administered with or up to two hours after a standardized breakfast. Concomitant administration of alendronate with coffee or orange juice reduced bioavailability by approximately 60%.

In healthy subjects, oral prednisone (20 mg three times daily for five days) did not produce a clinically meaningful change in the oral bioavailability of alendronate (a mean increase ranging from 20 to 44%).

Distribution: Preclinical studies (in male rats) show that alendronate transiently distributes to soft tissues following 1 mg/kg IV administration but is then rapidly redistributed to bone or excreted in the urine. The mean steady-state volume of distribution, exclusive of bone, is at least 28 L in humans. Concentrations of drug in plasma following therapeutic oral doses are too low (less than 5 ng/mL) for analytical detection. Protein binding in human plasma is approximately 78%.

Metabolism: There is no evidence that alendronate is metabolized in animals or humans.

Excretion: Following a single IV dose of [^{14}C]alendronate, approximately 50% of the radioactivity was excreted in the urine within 72 hours and little or no radioactivity was recovered in the feces. Following a single 10 mg IV dose, the renal clearance of alendronate was 71 mL/min and systemic clearance did not exceed 200 mL/min. Plasma concentrations fell by more than 95% within 6 hours following IV administration. The terminal half-life in humans is estimated to exceed 10 years, probably reflecting release of alendronate from the skeleton. Based on the above, it is estimated that after 10 years of oral treatment with FOSAMAX (10 mg daily) the amount of alendronate released daily from the skeleton is approximately 25% of that absorbed from the gastrointestinal tract.

Special Populations and Conditions: Pediatrics: The oral bioavailability in children (4 to 16 years of age) with osteogenesis imperfecta (OI) was similar to that observed in adults; however, FOSAMAX is not indicated for use in children (see Warnings and Precautions, Special Populations, Pediatrics (<18 years of age)).

Geriatrics: Bioavailability and disposition (urinary excretion) were similar in elderly (≥65 years of age) and younger patients. No dosage adjustment is necessary (see Dosage and Administration).

Gender: Bioavailability and the fraction of an IV dose excreted in urine were similar in men and women.

Race: Pharmacokinetic differences due to race have not been studied.

Hepatic Insufficiency: As there is evidence that alendronate is not metabolized or excreted in the bile, no studies were conducted in patients with hepatic insufficiency. No dosage adjustment is necessary.

Renal Insufficiency: Preclinical studies show that, in rats with kidney failure, increasing amounts of drug are present in plasma, kidney, spleen, and tibia. In healthy controls, drug that is not deposited in bone is rapidly excreted in the urine. No evidence of saturation of bone uptake was found after 3 weeks dosing with cumulative IV doses of 35 mg/kg in young male rats. Although no clinical information is available, it is likely that, as in animals, elimination of alendronate via the kidney will be reduced in patients with impaired renal function. Therefore, somewhat greater accumulation of alendronate in bone might be expected in patients with impaired renal function.

No dosage adjustment is necessary for patients with mild-to-moderate renal insufficiency (creatinine clearance 0.58 to 1 mL/s [35 to 60 mL/min]). FOSAMAX is not recommended for patients with more severe renal insufficiency (creatinine clearance <0.58 mL/s [<35 mL/min]) due to lack of experience.

STORAGE AND STABILITY: Tablets: Store at room temperature (15-30°C).
Oral Solution: Store at 25°C, excursions permitted to 15-30°C. Do not freeze.

INFORMATION FOR THE PATIENT: Published in e-CPS, available by subscription at www.e-cps.ca.

DOSAGE FORMS, COMPOSITION AND PACKAGING: Oral Solution: Each bottle of clear, colorless oral solution with a raspberry flavor contains: alendronate monosodium salt trihydrate 91.35 mg, which is the molar equivalent to 70 mg of free acid. Nonmedicinal ingredients: artificial raspberry flavor, citric acid anhydrous, purified water, sodium citrate dihydrate and sodium saccharin. Added as preservatives are sodium propylparaben and sodium butylparaben. Gluten-free. Single-dose bottles, cartons of 4.

Tablets: 5 mg: Each white, round, uncoated tablet, with an outline of a bone image on one side and MRK 925 on the other, contains: alendronate monosodium salt trihydrate 6.53 mg, which is the molar equivalent to 5 mg of free acid. Nonmedicinal ingredients: anhydrous lactose, croscarmellose sodium, magnesium stearate and microcrystalline cellulose. Gluten-free. Blister packages of 28.

10 mg: Each white, oval, wax-polished tablet, with MRK engraved on one side and 936 on the other, contains: alendronate monosodium salt trihydrate 13.05 mg, which is the molar equivalent to 10 mg of free acid. Nonmedicinal ingredients: anhydrous lactose, carnauba wax, croscarmellose sodium, magnesium stearate and microcrystalline cellulose. Gluten-free. Blister packages of 28.

40 mg: Each white, triangle-shaped, uncoated tablet, with FOSAMAX on one side and MSD 212 on the other, contains: alendronate monosodium salt trihydrate 52.21 mg, which is the molar equivalent to 40 mg of free acid. Nonmedicinal ingredients: anhydrous lactose, croscarmellose sodium, magnesium stearate and microcrystalline cellulose. Gluten-free. Blister packages of 28.

70 mg: Each white, oval, uncoated tablet, with an outline of a bone image on one side and 31 on the other, contains: alendronate monosodium salt trihydrate 91.37 mg, which is the molar equivalent to 70 mg of free acid. Nonmedicinal ingredients: anhydrous lactose, croscarmellose sodium, magnesium stearate and microcrystalline cellulose. Gluten-free. Blister packages of 4.

(Shown in Product Identification Section)

The reader is invited to consult CPhA's monograph **Bisphosphonates: Oral.**

Fosavance® Pr

alendronate sodium—cholecalciferol

Bone Metabolism Regulator and Vitamin D

Merck Frosst

Date of Revision: October 8, 2009

SUMMARY PRODUCT INFORMATION:

Route of Administration	Dosage Form/ Strength	Clinically Relevant Nonmedicinal Ingredients
Oral	Tablet Alendronate 70 mg Cholecalciferol 70 µg (2800 IU vitamin D_3) or Alendronate 70 mg Cholecalciferol 140 µg (5600 IU vitamin D_3)	Gelatin, lactose anhydrous and sucrose For a complete listing see Dosage Forms, Composition and Packaging.

INDICATIONS AND CLINICAL USE: FOSAVANCE (alendronate sodium/cholecalciferol) is indicated for:

- The treatment of osteoporosis in postmenopausal women.
- The treatment of osteoporosis in men.
  - For the treatment of osteoporosis, the alendronate sodium component of FOSAVANCE increases bone mass and can prevent fractures, including those of the hip and spine (vertebral compression fractures).
  - Osteoporosis may be confirmed by the finding of low bone mass (for example, at least 2.5 standard deviations below the premenopausal mean) or by the presence or history of osteoporotic fracture.

Patients suffering from osteoporosis are at an increased risk for vitamin D insufficiency, especially those over the age of 70 years, home bound, or chronically ill, and may need to receive vitamin D supplementation in addition to that provided in FOSAVANCE (see Dosage and Administration, Administration). Those living in high latitudes (including most of Canada) may also need additional supplementation.

An adequate calcium intake is also required.

Patients with gastrointestinal malabsorption may not adequately absorb vitamin D_3 and will also require further supplementation.

FOSAVANCE alone should not be used to treat vitamin D deficiency (commonly defined as 25-hydroxyvitamin D <22.5 nmol/L or 9 ng/mL).

CONTRAINDICATIONS:

- Patients who are hypersensitive to this drug or to any ingredient in the formulation. For a complete listing, see Dosage Forms, Composition and Packaging.
- Abnormalities of the esophagus which delay esophageal emptying such as stricture or achalasia.
- Inability to stand or sit upright for at least 30 minutes.
- Hypocalcemia (see Warnings and Precautions).
- Renal insufficiency with creatinine clearance <0.58 mL/s [<35 mL/min] (see Dosage and Administration).

WARNINGS AND PRECAUTIONS: General: To facilitate delivery to the stomach and thus reduce the potential for esophageal irritation, patients should be instructed to swallow each tablet of FOSAVANCE with a **full** glass of water (200-250 mL) and not to lie down for at least 30 minutes **and** until after their first food of the day. Patients should not chew or suck on the tablet because of a potential for oropharyngeal ulceration. Patients should be specifically instructed not to take FOSAVANCE at bedtime or before arising for the day. Patients should be informed that failure to follow these instructions may increase their risk of esophageal problems. Patients should be instructed that if they develop symptoms of esophageal disease (such as difficulty or pain upon swallowing, retrosternal pain or new or worsening heartburn) they should stop taking FOSAVANCE immediately and consult their physician.

Causes of osteoporosis other than estrogen deficiency, aging and glucocorticoid use should be considered.

Osteonecrosis of the Jaw: Osteonecrosis of the jaw (ONJ) has been reported in patients with cancer receiving treatment regimens including bisphosphonates. The majority of reports occurred following tooth extractions with delayed healing and involved cancer patients treated with intravenous bisphosphonates. Many of these patients were also receiving chemotherapy and corticosteroids. However, some cases have also occurred in patients receiving oral bisphosphonate treatment for postmenopausal osteoporosis and other diagnoses. The majority of reported cases have been associated with dental procedures such as tooth extraction. Many had signs of local infection, including osteomyelitis.

A dental examination with appropriate preventive dentistry should be considered prior to treatment with bisphosphonates in patients with concomitant risk factors. Known risk factors for osteonecrosis of the jaw include a diagnosis of cancer, concomitant therapies (e.g., chemotherapy, radiotherapy, corticosteroids, immunosuppressive drugs), poor oral hygiene, co-morbid disorders (e.g., periodontal and/or other pre-existing dental disease, anemia, coagulopathy, infection, diabetes mellitus), smoking, and heavy alcohol use.

Patients who develop osteonecrosis of the jaw should receive appropriate antibiotic therapy and/or oral surgery and discontinuation of bisphosphonate therapy should be considered based on individual benefit/risk assessment. Dental surgery may exacerbate the condition. For patients requiring dental procedures (e.g. tooth extraction, dental implants), there are no definitive data available to establish whether discontinuation of bisphosphonate treatment reduces the risk of ONJ.

Clinical judgment of the treating physician and/or oral surgeon should guide the management plan, including bisphosphonate treatment, of each patient based on individual benefit/risk assessment.

Musculoskeletal: In post-marketing experience, severe and occasionally incapacitating bone, joint, and/or muscle pain has been reported in patients taking bisphosphonates that are approved for the prevention and treatment of osteoporosis (see Adverse Reactions). However, such reports have been infrequent. This category of drugs includes FOSAMAX (alendronate sodium). Most of the patients were postmenopausal women. The time to onset of symptoms varied from one day to several months after starting the drug. Most patients had relief of symptoms after stopping the medication. A subset had recurrence of symptoms when rechallenged with the same drug or another bisphosphonate.

In placebo-controlled clinical studies of FOSAMAX, the percentages of patients with these symptoms were similar in the FOSAMAX and placebo groups.

Low-energy fractures of the subtrochanteric and proximal femoral shaft have been reported in some alendronate-treated patients. Some were stress fractures (also known as insufficiency fractures) occurring in the absence of trauma. Some patients experienced prodromal pain in the affected area, often associated with imaging features of stress fracture, weeks to months before a complete fracture occurred. Patients with suspected stress fractures should be evaluated, including evaluation for causes of stress fractures (e.g., vitamin D deficiency, malabsorption, glucocorticoid use, lower extremity arthritis or fracture, extreme or increased exercise, diabetes mellitus, chronic alcohol abuse), and receive appropriate orthopedic care. Interruption of alendronate therapy in patients with stress fractures should be considered based on individual benefit/risk assessment.

Endocrine and Metabolism: Alendronate Sodium: Hypocalcemia must be corrected before initiating therapy with FOSAVANCE (see Contraindications). Other disorders affecting mineral metabolism (such as vitamin D deficiency) should be treated. In patients with these conditions, serum calcium and symptoms of hypocalcemia should be monitored during therapy with FOSAVANCE. Symptomatic hypocalcemia has been reported rarely, both in patients with predisposing conditions and patients without known predisposing conditions. Patients should be advised to report to their physicians any symptoms of hypocalcemia, such as paresthesias or muscle spasms. Physicians should carefully evaluate patients who develop hypocalcemia during therapy with FOSAVANCE for predisposing conditions.

Due to the positive effects of alendronate in increasing bone mineral, small, asymptomatic decreases in serum calcium and phosphate may occur.

Cholecalciferol: FOSAVANCE alone should not be used to treat vitamin D deficiency (commonly defined as 25-hydroxyvitamin D <22.5 nmol/L or 9 ng/mL).

Patients suffering from osteoporosis are at an increased risk for vitamin D insufficiency, especially those over the age of 70 years, home bound, or chronically ill, and may need to receive vitamin D supplementation in addition to that provided in FOSAVANCE (see Dosage and Administration, Administration). Those living in high latitudes (including most of Canada) may also need additional supplementation.

Patients with gastrointestinal malabsorption syndromes may also require higher doses of vitamin D supplementation and measurement of 25-hydroxyvitamin D should be considered.

Vitamin D_3 supplementation may worsen hypercalcemia and/or hypercalciuria when administered to patients with diseases associated with unregulated overproduction of 1,25-dihydroxyvitamin D (e.g., leukemia, lymphoma, sarcoidosis). Urine and serum calcium should be monitored in these patients.

Gastrointestinal: FOSAVANCE, like other bisphosphonate-containing products, may cause local irritation of the upper gastrointestinal mucosa.

Esophageal adverse experiences, such as esophagitis, esophageal ulcers and esophageal erosions, rarely followed by esophageal stricture or perforation, have been reported in patients receiving treatment with alendronate. In some cases these have been severe and required hospitalization. Physicians should therefore be alert to any signs or symptoms signaling a possible esophageal reaction and patients should be instructed to discontinue FOSAVANCE immediately and seek medical attention if they develop dysphagia, odynophagia, retrosternal pain or new or worsening heartburn.

The risk of severe esophageal adverse experiences appears to be greater in patients who lie down after taking FOSAVANCE and/or who fail to swallow it with a full glass (200-250 mL) of water, and/or who continue to take FOSAVANCE after developing symptoms suggestive of esophageal irritation. Therefore, it is very important that the full dosing instructions are provided to, and understood by, the patient (see Dosage and Administration).

Because of possible irritant effects of alendronate on the upper gastrointestinal mucosa and a potential for worsening of the underlying disease, caution should be used when FOSAVANCE is given to patients with active upper gastrointestinal problems, such as dysphagia, esophageal diseases (including known Barrett's esophagus), gastritis, duodenitis, or ulcers.

While no increased risk was observed in extensive clinical trials, there have been rare (post-marketing) reports of gastric and duodenal ulcers with alendronate, some severe and with complications.

Special Populations: Pregnant Women: FOSAVANCE has not been studied in pregnant women and should not be given to them.

Nursing Women: FOSAVANCE has not been studied in nursing mothers and should not be given to them.

Pediatrics (<18 years of age): FOSAVANCE has not been studied in patients <18 years of age and should not be given to them.

Geriatrics: Alendronate Sodium: In clinical studies, there was no age-related difference in the efficacy or safety profiles of FOSAMAX.

Cholecalciferol: Daily requirements of vitamin D_3 may be increased in the elderly.

Monitoring and Laboratory Tests: Not applicable.

ADVERSE REACTIONS: Clinical Trial Adverse Drug Reactions: Because clinical trials are conducted under very specific conditions the adverse reaction rates observed in the clinical trials may not reflect the rates observed in practice and should not be compared to the rates in the clinical trials of another drug. Adverse drug reaction information from clinical trials is useful for identifying drug-related adverse events and for approximating rates.

FOSAMAX: In clinical studies, FOSAMAX was generally well tolerated. In studies of up to five years in duration, side effects, which usually were mild, generally did not require discontinuation of therapy.

FOSAMAX has been evaluated for safety in clinical studies in approximately 7200 postmenopausal women.

Treatment of Osteoporosis: Postmenopausal Women: In two, three-year, placebo-controlled, double-blind, multicenter studies (United States and Multinational) of virtually identical design, with a total of 994 postmenopausal women, the overall safety profiles of FOSAMAX 10 mg/day and placebo were similar. Discontinuation of therapy due to any clinical adverse experience occurred in 4.1% of 196 patients treated with FOSAMAX 10 mg/day and 6.0% of 397 patients treated with placebo.

Adverse experiences considered by the investigators as possibly, probably, or definitely drug-related in ≥1% of patients treated with either FOSAMAX 10 mg/day or placebo are presented in Table 1.

Table 1: FOSAVANCE

Drug-Related[a] Adverse Experiences Reported in ≥1% of Patients Treated for Osteoporosis

	FOSAMAX 10 mg/day % (n=196)	Placebo % (n=397)
Gastrointestinal		
Abdominal Pain	6.6	4.8
Nausea	3.6	4.0
Dyspepsia	3.6	3.5
Constipation	3.1	1.8
Diarrhea	3.1	1.8
Flatulence	2.6	0.5
Acid Regurgitation	2.0	4.3
Esophageal Ulcer	1.5	0.0
Vomiting	1.0	1.5
Dysphagia	1.0	0.0
Abdominal Distention	1.0	0.8
Gastritis	0.5	1.3
Musculoskeletal		
Musculoskeletal (bone, muscle or joint) Pain	4.1	2.5
Muscle Cramp	0.0	1.0
Nervous System/Psychiatric		
Headache	2.6	1.5
Dizziness	0.0	1.0
Special Senses		
Taste Perversion	0.5	1.0

[a] Considered possibly, probably, or definitely drug-related as assessed by the investigators.

One patient treated with FOSAMAX (10 mg/day), who had a history of peptic ulcer disease and gastrectomy and who was taking concomitant acetylsalicylic acid (ASA) developed an anastomotic ulcer with mild hemorrhage, which was considered drug-related. ASA and FOSAMAX were discontinued and the patient recovered.

In the two-year extension (treatment years 4 and 5) of the above studies, the overall safety profile of FOSAMAX 10 mg/day was similar to that observed during the three-year placebo-controlled period. Additionally, the proportion of patients who discontinued FOSAMAX 10 mg/day due to any clinical adverse experience was similar to that during the first three years of the study.

In the Fracture Intervention Trial, discontinuation of therapy due to any clinical adverse experience occurred in 9.1% of 3236 patients treated with FOSAMAX 5 mg/day for two years and 10 mg/day for either one or two additional years and 10.1% of 3223 patients treated with placebo. Discontinuations due to upper gastrointestinal adverse experiences were: FOSAMAX, 3.2%; placebo, 2.7%. The overall adverse experience profile was similar to that seen in other studies with FOSAMAX 5 or 10 mg/day.

In a one-year, double-blind multicenter study, the overall safety and tolerability profiles of FOSAMAX 70 mg once weekly and FOSAMAX 10 mg daily were similar. The adverse experiences considered by the investigators as possibly, probably, or definitely drug-related in ≥1% of patients in either treatment group are presented in Table 2.

Table 2: FOSAVANCE

Drug-Related[a] Adverse Experiences Reported in ≥1% of Patients Treated for Osteoporosis

	FOSAMAX 70 mg Once Weekly % (n=519)	FOSAMAX 10 mg/day % (n=370)
Gastrointestinal		
Abdominal Pain	3.7	3.0
Dyspepsia	2.7	2.2
Acid Regurgitation	1.9	2.4
Nausea	1.9	2.4
Abdominal Distention	1.0	1.4
Constipation	0.8	1.6
Flatulence	0.4	1.6
Gastritis	0.2	1.1
Gastric Ulcer	0.0	1.1
Musculoskeletal		
Musculoskeletal (bone, muscle, joint) Pain	2.9	3.2
Muscle Cramp	0.2	1.1

[a] Considered possibly, probably, or definitely drug-related as assessed by the investigators.

Men: In two placebo-controlled, double-blind, multicenter studies in men (a two-year study of FOSAMAX 10 mg/day [n=146] and a one-year study of FOSAMAX 70 mg once weekly [n=109]), the safety profile of FOSAMAX was generally similar to that seen in postmenopausal women. The rates of discontinuation of therapy due to any clinical adverse experience were 2.7% for FOSAMAX 10 mg/day vs. 10.5% for placebo, and 6.4% for FOSAMAX 70 mg once weekly vs. 8.6% for placebo.

Other Studies in Men and Women: In a ten-week endoscopy study in men and women (n=277; mean age: 55) no difference was seen in upper gastrointestinal tract lesions between FOSAMAX 70 mg once weekly and placebo.

In an additional one-year study in men and women (n=335; mean age: 50) the overall safety and tolerability profiles of FOSAMAX 70 mg once weekly were similar to that of placebo and no difference was seen between men and women.

Other Studies with FOSAMAX: Prevention of Osteoporosis in Postmenopausal Women: The safety of FOSAMAX 5 mg/day in postmenopausal women 40-60 years of age has been evaluated in three double-blind, placebo-controlled studies involving over 1400 patients randomized to receive FOSAMAX for either two or three years. In these studies the overall safety profiles of FOSAMAX 5 mg/day and placebo were similar. Discontinuation of therapy due to any clinical adverse experience occurred in 7.5% of 642 patients treated with FOSAMAX 5 mg/day and 5.7% of 648 patients treated with placebo. Adverse experiences reported by the investigators as possibly, probably or definitely drug-related in ≥1% of patients treated with either FOSAMAX 5 mg/day or placebo are presented in Table 3.

Table 3: FOSAVANCE

Drug-Related [a] Adverse Experiences Reported in ≥1% of Patients Prevention of Osteoporosis

	FOSAMAX 5 mg/day % (n=642)	Placebo % (n=648)
Gastrointestinal		
Abdominal Pain	1.7	3.4
Acid Regurgitation	1.4	2.5
Diarrhea	1.1	1.7
Dyspepsia	1.9	1.7
Nausea	1.4	1.4

[a] Considered possibly, probably, or definitely drug-related as assessed by the investigators.

Concomitant Use with Estrogen/Hormone Replacement Therapy: In two studies (of one and two years' duration) of postmenopausal osteoporotic women (total: n=853), the safety and tolerability profile of combined treatment with FOSAMAX 10 mg once daily and estrogen±progestin (n=354) was consistent with those of the individual treatments.

Treatment and Prevention of Glucocorticoid-Induced Osteoporosis: In two, one-year, placebo-controlled, double-blind, multicenter studies in patients receiving glucocorticoid treatment, the overall safety and tolerability profiles of FOSAMAX 5 or 10 mg/day were generally similar to that of placebo. Adverse experiences reported by the investigators as possibly, probably or definitely drug-related in ≥1% of patients treated with either FOSAMAX 5 or 10 mg/day or placebo are presented in Table 4.

Table 4: FOSAVANCE

Drug-Related[a] Adverse Experiences Reported in ≥1% of Patients Treatment and Prevention of Glucocorticoid-Induced Osteoporosis

	FOSAMAX 10 mg/day % (n=157)	FOSAMAX 5 mg/day % (n=161)	Placebo % (n=159)
Gastrointestinal			
Abdominal Pain	3.2	1.9	0.0
Acid Regurgitation	2.5	1.9	1.3
Constipation	1.3	0.6	0.0
Melena	1.3	0.0	0.0
Nausea	0.6	1.2	0.6
Diarrhea	0.0	0.0	1.3
Nervous System/Psychiatric			
Headache	0.6	0.0	1.3

[a] Considered possibly, probably, or definitely drug-related as assessed by the investigators.

The overall safety and tolerability profile in the glucocorticoid-induced osteoporosis population that continued therapy for the second year of the studies was consistent with that observed in the first year.

Paget's Disease of Bone: In clinical studies (Paget's disease and osteoporosis), adverse experiences reported in 175 patients taking FOSAMAX 40 mg/day for 3-12 months were similar to those in postmenopausal women treated with FOSAMAX 10 mg/day. However, there was an apparent increased incidence of upper gastrointestinal adverse experiences in patients taking FOSAMAX 40 mg/day (17.7% FOSAMAX vs. 10.2% placebo). Isolated cases of esophagitis and gastritis resulted in discontinuation of treatment.

Additionally, musculoskeletal pain (bone, muscle or joint), which has been described in patients with Paget's disease treated with other bisphosphonates, was reported by the investigators as possibly, probably, or definitely drug-related in approximately 6% of patients treated with FOSAMAX 40 mg/day versus approximately 1% of patients treated with placebo, but rarely resulted in discontinuation of therapy. Discontinuation of therapy due to any clinical adverse experience occurred in 6.4% of patients with Paget's disease treated with FOSAMAX 40 mg/day and 2.4% of patients treated with placebo.

FOSAVANCE: In a fifteen week double-blind, multinational study in osteoporotic postmenopausal women (n=682) and men (n=35), the safety profile of FOSAVANCE (70 mg/2800 IU) was similar to that of FOSAMAX 70 mg once weekly. In the 24-week double-blind extension study in women (n=619) and men (n=33), the safety profile of FOSAVANCE (70 mg/2800 IU) administered with an additional 2800 IU vitamin D_3 was similar to that of FOSAVANCE (70 mg/2800 IU).

Less Common Clinical Trial Adverse Drug Reactions (<1%): Skin: Rarely, rash and erythema have occurred.

Abnormal Hematologic and Clinical Chemistry Findings: Laboratory Tests: In double-blind, multicenter, controlled studies, asymptomatic, mild, and transient decreases in serum calcium and phosphate were observed in approximately 18 and 10%, respectively, of patients taking FOSAMAX versus approximately 12 and 3% of those taking placebo. However, the incidences of decreases in serum calcium to <8.0 mg/dL (2.0 mM) and serum phosphate to ≤2.0 mg P*/dL (0.65 mM) were similar in both treatment groups.

In a small, open-label study, at higher doses (80 mg/day) some patients had elevated transaminases. However, this was not observed at 40 mg/day. No clinically significant toxicity was associated with these laboratory abnormalities.

Rare cases of leukemia have been reported following therapy with other bisphosphonates. Any causal relationship to either the treatment or to the patients' underlying disease has not been established.

Post-Market Adverse Drug Reactions: Post-Marketing Experience: The following adverse reactions have been reported in post-marketing use with alendronate:

Body as a Whole: hypersensitivity reactions including urticaria and rarely angioedema. As with other bisphosphonates, transient symptoms as in an acute-phase response (myalgia, malaise, asthenia and rarely, fever) have been reported with alendronate, typically in association with initiation of treatment. Rarely, symptomatic hypocalcemia has occurred, both in association with predisposing conditions and in patients without known predisposing conditions. Rarely, peripheral edema.

Dental: Localized osteonecrosis of the jaw (ONJ) has been reported rarely with oral bisphosphonate treatment. ONJ is generally associated with local infection (including osteomyelitis), tooth extraction with delayed healing (see Warnings and Precautions, General).

Gastrointestinal: esophagitis, esophageal erosions, esophageal ulcers, rarely esophageal stricture or perforation, and oropharyngeal ulceration. Some of these have been serious and required hospitalization. Rarely, gastric or duodenal ulcers, some severe and with complications (see Warnings and Precautions and Dosage and Administration).

Musculoskeletal: bone, joint, and/or muscle pain, rarely severe and/or incapacitating (see Warnings and Precautions); joint swelling; low-energy femoral shaft fracture (see Warnings and Precautions).

* P: Elemental phosphorus.

Nervous System: dizziness, vertigo, dysgeusia.

Skin: rash (occasionally with photosensitivity), pruritus, alopecia, rarely severe skin reactions, including Stevens-Johnson syndrome and toxic epidermal necrolysis.

Special Senses: rarely uveitis, scleritis or episcleritis.

DRUG INTERACTIONS: Overview: Animal studies have demonstrated that alendronate is highly concentrated in bone and is retained only minimally in soft tissue. No metabolites have been detected. Although alendronate is bound approximately 78% to plasma protein in humans, its plasma concentration is so low after oral dosing that only a small fraction of plasma-binding sites is occupied, resulting in a minimal potential for interference with the binding of other drugs. Alendronate is not excreted through the acidic or basic transport systems of the kidney in rats, and thus it is not anticipated to interfere with the excretion of other drugs by those systems in humans. In summary, alendronate is not expected to interact with other drugs based on effects on protein binding, renal excretion, or metabolism of other drugs.

Drug-Drug Interactions: Alendronate Sodium: If taken at the same time it is likely that calcium supplements, antacids, other multivalent cations and other oral medications will interfere with absorption of alendronate. Therefore, patients must wait at least one-half hour after taking FOSAVANCE before taking any other oral medication.

Intravenous ranitidine was shown to double the bioavailability of oral alendronate. The clinical significance of this increased bioavailability and whether similar increases will occur in patients given oral H_2-antagonists is unknown; no other specific drug interaction studies were performed.

Concomitant use of hormone replacement therapy (HRT [estrogen±progestin]) and FOSAMAX was assessed in two clinical studies of one or two years' duration in postmenopausal osteoporotic women. Combined use of FOSAMAX and HRT resulted in greater increases in bone mass, together with greater decreases in bone turnover, than seen with either treatment alone. In these studies, the safety and tolerability profile of the combination was consistent with those of the individual treatments (see Adverse Reactions, Clinical Trial Adverse Drug Reactions, Concomitant Use with Estrogen/Hormone Replacement Therapy). The studies were too small to detect antifracture efficacy, and no significant differences in fracture incidence among the treatment groups were found.

Specific interaction studies were not performed. FOSAMAX was used in osteoporosis studies in men, postmenopausal women, and glucocorticoid users, with a wide range of commonly prescribed drugs without evidence of clinical adverse interactions.

In clinical studies, the incidence of upper gastrointestinal adverse events was increased in patients receiving daily therapy with dosages of FOSAMAX greater than 10 mg and ASA-containing products. This was not observed in a study with FOSAMAX 70 mg once weekly.

FOSAVANCE may be administered to patients taking nonsteroidal anti-inflammatory drugs (NSAIDs). In a three-year, controlled, clinical study (n=2027) during which a majority of patients received concomitant NSAIDs, the incidence of upper gastrointestinal adverse events was similar in patients taking FOSAMAX 5 or 10 mg/day compared to those taking placebo. However, since NSAID use is associated with gastrointestinal irritation, caution should be used during concomitant use with FOSAVANCE.

Cholecalciferol: Drugs That May Impair the Absorption of Cholecalciferol: Olestra, mineral oils, orlistat, and bile acid sequestrants (e.g. cholestyramine, colestipol) may impair the absorption of vitamin D.

Drugs That May Increase the Catabolism of Cholecalciferol: Anticonvulsants, cimetidine, and thiazides may increase the catabolism of vitamin D.

Drug-Food Interactions: Food and beverages other than **plain water** may markedly reduce the absorption and effectiveness of alendronate. FOSAVANCE must be taken at least one-half hour before the first food, beverage, or medication of the day with plain water only (see Dosage and Administration, Administration).

Drug-Herb Interactions: Herbal products may interfere with the absorption of alendronate. FOSAVANCE must be taken at least one-half hour before any herbal products.

Drug-Laboratory Test Interactions: Interactions with laboratory tests have not been established.

Drug-Lifestyle Interactions: No studies on the effects on the ability to drive and use machines have been performed. However, certain adverse reactions that have been reported with FOSAVANCE (e.g., dizziness, vertigo, visual disturbances, and severe bone, muscle or joint pain) may affect some patients' ability to drive or operate machinery. Individual responses to FOSAVANCE may vary.

DOSAGE AND ADMINISTRATION: Recommended Dose: Treatment of Osteoporosis in Postmenopausal Women/Treatment of Osteoporosis in Men: The recommended dosage is one tablet of FOSAVANCE (70 mg/2800 IU) or FOSAVANCE (70 mg/5600 IU) once weekly. The appropriate dosage of FOSAVANCE must be determined by the physician based on the patient's vitamin D requirement.

All patients must receive supplemental calcium and/or vitamin D, if intake is inadequate (see Warnings and Precautions).

Dosage Adjustment: No dosage adjustment is necessary for the elderly or for patients with mild-to-moderate renal insufficiency (creatinine clearance 0.58 to 1 mL/s [35 to 60 mL/min]). FOSAVANCE is not recommended for patients with more severe renal insufficiency (creatinine clearance <0.58 mL/s [<35 mL/min]) due to lack of experience.

Missed Dose: Patients should be instructed that if they miss a dose of FOSAVANCE, they should take one tablet on the morning after they remember. They should not take two tablets on the same day but should return to taking one tablet once a week, as originally scheduled on their chosen day.

Administration: FOSAVANCE must be taken at least one-half hour before the first food, beverage, or medication of the day with plain water only. Other beverages (including mineral water), food, and some medications are known to reduce the absorption of alendronate (see Drug Interactions). Waiting less than 30 minutes will lessen the effect of FOSAVANCE by decreasing its absorption into the body.

To facilitate delivery to the stomach and thus reduce the potential for esophageal irritation, FOSAVANCE should only be swallowed upon arising for the day with a **full** glass of water (200-250 mL) and patients should not lie down for at least 30 minutes **and** until after their first food of the day. FOSAVANCE should not be taken at bedtime or before arising for the day. Failure to follow these instructions may increase the risk of esophageal adverse experiences (see Warnings and Precautions).

All patients must receive supplemental calcium and/or vitamin D, if intake is inadequate. Physicians should consider the vitamin D intake from vitamins and dietary supplements. Patients at increased risk for vitamin D insufficiency (e.g. over the age of 70 years, home bound, or chronically ill) should receive FOSAVANCE (70 mg/5600 IU) and may also need additional vitamin D supplementation. For patients fifty years and over, the recommended dose is at least 800 IU per day. Those living in high latitudes (including most of Canada) may also need additional supplementation.

Although no specific studies have been conducted on the effects of switching patients on another therapy for osteoporosis to FOSAVANCE, there are no known or theoretical safety concerns related to FOSAVANCE in patients who previously received any other antiosteoporotic therapy.

OVERDOSAGE:

Alendronate Sodium: No specific information is available on the treatment of overdosage with alendronate. Hypocalcemia, hypophosphatemia, and upper gastrointestinal adverse events, such as upset stomach, heartburn, esophagitis, gastritis, or ulcer, may result from oral overdosage. Milk or antacids should be given to bind alendronate. Due to the risk of esophageal irritation, vomiting should not be induced and the patient should remain fully upright.

Dialysis would not be beneficial.

Cholecalciferol: Vitamin D toxicity has not been documented during chronic therapy in generally healthy adults at a dose less than 10 000 IU/day. In a clinical study of healthy adults, a 4000 IU daily dose of vitamin D^3 for up to five months was not associated with hypercalciuria or hypercalcemia.

For management of a suspected drug overdose, contact your regional Poison Control Centre. See the *CPS* Directory section for a list of Poison Control Centres.

ACTION AND CLINICAL PHARMACOLOGY: Mechanism of Action: FOSAVANCE contains alendronate sodium, a bisphosphonate, and cholecalciferol (vitamin D_3).

Alendronate sodium is a bisphosphonate that acts as a potent, specific inhibitor of osteoclast-mediated bone resorption. Bisphosphonates are synthetic analogs of pyrophosphate that bind to the hydroxyapatite found in bone.

Cholecalciferol (vitamin D_3) is a secosterol that is the natural precursor of the calcium-regulating hormone calcitriol (1,25-dihydroxyvitamin D_3).

Pharmacodynamics: Alendronate Sodium: Alendronate is a bisphosphonate that binds to bone hydroxyapatite and specifically inhibits the activity of osteoclasts, the bone-resorbing cells. Alendronate reduces bone resorption with no direct effect on bone formation, although the latter process is ultimately reduced because bone resorption and formation are coupled during bone turnover.

Osteoporosis in Postmenopausal Women: Osteoporosis is characterized by low bone mass that leads to an increased risk of fracture. The diagnosis can be confirmed by the finding of low bone mass, evidence of fracture on x-ray, a history of osteoporotic fracture, or height loss or kyphosis, indicative of vertebral fracture. Osteoporosis occurs in both males and females but is most common among women following the menopause, when bone turnover increases and the rate of bone resorption exceeds that of bone formation. Increased bone turnover is an independent risk factor of fractures. These changes result in progressive bone loss and lead to osteoporosis in a significant proportion of women over age 50. Fractures, usually of the spine, hip, and wrist, are the common consequences. From age 50 to age 90, the risk of hip fracture in white women increases 50-fold and the risk of vertebral fracture 15- to 30-fold. It is estimated that approximately 40% of 50-year-old women will sustain one or more osteoporosis-related fractures of the spine, hip, or wrist during their remaining lifetimes. Hip fractures, in particular, are associated with substantial morbidity, disability, and mortality.

Daily oral doses of alendronate (5, 20, and 40 mg for six weeks) in postmenopausal women produced biochemical changes indicative of dose-dependent inhibition of bone resorption, including decreases in urinary calcium and urinary markers of bone collagen degradation (such as deoxypyridinoline and cross-linked N-telopeptides of type I collagen). These biochemical changes tended to return toward baseline values as early as 3 weeks following the discontinuation of therapy with alendronate and did not differ from placebo after 7 months.

Long-term treatment of osteoporosis with FOSAMAX 10 mg/day (for up to five years) reduced urinary excretion of markers of bone resorption, deoxypyridinoline and cross-linked N-telopeptides of type I collagen, by approximately 50% and 70%, respectively, to reach levels similar to those seen in healthy premenopausal women. The decrease in the rate of bone resorption indicated by these markers was evident as early as one month and at three to six months reached a plateau that was maintained for the entire duration of treatment with FOSAMAX. In osteoporosis treatment studies, FOSAMAX 10 mg/day decreased the markers of bone formation, osteocalcin and bone specific alkaline phosphatase by approximately 50%, and total serum alkaline phosphatase, by approximately 25 to 30%, to reach a plateau after 6 to 12 months. Similar reductions in the rate of bone turnover were observed in postmenopausal women during a one-year study with FOSAMAX 70 mg once weekly for the treatment of osteoporosis. These data indicate that the rate of bone turnover reached a new steady-state, despite the progressive increase in the total amount of alendronate deposited within bone.

As a result of inhibition of bone resorption, asymptomatic reductions in serum calcium and phosphate concentrations were also observed following treatment with FOSAMAX. In the long-term studies, reductions from baseline in serum calcium (approximately 2%) and phosphate (approximately 4 to 6%) were evident the first month after the initiation of FOSAMAX 10 mg. No further decreases in serum calcium were observed for the five-year duration of treatment, however, serum phosphate returned toward pre-study levels during years three through five. In a one-year study with FOSAMAX 70 mg once weekly, similar reductions were observed at 6 and 12 months. The reduction in serum phosphate may reflect not only the positive bone mineral balance due to FOSAMAX but also a decrease in renal phosphate reabsorption.

Osteoporosis in Men: Even though osteoporosis is less prevalent in men than in postmenopausal women, a significant proportion of osteoporotic fractures occur in men. The prevalence of vertebral deformities appears to be similar in men and women. Treatment of men with osteoporosis with FOSAMAX 10 mg/day for two years reduced urinary excretion of cross-linked N-telopeptides of type I collagen by approximately 60% and bone-specific alkaline phosphatase by approximately 40%. Similar reductions were observed in a one-year study in men with osteoporosis receiving FOSAMAX 70 mg once weekly.

Pharmacokinetics: See Table 5.

Table 5: FOSAVANCE

Summary of Pharmacokinetic Parameters of Alendronate in the Normal Population

	Mean	90% Confidence Interval
Absolute bioavailability of 5 mg tablet, taken 2 hours before first meal of the day	0.63% (females)	(0.48, 0.83)
Absolute bioavailability of 10 mg tablet, taken 2 hours before first meal of the day	0.78% (females)	(0.61, 1.04)
	0.59% (males)	(0.43, 0.81)
Absolute bioavailability of 40 mg tablet, taken 2 hours before first meal of the day	0.60% (females)	(0.46, 0.78)
Absolute bioavailability of 70 mg tablet, taken 2 hours before first meal of the day	0.57% (females)	(0.44, 0.73)
Renal clearance mL/s (mL/min) (n=6)	1.18 (71)	(1.07, 1.3) (64,78)

Absorption: Alendronate Sodium: Relative to an intravenous (IV) reference dose, the mean oral bioavailability of alendronate in women was 0.64% for doses ranging from 5 to 70 mg when administered after an overnight fast and two hours before a standardized breakfast. Oral bioavailability of the 10 mg tablet in men was 0.59%.

The alendronate in the FOSAVANCE (70 mg/2800 IU) and FOSAVANCE (70 mg/5600 IU) tablets and the FOSAMAX (alendronate sodium) 70 mg tablet were found to be equally bioavailable.

A study examining the effect of timing of a meal on the bioavailability of alendronate was performed in 49 postmenopausal women. Bioavailability was decreased (by approximately 40%) when 10 mg alendronate was administered either 0.5 or 1 hour before a standardized breakfast, when compared to dosing 2 hours before eating. In studies of treatment and prevention of osteoporosis, alendronate was effective when administered at least 30 minutes before breakfast.

Bioavailability was negligible whether alendronate was administered with or up to two hours after a standardized breakfast. Concomitant administration of alendronate with coffee or orange juice reduced bioavailability by approximately 60%.

In healthy subjects, oral prednisone (20 mg three times daily for five days) did not produce a clinically meaningful change in the oral bioavailability of alendronate (a mean increase ranging from 20 to 44%).

Cholecalciferol: Following administration of FOSAVANCE (70 mg/2800 IU) after an overnight fast and two hours before a standard meal, the mean area under the serum-concentration-time curve ($AUC_{0\text{-}120\ hrs}$) for vitamin D_3 (unadjusted for endogenous vitamin D_3 levels) was 296.4 ng-hr/mL. The mean maximal serum concentration (C_{max}) of vitamin D_3 was 14.8 nmol/L or 5.9 ng/mL, and the median time to maximal serum concentration (T_{max}) was 12 hrs. Following administration of FOSAVANCE (70 mg/5600 IU) after an overnight fast and two hours before a meal, the mean area under the serum-concentration-time curve ($AUC_{0\text{-}80\ hrs}$) for vitamin D_3 (unadjusted for endogenous vitamin D_3 levels) was 490.2 ng·hr/ml. The mean maximal serum concentration (C_{max}) of vitamin D_3 was 30.5 nmol/L or 12.2 ng/mL and the median time to maximal serum concentration (T_{max}) was 10.6 hours. The bioavailability of the vitamin D_3 in FOSAVANCE (70 mg/2800 IU) and FOSAVANCE (70 mg/5600 IU) is similar to an equal dose of vitamin D_3 administered alone.

Distribution: Alendronate Sodium: Preclinical studies (in male rats) show that alendronate transiently distributes to soft tissues following 1 mg/kg IV administration but is then rapidly redistributed to bone or excreted in the urine. The mean steady-state volume of distribution, exclusive of bone, is at least 28 L in humans. Concentrations of drug in plasma following therapeutic oral doses are too low (less than 5 ng/mL) for analytical detection. Protein binding in human plasma is approximately 78%.

Cholecalciferol: Following absorption, vitamin D_3 enters the blood as part of chylomicrons. Vitamin D_3 is rapidly distributed mostly to the liver where it undergoes metabolism to 25-hydroxyvitamin D_3, the major storage form. Lesser amounts are distributed to adipose and muscle tissue and stored as vitamin D_3 at these sites for later release into the circulation. Circulating vitamin D_3 is bound to vitamin D-binding protein.

Metabolism: Alendronate Sodium: There is no evidence that alendronate is metabolized in animals or humans.

Cholecalciferol: Vitamin D_3 is rapidly metabolized by hydroxylation in the liver to 25-hydroxyvitamin D_3, and subsequently metabolized in the kidney to 1,25-dihydroxyvitamin D_3, which represents the biologically active form. Further hydroxylation occurs prior to elimination. A small percentage of vitamin D_3 undergoes glucuronidation prior to elimination.

Excretion: Alendronate Sodium: Following a single IV dose of [^{14}C]alendronate, approximately 50% of the radioactivity was excreted in the urine within 72 hours and little or no radioactivity was recovered in the feces. Following a single 10 mg IV dose, the renal clearance of alendronate was 71 mL/min and systemic clearance did not exceed 200 mL/min. Plasma concentrations fell by more than 95% within 6 hours following IV administration. The terminal half-life in humans is estimated to exceed 10 years, probably reflecting release of alendronate from the skeleton. Based on the above, it is estimated that after 10 years of oral treatment with FOSAMAX (10 mg daily) the amount of alendronate released daily from the skeleton is approximately 25% of that absorbed from the gastrointestinal tract.

Cholecalciferol: When radioactive vitamin D^3 was administered to healthy subjects, the mean urinary excretion of radioactivity after 48 hours was 2.4%, and the mean fecal excretion of radioactivity after 4 days was 4.9%. In both cases, the excreted radioactivity was almost exclusively as metabolites of the parent. The mean half-life of vitamin D^3 in the serum following an oral dose of FOSAVANCE (70 mg/2800 IU) is approximately 24 hours.

Special Populations and Conditions: Pediatrics: Alendronate pharmacokinetics have not been investigated in patients <18 years of age.

Geriatrics: Alendronate Sodium: Bioavailability and disposition of alendronate (urinary excretion) were similar in elderly (≥65 years of age) and younger patients. No dosage adjustment of alendronate is necessary (see Dosage and Administration).

Cholecalciferol: Dietary requirements of vitamin D_3 may be increased in the elderly.

Gender: Bioavailability and the fraction of an IV dose of alendronate excreted in urine were similar in men and women.

Race: Pharmacokinetic differences due to race have not been studied.

Hepatic Insufficiency: Alendronate Sodium: As there is evidence that alendronate is not metabolized or excreted in the bile, no studies were conducted in patients with hepatic insufficiency. No dosage adjustment is necessary.

Cholecalciferol: Vitamin D_3 may not be adequately absorbed in patients who have malabsorption due to inadequate bile production.

Renal Insufficiency: Alendronate Sodium: Preclinical studies show that, in rats with kidney failure, increasing amounts of drug are present in plasma, kidney, spleen, and tibia. In healthy controls, drug that is not deposited in bone is rapidly excreted in the urine. No evidence of saturation of bone uptake was found after 3 weeks dosing with cumulative IV doses of 35 mg/kg in young male rats. Although no clinical information is available, it is likely that, as in animals, elimination of alendronate via the kidney will be reduced in patients with impaired renal function. Therefore, somewhat greater accumulation of alendronate in bone might be expected in patients with impaired renal function.

No dosage adjustment is necessary for patients with mild-to-moderate renal insufficiency (creatinine clearance 0.58 to 1 mL/s [35 to 60 mL/min]). FOSAVANCE is not recommended for patients with more severe renal insufficiency (creatinine clearance <0.58 mL/s [<35 mL/min]) due to lack of experience.

STORAGE AND STABILITY: Store at 25°C, excursions permitted to 15-30°C. Protect from moisture and light. Store tablets in the original blister package until use.

INFORMATION FOR THE PATIENT: Published in e-CPS, available by subscription at www.e-cps.ca.

DOSAGE FORMS, COMPOSITION AND PACKAGING: 70 mg/2800 IU: Each white to off-white, modified capsule-shaped tablet, with code 710 on one side and an outline of a bone image on the other, contains: alendronate monosodium salt trihydrate 91.37 mg, the molar equivalent of 70 mg of free acid and cholecalciferol 70 µg (equivalent to 2800 IU Vitamin D_3). Nonmedicinal ingredients: butylated hydroxytoluene, colloidal silicon dioxide, croscarmellose sodium, gelatin, lactose anhydrous, magnesium stearate, medium chain triglycerides, microcrystalline cellulose, modified food starch (corn), sodium aluminum silicate and sucrose. Gluten-free. Blister packages of 4.

70 mg/5600 IU: Each white to off-white, modified rectangle-shaped tablet, with code 270 on one side and an outline of a bone image on the other, contains: alendronate monosodium salt trihydrate 91.37 mg, the molar equivalent of 70 mg of free acid and cholecalciferol 140 µg (equivalent to 5600 IU Vitamin D_3). Nonmedicinal ingredients: butylated hydroxytoluene, colloidal silicon dioxide, croscarmellose sodium, gelatin, lactose anhydrous, magnesium stearate, medium chain triglycerides, microcrystalline cellulose, modified food starch (corn), sodium aluminum silicate and sucrose. Gluten-free. Blister packages of 4.

(Shown in Product Identification Section)

Fosinopril

CPhA Monograph

see *ACE Inhibitors*

Fosrenol®

lanthanum carbonate

Phosphate Binder

Shire

Date of Revision: February 3, 2010

SUMMARY PRODUCT INFORMATION:

Route of Administration	Dosage Form/ Strength	Clinically Relevant Nonmedicinal Ingredients
Oral	Chewable tablets/250, 500, 750 and 1000 mg	For a complete listing see Dosage Forms, Composition and Packaging.

INDICATIONS AND CLINICAL USE: FOSRENOL (lanthanum carbonate hydrate) is indicated as a phosphate binding agent in patients with end stage renal disease on dialysis. Experience with therapy beyond 2 years is limited. The risk versus benefit from administration beyond two years should be carefully considered (see Warnings and Precautions, Bone and Action and Clinical Pharmacology, Pharmacokinetics, Distribution).

Geriatrics (>65 years of age): Of the total number of patients in clinical studies of FOSRENOL, 32% (538) were ≥65 years of age while 9.3% (159) were ≥75 years of age. No overall differences in safety or efficacy were observed between patients ≥65 years of age and younger patients.

Pediatrics (<18 years of age): The safety and efficacy of FOSRENOL have not been established in children (see Warnings and Precautions).

CONTRAINDICATIONS:

- FOSRENOL (lanthanum carbonate hydrate) is contraindicated in patients with hypophosphatemia.
- Patients who are hypersensitive to lanthanum carbonate or to any ingredient in the formulation or component of the container. For a complete listing, see Dosage Forms, Composition and Packaging.

WARNINGS AND PRECAUTIONS: Gastrointestinal: The safety of FOSRENOL (lanthanum carbonate hydrate) in patients with acute peptic ulcer, ulcerative colitis, Crohn's disease or bowel obstruction has not been established. Caution should be used in patients with these conditions.

Hepatic/Biliary/Pancreatic: No data are available in patients with severe hepatic impairment. Caution should be exercised in these patients, as elimination of absorbed lanthanum may be reduced.

Bone: Tissue Deposition: Tissue deposition of lanthanum has been shown with FOSRENOL in animal and human studies. In bone biopsies of patients treated with FOSRENOL for up to 4.5 years, rising levels of lanthanum were noted over time (see Action and Clinical Pharmacology, Pharmacokinetics, Distribution). There is no information on the re-distribution of lanthanum eliminated from bone into other tissues upon termination of lanthanum carbonate therapy.

The effect of iron or aluminum chelation on serum lanthanum released from bone has not been studied. Patients requiring chelation treatment who are taking FOSRENOL should be monitored closely.

Safety data exceeding 24 months are currently limited. The risk/benefit from longer-term administration should be carefully considered.

Long-term effects: There were no differences in the rates of fracture in patients treated with FOSRENOL compared to Standard Therapy* for up to 3 years. The duration of treatment exposure and time of observation in the clinical program is too short to conclude that FOSRENOL does not adversely affect bone quality or the risk for fracture or mortality beyond 3 years.

Special Populations: Pregnant Women: No adequate and well-controlled studies have been conducted in pregnant women. The effect of FOSRENOL on the absorption of vitamins and other nutrients has not been studied in pregnant women. FOSRENOL is not recommended for use during pregnancy.

Nursing Women: The excretion of lanthanum in milk has not been studied in animals. It is not known whether lanthanum is excreted in human breast milk. Therefore, the use of FOSRENOL in women who are breastfeeding is not recommended.

* Standard Therapy: Patients randomized to Standard Therapy continued to take their prescribed binder at the optimal dose required to control their phosphate levels at ≤5.9 mg/dL. Patients were allowed to switch phosphate binders throughout the study and could also take a combination of binders in order to achieve optimal phosphate control.

Pediatrics (<18 years of age) : While growth abnormalities were not identified in long-term animal studies, lanthanum was deposited into developing bone including growth plate. The consequences of such deposition in developing bone in pediatric patients are unknown. The safety and efficacy of FOSRENOL has not been established in patients below the age of 18 years.
Geriatrics (>65 years of age) : Of the total number of patients in clinical studies of FOSRENOL, 32% (538) were ≥65 years of age while 9.3% (159) were ≥75 years of age. No overall differences in safety or efficacy were observed between patients ≥65 years of age and younger patients.
Monitoring and Laboratory Tests: Patients should adhere to recommended diets in order to control phosphate and fluid intake. FOSRENOL is presented as a chewable tablet therefore avoiding the need to take additional fluid. Serum phosphate levels should be monitored and the dose of FOSRENOL titrated every 2-3 weeks until an acceptable serum phosphate level is reached, with regular monitoring thereafter.

ADVERSE REACTIONS: Adverse Drug Reaction Overview: Gastrointestinal symptoms including, but not limited to; nausea, vomiting, abdominal cramps and diarrhea were observed in patients taking FOSRENOL. These symptoms were less frequent when taking FOSRENOL with or immediately after food.
Clinical Trial Adverse Drug Reactions: Because clinical trials are conducted under very specific conditions the adverse reaction rates observed in the clinical trials may not reflect the rates observed in practice and should not be compared to the rates in the clinical trials of another drug. Adverse drug reaction information from clinical trials is useful for identifying drug-related adverse events and for approximating rates.

In three placebo-controlled studies in end stage renal disease (ESRD) patients, the most common adverse events for FOSRENOL were gastrointestinal events, such as nausea and vomiting and they generally abated over time with continued dosing. Adverse events that were more frequent (≥5% difference) in the FOSRENOL group are presented in Table 1.

Table 1: FOSRENOL

Adverse Events that Were More Common to FOSRENOL in Placebo-controlled, Double-blind Studies with Treatment Periods of 4-6 Weeks

Body System Preferred Terminology (WHOART)	FOSRENOL (N=180) %	Placebo (N=95) %
Dialysis Complication-NW		
Dialysis Graft Occlusion	7.8	1.1
Gastrointestinal System Disorders		
Abdominal Pain	5.0	0.0
Nausea	10.6	5.3
Vomiting	9.4	4.2

Legend: WHOART=World Health Organization Adverse Reactions Thesaurus; NW=non-WHOART term developed by Sponsor for the clinical development program.

The safety of FOSRENOL was studied in two long-term clinical trials that included 1215 patients treated with FOSRENOL and 944 with alternative therapy. Sixteen percent (16%) of patients in these comparative, open-label studies discontinued in the FOSRENOL-treated group due to adverse events. Gastrointestinal adverse events, such as nausea, diarrhea and vomiting, were the most common type of event leading to discontinuation.

The number of withdrawals and the most common adverse events (≥5% in either treatment group) in both the long-term (2 year), open-label, active controlled, study of FOSRENOL vs. alternative therapy (Study A) and the 6-month, comparative study of FOSRENOL vs. calcium carbonate (Study B) are shown in Table 2 and Table 3, respectively. In Table 3, Study A events have been adjusted for mean exposure differences between treatment groups (with a mean exposure of 1.0 year on lanthanum and 1.4 years on alternative therapy). The adjustment for mean exposure was achieved by multiplying the observed adverse event rates in the alternative therapy group by 0.74.

Table 2: FOSRENOL

Number of Withdrawals/Phosphate Levels Achieved by Study Phase

	Study A[a]		Study B[b]	
	FOSRENOL	Alternative Therapy	FOSRENOL	Calcium Carbonate
Withdrawals				
Titration Phase	98/668 (14.67%)	38/670 (5.67%)	60/510 (11.96%)	41/257 (15.95%)
Maintenance Phase	374/570 (65.61%)	311/632 (49.21%)	188/450 (41.78%)	103/207 (49.76%)
Mean serum phosphate level achieved				
Titration Phase	6.43 mg/dL[a] (2.06 mmol/L)	5.71 mg/dL[a] (1.85 mmol/L)	1.87 mmol/L[b]	1.66 mmol/L[b]
Maintenance Phase	6.17 mg/dL (1.97 mmol/L)	6.05 mg/dL (1.94 mmol/L)	1.73 mmol/L	1.73 mmol/L

[a] Study A: Patients in the FOSRENOL group were titrated over a six-week period starting from a dose of 750 mg/day and then maintained on doses up to 3000 mg/day.The alternative therapy group started the titration phase at their optimal dose and were subsequently maintained at their optimal dose with the allowance of switching/adding phosphate binders if they wished.
[b] Study B: Patients in the FOSRENOL group were titrated from 375 mg/day up to their optimal dose and then maintained on doses up to 3000 mg/day. The calcium carbonate group started the titration phase at their optimal dose and were maintained on doses up to 9000 mg/day.

Table 3: FOSRENOL

Incidence of Treatment-Emergent Adverse Events that Occurred in ≥5% of Patients (in Either Treatment Group) and in Both

	Comparative Studies A and B			
	Study A %		Study B %	
	FOSRENOL (N=682)	Alternative[a] Therapy Adjusted Rates (N=677)	FOSRENOL (N=533)	Calcium Carbonate (N=267)
Nausea	37	29	16	13
Vomiting	27	22	18	11
Dialysis graft complication	25	24	3	5
Diarrhea	24	24	13	10
Headache	22	21	5	6
Dialysis graft occlusion	21	21	4	6
Abdominal pain	17	18	5	3
Hypotension	16	18	8	9
Constipation	15	14	6	7
Bronchitis	5	6	5	6
Rhinitis	4	6	7	6
Hypercalcemia	4	8	0	20

[a] Alternative Therapy: Patients randomized to alternative therapy continued to take their prescribed binder at the optimal dose required to control their phosphate levels at ≤5.9 mg/dL. Patients were allowed to switch phosphate binders throughout the study and could also take a combination of binders in order to achieve optimal phosphate control.
The dose range used in Study B was FOSRENOL 375 mg-3000 mg as elemental lanthanum and calcium carbonate 1500 mg-9000 mg elemental calcium.

Less Common Clinical Trial Adverse Drug Reactions: In clinical studies, the following other, less common (>0.1%), adverse drug reactions were reported:
Infections and Infestations: gastroenteritis, laryngitis.
Blood and Lymphatic System Disorders: eosinophilia.
Endocrine Disorders: hyperparathyroidism.
Metabolism and Nutrition Disorders: hypocalcemia, hyperglycemia, hyperphosphatemia, hypophosphatemia, anorexia, appetite increased.
Nervous System Disorders: dizziness, taste alteration.
Ear and Labyrinth Disorders: vertigo.
Gastrointestinal Disorders: dyspepsia, flatulence, eructation, indigestion, irritable bowel syndrome, dry mouth, esophagitis, stomatitis, loose stools, tooth disorder, gastrointestinal disorder NOS (not otherwise specified).
Skin and Subcutaneous Tissue Disorders: alopecia, itching, pruritus, erythematous rash, sweating increased.
Musculoskeletal and Connective Tissue Disorders: arthralgia, myalgia, osteoporosis.
General Disorders: asthenia, chest pain, fatigue, malaise, peripheral edema, pain, thirst.
Investigations: blood aluminum increased, GGT increased, hepatic transaminases increased, alkaline phosphatase increased, weight decrease.

Although there have been a number of additional isolated events reported, none of these were considered unexpected in this patient population.

In a comparative clinical study, patients on FOSRENOL had a lower incidence of hypercalcemic episodes relative to patients on calcium-based phosphate binder (p<0.001).

DRUG INTERACTIONS: Overview: Lanthanum carbonate hydrate is not a substrate for cytochrome P450 and does not significantly inhibit the activities of the major human cytochrome P450 isoenzymes, CYP1A2, CYP2D6, CYP3A4, CYP2C9 or CYP2C19 in vitro.
Drug-Drug Interactions: In Vitro-Drug Interactions: Gastric Fluid: The potential for a physico-chemical interaction (precipitation) between lanthanum and six commonly used medications (warfarin, digoxin, furosemide, phenytoin, metoprolol and enalapril) was investigated in simulated gastric fluid. The results suggest that precipitation in the stomach of insoluble complexes of these drugs with lanthanum is unlikely.
In Vivo-Drug Interactions: No effects of lanthanum were found on the absorption of digoxin (0.5 mg), metoprolol (100 mg), or warfarin (10 mg) in healthy subjects co-administered lanthanum carbonate (three doses of 1000 mg on the day prior to exposure and one dose of 1000 mg on the day of co-administration). Potential pharmacodynamic interactions between lanthanum and these drugs (e.g. bleeding time or prothrombin time) were not evaluated. None of the drug interaction studies were done with the maximum recommended therapeutic dose of lanthanum carbonate.

In healthy subjects, the absorption and pharmacokinetics of a single dose of 1000 mg of FOSRENOL was unaffected by co-administration of citrate.

No effects of FOSRENOL on serum levels of 25-dihydroxy vitamin D_3, vitamin A, vitamin B_{12}, vitamin E and vitamin K were observed in patients who were monitored for 6 months.

Co-administration of FOSRENOL with quinolone antibiotics may reduce the extent of their absorption as a result of complex formation. The bioavailability of oral ciprofloxacin was decreased by approximately 50% when taken with FOSRENOL in a single dose study in healthy volunteers. FOSRENOL should not be taken simultaneously with oral quinolone antibiotics.

The bioavailability of levothyroxine was decreased by approximately 40% when taken together with FOSRENOL. FOSRENOL should not be taken simultaneously with thyroid hormones replacement therapy and closer monitoring of TSH levels is recommended in patients receiving both medicinal products.
Other Possible Interactions: Interactions with drugs such as tetracycline and doxycycline are theoretically possible. If these compounds are to be co-administered, it is recommended that they not be taken within 2 hours of dosing with FOSRENOL.

Lanthanum carbonate hydrate may increase gastric pH. It is recommended that compounds known to interact with antacids should not be taken within 2 hours of dosing with FOSRENOL (e.g. chloroquine, hydroxychloroquine and ketoconazole).

No drug interaction studies assessed the effects of drugs on phosphate binding by lanthanum carbonate.

The drug interactions profile of FOSRENOL is characterized by the potential of lanthanum to bind to drugs with anionic functions (e.g., carboxyl, carbonyl and hydroxyl groups). When administering any such medications where a reduction in the bioavailability of that medicine would have a clinically significant effect on safety or efficacy, the physician should consider dosing that medicine apart from FOSRENOL or monitoring blood levels.
Drug-Herb Interactions: Interactions of FOSRENOL with herbs have not been established.
Drug-Laboratory Test Interactions: Abdominal x-rays of patients taking lanthanum carbonate may have a radio-opaque appearance typical of an imaging agent.
Drug-Lifestyle Interactions: Interactions of FOSRENOL with lifestyle have not been established.

DOSAGE AND ADMINISTRATION: Dosing Considerations: Serum phosphorus levels should be monitored as needed during titration until an optimal serum phosphorus level is reached, and then on a regular basis thereafter.

Recommended Dose and Dosage Adjustment: The recommended initial daily dose of FOSRENOL (lanthanum carbonate hydrate) for adults is 750 mg-1500 mg. The dose should be titrated every 2-3 weeks to a level that achieves maintenance of acceptable serum phosphorus levels. The daily dose should be divided and taken with or immediately after meals. Patients should adhere to recommended diets in order to control phosphate and fluid intake. FOSRENOL is presented as a chewable tablet therefore avoiding the need to take additional fluid.

In clinical studies in ESRD patients, FOSRENOL doses up to 3750 mg were evaluated. Most patients required a total daily dose between 1500 and 3000 mg of FOSRENOL to reduce serum phosphorus levels to less than 6.0 mg/dL (1.92 mmol/L). Doses were generally titrated in increments of 750 mg/day.

Missed Dose: A missed dose should be taken at the next scheduled dose with a meal. Taking a dose at a time other than mealtime may lead to nausea and vomiting. Patients should not double-up the dose to catch up.

Administration: Tablets should be chewed completely before swallowing. Intact tablets should not be swallowed.

OVERDOSAGE:

No case of overdose of FOSRENOL has been reported. Lanthanum carbonate hydrate was not acutely toxic in animals by the oral route. No deaths and no adverse effects occurred in mice, rats or dogs after single oral doses of 2000 mg/kg The highest daily dose of lanthanum administered to healthy adult subjects during Phase I studies was 4718 mg/day for 3 days. The adverse events observed were mild to moderate and included gastrointestinal symptoms and headache. Given the local activity of FOSRENOL in the gut, and the excretion in feces of the majority of the dose, supportive therapy is recommended in case of overdosage.

For management of a suspected drug overdose, CPhA recommends that you contact your **regional Poison Control Centre**. See the *CPS* Directory section for a list of Poison Control Centres.

ACTION AND CLINICAL PHARMACOLOGY: Patients with end stage renal disease (ESRD) can develop hyperphosphatemia as a result of phosphorus retention, which may be associated with secondary hyperparathyroidism and elevated calcium phosphate product.

Treatment of hyperphosphatemia usually includes all of the following: reduction in dietary intake of phosphate, removal of phosphate by dialysis and inhibition of intestinal phosphate absorption with phosphate binders.

Mechanism of Action: FOSRENOL (lanthanum carbonate hydrate) acts in the lumen of the gut to bind dietary phosphorus released from food during digestion. Lanthanum carbonate hydrate inhibits the absorption of phosphorus by the formation of highly insoluble lanthanum phosphate complexes that cannot easily pass through the wall of the gastrointestinal tract, and are excreted in the feces.

Pharmacodynamics: Lanthanum carbonate dissociates in the acid environment of the upper GI tract to release lanthanum ions that bind dietary phosphate released from food during digestion. FOSRENOL inhibits absorption of phosphate by forming highly insoluble lanthanum phosphate complexes, consequently reducing both serum phosphate and calcium phosphate product.

In vitro studies have shown that in the physiologically relevant pH range of 3 to 5 in gastric fluid, lanthanum binds approximately 97% of the available phosphate when lanthanum is present in a two-fold molar excess to phosphate. In order to bind dietary phosphate efficiently, lanthanum should be administered with or immediately after a meal.

Pharmacokinetics: Since the binding of dietary phosphorus occurs in the lumen of the stomach and upper small intestine, plasma lanthanum concentrations are not predictive of lanthanum carbonate hydrate's efficacy.

Absorption: Following single or multiple dose oral administration of FOSRENOL to healthy subjects, the concentration of lanthanum in plasma was very low, with oral bioavailability estimated to be <0.002%.

In healthy subjects, plasma AUC and C_{max} increased as a function of dose, but in a less than proportional manner, after single oral doses of 250 to 1000 mg lanthanum, consistent with dissolution-limited absorption. The apparent plasma elimination half-life in healthy subjects was 36 hours.

In renal dialysis patients dosed for 10 days with 1000mg lanthanum carbonate hydrate three times daily, the mean (±sd) lanthanum C_{max} was 1.06 (±1.04) ng/mL, and the mean AUC_{last} was 31.1 (±40.5) ng·h/mL. During long-term administration (52 weeks) in renal dialysis patients, the mean lanthanum concentration in plasma was approximately 0.6 ng/mL. Regular blood level monitoring in renal dialysis patients taking lanthanum carbonate hydrate (with increasing doses within the therapeutic dose range) for up to 2 years showed minimal increase in plasma lanthanum concentrations over this time period.

The effect of food on the bioavailability of FOSRENOL has not been evaluated, but the timing of food intake relative to lanthanum administration (during and 30 minutes after food intake) has a negligible effect on the systemic level of lanthanum.

Distribution: Lanthanum is present in the environment. Measurement of background levels in non-lanthanum carbonate treated ESRD patients on dialysis during Phase III clinical trials revealed concentration of <0.05 to 0.90 ng/mL in plasma, and <0.0006 to 1.0 μg/g in bone biopsy samples.

In vitro, lanthanum is highly bound (>99%) to human plasma proteins, including human serum albumin, α1-acid glycoprotein, and transferrin. Binding to erythrocytes in vivo is negligible in rats.

In long-term studies in mice, rats and dogs, absorbed lanthanum was widely distributed to systemic tissues, predominantly bone, liver and the gastrointestinal tract, including the mesenteric lymph nodes. Lanthanum concentrations in several tissues, including the GI tract, bone and liver, increased over time and were several orders of magnitude higher than plasma concentrations. Changes in tissue lanthanum levels after withdrawal of treatment varied between tissues. A relatively high proportion of lanthanum was retained in tissues for longer than 6 months after cessation of dosing [median percent retained in bone ≤100% (rat) and ≤87% (dog) and in the liver ≤6% (rat) and ≤82% (dog)]. There is no evidence from animal studies that lanthanum crosses the blood-brain barrier.

In 105 bone biopsies from patients treated with FOSRENOL for up to 4.5 years, rising levels of lanthanum were noted over time. Steady state bone concentrations were not reached during the period studied. No clinical data are available on deposition of lanthanum in other tissues in humans, including liver and gastrointestinal tract.

Metabolism: Lanthanum carbonate is not metabolized and is not a substrate of CYP450. In vitro metabolic inhibition studies showed that lanthanum at concentrations of 10 and 40μg/mL does not have relevant inhibitory effects on any of the CYP450 isoenzymes tested (1A2, C9, 2C19, 2D6 and 3A4).

Excretion: Lanthanum was cleared from plasma following discontinuation of therapy with an elimination half-life of 53 hours.

No information is available regarding the mass balance of lanthanum in humans after oral administration. In healthy subjects the majority of an orally administered dose was excreted in the feces with only around 0.000031% of the oral dose excreted in the urine (representing <2% of total plasma clearance).

Studies in chronic renal failure patients with hepatic impairment have not been conducted. In patients with co-existing hepatic disorders at the time of entry into Phase III clinical studies, there was no evidence of increased plasma exposure to lanthanum or worsening hepatic function after treatment with FOSRENOL for periods up to 2 years.

Paired bone biopsies from 11 patients were collected after 12 months of lanthanum carbonate treatment and 24-26 months after stopping lanthanum carbonate treatment. The mean bone lanthanum concentration at the end of the treatment period was 2806 μg/kg (range 530 to 5513 μg/kg) and the mean concentration was 1903 μg/kg (range 543 to 5683 μg/kg) after 24-26 months off-treatment. This limited data demonstrated that lanthanum is slowly cleared from bone. Its clearance showed considerable variability between individuals.

STORAGE AND STABILITY: Store between 15-25°C; excursions permitted up to 30°C. Protect from moisture. Keep in a safe place out of the reach of children and pets.

INFORMATION FOR THE PATIENT: Published in e-CPS, available by subscription at www.e-cps.ca.

DOSAGE FORMS, COMPOSITION AND PACKAGING: 250 mg: Each white to off-white, round chewable tablet, flat with a beveled edge, and embossed on one side with 'S405' and the dosage strength corresponding to the content of the elemental lanthanum contains: elemental lanthanum 250 mg (as lanthanum carbonate hydrate). Nonmedicinal ingredients: colloidal silicon dioxide, dextrates (hydrated) and magnesium stearate. Bottles of 90 and 400.

500 mg: Each white to off-white, round chewable tablet, flat with a beveled edge, and embossed on one side with 'S405' and the dosage strength corresponding to the content of the elemental lanthanum contains: elemental lanthanum 500 mg (as lanthanum carbonate hydrate). Nonmedicinal ingredients: colloidal silicon dioxide, dextrates (hydrated) and magnesium stearate. Bottles of 45.

750 mg: Each white to off-white, round chewable tablet, flat with a beveled edge, and embossed on one side with 'S405' and the dosage strength corresponding to the content of the elemental lanthanum contains: elemental lanthanum 750 mg (as lanthanum carbonate hydrate). Nonmedicinal ingredients: colloidal silicon dioxide, dextrates (hydrated) and magnesium stearate. Bottles of 15.

1000 mg: Each white to off-white, round chewable tablet, flat with a beveled edge, and embossed on one side with 'S405' and the dosage strength corresponding to the content of the elemental lanthanum contains: elemental lanthanum 1000 mg (as lanthanum carbonate hydrate). Nonmedicinal ingredients: colloidal silicon dioxide, dextrates (hydrated) and magnesium stearate. Bottles of 10.

(Shown in Product Identification Section)

The reader is invited to consult CPhA's monograph **Heparins, Low Molecular Weight**.

Fragmin® ℞

dalteparin sodium

Anticoagulant—Antithrombotic

Pfizer

Date of Preparation: September 10, 2003
Date of Revision: July 19, 2010

SUMMARY PRODUCT INFORMATION:

Route of Administration	Dosage Form/ Strength	Clinically Relevant Nonmedicinal Ingredients
Parenteral	**Solution** Ampoule: 10 000 IU (anti-factor Xa)/1 mL; Multi-Dose Vial: 25 000 IU (anti-factor Xa)/mL 3.8 mL **Prefilled syringe with safety needle device** 2 500 IU (anti-factor Xa)/0.2 mL 5 000 IU (anti-factor Xa)/0.2 mL 7 500 IU (anti-factor Xa)/0.3 mL 10 000 IU (anti-factor Xa)/0.4 mL 12 500 IU (anti-factor Xa)/0.5 mL 15 000 IU (anti-factor Xa)/0.6 mL 18 000 IU (anti-factor Xa)/0.72 mL	Benzyl alcohol in vial only For a complete listing, see Dosage Forms, Composition and Packaging.

INDICATIONS AND CLINICAL USE: FRAGMIN (dalteparin sodium injection) is indicated for:

- Thromboprophylaxis in conjunction with surgery
- Treatment of acute deep venous thrombosis
- Unstable coronary artery disease (UCAD), i.e., unstable angina and non-Q-wave myocardial infarction
- Prevention of clotting in the extracorporeal system during hemodialysis and hemofiltration in connection with acute renal failure or chronic renal insufficiency
- Extended treatment of symptomatic venous thromboembolism to prevent recurrence of venous thromboembolism in patients with cancer
- Reduction of deep vein thrombosis (DVT) in hospitalized patients with severely restricted mobility during acute illness. Decreased mortality due to thromboembolic events and complications has not been demonstrated.

CONTRAINDICATIONS: FRAGMIN should not be used in patients who have the following:

- Hypersensitivity to FRAGMIN or any of its constituents, including benzyl alcohol (when using the 25 000 IU multi-dose vial) (see Warnings and Precautions, Special Populations, Pregnant Women), or to other low molecular weight heparins and/or heparin or pork products.
- History of confirmed or suspected immunologically-mediated heparin-induced thrombocytopenia (delayed-onset severe thrombocytopenia), and/or in patients in whom an in vitro platelet-aggregation test in the presence of FRAGMIN is positive
- Septic endocarditis (endocarditis lenta, subacute endocarditis)
- Uncontrollable active bleeding
- Major blood clotting disorders
- Acute gastroduodenal ulcer
- Cerebral hemorrhage
- Severe uncontrolled hypertension
- Diabetic or hemorrhagic retinopathy
- Other conditions or diseases involving an increased risk of hemorrhage
- Injuries to and operations on the central nervous system, eyes, and ears
- Spinal/epidural anesthesia is contraindicated where repeated high doses of FRAGMIN (100-120 IU/kg given twice daily or 200 IU/kg once daily) are required, due to an increased risk of bleeding

WARNINGS AND PRECAUTIONS:

Serious Warnings and Precautions
The multi-dose vial of FRAGMIN (25 000 IU/mL) contains benzyl alcohol (14 mg/mL) as a preservative. Benzyl alcohol has been associated with a potentially fatal "Gasping Syndrome" in neonates. Because benzyl alcohol may cross the placenta, FRAGMIN preserved with benzyl alcohol should not be used in pregnant women (see Special Populations, Pregnant Women).

General: FRAGMIN should NOT be administered intra-muscularly.

FRAGMIN cannot be used interchangeably (unit for unit) with unfractionated heparin (UFH) or other low molecular weight heparins (LMWHs) as they differ in their manufacturing process, molecular weight distribution, anti-Xa and anti-IIa activities, units and dosages. Special attention and compliance with instructions for use of each specific product are required during any change in treatment.

Cardiovascular: Use in Patients with Prosthetic Heart Valves: Cases of prosthetic valve thrombosis have been reported in these patients who have received low molecular weight heparins for thromboprophylaxis. Some of these patients were pregnant women in whom thrombosis led to maternal and/or fetal deaths. Pregnant women are at higher risk of thromboembolism (see Warnings and Precautions, Special Populations, Pregnant Women).

Use in Unstable Coronary Artery Disease: When thrombolytic treatment is considered appropriate in patients with unstable angina and non-Q-wave myocardial infarction, concomitant use of an anticoagulant such as FRAGMIN may increase the risk of bleeding.

Gastrointestinal: FRAGMIN should be used with caution in patients a history of gastrointestinal ulceration.

Hematologic: Hemorrhage: Bleeding may occur in conjunction with unfractionated heparin or low molecular weight heparin use. As with other anticoagulants, FRAGMIN should be used with extreme caution in patients at increased risk of hemorrhage. Bleeding can occur at any site during therapy with FRAGMIN. An unexpected drop in hematocrit or blood pressure should lead to a search for a bleeding site (see Adverse Reactions, Clinical Trial Adverse Drug Reactions, Bleeding, Post-Market Adverse Drug Reactions).

Platelets/Thrombocytopenia: Platelet counts should be determined prior to the start of treatment with FRAGMIN and, subsequently, twice weekly for the duration of treatment. Thrombocytopenia of any degree should be monitored closely. Heparin-induced thrombocytopenia can occur with the administration of FRAGMIN. Its incidence is unknown at present.

Caution is recommended when administering FRAGMIN to patients with congenital or drug induced thrombocytopenia or platelet defects.

During FRAGMIN administration, special caution is necessary in rapidly developing thrombocytopenia and severe thrombocytopenia (<100 000/μL). A positive or unknown result obtained from in vitro tests for antiplatelet antibody in the presence of FRAGMIN or other low molecular weight heparins and/or heparins would contraindicate FRAGMIN.

Hepatic/Biliary/Pancreatic: FRAGMIN should be used with caution in patients with hepatic insufficiency, as these patients may have potentially higher risk of hemorrhage.

Hyperkalemia: Heparin and low molecular weight Heparin can suppress adrenal secretion of aldosterone leading to hyperkalaemia, particularly in patients such as those with diabetes mellitus, chronic renal failure, pre-existing metabolic acidosis, raised plasma potassium or taking potassium sparing drugs. Plasma potassium should be measured in patients at risk.

Osteoporosis: Long-term treatment with heparin has been associated with a risk of osteoporosis. Although this has not been observed with dalteparin the risk of osteoporosis cannot be excluded.

Peri-Operative Considerations: Spinal/Epidural Hematomas: When neuraxial anesthesia (epidural/spinal anesthesia) or spinal puncture is employed, patients anticoagulated or scheduled to be anticoagulated with low molecular weight heparins or heparinoids for prevention of thromboembolic complications are at risk of developing an epidural or spinal hematoma which can result in long-term or permanent paralysis.

The risk of these events is increased by the use of indwelling epidural catheters for administration of analgesia or by the concomitant use of drugs affecting hemostasis such as non steroidal anti-inflammatory drugs (NSAIDs), platelet inhibitors, or other anticoagulants. The risk also appears to be increased by traumatic or repeated epidural or spinal puncture.

Patients should be frequently monitored for signs and symptoms of neurological impairment. If neurological compromise is noted, urgent treatment is necessary.

The physician should consider the potential benefit versus risk before neuraxial intervention in patients anticoagulated or to be anticoagulated for thromboprophylaxis (see Contraindications and Adverse Reactions).

When a higher dose (5000 IU s.c.) of FRAGMIN is administered for thromboprophylaxis in conjunction with surgery, no spinal/epidural invasion should be performed for at least 12 hours following the last dose of FRAGMIN and the next dose should be held until at least 12 hours after the anaesthetic procedure. Alternatively, when a lower dose (2500 IU s.c.) of FRAGMIN is administered, the dose can be initiated 1-2 hours prior to surgery. FRAGMIN injection should be given after spinal/epidural anaesthesia and only if the anaesthesiologist considers the spinal/epidural puncture as uncomplicated. Indwelling catheters should not be removed or manipulated for at least 10-12 hours following the last dose of FRAGMIN.

Use in Knee Surgery: The risk of bleeding in knee surgery patients receiving low molecular weight heparins may be greater than in other orthopedic surgical procedures. It should be noted that hemarthrosis is a serious complication of knee surgery. The frequency of bleeding events observed with FRAGMIN in orthopedic surgery patients is derived from clinical trials in hip replacement surgery patients. The physician should weigh the potential risks with the potential benefits to the patient in determining whether to administer a low molecular weight heparin in this patient population.

Selection of General Surgery Patients: Risk factors associated with postoperative venous thromboembolism following general surgery include history of venous thromboembolism, varicose veins, obesity, heart failure, malignancy, previous long bone fracture of a lower limb, bed rest for more than 5 days prior to surgery, predicted duration of surgery of more than 30 minutes, and age 60 years or above.

Renal: FRAGMIN should be used with caution in patients with renal insufficiency.

Patients with impaired renal function should be carefully monitored because the half-life for anti-Xa activity after administration of low molecular weight heparin may be prolonged in this patient population (see Action and Clinical Pharmacology, and Dosage and Administration, Use in Patients with Renal Impairment). Dose reduction should be considered in patients with severe renal impairment.

Meanwhile, emerging data from **one single publication** suggests that in critically ill patients with severe renal insufficiency, thromboprophylaxis with FRAGMIN at 5000 IU once daily, does not appear to be associated with an excessive anticoagulant effect due to drug bioaccumulation and is unlikely to contribute to bleeding (see Action and Clinical Pharmacology, Special Populations and Conditions, Renal Insufficiency).

Special Populations: Pregnant Women: The multi-dose vial of FRAGMIN (25 000 IU/mL) contains benzyl alcohol (14 mg/mL) as a preservative. Benzyl alcohol has been associated with a potentially fatal "Gasping Syndrome" in neonates. Cases of Gasping Syndrome have been reported in neonates when benzyl alcohol has been administered in amounts of 99-404 mg/kg/day. Manifestations of the disease include: metabolic acidosis, respiratory distress, gasping respirations, central nervous system dysfunction, convulsions, intracranial hemorrhages, hypoactivity, hypotonia, cardiovascular collapse and death. Because benzyl alcohol may cross the placenta, FRAGMIN preserved with benzyl alcohol should not be used in pregnant women.

There are also postmarketing reports of prosthetic valve thrombosis in pregnant women with prosthetic heart valves while receiving low molecular weight heparins for thromboprophylaxis. These events led to maternal death or surgical interventions.

Pregnant women with prosthetic heart valves appear to be at exceedingly high risk of thromboembolism. An incidence of thromboembolism approaching 30% has been reported in these patients, in some cases even with apparent adequate anticoagulation at treatment doses of low molecular weight heparins or unfractionated heparin. Any attempt to anticoagulate such patients should normally only be undertaken by medical practitioners with documented expertise and experience in this clinical area.

Data from one single publication suggests that ante partum thromboprophylaxis is warranted in pregnant women with idiopathic thrombosis or symptomatic thrombophilia (see Action and Clinical Pharmacology, Special Populations and Conditions, Pregnant Women).

Teratogenic Effects: As with other low molecular weight heparins (LMWH), FRAGMIN should not be used in pregnant women unless the therapeutic benefits to the patients outweigh the possible risks. There have been reports of congenital anomalies in infants born to women who received LMWHs during pregnancy, including cerebral anomalies, limb anomalies, hypospadias, peripheral vascular malformation, fibrotic dysplasia and cardiac defects. A causal relationship has not been established nor has the incidence been shown to be higher than in the general population.

Non-teratogenic Effects: There have been postmarketing reports of fetal death when pregnant women received low molecular weight heparins. Causality for these cases has not been established. Pregnant women receiving anticoagulants, including FRAGMIN, are at increased risk for bleeding. Hemorrhage can occur at any site and may lead to death of mother and/or fetus. Pregnant women receiving FRAGMIN should be carefully monitored. Pregnant women and women of child-bearing potential should be informed of the potential hazard to the fetus and the mother if FRAGMIN is administered during pregnancy.

Nursing Women: It is not known whether FRAGMIN is excreted in human milk. Because many drugs are excreted in human milk, caution should be exercised when FRAGMIN is administered to nursing women.

Pediatrics: The safety and effectiveness of FRAGMIN in children have not been established.

Geriatrics: Elderly patients receiving low molecular weight heparins are at increased risk of bleeding. Careful attention to dosing intervals and concomitant medications, especially anti-platelet preparations, is advised. Close monitoring of elderly patients with low body weight (e.g., <45 kg) and those predisposed to decreased renal function is recommended.

Patients with Extreme Body Weight: Safety and efficacy of low molecular weight heparins in high weight (e.g., >120 kg) and low weight (e.g., <46 kg) patients have not been fully determined. Individualized clinical and laboratory monitoring are recommended in these patients.

However, data from **one single publication** suggests that in the thrombosis treatment setting, a weight-adjusted dose **beyond the recommended maximum dose of 18 000 International Units/day (the largest patient weighed 190 kg and received a daily dose of 38 000 IU)** results in mean peak anti-Xa levels that are within the therapeutically acceptable range (see Action and Clinical Pharmacology, Special Populations and Conditions, Overweight Population).

Monitoring and Laboratory Tests: Monitoring FRAGMIN Activity: Determination of anti-factor Xa levels in plasma is the only method available for monitoring FRAGMIN activity. Routine clotting assays are unsuitable for monitoring its anticoagulant activity. Only at very high plasma FRAGMIN levels is activated partial thromboplastin time (APTT) prolongation observed. Prolongation of APTT during hemodialysis and treatment of acute deep venous thrombosis should only be used as a criterion of overdose. Dose increases aimed at prolonging APTT could cause overdosing and bleeding.

Measurement of peak anti-Xa levels at about 4 hours post-dose should be considered in patients at higher risk of bleeding and receiving FRAGMIN, such as the elderly, patients with renal impairment or the extremes of body weight, during pregnancy, or for children. At treatment doses of 100 IU/kg s.c. twice daily, peak anti-Xa levels should generally be maintained at no more than 1.0 IU/mL in these patients.

When FRAGMIN is administered subcutaneously, the individual patient's anti-Xa activity level will not remain within the range that would be expected with unfractionated heparin by continuous i.v. infusion throughout the entire dosing interval. FRAGMIN should be administered as directed (see Dosage and Administration). See Table 1.

Table 1: FRAGMIN

Peak Plasma Anti-Xa Levels

Dosage	Anti-Xa Levels (IU/mL) at Peak 3–4 Hours Post s.c. Injections[a] Mean±SD
2500 IU	0.20±0.08
5000 IU	0.49±0.13
100 IU/kg	0.61±0.17
120 IU/kg	0.91±0.32
200 IU/kg	1.2±0.43

[a] For 2500 IU and 5000 IU (given as single doses), peak levels were obtained from populations of healthy volunteers; for multiple doses of 100 IU/kg twice daily, 120 IU/kg twice daily and 200 IU/kg once daily, peak levels were obtained from patient populations treated for acute DVT.

As with all antithrombotic agents, there is a risk of systemic bleeding with FRAGMIN administration. Care should be taken with FRAGMIN use in high dose treatment of newly operated patients. After treatment is initiated patients should be carefully monitored for bleeding complications. This may be done by regular physical examination of the patients, close observation of the surgical drain and periodic measurements of hemoglobin, and anti-Xa determinations.

At higher doses, increases in APTT may occur. With normal prophylactic doses, FRAGMIN does not modify global clotting tests of APTT, prothrombin time (PT) and thrombin clotting time (TT). Therefore, treatment cannot be monitored with these tests.

Liver Function Tests: Since FRAGMIN use may be associated with a rise in hepatic transaminases, this observation should be considered when liver function tests are assessed.

ADVERSE REACTIONS: Adverse Drug Reaction Overview: Clinically significant adverse reactions observed with use of FRAGMIN and other low molecular weight heparins include bleeding events and local reactions, with a low incidence of thrombocytopenia and allergic reactions.

Clinical Trial Adverse Drug Reactions: Bleeding: As with any antithrombotic treatment, hemorrhagic manifestations can occur. Injection site hematomas are a common side effect with FRAGMIN (dalteparin sodium), occurring at a frequency of less than 5% with lower (prophylaxis) doses and less than 10% with higher (treatment) doses.

The incidence of major hemorrhagic complications during FRAGMIN treatment has been low and generally did not differ from that observed with unfractionated heparin. Patients taking FRAGMIN are at risk for major bleeding complications when plasma anti-Xa levels approach 2.0 IU/mL. Other risk factors associated with bleeding on therapy with heparins include serious concurrent illness, chronic heavy consumption of alcohol, use of platelet inhibiting drugs, renal failure, age and, possibly, female gender. Petechiae or easy bruising may precede frank hemorrhage. Bleeding may range from minor local hematomas to major hemorrhage. The early signs of bleeding may include epistaxis, hematuria, or melena. Bleeding may occur at any site and be difficult to detect, for example, retroperitoneal bleeding. Bleeding may also occur at surgical sites. Major hemorrhage, including retroperitoneal or intracranial bleeding, has been reported in association with FRAGMIN use, in some cases leading to fatality. Spinal or epidural hematomas have been reported with the concurrent use of FRAGMIN and spinal/epidural anaesthesia.

Thromboprophylaxis in Conjunction with Surgery: Table 2 summarizes major bleeding events that occurred in pivotal trials of FRAGMIN for thromboprophylaxis in general surgery associated with thromboembolic complications.

Table 2: FRAGMIN

Bleeding Events for Thromboprophylaxis in General Surgery Associated with Thromboembolic Complications

	FRAGMIN[a] N=385 n (%)	Heparin[b] N=265 n (%)	Placebo N=108 n (%)
Major Bleeding	11 (2.9)	3 (1.1)	4 (3.7)
Wound or Perioperative Bleed	10 (2.6)	2 (0.8)	4 (3.7)
Wound Hematoma	1 (0.3)	1 (0.4)	0 (0.0)

[a] 2500 IU s.c. 2 hours before surgery, then 2500 IU daily.
[b] Heparin 5000 IU s.c. 2 hours before surgery, then 12 hours later and once daily thereafter.
Treatment for at least 5-7 days.

Table 3 summarizes major bleeding events that occurred in pivotal trials of FRAGMIN for thromboprophylaxis in general surgery associated with other risk factors (e.g., malignancy) and trials of elective hip surgery.

Table 3: FRAGMIN

Bleeding Events for Thromboprophylaxis in General Surgery Associated with Other Risk Factors and Elective Hip Surgery

	General Surgery Associated with Other Risk Factors[a]		Elective Hip Surgery				
			FRAGMIN vs Warfarin Sodium[b]			FRAGMIN vs Heparin[a]	
	FRAGMIN[c] N=543 n (%)	Heparin[d] N=533 n (%)	FRAGMIN Started Before Surgery[e] N=496 n (%)	FRAGMIN Started After Surgery[f] N=487 n (%)	Warfarin Sodium[g] N=489 n (%)	FRAGMIN[c] N=69 n (%)	Heparin[d] N=97 n (%)
Major Bleeding	11 (2.0)	10 (1.9)	18 (3.6)	12 (2.5)	15 (3.1)	0 (0.0)	3 (4.3)

[a] Treatment for at least 5-10 days.
[b] Treatment for 6±2 days.
[c] 5000 IU s.c. once daily after surgery with the initial dose given 8 hours before surgery; or 2500 IU 2 hours before surgery and 2500 IU 12 hours later, then 5000 IU once daily.
[d] Heparin 5000 IU s.c. 2 hours before surgery, 5000 IU s.c. evening of surgery, then 5000 IU s.c. twice daily; or 5000 IU s.c. three times daily.
[e] 2500 IU s.c. ≤2 hours before surgery, 2500 IU s.c. at least 4 hours after surgery, then 5000 IU s.c. once daily.
[f] 2500 IU s.c. at least 4 hours after surgery, then 5000 IU s.c. once daily.
[g] Warfarin sodium 10 mg evening of day of surgery, then dose adjustment to maintain an INR from 2.0 to 3.0.

In a third hip replacement surgery clinical trial in which patients were randomized to FRAGMIN 2500 IU administered 2 hours before surgery, followed by 2500 IU at least 6 hours later and maintained on 5000 IU daily or warfarin 5-7.5 mg beginning the night before surgery, the incidence of major bleeding events was 2.6% (7/274) for patients treated with FRAGMIN and 0.4% (1/279) for patients treated with warfarin.

Treatment of Acute Deep Vein Thrombosis: In 3 pivotal studies of patients with deep vein thrombosis treated with FRAGMIN 100-120 IU/kg s.c. twice daily or 120-240 IU/kg continuous infusion over 12 hours vs. heparin 240 U/kg continuous infusion over 12 hours, 2/103 (1.9%) and 1/119 (0.8%) of patients treated with FRAGMIN and heparin, respectively, experienced major bleeding. The corresponding percentages from pivotal studies of patients treated with FRAGMIN 200 IU/kg given s.c. once daily vs. heparin given in a dose of 20 000-40 000 U/24 hour i.v. infusion were 4/328 (1.2%) and 5/353 (1.4%), respectively.

Unstable Angina and Non-Q-Wave Myocardial Infarction: Table 4 summarizes major bleeding events that occurred with FRAGMIN, heparin, and placebo in clinical trials of unstable angina and non-Q-wave myocardial infarction.

Table 4: FRAGMIN

Major Bleeding Events in Unstable Angina and Non-Q-Wave Myocardial Infarction

	FRAGMIN 120 IU/kg/12 hr. s.c.[a] N=1497 n (%)	Heparin i.v. and s.c[b] N=731 n (%)	Placebo q 12 hr. s.c. N=760 n (%)
Major Bleeding Events[c,d]	15 (1.0%)	7 (1.0%)	4 (0.5%)

[a] Treatment was administered for 5 to 8 days.
[b] Heparin i.v. infusion for at least 48 hours, APPT 1.5 to 2 times control, then 12 500 U s.c. every 12 hours for 5 to 8 days.
[c] Aspirin (75 to 165 mg per day) and beta blocker therapies were administered concurrently.
[d] Bleeding events were considered major if: 1) accompanied by a decrease in hemoglobin of ≥2 g/dL in connection with clinical symptoms; 2) a transfusion was required; 3) bleeding led to interruption of treatment or death; or 4) intracranial bleeding.

Extended Treatment of Symptomatic Venous Thromboembolism (VTE) to Prevent Recurrence of VTE in Patients with Cancer: Table 5 summarizes major bleeding events that occurred in the pivotal trial of FRAGMIN in patients with cancer treated for symptomatic VTE to prevent recurrence of VTE.

Table 5: FRAGMIN

Bleeding Events for Extended Treatment of Symptomatic VTE to Prevent Recurrence of VTE in Patients with Cancer

	FRAGMIN[a] N=338 n (%)	Oral Anticoagulant[b] N=335 n (%)	p-value[c]
Major Bleeding	19 (5.6)	12 (3.6)	0.270

[a] FRAGMIN 200 IU/kg s.c. administered once daily for the first month, then approximately 150 IU/kg s.c. for months 2-6.
[b] FRAGMIN 200 IU/kg s.c. for ≥5 days plus oral anticoagulant for 6 months dose adjusted to an INR of 2.0-3.0.
[c] Fisher's Exact Test.

Deep Vein Thrombosis in Hospitalized Patients with Severely Restricted Mobility: Table 6 summarizes the adverse events from the clinical trial of hospitalized patients with severely restricted mobility during acute illness.

Table 6: FRAGMIN

Adverse Events in Hospitalized Patients with Restricted Mobility

	Dalteparin, N=1848 n (%)	Placebo, N=1833 n (%)
Mortality		
Day 14	8 (0.43)	7 (0.38)
Day 21	43 (2.35)	42 (2.32)
Day 90	107 (6.12)	103 (6.01)
Hemorrhage[a]		
Fatal, day 21	2 (0.11)	1 (0.05)
Major, day 14	8 (0.43)	0 (0.00)
Major, day 21	9 (0.49)	3 (0.16)
Minor, day 14	16 (0.87)	5 (0.27)
Minor, day 21	19 (1.03)	10 (0.55)
Thrombocytopenia		
Day 14	10 (0.54)	6 (0.33)
Day 21	10 (0.54)	8 (0.44)

[a] A bleeding event was considered major if: 1) was accompanied by a decrease in hemoglobin of ≥2 g/dL in connection with clinical symptoms; 2) intraocular, spinal/epidural, intracranial, or retroperitoneal bleeding; 3) required transfusion of ≥2 units of blood products; 4) required significant medical or surgical intervention; or 5) led to death.

Three of the major bleeding events that occurred by Day 21 were fatal, all due to gastrointestinal hemorrhage (2 patients in the group treated with FRAGMIN and 1 in the group receiving placebo). Two deaths occurred after Day 21: 1 patient in the placebo group died from a subarachnoid hemorrhage that started on Day 55, and 1 patient died on day 71 (2 months after receiving the last dose of FRAGMIN) from a subdural hematoma.

Table 7: FRAGMIN

Adverse Drug Reactions

MedDRA System Organ Class	Adverse Drug Reactions	Frequency
Blood and Lymphatic System Disorders	Mild, reversible non-immunological thrombocytopenia	Common
	Angioedema	Rare
Hepato-biliary Disorders	Transient elevation of liver transaminases (ASAT, ALAT)[a]	Common
Immune System Disorders	Anaphylactoid reactions[b]	Rare
Skin and Subcutaneous Tissue Disorders	Skin rash, allergic reactions and skin necrosis	Rare
General Disorders and Administration Site Conditions	Pain at injection site	Common
Injury, Poisoning and Procedural Complications		

(cont'd)

Table 7: FRAGMIN (cont'd)

[a] Has not been correlated to any long-term effect on liver function.
[b] FRAGMIN therapy should be discontinued in patients showing local or systemic allergic responses.

Skeletal Effects: Use of low molecular weight heparins over extended periods has been reported to be associated with development of osteopenia.

Post-Market Adverse Drug Reactions: In post-marketing experience, the following undesirable effects have been reported:

Table 8: FRAGMIN

Post-Market Adverse Drug Reactions

MedDRA System Organ Class	Adverse Drug Reactions	Frequency
Blood and Lymphatic System Disorders	Severe immunologically-mediated heparin-induced thrombocytopenia (type II, with or without associated thrombotic complications), see Warnings and Precautions, Hematologic, Platelets/Thrombocytopenia	Rare
	Thrombocytopenia	Unknown
	Thrombocythemia	Unknown
Immune System Disorders	Anaphylactic reactions	Rare
Skin and Subcutaneous Tissue Disorders	Skin necrosis	Very rare
	Alopecia	Common
	Rash	Unknown
General Disorders and Administration Site Conditions	Retroperitoneal hemorrhage	Very rare
	Gastrointestinal hemorrhage[a]	Unknown
	Intracranial hemorrhage	Unknown
	Hemorrhage (bleeding at any site)[a]	
Injury, Poisoning and Procedural Complications	Spinal or epidural hematoma	Unknown

[a] Occasionally leading to fatality.

DRUG INTERACTIONS: Drug-Drug Interactions: FRAGMIN should be used with caution in patients receiving oral anticoagulants, platelet inhibitors, non-steroidal anti-inflammatories, thrombolytic agents and dextran because of increased risk of bleeding. Acetylsalicylic acid (ASA), unless contraindicated, is recommended in patients treated for unstable angina or non-Q-wave myocardial infarctions (see Dosage and Administration, Adverse Reactions).

Because NSAIDs and ASA analgesic/anti-inflammatory doses reduce production of vasodilatatory prostaglandins, and thereby renal blood flow and the renal excretion, particular care should be taken when administering dalteparin concomitantly with NSAIDs or high dose ASA in patients with renal failure.

Drug-Food Interactions: Interactions with food have not been established.
Drug-Herb Interactions: Interactions with herbs have not been established.
Drug-Laboratory Test Interactions: Interactions with lab tests have not been established.
Drug-Lifestyle Interactions: Interactions with lifestyle have not been established.

DOSAGE AND ADMINISTRATION: FRAGMIN may be given by subcutaneous (s.c.) injection or by intermittent or continuous intravenous (i.v.) infusion, depending upon the circumstances. **FRAGMIN must NOT be administered intramuscularly** (see Warnings and Precautions). Clinical trials conducted in support of clinical uses outlined below generally used subcutaneous dosing.

Dosing Considerations: Thromboprophylaxis in Conjunction with Surgery: The dose of FRAGMIN required for adequate prophylaxis without substantially increasing bleeding risk varies depending on patient risk factors.

General Surgery with Associated Risk of Thromboembolic Complications: 2500 IU s.c. administered 1-2 hours before the operation, and thereafter 2500 IU s.c. each morning until the patient is mobilized, in general 5-7 days or longer.

General Surgery Associated with Other Risk Factors: (See Warnings and Precautions, Peri-Operative Considerations, Selection of General Surgery Patients): 5000 IU s.c. is given the evening before the operation and then 5000 IU s.c. the following evenings. Treatment is continued until the patient is mobilized, in general for 5-7 days or longer.

As an alternative, 2500 IU s.c. is given 1-2 hours before the operation, with 2500 IU s.c. given again no sooner than 4 hours after surgery, but at least 8 hours after the previous dose, provided primary hemostasis is obtained. Starting on the day after surgery, 5000 IU s.c. is given each morning, in general for 5-7 days or longer.

Elective Hip Surgery: 5000 IU s.c. is given the evening before the operation and then 5000 IU s.c. the following evenings. Treatment is continued until the patient is mobilized, in general for 5-7 days or longer.

As an alternative 2500 IU s.c. is given 1-2 hours before the operation and 2500 IU s.c. 4-8 hours after surgery, provided primary hemostasis is obtained. Starting on the day after surgery, 5000 IU s.c. is given each morning, in general for 5-7 days or longer.

The pre-operative dose may be omitted and an initial dose of 2500 IU s.c. administered 4-8 hours after the operation, provided primary hemostasis is obtained. Starting on the day after surgery, 5000 IU s.c. is given each morning, in general for 5-7 days or longer. Omission of the pre-operative dose may reduce risk of peri-operative bleeding, however increased risk of venous thromboembolic events is possible. This option is based on the results of the North American Fragmin Trial (NAFT), which excluded patients at high risk of bleeding, i,e., documented cerebral or gastrointestinal bleeding within 3 months prior to surgery, defective hemostasis, e.g., thrombocytopenia (<100×10⁹/L), ongoing anticoagulant treatment.

Treatment of Acute Deep Vein Thrombosis: The following dosage is recommended: 200 IU/kg body weight given s.c. once daily. The expected plasma anti-Xa levels during subcutaneous treatment would be <0.3 IU anti-Xa/mL before injection and <1.7 IU anti-Xa/mL 3-4 hours after injection. In order to individualize the dose, a functional anti-Xa assay should be performed 3-4 hours post-injection. The single daily dose should not exceed 18 000 IU. The following weight intervals are recommended to be adapted to the single-dose prefilled syringes as in Table 9.

For patients with increased risk of bleeding, a dose of 100 IU/kg body weight given s.c. twice daily or 100 IU/kg body weight administered over a period of 12 hours as continuous i.v. infusion, can be used . The expected plasma anti-Xa levels during subcutaneous treatment would be >0.1 IU anti-Xa/mL before injection and <1.0 IU anti-Xa/mL 3-4 hours after injection.

Normally concomitant treatment with vitamin K antagonists is started immediately. Treatment with FRAGMIN should be continued until the levels of the prothrombin complex factors (FII, FVII, FIX, FX) have decreased to a therapeutic level, in general for approximately 5 days.

Table 9: FRAGMIN

Dosage and Weight Intervals

Weight (kg)	Dosage (IU)
46–56	10 000
57–68	12 500
69–82	15 000
83 and above[a]	18 000

[a] For patient weighing (kg) 83 and above, data from **one single publication** suggests that in the thrombosis treatment setting, a weight-adjusted dose **beyond the recommended maximum dose of 18 000 International Units/day (the largest patient weighed 190 kg and received a daily dose of 38 000 IU)** results in mean peak anti-Xa levels that are within the therapeutically acceptable range (see Action and Clinical Pharmacology, Special Populations and Conditions, Overweight Population).

Extended Treatment of Symptomatic Venous Thromboembolism (VTE) to Prevent Recurrence of VTE in Patients with Cancer: Month 1: 200 IU/kg body weight given s.c. once daily for the first 30 days of treatment. The total daily dose should not exceed 18 000 IU daily.

Months 2-6: Approximately 150 IU/kg given s.c. once daily using Table 10.

Table 10: FRAGMIN

Dosage and Weight Intervals

Weight (kg)	Dosage (IU)
≤56	7500
57–68	10 000
69–82	12 500
83–98	15 000
≥99	18 000

Dose Reductions for Chemotherapy-induced Thrombocytopenia: In the case of chemotherapy-induced thrombocytopenia with platelet counts <50 000/mm³, FRAGMIN should be interrupted until the platelet count recovers above 50 000/mm³. For platelet counts between 50 000 and 100 000/mm³, FRAGMIN should be reduced by 17% to 33% of the initial dose (allowing for dosage adjustment using the pre-filled syringes), depending on the patient's weight (see Table 11). Once the platelet count recovers to ≥100 000/mm³, FRAGMIN should be re-instituted at full dose.

Table 11: FRAGMIN

Dose Reductions for Chemotherapy-induced Thrombocytopenia

Weight (kg)	Scheduled Dose (IU)	Reduced Dose (IU)	Mean Dose Reduction (%)
≤56	7500	5000	33
57–68	10 000	7500	25
69–82	12 500	10 000	20
83–98	15 000	12 500	17
≥99	18 000	15 000	17

Unstable Coronary Artery Disease (Unstable Angina and Non-Q-Wave Myocardial Infarction): 120 IU/kg body weight given s.c. twice daily with a maximum dose of 10 000 IU/12 hours. The expected plasma anti-Xa levels during subcutaneous treatment would be >0.1 IU anti-Xa/mL before injection and <1.6 IU anti-Xa/mL 3-4 hours after injection. These levels were obtained from another patient population. Treatment should be continued for up to 6 days. Concomitant therapy with ASA is recommended.

Deep Vein Thrombosis in Hospitalized Patients with Severely Restricted Mobility: In hospitalized patients with severely restricted mobility during acute illness, the recommended dose of FRAGMIN is 5000 IU administered by s.c. injection once daily. In clinical trials, the usual duration of administration was 12 to 14 days.

Use in Patients with Renal Impairment: All patients with renal impairment treated with low molecular weight heparins should be monitored carefully.

Administration of low molecular weight heparins to patients with renal impairment has been shown to result in prolongation of anti-Xa activity, especially in those with severe renal impairment (creatinine clearance <30 mL/min), which may lead to an increased risk of bleeding. This effect has not yet been determined for FRAGMIN. Consideration of dosage adjustment in patients with severe renal impairment should be undertaken (see Action and Clinical Pharmacology). However, emerging data from the literature suggests that in critically ill patients with severe renal insufficiency, thromboprophylaxis with FRAGMIN at 5000 IU once daily, does not appear to be associated with an excessive anticoagulant effect due to drug bioaccumulation and is unlikely to contribute to bleeding (see Action and Clinical Pharmacology, Special Populations and Conditions, Renal Insufficiency).

Anticoagulation for Hemodialysis and Hemofiltration: Chronic Renal Failure, Patients with No Other Known Bleeding Risk: Hemodialysis and hemofiltration for a maximum of 4 hours: dose as below, or only i.v. bolus injection of 5000 IU. Hemodialysis and hemofiltration for more than 4 hours: i.v. bolus injection of 30-40 IU/kg body weight followed by i.v infusion of 10-15 IU/kg body weight per hour. This dose normally produces plasma levels lying within the range of 0.5-1.0 IU anti-Xa/mL.

Acute Renal Failure, Patients with High Bleeding Risk: i.v. bolus injection of 5-10 IU/kg body weight, followed by i.v. infusion of 4-5 IU/kg body weight per hour. Plasma level should lie within the range of 0.2-0.4 IU anti-Xa/mL.

Dilution: FRAGMIN solution for injection may be mixed with isotonic sodium chloride or isotonic glucose infusion solutions in glass infusion bottles and plastic containers. **Post dilution concentration:** 20 IU/mL. See Table 12.

As with all parenteral drug products, intravenous admixtures should be inspected visually for clarity, particulate matter, precipitation, discolouration and leakage prior to administration, whenever solution and container permit.

Table 12: FRAGMIN

Dilution

	1 mL 10 000 IU
Isotonic NaCl Infusion (9 mg/mL) **or**	500 mL
Isotonic Glucose Infusion (50 mg/mL)	500 mL

The infusion rate is 10 mL/hour. The solution should be used within 24 hours.

OVERDOSAGE:
Accidental overdosage following administration of FRAGMIN may lead to hemorrhagic complications. FRAGMIN should be immediately discontinued, at least temporarily, in cases of significant excess dosage. In more serious cases, protamine should be administered.

The anticoagulant effect of FRAGMIN is inhibited by protamine. This effect may be largely neutralized by slow intravenous injection of protamine sulphate. The dose of protamine to be given should be 1 mg protamine per 100 anti-Xa IU of FRAGMIN administered. A second infusion of 0.5 mg protamine per 100 anti-Xa IU of FRAGMIN may be administered if the APTT measured 2 to 4 hours after the first infusion remains prolonged. However, even with higher doses of protamine, the APTT may remain prolonged to a greater extent than usually seen with unfractionated heparin. Anti-Xa activity is never completely neutralized (maximum about 60%).

Particular care should be taken to avoid overdosage with protamine sulphate. Administration of protamine sulphate can cause severe hypotensive and anaphylactoid reactions. Because fatal reactions, often resembling anaphylaxis, have been reported with protamine sulphate, it should be given only when resuscitation equipment and treatment of anaphylactic shock are readily available. Refer to the protamine sulphate Product Monograph for further directions for use.

For management of a suspected drug overdose, contact your regional Poison Control Centre. See the *CPS* Directory section for a list of Poison Control Centres.

ACTION AND CLINICAL PHARMACOLOGY: Mechanism of Action: FRAGMIN is a low molecular weight heparin with antithrombotic properties.

Dalteparin sodium is produced through controlled nitrous acid depolymerization of sodium heparin from porcine intestinal mucosa. It is composed of strongly acidic sulphated polysaccharide chains with an average molecular weight of 5000 and about 90% of the material within the range 2000-9000. Dalteparin sodium is composed of molecules with and without a specially characterized pentasaccharide, the antithrombin binding site that is essential for high affinity binding to the plasma protein antithrombin (AT III).

Pharmacodynamics: FRAGMIN acts by potentiating the activity of antithrombin III, inhibiting formation of both Factor Xa and thrombin. However, it preferentially potentiates inhibition of Factor Xa, resulting in only slight increases of clotting time, i.e., activated partial thromboplastin time (APTT).

Effects of unfractionated heparin are monitored by assessing APTT and anti-factor Xa (anti-Xa) activity. For FRAGMIN, however, only high doses lead to noticeable increases in the APTT; therefore, measurement of APTT can be used only as an indicator of overdosage. In the case of FRAGMIN, anti-Xa activity of plasma is used both as an estimate of clotting activity , and as a basis to determine dosage. FRAGMIN potency is described in international anti-Xa units (IU).

The specific activity of FRAGMIN on factor Xa (by measurement of anti-factor Xa IU/mg) is 130, and its specific activity on factor IIa (by measurement of anti-factor IIa IU/mg) is 58. The ratio of anti-Xa/anti-IIa activity for FRAGMIN is 2.2 (for unfractionated heparin the anti Xa/anti IIa is equal to 1).

Dalteparin sodium has a smaller effect on platelet function and platelet adhesion than heparin, and thus has only a small effect on primary hemostasis. Heparin treatment depletes the pool of platelet factor 4, while dalteparin sodium has much less of an effect.

Pharmacokinetics: Absorption: The half-life of FRAGMIN has been shown to be 2 hours after intravenous injection and 3-4 hours after subcutaneous injection. The bioavailability after subcutaneous injection is approximately 90% and the pharmacokinetics are not dose-dependent. The plasma concentration of FRAGMIN following subcutaneous administration correlates directly with the administered dose and anti-Xa activity in plasma, as measured by the area under the activity curve. For the twice daily dosing regimen (100 IU/kg/12 hours) of FRAGMIN, the steady state level is attained after 2-4 s.c. injections (24-48 hours).

Distribution: The volume of distribution was found to be approximately 3 litres.

Animal studies using radioactively labelled drug have shown that the distribution of FRAGMIN is similar, whether the dose is administered intravenously or subcutaneously (i.v. or s.c.).

Excretion: After 4 hours about 20% is seen in the urine, with most of the remainder found in the liver, GI tract and kidney. After 72 hours, 70% of a radioactive FRAGMIN dose has been excreted. Less FRAGMIN is found in the liver than standard heparin; the kidneys are the major site of FRAGMIN excretion (approximately 70% based on animal studies). Dalteparin sodium, in contrast to heparin, is not cleared by a saturable mechanism; low doses are expressed in plasma and increasing the dose does not modify its clearance.

Special Populations and Conditions: Renal Insufficiency: In a study of 8 patients with chronic renal failure undergoing hemodialysis administered FRAGMIN 5000 IU intravenously, a half-life of about 5.7 hours was observed, compared to that of about 2 hours as previously reported in healthy volunteers receiving FRAGMIN intravenously (see Warnings and Precautions, Renal, and Dosage and Administration, Use in Patients with Renal Impairment).

In a multicenter, open-label, prospective cohort study (DIRECT study) of critically ill patients with severe acute or chronic renal insufficiency or dialysis (mean creatinine clearance of 18.9 ml/min), 138 evaluable patients received at least one dose of subcutaneous dalteparin 5000 IU once daily as thromboprophylaxis. The median duration of dalteparin administration was 7 days. Trough anti-Xa levels were measured twice weekly, 20 hours after the prior dalteparin dose, to assess for dalteparin bioaccumulation (defined as anti-Xa levels >0.40 IU/mL). No patient (0%; 95% CI: 0, 3.0) had bioaccumulation, during the study. The median (inter-quartile range [IQR]) trough anti-Xa level was <0.10 IU/mL (<0.10, <0.10). Serial anti-Xa levels were measured at approximately 3, 10, and 17 days after the start of dalteparin; Peak levels were between 0.29 IU/mL and 0.34 IU/mL and trough levels were below the lower limit of detection (<0.06 IU/mL) irrespective of the duration of treatment. These peak anti-Xa levels achieved with prophylactic dose dalteparin were consistent with peak prophylactic levels of anticoagulation of 0.20-0.40 IU/mL observed in other hospitalized medical and surgical patients.

Pregnant Women: In a prospective trial, the EThIG study, 810 pregnant women were assigned to one of three management strategies according to pre-defined risk factors related to history of VTE and thrombophilic profile. Low-risk women (group I), received 50-100 IU dalteparin/kg body weight/day for 14 days postpartum, or earlier when additional risk factors occurred. Women at high (group II) or very high risk (group III) received dalteparin from enrolment until six weeks postpartum (50-100 IU and 100-200 IU/ kg/ day, respectively). Risk-stratified heparin prophylaxis was associated with a low incidence of symptomatic VTE and few clinically important adverse events. Symptomatic VTE occurred in five women (0.6 %; 95% CI 0.2, 1.5%). There were no events in group I; three women in group II suffered an event (2 antepartum, 1 postpartum) and two in group III (both postpartum). Bleeding was classified as serious in 24 episodes (3.0% 95% CI: 1.9, 4.4 %) in 22 women (2.7% 95% CI: 1.8, 4.2 %), and no cases of fatal bleeding occurred. Thrombocytopenia occurred in 18 women (2.2%; 95% CI: 1.4, 3.6%), with no cases with clinical or laboratory features of heparin-induced thrombocytopenia (HIT).

Overweight Population: In a prospective, cohort study, 37 overweight patients were a priori stratified into three weight classes: (A) within 20 % of ideal body weight (IBW) (N=13), (B) 20-40% of IBW (n=14), and (C) greater than 40% of IBW (n=10). All patients, with serum creatinine levels <150 µmol/L, received dalteparin sodium 200 IU/kg based on actual body weight subcutaneously once daily for the treatment of DVT or pulmonary embolism for a minimum of 5 days. All patients had peak anti-Xa levels measured 3-4 h following their Day 3 injection and trough anti-Xa levels measured immediately prior to injections on Day 3 and Day 5. The largest patient weighted 190 kg with a BMI of 58. Patients were stratified per weight in three different groups: A, B, C with mean daily doses of dalteparin respectively of 14 030 IU, 17 646 IU, and 23 565 IU. Mean (SD) trough anti-Xa levels on Day 3 were 0.12 (0.05) anti-Xa IU/mL for group A, 0.11 (0.03) anti-Xa IU/mL for group B and 0.11 (0.03) anti-Xa IU/mL for group C (p>0.2). Similar trough anti-Xa levels were observed on Day 5. Mean (SD) peak anti-Xa levels on Day 3 were 1.01 (0.20), anti-Xa IU/mL, 0.97 (0.21) anti-Xa IU/mL and 1.12 (0.22) anti-Xa IU/mL for groups A, B and C respectively. No thromboembolic or bleeding complications occurred during dalteparin therapy in any patients.

STORAGE AND STABILITY: Store at room temperature, (15-30°C). The 25 000 IU/mL multi-dose vial must be used within 2 weeks after initial penetration.

SPECIAL HANDLING INSTRUCTIONS: No special handling required.

INFORMATION FOR THE PATIENT: Published in e-CPS, available by subscription at www.e-cps.ca.

DOSAGE FORMS, COMPOSITION AND PACKAGING: Potency is described in International anti-Xa units (IU). One unit (anti-Xa) of dalteparin sodium, average molecular weight 5000, corresponds to the activity of one unit of the 1st International Standard for Low Molecular Weight Heparin with respect to inhibition of coagulation Factor Xa in plasma utilizing the chromogenic peptide substrate S-2765 (N-α-Benzyloxycarbonyl-D-arginyl-glycyl-arginine-pNA·2HCl).

Ampoules: Each mL of solution for injection contains: dalteparin sodium 10 000 IU (anti-Xa). Nonmedicinal ingredients: hydrochloric acid, sodium chloride, sodium hydroxide and water for injection. Packages of 10×1 mL ampoules.

Prefilled Syringes with Safety Needle Device: 2500 IU/0.2 mL: Each single dose syringe contains: dalteparin sodium 2500 IU (anti-Xa). Nonmedicinal ingredients: hydrochloric acid, sodium chloride, sodium hydroxide and water for injection. Prefilled syringes of 0.2 mL, packages of 10.

5000 IU/0.2 mL: Each single dose syringe contains: dalteparin sodium 5000 IU (anti-Xa). Nonmedicinal ingredients: hydrochloric acid, sodium hydroxide and water for injection. Prefilled syringes of 0.2 mL, packages of 10.
7500 IU/0.3 mL: Each single dose syringe contains: dalteparin sodium 7500 IU (anti-Xa). Nonmedicinal ingredients: hydrochloric acid, sodium hydroxide and water for injection. Prefilled syringes of 0.3 mL, packages of 5.
10 000 IU/0.4 mL: Each single dose syringe contains: dalteparin sodium 10 000 IU (anti-Xa). Nonmedicinal ingredients: hydrochloric acid, sodium hydroxide and water for injection. Prefilled syringes of 0.4 mL, packages of 5.
12 500 IU/0.5 mL: Each single dose syringe contains: dalteparin sodium 12 500 IU (anti-Xa). Nonmedicinal ingredients: hydrochloric acid, sodium hydroxide and water for injection. Prefilled syringes of 0.5 mL, packages of 5.
15 000 IU/0.6 mL: Each single dose syringe contains: dalteparin sodium 15 000 IU (anti-Xa). Nonmedicinal ingredients: hydrochloric acid, sodium hydroxide and water for injection. Prefilled syringes of 0.6 mL, packages of 5.
18 000 IU/0.72 mL: Each single dose syringe contains: dalteparin sodium 18 000 IU (anti-Xa). Nonmedicinal ingredients: hydrochloric acid, sodium hydroxide and water for injection. Prefilled syringes of 0.72 mL, packages of 5.
Vials: Each mL of solution for injection contains: dalteparin sodium 25 000 IU (anti-Xa). Nonmedicinal ingredients: benzyl alcohol, hydrochloric acid, sodium chloride, sodium hydroxide and water for injection. Multidose vials of 3.8 mL. The 25 000 IU/mL multidose vial must be used within 2 weeks after initial penetration.

The reader is invited to consult CPhA's monograph **Heparins, Low Molecular Weight**.

Fraxiparine®

nadroparin calcium

Anticoagulant—Antithrombotic

GlaxoSmithKline

Fraxiparine® Forte

nadroparin calcium

Anticoagulant—Antithrombotic

GlaxoSmithKline

Date of Revision: September 16, 2008

SUMMARY PRODUCT INFORMATION:

Route of Administration	Dosage Form/ Strength	Clinically Relevant Nonmedicinal Ingredients
Injection	FRAXIPARINE (nadroparin calcium, 9500 anti-Xa IU/mL) single dose, prefilled glass syringes: 0.3 mL (ungraduated syringe), 2850 anti-Xa IU, green; 0.4 mL (ungraduated syringe), 3800 anti-Xa IU, orange; 0.6 mL (graduated syringe), 5700 anti-Xa IU, brown; 0.8 mL (graduated syringe), 7600 anti-Xa IU, green (teal); 1 mL (graduated syringe), 9500 anti-Xa IU, violet	Hydrochloric acid and/or calcium hydroxide For a complete listing see Dosage Forms, Composition and Packaging.
	FRAXIPARINE FORTE (nadroparin calcium, 19 000 anti-Xa IU/mL) single dose, prefilled glass syringes: 0.6 mL (graduated syringe), 11 400 anti-Xa IU, process blue; 0.8 mL (graduated syringe), 15 200 anti-Xa IU, magenta; 1 mL (graduated syringe), 19 000 anti-Xa IU, reflex blue	Hydrochloric acid and/or calcium hydroxide For a complete listing see Dosage Forms, Composition and Packaging.

INDICATIONS AND CLINICAL USE: FRAXIPARINE AND FRAXIPARINE FORTE (nadroparin calcium)

- Prophylaxis of thromboembolic disorders (particularly deep vein thrombosis and pulmonary embolism) in general surgery and in orthopaedic surgery.
- Treatment of deep vein thrombosis.
- Prevention of clotting during hemodialysis.
- Treatment of unstable angina and non-Q wave myocardial infarction.

FRAXIPARINE cannot be used interchangeably (unit for unit) with unfractionated heparin or other low molecular weight heparins (LMWHS) as they differ in their manufacturing process, molecular weight distribution, anti-Xa and anti-IIa activities, units and dosages. Special attention and compliance with instructions for use of each specific product is required during any change in treatment.

Geriatrics (>65 years of age): Elderly patients receiving low molecular weight heparins are at increased risk of bleeding. Careful attention to dosing and concomitant medications, especially anti-platelet preparations, is advised. Close monitoring of elderly patients with low body weight (e.g. <45 kg) and those predisposed to decreased renal function is recommended.
Pediatrics (<18 years of age): The safety and effectiveness of FRAXIPARINE in children has not been established.

CONTRAINDICATIONS:

- Hypersensitivity to FRAXIPARINE (nadroparin calcium) injection, or any of its constituents; or to other low molecular weight heparins and/or heparin.
- History of confirmed or suspected immunologically-mediated heparin-induced thrombocytopenia (delayed-onset severe thrombocytopenia), or in patients in whom an in vitro platelet-aggregation test in the presence of nadroparin is positive.
- Acute infective endocarditis.
- Active bleeding or increased risk of hemorrhage, in relation to hemostasis disorders.
- Major blood clotting disorders.
- Generalised hemorrhagic tendency or other conditions involving increased risk of bleeding.
- Organic lesions likely to bleed (such as active gastric or duodenal ulcers).
- Hemorrhagic cerebrovascular event (except if there are systemic emboli).
- Severe uncontrolled hypertension.
- Diabetic or hemorrhagic retinopathy.
- Injuries to and operations on the central nervous system, eyes and ears.
- Spinal/epidural anaesthesia is contraindicated where repeated high doses of FRAXIPARINE (171 IU/kg once daily or 86 IU/kg twice daily) are required, due to an increased risk of bleeding.
- Severe renal insufficiency (creatinine clearance less than 30 mL/min in patients receiving treatment for thromboembolic disorders, unstable angina and non-Q wave myocardial infarction).

WARNINGS AND PRECAUTIONS: General: FRAXIPARINE (nadroparin calcium) must NEVER be administered by the intramuscular route.

FRAXIPARINE cannot be used interchangeably (unit for unit) with unfractionated heparin or other low molecular weight heparins (LMWHS) as they differ in their manufacturing process, molecular weight distribution, anti-Xa and anti-IIa activities, units and dosages. Special attention and compliance with instructions for use of each specific product is required during any change in treatment.

Determination of anti-factor Xa levels in plasma is the only method available for monitoring nadroparin activity. Routine clotting assays are unsuitable for monitoring the anticoagulant activity, because APTT prolongation is generally observed only at very high plasma anti-Xa levels.

Measurement of peak anti-Xa levels at about 4 hours post-dose should be considered in patients at higher risk of bleeding and receiving FRAXIPARINE, such as the elderly, patients with renal insufficiency or the extremes of body weight, during pregnancy, or for children. At treatment doses, peak anti-Xa levels should generally be maintained at no more than 1.5 IU/mL in these patients (see Action and Clinical Pharmacology, and Warnings and Precautions, Monitoring and Laboratory Tests).

Latex Allergy: The needle guard of the pre-filled syringe contains dry natural latex rubber that has the potential to cause allergic reactions in latex sensitive individuals.

Cardiovascular: Use in Unstable Coronary Artery Disease: When thrombolytic treatment is considered appropriate in patients with unstable angina and non-Q wave myocardial infarction, concomitant use of an anticoagulant such as FRAXIPARINE may increase the risk of bleeding.

Use in Patients with Prosthetic Heart Valves: Cases of prosthetic valve thrombosis have been reported in patients who have received low molecular weight heparins for thromboprophylaxis. Some of these patients were pregnant women in whom thrombosis led to maternal and/or fetal deaths. Pregnant women are at higher risk of thromboembolism (see Warnings and Precautions, Pregnant Women).

Endocrine and Metabolism: Dosing in Patients with Extreme Body Weight: Safety and efficacy of low molecular weight heparins in high weight (e.g. >120 kg) and low weight (e.g. <45 kg) patients has not been fully determined. Individualised clinical and laboratory monitoring is recommended in these patients.

Hyperkalemia: Heparin can suppress adrenal secretion of aldosterone leading to hyperkalemia, particularly in patients with raised plasma potassium, or at risk of increased plasma potassium levels, such as patients with diabetes mellitus, chronic renal failure, pre-existing metabolic acidosis or those taking drugs that may cause hyperkalemia (e.g. ACE inhibitors, NSAIDs).

The risk of hyperkalemia appears to increase with duration of therapy but is usually reversible. Plasma potassium should be monitored in patients at risk.

Gastrointestinal: FRAXIPARINE should be used with caution in patients with/or a history of gastrointestinal ulceration.

Hematologic: Hemorrhage: Bleeding may occur in conjunction with unfractionated heparin or low molecular weight heparin use. As with other anticoagulants, FRAXIPARINE should be used with extreme caution in patients at increased risk of hemorrhage. Bleeding can occur at any site during therapy with FRAXIPARINE. An unexpected drop in hematocrit or blood pressure should lead to a search for a bleeding site (see Adverse Reactions, Bleeding).

In the prophylaxis or treatment of venous thromboembolic disorders and in the prevention of clotting during hemodialysis, the concomitant use of aspirin, other salicylates, non-steroidal anti-inflammatory drugs, and anti-platelet agents is not recommended, as they may increase the risk of bleeding. Where such combinations cannot be avoided, careful clinical and biological monitoring should be undertaken.

In clinical studies for the treatment of unstable angina and non-Q wave myocardial infarction, FRAXIPARINE was administered in combination with up to 325 mg aspirin per day (see Dosage and Administration).

Thrombocytopenia: Rare cases of thrombocytopenia, occasionally severe, have been reported, which may be associated with arterial or venous thrombosis. Such diagnosis should be considered in the following situations:

- thrombocytopenia
- any significant reduction in platelet level compared with baseline value
- worsening of the initial thrombosis while on therapy
- thrombosis occurring on treatment
- disseminated intra-vascular coagulation.

In this event, FRAXIPARINE treatment must be discontinued.

These effects are probably of an immuno-allergic nature and in the case of a first treatment are reported mainly between the 5th and the 21st day of therapy, but may occur much earlier if there is a history of heparin-related thrombocytopenia.

Thrombocytopenia of any degree should be monitored closely. Heparin-induced thrombocytopenia can occur with the administration of FRAXIPARINE. Its incidence is unknown at present.

When thrombocytopenia occurs with heparin (either standard or low molecular weight heparin), substitution with a different antithrombotic class should be considered. Cases of initial thrombocytopenia continuing after substitution of nadroparin with a different anti-thrombotic class have been reported.

In vitro platelet aggregation tests are only of limited value in the diagnosis of heparin-induced thrombocytopenia.

Platelets: Because of the possibility of heparin-induced thrombocytopenia, **platelet counts should be determined prior to the commencement of therapy with FRAXIPARINE and subsequently, twice weekly for the duration of therapy.**

Caution is recommended when administering FRAXIPARINE to patients with congenital or drug-induced thrombocytopenia, or platelet defects.

During FRAXIPARINE administration, special caution is necessary in rapidly developing thrombocytopenia and severe thrombocytopenia (<100 000/μL). A positive or indeterminate result obtained from in vitro tests for antiplatelet antibody in the presence of FRAXIPARINE or other low molecular weight heparins and/or heparin would contraindicate FRAXIPARINE.

Hepatic/Biliary/Pancreatic: FRAXIPARINE should be used with caution in patients with hepatic insufficiency.

There have been no studies conducted in patients with hepatic insufficiency.

Peri-Operative Considerations: Spinal/Epidural Hematomas: There have been cases of intra-spinal hematomas with the concurrent use of low molecular weight heparins and spinal/epidural anaesthesia resulting in long-term or permanent paralysis. The risk of these events may be higher with the use of post-operative indwelling epidural catheters or by the concomitant use of drugs affecting hemostasis: nonsteroidal anti-inflammatory drugs (NSAIDs), platelet inhibitors, or other drugs affecting coagulation. The risk also appears to be increased by traumatic or repeated epidural or spinal procedure. **FRAXIPARINE should only be used concurrently with spinal/epidural anaesthesia when the therapeutic benefits to the patients outweigh the possible risks (also see Contraindications).**

When used concurrently, no spinal invasion should be performed for 12 hours following the last dose of FRAXIPARINE, and the next dose should be held until at least 2 hours after the anaesthesia procedure. The same rules apply to the withdrawal or manipulation of the catheter. Careful vigilance for signs and symptoms of neurologic impairment is recommended with urgent diagnosis and treatment, if signs occur (see Adverse Reactions).

Use in Knee Surgery: The risk of bleeding in knee surgery patients receiving low molecular weight heparins may be greater than in other orthopaedic surgical procedures. It should be noted that hemarthrosis is a serious complication of knee surgery. The frequency of bleeding events observed with FRAXIPARINE in orthopaedic surgery patients is derived from clinical trials primarily in hip replacement surgery patients. The physician should weigh the potential risks with the potential benefits to the patient in determining whether to administer a low molecular weight heparin in this patient population.

Selection of General Surgery Patients: Risk factors associated with postoperative venous thromboembolism following general surgery include history of venous thromboembolism, varicose veins, obesity, heart failure, malignancy, previous long bone fracture of a lower limb, bed rest for more than 5 days prior to surgery, predicted duration of surgery of more than 30 minutes, age 60 years or above.

Renal: FRAXIPARINE should be used with caution in patients with renal insufficiency.

Reduced doses should be considered in patients with moderate to severe renal insufficiency receiving FRAXIPARINE for thromboprophylaxis, and in patients with moderate renal insufficiency receiving FRAXIPARINE for the treatment of thromboembolic disorders, angina and non-Q wave myocardial infarction (see Contraindications, Action and Clinical Pharmacology, Renal Insufficiency, and Dosage and Administration, Use in Renal Insufficiency).

Nadroparin is known to be mainly excreted by the kidney, which results in increased nadroparin exposure in patients with renal impairment (see Action and Clinical Pharmacology, Pharmacokinetics, Renal Insufficiency). Patients with impaired renal function are at increased risk of bleeding and should be treated with caution.

The decision on whether a dose reduction is appropriate for patients with creatinine clearance 30 to 50 mL/min should be based on the physician's assessment of an individual patient's risk of bleeding versus the risk of thromboembolism (see Dosage and Administration).

Patients with impaired renal function should be carefully monitored because half-life for anti-Xa activity after administration of low molecular weight heparin may be prolonged in this patient population (see Dosage and Administration).

Special Populations: Pregnant Women: Teratogenic Effects: Studies in animals have not shown any teratogenic or fetotoxic effects. However, there is only limited clinical data concerning transplacental passage of nadroparin in pregnant women. As with other low molecular weight heparins, FRAXIPARINE should not be used in pregnant women unless the therapeutic benefits to the patients outweigh the possible risks. There have been reports of congenital anomalies in infants born to women who received LMWHs during pregnancy, including cerebral anomalies, limb anomalies, hypospadias, peripheral vascular malformation, fibrotic dysplasia and cardiac defects. A causal relationship has not been established nor has the incidence been shown to be higher than in the general population.

Non-teratogenic Effects: There have been post-marketing reports of fetal death when pregnant women received LMWHs. Causality for these cases has not been established. Pregnant women receiving anticoagulants, including FRAXIPARINE, are at increased risk for bleeding. Hemorrhage can occur at any site and may lead to death of mother and/or fetus. Pregnant women receiving FRAXIPARINE should be carefully monitored.

Pregnant women and women of child-bearing potential should be informed of the potential hazard to the fetus and the mother if FRAXIPARINE is administered during pregnancy. There are also post-marketing reports of prosthetic valve thrombosis in pregnant women with prosthetic heart valves while receiving low molecular weight heparins for thromboprophylaxis. These events led to maternal death or surgical interventions.

Pregnant women with prosthetic heart valves appear to be at exceedingly high risk of thromboembolism. An incidence of thromboembolism approaching 30% has been reported in these patients, in some cases even with apparent adequate anticoagulation at treatment doses of low molecular weight heparins or unfractionated heparin. Any attempt to anticoagulate such patients should normally only be undertaken by medical practitioners with documented expertise and experience in this clinical area.

Nursing Women: It is not known whether nadroparin is excreted in human milk. Because many drugs are excreted in human milk, caution should be exercised when FRAXIPARINE is administered to nursing women.

Pediatrics (<18 years of age): The safety and effectiveness of FRAXIPARINE in children has not been established.

Geriatrics (>65 years of age): Geriatric patients receiving low molecular weight heparins are at increased risk of bleeding. Careful attention to dosing, and concomitant medications, especially anti-platelet preparations, is advised. Close monitoring of elderly patients with low body weight (e.g. <45 kg) and those predisposed to decreased renal function is recommended.

Caution should be exercised when FRAXIPARINE is administered in the following situations as they may be associated with an increased risk of bleeding:

- hepatic failure
- renal insufficiency
- severe arterial hypertension
- history of peptic ulcer or other organic lesion likely to bleed
- vascular disorder of the chorio-retina
- during the post-operative period following surgery of the brain, spinal cord or eye

Monitoring and Laboratory Tests: Since FRAXIPARINE use may be associated with a rise in hepatic transaminases, this observation should be considered when liver function tests are assessed (see Adverse Reactions, Hepatic/Biliary).

Nadroparin has only a moderate prolonging effect on clotting time assays such as APTT or thrombin time. For lab monitoring of effect, anti-Xa methods are recommended. Clinically meaningful prolongation of APTT during hemodialysis or treatment of acute deep vein thrombophlebitis with FRAXIPARINE should only be used as an indication of overdosage. Dose increases aimed at prolonging APTT to the same extent as with unfractionated heparin could cause overdose and bleeding.

FRAXIPARINE is administered subcutaneously, and therefore, the individual patient's anti-factor Xa activity level will not remain within the range that would be expected with unfractionated heparin by continuous intravenous infusion throughout the entire dosing interval. The peak plasma anti-factor Xa level occurs approximately 4 hours after subcutaneous administration. The peak level following a dose of 171 anti-Xa IU/kg is 1.2 to 1.8 IU/mL and following a dose of 86 anti-Xa IU/kg is 0.5 to 1.1 IU/mL. The steady state level is attained by Day 6. FRAXIPARINE should be administered as directed (see Dosage and Administration).

As with all antithrombotic agents, there is a risk of systemic bleeding with FRAXIPARINE administration. Care should be taken with FRAXIPARINE use in high dose treatment of newly operated patients.

After treatment is initiated patients should be carefully monitored for bleeding complications. This may be done by regular physical examination of the patients, close observation of the surgical drain and periodic measurements of hemoglobin, and anti-factor Xa determinations.

With normal prophylactic doses, FRAXIPARINE does not modify global clotting tests of activated partial thromboplastin (APTT), prothrombin time (PT) and thrombin clotting time (TT). Therefore, treatment can not be monitored with these tests.

At higher doses, increases in APTT and ACT may occur. Increases in APTT and ACT are not linearly correlated with increasing nadroparin antithrombotic activity and therefore are unsuitable and unreliable for monitoring FRAXIPARINE activity.

ADVERSE REACTIONS: Adverse Drug Reaction Overview: Bleeding: As with any antithrombotic treatment, hemorrhagic manifestations can occur. Small injection site hematomas are a very common side effect with FRAXIPARINE (nadroparin calcium), occurring at a frequency of less than 5% with lower (prophylaxis) doses and more than 10% with higher (treatment) doses. In some cases, the emergence of firm nodules which do not indicate an encystment of the heparin may be noted. These nodules usually disappear after a few days. Hemorrhagic manifestations at various sites are more frequent in patients with other risk factors.

The incidence of major hemorrhagic complications during FRAXIPARINE treatment has been low and generally did not differ from that observed with unfractionated heparin. Patients taking FRAXIPARINE are at a risk for major bleeding complications when plasma anti-factor Xa levels approach 2.0 IU/mL. Other risk factors associated with bleeding on therapy with heparins include serious concurrent illness, chronic heavy consumption of alcohol, use of platelet inhibiting drugs, renal failure, age, and possibly, female gender. Petechiae or easy bruising may precede frank hemorrhage. Bleeding may range from minor local hematoma to major hemorrhage. The early signs of bleeding may include epistaxis, hematuria, or melena. Bleeding may occur at any site and be difficult to detect, for example, retroperitoneal bleeding. Bleeding may also occur at surgical sites. Major hemorrhage, including retroperitoneal or intracranial bleeding, has been reported in association with FRAXIPARINE use, in some cases leading to fatality.

Hepatic/Biliary: A significant but transient elevation of liver transaminases (AST and ALT) has been commonly observed with FRAXIPARINE. This is a consistent finding with all members of the LMWHs class, as well as with unfractionated heparin. The mechanism associated with the increased levels of liver transaminases has not been elucidated. No consistent irreversible liver damage has been observed. The time for the transaminase levels to return to normal following the last dose of FRAXIPARINE varies depending on the dose and the individual patient.

Clinical Trial Adverse Drug Reactions: Because clinical trials are conducted under very specific conditions the adverse reaction rates observed in the clinical trials may not reflect the rates observed in practice and should not be compared to the rates in the clinical trials of another drug. Adverse drug reaction information from clinical trials is useful for identifying drug-related adverse events and for approximating rates.

The following rates of major bleeding have been reported during clinical trials with FRAXIPARINE. Major bleeding is defined as any of the following: overt bleeding associated with a decrease in Hb of 2 g/dL or more; requiring transfusion of one or more units of packed red cells; retroperitoneal or intracranial hemorrhage; leading to permanent discontinuation; leading to hemorrhagic death. See Table 1, Table 2, Table 3 and Table 4.

Table 1: FRAXIPARINE

Prophylaxis of Thromboembolic Disorders in General Surgery

	No. of Patients Evaluated	No. (%) of Patients with Major Hemorrhage
FRAXIPARINE	1076	9 (0.84%)
Unfractionated heparin	1006	9 (0.89%)

Table 2: FRAXIPARINE

Prophylaxis of Thromboembolic Disorders in Orthopaedic Surgery

	No. of Patients Evaluated	No. (%) of Patients with Major Hemorrhage
FRAXIPARINE	205	2 (0.99%)
Unfractionated heparin	204	4 (1.96%)

Skeletal: Use of low molecular weight heparins over extended periods has been reported to be associated with development of osteopenia.

Immune System: Severe immunologically-mediated thrombocytopenia has been observed rarely with FRAXIPARINE use, resulting in arterial and/or venous thrombosis or thromboembolism (see Warnings and Precautions, Thrombocytopenia and Platelets).

Thrombocytopenia (sometimes thrombogenic), thrombocytosis, skin rash, allergic reactions, and skin necrosis are rare, and occur with all LMWHs. Hypersensitivity reactions, including angioedema and anaphylactoid reactions, have been observed very rarely with unfractionated heparin and LMWHs. FRAXIPARINE should be discontinued in patients showing local or systemic allergic responses.

Table 3: FRAXIPARINE

Treatment of Deep Vein Thrombosis

	No. of Patients Evaluated	No. (%) of Patients with Major Hemorrhage
FRAXIPARINE	312	13 (4.17%)
Unfractionated heparin	272	11 (4.04%)

Table 4: FRAXIPARINE

Treatment of Unstable Angina & Non-Q-Wave Myocardial Infarction

	No. of Patients Evaluated	No. (%) of Patients with Major Hemorrhage
FRAXIPARINE	1164	8 (0.7%)
Unfractionated heparin	1146	12 (1.0%)

Blood and Lymphatic: Very rare cases of eosinophilia have been observed, however have been reversible following treatment discontinuation.

Skin and Subcutaneous Tissue: Very commonly, a small hematoma may occur at the injection site. In some cases, the emergence of firm nodules, which do not indicate an encasement of the heparin, may be noted. These nodules usually disappear after a few days. Injection site reactions are common.

Calcinosis occurs rarely at the injection site and is more frequent in patients with abnormal calcium phosphate product, such as in some cases of chronic renal failure.

Other infrequent serious side effects include cutaneous necrosis, usually occurring at the injection site. This has been reported both with unfractionated heparin and with low molecular weight heparins. It is preceded by purpura or infiltrated or painful erythematous blotches, which may or may not be manifested by systemic upset. In such cases, treatment should be immediately discontinued.

Endocrine: Reversible heparin-induced hypoaldosteronism which may be associated with hyperkalemia and/or hyponatremia, particularly in patients at risk (see Warnings and Precautions, Hyperkalemia).

Reproductive System: Very rare cases of priapism have been observed.

DRUG INTERACTIONS: Drug-Drug Interactions: FRAXIPARINE (nadroparin calcium) and FRAXIPARINE FORTE should be used with caution in patients receiving oral anticoagulants, dextrans, platelet inhibitors and thrombolytic agents because of increased risk of bleeding. Aspirin, unless contraindicated, is recommended in patients treated for unstable angina and/or non-Q wave myocardial infarction as concomitant therapy (see Dosage and Administration).

Drug-Food Interactions: Interactions with food have not been established.

Drug-Herb Interactions: Interactions with herbal products have not been established.

Drug-Laboratory Test Interactions: See Warnings and Precautions, Monitoring and Laboratory Tests.

DOSAGE AND ADMINISTRATION: Recommended Dose and Dosage Adjustment: Thromboprophylaxis in General Surgery: (FRAXIPARINE (nadroparin calcium) 9500 anti-Xa IU/mL): Single daily s.c. injections of 2850 anti-Xa IU (0.3 mL): The first dose should be given 2 to 4 hours before surgery. Treatment should continue for at least 7 days. In all cases, prophylaxis should continue throughout the risk period and at least until the patient is actively ambulant or is no longer at risk of deep vein thrombosis.

Thromboprophylaxis in Hip Replacement Surgery: (FRAXIPARINE (nadroparin calcium) 9500 anti-Xa IU/mL): Single daily s.c. doses should be adjusted according to the patient's body weight, as follows:

- 38 anti-Xa IU/kg administered 12 hours before surgery (if in the opinion of the physician the potential benefits outweigh the potential risks),
- 38 anti-Xa IU/kg administered 12 hours after the end of surgery,
- 38 anti-Xa IU/kg re-administered on a daily basis, up to and including post-operative Day 3,
- 57 anti-Xa IU/kg administered as of post-operative Day 4.

Treatment should continue for at least 10 days and should continue in all cases throughout the risk period and at least until the patient is actively ambulant.

As an example, the following dosages as a function of patient body weight are recommended: See Table 5.

Table 5: FRAXIPARINE

Recommended Dosages—Prophylaxis in Hip Replacement Surgery

Body Weight (kg)	FRAXIPARINE (9500 anti-Xa IU/mL), Volume per Injection, and per Day when Post-operative: Preoperatively, if so Used, and Daily Post-operative Doses Until Day 3 (mL)	As of Day 4 (mL)
<50	0.2	0.3
50–69	0.3	0.4
≥70	0.4	0.6

Treatment of Deep Vein Thrombosis: The following dosage is recommended: 171 anti-Xa IU/kg s.c. once daily. The expected plasma anti-Xa levels during s.c. treatment would be <0.2 anti-Xa IU/mL before injection and 1.2 to 1.8 anti-Xa IU/mL 3-4 hours post-injection. Monitoring of the activity of nadroparin is performed by a functional assay for anti-Xa 3-4 hours post-injection. The maximum daily dose should not exceed 17 100 IU.

As an example, the following dosages as a function of patient body weight are recommended: See Table 6.

Table 6: FRAXIPARINE FORTE

Recommended Dosages—Treatment of Thromboembolic Disorders

Body Weight (kg)	FRAXIPARINE FORTE (19 000 anti-Xa IU/mL), Volume per Injection, Once Daily (mL)
40–49	0.4
50–59	0.5
60–69	0.6

(cont'd)

Table 6: FRAXIPARINE FORTE *(cont'd)*

Recommended Dosages—Treatment of Thromboembolic Disorders

Body Weight (kg)	FRAXIPARINE FORTE (19 000 anti-Xa IU/mL), Volume per Injection, Once Daily (mL)
70–79	0.7
80–89	0.8
≥90	0.9

For patients at increased risk of bleeding, a dose of 86 anti-Xa IU/kg s.c. twice daily is recommended. The expected plasma anti-Xa levels during s.c. treatment would be 0.2-0.4 anti-Xa IU/mL before injection and 0.5 to 1.1 anti-Xa IU/mL 3-4 hours post-injection. Monitoring of the activity of nadroparin is performed by a functional assay for anti-Xa 3-4 hours post-injection.

As an example, the following dosages as a function of patient body weight are recommended: See Table 7.

Table 7: FRAXIPARINE

Recommended Dosages—Treatment of Thromboembolic Disorders in Patients at Increased Risk of Bleeding

Body Weight (kg)	FRAXIPARINE (9500 anti-Xa IU/mL), Volume per Injection, Twice Daily (mL)
40–49	0.4
50–59	0.5
60–69	0.6
70–79	0.7
80–89	0.8
≥90 kg	0.9

Monitoring of the activity of nadroparin is performed by a functional assay for anti-Xa 3-4 hours post-injection.

Concomitant therapy with vitamin K antagonists is usually started immediately. FRAXIPARINE therapy should continue until the INR ratio is within the therapeutic range, usually at least 5 days.

Treatment of Unstable Angina and Non-Q Wave Myocardial Infarction: (FRAXIPARINE 9500 anti-Xa IU/mL): FRAXIPARINE should be given subcutaneously twice daily (every 12 hours) in combination with ASA up to 325 mg per day. The initial dose should be given as an IV bolus of 86 anti-Xa IU/kg followed by subcutaneous injections of 86 anti- Xa IU/kg. The expected plasma anti-Xa levels during subcutaneous treatment would be <0.4 anti-Xa IU/mL before injection and <1.2 anti-Xa IU/mL 3-4 hours after injection. The usual treatment duration is 6 days with a dose adjusted to body weight as shown in Table 8.

Table 8: FRAXIPARINE

Treatment of Unstable Angina and Non-Q-Wave Myocardial Infarction

Body Weight (kg)	FRAXIPARINE (9500 anti-Xa IU/mL) Initial IV Bolus (mL)	Volume of SC Injections (every 12 hours) (mL)
<50	0.4	0.4
50–59	0.5	0.5
60–69	0.6	0.6
70–79	0.7	0.7
80–89	0.8	0.8
90–99	0.9	0.9
≥100	1.0	1.0

Prevention of Clotting During Hemodialysis: (FRAXIPARINE 9500 anti-Xa/mL): Only patients with chronic renal failure, without other risk factors for hemorrhage participated in the clinical trial, and the following dosage recommendations are for that patient population:

- Optimisation of dosage is required for each individual patient (different clotting stimuli are produced by different dialysis circuits and membranes, and there is inter-patient variability).
- In patients with no risk of hemorrhage: single dose of approximately 65 anti-Xa IU/kg into the arterial line at the start of each session, for a session lasting 4 hours or less. This dose normally produces plasma anti-Xa levels in the range 0.5-1.0 anti-Xa IU /mL.
- An additional dose may be given during sessions lasting longer than 4 hours.
- Doses in subsequent dialysis sessions should be adjusted as required.

As an example, the following dosages as a function of patient body weight are recommended: See Table 9.

Table 9: FRAXIPARINE

Recommended Dosages—Prevention of Clotting During Hemodialysis

Body Weight (kg)	FRAXIPARINE (9500 anti-Xa IU/mL), Volume of (mL)
<50	0.3
50–69	0.4
≥70	0.6

In patients at higher risk of hemorrhage: dialysis sessions may be carried out using halved doses. An additional smaller dose may be given during dialysis for sessions lasting longer than 4 hours. The dose in subsequent dialysis sessions should be adjusted as necessary to achieve plasma levels within the range of 0.2-0.4 anti-Xa IU/mL.

Dosing Considerations: Use in Renal Insufficiency: The risk of hemorrhage increases with renal failure. The benefit and risk should be carefully assessed before the administration of FRAXIPARINE to patients with renal insufficiency.

The administration of LMWHs to patients with renal insufficiency has been shown to result in prolongation of anti-Xa activity, especially in those with severe renal insufficiency (creatinine clearance <30 mL/min), leading to increased risk of bleeding (see Action and Clinical Pharmacology, Renal Insufficiency). All patients with renal insufficiency treated with LMWHs must be continuously monitored. The dose must be individualized and adjusted (see Table 5, Table 6, Table 7 and Table 8 for recommended doses as a function of body weight). Circulating anti-factor Xa activity must be closely monitored to adjust the dose administered.

Prophylaxis of Thromboembolic Disorders: Dose reduction is not required in patients with mild renal insufficiency (creatinine clearance greater than or equal to 50 mL/min).

Moderate and severe renal impairment is associated with increased exposure to nadroparin. These patients are at increased risk of thromboembolism and hemorrhage.

If a dose reduction is considered appropriate by the prescribing physician, taking into account the individual risk factors for hemorrhage and thromboembolism in patients with moderate renal impairment (creatinine clearance greater than or equal to 30 mL/min and less than 50 mL/min) the dose should be reduced by 25 to 33% (see Warnings and Precautions and Action and Clinical Pharmacology, Pharmacokinetics).

The dose should be reduced by 25 to 33% in patients with severe renal impairment (creatinine clearance less than 30 mL/min) (see Warnings and Precautions and Action and Clinical Pharmacology, Pharmacokinetics).

Treatment of Thromboembolic Disorders, Unstable Angina and Non-Q Wave Myocardial Infarction: Dose reduction is not required in patients with mild renal impairment (creatinine clearance greater than or equal to 50 mL/min).

Moderate and severe renal impairment is associated with increased exposure to nadroparin. These patients are at increased risk of thromboembolism and hemorrhage.

If a dose reduction is considered appropriate by the prescribing physician, taking into account the individual risk factors for hemorrhage and thromboembolism in patients with moderate renal impairment (creatinine clearance greater than or equal to 30 mL/min and less than 50 mL/min) the dose should be reduced by 25 to 33% (see Warnings and Precautions and Actions and Clinical Pharmacology, Pharmacokinetics).

FRAXIPARINE is contraindicated in patients with severe renal insufficiency (see Warnings and Precautions, and Actions and Clinical Pharmacology, Pharmacokinetics).

Hepatic Insufficiency: There have been no studies conducted in patients with hepatic insufficiency.

Administration: FRAXIPARINE (nadroparin calcium) and FRAXIPARINE FORTE are sterile solutions for subcutaneous injection into the anterolateral abdominal wall, with subsequent doses to be administered alternately, on the right and left sides of the abdominal wall. The thigh may be used as an alternative site. The needle should be fully inserted; perpendicularly into a pinched-up fold of skin.

FRAXIPARINE and FRAXIPARINE FORTE injection should be visually inspected for any particulate matter and discoloration before use. If any visual change is noted, the solution must be discarded.

Care should be taken to ensure use of the correct formulation, either FRAXIPARINE (9500 anti-Xa IU/mL) or FRAXIPARINE FORTE (19 000 anti-Xa IU/mL), when using these products.

Given the high degree of bioavailability of nadroparin calcium by the subcutaneous route (approximately 98%), the use of the intravascular route is not necessary except for hemodialysis. **FRAXIPARINE and FRAXIPARINE FORTE must not be administered intramuscularly (see Warnings and Precautions).**

OVERDOSAGE:

Accidental overdosage following administration of FRAXIPARINE (nadroparin calcium) may lead to hemorrhagic complications. FRAXIPARINE should be immediately discontinued, at least temporarily, in cases of significant excess dosage. In more serious cases, protamine should be administered.

The anticoagulant effect of FRAXIPARINE is inhibited by protamine. This effect may be largely neutralised by slow intravenous injection of protamine sulfate. The dose of protamine should be equal to the dose of FRAXIPARINE used, on a mg to mg basis. A second infusion of 0.5 mg protamine per 1 mg FRAXIPARINE may be administered if the APTT measured 2 to 4 hours after the first infusion remains prolonged. However, even with higher doses of protamine, the APTT may remain prolonged to a greater extent than usually seen with unfractionated heparin. Anti-factor Xa activity is never completely neutralized (maximum about 60%).

Particular care should be taken to avoid overdosage with protamine sulfate. Administration of protamine sulfate can cause severe hypotensive and anaphylactoid reactions. Because fatal reactions, often resembling anaphylaxis, have been reported with protamine sulfate, it should be given only when resuscitation equipment and treatment of anaphylactic shock are readily available.

For management of a suspected drug overdose, CPhA recommends that you contact your **regional Poison Control Centre**. See the *CPS* Directory section for a list of Poison Control Centres.

ACTION AND CLINICAL PHARMACOLOGY: Mechanism of Action: FRAXIPARINE (nadroparin calcium) is a low molecular weight heparin (LMWH). It is a heterogeneous mixture of sulphated polysaccharide glycosaminoglycan chains. Nadroparin calcium is obtained by the depolymerisation of porcine mucosal sodium heparin, followed by extraction/purification and conversion to the calcium salt. The mean molecular weight of nadroparin is approximately 4300 daltons; 75-95% of the glycosaminoglycan chains have molecular weights in the 2000 to 8000 dalton range. Nadroparin is composed of molecules with and without a specifically characterized pentasaccharide, which is the specific site for high affinity binding to the plasma protein antithrombin III (ATIII). This binding leads to an accelerated inhibition of factor Xa, which accounts for the majority of the antithrombotic effect of nadroparin. Other properties that are not dependent upon ATIII may contribute to the antithrombotic activity as well, but the relative contribution of these actions has not been determined. These include stimulation of tissue factor pathway inhibitor TFPI, activation of fibrinolysis via direct release of tissue plasminogen activator from endothelial cells, and modification of hemorreological parameters (decreased blood viscosity and increased platelet and granulocyte membrane fluidity).

Pharmacodynamics: The pharmacodynamic effect of nadroparin appears thus to be primarily related to its anti-Xa activity at approximately 90 IU/mg (range 85 to 110 IU/mg), with anti-IIa activity at approximately 27 IU/mg. The ratio of anti-Xa to anti-IIa activity for nadroparin is about 3.5:1, whereas it is 1:1 for heparin. The presence of nadroparin is not measured directly in the blood stream, but rather its effect on clotting mechanisms, e.g. level of anti-Xa activity.

Pharmacokinetics: The pharmacokinetics of nadroparin have been assessed by measuring anti-Xa activity. See Table 10.

Table 10: FRAXIPARINE

Summary of Mean (SD) Pharmacokinetics in Healthy Volunteers

Dose	AUC (anti-Xa IU·h/mL)	C_{max} (anti-Xa IU/mL)	T_{max} (h)	$T_{½}$ (h)
41 anti-Xa U/kg s.c.	5.08±1.22	0.61±0.15	3.42±1.17	3.79±1.49
166 anti-Xa U/kg once daily×10 days	15.1±2.3	1.34±0.15	4.67±1.1	11.2±8.0

Absorption: A linear relationship between nadroparin dose and plasma anti-Xa activity was observed in the pharmacokinetic studies. Peak concentrations of nadroparin are reached 3-6 hours after subcutaneous injection. Steady state is attained by Day 6. Following subcutaneous injection, the bioavailability of nadroparin is about 89%.

Maximal prolongation of APTT and thrombin time occurs at approximately 4 hours. After subcutaneous administration of prophylactic doses (2850 IU) of nadroparin in healthy volunteers, maximum APTT and thrombin time were increased by a negligible 2 seconds at 4 hours, and APTT returned to baseline by 8 hours. After administration of treatment doses, APTT was only slightly prolonged (1.2 times the control value; with unfractionated heparin, APTT values at curative dosage are aimed at obtaining 1.5-2.5 times the control value).

Distribution: The mean volume of distribution in humans is estimated to be 3.59 L.

Metabolism: The pharmacokinetics of nadroparin are linear over a wide range of doses. The mean half-life in healthy volunteers ranges between approximately 3.5 hours and 11.2 hours after subcutaneous administration.

Excretion: Although anti-Xa activity persists for at least 18 hours after injection, the elimination half-life is approximately 3.5 hours. Elimination of nadroparin is primarily by nonsaturable renal mechanisms, although recent data suggest that hepatic metabolism may occur prior to renal elimination.

Special Populations and Conditions: Pediatrics: The safety and effectiveness of FRAXIPARINE in children has not been established.

Geriatrics: In a small study in geriatric male and female subjects with normal renal function (n=6 per sex, age range 59-69), the mean anti-Xa peak and total exposure was 22 and 45% higher, respectively, than that observed in a similar study in healthy volunteers. The mean half-life values for anti-Xa activity were similar between the two studies. Renal function generally decreases with age so elimination of nadroparin anti-Xa activity may be slower in geriatric subjects (see Pharmacokinetics, Renal Insufficiency). The possibility of renal insufficiency in this age group must be considered and the dosage adjusted accordingly (see Warnings and Precautions).

Geriatric patients receiving low molecular weight heparins are at increased risk of bleeding. Careful attention to dosing and concomitant medications, especially anti-platelet preparations, is advised. Close monitoring of elderly patients with low body weight (e.g. <45 kg) and those predisposed to decreased renal function is recommended (see Dosage and Administration).

Renal Insufficiency: In a clinical study investigating the pharmacokinetics of nadroparin administered intravenously in patients with varying degrees of renal insufficiency (creatinine clearance values <10 mL/min, 10-20 mL/min, 30-50 mL/min and 75-200 mL/min), a correlation was found between nadroparin clearance and the creatinine clearance. In patients with moderate renal impairment (creatinine clearance 36-43 mL/min) both mean AUC and half-life were increased by 52 and 39% respectively compared with healthy volunteers. In these patients, mean plasma clearance of nadroparin was decreased to 63% of normal. Wide inter-individual variability was observed in the study. In subjects with severe renal insufficiency (creatinine clearance 10-20 mL/min) both mean AUC and half-life were increased by 95 and 112% respectively compared with healthy volunteers. Plasma clearance in patients with severe renal impairment was decreased to 50% of that observed in patients with normal renal function. In subjects with severe renal impairment (creatinine clearance 3-6 mL/min) on hemodialysis, both mean AUC and half-life were increased by 62 and 65% respectively compared with healthy volunteers. Plasma clearance in hemodialysis patients with severe renal impairment was decreased to 67% of that observed in patients with normal renal function (see Dosage and Administration and Warnings and Precautions).

Hepatic Insufficiency: The effects of hepatic insufficiency on the pharmacokinetics of nadroparin have not been studied. Because hepatic insufficiency is associated with an increased risk of bleeding, caution should be observed when administering nadroparin to such patients (see Warnings and Precautions).

Gender: In two studies of 12 healthy young or geriatric male and female volunteers, there was no clinically significant sex difference in the pharmacokinetics of nadroparin.

Race: The effect of race on the pharmacokinetics of nadroparin has not been studied.

Genetic Polymorphism: The effect of genetic polymorphisms on the pharmacokinetics of nadroparin has not been studied.

STORAGE AND STABILITY: Store between 15 to 30°C; do not freeze. Do not refrigerate, as cold injections may be painful. Syringes are intended for single use only—discard unused portion of each syringe. Do not mix with other preparations or re-dispense.

SPECIAL HANDLING INSTRUCTIONS: Keep out of reach of children.

INFORMATION FOR THE PATIENT: Published in e-CPS, available by subscription at www.e-cps.ca.

DOSAGE FORMS, COMPOSITION AND PACKAGING: FRAXIPARINE: Each mL of aqueous solution contains: nadroparin calcium 9500 anti-Xa IU. Single dose, disposable prefilled glass syringes of 0.3 mL (ungraduated green syringes) 2850 anti-Xa IU; 0.4 mL (ungraduated orange syringes) 3800 anti-Xa IU; 0.6 mL (graduated brown syringes) 5700 anti-Xa IU; 0.8 mL (graduated green [teal] syringes) 7600 anti-Xa IU; and 1 mL (graduated violet syringes) 9500 anti-Xa IU. Ungraduated 0.3 mL and 0.4 mL syringes are intended for administration of fixed dosages; 0.6 mL, 0.8 mL and 1 mL syringes are graduated so that adjusted dosages can be given. Cartons of 10.

FRAXIPARINE FORTE: Each mL of aqueous solution contains: nadroparin calcium 19 000 anti-Xa IU. Single dose, disposable prefilled glass syringes of 0.6 mL (graduated process blue syringes) 11 400 anti-Xa IU; 0.8 mL (graduated magenta syringes) 15 200 anti-Xa IU; and 1 mL (graduated reflex blue syringes) 19 000 anti-Xa IU. The 0.6 mL, 0.8 mL and 1 mL syringes are graduated so that adjusted dosages can be given. Cartons of 10.

Frova® Ⓟ

frovatriptan succinate

5-HT1 Receptor Subtype Agonist—Migraine Therapy

Teva Canada Innovation

Date of Preparation: May 11, 2007
Date of Revision: February 24, 2009

PHARMACOLOGY: Mechanism of Action: FROVA (frovatriptan succinate) is a 5-HT receptor agonist that binds with high affinity for 5-HT_{1B} and 5-HT_{1D} receptors. Frovatriptan has no significant effects on $GABA_A$ mediated channel activity and has no significant affinity for benzodiazepine binding sites.

Frovatriptan is believed to act on extracerebral, intracranial arteries and to inhibit excessive dilation of these vessels in migraine.

Pharmacokinetics: Mean maximum blood concentrations (C_{max}) in patients are achieved approximately 2-4 hours after administration of a single oral dose of frovatriptan 2.5 mg. The absolute bioavailability of an oral dose of frovatriptan 2.5 mg in healthy subjects is about 20% in males and 30% in females. Food has no significant effect on the bioavailability of frovatriptan, but delays t_{max} by one hour.

Binding of frovatriptan to serum proteins is low (approximately 15%). Reversible binding to blood cells at equilibrium is approximately 60%, resulting in a blood:plasma ratio of about 2:1 in both males and females. The mean steady state volume of distribution of frovatriptan following intravenous administration of 0.8 mg is 4.2 L/kg in males and 3.0 L/kg in females.

In vitro, cytochrome P450 1A2 appears to be the principal enzyme involved in the metabolism of frovatriptan. Following administration of a single dose of radiolabeled frovatriptan 2.5 mg to healthy male and female subjects, 32% of the dose was recovered in urine and 62% in feces. Radiolabeled compounds excreted in the urine were unchanged frovatriptan, hydroxylated frovatriptan, N-acetyl desmethyl frovatriptan, hydroxylated N-acetyl desmethyl frovatriptan and desmethyl frovatriptan, together with several other minor metabolites. Desmethyl frovatriptan has lower affinity for $5\text{-HT}1_{B/1D}$ receptors compared to the parent compound. The N-acetyl desmethyl metabolite has no significant affinity for 5-HT receptors. The activity of the other metabolites is unknown.

After an intravenous dose, mean clearance of frovatriptan was 220 and 130 mL/min in males and females, respectively. Renal clearance accounted for about 40% (82 mL/min) and 45% (60 mL/min) of total clearance in males and females, respectively. The mean terminal elimination half-life of frovatriptan in both males and females is approximately 26 hours.

The pharmacokinetics of frovatriptan are similar in migraine patients and healthy subjects.

Special Populations: Age: Mean AUC of frovatriptan was 1.5 to 2-fold higher in healthy elderly subjects (age 65-77 years) compared to those in healthy younger subjects (age 21-37 years). There was no difference in t_{max} or $t_{½}$ between the two populations.

Gender: There was no difference in the mean terminal elimination half-life of frovatriptan in males and females. Bioavailability was higher, and systemic exposure to frovatriptan was approximately 2-fold greater, in females than males, irrespective of age.

Renal Impairment: Since less than 10% of FROVA is excreted in urine after an oral dose, it is unlikely that the exposure to frovatriptan will be affected by renal impairment. The pharmacokinetics of frovatriptan following a single oral dose of 2.5 mg was not different in patients with renal impairment (5 males and 6 females, creatinine clearance 16-73 mL/min) and in subjects with normal renal function.

Hepatic Impairment: There is no clinical or pharmacokinetic experience with FROVA in patients with severe hepatic impairment. The AUC in subjects with mild (Child-Pugh 5-6) to moderate (Child-Pugh 7-9) hepatic impairment is about twice as high as the AUC in young, healthy subjects, but within the range found among normal elderly subjects.

Race: The effect of race on the pharmacokinetics of frovatriptan has not been examined.

Clinical Studies: The efficacy of FROVA (frovatriptan succinate) in the acute treatment of migraine headaches was demonstrated in five randomized, double-blind, placebo-controlled, outpatient trials. Two of these were dose-finding studies in which patients were randomized to receive doses of frovatriptan ranging from 0.5-40 mg. The three studies evaluating only one dose studied 2.5 mg. In these controlled short-term studies combined, patients were predominately female (88%) and Caucasian (94%) with a mean age of 42 years (range 18-69). Patients were instructed to treat a moderate or severe headache. Headache response, defined as a reduction in headache severity from moderate or severe pain to mild or no pain, was assessed for 24 hours after dosing. The associated symptoms nausea, vomiting, photophobia and phonophobia were also assessed. Maintenance of response was assessed for up to 24 hours post-dose. In two of the trials a second dose of FROVA was provided after the initial treatment, to treat recurrence of headache within 24 hours. Other medication, excluding other 5-HT_1 agonists and ergotamine-containing compounds was permitted from 2 hours after the first dose of FROVA. The frequency and time to use of additional medications were also recorded.

In all five placebo-controlled trials, the percentage of patients achieving a headache response 2 and 4 hours after treatment was significantly greater for those taking FROVA compared with those taking placebo (see Table 1).

Lower doses of frovatriptan (1 mg or 0.5 mg) were not effective at 2 hours. Higher doses (5 mg to 40 mg) of frovatriptan showed no added benefit over 2.5 mg but did cause a greater incidence of adverse events.

Table 1: FROVA

Percentage of Patients with Headache Response (Mild or No Headache) 2 and 4 Hours Following Treatment[a]

Trial	FROVA (frovatriptan 2.5 mg)		Placebo	
	2 hours	4 hours	2 hours	4 hours
1	42%[b] (n=90)	64%[c] (n=85)	22% (n=91)	38% (n=81)
2	38%[b] (n=121)	68%[c] (n=117)	25% (n=115)	33% (n=106)
3	39%[b] (n=187)	56%[c] (n=156)	21% (n=99)	31% (n=81)
4	46%[c] (n=672)	65%[c] (n=586)	27% (n=347)	38% (n=305)
5	37%[c] (n=438)	62%[c] (n=388)	23% (n=225)	32% (n=202)

[a] ITT observed data, excludes patients who had missing data or were asleep.
[b] $0.001 \leq p \leq 0.050$.
[c] $p < 0.001$ in comparison with placebo.

Comparisons of drug performance based upon results obtained in different clinical trials are never reliable. Because trials are conducted at different times, with different samples of patients, by different investigators, employing different criteria and/or different interpretations of the same criteria, under different conditions (dose, dosing regimen, etc.), quantitative estimates of treatment response and the timing of the response may be expected to vary considerably from study to study.

In patients with migraine-associated nausea, photophobia and phonophobia at baseline there was a decreased incidence of these symptoms in FROVA treated patients compared to placebo.

Following the treatment of migraine with FROVA tablets in controlled clinical trials, there was low recurrence of migraine headaches (7%-25%). This is postulated to be due to the long half-life of frovatriptan.

Efficacy was unaffected by a history of aura; gender; age; or concomitant medications commonly used by migraine patients.

INDICATIONS: FROVA (frovatriptan succinate) is indicated for the acute treatment of migraine attacks with or without aura in adults.

FROVA is not intended for the prophylactic therapy of migraine or for the use in the management of hemiplegic, ophthalmoplegic or basilar migraine (see Contraindications). The safety and effectiveness of FROVA have not been established for cluster headache, which is present in an older, predominantly male, population.

CONTRAINDICATIONS: FROVA (frovatriptan succinate) is contraindicated in patients with history, symptoms, or signs of ischemic cardiac, cerebrovascular or peripheral vascular syndromes, valvular heart disease or cardiac arrhythmias (especially tachycardia). In addition, patients with other significant underlying cardiovascular diseases (e.g., atherosclerotic disease, congenital heart disease) should not receive FROVA. Ischemic cardiac syndromes include, but are not limited to, angina pectoris of any type (e.g., stable angina of effort and vasospasm forms of angina such as the Prinzmetal's variant, all forms of myocardial infarction, and silent myocardial ischemia). Cerebrovascular syndromes include, but are not limited to, strokes of any type as well as transient ischemic attacks (TIAs). Peripheral vascular disease includes, but is not limited to, ischemic bowel disease, or Raynaud's syndrome (see Warnings).

Because FROVA may increase blood pressure, it is contraindicated in patients with severe or uncontrolled hypertension (see Warnings).

FROVA is contraindicated within 24 hours of treatment with another 5-HT_1 agonist, or an ergotamine-containing or ergot-type medication like dihydroergotamine or methysergide.

FROVA is contraindicated in patients with hemiplegic, ophthalmoplegic or basilar migraine.

Because there are no data available, FROVA is contraindicated in patients with severe hepatic impairment.

FROVA is contraindicated in patients who are hypersensitive to frovatriptan or any of the inactive ingredients in the tablets.

WARNINGS: FROVA (frovatriptan succinate) should only be used where a clear diagnosis of migraine has been established.

Risk of Myocardial Ischemia and/or Infarction and other Adverse Cardiac Events: FROVA has been associated with transient chest and/or neck pain and tightness which may resemble angina pectoris. Following the use of other 5-HT_1 agonists, in rare cases these symptoms have been identified as being the likely result of coronary vasospasm or myocardial ischemia. Rare cases of serious coronary events or arrhythmia have occurred following use of other 5-HT_1 agonists, and may therefore also occur with FROVA. Because of the potential of this class of compounds ($5\text{-HT}_{1B/1D}$ agonists) to cause coronary vasospasm, FROVA should not be given to patients with documented ischemic or vasospastic coronary artery disease (see Contraindications). It is strongly recommended that 5-HT_1 agonists (including FROVA) not be given to patients in whom unrecognized coronary artery disease (CAD) is predicted by the presence of risk factors such as: hypertension, hypercholesterolemia, smoker, obesity, diabetes, strong family history of CAD, female with surgical or physiological menopause, or male over 40 years of age, unless a cardiovascular examination provides satisfactory clinical evidence that the patient is reasonably free of coronary artery and ischemic myocardial disease or other significant underlying cardiovascular disease. The sensitivity of cardiac diagnostic procedures to detect cardiovascular diseases or predisposition to coronary artery vasospasm is modest at best. If, during the cardiovascular evaluation, the patient's medical history, electrocardiogram (ECG) or other evaluations reveal findings indicative of, or consistent with, coronary artery vasospasm, or myocardial ischemia, FROVA should not be administered (see Contraindications).

These evaluations, however, may not identify every patient who has cardiac disease, and in very rare cases, serious cardiac events, such as myocardial infarction or coronary ischemia have occurred in patients without evidence of underlying cardiovascular disease.

For patients with risk factors predictive of CAD, who are determined to have a satisfactory cardiovascular evaluation, it is strongly recommended that administration of the first dose of FROVA take place in a clinical setting, such as the physician's office or a similarly staffed medical facility, unless the patient has previously received frovatriptan. Because cardiac ischemia can occur in the absence of clinical symptoms, consideration should be given to obtaining an ECG during the interval immediately following the first use of FROVA in a patient with risk factors. However, an absence of drug-induced cardiovascular effects on the occasion of the initial dose does not preclude the possibility of such effects occurring with subsequent administrations.

If symptoms consistent with angina occur after the use of FROVA, ECG evaluation should be carried out to look for ischemic changes.

It is recommended that patients who are intermittent long-term users of FROVA and who have or acquire risk factors predictive of CAD as described above undergo periodic interval cardiovascular evaluation as they continue to use FROVA.

The systematic approach described above is intended to reduce the likelihood that patients with unrecognized cardiovascular disease are inadvertently exposed to FROVA.

Cardiac Events and Fatalities with 5-HT_1 Agonists: Serious adverse cardiac events including acute myocardial infarction, life-threatening disturbances of cardiac rhythm and death have been reported within a few hours following the administration of 5-HT_1 agonists. Considering the extent of use of 5-HT_1 agonists in patients with migraine, the incidence of these events is extremely low.

Premarketing Experience with Frovatriptan: Among more than 3000 patients with migraine who participated in premarketing clinical trials of FROVA, no deaths or serious cardiac events were reported which were related to the use of FROVA.

Post-marketing Experience with Frovatriptan: Rare reports of serious cardiovascular events have been reported in association with the use of FROVA, this includes chest tightness and tachycardia. There have been rare reports of serious allergic type reactions, including anaphylactic reactions. The uncontrolled nature of post-marketing surveillance, however, makes it impossible to definitely determine the proportion of the reported cases that were actually caused by frovatriptan or to reliably assess causation in individual cases.

Cerebrovascular Events and Fatalities with 5-HT_1 Agonists: Cerebral hemorrhage, subarachnoid hemorrhage, stroke and other cerebrovascular events have been reported in patients treated with other 5-HT_1 agonists, and some have resulted in fatalities. In a number of cases, it appears possible that the cerebrovascular events were primary, the agonist having been administered in the belief that the symptoms experienced were a consequence of migraine, when they were not. Before treating migraine headaches with FROVA in patients not previously diagnosed as migraineurs, and in migraineurs who present with atypical symptoms, care should be taken to exclude other potentially serious neurological conditions. If a patient does not respond to the first dose, the opportunity should be taken to review the diagnosis before a second dose is given. It should be noted, however, that patients who suffer from migraine may have an increased risk of certain cerebrovascular events such as stroke, hemorrhage or transient ischemic attack.

Special Cardiovascular Pharmacology Studies with Another 5-HT_1 Agonist: In subjects (n=10) with suspected coronary artery disease undergoing angiography, a 5-HT_1 agonist at a subcutaneous dose of 1.5 mg produced an 8% increase in aortic blood pressure, an 18% increase in pulmonary artery blood pressure, and an 8% increase in systemic vascular resistance. In addition, mild chest pain or tightness was reported by four subjects. Clinically significant increases in blood pressure were experienced by three of the subjects (two of whom also had chest pain/discomfort). Diagnostic angiogram results revealed that 9 subjects had normal coronary arteries and 1 had insignificant coronary artery disease.

In an additional study with this same drug, migraine patients (n=35) free of cardiovascular disease were subjected to assessments of myocardial perfusion by positron emission tomography while receiving a subcutaneous 1.5 mg dose in the absence of a migraine attack. Reduced coronary vasodilatory reserve (~10%), increased coronary resistance (~20%), and decreased hyperaemic myocardial blood flow (~10%) were noted. The relevance of these findings to the use of the recommended oral dose of this 5-HT_1 agonist is not known.

Similar studies have not been done with FROVA. However, owing to the common pharmacodynamic actions of 5-HT_1 agonists, the possibility of cardiovascular effects of the nature described above should be considered for any agent of this pharmacological class.

Hypersensitivity: Rare hypersensitivity (anaphylaxis/anaphylactoid) reactions have occurred in patients receiving other 5-HT_1 agonists. Such reactions can be life threatening or fatal. In general, hypersensitivity reactions to drugs are more likely to occur in individuals with a history of sensitivity to multiple allergens. Owing to the possibility of cross-reactive hypersensitivity reactions, FROVA should not be used in patients having a history of hypersensitivity to chemically-related 5-HT_1 receptor agonists (see Adverse Effects and Precautions).

Selective Serotonin Reuptake Inhibitors/Serotonin Norepinephrine Reuptake Inhibitors and Serotonin Syndrome: Cases of life-threatening serotonin syndrome have been reported during combined use of selective serotonin reuptake inhibitors (SSRIs)/serotonin norepinephrine reuptake inhibitors (SNRIs) and triptans. If concomitant treatment with FROVA and SSRIs (e.g., fluoxetine, fluvoxamine, paroxetine, sertraline) or SNRIs (e.g., venlafaxine) is clinically warranted, careful observation of the patient is advised, particularly during treatment initiation and dose increases. Serotonin syndrome symptoms may include mental status changes (e.g., agitation, hallucinations, coma), autonomic instability (e.g., tachycardia, labile blood pressure, hyperthermia), neuromuscular aberrations (e.g., hyperreflexia, incoordination) and/or gastrointestinal symptoms (e.g., nausea, vomiting, diarrhea) (see Precautions, Drug Interactions).

Other Vasospasm-Related Events: 5-HT_1 agonists may cause vasospastic reactions other than coronary artery vasospasm. Extensive post-market experience has shown the use of another 5-HT_1 agonist to be associated with rare occurrences of peripheral vascular ischemia and colonic ischemia with abdominal pain and bloody diarrhea.

Effects on Blood Pressure: Significant elevations in systemic blood pressure, including hypertensive crisis, have been reported on rare occasions in patients with and without a history of hypertension treated with other 5-HT_1 agonists. In young healthy subjects, there were statistically significant increases in systolic and diastolic blood pressure only at single doses of 80 mg frovatriptan (32 times the clinical dose) and above. These increases were transient, resolved spontaneously and were not clinically significant. FROVA is contraindicated in patients with severe or uncontrolled hypertension (see Contraindications). In patients with controlled hypertension, FROVA should be administered with caution, as transient increases in blood pressure and peripheral vascular resistance have been observed in a small portion of patients.

An 18% increase in mean pulmonary artery pressure was seen following dosing with another 5-HT_1 agonist in a study evaluating subjects undergoing cardiac catheterization.

PRECAUTIONS: General: FROVA (frovatriptan succinate) should be administered with caution to patients with diseases that may alter the absorption, metabolism, or excretion of drugs (see Pharmacology, Special Populations).

For a given attack, if a patient has no response to the first dose of FROVA, the diagnosis of migraine should be reconsidered before administration of a second dose.

Cardiovascular: Discomfort in the chest, neck, throat and jaw (including pain, tightness, pressure and heaviness) have been reported after treatment with FROVA. Because 5-HT_1 agonists may cause coronary vasospasm, patients who experience signs or symptoms suggestive of angina following dosing should be evaluated for the presence of CAD or a predisposition to variant angina before receiving additional doses, and should be monitored electrocardiographically if dosing is resumed and similar symptoms recur. Similarly, patients who experience other symptoms or signs suggestive of decreased arterial flow, such as ischemic bowel syndrome or Raynaud's syndrome following FROVA administration should be evaluated for atherosclerosis or predisposition to vasospasm (see Contraindications and Warnings).

Neurologic Conditions: Care should be taken to exclude other potentially serious neurologic conditions before treating headache in patients not previously diagnosed with migraine or who experience a headache that is atypical for them. There have been rare reports where patients received 5-HT_1 agonists for severe headache that were subsequently shown to have been secondary to an evolving neurological lesion. For newly diagnosed patients or patients presenting with atypical symptoms, the diagnosis of migraine should be reconsidered if no response is seen after the first dose of FROVA.

Seizures: Caution should be observed if FROVA is to be used in patients with a history of epilepsy or structural brain lesions which lower the convulsion threshold.

Hepatically Impaired Patients: Since there is no clinical or pharmacokinetic experience with FROVA in patients with severe hepatic impairment it is contraindicated in this population (see Contraindications and Dosage). FROVA can be used in patients with mild to moderate hepatic impairment (see Pharmacology, Pharmacokinetics, Special Populations).

Binding to Melanin-Containing Tissues: When pigmented rats were given a single oral dose of 5 mg/kg of radiolabelled frovatriptan, the radioactivity in the eye after 28 days was 87% of the value measured after 8 hours. This suggests that frovatriptan and/or its metabolites may bind to the melanin of the eye. Because there could be accumulation in melanin rich tissues over time, this raise the possibility that frovatriptan could cause toxicity in these tissues after extended use. However, no effects on the retina related to treatment with frovatriptan were noted in toxicity studies. Although no systemic monitoring of ophthalmologic function was undertaken in clinical trials, and no specific recommendations for ophthalmological monitoring are made, prescribers should be aware of the possibility of long-term ophthalmologic effects.

Carcinogenicity: The carcinogenic potential of frovatriptan was evaluated in an 84-week study in mice (4, 13 and 40 mg/kg/day), a 104-week study in rats (8.5, 27 and 85 mg/kg/day), and a 26-week study in p53(+/-) transgenic mice (20, 62.5, 200, and 400 mg/kg/day). Although the maximum tolerated dose (MTD) was not achieved in the 84-week mouse study and in female rats, exposures at the highest doses studied were many fold greater than those achieved at the maximum recommended daily human dose (MRHD) of 7.5 mg. There were no increases in tumor incidence in the 84-week mouse study at doses producing 140 times the exposure achieved at the MRHD based on blood AUC comparisons. In the rat study, there was a statistically significant increase in the incidence of pituitary adenomas in males only at 85 mg/kg/day, a dose that produced 250 times the exposure achieved at the MRHD based on AUC comparisons. In the 26-week p53 (+/-) transgenic mouse study, there was an increased incidence of subcutaneous sarcomas in females dosed at 200 and 400 mg/kg/day, or 390 and 630 times the human exposure based on AUC comparisons. The incidence of sarcomas was not increased at lower doses that achieved exposure 180 and 60 times the human exposure. These sarcomas were physically associated with subcutaneously implanted animal identification transponders. There were no other increases in tumor incidence of any type in any dose group. The relevance of these sarcomas to humans is unknown.

Mutagenicity: Frovatriptan was clastogenic in human lymphocyte cultures, in the absence of metabolic activation. In the bacterial reverse mutation assay (Ames test), frovatriptan produced an equivocal response in the absence of metabolic activation. No mutagenic or clastogenic activity were seen in an in vitro mouse lymphoma assay, an in vivo mouse bone marrow micronucleus test, or an ex vivo assay for unscheduled DNA synthesis in rat liver.

Impairment of Fertility: Male and female rats were dosed prior to and during mating, and up to implantation, at doses of 100, 500, and 1000 mg/kg/day (equivalent to approximately 130, 650 and 1300 times the MRHD on a mg/m^2 basis). At all dose levels, there was an increase in the number of females that mated on the first day of pairing compared to control animals. This occurred in conjunction with a prolongation of the estrous cycle. In addition females had a decreased mean number of corpora lutea, and consequently a lower number of live fetuses per litter, which suggested a partial impairment of ovulation. There were no other fertility-related effects.

When pregnant rats were administered frovatriptan during the period of organogenesis at oral doses of 100, 500 and 1000 mg/kg/day (equivalent to 130, 650 and 1300 times the MRHD) on a mg/m^2 basis) there were dose related increases in incidences of both litters and total numbers of fetuses with dilated ureters, unilateral and bilateral pelvic cavitation, hydronephrosis, and hydroureters. A no-effect dose for renal effects was not established. This signifies a syndrome of related effects on a specific organ in the developing embryo in all treated groups, which is consistent with a slight delay in fetal maturation. This delay was also indicated by a treatment related increased incidence of incomplete ossification of the sternebrae, skull and nasal bones in all treated groups. Slightly lower fetal weights and an increased incidence of early embryonic deaths in treated rats were observed; although not statistically significant compared to control, the latter effect occurred in both the embryo-fetal developmental study and in the prenatal-postnatal developmental study. There was no evidence of this latter effect at the lowest dose level studied, 100 mg/kg/day (equivalent to 130 times the MRHD on a mg/m^2 basis). When pregnant rabbits were dosed throughout organogenesis at doses up to 80 mg/kg/day (equivalent to 210 times the MRHD on a mg/m^2 basis) no effects on fetal development were observed.

Geriatrics: Mean blood concentrations of frovatriptan in elderly subjects were 1.5- to 2-times higher than those seen in younger adults (see Pharmacology, Special Populations). Because migraine occurs infrequently in the elderly, clinical experience with FROVA is limited in such patients.

Children: Safety and effectiveness of FROVA in pediatric patients have not been established; therefore, FROVA is not recommended for use in patients under 18 years of age. Post-marketing experience with other triptans includes a limited number of reports that describe pediatric patients who have experienced clinically serious adverse events that are similar in nature to those reported rarely in adults.

Lactation: It is not known whether frovatriptan is excreted in human milk. Frovatriptan and/or its metabolites are excreted in the milk of lactating rats with the maximum concentration being four-fold higher than that seen in blood. Therefore, caution should be exercised when considering the administration of FROVA to a nursing woman.

Pregnancy: There are no adequate and well-controlled trials in pregnant women. FROVA should be used during pregnancy only if clearly needed.

Dependence Liability: Although the abuse potential of FROVA has not been specifically assessed in clinical trials, no abuse of, tolerance to, withdrawal from, or drug-seeking behavior was observed in patients who received FROVA. The 5-HT_1 agonists, as a class, have not been associated with drug abuse.

Drug Interactions: Frovatriptan is not an inhibitor of human monoamine oxidase (MAO) enzymes or cytochrome P450 (isozymes 1A2, 2C9, 2C19, 2D6, 2E1, 3A4) in vitro at concentrations up to 250 to 500-fold higher than the highest blood concentrations observed in man at a dose of 2.5 mg. No induction of drug metabolizing enzymes was observed following multiple dosing of frovatriptan to rats or on addition to human hepatocytes in vitro. Although no clinical studies have been performed, it is unlikely that frovatriptan will affect the metabolism of co-administered drugs metabolized by these mechanisms.

Oral Contraceptives: Retrospective analysis of pharmacokinetic data from females across trials indicated that the mean C_{max} and AUC of frovatriptan are 30% higher in those subjects taking oral contraceptives compared to those not taking oral contraceptives. The effect of FROVA on the pharmacokinetics of oral contraceptives has not been studied.

Ergotamine and Ergot-Containing Drugs: The AUC and C_{max} of frovatriptan (2×2.5 mg dose) were reduced by approximately 25% when co-administered with ergotamine tartrate.

Ergot-containing drugs have been reported to cause prolonged vasospastic reactions. Due to a theoretical risk of a pharmacodynamic interaction, use of ergotamine-containing or ergot-type medications (like dihydroergotamine or methysergide) and FROVA within 24 hours of each other is contraindicated (see Contraindications).

Selective Serotonin Reuptake Inhibitors/Serotonin Norepinephrine Reuptake Inhibitors: Cases of life-threatening serotonin syndrome have been reported during combined use of selective serotonin reuptake inhibitors (SSRIs) or serotonin norepinephrine reuptake inhibitors (SNRIs) and triptans (see Warnings).

Propranolol: Propranolol increased the AUC of frovatriptan 2.5 mg in males by 60% and in females by 29%. The C_{max} of frovatriptan was increased 23% in males and 16% in females in the presence of propranolol. The t_{max} as well as half-life of frovatriptan, though slightly longer in the females, were not affected by concomitant administration of propranolol.

Moclobemide: The pharmacokinetic profile of frovatriptan was unaffected when a single oral dose of frovatriptan 2.5 mg was administered to healthy female subjects receiving the MAO-A inhibitor, moclobemide, at an oral dose of 150 mg bid for 8 days.

Other 5-HT_1 Agonists: The administration of FROVA with other 5-HT_1 agonists has not been evaluated in migraine patients. Because their vasospastic effects may be additive, coadministration of FROVA and other 5-HT_1 agonists within 24 hours of each other is contraindicated (see Contraindications).

Laboratory Tests: FROVA is not known to interfere with commonly employed clinical laboratory tests. No specific laboratory tests are recommended for monitoring patients prior to and/or after the treatment with FROVA.

Information to Be Provided to the Patient: Physicians should instruct their patients to read the patient package insert before taking FROVA. See Information for the Patient.

ADVERSE EFFECTS: Serious cardiac events, including some that have been fatal, have occurred following the use of other 5-HT_1 agonists. These events are extremely rare and most have been reported in patients with risk factors predictive of CAD. Events reported have included coronary artery vasospasm, transient myocardial ischemia, myocardial infarction, ventricular tachycardia and ventricular fibrillation (see Contraindications; Warnings and Precautions).

Incidence in Controlled Clinical Trials: Among 1554 patients treated with FROVA (frovatriptan succinate) in four placebo-controlled studies (Trials 1, 3, 4 and 5 in Table 1), only 1% (16) of the patients withdrew because of the treatment-emergent adverse events. In a long-term, open-label study where patients were allowed to treat multiple migraine attacks with FROVA for up to 1 year, 5% (26/496) patients discontinued due to treatment-emergent adverse events.

The treatment-emergent adverse events that occurred most frequently following the administration of frovatriptan 2.5 mg (i.e., in at least 1% of patients), and at an incidence ≥1% greater than with the placebo, in the four placebo-controlled trials, were dizziness, paresthesia, headache, dry mouth, fatigue, flushing, hot or cold sensation, chest pain, dyspepsia, dysesthesia, throat-tightness and skeletal pain.

Table 2 lists treatment-emergent adverse events reported within 48 hours of drug administration that occurred with frovatriptan 2.5 mg at an incidence rate of ≥1% and more than 1% more often than placebo, in the first attack in four placebo-controlled trials (Trials 1, 3, 4 and 5 in Table 1). These studies involved 2392 patients (1554 frovatriptan 2.5 mg and 838 placebo). The events cited reflect experience gained under closely monitored conditions of clinical trials in a highly selected patient population. In actual clinical practice or in other clinical trials, these incidence estimates may not apply, as the conditions of use, reporting behavior, and the kinds of patients treated may differ.

Table 2: FROVA

Treatment-Emergent Adverse Events (Incidence ≥1% and 1% Greater Than Placebo) of Patients in Four Placebo-Controlled Migraine Trials

Adverse Events	Frovatriptan 2.5 mg (n=1554)	Frovatriptan 5 mg (n=99)	Placebo (n=838)
Symptoms of Potentially Cardiac Origin			
Chest pain	2%	3%	1%
Throat tightness	2%	1%	0%
Central & Peripheral Nervous Systems			
Dizziness	8%	NR	5%
Headache	4%	NR	3%
Paresthesia	4%	NR	2%
Hypertonia	NR	4%	0%
Gastrointestinal System Disorders			
Mouth dry	3%	NR	1%
Dyspepsia	2%	3%	1%

(cont'd)

Table 2: FROVA *(cont'd)*

Treatment-Emergent Adverse Events (Incidence ≥1% and 1% Greater Than Placebo) of Patients in Four Placebo-Controlled Migraine Trials

Adverse Events	Frovatriptan 2.5 mg (n=1554)	Frovatriptan 5 mg (n=99)	Placebo (n=838)
Body as a Whole—General Disorders			
Fatigue	5%	4%	2%
Asthenia	NR	4%	1%
Hot or cold sensation[a]	3%	NR	2%
Rigors	NR	2%	1%
Dysesthesia	1%	NR	0%
Respiratory System Disorders			
Rhinitis	NR	3%	1%
Psychiatric Disorders			
Euphoria	NR	2%	0%
Musculoskeletal			
Skeletal pain	3%	NR	2%
Vascular			
Flushing	4%	NR	2%

[a] The term "sensation" encompasses adverse events described as pain, discomfort, pressure, constriction, numbness and tingling.
Legend: NR=No incidence rates of ≥1% and 1% greater than placebo.

FROVA is generally well tolerated. The incidence of adverse events in clinical trials did not increase when up to 2 doses were used within 24 hours. The majority of adverse events were mild or moderate and transient. The incidence of adverse events in four placebo-controlled clinical trials was not affected by gender, age or concomitant medications commonly used by migraine patients. There were insufficient data to assess the impact of race on the incidence of adverse events.

Other Events Observed in Association with FROVA: In the paragraphs that follow, the incidence of less commonly reported adverse events in four placebo-controlled trials are presented. The incidence of each adverse event is calculated as the number of patients reporting the event at least once divided by the number of patients who used FROVA. All adverse events reported within 48 hours of drug administration in the first attack in four placebo-controlled trials involving 2392 patients (1554 frovatriptan 2.5 mg and 838 placebo) are included, except those already listed in Table 2, those too general to be informative, those not reasonably associated with the use of the drug and those which occurred at the same or a greater incidence in the placebo group. Events are further classified within body system categories and enumerated in order of decreasing frequency using the following definitions: frequent adverse events are those occurring in at least 1/100 patients, infrequent adverse events are those occurring in between 1/100 and 1/1000 patients, and rare adverse events are those occurring in fewer than 1/1000 patients.

Central and Peripheral Nervous Systems: Frequent: dysesthesia and hypoesthesia. Infrequent: tremor, hyperesthesia, migraine aggravated, involuntary muscle contractions, vertigo, ataxia, abnormal gait and speech disorder. Rare: hypertonia, hypotonia, abnormal reflexes and tongue paralysis.

Gastrointestinal: Frequent: vomiting, abdominal pain and diarrhea. Infrequent: dysphagia, flatulence, constipation, anorexia, esophagospasm and increased salivation. Rare: change in bowel habits, cheilitis, eructation, gastroesophageal reflux, hiccup, peptic ulcer, salivary gland pain, stomatitis and toothache.

Body as Whole: Frequent: pain. Infrequent: asthenia, rigors, fever, hot flashes and malaise. Rare: feeling of relaxation, leg pain and edema mouth.

Psychiatric: Frequent: insomnia and anxiety. Infrequent: confusion, nervousness, agitation, euphoria, impaired concentration, depression, emotional lability, amnesia, thinking abnormal and depersonalization. Rare: depression aggravated, abnormal dreaming and personality disorder.

Musculoskeletal: Infrequent: myalgia, back pain, arthralgia, arthrosis, leg cramps and muscle weakness.

Respiratory: Frequent: sinusitis and rhinitis. Infrequent: pharyngitis, dyspnea, hyperventilation and laryngitis.

Vision Disorders: Frequent: abnormal vision. Infrequent: eye pain, conjunctivitis and abnormal lacrimation.

Skin and Appendages: Frequent: sweating increased. Infrequent: pruritus, and bullous eruption.

Hearing and Vestibular Disorders: Frequent: tinnitus. Infrequent: ear ache, and hyperacusis.

Heart Rate and Rhythm: Frequent: palpitation. Infrequent: tachycardia. Rare: bradycardia.

Metabolic and Nutritional Disorders: Infrequent: thirst and dehydration. Rare: hypocalcemia and hypoglycemia.

Special Senses, Other Disorders: Infrequent: taste perversion.

Urinary System Disorders: Infrequent: micturition frequency and polyuria. Rare: nocturia, renal pain and abnormal urine.

Cardiovascular Disorders, General: Infrequent: abnormal ECG.

Platelet, Bleeding and Clotting Disorders: Infrequent: epistaxis. Rare: purpura.

Autonomic Nervous System: Rare: syncope.

Long-Term Safety: The adverse events which occurred within 48 hours of drug administration in a long-term open-label safety study were similar to those that occurred in the placebo-controlled trials. The most frequent adverse events were: nausea, dizziness, fatigue, somnolence, headache, dyspepsia, skeletal pain, flushing and paresthesia.

Post-Marketing Experience with Frovatriptan: Rare reports of serious cardiovascular events have been reported in association with the use of FROVA, this includes chest tightness and tachycardia. There have been rare reports of serious allergic type reactions, including anaphylactic reactions. The uncontrolled nature of post-marketing surveillance, however, makes it impossible to definitely determine the proportion of the reported cases that were actually caused by frovatriptan or to reliably assess causation in individual cases.

OVERDOSE:

Symptoms: There is no direct experience of any patient taking an overdose of FROVA (frovatriptan succinate). The maximum single dose of frovatriptan given to male and female patients with migraine was 40 mg (16 times the clinical dose) and the maximum single dose given to healthy male subjects was 100 mg (40 times the clinical dose) without significant adverse events.

Treatment: As with other 5-HT_1 receptor agonists, there is no specific antidote for frovatriptan. The elimination half-life of frovatriptan is 26 hours, therefore if overdose occurs, the patient should be monitored closely for at least 48 hours and be given any necessary symptomatic treatment. The effects of hemo- or peritoneal dialysis on blood concentrations of frovatriptan are unknown.

> For management of a suspected drug overdose, contact your regional Poison Control Centre. See the *CPS* Directory section for a list of Poison Control Centres.

DOSAGE: Adults: The recommended dosage of FROVA (frovatriptan succinate) is a single tablet (frovatriptan 2.5 mg) taken orally with fluids for migraine headache with or without aura. FROVA is recommended only for the acute treatment of migraine attacks, and should not be used prophylactically.

If the headache recurs after initial relief, a second dose may be taken between 4 and 24 hours after the first dose. The total daily dose of FROVA should not exceed 2 tablets (2×2.5 mg per day).

There is no evidence that a second dose of frovatriptan is effective in patients who do not respond to a first dose of the drug for the same headache.

FROVA is contraindicated in patients with severe hepatic impairment (Child-Pugh grade C) due to the absence of clinical data. FROVA is contraindicated in patients with uncontrolled or severe hypertension. In patients with mild to moderate controlled hypertension, patients should be treated cautiously.

The safety of treating an average of more than 4 migraine attacks in a 30 day period has not been established.

INFORMATION FOR THE PATIENT: Published in e-CPS, available by subscription at www.e-cps.ca.

SUPPLIED: Each round, white, film-coated tablet, debossed with 2.5 on one side and "E" on the other side contains: frovatriptan (base) 2.5 mg as the succinate. Nonmedicinal ingredients: colloidal silicon dioxide NF, hydroxypropylmethylcellulose USP, lactose NF, magnesium stearate NF, microcrystalline cellulose NF, polyethylene glycol 3000 USP, sodium starch glycollate NF, triacetin USP, titanium dioxide USP and triacetin USP. Blister cards of 7 tablets, 1 blister card per carton. Store at controlled room temperature, 25°C, excursions permitted to 15-30°C. Protect from moisture.

(Shown in Product Identification Section)

Fucidin® Cream
fusidic acid
Antibiotic

LEO Pharma

Fucidin® Ointment
sodium fusidate
Antibiotic

LEO Pharma

PHARMACOLOGY: Fusidic acid inhibits bacterial protein synthesis by interfering with amino acid transfer from aminoacyl-tRNA to protein on the ribosomes. Fusidic acid may be bacteriostatic or bactericidal depending on inoculum size. Although bacterial cells stop dividing almost within 2 minutes after contact with the antibiotic in vitro, DNA and RNA synthesis continue for 45 minutes and 1 to 2 hours, respectively.

Fusidic acid is virtually inactive against Gram-negative bacteria. The differences in activity against Gram-negative and Gram-positive organisms are believed to be due to a difference in cell wall permeability.

Mammalian cells are much less susceptible to inhibition of protein synthesis by fusidic acid than sensitive bacterial cells. These differences are believed to be due primarily to a difference in cell wall permeability.

INDICATIONS: The treatment of primary and secondary skin infections caused by sensitive strains of *S. aureus*, Streptococcus species and *C. minutissimum*. Primary skin infections that may be expected to respond to treatment with fusidic acid topical include: impetigo contagiosa, erythrasma and secondary skin infections such as infected wounds and infected burns.

Appropriate culture and susceptibility studies should be performed. However, while waiting results of these studies and, if antibiotic therapy is considered to be necessary, fusidic acid topical may be administered to those patients in whom an infection caused by susceptible bacteria is suspected. This antibiotic treatment may subsequently require modification once these results become available.

In addition, local concentrations of fusidic acid topical are active against other Corynebacteria spp., Neisseria spp., Clostridia spp. and Bacteroides species. No cross-resistance has been observed to date between fusidic acid and other antibiotics presently in clinical use.

Resistance to fusidic acid has readily been induced in vitro. The development of resistance has also been shown to occur in the clinical setting.

CONTRAINDICATIONS: Sensitivity to fusidic acid and its salts, or lanolin in respect of Fucidin ointment.

PRECAUTIONS: Treatment of severe or refractory skin lesions should be supplemented with the administration of a systemic antibacterial agent. Use of topical antibiotics occasionally allows overgrowth of nonsusceptible organisms. If this occurs, or irritation or sensitization develop, treatment should be discontinued and appropriate therapy instituted. Fusidic acid topical preparations should not be used in or near the eye because of the possibility of conjunctival irritation.

Pregnancy: Safety in the treatment of infections during pregnancy has not been established. If administration of fusidic acid to pregnant patients is considered necessary, its potential benefits should be weighed against the possible hazards to the fetus.

Lactation: There is evidence to suggest that the drug can penetrate the placental barrier and is detectable in the milk of nursing mothers. Safety of fusidic acid for the treatment of infections in women who are breast-feeding has not been established.

ADVERSE EFFECTS: Mild irritation has occasionally been reported in patients with dermatoses treated with fusidic acid. It was not usually necessary to discontinue therapy. The application of fusidic acid to deep leg ulcers has been associated with pain. Reports of hypersensitivity reactions have been rare.

OVERDOSE:

Overdosage has not been known to occur during topical therapy with fusidic acid ointment or cream.

> For management of a suspected drug overdose, CPhA recommends that you contact your **regional Poison Control Centre**. See the *CPS* Directory section for a list of Poison Control Centres.

DOSAGE: Ointment and Cream: Apply a small amount to the lesion 3 or 4 times daily until favorable results are achieved. Whenever the lesion is to be covered with a gauze dressing, less frequent applications (1 or 2 daily) may be used. In impetigo contagiosa, it has not been shown necessary to remove the crusts before application.

When treating the face, care should be taken to avoid the eye.

SUPPLIED: Cream: Each tube contains: fusidic acid 2% in a cream base. Nonmedicinal ingredients: butylhydroxyanisole, cetanol, glycerin 85%, paraffin liquid, paraffin white soft, polysorbate 60, potassium sorbate and purified water. Tubes of 15 and 30 g. Store between 15 and 25°C.

Ointment: Each tube contains: sodium fusidate 2% (1.92% fusidic acid as the sodium salt) in an ointment base containing lanolin. Nonmedicinal ingredients: cetanol, lanolin anhydrous, liquid paraffin and white soft paraffin. Tubes of 15 and 30 g. Store between 15 and 30°C.

Fucidin® H
fusidic acid—hydrocortisone acetate
Topical Antibiotic—Corticosteroid

LEO Pharma

PHARMACOLOGY: Fucidin H combines the antibacterial activity of fusidic acid with the anti-inflammatory activity of the mild potency corticosteroid hydrocortisone acetate.

The antibacterial action of fusidic acid results from inhibition of bacterial protein synthesis. The drug interferes with amino acid transfer from aminoacyl-tRNA to protein on the ribosomes. The spectrum of antibacterial activity of fusidic acid is primarily toward gram positive organisms, demonstrating particularly high activity against *S. aureus*. Hydrocortisone has anti-inflammatory, antipruritic, and vasoconstrictive properties. The mechanism of the anti-inflammatory activity of topical corticosteroids is generally unclear. However, corticosteroids are thought to induce phospholipase A_2 inhibitor proteins, preventing arachidonic acid release and the biosynthesis of potent mediators of inflammation.

Skin penetration by fusidic acid is comparable to that of glucocorticoids. As much as 2% of the amount of topically applied fusidic acid penetrates intact skin. Dermal absorption of hydrocortisone is considered to be approximately 1 to 5% of the administered dose. Absorption of hydrocortisone may be higher in certain body areas such as the face, groin, axilla, or on injured or inflamed skin such as the lesions of atopic dermatitis.

The efficacy of Fucidin H in the treatment of mild to moderately severe atopic dermatitis has been compared with that of its individual components, fusidic acid and hydrocortisone, in clinical studies. For patients with *S. aureus* present on the lesions, Fucidin H was more effective than either hydrocortisone or fusidic acid based on a single efficacy criterion for alleviation of classical symptoms (erythema, scaling, edema, itch, serous discharge, and crusting) and bacteriological eradication at completion of 14 days of treatment. There is no data available regarding relapse rate.

INDICATIONS: For the treatment of mild to moderately severe atopic dermatitis where *S. aureus* is suspected as a contributing factor. The presence of *S. aureus* may be associated with crusting of lesions and/or erythema. Fucidin H has antibacterial activity which results in the eradication of *S. aureus* from the skin lesions of atopic dermatitis. In addition, Fucidin H also has anti-inflammatory activity.

CONTRAINDICATIONS: Patients with hypersensitivity to fusidic acid, hydrocortisone, or other components of the cream.

As with other topical antibiotic/corticosteroid combination preparations, Fucidin H is contraindicated in bacterial infections due to nonsusceptible organisms, fungal infections, tuberculosis of the skin, syphilitic skin infections, chicken pox, eruptions following vaccinations and viral diseases of the skin in general.

WARNINGS: When used under occlusive dressing, over extensive areas, or on the face, scalp, axillae and scrotum, sufficient absorption may occur giving rise to adrenal suppression and other systemic effects.

PRECAUTIONS: Fucidin H should not be used in or near the eye because of the possibility of conjunctival irritation by fusidic acid. Application of topical corticosteroids near the eye can potentially cause increased intraocular pressure, glaucoma or cataracts.

Steroid-antibiotic combinations should not be continued for more than 14 days in the absence of any clinical improvement, since occult extensions of the infection may occur due to masking by the steroid. Similarly, steroids may also mask hypersensitivity reactions.

As with all topical antibiotics, extended or recurrent application may allow overgrowth of nonsusceptible organisms, or increase the risk of contact sensitization and the development of antibiotic resistance. Sensitization and irritation due to dermal applications of topical corticosteroids have been noted in rare instances. Application to extensive areas, too frequent application, or application under occlusive dressings may result in systemic absorption with symptoms of adrenal suppression. Localized atrophy and striae, particularly on the flexor surfaces and on the face, may also develop.

Pregnancy: The safety of fusidic acid and/or topical hydrocortisone during pregnancy or lactation has not been established. The use of Fucidin H during pregnancy or lactation requires that the potential benefits be weighed against the risks to the fetus or nursing infant. Animal studies have not demonstrated teratogenicity with fusidic acid. Fusidic acid has been shown to penetrate the placental barrier following systemic administration, and fusidic acid has been detected in the milk of nursing mothers. Topical administration of corticosteroids to pregnant animals can cause abnormalities of fetal development, including cleft palate and intra-uterine growth retardation. There may, therefore, be a risk of such effects to the human fetus.

Lactation: See Pregnancy.

Children: Clinical trials with Fucidin H have not demonstrated any increased incidence of adverse effects in children 3 years and over. Pediatric patients may, however, demonstrate greater susceptibility to topical corticosteroid-induced hypothalamic-pituitary-adrenal axis suppression and to exogenous corticosteroid effects than mature patients because of greater absorption due to a larger skin surface area to body weight ratio. Therefore, excessive and prolonged use of Fucidin H, especially under occlusive conditions, should be avoided. There are no data from randomized, controlled clinical trials on the safety and efficacy of Fucidin H in children under 3 years of age.

ADVERSE EFFECTS: Clinical trials demonstrated that Fucidin H is well tolerated and associated with few adverse effects. In clinical trials, only 3.2% of patients experienced adverse effects. Adverse effects were not serious, consisting of irritation at the application site (1.6%) and flare up of dermatitis (1.6%).

Fusidic acid has been reported to cause mild irritation at the application site, but did not usually require discontinuation of therapy. Reports of hypersensitivity reactions have been rare.

Adverse effects are generally local and include: dryness, itching, burning, local irritation, striae, skin atrophy, atrophy of subcutaneous tissues, telangiectasia, hypertrichosis, change in pigmentation and secondary infection. If applied to the face, acne rosacea or perioral dermatitis can occur.

OVERDOSE:

Symptoms: Overdosage has not been known to occur during topical therapy with Fucidin H. However, adverse effects would be expected to be those associated with topical hydrocortisone.

> For management of a suspected drug overdose, CPhA recommends that you contact your **regional Poison Control Centre**. See the *CPS* Directory section for a list of Poison Control Centres.

DOSAGE: Fucidin H should be applied 3 times daily and gently massaged into the affected areas. In clinical trials the treatment period was 2 weeks. A shorter course should be considered if symptoms improve.

There are no data from randomized, controlled clinical trials on use of Fucidin H in children under 3 years of age (see Precautions).

INFORMATION FOR THE PATIENT: Published in e-CPS, available by subscription at www.e-cps.ca.

SUPPLIED: Each tube of white cream contains: fusidic acid (hemihydrate) 2% and hydrocortisone acetate 1%. Nonmedicinal ingredients: butylated hydroxyanisol, cetyl alcohol, glycerol, liquid paraffin, polysorbate 60, potassium sorbate, purified water and white soft paraffin. Lacquered aluminum tubes of 30 g. Store at room temperature (15 to 30°C).

Fucithalmic® Pr

fusidic acid

Topical Ophthalmic Antibiotic

LEO Pharma

PHARMACOLOGY: Fucithalmic viscous eye drops contain the antibiotic fusidic acid. The antibacterial action of fusidic acid results from the inhibition of bacterial protein synthesis. Fusidic acid interferes with amino acid transfer from aminoacyl-tRNA to protein on the ribosomes. Fusidic acid may be bacteriostatic or bactericidal depending on inoculum size. Although bacterial cells stop dividing almost within 2 minutes after contact with the antibiotic in vitro, DNA and RNA synthesis continue for 45 minutes and 1 to 2 hours, respectively. Fusidic acid has a steroid-like structure but does not exhibit any steroid-like pharmacological activity (i.e., hormonal or anti-inflammatory effects).

Pharmacokinetics: Fucithalmic is a 1% microcrystalline suspension of fusidic acid in a carbomer gel. The sustained release formulation of Fucithalmic provides prolonged contact with the eye. Pharmacokinetic studies in humans demonstrated that 1 hour following administration of a single drop of the product into the fornix of the eye, fusidic acid concentrations in lacrimal fluid ranged between 15.7 to 40 µg/mL. Fusidic acid concentrations ranged between 1.4 to 5.6 µg/mL 12 hours after administration. Median antibiotic levels of 0.3 µg/mL are maintained for 12 hours in aqueous humour. Since high ocular concentrations of fusidic acid are achieved after topical application, standardized susceptibility tests may not be appropriate to predict clinical effectiveness.

INDICATIONS: Treatment of superficial infections of the eye and its adnexa (i.e., conjunctivitis) caused by fusidic acid susceptible strains of the designated bacteria in adults and children (≥2 years of age): *S. aureus*, *S. pneumoniae* and *H. influenzae*.

Enterobacteriaciae and Pseudomonas are resistant to fusidic acid.

There are currently no NCCLS approved standards for testing in vitro susceptibility of conjunctival isolates toward topical ophthalmic antibiotics, including fusidic acid.

CONTRAINDICATIONS: In patients with hypersensitivity to fusidic acid or any of the other components of the preparations: multidose preserved preparation and unit-dose unpreserved preparation (see Supplied). The component benzalkonium chloride in the preserved preparation can be allergenic. A preservative-free unit-dose formulation is available for patients with known or suspected hypersensitivity to benzalkonium chloride.

WARNINGS: Not for injection into the eye.

PRECAUTIONS: Prolonged use of fusidic acid may result in overgrowth of nonsusceptible organisms, including fungi. If superinfection or drug resistance occurs, treatment should be discontinued and appropriate therapy should be initiated. Whenever clinical judgment dictates, the patient should be examined with the aid of magnification, such as slit lamp biomicroscopy and, where appropriate, fluorescein staining.

If irritation (other than transient stinging upon administration) or sensitization to any of the components of the product develops, then treatment should be discontinued.

Contact lenses (hard or soft) should not be worn during treatment with fusidic acid. Wearing contact lenses concomitant with an infection could cause eye damage. Treatment with Fucithalmic while wearing contact lenses has not been studied in clinical trials. In addition, the preservative benzalkonium chloride in Fucithalmic multidose vials may deposit in contact lenses.

Patients should be advised to avoid contaminating the tip of the multidose tube through contact with the eye, eyelid or any other objects during administration.

Pregnancy: There are no adequate and well-controlled studies in pregnant women. Therefore, the use of fusidic acid in pregnancy requires that the benefits be weighed against the potential risks to the fetus. Fusidic acid has been shown to penetrate the placental barrier of humans following systemic administration. Animal studies have not demonstrated teratogenicity with fusidic acid.

Lactation: Following systemic administration of fusidic acid, the drug has been detected in the milk of nursing mothers. The use of fusidic acid while nursing requires that the benefits be weighed against the potential risks to the nursing infant.

Children: Quantitative bacteriology studies have not been conducted in children <2 years of age and thus the efficacy of fusidic acid has not been established. The incidence and spectrum of adverse reactions in children <2 years is similar to children ≥2 years of age.

Neonates: Fusidic acid should not be used in the treatment of neonatal conjunctivitis. The etiology of bacterial conjunctivitis in neonates can be different as compared to adults and children. Fucithalmic has inadequate antibiotic activity toward pathogens associated with neonatal conjunctivitis (e.g., Chlamydia, Pseudomonas, *N. gonorrhea*, Coliforms etc.). Treatment of neonates should not be empirical but instead based on a diagnosis of conjunctivitis established following culture of conjunctival samples.

Drug Interactions: There is no clinical trial experience of concomitant use of fusidic acid with other ophthalmic preparations.

ADVERSE EFFECTS: Adverse drug reactions (events deemed possibly or probably related to fusidic acid viscous drops 1%) were reported for 6.4% of clinical trial patients (n=1214 patients studied) with 1.1% requiring discontinuation of treatment. The most frequent reaction was transient stinging or irritation upon administration (3.4% of patients). Severity was usually mild and discontinuation of therapy was not required.

In clinical trials, adverse drug reactions reported for <1% of patients include transient burning sensation and/or tearing, eye soreness, eyelid edema, eyelid stickiness, temporary blurring of vision immediately after administration, headache, and worsening of conjunctivitis. Reactions reported by ≤0.1% of patients include: localized allergic reaction, cobblestone appearance of the conjunctival sulcros, eyelid abscess, eye pain, tired eyes, skin rash, urticaria, oral candidiasis, chest infection, tonsillitis, enuresis, loss of appetite and vomiting.

Hypersensitivity reactions to fusidic acid viscous drops 1% are reported rarely and have been characterized by urticaria (localized or generalized). Cross-hypersensitivity between fusidic acid and other antibiotics has not been reported.

OVERDOSE:

There is no experience with overdosage of fusidic acid viscous drops 1%.

> For management of a suspected drug overdose, CPhA recommends that you contact your **regional Poison Control Centre**. See the *CPS* Directory section for a list of Poison Control Centres.

DOSAGE: Adults and Children (≥2 years): Instill 1 drop into the conjunctival sac of both eyes every 12 hours (i.e., twice daily application) for 7 days.

If clinical resolution has not been achieved after 7 days of treatment, the patient should be re-evaluated.

INFORMATION FOR THE PATIENT: Published in e-CPS, available by subscription at www.e-cps.ca.

SUPPLIED: Multidose Tubes: Each g of aqueous suspension, sterile viscous eye drop formulation contains: fusidic acid hemihydrate 10 mg (1%). Nonmedicinal ingredients: benzalkonium chloride (as a preservative), carbomer, disodium edetate, mannitol, sodium hydroxide (to adjust pH) and water. Multidose tubes of 5 g, boxes of 1. Store at 2 to 25°C. Discard 1 month after first opening the tube.

Unit-dose Droppers: Each g of aqueous suspension, sterile viscous eye drop formulation contains: fusidic acid hemihydrate 10 mg (1%). Nonmedicinal ingredients: carbomer, mannitol, sodium acetate trihydrate, sodium hydroxide (to adjust pH) and water. Preservative-free. Single unit-dose plastic droppers of 0.2 g, boxes of 12. Store at 2 to 25°C. Discard after single use.

Fungizone® Pr

amphotericin B

Antifungal

Bristol-Myers Squibb

Date of Preparation: September 16, 1980

Date of Revision: June 1, 2009

PHARMACOLOGY: Amphotericin B is fungistatic or fungicidal depending on the concentration obtained in body fluids and the susceptibility of the fungus. It has been shown to exhibit a high order of in vitro activity against a broad spectrum of yeast and fungi.

The drug probably acts by binding to sterols present in the membrane of sensitive fungi, with the resultant change in permeability allowing leakage of a variety of small molecules. Since mammalian cell membranes also contain sterols, it has been suggested that the damage to human cells and fungal cells may share common mechanisms.

Following i.v. infusion, the antibiotic is slowly excreted by the kidneys, and demonstrable blood levels persist for at least 18 hours after the infusion is discontinued.

INDICATIONS: FUNGIZONE (amphotericin B) is specifically intended for the treatment of disseminated mycotic infections, including coccidioidomycosis; cryptococcosis (torulosis); disseminated candidiasis, histoplasmosis, South American leishmaniasis, North and South American blastomycosis; mucormycosis (phycomycosis) caused by species of the genera Mucor, Rhizopus, Absidia, Entomophthora, and Basidiobolus, sporotrichosis (*S. schenckii*), and aspergillosis (*A. fumigatus*).

Other Clinical Uses: Limited studies have shown that amphotericin B powder for injection may be useful when administered by routes other than i.v. for the treatment of certain types of fungal infections.

1) Administration by Bladder Irrigation: The effective use of amphotericin B for fungal infections of the bladder has been reported in the literature.

The basic method used for bladder irrigation is as follows: 15 mg FUNGIZONE powder is dissolved in 100 to 400 mL of sterile water and injected via catheter after complete emptying of the bladder. The patient is then asked to retain the solution for as long as possible. An alkalizing mixture should be given every 4 hours. The treatment may be repeated until the culture is negative and the symptoms have disappeared.

2) Administration by Aerosol: Amphotericin B has also been administered by aerosol (nebulizer) for the treatment of pulmonary fungal infections. A preparation suitable for administration by aerosol is prepared as follows: Dissolve a 50 mg vial of FUNGIZONE in a bottle of Alevaire or in 10 mL of distilled or sterile water. Administer 1 to 2 mL of this solution (5 to 10 mg amphotericin B) 3 to 4 times daily for a period of 1 to 2 weeks.

3) Administration for Eye Infections: Several studies have been done using topical administration of amphotericin B for fungal infections of the eye. Such use has shown a low degree of efficacy after prolonged therapy and is not recommended unless there is no other alternative. It is unlikely to be of value except in superficial infections.

Reconstitute a 50 mg vial of amphotericin B by adding 10 mL of sterile water, giving a concentration of 5 mg/mL. Shake until the solution is clear. Further dilution of 1 mL of this solution to a concentration of 1 mg/mL using sterile water provides a solution suitable for use in the eye. Dosage varies from 2 drops every hour to 1 drop every 4 to 6 hours. Intervals between administration may be lengthened as improvement occurs. Amphotericin B has been reported in some instances to be toxic to the eye when applied locally and may cause local irritation and discomfort.

Solutions of 1.5 mg/mL up to 4.0 mg/mL have also been used. Normal (isotonic) saline is not recommended for dilution since it may cause precipitation of amphotericin B.

Higher concentrations can lead to serious damage to the eye and must not be used.

4) Administration for Ear Infections: There is little evidence to support the efficacy of such use.

CONTRAINDICATIONS: FUNGIZONE (amphotericin B) is contraindicated in those patients who have shown hypersensitivity to amphotericin B or any other component in the formulation, unless, in the opinion of the physician, the condition requiring therapy is life threatening and amenable only to amphotericin B therapy.

WARNINGS:

> **Serious Warnings and Precautions**
> Exercise caution to prevent inadvertent FUNGIZONE overdose. Verify the product name and dosage, pre-administration, especially if dose exceeds 1.5 mg/kg.

FUNGIZONE (amphotericin B) should be administered **primarily** to patients with progressive, potentially fatal infections and **should not** be used to treat nonserious fungal infections.

In the treatment of potentially fatal fungal diseases, the possible life-saving benefit of amphotericin B must be balanced against its untoward and dangerous side effects.

PRECAUTIONS: General: Prolonged therapy with amphotericin B is usually necessary. Adverse reactions are quite common when the drug is given parenterally at therapeutic dosage levels. Some of these reactions are potentially dangerous. Hence, FUNGIZONE (amphotericin B) should be used only in hospitalized patients or those under close clinical observation by medically trained personnel, and should be reserved for those patients in whom a diagnosis of the progressive, potentially fatal forms of susceptible mycotic infections has been firmly established, preferably by positive culture or histologic study.

Exercise caution to prevent inadvertent FUNGIZONE overdose, which can result in potentially fatal cardiac or cardiorespiratory arrest. **Verify the product name and dosage pre-administration especially if dose prescribed exceeds 1.5 mg/kg** (see Dosage and Symptoms and Treatment of Overdose).

Acute reactions including fever, shaking chills, hypotension, anorexia, nausea, vomiting, headache, and tachypnea are common 1 to 3 hours after starting an i.v. infusion.

Rapid i.v. infusion, over less than 1 hour, particularly in patients with renal insufficiency, has been associated with hyperkalemia and arrhythmias, and should, therefore, be avoided (see Dosage).

Leukoencephalopathy has been reported following use of amphotericin B in patients who received total body irradiation.

Laboratory Tests: Renal function should be monitored frequently during amphotericin B therapy. Serum creatinine should be monitored on a regular basis and discontinuation or marked dose reduction of amphotericin B should be considered if a significant increase from baseline value of serum creatinine occurs.

It is also advisable to monitor on a regular basis liver function, serum electrolytes (particularly magnesium and potassium), blood counts, and hemoglobin concentrations. Low serum magnesium levels have been noted during treatment with amphotericin B. Laboratory test results should be used as a guide to subsequent dosage adjustments.

Whenever medication is interrupted for a period longer than 7 days, therapy should be resumed by starting with the lowest dosage level, e.g., 0.25 mg/kg/day of body weight and increased gradually to an optimum level as outlined in Dosage.

Drug Interactions: Antineoplastic Agents: May enhance the potential for renal toxicity, bronchospasm and hypotension. Antineoplastic agents (e.g., nitrogen mustard, etc.) should be given concomitantly only with great caution.

Corticosteroids and Corticotropin (ACTH): May potentiate amphotericin B-induced hypokalemia and should not be administered concomitantly unless they are necessary to control drug reactions. Since deep fungal infections sometimes emerge in patients undergoing therapy with antibiotics and antineoplastic agents such as nitrogen mustard, they should not be given concomitantly with amphotericin B, if avoidable. Other nephrotoxic agents (e.g., cisplatin, pentamidine, aminoglycosides and cyclosporine) may enhance the potential for renal toxicity and should not be given concomitantly except with great caution.

Digitalis Glycosides: Amphotericin B-induced hypokalemia may potentiate digitalis toxicity. Serum potassium levels and cardiac function should be closely monitored and any deficit promptly corrected.

Flucytosine: Concomitant administration may increase the toxicity of flucytosine possibly by increasing its cellular uptake and/or impairing its renal excretion.

Imidazoles (e.g., ketoconazole, miconazole, clotrimazole, fluconazole, etc.): In vitro and animal studies with the combination of amphotericin B and imidazoles suggest that imidazoles may induce fungal resistance to amphotericin B. Combination therapy should be administered with caution, especially in immunocompromised patients.

Other Nephrotoxic Medications: Agents such as aminoglycosides, cyclosporine, and pentamidine may enhance the potential for drug-induced renal toxicity, and should be used concomitantly only with great caution. Intensive monitoring of renal function is recommended in patients requiring any combination of nephrotoxic medications (see Precautions, Laboratory Tests).

Leukocyte Transfusions: Though not observed in all studies, acute pulmonary reactions have been observed in patients given amphotericin B during or shortly after leukocyte transfusions, thus it is advisable to separate these infusions as far as possible and to monitor pulmonary function.

Skeletal Muscle Relaxants: Amphotericin B-induced hypokalemia may enhance the curariform effect of skeletal muscle relaxants (e.g., tubocurarine). Serum potassium levels should be monitored and deficiencies corrected.

Caution should be observed when agents whose effects or toxicity may be increased by hopokalemia (e.g., digitalis glycosides, skeletal muscle relaxants and antiarrhythmic agents) are administered concomitantly.

Pregnancy: Reproduction studies in animals have revealed no evidence of harm to the fetus due to amphotericin B for injection. Systemic fungal infections have been successfully treated in pregnant women with amphotericin B for injection without obvious effects to the fetus, but the number of cases reported has been small. Because animal reproduction studies are not always predictive of human response, and adequate and well-controlled studies have not been conducted in pregnant women, this drug should be administered during pregnancy with caution and only if the potential benefit to the mother outweighs the potential risk to the fetus.

Lactation: It is not known whether amphotericin B is excreted in human milk. Likewise, data are in conflict as to the extent of oral absorption, if any. Because many drugs are excreted in human milk and considering the potential toxicity of amphotericin B, it is prudent to advise a nursing mother to discontinue nursing.

Pediatric Use: Safety and effectiveness in pediatric patients have not been established through adequate and well-controlled studies. Systemic fungal infections have been treated in pediatric patients without reports of unusual side effects.

ADVERSE EFFECTS: While a few patients may tolerate full i.v. doses of amphotericin B without difficulty, most will exhibit some intolerance, often at less than the full therapeutic dosage. The adverse reactions most commonly observed are:

General (Body as a Whole): fever (sometimes accompanied by shaking chills occurring within 15 to 20 minutes after initiation of treatment), malaise and weight loss.

Digestive: anorexia, nausea, vomiting, diarrhea, dyspepsia and cramping epigastric pain.

Hematologic: normochromic and normocytic anemia.

Local: local venous pain at the injection site with or without phlebitis or thrombophlebitis.

Musculoskeletal : generalized pain, including muscle and joint pains.

Neurologic: headache.

Renal: decreased renal function and renal function abnormalities including azotemia, hyposthenuria, renal tubular acidosis and nephrocalcinosis, an increase in the serum creatinine level, a decrease in the serum creatinine clearance rate or a decrease in the phenol-sulfonphthalein (PSP) excretion is commonly observed. Hypokalemia with or without concomitant impairment of renal function has often been observed. Potassium replacement may be considered by oral or parenteral route. Concomitant diuretic therapy may be a predisposition for renal impairment whereas sodium repletion or supplementation may reduce the occurrence of nephrotoxicity.

Renal damage is often accompanied by the appearance of granular and hyaline casts, and sometimes by microhematuria. Renal dysfunction is usually reversible on discontinuation of therapy, but serious and permanent renal damage has been reported in patients given large doses for prolonged periods; especially in those receiving a total dose exceeding 5 g.

The following adverse reactions have also been reported:

General (Body as a Whole): flushing.

Allergic: anaphylactoid and other allergic reactions.

Cardiovascular: cardiac arrest, cardiovascular toxicity including arrhythmias, ventricular fibrillation, cardiac failure, hypertension, hypotension and shock.

Dermatologic: maculopapular rash and pruritus (without rash). Skin exfoliation, toxic epidermal necrolysis, and reports of Stevens-Johnson syndrome have been received during postmarketing surveillance.

Digestive: acute liver failure, jaundice, liver function test abnormalities, melena or hemorrhagic gastroenteritis and hepatotoxicity.

Hematologic: coagulation defects, thrombocytopenia, leukopenia, agranulocytosis, eosinophilia, leukocytosis.

Neurologic: hearing loss, tinnitus, transient vertigo, blurred vision or diplopia, peripheral neuropathy, encephalopathy, convulsions and other neurologic symptoms.

Pulmonary: dyspnea, bronchospasm, noncardiac pulmonary edema and hypersensitivity pneumonitis.

Renal: hypomagnesemia, hyperkalemia, acute renal failure, anuria and oliguria. Nephrogenic diabetes insipidus has been reported during postmarketing surveillance.

Fever, nausea, vomiting, headache and malaise sometimes subside with continued administration. Reactions to amphotericin B may be made less severe by administration of an antipyretic, e.g., ASA, an antihistaminic and/or an antiemetic prior to and concurrently with amphotericin B, or by modifying the rate of infusion. Meperidine (25 to 50 mg i.v.) has been shown in some patients to decrease the duration of shaking chills and fever that may accompany the infusion of amphotericin B. Addition of a small amount of heparin, rotation of the injection site, the use of a pediatric scalp-vein needle and alternate day therapy may lessen the incidence of thrombophlebitis and anorexia. Supplemental alkali medication may decrease renal tubular acidosis complications. Extravasation may cause chemical irritation.

I.V. or i.m. administration of small doses of adrenal corticosteroids just prior to, or during the amphotericin B infusion may decrease febrile reactions. The dosage and duration of such corticosteroid therapy should be kept to a minimum (see Precautions).

If a severe reaction occurs during the course of an infusion, therapy should be interrupted for about 15 minutes to allow the patient to recover. If the reaction recurs, therapy should be resumed at a lower dosage the next day. Blood transfusions may be required when reversible normocytic, normochromic anemia occurs during prolonged therapy.

OVERDOSE:

Symptoms : Amphotericin B overdoses can result in potentially fatal cardiac or cardiorespiratory arrest.

Treatment: If an overdose is suspected, discontinue therapy and monitor the patient's clinical status (e.g., cardiorespiratory, renal, and liver function, hematologic status, serum electrolytes) and administer supportive therapy as required. Amphotericin B is not hemodialyzable. Prior to reinstituting therapy, the patient's condition should be stabilized (including correction of electrolyte deficiencies, etc.).

> For management of a suspected drug overdose, CPhA recommends that you contact your **regional Poison Control Centre**. See the *CPS* Directory section for a list of Poison Control Centres.

DOSAGE: **Caution:** Under no circumstances should a total daily dose of 1.5 mg/kg be exceeded. Amphotericin B overdoses can result in potentially fatal cardiac or cardio-respiratory arrest (see Warnings and Precautions and Symptoms and Treatment of Overdose). Large total doses may cause significant and permanent renal impairment. Consideration must be given to the potential risk versus the expected benefit.

FUNGIZONE (Amphotericin B for Injection) should be administered by slow i.v. infusion. I.V. infusion should be given over a period of approximately 2 to 6 hours (depending on the dose) observing the usual precautions for i.v. therapy (see Precautions, General). The recommended concentration for i.v. infusion in 5% Dextrose is 0.1 mg/mL (1 mg/10 mL) (see Preparation of Solutions).

Since patient tolerance varies greatly, the dosage of amphotericin B must be individualized and adjusted according to the patient's clinical status (e.g., site and intensity of infection, etiologic agent, cardio-renal function, etc.).

Though not proven to be a reliable predictor of intolerance, a single i.v. test dose (1 mg in 20 mL of 5% dextrose solution) administered over 20 to 30 minutes may be preferred. The patient's temperature, pulse, respiration, and blood pressure should be recorded every 30 minutes for 2 to 4 hours.

In patients with good cardio-renal function and a well tolerated test dose, therapy is usually initiated with a daily dose of 0.25 mg/kg of body weight but, in those patients having severe and rapidly progressive fungal infection, therapy may be initiated with a daily dose of 0.3 mg/kg of body weight. However, the need for more aggressive therapy, which may include the need to attain full therapeutic dose within 24 hours, depends on the disease entity being treated, the etiologic agent involved, the patient's immune status as well as the patient's ability to tolerate the drug. It should be noted that amphotericin B does not penetrate well into certain tissues/fluids, such as CSF.

Depending on the patient's cardio-renal status (see Precautions, General), doses may gradually be increased by 5 to 10 mg/day to final daily dosage of 0.5 to 1 mg/kg. In patients with impaired cardio-renal function or a severe reaction to the test dose, therapy should be initiated with smaller daily doses (i.e., 5 to 10 mg).

There are insufficient data presently available to define total dosage requirements and duration of treatment necessary for eradication of specific mycoses. The optimal dose is unknown. Dosage may range up to 1 mg/kg per day when administered daily or up to 1.5 mg/kg body weight when given on alternate days.

Duration of therapy depends on such factors as the etiologic agent, anatomic locations of the lesions, stage and severity of the infection, ability of the patient to tolerate amphotericin B and the patient's response to therapy. Several months of therapy may be required; a shorter period of therapy may produce an inadequate response and lead to a relapse.

Sporotrichosis: Therapy with i.v. amphotericin B for sporotrichosis has ranged up to 9 months with a total dose up to 2.5 g.

Aspergillosis: Aspergillosis has been treated with amphotericin B administered i.v. for a period up to 11 months. Doses of 0.5 to 1 mg/kg/day or more, and cumulative doses of 2 to 4 g in adults may be required for serious infections (e.g., pneumonia or fungemia).

Rhinocerebral Phycomycosis: This fulminating disease, generally occurs in association with diabetic ketoacidosis. Therefore, it is imperative that rapid restoration of diabetic control be instituted in order to accomplish successful treatment with FUNGIZONE. In contradistinction, pulmonary phycomycosis, which is more common in association with hematologic malignancies, is often an incidental finding at autopsy. A cumulative dose of at least 3 g of amphotericin B is recommended. Although a total dose of 3 to 4 g will sometimes cause lasting renal impairment, this would seem a reasonable minimum where there is clinical evidence of invasion of the deep tissues. Since rhinocerebral phycomycosis usually follows a rapidly fatal course, the therapeutic approach which often includes surgical intervention must necessarily be more aggressive than that used in more indolent mycoses.

The duration of treatment for deep-seated mycoses may be 6 to 12 weeks or longer.

Candidiasis: In disseminated and/or deep-seated Candida infections, usual doses of amphotericin B range from 0.4 to 0.6 mg/kg/day for 4 or more weeks. Doses up to 1 mg/kg/day may need to be employed depending upon the severity of infection. Treatment is given until obvious clinical improvement is seen and total cumulative doses up to 2 to 4 g in adults may need to be administered. Lower doses (0.3 mg/kg/day) may be employed in special circumstances, e.g., Candida esophagitis that is resistant to local therapy or when amphotericin B is used in combination with other antifungal agents.

Cryptococcosis: Therapy with FUNGIZONE in cryptococcosis in nonimmunosuppressed patients typically may require doses of 0.3 mg/kg/day for periods approximating 4 to 6 weeks or until cultures demonstrate evidence of eradication. In immunosuppressed patients and/or in those with meningitis, amphotericin B may be given in combination with other antifungal agents for 6 weeks. Daily doses of amphotericin B may need to be increased in severely ill patients or in patients receiving amphotericin B alone.

In patients with cryptococcal meningitis and acquired immune deficiency syndrome (AIDS), higher doses (0.7 to 0.8 mg/kg/day) may need to be employed, and treatment courses may extend to 12 weeks. In AIDS patients who are culture negative after a standard course of therapy, chronic suppressive therapy, e.g., 1 mg/kg weekly should be considered.

Coccidioidomycosis: In primary coccidioidomycosis requiring treatment, FUNGIZONE in doses to a maximum of 1.5 mg/kg/day is given to total cumulative doses of 0.5 to 2.5 g in adults depending on the severity and site of infection. In coccidiodal meningitis, due to the poor penetration of amphotericin B into the CSF, alternative antifungal therapy or alternate route of administration should be considered.

Blastomycosis: In seriously ill patients with blastomycosis, FUNGIZONE in doses of 0.3 to 1 mg/kg/day to a total cumulative dose of 1.5 to 2.5 g in adults are recommended.

Histoplasmosis: In chronic pulmonary or disseminated histoplasmosis, doses approximating 0.5 to 1 mg/kg/day to a total cumulative dose of 2 to 2.5 g in adults are generally recommended.

Preparation of Solutions: Reconstitute the dry powder as follows: An initial concentrate of 5 mg amphotericin B/mL is first prepared by adding 10 mL Sterile Water for Injection USP without a bacteriostatic agent to the vial of dry powder and shaking the vial until the liquid is clear.

The infusion liquid, providing 0.1 mg amphotericin B/mL is then obtained by further dilution (1:50) with 5% Dextrose Injection USP **of pH above 4.2** to a volume of 500 mL. The pH of each container of Dextrose Injection should be ascertained before use. Commercial Dextrose Injection usually has a pH above 4.2; however, if it is below 4.2, 1 or 2 mL of sterile buffer should be added to the Dextrose Injection before it is used to dilute the concentrated solution of amphotericin B. The Dextrose Injection should then be retested to ascertain that the pH has been adjusted to the required range.

The recommended buffer has the following composition: dibasic sodium phosphate (anhydrous) 1.59 g, monobasic sodium phosphate (anhydrous) 0.96 g, water for injection USP q.s. 100 mL.

The buffer should be sterilized before it is added to the Dextrose Injection, either by filtration through a bacterial retentive stone, mat or membrane (maximum pore size of 0.45 microns), or by autoclaving for 30 minutes at 15 pounds pressure (121°C).

Caution: Aseptic technique must be strictly observed in all handling, since no preservative or bacteriostatic agent is present in the antibiotic or in materials used to prepare it for administration. Entry into the single use vial or into the diluents must be made with a sterile needle. Do not reconstitute with saline solutions. Single use. Discard unused portion.

The use of any diluent other than the ones recommended or the presence of a bacteriostatic agent (e.g., benzyl alcohol) in the diluent may cause precipitation of the antibiotic. Do not use the initial concentrate or the infusion solution if there is any evidence of precipitation or foreign matter in either one.

An in-line membrane filter may be used for i.v. infusion of amphotericin B; however, the mean pore diameter of the filter should not be less than 1.0 micron in order to assure passage of the antibiotic dispersion.

Stability and Storage Recommendations: Prior to reconstitution, FUNGIZONE (amphotericin B) should be stored in the refrigerator (2 to 8°C), protected against exposure to light. The concentrate (5 mg amphotericin B per mL after reconstitution with 10 mL of sterile water for injection USP) may be stored in the dark at room temperature for 24 hours, or in the refrigerator (2 to 8°C) for 1 week with minimal loss of potency and clarity. Any unused material should then be discarded. Solutions prepared for i.v. infusion (0.1 mg or less amphotericin B/mL) should be used promptly after preparation and should be protected from light during administration.

SUPPLIED: Each vial of sterile, lyophilized powder contains: amphotericin B 50 mg and 38.75 mg desoxycholic acid with 10.9 mg sodium phosphate as a buffer. Vials of 20 mL.

Furosemide Injection USP ℞

furosemide

Diuretic

Sandoz

Furosemide Special ℞

furosemide

Diuretic

Sandoz

SUPPLIED: Furosemide Injection USP: Each mL contains: furosemide 10 mg, sodium hydroxide to adjust pH and water for injection. Preservative-free. Amber ampuls of 2 mL, boxes of 10. Single-use amber vials of 4 mL, boxes of 10.

Furosemide Special: Each mL contains: furosemide 10 mg, sodium hydroxide to adjust pH and water for injection. Preservative-free. Single-use amber vials of 25 mL, boxes of 10.

Store between 15 and 30°C. Discard unused portion.

Fuzeon® ℞

enfuvirtide

Antiviral Agent (HIV-1 Fusion Inhibitor)

Roche

Date of Preparation: July 2, 2003
Date of Revision: June 16, 2008

SUMMARY PRODUCT INFORMATION:

Route of Administration	Dosage Form/ Strength	Clinically Relevant Nonmedicinal Ingredients
Subcutaneous Injection	Single-use vial/108 mg/vial	Mannitol For a complete listing of nonmedicinal ingredients see Dosage Forms, Composition and Packaging.

INDICATIONS AND CLINICAL USE: FUZEON (enfuvirtide) in combination with other antiretroviral agents is indicated for:

- the treatment of HIV-1 infection in treatment-experienced patients with evidence of HIV-1 replication despite ongoing antiretroviral therapy.

This indication is based on analysis of plasma HIV-1 RNA levels and CD4 cell counts from 2 controlled studies of FUZEON of 48 weeks duration. Subjects were treatment-experienced adults. Background therapy was selected on the basis of the patients' prior treatment history as well as genotypic and phenotypic viral resistance measurements. Information from these studies indicate that when antiretrovirals are changed due to loss of virologic response FUZEON should be paired with other active antiretrovirals and optimally should not be used as a single agent.

There are no studies of FUZEON in antiretroviral naive patients.

Geriatrics (>65 years of age): Clinical studies of FUZEON did not include sufficient numbers of subjects aged 65 and over to determine whether they respond differently from younger subjects.

Pediatrics: The safety and pharmacokinetics of FUZEON have not been established in pediatric patients below 6 years of age. Limited data are available in pediatric patients 6 years and older.

CONTRAINDICATIONS:

- FUZEON (enfuvirtide) is contraindicated in patients who are hypersensitive to this drug or to any ingredient in the formulation or component of the container. For a complete listing, see Dosage Forms, Composition and Packaging.

WARNINGS AND PRECAUTIONS:

> **Serious Warnings and Precautions**
> Hypersensitivity reactions have been associated with the use of FUZEON (enfuvirtide) in clinical trials (<1%). See Hypersensitivity Reactions.

General: FUZEON should always be used in combination with other antiretroviral agents.

Non HIV Infected Individuals: There is a theoretical risk that FUZEON use may lead to the production of anti-enfuvirtide antibodies which cross react with HIV gp41. This could result in a false positive HIV test with an ELISA assay; a confirmatory western blot test would be expected to be negative. FUZEON has not been studied in non HIV-infected individuals.

Carcinogenesis and Mutagenesis: Animal carcinogenicity studies of enfuvirtide are ongoing. Enfuvirtide was neither mutagenic nor clastogenic in a series of in vivo and in vitro assays.

Hypersensitivity Reactions: Hypersensitivity reactions have been associated with therapy with FUZEON and may recur on re-challenge. Hypersensitivity reactions have occurred in <1% of patients studied and have included individually and in combination: rash, fever, nausea and vomiting, chills, rigors, hypotension, and elevated serum liver transaminases. Other adverse events that may be immune mediated and have been reported in subjects receiving FUZEON include primary immune complex reaction, respiratory distress, glomerulonephritis, and Guillain-Barre syndrome. Patients developing signs and symptoms suggestive of a systemic hypersensitivity reaction should discontinue FUZEON and should seek medical evaluation immediately. Therapy with FUZEON should not be restarted following systemic signs and symptoms consistent with a hypersensitivity reaction. Risk factors that may predict the occurrence or severity of hypersensitivity to FUZEON have not been identified (see Adverse Reactions).

Immune: Immune Reconstitution: Immune Reconstitution Syndrome has been reported in patients treated with combination antiretroviral therapy, including FUZEON. During the initial phase of combination antiretroviral treatment, a patient whose immune system responds to therapy may develop an inflammatory response to indolent or residual opportunistic infections (such as MAC, CMV, PCP and TB) which may necessitate further evaluation and treatment.

Respiratory: Pneumonia: An increased rate of bacterial pneumonia was observed in patients treated with FUZEON in the Phase III clinical trials compared to the control arm (see Adverse Reactions). It is unclear if the increased incidence of pneumonia is related to the use of FUZEON. Patients with HIV infection should be monitored for signs and symptoms of pneumonia especially if they have underlying conditions which may predispose them to pneumonia. Risk factors for pneumonia included low initial CD4 lymphocyte count, high initial viral load, intravenous drug use, smoking and prior history of lung disease.

Skin: Local Injection Site Reactions: Local injection site reactions were the most common adverse events associated with the use of FUZEON (98% of patients in Phase III clinical trials had at least one local injection site reaction). Manifestations may include pain and discomfort, induration, erythema, nodules and cysts, pruritus and ecchymosis. Local site reactions that required analgesics or limited usual activities were seen in 11% of patients (see Adverse Reactions). Patients must be familiar with the "FUZEON Injection Instructions" in order to know how to inject FUZEON appropriately and how to monitor carefully for signs or symptoms of cellulitis or local infection.

Special Populations: Pregnant Women: There are no adequate and well-controlled studies in pregnant women. Enfuvirtide produced no adverse effects on the developing conceptus in teratology studies conducted at exposures of up to 8.9 times higher in rats and 3.2 times higher in rabbits, than estimated human therapeutic exposures. FUZEON should be used during pregnancy only if the potential benefit justifies the potential risk to the fetus.

Antiretroviral Pregnancy Registry: To monitor maternal-fetal outcomes of pregnant women exposed to FUZEON and other antiretroviral drugs, an Antiretroviral Pregnancy Registry has been established. Physicians are encouraged to register patients by calling 1-800-258-4263.

Nursing Women: It is not known whether enfuvirtide is secreted in human milk. Studies where radio-labeled ^{3}H-enfuvirtide was administered to lactating rats indicated that a very low level of radioactivity was present in the milk. Because of both the potential for HIV transmission and any possible adverse effects in nursing infants, mothers should be instructed not to breast-feed if they are receiving FUZEON.

Pediatrics: The safety and pharmacokinetics of FUZEON have not been fully established in pediatric patients below 6 years of age, as there were too few patients studied in this age group. Limited efficacy data are available in pediatric patients 6 years of age and older.

Geriatrics (>65 years of age): Clinical studies of FUZEON did not include sufficient numbers of subjects aged 65 and over to determine whether they respond differently from younger subjects.

ADVERSE REACTIONS: Adverse Drug Reaction Overview: In clinical studies the most serious adverse reactions observed with FUZEON (enfuvirtide) were hypersensitivity reactions and pneumonia. Local injection site reactions were the most common adverse events associated with the use of FUZEON.

Clinical Trial Adverse Drug Reactions: Because clinical trials are conducted under very specific conditions the adverse reaction rates observed in the clinical trials may not reflect the rates observed in practice and should not be compared to the rates in the clinical trials of another drug. Adverse drug reaction information from clinical trials is useful for identifying drug-related adverse events and for approximating rates.

The overall safety profile of FUZEON (enfuvirtide) is based on 2120 patients who received at least 1 dose of FUZEON during various clinical trials. The safety population consisted of 2051 adults including 658 adults who have been exposed to the recommended dose for greater than 48 weeks and 69 pediatric patients.

Assessment of treatment-emergent adverse events is based on the pooled data from the two Phase III studies TORO-1 and TORO-2. In these studies FUZEON was administered subcutaneously at a dose of 90 mg bid in combination with a background regimen to 663 patients. A total of 334 patients received background antiretroviral agents alone as the control arm.

In the TORO-1 and TORO-2 studies, after study week 8, patients on background alone who met protocol defined criteria for virological failure were permitted to revise their background regimens and add FUZEON. At week 48 of the study the cumulative exposure to FUZEON+background was 557 patient-years, and to background alone 162 patient-years. Due to this difference in exposure, safety results are expressed as the number of patients with an adverse event per 100 patient-years of exposure.

Treatment-emergent adverse events, excluding injection site reactions, from the Phase III studies (TORO-1 and TORO-2) are summarized for adult patients, regardless of severity and causality in Table 1. Only events occurring at ≥2 per 100 patient-years and at a higher rate in patients treated with FUZEON are summarized in the table; events that occurred at a higher rate in the control arms are not displayed.

Table 1: FUZEON

Rates (per 100 patient-years of exposure) of Patients with Selected Treatment-emergent Adverse Events[a] Reported in ≥2 per 100 Patient-years for Adult Patients and Occurring More Frequently in Patients Treated with FUZEON (Pooled Studies TORO-1/TORO-2 at 48 Weeks)

Adverse Event (by System Organ Class)	FUZEON+ Background Regimen (N=663)	Background Regimen (N=334)
Total Exposure (patient years)	557	162
Blood and Lymphatic System Disorders		
Lymphadenopathy	5.9	1.2
Ear and Labyrinth Disorders		
Vertigo	3.6	0.6
Eye disorders		
Conjunctivitis	4.1	2.5
Gastrointestinal Disorders		
Pancreatitis	3.6	2.5
Gastro-oesophageal Reflux Disease	2.7	2.5
General Disorders and Administrative Site Conditions		
Influenza Like Illness	4.5	3.7
Weakness	2.7	0.6
Infections and Infestations		
Sinusitis	9.5	6.2
Influenza	6.5	6.2
Skin Papilloma	6.6	3.1
Pneumonia	3.6	0.6
Ear Infection	2.2	1.2
Immune System Disorders		
Hypersensitivity	2.0	1.9
Investigations		
Weight Decreased	11.1	10.5
Blood Triglycerides Increased	2.9	1.9

(cont'd)

Table 1: FUZEON *(cont'd)*

Rates (per 100 patient-years of exposure) of Patients with Selected Treatment-emergent Adverse Events[a] Reported in ≥2 per 100 Patient-years for Adult Patients and Occurring More Frequently in Patients Treated with FUZEON (Pooled Studies TORO-1/TORO-2 at 48 Weeks)

Adverse Event (by System Organ Class)	FUZEON+ Background Regimen (N=663)	Background Regimen (N=334)
Haematuria Present	2.2	1.9
Metabolism and Nutrition Disorders		
Appetite Decreased	8.6	4.9
Anorexia	3.8	3.1
Hypertriglyceridaemia	2.0	1.9
Diabetes Mellitus	2.0	0.6
Musculoskeletal, Connective Tissue and Bone Disorders		
Myalgia	7.0	5.6
Nervous System Disorders		
Peripheral Neuropathy	15.4	13.6
Hypoaesthesia	2.9	1.9
Disturbance in Attention	2.3	1.9
Tremor	2.2	1.9
Psychiatric Disorders		
Anxiety	7.5	6.8
Irritability	2.3	1.9
Nightmare	2.3	1.2
Renal and Urinary Disorders		
Calculus Renal	2.3	1.2
Respiratory, Thoracic and Mediastinal Disorders		
Nasal Congestion	3.1	2.5
Skin and Subcutaneous Tissue Disorders		
Dry Skin	5.0	4.3
Eczema Seborrhoeic	2.3	1.9
Erythema	2.2	1.2
Acne	2.0	0.6

[a] Excludes Injection Site Reactions.

Hypersensitivity reactions have been attributed to FUZEON (≤1%) and in some cases have recurred upon re-challenge (see Warnings and Precautions).

The events most frequently reported in patients receiving FUZEON+background regimen, excluding injection site reactions, were diarrhea (38 per 100 patient-years), nausea (27 per 100 patient-years), and fatigue (24 per 100 patient-years). All these events were seen at a lower incidence than in patients that received background regimen alone: diarrhea (73 per 100 patient-years), nausea (50 per 100 patient-years), and fatigue (38 per 100 patient-years). The addition of FUZEON to background antiretroviral therapy generally did not increase the frequency or severity of most adverse events.

Rates of adverse events for patients who switched to FUZEON after virological failure were similar. The only adverse events with a statistically significant risk ratio between the FUZEON regimen and the background regimen alone were pneumonia and lymphadenopathy. Most adverse events were of mild or moderate intensity.

The incidence of pneumonia was 3.6 events/100 patient-years in subjects on the FUZEON+background regimen. On analysis of all diagnoses of pneumonia (pneumonia, bacterial pneumonia, bronchopneumonia, and related terms) in the Phase 3 clinical trials, an increased rate of bacterial pneumonia was observed in subjects on FUZEON+background compared to background alone (6.6 pneumonia events per 100 patient-years versus 0.6 events per 100 patient-years). Approximately half of the study subjects with pneumonia required hospitalization. Three subject deaths in the FUZEON arm were attributed to pneumonia; all three had serious concomitant AIDS-related illnesses that contributed to their deaths. Risk factors for pneumonia included low initial CD4 lymphocyte count, high initial viral load, intravenous drug use, smoking and a prior history of lung disease. It is unclear if the increased incidence of pneumonia was related to the use of FUZEON. However, because of this finding patients with HIV infection should be carefully monitored for signs and symptoms of pneumonia, especially if they have underlying conditions which may predispose them to pneumonia (see Warnings and Precautions). In uncontrolled studies in which only safety events were monitored, a rate of 2.1 pneumonia events per 100 patient-years was reported. The safety population for these studies comprised 1166 patients with exposure to FUZEON of 522 patient-years. Three cases of pneumonia resulted in death; risk factors for pneumonia in two of these cases included low CD4 count at initiation of therapy and one of these cases also had a prior history of recurrent pneumonia.

Local Injection Site Reactions (ISRs): Local injection site reactions were the most frequent adverse events associated with the use of FUZEON. In the TORO-1 and TORO-2 studies combined, 98% of patients had at least 1 local injection site reaction and 4% of patients discontinued treatment with FUZEON because of injection site reactions (see Table 2). Injection site reactions were generally seen within the first week of initiating therapy with FUZEON, and for the majority were associated with either mild tenderness or moderate pain at the injection site without limitation of usual activities. The percentage of patients that required analgesics or limited usual activities was 11% (Grade 3 reactions). The severity of the pain and discomfort associated with injection site reactions did not increase with treatment duration. The signs/symptoms characterizing the injection site reactions generally lasted ≤7 days and the average number of injection site reactions evident at any given study visit was ≤5 (in the 72% of patients with injection site reactions evident). In 24% of subjects an individual injection site reaction lasted for longer than 7 days. Individual signs and symptoms characterizing local injection site reactions are summarized in Table 2. Infection at the injection site (including abscess and cellulitis) was reported in 2.4 per 100 patient-years.

Table 2: FUZEON

Summary of Individual Signs/Symptoms Characterizing Local Injection Site Reactions to Enfuvirtide in Studies TORO-1 and TORO-2 Combined (% of Subjects) through 48 Weeks

Withdrawal Rate Due to Injection Site Reactions	n=663 4%		
Event Category	**FUZEON+ Background Regimen[a] %**	**% of Events Comprising Grade 3 Reactions %**	**% of Events Comprising Grade 4 Reactions %**
Pain/Discomfort	96	11[b]	0[b]
Induration	90	44[c]	19[c]
Erythema	91	24[d]	11[d]
Nodules and Cysts	80	29[e]	0.2[e]
Pruritus	65	4[f]	NA[f]
Ecchymosis	52	9[g]	5[g]

[a] Any severity grade.
[b] Grade 3=severe pain requiring analgesics (or narcotic analgesics for ≤72 hours) and/or limiting usual activities; Grade 4=severe pain requiring hospitalization or prolongation of hospitalization, resulting in death, or persistent or significant disability/incapacity, or life threatening, or medically significant.
[c] Grade 3=≥25 mm but <50 mm average diameter; Grade 4=≥50 mm average diameter.
[d] Grade 3=≥50 mm but <85 mm average diameter; Grade 4=≥85 mm average diameter.
[e] Grade 3=≥3 cm; Grade 4=if draining.
[f] Grade 3=refractory to topical treatment or requiring oral or parenteral treatment; Grade 4=not defined.
[g] Grade 3=>3 cm but ≤5 cm; Grade 4=>5 cm.

A non-blinded, randomized, 4 cohort, crossover study (N=66) evaluated the effects of gentle manual massage, heated moist cloth, topical hydrocortisone (1% cream) and self vs partner injection on ISRs. The severity of ISR signs and symptoms with each intervention was compared with no intervention (control) based on patient recall and clinical assessments. In general, manual gentle massage, and partner injection appear to be interventions that may offer a slight benefit in some patients for reducing the severity of ISR signs and symptoms.

Adverse Events in Pediatric Patients: FUZEON has been studied in 69 pediatric patients 4 through 16 years of age with duration of exposure to FUZEON ranging from 1 dose to 134 weeks. Adverse reactions seen during clinical trials were similar to those observed in adult patients.

Less Common Clinical Trial Adverse Events: The following adverse events have been reported in 1 or more patients; however, a causal relationship to FUZEON has not been established.

Blood and Lymphatic Disorders: thrombocytopenia with neutropenia and fever.
Cardiac Disorders: unstable angina pectoris.
Endocrine and Metabolic: hyperglycemia.
Gastrointestinal Disorders: constipation; abdominal pain upper.
General: asthenia.
Hepato-biliary Disorders: toxic hepatitis; hepatic steatosis.
Immune System Disorders: worsening abacavir hypersensitivity reaction.
Infections: sepsis; herpes simplex.
Investigations: increased amylase; increased lipase; increased AST; increased GGT.
Nervous System Disorders: taste disturbance; Guillain-Barre syndrome (fatal); sixth nerve palsy.
Psychiatric Disorders: insomnia; depression.
Renal and Urinary Disorders: glomerulonephritis; tubular necrosis; renal insufficiency; renal failure (including fatal cases).
Respiratory, Thoracic, and Mediastinal Disorders: pneumopathy; respiratory distress; cough.
Skin and Subcutaneous Tissue Disorders: pruritus.
Abnormal Hematologic and Clinical Chemistry Findings: Table 3 shows the treatment-emergent laboratory abnormalities that occurred in at least 2 patients per 100 patient-years and more frequently in those receiving FUZEON+background regimen than background regimen alone, from the pooled studies TORO-1 and TORO-2.

Table 3: FUZEON

Percentage of Treatment-emergent Laboratory Abnormalities That Occurred in ≥2 per 100 Patient-years for Adult Patients and More Frequently in Patients Receiving FUZEON (pooled studies TORO-1 and TORO-2, 48 weeks)

Laboratory Parameters	Grading	FUZEON + Background Regimen N=663	Background Regimen N=334
ALT			
Gr. 3	>5–10×ULN	4.8	4.3
Gr. 4	>10×ULN	1.4	1.2
Creatine Phosphokinase (U/L)			
Gr. 3	>5–10×ULN	8.3	8.0
Gr. 4	>10×ULN	3.1	8.6
Eosinophilia			
1–2×ULN (0.7×10[9] cells/L)	0.7–1.4×10[9]/L	10.8	3.7
>2×ULN (0.7×10[9] cells/L)	>1.4×10[9]/L	2.2	1.8
Hemoglobin (g/dL)			
Gr. 3	6.5–7.9 g/dL	2.0	1.9
Gr. 4	<6.5 g/dL	0.7	1.2

DRUG INTERACTIONS: Overview: CYP450 Metabolized Drugs: Results from in vitro and in vivo studies suggest that enfuvirtide is unlikely to have significant drug interactions with concomitantly administered drugs metabolized by CYP450 enzymes.
Antiretroviral Agents: No drug interactions with other antiretroviral medications have been identified that would warrant alteration of either the enfuvirtide dose or the dose of the other antiretroviral medication.

Drug-Drug Interactions: Influence of FUZEON (enfuvirtide) on the Metabolism of Concomitant Drugs: Based on the results from an in vitro human microsomal study, enfuvirtide is not an inhibitor of CYP450 enzymes. In an in vivo human metabolism study (N=12), FUZEON at the recommended dose of 90 mg bid did not affect the metabolic activity of CYP3A4, CYP2D6 and N-acetyltransferase, increased the metabolic activity of CYP2C19 by 13% (90% CI: −2% to +28%) and of CYP2E1 by 8% (90% CI: −13% to +29%) and decreased the metabolic activity for CYP1A2 by 6% (90% CI: −29% to +17%).

Influence of Concomitant Drugs on the Metabolism of Enfuvirtide: In separate pharmacokinetic interaction studies, coadministration of ritonavir (N=12), saquinavir/ritonavir (N=12), and rifampin (N=12) did not result in clinically significant pharmacokinetic interactions with FUZEON (see Table 4).

Table 4: FUZEON

Effect of Ritonavir, Saquinavir/Ritonavir, and Rifampin on the Steady-State Pharmacokinetics of Enfuvirtide (90 mg bid)[a]

Coadministered Drug	Dose of Coadministered Drug	N	% Change of Enfuvirtide Pharmacokinetic Parameters[b,c] (90% CI)		
			C_{max}	AUC	C_{trough}
Ritonavir	200 mg, q12h, 4 days	12	↑24 (↑9 to ↑41)	↑22 (↑8 to ↑37)	↑14 (↑2 to ↑28)
Saquinavir/Ritonavir	1000/100 mg, q12h, 4 days	12	↔	↑14 (↑5 to ↑24)	↑26 (↑17 to ↑35)
Rifampin	600 mg, qd, 10 days	12	↔	↔	↓15 (↓22 to ↓7)

[a] All studies were performed in HIV 1+ subjects using sequential crossover design.
[b] ↑=increase; ↓=decrease; ↔=No Effect (↑ or ↓ <10%).
[c] No interactions were clinically significant.

DOSAGE AND ADMINISTRATION: Recommended Dose and Dosage Adjustment: Adults: The recommended dose of FUZEON (enfuvirtide) is 90 mg (1 mL) twice daily injected subcutaneously into the upper arm, anterior thigh or abdomen. The injection should be given at a site different from the preceding injection site and where there is no current injection site reaction from an earlier dose. Also, do not inject into moles, scar tissue, bruises, and navel (see Information for the Patient, FUZEON Injection Directions).

Pediatric Patients: No data are available to establish a dose recommendation of FUZEON in pediatric patients below the age of 6 years. Based on limited data in pediatric patients 6 through 16 years of age, it is expected that a dosage of 2.0 mg/kg twice daily up to a maximum dose of 90 mg bid injected subcutaneously into the upper arm, anterior thigh or abdomen will produce enfuvirtide plasma concentrations similar to those achieved in adult patients receiving 90 mg bid dosage. The injection should be given at a site different from the preceding injection site and where there is no current injection site reaction from an earlier dose. Do not inject into moles, scar tissue, bruises, and navel (see Information for the Patient, FUZEON Injection Directions). Table 5 contains dosing guidelines for FUZEON based on body weight. Weight should be monitored periodically and the dose of FUZEON adjusted accordingly.

Table 5: FUZEON

Pediatric Dosing Guidelines

Weight (kg)	Dose per bid Injection (mg/dose)	Injection Volume (90 mg enfuvirtide per mL)
11.0 to 15.5	27	0.3 mL
15.6 to 20.0	36	0.4 mL
20.1 to 24.5	45	0.5 mL
24.6 to 29.0	54	0.6 mL
29.1 to 33.5	63	0.7 mL
33.6 to 38.0	72	0.8 mL
38.1 to 42.5	81	0.9 mL
≥42.6	90	1.0 mL

Missed Dose: If a dose of FUZEON is missed, you should take the missed dose as soon as you can and then take the next dose as scheduled. If you have missed a dose of FUZEON and it is close to the time for your next dose, wait and take the next dose as regularly scheduled. Do not take two doses of FUZEON at the same time.

Administration: For more detailed instructions, see Information for the Patient, FUZEON Injection Directions.

FUZEON must only be reconstituted with 1.1 mL of Sterile Water for Injection. After adding the water, the vial should be gently tapped for 10 seconds and then allowed to stand until the powder goes completely into solution, which could take up to 45 minutes. Before the solution is withdrawn for administration, the vial should be inspected visually to ensure that the contents are fully in solution, and that the solution is clear, colourless and without bubbles or particulate matter. If there is evidence of particulate matter, the vial must not be used and should be discarded or returned to the pharmacy.

FUZEON contains no preservative. Once reconstituted, FUZEON should be injected immediately. If the reconstituted FUZEON cannot be injected immediately, it must be kept refrigerated in the vial until use and used within 24 hours. Refrigerated reconstituted solution should be brought to room temperature before injection and the vial should be inspected visually again to ensure that the contents are fully in solution and that the solution is clear, colourless and without bubbles or particulate matter.

The reconstituted solution should be injected subcutaneously in the upper arm, abdomen or anterior thigh. The injection should be given at a site different from the preceding injection site and where there is no current injection site reaction. Also, do not inject into moles, scar tissue, bruises, and navel. A vial is suitable for single use only; unused portions must be discarded.

Patients should contact their healthcare professional for any questions regarding the administration of FUZEON. Patients should be taught to recognize the signs and symptoms of injection site reactions and instructed when to contact their healthcare professional about these reactions.

Reconstitution:

FUZEON Vial Size	Volume of Diluent to be Added to FUZEON Vial	Approximate Available Volume	Nominal Concentration per mL
3 mL	1.1 mL	1.2 mL	90 mg/mL[a]

[a] 1 mL of the reconstituted solution contains the label claim of 90 mg enfuvirtide.

FUZEON must only be reconstituted with the diluent supplied, 1.1 mL of sterile water for injection. Once reconstituted, FUZEON solution should be injected immediately. If the reconstituted solution cannot be injected immediately it must be refrigerated until use and used within 24 hours.

OVERDOSAGE:

There are no reports of human experience of acute overdose with FUZEON (enfuvirtide). The highest dose administered to 12 patients in a clinical trial was 180 mg as a single dose subcutaneously. These patients did not experience any adverse events that were not seen with the recommended dose. There is no specific antidote for overdose with FUZEON. Treatment of overdose should consist of general supportive measures.

For management of a suspected drug overdose, CPhA recommends that you contact your **regional Poison Control Centre**. See the *CPS* Directory section for a list of Poison Control Centres.

ACTION AND CLINICAL PHARMACOLOGY: Mechanism of Action: FUZEON (enfuvirtide) is an inhibitor of HIV-1 gp41 mediated fusion derived from a naturally occurring motif, amino acid residues (643-678) within the gp41 transmembrane glycoprotein of human immunodeficiency virus type 1 strain LAI ($HIV\text{-}1_{LAI}$).

Enfuvirtide interferes with the entry of HIV-1 into cells by inhibiting fusion of viral and cellular membranes. Enfuvirtide binds to the first heptad-repeat (HR1) in the gp41 subunit of the viral envelope glycoprotein and prevents the conformational changes required for the fusion of viral and cellular membranes.

Antiviral Activity In Vitro: The in vitro antiviral activity of enfuvirtide was assessed by infecting different CD4+ cell types with laboratory and clinical isolates of HIV-1. The IC_{50} (50% inhibitory concentration) for enfuvirtide in laboratory and primary isolates representing HIV-1 clades A to G ranged from 4 to 280 nM (18 to 1260 ng/mL). The IC_{50} for baseline clinical isolates ranged from 0.089 to 107 nM (0.4 to 480 ng/mL) by the cMAGI assay (n=130). The relationship between the in vitro susceptibility of HIV-1 to enfuvirtide and inhibition of HIV-1 replication in humans has not been established.

Pharmacokinetics: The pharmacokinetic properties of enfuvirtide were evaluated in HIV-1 infected adult and pediatric patients (see Table 6).

Table 6: FUZEON

Summary of Pharmacokinetic Parameters in HIV-1 Infected Patients

C_{max} (µg/mL)	$t_{1/2}$ (h)	$AUC_{0-\infty}$ (µ· h/mL)	Clearance (L/h)	Volume of Distribution (L)[a]
4.59	3.8	55.8	1.7	5.5

[a] Intravenous administration of a 90 mg dose of FUZEON.

Absorption: After a 90 mg subcutaneous single dose of FUZEON in the abdomen in 12 HIV-1 infected patients, the mean (±SD) C_{max} was 4.59±1.5 µg/mL, AUC was 55.8±12.1 µg·h/mL and absolute bioavailability (using the 90 mg intravenous dose as a reference) was 84.3%±15.5%.

The subcutaneous absorption of enfuvirtide is basically proportional to the administered dose over the 45 mg to 180 mg dose range. Subcutaneous absorption at the 90 mg dose is comparable when injected into the abdomen, thigh or arm. In 4 separate studies (N=9 to 12) the mean steady-state trough plasma concentration ranged from 2.6 to 3.4 µg/mL.

Distribution: The mean (±SD) steady state volume of distribution after intravenous administration of a 90 mg dose of FUZEON (N=12) was 5.5±1.1 L. Enfuvirtide is 92% bound to plasma proteins in HIV infected plasma over a concentration range of 2 to 10 µg/mL. It is bound predominantly to albumin and to a lower extent to α-1 acid glycoprotein. Enfuvirtide was not displaced from its binding sites by saquinavir, nelfinavir, lopinavir, efavirenz, nevirapine, amprenavir, itraconazole, midazolam or warfarin. Enfuvirtide did not displace warfarin, midazolam, amprenavir or efavirenz from their binding sites.

Enfuvirtide levels in the cerebrospinal fluid measured in a small number of HIV infected patients were reported to be negligible. The molecule may be too large to pass the blood brain barrier.

Metabolism: As a peptide, enfuvirtide is expected to undergo catabolism, to its constituent amino acids, with subsequent recycling of the amino acids in the body pool.

In in vitro human microsomal and hepatocyte studies, hydrolysis of the amide group of the C-terminus amino acid, phenylalanine, results in a deamidated metabolite. This reaction is not NADPH dependent. This metabolite is detected in human plasma following administration of enfuvirtide, with an AUC ranging from 2.4% to 15% of the enfuvirtide AUC.

Excretion: Mass balance studies to determine elimination pathway(s) of enfuvirtide have not been performed in humans. However, such studies in rodents using 3H-enfuvirtide indicated incomplete recovery of the administered radioactivity in the excreta 7 days after the dose. Following a 90 mg subcutaneous dose of enfuvirtide (N=12) the mean±SD elimination half-life of enfuvirtide is 3.8±0.6 h and the mean±SD clearance is 1.7±0.4 L/h.

Special Populations and Conditions: Pediatrics: The pharmacokinetics of enfuvirtide have been studied in 25 pediatric patients aged 5 through 16 years (one 5 year old was studied) at a dose of 2 mg/kg. Data from one patient was excluded due to a very low AUC_{12h} value. In the remaining 24 pediatric patients receiving the 2 mg/kg bid dose, the mean ±SD steady-state AUC_{12} was 56.3±21.8 µg·h/mL, C_{max} was 6.3±2.3 µg/mL, C_{trough} was 3.0±1.5 µg/mL, and the apparent clearance was 40±16 mL/h/kg.

A dose of 2 mg/kg bid (maximum 90 mg bid) is expected to provide enfuvirtide plasma concentrations similar to those obtained in adult patients receiving 90 mg bid dosage.

Geriatrics: The pharmacokinetics of enfuvirtide have not been studied in patients over 65 years of age.

Gender and Weight: Analysis of plasma concentration data from patients in clinical trials indicated that the clearance of enfuvirtide is 20% lower in females than males and is increased with increased body weight irrespective of gender (20% higher in a 100 kg and 20% lower in a 40 kg body weight patient relative to a 70 kg reference patient). However, these changes are not clinically significant and no dose adjustment is required.

Race: Analysis of plasma concentration data from patients in clinical trials indicated that the clearance of enfuvirtide was not different in Blacks compared to Caucasians. Other pharmacokinetic studies suggest no difference between Asians and Caucasians after adjusting for body weight.

Hepatic Insufficiency: The pharmacokinetics of enfuvirtide have not been studied in patients with hepatic impairment.

Renal Insufficiency: Analysis of plasma concentration data from patients in clinical trials indicated that the clearance of enfuvirtide is not affected to any clinically relevant extent in patients with creatinine clearance above 35 mL/min. The results of a renal impairment study indicate clearance of enfuvirtide was reduced by 38% in patients with severe renal impairment (n=4) and by 14-28% in patients with end stage renal disease maintained on dialysis (n=8) compared to patients with normal renal function (n=8). The results were within the range seen in patients in the pivotal studies with normal renal function. Hemodialysis did not significantly alter enfuvirtide clearance. Thus, no dose adjustment is recommended for patients with impaired renal function including those receiving hemodialysis.

STORAGE AND STABILITY: Powder for solution: Store at 15-30°C.

Reconstituted solution: Store in refrigerator (2 to 8°C) for no longer than 24 hours.

Unused portions of FUZEON remaining in the single-use vial should be discarded.

INFORMATION FOR THE PATIENT: Published in e-CPS, available by subscription at www.e-cps.ca.

DOSAGE FORMS, COMPOSITION AND PACKAGING: Each single-use vial of white to off-white, sterile, lyophilized powder contains: enfuvirtide 108 mg. Reconstitution with sterile water for injection yields a 90 mg/mL solution of enfuvirtide. Nonmedicinal ingredients: hydrochloric acid, mannitol, sodium carbonate and sodium hydroxide. Institutional or convenience kits containing: 60 vials of FUZEON, 60 vials containing 2 mL of diluent (sterile water for injection), reconstitution-syringes, administration syringes, and alcohol wipes; 28 vials of FUZEON, 28 vials containing 2 mL of diluent (sterile water for injection), reconstitution-syringes, administration syringes, and alcohol wipes; 10 vials of FUZEON, 10 vials containing 2 mL of diluent (sterile water for injection), reconstitution-syringes, administration syringes, and alcohol wipes.

FXT Ⓟ

fluoxetine HCl

Antidepressant—Antiobsessional—Antibulimic

Sepracor

SUPPLIED: Each light blue and white capsule, printed with "Fluoxetine 40 mg" on cap and "SHN" on body, contains: fluoxetine HCl equivalent to fluoxetine 40 mg. Nonmedicinal ingredients: FD&C Blue No. 2, FD&C Red No. 40 on an aluminum substrate and pregelatinized starch; capsule shell: FD&C Blue No. 1, gelatin and titanium dioxide. White HDPE bottles of 30, 100 and 500. Store at 15-25°C. Keep tightly closed. Protect from light.

G
H

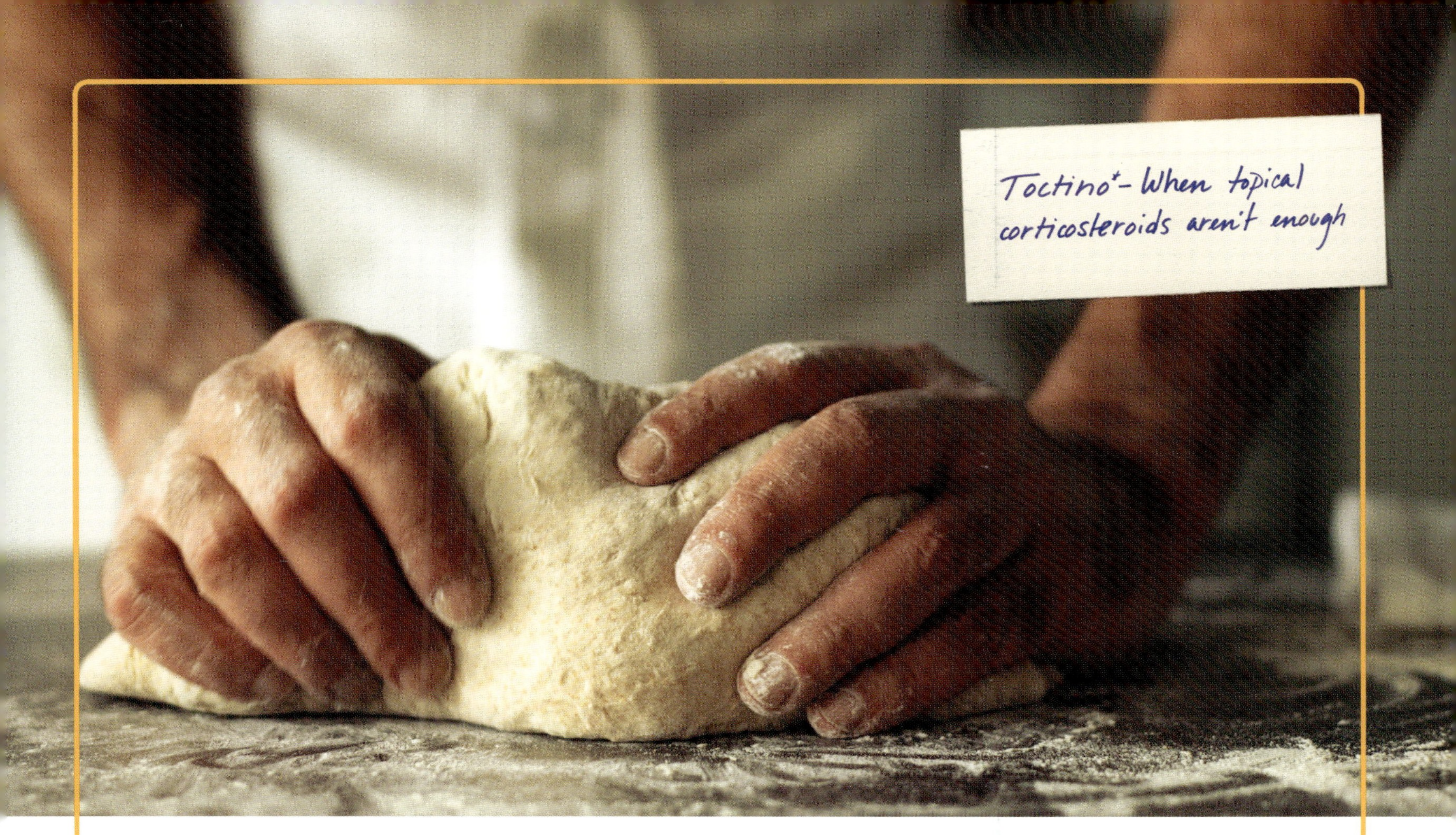

Toctino*. A new oral agent indicated for the treatment of severe **Chronic Hand Eczema** (CHE) refractory to high potency topical corticosteroids in adults.[1]

- Efficacy demonstrated in clearing severe CHE (PGA rating of clear/almost clear) at 12 to 24 weeks (48%‡, 28%△, and 17% for 30 mg, 10 mg, and placebo, respectively; ‡$p<0.001$ and △$p<0.004$ vs. placebo)[1,2†]

† Double-blind, placebo-controlled, parallel-group, multicentre study of 1,032 patients randomized in a 2:2:1 ratio to 30 mg, 10 mg, and placebo for the treatment of severe CHE refractory to high potency topical corticosteroids. PGA (Physician Global Assessment) detailed results: 30 mg (clear: 22%; almost clear: 25.7%; n=409); 10 mg (clear: 9.3%; almost clear: 18.2%; n=418); placebo (clear: 2.9%; almost clear: 13.7%; n=205).

TOCTINO* (alitretinoin) is contraindicated in pregnancy.

Females must not become pregnant while taking TOCTINO*, and for at least one month after its discontinuation. TOCTINO* can cause severe birth defects in infants born to women who become pregnant during treatment with TOCTINO* in any amount, even for a short period of time. Potentially any exposed fetus can be affected. There are no accurate means of determining whether an exposed fetus has been affected.

If pregnancy does occur during treatment with TOCTINO*, or within one month after its discontinuation, TOCTINO* treatment must be immediately stopped and the physician and patient should discuss the desirability of continuing the pregnancy.

TOCTINO* should only be prescribed by physicians knowledgeable in the use of retinoids systemically.

- Convenient once-daily oral dose[1]

Toctino* should only be prescribed by physicians knowledgeable in the use of retinoids systemically, who understand the risk of teratogenicity in females of childbearing potential.

Serious Warnings and Precautions

Pregnancy Prevention: TOCTINO* (alitretinoin) is a known teratogen contraindicated in pregnancy (see boxed CONTRAINDICATIONS). Physicians should only prescribe TOCTINO* to females of childbearing potential if ALL the conditions described below under "Conditions of use" are met. In addition, when prescribing this drug to female patients of childbearing potential, physicians must use the TOCTINO* Pregnancy Prevention Program, which includes comprehensive information about the potential risks of this drug, a checklist for criteria which must be met prior to prescribing this drug to female patients of childbearing potential, detailed information on birth control options, a patient informed consent for review and signature, and monthly pregnancy reminders for physicians to use at each patient visit during the treatment period.

Neurologic: Treatment with systemic retinoids, including alitretinoin, has been associated with the occurrence of benign intracranial hypertension, some of which involved concomitant use of tetracyclines (see CONTRAINDICATIONS AND WARNINGS AND PRECAUTIONS). Signs and symptoms of benign intracranial hypertension include headache, nausea and vomiting, visual disturbances and papilloedema. Patients who develop signs of benign intracranial hypertension should discontinue alitretinoin immediately (class effect).

TOCTINO*(alitretinoin) is indicated for the treatment of severe Chronic Hand Eczema (CHE) refractory to high potency topical corticosteroids in adults. The most frequent adverse drug reactions (ADRs) observed under alitretinoin therapy are headache (30 mg, 21%; 10 mg, 11.3%) and flushing (30 mg, 5.9%; 10 mg, 1.6%). TOCTINO* is contraindicated in patients with hepatic insufficiency, severe renal insufficiency, uncontrolled hypercholesterolemia, uncontrolled hypertriglyceridemia, uncontrolled hypothyroidism, hypervitaminosis A, hypersensitivity to retinoids or excipients, fructose intolerance, on tetracyclines, and breastfeeding women.

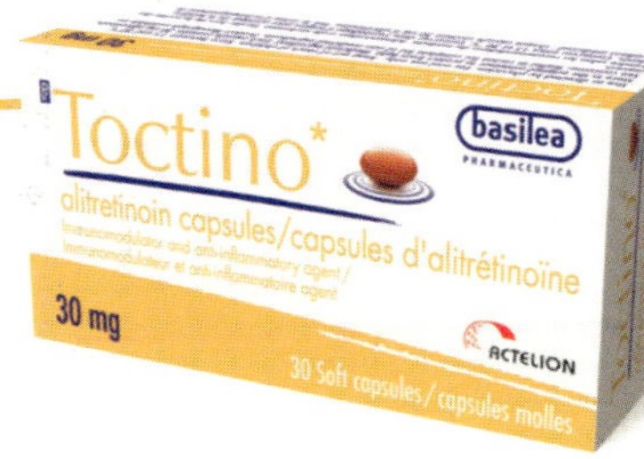

* Trademark of Basilea Pharmaceutica AG, Basel, Switzerland; used under licence.

Actelion Pharmaceuticals Canada Inc. Laval, Quebec H7T 2L1 Tel: 1-866-531-4885. www.toctino.ca

ACTELION

PAAB R&D

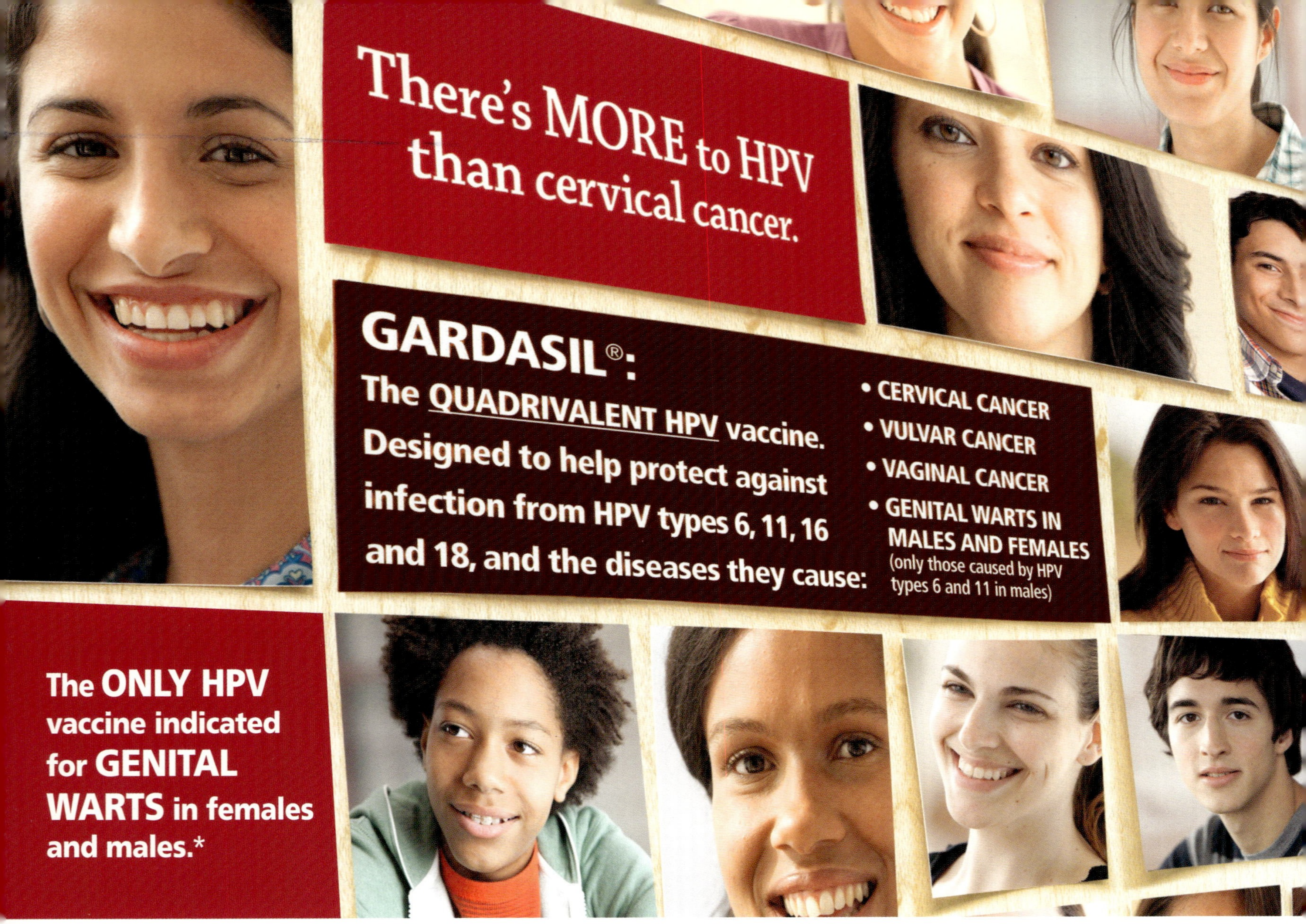

INDICATIONS AND CLINICAL USE

GARDASIL® is a vaccine indicated in girls and women 9-26 years of age, for the prevention of infection caused by the Human Papillomavirus (HPV) types 6,11,16 and 18, and the following diseases associated with these HPV types: cervical, vulvar and vaginal cancers, genital warts, cervical adenocarcinoma *in situ* (AIS), cervical intraepithelial neoplasia (CIN) grades 1, 2 and 3, and vulvar and vaginal intraepithelial neoplasia (VIN/VaIN) grades 2 and 3. GARDASIL® is indicated in boys and men 9-26 years of age for the prevention of infection caused by HPV types 6, 11, 16 and 18, and genital warts caused by HPV types 6 and 11.

SELECTED IMPORTANT SAFETY INFORMATION

The most commonly reported vaccine-related injection-site adverse experiences in clinical trials with GARDASIL® in females (n = 5,088), amorphous aluminum hydroxyphosphate sulfate (AAHS) adjuvant-containing placebo (n = 3,470) and saline placebo (n = 320), respectively, were pain (83.9%, 75.4%, 48.6%), swelling (25.4%, 15.8%, 7.3%), erythema (24.7%, 18.4%, 12.1%), and pruritus (3.2%, 2.8%, 0.6%). The most commonly reported vaccine-related systemic adverse experience in females was fever: 10.3% for GARDASIL® (n = 5,088) vs 8.6% for AAHS adjuvant- and non-AAHS adjuvant-containing placebo (n = 3,790). The most commonly reported vaccine-related injection-site adverse experiences in clinical trials with GARDASIL® in males (n = 3,092), AAHS adjuvant-containing placebo (n = 2,029) and saline placebo (n = 274), respectively, were pain (61.5%, 50.8%, 41.6%), erythema (16.7%, 14.1%, 14.5%) and swelling (13.9%, 9.6%, 8.2%). The most commonly reported vaccine-related systemic adverse experience in males was headache: 7.5% for GARDASIL® (n = 3,092) vs 6.7% for AAHS adjuvant- and non-AAHS adjuvant-containing placebo (n = 2,303).

This vaccine is not intended to be used for treatment of active external genital lesions; cervical, vulvar or vaginal cancers; CIN, VIN, or VaIN. This vaccine will not protect against diseases that are not caused by HPV. Routine monitoring and Pap test should continue to be performed as indicated, regardless of GARDASIL® administration. Pregnancy should be avoided during the vaccination regimen for GARDASIL®. As for any vaccine, vaccination with GARDASIL® may not result in protection in all vaccine recipients. Syncope (fainting) may follow any vaccination, especially in adolescents and young adults. Syncope, sometimes associated with falling, has occurred after vaccination with GARDASIL®. Therefore, vaccinees should be carefully observed for approximately 15 minutes after administration of GARDASIL®.

PLEASE CONSULT THE ENCLOSED PRESCRIBING INFORMATION FOR INDICATIONS, CONTRAINDICATIONS, WARNINGS, PRECAUTIONS AND DOSING GUIDELINES.

*Comparative clinical significance has not been established.

When you talk to your patients about **HPV**

SELECT GARDASIL® TO HELP PROTECT AGAINST HPV types 6, 11, 16 and 18, and the diseases they cause:

- CERVICAL CANCER
- VULVAR CANCER
- VAGINAL CANCER
- GENITAL WARTS IN MALES AND FEMALES (only those caused by HPV types 6 and 11 in males)

GARDASIL.

[Quadrivalent Human Papillomavirus (Types 6,11,16,18) Recombinant Vaccine]

The QUADRIVALENT HPV vaccine

MERCK

Merck Canada Inc., Kirkland, Quebec

Gardasil® is a Registered Trademark of Merck Sharp & Dohme Corp., a subsidiary of **Merck & Co., Inc.** Used under license. Please visit our website at www.merck.ca

PAAB

11-11-HPV-10-CDN-84140736-CPS/JA

G

Gadovist®1.0

gadobutrol

Contrast Enhancement Agent for Magnetic Resonance Imaging (MRI)

Bayer

Date of Revision: July 27, 2010

SUMMARY PRODUCT INFORMATION:

Route of Administration	Dosage Form/ Strength	Clinically Relevant Nonmedicinal Ingredients
Intravenous	Solution/604 mg/mL (1.0 mmol/L) gadobutrol injection	None. For a complete listing see Dosage Forms, Composition and Packaging.

INDICATIONS AND CLINICAL USE: GADOVIST 1.0 (gadobutrol) is a medicinal product for diagnostic use only.

GADOVIST 1.0 (gadobutrol) is indicated in adults, adolescents, and children aged 2 years and older for:

- contrast enhancement during cranial and spinal MRI investigations and for contrast-enhanced magnetic resonance angiography (CE-MRA). See Dosage and Administration, Recommended Dose and Dosage Adjustment for specific dosage recommendations.
- GADOVIST 1.0 is particularly suited for cases where the exclusion or demonstration of additional pathology may influence the choice of therapy or patient management, for detection of very small lesions and for visualization of tumors that do not readily take up contrast media.
- GADOVIST 1.0 is also suited for perfusion studies for the diagnosis of stroke, detection of focal cerebral ischemia and tumor perfusion.

Geriatrics: No special precautions are required in elderly patients unless renal function is impaired (see Warnings and Precautions, Serious Warnings and Precautions and Warnings and Precautions, Renal).

Pediatrics (2-17 years of age): The safety and efficacy of GADOVIST 1.0 at a dose of 0.1 mmol/kg have been established in adolescents and in children 2 years of age and older. (See Adverse Reactions, Clinical Trial Adverse Drug Reactions, Pediatric Population; Action and Clinical Pharmacology, Special Populations and Conditions, Pediatrics and Dosage and Administration.)

GADOVIST 1.0 is not recommended for use in children below 2 years of age due to a lack of data on safety and efficacy (see Warnings and Precautions, Special Populations).

CONTRAINDICATIONS:

- There are no absolute contraindications to the use of GADOVIST 1.0 (see Warnings and Precautions, Hypersensitivity).

WARNINGS AND PRECAUTIONS:

> **Serious Warnings and Precautions**
> **NEPHROGENIC SYSTEMIC FIBROSIS**
> Gadolinium-based contrast agents (GBCAs) increase the risk for Nephrogenic Systemic Fibrosis (NSF) in patients with:
> - acute or chronic severe renal insufficiency (glomerular filtration rate <30 mL/min/1.73m²), or
> - acute renal insufficiency of any severity due to the hepato-renal syndrome or in the perioperative liver transplantation period.
>
> In these patients, avoid use of GBCAs unless the diagnostic information is essential and not available with noncontrast-enhanced magnetic resonance imaging (MRI). NSF may result in fatal or debilitating systemic fibrosis affecting the skin, muscle, and internal organs. Screen all patients for renal dysfunction by obtaining a history and/or laboratory tests. When administering a GBCA, do not exceed the recommended dose (see Dosage and Administration, Recommended Dose and Dosage Adjustment) and allow a sufficient period of time for elimination of the agent from the body prior to any readministration (see Warnings and Precautions, General, Renal and Skin, and Adverse Reactions, Post-Market Adverse Drug Reactions).

General: Deoxygenated sickle erythrocytes have been shown in in vitro studies to align perpendicularly to a magnetic field which may result in vaso-occlusive complications in vivo. The enhancement of magnetic moment by gadobutrol may possibly potentiate sickle erythrocyte alignment. The use of gadobutrol in patients with sickle cell anemia and other hemoglobinopathies has not been studied.

MRI and MRA procedures which involve the use of gadobutrol should be carried out by medical staff who have the prerequisite training and a thorough knowledge of the particular procedure to be performed.

GADOVIST 1.0 is intended for intravenous administration only and may cause tissue irritation and pain if administered extravascularly.

Pronounced states of excitement, anxiety and pain may increase the risk of adverse reactions or intensify contrast medium-related reactions.

Nephrogenic Systemic Fibrosis (NSF): Gadolinium-based contrast agents (GBCAs) increase the risk for Nephrogenic Systemic Fibrosis (NSF) in patients with acute or chronic severe renal insufficiency (glomerular filtration rate <30 mL/min/1.73m²), and in patients with acute renal insufficiency of any severity due to the hepato-renal syndrome, or in the perioperative liver transplantation period. In these patients, avoid use of GBCAs unless the diagnostic information is essential and not available with noncontrast-enhanced magnetic resonance imaging (MRI). For patients receiving hemodialysis, healthcare professionals may consider prompt hemodialysis following GBCA administration in order to enhance the contrast agent's elimination. However, it is unknown if hemodialysis prevents NSF.

Among the factors that may increase the risk for NSF are repeated or higher than recommended doses of a GBCA and the degree of renal function impairment at the time of exposure.

NSF development is considered a potential class-related effect of all GBCAs.

Post-marketing reports have identified the development of NSF following single and multiple administrations of GBCAs. These reports have not always identified a specific agent. Where a specific agent was identified, the most commonly reported agent was gadodiamide (OMNISCAN), followed by gadopentetate dimeglumine (MAGNEVIST) and gadoversetamide (OPTIMARK). NSF has also developed following the sequential administration of gadodiamide with gadobenate dimeglumine (MULTIHANCE) or gadoteridol (PROHANCE). The number of postmarketing reports is subject to change over time and may not reflect the true proportion of cases associated with any specific GBCA.

The extent of risk for NSF following exposure to any specific GBCA is unknown and may vary among the agents. Published reports are limited and predominantly estimate NSF risks with gadodiamide. In one retrospective study of 370 patients with severe renal insufficiency who received gadodiamide, the estimated risk for development of NSF was 4%. The risk, if any, for the development of NSF among patients with mild to moderate renal insufficiency or normal renal function is unknown, and the cautious utilization of the lowest possible dose of GBCA is preferable.

Screen all patients for renal dysfunction by obtaining a history and/or laboratory tests. When administering a GBCA, do not exceed the recommended dose and allow a sufficient period of time for elimination of the agent from the body prior to any readministration (see Action and Clinical Pharmacology and Dosage and Administration, Recommended Dose and Dosage Adjustment).

A skin biopsy is necessary in order to exclude the diagnosis of similarly presenting skin disorders (e.g. scleromyxedema) (see Warnings and Precautions, Serious Warnings and Precautions, General and Skin and Adverse Reactions, Post-Market Adverse Drug Reactions).

Cardiovascular: In patients with severe cardiovascular disease, GADOVIST 1.0 should only be administered after careful risk-benefit assessment because only limited data are currently available.

Hypersensitivity: A particularly careful risk-benefit assessment is required in patients with known hypersensitivity to GADOVIST 1.0 or to any of its ingredients.

As with other contrast media, GADOVIST 1.0 can be associated with anaphylactoid/hypersensitivity or other idiosyncratic reactions, characterized by cardiovascular, respiratory or cutaneous manifestations, and ranging to severe reactions including shock.

Most of these reactions occur within 30 minutes of administration.

As with other contrast media, delayed allergoid reactions occurring hours or days after administration, have been observed, though rarely.

As with other contrast enhanced diagnostic procedures, post-procedure observation of the patient is recommended for at least 30 minutes after the administration of GADOVIST.

It is important to be familiar with the practice of emergency measures so that prompt action may be taken in the event of hypersensitivity reactions. To permit immediate countermeasures to be taken in emergencies, appropriate drugs and instruments, eg, endotracheal tube and ventilator, should be readily available.

The decision to use GADOVIST 1.0 should be made after careful evaluation of the risk-benefit ratio in patients with a history of previous reaction to contrast media, allergic disposition or bronchial asthma. Experience with contrast media in general shows that these patients suffer mork]e frequently from hypersensitivity reactions than others.

Neurologic: Convulsive States: While there is no evidence suggesting that gadobutrol directly precipitates convulsion, the possibility that it may decrease the convulsive threshold in susceptible patients cannot be ruled out. Precautionary measures should be taken with patients predisposed to seizure, eg, close monitoring and availability of injectable anticonvulsants.

Renal: Use of products of a similar class to GADOVIST has resulted in cases of acute renal failure.

- Exposure to GBCAs increase the risk for NSF in patients with:
  - acute or chronic severe renal insufficiency (glomerular filtration rate <30 mL/min/1.73m²), or
  - acute renal insufficiency of any severity due to the hepato-renal syndrome or in the perioperative liver transplantation period.
- Screen all patients for renal dysfunction by obtaining a history and/or laboratory tests.
- The risk, if any, for the development of NSF among patients with mild to moderate renal insufficiency or normal renal function is unknown, and the cautious utilization of the lowest possible dose of GBCA is preferable.

(See Warnings and Precautions, Serious Warnings and Precautions and Skin and Adverse Reactions, Post-Market Adverse Drug Reactions.)

In patients with severely impaired renal function, the benefits of gadobutrol must be weighed carefully against the risks, since elimination will be delayed in such patients. In very severe cases, gadobutrol should be removed from the body by hemodialysis. At least 3 dialysis sessions within 5 days of the injection are recommended (in which approximately 98% of GADOVIST 1.0 is removed from the body). However, it is unknown if hemodialysis prevents NSF.

Skin: NSF was first identified in 1997 and has, so far, been observed only in patients with renal disease. This is a systemic disorder with the most prominent and visible effects on the skin. Cutaneous lesions associated with this disorder are caused by excessive fibrosis and are usually symmetrically distributed on the limbs and trunk. Involved skin becomes thickened, which may inhibit flexion and extension of joints and result in severe contractures. The fibrosis associated with NSF can extend beyond dermis and involve subcutaneous tissues, striated muscles, diaphragm, pleura, pericardium, and myocardium. NSF may be fatal (see Warnings and Precautions, Serious Warnings and Precautions, General and Renal, and Adverse Reactions, Post-Market Adverse Drug Reactions).

Special Populations: Pregnant Women: The safe use of GADOVIST 1.0 during pregnancy has not been established. Animal studies indicate neither an embryotoxic nor teratogenic effects in diagnostic doses of GADOVIST 1.0. In animal studies, repeated dosing of gadobutrol only at maternally toxic dose levels (8 to 17 times the diagnostic dose) caused retardation of the embryonal development and embryolethality but no teratogenicity. The potential risk for humans is unknown. GADOVIST 1.0 should not be used unless the benefit outweighs the risk.

Nursing Women: Transfer of GADOVIST 1.0 into the milk of lactating mothers has not been investigated in humans, but there is evidence from animal studies that small amounts (less than 0.01% of the dose administered) enter breast milk. Breast-feeding should be interrupted for 24 hours following administration of gadobutrol and the milk discarded during this period.

Pediatrics (2–17 years of age): The safety and efficacy of GADOVIST 1.0 at a dose of 0.1 mmol/kg have been established in adolescents and in children 2 years of age and older (see Adverse Reactions – Clinical Trial Adverse Drug Reactions, Pediatric Population; Action and Clinical Pharmacology, Special Populations and Conditions, Pediatrics).

Pharmacokinetic parameters of GADOVIST 1.0 in healthy children ages 2 to 11 years and adolescents ages 12 to 17 years were comparable to those of healthy adult subjects (see Dosage and Administration, Recommended Dose and Dosage Adjustment and Action and Clinical Pharmacology, Special Populations and Conditions, Pediatrics). The use of GADOVIST 1.0 in these age groups is supported by evidence from adequate and well-controlled studies of GADOVIST 1.0 in adults, and pharmacokinetic studies in adults and children (see Action and Clinical Pharmacology, Special Populations and Conditions, Pediatrics).

GADOVIST 1.0 is not recommended for use in children below 2 years of age due to a lack of data on safety and efficacy.

Geriatrics: No special precautions are required in elderly patients unless renal function is impaired (see Warnings and Precautions, Serious Warnings and Precautions and Renal and Dosage and Administration).

ADVERSE REACTIONS: Adverse Drug Reaction Overview: Patients with a history of previous reaction to contrast media, allergic disposition or bronchial asthma suffer more frequently from hypersensitivity reactions than others. As with other contrast media, delayed allergoid reactions occurring hours or days after administration, have been observed, though rarely. Anaphylactoid reactions may occur (see Warnings and Precautions, Hypersensitivity).

Short lasting mild to moderate feelings of coldness, warmth or pain at the injection site have been uncommonly observed in association with the venous puncture or contrast medium injection.

Transient sensations of taste or smell perversion may occur during or immediately after injection of GADOVIST 1.0.

Upon accidental paravascular injection, GADOVIST 1.0 may cause tissue pain and irritation lasting several minutes. No other local tissue reactions have been observed.

Clinical Trial Adverse Drug Reactions: Because clinical trials are conducted under very specific conditions the adverse reaction rates observed in the clinical trials may not reflect the rates observed in practice and should not be compared to the rates in the clinical trials of another drug. Adverse drug reaction information from clinical trials is useful for identifying drug-related adverse events and for approximating rates.

Adult Population: Clinical Trials for Central Nervous System (CNS) Indications: The safety of GADOVIST was evaluated in 798 patients during clinical trials for CNS indications. Most adverse events reported developed soon after injection; however, the possibility of delayed reactions cannot be ruled out. No adverse drug reaction occurred at a rate greater than 1%.

Clinical Trials for CE-MRA Indication: The safety of GADOVIST 1.0 was evaluated in a total of 890 patients during clinical trials for CE-MRA. Of these, 708 patients were evaluated for efficacy. A total of 76 patients (8.5%) experienced 93 adverse events; in 31 cases (3.5%), the adverse event was assessed as at least possibly study drug-related.

Adverse events most often observed were short lasting thermal sensations (including paresthesia) (2.5%) and headache (1.1%). The majority of the adverse events were of mild or moderate intensity.

General: Where GADOVIST was administered in doses in excess of 0.3 mmol/kg in a small number of patients, the rate of adverse events was observed to increase to 25% (4 of 16 patients) compared to 9.5% for doses >0.2 mmol/kg to 0.3 mmol/kg (29 of 304 patients) and 7.9% for doses 0.1 mmol/kg to 0.2 mmol/kg (35 of 457 patients).

Transient sensations of taste or smell perversion may occur during or immediately after injection of GADOVIST.

Patients with an allergic disposition suffer more frequently than others from hypersensitivity reactions. As with all contrast media, delayed reactions occuring hours or days after administration, may occur. In very rare instances, anaphylactoid reactions may occur (see Warnings and Precautions, General).

Upon accidental paravascular injection, GADOVIST may cause tissue pain and irritation lasting several minutes. No other local tissue reactions have been observed.

Pediatric Population: The safety of GADOVIST 1.0 was evaluated in 138 pediatric patients (ages 2 to 17) in a clinical trial. A total of 8 patients (5.8%) experienced 10 adverse events considered as drug-related; those observed most often were dysgeusia (1.4%) and feeling hot (1.4%), and these were mild in severity.

Other Clinical Trials: Subsequent to market introduction, additional data from clinical trials with GADOVIST 1.0 (N>2900) has become available. No drug-related adverse event occurred at a rate greater than 1%.

Less Common Clinical Trial Adverse Drug Reactions: Adult Population: Clinical Trials for Central Nervous System (CNS) Indications: The most common adverse events reported following administration of GADOVIST were: headache (0.9%), vasodilatation (0.6%), nausea (0.5%), injection site pain (0.4%), dizziness (0.3%), rash (0.3%) and dyspnea (0.3%). These reactions were mild to moderate in severity.

The following other adverse events were reported, regardless of causality:

Body as a Whole: abdominal pain, allergic reaction, fever, infection.
Cardiovascular System: palpitation, postural hypotension.
Gastrointestinal System: diarrhea, vomiting.
Injection Site: pain at the injection site.
Nervous System: apathy, aphasia, convulsion, dry mouth, hot flashes, hypesthesia, insomnia, paresthesia, increased sweating, vertigo.
Special Senses: abnormal vision, parosmia.
Urogenital System: urinary urgency, urine abnormality.
Clinical Trials for CE-MRA Indication: Less common adverse events reported following administration of GADOVIST were nausea (0.9%) and vomiting, diarrhea, taste perversion and dizziness in 4 patients each (0.5%). All other events were observed in less than 0.5% of cases.
Pediatric Population: Less common adverse events considered as drug-related that were reported following administration of GADOVIST 1.0 in pediatric patients were: crystal urine (0.7%), headache (0.7%), nausea (0.7%), rash (0.7%), rash pruritic (0.7%) and pruritus (0.7%), occurring in one patient each; these were predominantly mild in severity.
Other Clinical Trials: Subsequent to market introduction, additional data from clinical trials with GADOVIST 1.0 (N>2900) has become available. Table 1 lists all adverse events considered as drug-related by the investigators; most were of mild to moderate intensity.

Table 1: GADOVIST 1.0

All Adverse Events Considered Drug-related by the Investigator and Reported by <1% of Patients During Clinical Trials (N>2900)[a]

System Organ Class	Uncommon (≥0.1% and <1%)	Rare (<0.1%)
Gastrointestinal disorders	nausea	vomiting
General disorders and administration site conditions	injection site pain, injection site reaction	—
Immune system disorders	—	anaphylactoid reaction
Nervous system disorders	headache, dizziness, dysgeusia, paresthesia	parosmia
Respiratory, thoracic and mediastinal disorders	—	dyspnea
Skin and subcutaneous tissue disorders	—	urticaria, rash
Vascular disorders	vasodilatation	hypotension

[a] Adverse reactions are classified by MedDRA system organ classes (MedDRA SOCs). The most appropriate MedDRA term is used to describe a certain reaction and its synonyms and related conditions. ADR term representation is based on MedDRA version 9.0.

Abnormal Hematologic and Clinical Chemistry Findings: All clinically significant changes in laboratory values observed in clinical trials in pediatric patients with GADOVIST have been summarized in Table 2.

Table 2: GADOVIST 1.0

Treatment-Emergent Laboratory Abnormalities in Clinical Trials in Pediatric Patients with GADOVIST

Laboratory Parameter	Number of Patients with Changes	Magnitude of Change From Baseline Values
Crystals in urine	1	one fold increase

Post-Market Adverse Drug Reactions: Nephrogenic Systemic Fibrosis (NSF): Postmarketing reports have identified the development of NSF following single and multiple administrations of GBCAs. These reports have not always identified a specific agent. Where a specific agent was identified, the most commonly reported agent was gadodiamide (OMNISCAN), followed by gadopentetate dimeglumine (MAGNEVIST) and gadoversetamide (OPTIMARK). NSF has also developed following the sequential administration of gadodiamide with gadobenate dimeglumine (MULTIHANCE) or gadoteridol (PROHANCE). The number of postmarketing reports is subject to change over time and may not reflect the true proportion of cases associated with any specific GBCA. The extent of risk for NSF following exposure to any specific GBCA is unknown and may vary among the agents. Published reports are limited and predominantly estimate NSF risks with gadodiamide. In one retrospective study of 370 patients with severe renal insufficiency who received gadodiamide, the estimated risk for development of NSF was 4%. The risk, if any for the development of NSF among patients with mild to moderate renal insufficiency or normal renal function is unknown, and the cautious utilization of the lowest possible dose of GBCA is preferable (see Warnings and Precautions, Serious Warnings and Precautions, General, Renal and Skin).
Additional Adverse Reactions: The following other drug-related adverse events were reported spontaneously post-marketing:
Cardiac Disorders: cardiac arrest, tachycardia.
Eye Disorders: conjunctivitis, eyelid edema.
General Disorders and Administration Site Conditions : feeling hot, malaise.
Immune System Disorders: anaphylactoid shock.
Nervous System Disorders: loss of consciousness, convulsion.
Respiratory, Thoracic and Mediastinal Disorders: bronchospasm, cough, cyanosis, respiratory arrest, sneezing, oropharyngeal swelling.
Skin and Subcutaneous Tissue Disorders: face edema, erythema, hyperhidrosis, pruritus.
Vascular Disorders: circulatory collapse, flushing.

The most appropriate MedDRA term is used to describe a certain reaction and its synonyms and related conditions. Adverse drug reaction term representation is based on MedDRA version 9.0.

DRUG INTERACTIONS: Overview: No specific drug interaction studies have been done for GADOVIST during the development of this product.
Drug-Drug Interactions: Interactions with specific drugs have not been established.
Drug-Food Interactions: Interactions with food have not been established.
Drug-Herb Interactions: Interactions with herbal products have not been established.
Drug-Laboratory Test Interactions: Interactions with laboratory tests have not been established.

DOSAGE AND ADMINISTRATION: Dosing Considerations: GADOVIST 1.0 is for intravenous administration only.

The administration of contrast media should, if possible, be done with the patient lying down. The patient should be kept under observation for at least 30 minutes following the administration of contrast media since experience shows that the majority of all severe adverse effects occur within this period.

GADOVIST 1.0 is not recommended for use in children below 2 years of age due to a lack of data on safety and efficacy (See Warnings and Precautions, Special Populations, Pediatrics (2–17 years of age)).

Recommended Dose and Dosage Adjustment: Dosage depends on the indication. A single intravenous injection of 0.1 mL GADOVIST 1.0/kg body weight is generally sufficient. A total amount of 0.3 mL GADOVIST 1.0/kg body weight may be administered at maximum.

The following dosages of GADOVIST 1.0 are recommended for cranial and spinal MRI examinations and in magnetic resonance angiography (CE MRA) in adults. See Table 3.

Table 3: GADOVIST 1.0

Dosages of GADOVIST in Adults

Type of Examination	GADOVIST 1.0
CNS Indications	
General	
-1st injection	0.1 mL/kg
-2nd injection (within 30 min of 1st injection) in cases where a strong clinical suspicion of a lesion persists despite a normal contrast-enhanced MRI or when more accurate information on the number, size or extent of lesions might influence the choice of therapy or management of the patient.	0.1 mL/kg to 0.2 mL/kg (corresponding to 0.1–0.2 mmol/kg of body weight)
Exclusion of Metastases or Recurrent Tumors	
Lesions with poor vascularization and/or small extracellular space or when relatively less heavily T_1-weighted scanning sequences are used.	0.3 mL/kg (corresponding to 0.3 mmol/kg of body weight)
Perfusion Studies[a]	
-T_2* -weighted gradient echo sequences are recommended for use in combination with cranial and spinal MRI for detection of mass lesions and for detection of focal ischemia without suspected mass lesions.	0.3 mL/kg (corresponding to 0.3 mmol/kg of body weight)
CE-MRA Indication	
Imaging of 1 field of view (FOV):	7.5 mL for body weight below 75 kg, 10 mL for body weight of 75 kg and higher; (corresponding to 0.1–0.15 mmol/kg of body weight).
Imaging of >1 field of view (FOV):	15 mL for body weight below 75 kg, 20 mL for body weight of 75 kg and higher (corresponding to 0.2–0.3 mmol/kg of body weight).

[a] For perfusion studies, the use of a non-magnetic, automatic injector is recommended at an infusion rate of 3–5 mL/sec.

Pediatric Patients (2-17 years of age): For adolescents and children aged 2 years and older, the recommended dose of GADOVIST 1.0 is 0.1 mL per kg body weight (corresponding to 0.1 mmol/kg), for all indications.
Renal Impairment: GADOVIST 1.0 should be used with caution in patients with renal insufficiency (see Warnings and Precautions, Serious Warnings and Precautions, General, Skin and Adverse Reactions, Post-Market Adverse Drug Reactions).
Administration: The required volume of GADOVIST 1.0 is administered intravenously as a bolus injection. Contrast-enhanced MRI can start shortly after the injection depending on the pulse sequences used and the protocol for the examination. Optimal opacification is generally observed during arterial first pass for CE-MRA and within a period of about 15 minutes after injection of GADOVIST 1.0 for CNS indications (time depending on type of lesion/tissue). Tissue enhancement is generally sustained up to 45 minutes after injection of GADOVIST 1.0. T_1-weighted scanning sequences are particularly suitable for contrast-enhanced examinations.

In the absence of compatibility studies, GADOVIST 1.0 must not be mixed with other medicinal products.

Parenteral Products: Use of vials: GADOVIST 1.0 should not be drawn into the syringe until immediately before use. The rubber stopper should never be pierced more than once. Any unused portion must be discarded upon completion of the procedure.
Use of prefilled syringes: The prefilled syringe must be taken from the pack and prepared for the injection immediately before the examination. The tip cap should be removed from the prefilled syringe immediately before use. Any unused portion must be discarded upon completion of the procedure.

OVERDOSAGE:
Single doses of GADOVIST as high as 1.5 mmol gadobutrol/kg of body weight have been tested in humans.

No signs of intoxication from an overdose have been observed during clinical use.

Cardiovascular monitoring and control of renal function are recommended as a measure of precaution.

It is recommended to contact the Poison Control Center in case of overdose.

Use of products of a similar class to GADOVIST has resulted in cases of acute renal failure. GADOVIST 1.0 should be used with caution in patients with renal insufficiency (see Warnings and Precautions, Renal and Dosage And Administration, Recommended Dose and Dosage Adjustment). In the event of inadvertent overdosage or in the case of severely impaired renal function, GADOVIST 1.0 can be removed from the body by hemodialysis. However, it is unknown if hemodialysis prevents NSF. (see Warnings and Precautions, Renal).

> For management of a suspected drug overdose, contact your regional Poison Control Centre. See the *CPS* Directory section for a list of Poison Control Centres.

ACTION AND CLINICAL PHARMACOLOGY: Mechanism of Action: GADOVIST is a non-ionic paramagnetic contrast agent for magnetic resonance imaging (MRI). The contrast-enhancing effect is mediated by gadobutrol, a neutral complex consisting of gadolinium (Gd^{3+}) and the macrocyclic compound dihydroxy-hydroxymethylpropyl-tetraazacyclododecane-triacetic acid (butrol).

Following injection of gadobutrol, improved diagnostic information compared to unenhanced MRI can be obtained in areas with a penetrable or missing blood-brain barrier as a result of altered perfusion or due to an enlarged extracellular space such as in cases of primary and secondary tumors, inflammatory or demyelinating diseases.

Pharmacodynamics: Gadobutrol produces a distinct shortening of the relaxation times even at low concentrations. The effect of gadobutrol on shortening of relaxation times at concentrations ranging from 0.25 mmol/L to 1.0 mmol/L was investigated in water and plasma at 0.47 Tesla and 2 Tesla; gadobutrol decreased both the spin-lattice (T_1) and the spin-spin (T_2) relaxation times. At pH 7 and 40°C the relaxivity, as determined from the shortening of the spin-lattice relaxation time (T_1) of protons in water, is about 3.58 L/mmol·sec and of the spin-spin relaxation time (T_2) is about 3.99 L/mmol·sec.

The relaxivity of gadobutrol in water at 0.47 Tesla and 2 Tesla was similar to that of gadopentetate dimeglumine.

The relaxivity displays only a slight dependency on the strength of the magnetic field.

Further evaluation of the relaxivity of gadobutrol at clinical relevant field strength and in blood and plasma show the following relaxivity values (see Table 4).

Table 4: GADOVIST 1.0

Relaxivities of GADOVIST 1.0 mmol/mL

	r_1 (r_2)
relaxivity in plasma at 37°, 1.5 Tesla	5.2 (6.1)

(cont'd)

Table 4: GADOVIST 1.0 *(cont'd)*

Relaxivities of GADOVIST 1.0 mmol/mL

	r_1 (r_2)
relaxivity in blood at 37°, 1.5 Tesla	5.3 (5.4)
relaxivity in plasma at 37°, 3.0 Tesla	5.0 (7.1)

The macrocyclic ligand forms a firm complex with the paramagnetic gadolinium ion with extremely high in vivo and in vitro stability. Gadobutrol is a highly water-soluble, extremely hydrophilic compound with a partition coefficient between n-butanol and buffer at pH 7.6 of about 0.006. Gadobutrol does not display any significant protein binding or inhibitory action on enzymes. Gadobutrol does not activate the complement system.

When a T_1-weighted spin-echo sequence is used in MRI, the shortening of the spin-lattice relaxation time resulting from the administration of gadobutrol leads to an increase in the signal intensity which appears as a positive contrast useful for tissue differentiation. For perfusion studies, a T_2*-weighted gradient echo sequence is recommended. The induction of local magnetic field fluctuations by the large magnetic moment of gadolinium leads to a signal decrease of tissues in such sequences.

Pharmacokinetics: The pharmacokinetics of gadobutrol in humans are dose proportional.

Distribution: After intravenous administration, gadobutrol is rapidly distributed in the extracellular space. Up to 0.4 mmol/kg body weight, plasma levels decline after an early distribution phase with a half life of about 90 minutes, identical to the renal elimination rate. Plasma levels measured at 2 and 60 minutes following injection of 0.1 mmol/kg were 0.59 and 0.3 mmol/L, respectively.

Metabolism: No gadobutrol metabolites are detected in plasma or urine.

Excretion: Gadobutrol is eliminated in an unchanged form via the kidneys by glomerular filtration. After intravenous administration, within 2 hours more than 50% of the dose was eliminated in the urine and within 12 hours more than 90% of the dose had been excreted. Extra-renal elimination is negligible; less than 0.1% of the dose was eliminated in the feces. The average renal clearance of gadobutrol was determined to be approximately 120 mL/min and was, therefore, comparable to that of other aqueous substances, such as inulin.

Special Populations and Conditions: Pediatrics: A single intravenous dose of 0.1 mmol/kg of GADOVIST was administered to 138 healthy subjects (85 males and 53 females) between the ages of 2 and 17 years. Pharmacokinetic parameters of GADOVIST for healthy children and adolescents age 2 to 17 years were comparable to those of healthy adult subjects. Individual differences in CL were accounted for by differences in body weight. Neither age nor gender were found to be additional independent parameters affecting the pharmacokinetics of gadobutrol in the pediatric population. (See Dosage And Administration, Recommended Dose and Dosage Adjustment.)

STORAGE AND STABILITY: GADOVIST 1.0 should be stored between 15 and 30°C. Protect from freezing.

INFORMATION FOR THE PATIENT: Published in e-CPS, available by subscription at www.e-cps.ca.

DOSAGE FORMS, COMPOSITION AND PACKAGING: Each mL of clear, sterile, aqueous solution, contains: gadobutrol 604.72 mg (1.0 mmol), trometamol 1.211 mg and calcium sodium butrol 0.513 mg in water for injection. The pH is adjusted to between 6.6 and 8.0 with hydrochloric acid. Single-dose vials of 7.5, 15 and 30 mL.

GamaSTAN™ S/D

immune globulin intramuscular (human)

Passive Immunizing Agent

Talecris

Date of Revision: November 14, 2005

SUMMARY PRODUCT INFORMATION:

Route of Administration	Dosage Form/Strength	Clinically Relevant Nonmedicinal Ingredients
Intramuscular Injection	Injectable solution, 15–18% protein	For a complete listing see Dosage Forms, Composition and Packaging.

DESCRIPTION: GamaSTAN S/D treated with solvent/detergent is a sterile solution of immune globulin for intramuscular administration; it contains no preservative. GamaSTAN S/D is prepared by cold ethanol fractionation from human plasma. The immune globulin is isolated from solubilized Cohn fraction II. The fraction II solution is adjusted to a final concentration of 0.3% tri-n-butyl phosphate (TNBP) and 0.2% sodium cholate. After the addition of solvent (TNBP) and detergent (sodium cholate), the solution is heated to 30°C and maintained at that temperature for not less than 6 hours. After the viral inactivation step, the reactants are removed by precipitation, filtration and finally ultrafiltration and diafiltration. GamaSTAN S/D is formulated as a 15-18% protein solution at a pH of 6.4-7.2 in 0.21-0.32 M glycine. The pH is adjusted with sodium carbonate. GamaSTAN S/D is then incubated in the final container for 21-28 days at 20-27°C.

INDICATIONS AND CLINICAL USE: Passive immunization should be considered when vaccines for active immunization are not available, or in situations when vaccine has not been used prior to exposure to the infective agent or is contraindicated. GamaSTAN S/D is indicated in the following situations.

Hepatitis A: The prophylactic value of GamaSTAN S/D is greatest when given before or soon after exposure to hepatitis A. GamaSTAN S/D is not indicated in persons with clinical manifestations of hepatitis A or in those exposed more than 2 weeks previously.

Measles (Rubeola): GamaSTAN S/D should be given to prevent or modify measles in susceptible person exposed fewer than 6 days previously. A susceptible person is one who has not been vaccinated and has not had measles previously. GamaSTAN S/D may be especially indicated for susceptible household contacts of measles patients, particularly contacts under 1 year of age, for whom the risk of complications is highest. GamaSTAN S/D and measles vaccine should not be given at the same time. If a child is older than 12 months and has received GamaSTAN S/D, he should be given measles vaccine about 5 months later when the measles antibody titer will have disappeared, provided there are no contraindications to the vaccine.

If a susceptible child exposed to measles is immunocompromised, GamaSTAN S/D should be given immediately. GamaSTAN S/D may also be considered for severely immunocompromised individuals exposed to measles regardless of immunization status. Children who are immunocompromised should not receive measles vaccine or any other live viral vaccine.

Varicella: Passive immunization against varicella in immunosuppressed patients is best accomplished by use of Varicella-Zoster Immune Globulin (Human) [VZIG]. If VZIG is unavailable, GamaSTAN S/D, promptly given, may also modify varicella.

Rubella: The routine use of GamaSTAN S/D for prophylaxis of rubella in early pregnancy is of dubious value and cannot be justified. Some studies suggest that the use of GamaSTAN S/D in exposed, susceptible women can lessen the likelihood of infection and fetal damage; therefore, GamaSTAN S/D may benefit those women who will not consider a therapeutic abortion.

Immunoglobulin Deficiency: In patients with immunoglobulin deficiencies, GamaSTAN S/D may prevent serious infection. However, GamaSTAN S/D may not prevent chronic infections of the external secretory tissues such as the respiratory and gastrointestinal tract.

Prophylactic therapy, especially against infections due to encapsulated bacteria, is effective in Bruton-type, sex-linked, congenital agammaglobulinemia, agammaglobulinemia associated with thymoma, and acquired agammaglobulinemia.

CONTRAINDICATIONS:

- GamaSTAN S/D should not be given to patients who are hypersensitive to this drug or to any ingredient in the formulation or component of the container. For a complete listing, see Dosage Forms, Composition and Packaging.
- GamaSTAN S/D should not be given to persons with isolated immunoglobulin A (IgA) deficiency. Such persons have the potential for developing antibodies to IgA and could have anaphylactic reactions to subsequent administration of blood products that contain IgA.
- GamaSTAN S/D should not be administered to patients who have severe thrombocytopenia or any coagulation disorder that would contraindicate intramuscular injections.

WARNINGS AND PRECAUTIONS:

Serious Warnings and Precautions

- For intramuscular injection only. Do not give intravenously (see Warnings and Precautions, General).
- Products made from human plasma may contain infectious agents such as viruses (see Warnings and Precautions, General).

General: GamaSTAN S/D should not be administered intravenously because of the potential for serious reactions. Injections should be made intramuscularly, and care should be taken to draw back on the plunger of the syringe before injection in order to be certain that the needle is not in a blood vessel.

Skin tests should not be done. In most human beings the intradermal injection of concentrated gamma globulin solution with its buffers causes a localized area of inflammation which can be misinterpreted as a positive allergic reaction. In actuality, this does not represent an allergy; rather, it is localized tissue irritation of a chemical nature. Misinterpretation of the results of such tests can lead the physician to withhold badly needed human immunoglobulin from a patient who is not actually allergic to this material. True allergic responses to human gamma globulin given in the prescribed intramuscular manner are rare.

Although systemic reactions to intramuscularly administered immunoglobulin preparations are rare, epinephrine should be available for treatment of acute allergic symptoms.

GamaSTAN S/D is made from human plasma. Products made from human plasma may contain infectious agents, such as viruses, that can cause disease. The risk that such products will transmit an infectious agent has been reduced by screening plasma donors for prior exposure to certain viruses, by testing for the presence of certain current virus infections, and by inactivating and/or removing certain viruses. Despite these measures, such products can still potentially transmit disease. There is also the possibility that unknown infectious agents may be present in such products. Individuals who receive infusions of blood or plasma products may develop signs and/or symptoms of some viral infections, particularly hepatitis C. All infections thought by a physician possibly to have been transmitted by this product should be reported by the physician or other healthcare provider to Talecris Biotherapeutics Ltd. at 1-866-482-5226.

The physician should discuss the risks and benefits of this product with the patient, before prescribing or administering to the patient.

Special Populations: Pregnant Women: There is no experience of exposure in pregnancy during clinical trials. Animal reproduction studies have not been conducted with GamaSTAN S/D. It is also not known whether GamaSTAN S/D can cause fetal harm when administered to a pregnant woman or can affect reproduction capacity. GamaSTAN S/D should be given to a pregnant woman only if clearly needed.

Nursing Women: Because of the potential for unknown effects from GamaSTAN S/D in infants being nursed by mothers taking GamaSTAN S/D, a decision should be made to either discontinue nursing or discontinue the administration of GamaSTAN S/D, taking into account the importance of GamaSTAN S/D therapy to the mother and the possible risk to the infant.

Pediatrics (<18 years of age): The safety and effectiveness of GamaSTAN S/D in the pediatric population have not been established.

Monitoring and Laboratory Tests: None required.

ADVERSE REACTIONS: Adverse Drug Reaction Overview: Local pain and tenderness at the injection site, urticaria, and angioedema may occur. Anaphylactic reactions, although rare, have been reported following the injection of human immune globulin preparations. Anaphylaxis is more likely to occur if GamaSTAN S/D is given intravenously; therefore, GamaSTAN S/D must be administered only intramuscularly.

Table 1: GamaSTAN S/D

Adverse Drug Reactions Associated with Immune Globulin (Human)

General Disorders and Administration Site Conditions	Local pain and injection site tenderness
Immune System Disorders	Angioedema Anaphylaxis Urticaria

DRUG INTERACTIONS: Drug-Drug Interactions: See Table 2.

Table 2: GamaSTAN S/D

Established or Potential Drug-Drug Interactions

Proper Name	Ref	Effect	Clinical Comment
Live Viral Vaccines	T	Antibodies in the globulin preparation may interfere with the response to live viral vaccines such as measles, mumps, polio and rubella.	Use of such vaccines should be deferred until approximately 5 months after GamaSTAN S/D administration

Legend:
C=Case Study.
CT=Clinical Trial.
T=Theoretical.

Drug-Food Interactions: No interactions are known.

Drug-Herb Interactions: No interactions are known.

Drug-Laboratory Test Interactions: No interactions are known.

DOSAGE AND ADMINISTRATION: Dosing Considerations: For intramuscular injection only. Do not give intravenously.

Recommended Dose and Dosage Adjustment: Hepatitis A: GamaSTAN S/D in a dose of 0.02 mL/kg is recommended for household and institutional hepatitis A case contacts.

The following doses of GamaSTAN S/D are recommended for persons who plan to travel in areas where hepatitis A is common, see Table 3.

Table 3: GamaSTAN S/D

Dosage Recommendations

Length of Stay	Dose Volume
Less than 3 months	0.02 mL/kg
3 months or longer	0.06 mL/kg (repeat every 4–6 months)

Measles (Rubeola): GamaSTAN S/D should be given in a dose of 0.25 mL/kg to prevent or modify measles in a susceptible person exposed fewer than 6 days previously. A susceptible child who is exposed to measles and who is immunocompromised should receive a dose of 0.5 mL/kg (maximum dose, 15 mL) of GamaSTAN S/D immediately. The dosage of Immune Globulin (Human) for exposed individuals who have underlying malignant disease should be 0.5 mL/kg or 15 mL maximum.

Varicella: If Varicella-Zoster Immune Globulin (Human) is unavailable, GamaSTAN S/D at a dose of 0.6 to 1.2 mL/kg, promptly given, may also modify varicella.

Rubella: Some studies suggest that the use of GamaSTAN S/D in exposed, susceptible women can lessen the likelihood of infection and fetal damage; therefore, GamaSTAN S/D at a dose of 0.55 mL/kg may benefit those women who will not consider a therapeutic abortion.

Immunoglobulin Deficiency: GamaSTAN S/D may prevent serious infection in patients with immunoglobulin deficiencies if circulating IgG levels of approximately 200 mg/100 mL plasma are maintained. The recommended dosage is 0.66 mL/kg (at least 100 mg/kg) given every 3 to 4 weeks. A double dose is given at onset of therapy; some patients may require more frequent injections.

Administration: GamaSTAN S/D is administered intramuscularly (see Warnings and Precautions, General), preferably in the anterolateral aspects of the upper thigh and the deltoid muscle of the upper arm. The gluteal region should not be used routinely as an injection site because of the risk of injury to the sciatic nerve. Doses over 10 mL should be divided and injected into several muscle sites to reduce local pain and discomfort. An individual decision as to which muscle is injected must be made for each patient based on the volume of material to be administered. If the gluteal region is used when very large volumes are to be injected or multiple doses are necessary, the central region **must** be avoided; only the upper, outer quadrant should be used.

Parenteral drug products should be inspected visually for particulate matter and discoloration prior to administration, whenever solution and container permit.

A number of factors beyond our control could reduce the efficacy of this product or even result in an ill effect following its use. These include improper storage and handling of the product after it leaves our hands, diagnosis, dosage, method of administration, and biological differences in individual patients. Because of these factors, it is important that this product be stored properly and that the directions be followed carefully during use.

Reconstitution: Not required.

OVERDOSAGE:

Although no data are available, clinical experience with other immunoglobulin preparations suggests that the only manifestations would be pain and tenderness at the injection site.

> For management of a suspected drug overdose, CPhA recommends that you contact your **regional Poison Control Centre**. See the *CPS* Directory section for a list of Poison Control Centres.

ACTION AND CLINICAL PHARMACOLOGY: Mechanism of Action: Passive immunization with GamaSTAN S/D modifies hepatitis A, prevents or modifies measles, and provides replacement therapy in persons with hypogammaglobulinemia or agammaglobulinemia. GamaSTAN S/D is not standardized with respect to antibody titers against hepatitis B surface antigen (HBsAg) and should not be used for prophylaxis of viral hepatitis type B. Prophylactic treatment to prevent hepatitis B can best be accomplished with use of Hepatitis B Immune Globulin (Human), often in combination with Hepatitis B Vaccine. GamaSTAN S/D is unlikely to be of benefit for post-exposure management of hepatitis C.

GamaSTAN S/D may be of benefit in women who have been exposed to rubella in the first trimester of pregnancy and who will not consider a therapeutic abortion. GamaSTAN S/D may also be considered for use in immunocompromised patients for passive immunization against varicella if Varicella-Zoster Immune Globulin (Human) is not available.

GamaSTAN S/D is not indicated for routine prophylaxis or treatment of rubella, poliomyelitis, mumps, or varicella. It is not indicated for allergy or asthma in patients who have normal levels of immunoglobulin.

Pharmacodynamics: See Mechanism of Action.

Pharmacokinetics: In a clinical study in healthy human adults receiving another hyperimmune immune globulin product treated with solvent/detergent, Rabies Immune Globulin (Human), prepared by the same manufacturing process, detectable passive antibody titers were observed in the serum of all subjects by 24 hours post injection and persisted through the 21 day study period. These results suggest that passive immunization with immune globulin products is not affected by the solvent/detergent treatment.

Duration of Effect: Peak levels of immunoglobulin G are obtained approximately 2 days after intramuscular injection of GamaSTAN S/D. The half-life of IgG in the circulation of individuals with normal IgG levels is 23 days.

STORAGE AND STABILITY: Store at 2-8°C. Do not freeze. Do not use after expiration date. The vials are single use. Once entered, discard any unused contents.

INFORMATION FOR THE PATIENT: Published in e-CPS, available by subscription at www.e-cps.ca.

DOSAGE FORMS, COMPOSITION AND PACKAGING: GamaSTAN S/D contains: 15-18% immune globulin (human). It also contains 0.21-0.32 M glycine, USP. Single use vials of 2, 5 and 10 mL.

Gammagard Liquid

immune globulin intravenous (human)

Replacement Therapy for Immunodeficiencies

Baxter

Date of Preparation: July 9, 2007

SUMMARY PRODUCT INFORMATION:

Route of Administration	Dosage Form/ Strength	Clinically Relevant Nonmedicinal Ingredients
Intravenous	Solution for infusion 1 g/10 mL 2.5 g/25 mL 5 g/50 mL 10 g/100 mL 20 g/200 mL	Glycine and water for injections

DESCRIPTION: GAMMAGARD LIQUID is a purified IgG liquid biologic product at 10% w/v protein concentration. This preparation is an isotonic solution containing a concentration of approximately 100 mg of protein per mL, of which at least 98% is gamma globulin, and has a pH of 4.6 to 5.1.* The stabilizing agent is glycine and is present in the amount of 0.25M (0.20 to 0.30M). The product contains no preservatives.

GAMMAGARD LIQUID is available in 5 pack sizes, i.e. 1 g in 10 mL, 2.5 g in 25 mL, 5 g in 50 mL, 10 g in 100 mL, and 20 g in 200 mL solution. The product is filled into containers of type I glass, which are closed with bromobutyl rubber stoppers.

The GAMMAGARD LIQUID manufacturing process employs a modified Cohn-Oncley cold alcohol fractionation procedure to isolate an intermediate immunoglobulin G (IgG) fraction, referred to as Precipitate G, from frozen human plasma pools. Precipitate G is further purified by a continuous process through the use of weak cation exchange chromatography (CM Sepharose Fast Flow) and weak anion exchange chromatography (ANX Sepharose 4 Fast Flow, low substitution), to final formulation. Three dedicated virus reduction steps are included in the downstream purification of Precipitate G, which are solvent/detergent (S/D) treatment, nanofiltration, and incubation at low pH and elevated temperature in the final formulation. The final formulation step is achieved at the ultra/diafiltration step against 0.25M glycine buffer at pH 4.2 to meet the final release criteria of an osmolality of 240 to 300 mOsmol/kg, a pH of 4.6 to 5.1*, and a protein concentration of human IgG of 9.0 to 11.0%.

This product is prepared from large pools of human plasma, which may contain the causative agents of hepatitis and viral diseases. (See Warnings and Precautions.)

GAMMAGARD LIQUID belongs to the pharmacotherapeutic group of immune sera and immunoglobulins, immunoglobulins, normal human, for intravascular administration, ATC code: J06BA02. The active ingredient of GAMMAGARD LIQUID is human polyvalent IgG. The native structure and function of the IgG molecules are not compromised throughout the manufacturing process. Therefore, the product retains the subclass distribution and the broad spectrum of antibody specificities present in human plasma, and exerts all the critical biological activities of polyvalent antibody molecules. The exact mechanism of action other than replacement therapy is not fully elucidated but includes immunomodulatory effects.

Intravenous immunoglobulins are indicated in primary immunodeficiency syndromes, and secondary antibody deficiencies such as in myeloma or chronic lymphocytic leukaemia (CLL) with severe secondary hypogammaglobulinemia, and in children with congenital AIDS or allogenic bone marrow transplantation. They are also recommended for immunomodulation in idiopathic thrombocytopenic purpura (ITP).

INDICATIONS AND CLINICAL USE: GAMMAGARD LIQUID IS indicated for:

* pH is measured after the solution is diluted to 1% protein with saline. The pH range of 4.6 to 5.1 corresponds to a range of 4.4 to 4.9 when the solution is measured undiluted. Measurement of the undiluted solution was performed during process and formulation development, and will be routinely performed in manufacturing to monitor the process.

Replacement therapy in:

- **Primary immunodeficiency syndromes (PID) Including:**
  - Congenital agammaglobulinaemia and hypogammaglobulinaemia
  - Common variable immunodeficiency
  - Severe combined immunodeficiency
  - Wiskott Aldrich syndrome
- **Secondary Immunodeficiency syndromes (SID), Including:**
  - B-cell chronic lymphocytic leukemia
  - Pediatric HIV infection
  - Allogeneic bone marrow transplantation
- **Idiopathic thrombocytopenic purpura (ITP)**

GAMMAGARD LIQUID should be administered under the supervision of a qualified health professional who is experienced in the use of immunoglobulins and in the management of PID, SID and ITP. Appropriate management of therapy and complications is only possible when adequate diagnostic and treatment facilities are readily available.

Geriatrics and Pediatrics (>24 months of age): Age inclusion criterion for Clinical Study No. 160101 was >24 months. However, no specific geriatric or pediatric studies were performed.

CONTRAINDICATIONS: Hypersensitivity to the active substance or to the excipient.

Hypersensitivity to homologous immunoglobulins, especially in very rare cases of IgA deficiency when the patient has antibodies against IgA. However, GAMMAGARD LIQUID contains only small amounts of IgA (≤0.14 mg per mL).

WARNINGS AND PRECAUTIONS:

> **Serious Warnings and Precautions**
>
> Immune Globulin Intravenous (Human) products have been reported to be associated with:
>
> - renal dysfunction,
> - acute renal failure,
> - osmotic nephrosis, and
> - death.
>
> Patients predisposed to acute renal failure include patients with any degree of pre-existing renal insufficiency, diabetes mellitus, age greater than 65, volume depletion, sepsis, paraproteinemia, or patients receiving known nephrotoxic drugs. Especially in such patients, IGIV products should be administered at the minimum concentration available and the minimum rate of infusion practicable. While these reports of renal dysfunction and acute renal failure have been associated with the use of many of the licensed IGIV products, those containing sucrose as a stabilizer accounted for a disproportionate share of the total number.
>
> GAMMAGARD LIQUID does not contain sucrose. Glycine, an amino acid, is used as a stabilizer.
>
> The physician should discuss the risks and benefits of this product with the patient.

General: GAMMAGARD LIQUID is made from human plasma. Products made from human plasma may contain infectious agents, such as viruses, that can cause disease. The risk that such products will transmit an infectious agent has been reduced by screening plasma donors for prior exposure to certain viruses, by testing for the presence of certain current virus infections, and by inactivating and/or removing certain viruses. Despite these measures, such products can still potentially transmit disease. There is also the possibility that unknown infectious agents may be present in such products. Individuals who receive infusions of blood or plasma products may develop signs and/or symptoms of some viral infections. **All** infections thought by a physician possibly to have been transmitted by this product should be reported by the physician or other healthcare provider to Baxter Corporation, 1-800-387-8399.

GAMMAGARD LIQUID should only be administered intravenously. Other routes of administration have not been evaluated.

Immediate anaphylactic and hypersensitivity reactions are a remote possibility. Epinephrine and antihistamines should be available for treatment of any acute anaphylactoid reactions.

Impaired Renal Function: Periodic monitoring of renal function tests and urine output is particularly important in patients judged to have a potential increased risk for developing acute renal failure. Assure that patients are not volume depleted prior to the initiation of infusion of GAMMAGARD LIQUID. Renal function, including measurement of blood urea nitrogen (BUN)/serum creatinine, should be assessed prior to the initial infusion of IGIV products and again at appropriate intervals thereafter. If renal function deteriorates, discontinuation of the product should be considered.

For patients judged to be at risk of developing renal dysfunction, it may be prudent to reduce the rate of infusion to less than 3.3 mg IgG/kg/min (<2 mL/kg/hr).

Hemolysis: IGIV products can contain blood group antibodies which may act as hemolysins and induce in vivo coating of red blood cells with immunoglobulin, causing a positive direct antiglobulin reaction and, rarely, hemolysis. Hemolytic anemia can develop subsequent to IGIV therapy due to enhanced red blood cells (RBC) sequestration (see Adverse Reactions). IGIV recipients should be monitored for clinical signs and symptoms of hemolysis (see Warnings and Precautions, Monitoring and Laboratory Tests).

Transfusion-Related Acute Lung Injury (TRALI): There have been reports of noncardiogenic pulmonary edema (Transfusion Related Acute Lung Injury [TRALI]) in patients administered IGIV. TRALI is characterized by severe respiratory distress, pulmonary edema, hypoxemia, normal left ventricular function, and fever, and typically occurs within 1-6 hours after transfusion. Patients with TRALI may be managed using oxygen therapy with adequate ventilatory support.

IGIV recipients should be monitored for pulmonary adverse reactions. If TRALI is suspected, appropriate tests should be performed for the presence of anti-neutrophil antibodies in both the product and patient serum (see Warnings and Precautions, Monitoring and Laboratory Tests).

Thrombotic Events: Thrombotic events have been reported in association with IGIV (see Adverse Reactions). Patients at risk may include those with a history of atherosclerosis, multiple cardiovascular risk factors, advanced age, impaired cardiac output, and/or known or suspected hyperviscosity, hypercoagulable disorders and prolonged periods of immobilization. The potential risks and benefits of IGIV should be weighed against those of alternative therapies for all patients for whom IGIV administration is being considered. Baseline assessment of blood viscosity should be considered in patients at risk for hyperviscosity, including those with cryoglobulins, fasting chylomicronemia/markedly high triacylglycerols (triglycerides), or monoclonal gammopathies (see Warnings and Precautions, Monitoring and Laboratory Tests).

Aseptic Meningitis Syndrome: An aseptic meningitis syndrome (AMS) has been reported to occur infrequently in association with IGIV treatment. Discontinuation of IGIV treatment has resulted in remission of AMS within several days without sequelae. The syndrome usually begins within several hours to two days following IGIV treatment. It is characterized by symptoms and signs including severe headache, nuchal rigidity, drowsiness, fever, photophobia, painful eye movements, and nausea and vomiting. Cerebrospinal fluid (CSF) studies are frequently positive with pleocytosis up to several thousand cells per cubic mm, predominantly from the granulocytic series, and elevated protein levels up to several hundred mg/dL. Patients exhibiting such symptoms and signs should receive a thorough neurological examination, including CSF studies, to rule out other causes of meningitis. AMS may occur more frequently in association with high dose (2 g/kg) IGIV treatment.

Special Populations: Pregnant Women and Nursing Women: The safety of this medicinal product for use in human pregnancy has not been established in controlled clinical trials and therefore it should only be given with caution to pregnant women and breast-feeding mothers. Clinical experience with immunoglobulins suggests that no harmful effects on the course of pregnancy, or on the foetus and the neonate are to be expected.

Monitoring and Laboratory Tests: If signs and/or symptoms of hemolysis are present after IGIV infusion, appropriate confirmatory laboratory testing should be done (see Warnings and Precautions).

If TRALI is suspected, appropriate tests should be performed for the presence of anti-neutrophil antibodies in both the product and patient serum (see Warnings and Precautions).

Because of the potentially increased risk of thrombosis, baseline assessment of blood viscosity should be considered in patients at risk for hyperviscosity, including those with cryoglobulins, fasting chylomicronemia/markedly high triacylglycerols (triglycerides), or monoclonal gammopathies (see Warnings and Precautions).

ADVERSE REACTIONS: General: Various mild and moderate reactions, such as headache, fever, fatigue, chills, flushing, dizziness, urticaria, wheezing or chest tightness, nausea, vomiting, rigors, back pain, chest pain, muscle cramps, and changes in blood pressure may occur with infusions of Immune Globulin Intravenous (Human). In general, reported adverse reactions to GAMMAGARD LIQUID in patients with Primary Immunodeficiency are similar in kind and frequency to those observed with other IGIV products. Slowing or stopping the infusion usually allows the symptoms to disappear promptly. Although hypersensitivity reactions have not been reported in the clinical studies with GAMMAGARD LIQUID immediate anaphylactic and hypersensitivity reactions are a remote possibility. Epinephrine and antihistamines should be available for treatment of any acute anaphylactic reactions (see Warnings and Precautions).

Cases of reversible aseptic meningitis, isolated cases of reversible haemolytic anaemia/haemolysis and rare cases of transient cutaneous reactions have been observed with human normal immunoglobulin.

Increase in serum creatinine level and/or acute renal failure have been observed.

Very rarely: Thromboembolic reactions such as myocardial infarction, stroke, pulmonary embolism,and deep vein thromboses.

Clinical Trial Adverse Drug Reactions: Because clinical trials are conducted under very special conditions, the adverse reaction rates observed in the clinical trials may not reflect the rates observed in practice and should not be compared to the rates in the clinical trials of another drug.

Adverse experiences were examined among a total of 61 enrolled subjects with Primary Immunodeficiency who received at least one infusion of GAMMAGARD LIQUID during the Phase 3 multicenter clinical study. For this study, temporally associated adverse events are defined by the FDA as those occurring during or within 72 hours of completion of an infusion. Adverse drug reactions (ADR's) are those adverse events that were deemed by the investigators as causally related to the infusion of GAMMAGARD LIQUID.

Of all adverse experiences, 15 events in 8 subjects were serious. Two serious events, two episodes of aseptic meningitis in one patient, were deemed to be possibly related to the infusion of GAMMAGARD LIQUID.

Among the 896 non-serious adverse experiences, 258 were judged by the investigator to be possibly or probably related to the infusion of GAMMAGARD LIQUID. Of these, 136 were mild, 106 were moderate, and 16 were severe. All of the severe non-serious adverse experiences were transient, did not lead to hospitalization, and resolved without complication. One subject withdrew from the study due to a non-serious adverse experience (papular rash).

Of the 345 temporally related adverse experiences, those occurring in >5% of subjects are shown in Table 1. Of these events, only headache occurred in association with more than 5% of infusions. All events were expected based on past experiences with intravenous gammaglobulin products.

Table 1: GAMMAGARD LIQUID

Adverse Events[a], Regardless of Causality, That Occurred Within 72 Hours of Infusion

Event	By Infusion Number	By Infusion Percentage	By Subject Number	By Subject Percentage
Headache	57	6.90	22	36.1
Fever	19	2.30	13	21.3
Fatigue	18	2.18	10	16.4
Vomiting	10	1.21	9	14.8
Chills	14	1.69	8	13.1
Infusion site events	8	0.97	8	13.1
Nausea	9	1.09	6	9.8
Dizziness	7	0.85	6	9.8
Pain in Extremity	7	0.85	5	8.2
Diarrhea	7	0.85	5	8.2
Cough	5	0.61	5	8.2
Pruritus	5	0.61	4	6.5
Pharyngeal Pain	5	0.61	4	6.5

[a] Excluding Infections.

The majority (227/258) of the non-serious adverse experiences deemed related to study product were considered expected based on previous experience with IGIV products and 31 were considered unexpected. In virtually every case, these unexpected events were either consistent with the subject's specific type of immunodeficiency or with the subject's medical history prior to entering the study. A total of 14 hospitalizations occurred during the study but none were related to infection.

Hematology and clinical chemistry parameters were monitored in all subjects prior to each infusion throughout the 12-month period of study. Mean values for all laboratory parameters remained consistent throughout the study period. Three of the hematology values in one subject were outside of the normal range and reported as non-serious adverse experiences that resolved completely. These were a red cell count of $3.9 \times 10^6/\mu L$, hematocrit of 31%, and white cell count of $3.88 \times 10^3/\mu L$. All spontaneously returned to baseline. Using the International Grading System only one decrease of hemoglobin to Grade 2 (on a 0-4 scoring system) was observed, a value of 9.5 g/dL. There were several patients who had hemoglobin levels of Grade 1 (>10 g/dL) that were below the lower limits of normal. There were no decreases in hemoglobin that required further evaluation or intervention in any of the three clinical trials. One subject had an elevated BUN (45 mg/dL) and creatinine (1.4 mg/dL) on one occasion that were reported as non-serious adverse experiences and resolved completely. These values improved to 30 mg/dL and 0.8 mg/dL, respectively, by the next infusion. Six of the patients had a single, transient elevation in serum transaminases. Two additional patients had persistent elevations in transaminases, ALT and AST, which were present at the initiation of the study, prior to the infusion of GAMMAGARD LIQUID. There was no other evidence of liver abnormalities. None of the hematology or chemistry laboratory abnormalities that occurred during the course of the study required clinical intervention and none had clinical consequences.

During the Phase 3 clinical study, viral safety was assessed by serological screening for HBsAg and antibodies to HCV and HIV-1 and HIV-2 prior to, during, and at the end of the study and by Polymerase Chain Reaction (PCR) tests for HBV, HCV, and HIV-1 genomic sequences prior to and at the end of the study. None of the 61 treated subjects were positive prior to study entry and none converted from negative to positive during the 12-month period of study.

In Europe, an additional Clinical Study (160001) in 22 patients with PID was performed. No serious adverse drug reactions were observed.

Table 2 is a list of the incidence of adverse drug reactions (ADRs) reported in the European Clinical Study (160001) in 22 PID subjects who received GAMMAGARD LIQUID for about 6 months. ADRs were all non-serious. ADR rates in the table correspond to the number of ADRs per hundred infusions.

Table 2: GAMMAGARD LIQUID

Adverse Drug Reactions in EU Study (160001) in Patients with PID

MedDRA System Organ Class	MedDRA Preferred Term	ADR Rate (%)	ADR Frequency[a] Category
Ear and labyrinth disorders	Vertigo	0.5	Uncommon
General disorders and administration site conditions	Infusion site pain	0.5	Uncommon
	Pyrexia	1.4	Common
Nervous system disorders	Headache	1.0	Common
Skin and subcutaneous tissue disorders	Pruritus	0.5	Uncommon
	Urticaria	3.0	Common
Vascular disorders	Flushing	0.5	Uncommon

(cont'd)

[a] Frequency has been evaluated using the following criteria: very common (>1/10), common (>1/100, <1/10), uncommon (>1/1 000, <1/100), rare (>1/10 000, <1/1 000), and very rare (<1/10 000).

Also in Europe, a Clinical Study (160002) in 23 patients with ITP was performed. No serious adverse drug reactions were observed. The total number of ADRs reported during the study is given in Table 3.

Table 3: GAMMAGARD LIQUID

Adverse Drug Reactions in EU Study 160002 in 23 Patients with ITP

MedDRA System Organ Class	MedDRA Preferred Term	No of ADRs	ADR Frequency Category[a]
Gastrointestinal disorders	Nausea	2	Common
General disorders and administration site conditions	Infusion site pain	1	Common
	Infusion site phlebitis	1	Common
	Pyrexia	7	Common
Investigations	Body temperature increased	2	Common
Musculoskeletal and connective tissue disorders	Back pain	1	Common
	Pain in extremity	2	Common
Nervous system disorders	Burning sensation	1	Common
	Headache	11	Very common
	Insomnia	2	Common
Psychiatric disorders	Anxiety	1	Common
Respiratory, thoracic and mediastinal disorders	Rhinorrhoea	1	Common
Skin and subcutaneous tissue disorders	Dermatitis	1	Common
	Rash	1	Common
	Urticaria	1	Common
Vascular disorders	Flushing	1	Common
	Hypertension	3	Common
	Phlebitis	1	Common

[a] Frequency has been evaluated using the following criteria: very common (>1/10), common (>1/100, <1/10), uncommon (>1/1 000, <1/100), rare (>1/10 000, <1/1 000), and very rare (<1/10 000).

Less Common Clinical Trial Adverse Drug Reactions (<1%): For less common clinical trial adverse drug reactions refer to tables above.

Post-Market Adverse Drug Reactions: During the first five months of use of GAMMAGARD LIQUID (approximately one million grams) sixteen adverse drug reactions were spontaneously reported. There was one serious reaction, hypotension secondary to an anaphylactic-like event. There were no episodes of fall in hemoglobin suggestive of hemolysis, and no episodes of thrombosis or aseptic meningitis.

Post-efficacy Observation Period: Following the 12 month efficacy period patients were permitted to continue receiving Gammagard Liquid to obtain additional safety data. A total of 51 patients received 985 infusions of Gammagard Liquid. Adverse events, regardless of causality, occurring within 72 hours of infusion in more than 5% of the subjects are listed in Table 4.

Table 4: GAMMAGARD LIQUID

Adverse Events, Regardless of Causality, That Occurred Within 72 Hours of Infusion (Study 160101)

Adverse Events, Regardless of Causality, That Occurred Within 72 Hours of Infusion Post Efficacy Study Period				
	By Infusion		By Subject	
Event	Number	Percent[a]	Number	Percent[b]
Headache	25	2.54	12	23.53
Chills	14	1.42	8	15.69
Fatigue	7	0.71	5	9.80
Nausea	7	0.71	5	9.80
Sinusitis	5	0.51	5	9.80
Dizziness	4	0.41	4	7.84
Oedema peripheral	4	0.41	4	7.84
Pyrexia	7	0.71	4	7.84
Upper respiratory tract infection	4	0.41	4	7.84

(cont'd)

Table 4: GAMMAGARD LIQUID *(cont'd)*

Adverse Events, Regardless of Causality, That Occurred Within 72 Hours of Infusion (Study 160101)

Adverse Events, Regardless of Causality, That Occurred Within 72 Hours of Infusion Post Efficacy Study Period				
	By Infusion		By Subject	
Event	Number	Percent[a]	Number	Percent[b]
Acne	3	0.30	3	5.88
Conjunctivitis	3	0.30	3	5.88
Erythema	4	0.41	3	5.88
Herpes simplex	3	0.30	3	5.88
Infusion site reaction	5	0.51	3	5.88
Myalgia	3	0.30	3	5.88
Oral candidiasis	3	0.30	3	5.88
Pain in extremity	5	0.51	3	5.88

[a] Percent of Infusions is based on total 985 post efficacy infusions.
[b] Percent of Subjects is based on total 51 subjects.

There were no episodes of hemolysis, thrombosis, or aseptic meningitis during this observation period. There were no instances of decreased haemoglobin that required further evaluation or therapy.

DRUG INTERACTIONS: Overview: Antibodies in IGIV products may interfere with patient responses to live vaccines, such as those for measles, mumps and rubella. The immunizing physician should be informed of recent therapy with IGIV products so that appropriate precautions can be taken.

Admixtures of GAMMAGARD LIQUID with other drugs and intravenous solutions have not been evaluated. It is recommended that GAMMAGARD LIQUID be administered separately from other drugs or medications that the patient may be receiving. Normal saline should not be used as a diluent. If dilution is preferred, GAMMAGARD LIQUID may be diluted with 5% dextrose in water. No other drug interactions or compatibilities have been evaluated.

Drug-Drug Interactions: Interactions with other drugs have not been established.
Drug-Food Interactions: Interactions with food have not been established.
Drug-Herb Interactions: Interactions with herbal products have not been established.
Drug-Laboratory Test Interactions: Interactions with laboratory tests have not been established.
Drug-Lifestyle Interactions: Interactions with lifestyle have not been established.

DOSAGE AND ADMINISTRATION:

Dosing Considerations: The dose and dosage regimen are dependent on the indication.

In replacement therapy the dosage may need to be individualized for each patient depending on the pharmacokinetic and clinical response. The dosage regimens are given as a guideline below.

Recommended Dose and Dosage Adjustment: GAMMAGARD LIQUID is intended for intravenous administration. Dosage will vary depending on condition and bodyweight. The following doses are in agreement with currently suggested dosing schedules: See Table 5.

Table 5: GAMMAGARD LIQUID

Recommended Dose and Dosage Adjustment

Indication	Dose	Frequency of Injections
Replacement therapy in primary immunodeficiency	- starting dose: 0.4–0.8 g/kg BW - thereafter: 0.2–0.8 g/kg BW	every 2–4 weeks to obtain IgG trough level of at least 4–6 g/L
Replacement therapy in secondary immunodeficiency		
Allogeneic bone marrow Transplantation	0.2–0.4 g/kg BW	every 3–4 weeks to obtain IgG trough level of at least 4–6 g/L
Treatment of infections and prophylaxis of graft-versus host disease	0.5 g/kg	every week from day -7 up to 3 months after transplantation
Persistent lack of antibody production	0.5 g/kg	every month until antibody levels return to normal
Idiopathic thrombocytopenic purpura	0.8–1 g/kg BW or 0.4 g/kg BW/d	on day 1, possibly repeated once within 3 days for 2–5 days

Missed Dose: Give product at the earliest available opportunity.

Administration: Human normal immunoglobulin should be infused intravenously at an initial rate of 0.5 mL/kg BW/hr for 30 minutes. If well tolerated, the rate of administration may gradually be increased to a maximum of 8 mL/kg BW/hr.

OVERDOSAGE:

Overdose may lead to fluid overload and hyperviscosity, particularly in patients at risk, including elderly patients or patients with renal impairment.

For management of a suspected drug overdose, CPhA recommends that you contact your **regional Poison Control Centre**. See the *CPS* Directory section for a list of Poison Control Centres.

ACTION AND CLINICAL PHARMACOLOGY: Mechanism of Action: Immunoglobulins are the main effector molecules of the humoral immune response. They have two separable functions: one is to bind specifically to the antigen of the pathogen that elicited the immune response via their antigen-binding region; the other is to engage the effector functions of the immune system that will dispose of the antigen via their constant Fc region.

Immunoglobulins can protect from pathogens or their toxic products in three distinct ways:

- By binding of immunoglobulin to the antigen, its access to cells is blocked, i.e. the antigen is neutralized.
- When pathogens or foreign particles are coated by immunoglobulins, a process known as opsonization, the Fc portion of the antibody engages specific receptors on phagocytic cells resulting in the removal and destruction of the pathogen.
- The Fc portion of antigen-antibody complexes can activate complement, which enhances engulfment of pathogens by phagocytes or direct damage of certain bacteria.

Pharmacodynamics: Pharmacotherapeutic group: immune sera and immunoglobulins: immunoglobulins, normal human, for intravascular administration, ATC code: J06BA02.

Human normal immunoglobulin contains mainly immunoglobulin G (IgG) with a broad spectrum of antibodies against infectious agents.

Human normal immunoglobulin contains the IgG antibodies present in the normal population. It is usually prepared from pooled plasma from not fewer than 1000 donations. It has a distribution of immunoglobulin G subclasses closely proportional to that in native human plasma. Adequate doses of this medicinal product may restore abnormally low immunoglobulin G levels to the normal range.

The mechanism of action in indications other than replacement therapy is not fully elucidated, but includes immunomodulatory effects.

Pharmacokinetics: Human normal immunoglobulin is immediately bioavailable in the recipient's circulation after intravenous administration. It is distributed relatively rapidly between plasma and extravascular fluid; after approximately 3-5 days equilibrium is reached between the intra- and extravascular compartments.

Pharmacokinetic parameters for GAMMAGARD LIQUID were determined in Clinical Study 160001 in 22 subjects with hypo- and agammaglobulinemia. In this study, doses of 300 to 450 mg/kg body weight were administered every 21 days for about 6 months. GAMMAGARD LIQUID has a half-life of about 30 days. This half-life may vary from patient to patient, in particular in primary immunodeficiency.

Pharmacokinetic parameters determined for total IgG are shown in Table 6.

Table 6: GAMMAGARD LIQUID

Summary of GAMMAGARD LIQUID Pharmacokinetic Parameters (Study 160001)

Parameter	N	Median	95% CI
$AUC_{0\text{-}21d}$ (g·h/dL)	22	545	(490; 603)
C_{max} (mg/dL)	22	1630	(1470; 1750)
C_{min} (mg/dL)	22	848	(772; 1000)
T_{max} (hours)	22	0.25	(0.25; 0.25)
Terminal half-life (days)	22	30.1	(27.1; 43.3)
Incremental recovery (mg/dL)/(mg/kg)	22	1.85	(1.71, 2.14)
In-vivo recovery (%)	22	89	(84;101)

Similar results (half-life of about 35 days) were obtained in the Clinical Study 160101. The values obtained are comparable to parameters reported for other human immunoglobulins.

Absorption: Median area under the curve ($AUC_{0\text{-}21d}$) observed in the clinical study 160001 was 545 g·h/dL and maximal concentration in the blood occurs shortly after the intravenous infusion.

Distribution and Metabolism: After equilibration between intravascular and extravascular body compartments, plasmaproteins are eliminated from the plasma at a constant rate, as usually illustrated by a hypothetical two-compartment model. IgG and IgG-complexes are broken down in cells of the reticuloendothelial system.

Excretion: Median half-lives determined in clinical studies 160001 and 160101 were about 30 and 35 days, respectively.

Special Populations and Conditions: Pharmacokinetic information was not established in distinct studies for special populations and conditions.

STORAGE AND STABILITY: Refrigeration storage: Store in a refrigerator (2-8°C) for up to **36 months**. Do not freeze.

Do not use after the expiry date stated on the label and carton. Keep the vial in the outer carton in order to protect from light.

"Room temperature storage: Within the first 24 months from the date of manufacture, GAMMAGARD LIQUID may be stored for a single period of up to 9 months at room temperature (below 25°C). After this period, unused product must be discarded. See below the detailed storage information.

The total storage time of GAMMAGARD LIQUID depends on the point of the time the vial is transferred to room temperature. Examples for storage times are illustrated in Figure 1. If GAMMAGARD LIQUID is stored at room temperature (below 25°C), the date on which carton is removed from refrigerated storage and the new expiry date must be recorded in the area provided on the carton.

The new expiry date will be the **shorter** of: 24 months from the date of manufacture (indicated on the carton); or 9 months from the date removed from refrigeration. Once removed from refrigeration and stored at room temperature GAMMAGARD LIQUID must be used or discarded and may not be returned to refrigerated storage."

Figure 1: GAMMAGARD LIQUID

Storage Guidelines for GAMMAGARD LIQUID Months from Date of Manufacture

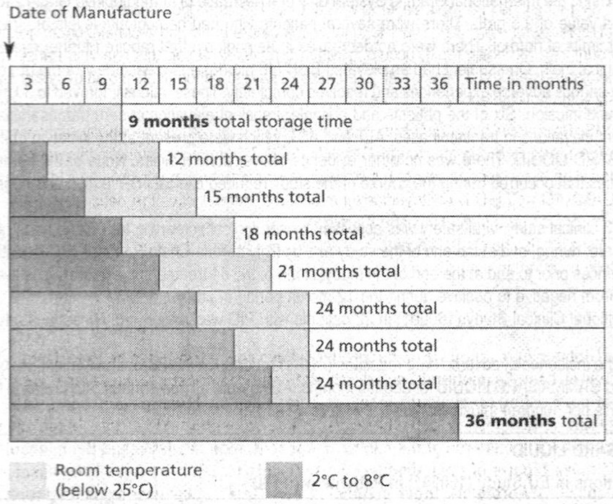

Example: If the product is taken out of the refrigerator after 3 months, it can be stored for 9 months at room temperature, and the total storage time is 12 months.

SPECIAL HANDLING INSTRUCTIONS: The product should be brought to room or body temperature before use.

If dilution to lower concentrations is warranted, 5% glucose is recommended.

The solution should be clear or slightly opalescent and colourless or pale yellow. Do not use solutions that are cloudy or have deposits.

GAMMAGARD LIQUID should only be administered intravenously. Other routes of administration have not been evaluated.

Any unused product or waste material should be disposed of in accordance with local requirements.

INFORMATION FOR THE PATIENT: Published in e-CPS, available by subscription at www.e-cps.ca.

DOSAGE FORMS, COMPOSITION AND PACKAGING: Solution for infusion administered intravenously.

The composition GAMMAGARD LIQUID is presented in Table 7.

Table 7: GAMMAGARD LIQUID
Target Composition of IGIV, 10%

Name of Component	Unit and/or Percentage Formula					Function
Protein (with at least 98% IgG)	1 g/vial	2.5 g/vial	5 g/vial	10 g/vial	20 g/vial	Active ingredient
Other Ingredients						
Glycine	0.25M	0.25M	0.25 M	0.25M	0.25M	Stabilizing agent
Water for injection	10 mL	25 mL	50 mL	100 mL	200 mL	Drug carrier

GAMMAGARD LIQUID is available in 1 g/10 mL, 2.5 g/25 mL, 5 g/50 mL, 10 g/100 mL, and 20 g/200 mL pack sizes. The product is filled into containers of type I glass, which are closed with bromobutyl rubber stoppers.

Gammagard® S/D

immune globulin intravenous (human)

Replacement Therapy for Immunodeficiencies

Baxter

Date of Preparation: November 12, 2003
Date of Revision: June 7, 2010

PHARMACOLOGY: GAMMAGARD S/D, Immune Globulin Intravenous (Human) [IGIV], Solvent/Detergent-Treated contains a broad spectrum of IgG antibodies against bacterial and viral agents that are capable of opsonization and neutralization of microbes and toxins.

Peak levels of IgG are reached immediately after infusion of IGIV, GAMMAGARD S/D. It has been shown that, after infusion, exogenous IgG is distributed relatively rapidly between plasma and extravascular fluid until approximately half is partitioned in the extravascular space. Therefore, a rapid initial drop in serum IgG levels is to be expected. As a class, IgG survives longer in vivo than other serum proteins. Studies show that the half life of IGIV, GAMMAGARD S/D, is approximately 37.7±15 days. Previous studies reported IgG half-life values of 21 to 25 days. The half-life of IgG can vary considerably from person to person, however. In particular, high concentrations of IgG and hypermetabolism associated with fever and infection have been seen to coincide with a shortened half-life of IgG.

INDICATIONS: GAMMAGARD S/D, Immune Globulin Intravenous (Human) [IGIV], Solvent/Detergent - Treated is contraindicated in patients with selective IgA deficiency where the IgA deficiency is the only abnormality of concern (see Contraindications and Warnings).

Primary Immunodeficiency Diseases: Immune Globulin Intravenous (Human) [IGIV], GAMMAGARD S/D, Solvent/Detergent-Treated is indicated for the treatment of primary immunodeficient states, such as: congenital agammaglobulinemias, common variable immunodeficiency, Wiskott-Aldrich syndrome, and severe combined immunodeficiencies. This indication was supported by a clinical trial of 17 patients with primary immunodeficiency who received a total of 341 infusions. IGIV, GAMMAGARD S/D, is especially useful when high levels or rapid elevation of circulating IgG are desired or when intramuscular injections are contraindicated (e.g., small muscle mass).

B-cell Chronic Lymphocytic Leukemia (CLL): IGIV, GAMMAGARD S/D, is indicated for prevention of bacterial infections in patients with hypogammaglobulinemia and/or recurrent bacterial infections associated with B-cell Chronic Lymphocytic Leukemia (CLL). In a study of 81 patients, 41 of whom were treated with IGIV, GAMMAGARD, bacterial infections were significantly reduced in the treatment group. In this study, the placebo group had approximately twice as many bacterial infections as the IGIV group. The median time to first bacterial infection for the IGIV group was greater than 365 days. By contrast, the time to first bacterial infection in the placebo group was 192 days. The number of viral and fungal infections, which were for the most part minor, was not statistically different between the two groups.

Idiopathic Thrombocytopenic Purpura (ITP): When a rapid rise in platelet count is needed to prevent and/or to control bleeding in a patient with Idiopathic Thrombocytopenic Purpura, the administration of IGIV, GAMMAGARD S/D, should be considered.

The efficacy of IGIV, GAMMAGARD, has been demonstrated in a clinical study involving 16 patients. Of these 16 patients, 13 had chronic ITP (11 adults, 2 children), and 3 patients had acute ITP (one adult, 2 children). All 16 patients (100%) demonstrated a clinically significant rise in platelet count to a level greater than 40 000/mm^3 following the administration of IGIV, GAMMAGARD. Ten of the 16 patients (62.5%) exhibited a significant rise to greater than 80 000 platelets/mm^3. Of these 10 patients, 7 had chronic ITP (5 adults, 2 children), and 3 patients had acute ITP (1 adult, 2 children).

The rise in platelet count to greater than 40 000/mm^3 occurred after a single 1 g/kg infusion of IGIV, GAMMAGARD in 8 patients with chronic ITP (6 adults, 2 children), and in 2 patients with acute ITP (one adult, one child). A similar response was observed after two 1 g/kg infusions in 3 adult patients with chronic ITP, and one child with acute ITP. The remaining 2 adult patients with chronic ITP received more than two 1 g/kg infusions before achieving a platelet count greater than 40 000/mm^3. The rise in platelet count was generally rapid, occurring within 5 days. However, this rise was transient and not considered curative. Platelet count rises lasted 2 to 3 weeks, with a range of 12 days to 6 months. It should be noted that childhood ITP may resolve spontaneously without treatment.

CONTRAINDICATIONS: Patients with IgA deficiency may experience severe hypersensitivity reactions or anaphylaxis in the setting of detectable IgA levels following infusion of GAMMAGARD S/D, Immune Globulin Intravenous (Human) [IGIV], Solvent/Detergent-Treated. The occurrence of severe hypersensitivity reactions or anaphylaxis should prompt consideration of an alternative therapy. GAMMAGARD S/D is contraindicated in patients with selective IgA deficiency where the IgA deficiency is the only abnormality of concern (see Indications and Warnings).

GAMMAGARD S/D should also be contraindicated in patients with a history of severe systemic or anaphylactic reactions to a human immune globulin preparation.

WARNINGS:

Warning: Immune Globulin Intravenous (Human) products have been reported to be associated with renal dysfunction, acute renal failure, osmotic nephrosis, and death. Patients predisposed to acute renal failure include patients with any degree of pre-existing renal insufficiency, diabetes mellitus, hypertension, age greater than 65, volume depletion, sepsis, paraproteinemia, or patients receiving known nephrotoxic drugs. Especially in such patients, IGIV products should be administered at the minimum concentration available and the minimum rate of infusion practicable. While these reports of renal dysfunction and acute renal failure have been associated with the use of many of the licensed IGIV products, those containing sucrose as a stabilizer accounted for a disproportionate share of the total number*.

See Precautions and Dosage for important information intended to reduce the risk of acute renal failure.

GAMMAGARD S/D, Immune Globulin Intravenous (Human) [IGIV], Solvent/Detergent-Treated, is made from human plasma. Products made from human plasma may contain infectious agents, such as viruses, that can cause disease. The risk that such products will transmit an infectious agent has been reduced by screening plasma donors for prior exposure to certain viruses, by testing for the presence of certain current virus infections, and by inactivating and/or removing certain viruses. (See Supplied). Despite these measures, such products can still potentially transmit disease. Because this product is made from human blood, it may carry a risk of transmitting infectious agents, e.g., viruses and theoretically, the Creutzfeldt-Jakob disease (CJD) and the variant Creutzfeldt-Jakob disease (vCJD) agents. All infections thought by a physician possibly to have been transmitted by this product should be reported by the physician or other healthcare provider to Baxter Corporation at 1-800-387-8399 (in Canada). The physician should discuss the risks and benefits of this product with the patient.

*** GAMMAGARD S/D does not contain sucrose.**

IGIV, GAMMAGARD S/D, should only be administered intravenously. Other routes of administration have not been evaluated.

Immediate anaphylactic and hypersensitivity reactions are a remote possibility. Epinephrine should be available for treatment of any acute anaphylactoid reactions.

IGIV, GAMMAGARD S/D, contains only trace amounts of IgA (≤2.2 µg/mL in a 5% solution). GAMMAGARD S/D is contraindicated in patients with selective IgA deficiency where the IgA deficiency is the only abnormality of concern and it should be given with caution to patients with antibodies to IgA or IgA deficiency, that is a component of an underlying primary immunodeficiency disease for which IGIV therapy is indicated. In such instances, a risk of anaphylaxis may exist despite the fact that GAMMAGARD S/D contains only trace amounts of IgA.

Physicians should report adverse reactions or any disease conditions which may occur concomitantly with the administration of this product to the manufacturer.

PRECAUTIONS: General: Some viruses, such as parvovirus B19 or hepatitis A, are particularly difficult to remove or inactivate at this time. Parvovirus B19 most seriously affects pregnant women, or immune-compromised individuals. Symptoms of parvovirus B19 infection include fever, drowsiness, chills, and runny nose followed about two weeks later by a rash and joint pain. Evidence of hepatitis A may include several days to weeks of poor appetite, tiredness, and low-grade fever followed by nausea, vomiting, and abdominal pain. Dark urine and a yellowed complexion are also common symptoms. Patients should be encouraged to consult their physician if such symptoms appear.

There is clinical evidence of a possible association between GAMMAGARD S/D, Immune Globulin Intravenous (Human) [IGIV], Solvent/Detergent-Treated administration and the potential for the development of thrombotic events. The exact cause of this is unknown; therefore, caution should be exercised in the prescribing and infusion of IGIV in patients with a history of and predisposing factors towards cardiovascular disease or thrombotic episodes, such as advanced age, restricted mobility, coagulation problems, gammopathies, diabetes, hypertension, cardiovascular problems or serious illness. Analysis of adverse events reports has indicated that a rapid rate of infusion may be a risk factor for vascular occlusive events.

For patients who are judged to be at risk for developing a thrombotic event the rate of infusion and percent of the solution concentrations should be targeted to the safety of the patient rather than convenience. Using a 5% concentration, the infusion rate should be initiated no faster than 0.5 mL/kg/h and advanced slowly, only if well tolerated, to a maximum rate of 4 mL/kg/h (<3.3 mg IgG/kg/min).

An aseptic meningitis syndrome (AMS) has been reported to occur infrequently in association with Immune Globulin Intravenous (Human) [IGIV] treatment. Discontinuation of IGIV treatment has resulted in remission of AMS within several days without sequelae. The syndrome usually begins within several hours to two days following IGIV treatment. It is characterized by symptoms and signs including severe headache, nuchal rigidity, drowsiness, fever, photophobia, painful eye movements, and nausea and vomiting. Cerebrospinal fluid (CSF) studies are frequently positive with pleocytosis up to several thousand cells per cu.mm., predominantly from the granulocytic series, and elevated protein levels up to several hundred mg/dL. Patients exhibiting such symptoms and signs should receive a thorough neurological examination, including CSF studies, to rule out other causes of meningitis. AMS may occur more frequently in association with high dose (2 g/kg) IGIV treatment.

Immunoglobulin administration may impair the efficacy of live attenuated virus vaccines such as measles, rubella, mumps, varicella and yellow fever for a period of at least six weeks and up to three months following infusion.

Assure that patients are not volume depleted prior to the initiation of the infusion of IGIV.

Periodic monitoring of renal function tests and urine output is particularly important in patients judged to have a potential increased risk for developing acute renal failure. Renal function, including measurement of blood urea nitrogen (BUN)/serum creatinine, should be assessed prior to the initial infusion of GAMMAGARD S/D and again at appropriate intervals thereafter. If renal function deteriorates, discontinuation of the product should be considered.

For patients judged to be at risk for developing renal dysfunction, it may be prudent to reduce the amount of product infused per unit time by infusing GAMMAGARD S/D at a rate less than 4 mL/kg/h (<3.3 mg IG/kg/min) for a 5% solution or at a rate less than 2 mL/kg/h (<3.3 mg IG/kg/min) for a 10% solution.

Certain components used in the packaging of this product contain natural rubber latex.

Information to Be Provided to the Patient: Patients should be instructed to immediately report symptoms of fluid retention/edema, decreased urine output, sudden weight gain, and/or shortness of breathe (which may suggest kidney damage) to their physician.

Drug Interactions: See Dosage.

Pregnancy: Category C: Animal reproduction studies have not been conducted with IGIV, GAMMAGARD S/D. It is also not known whether IGIV, GAMMAGARD S/D, can cause fetal harm when administered to a pregnant woman or can affect reproduction capacity. IGIV, GAMMAGARD S/D, should be given to a pregnant woman only if clearly needed.

ADVERSE EFFECTS: Increases in creatinine and blood urea nitrogen (BUN) have been observed as soon as one to two days following infusion. Progression to oliguria and anuria requiring dialysis has been observed, although some patients have improved spontaneously following cessation of treatment.

Types of severe renal adverse reactions that have been seen following IGIV therapy include: acute renal failure, acute tubular necrosis, proximal tubular nephropathy, osmotic nephrosis.

In general, reported adverse reactions to GAMMAGARD S/D, Immune Globulin Intravenous (Human) [IGIV], Solvent/Detergent-Treated in patients with either congenital or acquired immunodeficiencies are similar in kind and frequency. Various minor reactions, such as mild to moderate hypotension, headache, fatigue, chills, backache, leg cramps, lightheadedness, fever, urticaria, flushing, slight elevation of blood pressure, nausea and vomiting may occasionally occur. Slowing or stopping the infusion usually allows the symptoms to disappear promptly.

Immediate anaphylactic and hypersensitivity reactions are a remote possibility. Epinephrine should be available for treatment of any acute anaphylactoid reaction (see Warnings).

Primary Immunodeficiency Diseases: Twenty-one adverse reactions occurred in 341 infusions (6%), when using IGIV, GAMMAGARD (5% solution), in a clinical trial of 17 patients with primary immunodeficiency. Of the 17 patients, 12 (71%) were adults, and 5 (29%) were children (16 years or younger).

In a cross-over study comparing IGIV, GAMMAGARD, and IGIV, GAMMAGARD S/D (5% solutions), conducted in a small number (n=10) of primary immunodeficient patients, no unusual or unexpected adverse reactions were observed in the IGIV, GAMMAGARD S/D, group. The adverse reactions experienced in the IGIV, GAMMAGARD S/D, group were similar in frequency and nature to those observed in the control group consisting of patients receiving GAMMAGARD.

IGIV, GAMMAGARD, reconstituted to a concentration of 10%, was administered intravenously at rates varying from 2-11 mL/kg/h. Systemic reactions occurred in 23 (10.5%) of 219 infusions. This compares with an adverse reaction incidence of 6% (only systemic reactions reported) for primary immunodeficient patients previously treated with a 5% solution at infusion rates varying between 2 and 8 mL/kg/h, as described above. Local pain or irritation was experienced during 35 (16%) of 219 infusions. Application of a warm compress to the infusion site alleviated local symptoms. These local reactions tended to be associated with hand vein infusions and their incidence may be reduced by infusions via the antecubital vein.

B-cell Chronic Lymphocytic Leukemia (CLL): In the study of patients with B-cell Chronic Lymphocytic Leukemia, the incidence of adverse reactions associated with IGIV, GAMMAGARD infusions was approximately 1.3% while that associated with placebo (normal saline) infusions was 0.6%.

Idiopathic Thrombocytopenic Purpura (ITP): During the clinical study of IGIV, GAMMAGARD for the treatment of Idiopathic Thrombocytopenic Purpura, the only adverse reaction reported was headache, which occurred in 12 of 16 patients (75%). Of these 12 patients, 11 had chronic ITP (9 adults, 2 children), and one child had acute ITP. Oral antihistamines and analgesics alleviated the symptoms and were used as pretreatment for those patients requiring additional IGIV therapy. The remaining 4 patients did not report any side effects and did not require pretreatment.

OVERDOSE:

No overdosage has been reported for Gammagard S/D , Immune Globulin Intravenous (Human) [IGIV], Solvent/Detergent-Treated.

For management of a suspected drug overdose, CPhA recommends that you contact your **regional Poison Control Centre**. See the *CPS* Directory section for a list of Poison Control Centres.

DOSAGE: Primary Immunodeficiency Diseases: For patients with primary immunodeficiencies, monthly doses of at least 100 mg/kg are recommended. Initially, patients may receive 200-400 mg/kg. As there are significant differences in the half-life of IgG among patients with primary immunodeficiencies, the frequency and amount of immunoglobulin therapy may vary from patient to patient. The proper amount can be determined by monitoring clinical response. The minimum serum concentration of IgG necessary for protection has not been established.

B-cell Chronic Lymphocytic Leukemia (CLL): For patients with hypogammaglobulinemia and/or recurrent bacterial infections due to B-cell Chronic Lymphocytic Leukemia, a dose of 400 mg/kg every 3 to 4 weeks is recommended.

Idiopathic Thrombocytopenic Purpura (ITP): For patients with acute or chronic Idiopathic Thrombocytopenic Purpura, a dose of 1 g/kg is recommended. The need for additional doses can be determined by clinical response and platelet count. Up to three separate doses may be given on alternate days if required.

No prospective data are presently available to identify a maximum safe dose, concentration, and rate of infusion in patients determined to be at increased risk of acute renal failure. In the absence of prospective data, recommended doses should not be exceeded and the concentration and infusion rate selected should be the minimum level practicable. Reduction in dose, concentration, and/or rate of administration in patients at risk of acute renal failure has been proposed in the literature in order to reduce the risk of acute renal failure.

Reconstitution: The reconstituted product may be stored in either the original bottle or pooled into VIAFLEX bags. When reconstitution is performed aseptically in a sterile environment, the following storage guidelines are recommended: 24 hours at 5°C; or 12 hours at 25°C; or 12 hours at 25°C followed by 12 hours at 5°C.

Reconstitution: Use aseptic technique (see package insert for illustrations):

A. 5% Solution:

1. **Note: Reconstitute immediately before use.**
2. If refrigerated, warm the Sterile Water for Injection, USP (diluent) and GAMMAGARD S/D, Immune Globulin Intravenous (Human) [IGIV], Solvent/Detergent-Treated (freeze-dried concentrate), to room temperature.
3. Remove caps from concentrate and diluent bottles to expose central portion of rubber stoppers.
4. Cleanse stoppers with germicidal solution and allow to dry.

For 0.5 g Vials Only:

5. Remove protective covering from one end of the double-ended needle and insert exposed needle through diluent stopper at its **centre**.
6. Remove protective covering from other end of double-ended needle. Invert diluent bottle over upright concentrate bottle, then rapidly insert free end of the needle through the concentrate bottle stopper at its **centre**.
7. The vacuum in the concentrate bottle will draw in the diluent. When diluent transfer is complete, remove empty diluent bottle from needle and then needle from concentrate bottle. Discard needle after single use.
8. Thoroughly wet the dried material by tilting or inverting and gently rotating the bottle. **Do not shake. Avoid foaming.**
9. Repeat gentle rotation as long as undissolved product is observed.

For 2.5, 5 and 10 g Vials:

10. Remove spike cap from one end of transfer device. Do not touch spike.
11. Place diluent bottle on flat surface. Use exposed end of transfer device to spike diluent bottle through centre of the stopper. **CAUTION: Failure to insert spike into centre of the stopper may result in dislodging of the stopper.**
12. Ensure the collar collapses fully into the device by pushing down on the transfer device firmly. While holding onto transfer device, remove remaining spike cover. Do not touch spike.
13. Hold diluent bottle with attached transfer device at an angle to the concentrate bottle to prevent spilling the diluent. **Note: Do not hold diluent bottle upside down, for this can lead to diluent spillage.**
14. Spike concentrate bottle through centre of the stopper while **quickly inverting the diluent vial** to minimize spilling out diluent.
    CAUTION: Failure to insert the spike into the centre of the stopper may result in dislodging of the stopper and loss of vacuum.
15. Ensure that stopper collapses fully into the device by pushing down on the diluent bottle firmly.
16. After transfer of diluent is complete, remove transfer device and empty diluent bottle. Immediately swirl the concentrate bottle gently to thoroughly mix contents. Discard transfer device after single use per local guidelines. **CAUTION: Do not shake. Avoid foaming.**

B. 10% Solution: Follow steps 1 to 4 as previously described in **A**.

For 0.5 g Vials Only:

1. To prepare a 10% solution, reconstitute with the appropriate volume of diluent by using a sterile hypodermic syringe and needle. Table 1 indicates the volume of diluent required for 5 or 10% concentration. Using aseptic technique, draw required volume into a sterile hypodermic syringe and needle. The diluent is then injected into the concentrate bottle.
2. Discard any unused diluent after single use.
3. Thoroughly wet the dried material by tilting or inverting and gently rotating the bottle. **Do not shake. Avoid foaming.**
4. Repeat gentle rotation as long as undissolved product is observed.

For 2.5, 5 and 10 g Vials:

1. To prepare a 10% solution, it is necessary to remove half of the volume of diluent. Table 1 indicates the volume of diluent that should be removed from the vial before attaching the transfer device to produce a 10% concentration. Using aseptic technique, withdraw the necessary volume of diluent using a sterile hypodermic needle and syringe. Discard the filled syringe into a suitable puncture proof container.
2. Using the residual diluent in the diluent vial, follow steps 10 to 16 as previously described in **A**.

Table 1: GAMMAGARD S/D

Required Diluent Volume to be Removed

Concentration (%)	0.5 g Bottle (mL)	2.5 g Bottle (mL)	5 g Bottle (mL)	10 g Bottle (mL)
5	Do not remove any diluent for reconstitution of 5% solution			
10	5	25	48	96

Rate of Administration: It is recommended that initially a 5% solution be infused at a rate of 0.5 mL/kg/h. If infusion at this rate and concentration causes the patient no distress, the administration rate may be gradually increased to a maximum rate of 4 mL/kg/h. Patients who tolerate the 5% concentration at 4 mL/kg/h can be infused with the 10% concentration starting at 0.5 mL/kg/h. If no adverse effects occur, the rate can be increased gradually up to a maximum of 8 mL/kg/h.

For patients judged to be at risk for developing renal dysfunction, it may be prudent to reduce the amount of product infused per unit time by infusing GAMMAGARD S/D at a rate less than 4 mL/kg/h (<3.3 mg IG/kg/min) for a 5% solution or at a rate less than 2 mL/kg/h (<3.3 mg IG/kg/min) for a 10% solution.

For patients who are judged to be at risk for developing a thrombotic event the rate of infusion and percent of the solution concentrations should be targeted to the safety of the patient rather than convenience. Using a 5% concentration, the infusion rate should be initiated no faster than 0.5 mL/kg/h and advanced slowly, only if well tolerated, to a maximum rate of 4 mL/kg/h (<3.3 mg IgG/kg/min).

It is recommended that antecubital veins be used especially for 10% solutions, if possible. This may reduce the likelihood of the patient experiencing discomfort at the infusion site (see Adverse Effects).

A rate of administration which is too rapid may cause flushing and changes in pulse rate and blood pressure. Slowing or stopping the infusion usually allows the symptoms to disappear promptly.

Drug Interactions: Admixtures of GAMMAGARD S/D, with other drugs and intravenous solutions have not been evaluated. It is recommended that IGIV, GAMMAGARD S/D, be administered separately from other drugs or medications that the patient may be receiving. The product should not be mixed with IGIV from other manufacturers.

Antibodies in immune globulin preparations may interfere with patient responses to live vaccines, such as those for measles, mumps, and rubella. The immunizing physician should be informed of recent therapy with IGIV so that appropriate precautions can be taken.

Administration (see package insert for illustrations): **For intravenous use only.**

IGIV, GAMMAGARD S/D should be administered as soon after reconstitution as possible. The reconstituted material should be at room temperature during administration.

Parenteral drug products should be inspected visually for particulate matter and discoloration prior to administration, whenever solution and container permit. Reconstituted material should be a clear to slightly opalescent and colorless to pale yellow solution. Do not use if particulate matter and/or discoloration is observed.

For 0.5 g Bottles Only: Intravenous Syringe Injection:

1. Attach filter needle to a disposable syringe and draw back plunger to admit air into syringe.
2. Insert needle into reconstituted GAMMAGARD S/D.
3. Inject air into bottle and then withdraw the reconstituted material into the syringe.
4. Remove and discard the filter needle from the syringe; attach a suitable needle and inject i.v. as instructed under Rate of Administration.

For 2.5, 5 and 10 g Bottles: Follow directions for use which accompany the administration set provided. If another administration set is used, ensure that the set contains a similar filter.

SUPPLIED: GAMMAGARD S/D, Immune Globulin Intravenous (Human) [IGIV], is a solvent/detergent-treated, sterile, freeze-dried preparation of highly purified immunoglobulin G (IgG) derived from large pools of human plasma. The product is manufactured by the Cohn-Oncley cold ethanol fractionation process followed by ultrafiltration and ion exchange chromatography. The manufacturing process includes treatment with an organic solvent/detergent mixture, composed of tri(n-butyl) phosphate, octoxynol 9 and polysorbate 80. The IGIV, GAMMAGARD S/D, manufacturing process provides a significant viral reduction in in vitro studies. These studies, summarized in Table 2, demonstrate virus clearance during IGIV, GAMMAGARD S/D, manufacturing using infectious human immunodeficiency virus, Types 1 and 2 (HIV-1, HIV-2); Sindbis virus (SIN), a model virus for hepatitis C virus; pseudorabies virus (PRV), a model virus for lipid-enveloped DNA viruses such as herpes; and vesicular stomatitis virus (VSV), a model virus for lipid-enveloped RNA viruses. These reductions are achieved through a combination of process chemistry, partitioning and/or inactivation during cold ethanol fractionation and the solvent/detergent treatment.

Reduction factors (RFs) from the most recent and/or most comprehensive studies were used for this summary table. Only RFs for steps based on **different** mechanisms of virus removal/inactivation were used for calculation of the overall reduction factor (ORF). RFs used for calculation of the ORF are marked in bold. Study report numbers are provided in footnotes.

Table 2: GAMMAGARD S/D

In Vitro Virus Clearance During IGIV, GAMMAGARD S/D, Manufacturing

	Reduction Factor (log_{10})						
	Lipid Enveloped Viruses				Non-Enveloped Viruses		
Process Step Evaluated	HIV	BVDV	WNV	PRV	HAV	B19V	Parvo Model (PPV/MMV)
Step 1: From Cryo-Poor Plasma to Fraction I+II+III Precipitate	5.6[b]	0.6[c]	ND	1.0[d]	0.5[e]	ND	0.2[f]
Step 2 & 3 Combined: From Resuspended Precipitate A to Cuno 70 Filtrate	**>5.8**[g]	**2.7**[g]	**>5.8**[g]	**>5.7**[g]	**4.3**[h]	**>4.1**[i]	**>4.9 (PPV)**[j] **5.3 (MMV)**[g]
Step 4: S/D Treatment	**>3.7**[k]	**>8.4**[l]	**>6.0**[m]	**>4.1**[n]	NA	NA	NA
Overall log_{10} Reduction Factor (ORF)[a]	**>9.5**	**>11.1**	**>11.8**	**>9.8**	**4.3**	**>4.1**	**>4.9/5.3**

[a] Therefore, reduction factors for the steps 1 and (2&3 combined) were not added together for the ORF, as the mechanism of virus clearance is the same for all these steps (virus clearance by precipitation).
[b] Report 96002-CMC-017.
[c] Report 96002-CMC-015.
[d] Report 96002-CMC-012.
[e] Report 96002-CMC-018.
[f] Report 96002-CMC-016 (PPV Data).
[g] Report reg642e.
[h] Mean of 4.1 (report 94016-CMC-062) and >4.5 (reg642e).
[i] Report 94016-CMC-063.
[j] Report 94016-CMC-066.
[k] Report 94016-CMC-048.
[l] Report reg644e (for a more comprehensive investigation of the SD treatment, a high-volume assay was used for detection of BVDV).
[m] Report preg007e (investigational study) + Amendment AD1_PE0102.
[n] Report 94016-CMC-046.

Legend: ND=not done; NA=not applicable (SD treatment not effective against non-enveloped viruses); HIV=Human Immunodeficiency virus; BVDV=Bovine viral diarrhea virus; WNV=West Nile virus; PRV=Pseudorabies virus, HAV=Hepatitis A virus; B19V=Human Parvovirus B19; PPV=Porcine parvovirus; MMV=Mice minute virus.

When reconstituted with the total volume of diluent (Sterile Water for Injection, USP) supplied, this preparation contains approximately 50 mg of protein/mL (5%), of which at least 90% is gamma globulin.

The manufacturing process for IGIV, GAMMAGARD S/D, isolates IgG without additional chemical or enzymatic modification and the Fc portion is maintained intact. IGIV, GAMMAGARD S/D, contains all of the IgG antibody activities which are present in the donor population. On the average, the distribution of IgG subclasses present in this product is similar to that in normal plasma. IGIV, GAMMAGARD S/D, contains only trace amounts of IgA (≤2.2 µg/mL in a 5% solution). IgM is also present in trace amounts (<0.4 mg/mL in a 5% solution).

IGIV, GAMMAGARD S/D, contains no preservative.

IGIV, GAMMAGARD S/D, may be reconstituted with diluent (Water for Injection, USP) to a 5% (50 mg/mL) solution or a 10% (100 mg/mL) solution of protein of which at least 90% is gamma globulin. The product, reconstituted to 5%, contains a physiological concentration of sodium chloride (approximately 8.5 mg/mL) and has a pH of 6.8±0.4. Stabilizing agents and additional components are present in the following maximum amounts for a 5% solution: albumin (human) 3 mg/mL, glycine 22.5 mg/mL, glucose 20 mg/mL, polyethylene glycol 2 mg/mL, tri(n-butyl) phosphate 1 µg/mL, octoxynol 9 1 µg/mL and polysorbate 80, 100 µg/mL.

If it is necessary to prepare a 10% (100 mg/mL) solution for infusion, half the volume of diluent should be added as described in the Dosage section. In this case, the stabilizing agents and other components will be present at double the concentrations given for the 5% solution.

Bottles of 2.5, 5 and 10 g freeze-dried concentrate, which is packaged with Sterile Water for Injection, USP (diluent), 1 transfer device, 1 administration set and directions for use. The volume of sterile water for injection, USP (diluent) provided with each GAMMAGARD S/D package size is as follows: 2.5 g: 50 mL; 5 g: 96 mL; 10 g: 192 mL. Single dose bottles of 0.5 g of freeze-dried concentrate, which is packaged with a 10 mL bottle of sterile water for injection, USP (diluent), a double-ended needle, a filter spike, and directions for use.

The freeze-dried concentrate and diluent are provided in Type 1 USP clear glass, single dose bottles each with a rubber stopper and an aluminum cap with a twist-off centre.

Reconstituted Solutions: IGIV, GAMMAGARD S/D, should be administered intravenously after reconstitution with the appropriate volume of Water for Injection, USP (diluent) provided in each package. Refer to Table 1 under Dosage for the quantity of diluent required to produce both 5% and 10% concentrations of GAMMAGARD S/D.

Parenteral Solutions: GAMMAGARD S/D preparations should not be mixed with other pharmaceutical products. Administer separately from other medications.

Stability and Storage: Store at a temperature not to exceed 25°C. Freezing should be avoided to prevent the diluent bottle from breaking. Do not use after the expiration date. Any unused solution must be discarded due to the risk of bacterial contamination. Store out of reach of children.

Gamunex®

immune globulin intravenous (human)

Passive Immunizing Agent

Talecris

Date of Revision: May 13, 2010

SUMMARY PRODUCT INFORMATION:

Route of Administration	Dosage Form/ Strength	Clinically Relevant Nonmedicinal Ingredients
Intravenous or Subcutaneous	Injectable solution, 10%	Glycine For a complete list see Dosage Forms, Composition and Packaging.

DESCRIPTION: GAMUNEX (Immune Globulin Intravenous [Human], 10%) manufactured by a patented chromatography process is a ready-to-use sterile solution of human immune globulin protein for intravenous or subcutaneous administration. GAMUNEX consists of 9%-11% protein in 0.16-0.24 M glycine. GAMUNEX contains no preservative.

GAMUNEX is made from large pools of human plasma by a combination of cold ethanol fractionation, caprylate precipitation and filtration, and anion-exchange chromatography. The protein is stabilized during the process by adjusting the pH of the solution to 4.0-4.5. Isotonicity is achieved by the addition of glycine.

INDICATIONS AND CLINICAL USE: GAMUNEX (Immune Globulin Intravenous [Human], 10%) is indicated in:

Primary Immune Deficiency Syndromes (PID), including (Intravenous or Subcutaneous Administration):

- Congenital agammaglobulinaemia and hypogammaglobulinaemia
- Common variable immunodeficiency
- X-linked immunodeficiency with hyper IgM
- Severe combined immunodeficiency
- Wiskott Aldrich syndrome

Secondary Immune Deficiency Syndromes (SID), including (Intravenous or Subcutaneous Administration):

- Allogeneic bone marrow transplantation
- Pediatric HIV infection

Neurological and/or Autoimmune Conditions:

- Chronic inflammatory demyelinating polyneuropathy (CIDP) in adults, 18 years of age or older
- Idiopathic Thrombocytopenic Purpura (ITP)

Primary Immune Deficiency Syndromes (PID): GAMUNEX is indicated as replacement therapy of primary humoral immunodeficiency states in which severe impairment of antibody forming capacity has been shown, such as congenital agammaglobulinemia, common variable immunodeficiency, X-linked immunodeficiency with hyper IgM, Wiskott-Aldrich syndrome, and severe combined immunodeficiencies.

Secondary Immune Deficiency Syndromes (SID): Allogeneic Bone Marrow Transplantation: GAMUNEX is indicated for the reduction of septicemia and other infections, interstitial pneumonia and acute graft versus host disease in the first 100 days post-transplant in Allogeneic Bone Marrow Transplantation (BMT) patients of at least 20 years of age.

Shortly before, and for varying times after bone marrow transplantation, patients are immunosuppressed. The benefit of Immune Globulin Intravenous (Human) in these patients during the recovery period is similar to that of replacement therapy in PID. The utility of Immune Globulin Intravenous (Human) in BMT had been confirmed by long-term experience and in peer-reviewed published reports.

Graft-versus-host-disease (GvHD) is a frequent complication of BMT. Immune Globulin Intravenous (Human) has been demonstrated to significantly reduce the incidence of acute GvHD (see Action and Clinical Pharmacology).

Pediatric HIV Infection: GAMUNEX is indicated for the reduction of recurrent serious bacterial infections in those children who do not respond to or cannot tolerate antiretroviral combination therapy. Children with HIV infections, particularly when acquired through vertical transmission, are prone to recurrent serious bacterial infections, although they have apparently normal or supranormal IgG levels.

Neurological and/or Autoimmune Conditions: Chronic Inflammatory Demyelinating Polyneuropathy (CIDP): GAMUNEX is indicated for the treatment of CIDP to improve neuromuscular disability and impairment, and for maintenance therapy to prevent relapse. Patients treated in the pivotal trial with GAMUNEX for up to 48 weeks had improvements in neuromuscular disability scores and grip strength compared to placebo.

Idiopathic Thrombocytopenic Purpura: GAMUNEX is indicated in ITP to rapidly raise platelet counts to prevent bleeding or to allow a patient with ITP to undergo surgery.

Geriatrics (>65 years of age): No specific studies in elderly patients have been conducted. However, no evidence of a higher incidence of adverse events was observed in elderly patients.

Pediatrics (1-18 years of age): GAMUNEX is indicated for pediatric HIV infection. Pediatric patients were enrolled in the pivotal studies for primary humoral immunodeficiency and for idiopathic thrombocytopenic purpura. The clinical trial evaluating subcutaneous GAMUNEX in primary immune deficiency included three pediatric subjects (age range 13-15). Allogeneic bone marrow transplantation is not recommended for patients less than 20 years of age.

CONTRAINDICATIONS:

- GAMUNEX (Immune Globulin Intravenous [Human], 10%) is contraindicated in patients who are hypersensitive to this drug or to any ingredient in the formulation or component of the container. For a complete listing, see Dosage Forms, Composition and Packaging.
- GAMUNEX (Immune Globulin Intravenous [Human], 10%) is contraindicated in individuals with known anaphylactic or severe systemic response to human immune globulin. Individuals with severe, selective IgA deficiencies (serum IgA <0.05 g/L) who have known antibody against IgA (anti-IgA antibody) should only receive GAMUNEX with utmost cautionary measures. Recent reports claim that IgA exposure to individuals with severe, selective IgA deficiency and high levels of anti-IgA antibodies was not, or only in a few cases, associated with adverse reactions. Two groups have reported that human immune globulin intravenous preparations with an IgA content less than 50 mg/L could be given safely to patients with severe selective IgA deficiency despite a history of repeated severe infusion reactions to Immune Globulin Intravenous (Human). GAMUNEX has a markedly reduced IgA content (46 mg/L) compared to GAMIMUNE N, 10% (210 mg/L). However, no experience is available on tolerability of GAMUNEX in patients with selective IgA deficiency since they were excluded from participation in clinical trials with GAMUNEX.

WARNINGS AND PRECAUTIONS:

Serious Warnings and Precautions

- Immune Globulin Intravenous (Human) products have been reported to be associated with renal dysfunction, acute renal failure, osmotic nephrosis and death (see Renal, and Dosage and Administration, Recommended Dose and Dosage Adjustment)
- Hemolytic anemia, hemolysis, and hemolytic reaction have been reported in association with use of GAMUNEX and other Immune Globulin Intravenous (Human) products (see Hematologic)

General: On rare occasions, treatment with an immune globulin preparation may cause a precipitous fall in blood pressure and a clinical picture of anaphylaxis, even when the patient is not known to be sensitive to immune globulin preparations. Epinephrine should be available for the treatment of an acute anaphylactic reaction.

Any vial that has been punctured should be used promptly. Partially used vials should be discarded. Visually inspect each bottle before use. Do not use if turbid. If the solution has been frozen, it must not be used.

GAMUNEX is made from human plasma. Products made from human plasma may contain infectious agents, such as viruses, and theoretically, the Creutzfeldt-Jakob (CJD) agent that can cause disease. The risk that such products will transmit an infectious agent has been reduced by screening plasma donors for prior exposure to certain viruses, by testing for the presence of certain current virus infections, and by inactivating and/or removing certain viruses. Despite these measures, such products can still potentially transmit disease. There is also the possibility that unknown infectious agents may be present in such products. Individuals who receive infusions of blood or plasma products may develop signs and/or symptoms of some viral infections.

All infections thought by a physician possibly to have been transmitted by this product should be reported by the physician or other healthcare provider to Talecris Biotherapeutics Ltd. [1-866-482-5226]. The physician should discuss the risks and benefits of this product with the patient, before prescribing or administering it to the patient.

Cardiovascular: There is a possible association between thrombo-embolic (TE) events and administration of Immune Globulin Intravenous (Human) (IGIV) products. Caution should be exercised in administration of IGIV in patients with coagulopathies, cardiovascular disease, thrombophilia, restricted mobility, and the elderly. The etiology of TE events related to IGIV therapy is not clear and may reflect IGIV dose and hyperosmolality. GAMUNEX is an iso-osmolar solution. In clinical trials to date, no thromboembolic events were reported for any patient treated with GAMUNEX.

Hematologic: Immune Globulin Intravenous (Human) (IGIV) products can contain blood group antibodies which may act as hemolysins and induce in vivo coating of red blood cells with immunoglobulin, causing a positive direct antiglobulin reaction and, rarely, hemolysis (see Adverse Reactions, Post-Market Adverse Drug Reactions). Hemolytic anemia can develop subsequent to IGIV therapy due to enhanced RBC sequestration (see Drug Interactions, Drug-Laboratory Test Interactions). Risk factors for hemolytic anemia include use of certain antibiotics, renal transplant rejection, multiple or incompatible blood transfusions, and history of certain blood disorders. IGIV recipients should be monitored for clinical signs and symptoms of hemolysis (see Monitoring and Laboratory Tests).

Neurologic: An aseptic meningitis syndrome (AMS) has been reported to occur infrequently in association with Immune Globulin Intravenous (Human) treatment. The syndrome usually begins within several hours to two days following Immune Globulin Intravenous (Human) treatment. It is characterized by symptoms and signs including severe headache, nuchal rigidity, drowsiness, fever, photophobia, painful eye movements, nausea and vomiting. AMS may occur more frequently in association with high dose (2000 mg/kg) Immune Globulin Intravenous (Human) treatment. Discontinuation of Immune Globulin Intravenous (Human) treatment has resulted in remission of AMS within several days without sequelae.

Renal: Immune Globulin Intravenous (Human) (IGIV) products have been reported to be associated with renal dysfunction, acute renal failure, osmotic nephrosis and death. Patients predisposed to acute renal failure include patients with any degree of pre-existing renal insufficiency, diabetes mellitus, age greater than 65, volume depletion, sepsis, paraproteinemia, or patients receiving known nephrotoxic drugs. Especially in such patients, human immune globulin products should be administered at the minimum concentration available and the minimum rate of infusion practicable. While these reports of renal dysfunction and acute renal failure have been associated with the use of many of the licensed human immune globulin products, those containing sucrose as a stabilizer accounted for a disproportionate share of the total number. GAMUNEX (Immune Globulin Intravenous [Human], 10%) does not contain sucrose.

Respiratory: There have been reports of noncardiogenic pulmonary edema (Transfusion-Related Acute Lung Injury [TRALI]) in patients administered IGIV. TRALI is characterized by severe respiratory distress, pulmonary edema, hypoxemia, normal left ventricular function, and fever and typically occurs within 1-6 hrs after transfusion. Patients with TRALI may be managed using oxygen therapy with adequate ventilatory support.

IGIV recipients should be monitored for pulmonary adverse reactions. If TRALI is suspected, appropriate tests should be performed for the presence of anti-neutrophil antibodies in both the product and patient serum (see Monitoring and Laboratory Tests).

Special Populations: Pregnant Women: There is no experience of GAMUNEX in pregnancy during clinical trials. Animal reproduction studies have not been conducted with GAMUNEX. It is not known whether GAMUNEX can cause fetal harm when administered to a pregnant woman or can affect reproduction capacity. GAMUNEX should be given to a pregnant woman only if clearly needed.

Nursing Women: Immunoglobulins are excreted into the milk and may contribute to the transfer of protective antibodies to the neonate.

Pediatrics (1-18 years of age): GAMUNEX is indicated for pediatric patients in the treatment of primary humoral immunodeficiency, idiopathic thrombocytopenic purpura and pediatric HIV infection. The clinical trial evaluating subcutaneous GAMUNEX in primary immune deficiency included three pediatric subjects (age range 13-15).

Geriatrics (>65 years of age): See Renal. The clinical trial evaluating subcutaneous GAMUNEX in primary immune deficiency included four elderly subjects (age range 65-68).

Monitoring and Laboratory Tests: In some patients, administration of GAMUNEX results in a transitory rise of passively transferred antibodies which may produce misleading serological findings such as positive direct anti-globulin and anti-HBc results in the absence of viral transmission.

Periodic monitoring of renal function and urine output is particularly important in patients judged to have a potential increased risk for developing acute renal failure. Renal function, including measurements of blood urea nitrogen (BUN)/serum creatinine, should be assessed prior to the initial infusion of GAMUNEX and again at appropriate intervals thereafter.

If signs or symptoms of hemolysis are present after GAMUNEX infusion, appropriate confirmatory laboratory testing, such as unconjugated serum bilirubin, serum haptoglobulin, Direct Antiglobulin test (DAT) and serum LDH, should be done.

If TRALI is suspected, appropriate tests should be performed for the presence of anti-neutrophil antibodies in both the product and patient serum.

ADVERSE REACTIONS: Adverse Drug Reaction Overview: Increases in creatinine and blood urea nitrogen (BUN) have been observed as soon as one to two days following infusion, predominantly with other human immune globulin products, stabilized with sucrose. Progression to oliguria and anuria requiring dialysis has been observed, although some patients have improved spontaneously following cessation of treatment. GAMUNEX (Immune Globulin Intravenous [Human], 10%) does not contain sucrose. Glycine, a natural amino acid, is used as a stabilizer. In the studies undertaken to date with GAMUNEX, no increase in creatinine and blood urea nitrogen was observed.

Although not all adverse effects previously reported with intravenous and intramuscular immunoglobulin administration have been observed for GAMUNEX, adverse effects may be expected to be similar to those reported with these products. Potential reactions may include anxiety, flushing, wheezing, abdominal cramps, myalgias, arthralgia, dizziness, and rash. In addition, rare cases of hemolytic anemia/hemolysis which were moderate to severe in intensity have been reported with human immunoglobulins, including GAMUNEX (see Warnings and Precautions).

True allergic/anaphylactic reactions to GAMUNEX may occur in recipients with documented prior histories of severe allergic reactions to intramuscular immunoglobulin, but some patients may tolerate cautiously administered intravenous immunoglobulin without adverse effects. Very rarely an anaphylactic reaction may occur in patients with no prior history of severe allergic reactions to either intramuscular or intravenous immunoglobulin.

Clinical Trial Adverse Drug Reactions: Because clinical trials are conducted under very specific conditions the adverse reaction rates observed in the clinical trials may not reflect the rates observed in practice and should not be compared to the rates in the clinical trials of another drug. Adverse drug reaction information from clinical trials is useful for identifying drug-related adverse events and for approximating rates.

Primary Immune Deficiency (PID): Intravenous Administration: Adverse events were monitored in three randomized clinical trials, involving more than 200 primary immune deficiency patients receiving intravenous administration. In two trials, involving 18-20 patients each, patients received 100-600 mg/kg GAMUNEX or GAMIMUNE N, 10% for three subsequent infusions on a 3 or 4 week infusion interval and were then crossed over to three infusions of the alternate product. In the third trial, 172 patients were randomized to GAMUNEX or GAMIMUNE N, 10% for a nine-month double-blinded treatment with either of the two products at a dose between 100 and 600 mg/kg on a 3 or 4 week infusion interval. In a pooled analysis across the three studies, the infusion rate (0.08 mL/kg/min) was reduced for 11 of 210 exposed patients (7 GAMUNEX, 4 GAMIMUNE N, 10%) at 17 occasions. In most instances, mild to moderate hives/urticaria, itching, pain or reaction at infusion site, anxiety or headache was the main reason for reduction in infusion rate. There was one case of severe chills. There were no anaphylactic or anaphylactoid reactions.

In the pivotal clinical trial, the most frequently recorded drug related adverse events (≥0.5%) normalized per patient and infusion are given in Table 1.

Table 1: GAMUNEX

Most Frequently Recorded Drug Related Adverse Events (≥0.5%) Normalized per Patient and Infusion

Drug Related Adverse Events	GAMUNEX No. of Infusions: 825 n (%)	GAMIMUNE N, 10% No. of Infusions: 865 n (%)
Cough increased	14 (1.7%)	11 (1.3%)
Headache	7 (0.8%)	11 (1.3%)

(cont'd)

Table 1: GAMUNEX *(cont'd)*

Most Frequently Recorded Drug Related Adverse Events (≥0.5%) Normalized per Patient and Infusion

Drug Related Adverse Events	GAMUNEX No. of Infusions: 825 n (%)	GAMIMUNE N, 10% No. of Infusions: 865 n (%)
Fever	1 (0.1%)	9 (1.0%)
Pharyngitis	7 (0.8%)	9 (1.0%)
Nausea	4 (0.5%)	4 (0.5%)
Urticaria	4 (0.5%)	5 (0.6%)

At various time points after the infusion of Immune Globulin Intravenous (Human), 10%, serum samples were drawn to monitor the viral safety of the PID patients. Viral markers of hepatitis C, hepatitis B, HIV-1, and parvovirus B19 were monitored by nucleic acid testing (NAT, Polymerase Chain Reaction (PCR), and serological testing. There were no treatment related emergent findings of viral transmission.

Similar adverse reactions as for **PID** are expected for the Immune Globulin Intravenous (Human), 10% treatment of patients **with pediatric HIV infection** or **allogeneic bone marrow transplantation** due to the similar mechanism of action and dose schedule.

Subcutaneous Administration: Adverse events occurring in study 060001 (investigating subcutaneous infusion of GAMUNEX) were divided into 2 types: 1) Local infusion site reactions, and 2) Non-infusion site adverse events. Table 2 displays the most common drug-related adverse events, normalized per infusion, occurring with ≥0.5% of infusions during the subcutaneous phase of the study.

Table 2: GAMUNEX

Most Frequent Drug-Related Adverse Events, per Infusion (≥0.5%) by Subjects in the Subcutaneous Phase (study 060001)

Drug-related Adverse Event (≥0.5% of subjects)	Rate of Adverse Events Number of infusions: 725 n (%)
Local Infusion Site Reactions	427 (58.9%)
Non-infusion site adverse events	
Headache	21 (2.9%)
Arthralgia	4 (0.6%)

The most common drug-related adverse reactions with subcutaneous administration of GAMUNEX were infusion site reactions, consisting primarily of mild to moderate erythema, pain and swelling. The majority of local infusion site reactions resolved within 3 days. Among these local site reactions, 91.1% were classified as mild, 6.8% were moderate, and just 2.1% considered severe. No serious local infusion site reactions were observed. The number of subjects reporting these local infusion site reactions decreased substantially over time as subjects received continued weekly infusions (see Figure 1).

Figure 1: GAMUNEX

Percentages of Subjects Reporting Local Infusion Site Reactions After Repeated Infusions During the SC Phase (Safety Population)

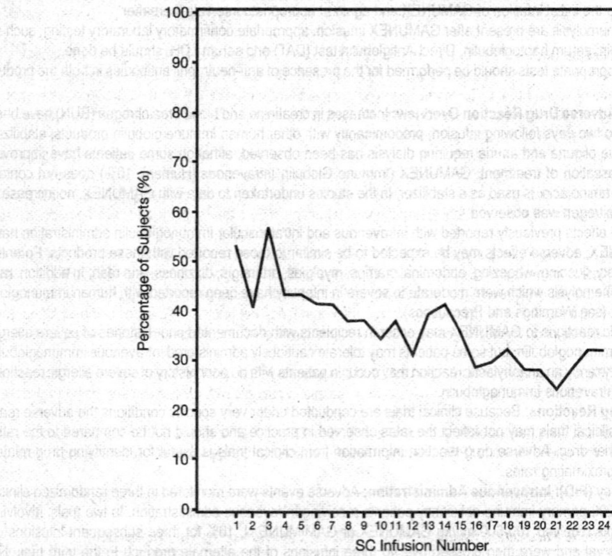

Idiopathic Thrombocytopenic Purpura (ITP): Adverse reactions were monitored in two randomized clinical trials with more than 100 patients with acute or chronic ITP.

In the first study (randomized and double-blind), 97 ITP patients were randomized to a single dose of 2000 mg/kg of GAMUNEX 10% or GAMIMUNE N, 10%. The total dose was divided into two 1000 mg/kg doses given on two consecutive days at a maximum infusion rate of 0.08 mL/kg/min.

As expected, the adverse event rate for Immune Globulin Intravenous (Human), 10% in this ITP trial was higher than observed in the replacement therapy for Primary Immune Deficiencies (PID), but was within the range reported earlier for Immune Globulin Intravenous (Human). It should be noted that the dose is 4-5 fold higher than in PID and that the total dose was given on two consecutive days rather than on five consecutive days, which is associated with a higher adverse event rate. Finally, no pre-medication with corticosteroids was permitted in the study protocol. More than 90% of the observed drug related adverse events were of mild to moderate severity and of transient nature.

The most frequently recorded drug related adverse events (≥2.0%) are given in Table 3.

The infusion rate was reduced for only 4 of the 97 treated patients (1 GAMUNEX, 3 GAMIMUNE N, 10%) on 4 occasions. Mild to moderate headache, nausea, and fever were the reported reasons. There were no anaphylactic or anaphylactoid reactions.

At various time points after the infusion of Immune Globulin Intravenous (Human), 10%, serum samples were drawn to monitor the viral safety of the ITP patients. Viral markers of hepatitis C, hepatitis B, HIV-1, and parvovirus B19 were monitored by nucleic acid testing (NAT), Polymerase Chain Reaction (PCR), and serological testing. There were no treatment related emergent findings of viral transmission.

Table 3: GAMUNEX

Most Frequently Recorded Drug Related Adverse Events (≥2.0%)

Drug Related Adverse Events	GAMUNEX No. of Patients: 48 n (%)	GAMIMUNE N 10% No. of Patients: 49 n (%)
Headache	24 (50%)	24 (49%)
Mild	25%	18%
Moderate	21%	20%
Severe	4%	12%
<Day 3	46%	49%
>Day 3	4%	0%
Vomiting	6 (13%)	8 (16%)
Mild	10%	10%
Moderate	2%	6%
Severe	0%	0%
<Day 3	10%	16%
>Day 3	2%	0%
Fever	5 (10%)	5 (10%)
Nausea	5 (10%)	4 (8%)
Rash	3 (6%)	0 (0%)
Back pain	3 (6%)	2 (4%)
Asthenia	2 (4%)	3 (6%)
Arthralgia	2 (4%)	0 (0%)
Pruritus	2 (4%)	0 (0%)
Dizziness	1 (2%)	3 (6%)
Neck pain	0 (0%)	2 (4%)

A second trial was carried out in 28 chronic ITP patients who received 1000 mg/kg GAMUNEX on three occasions for treatment of relapses to determine tolerability of various infusion rates. The maximum infusion rate on the three occasions was randomly assigned to 0.08, 0.11, or 0.14 mL/kg/min (8, 11 or 14 mg/kg/min) in which each patient was to receive Immune Globulin Intravenous (Human), 10%, at all 3 rates. No pre-medication with corticosteroids to alleviate infusion-related intolerability was permitted. Seven patients did not complete the study for the following reasons: one adverse event (hives) at the 0.08 mL/kg/min level, one patient withdrew because he refused to participate without a forbidden concomitant medication (prednisone) and five patients did not require additional treatment.

The number of patients who experienced at least one adverse event for the 0.08, 0.11, and 0.14 mL/kg/min infusion rates was 12 (46%), 13 (59%), and 11 (46%), respectively. The most commonly reported adverse event was headache, which occurred more frequently during the higher infusion rates (4% in 0.08 mL/kg/min patients vs 23% in 0.11 mL/kg/min patients vs 13% in 0.14 mL/kg/min patients). Importantly, all of the headaches were mild except for one severe headache at the 0.08 mL/kg/min rate. Otherwise, the incidence rates of adverse events and drug-related adverse events generally appeared to be similar among the three infusion groups. No patients experienced a drug related serious adverse event. There were no other abnormal safety results except for slightly decreased heart rates following all infusion rates.

Chronic Inflammatory Demyelinating Polyneuropathy (CIDP): In study 100538, 113 subjects were exposed to GAMUNEX and 95 were exposed to placebo. As a result of the study design, the drug exposure with GAMUNEX was almost twice that of placebo, with 1096 GAMUNEX infusions versus 575 placebo infusions. Therefore, adverse reactions are reported per infusion (represented as frequency) to correct for differences in drug exposure between the 2 groups. The majority of loading-dose infusions (2 g/kg), were administered over 2 days in both the GAMUNEX group (90 [87%] of 104 infusions) and placebo group (67 [83%] of 81 infusions). The majority of maintenance-dose infusions (1 g/kg) were administered over 1 day in both the GAMUNEX (698 [89%] of 783 infusions) and placebo (327 [91%] of 359 infusions) groups, and study drug infusions were administered in the mean over 2.7 hours among the two treatment groups.

Discontinuations due to adverse events during the Efficacy Period occurred in 1 subject in the GAMUNEX group (2%; urticaria) and 1 subject in the placebo group (2%; cerebrovascular accident). Two subjects (4%) treated with GAMUNEX discontinued due to adverse events (dyspnea, bronchopneumonia) during the rescue phase, and 1 subject (3%) treated with placebo discontinued due to an adverse event (deep vein thrombosis) during the Randomized Withdrawal Period.

The most frequently reported drug related adverse events (≥5%) are provided in Table 4.

Table 4: GAMUNEX

Most Frequent Drug-Related Treatment Emergent Adverse Events (TEAE) for all Study Periods Combined (safety population)

	GAMUNEX (N=113)—1096 Infusions			Placebo (N=95)—575 Infusions		
MedDRA PreferredTerm[a]	No. of Subjects (%)	No. of Adverse Events	Incidence Density[b]	No. of Subjects (%)	No. of Adverse Events	Incidence Density[b]
Any drug-related TEAE	62 (55)	194	0.177	16 (17)	25	0.043
Headache	31 (27)	44	0.04	6 (6)	7	0.012
Pyrexia	15 (13)	26	0.024	0	0	0
Hypertension	7 (6)	16	0.015	3 (3)	3	0.005
Influenza like illness	5 (4)	13	0.012	0	0	0
Chills	8 (7)	9	0.008	0	0	0

(cont'd)

Table 4: GAMUNEX *(cont'd)*

Most Frequent Drug-Related Treatment Emergent Adverse Events (TEAE) for all Study Periods Combined (safety population)

MedDRA PreferredTerm[a]	GAMUNEX (N=113)—1096 Infusions			Placebo (N=95)—575 Infusions		
	No. of Subjects (%)	No. of Adverse Events	Incidence Density[b]	No. of Subjects (%)	No. of Adverse Events	Incidence Density[b]
Rash	6 (5)	8	0.007	1 (1)	1	0.002
Nausea	6 (5)	7	0.006	3 (3)	3	0.005
Asthenia	6 (5)	6	0.005	0	0	0

[a] Reported in ≥5% of subjects in either treatment group.
[b] Calculated by the total number of TEAEs divided by the number of infusions received (1096 for GAMUNEX and 575 for placebo).

Abnormal Hematologic and Clinical Chemistry Findings: In some patients in the clinical trial program, administration with GAMUNEX resulted in a transitory decrease in RBC, hematocrit and hemoglobin with no evidence of hemolysis or significant clinical outcome.

Post-Market Adverse Drug Reactions: The following adverse reactions have been identified and reported during post-marketing use of GAMUNEX.

Very rare adverse events (<0.01%): aseptic meningitis; rare adverse events (<0.1%): hemolytic anemia. Some cases of hemolysis/hemolytic anemia, especially in association with pre-existing renal impairment, were severe and required blood component transfusion.

DRUG INTERACTIONS: Drug-Drug Interactions: Antibodies in GAMUNEX may interfere with the response to live viral vaccines such as measles, mumps and rubella. Therefore, use of such vaccines should be deferred until approximately 6 months after GAMUNEX administration.

GAMUNEX is not compatible with saline. If dilution is required, GAMUNEX may be diluted with 5% dextrose in water (D5W). No other drug interactions or compatibilities have been evaluated (see Dosage and Administration).

It is recommended to infuse GAMUNEX using a separate line by itself, without mixing with other intravenous fluids or medications the patient might be receiving. GAMUNEX should not be mixed with any other Immune Globulin Intravenous (Human) formulation.

Drug-Food Interactions: Interactions with food have not been established.

Drug-Herb Interactions: Interactions with herbal products have not been established.

Drug-Laboratory Test Interactions: Direct antiglobulin tests (DAT or direct Coombs tests), which are carried out in some centers as a safety check prior to red blood cell transfusions may show a positive result following treatment with GAMUNEX (Immune Globulin Intravenous [Human], 10%). This may be due to the fact that GAMUNEX may contain low levels of anti Blood Group A and B antibodies primarily of the IgG4 class. However, there was no evidence of hemolysis or significant clinical effect in association with positive DAT findings in clinical trials.

DOSAGE AND ADMINISTRATION: Recommended Dose and Dosage Adjustment: Clinical investigations indicate that Immune Globulin Intravenous (Human), 10% is well-tolerated and less likely to produce side effects when infused at the recommended rate. If side effects occur, the rate may be reduced, or the infusion interrupted until symptoms subside. The infusion may then be resumed at the rate which is comfortable for the patient.

Periodic monitoring of renal function and urine output is particularly important in patients judged to have a potential increased risk for developing acute renal failure. Renal function, including measurement of blood urea nitrogen (BUN)/serum creatinine, should be assessed prior to the initial infusion of GAMUNEX and again at appropriate intervals thereafter. If renal function deteriorates, discontinuation of the product should be considered.

For patients judged to be at increased risk for developing renal dysfunction, it may be prudent to reduce the amount of product infused per unit time by infusing GAMUNEX, (Immune Globulin Intravenous [Human], 10%) at a rate less than 8 mg/kg/min (0.08 mL/kg/min). No prospective data are presently available to identify a maximum safe dose, concentration, and rate of infusion in patients determined to be at increased risk of acute renal failure. In the absence of prospective data, recommended doses should not be exceeded and the concentration and infusion rate should be the minimum level practicable. Reduction in dose, concentration, and/or rate of administration in patients at risk of acute renal failure is suggested in order to reduce the risk of acute renal failure.

Assure that all patients are not volume depleted prior to the initiation of the infusion of Immune Globulin Intravenous (Human), 10%.

Intravenous Dosing: Primary Immune Deficiency: GAMUNEX doses between 100 and 600 mg/kg (1 and 6 mL/kg administered every 3 or 4 weeks) may be used for infection prophylaxis. The dose should be individualized taking into account dosing intervals (e.g., 3 or 4 weeks) and GAMUNEX dose (between 100 and 600 mg/kg). The goal should be to achieve serum IgG levels at trough (i.e., prior to the next infusion) of at least 5 g/L.

Idiopathic Thrombocytopenic Purpura: GAMUNEX may be administered at a total dose of 2000 mg/kg, divided into two doses of 1000 mg/kg (10 mL/kg) given on two consecutive days, or into five doses of 400 mg/kg (4 mL/kg) given on five consecutive days. If after administration of the first of two daily 1000 mg/kg (10 mL/kg) doses, an adequate increase in the platelet count is observed at 24 hours, the second dose of 1000 mg/kg body weight may be withheld.

The high dose regimen (1000 mg/kg×1-2 days) is not recommended for individuals with expanded fluid volumes or where fluid volume may be a concern.

Allogeneic Bone Marrow Transplantation (BMT): An equivalent dosage of 500 mg/kg GAMUNEX (5 mL/kg) is recommended beginning on days 7 and 2 prior to transplantation (or at the time conditioning therapy for transplantation begins), then weekly through 90 days after transplantation. GAMUNEX should be administered by itself through a Hickman line while it is in place, and thereafter through a peripheral vein.

Pediatric HIV Infection: An equivalent dosage of GAMUNEX is recommended in doses of 400 mg/kg (4 mL/kg) body weight every 28 days.

Chronic Inflammatory Demyelinating Polyneuropathy (CIDP): GAMUNEX may be initially administered as a total loading dose of 2 g/kg (20 mL/kg) given in divided doses over two to four consecutive days. GAMUNEX may be administered as a maintenance infusion of 1 g/kg administered over 1 day (10 mL/kg) or divided into two doses of 0.5 g/kg (5 mL/kg) given on two consecutive days, every 3 weeks.

Subcutaneous Dosing: Primary Immune Deficiency: GAMUNEX may be administered via subcutaneous infusion for replacement therapy in primary immune deficiency. The initial weekly subcutaneous GAMUNEX dose can be calculated by multiplying the previous intravenous dose by 1.37, then dividing this dose into weekly doses based on the patient's previous IGIV treatment interval; for example, if IGIV was administered every three weeks, divide by 3. This dose of GAMUNEX will provide a systemic IgG exposure (AUC) comparable to that of the previous IGIV treatment.

Secondary Immune Deficiencies : GAMUNEX may also be administered subcutaneously for the treatment of patients with secondary immune deficiencies. This approval is based on data collected in patients with Primary Immune Deficiency, and mechanistic similarities between Primary and Secondary Immune Deficiencies. Where applicable, the initial weekly subcutaneous GAMUNEX dose can be calculated by multiplying the previous intravenous dose by 1.37, then dividing this dose into weekly doses based on the patient's previous IGIV treatment interval; for example, if IGIV was administered every three weeks, divide by 3. This dose of GAMUNEX will provide a systemic IgG exposure (AUC) comparable to that of the previous IGIV treatment.

Administration: General: Prior to use, allow the solution to reach ambient room temperature. As with all parenteral drug products, GAMUNEX should be inspected visually for discoloration and particulate matter prior to administration. **Do not shake.** Do not use if the solution is cloudy or has particulates. Check the product expiration date on the vial. Do not use beyond the expiration date.

For intravenous use only: It is recommended that intravenously administered GAMUNEX should initially be infused at a rate of 0.01 to 0.02 mL/kg per minute (1 to 2 mg/kg per minute) for the first 30 minutes. If well-tolerated, the rate may be gradually increased to a maximum of 0.14 mL/kg per minute (14 mg/kg per minute). If side effects occur, the rate may be reduced, or the infusion interrupted until symptoms subside. The infusion may then be resumed at the rate, which is comfortable for the patient.

In a clinical trial with 28 chronic adult ITP patients receiving 1000 mg/kg GAMUNEX to treat relapses, the infusion rate could be safely increased up to 0.14 mL/kg per minute (14 mg/kg per minute). Caution should be exercised when an infusion rate higher than 0.08 mL/kg per minute (8 mg/kg per minute) is administered for the first time.

For subcutaneous use: Dosages for specific indications are provided above, but in general, it is recommended that subcutaneously administered GAMUNEX be infused by itself at a rate of 20 mL/hr per infusion site. In clinical study 060001, the mean volume administered per infusion site was 34 mL (17-69 mL) and the majority of infusions were administered at a rate of 20 mL/hr per site. Multiple simultaneous infusion sites were enabled by administration tubing and Y-site connection tubing. Most administrations (95.9%) involved 4 or more infusion sites with abdomen and thighs being the most commonly used sites.

1. Use aseptic technique when preparing and administering GAMUNEX for injection.
2. Remove the protective cap from the vial to expose the central portion of the rubber stopper.
3. Wipe the rubber stopper with alcohol and allow to dry.
4. Using a sterile syringe and needle, prepare to withdraw GAMUNEX by first injecting air into the vial that is equivalent to the amount of GAMUNEX to be withdrawn. Then withdraw the desired volume of GAMUNEX. If multiple vials are required to achieve the desired dose, repeat this step.
5. If using a pump, follow the manufacturer's instructions for filling the pump reservoir and preparing the pump, administration tubing and Y-site connection tubing, if needed. Be sure to prime the administration tubing to ensure that no air is left in the tubing or needle by filling the tubing/needle with GAMUNEX.
6. Select the number and location of injection sites.
7. Cleanse the injection site(s) with antiseptic solution using a circular motion working from the center of the site and moving to the outside. Sites should be clean, dry, and at least two inches apart.
8. Grasp the skin between two fingers and insert the needle into the subcutaneous tissue.
9. Repeat priming and needle insertion steps using a new needle, administration tubing and a new infusion site. Secure the needle in place by applying sterile gauze or transparent dressing over the site.
10. If using multiple, simultaneous injection sites, use Y-site connection tubing and secure to the administration tubing.
11. If a pump is being used, infuse GAMUNEX following the manufacturer's instructions for the pump.

Only 18 gauge needles should be used to penetrate the stopper for dispensing product from 10 mL vial sizes; 16 gauge needles or dispensing pins should only be used with 20 mL vial sizes and larger. Needles or dispensing pins should only be inserted within the stopper area delineated by the raised ring. The stopper should be penetrated perpendicular to the plane of the stopper within the ring.

Content of vials may be pooled under aseptic conditions into sterile infusion bags and infused within 8 hours after pooling.

It is recommended to infuse GAMUNEX using a separate line by itself, without mixing with other intravenous fluids or medications the patient might be receiving. GAMUNEX should not be mixed with any other Immune Globulin Intravenous (Human) formulation.

A number of factors beyond our control could reduce the efficacy of this product or even result in an ill effect following its use. These include improper storage and handling of the product after it leaves our hands, diagnosis, dosage, method of administration, and biological differences in individual patients. Because of these factors, it is important that this product be stored properly and that the directions be followed carefully during use.

OVERDOSAGE:

Overdosage may lead to fluid overload and hyperviscosity, particularly in the elderly and in patients with renal impairment.

For management of a suspected drug overdose, contact your regional Poison Control Centre. See the *CPS* Directory section for a list of Poison Control Centres.

ACTION AND CLINICAL PHARMACOLOGY: Mechanism of Action: Primary Immune Deficiency: Immune Globulin Intravenous (Human), 10% supplies a broad spectrum of opsonic and neutralizing IgG antibodies against bacteria, viruses or their toxins that have been demonstrated to be effective in the prevention or attenuation of lethal infections in animal models. Immune Globulin Intravenous (Human), 10% has proven to be effective in preventing infections in patients with Primary Immune Deficiency (PID). In randomized pharmacokinetic trials, GAMUNEX has demonstrated bioequivalence to GAMIMUNE N, 10% (Immune Globulin Intravenous [Human], 10%-Solvent/ Detergent Treated).

Idiopathic Thrombocytopenic Purpura: The mechanism of action of high doses of immunoglobulins in the treatment of Idiopathic Thrombocytopenic Purpura (ITP) has not been fully elucidated. It is postulated that the mechanisms of action may be the Fc-receptor blockade of phagocytes as well as the down regulation of auto-reactive B-cells by antiidiotypic antibodies provided by human immune globulin.

Allogeneic Bone Marrow Transplantation: The mechanism of action of Immune Globulin Intravenous (Human), 10% in protecting immune-compromised patients with Allogenic Bone Marrow Transplantation (BMT) from serious bacterial infections is similar to the anti-infective mechanism of action in PID. The immunomodulatory mechanism of action of Immune Globulin Intravenous (Human), 10% in suppressing acute graft versus host reaction in patients with immune cells involving Fab and Fc functions of the immunoglobulin molecules is similar to the discussed mode of action in ITP.

Pediatric HIV Infection: Children with HIV infections, particularly when acquired through vertical transmission, are prone to recurrent serious bacterial infections. Types of infection seen in these children are similar to those with primary hypogammaglobulinemia. The replacement of opsonic and neutralizing IgG antibodies has been shown to be effective in pediatric HIV infections. The anti-infective mechanism of action of Immune Globulin Intravenous (Human), 10% in the Pediatric HIV is comparable to that in PID.

Chronic Inflammatory Demyelinating Polyneuropathy (CIDP): The mechanism of action of GAMUNEX in the treatment of CIDP has not been fully elucidated. Immunoglobulins have multiple actions, which often operate in concert with each other. The main mechanisms of action which are likely relevant to the efficacy of the GAMUNEX in autoimmune neuromuscular disorders include effects on autoantibodies, inhibition of complement binding and prevention of membraneolytic attack complex formation, modulation or blockade of Fc receptors on macrophages, and suppression of pathogenic cytokines and other immunoregulatory molecules.

Pharmacodynamics: GAMUNEX is a passive immunizing agent, and by replacing IgG in immunosuppressed patients, prevents and treats infections in this population. GAMUNEX also raises platelet counts in patients with idiopathic thrombocytopenic purpura.

Pharmacokinetics: Intravenous: The pharmacokinetic parameters AUC and C_{max} of intravenous GAMUNEX in a randomized clinical trial involving Primary Immune Deficiency (PID) patients were determined to be approximately 6746 mg·h/mL and 19 mg/mL respectively.

Table 5: GAMUNEX

Summary of the Pharmacokinetic Parameters for intravenous GAMUNEX in Primary Immune Deficiency

	C_{max} (mg/mL)	$t_{½}$ (days)	$AUC_{0-tn,\ partial}$ (mg·h/mL)
Study 100152	19.04	35.74	6746.48

Absorption: The IgG concentration time curve follows a biphasic slope.

Distribution: The distribution phase of about 5 days is characterized by a fall in serum IgG levels to about 65-75% of the peak levels achieved immediately post-infusion.

Excretion: The elimination phase has a half-life of approximately 35 days.

Subcutaneous: The C_{max} of subcutaneous GAMUNEX in a randomized clinical trial involving Primary Immune Deficiency (PID) patients dosed at 137% of their previous intravenous dose, was determined to be approximately 12 mg/mL. Mean AUC for the weekly subcutaneous infusions was 1947 mg·h/mL. When this was adjusted to reflect the previous 3 or 4 week IV dosing schedules of the subjects, the AUC was calculated to be 6858 mg·h/mL.

Special Populations and Conditions: No specific studies were performed for the following: Gender, Race, Hepatic Insufficiency, Renal Insufficiency.

STORAGE AND STABILITY: GAMUNEX may be stored for 36 months at 2-8°C, and product may be stored at room temperature not to exceed 25°C for up to 6 months anytime during the 36 month shelf life, after which the product must be immediately used or discarded. Do not freeze. Do not use after expiration date.

INFORMATION FOR THE PATIENT: Published in e-CPS, available by subscription at www.e-cps.ca.

DOSAGE FORMS, COMPOSITION AND PACKAGING: GAMUNEX (Immune Globulin Intravenous [Human], 10%) manufactured by a patented Chromatography Process is a ready-to-use sterile solution of human immune globulin protein for intravenous administration. GAMUNEX consists of 9%-11% protein in 0.16-0.24 M glycine. Not less than 98% of the protein has the electrophoretic mobility of gamma globulin. GAMUNEX typically has low levels of IgA (average of 0.046 g/L) and trace levels of IgM. The distribution of IgG subclasses is similar to that found in normal serum. The measured buffer capacity is 35 mEq/L and the osmolality is 258 mOsmol/kg solvent, which is close to physiological osmolality (285-295 mOsmol/kg). GAMUNEX contains no preservative.

Table 6: GAMUNEX

Summary of the Pharmacokinetic Parameters for GAMUNEX in Primary Immune Deficiency (Study 060001)

Route of Administration	C_{max} (mg/mL)	$AUC_{0-\tau,IV}$ (mg·h/mL)	$AUC_{0-\tau,SC}$ (mg·h/mL)	Adj._$AUC_{0-\tau,SC}$[a] (mg·h/mL)
Intravenous	21.1	7640	NA	NA
Subcutaneous	12.2	NA	1947	6858

[a] Adj._ $AUC_{0-\tau,SC}$: Adjusted steady-state area under the concentration vs. time curve following SC administration based on IV dosing schedule, calculated as $AUC_{0-\tau,SC}$ multiplied by 3 or 4 for subjects on every-3-week or every-4-week IV dosing schedule, respectively.
Legend: NA: not applicable.

GAMUNEX (Immune Globulin Intravenous [Human], 10%) is supplied in the sizes listed in Table 7.

Table 7: GAMUNEX

Available Dosage Forms for GAMUNEX

Size	Protein (g)
25 mL	2.5
50 mL	5.0
100 mL	10.0
200 mL	20.0

Garamycin® Ophthalmic Drops ℞

gentamicin sulfate

Topical Antibiotic

Schering-Plough

Garamycin® Ophthalmic Ointment ℞

gentamicin sulfate

Topical Antibiotic

Schering-Plough

Garamycin® Otic Drops ℞

gentamicin sulfate

Topical Antibiotic

Schering-Plough

PHARMACOLOGY: Gentamicin, an aminoglycoside antibiotic, is active against the gram-positive bacteria commonly found in eye-ear infections: coagulase-positive and coagulase-negative Staphylococci, Group A beta-hemolytic and nonhemolytic Streptococci; and *D. pneumoniae*. Gentamicin is also active against gram-negative bacteria including *P. aeruginosa*, indole-positive and indole-negative Proteus species, *E. coli*, species of the Klebsiella-Enterobacter-Serratia group, Citrobacter species, Salmonella and Shigella, Moraxella species, Providencia species, *H. vaginicola* and Neisseria species, especially the gonococcus.

INDICATIONS: Ophthalmic: The treatment of superficial bacterial infections of the conjunctiva, cornea, eyelids, tear ducts and skin adjacent to the eye. Such infections include conjunctivitis, blepharitis, blepharoconjunctivitis, keratitis, keratoconjunctivitis, episcleritis, dacryocystitis, corneal ulcers and infected eye sockets. Also for the prevention of ocular infection if injury makes the eye or adjacent area vulnerable to infections: after removal of foreign bodies, after burns or laceration to the lids or conjunctivae or after damage from chemical or physical agents and before and after eye surgery.
Otic: May be used for the topical treatment of otitis externa caused by susceptible bacteria.

CONTRAINDICATIONS: Sensitivity to any of the components in Garamycin.
Ophthalmic Use: As with all Garamycin preparations containing benzalkonium chloride, patients are advised not to wear soft contact lenses during treatment.
Otic Use: Garamycin Otic preparations are contraindicated in patients with absent or perforated tympanic membranes.

WARNINGS: Otic Use: When gentamicin is used locally in the ear, potential eight cranial nerve toxicity should be considered. Animal studies have shown that gentamicin applied topically to the external ear canal may be absorbed since the drug has been detected in the serum and urine after this route of administration.

PRECAUTIONS: General: Use of topical antibiotics occasionally allows overgrowth of nonsusceptible microorganisms such as fungi. If irritation, sensitization or superinfection develop, treatment with gentamicin should be discontinued and appropriate therapy initiated. To avoid possible contamination of the drops or ointment, do not touch the dropper tip or the ointment tube to any surface.

Clinical studies have shown that organisms previously sensitive to gentamicin have become resistant during therapy. Although this has occurred infrequently, the possibility should nevertheless be considered. There is evidence that cross-resistance between gentamicin and the aminoglycoside antibiotics may occur since bacteria made resistant to aminoglycoside antibiotics artificially in the laboratory are also resistant to gentamicin; however, gentamicin may be active against clinical isolates of bacteria resistant to other aminoglycosides. Conversely, organisms resistant to gentamicin may be sensitive to other aminoglycoside antibiotics.
Otic Use: To minimize the risk of ototoxicity, the following precautions are suggested: the gentamicin drops should be used for the shortest duration possible; the patient should be instructed precisely regarding the dosage and duration of therapy. Treatment should be discontinued if hearing loss, tinnitus, vertigo, or imbalance is noted. The use of gentamicin eardrops should be reassessed, with respect to ototoxicity, 5 to 7 days after start of treatment and thereafter on a regular basis.
Pregnancy: The safety of gentamicin for use during pregnancy has not been established.
Lactation: Since it is not known whether components of gentamicin ophthalmic/otic solution are excreted in human milk, caution should be exercised when administered to a nursing woman.
Children: Safety and effectiveness in children below the age of 6 years have not been established.

ADVERSE EFFECTS: Ophthalmic Use: Eye and ear medications may sting briefly on application and gentamicin ophthalmic and otic preparations are no exception. The most frequently reported adverse reactions at least possibly related to gentamicin are ocular burning and irritation upon drug instillation, nonspecific conjunctivitis, conjunctival epithelial defects and conjunctival hyperemia.
Otic Use: The possibility of ototoxicity following otic application should be kept in mind, and the patient monitored accordingly on a regular basis (see Contraindications, Warnings and Precautions).

During the postmarketing of gentamicin containing otic preparations, rare cases of ototoxicity (hearing loss, tinnitus, vertigo, imbalance, ataxia or oscillopcia) in the presence of tympanic membrane perforation or tympanoplasty tubes have been reported. Ototoxicity was primarily vestibular and was generally associated with prolonged treatment duration. However, ototoxicity with treatment durations of 5 to 7 days has also been reported. In some instances, patients have not recovered from their symptoms (hearing loss, tinnitus, vertigo, imbalance, ataxia or oscillopcia).

OVERDOSE:

Symptoms: A single overdose of gentamicin would not be expected to produce symptoms.

Treatment: Although a single overdose is not expected to require treatment, gentamicin can be removed from the blood by hemodialysis or peritoneal dialysis.

For management of a suspected drug overdose, CPhA recommends that you contact your **regional Poison Control Centre**. See the *CPS* Directory section for a list of Poison Control Centres.

DOSAGE: Ophthalmic Drops: Instil 2 drops into the conjunctival sac of the affected eye 3 to 4 times daily. Dosage may be increased in severe infections and reduced at the end of treatment. In the infections that may develop intermittently in the immature tear ducts of children (dacryocystitis), hot compresses and massage of the area over the tear duct may be useful as adjunct to the solution. In the treatment of acute pseudomonal corneal ulcer, 1 to 2 drops every 15 minutes in the daytime hours can be supplemented with the ophthalmic ointment at bedtime. For prophylaxis, such as after removal of a foreign body or following physical or chemical trauma, instil 1 to 2 drops 3 to 4 times daily until signs of inflammation have subsided. For prophylaxis before intraocular surgery, 1 to 2 drops should be instilled 4 to 5 times, preferably within 8 hours prior to surgery. Gentamicin ophthalmic/otic solution may be administered as part of the routine postoperative daily dressing of the eye, until recovery from postsurgical inflammation is evident.
Ophthalmic Ointment: Apply ophthalmic ointment to the affected areas in or near the eye 3 to 4 times a day. If ophthalmic drops are used during the day, the ointment can be used at bedtime to continue treatment during the night.
Otic Drops: Thoroughly clean the ear canal of cerumen or debris. Instil 3 or 4 drops in the infected ear 3 times daily. The patient should lie with the affected ear upward; instil the solution and let the patient remain in this position for several minutes to insure penetration of the medication into the ear canal. The need for gentamicin eardrops should be reassessed 5 to 7 days after start of treatment and thereafter on a regular basis (see Contraindications, Warnings and Precautions).

INFORMATION FOR THE PATIENT: Published in e-CPS, available by subscription at www.e-cps.ca.

SUPPLIED: Ophthalmic: Drops: Each mL of sterile aqueous solution buffered to approximately pH 7 contains: gentamicin sulfate USP, equivalent to 3 mg (0.3%) gentamicin base. Nonmedicinal ingredients: benzalkonium chloride, purified water, sodium chloride, sodium phosphate dibasic anhydrous and sodium phosphate monobasic monohydrate. Plastic dropper bottles of 5 mL.
Ointment: Each g of sterile ointment contains: gentamicin sulfate USP, equivalent to 3 mg (0.3%) gentamicin base. Nonmedicinal ingredients: methylparaben, mineral oil, propylparaben and white petrolatum. Tubes of 3.5 g with applicator tip.
Otic: Drops: Each mL of sterile aqueous solution buffered to approximately pH 7 contains: gentamicin sulfate USP, equivalent to 3 mg (0.3%) gentamicin base. Nonmedicinal ingredients: benzalkonium chloride, purified water, sodium chloride, sodium phosphate dibasic anhydrous and sodium phosphate monobasic monohydrate. Plastic dropper bottles of 7.5 mL.
Store between 15 to 30°C.

Garasone® Ophthalmic/Otic Solution ℞

betamethasone sodium phosphate—gentamicin sulfate

Topical Corticosteroid—Antibiotic

Schering-Plough

Garasone® Ophthalmic Ointment ℞

betamethasone sodium phosphate—gentamicin sulfate

Topical Corticosteroid—Antibiotic

Schering-Plough

PHARMACOLOGY: In Garasone, the anti-inflammatory and antiallergic activity of betamethasone sodium phosphate is combined with the broad spectrum bactericidal activity of gentamicin sulfate. Betamethasone sodium phosphate inhibits the inflammatory response of the eye and ear to irritating agents of a mechanical, chemical or immunological nature, while gentamicin sulfate is active in vitro against a wide range of pathogenic gram-negative and gram-positive bacteria.

INDICATIONS: Ophthalmic Use: Garasone ophthalmic/otic solution and Garasone ophthalmic ointment are indicated for ocular inflammation when concurrent use of an antimicrobial is judged necessary, e.g., staphylococcal blepharoconjunctivitis. Garasone is indicated for the treatment of nonpurulent bacterial infections of the anterior segment of the eye due to organisms sensitive to the antibiotic and when the anti-inflammatory action of betamethasone sodium phosphate is indicated, as in allergic vernal and phlyctenular conjunctivitis; nonpurulent blepharitis; interstitial sclerosing postoperative keratitis; superficial chemical and thermal burns of the cornea.

In stubborn cases of anterior segment eye disease or in deep-seated ocular diseases, systemic therapy may be required. However, in these diseases Garasone ophthalmic/otic solution may be used as adjunctive therapy.
Otic Use: Garasone ophthalmic/otic solution may also be used for the treatment of lesions in the external ear canal, such as acute otitis externa, eczematoid-dermatitis, seborrheic dermatitis and contact dermatitis secondarily infected with susceptible organisms.

CONTRAINDICATIONS: In those individuals who have shown hypersensitivity to any of the components and to other aminoglycosides or to other corticosteroids.
Ophthalmic Use: Ophthalmic use is contraindicated in epithelial herpes simplex keratitis (dendritic keratitis), vaccinia, varicella, and many other viral diseases of the cornea and conjunctiva, mycobacterial infections of the eye or ear, trachoma, fungal diseases of ocular structures.

Use of corticosteroid/antibiotic combinations is contraindicated after removal of a corneal foreign body or in the presence of acute local viral lesions, e.g., herpes, and in patients with absent or perforated tympanic membranes. As with all ophthalmic products containing benzalkonium chloride, patients are advised not to wear soft contact lenses during treatment with Garasone ophthalmic/otic solution.
Otic Use: Garasone ophthalmic/otic drops are contraindicated in patients with absent or perforated tympanic membranes.

WARNINGS: General: If prompt clinical response is not obtained with the use of Garasone ophthalmic/otic solution or Garasone ophthalmic ointment, further evaluation is advised.
Ophthalmic Use: Garasone ophthalmic solution is for topical use only. It should never be injected subconjunctivally, nor should it be introduced directly into the anterior chamber of the eye.

Prolonged ophthalmic use may result in increased intraocular pressure in some individuals with a family history of open-angle glaucoma, with a high degree of myopia and with diabetes. If used for 10 days or longer, intraocular pressure should be routinely monitored. In diseases causing thinning of the cornea or sclera, perforation has been known to occur with the use of topical preparations containing corticosteroids. Protracted use of topical corticosteroids in the eye may result in the development of posterior subcapsular cataracts. Acute anterior uveitis may occur in susceptible individuals, primarily blacks. Prolonged use may suppress the host response and thus increase the hazard of secondary ocular infections. In acute purulent conditions of the eye, steroids may mask infection or enhance existing infection.

Although corticosteroids are contraindicated in acute viral infection of the cornea caused by herpes simplex, there may be occasion to employ steroids in the healing stage to prevent scarring; however, this must only be done with great caution and close observation. In patients with a history of herpetic infection of the cornea, reactivation of the disease may occur with the use of topical ophthalmic or otic corticosteroids.

The use of steroids after cataract surgery may delay healing and increase the incidence of filtering blebs.
Otic Use: When Garasone otic solution is used locally in the ear, potential 8th cranial nerve toxicity should be considered. Animal studies have shown that gentamicin applied topically to the external ear canal may be absorbed since the drug has been detected in the serum and urine after this route of administration.

PRECAUTIONS: General: During long-term use of preparations containing corticosteroids, such as Garasone, the possibility of overgrowth of nonsusceptible microorganisms such as fungi must be considered, especially in the presence of a persistent corneal ulceration that fails to respond to conventional therapy. By reducing inflammation, steroids may mask the symptoms of serious disease or enhance existing infection due to organisms resistant to gentamicin. Should this occur, or if irritation or hypersensitivity to Garasone ophthalmic/otic solution develops, discontinue use of this preparation and institute appropriate therapy.

Clinical studies have shown that organisms previously sensitive to gentamicin have become resistant during therapy. Although this has occurred infrequently, the possibility should nevertheless be considered. There is evidence that cross-resistance between gentamicin and other aminoglycoside antibiotics may occur since bacteria made resistant to aminoglycoside antibiotics artificially in the laboratory are also resistant to gentamicin. However, gentamicin may be active against clinical isolates of bacteria resistant to other aminoglycosides. Conversely, organisms resistant to gentamicin may be sensitive to other aminoglycoside antibiotics.

If irritation occurs with the use of Garasone, hypersensitivity to a component of the preparation is a possibility and use should be discontinued. Cross-allergenicity among aminoglycosides and corticosteroids has been demonstrated (see Contraindications).

To avoid possible contamination and cross-infection, avoid the use of the same bottle of medication for the treatment of otic and ocular infections. The use of this dispenser by more than one person may spread infection. Contamination may occur if the dropper tip touches any surface. Do not allow dispenser tip to touch the surface of the eye.

Ophthalmic Use: In ophthalmic use, intraocular pressure should be checked frequently (tonometry) (see Warnings). Slit-lamp examination should be done for dendritic keratitis.

It is not advisable to treat bacterial corneal ulcers, which may be due to *P. aeruginosa*, with a combination antibiotic-anti-inflammatory product as initial therapy. It is prudent to use an anti-infective agent alone initially. For ulcers caused by Pseudomonas, Garamycin ophthalmic ointment would be indicated. If the infection responds to the anti-infective treatment, then the addition of an anti-inflammatory agent to minimize the fibrous reaction and scarring of the cornea is suggested.

Eyelid cultures and tests to determine the susceptibility of infecting organisms may be indicated if signs/symptoms persist or recur in spite of recommended course of treatment with this product.

Otic Use: To minimize the risk of ototoxicity, the following precautions are suggested: Garasone drops should be used for the shortest duration possible; the patient should be precisely instructed regarding the dosage and duration of therapy. Treatment should be discontinued if hearing loss, tinnitus, vertigo, or imbalance is noted. The use of Garasone eardrops should be reassessed, with respect to ototoxicity, 5 to 7 days after start of treatment and thereafter, on a regular basis.

Pediatrics: Safety and effectiveness of Garasone in children below the age of 8 years have not been established.

Pregnancy: Safety of topical corticosteroid/antibiotic preparations during pregnancy has not been established, therefore, drugs of this class should be used during pregnancy only if the potential benefit justifies the potential risk to the fetus.

Lactation: Since it is not known whether topical administration of corticosteroids can result in sufficient systemic absorption to produce detectable quantities in breast milk, a decision should be made to discontinue nursing or to discontinue the drug, taking into account the importance of the drug to the mother.

ADVERSE EFFECTS: Ophthalmic Use: Adverse reactions reported after the use of Garasone include: increased ocular pressure; ocular hypersensitivity manifested by increased ocular hyperemia, edema and burning/stinging sensation.

Adverse reactions reported with other steroid-anti-infective combinations include: allergic sensitization due to the antibiotic component; elevation of intraocular pressure with possible development of glaucoma and infrequent optic nerve damage, posterior subcapsular cataract formation, filtering blebs following cataract surgery, secondary ocular infection from pathogens including herpes simplex and delayed wound healing due to the steroid component.

Corticosteroid-containing preparations can also cause anterior uveitis or perforation of the globe. Mydriasis, defects in visual acuity and visual fields, loss of accommodation and ptosis have also been reported following corticosteroid therapy.

Transient eye irritation has been reported with ophthalmic gentamicin sulfate. Ophthalmic preparations may sting briefly upon application.

Otic Use: The possibility of ototoxicity should be kept in mind and the patient monitored accordingly on a regular basis (see Contraindications, Warnings and Precautions).

During the postmarketing of gentamicin containing otic preparations, rare cases of ototoxicity (hearing loss, tinnitus, vertigo, imbalance, ataxia or oscillopsia) in the presence of tympanic membrane perforation or tympanoplasty tubes have been reported. Ototoxicity was primarily vestibular and was generally associated with prolonged treatment duration. However, ototoxicity with treatment durations of 5 to 7 days has also been reported. In some instances, patients have not recovered from their symptoms (hearing loss, tinnitus, vertigo, imbalance, ataxia or oscillopsia).

OVERDOSE:

Symptoms: Excessive prolonged use of topical corticosteroids can suppress pituitary-adrenal function resulting in secondary adrenal insufficiency, and produce manifestations of hypercorticism, including Cushing's disease.

A single overdosage of gentamicin would not be expected to produce symptoms.

Treatment: Appropriate symptomatic treatment of corticosteroid overdosage is indicated. Acute hypercorticoid symptoms are virtually reversible. Treat electrolyte imbalance, if necessary. In cases of chronic toxicity, slow withdrawal of corticosteroids is advised.

Although a single overdose is not expected to require treatment, gentamicin can be removed from the blood by hemodialysis or peritoneal dialysis. Approximately 80 to 90% is removed from the circulatory system during 12 hours of hemodialysis. Peritoneal dialysis appears to be less effective.

For management of a suspected drug overdose, CPhA recommends that you contact your **regional Poison Control Centre**. See the *CPS* Directory section for a list of Poison Control Centres.

DOSAGE: Garasone Ophthalmic/Otic Solution: Ophthalmic Drops: Instil 2 drops into the conjunctival sac of the affected eye 3 or 4 times daily. During the acute stage, 2 drops may be administered every 2 hours.

Garasone Ophthalmic Ointment: Apply a thin film to the affected eye area 3 or 4 times/day. When a favorable response is observed, the number of daily applications may be reduced. The ointment form is also indicated for application at bedtime in conjunction with daytime use of the drops.

Improvement usually occurs within 48 hours, with clearing of the signs and symptoms usually within 2 weeks. In chronic conditions, withdrawal of treatment should be carried out by gradually decreasing the frequency of application.

Garasone Ophthalmic/Otic Solution: Otic Use: Thoroughly clean the ear canal of cerumen and debris. Instil 3 or 4 drops into the affected ear 3 times daily or as directed by the physician. The patient should lie with the affected ear turned upward; instil the solution and let the patient remain in this position for several minutes to insure penetration of the medication into the ear canal. If preferred, a cotton wick may be inserted into the canal and then saturated with the solution. The wick should be kept moist by adding further solution every 4 hours. The wick should be replaced once every 24 hours.

After a favorable response is obtained, reduce dosage gradually and discontinue once a cure is achieved.

The need for Garasone eardrops should be reassessed, with respect to ototoxicity, 5 to 7 days after start of treatment and, thereafter, on a regular basis.

INFORMATION FOR THE PATIENT: Published in e-CPS, available by subscription at www.e-cps.ca.

SUPPLIED: Ophthalmic/Otic Solution: Each mL of sterile aqueous solution contains: gentamicin sulfate USP equivalent to 3.0 mg (0.3%) gentamicin base, and betamethasone sodium phosphate USP equivalent to 1 mg (0.1%) betamethasone USP. Nonmedicinal ingredients: benzalkonium chloride, disodium edetate, purified water, sodium borate, sodium chloride, sodium citrate dihydrate, sodium phosphate dibasic and sodium phosphate monobasic. Dropper bottles of 7.5 mL. Store between 15 and 30°C, away from light.

Ophthalmic Ointment: Each g of sterile ointment contains: gentamicin sulfate USP equivalent to 3.0 mg (0.3%) gentamicin base and betamethasone sodium phosphate USP equivalent to 1 mg (0.1%) betamethasone USP. Nonmedicinal ingredients: mineral oil and white petrolatum. Tubes of 3.5 g. Store between 15 and 30°C.

Gardasil®

quadrivalent human papillomavirus (types 6, 11, 16, 18) recombinant vaccine

Active Immunizing Agent

Merck Frosst

Date of Preparation: July 10, 2006
Date of Revision: May 20, 2010

SUMMARY PRODUCT INFORMATION:

Route of Administration	Dosage Form/ Strength	Clinically Relevant Nonmedicinal Ingredients
Intramuscular injection	Each 0.5 mL dose contains approximately: 20 µg of HPV 6 L1 protein, 40 µg of HPV 11 L1 protein, 40 µg of HPV 16 L1 protein, 20 µg of HPV 18 L1 protein.	For a complete listing see Dosage Forms, Composition and Packaging.

DESCRIPTION: GARDASIL [Quadrivalent Human Papillomavirus (Types 6, 11, 16, 18) Recombinant Vaccine] is a recombinant, quadrivalent vaccine that protects against Human Papillomavirus (HPV). It is a sterile liquid suspension prepared from the highly purified virus-like particles (VLPs) of the recombinant major capsid (L1) protein of HPV Types 6, 11, 16, and 18. The L1 proteins are produced by separate fermentations in recombinant *S. cerevisiae* (yeast) CANADE 3C-5 (Strain 1895) and self-assembled into VLPs.

INDICATIONS AND CLINICAL USE: GARDASIL is a vaccine indicated in girls and women 9- through 26 years of age for the prevention of infection caused by the Human Papillomavirus (HPV) types 6, 11, 16, and 18 and the following diseases associated with these HPV types:

- Cervical cancer
- Vulvar and vaginal cancers
- Genital warts (condyloma acuminata)
- Cervical adenocarcinoma in situ (AIS)
- Cervical intraepithelial neoplasia (CIN) grade 2 and grade 3
- Vulvar intraepithelial neoplasia (VIN) grade 2 and grade 3
- Vaginal intraepithelial neoplasia (VaIN) grade 2 and grade 3
- Cervical intraepithelial neoplasia (CIN) grade 1

GARDASIL is indicated in boys and men 9 through 26 years of age for the prevention of infection caused by HPV types 6, 11, 16, and 18 and genital warts caused by HPV types 6 and 11.

Pediatrics (<9 years of age): The safety and efficacy of GARDASIL have not been evaluated in children younger than 9 years.

Geriatrics (>65 years of age): The safety and efficacy of GARDASIL have not been evaluated in adults above the age of 26 years.

CONTRAINDICATIONS:

- Patients who are hypersensitive to the active substances or to any of the excipients of the vaccine. For a complete listing, see Dosage Forms, Composition and Packaging.
- Individuals who develop symptoms indicative of hypersensitivity after receiving a dose of GARDASIL should not receive further doses of GARDASIL.

WARNINGS AND PRECAUTIONS: General: As for any vaccine, vaccination with GARDASIL may not result in protection in all vaccine recipients.

This vaccine is not intended to be used for treatment of active external genital lesions; cervical, vulvar and vaginal cancers; CIN; VIN; or VaIN.

This vaccine will not protect against diseases that are not caused by HPV.

GARDASIL has not been shown to protect against diseases due to all HPV types.

As with all injectable vaccines, appropriate medical treatment should always be readily available in case of rare anaphylactic reactions following the administration of the vaccine.

Syncope (fainting) may follow any vaccination, especially in adolescents and young adults. Syncope, sometimes associated with falling, has occurred after vaccination with GARDASIL. Therefore, vaccinees should be carefully observed for approximately 15 minutes after administration of GARDASIL (see Adverse Reactions, Post-Market Adverse Drug Reactions).

Routine monitoring and Pap test should continue to be performed as indicated, regardless of GARDASIL administration.

Febrile Illness: The decision to administer or delay vaccination because of a current or recent febrile illness depends largely on the severity of the symptoms and their etiology. Low-grade fever itself and mild upper respiratory infection are not generally contraindications to vaccination.

Immunocompromised Individuals: Individuals with impaired immune responsiveness, whether due to the use of immunosuppressive therapy, a genetic defect, Human Immunodeficiency Virus (HIV) infection, or other causes, may have reduced antibody response to active immunization (see Drug Interactions). No specific data are available from the use of GARDASIL in these individuals.

Individuals with Bleeding Disorders: This vaccine should be given with caution to individuals with thrombocytopenia or any coagulation disorder only if the benefit clearly outweighs the risk of bleeding following an intramuscular administration in these individuals.

Special Populations: The safety, immunogenicity, and efficacy of GARDASIL have not been evaluated in HIV-infected individuals.

Pregnant Women: Studies in Female Rats: Animal studies do not indicate direct or indirect harmful effects with respect to pregnancy, embryonic/fetal development, parturition or postnatal development. GARDASIL induced a specific antibody response against HPV Types 6, 11, 16, and 18 in pregnant rats following one or multiple intramuscular injections. Antibodies against all 4 HPV types were transferred to the offspring during gestation and possibly during lactation.

Clinical Studies in Humans: There are, however, no adequate and well-controlled studies in pregnant women. Because animal reproduction studies are not always predictive of human response, pregnancy should be avoided during the vaccination regimen for GARDASIL.

In clinical studies, women underwent urine pregnancy testing prior to administration of each dose of GARDASIL. Women who were found to be pregnant before completion of a 3-dose regimen of GARDASIL were instructed to defer completion of their vaccination regimen until resolution of the pregnancy. Such non-standard regimens resulted in Postdose 3 anti-HPV 6, anti-HPV 11, anti-HPV 16, and anti-HPV 18 responses that were comparable to those observed in women who received a standard 0, 2 and 6 month vaccination regimen (see Dosage and Administration).

Merck Frosst Canada Ltd. maintains a Pregnancy Registry to monitor fetal outcomes of pregnant women exposed to GARDASIL vaccine. Patients and health-care providers are encouraged to report any exposure to GARDASIL vaccine during pregnancy by calling 1-800-567-2594.

During clinical trials, 3315 women (vaccine N=1657 vs placebo N=1658) reported at least one pregnancy. The overall proportions of pregnancies that resulted in an adverse outcome, defined as the combined numbers of spontaneous abortion, late fetal death, and congenital anomaly cases out of the total number of pregnancy outcomes for which an outcome was known (and excluding elective terminations), were 23.2% (393/1693) in individuals who received GARDASIL and 23.8% (403/1692) in individuals who received placebo.

Overall, 51 and 58 individuals in the group that received GARDASIL or placebo, respectively (3.1% and 3.5% of all individuals who reported a pregnancy in the respective vaccination groups), experienced a serious adverse experience during pregnancy. The most common events reported were conditions that can result in Caesarean section (e.g., failure of labor, malpresentation, cephalopelvic disproportion), premature onset of labor (e.g., threatened abortions, premature rupture of membranes), and pregnancy-related medical problems (e.g., preeclampsia, hyperemesis). The proportions of pregnant individuals who experienced such events were comparable between the groups receiving GARDASIL and placebo.

There were 37 cases of congenital anomaly in pregnancies that occurred in individuals who received GARDASIL and 27 cases of congenital anomaly in pregnancies that occurred in individuals who received placebo.

Further sub-analyses were done to evaluate pregnancies with estimated onset within 30 days or more than 30 days from administration of a dose of GARDASIL or placebo. For pregnancies with estimated onset within 30 days of vaccination, 5 cases of congenital anomaly were observed in the group that received GARDASIL compared to 0 cases of congenital anomaly in the group that received placebo. Conversely, in pregnancies with onset more than 30 days following vaccination, 32 cases of congenital anomaly were observed in the group that received GARDASIL compared with 27 cases of congenital anomaly in the group that received placebo. The types of anomalies observed were consistent (regardless of when pregnancy occurred in relation to vaccination) with those generally observed in pregnancies in women aged 16 through 26 years.

Nursing Women: It is not known whether vaccine antigens or antibodies induced by the vaccine are excreted in human milk.

GARDASIL may be administered to lactating women.

A total of 995 nursing mothers (vaccine N=500, placebo N=495) were given GARDASIL or placebo during the vaccination period of the clinical trials. In these studies, the rates of adverse experiences in the mother and the nursing infant were comparable between vaccination groups. In addition, vaccine immunogenicity was comparable among nursing mothers and women who did not nurse during the vaccine administration.

The Month 7 Geometric Mean Titers (GMTs) in nursing mothers were 595.9 (95% Confidence Interval [CI]: 522.5, 679.5) for anti-HPV 6, 864.3 (95% CI: 754.0, 990.8) for anti-HPV 11, 3056.9 (95% CI: 2594.4, 3601.8) for anti-HPV 16, and 527.2 (95% CI: 450.9, 616.5) for anti-HPV 18. The GMTs for women who did not nurse during vaccine administration were 540.1 (95% CI: 523.5, 557.2) for anti-HPV 6, 746.3 (95% CI: 720.4, 773.3) for anti-HPV 11, 2290.8 (95% CI: 2180.7, 2406.3) for anti-HPV 16, and 456.0 (95% CI: 438.4, 474.3) for anti-HPV 18.

Overall, 21 and 10 infants of individuals who received GARDASIL or placebo, respectively (representing 4.2% and 2.0% of the total number of individuals who were breast-feeding during the period in which they received GARDASIL or placebo, respectively), experienced a serious adverse experience. None was judged by the investigator to be vaccine-related.

In clinical studies, a higher number of breast-fed infants (n=6) whose mothers received GARDASIL had acute respiratory illnesses within 30 days post-vaccination of the mother as compared to infants (n=2) whose mothers received placebo. In these studies, the rates of other adverse experiences in the mother and the nursing infant were comparable between vaccination groups.

Pediatrics (<9 years of age): The safety and efficacy of GARDASIL have not been evaluated in children younger than 9 years.

Geriatrics (>65 years of age): The safety and efficacy of GARDASIL have not been evaluated in adults above the age of 26 years.

ADVERSE REACTIONS: Adverse Drug Reaction Overview: In clinical trials, GARDASIL was generally well tolerated when compared to placebo (Amorphous Aluminum Hydroxyphosphate Sulfate (AAHS) Adjuvant or saline).

Clinical Trial Adverse Drug Reactions: Because clinical trials are conducted under very specific conditions the adverse reaction rates observed in the clinical trials may not reflect the rates observed in practice and should not be compared to the rates in the clinical trials of another vaccine. Adverse drug reaction information from clinical trials is useful for identifying vaccine-related adverse events and for approximating rates.

In 6 clinical trials (5 placebo-controlled), individuals were administered GARDASIL or placebo on the day of enrollment, and approximately 2 and 6 months thereafter. In those clinical trials, a total of 13 798 individuals received GARDASIL and 11 715 individuals received placebo. GARDASIL demonstrated a favorable safety profile when compared with placebo (AAHS Adjuvant or saline). Few individuals (0.2%) discontinued due to adverse experiences. In all except one of the clinical trials, safety was evaluated using vaccination report card (VRC)-aided surveillance for 14 days after each injection of GARDASIL or placebo. The individuals who were monitored using VRC-aided surveillance included 8180 individuals (5088 girls and women 9 through 26 years of age and 3092 boys and men 9 through 26 years of age at enrollment) who received GARDASIL and 6093 individuals who received placebo.

The vaccine-related adverse experiences that were observed among 9- through 26-year-old recipients of GARDASIL at a frequency of at least 1.0% and also at a greater frequency than that observed among placebo recipients are shown in Table 1 and Table 2.

Table 1: GARDASIL

Vaccine-Related Injection-Site and Systemic Adverse Experiences in 9- Through 26-Year-Old Girls and Women[a]

Adverse Experience (1 to 5 Days Postvaccination)	GARDASIL (N=5088) %	AAHS[b] Adjuvant-Containing Placebo (N=3470) %	Saline Placebo (N=320) %
Injection Site			
Pain	83.9	75.4	48.6
Swelling	25.4	15.8	7.3
Erythema	24.7	18.4	12.1
Pruritus	3.2	2.8	0.6
Bruising	2.8	3.2	1.6
Adverse Experience (1 to 15 Days Postvaccination)	**GARDASIL (N=5088) %**	**Placebo (N=3790) %**	
Systemic			
Fever	10.3	8.6	
Nausea	4.2	4.1	
Dizziness	2.8	2.6	

[a] The vaccine-related adverse experiences that were observed among recipients of GARDASIL at a frequency of at least 1.0% and also at a greater frequency than that observed among placebo recipients.
[b] Amorphous Aluminum Hydroxyphosphate Sulfate.

Of those girls and women who reported an injection site reaction, 94.3% judged their injection-site adverse reaction to be mild or moderate in intensity.

In addition, bronchospasm was reported very rarely as a serious adverse experience.

Table 2: GARDASIL

Vaccine-Related Injection-Site and Systemic Adverse Experiences in 9- Through 26-Year-Old Boys and Men[a]

Adverse Experience (1 to 5 Days Postvaccination)	GARDASIL (N=3092) %	AAHS[b] Adjuvant-Containing Placebo (N=2029) %	Saline Placebo (N=274) %
Injection Site			
Pain	61.5	50.8	41.6
Erythema	16.7	14.1	14.5
Swelling	13.9	9.6	8.2
Adverse Experience (1 to 15 Days Postvaccination)	**GARDASIL (N=3092) %**	**Placebo (N=2303) %**	
Systemic			
Headache	7.5	6.7	

(cont'd)

Table 2: GARDASIL *(cont'd)*

Vaccine-Related Injection-Site and Systemic Adverse Experiences in 9- Through 26-Year-Old Boys and Men[a]

Fever	6.2	5.1

[a] The vaccine-related adverse experiences that were observed among recipients of GARDASIL at a frequency of at least 1.0% and also at a greater frequency than that observed among placebo recipients.
[b] Amorphous aluminum hydroxyphosphate sulfate.

Of those boys and men who reported an injection site reaction, 96.4% judged their injection-site adverse reaction to be mild or moderate in intensity.

All-Cause Common Systemic Adverse Experiences: All-cause systemic adverse experiences for 9- through 26-year-old recipients of GARDASIL, that were observed at a frequency of greater than or equal to 1% where the incidence in the vaccine group was greater than or equal to the incidence in the placebo group, are shown in Table 3 and Table 4.

Table 3: GARDASIL

All-Cause Common Systemic Adverse Experiences in Girls and Women 9 Through 26 Years of Age (GARDASIL ≥ Control)[a]

Adverse Reactions (1 to 15 Days Postvaccination)	GARDASIL (N=5088) %	AAHS Control[b] or Saline Placebo (N=3790) %
Pyrexia	13.0	11.2
Nausea	6.7	6.5
Dizziness	4.0	3.7
Diarrhea	3.6	3.5
Vomiting	2.4	1.9
Cough	2.0	1.5
Toothache	1.5	1.4
Upper Respiratory Tract Infection	1.5	1.5
Malaise	1.4	1.2
Arthralgia	1.2	0.9
Insomnia	1.2	0.9
Nasal Congestion	1.1	0.9

[a] The adverse reactions in this table are those that were observed among recipients of GARDASIL at a frequency of at least 1.0% and greater than or equal to those observed among AAHS control or saline placebo recipients.
[b] AAHS Control=Amorphous Aluminum Hydroxyphosphate Sulfate.

Table 4: GARDASIL

All-Cause Common Systemic Adverse Experiences in Boys and Men 9 Through 26 Years of Age (GARDASIL ≥ Control)[a]

Adverse Reactions (1 to 15 Days Postvaccination)	GARDASIL (N=3092) %	AAHS Control[b] or Saline Placebo (N=2303) %
Headache	12.3	11.2
Pyrexia	8.2	6.5
Pharyngolaryngeal Pain	2.8	2.1
Diarrhea	2.7	2.2
Nasopharyngitis	2.6	2.6
Nausea	2.0	1.0
Upper Respiratory Tract Infection	1.5	1.0
Abdominal Pain Upper	1.4	1.4
Myalgia	1.3	0.7
Dizziness	1.2	0.9
Vomiting	1.0	0.8

[a] The adverse reactions in this table are those that were observed among recipients of GARDASIL at a frequency of at least 1.0% and greater than or equal to those observed among AAHS control or saline placebo recipients.
[b] AAHS Control=Amorphous Aluminum Hydroxyphosphate Sulfate.

Serious Adverse Experiences in the Entire Study Population: A total of 229 individuals out of 25 513 total individuals (9- through 26-year-old girls and women and 9- through 26-year-old boys and men) who received both GARDASIL and placebo reported a serious systemic adverse experience following any vaccination visit during the clinical trials for GARDASIL. Out of the entire study population (25 513 individuals), only 0.04% of the reported serious systemic adverse experiences were judged to be vaccine related by the study investigator. The most frequently reported serious systemic adverse experiences for GARDASIL compared to placebo and regardless of causality were:
Headache [0.02% GARDASIL (3 cases) vs. 0.02% Placebo (2 cases)],
Gastroenteritis [0.02% GARDASIL (3 cases) vs. 0.01% Placebo (1 case)],
Appendicitis [0.04% GARDASIL (5 cases) vs. 0.01% Placebo (1 case)],
Pelvic inflammatory disease [0.01% GARDASIL (2 cases) vs. 0.02% Placebo (2 cases)],
Urinary tract infection [0.01% GARDASIL (2 cases) vs. 0.02% Placebo (2 cases)].

One case (0.01% GARDASIL: 0.0% Placebo) of bronchospasm and 2 cases (0.01% GARDASIL: 0.0% Placebo) of asthma were reported as serious systemic adverse experiences that occurred following any vaccination visit.

In addition, there was 1 individual in the clinical trials, in the group that received GARDASIL, who reported two injection-site serious adverse experiences (injection-site pain and injection-site joint movement impairment).

Deaths: Across the clinical studies, 31 deaths were reported in 25 513 (GARDASIL N=13 798; Placebo N=11 715) male and female individuals 9 through 26 years of age. The events reported were consistent with events expected in healthy adolescent and adult populations. The most common cause of death was motor vehicle accident (5 individuals who received GARDASIL and 4 individuals who received placebo), followed by drug overdose/suicide (2 individuals who received GARDASIL and 6 individuals who received placebo), gun shot wound (1 individual who received GARDASIL and 3 individuals who received placebo), and pulmonary embolus/deep vein thrombosis (1 individual who received GARDASIL and 1 individual who received placebo). In addition, there were 2 cases of sepsis, 1 case of pancreatic cancer, 1 case of arrhythmia, and 1 case of traumatic brain injury/cardiac arrest in the group that received GARDASIL; and 1 case of asphyxia, 1 case of chemical poisoning, and 1 case of myocardial ischaemia in the placebo group.

Systemic Autoimmune Disorders: In the clinical studies, male and female individuals ages 9 through 26, were evaluated for new medical conditions that occurred over the course of follow up. New medical conditions potentially indicative of a systemic autoimmune disorder seen in the group that received GARDASIL or placebo are shown in Table 5 and Table 6. This population includes all individuals who received at least one dose of GARDASIL or placebo, and had safety data available.

Table 5: GARDASIL

Summary of Girls and Women 9 Through 26 Years of Age Who Reported an Incident Condition Potentially Indicative of Systemic Autoimmune Disorder After Enrollment in Clinical Trials of GARDASIL Regardless of Causality

	GARDASIL (N=10 706)	AAHS Control[a] or Saline Placebo (N=9412)
Conditions	**n (%)**	**n (%)**
Arthralgia/Arthritis/Arthropathy[b]	120 (1.1)	98 (1.0)
Autoimmune Thyroiditis	4 (0.0)	1 (0.0)
Coeliac Disease	10 (0.1)	6 (0.1)
Diabetes Mellitus Insulin-dependent	2 (0.0)	2 (0.0)
Erythema Nodosum	2 (0.0)	4 (0.0)
Hyperthyroidism[c]	27 (0.3)	21 (0.2)
Hypothyroidism[d]	35 (0.3)	38 (0.4)
Inflammatory Bowel Disease[e]	7 (0.1)	10 (0.1)
Multiple Sclerosis	2 (0.0)	4 (0.0)
Nephritis[f]	2 (0.0)	5 (0.1)
Optic Neuritis	2 (0.0)	0 (0.0)
Pigmentation Disorder[g]	4 (0.0)	3 (0.0)
Psoriasis[h]	13 (0.1)	15 (0.2)
Raynaud's Phenomenon	3 (0.0)	4 (0.0)
Rheumatoid Arthritis[i]	6 (0.1)	2 (0.0)
Scleroderma/Morphea	2 (0.0)	1 (0.0)
Stevens-Johnson Syndrome	1 (0.0)	0 (0.0)
Systemic Lupus Erythematosus	1 (0.0)	3 (0.0)
Uveitis	3 (0.0)	1 (0.0)
All Conditions	245 (2.3)	218 (2.3)

[a] AAHS Control=Amorphous Aluminum Hydroxyphosphate Sulfate.
[b] Arthralgia/Arthritis/Arthropathy includes the following terms: arthralgia, arthritis, arthritis reactive, and arthropathy.
[c] Hyperthyroidism includes the following terms: Basedow's disease, goitre, toxic nodular goitre, and hyperthyroidism.
[d] Hypothyroidism includes the following terms: hypothyroidism and thyroiditis.
[e] Inflammatory bowel disease includes the following terms: colitis ulcerative, Crohn's disease, and inflammatory bowel disease.
[f] Nephritis includes the following terms: nephritis, glomerulonephritis minimal lesion, glomerulonephritis proliferative.
[g] Pigmentation disorder includes the following terms: pigmentation disorder, skin depigmentation, and vitiligo.
[h] Psoriasis includes the following terms: psoriasis, pustular psoriasis, and psoriatic arthropathy.
[i] Rheumatoid arthritis includes juvenile rheumatoid arthritis. One individual counted in the rheumatoid arthritis group reported rheumatoid arthritis as an adverse experience at Day 130.

Legend: N=Number of individuals enrolled; n=Number of individuals with specific new medical conditions.

Note: Although an individual may have had two or more new medical conditions, the individual is counted only once within a category. The same individual may appear in different categories.

Table 6: GARDASIL

Summary of Boys and Men 9 Through 26 Years of Age Who Reported an Incident Condition Potentially Indicative of Systemic Autoimmune Disorder After Enrollment in Clinical Trials of GARDASIL Regardless of Causality

	GARDASIL (N=3092)	AAHS Control[a] or Saline Placebo (N=2303)
Conditions	**n (%)**	**n (%)**
Alopecia Areata	1 (0.0)	0 (0.0)
Ankylosing Spondylitis	1 (0.0)	2 (0.1)
Arthralgia/Arthritis/Reactive Arthritis	30 (1.0)	17 (0.7)
Autoimmune Thrombocytopenia	1 (0.0)	0 (0.0)
Diabetes Mellitus Type 1	3 (0.1)	2 (0.1)
Hyperthyroidism	0 (0.0)	1 (0.0)
Hypothyroidism[b]	3 (0.1)	0 (0.0)
Inflammatory Bowel Disease[c]	0 (0.0)	2 (0.1)
Myocarditis	1 (0.0)	1 (0.0)
Proteinuria	1 (0.0)	0 (0.0)

(cont'd)

Table 6: GARDASIL (cont'd)

Summary of Boys and Men 9 Through 26 Years of Age Who Reported an Incident Condition Potentially Indicative of Systemic Autoimmune Disorder After Enrollment in Clinical Trials of GARDASIL Regardless of Causality

	GARDASIL (N=3092)	AAHS Control[a] or Saline Placebo (N=2303)
Conditions	**n (%)**	**n (%)**
Psoriasis	0 (0.0)	2 (0.1)
Vitiligo	2 (0.1)	5 (0.2)
All Conditions	43 (1.4)	32 (1.4)

[a] AAHS Control=Amorphous Aluminum Hydroxyphosphate Sulfate.
[b] Hypothyroidism includes the following terms: hypothyroidism and autoimmune thyroiditis.
[c] Inflammatory bowel disease includes the following terms: colitis ulcerative and Crohn's disease.

Legend: N=Number of individuals who received at least one dose of either vaccine or placebo; n=Number of individuals with specific new medical conditions.

Note: Although an individual may have had two or more new medical conditions, the individual is counted only once within a category. The same individual may appear in different categories.

Post-Market Adverse Drug Reactions: The following adverse experiences have been spontaneously reported during post-approval use of GARDASIL. Because these experiences were reported voluntarily from a population of uncertain size, it is not possible to reliably estimate their frequency or to establish a causal relationship to vaccine exposure.

Blood and Lymphatic System Disorders: autoimmune hemolytic anemia, idiopathic thrombocytopenic purpura, lymphadenopathy.

Nervous System Disorders: acute disseminated encephalomyelitis, dizziness, Guillain-Barré syndrome, headache, motor neuron disease, paralysis, syncope sometimes accompanied by tonic-clonic movements, transverse myelitis.

Gastrointestinal Disorders: nausea, pancreatitis, vomiting.

Musculoskeletal and Connective Tissue Disorders: arthralgia, myalgia.

General Disorders and Administration Site Conditions: asthenia, chills, death, fatigue, malaise.

Immune System Disorders: hypersensitivity reactions including anaphylactic/anaphylactoid reactions, bronchospasm, and urticaria.

DRUG INTERACTIONS: Drug-Drug Interactions: Use with Other Vaccines: Results from clinical studies indicate that GARDASIL may be administered concomitantly (at a separate injection site) with Menactra [Meningococcal (Groups A, C, Y and W-135) Polysaccharide Diphtheria Toxoid Conjugate Vaccine], Adacel [Tetanus Toxoid, Reduced Diphtheria Toxoid and Acellular Pertussis Vaccine Adsorbed (Tdap)], and RECOMBIVAX HB [hepatitis B vaccine (recombinant)].

The frequency of adverse experiences observed, in a placebo-controlled study with concomitant administration with hepatitis B vaccine (recombinant), was similar to the frequency when GARDASIL was administered alone.

In another placebo-controlled study, there was an increase in injection-site swelling when GARDASIL was given concomitantly with Meningococcal (Groups A, C, Y and W-135) Polysaccharide Diphtheria Toxoid Conjugate Vaccine and Tetanus Toxoid, Reduced Diphtheria Toxoid and Acellular Pertussis Vaccine Adsorbed (Tdap). The majority of injection-site swelling adverse experiences were reported as being mild to moderate in intensity.

Use with Common Medications: In clinical studies for girls and women (aged 16 to 26 years), 11.9%, 9.5%, 6.9%, and 4.3% of individuals used analgesics, anti-inflammatory drugs, antibiotics, and vitamin preparations, respectively. Conversely in a clinical study in boys and men (aged 16 to 26 years), 10.3%, 7.8%, 6.8%, 3.4% and 2.6% of individuals used analgesics, anti-inflammatory drugs, antibiotics, antihistamines, and vitamin preparations, respectively. The efficacy, immunogenicity, and safety of the vaccine were not impacted by the use of these medications.

Use with Hormonal Contraceptives: In clinical studies, 57.5% of women (aged 16 to 26 years) who received GARDASIL used hormonal contraceptives. Use of hormonal contraceptives did not appear to affect the immune responses to GARDASIL.

Use with Steroids: In clinical studies for girls and women (aged 16 to 26 years), 1.7% (n=158), 0.6% (n=56), and 1.0% (n=89) of individuals used inhaled, topical, and parenteral immunosuppressants, respectively. In a clinical study in boys and men (aged 16 to 26 years), 1.0% (n=21) used corticosteroids for systemic use. The corticosteroids for all individuals were administered close to the time of administration of a dose of GARDASIL. These medicines did not appear to affect the immune responses to GARDASIL. Very few individuals in the clinical studies were taking steroids, and the amount of immunosuppression is presumed to have been low.

Use with Systemic Immunosuppressive Medications: There are no data on the concomitant use of potent immunosuppressants with GARDASIL. Individuals receiving therapy with immunosuppressive agents (systemic doses of corticosteroids, antimetabolites, alkylating agents, cytotoxic agents) may not respond optimally to active immunization (see Warnings and Precautions, General).

Drug-Food Interactions: Interactions with food have not been established.

Drug-Herb Interactions: Interactions with herbal products have not been established.

Drug-Laboratory Test Interactions: Interactions with laboratory tests have not been established. There was no evidence from the clinical studies database of impact of GARDASIL administration on the performance characteristics of the Pap test and some commercially available HPV tests.

DOSAGE AND ADMINISTRATION: Recommended Dose and Dosage Adjustment: GARDASIL should be administered intramuscularly as 3 separate 0.5 mL-doses according to the following schedule:

First dose: at elected date
Second dose: 2 months after the first dose
Third dose: 6 months after the first dose

Individuals are encouraged to adhere to the 0, 2, and 6 months vaccination schedule. However, in clinical studies, efficacy has been demonstrated in individuals who have received all 3 doses within a 1-year period. If an alternate vaccination schedule is necessary, the second dose should be administered at least 1 month after the first dose, and the third dose be administered at least 3 months after the second dose.

Administration: GARDASIL should be administered intramuscularly in the deltoid region of the upper arm or in the higher anterolateral area of the thigh.

GARDASIL must not be injected intravascularly. Neither subcutaneous nor intradermal administration has been studied. These methods of administration are not recommended.

The prefilled syringe is for single use only and should not be used for more than one individual. For single-use vials, a separate sterile syringe and needle must be used for each individual.

The vaccine should be used as supplied; no dilution or reconstitution is necessary. The full recommended dose of the vaccine should be used.

Shake well before use. Thorough agitation immediately before administration is necessary to maintain suspension of the vaccine.

After thorough agitation, GARDASIL is a white, cloudy liquid. Parenteral drug products should be inspected visually for particulate matter and discoloration prior to administration. Discard the product if particulates are present or if it appears discolored.

Instructions for Use: Single-Dose Vial Use: Withdraw the 0.5 mL dose of vaccine from the single-dose vial using a sterile needle and syringe free of preservatives, antiseptics, and detergents. Once the single-dose vial has been penetrated, the withdrawn vaccine should be used promptly, and the vial must be discarded.

Prefilled Syringe Use: Inject the entire contents of the syringe.

Instructions for Using the Prefilled Single-Dose Syringes Preassembled with Needle Guard (safety) Device: Note: Please use the enclosed needle for administration. If a different needle is chosen, it should fit securely on the syringe and be no longer than 1 inch to ensure proper functioning of the needle guard device. Two detachable labels are provided which can be removed after the needle is guarded.

At any of the following steps, avoid contact with the Trigger Fingers to keep from activating the safety device prematurely.

Shake well before use. Thorough agitation immediately before administration is necessary to maintain suspension of the vaccine.

Remove Syringe Tip Cap and Needle Cap. Attach Luer Needle by pressing both Anti-Rotation Tabs to secure syringe and by twisting the Luer Needle in a clockwise direction until secured to the syringe. **Remove Needle Sheath. Administer injection** per standard protocol as stated above under Dosage and Administration. Depress the Plunger while grasping the Finger Flange **until the entire dose has been given**. The Needle Guard Device will **not** activate to cover and protect the needle unless the **entire** dose has been given. While the Plunger is still depressed, remove needle from the vaccine recipient. Slowly release the Plunger and allow syringe to move up until the entire needle is guarded. For documentation of vaccination, remove detachable labels by pulling slowly on them. **Dispose in approved sharps container.**

OVERDOSAGE:
There have been occasional reports of administration of higher than recommended doses of GARDASIL.

In general, the adverse event profile reported with overdose was comparable to recommended single doses of GARDASIL.

> For management of a suspected drug overdose, contact your regional Poison Control Centre. See the *CPS* Directory section for a list of Poison Control Centres.

ACTION AND CLINICAL PHARMACOLOGY: Disease Burden: Cervical cancer is caused by different types of Human Papillomavirus (HPV) infection. HPV causes squamous cell cervical cancer (and its histologic precursor lesions Cervical Intraepithelial Neoplasia [CIN] 1 or low grade dysplasia and CIN 2/3 or moderate to high grade dysplasia) and cervical adenocarcinoma (and its precursor lesion adenocarcinoma in situ [AIS]). HPV also causes approximately 35-50% of vulvar and vaginal cancers. Vulvar Intraepithelial Neoplasia (VIN) Grade 2/3 and Vaginal Intraepithelial Neoplasia (VaIN) Grade 2/3 are immediate precursors to these cancers.

HPV infection is very common. Most HPV infections clear without sequelae but some progress to cervical cancer and/or other HPV-related diseases. It is estimated that 75% of sexually active Canadians will have at least one HPV infection during their lifetime, with the highest prevalence observed in women aged 20-24 years. Men play an important role in transmission of HPV to their sexual partners. Several prospective studies have shown a high level of HPV concordance between couples who recently became infected, indicating transmission of HPV between the couples (male to female, and female to male). These data consistently support the sexually transmitted nature of HPV and the role of men in infecting women, who subsequently can develop HPV-related anogenital cancers and warts. Based on these various lines of evidence it is expected that decreasing the risk of HPV infection in men through vaccination should decrease the risk of infection in their sexual partners, thereby providing additional public health benefit.

Cervical cancer prevention focuses on routine screening and early intervention. This strategy has reduced cervical cancer rates by approximately 75% in compliant individuals by monitoring and removing premalignant dysplastic lesions. In 2001, more than 1350 Canadian women were diagnosed with cervical cancer and 400 women died from it. After breast cancer, cervical cancer is the most common cancer in Canadian women between the ages of 20 and 44.

HPV also causes genital warts (condyloma acuminata) which are growths of the cervicovaginal, vulvar, perianal and intra-anal mucosa, and the external genitalia that rarely progress to cancer, but cause significant psychosocial impact and disease recurrence. The lifetime risk for acquisition of genital warts has been estimated to exceed 10%.

Based on two recent epidemiologic studies from BC and Manitoba, anogenital warts (AGWs) are associated with a significant burden of illness and costs to the Canadian healthcare system. Of note is the similarity in findings between the two studies with respect to the incidence of genital warts. In BC overall incidence was found to be 1.26 per 1000 population, at an average cost of $190 per episode for treatment which, translates into approximately $1 million in annual, direct medical costs. Similarly, in Manitoba the incidence of genital warts in males was found to be 1.54 per 1000, whilst for females it was 1.23 per 1000, resulting in an average cost of $200 per individual treated. If the Manitoba rates are generalizable to Canada, then in 2006 (based 2004 Manitoba rates and the 2006 Canadian census population) there would have been 41 450 incident cases, 48 600 prevalent cases, and 617 950 people who had been diagnosed with AGWs since 1985.

HPV infection is strongly associated with anal cancer. The great majority of anal cancers are squamous cell carcinoma (SCC). Anal canal SCC are HPV positive in 84% of cases in men and women. HPV 16 (73%) and HPV 18 (5%) are the most common associated types.

Approximately 560 000 new cases of head and neck squamous cell cancers (HNSCC) and 250 000 deaths due to HNSCC are reported annually worldwide. Overall, 2/3 of HNSCC cases occur in men. Oropharyngeal squamous cell carcinomas (OPSCC) are a type of HNSCC. OPSCCs that tend to occur in young, non-smoker/non-drinker men account for approximately 24-36% of OPSCCs worldwide. Oral HPV 16 infection has been associated with a significantly elevated risk for development of HNSCC. HPV 16 is detected in >90% of HPV-positive OPSCC cases.

HPV 6, 11, 16, and 18 are common HPV types.

HPV types 16 and 18 cause approximately:
- 70% of cervical cancer, AIS, and CIN 3, cases;
- 50% of CIN 2 cases;
- 70% of HPV-related vulvar and vaginal cancer, VIN 2/3, and VaIN 2/3 cases;
- 90% of HPV-related anal cancers and their precursor lesions; and
- 60% of HPV-related penile cancers.

HPV types 6, 11, 16, and 18 cause approximately:
- 35 to 50% of all CIN 1, VIN 1, and VaIN 1 cases.

HPV types 6 and 11 cause approximately:
- 90% of genital wart cases; and
- 9 to 12% of CIN 1 cases.

HPV type 16 causes approximately:
- 90% of oropharyngeal squamous cell carcinomas.

HPV 31, 33, 52, 56, 58, and 59 are high-risk HPV types. These types are responsible for:
- 11.6% of cervical cancer cases;
- 32.2% of CIN 1 cases;
- 39.3% of CIN 2 cases; and
- 24.3% of CIN 3 or AIS cases.

A recent Canadian study evaluated the prevalence of HPV in liquid-based specimens from a sample of 8700 women throughout British Columbia who were attending for routine cytology screening at high-volume primary care screening sites. This study found that HPV types 31, 33, 52 and 58 were responsible for:
- 9.8% of LSILs (Low grade Squamous Intraepithelial Lesion, encompassing: HPV/mild dysplasia/CIN I);
- 18.8% of HSILs (High grade Squamous Intraepithelial Lesion, encompassing: moderate and severe dysplasia, carcinoma in situ, CIN II and CIN III).

Mechanism of Action: GARDASIL contains L1 VLPs, which are proteins that resemble wild-type virions. Because the virus-like particles contain no viral DNA, they cannot infect cells or reproduce.

HPV only infects humans, but animal studies with analogous animal papillomaviruses suggest that the efficacy of L1 VLP vaccines is mediated by the development of humoral immune responses.

In preclinical studies, induction of anti-papillomavirus antibodies with L1 VLP vaccines resulted in protection against infection. Administration of serum from vaccinated to unvaccinated animals resulted in the transfer of protection against HPV to the unvaccinated animals. These data suggest that the efficacy of L1 VLP vaccines is mediated by the development of humoral immune responses.

STORAGE AND STABILITY: Store refrigerated at 2 to 8°C. Do not freeze. Protect from light. GARDASIL should be administered as soon as possible after being removed from refrigeration. GARDASIL can be administered provided total time out of refrigeration (at temperatures at or below 25°C) does not exceed 72 hours.

INFORMATION FOR THE PATIENT: Published in e-CPS, available by subscription at www.e-cps.ca.

DOSAGE FORMS, COMPOSITION AND PACKAGING: GARDASIL is a sterile preparation for intramuscular administration supplied as a 0.5 mL single-dose vial or a 0.5 mL single-dose prefilled Luer Lock syringe, with or without safety device. After thorough agitation, GARDASIL is a white, cloudy liquid. Each 0.5 mL dose of sterile preparation for intramuscular administration contains: approximately 20 µg of HPV 6 L1 protein, 40 µg of HPV 11 L1 protein, 40 µg of HPV 16 L1 protein, and 20 µg of HPV 18 L1 protein. Nonmedicinal ingredients: aluminum (as amorphous aluminum hydroxyphosphate sulfate [AAHS] adjuvant), L-histidine, polysorbate 80, sodium borate, sodium chloride and water for injection. Preservative- and antibiotic-free. Vials and prefilled syringes components are latex free.

Vials: GARDASIL is supplied in 3 mL single-dose Type I glass vials containing one 0.5 mL dose of liquid vaccine. Packages of 1 and 10 single-dose vials.

Syringes: GARDASIL is supplied in 1.5 mL single-dose Type I glass prefilled Luer Lock syringes, preassembled with an Ultra-Safe Passive delivery system, containing one 0.5 mL dose of liquid vaccine in a carton. One needle is provided separately in the carton.

GARDASIL is supplied in 1.5 mL single-dose Type I glass prefilled Luer Lock syringes, **without** safety device, containing one 0.5 mL dose of liquid vaccine in a carton. One needle is provided separately in the carton.

Gastrolyte®
electrolytes—dextrose
Diarrhea Therapy

sanofi-aventis

Date of Revision: December 31, 2009

INDICATIONS: For the management of watery diarrhea of varying types, including gastroenteritis and oral correction of fluid and electrolyte loss in infants, children and adults.

Maintenance of fluid and electrolyte balance in situations such as post-operative when the oral route is available.

CONTRAINDICATIONS: There are no known contraindications to this product.

WARNINGS: Cow's milk and artificial milk feeds in infants should be stopped for 24 hours and gradually introduced when the diarrhea has lessened. However, breast feeding should be continued.

PRECAUTIONS: For oral administration only. GASTROLYTE should not be reconstituted in diluents other than water. Each sachet should always be dissolved in 200 mL of water. A weaker solution than recommended will not contain the optimal dextrose and electrolyte concentration while a stronger solution than recommended may give rise to electrolyte imbalance.

With intractable vomiting, adynamic ileus (inhibition of bowel motility), intestinal obstruction of perforated bowel, nothing should be administered orally.

If the diarrhea does not improve promptly, the patient should be reassessed.

OVERDOSE:

> For management of a suspected drug overdose, CPhA recommends that you contact your **regional Poison Control Centre**. See the *CPS* Directory section for a list of Poison Control Centres.

DOSAGE: Reconstitution: The contents of each sachet should be dissolved in sufficient drinking water to make 200 mL (approximately 7 fluid ounces). An infant's feeding bottle is a convenient measure of this volume. The solution should be made up immediately prior to feeding and any solution remaining an hour after reconstitution should be discarded. However, the solution may be used for up to 24 hours if stored in a refrigerator immediately after reconstitution. The reconstituted solution must not be boiled.

For oral administration only. A basic principle of treatment of diarrhea is to replace fluid loss and then to maintain sufficient fluid intake to replace further loss from stools.

For toddlers, older children and adults, GASTROLYTE solution may be given freely until the thirst is satisfied.

For infants, a number of different regimens are used by different physicians, but the basic principle is to omit milk feeds or solids initially, while maintaining adequate fluid intake. Milk can then be reintroduced to provide calories, but to avoid worsening or prolonging the diarrhea, this should be gradual.

The following dosage and regrading scheme are only a general guide and the volume of the product given and the speed of re-introduction of the normal feeds is at the discretion of the physician.

General Dosage Guide: 150 mL of GASTROLYTE solution per kg of body weight per day or 70 mL (2½ fluid ounces) per pound per day.

In those patients who are vomiting at the start of treatment, it may be advisable to give very small volumes initially until vomiting is under control. Infantile diarrhea is uncommon in breast-fed infants. However, if treatment with this product becomes necessary, it is suggested that for each feeding the chosen regimen be followed and the infant be given the appropriate volume of the solution for that feeding and then breast-fed until satisfied.

SUPPLIED: The composition of GASTROLYTE stimulates intestinal water absorption.

GASTROLYTE Fruit: Each sachet contains: dextrose monohydrate 3.56 g, disodium citrate 0.53 g, sodium chloride 0.47 g, potassium chloride 0.30 g. A liter made up of 5 sachets×200 mL contains: sodium 60 mmol, potassium 20 mmol, chloride 60 mmol, bicarbonate 10 mmol and dextrose (anhydrous) 90 mmol. Nonmedicinal ingredients: aspartame (as sweetening agent), grapefruit flavour, pineapple flavour and silicon dioxide. Boxes of 10 foil/laminate sachets. Store sachets in cool, dry place and avoid exposure to temperature in excess of 30°C. Keep unused solution in refrigerator for a maximum of 24 hours.

GASTROLYTE Regular: Each sachet contains: dextrose monohydrate 3.56 g, disodium citrate 0.53 g, sodium chloride 0.47 g, potassium chloride 0.30 g. A liter made up of 5 sachets×200 mL contains: sodium 60 mmol, potassium 20 mmol, chloride 60 mmol, bicarbonate 10 mmol and dextrose (anhydrous) 90 mmol. Nonmedicinal ingredients: aspartame (as sweetening agent) and silicon dioxide. Boxes of 10 foil/laminate sachets. Store sachets in cool, dry place and avoid exposure to temperature in excess of 30°C. Keep unused solution in refrigerator for a maximum of 24 hours.

Gatifloxacin Ⓟ
CPhA Monograph

see *Fluoroquinolones*

Gaviscon® Heartburn & Acid Reflux Relief Formula Tablets
alginic acid—magnesium carbonate
Gastroesophageal Reflux Disease Therapy

GlaxoSmithKline Consumer Healthcare

Gaviscon® Heartburn & Acid Reflux Relief Formula Liquid
sodium alginate—aluminum hydroxide
Gastroesophageal Reflux Disease Therapy

GlaxoSmithKline Consumer Healthcare

Gaviscon® MAXRELIEF™ Heartburn & Acid Reflux Formula Tablets
alginic acid—magnesium carbonate
Gastroesophageal Reflux Disease Therapy

GlaxoSmithKline Consumer Healthcare

PHARMACOLOGY: The liquid, or tablets when chewed, form a viscous foam barrier (alginate raft) which floats on stomach contents, acting as a physical barrier that prevents gastric acid from reaching the esophagus, preventing acid reflux.

INDICATIONS: For day and nighttime relief of heartburn and GERD (gastroesophageal reflux disease). Suitable for concomittant use with proton pump inhibitors and H_2 receptor antagonists for the treatment of breakthrough symptoms.

CONTRAINDICATIONS: No data supplied by the manufacturer.

WARNINGS: No data supplied by the manufacturer.

PRECAUTIONS: For patients on severely restricted sodium diets it should be noted that each 5 mL of liquid contains approximately 53 mg of Na^+, each regular strength tablet contains approximately 22 mg of Na^+, and each extra strength tablet contains approximately 35 mg of Na^+.

The cations of magnesium and aluminum interfere with the absorption of tetracycline, iron and phosphate. In addition, oral magnesium may accumulate in the plasma of patients with impaired renal function, thus individuals with kidney ailments should consult a physician prior to taking this product. A physician should be consulted if symptoms persist for more than two weeks or recur.

ADVERSE EFFECTS: Nausea, vomiting, eructation, flatulence.

Do not take if you suffer from kidney disease or within 2 hours of another medicine because effectiveness may be altered.

Pregnancy: While Gaviscon has not been studied for use during pregnancy, ingredients in this product (alginates) have been shown to be safe for use during pregnancy. There have been no reported adverse effects of Gaviscon on fetal development.

OVERDOSE:

Symptoms: Should overdosage occur, gastric distention may result and is best treated conservatively.

Treatment: See Symptoms.

For management of a suspected drug overdose, CPhA recommends that you contact your **regional Poison Control Centre**. See the *CPS* Directory section for a list of Poison Control Centres.

DOSAGE: Liquid: Adults: 10 or 20 mL (2 to 4 teaspoons) when symptoms occur. Maximum 80 mL/day (16 teaspoons/day).

Tablets (Aluminum-free): Regular Strength: Adults: 2 to 4 tablets chewed thoroughly, when symptoms occur. Maximum 16 tablets/day.

Extra Strength: Adults: 2 to 4 tablets chewed thoroughly, when symptoms occur. Maximum 12 tablets/day.

MAXRELIEF: Adults: 2 to 4 tablets chewed thoroughly when symptoms occur. Maximum 11 tablets/day.

Administration should be followed by a drink of water or milk if desired. **Do not swallow tablets whole.**

SUPPLIED: Liquid: Each 5 mL of a light tan-colored, pleasantly fruit-flavored suspension or cream-colored, mint-flavored suspension contains: sodium alginate 250 mg and aluminum hydroxide 100 mg. Plastic bottles of 340 and 600 mL.

Tablets (Aluminum-free): Regular Strength: Each round, creamy-white, peppermint, fruit, or butterscotch-flavored tablet contains: alginic acid 200 mg and magnesium carbonate 40 mg. Bottles of 100. Fruit-flavor also in bottles of 40.

Extra Strength: Each round, creamy-white, peppermint, fruit, butterscotch, strawberry, orange burst, and milk chocolate-flavored tablet contains: alginic acid 313 mg and magnesium carbonate 63 mg. Bottles of 60. Fruit-flavor also in bottles of 25 and 120.

MAXRELIEF: Each round, creamy-white, Icy Mint with cooling action or Berry-flavored tablet contains: alginic acid 360 mg and magnesium carbonate 72 mg. Cartons of 18 tablets in Single-Dose Portable Packs.

The reader is invited to consult CPhA's monograph **Calcium Channel Blockers**.

GD-amlodipine™ ℞

amlodipine besylate

Antihypertensive—Antianginal

GenMed, a division of Pfizer

Date of Preparation: May 9, 2006
Date of Revision: December 1, 2008

PHARMACOLOGY: GD-amlodipine (amlodipine besylate) is a calcium ion influx inhibitor (calcium entry blocker or calcium ion antagonist). Amlodipine is a member of the dihydropyridine class of calcium antagonists.

Mechanism of Action: The therapeutic effect of this group of drugs is believed to be related to their specific cellular action of selectively inhibiting transmembrane influx of calcium ions into vascular smooth muscle and cardiac muscle. The contractile processes of these tissues are dependent upon the movement of extracellular calcium ions into these cells through specific ion channels. Amlodipine inhibits calcium ion influx across cell membranes selectively, with a greater effect on vascular smooth muscle cells than on cardiac muscle cells. Serum calcium concentration is not affected by amlodipine. Within the physiologic pH range, amlodipine is an ionized compound and its kinetic interaction with the calcium channel receptor is characterized by the gradual association and dissociation with the receptor binding site. Experimental data suggest that amlodipine binds to both dihydropyridine and nondihydropyridine binding sites.

Hypertension: The mechanism by which amlodipine reduces arterial blood pressure involves direct peripheral arterial vasodilation and reduction in peripheral vascular resistance.

Angina: The precise mechanism by which amlodipine relieves angina has not been fully delineated. Amlodipine is a dilator of peripheral arteries and arterioles which reduces the total peripheral resistance and, therefore, reduces the workload of the heart (afterload). The unloading of the heart is thought to decrease ischemia and relieve effort angina by reducing myocardial energy oxygen consumption and oxygen requirements.

Pharmacokinetics: Pharmacokinetics and Metabolism: After oral administration of therapeutic doses of amlodipine, absorption occurs gradually with peak plasma concentration reached between 6 and 12 hours. Absolute bioavailability has been estimated to be between 64 and 90%. The bioavailability of amlodipine is not altered by the presence of food.

Amlodipine is metabolized through the cytochrome P450 system, mainly via CYP 3A4 isoenzyme. Amlodipine is extensively (about 90%) converted to inactive metabolites (via hepatic metabolism) with 10% of the parent compound and 60% of the metabolites excreted in the urine. Ex vivo studies have shown that approximately 93% of the circulating drug is bound to plasma proteins in hypertensive patients. Elimination from the plasma is biphasic with a terminal elimination half-life of about 35-50 hours. Steady state plasma levels of amlodipine are reached after 7 to 8 days of consecutive daily dosing.

The pharmacokinetics of amlodipine are not significantly influenced by renal impairment. Plasma concentrations in the patients with moderate to severe renal failure were higher than in the normal subjects. Accumulation and mean elimination half-life in all patients were within the range of those observed in other pharmacokinetic studies with amlodipine in normal subjects.

In elderly hypertensive patients (mean age 69 years) there was a decrease in clearance of amlodipine from plasma as compared to young volunteers (mean age 36 years) with a resulting increase in the area under the curve (AUC) of about 60%.

Following single oral administration of 5 mg of amlodipine, patients with chronic mild-moderate hepatic insufficiency showed about 40% increase in AUC of amlodipine as compared to normal volunteers. This was presumably due to a reduction in clearance of amlodipine as the terminal elimination half-life was prolonged from 34 hrs in young normal subjects to 56 hrs in the elderly patients with hepatic insufficiency.

Following oral administration of 10 mg amlodipine to 20 male volunteers, pharmacokinetics of amlodipine were similar when amlodipine was administered with and without grapefruit juice. Geometric mean C_{max} of amlodipine was 6.2 ng/mL when the drug was administered with grapefruit juice and 5.8 ng/mL when administered with water. Mean T_{max} of amlodipine was 7.6 hours with grapefruit juice and 7.9 hours with water. Geometric mean $AUC_{0-\infty}$ was 315 ng/hr/mL with grapefruit juice and 293 ng/hr/mL with water. Geometric mean bioavailability of amlodipine was 85% when administered with grapefruit juice and 81% when administered with water.

Pediatric Patients: Two studies were conducted to evaluate the use of GD-amlodipine in a pediatric population.

In one study (pharmacokinetic), sixty-two hypertensive patients aged greater than 6 years received doses of GD-amlodipine between 1.25 mg and 20 mg. Weight-adjusted clearance and volume of distribution were similar to values in adults (see Dosage). The mean absorption rate constant (K_a) in children (0.85 hr^{-1}) is approximately 50% higher than that in healthy adults (0.55 hr^{-1}, range of 0.28-1.09 hr^{-1}).

Gender effect: In a second trial (clinical), a pattern of greater reductions in both systolic and diastolic blood pressure in females than in males was observed. Mean change in systolic blood pressure from baseline to end of study: amlodipine 2.5 mg: males, −6.9 mmHg (n=51); females, −8.9 mmHg (n=32); amlodipine 5.0 mg: males, −6.6 mmHg (n=63); females, −14.0 mmHg (n=23); placebo males, −2.5 mmHg (n=54), females, −3.8 mmHg (n=33).

Pharmacodynamics: Hemodynamics: Following administration of recommended doses to patients with hypertension, amlodipine produces vasodilation resulting in a reduction of supine and standing blood pressures. These decreases in blood pressure are not accompanied by any significant change in heart rate or plasma catecholamine levels with chronic dosing. With chronic once daily oral administration (5 and 10 mg once daily), antihypertensive effectiveness is maintained throughout the 24 hours dose interval with minimal peak to trough differences in blood pressure reduction. Since the vasodilation induced by amlodipine is gradual in onset, acute hypotension has rarely been reported after oral administration of amlodipine. In normotensive patients with angina amlodipine has not been associated with any clinically significant reductions in blood pressure or changes in heart rate.

Negative inotropic effects have not been observed when amlodipine was administered at the recommended doses to man, but has been demonstrated in animal models. Hemodynamic measurements of cardiac function at rest and during exercise (or pacing) in angina patients with normal ventricular function have generally demonstrated a small increase in cardiac index without significant influence on dP/dt or on left ventricular end diastolic pressure or volume.

In hypertensive patients with normal renal function, therapeutic doses of amlodipine resulted in a decrease in renal vascular resistance and an increase in glomerular filtration rate and effective renal plasma flow without change in filtration fraction.

Electrophysiologic Effects: Amlodipine does not change sinoatrial nodal function or atrioventricular conduction in intact animals, or man. In patients with chronic stable angina, intravenous administration of 10 mg of amlodipine and a further 10 mg of amlodipine after a 30 min. interval produced peripheral vasodilation and afterload reduction, but did not significantly alter A-H and H-V conduction and sinus node recovery time after pacing. Similar results were obtained in patients receiving amlodipine and concomitant beta-blockers. In clinical studies in which amlodipine was administered in combination with beta-blockers to patients with either hypertension or angina, no adverse effects on electrocardiographic parameters were observed. In clinical trials with angina patients, amlodipine as monotherapy did not alter electrocardiographic intervals.

Effects in Hypertension: Pediatric Patients: Two hundred sixty-eight hypertensive patients aged 6 to 17 years were randomized first to GD-amlodipine 2.5 or 5 mg once daily for 4 weeks and then randomized again to the same dose or to placebo for another 4 weeks. Patients receiving 5 mg at the end of 8 weeks had lower blood pressure than those secondarily randomized to placebo. The magnitude of the treatment effect is difficult to interpret, but it is probably less than 5 mmHg systolic on the 5 mg dose. Adverse events were similar to those seen in adults.

Pediatric safety and efficacy studies beyond 8 weeks of duration have not been conducted. In addition, the long-term effect of amlodipine on growth and development, myocardial growth and vascular smooth muscles has not been studied.

INDICATIONS: Hypertension: GD-amlodipine (amlodipine besylate) is indicated in the treatment of mild to moderate essential hypertension.

Combination of GD-amlodipine with a diuretic, a beta-blocking agent, or an angiotensin converting enzyme inhibitor has been found to be compatible and showed additive antihypertensive effect.

Chronic Stable Angina: GD-amlodipine is indicated for the management of chronic stable angina (effort-associated angina) in patients who remain symptomatic despite adequate doses of beta-blockers and/or organic nitrates or who cannot tolerate those agents.

GD-amlodipine may be tried in combination with beta-blockers in chronic stable angina in patients with normal ventricular function. When such concomitant therapy is introduced, care must be taken to monitor blood pressure closely since hypotension can occur from the combined effects of the drugs.

CONTRAINDICATIONS: GD-amlodipine (amlodipine besylate) is contraindicated in patients with hypersensitivity to the drug or other dihydropyridines and in patients with severe hypotension (less than 90 mmHg systolic).

WARNINGS: Increased Angina and/or Myocardial Infarction: Rarely, patients, particularly those with severe obstructive coronary artery disease, have developed documented increased frequency, duration and/or severity of angina or acute myocardial infarction on starting calcium channel blocker therapy or at the time of dosage increase. The mechanism of this effect has not been elucidated.

Outflow Obstruction (Aortic Stenosis): GD-amlodipine should be used with caution in a presence of fixed left ventricular outflow obstruction (aortic stenosis).

Use in Patients with Impaired Hepatic Function: There are no adequate studies in patients with liver dysfunction and dosage recommendations have not been established. In a small number of patients with mild to moderate hepatic impairment given single dose of 5 mg, amlodipine half-life has been prolonged (see Pharmacology, Pharmacokinetics and Metabolism). GD-amlodipine should, therefore, be administered with caution in these patients and careful monitoring should be performed. A lower starting dose may be required (see Dosage).

Beta-blocker Withdrawal: GD-amlodipine gives no protection against the dangers of abrupt beta-blocker withdrawal and such withdrawal should be done by the gradual reduction of the dose of beta-blocker.

PRECAUTIONS: Use in Patients with Congestive Heart Failure: Although generally calcium channel blockers should only be used with caution in patients with heart failure, it has been observed that GD-amlodipine had no overall deleterious effect on survival and cardiovascular morbidity in both short-term and long-term clinical trials in these patients. While a significant proportion of the patients in these studies had a history of ischemic heart disease, angina or hypertension, the studies were not designed to evaluate the treatment of angina or hypertension in patients with concomitant heart failure.

Hypotension: GD-amlodipine (amlodipine besylate) may occasionally precipitate symptomatic hypotension. Careful monitoring of blood pressure is recommended, especially in patients with a history of cerebrovascular insufficiency, and those taking medications known to lower blood pressure.

Peripheral Edema: Mild to moderate peripheral edema was the most common adverse event in the clinical trials (see Adverse Effects). The incidence of peripheral edema was dose-dependent and ranged in frequency from 3.0 to 10.8% in 5 to 10 mg dose range. Care should be taken to differentiate this peripheral edema from the effects of increasing left ventricular dysfunction.

Pregnancy: Although amlodipine was not teratogenic in the rat and rabbit some dihydropyridine compounds have been found to be teratogenic in animals. In rats, amlodipine has been shown to prolong both the gestation period and the duration of labor. There is no clinical experience with GD-amlodipine in pregnant women. GD-amlodipine should be used during pregnancy only if the potential benefit outweighs the potential risk to the mother and fetus.

Lactation: It is not known whether amlodipine is excreted in human milk. Since amlodipine safety in newborns has not been established, GD-amlodipine should not be given to nursing mothers.

Children: The use of GD-amlodipine is not recommended in patients less than 6 years of age since safety and efficacy have not been established in that population. Pediatric safety and efficacy studies beyond 8 weeks of duration have not been conducted.

The effect of GD-amlodipine on blood pressure in patients less than 6 years of age is not known. The pediatric administration should be based on a careful risk/benefit assessment of the limited available information. The risk/benefit assessment should be conducted by a qualified physician.

Geriatrics: In elderly patients (≥65 years) clearance of amlodipine is decreased with a resulting increase in AUC (see Pharmacology, Pharmacokinetics and Metabolism). In clinical trials the incidence of adverse reactions in elderly patients was approximately 6% higher than that of younger population (<65 years). Adverse reactions include edema, muscle cramps and dizziness. GD-amlodipine should be used cautiously in elderly patients. Dosage adjustment is advisable (see Dosage).

Interaction with Grapefruit Juice: Published data indicate that through inhibition of the cytochrome P450 system, grapefruit juice can increase plasma levels and augment pharmacodynamic effects of some dihydropyridine calcium channel blockers. Following oral administration of 10 mg amlodipine to 20 male volunteers, pharmacokinetics of amlodipine were similar when amlodipine was administered with and without grapefruit juice. (See Pharmacology, Pharmacokinetics.)

Drug Interactions: As with all drugs, care should be exercised when treating patients with multiple medications. Dihydropyridine calcium channel blockers undergo biotransformation by the cytochrome P450 system, mainly via CYP 3A4 isoenzyme. Coadministration of amlodipine with other drugs which follow the same route of biotransformation may result in altered bioavailability of amlodipine or these drugs. Dosages of similarly metabolized drugs, particularly those of low therapeutic ratio, and especially in patients with renal and/or hepatic impairment, may require adjustment when starting or stopping concomitantly administered amlodipine to maintain optimum therapeutic blood levels.

Drugs known to be inhibitors of the cytochrome P450 system include: azole antifungals, cimetidine, cyclosporine, erythromycin, quinidine, terfenadine, warfarin.

Drugs known to be inducers of the cytochrome P450 system include: phenobarbital, phenytoin, rifampin.

Drugs known to be biotransformed via P450 include: benzodiazepines, flecainide, imipramine, propafenone, theophylline.

Amlodipine has a low (rate of first-pass) hepatic clearance and consequent high bioavailability, and thus, may be expected to have a low potential for clinically relevant effects associated with elevation of amlodipine plasma levels when used concomitantly with drugs that compete for or inhibit the cytochrome P450 system.

Cimetidine, Warfarin, Cyclosporin, Digoxin: Pharmacokinetic interaction studies with amlodipine in healthy volunteers have indicated:

- **cimetidine** did not alter the pharmacokinetics of amlodipine.
- amlodipine did not change **warfarin**-induced prothrombin response time.
- amlodipine does not significantly alter the pharmacokinetics of **cyclosporin**.
- amlodipine did not change serum **digoxin** levels or **digoxin** renal clearance.

Antacids: Concomitant administration of Maalox (magnesium hydroxide and aluminum hydroxide) had no effect on the disposition of a single 5 mg dose of amlodipine in 24 subjects.

Beta-blockers: When beta-adrenergic receptor blocking drugs are administered concomitantly with GD-amlodipine, patients should be carefully monitored since blood pressure lowering effect of beta-blockers may be augmented by amlodipine's reduction in peripheral vascular resistance.

Sildenafil: A single 100 mg dose of sildenafil (VIAGRA) in subjects with essential hypertension had no effect on AUC_t or C_{max} of amlodipine. When sildenafil (100 mg) was coadministered with amlodipine, 5 or 10 mg in hypertensive patients, the mean additional reduction of supine blood pressure was 8 mmHg systolic and 7 mmHg diastolic.

Special Studies: Effect of GD-amlodipine on other agents:

Atorvastatin: In healthy volunteers, coadministration of multiple 10 mg doses of GD-amlodipine with 80 mg of atorvastatin resulted in no significant change in the AUC_t or C_{max} or T_{max} of atorvastatin.

ADVERSE EFFECTS: GD-amlodipine (amlodipine besylate) has been administered to 1714 patients (805 hypertensive and 909 angina patients) in controlled clinical trials (vs placebo alone and with active comparative agents). Most adverse reactions reported during therapy were of mild to moderate severity.

Hypertension: In the 805 hypertensive patients treated with GD-amlodipine in controlled clinical trials, adverse effects were reported in 29.9% of patients and required discontinuation of therapy due to side effects in 1.9% of patients. The most common adverse reactions in controlled clinical trials were: edema (8.9%), and headache (8.3%).

The following adverse reactions were reported with an incidence of ≥0.5% in the controlled clinical trials program (n=805):
Cardiovascular: edema (8.9%), palpitations (2.0%), tachycardia (0.7%), postural dizziness (0.5%).
Skin and Appendages: pruritus (0.7%).
Musculoskeletal: muscle cramps (0.5%).
Central and Peripheral Nervous Systems: headache (8.3%), dizziness (3.0%), paresthesia (0.5%).
Autonomic Nervous System: flushing (3.1%), increased sweating (0.9%), dry mouth (0.7%).
Psychiatric: somnolence (1.4%).
Gastrointestinal: nausea (2.4%), abdominal pain (1.1%), dyspepsia (0.6%), constipation (0.5%).
General: fatigue (4.1%), pain (0.5%).

Angina: In the controlled clinical trials in 909 angina patients treated with GD-amlodipine, adverse effects were reported in 30.5% of patients and required discontinuation of therapy due to side effects in 0.6% of patients. The most common adverse reactions reported in controlled clinical trials were: edema (9.9%) and headache (7.8%).

The following adverse reactions occurred at an incidence of ≥0.5% in the controlled clinical trials program (n=909):
Cardiovascular: edema (9.9%), palpitations (2.0%), postural dizziness (0.6%).
Skin and Appendages: rash (1.0%), pruritus (0.8%).
Musculoskeletal: muscle cramps (1.0%).
Central and Peripheral Nervous Systems: headache (7.8%), dizziness (4.5%), paresthesia (1.0%), hypoesthesia (0.9%).
Autonomic Nervous System: flushing (1.9%).
Psychiatric: somnolence (1.2%), insomnia (0.9%), nervousness (0.7%).
Gastrointestinal: nausea (4.2%), abdominal pain (2.2%), dyspepsia (1.4%), diarrhea (1.1%), flatulence (1.0%), constipation (0.9%).
Respiratory System: dyspnea (1.1%).
Special Senses: vision abnormal (1.3%), tinnitus (0.6%).
General: fatigue (4.8%), pain (1.0%), asthenia (1.0%).

GD-amlodipine has been evaluated for safety in about 11 000 patients with hypertension and angina. The following events occurred in <1% but >0.1% of patients in comparative clinical trials (double-blind comparative vs placebo or active agents; n=2615) or under conditions of open trials or marketing experience where a causal relationship is uncertain.
Cardiovascular: arrhythmia (including ventricular tachycardia and atrial fibrillation), bradycardia, hypotension, peripheral ischemia, syncope, tachycardia, postural dizziness, postural hypotension, vasculitis.
Central and Peripheral Nervous Systems: hypoesthesia, peripheral neuropathy, tremor, vertigo.
Gastrointestinal: anorexia, constipation, dysphagia, vomiting, gingival hyperplasia.
General: allergic reaction, asthenia*, back pain, hot flushes, malaise, rigors, weight gain.
Musculoskeletal System: arthralgia, arthrosis, myalgia.
Psychiatric: sexual dysfunction (male* and female), insomnia, nervousness, depression, abnormal dreams, anxiety, depersonalization.
Respiratory System: epistaxis.
Skin and Appendages: pruritus*, rash erythematous, rash maculopapular, erythema multiforme.
Special Senses: conjunctivitis, diplopia, eye pain, tinnitus.
Urinary System: micturition frequency, micturition disorder, nocturia.
Autonomic Nervous System: dry mouth, sweating increased.
Metabolic and Nutritional: hyperglycemia, thirst.
Hemopoietic: leucopenia, purpura, thrombocytopenia.

The following events occurred in ≤0.1% of patients: cardiac failure, skin discoloration, urticaria, skin dryness, Stevens-Johnson syndrome, alopecia, twitching, ataxia, hypertonia, migraine, apathy, amnesia, gastritis, pancreatitis, increased appetite, coughing, rhinitis, parosmia, taste perversion, and xerophthalmia.

Isolated cases of angioedema have been reported. Angioedema may be accompanied by breathing difficulty.

In postmarketing experience, jaundice and hepatic enzyme elevations (mostly consistent with cholestasis or hepatitis) in some cases severe enough to require hospitalization have been reported in association with use of amlodipine.

OVERDOSE:

Symptoms: Overdosage can cause excessive peripheral vasodilation with marked and probably prolonged hypotension and possibly a reflex tachycardia. In humans, experience with overdosage of GD-amlodipine (amlodipine besylate) is limited. When amlodipine was ingested at doses of 105-250 mg some patients remained normotensive with or without gastric lavage while another patient experienced hypotension (90/50 mmHg) which normalized following plasma expansion. A patient who took 70 mg of amlodipine with benzodiazepine developed shock which was refractory to treatment and died. In a 19 month old child who ingested 30 mg of amlodipine (about 2 mg/kg) there was no evidence of hypotension but tachycardia (180 bpm) was observed. Ipecac was administered 3.5 hrs after ingestion and on subsequent observation (overnight) no sequelae were noted.

Treatment: Clinically significant hypotension due to overdosage requires active cardiovascular support including frequent monitoring of cardiac and respiratory function, elevation of extremities, and attention to circulating fluid volume and urine output. A vasoconstrictor (such as norepinephrine) may be helpful in restoring vascular tone and blood pressure, provided that there is no contraindication to its use. As GD-amlodipine is highly protein bound, hemodialysis is not likely to be of benefit. Intravenous calcium gluconate may be beneficial in reversing the effects of calcium channel blockade. Clearance of amlodipine is prolonged in elderly patients and in patients with impaired liver function. Since amlodipine absorption is slow, gastric lavage may be worthwhile in some cases.

> For management of a suspected drug overdose, CPhA recommends that you contact your **regional Poison Control Centre**. See the CPS Directory section for a list of Poison Control Centres.

DOSAGE: Dosage should be individualized depending on patient's tolerance and responsiveness.

For both hypertension and angina, the recommended initial dose of GD-amlodipine (amlodipine besylate) is 5 mg once daily. If necessary, dose can be increased after 1-2 weeks to a maximum dose of 10 mg once daily.

Use in the Elderly or in Patients with Impaired Renal Function: The recommended initial dose in patients over 65 years of age or patients with impaired renal function is 5 mg once daily. If required, increasing in the dose should be done gradually and with caution (see Precautions).

Use in Patients with Impaired Hepatic Function: Dosage requirements have not been established in patients with impaired hepatic function. When GD-amlodipine is used in these patients, the dosage should be carefully and gradually adjusted depending on patients tolerance and response. A lower starting dose of 2.5 mg once daily should be considered (see Warnings).

Children: The effective antihypertensive oral dose in pediatric patients ages 6-17 years is 2.5 mg to 5 mg once daily. Doses in excess of 5 mg daily have not been studied; dose should be determined based upon the medical need of the patients. See Pharmacology.

SUPPLIED: 5 mg: Each white, octagonal tablet, engraved "GD" on one side and "AML 5" on the scored side, contains: amlodipine besylate equivalent to amlodipine 5 mg. Nonmedicinal ingredients: dibasic calcium phosphate anhydrous, magnesium stearate, microcrystalline cellulose and sodium starch glycolate. White plastic (high density polyethylene) bottles of 250. Store at 15-30°C. Protect from light.

10 mg: Each white, octagonal tablet, engraved "GD" on one side and "AML-10" on the other side, contains: amlodipine besylate equivalent to amlodipine 10 mg. Nonmedicinal ingredients: dibasic calcium phosphate anhydrous, magnesium stearate, microcrystalline cellulose and sodium starch glycolate. White plastic (high density polyethylene) bottles of 250. Store at 15-30°C. Protect from light.

(Shown in Product Identification Section)

* These events occurred in less than 1% in placebo controlled trials, but the incidence of these side effects was between 1% and 2% in all multiple dose studies.

Gelfoam® Powder

gelatin

Hemostatic Agent

Pfizer

Date of Revision: September 2004

DESCRIPTION: GELFOAM is a medical device intended for application to bleeding surfaces as a hemostatic. It is a water-insoluble, off-white, nonelastic, porous, pliable product prepared from purified pork Skin Gelatin USP Granules and Water for Injection, USP and is able to absorb and hold within its interstices, many times its weight of blood and other fluids. GELFOAM Sterile Powder is a fine, dry, heat-sterilized light powder prepared by milling absorbable gelatin sponge.

PHARMACOLOGY: GELFOAM has hemostatic properties. While its mode of action is not fully understood, its effect appears to be more physical than the result of altering the blood clotting mechanism.

When not used in excessive amounts, GELFOAM is absorbed completely, with little tissue reaction. This absorption is dependent on several factors, including the amount used, degree of saturation with blood or other fluids, and the site of use. When placed in soft tissues, GELFOAM is usually absorbed completely in from four to six weeks, without inducing excessive scar tissue. When applied to bleeding nasal, rectal or vaginal mucosa, it liquefies within two to five days.

INDICATIONS: Hemostatis: GELFOAM Sterile Powder, saturated with sterile sodium chloride solution, is indicated in surgical procedures, including those involving cancellous bone bleeding, as a hemostatic device, when control of capillary, venous, and arteriolar bleeding by pressure, ligature, and other conventional procedures is either ineffective or impractical.

CONTRAINDICATIONS: GELFOAM should not be used in closure of skin incisions because it may interfere with healing of the skin edges. This is due to mechanical interposition of gelatin and is not secondary to intrinsic interference with wound healing.

GELFOAM should not be placed in intravascular compartments, because of the risk of embolization.

Do not use GELFOAM Sterile Powder in patients with known allergies to porcine collagen.

WARNINGS: GELFOAM is not intended as a substitute for meticulous surgical technique and the proper application of ligatures, or other conventional procedures for hemostasis.

GELFOAM is supplied as a sterile product and cannot be resterilized. Unused, opened envelopes of GELFOAM should be discarded.

To prevent contamination, employ aseptic procedure in opening envelope and withdrawing GELFOAM. If the envelope is torn or punctured, the contained GELFOAM should not be used.

Only the minimum amount of GELFOAM necessary to achieve hemostasis should be used. Once hemostasis is attained, excess GELFOAM should be carefully removed.

The use of GELFOAM is not recommended in the presence of infection. GELFOAM should be used with caution in contaminated areas of the body. If signs of infection or abscess develop where GELFOAM has been positioned, reoperation may be necessary in order to remove the infected material and allow drainage.

The safety and efficacy of the combined use of GELFOAM with other agents such as topical thrombin has not been evaluated in controlled clinical trials and therefore cannot be recommended. If in the physician's judgment concurrent use of topical thrombin or other agents are medically advisable, the product literature for that agent should be consulted for complete prescribing information.

While packing a cavity for hemostasis is sometimes surgically indicated, GELFOAM should not be used in this manner unless excess product not needed to maintain hemostasis is removed.

Whenever possible, it should be removed after use in laminectomy procedures and from foramina in bone, once hemostasis is achieved. This is because GELFOAM may swell on absorbing fluids, and produce nerve damage by pressure within confined bony spaces.

The packing of GELFOAM, particularly within bony cavities, should be avoided, since swelling may interfere with normal function and/or possibly result in compression necrosis of surrounding tissues.

PRECAUTIONS: The minimum amount of GELFOAM Sterile Powder needed for hemostasis should be applied together with pressure until the bleeding stops. The excess should then be removed.

GELFOAM should not be used for controlling postpartum hemorrhage or menorrhagia.

It has been demonstrated that fragments of another hemostatic agent, microfibrillar collagen, pass through the 40μ transfusion filters of blood scavenging systems. GELFOAM should not be used in conjunction with autologous blood salvage circuits since the safety of this use has not been evaluated in controlled clinical trials.

Microfibrillar collagen has been reported to reduce the strength of methylmethacrylate adhesives used to attach prosthetic devices to bone surfaces. As a precaution, GELFOAM should not be used in conjunction with such adhesives.

GELFOAM is not recommended for the primary treatment of coagulation disorders.

It is not recommended that GELFOAM be saturated with an antibiotic solution or dusted with antibiotic powder.

ADVERSE EFFECTS: There have been reports of fever associated with the use of GELFOAM, without demonstrable infection. GELFOAM may serve as a nidus for infection and abscess formation, and has been reported to potentiate bacterial growth. Giant-cell granuloma has been reported at the implantation site of absorbable gelatin product in the brain, as has compression of the brain and spinal cord resulting from the accumulation of sterile fluid.

Foreign body reactions, "encapsulation" of fluid and hematoma have also been reported.

When GELFOAM was used in laminectomy operations, multiple neurologic events were reported, including but not limited to cauda equina syndrome, spinal stenosis, meningitis, arachnoiditis, headaches, paresthesias, pain, bladder and bowel dysfunction, and impotence.

Excessive fibrosis and prolonged fixation of a tendon have been reported when absorbable gelatin products were used in severed tendon repair.

Toxic shock syndrome has been reported in association with the use of GELFOAM in nasal surgery.

Fever, failure of absorption, and hearing loss have been reported in association with the use of GELFOAM during tympanoplasty.

Adverse Reactions Reported From Unapproved Uses: GELFOAM is not recommended for use other than as an adjunct for hemostasis.

While some adverse medical events following the unapproved use of GELFOAM have been reported to Pharmacia & Upjohn Company (see Adverse Effects), other hazards associated with such use may not have been reported.

When GELFOAM has been used during intravascular catheterization for the purpose of producing vessel occlusion, the following adverse events have been reported; fever, duodenal and pancreatic infarct, embolization of lower extremity vessels, pulmonary embolization, splenic abscess, necrosis of specific anatomic areas, asterixis, and death.

These adverse medical events have been associated with the use of GELFOAM for repair of dural defects encountered during laminectomy and craniotomy operations: fever, infection, leg paresthesias, neck and back pain, bladder and bowel incontinence, cauda equina syndrome, neurogenic bladder, impotence, and paresis.

Adverse Events Associated With Bone Hemostasis: In a clinical study, 108 patients received GELFOAM Sterile Powder on the cut surface of the sternum during cardiopulmonary bypass surgery, while 107 patients received no treatment on the cut surface of the bone. Table 1 is a summary of medical events reported by at least 1.0% of patients in a treatment group. The most frequently reported events were atrial fibrillation, perioperative event, and wound infection. Events occurring in less than 1.0% of the patients were as follows: anaphylaxis, cardiogenic shock, delirium tremens, infection at the vascular catheter site, unevaluable reaction, sepsis, angina pectoris, atrial arrhythmia, nodal arrhythmia, arteriosclerosis, cardiac insufficiency, cardiac tamponade, cardiomyopathy, deep vein thrombosis, mitral valve disorder, endocarditis, ventricular extrasystoles, heart arrest, hypotension, mesenteric occlusion, superventricular tachycardia, thrombophlebitis, thrombosis, gastrointestinal disorder, gastrointestinal bleeding, increased serum creatinine, dehydration, anemia, thrombocytopenia, abnormal healing, hypovolemia, hypoxia, metabolic acidosis, cerebral infarction, visual hallucinations, stupor, aspiration pneumonia, chest congestion, pleural effusion, pulmonary infiltration, retinal artery occlusion, anuria, UG disorder, abnormal kidney function and menorrhagia.

Table 1: GELFOAM

Summary of Medical Events for GELFOAM Sterile Powder When Used as a Bone Hemostatic Agent During Cardiopulmonary Bypass Surgery

	GELFOAM N=108		Control N=107		Total N=215	
Medical Event	n	%	n	%	n	%
Atrial Fibrillation	14	(13.0)	12	(11.2)	26	(12.1)
Wound Infection	6	(5.6)	1	(0.9)	7	(3.3)
Perioperative Event	4	(3.7)	5	(4.7)	9	(4.2)
Congestive Heart Failure	4	(3.7)	0	(0.0)	4	(1.9)
Ventricular Tachycardia	2	(1.9)	3	(2.8)	5	(2.3)
Atrial Flutter	2	(1.9)	0	(0.0)	2	(0.9)
Peripheral Vascular Disorder	2	(1.9)	0	(.0.0)	2	(0.9)
Pneumothorax	2	(1.9)	3	(2.8)	5	(2.3)
Respiratory Failure	2	(1.9)	2	(1.9)	4	(1.9)
Respiratory Arrest	2	(1.9)	1	(0.9)	3	(1.4)
Fever	1	(0.9)	2	(1.9)	3	(1.4)
Heart Block	1	(0.9)	2	(1.9)	3	(1.4)
Prolonged Wound Drainage	0	(0.0)	1	(0.9)	1	(0.5)
Cellulitis	0	(0.0)	2	(1.9)	2	(0.9)
Dyspnea	0	(0.0)	2	(1.9)	2	(0.9)
Pneumonia	0	(0.0)	2	(1.9)	2	(0.9)

In general, the following adverse events have been reported with the use of absorbable porcine gelatin-based hemostatic agents:

- Gelatin-based hemostatic agents may serve as a nidus for infection and abscess formation and have been reported to potentiate bacterial growth.
- Giant cell granulomas have been observed at implant sites when used in the brain.
- Compression of the brain and spinal cord resulting from the accumulation of sterile fluid has been observed.
- Multiple neurologic events were reported when absorbable gelatin-based hemostatic agents were used in laminectomy operations, including cauda equina syndrome, spinal stenosis, meningitis, arachnoiditis, headaches, paresthesias, pain, bladder and bowel dysfunction, and impotence and paresis.
- The use of absorbable gelatin-based hemostatic agents have been associated with paralysis, due to device migration into foramina in the bone around the spinal cord, and blindness due to device migration in the orbit of the eye, during lobectomy, laminectomy and repair of a frontal skull fracture and lacerated lobe.
- Foreign body reactions, "encapsulation" of fluid, and hemotoma have been observed at implant sites.
- Excessive fibrosis and prolonged fixation of a tendon have been reported when absorbable gelatin-based sponges were used in severed tendon repair.
- Toxic shock syndrome was reported in association with the use of absorbable gelatin-based hemostats in nasal surgery.
- Fever, failure of absorption, and hearing loss have been observed when absorbable hemostatic agents were used during tympanoplasty.

Clinical Studies: GELFOAM Sterile Powder is a water-insoluble, hemostatic device prepared from purified skin gelatin, and capable of absorbing up to 45 times its weight of whole blood. The absorptive capacity of GELFOAM is a function of its physical size, increasing as the amount of the gelatin powder increases.

The mechanism of action of surface-mediated hemostatic devices is supportive and mechanical. Surface acting devices, when applied directly to bleeding surfaces, arrest bleeding by the formation of an artificial clot and by producing a mechanical matrix that facilitates clotting. Jenkins et al have theorized that the clotting effect of GELFOAM may be due to release of thromboplastin from platelets, occurring when platelets entering the sponge become damaged by contact with the walls of its myriad of interstices. Thromboplastin interacts with prothrombin and calcium to produce thrombin, and this sequence of events initiates the clotting reaction. The authors suggest that the physiologic formation of thrombin in the sponge is sufficient to produce formation of a clot, by its action on the fibrinogen in blood. The spongy physical properties of the gelatin sponge hasten clot formation and provide structural support for the forming clot.

Several investigators have claimed that GELFOAM becomes liquefied within a week or less and is completely absorbed in four to six weeks, without inducing excessive scar formation. Barnes reviewed experiences with GELFOAM in gynecologic surgery. No excessive scar tissue, attributable to the absorption of GELFOAM, could be palpated at postoperative examination.

Bone Hemostasis Study: The efficacy of GELFOAM Sterile Powder as a bone hemostatic agent during cardiopulmonary bypass surgery was evaluated.

Study Design: Two randomized open-label clinical studies were conducted at separate investigative sites. The objectives were as follows: to evaluate the effectiveness of GELFOAM Sterile Powder as a hemostatic agent in the treatment of sternal bone bleeding during cardiopulmonary bypass surgery; to identify any deleterious effects of GELFOAM Sterile Powder on interference with bone healing; to determine any systemic or local wound side effects from leaving GELFOAM Sterile Powder in situ.

Patients between the ages of 18 to 74 years old undergoing cardiopulmonary bypass surgery were randomly assigned to either a GELFOAM group or a Control group. The GELFOAM group (composed of 108 patients) had a paste made up of sterile saline solution and GELFOAM Sterile Powder applied to the cut sternal surface immediately following sternotomy. The Control group (composed of 107 patients) received no treatment applied to the cut surface.

Blood loss was monitored both during surgery and postoperatively. Blood loss during surgery was determined by measuring the weight of the powder before and after application to the cut edge of the sternum. Postoperative blood loss was collected from the mediastinal drainage tubes. The total blood loss (in milligrams) over 72 hours was determined for each patient.

Study Endpoints: Patients were evaluated upon admission (preoperative), during surgery (intraoperative), after surgery (postoperative), upon hospital discharge (7 to 10 days after surgery), and at the 3-month follow-up visit. An additional poststudy follow-up was required if a patient reported an ongoing medical event at the 3-month follow-up visit.

Study Results: In both studies, the amount of blood loss was significantly less in the GELFOAM group than in the Control group. In Study 001, the mean blood loss in the GELFOAM group was 13727.7 mg while the mean blood loss in the Control group was more than double at 27712.0 mg. Similar results were found in Study 002, where the mean blood loss in the GELFOAM group was 9514.8 mg while the mean blood loss in the Control group was 22687.5 mg. See Table 2.

Patients in the GELFOAM and Control groups were similar with regard to sternal bone healing. At hospital discharge, normal bone healing was reported for 105 patients (97%) in the GELFOAM group and 104 patients (97%) in the Control group. At the 3-month follow-up, 103 patients (95%) in the GELFOAM group and 100 patients (93%) in the Control group were healed.

Few patients in either treatment group had sternotomy infection or other post-operative infection complications related to sternotomy. At hospital discharge, two patients treated with GELFOAM had mediastinitis. No Control patients had any infections at hospital discharge. One patient treated with GELFOAM had a non-infection-related complication.

At the 3-month follow-up, one of the original patients treated with GELFOAM who had mediastinitis still showed signs of infection. In addition, two additional patients treated with GELFOAM developed mediastinitis at the 3-month follow-up.

Table 2: GELFOAM

Blood Loss in Sternotomy Patients

	Site 001		Site 002	
	GELFOAM	Control	GELFOAM	Control
Mean Blood Loss (mg)	13 727.7	27 712.0	9514.8	22 687.5
Median Blood Loss (mg)	11 561.0	24 798.0	6950.0	16 900.0
Minimum Blood Loss (mg)	2922.0	10 748.0	800.0	900.0
Maximum Blood Loss (mg)	87 448.0	61 535.0	46 000.0	89 800.0

One patient in the Control group experienced sternal osteomyelitis at the 3-month follow-up but recovered with no residual effects. No patients from the GELFOAM arm of the study had reported complications of sternal osteomyelitis.

There was a total of four Control patients who had non-infection-related complications. One Control patient had serous/sanguineous wound drainage from the left leg and sternum incisions at hospital discharge. This complication was non-infectious and the patient recovered with no residual side effects.

Three Control patients all experienced chronic pain syndrome, a symptom which can occur following thoracic/cardiac surgery. Evaluation sternal bone healing at the 3-month follow-up for these patients showed no evidence of non-union of the sternum. In all three cases, bone healing at the 3-month follow-up was reported as being normal. A summary of sternotomy infection information is located in Table 3.

Table 3: GELFOAM

Summary of Postoperative Infection Complications

	Hospital Discharge				3-Month Follow-up			
	GELFOAM		Control		GELFOAM		Control	
	N	%	N	%	N	%	N	%
Any Infection								
Yes	1	(1)	0	(0)	5	(5)	0	(0)
No	104	(99)	106	(100)	95	(95)	105	(100)
Superficial Wound								
Yes	0	(0)	0	(0)	2	(2)	0	(0)
No	105	(100)	106	(100)	98	(98)	105	(100)
Sternal Osteomyelitis								
Yes	0	(0)	0	(0)	1	(1)	1	(1)
No	105	(100)	106	(100)	99	(99)	105	(99)
Mediastinitis								
Yes	1	(1)	0	(0)	2	(2)	0	(0)
No	104	(99)	106	(100)	98	(98)	105	(100)
Complication Related to Sternotomy								
Yes	0	(0)	0	(0)	1	(1)	3	(3)
No	105	(100)	106	(100)	99	(99)	102	(97)

Study Conclusions: These studies demonstrate that a paste made from GELFOAM Sterile Powder is safe and effective in treating intraoperative bleeding when applied to the cut surface of cancellous bone and has shown superior hemostasis versus no treatment at all to the cut bone surface. The benefit to patients is that a reduction in bleeding will make surgery easier to perform by reducing the time the surgeon needs to revisit cut bone surfaces to clean up the bleeding. This study also demonstrated that GELFOAM Sterile Powder could be left in situ without increased risk of bone infection or non-union of the sternum.

DOSAGE: Sterile technique should always be used. The minimum amount of GELFOAM should be applied to the bleeding site (see Directions for Use) with pressure until hemostasis is observed. Opened envelopes of unused GELFOAM should always be discarded.

Directions for Use: GELFOAM Sterile Powder can be saturated with sterile, isotonic sodium chloride solution (sterile saline), before use as an adjunct to hemostasis. The envelope of GELFOAM Sterile Powder should be opened and the contents (1 g) poured carefully into a sterile beaker, avoiding contamination. Using sterile technique, a putty-like paste is prepared by adding a total of approximately 3-4 mL of sterile saline to the GELFOAM. Dispersion of the powder can be avoided by initially compressing it with the gloved fingers into the bottom of the beaker and then kneading it into the desired consistency. The resulting doughy paste may be smeared or pressed against the bleeding surface to control bleeding. When bleeding stops the excess should be removed.

Use only the minimum amount of GELFOAM, necessary to produce hemostasis. The GELFOAM may be left in place at the bleeding site, when necessary. Since GELFOAM causes little more cellular reaction than does the blood clot, the wound may be closed over it. GELFOAM may be left in place when applied to mucosal surfaces until it liquefies.

SUPPLIED: Each envelope contains: absorbable gelatin powder 1 g. Store at controlled room temperature 15-30°C. Once the envelope is opened, contents are subject to contamination. It is recommended that GELFOAM be used as soon as the envelope is opened and unused contents discarded.

SYMBOLS:
℞ = Prescription required
Ⓒ = Controlled Drug
Ⓝ = Narcotic
TC = Targeted Controlled Substance

Gelfoam® Sponge

gelatin

Hemostatic Agent

Pfizer

Date of Revision: September 2004

DESCRIPTION: GELFOAM Sterile Sponge is a medical device intended for application to bleeding surfaces as a hemostatic. It is a water insoluble, off-white, nonelastic, porous, pliable product prepared from purified pork Skin Gelatin USP Granules and Water for Injection, USP. It may be cut without fraying and is able to absorb and hold within its interstices, many times its weight of blood and other fluids.

PHARMACOLOGY: GELFOAM Sterile Sponge has hemostatic properties. While its mode of action is not fully understood, its effect appears to be more physical than the result of altering the blood clotting mechanism.

When not used in excessive amounts, GELFOAM is absorbed completely, with little tissue reaction. This absorption is dependent on several factors, including the amount used, degree of saturation with blood or other fluids, and the site of use. When placed in soft tissues, GELFOAM is usually absorbed completely in from four to six weeks, without inducing excessive scar tissue. When applied to bleeding nasal, rectal or vaginal mucosa, it liquefies within two to five days.

INDICATIONS: Hemostasis: GELFOAM Sterile Sponge, used dry or saturated with sterile sodium chloride solution, is indicated in surgical procedures as a hemostatic device, when control of capillary, venous, and arteriolar bleeding by pressure, ligature, and other conventional procedures is either ineffective or impractical. However, in case of brisk arterial bleeding, the pressure of the flow may prevent the sponge from remaining securely anchored, and bleeding is likely to continue.

CONTRAINDICATIONS: GELFOAM Sterile Sponge should not be used in closure of skin incisions because it may interfere with the healing of skin edges.

WARNINGS: GELFOAM Sterile Sponge should not be resterilized by heat, because heating may change absorption time. Ethylene oxide is not recommended for resterilization because it may be trapped in the interstices of the foam. Although, not reported for GELFOAM, the gas is toxic to tissue, and in trace amounts may cause burns or irritation.

GELFOAM should not be used intravascularly due to the risk of embolization.

The safety and efficacy of the combined use of GELFOAM with other agents such as topical thrombin has not been evaluated in controlled clinical trials and therefore cannot be recommended. If the physician determines that concurrent use of GELFOAM with topical thrombin or other agents is medically advisable, the product labeling for the other agent should be consulted for complete prescribing information.

PRECAUTIONS: Use of GELFOAM Sterile Sponge is not recommended in the presence of infection. GELFOAM should be used with caution in contaminated areas of the body. If signs of infection or abscess develop in an area where GELFOAM has been used, it may be necessary to remove the infected material and allow drainage.

GELFOAM should not be used to control postpartum bleeding or menorrhagia. Because GELFOAM absorbs fluid, it may expand and impinge on neighboring structures. Therefore, when placed into cavities or closed tissue spaces, minimal preliminary compression is advised and care should be taken to avoid overpacking.

ADVERSE EFFECTS: GELFOAM Sterile Sponge may form a nidus of infection and abscess. Fever, without a proven site of infection, has been reported with the use of GELFOAM. Toxic shock syndrome has been reported with the use of GELFOAM during nasal surgery. Fever, failure of absorption, and hearing loss have been reported with the use of GELFOAM during tympanoplasty.

Foreign body reactions, encapsulation of fluid and hematoma formation have been reported with the use of GELFOAM. Giant-cell granuloma has been reported at the implantation site of absorbable gelatin product in the brain, as well as compression of the brain and spinal cord resulting from the accumulation of sterile fluid. Multiple neurologic events have been reported when GELFOAM is used during laminectomy operations.

Excessive fibrosis and prolonged fixation of a tendon have been reported when absorbable gelatin products were used to repair severed tendons.

DOSAGE: Directions for use: To open envelope:

1. With the hands folded into fists, grasp each flap between the thumb and index finger.
2. With a slow, rolling motion, carefully peel back the envelope sides until the sterile inner envelope is exposed.
3. Employing sterile technique, remove sterile inner envelope and sterile sponge.

Always use sterile technique when handling GELFOAM Sterile Sponge.

GELFOAM should be cut to the minimum size required to attain hemostasis. GELFOAM may be applied dry or saturated with a physiologic saline solution.

When applied dry, GELFOAM should be manually compressed before application to the bleeding site. When used with saline, GELFOAM should be soaked in the solution, then withdrawn, squeezed between gloved fingers to expel air bubbles present in the interstices, replaced in saline, and kept there until needed. GELFOAM should immediately return to its original size and shape when returned to the solution. If it does not swell, it should be removed and kneaded vigorously until all air is expelled and it does expand to its original shape when dropped into the solution. GELFOAM can be used wet or blotted to dampness on gauze before application to the bleeding site.

GELFOAM should be applied to the bleeding surface and held in place with moderate pressure until hemostasis is attained. It is not necessary to apply suction to GELFOAM, since GELFOAM will draw up blood into its interstices by capillary action.

Usually, the first application of GELFOAM will control bleeding, but if not, additional applications may be made, using fresh pieces of GELFOAM. When bleeding is controlled, the pieces of GELFOAM may be left in place; otherwise, bleeding may start again. Since GELFOAM causes little more cellular infiltration than the blood clot, the wound may be closed over it. When applied to bleeding mucosa, GELFOAM will stay in place until it liquefies.

SUPPLIED: Size 12: 20 mm×60 mm (12 cm sq.)×7 mm in boxes of 4 sponges in individual envelopes.
Size 100: 80 mm×125 mm (100 cm sq.)×10 mm in boxes of 6 sponges in individual envelopes.
Dental Pack Size 4: 20 mm×20 mm (4 cm sq.)×7 mm in boxes of 12 sponges, 2 sponges per envelope.

GELFOAM Sterile Sponge should be stored at controlled room temperature 15 to 30°C. Once the package is opened, contents are subject to contamination. It is recommended that GELFOAM be used as soon as the package is opened and unused contents be discarded.

Gemcitabine for Injection, USP ℞

gemcitabine HCl

Antineoplastic

Hospira

SUPPLIED: 200 mg: Each vial contains: gemcitabine 200 mg (as the hydrochloride salt), mannitol 200 mg and sodium acetate 12.5 mg. Sodium hydroxide and hydrochloric acid are used for pH adjustments. Vials of 10 mL. Store in glass vials, at 15 to 30°C. Do not refrigerate.
1 g: Each vial contains: gemcitabine 1 g (as the hydrochloride salt), mannitol 1 g and sodium acetate 62.5 mg. Sodium hydroxide and hydrochloric acid are used for pH adjustments. Vials of 50 mL. Store in glass vials, at 15 to 30°C. Do not refrigerate.
2 g: Each vial contains: gemcitabine 2 g (as the hydrochloride salt), mannitol 2 g and sodium acetate 125 mg. Sodium hydroxide and hydrochloric acid are used for pH adjustments. Vials of 100 mL. Store in glass vials, at 15 to 30°C. Do not refrigerate.

Parenteral drugs should be inspected visually for particulate matter and discoloration, prior to administration, whenever solution and container permit. The reconstituted solution is stable for 24 hours at 15 to 30°C. Any unused solution should be discarded. Solutions of reconstituted Gemcitabine for Injection, USP should not be refrigerated, as crystallization may occur.

Gemcitabine Hydrochloride for Injection ℞

gemcitabine HCl

Antineoplastic

Sandoz

SUPPLIED: 200 mg: Each vial of sterile lyophilized powder contains: gemcitabine 200 mg (as the hydrochloride salt). Nonmedicinal ingredients: mannitol 200 mg and sodium acetate 12.5 mg. Hydrochloric acid and/or sodium hydroxide may have been added for pH adjustment. Colourless glass vials, boxes of 1. Store between 15 and 30°C. Any unused solution should be discarded. Reconstituted solutions should not be refrigerated, as crystallization may occur.
1 g: Each vial of sterile lyophilized powder contains: gemcitabine 1 g (as the hydrochloride salt). Nonmedicinal ingredients: mannitol 1 g and sodium acetate 62.5 mg. Hydrochloric acid and/or sodium hydroxide may have been added for pH adjustment. Colourless glass vials, boxes of 1. Store between 15 and 30°C. Any unused solution should be discarded. Reconstituted solutions should not be refrigerated, as crystallization may occur.

Gemzar® ℞

gemcitabine HCl

Antineoplastic

Lilly

Date of Revision: February 2, 2006

SUMMARY PRODUCT INFORMATION:

Route of Administration	Dosage Form/Strength	Clinically Relevant Nonmedicinal Ingredients
Intravenous	200 mg and 1 g vial	Mannitol and sodium acetate For a complete listing see Dosage Forms, Composition and Packaging.

INDICATIONS AND CLINICAL USE: GEMZAR is indicated for the:

- Treatment of patients with locally advanced (nonresectable Stage II or Stage III) or metastatic (Stage IV) adenocarcinoma of the pancreas to achieve a Clinical Benefit Response (a composite measure of clinical improvement).
- Treatment of patients with locally advanced or metastatic non-small cell lung cancer (NSCLC) as either a single agent or in combination with cisplatin.
- Treatment of patients with Stage IV (locally advanced or metastatic) transitional cell carcinoma (TCC) of the bladder in combination with cisplatin.
- Treatment, in combination with paclitaxel, of patients with unresectable, locally recurrent or metastatic breast cancer, who have good performance status and have relapsed following adjuvant anthracycline-based chemotherapy.

GEMZAR should be used only under the supervision of a qualified healthcare professional who is experienced in the use of chemotherapeutic agents and in the management of patients with cancer. Appropriate management of therapy and complications is only possible when adequate diagnostic and treatment facilities are readily available.

Geriatrics (>65 years of age): GEMZAR has been well tolerated in patients over the age of 65. Although clearance is affected by age (see Action and Clinical Pharmacology), there is no evidence that further dose adjustments, (i.e. other than those already recommended in Dosage and Administration) are necessary in patients over the age of 65.

Pediatrics (<17 years of age): Safety and effectiveness in children have not been established.

CONTRAINDICATIONS: GEMZAR is contraindicated in patients who are hypersensitive to this drug or to any ingredient in the formulation or component of the container. For a complete listing, see Dosage Forms, Composition and Packaging.

WARNINGS AND PRECAUTIONS:

Serious Warnings and Precautions

- GEMZAR is a cytotoxic drug and should be used only by physicians experienced with chemotherapeutic drugs. Patients should be informed of the risks associated with GEMZAR therapy.
- Prolongation of the infusion time beyond 60 minutes and more frequent than weekly dosing have been shown to increase toxicity (see Dosage and Administration).
- GEMZAR should be used with extreme caution in patients whose bone marrow reserve may have been compromised by prior irradiation or chemotherapy, or whose marrow function is recovering from previous chemotherapy.
- GEMZAR can suppress bone marrow function manifested by leucopenia, thrombocytopenia and anemia. Patients should be closely monitored prior to each dose for granulocyte and platelet counts. The dosage should be reduced, omitted, or the drug discontinued upon evidence of abnormal suppression of the bone marrow (see Dosage and Administration).
- Periodic physical examination and checks of renal and hepatic function should be made to detect non-hematologic toxicity. Doses may be reduced or withheld based upon the level of toxicity.
- Administration of GEMZAR in patients with concurrent liver metastases or a pre-existing medical history of hepatitis, alcoholism, or liver cirrhosis may lead to exacerbation of the underlying hepatic insufficiency (see Dosage and Administration).
- Acute shortness of breath with a temporal relationship to GEMZAR administration may occur (see Adverse Reactions and Dosage and Administration).
- This preparation is for intravenous administration only.

General: In all instances where the use of GEMZAR is considered for chemotherapy, the physician must evaluate the need and usefulness of the drug against the risk of adverse events. If severe adverse events occur, the drug should be reduced in dosage, omitted, or discontinued and appropriate corrective measures should be taken based on the clinical judgement of the physician (see Dosage and Administration).

Most drug-related adverse reactions observed with GEMZAR therapy are reversible (see Adverse Reactions).

Carcinogenesis and Mutagenesis: Information available is based upon preclinical studies.

Cardiovascular: Heart failure has been reported very rarely (<0.01%). Arrhythmias, predominantly supraventricular in nature, have been reported signaling awareness of the possibility of cardiovascular events (see Adverse Reactions, Clinical Trial Adverse Drug Reactions and Post-Market Adverse Drug Reactions).

Fever and Flu-Like Symptoms: GEMZAR may cause fever, with or without flu-like symptoms, in the absence of clinical infection (see Adverse Reactions). The administration of acetaminophen may provide symptomatic relief.

Hematologic: GEMZAR can suppress bone marrow function as manifested by leukopenia, thrombocytopenia and anemia. Blood counts should be taken prior to each dose (see Dosage and Administration for dose reduction guidelines).

Hepatic/Biliary/Pancreatic: Cases of serious hepatotoxicity including liver failure and death have been very rarely reported in patients receiving GEMZAR alone or in combination with other potentially hepatotoxic drugs. A causal relationship between GEMZAR and severe hepatotoxicity including liver failure and death has not been established (see Warnings and Precautions, Special Populations; Adverse Reactions, Clinical Trial Adverse Drug Reactions and Post-Market Adverse Drug Reactions).

Radiosensitizing Effect: In a single trial where GEMZAR at a dose of 1000 mg/m² was administered once weekly for up to six (6) consecutive weeks concurrently with therapeutic thoracic radiation to patients with NSCLC, significant toxicity was observed in the form of severe, and potentially life-threatening mucositis, especially esophagitis and pneumonitis, particularly in patients receiving large volumes of radiotherapy [median treatment volumes 4795 cm³] (see Drug Interactions). The optimum regimen for safe administration of GEMZAR with therapeutic doses of radiation has not yet been determined.

Renal: There have been cases of histologically confirmed Hemolytic Uremic Syndrome (HUS) reported in patients treated with GEMZAR. Renal failure leading to death or requiring dialysis despite discontinuation of therapy has been reported rarely. The majority of cases of renal failure leading to death were due to HUS (see Warnings and Precautions, Special Populations; Adverse Reactions, Clinical Trial Adverse Drug Reactions and Post-Market Adverse Drug Reactions).

GEMZAR should be discontinued at the first signs of any evidence of microangiopathic hemolytic anemia such as rapidly falling hemoglobin with concomitant thrombocytopenia, elevation of serum bilirubin, serum creatinine, blood urea nitrogen, or LDH. Renal failure may not be reversible even with discontinuation of therapy, and dialysis may be required.

Respiratory: Acute shortness of breath in association with GEMZAR administration may occur. Bronchodilators, corticosteroids, and/or oxygen produce symptomatic relief.

Pulmonary effects, sometimes severe (such as pulmonary edema, interstitial pneumonitis, or adult respiratory distress syndrome (ARDS)) have been reported rarely (<0.1%) in association with GEMZAR therapy. The etiology of these effects is unknown. If such effects develop, patients should discontinue therapy with GEMZAR and not be re-challenged with the drug. See Adverse Reactions, Pulmonary and Dosage and Administration.

Skin: GEMZAR administration has been associated with rash (see Adverse Reactions). Topical corticosteroids may provide symptomatic relief.

Severe skin reactions, including desquamation and bullous skin eruptions such as toxic epidermal necrolysis (TEN) and Stevens Johnson syndrome (SJS), have been reported very rarely (<0.01%).

Vascular: Clinical signs of peripheral vasculitis and gangrene have been reported very rarely (<0.01%) in association with GEMZAR therapy.

Special Populations: Gender: GEMZAR clearance is affected by gender (see Action and Clinical Pharmacology). There is no evidence, however, that further dose adjustments (i.e. other than those already recommended in Dosage and Administration) are necessary in women.

Renal and Hepatic Impairment: GEMZAR should be used with caution in patients with pre-existing renal or hepatic insufficiency, as there is insufficient information from clinical studies to allow clear dose recommendations for this patient population. All combination studies involving GEMZAR and cisplatin have been performed in patients with creatinine clearance of ≥60 mL/minute.

Administration of GEMZAR in patients with compromised liver function due to liver metastasis or a pre-existing medical history of hepatitis, alcoholism, or liver cirrhosis may lead to exacerbation of the underlying hepatic insufficiency (see Dosage and Administration).

Pregnant Women: The use of GEMZAR should be avoided in pregnant women because of the potential hazard to the fetus. Evaluation of experimental animal studies has shown reproductive toxicity, e.g. birth defects or other effects on the development of the embryo or fetus, the course of gestation or peri-and postnatal development.

Nursing Women: The use of GEMZAR should be avoided in nursing women because of the potential hazard to the infant.

Pediatrics (<17 years of age): Safety and effectiveness in children have not been established.

Geriatrics (>65 years of age): GEMZAR has been well tolerated in patients over the age of 65. Although clearance is affected by age (see Action and Clinical Pharmacology), there is no evidence that further dose adjustments, (i.e. other than those recommended under Dosage and Administration) are necessary in patients over the age of 65.

ADVERSE REACTIONS: Clinical Trial Adverse Drug Reactions: Because clinical trials are conducted under very specific conditions the adverse reaction rates observed in the clinical trials may not reflect the rates observed in practice and should not be compared to the rates in the clinical trials of another drug. Adverse drug reaction information from clinical trials is useful for identifying drug-related adverse events and for approximating rates.

GEMZAR (gemcitabine hydrochloride) has been used, both as a single agent and in combination with other cytotoxic drugs.

Single-Agent Use: Data in Table 1 are based on 22 clinical studies (N=979) of GEMZAR administered as a single agent, using starting doses in the range of 800 to 1250 mg/m² administered weekly as a 30-minute infusion for the treatment of a wide variety of malignancies. Of the 979 patients only 10.4% (102) were discontinued due to an adverse event regardless of causality. WHO grade 3 or 4 toxicity of non-laboratory events, was less than 1% for all parameters except nausea and vomiting, pulmonary toxicity, infection and pain.

All WHO-graded laboratory toxicities for a total of 979 patients are listed in Table 1, regardless of causality. Non-laboratory WHO-toxicities were available for 565 patients. They are listed in Table 1 (for parameters that occurred in ≥5% of patients), or discussed below. Edema, extravasation and flu-like symptoms were reported regardless of causality as treatment emergent signs and symptoms (TESS*; N=979).

Data are also shown (Table 1) for the subset of patients (N=360) with non-small cell lung cancer treated in 4 clinical studies (2 studies WHO laboratory toxicities; 2 studies non-laboratory WHO-toxicities) and the subset of patients (N=159) with pancreatic cancer treated in 5 clinical studies (WHO laboratory and non-laboratory toxicities). The frequency of all grades were generally similar for the overall safety database and the subsets of patients with non-small cell lung cancer and pancreatic cancer.

* TESS: An event was considered treatment-emergent, if it occurred for the first time or worsened while receiving therapy following baseline evaluation. It is important to emphasize that although the events were reported during therapy, they were not necessarily caused by the therapy.

Table 1: GEMZAR

WHO-Graded Toxicities Occurring with a ≥5% Frequency in Patients Receiving GEMZAR (WHO Grades [in % Frequency] are Rounded to the Closest Integer)

	All Patients			Non Small Cell Lung Cancer Patients			Pancreatic Cancer Patients			Discontinuations (%)
	All Grades	Grade 3	Grade 4	All Grades	Grade 3	Grade 4	All Grades	Grade 3	Grade 4	All Patients
Laboratory		(N=979)			(N=360)			(N=244)		(N=979)
Hematologic										
Anemia	68	7	1	65	5	<1	73	8	3	<1
Neutropenia	63	19	6	61	20	5	61	17	7	
Leukopenia	62	9	<1	55	7	<1	63	8	1	<1
Thrombocytopenia	24	4	1	16	1	1	36	7	<1	<1
Hepatic										
ALT	68	8	2	70	9	3	72	10	1	<1
AST	67	7	2	67	5	1	78	12	5	
Alkaline Phosphatase	55	7	2	48	2	0	77	16	4	
Bilirubin	13	2	<1	8	<1	<1	26	6	3	
Renal										
Proteinuria	36	<1	0	52	<1	0	15	<1	0	
Hematuria	31	<1	0	43	2	0	14	0	0	
BUN	16	0	0	16	0	0	15	0	0	<1
Creatinine	7	<1	0	6	<1	0	6	0	0	
Non-laboratory		(N=565)			(N=243)			(N=159)		(N=979)
Gastrointestinal Disorders										
Nausea and Vomiting	64	17	1	69	19	<1	62	12	2	<1
Diarrhea	12	<1	0	6	<1	0	24	2	0	0
Constipation	8	<1	0	7	<1	0	13	2	0	0
Stomatitis	8	<1	0	7	<1	0	10	0	0	<1
General Disorders and Administration Site Conditions										
Fever	37	<1	0	46	<1	0	28	<1	0	<1
Pain	16	1	0	16	1	0	12	2	0	<1
Infections										
Infection	9	1	<1	10	0	0	8	1	0	<1
Nervous System Disorders										
State of Consciousness/Somnolence	9	<1	0	6	0	0	10	3	0	<1
Respiratory Disorders										
Dyspnea	8	1	<1	8	2	0	6	0	0	<1
Skin and Subcutaneous Tissue Disorders										

(cont'd)

Table 1: GEMZAR *(cont'd)*

WHO-Graded Toxicities Occurring with a ≥5% Frequency in Patients Receiving GEMZAR (WHO Grades [in % Frequency] are Rounded to the Closest Integer)

	All Patients			Non Small Cell Lung Cancer Patients			Pancreatic Cancer Patients			Discontinuations (%)
	All Grades	Grade 3	Grade 4	All Grades	Grade 3	Grade 4	All Grades	Grade 3	Grade 4	All Patients
Skin Rash	25	<1	0	30	0	0	22	0	0	<1
Alopecia	14	<1	0	14	<1	0	14	0	0	0

Grade based on criteria from the World Health Organization (WHO).

Alopecia: Hair loss (alopecia), usually minimal, was reported for any WHO grade in only 13.7% of patients. No grade 4 toxicity (non-reversible alopecia) was reported, and only 0.4% of patients reported grade 3 toxicity (complete but reversible alopecia).

Cardiac Toxicity: Less than two percent of patients discontinued therapy with GEMZAR due to cardiovascular events such as myocardial infarction, arrhythmia, chest pain, heart failure, pulmonary edema and hypertension. Many of these patients had a prior history of cardiovascular disease.

Cutaneous Toxicity: A rash was seen in 24.8% of patients, was usually mild, not dose limiting and responded to local therapy (see Warnings and Precautions). The rash was typically a macular or finely granular maculopapular pruritic eruption of mild to moderate severity involving the trunk and extremities.

Edema: The occurrence of Edema is reported regardless of causality, as a treatment emergent event (TESS). Edema (13%), peripheral edema (20%) and facial edema (<1%) were reported. Overall, edema was usually mild to moderate and reversible. Less than 1% of patients (N=979) discontinued due to edema.

Extravasation: GEMZAR is well tolerated during the infusion with only a few cases (4%) of injection site reaction reported. GEMZAR does not appear to be a vesicant (see Dosage and Administration). There have been no reports of injection site necrosis.

Fever and Infection: Fever of any severity was reported in 37.3% of patients. Fever was frequently associated with other flu-like symptoms and was usually mild and clinically manageable. Less than 1% of patients were discontinued for fever. The incidence of fever contrasts with the incidence of infection (8.7%) and indicates that GEMZAR may cause fever in the absence of clinical infection (see Warnings and Precautions).

Flu-Like Symptoms: "Flu-syndrome" was reported regardless of causality (TESS) for 18.9% of patients (N=979). Individual symptoms of headache, anorexia, fever, chills, myalgia and asthenia were the most commonly reported symptoms. Cough, rhinitis, malaise, sweating and insomnia were also commonly reported. Less than 1% of patients discontinued due to flu-like symptoms.

Gastrointestinal: Mild or moderate nausea and vomiting (WHO toxicity grade 1 and 2) was reported in 64% of all patients. WHO grade 3 toxicity, defined as vomiting requiring therapy, was reported in 17.1% of patients. Any patient who received prophylactic antiemetics, was automatically graded ≥WHO grade 3, even if they only developed mild nausea. Diarrhea and stomatitis were usually mild and occurred in less than 13% of patients. WHO toxicity for constipation was mild (WHO grade 1) in the majority of cases and was reported for 7.8% of patients.

† WHO grade 1 peripheral neurotoxicity is defined as paresthesia and/or decreased tendon reflexes and WHO grade 2 toxicity is defined as severe paresthesia and/or mild weakness.

Hematologic: Myelosuppression is the major dose-limiting toxicity with GEMZAR; it was usually of short duration, reversible and not cumulative over time. Less than 1% of patients discontinued therapy for either anemia, leukopenia, or thrombocytopenia. Red blood cell transfusions were received by 19% of patients and less than 1% of patients received platelet transfusions. The incidence of major infection (WHO grade toxicity of 3) was only 1.1% and only one grade 4 toxicity for infection occurred.

Hepatic: GEMZAR was associated with transient elevations of serum transaminases (predominantly WHO grades 1 and 2) in approximately two-thirds of patients, but there was no evidence of increasing hepatic toxicity with either longer duration of treatment with GEMZAR or with greater total cumulative dose.

Neurotoxicity: WHO grade 1 or 2 peripheral neurotoxicity† was reported for 3.3% of patients. No patient reported WHO grade 3 or 4 toxicity.

State of consciousness toxicity was usually mild to moderate (WHO grades 1 and 2); somnolence was reported for 4.6% of patients.

Pulmonary and Allergic: GEMZAR should not be administered to patients with a known hypersensitivity to this drug. One case of anaphylactoid reaction has been reported.

The administration of GEMZAR has been infrequently associated with shortness of breath (Dyspnea; see Warnings and Precautions). Dyspnea when graded by WHO-toxicity criteria (Table 1), was reported in 8%, and severe dyspnea (WHO grades 3 and 4) was reported in 1.4% of patients.

Dyspnea, regardless of causality (TESS) was reported in 23% of patients and serious dyspnea was reported in 3% of patients. It should be noted that in both of these analyses, the occurrence of dyspnea may have been due to underlying disease such as lung cancer (40% of study population) or pulmonary manifestations of other malignancies. Dyspnea was occasionally accompanied by bronchospasm (<1% of patients).

Renal: Mild proteinuria and hematuria were commonly reported. Clinical findings consistent with the hemolytic uremic syndrome (HUS) were reported in 6 out of 2429 patients (0.25%) receiving GEMZAR in clinical trials (see Warnings and Precautions). Renal failure associated with HUS, may not be reversible even with discontinuation of therapy and dialysis may be required.

Combination Use with Cisplatin in Non-Small Cell Lung Cancer: This section focuses on adverse events that were increased in frequency and/or severity with the addition of cisplatin to GEMZAR. GEMZAR plus cisplatin was compared to single-agent cisplatin in a randomized trial, and safety data were collected using NCI Common Toxicity Criteria (CTC). In a second randomized trial, GEMZAR plus cisplatin was compared to the combination of cisplatin plus etoposide, and World Health Organization (WHO) criteria were used to grade adverse reactions. All CTC- and WHO-graded adverse events that occurred in ≥10% of patients are listed in Table 2. Toxicity grades for laboratory parameters are reported regardless of causality.

Table 2: GEMZAR

CTC- and WHO-Graded Toxicities Occurring with a ≥10% Frequency in NSCLC Patients Receiving GEMZAR plus Cisplatin (CTC and WHO Grades [in % frequency] are Rounded to the Closest Integer)

NCI Common Toxicity Criteria	GEMZAR plus Cisplatin (n=260)[a] vs Cisplatin (n=262) (% incidence)		
	All Grades	Grade 3	Grade 4
Laboratory[c]			
Hematologic			
Anemia	89	22	3
Thrombocytopenia	85	25	25
Leukopenia	82	35	11
Neutropenia	79	22	35
Lymphocytes	75	25	18
Hepatic			
Transaminase	22	2	1
Alkaline Phosphatase	19	1	0
Renal			
Creatinine	38	4	<1
Proteinuria	23	0	0
Hematuria	15	0	0
Other Laboratory			
Hypomagnesemia	30	4	3
Hyperglycemia	30	4	0
Hypocalcemia	18	2	0
Non-laboratory[d]			
Blood			
Hemorrhage	14	1	0
Gastrointestinal Disorders			
Nausea	93	25	2
Vomiting	78	11	12
Constipation	28	3	0

World Health Organization Criteria	GEMZAR plus Cisplatin (n=69)[b] vs Cisplatin plus Etoposide (n=66) (% incidence)		
	All Grades	Grade 3	Grade 4
Laboratory[c]			
Hematologic			
Anemia	88	22	0
Thrombocytopenia	81	39	16
Leukopenia	86	26	3
Neutropenia	88	36	28
Hepatic			
Alkaline Phosphatase	16	0	0
Renal			
Proteinuria	12	0	0
Hematuria	22	0	0
Non-laboratory[d]			
Gastrointestinal Disorders			
Nausea and Vomiting	96	35	4
Constipation	17	0	0

(cont'd)

Table 2: GEMZAR *(cont'd)*

CTC- and WHO-Graded Toxicities Occurring with a ≥10% Frequency in NSCLC Patients Receiving GEMZAR plus Cisplatin (CTC and WHO Grades [in % frequency] are Rounded to the Closest Integer)

NCI Common Toxicity Criteria	GEMZAR plus Cisplatin (n=260)[a] vs Cisplatin (n=262) (% incidence)			World Health Organization Criteria	GEMZAR plus Cisplatin (n=69)[b] vs Cisplatin plus Etoposide (n=66) (% incidence)		
	All Grades	Grade 3	Grade 4		All Grades	Grade 3	Grade 4
Diarrhea	24	2	2	Diarrhea	14	1	1
Stomatitis	14	1	0	Stomatitis	20	4	0
General Disorders and Administration Site Conditions							
Fever	16	0	0				
Local	15	0	0				
Infections				**Infections**			
Infections	18	3	2	Infection	28	3	1
Nervous System Disorders				**Nervous System Disorders**			
Neuro-Motor	35	12	0	Paresthesias	38	0	0
Neuro-Hearing	25	6	0				
Neuro-Sensory	23	1	0				
Neuro-Cortical	16	3	1				
Neuro-Mood	16	1	0				
Neuro-Headache	14	0	0				
Respiratory Disorders							
Dyspnea	12	4	3				
Skin and Subcutaneous Tissue Disorders				**Skin and Subcutaneous Tissue Disorders**			
Alopecia	53	1	0	Alopecia	77	13	0
Rash	11	0	0	Rash	10	0	0
Vascular Disorders							
Hypotension	12	1	0				

a GEMZAR plus cisplatin patients with laboratory or non-laboratory data, N=217-253. GEMZAR at 1000 mg/m² on Days 1, 8, and 15, and cisplatin at 100 mg/m² on Day 1 every 28 days.
b GEMZAR plus cisplatin patients with laboratory or non-laboratory data, N=67-69. GEMZAR at 1250 mg/m² on Days 1 and 8, and cisplatin at 100 mg/m² on Day 1 every 21 days.
c Regardless of causality.
d Non-laboratory events were graded only if assessed to be possibly drug-related.

Alopecia: In comparison with single-agent GEMZAR therapy, the incidence of alopecia with GEMZAR plus cisplatin combination therapy was increased; 14% with GEMZAR alone versus 53% and 77% with GEMZAR plus cisplatin. Hair loss was usually minimal (CTC/WHO Grade 1 or 2). However, 0.8% of patients that received GEMZAR plus cisplatin on the 4-week schedule experienced CTC Grade 3 alopecia, and 13% of patients who were on the 3-week schedule experienced WHO Grade 3 alopecia. No irreversible (i.e. Grade 4) hair loss was reported.

Fever and Infection: The majority of patients that received GEMZAR plus cisplatin did not develop fever and only one patient (4-week cycle) experienced CTC Grade 3 fever. On the 4-week GEMZAR plus cisplatin schedule, CTC Grade 3 and 4 infection was seen in 2.8% and 1.6% of patients, respectively. On the 3-week schedule, WHO Grade 3 and 4 infection was seen in 2.9% and 1.4% of patients, respectively.

Gastrointestinal: The incidence of nausea and vomiting was higher for combination therapy with GEMZAR plus cisplatin (~90%) than it was for single agent GEMZAR (50-70%). On the 4 week cycle, 23% of patients in the GEMZAR plus cisplatin arm experienced CTC Grade 3 or Grade 4 nausea and vomiting, and on the 3 week cycle, the incidence of WHO Grade 3 or 4 nausea and vomiting was 39.1% in the GEMZAR plus cisplatin arm, despite the use of antiemetics. Although nausea and vomiting were frequent, they were rarely dose-limiting and were seldom reasons for discontinuation from the study. Diarrhea, stomatitis and constipation were usually mild and occurred in 14-28% of patients that received GEMZAR plus cisplatin.

Hematologic: As expected, myelosuppression occurred more frequently with GEMZAR plus cisplatin treatment (~90%) than with GEMZAR monotherapy (~60%), and GEMZAR dosage adjustments for hematologic toxicity were required more often with combination therapy. Although myelosuppression was common, early study discontinuation due to bone marrow suppression occurred in only 3.1% and 4.3% of patients receiving GEMZAR plus cisplatin in the two randomized trials. Platelet transfusions were required by 3% and 21% of patients that received GEMZAR plus cisplatin on a 3-week or 4-week cycle, respectively, and red blood cell transfusions were required by approximately 30-40% of patients. Less than 8% of patients treated with GEMZAR plus cisplatin were hospitalized for febrile neutropenia. Sepsis and severe hemorrhagic events were rare.

Neurotoxicity: CTC Grade 3 neurohearing toxicity (hearing loss interfering with function but correctable with hearing aid) was experienced by 5.6% and 2.9% of GEMZAR plus cisplatin patients on 4-week and 3-week schedules, respectively. CTC Grade 3 neuromotor toxicity was experienced by 11.5% of GEMZAR plus cisplatin patients on the 4-week schedule, and 38% of patients on the 3-week schedule experienced peripheral neurotoxicity (WHO Grade 1 or 2 only).

Renal: On the 4-week GEMZAR plus cisplatin schedule, CTC Grade 3 creatinine toxicity was observed in 4.4% of patients, and one patient experienced Grade 4 creatinine toxicity. On the 3-week schedule, no WHO Grade 2, 3 or 4 BUN or creatinine toxicity were observed.

Combination Use with Cisplatin in Bladder Cancer [Transitional Cell Carcinoma (TCC) of the Urothelium]: The following information presents adverse events seen with GEMZAR in combination with cisplatin for treatment of bladder cancer. GEMZAR plus cisplatin (GC) was compared to MVAC in a pivotal, randomized trial.

Safety data were collected using the WHO toxicity criteria with the exception of Neuro-Hearing event which was graded using the NCI Common Toxicity Criteria. All WHO- and CTC graded adverse events that occurred in ≥10% of patients are listed in Table 3.

Alopecia: Grade 3 and 4 alopecia occurred significantly less often in GEMZAR plus cisplatin patients than in MVAC patients (GC 10.5% vs 55.2%).

Cardiac: Grade 3 and 4 cardiovascular events such as myocardial function, arrhythmia, chest pain, heart failure, pulmonary edema and hypertension were rare; Grade 3 events occurred in 4.1% of patients on GEMZAR plus cisplatin. There were no Grade 4 events. In the MVAC arm 2.2% of patients experienced Grade 3 events and 0.5% of patients experience Grade 4 events.

Gastrointestinal: The incidence of diarrhea was higher in the MVAC treatment arm than it was for the GEMZAR plus cisplatin. In the MVAC arm, 8% of patients experienced Grade 3 or Grade 4 diarrhea compared to 3% of patients in the GEMZAR plus cisplatin arm. Nausea and vomiting occurred in similar frequencies among the GEMZAR plus cisplatin (22%) and the MVAC arms (21%).

Hematologic: Hematologic toxicity was the most frequent laboratory toxicity seen on both treatment arms in this pivotal trial. Grade 3 and 4 neutropenia occurred less often in GEMZAR plus cisplatin patients than in MVAC patients (GC 71% vs MVAC 82%). Grade 3 and 4 anemia was more common on the GEMZAR plus cisplatin arm versus MVAC arm (27% vs 18%). Grade 3 and 4 thrombocytopenia was more common on the GEMZAR plus cisplatin arm versus MVAC arm (GC 57% vs MVAC 21%). In patients with Grade 3 or 4 thrombocytopenia there was no Grade 4 bleeding and only infrequent Grade 3 bleeding (<2%) on either arm. On the GEMZAR plus cisplatin arm, for every 100 cycles of chemotherapy, 13 patients received whole blood or red blood cell transfusion. On the MVAC arm, for every 100 cycles of chemotherapy, 13 patients received whole blood or red blood cell transfusion. On the GEMZAR plus cisplatin arm, for every 100 cycles of chemotherapy, 4 patients received platelet transfusion. On the MVAC arm, for every 100 cycles of chemotherapy, 2 patients received platelet transfusion.

Neurotoxicity: Of the 191 patients assessed in the GEMZAR plus cisplatin arm, CTC Grade 3 neurohearing toxicity occurred in 3 patients (2%). No patient experienced Grade 4 neurohearing toxicity. By comparison, out of 173 patients assessed in the MVAC arm, CTC Grade 3 neurohearing toxicity occurred in 3 patients. Grade 4 neurohearing toxicity occurred in 1 patient.

Pulmonary: Grade 3 and 4 dyspnea occurred in 2.5% and 0.5% of patients on the GEMZAR plus cisplatin respectively, while compared to 2.6% Grade 3 and 3.1% Grade 4 dyspnea in the MVAC arm.

Renal: No patients on the GEMZAR plus cisplatin arm experienced Grade 3 or 4 renal toxicity, while Grade 3 renal toxicity was observed in 0.5% of patients in the MVAC arm. Renal toxicity was measured by serum creatinine levels.

Table 3: GEMZAR

Selected WHO-Graded Adverse Events from Comparative Trial of GEMZAR plus Cisplatin versus MVAC in TCC of the Bladder (WHO Grades [% incidence])

	GEMZAR plus Cisplatin[a]			MVAC[b]		
	All Grades	Grade 3	Grade 4	All Grades	Grade 3	Grade 4
Laboratory[c]						
Hematologic						
Anemia	94	24	4	86	16	2
Leukopenia	92	44	7	93	46	18
Neutropenia	91	41	30	89	17	65
Thrombocytopenia	86	29	29	46	8	13
Platelet Transfusions[d]	18			8		
Hepatic						
AST	30	1	0	28	2	0
ALT	29	1	0	28	2	0
Alkaline Phosphatase	17	2	1	19	1	0
Renal						
BUN	36	1	0	37	0	0

(cont'd)

Table 3: GEMZAR *(cont'd)*

Selected WHO-Graded Adverse Events from Comparative Trial of GEMZAR plus Cisplatin versus MVAC in TCC of the Bladder (WHO Grades [% incidence])

	GEMZAR plus Cisplatin[a]			MVAC[b]		
	All Grades	Grade 3	Grade 4	All Grades	Grade 3	Grade 4
Creatinine	24	0	0	23	1	0
Hematuria	18	5	0	21	2	0
Proteinuria	9	0	0	14	1	0
Non-laboratory[e]						
Blood						
Hemorrhage	23	2	0	15	2	0
Gastrointestinal Disorders						
Nausea and Vomiting	78	22	0	86	19	2
Constipation	38	2	0	39	3	1
Diarrhea	24	3	0	34	8	1
Stomatitis	20	1	0	66	18	4
General Disorders and Administration Site Conditions						
Fever	21	0	0	30	3	0
Infections						
Infection	24	2	1	47	10	5
Nervous System Disorders						
Paresthesias	26	1	0	25	1	0
Neuro-Hearing[f]	19	2	0	14	2	1
Somnolence	17	1	0	30	3	1
Respiratory Disorders						
Dyspnea	28	3	1	21	3	3
Skin						
Alopecia	61	11	0	89	54	1
Rash	23	0	0	16	0	1

[a] N=191-200; all patients on GEMZAR plus cisplatin with laboratory or non-laboratory data; GEMZAR 1000 mg/m² on Days 1, 8, and 15, and cisplatin 70 mg/m² on Day 2 of each 28-day cycle.
[b] N=186-194: all patients on MVAC with laboratory or non-laboratory data: methotrexate 30 mg/m² on Days 1, 15, and 22, vinblastine 3 mg/m² on Days 2, 15, and 22, doxorubicin 30 mg/m² on Day 2, and cisplatin 70 mg/m² on Day 2 of each 28-day cycle.
[c] Regardless of causality.
[d] Percent of patients requiring transfusion.
[e] Non-laboratory events were graded only if assessed to be possibly treatment-related.
[f] Grade based on NCI Common Toxicity Criteria.
Grade based on criteria from the World Health Organization (WHO).

Combination Use with Paclitaxel in Breast Cancer: The following information presents adverse events seen with GEMZAR in combination with paclitaxel for the treatment of patients with unresectable, locally recurrent or metastatic breast cancer who have relapsed following anthracycline-based chemotherapy. GEMZAR plus paclitaxel was compared to paclitaxel in Study JHQG, an unblinded, multicentre, randomized Phase 3 study.

In the GEMZAR plus paclitaxel arm, 7% of patients discontinued treatment because of an adverse event compared to 5% on the paclitaxel arm. In the GEMZAR plus paclitaxel arm, 7% of GEMZAR doses were omitted and 8% were reduced, and 0.9% of paclitaxel doses were omitted and 5% were reduced. In the paclitaxel alone arm, 0.1% of paclitaxel doses were omitted and 2% were reduced. There were 12 deaths in the GEMZAR plus paclitaxel arm, and 8 in the paclitaxel alone arm on study or within 30 days after study drug discontinuation. One death on each arm of the study was possibly drug-related, while the rest of the deaths were attributed to progressive disease and a single death attributed to a traffic accident.

The hospitalization of patients in the GEMZAR plus paclitaxel arm and in the paclitaxel alone arm were similar and not statistically significant (8.8 % and 7.3%, respectively). Median number of cycles given in the GEMZAR plus paclitaxel arm was 6, compared with 5 cycles given in the paclitaxel alone arm.

Table 4 presents a summary of Grade 3 and 4 toxicities reported in the pivotal clinical study JHQG.

Table 4: GEMZAR

Percentages of Patients with Grade 3 and 4 Toxicities Reported in the Clinical Study of GEMZAR in Combination with Paclitaxel in Patients with Metastatic Breast Cancer (CTC Grades [% Incidence, Rounded to the Closest Integer])[a]

	GEMZAR plus Paclitaxel (N=262)			Paclitaxel alone (N=259)		
	All Grades	Grade 3	Grade 4	All Grades	Grade 3	Grade 4
Laboratory[b]						
Hematologic Events						
Neutropenia	69	31	17	31	4	7
Anemia	69	6	1	51	3	<1

(cont'd)

Table 4: GEMZAR *(cont'd)*

Percentages of Patients with Grade 3 and 4 Toxicities Reported in the Clinical Study of GEMZAR in Combination with Paclitaxel in Patients with Metastatic Breast Cancer (CTC Grades [% Incidence, Rounded to the Closest Integer])[a]

	GEMZAR plus Paclitaxel (N=262)			Paclitaxel alone (N=259)		
	All Grades	Grade 3	Grade 4	All Grades	Grade 3	Grade 4
Thrombocytopenia	26	5	<1	7	<1	<1
Leukopenia	21	10	1	12	2	0
Liver Abnormalities						
ALT	18	5	<1	6	<1	0
AST	16	2	0	5	<1	0
Metabolic						
Hyperglycemia	6	3	0	5	3	0
Non-laboratory[c]						
Cardiac Disorders						
Arrhythmia	<1	<1	0	0	0	0
Gastrointestinal Disorders						
Nausea	50	1	0	31	2	0
Vomiting	29	2	0	15	2	0
Diarrhea	20	3	0	13	2	0
Stomatitis/Pharyngitis	13	1	<1	8	<1	0
General Disorders						
Fatigue	40	6	<1	28	1	<1
Febrile Neutropenia (drug-related)	6	5	<1	2	1	0
Immune System Disorder						
Allergic Reaction/Hypersensitivity	5	0	0	3	<1	0
Musculoskeletal and Connective tissue Disorders						
Myalgia	33	4	0	33	3	<1
Arthralgia	24	3	0	22	2	<1
Peripheral Nervous System Disorders						
Neuropathy—sensory	64	5	<1	58	3	0
Neuropathy—motor	15	2	<1	10	<1	0
Respiratory Disorders						
Dyspnea	9	2	<1	3	0	0
Hypoxia	<1	0	0	<1	<1	0
Skin						
Alopecia	90	14	4	92	19	3

[a] The toxicities above are as measured by the CTC scale, Version 2.0 (Study JHQG).
[b] Regardless of causality.
[c] Non-laboratory events were graded only if assessed to be possibly drug-related.
Legend:
N=number of patients.
ALT=alanine aminotransferase.
AST=aspartate aminotransferase.

Hematologic: In Study JHQG, more Grade 3 and 4 hematologic toxicities were reported with GEMZAR plus paclitaxel than paclitaxel alone. There was an increased incidence of red blood cell and/or whole blood transfusions (10% versus 4%), erythropoietin use (8% versus 3.5%), and granulocyte colony-stimulating factor use (7.6% versus 1.2%) in the GEMZAR plus paclitaxel arm than in the paclitaxel alone arm, respectively. There was a higher incidence of febrile neutropenia in the GEMZAR plus paclitaxel arm than in the paclitaxel alone arm (5% versus 1%; p<0.05); however, there was not an increased incidence of Grade 3 and 4 infections (<1%) or hemorrhagic events (0%). Of the patients experiencing febrile neutropenia (5%) in the GEMZAR plus paclitaxel arm, the majority of patients required hospitalization and dose adjustments.
Hepatic: Grade 3 and 4 liver enzyme elevation (ALT/AST) occurred in 8% of the patients treated with GEMZAR plus paclitaxel, and in 2% of the patients treated with paclitaxel alone.
Neurotoxicity: Eleven patients in the GEMZAR plus paclitaxel arm and 4 patients in the paclitaxel alone arm discontinued study due to neuropathy. In the GEMZAR plus paclitaxel arm, the majority of patients with neuropathy reported the onset after Cycle 2, while in the paclitaxel alone arm, most patients with neuropathy reported the onset after Cycle 4. Nearly half of the patients on each treatment arm reported Grade 3 or 4 neuropathy that lasted for more than one cycle.
Pulmonary: Grade 3 and 4 pulmonary toxicity characterized as dyspnea or hypoxia (2% versus <1%), were more common in the GEMZAR plus paclitaxel arm compared with the paclitaxel alone arm. Dyspnea was reported as worsening at the time of disease progression in patients who had this symptom reported at the time of study entry. All patients who reported dyspnea as Grade 3 or 4 toxicity and most who reported it as a serious adverse event had metastatic disease in the lungs and/or pleural effusion. No patients discontinued from the study because of grade 3 or 4 dyspnea.
Other Grade 3 or 4 Toxicities: Grade 3 and 4 nonlaboratory toxicities were more common in the GEMZAR plus paclitaxel arm.

The incidence of Grade 3 and 4 fatigue was 6% in the GEMZAR plus paclitaxel arm and 2% in the paclitaxel alone arm ($p<0.05$); however, there were no discontinuations due to Grade 3 or 4 fatigue. Grade 3 and 4 fatigue was reported for only one cycle in most patients on both treatment arms and was not associated with anemia.

Alopecia was common and was noted in both treatment arms (18% Grade 3/4 alopecia in the GEMZAR plus paclitaxel arm, and 22% Grade 3/4 alopecia in the paclitaxel alone arm).

Post-Market Adverse Drug Reactions: Cardiovascular: Heart failure has been reported very rarely (<0.01%). Arrhythmias, predominantly supraventricular in nature, have been reported signaling awareness of the possibility of cardiovascular events.

Genito-Urinary System: Clinical findings consistent with the hemolytic uremic syndrome (HUS) were rarely (<0.1%) reported in patients receiving GEMZAR. GEMZAR should be discontinued at the first signs of any evidence of microangiopathic hemolytic anemia such as rapidly falling hemoglobin with concomitant thrombocytopenia, elevation of serum bilirubin, serum creatinine, blood urea nitrogen, or LDH. Renal failure may not be reversible even with discontinuation of therapy, and dialysis may be required.

Hepatobiliary: Increased liver function tests including elevations in aspartate aminotransferase (AST), alanine aminotransferase (ALT), gamma-glutamyl transferase (GGT), alkaline phosphatase, and bilirubin levels have been reported rarely (<0.1%). These increases were not all transient, mild or non-progressive (see Warnings and Precautions, Hepatic/Biliary/Pancreatic).

Injury, Poisoning, and Procedural Complications: Radiation toxicity and radiation recall reactions have been reported (see Drug Interactions).

Respiratory: Pulmonary effects, sometimes severe (such as pulmonary edema, interstitial pneumonitis, or adult respiratory distress syndrome (ARDS)) have been reported rarely (<0.1%) in association with GEMZAR therapy. The etiology of these effects is unknown. If such effects develop, consideration should be given to discontinuing GEMZAR. Early use of supportive care measures may help ameliorate the condition.

Skin and Appendages: Severe skin reactions, including desquamation and bullous skin eruptions, have been reported very rarely (<0.01%).

Vascular: Clinical signs of peripheral vasculitis and gangrene have been reported very rarely (<0.01%).

DRUG INTERACTIONS: Overview: The radiosensitizing effects of GEMZAR are reviewed below.

Drug-Drug Interactions: Interactions with other drugs have not been established.

Drug-Food Interactions: Interactions with food have not been established.

Drug-Herb Interactions: Interactions with herbal products have not been established.

Drug-Laboratory Test Interactions: Interactions with laboratory tests have not been established.

Drug-Radiation Interactions: Concurrent radiotherapy (given together or ≤7 days apart): Toxicity associated with this multimodality therapy is dependent on many different factors, including dose of GEMZAR, frequency of gemcitabine administration, dose of radiation, radiotherapy planning technique, the target tissue, and target volume. Pre-clinical and clinical studies have shown that gemcitabine has radiosensitizing activity. In a single trial where GEMZAR at a dose of 1000 mg/m² was administered once weekly for up to six (6) consecutive weeks concurrently with therapeutic thoracic radiation to patients with NSCLC, significant toxicity was observed in the form of severe, and potentially life-threatening mucositis, especially esophagitis and pneumonitis, particularly in patients receiving large volumes of radiotherapy [median treatment volumes 4795 cm³]. The optimum regimen for safe administration of GEMZAR with therapeutic doses of radiation has not yet been determined.

Radiation injury has been reported on targeted tissues (e.g. esophagitis, colitis, and pneumonitis) in association with both concurrent and non-concurrent use of GEMZAR. In addition, radiation recall has been seen with non-concurrent use.

DOSAGE AND ADMINISTRATION: Dosing Considerations:

- This preparation is for intravenous use only.
- GEMZAR should be administered by healthcare professionals experienced in the administration of chemotherapeutic drugs.
- Patients should be monitored prior to each dose for granulocyte and platelet counts.
- Periodic physical examination and checks of renal and hepatic function should be made to detect non-hematologic toxicity.
- Dosage escalation or reduction should be based upon the degree of toxicities experienced by the patient.

Treatment Discontinuation: Acute shortness of breath in association with GEMZAR administration may occur. Bronchodilators, corticosteroids and/or oxygen produce symptomatic relief. Some reports of parenchymal lung toxicity were consistent with drug induced pneumonitis in association with the use of GEMZAR (see Adverse Reactions). The mechanism of this toxicity is not known. Patients suspected of experiencing drug-induced pneumonitis should be discontinued and not be re-challenged with the drug.

Recommended Dose and Dosage Adjustment: Pancreatic Cancer: GEMZAR (gemcitabine hydrochloride) should be used by IV infusion at a dose of 1000 mg/m² over 30 minutes once weekly for up to 7 weeks (or until toxicity necessitates reducing or holding a dose), followed by one week of rest from treatment. Subsequent cycles should consist of infusions once weekly for 3 consecutive weeks out of every 4 weeks.

For dose adjustment guidelines, see Dose Adjustment, Dose Modifications for Pancreatic Cancer, Non-Small Cell Lung Cancer, and TCC of the Bladder Patients.

Non-Small Cell Lung Cancer: Single-agent GEMZAR should be administered by IV infusion at a dose of 1000 mg/m² over 30 minutes once weekly for three consecutive weeks, followed by a one week rest period. This 4 week cycle is repeated.

GEMZAR has been given in combination with cisplatin on either a 4-week or a 3-week schedule. With the 4-week schedule, GEMZAR should be administered intravenously at 1000 mg/m² over 30 minutes on days 1, 8, and 15 of each 28-day cycle. Cisplatin should be administered intravenously at 100 mg/m² on day 1 after the infusion of GEMZAR. With the 3-week schedule, GEMZAR should be administered intravenously at 1250 mg/m² over 30 minutes on days 1 and 8 of each 21-day cycle. Cisplatin at a dose of 100 mg/m² should be administered intravenously after the infusion of GEMZAR on day 1. See cisplatin prescribing information for administration and hydration guidelines.

For dose adjustment guidelines, see Dose Adjustment, Dose Modifications for Pancreatic Cancer, Non-Small Cell Lung Cancer, and TCC of the Bladder Patients.

TCC of the Bladder: GEMZAR should be administered by IV infusion at a dose of 1000 mg/m² over 30 minutes on Days 1, 8 and 15 of each 28-day cycle. Cisplatin should be administered intravenously at 70 mg/m² on Day 1 of each 28-day cycle. This 4-week schedule is then repeated. See cisplatin prescribing information for administration and hydration guidelines. A clinical trial showed more myelosuppression when cisplatin was used in doses of 100 mg/m².

For dose adjustment guidelines, see Dose Adjustment, Dose Modifications for Pancreatic Cancer, Non-Small Cell Lung Cancer, and TCC of the Bladder Patients.

Breast Cancer: GEMZAR has been given in combination with paclitaxel. It is recommended to administer paclitaxel (175 mg/m²) on Day 1 over approximately 3 hours as an intravenous infusion, followed by GEMZAR (1250 mg/m²) as a 30-minute intravenous infusion on Days 1 and 8 of each 21-day cycle. Patients should have an absolute granulocyte count ≥1500×10⁶/L and a platelet count ≥100 000×10⁶/L prior to each cycle. See paclitaxel prescribing information for administration guidelines.

For dose adjustment guidelines, see Dose Adjustment, Dose Modifications for Breast Cancer Patients.

Dosage Adjustment: Dose Modifications for Pancreatic Cancer, Non-Small Cell Lung Cancer, and TCC of the Bladder Patients: Patients receiving GEMZAR should be monitored prior to each dose for granulocyte and platelet counts and, if necessary, the dose of GEMZAR may be either reduced or withheld in the presence of hematological toxicity according to the guidelines in Table 5.

Table 5: GEMZAR

Dose Adjustments Based on Granulocyte and Platelet Counts

Absolute Granulocyte Count (×10⁶/L)		Platelet Count (×10⁶/L)	% of Full Dose
>1000	and	>100 000	100
500–1000	or	50 000–100 000	75
<500	or	<50 000	hold

Periodic physical examination and checks of renal and hepatic function should be made to detect non-hematologic toxicity. Doses may be reduced or withheld based upon the level of toxicity.

Doses should be reduced or withheld until toxicity has resolved in the opinion of the physician.

Dose Modifications for Breast Cancer Patients: Patients should be monitored prior to each dose with a complete blood count, including differential counts.

GEMZAR dosage adjustments for hematological toxicity are based on the granulocyte and platelet counts taken on Day 8 of therapy. If marrow suppression is detected, GEMZAR dosage should be modified according to the guidelines in Table 6.

Table 6: GEMZAR

Day 8 Dosage Reduction Guidelines for GEMZAR in Combination with Paclitaxel

Absolute Granulocyte Count (×10⁶/L)		Platelet Count (×10⁶/L)	% of Full Dose
≥1200	and	>75 000	100
1000–1199	or	50 000–75 000	75
700–999	and	≥50 000	50
<700	or	<50 000	hold

Periodic physical examination and checks of renal and hepatic function should be made to detect non-hematologic toxicity. Doses may be reduced or withheld based upon the level of toxicity.

Doses should be reduced or withheld until toxicity has resolved in the opinion of the physician.

For severe (Grade 3 or 4) non-hematological toxicity, therapy should be held or decreased by 50% depending on the judgement of the treating physician.

Administration: GEMZAR is well tolerated during the infusion, with only a few cases of injection site reaction reported. There have been no reports of injection site necrosis. GEMZAR also does not appear to act as a vesicant in a case of extravasation. GEMZAR may be administered on an outpatient basis.

As with other toxic compounds, caution should be exercised in handling and preparing solutions with GEMZAR. The use of gloves is recommended. If the solution of GEMZAR contacts the skin or mucosa, immediately wash the skin or mucosa thoroughly with soap and water or rinse the mucosa with copious amounts of water.

Reconstitution:

Vial Size	Volume of Diluent to be Added to Vial	Approximate Available Volume	Nominal Concentration per mL
200 mg	5.0 mL of 0.9% NaCl Injection	5 mL	38 mg/mL
1 g	25 mL of 0.9% NaCl Injection	25 mL	38 mg/mL

To reconstitute, add at least 5 mL of 0.9% Sodium Chloride Injection to the 200 mg vial or at least 25 mL of 0.9% Sodium Chloride Injection to the 1 g vial. Invert to dissolve. These dilutions each yield a GEMZAR concentration of 38 mg/mL. The appropriate amount of drug may be administered as prepared or further diluted with 0.9% Sodium Chloride Injection to concentrations as low as 0.1 mg/mL.

Reconstitution of concentrations greater than 40 mg/mL may result in incomplete dissolution, and should not be attempted.

Sterile isotonic saline (0.9% sodium chloride injection) without added preservatives should be used as a diluent.

Parenteral drugs should be inspected visually for particulate matter and discoloration, prior to administration, whenever solution and container permit.

See Storage and Stability for more details.

OVERDOSAGE:

There is no known antidote for overdoses of GEMZAR (gemcitabine hydrochloride). Myelosuppression, and paresthesiae were the principal toxicities seen when a single dose as high as 5700 mg/m² was administered by IV infusion over 30 minutes every 2 weeks to several patients in a Phase I study. In the event of a suspected overdose, the patient should be monitored with appropriate blood counts and should receive supportive therapy, as necessary.

For management of a suspected drug overdose, CPhA recommends that you contact your **regional Poison Control Centre**. See the *CPS* Directory section for a list of Poison Control Centres.

ACTION AND CLINICAL PHARMACOLOGY: Mechanism of Action: GEMZAR (gemcitabine hydrochloride) is a cell-cycle dependent oncolytic agent of the "antimetabolite" class. It is a deoxycytidine analog (difluoro-deoxycytidine; dFdC) that is metabolized intracellularly to the active diphosphate (dFdCDP) and triphosphate (dFdCTP) nucleosides. The cytotoxic effects of gemcitabine are exerted through dFdCDP-assisted incorporation of dFdCTP into DNA, resulting in inhibition of DNA synthesis and induction of apoptosis.

Pharmacokinetics: Gemcitabine disposition was studied in five patients who received a single 1000 mg/m²/30 minute infusion of radiolabeled drug. Within one (1) week, 92% to 98% of the dose was recovered, almost entirely in the urine. Gemcitabine (<10%) and the inactive uracil metabolite, 2'-deoxy-2',2'-difluorouridine (dFdU), accounted for 99% of the excreted dose. The metabolite dFdU is also found in plasma. Gemcitabine plasma protein binding is negligible.

The pharmacokinetics of gemcitabine were examined in 353 patients, about 2/3 men, with various solid tumours. Pharmacokinetic parameters were derived using data from patients treated for varying durations of therapy given weekly with periodic rest weeks and using both short infusions (<70 minutes) and long infusions (70-285 minutes). The total gemcitabine dose varied from 500 to 3600 mg/m².

Gemcitabine pharmacokinetics are linear and are described by a 2-compartment model. Population pharmacokinetic analyses of combined single and multiple dose studies showed that the volume of distribution of gemcitabine was significantly influenced by duration of infusion and gender. Clearance was affected by age and gender. Differences in either clearance or volume of distribution based on patient characteristics or the duration of infusion result in changes in half-life and plasma concentrations. Table 7 shows plasma clearance and half-life of gemcitabine following short infusions for typical patients by age and gender.

Table 7: GEMZAR

Gemcitabine Clearance and Half-Life for the "Typical" Patient

Age	Clearance Men (L/h/m²)	Clearance Women (L/h/m²)	Half-Life[a] Men (min)	Half-Life[a] Women (min)
29	92.2	69.4	42	49
45	75.7	57.0	48	57
65	55.1	41.5	61	73
79	40.7	30.7	79	94

[a] Half-life for patients receiving a short infusion (<70 min).

Gemcitabine half-life for short infusions ranged from 32 to 94 minutes, and the value for long infusions varied from 245 to 638 minutes, depending on age and gender, reflecting a greatly increased volume of distribution with longer infusions. The lower clearance in women and the elderly results in higher concentrations of gemcitabine for any given dose.

The volume of distribution was increased with infusion length. Volume of distribution of gemcitabine was 50 L/m² following infusions lasting <70 minutes, indicating that gemcitabine, after short infusions, is not extensively distributed into tissues. For long infusions, the volume of distribution rose to 370 L/m², reflecting slow equilibration of gemcitabine within the tissue compartment.

The maximum plasma concentrations of dFdU (inactive metabolite) were achieved up to 30 minutes after discontinuation of the infusions. The metabolite was excreted in urine without undergoing further biotransformation and did not accumulate with weekly dosing. Its elimination is dependent on renal excretion and the metabolite could accumulate with decreased renal function.

In patients with NSCLC or bladder cancer receiving combination therapy with gemcitabine plus cisplatin, the plasma concentrations of gemcitabine and its major metabolite, dFdU, did not differ significantly from those observed in patients receiving single-agent gemcitabine.

The effects of significant renal or hepatic insufficiency on the disposition of gemcitabine have not been assessed.

The active metabolite, gemcitabine triphosphate, can be extracted from peripheral blood mononuclear cells. The half-life of the terminal phase for gemcitabine triphosphate from mononuclear cells ranges from 1.7 to 19.4 hours.

STORAGE AND STABILITY: GEMZAR should be stored in glass vials, at 15 to 30°C.

Parenteral drugs should be inspected visually for particulate matter and discoloration, prior to administration, whenever solution and container permit. The reconstituted solution is stable for 24 hours at 15 to 30°C. Any unused solution should be discarded. Solutions of reconstituted GEMZAR should not be refrigerated, as crystallization may occur.

SPECIAL HANDLING INSTRUCTIONS: Procedures for proper handling and disposal of anti-cancer drugs should be considered. Several guidelines on this subject have been published.

INFORMATION FOR THE PATIENT: Published in e-CPS, available by subscription at www.e-cps.ca.

DOSAGE FORMS, COMPOSITION AND PACKAGING: 200 mg: Each vial of sterile lyophilized powder contains: gemcitabine 200 mg (as the hydrochloride salt). Nonmedicinal ingredients: mannitol and sodium acetate. Hydrochloric acid and/or sodium hydroxide may have been added for pH adjustment. Vials of 10 mL.

1 g: Each vial of sterile lyophilized powder contains: gemcitabine 1 g (as the hydrochloride salt). Nonmedicinal ingredients: mannitol and sodium acetate. Hydrochloric acid and/or sodium hydroxide may have been added for pH adjustment. Vials of 50 mL.

For intravenous use only.

Gen-Clozapine

clozapine

Antipsychotic

Mylan

Date of Preparation: February 14, 2003
Date of Revision: July 28, 2009

PHARMACOLOGY: GEN-CLOZAPINE (clozapine), a dibenzodiazepine derivative, is an atypical antipsychotic drug because its profile of binding to dopamine receptors and its effects on various dopamine-mediated behaviours differ from those exhibited by conventional antipsychotics. In contrast to conventional antipsychotics, clozapine produces little or no prolactin elevation. Clozapine exerts potent anticholinergic, adrenolytic, antihistaminic and antiserotoninergic activity.

Controlled clinical trials indicate that clozapine improves both positive and negative symptoms.

Patients on rare occasions may report an intensification of dream activity during clozapine therapy. Rapid eye movement (REM) sleep was found to be increased to 85% of the total sleep time. In these patients, the onset of REM sleep occurred almost immediately after falling asleep.

As is true of more typical antipsychotic drugs, clinical EEG studies have shown that clozapine increases delta and theta activity and slows dominant alpha frequencies. Enhanced synchronization occurs, and sharp wave activity and spike and wave complexes may also develop.

Pharmacokinetics: The absorption of orally administered clozapine is 90 to 95%. Food does not affect either the rate or the extent of absorption. Clozapine is subject to first-pass metabolism, resulting in an absolute bioavailability of 50 to 60%.

Plasma concentrations show large inter-individual differences, with peak concentrations occurring approximately 2.5 hours (range: 1 to 6 hours) after dosing. In a dose range of 37.5 mg bid to 150 mg bid, the area under the curve (AUC) and the peak plasma concentration (C_{max}) increase linearly in a dose-related fashion.

Clozapine is approximately 95% bound to plasma proteins. The elimination of clozapine is biphasic with a mean terminal half-life of 12 hours (range: 6 to 30 hours, calculated from three steady-state in vivo studies). After single doses of 75 mg, the mean terminal half-life was 7.9 hours; it increased to 14.2 hours when steady-state conditions were reached by administering daily doses of 75 mg for at least 7 days. Clozapine is almost completely metabolized prior to excretion. Only trace amounts of unchanged drug are detected in the urine and feces. Approximately 50% of the administered dose is excreted as metabolites in the urine and 30% in the feces.

Recent studies suggest that there is a significant correlation between clozapine plasma levels and clinical response. The concentrations of clozapine, and its major metabolite norclozapine, were significantly higher in responders than in nonresponders although the mean doses of clozapine did not differ between the two groups. Of the main metabolites, only norclozapine was found to be active. In patients who responded to treatment, plasma clozapine levels reached at least 350 to 370 ng/mL.

Clinical Trial Data on Suicidal Behaviour (InterSePT Study): The International Suicide Prevention Study (InterSePT) Study ABA 451 was a prospective, open-label randomized, international, parallel-group comparison of Clozapine vs. Zyprexa (olanzapine) of two years duration, with approximately 490 patients per treatment group.

Trial Design: Patients were diagnosed with schizophrenia or schizoaffective disorder using DSM-IV criteria, and meeting at least one of the following criteria in order to be deemed at high risk for suicide: a) a suicide attempt, or hospitalization to prevent an attempt, within the last three years; or b) moderate to severe suicidal ideation with either a depressive component or command hallucinations, within the last week. One fourth (27%) of the patient population was considered "treatment-resistant".

Due to the high-risk nature of the study population, the principle investigators (PIs) were permitted to treat patients as they judged necessary, including concomitant medications, non-drug treatments, and hospitalizations. Both the PIs and the patients were aware of the treatment group assignment.

Efficacy Measures: The primary efficacy measure was time to the first occurrence of either a Type I or Type II event.

The unblinded PIs were responsible for identifying Type I events: a suicide attempt, or the judgement of need for hospitalization/increased surveillance to prevent an attempt. In the case of the Type I events, all relevant information from the PIs was blinded and forwarded to a blinded group of experts (the Suicide Monitoring Board) for final confirmation of each potential Type I event. Blinded psychiatrists, who assessed the patients at pre-determined intervals, were responsible for identifying Type II events: "much worsening" or "very much worsening" from baseline in the Clinical Global Impression of Severity of Suicidality-Blinded Psychiatrist (CGI-SS-BP) scale.

Results: Analysis using the Cox's proportional hazard regression model demonstrates that within the context of the InterSePT trial there was a 26% reduced risk for a suicide attempt or hospitalization to prevent suicide (Type 1 event) for Clozapine-treated patients compared to Zyprexa treated-patients (p=0.02, hazard ratio 0.74 [95% C.I.: 0.57,0.96].

Factors that preclude regulatory endorsement of an indication for Clozapine for the risk of recurrent suicidal behaviour in patients with schizophrenia or schizoaffective disorder:

1. The heavy reliance of the endpoints on clinical judgement, when combined with the fact that the principle investigators were not blinded to the treatment group, creates the potential for bias in the results.
2. Separate indications for the domain of recurrent suicidal behaviour versus that of psychosis require a conclusion that the two domains are independent; currently, there is insufficient evidence to allow such a conclusion.
3. The usual concerns with generalizability of study results to individual patients in clinical practice are magnified in this therapeutic area. Given that schizophrenia is associated with long-term increased risk of suicide, the two year duration of the study limits generalizability. Many patients in this study had multiple suicide risk factors; the variable and dynamic nature of risk and protective factors, and the unpredictability of interaction with unique life circumstances also limit generalizability, as do the unusual efforts made in the study to prevent a suicide attempt, including frequent patient-clinician contact.
4. Because decisions about concomitant treatment were made by unblinded PIs, the post-doc finding that the Clozapine group received significantly less psychotropic medication than did the ZYPREXA group is not readily interpretable.
5. This is the sole prospective randomized trial.

Conclusion: Under the currently approved Canadian indication, Clozapine is already available to a substantial percentage of psychotic patients at risk of suicide, given the frequency of tolerability issues and the fact that a complete response to an antipsychotic is rare. The InterSePT study is a source of further information with regards to these patients.

While the InterSePT results are hypothesis-generating, they fail to provide sufficient evidence to support the safety and efficacy of the use of Clozapine in patients who are naive to anti-psychotics, or have schizoaffective disorder.

A two-way, single-dose, fasting bioequivalence study and a two-way, single-dose, fed bioequivalence study were conducted to compare the bioavailability of a single 12.5 mg dose (one-half 25 mg clozapine tablet) of the test product, GEN-CLOZAPINE (Genpharm ULC, Canada) to that of the Canadian reference product, Clozaril (Novartis Canada Inc., Canada). The results of the two studies are summarized in Table 1 and Table 2.

Table 1: GEN-CLOZAPINE
Summary Tables of the Comparative Bioavailability Data Two-Way, Single Dose, Fasting Study (one-half × 25 mg) From Measured Data

Parameter	Geometric Mean Arithmetic Mean (CV%)		
	GEN-CLOZAPINE One-half 25 mg tablet	Clozaril[a] One-half 25 mg tablet	Ratio (%) of Geometric Means
AUC_{0-t} (ng·h/mL)	225.4 272.6 (61.4)	221.5 263.2 (56.5)	102
AUC_{inf} (ng·h/mL)	235.9 293.1 (67.7)	234.8 294.6 (59.7)	100
C_{max} (ng/mL)	21.16 23.61 (35.9)	19.64 21.60 (37.0)	108
T_{max} (h)[b]	2.26 (65.9)	2.37 (59.4)	Not applicable
$T_{½}$ (h)[b]	16.57 (29.8)	16.89 (26.0)	Not applicable

[a] Novartis Canada Inc. Purchased in Canada.
[b] Expressed as arithmetic mean (CV%).

Table 2: GEN-CLOZAPINE
Summary Tables of the Comparative Bioavailability Data Two-Way, Single Dose, Fed Study (one-half × 25 mg) From Measured Data

Parameter	Geometric Mean Arithmetic Mean (CV%)		
	GEN-CLOZAPINE One-half 25 mg tablet	Clozaril[a] One-half 25 mg tablet	Ration (%) of Geometric Means
AUC_{0-t} (ng·h/mL)	233.8 262.8 (42.1)	232.0 261.0 (39.2)	101
AUC_{inf} (ng·h/mL)	241.2 271.7 (44.3)	238.9 274.0 (42.9)	101
C_{max} (ng/mL)	20.92 23.08 (41.6)	20.10 22.39 (41.4)	104
T_{max} (h)[b]	2.36 (53.9)	2.74 (53.2)	Not applicable
$T_{½}$ (h)[b]	13.94 (26.6)	14.30 (27.8)	Not applicable

[a] Novartis Canada Inc. Purchased in Canada.
[b] Expressed as arithmetic mean (CV%).

INDICATIONS: GEN-CLOZAPINE (clozapine) is indicated in the management of symptoms of treatment-resistant schizophrenia. In controlled clinical trials, clozapine was found to improve both positive and negative symptoms.

Due to the significant risk of agranulocytosis and seizure associated with its use, clozapine should be limited to treatment-resistant schizophrenic patients who are non-responsive to, or intolerant of, conventional antipsychotic drugs. Non-responsiveness is defined as the lack of satisfactory clinical response, despite treatment with appropriate courses of at least two marketed chemically-unrelated antipsychotic drugs. Intolerance is defined as the inability to achieve adequate benefit with conventional antipsychotic drugs because of dose-limiting, intolerable adverse effects.

Because of the significant risk of agranulocytosis and seizure, events which both present a continuing risk over time, the extended treatment of patients failing to show an acceptable level of clinical response to clozapine should ordinarily be avoided. In addition, the need for continuing treatment in patients exhibiting beneficial clinical responses should be periodically reevaluated.

Clozapine can be used only if regular hematological examinations can be guaranteed, as specified under Warnings and Dosage.

GEN-CLOZAPINE is available only through a distribution system (GenCAN) that ensures weekly, every two-week or every-four-week hematological testing prior to the dispensing of the next period's supply of GEN-CLOZAPINE (see Warnings).

This requires:

- registration of the patient, their current location, treating physician, testing laboratory and dispensing pharmacist in the GenCAN system.
- maintenance of a national Genpharm ULC-specific database that enables the monitoring of the hematological results of all patients on GEN-CLOZAPINE and provides timely feedback (within 24 hours of receipt of the blood test results) to the treating physician and dispensing pharmacist/or pharmacy.
- the ability to identify patients who have been assigned "Non-rechallengeable Status" (see Warnings). This requires that Genpharm ULC both provide to, and obtain from all other approved suppliers* of clozapine, the Non-rechallengeable Status/Hematological Status of all patients (see Dosage). Genpharm ULC must be able to provide this information within 24 hours of receiving a written request.

Physicians should not prescribe GEN-CLOZAPINE until the non-rechallengeable status and the hematological status of the patient has been verified.

For the distribution system to be effective, treating physicians must ensure that the hematological testing is performed at the required frequency (see Warnings) and that arrangements are made for the hematological results to be sent to GenCAN.

Physicians may obtain details on the GenCAN distribution system by calling a toll-free phone number (1-866-501-3338).

Other Monitoring and Distribution Systems: Between 1991 and 2003, clozapine was distributed by a single manufacturer, and patients were monitored by this manufacturer's specific registry and distribution system. The introduction of clozapine from other manufactures has now resulted in the establishment of manufacturer-specific registry and distribution systems.

In order to ensure the safe use and continued monitoring of all patients taking clozapine, the physician must have obtained consent from the patient for the potential sharing of hematological and other safety data between clozapine registries.

Patients may not be switched from one brand of clozapine to another without the completion of a new registry-specific patient registration form signed by the prescribing physician.

If a patient is switched from one brand of clozapine to another, the frequency of hematological monitoring may continue unaltered unless a change is clinically indicated.

CONTRAINDICATIONS: GEN-CLOZAPINE (clozapine) is contraindicated in patients with myeloproliferative disorders, a history of toxic or idiosyncratic agranulocytosis or severe granulocytopenia (with the exception of granulocytopenia/agranulocytosis from previous chemotherapy). [Clozapine should not be used simultaneously with other agents known to suppress bone marrow function.]

GEN-CLOZAPINE is also contraindicated in patients with active liver disease associated with nausea, anorexia, or jaundice; progressive liver disease; hepatic failure.

* "Approved supplier" is a manufacturer who holds a valid Notice of Compliance (NOC) for clozapine

Other contraindications include severe central nervous system depression or comatose states, severe renal or cardiac disease (e.g. myocarditis), paralytic ileus, uncontrolled epilepsy, and previous hypersensitivity to clozapine or any other components of GEN-CLOZAPINE.

GEN-CLOZAPINE is also contraindicated in patients unable to undergo blood tests.

WARNINGS: Elderly Patients with Dementia: Elderly patients with dementia treated with atypical antipsychotic drugs are at an increased risk of death compared to placebo. Analyses of thirteen placebo-controlled trials with various atypical antipsychotics (modal duration of 10 weeks) in these patients showed a mean 1.6 fold increase in the death rate in the drug-treated patients. Although the causes of death were varied, most of the deaths appeared to be either cardiovascular (e.g., heart failure, sudden death) or infectious (e.g., pneumonia) in nature. Clozapine has not been studied in elderly patients with dementia and therefore no such data were included in this analysis.

GEN-CLOZAPINE (clozapine) is not recommended in elderly patients with dementia (see Precautions, Geriatics, Use in Geriatric Patients with Dementia).

Agranulocytosis: Because of the significant risk of granulocytopenia and agranulocytosis, a potentially life-threatening adverse event (see below), GEN-CLOZAPINE clozapine) should be reserved for use in the treatment of schizophrenic patients who fail to show an acceptable response to adequate courses of conventional antipsychotic drug treatment, either because of insufficient effectiveness or the inability to achieve an effective dose due to intolerable adverse effects.

Patients must have a normal white blood cell (WBC) count and differential count prior to starting clozapine therapy. Subsequently, a WBC count and differential count must be carried out at least weekly for the first 26 weeks of treatment with clozapine. Thereafter, if acceptable WBC counts and absolute neutrophil counts (ANC) (WBC ≥3500/mm³ and ANC ≥2000/mm³) have been maintained during the first 26 weeks of continuous therapy, the WBC count and differential count can be performed at least at two-week intervals for the next 26 weeks. Thereafter, if acceptable WBC counts and ANCS (WBC ≥3500/mm³ and ANC ≥2000/mm³) have been maintained during the second 26 weeks of continuous therapy, the wbc count and differential count can be performed at least every four weeks throughout treatment.

The change from a weekly to a "once every two weeks", or from a "once every two weeks" to a "once every four weeks" schedule should be evaluated on an individual patient basis after 26 and 52 weeks of treatment, respectively. This decision should be made based upon the hematological profile of the patient during the first 26 or 52 weeks of treatment (as appropriate), as well as on the clinical judgement of the treating physician, and if he/she deems it appropriate, a consulting hematologist, and on the patient's willingness to pursue a given frequency of blood monitoring. In turn, the clinical evaluation should take into consideration possible factors that would place the patient in a higher risk group.

Monitoring must continue for as long as the patient is on the drug. Monitoring frequency does not have to be modified if therapy is interrupted for 3 days or less. However, weekly hematological testing should be resumed for an additional 6 weeks if therapy is disrupted for more than 3 days (see Figure 1). Furthermore, monitoring should occur at least weekly for a period of 4 weeks following discontinuation of clozapine therapy, irrespective of the cause of discontinuation.

GEN-CLOZAPINE is available only through a distribution system (GenCan) that requires weekly, every-two-week or every-four-week hematological testing prior to the dispensing of the next period's supply of GEN-CLOZAPINE (see Indications).

Granulocytopenia (defined as a granulocyte count of less than 1.5×10⁹/L) and agranulocytosis (defined as a granulocyte count of less than 0.5×10⁹/L, including polys + bands) have been shown to occur in association with clozapine use at an incidence of 3% and 0.7%, respectively. These incidences are derived from post-marketing data as per June 1993, covering over 60 000 patients treated with clozapine for up to 3 years in USA, Canada and UK. Approximately 88% of the cases of agranulocytosis have occurred during the first 26 weeks of therapy.

A fatality rate of 32% for clozapine-induced agranulocytosis had been reported in association with clozapine use as of December 31, 1989. However, more than half of these deaths occurred before 1977, prior to the recognition of the risk of agranulocytosis and the need for routine blood monitoring. From February 1990 to August 21, 1997, among approximately 150 409 patients treated with clozapine in the U.S.A., 585 new cases of agranulocytosis have been reported, of which 19 (3.2%) had a fatal outcome.

Fatalities occurring in association with clozapine-induced granulocytopenia/agranulocytosis have generally resulted from infections due to compromised immune system responses.

Therefore, patients should be advised to report immediately the appearance of lethargy, weakness, fever, sore throat, flu-like complaints or any other signs of infection.

All patients must be screened to ensure that they do not have a history of neutropenia/agranulocytosis associated with clozapine use (i.e., are not in the Non-rechallengeable databases of any of the current approved suppliers of clozapine).

GEN-CLOZAPINE treatment should be initiated and carried out according to the following guidelines:

- Treatment should not be initiated if the WBC count is less than 3.5×10⁹/L and/or the (ANC) count is less than 2.0×10⁹/L, or if the patient has a history of a myeloproliferative disorder, or toxic or idiosyncratic agranulocytosis or severe granulocytopenia (with the exception of granulocytopenia/agranulocytosis from previous chemotherapy).
- Independently of the frequency of their blood monitoring regimen (weekly, at two-week, or at four-week intervals), patients should be evaluated immediately and WBC and differential counts checked at least **twice weekly** if after the initiation of treatment:
  i) the total WBC count falls to between 2.0×10⁹/L and 3.5×10⁹/L,
  ii) the ANC falls to between 1.5×10⁹/L and 2.0×10⁹/L,
  iii) a single fall or sum of falls in WBC count of 3.0×10⁹/L or more is measured in the last four weeks, reaching a value below 4.0×10⁹/L,
  iv) a single fall or sum of falls in ANC of 1.5×10⁹/L or more is measured in the last four weeks, reaching a value below 2.5×10⁹/L,
  and/or
  v) flu-like complaints or other symptoms appear which might suggest infection.

In the event of a fall in total WBC to below 2.0×10⁹/L or in ANC to below 1.5×10⁹/L, GEN-CLOZAPINE therapy must be immediately withheld and the patient closely monitored. **The patient is to be assigned "non-rechallengeable" status upon confirmation of fall in WBC and neutrophil counts. GEN-CLOZAPINE therapy must not be resumed.** Particular attention should be paid to any flu-like complaints or other symptoms which might suggest infection. If the patient should develop a further fall in the WBC count to below 1.0×10⁹/L, or a decrease in ANC to below 0.5×10⁹/L, it is recommended that patients be placed in protective isolation with close observation and be watched for signs of infection by their physician. Should evidence of infection develop, the appropriate cultures should be performed and an appropriate antibiotic regimen instituted.

The development of granulocytopenia and agranulocytosis does not appear to be dose dependent, nor is duration of treatment a reliable predictor. Approximately 88% of the cases have occurred in the first twenty-six weeks of treatment, but some cases have developed after years of clozapine use. The incidence of neutropenia and agranulocytosis associated with the use of clozapine increases as a function of age. Experience in the U.S. (approx. 58 000 patients, as per June 1993) reveals that patients over 50 years old would present an approximately two to three times higher incidence of agranulocytosis when compared with the overall incidence in patients treated with clozapine.

Patients who have shown hematopoietic reactions to other medications may also be more likely to demonstrate such reactions with clozapine. A disproportionate number of the U.S. cases of agranulocytosis occurred in patients of Jewish origin compared to the overall proportion of such patients exposed to the drug in pre-marketing clinical experience in the United States.

Agranulocytosis associated with other antipsychotic drugs has been reported to occur with a greater frequency in patients who are cachectic or have a serious underlying medical illness.

Figure 1: GEN-CLOZAPINE

Resuming Monitoring Frequency after Interruption in Therapy

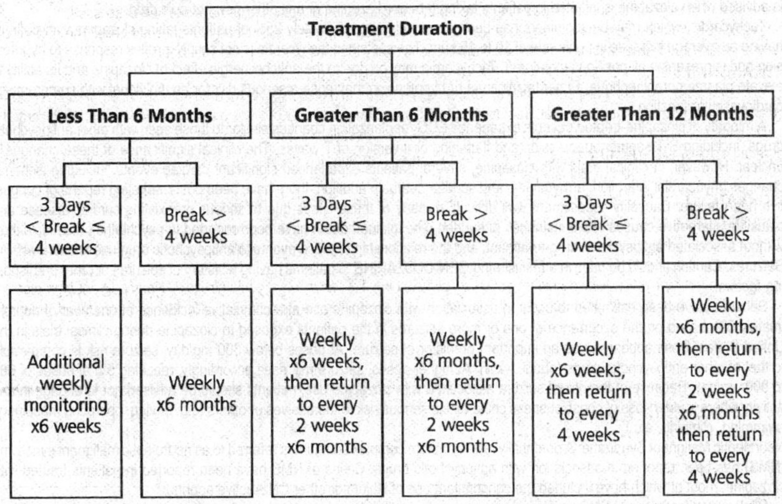

Cardiotoxicity: Important safety information regarding a constellation of cardiovascular events reported in patients treated with clozapine:

Cardiovascular Toxicity: Analysis of safety databases suggests that the use of clozapine is associated with an increased risk of myocarditis especially during, but not limited to, the first month of therapy. Myocarditis has been reported in patients 19 years of age and older, at dosages within the approved dosage range and during titration of clozapine. In Canada, there have been 9 reported cases of myocarditis. Of these, three have been fatal. Given the estimated 15 600 Canadian clozapine-treated patients as of August 2001, this represents an estimated incidence of 0.06% for all reports of myocarditis (or 1/1667 patients) and 0.02% for myocarditis fatalities (or 1/5200).

Pericarditis, pericardial effusion and cardiomyopathy have also been reported in association with clozapine use, as have heart failure, myocardial infarction and mitral insufficiency; these reports include fatalities.

In patients who develop persistent tachycardia at rest accompanied by other signs and symptoms of heart failure (e.g. chest pain, tachypnoea (shortness of breath), or arrhythmias), the possibility of myocarditis, cardiomyopathy and/or other cardiovascular dysfunction must be considered. Other symptoms which may be present in addition to the above include fatigue, flu-like symptoms, fever that is otherwise unexplained, hypotension and/or raised jugular venous pressure.

The occurrence of such signs and symptoms necessitates an urgent diagnostic evaluation for myocarditis, cardiomyopathy and/or other cardiovascular dysfunction by a cardiologist. Patients with a family history of heart failure should have a cardiac evaluation prior to commencing treatment; clozapine is contraindicated in patients with severe cardiac disease.

In patients in whom myocarditis is suspected, clozapine treatment should be promptly discontinued. Patients with clozapine-induced myocarditis should not be re-exposed to clozapine.

If cardiomyopathy and/or other cardiovascular dysfunction is diagnosed, discontinuation of clozapine, based on clinical grounds, should be considered.

Background Information for Cardiotoxicity Boxed Warning (as of early 2002): A) Myocarditis, pericarditis and pericardial effusion: Canadian Reports: In Canada, a total of 16 post-marketing surveillance spontaneous reports of myocarditis/pericarditis/pericardial effusion have been received by Health Canada since marketing in 1991 (see also boxed Warnings regarding myocarditis cases). Information additional to the Boxed Warnings: the age range was 19-37 years; the shortest known clozapine treatment duration was 2 weeks.

International Reports: Reporting incidences for myocarditis can be reliably calculated from the four countries with CLOZARIL national registries (USA, United Kingdom, Canada, Australia). The lowest rate is reported in the U.S. (1/20 000 person years) and the highest in Australia (1/800 person years). Of these 81 cases, 37% were fatal, with 80% of fatal cases showing evidence of myocarditis at autopsy. When all international reports of myocarditis are included (n=213 cases), the myocarditis rate is 1/14 000 patient years; 23% of cases had a fatal outcome and 85% occurred within the first two months of initiation of clozapine therapy. Recurrences of myocarditis upon rechallenge with clozapine have been documented.

Another analysis of clozapine and myocarditis revealed that 70% of patients were under 50 years of age; thus, clozapine-associated myocarditis can occur in younger patients. Dosages were mostly in accordance with current labelled dosage recommendations, with a third of patients taking less than therapeutic doses; this likely reflects the occurrence of myocarditis during dose titration.

There are also reports of pericarditis/pericardial effusion, some of which have been fatal. Eosinophilia has been co-reported in some cases, which may indicate that the carditis is a hypersensitivity reaction to clozapine; however, it is not known whether eosinophilia is a reliable predictor of carditis.

B) Cardiomyopathy/heart failure/mitral insufficiency: Canadian Reports: In Canada, seven cases of cardiomyopathy and 3 cases of heart failure/mitral insufficiency have been reported to Health Canada, with individual cases reported to have concomitant myo/endo carditis. The age range is 19-55 years; Two of the reports of heart failure are known to have been fatal (61y male, 46y male).

International Reports: A total of 178 cardiomyopathy reports (18% fatal), have been received by Novartis. Analysis of the reports revealed that four times as many men as women were diagnosed with cardiomyopathy. About 80% of the cases occurred in patients under the age of 50; the incidence rate of spontaneous reports of cardiomyopathy for this age range was greater in clozapine-treated patients than in the general population in established international market economies.

Diagnosis was confirmed (by echocardiography or autopsy) in 44% of the cases. Typically, the clozapine dose was within therapeutic range, with the duration of treatment more than 6 months in 65% of the patients. There was no other apparent cause of the cardiomyopathy in about 50% of all reported cases of cardiomyopathy and in 28% of fatalities including history, concomitant medications, comorbidities, with an average age of approximately 37 years. Terms most commonly co-reported with cardiomyopathy were: congestive heart failure (21%), heart rate and rhythm disorders (10%), cardiomegaly (8%). In the 4 cases where follow-up was reported after withdrawal of clozapine, there was improvement of the cardiomyopathy.

C) Myocardial infarction: In Canada, 30 reports of myocardial infarction in patients receiving clozapine have been received by Health Canada with 50% of cases known to be fatal.

Other Adverse Cardiovascular and Respiratory Effects: GEN-CLOZAPINE should be used with caution in patients with known cardiovascular and/or pulmonary disease, particularly in those with cardiac arrhythmias and conduction disturbances, and the recommendation for gradual titration of dose should be carefully observed.

Orthostatic hypotension, with or without syncope, can occur with GEN-CLOZAPINE treatment and may represent a continuing risk in some patients. Rarely (approximately 1 case per 3000 patients in the United States), collapse can be profound and can be accompanied by respiratory and/or cardiac arrest. Orthostatic hypotension is more likely to occur during initial titration in association with rapid dose escalation and may even occur on first dose. In one report, initial doses as low as 12.5 mg were associated with collapse and respiratory arrest. When restarting patients who have had even a brief interval of GEN-CLOZAPINE (clozapine), i.e. 2 days or more since the last dose, it is recommended that treatment be reinitiated with one-half of a 25 mg tablet (12.5 mg) once or twice daily (see Dosage).

Cases of collapse/respiratory arrest/cardiac arrest during initial clozapine treatment occurred in patients administered clozapine by itself and in patients administered clozapine in combination with benzodiazepines or other psychotropic drugs. Although it has not been established that there is an interaction between clozapine and benzodiazepines or other psychotropics, caution is advised when clozapine is initiated in patients taking a benzodiazepine or any other psychotropic drug.

Tachycardia, which may be sustained, has been observed in approximately 25% of patients taking clozapine with patients having an average increase in pulse rate of 10 to 15 bpm. The sustained tachycardia is not simply a reflex response to hypotension and is present in all positions monitored. Tachycardia may be due to the anticholinergic effect of clozapine and its ability to elevate plasma norepinephrine. Either tachycardia or hypotension may pose a serious risk for an individual with compromised cardiovascular function.

A minority of clozapine-treated patients experience ECG repolarization changes similar to those seen with other antipsychotic drugs, including S-T segment depression and flattening or inversion of T waves. The clinical significance of these changes is unclear. However, in clinical trials with clozapine, several patients experienced significant cardiac events, including ischemic changes, myocardial infarction, arrhythmias, and sudden death. In addition, there have been post-marketing reports of congestive heart failure. Causality assessment was difficult in many of these cases due to serious preexisting cardiac disease and plausible alternative causes. Rare instances of sudden, unexplained death have been reported in psychiatric patients, with or without associated antipsychotic drug treatment, and the relationship of these events to antipsychotic drug use is unknown.

Seizures: Caution should be used in administering GEN-CLOZAPINE to patients having a history of seizures or other predisposing factors.

Seizures have been estimated to occur in association with clozapine use at a cumulative incidence at one year of approximately 5%, based on the occurrence of one or more seizures in the patients exposed to clozapine during clinical trials in the United States. Dose appears to be an important predictor of seizure. At doses below 300 mg/day, seizure risk is comparable to that of other antipsychotic drugs (about 1-2%). At higher doses, seizure risk rises accordingly, reaching 5% at doses of 600 to 900 mg/day. Because of the risk of seizure associated with clozapine use, patients should be advised not to engage in any activity where sudden loss of consciousness could cause serious risk to themselves or others (e.g. driving, operating machinery, swimming, climbing, etc.)

Neuroleptic Malignant Syndrome: A potentially fatal symptom complex sometimes referred to as neuroleptic malignant syndrome (NMS) has been reported in association with antipsychotic drugs. Cases of NMS have been reported in patients treated with clozapine, most of which have included the concomitant use of lithium or other CNS-active agents.

Clinical manifestations of NMS are hyperpyrexia, muscle rigidity, altered mental status (including catatonic signs) and evidence of autonomic instability (irregular pulse or blood pressure, tachycardia, diaphoresis, and cardiac dysrhythmias). Additional signs may include elevated creatine phosphokinase, myoglobinuria (rhabdomyolysis), and acute renal failure.

The diagnostic evaluation of patients with this syndrome is complicated. In arriving at a diagnosis, it is important to identify cases where the clinical presentation includes both serious medical illness (e.g., pneumonia, systemic infection, etc.) and untreated or inadequately treated extrapyramidal signs and symptoms (EPS). Other important considerations in the differential diagnosis include central anticholinergic toxicity, heat stroke, drug fever and primary central nervous system (CNS) pathology.

The management of NMS should include: (1) immediate discontinuation of antipsychotic drugs and other drugs not essential to concurrent therapy; (2) intensive symptomatic treatment and medical monitoring; and (3) treatment of any concomitant serious medical problems for which specific treatments are available. There is no general agreement about specific pharmacological treatment regimens for uncomplicated NMS.

If a patient requires antipsychotic drug treatment after recovery from NMS, the potential reintroduction of drug therapy should be carefully considered. The patient should be carefully monitored, since recurrences of NMS have been reported.

Tardive Dyskinesia: A syndrome consisting of potentially irreversible, involuntary, dyskinetic movements may develop in patients treated with conventional antipsychotic drugs. Although the prevalence of tardive dyskinesia with conventional antipsychotics appears to be highest among the elderly, especially elderly women, it is impossible to rely upon prevalence estimates to predict, at the beginning of treatment, which patients are likely to develop the syndrome.

Both the risk of developing tardive dyskinesia and the likelihood that it will become irreversible are believed to increase as the duration of treatment and the total cumulative dose of antipsychotic drugs administered to the patient increase. However, the syndrome can develop, although much less commonly, after relatively brief treatment periods at low doses. There is no known treatment for established cases of tardive dyskinesia, although the syndrome may remit, partially or completely, if antipsychotic drug treatment is withdrawn. Antipsychotic drug treatment itself, however, may suppress (or partially suppress) the signs and symptoms of tardive dyskinesia and thereby may possibly mask the underlying process. The effect that symptom suppression has upon the long-term course of the syndrome is unknown.

There are several reasons for predicting that GEN-CLOZAPINE may be different from other antipsychotic drugs in its potential for inducing tardive dyskinesia. These include the preclinical finding that it has a relatively weak dopamine receptor blocking effect and the clinical finding that it is associated with a low incidence of extrapyramidal symptoms. Very rarely tardive dyskinesia has been reported in patients on clozapine who had been previously treated with other antipsychotic agents, so that a causal relationship cannot be established. Nevertheless, it cannot be concluded, without more extended experience, that GEN-CLOZAPINE will not induce this syndrome.

Given this consideration, GEN-CLOZAPINE should be prescribed in a manner that is most likely to minimize the risk of the occurrence of tardive dyskinesia. As with any antipsychotic drug, chronic GEN-CLOZAPINE use should be reserved for patients who appear to be obtaining substantial benefit from the drug. In such patients, the smallest dose and the shortest duration of treatment should be sought. The need for continued treatment should be reassessed periodically.

Patients in whom tardive dyskinesia developed with other neuroleptics have improved on clozapine.

If signs and symptoms of tardive dyskinesia appear in a patient on GEN-CLOZAPINE, drug discontinuation should be considered. However, some patients may require treatment with GEN-CLOZAPINE despite the presence of the syndrome.

PRECAUTIONS: Because of the significant risk of agranulocytosis and seizure, events which both present a continuing risk over time, the extended treatment of patients failing to show an acceptable level of clinical response to GEN-CLOZAPINE (clozapine) should ordinarily be avoided. In addition, the need for continuing treatment in patients exhibiting beneficial clinical responses should be reassessed periodically.

Patients with a history of primary bone marrow disorders may be treated only if the benefit outweighs the risk. They should be carefully evaluated by a hematologist prior to starting GEN-CLOZAPINE.

Patients who have low WBC counts because of benign ethnic neutropenia should be given special consideration and may be started on GEN-CLOZAPINE after agreement of a hematologist.

Fever: During GEN-CLOZAPINE therapy, patients may experience transient temperature elevations above 38°C with the peak incidence within the first three weeks of treatment. This fever is generally benign and self-limiting; however, on occasion there may be an associated increase or decrease in the white blood cell count. Patients should be carefully evaluated to rule out the possibility of an underlying infectious process or the development of blood dyscrasia. In the presence of high fever, the possibility of neuroleptic malignant syndrome must be considered (see Warnings). Fever that is otherwise unexplained can accompany myocarditis (see Warnings).

Occupational Hazards: Interference with Cognitive and Motor Performance: Because of the potential for initial sedation, GEN-CLOZAPINE may impair mental and/or physical abilities especially during the first few days of therapy. The recommendation for gradual dose escalation should be carefully adhered to and patients should be cautioned about activities requiring alertness (e.g., driving, operating machinery, swimming, climbing, etc.). (See Dosage.)

Drug Interactions: GEN-CLOZAPINE may enhance the central effects of alcohol, MAO inhibitors, CNS depressants including narcotics, antihistamines, and benzodiazepines, as well as the effects of anticholinergic and antihypertensive agents.

Caution is advised with patients who are receiving (or have recently received) benzodiazepines or other psychotropic drugs, as these patients may have an increased risk of circulatory collapse accompanied by respiratory and/or cardiac arrest.

Owing to its anti-alpha-adrenergic properties, GEN-CLOZAPINE may reduce the blood pressure increasing effect of norepinephrine or other predominantly alpha-adrenergic agents and reverse the pressor effect of epinephrine.

GEN-CLOZAPINE should not be used with other agents, such as carbamazepine, having a known potential to suppress bone marrow function. In particular, the concomitant use of long-acting depot antipsychotic drugs should be avoided because these medications, which may have the potential to be myelosuppressive, cannot be rapidly removed from the body.

Concomitant use of valproic acid with GEN-CLOZAPINE may alter the plasma levels of clozapine. Rare but serious reports of seizures, including onset of seizures in non-epileptic patients, and isolated cases of delirium where GEN-CLOZAPINE was co-administered with valproic acid have been reported. These effects are possibly due to a pharmacodynamic interaction, the mechanism of which has not been determined.

Clozapine is a substrate for many CYP 450 isoenzymes, in particular 1A2 and 3A4. Caution is called for in patients receiving concomitant treatment with other drugs which are either inhibitors or inducers of these enzymes.

Concomitant administration of drugs known to inhibit the activity of cytochrome P450 isozymes may increase the plasma levels of clozapine:

- Drugs known to inhibit the activity of the major isozymes involved in the metabolism of clozapine and with reported interactions include, cimetidine (2D6, 3A4), and erythromycin (3A4). Other potent inhibitors of CYP3A, such as azole antimycotics and protease inhibitors, could potentially also increase clozapine plasma concentrations; however, no interactions have been reported to date.
- Substantial elevation of the plasma concentration of clozapine has been reported in patients receiving the drug in combination with fluvoxamine (1A2). Smaller elevations in clozapine plasma concentrations have also been reported in patients receiving the drug in combination with other selective serotonin re-uptake inhibitors (SSRIs) such as paroxetine, sertraline, fluoxetine and citalopram (possibly a weak inhibitor of CYP1A2 and possibly the least likely among SSRIs to cause a clinically significant interaction with clozapine).
- The plasma concentration of clozapine is increased by caffeine (1A2) intake and decreased by nearly 50% following a 5-day caffeine-free period.

No clinically relevant interactions have been observed thus far with tricyclic antidepressants, phenothiazines or type 1_c antiarrhythmics, known to bind to cytochrome P450 2D6.

Concomitant administration of drugs known to induce cytochrome P450 enzymes may decrease the plasma levels of clozapine:

- Drugs known to induce the activity of 3A4 and with reported interactions with clozapine include, for instance, carbamazepine, phenytoin and rifampicin.
- Known inducers of 1A2 include, for instance, omeprazole and cigarette smoking. In cases of sudden smoking cessation, the plasma clozapine concentration may be increased, thus leading to an increase in adverse effects.

Anticholinergic Activity: GEN-CLOZAPINE has potent anticholinergic effects, which may produce undesirable effects throughout the body. Great care should be exercised in using the drug in the presence of prostatic enlargement, narrow-angle glaucoma or paralytic ileus. Probably on account of its anticholinergic properties, clozapine has been associated with varying degrees of impairment of intestinal peristalsis, ranging from constipation to intestinal obstruction, faecal impaction and paralytic ileus. On rare occasions, these cases have been fatal.

Deep Vein Thrombosis and Pulmonary Embolism: Deep vein thrombosis has been observed in association with clozapine. Since clozapine may cause sedation and weight gain, thereby increasing the risk of thromboembolism, immobilization of patients should be avoided.

Whether pulmonary embolism can be attributed to GEN-CLOZAPINE or some characteristic(s) of its users is not clear. However, the possibility of pulmonary embolism should be considered in patients receiving GEN-CLOZAPINE who present with deep vein thrombosis, acute dyspnea, chest pain, or other respiratory symptoms.

Eosinophilia: In the event of eosinophilia, it is recommended to discontinue GEN-CLOZAPINE if the eosinophil count rises above 3.0×10^9/L, and to re-start therapy only after the eosinophil count has fallen below 1.0×10^9/L. Eosinophilia has been co-reported in some cases of myocarditis and thus such cardiovascular adverse events associated with clozapine use may represent hypersensitivity reactions to clozapine.

Patients with both eosinophilia and clozapine-induced myocarditis should not be re-exposed to clozapine.

Thrombocytopenia: In the event of thrombocytopenia, it is recommended to discontinue GEN-CLOZAPINE therapy if the platelet count falls below 50.0×10^9/L.

Hepatitis: Patients with stable pre-existing liver disorders may receive GEN-CLOZAPINE, but need regular liver function tests. In patients in whom, during GEN-CLOZAPINE treatment, symptoms of possible liver dysfunction such as nausea, vomiting and/or anorexia develop, liver function tests should be performed immediately. If the elevation of these values is clinically relevant or if symptoms of jaundice occur, treatment with GEN-CLOZAPINE must be discontinued. It may be resumed (see Dosage, Re-Initiation of Treatment in Patients Previously Discontinued) only when the liver function tests have returned to normal values. In such cases, liver function should be closely monitored after the re-introduction of the drug.

Hyperglycemia: On rare occasions, severe hyperglycemia, sometimes leading to ketoacidosis/hyperosmolar coma including some fatal cases, has been reported during clozapine treatment in patients with no prior history of hyperglycemia. While a causal relationship to clozapine use has not been definitely established, glucose levels returned to normal in most patients after discontinuation of clozapine, and rechallenge produced a recurrence of hyperglycemia in a few cases. The effect of clozapine on glucose metabolism in patients with diabetes mellitus has not been studied. Impaired glucose tolerance, severe hyperglycemia, ketoacidosis and hyperosmolar coma have been reported in patients with no prior history of hyperglycaemia. In patient receiving clozapine who developed symptom of hyperglycaemia, such as polydipsia, polyuria, polyphagia or weakness discontinuation should be considered.

There is a risk of altering the metabolic balance resulting in slight impairment of glucose homeostasis and a possibility of unmasking a pre-diabetic condition or aggravating pre-existing diabetes.

Assessment of the relationship between atypical antipsychotic use and glucose abnormalities is complicated by the possibility of an increased background risk of diabetes mellitus in patients with schizophrenia and the increasing incidence of diabetes mellitus in the general population. Given these confounders, the relationship between atypical antipsychotic use and hyperglycemia-related adverse events is not completely understood. However, epidemiological studies suggest an increased risk of treatment-emergent hyperglycemia-related adverse events in patients treated with the atypical antipsychotics. Precise risk estimates for hyperglycemia-related adverse events in patients treated with atypical antipsychotics are not available.

Any patient treated with atypical antipsychotics should be monitored for symptoms of hyperglycemia including polydipsia, polyuria, polyphagia, and weakness. Patients who develop symptoms of hyperglycemia during treatment with atypical antipsychotics should undergo fasting blood glucose testing. In some cases, hyperglycemia has resolved when the atypical antipsychotic was discontinued; however, some patients required continuation of anti-diabetic treatment despite discontinuation of the suspect drug. Patients with risk factors for diabetes mellitus (e.g., obesity, family history of diabetes) who are starting treatment with atypical antipsychotics should undergo fasting blood glucose testing at the beginning of treatment and periodically during treatment. Patients with an established diagnosis of diabetes mellitus who are started on atypical antipsychotics should be monitored regularly for worsening of glucose control.

Dysphagia: Esophageal dysmotility and aspiration have been associated with antipsychotic drug use. Aspiration pneumonia is a common cause of morbidity and mortality in elderly patients, in particular those with advanced Alzheimer's dementia. GEN-CLOZAPINE and other antipsychotic drugs should be used cautiously in patients at risk for aspiration pneumonia.

Use in Patients with Concomitant Illness: Clinical experience with clozapine in patients with concomitant systemic diseases is limited. Nevertheless, caution is advised when using GEN-CLOZAPINE in patients with hepatic, renal, or cardiac disease. For severe cases, see Contraindications.

Pregnancy: Reproduction studies, performed in rats and rabbits at doses of approximately 2 to 4 times the human dose, have revealed no evidence of impaired fertility or harm to the fetus due to clozapine. However, there have not been any adequate and well-controlled studies in pregnant women. Because animal reproduction studies are not always predictive of human response and in view of the desirability of keeping the administration of all drugs to a minimum during pregnancy, GEN-CLOZAPINE should be used only if the benefits clearly outweigh the risks.

Lactation: Animal studies suggest that clozapine may be excreted in breast milk and have an effect on the nursing infant. Therefore, women receiving GEN-CLOZAPINE should not breast-feed.

Women of Childbearing Potential: Some female patients treated with antipsychotics other than GEN-CLOZAPINE may become amenorrheic. A return to normal menstruation may occur as a result of switching from other antipsychotics to GEN-CLOZAPINE. Adequate contraceptive measures must therefore be ensured in women of childbearing potential.

Children: Safety and efficacy in children below age 18 have not been established.

Geriatics: Use in Geriatric Patients with Dementia: Overall Mortality: Elderly patients with dementia treated with atypical antipsychotic drugs are at an increased risk of death compared to placebo. Clozapine has not been studied in elderly patients with dementia. GEN-CLOZAPINE (clozapine) is not recommended for the treatment of patients with dementia (see Warnings).

Orthostatic hypotension can occur with GEN-CLOZAPINE treatment and there have been rare reports of tachycardia, which may be sustained, in patients taking clozapine. Elderly patients, particularly those with compromised cardiovascular function, may be more susceptible to these effects.

Elderly patients may also be particularly susceptible to the anticholinergic effects of GEN-CLOZAPINE, such as urinary retention and constipation.

Information to Be Provided to the Patient: Physicians are advised to discuss the following issues with patients (and/or their guardians) for whom they prescribe GEN-CLOZAPINE:

Patients who are to receive GEN-CLOZAPINE should be warned about the significant risk of developing agranulocytosis, a potentially life-threatening adverse event. They should be informed that regular blood tests are required to monitor for the occurrence of agranulocytosis, and that GEN-CLOZAPINE tablets will be made available only through a special program designed to ensure the required blood monitoring. They should also be informed that the blood tests will be performed according to the following monitoring schedule:

- Weekly blood tests will be required for the first 26 weeks of their treatment with clozapine.

- Following this initial higher risk period, they could be allowed to change to a "once every two weeks" schedule, provided that acceptable WBC counts and ANCs (WBC ≥3500/mm³ and ANC ≥2000/mm³) have been maintained during the first 26 weeks of continuous therapy, and that their clinical condition is permitting such a change in monitoring regimen.
- Thereafter, if acceptable WBC counts and ANCs have been maintained during the second 26 weeks of continuous therapy, blood tests could be performed every four weeks.

Patients should be advised to report immediately the appearance of lethargy, weakness, fever, sore throat, malaise, mucous membrane ulceration or other possible signs of infection. Particular attention should be paid to any flu-like complaints or other symptoms that might suggest infection.

- Patients should be advised to contact their physician immediately if they develop persistent tachycardia (rapid heart rate) at rest accompanied by other signs and symptoms of heart failure (e.g. chest pain, shortness of breath, swelling of the ankles and feet, or arrhythmias (abnormal heart rhythms)). Other symptoms which may be present in addition to the above include fatigue, flu-like symptoms, fever that is otherwise unexplained, hypotension (low blood pressure) and/or raised jugular venous pressure (bulging neck veins when sitting or standing). Patients are advised to contact their physician before discontinuing any medication.
- Patients should be informed of the significant risk of seizure during GEN-CLOZAPINE treatment and should be advised to avoid activities that require alertness (e.g. driving, operating machinery, swimming, climbing, etc.).
- Patients should be advised of the risk of orthostatic hypotension, especially during the period of initial dose titration.
- Patients should be informed that if they stop taking GEN-CLOZAPINE for 2 days or more, they should not restart their medication at the same dosage, but should contact their physician for dosage instructions.
- Patients should notify their physician if they are taking, or plan to take, any prescription or over-the-counter drugs or alcohol.
- Patients should notify their physician if they become pregnant or intend to become pregnant during therapy.
- Patients should not breast feed an infant if they are taking GEN-CLOZAPINE.

ADVERSE EFFECTS: The most serious adverse reactions experienced with clozapine are agranulocytosis, seizure, cardiovascular effects and fever (see Warnings and Precautions). The most common side effects are drowsiness, hypersalivation, tachycardia and sedation.

Adverse Reactions Associated with Discontinuation of Treatment: Sixteen percent of 1080 patients who received clozapine in premarketing clinical trials discontinued treatment due to an adverse event, including both those that could be reasonably attributed to clozapine treatment and those that might more appropriately be considered intercurrent illness. The more common events considered to be causes of discontinuation included: CNS, primarily drowsiness/sedation, seizures, dizziness/syncope; cardiovascular, primarily tachycardia, hypotension and ECG changes; gastrointestinal, primarily nausea/vomiting; hematologic, primarily leukopenia/granulocytopenia/agranulocytosis; and fever. None of the events enumerated accounts for more than 1.7% of all discontinuations attributed to adverse clinical events.

Commonly Observed Adverse Reactions: Adverse events observed in association with the use of clozapine in clinical trials at an incidence of greater than 5% were: central nervous system complaints, including drowsiness/sedation, dizziness/vertigo, headache and tremor; autonomic nervous system complaints, including salivation, sweating, dry mouth and visual disturbances; cardiovascular findings, including tachycardia, hypotension and syncope; and gastrointestinal complaints, including constipation and nausea; and fever. Complaints of drowsiness/sedation tend to subside with continued therapy or dose reduction. Salivation may be profuse, especially during sleep, but may be diminished with dose reduction.

Incidence in Clinical Trials: Table 3 enumerates adverse events that occurred at a frequency of 1% or greater among clozapine patients who participated in clinical trials. These rates are not adjusted for duration of exposure.

Table 3: GEN-CLOZAPINE

Treatment-Emergent Adverse Experience Incidence Among Patients Taking Clozapine in Clinical Trials (N=842) (Percentage of Patients Reporting)

Body System Adverse Events[a]	Percent
Central Nervous System	
Drowsiness/Sedation	39
Dizziness/Vertigo	19
Headache	7
Tremor	6
Syncope	6
Disturbed sleep/Nightmares	4
Restlessness	4
Hypokinesia/Akinesia	4
Agitation	4
Seizures (convulsions)	3[b]
Rigidity	3
Akathisia	3
Confusion	3
Fatigue	2
Insomnia	2
Hyperkinesia	1
Weakness	1
Lethargy	1
Ataxia	1
Slurred speech	1
Depression	1
Epileptiform movements/Myoclonic jerks	1
Anxiety	1
Cardiovascular	
Tachycardia	25[b]
Hypotension	9
Hypertension	4
Chest pain/Angina	1
ECG change/Cardiac abnormality	1
Gastrointestinal	
Constipation	14
Nausea	5
Abdominal discomfort/Heartburn	4
Nausea/Vomiting	3
Vomiting	3
Diarrhea	2
Liver test abnormality	1
Anorexia	1
Urogenital	
Urinary abnormalities	2
Incontinence	1
Abnormal ejaculation	1
Urinary urgency/frequency	1
Urinary retention	1
Autonomic Nervous System	
Salivation	31
Sweating	6
Dry mouth	6
Visual disturbances	5
Integumentary (Skin)	
Rash	2
Musculoskeletal	
Muscle weakness	1
Pain (back, neck, legs)	1
Muscle spasm	1
Muscle pain, ache	1
Respiratory	
Throat discomfort	1
Dyspnea, shortness of breath	1
Nasal congestion	1
Hemic/Lymphatic	
Leukopenia/Decreased WBC/Neutropenia	3
Agranulocytosis	1[b]
Eosinophilia	1
Miscellaneous	
Fever	5
Weight gain	4
Tongue numb/sore	1

[a] Events reported by at least 1% of clozapine patients are included.
[b] Rate based on population of approximately 1700 exposed during premarket clinical evaluation of clozapine.

Adverse Events Observed During the InterSePT Study: Adverse events reported during the InterSePT study were consistent with the known safety profiles for clozapine and olanzapine. The ten most frequently reported adverse events in the Clozapine treatment group were: salivary hypersecretion, somnolence, weight increase, anxiety, depression, dizziness (excluding vertigo), psychotic disorder, suicidal ideation, constipation, and insomnia.

Other Events Observed During the Premarketing Evaluation of Clozapine: This section reports additional, less frequent adverse events which occurred among the patients taking clozapine in clinical trials. Various adverse events were reported as part of the total experience in these clinical studies; a causal relationship to clozapine treatment cannot be determined in the absence

of appropriate controls in some of the studies. Table 3 enumerates adverse events that occurred at a frequency of at least 1% of patients treated with clozapine. The list below includes all additional adverse experiences reported as being temporally associated with the use of the drug which occurred at a frequency less than 1%, enumerated by organ system:
Central Nervous System: loss of speech, amentia, tics, poor coordination, delusions/hallucinations, involuntary movement, stuttering, dysarthria, amnesia/memory loss, histrionic movements, libido increase or decrease, paranoia, shakiness, Parkinsonism, and irritability.
Cardiovascular System: edema, palpitations, phlebitis/thrombophlebitis, cyanosis, premature ventricular contraction, bradycardia, and nose bleed; ischemic changes, arrhythmias, myocardial infarction, and sudden death.
Gastrointestinal System: abdominal distention, gastroenteritis, rectal bleeding, nervous stomach, abnormal stools, hematemesis, gastric ulcer, bitter taste, and eructation.
Urogenital System: dysmenorrhea, impotence, breast pain/discomfort, and vaginal itch/infection.
Automatic Nervous System: numbness, polydypsia, hot flashes, dry throat, and mydriasis.
Integumentary (Skin): pruritus, pallor, eczema, erythema, bruise, dermatitis, petechiae, and urticaria.
Musculoskeletal System: twitching and joint pain.
Respiratory System: coughing, pneumonia/pneumonia-like symptoms, rhinorrhea, hyperventilation, wheezing, bronchitis, laryngitis, and sneezing.
Hemic and Lymphatic System: anemia and leukocytosis.
Miscellaneous: chills/chills with fever, malaise, appetite increase, ear disorder, hypothermia, eyelid disorder, bloodshot eyes, and nystagmus.
Postmarketing Clinical Experience: Postmarketing experience has shown an adverse experience profile similar to that presented above. Voluntary reports of adverse events temporally associated with clozapine not mentioned above that have been received since market introduction and that may have no causal relationship with the drug include the following:
Central Nervous System: delirium; EEG abnormal; exacerbation of psychosis; myoclonus; overdose; paresthesia; possible mild cataplexy; and status epilepticus.
Cardiovascular System: Analysis of safety databases suggests that the use of clozapine is associated with an increased risk of myocarditis especially during, but not limited to, the first month of therapy (see Warnings); atrial or ventricular fibrillation, periorbital edema, pericarditis, pericardial effusion, cardiomyopathy, heart failure, mitral insufficiency and myocardial infarction.
Gastrointestinal System: acute pancreatitis; dysphagia; fecal impaction; intestinal obstruction/paralytic ileus; and salivary gland swelling.
Hepatobiliary System: cholestasis; hepatitis; jaundice.
Hepatic System: cholestasis.
Urogenital System: acute interstitial nephritis and priapism.
Integumentary (Skin): hypersensitivity reactions: photosensitivity, vasculitis, erythema multiforme, and Stevens-Johnson Syndrome.
Metabolic and Nutritional Disorders: hyperglycemia, ketoacidosis/hyperosmolar coma, hyperuricemia, hyponatremia, weight loss, impaired glucose tolerance, diabetes aggravated, hypercholesterolemia, and hypertriglyceridemia.
Musculoskeletal System: myasthenic syndrome and rhabdomyolysis.
Respiratory System: aspiration, pleural effusion and respiratory arrest.
Hemic and Lymphatic System: deep vein thrombosis; elevated hemoglobin/hematocrit; ESR increased; pulmonary embolism; sepsis; thrombocytosis; and thrombocytopenia; and thombocythaemia.
Vision Disorders: narrow angle glaucoma.
Miscellaneous: CPK elevation.

OVERDOSE:

Symptoms: The signs and symptoms associated with clozapine overdose are: drowsiness, lethargy, coma, areflexia, confusion, agitation, delirium, hyperreflexia, convulsions, hypersalivation, mydriasis, blurred vision, thermolability, tachycardia, hypotension, collapse, cardiac arrhythmias, heart block, respiratory depression or failure, hallucinations, extrapyramidal symptoms, aspiration pneumonia and dyspnea.

In cases of acute intentional or accidental clozapine overdosage, for which information on the outcome is available, to date the mortality is about 12%. Most of the fatalities were associated with cardiac failure or pneumonia caused by aspiration and occurred at doses above 2000 mg. There have been reports of patients recovering from an overdose in excess of 10 000 mg. However, in a few adult individuals, primarily those not previously exposed to clozapine, the ingestion of doses as low as 400 mg led to life-threatening comatose conditions and, in one case, to death. In young children, the intake of 50 mg to 200 mg resulted in strong sedation or coma without being lethal.

Treatment: Establish and maintain an airway; ensure adequate oxygenation and ventilation. Perform gastric lavage and/or the administration of activated charcoal within the first 6 hours after the ingestion of the drug. Activated charcoal, which may be used with sorbitol, may be as or more effective than emesis or lavage, and should be considered in treating overdosage. Cardiac and vital signs monitoring is recommended along with general symptomatic and supportive measures. Surveillance should be continued for several days because of the risk of delayed effects. Avoid epinephrine when treating hypotension, and quinidine and procainamide when treating cardiac arrhythmia.

There are no specific antidotes for GEN-CLOZAPINE. Forced diuresis, dialysis, hemoperfusion and exchange transfusion are unlikely to be of benefit.

In managing overdosage, the physician should consider the possibility of multiple drug involvement.

> For management of a suspected drug overdose, contact your regional Poison Control Centre. See the *CPS* Directory section for a list of Poison Control Centres.

DOSAGE: GEN-CLOZAPINE (clozapine) treatment must be initiated on an in-patient basis or in an out-patient setting where medical supervision is available and vital signs can be monitored for a minimum of 6 to 8 hours after the initial 2 to 3 doses.

When treatment is initiated in out-patients, special caution is advised in patients who are receiving benzodiazepines or other psychotropic drugs as these patients may have an increased risk of circulatory collapse accompanied by respiratory and/or cardiac arrest (see Precautions, Drug Interactions). Extra caution is advised in patients with cardiovascular disease or a history of seizures (see Warnings).

GEN-CLOZAPINE is restricted to patients who have a normal white blood cell (WBC) count and differential cell (DC) count and in whom a WBC count and DC count can be carried out at least weekly for the first 26 weeks of treatment with clozapine, at least at two-week intervals for the next 26 weeks, and at least at four-week intervals thereafter. Monitoring must continue for as long as the patient is on the drug, as well as for at least four weeks after discontinuation of treatment.

> The change from a weekly to a "once every two weeks", or from a "once every two weeks" to a "once every four weeks" schedule should be evaluated on an individual patient basis after 26 and 52 weeks of treatment, respectively. This decision should be made based upon the hematological profile of the patient during the first 26 or 52 weeks of treatment (as appropriate) (see Warnings), the clinical judgement of the treating physician, and if he/she deems it appropriate, a consulting hematologist, as well as the patient's willingness to pursue a given frequency of blood monitoring. In turn, the clinical evaluation should take into consideration possible factors that would place the patient in a higher risk group. Weekly hematological testing should be resumed for an additional 6 weeks if therapy is disrupted for more than 3 days. If clozapine is interrupted for 4 weeks or longer, weekly monitoring is required for an additional 26 weeks.

GEN-CLOZAPINE is available only through a distribution system that requires weekly, every-two-week or every-four-week hematological testing prior to the dispensing of the next period's supply of medication (see Indications).

Genpharm ULC will provide the Non-rechallengeable Status/Hematological Status of patients to the requesting approved suppliers† of clozapine within 24 hours of receipt of a written request (see Indications).

The dosage of GEN-CLOZAPINE must be adjusted individually. For each patient the lowest effective dose should be used.
Other Monitoring and Distribution Systems: The introduction of clozapine from other manufacturers has resulted in the establishment of manufacturer-specific registry and distribution systems.

In order to ensure the safe use and continued monitoring of all patients taking clozapine, the physician must have obtained consent from the patient for the potential sharing of hematological and other safety data between clozapine registries.

Patients may not be switched from one brand of clozapine to another without the completion of a new registry-specific patient registration form signed by the prescribing physician.

† "approved supplier" is a manufacturer who holds a valid Notice of Compliance (NOC) for clozapine.

If a patient is switched from one brand of clozapine to another, the frequency of hematological monitoring may continue unaltered unless a change is clinically indicated.
Initial Dose: On the first day, GEN-CLOZAPINE (clozapine) should be given at a 12.5 mg dose (one-half of a 25 mg tablet) once or twice, followed by one or two 25 mg tablets on the second day. If well tolerated, the dosage may be increased in daily increments of 25 mg to 50 mg, achieving a target dose of 300-450 mg/day by the end of two weeks. Subsequent dosage increases should be made no more than once or twice weekly, in increments not to exceed 100 mg. Cautious titration and a divided dosage schedule are necessary to minimize the risks of hypotension, seizure and sedation.
Switching from Previous Neuroleptics: When GEN-CLOZAPINE therapy is initiated in a patient undergoing oral neuroleptic therapy, it is generally recommended that the other neuroleptic should first be discontinued by tapering the dosage downwards. Once the neuroleptic is completely discontinued for at least 24 hours, GEN-CLOZAPINE treatment can be started as described above. It is generally recommended that GEN-CLOZAPINE should not be used in combination with other neuroleptics.
Therapeutic Dose Range: In most patients, antipsychotic efficacy can be expected within the therapeutic range of 300-600 mg/day in divided doses. The total daily dose may be divided unevenly, with the larger portion at bedtime.

Since improvement may be gradual, continued therapeutic response can be expected beyond the first month of treatment.
Maximum Dose: Occasionally, patients may require doses higher than 600 mg/day to obtain an acceptable therapeutic response. Because of the possibility of increased adverse reactions (particularly seizures) at daily doses of 600 mg and higher, the decision to treat in the range of 600-900 mg/day must be taken prudently. Patients must be given adequate time to respond to a given dose level before escalation to a higher dose is contemplated. **The maximum dose of 900 mg/day should not be exceeded.**
Maintenance Dose: After achieving maximum therapeutic benefit, many patients can be maintained effectively at lower doses. Careful downward titration is recommended to the level of 150-300 mg/day in divided doses. At daily doses not exceeding 200 mg, a single administration in the evening may be appropriate.
Discontinuation of Therapy: In the event of planned termination of GEN-CLOZAPINE therapy, gradual reduction in dose is recommended over a 1 to 2 week period. However, should a patient's medical condition require abrupt discontinuation (e.g. severe leukopenia, cardiovascular toxicity), the patient should be carefully observed for the recurrence of psychotic symptoms and symptoms related to cholinergic rebound such as headache, nausea, vomiting and diarrhea.
Re-Initiation of Treatment in Patients Previously Discontinued: **GEN-CLOZAPINE therapy must not be resumed in:**

- **Patients who have been discontinued from treatment due to neutropenia (ANC <1.5×10⁹/L) or severe leukopenia (WBC <2.0×10⁹/L, i.e. Non-rechallengeable Status)**
- **Patients with clozapine-induced myocarditis**

When restarting patients who have had even a brief interval off GEN-CLOZAPINE i.e. two days or more since the last dose, it is recommended that treatment be re-initiated with 12.5 mg (one half of a 25 mg tablet) once or twice on the first day (see Dosage for hematological testing conditions). If that dose is well tolerated, it may be feasible to titrate patients back to a therapeutic dose more quickly than is recommended for initial treatment.

Certain additional precautions seem prudent when re-initiating treatment. The mechanisms underlying some of the GEN-CLOZAPINE-induced adverse reactions are unknown. It is conceivable that re-exposure of a patient might enhance the risk of an untoward event's occurrence and increase its severity. Such phenomena, for example, occur when immune mediated mechanisms are responsible. Therefore, any patient who has previously experienced respiratory or cardiac arrest with initial dosing, but was then able to be successfully titrated to a therapeutic dose, should be re-titrated with extreme caution after even 24 hours of discontinuation.

INFORMATION FOR THE PATIENT: Published in e-CPS, available by subscription at www.e-cps.ca.

SUPPLIED: 25 mg: Each pale yellow, round, bevelled-edge tablet with 'cz'/25 on one side and G/G (pressure sensitive bisect) on the other side, contains: clozapine 25 mg. Nonmedicinal ingredients: colloidal silicon dioxide, corn starch, lactose monohydrate, magnesium stearate, povidone and talc. PVC/PVDC & foil unit dose strips in cartons of 100 tablets (10 tablets/blister strip × 10 blister strips). Bottles of 100 tablets. Store at room temperature (between 15 and 30°C).
50 mg: Each pale yellow, round, flat bevelled-edge tablet with "CZ"/50 on one side and G/G (pressure sensitive bisect) on the other side, contains: clozapine 50 mg. Nonmedicinal ingredients: colloidal silicon dioxide, corn starch, lactose monohydrate, magnesium stearate, povidone and talc. Bottles of 100 tablets. Store at room temperature (between 15 and 30°C).
100 mg: Each pale yellow, round, bevelled-edge tablet with 'cz'/100 on one side and G/G (pressure sensitive bisect) on the other side, contains: clozapine 100 mg. Nonmedicinal ingredients: colloidal silicon dioxide, corn starch, lactose monohydrate, magnesium stearate, povidone and talc. PVC/PVDC & foil unit dose strips in cartons of 100 tablets (10 tablets/blister strip × 10 blister strips). Bottles of 100 tablets. Store at room temperature (between 15 and 30°C).
200 mg: Each pale yellow, oblong, normal convex with "CZ"/200 on one side and G/G on the other side, contains: clozapine 200 mg. Nonmedicinal ingredients: colloidal silicon dioxide, corn starch, lactose monohydrate, magnesium stearate, povidone and talc. Bottles of 100 tablets. Store at room temperature (between 15 and 30°C).

GEN-CLOZAPINE is available only through a distribution system that requires weekly, every-two-week or every-four-week hematological testing prior to the delivery of the next period's supply of medication (see Indications).

Gentamicin Ⓟ
Antibacterial

CPhA Monograph

Date of Preparation: August 2006
Date of Revision: November 2007

> This monograph has been compiled by CPhA and reviewed by experts. It may contain information different from that found in Health Canada-approved Product Monographs. The reader is referred to the *CPS* Editorial Policy for more information.

SUMMARY PRODUCT INFORMATION:

Drug	Route of Administration	Dosage Form	Strength
Gentamicin	Injectable (IV, IM)	Solution	0.8 mg/mL (100 mL); 1 mg/mL (100 mL); 1.2 mg/mL (50 mL, 100 mL); 1.4 mg/mL (50 mL); 1.6 mg/mL (50 mL); 9 mg/mL (50 mL, 100 mL); 10 mg/mL (2 mL); 40 mg/mL (2 mL, 20 mL)
Gentamicin	Ophthalmic	Solution	0.3% (0.3 mL, 5 mL); 3 mg/mL (5 mL, 7.5 mL); 5 mg/mL (5 mL)
Gentamicin	Ophthalmic	Ointment	3 mg/g (3.5 g); 0.3% (3.5 g)
Gentamicin	Ophthalmic/Otic	Solution	1 mg/mL (7.5 mL); 3 mg/mL (7.5 mL)
Gentamicin	Otic	Solution	3 mg/mL (5 mL, 7.5 mL)
Gentamicin	Topical	Cream	1 mg/g (15 g); 0.1% (15 g, 450 g)
Gentamicin	Topical	Ointment	1 mg/g (15 g, 450 g); 0.1% (15 g)
Gentamicin	Orthopedic	Polymethylmethacrylate (PMMA) beads for surgical implantation	4.5 mg/bead (chains of 10 beads, 30 beads or 60 beads)

Drug	Route of Administration	Dosage Form	Strength
Gentamicin/ betamethasone	Topical	Cream	Gentamicin 0.1%/ betamethasone 0.1% (15 g, 30 g); gentamicin 1.67 mg/g plus betamethasone 0.64 mg/g (30 g)
Gentamicin/ betamethasone	Topical	Ointment	Gentamicin 0.1%/ betamethasone 0.1% (15 g, 30 g); gentamicin 1 mg/g plus betamethasone 1 mg/g (15 g, 30 g); Gentamicin 1.67 mg/g plus betamethasone 0.64 mg/g (30 g)
Gentamicin/ betamethasone	Ophthalmic	Ointment	Gentamicin 3 mg/g plus betamethasone 1 mg/g (3.5 g)

INDICATIONS AND CLINICAL USE: Gentamicin is an aminoglycoside antibacterial agent. The spectrum of activity of gentamicin includes primarily aerobic gram-negative bacteria including nosocomial pathogens. Gentamicin has some activity against aerobic, gram-positive cocci; however, when the drug is used in the setting of a gram-positive infection it is intended to complement the antibacterial activity of other agents such as ampicillin, penicillin or vancomycin.

Gentamicin is indicated for:

- treatment of uncomplicated or complicated urinary tract infections
- treatment of intra-abdominal infections in combination with other antibacterial agents
- treatment of pelvic inflammatory disease
- treatment of nosocomial infections due to susceptible aerobic gram-negative bacteria
- use in synergistic antibacterial combination regimens for treatment of certain pathogens, including:
  - use with ampicillin against *L. monocytogenes*
  - use with an extended spectrum penicillin against *P. aeruginosa* and susceptible Enterobacter species
  - use with doxycycline for brucellosis
  - treatment of endocarditis caused by viridans streptococci, staphylococci, or enterococci [*Circulation* 2005;111(23):e394-433]
- empiric treatment of infection in febrile neutropenic patients in combination with another agent
- use in combination with other antibacterial agents (i.e., ampicillin or cefotaxime) for empiric treatment of suspected bacterial meningitis in neonates
- prophylaxis of surgical site infections
- treatment of chronic recurrent osteomyelitis as an adjunct to surgical debridement (PMMA beads)
- topical treatment of superficial skin infections
- topical treatment of superficial eye infections
- topical treatment of otitis externa

Aminoglycosides are generally active against *P. aeruginosa*; however, gentamicin is considered to have 2 to 4 times less activity against this pathogen than tobramycin (on the basis of minimum inhibitory concentration). In contrast, gentamicin is preferred for synergistic use in combination with a beta-lactam for enterococcal infections, because tobramycin (and amikacin) is relatively inactive in this setting.

Among aerobic gram-negative bacteria, *S. maltophilia* and *B. cepacia* are unusual in that they are not considered to be susceptible to aminoglycosides.

Anaerobic bacteria are not susceptible to aminoglycosides.

Acquired resistance to aminoglycosides is mediated via numerous aminoglycoside-modifying enzymes produced by bacteria that alter specific amino or hydroxyl functions on the drug. Acquired resistance to one aminoglycoside does not necessarily confer resistance to other agents in the class.

Gentamicin is eliminated almost exclusively by renal excretion and is associated with nephrotoxicity. For this reason the drug must be used with caution and the dose must be individualized in patients with renal impairment. Monitoring of renal function (i.e., BUN and serum creatinine) is recommended during treatment.

Gentamicin is also associated with ototoxicity, which is usually not reversible. Some individuals are predisposed to aminoglycoside-associated ototoxicity because of a maternally inherited mutation in mitochondrial DNA that makes the human mitochondrial ribosome more closely resemble the bacterial ribosome, which is the site of action for these drugs [*BMJ* 2007;335(7624):784-5].

Geriatrics: Elderly patients may be more susceptible to aminoglycoside-associated nephrotoxicity due to the age-related decline in renal function. The dosage regimen of gentamicin must be tailored to renal function.

Pediatrics: Aminoglycoside antibiotics have been used extensively in pediatric patients including neonates. Changes in renal function during the neonatal period (see Warnings and Precautions, Special Populations, Pediatrics) must be considered when selecting a dosing regimen for gentamicin or another aminoglycoside antibiotic.

CONTRAINDICATIONS:

- Patients who are hypersensitive to gentamicin, or other aminoglycoside antibiotics, or to any ingredient in the formulation.

WARNINGS AND PRECAUTIONS:

Serious Warnings and Precautions

- Nephrotoxicity and ototoxicity are serious adverse effects associated with gentamicin and other aminoglycosides. These effects may be seen in any patient treated with these drugs, but are more likely to occur in the following settings: pre-existing renal, vestibular or auditory impairment, older individuals, dehydration, concomitant therapy with other nephrotoxic or ototoxic agents, or prolonged therapy.
- Neuromuscular blockade has been associated with aminoglycoside antibiotics.

Neurologic: Aminoglycosides are associated with eighth cranial nerve toxicity, which may affect the vestibular and the auditory senses. Symptoms of vestibular toxicity include nausea, vomiting, dizziness, nystagmus, vertigo and ataxia. Symptoms of cochlear (auditory) toxicity include tinnitus, roaring in the ears and hearing impairment. Loss of high frequency auditory perception, which may be detected by audiometric testing, usually precedes clinically detectable hearing loss. Some individuals have a genetic predisposition to aminoglycoside-induced ototoxicity. Ototoxicity has occurred within the recommended target serum concentration range. Patients receiving high cumulative doses of gentamicin or therapy for protracted periods are at increased risk of developing ototoxicity. In patients receiving protracted therapy, consideration should be given to performing regular audiograms (e.g., weekly) to detect signs of ototoxicity before it becomes clinically significant.

Neuromuscular blockade associated with aminoglycosides is dose-related and generally self-limiting, but may rarely lead to respiratory muscle paralysis. Clinical manifestations include flaccid paralysis, dilated pupils and weakness of the respiratory musculature. Neuromuscular effects occur more commonly after application to serosal surfaces (e.g., after intrapleural injection or peritoneal instillation), after administration to patients with neuromuscular disease (e.g., myasthenia gravis), hypocalcemia or hypomagnesemia, or after concomitant administration with neuromuscular blocking agents. Rapid injection of aminoglycoside antibiotics is a risk factor for neuromuscular blockade; therefore, these drugs should be infused over at least 30 minutes.

Perioperative Considerations: Aminoglycosides may produce neuromuscular blockade when used in combination with neuromuscular blocking agents (e.g., succinylcholine, tubocurarine).

Renal: Aminoglycosides are associated with renal tubular necrosis, which decreases the glomerular filtration rate and is reflected in increased concentrations of BUN and serum creatinine. Aminoglycoside-associated nephrotoxicity is most often evident as nonoliguric azotemia; oliguria is rare. Changes in renal function are usually reversible when the drug is discontinued.

Patient-related factors associated with an increased risk of aminoglycoside-associated nephrotoxicity include older age, pre-existing renal disease, volume depletion, hypotension, hepatic dysfunction and recent treatment with an aminoglycoside antibiotic. Concomitant administration of nephrotoxic drugs may increase the clinical risk of aminoglycoside-associated nephrotoxicity.

Factors that decrease the risk of aminoglycoside-associated nephrotoxicity include younger age, normal renal and hepatic function, use of smaller cumulative doses and treatment for less than 3 days, and use of extended interval ("once daily") dosing regimens (see Dosage and Administration).

Nephrotoxicity has occurred within the recommended target serum concentration range. Peak serum aminoglycoside levels are not a clinical risk factor for aminoglycoside-associated nephrotoxicity. In contrast, nephrotoxicity is associated with persistently elevated trough serum concentrations.

Special Populations: Pregnant Women: Gentamicin crosses the placenta and is distributed into the fetal circulation and amniotic fluid; it is not considered to be teratogenic and has been used to treat serious infections in pregnancy.

Nursing Women: Gentamicin is excreted in breast milk, but is considered to be compatible with breast-feeding because it is minimally absorbed from the gastrointestinal tract.

Pediatrics: Gentamicin is used extensively in the pediatric setting including treatment of suspected or confirmed infections in neonates. The pharmacokinetics of gentamicin differs in neonates compared with older children in that renal clearance of the drug is prolonged in infants. Specific dosage guidelines for neonates and children should be consulted.

Geriatrics: Elimination of gentamicin is prolonged in elderly patients because of the age-related decline in glomerular filtration rate. Renal function should be determined at baseline and monitored during therapy with gentamicin. Specific dosage guidelines should be consulted and the dosage regimen should be adjusted according to renal function.

Monitoring and Laboratory Tests: Renal function (BUN and serum creatinine) should be monitored before and during therapy with gentamicin.

When extended interval ("once daily") dosing (Table 6) of gentamicin is done with a dosing nomogram, it is often not necessary to monitor peak serum drug levels. However, some extended interval dosing protocols require measurement of the serum concentration.

It is necessary to measure serum drug concentrations and individualize the dose of gentamicin if achievement of specific peak and trough serum concentrations is desired. Some authors have argued that dose individualization is preferred to the use of dosing nomograms because of the wide interindividual variation in aminoglycoside pharmacokinetics [*Clin Pharmacokinet* 1999;36(2):89-98 and *Pharmacotherapy* 2002;22(9):1077-83].

If gentamicin is dosed in the conventional manner (Table 6), monitoring of peak and trough gentamicin serum levels is recommended in patients receiving prolonged courses of therapy, and in those with renal dysfunction or serious infections. Calculation of pharmacokinetic parameters is done with steady state versions of one-compartment equations. Serum concentrations should be measured at steady state, which is achieved after 3 to 5 half-lives have elapsed. If no loading dose is administered, steady state will usually be achieved after the third or fourth dose (this is also the case after each dose adjustment). Peak concentrations should be measured after the distribution phase is complete; ideally 30 to 60 minutes after the end of the infusion. Trough concentrations may be measured 30 minutes before infusion of the next dose. Specific target peak and trough concentrations are provided in Table 7. If a higher peak concentration is desired, the dose of gentamicin should be increased. If a lower trough concentration is desired, prolonging the dosing interval is preferred. Determination of peak and trough levels should be repeated after dosage adjustments to ensure the desired results have been obtained.

ADVERSE REACTIONS: More Common Adverse Drug Reactions: See Table 1.

Table 1: Gentamicin

More Common Adverse Drug Reactions (>1%)

Body System	Effect	Clinical Comment
Renal	Nephrotoxicity. Damage to proximal tubule marked by elevated BUN, elevated serum creatinine and decreased urine specific gravity. May involve proteinuria, nonoliguric azotemia, aminoaciduria and metabolic acidosis, electrolyte wasting and renal failure.	Monitor renal function at baseline and during treatment. Individualize dose based on renal function and adjust the dose based on changes in renal function and or serum drug levels. Consider alternative antibiotics in patients at risk.

Less Common Adverse Drug Reactions (<1%): Cardiovascular: tachycardia, hypotension, hypertension.

Central Nervous System: headache, dizziness, nystagmus, vertigo, ataxia, tinnitus, roaring in the ears, hearing impairment, loss of high frequency hearing perception.

Dermatologic: local irritation, phlebitis, rash, urticaria, stomatitis, pruritus, fever, toxic epidermal necrolysis, erythema multiforme, Stevens-Johnson syndrome. Hypersensitivity reactions are rare with aminoglycosides. Cross-allergenicity with aminoglycosides has been reported.

Gastrointestinal: anorexia, weight loss, nausea and vomiting.

Hematologic: anemia, leukopenia, granulocytopenia, thrombocytopenia.

Hepatic/Biliary/Pancreatic: hepatic necrosis, hepatomegaly, splenomegaly, transient increase in serum transaminase, alkaline phosphatase and bilirubin levels.

Neurologic: peripheral neuropathy, numbness, tingling, muscle twitching, seizures, myasthenia gravis-like syndrome, tremor.

Abnormal Hematologic and Clinical Chemistry Findings: See Table 2.

Table 2: Gentamicin

Abnormal Hematologic and Clinical Chemistry Findings

Test	Effect	Clinical Comment
BUN	Increased	An increase in BUN and serum creatinine over baseline is an indication of nephrotoxicity. In patients with a serum creatinine in the normal range before therapy, an increase to >133 µmol/L or an absolute increase of >35 µmol/L may indicate nephrotoxicity. In patients with a baseline serum creatinine concentration >133 µmol/L, an increase of >44 µmol/L is indicative of nephrotoxicity; in those with a baseline serum creatinine concentration >265 µmol/L, an increase of >88 µmol/L is indicative of nephrotoxicity. If nephrotoxicity occurs during treatment with gentamicin, the preferred strategy is discontinuation of the drug and substitution with an alternative non-nephrotoxic agent. If discontinuation is not possible, then the dosage should be adjusted accordingly and renal function monitored.
Serum creatinine	Increased	

DRUG INTERACTIONS:

Serious Drug Interactions

- Concomitant administration of nephrotoxic drugs may increase the clinical risk of aminoglycoside-associated nephrotoxicity.
- Concomitant administration of gentamicin with neuromuscular blocking agents may result in an increased risk of neuromuscular blockade.

Overview: Because potential drug interactions involving gentamicin generally involve combinations that result in additive nephrotoxicity or ototoxicity, it is best to avoid combined use of gentamicin with any agent that is known to be nephrotoxic or ototoxic. If combined use cannot be avoided, monitoring of renal function and serum gentamicin levels and adjustment of the dosage of gentamicin are recommended. Gentamicin does not alter the pharmacokinetics of other drugs.

Drug-Drug Interactions: See Table 3.

Table 3: Gentamicin

Drug-Drug Interactions

Interacting Drug	Effect	Clinical Comment
Amphotericin B	Additive nephrotoxicity	Monitor renal function and adjust the dose of gentamicin if BUN or SCr increases.
Botulinum toxin	Additive neuromuscular blockade	Avoid concurrent use. If given together, monitor respiratory function.

(cont'd)

Table 3: Gentamicin (cont'd)

Drug-Drug Interactions

Interacting Drug	Effect	Clinical Comment
Cisplatin	Additive nephrotoxicity	Monitor renal function and adjust the dose of gentamicin if BUN or SCr increases.
Cyclosporine	Additive nephrotoxicity	Monitor renal function and adjust the dose of gentamicin if BUN or SCr increases.
Ethacrynic acid	Additive ototoxicity	Avoid combination use. Monitor for signs and symptoms of ototoxicity.
Furosemide or bumetanide	Increased risk of nephrotoxicity or ototoxicity	Monitor renal function and adjust the dose of gentamicin if BUN or SCr increases. Monitor for signs of ototoxicity.
Indomethacin	Increased gentamicin serum levels in infants	Monitor renal function and serum levels of gentamicin and adjust the dose of gentamicin accordingly.
Neuromuscular blocking agents	Additive neuromuscular blockade	Monitor respiratory function. Provide supportive care if an interaction occurs. May respond to neostigmine.
Vancomycin	Additive nephrotoxicity	Monitor renal function and adjust the dose of gentamicin if BUN or SCr increases.

DOSAGE AND ADMINISTRATION: Dosing Considerations: Gentamicin may be administered by iv or im injection. In addition, commercial preparations are available for ophthalmic, otic, orthopedic and dermal application.

In contemporary clinical practice there are two broad strategies used to dose gentamicin. Extended interval ("once daily") administration involves administration of single large iv doses of gentamicin at prolonged intervals (i.e., 24 hours or longer). The alternative (conventional) approach involves administering lower doses of the drug at more frequent intervals (e.g., q8h) with monitoring of peak and trough serum concentrations.

Whichever strategy is used, the dose of gentamicin should be individualized according to patient weight and renal function. Specialized references for pediatric patients should be consulted when prescribing gentamicin for neonates or children.

Several sources of evidence suggest that extended interval iv administration of aminoglycosides may be less toxic than conventional three-times-daily administration. The principles underlying extended interval administration include concentration-dependent killing of susceptible bacteria, the post-antibiotic effect, and time-dependent nephrotoxicity and ototoxicity. High peak serum concentrations of aminoglycoside antibiotics are not associated with an increased incidence of adverse events. Thus, extended interval administration of aminoglycosides may be preferred to administration of multiple daily doses for some but not all indications.

Situations in which extended interval dosing of aminoglycosides should not be considered are presented in Table 5.

There are several protocols for extended interval dosing of aminoglycosides. One approach is presented in Table 6. The Hartford method is an alternative in which the dose of gentamicin is 7 mg/kg. The serum concentration is determined 6 to 14 hours after the start of an infusion and the measured serum level is plotted on the nomogram to determine the dosage interval [*Antimicrob Agents Chemother* 1995;39(3):650-5]. The Hartford nomogram and more information on the use of this method is available online at www.bugsanddrugs.ca.

Ophthalmic: For the treatment of superficial ophthalmologic infections caused by susceptible bacteria, 1 or 2 drops in the affected eye(s) 4 times daily for 5 days. In severe infections instil 2 drops per hour.

Alternatively, a strip of ointment may be placed in the affected eye(s) 2 or 3 times daily.

Otic: For the treatment of otitis externa caused by susceptible bacteria, 3 or 4 drops placed in the affected ear(s) 3 times daily for 7 days. Avoid use in the setting of perforated tympanic membrane.

Orthopedic: The number of gentamicin-containing PMMA beads to be placed is determined by the size of the wound. Up to 540 beads have been implanted without toxicity. The last bead of the chain(s) should be left protruding above the skin so that the chains can be withdrawn starting on the fourth or fifth day. Chains should be completely removed by the 10th to 14th day to avoid encapsulation by connective tissue.

Dermatologic: For superficial skin infections, apply cream (moist lesions) or ointment (dry lesions) to affected area 3 times daily. Not for use on burns.

Recommended Dose and Dosage Adjustments: See Table 4, Table 5, Table 6, Table 7, Table 8, Table 9 and Table 10.

Table 5: Gentamicin

Situations in which Extended Interval ("Once Daily") Dosing of Gentamicin is Not Recommended in Adults

Extensive burns (>20% body surface area)
Ascites (altered volume of distribution)
Pregnancy/postpartum (altered volume of distribution)
Patients with gram-positive infections for which gentamicin is used for synergy (exception: endocarditis due to viridans group streptococci)
Surgical prophylaxis

Table 4: Gentamicin

Indications and Recommended Regimens in Adults

Indication	Route	Recommended Regimen (see also Table 5, Table 6, Table 7, Table 8)	Duration of Treatment	Clinical Comment
Treatment of Acute Infection				
Urinary tract infections	IV/IM	Extended interval ("once daily") iv dosing Alternative: conventional divided daily dosing	Dependent upon susceptibility of organisms and response to therapy. For uncomplicated infections treat for a total of 3 to 7 days with parenteral and oral therapy. For complicated infections treat with parenteral and oral therapy for a total of 14 days.	Switch to a suitable oral antibiotic as soon as feasible. Administer with ampicillin or vancomycin to cover enterococci.
Intra-abdominal infection	IV/IM	Extended interval ("once daily") iv dosing Alternative: conventional divided daily dosing	Dependent upon susceptibility of organisms and response to therapy. A total of 10 to 14 days of parenteral and oral therapy may be necessary.	Not recommended as first-line therapy for uncomplicated infections. An aminoglycoside is indicated when: resistant gram-negative bacteria are suspected to be involved; a broad spectrum antibiotic has been used in the last month; prolonged hospitalization preceded the onset of infection. Administer in combination with other agents to ensure broad spectrum coverage. Switch to a suitable oral antibiotic as soon as feasible.
Endocarditis	IV/IM	3 mg/kg per 24 h administered either extended interval or in 2 or 3 divided doses (if normal renal function) in combination with other antimicrobial agents as per current recommendations.	Dependent upon the identity and susceptibility of the organisms and response to therapy. Consult current guidelines for duration of therapy [*Circulation* 2005;111(23):e394-434].	Extended interval dosing is recommended only for viridans group streptococci [*Circulation* 2005;111(23):e394-434]. Monitor renal function.
Pelvic inflammatory disease	IV/IM	Extended interval ("once daily") iv dosing Alternative: conventional divided daily dosing	Dependent upon susceptibility of organisms and response to therapy. Continue iv antibiotics until defervescence then administer oral antibiotics to complete 14 days of therapy.	Administer in combination with an agent with anaerobic activity (e.g., clindamycin).
Tularemia	IV/IM	Extended interval ("once daily") iv dosing Alternative: conventional divided daily dosing	10 to 14 days	Alternative to streptomycin
Plague	IV/IM	Extended interval ("once daily") iv dosing Alternative: conventional divided daily dosing	10 to 14 days	Alternative to streptomycin
Empiric treatment of febrile neutropenic patients	IV/IM	Extended interval ("once daily") iv dosing Alternative: conventional divided daily dosing	Dependent upon susceptibility of organisms and response to therapy.	Administer in combination with a broad spectrum antipseudomonal agent (i.e., cephalosporin, antipseudomonal penicillin, carbapenem). Monitor renal function and adjust dosage (as per Table 8 recommendations).
Prophylaxis of Infection				
Surgical Prophylaxis (30 minutes to 1 hour prior to incision)				
Biliary tract surgery in high-risk patients (>60 yr, obstructive jaundice, acute cholecystitis, cholangitis, common duct stone, previous biliary surgery, nonfunctioning gall bladder)	IV	1.7 mg/kg q8h × 1 or 2 doses	1 or 2 doses	As an alternative to cefazolin
Gastrointestinal procedures	IV	1.7 mg/kg q8h × 1 or 2 doses	1 or 2 doses	Give in combination with metronidazole 500 mg iv (other regimens are also used).

Table 6: Gentamicin

Extended Interval ("Once Daily") Administration in Adults[a]

Estimated ClCr (mL/min)[b]	Dosage Interval (h)	Dose (mg/kg IBW)[c]
100	24	5.0
90	24	5.0
80	24	5.0
70	24	4.0
60	24	4.0
50	24	3.5
40	24	2.5
30	24	2.5
20	48	4.0
10	48	3.0
Hemodialysis	48 (give after dialysis)	2.0

[a] Measure trough level prior to third dose. Desired trough level is <1 µg/mL.
[b] ClCr=creatinine clearance (estimate using Cockcroft-Gault equation).

$$\text{ClCr (mL/min)} = \frac{1.2\ (140\text{–age})\ (\text{wt in kg})}{\text{serum creatinine (µmol/L)}}$$

For females, multiply result by 0.85.
[c] IBW = ideal body weight.
IBW (kg; males) = 50 + (2.3 × height in inches over 5 feet).
IBW (kg; females) = 45.5 + (2.3 × height in inches over 5 feet).
Adjusted body weight (ABW) has been recommended for dosing aminoglycosides in obese individuals (i.e. if total body weight is >25% above the IBW [*Br J Clin Pharmacol* 2004;58(2):119-33 and *Antimicrob Agents Chemother* 1995;39(2):545-8].
ABW=IBW + 0.4 × (total body weight–IBW).

Table 7: Gentamicin

Conventional Dosing in Adults with ClCr >90 mL/min (as an alternative to extended interval dosing)

Route	Loading Dose	Maintenance Dose	Desired Serum Concentration	
			Peak	Trough
IV/IM	2.0 mg/kg (IBW[a])	1.7 mg/kg (IBW[a]) q8h	5–10 µg/mL	0.5–2 µg/mL
Peak concentration is measured 30 to 60 minutes after infusion to allow for distribution. Trough concentration is measured ≤30 minutes prior to infusion of the next dose.				

[a] IBW = ideal body weight.
IBW (kg; males) = 50 + (2.3 × height in inches over 5 feet).
IBW (kg; females) = 45.5 + (2.3 × height in inches over 5 feet).
Adjusted body weight (ABW) has been recommended for dosing aminoglycosides in obese individuals (i.e. if total body weight is >25% above the IBW [*Br J Clin Pharmacol* 2004;58(2):119-33 and *Antimicrob Agents Chemother* 1995;39(2):545-8].
ABW=IBW + 0.4 × (total body weight–IBW).

Table 8: Gentamicin

Conventional Dose in Adults with Renal Dysfunction (as an alternative to extended interval dosing)

Route	ClCr[a] (mL/min)	Dose	Clinical Comment
IV/IM	>50–90	60–90% of recommended dose q8–12h (see Table 7)	Monitor serum concentration and adjust dosage regimen to achieve desired peak and trough serum levels.
IV/IM	10–50	30–70% of recommended dose q12h (see Table 7)	
IV/IM	<10	20–30% of recommended dose q24–48h (see Table 7)	
IV/IM	Hemodialysis	Dose as for ClCr <10 mL/min; give supplemental 1/2 dose after dialysis	

[a] ClCr=creatinine clearance (estimate using Cockcroft-Gault equation).

$$\text{ClCr (mL/min)} = \frac{1.2\ (140\text{–age})\ (\text{wt in kg})}{\text{serum creatinine (µmol/L)}}$$

For females, multiply result by 0.85.

Dosage in Continuous Ambulatory Peritoneal Dialysis: In adult patients receiving continuous ambulatory peritoneal dialysis it is estimated that 3 to 4 mg of gentamicin will be lost per litre of dialysate each day. The drug lost in dialysate may be replaced intravenously. Thus in a patient receiving 8 L of dialysate per day a total of 24 to 32 mg will be lost daily and may be replaced intravenously.

Gentamicin may be added directly to peritoneal dialysis fluid for the treatment of peritonitis. In patients receiving continuous ambulatory peritoneal dialysis the recommended dose of gentamicin is 0.6 mg/kg in one exchange per day. In patients receiving automated peritoneal dialysis a loading dose of 1.5 mg/kg on day 1 is followed by 0.5 mg/kg once daily added to the first or second ambulatory dwell. The duration of treatment is determined by the clinical response. Systemic toxicity can occur when gentamicin is given by the intraperitoneal route. Thus patients should be closely monitored.

Dosage in Hemodialysis: See Table 6 and Table 8.

Hepatic Impairment: Gentamicin is not eliminated by hepatic metabolism; hence no dosage adjustments are required in patients with hepatic dysfunction. However, patients with severe hepatic dysfunction are at increased risk of nephrotoxicity, and careful monitoring of renal function is advised in these individuals.

Pediatrics: Regimens recommended in the SickKids Drug Handbook and Formulary 2007-2008 are presented in Table 9 for neonates and inTable 10 for older infants and children.

There have been numerous studies of extended interval dosing of aminoglycosides in children. A meta-analysis of 24 studies concluded that this approach simplifies administration and provides similar or better efficacy and safety compared with conventional multiple daily dose regimens [*Pediatrics* 2004;114(1):e111-8]. Gentamicin was administered at dosages ranging from 4 to 7.5 mg/kg once daily in the studies that were considered in the analysis.

Table 9: Gentamicin

Dose in Neonates

Route	Age and Weight	Dose
IV	Neonates ≤7 days (PCA <34 weeks)[a]	3 mg/kg/dose q24h
IV	Neonates ≤7 days (PCA ≥34 weeks)[a]	3 mg/kg/dose q18h
IV	Neonates >7 days and ≤1 kg[a]	3.5 mg/kg/dose q24h
IV	Neonates >7 days (PCA <37 weeks) and >1 kg[a]	2.5 mg/kg/dose q12h
IV	Neonates >7 days (PCA ≥37 weeks) and >1 kg[a]	2.5 mg/kg/dose q8h
The peak concentration is measured 30 to 60 minutes after infusion to allow for distribution. The desired peak is 5–9 µg/mL. The trough concentration is measured 30 minutes prior to infusion of the next dose. The desired trough level is 0.5–2 µg/mL.		

[a] Applies to neonates until a PCA of >38 weeks and a postnatal age of 28 days is achieved [*SickKids Drug Handbook and Formulary* 2007-2008].
Abbreviations: PCA=postconceptional age.

Table 10: Gentamicin

Dose in Pediatric Patients

Route	Age and Weight	Dose
IM/IV	Infants >28 days and children	7.5 mg/kg/day divided q8h (maximum 120 mg/dose prior to measuring serum levels)
IV	Infants and children >28 days and <9 years[a]	10 mg/kg/day q24h (no dose limit)
IV	Children 9 to <12 years[a]	8 mg/kg/day q24h (no dose limit)
IV	Adolescents ≥12 years[a]	6 mg/kg/day q24h (no dose limit)
If given q8h the peak concentration is measured 30 to 60 minutes after infusion to allow for distribution. The desired peak is 5–9 µg/mL. If given q8h the trough concentration is measured 30 minutes prior to infusion of the next dose. The desired trough level is 0.5–2 µg/mL.		

[a] This regimen is used in hematology and oncology patients and in recipients of hematopoietic progenitor cell transplants with fever and neutropenia [*SickKids Drug Handbook and Formulary* 2007-2008].

Administration: Gentamicin may be administered by iv or im injection. It is impractical to administer large injection volumes, such as those required in extended interval regimens, by im injection. When large doses are given by iv infusion the drug should be infused over at least 30 minutes to minimize the possibility of neuromuscular blockade.

OVERDOSAGE:

For management of a suspected drug overdose, CPhA recommends that you contact your **regional Poison Control Centre**. See the *CPS* Directory section for a list of Poison Control Centres.

ACTION AND CLINICAL PHARMACOLOGY: Mechanism of Action: Gentamicin is highly water soluble, a property that limits its ability to cross lipid-rich cellular membranes. The drug is also positively charged, such that activity is enhanced at alkaline pH and decreased at acidic pH. Transport of aminoglycosides across bacterial cytoplasmic membranes is an energy-dependent process. Gentamicin binds to the 30S subunit of prokaryotic ribosomes. This results in a conformational change in the structure of the ribosomal subunit and impairs messenger RNA translation and translocation. The drug also binds electrostatically to the lipopolysaccharide layer of gram-negative bacteria, an effect that ultimately disrupts the permeability of the bacterial cell wall.

Aminoglycosides are bactericidal antibiotics that are characterized by concentration-dependent killing of susceptible bacteria. As the rate of killing increases in proportion to the serum concentration, achievement of higher serum concentrations may enhance efficacy. This phenomenon contributes to the rationale for extended interval dosing regimens.

Aminoglycosides are associated with a significant post-antibiotic effect. This phenomenon results in persistent suppression of bacterial growth after exposure to the antibiotic. The duration of the post-antibiotic effect is prolonged after exposure to high drug concentrations and persists after the concentration falls below the minimal inhibitory concentration of the organism. The post-antibiotic effect also contributes to the rationale for extended interval dosing of aminoglycosides.

The uptake of aminoglycosides by gram-positive cocci is enhanced by concomitant exposure to cell-wall active agents, a phenomenon which forms the basis for the clinical use of aminoglycosides and penicillins as a synergistic combination against certain pathogens.

The antibacterial efficacy of aminoglycosides is not affected by the size of the inoculum.

Pharmacokinetics: Adults: Absorption: Aminoglycosides are minimally absorbed from the gastrointestinal tract and thus must be administered intravenously or intramuscularly in order to treat systemic infections. When administered as a 1 mg/kg im dose, gentamicin was completely absorbed with maximal serum concentrations of 4.0 to 7.6 µg/mL occurring within 30 to 90 minutes of injection. Absorption may be delayed in patients with hypotension or poor tissue perfusion.

Topical administration on inflamed skin results in minimal absorption. In contrast, substantial amounts of drug may be absorbed into the systemic circulation when aminoglycosides are applied topically to patients with extensive burns.

Aminoglycoside antibiotics are rapidly absorbed into the systemic circulation after instillation into the peritoneal cavity or the pleural space. In contrast, detectable serum concentrations are not achieved after inhalation or bladder irrigation.

Serum levels of gentamicin did not exceed 1 µg/mL within 24 hours after surgical implantation of gentamicin 4.5 mg beads.

Distribution: Aminoglycoside antibiotics are minimally bound to plasma proteins (~10%) and, given their high water solubility, are distributed in the vascular space and interstices of most tissues. Drug concentrations in interstitial fluids at steady state approximate those of plasma. The volume of distribution is typically on the order of 0.2 to 0.3 L/kg. However, the volume of distribution increases in certain clinical situations including extensive burns, ascites, pregnancy and the postpartum state.

Aminoglycosides accumulate in the cells of the proximal convoluted tubule to concentrations that exceed those in plasma. Nephrotoxicity is probably due to time-dependent accumulation of drug within cells of the proximal convoluted tubule. Thus, minimizing exposure to the drug, as with extended interval administration, may minimize the risk of nephrotoxicity. This reasoning supports the concept of extended interval administration of aminoglycosides.

Concentrations of aminoglycosides in vitreous humor are approximately 40% of serum levels. Aminoglycosides have poor penetration across the blood-brain barrier and into bronchial secretions, the biliary tract and abscesses.

Gentamicin crosses the placenta and is distributed into fetal circulation and amniotic fluid. Gentamicin is excreted in breast milk and achieves detectable levels in the circulation of breast-fed infants.

Excretion: Gentamicin is not metabolized, but rather is eliminated almost exclusively (~99%) by renal excretion. In adults and infants over the age of 6 months with normal renal function, the elimination half-life of gentamicin typically ranges from 1.5 to 3.5 hours. In adults with normal renal function, >90% of an administered dose is recoverable in urine within 24 hours.

The elimination half-life may be shortened in patients with febrile conditions and is prolonged in elderly patients and in those with renal dysfunction in proportion to the extent of the impairment in glomerular filtration rate.

Special Populations: Pediatrics: The elimination half-life of aminoglycoside antibiotics is prolonged in neonates. In low birth-weight infants and premature neonates the half-life may be as long as 8 to 11 hours. In neonates weighing >2 kg the elimination half-life may be around 5 hours. Specific dosing guidelines should be consulted when prescribing gentamicin for newborns.
Geriatrics: Due to the age-related decline in glomerular filtration rate, the terminal elimination half-life of gentamicin is prolonged in elderly patients. The dose must be individualized according to renal function.

Gentamicin Injection USP Pr

gentamicin sulfate

Antibiotic

Sandoz

SUPPLIED: 10 mg/mL: Each mL contains: gentamicin (as sulfate) 10 mg. Nonmedicinal ingredients: disodium edetate, sodium bisulfite, sodium hydroxide and/or sulfuric acid to adjust pH and water for injection. Single use vials of 2 mL, boxes of 10. Store between 15 and 30°C. Protect from light. Discard unused portion.
40 mg/mL: Each mL contains: gentamicin (as sulfate) 40 mg. Nonmedicinal ingredients: disodium edetate, methylparaben, propylparaben, sodium bisulfite, sodium hydroxide and/or sulfuric acid to adjust pH and water for injection. Multidose vials of 2 mL, boxes of 10. Multidose vials of 20 mL, boxes of 1. Discard 28 days after initial use. Store between 15 and 30°C. Protect from light.

Gentamicin Sulfate in 0.9% Sodium Chloride Injection Pr

gentamicin sulfate—sodium chloride

Antibiotic

Hospira

SUPPLIED: Each flexible (PVC) container of sterile nonpyrogenic solution contains: gentamicin (as sulfate) 0.8 mg/mL (80 mg/100 mL) in 0.9% sodium chloride injection. May contain sulfuric acid and sodium hydroxide for pH adjustment. Also contains water for injection. The pH is approximately 4 and the osmolarity is approximately 284 mOsm/L. Store at controlled room temperature (20 to 25°C). Avoid excessive heat. Protect from freezing.

Flexible containers contain no preservative, and are intended only for use as a single dose injection. Unused portion must be discarded.

Parenteral drug products should be inspected visually for particulate matter and discoloration prior to administration, whenever solution and container permit. Note: Gentamicin Sulfate should not be physically mixed with other drugs (except, Normal saline and 5% Dextrose injection) to avoid chemical incompatibilities.

Cautions: **Do not use** in series connections. **Do not** administer unless solution is clear and container undamaged.

Gentamicin Sulfate Injection in 0.9% Sodium Chloride Pr

gentamicin sulfate—sodium chloride

Antibiotic

Baxter

SUPPLIED: Each mL of sterile, isotonic solution contains: gentamicin sulfate in 0.9% sodium chloride. Viaflex Plus plastic (polyvinyl chloride) containers in the following sizes and concentrations: see Table 1.

Table 1: Gentamicin Sulfate Injection in 0.9% Sodium Chloride Supplied

Total Volume (mL)	Total Gentamicin Sulfate Content (mg)	Gentamicin Sulfate Concentration (mg/mL)
50	60	1.2
50	80	1.6
100	100	1
100	120	1.2

pH ranges from 3 to 5.5. Store at controlled room temperature 15 to 30°C.

Genteal®

hypromellose

Artificial Tears

Novartis Pharmaceuticals

SUPPLIED: Eye Drops: Each bottle contains: hypromellose 3 mg/g. Nonmedicinal ingredients: boric acid, GenAqua (sodium perborate) as preservative, phosphonic acid, potassium chloride, purified water, sodium chloride and sodium hydroxide and/or hydrochloric acid (to adjust pH). Dropper-tipped, plastic squeeze bottles of 15 and 25 mL. Store at controlled room temperature (15 to 30°C).
Gel: Each tube contains: hypromellose 3 mg/g (0.3% w/v). Nonmedicinal ingredients: carbopol 980, GenAqua (sodium perborate) as preservative, phosphonic acid, purified water and sorbitol. Dropper-tipped, plastic squeeze tubes of 10 mL. Store between 15 and 30°C.

Genteal® Gel Drops

hypromellose—carboxymethylcellulose sodium

Artificial Tears

Novartis Pharmaceuticals

SUPPLIED: Each bottle contains: hypromellose 0.3% (w/v), carboxymethylcellulose sodium 0.25% (w/v). Nonmedicinal ingredients: boric acid, calcium chloride dihydrate, citric acid monohydrate, magnesium chloride hexahydrate, phosphonic acid, potassium chloride, purified water, sodium chloride and GenAqua (sodium perborate) added as a preservative. Dropper-tipped, plastic squeeze bottles of 15 mL solution. Store between 15 and 30°C.

Glaxal® Base

dermatological preparation

Dermatological Base—Moisturizer

WellSpring

SUPPLIED: Cream: Ingredients: aqua, petrolatum, cetearyl alcohol, paraffinum liquidum, ceteareth-20, sodium phosphate, p-chloro-m-cresol. Tubes of 50 g. Jars of 100 and 450 g.
Lotion: Ingredients: aqua, propylene glycol, paraffinum liquidum, petrolatum, cetearyl alcohol, hydroxyethylcellulose, carbomer, ceteareth-20, p-chloro-m-cresol, sodium hydroxide. Tubes of 100 and 227 g.
Lotion with Vitamin E: Ingredients: aqua, propylene glycol, paraffinum liquidum, petrolatum, cetearyl alcohol, hydroxyethylcellulose, carbomer, ceteareth-20, p-chloro-m-cresol, sodium hydroxide, tocopheryl acetate. Tubes of 227 g.

Gleevec® Pr

imatinib mesylate

Protein Kinase Inhibitor

Novartis Pharmaceuticals

Date of Preparation: September 19, 2001
Date of Revision: June 17, 2010

GLEEVEC, indicated for:
- the treatment of pediatric patients with newly diagnosed, Philadelphia chromosome-positive, chronic myeloid leukemia (CML) in chronic phase.
- the treatment of adult patients with Kit (CD117) positive unresectable and/or metastatic malignant gastrointestinal stromal tumours (GIST).
- the adjuvant treatment of adult patients who are at intermediate to high risk of relapse following complete resection of Kit (CD117) positive GIST.

has been issued marketing authorization with conditions, pending the results of studies to verify its clinical benefit. Patients should be advised of the nature of the authorization.
GLEEVEC has been issued non-conditional approval for the indications of:
- adult patients with newly diagnosed, Philadelphia-chromosome-positive, chronic myeloid leukemia (CML) in chronic phase.
- adult patients with Philadelphia chromosome-positive CML in blast crisis, accelerated phase or chronic phase (after failure of interferon-alpha therapy).
- for use as a single agent for induction phase therapy in adult patients with newly diagnosed Philadelphia chromosome-positive acute lymphoblastic leukemia (Ph+ALL).
- adult patients with relapsed or refractory Ph+ ALL as monotherapy.
- adult patients with myelodysplastic/myeloproliferative diseases (MDS/MPD) associated with platelet-derived growth factor receptor (PDGFR) gene re-arrangements.
- adult patients with aggressive sub-types of systemic mastocytosis (ASM and SM-AHNMD*) without the D816V c-Kit mutation. If c-Kit mutational status in patients with ASM or SM-AHNMD* is not known or unavailable, treatment with GLEEVEC may be considered if there is no satisfactory response to other therapies.
- adult patients with advanced hypereosinophilic syndrome (HES) and/or chronic eosinophilic leukemia (CEL) with FIP1L1-PDGFRα rearrangement.
- adult patients with unresectable, recurrent and/or metastatic dermatofibrosarcoma protuberans (DFSP).

SUMMARY PRODUCT INFORMATION:

Route of Administration	Dosage Form/ Strength	Clinically Relevant Nonmedicinal Ingredients
Oral	Tablets 100 mg and 400 mg	Coating: ferric oxide (red), ferric oxide (yellow) For a complete listing see Dosage Forms, Composition and Packaging.

INDICATIONS AND CLINICAL USE:
- GLEEVEC (imatinib mesylate) is indicated for the treatment of adult patients with newly diagnosed, Philadelphia chromosome-positive, chronic myeloid leukemia (CML) in chronic phase.
  Non-conditional approval in newly diagnosed CML, was based on hematologic and cytogenetic response rates (surrogate endpoints) that are reasonably likely to predict clinical benefit.
- GLEEVEC (imatinib mesylate) is indicated for the treatment of pediatric patients with newly diagnosed, Philadelphia chromosome-positive, chronic myeloid leukemia (CML) in chronic phase.
  Conditional approval in newly diagnosed CML, was based on hematologic and cytogenetic response rates (surrogate endpoints) that are reasonably likely to predict clinical benefit. There are no controlled trials that demonstrate clinical benefit in pediatric patients.
- GLEEVEC is also indicated for the treatment of adult patients with Philadelphia chromosome-positive chronic myeloid leukemia (CML) in blast crisis, accelerated phase, or in chronic phase (after failure of interferon-alpha therapy).
  Non-conditional approval in Philadelphia chromosome-positive chronic myeloid leukemia in blast crisis, accelerated phase or chronic phase (after failure of interferon-alpha therapy) was based on hematologic and cytogenetic response rates (surrogate endpoints), which have shown to be sustained for at least two years.
- GLEEVEC is also indicated for use as a single agent for induction phase therapy in adult patients with newly diagnosed Philadelphia chromosome-positive acute lymphoblastic leukemia (Ph+ALL).
  Non-conditional approval for use as a single agent for induction phase therapy in adult patients with newly diagnosed Philadelphia chromosome-positive acute lymphoblastic leukemia (Ph+ALL) was based on hematologic response rates (surrogate endpoints).
- GLEEVEC is also indicated for the treatment of adult patients with relapsed or refractory Ph+ ALL as monotherapy.
  Non-conditional approval in adult patients with relapsed or refractory Ph+ ALL as monotherapy was based on hematologic and cytogenetic response rates (surrogate endpoints).
- GLEEVEC is also indicated for the treatment of adult patients with myelodysplastic/myeloproliferative diseases (MDS/MPD) associated with platelet-derived growth factor receptor (PDGFR) gene re-arrangements.
  Non-conditional approval in adult patients with myelodysplastic/myeloproliferative diseases (MDS/MPD) associated with platelet-derived growth factor receptor (PDGFR) gene re-arrangements was based on hematologic and cytogenetic response rates (surrogate endpoints).
- GLEEVEC is also indicated for the treatment of adult patients with aggressive sub-types of systemic mastocytosis (ASM and SM-AHNMD*) without the D816V c-Kit mutation. If c-Kit mutational status in patients with ASM or SM-AHNMD* is not known or unavailable, treatment with GLEEVEC may be considered if there is no satisfactorily response to other therapies.
  Non-conditional approval in adult patients with aggressive sub-types of systemic mastocytosis (ASM and SM-AHNMD*) without the D816V c-Kit mutation and in adult patients with ASM or SM-AHNMD* where c-Kit mutational status is not known or unavailable, and if there is no satisfactory response to other therapies was based on hematologic response rates (surrogate endpoints).
- GLEEVEC is also indicated for the treatment of adult patients with advanced hypereosinophilic syndrome (HES) and/or chronic eosinophilic leukemia (CEL) with FIP1L1-PDGFRα rearrangement.
  Non-conditional approval in adult patients with advanced hypereosinophilic syndrome (HES) and/or chronic eosinophilic leukemia (CEL) with FIP1L1-PDGFRα rearrangement was based on hematologic and cytogenetic response rates (surrogate endpoints).
- GLEEVEC is also indicated for the treatment of adult patients with unresectable, recurrent and/or metastatic dermatofibrosarcoma protuberans (DFSP).

* ASM: Aggressive systemic mastocytosis; SM-AHNMD: Systemic mastocytosis with an associated clonal hematological non-mast-cell disorder.

Non-conditional approval in adult patients with unresectable, recurrent and/or metastatic dermatofibrosarcoma protuberans (DFSP) was based on objective response rate (surrogate endpoints).

- GLEEVEC is also indicated for the treatment of adult patients with Kit (CD117) positive unresectable and/or metastatic malignant gastrointestinal stromal tumors (GIST).

Conditional approval in gastrointestinal stromal tumors (GIST) was based on objective response rates (surrogate endpoints) that are reasonably likely to predict clinical benefit. There are no controlled trials demonstrating clinical benefit such as improvement in disease-related symptoms or increased survival.

- GLEEVEC is also indicated for the adjuvant treatment of adult patients who are at intermediate to high risk of relapse following complete resection of Kit (CD117) positive GIST.

Conditional approval in the adjuvant GIST indication was based on recurrence free survival after one year of adjuvant therapy. The optimal treatment duration with GLEEVEC is not known. Overall survival data are not available.

CONTRAINDICATIONS: GLEEVEC (imatinib mesylate) is contraindicated in patients with hypersensitivity to imatinib or to any other component of GLEEVEC.

WARNINGS AND PRECAUTIONS:

Serious Warnings and Precautions

- Severe congestive heart failure (CHF) and reduction of left ventricular ejection fraction (LVEF) have been observed (see Warnings and Precautions, Cardiovascular).
- Rhabdomyolysis has been rarely observed (see Adverse Reactions, Post-Market Adverse Drug Reactions).
- Severe hemorrhages may occur (see Warnings and Precautions, Hemorrhage).
- Fluid retention may occur (see Warnings and Precautions, Fluid Retention and Edema).
- Liver failure (in some cases, fatal) may occur (see Warnings and Precautions, Hepatic/Biliary/Pancreatic).
- Gastrointestinal perforation (in some cases, fatal) may occur (see Warnings and Precautions, Gastrointestinal).

GLEEVEC should only be administered under the supervision of a physician experienced with the use of chemotherapy and with treatment of hematological malignancies and/or malignant sarcomas including gastrointestinal stromal tumors (GISTs) and dermatofibrosarcoma protuberans (DFSP).

Carcinogenesis and Mutagenesis: A 2-year preclinical carcinogenicity study conducted in rats demonstrated renal adenomas/carcinomas, urinary bladder and urethra papillomas, papillomas/carcinomas of the preputial and clitoral gland, adenocarcinomas of the small intestine, adenomas of the parathyroid glands, benign and malignant tumors of the adrenal medulla and papillomas/carcinomas of the nonglandular stomach.

Long-term, non-neoplastic histological changes identified in the preclinical carcinogenicity study in rats include cardiomyopathy.

The relevance of these findings in the rat carcinogenicity study for humans is not known. An analysis of the clinical safety data from clinical trials and spontaneous adverse event reports did not provide evidence of an increased overall incidence of malignancies in patients treated with imatinib mesylate compared to that of the general population.

However, adverse events in cancer patients are significantly under reported and a large proportion of patients treated with GLEEVEC have had limited follow-up thus not permitting a final analysis of the potential for an increased incidence of a secondary malignancy in patients treated with GLEEVEC.

Cardiovascular: Severe congestive heart failure (CHF) and reduction of left ventricular ejection fraction (LVEF) have been reported in patients taking GLEEVEC. Although several of these patients had pre-existing conditions including hypertension, diabetes and prior coronary artery disease, they were subsequently diagnosed with CHF. Patients with known cardiac disease or risk factors for cardiac failure should be monitored carefully and those with symptoms or signs consistent with CHF should be evaluated and treated. In patients with history of cardiac disease or in elderly patients, a baseline evaluation of LVEF is recommended prior to initiation of GLEEVEC therapy.

In patients with hypereosinophilic syndrome (HES) and cardiac involvement, isolated cases of cardiogenic shock/left ventricular dysfunction have been associated with the initiation of GLEEVEC therapy. The condition was reported to be reversible with the administration of systemic steroids, circulatory support measures and temporarily withholding GLEEVEC. Myelodysplastic/myeloproliferative diseases (MDS/MPD) and systemic mastocytosis (SM) might be associated with high eosinophil levels. Performance of an echocardiogram and determination of serum troponin should therefore be considered in patients with HES/CEL and in patients with MDS/MPD or ASM and SM-AHNMD associated with high eosinophil levels. These patients with HES/CEL or ASM, SM-AHNMD and MDS/MPD must be also on 1- to 2 mg/kg of prednisone equivalent oral steroids for one to two weeks, initiated at least 2 days prior to beginning GLEEVEC therapy.

Endocrine and Metabolism: Clinical cases of hypothyroidism have been reported in thyroidectomy patients undergoing levothyroxine replacement during treatment with GLEEVEC. Thyroid-Stimulating Hormone (TSH) levels should be closely monitored in such patients.

Fluid Retention and Edema: GLEEVEC (imatinib mesylate) is often associated with edema and occasionally serious fluid retention (see Adverse Reactions Table 1 and Table 2). All Grades of fluid retention/edema were reported in up to 61.7% for newly diagnosed CML patients, up to 76.2% for other CML patients across all clinical trials, and up to 80.3% for GIST patients. Patients should be weighed and monitored regularly for signs and symptoms of fluid retention as fluid retention can occur after months of treatment. An unexpected rapid weight gain should be carefully investigated and appropriate treatment provided. The probability of edema was increased with higher imatinib dose and age >65 years. Severe superficial edema was reported in 1.5% of newly diagnosed CML patients taking GLEEVEC and in 2.1% to 5.8% of other adult CML patients taking GLEEVEC. In addition, other severe fluid retention events (e.g., pleural effusion, pericardial effusion, pulmonary edema, and ascites) were reported in 1.3% of newly diagnosed CML patients taking GLEEVEC and in 1.7% to 6.2% of other adult CML patients taking GLEEVEC.

Gastrointestinal: Hemorrhage: See Hemorrhage.

GLEEVEC is sometimes associated with GI irritation. GLEEVEC should be taken with food and a large glass of water to minimize this problem. There have been rare reports, including fatalities, of gastrointestinal perforation.

Hematologic: Hematologic Toxicity: Treatment with GLEEVEC is often associated with neutropenia or thrombocytopenia (see Adverse Reactions, Table 8, Table 9, Table 10 and Table 11). Complete blood counts should be performed weekly for the first month, biweekly for the second month, and periodically thereafter as clinically indicated (for example every 2-3 months). The occurrence of these cytopenias is dependent on the stage of disease and is more frequent in patients with accelerated phase CML or blast crisis than in patients with chronic phase CML. In pediatric CML patients the most frequent toxicities observed were Grade 3 or 4 cytopenias involving neutropenia (31%), thrombocytopenia (16%) and anemia (14%). These generally occur within the first several months of therapy (see Dosage and Administration).

An increased rate of opportunistic infections was observed in a monkey study with chronic imatinib treatment. In a 39-week monkey study, treatment with imatinib resulted in worsening of normally suppressed malarial infections in these animals. Lymphopenia was observed in animals (as in humans, where all grades of lymphopenia were observed in 0.3% patients).

Hemorrhage: All Grades of hemorrhage were reported in up to 28.9% for newly diagnosed CML patients, up to 53% for other CML patients across all clinical trials, and up to 29.9% for GIST patients.

In the newly diagnosed CML trial, 1.8% of patients had Grades 3/4 hemorrhage. In the unresectable and/or metastatic malignant GIST clinical trial (B2222) eight patients (5.4%, five patients in the 600 mg dose group and three patients in the 400 mg dose group) were reported to have had gastrointestinal (GI) bleeds or intra-tumoral bleeds. Four patients with intra-tumoral bleeds had either intra-abdominal or intra-hepatic, depending on the anatomical location of the tumor lesions. One patient, who had a history of GI bleeding prior to the study, died due to gastrointestinal bleeding. Caution should be exercised with the concomitant use of antiplatelet agents or warfarin.

Hepatic/Biliary/Pancreatic: Liver Failure: There have been cases of cytolytic and cholestatic hepatitis and hepatic failure; in some cases the outcome was fatal.

Hepatotoxicity: Hepatotoxicity, occasionally severe, may occur with GLEEVEC (see Adverse Reactions, Table 1, Table 2 and Table 5). Liver function (transaminases, bilirubin, and alkaline phosphatase) should be monitored before initiation of treatment and monthly or as clinically indicated. Laboratory abnormalities should be managed with interruption and/or dose reduction of the treatment with GLEEVEC. (See Dosage and Administration.) Patients with hepatic impairment should be closely monitored. Although pharmacokinetic analysis results showed there is considerable inter-subject variation, the mean exposure to imatinib did not differ significantly between patients with mild and moderate liver dysfunction (as measured by dose normalized AUC) and patients with normal liver function. Patients with severe liver dysfunction demonstrated increased exposure to imatinib and its active metabolite CGP 74588. Liver function monitoring remains crucial as no long term toxicity and tolerability have been established (see Action and Clinical Pharmacology).

In GIST patients with liver metastases, exposure to GLEEVEC may be higher than in CML patients, due to impaired liver function (see Adverse Reactions).

Hepatotoxicity has been observed in patients treated with GLEEVEC. All Grades of liver toxicity (including liver failure) were reported in up to 11.6% for newly diagnosed CML patients, up to 12% for other CML patients across all clinical trials, and up to 12.2% for unresectable and/or metastatic malignant GIST patients.

Toxicities From Long-Term Use: It is important to consider potential toxicities suggested by animal studies, specifically, **liver, kidney and cardiac toxicity, and immunosuppression**. Liver toxicity was observed in rats, dogs and cynomolgus monkeys in repeated dose studies. Most severe toxicity was noted in dogs and included elevated liver enzymes, hepatocellular necrosis, bile duct necrosis, and bile duct hyperplasia.

Renal: Renal toxicity was observed in monkeys treated for 2 weeks, with focal mineralization and dilation of the renal tubules and tubular nephrosis. Increased BUN and creatinine were observed in several of these animals.

GLEEVEC and its metabolites are not excreted via the kidney to a significant extent. Creatinine clearance (CrCL) is known to decrease with age, and age did not significantly affect imatinib kinetics.

In patients with impaired renal function, GLEEVEC plasma exposure is higher (1.5- to 2-fold increase) than in patients with normal renal function, probably due to an elevated plasma level of alpha-acid glycoprotein (AGP), a GLEEVEC-binding protein, in patients with renal dysfunction. As well, there is a significant correlation in the incidence of serious adverse events with decreased renal function (p=0.0096). Patients with mild or moderate renal impairment should be treated with **caution** (see Dosage and Administration). Since the effect of GLEEVEC treatment on patients with severe renal dysfunction or on dialysis has not been sufficiently assessed, recommendations on the treatment of these patients with GLEEVEC cannot be made.

Respiratory: Pulmonary Events: Rare cases of pulmonary fibrosis and interstitial pneumonitis have been reported in patients who have received GLEEVEC. However, no definitive relationship has been established between the occurrence of these pulmonary events and treatment with GLEEVEC.

Skin: Skin and Mucosa: Although rare, **Erythema multiforme** and **Stevens-Johnson** syndrome have been reported in patients who have received GLEEVEC. Skin biopsies in some cases of exfoliative skin rash associated with GLEEVEC use have shown a mixed cellular infiltrate characteristic of a toxic drug reaction. Severe cases of exfoliative rash may require treatment interruption or discontinuation.

Special Populations: Pregnant Women: There are no adequate and well-controlled studies in pregnant women. The potential risk for the fetus is unknown. There have been post-market reports of spontaneous abortions and infant congenital anomalies from women who have taken GLEEVEC. Imatinib is teratogenic in animals, therefore, GLEEVEC should not be administered to pregnant women unless clearly necessary. If used during pregnancy the patient should be apprised of the potential risk to the fetus. Women of childbearing potential must be advised to use effective birth control during treatment.

Nursing Women: In animals, imatinib and/or its metabolites were extensively excreted in milk. Both imatinib and its active metabolite can be distributed into human milk. There are two known cases of imatinib exposure during lactation. Their analysis shows the following results: the milk: plasma ratio was determined to be 0.5 for imatinib and 0.9 for the metabolite. Since the effects of exposure of the infant to imatinib are potentially serious, women taking GLEEVEC should not breast feed.

Men: Stem cell factor and c-Kit genes are known to be important for germ cell development. Human studies on male patients receiving GLEEVEC and its effect on male fertility and spermatogenesis have not been performed. However, clinical evidence of profound oligospermia with GLEEVEC use has been reported in the literature as has clinical evidence for maintained male fertility. There is also pre-clinical evidence of impaired spermatogenesis without a reduction in fertility. Therefore, physicians should advise and counsel their male patients as appropriate.

Pediatrics: There is no experience with the use of GLEEVEC in pediatric patients with CML under 2 years of age. There is very limited experience with the use of GLEEVEC in children under 3 years of age in other indications.

Geriatrics: In the CML phase II studies, approximately 20% of patients were older than 65 years. There was a higher frequency of mild to moderate superficial edema in patients older than 65 years of age as compared to younger patients. No other age associated differences in safety profile were observed. The efficacy of GLEEVEC was similar in all age groups studied.

In the adjuvant GIST study, 221 patients (31%) were older than 65 years. No difference was observed in the safety profile in patients older than 65 years as compared to younger patients, with the exception of a higher frequency of edema. The efficacy of GLEEVEC was similar in patients older than 65 years and younger patients.

Monitoring and Laboratory Tests: Patients with known cardiac disease or risk factors for cardiac failure should be monitored carefully and those with symptoms or signs consistent with CHF should be evaluated and treated. In patients with history of cardiac disease or in elderly patients, a baseline evaluation of LVEF is recommended prior to initiation of GLEEVEC therapy (see Warnings and Precautions).

For patients receiving GLEEVEC, complete blood counts should be performed weekly for the first month, biweekly for the second month, and periodically thereafter as clinically indicated (for example every 2-3 months) (see Warnings and Precautions and Dosage and Administration).

Liver function (transaminases, bilirubin, and alkaline phosphatase) should be monitored before initiation of treatment and monthly or as clinically indicated (see Warnings and Precautions and Dosage and Administration).

Patients should be weighed and monitored regularly for signs and symptoms of fluid retention as fluid retention can occur after months of treatment with GLEEVEC (see Warnings and Precautions).

Thyroid-Stimulating Hormone (TSH) levels should be closely monitored in thyroidectomy patients undergoing levothyroxine replacement during treatment with GLEEVEC (see Warnings and Precautions).

During treatment with GLEEVEC serum electrolytes should be regularly monitored for possible hypophosphatemia, hyperkalemia, and hyponatremia in all patients as well as glucose, blood urea nitrogen (BUN) and creatinine. In addition, in pediatric patients, serum calcium and albumin should also be regularly monitored. Grades 3/4 hypophosphatemia have been observed in 16.5% (15% Grade 3 and 1.5% Grade 4) of patients in a phase I dose finding study 03001 (N=143) and a phase II study 0102 (N=260) of chronic myeloid leukemia in blast crisis.

ADVERSE REACTIONS: Adverse Drug Reaction Overview: GLEEVEC (imatinib mesylate) was generally well tolerated across all studies in CML and GIST. Complications of advanced malignancies and co-administered medications make causality of adverse events difficult to assess in single arm studies. The majority of GLEEVEC-treated patients experienced adverse events at some time.

Clinical Trial Adverse Drug Reactions: Chronic Myeloid Leukemia: GLEEVEC was generally well tolerated with chronic oral daily dosing in patients with CML including pediatric patients. The majority of patients experienced adverse events at some point in time, however, most events were of mild to moderate Grade. In adult clinical trials, drug discontinuation for drug-related adverse events was observed in 2.4% of newly diagnosed patients, in 5 % of patients in chronic phase, 8% in accelerated phase and 9% in blast crisis.

The most frequently reported drug-related adverse events were fluid retention (superficial edema and other fluid retention events), nausea, vomiting, diarrhea, muscle cramps, fatigue and rash (refer to Table 1 and Table 2 for newly diagnosed CML and other CML patients, respectively). Superficial edemas were a common finding in all studies described primarily as periorbital edemas or lower limb edemas. However, these edemas were rarely severe and may be managed with diuretics, other supportive measures, or by reducing the dose of GLEEVEC. (See Dosage and Administration.)

Other adverse events such as pleural effusion, ascites, pulmonary edema and rapid weight gain with or without superficial edema may be collectively described as "other fluid retention events". These events were usually managed by withholding GLEEVEC treatment temporarily and/or with diuretics and/or other appropriate supportive care measures. However, a few of these events may be serious or life threatening and several patients with blast crisis died with a complex clinical history of pleural effusion, congestive heart failure and renal failure. The following tables list the adverse experiences which occurred in ≥10% of patients in the clinical trials, regardless of relationship to therapy.

Table 1: GLEEVEC

Adverse Experiences Reported in Newly Diagnosed CML (≥10% of all patients)[a]

Adverse Event (preferred term)	All Grades		CTC Grades 3/4	
	GLEEVEC N=551 (%)	IFN+Ara-C N=533 (%)	GLEEVEC N=551 (%)	IFN+Ara-C N=533 (%)
Any Event	99.1	99.6	57.2	77.3
Gastrointestinal Disorders				
Nausea	49.5	61.5	1.3	5.1
Diarrhea	45.4	43.3	3.3	3.2

(cont'd)

Table 1: GLEEVEC *(cont'd)*

Adverse Experiences Reported in Newly Diagnosed CML (≥10% of all patients)[a]

Adverse Event (preferred term)	All Grades GLEEVEC N=551 (%)	All Grades IFN+Ara-C N=533 (%)	CTC Grades 3/4 GLEEVEC N=551 (%)	CTC Grades 3/4 IFN+Ara-C N=533 (%)
Abdominal pain	36.5	25.9	4.2	3.9
Vomiting	22.5	27.8	2.0	3.4
Dyspepsia	18.9	8.3	0	0.8
Constipation	11.4	14.4	0.7	0.2
Dry mouth	2.9	10.9	0	0.2
General Disorders and Administration Site Conditions				
Fluid retention	61.7	11.1	2.5	0.9
Superficial edema	59.9	9.6	1.5	0.4
Other fluid retention events	6.9	1.9	1.3	0.6
Fatigue	38.8	67.0	1.8	25.1
Pyrexia	17.8	42.6	0.9	3.0
Rigors	9.3	34.0	0.2	0.8
Asthenia	8.0	16.9	0.2	3.8
Influenza like illness	7.3	15.9	0	0.9
Mucosal inflammation	1.1	10.3	0	3.2
Hepatobiliary Disorders				
Liver toxicity (including liver failure)	11.6	17.3	4.0	5.1
Infections and Infestations				
Nasopharyngitis	30.5	8.8	0	0.4
Upper respiratory tract infection	21.2	8.4	0.2	0.4
Influenza	13.8	6.2	0.2	0.2
Sinusitis	11.4	6.0	0.2	0.2
Investigations				
Weight increased	15.6	2.6	2.0	0.4
Weight decreased	5.1	17.3	0.4	1.3
Metabolic and Nutritional Disorders				
Anorexia	7.1	31.7	0	2.4
Musculoskeletal & Connective Tissue Disorders				
Muscle cramps	49.2	11.8	2.2	0.2
Musculoskeletal pain	47.0	44.8	5.4	8.6
Joint pain	31.4	38.1	2.5	7.7
Myalgia	24.1	38.8	1.5	8.3
Bone pain	11.3	15.6	1.6	3.4
Nervous System Disorders				
Headache	37.0	43.3	0.5	3.8
Dizziness	19.4	24.4	0.9	3.8
Psychiatric Disorders				
Depression	14.9	35.8	0.5	13.1
Insomnia	14.7	18.6	0	2.3
Anxiety	9.6	11.8	0.5	2.6
Respiratory Disorders				
Cough	20.0	23.1	0.2	0.6
Pharyngolaryngeal pain	18.1	11.4	0.2	0
Dyspnea	9.3	14.4	1.8	1.7
Skin and Subcutaneous Disorders				
Rash and related terms	40.1	26.1	2.9	2.4

(cont'd)

Table 1: GLEEVEC *(cont'd)*

Adverse Experiences Reported in Newly Diagnosed CML (≥10% of all patients)[a]

Adverse Event (preferred term)	All Grades GLEEVEC N=551 (%)	All Grades IFN+Ara-C N=533 (%)	CTC Grades 3/4 GLEEVEC N=551 (%)	CTC Grades 3/4 IFN+Ara-C N=533 (%)
Night sweats	9.8	15.8	0.2	0.4
Pruritus	9.8	11.8	0.2	0.2
Sweating increased	5.8	14.8	0.2	0.4
Alopecia	4.9	22.3	0	0.6
Vascular Disorders				
Hemorrhage	28.9	21.2	1.8	1.7
GI hemorrhages	1.6	1.1	0.5	0.2
CNS hemorrhages	0.2	0.4	0	0.4

[a] All adverse events occurring in ≥10% of patients are listed regardless of suspected relationship to treatment.

Table 2: GLEEVEC

Adverse Experiences Reported in Other CML Clinical Trials (≥10% of All patients in any trial)[b]

System Affected	Myeloid Blast Crisis N=260 (%) All Grades	Myeloid Blast Crisis N=260 (%) CTC Grades 3/4	Accelerated Phase N=235 (%) All Grades	Accelerated Phase N=235 (%) CTC Grades 3/4	Chronic Phase IFN Failure N=532 (%) All Grades	Chronic Phase IFN Failure N=532 (%) CTC Grades 3/4
Gastrointestinal Disorders						
Nausea	71	5	73	5	63	3
Vomiting	54	4	58	3	36	2
Diarrhea	43	4	57	5	48	3
Abdominal pain[a]	30	6	33	4	32	1
Constipation	16	2	16	0.9	9	0.4
Dyspepsia	12	0	22	0	27	0
General Disorders and Administration Site Conditions						
Fluid retention[a]	72	11	76	6	69	4
Superficial edemas[a]	66	6	74	3	67	2
Other fluid retention events[c,a]	22	6	15	4	7	2
Pyrexia	41	7	41	8	21	2
Fatigue	30	4	46	4	48	1
Asthenia	18	5	21	5	15	0.2
Rigors	10	0	12	0.4	10	0
Chest pain	7	2	10	0.4	11	0.8
Hepatobiliary Disorders						
Liver toxicity (including liver failure)	10	5	12	6	6	3
Infections and Infestations						
Nasopharyngitis	10	0	17	0	22	0.2
Pneumonia NOS	13	7	10	7	4	1
Upper respiratory tract infection NOS	3	0	12	0.4	19	0
Sinusitis NOS	4	0.4	11	0.4	9	0.4
Influenza	0.8	0.4	6	0	11	0.2
Investigations						
Weight increase	5	1	17	5	32	7
Metabolic and Nutritional Disorders						
Anorexia	14	2	17	2	7	0
Hypokalemia	13	4	9	2	6	0.8
Musculoskeletal & Connective Tissue Disorders						

(cont'd)

Table 2: GLEEVEC *(cont'd)*

Adverse Experiences Reported in Other CML Clinical Trials (≥10% of All patients in any trial)[b]

System Affected	Myeloid Blast Crisis N=260 (%) All Grades	Myeloid Blast Crisis CTC Grades 3/4	Accelerated Phase N=235 (%) All Grades	Accelerated Phase CTC Grades 3/4	Chronic Phase IFN Failure N=532 (%) All Grades	Chronic Phase IFN Failure CTC Grades 3/4
Musculoskeletal pain[a]	42	9	49	9	38	2
Muscle cramps[a]	28	1	47	0.4	62	2
Joint pain (arthralgia)[a]	25	5	34	6	40	1
Myalgia	9	0	24	2	27	0.2
Nervous System Disorders						
Headache	27	5	32	2	36	0.6
Dizziness	12	0.4	13	0	16	0.2
Psychiatric Disorders						
Insomnia	10	0	14	0	14	0.2
Anxiety	8	0.8	12	0	8	0.4
Respiratory Disorders						
Dyspnea NOS	15	4	21	7	12	0.9
Cough	14	0.8	27	0.9	20	0
Pharyngitis	10	0	12	0	15	0
Skin and Subcutaneous Disorders						
Rash and related terms[a]	36	5	47	5	47	3
Night sweats	13	0.8	17	1	14	0.2
Pruritus	8	1	14	0.9	14	0.8
Vascular Disorders						
Hemorrhages[a]	53	19	49	11	30	2
CNS hemorrhages[a]	9	7	3	3	2	1
GI hemorrhages[a]	8	4	6	5	2	0.4

[a] Grouped events.
[b] All adverse events occurring in ≥10% of patients are listed regardless of suspected relationship to treatment.
[c] Other fluid retention events include pleural effusion, ascites, pulmonary edema, pericardial effusion, anasarca, edema aggravated, and fluid retention not otherwise specified.

Adverse Reactions in the Pediatric Population: The overall safety profile of GLEEVEC treatment in 93 pediatric patients was similar to that observed in studies with adult patients. Nausea, vomiting were the most commonly reported individual adverse events with an incidence similar to that seen in adult patients. Although most patients experienced adverse events at some time during the studies, the incidence of Grade 3/4 adverse events was low.

Significantly higher frequencies of hypocalcemia (23.5 vs 1.1%), hyperglycemia (19.6 vs 2.9%), hypoglycemia (21.6 vs 1.5%), hypophosphatemia (19.6 vs 3.3%), hypoalbuminemia (13.7 vs 0.2%) and hyponatremia (13.7 vs 0.2%) were observed in pediatric patients compared to adult patients.

Acute Lymphoblastic Leukemia: The adverse reactions were similar for Ph+ ALL as for CML. The most frequently reported non-hematologic drug-related adverse events were fluid retention (superficial edema and other fluid retention events), nausea, vomiting, diarrhea, muscle cramps, fatigue and rash. Superficial edemas were a common finding in all studies described primarily as periorbital edemas or lower limb edemas. However, these edemas were rarely severe and may be managed with diuretics, other supportive measures, or by reducing the dose of GLEEVEC (see Dosage and Administration).

Myelodysplastic/Myeloproliferative Diseases: Adverse events, regardless of relationship to study drug, that were reported in at least 10% of the patients treated with GLEEVEC for MDS/MPD in Trial B2225, are shown in Table 3.

Table 3: GLEEVEC

Adverse Experiences Reported (more than one patient) in MDS/MPD Patients in Trial B2225 (≥10% all patients) all Grades

Preferred Term	N=7 n (%)
Nausea	4 (57.1)
Diarrhea	3 (42.9)
Anemia	2 (28.6)
Fatigue	2 (28.6)
Muscle cramp	3 (42.9)
Arthralgia	2 (28.6)
Periorbital edema	2 (28.6)

Aggressive Sub-types of Systemic Mastocytosis (ASM and SM-AHNMD): All ASM patients experienced at least one adverse event at some time. The most frequently reported adverse events were diarrhea, nausea, ascites, muscle cramps, dyspnea, fatigue, peripheral edema, anemia, pruritus, rash and lower respiratory tract infection. None of the 5 patients in Study B2225 with ASM discontinued GLEEVEC due to drug-related adverse events or abnormal laboratory values.

Hypereosinophilic Syndrome and Chronic Eosinophilic Leukemia: The overall safety profile in this HES/CEL small patient population does not seem different from the known safety profile of GLEEVEC observed in other larger populations of hematologic malignancies, such as CML. However, in patients with HES and cardiac involvement, isolated cases of cardiogenic shock/left ventricular dysfunction have been associated with the initiation of GLEEVEC therapy. The condition was reported to be reversible with the administration of systemic steroids, circulatory support measures and temporarily withholding GLEEVEC (see Warnings and Precautions). All patients experienced at least one adverse event, the most common being gastrointestinal, cutaneous and musculoskeletal disorders. Hematologic abnormalities were also frequent, with instances of CTC Grade 3 leukopenia, neutropenia, lymphopenia and anemia.

Dermatofibrosarcoma Protuberans: Adverse events, regardless of relationship to study drug, that were reported in at least 10% of the 12 patients treated with GLEEVEC for DFSP in Trial B2225 are shown in Table 4.

Table 4: GLEEVEC

Adverse Experiences Reported in DFSP Patients in Trial B2225 (≥10% all patients) all Grades

Preferred Term	N=12 n (%)
Nausea	5 (41.7)
Diarrhea	3 (25.0)
Vomiting	3 (25.0)
Periorbital edema	4 (33.3)
Face edema	2 (16.7)
Rash	3 (25.0)
Fatigue	5 (41.7)
Edema peripheral	4 (33.3)
Pyrexia	2 (16.7)
Eye edema	4 (33.3)
Lacrimation increased	3 (25.0)
Dyspnea exertional	2 (16.7)
Anemia	3 (25.0)
Rhinitis	2 (16.7)
Anorexia	2 (16.7)

Gastrointestinal Stromal Tumors: Unresectable and/or Metastatic Malignant GIST: GLEEVEC was generally well tolerated in patients with unresectable and/or metastatic malignant GIST. Most events were of mild to moderate severity. Drug was discontinued for adverse events in 7 (4.7%) patients in both treatment groups. The most frequently reported adverse events were edema, nausea, diarrhea, abdominal pain, muscle cramps, fatigue and rash.

Adverse events, regardless of relationship to study drug, that were reported in at least 10% of the patients treated with GLEEVEC are shown in Table 5. No major differences were seen in the incidence or severity of adverse events between the 400 mg or 600 mg dose groups.

Table 5: GLEEVEC

Adverse Experiences Reported in the Unresectable and/or Metastatic Malignant GIST (B2222) Trial (≥10%) of all Patients[a]

Preferred Term	All Doses (n=147) 600 mg n=73 All Grades (%)	Grades 3/4 (%)
Blood and Lymphatic System Disorders		
Anemia	19.7	5.4
Eye Disorders		
Lacrimation increased	17.0	0
Gastrointestinal Disorders		
Nausea	68.7	4.8
Diarrhea	64.6	4.8
Abdominal pain	57.1	8.8
Vomiting	36.7	4.1
Flatulence	32.0	0
Dyspepsia	15.0	0
Constipation	10.2	0.7
General Disorders and Administration Site Conditions		
Any fluid retention	80.3	9.5
Superficial edema	78.9	5.4
Other fluid retention events[b]	13.6	5.4
Fatigue	50.3	1.4

(cont'd)

Table 5: GLEEVEC *(cont'd)*

Adverse Experiences Reported in the Unresectable and/or Metastatic Malignant GIST (B2222) Trial (≥10%) of all Patients[a]

Preferred Term	All Doses (n=147) 600 mg n=73 All Grades (%)	Grades 3/4 (%)
Pyrexia	20.4	1.4
Other hemorrhage	24.5	2.7
Hepatobiliary Disorders		
Liver toxicity	12.2	6.8
Infections and Infestations		
Nasopharyngitis	23.8	0
Upper respiratory tract infection	15.6	0
Musculoskeletal & Connective Tissue Disorders		
Muscle cramps	52.4	0
Musculoskeletal pain	33.3	3.4
Back pain	24.5	0
Joint pain	12.9	0.7
Nervous System Disorders		
Headache	36.1	0
Dizziness	11.6	0
Peaces Abnormal		
Loose stools	10.9	0
Psychiatric Disorders		
Insomnia	18.4	0.7
Anxiety	8.8	0
Respiratory Disorders		
Pharyngolaryngeal pain	9.5	0
Skin and Subcutaneous Disorders		
Rash and related terms	45.6	3.4
Surgical and Medical Procedures		
Operation	10.2	4.8
Vascular Disorders		
Any hemorrhage	29.9	8.2
Upper GI tract bleeding/perforation	4.1	3.4
Tumor hemorrhage	2.7	2.7

[a] All adverse events occurring in ≥10% of patients are listed regardless of suspected relationship to treatment.
[b] Other fluid retention events included pleural effusion and ascites.

Adjuvant Treatment of GIST: The majority of both GLEEVEC and placebo treated patients experienced at least one adverse reaction at some time. The most frequently reported adverse reactions were similar to those reported in other clinical studies in other patient populations and include diarrhea, fatigue, nausea, edema, decreased hemoglobin, rash, vomiting and abdominal pain. No new adverse reactions were reported in the adjuvant GIST treatment setting that had not been previously reported in other patient populations including patients with unresectable and/or malignant metastatic GIST. Drug was discontinued for adverse reactions in 57 patients (17%) and 11 patients (3%) of the GLEEVEC and placebo treated patients respectively. Edema, gastrointestinal disturbances (nausea, vomiting, abdominal distension and diarrhea), fatigue, low hemoglobin and rash were the most frequently reported adverse reactions at the time of discontinuation.

Adverse reactions, regardless of relationship to study drug, that were reported in at least 5% of the patients treated with GLEEVEC are shown in Table 6.

Table 6: GLEEVEC

Adverse Reactions Reported in the Adjuvant GIST Trial (≥5% of GLEEVEC Treated Patients)[a]

Preferred Term	All CTC Grades GLEEVEC (n=337) %	All CTC Grades Placebo (n=345) %	CTC Grade 3 and Above GLEEVEC (n=337) %	CTC Grade 3 and Above Placebo (n=345) %
Blood and Lymphatic System Disorders				
Leukopenia	5.0	2.6	0.3	0
Eye Disorders				
Lacrimation increased	9.8	3.8	0	0
Vision blurred	5.0	2.3	0	0
Gastrointestinal Disorders				
Diarrhea	59.3	29.3	3.0	1.4
Nausea	53.1	27.8	2.4	1.2
Vomiting	25.5	13.9	2.4	0.6
Abdominal pain	21.1	22.3	3.0	1.4
Dyspepsia	17.2	13.0	0.9	0
Constipation	12.8	17.7	0	0.3
Abdominal distension	7.4	6.4	0.3	0.3
Flatulence	8.9	9.6	0	0
Abdominal pain upper	6.2	6.4	0.3	0
Stomatitis	5.0	1.7	0.6	0
General Disorders and Administration Site Conditions				
Fatigue	57.0	40.9	2.1	1.2
Peripheral edema	26.7	14.8	0.3	0
Facial edema	6.8	1.2	0.3	0
Hepatobiliary Disorders				
Liver enzymes (ALT) increased	16.6	13.0	2.7	0
Liver enzymes (AST) increased	12.2	7.5	2.1	0
Investigations				
Hemoglobin decreased	46.9	27.0	0.6	0
Weight increased	16.9	11.6	0.3	0
Neutrophil count decreased	16.0	6.1	3.3	0.9
White blood cell count decreased	14.5	4.3	0.6	0.3
Blood creatinine increased	11.6	5.8	0	0.3
Weight decreased	10.1	5.2	0	0
Blood alkaline phosphatase increased	6.5	7.5	0	0
Platelet count decreased	5.0	3.5	0	0
Metabolic and Nutritional Disorders				
Anorexia	16.9	8.7	0.3	0
Hyperglycemia	9.8	11.3	0.6	1.7
Hypokalemia	7.1	2.0	0.9	0.6
Hypocalcemia	5.6	1.7	0.3	0
Musculoskeletal & Connective Tissue Disorders				
Muscle spasms	16.3	3.3	0	0
Myalgia	12.2	11.6	0	0.3
Arthralgia	15.1	14.5	0	0.3
Back pain	7.4	8.1	0.6	0
Pain in extremity	7.4	7.2	0.3	0
Nervous System Disorders				
Headache	19.3	20.3	0.6	0
Dizziness	12.5	10.7	0	0.3
Insomnia	9.8	7.2	0.9	0
Depression	6.8	6.4	0.9	0.6

(cont'd)

Table 6: GLEEVEC *(cont'd)*

Adverse Reactions Reported in the Adjuvant GIST Trial (≥5% of GLEEVEC Treated Patients)[a]

	All CTC Grades		CTC Grade 3 and Above	
Preferred Term	**GLEEVEC (n=337) %**	**Placebo (n=345) %**	**GLEEVEC (n=337) %**	**Placebo (n=345) %**
Dysgeusia	6.5	2.9	0	0
Neuropathy peripheral	5.9	6.4	0	0
Respiratory Disorders				
Cough	11.0	11.3	0	0
Upper respiratory tract infection	5.0	3.5	0	0
Skin and Subcutaneous Disorders				
Periorbital edema	47.2	14.5	1.2	0
Rash (exfoliative)	26.1	12.8	2.7	0
Pruritus	11.0	7.8	0.9	0
Alopecia	9.5	6.7	0	0
Rash	8.9	5.2	0.9	0
Dry skin	6.5	5.2	0	0

[a] All adverse reactions occurring in ≥5% of patients are listed regardless of suspected relationship to treatment.
A patient with multiple occurrences of an adverse reaction is counted only once in the adverse reaction category.

Adverse Drug Reactions in Clinical Studies for CML and Unresectable and/or Metastatic Malignant GIST: The following adverse reactions as applicable are ranked under headings of frequency, the most frequent first, using the following convention: Very common (≥1/10); common (≥1/100, <1/10); uncommon (≥1/1000, <1/100); rare (≥1/10 000, <1/1000); very rare (<1/10 000), including isolated reports. Adverse reactions reported below are based on the registration studies for CML and GIST. Frequencies are determined by reported related events according to the investigator.

Cardiovascular: Common: flushing†. Uncommon: palpitations, cardiac failure congestive (on a patient-year basis, cardiac events including congestive heart failure were more commonly observed in patients with transformed CML than in patients with chronic CML), pulmonary edema, tachycardia, hypertension†, hematoma†, hypotension†, peripheral coldness†, Raynaud's phenomenon†. Rare: arrhythmia, atrial fibrillation, cardiac arrest, myocardial infarction, angina pectoris, pericardial effusion.

Clinical Laboratory Tests: (See Table 8, Table 9 and Table 11.)
Uncommon: blood CPK increased, blood LDH increased. Rare: blood amylase increased.

Dermatologic: Common: pruritus, face edema, dry skin, erythema, alopecia, photosensitivity reaction. Uncommon: rash pustular, sweating increased, urticaria, increased tendency to bruise, exfoliative dermatitis, onychoclasis, folliculitis, petechie, psoriasis, bullous eruption, nail disorder, skin pigmentation changes, purpura, palmar-plantar erythrodysaesthesia syndrome. Rare: nail discolouration, vesicular rash, erythema multiforme, leucocytoclastic vasculitis, Stevens-Johnson syndrome, acute generalized exanthematous pustulosis (AGEP), acute febrile neutrophilic dermatosis (Sweet's syndrome).

Digestive: Common: flatulence, abdominal distension, gastroesophageal reflux, dry mouth, gastritis. Uncommon: stomatitis, mouth ulceration, eructation, malaena, oesophagitis, ascites, gastric ulcer, hematemesis, cheilitis, dysphagia, pancreatitis. Rare: colitis, ileus, inflammatory bowel disease.

General Disorders and Administration Site Conditions: Common: weakness, anasarca, chills, rigors. Uncommon: chest pain, malaise.

Hematologic: (See Table 8, Table 9 and Table 11.)
Common: pancytopenia, febrile neutropenia. Uncommon: thrombocythemia, lymphopenia, eosinophilia, lymphadenopathy. Rare: aplastic anemia, hemolytic anemia.

Hepatobiliary Disorders: Uncommon: jaundice, hepatitis, hyperbilirubinemia. Rare: hepatic failure, hepatic necrosis (some fatal cases of hepatic necrosis have been reported).

Hypersensitivity: Rare: angioedema.

Infections: Uncommon: sepsis, herpes simplex, herpes zoster, sinusitis, cellulitis, influenza, urinary tract infection, gastroenteritis. Rare: fungal infection.

Metabolic and Nutritional: Common: anorexia, weight decreased. Uncommon: hypophosphatemia, dehydration, gout, appetite disturbances, hyperuricemia, hypercalcemia, hyperglycemia, hyponatremia. Rare: hyperkalemia, hypomagnesemia.

Musculoskeletal: Common: joint swelling. Uncommon: joint and muscle stiffness. Rare: muscular weakness, arthritis.

Nervous System/Psychiatric: Common: paresthesia, taste disturbance, hypoesthesia. Uncommon: depression‡, libido decrease, syncope, peripheral neuropathy, somnolence, migraine, memory impairment, sciatica, restless leg syndrome, tremor. Rare: increased intracranial pressure, confusion, convulsions, optic neuritis.

Renal: Uncommon: renal pain, renal failure acute, urinary frequency increased, hematuria.

Reproductive: Uncommon: erectile dysfunction, breast enlargement, menorrhagia, menstruation irregular, sexual dysfunction, nipple pain, scrotal edema.

Respiratory: Common: dyspnea, epistaxis, cough. Uncommon: pleural effusion (pleural effusion was reported more commonly in patients with GIST and in patients with transformed CML (CML-AP and CML-BC) than in patients with chronic CML), pharyngolaryngeal pain, pharyngitis. Rare: pleuritic pain, pulmonary fibrosis, pulmonary hypertension, pulmonary hemorrhage.

Special Senses: Common: eyelid edema, lacrimation increased, conjunctival hemorrhage, conjunctivitis, dry eye, vision blurred. Uncommon: eye irritation, eye pain, orbital edema, scleral hemorrhage, retinal hemorrhage, blepharitis, macular edema, vertigo, tinnitus, hearing loss. Rare: cataract, papilledema, glaucoma.

Second Malignancies in GLEEVEC-Treated Patients: See Table 7.

Table 7: GLEEVEC

Observed and Expected Numbers of Cases of Second Malignancies (excluding non-melanoma skin cancer) in Clinical Trials

Cancer Type	Person-Years	Number of Cases Observed	Expected[a]	SIR (95% CI)
Cancer any type	10 967.03	79	91.16	0.87 (0.69–1.08)
Prostate	6106.54	16	18.70	0.86 (0.49–1.39)
Kidney	10 769.60	3	2.26	1.33 (0.27–3.88)
Urinary bladder	10 766.46	2	3.72	0.54 (0.06–1.94)

[a] Expected in the general population.
Legend: SIR: Standardized incidence ratio.

† Vascular disorders (flushing was most common in GIST patients and hematoma was most common in patients with GIST and transformed CML (CML-AP and CML-BC).

‡ Depression may lead to suicide ideation and/or suicide attempts.

The numbers of cancers reported in the clinical trials were similar to those expected in the general population. The observed numbers of cases for all cancers, prostate cancer and urinary bladder cancer were slightly lower than those expected in the general population, while the number of observed kidney cancer cases was slightly higher (3 compared to 2.26 expected cases respectively). In all cases, the differences were not statistically significant.

Abnormal Hematologic and Clinical Chemistry Findings: Laboratory Test Abnormalities in CML Clinical Trials: Cytopenias, and particularly neutropenia and thrombocytopenia, have been a consistent finding in all studies, with the suggestion of a higher frequency at doses ≥750 mg (phase I study). However, the occurrence of cytopenias was also clearly dependent on the stage of the disease.

In patients with newly diagnosed CML, cytopenias were less frequent than in other CML patients (see Table 8 and Table 9). The frequency of Grade 3 or 4 neutropenia (ANC $<1.0\times10^9$/L) and thrombocytopenia (platelet count $<50\times10^9$/L) were higher in blast crisis and accelerated phase (36-48% and 32-33% for neutropenia and thrombocytopenia, respectively, Table 9) as compared to chronic phase CML (27% neutropenia and 21% thrombocytopenia). In chronic phase CML a Grade 4 neutropenia (ANC $<0.5\times10^9$/L) and thrombocytopenia (platelet count $<10\times10^9$/L) were observed in 9% and <1% of patients, respectively. The median duration of the neutropenic and thrombocytopenic episodes ranged usually from 2 to 3 weeks, and from 3 to 4 weeks, respectively. These events can usually be managed with either a reduction of the dose or an interruption of treatment with GLEEVEC, but can, in rare cases, lead to permanent discontinuation of treatment (see Warnings and Precautions, Hematologic for Hematologic Toxicity).

Severe elevation of transaminases or bilirubin was seen in <5% CML patients and were usually managed with dose reduction or interruption (the median duration of these episodes was approximately one week). Treatment was discontinued permanently because of liver laboratory abnormalities in less than 1.0% of CML patients. There have been cases of hepatic necrosis and cholestatic hepatitis and hepatic failure; in some of them outcome was fatal (see Drug Interactions).

Table 8: GLEEVEC

Newly Occurring Grade 3/4 Biochemical Toxicities in Newly Diagnosed CML Patients

	GLEEVEC n=551 %		IFN+Ara-C n=533 %	
Parameter	**Grade 3**	**Grade 4**	**Grade 3**	**Grade 4**
Hematologic				
Leucopenia	9.3	0.5	12.9	0.8
Neutropenia[a]	13.1	3.6	20.8	4.5
Thrombocytopenia[a]	8.5	0.4	15.9	0.6
Anemia	3.3	1.1	4.1	0.2
Biochemistry				
Elevated creatinine	0	0	0.4	0
Elevated bilirubin	0.9	0.2	0.2	0
Elevated alkaline phosphatase	0.2	0	0.8	0
Elevated AST/ALT	4.7	0.5	7.1	0.4

[a] p<0.001 (Difference in Grade 3+Grade 4 abnormalities between the two treatment groups).

Table 9: GLEEVEC

Laboratory Test Abnormalities in Other CML Clinical Trials

	Myeloid Blast Crisis n=260 (%)		Accelerated Phase n=235 (%)		Chronic Phase, IFN Failure n=532 (%)	
	Grade 3	**Grade 4**	**Grade 3**	**Grade 4**	**Grade 3**	**Grade 4**
Hematology Parameters						
Neutropenia	16	48	23	36	27	9
Thrombocytopenia	30	33	32	13	21	<1
Anemia	42	11	34	7	6	1
Biochemistry Parameters						
Elevated creatinine	1.5	0	1.3	0	0.2	0
Elevated bilirubin	3.8	0	2.1	0	0.6	0
Elevated alkaline phosphatase	4.6	0	5.5	0.4	0.2	0
Elevated AST	1.9	0	3	0	2.3	0
Elevated ALT	2.3	0.4	4.3	0	2.1	0

CTC grades: neutropenia (grade 3 $\geq0.5\text{-}1.0\times10^9$/L), grade 4 $<0.5\times10^9$/L), thrombocytopenia (grade 3 $\geq10\text{-}50\times10^9$/L, grade 4 $<10\times10^9$/L), anemia (hemoglobin ≥65-80 g/L, grade 4 <65 g/L), elevated creatinine (grade 3 >3-6 × upper limit normal range (ULN), grade 4 >6×ULN), elevated bilirubin (grade 3 >3-10×ULN, grade 4 >10×ULN), elevated alkaline phosphatase (grade 3 >5-20×ULN, grade 4 >20×ULN), elevated AST or ALT (grade 3 >5-20×ULN, grade 4 >20×ULN).

Clinically relevant or severe abnormalities of the 12 patients treated with GLEEVEC for DFSP in Trial B2225 are presented in Table 10.

In unresectable and/or metastatic malignant GIST patients (study B2222), 6.8% Grade 3 or 4 ALT (alanine transferase) elevations and 4.8% Grade 3 or 4 AST (aspartate transferase) elevations were observed. Bilirubin elevation was below 3%.

Clinically relevant or severe abnormalities of routine hematologic or biochemistry laboratory values were rare (Table 11).

The following types of reactions have been reported from post-marketing experience and from additional clinical studies with GLEEVEC. They include spontaneous case reports as well as serious adverse events from smaller or ongoing clinical studies and the expanded access programmes. Because these reactions are reported from a population of uncertain size, it is not always possible to reliably estimate their frequency or establish a causal relationship to imatinib exposure.

Post-Market Adverse Drug Reactions: The following additional adverse reactions have been identified during post approval use of GLEEVEC. Because these reactions are reported voluntarily from a population of uncertain size, it is not always possible to reliably estimate their frequency or establish a causal relationship to drug exposure.

Cardiovascular: thrombosis/embolism¶, pericarditis, cardiac tamponade, anaphylactic shock¶.

¶ Vascular disorders.

Dermatology: lichenoid keratosis, lichen planus, toxic epidermal necrolysis.
Digestive: ileus/intestinal obstruction, tumor hemorrhage/tumor necrosis, gastrointestinal perforation (some fatal cases of gastrointestinal perforation have been reported) diverticulitis.

Table 10: GLEEVEC

Laboratory Abnormalities Reported in DFSP Patients in Trial B2225

	N=12	
CTC Grades	**Grade 3**	**Grade 4**
Hematology Parameters		
Anemia	17%	0%
Thrombocytopenia	17%	0%
Neutropenia	0%	8%
Biochemistry Parameters		
Elevated creatinine	0%	8%

CTC Grades: neutropenia (Grade 3 ≥0.5-1.0×10^9/L, Grade 4 <0.5×10^9/L), thrombocytopenia (Grade 3 ≥10-50×10^9/L, Grade 4 <10×10^9/L), anemia (Grade 3 ≥65-80 g/L, Grade 4 <65 g/L), elevated creatinine (Grade 3 >3-6 × upper limit normal range [ULN], Grade 4 >6×ULN).

Table 11: GLEEVEC

Laboratory Abnormalities in the Unresectable and/or Metastatic Malignant GIST B2222 Trial

	All Doses (n=147) 400 mg n=73 600 mg n=74 n (%)		
Parameter	**Baseline[a]**	**New or Worsening Highest CTC Grade During Treatment**	
CTC Grading	**All Grades (1-4)**	**Grade 3**	**Grade 4**
Hematology Parameters			
Anemia	70 (47.6)	8 (5.4)	1 (0.7)
Thrombocytopenia	7 (4.8)	1 (0.7)	0
Neutropenia	10 (6.8)	11 (7.5)	4 (2.7)
Biochemistry Parameters			
Elevated creatinine	8 (5.4)	2 (1.4)	0
Reduced albumin	60 (40.8)	5 (3.4)	0
Elevated bilirubin	5 (3.4)	2 (1.4)	2 (1.4)
Elevated alkaline phosphatase	58 (39.5)	2 (1.4)	0
Elevated AST	32 (21.8)	5 (3.4)	2 (1.4)
Elevated ALT	19 (13.0)	9 (6.1)	1 (0.7)

[a] **New or worsening of CTC Grade for any individual patient for whom data is included in the All Grade (1-4) Baseline data cannot be inferred from this table.**
CTC grades: neutropenia (grade 1 = 1.5-<2.0×10^9/L, grade 2 = 1.0-<1.5×10^9/L, grade 3 = 0.5-<1.0×10^9/L, grade 4 <0.5×10^9/L), thrombocytopenia (grade 1 <LLN-75.0×10^9/L, grade 2 = 50.0-<75.0×10^9/L, grade 3 = 10.0-<50.0×10^9/L, grade 4 <10.0×10^9/L), anemia (hemoglobin: grade 1 <LLN-100 g/L, grade 2 = 80-<100 g/L, grade 3 = 65-<80 g/L, grade 4 <65 g/L), elevated creatinine (grade 1 >ULN-1.5×ULN, grade 2 >1.5-3.0×ULN, grade 3 >3.0-6.0×upper limit normal range (ULN), grade 4 >6.0×ULN), reduced albumin (grade 1 <LLN-30 g/L, grade 2 = 20-<30 g/L, grade 3 <20 g/L, grade 4 -), elevated bilirubin (grade 1 >ULN-1.5×ULN, grade 2 >1.5-3×ULN, grade 3 >3-10×ULN, grade 4 >10×ULN), elevated alkaline phosphatase (grade 1 >ULN-2.5×ULN, grade 2 >2.5-5×ULN, grade 3 >5-20×ULN, grade 4 >20×ULN), elevated AST or ALT (grade 1 >ULN-2.5×ULN, grade 2 >2.5-5.0×ULN, grade 3 >5-20×ULN, grade 4 >20×ULN).

Musculoskeletal: avascular necrosis/hip osteonecrosis, rhabdomyolysis/myopathy.
Nervous system/psychiatric: cerebral edema (including fatalities).
Reproductive: hemorrhagic corpus luteum/hemorrhagic ovarian cyst.
Respiratory: acute respiratory failure (fatal cases have been reported in patients with advanced disease, severe infections, severe neutropenia and other serious concomitant conditions), interstitial lung disease.
Special Senses: vitreous hemorrhage.

DRUG INTERACTIONS: Drug-Drug Interactions: Drugs That May Alter Imatinib Plasma Concentrations: Drugs that may **increase** imatinib plasma concentrations:
Substances that inhibit the cytochrome P450 isoenzyme (CYP3A4) activity may decrease metabolism and increase imatinib concentrations. There was a significant increase in exposure to imatinib (mean C_{max} and AUC of imatinib increased by 26% and 40%, respectively) in healthy subjects when GLEEVEC was co-administered with a single dose of ketoconazole (CYP3A4 inhibitor). Caution is recommended when administering GLEEVEC with inhibitors of the CYP3A4 family (e.g. ketoconazole, erythromycin, clarithromycin, itraconazole, grapefruit juice).
Drugs that may **decrease** imatinib plasma concentrations:
Substances that are inducers of CYP3A4 activity may increase metabolism and decrease imatinib plasma concentrations. Co-medications that induce CYP3A4 (e.g., dexamethasone, phenytoin, carbamazepine, rifampicin, phenobarbital or St. John's Wort) may significantly reduce exposure to GLEEVEC.

Administration of rifampin 600 mg daily for eight days to 14 healthy adult volunteers, followed by a single 400 mg dose of GLEEVEC increased imatinib oral dose clearance by 3.8-fold (90% CI 3.5- to 4.3-fold). Mean C_{max}, AUC_{0-24} and $AUC_{0-\infty}$ decreased by 54%, 68% and 74%, respectively compared to treatment without rifampin.

Similar results were observed in patients with malignant gliomas treated with GLEEVEC while taking enzyme-inducing anti-epileptic drugs (EIAEDs) such as carbamazepine, oxcarbazepine, phenytoin, fosphenytoin, phenobarbital, and primidone. The plasma AUC for imatinib decreased by 73% compared to patients not on EIADs.

In two published studies, concomitant administration of imatinib and a product containing St. John's wort led to a 30 to 32% reduction in the AUC of GLEEVEC. In patients in whom rifampin or other CYP3A4 inducers are indicated, alternate therapeutic agents with less enzyme induction potential should be considered.
Drugs That May Have Their Plasma Concentration Altered by GLEEVEC: There is limited data on drug interactions. Since the major metabolic pathway is CYP3A4 mediated and GLEEVEC is an inhibitor of CYP2D6, precaution should be exercised with the co-administration of the following classes of drugs. See Table 12.

Table 12: GLEEVEC

Common Classes of Drugs Used in Patients with CML

CYP3A4			CYP2D6	
Inhibitors	**Inducers**	**Substrates**	**Inhibitors**	**Substrates**
Cyclosporine Imidazole antifungals Macrolide antibiotics Metronidazole	Antiepileptics Glucocorticoids Rifampicin St. John's wort	Busulphan Calcium-channel blockers Cyclophosphamide Cyclosporine Doxorubicin Epipodophyllotoxins Glucocorticoids Ifosphamide Imidazole antifungals Macrolide antibiotics (Azithromycin, Clarithromycin, Erythromycin) PPIs Retinoic acid Rifampicin Serotonin-H_3 antagonist Vinca alkaloids	Dextropropoxyphene Doxorubicin Quinidine Vinca alkaloids	Cyclophosphamide Beta blockers Morphine Oxycodone Serotonin-H_3 antagonists

Imatinib increases the mean C_{max} and AUC of simvastatin (CYP3A4 substrate) 2- and 3.5-fold, respectively, suggesting an inhibition of the CYP3A4 by imatinib. Therefore, caution is recommended when administering GLEEVEC with CYP3A4 substrates with a narrow therapeutic window (e.g. cyclosporine, pimozide). (See Adverse Reactions.)

In vitro, GLEEVEC inhibits the cytochrome P450 isoenzyme CYP2D6 activity at similar concentrations that affect CYP3A4 activity. Imatinib at 400 mg twice daily had a weak inhibitory effect on CYP2D6-mediated metoprolol metabolism, with metoprolol C_{max} and AUC being increased by approximately 23%. Caution is advised for CYP2D6 substrates with a narrow therapeutic window such as metoprolol. In patients treated with imatinib and metoprolol clinical monitoring should be considered.

In vitro data suggest that imatinib has some capacity to act as an inhibitor of CYP2C9, although at concentrations higher than would be expected in plasma with recommended doses. However, caution should be exercised with the concomitant use of drugs metabolized by CYP2C9 (e.g. warfarin).

In view of the potential interaction between GLEEVEC and warfarin, the international normalised ratio (INR) of patients who require anticoagulation with warfarin should be monitored closely, especially when GLEEVEC dose adjustments are necessary. Consideration should be given to anticoagulation with low-molecular weight heparin or unfractionated heparin.

In vitro, GLEEVEC inhibits acetaminophen O-glucuronidation (Ki value of 58.5 µmol/L) at therapeutic levels. Systemic exposure to acetaminophen is expected to be increased when co administered with GLEEVEC. No specific studies in humans have been performed and caution is recommended.
Drug-Food Interactions: There were no clinically relevant differences in absorption when GLEEVEC was administered either with food or in the fasting state. The concomitant use of grapefruit juice should be avoided.

DOSAGE AND ADMINISTRATION: Dosing Considerations: Therapy should be administered under the supervision of a physician experienced in the treatment of patients with hematological malignancies and/or malignant sarcomas.

The prescribed dose should be administered orally, during a meal and with a large glass of water. Doses of 400 mg or 600 mg should be administered once daily, whereas a dose of 800 mg should be administered as 400 mg twice a day in the morning and in the evening. Efficacy data for the 800 mg/day dose are limited.

Dosing in pediatric patients should be on the basis of body surface area (mg/m²). Treatment can be given as a once daily dose or alternatively the daily dose may be split into two administrations—one in the morning and one in the evening. The dose recommendation is currently based on a small number of pediatric patients. (See Action and Clinical Pharmacology.) There is no experience with the use of GLEEVEC in pediatric patients under 2 years of age.

For patients unable to swallow the film-coated tablets, the tablets may be dispersed in a glass of water or apple juice. The required number of tablets should be placed in the appropriate volume of beverage (approximately 50 mL for a 100 mg tablet, and 200 mL for a 400 mg tablet) and stirred with a spoon. The suspension should be administered immediately after complete disintegration of the tablet(s). Traces of the disintegrated tablet left in the glass after drinking should also be consumed.

Treatment should be continued as long as the patient continues to benefit.

For daily dosing of 800 mg, GLEEVEC should be administered using the 400 mg tablet twice a day to reduce exposure to iron.
Recommended Dose and Dosage Adjustment: Chronic Myeloid Leukemia (CML): The recommended dosage of GLEEVEC is 400 mg/day for adult patients with newly diagnosed CML or in chronic phase CML. The recommended dosage for adult patients in accelerated phase or blast crisis is 600 mg/day. The recommended dosage of GLEEVEC for pediatric patients with newly diagnosed Ph+ CML is 340 mg/m²/day (rounded to the nearest 100 mg, i.e. not to exceed 600 mg).

In CML, a dose increase from 400 mg to 600 mg or to 800 mg/day in adult patients with chronic phase disease, or from 600 mg to 800 mg (given as 400 mg twice daily) in adult patients in accelerated phase or blast crisis may be considered in the absence of severe adverse drug reactions and severe non-leukemia related neutropenia or thrombocytopenia in the following circumstances: disease progression (at any time); failure to achieve a satisfactory hematologic response after at least 3 months of treatment; failure to achieve a cytogenetic response after 12 months of treatment; or loss of a previously achieved hematologic and/or cytogenetic response.
Ph+ Acute Lymphoblastic Leukemia (Ph+ALL): The recommended dose of GLEEVEC for use as a single-agent for induction phase therapy in adult patients with newly diagnosed Ph+ALL, or for adult patients with relapsed or refractory Ph+ ALL is 600 mg/day.
Myelodysplastic/Myeloproliferative Diseases (MDS/MPD): The recommended dose of GLEEVEC is 400 mg/day for adult patients with MDS/MPD.
Aggressive Sub-types of Systemic Mastocytosis (ASM and SM-AHNMD): The recommended dose of GLEEVEC is 400 mg/day for adult patients with ASM or SM-AHNMD without the D816V c-Kit mutation. If c-Kit mutational status is not known or unavailable, treatment with GLEEVEC 400 mg/day may be considered for patients with ASM or SM-AHNMD not responding satisfactory to other therapies.

For patients with ASM or SM-AHNMD associated with eosinophilia, a clonal hematological disease related to the fusion kinase FIP1L1-PDGFRα, a starting dose of 100 mg/day is recommended. A dose increase from 100 mg to 400 mg for these patients may be considered in the absence of adverse drug reactions if assessments demonstrate an insufficient response to therapy.
Hypereosinophilic Syndrome (HES) and/or Chronic Eosinophilic Leukemia (CEL): The recommended dose of GLEEVEC is 100 mg/day for adult patients with HES/CEL.

For HES/CEL patients, a dose increase from 100 mg to 400 mg may be considered in the absence of adverse drug reactions if assessments demonstrate an insufficient response to therapy.

Treatment should be continued as long as the patient continues to benefit.
Dermatofibrosarcoma Protuberans (DFSP): The recommended dose of GLEEVEC is 800 mg/day for adult patients with DFSP.
Gastrointestinal stromal tumors (GIST): Unresectable and/or Metastatic Malignant GIST: The recommended dose of GLEEVEC is 400 mg/day or 600 mg/day for adult patients with unresectable and/or metastatic malignant GIST, depending on the stage and the progression of the disease. In GIST, a dose increase from 400 mg/day to 600 mg/day or to 800 mg/day for adult patients may be considered in the absence of adverse drug reactions if assessments demonstrate an insufficient response to therapy.
Adjuvant Treatment of GIST: The recommended dose of GLEEVEC is 400 mg/day for the adjuvant treatment of adult patients at intermediate to high risk of relapse following complete resection of Kit (CD117) positive GIST. In the clinical study, GLEEVEC was administrated for one year. The optimal treatment duration with GLEEVEC is not known.

No dose adjustment of the initial 400 mg a day dose was made in patients with GIST with mild liver function abnormalities.

Patients with mild, and moderate liver dysfunction should be dosed at the minimum effective dose of 400 mg daily and patients with severe liver dysfunction should start at 200 mg daily. In the absence of severe toxicity, a dose increase up to 300 mg daily may be considered. The dose should be reduced if the patient develops unacceptable toxicity (see Action and Clinical Pharmacology).

Dose Adjustment for Hepatotoxicity and Other Non-Hematologic Adverse Reactions: If a severe non-hematologic adverse reaction develops (such as severe hepatotoxicity or severe fluid retention), GLEEVEC should be withheld until the event has resolved. Thereafter, treatment can be resumed as appropriate depending on the initial severity of the event.

If elevations in bilirubin >3× institutional upper limit of normal (IULN) or in liver transaminases >5×IULN occur, GLEEVEC should be withheld until bilirubin levels have returned to a <1.5×IULN and transaminase levels to <2.5×IULN. In adults, treatment with GLEEVEC may then be continued at a reduced daily dose (i.e., from 400 mg to 300 mg or from 600 mg to 400 mg, or from 800 mg to 600 mg). In children, daily doses can be reduced under the same circumstances from 340 mg/m²/day to 260 mg/m²/day.

Dose Adjustment for Patients with Renal Impairment: GLEEVEC and its metabolites are not excreted via the kidney to a significant extent. However, it has been shown that exposure to imatinib is increased up to 2-fold in patients with mild (CrCL: 40-59 mL/min) and moderate (CrCL: 20-39 mL/min) renal dysfunction, and that there is a significant correlation in the incidence of serious adverse events with decreased renal function.

In clinical trials to date, the safety and efficacy of GLEEVEC in patients with renal impairment has not been established. Patients with mild or moderate renal dysfunction should be treated with **caution**, and be given the minimum recommended effective dose of 400 mg daily as starting dose. The dose should be reduced if not tolerable, or increased for lack of efficacy (see Warnings and Precautions). Treatment of patients with moderate renal insufficiency at 800 mg cannot be recommended as this dose has not been investigated in these patients. The effect of GLEEVEC treatment on patients with severe renal dysfunction (CrCL: <20 mL/min) and on hemodialysis has not been assessed, so treatment of these patients with imatinib cannot be recommended.

Hematologic Adverse Reactions: Dose reduction or treatment interruptions for severe neutropenia and thrombocytopenia are recommended as indicated in Table 13.

Table 13: GLEEVEC

Dose Adjustments for Neutropenia and Thrombocytopenia

ASM or SM-AHNMD associated with eosinophilia and HES/CEL with FIP1L1-PDGFRα fusion kinase (starting dose 100 mg)	ANC <1.0×10⁹/L and/or platelets <50×10⁹/L	1. Stop GLEEVEC until ANC ≥1.5×10⁹/L and platelets ≥75×10⁹/L. 2. Resume treatment with GLEEVEC at previous dose (i.e. before severe adverse reaction).
Chronic phase CML (starting at dose 400 mg) MDS/MPD, ASM/SM-AHNMD, HES/CEL (at 400 mg dose) or GIST (starting dose either 400 mg or 600 mg)	ANC <1.0×10⁹/L and/or Platelets <50×10⁹/L	1. Stop GLEEVEC until ANC ≥1.5×10⁹/L and platelets ≥75×10⁹/L. 2. Resume treatment with GLEEVEC at the original dose of 400 mg or 600 mg (i.e. before severe adverse reaction). 3. If recurrence of ANC <1.0×10⁹/L and/or Platelets <50×10⁹/L, repeat step 1 and resume GLEEVEC at a reduced dose of 300 mg (if starting dose was 400 mg, 400 mg if starting dose was 600 mg).
Newly diagnosed pediatric chronic phase CML (at dose 340 mg/m²/day)	ANC <1.0×10⁹/L and/or platelets <50×10⁹/L	1. Stop GLEEVEC until ANC ≥1.5×10⁹/L and platelets ≥75×10⁹/L. 2. Resume treatment with GLEEVEC at previous dose (i.e. before severe adverse reaction). 3. In the event of recurrence of ANC <1.0×10⁹/L and/or platelets <50×10⁹/L, repeat step 1 and resume GLEEVEC at reduced dose of 260 mg/m²/day.
Accelerated phase CML and blast crisis and Ph+ALL (starting dose 600 mg)	[a]ANC <0.5×10⁹/L and/or Platelets <10×10⁹/L	1. Check if cytopenia is related to leukemia (marrow aspirate or biopsy). 2. If cytopenia is unrelated to leukemia, reduce dose of GLEEVEC to 400 mg. 3. If cytopenia persists for 2 weeks, reduce further to 300 mg. 4. If cytopenia persists for 4 weeks and is still unrelated to leukemia, stop GLEEVEC until ANC ≥1×10⁹/L and platelets ≥20×10⁹/L and then resume treatment at 300 mg.
DFSP (at 800 mg dose)	ANC <1.0×10⁹/L and/or platelets <50×10⁹/L	1. Stop GLEEVEC until ANC ≥1.5 ×10⁹/L and platelets ≥75×10⁹/L. 2. Resume treatment with GLEEVEC at 600 mg. 3. In the event of recurrence of ANC <1.0×10⁹/L and/or platelets <50×10⁹/L, repeat step 1 and resume GLEEVEC at reduced dose of 400 mg.

[a] Occurring after at least 1 month of treatment.
Legend: ANC=absolute neutrophil count.

OVERDOSAGE:

Experience with higher than therapeutic doses is limited. Isolated cases of GLEEVEC overdosage have been reported spontaneously and in the literature. Generally the reported outcome in these cases was improvement or recovery. In the event of overdosage the patient should be observed and appropriate symptomatic treatment should be given.

Events that have been reported at different dose ranges are as follows:

Adult Overdose: 1200 to 1600 mg (duration varying between 1 to 10 days): Nausea, vomiting, diarrhea, rash, erythema, oedema, swelling, fatigue, muscle spasms, thrombocytopenia, pancytopenia, abdominal pain, headache, decreased appetite, increased bilirubin and liver transaminase level. 1800 to 3200 mg (as high as 3200 mg daily for 6 days): Weakness, myalgia, increased CPK, increased bilirubin, gastrointestinal pain. 6400 mg (single dose): A case report in the literature about one patient who experienced nausea, vomiting, abdominal pain, pyrexia, facial swelling, neutrophil count decreased, increased transaminases. 8 to 10 g (single dose): Vomiting and gastrointestinal pain have been reported.

Pediatric Overdose: One 3 year-old male exposed to a single dose of 400 mg experienced vomiting, diarrhoea and anorexia and another 3 year old male exposed to a single dose of 980 mg dose experienced decreased white blood cell count and diarrhea.

> For management of a suspected drug overdose, contact your regional Poison Control Centre. See the *CPS* Directory section for a list of Poison Control Centres.

ACTION AND CLINICAL PHARMACOLOGY: Mechanism of Action: GLEEVEC (imatinib mesylate) is a protein tyrosine kinase inhibitor, which inhibits the Bcr-Abl tyrosine kinase at the in vitro, cellular, and in vivo levels. The compound selectively inhibits proliferation and induces apoptosis in Bcr-Abl positive cell lines as well as fresh leukemic cells from Philadelphia chromosome-positive chronic myeloid leukemia (CML) and acute lymphoid leukemia (ALL) patients. In colony formation assays using ex vivo peripheral blood and bone marrow samples, imatinib shows selective inhibition of Bcr-Abl positive colonies from CML patients.

In vivo, it inhibits tumor growth of Bcr-Abl transfected murine myeloid cells as well as Bcr-Abl positive leukemia lines derived from CML patients in blast crisis.

In addition, imatinib is an inhibitor of the receptor tyrosine kinases for platelet-derived growth factor (PDGF) and stem cell factor (SCF), c-Kit, and inhibits PDGF- and SCF-mediated cellular events. In vitro, imatinib inhibits proliferation and induces apoptosis in gastrointestinal stromal tumor (GIST) cells, which express an activating kit mutation.

Constitutive activation of the PDGFR or the Abl protein tyrosine kinases as a consequence of fusion to diverse partner proteins or constitutive production of PDGF have been implicated in the pathogenesis of several conditions including MDS/MPD, HES/CEL and DFSP. In addition, constitutive activation of c-Kit or the PDGFR has been implicated in the pathogenesis of SM. Imatinib inhibits signaling and proliferation of cells driven by dysregulated PDGFR, Kit and Abl kinase activity.

Several mechanisms of resistance have been identified from in vitro studies of Bcr-Abl positive cell lines. Mechanisms include amplification of the Bcr-Abl gene and overexpression of the multidrug resistance P-glycoprotein. Mutation or amplification of the Bcr-Abl gene has been described in relapsed patients with advanced stage CML.

Prevalence of Abl kinase domain mutations among samples of resistant CML patients varies across studies, likely reflecting variations in time frames for testing, the duration of imatinib exposure, patient selection differences, and perhaps differences in techniques and sensitivity.

The specific clinical relevance of Abl kinase domain mutations in the prognosis and management of patients with CML requires further study. It is likely that mutations will have different clinical phenotypes, with some being subject to higher-dose imatinib therapy, depending on the IC_{50} of the mutation, and others requiring alternative treatment strategies.

Recent in vitro experiments have indicated that some mutations remain sensitive to GLEEVEC at high concentrations, other mutants remain unresponsive to dose escalation, which may indicate a kinase independent, or even Bcr-Abl independent mechanisms of resistance.

Currently identified possible mechanisms of resistance to GLEEVEC can be categorized in two main groups: the mechanisms where Bcr-Abl is reactivated and cell proliferation remains dependent on Bcr-Abl signaling, and mechanisms where the Bcr-Abl protein remains inactivated by GLEEVEC but alternative signalling pathways become activated. Whereas the primary resistance to GLEEVEC seems mostly associated with amplification of the Bcr-Abl gene, secondary resistance (i.e. loss of response or progression) appears to be associated with the emergence of mutations of the Bcr-Abl gene (see Table 14).

Table 14: GLEEVEC

Currently Identified Mechanisms of Resistance to Imatinib

Bcr-Abl Dependent Mechanisms (cells remain dependent of Bcr-Abl signaling)	Bcr-Abl Independent Mechanisms (Bcr-Abl is inactivated)
Amplification of Bcr-Abl gene	Activation of signaling pathways downstream of Bcr-Abl
Mutations of Bcr-Abl preventing correct Bcr-Abl imatinib binding	Clonal evolution with appearance of new chromosomal abnormalities
Efflux of imatinib by PgP associated MDR protein	Activation of leukemogenic pathways unrelated to Bcr-Abl
Protein binding of imatinib (eg. to circulating AGP)	

Legend: P-gP=Protein–glyco-Protein; MDR=Multidrug Resistance; AGP=Alpha 1-acid glycoprotein.

The clinical utility of detecting mutations remains to be demonstrated, since mutations have been described among GLEEVEC treated patients without evidence of disease progression. In addition, the approach to managing resistance will differ by CML disease stage, irrespective of treatment. Clinical and molecular resistance is much more prevalent among patients with blast crisis and accelerated phase CML, than among patients with chronic phase CML.

Pharmacokinetics: The pharmacokinetics (PK) of GLEEVEC have been evaluated in 591 patients and 33 healthy subjects over a dosage range of 25 to 1000 mg.

Absorption: Mean absolute bioavailability for the capsule formulation is 98%. The coefficient of variation for plasma imatinib AUC is in the range of 40-60% after an oral dose. When given with a high fat meal the rate of absorption of imatinib was reduced (11% decrease in C_{max} and prolongation of t_{max} by 1.5 h), with a small reduction in AUC (7.4%) compared to fasting conditions.

Distribution: At clinically relevant concentrations of imatinib, binding to plasma proteins is approximately 95% on the basis of in vitro experiments, mostly to albumin and α_1-acid glycoprotein, with little binding to lipoproteins.

In in vitro experiments, the active metabolite, CGP74588, exhibited similar protein binding behaviour to imatinib at clinically relevant concentrations

Metabolism: CYP3A4 is the major enzyme responsible for metabolism of imatinib. Other cytochrome P450 enzymes, such as CYP1A2, CYP2D6, CYP2C9, and CYP2C19, play a minor role in its metabolism.

The main circulating active metabolite in humans is the N-demethylated piperazine derivative, formed predominantly by CYP3A4. It shows in vitro potency similar to the parent imatinib. The plasma AUC for this metabolite is about 15% of the AUC for imatinib and the terminal half-life is approximately 40 h at steady state. The plasma protein binding of the N-demethylated metabolite CGP74588 was shown to be similar to that of the parent compound in both healthy volunteers and Acute Myeloid Leukemia (AML) patients although there were variabilities in blood distribution and protein binding between AML patients. Some of the AML patients showed a significantly higher unbound fraction of both compounds which led to a higher blood cell uptake.

A phase I study has shown a 4- to 7-fold accumulation of the metabolite CGP74588 at steady state following once daily dosing, which was greater than the parent drug (see Plasma Pharmacokinetics). This might be due to the fact that CGP74588 is metabolized at a 53% lower metabolic conversion rate compared to GLEEVEC in human hepatocytes. The reduced metabolic clearance of CGP74588 is further implied by in vitro experiments which showed a lower infinity of CGP74588 to CYP3A4 in comparison to STI571.

Excretion: Based on the recovery of compound(s) after an oral ^{14}C-labelled dose of imatinib, approximately 81% of the dose was eliminated within 7 days in feces (68% of dose) and urine (13% of dose). Unchanged imatinib accounted for 25% of the dose (5% urine, 20% feces), the remainder being metabolites.

Plasma Pharmacokinetics: Following oral administration in healthy volunteers, the $t_{½}$ was approximately 18 hours suggesting that once daily dosing is appropriate. Plasma pharmacokinetic profiles were analyzed in CML patients on Day 1 and on either Day 7 or 28, by which time plasma concentrations had reached steady state. The increase in mean imatinib AUC with increasing dose was linear and dose proportional in the range 25-1000 mg after oral administration. There was no change in the kinetics of imatinib on repeated dosing, and accumulation is 1.5-2.5 fold at steady state when GLEEVEC is dosed once daily.

The effect of body weight on the clearance of imatinib is such that for a patient weighing 50 kg the mean clearance is expected to be 8.5 L/h, while for a patient weighing 100 kg the clearance will rise to 11.8 L/h. These changes are not considered sufficient to warrant dose adjustment based on body weight. There is no effect of gender on the kinetics of imatinib.

Special Populations and Conditions: Pediatrics: A total of 31 pediatric patients with either chronic phase CML (n=15), CML in blast crisis (n=4) or acute leukemias (n=12) have been enrolled in a dose-escalation phase I trial. In this trial the effective dose in pediatric patients was not identified. This was a population of heavily pretreated patients; 45% had received prior BMT and 68% prior multi-agent chemotherapy. Newly diagnosed patients or those eligible for bone marrow transplantation were not studied. The median age was 14 years (range 3 to 20 years). Of the 31 patients, n=12 were three to 11 years old at the start of the study, n=17 were between 12 and 18 years, and only two were more than 18 years old. Patients were treated with doses of GLEEVEC of 260 mg/m²/day (n=6), 340 mg/m²/day (n=11), 440 mg/m²/day (n= 8) and 570 mg/m²/day (n=6). Dosing based upon body surface area resulted in some patients receiving higher than the adult therapeutic dose, and the effect of this on pediatric patient safety is limited.

As in adult patients, imatinib was rapidly absorbed after oral administration in pediatric patients in both phase I and phase II studies. Dosing in children at 260 and 340 mg/m²/day achieved similar exposure, respectively, as doses of 400 mg and 600 mg in adult patients, although this was based upon a small sample size. The comparison of $AUC_{0\text{-}24}$ on Day 8 versus Day 1 at the 340 mg/m²/day dose level revealed a 1.7- fold drug accumulation after repeated once daily dosing. As in adults, there was considerable inter-patient variability in the pharmacokinetics, and the coefficient of variation for $AUC_{0\text{-}24}$ ranged from 21% (260 mg/m²/day) to 68% (570 mg/m²/day). The AUC did not increase proportionally with dose within the range of doses examined. The active metabolite, GCP 74588, contributed about 20% of the AUC for imatinib. Total plasma clearance is about 8-10 L/h at steady state. The plasma AUC of imatinib is significantly lower (p=0.02) in children at ages between 2 and <12 years old (29.3 μg*hr/mL) than those at ages between 12 and <20 years old (34.6 μg*hr/mL). However, the difference between the two age groups does not seem to be clinically significant, only 15% of difference (geometric mean of 29.3 in children compared to 34.6 in adolescents). The AUC exposure in both age groups falls within the adult $AUC_{(0\text{-}24\,h)}$ range, between 24.8 and 39.7 μg*h/mL, achieved at 400 mg and 600 mg daily doses, respectively.

Geriatrics: Based on population PK analysis, there was an effect of age on the volume of distribution (12% increase in patients >65 years old). This change is not thought to be clinically significant.

Hepatic Insufficiency: In a study of patients with mild and moderate hepatic dysfunction (Table 15), the mean exposure to imatinib (dose normalized AUC) did not differ significantly compared with patients with normal liver function. There was a tendency toward an increased exposure in patients with severe liver dysfunction (approximately 45% increase compared with patients with normal liver function). In this study up to 500 mg daily was used in patients with mild liver dysfunction, up to 400 mg daily in patients with moderate, and up to 300 mg daily in patients with severe liver dysfunction.

In the severe liver dysfunction group 29% of patients experienced serious adverse events at the 100 mg dose level, 60% at the 200 mg and 50% of patients treated at the 300 mg dose levels. (See Warnings and Precautions and Dosage and Administration.)

Table 15: GLEEVEC

Liver Dysfunction Classification

Liver Dysfunction	Liver Dysfunction Tests
Mild	Total bilirubin: =1.5 ULN AST: >ULN (can be normal or <ULN if Total bilirubin is >ULN)
Moderate	Total bilirubin: >1.5–3.0 ULN AST: any
Severe	Total bilirubin: >3–10 ULN AST: any

Legend: ULN=upper limit of normal for the institution; AST=aspartate transferase.

Renal Insufficiency: Imatinib and its metabolites are not excreted via the kidney to a significant extent.

In a study of patients with varying degrees of renal dysfunction (mild, moderate and severe—see Table 16 for renal function classification), the mean exposure to imatinib (dose normalized AUC) increased 1.5- to 2-fold compared to patients with normal renal function, which corresponded to an elevated plasma level of AGP, a protein to which imatinib binds strongly. There was a correlation with the incidence of serious adverse events and decreasing renal function (p=0.0096). In this study, 800 mg daily was used in patients with mild renal dysfunction and 600 mg daily was used in patients with moderate renal dysfunction. The 800 mg dose was not tested in patients with moderate renal dysfunction due to the limited number of patients enrolled. Similarly, only 2 patients with severe renal dysfunction were enrolled at the low (100 mg) dose, and no higher doses were tested. No patients on hemodialysis were enrolled in the study. Since the effect of GLEEVEC treatment on patients with severe renal dysfunction and on hemodialysis has not been sufficiently assessed, treatment of these patients with imatinib cannot be recommended. Patients with mild or moderate renal dysfunction should be treated with **caution**, and be given the minimum recommended dose of 400 mg daily as starting dose. The dose should be reduced if not tolerable, or increased for lack of efficacy. Dosing of patients with moderate renal insufficiency at 800 mg cannot be recommended as this has not been investigated (see Dosage and Administration and Warnings and Precautions).

Table 16: GLEEVEC

Renal Function Classification

Renal Dysfunction	Renal Function Tests
Mild	CrCL = 40–59 mL/min
Moderate	CrCL = 20–39 mL/min
Severe	CrCL = <20 mL/min

Legend: CrCL=creatinine clearance.

Drug-Drug Interactions: CYP3A4 Inhibitors: There was a significant increase in exposure to imatinib (mean C_{max} and AUC increased by 26% and 40%, respectively) in healthy subjects when GLEEVEC was co-administered with a single dose of ketoconazole (a CYP3A4 inhibitor). (See Drug Interactions.)

CYP3A4 Substrates: Imatinib increased the mean C_{max} and AUC of simvastatin (CYP3A4 substrate) by 2- and 3.5- fold, respectively, indicating an inhibition of CYP3A4 by imatinib. (See Drug Interactions.)

CYP3A4 Inducers: Administration of rifampin 600 mg daily for eight days to 14 healthy adult volunteers, followed by a single 400 mg dose of GLEEVEC increased imatinib oral dose clearance by 3.8-fold (90% CI 3.5- to 4.3-fold). Mean C_{max}, AUC_{0-24} and $AUC_{0-\infty}$ decreased by 54%, 68% and 74%, respectively compared to treatment without rifampin. In patients in whom rifampin or other CYP3A4 inducers are indicated, alternate therapeutic agents with less enzyme induction potential should be considered. (See Drug Interactions.)

In Vitro Studies of CYP Enzyme Inhibition: Human liver microsome studies demonstrated that imatinib is a potent competitive inhibitor of CYP2C9, CYP2D6, and CYP3A4/5 with K_i values of 27, 7.5, and 8 μM, respectively. Imatinib is likely to increase the blood level of drugs that are substrates of CYP2C9, CYP2D6 and CYP3A4/5. (See Drug Interactions.)

STORAGE AND STABILITY: Store GLEEVEC at room temperature (15-30°C). Protect tablets from moisture.

INFORMATION FOR THE PATIENT: Published in e-CPS, available by subscription at www.e-cps.ca.

DOSAGE FORMS, COMPOSITION AND PACKAGING: 100 mg: Each scored tablet contains: imatinib 100 mg (as mesylate). Nonmedicinal ingredients: cellulose (microcrystalline), colloidal silicon dioxide, crospovidone, hydroxypropyl methylcellulose and magnesium stearate; coating: ferric oxide (red), ferric oxide (yellow), hydroxypropyl methylcellulose, polyethylene glycol and talc. Blister strips of 10, cartons of 6, 12 and 18.

400 mg: Each scored or unscored tablet contains: imatinib 400 mg (as mesylate). Nonmedicinal ingredients: cellulose (microcrystalline), colloidal silicon dioxide, crospovidone, hydroxypropyl methylcellulose and magnesium stearate; coating: ferric oxide (red), ferric oxide (yellow), hydroxypropyl methylcellulose, polyethylene glycol and talc. Blister strips of 10, cartons of 1, 3 and 9.

(Shown in Product Identification Section)

Gliclazide

CPhA Monograph

see *Sulfonylureas*

Glimepiride

CPhA Monograph

see *Sulfonylureas*

GlucaGen®

glucagon

Hyperglycemic Agent

Novo Nordisk

GlucaGen® HypoKit

glucagon

Hyperglycemic Agent

Novo Nordisk

Date of Preparation: September 15, 2009

SUMMARY PRODUCT INFORMATION:

Route of Administration	Dosage Form/ Strength	Clinically Relevant Nonmedicinal Ingredients
Intramuscularly	Intramuscularly, lyophilized powder for injection/1 mg	Lactose For a complete listing see Dosage Forms, Composition and Packaging.

INDICATIONS AND CLINICAL USE: GlucaGen/GlucaGen HypoKit, is indicated for:

- the treatment of severe hypoglycemic reactions which may occur in the management of insulin treated persons with diabetes mellitus, when unconsciousness precludes oral carbohydrates.

The use of GlucaGen is approved when administered by i.m. injection.

Geriatrics: No data available.

Pediatrics: Pediatrics between birth and 16 years of age were not studied in the clinical studies (see Warnings and Precautions, Special Populations).

CONTRAINDICATIONS:

- Patients who are hypersensitive to this drug, lactose or any component of the container. For a complete listing, see Dosage Forms, Composition and Packaging.
- GlucaGen is contraindicated in phaeochromocytoma.

WARNINGS AND PRECAUTIONS:

> **Serious Warnings and Precautions**
> **GlucaGen should be given only if patients are unconscious or unresponsive and unable to ingest oral glucose. After intramuscular injection the patient will normally respond within 10 minutes. If the patient does not respond within 10 minutes, intravenous glucose must be administered as soon as an IV access can be established.**
> **Because glucagon is of little or no help in states of starvation, adrenal insufficiency, or chronic hypoglycemia, intravenous glucose should be used for the treatment of hypoglycemia in these conditions.**

General: GlucaGen for injection, rDNA origin, is helpful in treating hypoglycemia only if sufficient liver glycogen is present.

Glucagon reacts antagonistically towards insulin and caution should be observed if GlucaGen is used in patients with insulinoma. Caution should also be observed in patients with glucagonoma.

To prevent relapse of hypoglycemia, oral carbohydrates should be given to restore the liver glycogen when the patient has responded to the treatment.

Exogenous glucagon also stimulates the release of catecholamines. In the presences of pheochromocytoma, glucagon can cause the tumour to release catecholamines, which results in a sudden and marked increase in blood pressure (see Contraindications).

If fibril formation (viscous appearance) or solid particles are present in the solution, it must not be used.

Do not give GlucaGen via intravenous infusion.

Carcinogenesis and Mutagenesis: No carcinogenicity studies have been conducted.

The potential for genotoxicity of glucagon (rDNA origin) has been evaluated using a series of recognized in vitro and in vivo assays for mutagenic-genotoxic activity and results indicate that glucagon (rDNA origin) should be considered non mutagenic.

Cardiovascular: In high concentrations, glucagon exerts positive inotropic and chronotropic effect and may therefore cause tachycardia and acute hypertensive reactions (see Contraindications).

Information to Be Provided to the Patient: Because GlucaGen HypoKit is designed to be administered to the patient by relative(s) in emergency situations, in which a high level of stress will likely be involved, it is imperative that the kits be easy to find and easy to use. It is therefore important that the patient be instructed to make sure that family, friends and co-workers know when and how to use GlucaGen HypoKit. Specific directions for reconstitution and use should also be provided along with the GlucaGen HypoKit.

Specific instructions on the use of GlucaGen should be given to patients at risk of hypoglycemia unawareness, including elderly.

Sensitivity/Resistance: Glucagon is a protein in which hypersensitivity reactions may occur in rare events. Generalized allergic reactions including urticaria, respiratory distress, and hypotension (anaphylactic reaction/shock), have been reported in patients who received glucagon.

Special Populations: Patients with Type 2 Diabetes: When deciding about the use of glucagon for the patient with type 2 diabetes, consider those with a long duration of diabetes and/or insulin treatment. Those with advanced type 2 diabetes have a similar decline in counter-regulatory hormones as do those with type 1 diabetes.

Pregnant Women: Well-controlled studies in pregnant women have not been performed with recombinant glucagon. GlucaGen should be used during pregnancy only if oral carbohydrates cannot be administered (see Action and Clinical Pharmacology). Glucagon does not cross the human placenta barrier. The use of glucagon has been reported in pregnant women with diabetes and no harmful effects are known with respect to the course of pregnancy and the health of the fetus and neonate.

Nursing Women: It is not known whether GlucaGen is excreted in human milk. Glucagon is quickly cleared from the bloodstream by the liver ($T_{½}$=3-6 min); thus the amount excreted in the milk of nursing mothers following treatment of severe hypoglycemic reactions will be extremely small. As glucagon is degraded in the digestive tract and cannot be absorbed in its intact form, it will not exert any metabolic effect in the child.

Pediatrics: The use of GlucaGen in pediatric patients (>25 kg or older than 6-8 years) has been reported to be safe and effective (see Indications and Clinical Use).

Geriatrics: No data available. Elderly patients on insulin may also be candidates for glucagon, as they may have hypoglycemic unawareness simply because of the aging process.

Use with Alcohol: Alcohol can suppress hepatic gluconeogenesis and chronic alcoholism can deplete liver glycogen stores. Therefore glucagon may be less effective in presence of acute or chronic alcohol ingestion.

Monitoring and Laboratory Tests: Blood glucose determinations should be obtained to follow the patient with hypoglycemia until the patient is asymptomatic.

Occupational Hazards: No studies on the effects on the ability to drive and use machines have been performed.

ADVERSE REACTIONS: Adverse Drug Reaction Overview: The safety profile of GlucaGen has been assessed in six clinical studies after up to 3 doses of glucagon.

Adverse reactions are very rare except for occasional nausea and vomiting which may also occur with hypoglycemia.

Generalized allergic reactions including urticaria, respiratory distress, and hypotension (anaphylactic reaction/shock), have been reported in patients who received glucagon (see Warnings and Precautions).

Clinical Trial Adverse Drug Reactions: Because clinical trials are conducted under very specific conditions the adverse reaction rates observed in the clinical trials may not reflect the rates observed in practice and should not be compared to the rates in the clinical trials of another drug. Adverse drug reaction information from clinical trials is useful for identifying drug-related adverse events and for approximating rates.

Common Clinical Trial Adverse Drug Reactions: For summary of the most frequently reported (>1% of subjects) adverse events, see Table 1.

Less Common Clinical Trial Adverse Drug Reactions (<1%): Body as a Whole—General Disorders: anxiety, blurred vision, dry mouth, generally unwell, hungry, leg pain, malaise, reactive hypoglycemia, slightly apathetic, thirsty, trembling, tremor, very hungry, very tired, weakness.

Gastrointestinal System Disorders: slightly troubled stomach.

Cardiovascular Disorders: arrhythmia, myocarditis, pericarditis, pulmonary embolism, slight palpitation, tachycardia, unrest and palpitation, vasovagal.

Respiratory Disorders/Infections and Infestations: bronchospasm, pneumonia.

Abnormal Hematologic and Clinical Chemistry Findings: There were no abnormal hematologic and/or clinical chemistry findings considered related to GlucaGen treatment.

Table 1: GlucaGen

Number of Common Adverse Events in all Clinical Studies

Body System AE Preferred Term	1 mg GlucaGen N=187 N (%)	1 mg Pancreatic Glucagon[a] N=102 N (%)
Body as a Whole—General Disorders		
Tired	2 (1.1)	4 (3.92)
Sweating	2 (1.1)	—
Trembling (tremor)	2 (1.1)	—
Central & Peripheral Nervous System Disorders		
Headache	5 (2.7)	3 (2.9)
Dizziness	26 (13.9)	17(16.7)
Gastrointestinal System Disorders		
Nausea	49 (26.2)	27 (26.5)
Vomiting	7 (3.7)	6 (5.9)

[a] Adverse events reported form 6 different clinical trials, some of which had a pancreatic glucagon control group.

Post-Market Adverse Drug Reactions: Frequencies of undesirable effects considered related to treatment with GlucaGen during clinical trials and/or post-marketing surveillance survey is presented in Table 2. Undesirable effects which have not been observed in clinical trials, but have been reported spontaneously are presented as "very rare". During marketed use reporting of adverse drug reactions is very rare (≤1/10 000). However, post-marketing experience is subject to under-reporting and this reporting rate should be interpreted in that light. The estimated number of treatment episodes is 46.9 millions over a 16 year period.

Table 2: GlucaGen

Post-Marketing Experience

Body System	Subject Incidence	Adverse Drug Reaction
Immune System Disorders	Very rare ≤1/10 000	Hypersensitivity reactions including anaphylactic reaction/shock
Gastrointestinal Disorders	Common >1/100 and <1/10	Nausea
	Uncommon >1/1000 and ≤1/100	Vomiting
	Rare >1/10 000 and ≤1/1000	Abdominal pain

DRUG INTERACTIONS: Overview: Interactions between GlucaGen (glucagon) and other drugs are not known, when GlucaGen is used in diabetes.

Published literature has shown the following interactions:
Insulin: Reacts antagonistically towards glucagon.
Indomethacin: Glucagon may lose its ability to raise blood glucose or paradoxically may even produce hypoglycemia.
Warfarin: Glucagon may increase the anticoagulant effect of warfarin.

Alcohol induced hypoglycemia is associated with a failure of blood glucose levels to rise normally after the administration of glucagon.

Drug-Drug Interactions: Drug-drug interactions supported by animal or in vitro studies have not been established.
Sulfonylurea: Although the use of glucagon in patients taking a sulfonylurea should work acutely, the pharmacokinetic characteristics of sulfonylurea will result in remaining systemic concentrations for a long time and thus can cause significant and prolonged hypoglycemia. The preferred treatment of severe hypoglycemia in patients taking sulfonylurea is therefore the administration of glucose by i.v. bolus injection followed by continuous i.v. infusion until the end of the pharmacologic effects of the sulfonylurea.
Drug-Food Interactions: Interactions with food have not been established.
Drug-Herb Interactions: Interactions with herbs have not been established.
Drug-Laboratory Test Interactions: Interactions with laboratories have not been established.

DOSAGE AND ADMINISTRATION: Dosing Considerations: GlucaGen and GlucaGen HypoKit should be reconstituted with the accompanying diluent following the detailed directions contained within the section Administration.
Recommended Dose and Dosage Adjustment: GlucaGen and GlucaGen HypoKit: Dosage for Adult Patients: Administer 1 mg.
Dosage for Paediatric Patients: Administer 1 mg (children above 25 kg or older than 6-8 years) or 0.5 mg (children below 25 kg or younger than 6-8 years).

Administer by intramuscular injection. The patient will normally respond within 10 minutes. When the patient has responded to the treatment, give oral carbohydrate to restore the liver glycogen and prevent relapse of hypoglycemia. If the patient does not respond within 10 minutes, intravenous glucose should be given.

Medical consultation is required for all patients with severe hypoglycemia.

Caution: Although glucagon may be used for the treatment of hypoglycemia for the patient during an emergency, the physician must still be notified when hypoglycaemic reactions occur so that the dose of insulin and oral antidiabetic medication may be adjusted more accurately.
Missed Dose: Not applicable.
Administration: Reconstitution of the Parenteral GlucaGen Product:

Vial Size	Volume of Diluent to be Added to Vial	Approximate Available Volume	Nominal Concentration per mL
2.0 mL	1.1 mL	1.0 mL	1 mg/mL

Before reconstitution the powder should be a white or nearly white powder. The solvent should be clear and colourless without particles.
GlucaGen (glucagon): Draw up the Water for Injection (1.1 mL) in a disposable syringe. inject the Water for Injections into the vial containing the freeze-dried glucagon. Shake the vial gently until the glucagon is completely dissolved and the solution is clear. Withdraw the solution back into the syringe.

The reconstituted solution forms an injection of 1 mg (1 IU) per mL to be administered by intramuscular injection.

Any unused product or waste material should be disposed of in accordance with local requirements.

GlucaGen HypoKit (glucagon): Inject the Water for Injections (1.1 mL) into the vial containing the freeze-dried glucagon. Shake the vial gently until the glucagon is completely dissolved and the solution is clear. Withdraw the solution back into the syringe.

The reconstituted solution forms an injection of 1 mg (1 IU) per mL to be administered by intramuscular injection.

OVERDOSAGE:
Glucagon has a short half-life of approximately 3-6 minutes. Therefore, treatment of overdose is symptomatic—primarily for nausea, vomiting and hypokalemia.

Hyperglycemia may also be a symptom of overdose.

In case of suspected overdosing (i.e. above therapeutic dosages), the serum potassium may decrease and should be monitored and corrected, if needed.

> For management of a suspected drug overdose, CPhA recommends that you contact your **regional Poison Control Centre**. See the *CPS* Directory section for a list of Poison Control Centres.

ACTION AND CLINICAL PHARMACOLOGY: GlucaGen is a polypeptide hormone identical to human glucagon, which is manufactured by recombinant DNA technology and has the same molecular structure as animal-sources glucagon.
Mechanism of Action: Glucagon acts to increase the concentration of glucose in the blood by releasing glucose from storage in the liver. Parenteral administration of glucagon relaxes also smooth muscle of the stomach, duodenum, small bowel, and colon.
Pharmacodynamics: The pharmacodynamics of GlucaGen (glucagon) has been determined in a two part crossover, double-blind comparative bioavailability study in 12 healthy male adult subjects (Study 1). Plasma glucagon, insulin, blood glucose and C-peptide levels after were measured after i.m. injection of 1 mg GlucaGen (glucagon) and 1 mg pancreatic glucagon formulations.

Study 1 showed a rapid rise in circulating glucagon levels following an i.m. injection of 1 mg glucagon with a mean plasma level of 3612.6 pg/mL at 0.167 hr after pancreatic glucagon and 3975.38 pg/mL at 0.167 hr after GlucaGen.

The plasma levels of insulin increased in parallel with c-peptides to achieve a mean plasma level of 62.25 (±53.63) mU/L at a median time of 0.417 hr following injection of pancreatic glucagon. After GlucaGen administration, the plasma insulin concentration level increased to 85.79 (±101.46) mU/L at a median time of 0.5 hr.

The plasma glucose levels increased rapidly after injection of both formulations to a maximum of 9.06 mmol/L (±1.29) and 8.62 mmol/L (±0.90) following pancreatic glucagon and GlucaGen injections, respectively.

The c-peptide plasma levels increased, from a mean pre-dose value of 780.42 pmoles/L to a mean value of 2444.55 pmoles/L at 0.5 hr after pancreatic glucagon and from a mean pre-dose value of 575.83 pmoles/L to a mean value of 2289.09 pmoles/L at 0.833 hr after GlucaGen.

The plasma levels of glucose, c-peptide and insulin returned to pre-dose values at about 1.5 hr after injection of both pancreatic glucagon and GlucaGen.

Pharmacokinetics: A pharmacokinetic open-labelled study was performed to provide C_{max} and $AUC_{0\text{-}4hrs}$ for GlucaGen after a single i.m. dose in 12 healthy adult males for pharmacokinetic properties and in 20 subjects for safety evaluation (Study 2A).

A summary of the pharmacokinetic results for study 2A is presented in Table 3.

Table 3: GlucaGen

Summary of Glucagon Pharmacokinetic Parameters Following the I.M. Administration of GlucaGen to Healthy Volunteers

Study	Dose	C_{max} (mg/min) Mean (SD)	T_{max} (min) Mean (SD)	$AUC_{0\text{-}360}$ (mg) Mean (SD)	$AUC_{0\text{-}4\ hrs}$ (pg·min/mL) Mean (SD)
2A[a]	1 mg GlucaGen	1627.5 (730.4)	17.9 (23.4)	—	93 992.4 (43 682.0)

[a] Values for study 2A =average of 3 baseline readings subtracted from all samples.

Distribution: The volume of distribution of glucagon is approximately 0.2 L/kg.
Metabolism: Metabolic clearance rate of glucagon in humans is approximately 10 mL/kg/min. It is degraded enzymatically in the blood plasma and in the organs to which it is distributed. The liver and kidney are major sites of glucagon clearance, each organ contributing about 30% to the overall metabolic clearance rate.
Excretion: Following a 1 mg i.m. injection of GlucaGen, the half-life was approximately 3-6 minutes. The clearance of glucagon is approximately 19 mL/min·kg. Glucagon is eliminated in tissues, plasma, liver, and the kidneys however; the main route of elimination has not yet been determined.

STORAGE AND STABILITY: GlucaGen (glucagon): Prior to reconstitution, the shelf life of the product is 3 years. GlucaGen should be stored at a temperature not exceeding 2-8°C. The sealed container should be protected from light and freezing should be avoided.

The reconstituted GlucaGen should be used immediately after preparation. Any unused product or waste material should be disposed of in accordance with local requirements.

If, in rare cases, the reconstituted solution shows any signs of fibril formation (viscous appearance) or insoluble matter, it should be discarded.

GlucaGen HypoKit (glucagon): Prior to reconstitution, the shelf life of the product is 3 years at a temperature of 2-8°C. During this period, GlucaGen HypoKit can be stored at a temperature not exceeding 25°C for 18 months provided that the expiry date is not exceeded. The sealed container should be protected from light and freezing should be avoided.

The reconstituted GlucaGen HypoKit should be used immediately after preparation. Any unused product or waste material should be disposed of in accordance with local requirements.

If, in rare cases, the reconstituted solution shows any signs of fibril formation (viscous appearance) or insoluble matter, it should be discarded.

SPECIAL HANDLING INSTRUCTIONS: Not applicable.

INFORMATION FOR THE PATIENT: Published in e-CPS, available by subscription at www.e-cps.ca.

DOSAGE FORMS, COMPOSITION AND PACKAGING: GlucaGen : Each stoppered glass vial contains: glucagon 1 mg corresponding to 1 mg glucagon/mL after reconstitution. The vials are provided with a tamperproof plastic cap, which must be removed before use. GlucaCen 1 mg/mL vial is supplied as a sterile, freeze-dried white powder of glucagon in a 2 mL vial and accompanying solvent also in a 2 mL vial. Glucagon powder is reconstituted with 1.0 mL of water for injections (WFI), forming a solution of 1 mg (1 IU) glucagon and 107 mg of lactose monohydrate in each mL prior to use. It is to be administered intramuscularly (into the muscle). Nonmedicinal ingredients: hydrochloric acid and/or sodium hydroxide (pH adjusters), lactose monohydrate and water for injection.
GlucaGen HypoKit : GlucaGen HypoKit 1 mg/mL vial is supplied as a sterile, freeze-dried white powder of glucagon in a 2 mL vial and accompanying solvent in a 1.5 mL disposable syringe. Glucagon powder is reconstituted with 1.0 mL of water for injections (WFI), forming a solution of 1 mg (1 IU) glucagon and 107 mg of lactose monohydrate in each mL prior to use. It is to be administered intramuscularly (into the muscle). Nonmedicinal ingredients: hydrochloric acid and/or sodium hydroxide (pH adjusters), lactose monohydrate and water for injection.

Glucagon Injection
glucagon
Hyperglycemic Agent

Lilly

PHARMACOLOGY: Glucagon for injection, rDNA origin is a polypeptide hormone identical to human glucagon, which is manufactured by recombinant DNA technology and has the same molecular structure as animal-sourced glucagon. Glucagon causes an increase in blood glucose concentration. Glucagon acts only on liver glycogen, converting it to glucose. Parenteral administration of glucagon relaxes smooth muscle of the stomach, duodenum, small bowel, and colon.

Pharmacodynamics: In a study of 29 healthy volunteers, a s.c. dose of 1 mg glucagon resulted in a mean peak glucose concentration of 136 mg/dL 30 minutes after injection for the 25 evaluable patients. Similarly, following i.m. injection, the mean peak glucose level was 138 mg/dL, which occurred at 26 minutes after injection. No difference in glucodynamic activity between animal-sourced and rDNA glucagon was observed after s.c. and i.m. injection.

Pharmacokinetics: Glucagon has been studied following i.m., s.c., and i.v. administration in adult volunteers. Administration of the i.v. glucagon showed dose proportionality of the pharmacokinetics between 0.25 and 2.0 mg. Calculations from a 1 mg dose showed a small volume of distribution (mean, 0.25 L/kg) and a moderate clearance (mean, 13.5 mL/min/kg). The half-life ranged from 8 to 18 minutes.

Maximum plasma concentrations of 7.9 ng/mL were achieved approximately 20 minutes after s.c. administration. With i.m. dosing, maximum plasma concentrations of 6.9 ng/mL were attained approximately 13 minutes after dosing.

Glucagon is extensively degraded in liver, kidney, and plasma. Urinary excretion of intact glucagon has not been measured.

INDICATIONS: For the Treatment of Hypoglycemia: For emergency treatment of severe hypoglycemia in patients treated with insulin when unconsciousness precludes oral carbohydrates. Severe hypoglycemia should be treated with i.v. glucose if possible.
For Use as a Diagnostic Aid: As a diagnostic aid in the radiologic examination of the stomach, duodenum, small bowel, and colon when diminished intestinal motility would be advantageous.

CONTRAINDICATIONS: In patients with known hypersensitivity to it or in patients with pheochromocytoma.

WARNINGS: Glucagon for injection, rDNA origin should be administered cautiously to patients with a history suggestive of insulinoma, pheochromocytoma, or both.
Insulinoma: In patients with insulinoma, i.v. administration of glucagon will produce an initial increase in blood glucose; however, because of glucagon's insulin-releasing effect, it may cause the insulinoma to release its insulin and subsequently cause hypoglycemia. A patient developing symptoms of hypoglycemia after a dose of glucagon should be given glucose orally, intravenously, or by gavage, whichever is more appropriate.
Pheochromocytoma: Exogenous glucagon also stimulates the release of catecholamines. In the presence of pheochromocytoma, glucagon can cause the tumor to release catecholamines, which results in a sudden and marked increase in blood pressure. If a patient suddenly develops a marked increase in blood pressure, 5 to 10 mg of phentolamine mesylate may be administered i.v. in an attempt to control the blood pressure.
Allergic Reactions: Generalized allergic reactions, including urticaria, respiratory distress, and hypotension, have been reported in patients who received glucagon.

PRECAUTIONS: General: Glucagon for injection, rDNA origin is helpful in treating hypoglycemia only if sufficient liver glycogen is present. Because glucagon is of little or no help in states of starvation, adrenal insufficiency, or chronic hypoglycemia, glucose should be considered for the treatment of hypoglycemia in these conditions.

The patient with Type 1 diabetes does not have as great response in blood glucose levels upon administration of glucagon as does the person with stable Type 2 diabetes; therefore supplementary carbohydrate should be given as soon as possible, especially to a child or adolescent patient.
Laboratory Tests: Blood glucose determinations should be obtained to follow the patient with hypoglycemia until the patient is asymptomatic.
Pregnancy: Reproduction studies have not been performed with recombinant glucagon; however studies with animal sourced glucagon have been performed in rats at doses up to 2 mg/kg b.i.d. (up to 120 times the human dose), and have revealed no evidence of harm to the fetus due to glucagon. There are, however, no adequate and well-controlled studies in pregnant women. Because animal reproduction studies are not always predictive of human response, this drug should be used during pregnancy only if oral carbohydrates cannot be administered.
Lactation: It is not known whether this drug is excreted in human milk.
Use with Alcohol: Alcohol can suppress hepatic gluconeogenesis and chronic alcoholism can deplete liver glycogen stores. Therefore glucagon may be less effective in presence of acute or chronic alcohol ingestion.

ADVERSE EFFECTS: Severe adverse reactions are very rare, although nausea, vomiting and hypokalemia may occur occasionally. Generalized allergic reactions, including urticaria, respiratory distress, and hypotension have been reported in patients who received glucagon (see Warnings). In the event of lack of response to the administration of glucagon, i.v. glucose should be administered to the patient.

OVERDOSE:
Symptoms: Glucagon for injection, rDNA origin is generally well-tolerated. If overdosage occurred, it would not be expected to cause consequential toxicity, but would be expected to be associated with nausea, vomiting, gastric hypotonicity, and diarrhea.

I.V. administration of glucagon has been shown to have a positive inotropic and chronotropic effect. A transient increment in both blood pressure and pulse rate may occur following the administration of glucagon. Patients taking β-blockers might be expected to have a greater increment in both pulse rate and blood pressure. This increase will be transient because of glucagon's short half-life. The increase in blood pressure and pulse rate may require therapy in patients with pheochromocytoma or coronary artery disease.

When glucagon was given in large doses to patients with cardiac disease, investigators reported a positive inotropic effect. These investigators administered glucagon in doses of 0.5 to 16 mg/hour by continuous infusion for periods of 5 to 166 hours. Total doses ranged from 25 to 996 mg, and a 21-month-old infant received approximately 8.25 mg in 165 hours. Side effects included nausea, vomiting, and decreasing serum potassium concentration. Serum potassium concentration could be maintained within normal limits with supplemental potassium.

The i.v. median lethal dose for glucagon in mice and rats is approximately 300 mg/kg and 38.6 mg/kg, respectively.

Because glucagon is a polypeptide, it would be rapidly destroyed in the GI tract if it were to be accidentally ingested.

Treatment: In managing overdosage, consider the possibility of multiple drug overdoses, interaction among drugs, and unusual drug kinetics in your patient.

In view of the extremely short half-life of glucagon and its prompt destruction and excretion, the treatment of overdosage is symptomatic, primarily for nausea, vomiting, and possible hypokalemia.

If the patient develops a dramatic increase in blood pressure, 5 to 10 mg of phentolamine has been shown to be effective in lowering blood pressure for the short time that control would be needed.

Forced diuresis, peritoneal dialysis, hemodialysis, or charcoal hemoperfusion have not been established as beneficial for an overdose of glucagon; it is extremely unlikely that one of these procedures would ever be indicated.

All of the results mentioned above have been obtained with animal-sourced glucagon rather than recombinant glucagon. Since the structure of recombinant glucagon is identical to the animal-sourced glucagon, the results obtained from the animal-sourced glucagon studies are applicable to recombinant glucagon.

For management of a suspected drug overdose, CPhA recommends that you contact your **regional Poison Control Centre**. See the *CPS* Directory section for a list of Poison Control Centres.

DOSAGE: For the Treatment of Hypoglycemia: The diluent is provided for use only in the preparation of glucagon for injection, rDNA origin for intermittent parenteral injection and for no other use.

Glucagon should be reconstituted with the accompanying diluent following the detailed directions contained within the Directions for the User package insert.

Glucagon should be used immediately after reconstitution. **Discard any unused portion.**
Directions for Use of Glucagon:

1. Dissolve the lyophilized glucagon in the accompanying diluent.
2. Glucagon should not be used at concentrations greater than 1 mg/mL (1 unit/mL).
3. Glucagon solutions should not be used unless they are clear and of a water-like consistency.
4. For adults and for children weighing more than 20 kg, give 1 mg (1 unit) by s.c., i.m., or i.v. injection.
5. For children weighing less than 20 kg, give 0.5 mg (0.5 unit) or a dose equivalent to 20 to 30 μg/kg.
6. The patient will usually awaken within 15 minutes. If the response is delayed, there is no contraindication to the administration of 1 or 2 additional doses of glucagon; however, in view of the deleterious effects of cerebral hypoglycemia and depending on the duration and depth of coma, the use of parenteral glucose must be considered by the physician.
7. I.V. glucose **must** be given if the patient fails to respond to glucagon.
8. When the patient responds, give supplemental carbohydrate to restore the liver glycogen and prevent secondary hypoglycemia.

Instructions to the Family: Instructions describing the method of using this preparation are included in the literature that accompanies the patient's package. It is advisable for the patient and family members to become familiar with the technique of preparing Glucagon for injection before an emergency arises. Patients are instructed to use 1 mg (1 unit) for adults and, if recommended by a doctor, 1/2 the adult dose (0.5 mg [0.5 unit]) for children weighing less than 20 kg.
General Management of Hypoglycemia: The following are helpful measures in the prevention of hypoglycemic reactions due to insulin:

1. Reasonable uniformity from day to day with regard to diet, insulin, and exercise.
2. Careful adjustment of the insulin program so that the type (or types) of insulin, dose, and time (or times) of administration are suited to the individual patient.
3. Frequent testing of the blood glucose so that a change in insulin requirements can be foreseen.
4. Routine carrying of sugar, candy, or other readily absorbable carbohydrate by the patient so that it may be taken at the first warning of an oncoming reaction.

If the patient is unaware of the symptoms of hypoglycemia, he/she may lapse into insulin shock; therefore, the physician should instruct the patient in this regard when feasible.

It is important that the patient be aroused as quickly as possible, because prolonged hypoglycemic reactions may result in cortical damage. Glucagon or i.v. glucose will awaken the patient sufficiently so that oral carbohydrates may be taken.
Caution: Although glucagon may be used for the treatment of hypoglycemia for the patient during an emergency, the physician must still be notified when hypoglycemic reactions occur so that the dose of insulin or oral antidiabetic medication may be adjusted more accurately.
For Use as a Diagnostic Aid: Dissolve the lyophilized glucagon in the accompanying diluting solution. Glucagon should not be used at concentrations greater than 1 mg/mL (1 unit/mL).

The doses of glucagon listed in Table 1 may be administered for relaxation of the stomach, duodenum, and small bowel, depending on the onset and duration of effect required for the examination. Since the stomach is less sensitive to the effect of glucagon, 0.5 mg (0.5 units) i.v. or 2 mg (2 units) i.m. are recommended.

For examination of the colon, it is recommended that a 2 mg (2 unit) dose be administered i.m. approximately 10 minutes prior to initiation of the procedure. Relaxation of the colon and reduction of discomfort to the patient will allow the radiologist to perform a more satisfactory examination.

Table 1: Glucagon Injection

Dosage as a Diagnostic Aid

Dose	Route of Administration	Time of Onset of Action	Approximate Duration of Effect
0.25-0.5 mg[b]	I.V.	1 minute	9–17 minutes
1 mg[b]	I.M.	8-10 minutes	12–27 minutes
2 mg[a,b]	I.V.	1 minute	22–25 minutes
2 mg[a,b]	I.M.	4-7 minutes	21–32 minutes

[a] Administration of 2 mg (2 units) doses produces a higher incidence of nausea and vomiting than do lower doses.
[b] 1 mg equals 1 unit.

Stability and Storage: Do not use past expiry date.
Before Reconstitution: Prior to reconstitution, vials and prefilled Hyporets of diluting solution may be stored at controlled room temperature, 15 to 30°C.
Reconstituted Solutions: Glucagon should be reconstituted with the accompanying diluent following the detailed directions contained within the Directions for the User package insert.

Glucagon should be used immediately after reconstitution. **Discard any unused portion.**

INFORMATION FOR THE PATIENT: Published in e-CPS, available by subscription at www.e-cps.ca.

SUPPLIED: Each kit contains: 1 rubber-stoppered vial of lyophilized powder containing glucagon for injection USP 1 unit (1 mg) and 1 prefilled Hyporet of diluting solution. Nonmedicinal ingredients: vial of lyophilized glucagon: lactose 49 mg; diluting solution: glycerin. May contain hydrochloric acid for pH adjustment. Vials of 1 mL.

Glucobay™ Ⓟ

acarbose

Oral Antidiabetic—Alpha-glucosidase Inhibitor

Bayer

Date of Preparation: June 3, 1996
Date of Revision: June 10, 2010

SUMMARY PRODUCT INFORMATION:

Route of Administration	Dosage Form/ Strength	Clinically Relevant Nonmedicinal Ingredients
Oral	Tablet 50 mg, 100 mg	See Dosage Forms, Composition and Packaging.

INDICATIONS AND CLINICAL USE:

- GLUCOBAY (acarbose), as monotherapy, is indicated as an adjunct to prescribed diet for the management of blood glucose levels in patients with type 2 diabetes mellitus who are inadequately controlled by diet alone.
- GLUCOBAY may also be used in combination with either a sulfonylurea, metformin or insulin to improve glycemic control in patients with type 2 diabetes mellitus, who are inadequately controlled on diet, exercise and either a sulfonylurea, metformin or insulin alone. The effect of GLUCOBAY in enhancing glycemic control is additive to that of sulfonylureas, metformin or insulin when used in combination, because of its different mechanism of action.

In initiating treatment for type 2 diabetes mellitus, diet should be emphasized as the primary form of treatment. Caloric restriction and weight loss are essential in the obese diabetic patient. Proper dietary management alone may be effective in controlling blood glucose and symptoms of hyperglycemia. The importance of regular physical activity when appropriate should also be stressed. If this treatment program fails to result in adequate glycemic control, the use of GLUCOBAY should be considered. The use of GLUCOBAY must be viewed by both the physician and patient as a treatment in addition to diet, and not as a substitute for diet or as a convenient mechanism for avoiding dietary restraint. GLUCOBAY should be considered as complementary to dietary therapy and physical exercise before resorting to other forms of treatment, such as oral hypoglycemics.
Geriatrics: Elderly patients receiving GLUCOBAY may require more intensive supervision and follow-up.
Pediatrics (<18 years of age): Safety and effectiveness of GLUCOBAY in patients <18 years of age have not been established.

CONTRAINDICATIONS:

- Patients who are hypersensitive to acarbose or to any ingredient in the formulation or component of the container. For a complete listing, see Dosage Forms, Composition and Packaging.
- GLUCOBAY is contraindicated in patients with diabetic ketoacidosis.
- It is also contraindicated in patients with inflammatory bowel disease, colonic ulceration, partial intestinal obstruction or in patients predisposed to intestinal obstruction.
- In addition, GLUCOBAY should not be used in patients who have chronic intestinal diseases associated with marked disorders of digestion or absorption and in patients who suffer from states which may deteriorate as a result of increased gas formation in the intestine, e.g., larger hernias.

WARNINGS AND PRECAUTIONS: General: GLUCOBAY delays glucose absorption and lowers hyperglycemia following meals. Regular intake of GLUCOBAY should not be interrupted without the physician's knowledge, since such interruption can cause a rise in blood glucose.
Carcinogenesis and Mutagenesis: There is no evidence from preclinical data that GLUCOBAY is carcinogenic or mutagenic.
Endocrine and Metabolism: Hypoglycemia: Because of its mechanism of action, GLUCOBAY when administered alone will not cause hypoglycemia in the fasted or postprandial state. Sulfonylurea agents or insulin may cause hypoglycemia. Because GLUCOBAY given with a sulfonylurea, metformin or insulin may cause a further lowering of blood glucose, the potential for hypoglycemia may be increased. A fall of the blood glucose into the hypoglycemic range may necessitate a suitable decrease in the sulphonylurea, metformin or insulin dose. In individual cases, hypoglycemic shock may occur.

Oral glucose (dextrose), whose absorption is not inhibited by GLUCOBAY, should be used instead of sucrose (cane sugar) in the treatment of mild to moderate hypoglycemia. Sucrose, whose hydrolysis to glucose and fructose is inhibited by GLUCOBAY, is unsuitable for the rapid correction of hypoglycemia. Severe hypoglycemia may require the use of either intravenous glucose infusion or glucagon injection.
Loss of Control of Blood Glucose: When diabetic patients are exposed to stress such as fever, trauma, infection, or surgery, a temporary loss of control of blood glucose may occur. At such times, temporary insulin therapy may be necessary.

Gastrointestinal: Increased use of sucrose (cane sugar) and food that contains sucrose can lead to gastrointestinal symptoms (e.g., flatulence and bloating) and also loose stools and occasionally diarrhea as a result of increased carbohydrate fermentation in the colon during GLUCOBAY treatment.

If the prescribed diet is not observed, the intestinal side effects may be intensified. If strongly distressing symptoms develop in spite of adherence to the diabetic diet prescribed, the doctor must be consulted and the dose temporarily or permanently reduced.

Hepatic: In postmarketing experience with GLUCOBAY, reports of hepatic adverse events have been received, including reports of liver failure, liver transplant, and fulminant hepatitis, with and without fatal outcome. The mechanism is unknown, but GLUCOBAY may contribute to a multifactorial pathophysiology of liver injury, particularly in combination with impaired metabolic control and/or concomitant antidiabetic medications (see Adverse Reactions, Post-Market Adverse Drug Reactions).

GLUCOBAY may give rise to elevations of serum transaminases and, in rare instances, hyperbilirubinemia. If elevations are observed, a reduction in dosage or withdrawal of therapy may be indicated, particularly if the elevations persist. Liver enzyme monitoring should be considered during the first 6 to 12 months of treatment.

In patients with a known history of liver impairment or liver disease, liver enzymes should be measured prior to the start of GLUCOBAY therapy and monitored on a regular basis during the first year. If a clinical deterioration or increases in levels of hepatic enzymes are detected, discontinuation of treatment with GLUCOBAY should be considered.

Renal: Plasma concentrations of GLUCOBAY in renally impaired volunteers were proportionally increased relative to the degree of renal dysfunction. Long-term clinical trials in diabetic patients with severe renal dysfunction (creatinine clearance <25 mL/min) have not been conducted. Treatment of patients with severe renal dysfunction (creatinine clearance <25 mL/min) with GLUCOBAY is not recommended.

Special Populations: Pregnant Women: There are no adequate and well-controlled studies of GLUCOBAY in pregnant women and its use in these patients is not recommended.

Nursing Women: A small amount of radioactivity has been found in the milk of lactating rats after administration of radiolabelled acarbose. It is not known whether this drug is excreted in human milk. Because many drugs are excreted in human milk, GLUCOBAY should not be administered to a nursing woman.

Pediatrics (<18 years of age): Safety and effectiveness of GLUCOBAY in patients <18 years of age have not been established.

Geriatrics: Elderly patients receiving GLUCOBAY may require more intensive supervision and followup.

Monitoring and Laboratory Tests: Liver enzyme monitoring should be considered during the first 6 to 12 months of treatment. In patients with a known history of liver impairment or liver disease, liver enzymes should be measured prior to the start of GLUCOBAY therapy and monitored on a regular basis during the first year (see Warnings and Precautions, Hepatic).

Digoxin: In individual cases, GLUCOBAY may affect digoxin bioavailability, which may require dose adjustment of digoxin.

ADVERSE REACTIONS: Adverse Drug Reaction Overview: GLUCOBAY was administered to over 17 300 patients in clinical trials worldwide, including over 8500 in placebo-controlled trials. The most common adverse events occurring with use in placebo-controlled trials include flatulence, diarrhea, and gastrointestinal and abdominal pains.

Clinical Trial Adverse Drug Reactions: Because clinical trials are conducted under very specific conditions the adverse reaction rates observed in the clinical trials may not reflect the rates observed in practice and should not be compared to the rates in the clinical trials of another drug. Adverse drug reaction information from clinical trials is useful for identifying drug-related adverse events and for approximating rates.

In placebo controlled pivotal studies of ≥6 months duration where acarbose was used as monotherapy or in combination with a sulfonylurea, adverse experiences were reported in 53% of patients receiving placebo and in 77% of patients treated with GLUCOBAY. The majority of adverse experiences were gastrointestinal symptoms which result from the pharmacodynamic action of the drug. The majority of symptoms were of mild or moderate intensity and were dose-dependent. The symptoms occurred early (within 1-2 months of treatment) and improved tolerability with longer duration of treatment was observed. Therapy was discontinued prematurely due to adverse events in 14% of GLUCOBAY-treated patients and 5% of placebo-treated patients.

Adverse drug reactions (ADRs) based on placebo-controlled studies withGLUCOBAY sorted by CIOMS III categories of frequency (placebo-controlled studies in clinical trial database: GLUCOBAY N=8595; placebo N=7278) are listed in Table 1.

Table 1: GLUCOBAY

Incidence of Adverse Drug Reactions in Placebo-Controlled Studies (%)

Clinical Description	Very Common >10%	Common ≥1%
Gastrointestinal Disorders		
Gastrointestinal symptoms	Flatulence	Diarrhea Gastrointestinal and abdominal pains

The only significant difference in the incidence of adverse events between GLUCOBAY and placebo were gastrointestinal symptoms (e.g., flatulence, diarrhea, gastrointestinal and abdominal pain) which can be minimized by starting on a low dose and titrating slowly (see Dosage and Administration, Recommended Dose and Dosage Adjustment). Adverse events seen when GLUCOBAY is used concomitantly with other antidiabetic agents are generally similar to those seen during GLUCOBAY monotherapy. If GLUCOBAY tablets are prescribed in addition to sulphonylureas, metformin, or insulin, a fall of the blood glucose values into the hypoglycemic range may necessitate a decrease in the sulphonylurea, metformin or insulin dosage. In individual cases, hypoglycemic shock may occur.

Less Common Clinical Trial Adverse Drug Reactions: The following additional adverse events occurred in ≥0.1% to <1% of patients receiving GLUCOBAY in all clinical trials:

Gastrointestinal: nausea, vomiting, dyspepsia.

Hepatic: increase in liver enzymes.

The following additional adverse events occurred in ≥0.01% to <0.1% of patients receiving GLUCOBAY in all clinical trials:

Vascular: oedema.

Hepatic: jaundice.

Abnormal Hematologic and Clinical Chemistry Findings: In clinical trials, in patients receiving the recommended daily dose of 150 to 300 mg acarbose per day, rarely clinically relevant abnormal liver function tests (three times above upper limit of normal range) were observed. Abnormal values may be transient under ongoing acarbose therapy.

The incidence of serum transaminase elevations with GLUCOBAY was the same as with placebo.

Post-Market Adverse Drug Reactions: Very rarely (<0.01%), cases of hepatitis, thrombocytopenia and/or jaundice and associated liver damage have been reported. In addition, cases of serum transaminase levels >10 x ULN have been reported, some of which were associated with jaundice. In most cases where follow-up was reported, hepatic dysfunction improved or resolved upon discontinuation of GLUCOBAY. Reports of liver failure and liver transplant, with and without fatal outcome, have been received. Events reported as liver disorder, hepatic function abnormal, and liver injury have been received, especially from Japan. Individual cases of fulminant hepatitis with fatal outcome have also been reported in Japan. Other, as yet undefined, patient populations may be similarly susceptible. (See Warnings and Precautions, Hepatic.)

Very rarely (<0.01%), cases of subileus/ileus, pneumatosis cystoidis intestinalis, and hypersensitive skin reactions, such as rash, erythema, exanthema and urticaria, have been reported.

Rarely (≥0.01% and <0.1%), edema has been observed.

DRUG INTERACTIONS: Overview: Certain drugs tend to produce hyperglycemia and may lead to loss of blood glucose control. These drugs include diuretics (thiazides, furosemide), corticosteroids, phenothiazines, thyroid products, estrogens, oral contraceptives, phenytoin, nicotinic acid, sympathomimetics and isoniazid. When such drugs are administered to a patient receiving GLUCOBAY, the patient should be closely observed for loss of blood glucose control. When such drugs are withdrawn from patients receiving GLUCOBAY in combination with sulfonylureas or insulin, patients should be observed closely for evidence of hypoglycemia.

Drug-Drug Interactions: Intestinal Absorbents: Intestinal absorbents (e.g., charcoal) and digestive enzyme preparations containing carbohydrate-splitting enzymes (amylase, pancreatin) may reduce the effect of GLUCOBAY and should not be taken concomitantly. No interaction was observed with dimethicone/simethicone.

Antacids: The concomitant administration of GLUCOBAY and an antacid does not alter the effect of GLUCOBAY. The administration of antacid preparations is unlikely to ameliorate the gastrointestinal symptoms of GLUCOBAY and therefore should not be recommended to patients for this purpose.

Cholestyramine: The concomitant administration of cholestyramine may enhance the effects of GLUCOBAY, particularly with respect to reducing postprandial insulin levels. In healthy volunteers, a rebound phenomenon with respect to the postprandial insulin response was observed when both GLUCOBAY and cholestyramine therapy were withdrawn simultaneously.

Digoxin: In individual cases, GLUCOBAY may affect digoxin bioavailability, which may require dose adjustment of digoxin.

Metformin: The amount of metformin absorbed while taking GLUCOBAY was bioequivalent to the amount absorbed when taking placebo, as indicated by the plasma AUC values. However, the peak plasma level of metformin was reduced by approximately 20% when taking GLUCOBAY due to a slight delay in the absorption of metformin. There is little, if any, clinically significant interaction between GLUCOBAY and metformin. Therefore, no dose modification of either agent is necessary.

Other Drugs: Studies in healthy volunteers have shown that GLUCOBAY has no effect on either the pharmacokinetics or pharmacodynamics of nifedipine, propranolol or ranitidine.

Drug-Food Interactions: Not applicable.

Drug-Herb Interactions: Drug-Herb interactions have not been established.

Drug-Laboratory Test Interactions: Drug-laboratory interactions have not been established.

Drug-Lifestyle Interactions: Drug-Lifestyle interactions have not been established.

DOSAGE AND ADMINISTRATION: Dosing Considerations: During treatment initiation and dose titration (see Dosage and Administration, Recommended Dose and Dosage Adjustment), two-hour postprandial plasma glucose should be used to determine the therapeutic response to GLUCOBAY and identify the minimum effective dose for the patient. Thereafter, glycosylated hemoglobin should be measured at intervals of approximately three months. The therapeutic goal should be to decrease both postprandial plasma glucose and glycosylated hemoglobin levels to optimal or near optimal by using the lowest effective dose of GLUCOBAY, either as monotherapy or in combination with sulfonylureas, metformin or insulin.

Patients Receiving Sulfonylureas or Insulin: Sulfonylurea agents or insulin may cause hypoglycemia. Therefore, GLUCOBAY given in combination with a sulfonylurea or insulin may also cause hypoglycemia. If hypoglycemia occurs, appropriate adjustment in the sulfonylurea or insulin dosage should be made.

Recommended Dose and Dosage Adjustment: Initial Dosage: Dosage of GLUCOBAY must be individualized on the basis of both effectiveness and tolerance while not exceeding 100 mg t.i.d. GLUCOBAY should be started at a low dose, with gradual dose escalation as described below, both to reduce gastrointestinal side effects and to permit identification of the minimum dose required for adequate glycemic control of the patient.

The usual starting dosage of GLUCOBAY is 50 mg given orally once daily. After 1-2 weeks, the dosage should be increased to 50 mg b.i.d. with a subsequent increase to 50 mg t.i.d. after a further 1-2 weeks. Each dose should be taken with the first bite of a main meal. GLUCOBAY must always be taken together with food.

Once a maintenance dose of 50 mg t.i.d. has been reached, some patients may benefit from further increasing the dosage to 100 mg t.i.d. The maintenance dose ranges from 50 mg t.i.d. to 100 mg t.i.d. The dosage of GLUCOBAY should be adjusted at 4-8 week intervals based on two-hour postprandial glucose levels and on tolerance. Consideration should be given to lowering the dose if no further reduction in postprandial glucose or glycosylated hemoglobin levels is observed after titration to 100 mg t.i.d. Once an effective and tolerated dosage is established, it should be maintained.

Maximum Dosage: Dosages above 100 mg t.i.d. are not recommended.

Missed Dose: GLUCOBAY has to be taken at the beginning of a meal. If a dose has been missed, no effect on blood glucose and serum insulin can be expected. Should a dose be missed, the patient should not take a tablet until their next meal.

OVERDOSAGE:

Unlike sulfonylureas or insulin, an overdose of GLUCOBAY will not result in hypoglycemia. When GLUCOBAY is taken with drinks and/or meals containing carbohydrates (polysaccharides, oligosaccarides, or disaccharides), overdosage can lead to abdominal distention, flatulence, and diarrhea. In the event of GLUCOBAY being taken in an overdose independent of food, excessive intestinal symptoms need not be anticipated.

In cases of overdosage, the patient should not be given drinks or meals containing carbohydrates (polysaccharides, oligosaccharides, and disaccharides) for the next 4 to 6 hours.

> For management of a suspected drug overdose, contact your regional Poison Control Centre. See the *CPS* Directory section for a list of Poison Control Centres.

ACTION AND CLINICAL PHARMACOLOGY: Mechanism of Action: Acarbose has been shown in animal studies to be a competitive inhibitor of intestinal brush-border α-glucosidase enzymes. The inhibitory potency follows a rank order of glucoamylase > sucrase > maltase > isomaltase. Acarbose has little or no effect on lactase and trehalase. Studies in healthy volunteers demonstrated that oral doses of 75 to 300 mg acarbose taken together with a meal reduced elevated concentrations of blood glucose and serum insulin in a dose-dependent manner. A clear dose-proportionality of single oral doses of 50, 100 and 200 mg acarbose was shown in respect to an increase in blood glucose and serum insulin after simultaneous ingestion of 75 g sucrose. The inhibition of the postprandial insulin response was identical following oral administration of 1×100 mg and 2×50 mg acarbose, thus demonstrating pharmacological bioequivalence. The reduction in postprandial insulin concentrations was also found to be dose dependent in obese subjects, in whom insulin resistance is often present.

After oral administration of 200 mg acarbose, the area under the blood glucose concentration time curve was reduced by 89% after sucrose loading, and by 80% after starch loading and by 19% after maltose loading. There was no effect of acarbose observed after oral administration of lactose and glucose or after intravenous administration of glucose.

Pharmacodynamics: Acarbose is a complex oligosaccharide that inhibits α-glucosidase activity in the brush border membrane of the small intestine. This delays the digestion of ingested carbohydrates, thereby resulting in a smoothing and lowering of blood glucose concentration following meals (postprandial). As a consequence of decreases in plasma glucose postprandial increases, acarbose reduces levels of glycosylated hemoglobin in patients with type 2 diabetes mellitus. Systemic nonenzymatic protein glycosylation, as reflected by levels of glycosylated hemoglobin, is a function of average blood glucose concentration over time.

Acarbose does not enhance insulin secretion. The antihyperglycemic action of acarbose results from a competitive, reversible inhibition of pancreatic α-amylase and membrane bound intestinal α-glucoside hydrolase enzymes. Pancreatic α-amylase hydrolyzes complex starches to oligosaccharides in the lumen of the small intestine, while the membrane-bound intestinal α-glucosidases hydrolyze oligosaccharides, trisaccharides, and disaccharides to glucose and other monosaccharides in the brush border of the small intestine. In diabetic patients, this enzyme inhibition results in a delayed glucose absorption and a smoothing and lowering of postprandial hyperglycemia, resulting in improved glycemic control.

Because its mechanism of action is different, the effect of acarbose in enhancing glycemic control is additive to that of sulfonylureas, metformin or insulin when used in combination. In addition, acarbose diminishes the insulinotropic and weight-increasing effects of sulfonylureas.

Acarbose has no inhibitory activity against lactase and consequently does not induce lactose intolerance.

Pharmacokinetics: Absorption: One to 2% of an oral dose of acarbose is absorbed from the gastrointestinal tract as unchanged drug. When ^{14}C-labelled acarbose was administered orally, approximately 35% of the total radioactivity (changed and unchanged drug) was absorbed. An average of 51% of an oral dose was excreted in the feces as unabsorbed drug-related radioactivity within 96 hours of ingestion. Because acarbose acts locally within the gastrointestinal tract, this low systemic bioavailability of parent compound is therapeutically desired. Following oral dosing of healthy volunteers with ^{14}C-labelled acarbose, peak plasma concentrations of radioactivity were attained 14-24 hours after dosing, while peak plasma concentrations of active drug were attained at approximately 1 hour. The delayed absorption of acarbose-related radioactivity reflects the absorption of metabolites that may be formed by either intestinal bacteria or intestinal enzymatic hydrolysis.

Distribution: Only 1-2% of an oral dose of acarbose is absorbed into the central circulation.

Metabolism: Acarbose is metabolized exclusively within the gastrointestinal tract, principally by intestinal bacteria, but also by digestive enzymes. A fraction of these metabolites (approximately 34% of the dose) is absorbed and subsequently excreted in the urine. At least 13 metabolites have been separated chromatographically from urine specimens. The major metabolites have been identified as 4-methylpyrogallol derivatives (i.e., sulfate, methyl, and glucuronide conjugates). One metabolite (formed by cleavage of a glucose molecule from acarbose) also has α-glucosidase inhibitory activity. This metabolite, together with the parent compound, recovered from the urine, accounts for less than 2% of the total administered dose.

Excretion: The fraction of acarbose that is absorbed as intact drug is almost completely excreted by the kidneys. When acarbose was given intravenously, 89% of the dose was recovered in the urine as active drug within 48 hours. In contrast, less than 2% of an oral dose was recovered in the urine as active (i.e., parent compound and active metabolite) drug. This is consistent with the low bioavailability of the parent drug. The plasma elimination half-life of acarbose activity is approximately 2 hours in healthy volunteers. Consequently, drug accumulation does not occur with three times a day (t.i.d.) oral dosing.

Special Populations and Conditions: Renal Insufficiency: Patients with severe renal impairment (creatinine clearance <25 mL/min/1.73 m^2) attained about 5 times higher peak plasma concentrations of acarbose and 6 times larger AUCs than volunteers with normal renal function.

STORAGE AND STABILITY: Storage should be between 15 and 25°C.

At storage conditions up to 25°C and below 60% relative humidity, the unpacked tablets can be stored for up to two weeks. At higher temperatures and/or relative humidity, discoloration can occur in tablets that are not in the pack. The tablets should therefore not be removed from the foil until immediately before use.

INFORMATION FOR THE PATIENT: Published in e-CPS, available by subscription at www.e-cps.ca.

DOSAGE FORMS, COMPOSITION AND PACKAGING: 50 mg: Each round, white to yellow-tinged, scored tablet, marked with "G50" on one side and the Bayer cross on the other, with a 7 mm diameter and a 10 mm radius of curvature, contains: acarbose 50 mg. Nonmedicinal ingredients: cornstarch, magnesium stearate, microcrystalline cellulose and silicon dioxide. Preservative- and coloring agent-free. Blister packs in cartons of 120 tablets.

100 mg: Each round, white to yellow-tinged, scored tablet, marked with "G100" on one side and the Bayer cross on the other, with a 9 mm diameter and a 15 mm radius of curvature, contains: acarbose 100 mg. Nonmedicinal ingredients: cornstarch, magnesium stearate, microcrystalline cellulose and silicon dioxide. Preservative- and coloring agent-free. Blister packs in cartons of 120 tablets.

(Shown in Product Identification Section)

Glucodex

glucose

Diagnostic Agent for Diabetes

Rougier Pharma

INDICATIONS: Glucose tolerance test. Diagnostic agent for diabetes and glucose tolerance test in children. Also for screening of glucose intolerance in pregnant women. This test is generally performed between the 24th and 28th week of pregnancy.

CONTRAINDICATIONS: In patients with the glucose-galactose malabsorption syndrome.

PRECAUTIONS: Glucose should be administered with care to patients with diabetes insipides. Concentrated glucose solutions given by mouth may cause nausea and vomiting.

Drug Interactions: Purgatives may inhibit the intestinal absorption of glucose.

ADVERSE EFFECTS: Concentrated glucose solution given by mouth may cause nausea and vomiting.

OVERDOSE:

> For management of a suspected drug overdose, CPhA recommends that you contact your **regional Poison Control Centre**. See the *CPS* Directory section for a list of Poison Control Centres.

DOSAGE: Glucose tolerance test: Adults (except pregnant women): 75 g. Children: 1.75 g/kg of ideal body weight. Pregnant women: 100 g or according to physician's advice. Serve cold.

SUPPLIED: 50 g: Each mL of orange-flavored, yellow to pale orange clear liquid, contains: glucose USP 166.6 mg. Nonmedicinal ingredients: citric acid, FD&C Yellow #6, natural flavoring, purified water and sodium benzoate. Bottles of 300 mL.

75 g: Each mL of orange-flavored, orange clear liquid, contains: glucose USP 250 mg. Nonmedicinal ingredients: citric acid, FD&C Yellow #6, natural flavoring, purified water and sodium benzoate. Bottles of 300 mL.

100 g: Each mL of orange-flavored, dark orange clear liquid, contains: glucose USP 333.3 mg. Nonmedicinal ingredients: citric acid, FD&C Yellow #6, natural flavoring, purified water and sodium benzoate. Bottles of 300 mL.

GlucoNorm® Ⓟ

repaglinide

Oral Antidiabetic

Novo Nordisk

Date of Revision: June 30, 2010

SUMMARY PRODUCT INFORMATION:

Route of Administration	Dosage Form/ Strength	Clinically Relevant Nonmedicinal Ingredients
Oral	0.5 mg, 1 mg and 2 mg tablet	Microcrystalline cellulose (E460), calcium hydrogen phosphate anhydrous, maize starch, amberlite (polacrilin potassium), povidone (polyvidone), glycerol 85%, magnesium stearate, meglumine, poloxamer (0.5 mg), yellow iron oxide (1 mg), or red iron oxide (2 mg). For a complete listing see Dosage Forms, Composition and Packaging.

INDICATIONS AND CLINICAL USE: GlucoNorm (repaglinide) is indicated:

- as an adjunct to diet and exercise to lower the blood glucose in patients with type 2 diabetes mellitus whose hyperglycemia cannot be controlled satisfactorily by diet and exercise alone.
- in combination therapy with metformin to lower blood glucose in patients whose hyperglycemia cannot be controlled by diet and exercise plus metformin monotherapy.
- in combination with rosiglitazone in patients who show intolerance to metformin or for whom metformin is contraindicated, when diet and exercise plus rosiglitazone or GlucoNorm monotherapy do not result in adequate glycemic control.

If glucose control has not been achieved after a suitable trial of combination therapy, consideration should be given to discontinuing these drugs and other antihyperglycemic agents including insulin should be considered. Judgments should be based on regular clinical and laboratory evaluations.

In initiating treatment for type 2 diabetes, diet and exercise should be emphasized as the primary form of treatment. Caloric restriction, weight loss and exercise are essential in the obese diabetic patient. Proper dietary management and exercise alone may be effective in controlling the blood glucose and symptoms of hyperglycemia. In addition to regular physical activity, cardiovascular risk factors should be identified and corrective measures taken where possible.

If this treatment program fails to reduce symptoms and/or blood glucose GlucoNorm should be discontinued. The use of other oral blood glucose-lowering agent or insulin should be considered. Use of GlucoNorm must be viewed by both the physician and patient as a treatment in addition to diet, and not as a substitute for diet or as a convenient mechanism for avoiding dietary restraint. Furthermore, loss of blood glucose control on diet alone may be transient, thus requiring only short-term administration of GlucoNorm.

Geriatrics: GlucoNorm can be used in elderly above 65 years of age without further monitoring or special care except in those with renal, hepatic or other problems as described in Warnings and Precautions. GlucoNorm is not recommended for use in elderly above 75 years of age due to lack of data on safety and/or efficacy. Please see Warnings and Precautions, Special Populations; Action and Clinical Pharmacology and Monitoring and Laboratory Tests.

Pediatrics: No specific clinical studies have been conducted in patients below age of 18. Please see Warnings and Precautions.

CONTRAINDICATIONS: GlucoNorm (repaglinide) is contraindicated:

- In patients with known hypersensitivity to the drug or any of its components. For a complete listing, see Dosage Forms, Composition and Packaging.
- In patients with diabetic ketoacidosis, with or without coma. This condition should be treated with insulin.
- In patients with Type 1 diabetes.
- In patients with severe liver disease.
- In patients who are using gemfibrozil (see Drug Interactions).

WARNINGS AND PRECAUTIONS: General: GlucoNorm (repaglinide) is effective as a prandial glucose regulator and should be taken before meals (2, 3 or 4 times a day preprandially). Therefore, if a meal is missed or delayed, the dose of GlucoNorm should be skipped or delayed as appropriate.

Cardiovascular: The administration of insulin secretagogues in general has been reported to be associated with increased cardiovascular mortality as compared to treatment with diet alone or diet plus insulin. In controlled clinical trials comparing GlucoNorm (repaglinide) with glyburide and other sulfonylureas, there was no excess mortality with GlucoNorm use. The overall incidence of serious CV events including death was 4.2 per 100 patients years.

In clinical trials, the incidence of serious cardiovascular treatment emergent adverse events was higher for repaglinide than for glyburide but lower than that for glipizide. Please see Adverse Reactions.

Endocrine and Metabolism: Hypoglycemia: GlucoNorm is capable of inducing hypoglycemia. Proper patient selection, dosage, and instructions to the patient are important to avoid hypoglycemic episodes. Hepatic insufficiency may cause elevated repaglinide levels in the blood and may also diminish gluconeogenic capacity, both of which increase the risk of serious hypoglycemic reactions.

Elderly, debilitated or malnourished patients, and those with adrenal, pituitary or hepatic insufficiency are particularly susceptible to the hypoglycemic action of glucose-lowering drugs.

Hypoglycemia may be difficult to recognize in the elderly, and in people who are taking betaadrenergic blocking drugs.

Hypoglycemia is more likely to occur when caloric intake is deficient or when meals are skipped. Given the preprandial dosing regimen, patients taking GlucoNorm can adjust dosing according to their changing meal patterns, thereby reducing the risk of hypoglycemia when meals are missed.

Hypoglycemia is also more likely to occur after strenuous or prolonged exercise, when alcohol is ingested, or when more than one glucose-lowering drug is used.

Loss of Control of Blood Glucose: When a patient, stabilized on GlucoNorm is exposed to stress such as fever, trauma, infection, or surgery, a loss of control of blood glucose may occur. At such times, it may be necessary to temporarily discontinue GlucoNorm and administer insulin.

Hepatic/Biliary/Pancreatic: Patients with impaired liver function may be exposed to higher concentrations of repaglinide than would patients with normal liver functions receiving usual doses. GlucoNorm should be used cautiously in patients with impaired liver function. Longer intervals between dose adjustments should be utilized to allow full assessment of response (see Action and Clinical Pharmacology, Pharmacokinetics). GlucoNorm is contraindicated in patients with severe liver disease.

Neurologic: Severe hypoglycemic reactions with coma, seizure, or other neurological impairment occur infrequently, but constitute medical emergencies requiring immediate hospitalization. If hypoglycemic coma is diagnosed or suspected, the patient should be given a rapid intravenous injection of glucose solution, followed by a continuous infusion, according to standard medical practice.

Renal: Renal Insufficiency: Typically, GlucoNorm does not require initial dose adjustment in patients with reduced kidney function. However, subsequent increases in GlucoNorm should be made carefully in patients with type 2 diabetes who have renal function impairment or renal failure requiring hemodialysis (see Action and Clinical Pharmacology, Pharmacokinetics).

Pre-Operative Considerations: Please see Endocrine and Metabolism, Loss of Control of Blood Glucose.

Special Populations: Pregnant Women: GlucoNorm is not recommended for use during pregnancy. The safety of GlucoNorm in pregnant women has not been established.

Nursing Women: The safety of GlucoNorm in nursing women has not been established. In rat reproduction studies, measurable levels of repaglinide were detected in the breast milk of the dams and lowered blood glucose levels were observed in the pups. It is not known whether GlucoNorm is excreted in human milk. GlucoNorm is not recommended in nursing women because the potential for hypoglycemia in nursing infants may exist. Insulin therapy should be considered.

Pediatrics: The use of GlucoNorm is not recommended in pediatrics. The safety in pediatrics has not been established. No studies of GlucoNorm have been performed in pediatric patients.

Geriatrics (>65 years of age): No special dose titration is necessary in elderly patients. In repaglinide clinical studies of 24 weeks or greater duration, 415 patients were over 65 years of age. In one-year, active-controlled trials, no differences were seen in effectiveness or adverse events between these subjects and those less than 65 other than the expected age-related increase in cardiovascular events observed for GlucoNorm and comparator drugs. There was no increase in frequency or severity of hypoglycemia in older subjects. Other reported clinical experience has not identified differences in responses between the elderly and younger patients, but greater sensitivity of some older individuals to GlucoNorm therapy cannot be ruled out.

No specific clinical studies have been conducted in type 2 patients >75 years of age.

Monitoring and Laboratory Tests: In addition to self-monitoring of blood and/or urinary glucose, the patient's blood glucose should be monitored by the physician to determine the minimum effective dose for the patient. Periodic monitoring is necessary to detect primary failure (inadequate lowering of blood glucose at the maximum recommended dose of medication), and to detect secondary failure (loss of adequate blood glucose-lowering after an initial period of effectiveness). For patients with an increased risk of hypoglycemia, or at risk of losing blood glucose control (see Warnings and Precautions, Endocrine and Metabolism), a closer glucose monitoring should be considered. Glycosylated hemoglobin levels (HbA_{1C}) are of value in monitoring the patient's longer term response to therapy.

Hepatic function should be assessed before initiating the therapy and periodically in patients with impaired hepatic function.

ADVERSE REACTIONS: Adverse Drug Reaction Overview: The most frequently reported Adverse Drug Reaction (ADR) is hypoglycemia. The occurrence of such reactions depends, as for every diabetes therapy, on individual factors, such as dietary habits, dosage, exercise and stress.

In one-year comparator trials, the incidence of individual events was not greater than 1% except for chest pain (1.8%) and angina (1.8%). The overall incidence of other cardiovascular events (hypertension, abnormal EKG, myocardial infarction, arrhythmias, and palpitations) was $\leq$1% and not different for GlucoNorm and the comparator drugs.

The incidence of serious cardiovascular adverse events added together, including ischemia, was slightly higher for repaglinide (4%) than for sulfonylurea drugs (3%) in controlled comparator clinical trials. In 1-year controlled trials, GlucoNorm treatment was not associated with excess mortality rates compared to rates observed with other oral hypoglycemic agent therapies. See Table 1.

Table 1: GlucoNorm

Summary of Serious Cardiovascular Events (% of total patients with events)

	GlucoNorm	SU[a]
Total Exposed	1228	498
Serious CV Events	4%	3%
Cardiac Ischemic Events	2%	2%
Deaths due to CV Events	0.5%	0.4%

[a] Glyburide and glipizide.

Clinical Trial Adverse Drug Reactions: Because clinical trials are conducted under very specific conditions the adverse reaction rates observed in the clinical trials may not reflect the rates observed in practice and should not be compared to the rates in the clinical trials of another drug. Adverse drug reaction information from clinical trials is useful for identifying drug-related adverse events and for approximating rates.

GlucoNorm (repaglinide) has been administered to 2931 individuals worldwide during clinical trials. Approximately 1500 of these individuals with type 2 diabetes have been treated for at least 3 months, 1000 for at least 6 months, and 800 for at least 1 year. The majority of these individuals (1228) received GlucoNorm in one of five 1-year, active-controlled trials, where GlucoNorm was administered three times a day with meals in doses of 0.5-4 mg per meal. The comparator drugs in these 1-year trials were oral sulfonylurea drugs (SU).

GlucoNorm was well tolerated in these clinical trials and analysis of adverse events shows no dose relationship to rate of occurrence. The adverse event profile for the GlucoNorm and SU groups in these trials were generally comparable over one year. The rate of withdrawals due to adverse events was 13% among GlucoNorm treated patients and 14% among SU-treated patients. The most common adverse events leading to withdrawal were hyperglycemia, hypoglycemia, and related symptoms. Mild or moderate hypoglycemia occurred in 16% of GlucoNorm patients and 20% of sulfonylurea patients.

Table 2 lists common clinical trial adverse drug reactions for GlucoNorm patients compared to both placebo (in trials less than 6 months duration) and to glyburide, gliclazide and glipizide in one year trials. The clinical trial adverse drug reactions profile of GlucoNorm was generally comparable to that for sulfonylurea drugs (SU).

Table 2: GlucoNorm

Treatment-Emergent Adverse Events with Possible or Probable Relationship Reported at a Frequency of ≥1% with GlucoNorm

	GlucoNorm n=1228	SU n=597	GlucoNorm n=352	Placebo n=108
	Active Controlled Studies		Placebo Controlled Studies	
Event	n (%)	n (%)	n (%)	n (%)
Eye Disorders				
Vision abnormal	5 (<1.0)	2 (<1.0)	7 (2.0)	1 (<1.0)
General Disorders				
Fatigue	21 (1.7)	4 (<1.0)	9 (2.6)	3 (2.8)
Gastrointestinal Disorders				
Diarrhoea	11 (<1.0)	7 (1.2)	6 (1.7)	—[a]
Constipation	7 (<1.0)	6 (1.0)	4 (1.1)	—[a]
Abdominal pain	12 (1.0)	6 (1.0)	4 (1.1)	1 (<1.0)
Flatulence	7 (<1.0)	2 (<1.0)	4 (1.1)	—[a]
Nausea	12 (1.0)	7 (1.2)	4 (1.1)	2 (1.9)
Dyspepsia	13 (1.1)	5 (<1.0)	—[a]	—[a]
Nervous System Disorders				
Headache	28 (2.3)	12 (2.0)	9 (2.6)	1 (<1.0)
Dizziness	16 (1.3)	9 (1.5)	8 (2.3)	3 (2.8)
Tremor	14 (1.1)	6 (1.0)	1 (<1.0)	—[a]
Metabolism and Nutrition Disorders				
Hypoglycemia	179 (14.6)	102 (17.1)	24 (6.8)	2 (1.9)
Hyperglycaemia	35 (2.9)	18 (3.0)	4 (1.1)	5 (4.6)
Skin and Subcutaneous Tissue Disorders				
Sweating increased	13 (1.1)	4 (<1.0)	—[a]	—[a]

[a] No events observed.

Less Common Clinical Trial Adverse Drug Reactions (<1%): Cardiovascular Disorders: In one-year comparator trials, the incidence of individual cardiovascular events considered possibly or probably related to trial drug was less than 1%.

The incidence of all observed serious cardiovascular adverse events (i.e. including events not considered possible or probable related to trial drug) added together, including ischemia, was slightly higher for repaglinide (4%) than for sulfonylurea drugs (3%) in controlled comparator clinical trials. In 1-year controlled trials, GlucoNorm treatment was not associated with excess mortality rates compared to rates observed with other oral hypoglycemic agent therapies.

Table 3: GlucoNorm

Summary of Serious Cardiovascular Events (% of total patients with events)

	GlucoNorm	SU[a]
Total Exposed	1228	498
Serious CV Events	4%	3%
Cardiac Ischemic Events	2%	2%
Deaths due to CV Events	0.5%	0.4%

[a] Glyburide and glipizide.

Eye Disorders: Very rare visual disturbance.

Such disturbances have only been reported in very few cases, after initiation of repaglinide treatment. No such cases have led to discontinuation of repaglinide treatment in clinical trials.

Gastrointestinal Disorders: vomiting.

Hepatobiliary Disorders: Severe hepatic dysfunction.

In very rare cases, severe hepatic dysfunction has been reported. However, other causes were implicated in these cases and causal relationship with repaglinide has not been established.

Immune System Disorders: allergy.

Generalized hypersensitivity reactions or immunological reactions such as vasculitis may occur very rarely.

Skin and Subcutaneous Tissue Disorders: Hypersensitivity reactions of skin may occur as erythema, itching, rashes and urticaria.

Abnormal Hematologic and Clinical Chemistry Findings: Less common adverse clinical and laboratory events observed in clinical trials, including events not considered possibly or probably related to trial drug included elevated liver enzymes, bilirubinaemia, thrombocytopenia and leukopenia.

Isolated cases of increase in liver enzymes have been reported during treatment with repaglinide. Most cases were mild and transient, and very few patients discontinued treatment due to increase in liver enzymes.

Post-Market Adverse Drug Reactions: The following events have been spontaneously reported during ten years experience (i.e. 1998-2008) with GlucoNorm in clinical practice representing a total of 7 979 136 patient-years.

Eye Disorders: visual disturbance.

Gastrointestinal Disorders: abdominal pain, diarrhoea, vomiting, constipation, nausea.

Hepato-bilary Disorders: hepatic function abnormal, hepatic enzymes increased.

Immune System Disorders: allergy, anaphylactic reactions have been observed in very few cases.

Metabolism and Nutrition Disorders: hypoglycemia, hypoglycemic coma, hypoglycemic unconsciousness.

In post-market experience, there have been rare spontaneous reports of serious hypoglycemic episodes in patients co-administered repaglinide and gemfibrozil.

Skin and Subcutaneous Disorders: hypersensitivity (erythema, itching, rash, urticaria).

DRUG INTERACTIONS:

Serious Drug Interactions

The concomitant use of gemfibrozil and repaglinide is contraindicated (see Contraindications and Table 4).

Overview: Drug interaction studies performed in healthy volunteers show that repaglinide had no clinically relevant effect on the pharmacokinetic properties of digoxin, theophylline, or warfarin at steady state. Dosage adjustment of these compounds when co-administered with GlucoNorm is therefore not necessary. Co-administration of cimetidine, nifedipine, estrogen, or simvastatin with GlucoNorm did not significantly alter the absorption and disposition of repaglinide.

Additionally, the following drugs were studied in healthy volunteers with co-administration of repaglinide. The following are the study results:

Drug-Drug Interactions: The drugs listed in this table are based on either drug interaction case reports or studies, or potential interactions due to the expected magnitude and seriousness of the interaction (i.e., those identified as contraindicated).

Table 4: GlucoNorm

Established or Potential Drug-Drug Interactions

Drug Class	Ref	Effect	Clinical Comment
Gemfibrozil	CT	↑ AUC by 8.1 fold ↑ C_{max} by 2.4 fold ↑ t½ from 1.3 to 3.7 hours	Co-administration of gemfibrozil (600 mg), an inhibitor of CYP2C8 and OATP1B1, and a single dose of 0.25 mg repaglinide (after 3 days of twice-daily 600 mg gemfibrozil) resulted in an 8.1 fold higher repaglinide AUC and prolonged repaglinide half-life from 1.3 to 3.7 hr. The concomitant use of gemfibrozil and repaglinide is contraindicated (see Contraindications).
Itraconazole	CT	↑ AUC by 1.4 fold	Co-administration of itraconazole, a CYP3A4 inhibitor, and a single dose of 0.25 mg repaglinide (on the third day of a regimen of 200 mg initial dose, twice-daily 100 mg itraconazole) resulted in a 1.4-fold higher repaglinide AUC.
Gemfibrozil and itraconazole	CT	↑ AUC by 19 fold ↑ t½ from 1.3 to 6.1 hours	Co-administration of both gemfibrozil and itraconazole with repaglinide, resulted in a 19-fold higher repaglinide AUC and prolonged repaglinide half-life from 1.3 to 6.1 hr. Plasma repaglinide concentration at 7 h increased 28.6-fold with gemfibrozil co-administration and 70.4 fold with the gemfibrozil-itraconazole combination.
Ketoconazole	CT	↑ AUC by 1.2 fold ↑ C_{max} by 1.2 fold	Co-administration of 200 mg ketoconazole, a potent and competitive inhibitor of CYP3A4, and a single dose of 2 mg repaglinide in healthy subjects (after 4 days of once daily ketoconazole 200 mg) resulted in a 15% and 16% increase in repaglinide. The increases were from 20.2 ng/mL to 23.5 ng/mL for C_{max} and from 38.9 ng/mL·hr to 44.9 ng/mL·hr for AUC.
Rifampicin	CT	Co-administration: ↓ AUC by 32%–48% ↓ C_{max} by 26%–17% Monoadministration of repaglinide after 6 days of rifampicin: ↓AUC by 80% ↓ C_{max} by 79%	Co-administration of 600 mg rifampicin, and a single dose of 4 mg repaglinide (after 6 days of once daily rifampicin 600 mg) resulted in a 32% and 26% decrease in repaglinide AUC and C_{max} respectively. The decreases were from 40.4 ng/mL to 29.7 ng/mL for C_{max} and from 56.8 ng/mL·hr to 38.7 ng/mL·hr for AUC. In another study co-administration of 600 mg rifampicin and a single dose of 4 mg repaglinide (after 6 days of once daily rifampicin 600 mg) resulted in a 48% and 17% decrease in repaglinide AUC and C max respectively. The decreases were from 54 ng/mL·hr to 28 ng/mL·hr for AUC and from 35 ng/mL to 29 ng/mL for C_{max}. Repaglinide administered by itself (after 7 days of once daily rifampicin 600 mg) resulted in an 80% and 79% decrease in repaglinide AUC and C_{max} respectively. The decreases were from 54 ng/mL·hr to 11 ng/mL·hr for AUC and from 35 ng/mL to 7.5 ng/mL for C_{max}.
Clarithromycin	CT	↑ AUC by 1.4 fold ↑ C_{max} by 1.7 fold	Co-administration of 250 mg clarithromycin, a potent CYP3A4 inhibitor, and a single dose of 0.25 mg repaglinide (after 4 days of twice daily clarithromycin 250 mg resulted in a 40% and 67% increase in repaglinide AUC and C_{max}, respectively. The increase in repaglinide AUC was from 5.3 ng/mL·hr to 7.5 ng/mL·hr and the increase in C_{max} was from 4.4 ng/mL to 7.3 ng/mL.
Cyclosporine	CT	↑ AUC by 2.5 fold ↑ C_{max} by 1.8 fold	Co-administration of cyclosporine, an inhibitor of CYP3A4 and strong OATP1B1 inhibitor, caused an increase in repaglinide (0.25 mg) mean peak plasma concentrations of 175% and the total area under the plasma concentration-time curve was 244% of that in the placebo phase.
Trimethoprim	CT	↑ AUC by 1.6 fold ↑ C_{max} by 1.4 fold	Co-administration of trimethoprim, 160 mg and a single dose of 0.25 mg repaglinide (after 2 days of twice daily and one dose on the third day of trimethoprim 160 mg) resulted in a 61% and 41% increase in repaglinide AUC and C_{max}, respectively. The increase in AUC was from 5.9 ng/mL·hr to 9.6 ng/mL·hr and the increase in C_{max} was from 4.7 ng/mL to 6.6 ng/mL. The concomitant use of trimethoprim with repaglinide should be avoided.
Oral contraceptives (ethinyl estradiol/levon orgestrel)	CT		A pharmacokinetic clinical trial in healthy volunteers demonstrated that concomitant oral contraceptive administration (ethinyl estradiol/levonorgestrel) did not alter repaglinide's total bioavailability to a clinically relevant degree, although peak levels of repaglinide occurred earlier. Repaglinide had no clinically meaningful effect upon bioavailability of levonorgestrel but effects on ethinyl estradiol bioavailability cannot be excluded.

(cont'd)

Table 4: GlucoNorm *(cont'd)*

Established or Potential Drug-Drug Interactions

Drug Class	Ref	Effect	Clinical Comment
Monoamine Oxidase inhibitors (MAOI)	T	May potentiate the hypoglycemic effect of repaglinide	The patient should be observed for hypoglycemia. When these drugs are either administered or withdrawn from a patient receiving GlucoNorm, the patient should be observed for loss of glycemic control.
Beta blockers	T	May potentiate the hypoglycemic effect of repaglinide. Beta blockers may also mask the symptoms of hypoglycemia	The patient should be observed for hypoglycemia. When these drugs are either administered or withdrawn from a patient receiving GlucoNorm, the patient should be observed for loss of glycemic control.
ACE inhibitors	T	May potentiate the hypoglycemic effect of repaglinide	The patient should be observed for hypoglycemia.
Other antidiabetic agents	T	May potentiate the hypoglycemic effect of repaglinide	The patient should be observed for hypoglycemia.
Salicylates e.g. aspirin and non steroidal anti-inflammatory agents (NSAIDs)	T	May potentiate the hypoglycemic effect of repaglinide	The patient should be observed for hypoglycemia. When these drugs are either administered or withdrawn from a patient receiving GlucoNorm, the patient should be observed for loss of glycemic control.
Octreotide	T	May potentiate the hypoglycemic effect of repaglinide	The patient should be observed for hypoglycemia. When these drugs are either administered or withdrawn from a patient receiving GlucoNorm, the patient should be observed for loss of glycemic control.
Anabolic steroids	T	May potentiate the hypoglycemic effect of repaglinide	The patient should be observed for hypoglycemia. When these drugs are either administered or withdrawn from a patient receiving GlucoNorm, the patient should be observed for loss of glycemic control.
Thiazides	T	May reduce the hypoglycemic effect of repaglinide and potentiate hyperglycemia.	The patient should be observed for hyperglycaemia. When these drugs are either administered or withdrawn from a patient receiving GlucoNorm, the patient should be observed for loss of glycemic control.
Danazol	T	May reduce the hypoglycemic effect of repaglinide and potentiate hyperglycemia.	The patient should be observed for hyperglycaemia. When these drugs are either administered or withdrawn from a patient receiving GlucoNorm, the patient should be observed for loss of glycemic control.
Thyroid hormones	T	May reduce the hypoglycemic effect of repaglinide and potentiate hyperglycemia.	The patient should be observed for hyperglycaemia.
Sympathomimetics	T	May reduce the hypoglycemic effect of repaglinide and potentiate hyperglycemia.	The patient should be observed for hyperglycaemia. When these drugs are either administered or withdrawn from a patient receiving GlucoNorm, the patient should be observed for loss of glycemic control.
Phenytoin, carbamazepine and phenobarbital	T	May reduce the hypoglycemic effect of repaglinide and potentiate hyperglycemia.	The patient should be observed for hypoglycemia. When these drugs are either administered or withdrawn from a patient receiving GlucoNorm, the patient should be observed for loss of glycemic control.
Corticosteroids	T	May reduce the hypoglycemic effect of repaglinide and potentiate hyperglycemia.	The patient should be observed for hypoglycemia. When these drugs are either administered or withdrawn from a patient receiving GlucoNorm, the patient should be observed for loss of glycemic control.

Legend: C=case study; CT=clinical trial; T=theoretical.

Drug-Food Interactions: Grapefruit may increase the plasma concentration of repaglinide. In a study with healthy volunteers where grapefruit juice was consumed 2 hours prior to repaglinide intake, a 13% increase in AUC was observed. No other interactions with food have been established.

Drug-Herb Interactions: Interactions with herbal products have not been established.

Drug-Laboratory Test Interactions: Interactions with laboratory tests have not been established.

Drug-Lifestyle Interactions: Alcohol may enhance and/or prolong the hypoglycemic effect of repaglinide. The patient's ability to concentrate and react may be impaired as a result of hypoglycemia. This may constitute a risk in situations where these abilities are of special importance (e.g. driving a car or operating machinery).

Patients should be advised to take precautions to avoid hypoglycemia while driving. This is particularly important in those who have reduced or absent awareness of the warning signs of hypoglycemia or have frequent episodes of hypoglycemia. The advisability of driving should be considered in these circumstances.

DOSAGE AND ADMINISTRATION:

Dosing Considerations: There is no fixed dosage regimen for the management of type 2 diabetes with GlucoNorm (repaglinide).

GlucoNorm doses are usually taken within 15 minutes of the meal but time may vary from immediately preceding the meal to as long as 30 minutes before the meal. Patients who skip a meal (or add an extra meal) should be instructed to skip (or add) a dose for that meal.

Short-term administration of GlucoNorm may be sufficient during periods of transient loss of control in patients usually controlled by their diet.

Recommended Dose and Dosage Adjustment: Initiation Dose: For patients not previously treated with antidiabetic agents or whose HbA_{1c} <8% the starting dose should be 0.5 mg.

For patients previously treated with blood glucose-lowering drugs or whose HbA_{1c} is ≥8%, the initial dose is 1 or 2 mg with each meal preprandially.

Transfer from Other Therapies: When GlucoNorm is used to replace therapy with other oral hypoglycemic agents, GlucoNorm may be started on the day after the final dose is given. Patients should then be observed carefully for hypoglycemia due to potential overlapping of drug effects. When transferred from longer half-life sulfonylurea agents (e.g., chlorpropamide) to GlucoNorm, close monitoring may be indicated for up to one week or longer.

Titration: Dosing adjustments should be determined by blood glucose response, usually fasting blood glucose. The preprandial dose should be doubled up to 4 mg until satisfactory blood glucose response is achieved. A minimum of one week should elapse between titration steps to assess response after each dose adjustment.

Maintenance: The recommended dose range is 0.5 mg to 4.0 mg taken with meals. GlucoNorm offers flexible dietary options and may be dosed preprandially 2, 3 or 4 times a day in response to changes in the patient's meal pattern. The recommended maximum daily dose is 16 mg.

Long-term efficacy should be monitored by measurement of HbA_{1C} levels every 3 months. Failure to follow an appropriate dosage regimen may precipitate hypoglycemia or hyperglycemia. Patients who do not adhere to their prescribed dietary and drug regimen are more prone to exhibit unsatisfactory response to therapy, including hypoglycemia.

For patients maintained in tight glucose control, GlucoNorm treatment has less associated risk of hypoglycemia when meals are missed than does treatment with agents with a longer half life.

Combination Therapy: If GlucoNorm monotherapy does not result in adequate glycemic control, metformin or rosiglitazone may be added. Or, if metformin or rosiglitazone monotherapy does not provide adequate control, GlucoNorm may be added. The starting dose and dose adjustments for GlucoNorm combination therapy is the same as for GlucoNorm monotherapy. The dose of each drug should be carefully adjusted to determine the minimal dose required to achieve the desired pharmacologic effect. Failure to do so could result in an increase in the incidence of hypoglycemic episodes. Appropriate monitoring of FPG and HbA_{1C} measurements should be used to ensure that the patient is not subjected to excessive drug exposure or increased probability of secondary drug failure.

Missed Dose: If a dose is missed the next dose should be taken as usual. The dose should not be doubled.

OVERDOSAGE:

In a clinical trial, patients received increasing doses of GlucoNorm (repaglinide) up to 80 mg a day for 14 days. There were few adverse effects other than those associated with the intended pharmacodynamic effect of lowering blood glucose. Hypoglycemia did not occur when meals were given with these high doses.

Hypoglycemic symptoms without loss of consciousness or neurologic findings should be treated aggressively with oral glucose and adjustments in drug dosage and/or meal patterns. Close monitoring should continue until the physician is assured that the patient is out of danger. Patients should be closely monitored for a minimum of 24 to 48 hours, since hypoglycemia may recur after apparent clinical recovery. There is no evidence that repaglinide is dialyzable using hemodialysis.

> For management of a suspected drug overdose, contact your regional Poison Control Centre. See the *CPS* Directory section for a list of Poison Control Centres.

ACTION AND CLINICAL PHARMACOLOGY: Mechanism of Action: GlucoNorm (repaglinide) is an oral blood glucose-lowering drug used in the management of type 2 diabetes mellitus. Repaglinide is a short-acting insulin secretagogue which lowers blood glucose levels (as measured by HbA_{1C} and fasting plasma glucose) and is effective in regulating meal-related (prandial) glucose loads. Repaglinide lowers blood glucose levels by stimulating the release of insulin from the pancreas. This action is dependent upon functioning beta cells in the pancreatic islets. Insulin release is glucose-dependent and diminishes at low glucose concentrations.

Repaglinide is chemically unrelated to oral sulfonylurea insulin secretagogues used in the treatment of type 2 diabetes.)

Repaglinide closes ATP-dependent potassium channels in the β-cell membrane by binding at characterizable sites. This potassium channel blockade depolarizes the β-cell which leads to an opening of calcium channels. The resulting increased calcium influx induces insulin secretion. The ion channel mechanism is highly tissue selective with low affinity for heart and skeletal muscle.

Pharmacokinetics: Absorption: After oral administration, repaglinide is rapidly and completely absorbed from the gastrointestinal tract. After single and multiple oral doses in healthy subjects or in patients, peak drug levels (C_{max}) occur within 1 hour (T_{max}). Repaglinide is rapidly eliminated from the blood stream with a half-life of approximately 1 hour. The mean absolute bioavailability is 56%. When repaglinide was given with food, the mean T_{max} was not changed, but the mean C_{max} and AUC (area under the time/plasma concentration curve) were decreased 20% and 12.4%, respectively.

Distribution: After intravenous (IV) dosing in healthy subjects, the volume of distribution at steady state (VSS) was approximately 31 L, and the total body clearance (CL) was 38 L/h. Protein binding and binding to human serum albumin was greater than 98%.

Metabolism: Repaglinide is completely metabolized by oxidative biotransformation and direct conjugation with glucuronic acid after either an IV or oral dose. The major metabolites are an oxidized dicarboxylic acid (M_2), the aromatic amine (M_1) and the acyl glucuronide (M_7). The cytochrome P-450 enzyme system, specifically 2C8 and 3A4 has been shown to be involved in the N-dealkylation of repaglinide to M_2 and the further oxidation to M_1. Metabolites do not contribute to the glucose-lowering effect of repaglinide.

Excretion: Within 96 hours after dosing with ^{14}C-repaglinide as a single oral dose, approximately 90% of the radiolabel was recovered in the feces and 8% in the urine. Only 0.1% of the dose is cleared in the urine as parent compound. The major metabolite (M_2) accounted for 60% of the administered dose. Less than 2% of parent drug was recovered in feces.

Pharmacokinetic Parameters: Data indicate that repaglinide did not accumulate in serum. Repaglinide demonstrated pharmacokinetic linearity over the 0.5-4 mg dose range.

The pharmacokinetic parameters of repaglinide obtained from a single-dose, crossover study in healthy subjects and from a multiple-dose, parallel, dose-proportionality (0.5, 1, 2 and 4 mg) study in patients with Type 2 diabetes are summarized in Table 5.

Table 5: GlucoNorm

Pharmacokinetic Parameters of GlucoNorm

Parameter	Patients with Type 2 Diabetes[a]
$AUC_{0\text{-}24\ hr}$ (ng/mL×h):	**Mean (SD):**
0.5 mg	68.9 (154.4)
1.0 mg	125.8 (129.8)
2.0 mg	152.4 (89.6)
4.0 mg	447.4 (211.3)
$Cmax_{0\text{-}5\ hr}$ (ng/mL):	**Mean (SD):**
0.5 mg	9.8 (10.2)
1.0 mg	18.3 (9.1)
2.0 mg	26.0 (13.0)
4.0 mg	65.8 (30.1)
$Tmax_{0\text{-}5\ hr}$ (h): 0.5 to 4 mg	**Means (SD range):** 1.0 to 1.4 (0.3 to 0.5)
T½ (h): 0.5 to 4 mg	**Means (Indiv. Range):** 1.0 to 1.4 (0.4 to 8.0)
CL based on i.v. (L/h)	38 (16)
V_{SS} based on i.v. (L)	31 (12)
AbsBio (%)	56 (9)

[a] Dose preprandially three times daily.
Legend: CL=total body clearance; V_{ss}=volume of distribution at steady state; AbsBio=absolute bioavailability.

Variability: The intra-individual and inter-individual variabilities (coefficient of variation) in AUC were 36% and 69%, respectively after multiple dosing of repaglinide tablets (0.25 to 4 mg with each meal) in patients.

Special Populations and Conditions: Geriatrics: Healthy volunteers were treated with a regimen of 2 mg taken before each of 3 meals. There were no significant differences in repaglinide pharmacokinetics between the group of patients <65 years of age and a comparably sized group of patients ≥65 years of age.

Gender: A comparison of pharmacokinetics in males and females showed the AUC over the 0.5 mg to 4 mg dose range to be 15% to 70% higher in females with type 2 diabetes. This difference was not reflected in the frequency of hypoglycemic episodes (male: 16%; female: 17%) or other adverse events. With respect to gender, no change in general dosage recommendation is indicated since dosage for each patient should be individualized to achieve optimal clinical response.

Race: No pharmacokinetic studies to assess the effects of race have been performed, but in a U.S. 1-year study in patients with type 2 diabetes, the blood glucose-lowering effect was comparable between Caucasians (n=297) and African-Americans (n=33). In a U.S. doseresponse study, there was no apparent difference in exposure (AUC) between Caucasians (n=74) and Hispanics (n=33).

Hepatic Insufficiency: A single-dose, open-label study was conducted in 12 healthy subjects and 12 patients with chronic liver disease (CLD) classified by caffeine clearance. Patients with moderate to severe impairment of liver function had higher and more prolonged serum concentrations of both total and unbound repaglinide than healthy subjects ($AUC_{healthy}$: 91.6 ng/mL·h; AUC_{CLD} patients: 368.9 ng/mL·h; $C_{max, healthy}$: 46.7 ng/mL: $C_{max, CLD\ patients}$: 105.4 ng/mL). AUC was statistically correlated with caffeine clearance. No difference in glucose profiles was observed across patient groups. Patients with impaired liver function may be exposed to higher concentrations of repaglinide and its associated metabolites than would patients with normal liver function receiving the same doses.

Renal Insufficiency: Single-dose and steady state pharmacokinetics of repaglinide have been evaluated in patients with various degrees of renal impairment. Repaglinide was found to be well tolerated in all groups. Measures of AUC and C_{max} after multiple dosing of 2 mg repaglinide were found to be higher in three groups of patients with reduced renal function ($AUC_{mild/moderate\ impairment}$: 90.8 ng/mL·hr to $AUC_{severe\ impairment}$:137.7 ng/mL·hr versus $AUC_{healthy}$: 29.1 ng/mL·hr; $C_{max, mild/moderate\ impairment}$: 46.7 ng/mL to ; $C_{max, severe\ impairment}$: 44.0 ng/mL versus $C_{max, healthy}$: 20.6 ng/mL). Repaglinide AUC is only weakly correlated to creatinine clearance.

Genetic Polymorphism: In healthy subjects, polymorphism in the SLCO1B1 gene (c.521T>C) encoding for the OATP1B1 transporter has been observed to lead to approximately 72% higher exposure (AUC). Polymorphism in CYP2C8 (CYP2C8*3) has been studied in different studies in healthy subjects. The CYP2C8*3 allele has been found to have either no effect or been associated with an approximately 50% lower exposure (AUC). The observed effects are explaining factors for the observed inter individual variability together with the variability in the expression of metabolizing enzymes.

STORAGE AND STABILITY: GlucoNorm (repaglinide) should be stored at 15-25°C. Protect from moisture.

Keep out of reach of children.

Unused medication should not be disposed of down the drain or in household garbage.

INFORMATION FOR THE PATIENT: Published in e-CPS, available by subscription at www.e-cps.ca.

DOSAGE FORMS, COMPOSITION AND PACKAGING: 0.5 mg: Each white unscored, biconvex tablet, embossed with the Novo Nordisk (Apis) bull symbol and coloured to indicate strength contains: repaglinide 0.5 mg. Nonmedicinal ingredients: amberlite (polacrilin potassium), calcium hydrogen phosphate anhydrous, glycerol 85%, magnesium stearate, maize starch, meglumine, microcrystalline cellulose (E460), poloxamer and povidone (polyvidone). Bottles of 100.

1 mg: Each yellow unscored, biconvex tablet, embossed with the Novo Nordisk (Apis) bull symbol and coloured to indicate strength contains: repaglinide 1 mg. Nonmedicinal ingredients: amberlite (polacrilin potassium), calcium hydrogen phosphate anhydrous, glycerol 85%, magnesium stearate, maize starch, meglumine, microcrystalline cellulose (E460), povidone (polyvidone) and yellow iron oxide. Bottles of 100.

2 mg: Each peach unscored, biconvex tablet, embossed with the Novo Nordisk (Apis) bull symbol and coloured to indicate strength contains: repaglinide 2 mg. Nonmedicinal ingredients: amberlite (polacrilin potassium), calcium hydrogen phosphate anhydrous, glycerol 85%, magnesium stearate, maize starch, meglumine, microcrystalline cellulose (E460), povidone (polyvidone) and red iron oxide. Bottles of 100.

Glucophage® Ⓟ

metformin HCl

Oral Antihyperglycemic Agent

sanofi-aventis

Date of Revision: October 28, 2009

SUMMARY PRODUCT INFORMATION:

Route of Administration	Dosage Form/ Strength	Clinically Relevant Nonmedicinal Ingredients
Oral	Tablet 500 mg, 850 mg	For a complete listing see Dosage Forms, Composition and Packaging.

INDICATIONS AND CLINICAL USE: GLUCOPHAGE (metformin HCl) is indicated to control hyperglycemia in responsive, stable, mild, non-ketosis prone, maturity onset type of diabetes (Type II) which cannot be controlled by proper dietary management, exercise and weight reduction or when insulin therapy is not appropriate.

GLUCOPHAGE can be of value for the treatment of obese diabetic patients.

CONTRAINDICATIONS:

- Unstable and/or insulin-dependent (Type I) diabetes mellitus.
- Acute or chronic metabolic acidosis, including diabetic ketoacidosis, with or without coma, history of ketoacidosis with or without coma. Diabetic ketoacidosis should be treated with insulin.
- In patients with a history of lactic acidosis, irrespective of precipitating factors.
- In the presence of renal impairment or when renal function is not known, and also in patients with serum creatinine levels above the upper limit of normal range. Renal disease or renal dysfunction (e.g., as suggested by serum creatinine levels ≥136 µmol/L (males), ≥124 µmol/L (females) or abnormal creatinine clearance <60 mL/min)) which may result from conditions such as cardiovascular collapse (shock), acute myocardial infarction, and septicemia (see also Warnings and Precautions).
- In excessive alcohol intake, acute or chronic.

In patients suffering from severe hepatic dysfunction, since severe hepatic dysfunction has been associated with some cases of lactic acidosis, GLUCOPHAGE should generally be avoided in patients with clinical or laboratory evidence of hepatic disease.

GLUCOPHAGE should be temporarily discontinued in patients undergoing radiologic studies involving intravascular administration of iodinated contrast materials, because use of such products may result in acute alteration of renal function (see Warnings and Precautions).

- In cases of cardiovascular collapse and in disease states associated with hypoxemia such as cardiorespiratory insufficiency, which are often associated with hyperlactacidemia.
- During stress conditions, such as severe infections, trauma or surgery and the recovery phase thereafter.
- In patients suffering from severe dehydration.
- Known hypersensitivity or allergy to metformin HCl or any of the excipients. For a complete listing, see Dosage Forms, Composition and Packaging.
- During pregnancy and breastfeeding.

WARNINGS AND PRECAUTIONS:

Serious Warnings and Precautions

- Lactic acidosis is a rare, but serious, metabolic complication that occurs due to metformin accumulation during treatment with GLUCOPHAGE (see Endocrine and Metabolism, Lactic Acidosis).
- Patients should be cautioned against excessive alcohol intake, either acute or chronic, when taking GLUCOPHAGE, since alcohol intake potentiates the effect of metformin on lactate metabolism (see Endocrine and Metabolism, Lactic Acidosis).

General: Patient Selection and Follow-up: Careful selection of patients is important. It is imperative that there be rigid attention to diet and careful adjustment of dosage. Regular thorough follow-up examinations are necessary.

If vomiting occurs, withdraw drug temporarily, exclude lactic acidosis, then resume dosage cautiously (see Adverse Reactions).

Particular attention should be paid to short range and long range complications which are peculiar to diabetes. Periodic cardiovascular, ophthalmic, hematological, hepatic and renal assessments are advisable.

Use of GLUCOPHAGE must be considered as treatment in addition to proper dietary regimen and not as a substitute for diet.

Care should be taken to ensure that GLUCOPHAGE is not given when a contraindication exists.

If during GLUCOPHAGE therapy the patient develops acute intercurrent disease such as: clinically significant hepatic dysfunction, cardiovascular collapse, congestive heart failure, acute myocardial infarction, or other conditions complicated by hypoxemia, the drug should be discontinued.

Change in Clinical Status of Previously Controlled Diabetes Patients: A diabetic patient previously well controlled on GLUCOPHAGE who develops laboratory abnormalities or clinical illness (especially vague and poorly defined illness) should be evaluated promptly for evidence of ketoacidosis or lactic acidosis. Evaluation should include serum electrolytes and ketones, blood glucose and, if indicated, blood pH, lactate, pyruvate and metformin levels. If acidosis of either form occurs, GLUCOPHAGE must be stopped immediately and appropriate corrective measures initiated.

Hypoxic States: Cardiovascular collapse (shock) from whatever cause, acute congestive heart failure, acute myocardial infarction and other conditions characterized by hypoxemia have been associated with lactic acidosis and may also cause prerenal azotemia. When such event occur in patients on GLUCOPHAGE therapy, the drug should be promptly discontinued.

Endocrine and Metabolism: Lactic Acidosis: Lactic acidosis is a rare, but serious, metabolic complication that occurs due to metformin accumulation during treatment with GLUCOPHAGE. When it occurs, it is fatal in approximately 50% of cases. Lactic acidosis may also occur in association with a number of pathophysiologic conditions, including diabetes mellitus, and whenever there is significant tissue hypoperfusion and hypoxemia. Lactic acidosis is characterized by elevated blood lactate levels (>5 mmol/L), decreased blood pH, electrolyte disturbances with an increased anion gap, and an increased lactate/pyruvate ratio. When metformin is implicated as the cause of lactic acidosis, metformin plasma levels >5 µg/mL are generally found.

The reported incidence of lactic acidosis in patients receiving metformin HCl is very low (approximately 0.03 cases/1000 patient-years, with approximately 0.015 fatal cases/1000 patient-years) and occurs primarily in diabetic patients with significant renal insufficiency, including both intrinsic renal disease and renal hypoperfusion, often in the setting of multiple concomitant medical/surgical problems and multiple concomitant medications. Patients with congestive heart failure requiring pharmacologic management, in particular those with unstable or acute congestive heart failure who are at risk of hypoperfusion and hypoxemia, are at increased risk of lactic acidosis. In particular, treatment of the elderly should be accompanied by careful monitoring of renal function. GLUCOPHAGE treatment should not be initiated in patients ≥80 years of age, unless measurement of creatinine clearance demonstrates that renal function is not reduced, as the patients are more susceptible to developing lactic acidosis. The risk of lactic acidosis increases with the degree of renal dysfunction and the patient's age. The risk of lactic acidosis may, therefore, be significantly decreased by regular monitoring of renal function in patients taking GLUCOPHAGE and by use of the minimum effective dose of GLUCOPHAGE. In addition, GLUCOPHAGE should be promptly withheld in the presence of any condition associated with hypoxemia, dehydration or sepsis. Because impaired hepatic function may significantly limit the ability to clear lactate, GLUCOPHAGE should generally be avoided in patients with clinical or laboratory evidence of hepatic disease. Patients should be cautioned against excessive alcohol intake, either acute or chronic, when taking GLUCOPHAGE (metformin HCl), since alcohol intake potentiates the effect of metformin HCl on lactate metabolism. In addition, GLUCOPHAGE should be temporarily discontinued prior to any intravascular radiocontrast study and for any surgical procedure. The onset of lactic acidosis often is subtle, and accompanied only by nonspecific symptoms such as malaise, myalgias, respiratory distress, increasing somnolence and non-specific abdominal distress. There may be associated hypothermia, hypotension and resistance bradyarrhythmias with more marked acidosis. The patient and the patient's physician must be aware of the possible importance of such symptoms and the patient should be instructed to notify the physician immediately if they occur. GLUCOPHAGE should be withdrawn until the situation is clarified. Serum electrolytes, ketones, blood glucose and, if indicated, blood pH, lactate levels and even blood metformin levels may be useful. Once a patient is stabilized on any dose level of GLUCOPHAGE, gastrointestinal symptoms, which are common during initiation of therapy, are unlikely to be drug related. Later occurrence of gastrointestinal symptoms could be due to lactic acidosis or other serious disease. Levels of fasting venous plasma lactate above the upper limit of normal but less than 5 mmol/L in patients taking GLUCOPHAGE do not necessarily indicate impending lactic acidosis and may be explainable by other mechanisms, such as poorly controlled diabetes or obesity, vigorous physical activity or technical problems in sample handling. Lactic acidosis should be suspected in any diabetic patient with metabolic acidosis lacking evidence of ketoacidosis (ketonuria and ketonemia).

Lactic acidosis is a medical emergency that must be treated in a hospital setting. In a patient with lactic acidosis who is taking GLUCOPHAGE, the drug should be discontinued immediately and general supportive measures promptly instituted. Because metformin HCl is dialysable (with clearance of up to 170 mL/min under good hemodynamic conditions), prompt hemodialysis is recommended to correct the acidosis and remove the accumulated metformin. Such management often results in prompt reversal of symptoms and recovery (see Contraindications).

Note: When used as indicated, there has not been a single case of lactic acidosis in Canada. GLUCOPHAGE should be immediately discontinued in the presence of acidosis.

Physicians should instruct their patients to recognize the symptoms which could be signal onset of lactic acidosis. If acidosis of any kind develops, GLUCOPHAGE should be discontinued immediately.

Loss of Control of Blood Glucose: When a patient stabilized on any diabetic regimen is exposed to stress such as fever, trauma, infection, or surgery, a temporary loss of glycemic control may occur. At such times, it may be necessary to withhold GLUCOPHAGE and temporarily administer insulin. GLUCOPHAGE may be reinstituted after the acute episode is resolved.

The effectiveness of oral antidiabetic drugs in lowering blood glucose to a targeted level decreases in many patients over a period of time. This phenomenon, which may be due to progression of the underlying disease or to diminished responsiveness to the drug, is known as secondary failure, to distinguish it from primary failure in which the drug is ineffective during initial therapy.

Should secondary failure occur with GLUCOPHAGE, therapeutic alternatives should be considered.

Vitamin B_{12} Levels: Impairment of vitamin B_{12} absorption has been reported in some patients. Therefore, measurements of serum vitamin B_{12} are advisable at least every one to two years in patients on long-term treatment with GLUCOPHAGE.

A decrease to subnormal levels of previously normal serum Vitamin B_{12} levels, without clinical manifestations, is observed in approximately 7% of patients receiving GLUCOPHAGE in controlled clinical trials of 28 weeks duration. Such decrease, possibly due to interference with B_{12} absorption from B_{12}-intrinsic factor complex is, however, very rarely associated with anemia and appears to be rapidly reversible with discontinuation of GLUCOPHAGE or vitamin B_{12} supplementation. Measurement of hematologic parameters on an annual basis is advised in patients on GLUCOPHAGE and any apparent abnormalities should be appropriately investigated and managed (see Monitoring and Laboratory Tests). Certain individuals (those with inadequate vitamin B_{12} or calcium intake or absorption) appear to be predisposed to developing subnormal vitamin B_{12} levels.

Hepatic/Biliary/Pancreatic: Since impaired hepatic function has been associated with some cases of lactic acidosis, GLUCOPHAGE should generally be avoided in patients with clinical or laboratory evidence of hepatic disease.

Hypoglycemia: Hypoglycemia does not occur in patients receiving GLUCOPHAGE alone under usual circumstances of use, but could occur when caloric intake is deficient, when strenuous exercise is not compensated by caloric supplementation, or during concomitant use with other glucose lowering agents or ethanol.

Elderly, debilitated or malnourished patients, and those with adrenal or pituitary insufficiency or alcohol intoxication are particularly susceptible to hypoglycemic effects. Hypoglycemia may be difficult to recognize in the elderly, and in people who are taking beta-adrenergic blocking drugs.

The patient should be warned about driving a vehicle or operating machinery under these conditions where risk of hypoglycaemia is present.

Peri-Operative Considerations: GLUCOPHAGE therapy should be temporarily suspended for any surgical procedure (except minor procedures not associated with restricted intake of food and fluids). GLUCOPHAGE should be discontinued 2 days before surgical intervention and should not be restarted until the patient's oral intake has resumed and renal function has been evaluated as normal.

Renal: GLUCOPHAGE is known to be substantially excreted by the kidney, and the risk of metformin accumulation and lactic acidosis increases with the degree of impairment of renal function. Thus, patients with serum creatinine levels above the upper limit of the normal range for their age should not receive GLUCOPHAGE. In patients with advanced age, GLUCOPHAGE should be carefully titrated to establish the minimum dose for adequate glycemic effect, because aging is associated with reduced renal function. In elderly patients, renal function should be monitored regularly and generally, GLUCOPHAGE should not be titrated to the maximum dose (see Dosage and Administration).

Before initiation of GLUCOPHAGE therapy and every 6 months while on GLUCOPHAGE therapy, renal function should be assessed and verified as being within normal range.

In patients in whom development of renal dysfunction is anticipated, renal function should be assessed more frequently and GLUCOPHAGE discontinued if evidence of renal impairment is present.

Special caution should be exercised in situations where renal function may become impaired, for example when initiating antihypertensive therapy or diuretic therapy and when starting therapy with an NSAID.

Use of Concomitant Medications That May Affect Renal Function or Metformin Disposition: Concomitant medication(s) that may affect renal function or result in significant hemodynamic change or may interfere with disposition of GLUCOPHAGE, such as cationic drugs that are eliminated by renal tubular secretion (see Drug Interactions), should be used with caution.

Radiological studies involving the use of intravascular iodinated contrast materials (for example, intravenous urogram, intravenous cholangiography, angiography, and computed tomography (CT) scans with intravascular contrast material.

Intravascular contrast studies with iodinated materials can lead to acute alteration of renal function and have been associated with lactic acidosis in patients receiving metformin (see Contraindications). Therefore, in patients in whom any such study is planned, GLUCOPHAGE should be temporarily discontinued at the time of or prior to the procedure, and withheld for 48 hours subsequent to the procedure and reinstituted only after renal function has been re-evaluated and found to be normal.

Special Populations: Pregnant Women: Safety in pregnant women has not been established. Metformin was not teratogenic in rats and rabbits at doses up to 600 mg/kg/day, or about two times the maximum recommended human daily dose on a body surface area basis. Determination of fetal concentrations demonstrated a partial placental barrier to metformin. Because animal reproduction studies are not always predictive of human response, the use of GLUCOPHAGE is not recommended during pregnancy.

Because recent information suggests that abnormal blood glucose levels during pregnancy are associated with a higher incidence of congenital abnormalities, there is a consensus among experts that insulin be used during pregnancy to maintain blood glucose levels as close to normal as possible.

Nursing Women: Studies in lactating rats show that metformin is excreted into milk and reaches levels comparable to those in plasma. Similar studies have not been conducted in nursing mothers, but caution should be exercised in such patients, and a decision should be made whether to discontinue nursing or to discontinue the drug, taking into account the importance of the drug to the mother.

Pediatrics: Safety and effectiveness in pediatric patients have not been established.

Geriatrics: Controlled clinical studies of GLUCOPHAGE (metformin HCl) did not include sufficient numbers of elderly patients to determine whether they respond differently from younger patients, although other reported clinical experience has not identified differences in responses between the elderly and younger patients. GLUCOPHAGE is known to be substantially excreted by the kidney and because the risk of serious adverse reactions to the drug is greater in patients with impaired renal function, it should only be used in patients with normal renal function (see Contraindications and Warnings and Precautions). Because aging is associated with reduced renal function, GLUCOPHAGE should be used with caution as age increases. Care should be taken in dose selection and should be based on careful and regular monitoring or renal function. Generally, elderly patients should not be titrated to the maximum dose of GLUCOPHAGE.

Monitoring and Laboratory Tests: Response to all diabetic therapies should be monitored by periodic measurements of fasting blood glucose and glycosylated hemoglobin levels, with a goal of decreasing these levels toward the normal range. During initial dose titration, fasting glucose can be used to determine the therapeutic response. Thereafter, both glucose and glycosylated hemoglobin should be monitored. Measurements of glycosylated hemoglobin may be especially useful for evaluating long-term control (see Dosage and Administration).

Initial and periodic monitoring of hematologic parameters (e.g., hemoglobin/hematocrit and red blood cell indices) and renal function (serum creatinine) should be performed, at least on an annual basis. While megaloblastic anemia has rarely been seen with GLUCOPHAGE (metformin HCl) therapy, if this is suspected, vitamin B_{12} deficiency should be excluded.

ADVERSE REACTIONS: Adverse Drug Reaction Overview: The adverse events most commonly associated with GLUCOPHAGE (metformin HCl) are diarrhea, nausea, and upset stomach. Lactic acidosis is a rare, but serious side effect. Lactic acidosis is fatal in approximately 50% of cases.

Lactic Acidosis: very rare (<1/10 000 and isolated reports). See Warnings and Precautions and Overdosage.

Gastrointestinal Reactions: very common: (>1/10). Gastrointestinal symptoms (diarrhea, nausea, vomiting, abdominal bloating, flatulence, and anorexia) are the most common reactions to GLUCOPHAGE and are approximately 30% more frequent in patients on GLUCOPHAGE monotherapy than in placebo-treated patients, particularly during initiation of GLUCOPHAGE therapy. These symptoms are generally transient and resolve spontaneously during continued treatment. Occasionally, temporary dose reduction may be useful.

Because gastrointestinal symptoms during therapy initiation appear to be dose-related, they may be decreased by gradual dose escalation and by having patients take GLUCOPHAGE (metformin HCl) with meals (see Dosage and Administration).

Because significant diarrhea and/or vomiting can cause dehydration and prerenal azotemia, GLUCOPHAGE should be temporarily discontinued, under such circumstances.

For patients who have been stabilized on GLUCOPHAGE, nonspecific gastrointestinal symptoms should not be attributed to therapy unless intercurrent illness or lactic acidosis have been excluded.

Special Senses: common (≥1/100). During initiation of GLUCOPHAGE therapy complaints of taste disturbance are common, i.e. metallic taste.

Dermatologic Reactions: very rare (<1/10 000 and isolated reports). The incidence of rash/dermatitis in controlled clinical trials was comparable to placebo for GLUCOPHAGE monotherapy and to sulfonylurea for GLUCOPHAGE/sulfonylurea therapy. Reports of skin reactions such as erythema, pruritus, and urticaria are very rare.

Hematologic: During controlled clinical trials of 29 weeks duration, approximately 9% of patients on GLUCOPHAGE monotherapy and 6% of patients on GLUCOPHAGE/sulfonylurea therapy developed asymptomatic subnormal serum vitamin B_{12} levels; serum folic acid levels did not decrease significantly. However, only five cases of megaloblastic anemia have been reported with metformin administration (none during U.S. clinical studies) and no increased incidence of neuropathy has been observed (see also Warnings and Precautions).

Decrease of vitamin B_{12} absorption with decrease of serum levels during long-term use of metformin is rare (≥1/10 000 and <1/1000). Consideration of such aetiology is recommended if a patient presents with megaloblastic anemia.

Hepatic: very rare (<1/10 000 and isolated reports). Liver function tests abnormalities or hepatitis resolving upon metformin discontinuation has been documented in isolated reports.

DRUG INTERACTIONS: Overview: Certain drugs may potentiate the effect of GLUCOPHAGE, particularly sulfonylurea type of drugs in the treatment of diabetes. The simultaneous administration of these two types of drugs could produce a hypoglycemic reaction, especially if they are given in patients already receiving other drugs which, themselves, can potentiate the effect of sulfonylureas. These drugs can be: long-acting sulfonamides, tubercolostatics, phenylbutazone, clofibrate, monoamine oxidase inhibitors, salicylates, probenecid and propanolol.

In healthy volunteers, the pharmacokinetics of propranolol and ibuprofen were not affected by metformin when co-administered in single-dose interaction studies.

Metformin is negligibly bound to plasma proteins and is, therefore, less likely to interact with highly protein-bound drugs such as salicylates, sulfonamides, chloramphenicol, and probenecid, as compared to sulfonylureas, which are extensively bound to serum proteins.

Drug-Drug Interactions: Glyburide: In a single-dose interaction study in NIDDM subjects, co-administration of metformin and glyburide did not result in any changes in either metformin pharmacokinetics or pharmacodynamics. Decreases in glyburide AUC and C_{max} were observed, but were highly variable. The single-dose nature of this study and the lack of correlation between glyburide blood levels and pharmacodynamics effects, makes the clinical significance of this interaction uncertain.

Furosemide: A single-dose study, metformin-furosemide drug interaction study in healthy subjects demonstrated that pharmacokinetic parameters of both compounds were affected by co-administration. Furosemide increased the metformin plasma and blood C_{max} by 22% and blood AUC by 15%, without any significant change in metformin renal clearance. When administered with metformin, the C_{max} and AUC of furosemide were 31% and 12% smaller, respectively, than when administered alone, and the terminal half-life was decreased by 32%, without any significant change in furosemide renal clearance. No information is available about the interaction of metformin and furosemide when co-administered chronically.

Nifedipine: A single-dose, metformin-nifedipine drug interaction study in healthy volunteers demonstrated that co-administration of nifedipine increased plasma metformin C_{max} and AUC by 20% and 9%, respectively, and increased the amount excreted in the urine. T_{max} and half-life were unaffected. Nifedipine appears to enhance the absorption of metformin. Metformin had minimal effects on nifedipine.

Cationic Drugs: Cationic drugs (e.g., amiloride, digoxin, morphine, procainamide, quinidine, quinine, ranitidine, triamterene, trimethoprim, and vancomycin) that are eliminated by renal tubular secretion, theoretically have the potential for interaction with metformin by competing for common renal tubular transport systems. Such an interaction has been observed between metformin and oral cimetidine in normal healthy volunteers in both single and multiple-dose, metformin-cimetidine drug interaction studies, with a 60% increase in peak metformin plasma and whole blood concentrations and a 40% increase in plasma and whole blood metformin AUC was observed. There was no change in elimination half-life in the single-dose study. Metformin had no effect on cimetidine pharmacokinetics. Therefore, careful patient monitoring and dose adjustment of GLUCOPHAGE or the interfering drug is recommended in patients who are taking cationic medications that are excreted via renal tubular secretion.

Other: Other drugs tend to produce hyperglycemia and may lead to a loss of blood sugar control. These include thiazide and other diuretics, corticosteroids, phenothiazines, thyroid products, estrogens, estrogen plus progestogen, oral contraceptives, phenytoin, nicotinic acid, sympathomimetics, calcium channel blocking drugs, isoniazid, and beta-2-agonists. ACE-inhibitors may decrease the blood glucose levels. When such drugs are administered to patients receiving GLUCOPHAGE, the patient should be closely observed to maintain adequate glycemic control.

Elimination rate of the anticoagulant phenprocoumon has been reported to be increased by 20% when used concurrently with GLUCOPHAGE. Therefore, patients receiving phenprocoumon or other antivitamin K anticoagulants should be monitored carefully when both types of drugs used simultaneously. In such cases, an important increase of prothrombin time may occur upon cessation of GLUCOPHAGE therapy, with an increased risk of hemorrhage.

Drug-Food Interactions: Interactions with food have not been established.

Drug-Herb Interactions: Interactions with herbal products have not been established.

Drug-Laboratory Test Interactions: Intravascular contrast studies with iodinated materials can lead to acute alteration of renal function and have been associated with lactic acidosis in patients receiving metformin (see Contraindications and Warnings and Precautions).

Drug-Lifestyle Interactions: Patients should be cautioned against excessive alcohol intake, either acute or chronic, when taking GLUCOPHAGE, since alcohol intake potentiates the effect of metformin on lactate metabolism (see Contraindications).

DOSAGE AND ADMINISTRATION: Dosing Considerations: In diabetic patients, individual determination of the minimum dose that will lower blood glucose adequately should be made, aiming for glycemic targets as close to normal as possible. A lower recommended starting dose and gradually increased dosage is advised to minimize gastrointestinal symptoms.

Over a period of time, patients may become progressively less responsive to therapy with oral hypoglycemic agents because of deterioration of their diabetic state. Patients should therefore be monitored with regular clinical and laboratory evaluations, including blood glucose and glycosylated hemoglobin (A_{1C}) determinations, to determine the minimum effective dosage and to detect primary failure or secondary failure (see Warnings and Precautions).

In patients in whom the maximum dose fails to lower the blood glucose adequately, therapeutic alternatives should be considered.

The usual dose is 500 mg three or four times a day, or 850 mg two or three times a day. Maximal dose should not exceed 2.55 g a day. To minimize gastric intolerance such as nausea and vomiting GLUCOPHAGE (metformin HCl) should be taken with food whenever possible.

Transfer from Other Antidiabetic Therapy: When transferring patients from standard oral hypoglycaemic agents, other than chlorpropamide, to GLUCOPHAGE, no transition period generally is necessary. When transferring patients from chlorpropamide, care should be exercised during the first two weeks because of the prolonged retention of chlorpropamide in the body, leading to overlapping drug effects and possible hypoglycaemia.

Missed Dose: In case the patient forgets to take GLUCOPHAGE tablets, he/she should wait for the next dose at the usual time. He/she should not double the dose to make up the forgotten dose.

OVERDOSAGE:
Available information concerning treatment of a massive overdosage of GLUCOPHAGE (metformin HCl) is very limited. It would be expected that adverse reactions of a more intense character including epigastric discomfort, nausea and vomiting followed by diarrhea, drowsiness, weakness, dizziness, malaise and headache might be seen. Should those symptoms persist, lactic acidosis should be excluded. The drug should be discontinued and proper supportive therapy instituted.

Overdose of metformin hydrochloride has occurred, including ingestion of amounts greater than 50 grams. Hypoglycemia was reported in approximately 10% of cases, but no causal association with metformin hydrochloride has been established. Lactic acidosis has been reported in approximately 32% of metformin overdose cases (see Warnings and Precautions). Metformin is dialyzable with a clearance of up to 170 mL/min under good hemodynamic conditions. Therefore, hemodialysis may be useful for removal of accumulated drug from patients in whom metformin overdosage is suspected.

> For management of a suspected drug overdose, CPhA recommends that you contact your **regional Poison Control Centre**. See the *CPS* Directory section for a list of Poison Control Centres.

ACTION AND CLINICAL PHARMACOLOGY: Mechanism of Action: GLUCOPHAGE (metformin HCl) is a biguanide derivative producing an antihyperglycemic effect which can only be observed in man or in the diabetic animal and only when there is insulin secretion. Metformin, at therapeutic doses, does not cause hypoglycemia when used alone in man or in the non-diabetic animal, except when using a near lethal dose. Metformin has no effects on the pancreatic beta cells. The mode of action of metformin is not fully understood. It has been postulated that metformin might potentiate the effect of insulin or that it might enhance the effect of insulin on the peripheral receptor site. This increased sensitivity seems to follow an increase in the number of insulin receptors on cell surface membranes.

Metformin absorption is relatively slow and may extend over about 6 hours. The drug is excreted in urine at high renal clearance rate of about 450 mL/min. The initial elimination of metformin is rapid with a half-life varying between 1.7 and 3 hours. The terminal elimination phase accounting for about 4 to 5% of the absorbed dose is slow with a half-life between 9 and 17 hours. Metformin is not metabolized. Its main sites of concentration are the intestinal mucosa and the salivary glands. The plasma concentration at steady-state ranges about 1 to 2 μg/mL. Certain drugs may potentiate the effects of metformin (see Warnings and Precautions and Drug Interactions).

STORAGE AND STABILITY: Store at room temperature (15 to 30°C) in well closed containers.

INFORMATION FOR THE PATIENT: Published in e-CPS, available by subscription at www.e-cps.ca.

DOSAGE FORMS, COMPOSITION AND PACKAGING: 500 mg: Each white, round, biconvex tablet, scored on one face and debossed with "HMR" on the other, contains: metformin hydrochloride 500 mg. Nonmedicinal ingredients: magnesium stearate and povidone; coating: hydroxylpropyl methylcellulose, polyethylene glycol and titanium dioxide. Bottles of 100 and 500.

850 mg: Each white, oblong tablet, debossed with "HMR" on one face and "850" on the other, contains: metformin hydrochloride 850 mg. Nonmedicinal ingredients: magnesium stearate and povidone. Bottles of 100.

(Shown in Product Identification Section)

Glumetza® ℞
metformin HCl
Oral Antihyperglycemic Agent

Biovail Pharmaceuticals

Date of Revision: September 9, 2009

SUMMARY PRODUCT INFORMATION:

Route of Administration	Dosage Form/ Strength	Nonmedicinal Ingredients
Oral	Extended-release Tablet 500 mg	Hypromellose, microcrystalline cellulose, magnesium stearate, polyethylene glycol, polysorbate, titanium dioxide, polyethylene oxide For complete information see Dosage Forms, Composition and Packaging.
	Extended-release Tablet 1000 mg	Colloidal silicon dioxide, crospovidone, glyceryl behenate, polyvinyl alcohol, polyacrylate dispersion, hypromellose, talc, polyethylene glycol, titanium dioxide, simethicone emulsion, polysorbate, shellac glaze, iron oxide black, macrogol, n-butyl alcohol, propylene glycol, FD&C blue #2, FD&C yellow #6 and FD&C red #40 For complete information see Dosage Forms, Composition and Packaging.

INDICATIONS AND CLINICAL USE: GLUMETZA (metformin hydrochloride) extended-release tablets are indicated for the control of hyperglycemia in adult patients with type 2 (non-insulin-dependent, mature onset) diabetes, as an adjunct to dietary management, exercise, and weight reduction, or when insulin therapy is not appropriate.

GLUMETZA may be used as monotherapy, or concomitantly with a sulfonylurea. GLUMETZA is a once-daily formulation, which must be taken with food to ensure optimum delivery of metformin to the systemic circulation. Clinical data demonstrates that administration of GLUMETZA in the fed state significantly increases the systemic delivery of metformin when compared to the fasted state. Metformin can be of value in the treatment of obese diabetic patients.

Geriatrics: Limited data from controlled pharmacokinetic studies of metformin hydrochloride in healthy elderly subjects suggest that total plasma clearance of meformin is decreased, the half-life is prolonged and C_{max} is increased, compared to healthy young subjects. From these data, it appears that the change in metformin pharmacokinetics with aging is primarily accounted for by a change in renal function. Metformin treatment should not be initiated in patients greater than 80 years of age, unless measurement of creatinine clearance demonstrates that renal function is not significantly reduced. In patients with advanced age, metformin should be carefully titrated to establish the minimum dose for adequate glycemic effect, because aging is associated with reduced renal function (see Warnings and Precautions).

Pediatrics: The safety and efficacy of GLUMETZA in pediatric patients has not been established and no dosage regimen can be recommended in these patients.

CONTRAINDICATIONS:

- Patients who are hypersensitive to this drug or to any ingredient in the formulation or component of the container. For a complete listing, see Dosage Forms, Composition and Packaging.
- Unstable and/or type 1 (insulin-dependent) diabetes mellitus.
- Acute or chronic metabolic acidosis, including diabetic ketoacidosis, with or without coma; history of ketoacidosis with or without coma. Diabetic ketoacidosis should be treated with insulin.
- In patients with a history of lactic acidosis, irrespective of precipitating factors.
- In the presence of renal impairment or when renal function is not known, and also in patients with serum creatinine levels above the upper limit of normal range. Renal disease or renal dysfunction (e.g., as suggested by serum creatinine levels ≥136 μmol/L (males), ≥124 μmol/L (females) or abnormal creatinine clearance) which may result from conditions such as cardiovascular collapse (shock), acute myocardial infarction, and septicemia (see Warnings and Precautions).
- In excessive alcohol intake, acute or chronic.
- In patients suffering from severe hepatic dysfunction. Since severe hepatic dysfunction has been associated with some cases of lactic acidosis, metformin hydrochloride should generally be avoided in patients with clinical or laboratory evidence of hepatic disease.
- Metformin should be temporarily discontinued in patients undergoing radiologic studies involving intravascular administration of iodinated contrast materials, because use of such products may result in acute alteration of renal function (see Warnings and Precautions).
- In cases of cardiovascular collapse and in disease states associated with hypoxemia such as cardiorespiratory insufficiency, which are often associated with hyperlactacidemia.
- During stressful conditions, such as severe infections, trauma or surgery and the recovery phase thereafter.
- In patients suffering from severe dehydration.
- During pregnancy.

WARNINGS AND PRECAUTIONS:

Serious Warnings and Precautions

- Lactic acidosis is a rare, but serious, metabolic complication that may occur during treatment with GLUMETZA (see Endocrine and Metabolism, Lactic Acidosis).
- Patients should be cautioned against excessive alcohol intake, either acute or chronic, when taking GLUMETZA, since alcohol intake potentiates the effect of metformin on lactate metabolism (see Endocrine and Metabolism, Lactic Acidosis).

General: Use of GLUMETZA must be considered as treatment in addition to proper dietary and exercise regimen, and not as a substitute for either. Care should be taken to ensure that GLUMETZA is not given when a contraindication exists. If during metformin therapy the patient develops acute intercurrent disease such as clinically significant hepatic dysfunction, cardiovascular collapse, congestive heart failure, acute myocardial infarction, or other conditions complicated by hypoxemia which may also cause prerenal azotemia, the drug should be discontinued.

Endocrine and Metabolism: Lactic Acidosis: Lactic Acidosis is a rare, but serious, metabolic complication that may occur during treatment with GLUMETZA. When it occurs, it is fatal in approximately 50% of cases. Lactic acidosis may also occur in association with a number of pathophysiologic conditions, including diabetes mellitus, and whenever there is significant tissue hypoperfusion and hypoxemia. Lactic Acidosis is characterized by elevated blood lactate levels, decreased blood pH, electrolyte disturbances with an increased anion gap, and an increased lactate/pyruvate ratio. When metformin has been implicated in lactic acidosis, metformin plasma levels >5 μg/mL have been generally found.

The reported incidence of lactic acidosis in patients receiving metformin hydrochloride is very low (0.03 cases/1000 patient years) with approximately half of those cases being fatal. Reported cases have occurred primarily in diabetic patients with significant renal insufficiency, including both intrinsic renal disease and renal hypoperfusion. Patients with congestive heart failure requiring pharmacologic management are at increased risk of lactic acidosis. In particular, treatment of the elderly should be accompanied by careful monitoring of renal function. The risk of lactic acidosis increases with the degree of renal dysfunction and the patient's age. The risk of lactic acidosis may therefore, be significantly decreased by regular monitoring of renal function in patients taking GLUMETZA, and by use of the minimum effective dose of GLUMETZA. In addition, GLUMETZA should be promptly withheld in the presence of any condition associated with hypoxemia, dehydration or sepsis. Because impaired hepatic function may significantly limit the ability to clear lactate, GLUMETZA should generally be avoided in patients with clinical or laboratory evidence of hepatic disease. Patients should be cautioned against excessive alcohol intake when taking GLUMETZA, since alcohol intake potentiates the effect of metformin hydrochloride on lactate metabolism. The onset of lactic acidosis often is subtle, and accompanied only by non-specific symptoms such as malaise, myalgias, respiratory distress, increasing somnolence and non-specific abdominal distress. Lactic acidosis is a medical emergency that must be treated in a hospital setting. In a patient with lactic acidosis who is taking GLUMETZA, the drug should be discontinued immediately. Because metformin hydrochloride is dialysable, prompt hemodialysis is recommended to correct the acidosis and remove the accumulated metformin.

Hepatic/Biliary/Pancreatic: Since impaired hepatic function has been associated with some cases of lactic acidosis, GLUMETZA should generally be avoided in patients with clinical or laboratory evidence of hepatic disease.

Peri-operative Considerations: Metformin therapy should be temporarily suspended for any surgical procedure (except minor procedures not associated with restricted intake of food and fluids). Metformin should be discontinued 2 days before surgical intervention and should not be restarted until the patient's oral intake has resumed and renal function has been evaluated as normal.

Renal: Metformin hydrochloride is excreted by the kidney, and the risk of metformin accumulation and lactic acidosis increases with the degree of impairment of renal function. Patients with serum creatinine levels above the upper limit of normal for their age should not receive metformin. In patients with advanced age, metformin should be carefully titrated to establish the minimum dose for adequate glycemic effect, because aging is associated with reduced renal function. In elderly patients, renal function should be monitored regularly and generally should not be titrated to the maximum dose. Before initiation of metformin therapy and at least annually thereafter, renal function should be assessed and verified as normal. In patients in whom development of renal dysfunction is anticipated, renal function should be assessed more frequently and GLUMETZA discontinued if evidence of renal impairment is present (see Boxed Warning on Lactic Acidosis).

Radiologic studies involving the use of iodinated contrast materials can lead to acute renal failure, and have been associated with lactic acidosis in patients receiving metformin. Metformin should be discontinued 2 days before radiologic studies and should not be restarted until the patient's oral intake has resumed and renal function has been evaluated as normal.

Sexual Function/Reproduction: There are no adequate and well-controlled studies in pregnant women. Reproduction studies have been conducted in rats at doses up to and including 900 mg/kg/day (approximately 33-fold and 26-fold higher than humans), and have revealed no evidence of harm to the fetus due to metformin. The NOAEL in rabbits was >90 mg/kg/day, however, there were no toxicokinetic studies performed in rabbits and a relative exposure could not be determined.

Carcinogenesis and Mutagenesis: A long-term carcinogenicity study was performed in rats (dosing duration of 104 weeks) at metformin doses up to and including 450 mg/kg/day for male rats and 1200 mg/kg/day for female rats. These doses are approximately two and five times the maximum recommended human daily dose of 2000 mg based on body surface area comparisons. No evidence of carcinogenicity with metformin was found in either male or female rats. There was however, an increased incidence of adenomas and diffuse hyperplasia in the parathyroids of treated males. A carcinogenicity study was also performed in Tg.AC transgenic mice (dosing duration of 26 weeks) at doses up to 2000 mg/kg/day applied dermally. No evidence of carcinogenicity was observed in male or female mice. There was no evidence of mutagenic potential of metformin in the following in vitro tests: Ames test (*S. typhimurium* and *E. coli*), and gene mutation test (mouse lymphoma cells). Results of the in vivo mouse micronucleus test were also negative. Fertility of male and female rats was unaffected by metformin when administered at doses as high as 900 mg/kg/day, which is approximately four times the recommended human daily dose based on body surface area comparisons.

Special Populations: Pregnant Women: Safety of metformin in pregnant women has not been established. There are no adequate and well-controlled studies in pregnant women. Recent information strongly suggests that abnormal blood glucose levels during pregnancy are associated with a higher incidence of congenital abnormalities. Most experts recommend that insulin be used during pregnancy to maintain blood glucose levels as close to normal as possible.

The GLUMETZA nonclinical toxicology program included a complete battery of reproductive toxicity studies (fertility and early embryonic development, embryofetal development, and pre- and postnatal development). The combined fertility and developmental toxicity study in rats, (0, 150, 450, or 900 mg/kg/day orally) showed no adverse effects on fertility or embryofetal development, although a decrease in male reproductive organ weights was observed at a dose of 900 mg/kg/day. An embryofetal development study in rabbits revealed no effects on gross external, soft tissue, or skeletal malformation or variations at dose up to 90 mg/kg/day. A perinatal/postnatal toxicity study in rats demonstrated few findings, except that there was an increased latency in the passive avoidance test for F1 males in the 300 and 600 mg/kg/day groups and a decrease in body weight and feed consumption for F1 females during the precohabitation period in the 300 and 600 mg/kg/day groups. Therefore, the viability and growth NOAEL for this study was 150 mg/kg/day. Mating performance of F1 rats and caesarean-sectioning and litter parameters were unaffected at the highest dose of 600 mg/kg/day.

Based on the results of these studies, it was concluded that metformin produced no biologically significant, reproductive toxicity effects.

Nursing Women: It is not known whether metformin hydrochloride is excreted in human milk, however, studies in lactating rats have shown that metformin is excreted into milk and reaches levels comparable to those in plasma. Caution should be exercised in nursing mothers, and a decision should be made whether to discontinue nursing, or to discontinue treatment with GLUMETZA, taking into account the importance of the drug to the mother.

Pediatrics (<18 years of age): The safety and efficacy in pediatric patients have not been established and no dosage regimen can presently be recommended in these patients.

Geriatrics (>80 years of age): Metformin treatment should not be initiated in patients greater than 80 years of age, unless measurement of creatinine clearance demonstrates that renal function is not significantly reduced. In patients with advanced age, metformin should be carefully titrated to establish the minimum dose for adequate glycemic effect, because aging is associated with reduced renal function.

Vitamin B_{12} Levels: Impairment of vitamin B_{12} and folic acid absorption has been reported in some patients treated with metformin. Therefore, measurements of serum vitamin B_{12} and folic acid are advisable in patients on long-term treatment with GLUMETZA.

Monitoring and Laboratory Tests: Periodic monitoring of fasting blood glucose and glycosylated hemoglobin levels may be useful in the long term management of patients with type 2 diabetes. During initial dose titration, fasting glucose can be used to determine the therapeutic dose response.

Initial and periodic monitoring of hematologic parameters (e.g. hemoglobin/hematocrit and red blood cell indices) and renal function (serum creatinine) should be performed, at least on an annual basis. While megaloblastic anemia has rarely been seen with metformin hydrochloride therapy, if this is suspected, vitamin B_{12} deficiency should be excluded.

Particular attention should be paid to short range and long range complications which are peculiar to diabetes. Periodic cardiovascular, ophthalmic, hematological, hepatic and renal assessments are advisable (see Warnings and Precautions).

Hypoglycemia: Hypoglycemia does not occur in patients receiving metformin hydrochloride alone under usual circumstances of use, but could occur when caloric intake is deficient, when strenuous exercise is not compensated by caloric supplementation, or during concomitant use with other glucose-lowering agents or alcohol. Elderly, debilitated or malnourished patients and those with adrenal or pituitary insufficiency are particularly susceptible to hypoglycemic effect. Hypoglycemia may be difficult to recognize in the elderly and in people who are taking beta-adrenergic blocking drugs.

Change in Clinical Status of Previously Controlled Type 2 Diabetes Patient: A diabetic patient previously well controlled on GLUMETZA who develops laboratory abnormalities or clinical illness (especially vague and poorly defined illness) should be evaluated promptly for evidence of ketoacidosis or lactic acidosis. Evaluation should include serum electrolytes and ketones, blood glucose, and if indicated, blood pH, lactate, pyruvate and metformin levels. If acidosis of either form occurs GLUMETZA must be stopped immediately and appropriate corrective measures initiated (see Warnings and Precautions).

ADVERSE REACTIONS: Adverse Drug Reaction Overview: Gastrointestinal symptoms (GI) (diarrhea, nausea, vomiting) are common reactions to metformin hydrochloride treatment. These symptoms are generally transient and resolve spontaneously during continued treatment.

Additionally, as GI symptoms during therapy initiation appear to be dose-related, they may be decreased by gradual dose escalation and by having patients take their medication with meals.

Clinical Trial Adverse Drug Reactions: Because clinical trials are conducted under very specific conditions the adverse reaction rates observed in the clinical trials may not reflect the rates observed in practice and should not be compared to the rates in the clinical trials of another drug. Adverse drug reaction information from clinical trials is useful for identifying drug-related adverse events and for approximating rates.

In clinical trials conducted in the U.S., over 1000 patients with type 2 diabetes mellitus have been treated with GLUMETZA 1500-2000 mg/day in active-controlled and placebo-controlled studies.

Gastrointestinal disorders were the most frequently occurring events in all trials. Table 1 shows the combined incidence of gastrointestinal adverse events occurring in one Phase 2 study and one Phase 3 study comparing GLUMETZA to immediate-release metformin, coupled with the open label extension of the Phase 3 study.

Table 1: GLUMETZA

Combined Gastrointestinal Adverse Events Occurring in at least 5% of Patients, in Three Clinical Trials[a]

System Organ Class/ Preferred Term	GLUMETZA 1500 mg QD N=176 (%)	GLUMETZA 2000 mg QD N=279 (%)	Metformin IR 1500 mg am/pm N=174 (%)
Patients with at least one AE	133 (75.6)	222 (79.6)	136 (78.2)
Gastrointestinal Disorders	85 (48.3)	134 (48.0)	73 (42.0)
Diarrhea NOS	32 (18.2)	63 (22.6)	30 (17.2)
Nausea	30 (17)	41 (14.7)	24 (13.8)
Dyspepsia	15 (8.5)	35 (12.5)	13 (7.5)
Vomiting NOS	14 (8.0)	15 (5.4)	6 (3.5)
Abdominal Distention	5 (2.8)	22 (7.9)	1 (0.6)
Constipation	8 (4.5)	14 (5)	5 (2.9)
Abdominal Pain	13 (7.4)	12 (4.3)	7 (4.0)

[a] Combined data is from one Phase 2 study and one Phase 3 study comparing GLUMETZA to immediate-release metformin, coupled with the open label extension of the Phase 3 study.

In the Phase 3 trial comparing the safety and efficacy of GLUMETZA to metformin immediate-release tablets, all four treatment regimens (GLUMETZA at 1500 mg QD, 1500 mg BID, 2000 mg QD and Metformin IR 1500 mg BID) had comparable safety profiles. Patients in the once-daily treatment groups did not report any higher occurrence of adverse events than the twice daily treatment groups. The occurrence of GI adverse events was comparable between all treatment groups. All GLUMETZA treatment groups reported fewer occurrences of diarrhea and nausea than did the immediate-release treatment group during the first week of the titration period (1000 mg dose).

In the placebo-controlled study, patients receiving background glyburide (SU; sulfonylurea) therapy were randomized to receive add-on treatment of either one of three different regimens of GLUMETZA or placebo. In total, 431 patients received GLUMETZA+SU and 144 patients placebo+SU. Adverse events reported in greater than 5% of patients treated with GLUMETZA, that were more common in the combined GLUMETZA+SU group, than in the placebo+SU group, are shown in Table 2.

In 0.7% of patients treated with GLUMETZA+SU, diarrhea was responsible for discontinuation of study medication compared to zero in the placebo+SU group.

Table 2: GLUMETZA

Treatment-Emergent Adverse Events Reported By >5%[a] of Patients for the Combined GLUMETZA Group Versus Placebo Group

Adverse Event (Medra Preferred Term)	GLUMETZA+SU (n=431)	Placebo+SU (n=144)
Hypoglycemia NOS	13.7%	4.9%
Diarrhea	12.5%	5.6%
Nausea	6.7%	4.2%

[a] AE's that were more common in the GLUMETZA-treated than in the placebo-treated patients.

In the same study, the following adverse events were reported by 1-5% of patients for the combined GLUMETZA group and these events occurred more commonly in the GLUMETZA-treated than in the placebo-treated patients:
Ear and Labyrinth Disorders: ear pain.
Gastrointestinal Disorders: vomiting NOS, dyspepsia, flatulence, abdominal pain upper, abdominal distension, abdominal pain NOS, toothache, loose stools.
General Disorders and Administration Site Conditions: asthenia, chest pain.
Immune System Disorders: seasonal allergy.
Infections and Infestations: gastroenteritis viral NOS, tooth abscess, tonsillitis, fungal infection NOS.
Injury, Poisoning and Procedural Complications: muscle strain.
Musculoskeletal and Connective Tissue Disorders: pain in limb, myalgia, muscle cramp.
Nervous System Disorders: dizziness, tremor, sinus headache, hypoaesthesia.
Respiratory, Thoracic and Mediastinal Disorders: nasal congestion.
Skin and Subcutaneous Tissue Disorders: contusion.
Vascular Disorders: hypertension NOS.
Uncommon Clinical Trial Adverse Drug Reactions (<1%): The following adverse drug reactions were reported with <1% incidence in patients in any GLUMETZA treatment group in the placebo-controlled trial:
Blood Disorders: thrombocytopenia, neutropenia.
Eye Disorders: vision blurred.
Gastrointestinal Disorders: flatulence, gastric NOS, gastrointestinal upset, loose stools, vomiting NOS.
General Disorders and Administration Site Conditions: adverse drug reaction NOS, asthenia, chest pain, fatigue, lethargy, oedema aggravated, oedema peripheral, rigors.
Infection and Infestations: gastroenteritis viral NOS.
Investigations: blood glucose decreased, liver function test abnormal NOS, muscle cramp, white blood cell count increased.
Metabolism and Nutrition Disorders: hyperglycemia NOS.
Nervous System Disorders: dizziness, migraine NOS, parasthesia, syncope, tremor.
Reproductive System and Breast Disorders: sexual dysfunction NOS.
Respiratory Disorders: rhinorrhea, sinus congestion.

DRUG INTERACTIONS: Overview: Certain drugs may potentiate the effect of metformin in the treatment of diabetes, particularly sulfonylureas, and the "glitazones" rosiglitazone and pioglitazone. This potentiating effect has expanded the number of combination drug therapies for type 2 diabetes, and improved HbA_{1c} control. The simultaneous administration of potentiating drugs must be carefully monitored to prevent hypoglycemic reaction, especially if they are given to patients also receiving other drugs which can potentiate their effect. For example the effect of sulfonylureas can be potentiated by long-acting sulfonamides, tuberculostatics, phenylbutazone, clofibrate, monoamine oxidase inhibitors, salicylates, probenecid and propranolol. Metformin also potentiates the effect of insulin.

GLUMETZA and Sulfonylurea: With concomitant GLUMETZA and sulfonylurea (SU) therapy, the desired control of blood glucose may be obtained by adjusting the dose of each drug. The influence of glyburide on GLUMETZA pharmacokinetics was assessed in a single-dose interaction study in healthy subjects. Co-administration of GLUMETZA and glyburide did not result in any changes in metformin pharmacokinetics, as AUC, C_{max}, and T_{max}, were unchanged. Changes in pharmacodynamics were not evaluated in this study (see Dosage and Administration, Concomitant GLUMETZA and Oral Sulfonylurea Therapy in Adult Patients). In a clinical trial of patients with type 2 diabetes and prior treatment with glyburide, GLUMETZA plus glyburide combined therapy yielded a significant decrease from baseline to endpoint in mean HbA_{1c}, relative to SU treatment alone. With concomitant GLUMETZA and sulfonylurea therapy, the risk of hypoglycemia associated with sulfonylurea therapy exists. Appropriate precautions should be taken. If patients have not satisfactorily responded to one to three months of concomitant therapy with the maximum dose of GLUMETZA and the maximum dose of an oral sulfonylurea, consider therapeutic alternatives including switching to insulin.

Metformin is negligibly bound to plasma proteins and is, therefore, less likely to interact with highly protein-bound drugs such as salicylates, sulfonamides, chloramphenicol, and probenecid, as compared to sulfonylureas, which are extensively bound to serum proteins.

In healthy volunteers, the pharmacokinetics of propranolol and ibuprofen were not affected by metformin when co-administered in single-dose interaction studies.

Drugs that have a tendency to produce hyperglycemia and may lead to a loss of blood sugar control include thiazide and other diuretics, corticosteroids, phenothiazines, thyroid products, estrogens, estrogen plus progestrogen, oral contraceptives, phenytoin, nicotinic acid, sympathomimetics, calcium channel blocking drugs and isoniazid. When such drugs are administered to patients receiving GLUMETZA, the patient should be closely observed to maintain adequate glycemic control.

Furosemide: A single dose metformin-furosemide drug interaction study in healthy subjects demonstrated that pharmacokinetic parameters of both compounds were affected by co-administration. Furosemide increased the metformin plasma and blood C_{max} by 22% and blood AUC by 15%, without any significant change in metformin renal clearance. When administered with metformin, the C_{max} and AUC of furosemide were 31% and 12% smaller, respectively, than when administered alone, and the terminal half-life was decreased by 32%, without any significant change in furosemide renal clearance. No information is available about the interaction of metformin when co-administered chronically.

Nifedipine: A single dose metformin-nifedipine drug interaction study in healthy subjects demonstrated that co-administration of nifedipine increased plasma metformin C_{max} and AUC by 20% and 9%, and increased the amount excreted in the urine. T_{max} and half-life were unaffected.

Cationic Drugs: (amiloride, cimetidine, digoxin, morphine, procainamide, quinidine, quinine, ranitidine, triamterene, trimethoprim, vancomycin.) These drugs theoretically have the potential for interaction with metformin by competing for common renal tubular transport systems. Such interaction has been observed between metformin and oral cimetidine in normal healthy volunteers in both single and multiple-dose, metformin-cimetidine drug interaction studies, with a 60% increase in peak metformin plasma and whole blood concentrations and a 40% increase in plasma and whole blood metformin AUC was observed. The H_2-blocker cimetidine competitively inhibits renal tubular secretion of metformin, significantly decreasing its clearance and increasing its bioavailability. There was no change in elimination half-life in the single-dose study. Metformin had no effect on cimetidine pharmacokinetics. Therefore, careful patient monitoring and dose adjustment of metformin or the interfering drug is recommended in patients who are taking cationic medications that are excreted via renal tubular secretion.

Anticoagulant Phenprocoumon: Elimination rate of the anticoagulant phenprocoumon has been reported to be increased by 20% when used concurrently with metformin. Patients receiving phenprocoumon or other antivitamin K anticoagulants should be monitored carefully when both types of drugs are used simultaneously. In such cases, an important increase of prothrombin time may occur upon cessation of metformin therapy, with an increased risk of hemorrhage.

Drug-Food Interactions: GLUMETZA extended-release tablets have been formulated to be dosed with food. GLUMETZA extended-release tablets must be taken with food to ensure complete release and absorption of the metformin dose. In a single-dose study with the 500 mg tablet, when the product was given to healthy volunteers while fasting or with a high fat, or a AHA 30% low fat meal, AUC was increased significantly and a delay in T_{max} was observed when compared to the fasted state. The increase in AUC was significantly greater when the product was given with the high fat meal. There was no significant difference in C_{max}. In an open label pharmacoscintigraphic pharmacokinetic study in healthy volunteers, GLUMETZA 500 mg dosed with different fat content meals was evaluated. Both the gastric retention time and the systemic exposure of metformin were higher following the high fat meal than following the AHA 30% fat meal, demonstrating that prolonged gastric retention enables extended delivery of metformin.

Drug-Herb Interactions: Interactions with herbal products have not been established.

Drug-Laboratory Interactions: Interactions with laboratory tests have not been established.

Drug-Lifestyle Interactions: Patients should be cautioned against excessive alcohol intake, either acute or chronic, when taking GLUMETZA, since alcohol intake potentiates the effect of metformin hydrochloride on lactate metabolism (see Contraindications).

DOSAGE AND ADMINISTRATION: Dosing Considerations: GLUMETZA extended-release tablets must be taken with food to ensure optimum delivery of the metformin dose to the systemic circulation. (See Drug Interactions, Drug-Food Interactions and Action and Clinical Pharmacology, Pharmacokinetics). In adult type 2 diabetic patients, individual determination of the minimum GLUMETZA dose that will adequately lower blood glucose should be made. There is no fixed metformin hydrochloride dosage regimen for the management of hyperglycemic patients.

In patients in whom the maximum recommended dose fails to lower the blood glucose adequately, the drug should be discontinued. In some diabetic subjects, short-term administration of the drug may be sufficient during periods of transient loss of blood sugar control.

Recommended Dose and Dosage Adjustment: GLUMETZA therapy should usually be initiated at 1000 mg once-daily, taken with the evening meal. GLUMETZA extended-release tablets must be taken with food to ensure optimum delivery of the metformin dose to the systemic circulation. Gradual dose escalation in increments of 500 mg weekly are recommended, to reduce gastrointestinal side effects, and to permit identification of the minimum dose required for adequate glycemic control.

The maximum recommended dose is 2000 mg once daily, taken with the evening meal. Tablets should be taken whole, with a glass of water. During treatment initiation and dose titration, fasting plasma glucose should be used to determine the therapeutic response to GLUMETZA, and to identify the minimum effective dose for the patients. Care should be taken in dose selection for the elderly, and should be based on careful and regular monitoring of renal function. Generally, elderly patients should not be titrated to the maximum dose of metformin.

Transfer Other Therapy: When transferring patients from standard oral hypoglycemic agents, other than chlorpropamide, to GLUMETZA, no transition period generally is necessary. Patients treated with immediate release metformin have been switched to GLUMETZA once daily without incident. Following switching, from the IR formulation to GLUMETZA, glycemic control should be closely monitored and dosage adjustments made accordingly. When transferring patients from chlorpropamide, care should be exercised during the first two weeks because of the prolonged retention of chlorpropamide in the body, leading to overlapping drug effects and possible hypoglycemia.

Concomitant GLUMETZA and Oral Sulfonylurea Therapy in Adult Patients: If patients have not responded to four weeks of the maximum dose of GLUMETZA monotherapy, consideration should be given to gradual addition of oral sulfonylurea while continuing GLUMETZA at the maximum dose, even if prior primary or secondary failure to a sulfonylurea has occurred. With concomitant metformin and sulfonylurea therapy, the desired control of blood glucose may be obtained by adjusting the dose of each drug. In a clinical trial of patients with type 2 diabetes and prior treatment with glyburide, 15 mg/day, the efficacy of GLUMETZA in combination with glyburide was compared to the efficacy of glyburide alone (placebo), to achieve glycemic control as measured by significant reductions from baseline in FPG, HbA_{1c}, fructosamine and blood glucose response. The minimum effective dose of each drug should be identified. With concomitant GLUMETZA and sulfonylurea therapy, there is risk of hypoglycemia. Appropriate precautions should be taken (see Package Insert of the respective sulfonylurea). If patients have not satisfactorily responded to one to three months of concomitant therapy with the maximum dose of GLUMETZA and the maximum dose of an oral sulfonylurea, consider therapeutic alternatives including switching to insulin.

Missed Dose: If a dose of GLUMETZA is missed, it should be taken as soon as possible, with food. However, if it is less than ten hours before the next dose, skip the missed dose and go back to the regular dosing schedule. Do not double doses. If patients do not feel well, or home glucose testing shows elevated levels, a physician should be contacted.

Administration: GLUMETZA extended-release tablets must be taken with food, and should be taken whole, with a glass of water.

Do not break or crush tablets.

OVERDOSAGE:
Overdose with GLUMETZA has not been reported. It would be expected that adverse reactions of a more intense character, including epigastric discomfort, nausea, and vomiting followed by diarrhea, drowsiness, weakness, dizziness, malaise and headache might be seen. Should those symptoms persist, the presence of lactic acidosis should be excluded. Immediate contact with a physician should be made, to determine if treatment should be stopped and proper supportive therapy instituted.

Overdose of metformin hydrochloride has been reported, including ingestion of amounts greater than 50 grams. Hypoglycemia was reported in approximately 10% of cases, but no causal association with metformin hydrochloride has been established. Lactic acidosis has been reported in approximately 32% of metformin overdose cases (see Warnings and Precautions). Metformin is dialyzable with clearance of up to 170 mL/min under good hemodynamic conditions. Therefore, hemodialysis may be useful for removal of accumulated drug from patients in whom metformin overdosage is suspected.

For management of a suspected drug overdose, contact your regional Poison Control Centre. See the *CPS* Directory section for a list of Poison Control Centres.

ACTION AND CLINICAL PHARMACOLOGY: Pharmacodynamics: Metformin hydrochloride is a biguanide anti-hyperglycemic agent, which is widely used for the treatment of type 2 diabetes mellitus (non-insulin-dependent diabetes mellitus [NIDDM]. Metformin improves glycemic control by enhancing insulin sensitivity in liver and muscle, and reducing gastrointestinal glucose absorption and hepatic glucose production. However it does not stimulate insulin secretion and, therefore, is not associated with hypoglycemia. Improved metabolic control with metformin does not induce weight gain and may cause weight loss. It has been demonstrated that the favorable effects of metformin also include improvements in factors associated with cardiovascular risk including lipids, fibrinolysis and body weight.

Mechanism of Action: Metformin is an antihyperglycemic agent, which improves glucose tolerance in patients with type 2 diabetes, lowering both basal and postprandial plasma glucose. Its pharmacologic mechanisms of action are different from other classes of oral antihyperglycemic agents. Metformin decreases hepatic glucose production, decreases intestinal absorption of glucose, and improves insulin sensitivity by increasing peripheral glucose uptake and utilization. Unlike sulfonylureas, metformin does not produce hypoglycemia in either patients with type 2 diabetes or normal subjects (except in special circumstances, see Warnings and Precautions) and does not cause hyperinsulinemia. With metformin therapy, insulin secretion remains unchanged while fasting insulin levels and daylong plasma insulin response may actually decrease.

At therapeutic doses, metformin does not lower plasma glucose levels in non-diabetic animals or humans. Oral administration of metformin was demonstrated to effectively lower plasma glucose levels in streptozocine-induced diabetic mice, genetically diabetic KK mice, obese female fa/fa rats, and alloxan-induced diabetic rats. In addition to its antihyperglycemic effects, metformin has been shown to have hypolipidemic effects and to significantly improve the progression and regression of atherosclerotic lesions. Metformin has also been shown to reduce blood pressure in spontaneously hypertensive rats, either through sympathoinhibitory effects, a direct effect on vascular smooth muscle responsiveness to norepinephrine, and/or attenuation of hyperinsulinemia.

The antihyperglycemic effect of metformin does not appear to be due to effects on plasma insulin or glucagon concentrations. While some studies have demonstrated that metformin produces an increase in insulin receptor binding or an increase in low-affinity receptor number, it is generally accepted that the antihyperglycemic effects of metformin are poorly correlated with insulin binding and its effects on receptor binding and number are not directly related to its metabolic and clinical effects. A direct effect of metformin on insulin secretion has been ruled out as a mechanism for the antihyperglycemic effects because metformin does not increase circulating levels of insulin nor has it been shown experimentally to stimulate insulin secretion. Although the precise mechanism of hypoglycemic action of metformin remains unclear, it likely interrupts mitochondrial oxidative processes in the liver and corrects abnormalities of intracellular calcium metabolism in insulin-sensitive tissues (liver, skeletal muscle, and adipocytes) and cardiovascular tissue.

Pharmacokinetics: GLUMETZA pharmacokinetics have been characterized after oral administration of single and multiple doses to adult healthy volunteers, in eleven separate studies.

Absorption: Following a single oral dose of GLUMETZA 1000 mg extended-release tablets once-daily after a meal, the time to reach maximum plasma metformin concentration (T_{max}) is approximately 7-8 hours. In both single and multiple dose studies in healthy subjects, once daily 1000 mg dosing provides equivalent systemic exposure, as measured by area-under-the-curve (AUC), of metformin relative to the immediate release given as 500 mg twice daily.

Once daily oral doses of GLUMETZA 500 mg to 2500 mg doses resulted in less than proportional increases in both AUC and C_{max}. The mean C_{max} values were 473±145, 868±223, 1171±297, and 1630±399 ng/mL for once daily doses of 500, 1000, 1500, and 2500 mg, respectively. For AUC, the mean values were 3501±796, 6705±1918, 9299±2833, and 14161±4432 ng·hr/mL for once daily doses of 500, 1000, 1500, and 2500 mg, respectively.

Low-fat and high-fat meals increased the systemic exposure (as measured by AUC) from GLUMETZA extended-release tablets by about 38% and 73%, respectively, relative to fasting. Both meals prolonged metformin T_{max} by approximately 3 hours, but C_{max} was not affected. In an open label pharmacoscintigraphic pharmacokinetic study in healthy volunteers, GLUMETZA 500 mg dosed with different fat content meals was evaluated. Both the gastric retention time and the systemic exposure of metformin were higher following the high fat meal than following the AHA 30% fat meal, demonstrating that extended gastric retention enables extended delivery of metformin. For transit times less than 7 hours as sometimes seen in AHA 30% fat meal administration, absorption of metformin may be decreased almost linearly with decreasing upper GI transit time.

Distribution: The apparent volume of distribution (V/F) of metformin, following single oral doses of 850 mg immediate-release metformin hydrochloride averaged 654±358 L. At doses of 500 to 1500 mg, metformin has an absolute oral bioavailability of 50% to 60%. The drug is not protein bound and therefore has a wide volume of distribution, with maximal accumulation in the small intestine wall. Metformin partitions into erythrocytes, most likely as a function of time. At usual clinical doses and dosing schedules of metformin, steady state plasma concentrations of metformin are reached within 24-48 hours and are generally <1 μg/mL.

Metabolism: Intravenous single-dose studies in normal subjects demonstrate that metformin is excreted unchanged in the urine and does not undergo hepatic metabolism (no metabolites have been identified in humans) nor biliary excretion. Renal clearance is approximately 3.5 times greater than creatinine clearance, which indicates that tubular secretion is the major route of metformin elimination. Following oral administration, approximately 90% of the absorbed drug is eliminated via the renal route within the first 24 hours, with a plasma elimination half-life of approximately 6.2 hours. In blood, the elimination half-life is approximately 17.6 hours, suggesting that the erythrocyte mass may be a compartment of distribution.

Excretion: Metformin undergoes no modifications in the body and is secreted unchanged by rapid kidney excretion (through glomerular filtration and, possibly, tubular secretion). Impaired kidney function slows elimination, and may cause metformin accumulation.

The apparent plasma elimination half-life of metformin following a single dose of GLUMETZA tablets is approximately 8 hours. Results from a dose proportionality study involving once daily oral doses of GLUMETZA 500 mg to 2500 mg, indicate a lack of dose proportionality with increasing doses, as both AUC and C_{max} increased nonlinearly within the investigated dose range. Concomitant administration with glyburide (Diaβeta) does not lead to a change in the peak and systemic exposures of metformin.

Special Populations and Conditions: Pediatrics: No pharmacokinetic studies of GLUMETZA in pediatric subjects were conducted.

Geriatrics: Limited data from controlled pharmacokinetic studies of metformin hydrochloride in healthy elderly subjects suggest that total plasma clearance of meformin is decreased, the half-life is prolonged and C_{max} is increased, compared to healthy young subjects. From these data, it appears that the change in metformin pharmacokinetics with aging is primarily accounted for by a change in renal function (see Warnings and Precautions, Special Populations).

Gender: In the pharmacokinetic studies in healthy volunteers, there were no important differences between male and female subjects with respect to metformin AUC (males=268, females=293) and $t_{½}$ (males=229, females=260). However, C_{max} for metformin were somewhat higher in female subjects (Female/Male C_{max} Ratio=1.4). The gender differences for C_{max} are unlikely to be clinically important.

Race: There were no definitive conclusions on the differences between the races with respect to the pharmacokinetics of GLUMETZA because of the imbalance in the respective sizes of the racial groups. However, the data suggest a trend towards higher metformin C_{max} and AUC values for metformin are obtained in Asian subjects when compared to Caucasian, Hispanic and Black subjects. The differences between the Asian and Caucasian groups are unlikely to be clinically important.

Hepatic Insufficiency: No pharmacokinetic studies of GLUMETZA have been conducted in patients with hepatic insufficiency.

Renal Insufficiency: In patients with decreased renal function (based on measured serum creatinine) the blood half-life of metformin is prolonged and the renal clearance is decreased in proportion to the decrease in creatinine clearance.

STORAGE AND STABILITY: GLUMETZA (metformin hydrochloride extended-release) tablets are to be stored at 15-30°C.

INFORMATION FOR THE PATIENT: Published in e-CPS, available by subscription at www.e-cps.ca.

DOSAGE FORMS, COMPOSITION AND PACKAGING: 500 mg: Each white, film-coated, oval-shaped extended-release tablet, debossed with "M 500" contains: metformin HCl 500 mg. Nonmedicinal ingredients: hypromellose, magnesium stearate, microcrystalline cellulose, polyethylene glycol, polyethylene oxide, polysorbate and titanium dioxide. Bottles of 100 and 500.

1000 mg: Each white, oval-shaped extended-release tablet, printed with "M 1000" contains: metformin HCl 1000 mg. Nonmedicinal ingredients: colloidal silicon dioxide, crospovidone, FD&C blue #2, FD&C red #40, FD&C yellow #6, glyceryl behenate, hypromellose, iron oxide black, macrogol, n-butyl alcohol, polyacrylate dispersion, polyethylene glycol, polysorbate, polyvinyl alcohol, propylene glycol, shellac glaze, simethicone emulsion, talc and titanium dioxide. Bottles of 90.

(Shown in Product Identification Section)

Glyburide Ⓟ

CPhA Monograph

see Sulfonylureas

Glycerin Suppositories

glycerin

Laxative

Rougier Pharma

INDICATIONS: Laxative for rapid relief of occasional constipation.

CONTRAINDICATIONS: Use of this medication is contraindicated in the presence of anal fissures, fistula, ulcerous hemorrhoids and proctitis.

WARNINGS: No data supplied by the manufacturer.

PRECAUTIONS: Overuse or extended use may cause dependence for bowel function. Do not use in presence of fever, nausea, vomiting or abdominal pain. Adults: Do not take for more than 1 week unless directed by a physician. Infant/Child: Do not take for more than 3 days unless directed by a physician.

ADVERSE EFFECTS: No data supplied by the manufacturer.

OVERDOSE:
No data supplied by the manufacturer.

> For management of a suspected drug overdose, CPhA recommends that you contact your **regional Poison Control Centre**. See the *CPS* Directory section for a list of Poison Control Centres.

DOSAGE: Adults: Insert 1 suppository (adult size) into the rectum for effective relief of constipation.
Infant/Child: Children 2 years of age and older: 1 suppository daily (infant/child size) into the rectum for effective relief of constipation. **Children under the age of 2 according to the advice of a physician.**

For rectal use only. Insert 1 suppository into the rectum and allow to remain for 15 to 30 minutes. One suppository usually releases enough glycerin in 20 minutes to produce an easy bowel movement and need not have melted entirely.

SUPPLIED: Adults: Each 2.65 g suppository contains: glycerin USP 90%. Nonmedicinal ingredients: purified water, sodium hydroxide and stearic acid. Boxes of 12, 24, 48 and 100.

Infant/Child: Each 1.8 g suppository contains: glycerin USP 90%. Nonmedicinal ingredients: purified water, sodium hydroxide and stearic acid. Boxes of 12.

Protect from heat. Store between 15-30°C.

Glycopyrrolate Injection USP

glycopyrrolate

Anticholinergic

Sandoz

SUPPLIED: Single Use Vials: Each mL contains: glycopyrrolate 0.2 mg, sodium chloride, hydrochloric acid and/or sodium hydroxide to adjust pH, and water for injection. Single use vials of 1 and 2 mL, boxes of 10. Discard unused portion. Store between 15 and 30°C.

Multidose Vials: Each mL contains: glycopyrrolate 0.2 mg, sodium chloride, benzyl alcohol 0.9% (as preservative), hydrochloric acid and/or sodium hydroxide to adjust pH, and water for injection. Multidose vials of 20 mL, boxes of 1. Store between 15 and 30°C.

Glyquin® XM

hydroquinone—octocrylene—oxybenzone—avobenzone

Depigmenting Agent—Moisturizer

Valeant

PHARMACOLOGY: Hyperpigmentation refers to the brown skin spots caused by an excess of the skin pigment melanin in certain areas. It can be hereditary as are freckles, caused by sun damage, occur with increasing age, or be related to pregnancy or the use of oral contraceptives. Hyperpigmentation usually develops gradually and increases with sun exposure. Skin lightening can be achieved by using a hydroquinone cream (such as Glyquin XM) on small dark areas of skin.

INDICATIONS: Glyquin XM helps fade or lighten skin discolouration due to excessive sun exposure, freckles, or skin discolouration that may occur in pregnancy or due to the use of oral contraceptives.

CONTRAINDICATIONS: Prior history of sensitivity or allergic reaction to this product or any of its ingredients. The safety of topical hydroquinone use during pregnancy or in children (12 years and under) has not been established.

WARNINGS: Caution: Hydroquinone is a skin bleaching agent which may produce unwanted cosmetic effects if not used as directed.

Do not use on broken or irritated skin.

Test for skin sensitivity before using Glyquin XM by applying a small amount to an unbroken patch of skin behind the ear or inner upper arm and check in 24 hours. Minor redness is not a contraindication, but where there is itching or blister formation or excessive inflammatory response further treatment is not advised. Discontinue use if severe irritation or rash occurs. Some users of this product may experience mild skin irritation. Medication should be discontinued if mild irritation persists. Do not use near eyes or mucous membranes: in case of accidental contact rinse thoroughly with water. If no bleaching or lightening effect is noted after 2 months of use, Glyquin XM should be discontinued. Glyquin XM is formulated for use as a skin bleaching agent and **should not be used for the prevention of sunburn.**

Sunscreen use is an essential aspect of hydroquinone therapy because even minimal sunlight increases pigmentation. The sunscreens in Glyquin XM provides the necessary sun protection during skin bleaching therapy. After clearing and during maintenance therapy, sun exposure should be avoided on bleached skin by application of a sunscreen or sunblock agent or protective clothing to prevent repigmentation.

Keep out of reach of children. In case of accidental ingestion, call a physician or a Poison Control Centre immediately.

PRECAUTIONS: See Warnings.

Lactation: It is not known whether topical hydroquinone is absorbed or excreted in human milk. Caution is advised when topical hydroquinone is used by a nursing mother.

ADVERSE EFFECTS: Occasional hypersensitivity (localized contact dermatitis) may occur in which case the medication should be discontinued and a physician notified immediately.

OVERDOSE:
Treatment should be limited to relatively small areas of the body at one time since some patients experience a transient skin reddening and a mild burning sensation which does not preclude treatment.

> For management of a suspected drug overdose, CPhA recommends that you contact your **regional Poison Control Centre**. See the *CPS* Directory section for a list of Poison Control Centres.

DOSAGE: Glyquin XM should be applied to the affected area and rubbed in well twice daily or as directed by a physician. Children: Do not use in children under 12 years of age except on the advice of a physician.

SUPPLIED: Each g of cream contains: hydroquinone USP 40 mg, octocrylene USP 80 mg, oxybenzone USP 40 mg and avobenzone USP 30 mg. Nonmedicinal ingredients: ascorbyl palmitate, benzalkonium chloride, disodium edetate, glycerol monostearate, glycolic acid (AHA), hyaluronic acid, lemon extract, methylparaben, poloxamer 407, poloxyl 4 lauryl ether, propyl gallate, propylene glycol, dl-tocopherol (vitamin E), triethanolamine and purified water. Jars of 28 g.

Gonal-f® Ⓟ

follitropin alpha (rDNA origin)

Gonadotropin

EMD Canada

Date of Revision: February 22, 2007

SUMMARY PRODUCT INFORMATION:

Route of Administration	Dosage Form/ Strength	Clinically Relevant Nonmedicinal Ingredients
Subcutaneous injection or Intramuscular injection	Lyophilized powder for reconstitution/ 37.5 IU (2.8 μg), 75 IU (5.5 μg), 150 IU (11 μg), 450 IU (33 μg) and 1050 IU (77 μg)	For a complete listing of the nonmedicinal ingredients see Dosage Forms, Composition and Packaging.

DESCRIPTION: GONAL-f (follitropin alpha for injection) is a gonadotropin preparation of recombinant DNA origin. The active ingredient, recombinant human Follicle Stimulating Hormone (r-hFSH), is a human glycoprotein hormone which consists of two non-covalently linked, non-identical protein components designated as the α- and β-subunits. The physicochemical, immunological, and biological activities of r-hFSH are similar to those of human menopausal urine-derived hFSH, but free of urinary protein and of any luteinizing hormone (LH) component.

INDICATIONS AND CLINICAL USE: GONAL-f (follitropin alpha for injection) is indicated for the stimulation of multiple follicular development in ovulatory patients undergoing Assisted Reproductive Technologies (ART) such as in vitro fertilization. To complete follicular maturation in the absence of an endogenous LH surge, human chorionic gonadotropin (hCG) is given.

GONAL-f is also indicated for the stimulation of follicular development in patients with hypothalamic-pituitary dysfunction who present either oligomenorrhoea or amenorrhoea (WHO Group II). To complete follicular maturation and effect ovulation, hCG is given.

Selection of Patients:

1. Before treatment with GONAL-f is instituted, a thorough gynaecologic and endocrinologic evaluation must be performed. This should include an assessment of pelvic anatomy.
2. Primary ovarian failure should be excluded by the determination of gonadotropin levels.
3. Appropriate evaluation should be performed to exclude pregnancy.
4. Patients in late reproductive life have a greater predisposition to endometrial carcinoma as well as a higher incidence of anovulatory disorders. A thorough diagnostic evaluation should always be performed in patients who demonstrate abnormal uterine bleeding or other signs of endometrial abnormalities before starting GONAL-f therapy.
5. Evaluation of the partner's fertility potential should be included in the initial evaluation.

CONTRAINDICATIONS: GONAL-f (follitropin alpha for injection) is contraindicated in women who exhibit:

1. High levels of FSH indicating primary ovarian failure.
2. Uncontrolled thyroid or adrenal dysfunction.
3. An organic intracranial lesion such as pituitary or hypothalamus tumours.

4. The presence of any cause of infertility other than anovulation, as stated in Indications and Clinical Use, unless the women are candidates for Assisted Reproductive Technologies.
5. Abnormal uterine bleeding of unknown aetiology (see Indications and Clinical Use, Selection of Patients).
6. Ovarian cyst or enlargement of undetermined origin (see Indications and Clinical Use, Selection of Patients).
7. Sex hormone dependent tumours of the reproductive organs and breasts.
8. Pregnancy/lactation.
9. Hypersensitivity to or history of previous allergic reaction to follitropin alpha, FSH or to any of the excipients of GONAL-f.

WARNINGS AND PRECAUTIONS: General: Careful attention should be given to diagnosis in candidates for GONAL-f (follitropin alpha for injection) therapy (see Indications and Clinical Use, Selection of Patients).

GONAL-f should only be used by physicians who are thoroughly familiar with infertility problems and their management. GONAL-f is a potent gonadotropic substance capable of causing mild to severe adverse reactions. Gonadotropin therapy requires a certain time commitment by physicians and supportive health professionals, and requires the availability of appropriate monitoring facilities (see Monitoring and Laboratory Tests). Safe and effective use of GONAL-f requires monitoring of ovarian response with ultrasound, alone or in combination with measurement of serum estradiol levels, on a regular basis.

Prior to therapy with GONAL-f, patients should be informed of the duration of treatment and monitoring of their condition that will be required. Possible adverse reactions (see Adverse Reactions) and the risk of multiple births should also be discussed.

Before starting treatment, the couple's infertility should be assessed as appropriate and putative contraindications for pregnancy evaluated. In particular, patients should be evaluated for hypothyroidism, adrenocortical deficiency, hyperprolactinemia and pituitary or hypothalamus tumours, and appropriate specific treatment given.

During training of the patient for self-administration, special attention should be given to specific instructions for the use of the multidose and/or monodose preparations.

Overstimulation of the Ovary During FSH Therapy: Ovarian Enlargement: Use of FSH therapy to stimulate follicular development may result in the recruitment of a number of follicles. This may result in mild to moderate uncomplicated ovarian enlargement which may be accompanied by abdominal distention and/or abdominal pain. This degree of enlargement has been reported to occur in approximately 20% of those treated with urofollitropin and hCG, and generally regresses without treatment within two or three weeks.

To minimize the hazard associated with the occasional abnormal ovarian enlargement which may occur with GONAL-f therapy, the lowest dose consistent with the expectation of good results should be used. Careful monitoring of ovarian response can further minimize the risk of ovarian enlargement.

If there is clinical evidence of excessive ovarian response (see Monitoring and Laboratory Tests), treatment should be discontinued and hCG should not be administered. This will reduce the chances of development of the Ovarian Hyperstimulation Syndrome (OHSS).

Ovarian Hyperstimulation Syndrome (OHSS): OHSS is a medical event distinct from uncomplicated ovarian enlargement. OHSS may progress rapidly (within 24 hours to several days) to become a serious medical event. It is characterized by an apparent dramatic increase in vascular permeability which can result in an accumulation of fluid in the peritoneal, pleural and, rarely, in the pericardial cavities. The early warning signs of development of OHSS are severe pelvic pain, nausea, vomiting, and weight gain. The following symptomatology has been seen with cases of OHSS: abdominal pain, abdominal distention, severe ovarian enlargement, weight gain, dyspnea, oliguria and gastrointestinal symptoms including nausea, vomiting and diarrhoea. Clinical evaluation may reveal hypovolemia, hemoconcentration, electrolyte imbalances, ascites, hemoperitoneum, pleural effusions, hydrothorax, acute pulmonary distress, and thromboembolic events (see Cardiovascular and Respiratory). Transient liver function test abnormalities suggestive of hepatic dysfunction, which may be accompanied by morphologic changes on liver biopsy, have been reported in association with the OHSS.

Severe OHSS occurred in approximately 6.0% of patients treated with urofollitropin therapy in the initial clinical trials, in patients treated for anovulation due to polycystic ovarian syndrome. In these studies, prospective monitoring of ovarian response using serum estradiol determination or ultrasonographic visualizations was not routinely employed.

In the clinical trials in oligo-anovulatory infertile women treated with GONAL-f in which both estradiol and ultrasound measurements were utilized to monitor follicular development, the incidence of severe OHSS was 1 in 513 treatment cycles (0.2%).

In the clinical trials in ovulatory infertile women treated with GONAL-f for induction of multiple follicular induction for IVF/ET in which both estradiol and ultrasound measurements were utilized to monitor follicular development, there was no incident of severe OHSS.

To minimize the risk of OHSS or of multiple pregnancy, ultrasound scans, as well as serum oestradiol measurements are recommended.

When risk of OHSS or multiple pregnancies is assumed, treatment discontinuation should be considered.

OHSS may be more severe and more protracted if pregnancy occurs. OHSS develops rapidly; therefore, patients should be followed for at least two weeks after hCG administration. Most often, OHSS occurs after treatment has been discontinued and reaches its maximum at about seven to ten days following treatment. Usually, OHSS resolves spontaneously with the onset of menses. If there is evidence that OHSS may be developing prior to hCG administration (see Monitoring and Laboratory Tests), the hCG should not be administered.

If severe OHSS occurs, treatment should be stopped and the patient should be hospitalized. A physician experienced in the management of this syndrome, or who is experienced in the management of fluid and electrolyte imbalances should be consulted.

Carcinogenesis and Mutagenesis: Long-term studies in animals have not been performed to evaluate the carcinogenic potential of GONAL-f. However, r-hFSH showed no mutagenic activity in a series of tests performed to evaluate its potential genetic toxicity including, bacterial and mammalian cell mutation tests, a chromosome aberration test and a micronucleus test.

There have been reports of ovarian and other reproductive system neoplasms, both benign and malignant, in women who have undergone multiple drug regimens for infertility treatment. The causality of these neoplasms has not been established. Although, to date, the results of recent epidemiological studies do not suggest a causal relationship between the use of gonadotropins in ART and the occurrence of neoplasms, long term follow-up studies are still ongoing.

Cardiovascular and Respiratory: The following paragraph describes serious medical events reported following gonadotropin therapy. Serious pulmonary conditions (e.g., atelectasis, acute respiratory distress syndrome and exacerbation of asthma) have been reported. In addition, thromboembolic events both in association with, and separate from Ovarian Hyperstimulation Syndrome have been reported. Intravascular thrombosis and embolism can result in reduced blood flow to critical organs or the extremities. Sequelae of such events have included venous thrombophlebitis, pulmonary embolism, pulmonary infarction, cerebral vascular occlusion (stroke), and arterial occlusion resulting in loss of limb. In rare cases, pulmonary complications and/or thromboembolic events have resulted in death.

In women with generally recognized risk factors for thrombo-embolic events, such as personal or family history, treatment with gonadotropins may further increase the risk. In these women, the benefits of gonadotropin administration need to be weighed against the risks. It should be noted however, that pregnancy itself also carries an increased risk of thrombo-embolic events.

Dependence/Tolerance: There have been no reports of abuse or dependence with GONAL-f.

Sexual Function/Reproduction: In patients undergoing ovarian stimulation, the incidence of multiple pregnancies is increased as compared with natural conception. Reports of multiple births have been associated with GONAL-f treatment. The risk of multiple births in patients undergoing ART procedures is related to the number of embryos replaced. In other patients, the incidence of multiple births may be increased by GONAL-f, as has been observed with other gonadotropin preparations. The patient and her partner should be advised of the potential risk of multiple births before starting treatment.

Since women with infertility undergoing assisted reproduction, and particularly IVF, often have tubal abnormalities, the incidence of ectopic pregnancies might be increased. The prevalence of ectopic pregnancies after IVF was reported to be 2 to 5%, as compared to 1 to 1.5% in the general population. Early ultrasound confirmation that a pregnancy is intrauterine is therefore important.

The incidence of pregnancy wastage by miscarriage or abortion may be higher in patients undergoing stimulation of follicular growth for ovulation induction or ART than in the normal population.

The prevalence of congenital malformations after ART may be slightly higher than after spontaneous conception. This is thought to be due to differences in parental characteristics (e.g. maternal age, sperm characteristics) and multiple pregnancies.

Impaired fertility has been reported in rats exposed to pharmacological doses of r-hFSH (40 IU/kg/day) for extended periods through reduced fecundity.

Special Populations: Pregnant Women: There are no adequate and well-controlled studies in pregnant women. Given in high doses (>5 IU/kg/day) GONAL-f caused an increase in deaths, fetal effects and dystocia in pregnant rats and rabbits, but without being a teratogen. However, since GONAL-f is not indicated in pregnancy, these data are of limited clinical relevance. To date, no particular malformative effect has been reported. No teratogenic effect has been observed in animal studies.

Nursing Women: It is not known whether this drug is excreted in human milk, although animal studies have shown that r-hFSH is excreted in milk. Therefore, GONAL-f is contraindicated in lactating mothers. During lactation, the secretion of prolactin can entail a poor response to ovarian stimulation.

Pediatrics: Not indicated for treatment in pediatric population.

Geriatrics: Not indicated for treatment in the geriatric population.

Monitoring and Laboratory Tests: In most instances, treatment with GONAL-f results only in follicular recruitment and development. In the absence of an endogenous LH surge, hCG is given when monitoring of the patient indicates that sufficient follicular development has occurred. This may be estimated by ultrasound alone or in combination with measurement of serum estradiol levels. The combination of both ultrasound and serum estradiol measurement are useful for monitoring the development of follicles, for timing of the ovulatory trigger, as well as for detecting ovarian enlargement and minimizing the risk of the Ovarian Hyperstimulation Syndrome and multiple gestation. It is recommended that the number of growing follicles be confirmed using ultrasonography because plasma estrogens do not give an indication of the size or number of follicles.

The clinical confirmation of ovulation, with the exception of pregnancy, is obtained by direct and indirect indices of progesterone production. The indices most generally used are as follows: a rise in basal body temperature, increase in serum progesterone, and menstruation following a shift in basal body temperature.

When used in conjunction with the indices of progesterone production, sonographic visualization of the ovaries will assist in determining if ovulation has occurred. Sonographic evidence of ovulation may include the following: fluid in the cul-de-sac, ovarian stigmata, collapsed follicle, and secretory endometrium.

Accurate interpretation of the indices of follicle development and maturation require a physician who is experienced in the interpretation of these tests.

For patients undergoing extended cycles of treatment, PTT and liver enzymes should be monitored.

Occupational Hazards: No studies on the effects on the ability to drive and use machines have been performed.

ADVERSE REACTIONS: Adverse Drug Reaction Overview: Safety data on GONAL-f (follitropin alpha for injection) stem from clinical studies, as well as 10 years of post-marketing surveillance.

The most commonly reported adverse reactions with GONAL-f in clinical studies were ovarian cysts, injection site reaction of any severity, headache, mild to moderate OHSS manifesting with symptoms such as abdominal swelling and pain, ovarian enlargement, as well as gastrointestinal symptoms such as nausea, vomiting, and diarrhoea.

The most frequently reported adverse reactions resulting in clinical intervention (e.g., discontinuation of GONAL-f, adjustment in dosage, or the need for concomitant medication to treat an adverse reaction symptom) was severe OHSS and its associated complications, such as adnexal torsion, thromboembolic events, haemoperitoneum and acute pulmonary distress (see Warnings and Precautions).

Severe OHSS was also the most frequently reported serious adverse reaction (see Warnings and Precautions). Complications of severe OHSS have been reported both in clinical studies and from spontaneous sources.

Clinical Trial Adverse Drug Reactions: Because clinical trials are conducted under very specific conditions the adverse reaction rates observed in the clinical trials may not reflect the rates observed in practice and should not be compared to the rates in the clinical trials of another drug. Adverse drug reaction information from clinical trials is useful for identifying drug-related adverse events and for approximating rates.

Summary of Adverse Drug Reactions Reported During Clinical Trials and in Post-Market Experience: More than 1000 patients were exposed to r-hFSH during the clinical development programme of GONAL-f. In addition to the clinical trial patient population, it is estimated that 580 000 to 1 700 000 patients have been exposed to r-hFSH during the post-marketing phase. The following summary presents the adverse drug reactions that have been reported with the use of r-hFSH during clinical trials and during post-market use. These data provide a comprehensive description of the safety profile of GONAL-f.

≥1% (Common and Very Common): Reproductive Disorders, Female: ovarian cysts, mild to moderate ovarian enlargement, breast tenderness, mild to moderate OHSS.

Application Site Disorders: mild to severe injection site reaction (e.g. pain, redness, bruising, swelling and/or irritation at the site of injection).

Body as a Whole, General Disorders: headache.

Gastrointestinal System Disorders: abdominal pain, nausea, vomiting, diarrhea, abdominal cramps, bloating.

<1% (Uncommon, Rare and Very Rare): Reproductive Disorders, Female: severe OHSS, complications of severe OHSS (adnexal torsion, hemoperitoneum).

Vascular (Extracardiac) Disorders: thromboembolism.

Respiratory System Disorders: acute pulmonary distress.

Body as a Whole, General Disorders: mild systemic allergic reactions (e.g. erythema, rash or facial swelling), anaphylactic-like reactions, which can manifest by one or more of the following signs/symptoms: urticaria, diffuse edema and erythema, facial swelling, difficulty in breathing.

The common and very common ADRs have been reported from clinical studies, as well as in post-marketing surveillance. Severe OHSS has been reported from clinical studies, as well as in post-marketing surveillance. However, the rare and very rare ADRs, such as complications of severe OHSS and allergic reactions, have generally been reported from post-marketing sources.

The following adverse reactions reported during gonadotropin therapy are listed in decreasing order of potential severity: pulmonary and vascular complications (see Warnings and Precautions); ovarian hyperstimulation syndrome (see Warnings and Precautions); adnexal torsion (as a complication of ovarian enlargement); hemoperitoneum; mild to moderate ovarian enlargement; abdominal pain; ovarian cysts; gastrointestinal symptoms (nausea, vomiting, diarrhea, abdominal cramps, bloating); pain, rash, swelling, and/or irritation at the site of injection; breast tenderness; headache; dermatological symptoms (dry skin, body rash, hair loss, hives).

The following medical events have been reported subsequent to pregnancies resulting from GONAL-f therapy in controlled clinical trials: spontaneous abortion, ectopic pregnancy, premature labour, postpartum fever; congenital abnormalities.

Two incidents of congenital cardiac malformations have been reported in children born following pregnancies resulting from treatment with GONAL-f and hCG in clinical studies. In addition, a pregnancy occurring in a study following treatment with GONAL- f and hCG was characterized by apparent failure of intrauterine growth and terminated for a suspected syndrome of congenital abnormalities. No specific diagnosis was made.

Three incidents of chromosomal abnormalities and four birth defects have been reported following urofollitropin-hCG or urofollitropin, Pergonal (menotropins for injection, USP)-hCG therapy in clinical trials for stimulation prior to in vitro fertilization. The aborted pregnancies included one Trisomy 13, one Trisomy 18, and one fetus with multiple congenital anomalies (hydrocephaly, omphalocele, and meningocele). One meningocele, one external ear defect, one dislocated hip and ankle, and one dilated cardiomyopathy in presence of maternal Systemic Lupus Erythematosus were reported. None of these events were thought to be drug-related. The incidence does not exceed that found in the general population.

There have been infrequent reports of ovarian neoplasms, both benign and malignant, in women who have undergone multiple drug regimens for ovulation induction; however, a causal relationship has not been established.

GONAL-f multi-dose was examined in twenty-five healthy volunteers who received 300 IU (22 µg) each of GONAL-f from single-dose ampoules and multi-dose vials. Overall, both presentations were well tolerated and local tolerability between the two groups was comparable.

Injection site inspections revealed very rare local reactions (mild redness in one patient after single-dose injection and mild bruising in two subjects after multi-dose injection). Subjective assessments indicated minimal or mild transient pain in two and five subjects who received GONAL-f single-dose and GONAL-f Multi-Dose, respectively.

DRUG INTERACTIONS: Clomiphene citrate, LH and hCG used with GONAL-f may enhance follicular response, and caution is indicated when using these drugs together.

Use of GnRH agonist or antagonist to induce pituitary desensitisation may alter the dosage of GONAL-f needed.

No other clinically significant drug/drug or drug/food interactions have been reported during GONAL-f therapy.

DOSAGE AND ADMINISTRATION: Dosing Considerations: Treatment with GONAL-f (follitropin alpha for injection) should be initiated under the supervision of a physician experienced in the treatment of fertility problems.

Recommended Dose and Dosage Adjustment: The dose of GONAL-f to stimulate development of the follicle must be individualized for each patient and the particular indication. To minimize the hazard associated with the occasional abnormal ovarian enlargement which may occur with GONAL-f therapy, the lowest dose consistent with the expectation of good results should be used. GONAL-f should be administered subcutaneously or intramuscularly until adequate follicular development is indicated by ultrasound alone or in combination with measurement of serum estradiol levels.

The dosage recommendations given for GONAL-f are those in use for urinary FSH. Clinical assessment of GONAL-f indicates that its daily doses, regimens of administration, and treatment monitoring procedures should not be different from those currently used for urinary FSH-containing preparations. However, when these doses were used in a clinical study comparing GONAL-f and urinary FSH, GONAL-f was more effective than urinary FSH in terms of a lower total dose and a shorter treatment period needed to achieve pre-ovulatory conditions.

Over the course of treatment, doses may range between 75 to 450 IU (5.5 to 33 µg) depending on the indication and the individual patient response. To complete follicular development and effect ovulation in the absence of an endogenous LH surge, hCG is given when monitoring of the patient indicates that sufficient follicular development has occurred. If the ovaries are abnormally enlarged or significant abdominal pain occurs, GONAL-f treatment should be discontinued, hCG should not be administered, and the patient should be advised to refrain from intercourse until resolution of the cycle; this will reduce the chances of development of the Ovarian Hyperstimulation Syndrome and, should spontaneous ovulation occur, reduce the chances of multiple gestation. While individual dosing regimens will differ between patients, typical treatment regimens are presented below.

Assisted Reproductive Technologies: In patients undergoing Assisted Reproductive Technologies (ART) whose endogenous gonadotropin levels are not suppressed, GONAL-f should be initiated in the early follicular phase (cycle day 2 or 3) at a dose of 150 IU (11 µg) per day, administered subcutaneously or intramuscularly. Treatment should be continued until adequate follicular development is indicated as determined by either ultrasound alone or in combination with measurement of serum estradiol levels. Adjustments to dose, based on the patient's response, should only be considered after the first five days of treatment; subsequently dosage should be adjusted no more frequently than every 3-5 days and by no more than 37.5-150 IU (2.8-11 µg) additionally at each adjustment. Treatment should be continued until adequate follicular development is indicated. Once adequate follicular development is evident, hCG (5000 to 10 000 USP units) should be administered to induce final follicular maturation in preparation for oocyte retrieval.

In patients undergoing ART, whose endogenous gonadotropin levels are suppressed indicating a hypogonadotropic state, GONAL-f should be initiated at a dose of 225 IU (16.5 µg) per day, administered subcutaneously or intramuscularly. Treatment should be continued until adequate follicular development is indicated as determined by either ultrasound alone or in combination with measurement of serum estradiol levels. Adjustments to dose may be considered after five days based on the patient's response; subsequently dosage should be adjusted no more frequently than every 3-5 days and by no more than 37.5-150 IU (2.8-11 µg) additionally at each adjustment. Doses greater than 450 IU (33 µg) per day are not generally recommended. As before, once adequate follicular development is evident, hCG (5000 to 10 000 USP units) should be administered to induce final follicular maturation in preparation for oocyte retrieval.

Ovulation Induction: The majority of patients who require ovulation induction are patients with Polycystic Ovarian Syndrome (PCO). Patients with PCO tend to show a more rapid and exaggerated response to treatment. Therefore, in this patient population, particular care should be employed to ensure that patients are adequately monitored and that the lowest dose consistent with the expectation of good results is employed.

It is recommended that treatment of any patient be initiated at a dose of 75 IU (5.5 µg) GONAL-f per day, administered subcutaneously or intramuscularly. An incremental adjustment in dose of up to 37.5 IU (2.8 µg) may be considered after 14 days. Further dose increases of the same magnitude could be made, if necessary, every seven days. Treatment duration should not exceed 35 days unless an estradiol rise indicates imminent follicular development. Once adequate follicular development is evident, hCG (5000 to 10 000 USP units) should be administered to induce final follicular maturation and effect ovulation. The patient should attempt to have intercourse at a consistent frequency of at least three times/week from the day prior to administration of hCG until ovulation becomes apparent.

If there is evidence of ovulation but pregnancy does not ensue, this regimen should be repeated for at least two more courses before increasing the dose of GONAL-f to 150 IU (11 µg) per day for 7 to 12 days. As before, this dose should be followed by the administration of hCG (5000 to 10 000 USP units) when adequate follicular development is evident. If evidence of ovulation is present but pregnancy does not ensue, repeat the same dose for two more courses. Doses larger than this are not routinely recommended.

Missed Dose: For patients who miss a dose, it is not recommended to double the next dose. The patient should be reminded to contact the physician monitoring their treatment.

Administration: GONAL-f is intended for subcutaneous or intramuscular administration.

GONAL-f Single Dose: GONAL-f [37.5 IU (2.8 µg), 75 IU (5.5 µg), 150 IU (11 µg)] should be administered subcutaneously or intramuscularly immediately after reconstitution with Sterile Water for Injection, Ph.Eur./USP. One or more vials of GONAL-f may be dissolved in 0.5-1 mL of Sterile Water for Injection, Ph.Eur./USP (concentration should not exceed 225 IU (16.5 µg)/0.5 mL). Any unused reconstituted material should be discarded.

Parenteral drug products should be inspected visually for particulate matter and discoloration prior to administration, whenever solution and container permit.

GONAL-f Multi-Dose: If prescribed GONAL-f 450 IU (33 µg) or 1050 IU (77 µg) Multi-Dose preparations, the injection can be administered subcutaneously and/or intramuscularly after reconstitution of the vial with the solvent in the pre-filled syringe. Patients should be instructed to use the accompanying syringes, calibrated in FSH units, for injection of the reconstituted GONAL-f 450 IU (33 µg) or 1050 IU (77 µg) Multi-Dose.

The 27-gauge injection syringe has unit dose markings from 37.5-600 IU FSH (2.8- 44 µg) for use with GONAL-f 450 IU (33 µg) or 1050 IU (77 µg) Multi-Dose.

Patients should be instructed to take a specific dose of GONAL-f 450 IU (33 µg) or 1050 IU (77 µg) Multi-Dose. The doctor, nurse, or pharmacist should show the patient how to locate the syringe marking that corresponds to the prescribed dose.

The 450 IU (33 µg) and 1050 IU (77 µg) reconstituted solutions can be kept for 28 days, when stored at room temperature (at or below 25°C).

OVERDOSAGE:

Aside from possible ovarian hyperstimulation and multiple gestations (see Warnings and Precautions), little is known concerning the consequences of acute overdosage with GONAL-f (follitropin alpha for injection). Apart from expected ovarian and endometrial effects, no acute toxicity was seen in animals given doses of r-hFSH up to 1000-fold the human dose.

For management of a suspected drug overdose, CPhA recommends that you contact your **regional Poison Control Centre**. See the *CPS* Directory section for a list of Poison Control Centres.

ACTION AND CLINICAL PHARMACOLOGY: Mechanism of Action: GONAL-f (follitropin alpha for injection) stimulates ovarian follicular growth in women who do not have primary ovarian failure. FSH is the primary hormone responsible for follicular recruitment and development. To complete follicular maturation and effect ovulation in the absence of an endogenous LH surge, hCG is given when monitoring of the patient indicates that sufficient follicular development has occurred. There may be a degree of interpatient variability in response to FSH administration, with lack of response to FSH in some patients.

Pharmacodynamics: One main pharmacodynamics study has been performed in healthy female volunteers down-regulated with a GnRH agonist (Study 5117). The aim of this study was to assess pharmacodynamic characteristics of r-hFSH administered subcutaneously daily for one week. After subcutaneous administration over one week, the first pharmacodynamic marker of ovarian response to FSH was serum inhibin, followed by plasma E2 and follicular growth. When FSH administration was stopped, inhibin levels dropped, while E2 continued to rise for one day and follicle size further increased during four days.

Two thirds of the volunteers developed significant follicular growth followed by corresponding decreasing levels of inhibin and increasing levels of E2 secretion. Moreover, no correlation was found between maximal serum FSH concentrations during administration and the maximal E2 responses, inhibin responses and follicular growth responses.

Pharmacokinetics: Single dose pharmacokinetics of r-hFSH were determined following intravenous administration of 150 IU and 300 IU of GONAL-f to 12 healthy, down-regulated female volunteers (Study 5007). Single dose pharmacokinetics of r-hFSH were also determined following intravenous, subcutaneous and intramuscular administration of 150 IU GONAL-f to 12 healthy, down-regulated female volunteers. Steady-state pharmacokinetics were also determined in the same 12 healthy down-regulated female volunteers who were administered a single daily dose of 150 IU for seven days (Study 5117). The pharmacokinetic parameters from these studies are included in Table 1 and Table 2.

Table 1: GONAL-f

Summary of r-hFSH Pharmacokinetic Parameters in Healthy Female Volunteers (Study 5007)

	C_{max} (IU/L)	$t_{½}$ (h)	$AUC_{0-\infty}$ (IU·h/L)	Clearance (L/h)	Volume of distribution V_{ss} (L)
Single dose IV (150 IU)	32±10	14±7	274±71	0.6±0.2	10±6
Single dose IV (300 IU)	59±18	17±3	598±126	0.6±0.1	11±6

Following intravenous administration, GONAL-f is distributed to the extracellular fluid space with an initial half-life of approximately 2 hours and eliminated from the body with a terminal half-life of approximately 1 day. The steady-state volume of distribution and total clearance are 10 L and 0.6 L/h, respectively. One-eighth of the GONAL-f dose is excreted in the urine.

Following subcutaneous or intramuscular administration, the absolute bioavailability is 70%. Following repeated administration, GONAL-f accumulates 3-fold at steady-state within 3-4 days. In women whose endogenous gonadotropin secretion is suppressed, GONAL-f has been shown to effectively stimulate follicular development and steroidogenesis, despite unmeasurable LH levels.

Special Populations and Conditions: No studies have been conducted with special populations and conditions.

Table 2: GONAL-f

Summary of r-hFSH Pharmacokinetic Parameters in Healthy Female Volunteers (Study 5117)

	C_{max} (IU/L)	$t_{½}$ (h)	AUC (IU·h/L)	Clearance (L/h)	Volume of distribution V_{ss} (L)
Single dose IV (150 IU)	33±9	15±5	286±78	0.6±0.2	9±3
Single dose IM (150 IU)	3±1	50±27	206±66	—	—
Single dose SC (150 IU)	3±1	24±11	176±87		
Multiple dose SC (7×150 IU)	4±1[b] 9±3[c]	24±8	187±61[a]		

[a] Steady-state $AUC_{144-168}$ (after the 7th daily SC dose).
[b] After the first dose.
[c] After the last dose.

STORAGE AND STABILITY: Vials of GONAL-f lyophilized powder for reconstitution are stable when stored at or below room temperature (25°C) and protected from light.

Do not freeze.

Do not use the product after the expiry date indicated on the label.

SPECIAL HANDLING INSTRUCTIONS: The GONAL-f (follitropin alpha for injection) solution should not be administered if it contains particles or is not clear.

Any unused product or waste material should be disposed of in accordance with local requirements.

INFORMATION FOR THE PATIENT: Published in e-CPS, available by subscription at www.e-cps.ca.

DOSAGE FORMS, COMPOSITION AND PACKAGING: 37.5 IU (2.8 µg): Each single dose vial of sterile, lyophilized powder, intended for s.c. or i.m. injection after reconstitution, contains: FSH activity 37.5 IU. Diluent provided for reconstitution is Sterile Water for Injection PhEur/USP. Nonmedicinal ingredients: disodium phosphate dehydrate, methionine, polysorbate 20, sodium dihydrogen phosphate monohydrate and sucrose. O-phosphoric acid and/or sodium hydroxide may be used for pH adjustment prior to lyophilization. Single dose vials of 3 mL (nominal capacity). Packages of 1 vial accompanied by 1 glass vial (2 mL) of Sterile Water for Injection USP or 1 mL pre-filled syringe WFI, Ph.Eur., 1×27-gauge injection needle and 1 mixing needle.

75 IU (5.5 µg): Each single dose vial of sterile, lyophilized powder, intended for s.c. or i.m. injection after reconstitution, contains: FSH activity 75 IU. Diluent provided for reconstitution is Sterile Water for Injection USP. Nonmedicinal ingredients: disodium phosphate dehydrate, methionine, polysorbate 20, sodium dihydrogen phosphate monohydrate and sucrose. O-phosphoric acid and/or sodium hydroxide may be used for pH adjustment prior to lyophilization. Single dose vials of 3 mL (nominal capacity). Packages of 1 vial accompanied by 1 glass vial (2 mL) Sterile Water for Injection USP or 1 mL pre-filled syringe WFI, Ph.Eur., 1×27-gauge injection needle and 1 mixing needle.

150 IU (11 µg): Each single dose vial of sterile, lyophilized powder, intended for s.c. or i.m. injection after reconstitution, contains: FSH activity 150 IU. Diluent provided for reconstitution is Sterile Water for Injection USP. Nonmedicinal ingredients: disodium phosphate dehydrate, methionine, polysorbate 20, sodium dihydrogen phosphate monohydrate and sucrose O-phosphoric acid and/or sodium hydroxide may be used for pH adjustment prior to lyophilization. Single dose vials of 3 mL (nominal capacity). Packages of 1 vial accompanied by 1 glass vial (2 mL) Sterile Water for Injection USP or 1 mL pre-filled syringe WFI, Ph.Eur., 1×27-gauge injection needle and 1 mixing needle.

450 IU (33 µg): Each multidose vial of sterile, lyophilized powder contains: FSH activity 450 IU. Diluent provided for reconstitution is Bacteriostatic Water for Injection USP (0.9% benzyl alcohol). Nonmedicinal ingredients: disodium phosphate dihyrate, sodium dihydrogen phosphate monohydrate and sucrose. O-phosphoric acid and/or sodium hydroxide may be used for pH adjustment prior to lyophilization. Multidose vials of 3 mL (nominal capacity). Packages of 1 vial accompanied by 1 mL pre-filled BWFI syringe, 6 injection syringes with attached 27G×0.5 inch needle and calibrated in FSH units (IU FSH).

1050 IU (77 µg): Each multidose vial of sterile, lyophilized powder contains: FSH activity 1050 IU. Diluent provided for reconstitution is Bacteriostatic Water for Injection USP (0.9% benzyl alcohol). Nonmedicinal ingredients: disodium phosphate dihyrate, sodium dihydrogen phosphate monohydrate and sucrose. O-phosphoric acid and/or sodium hydroxide may be used for pH adjustment prior to lyophilization. Multidose vials of 3 mL (nominal capacity). Packages of 1 vial accompanied by 2 mL pre-filled BWFI syringe, 15 injection syringes with attached 27G×0.5 inch needle and calibrated in FSH units (IU FSH).

Gonal-f® Pen Ⓟ

follitropin alpha

Gonadotropin

EMD Canada

Date of Revision: June 29, 2007

SUMMARY PRODUCT INFORMATION:

Route of Administration	Dosage Form/ Strength	Clinically Relevant Nonmedicinal Ingredients
Subcutaneous Injection	Liquid in prefilled pen 300 IU/0.5 mL (22 µg/0.5 mL), 450 IU/0.75 mL (33 µg/0.75 mL), and 900 IU/1.5 mL (66 µg/1.5 mL)	Not applicable For a complete listing of the nonmedicinal ingredients see Dosage Forms, Composition and Packaging.

INDICATIONS AND CLINICAL USE: GONAL-f (follitropin alpha for injection) is indicated for the stimulation of multiple follicular development in ovulatory patients undergoing Assisted Reproductive Technologies (ART) such as in vitro fertilization. To complete follicular maturation in the absence of an endogenous lutenizing hormone (LH) surge, human chorionic gonadotropin (hCG) is given.

GONAL-f is also indicated for the stimulation of follicular development in patients with hypothalamic-pituitary dysfunction who present either oligomenorrhoea or amenorrhoea (WHO Group II). To complete follicular maturation and effect ovulation, hCG is given.

Selection of Patients:

1. Before treatment with GONAL-f is instituted, a thorough gynaecologic and endocrinologic evaluation must be performed. This should include an assessment of pelvic anatomy.
2. Primary ovarian failure should be excluded by the determination of gonadotropin levels.
3. Appropriate evaluation should be performed to exclude pregnancy.
4. Patients in late reproductive life have a greater predisposition to endometrial carcinoma as well as a higher incidence of anovulatory disorders. A thorough diagnostic evaluation should always be performed in patients who demonstrate abnormal uterine bleeding or other signs of endometrial abnormalities before starting GONAL-f therapy.
5. Evaluation of the partner's fertility potential should be included in the initial evaluation.

CONTRAINDICATIONS: GONAL-f (follitropin alpha for injection) is contraindicated in women who exhibit:

1. High levels of Follicle Stimulating Hormone (FSH) indicating primary ovarian failure.
2. Uncontrolled thyroid or adrenal dysfunction.
3. An organic intracranial lesion such as a pituitary tumour or tumours of the hypothalamus.

4. The presence of any cause of infertility other than anovulation, as stated in Indications and Clinical Use unless the women are candidates for Assisted Reproductive Technologies.
5. Abnormal uterine bleeding (see Indications and Clinical Use, Selection of Patients).
6. Ovarian cyst or enlargement of undetermined origin (see Indications and Clinical Use, Selection of Patients).
7. Sex hormone dependent tumours of the reproductive organs and breasts.
8. Pregnancy/lactation.
9. Hypersensitivity to or history of previous allergic reaction to follitropin alpha, FSH or to any of the excipients.

WARNINGS AND PRECAUTIONS: General: Careful attention should be given to diagnosis in candidates for GONAL-f (follitropin alpha for injection) therapy (see Indications and Clinical Use, Selection of Patients).

GONAL-f should only be used by physicians who are thoroughly familiar with infertility problems and their management. GONAL-f is a potent gonadotrophic substance capable of causing mild to severe adverse reactions. Gonadotropin therapy requires a certain time commitment by physicians and supportive health professionals, and requires the availability of appropriate monitoring facilities (see Monitoring and Laboratory Tests). Safe and effective use of GONAL-f requires monitoring of ovarian response with ultrasound, alone or in combination with measurement of serum estradiol levels, on a regular basis.

Prior to therapy with GONAL-f, patients should be informed of the duration of treatment and monitoring of their condition that will be required. Possible adverse reactions (see Adverse Reactions) and the risk of multiple births should also be discussed.

Overstimulation of the Ovary During FSH Therapy: Ovarian Enlargement: Use of FSH therapy to stimulate follicular development may result in the recruitment of a number of follicles. This may result in mild to moderate uncomplicated ovarian enlargement which may be accompanied by abdominal distention and/or abdominal pain. This degree of enlargement has been reported to occur in approximately 20% of those treated with urofollitropin and hCG, and generally regresses without treatment within two or three weeks.

To minimize the hazard associated with the occasional abnormal ovarian enlargement which may occur with GONAL-f therapy, the lowest dose consistent with the expectation of good results should be used. Careful monitoring of ovarian response can further minimize the risk of ovarian enlargement.

If there is clinical evidence of excessive ovarian response (see Monitoring and Laboratory Tests), treatment should be discontinued and hCG should not be administered. This will reduce the chances of development of the Ovarian Hyperstimulation Syndrome.

Ovarian Hyperstimulation Syndrome (OHSS): OHSS is a medical event distinct from uncomplicated ovarian enlargement. OHSS may progress rapidly (within 24 hours to several days) to become a serious medical event. It is characterized by an apparent dramatic increase in vascular permeability which can result in an accumulation of fluid in the peritoneal, pleural and, rarely, in the pericardial cavities. The early warning signs of development of OHSS are severe pelvic pain, nausea, vomiting, and weight gain. The following symptomatology has been seen with cases of OHSS: abdominal pain, abdominal distention, severe ovarian enlargement, weight gain, dyspnea, oliguria and gastrointestinal symptoms including nausea, vomiting and diarrhea. Clinical evaluation may reveal hypovolemia, hemoconcentration, electrolyte imbalances, ascites, hemoperitoneum, pleural effusions, hydrothorax, acute pulmonary distress, and thromboembolic events (see Respiratory and Cardiovascular). Transient liver function test abnormalities suggestive of hepatic dysfunction, which may be accompanied by morphologic changes on liver biopsy, have been reported in association with the Ovarian Hyperstimulation Syndrome (OHSS).

Severe OHSS occurred in approximately 6.0% of patients treated with urofollitropin therapy in the initial clinical trials, in patients treated for anovulation due to polycystic ovarian syndrome. In these studies, prospective monitoring of ovarian response using serum estradiol determination or ultrasonographic visualizations was not routinely employed.

In the clinical trials in oligo-anovulatory infertile women treated with GONAL-f in which both estradiol and ultrasound measurements were utilized to monitor follicular development, the incidence of severe OHSS was 1 in 513 treatment cycles (0.2%).

In the clinical trials in ovulatory infertile women treated with GONAL-f for induction of multiple follicular induction for IVF/ET in which both estradiol and ultrasound measurements were utilized to monitor follicular development, there was no incident of severe OHSS.

OHSS may be more severe and more protracted if pregnancy occurs. OHSS develops rapidly; therefore, patients should be followed for at least two weeks after hCG administration. Most often, OHSS occurs after treatment has been discontinued and reaches its maximum at about seven to ten days following treatment. Usually, OHSS resolves spontaneously with the onset of menses. If there is evidence that OHSS may be developing prior to hCG administration (see Monitoring and Laboratory Tests), the hCG must be withheld.

If severe OHSS occurs, treatment should be stopped and the patient should be hospitalized. A physician experienced in the management of this syndrome, or who is experienced in the management of fluid and electrolyte imbalances should be consulted.

Carcinogenesis and Mutagenesis: Long-term studies in animals have not been performed to evaluate the carcinogenic potential of GONAL-f. However, r-hFSH showed no mutagenic activity in a series of tests performed to evaluate its potential genetic toxicity including, bacterial and mammalian cell mutation tests, a chromosome aberration test and a micronucleus test.

There have been reports of ovarian and other reproductive system neoplasms, both benign and malignant, in women who have undergone multiple drug regimens for infertility treatment. It is not yet established whether or not treatment with gonadotropins increases the baseline risk of these tumours in infertile women.

Respiratory and Cardiovascular: The following paragraph describes serious medical events reported following gonadotropin therapy. Serious pulmonary conditions (e.g., atelectasis, acute respiratory distress syndrome and exacerbation of asthma) have been reported. In addition, thromboembolic events both in association with, and separate from Ovarian Hyperstimulation Syndrome have been reported. Intravascular thrombosis and embolism can result in reduced blood flow to critical organs or the extremities. Sequelae of such events have included venous thrombophlebitis, pulmonary embolism, pulmonary infarction, cerebral vascular occlusion (stroke), and arterial occlusion resulting in loss of limb. In rare cases, pulmonary complications and/or thromboembolic events have resulted in death.

Dependence/Tolerance: There have been no reports of abuse or dependence with GONAL-f.

Sexual Function/Reproduction: Reports of multiple births have been associated with GONAL-f treatment. The risk of multiple births in patients undergoing ART procedures is related to the number of embryos replaced. In other patients, the incidence of multiple births may be increased by GONAL-f, as has been observed with other gonadotropin preparations. The patient and her partner should be advised of the potential risk of multiple births before starting treatment.

Since women with infertility undergoing assisted reproduction, and particularly IVF, often have tubal abnormalities, the incidence of ectopic pregnancies might be increased. Early ultrasound confirmation that a pregnancy is intrauterine is therefore important.

The incidence of pregnancy wastage by miscarriage or abortion may be higher in patients undergoing stimulation of follicular growth for ovulation induction or ART than in the normal population.

The prevalence of congenital malformations after ART may be slightly higher than after spontaneous conception. This is thought to be due to differences in parental characteristics (e.g. maternal age, sperm characteristics) and multiple pregnancies.

Impaired fertility has been reported in rats exposed to pharmacological doses of r-hFSH (40 IU/kg/day) for extended periods through reduced fecundity.

Special Populations: Pregnant Women: There are no adequate and well-controlled studies in pregnant women. Given in high doses (>5 IU/kg/day), GONAL-f caused an increase in deaths, fetal effects and dystocia in pregnant rats and rabbits, but without being a teratogen. However, since GONAL-f is not indicated in pregnancy, these data are of limited clinical relevance.

Nursing Women: It is not known whether this drug is excreted in human milk, although animal studies have shown that r-hFSH is excreted in milk. Therefore, GONAL-f is contraindicated in lactating mothers. During lactation, the secretion of prolactin can entail a poor prognosis to ovarian stimulation.

Pediatrics: Not indicated for treatment in pediatric population.

Geriatrics: Not indicated for treatment in the geriatric population.

Monitoring and Laboratory Tests: In most instances, treatment with GONAL-f results only in follicular recruitment and development. In the absence of an endogenous LH surge, hCG is given when monitoring of the patient indicates that sufficient follicular development has occurred. This may be estimated by ultrasound alone or in combination with measurement of serum estradiol levels. The combination of both ultrasound and serum estradiol measurement are useful for monitoring the development of follicles, for timing of the ovulatory trigger, as well as for detecting ovarian enlargement and minimizing the risk of the Ovarian Hyperstimulation Syndrome and multiple gestation. It is recommended that the number of growing follicles be confirmed using ultrasonography because plasma estrogens do not give an indication of the size or number of follicles.

The clinical confirmation of ovulation, with the exception of pregnancy, is obtained by direct and indirect indices of progesterone production. The indices most generally used are as follows: a rise in basal body temperature, increase in serum progesterone, and menstruation following a shift in basal body temperature.

When used in conjunction with the indices of progesterone production, sonographic visualization of the ovaries will assist in determining if ovulation has occurred. Sonographic evidence of ovulation may include the following: fluid in the cul-de-sac, ovarian stigmata, collapsed follicle, and secretory endometrium.

Accurate interpretation of the indices of follicle development and maturation require a physician who is experienced in the interpretation of these tests.

For patients undergoing extended cycles of treatment, PTT and liver enzymes should be monitored.

Occupational Hazards: No studies on the effects on the ability to drive and use machines have been performed.

ADVERSE REACTIONS: Adverse Drug Reaction Overview: Safety data on GONAL-f (follitropin alpha for injection) stem from clinical studies, as well as 10 years of post-marketing surveillance.

The most commonly reported adverse reactions with GONAL-f in clinical studies were ovarian cysts, injection site reaction of any severity, headache, mild to moderate ovarian hyperstimulation syndrome (OHSS) manifesting with symptoms such as abdominal swelling and pain, ovarian enlargement, as well as gastrointestinal symptoms such as nausea, vomiting, and diarrhoea.

The most frequently reported adverse reactions resulting in clinical intervention (e.g., discontinuation of GONAL-f, adjustment in dosage, or the need for concomitant medication to treat an adverse reaction symptom) was severe OHSS and its associated complications, such as ovarian torsion, thromboembolic events, haemoperitoneum and pulmonary conditions (see Warnings and Precautions).

Severe OHSS was also the most frequently reported serious adverse reaction. (see Warnings and Precautions). Complications of severe OHSS have been reported both in clinical studies and from spontaneous sources.

Summary of Adverse Drug Reactions Reported during Clinical Trials and in Post-Market Experience: More than 1000 patients were exposed to r-hFSH during the clinical development programme of GONAL-f. In addition to the clinical trial patient population, it is estimated that 580 000 to 1 700 000 patients have been exposed to r-hFSH during the post-marketing phase. The following summary presents the adverse drug reactions that have been reported with the use of r-hFSH during clinical trials and during post-market use. These data provide a comprehensive description of the safety profile of GONAL-f.

≥1% (Common and Very Common): Reproductive Disorders, Female: ovarian cysts, mild to moderate ovarian enlargement, breast tenderness, mild to moderate OHSS.

Application Site Disorders: mild to severe injection site reaction (e.g. pain, redness, bruising, swelling and/or irritation at the site of injection).

Body as a Whole, General Disorders: headache.

Gastrointestinal System Disorders: abdominal pain, nausea, vomiting, diarrhea, abdominal cramps, bloating.

<1% (Uncommon, Rare and Very Rare): Reproductive Disorders, Female: severe OHSS, complications of severe OHSS (adnexal torsion, hemoperitoneum).

Vascular (extracardiac) Disorders: thromboembolism.

Respiratory System Disorders: acute pulmonary distress.

Body as a Whole, General Disorders: mild systemic allergic reactions (e.g. erythema, rash or facial swelling).

Common and very common ADR have been reported from clinical studies, as well as in post-marketing surveillance. Severe OHSS has been reported from clinical studies, as well as in post-marketing surveillance. However, rare and very rare ADRs such as complications of severe OHSS and allergic reactions have generally been reported from post-marketing sources.

The following adverse reactions reported during gonadotropin therapy are listed in decreasing order of potential severity: pulmonary and vascular complications (see Warnings and Precautions); Ovarian Hyperstimulation Syndrome (see Warnings and Precautions); adnexal torsion (as a complication of ovarian enlargement); hemoperitoneum; mild to moderate ovarian enlargement; abdominal pain; ovarian cysts; gastrointestinal symptoms (nausea, vomiting, diarrhea, abdominal cramps, bloating); pain, rash, swelling, and/or irritation at the site of injection; breast tenderness; headache; dermatological symptoms (body rash, hives/urticaria).

Subjective assessments indicated minimal or mild transient pain in two and five subjects who received GONAL-f single-dose and GONAL-f multi-dose, respectively.

The following medical events have been reported subsequent to pregnancies resulting from GONAL-f therapy in controlled clinical trials: spontaneous abortion; ectopic pregnancy; premature labour; postpartum fever; congenital abnormalities.

Two incidents of congenital cardiac malformations have been reported in children born following pregnancies resulting from treatment with GONAL-f and hCG in clinical studies. In addition, a pregnancy occurring in a study following treatment with GONAL-f and hCG was characterized by apparent failure of intrauterine growth and terminated for a suspected syndrome of congenital abnormalities. No specific diagnosis was made.

Three incidents of chromosomal abnormalities and four birth defects have been reported following urofollitropin-hCG or urofollitropin, Pergonal (menotropins for injection, USP)-hCG therapy in clinical trials for stimulation prior to in vitro fertilization. The aborted pregnancies included one Trisomy 13, one Trisomy 18, and one fetus with multiple congenital anomalies (hydrocephaly, omphalocele, and meningocele). One meningocele, one external ear defect, one dislocated hip and ankle, and one dilated cardiomyopathy in presence of maternal Systemic Lupus Erythematosus were reported. None of these events were thought to be drug-related. The incidence does not exceed that found in the general population.

There have been infrequent reports of ovarian neoplasms, both benign and malignant, in women who have undergone multiple drug regimens for ovulation induction; however, a causal relationship has not been established.

DRUG INTERACTIONS: Clomiphene citrate, LH and hCG used with GONAL-f (follitropin alpha for injection) may enhance follicular response, and caution is indicated when using these drugs together.

Use of GnRH agonist or antagonist to induce pituitary desensitisation may alter the dosage of GONAL-f needed.

No other clinically significant drug/drug or drug/food interactions have been reported during GONAL-f therapy.

DOSAGE AND ADMINISTRATION: Dosing Considerations: Treatment with GONAL-f Pen (follitropin alpha for injection) should be initiated under the supervision of a physician experienced in the treatment of fertility problems.

GONAL-f Pen is intended for subcutaneous administration.

Recommended Dose and Dosage Adjustment: The dose of GONAL-f to stimulate development of the follicle must be individualized for each patient and the particular indication. To minimize the hazard associated with the occasional abnormal ovarian enlargement which may occur with GONAL-f therapy, the lowest dose consistent with the expectation of good results should be used. GONAL-f should be administered subcutaneously until adequate follicular development is indicated by ultrasound alone or in combination with measurement of serum estradiol levels.

The dosage recommendations given for GONAL-f are those in use for urinary FSH. Clinical assessment of GONAL-f indicates that its daily doses, regimens of administration, and treatment monitoring procedures should not be different from those currently used for urinary FSH-containing preparations. However, when these doses were used in a clinical study comparing GONAL-f and urinary FSH, GONAL-f was more effective than urinary FSH in terms of a lower total dose and a shorter treatment period needed to achieve pre-ovulatory conditions.

Over the course of treatment, doses may range between 75 to 450 IU depending on the indication and the individual patient response. To complete follicular development and effect ovulation in the absence of an endogenous LH surge, hCG is given when monitoring of the patient indicates that sufficient follicular development has occurred. If the ovaries are abnormally enlarged or significant abdominal pain occurs, GONAL-f treatment should be discontinued, hCG should not be administered, and the patient should be advised to refrain from intercourse until resolution of the cycle; this will reduce the chances of development of the Ovarian Hyperstimulation Syndrome and, should spontaneous ovulation occur, reduce the chances of multiple gestation. While individual dosing regimens will differ between patients, typical treatment regimens are presented below.

Assisted Reproductive Technologies: In patients undergoing Assisted Reproductive Technologies (ART) whose endogenous gonadotropin levels are not suppressed, GONAL-f should be initiated in the early follicular phase (cycle day 2 or 3) at a dose of 150 IU per day, administered subcutaneously. Treatment should be continued until adequate follicular development is indicated as determined by either ultrasound alone or in combination with measurement of serum estradiol levels. Adjustments to dose, based on the patient's response, should only be considered after the first five days of treatment; subsequently dosage should be adjusted no more frequently than every 3-5 days and by no more than 37.5-150 IU additionally at each adjustment. Treatment should be continued until adequate follicular development is indicated. Once adequate follicular development is evident, hCG should be administered to induce final follicular maturation in preparation for oocyte retrieval.

In patients undergoing ART, whose endogenous gonadotropin levels are suppressed indicating a hypogonadotrophic state, GONAL-f should be initiated at a dose of 225 IU per day, administered subcutaneously. Treatment should be continued until adequate follicular development is indicated as determined by either ultrasound alone or in combination with measurement of serum estradiol levels. Adjustments to dose may be considered after five days based on the patient's response; subsequently dosage should be adjusted no more frequently than every 3-5 days and by no more than 37.5-150 IU additionally at each adjustment. Doses greater than 450 IU per day are not generally recommended. As before, once adequate follicular development is evident hCG should be administered to induce final follicular maturation in preparation for oocyte retrieval.

Ovulation Induction: The majority of patients who require ovulation induction are patients with Polycystic Ovarian Syndrome (PCO). Patients with PCO tend to show a more rapid and exaggerated response to treatment. Therefore, in this patient population, particular care should be employed to ensure that patients are adequately monitored and that the lowest dose consistent with the expectation of good results is employed.

It is recommended that treatment of any patient be initiated at a dose of 75 IU GONAL-f per day, administered subcutaneously. An incremental adjustment in dose of up to 37.5 IU may be considered after 14 days. Further dose increases of the same magnitude could be made, if necessary, every seven days. Treatment duration should not exceed 35 days unless an estradiol rise indicates imminent follicular development. Once adequate follicular development is evident, hCG should be administered to induce final follicular maturation and effect ovulation. The patient should attempt to have intercourse at a consistent frequency of at least three times/week from the day prior to administration of hCG until ovulation becomes apparent.

If there is evidence of ovulation but pregnancy does not ensue, this regimen should be repeated for at least two more courses before increasing the dose of GONAL-f to 150 IU per day for 7 to 12 days. As before, this dose should be followed by the administration of hCG when adequate follicular development is evident. If evidence of ovulation is present but pregnancy does not ensue, repeat the same dose for two more courses. Doses larger than this are not routinely recommended.

Missed Dose: For patients who miss a dose, it is not recommended to double the next dose. The patients should be reminded to contact the physician monitoring their treatment.

Administration: Each GONAL-f Pen is designed to administer multiple doses liquid solution of GONAL-f subcutaneously.

OVERDOSAGE:

Aside from possible ovarian hyperstimulation and multiple gestations (see Warnings and Precautions), little is known concerning the consequences of acute overdosage with GONAL-f (follitropin alpha for injection). Apart from expected ovarian and endometrial effects, no acute toxicity was seen in animals given doses of r-hFSH up to 1000-fold the human dose.

For management of a suspected drug overdose, CPhA recommends that you contact your **regional Poison Control Centre**. See the *CPS* Directory section for a list of Poison Control Centres.

ACTION AND CLINICAL PHARMACOLOGY: Mechanism of Action: GONAL-f (follitropin apha for injection) stimulates ovarian follicular growth in women who do not have primary ovarian failure. FSH is the primary hormone responsible for follicular recruitment and development. To complete follicular maturation and effect ovulation in the absence of an endogenous LH surge, hCG is given when monitoring of the patient indicates that sufficient follicular development has occurred. There may be a degree of interpatient variability in response to FSH administration, with lack of response to FSH in some patients.

Pharmacodynamics: One main PD study has been performed in healthy female volunteers down-regulated with a GnRH agonist (Study 5117). The aim of this study was to assess PD characteristics of r hFSH administered sc daily for one week. After sc administration over one week, the first PD marker of ovarian response to FSH was serum inhibin, followed by plasma E2 and follicular growth. When FSH administration was stopped, inhibin levels dropped, while E2 continued to rise for one day and follicle size further increased during four days.

Two thirds of the volunteers developed significant follicular growth followed by corresponding decreasing levels of inhibin and increasing levels of E2 secretion. Moreover, no correlation was found between maximal serum FSH concentrations during administration and the maximal E2 responses, inhibin responses and follicular growth responses.

Pharmacokinetics: Single dose pharmacokinetics of r-hFSH were determined following intravenous, administration of 150 IU and 300 IU of GONAL-f to 12 healthy, down-regulated female volunteers (Study 5007). Single pharmacokinetics of r-hFSH were determined following intravenous, subcutaneous and intramuscular administration of 150 IU GONAL-f to 12 healthy, down-regulated female volunteers. Steady-state pharmacokinetics were also determined in the same 12 healthy down-regulated female volunteers who were administered a single daily dose of 150 IU for seven days (Study 5117). The pharmacokinetic parameters from these studies are included in Table 1 and Table 2.

Table 1: GONAL-f Pen

Summary of r-hFSH Pharmacokinetic Parameters in Healthy Female Volunteers (Study 5007)

	C_{max} (IU/L)	$t_{½}$ (h)	$AUC_{0-\infty}$ (IU·h/L)	Clearance (L/h)	Volume of distribution V_{ss} (L)
Single dose IV (150 IU)	32±10	14±7	274±71	0.6±0.2	10±6
Single dose IV (300 IU)	59±18	17±3	598±126	0.6±0.1	11±6

Table 2: GONAL-f Pen

Summary of r-hFSH Pharmacokinetic Parameters in Healthy Female Volunteers (Study 5117)

	C_{max} (IU/L)	$t_{½}$ (h)	$AUC_{0-\infty}$ (IU·h/L)	Clearance (L/h)	Volume of distribution V_{ss} (L)
Single dose IV (150 IU)	33±9	15±5	286±78	0.6±0.2	9±3
Single dose IM (150 IU)	3±1	50±27	206±66	—	—
Single dose SC (150 IU)	3±1	24±11	176±87	—	—
Multiple dose SC (7×150 IU)	4 ±1[b] 9±3[c]	24±8	187±61[a]	—	—

[a] Steady-state $AUC_{144-168}$ (after the 7th daily SC dose).
[b] After the first dose.
[c] After the last dose.

Following intravenous administration, GONAL-f is distributed to the extracellular fluid space with an initial half-life of approximately 2 hours and eliminated from the body with a terminal half-life of approximately 1 day. The steady-state volume of distribution and total clearance are 10 L and 0.6 L/h, respectively. One-eighth of the GONAL-f dose is excreted in the urine.

Following subcutaneous or intramuscular administration, the absolute bioavailability is 70%. Following repeated administration, GONAL-f accumulates 3-fold at steady-state within 3-4 days. In women whose endogenous gonadotrophin secretion is suppressed, GONAL-f has been shown to effectively stimulate follicular development and steroidogenesis, despite unmeasurable LH levels.

Special Populations and Conditions: No studies have been conducted with special populations and conditions.

STORAGE AND STABILITY: Pharmacy: Store at 2-8°C (in a refrigerator) for up to 2 years.

Patient: Store at 2-8°C (in a refrigerator) or store for a single period between 2-25°C (in the refrigerator or at room temperature) for a maximum of 3 months. After first use, the pen may be stored at 25°C (room temperature) for a maximum of 28 days.

Do not use the GONAL-f prefilled pen if the solution contains particles or is not clear.

Do not freeze. Protect from light.

Keep in a safe place out of the reach of children.

Do not use after the expiry date.

SPECIAL HANDLING INSTRUCTIONS: The GONAL-f (follitropin alpha for injection) solution should not be administered if it contains particles or is not clear.

GONAL-f Pen is not designed to allow the cartridge to be removed or any other drug to be mixed in the cartridge.

Discard used needles immediately after injection.

Any unused product or waste material should be disposed of in accordance with local requirements.

INFORMATION FOR THE PATIENT: Published in e-CPS, available by subscription at www.e-cps.ca.

DOSAGE FORMS, COMPOSITION AND PACKAGING: GONAL-f (follitropin alpha for injection) Pen is presented as solution for injection in 3 mL cartridge (Type I glass), with a plunger stopper (halobutyl rubber) and a rubber crimp cap (halobutyl rubber). The cartridge is preassembled with the prefilled pen. GONAL-f Pen is shatterproof per EN ISO 11608-1:2000 standards.

300 IU/0.5 mL (22 µg/0.5 mL) Filled by Mass: 1 prefilled pen and 5 needles to be used with the pen for subcutaneous administration. Nonmedicinal ingredients: disodium phosphate dihydrate, L-methionine, m-cresol, phosphoric acid, poloxamer 188, sodium dihydrogen phosphate monohydrate, sodium hydroxide, sucrose and water for injection.

450 IU/0.75 mL (33 µg/0.75 mL) Filled by Mass: 1 prefilled pen and 7 needles to be used with the pen for subcutaneous administration. Nonmedicinal ingredients: disodium phosphate dihydrate, L-methionine, m-cresol, phosphoric acid, poloxamer 188, sodium dihydrogen phosphate monohydrate, sodium hydroxide, sucrose and water for injection.

900 IU/1.5 mL (66 µg/1.5 mL) Filled by Mass: 1 prefilled pen and 14 needles to be used with the pen for subcutaneous administration. Nonmedicinal ingredients: disodium phosphate dihydrate, L-methionine, m-cresol, phosphoric acid, poloxamer 188, sodium dihydrogen phosphate monohydrate, sodium hydroxide, sucrose and water for injection.

There is no latex in the components of the prefilled pen.

Granisetron Hydrochloride Injection Ⓟ

granisetron HCl

Antiemetic—5-HT3 Receptor Antagonist

Sandoz

SUPPLIED: Each mL of sterile injectable solution contains: granisetron 1 mg (as hydrochloride). Nonmedicinal ingredients: citric acid (monohydrate), hydrochloric acid and/or sodium hydroxide (to adjust pH), methylparaben and propylparaben (as preservatives), sodium chloride and water for injection. Clear multidose vials of 1 mL, boxes of 10. Clear multidose vials of 4 mL, boxes of 1. Store between 15 and 30°C. Protect from light. Discard 28 days after initial use.

Gravol® - Ginger - Natural Source

ginger root (Zingiber officinale Roscoe)

Herbal Medicine

Church & Dwight

PHARMACOLOGY: Ginger is the fresh or dried rhizome of Zingiber officinale Roscoe. The mechanism of action of ginger in humans is not known. Traditionally, ginger belongs to the group of acrid, pungent, medicinal plants that include garlic, cayenne, cinnamon and angelica. These medicinal plants presumably act by a mild irritation of mucous membranes and epithelia, leading to vasodilatation, warmth and stimulation of function in affected areas, including the digestive system. The mechanism is believed to be the involvement of prostaglandins, kinins and local hormones. Studies in humans have found that ginger had no effect on nystagmus response, either to vestibular or optokinetic stimulation. Another study found that ginger had no effect on gastric emptying. Ginger is believed to exert its antiemetic effect by some mechanism other than central nervous system stimulation.

Pharmacological data support the concept of a dual carminative and stimulating role on the digestive system, helping to explain the anti-nausea effects. Gingerols have been found to stimulate bile acids, which may be responsible for improved digestion and absorption, and may improve peristalsis. It is not exactly known which components of ginger exert a therapeutic effect. However, it is believed that the gingerols and possibly the shogaols are responsible.

INDICATIONS: For the prevention and treatment of nausea and vomiting.

CONTRAINDICATIONS: Ginger is contraindicated in patients with renal disease and in patients with gallstones.

WARNINGS: General: Ginger possesses both cardiotonic and antiplatelet activity in vitro and hypoglycemic activity in vivo studies, excessive doses may interfere with existing cardiac, antidiabetic or anticoagulant therapy.

Pregnancy: Ginger has been used in small doses for nausea and vomiting of pregnancy without problem, however, due to the lack of sufficient controlled studies on safety and efficacy, the product is not recommended to be used in pregnancy.

Lactation: It has been reported that ginger can reduce a lactating mother's milk flow. Ginger's effect on nursing infants has not been studied; the use is not recommended during breast-feeding.

Geriatrics: Ginger should not be used in the elderly with acute renal disease.

Children: Ginger should not be used in children with acute renal disease. Ginger is not recommended for children under 12 years.

PRECAUTIONS: No data supplied by the manufacturer.

ADVERSE EFFECTS: Ginger has been reported to exacerbate symptoms in patients with acute inflammatory skin diseases and can cause contact dermatitis.

No drowsiness has been reported.

OVERDOSE:

Symptoms: There are no reports of severe toxicity in humans. However, large overdoses may cause CNS depression or stimulation and cardiac arrhythmia.

Treatment: No specific antidote is presented in the literature.

For management of a suspected drug overdose, CPhA recommends that you contact your **regional Poison Control Centre**. See the *CPS* Directory section for a list of Poison Control Centres.

DOSAGE: Adults and Children over 12 years of Age: 2 tablets or lozenges every 4 hours 1 to 3 times a day. Do not exceed 6 tablets or lozenges a day. For the prevention of motion sickness, take 2 tablets or lozenges at least 30 minutes before departure. Consult a physician if symptoms of nausea and/or vomiting persist.

SUPPLIED: Filmkote Tablets: Each yellow, Filmkote tablet, intagliated "Gravol NS" on one side, and "20" on the other side, contains: ginger root extract (1:25) 20 mg equivalent to dried root 500 mg. Nonmedicinal ingredients: cellulose, cornstarch, oleic acid, polyethylene glycol, povidone, silicon dioxide, stearic acid and triglyceride. Artificial colours-, gluten-, preservatives- and sugar-free. Tablets have a smooth coating to mask any pungent or bitter aftertaste and facilitate swallowing. Bottles of 20. Store at controlled room temperature between 15 and 30°C. Do not freeze.

Lozenges: Each soft chewable lozenge contains: ginger root extract (1:25) 20 mg equivalent to ginger dried root 500 mg. Nonmedicinal ingredients: acacia, acesulfame potassium, aspartame, beeswax, cyclodextrin, D&C yellow No.10, glycerin, lactose, liquid paraffin, maltitol, natural flavours and xanthan gum. Artificial flavours-, gluten- and preservatives-free. Packs of 20.

(Shown in Product Identification Section)

Gravol® Preparations

dimenhydrinate

Antiemetic—Antivertigo Agent

Church & Dwight

INDICATIONS: Prevention or relief of motion sickness, radiation sickness, postoperative vomiting, and drug induced nausea and vomiting; it has also been used for the symptomatic relief of nausea and vertigo due to Ménière's disease and other labyrinthine disturbances.

CONTRAINDICATIONS: Glaucoma, chronic lung disease, difficulty in urination due to prostatic hypertrophy.

WARNINGS: As dimenhydrinate has a CNS depressant effect, the concomitant use of alcohol should be avoided.

If Gravol I.M. is required for i.v. use, it must be diluted at least 1:10 with a compatible physiological solution such as sterile saline or 5% dextrose in water, to prevent propylene glycol-associated serious adverse reactions, and should be injected slowly over 2 to 3 min.

Occupational Hazards: Patients receiving dimenhydrinate should be cautioned against operating automobiles or dangerous machinery because of drowsiness associated with the drug. If drowsiness is excessive, dosage should be reduced.

It should be borne in mind that antiemetics should be used with caution since they may mask the presence of underlying organic abnormalities or the toxic effects of other drugs.

Patients in whom anticholinergics may aggravate other clinical conditions, should use dimenhydrinate with caution, and preferably on a physician's advice. Patients should not take dimenhydrinate with other antihistamines, tranquilizers or any other sedative drugs without first consulting their physician.

Pregnancy: The use of dimenhydrinate by women who are pregnant or may become pregnant, or nursing mothers, require that potential benefits be weighed against the potential risks.

Lactation: The use of dimenhydrinate by women who are pregnant or may become pregnant, or nursing mothers, require that potential benefits be weighed against the potential risks.

PRECAUTIONS: No data supplied by the manufacturer.

ADVERSE EFFECTS: Drowsiness may be experienced by some patients, especially at high dosages. Dizziness may also occur. Symptoms of dry mouth, lassitude, excitement (especially in children) and nausea have been reported.

OVERDOSE:
Children are susceptible to the convulsant action of antihistamines. Cases of convulsions and eventually coma have been reported in children 1.5 to 3 years (especially in the presence of dehydration) having received large doses of 150 to 800 mg diphenhydramine HCl (equivalent to 260 to 1 400 mg dimenhydrinate). There have been reports of hallucinations after the ingestion of 500 and 700 mg dimenhydrinate.

Symptoms: Drowsiness, ataxia, disorientation, nystagmus, convulsions, stupor, coma and respiratory depression.

Treatment: No specific antidote. Gastric lavage. If coma and respiratory depression are present, use resuscitative measures, not stimulants. Maintain blood pressure with dopamine or levarterenol bitartrate. It has been reported that anticholinergic induced delirium, confusion, hallucinations, agitation, ataxia, dysarthria and somnolence are reversed by i.v. or s.c. administration of 1 to 2 mg physostigmine salicylate.

> For management of a suspected drug overdose, CPhA recommends that you contact your **regional Poison Control Centre**. See the *CPS* Directory section for a list of Poison Control Centres.

DOSAGE: Motion Sickness: Initial dose should be taken at least ½ hour and preferably 1 to 2 hours before departure.
Adults: For the treatment of motion sickness, nausea, vomiting, dizziness and vertigo: 50 to 100 mg every 4 hours if necessary to a maximum of 400 mg in 24 hours. For extended relief: 1 to 2 Gravol 75 mg long acting capsules every 8 hours to a maximum of 5 capsules in 24 hours, or 1 Gravol 75 mg long acting caplet every 8 to 12 hours up to a maximum of 3 caplets in 24 hours or 1 Gravol 100 mg long acting caplet every 8 to 12 hours up to a maximum of 3 caplets in 24 hours. Rectal: 50 to 100 mg suppository every 6 to 8 hours as necessary. (For ease and comfort smooth any edges on suppository prior to use.)
Radiation Sickness: 50 to 100 mg administered rectally or parenterally, 30 to 60 minutes before treatment. This dose is repeated as necessary to a maximum of 400 mg in 24 hours.
To control postoperative nausea and vomiting: 50 to 100 mg may be administered orally or 50 mg i.m. as a preoperative dose to be followed postoperatively by similar doses as needed to a maximum of 400 mg in 24 hours.
Children: Under 1 year: Not recommended.
Children: Under 2 years: As directed by a physician.
2 to 6 years: Oral: 15 to 25 mg every 6 to 8 hours as necessary to a maximum of 75 mg in 24 hours. Rectal: 12.5 to 25 mg not to be repeated except on the advice of a physician.
6 to 8 years: Oral: 25 to 50 mg every 6 to 8 hours as necessary to a maximum of 150 mg in 24 hours. Rectal: 12.5 to 25 mg every 8 to 12 hours as necessary.
8 to 12 years: Oral: 25 to 50 mg every 6 to 8 hours as necessary to a maximum of 150 mg in 24 hours. Rectal: 25 to 50 mg every 8 to 12 hours as necessary.
12 years and over: Oral: 50 mg every 4 to 6 hours as necessary to a maximum of 300 mg in 24 hours. Rectal: 50 mg every 8 to 12 hours as necessary.

SUPPLIED: I.V. Ampuls: Each single dose ampul of clear solution contains: dimenhydrinate 50 mg and must be administered by slow i.v. injection only. Nonmedicinal ingredients: alcohol 17%. Tartrazine-free. Ampuls of 5 mL, boxes of 10. Store at controlled room temperature (15 to 30°C). Protect from freezing.
I.M. Injection: Each mL contains: dimenhydrinate 50 mg. This dosage form is for i.m use only, unless diluted at least 1:10 with a compatible physiological solution, i.e., sterile saline or 5% dextrose in water. Nonmedicinal ingredients: methylparaben (multidose vials only), propylene glycol and propylparaben (multidose vials only). Tartrazine-free. Multidose vials of 5 mL, boxes of 3. Unit dose ampuls of 1 mL (preservative-free), boxes of 10. Store at controlled room temperature (15 to 30°C). Protect from freezing.
L/A Caplets 100 mg: Each red-white bi-layer film coated caplet, intagliated GRAVOL on one side, contains: dimenhydrinate 25 mg for immediate release and dimenhydrinate 75 mg for sustained release. Nonmedicinal ingredients: butyl hydroxytoluene, calcium carbonate, calcium phosphate, FD&C Red No. 40, hydroxypropyl cellulose, hypromellose, magnesium stearate, microcrystalline cellulose, polyethylene glycol, polyethylene oxide and starch. Push through packages of 8 and 24.
Liquid: Each 5 mL of yellow, transparent, viscous liquid with a bittersweet mixed fruit flavor, contains: dimenhydrinate 15 mg. Nonmedicinal ingredients: citric acid, D&C Yellow No. 10, FD&C Yellow No. 6, flavor, propylene glycol, sodium benzoate, sorbitol and sucrose. Energy: 61.5 kJ (14.7 kcal)/5 mL. Sodium: <1 mmol (0.8 mg). Gluten- and tartrazine-free. Bottles of 75 mL.
Suppositories: Each white, opaque suppository contains: dimenhydrinate 25 mg children, 50 mg junior or 100 mg adult. Nonmedicinal ingredients: polyethylene glycol, silicon dioxide and titanium dioxide. Gluten- and tartrazine-free. Gravol 25 mg and 50 mg: boxes of 10. Gravol 100 mg: boxes of 10 and 100. Individually sealed in foil. Store in a cool place.
Filmkote Tablets 25 mg (Junior Strength): Each round, biconvex, pale yellow tablet, intagliated GRAVOL on one side, contains: dimenhydrinate 25 mg. Nonmedicinal ingredients: alumina, cellulose, D&C Yellow No. 10, FD&C Yellow No. 6 and Blue No. 2, lactose, magnesium stearate, polyethylene glycol, povidone, silicon dioxide, starch (corn), talc and tianium dioxide. Energy: 1.3 kJ (0.3 kcal). Gluten- and tartrazine-free. Push through packages of 10.
Filmkote Tablets 50 mg: Each round, biconvex, peach coral tablet, intagliated GRAVOL on one side and quadrisected on the other, contains: dimenhydrinate 50 mg. Nonmedicinal ingredients: alumina, cellulose, FD&C Yellow No. 6, lactose, magnesium stearate, polyethylene glycol, silicon dioxide, starch (corn), talc and titanium dioxide. Energy: 1.3 kJ (0.3 kcal). Gluten- and tartrazine-free. Push through packages of 10 and 30; bottles of 100 and 1 000, unit dose cartons of 5×20 and unit dose tins of 1 000.
Chewable Tablets for Children: Each round, flat, light purple, cherry-flavored tablet with bevelled edge intagliated GRAVOL 15 on one side, plain on the other side, contains: dimenhydrinate 15 mg. Nonmedicinal ingredients: alumina, aspartame, cellulose, citric acid, FD&C Red No. 40, flavors, magnesium stearate, methacrylic acid copolymer, monoglycerides, polyethylene glycol, sorbitol and starch (corn). Energy: 5.8 kJ (1.4 kcal). Gluten- and tartrazine-free. Push through packages of 12.
Chewable Tablets for Adults: Each round, flat, light pink, orange-flavored tablet with bevelled edge, intagliated GRAVOL 50 on one side, bisected on the other side, contains: dimenhydrinate 50 mg. Nonmedicinal ingredients: alumina, aspartame, cellulose, citric acid, FD&C Yellow No. 6, flavors, magnesium stearate, methacrylic acid copolymer, monoglycerides, polyethylene glycol, sorbitol and starch (corn). Energy: 10.9 kJ (2.6 kcal). Gluten- and tartrazine-free. Push through packages of 8.
Softgel Capsules: Each pink translucent softgel capsule printed in white "Gravol" contains: dimenhydrinate 50 mg. Nonmedicinal ingredients: D&C red No. 33, gelatin, glycerin, mannitol, methylparaben, polyethylene glycol, povidone, propylparaben, sorbitol, water. Push through packages of 8.

(Shown in Product Identification Section)

Guaifenesin
Expectorant

CPhA Monograph

Date of Revision: November 2008

> This monograph has been compiled by CPhA and reviewed by experts. It may contain information different from that found in Health Canada-approved Product Monographs. The reader is referred to the *CPS* Editorial Policy for more information.

PHARMACOLOGY: Guaifenesin, an expectorant, is believed to produce its effect through a local or reflex irritant action on the gastric mucosa that activates the vagus nerve to stimulate secretion of respiratory tract fluid. This is thought to increase sputum volume, decrease its viscosity, enhance the flow of less viscid secretions and promote mucociliary clearance.
Pharmacokinetics: The drug is rapidly and well absorbed from the gastrointestinal tract and excreted in the urine.

INDICATIONS: Guaifenesin may be used in the symptomatic relief of respiratory conditions associated with productive cough, with the presence of mucus in the respiratory tract. May also be useful in the management of dry, unproductive cough by easing expectoration of thick, viscous secretions.

Evidence suggests guaifenesin has no effect on cough frequency related to chronic bronchitis and acute cough related to the common cold [*Chest* 2006;129(1 Suppl):238S-49S].

CONTRAINDICATIONS: Patients who are hypersensitive to guaifenesin or to any ingredient in the formulation or component of the container.

WARNINGS: See Precautions.

PRECAUTIONS: A physician should be consulted if cough persists for longer than 7 days or if high fever, hemoptysis, skin rash, persistent headache, or severe sore throat is present with cough.

Guaifenesin may cause a color interference with certain laboratory determinations of 5 hydroxyindoleacetic acid and vanillylmandelic acid.

Special Populations: *Pregnant Women:* Pregnancy Category C. Guaifenesin use during pregnancy may be associated with inguinal hernias in newborn infants but evidence is weak. An increased risk of major malformations was not seen in several studies. Products containing guaifenesin may contain high alcohol content. The use of guaifenesin during pregnancy requires the potential benefits be weighed against the possible risks to the mother and the fetus.
Nursing Women: It is not known if guaifenesin passes into breast milk. Products containing guaifenesin may contain high alcohol content. The use of guaifenesin during nursing requires that potential benefits be weighed against the possible risks to the mother and infant.
Pediatrics: Evidence to support the efficacy of oral cough and cold products in children younger than 6 years of age is lacking. Serious adverse effects such as death due to unintentional overdose, although rare, have been reported. Instruct parents and caregivers to consult health care practitioners in children under 6 years of age prior to using cough and cold products. Little evidence, if any, exists for the management of productive cough in children under the age of 6 years.

ADVERSE EFFECTS: Nausea, gastrointestinal upset, dizziness, headache, rash, diarrhea and drowsiness occur infrequently. Kidney stone formation (large doses).

OVERDOSE:

> For management of a suspected drug overdose, CPhA recommends that you contact your **regional Poison Control Centre**. See the *CPS* Directory section for a list of Poison Control Centres.

DOSAGE: See Table 1. Administer with sufficient oral fluid to ensure therapeutic effect.

Table 1: Guaifenesin Dosage

Age (years)	Dose	Maximum Daily Dose (mg)	Comment
2 to 5	50 to 100 mg Q4H	600	Guaifenesin is not recommended in children under the age of 6 years. Use only under the advice of health care practitioner.
6 to 11	100 to 200 mg Q4H	1200	
≥12	200 to 400 mg Q4H	2400	

Gynazole•1®
butoconazole nitrate
Antifungal

Ferring

Date of Preparation: December 18, 2003
Date of Revision: June 21, 2004

PHARMACOLOGY: GYNAZOLE•1 (butoconazole nitrate) vaginal cream 2%, contains butoconazole nitrate 2%, an imidazole derivative with antifungal activity.

Like other imidazole derivatives, butoconazole nitrate presumably exerts its antifungal activity by altering cellular membranes, resulting in increased membrane permeability, secondary metabolic effects, and growth inhibition. Although the exact mechanism of action of butoconazole nitrate has not been fully determined, it has been suggested that the fungistatic activity of the drug may result from interference with ergosterol synthesis, probably via inhibition of C-14 demethylation of sterol intermediates (e.g. lanosterol). Like some other imidazole derivatives (e.g. miconazole), the fungicidal activity of butoconazole at high concentrations may result from a direct physicochemical effect of the drug on the fungal cell. This effect may involve hydrophobic interactions between the drug and unsaturated fatty acid components of the membrane.

Butoconazole has some antibacterial activity against gram-positive organisms, but this effect cannot be explained on the basis of inhibition of ergosterol synthesis since bacteria generally do not contain membrane sterols. It has been suggested that the antibacterial effect of butoconazole and other imidazole derivatives may be similar to the physicochemical effect of these agents on fungi or may involve other metabolic sites.

INDICATIONS: GYNAZOLE•1 (butoconazole nitrate) vaginal cream 2%, is indicated for the local treatment of vulvovaginal infections caused by *C. albicans*. The diagnosis should be confirmed by KOH smears and/or cultures.
Note: GYNAZOLE•1 is safe and effective in non-pregnant women; however, the safety and effectiveness of this product in pregnant women has not been established (see Precautions).

CONTRAINDICATIONS: GYNAZOLE•1 is contraindicated in patients with a history of hypersensitivity to any of the components of the product.

WARNINGS: This cream contains mineral oil. Mineral oil may weaken latex or rubber products such as condoms or vaginal contraceptive diaphragms; therefore, use of such products within 72 hours following treatment with GYNAZOLE•1 is not recommended.

Recurrent vaginal yeast infections, especially those that are difficult to eradicate, can be an early sign of infection with the human immunodeficiency virus (HIV) in women who are considered at risk for HIV infection.

PRECAUTIONS: General: If clinical symptoms persist, tests should be repeated to rule out other pathogens, to confirm the original diagnosis, and to rule out other conditions that may predispose a patient to recurrent vaginal fungal infections.

Appropriate microbiologic studies should be performed to confirm the diagnosis and rule out infection caused by non-susceptible pathogens when an adequate response is not achieved following a course of butoconazole therapy. Patients should be instructed not to rely on condoms or diaphragms to prevent sexually transmitted diseases or pregnancy during butoconazole nitrate therapy, since the cream may damage these devices and result in protective failure. Alternative methods of birth control should be used. Patients also should be instructed not to use tampons while using intravaginal butoconazole nitrate vaginal cream.

Butoconazole nitrate vaginal cream should not be applied to the eye nor administered orally. Patients receiving butoconazole nitrate vaginal cream should be instructed to contact their physician or local poison control centre immediately if they accidentally ingest the vaginal cream.

Patients also should be advised to consult a clinician if manifestations of vulvovaginitis recur within 2 months of therapy, or if they think that they may have been exposed to HIV. Recurrent infection may be a sign of pregnancy or a serious underlying condition such as AIDS or diabetes mellitus.

Women with diabetes mellitus, or who are HIV positive or have AIDS, or possible pelvic inflammatory disease (abdominal pain, fever, or a foul-smelling vaginal discharge) should only be treated with butoconazole nitrate while under the care of a physician familiar with their medical history.
Lactation: It is not known whether this drug is excreted in human milk. Because many drugs are excreted in human milk, caution should be exercised when butoconazole nitrate is administered to a nursing woman.
Pediatrics: Safety and effectiveness in children have not been established.

Carcinogenesis, Mutagenesis, Impairment of Fertility: Carcinogenesis: Long term studies in animals have not been performed to evaluate the carcinogenic potential of this drug.

Mutagenicity: Butoconazole nitrate was not mutagenic when tested in the Ames bacterial test, yeast gene conversion, chromosomal aberration assay in CHO cells, CHO/HGPRT point mutation assay, mouse micronucleus, and rat dominant lethal assays.

Impairment of Fertility: No impairment of fertility was seen in rabbits or rats administered butoconazole nitrate in oral doses up to 30 mg/kg/day (3 times the human dose based on mg/m^2) or 100 mg/kg/day (10 times the human dose based on mg/m^2), respectively.

Pregnancy: In pregnant rats administered 6 mg/kg/day of butoconazole nitrate intravaginally during the period of organogenesis, there was an increase in resorption rate and decrease in litter size; however, no teratogenicity was noted. This dose represents a 130- to 353-fold margin of safety based on serum levels achieved in rats following intravaginal administration compared to the serum levels achieved in humans following intravaginal administration of the recommended therapeutic dose of butoconazole nitrate.

Butoconazole nitrate has no apparent adverse effect when administered orally to pregnant rats throughout organogenesis at dose levels up to 50 mg/kg/day (5 times the human dose based on mg/m^2). Daily oral doses of 100, 300 or 750 mg/kg/day (10, 30 or 75 times the human dose based on mg/m^2 respectively) resulted in fetal malformations (abdominal wall defects, cleft palate), and maternal stress was also evident at these higher dose levels. There were, however, no adverse effects on litters of rabbits who received butoconazole nitrate orally, even at maternally stressful dose levels (e.g., 150 mg/kg, 24 times the human dose based on mg/m^2).

Butoconazole nitrate, like other azole anti-fungal agents, causes dystocia in rats when treatment is extended through parturition. However, this effect was not apparent in rabbits treated with as much as 100 mg/kg/day orally (16 times the human dose based on mg/m^2). There are, however, no adequate and well-controlled studies in pregnant women. GYNAZOLE•1 should be used during pregnancy only if the potential benefit justifies the potential risk to the fetus.

ADVERSE EFFECTS: Of the 314 patients treated with GYNAZOLE•1 for 1 day in controlled clinical trials, 18 patients (5.7%) reported complaints such as vulvar/vaginal burning, itching, soreness and swelling, pelvic or abdominal pain or cramping, or a combination of two or more of these symptoms. In 3 patients (1%) these complaints were considered treatment-related. Five of the 18 patients reporting adverse events discontinued the study because of them.

Although hepatocellular dysfunction has occurred during systemic treatment with imidazole-derived antifungal agents (e.g. ketoconazole), this adverse event has not been reported to date following intravaginal butoconazole nitrate therapy.

OVERDOSE:

Treatment: There is no specific treatment for butoconazole overdose; therefore, management of the patient should consist of symptomatic and supportive therapy.

For management of a suspected drug overdose, CPhA recommends that you contact your **regional Poison Control Centre**. See the *CPS* Directory section for a list of Poison Control Centres.

DOSAGE: The recommended dose of GYNAZOLE•1 is one applicator of cream (approximately 5 g of the cream) intravaginally as a single dose treatment. This amount of cream contains approximately 100 mg of butoconazole nitrate.

Butoconazole nitrate vaginal cream is for intravaginal administration only and should not be administered orally; contact with the eyes should be avoided.

INFORMATION FOR THE PATIENT: Published in e-CPS, available by subscription at www.e-cps.ca.

SUPPLIED: Each g of cream contains: butoconazole nitrate 2%. Nonmedicinal ingredients: colloidal silicon dioxide, edetate disodium, glyceryl monoisostearate, methylparaben, microcrystalline wax, mineral oil, polyglyceryl-3 oleate, propylene glycol, propylparaben, purified water and sorbitol solution. Cartons of 1 single-dose prefilled disposable applicator (approximately 5 g of the cream). Store at room temperature 15 to 30°C. Avoid heat above 30°C.

H

Habitrol®

nicotine transdermal system

Smoking Cessation Aid

Novartis Consumer Health

Date of Preparation: July 1997
Date of Revision: March 29, 2005

PHARMACOLOGY: HABITROL (S(-)-nicotine) delivers S(-)-nicotine, the active component of tobacco smoke, transdermally into the systemic circulation, continuously over 24 hours. HABITROL releases S(-)-nicotine in controlled amounts at a rate sufficient to produce plasma nicotine concentrations comparable to trough levels observed in smokers before smoking a cigarette. Because of the low, continuous delivery of S(-)-nicotine through the skin, HABITROL does not produce the rapid increases in plasma nicotine concentrations that occur with cigarette smoking and which are primarily responsible for smoking's addictive effects. HABITROL has been shown to increase rates of cessation in smokers who are motivated to quit.

INDICATIONS: HABITROL (S(-)-nicotine) is indicated as a temporary aid used to facilitate smoking cessation in smokers who strongly desire to give up their smoking habit. HABITROL is intended to be used as part of a smoking cessation strategy, and should, whenever possible, be combined with behavior modification therapy.

CONTRAINDICATIONS: HABITROL (S(-)-nicotine) is contraindicated in: non-smokers, occasional smokers, and children under 18 years of age (see Warnings); known hypersensitivity of the skin, allergy to nicotine or HABITROL components; generalized skin disorders; recovery phase of acute myocardial infarction, unstable or worsening angina pectoris, severe cardiac arrhythmias, and recent cerebrovascular accident.

Any form of nicotine administration is contraindicated in pregnant and breast-feeding women.

WARNINGS: In view of its pharmacological effects, HABITROL (S(-)-nicotine) should not be used in smokers with the following conditions unless there has been careful consideration of the risks and benefits of therapy: hypertension, stable angina pectoris, variant (Prinzmetal's) angina, cerebrovascular disease, occlusive peripheral arterial and vasospastic diseases, heart failure, hyperthyroidism, diabetes mellitus, renal and hepatic insufficiency, peptic ulcer. Use of HABITROL in these smokers should only be considered if tobacco withdrawal with psychological support alone has been unsuccessful. If these smokers continue to smoke while wearing HABITROL, excessive nicotine levels could be produced that can exacerbate pre-existing diseases and can cause serious adverse reactions (see Adverse Effects).

Adult smokers tolerate doses of nicotine that can be poisonous or fatal to children and pets. Both new and used HABITROL systems contain enough nicotine to cause serious harm if applied or ingested. Therefore it is important that smokers keep both new and used systems out of the reach of children and pets (see Information for the Patient for the recommended disposal procedure).

Treatment with HABITROL should be discontinued in cases of severe or persistent skin reactions.

No experience is available on treatment with HABITROL in smokers under 18 years of age, and is limited in ages 65 years and above.

PRECAUTIONS: Continued Smoking and Adverse Reactions: If the user continues to smoke while wearing HABITROL (S(-)-nicotine), adverse reactions consistent with excessive nicotine exposure, including cardiovascular effects, may be more frequent and more pronounced.

Strenuous Exercise: Preliminary evidence suggests that wearing a nicotine transdermal patch during periods of strenuous exercise may lead to nicotine toxicity as a result of increased absorption of nicotine from the depot of nicotine in the skin under the patch, due to increase skin temperature and increased cutaneous vasodilation and perfusion from exercising. Three cases illustrating this phenomenon were described in Health Canada Adverse Reaction Newsletter, Volume 6, No. 1, Jan. 1996. Advice to remove the nicotine patch before engaging in strenuous exercise was recommended by: W. Dafoe and P. Huston, *Current Trends In Cardiac Rehabilitation*, Canadian Medical Association Journal, Feb 15, 1997;156 (14):527-532. Until definitive studies have been undertaken to clarify this hazard, it is advisable to remove the nicotine patch prior to engaging in strenuous activity.

Occupational Hazards: Effects on ability to drive or use machines: Nicotine acts as a central nervous stimulant agent. While no direct effect on reaction time is to be expected, the smoker should be cautioned that sleep disturbance, irritability and nervousness may occur during smoking cessation, and could affect performance.

Drug Interactions: To date, no information is available on interactions between HABITROL and any other drugs. Experience with other forms of nicotine replacement therapy has shown that there are no pharmacodynamic or pharmacokinetic interactions of clinical relevance with various concomitant treatments.

Tobacco withdrawal, with or without nicotine substitution, may alter the response to concomitant medication in ex-smokers. Through enzyme induction, smoking is thought to increase the metabolism—and thus lower the blood levels—of drugs such as antipyrine, caffeine, phenacetin, imipramine, lidocaine, pentazocine, warfarin, theophylline, oxazepam, lorazepam, desmethyldiazepam, and estrogens. Smoking cessation may result in increased blood levels of these drugs, therefore requiring appropriate adaptation of dose. Smoking reduces the analgesic efficacy of propoxyphene. Absorption of subcutaneous insulin may be increased upon cessation of smoking.

Although the relevance to transdermal nicotine therapy is unknown, reported drug interactions with smoking which do not involve alteration of pharmacokinetics (e.g., enzyme induction) include: increased cortisol concentrations; increased circulating levels of catecholamines necessitating dose adjustments for adrenergic agonists (e.g., phenylephrine, isoproterenol), adrenergic α- and β- receptor antagonists, (e.g., prazosin and propranolol, respectively) and calcium channel blockers (e.g., nifedipine); reduced diuretic response to furosemide, and reduced clinical efficacy of H_2-antagonists.

Cessation of smoking may reverse these actions.

Contact Sensitization to Nicotine: Contact sensitization to nicotine has been reported in transdermal nicotine users. Smokers developing this contact sensitization should be cautioned against using nicotine-containing products. Delayed type hypersensitivity reactions (e.g., generalized urticaria, edema) or severe allergic reactions could result.

MRI Procedures: Habitrol patches should be removed prior to undergoing Magnetic Resonance Imaging (MRI) studies and/or MRI-guided procedures. Patches should be removed, regardless of the location of the patch, the anatomy being scanned, or the MRI device being used, in order to avoid the possibility of application site thermal burns, however infrequent or minor they may be.

ADVERSE EFFECTS: In principle, HABITROL (S(-)-nicotine) can cause adverse reactions similar to those associated with nicotine administered by smoking, or those that accompany tobacco withdrawal, especially in the GI and CNS systems. However, since the plasma S(-) nicotine concentrations reached with HABITROL are substantially lower and fluctuate less than those produced by smoking, nicotine related adverse reactions occurring during treatment with HABITROL can be expected to be less marked. If the user continues to smoke while wearing HABITROL, adverse reactions consistent with excessive nicotine exposure may be more frequent and more pronounced. Severe and fatal adverse reactions have occurred in smokers that continued to smoke while using nicotine transdermal systems. Smokers are strongly advised to stop smoking during HABITROL therapy, especially high risk smokers, as described in Warnings.

The most commonly reported adverse effect associated with HABITROL in clinical trials was skin reaction at the application site. This was responsible for about 6% of premature discontinuations and included symptoms such as erythema, pruritus, edema, burning sensation, blisters, rash and pinching. Most cases were mild in severity, usually resolving within 48 hours, but in more severe cases erythema and infiltration lasted 1 to 3 weeks. The majority of cases with notable symptoms of erythema (severity: well-defined, moderate or severe) and edema (severity: very slight, slight or moderate) occurred within 3-8 weeks. There have been isolated reports of skin reactions beyond the application site. The incidence of cutaneous hypersensitivity is 1.5-2.0%.

The most commonly reported adverse reactions/withdrawal symptoms reported (considered possibly related to HABITROL) in three double-blind trials, irrespective of causal association, were as follows: see Table 1.

Table 1: HABITROL

Most Commonly Reported Adverse Reactions/Withdrawal Symptoms

Body System	Adverse Event	HABITROL % (N=401)	Placebo % (N=391)
Central Nervous System	Headache	29.7	29.2
	Dizziness	6.0	5.9
	Insomnia	6.5	5.4
	Anxiety	3.7	4.6
	Emotional lability	2.2	2.8
	Irritability	2.2	2.8
	Abnormal dreaming	2.0	1.0
Respiratory, Ears, Nose and Throat	Cold and flu-like symptoms	12.0	8.4
	Pharyngitis	4.0	3.6
	Sinusitis	3.2	2.8
	Coughing	2.7	1.5
	Rhinitis	2.5	3.1
	Upper respiratory symptoms	2.2	2.3
Gastrointestinal System	Nausea	6.2	4.6
	Diarrhea	4.5	5.1
	Dyspepsia	5.2	4.4
	Abdominal pain	3.5	1.5
	Constipation	2.2	3.3
Musculoskeletal System	Myalgia	6.1	4.0
	Back pain	4.7	5.6
	Arthralgia	3.5	4.1
	Arthritis	2.0	1.0
Dermatological	Application site reaction	34.9	17.6
Miscellaneous	Dysmenorrhea	6.6	8.8
	Toothache	3.5	3.6
	Allergy	2.7	1.5

Adverse Events having an incidence of <2% (causality not established) were also reported as follows: see Table 2.

Incidence Rates: A - Incidence between 1-2%. B - Incidence ≤1%.

Table 2: HABITROL

Adverse Events Having an Incidence of <2%

Body System	A	B
CNS	Somnolence, impaired concentration	Taste perversion, abnormal vision, paresthesia, memory impairment, confusion, agitation, twitching
Respiratory, Ears, Nose and Throat	Bronchitis, earache	Dyspnea
Gastrointestinal System	Vomiting	Gastric ulcer, flatulence, abnormal stool, dysphagia
Cardiovascular System	Chest pain, blood pressure changes	Hot flushes, local edema, extra-systoles, palpitations, hypertension
Dermatological	Rash, herpetic rash	Pruritus, urticaria, acne
Oral Cavity		Dry mouth, gingivitis
Musculoskeletal System		Leg cramps
Miscellaneous	Fatigue	Angioneurotic edema, thyroid disorders, lymph gland tenderness, cytosis, increased appetite, increased sweating, migraine

OVERDOSE:

The toxicity of nicotine cannot be directly compared to that of smoking, since tobacco smoke contains additional toxic substances (e.g., carbon monoxide and tar).

Acute Toxic Effects:

The acute lethal oral dose of nicotine in non-smoking adults is about 40-60 mg. In children the following signs and symptoms have been reported after ingestion of tobacco products: vomiting, agitation, nausea, diarrhea, pallor, weakness, absence of reaction, and twitching of the extremities. In non-smoking adults the following signs and symptoms have been reported in cases of severe nicotine poisoning: pallor, sweating, nausea, salivation, vomiting, abdominal cramps, diarrhea, headache, dizziness, tremor, mental confusion, hearing and visual disturbances, muscular weakness, convulsions, prostration, absence of neurological reaction, and respiratory failure. Lethal doses quickly produce convulsions, and death follows as a result of cardiac failure or (more frequently) peripheral or central respiratory paralysis.

Chronic smoking causes the development of tolerance, which means that chronic smokers can tolerate acute, highly toxic doses of nicotine.

The application of several HABITROL (S(-)-nicotine) systems simultaneously, could result in serious overdosage. The effects of chewing and swallowing HABITROL are unknown.

Chronic Toxic Effects:
No experience has been obtained with HABITROL treatment longer than 3 months duration.

Management of Excessive Topical Exposure:
If the smoker shows signs of overdosage, HABITROL should be removed immediately. The skin may be washed with water only, as soap may facilitate absorption. Owing to a depot of nicotine in the skin, delivery of nicotine to the bloodstream will continue for several hours afterward.

Management of Nicotine Poisoning:
In cases of severe poisoning, the following measures are recommended: supportive measures for seizure control, warming the body to normal temperature, artificial respiration in respiratory failure, atropine for excessive bronchial secretions, and vigorous fluid support for pronounced hypotension or cardiovascular collapse.

> For management of a suspected drug overdose, CPhA recommends that you contact your **regional Poison Control Centre**. See the *CPS* Directory section for a list of Poison Control Centres.

DOSAGE: When starting treatment with HABITROL (S(-)-nicotine), the smoker should stop smoking completely.

One HABITROL system should be applied daily and left on the skin for 24 hours.

If the smoker has been unable to maintain or otherwise re-establish initial abstinence with the aid of HABITROL after one month, the treatment should be discontinued.

Prolonged continuous use of HABITROL should not exceed 3 months.

Treatment is divided into three components: selection and evaluation of an initial dosage strength, a maintenance phase and a weaning phase. Treatment should be completed in 8 weeks.

The dosage strengths employed, and the duration of use of each, depend upon the individual smoker's response. Tobacco withdrawal must be accompanied with behavioral support at all times.

Selection and Evaluation: Treatment is initiated with HABITROL 21 mg/day or 14 mg/day, depending on the number of cigarettes smoked per day. HABITROL 21 mg/day is usually recommended for smokers with a consumption of more than 10 cigarettes a day. HABITROL 14 mg/day is usually sufficient for smokers with a consumption of up to 10 cigarettes daily. The dosage strength may be adjusted early in the maintenance phase in response to either the appearance of side effects or difficulty in maintaining abstinence.

Maintenance (4 or 6 weeks): If the initial dosage selected was HABITROL 21 mg/day, these patches should be worn for a period of 4 weeks. If the initial dosage selected was HABITROL 14 mg/day, these should be used for a period of 6 weeks.

Weaning (2 or 4 weeks): The goal of a stepwise reduction from HABITROL 21 mg/day to the lowest dosage strength is accomplished by an intermediate step employing HABITROL 14 mg/day for 2 weeks, whereas HABITROL 7 mg/day is employed directly after maintenance on HABITROL 14 mg/day. HABITROL 7 mg/day, designed to reduce nicotine substitution towards the end of therapy and consolidate abstinence, should be worn for 2 weeks.

After completing treatment with HABITROL it is advisable for behavioral therapy to be continued.

No experience is available on treatment with HABITROL in smokers below the age of 18, and is limited in ages 65 years and above (see Warnings).

Administration: To avoid evaporative loss of nicotine, and as a matter of safety concerning accidental exposure of children and pets, the system should be applied promptly after its removal from the protective pouch. After removing the release liner (first the smaller strip and then the larger portion), the HABITROL system should be applied to a clean, oil-free, non-hairy, dry, intact area of skin on the trunk, or the upper outer arm. A different site of application should be chosen each day, and no site should be re-used within 1 week. The smoker should be advised that the system not be worn for longer than 24 hours, and to dispose of used systems out of the reach of children and pets. For detailed instructions, see Information for the Patient.

Note: Dosage adjustment cannot be achieved by cutting a transdermal system. This will cause the nicotine to evaporate rapidly, and render the pieces ineffective.

INFORMATION FOR THE PATIENT: Published in e-CPS, available by subscription at www.e-cps.ca.

SUPPLIED: See Table 3. Nonmedicinal ingredients: acrylate vinylacetate copolymers, fractionated coconut oil, methacrylic acid esters copolymers. Store below 25°C. Do not store unpouched. Apply immediately upon removal from the protective pouch.

Table 3: HABITROL

Dosage Forms

	HABITROL 7 mg/day	HABITROL 14 mg/day	HABITROL 21 mg/day
Average dose (mg) of S(-)-nicotine delivered in vivo during 24 hours	7	14	21
Content of S(-)nicotine (mg)	17.5	35	52.5
Drug releasing area (cm^2)	10	20	30
Printed code (on backing film)	Habitrol® 7MG	Habitrol® 14MG	Habitrol® 21MG

The total amount of S(-)-nicotine in the reservoir is needed to maintain the delivery pattern as required while the system is being worn.

Since the amount of S(-)-nicotine released from HABITROL per cm^2 is constant, the dose administered is determined solely by the size of the contact area of the system.

Safety Note Concerning Children: Nicotine is a highly toxic substance. Doses of nicotine that are tolerated by adults during treatment with HABITROL can produce severe symptoms of poisoning in small children (see Warnings). Even after use, HABITROL contains more than half its initial nicotine content. Therefore smokers must be cautioned that new and used systems must not be handled casually or left where they may be misused (by application), or ingested.

Similarly, care must also be taken when disposing of used systems (for detailed instructions see Information for the Patient).

Halcinonide ℞

CPhA Monograph

see *Corticosteroids: Topical*

Halobetasol ℞

CPhA Monograph

see *Corticosteroids: Topical*

Haloperidol ℞

haloperidol
haloperidol decanoate

Antipsychotic

CPhA Monograph

Date of Revision: October 2009

> This monograph has been compiled by CPhA and reviewed by experts. It may contain information different from that found in Health Canada-approved Product Monographs. The reader is referred to the *CPS* Editorial Policy for more information.

SUMMARY PRODUCT INFORMATION:

Route of Administration	Dosage Form	Strength
Oral	Tablet	0.5 mg, 1 mg, 2 mg, 5 mg, 10 mg
	Liquid	2 mg/mL
IM, IV	Immediate-acting injection	5 mg/mL
IM	Long-acting injection	50 mg/mL, 100 mg/mL

PHARMACOLOGY: Haloperidol is a butyrophenone derivative, classified as a high-potency first-generation antipsychotic agent. Haloperidol exhibits high affinity for dopamine D_2 receptors, which is the theoretical basis for its antipsychotic activity and extrapyramidal side effects. Haloperidol exhibits weak anticholinergic activity; its antiemetic effect has been attributed to dopamine blockade in the chemoreceptor trigger zone.

Pharmacokinetics: Haloperidol is well absorbed after oral administration. Peak plasma concentrations are achieved within 2 to 6 hours. Its elimination half-life is approximately 20 hours. Following im injection, peak concentrations occur within 10 to 20 minutes, with full pharmacologic effect in 30 to 45 minutes. Intramuscular injection of haloperidol decanoate is followed by gradual release of the drug from fatty tissues, prolonging its duration of action. Peak concentrations are reached in approximately one week. The apparent half-life of the decanoate injection is 3 weeks.

Haloperidol is approximately 92% bound to albumin and is metabolized mainly in the liver. It is a substrate and inhibitor of CYP3A4 and a substrate of CYP2D6. Haloperidol and its metabolites are excreted slowly in the urine and feces.

INDICATIONS: Haloperidol is indicated for:

- Management of psychotic disorders (e.g., schizophrenia)
- Management of Tourette's disorder
- Management of manic states

Haloperidol is also used in the management of acute agitation and delirium. It has also been used as an antiemetic, in the treatment of intractable hiccoughs and in the management of severe agitation in patients with acute alcohol withdrawal, although this use is not evidence-based and sedative-hypnotics such as benzodiazepines are preferred.

CONTRAINDICATIONS: Haloperidol is contraindicated in patients with hypersensitivity to haloperidol or any component of the formulation, and in patients with severe CNS depression, Parkinson's disease or coma.

WARNINGS: Tardive Dyskinesia: The use of haloperidol has been associated with the chronic, potentially irreversible movement disorder, tardive dyskinesia. Duration of use, daily dose and possibly total cumulative dose are important risk factors for the development of tardive dyskinesia, although it has occurred following as little as 6 months of continuous therapy. Other risk factors include age, history of acute extrapyramidal side effects, poor antipsychotic response to the drug and female gender. There is no standard treatment for tardive dyskinesia, although discontinuing the antipsychotic, when possible, may lead to remission of symptoms. Fine vermicular movements of the tongue may be an early sign of tardive dyskinesia. Discontinuing the drug when this occurs may prevent full onset of the syndrome.

Neuroleptic Malignant Syndrome: This potentially fatal syndrome characterized by muscle rigidity, fever/hyperthermia, labile blood pressure and fluctuating levels of consciousness, can occur in patients taking haloperidol and other antipsychotics. Dehydration is an additional risk factor. Patients need to be aware of the importance of adequate hydration, particularly in situations involving environmental exposure to extreme heat.

Sedation: Although haloperidol is less sedating than many first-generation antipsychotics, patients should be warned of potential sedative effects that could impair their ability to perform tasks requiring mental alertness.

PRECAUTIONS: Because of its potential to cause orthostatic hypotension through alpha adrenergic blockade, haloperidol should be used with caution in patients with cardiovascular disease. Orthostasis can occur in any patient, but older individuals, patients with diabetes and those with pre-existing cardiovascular disease may be more susceptible.

Haloperidol may lower the seizure threshold and should be used with caution in patients with a seizure disorder or a history of drug-induced seizures, abnormal EEG or head trauma.

Haloperidol should be used with caution in patients with thyrotoxicosis as severe neurotoxicity has occurred with antipsychotic therapy in these patients.

The need for continued therapy should be frequently re-evaluated, particularly when haloperidol is used in elderly patients for behavioral symptoms. Long-term use of haloperidol is more likely than short-term use to be associated with onset of dyskinesias, sometimes indistinguishable from tardive dyskinesia, on abrupt withdrawal of the drug. Gradual discontinuation of the drug is recommended when possible, although it has not been proven to prevent withdrawal emergent dyskinetic movements.

Haloperidol should be used with caution in patients with severe hepatic or renal impairment.

Drug Interactions: Additive sedative effects may occur if haloperidol is used concurrently with other CNS depressants such as alcohol, benzodiazepines or opioids.

Concomitant therapy with inducers of CYP3A4 (such as phenytoin or rifampin) may increase the clearance and decrease the effect of haloperidol.

Inhibitors of CYP2D6 or CYP3A4 (e.g., erythromycin, fluoxetine, fluvoxamine, itraconazole, ketoconazole, paroxetine, quinidine) may decrease the clearance of haloperidol and potentiate its pharmacologic and adverse effects.

Some patients have experienced neurotoxicity (e.g., delirium, seizures) during concomitant therapy with haloperidol and lithium, especially when higher than usual doses were used. Patients should be monitored for signs of neurotoxicity if the two drugs are used concurrently.

Haloperidol may antagonize the effects of dopamine agonists such as levodopa.

Food Interactions: Oral liquid formulations should not be mixed with coffee or tea as a precipitate may form.

Children: Safety and efficacy have not been established for children under 3 years of age.

Pregnancy: There have been some reports of limb defects in infants exposed to haloperidol in the first trimester. Infants exposed at any point during gestation should be observed for possible extrapyramidal effects. The decision to use haloperidol during pregnancy should be based on whether the expected benefit of therapy justifies the potential risk to the exposed fetus.

Lactation: Haloperidol is excreted in breast milk, with a milk to plasma concentration ratio of approximately 0.65. Cases of decline in mental and psychomotor development at 12-18 mos have been reported in babies whose mothers took 20-40 mg/day while breast-feeding. Caution is recommended when haloperidol is used in breast-feeding mothers; use the lowest effective dose, monitor infant's developmental progress and watch for adverse effects such as drowsiness or lethargy. It may be advisable not to breast-feed when taking high doses.

Occupational Hazards: See Warnings.

ADVERSE EFFECTS: Cardiovascular: Many antipsychotics, including haloperidol, can cause prolongation of the QTc interval which is associated with the potentially lethal arrhythmia, torsades de pointes. Recurrent syncope, ventricular fibrillation and sudden cardiac death can occur with torsades de pointes. Risk factors for drug-induced QTc prolongation include interaction with other drugs that can prolong the QTc, diabetes, obesity, hypokalemia and congenital long QT syndrome.

CNS: (See also Warnings, Neuroleptic Malignant Syndrome): Haloperidol, like other high-potency first-generation antipsychotics, has a relatively high propensity to cause extrapyramidal side effects such as dystonias (briefly sustained or fixed abnormal movements), akathisia (restlessness) or parkinsonism (e.g., tremor, muscle rigidity, slow movement, blunted or flat affect).

Although haloperidol has a lower propensity than many other antipsychotics to cause anticholinergic side effects such as dry mouth, constipation and urinary retention, these symptoms can emerge when haloperidol is used concurrently with other drugs that have anticholinergic activity.

Haloperidol may lower the seizure threshold, although this occurs more commonly with low-potency antipsychotics.

Hematologic: Mild and transient leukopenia can occur with haloperidol and other antipsychotics. Agranulocytosis is a rare side effect of antipsychotics. If patients taking haloperidol present with sore throat, leukoplakia, erythema, ulcerations of the pharynx, usually within the first 8 weeks of therapy, a white blood cell count should be obtained.

Endocrine: Haloperidol can cause hyperprolactinemia, leading to symptoms such as breast engorgement and lactation, sexual dysfunction, mastalgia or gynecomastia in some patients. Hypoglycemia is a rare side effect.

Ophthalmologic: Although haloperidol has a mild anticholinergic effect, the possibility of increased intraocular pressure should be considered when haloperidol is used with other drugs with anticholinergic properties.

OVERDOSE:

Symptoms: Symptoms of haloperidol overdose can include extrapyramidal symptoms such as akathisia, dystonic reactions or parkinsonian effects, seizures, hypotension, hypokalemia, altered temperature regulation, arrhythmias, respiratory depression and coma. Neuroleptic malignant syndrome can occur at therapeutic or toxic doses (see Warnings).

Treatment: Do not induce vomiting as the gag reflex may be impaired. Management includes administration of activated charcoal and supportive measures such as maintaining ventilation and monitoring vital signs and renal function. Acute extrapyramidal reactions may respond to the iv administration of an anticholinergic agent such as benztropine or diphenhydramine. Lorazepam, propranolol or an anticholinergic agent may be useful for akathisia. Seizures may be treated with a benzodiazepine such as diazepam. Hypotension can be managed with vasopressors such as norepinephrine, if unresponsive to iv fluids and positioning. Ventricular arrhythmias may respond to sodium bicarbonate and/or lidocaine. If torsades de pointes is present, magnesium or a pacemaker may be effective. Neuroleptic malignant syndrome is usually managed with cooling blankets, cool mist and/or fans for hyperthermia, benzodiazepines and/or dantrolene for muscle rigidity, and hydration.

Hemodialysis, peritoneal dialysis and forced diuresis are not effective in enhancing elimination of haloperidol.

> For management of a suspected drug overdose, CPhA recommends that you contact your **regional Poison Control Centre**. See the *CPS* Directory section for a list of Poison Control Centres.

DOSAGE: Oral: Adults: Psychosis or Tourette's disorder: Initial daily dose is 1.5 to 3 mg, increasing gradually to a usual maintenance dose of 4 to 12 mg daily, in 1 to 2 divided doses. The usual maximum daily dose is 20 mg. In elderly patients, a starting dose of 0.5 to 1 mg daily is recommended.

For behavioral symptoms in elderly patients with dementia, an initial dose of 0.25 to 0.5 mg once or twice daily has been suggested.

Children: 3-12 years (15-40 kg): Initial dose is 0.25 to 0.5 mg/day in 2 to 3 divided doses, increasing by 0.25 to 0.5 mg daily, at intervals of 5 to 7 days, to a maximum of 0.15 mg/kg/day. Usual maintenance dose for psychotic disorders is 0.05 to 0.15 mg/kg/day in 2 to 3 divided doses; for Tourette's disorder, 0.05 to 0.075 mg/kg/day in 2 to 3 divided doses.

Oral haloperidol should be administered with food or milk to avoid GI irritation; the oral concentrate can be mixed with water or an acidic beverage such as juice but should not be mixed with tea or coffee.

IM: Adults: For acute psychosis with agitation/aggression, haloperidol can be administered im at a dose of 2 to 5 mg, in combination with lorazepam. The two drugs can be administered in the same syringe and given as often as every hour, until the patient responds. The usual daily maximum dose of 20 mg applies. For elderly patients, begin with 0.5 to 1 mg haloperidol per dose; it is rarely necessary to go beyond a total of 5 mg.

Long-acting haloperidol decanoate injection is usually administered every 4 weeks in the management of chronic psychotic disorders. The initial dose is approximately 10 to 15 times the previous daily oral dose, with subsequent titration to determine the lowest effective and tolerated dose. The usual range is 50 to 200 mg every 4 weeks. Short-acting preparations may be required for supplementation while dosage titration is taking place.

IV: Adults: Haloperidol has been administered iv in patients with delirium, at a dose of 1 to 2 mg every 2 to 4 hours. In elderly patients a lower dose of 0.25 to 0.5 mg is suggested. Haloperidol decanoate is **not** to be administered iv.

Haloperidol Injection USP ℞
haloperidol
Antipsychotic

Sandoz

Haloperidol LA ℞
haloperidol decanoate
Antipsychotic

Sandoz

SUPPLIED: Haloperidol Injection USP: Each mL contains: haloperidol 5 mg, lactic acid to adjust pH and water for injection USP. Preservative-free. Ampoules of 1 mL, boxes of 10. Store below 40°C, preferably between 15 and 30°C. Protect from light. Protect from freezing.

Haloperidol LA: 50 mg/mL: Each mL of slightly amber, slightly viscous solution contains: haloperidol decanoate 70.52 mg equivalent to haloperidol 50 mg, benzyl alcohol 1.2% v/v as preservative and sesame oil. Multidose vials of 5 mL, boxes of 1.

100 mg/mL: Each mL of slightly amber, slightly viscous solution contains: haloperidol decanoate 141.04 mg equivalent to haloperidol 100 mg, benzyl alcohol 1.2% v/v as preservative and sesame oil. Ampoules of 1 mL, boxes of 3. Multidose vials of 5 mL, boxes of 1.

Store between 15 and 30°C. Protect from light. As with other depot neuroleptics, precipitation may occur if the drug is stored for long periods in the cold. The precipitate should clear on storage at room temperature.

Havrix®
hepatitis A vaccine inactivated
Active Immunization Agent against infection by Hepatitis A virus

GlaxoSmithKline

Date of Revision: October 15, 2008

SUMMARY PRODUCT INFORMATION:

Route of Administration	Dosage Form/ Strength	Clinically Relevant Nonmedicinal Ingredients
Intramuscular Injection	Sterile suspension for injection/HAVRIX 1440 contains: 1440 ELISA units per 1.0 mL of formaldehyde-inactivated hepatitis A virus (HM175 hepatitis A virus strain); HAVRIX 720 Junior contains: 720 ELISA units per 0.5 mL of formaldehyde-inactivated hepatitis A virus (HM175 hepatitis A virus strain).	Aluminum hydroxide, amino acids for injection, disodium phosphate, monopotassium phosphate, neomycin sulphate, polysorbate 20, potassium chloride, sodium chloride and water for injection

DESCRIPTION: HAVRIX (hepatitis A vaccine, inactivated) is a sterile suspension containing formaldehyde-inactivated hepatitis A virus (HM175 hepatitis A virus strain) adsorbed onto aluminum hydroxide.

INDICATIONS AND CLINICAL USE: HAVRIX (hepatitis A vaccine, inactivated) is indicated for:

- active immunization against hepatitis A virus (HAV) infection in subjects at risk of exposure to HAV.

HAVRIX will not prevent hepatitis infection caused by other agents such as hepatitis B virus, hepatitis C virus, hepatitis E virus or other pathogens known to infect the liver.

In areas of **low to intermediate prevalence** of hepatitis A, immunization with HAVRIX is particularly recommended in subjects who are, or will be, at increased risk of infection such as:

Travelers: Persons traveling to areas where the prevalence of hepatitis A is high. These areas include Africa, Asia, the Mediterranean basin, the Middle East, Central and South America.

Armed Forces: Armed Forces personnel who travel to higher endemicity areas or to areas where hygiene is poor have an increased risk of HAV infection. Active immunization is indicated for these individuals.

Persons for whom Hepatitis A is an Occupational Hazard: These include employees in day-care centres, nursing, medical and paramedical personnel in hospitals and institutions, especially gastroenterology and pediatric units, sewage workers, and food handlers, among others.

Persons for whom there is an Increased Risk of Transmission of Hepatitis A: e.g. homosexuals, persons with multiple sexual partners, abusers of injectable drugs, hemophiliac patients.

Contacts of Infected Persons: Since virus shedding of infected persons may occur for a prolonged period, active immunization of close contacts is recommended.

Specific Population Groups known to have Higher Incidence of Hepatitis A: e.g. North American Indians, Inuits, recognized community-wide HAV epidemics.

Subjects with chronic liver disease or who are at risk of developing chronic liver disease: e.g. Hepatitis B (HB) and Hepatitis C (HC) chronic carriers and alcohol abusers. Hepatitis A tends to compromise the outcome of chronic liver disease.

In areas of **intermediate to high prevalence** of hepatitis A (e.g. Africa, Asia, the Mediterranean basin, the Middle East, Central and South America) susceptible individuals may be considered for active immunization.

CONTRAINDICATIONS: HAVRIX (hepatitis A vaccine, inactivated) should not be administered:

- to subjects with known hypersensitivity to any component of the vaccine preparation or component of the container, or to subjects having shown signs of hypersensitivity after previous HAVRIX administration. For a complete listing, see Dosage Forms, Composition and Packaging.

As with other vaccines, the administration of HAVRIX should be postponed in subjects with severe febrile illness. The presence of a minor infection however, is not a contraindication.

WARNINGS AND PRECAUTIONS: General: As with other injectable vaccines, appropriate medication (e.g. adrenaline) should be readily available for immediate use in case of anaphylaxis or anaphylactoid reactions following administration of the vaccine. For this reason, the vaccinee should remain under medical supervision for 30 minutes after immunization.

Hematologic: HAVRIX (hepatitis A vaccine, inactivated) should be administered with caution to subjects with thrombocytopenia or a bleeding disorder since bleeding may occur following an intramuscular administration to these subjects.

Immune: It is possible that subjects may be in the incubation period of hepatitis A infection at the time of immunization. It is not known whether HAVRIX will prevent hepatitis A in such cases.

Since there is a possibility that the vaccine may contain trace amounts of neomycin, the possibility of an allergic reaction in individuals sensitive to this substance should be kept in mind when considering the use of this vaccine (see Dosage Forms, Composition and Packaging).

As with other vaccines, subjects with an impaired immune system may not obtain adequate antibody titres after the primary immunization course. Such patients may require administration of additional doses of HAVRIX. However, no specific dosing recommendations can be made at this time.

Renal: As with other vaccines, hemodialysis patients may not obtain adequate antibody titres after the primary immunization course. Such patients may require administration of additional doses of HAVRIX. However, no specific dosing recommendations can be made at this time.

Special Populations: Pregnant Women: Animal reproduction studies and adequate human data on use during pregnancy are not available. However, as with all inactivated viral vaccines, the risks to the fetus are considered to be negligible. HAVRIX should be used during pregnancy only when clearly needed.

Nursing Women: Animal reproduction studies and adequate human data on use during lactation are not available. Therefore, caution should be exercised if HAVRIX is to be administered to breast feeding women.

ADVERSE REACTIONS: Clinical Trial Adverse Drug Reactions: Because clinical trials are conducted under very specific conditions the adverse reaction rates observed in the clinical trials may not reflect the rates observed in practice and should not be compared to the rates in the clinical trials of another drug. Adverse drug reaction information from clinical trials is useful for identifying drug-related adverse events and for approximating rates.

The safety profile presented in Table 1 is based on data from more than 5300 subjects.

Table 1: HAVRIX

Safety Profile

Frequency of doses	Adverse Event	System/Organ Class
Very Common ≥10%	Irritability	Psychiatric disorders
	Headache	Nervous system disorders
	Pain and redness at the injection site, fatigue	General disorders and administration site conditions
Common ≥1% and <10%	Appetite loss	Metabolism and nutrition disorders
	Drowsiness	Nervous system disorders
	Gastrointestinal symptoms (such as nausea, vomiting, diarrhea)	Gastrointestinal disorders
	Swelling at the injection site, malaise, injection site reaction (such as induration), fever (≥37.5°C)	General disorders and administration site conditions
Uncommon ≥0.1% and <1%	Upper respiratory tract infection, rhinitis	Infections and infestations
	Dizziness	Nervous system disorders
	Rash	Skin and subcutaneous tissue disorders
	Myalgia, musculoskeletal stiffness	Musculoskeletal and connective tissue disorders
	Influenza-like illness	General disorders and administration site conditions
Rare ≥0.01% and <0.1%	Hypoaesthesia, paraesthesia	Nervous system disorders
	Pruritus	Skin and subcutaneous tissue disorders
	Chills	General disorders and administration site conditions

Post-Market Adverse Drug Reactions: The following adverse reactions have been reported with HAVRIX (see Table 2).

DRUG INTERACTIONS: Overview: Since HAVRIX is an inactivated vaccine, its concomitant use with other inactivated vaccines is unlikely to result in interference with immune responses. When concomitant administration of other vaccines is considered necessary, the vaccines must be given with different syringes and at different injection sites.

Clinical experiences with the concomitant administration of HAVRIX and the recombinant hepatitis B virus vaccine, ENGERIX-B, has been satisfactory. No interference in the respective immune responses to both antigens has been observed.

Concomitant administration of typhoid, yellow fever, cholera (injectable) or tetanus does not interfere with HAVRIX immune response.

HAVRIX must not be mixed with other vaccines.

Drug-Drug Interactions: The concomitant administration of HAVRIX (hepatitis A vaccine, inactivated) and immune globulin (human) does not influence the seroconversion rate, but may result in a relatively lower anti-HAV antibody titre than when the vaccine is given alone. HAVRIX and immune globulin (human) should be administered at separate injection sites.

Drug-Food Interactions: Interactions with food have not been established.

Drug-Herb Interactions: Interactions with herbal products have not been established.

Drug-Laboratory Test Interactions: Interactions with laboratory tests have not been established.

Table 2: HAVRIX

Post-Market Adverse Reactions

Immune System Disorders	Anaphylaxis, allergic reactions including anaphylactoid reactions and mimicking serum sickness
Nervous System Disorders	Convulsions
Vascular Disorders	Vasculitis
Skin and Subcutaneous Tissue Disorders	Angioneurotic oedema, urticaria, erythema multiforme
Musculoskeletal and Connective Tissue Disorders	Arthralgia

DOSAGE AND ADMINISTRATION: Recommended Dose and Dosage Adjustment: Primary Immunization: Adults from 19 years onwards: A single dose of HAVRIX 1440 (hepatitis A vaccine, inactivated) (1.0 mL suspension) is used for primary immunization.

Children and adolescents from 1 year up to and including 18 years of age: A single dose of HAVRIX 720 Junior (0.5 mL suspension) is used for primary immunization. If a pediatric vial is not available, a pediatric dose of 0.5 mL may be withdrawn from the HAVRIX 1440 vial.

Booster Dose: A booster dose is recommended at any time between 6 and 12 months after a single dose of HAVRIX 1440 or HAVRIX 720 Junior in order to ensure long-term protection.

Long-term persistence of serum antibodies to hepatitis A virus after vaccination with HAVRIX is under evaluation. Nevertheless, data available after 5 years show persistence of antibodies which is consistent with a projected 20 years persistence (based on mathematical calculations).

Concomitant Administration with Immune Globulin (human): Concomitant administration of HAVRIX and immune globulin (human) may be considered when a subject is at risk of being exposed to hepatitis A before adequate anti-HAV antibody titres can be reached.

Administration: HAVRIX should be injected **intramuscularly** in the deltoid region in adults and children, in the antero-lateral part of the thigh in young children up to 2 years of age. The vaccine **should not** be administered intramuscularly in the gluteal region or subcutaneously/intradermally since administration by these routes may result in a less than optimal anti-HAV antibody response.

As with all parenterals, vaccine products should be inspected visually for any foreign particulate matter and/or discolouration prior to administration. Before use of HAVRIX, the vial/syringe should be well shaken to obtain a slightly opaque, white suspension. Discard the vaccine if the contents of the vial/syringe appear otherwise.

The vaccine must be used as supplied.

Syringe Instructions: Do not remove the white back-stop from the syringe. Prior to administration, ensure that the plunger rod is firmly attached to the rubber stopper by turning the plunger clockwise until slight resistance is felt. Do not over tighten. Remove syringe LUER Tip-cap and needle cap. Attach needle by pressing and twisting in a clockwise rotation until secured to the syringe.

HAVRIX should never be administered intravenously.

OVERDOSAGE:

Cases of overdose have been reported during post-marketing surveillance. Adverse events reported following overdosage were similar to those reported with normal vaccine administration.

> For management of a suspected drug overdose, CPhA recommends that you contact your **regional Poison Control Centre**. See the *CPS* Directory section for a list of Poison Control Centres.

ACTION AND CLINICAL PHARMACOLOGY: Mechanism of Action: HAVRIX (hepatitis A vaccine, inactivated) confers immunity against hepatitis A virus (HAV) infection by inducing the production of specific anti-HAV antibodies.

In clinical studies involving subjects of 18-50 years of age, specific humoral antibodies against HAV were detected in more than 88% of vaccinees at day 15 and 99% at month 1 following administration of a single dose of HAVRIX 1440 (hepatitis A vaccine, inactivated).

In clinical studies involving subjects of 1-18 years of age, specific humoral antibodies against HAV were detected in more than 93% of vaccinees at day 15 and 99% of vaccines one month following administration of HAVRIX 720 Junior.

Results of hepatitis A outbreak control program showed a substantial drop in symptomatic cases in 4930 vaccinees within 3 weeks of receiving 1 dose of hepatitis A vaccine. In villages where more than 70% of estimated susceptible individuals were vaccinated, a dramatic drop in the number of symptomatic cases of disease was observed within 8 weeks of vaccination.

The mean titre of anti-HAV antibodies induced by HAVRIX is at least 3 times higher than the maximum observed after passive immunization using immune globulin (human). In a randomly selected subset of subjects, vaccine induced anti-HAV antibodies were shown to be qualitatively indistinguishable from immune globulin (human) anti-HAV antibodies.

To obtain long-term immunity a booster dose is recommended at any time between 6 and 12 months after primary vaccination with HAVRIX 1440 Adult or HAVRIX 720 Junior, to induce long-term antibody titres.

Long-term persistence of serum antibodies to hepatitis A virus after vaccination with HAVRIX is under evaluation. Nevertheless, data available after 5 years show persistence of antibodies which is consistent with a projected 20 years persistence (based on mathematical calculations).

Primates exposed to the virulent heterologous hepatitis A strain were vaccinated 2 days after exposure. This post exposure vaccination resulted in total protection of the animals.

STORAGE AND STABILITY: The vaccine should not be used beyond the expiry date stamped on the vial or syringe.

HAVRIX (hepatitis A vaccine, inactivated) must be stored at 2 to 8°C.

Do not freeze; discard if vaccine has been frozen.

INFORMATION FOR THE PATIENT: Published in e-CPS, available by subscription at www.e-cps.ca.

DOSAGE FORMS, COMPOSITION AND PACKAGING: HAVRIX (hepatitis A vaccine, inactivated) is available as HAVRIX 1440 (1440 ELISA Units/mL) and HAVRIX 720 Junior (720 ELISA Units/0.5 mL) suspension for injection.

HAVRIX is a sterile suspension containing formaldehyde-inactivated hepatitis A virus (HM175 hepatitis A virus strain) adsorbed onto aluminum hydroxide.

The virus is propagated in MRC5 human diploid cells. Before viral extraction, the cells are extensively washed to remove culture medium constituents. A virus suspension is then obtained by lysis of the cells followed by purification using ultrafiltration techniques and gel chromatography. Inactivation of the virus is assured by treatment with formalin. The viral antigen content of HAVRIX is determined by an ELISA test.

The virus is adsorbed on aluminum (0.5 mg/1.0 mL adult dose, 0.25 mg/0.5 mL pediatric dose) in the form of aluminum hydroxide. Nonmedicinal ingredients: aluminum hydroxide, amino acids for injection, disodium phosphate, monopotassium phosphate, neomycin sulphate (less than 10 ng for HAVRIX 720 Junior; less than 20 ng for HAVRIX 1440), polysorbate 20, potassium chloride, sodium chloride, water for injection.

HAVRIX meets the World Health Organization requirement for biological substances including those for final vaccine residual bovine serum albumin.

Havrix 720 Junior: single dose vials of 0.5 mL, packages of 1 and 10. Single dose prefilled syringes of 0.5 mL, packages of 1.
Havrix 1440: single dose vials of 1 mL, packages of 1, 10 and 25. Single dose prefilled syringes of 1 mL, packages of 1.

Helixate® FS

antihemophilic factor (recombinant)

Coagulation Factor

CSL Behring

Date of Revision: January 27, 2010

SUMMARY PRODUCT INFORMATION:

Route of Administration	Dosage Form/ Strength	Clinically Relevant Nonmedicinal Ingredients
Intravenous	Lyophilized powder for injection 250, 500, 1000, 2000, 3000 IU/vial	Sucrose, glycine, histidine, calcium chloride, sodium, chloride, polysorbate 80 For a complete listing see Dosage Forms, Composition and Packaging.

DESCRIPTION: HELIXATE FS is a sterile, stable, purified, nonpyrogenic, dried product, which has been manufactured by recombinant DNA technology.

INDICATIONS AND CLINICAL USE: HELIXATE FS (Antihemophilic Factor [Recombinant]) is indicated for the treatment of classical hemophilia (hemophilia A), in which there is a demonstrated deficiency of activity of the plasma clotting factor, factor VIII (FVIII). HELIXATE FS provides a means of temporarily replacing the missing clotting factor in order to correct or prevent bleeding episodes, or in order to perform emergency or elective surgery in hemophiliacs.

When used as a regular prophylactic treatment, HELIXATE FS is also indicated to prevent the occurrence of spontaneous hemorrhagic episodes and to prevent joint damage in children with no pre-existing joint damage.

Because HELIXATE FS showed comparable biological activity to other FVIII preparations, it should be used in the same manner as HELIXATE (Antihemophilic Factor [Recombinant]). This includes treatment of bleeding in certain patients with inhibitors to FVIII. In clinical studies of HELIXATE, some patients who developed inhibitors on study continued to manifest a clinical response when inhibitor titres were less than 10 Bethesda Units (B.U.) per mL. When an inhibitor is present, the dosage requirement for FVIII is variable. The dosage can be determined only by clinical response and by monitoring of circulating FVIII levels after treatment (see Dosage and Administration).

HELIXATE FS does not contain von Willebrand Factor and therefore, is not indicated for the treatment of von Willebrand disease.

Geriatrics (>65 years of age): Clinical studies with HELIXATE FS did not include sufficient numbers of patients aged 65 and over to be able to determine whether they respond differently from younger patients. However, clinical experience with HELIXATE and other FVIII products has not identified differences between the elderly and younger patients. As with any patient receiving HELIXATE FS, dose selection for an elderly patient should be individualized.

Pediatrics (<18 years of age): HELIXATE FS is appropriate for use in pediatric patients. Safety and efficacy studies have been performed in two studies (n=60) in less than 4 year old previously untreated and minimally treated pediatric patients.

HELIXATE FS is comparable to HELIXATE (Antihemophilic Factor [Recombinant]) in its biological activity and should be used in the same manner as HELIXATE.

CONTRAINDICATIONS:

- Patients who are hypersensitive to this drug or to any ingredient in the formulation or component of the container. For a complete listing, see Dosage Forms, Composition and Packaging.
- Known hypersensitivity to mouse or hamster protein.

WARNINGS AND PRECAUTIONS:

> **Serious Warnings and Precautions**
> The development of circulating neutralizing antibodies to FVIII may occur during the treatment of patients with hemophilia A (see Warnings and Precautions, Immune).

General: HELIXATE FS (Antihemophilic Factor [Recombinant]) is intended for the treatment of bleeding disorders arising from a deficiency in FVIII. This deficiency should be proven prior to administering HELIXATE FS.

Reconstitution, product administration, and handling of the administration set and needles must be done with caution. Percutaneous puncture with a needle contaminated with blood can transmit infectious viruses including HIV (AIDS) and hepatitis. Obtain immediate medical attention if injury occurs. Place needles in a sharps container after single use. Discard all equipment, including any reconstituted HELIXATE FS product in accordance with biohazard procedures.

Immune: The development of circulating neutralizing antibodies to FVIII may occur during the treatment of patients with hemophilia A. Inhibitor formation is especially common in young children with severe hemophilia during their first years of treatment or in patients of any age who have received little previous treatment with FVIII. Nonetheless, inhibitor formation may occur at any time in the treatment of a patient with hemophilia A. Patients treated with any rFVIII preparation, including rFVIII-FS, should be carefully monitored for the development of antibodies to rFVIII by appropriate clinical observation and laboratory tests, according to the recommendation of the patient's hemophilia treatment centre. In a clinical study about the use of continuous infusion in surgeries, heparin was used to prevent thrombophlebitis at the infusion site, as with any other long-term intravenous infusions.

Among patients treated with antihemophilic factor products, cases of hypotension, urticaria, and chest tightness in association with hypersensitivity reactions have been reported in the literature. Very rare cases of allergic and anaphylactic reactions have been reported with the predecessor product HELIXATE (Antihemophilic Factor [Recombinant]), particularly in very young patients or patients who have previously reacted to other FVIII products (see Adverse Reactions, Post-Market Adverse Drug Reactions). Serious anaphylactic reactions require immediate emergency treatment with resuscitative measures such as the administration of epinephrine and oxygen.

In clinical studies, HELIXATE FS has been used in the treatment of bleeding episodes in 37 previously untreated patients (PUPs) and 23 minimally treated pediatric patients ([MTP], defined as having equal to or less than 4 exposure days). Bleeding episodes were treated effectively with 1 or 2 infusions of rFVIII-FS. Overall, 9 out of 60 (15%) patients developed inhibitors. This included 5 out of 37 (14%) PUP and 4 out of 23 (17%) MTP patients treated with HELIXATE FS: overall 6 out of 60 (10%) with a titer above 10 BU and 3 out of 60 (5%) with a titer below 10 BU. The median number of exposure days at the time of inhibitor detection in these patients was 9 days (range: 3-18 days).

The median number of exposure days in the clinical studies was 114 (range: 4-478). Four of the five patients, who had not achieved 20 exposure days at the end of the study, ultimately achieved more than 20 exposure days in poststudy follow-up and 1 of them developed a low titer inhibitor. The fifth patient was lost to follow-up.

Formation of Antibodies to Mouse and Hamster Protein: Assays to detect seroconversion to mouse and hamster protein were conducted on all patients in clinical studies. None of the patients developed specific antibodies to these proteins following study enrollment and no animal protein associated serious allergic reactions have been observed with rFVIII-FS infusions. Although no such reactions were observed, patients should be made aware of the possibility of a hypersensitivity reaction to mouse and/or hamster protein and alerted to the early signs of such a reaction (e.g., hives, localized or generalized urticaria, wheezing and hypotension). Patients should be advised to discontinue use of the product and contact their physician if such symptoms occur.

Special Populations: Pregnant Women: Animal reproduction studies have not been conducted with HELIXATE FS. It is also not known whether HELIXATE FS can cause fetal harm when administered to a pregnant woman or whether it affects reproduction capacity. HELIXATE FS should not be used during pregnancy unless the benefits clearly outweigh any potential risks.

Nursing Women: HELIXATE FS should not be used during lactation unless the benefits clearly outweigh any potential risks.

Pediatrics (<18 years of age): HELIXATE FS is appropriate for use in pediatric patients. Safety and efficacy studies have been performed in two studies (n=60) in less than 4 year old previously untreated and minimally treated pediatric patients.

HELIXATE FS is comparable to HELIXATE (Antihemophilic Factor [Recombinant]) in its biological activity and should be used in the same manner as HELIXATE.

Geriatrics (>65 years of age): Clinical studies with HELIXATE FS did not include sufficient numbers of patients aged 65 and over to be able to determine whether they respond differently from younger patients. However, clinical experience with HELIXATE and other FVIII products has not identified differences between the elderly and younger patients. As with any patient receiving HELIXATE FS, dose selection for an elderly patient should be individualized.

Monitoring and Laboratory Tests: The clinical effect of HELIXATE FS is the most important element in evaluating the effectiveness of treatment. It may be necessary to administer more HELIXATE FS than would be estimated in order to attain satisfactory clinical results. If the calculated dose fails to attain the expected FVIII levels or if bleeding is not controlled after administration of the calculated dosage, the presence of a circulating inhibitor in the patient should be suspected. Its presence should be substantiated and the inhibitor level quantitated by appropriate laboratory tests. When an inhibitor is present, the dosage requirement for rFVIII-FS is extremely variable and the dosage can be determined only by the clinical response.

ADVERSE REACTIONS: Adverse Drug Reaction Overview: During the clinical studies conducted in previously treated patients, 109 adverse events were reported out of a total 73 patients infused. Only 13 events were considered to be at least remotely related to rFVIII-FS administration; the relationship of another 7 events to rFVIII-FS administration was non-assessable. Thus, 20 events in 11 patients were considered to be either non-assessable or at least remotely related to rFVIII-FS administration for an incidence of 0.5% relative to the number of infusions administered. Events which were at least remotely drug-related included local site reactions (2), dizziness (2), rash (2), unusual taste in the mouth (2), increased blood pressure (1), pruritus (1), depersonalization/"feeling funny" (1), nausea (1) and rhinitis (1). In clinical studies with 73 previously-treated patients ([PTP], defined as having more than 100 exposure days) followed over four years, no de novo inhibitors were observed.

In clinical studies with previously untreated patients (PUPs) and minimally treated (MTP) pediatric patients, 18 adverse events were reported by the clinical investigators as at least possibly related to the study drug including the expected complication of inhibitor development in 8 patients (included in the 9 patients above), a forearm bleed following venipuncture, constipation, adenopathy, rash, anemia and pallor in one inhibitor patient with gastroenteritis, and serous otitis media. See Table 1.

Table 1: HELIXATE FS

Adverse Drug Reactions

Blood and Lymphatic System Disorders	Factor VIII inhibition
Gastrointestinal Disorders	Dysgeusia
	Nausea
General Disorders and Administration Site Conditions	Injection site reaction
Immune System Disorders	Allergic/anaphylactic reaction
Investigations	Blood pressure abnormal
Nervous System Disorders	Dizziness
Skin and Subcutaneous Tissue Disorders	Rash
	Pruritus

Post-Market Adverse Drug Reactions: The following events are principally derived from post-marketing experience and publications and accurate rate estimates are generally not possible. Among patients treated with its predecessor product HELIXATE (Antihemophilic Factor [Recombinant]), very rare cases of serious allergic reactions and anaphylactic reactions have been reported, particularly in very young patients or patients who have previously reacted to other FVIII products. Individual cases of hypotension have been very rarely reported. Rare cases of urticaria have also been reported. Although such serious reactions have not been reported with the use of HELIXATE FS, it is likely that these may also occur. Rare cases of dyspnea have been reported with HELIXATE FS.

In extensive postregistration studies with HELIXATE FS involving more than 1000 patients, the following was observed: less than 0.2% PTPs developed de novo inhibitors. In a subset defined as having less than 20 exposure days at study entry, less than 11% developed de novo inhibitors.

DRUG INTERACTIONS: Drug-Drug Interactions: HELIXATE FS is a recombinant version of FVIII, a physiological human protein. Besides the known interactions of FVIII with other coagulation proteins, no other interactions with other drugs have been established.

Drug-Food Interactions: Interactions with food have not been established.

Drug-Herb Interactions: Interactions with herbal preparations have not been established.

Drug-Laboratory Test Interactions: There are no known laboratory interactions.

DOSAGE AND ADMINISTRATION: Dosing Considerations: Each bottle of HELIXATE FS (Antihemophilic Factor [Recombinant]) has the rFVIII-FS potency in international units stated on the label based on the one-stage assay methodology.

The reconstituted product must be administered intravenously by direct syringe injection. The product must be administered within 3 hours after reconstitution. It is recommended to use a microbore tubing administration set to minimize losses of product due to adsorption and volume retention. HELIXATE FS should not be mixed with other medicinal products or infusion solutions.

Recommended Dose and Dosage Adjustment: The dosages described below are presented as general guidance. It should be emphasized that the dosage of HELIXATE FS required for hemostasis must be individualized according to the needs of the patient, the severity of the deficiency, the severity of the hemorrhage, the presence of inhibitors and the FVIII level desired. It is often critical to follow the course of therapy with FVIII level assays.

The clinical effect of HELIXATE FS is the most important element in evaluating the effectiveness of treatment. It may be necessary to administer more HELIXATE FS than would be estimated in order to attain satisfactory clinical results. It has been shown in a clinical study performed in 14 adults with severe hemophilia A (≤1% FVCIII:C) undergoing a major surgery that HELIXATE FS can be used for continuous infusion in surgeries (pre-and postoperative). In this study, heparin was used to prevent thrombophlebitis at the infusion site, as with any other long-term intravenous infusions. For the calculation of the initial infusion rate, clearance can be obtained by performing a presurgery decay curve, or by starting from an average population value (3-3.5 mL/h/kg) and then adjusting accordingly.

Infusion rate (in IU/kg/h)=Clearance (in mL/h/kg) x desired factor VIII level (in IU/mL).

Continuous infusion, clinical, and in vitro stability has been demonstrated using ambulatory pumps with a polyvinyl chloride (PVC) reservoir. HELIXATE FS contains low levels of polysorbate 80 as an excipient, which in known to increase the rate of di-(2-ethylhexyl)phthalate (DHEP) extraction from PVC materials. This should be considered for a continuous infusion administration (see Reconstitution, For Continuous Infusion).

If the calculated dose fails to attain the expected FVIII levels or if bleeding is not controlled after administration of the calculated dosage, the presence of a circulating inhibitor in the patient should be suspected. Its presence should be substantiated and the inhibitor level quantitated by appropriate laboratory tests. When an inhibitor is present, the dosage requirement for rFVIII-FS is extremely variable and the dosage can be determined only by the clinical response.

Some patients with low titre inhibitors (<10 B.U.) can be successfully treated with rFVIII-FS without a resultant anamnestic rise in inhibitor titre. Factor VIII levels and clinical response to treatment must be assessed to ensure adequate response. Use of alternative treatment products, such as Factor IX Complex products, Antihemophilic Factor (Porcine), recombinant Factor VIIa or Anti-Inhibitor Coagulant Complex may be necessary for patients with anamnestic responses to FVIII treatment and/or high titre inhibitors.

Calculation of Dosage: The in vivo percent increase in FVIII level can be estimated by multiplying the dose of rFVIII-FS per kilogram of body weight (IU/kg) by 2%. This method of calculation is based on clinical findings by Abildgaard et al. and is illustrated in the following examples.

Equation 1: Calculation of HELIXATE FS Dosage (Expected % FVIII Increase)

$$\text{Expected \% FVIII increase} = \frac{(\text{\# units administered})\times 2\%/\text{IU/kg}}{\text{body weight (kg)}}$$

$$\text{Example for a 70 kg adult:} \quad \frac{1400\ \text{IU}\times 2\%/\text{IU/kg}}{70\ \text{kg}} = 40\%$$

Equation 2: Calculation of HELIXATE FS Dosage (Dosage Required)

$$\text{Dosage required (IU)} = \frac{(\text{body weight [kg]})\times(\text{desired \% FVIII})\ \text{increase}}{2\%/\text{IU/kg}}$$

$$\text{Example for a 15 kg child:} \quad \frac{15\ \text{kg}\times 100\%}{2\%/\text{IU/kg}} = 750\ \text{IU required}$$

The dosage necessary to achieve hemostasis depends upon the type and severity of the bleeding episode, according to the following general guidelines. See Table 2.

Table 2: HELIXATE FS

Dosage Necessary to Achieve Hemostasis

Hemorrhagic Event	Therapeutically Necessary Plasma Level of FVIII Activity	Dosage Necessary to Maintain the Therapeutic Plasma Level
Minor Hemorrhage (superficial, early hemorrhages, hemorrhages into joints)	20–40%	10–20 IU per kg Repeat dose if evidence of further bleeding.
Moderate to Major Hemorrhage (hemorrhages into muscles, hemorrhages into the oral cavity, definite hemarthroses, known trauma)	30–60%	15–30 IU per kg Repeat one dose at 12–24 hours if needed.
Surgery (minor surgical procedures)		
Major to Life-Threatening Hemorrhage (intracranial, intra-abdominal or intrathoracic hemorrhages, gastrointestinal bleeding, central nervous system bleeding, bleeding in the retro pharyngeal or retro peritoneal spaces or iliopsoas sheath)	80–100%	Initial dose 40–50 IU per kg Repeat dose 20–25 IU per kg every 8–12 hours.
Fractures		
Head Trauma		
Surgery (major surgical procedures)	~100%	a) By bolus infusions: Preoperative dose 50 IU/kg Verify ~100 % activity prior to surgery. Repeat as necessary after 6 to 12 hours initially and for 10 to 14 days until healing is complete. b) By continuous infusion: Raise factor VIII activity presurgery with an initial bolus infusion (in IU/h/kg) adjusting according to patient's daily clearance and desired factor VIII levels for at least 7 days.

Prophylaxis: FVIII products may also be administered on a regular schedule for prophylaxis of bleeding, as reported by Nilsson et al. In children, the recommended dose for a regular prophylaxis schedule is 25 IU/kg of body weight every other day.

Immune Tolerance: FVIII products have been administered to patients on a high dose schedule in order to induce immune tolerance to FVIII, which resulted in disappearance of the inhibitor activity. There is currently no consensus among treaters to the optimal treatment schedule.

Administration: For details on precautions associated with administration, see Warnings and Precautions, General.

Rate of Administration: The rate of administration should be adapted to the response of the individual patient but administration of the entire dose in 5 to 10 minutes or less is well-tolerated. HELIXATE FS can be infused by continuous infusion. The infusion rate should be calculated based on the clearance and the desired FVIII level. In a clinical study performed in 14 adults with severe hemophilia A (≤1% FVIII:C) who underwent a major surgery, the range of infusion rates for HELIXATE FS was 0.2 to 3.6 mL/h.

Example: For a 75 kg patient with a clearance of 3 mL/h/kg, the initial infusion rate would be 3 IU/h/kg to achieve a FVIII level of 100 %. For calculation of mL/h, multiply infusion rate in IU/h/kg by kg b.w./concentration of solution (IU/mL).

Higher infusion rates may be required in conditions with accelerated clearance during major bleeds and extensive tissue damage during surgical interventions. Subsequent infusion rates should be calculated based on the actual FVIII levels and recalculated clearance for each day post surgery based on the equation: Clearance = infusion rate/actual FVIII level.

Table 3: HELIXATE FS

Calculation of Infusion Rate Based on Clearance and the Desired FVIII Level

Clearance: 3 mL/h/kg	Desired Plasma FVIII Level	Infusion Rate (IU/h/kg)	Infusion Rate for 75 kg Patient, mL/h		
			Concentrations of rFVIII Solution		
			100 IU/mL	200 IU/mL	400 IU/mL
	100% (1 IU/mL)	3.0	2.25	1.125	0.56
	60% (0.6 IU/mL)	1.8	1.35	0.68	0.34
	40% (0.4 IU/mL)	1.2	0.9	0.45	0.225

Reconstitution: Parenteral Products: HELIXATE FS powder should only be reconstituted with the supplied diluent (2.5 mL or 5.0 mL Sterile Water for Injection) using the supplied sterile transfer device. Reconstitution and dilution should be performed in accordance with good practices rules, particularly with attention to asepsis. Always work on a clean surface and wash your hands before performing the following procedures. (See package insert for illustrations.)

1. Warm the unopened diluent and the product to room temperature (no more than 37°C).
2. Place the product vial, diluent vial and Mix2Vial on a flat surface.
3. Ensure product and diluent vial flip caps are removed and the stoppers are treated with an aseptic solution and allowed to dry prior to opening the Mix2Vial package.
4. Open the Mix2Vial package by peeling away the lid. Leave the Mix2Vial in the clear package. Place the diluent on an even surface and hold the vial tight. Grip the Mix2Vial together with the package and snap the blue end onto the diluent stopper.
5. Carefully remove the clear package from the Mix2Vial set. Make sure that you only pull up the package and not the Mix2Vial set.
6. With the product vial firmly on a surface, invert the diluent vial with the set attached and snap the transparent adapter onto the product vial stopper. The diluent will automatically transfer into the product vial.

7. With the diluent and product vial still attached, gently swirl the product vial to ensure the product is fully dissolved. Do not shake vial.
8. With one hand grasp the product-side of the Mix2Vial set and with the other hand grasp the blue diluent-side of the Mix2Vial set and unscrew the set into two pieces.
9. Draw air into an empty, sterile syringe. While the product vial is upright, screw the syringe to the Mix2Vial set. Inject air into the product vial. While keeping the syringe plunger pressed, invert the system upside down and draw the concentrate into the syringe by pulling the plunger back slowly.
10. Now that the concentrate has been transferred into the syringe, firmly grasp the barrel of the syringe (keeping the syringe plunger facing down) and unscrew the syringe from the Mix2Vial set.

For Bolus Injection:

11. Attach the syringe to an administration set made with microbore tubing. Use of other administration sets without microbore tubing may result in a larger retention of the solution within the administration set.
12. If the same patient is to receive more than one bottle, the contents of two bottles may be drawn into the same syringe through a separate unused Mix2Vial set before attaching the vein needle.
13. Parenteral drug products should be inspected visually for particulate matter and discolouration prior to administration, whenever solution and container permit.

Table 4: HELIXATE FS

Reconstitution of Parenteral Products

Vial Size	Volume of Diluent to be Added to Vial	Approximate Available Volume	Nominal Concentration per mL
250 IU	2.5 mL	2.5 mL	100 IU/ mL
500 IU	2.5 mL	2.5 mL	200 IU/mL
1000 IU	2.5 mL	2.5 mL	400 IU/mL
2000 IU	5.0 mL	5.0 mL	400 IU/mL
3000 IU	5.0 mL	5.0 mL	600 IU/mL

For Continuous Infusion: Reconstitute HELIXATE FS according to Steps 1-10 above. Continuous infusion of HELIXATE FS must employ an infusion pump that can provide continuous delivery, deal with low volumes and low infusion speeds. Technical instructions of the pump manufacturer, including the devices to be used, should be followed. The reservoir of the pump should be filled under aseptic conditions and the reservoir and the tubing should be changed at least every 24 hours. In a clinical study performed in 14 adults with severe hemophilia A (≤1% FVIII:C) undergoing a major surgery, a minute amount of heparin was added to the infusion solution (final concentration of 5 IU/mL) in order to prevent local thrombophlebitis at the site of the infusion. Refer to Table 3 for infusion rates.

Note: HELIXATE FS reconstituted with 2.5 mL or 5.0 mL Sterile Water for Injection should not be further diluted.

OVERDOSAGE:

No symptoms of overdose have been reported.

For management of a suspected drug overdose, CPhA recommends that you contact your **regional Poison Control Centre**. See the *CPS* Directory section for a list of Poison Control Centres.

ACTION AND CLINICAL PHARMACOLOGY: Mechanism of Action: See Indications and Clinical Use.

Pharmacodynamics: The activated partial thromboplastin time (aPTT) shortened appropriately with both HELIXATE (Antihemophilic Factor [Recombinant]) (rFVIII) and rFVIII-FS.

Pharmacokinetics: Initial pharmacokinetic studies were conducted in 35 patients, with severe hemophilia A.

Absorption: Not applicable. HELIXATE FS is administered directly into the blood stream by IV injection.

Distribution: No specific distribution studies have been performed, **however** after administration of HELIXATE FS (Antihemophilic Factor [Recombinant]), peak factor VIII activity decreases by a two-phase exponential decay. This is similar to that of plasma-derived factor VIII. HELIXATE FS binds to its natural protein carrier vWF and is mostly confined into the vascular space.

Metabolism: HELIXATE FS is metabolized as it produces its biological activity during the activation of the coagulation cascade.

Excretion: After administration of HELIXATE FS (Antihemophilic Factor [Recombinant]), peak factor VIII activity decreased by a two-phase exponential decay with a mean terminal half-life of about 15 hours. This is similar to that of plasma-derived factor VIII which has a mean terminal half-life of approximately 13 hours. The half-life data for rFVIII-FS were unchanged after 24 weeks of exclusive treatment, indicating continued efficacy and no evidence of FVIII inhibition.

Duration of Effect: The duration of effect is variable and dependent on the individual patient, the severity of the bleed and the clinical situation.

STORAGE AND STABILITY: HELIXATE FS (Antihemophilic Factor [Recombinant]) should be stored under refrigeration (2-8°C). Storage of lyophilized powder at room temperature (up to 25°C) for 3 months, such as in home storage situations, may be done. If the product is stored outside the refrigerator, please add the date removed from refrigeration and note a new expiry date on the carton and vial. The new expiry date should be 3 months from the date product is removed from the refrigerator, or the previously stamped expiry date, whichever is shorter. Once product is removed from refrigeration, it cannot be returned to the refrigerator. Freezing must be avoided. Protect from extreme exposure to light and store the lyophilized powder in the carton prior to use. After reconstitution, the product should be used immediately. For continuous infusion, stability has been demonstrated for 48 hours at 30°C.

SPECIAL HANDLING INSTRUCTIONS: Not applicable.

INFORMATION FOR THE PATIENT: Published in e-CPS, available by subscription at www.e-cps.ca.

DOSAGE FORMS, COMPOSITION AND PACKAGING: HELIXATE FS (Antihemophilic Factor [Recombinant]) is supplied in the following single use bottles. A suitable volume of Sterile Water for Injection, USP and a Mix2Vial filter transfer set are provided. The actual potency is printed on the label and the carton.

Table 5: HELIXATE FS

Vial Sizes

Approximate Factor VIII Activity	Dosage	Diluent
250 IU	L-Low	2.5 mL
500 IU	M-Mid	2.5 mL
1000 IU	H-High	2.5 mL
2000 IU	U-Ultra-High	5.0 mL
3000 IU	MH-Max-High	5.0 mL

Each vial of HELIXATE FS contains the labelled amount of rFVIII in international units (IU). One IU, as defined by the World Health Organization standard for blood coagulation FVIII, human, is approximately equal to the level of FVIII activity found in 1 mL of fresh pooled human plasma. The final product, when reconstituted as directed contains the following nonmedicinal ingredients: calcium chloride, chloride, glycine, histidine, polysorbate 80, sodium and sucrose. The product contains no preservative. HELIXATE FS must be administered by the intravenous route.

Hemabate™ Ⓟ

carboprost tromethamine

Prostaglandin

Pfizer

Date of Preparation: September 17, 2003

PHARMACOLOGY: Carboprost tromethamine given intramuscularly during the immediate postpartum period stimulates myometrial contractions. The result of postpartum contractions provides effective hemostasis at the site of placentation. The mechanism of action of these contractions has not been determined.

Uterine atony is the leading cause of postpartum hemorrhage. Extensive clinical experience with prostaglandins in term labour induction trials and pregnancy termination has established them as effective uterotonic agents. Prostaglandins appear to be involved in postpartum hemostatic mechanisms by virtue of their pharmacodynamic properties relative to myometrial stimulation, vasoactive effects and platelet function. Carboprost tromethamine, a methylated analogue of $PGF_{2\alpha}$, has been shown to be a more potent uterotonic agent with longer duration of action than the parent compound.

Carboprost tromethamine also stimulates the smooth muscle of the human gastrointestinal tract. This activity may produce the vomiting and/or diarrhea that is common when carboprost tromethamine is used. In laboratory animals and humans, carboprost tromethamine can elevate body temperature. With the clinical doses of carboprost tromethamine, some patients do experience transient temperature increases.

In laboratory animals, and in humans, large doses of carboprost tromethamine can raise blood pressure, probably by contracting the vascular smooth muscle. With the doses of carboprost tromethamine used for terminating pregnancy, this effect has not been clinically significant. In some patients, carboprost tromethamine may cause transient bronchoconstriction.

Five women who had spontaneous vaginal deliveries (at term) were treated immediately postpartum with a single intramuscular injection of 250 µg carboprost tromethamine. Peripheral blood samples were collected at several times during the four hours following treatment and carboprost tromethamine plasma levels were determined by radioimmunoassay. The highest plasma concentration of carboprost tromethamine was observed at 15 minutes in two patients (3009 and 2916 picograms/mL); at 30 minutes in two patients (3097 and 2792 picograms/mL); and at 60 minutes in one patient (2718 picograms/mL).

INDICATIONS: HEMABATE (carboprost tromethamine) is indicated for the treatment of postpartum hemorrhage due to uterine atony which has not responded to conventional methods of management. Prior treatment should include the use of intravenously administered oxytocin, manipulative techniques such as uterine massage and, unless contraindicated, intramuscular ergot preparations. Studies have shown that in such cases, the use of HEMABATE has resulted in satisfactory control of hemorrhage, although it is unclear whether or not ongoing or delayed effects of previously administered ecbolic agents have contributed to the outcome. In a high proportion of cases, HEMABATE used in this manner has resulted in the cessation of life threatening bleeding and the avoidance of emergency surgical intervention.

CONTRAINDICATIONS:

1. Hypersensitivity to any of the components of the preparation (carboprost, tromethamine, sodium chloride, benzyl alcohol).
2. Patients with known active cardiac, pulmonary, renal, or hepatic disease.
3. Acute pelvic inflammatory disease.

WARNINGS: HEMABATE (carboprost tromethamine), like other potent oxytocic agents, should be used with strict adherence to recommended dosages, by medically trained personnel in hospital surroundings with appropriate intensive care and acute surgical facilities.

Use of HEMABATE is associated with transient pyrexia that may be due to hypothalamic thermoregulation. Fever was reported by 8 of 115 (7%) patients treated in an open-label clinical trial of patients with postpartum hemorrhage due to uterine atony who had not responded to conventional non-surgical treatment of fundal massage, intravenous oxytocin and/or intramuscular methylergonovine.

On rare occasions, cardiovascular collapse has been reported with some of the prostaglandins, so this should always be considered when using HEMABATE.

Bronchoconstriction has been reported after exposure to HEMABATE, but it is rarely clinically important except in asthmatic patients.

PRECAUTIONS: General: Animal studies lasting several weeks at high doses have shown that prostaglandins of the E and F series can induce proliferation of bone. Such effects have also been noted in newborn infants who have received prostaglandin E_1 during prolonged treatment. There is no evidence that short term administration of HEMABATE (carboprost tromethamine) can cause similar bone effects.

Prostaglandins in general affect platelet aggregation by inhibiting it. Clinical experience on the effect of HEMABATE on human coagulation factors is limited. Due to this lack of information, it is advised that coagulation parameters be measured.

HEMABATE should be used cautiously in patients with a history of asthma, hypo- or hypertension, cardiovascular, renal, or hepatic disease, anemia, jaundice, diabetes, or epilepsy; or patients with previously compromised (scarred) uteri.

Table 1: HEMABATE

Medical Events of 248 Patients Who Received HEMABATE

	Medical Events N=248 patients (all routes)[a]		
Body System	Event	N	%
Gastrointestinal	Nausea	25	10.1
	Diarrhea	21	8.5
	Vomiting	19	7.7
	Abdominal Pain/Cramp	1	0.4
Cardiovascular	Increased Blood Pressure	9	3.6
	Flushing	5	2.0
	Tachycardia	2	0.8
Allergic	Fever	16	6.4
	Chills	1	0.4
Central Nervous System	Headache	4	1.6
Other	Dyspnea	1	0.4
	Erythema at Injection Site	1	0.4
	Sweating	1	0.4

[a] Most patients received HEMABATE intramuscularly. There were some patients who received HEMABATE intramyometrially (IMM) or intravenously (IV). The safety of the IMM and IV route has not been fully established at this time.

Nine of 248 patients (4%) treated for postpartum hemorrhage had an increase of blood pressure reported as a side effect. The degree of hypertension was moderate and it is not certain as to whether this was in fact due to a direct effect of HEMABATE or a return to a status of pregnancy-associated hypertension manifest by the correction of hypovolemic shock. In any event, the cases reported did not require specific therapy for the elevated blood pressure.

In a post-marketing trial of 333 cases of postpartum hemorrhage, investigator's considered 17 cases (5%) of increased blood pressure to be drug related.

Chorioamnionitis was identified as a complication contributing to postpartum uterine atony and hemorrhage in eight of 115 patients, 3 of which failed to respond to HEMABATE. This complication during labour may have an inhibitory effect on the uterine response to HEMABATE similar to what has been reported for other oxytocic agents.

Lactation: Human pharmacokinetics studies were not conducted on the excretion of HEMABATE in breast milk. However based on plasma clearance rates it is recommended that breast feeding not occur for at least 6 hours after administration.

Drug Interactions: Concomitant use with other oxytocic agents is not recommended. However, 578 (92%) out of 628 patients who received HEMABATE had prior treatment with conventional oxytocics such as oxytocin and ergometrine (ergonovine) maleate. It must be considered that HEMABATE may augment the activity of these oxytocic agents.

ADVERSE EFFECTS: The adverse effects of HEMABATE (carboprost tromethamine) are generally transient and reversible when therapy ends. The most frequent adverse reactions are related to its contractile effect on smooth muscle. Table 1 lists the medical events of 248 patients who received HEMABATE.

OVERDOSE:

Symptoms: Overdosage with HEMABATE (carboprost tromethamine) should result in the accentuation of expected side effects such as nausea, vomiting and diarrhea. Elevated blood pressure and body temperature may occur.

Treatment: Supportive therapy, particularly fluid replacement, should be given if serious vomiting and diarrhea occur.

Although prostaglandin antagonists are known to exist, no experience has been obtained at the present time with their usage in overdosage. Therefore, no specific therapy for overdosage is available.

For management of a suspected drug overdose, CPhA recommends that you contact your **regional Poison Control Centre**. See the *CPS* Directory section for a list of Poison Control Centres.

DOSAGE: HEMABATE (carboprost tromethamine) is administered by deep intramuscular injection. Initially a 250 µg (1 mL, the entire contents of the ampoule) dose of HEMABATE is given. In clinical trials, 80% of successful cases responded to ≤250 µg and 95% of successful cases responded to ≤500 µg. In some cases, multiple dosing of 250 µg at intervals of 15 to 90 minutes was carried out with successful outcome. The need for additional injections and the interval at which these should be given can be determined only by the attending physician as dictated by the course of clinical events. The total dose of HEMABATE (carboprost tromethamine) should not exceed 2 mg (8 doses).

Parenteral drug products should be inspected visually for particulate matter and discoloration prior to administration, whenever solution and container permit.

SUPPLIED: Each mL contains: carboprost tromethamine 332 µg (equivalent to 250 µg carboprost), tromethamine 83 µg, sodium chloride 9 mg and benzyl alcohol 9.45 mg. When necessary, pH was adjusted with sodium hydroxide and/or hydrochloric acid. Ampoules of 1 mL (250 µg/mL), cartons of 10. Refrigerate at 2 to 8°C.

HepaGam B™

hepatitis B immune globulin (human)

Passive Immunizing Agent

Cangene

Date of Preparation: May 29, 2007

HepaGam B, indicated for the prevention of hepatitis B recurrence following liver transplantation, has been issued marketing authorization with conditions, pending the results of studies to verify its clinical benefit. Patients should be advised of the nature of the authorization.

SUMMARY PRODUCT INFORMATION:

Route of Administration	Dosage Form/ Strength	Clinically Relevant Nonmedicinal Ingredients
Intravenous	Liquid/>312 IU/mL Hepatitis B Immune Globulin (Human)	For a complete listing see Dosage Forms, Composition and Packaging.

DESCRIPTION: HepaGam B (Hepatitis B Immune Globulin (Human) Injection), is a sterile solution of purified gamma globulin (IgG) fraction of human plasma containing antibodies to hepatitis B surface antigen (anti-HBs). HepaGam B, is manufactured from plasma collected from healthy, screened donors with high titres of anti-HBs which is purified by an anion-exchange column chromatography method.

HepaGam B is prepared from pools of human plasma which may contain the causative agents of hepatitis and other viral diseases. The manufacturing process includes both a Planova 20 nm virus filter that effectively removes lipid-enveloped and non-enveloped viruses based on size and a solvent/detergent treatment step (using tri-n-butyl phosphate and Triton X-100) that effectively inactivates lipid-enveloped viruses. These two processes are designed to increase product safety by reducing the risk of viral transmission of several viruses including human immunodeficiency virus (HIV), hepatitis B and hepatitis C. However, despite these measures, such products can still potentially transmit disease. There is also the possibility that unknown infectious agents may be present in such products (see Warnings and Precautions).

The product potency is expressed in international units (IU) by comparison to the World Health Organization (WHO) international Hepatitis B Immune Globulin reference preparation. Each vial contains greater than 312 IU/mL of anti-HBs.

HepaGam B is stabilized with 10% maltose and 0.03% polysorbate 80. The product contains no preservative.

INDICATIONS AND CLINICAL USE: HepaGam B (Hepatitis B Immune Globulin (Human) Injection) is used in the prevention of hepatitis B recurrence following liver transplantation, in adult patients with Hepatitis B who have no or low levels of HBV replication. The efficacy of HepaGam B in conjunction with antivirals such as lamivudine will be assessed in a Phase III confirmatory study.

Geriatrics: No data is available.

Pediatrics: No data is available.

CONTRAINDICATIONS:

- Patients with a history of anaphylactic or severe system reaction to any component of the product.
- Patients who are deficient in IgA. While HepaGam B contains less than 40 µg/mL IgA, individuals who are deficient in IgA may have the potential to develop IgA antibodies and have an anaphylactoid reaction.

WARNINGS AND PRECAUTIONS:

Serious Warnings and Precautions

HepaGam B is prepared from pools of human plasma which may contain the causative agents of hepatitis and other viral diseases. The risk that such products will transmit an infectious agent has been reduced by screening plasma donors for prior exposure to certain viruses, by testing for the presence of certain current virus infections, and by inactivating and/or removing certain viruses during manufacturing. Despite these measures, such products can still potentially transmit disease. There is also the possibility that unknown infectious agents may be present in such products.

True hypersensitivity reactions are rare. These reactions can occur in very rare cases of IgA deficiency or hypersensitivity to human globulin. In case of allergic or anaphylactic reaction, the infusion should be stopped immediately. In case of shock, the current medical standards for treatment of shock should be observed.

The physician should discuss the risks and benefits of this product with the patient, before prescribing or administering to the patient (see Warnings and Precautions, General).

General: Although HepaGam B is formulated for intravenous or intramuscular administration, HepaGam B should only be administered intravenously for the prevention of hepatitis B recurrence following liver transplantation. Intravenous administration is required due to the large volume required per dose (35 mL) and because many liver transplant patients will have thrombocytopenia or coagulation disorders following transplantation, which may contraindicate intramuscular administration.

Certain adverse drug reactions may be related to the rate of infusion. The recommended infusion rate given under Administration must be closely followed. Patients must be closely monitored and carefully observed for any symptoms throughout the infusion period and immediately following an infusion.

If patients develop treatment-related adverse events due to immune complex formation between HBIG and circulating HBsAg, dose adjustments may be required. Symptoms related to immune complexes should be treated with antihistamines or analgesic agents and the HepaGam B infusion rate should be decreased (see Administration).

HepaGam B is made from human plasma. Products made from human plasma may contain infectious agents, such as viruses and theoretically, the Creutzfeldt-Jakob disease agent. The risk that such products will transmit an infectious agent has been reduced by screening plasma donors for prior exposure to certain viruses, by testing for the presence of certain current virus infections, and by inactivating and/or removing certain viruses. The manufacturing process includes both a Planova 20 nm virus filter that effectively removes lipid-enveloped and nonenveloped viruses based on size and a solvent/detergent treatment step (using tri-n-butyl phosphate and Triton X-100) that effectively inactivates lipid-enveloped viruses by irreversibly destroying the lipid coat. These two processes are designed to increase product safety by reducing the risk of viral transmission of several viruses including human immunodeficiency virus (HIV), hepatitis B and hepatitis C. However, despite these measures, such products can still potentially transmit disease. There is also the possibility that unknown infectious agents may be present in such products. Individuals who receive infusions of blood or plasma products may develop signs and/or symptoms of some viral infections. All infections thought to have been possibly transmitted by this product should be reported by the physician or other health care provider to Cangene Corporation at 1-877-CANGENE (226-4363).

Renal: Intravenous immune globulin (human) products have been reported to produce renal dysfunction in patients that are predisposed to acute renal failure or those that have renal insufficiency. In such patients, it has been recommended that intravenous immune globulin (human) products be administered at a minimum practical concentration and infusion rate. While renal dysfunction has been reported with various intravenous immune globulin (human) products, the vast majority of these reports have involved products that utilize sucrose as a stabilizer. **HepaGam B does not contain sucrose as a stabilizer.** Regardless, it is recommended that renal function be assessed prior to administration of HepaGam B and at appropriate intervals following administration, especially for patients at risk of developing acute renal failure. If renal dysfunction occurs, clinical judgment should be used to determine whether the infusion rate of HepaGam B should be decreased or the product should be discontinued.

Sensitivity/Resistance: Although allergic reactions have not been reported following HepaGam B administration (see Adverse Drug Reaction Overview), epinephrine and diphenhydramine should be available for the treatment of any allergic reactions.

Special Populations: Pregnant Women: Animal reproduction studies have not been conducted with HepaGam B. It is also not known whether HepaGam B can cause fetal harm when administered to a pregnant woman or can affect reproductive capacity. However, immune globulins have been widely used during pregnancy for many years without any apparent negative reproductive effects. The risk/benefit of HepaGam B administration should be assessed for each individual case.

Extent of exposure in pregnancy during clinical trials: No experience.

Nursing Women: It is not known whether HepaGam B is excreted in human milk. Because many drugs are excreted in human milk, caution should be exercised when HepaGam B is administered to a nursing mother.

Pediatrics (<18 years of age): Safety and effectiveness in the pediatric population have not been established for HepaGam B.

Geriatrics (>65 years of age): Safety and effectiveness in the geriatric population have not been established for HepaGam B.

Monitoring and Laboratory Tests: Patients should be monitored regularly for serum anti-HBs antibody levels.

Blood Glucose Testing: The maltose contained in HepaGam B can interfere with some types of blood glucose monitoring systems, i.e., those based on the glucose dehydrogenase pyrroloquinequinone (GDH-PQQ) method. This can result in falsely elevated glucose readings and, consequently, in the inappropriate administration of insulin, resulting in life-threatening hypoglycemia. Cases of true hypoglycemia may go untreated if the hypoglycemic state is masked by falsely elevated results.

ADVERSE REACTIONS: Adverse Drug Reaction Overview: The most common expected adverse drug reactions for intravenous immune globulins like HepaGam B are chills, fever, headaches, vomiting, allergic reactions, nausea, arthralgia and moderate low back pain. In a clinical trial in liver transplant patients, 2 adverse drug reactions of tremor and hypotension were reported in 2 of 14 patients who received intravenous infusions of HepaGam B. In studies with healthy volunteers, only 1 adverse drug reaction of nausea was been reported in the 70 adult subjects who received an intramuscular administration of HepaGam B.

Although no anaphylactic reactions have been reported following HepaGam B administration, anaphylactic reactions have been reported following the administration of intravenous immune globulin (human) products on rare occasions (see Warnings and Precautions, General).

Clinical Trial Adverse Drug Reactions: Because clinical trials are conducted under very specific conditions the adverse reaction rates observed in the clinical trials may not reflect the rates observed in practice and should not be compared to the rates in the clinical trials of another drug. Adverse drug reaction information from clinical trials is useful for identifying drug-related adverse events and for approximating rates.

Hepatitis B-Related Liver Transplantation: In an ongoing clinical trial, only 2 adverse drug reactions occurred following the 313 (<1%) HepaGam B infusions in 14 liver transplant patients. These adverse events were reported in an interim analysis from a Phase III clinical trial examining HepaGam B for the prevention of hepatitis B recurrence following liver transplantation. This study utilized the recommended dosing regimen outlined in Table 2. The 2 adverse drug reactions of tremor and hypotension were reported in 2 patients. All reactions were associated with a single HepaGam B infusion during the first week post-transplant. All reactions resolved on the same day and did not recur with subsequent HepaGam B infusions.

Healthy Volunteer Studies: Seventy healthy male and female volunteers received a single dose of HepaGam B, Hepatitis B Immune Globulin (Human), intramuscularly in clinical trials. Seventeen (17) subjects reported 30 adverse events following administration of HepaGam B. The most frequently reported adverse events included 4 subjects (6%) who experienced headache, 7 subjects (10%) who had cold symptoms or flu and 2 subjects (3%) who experienced lightheadeness/fainted. The majority of events were reported as mild. One adverse event, an episode of nausea, was considered to be drug related. There were no serious adverse events reported. A similar number of subjects in the comparator groups reported adverse events.

Abnormal Hematologic and Clinical Chemistry Findings: There have been no abnormal hematology or clinical chemistry values reported to be related to HepaGam B administration.

Post-Market Adverse Drug Reactions: There is no post-marketing experience.

DRUG INTERACTIONS:

Serious Drug Interactions

- Live attenuated virus vaccines: immune globulin administration may impair the efficacy of live attenuated virus vaccines for a period of 3 months or more (see Drug Interactions, Overview).

Overview: Immune globulin administration may impair the efficacy of live attenuated virus vaccines such as measles, rubella, mumps and varicella. Vaccination with live virus vaccines should be deferred until approximately three months after administration of HepaGam B (Hepatitis B Immune Globulin (Human) Injection). Persons who received HepaGam B less than 14 days after live virus vaccination, should be revaccinated 3 months after the administration of the immune globulin, unless serologic test results indicate that antibodies were produced.

There are no available data on concomitant use of HepaGam B and other medications.

Antibodies present in HepaGam B may interfere with some serological tests (see Drug-Laboratory Test Interactions).

Drug-Drug Interactions: See Table 1.

Table 1: HepaGam B

Established or Potential Drug-Drug Interactions

Hepatitis B Immune Globulin (Human)	Reference	Effect	Clinical Comment
Live attenuated virus vaccines (e.g. measles, rubella, mumps, varicella)	T	Immune globulin may impair efficacy	If hepatitis B immune globulin is given less than 14 days after live virus vaccination, revaccination should be considered.

Legend:
T=theoretical.

The use of live virus vaccination before or after HepaGam B administration should follow the recommendations by the Canadian National Advisory Committee on Immunization.

Interactions with other drugs have not been established.

Drug-Food Interactions: Interactions with food have not been established.

Drug-Herb Interactions: Interactions with herbal products have not been established.

Drug-Laboratory Test Interactions: After administration of hepatitis B immune globulin (human), a transitory increase of passively transferred antibodies in the patients blood may result in misleading positive results in serological testing (e.g. Coombs' test).

HepaGam B contains maltose which can interfere with certain types of blood glucose testing and monitoring systems, i.e., those based on the GDH-PQQ (see Warnings and Precautions, Blood Glucose Testing). Even though HepaGam B is administered intravenously, due to the potential for falsely elevated glucose readings, only testing systems that are glucose-specific should be used to test or monitor blood glucose levels in patients receiving maltose-containing parenteral products, including HepaGam B.

The product information of the blood glucose testing system, including that of the test strips, should be carefully reviewed to determine if the system is appropriate for use with maltose-containing parenteral products. If any uncertainty exists, contact the manufacturer of the testing system to determine if the system is appropriate for use with maltose-containing parenteral products.

DOSAGE AND ADMINISTRATION: Dosing Considerations: For the prevention of hepatitis B recurrence following liver transplantation in adult patients with hepatitis B, HepaGam B (Hepatitis B Immune Globulin (Human) Injection), should be administered intravenously to attain serum anti-HBs levels greater than 500 mIU/mL as described below.

These dosing recommendations are based on a systematic review of the clinical trial literature and meta-analysis undertaken by Cangene Corporation. This report found that hepatitis B Immune globulin (HBIG) prophylaxis was most effective when administered in high doses (to achieve anti-HBs levels of greater than 500 mIU/mL) over longer time periods (greater than 6 months). The recommended dosing schedule described below is designed to achieve anti-HBs levels of greater than 500 mIU/mL. This regimen is based on that published in Terrault et al., 1996 and reviewed by Shouval & Samuel, 2000. This regimen is currently being evaluated in a Phase III clinical trial. Recommendations for dose adjustments are based on McGory et al., 1996, using a similar dosing regimen.

Recommended Dose and Dosage Adjustment: Each dose of HepaGam B should be administered as an intravenous dose of 35 mL (10,920 IU anti-HBs). The first dose should be administered concurrently with the grafting of the transplanted liver (the anhepatic phase) with subsequent dosing as recommended in Table 2. Anti-HBs levels should be measured after the first week of treatment, to allow for initial adjustment of dosage.

Table 2: HepaGam B

Dosing Regimen

Anhepatic Phase[a]	Week 1 Post-Operative[a]	Months 1–3 Post-Operative	Month 4 onwards
First dose	Daily from Day 1–7	Biweekly from Day 14	Monthly

[a] Anti-HBs levels should be measured after the first week of treatment, to allow for initial adjustment of dosage.

HepaGam B dose adjustments may be required in patients who fail to reach anti-HBs levels of 500 mIU/mL within the first week post-liver transplantation. Patients who have surgical bleeding or abdominal fluid drainage (>500 mL) or patients who undergo plasmapheresis are particularly susceptible to extensive loss of circulated anti-HBs. The following dose adjustment is recommended:

- the dosing regimen should be increased to 5460 IU (17.5 mL IV) every 6 hours until the target anti-HBs is reached.

Regular monitoring of serum HBsAg, HBV-DNA and HBeAg as well as anti-HBs antibody levels should be performed to decide on the continuation of HepaGam B treatment and/or treatment adjustment.

In patients who develop treatment-related adverse events, especially during early post-operative period when immune complexes may develop from the large amounts of hepatitis B immune globulin immunoprecipitating with HBsAg, the HepaGam B infusion rate should be decreased. Symptoms related to immune complex formation should be treated with antihistamines or analgesic agents.

Missed Dose: If a scheduled dose is missed, HepaGam B should be administered as soon as possible after the missed dose(s). Scheduling of subsequent doses should be determined by the treating physician and the HepaGam B dosing regimen (see Recommended Dose and Dosage Adjustment).

Administration: HepaGam B should be prepared for IV administration under aseptic conditions. **Do not shake vial; avoid foaming.** Parenteral drugs should be visually assessed for particulate matter and discolouration prior to administration.

- HepaGam B should be administered as provided through a separate IV line using an intravenous administration set containing an in-line filter and a constant infusion pump.
- Rate of administration should be set at 2 mL per minute.
- The rate of infusion should be decreased to 1 mL per minute or slower if the patient develops discomfort or there is concern about the speed of infusion.

OVERDOSAGE:

Consequences of an overdose are not known.

For management of a suspected drug overdose, CPhA recommends that you contact your **regional Poison Control Centre**. See the *CPS* Directory section for a list of Poison Control Centres.

ACTION AND CLINICAL PHARMACOLOGY: Mechanism of Action: Hepatitis B virus reinfection is the consequence of an immediate reinfection of the graft due to circulating HBV particles, a reinfection of the graft from HBV particles coming from extrahepatic sites or both.

The mechanism whereby hepatitis B Immune globulin (HBIG) protects the transplanted liver against HBV reinfection is not well understood. One hypothesis is that HBIG protects naive hepatocytes against HBV release from extrahepatic sites through blockage of a putative HBV receptor. Alternatively, HBIG may neutralize circulating virions through immune precipitation and immune complex formation or trigger an antibody-dependent cell-mediated cytotoxicity response resulting in target cell lysis. In addition, HBIG has been reported to bind to hepatocytes and interact with HBsAg within cells.

Regardless of the mechanism, there is evidence of a dose-dependent response to HBIG treatment.

Pharmacodynamics: Hepatitis B immune globulin products provide passive immunization to the hepatitis B virus and significantly decrease hepatitis B recurrence and increase graft and patient survival following liver transplantation in hepatitis B surface antigen (HBsAg) positive patients.

The clinical effectiveness of HBIG prophylaxis in the prevention of Hepatitis B recurrence following liver transplantation is dependent on the dose, length of administration and the viral replication status of the patient at the time of transplant.

HBIG is most effective when administered in high doses (to achieve anti-HBs levels greater than 500 mIU/mL), over long time periods (greater than 6 months). A meta-analysis of the literature data showed that patients treated with long-term high-dose HBIG had a hepatitis B recurrence rate of 15.2%, compared to a 40.4% recurrence rate in subjects treated with long-term, low-dose HBIG. Short-term immunoprophylaxis with HBIG may delay hepatitis B recurrence, but the overall rate of reinfection is similar to untreated patients. Therefore, it is important that treatment be continued long-term.

The absence of viral replication (absence of HBeAg and/or HBV DNA in serum) at the time of liver transplant is associated with an increase in the effectiveness of HBIG. As a result, HepaGam B is recommended in patients who have no or low levels of viral replication at the time of liver transplantation.

Pharmacokinetics: Currently there are no pharmacokinetic data available for HepaGam B IV administration in liver transplant patients. The ability of the described dosing regimen (see Table 2) to maintain anti-HBs levels was examined in an interim analysis of 14 hepatitis B-related liver transplant patients from an ongoing clinical trial. Anti-HBs levels taken before and after each dose showed that the target trough of 500 mIU/mL was achieved after the first few HepaGam B doses and maintained in the first year post-transplant in 12 of the 14 patients. As described above under Dosing Considerations, these levels have been associated with efficacy.

The pharmacokinetic profile of HepaGam B after intramuscular injection of 0.06 mL/kg is summarized in Table 3.

Table 3: HepaGam B

Summary of Pharmacokinetic Parameters of Intramuscular Hepatitis B Immune Globulin (Human) in Healthy Volunteers

	C_{max}	$t_{½}$	$AUC_{0-\infty}$	Volume of Distribution
Single dose mean	211.6 mIU/mL	24.5 days	8253.9 mIU*day/mL	7.0±1.5 L

Absorption: A pharmacokinetics trial of HepaGam B (Hepatitis B Immune Globulin (Human) Injection), given intramuscularly to 30 healthy male and female volunteers demonstrated pharmacokinetic parameters similar to those reported in the literature by Scheiermann and Kuwert. The volume of distribution was 7.0±1.5 L. Maximum concentration of HepaGam B was 215.6 mIU/mL, which was reached 5.4±2.4 days following administration. The maximum concentration of anti-HBs achieved by HepaGam B was consistent with that of a commercially available HBIG when compared in the same comparative pharmacokinetics trial. There is an immediate time to the onset of HepaGam B action and the time to steady state between intravascular and extravascular spaces is approximately 5 days.

Distribution: The bioavailability of hepatitis B immune globulin (human) for intravenous use is complete and immediate. IgG is quickly distributed between plasma and extravascular fluid. Immune globulin products have been demonstrated to poorly penetrate across an intact blood brain barrier.

Metabolism: Immune globulins and immune complexes are broken down in the reticuloendothelial system.

Excretion: The elimination half-life of HepaGam B is 24.5 days following intramuscular administration. Based on studies with other immune globulin products, a slightly decreased half-life is expected following intravenous administration.

STORAGE AND STABILITY: Store under refrigeration (2 to 8°C). Do not freeze. Do not use after expiration date indicated on the label.

SPECIAL HANDLING INSTRUCTIONS: The product should be brought to room or body temperature before use.

The solution should be clear or slightly opalescent. Do not use solutions that are cloudy or have deposits.

INFORMATION FOR THE PATIENT: Published in e-CPS, available by subscription at www.e-cps.ca.

DOSAGE FORMS, COMPOSITION AND PACKAGING: Each vial of sterile solution contains: a purified gamma globulin (5 % or 50 mg/mL) fraction containing antibodies to hepatitis B surface antigen (anti-HBs). Preservative-free. Nonmedicinal ingredients: human plasma protein (≥96% Human IgG), maltose, polysorbate 80. May contain trace amounts of tri-n-butyl phosphate and Triton X-100. Cartons containing a 1 mL single dose (>312 IU/mL) in a 3 mL glass vial with a plastic flip off seal and a package insert. Cartons containing a 5 mL single dose (>312 IU/mL) in a 6 mL glass vial with a plastic flip off seal and a package insert.

Hepalean®

heparin sodium

Anticoagulant

Schering-Plough

PHARMACOLOGY: Hepalean is a sterile, pyrogen-free solution of a highly purified sodium salt of heparin, a high molecular weight polysaccharide derived from porcine intestinal mucosa. It is standardized in vitro according to the method of USP and is labelled in terms of USP units for use as an anticoagulant. It acts very rapidly and, even in large doses, is metabolized in the body and eliminated within 24 hours. It will not lyse existing thrombi or emboli.

Hepalean, being of intestinal mucosal origin, offers 2 advantages over that derived from lung tissue, namely, the potency of USP units per unit weight is higher and the amount of protamine sulfate required for neutralization of the heparin is much less.

Heparin inhibits the clotting of blood and the formation of fibrin clots both in vitro and in vivo. In combination with a cofactor, it inactivates thrombin thus preventing the conversion of fibrinogen to fibrin. Heparin also prevents the formation of a stable fibrin clot by inhibiting the activation of the fibrin-stabilizing factor.

Heparin sodium inhibits reactions which lead to clotting but does not alter the normal components of the blood. Although clotting time is prolonged by therapeutic doses, bleeding time is usually unaffected. Heparin sodium does not have fibrinolytic activity; therefore, it will not lyse existing clots.

INDICATIONS: Used in the treatment of thrombophlebitis, phlebothrombosis, and cerebral, coronary, and retinal vessel thrombosis to prevent extension of clots and thromboembolic phenomena. Also used prophylactically to prevent the occurrence of thromboembolism, and to prevent clotting during dialysis and other surgical procedures, particularly vascular surgery.

When using in conjuction with dialysis machines or where heparin is added to glucose or saline it is most important that the pH is not less than 5 for heparin to act as an effective anticoagulant. Under pH 5 degradation sets in and with a pH around 4 or less there is very little activity. Likewise, with pH over 8.5 there will be some degradation. Recent work has indicated that early hemodialysis is of value in cases of multiple trauma.

Heparin has also been used as an anticoagulant in blood transfusion samples, particularly when the presence of citrates, oxalates, or fluorides might interfere with laboratory tests, such as electrolyte determination. Anti-inflammatory and diuretic activity have been obtained with heparin. However, these properties have not yet been put to any widespread clinical use.

Low Dose S.C. Heparin: For the prevention of serious venous thromboembolic complications in high risk surgical patients.

CONTRAINDICATIONS: Hemophilia and severe clotting disorders; shock; hypersensitivity to heparin; severe liver damage. Active bleeding from a local lesion such as an acute ulcer or ulcerating carcinoma. Recent neurosurgery or spinal surgery.

WARNINGS: Administration of large doses of heparin should be delayed 4 hours postoperatively.

When any of the conditions mentioned under Precautions are present the advantages of heparin therapy must be carefully weighed against the possibility of deleterious results.

PRECAUTIONS: Purpura, and other blood dyscrasias with bleeding tendencies; active ulcerative diseases of the gastrointestinal tract; jaundice; subacute bacterial endocarditis; increased capillary fragility; threatened abortion; postoperative disease, following brain or spinal cord surgery; malignant hypertension.

Heparin should be used with caution in the immediate postoperative period. Bleeding may be concealed, as in the case of hemothorax.

Pregnancy: Heparin should be used with caution in pregnancy although it does not cross the placental barrier and is the safest and most useful form of therapy in thromboembolic disorders of pregnancy.

For these reasons strict laboratory control of dosage is necessary. Heparin should be used with caution in patients with allergy. Patients on long-term daily administration should be observed for the possible development of osteoporosis and spontaneous fractures of ribs and/or vertebrae.

Care must be taken where large doses of antibiotics and/or drugs containing amino groups are administered along with or prior to heparin administration.

Drugs such as codeine phosphate, pethidine HCl, streptomycin, erythromycin, kanamycin, neomycin, novobiocin, tetracyclines, ampicillin, penicillin G, polymyxin B, vancomycin, hydrocortisone sodium succinate, pentobarbitone, promazine HCl, vitamin B complex and vitamin C may complex with heparin. This complex may be reversible (heparin rebound) and may result in excess bleeding at the surgical site. Extra protamine sulfate may then be indicated.

Please also refer to the pH requirements in hemodialysis under Indications.

Incompatibilities: Heparin has not been reported to interact pharmacologically in vivo with any other drugs. An increased bleeding tendency may be seen when heparin is used in combination with ethacrynic acid, ASA and dextran. Although digitalis, quinine, tetracycline, antihistamines, and nicotine have been stated to interfere with the anticoagulant activity of heparin, there is no substantial literature support for such interactions. The chemical interaction occurring between heparin and protamine is well known. This interaction is used clinically to antagonize the anticoagulant effect of heparin.

Ethacrynic Acid: I.V. administered ethacrynic acid can cause gastrointestinal bleeding. However, a significantly higher incidence of gastrointestinal bleeding has been attributed to the concurrent use of i.v. ethacrynic acid and heparin. Furosemide may be a safer alternative when such diuretic therapy is indicated in the patient receiving heparin.

ASA: In a review article of heparin therapy, it was advocated that concurrent ASA administration be scrupulously avoided. While documentation to support this interaction is incomplete, it would be prudent to avoid concurrent therapy. ASA impairs the platelet release reaction and this platelet function defect combined with the anticoagulant effect of heparin may produce a hemorrhagic tendency.

Dextran: Limited data suggest that dextran and heparin may act synergistically when administered concurrently. Although the data are inadequate to document the clinical significance of this interaction, baseline laboratory measurements of anticoagulant activity should be obtained upon initiation of concurrent therapy as well as at frequent intervals during such therapy.

ADVERSE EFFECTS: Hemorrhage is the chief complication which may result from heparin therapy. Please refer to Overdose, Treatment, Heparin Neutralization with Protamine.

Hypersensitivity reactions, such as fever, skin eruptions, naso-pharyngeal congestion, bronchial asthma, anaphylactic shock, and osteoporosis, have been reported in some patients following heparin injection. Alopecia, affecting the entire scalp or confined to the temple, has been reported with the use of heparin; the mechanism is unknown.

Thrombocytopenia has also been described with heparin treatment. Heparin Induced Thrombocytopenia (HIT) is an allergic reaction. It has been reported to occur in 1 to 30% of patients treated with standard heparin. It has also occurred with the use of LMWHs, both in patients with a history of HIT and patients with no previous exposure to heparin. The risk of developing HIT may be lower with LMWHs, but cannot be reliably estimated until more patients have been exposed. It is thought to be more common with heparin derived from bovine lung (5 to 10%) than from porcine gut (2 to 5%). Two types of acute, reversible thrombocytopenia have been described. Mild thrombocytopenia most commonly occurs between 5 and 12 days after initiation of full dose therapy. Platelet count usually remains above 100×10^9/L, and heparin therapy does not necessarily have to be withdrawn. Platelet count may remain stable or even increase despite continued therapy; however, it should still be monitored. The more severe, delayed form of thrombocytopenia (platelets $<100\times10^9$/L) is much less frequent, usually appearing 5 to 12 days after starting heparin therapy, and recurs rapidly on rechallenge. It has occurred with low dosages and is not dose related. It is generally reversible, platelet counts usually begin to return to normal within 4 days of stopping heparin. Paradoxically, patients may develop thrombotic complications including arterial thrombosis, gangrene, stroke, myocardial infarction and disseminated intravascular coagulation. Thrombosis is due to "white clots" composed of platelets and fibrin that result from marked in vivo platelet aggregation. Patients receiving heparin acutely should have platelet counts monitored at least every 2 or 3 days.

OVERDOSE:

Treatment: Heparin Neutralization with Protamine: Bleeding which may occur during therapy with heparin can usually be corrected by withdrawal. Clotting time should then return to normal in 30 to 60 minutes provided venous clotting time is not longer than 15 minutes when the infusion is interrupted. Should withdrawal of heparin fail to control bleeding, fresh, matched blood (not more than 3 days old) may be administered in quantities of 250 to 500 mL.

The most rapid means of counteracting the effects of heparin is i.v. administration of protamine sulfate. However, protamine is by itself an anticoagulant and, therefore, excess must be avoided. The amount of heparin neutralized by protamine varies with the organ from which it is derived, method of manufacture and specific activity of heparin. The amount of protamine required to neutralize 1000 units of each lot of heparin used in the preparation of Hepalean is therefore accurately determined and is stated on the label as the number of mg of protamine sulfate required to neutralize 1000 units of Hepalean.

Allowance should be made for the rapid removal of heparin from circulation. The rate of heparin removal from plasma is dose-dependent. However, it may be assumed that about 30 minutes after an i.v. injection, about 50% of the heparin is removed from circulation.

So the amount of protamine sulfate required to neutralize the heparin will be approximately half of that required for the original dose. For example if 1000 units required 8.4 mg of protamine sulfate for neutralization, half an hour after i.v. administration of a 5000 unit dose, the amount of protamine sulfate required will only be approximately:

$$5/2\times8.4=21 \text{ mg}$$

Do not administer more than 50 mg protamine sulfate at any one time.

> For management of a suspected drug overdose, CPhA recommends that you contact your **regional Poison Control Centre**. See the *CPS* Directory section for a list of Poison Control Centres.

DOSAGE: I.M. injection (especially in the arm or thigh) and shallow s.c. injection are not recommended. The duration of effect is shortened and it is more likely to produce pain and hematoma.

Heparin activity is expressed in USP units and should be prescribed in units only.

The route of administration may be i.v. or s.c., depending upon the situation and the choice of the prescriber (see Table 1). Adequate heparin-induced anti-coagulant therapy is present when the clotting time is elevated from 2 to 3 times normal as measured by the Lee-White method. Two types of dosage schedules are suggested: heparin may be administered i.v. in a dose of 5000 USP units every 4 hours or in a dose of 10 000 USP units every 6 hours, depending upon the results of a whole blood clotting time test performed at the bedside just prior to each additional dose. If the clotting time is less than twice normal, the next dose is increased by one-third to one-half. If the clotting time is more than 2 ½ times normal, the next dose is decreased by one-third to one-half. If the clotting time is between 2 and 2½ times normal, the regular dose is repeated.

S.C. Injection Technique: Use of a 1 mL tuberculin syringe with a No. 25 or No. 26, ½ inch needle is recommended.

Disinfect area with alcohol then apply pressure between finger and thumb to the dermal fold until the injection site is blanched. Insert the needle into the raised, blanched area. Reduce the pressure on the skin and inject slowly. Withdraw the needle quickly and apply alcohol swab with pressure to the site of injection for 5 to 10 seconds to prevent loss of the heparin.

Table 1: Hepalean

Hepalean Dosage

Administration		
Method	**Frequency**	**Recommended dosage[a]**
Low-dose s.c.[b]	Every 8 to 12 hours	5000 units
S.C.	Every 8 hours	10 000 to 20 000 units initially[c] then 8000 to 10 000 units 3 times a day.
Intermittent i.v.	Every 4 to 6 hours	10 000 units initially, then 5000 to 10 000 units 4 to 6 times a day.
I.V. infusion	Continuous or intermittent	20 000 to 40 000 units per L at a rate of 15 to 30 units per minute.
Dialysis	See below	See below
Usual pediatric dose	Every 4 hours	By i.v. infusion 50 units per kg of body weight initially, followed by 100 units per kg or 3333 units per m² of body surface, 6 times a day.

[a] Based on 68 kg of body weight.
[b] It is not necessary to monitor low-dose prophylactic heparin.
[c] Following immediately after an initial dose of 5000 units i.v.

Therapy Required: Low Dose S.C. Heparin: There is now good evidence that low dose heparin is effective in preventing serious venous thromboembolic complications in high risk surgical patients. The usually recommended dose is 5000 units s.c. 2 hours before surgery and then 5000 units given either 12 hourly or 8 hourly after surgery with the first dose given at approximately 12 hours after surgery. It is not necessary to monitor low dose prophylactic heparin.

Therapeutic Anticoagulant Action (Immediate and Short-term): The dose should be adjusted in keeping with the patient's clotting time which should be determined just prior to the injection during the first day of treatment. It is also recommended that, in order to help regulate dosage, the clotting time be determined on the second and third day of treatment. (The recommended method is the Lee-White whole blood method.)

Anticoagulation is adequate when the clotting time is 2 to 3 times the normal value.

S.C. administration is usually employed for maintenance therapy after initial regulation.

Long-term Protective Anticoagulant Action: S.C. administration of 15 000 units every 12 hours is usually employed. Daily injections of 20 000 to 30 000 units have also been employed with success. After initial regulation the dosage should be adjusted according to weekly to monthly clotting time determinations. Anticoagulant therapy should not be terminated abruptly but should be gradually reduced over 3 to 4 days.

Deep Venous Thrombosis and Pulmonary Emoblism: Dosage of 20 000 units daily for 6 to 10 days has been of value.

Hemodialysis: (a) Multiple trauma: Recent literature has suggested the use of early hemodialysis in multiple trauma. (b) Chronic renal failure: The use of hemodialysis in this area has increased dramatically in recent years and may be in hospital or home dialysis.

It is most important to stress that the instructions for each manufacturer's equipment unit must be followed scrupulously.

The following is merely intended as an overall summary of possible general procedures: 3000 units of heparin is added to 1000 mL of sterile saline as a dialyser flush prior to connection. Initial dosage: 5000 units of heparin into the venous shunt or 2500 units into the arterial fistula needle. With the shunt type the usual continuing dosage is 2000 units per hour, with the fistula type, 1500 units per hour by means of a suitable syringe and a pump to allow continuing infusion. Heparin reversal with protamine will be decided by the individual physician. Usually this is not done unless dialysis is being performed soon after surgery.

Coronary and Vascular Surgery: Patients undergoing total body perfusion for open heart surgery should receive an initial dose of not less than 150 units of heparin/kg. Frequently a dose of 300 units of heparin/kg is used for procedures estimated to last less than 60 minutes; or 400 units/kg for those estimated to last longer than 60 minutes.

SUPPLIED: Aqueous solutions, containing sodium chloride, hydrochloric acid and/or sodium hydroxide and 1% benzyl alcohol as preservative, color coded labels: heparin sodium 1000 USP units/mL in 10 or 30 mL vials; heparin sodium 10 000 USP units/mL in 5 mL vials; heparin sodium 25 000 USP units/mL in 2 mL vials. Cartons of 10 (2, 5, 10 and 30 mL).

Aqueous solution without preservative containing sodium chloride, hydrochloric acid and/or sodium hydroxide and heparin sodium 1000 USP units/mL in 1 mL vial and heparin sodium 10 000 USP units/mL in 1 mL vial. Cartons of 100 (1 mL).

Source: Porcine intestinal mucosa.

Heparin LEO®

heparin sodium

Anticoagulant

LEO Pharma

PHARMACOLOGY: Heparin is an anticoagulant which prevents the formation of thrombin by accelerating the neutralization of activated coagulation factors by naturally occurring inhibitors.

INDICATIONS: For the prophylaxis and management of intravascular clotting and embolism in susceptible patients.

It is also used in extra-corporeal circulation, i.e. heart-lung and renal dialysis machines and blood transfusions.

CONTRAINDICATIONS: Hemorrhagic disorders and patients with an actual or potential bleeding site, e.g. peptic ulcer.

Low doses of heparin, administered as recommended, do not cause alterations in clotting times in most patients, but occasionally local hematomata may occur at injection sites.

Pregnancy: Menstruation and pregnancy are not contraindications to heparin therapy since heparin does not cross placenta or appear in breast milk.

Lactation: See Pregnancy.

WARNINGS: Patients with hemorrhagic disorders may experience bleeding, especially from surgical wounds. The relative risks and benefits of heparin administration in these patients should be assessed carefully.

Oral anticoagulants or drugs which interfere with platelet function, e.g. ASA and dextran solutions, should be administered with caution.

OVERDOSE:

Treatment: If bleeding should occur, the effect of heparin can be reversed immediately by i.v. administration of a 1% protamine sulfate solution (1 mg for every 100 IU of heparin to be neutralized). The precise dose of protamine sulfate required for neutralization should be determined accurately by titrating with the patient's plasma.

> For management of a suspected drug overdose, CPhA recommends that you contact your **regional Poison Control Centre**. See the *CPS* Directory section for a list of Poison Control Centres.

DOSAGE: Low dose for prophylaxis (by s.c. injection only): Patients undergoing surgery: 5000 IU should be given 2 to 6 hours pre-operatively and every 8 to 12 hours post-operatively for 10 to 14 days or until ambulation, whichever is the longer.

Other Patients: 5000 units every 8 to 12 hours.

Therapeutic dose (by i.v. or s.c. injection): Average daily dose: 20 000 to 40 000 IU daily. However, the dose should be monitored with coagulation tests and varied according to individual response. The treatment period varies and can be as long as 6 weeks in patients with established thrombosis.

Stability in Infusion Fluids: Heparin LEO is stable for 24 hours at room temperature in the following infusion fluids: sodium chloride 0.9%, dextrose solutions (55 and 100 g/L), invertose (100 mg/L), Ringer solution, Ringer glucose, Ringer acetate, sodium bicarbonate 8.4%, Vamin with glucose. Stability tests were carried out using heparin concentrations of 10 and 200 units/mL.

SUPPLIED: 100 IU/mL: Each mL of solution contains: heparin sodium 100 IU. Nonmedicinal ingredients: benzyl alcohol, methyl parahydroxybenzoate, propyl parahydroxybenzoate, sodium chloride, sodium citrate dihydrate and water for injection. Ampuls (with preservative) of 2 mL. Multidose vials (with preservative) of 10 mL.

1000 IU/mL: Each mL of solution contains: heparin sodium 1000 IU. Nonmedicinal ingredients: benzyl alcohol, methyl parahydroxybenzoate, propyl parahydroxybenzoate, sodium chloride, sodium citrate dihydrate and water for injection. Multidose vials (with preservative) of 10 mL.

10 000 IU/mL: Ampuls (preservative-free) of 1 mL: Each mL of solution contains: heparin sodium 10 000 IU. Nonmedicinal ingredients: water for injection. Multidose vials (with preservative) of 5 mL: Each mL of solution contains: heparin sodium 10 000 IU. Nonmedicinal ingredients: benzyl alcohol, methyl parahydroxybenzoate, propyl parahydroxybenzoate, sodium chloride, sodium citrate dihydrate and water for injection.

25 000 IU/mL: Multidose vials (with preservative) of 2 mL: Each mL of solution contains: heparin sodium 25 000 IU. Nonmedicinal ingredients: benzyl alcohol, methyl parahydroxybenzoate, propyl parahydroxybenzoate, sodium citrate dihydrate and water for injection.

Store below 25°C. Admixture of heparin with solutions of other medicinal products may result in precipitation or loss of potency.

Heparin LEO multi-dose vials for injection are not affected significantly chemically, physically or microbiologically following multiple puncture (7 times) over a 28 day period when stored at 25°C±2°C.

Heparin Lock Flush

heparin sodium

Heparin Lock Flush

Hospira

SUPPLIED: Each mL of sterile, nonpyrogenic solution contains: heparin sodium 10 or 100 USP units (derived from porcine intestinal mucosa), sodium chloride, edetate disodium anhydrous as a stabilizer and water for injection. Also contains benzyl alcohol and sodium hydroxide. Multidose vials of 10 mL. Boxes of 25.

Heparin Sodium and 0.9% Sodium Chloride Injection

heparin sodium—sodium chloride

Anticoagulant

Baxter

SUPPLIED: Each mL of sterile, nonpyrogenic solution contains: heparin sodium USP in 0.9% sodium chloride injection. Viaflex Plus plastic (polyvinylchloride) containers in the following sizes and concentrations: see Table 1.

Table 1: Heparin Sodium and 0.9% Sodium Chloride Injection Supplied

Total Volume (mL)	USP Heparin Units	Heparin Concentration (U/mL)
500	1000	2
1000	2000	2

Do not store above 30°C. Protect from freezing.

Heparin Sodium in 5% Dextrose Injection
heparin sodium—dextrose
Anticoagulant

Baxter

SUPPLIED: Each mL of sterile, nonpyrogenic solution contains: heparin sodium USP in 5% dextrose injection. Viaflex Plus plastic (polyvinyl chloride) containers in the following sizes and concentrations: see Table 1.

Table 1: Heparin Sodium in 5% Dextrose Injection Supplied

Total Volume (mL)	USP Heparin Units	Heparin Concentration (U/mL)
500	20 000	40
500	25 000	50
250	25 000	100

Exposure of pharmaceutical products to heat should be minimized. Avoid excessive heat. It is recommended the products be stored at room temperature (25°C); brief exposure up to 40°C does not adversely affect the product.

Heparin Sodium in 5% Dextrose Injection
heparin sodium—dextrose
Anticoagulant

Hospira

SUPPLIED: Each mL of sterile, nonpyrogenic fluid for i.v. administration contains: heparin sodium (derived from porcine intestinal mucosa) 40 units (20 000 units/500 mL) or 50 units (25 000 units/500 mL) and 0.05 g of dextrose, anhydrous. Nonmedicinal ingredients: citric acid anhydrous, sodium metabisulfite, sodium phosphate dibasic anhydrous and water for injection. Single dose flexible plastic containers, cases of 20.

Heparin Sodium Injection USP
heparin sodium
Anticoagulant

Sandoz

SUPPLIED: 1000 USP units/mL (multidose): Each mL of sterile solution contains: heparin sodium 1000 USP units. Nonmedicinal ingredients: benzyl alcohol 10 mg (as a preservative), sodium chloride 5.8 mg, sodium hydroxide and/or hydrochloric acid to adjust the pH, water for injection. Vials of 10 and 30 mL, boxes of 10. Store between 15 and 30°C. Protect from light. Protect from freezing. Discard unused portion 28 days after initial puncture.

10 000 USP units/mL (multidose): Each mL of sterile solution contains: heparin sodium 10 000 USP units. Nonmedicinal ingredients: benzyl alcohol 10 mg (as a preservative), sodium chloride 2.2 mg, sodium hydroxide and/or hydrochloric acid to adjust the pH, water for injection. Vials of 5 mL, boxes of 10. Store between 15 and 30°C. Protect from light. Protect from freezing. Discard unused portion 28 days after initial puncture.

10 000 USP units/mL (single dose): Each mL of preservative-free sterile solution contains: heparin sodium 10 000 USP units. Nonmedicinal ingredients: sodium chloride 5.0 mg, sodium hydroxide and/or hydrochloric acid to adjust the pH, water for injection. Vials of 1 mL, boxes of 10. Store between 15 and 30°C. Protect from light. Protect from freezing. Discard unused portion.

Heparin: Unfractionated
heparin sodium
Anticoagulant

CPhA Monograph

Date of Revision: February 2010

This monograph has been compiled by CPhA and reviewed by experts. It may contain information different from that found in Health Canada-approved Product Monographs. The reader is referred to the *CPS* Editorial Policy for more information.

SUMMARY PRODUCT INFORMATION:

Route of Administration	Dosage Form	Strength
Intravenous, subcutaneous	Vials	1000 IU/mL, 10 000 IU/mL, 25 000 IU/mL
Intravenous	Vials	10 IU/mL, 100 IU/mL
	Solution	2 IU/mL, 40 IU/mL, 50 IU/mL, 100 IU/mL

PHARMACOLOGY: Heparin is a heterogeneous preparation of sulfated mucopolysaccharide polymers whose molecular weights range from 3000 to 30 000 daltons, averaging between 12 000 and 15 000 daltons. Heparin exerts its anticoagulant activity by reversibly binding to antithrombin (AT), accelerating the ability of AT to neutralize thrombin (factor IIa) and activated coagulation factor X (Xa). The heparin-AT complex also inactivates activated coagulation factors IX, XI, XII and plasmin. Thrombin and factor Xa are the most sensitive to inactivation by the heparin-AT complex.

Heparin is not a thrombolytic agent. It does not directly cause clot lysis, but prevents progression of an existing clot by inhibiting any further clotting processes, allowing naturally occurring thrombolytics to slowly effect clot lysis.

At therapeutic doses, heparin prolongs several coagulation tests including activated coagulation time, activated partial thromboplastin time (APTT, used clinically), plasma recalcification time, prothrombin time (minimally), thrombin time and whole blood clotting time.

Pharmacokinetics: Heparin is not absorbed through the gastrointestinal mucosa and must be given parenterally, usually by iv infusion or deep sc injection. The onset of action is immediate after iv injection but can be delayed 20 to 60 minutes following sc injection. Heparin is extensively bound to plasma proteins. Heparin does not cross the placental barrier and is not distributed into breast milk. Heparin is not removed by hemodialysis.

The dose-response relationship of heparin is not linear. Anticoagulant effect increases disproportionately in intensity and duration as the dose is increased. The plasma half-life of heparin increases from approximately 60 minutes with a 100 unit/kg dose to about 150 minutes with a 400 unit/kg dose. Clinically a half-life of approximately 90 minutes is used.

Heparin is cleared via a dual mechanism. At low doses, clearance is predominantly through a saturable mechanism by the reticuloendothelial system. At higher doses, renal clearance through a nonsaturable mechanism also occurs. The rapid saturable mechanism predominates at therapeutic heparin concentrations.

The clearance of heparin from plasma is accelerated in patients with pulmonary embolism and may be reduced in patients with cirrhosis or severe renal impairment.

INDICATIONS: Health Canada-approved indications include:

- treatment of venous thrombosis and thromboembolic phenomena.
- prevention of venous thromboembolism.
- prevention of clotting during dialysis and surgical procedures.
- maintaining the patency of iv injection devices.

CONTRAINDICATIONS: Patients with a generalized clotting disorder such as hemophilia, Christmas disease, idiopathic thrombocytopenic purpura and patients with active bleeding from a local lesion such as an acute ulcer or ulcerating carcinoma; patients who have had recent cranial, spinal, eye or ear surgery or trauma; hypersensitivity to heparin, including thrombocytopenia; severe liver damage; shock.

WARNINGS: Administration of large doses of heparin should be delayed at least 4 hours postoperatively.

PRECAUTIONS: The use of iv heparin in the treatment of ischemic stroke is controversial. Clinical trials investigating the benefits of heparin in ischemic stroke have been inconclusive. Heparin may increase the risk of clinically significant cerebral bleeding. Administration of an iv bolus of heparin is not recommended in the treatment of stroke. If heparin is used, brain imaging should be performed prior to initiation of therapy to exclude hemorrhage and estimate infarct size.

When considered for use in any of the following conditions, the advantages of heparin therapy must be carefully weighed against the risks: subacute bacterial endocarditis; increased capillary permeability; dissecting aneurysm; severe hypertension; during and immediately following major surgery, especially of the brain, spinal cord, eye or ear; conditions associated with increased bleeding tendencies such as hemophilia, thrombocytopenia and some purpuras; inaccessible gastrointestinal ulcers; ulcerative colitis; continuous tube drainage of stomach or small intestine; threatened abortion; menstruation.

In patients with a history of heparin-induced thrombocytopenia (HIT), heparinoids (e.g., danaparoid), lepirudin and argatroban are considered appropriate alternatives to heparin.

When used in therapeutic doses, heparin should be regulated by frequent blood coagulation indicators, particularly the APTT. If the indicator is unduly prolonged or if hemorrhage occurs, heparin should be at least temporarily discontinued (see Overdose). Dosing can be effectively guided using a weight-based heparin dose adjustment nomogram (see Table 2 for an example).

Heparin can prolong the prothrombin time.

Apparent resistance to heparin may be encountered in patients with acquired or familial AT deficiency, because adequate levels of AT are required for heparin's anticoagulant effect. Larger doses of heparin may be required initially in patients with various disease states due to alterations in their physiology, the pharmacokinetics of the drug, or elevations in levels of acute phase heparin binding proteins. Among these are febrile illness, infections associated with thrombosing tendencies, pulmonary embolism, myocardial infarction, extensive thrombotic disorders especially those associated with neoplastic disease and following surgery.

Heparin should be used with caution in the presence of severe hepatic or renal disease, or in patients with indwelling catheters. A higher incidence of bleeding may be seen in women over 60 years of age.

Patients on long-term daily administration of heparin should be observed for the possible development of osteoporosis and spontaneous fracture of ribs and/or vertebrae.

IM injections of other drugs should be avoided during heparin therapy to reduce the risk of hematoma formation and bleeding from the site. Most drugs can be given by another route (iv or sc).

Drug Interactions: Oral anticoagulants (e.g., warfarin) can contribute to a small extent to an increase in APTT. Heparin can contribute to an increase in PT. While these two drugs are given together, the fact that each may contribute to an increase in PT and APTT should be taken into account (see Precautions).

Heparin is often started with or several hours after thrombolytic therapy (e.g., alteplase) for acute myocardial infarction. Close patient monitoring for clinical signs of bleeding is indicated. The APTT should also be monitored closely (see Dosage, Acute MI). In acute ischemic stroke, alteplase administration is contraindicated within 48 hours of heparin use.

Salicylates, other nonsteroidal anti-inflammatory agents, dipyridamole, clopidogrel, ticlopidine and GPIIb-IIIa antagonists (e.g., abciximab) interfere with platelet aggregation which increases the risk of bleeding. They should be used cautiously with monitoring for signs of hemorrhage. In addition, in some situations, when heparin is used in conjunction with GPIIb-IIIa antagonists the dose of heparin may need to be modified (see Dosage, Coronary Surgery).

IV nitroglycerin may reduce heparin's anticoagulant effect and necessitate higher doses. This interaction has been reported to occur regardless of whether or not propylene glycol is used as a solvent for the nitroglycerin. The mechanism has not been conclusively documented. When iv nitroglycerin therapy is initiated, patients should be closely monitored to ensure anticoagulation remains adequate. Likewise, when nitroglycerin therapy is stopped, a decrease in heparin dosage may be necessary and patients should be monitored for signs of excessive anticoagulation.

Pregnancy: Heparin does not cross the placenta and has not been associated with congenital defects. However, its use during pregnancy has been associated with a 13% to 22% risk of fetal mortality or prematurity. It is not clear whether severity of maternal disease or an indirect effect of heparin is responsible. Coumarin anticoagulants have been associated with a 31% incidence of unfavorable outcome and a definite drug-induced pattern of malformations has been demonstrated (fetal warfarin syndrome). However, the incidence of warfarin-induced fetopathic effects in the second and third trimesters is very low. In general, heparin is considered to be the anticoagulant of choice in pregnancy. Long-term usage (>3 to 5 months) of therapeutic doses of heparin during pregnancy increases the risk of osteoporosis and warrants careful monitoring of patients. Heparin therapy during the last trimester and immediate postpartum period is associated with a risk of maternal hemorrhage. Changes in pharmacokinetics during pregnancy require caution and close patient monitoring if heparin is used.

Reports of therapeutic failure with adjusted-dose heparin therapy in pregnant patients with prosthetic heart valves may have been due to inadequate dosing and/or monitoring or to an inherent lack of efficacy in these patients. The American College of Chest Physicians recommends that if subcutaneous heparin is used in pregnant patients with mechanical heart valves, it be administered every 12 hours and the dose adjusted to keep the mid-interval APTT at least twice the control, or an anti-Xa heparin level of 0.35 to 0.7 U/mL [*Chest* 2008;133(6 Suppl):844S-886S]. In addition, some clinicians suggest an initial dose of 17 500 to 20 000 units sc every 12 hours.

Lactation: Heparin is not excreted in breast milk because of its high molecular weight.

ADVERSE EFFECTS: Bone and Joint: Therapeutic doses of heparin administered for longer than 3 months have been associated with osteoporosis and spontaneous vertebral fractures. Osteoporosis may be reversible after discontinuation of heparin.

Hematologic: Bleeding is the most common side effect of heparin and is an extension of its pharmacologic effect. The rate of occurrence is approximately 10% overall but may increase up to 20% in patients treated with high dose therapy. Risk of bleeding likely increases with APTT ratios above the recommended target range. Other risk factors associated with bleeding are: a serious concurrent illness, chronic heavy consumption of alcohol, use of platelet-inhibiting drugs, renal failure, age and female sex. Bleeding may range from minor local ecchymoses to major hemorrhagic events. Often the first sign of bleeding may be epistaxis, hematuria or melena. Bleeding may be from any site and can be difficult to detect, e.g., retroperitoneal bleeds. Bleeding may also occur from surgical sites. Petechiae or easy bruising may precede frank hemorrhage. A supratherapeutic APTT or minor bleeding during therapy can usually be controlled by adjusting the dosage or withdrawing the drug (see Overdose).

Heparin is associated with two types of thrombocytopenia. Type 1 is most common, occurring in up to 10% of patients. The platelet count drops within the first several days of therapy, but usually remains above 100×10^9/L. This form of thrombocytopenia is not associated with thrombosis, and heparin therapy does not necessarily have to be withdrawn. The platelet count may remain stable or even increase despite continued therapy; however, it should be monitored closely. This form of heparin-induced thrombocytopenia (HIT) is not immune-mediated, but appears to result from a direct action of heparin on platelets.

Type 2 HIT (HIT-2) is much less common but is a more serious complication than Type 1 HIT. It is an immune-mediated reaction, and the platelet count does not usually fall until between day 5 and day 12 of heparin therapy. Exceptions occur in patients who have received a previous course of heparin within the past 3 months; these patients may experience onset of thrombocytopenia within 24 hours of being reexposed to heparin. HIT-2 has occurred with low doses of heparin and is not dose-related.

The thrombocytopenia seen in HIT-2 is often severe (platelet count <100×10⁹/L). Up to 50% of patients with HIT-2 will go on to develop thrombotic complications such as arterial thrombosis, gangrene, stroke, MI and disseminated intravascular coagulation. Thrombosis is due to "white clots" composed of platelets and fibrin that result from marked in vivo platelet aggregation. Treatment of HIT-2 includes immediate cessation of all forms of heparin therapy, including heparin used to flush iv lines. Other treatment options include danaparoid, lepirudin and argatroban. LMWHs should not be used in patients with a history of HIT-2, since there is a high degree of cross-reactivity. The thrombocytopenia itself usually reverses within 3 to 7 days of stopping heparin, but the risk of thrombosis persists for up to 30 days. Patients receiving heparin acutely should have platelet counts monitored at least every 2 or 3 days to screen for the development of HIT.

Hepatic: Heparin has been reported to cause elevations of AST and ALT in approximately 27% and 59% of patients, respectively. Transient increases in serum LDH levels have also occurred. No clinical signs of liver dysfunction have been reported and the significance is not known, except that interpretation of liver enzymes for other purposes (i.e., liver disease) must take into consideration the possible contribution of heparin.

Hypersensitivity: Heparin-induced thrombocytopenia (see Adverse Effects, Hematologic). Other allergic reactions to heparin are rare. The most common manifestations of hypersensitivity are chills, fever and urticaria. Asthma, rhinitis, tearing, headache, nausea, vomiting, shock and anaphylactoid reactions have also occurred. Vasospasm has been reported 6 to 10 days after starting heparin; the etiology is thought to be allergic. Vasospasm often appears in a limb where an artery has recently been catheterized. The affected limb is usually painful, ischemic and cyanotic. Protamine sulfate is of no use in hypersensitivity reactions.

Miscellaneous: Alopecia, affecting the entire scalp or confined to the temple, may occur. Itching and burning of the plantar surfaces of the feet, suppression of aldosterone production, hyperkalemia (due to aldosterone suppression), priapism and rebound hyperlipidemia have also been reported.

OVERDOSE:

Symptoms: Overdose may be manifested by excessive prolongation of the APTT or by bleeding. Bleeding may be internal or external, major or minor.

Treatment: If the APTT is excessively high but bleeding is not apparent or is minor, heparin infusion may be stopped temporarily and then restarted if desired, at a reduced rate. The heparin antagonist, protamine sulfate, can be considered for severe bleeding, especially if the APTT is greater than 3 times control.

If immediate reversal of heparinization is desired, 1 mg of protamine sulfate can be used to neutralize approximately 115 units of porcine intestinal mucosa source heparin. The amount of heparin neutralized by protamine varies not only with the organ from which it is derived but also with the method of manufacture and the specific activity of heparin. The amount of protamine required to neutralize 1000 units of an individual lot of heparin can be determined and may be listed on individual product labels.

Too rapid administration of protamine can cause severe hypotensive and anaphylactoid reactions. Facilities to treat shock should be readily available when administering protamine. The rate of protamine administration should not exceed 20 mg/min and no more than 50 mg should be given in any 10 minute period. Doses exceeding 100 mg in a short period of time should be avoided, unless there is certain knowledge of larger protamine requirements. Any excess protamine sulfate, not complexed to heparin, has its own intrinsic anticoagulant effect. However, one study found overdose of protamine up to 600 to 800 mg iv to have only minor, transient effects on blood coagulation.

Due to the relatively short half-life of heparin (approximately 90 minutes), decreasing amounts of protamine sulfate are required as time from the last heparin injection increases. Some clinicians recommend that protamine dosage be based on sequential coagulation tests which correlate with the amount of heparin remaining in the body.

If heparin is given by continuous infusion, 25 to 50 mg of protamine sulfate may be given slowly after stopping the infusion. If heparin was given by deep sc injection, protamine dosage should be determined according to the amount given.

For management of a suspected drug overdose, CPhA recommends that you contact your **regional Poison Control Centre**. See the *CPS* Directory section for a list of Poison Control Centres.

DOSAGE: Heparin may be given by intermittent or continuous iv infusion or by deep (intrafat) sc injection, depending upon the situation and the prescriber's choice. Avoid im injection of heparin (see Precautions). Continuous infusion is the preferred method for administration of full-dose heparin therapy, but requires the use of a constant rate infusion pump. Intermittent infusions are not recommended, having been associated with a higher incidence of bleeding, likely due to higher total dosages required. Undesirable fluctuations of over- and under-coagulation also occur with intermittent infusions due to the short half-life of heparin. The sc route is usually reserved for prophylactic administration of heparin; however, it can also be used for dosages sufficient to treat thromboembolism. Ideally, the dose of heparin should be adjusted to prolong the APTT to a targeted therapeutic range based on a "gold standard" heparin assay. An APTT ratio of 1.5 to 2.5 times control corresponds to a whole blood heparin concentration of 0.2 to 0.4 units/mL by protamine sulfate titration or a plasma heparin concentration of 0.35 to 0.7 units/mL by inhibition of factor Xa.

Dosage requirements for full-dose heparin therapy vary widely between individuals. Body weight is a relatively good predictor of heparin dosage requirements and initial dosages may often be calculated on a unit/kg basis (see Table 1).

An initial APTT should be obtained 6 hours after commencement of heparin therapy and after every change in infusion rate. In children, an APTT should be obtained 4 hours after the loading dose and every 4 hours following each change in infusion rate. It is desirable to obtain 2 or 3 APTT determinations in the first 24 hours to stabilize the dose, and then one each day for the remainder of heparin therapy. Further dosage changes should reflect both laboratory and clinical findings.

The use of heparin in the treatment of ischemic stroke is controversial. If used during stroke, heparin should be used only if hemorrhage has been ruled out (see Precautions). It should be noted that the use of heparin in this situation might preclude the use of alteplase.

When used during coronary angioplasty, coronary stenting or cardiopulmonary bypass, heparin is used at doses above the sensitivity limit of the APTT. In these situations, the activated clotting time (ACT) is used to guide dosage adjustments.

Table 1: Heparin: Unfractionated

Initial Heparin Dosage for Treatment and Prevention of DVT/PE

Indication	Route	Dosage
Treatment (Full-Dose Therapy) Adults	Continuous IV	Bolus: 5000 units, then 1300 units/hour OR Bolus: 80 units/kg then 18 units/kg/hour
	Subcutaneous	Monitored: 17 500 units or 250 units/kg Q12H OR Unmonitored: 333 units/kg first dose then 250 units/kg Q12H
Children	Continuous IV	Initial bolus of 75 to 100 units/kg then 28 units/kg/h for infants, 20 units/kg/h for children older than 1 year, 18 units/kg/h for older children
Prophylaxis (Fixed-Dose Therapy) Adults	Low Dose Subcutaneous	5000 units sc every 8 to 12 hours

Treatment of Venous Thrombosis (DVT) and Pulmonary Embolism (PE) (see Treatment, Table 1): Adults: The following regimens have been recommended: IV: Initial bolus of 5000 units, followed by 1300 units/hour by continuous infusion, adjusted to maintain a therapeutic APTT or anti-Xa activity OR Initial bolus of 80 units/kg, followed by continuous infusion of 18 units/kg/hour, adjusted according to body weight to maintain a therapeutic APTT (see Table 2) or anti-Xa activity.

SC: If plasma monitoring is planned, the starting dose should be 17 500 units (or 250 units/kg) sc every 12 hours. The dose should then be adjusted to maintain a therapeutic APTT or anti-Xa activity measured 6 hours after a dose. The unmonitored option uses a first dose of 333 units/kg sc followed by 250 units/kg sc every 12 hours.

Duration of Therapy (IV or SC): In adult patients in whom subsequent warfarin therapy is planned, warfarin can be started as early as day 1. Heparin therapy should be continued concomitantly with warfarin therapy for at least 5 days, and should not be discontinued until the INR is in the therapeutic range for 24 hours [*Chest* 2008;133(6 Suppl):454S-545S].

Children: IV: Initial bolus of 75 units/kg over 10 min followed by continuous infusion of 28 units/kg/h for infants, 20 units/kg/h for children older than 1 year of age and 18 units/kg/h for older children. The infusion rate should be adjusted to achieve a target APTT of 60 to 85 seconds (anti-Xa activity 0.3-0.7units/mL).

In children over 2 months of age in whom subsequent warfarin therapy is planned, warfarin can be started as early as day 1. Heparin treatment should continue concomitantly with warfarin therapy for at least 6 days, and should not be discontinued until the INR is above 2.0 [*Chest* 2008;133(6 Suppl):887S-968S].

Prevention of Venous Thromboembolism (Fixed-Dose Therapy) (see Prophylaxis, Table 1): The usual prophylactic dose for general surgical and medical patients at risk for thromboembolism is 5000 units sc every 8 to 12 hours. Prophylaxis should begin on hospital admission if indicated, or 1 to 2 hours preoperatively. Heparin should continue until the patient is fully ambulatory, or until hospital discharge [*Chest* 2008;133(6 Suppl):381S-453S]. The APTT is usually not prolonged by this dose and it is not necessary to monitor the APTT. The patient must still be assessed clinically for signs of thrombotic events (i.e., failure of prophylaxis) and full-dose heparin initiated if this occurs.

Table 2: Heparin: Unfractionated

Body Weight-Based Heparin Dosage Adjustment for Treatment of DVT/PE in Adults[a,b]

APTT (seconds)	Dose Change (units/kg/h)	Additional Action	Next APTT (h)
<35 (<1.2×mean normal)	+4	Rebolus with 80 units/kg	6
35–45 (1.2–1.5×mean normal)	+2	Rebolus with 40 units/kg	6
46–70[c] (1.5–2.3×mean normal)	0	None	6[d]
71–90 (2.3–3.0×mean normal)	−2	None	6
>90 (>3×mean normal)	−3	Stop infusion for 1 h	6

[a] Adapted with permission from: Hirsh J. Guidelines for Antithrombotic Therapy. 4th ed., B.C. Decker Inc. 2001.

[b] Initial dosing: 80 units/kg; maintenance infusion of heparin, at a rate dictated by body weight through an infusion apparatus calibrated for low flow rates: 18 units/kg/h (APTT in 6 hours).

[c] The therapeutic range in seconds should correspond to a plasma heparin level of 0.2 to 0.4 units/mL by protamine sulfate titration. When APTT is checked at 6 hours or longer, steady-state kinetics can be assumed.

[d] During the first 24 hours, repeat APTT every 6 hours. Thereafter, monitor APTT once every morning unless it is outside the therapeutic range.

Long-Term Therapy: Low dose sc heparin has been used for prevention of venous thrombosis or for follow-up treatment of deep vein thrombosis in patients in whom the use of oral anticoagulants is not feasible (e.g., pregnancy). Dosages have ranged from 5000 units every 8 to 12 hours over 6 weeks to 6 months. When used as follow-up treatment of DVT, dosage of sc heparin may be adjusted following APTT or anti-Xa activity testing.

Disseminated Intravascular Coagulation: Heparin therapy for the treatment of DIC is controversial. For adults, 50 to 100 units/kg and for children 25 to 50 units/kg by iv infusion over 4 hours or by iv injection every 4 hours has been recommended. If no improvement is apparent by 4 to 8 hours, heparin should be discontinued.

Hemodialysis: For patients with multiple trauma or chronic renal failure, follow the equipment manufacturer's operating instructions carefully.

Coronary Surgery: Weight-adjusted boluses (60 to 100 units/kg) should be given immediately prior to angioplasty or coronary stent placement to achieve a target activated coagulation time (ACT) of 250 to 300 seconds with the Hemotec device and 300 to 350 seconds with the Hemochron device. If the target ACT is not achieved, additional boluses of 2000 to 5000 units can be administered. Many experts do not recommend routine post-procedural heparin infusions after uncomplicated procedures.

When glycoprotein IIb/IIIa (GPIIb/IIIa) inhibitors such as abciximab are used, the initial bolus may be reduced to 50 to 70 units/kg to achieve a target ACT of 200 seconds with either the Hemotec or Hemochron device. Many experts do not recommend post-procedural heparin infusions during GPIIb/IIIa therapy.

The femoral sheath may be removed once the ACT falls to <150 to 180 seconds, regardless of whether or not GPIIb/IIIa inhibitors were employed.

Peripheral Arterial Surgery: Heparin in doses of 100 to 150 units/kg iv is usually administered prior to cross-clamping and supplemented with doses of 50 units/kg iv every 45 to 50 minutes until flow is restored. Alternatively, some surgeons routinely obtain a baseline ACT in the operating room and adjust heparin to maintain a twofold prolongation of the ACT. The administration of protamine sulfate is recommended at the end of the procedure.

Heparin Lock Flush: Heparin lock flush solution in a concentration of 10 to 100 units/mL can be used to maintain the patency of indwelling peripheral or central venipuncture devices. Current evidence suggests that normal saline is as effective as heparin lock solution in maintaining patency of peripheral venous lines, when blood is not aspirated into the venipuncture device. It is also suggested that heparin lock solution is more effective than saline for use in arterial lines or when peripheral lines are used to obtain blood samples.

Acute MI: Patients who receive alteplase or reteplase should receive iv heparin in conjunction with low dose oral ASA as follows: bolus 60 units/kg (maximum 4000 U) then approximately 12 units/kg/hour by infusion (maximum 1000 units/hour), adjusted to maintain an APTT of 50 to 70 seconds, for 48 hours. Heparin should be initiated at the same time as thrombolytic therapy. If the patient is at high risk of systemic or venous thromboembolism (anterior Q-wave infarction, severe LV dysfunction, heart failure, history of systemic or pulmonary embolus, 2-dimensional echocardiographic evidence of mural thrombosis, atrial fibrillation) the iv regimen may be continued and the patient switched to another anticoagulant as appropriate.

Patients who receive a nonselective thrombolytic (streptokinase or urokinase) should also receive iv heparin as follows: Initial iv bolus of 5000 units, followed by 1000 units/hour (patients >80 kg) or 800 units/hour (patients <80 kg) adjusted to maintain an APTT of 50 to 70 seconds or 12 500 units sc every 12 hours [*Chest* 2008;133(6 Suppl):708S-775S]. Heparin should be continued for 48 hours and then switched to another anticoagulant if appropriate.

Patients who do not receive a thrombolytic should be considered for iv heparin. These patients should be given an iv bolus of 60 units/kg (maximum 4000 U) then approximately 12 units/kg/hour by infusion (maximum 1000 units/hr), adjusted to maintain an APTT of 50 to 70 seconds. Heparin should be continued for 48 hours and then followed by another anticoagulant if appropriate.

All patients with **acute MI** should at least be given low-dose heparin therapy or low molecular weight heparin therapy until ambulatory to prevent DVT/PE.

Unstable Angina or Non-ST-Segment Elevation MI: Initial iv bolus of 60 to 70 units/kg (maximum 5000 U) followed by an initial infusion of 12 to 15 units/kg/hour (maximum 1000 units/hr). The infusion rate should be adjusted to maintain the APTT in the target range of 1.5 to 2.5 times control. Duration of therapy is controversial, but many clinicians recommend that it be continued for at least 48 hours.

Heparins: Low Molecular Weight 🅿

dalteparin sodium
enoxaparin sodium
nadroparin calcium
tinzaparin sodium

Anticoagulant

CPhA Monograph

Date of Revision: October 2006

This monograph has been compiled by CPhA and reviewed by experts. It may contain information different from that found in Health Canada-approved Product Monographs. The reader is referred to the *CPS* Editorial Policy for more information.

PHARMACOLOGY: Low molecular weight heparins (LMWHs) are fragments of heparin produced by enzymatic or chemical depolymerization. They have an average molecular weight of 4000 to 5000 daltons (range 1000 to 10 000 daltons) which is approximately one-third that of unfractionated heparin.

Most heparin molecules with molecular weights smaller than 5400 daltons are unable to bind thrombin and antithrombin simultaneously, as can unfractionated heparin. Therefore, LMWHs are less able to accelerate the inactivation of thrombin (factor IIa) but retain the ability to catalyze the inhibition of factor Xa. The anti-factor Xa to anti-factor IIa ratio of LMWHs ranges from 2:1 to 4:1, compared to 1:1 for unfractionated heparin (see Table 1). These ratios are based on in vitro testing and may not reflect the relative anticoagulant activity in humans.

Pharmacokinetics: Unlike unfractionated heparin, LMWHs do not bind significantly to plasma proteins. This accounts for the different pharmacokinetic properties, dosing regimens and laboratory monitoring requirements of these two classes of heparins. Furthermore, LMWHs do not bind to endothelial cells and macrophages, which is felt to partially account for their longer plasma half-lives in comparison with unfractionated heparin.

The biological half-life of LMWHs is not dose-dependent and is about 2 to 4 times longer than that of unfractionated heparin at therapeutic doses. In contrast, unfractionated heparin exhibits a dose-dependent biological half-life due to a rapid phase of saturable intracellular elimination followed by nonsaturable renal elimination.

LMWHs are cleared primarily by the renal route. This process is not saturable. The half-life is extended in patients with renal failure. Table 2 compares the pharmacokinetics of LMWHs and unfractionated heparin.

Table 1: Heparins: Low Molecular Weight

Pharmacologic Comparison, including Unfractionated Heparin

	Anti-Xa to Anti-IIa Activity Ratio	Average Molecular Weight (daltons)
Dalteparin	2.2 : 1.0	5000
Enoxaparin	> 4.0 : 1.0	4500
Nadroparin	2.5 to 4.0 : 1.0	4300
Tinzaparin	1.9 : 1.0	4500
Unfractionated heparin	1.0 : 1.0	15 000

Compared to unfractionated heparin, LMWHs exhibit a more predictable dose-response relationship and generally require less monitoring. This is due to their better bioavailability, longer half-life and dose-independant clearance.

Table 2: Heparins: Low Molecular Weight

Pharmacokinetic Comparison of Low Molecular Weight Heparins vs Unfractionated Heparin

Pharmacokinetic Property	Low Molecular Weight Heparins	Unfractionated Heparin
Plasma protein binding	minimal	significant
Endothelial cell/macrophage binding	no	yes
Dose-dependent clearance	no	yes
Bioavailability at low-dose (subcutaneous)	> 90%	10-30%
Bioavailability at high-dose	> 90%	90%
Elimination	renal (nonsaturable)	low-dose cellular uptake (saturable) high-dose renal (nonsaturable)
Half-life	dose-independent (2 to 4 hours)	dose-dependent (0.5 to 4 hours)

INDICATIONS: Currently, no data are available which directly compare the efficacy of different LMWHs for a given indication using recommended doses; therefore, the available agents cannot be used interchangeably.

Table 3 lists the current labeled indications for the available LMWHs.

Table 3: Heparins: Low Molecular Weight

Labeled Indications

Indication	Dalteparin	Enoxaparin	Nadroparin	Tinzaparin
Prophylaxis of deep vein thrombosis in:				
Selected medical patients[a]	Yes	Yes		
General surgery	Yes	—	Yes	Yes[b]
Orthopedic surgery	—	—	Yes	Yes
Orthopedic surgery, specifically of knee or hip	Yes[c]	Yes	—	—
High-risk abdominal, gynecological or urological surgery	—	Yes	—	—
Colorectal surgery	—	Yes	—	—
Treatment of deep vein thrombosis	Yes	Yes	Yes	Yes
Prevention of clotting in the extracorporeal system during hemodialysis and hemoperfusion in patients with chronic renal failure	Yes	—	Yes	Yes
Treatment of unstable angina or non-Q-wave MI, concurrently with ASA	Yes	Yes	Yes	—

a In patients at moderate risk of DVT who are bedridden or have severely restricted mobility, and require short-term prophylaxis of DVT (see product monographs for details).

b In patients at high risk for developing postoperative venous thromboembolism.

c Elective hip surgery.

CONTRAINDICATIONS: LMWHs should not be used when the following medical problems exist: uncontrolled active bleeding, severe hypertension (because of increased risk of cerebral hemorrhage), hemorrhagic stroke, allergy or hypersensitivity to heparin, pork products or to the LMWH, a history of thrombocytopenia with the specific LMWH, or a positive in vitro platelet aggregation test in the presence of the specific LMWH.

LMWHs should be avoided in patients with a history of heparin-induced thrombocytopenia (HIT). Alternatives include heparinoids, lepirudin and ancrod.

WARNINGS: LMWHs should not be injected by the i.m. route because of the risk of hematoma.

There have been reports of intraspinal hematoma resulting in long-term or permanent paralysis in patients undergoing spinal or epidural anesthesia while on LMWH therapy. The risk may be higher with repeated or traumatic catheter insertion, with use of indwelling epidural catheters for administration of anesthesia, or with concurrent use of other drugs affecting hemostasis. Caution is advised if concurrent LMWH therapy and spinal or epidural anesthesia is considered. If concurrent treatment is undertaken, patients must be monitored frequently for signs and symptoms of neurological compromise. If neurological impairment is noted, urgent treatment is necessary. The reader is referred to the relevant individual product monograph for specific precautions pertinent to each product.

LMWHs, like other anticoagulants, should be used with extreme caution in any medical procedure or condition in which the risk of bleeding or hemorrhage is present such as: septic endocarditis, major blood clotting disorders, blood dyscrasias, active gastric or duodenal ulceration, injuries to or surgery involving the CNS, eyes or ears, diabetic or hemorrhagic retinopathy, or severe hepatic or renal insufficiency.

Doses of LMWHs recommended for prophylaxis are lower and not appropriate for the treatment of acute thrombosis.

The official product monographs for LMWH warn against the use of LMWH for prevention of thromboembolism in patients with prosthetic heart valves, including those who are pregnant. The use of LMWH in pregnant patients with mechanical valves is controversial. Some clinicians say it cannot be recommended at this time; others consider it a valid option. Also see Precautions, Pregnancy.

PRECAUTIONS: Periodic complete blood counts including platelet counts and stool occult blood tests are recommended during the course of treatment. Physical examinations should be performed to monitor for bleeding complications.

With usual dosing, LMWHs do not consistently modify global clotting tests of activated partial thromboplastin time (APTT), prothrombin time (PT) and thrombin clotting time (TT); therefore, treatment cannot be monitored with these tests. Anti-factor Xa activity has been used for assessing the activity of LMWHs. However, it does not correlate directly with therapeutic efficacy. In the majority of cases monitoring of anti-factor Xa levels is not required. Exceptions include cases where the patient is a child, is pregnant, is morbidly obese or has renal insufficiency. Some experts state that the target range for treatment of venous thrombosis should be 0.6 to 1 anti-Xa IU/mL 4 hours after a twice-daily dose and 1 to 2 anti-Xa IU/mL 4 hours after a once-daily dose. Risk of major bleeding appears to be increased if the anti-factor Xa level is 2 IU/mL or higher.

Except under special circumstances, LMWHs should not be used when abortion is imminent or threatened. They may be used in such cases only when, in the opinion of the physician, the increased risk of bleeding is outweighed by the risk of thrombosis or thromboembolism.

Multidose vials of tinzaparin may contain sodium metabisulfite. This agent may cause allergic-type reactions including anaphylactic symptoms and possibly life-threatening asthmatic episodes in susceptible individuals. The exact prevalence of sulfite sensitivity in the general population is not known but is probably low. Asthmatic persons are at higher risk than non-asthmatics.

Drug Interactions: Caution should be exercised when using LMWHs together with oral anticoagulants or platelet inhibitors because of an increased risk of bleeding.

Pregnancy: LMWHs are relatively large molecules and are not expected to cross the placenta. There have been reports of congenital anomalies in infants born to women who received low molecular weight heparin during pregnancy including cerebral anomalies, limb anomalies, hypospadias, peripheral vascular malformation, fibrotic dysplasia and cardiac defects. However, a causal relationship has not been established nor has the incidence been shown to be higher than in the general population. While product monographs include this warning, some clinicians have stated that the potential of these agents for teratogenecity lacks biological plausibility.

As with heparin, there have been post-marketing reports of fetal death when pregnant women received LMWHs. Causality for these cases has not been established.

Multidose vials of dalteparin or enoxaparin may contain benzyl alcohol. This agent has been associated with a fatal toxic syndrome when administered to premature infants. The manufacturer of dalteparin therefore recommends against the use of these multidose vials in pregnant women, even though it is not known if benzyl alcohol crosses the placenta and the amount of benzyl alcohol received by the pregnant woman is small compared to amounts implicated in published case reports of the toxic syndrome.

Also see Warnings regarding the use of LMWH in patients with prosthetic heart valves.

Lactation: Because of the relatively high molecular weight of LMWHs and because they are inactivated in the gastrointestinal tract, their passage into breast milk and subsequent risk to a nursing infant should be considered negligible.

Children: Safety and efficacy have not been established. Risks to the child must be balanced against expected benefits on a case-by-case basis.

ADVERSE EFFECTS: The incidence of hemorrhagic complications during treatment with LMWHs has been low. The incidence of bleeding may increase with higher doses. The risk of bleeding does not appear to differ substantially from that of unfractionated heparin. Risk factors for bleeding during therapy with heparins in general include serious concurrent illness, chronically heavy alcohol consumption, use of platelet inhibiting drugs, renal failure, advanced age and possibly female gender.

The most commonly reported side effect is hematoma at the injection site. Mild local irritation, pain and erythema following s.c. injection are reported less frequently.

The following side effects have been reported rarely: allergic reactions (e.g., pruritus, rash, fever, injection site reaction, hives), skin necrosis, anaphylactoid reactions and thrombocytopenia. To date, LMWHs have been associated with a lower risk of thrombocytopenia than standard heparin; however, until a greater number of patients have been exposed, the exact incidence cannot be reliably estimated.

Slight to moderate elevations of liver transaminases (AST, ALT) have been reported but have not been correlated with any long-term effect on liver function. Transaminase determinations are important in the differential diagnosis of myocardial infarction, liver disease or pulmonary embolism; elevations should be interpreted carefully.

Bleeding complications associated with overdose may include: hematuria, bloody or black tarry stools, bruising, hemoptysis, hematemesis, ecchymosis, hematoma, hypochromic anemia, nosebleed, persistent bleeding or oozing from mucous membranes or surgical wounds, shortness of breath, vomiting of material that resembles coffee grounds.

Osteoporosis has been reported with prolonged use of LMWHs.

OVERDOSE:

Symptoms: Overdosage with LMWHs may lead to bleeding. Monitor platelet counts, hematocrit and coagulation parameters, including APTT.

Treatment: Minor bleeding usually requires reduction or delay of subsequent doses. In the case of major bleeding, discontinue the LMWH. Consider the use of protamine in serious cases of bleeding only. To avoid overdosage of protamine, the half-life and rate of absorption of the LMWH in question should be taken into account when calculating the neutralizing dose. A dose of 1 mg of protamine sulfate is administered for every 100 anti-Xa IU of dalteparin or tinzaparin, for each 158 anti-Xa IU of nadroparin, or for each 1 mg of enoxaparin. If the APTT measured 2 to 4 hours after the first infusion remains prolonged, a second infusion of 0.5 mg protamine sulfate per 100 anti-Xa IU of dalteparin or tinzaparin or per mg of enoxaparin may be administered. Even after an additional dose of protamine, the APTT may remain more prolonged following administration of a LMWH than after standard heparin. Protamine sulfate should completely neutralize the anti-IIa effect but not the anti-Xa effect which is neutralized to a maximum of only 60 to 75%, depending on the particular LMWH.

Protamine should be administered by slow i.v. injection, no faster than 20 mg/min. Too rapid administration of protamine can cause severe hypotensive and anaphylactoid reactions. It should only be administered when treatment for anaphylactic shock and resuscitation techniques are readily available. A maximum of 50 mg of protamine should be administered in any 10-minute period. Protamine doses exceeding 100 mg in a short period of time should be avoided unless there is certain knowledge of larger protamine requirements. Protamine should be administered with caution to patients with a history of fish allergy.

Fresh frozen plasma may also be helpful in cases of serious hemorrhage requiring transfusion.

For management of a suspected drug overdose, CPhA recommends that you contact your **regional Poison Control Centre**. See the *CPS* Directory section for a list of Poison Control Centres.

DOSAGE: In general, LMWHs are administered by deep s.c. injection once or twice daily as recommended by the manufacturer. They should not be injected by the i.m. route (see Warnings). Dalteparin may also be administered by intermittent or continuous i.v. infusion; however, the manufacturer suggests that s.c. administration may be the route of choice because of the long half-life, high bioavailability, low incidence of side effects and ease of administration.

Depending on the product, injection sites include: a U-shaped area around the navel, the upper outer aspect of the thigh, or upper outer quadrangle of the buttock. The site should be varied daily. The patient should be sitting or lying down during injection. If giving the injection around the navel or the thigh, a fold of skin must be lifted up with thumb and forefinger and the entire length of the needle inserted at a 45- to 90-degree angle.

Though LMWHs have a relatively predictable dose-response relationship, some experts recommend periodic monitoring of anti-Xa levels in specific patient populations (see Precautions).

LMWHs cannot be used interchangeably (unit for unit) with unfractionated heparin or with other LMWHs since they differ in their relative inhibition of factor Xa and factor IIa.

Table 4 lists the dosage recommendations for the labeled indications of the available LMWHs. It is not meant to be exhaustive; consult product monographs for specific dosage recommendations, including those regarding dosage adjustment in renal failure.

Table 4: Heparins: Low Molecular Weight
Dosage in Adults

Indication	Dalteparin	Enoxaparin	Nadroparin	Tinzaparin
Prophylaxis of deep vein thrombosis in:				
Selected medical patients	5000 anti-Xa IU s.c. once daily	40 mg s.c. once daily for 6 to 11 days.		
General surgery	2500 anti-Xa IU s.c. 1 to 2 hours before surgery, then each morning for at least 5 to 7 days.[a]	See below.	2850 anti-Xa IU s.c. 2 to 4 hours before surgery then daily for at least 7 days.	3500 anti-Xa IU s.c. 2 hours before surgery,[b] then 3500 anti-Xa IU s.c. daily for 7 to 10 days.
Orthopedic surgery	See below.	—	38 anti-Xa IU/kg s.c. 12 hours before surgery, 12 hours after surgery and daily for 3 days, then 57 anti-Xa IU/kg s.c. daily for at least 7 additional days.[d]	See below.
Orthopedic surgery, specifically of knee or hip	Hip Surgery: 5000 anti-Xa IU s.c. the evening before surgery, then every evening for at least 5 to 7 days[c] **OR** 2500 anti-Xa IU s.c. 1 to 2 hours before surgery and again 8 to 12 hours later, then 5000 anti-Xa IU each morning for at least 5 to 7 days.	30 mg s.c. every 12 hours starting 12 to 24 hours after surgery, for 7 to 14 days.	—	Hip Surgery: 50 anti-Xa IU/kg s.c. 2 hours before surgery, then 50 anti-Xa IU/kg daily for 7 to 10 days **OR** 75 anti-Xa IU/kg s.c. daily postoperatively for 7 to 10 days. Knee Surgery: 75 anti-Xa IU/kg s.c. daily postoperatively, for 7 to 10 days.
Colorectal surgery or high-risk abdominal, gynecological or urological surgery	—	40 mg s.c. 2 hours before surgery, then daily for 7 to 10 days.	—	—
Treatment of deep vein thrombosis	200 anti-Xa IU/kg s.c. daily. Single daily dose should not exceed 18 000 IU. For patients at increased risk of bleeding: 100 anti-Xa IU/kg s.c. twice daily **OR** 100 anti-Xa IU/kg over 12 hours i.v. as a continuous infusion.[e]	1.5 mg/kg s.c. daily **OR** 1 mg/kg s.c. every 12 hours. Single daily dose should not exceed 180 mg.[e]	171 anti-Xa IU/kg s.c. once daily. Single daily dose should not exceed 17 100 IU. For patients at higher risk of bleeding: 86 anti-Xa IU/kg s.c. twice daily.[e]	175 anti-Xa IU/kg s.c. daily.[e]
Prevention of clotting in the extracorporeal system during hemodialysis and hemoperfusion in patients with chronic renal failure with no known bleeding risk	30 to 40 anti-Xa IU/kg i.v. bolus at start of session then i.v. infusion of 10 to 15 anti-Xa IU/kg/hour. Alternatively, for sessions lasting 4 hours or less, may give one i.v. bolus injection of 5000 anti-Xa IU.[f]	—	65 anti-Xa IU/kg into the arterial line at start of each session; if session longer than 4 hours, may give a repeat dose.[f]	4500 anti-Xa IU into the arterial side of dialyser (or i.v.) at start of session lasting 4 hours or less. Adjustment of dose for subsequent sessions may be achieved in steps of 500 anti-Xa IU, up or down.[f,g]
Treatment of unstable angina and non-Q-wave MI, concurrently with ASA	120 anti-Xa IU/kg s.c. twice daily, with a maximum of 10 000 IU/dose, for up to 6 days.[h]	1 mg/kg s.c. every 12 hours, with a maximum of 100 mg/dose, for 2 to 8 days.[h]	86 anti-Xa IU/kg i.v. bolus initially, then 86 anti-Xa IU/kg s.c. q12h. Usual treatment duration is 6 days.[h]	—

[a] Patients with higher risk of thromboembolic complications may receive the dosage regimen indicated in the table for dalteparin in hip surgery. Prophylaxis should continue until patient is well-mobilized.
[b] General surgery in patients at high risk for developing postoperative venous thromboembolism.
[c] This dosing regimen may also be used for patients with other risk factors for thromboembolic complications undergoing general surgery.
[d] Treatment should continue until patient is actively ambulated.
[e] Treatment with warfarin is normally started immediately. LMWH therapy should continue concomitantly with warfarin therapy for at least 5 days, and should not be discontinued until the INR is in the therapeutic range for 2 consecutive days.
[f] Consult individual product monographs for recommendations pertaining to hemodialysis in patients with acute renal failure or high risk of bleeding.
[g] A larger starting dose may be given for dialysis sessions lasting longer than 4 hours.
[h] Concomitant therapy with ASA (100 to 325 mg daily) is recommended.

Children: Therapeutic doses of LMWHs recommended by the Seventh ACCP Conference on Antithrombotic and Thrombolytic Therapy were extrapolated from adults and are based on anti-FXa levels (Table 5). Dosage adjustment should be based on measurement of anti-FXa levels 2 to 6 hours after a subcutaneous injection (target 0.5-1.0 U/mL).

Table 5: Heparins: Low Molecular Weight
Dosage in Children[a]

Indication	Dalteparin	Enoxaparin	Tinzaparin
Initial Treatment Dose	All ages: 129±43 U/kg q24h	<2 mo: 1.5 mg/kg q12h >2 mo: 1.0 mg/kg q12h	0–2 mo: 275 U/kg daily 2–12 mo: 250 U/kg daily 1–5 yr: 240 U/kg daily 5–10 yr: 200 U/kg daily 10–16 yr: 275 U/kg daily
Initial Prophylactic Dose	All ages: 92±52 U/kg q24h	<2 mo: 0.75 mg/kg q12h >2mo: 0.5 mg/kg q12h	

[a] Monagle P et al. Antithrombotic Therapy in Children. The Seventh ACCP Conference on Antithrombotic and Thrombolytic Therapy. Chest 2004;3 (suppl):645S–687S.

SUPPLIED: Not currently available for CPhA monographs. Please consult individual product monographs.

Hepsera® 🅿
adefovir dipivoxil
Antiviral Agent

Gilead Sciences

Date of Revision: May 25, 2009

SUMMARY PRODUCT INFORMATION:

Route of Administration	Dosage Form/ Strength	Clinically Relevant Nonmedicinal Ingredients
Oral	Tablet 10 mg	Pregelatinized starch (gluten-free), lactose monohydrate For a complete listing, see Dosage Forms, Composition and Packaging.

INDICATIONS AND CLINICAL USE: HEPSERA (adefovir dipivoxil) is indicated for the treatment of chronic hepatitis B in adults with compensated and decompensated liver disease with evidence of active viral replication, and either evidence of histologically active disease or elevation in serum aminotransferases (ALT or AST).

This indication is based on data from:
- two randomized, double-blind, placebo-controlled studies in adult patients with HBeAg+ and HBeAg− chronic hepatitis B with compensated liver function evaluating histological response
- and a non-placebo controlled study in pre- and post-liver transplantation patients, with either compensated or decompensated liver function, and an active-controlled study in patients with lamivudine-resistant hepatitis B and compensated liver function, evaluating virological response. The clinical significance of a reduction in serum HBV DNA with respect to histological improvement could not be evaluated.

CONTRAINDICATIONS: HEPSERA is contraindicated in patients with previously demonstrated hypersensitivity to any of the components of the product. For a complete listing, see Dosage Forms, Composition and Packaging.

WARNINGS AND PRECAUTIONS:

Serious Warnings and Precautions
- **Severe acute exacerbations of hepatitis have been reported in patients who have discontinued anti-hepatitis B therapy, including therapy with HEPSERA (adefovir dipivoxil). Hepatic function should be monitored closely in patients who discontinue anti-hepatitis B therapy. If appropriate, resumption of anti-hepatitis B therapy may be warranted (see Warnings and Precautions).**
- **Chronic administration of HEPSERA may result in nephrotoxicity. It is important to monitor renal function before and during treatment with HEPSERA (see Warnings and Precautions). Patients at risk for or having underlying renal dysfunction and patients taking nephrotoxic agents are particularly at risk and should be monitored closely. Patients with renal insufficiency at baseline or during treatment may require dose adjustment (see Dosage and Administration).**
- **HIV resistance may emerge in chronic hepatitis B patients with unrecognized or untreated human immunodeficiency virus (HIV) infection treated with anti-hepatitis B therapies, such as therapy with HEPSERA, that may have activity against HIV (see Warnings and Precautions).**
- **Lactic acidosis and severe hepatomegaly with steatosis, including fatal cases, have been reported with the use of nucleoside analogs alone or in combination with other antiretrovirals (see Warnings and Precautions).**

General: HEPSERA should not be administered concurrently with VIREAD (tenofovir disoproxil fumarate) or tenofovir disoproxil fumarate-containing products including TRUVADA (emtricitabine/tenofovir disoproxil fumarate combination tablet) and ATRIPLA (efavirenz/emtricitabine/tenofovir disoproxil fumarate combination tablet).

Patients should be advised that therapy of chronic hepatitis B with HEPSERA has not been proven to reduce the risk of transmission of hepatitis B virus to others through sexual contact or blood contamination and therefore, appropriate precautions should still be taken.

Exacerbations of Hepatitis after Discontinuation of Treatment: Severe acute exacerbation of hepatitis has been reported in patients who have discontinued anti-hepatitis B therapy, including therapy with HEPSERA. Patients who discontinue HEPSERA should be monitored at repeated intervals for hepatic function. If appropriate, resumption of anti-hepatitis B therapy may be warranted.

In clinical trials of HEPSERA, exacerbations of hepatitis (ALT elevations 10 times the upper limit of normal or greater) occurred in up to 25% of patients after discontinuation of HEPSERA. Most of these events occurred within 12 weeks of drug discontinuation. These exacerbations generally occurred in the absence of HBeAg seroconversion, and presented as serum ALT elevations in addition to re-emergence of viral replication. In the HBeAg-positive and HBeAg-negative studies in patients with compensated liver function, the exacerbations were not generally accompanied by hepatic decompensation. However, patients with advanced liver disease or cirrhosis may be at higher risk for hepatic decompensation. Although most events appear to have been self-limited or resolved with re-initiation of treatment, severe hepatitis exacerbations, including fatalities, have been reported. Therefore, patients should be closely monitored after stopping treatment.

Nephrotoxicity: Chronic administration of HEPSERA (10 mg once daily) may result in nephrotoxicity.

Nephrotoxicity characterized by a delayed onset of gradual increases in serum creatinine and decreases in serum phosphorus was historically shown to be the treatment-limiting toxicity of adefovir dipivoxil therapy at substantially higher doses in HIV-infected patients (60 mg and 120 mg daily) and in chronic hepatitis B patients (30 mg daily). Patients at risk of or having underlying renal dysfunction and patients taking concomitant nephrotoxic agents such as cyclosporine, tacrolimus, aminoglycosides, vancomycin and non-steroidal anti-inflammatory drugs are at risk for nephrotoxicity (see Adverse Reactions). It is recommended that creatinine clearance is calculated in all patients prior to initiating therapy with HEPSERA.

It is important to monitor renal function in all patients before and during treatment with HEPSERA, particularly for those with pre-existing or other risks for renal impairment. There is limited safety and efficacy data in patients with renal impairment. HEPSERA is not recommended for these patients unless the potential benefit outweighs the potential risk. Patients with renal impairment at baseline or during treatment may require dose adjustment (see Dosage and Administration). The risks and benefits of HEPSERA treatment should be carefully evaluated prior to discontinuing HEPSERA in a patient with treatment-emergent nephrotoxicity.

HIV Resistance: Prior to initiating HEPSERA therapy, HIV antibody testing should be offered to all patients. Treatment with anti-hepatitis B therapies, such as HEPSERA, that have activity against HIV in a chronic hepatitis B patient with unrecognized or untreated HIV infection may result in emergence of HIV resistance. HEPSERA has not been shown to suppress HIV RNA in patients, however, there are limited data on the use of HEPSERA to treat patients with chronic hepatitis B co-infected with HIV.
Lactic Acidosis/Severe Hepatomegaly with Steatosis: Lactic acidosis and severe hepatomegaly with steatosis, including fatal cases, have been reported with the use of nucleoside analogs alone or in combination with antiretrovirals.

A majority of these cases have been in women. Obesity and prolonged nucleoside exposure may be risk factors. Particular caution should be exercised when administering nucleoside analogs to any patient with known risk factors for liver disease; however, cases have also been reported in patients with no known risk factors. Treatment with HEPSERA should be suspended in any patient who develops clinical or laboratory findings suggestive of lactic acidosis or pronounced hepatotoxicity (which may include hepatomegaly and steatosis even in the absence of marked transaminase elevations).
Duration of Treatment: The optimal duration of treatment with HEPSERA has not been established. The relationship between treatment with HEPSERA and long-term outcomes such as hepatocellular carcinoma or decompensated cirrhosis is not known.
HBV Resistance: Long-term use of adefovir dipivoxil may result in emergence of HBV resistance. Resistance to adefovir dipivoxil can result in viral load rebound which may result in exacerbation of hepatitis B and, particularly in the setting of diminished hepatic function, lead to liver decompensation and possible fatal outcome. In order to reduce the risk of resistance, serum HBV virus level should be monitored during adefovir dipivoxil treatment and a change of treatment should be considered if serum HBV DNA remains above 1000 copies/mL after 48 weeks of treatment.
Special Populations: Pregnant Women: There are no adequate and well-controlled studies in pregnant women. HEPSERA should be used in pregnant women only if the potential benefits outweigh the potential risks to the fetus. For patients who are on HEPSERA and subsequently become pregnant, consideration should be given to the possibility of a recurrence of hepatitis on discontinuation of HEPSERA.
Pregnancy Registry: To monitor fetal outcomes of pregnant women exposed to HEPSERA, a pregnancy registry has been established. Healthcare providers are encouraged to register patients by calling 1-800-258-4263.
Labor and Delivery: There are no studies in pregnant women and no data on the effect of HEPSERA on transmission of HBV from mother to infant. Therefore appropriate infant immunizations should be used to prevent neonatal acquisition of HBV.
Nursing Women: It is not known whether adefovir is excreted in human milk. Mothers should be instructed not to breast-feed if they are taking HEPSERA.
Pediatrics: Safety and efficacy of HEPSERA in pediatric patients have not been established.
Geriatrics: Clinical studies of HEPSERA did not include sufficient numbers of subjects aged 65 and over to determine whether they respond differently from younger subjects. In general, caution should be exercised when prescribing to elderly patients, since they have a greater frequency of decreased renal or cardiac function due to concomitant disease or other drug therapy.

ADVERSE REACTIONS: Clinical Trial Adverse Drug Reactions: Experience in Patients with Compensated Liver Disease: Assessment of adverse reactions is based on two placebo-controlled studies (437 and 438) in which 522 patients with chronic hepatitis B and compensated liver disease received double-blind treatment with HEPSERA (N=294) or placebo (N=228) for 48 weeks. The most common treatment related adverse events in patients receiving HEPSERA were asthenia, headache, and abdominal pain.

In addition to specific adverse events described under Warnings and Precautions, all treatment-related clinical adverse events that occurred in 3% or greater of HEPSERA-treated patients compared with placebo are listed in Table 1. Patients who received HEPSERA up to 240 weeks in Study 438 reported adverse reactions similar in nature and severity to those reported in the first 48 weeks.

Table 1: HEPSERA

Treatment-Related Adverse Events (Grades 1-4) Reported in ≥3% of ADV-Treated Patients in the Pooled 437-438 Studies (0–48 Weeks)

	HEPSERA N=294 %	Placebo N=228 %
Body as a Whole		
Asthenia	13	14
Headache	9	10
Abdominal Pain	9	11
Digestive		
Nausea	5	8
Flatulence	4	4
Diarrhea	3	4
Dyspepsia	3	2

In addition, the following selected adverse events were reported in less than 3% of patients treated with HEPSERA:
Body as a Whole: back pain, chest pain.
Digestive: anorexia.
Hematologic and Lymphatic: anemia, thrombocytopenia.
Metabolic and Nutritional: weight loss.
Respiratory: pharyngitis.
Skin and Appendages: rash.
Abnormal Hematologic and Clinical Chemistry Findings: Laboratory abnormalities observed in these studies occurred with similar frequency in the HEPSERA and placebo treated groups with the exception of hepatic transaminase elevations which occurred more frequently in the placebo group. Increased liver transaminases were the most common post-treatment laboratory abnormality in the HEPSERA treated group (see Warnings and Precautions). In addition, increased creatinine was identified as an adverse reaction with extended open-label treatment.

A summary of Grade 3 and 4 laboratory abnormalities is provided in Table 2.

Table 2: HEPSERA

Grade 3-4 Laboratory Abnormalities Reported in ≥1% of All HEPSERA-Treated Patients in the Pooled 437-438 Studies (0-48 Weeks)

	HEPSERA N=294 %	Placebo N=228 %
ALT (>5×ULN)	20	41
Hematuria (≥3+)	11	10
AST (>5×ULN)	8	23
CK (>4×ULN)	7	7
Amylase (>2×ULN)	4	4
Glycosuria (≥3+)	1	3

No patients with adequate renal function treated with HEPSERA developed a serum creatinine increase ≥44 µmol/L (≥0.5 mg/dL) from baseline by Week 48. By Week 96, 10% and 2% of HEPSERA-treated patients, by Kaplan-Meier estimate, had increases in serum creatinine ≥27 µmol/L (≥0.3 mg/dL) and ≥44 µmol/L from baseline, respectively (no placebo-controlled results were available for comparison beyond Week 48). Of the 29 of 492 patients with elevations in serum creatinine ≥27 µmol/L from baseline, 20 out of 29 resolved on continued treatment (≤18 µmol/L or ≤0.2 mg/dL), 8 of 29 remained unchanged and 1 of 29 resolved on discontinuing treatment. Patients who received placebo during the first 48 weeks and HEPSERA during the second 48 weeks and patients who received HEPSERA during the first and second 48 weeks in Study 438 continued on HEPSERA for a median duration of 226 weeks (n=125); 4/125 patients (3%) had elevations in serum creatinine ≥44 µmol/L from baseline which resolved in 1 patient who permanently discontinued treatment and remained stable in 3 patients who continued treatment. In Study 437, 65 patients continued HEPSERA for a median duration of 234 weeks. Six patients had a confirmed increase of ≥44 µmol/L (≥0.5 mg/dL) from baseline with 2 patients discontinuing from the study due to the elevated serum creatinine concentration (see Laboratory Abnormalities—Special Risk Patients).
Experience in Pre- and Post-liver Transplantation Patients with Lamivudine-Resistant HBV: Pre- (N=226) and post-liver transplantation patients (N=241) with chronic hepatitis B and clinical evidence of lamivudine-resistant hepatitis B virus were treated in an open-label study with HEPSERA for up to 203 weeks, with a median time on treatment of 51 and 99 weeks, respectively.

The most common treatment-related adverse events reported in pre- and post-liver transplantation patients treated with HEPSERA with a 2% frequency or higher are shown in Table 3.

Table 3: HEPSERA

Treatment-Related Adverse Events Reported in ≥2% of Pre- or Post-liver Transplantation Patients

	Pre-liver Transplantation N=226 %	Post-liver Transplantation N=241 %
Body as a Whole		
Asthenia	4	6
Abdominal Pain	2	5
Headache	<1	4
Digestive		
Nausea	1	5
Vomiting	1	3
Diarrhea	2	4
Jaundice	<1	2
Metabolic and Nutritional		
ALT increase	1	4
AST increase	1	3
Hyperkalemia	0	2
Hypophosphatemia	2	2
Liver Function Tests Abnormal	1	2
Musculoskeletal		
Myalgia	0	3
Skin and Appendages		
Pruritus	1	5
Rash	1	2
Urogenital		
Abnormal kidney function	1	3
Creatinine Increase	2	12
Renal Failure	1	2

Fever, flatulence, hepatic failure, cough increase, pharyngitis and sinusitis occurred in less than 2% of patients.
Laboratory Abnormalities—Special Risk Patients: Pre- (N=226) and post-liver transplantation patients (N=241) with chronic hepatitis B and clinical evidence of lamivudine-resistant hepatitis B virus were treated in an open-label study with HEPSERA for up to 203 weeks, with a median time on treatment of 51 and 99 weeks, respectively. Changes in renal function occurred in pre- and post-liver transplantation patients with risk factors for renal dysfunction including concomitant use of cyclosporine and tacrolimus, renal insufficiency at baseline, hypertension, diabetes, and on-study transplantation. Increases in serum creatinine ≥44 µmol/L (≥0.5 mg/dL) from baseline were observed in 18%, 35%, and 35% of pre-liver transplantation patients by Weeks 48, 96, and 144, respectively, by Kaplan-Meier estimates. Increases in serum creatinine ≥44 µmol/L from baseline were observed in 12%, 28%, and 30% of post-liver transplantation patients by Weeks 48, 96, and 144, respectively, by Kaplan-Meier estimates. Elevations in serum creatinine ≥44 µmol/L from baseline resolved (≤27 µmol/L or ≤0.3 mg/dL increase from baseline) in 8 of 39 (21%) patients in the pre-liver transplantation cohort and in 14 of 43 (33%) patients in the post-liver transplantation cohort by the last study visit. Among patients who were assessed for serum phosphorus, values <0.65 mmol/L were observed in 3/186 (1.6%) of pre-liver transplantation patients and in 6/208 (2.9%) of post-liver transplantation patients by last study visit. Four percent (19 of 467) of pre- and post-liver transplantation patients discontinued HEPSERA due to renal events.

Due to the presence of multiple concomitant risk factors for renal dysfunction in these patients, the contributory role of HEPSERA to these changes in serum creatinine and serum phosphorus is difficult to assess.
Post-Market Adverse Drug Reactions: In addition to adverse reaction reports from clinical trials the following possible adverse reactions have also been identified during post-approval use of adefovir dipivoxil. Because these events have been reported voluntarily from a population of unknown size, estimates of frequency cannot be made.
Metabolism and Nutrition Disorders: hypophosphatemia.
Gastrointestinal Disorders: pancreatitis.
Musculoskeletal System and Connective Tissue Disorders: myopathy, osteomalacia (both associated with proximal renal tubulopathy).
Renal and Urinary Disorders: renal failure, Fanconi syndrome, proximal renal tubulopathy.

DRUG INTERACTIONS: Since adefovir is eliminated by the kidney, coadministration of HEPSERA (adefovir dipivoxil) with drugs that reduce renal function or compete for active tubular secretion may increase serum concentrations of either adefovir and/or renally eliminated coadministered drugs.

At concentrations substantially higher (>4000 fold) than those observed in vivo, adefovir did not inhibit any of the following human CYP450 isoforms, CYP1A2, CYP2C9, CYP2C19, CYP2D6 and CYP3A4. The potential for adefovir to induce CYP450 enzymes is unknown. Based on the results of these in vitro experiments and the known elimination pathway of adefovir, the potential for CYP450 mediated interactions involving adefovir with other medicinal products is low.

HEPSERA has been evaluated in healthy volunteers in combination with lamivudine, trimethoprim/sulfamethoxazole, acetaminophen and ibuprofen and in post-liver transplantation patients in combination with tacrolimus.

The pharmacokinetics of lamivudine, trimethoprim/sulfamethoxazole, acetaminophen, tacrolimus, and ibuprofen were unaltered when coadministered with HEPSERA.

The pharmacokinetics of adefovir were unaltered when HEPSERA was coadministered with lamivudine, acetaminophen, tacrolimus, and trimethoprim/sulfamethoxazole. When HEPSERA was coadministered with ibuprofen (800 mg TID) increases in adefovir C_{max} (33%), AUC (23%) and urinary recovery were observed. This increase appears to be due to higher relative oral bioavailability, not a reduction in renal clearance of adefovir. This increase was not considered to be of a sufficient magnitude to warrant a change in dosing of HEPSERA.

DOSAGE AND ADMINISTRATION: The recommended dose of HEPSERA (adefovir dipivoxil) in chronic hepatitis B patients with adequate renal function is 10 mg, once daily, taken orally, without regard to food. The optimal duration of treatment is unknown (see Warnings and Precautions, Exacerbations of Hepatitis after Discontinuation of Treatment). Therapy should be initiated and monitored by a physician experienced in the management of chronic hepatitis B.

Discontinuation of HEPSERA treatment and a change in treatment should be considered in case of evidence of ineffectiveness or efficacy loss.

Recommended Dose and Dosage Adjustment: Dosage Adjustment in Renal Impairment: Adefovir is eliminated by renal excretion, therefore adjustments in the dosing interval of HEPSERA are required in patients with creatinine clearance <50 mL/min.

The dosing frequency according to renal function must not exceed the recommended scheduled based on a pharmacokinetic study (see Table 4). Clinical response to treatment and renal function should be closely monitored in these patients.

Table 4: HEPSERA

Dosing Interval Adjustments of HEPSERA in Patients with Renal Impairment

	Creatinine Clearance (mL/min)[a]			
	≥50	30–49	10–29	Hemodialysis Patients
Recommended Dose and Dosing Interval	10 mg every 24 hours	10 mg every 48 hours	10 mg every 72 hours	10 mg every 7 days following dialysis

[a] Creatinine clearance calculated by Cockcroft-Gault method using lean or ideal body weight.

Hepatic Impairment: No dose adjustment is required in patients with hepatic impairment (see Actions and Clinical Pharmacology, Special Populations and Conditions).

Missed Dose: If a patient misses a dose at the regularly scheduled time, but then remembers it that same day, the patient should take the missed dose immediately. The next dose should be taken at the regularly scheduled time the following day. The patient should not take two doses of HEPSERA at once to make up for missing a dose.

OVERDOSAGE:

If overdose occurs, activated charcoal may be used to remove unabsorbed drug. The patient should be monitored for evidence of toxicity, and standard supportive treatment should be applied as necessary.

Following a single 10 mg dose of HEPSERA (adefovir dipivoxil), a four-hour hemodialysis session removed approximately 35% of the adefovir dose.

Daily doses of adefovir dipivoxil 500 mg for 2 weeks and 250 mg for 12 weeks have been associated with gastrointestinal side effects (see Warnings and Precautions, Nephrotoxicity).

> For management of a suspected drug overdose, contact your **regional Poison Control Centre**. See the *CPS* Directory section for a list of Poison Control Centres.

ACTION AND CLINICAL PHARMACOLOGY: HEPSERA is an oral prodrug of adefovir, a nucleoside phosphonate analog of adenosine monophosphate, which is actively transported into mammalian cells where it is converted into the active metabolite, adefovir diphosphate, by host enzymes. Adefovir diphosphate has an intracellular half-life of 12 to 36 hours in activated and resting lymphocytes. Adefovir diphosphate inhibits viral polymerases by direct binding competition with the natural substrate (deoxyadenosine triphosphate) and, after incorporation into viral DNA, results in DNA chain termination. The inhibition constant (Ki) for adefovir diphosphate for recombinant HBV DNA polymerase was 0.1 µM. Adefovir diphosphate selectively inhibits HBV DNA polymerases at concentrations 12-, 700-, and 10-fold lower than those needed to inhibit human DNA polymerases α, β, and γ, respectively.

Adefovir has in vitro antiviral activity against hepadnaviruses. The in vitro IC_{50} (concentration of drug which inhibits viral replication by 50%) of adefovir against wild-type HBV varied from 0.2 µM to 1.2 µM in human hepatic cell lines (0.2-1.2 µM in HB611, and 0.7-1.2 µM in HepG2 hepatoma cell lines).

Pharmacokinetics: The pharmacokinetics of adefovir have been evaluated in healthy volunteers and patients with chronic hepatitis B. Adefovir pharmacokinetics are similar between these populations. The pharmacokinetics of adefovir has also been investigated in patients with hepatic and renal impairment.

Absorption: Adefovir dipivoxil is a dipivaloyloxymethyl ester prodrug of the active ingredient adefovir. The oral bioavailability of adefovir is approximately 59%.

Following oral administration of a single dose of HEPSERA to chronic hepatitis B patients, the median (range) peak serum concentration (C_{max}) was achieved after 1.75 h (0.58-4.00). C_{max} and area under the curve (AUC) values were 16.70 (9.66-30.56) ng/mL and 204 (110-356) ng· hr/mL, respectively. The median (range) oral clearance of adefovir was 304.90 (173.07-490.62) mL/hr/kg. Plasma adefovir concentrations declined in a biexponential manner with a median terminal elimination half-life of 7.22 hours (4.72-10.70 hours).

The pharmacokinetics of adefovir in subjects with adequate renal function were not affected following 10 mg once daily dose of HEPSERA over 7 days. The effect of long term once daily administration of HEPSERA on adefovir pharmacokinetics has not been studied.

Distribution: In vitro binding of adefovir to human plasma or human serum proteins is ≤4 % over the adefovir concentration range of 0.1 to 25 µg/mL. The volume of distribution at steady-state following intravenous administration of 1.0 or 3.0 mg/kg/day is 392±75 and 352±9 mL/kg, respectively.

Metabolism: Following oral administration, HEPSERA is rapidly converted to adefovir. Forty-five percent of the dose is recovered as adefovir in the urine over 24 hours after multiple doses of HEPSERA.

Excretion: Adefovir is renally excreted by a combination of glomerular filtration and active tubular secretion. The pharmacokinetics of HEPSERA have been evaluated with a number of drugs that also undergo tubular secretion (see Drug Interactions). Coadministration of HEPSERA with other drugs that are eliminated by, or alter tubular secretion may increase serum concentrations of either adefovir or the administered drug.

Effects of Food on Oral Absorption: HEPSERA may be taken without regard to food. Adefovir exposure was unaffected when HEPSERA was administered with food (~1000 kcal high-fat meal).

Special Populations and Conditions: Pediatrics: Pharmacokinetic studies have not been conducted in children.

Geriatrics: Pharmacokinetic studies have not been conducted in the elderly.

Gender: The pharmacokinetics of adefovir were similar in male and female patients.

Race: No definitive studies have been performed. Results from two pharmacokinetic studies in healthy Chinese volunteers (N=12 in single dose study and N=20 in 7-day multiple dose study) reported similar pharmacokinetic results to historical data from various studies in healthy and chronic hepatitis B Caucasian volunteers and patients.

Renal Insufficiency: In subjects with moderately or severely impaired renal function or with end-stage renal disease (ESRD) requiring hemodialysis, C_{max}, AUC, and half-life ($T_{1/2}$) were increased. It is recommended that the dosing interval of HEPSERA is modified in these patients (see Dosage and Administration).

In Table 5, the pharmacokinetics of adefovir in patients with varying degrees of renal impairment without chronic hepatitis B are described.

Table 5: HEPSERA

Pharmacokinetic Parameters (Median) of Adefovir in Patients with Varying Degrees of Renal Function

Renal Function Group	Unimpaired N=7	Mild N=8	Moderate N=7	Severe N=10	ESRD N=8
Baseline Creatinine Clearance (mL/min)	>80	50–80	30–49	<30	NA
C_{max} (ng/mL)	18.7	21.7	27.1	53.7	56.7
$AUC_{0-\infty}$(ng· hr/mL)	200	281	466	1300	NA
CL/F (mL/min)	454	324	195	70	NA
CL_{renal} (mL/min)	211	149	86	35	NA

Legend: NA=not applicable.

Hepatic Insufficiency: The pharmacokinetics of adefovir have been studied in patients with hepatic impairment without chronic hepatitis B. There were no substantial alterations in adefovir pharmacokinetics in patients with moderate and severe hepatic impairment compared to unimpaired patients. No change in dosing is required in patients with hepatic impairment.

STORAGE AND STABILITY: Store HEPSERA (adefovir dipivoxil) tablets in original container at 25°C, excursions permitted to 15-30°C (see USP Controlled Room Temperature).

Do not use if seal over bottle opening is broken or missing.

SPECIAL HANDLING INSTRUCTIONS: There are no special handling instructions.

INFORMATION FOR THE PATIENT: Published in e-CPS, available by subscription at www.e-cps.ca.

DOSAGE FORMS, COMPOSITION AND PACKAGING: Each white, flat-faced tablet, debossed with "10" and "GILEAD" on one side and the stylized figure of a liver on the other side, contains: adefovir dipivoxil 10 mg. Nonmedicinal ingredients: croscarmellose sodium, lactose monohydrate, magnesium stearate, pregelatinized starch and talc. Bottles of 30 with desiccant (silica gel), closed with a child-resistant closure.

Heptovir® Ⓟ

lamivudine

Antiviral Agent

GlaxoSmithKline Shire Canada

Date of Revision: December 19, 2008

SUMMARY PRODUCT INFORMATION:

Route of Administration	Dosage Form/ Strength	Clinically Relevant Nonmedicinal Ingredients
Oral	Tablets/100 mg	Hydroxypropyl methylcellulose, magnesium stearate, microcrystalline cellulose, polyethylene glycol 400, polysorbate 80, sodium starch glycolate, synthetic yellow and red iron oxides, titanium dioxide
	Solution/5 mg/mL	Artificial strawberry and banana flavors, citric acid (anhydrous), methylparaben, propylene glycol, propylparaben, sodium citrate, and sucrose

INDICATIONS AND CLINICAL USE: HEPTOVIR (lamivudine) is indicated for:

- the treatment of patients with chronic hepatitis B and evidence of hepatitis B virus (HBV) replication.

This indication is based on the analysis of histologic and serologic endpoints in patients with compensated chronic hepatitis B, which were mainly derived from studies of one year duration. Data beyond one year are limited. The safety and efficacy of HEPTOVIR have not been established in patients with decompensated liver disease in placebo controlled studies.

Studies in patients with chronic hepatitis B have shown that compared to placebo, HEPTOVIR therapy can produce improvements in liver necro-inflammatory activity, increased HBeAg seroconversion, suppression of HBV DNA, and/or normalisation of serum aminotransferase.

CONTRAINDICATIONS: HEPTOVIR (lamivudine) is contraindicated in patients previously demonstrated clinically significant hypersensitivity to any of the components of the products (see Dosage Forms, Composition and Packaging).

WARNINGS AND PRECAUTIONS:

> **Serious Warnings and Precautions**
>
> - HIV resistance may emerge in chronic hepatitis B patients with unrecognized or untreated human immunodeficiency virus (HIV) infection when treated with HEPTOVIR. HEPTOVIR contains lower doses of the same active ingredient (lamivudine) as 3TC, which has activity against HIV (see Warnings and Precautions).
> - **Lactic Acidosis and Severe Hepatomegaly with Steatosis:** Lactic acidosis and sever hepatomegaly with steatosis, including fatal cases, have been reported with the use of nucleoside analogues alone or in combination, including HEPTOVIR and other anti-retrovirals.
>
>   A majority of these cases have been in women. Obesity and prolonged nucleoside exposure may be risk factors. However, cases have also been reported in patients with no known risk factors. Treatment with HEPTOVIR should be suspended in any patient who develops clinical or laboratory findings suggestive of lactic acidosis or pronounced hepatotoxicity (which may include hepatomegaly and steatosis even in the absence of marked transaminase elevations.
> - **Post-Treatment Exacerbation of Hepatitis:** Severe acute exacerbations of hepatitis have been reported in patients who have discontinued anti-hepatitis B therapy, including therapy with HEPTOVIR (lamivudine). Hepatic function should be monitored closely in patients who discontinue anti-hepatitis B therapy. If appropriate, resumption of anti-hepatitis B therapy may be warranted.
>
>   Patients co-infected with HIV and HBV should be closely monitored with both clinical and laboratory follow-up for at least several months after stopping treatment with HEPTOVIR.

General: Patients should be monitored regularly during treatment by a physician experienced in the management of chronic hepatitis B.

Optimum duration of therapy has not been established.

The efficacy of lamivudine has not been established in patients not responding to alpha-interferon therapy.

Chronic hepatitis B is a highly variable condition and it is possible the patient may experience re-bound during therapy (i.e., viral load increase or increase in liver enzyme levels) or other discordant results (e.g. increased HBV DNA and improved liver histology). Since, there are no strong correlations between serological and histological markers of response, the decision on whether or not to continue HEPTOVIR (lamivudine) therapy should be based on clinical status and serological marker trends rather than a single result.

Patients should be advised that therapy of chronic hepatitis B, with HEPTOVIR has not been proven to reduce the risk of transmission of hepatitis B virus to others through sexual contact or blood contamination and therefore, appropriate precautions should still be taken.

Several serious adverse events have been reported with use of lamivudine in HIV-infected patients. Reports of anaphylaxis, rhabdomyolysis and peripheral neuropathy have been rare (<1 in 1000).

Endocrine and Metabolism: Diabetic patients should be advised that each dose of HEPTOVIR oral solution (100 mg=20 mL) contains 4 g of sucrose.

Hematologic: Lamivudine use at higher doses in HIV disease, has resulted in very rare occurrences of pure red cell aplasia. To date no definitive occurrences have been seen in hepatitis B patients at the recommended dose.

Hepatic/Biliary/Pancreatic: The safety and efficacy of HEPTOVIR have not been established in patients with decompensated liver disease.

Patients with marginal liver function are at greater risk from active viral replication. In these patients, hepatitis reactivation at discontinuation of lamivudine or loss of efficacy during treatment may induce severe and even fatal decompensation. It is recommended that these patients are monitored for parameters associated with hepatitis B, for liver and renal functions, and for antiviral response during treatment. If treatment is discontinued for any reason, it is recommended that these patients are monitored closely for at least 6 months post cessation of treatment.

Lactic Acidosis/Severe Hepatomegaly with Steatosis: Lactic acidosis and severe hepatomegaly with steatosis, including fatal cases, have been reported with the use of antiretroviral nucleoside analogues alone or in combination, including lamivudine, in the treatment of HIV infection. A majority of these cases have been in women. Obesity and prolonged nucleoside exposure may be risk factors. Most of these reports have described patients receiving nucleoside analogues for the treatment of HIV infection, but there have been rare reports of lactic acidosis in patients receiving lamivudine for hepatitis B. Particular caution should be exercised when administering 3TC or HEPTOVIR to any patient with known risk factors for liver disease (other than hepatitis B). However, cases have been reported in patients with no known risk factors. Treatment with HEPTOVIR should be suspended in any patient who develops clinical or laboratory findings suggestive of lactic acidosis or pronounced hepatotoxicity.

Pancreatitis: Pancreatitis has been reported in patients receiving 3TC (lamivudine), particularly in HIV-infected pediatric patients with prior nucleoside exposure.

Immune: HBV viral subpopulations (YMDD variant HBV) with reduced susceptibility to lamivudine have been identified during extended therapy. In a minority of cases this variant can lead to recurrent hepatitis.

If HEPTOVIR is discontinued or there is a loss of efficacy, some patients may experience clinical or laboratory evidence of recurrent hepatitis. Exacerbation of hepatitis has primarily been detected by serum ALT elevations, in addition to the re-emergence of HBV DNA. Most events appear to have been self-limited. Fatalities due to exacerbation of hepatitis after discontinuation of HEPTOVIR are uncommon.

Some chronic hepatitis B patients may be co-infected with HIV. The possibility of such co-infection should be considered prior to initiating HEPTOVIR therapy. Co-infected patients receiving or requiring an antiretroviral treatment regimen including lamivudine for HIV should be treated with the dose of lamivudine usually recommended for HIV infection. For co-infected patients not requiring antiretroviral therapy, the benefit of using lamivudine for treating chronic hepatitis B needs to be weighed against the potential compromise of a therapeutic option to subsequent progressive HIV and the possible emergence of drug-resistant HIV.

There is no clinical data on the efficacy of lamivudine in patients <16 years of age or co-infected with Delta hepatitis.

Renal: Patients with Impaired Renal Function: In patients with moderate to severe renal impairment, serum lamivudine concentrations are increased due to decreased renal clearance, therefore the dose should be reduced for patients with a creatinine clearance of <50 mL/minute (see Dosage and Administration).

Special Populations: Pregnant Women: There are no adequate and well-controlled studies in pregnant women.

There are limited data on the use of lamivudine in pregnancy. In the phase III clinical studies, 15 pregnancies have been reported in patients receiving lamivudine for chronic hepatitis B: 2 were terminated in elective abortions, 11 were normal live births, and the outcome is unknown in 2. One of the 11 normal births was later found to have a mitral valve prolapse, which was not regarded as related to lamivudine by the investigator.

Reproductive studies in animals have not shown evidence of teratogenicity, and showed no effect on male or female fertility. Lamivudine induced early embryolethality when administered to pregnant rabbits, at exposure levels comparable to those achieved in man. Consistent with passive transmission of the drug across the placenta, lamivudine concentrations in infant serum at birth were similar to those in maternal and cord serum. However, there was no evidence of embryonic loss in rats at exposure levels of approximately 60 times the clinical exposure (based on C_{max}).

Use in pregnancy should be considered only if the benefit outweighs the risk. Although the results of animal studies are not always predictive of human response, the findings in the rabbit suggest a potential risk of early embryonic loss. Consequently, HEPTOVIR administration is not recommended during the first three months of pregnancy.

For patients who are on treatment with HEPTOVIR and subsequently become pregnant, consideration should be given to the possibility of a recurrence of hepatitis on discontinuation of HEPTOVIR.

There is no information available on maternal-fetal transmission of hepatitis B virus in pregnant women receiving treatment with HEPTOVIR. The standard recommended procedures for hepatitis B virus immunization in infants should be followed.

Pregnancy Registry: To monitor maternal-fetal outcomes of pregnant women exposed to lamivudine, a Pregnancy Registry has been established. Physicians are encouraged to register patients by calling GlaxoSmithKline's Drug Surveillance Department via the Customer Service Unit at 1-800-387-7374.

Nursing Women: Following oral administration, lamivudine was excreted in breast milk at similar concentrations to those found in serum. It is recommended that mothers taking lamivudine do not breast feed to avoid potential adverse effects from lamivudine in nursing infants.

Pediatrics (<16 years of age): There is no clinical data on the efficacy of lamivudine in patients <16 years of age or co-infected with Delta hepatitis.

Monitoring and Laboratory Tests: If HEPTOVIR is discontinued, patients should be periodically monitored both clinically and by assessment of serum liver function tests (ALT and bilirubin levels), for at least four months for evidence of recurrent hepatitis; patients should then be followed as clinically indicated. For patients who develop evidence of recurrent hepatitis post-treatment, there are insufficient data on the benefits of re-initiation of HEPTOVIR treatment.

ADVERSE REACTIONS: Clinical Trial Adverse Drug Reactions: Because clinical trials are conducted under very specific conditions the adverse reaction rates observed in the clinical trials may not reflect the rates observed in practice and should not be compared to the rates in the clinical trials of another drug. Adverse drug reaction information from clinical trials is useful for identifying drug-related adverse events and for approximating rates.

In clinical studies of patients with chronic hepatitis B, HEPTOVIR (lamivudine) was well tolerated. The incidence of adverse events was similar between placebo and HEPTOVIR treated patients. The most common adverse events reported were malaise and fatigue, respiratory tract infections, headache, abdominal discomfort and pain, nausea, vomiting and diarrhea. The most common adverse events (≥5%), reported in three pivotal trials (NUCB3009, NUCA3010 and NUCB3010) during treatment are summarised in Table 1.

Table 1: HEPTOVIR

Most Common Adverse Events (≥5%) Reported in 3 Pivotal Trials During Treatment

Most Common Adverse Events During Treatment	No. (%) of Patients PLA n=144	LAM 100 mg n=297
Malaise and Fatigue	36 (25%)	73 (25%)
Headache	30 (21%)	63 (21%)
Viral Respiratory Infection	26 (18%)	61 (21%)
Abdominal Discomfort and Pain	25 (17%)	41 (14%)
Diarrhea	18 (13%)	41 (14%)
Cough	14 (10%)	35 (12%)
ENT Infections	15 (10%)	35 (12%)
Nausea and Vomiting	20 (14%)	43 (14%)

(cont'd)

Table 1: HEPTOVIR *(cont'd)*

Most Common Adverse Events (≥5%) Reported in 3 Pivotal Trials During Treatment

Most Common Adverse Events During Treatment	No. (%) of Patients PLA n=144	LAM 100 mg n=297
Throat and Tonsil Discomfort and Pain	12 (8%)	35 (12%)
Viral Ear Nose and Throat Infections	15 (10%)	29 (10%)
Musculoskeletal Pain	14 (10%)	23 (8%)
Nasal Signs and Symptoms	10 (7%)	23 (8%)
Dizziness	10 (7%)	22 (7%)
Sleep Disorders	11 (8%)	20 (7%)
Temperature Regulation Disturbances	10 (7%)	15 (5%)
Abnormal Enzyme Levels	8 (6%)	16 (5%)

Legend: LAM=Lamivudine; PLA=Placebo.

The incidence of laboratory abnormalities in chronic hepatitis B patients were similar in the HEPTOVIR and placebo treated groups with the exception of ALT elevations which were more common post-treatment in patients treated with HEPTOVIR. In controlled trials however, there was no appreciable difference post-treatment in clinically severe ALT elevations, associated with bilirubin elevations and/or signs of hepatic insufficiency, between HEPTOVIR and placebo treated patients. The relationship of these recurrent hepatitis events to HEPTOVIR treatment or to the previous underlying disease is uncertain (see Warnings and Precautions).

In patients with HIV infection, cases of pancreatitis and peripheral neuropathy (or paraesthesia) have been reported, although no relationship to treatment with lamivudine (3TC) has been clearly established. In patients with chronic hepatitis B there was no observed difference in incidence of these events between placebo and HEPTOVIR treated patients.

Cases of lactic acidosis, usually associated with severe hepatomegaly and hepatic steatosis, have been reported with the use of combination nucleoside analogue therapy in patients with HIV. There have been occasional reports of these adverse events in hepatitis B patients with decompensated liver disease, however, the association of HEPTOVIR with these events has not been established.

Post-Market Adverse Drug Reactions: The following events have been reported during therapy for HIV disease with lamivudine alone and in combination with other antiretroviral agents. With many it is unclear whether they are related to the medicinal products or are as a result of the underlying disease process.

The following convention has been utilised for the classification of undesirable effects: Very common (>1/10), common (>1/100, <1/10), uncommon (>1/1000, <1/100), rare (>1/10 000, <1/1000), very rare (<1/10 000).

Blood and Lymphatic Systems Disorders: Uncommon: neutropenia, anaemia, thrombocytopenia. Very rare: pure red cell aplasia.

Metabolism and Nutrition Disorders: Common: hyperlactataemia. Rare: lactic acidosis (see Warnings and Precautions).

Redistribution/accumulation of body fat. The incidence of this event is dependent on multiple factors including the particular antiretroviral drug combination.

Nervous System Disorders: Common: headache. Very rare: paraesthesia. Peripheral neuropathy has been reported although a causal relationship to treatment is uncertain.

Gastrointestinal Disorders: Common: nausea, vomiting, upper abdominal pain, diarrhea. Rare: pancreatitis, although a causal relationship to treatment is uncertain. Rises in serum amylase.

Hepatobiliary Disorders: Uncommon: transient rises in liver enzymes (AST, ALT).

Skin and Subcutaneous Tissue Disorders: Common: rash, alopecia.

Musculoskeletal and Connective Tissue Disorders: Common: arthralgia, muscle disorders. Rare: rhabdomyolysis.

General Disorders and Administration Site Conditions: Common: fatigue, malaise, fever.

DRUG INTERACTIONS: Overview: The likelihood of metabolic interactions is low due to limited metabolism and plasma protein binding and almost complete renal elimination of unchanged drug.

Lamivudine is predominantly eliminated by active organic cationic secretion. The possibility of interactions with other drugs administered concurrently should be considered, particularly when their main route of elimination is active renal secretion via the organic cationic transport system (e.g. trimethoprim). Other drugs (e.g. ranitidine, cimetidine) are eliminated only in part by this mechanism and were shown not to interact with lamivudine.

Drugs shown to be predominately excreted either via the active organic anionic pathway, or by glomerular filtration are unlikely to yield clinically significant interactions with lamivudine.

Drug-Drug Interactions: (See Table 2.)

Table 2: HEPTOVIR

Established or Potential Drug-Drug Interactions

Proper name	Effect	Clinical Comment
Trimethoprim/Sulphamethoxazole 160 mg/800 mg	Increased lamivudine exposure by about 40%.	Lamivudine had no effect on the pharmacokinetics of trimethoprim or sulphamethoxazole. However, unless the patient has renal impairment, no dosage adjustment of lamivudine is necessary.
Zidovudine	A modest increase in C_{max} (28%) for zidovudine when administered with lamivudine.	Overall exposure (AUC) was not significantly altered. Zidovudine had no effect on the pharmacokinetics of lamivudine.
alpha-interferon	Lamivudine has no pharmacokinetic interaction with alpha-interferon when the two drugs are concurrently administered.	Formal interaction studies have not been performed.
Immunosuppressant Drugs	There were no observed clinically significant adverse interactions in patients taking HEPTOVIR (lamivudine) concurrently with commonly used immunosuppressant drugs (e.g. cyclosporin A).	Formal interaction studies have not been performed.
Zalcitabine	Lamivudine may inhibit the intracellular phosphorylation of zalcitabine when the two medicinal products are used concurrently.	HEPTOVIR is therefore not recommended to be used in combination with zalcitabine.

DOSAGE AND ADMINISTRATION: Dosing Considerations: Discontinuation of HEPTOVIR (lamivudine) may be considered in immunocompetent patients when HBeAg and/or HBsAg seroconversion occurs and when loss of efficacy occurs as indicated by recurrent signs of hepatitis. There are limited data regarding the maintenance of seroconversion long term after stopping treatment with HEPTOVIR. If HEPTOVIR is discontinued, patients should be periodically monitored for evidence of recurrent hepatitis (see Warnings and Precautions).

The formulation and dosage of lamivudine in HEPTOVIR are not appropriate in patients dually infected with Hepatitis B and HIV. If lamivudine is administered to such patients, the higher dosage indicated for HIV therapy should be used as part of a combination treatment regimen and the Product Monographs for 3TC and HEPTOVIR should be consulted.

Recommended Dose and Dosage Adjustment: The recommended dose of HEPTOVIR for adults and adolescents who are at least 16 years old is 100 mg once daily. Optimum duration of therapy has not been established.

Renal Impairment: Lamivudine serum concentrations are increased in patients with moderate to severe renal impairment due to decreased renal clearance. The dosage should therefore be reduced for patients with a creatinine clearance of <50 mL/minute. When doses below 100 mg are required HEPTOVIR oral solution should be used (see Table 3).

Table 3: HEPTOVIR

Dosage in Patients with Renal Impairment

Creatinine Clearance mL/min	First Dose of Lamivudine Oral Solution[a]	Maintenance Dose Once Daily
30 to <50	20 mL (100 mg)	10 mL (50 mg)
15 to <30	20 mL (100 mg)	5 mL (25 mg)
5 to <15	7 mL (35 mg)	3 mL (15 mg)
<5	7 mL (35 mg)	2 mL (10 mg)

[a] HEPTOVIR Oral Solution containing 5 mg/mL lamivudine.

Data available in patients undergoing intermittent haemodialysis (≤4 hours dialysis 2-3 times weekly), indicate that following the initial dosage reduction of HEPTOVIR to correct for the patient's creatinine clearance, no further dosage adjustments are required while undergoing dialysis.

Missed Dose: If the patients forget to take their medicine, they should take it as soon as they remember, then continue as before.

Administration: HEPTOVIR can be taken with or without food.

OVERDOSAGE:

Limited data are available on the consequences of ingestion of acute overdoses in humans. No fatalities occurred, and the patients recovered. No specific signs or symptoms have been identified following such overdosage.

If overdose occurs the patient should be monitored and standard supportive treatment applied. Although no data is available, administration of activated charcoal may be used to aid in removal of unabsorbed drug. Since lamivudine is dialysable, continuous hemodialysis could be used in the treatment of overdose, although this has not been studied.

For management of a suspected drug overdose, CPhA recommends that you contact your **regional Poison Control Centre**. See the *CPS* Directory section for a list of Poison Control Centres.

ACTION AND CLINICAL PHARMACOLOGY: Mechanism of Action: Lamivudine is an antiviral agent which is active against hepatitis B virus (HBV) in all cell lines tested and in experimentally infected animals.

Pharmacodynamics: Lamivudine is metabolised by both infected and uninfected cells to the triphosphate (TP) derivative which is the active form of the parent compound. The intracellular half-life of the triphosphate in hepatocytes is 17-19 hours in vitro. Lamivudine-TP acts as a substrate for the HBV viral polymerase. The formation of further viral DNA is blocked by incorporation of lamivudine- MP into the chain and subsequent chain termination.

Lamivudine-TP is also a substrate for mammalian DNA polymerases, with the subsequent incorporation into mammalian DNA. However, incorporated lamivudine is removed from mammalian DNA by 3'-5' exonuclease DNA repair enzymes. Viral polymerases do not possess such a DNA repair function. Consequently, at concentrations in vitro which inhibit replication of HBV DNA in infected cells, lamivudine has no effect on mammalian mitochondrial DNA synthesis and has no cytotoxicity. In vitro concentrations of lamivudine which cause reductions of mammalian DNA and cytotoxicity are approximately 1000 times or greater than those which inhibit HBV replication. Thus, lamivudine has a high therapeutic index.

Pharmacokinetics: Absorption: Lamivudine is well absorbed from the gastrointestinal tract.

Distribution: The bioavailability of oral lamivudine in adults is normally between 80 and 85%. Following oral administration, the mean time (t_{max}) to maximal serum concentrations (C_{max}) is about an hour. At therapeutic dose levels i.e. 100 mg once daily, C_{max} is in the order of 1.1-1.5 µg/mL.

Co-administration of lamivudine with food resulted in a delay of t_{max} and a lower C_{max} (decreased by up to 47%). However, the extent (based on the AUC) of lamivudine absorbed was not influenced, therefore HEPTOVIR (lamivudine) can be administered with or without food.

STORAGE AND STABILITY: HEPTOVIR (lamivudine) tablets should be stored between 2 and 30°C.

HEPTOVIR oral solution should be stored between 15 and 25°C.

SPECIAL HANDLING INSTRUCTIONS: Not applicable.

INFORMATION FOR THE PATIENT: Published in e-CPS, available by subscription at www.e-cps.ca.

DOSAGE FORMS, COMPOSITION AND PACKAGING: Oral Solution: Each mL of oral solution, colorless to pale yellow, strawberry-banana flavored, clear liquid, contains: lamivudine 5 mg. Nonmedicinal ingredients: artificial strawberry and banana flavors, citric acid (anhydrous), methylparaben, propylene glycol, propylparaben, sodium citrate, and sucrose. Plastic bottles of 240 mL.

Tablets: Each butterscotch-colored, film-coated, capsule-shaped tablet, engraved "GXCG5" on one face, contains: lamivudine 100 mg. Nonmedicinal ingredients: hydroxypropyl methylcellulose, magnesium stearate, microcrystalline cellulose, polyethylene glycol 400, polysorbate 80, sodium starch glycolate, synthetic red iron oxide, synthetic yellow iron oxide and titanium dioxide. Bottles of 60.

(Shown in Product Identification Section)

Herceptin® P

trastuzumab

Antineoplastic

Roche

Date of Preparation: August 13, 1999
Date of Revision: August 4, 2010

SUMMARY PRODUCT INFORMATION:

Route of Administration	Dosage Form/ Strength	Clinically Relevant Nonmedicinal Ingredients
IV Infusion	Vial/440 mg	None **Note:** The Bacteriostatic Water for Injection (BWFI) supplied with HERCEPTIN (trastuzumab) contains 1.1% benzyl alcohol (see Warnings and Precautions). For a complete listing of nonmedicinal ingredients see Dosage Forms, Composition and Packaging.

INDICATIONS AND CLINICAL USE: Early Breast Cancer (EBC): HERCEPTIN (trastuzumab) is indicated for the treatment of patients with early stage breast cancer, whose tumours overexpress HER2, following surgery and after chemotherapy.

Metastatic Breast Cancer (MBC): HERCEPTIN (trastuzumab) is indicated for the treatment of patients with metastatic breast cancer whose tumours substantially overexpress HER2.

The benefits of treatment with HERCEPTIN in patients who do not overexpress HER2, or who exhibit lower-level overexpression, are unclear (see Warnings and Precautions, Selection of Patients/Diagnostic Tests).

Based on the analysis of the HERA trial, the benefit of the adjuvant treatment with HERCEPTIN for low risk patients not given adjuvant chemotherapy are unknown.

Metastatic Gastric Cancer (MGC): HERCEPTIN in combination with capecitabine or intravenous 5-fluorouracil and cisplatin is indicated for the treatment of patients with HER2-positive metastatic adenocarcinoma of the stomach or gastro-esophageal junction who have not received prior anti-cancer treatment for their metastatic disease.

HERCEPTIN should only be administered to patients with metastatic gastric cancer whose tumours have HER2 overexpression as defined by IHC2+ confirmed by FISH+, or IHC 3+ as determined by an accurate and validated assay.

CONTRAINDICATIONS:

- HERCEPTIN (trastuzumab) is contraindicated in patients with known hypersensitivity to trastuzumab, Chinese Hamster Ovary (CHO) cell proteins, or any component of this product.

WARNINGS AND PRECAUTIONS:

Serious Warnings and Precautions

Cardiotoxicity: HERCEPTIN can result in the development of ventricular dysfunction and congestive heart failure. In the adjuvant treatment setting, the incidence of cardiac dysfunction was higher in patients who received HERCEPTIN plus chemotherapy versus chemotherapy alone. In the metastatic setting, the incidence and severity of cardiac dysfunction was particularly high in patients who received HERCEPTIN concurrently with anthracyclines and cyclophosphamide (see Warnings and Precautions, Cardiovascular).

Evaluate left ventricular function in all patients prior to and during treatment with HERCEPTIN (see Warnings and Precautions, Cardiovascular).

Infusion Reactions; Pulmonary Toxicity: HERCEPTIN administration can result in serious infusion reactions and pulmonary toxicity. Fatal infusion reactions have been reported. In most cases, symptoms occurred during or within 24 hours of administration of HERCEPTIN. HERCEPTIN infusion should be interrupted for patients experiencing dyspnea or clinically significant hypotension. Patients should be monitored until signs and symptoms completely resolve. Discontinue HERCEPTIN for infusion reactions manifesting as anaphylaxis, angioedema, interstitial pneumonitis, or acute respiratory distress syndrome (see Warnings and Precautions).

General: Therapy with HERCEPTIN (trastuzumab) should only be initiated under supervision of a physician experienced in the treatment of cancer patients.

Early Breast Cancer: The safety of the various combination chemotherapy regimens prior to HERCEPTIN therapy was not separately analyzed in the HERA trial. The data provided in the Product Monograph reflects the safety and efficacy of HERCEPTIN for 1 year of treatment.

Benzyl Alcohol: Benzyl alcohol, used as a preservative in BWFI, has been associated with toxicity in neonates and children up to 3 years old. For patients with a known hypersensitivity to benzyl alcohol (the preservative in BWFI), reconstitute HERCEPTIN with Sterile Water for Injection (SWFI). **Use SWFI-reconstituted HERCEPTIN immediately and discard the vial** (see Dosage and Administration).

Cardiovascular: Cardiotoxicity: Administration of HERCEPTIN can result in the development of ventricular dysfunction and congestive heart failure. In the adjuvant treatment setting, the incidence of cardiac dysfunction was higher in patients who received HERCEPTIN plus chemotherapy versus chemotherapy alone. In the metastatic setting, the incidence and severity of cardiac dysfunction was particularly high in patients who received HERCEPTIN concurrently with anthracyclines and cyclophosphamide.

Because the half-life of trastuzumab, using a population pharmacokinetic method, is approximately 28.5 days (95% CI, 25.5-32.8 days), trastuzumab may persist in the circulation for approximately 24 weeks (range: 22-28 weeks) after stopping treatment with HERCEPTIN. Since the use of an anthracycline during this period could possibly be associated with an increased risk of cardiac dysfunction, a thorough assessment of the risks versus the potential benefits is recommended in addition to careful cardiac monitoring.

Patients who receive HERCEPTIN either as a component of adjuvant treatment or as a treatment for metastatic HER2 positive breast cancer may experience signs and symptoms of cardiac dysfunction such as dyspnea, increased cough, paroxysmal nocturnal dyspnea, peripheral edema, S_3 gallop, or reduced ejection fraction. Cardiac dysfunction associated with therapy with HERCEPTIN may be severe and has been associated with disabling cardiac failure, death, and mural thrombosis leading to stroke.

Left ventricular function should be evaluated in all patients prior to and during treatment with HERCEPTIN. If LVEF drops 10 ejection points from baseline and/or to below 50%, HERCEPTIN should be withheld and a repeat LVEF assessment performed within approximately 3 weeks. If LVEF has not improved, or declined further, discontinuation of HERCEPTIN should be strongly considered, unless the benefits for the individual patient are deemed to outweigh the risks. The scientific basis of cardiotoxicity has been incompletely investigated in pre-clinical studies.

Extreme caution should be exercised in treating patients with pre-existing cardiac dysfunction, and in early breast cancer, in those patients with an LVEF of 55% or less. Candidates for treatment with HERCEPTIN as part of adjuvant treatment for operable breast cancer or for metastatic breast cancer, especially those with prior anthracycline and cyclophosphamide (AC) exposure, should undergo thorough baseline cardiac assessment including history and physical exam and one or more of the following: EKG, echocardiogram and MUGA scan. A careful risk-benefit assessment should be made before deciding to treat with HERCEPTIN. Cardiac function, including LVEF, should be further monitored during treatment (e.g. every three months) and if patients are treated with anthracyclines after treatment with HERCEPTIN. Monitoring may help to identify patients who develop cardiac dysfunction. Patients who develop asymptomatic cardiac dysfunction may benefit from more frequent monitoring (e.g. every 6-8 weeks). If patients have a continued decrease in left ventricular function, but remain asymptomatic, the physician should consider discontinuing therapy if no clinical benefit of therapy with HERCEPTIN has been seen.

If symptomatic cardiac failure develops during therapy with HERCEPTIN, it should be treated with the standard medications for this purpose. Discontinuation of HERCEPTIN should be strongly considered in patients who develop clinically significant congestive heart failure. In the metastatic breast cancer clinical trials, approximately two-thirds of patients with cardiac dysfunction were treated for cardiac symptoms, most patients responded to appropriate medical therapy (diuretics, cardiac glycosides, and/or angiotensin-converting enzyme inhibitors) often including discontinuation of HERCEPTIN. The safety of continuation or resumption of HERCEPTIN in patients who have previously experienced cardiac toxicity has not been prospectively studied.

Early Breast Cancer: In EBC, the following patients were excluded from the HERA trial, there are no data about the benefit:risk balance, and therefore treatment can not be recommended in such patients:

- History of documented CHF
- High-risk uncontrolled arrhythmias
- Angina pectoris requiring medication
- Clinically significant valvular disease
- Evidence of transmural infarction on ECG
- Poorly controlled hypertension

The safety of continuation or resumption of HERCEPTIN in patients who have previously experienced cardiac toxicity has not been prospectively studied. According to the narrative reports of cardiac events, about half of the events had resolved completely by the time of the interim analysis. Please see Table 2.

At a minimum, patients need to be screened at baseline, and have their LVEF re-checked after any anthracycline based chemotherapy, and again during HERCEPTIN therapy (e.g. 6 months). A high index of clinical suspicion is warranted for discontinuing treatment in the setting of cardiopulmonary symptoms. Close monitoring of cardiac function should be carried out for all patients and adequate treatment for CHF should be administered regardless of the discontinuation of HERCEPTIN therapy. Please see Figure 1 in Dosage and Administration: Monitoring of Cardiac Function, for the algorithm for continuation and discontinuation of HERCEPTIN based on interval LVEF assessments as described in the HERA protocol.

HERA: In the HERA trial, NYHA class III-IV heart failure was observed in 0.6% of patients in the one-year arm. See Table 1.

Joint Analysis: NSABP B-31 and NCCTG N9831: Cardiac dysfunction adverse events, defined in both B-31 and N9831 as symptomatic congestive heart failure, death due to cardiac causes, and probable cardiac death, were observed in studies of HERCEPTIN for patients with early stage breast cancer. In all analyses the rate of cardiac dysfunction was higher in patients in the HERCEPTIN + chemotherapy arm compared with those in the chemotherapy alone arm. From the paclitaxel baseline to the six month assessment, the average change in LVEF was more pronounced in the HERCEPTIN + chemotherapy arm (−3.9% in the HERCEPTIN + chemotherapy alone arm versus −0.9% in the chemotherapy alone arm). The cardiac event rates at 3 years for each study are presented in Table 4.

Table 1: HERCEPTIN

Absolute Numbers and Rates of Cardiac Endpoints in HERA

HERA Study	Observation n (%) N=1708	HERCEPTIN n (%) N=1678
Primary cardiac endpoint	1 (0.1)	10 (0.6)
Cardiac death	1 (0.1)	0
NYHA class IV+III	0	10 (0.6)
Secondary cardiac endpoint	9 (0.5)	51 (3.0)
NYHA class II+I	9 (0.5)	51 (3.0)
Total "cardiac endpoints"	10 (0.6)	61 (3.6)

Table 2: HERCEPTIN

Median Time to Return to Baseline LVEF/Stabilizations of LVEF in the HERA Trial

HERA Study	Primary Cardiac Endpoint[a]	Secondary Cardiac Endpoint	
	HERCEPTIN (n=10)	Observation (n=9)	HERCEPTIN (n=51)
Return to baseline LVEF	6 (60%)	6 (67%)	35 (69%)
Median time to return to baseline LVEF	121 d	204 d	189 d
Stabilisation of LVEF	4 (40%)	2 (22%)	11 (22%)

[a] Only one patient reached a primary cardiac endpoint in the observation arm which was cardiac death.
A **primary cardiac endpoint** was defined as the occurrence at any time after randomization but prior to any new therapy for recurrent disease of symptomatic congestive heart failure of NYHA class III or IV, confirmed by a cardiologist and a drop in LVEF of at least 10 EF points from baseline and to below 50%, or cardiac death defined as definite or probable cardiac death.
A **secondary cardiac endpoint** was cardiac dysfunction defined as a significant asymptomatic (NYHA class I) or mildly symptomatic (NYHA class II) LVEF drop measured by MUGA scan or echocardiogram, unless the following assessment of LVEF indicated a return to levels which did not meet the definition of a significant LVEF drop. A significant LVEF drop was defined as an absolute decrease of 10 EF points or more from baseline and to below 50%. In addition events which did not meet the above criteria for a secondary cardiac endpoint but which in the opinion of the Cardiac Advisory Board should be classed as secondary cardiac endpoints were included.

Table 3: HERCEPTIN

The Incidence and Type of Cardiac Events Seen in the Joint Analysis

	B-31		N9831		B-31+N9831	
	AC→T (n=972)	AC→T+H (n=992)	AC→T (n=803)	AC→T+H (n=807)	AC→T (n=1775)	AC→T+H (n=1799)
Type						
Any events	10 (1.0 %)	32 (3.2 %)	1 (0.1 %)	21 (2.6 %)	11 (0.6 %)	53 (2.9 %)
Symptomatic CHF (non-death)	9 (0.9 %)	31 (3.1 %)	1 (0.1 %)	19 (2.4 %)	10 (0.6 %)	50 (2.8 %)
Cardiac death	1 (0.1 %)	1 (0.1 %)	0 (0.0 %)	2 (0.2 %)	1 (0.1 %)	3 (0.2 %)
Death due to CHF, MI, or primary arrhythmia	0 (0.0 %)	0 (0.0 %)	0 (0.0 %)	1 (0.1 %)	0 (0.0 %)	1 (0.1 %)
Sudden death w/out documented etiology	1 (0.1 %)	1 (0.1 %)	0 (0.0 %)	1 (0.1 %)	1 (0.1 %)	2 (0.1 %)

Legend: A=doxorubicin; C=cyclophosphamide; CHF=congestive heart failure; H=HERCEPTIN; MI=myocardial infarction; T=paclitaxel.

Table 4: HERCEPTIN

3 Year Cumulative Incidence Rate in Subjects in the Joint Analysis: NSABP B-31 and NCCTG N9831 who Experienced Cardiac Dysfunction from the Start of Paclitaxel Treatment

	AC→T	AC→T+HERCEPTIN
ACREC (B-31+N9831)	0.43%	2.07%
Pooled studies[a] (B-31+N9831)	0.69%	3.49%
NSABP B-31	1.14%	3.77%
NCCTG N9831	0%	3.03%

[a] As determined by individual study cardiac review committees.

An independent clinical review was performed on 36 patients with symptomatic congestive heart failure in the HERCEPTIN + chemotherapy arm to assess treatment and resolution status. Most patients were treated with oral medications commonly used to manage congestive heart failure, and complete or partial functional left ventricular recovery was documented in 29 patients.

Risk factors for a cardiac event included HERCEPTIN treatment, increased age, prior or current use of anti-hypertensive medications and low LVEF prior to or following the initiation of paclitaxel treatment. In the HERCEPTIN + chemotherapy arm, the risk of a cardiac event increased with the number of these risk factors present. In Study B-31, there was no association between the incidence of cardiac events and either radiation to the left side or smoking.

* New York Heart Association Functional Classification. Class I: Patients with cardiac disease but without resulting limitations of physical activity. Ordinary physical activity does not cause undue fatigue, palpitation, dyspnea or anginal pain. Class II: Patients with cardiac disease resulting in slight limitation of physical activity. They are comfortable at rest. Ordinary physical activity results in fatigue, palpitation, dyspnea or anginal pain. Class III: Patients with cardiac disease resulting in marked limitation of physical activity. They are comfortable at rest. Less than ordinary physical activity causes fatigue, palpitation, dyspnea or anginal pain. Class IV: Patients with cardiac disease resulting in inability to carry on any physical activity without discomfort. Symptoms of cardiac insufficiency or of the anginal syndrome may be present even at rest. If any physical activity is undertaken, discomfort is increased.

Metastatic Breast Cancer: In particular, moderate to severe cardiac dysfunction has been observed in metastatic breast cancer patients treated with HERCEPTIN in combination with an anthracycline (doxorubicin or epirubicin) and cyclophosphamide (see Adverse Reactions). The clinical status of patients in the trials who developed congestive heart failure were classified for severity using the New York Heart Association classification system (I-IV* where IV is the most severe level of cardiac failure). (See Table 5.)

Table 5: HERCEPTIN

Incidence and Severity of Cardiac Dysfunction in Metastatic Breast Cancer Patients

	HERCEPTIN + Anthracycline + Cyclophosphamide[b] (n=143)	Anthracycline + Cyclophosphamide[b] (n=135)	HERCEPTIN + Paclitaxel[b] (n= 91)	Paclitaxel[b] (n= 95)	HERCEPTIN[a] Alone (n= 338)
Any cardiac dysfunction	27%	7%	12%	1%	4%
Class III-IV	16%	3%	2%	1%	3%

[a] Single agent studies H0551g, H0649g and H0650g.
[b] Randomized Phase III study comparing chemotherapy plus HERCEPTIN to chemotherapy alone, where chemotherapy is either anthracycline/cyclophosphamide or paclitaxel.

In a subsequent trial with prospective monitoring of cardiac function, the incidence of symptomatic heart failure was 2.2% in patients receiving HERCEPTIN and docetaxel, compared with 0% in patients receiving docetaxel alone.

In the metastatic breast cancer trials, the probability of cardiac dysfunction was highest in patients who received HERCEPTIN concurrently with anthracyclines. The metastatic breast cancer data suggest that advanced age may increase the probability of cardiac dysfunction.

Pre-existing cardiac disease or prior cardiotoxic therapy (e.g., anthracycline or radiation therapy) to the chest may decrease the ability to tolerate therapy with HERCEPTIN; however, the data is not adequate to evaluate correlation between cardiotoxicity observed with HERCEPTIN and these factors in patients with HER2 positive metastatic breast cancer.

Hematologic: Exacerbation of Chemotherapy-Induced Neutropenia: In randomized, controlled clinical trials in both adjuvant and metastatic breast cancer designed to assess the impact of the addition of HERCEPTIN on chemotherapy, the per-patient incidences of moderate to severe neutropenia and of febrile neutropenia were higher in patients receiving HERCEPTIN in combination with myelosuppressive chemotherapy compared with those receiving chemotherapy alone.

Using NCI-CTC criteria, in the adjuvant HERA trial, 0.4% of patients treated with HERCEPTIN experienced a shift of 3 or 4 grades from baseline, compared with 0.6% in the observation arm.

In the adjuvant studies, NSABP B-31 and NCCTG N9831, there were 6 deaths due to septicemia or severe neutropenia. Five deaths occurred on the chemotherapy alone arm: 2 patients died of pneumonia with febrile neutropenia and 3 patients died of septicemia. One death occurred on the HERCEPTIN + chemotherapy arm and the patient died of infection/neutropenic fever with pulmonary infiltrates. All except 2 septicemia deaths occurred during protocol treatment period.

In the postmarketing setting in metastatic breast cancer, deaths due to sepsis in patients with severe neutropenia have been reported in patients receiving HERCEPTIN and myelosuppressive chemotherapy, although in controlled metastatic breast cancer clinical trials (pre- and postmarketing), the incidence of septic death was not significantly increased. The pathophysiologic basis for exacerbation of neutropenia has not been determined; the effect of HERCEPTIN on the pharmacokinetics of chemotherapeutic agents has not been fully evaluated. If neutropenia occurs, the appropriate management should be instituted as per local practice/guidelines and the labelled instructions for chemotherapy agents should be followed with regard to dose interruption or dose reduction (see Dosage and Administration, Recommended Dose and Dosage Adjustment, Dose Reduction).

Hypersensitivity Reactions Including Anaphylaxis, Infusion-Associated Reactions and Pulmonary Events: Administration of HERCEPTIN can result in severe hypersensitivity reactions (including anaphylaxis), infusion reactions and pulmonary events. In rare cases, these reactions have been fatal. See discussion below.

There are no data regarding the most appropriate method of identification of patients who may safely be retreated with HERCEPTIN after experiencing a severe reaction. HERCEPTIN has been readministered to some patients who fully recovered from a previous severe reaction. Prior to readministration of HERCEPTIN the majority of these patients were prophylactically treated with pre-medications including antihistamines and/or corticosteroids. While some of these patients tolerated retreatment, others had severe reactions again despite the use of prophylactic pre-medications.

Hypersensitivity Reactions Including Anaphylaxis: Severe hypersensitivity reactions have been infrequently reported in patients treated with HERCEPTIN. Signs and symptoms include anaphylaxis, urticaria, bronchospasm, angioedema, and/or hypotension. In some cases, the reactions have been fatal. The onset of symptoms generally occurred during an infusion, but there have also been reports of symptom onset after the completion of an infusion. Reactions were most commonly reported in association with the initial infusion. In HERA 1 observation and 10 HERCEPTIN treated patients experienced hypersensitivity. Eight out of the 10 events were considered related to HERCEPTIN treatment. The incidence of allergic reactions in the Joint analysis (chemotherapy alone versus HERCEPTIN + chemotherapy: 3.2% versus 3.2% in Study B-31 and 0.9% versus 0.4% in Study N9831) was comparable between the two treatment arms in both studies.

In the two adjuvant studies, B-31 and N9831, the incidence of allergic reaction was comparable between the HERCEPTIN + chemotherapy and chemotherapy alone.

Infusional administration of HERCEPTIN should be interrupted in all patients with severe hypersensitivity reactions. In the event of a hypersensitivity reaction, appropriate medical therapy should be administered, which may include epinephrine, corticosteroids, diphenhydramine, bronchodilators, and oxygen. Patients should be evaluated and carefully monitored until complete resolution of signs and symptoms.

Infusion-Associated Reactions: Serious adverse reactions to infusions of HERCEPTIN including dyspnea, hypotension, hypertension, wheezing, bronchospasm, tachycardia, reduced oxygen saturation and respiratory distress have been reported infrequently. The infusion should be discontinued and the patient monitored until resolution of any observed symptoms. Serious reactions have been treated successfully with supportive therapy such as oxygen, beta-agonists and corticosteroids (see Adverse Reactions). The appropriate management of patients with uncontrolled hypertension or history of hypertension should be considered prior to infusion with HERCEPTIN.

These severe reactions were usually associated with the first infusion of HERCEPTIN and generally occurred during or immediately following the infusion. For some patients, symptoms later worsened and led to further pulmonary complications. Initial improvement followed by clinical deterioration and delayed reactions with rapid clinical deterioration have also been reported. Fatalities have occurred within hours and up to one week following infusion. On very rare occasions, patients have experienced the onset of infusion symptoms or pulmonary symptoms more than six hours after the start of the infusion of HERCEPTIN. Patients should be warned of the possibility of such a late onset and should be instructed to contact their physician if those symptoms occur. In rare cases, these reactions are associated with a clinical course culminating in a fatal outcome. Patients who are experiencing dyspnea at rest due to complications of advanced malignancy and comorbidities may be at increased risk of a fatal infusion reaction. Therefore, these patients should be treated with extreme caution and the risk versus benefit be considered for each patient.

Pulmonary Events: Severe pulmonary events leading to death have been reported rarely with the use of HERCEPTIN in the adjuvant breast cancer clinical studies and the postmarketing metastatic breast cancer setting. Signs, symptoms, and clinical findings include dyspnea, pulmonary infiltrates, pneumonitis, pleural effusions, non-cardiogenic pulmonary edema, pulmonary insufficiency and hypoxia and acute respiratory distress syndrome. These events may or may not occur as sequelae of infusion reactions (see Warnings and Precautions, Infusion-Associated Reactions), and were reported to occur at varying onset latencies, from within 24 hours to over 30 days, since the start of treatment with HERCEPTIN. Patients with symptomatic intrinsic lung disease or with extensive tumour involvement of the lungs, resulting in dyspnea at rest, may be at greater risk of severe reactions.

Others severe events reported rarely in the postmarketing metastatic breast cancer setting include pneumonitis and pulmonary fibrosis. All of the confirmed cases of pulmonary fibrosis received to date are characterized by one or more significant confounding factors including pre-existing lung disease and prior/concomitant chemotherapy such as cyclophosphamide. However, a causal relationship between HERCEPTIN and pulmonary fibrosis cannot be excluded.

Immune: Immunogenicity: In N9831 and B-31, the incidence of human anti-human antibody (HAHA) to trastuzumab is unknown. Of 903 patients that have been evaluated in the metastatic breast cancer trials, human anti-human antibody (HAHA) to trastuzumab was detected in 1 patient, who had no allergic manifestations.

Respiratory: Refer to Pulmonary Events of Warnings and Precautions.

Thrombosis/Embolism: Thrombosis/embolism has been observed in patients who receive HERCEPTIN + chemotherapy in both the adjuvant and metastatic treatment setting, and in rare cases, has been fatal (see Adverse Reactions).

Special Populations: Pregnant Women: Reproduction studies have been conducted in cynomolgus monkeys at doses up to 25 times the weekly human maintenance dose of 2 mg/kg HERCEPTIN and have revealed no evidence of impaired fertility or harm to the fetus. However, when assessing the risk of reproductive toxicity in humans, it is important to consider the significance of the rodent form of the HER2 receptor in normal embryonic development and the embryonic death in mutant mice lacking this receptor. Placental transfer of HERCEPTIN during the early (days 20-50 of gestation) and late (days 120-150 of gestation) fetal development period was observed. There are, however, no adequate and well-controlled studies in pregnant women and it is not known whether HERCEPTIN can cause fetal harm when administered to a pregnant woman or whether it can affect reproductive capacity. In the post-marketing setting, cases of oligohydramnios during the second and third trimesters have been reported in pregnant women receiving HERCEPTIN.

Because animal reproduction studies are not always predictive of human response, HERCEPTIN should not be used during pregnancy unless the potential benefit for the mother outweighs the potential risk to the fetus.

Nursing Women: A study conducted in lactating cynomolgus monkeys at doses 25 times the weekly human maintenance dose of 2 mg/kg HERCEPTIN demonstrated that trastuzumab is secreted in the milk. The presence of trastuzumab in the serum of infant monkeys was not associated with any adverse effects on their growth or development from birth to 1 month of age. It is not known whether HERCEPTIN is excreted in human milk. As human IgG is excreted in human milk, and the potential for absorption and harm to the infant is unknown, women should be advised to discontinue nursing during therapy with HERCEPTIN.

Pediatrics: The safety and effectiveness of HERCEPTIN in pediatric patients have not been established.

Geriatrics (>65 years of age): HERCEPTIN has been administered to 394 patients who were 65 years of age or over (141 in the adjuvant studies B-31 and N9831, 120 in the HERA trial for a period of 1 year and 133 in the metastatic breast cancer setting). The risk of hematologic toxicities (leucopenia and thrombocytopenia) may be increased in geriatric patients. The risk of cardiac dysfunction may be increased in geriatric patients as compared to younger patients in both those receiving treatment for metastatic disease or adjuvant therapy.

The reported clinical experience is not adequate to determine whether older patients respond differently to HERCEPTIN treatment from younger patients.

Data suggest that the disposition of HERCEPTIN is not altered based on age (see Action and Clinical Pharmacology, Pharmacokinetics). In clinical studies, elderly patients did not receive reduced doses of HERCEPTIN.

Selection of Patients/Diagnostic Tests: Early Breast Cancer (EBC)/Metastatic Breast Cancer (MBC): HERCEPTIN should only be used in patients whose tumours overexpress HER2 as determined by immunohistochemistry. CICH or FISH testing for HER2 status also may be used, provided that the testing is done in experienced laboratories that have validated the test.

To ensure accurate and reproducible results, the protocol described in the package insert of an appropriate diagnostic test needs to be strictly followed. However, based on the current scientific knowledge, no standard test can be recommended at this time. There is no standard method of staining and no standard for the type of antibodies used. The grading for overexpression is subjective, and the signal may fade with time on stored slides.

The test method for HER2 overexpression used to determine eligibility of patients for inclusion in the metastatic breast cancer clinical trials employed immunohistochemical staining for HER2 of fixed material from tissue biopsy using the murine monoclonal antibodies CB11 and 4D5. Patients classified as staining 2+ or 3+ were included, while those staining 0 or 1+ were excluded. Greater than 70% of patients enrolled exhibited 3+ overexpression. The data suggest that beneficial effects were greater among those patients with higher levels of overexpression of HER2.

In the studies, an investigative clinical trial assay was employed which utilized a 0 to 3+ scale. The degree of HER2 overexpression indicated by different test methods may not correlate with that used as the eligibility criterion for inclusion in the clinical trials. **For example, the HercepTest kit (registered Trade-Mark of Genentech, Inc.) also utilizes a scale of 0 to 3+. A reading of 3+ with HercepTest is likely to correspond to that of a 2+ or 3+ with the investigative clinical trial assay. A 2+ reading with the HercepTest would likely incorporate a significant number of patients who were scored as 1+ by the investigative clinical trial assay. These patients (1+) would not have met the inclusion criteria.** Test methods having increased sensitivity, relative to the investigative clinical trial assay, may alter the benefit-to-risk ratio compared to that seen in the clinical trials. In deciding which patients should receive HERCEPTIN, the risk of cardiotoxicity (see Warnings and Precautions) must be weighed against the potential benefits of treatment, especially for those not in the high range of HER2 overexpression.

Metastatic Gastric Cancer (MGC): HERCEPTIN should only be administered to patients with metastatic gastric cancer whose tumours have HER2 overexpression as determined by a validated immunohistochemistry (IHC) and FISH testing. The testing should be done in experienced laboratories that have validated the test.

Patients are eligible for HERCEPTIN treatment if they demonstrate strong HER2 protein overexpression, defined by a 3+ score by IHC, or a 2+ score by IHC and a positive FISH result.

ADVERSE REACTIONS: Clinical Trial Adverse Drug Reactions: Because clinical trials are conducted under very specific conditions the adverse reaction rates observed in the clinical trials may not reflect the rates observed in practice and should not be compared to the rates in the clinical trials of another drug. Adverse drug reaction information from clinical trials is useful for identifying drug-related adverse events and for approximating rates.

The following information is relevant to all indications.

Cardiac: For a description of cardiac toxicities, see Warnings and Precautions.

Metastatic Gastric Cancer: In the ToGA (BO18255) study, at screening, the median LVEF value was 64% (range 48%-90%) in the FP arm and 65% (range 50%-86%) in the FP+H arm. At baseline, a LVEF value of 50% or more (measured by ECHO or MUGA) was required at study entry.

The majority of the LVEF decreases noted in ToGA were asymptomatic, with the exception of one patient in the HERCEPTIN-containing arm whose LVEF decrease coincided with cardiac failure.

Table 6: HERCEPTIN

Summary of LVEF Change from Screening

LVEF Decrease: Lowest Post-Screening Value	Fluoropyrimidine/Cisplatin (N=290) (% of patients in each treatment arm)	Trastuzumab/Fluoropyrimidine/ Cisplatin (N=294) (% of patients in each treatment arm)
[a]LVEF decrease of ≥10% to a value of <50%	1.10%	4.60%
Absolute value <50%	1.10%	5.90%
[a]LVEF decrease of ≥10% to a value of ≥50%	11.80%	16.50%

[a] Only includes patients whose method of assessment at that visit is the same as at their initial assessments (F+C, n=187 and H+FC, n=237).

Cardiac Adverse Events: See Table 7.

Table 7: HERCEPTIN

Cardiac Adverse Events

	Fluoropyrimidine/Cisplatin (N=290) (% of patients in each treatment arm)	Trastuzumab/Fluoropyrimidine/ Cisplatin (N=294) (% of patients in each treatment arm)
Total cardiac events	6%	6%
≥Grade 3 NCI CTCAE V3.0	[a]3%	[b]1%

[a] 9 patients experienced 9 events.
[b] 4 patients experienced 5 events.

Infusion-Associated Symptoms: During the first infusion with HERCEPTIN (trastuzumab), chills and/or fever are observed commonly in patients. Other signs and/or symptoms may include nausea, vomiting, pain, rigors, headache, cough, dizziness, rash, asthenia and hypertension. The symptoms are usually mild to moderate in severity, and occur infrequently with subsequent infusions of HERCEPTIN. The symptoms can be treated with an analgesic/antipyretic such as meperidine or acetaminophen, or an antihistamine such as diphenhydramine (see Dosage and Administration). Interruption of the infusion was infrequent. Some adverse reactions to infusions of HERCEPTIN including dyspnea, hypotension, wheezing, bronchospasm, tachycardia, reduced oxygen saturation and respiratory distress can be serious and potentially fatal (see Warnings and Precautions).

Adverse reactions are described separately for HERCEPTIN administered in the adjuvant versus metastatic setting.

Early Breast Cancer: HERA: Please see Warnings and Precautions, Cardiovascular/Cardiotoxicity/Early Breast Cancer—Table 1 and Table 2 for a description of the absolute numbers and rates of cardiac endpoints in HERA as well as the median time to return to baseline LVEF/stabilizations of LVEF in the HERA trial.

The HERA trial is a randomised, open label study in patients with HER2-positive early breast cancer. Table 8 displays adverse events which were reported at 1 year in ≥1% of patients, by study treatment.

In HERA, 1 observation and 10 HERCEPTIN treated patients experienced hypersensitivity. Eight out of the 10 events were considered related to HERCEPTIN treatment.

Long term follow-up data on all patients with heart failure or drop in LVEF are being monitored.

Joint Analysis—NSABP Study B-31 and NCCTG Study N9831: Cardiac failure/dysfunction, pulmonary events, and exacerbation of chemotherapy-induced neutropenia were the most serious adverse reactions in the two randomized, controlled adjuvant breast cancer studies (NSABP Study B-31 and NCCTG Study N9831). Please refer to Warnings and Precautions for detailed description of these reactions and Table 3 for a description of the incidence and type of cardiac events seen in the Joint Analysis.

Anemia and Leucopenia: In Study B-31, the per patient incidences of anemia (19.6% versus 17.0%) and leucopenia (19.9% versus 17.4%) were higher in patients randomized to HERCEPTIN + chemotherapy compared with those randomized to chemotherapy alone.

In Study N9831, the incidences of anemia (0% chemotherapy alone versus 0.2% HERCEPTIN + chemotherapy) and leucopenia (7.7% chemotherapy alone versus 8.2% HERCEPTIN + chemotherapy) were comparable between the two treatment arms.

Table 8: HERCEPTIN

Adverse Events Reported at 1 year in ≥1% of Patients, by Study Treatment

Body System	Adverse Event	Observation Only N=1708 No. (%)	HERCEPTIN 1 year N=1678 No. (%)
Total Pts with at least one AE		**792 (46)**	**1179 (70)**
Total number of AEs		**2251**	**5248**
Cardiac Disorders	Cardiac failure congestive	5 (0.3)	30 (1.8)
	Palpitations[a]	12 (0.7)	48 (2.9)
	Tachycardia	5 (0.3)	20 (1.2)
Gastrointestinal Disorders	Abdominal pain	16 (0.9)	40 (2.4)
	Abdominal pain upper	15 (0.9)	29 (1.7)
	Constipation	17 (1.0)	33 (2.0)
	Diarrhea[a]	16 (0.9)	123 (7.3)
	Dyspepsia	9 (0.5)	30 (1.8)
	Gastritis	11 (0.6)	20 (1.2)
	Nausea[a]	19 (1.1)	108 (6.4)
	Stomatitis	1 (<0.1)	26 (1.5)
	Vomiting[a]	10 (0.6)	58 (3.5)
General Disorders and Administration Site Conditions	Asthenia[a]	30 (1.8)	75 (4.5)
	Chest discomfort	2 (0.1)	20 (1.2)
	Chest pain[a]	22 (1.3)	45 (2.7)
	Chills[a]	—	85 (5.1)
	Edema	7 (0.4)	18 (1.1)
	Edema peripheral	38 (2.2)	79 (4.7)
	Fatigue[a]	44 (2.6)	128 (7.6)
	Influenza illness	3 (0.2)	40 (2.4)
	Pyrexia[a]	6 (0.4)	100 (6.0)
Infections and Infestations[b]	Bronchitis	9 (0.5)	18 (1.1)
	Cystitis	11 (0.6)	19 (1.1)
	Herpes zoster	9 (0.5)	17 (1.0)
	Influenza[a]	9 (0.5)	69 (4.1)
	Nasopharyngitis[a]	43 (2.5)	135 (8.0)
	Pharyngitis	9 (0.5)	20 (1.2)
	Rhinitis	6 (0.4)	36 (2.1)
	Sinusitis	5 (0.3)	26 (1.5)
	Upper respiratory tract infection[a]	20 (1.2)	46 (2.7)
	Urinary tract infection	13 (0.8)	39 (2.3)

(cont'd)

Table 8: HERCEPTIN *(cont'd)*

Adverse Events Reported at 1 year in ≥1% of Patients, by Study Treatment

Body System	Adverse Event	Observation Only N=1708 No. (%)	HERCEPTIN 1 year N=1678 No. (%)
Investigations	Ejection fraction decreased[a]	11 (0.6)	58 (3.5)
	Weight increased	17 (1.0)	29 (1.7)
Musculoskeletal and Connective Tissue Disorders	Arthralgia[a]	98 (5.7)	137 (8.2)
	Back pain[a]	59 (3.5)	91 (5.4)
	Bone pain	26 (1.5)	49 (2.9)
	Chest wall pain	24 (1.4)	26 (1.5)
	Muscle spasms[a]	3 (0.2)	45 (2.7)
	Musculoskeletal pain	11 (0.6)	17 (1.0)
	Myalgia[a]	17 (1.0)	63 (3.8)
	Pain in extremity	45 (2.6)	60 (3.6)
	Shoulder pain	29 (1.7)	30 (1.8)
Nervous System Disorders	Dizziness[a]	29 (1.7)	60 (3.6)
	Headache[a]	49 (2.9)	161 (9.6)
	Paraesthesia	11 (0.6)	29 (1.7)
	Vertigo	7 (0.4)	25 (1.5)
Psychiatric	Anxiety	19 (1.1)	39 (2.3)
	Depression	34 (2.0)	51 (3.0)
	Insomnia	31 (1.8)	58 (3.5)
Renal and Urinary Disorders	Dysuria	2 (0.1)	17 (1.0)
Respiratory, Thoracic and Mediastinal Disorders	Cough[a]	34 (2.0)	81 (4.8)
	Dyspnea	26 (1.5)	56 (3.3)
	Dyspnea exertional	15 (0.9)	21 (1.3)
	Epistaxis	1 (<0.1)	24 (1.4)
	Pharyngolaryngeal pain	8 (0.5)	32 (1.9)
	Rhinorrhea	5 (0.3)	24 (1.4)

(cont'd)

Table 8: HERCEPTIN *(cont'd)*

Adverse Events Reported at 1 year in ≥1% of Patients, by Study Treatment

Body System	Adverse Event	Observation Only N=1708 No. (%)	HERCEPTIN 1 year N=1678 No. (%)
Reproductive System and Breast Disorders	Breast pain	19 (1.1)	24 (1.4)
Skin and Subcutaneous Tissue	Erythema	7 (0.4)	24 (1.4)
	Nail disorder[a]	—	43 (2.6)
	Onychorrhexis	1 (<0.1)	36 (2.1)
	Pruritus	10 (0.6)	40 (2.4)
	Rash[b]	10 (0.6)	70 (4.2)
Vascular Disorders	Hot flush	84 (4.9)	98 (5.8)
	Hypertension[a]	35 (2.0)	64 (3.8)
	Lymphoedema	40 (2.3)	42 (2.5)

[a] Adverse events that were reported at higher incidence (≥2% difference) in the HERCEPTIN group compared with the observation group and therefore may be attributable to HERCEPTIN.

[b] Serious adverse reactions of cellulitis and erysipelas were also reported in the HERA study.

Hypersensitivity Reactions Including Anaphylaxis: The incidence of allergic reactions (chemotherapy alone versus HERCEPTIN + chemotherapy: 3.2% versus 3.2% in Study B-31 and 0.9% versus 0.4% in Study N9831) was comparable between the two treatment arms in both studies.

Pulmonary Events: The incidence of pulmonary events in the adjuvant studies (16.1% versus 7.8% in Study B-31 and 4.1% versus 1.4% in Study N9831) was higher in patients randomized to HERCEPTIN + chemotherapy versus chemotherapy alone. The most common pulmonary event was dyspnea. The majority of these events were mild to moderate in intensity. Fatal pulmonary events were reported in 4 patients in the HERCEPTIN + chemotherapy arm. Only 1 of these patients actually received HERCEPTIN. The cause of death in these 4 patients was cardio-respiratory arrest, bronchopneumonia, respiratory insufficiency, and pneumonia accompanied by neutropenic fever. Pneumonitis/pulmonary infiltrates were reported in 20 patients who participated in either adjuvant clinical trial. Twelve of these 20 patients had received HERCEPTIN + chemotherapy. The etiology of pneumonitis/pulmonary infiltrates was possible hypersensitivity/inflammation reaction (n= 4), pneumonia (n=5), radiation therapy toxicity (n=1) and unknown etiology (n=2).

Thrombosis/Embolism: The incidence of thrombotic adverse events was higher in patients randomized to HERCEPTIN + chemotherapy versus chemotherapy alone in Study B-31, but not in Study N9831. In Study B-31, thrombotic adverse events were reported in 4.1% of patients randomized to HERCEPTIN + chemotherapy versus 2.5% of patients randomized to the chemotherapy alone arm. In Study N9831, thrombotic adverse events were reported in 1.9% of patients randomized to HERCEPTIN + chemotherapy versus 2.3% of patients randomized to chemotherapy alone.

Adverse events occurring at a frequency of ≥1% for NSABP-B31 and NCCTG N9831, are summarized in Table 9 and Table 10 respectively.

Metastatic Breast Cancer: In clinical trials conducted prior to marketing, a total of 958 patients received HERCEPTIN (trastuzumab) alone or in combination with chemotherapy. Data in Table 13 are based on the experience with the recommended dosing regimen for HERCEPTIN in the randomized controlled clinical trial in 234 patients who received HERCEPTIN in combination with chemotherapy and the open-label study of HERCEPTIN as a single agent in 213 patients with HER2-overexpressing metastatic breast cancer.

Metastatic Gastric Cancer: The ToGA trial (BO18255) is a randomised, open-label multicentre, phase III study of trastuzumab in combination with a fluoropyrimidine and cisplatin versus chemotherapy alone in patients with HER2 positive metastatic gastric cancer. There were only 3.4% of patients in each treatment group with locally advanced cancer. The majority of patients had metastatic disease.

The adverse drug reactions that occurred with the incidence of at least 1% in the ToGA (BO18255) study are presented in Table 11.

Table 9: HERCEPTIN

Adverse Events of Any Grade with Incidence ≥1% in the HERCEPTIN + Chemotherapy Arm in B-31

	AC→T (n=962)			AC→T+H (n=967)		
Adverse Event Term[b]	**Any Grade**	**Grades 3-4**	**Grade 5**	**Any Grade**	**Grades 3-4**	**Grade 5**
Abdominal pain or cramping	23 (2.4%)	11 (1.1%)	0	25 (2.6%)	8 (0.8%)	0
Allergic reaction[a]	31 (3.2%)	10 (1.0%)	0	31 (3.2%)	10 (1.0%)	0
Allergic rhinitis	11 (1.1%)	0.00%	0	22 (2.3%)	0.00%	0
Alopecia	313 (32.5%)	3 (0.3%)	0	325 (33.6%)	2 (0.2%)	0
Anorexia[a]	69 (7.2%)	11 (1.1%)	0	64 (6.6%)	12 (1.2%)	0
Any adverse events	883 (91.8%)	561 (58.3%)	3 (0.3%)	905 (93.6%)	573 (59.3%)	4 (0.4%)
Arthralgia (joint pain)[a]	273 (28.4%)	56 (5.8%)	0	292 (30.2%)	62 (6.4%)	0
Bone pain	52 (5.4%)	16 (1.7%)	0	50 (5.2%)	7 (0.7%)	0
Cardiac-left ventricular function[a]	28 (2.9%)	5 (0.5%)	0	132 (13.7%)	32 (3.3%)	0
Chest pain	11 (1.1%)	3 (0.3%)	0	34 (3.5%)	4 (0.4%)	0
Constipation[a]	87 (9.0%)	9 (0.9%)	0	111 (11.5%)	3 (0.3%)	0
Cough	9 (0.9%)	1 (0.1%)	0	26 (2.7%)	1 (0.1%)	0
Dehydration	22 (2.3%)	7 (0.7%)	0	24 (2.5%)	5 (0.5%)	0
Diarrhea without prior colostomy[a]	86 (8.9%)	25 (2.6%)	0	95 (9.8%)	25 (2.6%)	0
Dizziness/lightheadedness	29 (3.0%)	5 (0.5%)	0	33 (3.4%)	8 (0.8%)	0
Dyspepsia	49 (5.1%)	3 (0.3%)	0	47 (4.9%)	2 (0.2%)	0

(cont'd)

Table 9: HERCEPTIN *(cont'd)*

Adverse Events of Any Grade with Incidence ≥1% in the HERCEPTIN + Chemotherapy Arm in B-31

	AC→T (n=962)			AC→T+H (n=967)		
Adverse Event Term[b]	**Any Grade**	**Grades 3-4**	**Grade 5**	**Any Grade**	**Grades 3-4**	**Grade 5**
Dyspnea (shortness of breath)	62 (6.4%)	19 (2.0%)	0	126 (13.0%)	24 (2.5%)	0
Edema	27 (2.8%)	1 (0.1%)	0	43 (4.4%)	0.00%	0
Fatigue[a]	346 (36.0%)	54 (5.6%)	0	385 (39.8%)	57 (5.9%)	0
Febrile neutropenia[a]	53 (5.5%)	52 (5.4%)	1 (0.1%)	43 (4.4%)	43 (4.4%)	0
Fever (in the absence of neutropenia)[a]	18 (1.9%)	2 (0.2%)	0	29 (3.0%)	5 (0.5%)	0
GI-other	17 (1.8%)	2 (0.2%)	0	25 (2.6%)	5 (0.5%)	0
Headache[a]	82 (8.5%)	20 (2.1%)	0	106 (11.0%)	25 (2.6%)	0
Hemoglobin[a]	164 (17.0%)	29 (3.0%)	0	190 (19.6%)	29 (3.0%)	0
Hot flashes/flushes	171 (17.8%)	2 (0.2%)	0	179 (18.5%)	0.00%	0
Hyperglycemia	121 (12.6%)	46 (4.8%)	0	134 (13.9%)	47 (4.9%)	0
Hypertension	6 (0.6%)	3 (0.3%)	0	22 (2.3%)	16 (1.7%)	0
Hypoglycemia	8 (0.8%)	2 (0.2%)	0	13 (1.3%)	7 (0.7%)	0
Infection[a]	261 (27.1%)	127 (13.2%)	1 (0.1%)	295 (30.5%)	127 (13.1%)	1 (0.1%)
Insomnia	38 (4.0%)	2 (0.2%)	0	51 (5.3%)	5 (0.5%)	0
Irregular menses (change from baseline)	37 (3.8%)	29 (3.0%)	0	42 (4.3%)	35 (3.6%)	0
Joint, muscle, bone-other	10 (1.0%)	1 (0.1%)	0	14 (1.4%)	2 (0.2%)	0
Leukocytes (total WBC)	167 (17.4%)	104 (10.8%)	0	192 (19.9%)	101 (10.4%)	0
Lymphatics	10 (1.0%)	0.00%	0	22 (2.3%)	0.00%	0
Lymphopenia	43 (4.5%)	24 (2.5%)	0	49 (5.1%)	30 (3.1%)	0
Mood alteration-anxiety/agitation	48 (5.0%)	6 (0.6%)	0	40 (4.1%)	6 (0.6%)	0
Mood alteration-depression	64 (6.7%)	11 (1.1%)	0	57 (5.9%)	10 (1.0%)	0
Myalgia (muscle pain)[a]	304 (31.6%)	84 (8.7%)	0	318 (32.9%)	60 (6.2%)	0
Nail changes	13 (1.4%)	0.00%	0	24 (2.5%)	0.00%	0
Nausea[a]	331 (34.4%)	66 (6.9%)	0	340 (35.2%)	75 (7.8%)	0
Neuropathic pain	8 (0.8%)	4 (0.4%)	0	16 (1.7%)	4 (0.4%)	0
Neuropathy-motor[a]	43 (4.5%)	16 (1.7%)	0	44 (4.6%)	12 (1.2%)	0
Neuropathy-sensory[a]	211 (21.9%)	53 (5.5%)	0	205 (21.2%)	43 (4.4%)	0
Neutrophils/granulocytes	128 (13.3%)	105 (10.9%)	0	130 (13.4%)	104 (10.8%)	0
Pain-other	52 (5.4%)	8 (0.8%)	0	66 (6.8%)	10 (1.0%)	0
Platelets	21 (2.2%)	11 (1.1%)	0	24 (2.5%)	12 (1.2%)	0
Pruritus	17 (1.8%)	1 (0.1%)	0	16 (1.7%)	2 (0.2%)	0
Pulmonary-other	7 (0.7%)	2 (0.2%)	0	14 (1.4%)	5 (0.5%)	0
Radiation dermatitis	18 (1.9%)	3 (0.3%)	0	32 (3.3%)	10 (1.0%)	0
Rash/desquamation[a]	89 (9.3%)	12 (1.2%)	0	119 (12.3%)	8 (0.8%)	0
AST[a]	20 (2.1%)	6 (0.6%)	0	22 (2.3%)	6 (0.6%)	0
ALT[a]	35 (3.6%)	4 (0.4%)	0	24 (2.5%)	6 (0.6%)	0
Skin-other	18 (1.9%)	3 (0.3%)	0	22 (2.3%)	1 (0.1%)	0
Stomatitis/pharyngitis[a]	160 (16.6%)	6 (0.6%)	0	173 (17.9%)	8 (0.8%)	0
Sweating (diaphoresis)	9 (0.9%)	0.00%	0	13 (1.3%)	0.00%	0
Syncope (fainting)	8 (0.8%)	8 (0.8%)	0	11 (1.1%)	11 (1.1%)	0
Taste disturbance (dysgeusia)	14 (1.5%)	0.00%	0	22 (2.3%)	0.00%	0
Thrombosis/embolism[a]	21 (2.2%)	20 (2.1%)	0	35 (3.6%)	33 (3.4%)	0
Urinary frequency/urgency	8 (0.8%)	3 (0.3%)	0	10 (1.0%)	1 (0.1%)	0
Vaginal bleeding	5 (0.5%)	0.00%	0	17 (1.8%)	0.00%	0
Vaginal dryness	11 (1.1%)	0.00%	0	22 (2.3%)	1 (0.1%)	0
Vision-blurred vision	13 (1.4%)	0.00%	0	18 (1.9%)	0.00%	0

(cont'd)

Table 9: HERCEPTIN *(cont'd)*

Adverse Events of Any Grade with Incidence ≥1% in the HERCEPTIN + Chemotherapy Arm in B-31

	AC→T (n=962)			AC→T+H (n=967)		
Adverse Event Term[b]	**Any Grade**	**Grades 3-4**	**Grade 5**	**Any Grade**	**Grades 3-4**	**Grade 5**
Vomiting[a]	237 (24.6%)	65 (6.8%)	0	248 (25.6%)	69 (7.1%)	0
Weight gain	7 (0.7%)	2 (0.2%)	0	11 (1.1%)	2 (0.2%)	0
Wound-infectious	9 (0.9%)	4 (0.4%)	0	11 (1.1%)	6 (0.6%)	0

[a] Adverse event term is itemized on the Adverse Event CRF.
[b] NCIC CTC terminology.
Legend: A=doxorubicin; C=cyclophosphamide; GI=gastrointestinal; H=HERCEPTIN; AST=serum glutamic oxaloacetic transaminase; ALT=serum glutamic pyruvic transaminase; T=paclitaxel; WBC=white blood cell.
Note: Only Grade 3-5 events, treatment-related Grade 2 events, Grade 2-5 cardiac left ventricular dysfunction, and Grade 2-5 dyspnea were collected during and 3 months following protocol treatment. The term "febrile neutropenia" refers to febrile neutropenia with no evidence of infection; decreased neutrophils were not intended to be collected.

Table 10: HERCEPTIN

Adverse Events of Any Grade with Incidence ≥1% in the HERCEPTIN + Chemotherapy Arm in N9831

	AC→T (n=797)			AC→T+H (n=803)		
Adverse Event Term[b]	**Any Grade**	**Grades 3-4**	**Grade 5**	**Any Grade**	**Grades 3-4**	**Grade 5**
Any adverse events	466 (58.5%)	348 (43.7%)	2 (0.3%)	557 (69.4%)	420 (52.3%)	2 (0.2%)
Arthralgia (joint pain)[a]	75 (9.4%)	10 (1.3%)	0	90 (11.2%)	14 (1.7%)	0
Cardiac-left ventricular function[a]	48 (6.0%)	1 (0.1%)	0	157 (19.6%)	18 (2.2%)	0
Chest pain	5 (0.6%)	1 (0.1%)	0	11 (1.4%)	3 (0.4%)	0
Diarrhea without prior colostomy[a]	8 (1.0%)	8 (1.0%)	0	18 (2.2%)	18 (2.2%)	0
Dyspnea (shortness of breath)	3 (0.4%)	3 (0.4%)	0	24 (3.0%)	19 (2.4%)	0
Edema	7 (0.9%)	0.00%	0	9 (1.1%)	0.00%	0
Fatigue[a]	32 (4.0%)	32 (4.0%)	0	35 (4.4%)	35 (4.4%)	0
Febrile neutropenia[a]	29 (3.6%)	28 (3.5%)	1 (0.1%)	58 (7.2%)	58 (7.2%)	0
Hyperglycemia	17 (2.1%)	17 (2.1%)	0	9 (1.1%)	9 (1.1%)	0
Hypertension	7 (0.9%)	3 (0.4%)	0	10 (1.2%)	4 (0.5%)	0
Infection[a]	37 (4.6%)	37 (4.6%)	0	60 (7.5%)	59 (7.3%)	1 (0.1%)
Leukocytes (total WBC)[a]	61 (7.7%)	60 (7.5%)	1 (0.1%)	66 (8.2%)	66 (8.2%)	0
Myalgia (muscle pain)[a]	66 (8.3%)	8 (1.0%)	0	83 (10.3%)	9 (1.1%)	0
Nail changes[a]	56 (7.0%)	0.00%	0	70 (8.7%)	0.00%	0
Nausea[a]	44 (5.5%)	44 (5.5%)	0	49 (6.1%)	49 (6.1%)	0
Neuropathy-motor[a]	33 (4.1%)	6 (0.8%)	0	32 (4.0%)	9 (1.1%)	0
Neuropathy-sensory[a]	139 (17.4%)	30 (3.8%)	0	130 (16.2%)	34 (4.2%)	0
Neutrophils/granulocytes[a]	204 (25.6%)	203 (25.5%)	1 (0.1%)	258 (32.1%)	258 (32.1%)	0
Palpitations	12 (1.5%)	0.00%	0	9 (1.1%)	0.00%	0
Thrombosis/embolism[a]	16 (2.0%)	15 (1.9%)	1 (0.1%)	10 (1.2%)	9 (1.1%)	1 (0.1%)
Vomiting[a]	39 (4.9%)	39 (4.9%)	0	37 (4.6%)	37 (4.6%)	0

[a] Adverse event term is itemized on the Adverse Event CRF.
[b] NCIC CTC terminology.
Legend: A=doxorubicin; AE=adverse event; C=cyclophosphamide; H=HERCEPTIN; T=paclitaxel; WBC=white blood cell.
Note: Only treatment-related Grade 4 and 5 hematologic toxicities, Grade 3-5 non-hematologic toxicities, Grade 1-5 cardiac toxicities, as well as Grade 2-5 arthralgia, myalgia, nail changes, neuropathy-motor, and neuropathy-sensory adverse events were collected during the treatment period. During the post-treatment follow-up period, only Grade 3-5 cardiac ischemia/infarction, thrombosis/embolism, pneumonitis/pulmonary infiltrates, and lymphatic events were collected.

Table 11: HERCEPTIN

Adverse Drug Reactions with Incidence Rate ≥1% in ToGA (BO18255)

	Fluoropyrimidine/Cisplatin (FP) N=290 No. (%)	**Trastuzumab/Fluoropyrimidine/ Cisplatin (H+FP) N=294 No. (%)**
Blood and Lymphatic System Disorders		
Neutropenia	165 (57)	157 (53)
Anemia	61 (21)	81 (28)
Thrombocytopenia	33 (11)	47 (16)
Febrile neutropenia	8 (3)	15 (5)
Leukopenia	11 (4)	11 (4)
Cardiac Disorders		
Palpitations	2 (<1)	6 (2)

(cont'd)

Table 11: HERCEPTIN *(cont'd)*

Adverse Drug Reactions with Incidence Rate ≥1% in ToGA (BO18255)

	Fluoropyrimidine/Cisplatin (FP) N=290 No. (%)	**Trastuzumab/Fluoropyrimidine/ Cisplatin (H+FP) N=294 No. (%)**
Ear and Labyrinth Disorders		
Deafness	1 (<1)	8 (3)
Eye Disorders		
Lacrimation increased	2 (<1)	5 (2)
Gastrointestinal Disorders		
Nausea	184 (63)	197 (67)
Vomiting	134 (46)	147 (50)

(cont'd)

Table 11: HERCEPTIN *(cont'd)*

Adverse Drug Reactions with Incidence Rate ≥1% in ToGA (BO18255)

	Fluoropyrimidine/Cisplatin (FP) N=290 No. (%)	Trastuzumab/Fluoropyrimidine/ Cisplatin (H+FP) N=294 No. (%)
Diarrhea	80 (28)	109 (37)
Constipation	93 (32)	75 (26)
Stomatitis	43 (15)	72 (24)
Abdominal pain	42 (14)	46 (16)
Abdominal pain upper	15 (5)	27 (9)
Dyspepsia	16 (6)	18 (6)
Hemorrhoids	3 (1)	5 (2)
Abdominal discomfort	3 (1)	3 (1)
Dry mouth	2 (<1)	4 (1)
General Disorders and Administration Site Conditions		
Fatigue	82 (28)	102 (35)
Asthenia	53 (18)	55 (19)
Pyrexia	36 (12)	54 (18)
Mucosal inflammation	18 (6)	37 (13)
Edema	25 (9)	22 (7)
Edema peripheral	12 (4)	17 (6)
Chills	—	23 (8)
Chest pain	4 (1)	8 (3)
Malaise	6 (2)	6 (2)
Pain	4 (1)	5 (2)
Infusion related reaction	—	3 (1)
Hepatobiliary Disorders		
Hepatic function abnormal	3 (1)	3 (1)
Infections and Infestations		
Nasopharyngitis	17 (6)	37 (13)
Upper respiratory tract infection	10 (3)	15 (5)
Pneumonia	2 (<1)	9 (3)
Cystitis	1 (<1)	5 (2)
Pharyngitis	2 (<1)	4 (1)
Respiratory tract infection	3 (1)	3 (1)
Infection	2 (<1)	3 (1)
Influenza	1 (<1)	4 (1)
Immune System Disorders		
Hypersensitivity	3 (1)	6 (2)
Injury, Poisoning and Procedural Complications		
Contusion	2 (<1)	3 (1)
Investigations		
Weight decreased	40 (14)	69 (23)
Hemoglobin decreased	2 (<1)	7 (2)
Platelet count decreased	6 (2)	1 (<1)
Neutrophil count decreased	3 (1)	3 (1)
Metabolism and Nutrition Disorders		
Anorexia	133 (46)	135 (46)
Hyperkalaemia	3 (1)	—
Musculoskeletal and Connective Tissue Disorders		
Back pain	15 (5)	12 (4)

(cont'd)

Table 11: HERCEPTIN *(cont'd)*

Adverse Drug Reactions with Incidence Rate ≥1% in ToGA (BO18255)

	Fluoropyrimidine/Cisplatin (FP) N=290 No. (%)	Trastuzumab/Fluoropyrimidine/ Cisplatin (H+FP) N=294 No. (%)
Pain in extremity	7 (2)	4 (1)
Arthralgia	2 (<1)	7 (2)
Musculoskeletal pain	4 (1)	5 (2)
Myalgia	3 (1)	4 (1)
Muscular weakness	3 (1)	2 (<1)
Muscle spasms	1 (<1)	3 (1)
Musculoskeletal chest pain	3 (1)	1 (<1)
Neck pain	1 (<1)	3 (1)
Nervous System Disorders		
Dizziness	28 (10)	31 (11)
Peripheral sensory neuropathy	24 (8)	23 (8)
Neuropathy peripheral	21 (7)	24 (8)
Dysgeusia	14 (5)	28 (10)
Headache	19 (7)	14 (5)
Paraesthesia	9 (3)	9 (3)
Lethargy	8 (3)	6 (2)
Peripheral motor neuropathy	6 (2)	8 (3)
Tremor	5 (2)	3 (1)
Renal and Urinary Disorders		
Renal impairment	39 (13)	47 (16)
Nephropathy toxic	12 (4)	18 (6)
Renal failure acute	2 (<1)	3 (1)
Renal failure	1 (<1)	3 (1)
Respiratory, Thoracic and Mediastinal Disorders		
Cough	17 (6)	19 (6)
Dyspnea	16 (6)	9 (3)
Epistaxis	9 (3)	13 (4)
Rhinorrhea	2 (<1)	6 (2)
Psychiatric Disorders		
Insomnia	20 (7)	24 (8)
Depression	5 (2)	4 (1)
Anxiety	5 (2)	3 (1)
Sleep disorder	3 (1)	2 (<1)
Skin and Subcutaneous Tissue Disorders		
Alopecia	27 (9)	32 (11)
Rash	12 (4)	16 (5)
Nail disorder	6 (2)	13 (4)
Dry skin	4 (1)	10 (3)
Pruritus	3 (1)	8 (3)
Urticaria	3 (1)	3 (1)
Vascular Disorders		
Hypertension	7 (2)	11 (4)
Hypotension	6 (2)	6 (2)

Adverse Drug Reactions With Incidence Rate <1% in ToGA (BO18255): Cardiac Disorders: arrhythmia, atrial fibrillation, atrial flutter, bradycardia, cardiac failure, left ventricular dysfunction.
Eye Disorders: dry eye.
Gastrointestinal Disorders: abdominal pain lower, haemorrhoidal haemorrhage, lip swelling, pancreatitis acute.
General Disorders and Administration Site Conditions: influenza like illness, mucous membrane disorder.
Hepatobiliary Disorders: hepatic failure, hepatitis toxic, hepatotoxicity, jaundice.
Infections and Infestations: bronchitis, cellulitis, herpes zoster, lower respiratory tract infection, lung infection, neutropenic sepsis, paronychia, rhinitis, sepsis, sinusitis, urinary tract infection.

Investigations: alanine aminotransferase increased, aspartate aminotransferase increased, blood alkaline phosphatase increased, blood alkaline phosphatase increased, blood lactate dehydrogenase increased, blood potassium increased, blood pressure decreased, ejection fraction decreased, gamma-glutamyltransferase increased, transaminases increased, white blood cell count decreased.
Metabolism and Nutrition Disorders: decreased appetite, fluid retention.
Musculoskeletal and Connective Tissue Disorders: arthritis, joint swelling.
Nervous System Disorders: neurotoxicity, paresis, somnolence, toxic neuropathy.
Renal and Urinary Disorders: renal disorder.
Respiratory, Thoracic and Mediastinal Disorders: acute respiratory distress syndrome, hypoxia, pharyngeal edema, pleural effusion, pneumonitis.
Skin and Subcutaneous Tissue Disorders: acne, dermatitis, erythema, hyperhidrosis, rash macular, rash papular, rash pruritic.
Hematological Toxicity: Early Breast Cancer (EBC)/Metastatic Breast Cancer (MBC): WHO Grade 3 or 4† hematological toxicity was observed in 63% of patients treated with HERCEPTIN and an anthracycline plus cyclophosphamide compared to an incidence of 62% in patients treated with anthracycline/cyclophosphamide combination without HERCEPTIN. There was an increase in WHO Grade 3 or 4 hematological toxicity in patients treated with the combination of HERCEPTIN and paclitaxel compared with patients receiving paclitaxel alone (34% vs 21%).

In a randomized, controlled trial conducted in the post-marketing setting, hematological toxicity was also increased in patients receiving HERCEPTIN and docetaxel, compared with docetaxel alone (32% grade 3/4 neutropenia versus 22%, using NCI-CTC criteria). The incidence of febrile neutropenia/neutropenic sepsis was also increased in patients treated with HERCEPTIN plus docetaxel (23% versus 17% for patients treated with docetaxel alone), see Warnings and Precautions.

An increased incidence of anemia and leukopenia was observed in the treatment group receiving HERCEPTIN and chemotherapy, especially in the HERCEPTIN and AC subgroup, compared with the treatment group receiving chemotherapy alone. The majority of these cytopenic events were mild or moderate in intensity, reversible, and none resulted in discontinuation of therapy with HERCEPTIN.

Hematologic toxicity is infrequent following the administration of HERCEPTIN as a single agent, with an incidence of Grade 3 toxicities for WBC, platelets, hemoglobin all <1%. No Grade 4 toxicities were observed.
Metastatic Gastric Cancer (MGC):

Table 12: HERCEPTIN

Blood and Lymphatic System Disorders SOC: the Most Frequently Reported AEs of Grade ≥3 with Incidence Rate ≥1%

	Fluoropyrimidine/Cisplatin (N=290) (% of patients in each treatment arm)	Trastuzumab/Fluoropyrimidine/Cisplatin (N=294) (% of patients in each treatment arm)
Neutropenia	30%	27%
Anaemia	10%	12%
Febrile neutropenia	3%	5%
Thrombocytopenia	3%	5%
Leukopenia	<1%	2%

The total percentage of patients who experienced an AE of ≥grade 3 NCI CTCAE v3.0 that has been categorised under this SOC were 38% in the FP arm and 40% in the FP + H arm.
Diarrhea: Early Breast Cancer (EBC)/Metastatic Breast Cancer (MBC): Of patients treated with HERCEPTIN as a single agent, 27% experienced diarrhea. An increased incidence of diarrhea, primarily mild to moderate in severity, was observed in patients receiving HERCEPTIN in combination with chemotherapy.
Metastatic Gastric Cancer (MGC): In the ToGA study, 109 patients (37%) participating in the HERCEPTIN-containing treatment arm versus 80 patients (28%) in the comparator arm experienced any grade diarrhea. Using NCI-CTCAE v3.0 severity criteria, the percentage of patients experiencing grade ≥3 diarrhea was 4% in the FP arm vs 9% in the FP+ H arm.
Infection: Early Breast Cancer (EBC)/Metastatic Breast Cancer (MBC): An increased incidence of infections, primarily mild upper respiratory infections of minor clinical significance or catheter infections, was observed in patients receiving HERCEPTIN in combination with chemotherapy.
Metastatic Gastric Cancer (MGC): Infections and infestations were reported in 20 % of patients in the FP arm vs 32% in the FP+ H arm. The major contributors to the higher incidence of infections and infestations in the HERCEPTIN arm were nasopharyngitis (6% in the FP arm vs 13% in the FP+ H arm) and upper respiratory tract infection (3% vs 5%).
Hypersensitivity Reactions Including Anaphylaxis and Pulmonary Events: In the postmarketing setting, severe hypersensitivity reactions (including anaphylaxis), infusion reactions, and pulmonary adverse events have been reported. These events include anaphylaxis, angioedema, bronchospasm, hypotension, hypoxia, dyspnea, pulmonary infiltrates, pleural effusions, non-cardiogenic pulmonary edema, and acute respiratory distress syndrome (see Warnings and Precautions).
Hepatic and Renal Toxicity: Early Breast Cancer (EBC)/Metastatic Breast Cancer (MBC): WHO Grade 3 or 4‡ hepatic toxicity was observed in 6% of patients treated with HERCEPTIN and an anthracycline plus cyclophosphamide compared with an incidence of 8% in patients treated with anthracycline/cyclophosphamide combination without HERCEPTIN. Hepatic toxicity was less frequently observed among patients receiving HERCEPTIN and paclitaxel than among patients receiving paclitaxel (7% vs 15%).

WHO Grade 3 or 4 hepatic toxicity was observed in 12% of patients following administration of HERCEPTIN as a single agent. This toxicity was associated with progression of disease in the liver in 60% of these patients.

No WHO Grade 3 or 4 renal toxicity was observed in either the combination or single agent study.

Table 13: HERCEPTIN

Adverse Events Occurring in ≥10% of Patients or at Increased Incidence* in the HERCEPTIN Arm of the Randomized Study (Percent of Patients)

	Single Agent (n=213)	HERCEPTIN + Paclitaxel (n=91)	Paclitaxel Alone (n=95)	HERCEPTIN + AC (n=143)	AC Alone (n=135)
Body as a Whole					
Abdominal pain	22	34	22	23	18
Accidental injury	6	13*	3	9	4
Asthenia	47	62	57	54	55
Back pain	21	36	30	27*	16

† WHO Grade 3 Hematological Toxicity: Hemoglobin—6.5-7.9 g/100 mL, 65-79 g/L, 4.0-4.9 mmol/L, Leukocytes (1000/mm³)—1.0-1.9, Granulocytes (1000/mm³)—0.5-0.9, Platelets (1000/mm³)—25-49. WHO Grade 4 Hematological Toxicity: Hemoglobin—<6.5 g/100 mL, <65 g/L, <4.0 mmol/L, Leukocytes (1000/mm³)—<1.0, Granulocytes (1000/mm³)—<0.5, Platelets (1000/mm³)—<25.

‡ WHO Grade 3 Hepatic Toxicity: Bilirubin—5.1-10×N, Transaminases (ASAT/ALAT)—5.1-10×N, Alkaline Phosphatase—5.1-10×N, where N is the upper limit of normal of population under study. WHO Grade 4 Hepatic Toxicity: Bilirubin—>10×N, Transaminases (ASAT/ALAT)—>10×N, Alkaline Phosphatase—>10×N, where N is the upper limit of normal of population under study.

(cont'd)

Table 13: HERCEPTIN *(cont'd)*

Adverse Events Occurring in ≥10% of Patients or at Increased Incidence* in the HERCEPTIN Arm of the Randomized Study (Percent of Patients)

	Single Agent (n=213)	HERCEPTIN + Paclitaxel (n=91)	Paclitaxel Alone (n=95)	HERCEPTIN + AC (n=143)	AC Alone (n=135)
Chest pain	22	30	27	20	21
Chills	36	42*	4	35*	11
Fever	39	47*	23	56*	33
Flu syndrome	11	12	5	12	6
Headache	26	36	28	44*	31
Infection	20	46*	27	47*	30
Mucous membrane disorder	2	11	7	22	18
Neck pain	5	9	5	10	8
Pain	49	60	61	57*	42
Reaction unvaluable	<1	4	2	10	7
Cardiovascular					
Congestive heart failure	2	2	1	12*	2
Left heart failure	0	6	0	10	5
Tachycardia	6	12*	4	10	5
Vasodilation	8	22	20	18	16
Digestive					
Anorexia	13	24	16	31	26
Constipation	13	25	27	36	28
Diarrhea	27	45*	30	45*	25
Dyspepsia	8	18	16	22	20
Mouth ulceration	2	4	1	12	14
Nausea	37	50	48	76	79
Nausea and vomiting	8	14	12	18*	9
Stomatitis	4	10	7	30	31
Vomiting	28	37	28	53	49
Heme and Lymphatic					
Anemia	4	14	10	35	25
Leukopenia	3	24	17	52*	33
Thrombocytopenia	<1	3	3	11	9
Metabolic					
Dehydration	2	9	10	10*	4
Edema	8	10	8	11	5
Hypokalemia	4	2	3	13*	4
Peripheral edema	10	22	20	20	17
Musculoskeletal					
Arthralgia	6	37*	21	8	10
Bone pain	9	24	18	7	7
Myalgia	8	38	36	13	13
Nervous					
Anxiety	13	19	15	18	14
Depression	8	12	13	20	12
Dizziness	13	22	24	24	18
Hypertonia	4	11*	3	8*	2

(cont'd)

Table 13: **HERCEPTIN** *(cont'd)*

Adverse Events Occurring in ≥10% of Patients or at Increased Incidence* in the HERCEPTIN Arm of the Randomized Study (Percent of Patients)

	Single Agent (n=213)	HERCEPTIN + Paclitaxel (n=91)	Paclitaxel Alone (n=95)	HERCEPTIN + AC (n=143)	AC Alone (n=135)
Insomnia	16	25*	13	29*	16
Neuropathy	2	13	5	4	4
Paresthesia	9	47	39	17	11
Peripheral neuritis	2	23	16	2	2
Somnolence	7	10	10	10	15
Respiratory					
Cough increased	28	42*	22	43*	28
Dyspnea	23	28	26	42*	24
Epistaxis	6	18*	4	7	6
Pharyngitis	13	22	14	30*	18
Rhinitis	16	22*	5	22	16
Sinusitis	12	21*	7	13	6
Skin					
Acne	2	11*	3	3	<1
Alopecia	1	56	56	58	59
Herpes simplex	2	12*	3	7	8
Pruritus	11	14	13	8	6
Rash	14	38*	18	27	17
Special Senses					
Taste perversion	2	6	3	11	13
Urogenital					
Urinary tract infection	3	19	14	13	7

Metastatic Gastric Cancer (MGC): A higher incidence of renal impairment (13% in the FP arm vs 16% in the FP+ H arm) and toxic nephropathy (4% in the FP arm vs 6% in the FP+ H arm) was reported in ToGA trial. NCICTCAE (v 3.0) grade ≥3 renal toxicity was higher in patients receiving HERCEPTIN than those in the F+ P arm (3% and 2% respectively).

NCICTCAE (v 3.0) grade ≥3 adverse event in the Hepatobiliary Disorders SOC: Hyperbilirubinaemia was reported in 1% of patients receiving HERCEPTIN compared to <1% in patients in the F+ P arm.

Other Serious Adverse Events: The following other serious adverse events occurred in at least one of the 958 patients treated with HERCEPTIN in the metastatic breast cancer clinical trials conducted prior to market approval:

Body as a Whole: abdomen enlarged, allergic reaction, anaphylactoid reaction, ascites, carcinoma, cellulitis, chills and fever, death, dermatomyositis, hydrocephalus, necrosis, neoplasm, pelvic pain, radiation injury, sepsis.

Cardiovascular: atrial fibrillation, cardiomyopathy, cardiovascular disorder, cerebrovascular accident, deep thrombophlebitis, heart arrest, heart failure, hemorrhage, hypotension, pericardial effusion, pulmonary embolus, thrombophlebitis, thrombosis, syncope, shock, supraventricular tachycardia, vascular disorder, ventricular arrhythmia.

Digestive: colitis, dysphagia, esophageal hemorrhage, esophageal ulcer, gastritis, gastroenteritis, gastrointestinal disorder, gastrointestinal hemorrhage, hematemesis, hepatic coma, hepatic failure, hepatic neoplasia, hepatitis, hepatomegaly, ileus, intestinal obstruction, liver tenderness, pancreatitis, peptic ulcer hemorrhage, pseudomembranous colitis, rectal hemorrhage.

Endocrine: hypothyroidism.

Hematological: acute leukemia, coagulation disorder, lymphangitis, marrow depression, myeloid maturation arrest, pancytopenia.

Metabolic: bilirubinemia, growth retardation, hypercalcemia, hyponatremia, hypoglycemia, hypomagnesemia, weight loss.

Musculoskeletal: pathologic fracture, bone necrosis, myopathy.

Nervous: ataxia, CNS neoplasia, confusion, convulsion, grand mal convulsion, manic reaction, thinking abnormal.

Respiratory: apnea, asthma, hypoxia, laryngitis, lung disorder, lung edema, pleural effusion, pneumonia, pneumothorax, respiratory disorder.

Skin: herpes zoster, skin ulceration.

Special Senses: amblyopia, deafness, retinal artery occlusion.

Urogenital: breast carcinoma, breast neoplasm, cervical cancer, hematuria, hemorrhagic cystitis, hydronephrosis, kidney failure, kidney function abnormal, pyelonephritis, vaginal hemorrhage.

Post-Market Adverse Drug Reactions: The following additional serious adverse reactions have been reported in at least one patient during post marketing experience in the metastatic breast cancer setting:

Body as a Whole: infusion-related symptoms, peripheral edema, bone pain, coma, meningitis, cerebral edema, thinking abnormal.

Cardiovascular: cardiac failure, cardiogenic shock, pericarditis, hypertension.

Digestive: pancreatitis, hepatic failure, jaundice.

Heme and Lymphatic: anaemia, prothrombin decreased, febrile neutropenia, neutropenia.

Musculoskeletal: myalgia.

Renal: glomerulopathy, renal failure.

Respiratory: dyspnea, hypoxia, larynx edema, acute respiratory distress, adult respiratory distress syndrome, pleural effusion, pulmonary infiltrates, pneumonia, pneumonitis, pulmonary fibrosis.

Skin and Appendages: dermatitis, urticaria.

Special Senses: deafness.

DRUG INTERACTIONS: There have been no formal drug interaction studies performed with HERCEPTIN (trastuzumab) in humans. Strong evidence for clinically significant interactions with concomitant medications used in clinical studies has not been observed. However, administration of paclitaxel in combination with HERCEPTIN resulted in a two-fold decrease in clearance of HERCEPTIN in a non-human primate study. In one clinical study, an apparent 1.5-fold increase in serum levels of HERCEPTIN was seen when HERCEPTIN was administered with paclitaxel. However this observation was not confirmed using a population pharmacokinetic approach.

A population pharmacokinetic method using data from phase I, phase II and pivotal phase III studies, was used to estimate the steady state pharmacokinetics in patients administered trastuzumab at a loading dose of 4 mg/kg followed by a 2 mg/kg maintenance dose administered weekly. The administration of concomitant chemotherapy (either anthracycline/cyclophosphamide or paclitaxel) did not appear to influence the pharmacokinetics of trastuzumab.

Experience from phase III clinical trials suggests that there is a potential drug interaction between trastuzumab and anthracycline chemotherapy. However, the clinical pharmacokinetic profile of doxorubicin or epirubicin, in the presence of trastuzumab, has not been described to date, and the exact nature of this potential interaction has yet to be described.

DOSAGE AND ADMINISTRATION: Recommended Dose and Dosage Adjustment: Early Breast Cancer/Metastatic Gastric Cancer: 3-Weekly Schedule: The recommended initial loading dose is 8 mg/kg HERCEPTIN administered as a 90-minute infusion. The recommended maintenance dose is 6 mg/kg HERCEPTIN 3 weeks later and then 6 mg/kg repeated at 3-weekly intervals administered as infusions over approximately 90 minutes. If the prior dose was well tolerated, the dose can be administered as a 30-minute infusion. **Do not administer as an IV push or bolus** (see Preparation for Administration).

Metastatic Breast Cancer: Weekly Schedule: The recommended initial loading dose is 4 mg/kg HERCEPTIN (trastuzumab) administered as a 90-minute infusion. The recommended weekly maintenance dose is 2 mg/kg HERCEPTIN and can be administered as a 30-minute infusion if the initial loading dose was well tolerated. HERCEPTIN may be administered in an outpatient setting. **Do not administer as an IV push or bolus** (see Preparation for Administration).

Duration of Treatment: In clinical studies, patients with metastatic breast cancer or metastatic gastric cancer were treated with HERCEPTIN until progression of disease. Patients with early breast cancer should be treated for 1 year or until disease recurrence.

Dose Reduction: No reductions in the dose of HERCEPTIN were made during clinical trials. Patients may continue therapy with HERCEPTIN during periods of reversible, chemotherapy-induced myelosuppression, but they should be monitored carefully for complications of neutropenia during this time. The specific instructions to reduce or hold the dose of chemotherapy should be followed.

Missed Dose: Weekly Schedule: If the patient misses a dose of HERCEPTIN by one week or less, then the usual dose of trastuzumab (2 mg/kg) should be given as soon as possible (do not wait until the next planned cycle). Subsequent maintenance HERCEPTIN doses of 2 mg/kg should then be given every week, according to the previous schedule.

If the patient misses a dose of HERCEPTIN by more than one week, a re-loading dose of HERCEPTIN should be given (4 mg/kg over approximately 90 minutes). Subsequent maintenance HERCEPTIN doses of 2 mg/kg should then be given every week from that point.

3-Weekly Schedule: If the patient misses a dose of HERCEPTIN by one week or less, then the usual dose of trastuzumab (6 mg/kg) should be given as soon as possible (do not wait until the next planned cycle). Subsequent maintenance HERCEPTIN doses of 6 mg/kg should then be given every 3 weeks, according to the previous schedule.

If the patient misses a dose of HERCEPTIN by more than one week, a re-loading dose of HERCEPTIN should be given (8 mg/kg over approximately 90 minutes). Subsequent maintenance HERCEPTIN doses of 6 mg/kg should then be given every 3 weeks from that point.

Preparation for Administration: Use appropriate aseptic technique. Each vial of HERCEPTIN should be reconstituted with 20 mL of BWFI, containing 1.1% benzyl alcohol, as supplied, to yield a multi-dose solution containing 21 mg/mL trastuzumab. Immediately upon reconstitution with BWFI, the vial of HERCEPTIN must be labelled in the area marked "Do not use after:" with the future date that is 28 days from the date of reconstitution.

If the patient has a known hypersensitivity to benzyl alcohol, HERCEPTIN must be reconstituted with Sterile Water for Injection (see Warnings and Precautions). HERCEPTIN **which has been reconstituted with SWFI must be used immediately and any unused portion discarded. Use of other reconstitution diluents should be avoided.**

HERCEPTIN should be carefully handled during reconstitution. Causing excessive foaming during reconstitution or shaking the reconstituted HERCEPTIN may result in problems with the amount of HERCEPTIN that can be withdrawn from the vial.

Reconstitution:

1. Using a sterile syringe, slowly inject 20 mL of Bacteriostatic Water for Injection in the vial containing the lyophilized HERCEPTIN directing the stream into the lyophilized cake.
2. Swirl vial gently to aid reconstitution. **Do not shake.**

Slight foaming of the product upon reconstitution is not unusual. Allow the vial to stand undisturbed for approximately 5 minutes. The reconstituted HERCEPTIN results in a colorless to pale yellow transparent solution and should be essentially free of visible particles.

Determine the volume in mL of HERCEPTIN solution needed:

Weekly Schedule: based on a loading dose of 4 mg trastuzumab/kg body weight or a maintenance dose of 2 mg trastuzumab/kg body weight.

$$\textbf{Volume (mL)} = \frac{\textbf{[Body Weight (kg)} \times \textbf{Dose} \text{ (4 mg/kg for loading or 2 mg/kg for maintenance)]}}{\text{21 mg/mL (concentration of reconstituted solution)}}$$

3-Weekly Schedule: based on a loading dose of 8 mg trastuzumab/kg body weight, or a subsequent 3 weekly dose of 6 mg trastuzumab/kg body weight:

$$\textbf{Volume (mL)} = \frac{\textbf{[Body Weight (kg)} \times \textbf{Dose} \text{ (8 mg/kg for loading or 6 mg/kg for maintenance)]}}{\text{21 mg/mL (concentration of reconstituted solution)}}$$

Withdraw the appropriate volume of solution calculated from the vial and add it to an infusion bag containing 250 mL of 0.9% sodium chloride, USP. **Dextrose (5%) solution should not be used.** To mix the solution and avoid foaming, invert the bag gently. The reconstituted preparation results in a colourless to pale yellow transparent solution. Parenteral drug products should be inspected visually for particulates and discolouration prior to administration. No incompatibilities between HERCEPTIN and polyvinylchloride, polyethylene or polypropylene bags have been observed.

Administration: Weekly Schedule: Treatment may be administered in an outpatient setting by administration of a 4 mg/kg loading dose of HERCEPTIN by intravenous (IV) infusion over 90 minutes. **Do not administer as an IV push or bolus.** Patients should be observed for fever and chills or other infusion associated symptoms (see Adverse Reactions). Interruption of the infusion may help control such symptoms. The infusion may be resumed when symptoms abate.

If prior infusion was well tolerated, subsequent weekly doses of 2 mg/kg HERCEPTIN may be administered over 30 minutes. Patients should still be observed for fever and chills or other infusion-associated symptoms (see Adverse Reactions).

3-Weekly Schedule: Treatment may be administered in an outpatient setting by administration of a 8 mg/kg loading dose of HERCEPTIN by intravenous (IV) infusion over 90 minutes. **Do not administer as an IV push or bolus.** Patients should be observed for fever and chills or other infusion associated symptoms (see Adverse Reactions). Interruption of the infusion may help control such symptoms. The infusion may be resumed when symptoms abate.

If prior infusion was well tolerated, subsequent 3-weekly doses of 6 mg/kg HERCEPTIN may be administered over 30 minutes. Patients should still be observed for fever and chills or other infusion-associated symptoms (see Adverse Reactions).

HERCEPTIN should not be mixed or diluted with other drugs. Infusions of HERCEPTIN should not be administered or mixed with dextrose solutions.

Monitoring of Cardiac Function: Figure 1 describes the continuation and discontinuation of HERCEPTIN based on the LVEF assessments from the HERA trial.

OVERDOSAGE:

There is no experience with overdosage in human clinical trials. Single doses higher than 500 mg (10 mg/kg) have not been tested.

> For management of a suspected drug overdose, contact your regional Poison Control Centre. See the *CPS Directory* section for a list of Poison Control Centres.

ACTION AND CLINICAL PHARMACOLOGY: Mechanism of Action: Trastuzumab is a recombinant DNA-derived humanized monoclonal antibody that selectively targets the extracellular domain of the human epidermal growth factor receptor 2 protein (HER2). The antibody is an IgG1 that contains human framework regions with complementarity-determining regions of a murine anti-p185 HER2 antibody that binds to HER2. The HER2 (or c-erbB2) proto-oncogene or c-erbB2 encodes for a single transmembrane spanning, receptor-like protein of 185 kDa, which is structurally related to the epidermal growth factor receptor. HER2 protein overexpression is observed in 25%-30% of primary breast cancers. Studies of HER2-positivity rates in gastric cancer (GC) using immunohistochemistry (IHC) and fluorescence in situ hybridization (FISH) or chromogenic in situ hybridization (CISH) have shown that there is a broad variation of HER2-positivity ranging from 6.8% to 34.0% for IHC and 7.1% to 42.6% for FISH A consequence of HER2 gene amplification is an increase in HER2 protein expression on the surface of these tumour cells, which results in a constitutively-activated HER2 receptor. Studies indicate that patients whose tumours overexpress HER2 have a shortened disease-free survival compared to patients whose tumours do not overexpress HER2. HER2 protein overexpression can be determined using an immunohistochemistry-based assessment of fixed tumour blocks, ELISA techniques on tissue or serum samples or Fluorescence In Situ Hybridisation (FISH) technology. N.B., to date, only data derived from immunohistochemistry staining is relevant to treatment with trastuzumab (see Warnings and Precautions, Selection of Patients/Diagnostic Tests).

Figure 1: HERCEPTIN
Algorithm for Continuation and Discontinuation of HERCEPTIN Based on Interval LVEF Assessments

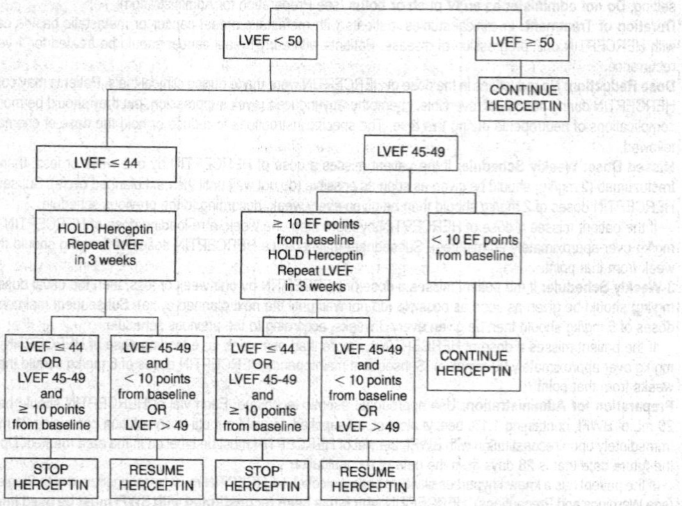

Note: LVEF assessment results must be available before/on the day of the next scheduled HERCEPTIN administrations, and a decision to give or hold that dose must be made based on this algorithm.

Trastuzumab has been shown, in both in vitro assays and in animals, to inhibit the proliferation of human tumour cells that overexpress HER2.

Trastuzumab is a mediator of antibody-dependent cell-mediated cytotoxicity (ADCC). In vitro, ADCC mediated by HERCEPTIN has been shown to be preferentially exerted on HER2 overexpressing cancer cells compared with cancer cells that do not overexpress HER2.

Pharmacokinetics: The pharmacokinetics of trastuzumab have been studied in breast cancer patients with metastatic disease. In phase I studies, short duration intravenous infusions of 10, 50, 100, 250 and 500 mg once weekly in patients demonstrated dose-dependent pharmacokinetics at doses below 100 mg. Mean half-lives increased and clearance decreased with increasing dose level. The half-life of trastuzumab averaged 1.7 and 12 days at the 10 and 500 mg dose levels, respectively.

Early Breast Cancer (EBC)/Metastatic Breast Cancer (MBC): A population pharmacokinetic method, using data from phase I, phase II and pivotal phase III studies, was used to estimate the steady state pharmacokinetics in patients administered trastuzumab at a loading dose of 4 mg/kg followed by a weekly maintenance dose of 2 mg/kg. In this assessment, the typical clearance of trastuzumab was 0.225 L/day and the typical volume of distribution was 2.95 L, with a corresponding terminal half-life of 28.5 days (95% confidence interval, 25.5-32.8 days). The inter-patient variability in clearance and volume of distribution was 43% and 29% (co-efficient of variation), respectively. These values are lower than those estimated from the base model. Steady state weekly AUC of 578 mg·day/L, peak concentrations of 110 mg/L and trough concentrations of 66 mg/L should be reached by 143 days, or approximately 20 weeks. It should be noted that these values represent free and dimer complexes of trastuzumab as the assay utilized was unable to detect the trimer complex. Trastuzumab may persist in the circulation for approximately 24 weeks (range: 22-28 weeks, based on a 6-fold terminal elimination half-life value). (See Warnings and Precautions, Cardiovascular, Cardiotoxicity.)

An assessment in early breast cancer patients administered HERCEPTIN (trastuzumab) at an initial loading dose of 8 mg/kg followed by a three weekly maintenance dose of 6 mg/kg achieved steady state trough concentrations of 63 mg/L, by cycle 13. The concentrations were comparable to those reported previously in patients with metastatic breast cancer.

Detectable concentrations of the circulating extracellular domain of the HER2 receptor (shed antigen) are found in the serum of some patients with HER2-overexpressing tumours. Patients with higher baseline shed antigen levels were more likely to have lower serum trough concentrations of trastuzumab, however, with weekly dosing, most patients with elevated shed antigen levels achieved target serum concentrations by week 6. Levels of shed antigen were only determined at baseline in the clinical trials. As a result, the available data are too limited to adequately characterize the interrelationship of HER2 overexpression and serum shed antigen concentrations.

Data suggest that the disposition of trastuzumab is not altered based on age or serum creatinine (up to 2.0 mg/dL or 176.8 µmol/L). No formal interaction studies have been performed.

Metastatic Gastric Cancer (MGC): A population pharmacokinetic method, using data from the Phase III study BO18255, was used to estimate the steady state pharmacokinetics in patients with metastatic gastric cancer administered trastuzumab 3-weekly at a loading dose of 8 mg/kg followed by a 3-weekly maintenance dose of 6 mg/kg. In this assessment, the typical clearance of trastuzumab was 0.378 L/day and the typical volume of distribution was 3.91 L, with a corresponding equilibrium half-life of 12.2 days. The median predicted steady-state AUC values (over a period of 3 weeks at steady state) is equal to 1030 mg·day/L, the median steady-state C_{max} is equal to 128 mg/L and the median steady-state C_{min} values is equal to 23 mg/L. Steady state concentrations should be reached by 49 days, (four equilibrium half lives) or approximately 7 weeks.

Trastuzumab clearance in MGC patients is higher than that in MBC patients, leading to lower AUC, C_{max} and C_{min} at steady-state.

The estimated equilibrium half-life of trastuzumab was 12.2 days in the ToGA (BO18255) trial and 26.3 days for studies BO15935 and WO16229 (in MBC). The lower value in the ToGA (BO18255) trial was due to the increase in clearance in the MGC patients.

Special Populations and Conditions: Detailed pharmacokinetic studies in the elderly and those with renal or hepatic impairment have not been carried out.

STORAGE AND STABILITY: Vials of HERCEPTIN (trastuzumab) are stable at 2-8°C prior to reconstitution. A vial of HERCEPTIN reconstituted with BWFI, containing 1.1% benzyl alcohol, as supplied, is stable for 28 days after reconstitution when stored refrigerated at 2-8°C, and the solution is preserved for multiple use. Discard any remaining multi-dose reconstituted solution after 28 days. If unpreserved SWFI (not supplied) is used, the reconstituted solution of HERCEPTIN should be used immediately and any unused portion must be discarded. **Do not freeze HERCEPTIN that has been reconstituted.**

The solution of HERCEPTIN for infusion diluted in polyvinylchloride, polyethylene or polypropylene bags containing 0.9% Sodium Chloride Injection, USP, has been shown to be stable for up to 24 hours at temperatures up to 30°C prior to use. However, since diluted HERCEPTIN contains no effective preservative, the reconstituted and diluted solution should be stored refrigerated (2-8°C). From a microbiological point of view, the infusion solution of HERCEPTIN should be used immediately. The product is not intended to be stored after dilution unless the dilution has taken place under controlled and validated aseptic conditions.

INFORMATION FOR THE PATIENT: Published in e-CPS, available by subscription at www.e-cps.ca.

DOSAGE FORMS, COMPOSITION AND PACKAGING: Each vial of a sterile, white to pale yellow lyophilized powder for i.v. administration, under vacuum, contains: trastuzumab 440 mg. Nonmedicinal ingredients: α,α-trehalose dihydrate, L-histidine HCl, L-histidine and polysorbate 20. Preservative-free. Bacteriostatic water for injection supplied as a 20 mL vial of sterile solution containing 1.1% benzyl alcohol (as antimicrobial preservative), yields 21 mL of a multi-dose solution containing 21 mg/mL of trastuzumab, at a pH of approximately 6. Cartons of 1 vial of HERCEPTIN 440 mg and 1 vial of bacteriostatic water for injection.

Hexit™ Lotion
lindane
Scabicide—Pediculicide

Odan

Hexit™ Shampoo
lindane
Scabicide—Pediculicide

Odan

SUPPLIED: Lotion: Each mL of white lotion contains: lindane USP (gamma benzene hexachloride) 1%. Nonmedicinal ingredients: butylene glycol, cetyl alcohol, dicaprylyl ether, glyceryl stearate and PEG 100 stearate, phenoxyethanol and methylparaben and ethylparaben and butylparaben and propylparaben, purified water, stearic acid, xanthan gum and triethanolamine. Plastic bottles of 50 and 500 mL with childproof safety caps. Keep away from heat and light. Store between 15 and 30°C. Protect from freezing.

Shampoo: Each mL of shampoo contains: lindane USP (gamma benzene hexachloride) 1% in a nonmedicinally scented, sudsing shampoo base. Nonmedicinal ingredients: acetone, citric acid, cocamide DEA, glycol distearate and sodium laureth sulfate and cocamide MEA and laureth-10, diazolidinyl urea, hydroxypropyl methylcellulose, methylparaben, perfume, polysorbate 60, propylparaben and purified water. Amber glass bottles of 50 and 250 mL with childproof safety caps. Store between 15 and 30°C.

HMG-CoA Reductase Inhibitors ℞
atorvastatin calcium
fluvastatin sodium
lovastatin
pravastatin sodium
rosuvastatin calcium
simvastatin

Statins—Lipid Metabolism Regulator

CPhA Monograph

Date of Preparation: January 2003
Date of Revision: May 2010

This monograph has been compiled by CPhA and reviewed by experts. It may contain information different from that found in Health Canada-approved Product Monographs. The reader is referred to the *CPS* Editorial Policy for more information.

SUMMARY PRODUCT INFORMATION:

Drug	Route of Administration	Dosage Form	Strength
Atorvastatin	Oral	Tablet	10 mg, 20 mg, 40 mg, 80 mg
Fluvastatin	Oral	Capsule	20 mg, 40 mg
		Tablet	80 mg extended release
Lovastatin	Oral	Tablet	20 mg, 40 mg
Pravastatin	Oral	Tablet	10 mg, 20 mg, 40 mg
Rosuvastatin	Oral	Tablet	5 mg, 10 mg, 20 mg, 40 mg
Simvastatin	Oral	Tablet	5 mg, 10 mg, 20 mg, 40 mg, 80 mg

ACTION AND CLINICAL PHARMACOLOGY: The first 3-hydroxy-3-methylglutaryl coenzyme A (HMG-CoA) reductase inhibitor (statin), was isolated from cultures of Penicillium species and was known initially as compactin, then as mevastatin. The first agent used clinically was lovastatin, isolated from *A. terreus* cultures and differing from mevastatin only in the presence of a methyl group. Pravastatin is derived from *P. citrium*; simvastatin is produced synthetically from a fermentation product of *A. terreus*. Atorvastatin, fluvastatin and rosuvastatin are completely synthetic.

Statins block hepatic synthesis of cholesterol by inhibiting HMG-CoA reductase-mediated conversion of HMG-CoA to mevalonic acid, an early precursor of cholesterol. This leads to a compensatory increase in the number of low-density lipoprotein (LDL) receptors, principally in the liver, that play a role in clearance of LDL from plasma and reduction of VLDL assembly and secretion, leading to a reduction in LDL production. Statins have a modest effect on elevated triglyceride levels and in raising high-density lipoprotein (HDL) levels, but their most pronounced effect is in lowering LDL. Effects on LDL and HDL vary among the different statins (see Dosage and Administration, Table 4).

The causal association between elevated LDL levels and cardiovascular risk is well established. Reducing elevated LDL levels has been shown to reduce the incidence of cardiovascular events, including transient ischemic attacks and stroke, and to reduce all-cause mortality. It is generally agreed that these benefits are conferred regardless of age or gender and in patients with or without pre-existing coronary artery disease (CAD), although the greatest benefit is seen with individuals at higher risk.

Pharmacokinetics: On first pass through the liver following absorption from the gastrointestinal tract, statins inhibit HMG-CoA reductase and are extensively metabolized. Most are transformed by the cytochrome P450 system to active and/or inactive metabolites. The amount reaching the systemic circulation is generally low and most statins are highly protein bound. Statins and their metabolites are eliminated mainly by biliary excretion (in the feces) and to a much lesser extent by the kidneys. Statins should not be used in patients with active liver disease (see Contraindications). In renal insufficiency, dosage adjustment is generally not required, although some manufacturers recommend starting with the lowest dose as a precaution in patients with severe renal disease.

Table 1 lists various pharmacokinetic properties of the statins. For information on the significance of these properties with respect to the potential for drug interactions and adverse effects, see Drug Interactions.

INDICATIONS AND CLINICAL USE: The specific Health Canada-approved indications vary between the HMG-CoA reductase inhibitors available. However, in general indications relate to control of lipid abnormalities and cardiovascular risk including:

- adjunct to diet and lifestyle changes for the reduction of elevated total cholesterol (TC), LDL-cholesterol, triglycerides and apolipoprotein B (apo B) where the response to diet and other nonpharmacologic measures is inadequate in patients with:
  - primary hypercholesterolemia (Type IIa)
  - combined (mixed) hyperlipidemia (Type IIb)
  - dysbetalipoproteinemia (Type III)

- hypertriglyceridemia (Type IV)
- familial hypercholesterolemia
- boys and postmenarchal girls aged 10 to 17 years for treatment of heterozygous familial hypercholesterolemia (atorvastatin and rosuvastatin).
- reducing the risk of myocardial infarction, ischemic stroke and death in patients with known coronary heart disease
- reducing the risk of myocardial infarction and ischemic stroke in patients without clinically evident coronary heart disease, but two or more risk factors (e.g., age, diabetes, hypertension).

Table 1: HMG-CoA Reductase Inhibitors

Pharmacokinetics

	Statin					
	Atorvastatin	Fluvastatin	Lovastatin	Pravastatin	Rosuvastatin	Simvastatin
First-pass Hepatic Extraction (%)	40 to 70	40 to 70	40 to 70	50 to 70		50 to 80
Systemic Bioavailability (%)	14	24	<5	17	20	<5
Known Metabolizing Enzyme(s)	CYP3A4	CYP2C9, 2C8, 3A4	CYP3A4	Not known[a]	CYP2C9	CYP3A4
Active Metabolites	Yes	No[b]	Yes	Yes	Yes	Yes
Protein Binding (%)	98	98	>95	50	90	95
Half-life (hours)	13 to 16	0.5 to 3	3 to 4	1.8	19	3
Renal Excretion (%)	<2	<6	<10	20	10	13

[a] Pravastatin is not extensively metabolized by the cytochrome P450 system. Its precise metabolic pathway is not known.
[b] Active metabolites formed but do not reach systemic circulation.

CONTRAINDICATIONS:
- Patients who are hypersensitive to statins or to any ingredient in the formulation or component of the container.
- Patients with active liver disease or persistent unexplained elevations in serum transaminases greater than 3 times the upper limit of normal.
- Patients who are pregnant or breastfeeding.

WARNINGS AND PRECAUTIONS: General: Statins should be used in conjunction with appropriate dietary, exercise, weight control and other lifestyle measures aimed at achieving target cholesterol levels. Prior to initiating statin therapy, patients should be thoroughly assessed to identify underlying conditions that might be contributing to the lipid abnormality such as poorly controlled diabetes mellitus, hypothyroidism, liver disease and nephrotic syndrome.

Hepatic: Statins have been associated with elevated transaminases in approximately 1% to 2% of recipients, usually occurring 3 to 12 months after initiation of treatment. It is recommended that liver function tests be performed at baseline, after 3, 6 and 12 months of therapy and then yearly, in all patients. If transaminase levels rise to 3 times the upper limit of normal and are sustained, the statin should be discontinued. Transaminase levels should slowly return to pretreatment levels after discontinuation. Statins should be used with caution in patients who regularly consume large quantities of alcohol and/or have a history of liver disease.

Musculoskeletal: Transient elevations in creatine phosphokinase (CK) are commonly seen in patients treated with statins. Usually, this is of no clinical consequence. Rarely, statin use has been associated with myopathy, characterized by muscle pain and weakness and grossly elevated CK levels (>10 times the upper limit of normal). Rhabdomyolysis defined as skeletal muscle necrosis with release of potentially toxic muscle cell components into the general circulation, has occurred rarely. Possible complications of rhabdomyolysis include myoglobinuric acute renal failure, disseminated intravascular coagulation, hyperkalemia and cardiac arrest.

The incidence of myopathy with the use of a statin alone is reported to be 0.1 to 0.2%. The risk of myopathy or rhabdomyolysis is increased by higher statin plasma levels (e.g., higher doses, decreased hepatic clearance) and by concomitant drug therapy that inhibits statin metabolism or has its own intrinsic ability to cause myopathy (see Drug Interactions).

Because statins can cause myopathy or rhabdomyolysis, especially in combination with certain drugs, patients should be advised to promptly report any unexplained muscle tenderness, pain or weakness to their physician and to inform their health care providers that they are taking a statin (see Drug Interactions).

Respiratory: There are case reports which suggest statins may rarely be associated with interstitial lung disease [*Chest* 2008;134(4):824-30]. The mechanism of this reaction is not known. Symptoms which could indicate this complication include dyspnea, nonproductive cough and deterioration in general health (e.g., fatigue, weight loss and fever).

Special Populations: Pregnant Women: There is limited experience with statin use in pregnant women and no proven association with an increased incidence of congenital anomalies. However, statins are generally contraindicated in pregnancy because cholesterol synthesis is thought to be essential for normal fetal development. Management of dyslipidemia is a chronic process, such that discontinuation of the statin during pregnancy poses no immediate risk to the mother. Appropriate dietary measures are used to manage dyslipidemia during pregnancy.

Breastfeeding Women: It is not known to what extent each statin is excreted in breast milk, but because of the theoretical potential for harmful effects from inhibiting cholesterol synthesis in neonates, statin use is not recommended in breastfeeding women.

Pediatrics: Statins reduced LDL-C levels and were generally well tolerated in clinical trials conducted in children.

Geriatrics: Elderly patients benefit from statin therapy similarly to younger patients and do not experience higher incidence of adverse effects. Dosage reduction based on advanced age alone is generally not required, although some manufacturers recommend starting with a lower initial dose as a precaution.

DRUG INTERACTIONS: Individual statins have been involved in drug interactions that have produced serious adverse effects, involving mainly skeletal muscle damage and its possible complications (e.g., myopathy, rhabdomyolysis; see Warnings and Precautions). Some cases have involved additive effects with other drugs that have an inherent potential to cause muscle damage (e.g., fibrates) and others have been associated with higher plasma levels of the statin because of a pharmacokinetic interaction resulting in inhibition of the statin's metabolism (e.g., protease inhibitors, particularly ritonavir) (see Table 2).

Pravastatin is not extensively metabolized by the cytochrome P450 enzyme system and is not expected to significantly interact with substrates, inhibitors or inducers of these enzymes. To date, this has been the case in clinical practice. However, caution should be exercised when pravastatin is used in conjunction with these drugs (see Table 2).

Because the theoretical potential for drugs to interact may or may not translate into clinically significant interactions, health care providers should exercise prudent judgement in managing the drug therapy of patients with dyslipidemias. Careful monitoring for early signs of muscle damage (e.g., otherwise unexplained weakness, tenderness or pain) is important for all patients taking statins.

Pharmacokinetic Interactions: The pharmacokinetic differences among the statins, particularly their principal metabolizing cytochrome P450 isoenzyme, play an important role in their potential to interact with specific other drugs. Pharmacokinetic interactions can involve displacement from protein binding sites, competition among multiple substrates for the same hepatic enzyme, or inhibition or induction of one drug's metabolism by another (see Table 2).

Drug-Food Interactions: As a potent inhibitor of intestinal CYP3A4, grapefruit juice can significantly increase the bioavailability of statins that are metabolized by this enzyme. The duration of enzyme inhibition is thought to be as long as 24 hours. Patients taking atorvastatin, lovastatin or simvastatin should avoid grapefruit juice. Patients who take one of these statins and consume grapefruit juice should be advised about the increased potential for adverse drug effects including myotoxicity and to monitor closely for them. Another option is to switch to a statin that is not metabolized by CYP3A4 (i.e., pravastatin). For more information on grapefruit juice interactions, see Drug Administration and Grapefruit Juice in the Clin-Info Section.

Table 2: HMG-CoA Reductase Inhibitors

Drug-Drug Interactions

Interacting Drug	Effect	Clinical Comment
Bile acid sequestrants (e.g., cholestyramine, colestipol)	Concurrent use may decrease bioavailability of statins, possibly due to adsorption of statins in the GI tract, resulting in decreased therapeutic effect.	Separate doses to minimize interaction. Administer bile acid sequestrants 1 hour before or 4–6 hours after statin, e.g., if using bile acid sequestrant before supper and statin at bedtime.
CYP3A4 inhibitors and substrates (e.g., amiodarone, clarithromycin, cyclosporine, diltiazem, erythromycin, grapefruit juice, itraconazole, ketoconazole, protease inhibitors)	Increased plasma concentrations of atorvastatin, lovastatin and simvastatin due to decreased metabolism resulting in myopathy with or without rhabdomyolysis.	In certain situations, it may be advisable to discontinue statin therapy during CYP3A4 substrate or inhibitor therapy. Statins not metabolized by CYP3A4 (i.e., pravastatin) could be used as alternative agents. If used concurrently, monitor for side effects such as unexplained muscle pain, muscle weakness and darkened urine.
CYP2C9 substrates (e.g., NSAIDs, phenytoin, warfarin)	Increased plasma concentrations of CYP2C9 substrates with concurrent use of fluvastatin, a CYP2C9 substrate and inhibitor. Reports of decreased plasma concentrations of atorvastatin and simvastatin with concurrent phenytoin use, possibly due to increased statin metabolism.	Monitor for increased pharmacologic and adverse effects of CYP2C9 substrates and adjust dose accordingly. Decreased therapeutic effects of statins.
Fibric acid derivatives (e.g., bezafibrate, fenofibrate, gemfibrozil)	Concurrent use may result in myopathy with or without rhabdomyolysis. Additive pharmacodynamic interaction between two drugs that possess inherent myotoxic potential.	Avoid combination when possible; however, benefit of additive lipid-lowering effects with combination may outweigh the risk in certain patient subgroups. Monitor for signs of muscle damage if used concurrently with statins. Educate patients to recognize symptoms of myopathy.
Niacin	Case reports of myopathy with or without rhabdomyolysis in patients taking niacin and lovastatin concurrently.	Monitor for side effects such as unexplained muscle pain, muscle weakness and darkened urine.
Rifampin	Decreased plasma levels of statins secondary to induction of CYP2C9 and CYP3A4.	Monitor therapeutic effect and clinical response in patient. Pravastatin could be used as an alternative.
Warfarin	Reports of increased hypoprothrombinemic response with fluvastatin, lovastatin, rosuvastatin and simvastatin. Inhibition of warfarin hepatic metabolism may result in increased anticoagulant effect and therefore increased risk of bleeding.	Close monitoring of INR is advised upon initiation, discontinuation or change in dose of statin.

In general, administration of statins with food does not affect their lipid-lowering effects. Most can be taken with or without a meal. Lovastatin, however, is better absorbed when taken with a meal.

ADVERSE REACTIONS: The most serious adverse effects of statins are myopathy/rhabdomyolysis, elevated hepatic enzymes and interstitial lung disease (see Warnings and Precautions).

Other adverse effects are generally mild and transient and seldom necessitate discontinuation of therapy. With few exceptions, the incidence of these less serious side effects has been similar among placebo groups and the different statins. Not every side effect has been reported with every agent. Table 3 lists the average incidences of the less serious side effects of statins.

Table 3: HMG-CoA Reductase Inhibitors

Adverse Reactions

Adverse Effect	Average Incidence Among Statins (%)
Gastrointestinal	
Abdominal Pain/Cramps	3.3
Constipation	2.7
Diarrhea	4.5
Dry Mouth	0.8
Flatulence	3.0
Heartburn	2.2
Nausea/Vomiting	3.3
Taste Perversion	0.8
CNS	
Dizziness	2.3
Headache	7.7
Insomnia	1.9
Paresthesia	1.0
Dermatologic	

(cont'd)

Table 3: HMG-CoA Reductase Inhibitors *(cont'd)*

Adverse Reactions

Adverse Effect	Average Incidence Among Statins (%)
Rash/Pruritus	3.0

OVERDOSAGE:

For management of a suspected drug overdose, CPhA recommends that you contact your **regional Poison Control Centre**. See the *CPS* Directory section for a list of Poison Control Centres.

DOSAGE AND ADMINISTRATION: Specific recommendations for the diagnosis and treatment of dyslipidemia and prevention of cardiovascular disease have been issued by the Canadian Cardiovascular Society [*Can J Cardiol* 2009;25(10):567-79]. The decision to start treatment is based on an assessment of the 10-year risk of coronary artery disease (CAD)-related death or non-fatal MI (an on-line calculator is available from: hp2010.nhlbihin.net/atpiii/calculator.asp?usertype=prof).

All patients at high risk (10-year risk of CAD ≥20%) are candidates for treatment. This category includes any patient with a diagnosis of CAD, peripheral artery disease or cerebrovascular disease, and most patients with type 1 or type 2 diabetes mellitus or chronic kidney disease. The primary target of therapy in patients at high risk is an LDL-C of <2 mmol/L or a 50% reduction in LDL-C.

Patients with a moderate 10-year risk of CAD (10-19% probability of CAD-related death or non-fatal MI) should be treated if their LDL-C level is >3.5 mmol/L or their TC/HDL-C ratio is ≥5.0. Those with a low 10-year risk (<10%) should be treated if their LDL-C level is >5.0 mmol/L or their TC/HDL-C ratio is ≥6.0

Statins should be used in conjunction with other appropriate lifestyle modifications such as diet (see Action and Clinical Pharmacology). The dose of the statin should be based mainly on target lipid levels. Generally, the lowest dose that produces and maintains the desired levels should be used.

Factors such as alcohol intake and concurrent drug therapy may influence the initial dose. When a statin is initiated, other drug therapy should be carefully evaluated to identify potential interactions and/or necessary dosing implications (see Drug Interactions). Advanced age is generally not a factor in determining initial doses of statins, although some manufacturers recommend starting with a lower initial dose as a precaution.

Statins are usually taken in one daily dose. Taking the dose in the evening may be preferred since cholesterol synthesis peaks in the early morning hours. Lovastatin is better absorbed in the presence of food and is recommended to be taken with meals. The other statins can be taken without regard to meals. Consumption of grapefruit juice should be avoided in patients taking statins metabolized by CYP3A4 (see Drug Interactions, Drug-Food Interactions).

Maximum therapeutic benefit is usually seen after 4 weeks of therapy at a given dose and is maintained during chronic therapy. Therefore, lipid level determinations and any necessary dosage adjustments should be made at intervals of no less than 4 weeks.

With respect to efficacy, the percentage reduction of elevated LDL and increase in HDL varies among the statins and is dose-related. Atorvastatin appears to have a greater effect on reducing elevated triglycerides than the other agents. Table 4 lists the dosage range for each statin and its effect on lipid levels, pooled from clinical trials to date.

Table 4: HMG-CoA Reductase Inhibitors

Adult Dosage and Effect on Lipids

Drug	Dose per Day[a]	LDL	HDL	Triglycerides
Atorvastatin	10 to 80 mg at any time	−39 to 60%	+5 to 9%	−19 to 52%
Fluvastatin	20[b] to 80 mg[c] with evening meal	−19 to 35%	+2 to 7%	−5 to 11%
Lovastatin	20 to 80 mg[d] with evening meal	−24 to 40%	+7 to 10%	−10 to 16%
Pravastatin	10[e] to 40 mg HS	−22 to 34%	+7 to 12%	−11 to 24%
Rosuvastatin	5[f] to 40 mg at any time	−52 to 63%	+8 to 14%	−10 to 28%
Simvastatin	10 to 80 mg with evening meal	−24 to 47%	+8 to 12%	−10 to 36%

[a] The lower number in the range is the usual starting dose. The higher number represents the maximum daily dose.
[b] The usual starting dose of fluvastatin is 20 to 40 mg daily.
[c] A daily dose of fluvastatin 80 mg should be given in 2 divided doses.
[d] A daily dose of lovastatin 80 mg can be given at once with supper or in 2 divided doses, with breakfast and supper.
[e] The usual starting dose of pravastatin is 10 to 20 mg daily.
[f] In Asian patients and in those with severe renal impairment, the initial dose of 5 mg daily is recommended.

Pediatrics: The recommended initial dose of atorvastatin is 10 mg/day and the maximum dose is 20 mg/day for boys and post-menarchal girls aged 10 to 17 years with heterozygous familial hypercholesterolemia. For rosuvastatin the recommended initial dose is 5 mg/day and the maximum dose is 10 mg/day.

Homatropine Hydrobromide

homatropine HBr

Mydriatic—Cycloplegic—Anticholinergic

CPhA Monograph

Date of Revision: April 2009

This monograph has been compiled by CPhA and reviewed by experts. It may contain information different from that found in Health Canada-approved Product Monographs. The reader is referred to the *CPS* Editorial Policy for more information.

SUMMARY PRODUCT INFORMATION:

Route of Administration	Dosage Form	Strength
Ophthalmic	Drops	2%, 5%

PHARMACOLOGY: Homatropine is a tertiary amine anticholinergic agent used topically to produce mydriasis and cycloplegia. It blocks the responses of the iris sphincter and ciliary muscle to cholinergic stimuli. Homatropine is less potent than atropine and has a shorter duration of action. Complete cycloplegia is not usually attainable. The maximum mydriatic effect occurs in about 10 to 30 minutes, and the maximum cycloplegic effect in about 30 to 90 minutes. Mydriasis may last 6 hours to 4 days and cycloplegia may persist 10 to 48 hours.

INDICATIONS: Homatropine is used to produce mydriasis and cycloplegia for refraction and in the treatment of acute inflammatory conditions of the uveal tract.

CONTRAINDICATIONS: Patients with primary glaucoma or a predisposition to glaucoma; patients whose intraocular pressures are unknown; patients with narrow angle or shallow anterior chambers because they are susceptible to acute angle-closure glaucoma; hypersensitivity to homatropine or any ingredient in the formulation.

PRECAUTIONS: Frequent, prolonged or excessive use of ophthalmic homatropine may cause systemic anticholinergic effects such as dry mouth, blurred vision, photophobia, tachycardia, headache, visual hallucinations and somnolence.

Children: Infants, young children and elderly patients may be more susceptible to the systemic effects of homatropine.

ADVERSE EFFECTS: Local effects can include increased intraocular pressure and transient burning or stinging. Prolonged use can be associated with allergic lid reactions, follicular conjunctivitis, vascular congestion, edema, exudate or eczematoid dermatitis.

For systemic effects, see Precautions.

OVERDOSE:

For management of a suspected drug overdose, CPhA recommends that you contact your **regional Poison Control Centre**. See the *CPS* Directory section for a list of Poison Control Centres.

DOSAGE: To minimize systemic absorption, finger pressure should be applied to the lacrimal sac for 1 to 2 minutes after instillation of drops. To produce mydriasis and cycloplegia for diagnostic purposes: Adults: Instil 1 drop of 2% or 5% solution in the eye(s) immediately prior to procedure; may be repeated at 5- to 10-minute intervals as needed.

Children: 1 drop of 2% solution instilled in the eye(s) immediately prior to procedure; may be repeated at 10-minute intervals as needed.

Treatment of Inflammatory Conditions of the Uveal Tract: Adults: 1 drop of 2% or 5% solution instilled in the eye(s) 2 or 3 times daily.

Children: 1 drop of 2% solution 2 or 3 times daily.

Hp-PAC® Ⓟ

lansoprazole—clarithromycin—amoxicillin trihydrate

H. pylori Eradication Therapy

Takeda

Date of Preparation: July 24, 1998
Date of Revision: September 25, 2008

Note: These products are intended only for use as described. The individual products contained in the Hp-PAC should not be used alone or in combination for other purposes. The information described in this product monograph concerns only the use of these products as indicated in this daily administration pack. For information on the use of the individual components when dispensed as individual medications outside this combined use for the eradication of *Helicobacter pylori* (*H. pylori*), the respective product monographs for these products should be consulted.

SUMMARY PRODUCT INFORMATION:

Route of Administration	Dosage Form/ Strength	Clinically Relevant Nonmedicinal Ingredients
Oral	Lansoprazole delayed-release capsules/30 mg	Cellulosic polymers, colloidal silicon dioxide, D&C Red No. 28, FD&C Blue No. 1, FD&C Red No. 40, gelatin, magnesium carbonate, methacrylic acid copolymer, starch, talc, sugar spheres, sucrose, polyethylene glycol, polysorbate 80, and titanium dioxide
	Clarithromycin film-coated tablets/500 mg	Cellulosic polymers, croscarmellose sodium, D&C Yellow No. 10, magnesium stearate, povidone, propylene glycol, silicon dioxide, sorbic acid, sorbitan monooleate, stearic acid, talc, titanium dioxide and vanillin
	Amoxicillin capsules/500 mg	Colloidal silicon dioxide, D&C Yellow No. 10, dry-flo starch, FD&C Blue No. 1, FD&C Red No. 3, FD&C Red No. 40, FD&C Yellow No. 6, gelatin, magnesium stearate, sodium lauryl sulfate, talc and titanium dioxide
		This is a complete listing of nonmedicinal ingredients.

INDICATIONS AND CLINICAL USE: The components of the Hp-PAC [PREVACID (lansoprazole delayed-release capsules)], in combination with clarithromycin film-coated tablets plus amoxicillin capsules as triple therapy, are indicated for:

- the treatment of patients with *Helicobacter pylori* (*H. pylori*) infection and active duodenal ulcer disease. Eradication of *H. pylori* has been shown to reduce the risk of duodenal ulcer recurrence (see Dosage and Administration).

In patients with a recent history of duodenal ulcers who are *H. pylori* positive, eradication therapy may reduce the rate of recurrence of duodenal ulcers. The optimal timing for eradication therapy for such patients remains to be determined.

In patients who fail a therapy combination containing clarithromycin, susceptibility testing should be done. If resistance to clarithromycin is demonstrated or susceptibility testing is not possible, an alternative therapy combination is recommended.

Resistance to amoxicillin has not been demonstrated in clinical studies with lansoprazole delayed-release capsules and amoxicillin.

Table 1 summarizes the eradication rates for the *H. pylori* Triple Therapy treatment regimens.

Table 1: Hp-PAC

Eradication Rates for the *H. pylori* Triple Therapy Treatment Regimens

Treatment Regimen	Days/Study No.	Evaluable (Per Protocol)[a] % (n/N)	ITT (All Data)[b] % (n/N)	ITT (Worst Case)[c] % (n/N)
PREVACID 30 mg/Clarithromycin 500 mg/Amoxicillin 1 g (all b.i.d.)	14/M93-131	92 (44/48)	94 (47/50)	86 (47/55)
	14/M95-392	86 (57/66)	87 (58/67)	83 (58/70)
PREVACID 30 mg/Clarithromycin 500 mg/Amoxicillin 1 g (all b.i.d.)	10/M95-399	84 (103/123)	86 (110/128)	81 (110/135)
PREVACID 30 mg/Clarithromycin 250 mg/Amoxicillin 1 g (all b.i.d.)	7/GB 94/110	90 (103/114)	90 (104/116)	86 (104/121)

[a] Based on evaluable patients with confirmed duodenal ulcer and/or gastritis and *H. pylori* infection at baseline defined as at least 2 of 3 positive endoscopic tests from CLOtest, histology and/or culture. Patients were included in the analysis if they completed the study. Additionally, if patients dropped out of the study due to an adverse event related to the study drug, they were included in the analysis as failures of therapy.
[b] Patients were included in the analysis if they had documented *H. pylori* infection at baseline as defined above and had a confirmed duodenal ulcer.
[c] "Worst case" included patients with no available data as failures.
Patients were included in the analysis if they had documented duodenal ulcer (active) and *H. pylori* infection at baseline defined as at least 2 of 3 positive endoscopic tests from CLOtest, histology and/or culture.
Legend: ITT=intent-to-treat patients.

CONTRAINDICATIONS:

- Patients with known hypersensitivity to any component of the formulations of PREVACID, any macrolide antibiotic or any penicillin. For a complete listing, see Dosage Forms, Composition and Packaging.

- Clarithromycin is contraindicated as concurrent therapy with astemizole, terfenadine, cisapride, pimozide, ergotamine or dihydroergotamine. There have been post-marketing reports of drug interactions when clarithromycin and/or erythromycin are coadministered with cisapride, astemizole, pimozide, or terfenadine resulting in cardiac arrhythmias (QT prolongation, ventricular tachycardia, ventricular fibrillation, and torsades de pointes) most likely due to inhibition of hepatic metabolism of these drugs by erythromycin and clarithromycin. Fatalities have been reported (see Drug Interactions).
- Amoxicillin is contraindicated in cases where infectious mononucleosis is either suspected or confirmed.

For information on the use of the individual components of the Hp-PAC when dispensed as individual medications outside the combined use for the treatment of *Helicobacter pylori* (*H. pylori*), the respective Product Monographs for these products should be consulted.

WARNINGS AND PRECAUTIONS:

Serious Warnings and Precautions

- **Clarithromycin should not be used in pregnancy except where no alternative therapy is appropriate, particularly during the first 3 months of pregnancy. If pregnancy occurs while taking the drug, the patient should be apprised of the potential hazard to the fetus. Clarithromycin has demonstrated adverse effects on pregnancy outcome and/or embryo-fetal development in monkeys, mice, rats and rabbits at doses that produced plasma levels 2 to 17 times the serum levels obtained in humans treated at the maximum recommended doses (see Warnings and Precautions section in the Clarithromycin Product Monograph).**
- **Serious and occasionally fatal hypersensitivity (anaphylactic) reactions have been reported in patients on penicillin therapy. These reactions are more apt to occur in individuals with a history of penicillin hypersensitivity and/or a history of sensitivity to multiple allergens.**
- **There have been well documented reports of individuals with a history of penicillin hypersensitivity reactions who have experienced severe hypersensitivity reactions when treated with a cephalosporin. Before initiating therapy with any penicillin, careful inquiry should be made concerning previous hypersensitivity reactions to penicillins, cephalosporins, and other allergens. If an allergic reaction occurs, amoxicillin should be discontinued and the appropriate therapy instituted.**

Serious anaphylactic reactions require immediate emergency treatment with epinephrine, oxygen, corticosteroids, and airway management, including intubation, as indicated.

General: *H. pylori* Eradication and Compliance: To avoid failure of the eradication treatment with a potential for developing antimicrobial resistance and a risk of failure with subsequent therapy, patients should be instructed to follow closely the prescribed regimen.

For the eradication of *H. pylori*, amoxicillin and clarithromycin should not be administered to patients with renal impairment since the appropriate dosage in this patient population has not yet been established.

The possibility of superinfections with fungal organisms or bacterial pathogens should be kept in mind during therapy. In such cases, discontinue Hp-PAC and substitute appropriate treatment.

PREVACID (lansoprazole delayed-release capsules): Symptomatic response to therapy with lansoprazole does not preclude the presence of gastric malignancy.

BIAXIN BID (clarithromycin tablets, USP, film-coated): Clarithromycin should be administered with caution to any patient who has demonstrated some form of drug allergy, particularly to structurally related-drugs. If an allergic reaction to clarithromycin occurs, administration of the drug should be discontinued. Serious hypersensitivity reactions may require epinephrine, antihistamines, or corticosteroids.

There have been post-marketing reports of colchicine toxicity with concurrent use of clarithromycin and colchicine. In patients with impaired renal function and/or who are elderly, colchicine and clarithromycin should not be used concurrently due to the risk of colchicine toxicity. Deaths have been reported in some such patients (see Drug Interactions, Table 5, Colchicine and Adverse Reactions).

AMOXICILLIN (amoxicillin trihydrate) Capsules: Periodic assessment of renal, hepatic and hematopoietic functions should be made during prolonged therapy with Amoxicillin (amoxicillin trihydrate).

If superinfections with mycotic or bacterial pathogens occur (usually involving Aerobacter, Pseudomonas or Candida) treatment with Amoxicillin should be discontinued and appropriate therapy instituted.

Carcinogenesis and Mutagenesis: PREVACID (lansoprazole delayed-release capsules): Safety concerns of long-term treatment relate to hypergastrinemia, possible enterochromaffin-like (ECL) effect and carcinoid formation. ECL cell hyperplasia and gastric carcinoid tumours were observed in four animal studies.

In two 24-month carcinogenicity studies, Sprague-Dawley rats were treated orally with doses of 5 to 150 mg/kg/day about 1 to 40 times the exposure on a body surface (mg/m^2) basis, of a 50 kg person of average height (1.46 m^2 body surface area) given the recommended human dose of 30 mg/day (22.2 mg/m^2). Lansoprazole produced dose-related gastric entero-chromaffin-like (ECL) cell hyperplasia and ECL cell carcinoids in both male and female rats. It also increased the incidence of intestinal metaplasia of the gastric epithelium in both sexes. In male rats, lansoprazole produced a dose related increase of testicular interstitial cell adenomas. The incidence of these adenomas in rats receiving doses of 15 to 150 mg/kg/day (4 to 40 times the recommended human dose based on body surface area) exceeded the low background incidence (range=1.4 to 10%) for this strain of rats. Testicular interstitial cell adenoma also occurred in 1 of 30 rats treated with 50 mg/kg/day (13 times the recommended human dose based on body surface area) in a one-year toxicity study.

In a 24-month carcinogenicity study, CD-1 mice were treated orally with doses of 15 to 600 mg/kg/day, 2 to 80 times the recommended human dose based on body surface area. Lansoprazole produced a dose-related increased incidence of gastric ECL cell hyperplasia. Lansoprazole also induced a low, non-dose-related incidence of carcinoid tumours in the gastric mucosa in several dose groups (one female mouse in the 15 mg/kg/day group, one male mouse in the 150 mg/kg/day group, and 2 males and 1 female in the 300 mg/kg/day group). It also produced an increased incidence of liver tumours (hepatocellular adenoma plus carcinoma). The tumour incidences in male mice treated with 300 and 600 mg/kg/day (40 to 80 times the recommended human dose based on body surface area) and female mice treated with 150 to 600 mg/kg/day (20 to 80 times the recommended human dose based on body surface area) exceeded the ranges of background incidences in historical controls for this strain of mice. Lansoprazole treatment produced adenoma of rete testis in male mice receiving 75 to 600 mg/kg/day (10 to 80 times the recommended human dose based on body surface area).

Analysis of gastric biopsy specimens from patients after short-term treatment of proton pump inhibitors have not detected ECL cell effects similar to those seen in animal studies. Longer term studies in humans revealed a slight increase in the mean ECL-cell density, although there was no microscopic evidence of cell hyperplasia. Similar results were seen in the maintenance treatment studies, where patients received up to 15 months of lansoprazole therapy. Serum gastrin values increased significantly from their baseline values but reached a plateau after two months of therapy. By one month post-treatment, fasting serum gastrin values returned to lansoprazole therapy baseline. Moreover, results from gastric biopsies from short-term, long-term and maintenance treatment studies indicate that there are no clinically meaningful effects on gastric mucosa morphology among lansoprazole-treated patients.

BIAXIN BID (clarithromycin tablets, USP, film-coated): Long-term studies in animals have not been performed to evaluate the carcinogenic potential of clarithromycin.

The following in vitro mutagenicity tests have been conducted with clarithromycin: Salmonella/mammalian microsome test, bacterial induced mutation frequency test, in vitro chromosome aberration test, rat hepatocyte DNA synthesis assay, mouse lymphoma assay, mouse dominant lethal study, mouse micronucleus test. All tests had negative results except the in vitro chromosome aberration test which was weakly positive in one test and negative in another. In addition, a Bacterial Reverse-Mutation Test (Ames Test) has been performed on clarithromycin metabolites with negative results.

AMOXICILLIN (amoxicillin trihydrate) Capsules: Long-term studies in animals have not been performed to evaluate the carcinogenic potential of amoxicillin. Studies to detect mutagenic potential of amoxicillin alone have not been conducted.

Gastrointestinal: PREVACID (lansoprazole delayed-release capsules): When gastric ulcer is suspected, the possibility of malignancy should be excluded before therapy with lansoprazole delayed-release capsules is instituted as treatment with this drug may alleviate symptoms and delay diagnosis.

BIAXIN BID (clarithromycin tablets, USP, film-coated): Pseudomembranous colitis has been reported with nearly all antibacterial agents, including macrolides, and may range in severity from mild to life threatening. Therefore, it is important to consider this diagnosis in patients who present with diarrhea subsequent to the administration of antibacterial agents, including clarithromycin.

Treatment with antibacterial agents alters the normal flora of the colon and may permit overgrowth of clostridia. Studies indicate that a toxin produced by *C. difficile* is a primary cause of "antibiotic-associated colitis".

After the diagnosis of pseudomembranous colitis has been established, therapeutic measures should be initiated. Mild cases of pseudomembranous colitis usually respond to discontinuation of the drug alone. In moderate to severe cases, consideration should be given to management with fluids and electrolytes, protein supplementation, and treatment with an antibacterial drug effective against *C. difficile*.

Genitourinary: PREVACID (lansoprazole delayed-release capsules): In the 24-month toxicology study in rats, after 18 months of treatment, Leydig cell hyperplasia increased above the concurrent and historical control level at dosages of 15 mg/kg/day or higher.

Testicular interstitial cell adenoma also occurred in 1 of 30 rats treated with 50 mg/kg/day (13 times the recommended human dose based on body surface area) in a one-year toxicity study.

These changes are associated with endocrine alterations which have not been, to date, observed in humans.

Hepatic/Biliary/Pancreatic: PREVACID (lansoprazole delayed-release capsules): It is recommended that the initial dosing regimen need not be altered for patients with mild or moderate liver disease, but for patients with moderate impairment, doses higher than 30 mg per day should not be administered unless there are compelling clinical indications. Dose reduction in patients with severe hepatic disease should be considered.

BIAXIN BID (clarithromycin tablets, USP, film-coated): Refer to Warnings and Precautions, Renal.

Immune: BIAXIN BID (clarithromycin tablets, USP, film-coated): Allergic reactions (including anaphylaxis) have been reported in patients receiving clarithromycin orally.

AMOXICILLIN (amoxicillin trihydrate) Capsules: A morbilliform rash following the use of ampicillin in patients with infectious mononucleosis has been well documented and has also been reported to occur following the use of amoxicillin.

Ophthalmologic: PREVACID (lansoprazole delayed-release capsules): Retinal Atrophy: In animal studies, retinal atrophy was observed in rats dosed orally for 2 years with lansoprazole at doses of 15 mg/kg/day and above. These changes in rats are believed to be associated with the effects of taurine imbalance and phototoxicity in a susceptible animal model.

Clinical data available from long-term lansoprazole delayed-release capsules studies are not suggestive of any drug-induced eye toxicity in humans. In humans, there are presently no concerns for ocular safety with short-term lansoprazole treatment and the risks associated with long-term use for nearly five years appear to be negligible.

The finding of drug-induced retinal atrophy in the albino rat is considered to be species-specific with little relevance for humans.

Renal: PREVACID (lansoprazole delayed-release capsules): No dosage modification of lansoprazole is required in patients with renal insufficiency.

BIAXIN BID (clarithromycin tablets, USP, film-coated): Clarithromycin is principally excreted by the liver and kidney (see Dosage and Administration).

For the eradication of *H. pylori*, amoxicillin and clarithromycin should not be administered to patients with renal impairment since the appropriate dosage in this patient population has not yet been established.

AMOXICILLIN (amoxicillin trihydrate) Capsules: Because amoxicillin is excreted mostly by the kidney, the dosage for patients with renal impairment should be reduced in proportion to the degree of loss of renal function.

Sensitivity/Resistance: BIAXIN BID (clarithromycin tablets, USP, film-coated): Antibiotic Resistance in Relation to *H. pylori* Eradication: Three patients 3/82 (3.7%) who had isolates susceptible to clarithromycin pretreatment and were treated with the triple therapy regimen remained *H. pylori* positive posttreatment. None of the isolates from these three patients had susceptibility results available after treatment with triple therapy; therefore, it is unknown whether or not these patients developed resistance to clarithromycin. Sixteen percent of the patients treated with the dual therapy regimen developed clarithromycin resistance post-treatment. Therefore, development of clarithromycin resistance should be considered as a possible risk.

AMOXICILLIN (amoxicillin trihydrate) Capsules: If superinfections with mycotic or bacterial pathogens occur (usually involving Aerobacter, Pseudomonas or Candida) treatment with Amoxicillin should be discontinued and appropriate therapy instituted.

Use in Women: Over 4000 women were treated with lansoprazole. Ulcer healing rates in females are similar to those in males. The incidence rates of adverse events are also similar to those seen in males.

Special Populations: Pregnant Women: PREVACID (lansoprazole delayed-release capsules): Reproductive studies conducted in pregnant rats at oral doses up to 150 mg/kg/day (40 times the recommended human dose based on body surface area), and in rabbits at oral doses up to 30 mg/kg/day (16 times the recommended human dose based on body surface area), did not disclose any evidence of a teratogenic effect. Maternal toxicity and a significant increase in fetal mortality were observed in the rabbit study at doses above 10 mg/kg/day. In rats, maternal toxicity and a slight reduction in litter survival and weights were noted at doses above 100 mg/kg/day.

There are no adequate or well-controlled studies in pregnant women. Therefore, lansoprazole should be used during pregnancy only if the potential benefit justifies the potential risk to the fetus.

BIAXIN BID (clarithromycin tablets, USP, film-coated): There are no adequate and well-controlled studies in pregnant women. The benefits against risk, particularly during the first 3 months of pregnancy should be carefully weighed by a physician (see Warnings and Precautions). Four teratogenicity studies in rats (three with oral doses and one with intravenous doses up to 160 mg/kg/day administered during the period of major organogenesis) and two in rabbits (at oral doses up to 125 mg/kg/day or intravenous doses of 30 mg/kg/day administered during gestation days 6 to 18) failed to demonstrate any teratogenicity from clarithromycin. Two additional oral studies in a different rat strain at similar doses and similar conditions demonstrated a low incidence of cardiovascular anomalies at doses of 150 mg/kg/day administered during gestation days 6 to 15. Plasma levels after 150 mg/kg/day were 2 times the human serum levels.

Four studies in mice revealed a variable incidence of cleft palate following oral doses of 1000 mg/kg/day during gestation days 6 to 15. Cleft palate was also seen at 500 mg/kg/day. The 1000 mg/kg/day exposure resulted in plasma levels 17 times the human serum levels. In monkeys, an oral dose of 70 mg/kg/day produced fetal growth retardation at plasma levels that were 2 times the human serum levels.

Embryonic loss has been seen in monkeys and rabbits.

AMOXICILLIN (amoxicillin trihydrate) Capsules: The safety of Amoxicillin in the treatment of infections during pregnancy has not been established. If the administration of Amoxicillin to pregnant patients is considered to be necessary, its use requires that the potential benefits be weighed against the possible hazards to the fetus.

Nursing Women: PREVACID (lansoprazole delayed-release capsules): Lansoprazole or its metabolites are excreted in the milk of rats. It is not known whether lansoprazole is excreted in human milk. Because drugs are excreted in human milk, lansoprazole should not be given to nursing mothers unless its use is considered essential.

BIAXIN BID (clarithromycin tablets, USP, film-coated): The safety of clarithromycin for use during breast-feeding of infants has not been established. Clarithromycin is excreted in human milk.

Preweaned rats, exposed indirectly via consumption of milk from dams treated with 150 mg/kg/day for 3 weeks, were not adversely affected, despite data indicating higher drug levels in milk than in plasma.

Pediatrics (1 to 17 years of age): Hp-PAC—Triple Therapy: PREVACID/clarithromycin/amoxicillin: The safety and effectiveness of Hp-PAC in pediatric patients infected with *H. pylori* have not been established.

Geriatrics: Hp-PAC—Triple Therapy: PREVACID/clarithromycin/amoxicillin: Elderly patients may suffer from asymptomatic renal and hepatic dysfunction. Care should be taken when administering Hp-PAC to this patient population. (See Warnings and Precautions, Hepatic/Biliary/Pancreatic and Renal.)

PREVACID (lansoprazole delayed-release capsules): Ulcer healing rates in elderly patients are similar to those in younger age groups. The incidence rates of adverse events and laboratory test abnormalities are also similar to those seen in other age groups. The initial dosing regimen need not be altered for elderly patients, but subsequent doses higher than 30 mg per day should not be administered unless additional gastric acid suppression is necessary.

BIAXIN BID (clarithromycin tablets, USP, film-coated): Dosage adjustment should be considered in elderly patients with severe renal impairment. In a steady-state study in which healthy elderly subjects (age 65 to 81 years old) were given 500 mg every 12 hours, the maximum concentrations of clarithromycin and 14-OH clarithromycin were increased. The AUC was also increased. These changes in pharmacokinetics parallel known age-related decreases in renal function. In clinical trials, elderly patients did not have an increased incidence of adverse events when compared to younger patients.

AMOXICILLIN (amoxicillin trihydrate) Capsules: There are no known specific precautions for the use of amoxicillin in the elderly.

ADVERSE REACTIONS: Adverse Drug Reaction Overview: Hp-PAC—Triple Therapy: PREVACID/clarithromycin/amoxicillin : The most frequently reported (≥3%) adverse events for patients who received triple therapy were diarrhea (7%), headache (6%), and taste perversion (5%).

PREVACID (lansoprazole delayed-release capsules): Worldwide, over 7000 patients have been treated with PREVACID (lansoprazole) Delayed-Release Capsules during Phase II-III short-term and long-term clinical trials involving various dosages and duration of treatment. In general, lansoprazole treatment has been well tolerated.

BIAXIN BID (clarithromycin tablets, USP, film-coated): The majority of side effects observed in clinical trials involving 3563 patients treated with BIAXIN BID were of a mild and transient nature. Fewer than 3% of adult patients without mycobacterial infections discontinued therapy because of drug-related side-effects. The most common drug-related adverse reactions in adults taking BIAXIN BID were nausea, diarrhea, abdominal pain, dyspepsia, headache, taste perversion and vomiting.

Clinical Trial Adverse Drug Reactions: Because clinical trials are conducted under very specific conditions the adverse reaction rates observed in the clinical trials may not reflect the rates observed in practice and should not be compared to the rates in the clinical trials of another drug. Adverse drug reaction information from clinical trials is useful for identifying drug-related adverse events and for approximating rates.

Hp-PAC—Triple Therapy: PREVACID/clarithromycin/amoxicillin: Patients in the 7-day triple therapy regimen reported fewer adverse events than those in the 10 and/or 14-day triple therapy regimens. There were no statistically significant differences in the frequency of reported adverse events between the 10- and 14-day triple therapy regimens. No treatment-emergent adverse events were observed at significantly higher rates with triple therapy than with any dual therapy regimen.

Combination Therapy with Clarithromycin and Amoxicillin: In clinical trials using combination therapy with PREVACID plus clarithromycin and amoxicillin, no adverse reactions related to these drug combinations were observed. Adverse reactions that have occurred have been limited to those that have been previously reported with PREVACID, clarithromycin, or amoxicillin.

For more information on adverse reactions with lansoprazole, clarithromycin or amoxicillin, refer to their respective Product Monographs, under Adverse Reactions.

PREVACID (lansoprazole delayed-release capsules): The following adverse events were reported to have a possible or probable relationship to drug as described by the treating physician in 1% or more of lansoprazole delayed-release capsules-treated patients who participated in placebo- and positive-controlled trials (Table 2 and Table 3, respectively). Numbers in parentheses indicate the percentage of the adverse events reported.

Table 2: Hp-PAC

Incidence of Possibly or Probably Treatment-related Adverse Events in Short-term, Placebo-controlled Studies in Takeda[a] Safety Database

Body System/Adverse Event[b]	PREVACID[c] (N=817), N(%)	Placebo (N=254), N(%)
Body as a Whole		
Headache	63 (7.7)	31 (12.2)
Abdominal Pain	19 (2.3)	3 (1.2)
Digestive System		
Diarrhea	29 (3.5)	6 (2.4)
Nausea	9 (1.1)	5 (2.0)
Vomiting	7 (0.9)	3 (1.2)
Liver Function Tests Abnormal	2 (0.2)	3 (1.2)
Nervous System		
Dizziness	8 (1.0)	2 (0.8)

[a] Takeda Pharmaceuticals America Inc.
[b] Events reported by at least 1% of patients on either treatment are included.
[c] Doses 15 mg, 30 mg and 60 mg q.d. for 4-8 weeks.

In the Takeda Safety Database, all short-term, Phase II/III studies, one or more treatment-emergent AEs were reported by 715/1359 (52.6%) PREVACID-treated patients; of those considered to be possibly or probably treatment-related AEs, one or more were reported by 276/1359 (20.3%) PREVACID-treated patients. In all short-term, Phase II/III studies, one or more treatment-emergent AEs were reported by 150/254 (59.1%) placebo-treated patients; of those considered to be possibly or probably treatment-related AEs, one or more were reported by 56/254 (22.0%).

The most frequent AEs reported in the European short-term studies were diarrhea (3.3%), laboratory test abnormal (2.3%), headache (1.5%), constipation (1.2%), asthenia (1.1%), dizziness (1.1%), and abdominal pain (1.0%). The most frequent AEs reported in the Asian short-term studies were unspecified laboratory test abnormalities (7.3%), eosinophilia (1.0%), and increased ALT (1.0%).

Table 3: Hp-PAC

Incidence of Possibly or Probably Treatment-related Adverse Events in Short-term, Positive-controlled Studies in Takeda[a] Safety Database

Body System/Adverse Event[b]	PREVACID[c] (N=647), N(%)	Ranitidine (N=393), N(%)
Body as a Whole		
Headache	26 (4.0)	14 (3.6)
Abdominal Pain	8 (1.2)	3 (0.8)
Digestive System		
Diarrhea	27 (4.2)	8 (2.0)
Nausea	7 (1.1)	4 (1.0)
Nervous System		
Dizziness	8 (1.2)	3 (0.8)
Skin and Appendages		
Rash	7 (1.1)	1 (0.3)

[a] Takeda Pharmaceuticals America Inc.
[b] Events reported by at least 1% of patients on either treatment are included.
[c] Doses 15 mg, 30 mg and 60 mg q.d. for 4-8 weeks.

Less Common Clinical Trial Adverse Drug Reactions: Hp-PAC—Triple Therapy: PREVACID/clarithromycin/amoxicillin: The additional adverse reactions which were reported as possibly or probably related to treatment (<3%) in clinical trials when all three components of this therapy were given concomitantly are listed below and divided by body system:

Body as a Whole: abdominal pain.

Digestive System: dark stools, dry mouth/thirst, glossitis, rectal itching, nausea, oral moniliasis, stomatitis, tongue discoloration, tongue disorder, vomiting.

Musculoskeletal System: myalgia.

Nervous System: confusion, dizziness.

Respiratory System: respiratory disorders.

Skin and Appendages: skin reactions.

Urogenital System: vaginitis, vaginal moniliasis.

PREVACID (lansoprazole delayed-release capsules): Additional adverse experiences occurring in <1% of patients or subjects in domestic and/or international trials, or occurring since the drug was marketed, are shown below within each body system:

Body as a Whole: asthenia, candidiasis, chest pain (not otherwise specified), edema, fever, flu syndrome, halitosis, infection (not otherwise specified), malaise, carcinoma, general pain.

Cardiovascular System: angina, cerebrovascular accident, hypertension/hypotension, myocardial infarction, palpitations, shock (circulatory failure), vasodilation.

Digestive System: melena, cholelithiasis, abnormal stools/melena, bezoar, constipation, dry mouth/thirst, flatulence, gastroenteritis, gastrointestinal hemorrhage, hematemesis, anorexia, increased appetite, increased salivation, rectal hemorrhage, cardiospasm, dyspepsia, dysphagia, eructation, esophageal stenosis, esophageal ulcer, esophagitis, stomatitis, fecal discoloration, tenesmus, ulcerative colitis, gastric nodules/fundic gland polyps, carcinoid.

Endocrine System: diabetes mellitus, goiter, hyperglycemia/hypoglycemia.

Hematologic and Lymphatic System*: agranulocytosis, anemia, aplastic anemia, hemolysis, hemolytic anemia, leukopenia, neutropenia, pancytopenia, thrombocytopenia, and thrombotic thrombocytopenic purpura.

Metabolic and Nutritional Disorders: gout, weight gain/loss, edema.

Musculoskeletal System: arthritis/arthralgia, musculoskeletal pain, myalgia.

Nervous System: agitation, amnesia, apathy, confusion, dizziness, syncope, hallucinations, hostility aggravated, libido decreased, depression, hemiplegia, insomnia, somnolence, thinking abnormality, anxiety, nervousness, paresthesia.

Respiratory System: asthma, bronchitis, cough increased, dyspnea, hemoptysis, hiccup, upper respiratory inflammation/infection, pneumonia, epistaxis.

Skin and Appendages: acne, pruritus, rash, urticaria, alopecia.

Special Senses: blurred vision, eye pain, visual field defect, tinnitus, ophthalmologic disorders, ear disorder, deafness, otitis media, taste perversion.

Urogenital System: abnormal menses, albuminuria, breast enlargement/gynecomastia, breast tenderness, glycosuria, impotence, kidney calculus, hematuria, urinary urgency.

BIAXIN BID (clarithromycin tablets, USP, film-coated): The following adverse reactions from the clarithromycin Product Monograph are provided for information:

The majority of side effects observed in clinical trials involving 3563 patients treated with BIAXIN BID were of a mild and transient nature. Fewer than 3% of adult patients without mycobacterial infections discontinued therapy because of drug related side-effects.

The following adverse reactions were reported during these clinical studies or during post-marketing surveillance:

Body as a Whole: headache (2%), asthenia, infection, back pain, pain and chest pain.

Cardiovascular System: As with other macrolides, QT prolongation, ventricular tachycardia, and torsades de pointes have rarely been reported with clarithromycin.

Digestive System: nausea (4%), diarrhea (3%), abdominal pain (2%), dyspepsia (2%), vomiting (1%), constipation, flatulence, dry mouth, glossitis, stomatitis, gastrointestinal disorder, anorexia, oral moniliasis, tongue discoloration, hepatomegaly and pseudomembranous colitis. There have been reports of tooth discoloration in patients treated with BIAXIN BID. Tooth discoloration is usually reversible with professional dental cleaning.

As with other macrolides, hepatic dysfunction, including increased liver enzymes, and hepatocellular and/or cholestatic hepatitis, with or without jaundice, has been infrequently reported with BIAXIN BID. This hepatic dysfunction may be severe and is usually reversible. In very rare instances, hepatic failure with fatal outcome has been reported and generally has been associated with serious underlying diseases and/or concomitant medications.

Metabolic: There have been rare reports of hypoglycemia, some of which have occurred in patients on concomitant oral hypoglycemic agents or insulin.

Nervous System: dizziness, vertigo, tinnitus, nervousness, anxiety, insomnia, nightmares, somnolence, depression, confusion, disorientation, depersonalization, hallucinations and psychosis.

Respiratory System: rhinitis, cough increased, dyspnea, pharyngitis and asthma.

Skin and Appendages: pruritus, rash, sweating; allergic reactions ranging from urticaria and mild skin eruptions to anaphylaxis and Stevens-Johnson Syndrome have occurred with orally administered clarithromycin.

Special Senses: taste perversion (2%), ear disorder, abnormal vision and conjunctivitis. There have been reports of hearing loss with clarithromycin which is usually reversible upon withdrawal of therapy. Reports of alteration of the sense of smell, usually in conjunction with taste perversion or taste loss have also been reported.

Urogenital System: hematuria, vaginal moniliasis, vaginitis and dysmenorrhea.

Hemic and Lymphatic System: eosinophilia, anemia, leukopenia and thrombocythemia. Isolated cases of thrombocytopenia have been reported.

Others: Central nervous system side effects (including seizures) have been occasionally reported with erythromycin, another macrolide.

In studies of adults with pneumonia comparing clarithromycin to erythromycin base or erythromycin stearate, there were significantly fewer adverse events involving the digestive system in patients treated with clarithromycin.

AMOXICILLIN (amoxicillin trihydrate) Capsules: As with other penicillins, it may be expected that untoward reactions will be related to sensitivity phenomena. They are more likely to occur in individuals who have previously demonstrated hypersensitivity to penicillins and cephalosporins and in those with a history of allergy, asthma, hay fever or urticaria.

The following adverse reactions have been reported as associated with the use of Amoxicillin.

Gastrointestinal: nausea, vomiting and diarrhea.

Hypersensitivity Reactions: Skin rashes and urticaria have been reported frequently. A few cases of exfoliative dermatitis and erythema multiforme have been reported. Anaphylaxis is the most serious reaction experienced and has usually been associated with the parenteral dosage form.

Note: Urticaria, other skin rashes, and serum sickness-like reactions may be controlled with antihistamines and if necessary, systemic corticosteroids. Whenever such reactions occur, Amoxicillin (amoxicillin trihydrate) should be discontinued unless, in the opinion of the physician, the condition being treated is life threatening and amenable only to amoxicillin therapy. Serious anaphylactic reactions require the immediate use of epinephrine, oxygen and intravenous steroids.

Liver: A moderate rise in serum glutamic oxaloacetic transaminase (SGOT) has been noted, particularly in infants, but the significance of this finding is not known. Transient increases in serum alkaline phosphatase and lactic dehydrogenase levels have also been observed but they returned to normal on discontinuation of amoxicillin.

Hematologic and Lymphatic Systems: anemia thrombocytopenia, thrombocytopenic purpura, eosinophilia, leukopenia, neutropenia and agranulocytosis have been reported during therapy with the penicillins. These reactions are usually reversible on discontinuation of therapy and are believed to be a hypersensitivity phenomena.

Digestive System: glossitis, black "hairy" tongue and stomatitis.

Nervous System: As with other penicillins, acute and chronic toxicity is not a clinical problem. At extremely high doses, convulsions can occur. When penicillin reaches a high concentration in the cerebrospinal fluid, neurotoxic symptoms consisting of myoclonia, convulsive seizures and depressed consciousness may occur. Unless administration of the drug is stopped or its dosage reduced, the syndrome may progress to coma and death. Although penicillins do not normally cross the blood-brain barrier to any substantial extent, if massive doses are given (several grams per day) to elderly patients, patients with inflamed meninges or patients with impaired renal function, the above toxic reactions are likely to occur.

Abnormal Hematologic and Clinical Chemistry Findings: PREVACID (lansoprazole delayed-release capsules): In addition, the following changes in laboratory parameters were reported as adverse events. Abnormal liver function tests, increased AST, increased ALT, increased creatinine, increased alkaline phosphatase, increased gamma globulins, increased GGTP, increased/decreased/abnormal WBC, abnormal AG ratio, abnormal RBC, bilirubinemia, eosinophilia, hyperlipemia, increased/decreased electrolytes, increased/decreased cholesterol, increased glucocorticoids, increased LDH, increased/decreased/abnormal platelets, and increased gastrin levels. Urine abnormalities such as albuminuria, glycosuria, and hematuria were also reported. Additional isolated laboratory abnormalities were reported.

In the placebo controlled studies, when AST and ALT were evaluated, 0.4% (4/978) placebo patients and 0.3% (11/2677) lansoprazole patients had enzyme elevations greater than three times the upper limit of normal range at the final treatment visit. None of these lansoprazole patients reported jaundice at any time during the study.

For more information on laboratory value changes with clarithromycin or amoxicillin, refer to their respective Product Monographs, under the Adverse Reactions section.

BIAXIN BID (clarithromycin tablets, USP, film-coated): In addition, changes in laboratory values with possible clinical significance were as follows:

Hepatic: elevated ALT <1%, AST <1%, GGT <1%, alkaline phosphatase <1%, LDH <1% and total bilirubin <1%.

Hematologic: decreased WBC <1% and elevated prothrombin time (1%).

Renal: elevated BUN (4%) and elevated serum creatinine <1%.

Post-Market Adverse Drug Reactions: These events were reported during post-marketing surveillance. Estimates of frequency cannot be made since such events are reported voluntarily from a population of unknown size. Due to the uncontrolled nature of spontaneous reports, a clear causal relationship to lansoprazole cannot be established.

PREVACID (lansoprazole delayed-release capsules): Body as a Whole: hypersensitivity reactions, including anaphylaxis; Digestive System: colitis, hepatotoxicity, pancreatitis, vomiting; Hematologic and Lymphatic System: agranulocytosis, aplastic anemia, hemolytic anemia, leukopenia, neutropenia, pancytopenia, thrombocytopenia, and thrombotic thrombocytopenic pur-

*** The majority of hematologic cases received were foreign-sourced and their relationship to lansoprazole was unclear.**

pura; Musculoskeletal System: myositis; Skin and Appendages: severe dermatologic reactions including erythema multiforme, Stevens-Johnson syndrome, toxic epidermal necrolysis (some fatal); Special Senses: speech disorder; Urogenital System: urinary retention, interstitial nephritis.

In an estimated exposure of 240 million patients worldwide (in both postmarketing surveillance and the clinical trials), the most commonly reported ophthalmic adverse events are amblyopia (13) and vision blurred (67) according to the MedDRA terminology. All the 13 cases of amblyopia had the reported term/verbatim "blurred or smeary vision". Only two of these 13 reports were considered serious, and both are foreign-sourced reports with very little information provided. Among the 67 reports with the "vision blurred," 10 were considered serious and might be related to optic neuritis/neuropathy, whether or not believed related to the drug. In two of these ten cases, one of the examining ophthalmologists proposed a diagnosis of AION. Eight out of the ten cases were foreign-sourced. Only two US-sourced serious cases involved the report of blurred vision. Both were consumer reports without any detailed information. No physician assessed any causality in either case.

BIAXIN BID (clarithromycin tablets, USP, film-coated): The following list (see Table 4) of adverse events is a compilation of adverse reactions from Post-marketing Surveillance and Post-marketing Clinical Studies for all clarithromycin formulations.

Table 4: Hp-PAC

Clarithromycin Post-market Adverse Drug Reactions

System Organ Class	Adverse Event
Blood and Lymphatic System Disorders	Leukopenia Thrombocytopenia
Investigations	Electrocardiogram QT prolonged Ventricular tachycardia
Cardiac Disorders	Torsades de pointes
Gastrointestinal Disorders	Dyspepsia Vomiting Glossitis Stomatitis
Infections and Infestations	Candidiasis
Gastrointestinal Disorders	Tongue discolouration Tooth discolouration Pancreatitis
Hepatobiliary Disorders	Hepatic function abnormal Hepatitis Hepatitis cholestatis Hepatic failure Jaundice
Investigations	Increased liver enzymes
Metabolism and Nutrition Disorders	Hypoglycemia
Nervous System Disorders	Dizziness Vertigo Alteration of sense of smell Convulsions
Psychiatric Disorders	Anxiety Insomnia Bad dreams Confusion Disorientation Hallucination Psychosis Depersonalization
Skin and Subcutaneous Tissue Disorders	Urticaria Mild skin eruptions Stevens-Johnson syndrome Toxic epidermal necrosis
Immune System Disorders	Anaphylaxis
Ear and Labyrinth Disorders	Tinnitus Hearing loss
Renal and Urinary Disorders	Interstitial nephritis

DRUG INTERACTIONS:

Serious Drug Interactions

- Concomitant administration of clarithromycin with astemizole, cisapride, pimozide, terfenadine, ergotamine, or dihydroergotamine is contraindicated (see Contraindications and Drug Interactions).
- Clarithromycin is an inhibitor of CYP3A4. The concomitant administration of clarithromycin and drugs metabolized by this enzyme (or enzyme system) may lead to an increase in the plasma concentrations of the coadministered drug which could result in clinically significant safety concerns.

Overview: PREVACID (lansoprazole delayed-release capsules): Lansoprazole is metabolized through the cytochrome P450 system, specifically through CYP3A and CYP2C19. Studies have shown that lansoprazole does not have clinically significant interactions with other drugs metabolized by the cytochrome P450 system such as warfarin, antipyrine, indomethacin, acetylsalicylic acid, ibuprofen, phenytoin, prednisone, antacids (Maalox and Riopan), diazepam, clarithromycin, propranolol, amoxicillin or terfenadine in healthy subjects. These compounds are metabolized through various cytochrome P450 isozymes including CYP1A2, CYP2C9, CYP2C19, CYP2D6, and CYP3A.

Lansoprazole causes a profound and long lasting inhibition of gastric acid secretion; therefore, it is theoretically possible that lansoprazole may interfere with the absorption of drugs where gastric pH is an important determinant of bioavailability (e.g., ketoconazole, ampicillin esters, iron salts, digoxin). Lansoprazole substantially decreases the systemic concentrations of the HIV protease inhibitor atazanavir, which is dependent upon the presence of gastric acid for absorption, and may result in a loss of therapeutic effect of atazanavir and the development of HIV resistance. Therefore, lansoprazole should not be coadministered with atazanavir. This appears to be a class effect. It is theoretically possible that lansoprazole may also interfere with the absorption of other drugs where gastric pH is an important determinant of bioavailability (e.g., ketoconazole, ampicillin esters, iron salts, digoxin).

In a study of healthy subjects neither the pharmacokinetics of warfarin enantiomers nor prothrombin time were affected following single or multiple 60 mg doses of lansoprazole. However, there have been reports of increased International Normalized Ratio (INR) and prothrombin time in patients receiving proton pump inhibitors, including lansoprazole, and warfarin concomitantly. Increases in INR and prothrombin time may lead to abnormal bleeding and even death. Patients treated with proton pump inhibitors and warfarin concomitantly may need to be monitored for increases in INR and prothrombin time.

BIAXIN BID (clarithromycin tablets, USP, film-coated): Many categories of drugs are metabolized by the cytochrome P450 3A4 enzyme located in the liver and in the intestine. Some drugs inhibit and others induce this enzyme. Coadministration of such drugs may impact upon each other's metabolism. In some cases serum concentration may be increased and in others decreased. Care must therefore be exercised when coadministering such drugs.

Clarithromycin is reported to be an inhibitor of the enzyme P450 3A4. This may lead to increased or prolonged serum levels of those drugs also metabolized by the enzyme when coadministered with clarithromycin. For such drugs the monitoring of their serum concentrations may be necessary.

Drug-Drug Interactions: PREVACID (lansoprazole delayed-release capsules): When lansoprazole was administered concomitantly with theophylline (CYP1A2, CYP3A), a minor increase (10%) in the clearance of theophylline was seen, which is unlikely to be of clinical concern. Nonetheless, individual patients may require adjustment of their theophylline dosage when lansoprazole is started or stopped to ensure clinically effective blood levels.

In a single-dose crossover study when 30 mg of lansoprazole was administered concomitantly with one gram of sucralfate in healthy volunteers, absorption of lansoprazole was delayed and its bioavailability was reduced. The value of lansoprazole AUC was reduced by 17% and that for C_{max} was reduced by 21%.

In a similar study when 30 mg of lansoprazole was administered concomitantly with 2 grams of sucralfate, lansoprazole AUC and C_{max} were reduced by 32% and 55%, respectively. When lansoprazole dosing occurred 30 minutes prior to sucralfate administration, C_{max} was reduced by only 28% and there was no statistically significant difference in lansoprazole AUC. Therefore, lansoprazole may be given concomitantly with antacids but should be administered at least 30 minutes prior to sucralfate.

BIAXIN BID (clarithromycin tablets, USP, film-coated): Some of the drug-drug interactions which have been reported between clarithromycin-macrolides and other drugs or drug categories are listed in Table 5. Like clarithromycin and omeprazole, most of the following drugs are metabolized by the P450 3A4 enzyme system.

Additional mechanisms, such as effects upon absorption, may also be responsible for interaction between drugs, including digoxin and clarithromycin.

The drugs listed in this table are based on either drug interactions case reports, clinical trials, or potential interactions due to the expected mechanism of the interaction.

Table 5: Hp-PAC

Established or Potential Drug-Drug Interactions

Clarithromycin	Ref.	Effect	Clinical Comments
Astemizole/Terfenadine	CT	terfenadine-acid metabolite concentrations increase	Macrolides have been reported to alter the metabolism of terfenadine resulting in increased serum levels of terfenadine which has occasionally been associated with cardiac arrhythmias such as QT prolongation, ventricular tachycardia, ventricular fibrillation and torsades de pointes (see Contraindications).
		↑ QT interval	In a study involving 14 healthy volunteers, the concomitant administration of BIAXIN BID tablets and terfenadine resulted in a two to three-fold increase in the serum levels of the acid metabolite of terfenadine, MDL 16, 455, and in prolongation of the QT interval. Similar effects have been observed with concomitant administration of astemizole and other macrolides.
Carbamazepine	C	↑ levels of carbamazepine	Clarithromycin administration in patients receiving carbamazepine has been reported to cause increased levels of carbamazepine. Blood level monitoring of carbamazepine may be considered.
Cisapride/Pimozide	C	↑ levels of cisapride ↑ levels of pimozide	Elevated cisapride levels have been reported in patients receiving clarithromycin and cisapride concomitantly. This may result in QT prolongation and cardiac arrhythmias including ventricular tachycardia, ventricular fibrillation and torsades de pointes. Similar effects have been observed in patients taking clarithromycin and pimozide concomitantly (see Contraindications).
Colchicine	C	Potential colchicines toxicity	Colchicine is a substrate for both CYP3A and the efflux transporter, P-glycoprotein (Pgp). Clarithromycin and other macrolides are known to inhibit CYP3A and Pgp. When clarithromycin and colchicine are administered together, inhibition of Pgp and/or CYP3A by clarithromycin may lead to increased exposure to colchicine. Patients should be monitored for clinical symptoms of colchicine toxicity (see Warnings and Precautions, General and Adverse Reactions).
Cyclosporine	C	↑ levels of cyclosporine	There have been reports of elevated cyclosporine serum concentrations when clarithromycin and cyclosporine are used concurrently. Cyclosporine levels should be monitored and the dosage should be adjusted as necessary. Patients should also be monitored for increased cyclosporine toxicity.
Didanosine	CT	No change in didanosine pharmacokinetics in HIV-infected patients (n=12)	Simultaneous administration of BIAXIN BID tablets and didanosine to 12 HIV-infected adult patients resulted in no statistically significant change in didanosine pharmacokinetics.
Digoxin	C	↑ levels of digoxin	Elevated digoxin serum concentrations have been reported in patients receiving BIAXIN BID tablets and digoxin concomitantly. In post-marketing surveillance some patients have shown clinical signs consistent with digoxin toxicity, including arrhythmias. Serum digoxin levels should be carefully monitored while patients are receiving digoxin and clarithromycin simultaneously.
Disopyramide/Quinidine	C	↑ levels of disopyramide, resulting ventr. Fibrillation & QT prolongation (rarely reported)	Increased disopyramide plasma levels, resulting in ventricular fibrillation and QT prolongation, coincident with the coadministration of disopyramide and clarithromycin has rarely been reported.
		Torsades de pointes	There have been post-marketed reports of torsades de pointes occurring with concurrent use of clarithromycin and quinidine or disopyramide. Serum levels of these medications should be monitored during clarithromycin therapy.

(cont'd)

Table 5: Hp-PAC (cont'd)
Established or Potential Drug-Drug Interactions

Clarithromycin	Ref.	Effect	Clinical Comments
Ergotamine/ Dihydroergotamine	C	Potential ischemic reactions Potential ergot toxicity	There are reports that ischemic reactions may occur when clarithromycin is given concurrently with ergotamine-containing drugs. Concurrent use of clarithromycin and ergot alkaloids has been associated in some patients with acute ergot toxicity characterized by severe peripheral vasospasm and dysesthesia (see Contraindications).
Fluconazole	CT	↑ clarithromycin C_{min} & AUC	Concomitant administration of fluconazole 200 mg daily and clarithromycin 500 mg twice daily to 21 healthy volunteers led to increases in the mean steady-state clarithromycin C_{min} and AUC of 33% and 18%, respectively. Steady-state concentrations of 14-OH clarithromycin were not significantly affected by concomitant administration of fluconazole.
Lansoprazole/ Omeprazole	CT	Mild change of lansoprazole and 14-OH clarithromycin concentrations	One study demonstrated that concomitant administration of clarithromycin and lansoprazole resulted in mild changes of serum concentrations of lansoprazole and 14-OH clarithromycin. However, no dosage adjustment is considered necessary based on these data.
		↑ omeprazole C_{max} & AUC_{0-24}	Clarithromycin 500 mg t.i.d. was given in combination with omeprazole 40 mg q.d. to healthy subjects. The steady-state plasma concentrations of omeprazole were increased (i.e., C_{max}, AUC_{0-24}, and $t_{1/2}$ increased by 30%, 89%, and 34%, respectively), by concomitant administration of clarithromycin. The mean 24-hour gastric pH value was 5.2 when omeprazole was administered alone and 5.7 when coadministered with clarithromycin.
		↑ levels of clarithromycin	To a lesser extent, omeprazole administration increases the serum concentrations of clarithromycin. Omeprazole administration also increases tissue and mucus concentrations of clarithromycin.
Lovastatin/Simvastatin	C	Rhabdomyolysis (rarely reported)	Rhabdomyolysis coincident with the coadministration of clarithromycin and the HMG-CoA reductase inhibitors, lovastatin and simvastatin, has rarely been reported.
Atorvastatin	C	Rhabdomyolysis (rarely reported)	Concurrent use of atorvastatin and clarithromycin may result in increased atorvastatin exposure and an increased risk of rhabdomyolysis.
Midazolam/Triazolam	C	↓ clearance of midazolam & triazolan	Clarithromycin has been reported to decrease the clearance of midazolam and triazolam and thus may increase the pharmacologic effect of these drugs.
Rifabutin/Rifampin	C	↓ levels of clarithromycin	Coadministration of rifabutin or rifampin and clarithromycin has resulted in decreased clarithromycin concentrations.
		↑ levels of rifabutin	Clarithromycin has been reported to increase serum and tissue concentration of rifabutin and thus may increase the risk of toxicity.
Ritonavir/Indinavir	CT	↑ clarithromycin C_{max}, C_{min} & AUC	A pharmacokinetic study demonstrated that the concomitant administration of ritonavir 200 mg q8h and clarithromycin 500 mg q12h resulted in a marked inhibition of the metabolism of clarithromycin. The clarithromycin C_{max} increased by 31%, C_{min} increased 182% and AUC increased by 77% with concomitant administration of ritonavir. An essentially complete inhibition of the formation of 14-[R]-hydroxy-clarithromycin was noted. Because of the large therapeutic window for clarithromycin, no dosage reduction should be necessary in patients with normal renal function. However, for patients with renal impairment, the following dosage adjustments should be considered: For patients with CLCR 30 to 60 mL/min the dose of clarithromycin should be reduced by 50%. For patients with CLCR <30 mL/min the dose of clarithromycin should be decreased by 75%. Doses of clarithromycin greater than 1 gm/day should not be coadministered with ritonavir.
		↑ indinavir AUC ↑ clarithromycin AUC	One study demonstrated that the concomitant administration of clarithromycin and indinavir resulted in a metabolic interaction; the clarithromycin AUC increased by 53% and the indinavir AUC was increased by 20%, but the individual variation was large. No dose adjustment is necessary with normal renal function.
Tacrolimus	P	Potential ↑ in tacrolimus concentrations	Concomitant administration of tacrolimus and clarithromycin may result in increased plasma levels of tacrolimus and increased risk of toxicity.
Theophylline	P	Potential ↑ in theophylline concentrations	Clarithromycin use in patients who are receiving theophylline may be associated with an increase of serum theophylline concentrations. Monitoring of serum theophylline concentrations should be considered for patients receiving high doses of theophylline or with baseline concentrations in the upper therapeutic range.
Warfarin/ Acenocoumarol	C	↑ anticoagulant effect	There have been reports of increased anticoagulant effect when clarithromycin and oral anticoagulants are used concurrently. Anticoagulant parameters should be closely monitored. Adjustment of the anticoagulant dose may be necessary. Clarithromycin has also been reported to increase the anticoagulant effect of acenocoumarol.
Zidovudine	C	Potential ↓ in zidovudine concentrations	Simultaneous oral administration of BIAXIN BID tablets and zidovudine to HIV-infected adult patients may result in decreased steady-state zidovudine concentrations. Clarithromycin appears to interfere with the absorption of simultaneously administered oral zidovudine, therefore this interaction can be largely avoided by staggering the doses of clarithromycin and zidovudine.
Others/Drugs Metabolized by Cytochrome P450 System	C/P	Potential change in serum concentration	Interactions with erythromycin and/or clarithromycin have been reported with a number of other drugs metabolized by the cytochrome P450 system, such as alfentanil, alprazolam, bromocriptine, cilostazol, hexobarbital, methylprednisolone, phenytoin, sildenafil, valproate or vinblastine. Serum concentrations of drugs metabolized by the cytochrome P450 system should be monitored closely in patients concurrently receiving erythromycin or clarithromycin.

Interactions with other drugs have not been established.
Legend: C=Case Study; CT=Clinical Trial; P=Potential.

Drug-Food Interactions: PREVACID (lansoprazole delayed-release capsules): Food reduces the peak concentration and the extent of absorption of lansoprazole by about 50% to 70%. Therefore, it is recommended that lansoprazole delayed-release capsules be administered in the morning prior to breakfast and another meal.
BIAXIN BID (clarithromycin tablets, USP, film-coated): BIAXIN BID (clarithromycin tablets, USP, film-coated) may be given with or without meals.
Drug-Herb Interactions: Interactions with herbal products have not been established.
Drug-Laboratory Test Interactions: Interactions with laboratory tests have not been established.

DOSAGE AND ADMINISTRATION: Dosing Considerations: PREVACID (lansoprazole delayed-release capsules): It is recommended that the initial dosing regimen need not be altered for patients with mild or moderate liver disease, but for patients with moderate impairment, doses higher than 30 mg per day should not be administered unless there are compelling clinical indications (see Warnings and Precautions, Hepatic/Biliary/Pancreatic and Renal).
BIAXIN BID (clarithromycin tablets, USP, film-coated): For the eradication of *H. pylori*, amoxicillin and clarithromycin should not be administered to patients with renal impairment since the appropriate dosage in this patient population has not yet been established.
Recommended Dose and Dosage Adjustment: *H. pylori* Eradication to Reduce the Risk of Duodenal Ulcer Recurrence: Hp-PAC—Triple Therapy: PREVACID/clarithromycin/amoxicillin: The recommended adult oral dose is 30 mg lansoprazole, 500 mg clarithromycin, and 1 g amoxicillin, all given twice daily for 7, 10 or 14 days (see Indications and Clinical Use). Daily doses should be taken before meals.
PREVACID (lansoprazole delayed-release capsules): PREVACID (lansoprazole delayed-release capsules) should be taken daily before breakfast. Where the product may be used twice daily, it should be taken prior to breakfast and another meal. PREVACID delayed-release capsules **should not be crushed or chewed.**
Patients with Hepatic Impairment: The daily dose of lansoprazole should not exceed 30 mg (see Warnings and Precautions).
Clarithromycin may be administered without dosage adjustment in the presence of hepatic impairment if there is normal renal function.
Patients with Renal Impairment: PREVACID (lansoprazole delayed-release capsules): No dosage modification of lansoprazole is necessary (see Warnings and Precautions).
BIAXIN BID (clarithromycin tablets, USP, film-coated): Refer to Warnings and Precautions, Renal.
Elderly Patients: The daily dose of lansoprazole should not exceed 30 mg (see Warnings and Precautions).
Concomitant Antacid Use: Simultaneous administration of lansoprazole with Maalox (aluminum and magnesium hydroxide) or Riopan (magaldrate) results in lower peak plasma levels, but does not significantly reduce bioavailability. Antacids may be used concomitantly if required. If sucralfate is to be given concomitantly, lansoprazole should be administered at least 30 minutes prior to sucralfate (see Action and Clinical Pharmacology, Absorption with Antacids). In clinical trials, antacids were administered concomitantly with lansoprazole delayed-release capsules; this did not interfere with its effect.
Missed Dose: If a dose of clarithromycin is missed, the patient should take the dose as soon as possible and then return to their normal scheduled dose. However, if a dose is skipped, the patient should not double the next dose.
Administration: PREVACID (lansoprazole delayed-release capsules): PREVACID (lansoprazole delayed-release capsules) should be taken daily before breakfast. Where the product may be used twice daily, it should be taken prior to breakfast and another meal. PREVACID delayed-release capsules **should not be crushed or chewed.**

OVERDOSAGE:
Hp-PAC—Triple Therapy: PREVACID/clarithromycin/amoxicillin: In case of an overdose, patients should contact a physician, poison control center, or emergency room. There is neither a pharmacologic basis nor any data suggesting an increase in the toxicity of the Hp-PAC combination compared to its individual components.
PREVACID (lansoprazole delayed-release capsules): As in all cases where overdosing is suspected, treatment should be supportive and symptomatic. Any unabsorbed material should be removed from the gastrointestinal tract, and the patient should be carefully monitored. Lansoprazole is not removed from the circulation by hemodialysis. In one reported case of overdose, the patient consumed 600 mg of lansoprazole with no adverse reaction.
Oral doses up to 5000 mg/kg in rats (approximately 1300 times the recommended human dose based on body surface area) and mice (about 675.7 times the recommended human dose based on body surface area) did not produce deaths or any clinical signs.
BIAXIN BID (clarithromycin tablets, USP, film-coated): Reports indicate that the ingestion of large amounts of clarithromycin can be expected to produce gastrointestinal symptoms. Adverse reactions accompanying overdosage should be treated by the prompt elimination of unabsorbed drug and supportive measures. Clarithromycin is protein bound (70%). No data are available on the elimination of clarithromycin by hemodialysis or peritoneal dialysis.
AMOXICILLIN (amoxicillin trihydrate) Capsules: Treatment of overdosage would likely be needed only in patients with severely impaired renal function, since patients with normal kidneys excrete penicillins at a fast rate. Hemodialysis would therefore represent the main form of treatment.

For management of a suspected drug overdose, CPhA recommends that you contact your **regional Poison Control Centre**. See the *CPS* Directory section for a list of Poison Control Centres.

ACTION AND CLINICAL PHARMACOLOGY: Mechanism of Action: PREVACID (lansoprazole delayed-release capsules): PREVACID (lansoprazole delayed-release capsules) inhibit inhibits the gastric H+, K+-ATPase (the proton pump) which catalyzes the exchange of H+ and K+. It is effective in the inhibition of both basal acid secretion and stimulated acid secretion.
BIAXIN BID (clarithromycin tablets, USP, film-coated): Clarithromycin exerts its antibacterial action by binding to the 50S ribosomal subunit of susceptible bacteria and suppressing protein synthesis.
Pharmacodynamics: Eradication of *H. pylori*: *H. pylori* is considered to be a major factor in the etiology of duodenal ulcer disease. The presence of *H. pylori* may damage the mucosal integrity due to the production of enzymes (catalase, lipases, phospholipases, proteases, and urease), adhesins and toxins; the inflammatory response generated in this manner contributes to mucosal damage.
The concomitant administration of an antimicrobial(s) such as clarithromycin and amoxicillin, and an antisecretory agent such as lansoprazole, improves the eradication of *H. pylori* as compared to individual drug administration. The higher pH resulting from antisecretory treatment, optimizes the environment for the pharmacologic action of the antimicrobial agent(s) against *H. pylori*.
PREVACID (lansoprazole delayed-release capsules): In healthy subjects, single and multiple doses of lansoprazole delayed-release capsules (15 mg to 60 mg) have been shown to decrease significantly basal gastric acid output and to increase significantly mean gastric pH and percent of time at pH >3 and 4. These doses have also been shown to reduce significantly

(cont'd)

meal-stimulated gastric acid output and gastric secretion volume. Single or multiple doses of lansoprazole delayed-release capsules (10 mg to 60 mg) reduced pentagastrin-stimulated acid output. In addition, lansoprazole delayed-release capsules have been demonstrated to reduce significantly basal and pentagastrin-stimulated gastric acid secretion among Duodenal Ulcer (DU) and hypersecretory patients, and basal gastric acid secretion among patients with Gastric Ulcer (GU) disease.

A dose-response effect was analyzed by considering the results from clinical pharmacology studies that evaluated more than one dose of lansoprazole delayed-release capsules. The results indicated that, in general, as the dose was increased from 7.5 mg to 30 mg, there was a decrease in mean gastric acid secretion and an increase in the average time spent at higher pH values (pH >4).

The results of pharmacodynamic studies with lansoprazole delayed-release capsules in normal subjects suggest that doses of 7.5 to 10 mg are substantially less effective in inhibiting gastric acid secretion than doses of 15 mg or greater. In view of these results, the doses of lansoprazole delayed-release capsules evaluated in the principal clinical trials ranged from 15 mg to 60 mg daily.

Pharmacokinetics: Hp-PAC—Triple Therapy: PREVACID/clarithromycin/amoxicillin: The pharmacokinetics of the drugs when all three components of the Hp-PAC (PREVACID capsules, clarithromycin tablets and amoxicillin capsules) were coadministered, has not been studied. Studies have shown no clinically significant interactions between PREVACID and amoxicillin or PREVACID and clarithromycin when coadministered. There is no information about the gastric mucosal concentrations of PREVACID, amoxicillin and clarithromycin after administration of these agents concomitantly. The systemic pharmacokinetic information presented below is based on studies in which each product was administered alone.

PREVACID (lansoprazole delayed-release capsules): Lansoprazole delayed-release capsules contain an enteric-coated granule formulation of lansoprazole to ensure that absorption of lansoprazole begins only after the granules leave the stomach (lansoprazole is acid-labile). Peak plasma concentrations of lansoprazole (C_{max}) and the area under the plasma concentration curve (AUC) of lansoprazole are approximately proportional in doses from 15 mg to 60 mg after single-oral administration. Lansoprazole pharmacokinetics are unaltered by multiple dosing and the drug does not accumulate.

Lansoprazole delayed-release capsules is highly bioavailable when administered orally. In a definitive absolute bioavailability study, the absolute bioavailability was shown to be 86% for a 15 mg capsule and 80% for a 30 mg capsule. First pass effect is apparently minimal.

Table 6 summarizes the pharmacokinetic parameters (T_{max}, $T_{½}$, AUC and C_{max}) of lansoprazole delayed-release capsules in healthy subjects).

Table 6: Hp-PAC

Pharmacokinetic Parameters of Lansoprazole Delayed-release Capsules Pooled Across Phase 1 Studies

Parameter	T_{max} (h)	$t_{1/2}$ (h)	AUC[a] (ng·h/mL)	C_{max}[a] (ng/mL)
Mean	1.68	1.53	2133	824
Median	1.50	1.24	1644	770
SD	0.80	1.01	1797	419
% CV	47.71	65.92	84.28	50.81
Min	0.50	0.39	213	27
Max	6.00	8.50	14 203	2440
N[b]	345	285	513	515

[a] Normalized to a 30 mg dose.
[b] Number of dosages associated with a parameter.

BIAXIN BID (clarithromycin tablets, USP, film-coated): A summary of clarithromycin pharmacokinetic parameters following the administration of clarithromycin film-coated tablets is provided in Table 7.

Table 7: Hp-PAC

Clarithromycin Pharmacokinetic Parameters Following the Administration of Clarithromycin Film-coated Tablets

	C_{max} (mg/L)	t_{max} (h)	$t_{½}$ (h)	AUC_{0-t} (mg·h/L)
Single Dose[a]				
250 mg Mean	1	1.5	2.7	5.47
500 mg Mean	1.77	2.2	—	11.66
Multiple Doses[b]				
250 mg b.i.d. Mean	1	—	3 to 4	6.34
500 mg b.i.d. Mean	3.38	2.1	5 to 7	44.19

[a] Single doses.
[b] Multiple doses.

Absorption: PREVACID (lansoprazole delayed-release capsules): The absorption of lansoprazole is rapid, with mean peak plasma levels of lansoprazole occurring at approximately 1.7 hours. Peak plasma concentrations of lansoprazole (C_{max}) and the area under the plasma concentration curve (AUC) are approximately proportional to dose throughout the range that has been studied (up to 60 mg).

Absorption with Food: Food reduces the peak concentration and the extent of absorption by about 50% to 70%. Moreover, the results of a pharmacokinetic study that compared the bioavailability of lansoprazole following a.m. dosing (fasting) versus p.m. dosing (three hours after a meal) indicated that both C_{max} and AUC values were increased by approximately two-fold or more with a.m. dosing. Therefore, it is recommended that lansoprazole delayed-release capsules be administered in the morning prior to breakfast.

Absorption with Antacids: Simultaneous administration of lansoprazole delayed-release capsules with Maalox (aluminum and magnesium hydroxide) or Riopan (magaldrate) resulted in lower peak serum levels, but did not significantly reduce the bioavailability of lansoprazole.

In a single-dose crossover study when 30 mg of lansoprazole was administered concomitantly with one gram of sucralfate in healthy volunteers, absorption of lansoprazole was delayed and its bioavailability was reduced. The value of lansoprazole AUC was reduced by 17% and that for C_{max} was reduced by 21%.

In a similar study when 30 mg of lansoprazole was administered concomitantly with 2 grams of sucralfate, lansoprazole AUC and C_{max} were reduced by 32% and 55%, respectively. When lansoprazole dosing occurred 30 minutes prior to sucralfate administration, C_{max} was reduced by only 28% and there was no statistically significant difference in lansoprazole AUC. Therefore, lansoprazole may be given concomitantly with antacids but should be administered at least 30 minutes prior to sucralfate.

BIAXIN BID (clarithromycin tablets, USP, film-coated): The absolute bioavailability of 250 mg and 500 mg clarithromycin tablets is approximately 50%. Food slightly delays the onset of clarithromycin absorption but does not affect the extent of bioavailability. Therefore, BIAXIN BID tablets may be given without regard to meals.

In fasting healthy human subjects, peak serum concentrations are attained within 2 hours after oral dosing. Steady-state peak serum clarithromycin concentrations, which are attained within 2 to 3 days, are approximately 1 mg/L with a 250 mg dose twice daily and 2 to 3 mg/L with a 500 mg dose twice daily. The elimination half-life of clarithromycin is about 3 to 4 hours with 250 mg twice daily dosing but increases to about 5 to 7 hours with 500 mg administered twice daily.

Clarithromycin displays non-linear pharmacokinetics at clinically relevant doses, producing greater than proportional increases in AUC with increasing dose. The degree of non-linearity is reduced on chronic clarithromycin administration (i.e., at steady state). The non-linearity of the pharmacokinetics of the principle metabolite, 14-OH clarithromycin, is slight at the recommended doses of 250 mg and 500 mg administered twice daily. With 250 mg twice daily, 14-OH clarithromycin attains a peak steady state concentration of about 0.6 mg/L and has an elimination half-life of 5 to 6 hours. With a 500 mg twice daily dose, the peak steady-state of 14-OH concentrations of clarithromycin are slightly higher (up to 1 mg/L) and its elimination half-life is about 7 hours. With either dose, the steady-state concentration of this metabolite is generally attained within 2 to 3 days.

Adult Patients with HIV: Steady-state concentrations of clarithromycin and 14-OH clarithromycin observed following administration of 500 mg doses of clarithromycin twice a day to adult patients with HIV infection were similar to those observed in healthy volunteers. However, at the higher clarithromycin doses which may be required to treat mycobacterial infections, clarithromycin concentrations can be much higher than those observed at 500 mg clarithromycin doses. In adult HIV-infected patients taking 2000 mg/day in two divided doses, steady-state clarithromycin C_{max} values ranged from 5 to10 mg/L. C_{max} values as high as 27 mg/L have been observed in HIV-infected adult patients taking 4000 mg/day in two divided doses of clarithromycin tablets.

Elimination half-lives appeared to be lengthened at these higher doses as well. The higher clarithromycin concentrations and longer elimination half-lives observed at these doses are consistent with the known non-linearity in clarithromycin pharmacokinetics.

Clarithromycin and Omeprazole: Clarithromycin 500 mg t.i.d. and omeprazole 40 mg q.d. were studied in fasting healthy adult subjects. When clarithromycin was given alone as 500 mg q8h, the mean steady state C_{max} value was approximately 3.8 µg/mL and the mean C_{min} value was approximately 1.8 µg/mL. The mean AUC_{0-8} for clarithromycin was 22.9 µg·h/mL. The T_{max} and half life were 2.1 hrs and 5.3 hrs, respectively, when clarithromycin was dosed at 500 mg t.i.d. When clarithromycin was administered with omeprazole, increases in omeprazole half-life and AUC_{0-24} were observed. For all subjects combined, the mean omeprazole AUC_{0-24} was 89% greater and the harmonic mean for omeprazole $t_{½}$ was 34% greater when omeprazole was administered with clarithromycin than when omeprazole was administered alone. When clarithromycin was administered with omeprazole, the steady state C_{max}, C_{min}, and AUC_{0-8} of clarithromycin were increased by 10%, 27%, and 15%, respectively over values achieved when clarithromycin was administered with placebo.

AMOXICILLIN (amoxicillin trihydrate) Capsules: Amoxicillin is stable in the presence of gastric acid and is well absorbed from the gastrointestinal tract and may be given with no regard to food. The half-life of amoxicillin is 61.3 minutes.

Orally administered doses of 500 mg amoxicillin capsules result in average peak blood levels 1 to 2 hours after administration in the range of 5.5 to 7.5 µg/mL.

Detectable serum levels are observed up to eight hours after an orally administered does of amoxicillin.

Distribution: PREVACID (lansoprazole delayed-release capsules): The apparent volume of distribution of lansoprazole is approximately 15.7 (±1.9) L, distributing mainly in extracellular fluid. Lansoprazole is 97% bound to plasma proteins. The mean total body clearance (CL) of lansoprazole was calculated at 31±8 L/h, and the volume of distribution (Vss) was calculated to be 29 (±4) L.

BIAXIN BID (clarithromycin tablets, USP, film-coated): Clarithromycin distributes readily into body tissues and fluids, and provides tissue concentrations that are higher than serum concentrations. Examples from tissue and serum concentrations are presented in Table 8.

Table 8: Hp-PAC

Representative Clarithromycin Tissue and Serum Concentrations Following the Administration of 250 mg b.i.d of Clarithromycin Film-coated Tablets

	Concentrations	
Tissue Type	Tissue (µg/g)	Serum (mg/L)
Tonsil	1.6	0.8
Lung	8.8	1.7
Leukocytes[a]	9.2	1.0

[a] In vitro data.

AMOXICILLIN (amoxicillin trihydrate) Capsules: Amoxicillin diffuses readily into most body tissues and fluids, with the exception of brain and spinal fluid, except when the meninges are inflamed. Amoxicillin Is not highly protein-bound. In serum, amoxicillin is approximately 20% protein-bound as compared to 60% for penicillin G.

Metabolism: PREVACID (lansoprazole delayed-release capsules): Lansoprazole is extensively metabolized in the liver. Two metabolites have been identified in measurable quantities in plasma; the hydroxylated sulfinyl and the sulfone derivatives of lansoprazole. These metabolites have very little or no antisecretory activity. Within the parietal cell canaliculus, lansoprazole is thought to be transformed into two active metabolites that inhibit acid secretion by H+,K+-ATPase, but these metabolites are not present in the systemic circulation. The plasma elimination half-life of lansoprazole does not reflect the duration of suppression of gastric acid secretion. Thus, the plasma elimination half-life is less than two hours while the acid inhibitory effect lasts over 24 hours.

BIAXIN BID (clarithromycin tablets, USP, film-coated): Clarithromycin is principally excreted by the liver and kidney. The major metabolite found in urine is 14-OH-clarithromycin.

Excretion: PREVACID (lansoprazole delayed-release capsules): Following single dose oral administration of lansoprazole, virtually no unchanged lansoprazole was excreted in the urine. After a 30 mg single oral dose of 14C-lansoprazole, approximately one-third of the dose was excreted in the urine and approximately two-thirds were recovered in the feces. This implies a significant biliary excretion of the metabolites of lansoprazole.

BIAXIN BID (clarithromycin tablets, USP, film-coated): At 250 mg twice daily, approximately 20% of an orally administered dose of clarithromycin film-coated tablet is excreted in the urine as the unchanged parent drug. The urinary excretion of unchanged clarithromycin is somewhat greater (approximately 30%) with 500 mg twice daily dosing. The renal clearance of clarithromycin is, however, relatively independent of the dose size and approximates the normal glomerular filtration rate. The major metabolite found in urine is 14-OH-clarithromycin which accounts for an additional 10 to 15% of the dose with twice daily dosing at either 250 mg or 500 mg. Most of the remainder of the dose is eliminated in the feces, primarily via the bile. About 5 to 10% of the parent drug is recovered from the feces. Fecal metabolites are largely products of N-demethylation, 14-hydroxylation or both.

AMOXICILLIN (amoxicillin trihydrate) Capsules: Most of the amoxicillin is excreted unchanged in urine; its excretion can be delayed by concurrent administration of probenecid.

Approximately 60% of an orally administered dose of amoxicillin is excreted in the urine within 6 to 8 hours.

Special Populations and Conditions: Pediatrics: Hp-PAC—Triple Therapy: PREVACID/clarithromycin/amoxicillin: The safety and effectiveness of Hp-PAC in pediatric patients infected with *H. pylori* have not been established.

Geriatrics: PREVACID (lansoprazole delayed-release capsules): The results from the studies that evaluated the pharmacokinetics of lansoprazole following oral administration in an older population revealed that in comparison with younger subjects, older subjects exhibited significantly larger AUCs and longer $t_{½}$. Lansoprazole did not accumulate in the older subjects upon multiple dosing since the longest mean $t_{½}$ in the studies was 2.9 hours, and lansoprazole is dosed once daily. C_{max} in the elderly was comparable to that found in adult subjects.

BIAXIN BID (clarithromycin tablets, USP, film-coated): In a steady-state study in which healthy elderly subjects (age 65 to 81 years old) were given 500 mg of clarithromycin every 12 hours, the maximum concentrations of clarithromycin and 14-OH clarithromycin were increased. The AUC was also increased. These changes in pharmacokinetics parallel known age-related decreases in renal function. In clinical trials, elderly patients did not have an increased incidence of adverse events when compared to younger patients (see Warnings and Precautions, Renal).

Gender: In a study comparing 12 male and six female subjects, no gender differences were found in pharmacokinetics or intragastric pH results (see Warnings and Precautions, Use in Women).

Race: The pooled pharmacokinetic parameters of oral administered lansoprazole from twelve U.S. Phase I studies (N=513) were compared to the mean pharmacokinetic parameters from two Asian studies (N=20). The mean AUCs of lansoprazole in Asian subjects are approximately twice that seen in pooled U.S. data, however, the inter-individual variability is high. The C_{max} values are comparable.

Hepatic Insufficiency: PREVACID (lansoprazole delayed-release capsules): As would be expected with a drug that is primarily metabolized by the liver, in patients with mild (Child-Pugh Class A) or moderate (Child-Pugh Class B) chronic hepatic disease, the plasma half-life of the drug after oral administration increased to 5.2 hours compared to the 1.5 hours half-life in healthy subjects. An increase in AUC of 3.4 fold was observed in patients with hepatic impairment versus healthy subjects (7096 versus 2645 ng·h/mL) which was due to slower elimination of lansoprazole; however, C_{max} was not significantly affected. Dose reduction in patients with severe hepatic disease should be considered.

BIAXIN BID (clarithromycin tablets, USP, film-coated): The steady-state concentrations of clarithromycin in subjects with impaired hepatic function did not differ from those in normal subjects; however, the 14-OH clarithromycin concentrations were lower in the hepatically impaired subjects. The decreased formation of 14-OH clarithromycin was at least partially offset by an increase in renal clearance of clarithromycin in subjects with impaired hepatic function when compared to healthy subjects (see Warnings and Precautions and Dosage and Administration).

Renal Insufficiency: PREVACID (lansoprazole delayed-release capsules): In patients with mild (Cl_{cr} 40 to 80 mL/min), moderate (Cl_{cr} 20 to 40 mL/min) and severe (Cl_{cr} <20 mL/min) chronic renal impairment, the disposition of lansoprazole after oral administration was very similar to that of healthy volunteers.

The impact of dialysis on lansoprazole was evaluated from a pharmacokinetic standpoint, and there were no significant differences in AUC, C_{max} or $t_{½}$ between dialysis day and dialysis-free day. Dialysate contained no measurable lansoprazole or metabolite. Lansoprazole is not significantly dialysed.

BIAXIN BID (clarithromycin tablets, USP, film-coated): The pharmacokinetics of clarithromycin was also altered in subjects with impaired renal function. The elimination of clarithromycin was impaired in patients with impaired renal function (see Warnings and Precautions, Renal and Dosage and Administration).

STORAGE AND STABILITY: Store the Hp-PAC blister cards between 15 and 25°C. Protect from light and moisture.

INFORMATION FOR THE PATIENT: Published in e-CPS, available by subscription at www.e-cps.ca.

DOSAGE FORMS, COMPOSITION AND PACKAGING: Hp-PAC—*H. pylori* Individual Daily Administration Blister Pack: Each triple therapy Hp-PAC (lansoprazole/amoxicillin/clarithromycin) daily administration blister pack contains:

PREVACID 30 mg (lansoprazole delayed-release capsules): 2 opaque, hard gelatin, pink and black capsules, with the TAP logo and "PREVACID 30" imprinted on the capsule, contains: lansoprazole 30 mg each. Nonmedicinal ingredients: cellulosic polymers, colloidal silicon dioxide, D&C Red No. 28, FD&C Blue No. 1, FD&C Red No. 40, gelatin, magnesium carbonate, methacrylic acid copolymer, polyethylene glycol, polysorbate 80, starch, sucrose, sugar spheres, talc and titanium dioxide.

BIAXIN BID 500 mg (clarithromycin tablets, USP, film-coated): 2 pale yellow, oval, film-coated tablets, with the Abbott logo printed on one side, contains: clarithromycin 500 mg each. Nonmedicinal ingredients: cellulosic polymers, croscarmellose sodium, D&C Yellow No. 10, magnesium stearate, povidone, propylene glycol, silicon dioxide, sorbic acid, sorbitan monooleate, stearic acid, talc, titanium dioxide and vanillin. Tartrazine-free.

AMOXICILLIN 500 mg (amoxicillin trihydrate) Capsules: 4 opaque, scarlet and yellow capsules, with the Abbott logo and "500" imprinted on the capsule, contains: amoxicillin trihydrate 500 mg each. Nonmedicinal ingredients: colloidal silicon dioxide, D&C Yellow No. 10, dry-flo starch, FD&C Blue No. 1, FD&C Red No. 3, FD&C Red No. 40, FD&C Yellow No. 6, gelatin, magnesium stearate, sodium lauryl sulfate, talc and titanium dioxide. Gluten- and tartrazine-free.

Hp-PAC daily administration blister packs are available in boxes containing (seven) 7 days of therapy.

Humalog®
insulin lispro
Antidiabetic

Lilly

Humalog® Mix25®
insulin lispro—insulin lispro protamine
Antidiabetic

Lilly

Humalog Mix50®
insulin lispro—insulin lispro protamine
Antidiabetic

Lilly

Date of Preparation: June 11, 2009

PHARMACOLOGY: Insulin lispro, the active pharmaceutical ingredient in Humalog (insulin lispro injection), Humalog Mix25 (25% insulin lispro injection, 75% insulin lispro protamine suspension), and Humalog Mix50 (50% insulin lispro injection, 50% insulin lispro protamine suspension) is created by inverting the natural Pro-Lys sequence in human insulin at positions 28 and 29 in the C terminal portion of the B-chain. This change in amino acid sequence slightly modifies the physicochemical properties of the molecule relative to native human insulin in such a manner that insulin lispro self-associates less avidly and dissociates into its monomeric form more rapidly than regular insulin. As a result, insulin lispro is absorbed more rapidly than regular soluble insulin from s.c. sites of injection and also has a shorter duration of action.

The reversed sequence of lysine and proline in insulin lispro, is identical to that on the B-chain of human IGF-1. The incidence of self-association with IGF-1 is known to be lower than observed with human insulin. Incorporating this IGF-1-like feature into the human insulin molecule markedly changes the physicochemical behavior of the resulting insulin lispro but does not significantly alter its pharmacodynamic action because the terminal part of the B-chain does not participate in insulin's interaction with the insulin receptor. In vitro experiments showed that insulin lispro interacts with the insulin receptor much like regular human insulin does. Although binding to the IGF-1 receptor is higher than for regular human insulin (1.5 times more), it is significantly less than that of IGF-1 itself (more than 1000 times less) and does not promote cell growth in biological assays to any greater extent than human insulin.

The primary activity of insulins, including Humalog, Humalog Mix25, and Humalog Mix50, is the regulation of glucose metabolism. In addition, all insulins have several anabolic and anticatabolic actions on many tissues in the body. In muscle and other tissues (except the brain), insulin causes rapid transport of glucose and amino acids intracellularly, promotes anabolism, and inhibits protein catabolism. In the liver, insulin promotes the uptake and storage of glucose in the form of glycogen, inhibits gluconeogenesis and promotes the conversion of excess glucose into fat.

Humalog: Humalog is absorbed more rapidly than regular soluble insulin from s.c. sites of injection and also has a shorter duration of action. Due to its quick onset of action, Humalog should be given within 15 minutes before a meal. When necessary, Humalog may be given shortly after a meal instead (within 20 minutes of the start of the meal).

S.C. injected regular insulin typically results in serum insulin concentrations that peak later and remain elevated for a longer time than those following normal pancreatic insulin secretion in non-diabetics. When regular insulin is used to control postprandial blood glucose, adequate control is often not achieved because the amount of regular insulin needed to normalize postprandial glucose excursion often leads to late hypoglycemia. By producing more rapid and higher serum insulin concentrations with a shorter duration of activity (2 to 5 hours), Humalog decreases glucose excursion during and after meals with less chance for hypoglycemia.

A glucose clamp study was performed, in healthy volunteers, in which a 10 U dose of Humalog was compared to Humulin R. Doses were given s.c.; an additional 10 U dose of i.v. regular insulin was given as an absolute reference.

Humalog showed statistically higher peak concentrations (C_{max}) which occurred earlier than Humulin R (t_{max}). Total absorption was comparable, with area under the curve (AUC) values of serum concentration vs time which were not statistically different (see Table 1 and Table 2).

Table 1: Humalog

Pharmacokinetics of Humalog Compared with Humulin R in Healthy Volunteers

Mean±SD	Humalog	Humulin R
t_{max} (min)	53±30	101±40
C_{max} (ng/mL)	3.20±1.33	1.79±0.77
AUC (ng.min/mL)	380±52.2	423±71.8

Table 2: Humalog

Pharmacodynamics of Humalog Compared with Humulin R in Healthy Volunteers

Mean±SD	Humalog	Humulin R
Duration of Action (h)[a]	3.5–4.75 h	5.0–7.5 h
Onset of Action (h)[a]	0.5–0.75 h	0.5–1.0 h
Time of Maximum Effect (h)[a]	0.75–2.5 h	0.75–4.5 h

[a] Results predicted from a pharmacokinetic-pharmacodynamic link model.

Subsequent pharmacokinetic studies in Type 1 patients confirmed that a significantly faster increase in serum insulin levels and a shorter plasma half-life resulted from an injection of Humalog when compared to Humulin R (see Figure 1).

Postprandial and Overall Glycemic Control: In clinical studies after 1 year, the decrease in glucose excursion during and after meals with Humalog was consistent, although not always significant, when compared to Humulin R. However, there was no significant difference in hemoglobin A1c levels between the two treatment groups. These studies were specifically designed to study meal time therapy without optimization of basal insulin regimens.

Subsequent clinical studies have demonstrated that in an intensive insulin treatment regimen with basal insulin optimization, Humalog controls postprandial glucose and contributes to lower hemoglobin A1c levels to a greater degree than regular human insulin, without increasing the risk of hypoglycemia.

Hypoglycemia: The frequency of hypoglycemia was not statistically significant in 1 year parallel studies (Humalog, n=543; Humulin R, n=561), but was significantly less with Humalog therapy in a 6-month crossover study in type 1 patients (n=1008) which also demonstrated a significant reduction in nocturnal hypoglycemia with Humalog.

Figure 1: Humalog

Mean Serum Insulin Concentrations in Type 1 Patients Following Injection of Humulin R and Humalog (basal 0.2 mU/min/kg insulin infusion)

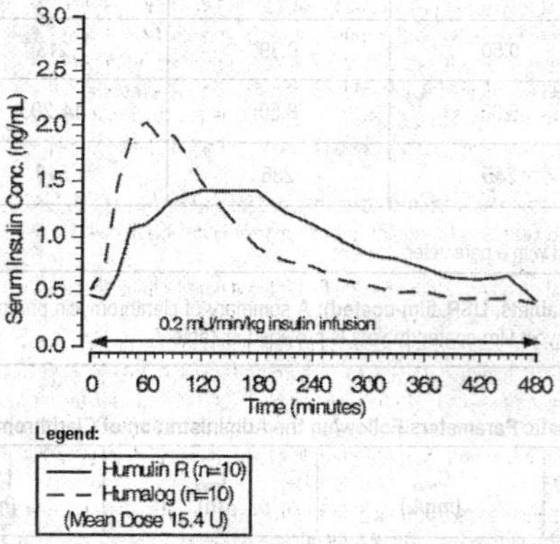

Use in Pumps: When used in subcutaneous insulin infusion pumps, treatment with Humalog has been shown to result in lower hemoglobin A1c levels compared to regular human insulin without increasing the risk of hypoglycemia. In clinical trials that compared Humalog with regular human insulin, Humalog consistently showed significant HbA1c improvement in the range of 0.33% to 0.65%.

Special Populations: Renal Impairment: Some studies with human insulin have shown increased circulating levels of insulin in patients with renal failure. In a study of 25 patients with type 2 diabetes and varying degrees of renal function (from normal to severe impairment, including endstage renal failure), the pharmacokinetic differences between Humalog and human regular insulin were generally maintained. However, the sensitivity of the patients to insulin did change, with an increased response to insulin as the renal function declined. Careful glucose monitoring and dose adjustments of insulin, including Humalog, may be necessary in patients with renal dysfunction.

Hepatic Impairment: Some studies with human insulin have shown increased circulating levels of insulin in patients with hepatic failure. In a study of 22 patients with type 2 diabetes, impaired hepatic function did not affect the s.c. absorption or general disposition of Humalog when compared to patients with no history of hepatic dysfunction. In that study, Humalog maintained its more rapid absorption and elimination when compared to human regular insulin. Careful glucose monitoring and dose adjustments of insulin, including Humalog, may be necessary in patients with hepatic dysfunction.

Humalog Mix25 and Humalog Mix50: Insulin lispro protamine suspension is an intermediate-acting protamine formulation of insulin lispro that displays absorption and activity profiles similar to those of Humulin N (insulin isophane). Fixed mixtures of insulin lispro injection and insulin lispro protamine suspension provide the rapid-acting blood glucose lowering activity associated with insulin lispro injection in combination with the intermediate-acting blood glucose lowering activity associated with the insulin lispro protamine suspension.

The Humalog family of insulins includes a fixed mixture of insulin lispro injection and insulin lispro protamine suspension that has been formulated in ratio of 25% insulin lispro injection, 75% insulin lispro protamine suspension (Humalog Mix25) and 50% insulin lispro injection, 50% insulin lispro protamine suspension (Humalog Mix50). The pharmacokinetic and pharmacodynamic profiles of various fixed mixtures were investigated in a glucose clamp study. The rapid activity of insulin lispro was maintained within each mixture. In addition, each mixture demonstrated a distinct pharmacokinetic and glucodynamic profile.

INDICATIONS: Humalog (insulin lispro injection), Humalog Mix25 (25% insulin lispro injection, 75% insulin lispro protamine suspension), and Humalog Mix50 (50% insulin lispro injection, 50% insulin lispro protamine suspension) are indicated for the treatment of patients with diabetes mellitus who require insulin for the maintenance of normal glucose homeostasis. Humalog insulins are also indicated for the initial stabilization of diabetes mellitus. Humalog (insulin lispro injection) is a short-acting insulin analogue and is for use in conjunction with a longer-acting human insulin, such as Humulin N except when used in a subcutaneous insulin infusion pump.

CONTRAINDICATIONS: The Humalog (insulin lispro) family of insulins are contraindicated during episodes of hypoglycemia (for details see Overdose, Symptoms and Treatment) and in patients sensitive to insulin lispro or any of the excipients they contain.

WARNINGS: Due to its quick onset of action, the Humalog family of insulins should be given within 15 minutes before a meal.

When necessary, Humalog (insulin lispro injection) may be given shortly after a meal instead (within 20 minutes of the start of the meal). When used in a subcutaneous insulin infusion pump, Humalog should not be diluted or mixed with any other insulin. Patients should carefully read and follow the insulin infusion pump manufacturer's instructions and the Information for the Patient insert before use.

Hypoglycemia is the most common adverse effect associated with insulins, including the Humalog family of insulins. As with all insulins, the timing of hypoglycemia may differ among various insulin formulations. Glucose monitoring is recommended for all patients with diabetes.

Any change of insulin or human insulin analogue should be made cautiously and only under medical supervision. Changes in purity, strength, brand (manufacturer), type (insulin lispro, regular, NPH, etc.), species (beef, pork, beef-pork, human), and/or method of manufacture (recombinant DNA vs animal source insulin) may result in the need for a change in dosage.

PRECAUTIONS: General: Humalog had a similar safety profile to Humulin R over the course of the clinical studies although its efficacy has not been studied in clinical trials beyond 1 year. Humalog has been shown to control hemoglobin A1c levels as effectively as human insulin in comparator studies specifically designed to study meal time therapy without optimization of basal insulin regimens. Once a patient is using Humalog, reassessment and adjustment, as necessary, of the basal insulin regimen (dosage and number of injections) has been shown to optimize overall glycemic control.

Visual disturbances in uncontrolled diabetes due to refractive changes are reversed during the early phase of effective management. However, since alteration in osmotic equilibrium between the lens and ocular fluids may not stabilize for a few weeks after initiating therapy, it is wise to postpone prescribing new corrective lenses for 3 to 6 weeks.

Additional adjustment of dosage may be required during intercurrent illness and/or emotional disturbances such as stress.

Any rapid- or short-acting insulin formulation should be used with caution in patients with gastroparesis. However, some patients with gastroparesis may benefit from postprandial administration of Humalog, which has been shown to provide postprandial glycemic control similar to that provided by human insulin injected 30 minutes pre-prandially. Using the postprandial dosing approach, the insulin dose can be adjusted according to the actual caloric intake and/or the observed rise in blood glucose following a meal.

Transferring Patients from Other Insulins: Patients taking a Humalog insulin may require a change in dosage from that used with their usual insulins. If an adjustment is needed, it may occur with the first dose or during the first several weeks or months.

A few patients who have experienced hypoglycemic reactions after transfer from animal-source insulin to human insulin have reported that the early warning symptoms of hypoglycemia were less pronounced or different from those experienced with their previous insulin. However, the counterregulatory and symptomatic (autonomic and neuroglycopenic) responses to hypoglycemia were studied and found to be superimposable for insulin lispro and regular human insulin.

Patients whose blood glucose is greatly improved, e.g., by intensified insulin therapy, may lose some or all of the warning symptoms of hypoglycemia and should be advised accordingly. Uncorrected hypoglycemic or hyperglycemic reactions can cause loss of consciousness, coma, or death.

Renal Impairment: The requirements for insulin may be reduced in patients with renal impairment.

Hepatic Impairment: Although impaired hepatic function does not affect the absorption or disposition of Humalog, careful glucose monitoring and dose adjustments of insulin, including Humalog, may be necessary.

Allergic Reaction: Prompt recognition and appropriate management of the allergic complications of insulin therapy are important for the safe and effective control of diabetes mellitus. Antibodies to insulin are frequently cross-reactive. Therefore, patients who have demonstrated an allergic reaction to other insulins may demonstrate an allergic reaction to a Humalog insulin. Local allergy in patients occasionally occurs as redness, swelling, and itching at the site of insulin injection. This condition usually resolves in a few days to a few weeks. In some instances, this condition may be related to factors other than insulin, such as irritants in the skin cleansing agent or poor injection technique. Systemic allergy may cause rash (including pruritus) over the whole body, shortness of breath, wheezing, reduction in blood pressure, fast pulse, or sweating. Severe cases of generalized allergy may be life-threatening (see Contraindications).

Pregnancy: Humalog can be used in pregnancy if clinically indicated. Data on a large number of exposed pregnancies do not indicate any adverse effect of Humalog on pregnancy or on the health of the foetus/newborn. It is essential to maintain good glucose control in both gestational diabetes and throughout pregnancy in Type 1 and 2 patients. Insulin requirements usually decrease during the first trimester and increase during the second and third trimesters.

Patients with diabetes should be advised to inform their doctor if they are pregnant or are contemplating pregnancy. Careful monitoring of glucose control, as well as general health is essential in pregnant patients with diabetes.

Lactation: The use of Humalog insulins in nursing mothers has not been studied. Diabetic patients who are nursing may require adjustments in insulin dose and/or diet.

Children: Clinical trials have been performed in children (61 patients aged 3 to 11) and children and adolescents (481 patients aged 9 to 18 years), comparing Humalog to regular human insulin. Humalog showed better postprandial blood glucose control while maintaining a similar safety profile.

As in adults, Humalog should be given within 15 minutes before a meal. When necessary, Humalog may be given shortly after a meal instead (within 20 minutes of the start of the meal).

The safety and effectiveness of Humalog Mix25 (25% insulin lispro injection, 75% insulin lispro protamine suspension) and Humalog Mix50 (50% insulin lispro injection, 50% insulin lispro protamine suspension) in children have not been established.

Drug Interactions: Drug interactions with insulin formulations including Humalog insulins may include the following: Insulin requirements may be decreased in the presence of agents such as oral antidiabetic agents, salicylates, sulfa antibiotics, certain antidepressants (monoamine oxidase inhibitors), beta-adrenergic blockers, alcohol, angiotensin converting enzyme inhibitors, and angiotensin II receptor blockers.

Insulin requirements may be increased by medications with hyperglycemic activity such as corticosteroids, isoniazid, certain lipid lowering drugs (e.g., niacin), estrogens, oral contraceptives, phenothiazines, and thyroid replacement therapy.

Hormones that tend to counteract the hypoglycemic effects of insulin include growth hormone, corticotropin, glucocorticoids, thyroid hormone and glucagon. Epinephrine not only inhibits the secretion of insulin, but also stimulates glycogen breakdown to glucose. Thus, the presence of such diseases as acromegaly, Cushing's syndrome, hyperthyroidism, and pheochromocytoma complicate the control of diabetes. The hypoglycemic action of insulin may also be antagonized by diphenylhydantoin.

Insulin requirements can be increased, decreased, or unchanged in patients receiving diuretics.

The physician should be consulted when using other medications in addition to a Humalog insulin.

ADVERSE EFFECTS: Rarely, administration of insulin s.c. can result in lipoatrophy (depression in the skin) or lipohypertrophy (enlargement or thickening of tissue). Patients should be advised to consult their doctors if they notice any of these conditions. A change in injection technique may help alleviate the problem.

OVERDOSE:

Symptoms: With the rapid onset of activity of the Humalog family of insulins, it is important that the insulin analogue be given close to mealtime (within 15 minutes before a meal). When necessary, Humalog (insulin lispro injection) may be given shortly after a meal instead (within 20 minutes of the start of the meal). A significant deviation could put the patient at risk of hypoglycemia.

Insulins have no specific overdose definitions because serum glucose concentrations are a result of complex interactions between insulin levels, glucose availability and other metabolic processes. Hypoglycemia may occur as a result of an excess of insulin or insulin lispro relative to food intake and energy expenditure or in patients who have an infection or become ill (especially with diarrhea or vomiting).

Symptoms are likely to appear anytime when the blood sugar concentration falls below 3 mmol/L (50 mg/100 mL) but may occur with a sudden drop in blood glucose even when the value remains above 3 mmol/L (50 mg/100 mL).

Hypoglycemia may be associated with listlessness, confusion, palpitations, headache, sweating and vomiting.

Treatment: Mild hypoglycemic episodes will respond to oral administration of glucose or sugar-containing foods.

Correction of moderately severe hypoglycemia can be accomplished by i.m. or s.c. administration of glucagon, followed by oral carbohydrate when the patient recovers sufficiently. Patients who fail to respond to glucagon must be given glucose solution i.v.

Patients who are unable to take sugar orally or who are unconscious should be treated with i.v. administration of glucose at a medical facility or should be given an injection of glucagon (either i.m. or s.c.). The patient should be given oral carbohydrates as soon as consciousness is recovered.

> For management of a suspected drug overdose, CPhA recommends that you contact your **regional Poison Control Centre**. See the *CPS* Directory section for a list of Poison Control Centres.

DOSAGE: The dosage of Humalog (insulin lispro injection), Humalog Mix25 (25% insulin lispro injection, 75% insulin lispro protamine suspension), or Humalog Mix50 (50% insulin lispro injection, 50% insulin lispro protamine suspension) is determined by a physician in accordance with the requirements of the patient.

Although Humalog insulins have a quicker onset of action and shorter duration of activity, dosing is comparable to regular human insulin. The dosage of a Humalog insulin, like all other insulin formulations, is dependent upon the individual patient requirements. The dose and number of insulin injections should be adjusted to maintain blood glucose concentrations as close to normal as possible.

Additional adjustment of dosage may be required in diabetes patients with renal impairment, during intercurrent illness and/or emotional disturbances.

Adjustment of dosage may also be necessary if patients undertake increased physical activity or change their usual diet.

New Patients: Patients receiving insulin for the first time can be started on a Humalog insulin in the same manner as they would be on animal-source or human insulin.

Patients should be monitored closely during the adjustment period.

Transfer Patients: When transferring patients to a Humalog insulin, use the same dose and dosage schedule. However, some patients transferring to a Humalog insulin may require a change in dosage from that used with their previous insulin. Analysis of a database of type 1 diabetic patients indicated that basal insulin requirements increased by 0.04 U/kg, while Humalog requirements decreased by 0.03 U/kg, after 1 year of treatment. For type 2 diabetic patients, both short acting and basal insulin requirements increased slightly after 1 year of treatment with both Humalog and Humulin R.

Optimizing Glycemic Control: In order to achieve optimal glycemic control, changes in total daily dosage, the number of injections per day, and/or timing of injections may be necessary when using a Humalog insulin.

Once a patient is using Humalog, reassessment and adjustment as necessary of the basal insulin regimen (dosage and number of injections) has been shown to optimize overall glycemic control.

Administration: Humalog is a clear, colorless solution. It is important to always examine the appearance of the vial or cartridge before withdrawing a dose. It should not be used it if it is cloudy, unusually viscous or gelled, precipitated, or even slightly colored; if there are clumps floating in the liquid, or if particles appear to be sticking to the sides or bottom of the vial or cartridge.

Humalog should be given by s.c. injection or by continuous s.c. insulin infusion pump and may, although not recommended, also be given by i.m. injection. It may also be administered i.v. under conditions where regular human insulin is given i.v. When used as a meal-time insulin, Humalog should be given within 15 minutes before a meal, or when necessary shortly after a meal instead (within 20 minutes of the start of the meal).

Humalog Mix25 (25% insulin lispro injection, 75% insulin lispro protamine suspension) and Humalog Mix50 (50% insulin lispro injection, 50% insulin lispro protamine suspension) are white suspensions. They should be administered by subcutaneous injection only and must not be administered intravenously. Humalog Mix25 and Humalog Mix50 start lowering blood glucose more quickly than regular human insulin, and should be given within 15 minutes before a meal.

S.C. administration, preferably by the patient, should be in the upper arms, thighs, buttocks or abdomen. When compared to Humulin R, Humalog retains its more rapid onset and shorter duration of action irrespective of the s.c. injection site used. Therefore, injection sites can be rotated so that the same site is not used more than approximately once a month.

Care should be taken to ensure that a blood vessel has not been entered. The injection site should not be massaged.

Mixing of Insulins: Mixing Humalog with Humulin N does not decrease the absorption rate or the total bioavailability of Humalog. Given alone or mixed with Humulin N, Humalog results in a more rapid absorption and glucose-lowering effect compared with human regular insulin.

If Humalog is mixed with a longer-acting insulin, Humalog should be drawn into the syringe first to prevent clouding of the Humalog by the longer-acting insulin. Injection should be made immediately after mixing. Mixtures should not be administered i.v. Humalog should not be diluted or mixed with any other insulin when used in a subcutaneous insulin infusion pump.

The effects of mixing Humalog, Humalog Mix25, or Humalog Mix50 with either animal-source insulins or human insulin preparations produced by other manufacturers have not been studied. This practice is not recommended.

INFORMATION FOR THE PATIENT: Published in e-CPS, available by subscription at www.e-cps.ca.

SUPPLIED: Humalog: Each mL of insulin lispro injection contains: human insulin analogue 100 units. Nonmedicinal ingredients: dibasic sodium phosphate, glycerin, m-cresol distilled, water for injection and zinc (as ion). Hydrochloric acid 10% and/or sodium hydroxide 10% may be added to adjust pH. Vials of 10 mL. Cartridges of 3 mL, boxes of 5. Stylo Humalog Pen (Turbo), prefilled pens of 3 mL, boxes of 5. KwikPen Humalog, prefilled pens of 3 mL, boxes of 5.

Humalog Mix25: Each mL of 25% insulin lispro injection and 75% insulin lispro protamine suspension contains: human insulin analogue 100 units and protamine sulfate 0.28 mg. Nonmedicinal ingredients: dibasic sodium phosphate, glycerin, liquified phenol, m-cresol distilled, water for injection and zinc oxide. Hydrochloric acid 10% and/or sodium hydroxide 10% may be added to adjust pH. Cartridges of 3 mL, boxes of 5. Stylo Humalog Mix25 Pen (Turbo), prefilled pens of 3 mL, boxes of 5. KwikPen Humalog Mix25, prefilled pens of 3 mL, boxes of 5.

Humalog Mix50 : Each mL of 50% insulin lispro injection and 50% insulin lispro protamine suspension contains: human insulin analogue 100 units and protamine sulfate 0.19 mg. Nonmedicinal ingredients: dibasic sodium phosphate, glycerin, liquified phenol, m-cresol distilled, water for injection and zinc oxide. Hydrochloric acid 10% and/or sodium hydroxide 10% may be added to adjust pH. Cartridges of 3 mL, boxes of 5. KwikPen Humalog Mix50, prefilled pens of 3 mL, boxes of 5.

Stability and Storage Recommendations: Prior to first use, Humalog preparations must be stored in a refrigerator between 2 and 8°C. They should not be frozen or exposed to excessive heat or sunlight. Cartridges, vials, and prefilled pens that are in current use, should be stored at room temperature (below 30°C and away from direct heat and light) and discarded after 28 days. Do not use after expiry date on label.

Cartridges are designed for use with Lilly injector systems. The cartridge containing Humalog, Humalog Mix25, or Humalog Mix50 is not designed to allow any other insulin to be mixed in the cartridge or for the cartridge to be reused.

(Shown in Product Identification Section)

Humate-P®

antihemophilic factor/von Willebrand factor complex (human), dried, pasteurized

Blood Coagulation Factor

CSL Behring

Date of Revision: October 9, 2009

SUMMARY PRODUCT INFORMATION:

Route of Administration	Dosage Form/ Strength	Clinically Relevant Nonmedicinal Ingredients
Intravenous injection	Factor VIII/von Willebrand Facor Activity 250/600 IU/Vial, 500/1200 IU/Vial, 1000/2400 IU/Vial Dried, pasteurized preparation to be reconstituted with diluent prior to injection.	Glycine, albumin (Human), sodium chloride and sodium citrate For a complete listing, see Dosage Forms, Composition and Packaging.

DESCRIPTION: Antihemophilic Factor/von Willebrand Factor Complex (Human), Dried, Pasteurized, Humate-P is a stable, purified, sterile, lyophilized concentrate of Antihemophilic Factor (Human) and von Willebrand Factor (vWF) (Human) to be administered in the treatment of patients with classical hemophilia (hemophilia A) and von Willebrand disease (VWD).

INDICATIONS AND CLINICAL USE: Antihemophilic Factor/von Willebrand Factor Complex (Human), Dried, Pasteurized, Humate-P is indicated (1) in adult patients for treatment and prevention of bleeding in hemophilia A (classical hemophilia) and (2) in adult and pediatric patients (see Warnings and Precautions, Pediatrics) for treatment of spontaneous and trauma-induced bleeding episodes in severe von Willebrand disease, and in mild and moderate von Willebrand disease where use of desmopressin is known or suspected to be inadequate and (3) to prevent excessive bleeding (i.e. bleeding that exceeds the expected blood loss under a given condition) during and after surgery in adult and pediatric patients.

CONTRAINDICATIONS: None known, caution is advised in patients with a known allergic reaction to constituents of the preparation.

WARNINGS AND PRECAUTIONS:

> **Serious Warnings and Precautions**
> - Serious thromboembolic events have been reported in patients with von Willebrand disease who are treated with coagulation factor replacement therapy (see Cardiovascular).
> - May potentially contain infectious agents (see General).

General: It is important to determine that the coagulation disorder is caused by factor VIII or VWF deficiency, since no benefit in treating other deficiencies can be expected.

Antihemophilic Factor/von Willebrand Factor Complex (Human), Dried, Pasteurized, Humate-P is made from human plasma. Products made from large pools of human plasma may contain infectious agents, including the causative agents of hepatitis and other viruses that can cause disease. The risk that such products will transmit an infectious agent has been reduced by screening plasma donors for prior exposure to certain viruses, by testing for the presence of certain current viral infections and by inactivating and/or removing certain viruses during manufacture. The manufacturing procedure for Humate-P includes processing steps designed to reduce further the risk of viral transmission. Stringent procedures, utilized at plasma collection centers, plasma testing laboratories, and fractionation facilities are designed to reduce the risk of viral transmission. The primary viral reduction step of the Humate-P manufacturing process is the heat treatment of the purified, stabilized aqueous solution at 60.0+/−1°C for 10 hours. In addition, the purification procedure (several precipitation steps) used in the manufacture of Humate-P also provides viral reduction capacity. Despite these measures, such products may still potentially contain human pathogenic agents, including those not yet known or identified. Thus the risk of transmission of infectious agents cannot be totally eliminated.

Some viruses, such as parvovirus B19 or hepatitis A, are particularly difficult to remove or inactivate at this time. Parvovirus B19 may most seriously affect pregnant women, or immune-compromised individuals and may induce red cell aplasia in some of these patients.

Although the overwhelming number of hepatitis A and parvovirus B19 cases are community acquired, there have been reports of these infections associated with the use of some plasma-derived products. Therefore, physicians should be alert to the potential symptoms of parvovirus B19 and hepatitis A infections and inform patients under their supervision receiving plasma-derived products to report potential symptoms promptly.

Symptoms of parvovirus B19 may include low-grade fever, rash, arthralgias and transient symmetric, nondestructive arthritis. Diagnosis is often established by measuring B19 specific IgM and IgG antibodies. Symptoms of hepatitis A include low grade fever, anorexia, nausea, vomiting, fatigue and jaundice. A diagnosis may be established by determination of specific IgM antibodies.

Because Humate-P is made from human blood; it may carry a risk of transmitting infectious agents, e.g. viruses, and theoretically, the Creutzfeldt-Jakob Disease (CJD) agent. Any infections thought by a physician possibly to have been transmitted by this product should be reported by the physician or other healthcare provider to CSL Behring at 1-613-783-1892. The physician should discuss the risks and benefits of this product with the patient.

Patients who are undergoing treatment using a therapeutic product derived from human blood or plasma should be appropriately vaccinated.

Other precautions are as follows:

- The administration equipment and any unused Humate-P should be discarded.

Cardiovascular: Serious thromboembolic events have been reported in VWD patients receiving coagulation factor replacement therapy, especially in the setting of known risk factors for thrombosis. In these patients caution should be exercised and antithrombotic measures and FVIII monitoring should be considered.

Hematologic: This Antihemophilic Factor/von Willebrand Factor (Human), Dried, Pasteurized, Humate-P preparation contains blood group isoagglutinins (anti-A and anti-B). When very large or frequently repeated doses are needed, as when inhibitors are present or when pre- and post- surgical care is involved, patients of blood groups A, B and AB should be monitored for signs of intravascular hemolysis and decreasing hematocrit values and be treated appropriately as required.

Special Populations: Pregnant Women: Animal reproduction studies have not been conducted with Antihemophilic Factor/von Willebrand Factor (Human). It is also not known whether Humate-P can cause fetal harm when administered to a pregnant woman or can affect reproduction capacity. Humate-P should be given to a pregnant woman only if clearly needed and the expected benefit outweighs any potential risks.

Pediatrics: Hemophilia A: Adequate and well-controlled studies with long term evaluation of joint damage have not been done in pediatric patients. Joint damage may result from suboptimal treatment of hemarthroses. For immediate control of bleeding for Hemophilia A, the general recommendations for dosing and administration for adults, found in the Dosage and Administration, may be referenced.

Von Willebrand Disease: The safety and effectiveness of Humate-P for the treatment of von Willebrand's disease was demonstrated in 26 pediatric patients, including infants, children and adolescents but has not yet been evaluated in neonates. The safety of Humate-P for the prevention of excessive bleeding during and after a surgery was demonstrated in 8 pediatric subjects (age 3-15) with VWD. Of the 34 pediatric studied for both treatment of von Willebrand disease and prevention of excessive bleeding during and after surgery, 4 were infants (1 month old to under 2 years of age), 23 were children (2 through 12 years old), and 7 were adolescents (13 through 15 years old). As in adults, pediatric patients should be dosed based upon weight (kg) in accordance to information in Dosage and Administration.

Monitoring and Laboratory Tests: Strong consideration should be given to monitoring vWF:RCof and F-VIII levels in VWD patients receiving Humate-P for the prevention of excessive bleeding during and after surgery. It is advisable to monitor trough vWF:RCof and FVIII:C levels at least once daily in order to adjust the dosage of Humate-P as needed, to avoid excessive accumulation of coagulation factors.

Interactions with Other Agents: There are no known interactions of Antihemophilic Factor/von Willebrand Factor Complex (Human), Dried, Pasteurized, Humate-P with other agents.

ADVERSE REACTIONS: Adverse Drug Reaction Overview: Antihemophilic Factor/von Willebrand Factor (Human), Dried, Pasteurized, Humate-P is usually tolerated without reaction. Cases of allergic reaction and rise in temperature have been observed. Anaphylactic reactions can occur in rare instances. If allergic/anaphylactic reactions occur, the infusion should be discontinued and appropriate treatment given as required.

In some cases, inhibitors of Factor VIII may occur.

Clinical Trial Adverse Drug Reactions: Because clinical trials are conducted under very specific conditions the adverse reaction rates observed in the clinical trials may not reflect the rates observed in practice and should not be compared to the rates in the clinical trials of another drug. Adverse drug reaction information from clinical trials is useful for identifying drug-related adverse events and for approximating rates.

Allergic symptoms, including allergic reaction, urticaria, chest tightness, rash, pruritus, and edema, were reported in 6 of 97 (6%) of patients in a Canadian retrospective study. Two of 97 (2%) experienced other adverse events that were considered to have a possible or probable relationship to the product. These included chills, phlebitis, vasodilatation, and paresthesia. All adverse events were mild or moderate in intensity.

In a study of 71 VWD patients, the safety of Humate-P was evaluated in 53 serious bleeding events and 42 surgical events. Nine (9/95, 9.5%) adverse events were considered to have a possible or probable relationship to the product and included mild allergic reaction, paresthesia, vasodilatation, peripheral edema, extremity pain, pseudothrombocytopenia and pruritus. Seven (7/95, 7.4%) serious adverse events were considered non-related and included menorrhagia, anemia, hemorrhage, abdominal pain, infection, abnormal wound healing and pneumonia.

VWD Subjects Undergoing Surgery: Among 63 VWD subjects who received Humate-P for prevention of excessive bleeding during and after surgery, including 1 subject who underwent colonoscopy without the planned polypectomy, the most common adverse events were postoperative bleeding (35 events in 19 subjects with five subjects experiencing bleeding at up to three different sites), postoperative nausea (15 subjects), and postoperative pain (11 subjects). Postoperative bleeding adverse events are shown in Table 1. Although these events were not considered by the investigators as the result of ineffective hemostasis, the lack of efficacy due to inadequate dosing or duration of treatment is a possible risk factor. Even though dosage values are given in Dosage and Administration, the clinical effect of Humate-P remains the single most important factor to determine adequacy of treatment, thus the dosage should be adjusted as needed.

Table 2 lists the non-hemorrhagic adverse events reported in at least two subjects, regardless of causality, and the adverse events that were possibly related to Humate-P. A pulmonary embolus that was considered possibly related to Humate-P occurred in one elderly subject who underwent bilateral knee replacement.

Eight subjects experienced 10 post-operative serious adverse events: one with subdural hematoma and intracerebral bleeding following intracranial surgery related to an underlying cerebrovascular abnormality; one with two occurrences of gastrointestinal bleeding following gastrojejunal bypass; and one each with sepsis, facial edema, infection, menorrhagia requiring hysteroscopy and dilatation and curettage, pyelonephritis, and pulmonary embolus.

Post-Market Adverse Drug Reactions: During post-marketing surveillance, especially in the setting of known risk factors for thrombosis, serious thromboembolic complications in VWD patients receiving coagulation factor replacement therapy have been reported (see Warnings and Precautions, Cardiovascular).

DOSAGE AND ADMINISTRATION: General: Physicians should strongly consider administration of hepatitis A and hepatitis B vaccines to individuals receiving plasma derivatives. Potential risks and benefits of vaccination should be carefully weighed by the physician and discussed with the patient.

Each vial of Humate-P contains the labeled amount of Factor VIII activity in IU for the treatment of hemophilia A. Additionally, each vial of Humate-P also contains VWF:RCo activity in IU for the treatment of VWD.

Recommended Dose and Dosage Adjustment: Therapy for Hemophilia A: As a general rule, 1 IU of Factor VIII activity per kg body weight will increase the circulating Factor VIII level by approximately 2 IU/dL. Adequacy of treatment must be judged by the clinical effects; thus, the dosage may vary with individual cases. Although dosage must be individualized according to the needs of the patient (weight, severity of hemorrhage, presence of inhibitors), the following general dosages are recommended for adult patients: see Table 3.

Table 1: Humate-P

Bleeding Adverse Events in 63 Surgical Subjects

Adverse Events	Surgical Procedure Category	Number of Subjects/ Events	Onset[a] (Number of Events)		Severity (Number of Events)		
			On	Post	Mild	Mod	Severe
Wound/injection site bleeding	Major	8/11	7	4	9	—	2
	Minor	2/2	2	—	1	1	—
	Oral	2/6	—	6	3	3	—
Epistaxis	Major	4/4	2	2	3	1	—
	Minor	1/1	1	—	1	—	—
Cerebral hemorrhage/subdural hematoma	Major	1/2	2[b]	—	—	2	—
Gastrointestinal bleeding	Major	1/3	32[c]	—	—	2	1
Menorrhagia	Major	1/1	1[d]	—	—	1	—
Groin bleed	Oral	1/1	—	1	1	—	—
Ear bleed	Major	1/1	1	—	1	—	—
Hemoptysis	Major	1/1	1	—	1	—	—
Hematuria	Major	1/1	1	—	1	—	—
Shoulder bleed	Major	1/1	1	—	1	—	—

[a] On=on-therapy; onset while receiving Humate-P or within 1 day of completing Humate-P administration. Post=post-therapy; onset at least one day after completing Humate-P administration.
[b] Reported as serious adverse events after intracranial surgery.
[c] Two of these events reported as serious adverse events occurring after gastrojejunal bypass.
[d] Reported as serious adverse events requiring hysterectomy after hysteroscopy and dilation and curettage.

Table 2: Humate-P

Non-Hemorrhagic and Possibly Related Adverse Events (AE) in 63 Surgical Subjects

Body System	Adverse Event	Number of Subjects with an AE Possibly Related to Humate-P	Number of Subjects with an AE Regardless of Causality[a]
Body as a whole	Pain	—	11
	Fever	—	4
	Abdominal pain	—	3
	Infection	—	3
	Surgery	—	3
	Back pain	—	2
	Facial edema	—	2
Cardiovascular	Chest pain	—	3
	Pulmonary embolus[b]	1	1
	Thrombophlebitis[b]	1	1
Digestive	Nausea	1	15
	Constipation	—	7
	Vomiting	1	3
	Sore throat	—	2
Hemic and lymphatic system	Anemia/decreased hemoglobin	—	2
Metabolic/nutritional	Increase ALT	1	1

(cont'd)

Table 2: Humate-P (cont'd)

Non-Hemorrhagic and Possibly Related Adverse Events (AE) in 63 Surgical Subjects

Body System	Adverse Event	Number of Subjects with an AE Possibly Related to Humate-P	Number of Subjects with an AE Regardless of Causality[a]
Nervous	Dizziness	1	5
	Headache	1	4
	Increase sweating	—	3
	Insomnia	—	2
Skin and appendages	Pruritus	—	3
	Rash	1	1
Urogenital	Urinary retention	—	4
	Urinary tract infection	—	2

[a] Occuring in two or more subjects.
[b] These events occurred in separate subjects.

Table 3: Humate-P

Dosage Recommendations for the Treatment of Hemophilia A

Hemorrhagic Event	Dosage (IU FVIII:C/kg body weight)
Minor hemorrhage: • Early joint or muscle bleed • Severe epistaxis	Loading dose 15 IU FVIII:C/kg to achieve FVIII:C plasma level of approximately 30% of normal; one infusion may be sufficient. If needed, half of the loading dose may be given once or twice daily for 1–2 days.
Moderate hemorrhage: • Advanced joint or muscle bleed • Neck, tongue or pharyngeal hematoma (without airway compromise) • Tooth extraction • Severe abdominal pain	Loading dose 25 IU FVIII:C/kg to achieve FVIII:C plasma level of approximately 50% of normal, followed by 15 IU FVIII:C/kg every 8–12 hours for first 1–2 days to maintain FVIII:C plasma level at 30% of normal, and then the same dose once or twice a day for a total of up to 7 days, or until adequate wound healing.
Life-threatening hemorrhage: • Major operations • Gastrointestinal bleeding • Neck, tongue or pharyngeal hematoma with potential for airway compromise • Intracranial, intraabdominal or intrathoracic bleeding • Fractures	Initially 40 to 50 IU FVIII:C/kg, followed by 20–25 IU FVIII:C/kg every 8 hours to maintain FVIII:C plasma level at 80–100% of normal for 7 days, then continue the same dose once or twice a day for another 7 days in order to maintain the FVIII:C level at 30–50% of normal.

In all cases, the dose should be adjusted individually by clinical judgement of the potential for compromise of a vital structure, and by frequent monitoring of factor VIII activity in the patient's plasma.

Pediatric Use for Hemophilia A: See Warnings and Precautions.

Therapy for von Willebrand Disease: The dosage should be adjusted according to the extent and location of bleeding. As a rule, 40-80 IU VWF:RCo per kg body weight are given every 8 to 12 hours. Repeat doses are administered for as long as needed based on repeat monitoring of appropriate clinical and laboratory measures. Expected levels of VWF:RCo are based on an expected in vivo recovery of 2.0 IU/dL rise per IU/kg VWF:RCo administered. The administration of 1 IU of Factor VIII per kg body weight can be expected to lead to a rise in circulating VWF:RCo of approximately 5 IU/dL.Table 4 provides dosing guidelines for pediatric and adult patients.

Table 4: Humate-P

Dosing Recommendations for the Treatment of von Willebrand Disease

Classification of VWD	Hemorrhage	Dosage (IU VWF:RCo/kg body weight)
Type 1		
• Mild, if desmopressin is inappropriate (Baseline VWF:RCo activity typically >30%)	Major (e.g. severe or refractory epistaxis, GI bleeding, CNS trauma, or traumatic hemorrhage)	40 to 50 IU/kg every 8 to 12 hours for 3 days to keep the nadir level of VWF:RCo >50%; then 40 to 50 IU/kg daily for a total of up to 7 days of treatment.
• Moderate or severe (Baseline VWF:RCo activity typically <30%)	Minor (e.g. epistaxis, oral bleeding, menorrhagia)	40 to 50 IU/kg (1 or 2 doses)
	Major (e.g. severe or refractory epistaxis, GI bleeding, CNS trauma, hemarthrosis or traumatic hemorrhage	40 to 60 IU/kg every 8 to 12 hours for 3 days to keep the nadir level of VWF:RCo >50%; then 40 to 60 IU/kg daily for a total of up to 7 days of treatment. Factor VIII:C levels should be monitored and maintained according to the guidelines for hemophilia A therapy, see Table 3.
Types 2 (all variants) and 3	Minor (clinical indications above)	40 to 50 IU/kg (1 or 2 doses)
	Major (clinical indications above)	40 to 80 IU/kg every 8 to 12 hours for 3 days to keep the nadir level of VWF:RCo >50%; then 40 to 60 IU/kg daily for a total of up to 7 days of treatment. Factor VIII:C levels should be monitored and maintained according to the guidelines for hemophilia A therapy, see Table 3.

For additional information, see the Clinical Practice Guidelines; Hemophilia and von Willebrand Disease; 2. Management by the Association of Hemophilia Clinic Directors of Canada, Edition 2, Update 2, July 7, 1999.

Prevention of Excessive Bleeding During and After Surgery in VWD: The following information provides guidelines for calculating loading and maintenance doses of Humate-P for patients undergoing surgery. However **in the case of emergency surgery**, administer a loading dose of 50 to 60 IU/kg and, subsequently, closely monitor the patient's through coagulation factor levels.

When possible, it is recommended that the incremental in vivo recovery (IVR) be measured and that baseline plasma vWF:RCof and FVIII:C be assessed in all patients prior a surgery. Measure IVR as follows:

1. Measure baseline plasma vWF:RCof.
2. Infuse 60 IU vWF:RCof/kg b.w. intravenously at time 0.
3. At time +30 minutes, measure plasma vWF:RCof.

IVR = (plasma $\text{vWF:RCof}_{\text{time+ 30 min}}$—plasma $\text{vWF:RCof}_{\text{baseline}}$)/60 IU/kg

Calculation of the loading dose requires four values: the target peak plasma vWF:RCof level, the baseline vWF:RCof level, body weight (bw) in kilograms, and IVR. When individual values are not available (e.g. in the case of emergency surgery), a standardized loading dose can be used based on an assumed vWF:RCof IVR of 2.0 IU/dL per IU/kg of vWF:RCof product administered. Table 5 provides dosing guidelines for adults and pediatric patients.

Table 5: Humate-P

vWF:RCof and FVIII:C Loading Dose Recommendations for the Prevention of Excessive Bleeding During and After Surgery

Type of Surgery	vWF:RCof Target Peak Plasma Level	FVIII:C Target Peak Plasma Level	Calculation of Loading Dose (to be administered 1 to 2 hours before surgery)
Major	100 IU/dL	80–100 IU/dL	Δ[a] vWF:RCof×BW (kg)/IVR[b]=IU vWF:RCof required If the incremental IVR is not available (e.g. in the case of emergency surgery), assume an IVR of 2 IU/dL per IU/kg and calculate the loading dose as follows: (100–baseline plasma vWF:RCof)×BW (in kg)/2.0
Minor/oral[c]	50–60 IU/dL	40–50 IU/dL	Δ[a] vWF:RCof×BW (kg)/IVR[b]=IU vWF:RCof required

[a] Δ=Target peak plasma vWF:RCof-baseline plasma vWF:RCof.
[b] IVR= Incremental recovery as measured in the patient.
[c] Oral surgery is defined as removal of fewer than three teeth, if the teeth are non-molars and have no bony involvement. Removal of more than one impacted wisdom tooth is considered major surgery due to the expected difficulty of the surgery and the expected blood loss, particularly in subjects with type 2A or type 3 VWD. Removal of more than two teeth is considered major surgery in all patients.

For example, the loading dose of Humate-P required assuming a target vWF:RCof level of 100 IU/dL, baseline vWF:RCof level 20 IU/dL, an IVR of 2.0 (IU/dL)/(IU/kg), Δ of 80 IU/dL, and a body weight of 70 kg would be calculated as follows: (80 IU/dL×70 kg)/2 (IU/dL)/(IU/kg) = 2800 IU vWF:RCof required.

For FVIII:C, attaining peak plasma level of 80 to 100 IU FVIII:C/dL for major surgery and 40 to 50 IU FVIII:C/dL for minor surgery or oral surgery might require additional dosing with Humate-P. Because the ratio of vWF:RCof to FVIII:C activity in Humate-P is approximately 2.4 to 1, any additional dosing will increase vWF:RCof proportionally more than FVIII:C. Assuming an incremental IVR of 2.0 IU vWF:RCof/dL per IU/kg infused, additional dosing to increase FVIII:C in plasma will also increase plasma vWF:RCof by approximately 5 IU/dL for each IU/kg of FVIII:C administered.

The initial maintenance dose for the prevention of excessive bleeding during and after surgery should be half the loading dose, irrespective of additional dosing required to meet FVIII:C targets. Table 6 provides recommendations for target through plasma levels (based on the type of surgery and the number of days following surgery) and minimum duration of treatment for subsequent maintenance doses. These recommendations apply to both adult and pediatric patients.

Based on individual pharmacokinetic-derived half-lives, the frequency of maintenance doses is generally every 8 to 12 hours; patients with shorter half-lives may require dosing every 6 hours. In the absence of pharmacokinetic data, it is recommended that Humate-P be administered initially every 8 hours with further adjustments determined by monitoring trough coagulation factor levels.

Table 6: Humate-P

vWF:RCof and FVIII:C Target Through Plasma Level and Minimum Duration of Treatment Recommendations for Subsequent Maintenance Doses for the Prevention of Excessive Bleeding During and After Surgery

	vWF:RCof Target Trough Plasma Levels[a]		FVIII:C Target Trough Plasma Levels[a]		
Type of Surgery	Up to 3 Days Following Surgery	After Day 3	Up to 3 Days Following Surgery	After Day 3	Minimum Duration of Treatment
Major	>50 IU/dL	>30 IU/dL	>50 IU/dL	>30 IU/dL	72 hours
Minor	≥30 IU/dL			>30 IU/dL	48 hours
Oral[b]	≥30 IU/dL			>30 IU/dL	8–12 hours[c]

[a] Trough levels for either coagulation factor should not exceed 100 IU/dL.
[b] Oral surgery is defined as removal of fewer than three teeth, if the teeth are non-molars and have no bony involvement. Removal of more than one impacted wisdom tooth is considered major surgery due to the expected difficulty of the surgery and the expected blood loss, particularly in subjects with type 2A or type 3 VWD. Removal of more than two teeth is considered major surgery in all patients.
[c] At least one maintenance dose following surgery based on individual pharmacokinetic values.

It is advisable to monitor trough vWF:RCof and FVIII:C levels at least once daily in order to adjust Humate-P dosing as needed to avoid excessive accumulation of coagulation factors. The duration of the treatment generally depends on the type of surgery performed, but must be assessed for individual patients based on their hemostatic response.

For use in pediatric VWD patients, see Warnings and Precautions, Special Populations, Pediatrics.

Administration: Antihemophilic Factor/von Willebrand Factor Complex (Human), Dried, Pasteurized, Humate-P is for **intravenous administration** only.

To assure product sterility, Humate-P should be administered within 3 hours after reconstitution.

Slowly inject the solution (maximally 4 mL/minute) intravenously with a venipuncture set or with another suitable injection set. Discard the administration equipment and any unused Humate-P after use.

Reconstitution: Plastic disposable syringes are recommended for withdrawal and administration of Humate-P solution. Protein solutions of this type tend to adhere to the ground glass surface of all-glass syringes.

1. Before infusion, ensure that Humate-P and diluent are at room temperature.
2. Remove caps from both vials to expose central portions of the rubber stoppers.
3. Treat surface of rubber stoppers with an antiseptic solution such as an alcohol swab and allow to dry prior to opening the Mix2Vial package.
4. Open the Mix2Vial package by peeling away the lid. To maintain sterility, leave the Mix2Vial in the clear outer packaging. Place the diluent vial on an even surface and hold the vial tight. Grip the Mix2Vial together with the clear packaging and firmly snap the blue end onto the diluent stopper.
5. While holding onto the diluent vial, carefully remove the clear outer packaging from the Mix2Vial set. Make sure that you only pull up the clear outer packaging and not the Mix2Vial set.

6. With the product vial firmly on a surface, invert the diluent vial with set attached and firmly snap the transparent adapter onto the product vial stopper. The diluent will automatically transfer into the product vial.
7. With the diluent and product vial still attached, gently swirl the product vial to ensure the product is fully dissolved. Do not shake vial.
8. With one hand grasp the product-side of the Mix2Vial set and with the other hand grasp the blue diluent-side of the Mix2Vial set and unscrew the set into two pieces.
9. Draw air into an empty, sterile syringe. While the product vial is upright, screw the syringe to the Mix2Vial set. Inject air into the product vial. While keeping the syringe plunger pressed, invert the system upside down and draw the concentrate into the syringe by pulling the plunger back slowly.
10. Now that the concentrate has been transferred into the syringe, firmly grasp the barrel of the syringe (keeping the syringe plunger facing down) and unscrew the syringe from the Mix2Vial. Attach the syringe to a venipuncture set.
11. If the same patient is to receive concentrate from more than one vial, the contents of two vials may be drawn into the same syringe through a separate unused Mix2Vial set before attaching the vein needle.
12. Parenteral drug products should be inspected visually for particulate matter and discoloration prior to administration, whenever solution and container permit. When the reconstitution procedure is precisely followed, it is not uncommon for a few small flakes or particles to remain. Mix2Vial set provided with Humate-P should remove those particles and this should not influence dosage calculations.

Do not refrigerate after reconstitution. To assure product sterility, Humate-P should be administered within three hours after reconstitution.

OVERDOSAGE:
No symptoms of overdose with Antihemophilic Factor/von Willebrand Factor Complex, (Human), Dried, Pasteurized, Humate-P are known so far.

For management of a suspected drug overdose, CPhA recommends that you contact your **regional Poison Control Centre**. See the *CPS* Directory section for a list of Poison Control Centres.

ACTION AND CLINICAL PHARMACOLOGY: Hemophilia A is a hereditary disorder of blood coagulation associated with a deficiency of antihemophilic factor VIII activity. It manifests most frequently in males and results in bleeding into joints, muscles or internal organs. Female carriers may also be at risk with surgery.

Factor VIII is essential to the intrinsic pathway of blood coagulation in the activation of factor X, ultimately leading to the conversion of prothrombin to thrombin, thus maintaining effective haemostasis.

VWD is caused by quantitative or qualitative abnormalities of the vWF, a protein present in plasma and platelets in the form of multimers of which the high molecular weight multimers support platelet adhesion to the subendothelium.

Pharmacodynamics: In severe forms of VWD and in these forms where the vWF is qualitatively abnormal (e.g. type II VWD), the use of plasma-derived products is a prerequisite for normalization of the bleeding time. Humate-P has been shown to contain vWF with a multimeric pattern similar to that of normal plasma. When administered to patients with VWD [types 1, 2 (A,B,C), 3] effective haemostasis was achieved, as evidenced by decreased bleeding time. This effect was correlated with the presence of a multimeric composition of vWF similar to that found in normal plasma.

Pharmacokinetics: Pharmacokinetics in Hemophilia A: After intravenous injection of Humate-P in humans, there is a rapid increase in the plasma level of antihemophilic factor followed by a rapid decrease in activity (time of equilibration with the extravascular compartment) and a subsequent slower rate of decrease in activity (biological half-life). Studies with Humate-P in hemophilic patients have demonstrated a mean initial half-disappearance time of 8 hours and a mean biological half-life of 12.2 hours (range: 8.4 to 17.4 hours).

Pharmacokinetics in von Willebrand Disease: Humate-P has been demonstrated in several studies to contain the high-molecular-weight multimers of vWF. This component is reported to be important for correcting the coagulation defect in patients with VWD.

When administered to patients with VWD (types 1, 2 [A, B, C], or 3), bleeding time decreased. This effect was correlated with the presence of a multimeric composition of vWF similar to that found in normal plasma.

Pharmacokinetic studies of Humate-P have been performed with cohorts of subjects in the non-bleeding state. Wide inter-subject variability was observed in pharmacokinetic values obtained from these studies.

The pharmacokinetics of Humate-P were evaluated in 41 subjects in a prospective US study in the non-bleeding state prior to a surgical procedure. Subjects received 60 IU vWF:RCof/kg body weight of Humate-P. Sixteen subjects had type 1 VWD, two had type 2A, four had type 2B, six had type 2M, and 13 had type 3. The median terminal half-life of vWF:RCof was 11 hours (range: 3.5 to 33.6 hours), excluding five subjects with a half-life exceeding the blood sampling time of 24 or 48 hours. The median clearance and volume of distribution at steady sate were 3.1 mL/hr/kg (range 1 to 16.6 mL/hr/kg) and 53 mL/kg (range 29 to 141 mL/kg), respectively. The median in vivo recovery for vWF:RCof activity was 2.4 IU/dL per IU/kg (range: 1.1 to 4.2). High molecular weight multimers were measured in 13 subjects with type 3 VWD; 11 had absent or barely detectable multimers at baseline. Of those 11 subjects, all had some high molecular weight multimers present 24 hours after infusion of Humate-P.

Pharmacokinetics were also evaluated in 28 subjects in a European study in the non-bleeding state prior to a surgical procedure. Subjects received 80 IU vWF:RCof/kg body weight of Humate-P. Ten subjects had type 1 VWD, 10 had type 2A, one had type 2M, and seven had type 3. The median terminal half-life of vWF:RCof was 10 hours (range: 2.8 to 28.3 hours) excluding one subject with a half-life exceeding the blood sampling time of 48 hours. The median clearance and volume of distribution at steady state were 4.8 mL/hr/kg (range: 2.1 to 53 mL/hr/kg) and 59 mL/kg (range: 32 to 290 mL/kg), respectively. The median in vivo recovery for vWF:RCof activity was 1.9 IU/dL per IU/kg (range: 0.6 to 4.5). Infusion of Humate-P corrected the defect of the multimer pattern in subjects with types 2A and 3 VWD. High molecular weight multimers were detectable until at least 8 hours after infusion.

Based on the small sample size evaluation, it appears that age, sex and types of VWD have no impact on the pharmacokinetics of vWF:RCof.

STORAGE AND STABILITY: When stored at room temperature, up to 25°C, Humate-P is stable for the period indicated by the expiration date on its label. Avoid freezing, which may damage the diluent container.

INFORMATION FOR THE PATIENT: Published in e-CPS, available by subscription at www.e-cps.ca.

DOSAGE FORMS, COMPOSITION AND PACKAGING: Humate-P is purified from the cold insoluble fraction of pooled human fresh-frozen plasma and contains highly purified and concentrated Antihemophilic Factor/von Willebrand Factor Complex (Human). Humate-P has a high degree of purity with a low amount of non-factor proteins. Fibrinogen is less than or equal to 0.2 mg/mL. Humate-P has a higher factor potency than cryoprecipitate preparations. Each vial of Humate-P contains the labeled amount of Factor VIII activity in international units. Additionally, each vial of Humate-P also contains the labeled amount of von Willebrand factor: Ristocetin Cofactor (vWF:RCof) activity expressed in IU (see Dosage and Administration). An international unit (IU) is defined by current international standards. One IU Factor VIII or 1 IU vWF:RCof is approximately equal to the level of Factor VIII or vWF:RCof found in 1.0 mL of fresh-pooled human plasma.

This product is prepared from pooled human plasma collected from U.S. licensed facilities in the U.S.

Antihemophilic Factor/von Willebrand Factor Complex (Human), Dried, Pasteurized, Humate-P is supplied in a single dose vial with a vial of diluent containing sterile water (meets USP chemistry requirements for Sterile Water for Injection, except for pH; pH 4.5-8.5), Mix2Vial, a needleless filter transfer device for reconstitution and withdrawal of the product. International unit activity of Factor VIII and VWF:RCo is stated on the carton and label of each vial.

The reconstituted preparations have the following antihemophilic factor and vWF:RCof activity per mL:

Vial size (IU/vial) (F VIII:C/ vWF:RCof)	Volume of Diluent to be Added to Vial	Approximate Available Volume	Concentration (IU/mL) (F VIII:C/vWF:RCof)
250/600	5 mL	5 mL	50/120
500/1200	10 mL	10 mL	50/120
1000/2400	15 mL	15 mL	67/160

Upon reconstitution with the volume of diluent provided [Diluent (sterile water)], each mL of Humate-P contains 40 to 80 IU Factor VIII activity, 72 to 224 IU vWF:RCof activity, 8 to 16 mg of Albumin (Human), 15 to 33 mg of glycine, 2 to 5.3 mg of sodium chloride, <0.1 µg aluminum, 3.5 to 9.3 mg of sodium citrate, 2 to 14 mg of other proteins, and 10 to 30 mg of total proteins. Humate-P contains no preservative. To assure product sterility, Humate-P should be administered within 3 hours after reconstitution.

Humatrope® Ⓟ
somatropin
Growth Stimulant

Lilly

Date of Revision: July 13, 2010

SUMMARY PRODUCT INFORMATION:

Route of Administration	Dosage Form/Strength (1 mg=3 IU)	Clinically Relevant Nonmedicinal Ingredients
Subcutaneous	Sterile lyophilized powder in: Vials: 2 mg (~6 IU), 5 mg (~15 IU) Cartridges: 6 mg (~18 IU), 12 mg (~36 IU) 24 mg (~72 IU)	Supplied with diluent that contains metacresol and glycerin. For a complete listing, see Dosage Forms, Composition and Packaging.

DESCRIPTION: HUMATROPE (somatropin for injection) is a polypeptide hormone of recombinant DNA origin. The amino acid sequence is identical to that of human growth hormone of pituitary origin. HUMATROPE is synthesized in a strain of *E. coli* which has been modified by the addition of the gene for human growth hormone.

INDICATIONS AND CLINICAL USE: Pediatrics: Growth Hormone Deficiency: HUMATROPE (somatropin for injection) is indicated for the long-term treatment of pediatric patients who have growth failure due to an inadequate secretion of normal endogenous growth hormone and whose epiphyses are not closed.

Turner Syndrome: HUMATROPE is indicated for the treatment of short stature associated with Turner syndrome in patients whose epiphyses are not closed.

Patients with Idiopathic Short Stature (ISS): HUMATROPE is indicated for the long-term treatment of idiopathic short stature defined by:
- normal birth weight,
- careful diagnostic evaluation that excludes other known causes of short stature that should be either observed or treated by other means,
- height at least 2.25 standard deviation scores (SDS) below the mean for age and sex,
- height velocity below the 25th percentile for bone age and sex over 12 months of observation and unlikely to permit attainment of adult height in the expected range.

HUMATROPE treatment for idiopathic short stature should be prescribed only for those patients whose epiphyses are not closed and should be managed by physicians who have sufficient knowledge of idiopathic short stature and the efficacy/safety profile of HUMATROPE.

Patients with Short Stature Homeobox-containing Gene (SHOX) Deficiency: HUMATROPE is indicated for the treatment of short stature or growth failure in children with SHOX (short stature homeobox-containing gene) deficiency whose epiphyses are not closed.

Small for Gestational Age (SGA): HUMATROPE is indicated for the treatment of growth failure in children born small for gestational age (birth weight and/or length below −2 SD) and who fail to achieve catch-up growth by 2 to 4 years or later.

Adult Patients: HUMATROPE is indicated for replacement of endogenous growth hormone in adults with growth hormone deficiency, who meet either of the following two criteria:
1. **Adult Onset:** Patients must have somatotropin deficiency syndrome, either alone or associated with multiple hormone deficiencies (hypopituitarism), as a result of pituitary disease, hypothalamic disease, surgery, radiation therapy, or trauma; **or**
2. **Childhood Onset:** Patients who were growth hormone-deficient during childhood as a result of congenital, genetic, acquired, or idiopathic causes.

Confirmation of the diagnosis of adult growth hormone deficiency in both groups by appropriate growth hormone stimulation test is usually required. However, confirmatory growth hormone stimulation testing may not be required in patients with congenital/genetic growth hormone deficiency or multiple pituitary hormone deficiencies due to organic disease.

CONTRAINDICATIONS: Somatropin should not be initiated to treat patients with acute critical illness due to complications following open heart or abdominal surgery, multiple accidental trauma, or to patients having acute respiratory failure (see Warnings and Precautions, General).

Somatropin is contraindicated in patients with Prader-Willi syndrome who are severely obese or have severe respiratory impairment (see Warnings and Precautions, General, Congenital Disorders). HUMATROPE (somatropin for injection) is not indicated for the long-term treatment of pediatric patients who have growth failure due to genetically confirmed Prader-Willi syndrome

HUMATROPE should not be used for growth promotion in pediatric patients with closed epiphyses.

HUMATROPE should not be used or should be discontinued when there is any evidence of active malignancy. Anti-malignancy treatment must be complete with evidence of remission prior to the institution of therapy.

HUMATROPE should not be used in patients with active intracranial tumour (see Warnings and Precautions).

For patients with a known sensitivity to either metacresol or glycerin, HUMATROPE should not be reconstituted with the supplied diluent for HUMATROPE (see Warnings and Precautions, Sensitivity/Resistance; Dosage and Administration, Reconstitution and Specific Precautions).

WARNINGS AND PRECAUTIONS: General: HUMATROPE (somatropin for injection) therapy should be directed by physicians experienced in the diagnosis and management of patients with growth hormone deficiency, Turner syndrome, idiopathic short stature, SHOX deficiency, children born small for gestational age, or adult patients with either childhood-onset or adult-onset growth hormone deficiency.

If home use is determined to be desirable by the physician, instructions on appropriate use should be given, including a review of the Information for the Patient.

It is recommended that insulin-like growth factor-I (IGF-I) concentrations be monitored regularly and maintained within the normal range for age and sex.

Pharmacologic glucocorticoid therapy and supraphysiologic glucocorticoid treatment may attenuate the growth promoting effects of somatropin in children. Therefore, glucocorticoid replacement dosing should be carefully adjusted in children receiving concomitant somatropin and glucocorticoid treatments to avoid both hypoadrenalism and an inhibitory effect on growth (see Drug Interations, Drug-Drug Interactions).

HUMATROPE should be administered by subcutaneous injection, with regular rotation of injection sites to prevent lipoatrophy.

Acute Critical Illnesses: In 2 placebo-controlled trials in non-growth hormone deficient adults (N=522), a significant increase in mortality was reported among somatropin treated patients with acute critical illnesses in intensive care units due to complications following open heart surgery or abdominal surgery, multiple accidental trauma or acute respiratory failure (41.9%), compared with those receiving placebo (19.3%). Doses of 5.3 to 8.0 mg/day were given (see Contraindications). The safety of continuing somatropin in patients receiving replacement doses for approved indications who concurrently develop these illnesses has not been established. Therefore, the potential benefit of treatment continuation with somatropin in patients having acute critical illnesses should be weighed against the potential risk.

Pre-existing Tumours or Growth Hormone Deficiency Secondary to an Intracranial Tumour: Patients with pre-existing tumours or with growth hormone deficiency secondary to an intracranial tumour should be examined routinely for progression or recurrence of the underlying disease process.
- In pediatric patients, clinical literature has demonstrated no relationship between somatropin therapy and CNS tumour recurrence.
- In adults, it is unknown whether there is any relationship between somatropin therapy and CNS tumour recurrence.

Carcinogenesis and Mutagenesis: Long-term animal studies for carcinogenicity with this human growth hormone (HUMATROPE) have not been performed. There has been no evidence to date of HUMATROPE-induced mutagenicity. Patients developing neoplasia should be reported to the Health Products and Food Branch (HPFB) by the treating physician.

Leukemia has been reported in a small number of children who have been treated with growth hormone, including growth hormone of pituitary origin as well as of recombinant DNA origin (somatrem and somatropin). The relationship, if any, between leukemia and somatropin therapy continues to be uncertain.

In childhood cancer survivors, an increased risk of a second neoplasm (benign and malignant) has been reported in patients treated with somatropin. Intracranial tumours, in particular meningiomas in patients treated with radiation to the head for their first neoplasm, were the most common of these second neoplasms. However, in childhood cancer survivors, no increased risk of primary cancer recurrence has been reported with somatropin treatment.

Congenital Disorders: Prader-Willi Syndrome (see Contraindications): There have been reports of sleep apnea and fatalities after initiating therapy with somatropin in pediatric patients with Prader-Willi syndrome who had one or more of the following risk factors:

- severe obesity,
- history of upper airway obstruction or sleep apnea, or
- unidentified respiratory infection.

Male patients with one or more of these factors may be at greater risk than females.

Patients with Prader-Willi syndrome should be evaluated for signs of upper airway obstruction and sleep apnea before initiation of treatment with somatropin. If during treatment with somatropin patients show signs of upper airway obstruction (including onset of or increased snoring) and/or new onset of sleep apnea treatment should be interrupted. All patients with Prader-Willi syndrome treated with somatropin should also have effective weight control and be monitored for signs of respiratory infection, which should be diagnosed as early as possible and treated aggressively (see Contraindications).

Unless patients with Prader-Willi syndrome also have a diagnosis of growth hormone deficiency, HUMATROPE is not indicated for the long-term treatment of pediatric patients who have growth failure due to genetically confirmed Prader-Willi syndrome.

Turner Syndrome (see Warnings and Precautions, General): Skeletal abnormalities including scoliosis are commonly seen in untreated Turner syndrome patients.

Patients with Turner syndrome may be at increased risk for development of intracranial hypertension.

Patients with Turner syndrome should be evaluated carefully for otitis media and other ear disorders since these patients have an increased risk of ear or hearing disorders (see Adverse Reactions).

Patients with Turner syndrome are at risk for cardiovascular disorders (e.g. stroke, aortic aneurysm, hypertension) and these conditions should be monitored closely.

Patients with Turner syndrome have an inherently increased risk of developing autoimmune thyroid disease. Therefore, patients should have periodic thyroid function tests and be treated as indicated (see Endocrine and Metabolism).

Endocrine and Metabolism: (See Warnings and Precautions, General): Treatment with somatropin may decrease insulin sensitivity, particularly at higher doses in patients with risk factors for diabetes mellitus, such as obesity, Turner syndrome, or a family history of diabetes mellitus, and patients with impaired glucose tolerance or pre-existing diabetes mellitus. As a result, previously undiagnosed impaired glucose tolerance and overt diabetes mellitus may be unmasked during somatropin treatment. Therefore, patients who receive somatropin should be monitored for evidence of abnormal glucose metabolism and/or diabetes mellitus. New-onset type 2 diabetes mellitus has been reported in children and adults receiving somatropin.

Patients who have pre-existing or treatment-emergent diabetes mellitus and who receive concomitant somatropin may require adjustment of their doses of insulin and/or other anti-hyperglycemic agents.

In patients with hypopituitarism (multiple hormonal deficiencies) standard hormonal replacement therapy should be monitored closely when somatropin therapy is administered. Hypothyroidism may develop during treatment with somatropin. Because inadequate treatment of hypothyroidism may prevent optimal response to somatropin, thyroid function should be monitored regularly during somatropin treatment.

Ophthalmologic: See Special Populations, Pediatrics.

Peri-Operative Considerations: See General, Acute Critical Illnesses.

Renal: Somatropin should be discontinued at the time of the renal transplantation until one year post-transplant.

Before instituting treatment with somatropin for growth retardation secondary to chronic renal insufficiency, patients should be followed for one year to verify growth disturbance.

Sensitivity/Resistance: Sensitivity to diluent (metacresol or glycerin): If patients are sensitive to the metacresol or if sensitivity to the diluent develops, the drug should be reconstituted with Water for Injection, USP (see Dosage and Administration, Reconstitution and Specific Precautions).

Resistance: As with all protein pharmaceuticals, a small percentage of patients may develop antibodies to the protein (see Adverse Reactions, Growth Hormone-Deficient Pediatric Patients).

In addition to an evaluation of compliance with the treatment program and of thyroid status, testing for antibodies to somatropin should be carried out in any patient who fails to respond to therapy.

Special Populations: Pregnant Women: Animal reproduction studies and animal studies for impairment of fertility with HUMATROPE have not been performed. HUMATROPE should be given to a pregnant woman only if clearly needed. It is not known whether HUMATROPE can cause fetal harm when administered to a pregnant woman or can affect reproduction capacity.

Nursing Women: There have been no studies conducted with HUMATROPE in nursing mothers. It is not known whether this drug is excreted in human milk. Because many drugs are excreted in human milk, caution should be exercised when HUMATROPE is administered to a nursing woman.

Pediatrics: (See Indications and Clinical Use): Patients with endocrine disorders, including growth hormone deficiency, may develop slipped capital femoral epiphyses more frequently. Any pediatric patient with onset of a limp during somatropin therapy should be evaluated.

Somatropin has not been shown to increase the incidence of scoliosis. Progression of scoliosis can occur in pediatric patients who experience rapid growth. Because growth hormone increases growth rate, patients with a history of scoliosis who are treated with somatropin should be monitored for progression of scoliosis.

Intracranial hypertension (IH) with papilledema, visual changes, headache, nausea and/or vomiting has been reported in a small number of patients treated with growth hormone products. Symptoms usually occurred within the first eight (8) weeks of the initiation of growth hormone therapy. In all reported cases, IH-associated signs and symptoms resolved after termination of therapy or a reduction of the growth hormone dose. Funduscopic examination of patients is recommended at the initiation and periodically during the course of growth hormone therapy.

Idiopathic Short Stature: HUMATROPE treatment for idiopathic short stature should be prescribed only for those patients whose epiphyses are not closed and should be managed by physicians who have sufficient knowledge of idiopathic short stature and the efficacy/safety profile of HUMATROPE.

Second Neoplasms in Survivors of Childhood Cancer: In childhood cancer survivors, an increased risk of a second neoplasm (benign and malignant) has been reported in patients treated with somatropin. Intracranial tumours, in particular meningiomas in patients treated with radiation to the head for their first neoplasm, were the most common of these second neoplasms. However, in childhood cancer survivors, no increased risk of primary cancer recurrence has been reported with somatropin treatment.

Pancreatitis in Children: Children treated with somatropin may have an increased risk of developing pancreatitis compared to adults treated with somatropin. Although rare, pancreatitis should be considered in somatropin-treated children who develop abdominal pain.

Adult Patients: Patients with epiphyseal closure who were treated with somatropin therapy in childhood should be re-evaluated according to the criteria in Indications and Clinical Use before continuation of somatropin therapy at the reduced dose level required for growth hormone-deficient adults.

Experience with prolonged treatment in adults is limited. Adverse events such as peripheral edema, myalgia, arthralgia, and paresthesiae were reported during post-marketing studies (see under Adverse Reactions). In addition, an assessment of clinical trial data, post-marketing data, and spontaneous reports found that carpal tunnel syndrome occurs more frequently in patients over 40 years of age, and in almost half of these cases the recommended maximum dose had been exceeded. In the majority of cases, the condition resolved with a decrease in dosage, interruption of treatment, discontinuation of treatment or spontaneously. The maximum recommended dosage should not be exceeded.

Geriatrics (≥65 years of age): The safety and effectiveness of HUMATROPE in patients aged ≥65 years have not been evaluated in clinical studies. Geriatric patients may be more sensitive to somatropin, and therefore may be more prone to adverse reactions. A lower starting dose and smaller dose increments should be considered for older patients.

Obese Patients: Obese individuals are more likely to manifest adverse effects when treated with a weight-based regimen (see Dosage and Administration).

Monitoring and Laboratory Tests: See General, Congenital Disorders, and Endocrine and Metabolism.

Serum concentrations of inorganic phosphorus, alkaline phosphatase, parathyroid hormone and IGF-I may increase during somatropin therapy. It is recommended that IGF-I concentrations be monitored regularly and maintained within the normal range. When these concentrations are higher than the normal range, a dose reduction should be considered.

ADVERSE REACTIONS: Adverse Drug Reaction Overview: The data presented below reflect the findings from clinical trials and post-marketing experience of treatment with HUMATROPE.

Clinical Trial Adverse Drug Reactions: Because clinical trials are conducted under very specific conditions the adverse reaction rates observed in the clinical trials may not reflect the rates observed in practice and should not be compared to the rates in the clinical trials of another drug. Adverse drug reaction information from clinical trials is useful for identifying drug-related adverse events and for approximating rates.

Table 1: HUMATROPE

Adverse Reactions from All Clinical Trial Sources by Body System

Body System	Adverse Reactions	Frequency
Body as a Whole	Injection site reaction	≥1% and <10%
	Hypersensitivity to diluent	≥1% and <10%
	Localized muscle pain	≥0.01% and <0.1% (pediatric) ≥1% and <10% (adults)
	Benign intracranial hypertension	≤0.1%
Endocrine	Hypothyroidism	≥10%
Metabolic	Edema	≥1% and <10% (pediatric); ≥10% (adults)
	Hyperglycemia	<1% (pediatric); ≥1% and <10% (adults)
Musculoskeletal	Arthralgia	≥10% (adults)
Nervous	Carpal Tunnel Syndrome	≥1% and <10% (adults)
	Paresthesias	≥1% and <10% (adults)

Growth Hormone-Deficient Pediatric Patients: As with all protein pharmaceuticals, a small percentage of patients may develop antibodies to the protein. During the first six months of HUMATROPE (somatropin for injection) therapy in 314 naive patients, only 1.6% developed specific antibodies to HUMATROPE (binding capacity ≥0.02 mg/L). None had antibody concentrations, which exceeded 2 mg/L. Throughout 8 years of this same study, 2 patients (0.6%) had binding capacity >2 mg/L. Neither patient demonstrated a decrease in growth velocity at or near the time of increased antibody production. It has been reported that growth attenuation from pituitary-derived growth hormone may occur when antibody concentrations are >1.5 mg/L.

In addition to an evaluation of compliance with the treatment program and of thyroid status, testing for antibodies to somatropin should be carried out in any patient who fails to respond to therapy (see Warnings and Precautions, Sensitivity/Resistance).

In studies with growth hormone-deficient pediatric patients, injection site pain was reported infrequently. Mild and transient edema, (either localized or generalized) was observed in 2.5% of patients during the course of treatment.

Leukemia has been reported in a small number of pediatric patients who have been treated with growth hormone, including growth hormone of pituitary origin, and recombinant somatrem and somatropin. The relationship, if any, between leukemia and growth hormone is uncertain.

Healthy Adult Volunteers: In clinical studies in which high doses of HUMATROPE were administered to healthy adult volunteers, the following events occurred infrequently: headache, localized muscle pain, weakness, mild hyperglycemia and glucosuria.

Adult Patients: In the first 6 months of controlled, blinded trials, adult-onset growth hormone deficient patients experienced a statistically significant increase in edema (HUMATROPE 17.3% vs placebo 4.4%, (p=0.043) and peripheral edema relative to patients receiving placebo (11.5% vs 0% respectively, (p=0.017).

In patients with adult-onset somatotropin deficiency, edema, muscle pain, and joint pain and disorder, were reported early in therapy and tended to be transient or responsive to dosage titration.

Two out of 113 adult onset patients developed carpal tunnel syndrome after beginning maintenance therapy without a low dose (0.00625 mg/kg/day) lead-in phase. Symptoms abated in these patients after dosage reduction.

In growth hormone-deficient adults, treatment-emergent adverse events reported after 18 months of therapy which are possibly related to replacement therapy but were not statistically significant during the first 6 months, include carpal tunnel syndrome, edema, arthralgia, paresthesia, hypesthesia, myalgia, peripheral edema, back pain, headache and joint disorder.

Adult patients treated with somatropin, following diagnosis of growth hormone deficiency in childhood, reported side effects less frequently than those with adult onset growth hormone deficiency.

Turner Syndrome: Patients with Turner syndrome have an increased risk of ear or hearing disorders. In a randomized, concurrent controlled clinical trial, there was a statistically significant increase, as compared to untreated controls, in otitis media, (43% vs 26%) ear disorders (18% vs 5%) and surgical procedures (45% vs 27%) in patients receiving HUMATROPE (see Warnings and Precautions, Congenital Disorders).

Patients with Idiopathic Short Stature: In the placebo-controlled study, there were no significant differences between the HUMATROPE-treated and placebo-treated groups for any of the nonserious clinically significant treatment-emergent adverse events (see Table 2). Mean serum glucose level did not change during HUMATROPE treatment. Mean fasting serum insulin levels increased 10% in the HUMATROPE treatment group at the end of treatment relative to baseline values but remained within the normal reference range. For the same duration of treatment the mean fasting serum insulin levels decreased by 2% in the placebo group. The occurrence of above-range values for glucose, insulin, and HbA_{1c} were similar in the HUMATROPE and placebo-treated groups. No patient developed diabetes mellitus. Consistent with the known mechanism of growth hormone action, HUMATROPE-treated patients (0.222 mg/kg/week) had greater mean increases, relative to baseline, in serum insulin-like growth factor-I (IGF-I) than placebo-treated patients at each study observation. However, there was no significant difference between the HUMATROPE and placebo treatment groups in the proportion of patients who had at least one serum IGF-I concentration more than 2.0 SD above the age- and gender-appropriate mean (HUMATROPE: 9 of 35 patients [26%]; placebo: 7 of 28 patients [25%]). There is no available information regarding IGF-I levels at the recommended dose of 0.37 mg/kg/week.

Table 2: HUMATROPE

Nonserious Clinically Significant Treatment-Emergent Adverse Events[a] by Treatment Group in Idiopathic Short Stature

	Treatment Group	
Adverse Event	**HUMATROPE**	**Placebo**
Total Number of Patients	37	31
Scoliosis	7 (18.9%)	4 (12.9%)
Otitis Media	6 (16.2%)	2 (6.5%)
Hyperlipidemia	3 (8.1%)	1 (3.2%)
Gynecomastia	2 (5.4%)	1 (3.2%)
Hypothyroidism	0	2 (6.5%)
Aching Joints	0	1 (3.2%)
Hip Pain	1 (2.7%)	0
Arthralgia	4 (10.8%)	1 (3.2%)
Arthosis	4 (10.8%)	2 (6.5%)
Myalgia	9 (24.3%)	4 (12.9%)

(cont'd)

Table 2: HUMATROPE *(cont'd)*

Nonserious Clinically Significant Treatment-Emergent Adverse Events[a] by Treatment Group in Idiopathic Short Stature

	Treatment Group	
Adverse Event	HUMATROPE	Placebo
Hypertension	1 (2.7%)	0

[a] Coding of adverse events was performed using the Medical Dictionary for Regulatory Activities (MedDRA).

The adverse events observed in the dose-response study (239 patients treated for 2 years) did not indicate a pattern suggestive of a somatropin dose effect. Among HUMATROPE dose groups, mean fasting blood glucose, mean glycosylated hemoglobin, and the occurrence rates of elevated fasting blood glucose concentrations were similar. One patient developed abnormalities of carbohydrate metabolism (glucose intolerance and slightly elevated HbA_{1c}) on treatment, which resolved when treatment was discontinued.

Five patients discontinued from the clinical trials because of adverse events. One patient discontinued from the placebo-controlled study following diagnosis of Stage 3B Hodgkin disease after 19 weeks of HUMATROPE treatment. It was subsequently determined on the basis of clinical, radiographic and laboratory findings that subclinical Hodgkin disease was likely present at study entry. One placebo-treated patient discontinued the study after an accidental injury. One patient in the dose-response study discontinued following diagnosis of a desmoplastic small round cell tumour after 6.4 years of HUMATROPE treatment and died 4 years later. It was subsequently determined that the tumour had an abnormal karyotype typically associated with this type of tumour. Neither case of neoplasia in the ISS studies was considered causally related to HUMATROPE exposure. Two additional patients discontinued from the dose-response study due to adverse events: one patient discontinued after diagnosis of a slipped capital femoral epiphysis following trauma; one patient was withdrawn from the study due to decreased glucose tolerance. Both events have been previously reported in patients receiving somatropin.

The impact of ethnicity was not evaluated in the clinical trials for idiopathic short stature.

Patients with SHOX Deficiency: Clinically significant adverse events (adverse events previously observed in association with growth hormone treatment in general) were assessed prospectively during the 2-year randomized, open-label study; those observed are presented in Table 3. In both treatment groups, the mean fasting plasma glucose concentration at the end of the first year was similar to the baseline value and remained in the normal range. No patient developed diabetes mellitus or had an above normal value for fasting plasma glucose at the end of one-year of treatment. During the 2 year study period, the proportion of patients who had at least one IGF-I concentration greater than 2.0 SD above the age- and gender-appropriate mean was 10 of 27 [37.0%] for the HUMATROPE-treated group vs. 0 of 24 patients [0.0%] for the untreated group. The proportion of patients who had at least one IGFBP-3 concentration greater than 2.0 SD above the age and gender appropriate mean was 16 of 27 [59.3%] for the HUMATROPE treated group vs. 7 of 24 [29.2%] for the untreated group. There were no discontinuations due to adverse events in this study. No serious adverse events were reported for subjects with SHOX Deficiency.

Table 3: HUMATROPE

Clinically Significant Treatment-Emergent Adverse Events[a,b] by Treatment Group and Patients with SHOX Deficiency

	Treatment Group	
Adverse Event	Untreated	HUMATROPE
Total Number of Patients	25	27
Patients with at least one event	2	5
Arthralgia	2 (8.0%)	3 (11.1%)
Gynecomastia[c]	0 (0.0%)	1 (8.3%)
Excessive number of cutaneous nevi	0 (0.0%)	2 (7.4%)
Scoliosis	0 (0.0%)	1 (3.7%)

[a] All events were non-serious.
[b] Events are included only if reported for a greater number of HUMATROPE-treated than Untreated patients.
[c] Percentage calculated for males only (1/12).

Patients Born Small for Gestational Age: The safety of Humatrope treatment in children born small for gestational age was assessed in 2 clinical trials (Study GDGB and Study 0908) and one observational study (Study GDFC).

In Study GDGB, 4 patients discontinued due to adverse events, 3 from the FHD group (1 patient each for impaired fasting glucose, mood alteration and pain in extremity) and 1 patient from the IAD group (focal glomerulosclerosis).

Adverse events possibly or probably related to HUMATROPE are provided in Table 4. The most frequently reported of these adverse drug reactions was headache, for which there was a suggestion of a modest dose-response (FHD, 9%; IAD, 3%). There were no clear cut cases of new-onset diabetes mellitus, no children treated for hyperglycemia, and no children whose fasting blood glucose exceeded 7 mmol/L at any time during the study. However, 6 children (4 in the FHD group and 2 in the IAD group whose dose was increased from 0.035 mg/kg/day to 0.067 mg/kg/day [one at Month 3 and one at Year 1]) manifested impaired fasting glucose at Year 2. Two of these six children had impaired fasting glucose during the study as well, and one of them was required to discontinue Humatrope at Month 15 as a consequence.

A modestly dose-dependent increase in mean serum IGF-I SDS concentrations within the reference range was observed; of note, at study completion, 22% of these children had serum IGF-I values more than 2 standard deviations above the mean for age and sex. Eight children in the FHD group and 2 in the IAD group required dose reduction due to high IGF-I or IGFBP-3.

Table 4 represents adverse drug reactions reported at a frequency of ≥1% in Study GDGB, listed in descending order of frequency within system organ class.

Table 4: HUMATROPE

Adverse Drug Reactions[a] with Frequency ≥1% in Study GDGB

System Organ Class	Preferred Term	FHD (N=99) n (%)	IAD (N=94) n (%)	Total (N=193) n (%)
Ear and Labyrinth Disorders	Vertigo	1 (1)	1 (1)	2 (1)
Endocrine Disorders	Hypothyroidism	2 (2)	2 (2)	4 (2)
General Disorders and Administration Site Conditions	Fatigue	2 (2)	1 (1)	3 (2)
	Injection site pain	2 (2)	1 (1)	3 (2)
	Edema	0 (0)	2 (2)	2 (1)
Investigations	Blood insulin increased	4 (4)	3 (3)	7 (4)
	Low density lipoprotein decreased	3 (3)	1 (1)	4 (2)
Musculoskeletal and Connective Tissue Disorders	Pain in extremity	3 (3)	6 (6)	9 (5)
	Arthralgia	1 (1)	2 (2)	3 (2)
	Limb deformity	2 (2)	0 (0)	2 (1)
Neoplasms Benign, Malignant and Unspecified (incl cysts and polyps)	Melanocytic naevus	2 (2)	0 (0)	2 (1)
Nervous System Disorders	Headache	9 (9)	3 (3)	12 (6)
	Psychomotor hyperactivity	1 (1)	3 (3)	4 (2)
Psychiatric Disorders	Aggression	1 (1)	1 (1)	2 (1)
Respiratory, Thoracic and Mediastinal Disorders	Adenoidal hypertrophy	0 (0)	3 (3)	3 (2)

[a] Terms designated by investigator as related to study drug in at least one patient.
Legend: N=total number in treatment group; n=number for whom event was reported; FHD=fixed high dosage (0.067 mg/kg/day); IAD=individually-adjusted dosage (0.035 to 0.067 mg/kg/day).

In Study 0908, treatment-emergent adverse events (TEAEs) were reported for 30/35 (86%) of study participants. Because of the size of this study, all events were reported at a frequency of >1%. The most frequently reported non-serious TEAEs were typical childhood illnesses, such as nasopharyngitis (29%) and bronchitis, gastroenteritis, influenza and vomiting (14% for each event). Gynecomastia was reported for 13% of males. In addition, the following events were each reported for 11% of study patients: arthralgia, headache, injection site pain, pyrexia; the following events were reported for 9% of patients: asthenia, cough, eczema, pharyngitis, pharyngolaryngeal pain, rhinitis; the following events were reported for 6% of patients: appendicitis, ear infection, hyperthermia, hypothyroidism, joint sprain, lymphadenopathy, tracheitis, tracheobronchitis. No patient was reported to have discontinued the study because of an adverse event.

In the observational study, GDFC, non-serious TEAEs were reported for 76 of 379 (20%) children with a study entry diagnosis of short stature due to small for gestational age birth, who were naïve to treatment at study entry and had at least one post-baseline visit. The majority of these events were typical childhood illnesses or injuries unlikely to have been related to HUMATROPE treatment.

Less Common Clinical Trial Adverse Drug Reactions (<1%): The following list provides the adverse events reported with a frequency of <1% in studies GDGB and GDFC that were designated by the investigators as possibly-related to the study drug, or for which no designation was made: abnormal behaviour, back pain, blood thyroid stimulating hormone increased, cardiovascular disorder, carpal tunnel syndrome, contusion, eyelid edema, epiphysiolysis (slipped capital femoral epiphysis), hyperinsulinemia, hypertension, impaired fasting glucose, injection site bruising, injection site hematoma, injection site induration, injection site pain, injection site vesicles, mood altered, muscle mass, nervousness, periorbital edema, precocious puberty, puberty, tonsillar hypertrophy, type 2 diabetes mellitus, and visual disturbance. In study 0908, there were no events reported with a frequency of <1%, due to study size (n=35).

Post-Market Adverse Drug Reactions: In addition to the Clinical Trial Adverse Reactions listed in Table 1, the Adverse Reactions shown in Table 5 have been noted in post-marketing studies.

Table 5: HUMATROPE

Adverse Reactions from Post-Marketing Studies by Body System

Body System	Adverse Reactions	Frequency
Respiratory	Dyspnea	≥1% and <10% (adults)
	Sleep apnea	≥1% and <10% (adults)
Vascular	Hypertension	≥1% and <10% (adults)
Metabolic	Type 2 diabetes mellitus	≥0.1% and <1% (pediatric)

[a] Adult cases of Type 2 diabetes mellitus were reported spontaneously.

DRUG INTERACTIONS: Drug-Drug Interactions: Potential drug interactions are tabulated in (Table 6).

Table 6: HUMATROPE

Established or Potential Drug-Drug Interactions with HUMATROPE (somatropin for injection)

Therapeutic Class	Effects	Clinical Comments
Glucocorticoids	Inhibition of 11β-hydroxysteroid dehydrogenase type 1 (11βHSD-1). Somatropin inhibits the liver enzyme 11β-HSD-1 which is required for conversion of administered cortisone and prednisone to their active metabolites, cortisol and prednisolone, respectively.	In patients treated with somatropin, previously undiagnosed secondary hypoadrenalism may be unmasked and may require glucocorticoid replacement therapy. If glucocorticoid replacement therapy is required for newly-diagnosed or preexisting hypoadrenalism, dosage and compliance should be monitored carefully to avoid either inhibition of growth promoting effects or adrenal insufficiency; increases in maintenance or stress doses of glucocorticoids may be required after initiation of somatropin.
Cytochrome P450 Metabolized Drugs	Somatropin can increase cytochrome P450 (CYP) liver enzyme activity in humans and may result in reduced plasma concentrations and decreased effectiveness of drugs metabolized by CYP3A such as sex steroids (for example, estrogen or oral contraceptives), cyclosporine and some anticonvulsants.	Limited published data indicate that somatropin treatment increases cytochrome P450 (CP450)-mediated antipyrine clearance in human. Careful monitoring is advised when somatropin is administered in combination with drugs metabolized by CP450 liver enzymes.
Insulin and Anti-hyperglycemic Agents	Patients with diabetes mellitus who receive concomitant somatropin may require adjustment of their doses of insulin and/or other anti-hyperglycemic agents.	Because somatropin may induce a state of insulin resistance, patients who receive somatropin should be monitored for evidence of abnormal glucose metabolism and/or diabetes mellitus. New-onset type 2 diabetes mellitus has been reported in children and adults receiving somatropin.

Drug-Food Interactions: Interactions with food have not been established.
Drug-Herb Interactions: Interactions with herbal products have not been established.
Drug-Laboratory Test Interactions: For interactions between HUMATROPE and laboratory tests, see Warnings and Precautions, Monitoring and Laboratory Tests.

DOSAGE AND ADMINISTRATION: **Dosing Considerations: Adult Patients:** Patients with epiphyseal closure who were treated with somatropin therapy in childhood should be re-evaluated according to the criteria in Indications and Clinical Use before continuation of somatropin therapy at the reduced dose level required for growth hormone-deficient adults. A lower starting dose may be necessary in older and obese patients.
Estrogen-Replete Women: Estrogen-replete women may need higher doses than men. Oral estrogen administration may increase the dose requirements in women.
Recommended Dose and Dosage Adjustment: The dosage and administration schedule for HUMATROPE (somatropin for injection) should be individualized for each patient (see Table 7). Clinicians should carefully monitor the growth response in all children, and adjust the somatropin dose as necessary.

Table 7: HUMATROPE

Recommended Dose and Administration Schedule for HUMATROPE

Indication	Recommended Dose (mg/kg body weight)	Route	Comments
GH-Deficient Pediatric Patients	0.18 mg/kg/week (0.54 IU[a]/kg/week) Maximum: 0.3 mg/kg/week (0.90 IU[a]/kg/week)	SC	Divide into equal doses given on: 3 alternate days **or** 6 times/week **or** daily
GH-Deficient Adult Patients	Initiate at not more than 0.006 mg/kg/day (0.018 IU[a]/kg/day) Maximum: 0.0125 mg/kg/day (0.375 IU[a]/kg/day)	SC	Should be titrated • based on adverse effects (increasing age or excessive body weight may require dose reductions) • to maintain IGF-I <ULN matched for age and sex
Patients with Turner Syndrome	Up to 0.375 mg/kg/week (1.125 IU[a]/kg/week)	SC	Divide into equal doses given: • daily **or** • on 3 alternate days
Patients with Idiopathic Short Stature	0.37 mg/kg/week (1.125 IU[a]/kg/week)	SC	Divided into equal doses given 6 to 7 times per week
Patients with SHOX Deficiency	0.35 mg/kg/week	SC	Divided into equal doses given 6 to 7 times per week
Patients Born Small for Gestational Age[b]	Up to 0.47 mg/kg/week	SC	Divided into equal doses given 6 to 7 times per week

[a] Based on a specific activity of 3 International Units/mg protein.
[b] It is recommended that treatment be initiated with larger doses of somatropin (e.g., 0.067 mg/kg/day), especially in very short children (i.e., height SDS ≤3) and/or older pubertal children. A reduction in dosage (e.g. to 0.035 mg/kg/day) should be considered if substantial catch-up growth is observed during the first few years of therapy.
In younger SGA children (approximately <4 years of age) with less severe short stature (i.e., baseline height SDS values between −2 and −3), consideration should be given to initiating treatment with a lower dose (e.g., 0.035 mg/kg/day), then titrating the dose as needed.

It is recommended that IGF-I concentrations be monitored regularly and maintained within the normal range for age and sex. When these concentrations are higher than the normal range, a dose reduction should be considered.
Administration: HUMATROPE should be administered subcutaneously and the injection site should be rotated to minimize the risk of lipoatrophy.
HUMATROPE treatment for improvement of linear growth in childhood should be administered to pediatric patients whose epiphyses have not closed. For patients whose height velocity in the first year of treatment does not improve by at least 50% above the pre-treatment height velocity, consideration should be given to the following:
- Is the patient receiving the correct dosage and frequency of the medication?
- Is the growth disorder diagnosis correct?
- Does the patient have a coexistent condition that may impair growth (such as hypothyroidism, a gastrointestinal disorder or severe psychological disturbance)?
- Is the patient receiving adequate nutrition?
- Is the patient receiving a concomitant medication that may impair response to GH (such as systemic corticosteroids or stimulant medications)?

If no underlying reason for a suboptimal response to HUMATROPE treatment can be found, discontinuation of treatment should be considered.
In pediatric patients receiving HUMATROPE for improvement of linear growth consideration should be given to discontinuation of treatment when growth is nearly complete, as evidenced by:
- Height velocity less than 2.0 cm per year
- Bone age of 14 years or greater in girls or 16 years or greater in boys.

Reconstitution and Specific Precautions: If home use is prescribed, a puncture resistant container for the disposal of used needles and syringes should be recommended to the patient. Patients and/or caregivers should be thoroughly instructed in the importance of proper needle disposal and cautioned against the reuse of needles and syringes.
HUMATROPE Vials: Reconstitute each vial of HUMATROPE with 1.5 to 5 mL of diluent for HUMATROPE. Inject the diluent for HUMATROPE (metacresol and glycerin solution) into the vial of HUMATROPE aiming the stream of liquid against the glass wall. Following reconstitution, swirl the vial with a **gentle rotary** motion until the contents are completely dissolved. **Do not shake.** The resulting solution should be clear, without particulate matter. If the solution is cloudy or contains particulate matter, the contents **must not** be injected.
Before and after injections, the septum of the vial should be wiped with rubbing alcohol or another alcoholic antiseptic solution to prevent contamination of the contents by repeated needle insertions. HUMATROPE should be administered using sterile, disposable syringes and needles. The syringes should be of small enough volume that the prescribed dose can be drawn from the vial with reasonable accuracy. The needle should be of sufficient length (usually 1 inch or more) to ensure that the injection reaches the muscular layer for intramuscular injections.
If sensitivity to the diluent should occur, HUMATROPE vials may be reconstituted with Sterile Water for Injection, USP. When reconstituting with water, use only once and discard the unused portion. The vial should be used immediately after reconstitution. Although not recommended, the solution can be stored refrigerated (2° to 8°C) but must be used within 24 hours.
HUMATROPE Cartridges: Each HUMATROPE cartridge (for use with the HumatroPen) should be reconstituted using the accompanying diluent syringe. To reconstitute, attach the cartridge to the pre-filled diluent syringe and then inject the entire contents of the pre-filled diluent syringe into the cartridge. The diluent needle aims the stream of liquid against the glass wall of the cartridge. Following reconstitution, gently invert the cartridge up and down 10 times until the contents are completely dissolved. **Do not shake.** The resulting solution should be clear, without particulate matter. If the solution is cloudy or contains particulate matter, the contents **must not** be injected. If the solution is clear, the cartridge is ready to be attached to the HumatroPen. For complete instructions on the reconstitution of HUMATROPE cartridges, please refer to the reconstitution instruction leaflet provided with all HUMATROPE cartridges.
The diluent syringe is for single use only. Discard it after use.

If sensitivity to the accompanying diluent occurs, Sterile Water for Injection, USP, may be used for reconstitution. The Sterile Water for Injection, USP, should be administered using a sterile, disposable syringe and needle. The syringe should be of small enough volume that 3.15 mL can be measured with reasonable accuracy. Before and after injections, the septum of the cartridge should be wiped with rubbing alcohol or another alcoholic antiseptic solution. Inject 3.15 mL of Sterile Water for Injection, USP, into the cartridge through the rubber septum, aiming the stream of liquid against the glass wall of the cartridge. Following reconstitution, the cartridge should be gently inverted up and down 10 times until the contents are completely dissolved. **Do not shake.** The resulting solution should be clear, without particulate matter. If the solution is cloudy or contains particulate matter, the contents **must not** be injected.
HUMATROPE reconstituted in this manner should be used immediately. Although not recommended, the solution can be stored refrigerated (2 to 8°C) but must be used within 24 hours. Discard any unused portion. However, to minimize waste, the smallest vials of HUMATROPE rather than cartridges are recommended.
HUMATROPE cartridges are designed for use only with the HumatroPen family of pens. A sterile needle should be used for each administration of somatropin.
For complete instructions on the use of the HumatroPen, see the relevant HumatroPen Instruction Manual.

OVERDOSAGE:
Acute overdosage could lead initially to hypoglycemia and subsequently to hyperglycemia. Long-term overdosage could result in signs and symptoms of gigantism/acromegaly, consistent with the known effects of excess human growth hormone. See Recommended Dose and Dosage Adjustments, Table 7.

For management of a suspected drug overdose, contact your regional Poison Control Centre. See the *CPS* Directory section for a list of Poison Control Centres.

ACTION AND CLINICAL PHARMACOLOGY: Mechanism of Action: The following actions have been demonstrated for HUMATROPE (somatropin for injection) and/or human growth hormone of pituitary origin.
Tissue Growth:
a. Skeletal Growth: HUMATROPE stimulates skeletal growth in pediatric patients with growth hormone deficiency. The measurable increase in body length after administration of either HUMATROPE or human growth hormone of pituitary origin results from an effect on the growth plates of long bones. Concentrations of IGF-I, which may play a role in skeletal growth, are low in the serum of growth hormone-deficient pediatric patients but increase during treatment with HUMATROPE. Elevations in mean serum alkaline phosphatase concentrations are also seen.
b. Cell Growth: It has been shown that there are fewer skeletal muscle cells in short-statured pediatric patients who lack endogenous growth hormone as compared to normal pediatric populations. Treatment with human growth hormone of pituitary origin results in an increase in both the number and the size of muscle cells.

Protein Metabolism: Linear growth is facilitated in part by increased cellular protein synthesis. Nitrogen retention as demonstrated by decreased urinary nitrogen excretion and serum urea nitrogen, follows the initiation of therapy with human growth hormone of pituitary origin. Treatment with HUMATROPE results in a similar decrease in serum urea nitrogen.
Carbohydrate Metabolism: Pediatric patients with hypopituitarism sometimes experience fasting hypoglycemia, which is improved by treatment with HUMATROPE. Large doses of somatropin may impair glucose tolerance. Untreated patients with Turner syndrome have an increased incidence of glucose intolerance. Administration of somatropin to healthy adults or patients with Turner syndrome resulted in increases in mean serum fasting and postprandial insulin levels although mean values remained in the normal range. In addition, mean fasting and postprandial glucose and hemoglobin A_{1c} levels remained in the normal range.
Lipid Metabolism: In growth hormone-deficient patients, long-term administration of human growth hormone of pituitary origin has resulted in lipid mobilization, reduction in body fat stores, and an increase in plasma fatty acids.
Mineral Metabolism: Retention of sodium, potassium and phosphorus is induced by human growth hormone of pituitary origin. Serum concentrations of inorganic phosphate increased in patients with growth hormone deficiency after therapy with HUMATROPE or human growth hormone of pituitary origin. Serum calcium is not significantly altered in patients treated with either human growth hormone of pituitary origin or HUMATROPE.
HUMATROPE stimulates linear growth in pediatric patients lacking adequate normal endogenous growth hormone. Treatment of growth hormone-deficient pediatric patients and patients with Turner syndrome with HUMATROPE produces increased growth rate and IGF-I (insulin-like growth factor-I/somatomedin C) concentrations similar to those seen in therapy with human growth hormone of pituitary origin.
As a result of replacement therapy in growth hormone deficient adults, body composition improved, HDL cholesterol values normalized, and health related quality of life measures concerning physical mobility and social isolation improved in placebo-controlled clinical trials. Exercise capacity improved as compared to placebo.
Pharmacokinetics: In vitro, preclinical, and clinical testing have demonstrated that HUMATROPE is therapeutically equivalent to human growth hormone of pituitary origin with equivalent pharmacokinetics in normal adults.
Absorption: HUMATROPE has been studied following intramuscular, subcutaneous and intravenous administration in adult volunteers. The absolute bioavailability of somatropin is 75% and 63% after subcutaneous and intramuscular administration respectively.
Distribution: The volume of distribution of somatropin after intravenous injection is about 0.07 L/kg.
Metabolism: Extensive metabolism studies have not been conducted. The metabolic fate of somatropin involves classical protein catabolism in both the liver and kidneys. In renal cells, at least a portion of the breakdown products of somatropin is returned to the systemic circulation. In normal volunteers, mean clearance is 0.14 L/hr/kg. The mean half-life of intravenous somatropin is 0.36 hours, whereas subcutaneously and intramuscularly administered somatropin have mean half-lives of 3.8 and 4.9 hours, respectively. The longer half-life observed after subcutaneous or intramuscular administration is due to slow absorption from the injection site.
Excretion: Urinary excretion of intact HUMATROPE has not been measured. Small amounts of somatropin have been detected in the urine of pediatric patients following replacement therapy.

STORAGE AND STABILITY: Before Reconstitution: Vials of HUMATROPE (somatropin for injection), HUMATROPE cartridges for use with the HumatroPen and the supplied diluent for HUMATROPE are stable when stored at (2 to 8°C). Avoid freezing the diluent for HUMATROPE. Expiration dates are stated on the labels.
After Reconstitution: When reconstituted with the supplied diluent and stored at 2 to 8°C:
- HUMATROPE vials are stable for up to 21 days and
- HUMATROPE cartridges for use with the HumatroPen are stable for up to 28 days
- Avoid freezing the reconstituted vials and cartridges of HUMATROPE.

If HUMATROPE vials or cartridges are reconstituted with Sterile Water for Injection, USP, they should be used immediately after reconstitution. Although not recommended, the solution can be stored refrigerated (2 to 8°C) but must be used within 24 hours. Discard any unused portion.
To minimize waste, the smallest vials of HUMATROPE rather than the cartridges are recommended.
Light: Protect from light.

INFORMATION FOR THE PATIENT: Published in e-CPS, available by subscription at www.e-cps.ca.

DOSAGE FORMS, COMPOSITION AND PACKAGING: HUMATROPE (somatropin for injection) is a sterile, white, lyophylized powder of highly purified rhGH, which is intended for subcutaneous or intramuscular use after reconstitution with the supplied diluent. HUMATROPE is available as vials and cartridges (see Table 8).

Table 8: HUMATROPE

Dosage Forms and Packaging

	Combination Packages			
Dosage Form	HUMATROPE	Vial #	Diluent	Vial #
Vials	2 mg (6 IU)	7332	2 mL	7333
	5 mg (~15 IU)	7335	5 mL	7336

(cont'd)

Table 8: HUMATROPE *(cont'd)*

Dosage Forms and Packaging

Dosage Form	Combination Packages			
	HUMATROPE	Vial #	Diluent	Vial #
Cartridges (for use with HumatroPen[a])	6 mg (~18 IU)	7554	3.15 mL	7616
	12 mg (~36 IU) 24 mg (~72 IU)	7555 7556	3.15 mL	7617

[a] The HumatroPen family of pens are available separately with a HumatroPen Instruction Manual.

Vials: Each vial of HUMATROPE contains: 2 mg (approximately 6 IU) or 5 mg (approximately 15 IU) of somatropin for injection, in addition to mannitol, glycine, and dibasic sodium phosphate. Phosphoric acid and/or sodium hydroxide may have been used for pH adjustment. Each vial of HUMATROPE is supplied in a combination pack with an accompanying vial of diluting solution. The diluent for HUMATROPE contains water for injection with 1.7% glycerin and 0.3% metacresol as a preservative. At a concentration of 2 mg HUMATROPE per mL diluent, the 1.7% glycerin makes the reconstituted product nearly isotonic. Reconstituted solutions have a pH of approximately 7.5.

Cartridges: Each cartridge of HUMATROPE (for use with the HumatroPen) contains: 6 mg (approximately 18 IU), 12 mg (approximately 36 IU), or 24 mg (approximately 72 IU) of somatropin for injection. The cartridge also contains mannitol, glycine, and dibasic sodium phosphate. Phosphoric acid and/or sodium hydroxide may have been added at the time of manufacture to adjust the pH. Each cartridge is supplied in a combination package with an accompanying syringe containing 3.15 mL of diluting solution. The diluent for 6 mg cartridges contains water for injection, 0.3% metacresol as a preservative; and 1.7% glycerin. The diluent for 12 and 24 mg cartridges contains water for injection, 0.3% metacresol, and 0.29% glycerin. Glycerin is added to the diluent to modify tonicity of the reconstituted solutions. Reconstituted solutions have a pH of approximately 7.5.

Humira® Pr

adalimumab

Biological Response Modifier

Abbott

Date of Preparation: September 24, 2004
Date of Revision: February 5, 2010

SUMMARY PRODUCT INFORMATION:

Route of Administration	Dosage Form/ Strength	Clinically Relevant Nonmedicinal Ingredients
Subcutaneous injection	**Pre-filled Syringe/Pre-filled Pen** Single-Dose, 1 mL Pre-filled Glass Syringe/40 mg adalimumab dissolved in 0.8 mL sterile solution (50 mg/mL).	Mannitol, sodium chloride, dibasic sodium phosphate dihydrate, citric acid monohydrate, polysorbate 80, monobasic sodium phosphate dihydrate and sodium citrate. For a complete listing see Dosage Forms, Composition and Packaging.

DESCRIPTION: HUMIRA (adalimumab) is a recombinant human immunoglobulin (IgG1) monoclonal antibody. Adalimumab was created using phage display technology resulting in fully human heavy and light chain variable regions, which confer specificity to human tumor necrosis factor (TNF), and human IgG1 heavy chain and kappa light chain sequences. Adalimumab binds with high affinity and specificity to soluble tumor necrosis factor (TNF-alpha) but not lymphotoxin (TNF-beta). Adalimumab is produced by recombinant DNA technology in a mammalian cell expression system. It consists of 1330 amino acids and has a molecular weight of approximately 148 kilodaltons.

INDICATIONS AND CLINICAL USE: HUMIRA (adalimumab) treatment should be initiated and supervised by specialist physicians experienced in the diagnosis and treatment of rheumatoid arthritis (RA), psoriatic arthritis (PsA), ankylosing spondylitis (AS), Crohn's Disease (CD), or psoriasis (Ps), and familiar with the HUMIRA efficacy and safety profile.

HUMIRA is indicated for:

Rheumatoid Arthritis:

- reducing the signs and symptoms, inducing major clinical response and clinical remission, inhibiting the progression of structural damage and improving physical function in adult patients with moderately to severely active rheumatoid arthritis. HUMIRA can be used alone or in combination with methotrexate (MTX) or other Disease-Modifying Anti-rheumatic Drugs (DMARDs).

When used as first-line treatment in recently diagnosed patients who have not been previously treated with methotrexate (MTX), HUMIRA should be given in combination with MTX. HUMIRA can be given as monotherapy in case of intolerance to MTX or when treatment with MTX is contraindicated.

Psoriatic Arthritis:

- reducing the signs and symptoms of active arthritis and inhibiting the progression of structural damage and improving the physical function in adult psoriatic arthritis patients. HUMIRA can be used in combination with methotrexate (MTX) in patients who do not respond adequately to methotrexate alone.

Ankylosing Spondylitis:

- reducing signs and symptoms in patients with active ankylosing spondylitis who have had an inadequate response to conventional therapy.

Crohn's Disease:

- reducing signs and symptoms and inducing and maintaining clinical remission in adult patients with moderately to severely active Crohn's disease who have had an inadequate response to conventional therapy, including corticosteroids and/or immunosuppressants. HUMIRA is indicated for reducing signs and symptoms and inducing clinical remission in these patients if they have also lost response to or are intolerant to infliximab.

Psoriasis:

- treatment of adult patients with chronic moderate to severe psoriasis who are candidates for systemic therapy. For patients with chronic moderate plaque psoriasis, HUMIRA should be used after phototherapy has been shown to be ineffective or inappropriate.

Geriatrics (>65 years of age): Evidence from clinical studies and experience suggests that use of adalimumab in the geriatric population is not associated with differences in safety or effectiveness. A brief discussion can be found under Warnings and Precautions, Special Populations, Geriatrics (>65 years of age).

Pediatrics: Safety and effectiveness in pediatric patients have not been established.

CONTRAINDICATIONS:

- Patients with known hypersensitivity to adalimumab or any of its components. For a complete listing, see Dosage Forms, Composition and Packaging.
- Patients with severe infections such as sepsis, tuberculosis and opportunistic infections (see Warnings and Precautions, Serious Warnings and Precautions, Infections).

WARNINGS AND PRECAUTIONS:

Serious Warnings and Precautions

Infections: SERIOUS INFECTIONS DUE TO BACTERIAL, MYCOBACTERIAL, INVASIVE FUNGAL (DISSEMINATED OR EXTRAPULMONARY HISTOPLASMOSIS, ASPERGILLOSIS, COCCIDIODOMYCOSIS), VIRAL, PARASITIC, OR OTHER OPPORTUNISTIC INFECTIONS HAVE BEEN REPORTED IN PATIENTS RECEIVING TNF-BLOCKING AGENTS. SEPSIS, RARE CASES OF TUBERCULOSIS, CANDIDIASIS, LISTERIOSIS, AND PNEUMOCYSTIS HAVE ALSO BEEN REPORTED WITH THE USE OF TNF-BLOCKING AGENTS, INCLUDING HUMIRA (ADALIMUMAB). OTHER SERIOUS INFECTIONS SEEN IN CLINICAL TRIALS INCLUDE PNEUMONIA, PYELONEPHRITIS, SEPTIC ARTHRITIS AND SEPTICEMIA. HOSPITALIZATION OR FATAL OUTCOMES ASSOCIATED WITH INFECTIONS HAVE BEEN REPORTED. MANY OF THE SERIOUS INFECTIONS HAVE OCCURRED IN PATIENTS ON CONCOMITANT IMMUNOSUPPRESSIVE THERAPY THAT, IN ADDITION TO THEIR UNDERLYING DISEASE, COULD PREDISPOSE THEM TO INFECTIONS.

TREATMENT WITH HUMIRA SHOULD NOT BE INITIATED IN PATIENTS WITH ACTIVE INFECTIONS, INCLUDING CHRONIC OR LOCALIZED INFECTIONS, UNTIL INFECTIONS ARE CONTROLLED. IN PATIENTS WHO HAVE BEEN EXPOSED TO TUBERCULOSIS, AND PATIENTS WHO HAVE TRAVELED IN AREAS OF HIGH RISK OF TUBERCULOSIS OR ENDEMIC MYCOSES, SUCH AS HISTOPLASMOSIS, COCCIDIOIDOMYCOSIS, OR BLASTOMYCOSIS, THE RISK AND BENEFITS OF TREATMENT WITH HUMIRA SHOULD BE CONSIDERED PRIOR TO INITIATING THERAPY (SEE Other Opportunistic Infections).

AS WITH OTHER TNF ANTAGONISTS, PATIENTS SHOULD BE MONITORED CLOSELY FOR INFECTIONS - INCLUDING TUBERCULOSIS -BEFORE, DURING AND AFTER TREATMENT WITH HUMIRA.

PATIENTS WHO DEVELOP A NEW INFECTION WHILE UNDERGOING TREATMENT WITH HUMIRA SHOULD BE MONITORED CLOSELY AND UNDERGO A COMPLETE DIAGNOSTIC EVALUATION. ADMINISTRATION OF HUMIRA SHOULD BE DISCONTINUED IF A PATIENT DEVELOPS A SERIOUS INFECTION OR SEPSIS, AND APPROPRIATE ANTIMICROBIAL OR ANTIFUNGAL THERAPY SHOULD BE INITIATED.

PHYSICIANS SHOULD EXERCISE CAUTION WHEN CONSIDERING THE USE OF HUMIRA IN PATIENTS WITH A HISTORY OF RECURRENT INFECTION OR WITH UNDERLYING CONDITIONS WHICH MAY PREDISPOSE THEM TO INFECTIONS, OR PATIENTS WHO HAVE RESIDED IN REGIONS WHERE TUBERCULOSIS AND HISTOPLASMOSIS ARE ENDEMIC (see WARNINGS AND PRECAUTIONS, Infections,Tuberculosis and ADVERSE REACTIONS, Adverse Drug Reaction Overview, Infections). THE BENEFITS AND RISKS OF TREATMENT WITH HUMIRA SHOULD BE CAREFULLY CONSIDERED BEFORE INITIATING THERAPY.

Hepatosplenic T-cell lymphoma: Very rare postmarketing reports of hepatosplenic T-cell lymphoma (HSTCL), a rare aggressive lymphoma that is often fatal, have been identified in patients treated with adalimumab. Most of the patients had prior infliximab therapy as well as concomitant azathioprine or 6-mercaptopurine use for Crohn's disease. The causal association of HSTCL with adalimumab is not clear.

Pediatric Malignancy: Lymphoma and other malignancies, some fatal, have been reported in children and adolescent patients treated with TNF-blockers, including HUMIRA. (See Warnings and Precautions, Malignancies.)

General: Use with Anakinra: Serious infections were seen in clinical studies with concurrent use of anakinra (an interleukin-1 antagonist) and another TNF blocking agent, etanercept, with no added benefit compared to etanercept alone. Because of the nature of the adverse events seen with the combination of etanercept and anakinra, similar toxicities may also result from the combination of anakinra and other TNF-blocking agents. Therefore, the combination of adalimumab and anakinra is not recommended (see Drug Interactions, Drug-Drug Interactions).

Switching Between Biological DMARDs: When switching from one biologic to another, patients should continue to be monitored for signs of infection.

Malignancies: In the controlled portions of clinical trials of some TNF-blocking agent, including HUMIRA, more cases of malignancies have been observed among patients receiving those TNF blockers compared to control patients.

In the controlled and uncontrolled open-label portions of clinical trials of HUMIRA, the more frequently observed malignancies, other than lymphoma and non-melanoma skin cancer, were breast, colon, prostate, lung and melanoma.

Malignancies, some fatal, have been reported among children and adolescents who received treatment with TNF-blocking agents. Approximately half the cases were lymphomas, including Hodgkin's and non-Hodgkin's lymphoma. The other cases represented a variety of different malignancies and included rare malignancies usually associated with immunosuppression. The malignancies occurred after a median of 30 months of therapy. Most of the patients were receiving concomitant immunosuppressants. These cases were reported post-marketing and are derived from a variety of sources including registries and spontaneous postmarketing reports.

Cases of acute and chronic leukemia have been reported in association with postmarketing TNF-blocker use in rheumatoid arthritis and other indications. Patients with rheumatoid arthritis may be at a higher risk (up to 2-fold) than the general population for the development of leukemia, even in the absence of TNF-blocking therapy.

Lymphoma: In the controlled portions of clinical trials of all the TNF-blocking agents, more cases of lymphoma have been observed among patients receiving TNF blockers compared to control patients.

However, for HUMIRA, the occurrence of lymphoma was rare, and the follow-up period of placebo patients was shorter than for patients receiving TNF-antagonist therapy. The size of the control group and limited duration of the controlled portions of studies precludes the ability to draw firm conclusions. Furthermore, there is an increased background lymphoma risk in rheumatoid arthritis patients with long-standing, highly active, inflammatory disease, which complicates the risk estimation.

In combining the controlled and uncontrolled open-label portions of these clinical trials with a median duration of approximately 1.7 years, including 6539 patients and over 16 000 patient-years of therapy, the observed rate of lymphomas is approximately 0.11/100 patient-years. This is approximately 3.0 fold higher than expected in the general population.

During the long-term open label trials with HUMIRA, the overall standard incidence ratio (SIR) of malignancies was 0.99 (95% CI; 0.81-1.20). With current knowledge in this area, a possible risk for development of lymphomas or other malignancies in patients treated with a TNF-antagonist cannot be excluded.

No studies have been conducted that include patients with a history of malignancy or that continue treatment in patients who develop malignancy while receiving HUMIRA. Additional caution should be exercised when considering HUMIRA treatment in these patients.

Non-lymphoma Malignancy: During the controlled portions of HUMIRA trials in patients with rheumatoid arthritis, psoriatic arthritis, ankylosing spondylitis, Crohn's disease, and psoriasis, malignancies, other than lymphoma and non-melanoma skin cancer, were observed at a rate (95% confidence interval) of 0.6 (0.4, 1.0)/100 patient-years among 3853 HUMIRA-treated patients versus a rate of 0.4 (0.2,1.0)/100 patient-years among 2183 control patients (median duration of treatment of 5.5 months for HUMIRA-treated patients and 3.9 months for control-treated patients).

During the controlled portions of HUMIRA rheumatoid arthritis, psoriatic arthritis, ankylosing spondylitis, Crohn's disease, and psoriasis trials, the rate (95% confidence interval) of non-melanoma skin cancers was 0.9 (0.57, 1.35)/100 patient-years among HUMIRA-treated patients and 0.3 (0.08, 0.80)/100 patient-years among control patients. Of these skin cancers, squamous cell carcinomas occurred at rates (95% confidence interval) of 0.2 (0.1, 0.6) per 100 patient-years among HUMIRA-treated patients and 0 per 100 patient-years among control patients. The rate (95% confidence interval) of lymphomas was 0.1 (0.02, 0.33) per 100 patient-years among HUMIRA treated patients and 0.1 (0.01, 0.61) per 100 patient-years among control patients.

The observed rate of malignancies, other than lymphoma and non-melanoma skin cancers, is approximately 8.3 per 1000 patient years in the controlled portion of clinical trials and ongoing open label extension studies. The observed rate of non-melanoma skin cancers is approximately 9.3 per 1000 patient years, and the observed rate of lymphomas is approximately 1.2 per 1000 patient years. The median duration of these studies is approximately 2.7 years and included 4767 patients who were on HUMIRA for at least 1 year or who developed a malignancy within a year of starting therapy, representing over 15 332 patient years of therapy.

All patients, and in particular psoriasis patients with a medical history of extensive immunosuppressant therapy or psoriasis patients with a history of Psoralen Ultra Violet A (PUVA) treatment should be examined for the presence of non-melanoma skin cancer prior to and during treatment with HUMIRA.

Hypersensitivity Reactions: Allergic reactions (e.g., allergic rash, anaphylactoid reaction, fixed drug reaction, non-specified drug reaction, urticaria) have been observed in approximately 1% of patients receiving HUMIRA in clinical trials (see Adverse Reactions). Serious allergic reactions, including anaphylaxis, have been reported very rarely following post-marketing HUMIRA administration. If an anaphylactic reaction or other serious allergic reactions occur, administration of adalimumab should be discontinued immediately and appropriate therapy initiated.

The needle cover of the syringe contains dry natural rubber (latex). This may cause severe allergic reactions in patients sensitive to this substance (see Dosage and Administration, Administration, Pre-filled Syringe or Pre-filled Pen).

Carcinogenesis and Mutagenesis: Long-term animal studies of adalimumab have not been conducted to evaluate the carcinogenic potential or its effect on fertility. No clastogenic or mutagenic effects of adalimumab were observed in the in vivo mouse micronucleus test or the *Salmonella-E. coli* (Ames) assay, respectively.

Immune: Immunosuppression: The possibility exists for TNF blocking agents, including HUMIRA, to affect host defences against infections and malignancies since TNF mediates inflammation and modulates cellular immune responses. In a study of 64 patients with rheumatoid arthritis who were treated with adalimumab, there was no evidence of depression of delayed-type hypersensitivity, depression of immunoglobulin levels, or change in enumeration of effector T- and B-cells and NK-cells, monocyte/macrophages, and neutrophils. The impact of treatment with adalimumab on the development and course of malignancies, as well as active and/or chronic infections, is not fully understood (see Warnings and Precautions and Adverse Reactions, Adverse Drug Reaction Overview, Infections and Malignancies).

Immunizations: In a randomized, double-blind, placebo-controlled study in 226 adult rheumatoid arthritis patients treated with HUMIRA, antibody responses to concomitant pneumococcal and influenza vaccines were assessed. Protective antibody levels to the pneumococcal antigens were achieved by 86% of patients in the HUMIRA group compared to 82% in the placebo group. A total of 37% of HUMIRA-treated subjects and 40% of placebo-treated subjects achieved at least a 2-fold increase in antibody titer to at least three out of five pneumococcal antigens. In the same study, 98% of patients in the HUMIRA group and 95% in the placebo group achieved protective antibody levels to the influenza antigens. A total of 52% of HUMIRA-treated subjects and 63% of placebo-treated subjects achieved at least a 4-fold increase in antibody titer to at least two out of three influenza antigens.

Patients on HUMIRA may receive concurrent vaccinations, except for live vaccines. No data are available on the secondary transmission of infection by live vaccines in patients receiving HUMIRA.

Autoimmunity: Treatment with adalimumab may result in the formation of autoantibodies, and rarely, in the development of a lupus-like syndrome. If a patient develops symptoms suggestive of a lupus-like syndrome following treatment with adalimumab, treatment should be discontinued (see Adverse Reactions, Adverse Drug Reaction Overview, Autoantibodies).

Neurologic Events: Use of TNF blocking agents, including HUMIRA, has been associated with rare cases with new onset or exacerbation of clinical symptoms and/or radiographic evidence of demyelinating disease, including multiple sclerosis. Prescribers should exercise caution in considering the use of adalimumab in patients with preexisting or recent-onset central nervous system demyelinating disorders.

Infections: Tuberculosis: As observed with other TNF blocking agents, tuberculosis (frequently disseminated or extrapulmonary at clinical presentation) associated with the administration of HUMIRA in clinical trials has been reported (see Warnings and Precautions, Serious Warnings and Precautions, Infections). While cases were observed at all doses, the incidence of tuberculosis reactivations was particularly increased at doses of HUMIRA that were higher than the recommended dose.

Before initiation, during and after treatment with HUMIRA, patients should be evaluated for active or latent tuberculosis infection with a tuberculin skin test. Treatment of latent tuberculosis infections should be initiated prior to therapy with HUMIRA. When tuberculin skin testing is performed for latent tuberculosis infection, an induration size of 5 mm or greater should be considered positive, even if vaccinated previously with Bacille Calmette-Guerin (BCG).

The possibility of undetected latent tuberculosis should be considered especially in patients who have immigrated from or traveled to countries with a high prevalence of tuberculosis or who had close contact with a person with active tuberculosis. If latent infection is diagnosed, appropriate prophylaxis in accordance with the Canadian Tuberculosis Standards and Centers for Disease Control and Prevention guidelines should be instituted. Anti-tuberculosis therapy prior to initiating HUMIRA should also be considered in patients who have a negative test for latent tuberculosis but have risk factors for TB infection. The decision to initiate anti-tuberculosis therapy in these patients should only be made after taking into account both the risk for latent tuberculosis infection and the risks of anti-tuberculosis therapy. If necessary, consultation should occur with a physician with expertise in the treatment of tuberculosis. Active tuberculosis has developed in patients receiving HUMIRA whose screening for latent tuberculosis infection was negative, and some patients who have previously received treatment for latent or active tuberculosis have developed active tuberculosis while being treated with TNF blocking agents.

Patients receiving HUMIRA should be monitored for signs and symptoms of active tuberculosis, particularly because tests for latent tuberculosis infection may be falsely negative. The risk of false negative tuberculin skin test results should be considered especially in patients who are severely ill or immunocompromised. Patients should be instructed to seek medical advice if signs/symptoms (e.g., persistent cough, wasting/weight loss, low grade fever) suggestive of a tuberculosis infection occur, and physicians should monitor for signs and symptoms of active tuberculosis, including patients who are tuberculosis skin test negative.

Other Opportunistic Infections: Opportunistic infections, including invasive fungal infections, have been observed in patients receiving HUMIRA. These infections are not consistently recognized in patients taking TNF-blockers and this has resulted in delays in appropriate treatment, sometimes resulting in fatal outcomes.

Patients taking TNF-blockers are more susceptible to serious fungal infections such as histoplasmosis, coccidioidomycosis, blastomycosis, aspergillosis, candidiasis, and other opportunistic infections. Those who develop fever, malaise, weight loss, sweats, cough, dyspnea, and/or pulmonary infiltrates, or other serious systemic illness with or without concomitant shock should promptly seek medical attention for a diagnostic evaluation.

For patients who reside or travel in regions where mycoses are endemic, invasive fungal infections should be suspected if they develop the signs and symptoms of possible systemic fungal infection. Patients are at risk of histoplasmosis and other invasive fungal infections and hence clinicians should consider empiric antifungal treatment until the pathogen(s) are identified. Antigen and antibody testing for histoplasmosis may be negative in some patients with active infection. When feasible, the decision to administer empiric antifungal therapy in these patients should be made in consultation with a physician with expertise in the diagnosis and treatment of invasive fungal infections and should take into account both the risk for severe fungal infection and the risks of antifungal therapy. Patients who develop a severe fungal infection are also advised to stop the TNF-blocker until infections are controlled.

Hepatitis B Virus (HBV) Reactivation: Very rare cases of Hepatitis B virus (HBV) reactivation have been associated with anti-TNF therapy. Clinically active HBV infection occurred following a latency period ranging from 3 to 20 months after initiation of therapy. In the majority of cases, patients were also taking other immunosuppressive drugs, including methotrexate, azathioprine, and/or corticosteroids. Hence, establishing a causal relationship to anti-TNF agents is confounded by the presence of these other medications. Where outcome information was provided, most patients were reported to have improved after antiviral treatment and/or discontinuation of the anti-TNF agent. However, fatal outcomes have also occurred in reported cases. Patients at risk of HBV infection should be evaluated for prior evidence of HBV infection before initiating anti-TNF therapy. Those identified as chronic carriers (i.e., surface antigen positive) should be monitored for signs and symptoms of active HBV infection throughout the course of therapy and for several months following discontinuation of therapy. Reactivation of HBV is not unique to anti-TNF-alpha agents and has been reported with other immunosuppressive drugs.

Hematologic Events: Rare reports of pancytopenia, including aplastic anemia, have been reported with TNF blocking agents. Adverse events of the hematologic system, including medically significant cytopenia (e.g., thrombocytopenia, leukopenia) have been infrequently reported with HUMIRA. The causal relationship of these reports to HUMIRA remains unclear. All patients should be advised to seek immediate medical attention if they develop signs and symptoms suggestive of blood dyscrasias (e.g., persistent fever, bruising, bleeding, pallor) while on HUMIRA. Discontinuation of HUMIRA therapy should be considered in patients with confirmed significant hematologic abnormalities.

Patients with Congestive Heart Failure: Cases of worsening congestive heart failure (CHF) and new onset CHF have been reported with TNF blockers. Cases of worsening CHF have also been observed with HUMIRA. HUMIRA has not been formally studied in patients with CHF; however, in clinical trials of another TNF blocker, a higher rate of serious CHF-related adverse events was observed. Physicians should exercise caution when using HUMIRA in patients who have heart failure and monitor them carefully.

Small Bowel Obstruction: Failure to respond to treatment for Crohn's disease may indicate the presence of fixed fibrotic stricture that may require surgical treatment. Available data suggest that HUMIRA does not worsen or cause strictures.

Special Populations: Pregnant Women: The extent of exposure in pregnancy during clinical trials is very limited, consisting only of individual cases.

An embryo-fetal perinatal developmental toxicity study has been performed in cynomolgus monkeys at dosages up to 100 mg/kg (266 times human AUC when given 40 mg adalimumab subcutaneously with methotrexate every week, or 373 times when given 40 mg adalimumab subcutaneously without methotrexate) and has revealed no evidence of harm to the fetuses due to adalimumab. There are, however, no adequate and well-controlled studies in pregnant women. Because animal reproduction and developmental studies are not always predictive of human response, HUMIRA should be used during pregnancy only if clearly needed.

Labor and Delivery: There are no known effects of adalimumab on labor or delivery.

Nursing Women: It is not known whether adalimumab is excreted in human milk or absorbed systemically after ingestion. Because many drugs and immunoglobulins are excreted in human milk, and because of the potential for serious adverse reactions in nursing infants from adalimumab, a decision should be made whether to discontinue nursing or to discontinue the drug, taking into account the importance of the drug to the mother.

Pediatrics: Safety and effectiveness in pediatric patients have not been established.

Renally and Hepatically Impaired: HUMIRA has not been studied in these patient populations.

Geriatrics (>65 years of age): A total of 519 rheumatoid arthritis patients 65 years of age and older, including 107 patients 75 years and older, received adalimumab in clinical studies RA I to RA IV. No overall differences in effectiveness were observed between these subjects and younger subjects. The frequency of serious infection and malignancy among adalimumab-treated subjects over age 65 was higher than for those under the age of 65. Because there is a higher incidence of infections and malignancies in the elderly population in general, caution should be used when treating the elderly.

Monitoring and Laboratory Tests: There is no known interference between adalimumab and laboratory tests.

ADVERSE REACTIONS: Adverse Drug Reaction Overview: The most serious adverse reactions were (see Warnings and Precautions): serious infections, neurologic events, malignancies.

The most common adverse reaction in rheumatoid arthritis patients treated with HUMIRA (adalimumab) was injection site reactions. In the fifteen controlled trials for rheumatoid arthritis, psoriatic arthritis, ankylosing spondylitis, Crohn's disease, and psoriasis, 14% of patients treated with adalimumab developed injection site reactions (erythema and/or itching, hemorrhage, pain or swelling), compared to 8% of patients receiving control treatment. Most injection site reactions were described as mild and generally did not necessitate drug discontinuation.

The proportion of rheumatoid arthritis patients who discontinued treatment due to adverse events during the double-blind, placebo-controlled portion of rheumatoid arthritis Studies RA I, RA II, RA III, and RA IV was 7.0% for patients taking adalimumab, and 4.0% for placebo-treated patients. The most common adverse events leading to discontinuation of HUMIRA were clinical flare reaction (0.7%), rash (0.3%) and pneumonia (0.3%).

Among patients with rheumatoid arthritis in placebo-controlled studies, deaths occurred in 8 of 1380 (0.58%) HUMIRA-treated patients compared to 1 of 690 (0.14%) placebo-treated patients. The rate of deaths in both treatment arms is less than expected in the normal population with a Standardized Mortality Ratio (SMR) of 0.87 (0.38, 1.72; 95% CI) in the adalimumab group and 0.25 (0.00, 1.37; 95% CI) in the placebo group.

HUMIRA has also been studied in 542 patients with early rheumatoid arthritis (disease duration less than 3 years) who were methotrexate (MTX) naïve (Study RA V). No new safety signals were seen in this patient population compared to the safety profile seen in HUMIRA Studies RA I to RA IV. In this study, deaths occurred in 5 of 542 (0.92%) HUMIRA-treated patients compared to 1 of 257 (0.39%) methotrexate-treated patients. The rate of deaths in both treatment arms is less than expected in the normal population with a Standardized Mortality Ratio of 0.57 (0.18, 1.32; 95% CI) in the adalimumab group and 0.22 (0.00, 1.23; 95% CI) in the methotrexate group.

HUMIRA has also been studied in 395 patients with psoriatic arthritis in two placebo-controlled studies and in an open-label extension study, in 393 patients with ankylosing spondylitis in two placebo-controlled studies and in over 1400 patients with Crohn's disease in four placebo controlled and two open-label extension studies. The safety profile for patients with psoriatic arthritis treated with HUMIRA 40 mg every other week was similar to the safety profile seen in patients with rheumatoid arthritis, HUMIRA Studies RA I to RA V. During the controlled period of the psoriatic arthritis studies, no deaths occurred in the HUMIRA-treated or placebo-treated patients. During the psoriatic arthritis open-label study 2 deaths occurred in 382 patients with 795.7 patient-years of exposure. The rate of deaths is less than expected in the normal population with a Standardized Mortality Ratio (SMR) of 0.39 (0.04, 1.43; 95% CI).

Injection Site Reactions: In the 15 controlled trials, 14% of patients treated with HUMIRA developed injection site reactions (erythema and/or itching, hemorrhage, pain or swelling), compared to 8% of patients receiving placebo or active control. Injection site reactions generally did not necessitate discontinuation of the medicinal product.

Infections: In the fifteen controlled trials for rheumatoid arthritis, psoriatic arthritis, ankylosing spondylitis, Crohn's disease, and psoriasis, the rate of infection was 1.56 per patient year in the adalimumab treated patients and 1.39 per patient year in the control-treated patients. The infections consisted primarily of nasopharyngitis, upper respiratory tract infection, sinusitis. Most patients continued on HUMIRA after the infection resolved.

The incidence of serious infections was 0.03 per patient year in HUMIRA-treated patients and 0.03 per patient year in placebo- and active control-treated patients.

In controlled and open-label studies with HUMIRA, serious infections (including fatal infections, which occurred rarely) have been reported, which include reports of tuberculosis (including miliary and extra-pulmonary locations) and invasive opportunistic infections (e.g., disseminated histoplasmosis, *P.carinii* pneumonia, aspergillosis and listeriosis). Most of the cases of tuberculosis occurred within the first eight months after initiation of therapy and may reflect recrudescence of latent disease.

Malignancies: More cases of malignancy have been observed in HUMIRA-treated patients compared to control-treated patients in clinical trials (see Warnings and Precautions, Malignancies).

Autoantibodies: Patients had serum samples tested for autoantibodies at multiple time points in studies RA I to RA V. In those rheumatoid arthritis controlled trials, 11.9% of patients treated with adalimumab and 8.1% of placebo- or active control-treated patients who had negative baseline antinuclear antibody (ANA) titers, developed positive titers at Week 24. Two patients out of 3441 treated with adalimumab developed clinical signs suggestive of new-onset lupus-like syndrome. The patients improved following discontinuation of therapy. No patients developed lupus nephritis or central nervous system symptoms. The impact of long-term treatment with adalimumab on the development of autoimmune diseases is unknown.

Psoriasis: New-onset and Worsening: Cases of new onset psoriasis, including pustular psoriasis and palmoplantar psoriasis, and cases of worsening of pre-existing psoriasis have been reported with the use of TNF-blockers, including HUMIRA. Many of these patients were taking concomitant immunosuppressants (e.g., MTX, corticosteroids). Some of these patients required hospitalization. Most patients had improvement of their psoriasis following discontinuation of their TNF-blocker. Some patients have had recurrences of the psoriasis when they were re-challenged with a different TNF-blocker. Discontinuation of HUMIRA should be considered for severe cases and those that do not improve or that worsen despite topical treatments.

Immunogenicity: Formation of anti-adalimumab antibodies is associated with increased clearance and reduced efficacy of adalimumab. There is no apparent correlation between the presence of anti-adalimumab antibodies and adverse events.

Rheumatoid arthritis patients in Studies RA I, RA II, and RA III were tested at multiple time points for antibodies to adalimumab during the 6- to 12-month period. Approximately 5% (58 of 1062) of adult rheumatoid arthritis patients receiving adalimumab developed low-titer antibodies to adalimumab at least once during treatment, which were neutralizing in vitro. Patients treated with concomitant methotrexate (MTX) had a lower rate of antibody development than patients on adalimumab monotherapy (1% versus 12 %). With monotherapy, patients receiving every-other-week dosing may develop antibodies more frequently than those receiving weekly dosing. In patients receiving the recommended dosage of 40 mg every other week as monotherapy, the ACR 20 response was lower among antibody-positive patients than among antibody-negative patients. The immunogenicity of adalimumab long-term is unknown.

In patients with psoriatic arthritis, adalimumab antibodies were identified in 38/376 subjects (10%) treated with adalimumab. In patients not given concomitant methotrexate, the incidence was 13.5 % (24/178 subjects), compared to 7 % (14 of 198 subjects) when adalimumab was used as add-on to methotrexate.

In patients with ankylosing spondylitis antibodies were identified in 17/204 subjects (8.3%) treated with adalimumab. In patients not given concomitant methotrexate, the incidence was 16/185 (8.6%), compared to 1/19 (5.3%) when adalimumab was used as add-on to methotrexate.

In patients with Crohn's disease, adalimumab antibodies were identified in 2.6% (7 of 269) of patients receiving adalimumab.

In patients with psoriasis, anti-adalimumab antibodies were identified in 77/920 subjects (8.4%) treated with adalimumab monotherapy.

The data reflect the percentage of patients whose test results were considered positive for antibodies to adalimumab in an ELISA assay, and are highly dependent on the sensitivity and specificity of the assay. Additionally, the observed incidence of antibody positivity in an assay may be influenced by several factors including sample handling, timing of sample collection, concomitant medications, and underlying disease. For these reasons, comparison of the incidence of antibodies to adalimumab with the incidence of antibodies to other products may be misleading.

Clinical Trial Adverse Drug Reactions: General Statement: Because clinical trials are conducted under very specific conditions, the adverse reaction rates observed in the clinical trials may not reflect the rates observed in practice and should not be compared to the rates in the clinical trials of another drug. Adverse drug reaction information from clinical trials is useful for identifying drug-related adverse events and for approximating rates.

Rheumatoid Arthritis Clinical Trials: Description of Data Sources: The data described below reflect exposure to HUMIRA (adalimumab) in 3046 patients, including more than 2000 patients exposed for 6 months, and more than 1500 exposed for more than one year (Studies RA I, RA II, RA III, RA IV, and RA V). Adalimumab was studied in placebo-controlled trials and in long-term follow-up studies for up to 60 months duration in patients with moderately to severely active rheumatoid arthritis who had failed previous DMARD therapy; the mean age was 54 years, 77% were female and 91% Caucasian (Studies RA I, RA II, RA III, RA IV). A further study (Study RA V) was in patients with recently diagnosed rheumatoid arthritis who had not previously been treated with methotrexate. Most patients received 40 mg adalimumab every other week.

Relative Frequency of Adverse Drug Reactions: Table 1 summarizes adverse drug reactions reported at a rate of at least 1% in patients treated with adalimumab 40 mg every other week (eow), as well as all doses of adalimumab tested, compared to placebo or methotrexate (Study RA V). Adverse reaction rates in patients treated with adalimumab 40 mg weekly were similar to rates in patients treated with adalimumab every other week. In Study RA III, the types and frequencies of adverse drug reactions in the 5-year open-label extension were similar to those observed in the one-year double-blind portion.

Table 1: HUMIRA

Number and Percentage of Subjects with ≥1% Treatment-emergent Adverse Events at Least Possibly Related to Study Drug During the Control Period in RA Studies (Studies RA I, RA II, RA III, RA IV, RA V)

System Organ Class (SOC)	Adalimumab 40 mg s.c. eow N=1247 N (%)	All Adalimumab N=1922 N (%)	Placebo (not DE013) N=690 N (%)	MTX (DE013) N=257 N (%)
Gastrointestinal Disorders				
Nausea	80 (6.4)	112 (5.8)	12 (1.7)	33 (12.8)
Diarrhea	47 (3.8)	60 (3.1)	17 (2.5)	18 (7.0)
Abdominal pain	22 (1.8)	29 (1.5)	5 (0.7)	3 (1.2)
Abdominal pain upper	20 (1.6)	25 (1.3)	0 (0.0)	13 (5.1)
Mouth ulceration	17 (1.4)	24 (1.2)	5 (0.7)	12 (4.7)
Dyspepsia	14 (1.1)	21 (1.1)	4 (0.6)	7 (2.7)
Vomiting	16 (1.3)	20 (1.0)	5 (0.7)	6 (2.3)
General Disorders and Administration Site Conditions				
Injection site irritation	74 (5.9)	122 (6.3)	61 (8.8)	3 (1.2)
Injection site reaction	49 (3.9)	67 (3.5)	3 (0.4)	2 (0.8)
Injection site pain	36 (2.9)	63 (3.3)	24 (3.5)	6 (2.3)
Injection site erythema	36 (2.9)	60 (3.1)	2 (0.3)	1 (0.4)
Fatigue	37 (3.0)	58 (3.0)	7 (1.0)	9 (3.5)
Injection site rash	17 (1.4)	22 (1.1)	2 (0.3)	0 (0.0)
Influenza like illness	15 (1.2)	21 (1.1)	2 (0.3)	8 (3.1)
Pyrexia	13 (1.0)	20 (1.0)	1 (0.1)	6 (2.3)
Infections and Infestations				
Nasopharyngitis	61 (4.9)	95 (4.9)	10 (1.5)	28 (10.9)
Upper respiratory infection	72 (5.8)	93 (4.8)	15 (2.2)	17 (6.6)
Sinusitis	46 (3.7)	55 (2.9)	17 (2.5)	4 (1.6)
Herpes simplex	33 (2.6)	48 (2.5)	6 (0.9)	5 (1.9)
Urinary tract infection	31 (2.5)	44 (2.3)	6 (0.9)	7 (2.7)
Bronchitis	19 (1.5)	29 (1.5)	8 (1.2)	9 (3.5)
Herpes zoster	17 (1.4)	23 (1.2)	8 (1.2)	2 (0.8)
Influenza	16 (1.3)	21 (1.1)	7 (1.0)	5 (1.9)
Pneumonia	17 (1.4)	21 (1.1)	3 (0.4)	1 (0.4)
Investigations				
Lymphocyte count decreased	11 (0.9)	38 (2.0)	11 (1.6)	1 (0.4)
Alanine aminotransferase increased	27 (2.2)	33 (1.7)	4 (0.6)	9 (3.5)
Liver function test abnormal	19 (1.5)	22 (1.1)	4 (0.6)	7 (2.7)
Musculoskeletal and Connective Tissue Disorders				
Rheumatoid arthritis	11 (0.9)	28 (1.5)	7 (1.0)	2 (0.8)
Nervous System Disorders				
Headache	75 (6.0)	124 (6.5)	14 (2.0)	14 (5.4)
Dizziness	23 (1.8)	32 (1.7)	6 (0.9)	3 (1.2)
Respiratory, Thoracic and Mediastinal Disorders				
Pharyngolaryngeal pain	33 (2.6)	44 (2.3)	9 (1.3)	7 (2.7)
Cough	31 (2.5)	42 (2.2)	4 (0.6)	9 (3.5)
Skin and Subcutaneous Tissue Disorders				
Rash	44 (3.5)	66 (3.4)	9 (1.3)	8 (3.1)
Pruritus	28 (2.2)	43 (2.2)	4 (0.6)	5 (1.9)
Alopecia	22 (1.8)	28 (1.5)	2 (0.3)	6 (2.3)

(cont'd)

Table 1: HUMIRA *(cont'd)*

Number and Percentage of Subjects with ≥1% Treatment-emergent Adverse Events at Least Possibly Related to Study Drug During the Control Period in RA Studies (Studies RA I, RA II, RA III, RA IV, RA V)

System Organ Class (SOC)	Adalimumab 40 mg s.c. eow N=1247 N (%)	All Adalimumab N=1922 N (%)	Placebo (not DE013) N=690 N (%)	MTX (DE013) N=257 N (%)
Rash pruritic	14 (1.1)	22 (1.1)	0 (0.0)	3 (1.2)

Psoriatic Arthritis Clinical Trials: Table 2 summarizes adverse drug reactions reported in placebo-controlled and open-label studies at a rate of at least 1% in psoriatic arthritis patients treated with adalimumab 40 mg every other week.

Table 2: HUMIRA

Number and Percentage of Subjects with ≥1% Treatment-emergent Adverse Events at Least Possibly Related to Study Drug During the Control and Open-label Periods in PsA Studies (Studies PsA I, PsA II, and PsA III)

	Double-blind Study		Open-label Study
System Organ Class (SOC)	Placebo N=211 n (%)	Adalimumab 40 mg s.c. eow N=202 n (%)	Adalimumab 40 mg s.c. eow N=382 n (%)
Gastrointestinal Disorders			
Nausea	2 (0.9)	2 (1.0)	3 (0.8)
General Disorders and Administration Site Conditions			
Injection site reaction	5 (2.4)	11 (5.4)	21 (5.5)
Injection site pain	8 (3.8)	8 (4.0)	2 (0.5)
Injection site erythema	0 (0.0)	4 (2.0)	2 (0.5)
Injection site burning	4 (1.9)	4 (2.0)	4 (1.0)
Fatigue	5 (2.4)	0 (0.0)	4 (1.0)
Infections and Infestations			
Upper respiratory infection	7 (3.3)	8 (4.0)	17 (4.5)
Herpes simplex	3 (1.4)	6 (3.0)	7 (1.8)
Skin fungal infection NOS	0 (0.0)	3 (1.5)	—
Pharyngitis	1 (0.5)	2 (1.0)	4 (1.0)
Sinusitis	4 (1.9)	2 (1.0)	12 (3.1)
Urinary tract infection	0 (0.0)	2 (1.0)	6 (1.6)
Bronchitis	1 (0.5)	1 (0.5)	5 (1.3)
Nasopharyngitis	2 (0.9)	1 (0.5)	8 (2.1)
Influenza	2 (0.9)	0 (0.0)	5 (1.3)
Investigations			
Liver function tests abnormal	1 (0.5)	2 (1.0)	5 (1.3)
Nervous System Disorders			
Headache	5 (2.4)	5 (2.5)	5 (1.3)
Paresthesia	1 (0.5)	3 (1.5)	2 (0.5)
Respiratory, Thoracic, and Mediastinal Disorders			
Rhinitis NOS	0 (0.0)	3 (1.5)	3 (0.8)
Skin and Subcutaneous Tissue Disorders			
Erythema	0 (0.0)	3 (1.5)	—

Ankylosing Spondylitis Clinical Trials: HUMIRA has been studied in 393 patients with ankylosing spondylitis in two placebo controlled studies. The safety profile for patients with ankylosing spondylitis treated with HUMIRA 40 mg every other week (eow) was similar to the safety profile seen in patients with rheumatoid arthritis, HUMIRA Studies RA I to RA IV. Table 3 summarizes adverse drug reactions reported at a rate of at least 1% in ankylosing spondylitis patients treated with adalimumab 40 mg every other week compared to placebo.

Table 3: HUMIRA

Number and Percentage of Subjects with ≥1% Treatment-emergent Adverse Events at Least Possibly Related to Study Drug During the Control Period in AS Studies (Studies AS I and AS II)

System Organ Class (SOC)	Adalimumab 40 mg s.c. eow N=246 N (%)	Placebo N=151 N (%)
General Disorders and Administration Site Conditions		
Fatigue	5 (2.0)	3 (2.0)
Injection site erythema	5 (2.0)	1 (0.7)

(cont'd)

Table 3: HUMIRA *(cont'd)*

Number and Percentage of Subjects with ≥1% Treatment-emergent Adverse Events at Least Possibly Related to Study Drug During the Control Period in AS Studies (Studies AS I and AS II)

System Organ Class (SOC)	Adalimumab 40 mg s.c. eow N=246 N (%)	Placebo N=151 N (%)
Injection site irritation	4 (1.6)	2 (1.3)
Injection site pain	6 (2.4)	3 (2.0)
Injection site reaction	8 (3.3)	1 (0.7)
Infections and Infestations		
Nasopharyngitis	8 (3.3)	0 (0.0)
Upper respiratory tract infection	5 (2.0)	2 (1.3)
Nervous System Disorders		
Dizziness	3 (1.2)	3 (2.0)
Headache	11 (4.5)	4 (2.6)
Skin and Subcutaneous Tissue Disorders		
Eczema	3 (1.2)	1 (0.7)
Pruritus	4 (1.6)	1 (0.7)
Pruritus generalized	3 (1.2)	0 (0.0)
Rash	4 (1.6)	1 (0.7)
Urticaria	3 (1.2)	0 (0.0)

Crohn's Disease Clinical Studies: HUMIRA has been studied in over 1400 patients with Crohn's disease in four placebo controlled and two open-label extension studies. The safety profile for patients with Crohn's disease treated with HUMIRA was similar to the safety profile seen in patients with rheumatoid arthritis.

Table 4 and Table 5 summarize adverse drug reactions reported at a rate of at least 1% in Crohn's Disease patients treated with HUMIRA in Induction and Maintenance studies, respectively.

Table 4: HUMIRA

Number and Percentage of Subjects with ≥1% Treatment-emergent Adverse Events at Least Possibly Related to Study Drug During Administration of Induction Study Medications in CD Studies

System Organ Class (SOC)	Adalimumab 160/80 mg N=235 N (%)	Adalimumab 80/40 mg N=75 N (%)	Placebo N=240 N (%)
Eye Disorders			
Corneal pigmentation	0 (0,0)	1 (1.3)	0 (0,0)
Visual disturbance	0 (0,0)	1 (1.3)	0 (0,0)
Gastrointestinal Disorders			
Abdominal pain	5 (2.1)	0 (0,0)	2 (0.8)
Abdominal pain lower	3 (1.3)	0 (0,0)	0 (0,0)
Change of bowel habit	0 (0,0)	1 (1.3)	0 (0,0)
Cheilitis	0 (0,0)	1 (1.3)	1 (0.4)
Constipation	2 (0.9)	1 (1.3)	3 (1.3)
Crohn's disease	2 (0.9)	1 (1.3)	3 (1.3)
Flatulence	3 (1.3)	0 (0,0)	0 (0,0)
Nausea	6 (2.6)	0 (0,0)	4 (1.7)
Vomiting	1 (0.4)	1 (1.3)	3 (1.3)
General Disorders and Administration Site Conditions			
Asthenia	0 (0,0)	1 (1.3)	1 (0.4)
Chills	0 (0,0)	2 (2.7)	1 (0.4)
Fatigue	2 (0.9)	1 (1.3)	10 (4.2)
Influenza like illness	0 (0,0)	2 (2.7)	2 (0.8)
Injection site bruising	5 (2.1)	1 (1.3)	1 (0.4)
Injection site erythema	4 (1.7)	0 (0,0)	0 (0,0)
Injection site irritation	19 (8.1)	8 (10.7)	14 (5.8)
Injection site pain	6 (2.6)	4 (5.3)	9 (3.8)
Injection site pruritus	3 (1.3)	0 (0,0)	0 (0,0)

(cont'd)

Table 4: HUMIRA *(cont'd)*

Number and Percentage of Subjects with ≥1% Treatment-emergent Adverse Events at Least Possibly Related to Study Drug During Administration of Induction Study Medications in CD Studies

System Organ Class (SOC)	Adalimumab 160/80 mg N=235 N (%)	Adalimumab 80/40 mg N=75 N (%)	Placebo N=240 N (%)
Injection site reaction	11 (4.7)	5 (6.7)	6 (2.5)
Pain	2 (0.9)	1 (1.3)	3 (1.3)
Pyrexia	3 (1.3)	3 (1.3)	3 (1.3)
Infections and Infestations			
Staphylococcal infection	0 (0,0)	1 (1.3)	0 (0,0)
Investigations			
Double stranded DNA antibody	0 (0,0)	1 (1.3)	0 (0,0)
White blood cell count increased	0 (0,0)	1 (1.3)	0 (0,0)
Metabolism and Nutrition Disorders			
Hypokalemia	0 (0,0)	1 (1.3)	0 (0,0)
Musculoskeletal and Connective Tissue Disorders			
Arthralgia	3 (1.3)	1 (1.3)	2 (0.8)
Back pain	0 (0,0)	1 (1.3)	0 (0,0)
Muscle spasms	0 (0,0)	1 (1.3)	1 (0.4)
Pain in extremity	0 (0,0)	1 (1.3)	0 (0,0)
Nervous System Disorders			
Dizziness	3 (1.3)	0 (0,0)	2 (0.8)
Headache	8 (3.4)	2 (2.7)	7 (2.9)
Restless legs syndrome	0 (0,0)	1 (1.3)	0 (0,0)
Reproductive System and Breast Disorders			
Genital pruritus female	0 (0,0)	1 (1.3)	0 (0,0)
Skin and Subcutaneous Tissue Disorders			
Eczema	1 (0.4)	1 (1.3)	0 (0,0)
Erythema	1 (0.4)	1 (1.3)	1 (0.4)
Hyperhidrosis	0 (0,0)	1 (1.3)	0 (0,0)
Onychorrhexis	0 (0,0)	1 (1.3)	0 (0,0)
Pruritus	1 (0.4)	0 (0,0)	4 (1.7)
Rash	2 (0.9)	2 (2.7)	1 (0.4)
Rash maculopapular	1 (0.4)	1 (1.3)	0 (0,0)
Rash pruritic	0 (0,0)	1 (1.3)	1 (0.4)

Table 5: HUMIRA

Number and Percentage of Subjects with ≥1% Treatment-emergent Adverse Events at Least Possibly Related to Study Drug During Administration of Blinded Study Maintenance Medications in CD Studies

System Organ Class (SOC)	Adalimumab 40 mg s.c. eow, 40 mg ew N=554 N (%)	Placebo N=279 N (%)
Gastrointestinal Disorders		
Abdominal pain	7 (1.3)	4 (1.4)
Crohn's disease	9 (1.6)	9 (3.2)
Diarrhoea	7 (1.3)	1 (0.4)
Nausea	9 (1.6)	5 (1.8)
General Disorders and Administration Site Conditions		
Fatigue	10 (1.8)	1 (0.4)
Injection site bruising	6 (1.1)	1 (0.4)
Injection site erythema	10 (1.8)	0 (0.0)
Injection site irritation	18 (3.2)	2 (0.7)
Injection site pain	8 (1.4)	2 (0.7)

(cont'd)

Table 5: HUMIRA *(cont'd)*

Number and Percentage of Subjects with ≥1% Treatment-emergent Adverse Events at Least Possibly Related to Study Drug During Administration of Blinded Study Maintenance Medications in CD Studies

System Organ Class (SOC)	Adalimumab 40 mg s.c. eow, 40 mg ew N=554 N (%)	Placebo N=279 N (%)
Injection site reaction	26 (4.7)	1 (0.4)
Pyrexia	7 (1.3)	5 (1.8)
Infections and Infestations		
Herpes simplex	6 (1.1)	4 (1.4)
Nasopharyngitis	8 (1.4)	2 (0.7)
Rhinitis	7 (1.3)	1 (0.4)
Musculoskeletal and Connective Tissue Disorders		
Arthralgia	9 (1.6)	2 (0.7)
Nervous System Disorders		
Headache	19 (3.4)	6 (2.2)
Skin and Subcutaneous Tissue Disorders		
Rash	11 (2.0)	5 (1.8)

Psoriasis: HUMIRA has been studied in 1696 patients with psoriasis in placebo-controlled and open-label extension studies. The safety profile for patients with psoriasis treated with HUMIRA was similar to the safety profile seen in patients with rheumatoid arthritis. Table 6 summarizes adverse drug reactions reported at a rate of at least 1% in psoriasis patients treated with an initial dose of adalimumab 80 mg followed by adalimumab 40 mg every other week compared to placebo or methotrexate.

Table 6: HUMIRA

Number and Percentage of Subjects ≥1% Reporting Treatment-emergent Adverse Events Possibly or Probably Related to Study Drug in Controlled Psoriasis Studies (Studies I, II and III)

System Organ Class (SOC)	Adalimumab 80 mg×1, then 40 mg s.c. eow N=966 N (%)	Placebo + MTX N=613 N (%)
Gastrointestinal Disorders		
Nausea	10 (1.0)	11 (1.8)
General Disorders and Administration Site Conditions		
Injection site reaction	29 (3.0)	9 (1.5)
Injection site irritation	16 (1.7)	6 (1.0)
Injection site pain	14 (1.5)	9 (1.5)
Fatigue	10 (1.0)	5 (0.8)
Infections and Infestations		
Upper respiratory infection	12 (1.2)	3 (0.5)
Musculoskeletal and Connective Tissue Disorders		
Arthralgia	10 (1.0)	3 (0.5)
Nervous System Disorders		
Headache	19 (2.0)	14 (2.3)

Other Common Clinical Trial Adverse Drug Reactions: Other clinical trial adverse reactions occurring at an incidence of ≥1% that were observed among the various indications include:
Eye Disorders: conjunctivitis, visual impairment.
Renal and Urinary Disorders: hematuria, renal impairment.
Less Common Clinical Trial Adverse Drug Reactions (<1%): Infrequent serious adverse drug reactions occurring at an incidence of less than 1% in patients treated with HUMIRA in Studies RA I to RA V, Studies PsA I and PsA II, Studies AS I and AS II, CD Maintenance Studies, and Ps Studies I to III:
Blood and Lymphatic System Disorders: lymphadenopathy, pancytopenia, agranulocytosis, eosinophilia, leukopenia, lymphocytosis, neutropenia, anemia.
Cardiac Disorders: arrhythmia superventricular, cardiac arrest, chest pain, palpitations.
Gastrointestinal Disorders: abdominal pain, Crohn's disease, anal fistula, frequent bowel movements hemorrhoidal hemorrhage, rectal hemorrhage, small intestine obstruction, pancreatitis.
General Disorders and Administration Site Conditions: death, non-cardiac chest pain, pyrexia.
Eye Disorders: blepharitis, diplopia, eye swelling.
Hepatobiliary Disorders: hepatic necrosis.
Immune System Disorders: hypersensitivity.
Infections and Infestations: pneumonia, arthritis bacterial, cellulitis, escherichia sepsis, perianal abscess, urinary tract infection, wound infection, sinusitis, bronchitis, cystitis, device related infection, diverticulitis, erysipelas, gastroenteritis, herpes virus infection, herpes zoster, histoplasmosis, infected skin ulcer, infection, lobar pneumonia, lower respiratory tract infection, meningitis viral, mycobacterium avium complex infection, necrotizing fasciitis, pneumonia pneumococcal, pyelonephritis, respiratory tract infection, sepsis, septic shock, tuberculosis, urosepsis, abscess, abscess limb.
Injury, Poisoning and Procedural Complications: postoperative wound complication.
Investigations: double stranded DNA antibody, hepatic enzyme increased.
Musculoskeletal and Connective Tissue Disorders: rheumatoid arthritis, arthritis, arthropathy, back pain, muscular weakness, musculoskeletal chest pain, osteitis, systemic lupus erythematosus.
Neoplasms Benign, Malignant and Unspecified (Including Cysts and Polyps): B-cell lymphoma, breast cancer, malignant melanoma in situ, metastases to liver, ovarian cancer, basal cell carcinoma, squamous cell carcinoma, testicular seminoma (pure).
Nervous System Disorders: hyperreflexia, clonus, hypertensive encephalopathy, intention tremor, multiple sclerosis, paresthesia, tremor.
Psychiatric Disorders: confusional state.
Renal and Urinary Disorders: nocturia.
Reproductive System Disorders: cervical dysplasia, endometrial hyperplasia.
Respiratory, Thoracic and Mediastinal Disorders: pleural effusion, pneumonitis, bronchospasm, lung infiltration, pleurisy, respiratory failure.
Skin and Subcutaneous Tissue Disorders: psoriasis, pustular psoriasis, rash.
Surgical and Medical Procedures: arthrodesis.
Vascular Disorders: circulatory collapse, rheumatoid vasculitis.
Abnormal Hematologic and Clinical Chemistry Findings: There are no known laboratory tests that may be helpful in following the patient's response or in identifying possible adverse reactions.
Rheumatoid Arthritis Clinical Trials: In controlled rheumatoid arthritis clinical trials (RA Studies I-IV), elevations of ALT were similar in patients receiving adalimumab or placebo. In patients with early rheumatoid arthritis (disease duration of less than 3 years) (RA Study V), elevations of ALT were more common in the combination arm (HUMIRA/methotrexate) compared to the methotrexate monotherapy arm or the HUMIRA monotherapy arm.
Psoriatic Arthritis Clinical Trials: Elevations in ALT were more common in psoriatic arthritis patients compared with patients in rheumatoid arthritis clinical studies.
Crohn's Disease Clinical Trials: In controlled clinical trials, elevations of ALT were similar in patients receiving adalimumab or placebo.

In all indications, patients with raised ALT were asymptomatic and in most cases, elevations were transient and resolved on continued treatment.

Post-Market Adverse Drug Reactions: The following post-market adverse drug reactions have been rarely reported:
Cardiac Disorders: myocardial infarction.
Hematologic Events: thrombocytopenia (see Warnings and Precautions, Hematologic Events).
Hypersensitivity Reactions: anaphylaxis, angioedema and angioneurotic edema (see Warnings and Precautions, Hypersensitivity Reactions).
Skin Reactions: cutaneous vasculitis, Stevens-Johnson Syndrome, erythema multiforme, new onset or worsening of psoriasis (including palmoplantar pustular psoriasis).
Respiratory Disorders: interstitial lung disease, including pulmonary fibrosis.
Infections: reactivation of hepatitis B virus (HBV). See Warnings and Precautions, Infections.
Gastrointestinal Disorders: intestinal perforation.
Musculoskeletal and Connective Tissue Disorders: lupus-like syndrome. See Warnings and Precautions, Immune, Autoimmunity and Adverse Reactions, Adverse Drug Reaction Overview, Autoantibodies).
Nervous System Disorders: demyelinating disorders (e.g., Guillain-Barré syndrome, optic neuritis), cerebrovascular accident.
Neoplasia: hepatosplenic T-cell lymphoma. See Warnings and Precautions.

DRUG INTERACTIONS:

> **Serious Drug Interactions**
> **Serious infections and sepsis, including fatalities, have been reported with the use of TNF blocking agents, including HUMIRA (adalimumab). Many of the serious infections have occurred in patients on concomitant immunosuppressive therapy that, in addition to their rheumatoid arthritis, could predispose them to infections. Tuberculosis and invasive opportunistic fungal infections have been observed in patients treated with TNF blocking agents, including adalimumab.**

Overview: Population pharmacokinetic analyses with data from over 1200 rheumatoid arthritis (RA) patients revealed that coadministration of methotrexate (MTX) had an intrinsic effect on the apparent clearance of adalimumab (CL/F) (see Drug Interactions, Drug-Drug Interactions). As expected, there was a trend toward higher apparent clearance of adalimumab with increasing body weight and in the presence of anti-adalimumab antibodies.

Other more minor factors were also identified: higher apparent clearance was predicted in RA patients receiving doses lower than the recommended dose, and in RA patients with high rheumatoid factor or CRP concentrations. These factors are not likely to be clinically important.

Adalimumab has been studied in rheumatoid arthritis patients taking concomitant MTX. The data do not suggest the need for dose adjustment of either adalimumab or methotrexate.

Drug-Drug Interactions: Methotrexate (MTX): When adalimumab was administered to 21 rheumatoid arthritis patients on stable MTX therapy, there were no statistically significant changes in the serum MTX concentration profiles. In contrast, after single and multiple dosing, MTX reduced adalimumab apparent clearances by 29% and 44% respectively, in patients with rheumatoid arthritis.
Anakinra: Concurrent administration of anakinra (an interleukin-1 antagonist) and another TNF blocking agent has been associated with an increased risk of serious infections, an increased risk of neutropenia and no additional benefit compared to these medicinal products alone. Therefore, the combination of anakinra with other TNF blocking agents, including HUMIRA, may also result in similar toxicities. (See Warnings and Precautions, Use with Anakinra.)
Abatacept: Concurrent administration of TNF antagonists and abatacept has been associated with an increased risk of infections including serious infections compared to TNF antagonists alone. This combination has not demonstrated increased clinical benefit. Thus the combined use of TNF antagonists and abatacept is not recommended.
Other: Interactions between HUMIRA and drugs other than methotrexate (MTX) have not been evaluated in formal pharmacokinetic studies. In rheumatoid arthritis clinical trials where HUMIRA was coadministered with commonly-used DMARDs (sulfasalazine, hydrochloroquine, leflunomide and parenteral gold), glucocorticoids, salicylates, nonsteroidal anti-inflammatory drugs or analgesics, no safety signals were seen.

There is no data on other DMARDs, and patients with prior treatment with alkylating agents (e.g., cyclophosphamide) were excluded.

Drug-Food Interactions: Adalimumab is administered as a subcutaneous injection. Interactions with food are therefore not applicable.
Drug-Herb Interactions: Interactions with herbal products have not been established.
Drug-Laboratory Test Interactions: There are no known laboratory tests that may be helpful in following the patient's response or in identifying possible adverse reactions.
Drug-Lifestyle Interactions: HUMIRA may have a minor influence on the ability to drive and use machines. Dizziness (including vertigo, vision disorder and fatigue) may occur following administration of HUMIRA.

DOSAGE AND ADMINISTRATION: Dosing Considerations: Pediatric Use: Safety and effectiveness in pediatric patients have not been established.
Geriatric Use: Evidence from clinical studies and experience suggests that use of HUMIRA (adalimumab) in the geriatric population is not associated with differences in safety or effectiveness. A brief discussion can be found under Warnings and Precautions, Special Populations, Geriatrics (>65 years of age).
Hepatic and Renal Insufficiency: No pharmacokinetic data are available in patients with hepatic or renal impairment. No dose recommendation can be made.
Disease States: Healthy volunteers and patients with rheumatoid arthritis displayed similar adalimumab pharmacokinetics.
Gender: No gender-related pharmacokinetic differences were observed after correction for a patient's body weight. Healthy volunteers and patients with rheumatoid arthritis displayed similar adalimumab pharmacokinetics.
Race: No differences in immunoglobulin clearance would be expected among races. From limited data in non-Caucasians, no important kinetic differences were observed for adalimumab. Dosage adjustment is not required.
Recommended Dose and Dosage Adjustment: Rheumatoid Arthritis: The recommended dose of HUMIRA (adalimumab) for adult patients with rheumatoid arthritis (RA) is 40 mg administered every other week as a subcutaneous (s.c.) injection.
Psoriatic Arthritis: The recommended dose of HUMIRA (adalimumab) for adult patients with psoriatic arthritis (PsA) is 40 mg administered every other week as a subcutaneous (s.c.) injection.

For the RA and PsA indications, available data suggest that the clinical response is usually achieved within 12 weeks of treatment. Continued therapy should be carefully reconsidered in a patient not responding within this time period.

Ankylosing Spondylitis: The recommended dose of HUMIRA (adalimumab) for patients with ankylosing spondylitis (AS) is 40 mg adalimumab administered every other week as a single dose via subcutaneous (s.c.) injection. Glucocorticoids, salicylates, nonsteroidal anti-inflammatory drugs, analgesics or disease modifying anti-rheumatic drugs can be continued during treatment with HUMIRA.

Crohn's Disease: The recommended HUMIRA (adalimumab) induction dose regimen for adult patients with Crohn's disease is 160 mg at Week 0 (dose can be administered as four subcutaneous (s.c.) injections in one day or as two subcutaneous (s.c.) injections per day for two consecutive days), followed by 80 mg at Week 2.

The recommended HUMIRA maintenance dose regimen for adult patients with Crohn's disease is 40 mg every other week beginning at Week 4.

During treatment with HUMIRA, other concomitant therapies (e.g., corticosteroids and/or immunomodulatory agents) should be optimized.

For patients who experience a disease flare, dose escalation may be considered.

Some patients who have not responded by Week 4 (induction period) may benefit from continued maintenance therapy through Week 12. Available data suggest that the clinical response is usually achieved at Week 4 of treatment. Continued therapy should be carefully reconsidered in a patient not responding within this time period.

The use of HUMIRA in Crohn's disease beyond one year has not been evaluated in controlled clinical studies.

Psoriasis: The recommended dose of HUMIRA (adalimumab) for adult patients with psoriasis (Ps) is an initial dose of 80 mg administered subcutaneously, followed by 40 mg subcutaneously given every other week starting one week after the initial dose.

Continued therapy beyond 16 weeks should be carefully reconsidered in a patient not responding within this time period.

Missed Dose: Patients who miss a dose of HUMIRA should be advised to inject this missed dose as soon as they become aware of it, and then follow with their next scheduled dose.

Administration: Administration of HUMIRA (adalimumab) Subcutaneous Injection: HUMIRA is intended for use under the guidance and supervision of a physician. Patients may self-inject HUMIRA if their physician determines that it is appropriate and with medical follow-up, as necessary, after proper training in subcutaneous injection technique.

Methotrexate (MTX), glucocorticoids, salicylates, nonsteroidal anti-inflammatory drugs (NSAIDs), analgesics or other DMARDs may be continued during treatment with adalimumab. When treated with HUMIRA as monotherapy, some rheumatoid arthritis patients who experience a decrease in their response to HUMIRA 40 mg every other week, may benefit from an increase in dose intensity to 40 mg HUMIRA every week.

Pre-filled Syringe or Pre-filled Pen: The solution in the syringe or Pen should be carefully inspected visually for particulate matter and discolouration prior to subcutaneous administration. If particulates and discolourations are noted, the product should not be used. HUMIRA does not contain preservatives; therefore, unused portions of drug remaining in the syringe should be discarded.

Note: The needle cover of the syringe contains a dry natural rubber (latex), which should not be handled by persons sensitive to this substance.

Patients using the pre-filled syringes should be instructed to inject the full amount in the syringe (0.8 mL), which provides 40 mg of HUMIRA, according to the directions provided in the Information for the Patient.

Injection sites should be rotated and injections should never be given into areas where the skin is tender, bruised, red or hard (see Information for the Patient).

OVERDOSAGE:

The maximum tolerated dose of HUMIRA (adalimumab) has not been established in humans. Multiple doses up to 10 mg/kg have been administered to patients in clinical trials without evidence of dose-limiting toxicities. In case of overdosage, it is recommended that the patient be monitored for any signs or symptoms of adverse reactions or effects and appropriate symptomatic treatment instituted immediately.

For management of a suspected drug overdose, CPhA recommends that you contact your **regional Poison Control Centre**. See the *CPS* Directory section for a list of Poison Control Centres.

ACTION AND CLINICAL PHARMACOLOGY: Mechanism of Action: Adalimumab binds specifically to TNF-alpha and blocks its interaction with the p55 and p75 cell surface TNF receptors. Adalimumab also lyses surface TNF-expressing cells in vitro in the presence of complement. Adalimumab does not bind or inactivate lymphotoxin (TNF-beta). TNF is a naturally-occurring cytokine that is involved in normal inflammatory and immune responses. Elevated levels of TNF are found in the synovial fluid of rheumatoid arthritis, psoriatic arthritis and ankylosing spondylitis patients and play an important role in both pathologic inflammation and joint destruction that are hallmarks of these diseases. Increased levels of TNF are also found in psoriasis plaques, which contribute to the inflammatory response, to the proliferation and decreased maturation of keratinocytes and to the associated vascular damages that are characteristic of the disease.

Adalimumab also modulates biological responses that are induced or regulated by TNF, including changes in the levels of adhesion molecules responsible for leukocyte migration (ELAM-1, VCAM-1, and ICAM-1 with an IC_{50} of $1\text{-}2\times10^{-10}$M).

Pharmacodynamics: After treatment with HUMIRA (adalimumab), a rapid decrease in levels of acute phase reactants of inflammation [C-reactive protein (CRP) and erythrocyte sedimentation rate (ESR)] and serum cytokines (IL-6) was observed compared to baseline in patients with rheumatoid arthritis. A rapid decrease in CRP levels was also observed in patients with Crohn's disease. Serum levels of matrix metalloproteinases (MMP-1 and MMP-3) that produce tissue remodeling responsible for cartilage destruction were also decreased after adalimumab administration.

The serum adalimumab concentration-efficacy relationship as measured by the American College of Rheumatology response criteria (ACR 20) appears to follow the Hill E_{max} equation as shown in Figure 1.

Figure 1: HUMIRA

Serum Adalimumab Concentration-efficacy Relationship as Measured by the American College of Rheumatology Response Criteria (ACR 20)

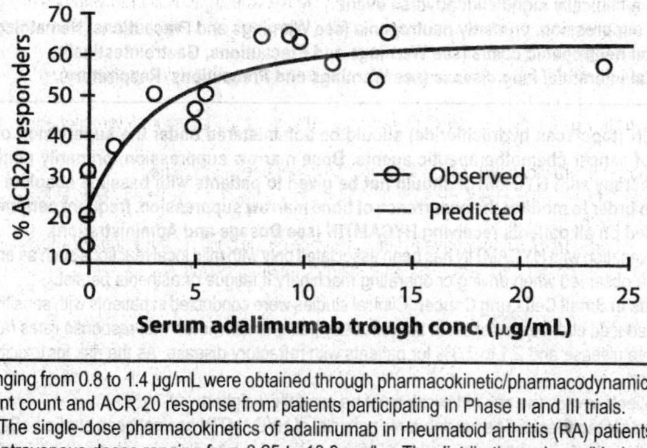

EC_{50} estimates ranging from 0.8 to 1.4 μg/mL were obtained through pharmacokinetic/pharmacodynamic modelling of swollen joint count, tender joint count and ACR 20 response from patients participating in Phase II and III trials.

Pharmacokinetics: The single-dose pharmacokinetics of adalimumab in rheumatoid arthritis (RA) patients were determined in several studies with intravenous doses ranging from 0.25 to 10.0 mg/kg. The distribution volume (Vss) ranged from 4.7 to 6.0 L. The systemic clearance of adalimumab is approximately 12 mL/hr. The mean terminal half-life was approximately 2 weeks, ranging from 10 to 20 days across studies. The pharmacokinetics of adalimumab were linear over the dose range of 0.5 to 10.0 mg/kg following a single intravenous dose.

Adalimumab mean steady-state trough concentrations of approximately 5 μg/mL and 8 to 9 μg/mL, were observed in rheumatoid arthritis patients without and with methotrexate (MTX), respectively. The serum adalimumab trough levels at steady-state increased approximately proportionally with dose following 20, 40 and 80 mg every other week and every week subcutaneous dosing. In long-term studies with dosing more than two years, there was no evidence of changes in clearance over time.

Population pharmacokinetic analyses in patients with rheumatoid arthritis revealed that there was a trend toward higher apparent clearance of adalimumab in the presence of anti-adalimumab antibodies.

In patients with psoriatic arthritis, adalimumab mean steady-state trough concentrations of adalimumab of 8.5-12 μg/mL and 6-10 μg/mL were observed in patients with and without methotrexate, respectively.

In patients with Crohn's disease, the loading dose of 160 mg HUMIRA on Week 0 followed by 80 mg HUMIRA on Week 2 achieves mean serum adalimumab trough concentrations of approximately 12 μg/mL at Week 2 and Week 4. Mean steady-state trough levels of approximately 7 μg/mL were observed at Week 24 and Week 56 in Crohn's disease patients who received a maintenance dose of 40 mg HUMIRA every other week.

Population pharmacokinetic analysis in patients with Crohn's disease revealed a lower apparent clearance of HUMIRA as compared to patients with RA.

In patients with psoriasis, the mean steady-state trough concentration was 5 μg/mL during adalimumab 40 mg every other week monotherapy treatment.

Absorption: The maximum serum concentration (C_{max}) and the time to reach the maximum concentration (T_{max}) were 4.7±1.6 μg/mL and 131±56 hours respectively, following a single 40 mg subcutaneous administration of adalimumab to healthy adult subjects. The average absolute bioavailability of adalimumab estimated from three studies following a single 40 mg subcutaneous dose was 64%. The pharmacokinetics of adalimumab were linear over the dose range of 0.5 to 10.0 mg/kg following a single intravenous dose.

Distribution: Adalimumab concentrations in the synovial fluid from five rheumatoid arthritis patients ranged from 31 to 96% of those in serum.

Metabolism and Excretion: No formal studies have been conducted to evaluate the metabolism and excretion of adalimumab. However, as adalimumab is an IgG1 antibody of entirely human sequences, it is expected that its metabolism and excretion would follow the course of other IgG molecules.

Special Populations and Conditions: Pediatrics: Adalimumab has not been studied in children.

Geriatrics: Population pharmacokinetic analyses in patients with rheumatoid arthritis revealed that there was a trend toward lower clearance with increasing age in patients aged 40 to >75 years.

Gender: Population pharmacokinetic analyses in patients with rheumatoid arthritis revealed that no gender-related pharmacokinetic differences were observed after correction for a patient's body weight.

Race: No differences in immunoglobulin clearance would be expected among races. From limited data in non-Caucasians, no important kinetic differences were observed for adalimumab.

Hepatic Insufficiency: No pharmacokinetic data are available in patients with hepatic impairment.

Renal Insufficiency: No pharmacokinetic data are available in patients with renal impairment.

Disease States: Healthy volunteers and patients with rheumatoid arthritis displayed similar adalimumab pharmacokinetics. Population pharmacokinetic analyses predicted minor increases in apparent clearance in patients receiving doses lower than the recommended dose and in patients with high rheumatoid factor or CRP concentrations. These increases are not likely to be clinically important.

Drug Interactions: Methotrexate (MTX) reduced adalimumab apparent clearance after single and multiple doses by 29% and 44%, respectively in patients with rheumatoid arthritis.

STORAGE AND STABILITY: HUMIRA (adalimumab) must be refrigerated between 2-8°C. Store in original carton until time of administration. **Do not freeze.** Protect from light. Do not use beyond the expiration date.

SPECIAL HANDLING INSTRUCTIONS: A puncture-resistant container for disposal of needles and syringes should be used. Patients or caregivers should be instructed in the handling technique as well as proper syringe and needle disposal, and be cautioned against reuse of these items.

A healthcare provider should be consulted for instructions on how to properly dispose of used needles and syringes. Special provincial or local laws regarding the proper disposal of needles and syringes should be followed. Needles or syringes should **never** be thrown in the household trash or recycled.

- Used needles and syringes should be placed in a container made specially for this purpose ("Sharps" container), or a hard plastic container with a screw-on cap or metal container with a plastic lid labelled "**Used Syringes**". Glass or clear plastic containers should not be used.
- Container should always be kept out of the reach of children.
- When the container is about two-thirds full, the cap or lid should be taped down so that it does not come off. The container should be disposed of as instructed by a healthcare professional (e.g., doctor, nurse or pharmacist). **Containers should never be thrown in the household trash or recycled.**
- Unless otherwise instructed by a healthcare professional (e.g., doctor, nurse or pharmacist), used alcohol pads may be placed in the trash. Dose trays and covers may be recyclable.

INFORMATION FOR THE PATIENT: Published in e-CPS, available by subscription at www.e-cps.ca.

DOSAGE FORMS, COMPOSITION AND PACKAGING: Pre-filled Syringes: Each mL of sterile solution for subcutaneous administration contains: adalimumab 50 mg. Nonmedicinal ingredients: citric acid monohydrate, dibasic sodium phosphate dihydrate, mannitol, monobasic sodium phosphate dihydrate, polysorbate 80, sodium citrate, sodium chloride, sodium hydroxide (added as necessary to adjust pH) and water for injection. Cartons containing two dose trays: in addition to one alcohol pad, each dose tray consists of a single-dose, 1 mL pre-filled glass syringe with a fixed 27 gauge ½ inch needle, providing 40 mg adalimumab dissolved in 0.8 mL sterile solution (50 mg/mL).

Pre-filled Pens: Each mL of sterile solution for subcutaneous administration contains: adalimumab 50 mg. Nonmedicinal ingredients: citric acid monohydrate, dibasic sodium phosphate dihydrate, mannitol, monobasic sodium phosphate dihydrate, polysorbate 80, sodium citrate, sodium chloride, sodium hydroxide (added as necessary to adjust pH) and water for injection. Cartons containing two dose trays and two alcohol pads. Each dose tray consists of a single-use pen containing 1 mL pre-filled glass syringe with a fixed 27 gauge ½ inch needle, providing 40 mg adalimumab dissolved in 0.8 mL sterile solution (50 mg/mL).

Humulin® (30/70)

insulin regular (human biosynthetic)—insulin NPH (human biosynthetic)

Antidiabetic

Lilly

Humulin®-N

insulin NPH (human biosynthetic)

Antidiabetic

Lilly

Humulin®-R

insulin regular (human biosynthetic)

Antidiabetic

Lilly

Date of Preparation: January 11, 1983
Date of Revision: May 4, 2010

PHARMACOLOGY: Insulin, human biosynthetic, is a polypeptide hormone consisting of a 21 amino acid A-chain and a 30 amino acid B-chain linked by 2 disulfide bonds. Insulin, human biosynthetic, is found to be chemically, physically, biologically and immunologically equivalent to pancreatic human insulin which differs slightly from porcine or bovine insulin in amino acid composition.

Studies indicate immunogenicity problems with biosynthetic human insulin (BHI) produced by recombinant DNA technology are less likely than with insulin derived from animal origin. Biosynthetic human insulin is devoid of all protein contaminants of pancreatic origin normally present in trace amounts in all insulins of pancreatic origin. The purification procedures used in the manufacture of biosynthetic human insulin result in a product which contains an insufficient quantity of *E. coli* polypeptides to be antigenic in deliberately sensitized animals. No antibodies to *E. coli* polypeptides have been detected in specifically designed radioimmunoassay methods examining patient serum samples.

The administration of suitable doses of insulin to patients with diabetes mellitus, along with controlled diet and exercise, temporarily restores their ability to metabolize carbohydrates, fats and proteins; to store glycogen in the liver; and to convert glucose to fat. When given in suitable doses at regular intervals to a patient with diabetes mellitus, the blood sugar is maintained within a reasonable range, the urine remains relatively free of sugar and ketone bodies, and diabetic acidosis and coma are prevented.

Insulin preparations differ in onset, peak and duration of action. Individual variations of blood glucose response profiles are dependent upon factors such as the size of dose, site of injection and physical activity of the patient (for all human insulin formulations). The addition of protamine to insulin, in the presence of zinc, produces a stable complex with less intense and more prolonged action, due to its slow dissolution.

Humulin-R, Regular, Insulin Injection, Human Biosynthetic, is a rapidly acting insulin with a relatively short duration of activity (6 to 8 hours).

Humulin-N, NPH, Insulin Isophane, Human Biosynthetic, is an intermediate-acting insulin with a slower onset of action than Regular insulin and a longer duration of activity of up to 24 hours.

Humulin Mixture (30/70 Insulin Injection, Human Biosynthetic and Insulin Isophane, Human Biosynthetic) is an intermediate-acting insulin with a more rapid onset of action than NPH alone and a duration of activity of up to 24 hours.

Humulin-N, may be mixed with Humulin-R to meet individual metabolic requirements of the patient as determined by the physician.

INDICATIONS: For the treatment of insulin-requiring diabetic patients.

Humulin-R **only** should be used for the treatment of emergencies such as diabetic coma and pre-coma, in diabetics undergoing surgery, but **not** Humulin-N or Humulin Mixtures.

In switching patients from animal source insulins to Humulin, it is possible that the patients will require a change in dosage; the adjustment may be made with the first dose or over a period of several weeks. Any change of insulin should be made cautiously and only under medical supervision.

Changes in refinement, purity, strength, brand, type and/or method of manufacture (recombinant DNA versus animal source insulin) may result in the need of a change in dosage.

CONTRAINDICATIONS: Hypoglycemia (see Overdose).

Humulin is contraindicated in patients with hypersensitivity to human insulin or any of its excipients contained in the formulation (unless used as part of a desensitization program).

Humulin-N, Humulin Mixtures, should not be given i.v. or used for treatment of diabetic coma.

WARNINGS: A few patients who experienced hypoglycemic reactions after being transferred to Humulin have reported that these early warning symptoms were less pronounced than they were with animal-source insulin.

Under no circumstances should any Humulin Mixture be given i.v.

Do not use the Humulin-N or Humulin Mixtures if you see lumps that float or that stick to the sides of the vial, or if the contents of the vial are clear and remain clear after the bottle is shaken or rotated. Note: The contents of the vial of Humulin-R should be clear. Do not use if cloudy.

PRECAUTIONS: General: Visual disturbances in uncontrolled diabetes due to refractive changes are reversed during the early phase of effective management. However, since alteration in osmotic equilibrium between the lens and ocular fluids may not stabilize for a few weeks after initiating therapy, it is wise to postpone prescribing new corrective lenses for 3 to 6 weeks.

Insulin requirements may be increased during illness or emotional disturbances or if the patient is receiving concurrent administration of drugs with hyperglycemic activity, e.g., oral contraceptives, corticosteroids or thyroid replacement therapy.

Insulin requirements may be decreased in the presence of renal or hepatic impairment or in the presence of agents such as oral antidiabetic agents, salicylates, sulfa antibiotics, certain antidepressants (monoamine oxidase inhibitors), beta-adrenergic blockers, alcohol, angiotensin converting enzyme inhibitors and angiotensin II receptor blockers.

The number and size of daily doses and the time of administration, as well as diet and exercise, are problems that require direct and continuous medical supervision. Usually, the most satisfactory injection time is before breakfast.

Prompt recognition and appropriate management of the allergic complications of insulin therapy are essential for the safe and effective control of diabetes mellitus.

Transferring from Other Insulins: A small number of patients transferring from insulins of animal source to insulins of recombinant DNA origin may require a reduced dosage, especially if they are tightly controlled and bordering on hypoglycemia. The dosage reduction may occur with the first dose or over a period of several weeks. There is a risk of hypoglycemia if the insulin requirement is decreased, and both the physician and the patient should be aware of this possibility. The risk can be considered to be minimal if the daily dose is less than 40 units.

Pregnancy: It is essential to maintain good control of the insulin-diabetic patient throughout pregnancy. Insulin requirements usually decrease during the first trimester and increase during the second and third trimesters.

Lactation: Diabetic patients who are nursing may require adjustments in insulin dose and/or diet.

Drug Interactions: Hormones that tend to counteract the hypoglycemic effects of insulin include growth hormone, corticotropin, glucocorticoids, thyroid hormone and glucagon. Epinephrine not only inhibits the secretion of insulin, but also stimulates glycogen breakdown to glucose. Thus, the presence of such diseases as acromegaly, Cushing's syndrome, hyperthyroidism, and pheochromocytoma complicate the control of diabetes.

The hypoglycemic action of insulin may also be antagonized by phenytoin. Insulin's hypoglycemic action can be increased in some patients by concomitant administration of anabolic steroids, MAO inhibitors, guanethidine, alcohol, propranolol (masking effect) or other drugs affecting beta-adrenergic receptors, or by daily doses of 1.5 to 6 g of salicylates.

Insulin requirements can be increased, decreased, or unchanged in patients receiving diuretics. Concomitant administration of oral contraceptives can cause a decrease in glucose tolerance in diabetic women possibly resulting in increased daily insulin requirements.

The physician should be consulted when using other medications in addition to human insulin.

ADVERSE EFFECTS: Since Humulin has been available worldwide, reports of local and systemic allergic reactions in patients receiving it have been received. As with all insulins, local inflammatory responses may result from improper cleansing of the skin, contamination of the injection site with alcohol, use of an antiseptic containing impurities or accidental intracutaneous rather than s.c. injection. Local reactions that result in skin sensitivity phenomena usually subside spontaneously.

Insulin lipohypertrophy has been reported with Humulin. This complication has been ascribed to the local pharmacologic effects of the s.c. injection of insulin. A few cases of lipoatrophy and serum sickness have also been reported.

OVERDOSE:

Hypoglycemia: Cause: Hypoglycemia (low blood glucose, also called "insulin reaction") can occur if the patient takes too much insulin, misses meals, exercises or works too hard just before a meal, or has an infection or becomes ill (especially with diarrhea or vomiting) or if his/her body's need for insulin changes for other reasons.

Symptoms: Hypoglycemia may occur in any patient receiving insulin and is most commonly manifested by hunger, nervousness, warmth and sweating, and palpitations. Patients also may experience headache, confusion, drowsiness, fatigue, anxiety, blurred vision, diplopia, or numbness of the lips, nose or fingers. The clinical manifestations of hypoglycemia can be masked by the concomitant administration of propranolol or other beta-adrenergic blockers.

Symptoms are likely to appear anytime when the blood sugar concentration falls below 2.2 mmol/L (40 mg/100 mL) but may occur with a sudden drop in blood glucose even when the value remains above 2.2 mmol/L (40 mg/100 mL).

Treatment: If a patient is unable to take soluble carbohydrate or fruit juice orally, hypoglycemia is treated with 10 to 20 g of dextrose i.v., or glucagon may be given s.c. or i.m.

> For management of a suspected drug overdose, CPhA recommends that you contact your **regional Poison Control Centre**. See the *CPS* Directory section for a list of Poison Control Centres.

DOSAGE: The dosage should be determined by the physician, according to the requirements of the patient.

New Patients: Patients receiving insulin for the first time can be started on Humulin in the same manner as they would be on animal-source insulin.

Patients should be monitored closely during the adjustment period.

Transfer Patients: When transferring patients from animal-source insulin to Humulin, use the same dose and dosage schedule.

Some patients transferring to Humulin will require a change in dosage from that used with animal-source insulin. If an adjustment is needed, it may be made with the first dose or over a period of several weeks.

Changes in total daily dosage, the number of injections per day, and/or timing of injections may be necessary to achieve maximum glycemic control.

When a patient on high doses of animal insulin is switched to Humulin, it may be appropriate to reduce the starting dosage and monitor the patient carefully.

Patients who have systemic allergy to pork or beef insulin may also react to human insulin. In such patients, appropriate procedures (intradermal testing and, if necessary, desensitization) should be undertaken before therapeutic doses of human insulin are administered.

A few patients who experienced hypoglycemic reactions after being transferred to Humulin have reported that the early warning symptoms, i.e., nervousness, sweating and palpitations, were less pronounced than they were with animal-source insulin.

Formulations of Humulin appear to produce a slightly faster onset and slightly shorter duration of action than the corresponding forms of animal-source insulins.

Humulin-R is a clear, colorless solution. It may be administered by s.c., i.m. or i.v. injection.

Humulin-N and Humulin Mixtures are suspensions. They should be administered by s.c. injection only.

S.C. administration, preferably by the patient, should be in the upper arms, thighs, buttocks or abdomen. Injection sites should be rotated so that the same site is not used more than approximately once a month.

Care should be taken to ensure that a blood vessel has not been entered. The injection site should not be massaged.

Mixing Instructions: The rapid action of Humulin-R is preserved when mixed with Humulin-N, independent of the time lag between mixing and administration, and independent of the proportion of regular insulin incorporated in the mixture.

The effects of mixing Humulin with animal-source insulins have not been studied. This practice is not recommended.

Stability and Storage: Prior to first use insulin should be stored in a cold place (2 to 8°C), preferably in a refrigerator, but not in a freezer. Do not let it freeze or leave it in direct sunlight. Expiration dates are stated on the labels.

When in current use, vials, cartridges and prefilled pens should be stored at room temperature and discarded after 28 days.

INFORMATION FOR THE PATIENT: Published in e-CPS, available by subscription at www.e-cps.ca.

SUPPLIED: Humulin 30/70: Each mL contains: 30 units Regular insulin and 70 units of NPH insulin. Nonmedicinal ingredients: dibasic sodium phosphate, glycerol, m-cresol, phenol, protamine sulfate and zinc. May contain: dimethicone, hydrochloric acid and sodium hydroxide. Cartridges of 3 mL, boxes of 5. Vials of 10 mL.

Humulin-N: Each mL contains: 100 units of NPH insulin. Nonmedicinal ingredients: dibasic sodium phosphate, glycerol, m-cresol, phenol, protamine sulfate and zinc. May contain: dimethicone, hydrochloric acid and sodium hydroxide. Cartridges of 3 mL, boxes of 5. Vials of 10 mL.

Humulin-N Pens: Each mL contains: 100 units of NPH insulin. Nonmedicinal ingredients: dibasic sodium phosphate, glycerol, m-cresol, phenol, protamine sulfate and zinc. May contain: dimethicone, hydrochloric acid and sodium hydroxide. Prefilled pens of 3 mL, boxes of 5.

Humulin N KwikPen: Each mL contains: 100 units of NPH insulin. Nonmedicinal ingredients: dibasic sodium phosphate, glycerol, m-cresol, phenol, protamine sulfate and zinc. May contain: dimethicone, hydrochloric acid and sodium hydroxide. Prefilled pens of 3 mL, boxes of 5.

Humulin-R: Each mL contains: 100 units of Regular insulin. Nonmedicinal ingredients: glycerol and m-cresol. May contain: dimethicone, hydrochloric acid and sodium hydroxide. Cartridges of 3 mL, boxes of 5. Vials of 10 mL.

Humulin cartridges are designed for use with Lilly injector systems.

(Shown in Product Identification Section)

Hycamtin® Ⓟ

topotecan HCl

Antineoplastic

GlaxoSmithKline

Date of Revision: July 9, 2009

SUMMARY PRODUCT INFORMATION:

Route of Administration	Dosage Form/ Strength	Clinically Relevant Nonmedicinal Ingredients
Intravenous infusion	Lyophilized powder Topotecan 4 mg per vial, incorporated as the hydrochloride for the reconstitution	Mannitol and tartaric acid

INDICATIONS AND CLINICAL USE: Adults: HYCAMTIN (topotecan hydrochloride) is indicated for the treatment of:

- metastatic carcinoma of the ovary after failure of initial or subsequent therapy.
- sensitive small cell lung cancer after failure of first line chemotherapy (defined as recurrence at least 60 days after first line chemotherapy).

Pediatrics: Safety and effectiveness in pediatric patients have not been established, therefore it is not recommended for use in this population.

CONTRAINDICATIONS: HYCAMTIN (topotecan hydrochloride) is contraindicated:

- in patients who have a history of hypersensitivity reactions to topotecan or to any of its other ingredients.
- in patients who are pregnant or breast-feeding.
- in patients who already have severe bone marrow depression prior to starting first course, as evidenced by baseline absolute neutrophils <1.5×10^9/L and/or a platelet count of <100×10^9/L
- in patients with severe renal impairment (creatinine clearance of <20 mL/min or <0.33 mL/sec).

WARNINGS AND PRECAUTIONS:

> **Serious Warnings and Precautions**
> **HYCAMTIN (topotecan hydrochloride) should be prescribed by a qualified health care professional who is experienced in the use of antineoplastic therapy agents.**
> **The following is a clinically significant adverse event:**
> - **Bone marrow suppression, primarily neutropenia (see Warnings and Precautions, Hematologic);**
> - **Potentially fatal neutropenic colitis (see Warnings and Precautions, Gastrointestinal);**
> - **Potentially fatal interstitial lung disease (see Warnings and Precautions, Respiratory).**

General: HYCAMTIN (topotecan hydrochloride) should be administered under the supervision of a physician experienced in the use of cancer chemotherapeutic agents. Bone marrow suppression, primarily neutropenia, is the dose limiting toxicity. Therapy with HYCAMTIN should not be given to patients with baseline absolute neutrophil counts of 1.5×10^9/L or less. In order to monitor the occurrence of bone marrow suppression, frequent peripheral blood cell counts should be performed on all patients receiving HYCAMTIN (see Dosage and Administration).

Inadvertent extravasation with HYCAMTIN has been associated only with mild local reactions such as erythema (and bruising).

Caution should be observed when driving or operating machinery if fatigue or asthenia persist.

Selection of Patients in Small Cell Lung Cancer: Clinical studies were conducted in patients with sensitive and refractory small cell lung cancer; a reduced chance for benefit in the refractory patients was noted with response rates ranging from 11-31% for patients with sensitive disease and 2.1 to 7.3% for patients with refractory disease. As the risk for toxicity is similar, the overall benefit/risk is reduced.

The benefit to patients versus the risk of toxicity must be carefully weighed.

Carcinogenesis and Mutagenesis: The carcinogenic potential of HYCAMTIN has not been studied. (See Special Populations, Pregnant Women.)

Topotecan hydrochloride has been shown to be genotoxic to mammalian cells (mouse lymphoma cells and human lymphocytes) in vitro, and mouse bone marrow cells in vivo, but is not mutagenic in bacterial cells (*S. typhimurium* and *E. coli*).

Gastrointestinal: Topotecan-induced neutropenia can cause neutropenic colitis (caecitis or typhlitis). Fatalities due to neutropenic colitis have been reported in clinical trials with topotecan. In patients presenting with fever, neutropenia, and a compatible pattern of abdominal pain, the possibility of neutropenic colitis should be considered.

Hematologic: Bone marrow suppression (primarily neutropenia) is the dose-limiting toxicity of topotecan. Neutropenia is not cumulative over time. Myelosuppression leading to sepsis and fatalities due to sepsis have been reported in patients treated with topotecan [2% fatalities across all SCLC studies (n=426 subjects), which includes 3% fatalities in one Phase III SCLC study (n=107 subjects, Table 4)] (see Adverse Reactions).

HYCAMTIN should not be administered to patients with baseline absolute neutrophil counts of less than 1.5×10^9/L. To monitor the occurrence of myelotoxicity, it is recommended that frequent peripheral blood cell counts be performed on all patients receiving HYCAMTIN. Patients should not be retreated with subsequent courses of HYCAMTIN until neutrophils recover to a level >1×10^9/L, platelets recover to a level >100×10^9/L and hemoglobin recovers to 90 g/L, using transfusion if necessary.

Neutropenia: Grade 4 neutropenia (<0.5×10^9/L) occurred in 78% of patients and in 39% of all courses, with a median duration of 7 days. The nadir neutrophil count occurred at a median of 12 days. Therapy-related sepsis or febrile neutropenia occurred in 23% of patients and sepsis was fatal in 1.3%.

Topotecan-induced neutropenia can cause neutropenic colitis (see Gastrointestinal).

In the case of severe neutropenia (<0.5×10^9/L for 7 days or more) during a course of HYCAMTIN, a reduction in dose of 0.25 mg/m² for subsequent courses of therapy is recommended.

Thrombocytopenia: Grade 4 thrombocytopenia (<25×10^9/L) occurred in 27% of patients and in 9% of courses, with a median duration of 5 days and platelet nadir at a median of 15 days. Platelet transfusions were given to 15% of patients in 4% of courses.

Anemia: Severe anemia (grade 3/4, <80 g/L) occurred in 37% of patients and in 14% of courses. Median nadir was at day 15. Transfusions were needed in 52% of patients in 22% of courses.

Monitoring of Bone Marrow Function: HYCAMTIN should only be administered in patients with adequate bone marrow reserves including baseline absolute neutrophil counts of at least 1.5×10^9/L and platelet count at least 100×10^9/L. Frequent monitoring of blood counts should be instituted during treatment with HYCAMTIN.

Respiratory: Topotecan has been associated with reports of interstitial lung disease (ILD), some of which have been fatal (see Adverse Reactions). Underlying risk factors include history of ILD, pulmonary fibrosis, lung cancer, thoracic exposure to radiation and use of pneumotoxic drugs and/or colony stimulating factors. Patients should be monitored for pulmonary symptoms indicative of ILD (e.g. cough, fever, dyspnea and/or hypoxia), and topotecan should be discontinued if a new diagnosis of ILD is confirmed.

Special Populations: Pregnant Women: HYCAMTIN may cause fetal harm when administered to a pregnant woman. Topotecan was shown to cause embryonic and fetal lethality when given to rats (0.59 mg/m²) and rabbits (1.25 mg/m²) at doses less than the human clinical intravenous dose (1.5 mg/m²). At maternally toxic doses (0.59 mg/m²), topotecan caused malformations, primarily of the eye, brain, skull, and vertebrae. The drug is contraindicated during pregnancy. Women of childbearing potential should be advised to avoid becoming pregnant during therapy with HYCAMTIN.

Nursing Women: HYCAMTIN is contraindicated during breast-feeding (see Contraindications).

Pediatrics: Safety and effectiveness of topotecan in pediatric patients have not been established, and therefore is not indicated for use in this population.

ADVERSE REACTIONS: Clinical Trial Adverse Drug Reactions: Data in the following section are based on the combined experience of 453 patients with metastatic ovarian carcinoma, and 426 patients with small cell lung cancer, treated with HYCAMTIN (topotecan hydrochloride). Table 1 lists the principal hematologic toxicities and Table 2 lists non-hematologic toxicities occurring in at least 15% of patients.

Table 1: HYCAMTIN

Summary of Hematologic Adverse Events in Patients Receiving HYCAMTIN

Hematologic Adverse Events	Patients n=879 % Incidence	Courses n=4124 % Incidence
Neutropenia		
<1.5×10^9/L	97	81
< 0.5×10^9/L	78	39
Leukopenia		
<3×10^9/L	97	80
<1×10^9/L	32	11
Thrombocytopenia		
<75×10^9/L	69	42
<25×10^9/L	27	9
Anemia		
<100 g/L	89	71
<80 g/dL	37	14
Sepsis or fever/infection with grade 4 neutropenia	23	7
Platelet transfusions	15	4
RBC transfusions	52	22

Table 2: HYCAMTIN

Summary of Non-hematologic Adverse Events in Patients Receiving HYCAMTIN

Non-hematologic Adverse Events	All Grades % Incidence n=879 Patients	All Grades % Incidence n=4124 Courses	Grade 3 % Incidence n=879 Patients	Grade 3 % Incidence n=4124 Courses	Grade 4 % Incidence n=879 Patients	Grade 4 % Incidence n=4124 Courses
Gastrointestinal						
Nausea	64	42	7	2	1	<1
Vomiting	45	22	4	1	1	<1
Diarrhea	32	14	3	1	1	<1
Constipation	29	15	2	1	1	<1
Abdominal Pain	22	10	2	1	2	<1
Stomatitis	18	8	1	<1	<1	<1
Anorexia	19	9	2	1	<1	<1
Body as a Whole						
Fatigue	29	22	5	2	0	0
Fever	28	11	1	<1	<1	<1
Pain[a]	23	11	2	1	1	<1

(cont'd)

Table 2: HYCAMTIN *(cont'd)*

Summary of Non-hematologic Adverse Events in Patients Receiving HYCAMTIN

Non-hematologic Adverse Events	All Grades % Incidence n=879 Patients	All Grades % Incidence n=4124 Courses	Grade 3 % Incidence n=879 Patients	Grade 3 % Incidence n=4124 Courses	Grade 4 % Incidence n=879 Patients	Grade 4 % Incidence n=4124 Courses
Asthenia	25	13	4	1	2	<1
Skin/Appendages						
Alopecia	49	54	NA	NA	NA	NA
Rash[b]	16	6	1	<1	0	0
Respiratory System						
Dyspnea	22	11	5	2	3	1
Coughing	15	7	1	<1	0	0
CNS/Peripheral Nervous System						
Headache	18	7	1	<1	<1	0

[a] Pain includes body pain, back pain and skeletal pain.

[b] Rash also includes pruritus, rash erythematous, urticaria, dermatitis, bullous eruption and rash maculo-papular.

Legend: NA=not applicable.

Hematologic: See Warnings and Precautions.

Gastrointestinal: The prophylactic use of anti-emetics was not routine in patients treated with HYCAMTIN. Gastrointestinal effects were usually mild at the recommended dose level. The incidence of nausea was 64% (8% grade 3/4) and vomiting occurred in 45% (6% grade 3/4) of patients (see Table 2).

Thirty-two percent of patients had diarrhea (4% grade 3/4), 29% constipation (2% grade 3/4) and 22% had abdominal pain (4% grade 3/4). Grade 3/4 abdominal pain was 6% in ovarian cancer patients and 2% in small cell lung cancer patients.

Skin/Appendages: Total alopecia (Grade 2) occurred in 31% of patients.

Central and Peripheral Nervous System: Headache (18%) was the most frequently reported neurologic toxicity. Paresthesia occurred in 7% of patients, but was generally Grade 1.

Liver/Biliary: Grade 1 transient elevations in hepatic enzymes (8%); Grade 3/4 elevated bilirubin elevations occurred in <2% of patients.

Respiratory: The incidence of grade 3/4 dyspnea was 3.8% in ovarian cancer patients and 12.2% in small cell lung cancer patients. Table 3 shows the grade 3/4 hematologic and major non-hematologic adverse events in the topotecan/paclitaxel comparator trial. Table 4 shows the grade 3/4 hematologic and major non-hematologic adverse events in the topotecan/CAV comparator trial in small cell lung cancer.

Note: All grading scales are based on National Cancer Institute criteria.

Table 3: HYCAMTIN

Comparative Toxicity Profiles for Ovarian Cancer Patients Randomized to Receive HYCAMTIN or Paclitaxel

Adverse Event	HYCAMTIN Patients n=112 %	HYCAMTIN Courses n=597 %	Paclitaxel Patients n=114 %	Paclitaxel Courses n=589 %
Hematologic Grade 3/4				
Grade 4 Neutropenia (<0.5×10^9/L)	80.2	35.8	21.4	8.6
Grade 3/4 Anemia (Hgb <80 g/L)	41.4	16.1	6.3	1.9
Grade 4 Thrombocytopenia (<25×10^9/L)	27.0	10.0	2.7	0.5
Fever/Grade 4 Neutropenia	23.2	6.0	4.0	1.0
Documented Sepsis	4.5	0.8	1.8	0.3
Death Related to Sepsis	1.8	N/A	0.0	N/A
Non-hematologic Grade 3/4				
Gastrointestinal				
Abdominal Pain	5.4	1.3	3.5	0.9
Constipation	5.4	1.0	0.0	0.0
Diarrhea	6.3	1.9	0.9	0.2
Intestinal Obstruction	4.5	1.0	4.4	0.8
Nausea	9.8	2.7	1.8	0.3
Stomatitis	0.9	0.2	0.9	0.2
Vomiting	9.9	1.9	2.7	0.5
Constitutional				
Anorexia	3.6	0.8	0.0	0.0
Dyspnea	6.3	1.8	5.4	1.2
Fatigue	7.1	1.8	6.1	2.2
Malaise	1.8	0.5	1.8	0.3

(cont'd)

Table 3: HYCAMTIN *(cont'd)*

Comparative Toxicity Profiles for Ovarian Cancer Patients Randomized to Receive HYCAMTIN or Paclitaxel

	HYCAMTIN		Paclitaxel	
Adverse Event	Patients n=112 %	Courses n=597 %	Patients n=114 %	Courses n=589 %
Neuromuscular				
A[illegible]	0.9	0.2	2.6	0.5
[illegible]	5.4	1.6	2.6	1.0
[illegible]	0.9	0.2	1.8	0.8
[illegible]	0.0	0.0	2.6	1.5
[illegible]	4.5	1.0	7.0	2.2
[illegible]	1.8	0.3	0.9	0.3
[illegible]ppendages				
[illegible]	0	0	0.9	0.2
[illegible]ry				
Increased Hepatic Enzymes[c]	0.9	0.2	0.9	0.2

a [illegible]ludes body pain, skeletal pain, and back pain.
b [illegible] includes pruritus, rash erythematous, urticaria, dermatitis, bullous eruption, and rash maculo-papular.
c [illegible]d hepatic enzymes includes Increased AST, Increased ALT and Increased Hepatic Enzymes.
Legend: NA=not available.

Table 4: HYCAMTIN

Comparative Toxicity Profiles for Small Cell Lung Cancer Patients Randomized to Receive HYCAMTIN or CAV

	HYCAMTIN		CAV	
[illegible] Event	Patients n=107 %	Courses n=446 %	Patients n=104 %	Courses n=359 %
[illegible]ogic Grade 3/4				
Grade 4 Neutropenia ([illegible]/L)	70	38	72	51
Grade 3/4 Anemia ([illegible]<80 g/L)	42	18	20	7
Grade 4 Thrombocytopenia (<25×10⁹/L)	29	10	5	1
Fever/Grade 4 Neutropenia	28	9	26	13
Documented Sepsis	5	1	5	1
Death Related to Sepsis	3	N/A	1	N/A
Non-hematologic Grade 3/4				
Gastrointestinal				
Abdominal Pain	6	1	4	2
Constipation	1	<1	0	0
Diarrhea	1	<1	0	0
Nausea	8	2	6	2
Stomatitis	2	<1	1	<1
Vomiting	3	<1	3	1
Constitutional				
Anorexia	3	1	4	2
Dyspnea	9	5	14	7
Fatigue	6	4	10	3
Neuromuscular				
Asthenia	9	4	7	2
Headache	0	0	2	<1
Pain[illegible]	5	2	7	4
Respiratory System				
Pneumonia	8	2	6	2
[illegible]g	2	1	0.0	0
[illegible]nd Appendages				

(cont'd)

Table 4: HYCAMTIN *(cont'd)*

Comparative Toxicity Profiles for Small Cell Lung Cancer Patients Randomized to Receive HYCAMTIN or CAV

	HYCAMTIN		CAV	
Adverse Event	Patients n=107 %	Courses n=446 %	Patients n=104 %	Courses n=359 %
Rash[b]	1	<1	1	<1
Liver/Biliary				
Increased Hepatic Enzymes[c]	1	<1	0	0

a Pain includes body pain, skeletal pain, and back pain.
b Rash also includes pruritus, rash erythematous, urticaria, dermatitis, bullous eruption, and rash maculo-papular.
c Increased hepatic enzymes includes Increased AST, Increased ALT and Increased Hepatic Enzymes.
Legend: NA=not available.

Premedications were not routinely used in patients randomized to HYCAMTIN, while patients receiving CAV received routine pretreatment with corticosteroids, diphenhydramine, and histamine receptor type 2 blockers.

Post-Market Adverse Drug Reactions: Reports of adverse events in patients taking HYCAMTIN after market introduction include the following:

Body as a Whole: allergic manifestations, angioedema, anaphylactoid reactions, extravasation*, pancytopenia.
Gastrointestinal: abdominal pain†.
Hematologic: severe bleeding (in association with thrombocytopenia).
Respiratory, Thoracic and Mediastinal Disorders: interstitial lung disease.
Skin/Appendages: severe dermatitis, severe pruritus.

DRUG INTERACTIONS: There are no adequate data to define a safe and effective regimen for HYCAMTIN in combination with other cytotoxic agents. Preliminary studies combining HYCAMTIN with platinum-containing agents (e.g. cisplatin or carboplatin) suggest a sequence-dependent interaction whereby greater myelosuppression is seen when the platinum-containing agent is given on day 1 compared to day 5 of the HYCAMTIN dosing. If topotecan is administered in combination with other cytotoxic agents, dose reduction may be necessary.

DOSAGE AND ADMINISTRATION: Dosing Considerations: Initial Dose: Prior to administration of the first course of HYCAMTIN (topotecan hydrochloride), patients must have:

- a baseline absolute neutrophil count of ≥1.5×10⁹/L
- a platelet count of ≥100×10⁹/L
- a hemoglobin level of ≥90 g/L

Recommended Dose and Dosage Adjustment: Initial Dose: The recommended dose of HYCAMTIN is 1.5 mg/m² by intravenous infusion over 30 minutes daily for 5 consecutive days, starting on day one of a 21-day course. Because median time to response in three clinical trials was 9 to 12 weeks and median time to response in four small cell lung cancer trials was 5 to 7 weeks, a minimum of four courses of HYCAMTIN is recommended.

Subsequent Doses: Topotecan should not be re-administered unless the absolute neutrophil count is more than or equal to 1×10⁹/L, the platelet count is more than or equal to 100×10⁹/L, and the hemoglobin level is more than or equal to 90 g/L (after transfusion if necessary).

Standard oncology practice for the management of neutropenia is either to administer topotecan with other medications (e.g. G-CSF) or to dose reduce to maintain neutrophil counts.

If dose reduction is chosen for patients who experience severe neutropenia (absolute neutrophil count less than or equal to 0.5×10⁹/L) for 7 days or more, or severe neutropenia associated with fever or infection, or who have had treatment delayed due to neutropenia, the dose should be reduced by 0.25 mg/m²/day to 1.25 mg/m²/day (or subsequently down to 1.0 mg/m²/day if necessary).

Doses should be similarly reduced if the platelet count falls below 25×10⁹/L.

Routine pre-medication for the prevention of non-hematological adverse events is not required with HYCAMTIN.

Hepatic Impairment: No dosage adjustment is required for treating patients with hepatic impairment (plasma bilirubin >1.5 to <10 mg/dL or (SI units) >25.7 to <171 µmol/L).

Renally Impaired Patients: No dosage adjustment is required for patients with mild renal impairment (CrCl 40 to 60 mL/min or 0.67 to 1 mL/sec). Dosage adjustment to 0.75 mg/m²/day is recommended for patients with moderate renal impairment (CrCl 20 to 39 mL/min or 0.33 to 0.65 mL/sec). Advice on dosing of topotecan for patients with moderate renal impairment (20 to 39 mL/min) is based on studies involving patients with advanced cancer. Treatment with HYCAMTIN in patients with severe renal impairment (CrCl <20 mL/min or 0.33 mL/sec) is not recommended (see Contraindications).

Pediatrics: Insufficient data are available in pediatric patients to provide a dosage recommendation (see Warnings and Precautions).

Geriatrics: No dosage adjustment appears to be needed in the elderly, other than adjustments related to renal function.

Dosage in Combination with Cytotoxic Agents: Dose adjustment may be necessary if topotecan is administered in combination with other cytotoxic agents (see Drug Interactions).

Administration: HYCAMTIN is a cytotoxic anticancer drug. As with other potentially toxic compounds, HYCAMTIN should be prepared under a vertical laminar flow hood while wearing gloves and protective clothing. If HYCAMTIN solution contacts the skin; wash the skin immediately and thoroughly with soap and water. If HYCAMTIN contacts mucous membranes, flush thoroughly with water.

Preparation for Intravenous Administration: Each HYCAMTIN 4 mg vial is reconstituted with 4 mL Sterile Water for Injection, giving a final concentration of 1 mg/mL.

Then the appropriate volume of the reconstituted solution is further diluted to an infusion concentration of 20-500 µg/mL in 50 to 100 mL of either 0.9% Sodium Chloride Intravenous Infusion or 5% Dextrose Intravenous Infusion prior to administration.

Since the vials contain no preservative, it is recommended that the product be used immediately after reconstitution. If not used immediately the reconstituted product should be stored in a refrigerator, for up to 24 hours.

As with all parenteral drug products, intravenous admixtures should be inspected visually for clarity and particulate matter, discoloration and leakage prior to administration, whenever solution and container permit.

OVERDOSAGE:
There is no known antidote for overdosage with HYCAMTIN (topotecan hydrochloride). The primary anticipated complication of overdosage would consist of bone marrow suppression. In a phase I study, one patient was incorrectly dosed at 35 mg/m² during course 9 of therapy and experienced hematologic toxicity associated with this increased dose.

The LD_{10} Rate in mice receiving single intravenous infusions of HYCAMTIN was 74.85 mg/m² (CI 95%: 47.22 to 97.41).

> For management of a suspected drug overdose, CPhA recommends that you contact your **regional Poison Control Centre**. See the *CPS* Directory section for a list of Poison Control Centres.

ACTION AND CLINICAL PHARMACOLOGY: Mechanism of Action: HYCAMTIN (topotecan hydrochloride) inhibits topoisomerase-I, an enzyme that functions in DNA replication to relieve the torsional strain introduced ahead of the moving replication fork. Topotecan inhibits topoisomerase-I by stabilizing the covalent complex of enzyme and strand-cleaved DNA, which is an intermediate of the catalytic mechanism, thereby inducing breaks in the protein-associated DNA single-strands, resulting in cell death.

Pharmacodynamics: The dose-limiting toxicity for topotecan is leukopenia. The relationship between decreased white blood count and either topotecan or total topotecan AUC can be described by a Sigmoid E_{max} Model.

Pharmacokinetics: Following intravenous administration of topotecan at doses of 0.5 to 1.5 mg/m² as a 30-minute infusion daily for 5 days, topotecan demonstrated a clearance of 1030 mL/min with a plasma half-life of 2 to 3 hours.

* Reactions associated with extravasation have been mild and have not generally required specific therapy.
† Neutropenic colitis, including fatal neutropenic colitis, has been reported to occur as a complication of topotecan-induced neutropenia (see Warning and Precautions).

Comparison of pharmacokinetic parameters did not suggest any change in pharmacokinetics over the dosing period. Area under the curve increased approximately in proportion to the increase in dose.

Distribution: Topotecan has a volume of distribution of 130 L. Binding of topotecan to plasma proteins is about 35%. Topotecan is evenly distributed between blood cells and plasma.

Metabolism: Topotecan undergoes pH dependent hydrolysis, with the equilibrium favoring the ring-opened hydroxy-acid form at physiologic pH.

Excretion: The renal clearance of topotecan could not be measured in humans due to the effect of urine pH on interconversion, although measurement of total topotecan (the lactone ring and the ring-opened hydroxy acid) in urine suggests that a variable fraction of the dose (generally 20 to 60%) is excreted in urine. Topotecan has also been measured in human bile samples indicating that topotecan is excreted by both biliary and urinary routes in humans.

Special Populations and Conditions: Pediatrics: The pharmacokinetics of topotecan were studied in 12 pediatric patients treated with topotecan at doses between 2.0 and 7.5 mg/m² as a 24-hour continuous infusion. Mean plasma clearance was 28.3 L/h/m² with a range of 18.1 to 44.2 L/h/m². These values are similar to plasma clearance values seen in adults (approx. 36 L/h/m²) who received 24-hour topotecan infusions.

Geriatrics: Topotecan pharmacokinetics has not been specifically investigated in elderly patients. However, a population pharmacokinetic analysis in female patients did not identify age as a significant factor. Renal clearance is likely to be a more important determinant of topotecan clearance than age in this patient population.

Gender: The overall mean topotecan plasma clearance in male patients was approximately 24% higher than in female patients, largely reflecting difference in body size.

Race: The effect of race on topotecan pharmacokinetics has not been determined.

Hepatic Insufficiency: Based on clinical data and total topotecan pharmacokinetics, no dosage adjustment is required in patients with hepatic impairment (serum bilirubin <10 mg/dL or 171 μmol/L). Plasma clearance in patients with hepatic impairment decreased to about 67% when compared with a control group of patients. Topotecan half-life was increased by about 30%, but no change in volume of distribution was observed. Total topotecan clearance in patients with hepatic impairment only decreased by about 10% compared with the control group of patients.

Renal Insufficiency: Plasma clearance of topotecan in patients with mild renal impairment (creatinine clearance [CrCl] of 40 to 60 mL/min or 0.67 to 1 mL/sec) decreased to about 67% compared with control patients. Volume of distribution was slightly decreased and thus half-life only increased by 14%.

In patients with moderate renal impairment (CrCl of 20 to 39 mL/min or 0.33 to 0.65 mL/sec), topotecan plasma clearance was reduced to 34% of the value in control patients. Volume of distribution also decreased by about 25%, which resulted in an increase in mean half-life from 1.9 hours to 4.9 hours. Total topotecan clearance also decreased by 57% in patients with moderate renal impairment and by 17% in patients with mild renal impairment. Based on clinical data and on total topotecan pharmacokinetics, no dosage adjustment is required for patients with mild renal impairment (CrCl 40 to 60 mL/min or 0.67 to 1 mL/sec). Dosage adjustment to 0.75 mg/m²/day is recommended for patients with moderate renal impairment. HYCAMTIN is not recommended for patients with a creatinine clearance of <20 mL/min (0.33 mL/min).

STORAGE AND STABILITY: Unopened vials of HYCAMTIN (topotecan hydrochloride) are stable until the date indicated on the package when stored between 15 and 30°C and protected from light in the original package.

Reconstituted Solutions: Vials which have been reconstituted with Water for Injection are stable for up to 24 hours when refrigerated at 5°C or stored at 30°C.

However, since the vials contain no preservative, it is recommended that the product should be used immediately after reconstitution. If not used immediately, the reconstituted solution should be stored in a refrigerator and discarded after 24 hours.

Diluted Solutions: Reconstituted vials of HYCAMTIN diluted for infusion are stable for up to 24 hours at approximately 20 to 25°C and ambient lighting conditions. If not used immediately, the diluted solution should be stored in a refrigerator in line with good pharmaceutical practice.

SPECIAL HANDLING INSTRUCTIONS: Handling and Disposal: Procedures for proper handling and disposal of anticancer drugs should be used. Several guidelines on this subject have been published.

INFORMATION FOR THE PATIENT: Published in e-CPS, available by subscription at www.e-cps.ca.

DOSAGE FORMS, COMPOSITION AND PACKAGING: Each single dose vial of a sterile lyophilized, buffered, light yellow to greenish powder contains: topotecan HCl equivalent to 4 mg of topotecan as free base. Nonmedicinal ingredients: mannitol and tartaric acid. Hydrochloric acid and sodium hydroxide may be used to adjust to a pH of 3. The solution pH ranges from 2.5 to 3.5. Single dose vials, packages of 5.

Hycodan® Ⓝ

hydrocodone bitartrate

Antitussive

Bristol-Myers Squibb

Date of Preparation: September 13, 1983
Date of Revision: November 5, 2001

PHARMACOLOGY: Clinical trials have proven hydrocodone bitartrate to be an effective antitussive agent which is pharmacologically 2 to 8 times as potent as codeine. At equi-effective doses, its sedative action is greater than that of codeine. The precise mechanisms of action of hydrocodone and other opiates are not known; however, hydrocodone is believed to act by directly depressing the cough centre. In excessive doses, hydrocodone, like other opium derivatives, can depress respiration. The effects of therapeutic doses of hydrocodone on the cardiovascular system are insignificant. The constipating effects of hydrocodone are much weaker than those of morphine and no stronger than those of codeine. Hydrocodone can produce miosis, euphoria, physical and psychological dependence. At therapeutic antitussive doses, it does exert analgesic effects. Following a 10 mg oral dose of hydrocodone administered to 5 male human subjects, the mean peak serum concentration was 23.6±5.2 ng/mL. Maximum serum levels were achieved at approximately 1.3±0.3 hours and the half-life was determined to be approximately 3.8±0.3 hours. Hydrocodone exhibits a complex pattern of metabolism including O-demethylation, N-demethylation and 6-keto reduction to the corresponding 6-α- and 6-β-hydroxymetabolites.

INDICATIONS: The control of exhausting, nonproductive cough.

CONTRAINDICATIONS: HYCODAN TABLETS and SYRUP should not be used in patients with hypersensitivity to any component of the drug. Patients known to be hypersensitive to other opioids may exhibit cross-sensitivity to hydrocodone. Hydrocodone is contraindicated in the presence of an intracranial lesion associated with increased intracranial pressure, and whenever ventilatory function is depressed.

WARNINGS: Drug Abuse and Dependence: Hydrocodone can produce drug dependence and, therefore, has the potential for being abused. Psychic dependence, physical dependence and tolerance may develop upon repeated administration of hydrocodone, and it should be prescribed and administered with the same degree of caution appropriate to the use of other narcotic drugs (see Adverse Effects, Drug Abuse and Dependence).

Respiratory Depression: Hydrocodone produces dose-related respiratory depression by directly acting on the brain stem respiratory centres. If respiratory depression occurs, it may be antagonized by the use of naloxone HCl and other supportive measures when indicated.

Occupational Hazards: Ambulatory Patients: Hydrocodone may impair the mental and/or physical abilities required for the performance of potentially hazardous tasks such as driving a car or operating machinery. Patients using HYCODAN TABLETS or SYRUP should be cautioned accordingly.

Head Injury and Increased Intracranial Pressure: The respiratory depressant effects of narcotics and their capacity to elevate cerebrospinal fluid pressure may be markedly exaggerated in the presence of head injury, other intracranial lesions or a pre-existing elevated intracranial pressure. Furthermore, narcotics may produce adverse reactions which can obscure the clinical course of patients with head injuries.

Acute Abdominal Conditions: The administration of hydrocodone or other opioids may obscure the diagnosis or clinical course in patients with acute abdominal conditions.

Interactions with Other CNS Depressants: Patients receiving other narcotic analgesics, general anesthetics, phenothiazines or other tranquilizers, tricyclic antidepressants, sedative-hypnotics or other CNS depressants (including alcohol) concomitantly with HYCODAN TABLETS or SYRUP may exhibit an additive CNS depression. When such combined therapy is contemplated, the dose of one or both agents should be reduced.

PRECAUTIONS: Before prescribing medication to suppress or modify cough, it is important to ascertain that the underlying cause of the cough is identified, that modification of the cough does not increase the risk of clinical or physiological complications, and that appropriate therapy for the primary disease is provided.

In young children the respiratory centre is especially susceptible to the depressant action of narcotic cough suppressants. Benefit to risk ratio should be carefully considered, especially in children with respiratory embarrassment, e.g., croup. Estimation of dosage relative to the child's age and weight is of great importance.

As hydrocodone may inhibit peristalsis, patients with chronic constipation should be given the drug only after weighing the potential therapeutic benefit against the hazards involved. In patients with asthma or pulmonary emphysema, indiscriminate use may precipitate respiratory insufficiency resulting from increased viscosity of bronchial secretions and suppression of the cough reflex.

Use with caution in sedated or debilitated patients, in patients who have undergone thoracotomies or laparotomies, since suppression of the cough reflex may lead to retention of secretions postoperatively in these patients.

Carcinogenesis, Mutagenesis, Impairment of Fertility: Carcinogenicity, mutagenicity and reproduction studies have not been conducted with HYCODAN TABLETS and SYRUP.

Pregnancy: Animal reproduction studies have not been conducted with HYCODAN TABLETS and SYRUP. It is not known whether HYCODAN TABLETS and SYRUP can cause fetal harm when administered to a pregnant woman or can affect reproductive capacity. Since hydrocodone crosses the placental barrier, HYCODAN TABLETS and SYRUP should be given to pregnant women only if clearly needed.

Nonteratogenic Effects: Babies born to mothers who have been taking opioids regularly prior to delivery will be physically dependent. The withdrawal signs include: irritability and excessive crying, tremors, hyperactive reflexes, increased respiratory rate, increased stools, sneezing, yawning, vomiting, and fever. Intensity of the syndrome does not always correlate with the duration of maternal opioids use or dose. There is no consensus on the best method of managing withdrawal. Chlorpromazine (0.7 to 1.0 mg/kg q6h), phenobarbital (2 mg/kg q6h), and paregoric (2 to 4 drops/kg q4h) have been used to treat withdrawal symptoms in infants. Duration of therapy is 4 to 28 days, with dosages decreased as tolerated.

Lactation: It is not known if this drug is excreted in human milk. Because many drugs are excreted in human milk and because of the potential for serious adverse reactions in nursing infants from HYCODAN TABLETS and SYRUP, a decision should be made whether to discontinue nursing or discontinue the drug taking into account the importance of the drug to the mother.

Drug Interactions: The central nervous system depressant effect of HYCODAN TABLETS and SYRUP may be additive with that of other central nervous system depressants. See Warnings.

ADVERSE EFFECTS: Respiratory: Hydrocodone produces dose-related respiratory depression by acting directly on brain stem respiratory centres.

Cardiovascular: Hypertension, postural hypotension and palpitations.

Genitourinary: Ureteral spasm, spasm of vesical sphincters and urinary retention have been reported with opiates.

Central Nervous System: Sedation, drowsiness, mental clouding, lethargy, impairment of mental and physical performance, anxiety, fear, dysphoria, dizziness, psychic dependence, mood changes and blurred vision.

Gastrointestinal: Nausea and vomiting occur more frequently in ambulatory than in recumbent patients. Constipation may also occur.

Drug Abuse and Dependence: Special care should be exercised in prescribing hydrocodone for emotionally unstable patients and for those with a history of drug misuse. Such patients should be closely supervised when long-term therapy is contemplated.

Psychic dependence, physical dependence, and tolerance may develop upon repeated administration of narcotics; therefore HYCODAN TABLETS and SYRUP should always be prescribed and administered with caution. Physical dependence is the condition in which continued administration of the drug is required to prevent the appearance of a withdrawal syndrome.

Patients physically dependent on opioids will develop an abstinence syndrome upon abrupt discontinuation of the opioid or following administration of a narcotic antagonist. The character and severity of the withdrawal symptoms are related to the degree of physical dependence. Manifestations of opioid withdrawal are similar to, but milder than that of morphine and include: lacrimation, rhinorrhea, yawning, sweating, restlessness, dilated pupils, anorexia, gooseflesh, irritability, and tremor. In more severe forms, nausea, vomiting, intestinal spasm and diarrhea, increased heart rate and blood pressure, chills, and pains in bones and muscles of the back and extremities may occur. Peak effects will usually be apparent at 48 to 72 hours.

Treatment of withdrawal is usually managed by providing sufficient quantities of an opioid to suppress severe withdrawal symptoms and then gradually reducing the dose of opioid over a period of several days.

OVERDOSE:

Symptoms: Serious overdosage with hydrocodone may be characterized by respiratory depression (a decrease in respiratory rate and/or tidal volume, Cheyne-Stokes respiration, cyanosis), extreme somnolence progressing to stupor or coma, skeletal muscle flaccidity, cold, clammy skin, and sometimes bradycardia and hypotension. In severe overdosage, apnea, circulatory collapse, cardiac arrest and death may occur.

Treatment: Primary attention should be given to the re-establishment of adequate respiratory exchange by providing a patent airway and the institution of assisted or controlled ventilation. The narcotic antagonist naloxone HCl is a specific antidote against respiratory depression which may result from overdosage or unusual sensitivity to narcotics, including hydrocodone. An appropriate dose of naloxone HCl should be administered preferably by the i.v. route, simultaneously with efforts at respiratory resuscitation. Since the duration of action of hydrocodone may exceed that of the antagonist, the patient should be kept under continued surveillance and repeated doses of the antagonist should be administered as needed to maintain adequate respiration. The instructions contained in the package insert should be carefully observed. Oxygen, i.v. fluids, vasopressors, and other supportive measures should be employed as indicated. Gastric emptying may be useful in removing unabsorbed drug. Activated charcoal may be of benefit.

For management of a suspected drug overdose, CPhA recommends that you contact your **regional Poison Control Centre**. See the *CPS* Directory section for a list of Poison Control Centres.

DOSAGE: Usual Adult Dosage: 5 mg (1 tablet or 5 mL (one teaspoonful) of syrup) not less than 4 hours apart, after meals and at bedtime with food or a glass of milk, not to exceed 30 mg (6 tablets or 30 mL (six teaspoonfuls) of syrup) in a 24-hour period. Maximum single dose 15 mg (3 tablets or 15 mL (three teaspoonfuls) of syrup).

Usual Children's Dosage: Over 12 yrs: 5 mg (1 tablet or 5 mL (one teaspoonful) of syrup) not less than 4 hours apart, after meals and at bedtime with food or a glass of milk, not to exceed 30 mg (6 tablets or 30 mL (six teaspoonfuls) of syrup) in a 24-hour period. Maximum single dose 10 mg (2 tablets or 10 mL (two teaspoonfuls) of syrup).

Age 2 to 12 yrs: 2.5 mg (one half tablet or 2.5 mL (½ teaspoonful) of syrup) not less than 4 hours apart, after meals and at bedtime with food or a glass of milk, not to exceed a total of 15 mg (3 tablets or 15 mL (three teaspoonfuls) of syrup) in a 24-hour period. Maximum single dose 5 mg (1 tablet or 5 mL (one teaspoonful) of syrup).

Age less than 2 yrs: 1.25 mg (one quarter tablet or 1.25 mL (¼ teaspoonful) of syrup) not less than 4 hours apart, after meals and at bedtime with food or a glass of milk, not to exceed a total of 7.5 mg (1.5 tablets or 7.5 mL (1½ teaspoonfuls) of syrup) in a 24-hour period. Maximum single dose 1.25 mg (one quarter tablet or 1.25 mL (¼ teaspoonful) of syrup).

SUPPLIED: Syrup: Each 5 mL of red, wild-cherry-flavored syrup contains: hydrocodone bitartrate 5 mg. Nonmedicinal ingredients: artificial cherry flavor, caramel syrup, FD&C Red No. 2, hydrochloric acid, methylparaben, propylparaben, purified water, sorbitol solution 70% and sucrose. Alcohol-, lactose-, sodium-, sulfite- and tartrazine-free. Bottles of 500 mL. Patients should be instructed to store HYCODAN SYRUP, as for any medication, well out of the reach of children. Keep tightly closed. Store at 15 to 30°C. Dispense syrup in a tight, light resistant container.

Tablets: Each white, biconvex tablet, bisected and embossed with "HYCODAN" on one side and the other side blank, contains: hydrocodone bitartrate 5 mg. Nonmedicinal ingredients: cornstarch, lactose, pregelatinized tapioca starch, stearic acid, talc and zinc stearate. Sodium- and tartrazine-free. Bottles of 100. Patients should be instructed to store HYCODAN TABLETS, as for any medication, well out of the reach of children. Keep tightly closed. Store at 15 to 30°C.

(Shown in Product Identification Section)

Hycomine® Ⓝ

hydrocodone bitartrate—pyrilamine maleate—phenylephrine HCl—ammonium chloride

Antitussive—Antihistaminic—Decongestant

Bristol-Myers Squibb

Hycomine®-S Ⓝ

hydrocodone bitartrate—pyrilamine maleate—phenylephrine HCl—ammonium chloride

Antitussive—Antihistaminic—Decongestant

Bristol-Myers Squibb

Date of Preparation: December 31, 1976
Date of Revision: November 5, 2001

PHARMACOLOGY: Clinical trials have proven hydrocodone bitartrate to be an effective antitussive agent which is pharmacologically two to eight times as potent as codeine. At equi-effective doses, its sedative action is greater than that of codeine. The precise mechanisms of action of hydrocodone and other opiates are not known; however, hydrocodone is believed to act by directly depressing the cough center. In excessive doses, hydrocodone, like other opium derivatives, can depress respiration. The effects of therapeutic doses of hydrocodone on the cardiovascular system are insignificant. The constipating effects of hydrocodone are much weaker than those of morphine and no stronger than those of codeine. Hydrocodone can produce miosis, euphoria, physical and psychological dependence. At therapeutic antitussive doses, it does exert analgesic effects. Following a 10 mg oral dose of hydrocodone administered to five male human subjects, the mean peak serum concentration was 23.6±5.2 ng/mL. Maximum serum levels were achieved at 1.3±0.3 hours and the half-life was determined to be 3.8±0.3 hours. Hydrocodone exhibits a complex pattern of metabolism including O-demethylation, N-demethylation and 6-keto reduction to the corresponding 6-α- and 6-β-hydroxymetabolites.

Pyrilamine maleate is a competitive H_1-receptor histamine-blocking drug, thereby counteracting the effects of histamine release associated with allergic manifestations of upper respiratory tract inflammatory disorders. H_1-blocking drugs inhibit the actions of histamine on smooth muscle, capillary permeability, and can both stimulate and depress the CNS.

Phenylephrine HCl effects its vasoconstrictor activity by releasing norepinephrine from sympathetic nerve endings, and from direct stimulation of α-adreno-receptors in blood vessels.

Ammonium chloride exerts an expectorant effect by virtue of a local action on the gastric mucosa.

INDICATIONS: To control cough, and to provide symptomatic relief of congestion in the upper respiratory tract due to the common cold, nasopharyngitis, tracheitis, and bronchitis, which do not respond to products of lesser potency.

CONTRAINDICATIONS: HYCOMINE SYRUP and HYCOMINE-S PEDIATRIC SYRUP should not be used in patients with hypersensitivity to any of the components of the drug. Patients known to be hypersensitive to other opioids, antihistamines or sympathomimetic amines may exhibit cross-sensitivity to hydrocodone, pyrilamine or phenylephrine. Should not be used in patients using monoamine oxidase inhibitors. Phenylephrine is contraindicated in patients with heart disease, hypertension, diabetes or hyperthyroidism. Hydrocodone is contraindicated in the presence of an intracranial lesion associated with increased intracranial pressure, and whenever ventilatory function is depressed.

WARNINGS: Drug Abuse and Dependence: Hydrocodone can produce drug dependence and, therefore, has the potential for being abused. Psychic dependence, physical dependence and tolerance may develop upon repeated administration of hydrocodone, and it should be prescribed and administered with the same degree of caution appropriate to the use of other narcotic drugs (see Adverse Effects, Drug Abuse and Dependence).

Respiratory Depression: Hydrocodone produces dose-related respiratory depression by directly acting on the brain stem respiratory centers. If respiratory depression occurs, it may be antagonized by the use of naloxone hydrochloride and other supportive measures when indicated.

Usage in Ambulatory Patients: Hydrocodone may impair the mental and/or physical abilities required for the performance of potentially hazardous tasks such as driving a car or operating machinery. Patients using HYCOMINE SYRUP and HYCOMINE-S PEDIATRIC SYRUP should be cautioned accordingly.

Head Injury and Increased Intracranial Pressure: The respiratory depressant effects of narcotics and their capacity to elevate cerebrospinal fluid pressure may be markedly exaggerated in the presence of head injury, other intracranial lesions or a pre-existing elevated intracranial pressure. Furthermore, narcotics may produce adverse reactions which can obscure the clinical course of patients with head injuries.

Acute Abdominal Conditions: The administration of hydrocodone or other opioids may obscure the diagnosis or clinical course in patients with acute abdominal conditions.

Interaction with Other CNS Depressants: Patients receiving other narcotic analgesics, general anesthetics, phenothiazines or other tranquilizers, tricyclic antidepressants, sedative-hypnotics or other CNS depressants (including alcohol) concomitantly with HYCOMINE SYRUP and HYCOMINE-S PEDIATRIC SYRUP may exhibit an additive CNS depression. When such combined therapy is contemplated, the dose of one or both agents should be reduced.

Phenylephrine: Hypersensitive crises can occur with concurrent use of phenylephrine and MAO inhibitors, indomethacin or with beta-blockers and methyldopa.

If a hypertensive crisis occurs, these drugs should be discontinued immediately and therapy to lower blood pressure should be instituted immediately. Fever should be managed by external cooling.

Pyrilamine: Antihistamines may produce drowsiness or excitation, particularly in children and elderly patients.

PRECAUTIONS: Before prescribing medication to suppress or modify cough, it is important to ascertain that the underlying cause of cough is identified, that modification of cough does not increase the risk of clinical or physiological complications, and that appropriate therapy for the primary disease is provided.

In young children the respiratory centre is especially susceptible to the depressant action of narcotic cough suppressants. Benefit-to-risk ratio should be carefully considered, especially in children with respiratory embarrassment, e.g., croup. Estimation of dosage relative to the child's age and weight is of great importance.

As hydrocodone may inhibit peristalsis, patients with chronic constipation should be given the drug only after weighing the potential therapeutic benefit against the hazards involved.

In patients with asthma or pulmonary emphysema, indiscriminate use may precipitate respiratory insufficiency resulting from increased viscosity of bronchial secretions and suppression of the cough reflex.

Use with caution in sedated or debilitated patients, in patients who have undergone thoracotomies or laparotomies, since suppression of the cough reflex may lead to retention of secretions postoperatively in these patients.

Use with caution in glaucoma, prostatic hypertrophy, urinary retention, and in the aged.

Special Risk Patients: HYCOMINE should be given with caution to certain patients such as the elderly or debilitated, and those with severe impairment of hepatic or renal functions, hypothyroidism, Addison's disease, prostatic hypertrophy or urethral stricture, asthma, narrow-angle glaucoma, and uncontrolled hypertension.

Carcinogenesis/Mutagenesis/Impairment of Fertility: Carcinogenicity, mutagenicity and reproduction studies have not been conducted with HYCOMINE SYRUP and HYCOMINE-S PEDIATRIC SYRUP.

Pregnancy: HYCOMINE-S PEDIATRIC SYRUP is only recommended for pediatric use. Animal reproduction studies have not been conducted. It is also not known whether HYCOMINE SYRUP or HYCOMINE-S PEDIATRIC SYRUP can cause fetal harm when administered to a pregnant woman or can affect reproductive capacity. Since hydrocodone crosses the placental barrier, HYCOMINE SYRUP and HYCOMINE-S PEDIATRIC SYRUP should be given to pregnant women only if clearly needed.

Nonteratogenic Effects: Babies born to mothers who have been taking opioids regularly prior to delivery will be physically dependent. The withdrawal signs include: irritability and excessive crying, tremors, hyperactive reflexes, increased respiratory rate, increased stools, sneezing, yawning, vomiting and fever. The intensity of the syndrome does not always correlate with the duration of maternal opioids use or dose. There is no consensus on the best method of managing withdrawal. Chlorpromazine (0.7 to 1.0 mg/kg q6h), phenobarbital (2 mg/kg q6h), and paregoric (2 to 4 drops/kg q4h), have been used to treat withdrawal symptoms in infants. The duration of therapy is 4 to 28 days, with the dosages decreased as tolerated.

Lactation: It is not known whether hydrocodone is excreted in human milk. Because many drugs are excreted in human milk and because of the potential for serious adverse reactions in nursing infants from HYCOMINE SYRUP, a decision should be made whether to discontinue nursing or discontinue the drug, taking into account the importance of the drug to the mother.

Drug Interactions: The CNS-depressant effect of HYCOMINE SYRUP and HYCOMINE-S PEDIATRIC SYRUP may be additive with that of other CNS depressants (see Warnings).

ADVERSE EFFECTS: Respiratory: Hydrocodone produces dose-related respiratory depression by acting directly on brain stem respiratory centers.

Cardiovascular: hypertension, postural hypotension, tachycardia and palpitations.

Genitourinary: Ureteral spasm, spasm of vesical sphincters and urinary retention have been reported with opiates.

CNS: sedation, drowsiness, mental clouding, lethargy, impairment of mental and physical performance, anxiety, fear, dysphoria, dizziness, psychic dependence, mood changes and blurred vision.

Gastrointestinal: Nausea and vomiting occur more frequently in ambulatory than in recumbent patients. Constipation may also occur.

Drug Abuse and Dependence: Special care should be exercised in prescribing hydrocodone for emotionally unstable patients and for those with a history of drug misuse. Such patients should be closely supervised when long-term therapy is contemplated.

Psychic dependence, physical dependence, and tolerance may develop upon repeated administration of narcotics, therefore HYCOMINE SYRUP and HYCOMINE-S PEDIATRIC SYRUP should always be prescribed and administered with caution. Physical dependence is the condition in which continued administration of the drug is required to prevent the appearance of a withdrawal syndrome.

Patients physically dependent on opioids will develop an abstinence syndrome upon abrupt discontinuation of the opioid or following the administration of a narcotic antagonist. The character and severity of the withdrawal symptoms are related to the degree of physical dependence. Manifestation of opioid withdrawal are similar to but milder than that of morphine and include lacrimation, rhinorrhea, yawning, sweating, restlessness, dilated pupils, anorexia, gooseflesh, irritability and tremor. In more severe forms, nausea, vomiting, intestinal spasm and diarrhea, increased heart rate and blood pressure, chills, and pains in bones and muscles of the back and extremities may occur. Peak effects will usually be apparent at 48 to 72 hours.

Treatment of withdrawal is usually managed by providing sufficient quantities of an opioid to suppress severe withdrawal symptoms and then gradually reducing the dose of opioid over a period of several days.

OVERDOSE:

The signs and symptoms of overdosage of the individual components of HYCOMINE SYRUP or HYCOMINE-S PEDIATRIC SYRUP may be modified in varying degrees by the presence of other active ingredients.

Symptoms: Serious overdosage with hydrocodone may be characterized by: respiratory depression (a decrease in respiratory rate and/or tidal volume, Cheyne-Stokes respiration, cyanosis), extreme somnolence progressing to stupor or coma, skeletal muscle flaccidity, cold and clammy skin, and sometimes bradycardia and hypotension. In severe overdosage, apnea, circulatory collapse, cardiac arrest, and death may occur.

Treatment: Primary attention should be given to re-establishing adequate respiratory exchange by providing a patent airway and instituting assisted or controlled ventilation. The narcotic antagonist naloxone HCl is a specific antidote against respiratory depression which may result from overdosage or unusual sensitivity to narcotics, including hydrocodone. Administer an appropriate dose of naloxone HCl, preferably by the i.v. route, simultaneously with efforts at respiratory resuscitation. Since the duration of action of hydrocodone may exceed that of the antagonist, the patient should be kept under continued surveillance and repeated doses of the antagonist should be administered as needed to maintain adequate respiration. The instructions contained in the package insert should be carefully observed.

Oxygen, i.v. fluids, vasopressors, and other supportive measures should be employed as indicated.

Gastric emptying may be useful in removing unabsorbed drug. Activated charcoal may be of benefit.

> For management of a suspected drug overdose, CPhA recommends that you contact your **regional Poison Control Centre**. See the *CPS* Directory section for a list of Poison Control Centres.

DOSAGE: HYCOMINE: Adults, 5 mL after meals and at bedtime with food or a glass of milk at intervals of not less than 4 hours not to exceed 30 mL in a 24-hour period. Maximum single dose 15 mL.

HYCOMINE-S: Children over 12 years: 10 mL after meals and at bedtime with food or a glass of milk at intervals of not less than 4 hours, not to exceed a total of 60 mL in a 24-hour period. Maximum single dose 20 mL.

Children 6 to 12 years: 5 mL after meals and at bedtime with food or a glass of milk at intervals of not less than 4 hours: not to exceed a total of 30 mL in a 24-hour period. Maximum single dose 10 mL.

Children 3 to 6 years: 2.5 mL after meals and at bedtime with food or a glass of milk, at intervals of not less than 4 hours, not to exceed a total of 15 mL in a 24-hour period. Maximum single dose 5 mL.

Children less than 2 years: According to weight on the basis of 300 µg (0.3 mg) hydrocodone bitartrate/kg body weight/day, divided into 4 equal doses taken after meals and at bedtime.

SUPPLIED: HYCOMINE: Each 5 mL of orange, cherry-flavored syrup contains: hydrocodone bitartrate 5 mg, pyrilamine maleate 12.5 mg, phenylephrine HCl 10 mg and ammonium chloride 60 mg. Nonmedicinal ingredients: casiline orange, cherry flavor, hydrochloric acid, methylparaben, propylparaben, purified water, sorbitol solution and sucrose. Alcohol-, lactose-, sodium-, sulfite- and tartrazine-free. Bottles of 500 mL. Keep out of the reach of children. Store at 15 to 30°C. Dispense in a tight, light-resistant container.

HYCOMINE-S: Each 5 mL of green, cherry-flavored pediatric syrup contains: hydrocodone bitartrate 2.5 mg, pyrilamine maleate 6.25 mg, phenylephrine HCl 5 mg and ammonium chloride 30 mg. Nonmedicinal ingredients: cherry flavor, hydrochloric acid, methylparaben, minoline green, propylparaben, purified water, sorbitol solution and sucrose. Alcohol-, lactose-, sodium-, sulfite- and tartrazine-free. Bottles of 100 and 500 mL. Keep out of the reach of children. Store at 15 to 30°C. Dispense in a tight, light-resistant container.

(Shown in Product Identification Section)

Hycort® Pr

hydrocortisone

Glucocorticoid

Valeant

SUPPLIED: Each retention enema contains: hydrocortisone, USP 100 mg. Nonmedicinal ingredients: carboxypolymethylene carbomer, methylparaben, polysorbate 80 and sodium hydroxide. Bottles of 60 mL. Packs of 7 bottles. Store away from heat and direct light. Keep from freezing.

Hydergine® Pr

ergoloid mesylates

Adjunctive Management of Idiopathic Dementia

SteriMax

SUPPLIED: Each round, white, compressed, 8 mm diameter, flat, beveled tablet, scored, with "VJ" on one side and "HYDERGINE" on the other, contains: ergoloid mesylates 1 mg. Nonmedicinal ingredients: cornstarch, lactose, povidone, stearic acid and talc. Bottles of 100.

The reader is invited to consult CPhA's monograph **Corticosteroids: Topical**.

Hyderm
hydrocortisone acetate
Topical Corticosteroid

Taro

SUPPLIED: 0.5%: Each g contains: hydrocortisone acetate 0.5% in a water-washable cream base of cetostearyl alcohol, propylene glycol, purified water, sodium lauryl sulfate and white petrolatum. Paraben-free. Tubes of 15 g. Store at room temperature (15-30°C).
1% Ⓟ: Each g contains: hydrocortisone acetate 1% in a water-washable cream base of cetostearyl alcohol, propylene glycol, purified water, sodium lauryl sulfate and white petrolatum. Paraben-free. Tubes of 15 g and jars of 500 g. Store at room temperature (15-30°C).

Hydralazine Ⓟ
Vasodilator—Antihypertensive

CPhA Monograph

Date of Preparation: October 2005
Date of Revision: December 2009

This monograph has been compiled by CPhA and reviewed by experts. It may contain information different from that found in Health Canada-approved Product Monographs. The reader is referred to the *CPS* Editorial Policy for more information.

SUMMARY PRODUCT INFORMATION:

Route of Administration	Dosage Form	Strength
Oral	Tablet	10 mg, 25 mg, 50 mg
Intravenous	Powder for solution	20 mg/mL

INDICATIONS AND CLINICAL USE: Health Canada-approved indications include:
- treatment of hypertension including hypertensive emergencies and hypertension in pregnancy

Uses Without Health Canada Approval: Hydralazine has been used in the treatment of heart failure when used in combination with isosorbide dinitrate.
Hypertension: For the management of hypertension, hydralazine is recommended only in patients who do not respond adequately to a combination of first-line antihypertensive agents (e.g., a thiazide diuretic and a β-blocker and/or an ACE inhibitor or calcium channel blocking agent or angiotensin II antagonist).
Hydralazine, in combination with isosorbide dinitrate, can be considered in patients with hypertension and heart failure if first line agents cannot be tolerated. Guidelines recommend that hydralazine should be avoided in patients with hypertension and left ventricular hypertrophy [*Can J Cardiol* 2008;24(6):465-75]. Hydralazine has not been shown to produce regression of left ventricular hypertrophy, therefore other agents are preferred.
Hydralazine is generally administered in combination with a thiazide diuretic and a β-blocker. This reduces the hydralazine-induced sodium and water retention and reflex tachycardia, permits use of lower dosages of each drug and minimizes the probability of adverse effects.
Heart Failure: The combination of a beta-blocking agent and an ACE inhibitor is considered to be first line treatment for heart failure. The combination of hydralazine and isosorbide dinitrate is recommended as an alternative in patients who cannot tolerate first line agents. In addition, hydralazine and isosorbide dinitrate in combination should be considered as additional therapy for black patients [*Can J Cardiol* 2006;22(1):23-45].

CONTRAINDICATIONS:
- Hypersensitivity to hydralazine or to any ingredient in the formulation or component of the container.
- Acute dissecting aortic aneurysm
- Cor pulmonale
- Mitral valve rheumatic heart disease
- Myocardial insufficiency due to mechanical obstruction (e.g., aortic or mitral stenosis or constrictive pericarditis)
- Severe tachycardia and heart failure with high cardiac output (i.e., thyrotoxicosis)
- Systemic lupus erythematosus (SLE)

Table 1: Hydralazine
Adverse Drug Reactions

Body System	Effect	Clinical Comment
Cardiovascular	Palpitations, tachycardia, flushing, sodium and water retention, hypotension, paradoxical hypertension, heart failure, angina	Often administered with a β-blocker to counteract reflex tachycardia, and a diuretic to counteract sodium and water retention.
Central Nervous System	Headache, dizziness, anxiety, disorientation, agitation, depression, hallucinations, sleep disturbances, cerebral ischemia or hypoperfusion	Mild CNS effects usually do not require medical attention and resolve over time.
Dermatologic	Rash, urticaria, pruritus	
Gastrointestinal	Anorexia, diarrhea, constipation, nausea, vomiting, gastrointestinal distress, paralytic ileus	Gastrointestinal effects usually do not require medical attention and resolve over time.
Genitourinary	Proteinuria, hematuria, uremia, glomerulonephritis, acute renal failure, urinary retention, difficult micturition, increased serum creatinine concentration	Microhematuria and/or proteinuria in the presence of elevated ANA titres may result from immune-complex glomerulonephritis and be associated with SLE-like syndrome.
Hematologic	Anemia, leukopenia (agranulocytosis and thrombocytopenia), Coomb's-test positive hemolytic anemia, leukocytosis, lymphadenopathy, pancytopenia, splenomegaly, antinuclear antibodies	A positive ANA does not correlate with the onset of the SLE-like syndrome; serial measurement of ANA titre is not recommended.
Hepatic	Jaundice, liver enlargement, elevated liver enzymes, hepatocellular necrosis and granulomatous hepatitis	Monitor transaminase levels.
Hypersensitivity	SLE-like syndrome, chills, eosinophilia, cutaneous and systemic vasculitis, pruritus, urticaria, hepatitis, fever, vascular collapse	Clinical manifestations of the syndrome are usually reversible upon stopping hydralazine.
Neuromuscular	Peripheral neuritis with paresthesia, numbness and tingling, polyneuritis, tremor, muscle cramps, weakness	Peripheral neuritis may respond to pyridoxine administration.
Ocular	Lacrimation, conjunctivitis, blurred vision	
Respiratory	Nasal congestion, dyspnea, pleural pain, pulmonary hemorrhage, pulmonary edema, pulmonary hypertension	Nasal congestion usually resolves with time. Pleuropulmonary symptoms occur in 30% of patients with SLE-like syndrome.
Other	Weight decrease, malaise, impotence, decreased libido, sweating	

Abbreviations: ANA=antinuclear antibodies; SLE=systemic lupus erythematosis.

Table 2: Hydralazine
Abnormal Hematologic and Clinical Chemistry Findings

Test	Effect	Clinical Comment
Antinuclear antibodies	Positive	Possible SLE-like syndrome (see Warnings and Precautions, Hypersensitivity)
Coomb's test	Positive	Hemolytic anemia
Serum liver enzymes	Elevated	Possible hepatotoxicity

Table 3: Hydralazine
Drug-Drug Interactions

Interacting Drug	Effect	Clinical Comment
β-blockers (i.e., metoprolol, propranolol)	Serum levels of extensively metabolized β-blockers may be increased by hydralazine	The bioavailability of metoprolol and propranolol are increased by hydralazine, likely because of reduced hepatic blood flow. Adverse events have not been reported. Monitor for increased effects of β-blocker.
Digoxin	Increased renal clearance and decreased serum levels of digoxin	Renal clearance of digoxin increased and serum levels decreased in patients with congestive heart failure who received intravenous hydralazine. It is not known if the effect is sustained during long-term administration or whether dosage adjustments of digoxin are required. Monitor digoxin levels in patients receiving intravenous hydralazine.
NSAIDs (e.g., indomethacin, diclofenac)	Decreased hypotensive effect	NSAIDs can cause sodium and water retention, which opposes the effects of antihypertensive agents such as hydralazine. Blood pressure should be closely monitored in patients receiving the combination of hydralazine plus an NSAID.

Table 4: Hydralazine
Dose in Adult Patients

Indication	Route	Initial Dose	Dose Titration	Usual Dose	Maximum Dose	Clinical Comment
Hypertension[a]	Oral	10 mg QID	After 2–4 days, may be increased to 25 mg QID for remainder of first week of therapy; then, may increase by 25 mg per day at 1-week intervals up to 50 mg QID	50 mg QID; has also been used at doses of 25 to 150 mg BID	Rarely, doses up to 300 to 400 mg daily may be required to control blood pressure	Patients with the slow acetylator phenotype should receive a daily dose of no more than 200 mg.

(cont'd)

Table 4: Hydralazine *(cont'd)*

Dose in Adult Patients

Indication	Route	Initial Dose	Dose Titration	Usual Dose	Maximum Dose	Clinical Comment
Acute Hypertension	IV	10 to 20 mg repeated as necessary at 20 to 30 minute intervals to achieve desired blood pressure response				May also be administered as a continuous infusion at an initial dose of 200 to 300 µg/min, titrated to achieve desired blood pressure; usual maintenance dose 50 to 150 µg/minute.[b]
Hypertensive Emergencies during Pregnancy	IV	5 to 10 mg initially, followed by 5 to 10 mg every 20 to 30 minutes as necessary				For severe hypertension, may be infused at a rate of 0.5 to 10 mg/hour.[b]
Heart Failure (Not an approved use in Canada)	Oral	50 to 100 mg Q8H		200 to 600 mg/day divided every 4 to 12 hours		Used in conjunction with isosorbide dinitrate.

[a] Canadian guidelines on the management of hypertension are published [*Can J Cardiol* 2008;24(6):465-75] or available from www.hypertension.ca.

[b] Patients started on intravenous hydralazine should be switched to oral therapy as soon as is practical; an intravenous dose of 25 to 50 mg has been reported to be equivalent to an oral dose of 75 to 100 mg.

Table 5: Hydralazine

Dose in Pediatric Patients

Indication	Route	Initial Dose	Dose Titration	Usual Dose	Maximum Dose	Clinical Comment
Hypertension (Not an approved use in Canada)	Oral	0.75 mg/kg/day in 4 divided doses; initial oral dose should not exceed 25 mg/dose	May be increased slowly to a dose of 7 mg/kg/day over a period of 3 to 4 weeks	0.75 to 7 mg/kg/day in 4 divided doses	200 mg/day	
Hypertension (Not an approved use in Canada)	IM/IV	1.7 to 3.5 mg/kg/day in 4 to 6 divided doses; not to exceed 20 mg/dose			20 mg/dose	When administered by continuous infusion the initial recommended dose is 1.5 µg/kg/min.

WARNINGS AND PRECAUTIONS:

Serious Warnings and Precautions
- SLE-like syndrome
- Peripheral neuritis possibly related to an antipyridoxine effect
- Hydralazine may precipitate angina pectoris or myocardial infarction and may produce ECG changes indicative of myocardial ischemia
- Blood dyscrasias have been reported in patients receiving hydralazine

Hypersensitivity: Hydralazine is associated with the development of antinuclear antibodies (ANA) and a potentially fatal SLE-like syndrome that manifests most often as fever, arthralgia, asthenia, myalgia, malaise, lymphadenopathy, splenomegaly, pleuritic chest pain and edema. Development of ANA does not necessarily predict the onset of the SLE-like syndrome, as approximately 30–60% of patients develop a positive ANA titre after 3 years of therapy with hydralazine. The SLE-like syndrome has been estimated to occur in 7-13% of patients taking hydralazine [*Ann N Y Acad Sci* 2007;1108:166-82]. It is thought to be a type of hypersensitivity reaction in which hydralazine-directed antibodies and anti-DNA antibodies arise.

The SLE-like syndrome most often develops with the use of doses >200 mg/day although it has been reported with lower doses. The onset usually is 1 month to 5 years after the start of therapy with hydralazine and usually manifests as arthralgia and arthritis (95% of patients), fever and myalgia (50%) and as pleuropulmonary symptoms (30% of patients; pleurisy, pleural effusions, pulmonary infiltrates). The clinical syndrome usually resolves after withdrawal of hydralazine.

Special Populations: Pregnant Women: Hydralazine readily crosses the placenta, and serum concentrations in the fetus are similar to maternal levels of the drug. Hydralazine has not been associated with any congenital defects and the drug is used to manage hypertension during pregnancy.

Nursing Women: The American Academy of Pediatrics considers hydralazine to be compatible with breast-feeding.

Monitoring and Laboratory Tests: The manufacturer recommends that prescribers obtain a complete blood count, ANA titre, lupus erythematosus cell preparation and urinalysis at baseline and after 6 months of treatment, and if arthralgia, fever, chest pain or malaise occur during treatment with hydralazine.

ADVERSE REACTIONS: Adverse Drug Reactions: See Table 1.

Abnormal Hematologic and Clinical Chemistry Findings: See Table 2.

DRUG INTERACTIONS:

Serious Drug Interactions
- Profound hypotension may occur when coadministered with other parenteral hypotensive agents

Overview: A clinically significant additive hypotensive effect may occur when hydralazine is used in combination with other drugs that cause hypotension. Fatalities have been reported in patients treated with the combination of hydralazine and diazoxide, so this combination should be avoided if possible, or used with extreme caution.

Drug-Drug Interactions: See Table 3.

DOSAGE AND ADMINISTRATION: Recommended Dose and Dosage Adjustment: Adults: See Table 4.

Dose in Geriatric Patients: No specific dosage adjustment recommended for older individuals. Use same dosage as for adult patients.

Pediatrics: See Table 5.

Dose in Adult Patients with Renal Impairment: In patients with creatinine clearance <10 mL/minute the dosage interval should be extended to 8 to 16 hours (12 to 24 hours in slow acetylators).

Dosage in Dialysis: No specific recommendations. It is not known whether hydralazine is dialyzable.

Hepatic Impairment: Reduce the dose in patients with hepatic dysfunction.

Genetic Polymorphism: Patients may be slow or fast acetylator phenotype; related to intestinal activity of N-acetyl transferase.

Missed Dose: Wait until next dose. Do not take a double dose.

OVERDOSE:

For management of a suspected drug overdose, CPhA recommends that you contact your **regional Poison Control Centre**. See the *CPS* Directory section for a list of Poison Control Centres.

ACTION AND CLINICAL PHARMACOLOGY: Mechanism of Action: Hydralazine has a direct vasodilatory effect that leads to a reduction in peripheral vascular resistance. The effect is greater in arterioles than in veins, results in a greater reduction in diastolic than systolic blood pressure and produces little orthostatic hypotension. The decrease in peripheral resistance is usually accompanied by reflex tachycardia with an accompanying increase in cardiac output and stroke volume. Sodium and water retention with an expansion of plasma volume occur and may be counteracted by administration of a diuretic.

Pharmacokinetics: Adults: Absorption: Hydralazine is rapidly absorbed from the gastrointestinal tract after oral administration. Peak plasma concentrations were achieved 2 hours after oral administration of a single 100 mg dose of ^{14}C-hydralazine in healthy adults. There are large interindividual differences in plasma concentrations, but plasma concentrations are generally fairly constant in individuals receiving a fixed dose. Acetylator phenotype is an important determinant of plasma concentrations. Higher concentrations occur in slow acetylators. Administration with food may increase oral absorption.

Distribution: Hydralazine is widely distributed in body tissues. Approximately 85% of the drug in circulation is bound to plasma proteins. Hydralazine crosses the placenta and is excreted in breast milk.

Metabolism: The serum elimination half-life is about 2 to 4 hours, but may range up to 8 hours. The plasma elimination half-life is the same in slow and fast acetylators. Hydralazine is metabolized in the gastrointestinal mucosa and the liver (including extensive first-pass metabolism). Metabolism occurs by acetylation, hydroxylation and conjugation with glucuronic acid. Four pharmacologically inactive metabolites have been identified. The extent of first-pass acetylation in the gastric mucosa and liver is affected by acetylator phenotype. Slow acetylation is an autosomal recessive trait and is attributable to a relative deficiency in N-acetyl transferase. Approximately 50% of black and white patients and the majority of East Asian and North American Aboriginal patients are fast acetylators.

Excretion: The major portion of a dose is rapidly eliminated in urine as inactive metabolites. Approximately 10% of an orally administered dose is excreted in feces. It is not known if the drug is dialyzable.

STORAGE AND STABILITY: Dry powder ampoules should be stored at room temperature (15 to 30°C). Tablets should be protected from heat and humidity, below 30°C.

hydraSense®
sea water
Nasal Cleanser

Schering-Plough

DESCRIPTION: The hydraSense family of products include clinically proven 100% natural-source nasal irrigators as well as an innovative nasal aspirator. They are intended to improve breathing impaired by excessive mucus accumulation, nasal dryness, colds and allergies. The hydraSense solutions are offered in isotonic or hypertonic formulations.

The hydraSense 135 mL bottles have a unique SteriFlo delivery system that ensures sterility of the product throughout its use. hydraSense is also available in convenient single-use Easydose and ToGo formats, and hydraSense Congestion Relief and Eucalyptus are also available in convenient 25 mL bottles. There is no mixing or other preparation required.

INDICATIONS: hydraSense Easydose, Ultra-Gentle Mist with Comfort Tip, Gentle Mist, Medium Stream and ToGo: hydraSense is a simple, ready-to-use and effective way of cleansing excessive mucus accumulation in congested nasal cavities and passages caused by allergies, colds and upper respiratory infections. It is clinically proven that hydraSense relieves cold symptoms such as nasal obstruction and secretion, related sinus pressure and sore throat. Contributes as well in reducing the duration of cold symptoms, the occurrence of complications such as sinusitis, medication use and the number of sick days. hydraSense also reduces excessive dryness due to dust or dry air.

hydraSense Full Stream: hydraSense Full Stream is a simple, ready-to-use and effective way of cleansing excessive mucus accumulation in congested nasal cavities and passages caused by allergies, colds, and upper respiratory infections such as sinusitis. hydraSense also reduces excessive dryness due to dust or dry air. hydraSense Full Stream is also recommended and clinically proven for postoperative care following endonasal surgery. hydraSense cleanses excessive secretion and encrustation, improves healing time of nasal mucosa and restores nasal function. It helps reduce the duration of endonasal postoperative follow-up and reduces the risk of infections following the surgery.

hydraSense Nasal Aspirator: The hydraSense Nasal Aspirator is a gentle way to relieve your baby's nasal congestion quickly and effectively. It helps to maintain clear breathing and thus facilitate eating and sleeping. Its soft nasal tip is specifically designed for babies' delicate noses, while the protective single-use filter traps excess mucus, providing hygienic aspiration.

hydraSense Congestion Relief, Congestion Relief Kids and Eucalyptus: hydraSense Congestion Relief is a 100% naturally-sourced clinically proven nasal spray that relieves nasal and sinus congestion caused by colds, allergies or sinusitis. It clears blocked nasal passages without causing dryness to help breathing. hydraSense Congestion Relief may reduce the use of medicated decongestant. It also cleanses nasal cavities, helping to eliminate mucus-trapped infectious agents and allergens.

hydraSense Congestion Relief Kids helps relieve nasal congestion in the more sensitive noses of children and adults, while hydraSense Eucalyptus provides effective relief of nasal and sinus congestion with a pleasant feeling of freshness and a long-lasting cooling sensation.

WARNING: hydraSense Congestion Relief, Congestion Relief Kids and Eucalyptus: You may experience a temporary tingling sensation if mucus membranes are highly irritated.

PRECAUTIONS: hydraSense Easydose and Ultra-Gentle Mist with Comfort Tip: hydraSense Easydose and Ultra-Gentle Mist with Comfort Tip are intended for Newborns and Infants.

hydraSense Gentle Mist, Medium Stream and ToGo: hydraSense Gentle Mist, Medium Stream and ToGo are intended for Adults and children 2 years and older.

hydraSense Full Stream : hydraSense Full Stream is intended for Adults and children 12 years and older.

hydraSense Congestion Relief and Congestion Relief Kids: hydraSense Congestion Relief Kids is specially designed for children 6+. It is non-habit forming.

hydraSense Eucalyptus: hydraSense Eucalyptus is intended for Adults and children 6 years and older. It should not be used in women who are pregnant, planning to become pregnant of breastfeeding.

OVERDOSE:

For management of a suspected drug overdose, CPhA recommends that contact your **regional Poison Control Centre**. See the *CPS* Directory section for a list of Poison Control Centres.

DOSAGE: hydraSense Easydose: Can be used at least 2 times/day (morning and evening) and 4 to 6 times/day when the symptoms of colds or allergies are present.

hydraSense Ultra-Gentle Mist with Comfort Tip, Gentle Mist, Medium Stream and ToGo: Gently apply hydraSense at least twice a day (morning and evening) and 4 to 6 times a day when cold or allergy symptoms are present.

hydraSense Full Stream: Gently apply at least twice a day (morning and evening) and 4 to 6 times a day when cold or allergy symptoms are present. Following endonasal surgery, apply hydraSense 2 to 6 times a day.

hydraSense Nasal Aspirator: Can be used when relief from nasal discharge is desired, even in newborns.

hydraSense Congestion Relief: Apply 1 to 3 sprays per nostril, 2-3 times daily or as often as needed, followed by blowing for desired relief.

hydraSense Congestion Relief Kids: Can be used up to 6 times daily, followed by blowing for desired relief.

hydraSense Eucalyptus: Apply 1 spray of hydraSense Eucalyptus in each nostril by depressing the nozzle for 1 or 2 seconds, up to 4 times daily, followed by blowing of the nose for desired relief.

Instructions: hydraSense Easydose:

1. Break off one Easydose from the strip and turn the tamper-proof tip to open.
2. Lay the child on his back with his head tilted towards the right. Carefully place the tip in the (upper) nostril, and apply 1 or 2 drops by pressing gently on the dose. Follow the same procedure in the opposite nostril after turning the child's head to the left.
3. Soak a tissue or cotton ball in hydraSense and use it to gently wipe the child's nostrils.

Do not reuse vials after opening.

If the child is still presenting or has nasal secretions, it is recommended to repeat the above steps until the airways are properly cleared.

Ultra-Gentle Mist with Comfort Tip:

1. Place the nasal applicator on top of the container.
2. Lay the child on his back with his head tilted towards the right. Carefully insert the applicator in the left (upper) nostril, parallel to his nose (septum). Press down on the applicator. Follow the same procedure in the right nostril after turning the child's head to the left.
3. Spray a tissue or cotton ball with hydraSense and gently wipe nostrils.
4. Rinse the nasal applicator with hot water after each use and dry thoroughly.

hydraSense Nasal Aspirator:

1. Rinse the aspirator with hot water before first use and dry thoroughly.
2. Place a clean filter in the filter chamber and reconnect the aspirator.
3. Place baby on his back in a stable and comfortable position.
4. Place the Nasal Aspirator soft tip at the entrance of baby's nostril and inhale through the mouthpiece to gently draw out the mucus. Mucus will be collected in the hygienic filter chamber and cannot pass through the inhalation tube.
5. Repeat in the other nostril.
6. Gently lift baby to allow any remaining mucus to drain out and gently wipe the child's nostrils.
7. After each use, unscrew the aspirator at its base, remove and discard the used filter, rinse the Nasal Aspirator with hot water and dry. Do not sterilize or boil the Nasal Aspirator.

hydraSense Gentle Mist, Medium Stream, Full Stream, hydraSense Congestion Relief, Congestion Relief Kids and Eucalyptus:

1. Place the nasal applicator on top of the container.
2. Bend the head forward over a wash basin and tilt the head horizontally and to the right. Place the applicator in the left (upper) nostril, parallel to your nose (septum). Press down on the applicator. Tilt the head horizontally and to the left. Place the applicator in the right (upper) nostril and press down.
3. Blow the nose.
4. Rinse the nasal applicator with hot water after each use and dry thoroughly.

hydraSense ToGo:

1. Break off one vial from the strip and turn the tamper-proof tip to open.
2. Bend the head forward over a wash basin and tilt the head horizontally and to the right. Place the applicator in the left (upper) nostril, parallel to your nose (septum). Press down on the applicator. Tilt the head horizontally and to the left. Place the applicator in the right (upper) nostril and press down.
3. Blow the nose.

Do not reuse vials after opening.

SUPPLIED: Each isotonic solution contains undiluted, sterile, 100% natural-source desalinated sea water extracted from the mineral-rich ocean tides off the shores of Saint-Malo, France. It contains more than 70 trace elements and minerals naturally-occurring in sea water.

hydraSense Congestion Relief and Congestion Relief Kids contain hypertonic, undiluted, sterile, 100% natural-source desalinated seawater to 22 g/L (2.2%) (1.8% for hydraSense Congestion Relief Kids). hydraSense Eucalyptus contains hypertonic, undiluted, 100% natural-source desalinated seawater to 22 g/L (2.2%) and eucalyptus and wild mint extracts.

hydraSense is hypoallergenic and contains no preservatives or propellant gases with the use of SteriFlo dispensing system. Store between 15 and 25°C.

Safety Information for health care professionals: If you are a health care professional and require additional information or have questions, please contact Schering-Plough Canada, now part of Merck, Medical Information at 1 800 463-5442, anytime between 8:00 a.m. and 6:00 p.m. Eastern time, Monday through Friday.

Hydrea® Ⓟ

hydroxyurea

Antineoplastic

Bristol-Myers Squibb

Date of Preparation: March 23, 1979

Date of Revision: January 18, 2008

HYDREA (hydroxyurea) should be administered under the supervision of a physician experienced in the use of cancer chemotherapeutic agents.

PHARMACOLOGY: Neoplastic Disease: The precise mechanism by which HYDREA (hydroxyurea) produces its antineoplastic effects cannot, at present, be described. However, the reports of various studies in rat and human tissue cultures lend support to the hypothesis that hydroxyurea causes an immediate inhibition of DNA synthesis, by acting as a ribonucleotide reductase inhibitor, without interfering with the synthesis of ribonucleic acid or of protein. Hydroxyurea probably acts by decreasing the rate of conversion of ribonucleotides and deoxyribonucleotides. This effect is particularly apparent in cells with a high rate of proliferation.

Potentiation of Irradiation Therapy: Three mechanisms have been postulated for the potentiation of the therapeutic effects of irradiation by hydroxyurea on squamous cell (epidermoid) carcinomas of the head and neck. In vitro studies utilizing Chinese hamster cells suggest that hydroxyurea is lethal to normally radioresistant S-stage cells and holds other cells of the cell cycle in the G1 or pre-DNA synthesis stage where they are most susceptible to the effects of irradiation. The third mechanism of action has been theorized on the basis of in vitro studies of HeLa cells: it appears that hydroxyurea, by inhibition of DNA synthesis, hinders the normal repair process of cells damaged but not killed by irradiation, thereby decreasing their survival rate; there is no alteration of RNA and protein syntheses.

Pharmacokinetics: Absorption: Hydroxyurea is readily absorbed after oral administration. Peak plasma levels are reached in 1 to 4 hours after an oral dose. With increasing doses, disproportionately greater mean peak plasma concentrations and area under the plasma concentration-time curve (AUC) are observed. There are no data on the effect of food on the absorption of hydroxyurea.

Distribution: Hydroxyurea distributes rapidly and widely in the body with an estimated volume of distribution approximating total body water. Plasma to ascites fluid ratios range from 2:1 to 7.5:1. Hydroxyurea concentrates in leukocytes and erythrocytes. Hydroxyurea crosses the blood-brain barrier.

Metabolism: Up to 50% of an oral dose undergoes conversion through metabolic pathways that are not fully characterized. In one minor pathway, hydroxyurea may be degraded to acetohydroxamic acid by urease found in intestinal bacteria.

Excretion: Excretion of hydroxyurea in humans is a nonlinear process occurring through 2 pathways: one is saturable, probably hepatic metabolism; the other is first-order renal excretion. In patients with malignancies, renal elimination ranged from 25 to 55% of the administered dose. The concentration in the serum at 24 hours is negligible when the usual dose is given as a single daily dose.

Special Populations: No information is available regarding pharmacokinetic differences due to age, gender, or race.

Renal Insufficiency: Since renal excretion is a pathway of elimination, consideration should be given to decreasing the dosage in this population. In adult patients with sickle cell disease, an open-label, non-randomized, single dose, multi-center study was conducted to assess the influence of renal function on the pharmacokinetics of hydroxyurea. Patients in the study with normal (creatinine clearance (CrCl) >80 mL/min), mild (CrCl 50-80 mL/min), or severe (CrCl <30 mL/min) renal impairment received hydroxyurea as a single oral dose of 15 mg/kg, achieved by using combinations of the 200 mg, 300 mg, or 400 mg capsules. Patients with end-stage renal disease (ESRD) received two doses of 15 mg/kg separated by 7 days, the first was given following a 4-hour hemodialysis session, the second prior to hemodialysis. In this study the mean exposure (AUC) in patients whose creatinine clearance was <60 mL/min (or ESRD) was approximately 64% higher than in patients with normal renal function. The results suggest that the initial dose of hydroxyurea should be reduced when used to treat patients with renal impairment. (See Precautions and Dosage.)

Hepatic Insufficiency: There are no data that support specific guidance for dosage adjustment in patients with impaired hepatic function. (See also Dosage.)

INDICATIONS: For concomitant use with irradiation therapy in the treatment of primary squamous cell (epidermoid) carcinomas of the head and neck, excluding the lip.

Tumor responses to HYDREA have been reported in melanoma and resistant chronic myelocytic leukemia.

CONTRAINDICATIONS: In patients with marked bone marrow depression, i.e., leukopenia (<2500 WBC/mm³) or thrombocytopenia (<100 000/mm³), or severe anemia; or in patients who have demonstrated a previous hypersensitivity to hydroxyurea or any other component of its formulation.

WARNINGS: HYDREA (hydroxyurea) should be administered under the supervision of a physician experienced in the use of cancer chemotherapeutic agents.

Treatment with HYDREA should not be initiated if bone marrow function is depressed (see Contraindications). HYDREA may produce bone marrow suppression; leukopenia is generally its first and most common manifestation. Thrombocytopenia and anemia occur less often and are seldom seen without a preceding leukopenia. The recovery from myelosuppression is rapid when HYDREA therapy is interrupted. Bone marrow depression is more likely in patients who have previously received radiotherapy or cytotoxic cancer chemotherapeutic agents; HYDREA should be used cautiously in such patients.

Severe anemia must be corrected before initiating therapy with HYDREA.

Erythrocytic Abnormalities: Megaloblastic erythropoiesis, which is self-limiting, is often seen early in the course of HYDREA therapy. The morphologic change resembles that seen in pernicious anemia, but is not related to vitamin B_{12} or folic acid deficiency. The macrocytosis may mask the incidental development of folic acid deficiency; thus, prophylactic administration of folic acid may be warranted. Hydroxyurea may also delay plasma iron clearance and reduce the rate of iron utilization by erythrocytes, but it does not appear to alter the red blood cell survival time.

Patients who have received irradiation therapy in the past may have an exacerbation of postirradiation erythema when HYDREA is given.

Geriatrics: Elderly patients may be more sensitive to the effects of HYDREA and may require a lower dose regimen.

Carcinogenesis, Mutagenesis, Impairment of Fertility: Hydroxyurea is unequivocally genotoxic and a presumed transspecies carcinogen which implies a carcinogenic risk to humans. In patients receiving long-term therapy with hydroxyurea for myeloproliferative disorders, such as polycythemia vera and thrombocytopenia, secondary leukemia has been reported. It is unknown whether this leukemogenic effect is secondary to hydroxyurea or is associated with the patients' underlying disease. Skin cancer has also been reported in patients receiving long-term hydroxyurea.

Pregnancy: Hydroxyurea has been demonstrated to be a potent teratogen in a wide variety of animal models, including mice, rats, hamsters, rabbits, cats, miniature swine, dogs, and monkeys. The spectrum of effects following prenatal exposure to hydroxyurea includes embryo-fetal death, numerous fetal malformations of the viscera and skeleton, growth retardation, and functional deficits.

HYDREA can cause fetal harm when administered to a pregnant woman. There are no adequate and well-controlled studies in pregnant women. If HYDREA is used during pregnancy or if the patient becomes pregnant while on HYDREA therapy, the patient should be apprised of the potential hazard to the fetus. Women of childbearing potential should be advised to avoid becoming pregnant while taking HYDREA.

HYDREA should not be used to treat males contemplating conception.

Other: Fatal and nonfatal pancreatitis has occurred in HIV-infected patients during therapy with hydroxyurea and didanosine, with or without stavudine. Hepatotoxicity and hepatic failure resulting in death were reported during postmarketing surveillance in HIV-infected patients treated with hydroxyurea and other retroviral agents. Fatal hepatic events were reported most often in patients treated with the combination of hydroxyurea, didanosine, and stavudine. This combination should be avoided. Peripheral neuropathy, which was severe in some cases, has been reported in HIV-infected patients receiving hydroxyurea in combination with antiretroviral agents, including didanosine, with or without stavudine (see Adverse Effects).

Cutaneous vasculitic toxicities including vasculitic ulcerations and gangrene have occurred in patients with myeloproliferative disorders during therapy with hydroxyurea. These vasculitic toxicities were reported most often in patients with a history of or currently receiving interferon therapy. Due to potentially severe clinical outcomes for the cutaneous vasculitic ulcers reported in patients with myeloproliferative disease, hydroxyurea should be discontinued if cutaneous vasculitic ulcerations develop and alternative cytoreductive agents should be initiated as indicated (see Adverse Effects, Dermatologic).

PRECAUTIONS: Renal Insufficiency: HYDREA should be used with caution in patients with renal dysfunction (see Dosage).

Children: Safety and effectiveness of HYDREA in children have not been established.

Lactation: Hydroxyurea is secreted in human milk. Because of the potential for serious adverse reactions in nursing infants from hydroxyurea, breast-feeding should be discontinued.

Drug Interactions: Prospective studies on the potential for hydroxyurea to interact with other drugs have not been performed.

Concurrent use of hydroxyurea and other myelosuppressive agents or radiation therapy may increase the likelihood of bone marrow depression or other adverse events (see Warnings and Adverse Effects).

Since hydroxyurea may raise the serum uric acid level, dosage adjustment of uricosuric medication may be necessary.

In vitro studies have shown a significant increase in cytarabine cytotoxic activity in hydroxyurea-treated cells. Whether this interaction will lead to synergistic toxicity in the clinical setting or the need to modify cytarabine doses has not been established.

Occupational Hazards: Driving/Operating Machinery: The effect of HYDREA on driving and operating machinery has not been studied. Since HYDREA may cause drowsiness and other neurologic effects (see Adverse Effects, Neurologic), alertness may be impaired.

Information to Be Provided to the Patient: Patients should be informed to maintain adequate fluid intake. The physician should be consulted regarding missed doses.

ADVERSE EFFECTS: Hematologic: bone marrow depression (leukopenia, anemia, and occasionally thrombocytopenia) (see Warnings).

Gastrointestinal : stomatitis, anorexia, nausea, vomiting, diarrhea, and constipation.

Dermatologic: maculopapular rash, facial erythema, peripheral erythema, skin ulceration and dermatomyositis-like skin changes. Alopecia occurs rarely. Hyperpigmentation, erythema, atrophy of skin and nails, scaling, violet papules, and alopecia have been observed in some patients after several years of long-term daily maintenance therapy with hydroxyurea. Skin cancer has also been reported rarely.

Cutaneous vasculitic toxicities including vasculitic ulcerations and gangrene have occurred in patients with myeloproliferative disorders during therapy with hydroxyurea. These vasculitic toxicities were reported most often in patients with a history of or currently receiving interferon therapy (see Warnings).

Neurologic: drowsiness, rare instances of headache, dizziness, disorientation, hallucinations, and convulsions. Their relationship to hydroxyurea administration is questionable because cerebral metastatic disease was not excluded.

Renal: elevated serum uric acid, BUN, and creatinine levels; rare instances of dysuria. Abnormal BSP retention has been reported.

Other: fever, chills, malaise, asthenia, and elevation of hepatic enzymes; rare instances of acute pulmonary reactions (diffuse pulmonary infiltrates/fibrosis, and dyspnea). Fatal and nonfatal pancreatitis and hepatotoxicity and severe peripheral neuropathy have been reported in HIV-infected patients who received hydroxyurea in combination with antiretroviral agents, in particular didanosine plus stavudine. Patients treated with hydroxyurea in combination with didanosine, stavudine, and indinavir in study ACTG 5025 showed a median decline in CD4 cells of approximately 100/mm³ (see Warnings).

Combined HYDREA and Irradiation Therapy: Adverse reactions observed with combined hydroxyurea and irradiation therapy were similar to those reported with the use of HYDREA alone, primarily bone marrow depression (leukopenia and anemia), and gastric irritation. Nearly all patients receiving an adequate course of combined HYDREA and irradiation therapy will develop leukopenia. Decreased platelet counts (<100 000 cells/mm³) have occurred rarely and usually in the presence of marked leukopenia. HYDREA may potentiate some adverse reactions usually seen with irradiation alone, such as gastric distress and mucositis.

OVERDOSE:

Symptoms: Acute mucocutaneous toxicity has been reported in patients receiving hydroxyurea at a dosage several times the therapeutic dose. Soreness, violet erythema, edema on palms and foot soles followed by scaling of hands and feet, severe generalized hyperpigmentation of skin, and stomatitis have also been observed.

For management of a suspected drug overdose, CPhA recommends that you contact your **regional Poison Control Centre**. See the *CPS* Directory section for a list of Poison Control Centres.

DOSAGE: Because of the rarity of carcinomas of the head and neck in children, dosage regimens have not been established.

Dosage regimens in the treatment of the neoplastic diseases should be based on the patient's actual or ideal weight, whichever is less.

Solid Tumors: Intermittent Therapy: 80 mg/kg administered orally as a **single** dose every **third** day.

This intermittent dosage schedule may offer the advantage of reduced toxicity over daily therapy (e.g., bone marrow depression).

Concomitant Therapy with Irradiation (Carcinoma of the head and neck): 80 mg/kg administered orally as a **single** dose every **third** day.

Administration of HYDREA should be started at least 7 days before initiation of irradiation, and continued during radiotherapy and continue indefinitely thereafter, provided the patient is kept under adequate observation and exhibits no unusual or severe toxicity.

Resistant Chronic Myelocytic Leukemia: Continuous Therapy: 20 to 30 mg/kg administered orally as a single daily dose.

An adequate trial period for determining the effectiveness of HYDREA is 6 weeks. When there is regression in tumor size or arrest in tumor growth, therapy should be continued indefinitely. Therapy should be interrupted if the white blood cell count drops below 2500/mm³, or the platelet count below 100 000/mm³. In these cases, the counts should be re-evaluated after 3 days, and therapy resumed when the counts return to acceptable levels. Hematopoietic rebound is usually rapid. If rapid rebound has not occurred during combined HYDREA and irradiation therapy, irradiation may also be interrupted. Anemia, even if severe can be managed without interrupting HYDREA therapy.

HYDREA should be administered cautiously to patients who have recently received extensive radiation therapy or chemotherapy with other cytotoxic drugs (see Warnings and Adverse Effects).

Pain or discomfort from inflammation of the mucous membranes at the irradiated site (mucositis) is usually controlled by measures such as topical anesthetics and orally administered analgesics. If the reaction is severe, HYDREA therapy may be temporarily interrupted; if it is extremely severe, irradiation dosage may, in addition, be temporarily postponed.

Severe gastric distress, such as nausea, vomiting, and anorexia, resulting from combined therapy may usually be controlled by interruption of HYDREA administration.

Dosage Adjustment: Concurrent use of HYDREA with other myelosuppressive agents may require adjustments of dosages.

Renal Insufficiency: There are no data that support specific guidance for dosage adjustment in patients with impaired renal function. Since renal excretion is a pathway of elimination, consideration should be given to decreasing the dosage in this population. Close monitoring of hematologic parameters is advised.

Hepatic Insufficiency: There are no data that support specific guidance for dosage adjustment in patients with impaired hepatic function. Close monitoring of hematologic parameters is advised.

Instructions for Use, Handling and Disposal: If the patient prefers, or is unable to swallow capsules, the contents of the capsules may be emptied into a glass of water and taken immediately (see Precautions, Information to Be Provided to the Patient). Some inert material used as a vehicle in the capsule may not dissolve and may float on the surface.

Patients who take the drug by emptying the contents of the capsule into water should be reminded that this is a potent medication that must be handled with care. Patients must be cautioned not to allow the powder to come in contact with the skin and mucous membranes, including avoidance of inhaling the powder when opening the capsules. People who are not taking HYDREA should not be exposed to it. To decrease the risk of exposure, wear disposable gloves when handling HYDREA or bottles containing HYDREA. Anyone handling HYDREA should wash their hands before and after contact with the bottle or capsules.

If the powder is spilled, it should be immediately wiped up with a damp disposable towel and discarded in a closed container, such as a plastic bag, as should the empty capsules. Hydroxyurea should be kept away from children and pets.

To minimize the risk of dermal exposure, always wear impervious gloves when handling bottles containing HYDREA capsules. This includes handling activities in clinical settings, pharmacies, storerooms, and home healthcare settings, including during unpacking and inspection, transport within a facility, and dose preparation and administration.

Procedures for proper handling and disposal of anticancer drugs should be considered. Several guidelines on this subject have been published. There is no general agreement that all of the procedures recommended in the guidelines are necessary or appropriate.

INFORMATION FOR THE PATIENT: Published in e-CPS, available by subscription at www.e-cps.ca.

SUPPLIED: Each capsule with opaque green cap and opaque pink body, printed with "BMS 303" in black ink on both body and cap, contains: hydroxyurea 500 mg. Nonmedicinal ingredients: citric acid, dibasic sodium phosphate, lactose and magnesium stearate; capsule shell: FD&C blue No. 2 and red No. 3, gelatin, sodium lauryl sulfate, titanium dioxide and yellow iron oxide. Bottles of 100. Store at room temperature (15 to 30°C). Protect from excessive heat and moisture.

(Shown in Product Identification Section)

Hydrochlorothiazide Ⓟ

CPhA Monograph

see *Thiazide Diuretics*

Hydrocodone Ⓝ

CPhA Monograph

see *Opioids*

Hydrocortisone Ⓟ

CPhA Monograph

see *Corticosteroids: Eye Ear Nose*

see *Corticosteroids: Systemic*

see *Corticosteroids: Topical*

Hydrocortisone 17-valerate Ⓟ

CPhA Monograph

see *Corticosteroids: Topical*

Hydromorph Contin® Ⓝ

hydromorphone HCl

Opioid Analgesic

Purdue Pharma

Date of Revision: August 25, 2009

PHARMACOLOGY: Hydromorphone, a semi-synthetic μ opioid agonist, is a hydrogenated ketone of morphine and shares the pharmacologic properties typical of opioid analgesics. Hydromorphone and related opioids produce their major effects on the central nervous system and gastrointestinal tract. These include analgesia, drowsiness, mental clouding, changes in mood, euphoria or dysphoria, respiratory depression, cough suppression, decreased gastrointestinal motility, nausea, vomiting, increased cerebrospinal fluid pressure, increased biliary pressure, pinpoint constriction of the pupils, increased parasympathetic activity and transient hyperglycemia.

Estimates of the relative analgesic potency of parenterally administered hydromorphone to morphine in acute pain studies in man range from approximately 7:1 to 11:1.

The relationship between plasma concentration of hydromorphone and analgesic effect has not been well established. In patients with chronic pain, hydromorphone should be titrated to the dose required to adequately relieve pain without unmanageable side effects.

There is no intrinsic limit to the analgesic effect of hydromorphone; like morphine, adequate doses will relieve even the most severe pain. Clinically however, dosage limitations are imposed by the adverse effects, primarily respiratory depression, nausea and vomiting, which can result from high doses.

Pharmacokinetics: After oral administration of conventional release hydromorphone tablets, the drug is rapidly absorbed and, like morphine, undergoes presystemic elimination (approximately 50%), presumably as a result of metabolism in the liver. The terminal elimination half-life after intravenous administration in humans is approximately 2.5-3.0 hours. The pharmacokinetics of hydromorphone have been shown to be linear over a range of intravenous doses from 10-40 μg/kg. The principal mode of elimination is by excretion in the urine as hydromorphone-3-glucuronide, which, at steady-state is present in plasma at concentrations approximately 26 times those of the parent drug. The pharmacologic activity of this and other hydromorphone metabolites in humans is not known.

HYDROMORPH CONTIN (hydromorphone hydrochloride controlled release capsules) administered 12 hourly provides equivalent analgesia to conventional release hydromorphone tablets (Dilaudid) administered every 4 hours in patients with cancer pain. Steady state pharmacokinetic studies demonstrate that maximum plasma concentration (C_{max}) of hydromorphone is achieved at a mean of 4.8 hours after administration of HYDROMORPH CONTIN, with maximum and minimum concentrations equivalent to those obtained with 4 hourly administration of the conventional release tablets. The extent of absorption of hydromorphone from HYDROMORPH CONTIN is equivalent to that from conventional tablets (Dilaudid) and is not significantly influenced when administered in the presence of food. In patients with chronic cancer pain receiving doses of HYDROMORPH CONTIN ranging from 6 mg to 216 mg/day there was a linear relationship between area under the plasma concentration-time curve (AUC) and dose.

Dilaudid is a product of Purdue Pharma.

INDICATIONS: HYDROMORPH CONTIN (hydromorphone hydrochloride controlled release capsules) is indicated for the relief of severe chronic pain requiring the prolonged use of an oral opioid preparation.

CONTRAINDICATIONS: HYDROMORPH CONTIN (hydromorphone hydrochloride controlled release capsules) should not be given to patients with: hypersensitivity to opioid analgesics, hydromorphone, or any other component of the product; acute asthma or other obstructive airway disease and acute respiratory depression; elevated carbon dioxide levels in the blood; cor pulmonale; acute alcoholism; delirium tremens; severe CNS depression; convulsive disorders; increased cerebrospinal or intracranial pressure; head injury; suspected surgical abdomen (e.g., paralytic ileus); concomitant MAO inhibitors (or within 14 days of such therapy).

WARNINGS: HYDROMORPH CONTIN (hydromorphone hydrochloride controlled release capsules) must be swallowed whole, or opened and the contents sprinkled on cold, soft food. The capsule contents should not be chewed, crushed or dissolved. Taking broken, chewed, dissolved or crushed capsules, or their contents, could lead to the rapid release and absorption of a potentially fatal dose of hydromorphone.

HYDROMORPH CONTIN 18 mg capsules and higher are for use in opioid tolerant patients only (see also Dosage). These strengths may cause fatal respiratory depression if administered to patients not previously exposed to daily hydromorphone equivalent dosages of 36 mg or more. Care should be taken in the prescribing of these capsule strengths.

Patients should be instructed not to give HYDROMORPH CONTIN to anyone other than for whom it was prescribed, as such, inappropriate use may have severe medical consequences, including death.

Patients should be cautioned not to consume alcohol while taking HYDROMORPH CONTIN, as it may increase the chance of experiencing dangerous side effects (see Precautions, Drug Interactions).

HYDROMORPH CONTIN is not recommended for preoperative use or postoperatively within the first 24 hours.

Abuse of Opioid Formulations: HYDROMORPH CONTIN capsules are intended for oral use only. Abuse can lead to overdose and death. This risk is increased when the capsules or contents are crushed, broken, dissolved or chewed, and with concurrent consumption of alcohol or other CNS depressants. With parenteral abuse, the capsule excipients can be expected to result in local tissue necrosis, infection, pulmonary granulomas, and increased risk of endocarditis and valvular heart injury.

Drug Dependence: As with other opioids, tolerance and physical dependence tend to develop upon repeated administration of hydromorphone and there is a potential for abuse of the drug and for development of psychological dependence. HYDROMORPH CONTIN should therefore be prescribed and handled with the high degree of caution appropriate to the use of a drug with strong abuse potential. Drug abuse is not usually a problem in patients with severe pain in which hydromorphone is appropriately indicated. However, in the absence of a clear indication for a strong opioid analgesic, drug-seeking behaviour must be suspected and resisted, particularly in individuals with a history of, or propensity for drug abuse. Withdrawal symptoms may occur following abrupt discontinuation of therapy or upon administration of an opioid antagonist. Therefore, patients on prolonged therapy should be withdrawn gradually from the drug if it is no longer required for pain control.

Use in Drug and Alcohol Addiction: HYDROMORPH CONTIN is an opioid with no approved use in the management of addictive disorders. Its proper usage in individuals with drug or alcohol dependence, either active or in remission is for the management of pain requiring opioid analgesia.

CNS Depression: Hydromorphone should be used only with caution and in reduced dosage during concomitant administration of other opioid analgesics, general anaesthetics, phenothiazines and other tranquilizers, sedative-hypnotics, antidepressants and other CNS depressants, including alcohol. Respiratory depression, hypotension and profound sedation or coma may result.

Severe pain antagonizes the subjective and respiratory depressant actions of hydromorphone. Should pain suddenly subside, these effects may rapidly become manifest. Patients who are scheduled for cordotomy or other interruption of pain transmission pathways should not receive HYDROMORPH CONTIN within 24 hours of the procedure.

Pregnancy: Animal studies with both morphine and hydromorphone have indicated the possibility of teratogenic effects on the fetus. While experience in humans has not identified this as a risk, HYDROMORPH CONTIN should be given to pregnant patients only when the anticipated benefits outweigh the potential risks to the fetus.

PRECAUTIONS: Respiratory Depression: Hydromorphone should be used with extreme caution in patients with substantially decreased respiratory reserve, pre-existing respiratory depression, hypoxia or hypercapnia. Such patients are often less sensitive to the stimulatory effects of carbon dioxide on the respiratory centre and the respiratory depressant effects of hydromorphone may reduce respiratory drive to the point of apnea.

Head Injury: The respiratory depressant effects of hydromorphone, and the capacity to elevate cerebrospinal fluid pressure, may be greatly increased in the presence of an already elevated intracranial pressure produced by trauma. Also, hydromorphone may produce confusion, miosis, vomiting and other side effects which obscure the clinical course of patients with head injury. In such patients, hydromorphone must be used with extreme caution and only if it is judged essential.

Hypotension: Hydromorphone administration may result in severe hypotension in patients whose ability to maintain adequate blood pressure is compromised by reduced blood volume, or concurrent administration of such drugs as phenothiazines or certain anaesthetics.
Acute Abdominal Conditions: Hydromorphone (and other morphine-like opioids) have been shown to decrease bowel motility. Hydromorphone may obscure the diagnosis or clinical course of patients with acute abdominal conditions.
Special Risk Groups: Hydromorphone should be administered with caution, and in reduced dosages, to elderly or debilitated, to patients with severely impaired pulmonary, hepatic or renal function, and in patients with adrenocortical insufficiency (e.g., Addison's disease), hypothyroidism, pancreatitis, prostatic hypertrophy, toxic psychosis or urethral stricture.

Hydromorphone should not be used where there is the possibility of paralytic ileus occurring.

Labor/Delivery: In view of the potential for opioids to cross the placental barrier and to be excreted in breast milk, hydromorphone should be used with caution during labor or in nursing mothers. Physical dependence or respiratory depression may occur in the infant.
Lactation: See Labor/Delivery.
Occupational Hazards: Driving and Operating Dangerous Machinery: Hydromorphone may impair the mental and/or physical abilities needed for certain potentially hazardous activities such as driving a car or operating machinery. Patients should be cautioned accordingly.

Patients should also be cautioned about the combined effects of hydromorphone with other CNS depressants, including other opioids, phenothiazines, sedative/hypnotics and alcohol.

Drug Interactions: CNS depressants, such as other opioids, anaesthetics (e.g., barbiturates), sedatives, antidepressants, hypnotics, tranquilizers, neuroleptics, (centrally acting) antiemetics, chloral hydrate and glutethimide may enhance the depressant effect of hydromorphone. Monoamine oxidase inhibitors (including procarbazine hydrochloride) should not be taken within two weeks of use. Pyrazolidone antihistamines, beta-blockers and alcohol may also enhance the depressant effect of hydromorphone. When combined therapy is contemplated, the dose of one or both agents should be reduced.
"In Vitro" Dissolution Studies of Interaction with Alcohol: Increasing concentrations of alcohol in the dissolution medium resulted in a decrease in the rate of release of hydromorphone from HYDROMORPH CONTIN capsules at lower alcohol concentrations (up to 20%) and more rapid release, only at the highest alcohol concentrations (35-40%). The clinical significance of these findings is unknown.

Mixed agonist/antagonist opioid analgesics (i.e., pentazocine, nalbuphine, butorphanol, and buprenorphine) should be administered with caution to a patient who has received or is receiving a course of therapy with a pure opioid agonist analgesic such as hydromorphone. In this situation, mixed agonist/antagonist analgesics may reduce the analgesic effect of hydromorphone and/or may precipitate withdrawal symptoms in these patients.

Hydromorphone may increase the anticoagulant activity of coumarin and other anticoagulants.

ADVERSE EFFECTS: Adverse effects of HYDROMORPH CONTIN (hydromorphone hydrochloride controlled release capsules) are similar to those of other opioid analgesics, and represent an extension of pharmacological effects of the drug class. The major hazards of hydromorphone include respiratory and central nervous system depression. To a lesser degree, circulatory depression, respiratory arrest, shock and cardiac arrest have occurred.

The most frequently observed adverse effects are asthenic conditions, confusion, constipation, dizziness, lightheadedness, nausea, sedation, sweating and vomiting.

Sedation: Some degree of sedation is experienced by most patients upon initiation of therapy. This may be at least partly because patients often recuperate from prolonged fatigue after the relief of persistent pain. Most patients develop tolerance to the sedative effects of opioids within three to five days and, if the sedation is not severe, will not require any treatment except reassurance. If excessive sedation persists beyond a few days, the dose of the opioid should be reduced and alternate causes investigated. Some of these are: concurrent CNS depressant medication, hepatic or renal dysfunction, brain metastases, hypercalcemia and respiratory failure. If it is necessary to reduce the dose, it can be carefully increased again after three or four days if it is obvious that the pain is not being well controlled. Dizziness and unsteadiness may be caused by postural hypotension particularly in elderly or debilitated patients and may be alleviated if the patient lies down.
Nausea and Vomiting: Nausea is a common side effect on initiation of therapy with opioid analgesics and is thought to occur by activation of the chemoreceptor trigger zone, stimulation of the vestibular apparatus and through delayed gastric emptying. The prevalence of nausea declines following continued treatment with opioid analgesics. When instituting prolonged therapy with an opioid for chronic pain, the routine prescription of an antiemetic should be considered. In the cancer patient, investigation of nausea should include such causes as constipation, bowel obstruction, uremia, hypercalcemia, hepatomegaly, tumor invasion of celiac plexus and concurrent use of drugs with emetogenic properties. Persistent nausea which does not respond to dosage reduction may be caused by opioid-induced gastric stasis and may be accompanied by other symptoms including anorexia, early satiety, vomiting and abdominal fullness. These symptoms respond to chronic treatment with gastrointestinal prokinetic agents.
Constipation: Practically all patients become constipated while taking opioids on a persistent basis. In some patients, particularly the elderly or bedridden, fecal impaction may result. It is essential to caution the patients in this regard and to institute an appropriate regimen of bowel management at the start of prolonged opioid analgesic therapy. Stool softeners, stimulant laxatives and other appropriate measures should be used as required.
Less Frequently Observed with Opioid Analgesics: General and CNS: agitation, alterations of mood (nervousness, apprehension, depression floating feelings, dreams), blurred vision, confusion, convulsions, drug dependence, drug tolerance, drug withdrawal syndrome, diplopia and miosis, dyskinesia, dysphoria, euphoria, headache, high dose hyperalgesia that will not respond to a further dose increase of hydromorphone (possibly dose reduction or change in opioid required), insomnia, increased intracranial pressure, muscle rigidity, muscle tremor, nystagmus, paresthesia, peripheral edema, hallucinations and disorientation, somnolence, tremor, uncoordinated muscle movements, visual disturbances and weakness.
Cardiovascular: bradycardia, chills, faintness, flushing of the face, hypertension, hypotension, palpitation, syncope and tachycardia.
Respiratory: bronchospasm, laryngospasm and respiratory depression.
Gastrointestinal: anorexia biliary tract spasm, cramps, diarrhea, dry mouth, hepatic enzymes increased, paralytic ileus and taste alterations.
Genitourinary: antidiuretic effects, urinary retention or hesitancy.
Dermatologic: diaphoresis, pruritus, other skin rashes and urticaria.
Immune: hypersensitivity reactions (including oropharyngeal swelling).
Withdrawal (Abstinence) Syndrome: Physical dependence with or without psychological dependence tends to occur with chronic administration. An abstinence syndrome may be precipitated when opioid administration is discontinued or opioid antagonists administered. The following withdrawal symptoms may be observed after opioids are discontinued: body aches, diarrhea, gooseflesh, loss of appetite, nausea, nervousness or restlessness, runny nose, sneezing, tremors or shivering, stomach cramps, tachycardia, trouble with sleeping, unusual increase in sweating, unexplained fever, weakness and yawning. In patients who are appropriately treated with opioid analgesics and who undergo gradual withdrawal from the drug, these symptoms are usually mild.

OVERDOSE:

Symptoms: Serious overdosage with hydromorphone may be characterized by respiratory depression (a decrease in respiratory rate and/or tidal volume, Cheyne-Stokes respiration, cyanosis), extreme somnolence progressing to stupor or coma, miotic pupils, skeletal muscle flaccidity, cold and clammy skin, and sometimes bradycardia and hypotension. In severe overdosage, apnea, circulatory collapse, cardiac arrest and death may occur.

Treatment: Primary attention should be given to the establishment of adequate respiratory exchange through the provision of a patent airway and controlled or assisted ventilation. The opioid antagonist naloxone hydrochloride is a specific antidote against respiratory depression due to overdosage or as a result of unusual sensitivity to hydromorphone. An appropriate dose of the antagonist should therefore be administered, preferably by the intravenous route. The usual initial i.v. adult dose of naloxone is 0.4 mg or higher. Concomitant efforts at respiratory resuscitation should be carried out. Since the duration of action of hydromorphone, particularly sustained release formulations, may exceed that of the antagonist, the patient should be under continued surveillance and doses of the antagonist should be repeated as needed to maintain adequate respiration.

An antagonist should not be administered in the absence of clinically significant respiratory or cardiovascular depression. Oxygen, intravenous fluids, vasopressors and other supportive measures should be used as indicated.

In individuals physically dependent on opioids, the administration of the usual dose of opioid antagonist will precipitate an acute withdrawal syndrome. The severity of this syndrome will depend on the degree of physical dependence and the dose of antagonist administered. The use of opioid antagonists in such individuals should be avoided if possible. If an opioid antagonist must be used to treat serious respiratory depression in the physically dependent patient, the antagonist should be administered with extreme care by using dosage titration, commencing with 10 to 20% of the usual recommended initial dose.

Evacuation of gastric contents may be useful in removing unabsorbed drug, particularly when a sustained release formulation has been taken.

For management of a suspected drug overdose, contact your **regional Poison Control Centre**. See the *CPS* Directory section for a list of Poison Control Centres.

DOSAGE: HYDROMORPH CONTIN (hydromorphone hydrochloride controlled release capsules) must be swallowed whole, or opened and the contents sprinkled on cold, soft food. The capsule contents should not be chewed, crushed or dissolved. Taking broken, chewed, dissolved or crushed capsules could lead to the rapid release and absorption of a potentially fatal dose of hydromorphone.

Capsule strengths of 18 mg and higher are for opioid tolerant patients only, requiring hydromorphone equivalent dosages of 36 mg or more per day. These doses may lead to severe medical consequences, including fatal respiratory depression, in patients not previously exposed to similar doses of opioids.

Adults: Individual dosing requirements vary considerably based on each patient's age, weight, severity and cause of pain, and medical and analgesic history.
Patients Not Receiving Opioids at the Time of Initiation of HYDROMORPH CONTIN Treatment: Patients who are opioid naive or receiving low, intermittent doses of weak opioid analgesics may be initiated on HYDROMORPH CONTIN 3 mg every 12 hours.
Patients Currently Receiving Opioids: Patients currently receiving other oral hydromorphone formulations may be transferred to HYDROMORPH CONTIN at the same total daily hydromorphone dosage, equally divided into two 12 hourly HYDROMORPH CONTIN doses.

For patients who are receiving an alternate opioid, the "oral hydromorphone equivalent" of the analgesic presently being used should be determined. Having determined the total daily dosage of the present analgesic, Table 1 can be used to calculate the approximate daily oral hydromorphone dosage that should provide equivalent analgesia. This total daily oral hydromorphone dose should then be equally divided into two 12 hourly HYDROMORPH CONTIN doses.

Dose Titration: Dose titration is the key to success with opioid analgesic therapy. **Proper optimization of doses scaled to the relief of the individual's pain should aim at regular administration of the lowest dose of controlled release hydromorphone (HYDROMORPH CONTIN) which will achieve the overall treatment goal of satisfactory pain relief with acceptable side effects. Dosage adjustments should be based on the patient's clinical response.**

In patients receiving HYDROMORPH CONTIN chronically, the dose should be titrated at intervals of 48 hours to that which provides satisfactory pain relief without unmanageable side effects. HYDROMORPH CONTIN is designed to allow 12 hourly dosing.

If breakthrough pain repeatedly occurs at the end of the dosing interval it is generally an indication for a dosage increase rather than more frequent administration of controlled release hydromorphone (HYDROMORPH CONTIN).

Adjustment or Reduction of Dosage: Following successful relief of severe pain, periodic attempts to reduce the opioid dose should be made. Smaller doses or complete discontinuation may become feasible due to a change in the patient's condition or mental state. If treatment discontinuation is required, the dose of opioid may be decreased as follows: one-half of the previous daily dose given q12h for the first two days, followed thereafter by a 25% reduction every two days.

Opioid analgesics may only be partially effective in relieving dysesthetic pain, postherpetic neuralgia, stabbing pains, activity-related pain and some forms of headache. That is not to say that patients with advanced cancer suffering from some of these forms of pain should not be given an adequate trial of opioid analgesics, but it may be necessary to refer such patients at an early time to other forms of pain therapy.

INFORMATION FOR THE PATIENT: Published in e-CPS, available by subscription at www.e-cps.ca.

SUPPLIED: 3 mg: Each green, controlled release capsule, imprinted with the letters PF and HYDROMORPH CONTIN, and the strength 3 mg, contains: hydromorphone HCl 3 mg. Nonmedicinal ingredients: colloidal silicon dioxide, dibutyl sebacate, ethyl cellulose, hydroxypropylmethyl cellulose, magnesium stearate and microcrystalline cellulose; capsule shell: D&C Yellow No. 10, FD&C Green No. 3, gelatin and titanium dioxide. Opaque plastic bottles of 50. Store at room temperature (15-25° C).
6 mg: Each pink, controlled release capsule, imprinted with the letters PF and HYDROMORPH CONTIN, and the strength 6 mg, contains: hydromorphone HCl 6 mg. Nonmedicinal ingredients: colloidal silicon dioxide, dibutyl sebacate, ethyl cellulose, hydroxypropylmethyl cellulose, magnesium stearate and microcrystalline cellulose; capsule shell: D&C Red No. 28, FD&C Blue No. 1, FD&C Red No. 40, gelatin and titanium dioxide. Opaque plastic bottles of 50. Store at room temperature (15-25° C).
12 mg: Each orange, controlled release capsule, imprinted with the letters PF and HYDROMORPH CONTIN, and the strength 12 mg, contains: hydromorphone HCl 12 mg. Nonmedicinal ingredients: colloidal silicon dioxide, dibutyl sebacate, ethyl cellulose, hydroxypropylmethyl cellulose, magnesium stearate and microcrystalline cellulose; capsule shell: D&C Red No. 28, D&C Yellow No. 10, FD&C Blue No. 1, FD&C Red No. 40, gelatin and titanium dioxide. Opaque plastic bottles of 50. Store at room temperature (15-25° C).

Table 1: HYDROMORPH CONTIN

Opioid Analgesics: Approximate Analgesic Equivalences[a]

Drug	Equivalent Dose (mg)[b] (compared to morphine 10 mg IM)		Duration of Action (hours)
	Parenteral	Oral	
Strong Opioid Agonists			
Morphine	10	60[c]	3–4
Oxycodone	15	30[d]	2–4
Hydromorphone	1.5	7.5[e]	2–4
Anileridine	25	75	2–3
Levorphanol	2	4	4–8
Meperidine[f]	75	300	1–3
Oxymorphone	1.5	5 (rectal)	3–4
Methadone[g]	—	—	—
Heroin	5–8	10–15	3–4
Weak Opioid Agonists			
Codeine	120	200	3–4
Propoxyphene	50	100	2–4
Mixed Agonist-Antagonists[h]			
Pentazocine[f]	60	180	3–4
Nalbuphine	10	—	3–6

(cont'd)

Table 1: HYDROMORPH CONTIN *(cont'd)*

Opioid Analgesics: Approximate Analgesic Equivalences[a]

Drug	Equivalent Dose (mg)[b] (compared to morphine 10 mg IM)		Duration of Action (hours)
	Parenteral	Oral	
Butorphanol	2	—	3–4

[a] References:
Expert Advisory Committee on the Management of Severe Chronic Pain in Cancer Patients, Health and Welfare Canada. Cancer pain: A monograph on the management of cancer pain. Ministry of Supplies and Services Canada, 1987. Cat. No. H42-2/5-1984E.
Foley KM. The treatment of cancer pain. N Engl J Med 1985;313(2):84-95.
Aronoff GM, Evans WO. Pharmacological management of chronic pain: A review. In: Aronoff GM, editor. Evaluation and treatment of chronic pain. 2nd ed. Baltimore (MD): Williams and Wilkins; 1992. p. 359-68.
Cherny NI, Portenoy RK. Practical issues in the management of cancer pain. In: Wall PD, Melzack R, editors. Textbook of pain. 3rd ed. New York: Churchill Livingstone; 1994. p. 1437-67.

[b] **Most of this data was derived from single-dose, acute pain studies and should be considered an approximation for selection of doses when treating chronic pain.**

[c] **For acute pain, the oral or rectal dose of morphine is six times the injectable dose. However, for chronic dosing, clinical experience indicates that this ratio is 2-3: 1 (i.e., 20-30 mg of oral or rectal morphine is equivalent to 10 mg of parenteral morphine).**

[d] Based on single entity oral oxycodone in acute pain.

[e] Clinical experience indicates that during chronic dosing the oral morphine/oral hydromorphone dose ratio is 5-7.5:1.

[f] Not recommended for the management of chronic pain.

[g] Extremely variable equianalgesic dose. Patients should undergo individualized titration starting at an equivalent to 1/10 of the morphine dose.

[h] Mixed agonist-antagonists can precipitate withdrawal in patients on pure opioid agonists.

18 mg: Each yellow, controlled release capsule, imprinted with the letters PF and HYDROMORPH CONTIN, and the strength 18 mg, contains: hydromorphone HCl 18 mg. Nonmedicinal ingredients: colloidal silicon dioxide, dibutyl sebacate, ethyl cellulose, hydroxypropylmethyl cellulose, magnesium stearate and microcrystalline cellulose; capsule shell: gelatin, titanium dioxide and yellow iron oxide. Opaque plastic bottles of 50. Store at room temperature (15-25° C).

24 mg: Each grey, controlled release capsule, imprinted with the letters PF and HYDROMORPH CONTIN, and the strength 24 mg, contains: hydromorphone HCl 24 mg. Nonmedicinal ingredients: colloidal silicon dioxide, dibutyl sebacate, ethyl cellulose, hydroxypropylmethyl cellulose, magnesium stearate and microcrystalline cellulose; capsule shell: gelatin, iron oxide and titanium dioxide. Opaque plastic bottles of 50. Store at room temperature (15-25° C).

30 mg: Each red, controlled release capsule, imprinted with the letters PF and HYDROMORPH CONTIN, and the strength 30 mg, contains: hydromorphone HCl 30 mg. Nonmedicinal ingredients: colloidal silicon dioxide, dibutyl sebacate, ethyl cellulose, hydroxypropylmethyl cellulose, magnesium stearate and microcrystalline cellulose; capsule shell: FD&C Blue No. 1, FD&C Red No. 40, gelatin and titanium dioxide. Opaque plastic bottles of 50. Store at room temperature (15-25° C).

(Shown in Product Identification Section)

Hydromorphone Ⓝ

CPhA Monograph

see *Opioids*

Hydromorphone HP® 10 Ⓝ

hydromorphone HCl

Opioid Analgesic

Sandoz

Hydromorphone HP® 20 Ⓝ

hydromorphone HCl

Opioid Analgesic

Sandoz

Hydromorphone HP® 50 Ⓝ

hydromorphone HCl

Opioid Analgesic

Sandoz

Hydromorphone HP® Forte Ⓝ

hydromorphone HCl

Opioid Analgesic

Sandoz

SUPPLIED: Hydromorphone HP 10: Each mL contains: hydromorphone HCl 10 mg, citric acid 2 mg, sodium citrate 2 mg, sodium chloride 5.68 mg, hydrochloric acid and/or sodium hydroxide to adjust pH, and water for injection. Single use vials of 1 mL, boxes of 10. Single use vials of 5 mL, boxes of 5. Single use vials of 50 mL, boxes of 1. Store between 15 and 30°C. Protect from light. Discard unused portion.

Hydromorphone HP 20: Each mL contains: hydromorphone HCl 20 mg, citric acid 2 mg, sodium citrate 2 mg, sodium chloride 4.08 mg, hydrochloric acid and/or sodium hydroxide to adjust pH, and water for injection. Single use vials of 50 mL, boxes of 1. Store between 15 and 30°C. Protect from light. Discard unused portion.

Hydromorphone HP 50: Each mL contains: hydromorphone HCl 50 mg, citric acid 2 mg, sodium citrate 2 mg, sodium chloride 0.5 mg, hydrochloric acid and/or sodium hydroxide to adjust pH, and water for injection. Single use vials of 1 mL, boxes of 10. Single use vials of 50 mL, boxes of 1. Store between 15 and 30°C. Protect from light. Discard unused portion.

Hydromorphone HP Forte: Each mL contains: hydromorphone HCl 100 mg, citric acid 2 mg, sodium citrate 2 mg, edetate disodium 0.5 mg, hydrochloric acid and/or sodium hydroxide to adjust pH, and water for injection. Single use vials of 10 mL, boxes of 1. Store between 15 and 30°C. Protect from light. Discard unused portion.

Hydromorphone Hydrochloride Injection USP Ⓝ

hydromorphone HCl

Opioid Analgesic

Sandoz

SUPPLIED: Each mL contains: hydromorphone HCl 2 mg. Nonmedicinal ingredients: citric acid 2 mg, hydrochloric acid and/or sodium hydroxide to adjust pH, sodium chloride 7.48 mg, sodium citrate 2 mg and water for injection. Single use vials and ampoules of 1 mL, boxes of 10. Store between 15 and 30°C. Protect from light. Discard unused portion.

The reader is invited to consult CPhA's monograph **Corticosteroids: Topical**.

Hydrosone

hydrocortisone

Topical Corticosteroid

Rougier Pharma

SUPPLIED: Each g of white homogeneous cream contains: hydrocortisone 5 mg (0.5%) USP. Nonmedicinal ingredients: caprylic/capric triglyceride, ceteareth-12, ceteareth-20, cetearyl alcohol, glycerin, methylparaben, propylparaben and purified water. Tube of 15 g. For external use only. Keep out of reach of children. Store between 15-30°C. Do not refrigerate.

The reader is invited to consult CPhA's monograph **Corticosteroids: Topical**.

HydroVal® Ⓟ

hydrocortisone 17-valerate

Topical Corticosteroid

TaroPharma

SUPPLIED: Cream: Each tube contains: hydrocortisone 17-valerate 0.2%. Nonmedicinal ingredients: carbomer 940, dibasic sodium phosphate, methylparaben, propylene glycol, purified water, sodium lauryl sulfate, stearyl alcohol, steareth-2, steareth-100 and white petrolatum. Tubes of 15, 45 and 60 g. Store at controlled room temperature (15 to 25°C).

Ointment: Each tube contains: hydrocortisone 17-valerate 0.2%. Nonmedicinal ingredients: carbomer 934P, dibasic sodium phosphate, methylparaben, mineral oil, propylene glycol, purified water, sodium lauryl sulfate, stearyl alcohol, steareth-2, steareth-100 and white petrolatum. Tubes of 15 and 60 g. Store at controlled room temperature (15 to 25°C).

Hydroxocobalamin

CPhA Monograph

see *Vitamin B12*

Hydroxyzine Ⓟ

Antihistamine

CPhA Monograph

Date of Preparation: July 2008

This monograph has been compiled by CPhA and reviewed by experts. It may contain information different from that found in Health Canada-approved Product Monographs. The reader is referred to the *CPS* Editorial Policy for more information.

SUMMARY PRODUCT INFORMATION:

Route of Administration	Dosage Form	Strength
Injectable (im)	Liquid	50 mg/mL
Oral	Capsule	10 mg, 25 mg, 50 mg
	Syrup	2 mg/mL

INDICATIONS AND CLINICAL USE: Hydroxyzine is indicated in the following clinical settings:

- The management of histamine-mediated pruritus due to allergic conditions such as atopic and contact dermatoses, and chronic urticaria.

  Few clinical studies support the effectiveness of hydroxyzine. Patients who experience pruritus from skin diseases or systemic conditions in which histamine is not the sole cause, may experience variable effects with hydroxyzine. In patients whose pruritus is worse at night, hydroxyzine may be suitable as its sedating properties may facilitate sleep.
- The management of anxiety and tension in the preparation for dental procedures, acute emotional problems and anxiety associated with organic disturbances.

  For management of anxiety in preparation of dental procedures, benzodiazepines are more effective. Hydroxyzine may be considered a treatment option in the management of generalized anxiety disorder (GAD) in some patients, excluding elderly patients or patients with GAD with depression or other anxiety disorders. Selective serotonin reuptake inhibitors (SSRIs) and serotonin norepinephrine reuptake inhibitors (SNRIs) are considered first-line drug treatments for GAD.
- As adjunctive treatment for alcoholism.

  Current practice for the management of acute alcohol withdrawal includes the use of benzodiazepines, barbiturates and vitamin B_1.
- As adjunctive treatment for allergic conditions.

  Antihistamines may aid in controlling symptoms of allergic rhinoconjunctivitis and/or eczema.
- The management of nausea and vomiting, except in pregnancy.

  Antihistamines may reduce opioid-induced vestibular sensitivity (a possible mechanism for opioid-induced nausea and vomiting) in ambulatory patients.

Hydroxyzine may be used to alleviate opioid-induced pruritus which is more likely to be an adverse effect than an allergic reaction. The pruritus associated with opioids may be related to the histamine release in the periphery or to a centrally mediated process.

Previously, hydroxyzine was the mainstay therapy to alleviate symptoms of interstitial cystitis/painful bladder syndrome; benefit was not seen in a recent controlled trial.

The intramuscular route is preferred in situations where the patient is acutely disturbed and hysterical or an acute or chronic alcoholic experiencing anxiety, withdrawal symptoms or delirium tremens, or as pre- and post-operative, post-partum adjunct to allay anxiety and to permit substantial reduction in narcotic dose and to control emesis, except in pregnancy.

Geriatrics: In general, avoid first-generation antihistamines in elderly patients (≥65 years) because of their increased susceptibility to cognitive impairment due to central anticholinergic effects, such as CNS stimulation and depression, and excessive daytime sedation (see Adverse Reactions). In elderly patients, hydroxyzine may increase the risk of complications, e.g., in patients with bladder outflow obstruction, hydroxyzine use may exacerbate urinary retention by decreasing urinary flow. Other complications

include worsening of narrow-angle glaucoma and symptoms of benign prostatic hyperplasia. If hydroxyzine is used in the elderly, start at a low dose; however, antihistamines which lack anticholinergic effects, such as loratadine or cetirizine, may be preferred in the elderly when treating allergic reactions.
Pediatrics: Caution is advised in young children as paradoxical excitement has been reported.

CONTRAINDICATIONS:
- Patients who are hypersensitive to hydroxyzine or to any ingredient in the formulation.
- Newborn or premature infants.

WARNINGS AND PRECAUTIONS:

Serious Warnings and Precautions
- Assess therapeutic benefits versus implications of various side effects (anticholinergic effects, drowsiness) when considering hydroxyzine as an option in the elderly and patients with renal or hepatic impairment. Drowsiness, confusion, syncope and dizziness due to hydroxyzine use may be more common in the elderly.
- Avoid driving or operating machinery as mental alertness or physical coordination may be impaired as a result of hydroxyzine administration.
- Extravasation causing pain, reddening and irritation at the site of intramuscular injection. Hydroxyzine should not be administered by intravenous, subcutaneous or intra-arterial injection.

Cardiovascular: Use with caution in patients with cardiovascular disease as hydroxyzine may cause hypotension.
Genitourinary: Use with caution in patients with benign prostatic hyperplasia and bladder neck obstruction as hydroxyzine may exacerbate urinary retention by reducing urine flow.
Ophthalmologic: Patients with angle-closure glaucoma should avoid using hydroxyzine, due to its ability to increase intraocular pressure.
Respiratory: The anticholinergic effects of hydroxyzine may dry salivary secretions.
Special Populations: Pregnant Women: Pregnancy Category C. Although neonatal withdrawal syndrome, including seizures, has been reported with high doses of hydroxyzine (600 mg/day) throughout pregnancy, seizures have also been reported with long term maternal administration of usual therapeutic doses of hydroxyzine (150 mg/day). A prospective, controlled, observational study found no statistically significant differences in rate of live births, spontaneous or therapeutic abortion or stillbirth between hydroxyzine or cetirizine groups versus placebo. The oral antihistamine of choice in pregnancy is chlorpheniramine and the injectable antihistamine of choice is diphenhydramine.
Nursing Women: There are no reports of the effects of hydroxyzine on the infant during breast-feeding. Because of its low molecular weight, excretion into breast milk is expected. Antihistamines given in relatively large doses by injection may decrease basal prolactin levels in women who are not lactating and in early postpartum women. Larger doses or prolonged use of hydroxyzine may cause drowsiness or paradoxical stimulation (irritability, restlessness) in the infant. Use hydroxyzine at bedtime after the last feeding of the day as this may minimize symptoms in the infant, or offer a nonsedating antihistamine that is compatible with breast-feeding, e.g., loratadine, fexofenadine.
Pediatrics: Avoid hydroxyzine in premature and newborn infants (see Contraindications). Paradoxical excitement may occur in young children. In one study looking at diphenhydramine and loratadine and their impact on school performance in children 8 to 10 years, no difference was seen in the verbal instruction score, reading test score, reaction time, or somnolence scale between these two antihistamines. However, hydroxyzine has been found to increase subjective somnolence. Thus, caution is advised.
Geriatrics: The elderly may be more susceptible to adverse effects of hydroxyzine such as drowsiness, anticholinergic effects and hypotension. Avoid hydroxyzine and other first-generation antihistamines in elderly patients (see Indications and Clinical Use).
Occupational Hazards: Because hydroxyzine causes sedation, use caution when performing tasks requiring alertness such as driving or operating machinery.

ADVERSE REACTIONS: Adverse Drug Reactions Overview: Most patients on hydroxyzine may experience dose-related adverse effects of which CNS and anticholinergic effects are the most prominent. Elderly patients and patients with renal and hepatic impairment may be more susceptible to these effects. See Table 1.

Table 1: Hydroxyzine
More Common Adverse Drug Reactions (≥1%)

Body System	Effect	Clinical Comment
CNS	Common: somnolence, dizziness, fatigue, lack of coordination	Avoid driving cars, other motorized vehicles or operating heavy machinery. One study reported significant sedation and slower brake reaction time while driving a car, which suggests slower hazard recognition and brake application. Patients with renal and hepatic impairment and the elderly may be more susceptible to these adverse effects. Sedative effects of hydroxyzine may be useful in patients who cannot sleep because of symptoms of pruritus; bedtime dosing may be beneficial. Drowsiness may abate or diminish with continued use. Consider a reduction in dose if drowsiness is an issue.
Ear/Nose/Throat	Dry mouth (especially at high doses)	
Gastrointestinal	Loss of appetite, nausea, vomiting, epigastric distress, constipation or diarrhea	
Genitourinary	Urinary retention, urinary frequency, dysuria, impotence	
Ophthalmologic	Blurred vision, increased intraocular pressure	See Warnings and Precautions.

Less Common Adverse Drug Reactions (<1%): Cardiovascular: supraventricular tachycardia in a nine-year-old child (case report), hypotension in an overdose situation.
Central Nervous System: increased reaction time, headache, paradoxical excitation in young children and infants, CNS stimulation (insomnia, irritability, restlessness, tremor, nightmares, hallucination, convulsions), tremor and seizures (rare; reported with higher than recommended doses of hydroxyzine).
Dermatologic: urticaria, livedoid dermatitis and severe necrosis with hydroxyzine im injection (Nicolau's syndrome), drug eruptions (including fixed drug eruption of the penis), generalized maculopapular eruption, systemic contact dermatitis.
Gastrointestinal: increased peristalsis of the intestinal tract, bitter taste.
Genitourinary: prolonged penile erections.
Neurologic: tardive dyskinesia (long-term use).
Other: im injection: local injection site discomfort, erythema, local irritation, tissue necrosis, localized subcutaneous tissue induration.

DRUG INTERACTIONS: Drug-Drug Interactions: See Table 2.
Drug-Food Interactions: Hydroxyzine may be taken with or without food.
Drug-Herb Interactions: Avoid combination with valerian and St. John's wort as this may increase CNS depression.
Drug-Laboratory Interactions: Hydroxyzine may cross-react with the carbamazepine particle-enhanced turbidimetric inhibition immunoassay or PETINIA, resulting in false interpretation of serum carbamazepine concentration (false elevation). Hydroxyzine may interfere with the measurement of total tricyclic antidepressants (false elevation) using the fluorescence polarization immunoassay.

Hydroxyzine may interfere with allergy skin test antigens by masking the response via histamine antagonism. Discontinue hydroxyzine approximately 3 to 5 days prior to an allergen skin test, as it may suppress the reaction.

Table 2: Hydroxyzine
Drug-Drug Interactions

Interacting Drug	Effect	Clinical Comment
Alcohol and other CNS depressants (e.g., benzodiazepines)	Additive CNS depressive effects	Avoid combination, as it may cause psychomotor and cognitive impairment. If used concomitantly, monitor for additive CNS depressive effects, e.g., confusion, drowsiness, respiratory depression and weakness.

DOSAGE AND ADMINISTRATION: Dosing Considerations: The intramuscular route is preferred over the oral route in certain situations:
- if the patient is acutely disturbed and hysterical
- if the patient is an acute or chronic alcoholic experiencing anxiety, withdrawal symptoms or delirium tremens
- as adjunctive therapy in pre- and post-operative and post-partum settings to permit substantial reduction in dose of opioids and to control emesis.

Recommended Dose and Dosage Adjustment: See Table 3, Table 4 and Table 5.

Table 3: Hydroxyzine
Dose in Adult Patients

Indication	Route	Usual Dose	Clinical Comment
Pruritus	PO	25 mg TID to QID	Regular administration of hydroxyzine may be needed if itch is severe.
Urticaria, acute or chronic	PO	25–50 mg every 6 hours	
Opioid-induced pruritus	PO	25–100 mg HS PRN	
Psychiatric and emotional emergencies including acute alcoholism	IM	50–100 mg STAT, then 50–100 mg every 4 to 6 hours PRN	May be used for relief of agitation during acute alcohol withdrawal. Current practice for the management of acute alcohol withdrawal includes the use of benzodiazepines, barbiturates and vitamin B_1.
Nausea and vomiting, except in pregnancy	IM	Initial dose: 25–100 mg, may administer every 4 to 6 hours PRN depending on individual requirements	
Anxiety	PO	50–100 mg QID, maximum 600 mg/day	
Pre-operative sedation	PO/IM	PO: 50–100 mg single dose IM: 25–100 mg single dose	Using hydroxyzine in this setting may reduce the opioid requirement by 50%.
Post-operative sedation	PO/IM	PO: 50–100 mg every 4 to 6 hours PRN IM: 25–100 mg every 4 to 6 hours PRN	
Pre-and post-partum adjunctive therapy	IM	25–100 mg every 4 to 6 hours PRN	

Table 4: Hydroxyzine
Dose in Pediatric Patients[a]

Indication	Route	Usual Dose
Pruritus	PO	≥6 years: 50–100 mg daily, divided TID to QID <6 years: 30–50 mg daily, divided TID to QID
Urticaria, chronic	PO	2–4 mg/kg daily, divided TID to QID, maximum 400 mg/day
Nausea and vomiting	IM	1 mg/kg every 4 to 6 hours PRN
Anxiety	PO	≥6 years: 50–100 mg daily, divided TID to QID <6 years: 30–50 mg daily, divided TID to QID
Pre-operative sedation	PO/IM	PO: 0.6 mg/kg single dose IM: 0.5–1.1 mg/kg single dose
Post-operative sedation	PO/IM	PO: 0.6 mg/kg every 6 hours PRN IM: 0.5–1.1 mg/kg every 4 to 6 hours PRN

[a] Infants and children excluding newborn infants, see Contraindications.

Table 5: Hydroxyzine
Dose in Adult Patients with Renal Impairment

Creatinine Clearance	Dosage Adjustment
>50 mL/min	Usual dose
≤50 mL/min	50% of usual dose

Dosage in Dialysis: Hydroxyzine accumulates in end-stage renal disease; dose as for GFR less than 10 mL/min.
Hepatic Impairment: In patients with primary biliary cirrhosis, administer hydroxyzine every 24 hours.

OVERDOSAGE:

For management of a suspected drug overdose, CPhA recommends that you contact your **regional Poison Control Centre**. See the *CPS* Directory section for a list of Poison Control Centres.

ACTION AND CLINICAL PHARMACOLOGY: Mechanism of Action: Hydroxyzine, a piperazine, is an H_1-receptor antagonist which reversibly competes with endogenous histamine for the H_1-receptor sites on effector cells in the gastrointestinal tract, blood vessels and respiratory tract, thereby preventing histamine binding and action. By acting on vascular smooth muscle cells and endothelial cells, histamine leads to vasodilation and an increase in vascular permeability. By blocking vasodilation and reducing capillary permeability, hydroxyzine reduces edema and wheal formation associated with histamine release. Hydroxyzine does not, however, inactivate or prevent histamine release from effector cells. In addition to antagonizing the effects of histamine, hydroxyzine may have effects on the adrenergic, serotonergic and cholinergic receptor and thus is more likely to cause anticholinergic side effects such as dry mouth, blurred vision, urinary retention and somnolence, due to penetration across the blood-brain barrier.

Pharmacokinetics: Adults: Absorption: Hydroxyzine is well absorbed after oral administration. Peak serum concentrations were reached in approximately 2 hours following a 0.7 mg/kg oral dose of hydroxyzine. Sedation corresponds to peak serum concentration; onset occurs within 15 to 30 minutes and lasts approximately 4 to 6 hours. Therapeutic effects of hydroxyzine do not correspond to peak serum concentration or half-life. Onset of action occurs within 1 hour and lasts about 36 hours.

Distribution: Hydroxyzine has a large volume of distribution; the apparent volume of distribution in adults ranges from 16 L/kg to 18.5 L/kg following a 0.7 mg/kg dose of hydroxyzine. Patients with primary biliary cirrhosis showed an increase in the apparent volume of distribution to 23 L/kg following a 0.7 mg/kg dose of hydroxyzine.

Metabolism: Hydroxyzine is metabolized in the liver to cetirizine, its major metabolite.

Excretion: Serum half-lives vary considerably between patients; elimination half-life of hydroxyzine ranges from 3 to 20 hours. Elimination half-life of cetirizine ranges from 7 to 10 hours; in patients with end-stage renal disease, the half-life increases to 20 to 30 hours. Cetirizine is mostly excreted unchanged in the urine with the remainder in the feces.

Special Populations: Pediatrics: The half-life increases with increasing age; 4 hours in 1-year-old patients and 11 hours in a 14-year-old patient.

Geriatrics: The apparent volume of distribution in the elderly is increased to 23 L/kg following a 0.7 mg/kg dose of the syrup. The mean serum elimination half-life was reported as 29.3 hours following administration of hydroxyzine syrup 0.7 mg/kg in fasting subjects.

Hyoscine Butylbromide Injection

hyoscine butylbromide

Antispasmodic

Sandoz

SUPPLIED: Each mL contains: hyoscine butylbromide 20 mg, sodium chloride 6.6 mg, hydrochloric acid and/or sodium hydroxide to adjust pH, and water for injection. Preservative-free. Single use, amber glass vials of 1 mL, boxes of 10. Discard any unused portion. Store between 15 and 30°C. Protect from light.

HyperHEP B™ S/D

hepatitis B immune globulin (human)

Passive Immunizing Agent

Talecris

Date of Revision: February 2, 2006

SUMMARY PRODUCT INFORMATION:

Route of Administration	Dosage Form/Strength	Clinically Relevant Nonmedicinal Ingredients
Intramuscular Injection	Injectable solution, ≥220 IU/mL	For a complete listing see Dosage Forms, Composition and Packaging.

DESCRIPTION: HyperHEP B S/D (Hepatitis B Immune Globulin [Human]) treated with solvent/detergent is a sterile solution of hepatitis B hyperimmune immune globulin for intramuscular administration; it contains no preservative. HyperHEP B S/D is prepared by cold ethanol fractionation from the plasma of donors with high titers of antibody to the hepatitis B surface antigen (anti-HBs). The immune globulin is isolated from solubilized Cohn fraction II. The fraction II solution is adjusted to a final concentration of 0.3% tri-n-butyl phosphate (TNBP) and 0.2% sodium cholate. After the addition of solvent (TNBP) and detergent (sodium cholate), the solution is heated to 30°C and maintained at that temperature for not less than 6 hours. After the viral inactivation step, the reactants are removed by precipitation, filtration and finally ultrafiltration and diafiltration. HyperHEP B S/D is formulated as a 15-18% protein solution at a pH of 6.4-7.2 in 0.21-0.32 M glycine. The pH is adjusted with sodium carbonate. HyperHEP B S/D is then incubated in the final container for 21-28 days at 20-27°C.

INDICATIONS AND CLINICAL USE: The Canadian Immunization Guide recommends that hepatitis B prevention should include programs for active immunization of children, pre-exposure vaccination of high risk groups, and post-exposure passive immunization for those exposed to disease, particularly infants born to HBV-carrier mothers. Recommendations on post-exposure prophylaxis are based on available efficacy data and on the likelihood of future HBV exposure for the person requiring treatment. In all exposures, a regimen combining Hepatitis B Immune Globulin (Human) with hepatitis B vaccine will provide both short- and long-term protection, will be less costly than the two-dose Hepatitis B Immune Globulin (Human) treatment alone and is the treatment of choice.

Administration of Hepatitis B Immune Globulin (Human) either preceding or concomitant with the commencement of active immunization with Hepatitis B vaccine provides for more rapid achievement of protective levels of hepatitis B antibody, than when the vaccine alone is administered. Rapid achievement of protective levels of antibody to hepatitis B virus may be desirable in certain clinical situations, as in cases of accidental inoculations with contaminated medical instruments. Administration of Hepatitis B Immune Globulin (Human) either 1 month preceding or at the time of commencement of a program of active vaccination with hepatitis B vaccine has been shown not to interfere with the active immune response to the vaccine.

HyperHEP B S/D is indicated for post-exposure prophylaxis in the following situations, unless it is known, by testing within the 24 previous months or can be established within 48 hours that the patient has levels of pre-existing antibodies to hepatitis B virus surface antigen at greater than or equal to 10 IU/L.

Acute Exposure to Blood Containing HBsAg: After either parenteral exposure, e.g., by accidental "needlestick" or direct mucous membrane contact (accidental splash), or oral ingestion (pipetting accident) involving HBsAg-positive materials such as blood, plasma or serum. For inadvertent percutaneous exposure in patients unwilling to take the hepatitis B vaccine regimen, a regimen of two doses of Hepatitis B Immune Globulin (Human), one given after exposure and one a month later, is about 75% effective in preventing hepatitis B in this setting.

Perinatal Exposure of Infants Born to HBsAg-positive Mothers: Infants born to HBsAg-positive mothers are at risk of being infected with hepatitis B virus and becoming chronic carriers. This risk is especially great if the mother is HBeAg-positive. For an infant with perinatal exposure to an HBsAg-positive and HBeAg-positive mother, a regimen combining one dose of Hepatitis B Immune Globulin (Human) at birth with the hepatitis B vaccine series started soon after birth is 85%-95% effective in preventing development of the HBV carrier state. Regimens involving either multiple doses of Hepatitis B Immune Globulin (Human) alone or the vaccine series alone have 70%-90% efficacy, while a single dose of Hepatitis B Immune Globulin (Human) alone has only 50% efficacy.

Sexual Exposure to an HBsAg-positive Person: Sex partners of HBsAg-positive persons are at increased risk of acquiring HBV infection. Sexual partners of an acute case of hepatitis B should begin a hepatitis B vaccine series. For sexual exposure to a person with acute hepatitis B, a single dose of Hepatitis B Immune Globulin (Human) is 75% effective if administered within 2 weeks of last sexual exposure. The Canadian Immunization Guide indicates that the administration of Hepatitis B Immune Globulin (Human) to a sexual assault victim should prevent the development of hepatitis B virus infection if the alleged assailant is HBsAg positive.

Household Exposure to Persons with Acute HBV Infection: Since infants have close contact with primary care-givers and they have a higher risk of becoming HBV carriers after acute HBV infection, prophylaxis of an infant less than 12 months of age with Hepatitis B Immune Globulin (Human) and hepatitis B vaccine is indicated if the mother or primary care-giver has acute HBV infection.

CONTRAINDICATIONS:

- HyperHEP B S/D should not be given to patients who are hypersensitive to this drug or to any ingredient in the formulation or component of the container. For a complete listing, see Dosage Forms, Composition and Packaging.
- In patients who have severe thrombocytopenia or any coagulation disorder that would contraindicate intramuscular injections, HyperHEP B S/D should be given only if the expected benefits outweigh the risks.

WARNINGS AND PRECAUTIONS:

Serious Warnings and Precautions

- For intramuscular injection only. Do not give intravenously (see Warnings and Precautions, General).
- Products made from human plasma may contain infectious agents such as viruses (see Warnings and Precautions, General).

General: HyperHEP B S/D should **not** be administered intravenously because of the potential for serious reactions. Injections should be made intramuscularly, and care should be taken to draw back on the plunger of the syringe before injection in order to be certain that the needle is not in a blood vessel.

Intramuscular injections are preferably administered in the anterolateral aspects of the upper thigh and the deltoid muscle of the upper arm. The gluteal region should not be used routinely as an injection site because of the risk of injury to the sciatic nerve. An individual decision as to which muscle is injected must be made for each patient based on the volume of material to be administered. If the gluteal region is used when very large volumes are to be injected or multiple doses are necessary, the central region **must** be avoided; only the upper, outer quadrant should be used.

HyperHEP B S/D is made from human plasma. Products made from human plasma may contain infectious agents, such as viruses, that can cause disease. The risk that such products will transmit an infectious agent has been reduced by screening plasma donors for prior exposure to certain viruses, by testing for the presence of certain current virus infections, and by inactivating and/or removing certain viruses. Despite these measures, such products can still potentially transmit disease. There is also the possibility that unknown infectious agents may be present in such products. Individuals who receive infusions of blood or plasma products may develop signs and/or symptoms of some viral infections, particularly hepatitis C. All infections thought by a physician possibly to have been transmitted by this product should be reported by the physician or other healthcare provider to Talecris Biotherapeutics Ltd. at 1-866-482-5226.

The physician should discuss the risks and benefits of this product with the patient, before prescribing or administering to the patient.

Hypersensitivity: HyperHEP B S/D should be given with caution to patients with a history of prior systemic allergic reactions following the administration of human immune globulin preparations. Epinephrine should be available.

Special Populations: Pregnant Women: There is no experience of exposure in pregnancy during clinical trials. Animal reproduction studies have not been conducted with HyperHEP B S/D. It is also not known whether HyperHEP B S/D can cause fetal harm when administered to a pregnant woman or can affect reproduction capacity. HyperHEP B S/D should be given to a pregnant woman only if clearly needed.

Pediatrics: With the exception of neonates and infants up to 12 months of age, safety and effectiveness in the pediatric population have not been established.

Monitoring and Laboratory Tests: None required.

ADVERSE REACTIONS: Adverse Drug Reaction Overview: Local pain and tenderness at the injection site, urticaria and angioedema may occur; anaphylactic reactions, although rare, have been reported following the injection of human immune globulin preparations.

DRUG INTERACTIONS: Drug-Drug Interactions: See Table 1.

Table 1: HyperHEP B S/D

Established or Potential Drug-Drug Interactions

Proper Name	Ref	Effect	Clinical Comment
Live viral vaccines	CT/T	Although administration of Hepatitis B Immune Globulin (Human) did not interfere with measles vaccination it is not known whether Hepatitis B Immune Globulin (Human) may interfere with other live virus vaccines.	Immunization with live vaccines, other than measles vaccination, should not be given within 3 months after HyperHEP B S/D administration.

Legend:
C=Case Study.
CT=Clinical Trial.
T=Theoretical.

Hepatitis B vaccine may be administered at the same time as HyperHEP B S/D, but at a different injection site, without interfering with the immune response. No interactions with other products are known.

Drug-Food Interactions: No interactions are known.

Drug-Herb Interactions: No interactions are known.

Drug-Laboratory Test Interactions: No interactions are known.

DOSAGE AND ADMINISTRATION: Dosing Considerations: The Canadian Immunization Guide recommends in general that Hepatitis B Immune Globulin (Human) be given along with a regimen of hepatitis B vaccine. Consult the hepatitis B vaccine package insert for dosage information concerning that product.

Recommended Dose and Dosage Adjustment: Acute Exposure to Blood Containing HBsAg: Table 2 summarizes prophylaxis for percutaneous (needlestick or bite), ocular, or mucous-membrane exposure to blood according to the source of exposure and vaccination status of the exposed person. For greatest effectiveness, passive prophylaxis with Hepatitis B Immune Globulin (Human) should be given as soon as possible after exposure (its value beyond 7 days of exposure is unclear). As soon as possible and within 48 hours of exposure, for adults, an injection of 0.06 mL/kg of body weight should be administered intramuscularly (see Warnings and Precautions, General). Treatment with Hepatitis B Immune Globulin (Human) is more effective if combined with a hepatitis B vaccine regimen given immediately but at a different site. Consult hepatitis B vaccine package insert for dosage information regarding that product. There is no established dosage for children.

Prophylaxis of Infants Born to HBsAg and HBeAg Positive Mothers: Efficacy of prophylactic Hepatitis B Immune Globulin (Human) in infants at risk depends on administering Hepatitis B Immune Globulin (Human) on the day of birth. It is therefore vital that HBsAg-positive mothers be identified before delivery.

Hepatitis B Immune Globulin (Human) (0.5 mL) should be administered intramuscularly (IM) to the newborn infant after physiologic stabilization of the infant and preferably within 12 hours of birth. Hepatitis B Immune Globulin (Human) efficacy decreases markedly if treatment is delayed beyond 48 hours. Hepatitis B vaccine should be administered as per the package insert of the manufacturer. Hepatitis B vaccine should be administered, starting the regimen within 7 days of birth, and may be given concurrently with Hepatitis B Immune Globulin (Human), but at a different site. If administration of the first dose of hepatitis B vaccine is delayed for as long as 3 months, then a 0.5 mL dose of Hepatitis B Immune Globulin (Human) should be repeated at 3 months. If hepatitis B vaccine is refused, the 0.5 mL dose of Hepatitis B Immune Globulin (Human) should be repeated at 3 and 6 months. Hepatitis B Immune Globulin (Human) administered at birth should not interfere with oral polio and diphtheria-tetanus-pertussis vaccines administered at 2 months of age.

Table 2: HyperHEP B S/D

Course of Action Following Percutaneous ("Needlestick") or Mucosal Exposure to Hepatitis B Virus

Exposed Person		Source[a]		
			Unknown Status	
Vaccination Status	Anti-HBs Level	HBsAg Positive	High Risk	Low Risk
Vaccinated	≥10 IU/L documented within the previous 2 years	no action necessary	no action necessary	no action necessary
	≥10 IU/L documented more than 2 years ago	assess anti-HBs level; if ≥10 IU/L, no action; if <10 IU/L, give single booster of vaccine	assess anti-HBs level; if ≥10 IU/L, no action; if <10 IU/L, give single booster of vaccine	no action necessary
	known non-responder (anti-HBs level <10 IU/L after vaccination)	HBIG[b,c,d]	HBIG[c,d]	no action necessary[d]
	level unknown and unable to be determined within 48 hours	HBIG[c] + single booster of vaccine	single booster of vaccine ± HBIG[c]	no action necessary
Unvaccinated	≥10 IU/L	no action necessary	no action necessary	no action necessary
	level unknown at 48 hours or <10 IU/L	HBIG[c] + full vaccine course	full vaccine course ± HBIG[c]	full vacine course

[a] If source is known to be HBsAg negative, no action is required unless exposed person requires initiation of vaccination series.
[b] Hepatitis B Immune Globulin (Human).
[c] Hepatitis B Immune Globulin (Human) 0.06 mL/kg preferably given within 48 hours of exposure. Efficacy decreases with time and is unknown after 7 days.
[d] If exposed person has received only three vaccine doses, an additional three-dose series may be administered.

Sexual Exposure to an HBsAg-positive Person: All susceptible persons whose sex partners have acute hepatitis B infection should receive a single dose of Hepatitis B Immune Globulin (Human) (0.06 mL/kg) and should begin the hepatitis B vaccine series if prophylaxis can be started within 14 days of the last sexual contact or if sexual contact with the infected person will continue (see Table 3). Administering the vaccine with Hepatitis B Immune Globulin (Human) may improve the efficacy of post-exposure treatment. The vaccine has the added advantage of conferring long-lasting protection.

Table 3: HyperHEP B S/D

Recommendations for Postexposure Prophylaxis for Sexual Exposure to Hepatitis B (adapted from 1)

HBIG[a]		Vaccine	
Dose	Recommended Timing	Dose	Recommended Timing
0.06 mL/kg IM[b]	Single dose within 14 days of last sexual contact	See package insert of that product for dosage and administration	First dose at time of HBIG[a] treatment[c]

[a] HBIG - Hepatitis B Immune Globulin (Human).
[b] Hepatitis B Immune Globulin (Human) 0.06 mL/kg preferably given within 48 hours of exposure. Efficacy decreases with time and is unknown after 7 days.
[c] The first dose can be administered the same time as the HBIG dose but at a different site; subsequent doses should be administered as recommended for specific vaccine.

Household Exposure to Persons with Acute HBV Infection: Prophylactic treatment with a 0.5 mL dose of Hepatitis B Immune Globulin (Human) and hepatitis B vaccine is indicated for infants 12 months of age who have been exposed to a primary caregiver who has acute hepatitis B. Prophylaxis for other household contacts of persons with acute HBV infection is not indicated unless they have had identifiable blood exposure to the index patient, such as by sharing toothbrushes or razors. Such exposures should be treated like sexual exposures. If the index patient becomes an HBV carrier, all household contacts should receive hepatitis B vaccine.

Administration: Hepatitis B Immune Globulin (Human) may be administered at the same time (but at a different site), or up to 1 month preceding hepatitis B vaccination without impairing the active immune response from hepatitis B vaccination.

Parenteral drug products should be inspected visually for particulate matter and discoloration prior to administration, whenever solution and container permit.

HyperHEP B S/D is to be administered intramuscularly. Do not inject intravenously. Discard any unused remaining material immediately into biohazardous waste. HyperHEP B S/D is supplied as single use syringe and vials.

Directions for Syringe Usage: HyperHEP B S/D is supplied with a syringe and an attached UltraSafe Needle Guard for your protection and convenience. Please follow instructions below for proper use of syringe and UltraSafe Needle Guard.

1. Remove the prefilled syringe from the package. Lift syringe by barrel, **not** by plunger.
2. Twist the plunger rod clockwise until the threads are seated.
3. With the rubber needle shield secured on the syringe tip, push the plunger rod forward a few millimeters to break any friction seal between the rubber stopper and the glass syringe barrel.
4. Remove the needle shield and expel air bubbles. (Do not remove the rubber needle shield to prepare the product for administration until immediately prior to the anticipated injection time.)
5. Proceed with hypodermic needle puncture.
6. Aspirate prior to injection to confirm that the needle is not in a vein or artery.
7. Inject the medication.
8. Keeping your hands behind the needle, grasp the guard with free hand and slide forward toward needle until it is completely covered and guard clicks into place. If audible click is not heard, guard may not be completely activated.
9. Place entire prefilled glass syringe with guard activated into an approved sharps container for proper disposal.

OVERDOSE:
Although no data are available, clinical experience with other immunoglobulin preparations suggests that the only manifestations would be pain and tenderness at the injection site.

For management of a suspected drug overdose, CPhA recommends that you contact your **regional Poison Control Centre**. See the *CPS* Directory section for a list of Poison Control Centres.

ACTION AND CLINICAL PHARMACOLOGY: Mechanism of Action: HyperHEP B provides passive immunization for individuals exposed to the hepatitis B virus (HBV) as evidenced by a reduction in the attack rate of hepatitis B following its use.

Cases of type B hepatitis are rarely seen following exposure to HBV in persons with preexisting anti-HBs. No confirmed instance of transmission of hepatitis B has been associated with this product.

Pharmacodynamics: See Action and Clinical Pharmacology, Mechanism of Action.

Pharmacokinetics: In a clinical study in healthy human adults receiving another hyperimmune immune globulin product treated with solvent/detergent, Rabies Immune Globulin (Human), prepared by the same manufacturing process, detectable passive antibody titers were observed in the serum of all subjects by 24 hours post injection and persisted through the 21 day study period. These results suggest that passive immunization with immune globulin products is not affected by the solvent/detergent treatment.

Duration of Effect: The administration of the usual recommended dose of this immune globulin generally results in a detectable level of circulating anti-HBs which persists for approximately 2 months or longer. Table 4 presents the highest antibody (IgG) serum levels were seen in subjects studied.

Table 4: HyperHEP B S/D

Highest Antibody (IgG) Serum Levels

Day	% of Subjects
3	38.9
7	41.7
14	11.1
21	8.3

Mean values for half-life were between 17.5 and 25 days, with the shortest being 5.9 days and the longest 35 days.

STORAGE AND STABILITY: Store at 2-8°C. Do not freeze. Do not use after expiration date. The vials are single use. Once entered, discard any unused contents.

INFORMATION FOR THE PATIENT: Published in e-CPS, available by subscription at www.e-cps.ca.

DOSAGE FORMS, COMPOSITION AND PACKAGING: Each vial contains HBs antibody equivalent to or exceeding the potency of anti-HBs (i.e. ≥220 IU/mL) in a U.S. reference hepatitis B immune globulin (Center for Biologics Evaluation and Research, FDA). The U.S. reference has been tested against the World Health Organization standard Hepatitis B Immune Globulin and found to be equal to 220 international units (IU) per mL. Neonatal single dose disposable syringes of 0.5 mL with attached needle. Single dose disposable syringes of 1 mL with attached needle. Single use vials of 5 mL.

HYPERRAB™ S/D

rabies immune globulin (human)

Passive Immunizing Agent

Talecris

Date of Preparation: June 8, 2005
Date of Revision: June 28, 2006

PHARMACOLOGY: The usefulness of prophylactic rabies antibody in preventing rabies in humans when administered immediately after exposure was dramatically demonstrated in a group of persons bitten by a rabid wolf in Iran. Similarly, beneficial results were later reported from the U.S.S.R. Studies coordinated by WHO helped determine the optimal conditions under which antirabies serum of equine origin and rabies vaccine can be used in man. These studies showed that serum can interfere to a variable extent with the active immunity induced by the vaccine, but could be minimized by booster doses of vaccine after the end of the usual dosage series.

Preparation of rabies immune globulin of human origin with adequate potency was reported by Cabasso et al. In carefully controlled clinical studies, this globulin was used in conjunction with rabies vaccine of duck-embryo origin (DEV). These studies determined that a human globulin dose of 20 IU/kg of rabies antibody, given simultaneously with the first DEV dose, resulted in amply detectable levels of passive rabies antibody 24 hours after injection in all recipients. The injections produced minimal, if any, interference with the subject's endogenous antibody response to DEV.

More recently, human diploid cell rabies vaccines (HDCV) prepared from tissue culture fluids containing rabies virus have received substantial clinical evaluation in Europe and the United States. In a study in adult volunteers, the administration of Rabies Immune Globulin (Human) did not interfere with antibody formation induced by HDCV when given in a dose of 20 IU per kilogram body weight simultaneously with the first dose of vaccine.

In a clinical study in healthy human adults receiving a 20 IU/kg intramuscular dose of Rabies Immune Globulin (Human) treated with solvent/detergent, Rabies Immune Globulin (Human) - HYPERRAB S/D, detectable passive rabies antibody titers were observed in the serum of all subjects by 24 hours post injection and persisted through the 21 day study period. These results are consistent with prior studies with non-solvent/detergent treated product.

INDICATIONS: Rabies vaccine and Rabies Immune Globulin (Human) - HYPERRAB S/D should be given to all persons suspected of exposure to rabies with one exception: persons who have been previously immunized with rabies vaccine and have a confirmed adequate rabies antibody titer should receive only vaccine. HYPERRAB S/D should be administered as promptly as possible after exposure, but can be administered up to the eighth day after the first dose of vaccine is given.

Recommendations for use of passive and active immunization after exposure to an animal suspected of having rabies have been detailed by the Health Canada National Advisory Committee on Immunization and the U.S. Public Health Service Immunization Practices Advisory Committee (ACIP).

Every exposure to possible rabies infection must be individually evaluated. The following factors should be considered before specific antirabies treatment is initiated:

1. **Species of Biting Animal:** The animals in Canada most often proven rabid and considered to pose a risk to humans are foxes, skunks, dogs, cats and bats. Carnivorous wild animals (especially skunks, foxes, coyotes, raccoons, and bobcats) and bats are the animals most commonly infected with rabies and have caused most of the indigenous cases of human rabies in the United States since 1960. Unless the animal is tested and shown not to be rabid, postexposure prophylaxis should be initiated upon bite or nonbite exposure to these animals (see item 3 below). If treatment has been initiated and subsequent testing in a competent laboratory shows the exposing animal is not rabid, treatment can be discontinued.

   In Canada and the United States, the likelihood that a domestic dog or cat is infected with rabies varies from region to region; hence, the need for postexposure prophylaxis also varies. However, in most of Asia and all of Africa and Latin America, the dog remains the major source of human exposure; exposures to dogs in such countries represent a special threat. Travelers to those countries should be aware that >50% of the rabies cases among humans in the United States result from exposure to dogs outside the United States.

   Rodents (such as squirrels, hamsters, guinea pigs, gerbils, chipmunks, rats, and mice) and lagomorphs (including rabbits and hares) are rarely found to be infected with rabies and have not been known to cause human rabies in the United States. However, from 1971 through 1988, woodchucks accounted for 70% of the 179 cases of rabies among rodents reported to CDC. In these cases, the local health department should be consulted before a decision is made to initiate postexposure antirabies prophylaxis.
2. **Circumstances of Biting Incident:** An unprovoked attack is more likely to mean that the animal is rabid. (Bites during attempts to feed or handle an apparently healthy animal may generally be regarded as provoked.)
3. **Type of Exposure:** Rabies is transmitted only when the virus is introduced into open cuts or wounds in skin or mucous membranes. If there has been no exposure (as described in this section), postexposure treatment is not necessary. Thus, the likelihood that rabies infection will result from exposure to a rabid animal varies with the nature and extent of the exposure. Two categories of exposure should be considered:

   Bite: any penetration of the skin by teeth. Bites to the face and hands carry the highest risk, but the site of the bite should not influence the decision to begin treatment.

   Bat-associated strains of rabies can be transmitted to humans either directly through a bat's bite or indirectly through the bite of an animal previously infected by a bat. Because some bat bites may be less severe, and therefore more difficult to recognize, than bites inflicted by larger mammalian carnivores, rabies postexposure treatment should be considered for any physical contact with bats when bite or mucous membrane contact cannot be excluded.

Nonbite: scratches, abrasions, open wounds or mucous membranes contaminated with saliva or any potentially infectious material, such as brain tissue, from a rabid animal constitute nonbite exposures. If the material containing the virus is dry, the virus can be considered noninfectious. Casual contact, such as petting a rabid animal and contact with the blood, urine, or feces (e.g., guano) of a rabid animal, does not constitute an exposure and is not an indication for prophylaxis. Instances of airborne rabies have been reported rarely. Adherence to respiratory precautions will minimize the risk of airborne exposure.

The only documented cases of rabies from human-to-human transmission have occurred in patients who received corneas transplanted from persons who died of rabies undiagnosed at the time of death. Stringent guidelines for acceptance of donor corneas have reduced this risk.

Bite and nonbite exposures from humans with rabies theoretically could transmit rabies, although no cases of rabies acquired this way have been documented.

4. **Vaccination Status of Biting Animal:** A properly immunized animal has only a minimal chance of developing rabies and transmitting the virus.
5. **Presence of Rabies in Region:** If adequate laboratory and field records indicate that there is no rabies infection in a domestic species within a given region, local health officials are justified in considering this in making recommendations on antirabies treatment following a bite by that particular species. Such officials should be consulted for current interpretations.

Rabies Postexposure Prophylaxis: The following recommendations are only a guide. In applying them, take into account the animal species involved, the circumstances of the bite or other exposure, the vaccination status of the animal, and presence of rabies in the region. Public health and Food Inspection Agency officials should be consulted if questions arise about the need for rabies prophylaxis. See Table 1.

Local Treatment of Wounds: Immediate and thorough washing of all bite wounds and scratches with soap and water is perhaps the most effective measure for preventing rabies. In experimental animals, simple local wound cleansing has been shown to reduce markedly the likelihood of rabies. Tetanus prophylaxis and measures to control bacterial infection should be given as indicated.

Active Immunization: Active immunization should be initiated as soon as possible after exposure (within 24 hours). Many dosage schedules have been evaluated for the currently available rabies vaccines and their respective manufacturers' literature should be consulted.

Passive Immunization: A combination of active and passive immunization (vaccine and immune globulin) is considered the acceptable postexposure prophylaxis except for those persons who have been previously immunized with rabies vaccine and who have documented adequate rabies antibody titer. These individuals should receive vaccine only. For passive immunization, Rabies Immune Globulin (Human) is preferred over antirabies serum, equine. It is recommended both for treatment of all bites by animals suspected of having rabies and for nonbite exposure inflicted by animals suspected of being rabid. Rabies Immune Globulin (Human) should be used in conjunction with rabies vaccine and can be administered through the seventh day after the first dose of vaccine is given. Beyond the seventh day, Rabies Immune Globulin (Human) is not indicated since an antibody response to cell culture vaccine is presumed to have occurred.

Table 1: HYPERRAB S/D

Rabies Post-exposure Prophylaxis Guide

Animal Species	Condition of animal at time of exposure/attack	Treatment of exposed person[a]
Dog and cat	Healthy and available for 10 days of observation	None, unless animal develops rabies[b]
	Rabid or suspected rabid	1. Local treatment of wound 2. RIGH (local and intramuscular)[c] and HDCV
	Unknown (escaped)	Consult public health officials
Skunk, bat, fox, coyote, racoon, bobcat, and other carnivores; woodchuck. Includes bat found in room when a person was sleeping unattended.	Regard as rabid unless geographic area is known to be free of rabies or proven negative by laboratory tests[d]	1. Local treatment of wound 2. RIGH (local and intramuscular)[c] and HDCV
Livestock, rodents and lagomorphs (rabbits and hares)	Consider individually. Consult appropriate public health and Food Inspection Agency officials. Bites of squirrels, hamsters, guinea pigs, gerbils, chipmunks, rats, mice, other rodents, rabbits, and hares may rarely warrant post-exposure rabies prophylaxis if the behaviour of the biting animal was highly unusual.	

[a] All bites and wounds should immediately be thoroughly cleansed with soap and water. If antirabies treatment is indicated, both Rabies Immune Globulin (Human) [RIGH] and human diploid cell rabies vaccine (HDCV) should be given as soon as possible, regardless of the interval from exposure.

[b] During the usual holding period of 10 days, begin treatment with RIGH and vaccine (HDCV) at first sign of rabies in a dog or cat that has bitten someone. The symptomatic animal should be killed immediately and tested.

[c] If RIGH is not available, use antirabies serum, equine (ARS). Do not use more than the recommended dosage.

[d] The animal should be killed and the brain be tested as soon as possible. Holding for observation is not recommended. Discontinue vaccine if immunofluorescence test results of the animal are negative.

CONTRAINDICATIONS: None known.

WARNINGS: Rabies Immune Globulin (Human) - HYPERRAB S/D is made from human plasma. Products made from human plasma may contain infectious agents, such as viruses, that can cause disease. The risk that such products will transmit an infectious agent has been reduced by screening plasma donors for prior exposure to certain viruses, by testing for the presence of certain current virus infections, and by inactivating and/or removing certain viruses. Despite these measures, such products can still potentially transmit disease. There is also the possibility that unknown infectious agents may be present in such products. Individuals who receive infusions of blood or plasma products may develop signs and/or symptoms of some viral infections, particularly hepatitis C. All infections thought by a physician possibly to have been transmitted by this product should be reported by the physician or other healthcare provider to Talecris Biotherapeutics Ltd. at 1-866-482-5226.

The physician should discuss the risks and benefits of this product with the patient, before prescribing or administering it to the patient.

Rabies Immune Globulin (Human) - HYPERRAB S/D should be given with caution to patients with a history of prior systemic allergic reactions following the administration of human immunoglobulin preparations.

The attending physician who wishes to administer HYPERRAB S/D to persons with isolated immunoglobulin A (IgA) deficiency must weigh the benefits of immunization against the potential risks of hypersensitivity reactions. Such persons have increased potential for developing antibodies to IgA and could have anaphylactic reactions to subsequent administration of blood products that contain IgA.

As with all preparations administered by the intramuscular route, bleeding complications may be encountered in patients with thrombocytopenia or other bleeding disorders.

PRECAUTIONS: General: Rabies Immune Globulin (Human) - HYPERRAB S/D should **not** be administered intravenously because of the potential for serious reactions. Although systemic reactions to immunoglobulin preparations are rare, epinephrine should be available for treatment of acute anaphylactoid symptoms.

Drug Interactions: Repeated doses of HYPERRAB S/D should not be administered once vaccine treatment has been initiated as this could prevent the full expression of active immunity expected from the rabies vaccine.

Other antibodies in the HYPERRAB S/D preparation may interfere with the response to live vaccines such as measles, mumps, polio or rubella. Therefore, immunization with live vaccines should not be given within 3 months after HYPERRAB S/D administration.

Pregnancy: Animal reproduction studies have not been conducted with HYPERRAB S/D. It is also not known whether HYPERRAB S/D can cause fetal harm when administered to a pregnant woman or can affect reproduction capacity. HYPERRAB S/D should be given to a pregnant woman only if clearly needed.

Children: Safety and effectiveness in the pediatric population have not been established.

ADVERSE EFFECTS: Soreness at the site of injection and mild temperature elevations may be observed at times. Sensitization to repeated injections has occurred occasionally in immunoglobulin-deficient patients. Angioneurotic edema, skin rash, nephrotic syndrome, and anaphylactic shock have rarely been reported after intramuscular injection, so that a causal relationship between immunoglobulin and these reactions is not clear.

OVERDOSE:

Symptoms: Although no data are available, clinical experience with other immunoglobulin preparations suggests that the only manifestations would be pain and tenderness at the injection site.

For management of a suspected drug overdose, CPhA recommends that you contact your **regional Poison Control Centre**. See the *CPS* Directory section for a list of Poison Control Centres.

DOSAGE: For intramuscular injection. Do not give intravenously. The recommended dose for Rabies Immune Globulin (Human) - HYPERRAB S/D is 20 IU/kg (0.133 mL/kg) of body weight given preferably at the time of the first vaccine dose. It may also be given through the seventh day after the first dose of vaccine is given. If anatomically feasible, up to one-half the dose of HYPERRAB S/D should be thoroughly infiltrated in the area around the wound and the rest should be administered intramuscularly in the gluteal area or lateral thigh muscle using a separate syringe and needle. Because of risk of injury to the sciatic nerve, the central region of the gluteal area **must** be avoided; only the upper, outer quadrant should be used. HYPERRAB S/D should never be administered in the same syringe or needle or in the same anatomical site as vaccine. Because of interference with active antibody production, the recommended dose should not be exceeded.

Parenteral drug products should be inspected visually for particulate matter and discoloration prior to administration, whenever solution and container permit.

Rabies Post-exposure Prophylaxis Schedule: See Table 2.

Table 2: HYPERRAB S/D

Rabies Post-exposure Prophylaxis Schedule

Vaccination Status	Treatment	Regimen[a]
Not previously vaccinated	Wound cleansing	All post-exposure treatment should begin with immediate thorough cleansing of all wounds with soap and water. If available, a virucidal agent such as a povidone-iodine solution should be used to irrigate the wounds.
	RIG	Administer 20 IU/kg body weight as soon as possible after exposure. If anatomically feasible, up to one-half the dose should be infiltrated around the wound(s) and any remaining volume should be administered IM into the gluteal area (upper outer quadrant only) or lateral thigh muscle (because of the large volume to be injected). When more than one wound exists, each should be locally infiltrated with a portion of the RIG. Also, RIG should not be administered in the same syringe as vaccine. Because RIG might partially suppress active production of the antibody, no more than the recommended dose should be given.
	Vaccine	HDCV started immediately (as soon as possible after exposure) 1.0 mL, IM (deltoid area[b]), one each on days 0[c], 3, 7, 14, and 28.
Previously vaccinated[d]	Wound cleansing	All post-exposure treatment should begin with immediate thorough cleansing of all wounds with soap and water. If available, a virucidal agent such as a povidone-iodine solution should be used to irrigate the wounds.
	RIG	RIG should **not** be administered.
	Vaccine	HDCV started immediately (as soon as possible after exposure) 1.0 mL, IM (deltoid area[b]), one each on days 0[c] and 3.

[a] These regimens are applicable for all age groups, including children.

[b] The deltoid area is the only acceptable site of vaccination for adults and older children. For younger children, the outer aspect of the thigh may be used. Vaccine should never be administered in the gluteal area.

[c] Day 0 is the day the first dose of vaccine is administered.

[d] Any person with a history of pre-exposure vaccination with HDCV; prior post-exposure prophylaxis with HDCV; or previous vaccination with other types of rabies vaccine or with HDCV according to unapproved schedules but in whom neutralizing rabies antibody is demonstrated in serum.

SUPPLIED: Rabies Immune Globulin (Human) - HYPERRAB S/D treated with solvent/detergent is a sterile solution of antirabies immune globulin for intramuscular administration; it contains no preservative. HYPERRAB S/D is prepared by cold ethanol fractionation from the plasma of donors hyperimmunized with rabies vaccine. The immune globulin is isolated from solubilized Cohn fraction II. The fraction II solution is adjusted to a final concentration of 0.3% tri-n-butyl phosphate (TNBP) and 0.2% sodium cholate. After the addition of solvent (TNBP) and detergent (sodium cholate), the solution is heated to 30°C and maintained at that temperature for not less than 6 hours. After the viral inactivation step, the reactants are removed by precipitation, filtration and finally ultrafiltration and diafiltration. HYPERRAB S/D is formulated as a 15-18% protein solution at a pH of 6.4-7.2 in 0.21-0.32 M glycine. The pH is adjusted with sodium carbonate. HYPERRAB S/D is then incubated in the final container for 21-28 days at 20-27°C.

The removal and inactivation of spiked model enveloped and non-enveloped viruses during the manufacturing process for HYPERRAB S/D has been validated in laboratory studies. Human Immunodeficiency Virus, Type 1(HIV-1), was chosen as the relevant virus for blood products; Bovine Viral Diarrhea Virus (BVDV) was chosen to model Hepatitis C virus; Pseudorabies virus (PRV) was chosen to model Hepatitis B virus and the Herpes viruses; and Reo virus type 3 (Reo) was chosen to model non-enveloped viruses and for its resistance to physical and chemical inactivation. Significant removal of model enveloped and non-enveloped viruses is seen in the Fraction II + IIIW to Effluent III step and significant removal of PRV and Reo virus is also seen in the Effluent III to Filtrate III step. Significant inactivation of enveloped viruses is achieved at the time of treatment of solubilized Cohn Fraction II with solvent/detergent.

Single use vials of 2 and 10 mL with an average potency value of 150 international units per mL (IU/mL) based on the U.S. Standard Rabies Immune Globulin. The 2 mL vial contains a total of 300 IU which is sufficient for a child weighing 15 kg. The 10 mL vial contains a total of 1500 IU which is sufficient for an adult weighing 75 kg. Store under refrigeration (2 to 8°C). Do not freeze. Solution that has been frozen should not be used. Do not use beyond the expiration date. The vials are single use. Once entered, discard any unused contents.

HYPERTET™ S/D

immune globulin, tetanus (human)

Passive Immunizing Agent

Talecris

Date of Preparation: June 8, 2005

PHARMACOLOGY: The occurrence of tetanus in the United States has decreased dramatically from 560 reported cases in 1947, when national reporting began, to a record low of 48 reported cases in 1987. The decline has resulted from widespread use of tetanus toxoid and improved wound management, including use of tetanus prophylaxis in emergency rooms.

Tetanus Immune Globulin (Human) - HYPERTET S/D supplies passive immunity to those individuals who have low or no immunity to the toxin produced by the tetanus organism, *C. tetani*. The antibodies act to neutralize the free form of the powerful exotoxin produced by this bacterium. Historically, such passive protection was provided by antitoxin derived from equine or bovine serum; however, the foreign protein in these heterologous products often produced severe allergic manifestations, even in individuals who demonstrated negative skin and/or conjunctival tests prior to administration. Estimates of the frequency of these foreign protein reactions following antitoxin of equine origin varied from 5%-30%.

If passive immunization is needed, human tetanus immune globulin (TIG) is the product of choice. It provides protection longer than antitoxin of animal origin and causes few adverse reactions.

Several studies suggest the value of human tetanus antitoxin in the treatment of active tetanus. In 1961 and 1962, Nation et al, using Tetanus Immune Globulin (Human) - HYPERTET S/D treated 20 patients with tetanus using single doses of 3000 to 6000 antitoxin units in combination with other accepted clinical and nursing procedures. Six patients, all over 45 years of age, died of causes other than tetanus. The authors felt that the mortality rate (30%) compared favourably with their previous experience using equine antitoxin in larger doses and that the results were much better than the 60% national death rate for tetanus reported from 1951 to 1954. Blake et al, however, found in a data analysis of 545 cases of tetanus reported to the Centers for Disease Control from 1965 to 1971 that survival was no better with 8000 units of human tetanus immune globulin (TIG) than with 500 units; however, an optimal dose could not be determined.

Serologic tests indicate that naturally acquired immunity to tetanus toxin does not occur in the United States. Thus universal primary vaccination, with subsequent maintenance of adequate antitoxin levels by means of appropriately timed boosters, is necessary to protect persons among all age groups. Tetanus toxoid is a highly effective antigen; a completed primary series generally induces protective levels of serum antitoxin that persist for ≥ 10 years.

Passive immunization with HYPERTET S/D may be undertaken concomitantly with active immunization using tetanus toxoid in those persons who must receive an immediate injection of tetanus antitoxin and in whom it is desirable to begin the process of active immunization. Based on the work of Rubbo, McComb and Dwyer, and Levine et al, the physician may thus supply immediate passive protection against tetanus, and at the same time begin formation of active immunization in the injured individual which upon completion of a **full toxoid series** will preclude future need for antitoxin.

Peak blood levels of IgG are obtained approximately 2 days after intramuscular injection. The half-life of IgG in the circulation of individuals with normal IgG levels is approximately 23 days.

In a clinical study in healthy human adults receiving another hyperimmune immune globulin product treated with solvent/detergent, Rabies Immune Globulin (Human), prepared by the same manufacturing process, detectable passive antibody titers were observed in the serum of all subjects by 24 hours post injection and persisted through the 21 day study period. These results suggest that passive immunization with immune globulin products is not affected by the solvent/detergent treatment.

INDICATIONS: Tetanus Immune Globulin (Human) - HYPERTET S/D is indicated for prophylaxis against tetanus following injury in patients whose immunization is incomplete or uncertain (see below). It is also indicated, although evidence of effectiveness is limited, in the regimen of treatment of active cases of tetanus.

A thorough attempt must be made to determine whether a patient has completed primary vaccination. Patients with unknown or uncertain previous vaccination histories should be considered to have had no previous tetanus toxoid doses. Persons who had military service since 1941 can be considered to have received at least one dose, and although most of them may have completed a primary series of tetanus toxoid, this cannot be assumed for each individual. When a contraindication of tetanus toxoid exists and a patient sustains a major or unclean wound, tetanus immune globulin should be given. Patients who have not completed a primary series may require tetanus toxoid and passive immunization at the time of wound cleaning and debridement.

Table 1 is a summary guide to tetanus prophylaxis in wound management:

Table 1: HYPERTET S/D

Guide to Tetanus Prophylaxis in Wound Management

History of Tetanus Immunization (Doses)	Clean, Minor Wounds		All Other Wounds[a]	
	Td[b]	TIG[c]	Td	TIG
Uncertain or less than 3	Yes	No	Yes	Yes
3 or more[d]	No[e]	No	No[f]	No

a Such as, but not limited to, wounds contaminated with dirt, feces, soil, and saliva; puncture wounds; avulsions; and wounds resulting from missiles, crushing, burns and frostbite.
b Adult type tetanus and diphtheria toxoids. If the patient is less than 7 years old, DT or DTP is preferred to tetanus toxoid alone. For persons ≥ 7 years of age, Td is preferred to tetanus toxoid alone (see Dosage).
c Tetanus Immune Globulin (Human).
d If only three doses of fluid tetanus toxoid have been received, a fourth dose of toxoid, preferably an adsorbed toxoid, should be given.
e Yes if more than 10 years since the last dose.
f Yes if more than 5 years since the last dose.

CONTRAINDICATIONS: None known.

WARNINGS: Tetanus Immune Globulin (Human) - HYPERTET S/D is made from human plasma. Products made from human plasma may contain infectious agents, such as viruses, that can cause disease. The risk that such products will transmit an infectious agent has been reduced by screening plasma donors for prior exposure to certain viruses, by testing for the presence of certain current virus infections, and by inactivating and/or removing certain viruses. Despite these measures, such products can still potentially transmit disease. There is also the possibility that unknown infectious agents may be present in such products. Individuals who receive infusions of blood or plasma products may develop signs and/or symptoms of some viral infections, particularly hepatitis C. All infections thought by a physician possibly to have been transmitted by this product should be reported by the physician or other healthcare provider to Talecris Biotherapeutics Ltd. [1-866-482-5226].

The physician should discuss the risks and benefits of this product with the patient, before prescribing or administering to the patient.

Tetanus Immune Globulin (Human) - HYPERTET S/D should be given with caution to patients with a history of prior systemic allergic reactions following the administration of human immunoglobulin preparations.

In patients who have severe thrombocytopenia or any coagulation disorder that would contraindicate intramuscular injections, HYPERTET S/D should be given only if the expected benefits outweigh the risks.

PRECAUTIONS: General: **Tetanus Immune Globulin (Human) - HYPERTET S/D should not be given intravenously.** Intravenous injection of immunoglobulin intended for intramuscular use can, on occasion, cause a precipitous fall in blood pressure, and a picture not unlike anaphylaxis. Injections should only be made **intramuscularly** and care should be taken to draw back on the plunger of the syringe before injection in order to be certain that the needle is not in a blood vessel. Intramuscular injections are preferably administered in the anterolateral aspects of the upper thigh and the deltoid muscle of the upper arm. The gluteal region should not be used routinely as an injection site because of the risk of injury to the sciatic nerve. If the gluteal region is used, the central region **must** be avoided; only the upper, outer quadrant should be used.

Chemoprophylaxis against tetanus is neither practical nor useful in managing wounds. Wound cleaning, debridement when indicated, and proper immunization are important. The need for tetanus toxoid (active immunization), with or without TIG (passive immunization), depends on both the condition of the wound and the patient's vaccination history. Rarely has tetanus occurred among persons with documentation of having received a primary series of toxoid injections. See Table 1 under Indications.

Skin tests should not be done. The intradermal injection of concentrated IgG solutions often causes a localized area of inflammation which can be misinterpreted as a positive allergic reaction. In actuality, this does not represent an allergy; rather, it is localized tissue irritation. Misinterpretation of the results of such tests can lead the physician to withhold needed human antitoxin from a patient who is not actually allergic to this material. True allergic responses to human IgG given in the prescribed intramuscular manner are rare.

Although systemic reactions to human immunoglobulin preparations are rare, epinephrine should be available for treatment of acute anaphylactic reactions.

Drug Interactions: Antibodies in immunoglobulin preparations may interfere with the response to live viral vaccines such as measles, mumps, polio, and rubella. Therefore, use of such vaccines should be deferred until approximately 3 months after HYPERTET S/D administration.

No interactions with other products are known.

Pregnancy: Animal reproduction studies have not been conducted with HYPERTET S/D. It is also not known whether HYPERTET S/D can cause fetal harm when administered to a pregnant woman or can affect reproduction capacity. HYPERTET S/D should be given to a pregnant woman only if clearly needed.

Children: Safety and effectiveness in the pediatric population have not been established.

ADVERSE EFFECTS: Slight soreness at the site of injection and slight temperature elevation may be noted at times. Sensitization to repeated injections of human immunoglobulin is extremely rare.

In the course of routine injections of large numbers of persons with immunoglobulin there have been a few isolated occurrences of angioneurotic edema, nephrotic syndrome, and anaphylactic shock after injection.

OVERDOSE:

Symptoms: Although no data are available, clinical experience with other immunoglobulin preparations suggests that the only manifestations would be pain and tenderness at the injection site.

For management of a suspected drug overdose, CPhA recommends that you contact your **regional Poison Control Centre**. See the *CPS* Directory section for a list of Poison Control Centres.

DOSAGE: For intramuscular injection only. Do not give intravenously.

Routine Prophylaxis Dosage Schedule: Adults and children 7 years and older: Tetanus Immune Globulin (Human) - HYPERTET S/D, 250 units should be given by deep intramuscular injection (see Precautions). At the same time, but in a different extremity and with a separate syringe, Tetanus and Diphtheria Toxoids Adsorbed (For Adult Use) (Td) should be administered according to the manufacturer's package insert. Adults with uncertain histories of a complete primary vaccination series should receive a primary series using the combined Td toxoid. To ensure continued protection, booster doses of Td should be given every 10 years.

Children less than 7 years old: In small children, the routine prophylactic dose of HYPERTET S/D may be calculated by the body weight (4.0 units/kg). However, it may be advisable to administer the entire contents of the vial or syringe of HYPERTET S/D (250 units) regardless of the child's size, since theoretically the same amount of toxin will be produced in the child's body by the infecting tetanus organism as it will in an adult's body. At the same time but in a different extremity and with a different syringe, Diphtheria and Tetanus Toxoids and Pertussis Vaccine Adsorbed (DTP) or Diphtheria and Tetanus Toxoids Adsorbed (For Pediatric Use) (DT), if pertussis vaccine is contraindicated, should be administered per the manufacturer's package insert.

Note: The single injection of tetanus toxoid only initiates the series for producing active immunity in the recipient. The physician must impress upon the patient the need for further toxoid injections in 1 month and 1 year. Without such, the active immunization series is incomplete. If a contraindication to using tetanus toxoid-containing preparations exists for a person who has not completed a primary series of tetanus toxoid immunization and that person has a wound that is neither clean nor minor, only passive immunization should be given using tetanus immune globulin (TIG). See Table 1 under Indications.

Available evidence indicate that complete primary vaccination with tetanus toxoid provides long-lasting protection ≥ 10 years for most recipients. Consequently, after complete primary tetanus vaccination, boosters — even for wound management — need be given only every 10 years when wounds are minor and uncontaminated. For other wounds, a booster is appropriate if the patient has not received tetanus toxoid within the preceding 5 years. Persons who have received at least two doses of tetanus toxoid rapidly develop antitoxin antibodies. The prophylactic dosage schedule for these patients and for those with incomplete or uncertain immunity is shown in Table 1 in Indications.

Since tetanus is actually a local infection, proper initial wound care is of paramount importance. The use of antitoxin is adjunctive to this procedure. However, in approximately 10% of recent tetanus cases, no wound or other breach in skin or mucous membrane could be implicated.

Treatment of Active Cases of Tetanus: Standard therapy for the treatment of active tetanus including the use of HYPERTET S/D must be implemented immediately. The dosage should be adjusted according to the severity of the infection.

Parenteral drug products should be inspected visually for particulate matter and discoloration prior to administration, whenever solution and container permit. They should not be used if particulate matter and/or discoloration are present.

HYPERTET S/D is supplied with a syringe and an attached UltraSafe Needle Guard for your protection and convenience. Please follow instructions below for proper use of syringe and UltraSafe Needle Guard.

Directions for Syringe Usage:

1. Remove the prefilled syringe from the package. Lift syringe by barrel, **not** by plunger.
2. Twist the plunger rod clockwise until the threads are seated.
3. With the rubber needle shield secured on the syringe tip, push the plunger rod forward a few millimeters to break any friction seal between the rubber stopper and the glass syringe barrel.
4. Remove the needle shield and expel air bubbles. (Do not remove the rubber needle shield to prepare the product for administration until immediately prior to the anticipated injection time.)
5. Proceed with hypodermic needle puncture.
6. Aspirate prior to injection to confirm that the needle is not in a vein or artery.
7. Inject the medication.
8. Keeping your hands behind the needle, grasp the guard with free hand and slide forward towards needle until it is completely covered and clicks into place. If audible click is not heard, guard may not be completely activated.
9. Place entire prefilled glass syringe with guard activated into an approved sharps container for proper disposal.

A number of factors beyond our control could reduce the efficacy of this product or even result in an ill effect following its use. These include improper storage and handling of the product after it leaves our hands, diagnosis, dosage, method of administration, and biological differences in individual patients. Because of these factors it is important that this product be stored properly and that the directions be followed carefully during use.

SUPPLIED: Tetanus Immune Globulin (Human) - HYPERTET S/D treated with solvent/detergent is a sterile solution of tetanus hyperimmune immune globulin for intramuscular administration; it contains no preservative and is supplied as a single dose syringe or single dose vial. HYPERTET S/D is prepared by cold ethanol fractionation from the plasma of donors immunized with tetanus toxoid. The immune globulin is isolated from solubilized Cohn fraction II. The fraction II solution is adjusted to a final concentration of 0.3% tri-n-butyl phosphate (TNBP) and 0.2% sodium cholate. After the addition of solvent (TNBP) and detergent (sodium cholate), the solution is heated to 30°C and maintained at that temperature for not less than 6 hours. After the viral inactivation step, the reactants are removed by precipitation, filtration and finally ultrafiltration and diafiltration. HYPERTET S/D is formulated as a 15-18% protein solution at a pH of 6.4-7.2 in 0.21-0.32 M glycine. The pH is adjusted with sodium carbonate. HYPERTET S/D is then incubated in the final container for 21-28 days at 20-27°C. The product is standardized against the U.S. Standard Antitoxin and the U.S. Control Tetanus Toxin and contains not less than 250 tetanus antitoxin units per container.

The removal and inactivation of spiked model enveloped and non-enveloped viruses during the manufacturing process for HYPERTET S/D has been validated in laboratory studies. Human Immunodeficiency Virus, Type 1 (HIV-1), was chosen as the relevant virus for blood products; Bovine Viral Diarrhea Virus (BVDV) was chosen to model Hepatitis C virus; Pseudorabies virus (PRV) was chosen to model Hepatitis B virus and the Herpes viruses; and Reo virus type 3 (Reo) was chosen to model non-enveloped viruses and for its resistance to physical and chemical inactivation.

Significant removal of model enveloped and non-enveloped viruses is seen in the Fraction II and IIIW to Effluent III step and significant removal of PRV and Reo-virus is seen in the Effluent III to Filtrate III step. Significant inactivation of enveloped viruses is achieved at the time of treatment of solubilized Cohn Fraction II with solvent/detergent.

Single dose prefilled disposable syringes of 250 units with attached needles and single dose vials of 250 units. Store at 2 to 8°C. Do not freeze. Solution that has been frozen should not be used. Do not use beyond expiration date.

Hypotears® Eye Ointment
mineral oil—white petrolatum
Ocular Lubricant

Novartis Pharmaceuticals

SUPPLIED: Each tube contains: white petrolatum 85% (w/w) and mineral oil 15% (w/w). Preservative-free. Tubes of 3.5 g. Store at 15 to 30°C. Keep tube tightly closed when not in use.

Hypotears® Ophthalmic Solution
polyvinyl alcohol
Artificial Tears

Novartis Pharmaceuticals

SUPPLIED: Each bottle contains: polyvinyl alcohol 1% (w/v). Nonmedicinal ingredients: benzalkonium chloride 0.01% (w/v) (preservative), dextrose, disodium edetate, polyethylene glycol and purified water. Plastic squeeze bottles of 15 and 30 mL with dropper tip. Store at 15 to 30°C. Keep bottle tightly closed when not in use.

Hytrin® Ⓟ
terazosin HCl
Antihypertensive—Symptomatic Treatment of Benign Prostatic Hyperplasia (BPH)

Abbott

Date of Preparation: May 15, 1997
Date of Revision: February 27, 2008

SUMMARY PRODUCT INFORMATION:

Route of Administration	Dosage Form/ Strength	Clinically Relevant Nonmedicinal Ingredients
Oral	Tablet/1 mg, 2 mg, 5 mg, 10 mg	Corn starch, lactose, magnesium stearate, povidone (for 1, 2, 5 mg only), pregelatinized starch (for 10 mg only) and talc. Also contains FD&C yellow No. 6 (for 2 mg), iron oxide (for 5 mg) and FD&C blue No. 2 (for 10 mg).

INDICATIONS AND CLINICAL USE: HYTRIN (terazosin hydrochloride) is indicated for:
- the treatment of mild to moderate hypertension.
- the treatment of symptoms of benign prostatic hyperplasia (BPH).

Hypertension: It is employed in a general treatment program in conjunction with a thiazide diuretic and/or other antihypertensive drugs as needed for proper patient response. HYTRIN may be tried as a sole therapy in those patients in whom other agents caused adverse effects or are inappropriate.

Benign Prostatic Hyperplasia (BPH): The onset of effect is rapid, with improvement in peak flow rate and symptoms observed at 2 weeks. The effect on these variables was well maintained throughout the study duration (18 months). HYTRIN does not retard or stop the progression of BPH. The long-term effects of HYTRIN on the incidence of surgery, acute urinary obstruction or other complications of BPH, are yet to be determined.

A number of clinical conditions can mimic symptomatic BPH (i.e. stricture of urethra, stricture of bladder neck, urinary bladder stones, neurogenic bladder dysfunction secondary to diabetes, Parkinsonism, etc.). These conditions should therefore be ruled out before terazosin hydrochloride therapy is initiated.

Geriatrics (>75 years of age): Patients over 75 years of age may have limited benefit from HYTRIN therapy.

Pediatrics (<18 years of age): HYTRIN has not been studied in children and therefore use in this age group is not recommended.

CONTRAINDICATIONS:
- Patients who are hypersensitive to HYTRIN (terazosin hydrochloride) or its analogs or to any ingredient in the formulation or component of the container. For a complete listing, see Dosage Forms, Composition and Packaging.

WARNINGS AND PRECAUTIONS:

Serious Warnings and Precautions
- Patients with a history of micturition syncope should not receive terazosin hydrochloride (see Warnings and Precautions, Cardiovascular, Syncope and "First dose" Effect)

General: HYTRIN (terazosin hydrochloride) therapy does not modify the natural history of benign protatic hyperplasia (BPH). It does not retard or stop the progression of BPH, nor does it improve urine flow sufficiently to significantly reduce the residual urine volume. However, significant reduction of the mean residual volume have been shown in patients with baseline residual volumes of >50 mL. The patient may continue to be at risk of developing urinary retention and other BPH complications during terazosin hydrochloride therapy.

Prostatic Cancer: Carcinoma of the prostate and BPH cause many of the same symptoms. These two diseases frequently coexist. Therefore, patients thought to have BPH should be examined prior to starting terazosin hydrochloride therapy to rule out the presence of carcinoma of the prostate.

Carcinogenesis and Mutagenesis: Terazosin hydrochloride was devoid of mutagenic potential when evaluated in vivo and in vitro.

Terazosin hydrochloride, administered in the feed to rats at doses of 8, 40, and 250 mg/kg/day for two years, was associated with a statistically significant increase in benign adrenal medullary tumors of male rats exposed to the 250 mg/kg dose. Female rats were unaffected. Terazosin hydrochloride was not oncogenic in mice when administered in feed for 2 years at a maximum tolerated dose of 32 mg/kg/day.

Cardiovascular: Syncope and "First dose" Effect: Terazosin hydrochloride can cause marked hypotension, especially postural hypotension, and syncope in association with the first dose or first few doses of therapy. A similar effect can occur if therapy is re-instated following interruption for more than a few doses. Syncope has also occurred in association with rapid dosage increases or the introduction of another antihypertensive agent into the regimen of a patient taking high doses of terazosin hydrochloride.

Syncope is believed to be due to an excessive postural hypotensive effect, although occasionally the syncopal episode has been preceded by a bout of severe supraventricular tachycardia with heart rates of 120 to 160 beats per minute.

In studies of terazosin hydrochloride the incidence of syncopal episodes was approximately 1% in hypertensive patients and 0.7% in patients with BPH.

The likelihood of syncopal episodes or excessive hypotension can be minimized by limiting the initial dose of the drug to 1 mg of terazosin hydrochloride given at bedtime, by increasing the dosage slowly, and by introducing any additional antihypertensive drugs into the patient's regimen with caution (see Dosage and Administration).

Patients should be advised of the possibility of syncopal and orthostatic symptoms, and to avoid driving or hazardous tasks for 12 hours after the initial dose of terazosin hydrochloride, after the dose is increased and after interruption of therapy when treatment is resumed. They should be cautioned to avoid situations where injury could result should syncope occur.

If syncope occurs, place the patients in the recumbent position and institute supportive measures as necessary.

Patients with a history of micturition syncope should not receive terazosin hydrochloride.

Concomitant administration of terazosin hydrochloride with verapamil to hypertensive patients may result in symptomatic hypotension and in some cases tachycardia (see Warnings and Precautions).

Use with Phosphodiesterase type 5 (PDE5) Inhibitors: Caution is advised when PDE5 inhibitors such as VIAGRA (sildenafil), CIALIS (tadalafil) and LEVITRA (vardenafil) are co-administered with alpha-blockers. Both PDE5 inhibitors and alpha-adrenergic blocking agents are vasodilators with blood pressure lowering effects. When vasodilators are used in combination, additive effects on blood pressure may be anticipated. In some patients, concomitant use of these two classes of drugs can lower blood pressure significantly, which may lead to symptomatic hypotension. Consideration should be given to the following:
- Patients should be stable on alpha-blocker therapy prior to initiating a PDE5 inhibitor. Patients who demonstrate hemodynamic instability on alpha-blocker therapy alone are at increased risk of symptomatic hypotension with concomitant use of PDE5 inhibitors.
- In patients who are stable on alpha-blocker therapy, PDE5 inhibitors should be initiated at the lowest dose.
- Safety of combined use of PDE5 inhibitors and alpha-blockers may be adversely affected by other factors, such as intravascular volume depletion and other antihypertensive therapy.

Orthostatic Hypotension: While syncope is the most severe orthostatic effect of terazosin hydrochloride (see Warnings and Precautions, Cardiovascular) other symptoms of lowered blood pressure, such as dizziness, lightheadedness and palpitations are more common with one or more of these occurring in 28% of patients in clinical trials of hypertension. In BPH clinical trials, 21% of the patients experienced one or more of the following: dizziness, hypotension, postural hypotension, syncope, and vertigo. Patients should be advised to lie down when these symptoms occur and then wait for a few minutes before standing to prevent their recurrence.

Patients with occupation in which such events represent potential problems should be treated with particular caution.

There is evidence that the orthostatic effect of terazosin hydrochloride is greater, even in chronic use, shortly after dosing.

Peripheral Edema: Fluid retention resulting in weight gain may occur during terazosin hydrochloride therapy. In placebo-controlled monotherapy trials, male and female patients receiving terazosin hydrochloride gained a mean 0.8 and 1 kg respectively, compared to losses of 0.1 and 0.5 kg respectively, in the placebo group. Both differences are significant.

Genitourinary: Concomitant Conditions: Terazosin hydrochloride should not be prescribed to patients with symptomatic BPH who have the following concomitant conditions: chronic urinary retention, high residual urine (over 200 mL), peak urine flow of 5 mL/sec or less, history of prior prostatic surgery, chronic fibrous or granulomatous prostatitis, urethral stricture, history of pelvic irradiation, presence of prostatic calculi, presence of large median lobe of prostate, presence of calculi in urinary bladder, recent history of epididymitis, gross hematuria, presence of neurogenic bladder dysfunction (diabetes mellitus, Parkinsonism, uninhibited neurogenic bladder, etc.), hydro-nephrosis, presence of carcinoma of the prostate, patients with clinically significant renal or hepatic impairment (i.e. serum creatinine >2 mg/dL or AST >1.5 times the upper limit of normal (or equivalent level on the international scale).

Hepatic/Biliary/Pancreatic: Use in Patients with Liver Impairment: No information is available on the use of terazosin hydrochloride in patients with impaired liver function.

Peri-Operative Considerations: Cataract Surgery: Intraoperative Floppy Iris Syndrome (IFIS) has been observed during cataract surgery in some patients on/or previously treated with alpha-1 blockers. This variant of small pupil syndrome is characterized by the combination of a flaccid iris that billows in response to intraoperative irrigation currents, progressive intraoperative miosis despite preoperative dilation with standard mydriatic drugs, and potential prolapse of the iris toward the phacoemulsification incisions. The patient's ophthalmologist should be prepared for possible modifications to their surgical technique, such as the utilization of iris hooks, iris dilator rings, or viscoelastic substances. There does not appear to be a benefit of stopping alpha-1 blocker therapy prior to cataract surgery.

Renal: The use of terazosin hydrochloride in patients with impaired renal function requires careful monitoring. Limited pharmacokinetic studies using low doses (1 mg) showed no difference in the pharmacokinetic of terazosin as compared to patients with normal renal function. Approximately 40% of oral terazosin dose is excreted by the kidney as parent drug or metabolites.

Sensitivity/Resistance: Anaphylactoid-like Reactions: Anaphylactoid-like reactions manifested by angioedema of the lips, tongue, pharynx, and/or laryngeal spasm have been rarely reported in patients treated with terazosin hydrochloride (see Adverse Reactions). In such cases, terazosin hydrochloride should be promptly discontinued and appropriate therapy and monitoring should be provided until complete and sustained resolution of signs and symptoms has occurred.

Sexual Function/Reproduction: Effect on fertility was assessed in a standard fertility/reproductive performance study in which male and female rats were administered oral doses of 8, 30 and 120 mg/kg/day. Four of 20 male rats given 30 mg/kg and five of 19 male rats given 120 mg/kg failed to sire a litter. Testicular weights and morphology were unaffected by treatment. Vaginal smears at 30 and 120 mg/kg, however, appeared to contain less sperm than smears from control matings and good correlation was reported between sperm count and subsequent pregnancy.

Oral administration of terazosin hydrochloride for one or two years elicited a statistically significant increase in the incidence of testicular atrophy in rats exposed to 40 and 250 mg/kg/day, but not in rats exposed to 8 mg/kg/day. Testicular atrophy was also observed in dogs dosed with 300 mg/kg/day for 3 months but not after one year when dosed with 20 mg/kg/day.

Special Populations: Pregnant Women: The safety of terazosin hydrochloride in pregnancy has not been established. Terazosin hydrochloride is not recommended during pregnancy unless potential benefits justifies potential risks to mother and fetus.

In animal studies there was no teratogenic effect. In peri- and post-natal development studies in rats, significantly more pups died in the group dosed with 120 mg/kg/day than in the control group during the three week postpartum period.

Nursing Women: It is not known whether terazosin is excreted in human milk. Because of possible adverse reactions in nursing infants an alternate method of infant feeding should be considered when the use of drug is essential.

Pediatrics (<18 years of age): The use of terazosin hydrochloride in children is not recommended since safety and efficacy have not been established.

Geriatrics (>65 years of age): Terazosin hydrochloride should be used cautiously in elderly patients because of the possibility of orthostatic hypotension. There was an age-related trend towards an increased incidence of dizziness, blurred vision and syncope in elderly patients treated with this drug. Patients over seventy-five years of age may have limited benefit from terazosin hydrochloride therapy.

Monitoring and Laboratory Tests: Long-term (6 months or longer) administration of terazosin hydrochloride has produced no pattern of clinically significant changes attributable to the drug in the following clinical laboratory measurements: glucose, uric acid, creatinine, BUN, liver function tests, and electrolytes.

Small but statistically significant decreases in hematocrit, hemoglobin, white blood cells, total protein and albumin were observed in controlled clinical trials. These laboratory findings suggested the possibility of hemodilution. Treatment with terazosin hydrochloride for up to 24 months had no significant effect on prostate specific antigen (PSA) levels.

ADVERSE REACTIONS: Adverse Drug Reaction Overview: Hypertension: The incidence of adverse reactions is derived from clinical trials involving 1986 hypertensive patients on terazosin hydrochloride monotherapy or combination therapy.

The most serious adverse reaction encountered with HYTRIN (terazosin hydrochloride) is syncope occurring in approximately 1% of patients.

The most common reactions were dizziness (18.9%), headache (14.1%), asthenia (11%), somnolence (4.8%), nasal congestion (4.6%) and palpitation (4.6%).

The most frequently reported adverse effects which resulted in termination of terazosin hydrochloride were dizziness (3.5%), asthenia (2.1%) and headache (1.8%).

Benign Prostatic Hyperplasia (BPH): In clinical trials involving 1171 patients with BPH, syncope was reported in 0.7% of patients following treatment with terazosin hydrochloride.

Clinical Trial Adverse Drug Reactions: Because clinical trials are conducted under very specific conditions the adverse reaction rates observed in the clinical trials may not reflect the rates observed in practice and should not be compared to the rates in the clinical trials of another drug. Adverse drug reaction information from clinical trials is useful for identifying drug-related adverse events and for approximating rates.

Most Common Adverse Drug Reactions (>1%): Hypertension: Adverse drug reactions occurring more commonly in 1% or more of hypertensive patients on terazosin hydrochloride monotherapy or combination therapy are shown in Table 1.

Table 1: HYTRIN

Adverse Drug Reactions in Clinical Trials Involving Hypertensive Patients on Terazosin Hydrochloride Monotherapy or Combination Therapy

	Terazosin hydrochloride n=1986 (%)
Body as a Whole	
Headache	14.1

(cont'd)

Table 1: HYTRIN *(cont'd)*

Adverse Drug Reactions in Clinical Trials Involving Hypertensive Patients on Terazosin Hydrochloride Monotherapy or Combination Therapy

	Terazosin hydrochloride n=1986 (%)
Asthenia	11.0
Peripheral Edema	3.6
Chest Pain	2.2
Abdominal Pain	1.5
Edema	1.3
Facial Edema	1.0
Cardiovascular System	
Palpitation	4.6
Tachycardia	2.9
Syncope	1.0
Digestive System	
Nausea	3.9
Dry Mouth	1.7
Diarrhea	1.3
Nervous System	
Dizziness	18.9
Somnolence	4.8
Nervousness	2.2
Paresthesia	1.5
Insomnia	1.2
Respiratory System	
Nasal Congestion	4.6
Dyspnea	2.8
Rhinitis	1.2
Skin and Appendages	
Sweating	1.1
Special Senses	
Blurred Vision	1.4
Eye Disorder	1.2
Urogenital System	
Impotence	1.1
Miscellaneous	
Pain in Extremities	1.8

Benign Prostatic Hyperplasia (BPH): In controlled and uncontrolled clinical trials involving 1171 patients with BPH, the most common reactions (≥1%) were dizziness (14.0%), asthenia (9.0%), headache (6.4%), somnolence (4.5%), postural hypotension (3.8%), impotence (3.5%), urinary tract infection (3.1%), pharyngitis (2.7%), dyspnea (2.5%), rhinitis (2.2%), dysuria (2%), back pain (1.8%), nausea (1.8%), flu syndrome (1.7%), rash (1.7%), sinusitis (1.7%), hypotension (1.5%), chest pain (1.5%), vertigo (1.3%), dyspepsia (1.1%), diarrhea (1%), palpitation (1%), abdominal pain (1%) and amblyopia (1.0%).

Less Common Clinical Trial Adverse Drug Reactions (<1%): Hypertension: The following events were reported in less than 1% of cases. The order of presentation corresponds within each heading to the relative frequency of occurrence.

Body as a Whole: back pain, weight gain, allergic reactions, malaise.

Cardiovascular System: postural hypotension, angina pectoris, arrhythmias, cerebrovascular accident, heart failure, hypotension (at times severe), migraine.

Digestive System: dyspepsia, vomiting, anorexia, gastritis, liver function abnormality, jaundice.

Nervous System: incoordination, abnormal dreams, confusion, speech disorder, tremor, vertigo, seizure, depression.

Respiratory System: sinusitis, cold symptoms, pharyngitis, asthma, increased cough, laryngeal spasm.

Skin and Appendages: pruritus, rash, photosensitivity.

Special Senses: tinnitus, taste perversion.

Urogenital System: urinary frequency, dysuria.

Miscellaneous: hypokalemia, hypophosphatemia, decreased libido.

Benign Prostatic Hyperplasia (BPH): Cardiovascular System: syncope, tachycardia.

Metabolic and Nutritional Disorders: peripheral edema, weight gain.

Nervous System: libido decrease.

Post-Market Adverse Drug Reactions: Body as a Whole: fever, neck pain, and shoulder pain, anaphylaxis has rarely been reported.

Cardiovascular System: vasodilation, atrial fibrillation has been reported; however, a cause and effect relationship has not been established.

Digestive System: constipation, and flatulence.

Nervous System: anxiety.

Respiratory System: bronchitis, epitaxis, and flu symptoms.

Special Senses: conjunctivitis.

Urogenital System: priapism, urinary tract infection, and urinary incontinence primarily reported in post-menopausal women.

Musculoskeletal System: arthralgia, arthritis, joint disorder, and myalgia.

Hematopoietic System: Thrombocytopenia has been reported.

Metabolic/Nutritional Disorders: gout.

During cataract surgery, a variant of small pupil syndrome known as Intraoperative Floppy Iris Syndrome (IFIS) has been reported in association with alpha-1 blocker therapy.

DRUG INTERACTIONS: Drug-Drug Interactions: Table 2 provides a list of potential drug interactions due to pharmacokinetic reasons:

Table 2: HYTRIN

Potential Drug Interactions Associated with Terazosin Hydrochloride

Concomitant Drug Class: Drug Name	Ref	Effect	Clinical Comment
Verapamil	P/CT	Significant increases in AUC, C_{max} and C_{min} of terazosin hydrochloride in hypertensive patients. The pharmacokinetics of verapamil were not altered.	Symptomatic hypotension, and in some cases tachycardia, were observed when terazosin hydrochloride was administered concomitantly with verapamil. Caution should therefore be exercised when these drugs are administered concomitantly (see Warnings and Precautions).
PDE5 Inhibitors e.g., VIAGRA (sildenafil), LEVITRA (vardenafil), and CIALIS (tadalafil)	P/C	Hypotension has been reported during the concomitant use of PDE5 inhibitors and HYTRIN (see Warnings and Precautions).	Symptomatic hypotension

Legend: C=Case Study; CT=Clinical Trials; P=Potential.

In controlled trials, terazosin hydrochloride has been added to diuretics and several beta-adrenergic blockers; except for the additive hypotensive effect, no unexpected interactions were observed. Terazosin hydrochloride has also been used in patients on a variety of concomitant therapies. While these were not formal interaction studies, no interactions were observed. Terazosin hydrochloride has been used concomitantly in at least 50 patients on the following drugs or drug classes: 1) analgesic/anti-inflammatory (e.g., acetaminophen, acetylsalicylic acid, codeine, ibuprofen, indomethacin); 2) antibiotics (e.g., erythromycin, trimethoprim and sulfamethoxazole); 3) anticholinergic/ sympathomimetics (e.g., phenylephrine hydrochloride, phenylpropanolamine hydrochloride, pseudoephedrine hydrochloride); 4) antigout (e.g., allopurinol); 5) antihistamines (e.g., chlorpheniramine); 6) cardiovascular agents (e.g., atenolol, hydrochlorothiazide, methyclothiazide, propranolol); 7) corticosteroids; 8) gastrointestinal agents (e.g., antacid); 9) hypoglycemics; 10) sedatives and tranquilizers (e.g. diazepam).

DOSAGE AND ADMINISTRATION:

Dosing Considerations: Hypertension: The dose and the dosing intervals (12 to 24 hours) of HYTRIN (terazosin hydrochloride) should be adjusted to the patient's individual blood pressure response.

When terazosin hydrochloride is being added to the existing antihypertensive therapy, the patient should be carefully monitored for the occurrence of hypotension. If a diuretic or other antihypertensive agent is being added to terazosin hydrochloride regimen, dosage reduction of terazosin hydrochloride and re-titration with careful monitoring may be necessary.

Benign Prostatic Hyperplasia (BPH): The dose of terazosin hydrochloride should be adjusted to the patient's individual response.

Recommended Dose and Dosage Adjustment: Hypertension: Initial Dose: 1 mg of terazosin hydrochloride at bedtime is the starting dose for all patients and this dose should not be exceeded; compliance with this initial dosage recommendation should be strictly observed to minimize the potential for acute hypotensive episodes.

Subsequent Doses: The dose may be slowly increased to achieve the desired blood pressure response. The usual dose range is 1 to 5 mg once-a-day. Some patients may benefit from doses up to 20 mg per day which is the maximum recommended daily dose.

The blood pressure should be monitored at the end of the dosing interval to assure that control is maintained. It is also helpful to measure the blood pressure two to three hours after dosing to see if the maximum and minimum responses are similar and to evaluate symptoms.

If response to terazosin hydrochloride is substantially diminished at 24 hours, patients may be tried on a larger dose or twice daily dosage regimen. The latter should also be considered if adverse effects such as dizziness, palpitations or orthostatic complaints are seen two to three hours after dosing.

Benign Prostatic Hyperplasia (BPH): Initial Dose: 1 mg of terazosin hydrochloride at bedtime is the starting dose for all patients, and this dose should not be exceeded for the first week. Compliance with this initial dosage should be strictly observed to minimize the potential for acute hypotensive episodes.

Subsequent Doses: The dose should be increased in a stepwise fashion at weekly intervals to 2 mg, 5 mg, or 10 mg once daily to achieve the desired improvement of symptoms and/or flow rates. Maintenance doses of 5 to 10 mg once daily are generally required for the clinical response. The duration and dosage of treatment should be carefully titrated. Four weeks of terazosin hydrochloride therapy may be required before statistically significant improvement in the objective parameters of flowmetry (peak urine flow) are obtained. Improvement in the symptoms may appear as early as 2 weeks, but may be delayed as late as six weeks or more. Some patients may not achieve a clinical response despite appropriate titration. Following 18 months of treatment, a complete re-evaluation of the patient's condition should be made.

Following the administration of the maximum recommended dosage, terazosin hydrochloride should be discontinued if improvement in uroflowmetry is not clinically significant from baseline level or improvement in the American Urology Association (AUA) scores are not translated into improvements in quality of life. Terazosin hydrochloride therapy should also be discontinued if terazosin hydrochloride side effects are more bothersome than BPH symptoms or if the patient develops a urinary complication while on terazosin hydrochloride therapy.

Missed Dose: If terazosin hydrochloride administration is discontinued for several days or longer, therapy should be reinstituted using the initial dosing regimen.

OVERDOSAGE:

Should administration of HYTRIN (terazosin hydrochloride) lead to hypotension, support of the cardiovascular system is of first importance. Restoration of blood pressure and normalization of heart rate may be accomplished by keeping the patient in the supine position. If this measure is inadequate, shock should first be treated with volume expanders. If necessary, vasopressors should then be used and the renal function should be monitored and supported as needed. Laboratory data indicate that terazosin hydrochloride is highly protein bound; therefore, dialysis may not be of benefit.

For management of a suspected drug overdose, CPhA recommends that you contact your **regional Poison Control Centre**. See the *CPS* Directory section for a list of Poison Control Centres.

ACTION AND CLINICAL PHARMACOLOGY: Mechanism of Action: Hypertension: The antihypertensive effect of HYTRIN (terazosin hydrochloride) is believed to be a direct result of peripheral vasodilation. Although the exact mechanism by which the lowering of blood pressure is achieved is not known, the relaxation of the vessels appears to be produced mainly by selective blockade of alpha-1-adrenoceptors.

Benign Prostatic Hyperplasia (BPH): The reduction in the symptoms associated with BPH following administration of terazosin hydrochloride may be related to the changes in muscle tone produced by a blockade of alpha-1 adrenoceptors in the smooth muscle of the bladder neck and prostate.

Pharmacodynamics: Hypertension: Systolic and diastolic blood pressure is lowered in both the supine and standing positions. In clinical trials, blood pressure responses were measured at the end of the dosing interval (24 hours), with the usual supine response 5 to 10 mmHg systolic and 3.5 to 8 mmHg diastolic. The response in the standing position tended to be larger by 1 to 3 mmHg.

Limited measurements of peak response (2 to 3 hours after dosing) during chronic terazosin hydrochloride administration indicate that this response is somewhat greater than the trough (24-hour) response, suggesting some attenuation of response at 24 hours, presumably due to a fall in blood terazosin concentrations at the end of the dose interval.

The greater blood pressure effect associated with peak plasma concentrations appears to be more position dependent (greater in the standing position) than the effect of terazosin hydrochloride at 24 hours; in the standing position there is also a 6 to 10 beat per minute increase in heart rate in the first few hours after dosing. During the first 3 hours after dosing 12.5% of patients had a systolic pressure fall of 30 mmHg or more from supine to standing, or standing systolic pressure below 90 mm Hg with a fall of at least 20 mmHg.

During controlled clinical studies, patients receiving terazosin hydrochloride monotherapy had a small but statistically significant decrease (a 3% fall) compared to placebo in total cholesterol and the combined low-density and very-low density lipoprotein fractions. No significant changes were observed in high-density lipoprotein fraction and triglycerides compared to placebo.

Benign Prostatic Hyperplasia (BPH): The symptoms associated with BPH are related to bladder outlet obstruction. The bladder outlet obstruction is comprised of a static obstruction due to the enlarged prostate and a dynamic obstruction which is dependent upon the sympathetically controlled tone of the smooth muscle in the prostate and the bladder neck. Stimulation of alpha-1 adrenoceptors in the smooth muscle of the bladder neck and the prostate causes smooth muscle contraction and an increase in muscle tone.

In three placebo-controlled studies in men with symptomatic BPH, symptom evaluation and uroflowmetric measurements were performed approximately 24 hours following dosing. Results from these studies indicated that terazosin hydrochloride significantly improved symptoms and peak urine flow rates over placebo.

In 30 to 70% of patients with symptomatic BPH, placebo has also shown a remarkable and sometimes dramatic effect in controlled short-term studies. The symptoms may subside or fade away without treatment in approximately 20% of patients.

Pharmacokinetics: See Table 3.

Table 3: HYTRIN

Summary of Terazosin's Pharmacokinetic Parameters

	C_{max}	$t_{½}$ (h)	AUC_{0-48}	Clearance	Volume of distribution
Single dose mean (intravenous)	—	12 h	—	Plasma: 80 mL/min Renal: 10 mL/min	25–30 L
Single dose mean (1 mg tablet)	21 ng/mL	—	202.8 ng·h/mL	—	—

Absorption: Orally administered terazosin hydrochloride is essentially completely absorbed in man. Nearly all of the circulating dose is in the form of parent drug. Food has little or no effect on the bioavailability. The plasma levels of the free base peak in about 1 hour and then decline with a $t_{½}$ of approximately 12 hours.

Metabolism: Approximately 90 to 94% of the drug is bound to plasma proteins and binding is constant over the clinically observed concentration range. Hepatic metabolism is extensive with major biliary elimination.

Excretion: Approximately 10% of an orally administered dose is excreted as parent drug in the urine and approximately 20% is excreted in the feces. The remainder is eliminated as metabolites. Overall approximately 40% of the administered dose is excreted in the urine and approximately 60% in the feces.

Special Populations and Conditions: Geriatrics: In a study that evaluated the effect of age on terazosin hydrochloride pharmacokinetics, the mean plasma half-lives were 14.0 and 11.4 hours for the age group ≥70 years and the age group 20 to 39 years, respectively. After oral administration, the plasma clearance was decreased by 31.7% in patients 70 years of age or older compared to that in patients 20 to 39 years of age.

Renal Insufficiency: Impaired renal function had no significant effect on the elimination of terazosin hydrochloride, and dosage adjustment of terazosin hydrochloride to compensate for the drug removal during hemodialysis (approximately 10%) does not appear to be necessary.

STORAGE AND STABILITY: HYTRIN (terazosin hydrochloride) tablets should be stored at controlled room temperature between 15 and 25°C.

INFORMATION FOR THE PATIENT: Published in e-CPS, available by subscription at www.e-cps.ca.

DOSAGE FORMS, COMPOSITION AND PACKAGING: 1 mg: Each white, round tablet contains: terazosin 1 mg (as terazosin HCl dihydrate). Nonmedicinal ingredients: cornstarch, lactose, magnesium stearate, povidone and talc. Alcohol-, gluten-, paraben-, sodium-, sucrose-, sulfite- and tartrazine-free. Plastic bottles of 100.

2 mg: Each orange round tablet contains: terazosin 2 mg (as terazosin HCl dihydrate). Nonmedicinal ingredients: cornstarch, FD&C yellow No. 6, lactose, magnesium stearate, povidone and talc. Alcohol-, gluten-, paraben-, sodium-, sucrose-, sulfite- and tartrazine-free. Plastic bottles of 100.

5 mg: Each tan, round tablet contains: terazosin 5 mg (as terazosin HCl dihydrate). Nonmedicinal ingredients: cornstarch, iron oxide, lactose, magnesium stearate, povidone and talc. Alcohol-, gluten-, paraben-, sodium-, sucrose-, sulfite- and tartrazine-free. Starter Pack - one strip (seven) of each 1 mg and 2 mg tablets and, two strips (two times seven) of 5 mg tablets in blisters. Plastic bottles of 100.

10 mg: Each blue, round tablet contains: terazosin 10 mg (as terazosin HCl dihydrate). Nonmedicinal ingredients: cornstarch, FD&C Blue No. 2, lactose, magnesium stearate, pregelatinized starch and talc. Alcohol-, gluten-, paraben-, sodium-, sucrose-, sulfite- and tartrazine-free. Plastic bottles of 100.

Starter Pack: One strip (seven) of each 1 mg and 2 mg tablets and, two strips (two times seven) of 5 mg tablets in blisters.

Hyzaar® ℞
losartan potassium—hydrochlorothiazide
Angiotensin II Receptor Antagonist—Diuretic

Merck Frosst

Hyzaar® DS ℞
losartan potassium—hydrochlorothiazide
Angiotensin II Receptor Antagonist—Diuretic

Merck Frosst

Date of Revision: May 3, 2010

SUMMARY PRODUCT INFORMATION:

Route of Administration	Dosage Form/ Strength	Nonmedicinal Ingredients
Oral	Tablet 50 mg/12.5 mg, 100 mg/12.5 mg, 100 mg/25 mg	Hydroxypropyl cellulose, hypromellose, lactose monohydrate, magnesium stearate, microcrystalline cellulose, pregelatinized starch, titanium dioxide, and may contain carnauba wax. HYZAAR 50 mg/12.5 mg and HYZAAR DS 100 mg/25 mg also contain quinoline yellow aluminium lake or D&C Yellow No. 10 aluminum lake. HYZAAR 50 mg/12.5 mg contains 4.24 mg (<1 mmol) of potassium and HYZAAR 100 mg/12.5 mg and HYZAAR DS 100 mg/25 mg contain 8.48 mg (<1 mmol) of potassium, as losartan potassium. See Dosage Forms, Composition and Packaging.

INDICATIONS AND CLINICAL USE: HYZAAR (losartan potassium and hydrochlorothiazide) is indicated for the treatment of essential hypertension in patients for whom combination therapy is appropriate.

HYZAAR is not indicated as the initial therapy for essential hypertension, except in patients with severe essential hypertension (Sitting DBP ≥110 mmHg) for whom the benefit of a prompt blood pressure reduction exceeds the risk of initiating combination therapy in these patients (see Dosage and Administration).

Geriatrics (>65 years of age): No overall differences in safety or effectiveness were observed between these patients and younger patients, but greater sensitivity of some older individuals cannot be ruled out (see Dosage and Administration).

Pediatrics (<18 years of age): No data are available.

CONTRAINDICATIONS:

- Patients who are hypersensitive to this drug or to any ingredient in the formulation. For a complete listing, see Dosage Forms, Composition and Packaging.
- Because of the hydrochlorothiazide component, HYZAAR is also contraindicated in patients with anuria, and in patients who are hypersensitive to other sulfonamide-derived drugs.

WARNINGS AND PRECAUTIONS:

> **Serious Warnings and Precautions**
> **When used in pregnancy, angiotensin receptor (AT_1) blockers (ARB) can cause injury or even death of the developing fetus. When pregnancy is detected, HYZAAR should be discontinued as soon as possible (see Special Populations).**

Cardiovascular: Hypotension: Occasionally, symptomatic hypotension has occurred after administration of losartan, in some cases after the first dose. It is more likely to occur in patients who are volume-depleted by diuretic therapy, dietary salt restriction, dialysis, diarrhea, or vomiting. In these patients, because of the potential fall in blood pressure, therapy should be started under close medical supervision. Similar considerations apply to patients with ischemic heart or cerebrovascular disease, in whom an excessive fall in blood pressure could result in myocardial infarction or cerebrovascular accident.

Valvular Stenosis: There is concern on theoretical grounds that patients with aortic stenosis might be at particular risk of decreased coronary perfusion when treated with vasodilators because they do not develop as much afterload reduction.

Endocrine and Metabolism: Metabolism: Hyperuricemia may occur or acute gout may be precipitated in certain patients receiving thiazide therapy.

Thiazides may decrease serum PBI levels without signs of thyroid disturbance.

Thiazides have been shown to increase excretion of magnesium; this may result in hypomagnesemia.

Thiazides may decrease urinary calcium excretion. Thiazides may cause intermittent and slight elevation of serum calcium in the absence of known disorders of calcium metabolism. Marked hypercalcemia may be evidence of hidden hyperparathyroidism. Thiazides should be discontinued before carrying out tests for parathyroid function.

Increases in cholesterol, triglyceride and glucose levels may be associated with thiazide diuretic therapy.

Hepatic/Biliary/Pancreatic: Patients with Liver Impairment: Based on pharmacokinetic data which demonstrate significantly increased plasma concentrations of losartan and its active metabolite in cirrhotic patients after administration of COZAAR (losartan potassium), a lower dose should be considered for patients with hepatic impairment, or a history of hepatic impairment (see Dosage and Administration).

Thiazides should be used with caution in patients with impaired hepatic function or progressive liver disease, since minor alterations of fluid and electrolyte balance may precipitate hepatic coma.

Renal: Renal Impairment: As a consequence of inhibiting the renin-angiotensin-aldosterone system, changes in renal functions have been reported in susceptible individuals. In patients whose renal function may depend on the activity of the renin-angiotensin-aldosterone system, such as patients with bilateral renal artery stenosis, unilateral renal artery stenosis to a solitary kidney, or severe congestive heart failure, treatment with agents that inhibit this system has been associated with oliguria, progressive azotemia, and rarely, acute renal failure and/or death. In susceptible patients, concomitant diuretic use may further increase risk.

Use of losartan should include appropriate assessment of renal function.

Thiazides should be used with caution.

Because of the hydrochlorothiazide component, HYZAAR is not recommended in patients with severe renal impairment (creatinine clearance ≤30 mL/min).

Azotemia: Azotemia may be precipitated or increased by hydrochlorothiazide. Cumulative effects of the drug may develop in patients with impaired renal function. If increasing azotemia and oliguria occur during treatment of severe progressive renal disease the diuretic should be discontinued.

Sensitivity/Resistance: Hypersensitivity Reactions: Sensitivity reactions to hydrochlorothiazide may occur in patients with or without a history of allergy or bronchial asthma.

The possibility of exacerbation or activation of systemic lupus erythematosus has been reported in patients treated with hydrochlorothiazide.

Special Populations: Pregnant Women: Drugs that act directly on the renin-angiotensin-aldosterone-system (RAAS) can cause fetal and neonatal morbidity and death when administered to pregnant women. When pregnancy is detected, HYZAAR should be discontinued as soon as possible.

The use of ARB is not recommended during pregnancy. Epidemiological evidence regarding the risk of teratogenicity following exposure to angiotensin converting enzyme inhibitors (another class of therapeutic products interfering with the RAAS) during the first trimester of pregnancy has not been conclusive; however a small increase in risk cannot be excluded. Given the current evidence available on the risk with ARB, similar risks may exist for this class of drugs. Patients planning pregnancy should be changed to alternative antihypertensive treatments which have an established safety profile for use in pregnancy. When pregnancy is diagnosed, treatment with angiotensin II antagonists should be stopped immediately, and, if appropriate, alternative therapy should be started.

The use of ARBs during the second and third trimesters is known to induce human fetotoxicity (decreased renal function; oligohydramnios, skull ossification retardation) and neonatal toxicity (renal failure, hypotension, hyperkalemia).

Infants with a history of in utero exposure to ARB should be closely observed for hypotension, oliguria, and hyperkalemia. If oliguria occurs, attention should be directed toward support of blood pressure and renal perfusion. Exchange transfusion or dialysis may be required as means of reversing hypotension and/or substituting for impaired renal function; however, limited experience with those procedures has not been associated with significant clinical benefit. Neither losartan nor the active metabolite can be removed by hemodialysis.

Thiazides cross the placental barrier and appear in cord blood. The routine use of diuretics in otherwise healthy pregnant women is not recommended and exposes mother and fetus to unnecessary hazard including fetal or neonatal jaundice, thrombocytopenia and possibly other adverse experiences which have occurred in the adult. Diuretics do not prevent development of toxemia of pregnancy and there is no satisfactory evidence that they are useful in the treatment of toxemia.

Animal data: Losartan potassium has been shown to produce adverse effects in rat fetuses and neonates, which include decreased body weight, mortality and/or renal toxicity. Significant levels of losartan and its active metabolite were shown to be present in rat milk. Based on pharmacokinetic assessments, these findings are attributed to drug exposure in late gestation and during lactation.

Nursing Women: It is not known whether losartan or its active metabolite are excreted in human milk, but significant levels of both of these compounds have been found in the milk of lactating rats. Thiazides appear in human milk. Because many drugs are excreted in human milk and because of their potential for affecting the nursing infant adversely, a decision should be made whether to discontinue nursing or discontinue the drug, taking into account the importance of the drug to the mother.

Pediatrics (<18 years of age): HYZAAR has not been studied in children, therefore use in this age group is not recommended.

Geriatrics (>65 years of age): No overall differences in safety were observed between elderly patients and younger patients, but appropriate caution should nevertheless be used when prescribing to the elderly, as increased vulnerability to drug effect is possible in this patient population.

ADVERSE REACTIONS: Adverse Drug Reaction Overview: HYZAAR has been evaluated for safety in 2498 patients treated for essential hypertension. Of these, 1088 were treated with HYZAAR monotherapy in controlled clinical trials. In open studies, 926 patients were treated with HYZAAR for a year or more.

The following potentially serious adverse reactions have been reported rarely with HYZAAR in controlled clinical trials: syncope, hypotension.

In controlled clinical trials, discontinuations of therapy due to clinical adverse experiences occurred in 2.4% and 2.1% of patients treated with HYZAAR and placebo, respectively.

Clinical Trial Adverse Drug Reactions: Because clinical trials are conducted under very specific conditions the adverse reaction rates observed in the clinical trials may not reflect the rates observed in practice and should not be compared to the rates in the clinical trials of another drug. Adverse drug reaction information from clinical trials is useful for identifying drug-related adverse events and for approximating rates.

In double-blind controlled clinical trials, the following adverse experiences were reported with losartan potassium-hydrochlorothiazide in ≥1% of patients, regardless of drug relationship: see Table 1.

Table 1: HYZAAR

Adverse Experiences Reported with Losartan Potassium-Hydrochlorothiazide in ≥1% of Patients

	Losartan Potassium-Hydrochlorothiazide (n=1088)	Losartan Alone (n=655)	Hydrochlorothiazide (n=272)	Placebo (n=187)
Body as a Whole				
Abdominal pain	1.3	0.9	1.8	1.1
Asthenia/fatigue	3.1	2.9	5.1	3.7
Edema/swelling	1.2	0.6	2.9	1.6
Cardiovascular				
Palpitation	1.6	1.5	1.1	0
Digestive				
Diarrhea	1.6	1.8	0.4	2.1
Nausea	1.5	1.2	0	2.1
Musculoskeletal				
Back pain	2.9	1.1	0	0.5
Nervous/Psychiatric				
Dizziness	5.8	3.7	3.7	3.2
Headache	8	10.5	14	15
Respiratory				
Bronchitis	1.1	1.2	0.4	1.6
Cough	2.2	2.1	1.1	2.1
Influenza	1.2	0.2	0.7	0.5
Pharyngitis	1.2	0.8	1.8	1.6
Sinusitis	1	0.9	2.2	0.5
Upper respiratory infection	5.8	4.6	5.5	4.8
Skin				
Rash	1.3	0.5	1.5	0.5

In these controlled clinical trials for essential hypertension, dizziness was the only adverse experience, occurring in more than 1% of cases, that was reported as drug-related, and that occurred at a greater incidence in losartan potassium-hydrochlorothiazide-treated (3.3%) than placebo-treated (2.1%) patients.

Severe Hypertension (SiDBP ≥110 mmHg): The adverse experience profile for patients with severe hypertension (SiDBP ≥110 mmHg) treated with losartan/hydrochlorothiazide as initial therapy was similar to the adverse experience profile in patients treated with losartan monotherapy at the time of first dose, at 4 weeks of therapy, and at 6 weeks of therapy. Additionally, the adverse experience rates for hypotension, syncope, dizziness, and increased serum creatinine (all of which are signs and symptoms of hypoperfusion) did not differ between the treatment groups.

Less Common Clinical Trial Adverse Drug Reactions (<1%): In double-blind, controlled clinical trials with losartan potassium alone, the following adverse experiences were reported at an occurrence rate of less than 1%, regardless of drug relationship: orthostatic effects, somnolence, vertigo, epistaxis, tinnitus, constipation, malaise, rash.

Abnormal Hematologic and Clinical Chemistry Findings: Liver Function Tests: Rarely, elevations of liver enzymes and/or serum bilirubin have occurred.

Hyperkalemia: In controlled hypertensive trials with losartan monotherapy and HYZAAR, a serum potassium >5.5 mEq/L occurred in 1.5% and 0.7% of patients, respectively. However, no patient discontinued losartan or HYZAAR therapy due to hyperkalemia.

Serum Creatinine, Blood Urea Nitrogen (BUN): Minor increases in blood urea nitrogen (1.0%) and serum creatinine (1.0%) were observed in patients with essential hypertension treated with HYZAAR. More marked increases have also been reported and were more likely to occur in patients with bilateral renal artery stenosis (see Warnings and Precautions).

Minor increases in blood urea nitrogen (BUN) or serum creatinine were observed in less than 0.1 percent of patients with essential hypertension treated with losartan potassium alone. In clinical studies, no patient discontinued taking losartan potassium alone due to increased BUN or serum creatinine.

No other adverse experiences have been reported with HYZAAR which have not been reported with losartan or hydrochlorothiazide individually.

Post-Market Adverse Drug Reactions: The following additional adverse reactions have been reported in post-marketing experience:

Thrombocytopenia and Adult Respiratory Distress Syndrome have been reported rarely in post-marketing experience.

Anaphylactic Reactions: Angioedema (involving swelling of the larynx and glottis causing airway obstruction and/or swelling of the face, lips, and/or tongue and pharynx, requiring therapeutic intervention in some cases) has been reported rarely in patients treated with losartan. Some patients previously experienced angioedema with ACE inhibitors. Vasculitis, including Henoch-Schoenlein purpura, has been reported rarely.

Other adverse reactions reported rarely with losartan potassium alone in open-label studies or post-marketing use, regardless of drug relationship, include anemia, hepatitis, liver function tests abnormalities, drug induced cough, asthenia, diarrhea, migraine, arthralgia, pruritus, dysgeusia, taste disorder, urticaria, erythroderma, vomiting, malaise and erectile dysfunction/impotence. Photosensitivity has been reported with both losartan potassium- and hydrochlorothiazide. Cases of muscle pain, muscle weakness, myositis and rhabdomyolysis have been reported in patients receiving angiotensin II receptor blockers.

DRUG INTERACTIONS: Drug-Drug Interactions: Diuretics: Patients on diuretics, and especially those in whom diuretic therapy was recently instituted, may occasionally experience an excessive reduction of blood pressure after initiation of therapy with losartan potassium. The possibility of symptomatic hypotension with losartan potassium can be minimized by discontinuing the diuretic or increasing the salt intake prior to initiation of treatment with losartan potassium (see Warnings and precautions, Cardiovascular,Hypotension and Dosage and Administration).

Agents Increasing Serum Potassium: Concomitant use of potassium-sparing diuretics (e.g., spironolactone, triamterene, amiloride), potassium supplements, or salt substitutes containing potassium may lead to increases in serum potassium.

Since losartan decreases the production of aldosterone, potassium-sparing diuretics or potassium supplements should be given only for documented hypokalemia and with frequent monitoring of serum potassium when losartan therapy is instituted. Potassium-containing salt substitutes should also be used with caution. Concomitant thiazide diuretic use may attenuate any effect that losartan may have on serum potassium.

Lithium Salts: As with other drugs which eliminate sodium, lithium clearance may be reduced in the presence of losartan. Therefore, serum lithium levels should be monitored carefully if lithium salts are to be administered with losartan.

Lithium generally should not be given with diuretics. Diuretic agents reduce the renal clearance of lithium and add a high risk of lithium toxicity.

Digitalis: In 9 healthy volunteers, when a single oral dose of 0.5 mg digoxin was administered to patients receiving losartan for 11 days, digoxin AUC and digoxin C_{max} ratios, relative to placebo, were found to be 1.06 (90% C.I. 0.98-1.14) and 1.12 (90% C.I. 0.97-1.28), respectively. The effect of losartan on steady-state pharmacokinetics of cardiac glycosides is not known.

Thiazide-induced electrolyte disturbances may predispose to digitalis-induced arrhythmias.

Warfarin: Losartan administered for 7 days did not affect the pharmacokinetics or pharmacodynamic activity of a single dose of warfarin. The effect of losartan on steady-state pharmacokinetics of warfarin is not known.

Drugs Affecting Cytochrome P450 System: Rifampin, an inducer of drug metabolism, decreases the concentrations of the active metabolite of losartan. In humans, two inhibitors of P450 3A4 have been studied. Ketoconazole did not affect the conversion of losartan to the active metabolite after intravenous administration of losartan, and erythromycin had no clinically significant effect after oral losartan administration. Fluconazole, an inhibitor of P450 2C9, decreased active metabolite concentration. The pharmacodynamic consequences of concomitant use of losartan and inhibitors of P450 2C9 have not been examined.

When losartan was administered to 10 healthy male volunteers as a single dose in steady-state conditions of phenobarbital, a cytochrome P450 inducer, losartan AUC, relative to baseline, was 0.80 (90% C.I. 0.72-0.88), while AUC of the active metabolite, E-3174, was 0.80 (90% C.I. 0.78-0.82).

When losartan was administered to 8 healthy male volunteers as a single dose in steady-state conditions of cimetidine, a cytochrome P450 inhibitor, losartan AUC, relative to baseline, was 1.18 (90% C.I. 1.10-1.27), while AUC of the active metabolite, E-3174, was 1.00 (90% C.I. 0.92-1.08).

d-Tubocurarine: Thiazide drugs may increase the responsiveness to tubocurarine.

Insulin: Insulin requirements in diabetic patients treated with diuretics may be increased, decreased or unchanged. Diabetes mellitus which has been latent may become manifest during thiazide administration.

Alcohol, Barbiturates, or Narcotics: Diuretic potentiation of orthostatic hypotension may occur.

Corticosteroids, ACTH: Intensified electrolyte depletion, particularly hypokalemia, may occur when given concomitantly with diuretics.

Cholestyramine and Colestipol Resins: Absorption of hydrochlorothiazide is impaired in the presence of anionic exchange resins. Single doses of either cholestyramine or colestipol resins bind the hydrochlorothiazide and reduce its absorption from the gastrointestinal tract by up to 85 and 43 percent, respectively.

Pressor Amines (e.g. norepinephrine): In the presence of diuretics possible decreased response to pressor amines may be seen but not sufficient to preclude their use.

Non-Steroidal Anti-inflammatory Drugs Including Cyclooxygenase-2 Inhibitors: In some patients, the administration of a non-steroidal anti-inflammatory agent including a selective cyclooxygenase-2 inhibitor can reduce the diuretic, natriuretic, and antihypertensive effects of loop, potassium-sparing and thiazide diuretics. Therefore, when HYZAAR and non-steroidal anti-inflammatory agents are used concomitantly, the patient should be observed closely to determine if the desired effect of the diuretic is obtained.

Non-steroidal anti-inflammatory drugs (NSAIDs) including indomethacin and selective cyclooxygenase-2 inhibitors (COX-2 inhibitors) may reduce the effect of diuretics and other antihypertensive drugs. Therefore, the antihypertensive effect of angiotensin II receptor antagonists or ACE inhibitors may be attenuated by NSAIDs including selective COX-2 inhibitors.

In some patients with compromised renal function (e.g., elderly patients or patients who are volume-depleted, including those on diuretic therapy) who are being treated with NSAIDS, including selective COX-2 inhibitors, the coadministration of angiotensin II receptor antagonists or ACE inhibitors may result in a further deterioration of renal function. Cases of acute renal failure, usually reversible, have been reported. Therefore, this combination should be administered with caution in this patient population.

DOSAGE AND ADMINISTRATION: Dosing Considerations:

- **Dosage must be individualized.**
- **The fixed combination is not for initial therapy, except for severe hypertension.**
- **The dose of HYZAAR should be determined by the titration of the individual components.**

Recommended Dose and Dosage Adjustment: Hypertension: Once the patient has been stabilized on the individual components as described below, either one tablet HYZAAR 50 mg/12.5 mg or 100 mg/12.5 mg, or one tablet HYZAAR DS 100 mg/25 mg once daily may be substituted if the doses on which the patient was stabilized are the same as those in the fixed combination. The maximum dose is one tablet HYZAAR DS 100 mg/25 mg once daily (see Indications and Clinical Use).

Severe Hypertension (SiDBP ≥110 mmHg): The starting dose of HYZAAR for initial treatment of severe hypertension is one tablet of HYZAAR 50 mg/12.5 mg once daily. For patients who do not respond adequately to HYZAAR 50 mg/12.5 mg after 2 to 4 weeks of therapy, the dosage may be increased to one tablet of HYZAAR DS 100 mg/25 mg once daily. The maximum dose is one tablet of HYZAAR DS 100 mg/25 mg once daily.

HYZAAR may be administered with or without food, however it should be taken consistently with respect to food intake.

Losartan Monotherapy: The usual starting dose of losartan monotherapy is 50 mg once daily.

Dosage should be adjusted according to blood pressure response. The maximal antihypertensive effect is attained 3-6 weeks after initiation of therapy.

The usual dose range for losartan is 50 to 100 mg once daily. A dose of 100 mg daily should not be exceeded, as no additional antihypertensive effect is obtained with higher doses.

In most patients taking losartan 50 mg once daily, the antihypertensive effect is maintained. In some patients treated once daily, the antihypertensive effect may diminish toward the end of the dosing interval. This can be evaluated by measuring the blood pressure just prior to dosing to determine whether satisfactory control is being maintained for 24 hours. If it is not, either twice daily administration with the same total daily dosage, or an increase in the dose should be considered. If blood pressure is not adequately controlled with losartan alone, a non-potassium-sparing diuretic may be administered concomitantly.

For patients with volume-depletion, a starting dose of 25 mg once daily should be considered (see Warnings and Precautions, Hypotension and Drug Interactions).

Diuretic Treated Patients: In patients receiving diuretics, losartan therapy should be initiated with caution, since these patients may be volume-depleted and thus more likely to experience hypotension following initiation of additional antihypertensive therapy. Whenever possible, all diuretics should be discontinued two to three days prior to the administration of losartan, to reduce the likelihood of hypotension (see Warnings and Precautions, Hypotension and Drug Interactions, Diuretics). If this is not possible because of the patient's condition, losartan should be administered with caution and the blood pressure monitored closely. Thereafter, the dosage should be adjusted according to the individual response of the patient.

Dosage Adjustment in Renal Impairment: No initial dosage adjustment in losartan is usually necessary for patients with renal impairment, including those requiring hemodialysis. However, appropriate monitoring of these patients is recommended.

The usual regimens of therapy with HYZAAR may be followed as long as the patient's creatinine clearance is >30 mL/min. In patients with more severe renal impairment, loop diuretics are preferred to thiazides, so HYZAAR is not recommended.

Patients with Liver Impairment: Since dosage adjustment of losartan is required in patients with liver impairment, and thiazide diuretics may precipitate hepatic coma, a fixed combination product such as HYZAAR is not advisable (see Warnings and Precautions, Patients with Liver Impairment).

Geriatrics (>65 years of age): No initial dosage adjustment is necessary for most elderly patients. Appropriate caution should nevertheless be used when prescribing to the elderly, as increased vulnerability to drug effect is possible in this patient population (see Warnings and Precautions, Geriatrics (>65 years of age)).

Missed Dose: If a dose is missed, an extra dose should not be taken. The usual schedule should be resumed.

OVERDOSAGE:

No specific information is available on the treatment of overdosage with HYZAAR. Treatment is symptomatic and supportive.

Losartan: Limited data are available in regard to overdosage in humans. The most likely manifestation of overdosage would be hypotension and tachycardia.

If symptomatic hypotension should occur, supportive treatment should be instituted.

Neither losartan nor its active metabolite can be removed by hemodialysis.

Hydrochlorothiazide: The most common signs and symptoms observed are those caused by electrolyte depletion (hypokalemia, hypochloremia, hyponatremia) and dehydration resulting from excessive diuresis. If digitalis has also been administered, hypokalemia may accentuate cardiac arrhythmias.

The degree to which hydrochlorothiazide is removed by hemodialysis has not been established.

For management of a suspected drug overdose, contact your regional Poison Control Centre. See the *CPS* Directory section for a list of Poison Control Centres.

ACTION AND CLINICAL PHARMACOLOGY: Mechanism of Action: HYZAAR combines the actions of losartan potassium, an angiotensin II receptor antagonist, and that of a thiazide diuretic, hydrochlorothiazide.

Losartan: Losartan potassium antagonizes angiotensin II by blocking the angiotensin type one (AT_1) receptor.

Angiotensin II is the primary vasoactive hormone of the renin-angiotensin system. Its effects include vasoconstriction and the stimulation of aldosterone secretion by the adrenal cortex.

Losartan, and its active metabolite, E-3174, block the vasoconstrictor and aldosterone-secreting effects of angiotensin II by selectively blocking the binding of angiotensin II to AT_1 receptors found in many tissues, including vascular smooth muscle. A second type of angiotensin II receptor has been identified as the AT_2 receptor, but it plays no known role in cardiovascular homeostasis to date. Both losartan and its active metabolite do not exhibit any agonist activity at the AT_1 receptor, and have much greater affinity, in the order of 1000-fold, for the AT_1 receptor than for the AT_2 receptor. In vitro binding studies indicate that losartan itself is a reversible, competitive antagonist at the AT_1 receptor, while the active metabolite is 10 to 40 times more potent than losartan, and is a reversible, non-competitive antagonist of the AT_1 receptor.

Neither losartan nor its active metabolite inhibits angiotensin converting enzyme (ACE), also known as kininase II, the enzyme that converts angiotensin I to angiotensin II and degrades bradykinin, nor do they bind to or block other hormone receptors or ion channels known to be important in cardiovascular regulation.

Hydrochlorothiazide: Hydrochlorothiazide is a diuretic and antihypertensive which interferes with the renal tubular mechanism of electrolyte reabsorption. It increases excretion of sodium and chloride in approximately equivalent amounts. Natriuresis may be accompanied by some loss of potassium and bicarbonate. While this compound is predominantly a saluretic agent, in vitro studies have shown that it has a carbonic anhydrase inhibitory action which seems to be relatively specific for the renal tubular mechanism. It does not appear to be concentrated in erythrocytes or the brain in sufficient amounts to influence the activity of carbonic anhydrase in those tissues.

Hydrochlorothiazide is useful in the treatment of hypertension. It may be used alone or as an adjunct to other antihypertensive drugs. Hydrochlorothiazide does not affect normal blood pressure.

Pharmacodynamics: Losartan: Losartan inhibits the pressor effect of angiotensin II. A dose of 100 mg inhibits this effect by about 85% at peak, with 25-40% inhibition persisting for 24 hours. Removal of the negative feedback of angiotensin II causes a 2-3 fold rise in plasma renin activity, and a consequent rise in angiotensin II plasma concentration, in hypertensive patients.

Maximum blood pressure lowering, following oral administration of a single dose of losartan, as seen in hypertensive patients, occurs at about 6 hours.

In losartan-treated patients during controlled trials, there was no meaningful change in heart rate.

There is no apparent rebound effect after abrupt withdrawal of losartan therapy.

Black hypertensive patients show a smaller average blood pressure response to losartan monotherapy than other hypertensive patients.

Hydrochlorothiazide: Onset of the diuretic action following oral administration occurs in 2 hours and the peak action in about 4 hours. Diuretic activity lasts about 6 to 12 hours.

Losartan-Hydrochlorothiazide: The components of HYZAAR have been shown to have an additive effect on blood pressure reduction, reducing blood pressure to a greater degree than either component alone.

The antihypertensive effect of HYZAAR is sustained for a 24-hour period. In clinical studies of at least one year's duration, the antihypertensive effect was maintained with continued therapy. Despite the significant decrease in blood pressure, administration of HYZAAR had no clinically significant effect on heart rate.

Pharmacokinetics: Absorption: Losartan: Following oral administration, losartan is well absorbed, with systemic bioavailability of losartan approximately 33%. About 14% of an orally-administered dose of losartan is converted to the active metabolite, although about 1% of subjects did not convert losartan efficiently to the active metabolite.

Mean peak concentrations of losartan occur at about one hour, and that of its active metabolite at about 3-4 hours. Although maximum plasma concentrations of losartan and its active metabolite are approximately equal, the AUC of the metabolite is about 4 times greater than that of losartan.

Hydrochlorothiazide: Hydrochlorothiazide is rapidly absorbed from the gastrointestinal tract with an oral bioavailability of about 65% to 75%. Peak concentrations of hydrochlorothiazide were reached approximately 2 hours after dosing.

Distribution: Losartan: Both losartan and its active metabolite are highly bound to plasma proteins, primarily albumin, with plasma free fractions of 1.3% and 0.2% respectively. Plasma protein binding is constant over the concentration range achieved with recommended doses. Studies in rats indicate that losartan crosses the blood-brain barrier poorly, if at all.

The volume of distribution of losartan is about 34 liters, and that of the active metabolite is about 12 liters.

Hydrochlorothiazide: Hydrochlorothiazide crosses the placental but not the blood-brain barrier and is excreted in breast milk.

Metabolism: Losartan: Losartan is an orally active agent that undergoes substantial first-pass metabolism by cytochrome P450 enzymes. It is converted, in part, to an active carboxylic acid metabolite, E-3174, that is responsible for most of the angiotensin II receptor antagonism that follows oral losartan administration.

Various losartan metabolites have been identified in human plasma and urine. In addition to the active carboxylic acid metabolite, E-3174, several inactive metabolites are formed. In vitro studies indicate that the cytochrome P450 isoenzymes 2C9 and 3A4 are involved in the biotransformation of losartan to its metabolites.

Hydrochlorothiazide: Hydrochlorothiazide is not metabolized.

Excretion: Losartan: The terminal half-life of losartan itself is about 2 hours, and that of the active metabolite, about 6-9 hours. The pharmacokinetics of losartan and this metabolite are linear with oral losartan doses up to 200 mg and do not change over time. Neither losartan nor its metabolite accumulate in plasma upon repeated once-daily administration.

Total plasma clearance of losartan is about 600 mL/min, with about 75 mL/min accounted for by renal clearance. Total plasma clearance of the active metabolite is about 50 mL/min, with about 25 mL/min accounted for by renal clearance. Both biliary and urinary excretion contribute substantially to the elimination of losartan and its metabolites.

Following oral ^{14}C-labeled losartan, about 35% of radioactivity is recovered in the urine and about 60% in the feces. Following an intravenous dose of ^{14}C-labeled losartan, about 45% of radioactivity is recovered in the urine and 50% in the feces.

Hydrochlorothiazide: Hydrochlorothiazide is eliminated rapidly by the kidney. The plasma half-life is 5.6-14.8 hours when the plasma levels can be followed for at least 24 hours. At least 61% of the oral dose is eliminated unchanged within 24 hours.

STORAGE AND STABILITY: Store at room temperature (15-30°C). Keep container tightly closed. Protect from light.

INFORMATION FOR THE PATIENT: Published in e-CPS, available by subscription at www.e-cps.ca.

DOSAGE FORMS, COMPOSITION AND PACKAGING: HYZAAR: 50 mg/12.5 mg: Each yellow, oval shaped, film-coated tablet, marked with code 717 on one side and plain on the other, contains: losartan potassium 50 mg and hydrochlorothiazide 12.5 mg. Nonmedicinal ingredients: hydroxypropylcellulose, hypromellose, lactose monohydrate, magnesium stearate, microcrystalline cellulose, pregelatinized starch, quinoline yellow aluminum lake or D&C Yellow No. 10 aluminum lake and titanium dioxide. May contain carnauba wax. Potassium as losartan potassium: 4.24 mg (<1 mmol). Push-through blister packages of 30. Bottles of 100.

100 mg/12.5 mg: Each white to off-white, oval shaped, film-coated tablet, with code 745 on one side and plain on the other, contains: losartan potassium 100 mg and hydrochlorothiazide 12.5 mg. Nonmedicinal ingredients: hydroxypropylcellulose, hypromellose, lactose monohydrate, magnesium stearate, microcrystalline cellulose, pregelatinized starch and titanium dioxide. May contain carnauba wax. Potassium as losartan potassium: 8.48 mg (<1 mmol). Push-through blister packages of 30. Bottles of 100.

HYZAAR DS 100 mg/25 mg : Each light yellow, oval shaped, film-coated tablet, with code 747 on one side and plain on the other, contains: losartan potassium 100 mg and hydrochlorothiazide 25 mg. Nonmedicinal ingredients: hydroxypropylcellulose, hypromellose, lactose monohydrate, magnesium stearate, microcrystalline cellulose, pregelatinized starch, quinoline yellow aluminum lake or D&C Yellow No. 10 aluminum lake and titanium dioxide. May contain carnauba wax. Potassium as losartan potassium: 8.48 mg (<1 mmol). Push-through blister packages of 30. Bottles of 100.

(Shown in Product Identification Section)

I

Idamycin® Pr
idarubicin HCl
Antineoplastic

Pfizer

Idamycin® PFS Pr
idarubicin HCl
Antineoplastic

Pfizer

Date of Revision: July 20, 2009

SUMMARY PRODUCT INFORMATION:

Route of Administration	Dosage Form/ Strength	Clinically Relevant Nonmedicinal Ingredients
Intravenous injection	Lyophilised Sterile Powder, 5 mg and 10 mg vials (1 mg/mL after reconstitution)	Lactose For a complete listing see Dosage Forms, Composition and Packaging.
Intravenous injection	Solution for injection 1 mg/mL (5 mL, 10 mL, and 20 mL vials)	For a complete listing see Dosage Forms, Composition and Packaging.

INDICATIONS AND CLINICAL USE: IDAMYCIN (idarubicin hydrochloride for injection, house std.) and IDAMYCIN PFS (idarubicin hydrochloride injection) alone or in combination chemotherapy regimens involving other cytotoxic agents are indicated in:
- Acute non-lymphocytic leukemia (ANLL); in adults for remission induction as front-line therapy or for remission induction in relapsed or refractory patients.
- Acute lymphocytic leukemia (ALL) as second line treatment in adults and children.

Pediatrics: IDAMYCIN and IDAMYCIN PFS are indicated in Acute lymphocytic leukemia (ALL) as second line treatment in children.

Geriatrics (>65 years of age): Patients over 60 years of age who were undergoing induction therapy experienced congestive heart failure, serious arrhythmias, chest pain, myocardial infarction, and asymptomatic declines in LVEF more frequently than younger patients (see Warnings and Precautions, Dosage and Administration and Adverse Reactions).

CONTRAINDICATIONS:
- Patients who are hypersensitive to idarubicin or to any ingredient in the formulation or component of the container. For a complete listing, see Dosage Forms, Composition and Packaging.
- Hypersensitivity to any other anthracyclines or anthracenediones such as PHARMORUBICIN (epirubicin hydrochloride), daunorubicin hydrochloride, mitoxantrone or mitomycin C;
- Uncontrolled infections;
- Marked persistent myelosuppression induced by prior treatment with other antitumour agents or by radiotherapy;
- Severe hepatic impairment;
- Severe renal impairment;
- Severe myocardial insufficiency;
- Recent myocardial infarction;
- Severe arrhythmias;
- History of severe cardiac disease;
- Previous treatment with maximum cumulative doses of idarubicin, doxorubicin, daunorubicin, epirubicin and/or other anthracyclines and anthracenediones (see Warnings and Precautions).

WARNINGS AND PRECAUTIONS:

> **Serious Warnings and Precautions**
> **IDAMYCIN and IDAMYCIN PFS are intended for use under the direction of physicians experienced in chemotherapy.**
> - **Myelosuppression (see Warnings and Precautions, Hematologic)**
> - **Cardiotoxicity (see Warnings and Precautions, Cardiovascular)**

General: Therapy with IDAMYCIN or IDAMYCIN PFS requires close observation of the patient and laboratory monitoring. Idarubicin may induce hyperuricemia as a consequence of the extensive purine catabolism that accompanies drug-induced rapid lysis of neoplastic cells ('tumour lysis syndrome'). Blood uric acid levels, potassium, calcium, phosphate, and creatinine should be evaluated after initial treatment. Hydration, urine alkalinization, and prophylaxis with allopurinol to prevent hyperuricemia may minimize potential complications of tumour lysis syndrome. Appropriate measures must be taken to control any systemic infection before beginning therapy.

Patients should recover from acute toxicities of prior cytotoxic treatment (such as stomatitis, neutropenia, thrombocytopenia, and generalized infections) before beginning treatment with idarubicin.

Extravasation of IDAMYCIN or IDAMYCIN PFS at the site of intravenous injection can cause severe local tissue necrosis. The risk of thrombophlebitis at the injection site may be minimized by following the recommended procedure for administration.

Carcinogenesis and Mutagenesis: Like most other cytotoxic agents, idarubicin has mutagenic properties.

Idarubicin was genotoxic in most of the in vitro or in vivo tests performed. Intravenous idarubicin was carcinogenic, toxic to the reproductive organs, and embryotoxic and teratogenic in rats.

Idarubicin can induce chromosomal damage in human spermatozoa. For this reason, males undergoing idarubicin treatment should use contraceptive measures.

Secondary leukemia, with or without a preleukemic phase, has been reported in patients treated with anthracyclines, including idarubicin. Secondary leukemia is more common when such drugs are given in combination with DNA-damaging antineoplastic agents. These leukemias can have a 1- to 3-year latency period.

Cardiovascular: Cardiotoxicity is a risk of anthracycline treatment that may be manifested by early (i.e., acute) or late (ie, delayed) events.

Early (i.e., Acute) Events: Early cardiotoxicity of idarubicin consists mainly of sinus tachycardia and/or ECG abnormalities, such as non-specific ST-T wave changes. Tachyarrhythmias, including premature ventricular contractions and ventricular tachycardia, bradycardia, as well as atrioventricular and bundle-branch block have also been reported. These effects do not usually predict subsequent development of delayed cardiotoxicity, are rarely of clinical importance, and are generally not a consideration for the discontinuation of idarubicin treatment. However acute life-threatening arrhythmias have been occasionally observed during therapy. Subacute effects such as pericarditis/myocarditis have also been reported.

Late (i.e., Delayed) Events: Delayed cardiotoxicity usually develops late in the course of therapy or within 2 to 3 months after completion of treatment, but later events, several months to years after completion of treatment have also been reported. Delayed cardiomyopathy is manifested by reduced left ventricular ejection fraction (LVEF) and/or signs and symptoms of congestive heart failure (CHF) such as dyspnea, pulmonary edema, dependent edema, cardiomegaly and hepatomegaly, oliguria, ascites, pleural effusion, and gallop rhythm. Subacute effects such as pericarditis/myocarditis have also been reported. Life-threatening CHF is the most severe form of anthracycline-induced cardiomyopathy and represents the cumulative dose-limiting toxicity of the drug.

Cumulative dose limits for i.v. or oral idarubicin have not been defined. **However, idarubicin-related cardiomyopathy was reported in 5% of patients who received cumulative i.v. doses of 150 to 290 mg/m².** Available data on patients treated with oral idarubicin total cumulative doses up to 400 mg/m² suggest a low probability of cardiotoxicity.

Cardiac function should be assessed before patients undergo treatment with idarubicin and must be monitored throughout therapy to minimize the risk of incurring severe cardiac impairment. The risk may be decreased through regular monitoring of LVEF during the course of treatment with prompt discontinuation of idarubicin at the first sign of impaired function. The appropriate quantitative method for repeated assessment of cardiac function (evaluation of LVEF) includes multi-gated radionuclide angiography (MUGA) or echocardiography (ECHO). A baseline cardiac evaluation with an ECG and either a MUGA scan or an ECHO is recommended, especially in patients with risk factors for increased cardiotoxicity. Repeated MUGA or ECHO determinations of LVEF should be performed, particularly with higher, cumulative anthracycline doses. The technique used for assessment should be consistent throughout follow-up.

Risk factors for cardiac toxicity include active or dormant cardiovascular disease, prior or concomitant radiotherapy to the mediastinal/pericardial area, previous therapy with other anthracyclines or anthracenediones, and concomitant use of drugs with the ability to suppress cardiac contractility or cardiotoxic drugs. Anthracyclines including idarubicin should not be administered in combination with other cardiotoxic agents unless the patient's cardiac function is closely monitored.

Patients receiving anthracyclines after stopping treatment with other cardiotoxic agents, especially those with long half-lives such as trastuzumab, may also be at an increased risk of developing cardiotoxicity. The half-life of trastuzumab is approximately 28.5 days and may persist in the circulation for up to 24 weeks. Therefore, physicians should avoid anthracycline-based therapy for up to 24 weeks after stopping trastuzumab when possible. If anthracyclines are used before this time, careful monitoring of cardiac function is recommended.

Cardiac function monitoring must be particularly strict in patients receiving high cumulative doses and in those with risk factors. However, cardiotoxicity with idarubicin may also occur at lower cumulative doses whether or not cardiac risk factors are present.

Cardiac toxicity of the type described for other anthracycline compounds, manifested by clinically evident CHF or by a decrease in LVEF may occur during therapy or several weeks after termination of therapy. Discontinuation of IDAMYCIN or IDAMYCIN PFS and treatment with vasodilators, diuretics, digitalis, sodium restriction and bed-rest are indicated.

In infants and children, there appears to be a greater susceptibility to anthracycline-induced cardiac toxicity, and a long-term periodic evaluation of cardiac function should be performed.

Extravasation and Vascular Effects: Extravasation of IDAMYCIN or IDAMYCIN PFS during intravenous administration can cause local pain, severe tissue lesions (vesication, severe cellulitis) and severe local tissue necrosis. Extravasation may occur with or without an accompanying stinging or burning sensation even if blood returns well on aspiration of the infusion needle. If signs or symptoms of extravasation occur, the injection or infusion should be immediately stopped (see Dosage and Administration).

Phlebosclerosis may result from an injection into a small vessel or from previous injections into the same vein. Following the recommended procedures may minimize the risk of phlebitis/thrombophlebitis at the injection site (see Dosage and Administration).

As with other cytotoxic agents, thrombophlebitis and thromboembolic phenomena, including pulmonary embolism, have been coincidentally reported with the use of idarubicin.

Gastrointestinal: Idarubicin is emetogenic. Mucositis (mainly stomatitis, less often esophagitis) generally appears early after drug administration and, if severe, may progress over a few days to mucosal ulcerations. Most patients recover from this adverse event by the third week of therapy.

Occasionally, episodes of serious gastrointestinal events (such as perforation or bleeding) have been observed in patients receiving oral idarubicin who had acute leukemia or a history of other pathologies or had received medications known to lead to gastrointestinal complications. In patients with active gastrointestinal disease with increased risk of bleeding and/or perforation, the physician must balance the benefit of oral idarubicin therapy against the risk.

Hematologic: IDAMYCIN and IDAMYCIN PFS are potent bone marrow suppressants. Myelosuppression primarily of leukocytes will therefore occur in all patients given a therapeutic dose of this agent. Hematologic profiles should be assessed before and during each cycle of therapy with idarubicin including differential white blood cell (WBC) counts. A dose-dependent reversible leukopenia and/or granulocytopenia (neutropenia) is the predominant manifestation of idarubicin hematologic toxicity and is the most common acute dose-limiting toxicity of this drug. Leukopenia and neutropenia are usually severe; thrombocytopenia and anemia may also occur. Neutrophil and platelet counts usually reach their nadir 10 to 14 days following administration; however cell counts generally return to normal levels during the third week. Clinical consequences of severe myelosuppression may be fever, infections, sepsis/septicemia, septic shock, hemorrhage, tissue hypoxia, or death. Facilities with laboratory and supportive resources adequate to monitor drug tolerability and protect and maintain a patient compromised by drug toxicity should be available. It must be possible to treat rapidly and completely a severe hemorrhagic condition and/or a severe infection.

Hepatic/Biliary/Pancreatic: IDAMYCIN or IDAMYCIN PFS therapy should not be administered in patients with severe liver impairment or in patients with uncontrolled infections unless the benefit outweighs the risk.

Since hepatic function impairment can affect the disposition of idarubicin, liver function should be evaluated with conventional clinical laboratory tests (using serum bilirubin as indicator) prior to, and during, treatment. In a number of Phase III clinical trials, treatment was not given if bilirubin serum levels exceeded 2 mg/dL. With other anthracyclines, a 50% dose reduction is generally employed if bilirubin levels exceed 40 µmol/L (2.35 mg/dL).

Renal: IDAMYCIN or IDAMYCIN PFS therapy should not be administered in patients with severe renal impairment.

Since renal function impairment can affect the disposition of idarubicin, kidney function should be evaluated with conventional clinical laboratory tests (using serum creatinine as indicator) prior to, and during, treatment. In a number of Phase III clinical trials, treatment was not given if creatinine serum levels exceeded 2 mg/dL. With other anthracyclines, a 50% dose reduction is generally employed if creatinine levels exceed 200 µmol/L (2.25 mg/dL).

Immunosuppressant Effects/Increased Susceptibility to Infections: Administration of live or live-attenuated vaccines in patients immunocompromised by chemotherapeutic agents including idarubicin, may result in serious or fatal infections. Vaccination with a live vaccine should be avoided in patients receiving idarubicin. Killed or inactivated vaccines may be administered; however, the response to such vaccines may be diminished.

Special Populations: Pregnant Women: The embryotoxic potential of idarubicin has been demonstrated in both in vitro and in vivo studies. However, there are no adequate and well-controlled studies in pregnant women. Therefore, women of child bearing potential should be prescribed effective contraceptive methods and counselled on the risks of pregnancy. Idarubicin should be used during pregnancy only if the potential benefit justifies the potential risk to the fetus. The patient should be informed of the potential hazard to the fetus if IDAMYCIN or IDAMYCIN PFS is to be used during pregnancy, or if the patient becomes pregnant during therapy.

Nursing Women: It is not known whether idarubicin or its metabolites are excreted in human milk. Mothers should be advised not to breastfeed while undergoing chemotherapy with IDAMYCIN or IDAMYCIN PFS.

Monitoring and Laboratory Tests: Therapy with IDAMYCIN or IDAMYCIN PFS requires close observation of the patient and laboratory monitoring (see Warnings and Precautions, General).

Cardiac function should be assessed before patients undergo treatment with idarubicin and must be monitored throughout therapy to minimize the risk of incurring severe cardiac impairment (see Warnings and Precautions, Cardiovascular).

Liver and kidney functions should be evaluated with conventional clinical laboratory tests (using serum bilirubin and serum creatinine as indicators) prior to, and during, treatment (see Warnings and Precautions, Hepatic/Biliary/Pancreatic and Warnings and Precautions, Renal).

Hematologic profiles should be assessed before and during each cycle of therapy with idarubicin including differential white blood cell (WBC) counts (see Warnings and Precautions, Hematologic).

ADVERSE REACTIONS: Cardiovascular: sinus tachycardia, ECG abnormalities, tachyarrhythmias, atrio-ventricular and bundle branch block, asymptomatic reductions in LVEF, CHF, pericarditis, myocarditis.

Hematologic: leukopenia, neutropenia, anemia, thrombocytopenia, hemorrhage.

Gastrointestinal: anorexia, nausea/vomiting, dehydration, mucositis/stomatitis, esophagitis, abdominal pain or burning sensation, erosions/ulceration, gastrointestinal tract bleeding, diarrhea, colitis, including severe enterocolitis/neutropenic enterocolitis with perforation.

Liver: elevation of liver enzymes and bilirubin.
Endocrine: hot flashes.
Skin: alopecia, local toxicity (see Warnings and Precautions), rash/itch, skin changes, skin and nail hyperpigmentation, hypersensitivity of irradiated skin ('radiation recall reaction'), urticaria, acral erythema.
Vascular: phlebitis, thrombophlebitis, thromboembolism.
Urological: red colour to the urine for 1-2 days after administration.
Other: anaphylaxis, infection, sepsis/septicemia, secondary leukemias (acute myeloid leukemia and myelodysplastic syndrome), fever, shock, hyperuricemia.

Severe and sometimes fatal infections have been associated with idarubicin alone or in combination with cytarabine. Acute toxicities such as nausea and vomiting, mucositis, diarrhea and liver dysfunction are comparable to those of daunorubicin.

IDARUBICIN appears to have a cardiac toxicity potential which is similar to that of daunorubicin. Overall, the incidence of serious cardiac events has been 2.0% out of 1204 patients receiving idarubicin via i.v. administration. If patients previously treated with anthracyclines are excluded, the overall incidence is 1.58%. When idarubicin was administered orally, the incidence of serious cardiac events (grade 3 only) was 3.2%.

DRUG INTERACTIONS: Drug-Drug Interactions: Idarubicin is a potent myelosuppressant and combination chemotherapy regimens that contain other agents with similar action (e.g. other anthracyclines, anthracenediones) may lead to additive toxicity, especially with regard to bone marrow/hematologic and gastrointestinal effects (see Warnings and Precautions). Combination chemotherapy regimens that contain other agents which may potentiate additive hematological toxicity may include alkylating agents (e.g. cyclophosphamide), antineoplastic agents (such as etoposide, cytarabine, fludarabine), and corticosteroids (e.g. dexamethasone). The use of idarubicin in combination chemotherapy with other potentially cardiotoxic drugs (e.g. cyclophosphamide, paclitaxel), as well as the concomitant use of other cardioactive compounds (e.g. calcium channel blockers such as amlodipine, diltiazem or verapamil), requires monitoring of cardiac function throughout treatment. Changes in hepatic or renal function induced by concomitant therapies may affect idarubicin metabolism, pharmacokinetics, and therapeutic efficacy and/or toxicity.

An additive myelosuppressant effect may occur when radiotherapy is given concomitantly or within 2-3 weeks prior to treatment with idarubicin.

Interactions with other drugs have not been established.

Precipitation occurs with heparin. Prolonged contact with any solution of an alkaline pH will result in degradation of the drug.
Drug-Food Interactions: Interactions with food have not been established.
Drug-Herb Interactions: Interactions with herbal products have not been established.
Drug-Laboratory Test Interactions: Interactions with laboratory tests have not been established.

DOSAGE AND ADMINISTRATION:

As with all parenteral products, intravenous solution should be inspected visually for clarity, particulate matter, precipitate, discolouration and leakage prior to administration. Solution showing haziness, particulate matter, precipitate, discolouration or leakage should not be used and **discard unused portions**.

Dosing Considerations:

- These dose schedules should take into account the hematological status of the patient and the dosage of the other cytotoxic drugs when used in combination.
- Hepatic or Renal Dysfunction. While no specific dose recommendation can be made based on the limited available data in patients with hepatic and/or renal impairment, dose reductions should be considered in patients with bilirubin and/or creatinine serum levels greater than 2 mg/dL (see Warnings and Precautions).
- The total dose of IDAMYCIN or IDAMYCIN PFS administered to a patient should take into account: prior or concomitant therapy with related compounds such as epirubicin and daunorubicin or anthracene derivatives, and/or radiotherapy to the mediastinal area.

Recommended Dose and Dosage Adjustment: Intravenous: Acute Non-Lymphocytic Leukemia (ANLL): In adults, for remission induction as front line therapy or for remission induction in relapsed or refractory patients, the following dose schedules are recommended:

a. 12 mg/m² daily by intravenous injection for 3 days in combination with cytarabine, or
b. 8 mg/m² daily by intravenous injection as a single agent for 5 days.

Acute Lymphocytic Leukemia (ALL): As a second line treatment, the following dose schedules are recommended:

a. in adults, 12 mg/m² daily by intravenous injection for 3 days as a single agent, or
b. in children, 10 mg/m² daily by intravenous injection for 3 days as a single agent.

Administration: IV administration: IDAMYCIN and IDAMYCIN PFS **must not** be administered by intramuscular or subcutaneous injection. Unless specific compatibility data are available, IDAMYCIN and IDAMYCIN PFS should not be mixed with other drugs. Precipitation occurs with heparin. Prolonged contact with any solution of an alkaline pH will result in degradation of the drug.

IDAMYCIN and IDAMYCIN PFS should be slowly administered into the tubing of a freely running intravenous infusion of Sodium Chloride injection, USP 0.9%. The tubing should be attached to a Butterfly needle or other suitable device and inserted preferably into a large vein. If possible, avoid veins over joints or in extremities with compromised venous or lymphatic drainage. The rate of administration is dependent on the size of the vein and the dosage. However, the dosage should be administered over 5 to 10 minutes. Local erythematous streaking along the vein as well as facial flushing may be indicative of too rapid administration. A burning or stinging sensation may be indicative of perivenous infiltration and the infusion should be immediately terminated and restarted in another vein. Perivenous infiltration may occur painlessly. A direct push injection is not recommended due to the risk of extravasation, which may occur even in the presence of adequate blood return upon needle aspiration (see Warnings and Precautions).

If it is known or suspected that subcutaneous extravasation has occurred, it is recommended that intermittent ice packs (½ hour immediately, then ½ hour 4 times per day for 3 days) be placed over the area of extravasation and that the affected extremity be elevated. Because of the progressive nature of extravasation reactions, the area of injection should be frequently examined and plastic surgery consultation obtained early if there is any sign of a local reaction such as pain, erythema, edema or vesication. If ulceration begins or there is severe persistent pain at the site of extravasation, early wide excision of the involved area should be considered.

Reconstitution: Parenteral Products:

Vial Size	Volume of Diluent to be Added to Vial	Approximate Available Volume	Nominal Concentration per mL
5 mg	5 mL Water for Injection USP	5 mL	1 mg/mL
10 mg	10 mL Water for Injection USP	10 mL	1 mg/mL

Preparation of the Solution: Caution in handling of the powder and preparation of the solution must be exercised as skin reaction associated with idarubicin may occur (see Special Handling Instructions).

IDAMYCIN 5 mg and 10 mg vials should be reconstituted with 5 mL and 10 mL respectively of Water for Injection USP to give a final concentration of 1 mg/mL of idarubicin hydrochloride. Diluents containing bacteriostatic agents are not recommended. The resulting solution is hypotonic and since the vial contents are under negative pressure, particular care should be taken when the needle is inserted to minimize aerosol formation during reconstitution. Inhalation of any aerosol produced during reconstitution must be avoided. The reconstituted solution is stable for 24 hours at room temperature and 48 hours under refrigeration at 2-8°C. The solution should be protected from exposure to direct light and any unused solution should be discarded.

OVERDOSAGE:

Very high doses of IDAMYCIN or IDAMYCIN PFS may be expected to cause acute myocardial toxicity within 24 hours and severe myelosuppression within 1 or 2 weeks. Treatment should aim to support the patient during this period and should utilize such measures as blood transfusions and reverse-barrier nursing. Delayed cardiac failure has been seen with the anthracyclines up to several months after the overdose. Patients should be observed carefully and if signs of cardiac failure arise, should be treated along conventional lines.

> For management of a suspected drug overdose, CPhA recommends that you contact your **regional Poison Control Centre**. See the *CPS* Directory section for a list of Poison Control Centres.

ACTION AND CLINICAL PHARMACOLOGY: Mechanism of Action: Idarubicin, either as a single agent or in combination, has been shown to be a potent antileukemic agent capable of inducing complete remission in previously untreated and in relapsed and refractory acute non-lymphocytic leukemia (ANLL) including resistant patients, and in adult and pediatric relapsed patients with acute lymphoblastic leukemia (ALL).

Idarubicin is a DNA-intercalating analog of daunorubicin which has an inhibitory effect on nucleic acid synthesis and interacts with the enzyme topoisomerase II. The modification, in position 4 of the anthracycline structure, gives the compound a high lipophilicity which results in an increased rate of cellular uptake compared with other anthracyclines.

Idarubicin has been shown to have a higher potency than daunorubicin and to be an effective agent against murine leukemias and lymphomas. In vitro studies on human and murine anthracycline resistant cells have revealed a lower degree of cross resistance for idarubicin in comparison with doxorubicin and daunorubicin.

Pharmacokinetics: Seven pharmacokinetic studies were carried out in 49 patients. The plasma concentrations of idarubicin fit a 2 or 3 compartment open models.

Studies of cellular (nucleated blood and bone marrow cells) drug concentrations in leukemic patients have shown that peak cellular idarubicin concentrations are reached a few minutes after injection. Idarubicin and idarubicinol concentrations in nucleated blood and bone marrow cells are more than 100 times the plasma concentrations. Idarubicin disappearance rates in plasma and cells were comparable with a terminal half-life of about 15 hours. The terminal half-life of idarubicinol in cells was about 72 hours.

Absorption: After oral administration to patients with normal renal and hepatic function, idarubicin is rapidly absorbed, with a peak time of 2-4 hours.

Distribution: The absolute bioavailability of idarubicin given orally has been shown to range between 18 and 39%, whereas that calculated from the data on the active metabolite, idarubicinol, is somewhat higher (29-58%). The effective bioavailability, calculated on the basis of the pharmacological response, is approximately 35%. Protein binding was studied in vitro by equilibrium dialysis at concentrations of idarubicin and idarubicinol similar to the maximum plasma level obtained in the pharmacokinetic studies. The percent of idarubicin and idarubicinol bound to human plasma proteins at the concentration of 100 ng/mL plasma is on the average 97% and 94%, respectively.

Metabolism: After intravenous administration to patient with normal and hepatic function, idarubicin is extensively metabolized to an active metabolite, idarubicinol.

Excretion: After intravenous administration to patients with normal renal and hepatic function, idarubicin is eliminated from systemic circulation with a terminal plasma half-life ranging between 11-25 hours. Active metabolite, idarubicinol, is more slowly eliminated with a plasma half-life ranging between 41-69 hours. The drug is eliminated by biliary and renal excretion, mostly in the form of active metabolite idarubicinol.

After oral administration to patients with normal renal and hepatic function, idarubicin is rapidly absorbed, with a peak time of 2-4 hours. It is rapidly eliminated from systemic circulation with a terminal plasma $t_{1/2}$ ranging between 10-35 hours and is extensively metabolized to an active metabolite, idarubicinol. Idarubicinol is more slowly eliminated with a plasma $t_{1/2}$ ranging between 33-60 hours.

STORAGE AND STABILITY: IDAMYCIN PFS (idarubicin hydrochloride injection) should be stored at 2-8°C and protected from light.

IDAMYCIN (idarubicin hydrochloride for injection, house std.) should be stored at 15-30°C and protected from light.

Stability of the Reconstituted Solution: Storage: The reconstituted solution is stable for 24 hours at room temperature or for 48 hours under refrigeration. The solution should be protected from exposure to direct light and any unused solution should be discarded.

Incompatibility: Unless specific compatibility data are available, IDAMYCIN and IDAMYCIN PFS should not be mixed with other drugs. Precipitation occurs with heparin. Prolonged contact with any solution of an alkaline pH will result in degradation of the drug.

SPECIAL HANDLING INSTRUCTIONS: Preparation and Handling:

1. Personnel should be trained in good techniques for reconstitution and handling. Pregnant staff should be excluded from working with this drug.
2. Preparation of antineoplastic solutions should be done in a vertical laminar flow hood (Biological Safety Cabinet—Class II). The work surface should be protected by disposable, plastic-backed, absorbent paper.
3. Personnel preparing idarubicin solutions should wear PVC gloves, safety glasses and protective clothing such as disposable gowns and masks. If idarubicin contacts the skin or mucosa, the area should be washed with soap and water immediately.
4. Personnel regularly involved in the preparation and handling of antineoplastics should have blood examinations on a regular basis.

Disposal:

1. Avoid contact with skin and inhalation of airborne particles by use of PVC gloves and disposable gowns and masks.
2. All needles, syringes, vials and other materials which have come in contact with IDAMYCIN and IDAMYCIN PFS should be segregated in plastic bags, sealed and marked as hazardous waste. Incinerate at 1000°C or higher. Sealed containers may explode if a tight seal exists.
3. If incineration is not available, IDAMYCIN and IDAMYCIN PFS may be detoxified by adding sodium hypochlorite solution (household bleach) to the vial, in sufficient quantity to decolourize the idarubicin, care being taken to vent the vial to avoid a pressure build-up of the chlorine gas which is generated. Dispose detoxified vials in a safe manner.

Needles, Syringes, Disposable and Non-Disposable Equipment: Rinse equipment with an appropriate quantity of sodium hypochlorite solution. Discard the solution in the sewer system with running water and discard disposable equipment in a safe manner. Thoroughly wash non-disposable equipment in soap and water.

Spillage/Contamination: Wear gloves, mask, protective clothing. Treat spilled powder or liquid with dilute sodium hypochlorite (1% available chlorine) solution. Carefully absorb solution with gauze or towels again and place in polyethylene bag; seal, double bag and mark as hazardous waste. Dispose waste by incineration or by other methods approved for hazardous materials. Personnel involved in cleanup should wash with soap and water.

INFORMATION FOR THE PATIENT: Published in e-CPS, available by subscription at www.e-cps.ca.

DOSAGE FORMS, COMPOSITION AND PACKAGING: IDAMYCIN: 5 mg: Each vial of sterile, red-orange lyophilized powder contains: idarubicin HCl 5 mg. Nonmedicinal ingredients: lactose 50 mg. Vials of 5 mg, cartons of 1.

10 mg: Each vial of sterile, red-orange lyophilized powder contains: idarubicin HCl 10 mg. Nonmedicinal ingredients: lactose 100 mg. Vials of 10 mg, cartons of 1.

IDAMYCIN PFS: Each vial of clear, red-orange, aqueous, preservative-free solution, free from visible particles contains: idarubicin HCl 1 mg/mL. Nonmedicinal ingredients: glycerol, hydrochloric acid and Water for Injection USP. The solution is filled in medical grade polypropylene vials. Vials of 5, 10 and 20 mL, cartons of 1.

Ifex® Ⓕ

ifosfamide

Antineoplastic

Baxter

Caution: Ifosfamide is a potent drug and should be used only by physicians experienced with cancer chemotherapeutic drugs (see Warnings and Precautions). In those patients who develop bacterial, fungal or viral infections, interruption or modification of dosage should be considered. Blood counts should be taken at regular intervals. Due to the urotoxic effect of oxazaphosphorines, ifosfamide should not be administered without the use of a uroprotective agent such as mesna (see Uromitexan product monograph for Dosage).

PHARMACOLOGY: Ifosfamide is activated by metabolism in the liver by the mixed-function oxidase system of the smooth endoplasmic reticulum. The activation is induced by hydroxylation at the ring carbon atom 4. Opening of the ring results in the formation of aldo-ifosfamide, the tautomer of 4-hydroxy-ifosfamide. Two stable metabolites, 4-keto-ifosfamide and 4-carboxy-ifosfamide, appear in the urine. However, they have no cytotoxic activity. N,N'-bis(2-chloroethyl)-phosphoric acid diamide and acrolein are also found. The enzymatic oxidation of the chloroethyl side chains and subsequent dealkylation may produce further metabolites.

DNA is one of the main target sites of ifosfamide. In vitro, incubation of DNA with activated ifosfamide produces phosphotriesters as the predominant reaction products. The treatment of intact cell nuclei may also result in the formation of DNA-DNA crosslinks. DNA repair occurs in G-1 and G-2 stage cells. Repair capacity is more marked in less sensitive tumors. An accumulation of cells in the G-1 phase is found in tumors that respond well.

INDICATIONS: Soft Tissue Sarcoma: First-line single agent therapy; second-line single agent therapy in patients who have failed to respond or who have relapsed on other chemotherapeutic regimens.
Pancreatic Carcinoma: Second-line single agent therapy in patients who have failed to respond or who have relapsed on other chemotherapeutic regimens.
Cervical Carcinoma: As a single agent or in combination with cisplatin and bleomycin in advanced or recurrent disease.
CONTRAINDICATIONS: In individuals with a known hypersensitivity to it. It is also contraindicated in patients having severe leukopenia, thrombocytopenia, severe renal and/or hepatic impairment, cystitis, obstructions to the urine flow, or active infections. Ifosfamide should not be administered to patients with advanced cerebral arteriosclerosis.
WARNINGS: Urotoxic side effects, especially hemorrhagic cystitis, have been frequently associated with the use of ifosfamide. Until recently these effects resulted in cessation of therapy. The therapeutic benefit of mesna as a uroprotective agent has been demonstrated in that the incidence of urinary tract complications was reduced from 40 to 3.5%. Thus ifosfamide should always be accompanied by uroprotective treatment with mesna (see Uromitexan product monograph for Dosage).

Patients, male or female, during the reproductive period of life, should be advised of the mutagenic potential of ifosfamide. Adequate methods of contraception are recommended for such patients (see Adverse Effects).
Pregnancy: **Ifosfamide can be teratogenic or cause fetal resorption in experimental animals. It should not be used in pregnancy, particularly in early pregnancy, unless in the judgment of the physician the potential benefits outweigh the possible risks.**
Lactation: **As is the case with the oxazaphosphorine class of alkylating agents, ifosfamide is excreted in breast milk and breast-feeding should be terminated prior to institution of drug therapy.**

Since the possibility of interference with normal wound healing has been reported with other oxazaphosphorines, therapy should not be initiated for at least 10 to 14 days after surgery.

Ifosfamide, like other alkylating agents, has been reported to have oncogenic activity in animals. Thus the possibility that it may have oncogenic potential in humans should be considered.
PRECAUTIONS: Ifosfamide should be given cautiously to patients with any of the following conditions: leukopenia, thrombocytopenia, tumor-cell infiltration of the bone marrow, prior radiotherapy, prior treatment with other antineoplastic agents, brain metastases and advanced cerebral arteriosclerosis, impaired renal function, impaired hepatic function, in the presence of known infections, abnormal serum creatinine and serum albumin levels.

Because ifosfamide may exert a suppressive action in immune mechanisms, the interruption or modification of dosage should be considered for patients who develop bacterial, fungal or viral infections. This is especially true for patients receiving concomitant steroid therapy, since infections in some of these patients have been fatal.

Ifosfamide may cause significant neurologic, renal and hematologic toxicities which may prove fatal despite careful monitoring prior to and during therapy.

Prior to initiating treatment, it is necessary to exclude or correct any obstruction of the efferent urinary tract, cystitis, infections, and electrolyte imbalances.

Urinary sediment should be examined at regular intervals. Extra care is required in unilaterally nephrectomized patients, in patients with impaired renal function, and in patients pretreated with nephrotoxic drugs (e.g., cisplatin) who obviously tolerate high-doses of ifosfamide less well. Ifosfamide should not be given until 3 months after the nephrectomy. Additional caution is also advisable in patients treated concomitantly with drugs having nephrotoxic potential (e.g., aminoglycosides and amphotericin B).

Careful monitoring is also required for patients with cerebral metastases, as ifosfamide has been associated with several CNS symptoms.

Leukocyte, erythrocyte and platelet counts should be carried out at regular intervals. There is normally a reduction in the leukocyte count beginning on approximately day 5. The nadir, depending on dosage and baseline count, tends to be reached after 8 to 10 days. Recovery occurs after 10 to 14 days and is usually complete after 2 to 3 weeks.

Neurologic manifestations consisting of somnolence, confusion, hallucinations and in some instances, coma have been reported following ifosfamide therapy. In the case of ifosfamide induced CNS symptoms, drugs acting on the CNS (e.g., antiemetics and narcotics) should be discontinued, if possible, or used with caution. The occurrence of these symptoms requires discontinuing ifosfamide therapy. These symptoms have usually been reversible and supporting therapy should be maintained until their resolution.
ADVERSE EFFECTS: Urinary: Hemorrhagic cystitis, manifested by the occurrence of hematuria, dysuria, urinary frequency and occasionally urinary incontinence or retention, develops frequently in patients treated with ifosfamide. The incidence, severity and persistence of ifosfamide-induced hemorrhagic cystitis increase as the dose of the drug increases. In most instances, the hematuria resolves spontaneously upon cessation of therapy.

The urinary tract toxicity of ifosfamide can be minimized by administering a uroprotective agent such as mesna (see Uromitexan product monograph for Dosage), and ensuring adequate hydration and maintenance of fluid balance.

Granular casts in the urinary sediment have occurred mainly after high doses of ifosfamide. The cylinduria generally resolves spontaneously a few days after the last injection.

Renal parenchymal and tubular necrosis, which could lead to death, have been reported. Disorders of glomerular renal function with an increase in serum creatinine, a decrease in creatinine clearance and proteinuria occasionally occur; more frequently, disorders of tubular renal function with hyperaminoaciduria, phosphaturia, acidosis, or proteinuria occur. Severe nephropathies are rare. Predisposing factors for nephrotoxicity include the presence of renal tumors, pre-existing renal impairment, prior treatment with platinum containing drugs, and concomitant treatment with potentially nephrotoxic agents (see Precautions).

Increases and decreases in creatinine clearance are usually reversible.

Metabolic acidosis was reported in 31% of patients in one study when ifosfamide was administered at doses of 2 to 2.5 g/m²/day for 4 days.

Renal tubular acidosis, Fanconi Syndrome and renal rickets have also been reported. Close clinical monitoring of serum and urine chemistries including phosphorus, potassium, alkaline phosphatase and other appropriate laboratory studies is recommended. Appropriate replacement therapy should be administered as indicated.
Hematopoietic: Leukopenia with the risk of life-threatening infection is an expected effect and ordinarily is used as a guide to therapy. Thrombocytopenia with the risk of hemorrhage and anemia have been known to occur in a few patients. These effects are almost always reversible when therapy is interrupted. Episodes of petechial bleeding due to severe thrombocytopenia have been reported.

When ifosfamide is used in combination with other myelosuppressive agents, adjustments in dosing may be necessary.
Gastrointestinal: Nausea and vomiting are dose-related and also depend on individual sensitivity. Other gastrointestinal adverse events include anorexia, diarrhea, constipation, and stomatitis.
Effects on Gonads: Gonadal suppression, resulting in amenorrhea or azoospermia, has been reported with other oxazaphosphorines and thus may occur with ifosfamide.
Integumentary: It is ordinarily advisable to inform patients in advance of possible alopecia, a frequent complication of ifosfamide therapy. Regrowth of hair can be expected although occasionally the new hair may be of a different color or texture. Nonspecific dermatitis and inflammation of mucous membranes have been reported to occur with ifosfamide.
Central Nervous System: Cerebral side effects consist mainly of somnolence, confusion, hallucinations and depressive psychosis. Other less frequent symptoms included dizziness, disorientation, cranial nerve dysfunction, and cerebellar symptoms. Seizures of the tonic-clonic type have been reported occasionally. Isolated cases of encephalitis, generalized seizure and seizures resulting in coma have also been observed.

It is possible that the severity and incidence of cerebral effects increase with the administration of high doses, the presence of brain metastases, or advanced cerebral arteriosclerosis. The incidence and extent of cerebral effects due to ifosfamide may also be affected by the age of the patient, impaired renal clearance, pretreatment with nephrotoxic drugs, and post-renal obstructions (e.g., pelvic tumors). Other possible risk factors may include decreased levels of serum albumin or hydrogen carbonate, or concurrent high-dose treatment with antiemetic drugs.
Cardiotoxicity: Although cardiotoxicity is rarely encountered, there have been reported cases of supraventricular or ventricular arrhythmias, ST segment changes and heart failure at high doses of ifosfamide, or after pretreatment or concomitant treatment with anthracyclines. Hypertension and hypotension have been reported rarely.
Respiratory: Interstitial pulmonary fibrosis has been reported in patients treated with large doses of alkylating agents for prolonged periods. Although not reported in patients treated with ifosfamide, physicians should be aware of its possible occurrence. Pulmonary toxicities, including reports of interstitial pneumonitis and pulmonary edema, have been reported from fewer than 1% of patients.
Other: Adverse reactions in addition to those mentioned above have been noted with ifosfamide. They include infection with or without fever, hematemesis, asthenia, thrombophlebitis, increase in liver enzymes and/or bilirubin, allergic reactions, polyneuropathy, impaired or blurred vision, and increased sensitivity to irradiation. In addition, in isolated cases, syndrome of inappropriate of antidiuretic hormone (SIADH) has been reported.

Pancreatitis has been reported in isolated cases.
Drug Interactions: The concurrent use of ifosfamide may enhance the anticoagulant effect of warfarin and thus raise the risk of hemorrhages.
OVERDOSE:
Treatment: No specific antidote is known. Management of overdosage would include general supportive measures to sustain the patient through any period of toxicity that might occur.

For management of a suspected drug overdose, CPhA recommends that you contact your **regional Poison Control Centre**. See the *CPS* Directory section for a list of Poison Control Centres.

DOSAGE: Chemotherapy with ifosfamide, as with other drugs used in cancer chemotherapy, is potentially hazardous and fatal complications can occur. It is recommended that it be administered only by physicians aware of the associated risks. Total dosage of 250 to 300 mg/kg per cycle is the usual standard. As a rule, 50 to 60 mg/kg are administered i.v., over a period of a minimum of 30 minutes, each day for 5 consecutive days. If the calculation of the dosage is based on body surface area, the recommended dosage is 2000 to 2400 mg/m² daily on 5 consecutive days. If a lower daily dosage or the total dosage over a longer period is indicated, ifosfamide can be given every other day (days 1, 3, 5, 7 and 9) or on 10 consecutive days in lower doses.

A treatment series should be repeated after an interval of not less than 3 to 4 weeks.

The therapeutic administration should invariably be accompanied by uroprotective treatment with mesna. Alternately, the administration of high single dose infusions is now feasible up to 5 to 8 g/m²/24 h under protection of continuous mesna infusion. The optimal use of ifosfamide in combination with other myelosuppressive agents requires dosage adjustments according to the regimen and schedule to be adopted.
Prevention of Cystitis: The concomitant administration of mesna helps to prevent the urotoxic side effects of ifosfamide which had previously limited the drug's therapeutic use. Every ifosfamide regimen should be accompanied by uroprotective treatment with mesna.

Mesna is usually given by i.v. injection concurrently with ifosfamide and 4 and 8 hours afterwards, each dose being 20% of the ifosfamide dose (see Uromitexan product monograph for Dosage).

Even with the administration of the uroprotector mesna, the daily fluid intake should be at least 2 L. If urinary excretion appears insufficient, a fast-acting diuretic such as furosemide may be administered.
Reconstitution: Preparation for I.V. Use: Reconstitute with Sterile Water for Injection as in Table 1.

Table 1: Ifex Reconstitution

Vial Size	Volume to be Added	Approximate Available Volume	Approximate Average Concentration
1 g	20 mL	20 mL	50 mg/mL
3 g	60 mL	60 mL	50 mg/mL

Shake well until dissolved. The prepared solution may be further diluted to achieve concentrations of 0.6 to 20 mg/mL with any of the solutions for i.v. infusion listed below.
Solutions for I.V. Infusion: 5% Dextrose Injection USP, 0.9% Sodium Chloride USP, Lactated Ringer's Injection USP.
Stability of Solutions: Reconstituted and further diluted solutions should be used within 24 hours from the time of the initial constitution or within 72 hours when refrigerated, when stored in glass bottles, viaflex bags or PAB bags.
Note: Product should be inspected visually for particulate matter and discoloration prior to administration.
Handling and Disposal: Preparation of ifosfamide should be done in a vertical laminar flow hood (Biological Safety Cabinet—Class II). Personnel preparing ifosfamide should wear PVC gloves, safety glasses, disposable gowns and masks. All needles, syringes, vials and other materials which have come in contact with ifosfamide should be segregated and incinerated at 1000°C or more. Sealed containers may explode. Intact vials should be returned to the manufacturer for destruction. Proper precautions should be taken in packaging these materials for transport.

Personnel regularly involved in the preparation and handling of ifosfamide should have bi-annual blood examinations.

SUPPLIED: Each vial of sterile powder contains: ifosfamide 1 g and 3 g. Nonmedicinal ingredients: none.

Ilaris™ Ⓟ

canakinumab

Immunomodulatory Agent

Novartis Pharmaceuticals

Date of Preparation: February 26, 2010
ILARIS should be used by physicians who have sufficient knowledge of Cryopyrin-Associated Periodic Syndromes (CAPS) and who have fully familiarized themselves with the efficacy/safety profile of ILARIS.

SUMMARY PRODUCT INFORMATION:

Route of Administration	Dosage Form/ Strength	Clinically Relevant Nonmedicinal Ingredients
Subcutaneous Injection	150 mg lyophilized powder for solution for injection; corresponding to a concentration of 150 mg/mL after reconstitution	Sucrose, L-histidine, L-histidine HCl monohydrate, polysorbate 80

DESCRIPTION: ILARIS (canakinumab) is a genetically engineered high-affinity human anti-human-IL-1β monoclonal antibody that belongs to the IgG1/κ isotype subclass. It is expressed in a murine Sp2/0-Ag14 cell line and comprised of two 447- (or 448-) residue heavy chains and two 214-residue light chains, with a molecular mass of 145 kDa. The mechanism of action of canakinumab is to bind to and inactivate IL-1β and thus to inhibit the downstream events of IL-1β signalling.

ILARIS is supplied in sterile, single-use, colorless 6 mL glass vial. Each vial contains 150 mg of canakinumab as a white, preservative-free, lyophilized powder, which is intended for delivery by subcutaneous injection after reconstitution with 1 mL of preservative-free sterile water.

INDICATIONS AND CLINICAL USE: ILARIS is indicated for the ongoing management of Cryopyrin-Associated Periodic Syndromes (CAPS), in adults and children aged 4 years and older, including:
- Familial Cold Autoinflammatory Syndrome (FCAS)/ Familial Cold Urticaria (FCU),
- Muckle-Wells Syndrome (MWS)

ILARIS may also be used in Neonatal-Onset Multisystem Inflammatory Disease (NOMID)/Chronic Infantile Neurological, Cutaneous, Articular Syndrome (CINCA). Clinical data to support the use of ILARIS in patients with this phenotype are still very limited.
Geriatrics (>65 years of age): Clinical studies of ILARIS did not include sufficient numbers of subjects aged 65 and over to determine whether they respond differently from younger subjects.
Pediatrics (<4 years of age): ILARIS is not recommended for use in children below age of 4 years or with body weight below 15 kg due to lack of clinical data.

CONTRAINDICATIONS: Patients who are hypersensitive to canakinumab or to any ingredient in the formulation of ILARIS or component of the container. For a complete listing, see Dosage Forms, Composition and Packaging. A risk for hypersensitivity reactions, which is not uncommon for injectable proteins, can not be excluded.

Patients who have active, severe infections (see Adverse Reactions, Serious Infections).

WARNINGS AND PRECAUTIONS: Serious Infections: ILARIS may be associated with an increased incidence of serious infections. Therefore patients should be monitored carefully for signs and symptoms of infections during and after treatment with ILARIS. Physicians should exercise caution when administering ILARIS to patients with infections, a history of recurring infections or underlying conditions which may predispose them to infections. Treatment with ILARIS should not be initiated or continued in patients with active infection requiring medical intervention.

Infections, predominantly of the upper respiratory tract, in some instances serious, have been reported more frequently with ILARIS than with placebo treatment. All infections responded to standard therapy. No unusual or opportunistic infections were reported with ILARIS.

In canakinumab-treated patients with serious and systemic infections, a physiological inflammatory response was maintained as evidenced by concomitant C-reactive protein (CRP) elevation and fever. A blunted inflammatory response to infections cannot be excluded and increased vigilance is therefore recommended.

Drugs that affect the immune system by blocking TNF have been associated with an increased risk of reactivation of latent tuberculosis (TB). It is possible that taking drugs such as ILARIS that block IL-1 increases the risk of TB or other atypical or opportunistic infections.

Prior to initiating immunomodulatory therapies, including ILARIS, patients should be tested for latent tuberculosis infection. ILARIS has not been studied in patients with a positive tuberculosis screen, and the safety of ILARIS in individuals with latent tuberculosis infection is unknown. Patients testing positive in tuberculosis screening should be treated by standard medical practice prior to therapy with ILARIS.

Concomitant use of ILARIS with tumour necrosis factor (TNF) inhibitors is not recommended because this may increase the risk of serious infections (see Drug Interactions).

Cardiovascular: In clinical trials for CAPS, notable changes from baseline in systolic and diastolic blood pressure values were more frequently seen in patients in the canakinumab group than in patients in the placebo group. Blood pressure should be monitored in patients on ILARIS treatment (see Adverse Reactions, Vital Signs and Physical Findings).

Neutropenia: Neutropenia (absolute neutrophil count [ANC] $<1.5\times10^9$/L) has been observed commonly with another medicinal product that inhibits IL-1 used in a patient population (rheumatoid arthritis) other than CAPS. Neutropenia was observed commonly in patients with rheumatoid arthritis (not an approved use) who were administered ILARIS subcutaneously in clinical studies. Treatment with ILARIS should not be initiated in patients with neutropenia. It is recommended that neutrophil counts be assessed prior to initiating treatment, after 1 to 2 months, and periodically thereafter while receiving ILARIS. If a patient becomes neutropenic the ANC should be monitored closely and treatment discontinuation should be considered.

Hypersensitivity Reactions : Cases suggestive of hypersensitivity reactions with ILARIS therapy have been reported in clinical trials (see Adverse Reactions).

Hepatic Function : Rare, mild, transient and asymptomatic cases of elevations of serum transaminases or bilirubin have been reported in clinical trials for CAPS (see Adverse Reactions, Hepatobiliary Events, and Abnormal Hematologic and Clinical Chemistry Findings).

Vaccinations: Live vaccines should not be given concurrently with ILARIS (see Drug Interactions).

Since ILARIS may interfere with normal immune response to new antigens, vaccinations may not be effective in patients receiving ILARIS. No data are available on the effectiveness of vaccinations with inactivated (killed) antigens in patients receiving ILARIS.

Prior to initiation of ILARIS therapy, adult and paediatric patients should receive all recommended vaccinations, as appropriate, including pneumococcal vaccine and inactivated influenza vaccine. In a dedicated study in healthy volunteers, a normal antibody-response to vaccination with meningococcal and influenza antigen was observed.

Lymphoid Organ Toxicity: Minimal to slight lymphoid hyperplasia of the spleen and lymph nodes has been infrequently observed in animal studies. Enlargement of lymphoid organs (lymph nodes, spleen), in patients treated with ILARIS, should be assessed for their etiology.

Malignancies: The risk for the development of malignancies with anti-interleukin (IL)-1 therapy is unknown. A potential risk cannot be excluded in patients treated with ILARIS.

Special Populations: Pregnant Women: There are no adequate and well-controlled studies of ILARIS in pregnant women. There is a limited amount of data from the use of ILARIS in this population. Women should use effective contraceptives during treatment with ILARIS and for up to 3 months after the last dose.

A significant shift in the litter size was observed in marmosets treated with 150 mg/kg of canakinumab. Singlet pregnancy that was seen in 0% of animals in the control group, increased to 21% in the treated group and triplet pregnancy in control vs treated group was down from 45% to 7%. This shift could be an indication of impaired fertility. Delayed ossification was seen in study 0680148 in a mouse model. Because animal reproduction studies are not always predictive of the human response, the risk for the foetus/mother is unknown, therefore, ILARIS should not be given to pregnant women or women who desire to become pregnant, unless clearly needed.

Nursing Women: It is not known whether canakinumab is excreted in human milk. Animal studies have shown that a murine anti-murine IL-1beta antibody had no undesirable effects on development in nursing mouse pups and that the antibody was transferred to them.

Breast-feeding is not recommended during ILARIS therapy.

Pediatrics (<4 years of age): ILARIS is not recommended for use in children below age of 4 years or with body weight below 15 kg due to lack of clinical data.

Geriatrics (>65 years of age): Clinical studies of ILARIS did not include sufficient numbers of subjects aged 65 and over to determine whether they respond differently from younger subjects.

Patients with Renal Impairment: No formal studies have been conducted to examine the pharmacokinetics of ILARIS administered subcutaneously in patients with renal impairment.

Patients with Hepatic Impairment: No formal studies have been conducted to examine the pharmacokinetics of ILARIS administered subcutaneously in patients with hepatic impairment.

Monitoring and Laboratory Tests: Annual monitoring for changes in lipid profile are recommended.

ADVERSE REACTIONS: Adverse Drug Reaction Overview: The data described herein reflect exposure to ILARIS in 104 adult and pediatric CAPS patients (20 FCAS, 72 MWS, 10 MWS/NOMID overlap, 1 NOMID, and 1 miss-classified with cold-induced urticaria) in placebo-controlled and uncontrolled clinical studies. Sixty-two (62) patients were exposed to ILARIS for at least 6 months, 56 for at least 1 year and 4 for at least 3 years. A total of 10 patients reported serious adverse drug reactions in CAPS, including vertigo (2 patients), infection (3 patients), and intra-abdominal abscess following appendectomy (1 patient). The most commonly reported adverse reaction associated with ILARIS treatment in the CAPS patients were upper respiratory tract infections and nasopharyngitis. No impact on the type or frequency of adverse drug reactions was seen with longer-term treatment. One (1) patient discontinued treatment due to potential infection.

Clinical Trial Adverse Drug Reactions: Because clinical trials are conducted under very specific conditions the adverse reaction rates observed in the clinical trials may not reflect the rates observed in practice and should not be compared to the rates in the clinical trials of another drug. Adverse drug reaction information from clinical trials is useful for identifying drug-related adverse events and for approximating rates.

To date, 833 subjects have received ILARIS in blinded and open-label clinical trials in CAPS and other diseases, including clinical trials in healthy volunteers.

The safety of ILARIS compared with placebo was investigated in a pivotal phase III trial (Study D2304) that consisted of an 8-week, open-label period (Part I), followed by a 24-week, randomized, double-blind and placebo-controlled withdrawal period (Part II), followed by a 16-week open-label period (Part III). All patients were treated with ILARIS 150 mg subcutaneously or 2 mg/kg if body weight was ≥15 kg and ≤40 kg (see Table 1).

In placebo-controlled period in Part II of Study D2304 (canakinumab; n=15 vs placebo; n=16), with a mean duration of 168.4 days (mean 3 doses) in ILARIS patients and 109.9 days (mean 2.3 doses) in placebo patients, there were more patients in the canakinumab treatment group reporting adverse events in the immune system disorders (13.3% vs 0), infections and infestations (80% vs 56.3%), injury, poisoning and procedural complications (26.7% vs 12.5%), nervous system disorders (26.7% vs 0), psychiatric disorders (20.0% vs 6.3%) and respiratory, thoracic and mediastinal disorders (33.3% vs 6.3%) in system organ classes than in the placebo group.

In 1 placebo-controlled and 2 uncontrolled clinical studies for CAPS, a total of 104 unique CAPS patients analysed for safety included 20 FCAS, 72 MWS, 10 MWS/NOMID, 1 NOMID and 1 mis-diagnosed patient with an overall exposure of 95.7 patient-years and a treatment duration of up to 4 years, with age ranging from 4 to 74 years of age at time of treatment-start with canakinumab. This includes 23 pediatric (4 to 17 years of age; median: 10 years) patients.

Adverse events (AEs) were reported in 88.2% in Study A2102, and in 82.9% (Part I), 100% in canakinumab group and 87.5% in placebo group (Part II) and 77.4% (Part III) of Study D2304. A total of 10 patients reported serious adverse drug reactions (that were considered by the investigators as related to treatment) during the clinical trial program in CAPS, including vertigo (2 patients), infection (3 patients), and intra-abdominal abscess following appendectomy (1 patient). The most commonly reported adverse events associated with ILARIS treatment in the CAPS patients were upper respiratory tract infections and nasopharyngitis. There were no deaths reported in any of the 3 clinical trials for CAPS.

Table 1: ILARIS

Number (%) of Patients with AEs by Primary System Organ Class and Preferred Terms, in Parts I, II and III and the Entire Study (Safety population)

	Part I	Part II		Part III	Entire Study
Primary System Organ Class Affected Preferred Term	**ACZ885 N=35 n (%)**	**ACZ885 N=15 n (%)**	**Placebo N=16 n (%)**	**ACZ885 N=31 n (%)**	**ACZ885 N=35 n (%)**
n % of patients with AEs	**29 (82.9)**	**15 (100)**	**14 (87.5)**	**24 (77.4)**	**35 (100)**
Ear and Labyrinth Disorders	2 (5.7)	1 (6.7)	0 (0.0)	6 (19.4)	8 (22.9)
Tinnitus	0 (0.0)	1 (6.7)	0 (0.0)	1 (3.2)	2 (5.7)
Vertigo	1 (2.9)	0 (0.0)	0 (0.0)	3 (9.7)	4 (11.4)
Gastrointestinal Disorders	6 (17.1)	6 (40.0)	5 (31.3)	8 (25.8)	18 (51.4)
Abdominal pain	0 (0.0)	0 (0.0)	0 (0.0)	2 (6.5)	2 (5.7)
Abdominal pain upper	2 (5.7)	0 (0.0)	0 (0.0)	0 (0.0)	2 (5.7)
Aphthous stomatitis	0 (0.0)	1 (6.7)	1 (6.3)	1 (3.2)	3 (8.6)
Diarrhea	0 (0.0)	1 (6.7)	2 (12.5)	5 (16.1)	7 (20.0)
Mouth ulceration	0 (0.0)	1 (6.7)	0 (0.0)	1 (3.2)	2 (5.7)
Nausea	3 (8.6)	1 (6.7)	1 (6.3)	1 (3.2)	5 (14.3)
Stomach discomfort	1 (2.9)	1 (6.7)	0 (0.0)	0 (0.0)	2 (5.7)
General Disorders and Administration Site Conditions	7 (20.0)	3 (20.0)	3 (18.8)	4 (12.9)	14 (40.0)
Asthenia	2 (5.7)	1 (6.7)	0 (0.0)	0 (0.0)	2 (5.7)
Influenza like illness	1 (2.9)	0 (0.0)	0 (0.0)	1 (3.2)	2 (5.7)
Infections and Infestations	12 (34.3)	12 (80.0)	9 (56.3)	10 (32.3)	27 (77.1)
Bronchitis	3 (8.6)	1 (6.7)	1 (6.3)	0 (0.0)	4 (11.4)
Gastroenteritis	0 (0.0)	2 (13.3)	1 (6.3)	2 (6.5)	4 (11.4)
Influenza	1 (2.9)	2 (13.3)	3 (18.8)	0 (0.0)	6 (17.1)
Nasopharyngitis	4 (11.4)	4 (26.7)	2 (12.5)	4 (12.9)	12 (34.3)
Oral herpes	1 (2.9)	0 (0.0)	2 (12.5)	0 (0.0)	3 (8.6)
Pharyngitis	0 (0.0)	1 (6.7)	1 (6.3)	2 (6.5)	4 (11.4)
Rhinitis	4 (11.4)	1 (6.7)	2 (12.5)	0 (0.0)	6 (17.1)
Upper respiratory tract infection	0 (0.0)	1 (6.7)	1 (6.3)	1 (3.2)	3 (8.6)
Urinary tract infection	0 (0.0)	2 (13.3)	0 (0.0)	1 (3.2)	2 (5.7)
Viral infection	0 (0.0)	2 (13.3)	0 (0.0)	0 (0.0)	2 (5.7)
Injury, Poisoning and Procedural Complications	1 (2.9)	4 (26.7)	2 (12.5)	3 (9.7)	9 (25.7)
Joint sprain	0 (0.0)	2 (13.3)	1 (6.3)	0 (0.0)	3 (8.6)
Investigations	3 (8.6)	0 (0.0)	1 (6.3)	2 (6.5)	6 (17.1)
Weight increased	3 (8.6)	0 (0.0)	0 (0.0)	1 (3.2)	4 (11.4)
Musculoskeletal and Connective Tissue Disorders	6 (17.1)	3 (20.0)	2 (12.5)	6 (19.4)	13 (37.1)
Back pain	1 (2.9)	0 (0.0)	0 (0.0)	2 (6.5)	3 (8.6)
Muscle contracture	0 (0.0)	0 (0.0)	1 (6.3)	1 (3.2)	2 (5.7)
Muscle spasms	2 (5.7)	0 (0.0)	0 (0.0)	0 (0.0)	2 (5.7)
Musculoskeletal pain	0 (0.0)	1 (6.7)	1 (6.3)	2 (6.5)	4 (11.4)
Pain in extremity	1 (2.9)	0 (0.0)	0 (0.0)	2 (6.5)	3 (8.6)
Nervous System Disorders	4 (11.4)	4 (26.7)	0 (0.0)	9 (29.0)	13 (37.1)
Headache	0 (0.0)	2 (13.3)	0 (0.0)	3 (9.7)	5 (14.3)
Memory impairment	0 (0.0)	0 (0.0)	0 (0.0)	2 (6.5)	2 (5.7)
Nystagmus	0 (0.0)	0 (0.0)	0 (0.0)	2 (6.5)	2 (5.7)
Sciatica	1 (2.9)	1 (6.7)	0 (0.0)	2 (6.5)	2 (5.7)
Tension headache	1 (2.9)	0 (0.0)	0 (0.0)	1 (3.2)	2 (5.7)
Psychiatric Disorders	1 (2.9)	3 (20.0)	1 (6.3)	2 (6.5)	6 (17.1)

(cont'd)

Table 1: ILARIS *(cont'd)*

Number (%) of Patients with AEs by Primary System Organ Class and Preferred Terms, in Parts I, II and III and the Entire Study (Safety population)

Primary System Organ Class Affected Preferred Term	Part I ACZ885 N=35 n (%)	Part II ACZ885 N=15 n (%)	Part II Placebo N=16 n (%)	Part III ACZ885 N=31 n (%)	Entire Study ACZ885 N=35 n (%)
Anxiety	0 (0.0)	1 (6.7)	1 (6.3)	0 (0.0)	2 (5.7)
Depression	0 (0.0)	1 (6.7)	0 (0.0)	1 (3.2)	2 (5.7)
Respiratory, Thoracic and Mediastinal Disorders	5 (14.3)	5 (33.3)	1 (6.3)	5 (16.1)	12 (34.3)
Cough	0 (0.0)	2 (13.3)	0 (0.0)	0 (0.0)	2 (5.7)
Epistaxis	1 (2.9)	0 (0.0)	1 (6.3)	1 (3.2)	3 (8.6)
Oropharyngeal pain	1 (2.9)	1 (6.7)	0 (0.0)	1 (3.2)	3 (8.6)
Respiratory tract congestion	1 (2.9)	0 (0.0)	0 (0.0)	1 (3.2)	2 (5.7)
Skin and Subcutaneous Tissue Disorders	4 (11.4)	1 (6.7)	0 (0.0)	7 (22.6)	10 (28.6)
Acne	0 (0.0)	0 (0.0)	0 (0.0)	2 (6.5)	2 (5.7)
Erythema	1 (2.9)	0 (0.0)	0 (0.0)	2 (6.5)	3 (8.6)
Hyperhidrosis	0 (0.0)	0 (0.0)	0 (0.0)	2 (6.5)	2 (5.7)
Pruritus	1 (2.9)	1 (6.7)	0 (0.0)	1 (3.2)	3 (8.6)
Vascular Disorders	2 (5.7)	2 (13.3)	1 (6.3)	0 (0.0)	5 (14.3)
Haematoma	1 (2.9)	0 (0.0)	1 (6.3)	0 (0.0)	2 (5.7)
Hot flush	1 (2.9)	1 (6.7)	0 (0.0)	0 (0.0)	2 (5.7)

Part I: AEs occurring from baseline up to Week 8.
Part II: AEs occurring from Week 8 up to the end of part II.
Part III: AEs occurring from Visit 11 up to the end of study. Entire study: AEs occurring from baseline up to the end of study. AEs preferred terms in each primary system organ class are presented alphabetically.

Vertigo: Vertigo has been reported in 9 to 14% of patients in CAPS studies, exclusively in MWS patients, and reported as a serious adverse event in two cases. All events resolved with continued treatment with ILARIS.

Hypersensitivity Reactions: Cases suggestive of hypersensitivity reactions with ILARIS therapy have been reported in patients treated with canakinumab in clinical trials. The majority of these events were mild in severity. No anaphylactoid or anaphylactic reactions have been reported (see Warnings and Precautions, Hypersensitivity Reactions).

Injection Site Reactions: In Study D2304, subcutaneous injection site reactions were observed in 9% of patients in Part 1 with mild tolerability reactions; in Part 2, one patient each (7%) had a mild or a moderate tolerability reaction and, in Part 3, one patient had a mild local tolerability reaction. No severe injection-site reactions were reported and none led to discontinuation of treatment. In the largest of 3 CAPS studies (98 patients), study D2306, injection site reactions were rare (5 patients) and all mild in severity.

Immunogenicity : A specific biosensor binding assay was used to detect antibodies directed against canakinumab in patients who received ILARIS. None of the 60 CAPS patients who had received ILARIS tested positive for treatment-emergent binding antibodies at the time points tested. Thirty-one (31) of 60 CAPS patients had a duration of exposure to canakinumab >48 weeks. The data obtained in an assay is highly dependent on several factors including assay sensitivity and specificity, assay methodology, sample handling, timing of sample collection, concomitant medications, underlying disease, and the number of patients tested. For these reasons, comparison of the incidence of antibodies to canakinumab with the incidence of antibodies to other products may be misleading.

Hepatobiliary Events: In 1 patient a transient and reversible elevation of liver function test (LFT) was reported as "toxic hepatitis" (see Warnings and Precautions, Hepatic Function).

Pediatric Population: Twenty-three (23) pediatric CAPS patients (4 to 17 years of age) demonstrated similar safety to adult patients. Specifically, the overall frequency and severity of infectious episodes in pediatric patients were comparable to that in the adult population. Infection of the upper respiratory tract was the most frequently reported infection.

Vital Signs and Physical Findings: In Part II of Study D2304, notable systolic and diastolic blood pressure values/change from baseline were more frequently seen in those patients randomized to canakinumab. Three (3) patients had notably high systolic blood pressure readings in Part III, and 1 a notably high diastolic pressure (see Table 2).

Table 2: ILARIS

Number (%) of Patients with Post-Baseline Vital Signs Abnormalities Newly Occurring in Part I, II and III (Safety population)

	Part I ACZ885 N=35 n (%)	Part II ACZ885 N=15 n (%)	Part II Placebo N=16 n (%)	Part III ACZ885 N=31 n (%)	Entire Study ACZ885 N=35 n (%)
Systolic Blood Pressure (mmHg)					
Decrease from baseline ≥25%	0 (0.0)	1 (6.7)	0 (0.0)	0 (0.0)	1 (2.9)
Increase from baseline ≥25%	1 (2.9)	2 (13.3)	0 (0.0)	0 (0.0)	3 (8.6)
Notable high systolic blood pressure value	3 (8.6)	4 (26.7)	2 (12.5)	3 (9.7)	8 (22.9)
Diastolic Blood Pressure (mmHg)					
Decrease from baseline ≥25%	0 (0.0)	1 (6.7)	0 (0.0)	2 (6.5)	3 (8.6)
Increase from baseline ≥25%	2 (5.7)	7 (46.7)	3 (18.8)	8 (25.8)	11 (31.4)
Notable high diastolic blood pressure value	2 (5.7)	3 (20.0)	2 (12.5)	1 (3.2)	7 (20.0)
Supine Pulse (bpm)					
Notable clinically significant decrease	0 (0.0)	0 (0.0)	0 (0.0)	0 (0.0)	0 (0.0)
Notable clinically significant increase	0 (0.0)	0 (0.0)	0 (0.0)	0 (0.0)	0 (0.0)

(cont'd)

Part I; notable abnormality occurring from baseline in Part I.
Part II; notable abnormality occurring from Week 8 in Part II.
Part III; notable abnormality occurring from baseline until the end of the study.
Entire study; notable abnormality occurring from baseline until the end of the study.
In Part II decrease is from baseline.
In Part III decrease is from baseline.

Abnormal Hematologic and Clinical Chemistry Findings: During clinical trials with canakinumab mean values for hemoglobin increased and decreased for white blood cell, neutrophils and platelets. These changes were potentially due to decrease in inflammation and not considered to be of clinical relevance.

Elevations of transaminases have been observed rarely in CAPS patients. Asymptomatic and mild elevations of serum bilirubin have been observed in CAPS patients treated with canakinumab without concomitant elevations of transaminases.

Table 3: ILARIS

Proportion of Patients with Post-Baseline AST/ALT and Bilirubin Elevations

	A2102 N=34	D2304 N=35
AST		
>1 to <3×ULN	6/34 (17.6%)	4/35 (11.4%)
≥3×ULN	2/34 (5.9%)	3/35 (8.6%)
≥5×ULN	1/34 (2.9%)	2/35 (5.7%)
ALT		
>1 to <3×ULN	7/34 (20.6%)	6/35 (17.1%)
≥3×ULN	2/34 (5.9%)	3/35 (8.6%)
≥5×ULN	2/34 (5.9%)	3/35 (8.6%)
Bilirubin (total)		
>ULN	4/34 (11.8%)	1 (2.9%)
≥1.5×ULN	0	0
≥3×ULN	0	0

Number of patients with post-treatment values.

Some patients experienced increased ALT and AST values in Part I of the Study D2304 after one dose of ILARIS. Two (2) patients had decreased values in Part II with placebo, 1 of them increased up to 5×ULN in Part III after re-treated with ILARIS (see Warnings and Precautions).

DRUG INTERACTIONS: Overview: Interactions between ILARIS and other medicinal products have not been investigated in formal studies.

Drug-Drug Interactions: Immunization: No data are available on either the effects of live vaccination or the secondary transmission of infection by live vaccines in patients receiving ILARIS. Therefore, live vaccines should not be given concurrently with ILARIS. It is recommended that, if possible, pediatric and adult patients should complete all immunizations in accordance with current immunization guidelines prior to initiating ILARIS therapy (see Warnings and Precautions, Vaccinations).

Cytochrome P450 Substrates : The formation of CYP450 enzymes is suppressed by increased levels of cytokines (e.g., IL-1) during chronic inflammation. Thus it is expected that for a molecule that binds to IL-1, such as canakinumab, the formation of CYP450 enzymes could be normalized. This is clinically relevant for CYP450 substrates with a narrow therapeutic index, where the dose is individually adjusted (e.g., warfarin). Upon initiation of canakinumab, in patients being treated with these types of medicinal products, therapeutic monitoring of the effect or drug concentration should be performed and the individual dose of the medicinal product may need to be adjusted as needed.

TNF-Blocker and IL-1 Blocking Agent: The concomitant administration of ILARIS with other drugs that block IL-1 has not been studied. Based upon the potential for pharmacological interactions between ILARIS and a recombinant IL-1ra, concomitant administration of ILARIS and other agents that block IL-1 or its receptors is not recommended.

An increased incidence of serious infections has been associated with administration of another IL-1 blocker in combination with TNF inhibitors. Use of ILARIS with TNF inhibitors is not recommended because this may increase the risk of serious infections.

Drug-Food Interactions: Since canakinumab is given as a subcutaneous injection no studies on oral food effects were performed.

Drug-Herb Interactions: The interaction of canakinumab with herbal medications or supplements has not been studied.

Drug-Laboratory Test Interactions: No evidence suggest that canakinumab interferes with laboratory tests.

Drug-Lifestyle Interactions: Specific drug-lifestyle interaction studies have not been conducted with canakinumab.

DOSAGE AND ADMINISTRATION: Dosing Considerations: Special populations: Renal Impairment: No dose adjustment is needed in patients with renal impairment. However, clinical experience in such patients is limited.

Hepatic Impairment: ILARIS has not been studied in patients with hepatic impairment.

Pediatric Patients: ILARIS is not recommended for use in children below age 4 years or with body weight below 15 kg due to a lack of clinical data.

Geriatric Patients: No dose adjustment is required in geriatric patients. However, clinical experience in such patients is limited.

Recommended Dose and Dosage Adjustment: The recommended dose of ILARIS is 150 mg for CAPS patients with body weight greater than 40 kg. For CAPS patients with body weight between 15 kg and 40 kg, the recommended dose is 2 mg/kg. For children 15 to 40 kg with an inadequate response, the dose can be increased to 3 mg/kg.

ILARIS is administered every eight weeks as a single dose via subcutaneous injection.

If a satisfactory clinical response (resolution of rash and other generalised inflammatory symptoms) has not been achieved 7 days after treatment start, a second dose of ILARIS at 150 mg or 2 mg/kg may be considered.

Discontinuation of drug should be considered if an unsatisfactory therapeutic effect persists.

Administration: Treatment should be initiated and supervised by a specialist physician experienced in the diagnosis and treatment of CAPS.

After proper training in injection technique, patients may self-inject ILARIS if their physician determines that it is appropriate and with medical follow-up as necessary.

Reconstitution: Parenteral Products:

Vial Size	Volume of Water for Injection to be Added to Vial	Approximate Available Volume	Nominal Concentration per mL
6 mL	1.0 mL	1.0 mL	150 mg/mL

Using aseptic technique, reconstitute each vial of ILARIS by slowly injecting 1 mL of preservative-free Sterile Water for Injection with a 1 mL syringe and an 18 G × 2" needle. Swirl the vial slowly at an angle of about 45° for approximately 1 minute and allow to stand for 5 minutes. Then gently turn the vial upside down and back again ten times. Avoid touching the rubber stopper with your fingers. Allow to stand for about 15 minutes at room temperature to obtain a clear solution. Do not shake. Do not use if particulate matter is present in the solution. Tap the side of the vial to remove any residual liquid from the stopper. The reconstituted solution should be free from particulates, and clear to opalescent. The solution should be colorless or may have a slight brownish-yellow tint. If the solution has a distinctly brown discoloration it should not be used. If not used within 60 minutes of reconstitution, the solution should be stored in the refrigerator at 2 to 8°C and used within 24 hours. Slight foaming of the product upon reconstitution is not unusual.

Using a sterile syringe and needle carefully withdraw the required volume depending on the dose to be administered (0.2 mL to 1 mL) and subcutaneously inject using a 27 G × 0.5" needle.

Injection into scar tissue should be avoided as this may result in insufficient exposure to ILARIS.

OVERDOSAGE:
No case of overdose has been reported.

> For management of a suspected drug overdose, contact your regional Poison Control Centre. See the *CPS* Directory section for a list of Poison Control Centres.

ACTION AND CLINICAL PHARMACOLOGY: Mechanism of Action: Canakinumab is a fully human monoclonal anti-human interleukin-1beta (IL-1β) antibody of the IgG1/k isotype. Canakinumab binds with high affinity specifically to human IL-1β and neutralizes its activity by blocking its interaction with IL-1 receptors, and thereby, prevents IL-1β-induced gene activation and the production of inflammatory mediators, such as interleukin-6 or cyclooxygenase-2.

Pharmacodynamics: Excess production of IL-1β in inflammatory diseases leads to local or systemic inflammation, increased production of the acute phase response markers such as C-reactive protein (CRP) or serum amyloid A (SAA), and fever. Elevated SAA has been associated with the development of systemic amyloidosis in patients with CAPS. The pharmacodynamic (PD) action of canakinumab is to bind to and inactivate IL-1β and thus to inhibit the down-stream events of IL-1 signaling, including IL-1β production, IL-1β pathway related gene activation, elevation of acute phase proteins such as SAA and CRP, and the mobilization of neutrophils and platelets from bone marrow.

CAPS patients who have an uncontrolled overproduction of IL-1β manifesting as fever, rash, fatigue, skin rash, arthritis, leukocytosis, high platelets counts, and acute phase protein response, show a rapid response to ILARIS therapy. Following ILARIS treatment, CRP and SAA levels, leukocytosis and high platelet count rapidly returned to normal within 8 days.

Pharmacokinetics: Absorption: The peak serum canakinumab concentration (C_{max}) of 16±3.5 μg/mL occurred approximately 7 days following single subcutaneous administration of 150 mg in adult CAPS patients. The mean terminal half-life was 26 days.

The absolute bioavailability of subcutaneous canakinumab was estimated to be 70%. Exposure parameters (such as AUC and C_{max}) increased in proportion to dose over the dose range of 0.30 to 10.0 mg/kg given as intravenous infusion or from 150 to 300 mg as subcutaneous injection.

Distribution: Canakinumab binds to serum IL-1β. The volume of distribution (Vss) of canakinumab varied according to body weight and were estimated to be 6.01 L, in a typical CAPS patient of body weight 70 kg. The expected accumulation ratio was 1.3-fold following 6 months of subcutaneous administration of 150 mg canakinumab every 8 weeks.

Excretion: Clearance (CL) of canakinumab varied according to body weight and was estimated to be 0.174 L/day in a typical CAPS patient weighing 70 kg. There was no indication of accelerated clearance or time-dependent change in the pharmacokinetic properties of canakinumab following repeated administration. No gender or age-related pharmacokinetic differences were observed after correction for body weight.

Special Populations and Conditions: Pediatrics: Peak concentrations of canakinumab occurred between 2 to 7 days following single subcutaneous administration of canakinumab 150 mg or 2 mg/kg in pediatric patients. The terminal half-life ranged from 22.9 to 25.7 days, similar to the pharmacokinetic properties observed in adults.

Geriatrics: Based on the pharmacokinetic-binding model, subject's age did not impact the key pharmacokinetic parameters (canakinumab clearance, volumes of distribution) after correction for the subject's body weight. It should also be noted that the number of patients aged 65 and over is not sufficient to determine whether the pharmacokinetics of canakinumab is truly different in elderly patients compared to the adult patients.

Race: Based on the population pharmacokinetic binding model, which included 175 Caucasians, 54 Asians (of which 48 were healthy Japanese and 6 non Japanese Asians), 1 black, 1 Native American, and 2 coded as "other", the pharmacokinetic parameters were comparable between CAPS patients who were predominantly Caucasians and the Japanese healthy volunteers.

Hepatic Insufficiency: No formal studies have been conducted to examine the pharmacokinetics of ILARIS administered subcutaneously in patients with hepatic impairment.

Renal Insufficiency: No formal studies have been conducted to examine the pharmacokinetics of ILARIS administered subcutaneously in patients with renal impairment.

STORAGE AND STABILITY: ILARIS unopened vial must be stored under refrigerated conditions, between 2 and 8°C. Do not freeze. Store in the original package in order to protect from light.

For the reconstituted preparation chemical and physical in-use stability has been demonstrated for 24 hours at 2-8°C. For microbiological reasons, the prepared solution should be used immediately after reconstitution. If this is not possible, duration and conditions of storage are the responsibility of the user and should not normally exceed 24 hours at 2-8°C. Reconstitution should be performed in accordance with the rules of good practice.

ILARIS must be kept out of the reach and sight of children.

SPECIAL HANDLING INSTRUCTIONS: ILARIS 150 mg/mL powder for solution for injection is supplied in a single-use vial. Any unused product or waste material should be disposed of in accordance with local requirements.

Note: Parenteral drug products should be inspected visually for particulate matter and discoloration prior to administration, whenever solution and container permit. The solution should be free of particles and should be colorless or may have a slight brownish yellow brownish tint.

INFORMATION FOR THE PATIENT: Published in e-CPS, available by subscription at www.e-cps.ca.

DOSAGE FORMS, COMPOSITION AND PACKAGING: Each vial of white, preservative-free, lyophilized powder contains: canakinumab 150 mg. Reconstitution with 1 mL of preservative-free sterile Water for injection is required prior to subcutaneous administration of the drug. The reconstituted canakinumab is a 150 mg/mL solution with colorless to slightly brownish-yellow tint, free of visible particles, and clear to slightly opalescent. A volume of up to 1 mL can be withdrawn, which is designed to deliver 150 mg for subcutaneous administration only. Each reconstituted vial contains 150 mg canakinumab (150 mg/1 mL after reconstitution), sucrose, L-histidine, L-histidine HCL monohydrate, polysorbate 80. Preservative-free. Sterile, single-use, colorless 6 mL glass vials with coated stopper and aluminium flip off cap.

Imdur®
isosorbide-5-mononitrate
Antianginal

AstraZeneca

Date of Preparation: June 26, 2000
Date of Revision: October 29, 2008

PHARMACOLOGY: As with other organic nitrates, the principal pharmacological action of isosorbide-5-mononitrate, the major active metabolite of isosorbide dinitrate (ISDN), is relaxation of vascular smooth muscle and consequent dilation of peripheral arteries and veins, especially the latter. Dilation of the veins promotes peripheral pooling of blood and decreases venous return to the heart, thereby reducing left ventricular end-diastolic pressure and pulmonary capillary wedge pressure (pre-load). Arteriolar relaxation reduces systemic vascular resistance, systolic arterial pressure, and mean arterial pressure (after-load). Dilation of the coronary arteries also occurs. The hemodynamic responses to isosorbide-5-mononitrate are similar to those produced by other nitrates.

Pharmacodynamics: Dosage regimens for most chronically used drugs are designed to provide plasma concentrations that are continuously greater than a minimally effective concentration. This strategy is inappropriate for organic nitrates. Prolonged administration of nitrate drugs according to traditionally recommended dosage regimens has been shown to produce tolerance. Tolerance results in a loss of efficacy. Several well-controlled clinical trials have used exercise testing to assess the antianginal efficacy of continuously delivered nitrates. In the large majority of these trials, nitrate effectiveness was indistinguishable from placebo after 24 hours (or less) of continuous therapy. Attempts to overcome tolerance by dose escalation, even to doses far in excess of those used acutely, have consistently failed. Only after nitrates have been absent from the body for several hours has their antianginal efficacy been restored. Drug-free intervals of 10 to 12 hours are known to be sufficient to restore response. The drug-free interval sufficient to avoid tolerance to isosorbide-5-mononitrate has not been completely defined. Imdur tablets during long-term use over 42 days dosed at 120 mg once daily continued to improve exercise performance at 4 hours and 12 hours after dosing but its effects (although better than placebo) are less than or at best equal to the effects of the first dose of 60 mg. Considering the pharmacokinetic profile of isosorbide-5-mononitrate and its long half-life (see Pharmacokinetics), clinical efficacy is consistent with that observed for other organic nitrates.

Pharmacokinetics: After oral administration of isosorbide-5-mononitrate as a solution or immediate-release tablets, maximum plasma concentrations of isosorbide-5-mononitrate are achieved in 30 to 60 minutes with an absolute bioavailability of approximately 100%. After i.v. administration, isosorbide-5-mononitrate is distributed into total body water in about 9 minutes with a volume of distribution of approximately 0.6 to 0.7 L/kg. Isosorbide-5-mononitrate is approximately 5% bound to human plasma proteins and is distributed into blood cells and saliva. Isosorbide-5-mononitrate is primarily metabolized by the liver, but unlike oral isosorbide dinitrate, it is not subject to first-pass metabolism. Isosorbide-5-mononitrate is cleared by denitration to isosorbide and glucuronidation as the mononitrate, with 96% of the administered dose excreted in the urine within 5 days and only about 1% eliminated in the feces. At least 6 different compounds have been detected in urine, with about 2% of the dose excreted as the unchanged drug and at least 5 metabolites. The metabolites are not pharmacologically active. Renal clearance accounts for only about 4% of total body clearance. The mean plasma elimination half-life of isosorbide-5-mononitrate is approximately 5 hours.

The disposition of isosorbide-5-mononitrate in patients with various degrees of renal insufficiency, liver cirrhosis or cardiac dysfunction was evaluated and found to be similar to that observed in healthy subjects.

The elimination half-life of isosorbide-5-mononitrate was not prolonged, and there was no drug accumulation in patients with chronic renal failure after multiple oral dosing.

Impaired liver or kidney function has no major influence on the pharmacokinetic properties.

Food intake may decrease the rate (increase in T_{max}) but not the extent (AUC) of absorption of isosorbide-5-mononitrate.

With the extended release formulation of Imdur, isosorbide-5-mononitrate is gradually released, independent of pH, over a 10 hour period, according to a first order process.

This prolongation of the absorption phase results in reduced and delayed peak plasma levels compared to conventional tablets of isosorbide-5-mononitrate. After administration of 60 mg of isosorbide-5-mononitrate extended release tablets, peak plasma levels of around 3000 nmol/L are usually obtained within approximately 4 hours. The plasma concentrations then gradually fall to around 500 nmol/L at the end of the dosage interval (24 hours after dose intake).

INDICATIONS: For the prevention of anginal attacks in patients with chronic stable angina pectoris associated with coronary artery disease.

Not intended for the immediate relief of acute attacks of angina pectoris.

CONTRAINDICATIONS: Known hypersensitivity to isosorbide-5-mononitrate or to other nitrates or nitrites. Acute circulatory failure associated with marked hypotension (shock and states of collapse). Postural hypotension. Myocardial insufficiency due to obstruction (e.g., in the presence of aortic or mitral stenosis or of constrictive pericarditis). Increased intracranial pressure. Severe anemia. Concomitant use of nitrates, either regularly and/or intermittently, with phosphodiesterase type 5 inhibitors (e.g. sildenafil, tadalafil, vardenafil) is absolutely contraindicated.

WARNINGS: The benefits and safety of isosorbide-5-mononitrate in anginal patients with acute myocardial infarction or congestive heart failure have not been established. Because the effects of isosorbide-5-mononitrate are difficult to terminate rapidly, this drug is not recommended in these settings.

Abrupt withdrawal may occasionally aggravate anginal symptoms. To avoid possible withdrawal effects, the administration of isosorbide-5-mononitrate should be gradually reduced and not abruptly discontinued.

Caution should be observed in patients with severe cerebral arteriosclerosis or severe hypotension.

PRECAUTIONS: Headaches or symptoms of severe hypotension, such as weakness or dizziness, particularly when arising suddenly from a recumbent position, may occur.

Caution should be exercised when using nitrates in patients prone to, or who might be affected by, hypotension. Isosorbide-5-mononitrate should therefore be used with caution in patients who may have volume depletion from diuretic therapy or in patients who have low systolic blood pressure (e.g., below 90 mmHg). Paradoxical bradycardia and increased angina pectoris may accompany nitrate-induced hypotension.

Nitrate therapy may aggravate the angina caused by hypertrophic cardiomyopathy.

In industrial workers who have had long-term exposure to unknown (presumably high) doses of organic nitrates, tolerance clearly occurs. There is, moreover, physical dependence since chest pain, acute myocardial infarction, and even sudden death have occurred during temporary withdrawal of nitrates from these workers. In clinical trials of angina patients, there are reports of anginal attacks being more easily provoked and of rebound in the hemodynamic effects soon after nitrate withdrawal. The importance of these observations to the routine, clinical use of oral isosorbide-5-mononitrate has not been fully elucidated.

Caution should be exercised in patients with arterial hypoxemia due to anemia (see Contraindications). Similarly, caution is called for in patients with hypoxemia and a ventilation/perfusion imbalance due to lung disease or ischemic heart failure. Patients with angina pectoris, myocardial infarction, or cerebral ischemia frequently suffer from abnormalities of the small airways (especially alveolar hypoxia). Under these circumstances vasoconstriction occurs within the lung to shift perfusion from areas of alveolar hypoxia to better ventilated regions of the lung. As a potent vasodilator, isosorbide-5-mononitrate could reverse this protective vasoconstriction and thus result in increased perfusion to poorly ventilated areas, worsening of the ventilation/perfusion imbalance, and a further decrease in the arterial partial pressure of oxygen.

Tolerance to isosorbide-5-mononitrate with cross tolerance to other nitrates or nitrites may occur (see Pharmacology). As tolerance to isosorbide-5-mononitrate develops, the effect of sublingual nitroglycerin on exercise tolerance, although still observable, is somewhat blunted.

Occupational Hazards: As patients may experience faintness and/or dizziness, reaction time when driving or operating machinery may be impaired, especially at the start of treatment.

Pregnancy: Teratogenic Effects: In studies designed to detect effects of isosorbide-5-mononitrate on embryo-fetal development, doses of up to 240 to 248 mg/kg/day, administered to pregnant rats and rabbits, were unassociated with evidence of such effects. No adverse effects on reproduction or fetal development were reported. These animal doses are about 100 times the maximum recommended human dose when comparison is based on body weight; when comparison is based on body surface area, the rat dose is about 17 times the human dose and the rabbit dose is about 38 times the human dose. There are no studies in pregnant women. Because animal reproduction studies are not always predictive of human response, isosorbide-5-mononitrate should be used during pregnancy only if the potential benefit justifies the potential risk to the fetus.

Nonteratogenic Effects: Neonatal survival and development and incidence of stillbirths were adversely affected when pregnant rats were administered oral doses of 750 (but not 300) mg isosorbide-5-mononitrate/kg/day during late gestation and lactation. This dose (about 312 times the human dose when comparison is based on body weight and 54 times the human dose when comparison is based on body surface area) was associated with decreases in maternal weight gain and motor activity and evidence of impaired lactation.

Lactation: It is not known whether isosorbide-5-mononitrate is excreted in human milk. Because many drugs are excreted in human milk, caution should be exercised when isosorbide-5-mononitrate is administered to a nursing mother.

Children: The safety and efficacy of isosorbide-5-mononitrate in children have not been established. Therefore, its use is not recommended.

Drug Interactions: Concomitant treatment with other vasodilators, calcium antagonists, ACE inhibitors, beta-blockers, diuretics, antihypertensives, tricyclic antidepressants, and major tranquilizers may potentiate the blood pressure lowering effect of isosorbide-5-mononitrate.

Marked symptomatic orthostatic hypotension has been reported when calcium channel blockers and organic nitrates were used in combination. Dose adjustments of either class of agents may be necessary.

Concomitant use of isosorbide-5-mononitrate and phosphodiesterase type 5 inhibitors (e.g. sildenafil, tadalafil, vardenafil) can potentiate the hypotensive effect of isosorbide-5-mononitrate. This could result in life-threatening hypotension with syncope or myocardial infarction and death. Therefore, phosphodiesterase type 5 inhibitors (e.g. sildenafil, tadalafil, vardenafil) should not be given to patients receiving isosorbide-5-mononitrate therapy.

Alcohol may enhance sensitivity to the hypotensive effects of nitrates.

ADVERSE EFFECTS: In 17 clinical trials, both controlled and uncontrolled, 861 patients were treated with isosorbide-5-mononitrate 30 to 240 mg once daily, alone or in combination with β-adrenergic blocking agents. Adverse events were reported in 71% of the patients. Discontinuation of therapy due to adverse reactions was required in 8% of the patients. Most of these were discontinued because of headache. Dizziness, myocardial infarction, nausea, and vertigo were also associated with withdrawal from these studies. The most common adverse events were headache, dizziness, fatigue, nausea and flushing.

The following adverse events were reported by >1 to 3% of patients: myocardial infarction, postural hypotension, tachycardia, angina pectoris, somnolence, coughing, paresthesia, vertigo, abdominal pain, diarrhea, flatulence, extra systoles, palpitation, aggravated angina, insomnia, dyspnea, respiratory infection, increased sweating, vasospasm, abnormal vision, back pain, musculoskeletal pain, dyspepsia, chest pain, rhinitis, constipation.

The following adverse events were reported in ≤1% of the patients:

Cardiovascular: bundle branch block, cardiac failure, circulatory failure, hypotension, hypertension, syncope, arrhythmia, AV block, bradycardia, atrial fibrillation, heart murmur, abnormal heart sound, Q-wave abnormality, T-wave changes, ECG abnormal.

Dermatological: rash, pruritus, eczema, acne, rash erythematous, rash psoriaform, abnormal hair texture, skin disorder.

Gastrointestinal: duodenal ulcer, eructation, hemorrhagic gastric ulcer, gastritis, hemorrhoids, intestinal obstruction, melena, dry mouth, pharynx disorder, tooth disorder, vomiting, loose stools, glossitis.

Genitourinary: atrophic vaginitis, prostatic disorder, renal calculus, urinary bladder diverticulum, urinary tract infection, polyuria.

Miscellaneous: allergic reaction, asthenia, female breast pain, edema, feeling of warmth, fever, flu-like symptoms, malaise, rigors, earache, biliary pain, cholecystitis, hepatomegaly, diabetes mellitus, gout, weight decrease, weight increase, peripheral edema, tinnitus, epistaxis, purpura, infection, bacterial infection, cerebrovascular disorder, intermittent claudication, leg ulcer, peripheral ischemia, varicose vein, amaurosis fugax, conjunctivitis, diplopia, photophobia, moniliasis, skin nodule, tympanic membrane perforation, allergy, pain.

Musculoskeletal: arthralgia, arthritis, arthropathy, arthrosis, frozen shoulder, muscle weakness, myalgia, myositis, torticollis, tendon disorder.

Neurological: hypoesthesia, migraine, neuritis, tremor, agitation, amnesia, impaired concentration, depression, decreased libido, nervousness, paroninia, confusion, anxiety, paresis, ptosis, impotence.

Respiratory: bronchitis, bronchospasm, pharyngitis, pneumonia, rales, respiratory disorder, pulmonary infiltration, increased sputum, sinusitis, nasal congestion.

Laboratory Changes: albuminuria, hematuria, gamma GT increased, AST increased, ALT increased, hypercholesterolemia, hyperlipemia, hyperuricemia, hypocalcemia, hypokalemia, increased non-protein nitrogen, thrombocytopenia, anemia, leukopenia, leukocytosis, glycosuria.

OVERDOSE:

Symptoms: Hemodynamic Effects: Symptoms of isosorbide-5-mononitrate overdose are generally the results of vasodilation, venous pooling, reduced cardiac output and hypotension. These hemodynamic changes may have protean manifestations, including increased intracranial pressure, with any or all of persistent throbbing headache, confusion, and moderate fever; vertigo; palpitations; visual disturbances; nausea and vomiting (possibly with colic and even bloody diarrhea); syncope (especially in the upright posture); air hunger and dyspnea, later followed by reduced ventilatory effort; diaphoresis, with the skin either flushed or cold and clammy; heart block and bradycardia; paralysis; coma; seizures and death.

No specific antagonist to the vasodilator effects of isosorbide-5-mononitrate is known, and no intervention has been subject to controlled study as a therapy of isosorbide-5-mononitrate overdose. Because the hypotension associated with isosorbide-5-mononitrate overdose is the result of venodilation and arterial hypovolemia, prudent therapy in this situation should be directed toward an increase in central fluid volume. Passive elevation of the patient's legs may be sufficient, but i.v. infusion of normal saline or similar fluid may also be necessary.

In patients with renal disease or congestive heart failure, therapy resulting in central volume expansion is not without hazard. Treatment of isosorbide-5-mononitrate overdose in these patients may be subtle and difficult, and invasive monitoring may be required.

The use of epinephrine or other vasoconstrictors is ineffective in reversing the severe hypotensive effects of overdose and is therefore contraindicated in this situation.

Dialysis is known to be ineffective in removing isosorbide-5-mononitrate from the body.

Methemoglobinemia: Methemoglobinemia has been reported in patients receiving other organic nitrates, and it may occur as a side effect of isosorbide-5-mononitrate. Nitrate ions liberated during metabolism of isosorbide-5-mononitrate can oxidize hemoglobin into methemoglobin. In patients totally without cytochrome b_5 reductase activity, about 2 mg/kg of isosorbide-5-mononitrate would be required before any of these patients manifests clinically significant (≥10%) methemoglobinemia. In patients with normal reductase function, significant production of methemoglobin would require even larger doses of isosorbide-5-mononitrate.

Methemoglobin levels are available from most clinical laboratories. The diagnosis should be suspected in patients who exhibit signs of impaired oxygen delivery despite adequate cardiac output and adequate arterial pO_2. Classically, methemoglobinemic blood is described as chocolate brown without color change on exposure to air. When methemoglobinemia is diagnosed, administration of methylene blue, 1 to 2 mg/kg i.v. may be required.

Treatment: See Symptoms.

> For management of a suspected drug overdose, CPhA recommends that you contact your **regional Poison Control Centre**. See the *CPS* Directory section for a list of Poison Control Centres.

DOSAGE: Isosorbide-5-mononitrate, administered once daily, provides efficacy for up to 12 hours. This formulation is designed to avoid or attenuate the development of tolerance.

The recommended starting dose, for those patients who are active during the day, is 60 mg (1 tablet) once daily to be taken in the morning on arising. The dose may be increased to 120 mg (2 tablets) once daily. Rarely 240 mg may be required. To minimize the possibility of headache the dose can be titrated by initiating treatment with 30 mg (½ a tablet) for the first 2 to 4 days.

Dosage adjustments are not necessary for elderly patients or patients with altered renal or hepatic function.

The tablet may be taken whole or as divided halves.

The tablets should not be chewed or crushed, and should be swallowed together with half a glass of water. Whole tablets may sometimes seem to appear in the stool; these will only be the matrices which have remained intact after the active substance has been leached out.

Note: Isosorbide-5-mononitrate is not indicated for the relief of acute anginal attacks; in these situations sublingual or buccal nitroglycerin should be used.

INFORMATION FOR THE PATIENT: Published in e-CPS, available by subscription at www.e-cps.ca.

SUPPLIED: Each oval, yellow, biconvex, film-coated, extended release tablet, scored on both sides and engraved $\frac{A}{ID}$ on one side, contains: isosorbide-5-mononitrate 60 mg. Nonmedicinal ingredients: tablet core: colloidal silicon dioxide, hydroxypropylcellulose, magnesium stearate, paraffin and sodium aluminum silicate; coating: hydroxypropylmethylcellulose, iron oxide yellow, paraffin, polyethylene glycol and titanium dioxide. Blister packs of 30. Bottles of 100. Store between 15 and 30°C.

(Shown in Product Identification Section)

Imitrex DF™ Tablets Ⓟ

sumatriptan succinate

5-HT1 Receptor Agonist—Migraine Therapy

GlaxoSmithKline

Imitrex® Injection/Autoinjector Ⓟ

sumatriptan succinate

5-HT1 Receptor Agonist—Migraine Therapy

GlaxoSmithKline

Imitrex® Nasal Spray Ⓟ

sumatriptan hemisulfate

5-HT1 Receptor Agonist—Migraine Therapy

GlaxoSmithKline

Date of Revision: April 8, 2009

SUMMARY PRODUCT INFORMATION:

Route of Administration	Dosage Form/ Strength	Clinically Relevant Nonmedicinal Ingredients
Oral	(sumatriptan succinate) Tablets 50 mg and 100 mg	No clinically relevant nonmedicinal ingredients. For a complete listing see Dosage Forms, Composition and Packaging.
Subcutaneous	(sumatriptan succinate) Subcutaneous Injection and Autoinjector 6 mg	
Intranasal	(sumatriptan hemisulphate) Nasal Spray 5 mg and 20 mg	

INDICATIONS AND CLINICAL USE: Adults: IMITREX DF (sumatriptan succinate) and IMITREX (sumatriptan succinate/sumatriptan hemisulphate) are indicated for the acute treatment of migraine attacks with or without aura.

IMITREX DF and IMITREX are not intended for the prophylactic therapy of migraine or for use in the management of hemiplegic, basilar, or ophthalmoplegic migraine (see Contraindications). Safety and efficacy have not been established for cluster headache which is present in an older, predominantly male population.

Pediatrics (<18 years of age): The safety and efficacy of IMITREX DF or IMITREX in children has not been established and its use in this age group is not recommended. (See Warnings and Precautions.)

Geriatrics (>65 years of age): Experience of the use of IMITREX DF or IMITREX in patients aged over 65 years is limited. Therefore the use of IMITREX DF or IMITREX in patients over 65 years is not recommended. (See Warnings and Precautions.)

CONTRAINDICATIONS: IMITREX DF and IMITREX are contraindicated in patients with history, symptoms, or signs of ischemic cardiac, cerebrovascular, or peripheral vascular syndromes, valvular heart disease or cardiac arrhythmias (especially tachycardias). In addition, patients with other significant underlying cardiovascular diseases (e.g., atherosclerotic disease, congenital heart disease) should not receive IMITREX DF or IMITREX. Ischemic cardiac syndromes include, but are not limited to, angina pectoris of any type (e.g., stable angina of effort and vasospastic forms of angina such as the Prinzmetal's variant), all forms of myocardial infarction, and silent myocardial ischemia. Cerebrovascular syndromes include, but are not limited to, strokes of any type as well as transient ischemic attacks (TIAs). Peripheral vascular disease includes, but is not limited to, ischemic bowel disease, or Raynaud's syndrome (see Warnings and Precautions).

Because IMITREX DF and IMITREX may increase blood pressure, they are contraindicated in patients with uncontrolled or severe hypertension.

Concurrent administration of MAO inhibitors or use within 2 weeks of discontinuation of MAO inhibitor therapy is contraindicated (see Action and Clinical Pharmacology and Drug Interactions).

Ergot-containing drugs have been reported to cause prolonged vasospastic reactions. Because IMITREX DF and IMITREX may also cause coronary vasospasm and these effects may be additive, the use of IMITREX DF and IMITREX within 24 hours before or after treatment with other 5-HT$_1$ receptor agonists, or ergotamine-containing drugs or their derivatives (eg. dihydroergotamine, methysergide) is contraindicated.

IMITREX DF and IMITREX should not be administered to patients with severe hepatic impairment.

IMITREX DF and IMITREX are contraindicated in patients with hemiplegic, basilar, or ophthalmoplegic migraine.

IMITREX DF and IMITREX are contraindicated in patients with hypersensitivity to sumatriptan or to any of the ingredients of the formulations, or component of the container. For a complete listing, see Dosage Forms, Composition and Packaging.

IMITREX Injection should not be given intravenously because of its potential to cause coronary vasospasm.

WARNINGS AND PRECAUTIONS: General: IMITREX DF and IMITREX should only be used where a clear diagnosis of migraine has been established.

Cluster Headache: There is insufficient information on the efficacy and safety of IMITREX DF and IMITREX in the treatment of cluster headache, which is present in an older, predominantly male population. The need for prolonged use and the demand for repeated medication in this condition renders the dosing information inapplicable for cluster headache.

Psychomotor Impairment: Patients should be cautioned that drowsiness may occur as a result of treatment with IMITREX DF and IMITREX. They should be advised not to perform skilled tasks (e.g. driving or operating machinery) if drowsiness occurs.

Medication Overuse Headache: Overuse of acute migraine treatments has been associated with the exacerbation of headache (medication overuse headache, MOH) in susceptible patients. Withdrawal of the treatment may be necessary.

Cardiovascular: Risk of Myocardial Ischemia and/or Infarction and Other Adverse Cardiac Events: IMITREX has been associated with transient chest and/or neck pain, pressure, heaviness and tightness which may resemble angina pectoris. In rare cases, the symptoms have been identified as being the likely result of coronary vasospasm or myocardial ischemia. Rare cases of serious coronary events or arrhythmia have occurred following use of IMITREX. IMITREX DF and IMITREX should not be given to patients who have documented ischemic or vasospastic coronary artery disease (CAD) (see Contraindications). It is strongly recommended that IMITREX DF and IMITREX not be given to patients in whom unrecognized CAD is predicted by the presence of risk factors (e.g., hypertension, hypercholesterolemia, smoking, obesity, diabetes, strong family history of CAD, female who is surgically or physiologically postmenopausal, or male who is over 40 years of age) unless a cardiovascular evaluation provides satisfactory clinical evidence that the patient is reasonably free of coronary artery and ischemic myocardial disease or other significant underlying cardiovascular disease. The sensitivity of cardiac diagnostic procedures to detect cardiovascular disease or predisposition to coronary artery vasospasm is unknown. If, during the cardiovascular evaluation, the patient's medical history or electrocardiographic investigations reveal findings indicative of, or consistent with, coronary artery vasospasm or myocardial ischemia, IMITREX DF or IMITREX should not be administered (see Contraindications).

For patients with risk factors predictive of CAD, who are considered to have a satisfactory cardiovascular evaluation, the first dose of IMITREX DF or IMITREX should be administered in the setting of a physician's office or similar medically staffed and equipped facility. Because cardiac ischemia can occur in the absence of clinical symptoms, consideration should be given to obtaining electrocardiograms in patients with risk factors during the interval immediately following IMITREX DF or IMITREX administration on the first occasion of use. However, an absence of drug-induced cardiovascular effects on the occasion of the initial dose does not preclude the possibility of such effects occurring with subsequent administrations.

Intermittent long term users of IMITREX DF or IMITREX, who have or acquire risk factors predictive of CAD as described above, should receive periodic interval cardiovascular evaluations over the course of treatment.

If symptoms consistent with angina occur after the use of IMITREX DF or IMITREX, ECG evaluation should be carried out to look for ischemic changes.

The systematic approach described above is intended to reduce the likelihood that patients with unrecognized cardiovascular disease will be inadvertently exposed to IMITREX DF or IMITREX.

Discomfort in the chest, neck, throat and jaw (including pain, pressure, heaviness, tightness, dyspnea) has been reported after administration of IMITREX. Because 5-HT$_1$ agonists may cause coronary vasospasm, patients who experience signs or symptoms suggestive of angina following IMITREX DF or IMITREX should be evaluated for the presence of CAD or a predisposition to variant angina before receiving additional doses, and should be monitored electrocardiographically if dosing is resumed and similar symptoms recur. Similarly, patients who experience other symptoms

or signs suggestive of decreased arterial flow, such as ischemic bowel syndrome or Raynaud's syndrome following IMITREX DF or IMITREX should be evaluated for atherosclerosis or predisposition to vasospasm (see Contraindications; Warnings and Precautions and Adverse Drug Reactions, Clinical Trial Adverse Drug Reactions).

Cardiac Events and Fatalities Associated with 5-HT$_1$ Agonists: IMITREX DF and IMITREX can cause coronary artery vasospasm. Serious adverse cardiac events, including acute myocardial infarction, life threatening disturbances of cardiac rhythm, and death have been reported within a few hours following the administration of 5-HT$_1$ agonists. Considering the extent of use of 5-HT$_1$ agonists in patients with migraine, the incidence of these events is extremely low. The fact that some of these events have occurred in patients with no prior cardiac disease history and with documented absence of CAD, and the close proximity of the events to IMITREX use support the conclusion that some of these cases were caused by the drug. In many cases, however, where there has been known underlying coronary artery disease, the relationship is uncertain.

Premarketing Experience with IMITREX: Of 6348 patients with migraine who participated in premarketing controlled and uncontrolled clinical trials of oral and IMITREX, two experienced clinical adverse events shortly after receiving oral IMITREX that may have reflected coronary vasospasm. Neither of these adverse events was associated with a serious clinical outcome.

Among the more than 1900 patients with migraine who participated in premarketing controlled clinical trials of subcutaneous IMITREX, there were eight patients who sustained clinical events during or shortly after receiving IMITREX that may have reflected coronary artery vasospasm. Six of these eight patients had ECG changes consistent with transient ischemia, but without accompanying clinical symptoms or signs. Of these eight patients, four had either findings suggestive of CAD or risk factors predictive of CAD prior to study enrollment.

Among approximately 4000 patients with migraine who participated in premarketing controlled and uncontrolled clinical trials of IMITREX nasal spray, one patient experienced an asymptomatic subendocardial infarction possibly subsequent to a coronary vasospastic event.

Postmarketing Experience with IMITREX: Serious cardiovascular events, some resulting in death, have been reported in association with the use of IMITREX Injection or IMITREX Tablets. The uncontrolled nature of postmarketing surveillance, however, makes it impossible to determine definitively the proportion of the reported cases that were actually caused by IMITREX or to reliably assess causation in individual cases. On clinical grounds, the longer the latency between the administration of IMITREX and the onset of the clinical event, the less likely the association is to be causative. Accordingly, interest has focused on events beginning within 1 hour of the administration of IMITREX.

Cardiac events that have been observed to have onset within 1 hour of IMITREX administration include: coronary artery vasospasm, transient ischemia, myocardial infarction, ventricular tachycardia and ventricular fibrillation, cardiac arrest, and death.

Some of these events occurred in patients who had no findings of CAD and appear to represent consequences of coronary artery vasospasm. However, among reports from the USA of serious cardiac events occurring within 1 hour of IMITREX administration, almost all of the patients had risk factors predictive of CAD and the presence of significant underlying CAD was established in most cases (see Contraindications).

Cerebrovascular Events and Fatalities with 5-HT$_1$ Agonists: Cerebral hemorrhage, subarachnoid hemorrhage, stroke, and other cerebrovascular events have been reported in patients treated with oral or subcutaneous IMITREX, and some have resulted in fatalities. The relationship of IMITREX to these events is uncertain. In a number of cases, it appears possible that the cerebrovascular events were primary, IMITREX having been administered in the incorrect belief that the symptoms experienced were a consequence of migraine when they were not. Before treating migraine headaches with IMITREX DF and IMITREX in patients not previously diagnosed as migraineurs, and in migraineurs who present with atypical symptoms, care should be taken to exclude other potentially serious neurological conditions. If a patient does not respond to the first dose, the opportunity should be taken to review the diagnosis before a second dose is given. It should also be noted that patients with migraine may be at increased risk of certain cerebrovascular events (e.g., stroke, hemorrhage, TIA).

Special Cardiovascular Pharmacology Studies: In subjects (n=10) with suspected coronary artery disease undergoing angiography, a 5-HT$_1$ agonist at a subcutaneous dose of 1.5 mg produced an 8% increase in aortic blood pressure, an 18% increase in pulmonary artery blood pressure, and an 8% increase in systemic vascular resistance. In addition, mild chest pain or tightness was reported by four subjects. Clinically significant increases in blood pressure were experienced by three of the subjects (two of whom also had chest pain/discomfort). Diagnostic angiogram results revealed that 9 subjects had normal coronary arteries and 1 had insignificant coronary artery disease.

In an additional study with this same drug, migraine patients (n=35) free of cardiovascular disease were subjected to assessments of myocardial perfusion by positron emission tomography while receiving a subcutaneous 1.5 mg dose in the absence of a migraine attack. Reduced coronary vasodilatory reserve (~10%), increase in coronary resistance (~20%), and decrease in hyperemic myocardial blood flow (~10%) were noted. The relevance of these finding to the use of the recommended oral doses of this 5-HT$_1$ agonist is not known.

Similar studies have not been done with IMITREX DF or IMITREX. However, owing to the common pharmacodynamic actions of 5-HT$_1$ agonists, the possibility of cardiovascular effects of the nature described above should be considered for any agent of this pharmacological class.

Other Vasospasm Related Events: 5-HT$_1$ agonists may cause vasospastic reactions other than coronary artery vasospasm. Extensive post-market experience has shown the use of IMITREX to be associated with rare occurrences of peripheral vascular ischemia and colonic ischemia with abdominal pain and bloody diarrhea, and in isolated cases there was no previous history or concomitant medications.

Increase in Blood Pressure: Significant elevation in blood pressure, including hypertensive crisis, has been reported on rare occasions in patients with and without a history of hypertension. IMITREX DF and IMITREX are contraindicated in patients with uncontrolled or severe hypertension (see Contraindications). In patients with controlled hypertension, IMITREX DF or IMITREX should be administered with caution, as transient increases in blood pressure and peripheral vascular resistance have been observed in a small portion of patients.

Hepatic: The effect of hepatic impairment on the efficacy and safety of IMITREX DF and IMITREX has not been evaluated, however, the pharmacokinetic profile of sumatriptan in patients with moderate* hepatic impairment shows that these patients, following an oral dose of 50 mg, have much higher plasma sumatriptan concentrations than healthy subjects (Table 1).

Table 1: IMITREX Tablets

Pharmacokinetic Parameters After Oral Administration of IMITREX 50 mg to Healthy Volunteers and Moderately Hepatically Impaired Patients

Parameter	Mean Ratio (hepatic impaired/healthy) n=8	90% CI	p-value
AUC_∞	181%	130 to 252%	0.009[a]
C_{max}	176%	129 to 240%	0.007[a]

[a] Statistically significant.
Legend: CI=confidence interval.

The pharmacokinetic parameters of 6 mg subcutaneous sumatriptan do not differ statistically between normal volunteers and moderately hepatically impaired subjects. However, sumatriptan should not be administered to patients with severe hepatic impairment (see Contraindications).

Immune: Rare hypersensitivity (anaphylaxis/anaphylactoid) reactions may occur in patients receiving 5-HT$_1$ agonists such as IMITREX DF or IMITREX. Such reactions can be life threatening or fatal. In general, hypersensitivity reactions to drugs are more likely to occur in individuals with a history of sensitivity to multiple allergens (see Contraindications). Owing to the possibility of cross-reactive hypersensitivity reactions, IMITREX DF and IMITREX should not be used in patients having a history of hypersensitivity to chemically-related 5-HT$_1$ receptor agonists. There have been reports of patients with known hypersensitivity to sulphonamides exhibiting an allergic reaction following administration of IMITREX. Reactions ranged from cutaneous hypersensitivity to anaphylaxis.

Neurologic: Care should be taken to exclude other potentially serious neurologic conditions before treating headache in patients not previously diagnosed with migraine headache or who experience a headache that is atypical for them. There have been rare reports where patients received 5-HT$_1$ agonists for severe headaches that were subsequently shown to have been secondary to an evolving neurologic lesion. For newly diagnosed patients or patients presenting with atypical symptoms, the diagnosis of migraine should be reconsidered if no response is seen after the first dose of IMITREX DF or IMITREX.

* Assessed by aminopyrine breath best (>0.2-0.4 scaling units).

Seizures: Caution should be observed if IMITREX DF or IMITREX is to be used in patients with a history of seizures or other risk factors, such as structural brain lesions, which lower the convulsion threshold. There have also been rare post-market reports of seizures following administration of IMITREX in patients without risk factors or previous history of seizures. (See Adverse Reactions, Post-Market Adverse Drug Reactions, Nervous System Disorders.)

Selective Serotonin Reuptake Inhibitors (SSRIs)/Serotonin Norepinephrine Reuptake Inhibitors (SNRIs) and Serotonin Syndrome: Cases of life-threatening serotonin syndrome have been reported during combined use of selective serotonin reuptake inhibitors (SSRIs)/serotonin norepinephrine reuptake inhibitors (SNRIs) and triptans. If concomitant treatment with IMITREX DF or IMITREX and SSRIs (e.g., fluoxetine, paroxetine, sertraline) or SNRIs (e.g., venlafaxine) is clinically warranted, careful observation of the patient is advised, particularly during treatment initiation and dose increases. Serotonin syndrome symptoms may include mental status changes (e.g., agitation, hallucinations, coma), autonomic instability (e.g., tachycardia, labile blood pressure, hyperthermia), neuromuscular aberrations (e.g., hyperreflexia, incoordination) and/or gastrointestinal symptoms (e.g., nausea, vomiting, diarrhea) (see Drug Interactions, Selective Serotonin Reuptake Inhibitors (SSRIs)/Serotonin Norepinephrine Reuptake Inhibitors (SNRIs)).

Ophthalmologic: Binding to Melanin Containing Tissues: In rats treated with a single subcutaneous dose (0.5 mg/kg) or oral dose (2 mg/kg) of radiolabeled sumatriptan, the elimination half life of radioactivity from the eye was 15 and 23 days, respectively, suggesting that sumatriptan and/or its metabolites bind to the melanin of the eye. Because there could be an accumulation in melanin rich tissues over time, this raises the possibility that sumatriptan could cause toxicity in these tissues after extended use. However, no effects on the retina related to treatment with sumatriptan were noted in any of the oral or subcutaneous toxicity studies. Although no systematic monitoring of ophthalmologic function was undertaken in clinical trials, and no specific recommendations for ophthalmologic monitoring are offered, prescribers should be aware of the possibility of long term ophthalmologic effects.

Renal: The effects of renal impairment on the efficacy and safety of IMITREX DF and IMITREX have not been evaluated. Therefore IMITREX DF and IMITREX are not recommended in this patient population.

Special Populations: Pregnant Women: Reproduction studies, performed in rats, have not revealed any evidence of impaired fertility, teratogenicity, or post-natal development due to IMITREX. Reproduction studies, performed in rabbits by the oral route, have shown increased incidence of variations in cervico-thoracic blood vessel configuration in the fetuses. These effects were only seen at the highest dose tested, which affected weight gain in the dams, and at which blood levels were in excess of 50 times those seen in humans after therapeutic doses. A direct association with IMITREX DF or IMITREX treatment is considered unlikely but cannot be excluded.

Post-marketing data from multiple prospective pregnancy registries have documented the pregnancy outcomes in approximately 1100 women exposed to sumatriptan. At this time, there is insufficient information to draw conclusions. Therefore, use of IMITREX DF and IMITREX is not recommended in pregnancy and it should be used only if the potential benefit to the mother justifies the potential risk to the fetus.

In a rat fertility study, oral doses of IMITREX resulting in plasma levels approximately 150 times those seen in humans after a 6 mg subcutaneous dose and approximately 200 times those seen in humans after a 100 mg oral dose were associated with a reduction in the success of insemination. This effect did not occur during a subcutaneous study where maximum plasma levels achieved approximately 100 times those in humans by the subcutaneous route and approximately 150 times those in humans by the oral route.

To monitor maternal fetal outcomes of pregnant women exposed to sumatriptan, a Pregnancy Registry has been established. Physicians are encouraged to register patients by calling 1-800-336-2176.

Nursing Women: Sumatriptan is excreted in human breast milk. Therefore, caution is advised when administering IMITREX DF or IMITREX to nursing women. Infant exposure can be minimised by avoiding breast feeding for 24 hours after treatment.

Pediatrics (<18 years of age): The safety and efficacy of IMITREX DF or IMITREX in children has not been established and its use in this age group is not recommended.

Geriatrics (>65 years of age): Experience of the use of IMITREX DF or IMITREX in patients aged over 65 years is limited. Therefore the use of IMITREX DF or IMITREX in patients over 65 years is not recommended.

Special Disease Conditions: IMITREX and IMITREX DF should be administered with caution to patients with diseases that may alter the absorption, metabolism, or excretion of drugs, such as impaired hepatic or renal function. (See Warnings and Precautions, Hepatic; Renal.)

Monitoring and Laboratory Tests: No specific laboratory tests are recommended for monitoring patients prior to and/or after treatment with IMITREX DF or IMITREX.

ADVERSE REACTIONS: Serious cardiac events, including some that have been fatal, have occurred following the use of 5-HT$_1$ agonists. These events are extremely rare and most have been reported in patients with risk factors predictive of CAD. Events reported have included coronary artery vasospasm, transient myocardial ischemia, myocardial infarction, ventricular tachycardia, and ventricular fibrillation (see Contraindications and Warnings and Precautions).

Clinical Trial Adverse Drug Reactions: Because clinical trials are conducted under very specific conditions the adverse reaction rates observed in the clinical trials may not reflect the rates observed in practice and should not be compared to the rates in the clinical trials of another drug. Adverse drug reaction information from clinical trials is useful for identifying drug-related adverse events and for approximating rates.

Experience in Controlled Clinical Trials with IMITREX: Typical 5-HT$_1$ Agonist Adverse Reactions: As with other 5-HT$_1$ agonists, IMITREX has been associated with sensations of heaviness, pressure, tightness or pain which may be intense. These may occur in any part of the body including the chest, throat, neck, jaw and upper limb.

Acute Safety: In placebo-controlled migraine trials, 7,668 patients received at least one dose of IMITREX (3095 oral, 1432 subcutaneous, 3141 intranasal). The following tables (Table 2, Table 3 and Table 4) list adverse events occurring in these trials at an incidence of 1% or more in any of the IMITREX dose groups and that occurred at a higher incidence than in the placebo groups.

Table 2: IMITREX Tablets

Treatment-Emergent Adverse Events in Oral Placebo-Controlled Clinical Trials Reported by at Least 1% of Patients with Migraine

	Placebo	IMITREX 25 mg	IMITREX 50 mg	IMITREX 100 mg[b]
Number of Patients	690	351	723	2021
Number of Migraine Attacks Treated	1187	945	1889	14 750
Symptoms of Potentially Cardiac Origin				
Chest Sensations[a]	0.6%	2.3%	2.6%	3.2%
Neck/Throat/Jaw Sensations[a]	1.4%	2.3%	3.5%	5.2%
Upper Limb Sensations[a]	1.2%	1.4%	2.5%	3.6%
Palpitations	0.6%	0.3%	1.0%	1.1%
Neurological				
Head/Face Sensations[a]	1.3%	2.3%	2.5%	4.7%
Dizziness	2.5%	3.1%	3.3%	6.2%
Headache	3.3%	4.0%	2.2%	3.3%
Vertigo	0.6%	1.1%	1.1%	1.0%
Drowsiness	1.6%	1.1%	1.2%	2.1%

(cont'd)

Table 2: IMITREX Tablets *(cont'd)*

Treatment-Emergent Adverse Events in Oral Placebo-Controlled Clinical Trials Reported by at Least 1% of Patients with Migraine

	Placebo	IMITREX 25 mg	IMITREX 50 mg	IMITREX 100 mg[b]
Tremor	0.4%	0.9%	0.4%	1.1%
Gastrointestinal				
Nausea	5.8%	2.8%	4.4%	11.0%
Hyposalivation	1.2%	1.4%	1.1%	1.2%
Vomiting	2.9%	4.3%	1.1%	4.4%
Gastrointestinal Discomfort and Pain	1.4%	1.1%	0.8%	2.0%
Abdominal Discomfort and Pain	0.3%	NR	0.4%	1.2%
Diarrhea	0.9%	0.3%	0.6%	1.1%
Musculoskeletal				
Musculoskeletal Pain	0.7%	2.3%	0.4%	1.4%
Muscle Pain	0.3%	0.9%	0.1%	1.0%
Muscle Atrophy Weakness and Tiredness	NR	0.6%	0.4%	1.4%
Ear, Nose and Throat				
Infections	0.6%	0.6%	1.1%	1.4%
Nasal Signs and Symptoms	0.7%	1.4%	0.8%	1.0%
Throat and Tonsil Symptoms	0.6%	NR	0.4%	2.3%
Respiratory				
Viral Infection	0.3%	1.1%	0.1%	1.0%
Non-Site Specific				
Limb Sensations[a]	0.4%	1.1%	0.4%	1.5%
Sensations[a] (body region unspecified)	4.5%	5.7%	8.0%	9.0%
Malaise/Fatigue	5.1%	3.7%	2.6%	9.5%
Sweating	0.4%	0.6%	0.6%	1.6%

[a] The term "sensations" encompasses adverse events described as pain and discomfort, pressure, heaviness, constriction, tightness, heat/burning or cold sensation, paresthesia, hypoesthesia, numbness, and strange sensations.
[b] Includes patients receiving up to 3 doses of 100 mg.
Legend: NR=not reported.

Table 3: IMITREX Injection

Treatment-Emergent Adverse Events in S.C. Placebo-Controlled Clinical Trials Reported by at Least 1% of Patients with Migraine

	Placebo	IMITREX 6 mg
Number of Patients	615	1432
Number of Migraine Attacks Treated	742	2540
Symptoms of Potentially Cardiac Origin		
Chest Sensations[a]	1.6%	5.7%
Neck/Throat/Jaw Sensations[a]	1.3%	12.0%
Upper Limb Sensations[a]	2.0%	6.8%
Neurological		
Head/Face Sensations[a]	3.7%	16.6%
Dizziness	3.7%	7.9%
Headache	0.7%	3.4%
Drowsiness	1.8%	2.9%
Gastrointestinal		
Nausea	5.9%	9.4%
Hyposalivation	2.8%	3.3%
Musculoskeletal		

(cont'd)

Table 3: IMITREX Injection *(cont'd)*

Treatment-Emergent Adverse Events in S.C. Placebo-Controlled Clinical Trials Reported by at Least 1% of Patients with Migraine

	Placebo	IMITREX 6 mg
Muscle Atrophy Weakness and Tiredness	NR	1.7%
Ear/Nose and Throat		
Throat and Tonsil Symptoms	0.3%	1.0%
Respiratory		
Breathing Disorders	0.8%	1.3%
Non-Site Specific		
Sensations[a] (body region unspecified)	15.9%	39.0%
Injection Site Reactions	10.4%	24.7%
Limb Sensations[a]	1.5%	6.0%
Malaise/Fatigue	2.3%	4.7%
Sweating	1.1%	1.7%
Trunk Symptoms[a]	0.5%	1.4%

[a] The term "sensations" encompasses adverse events described as pain and discomfort, pressure, heaviness, constriction, tightness, heat/burning or cold sensation, paresthesia, hypoesthesia, numbness, and strange sensations.
Legend: NR=not reported.

Table 4: IMITREX Nasal Spray

Treatment-Emergent Adverse Events in Intranasal Placebo-Controlled Clinical Trials Reported by at Least 1% of Patients with Migraine

	Placebo	IMITREX 5 mg	IMITREX 10 mg	IMITREX 20 mg[b]
Number of Patients	741	496	1007	1638
Number of Migraine Attacks Treated	1047	933	1434	2070
Symptoms of Potentially Cardiac Origin				
Chest Sensations[a]	0.3%	1.0%	0.7%	0.6%
Neck/Throat/Jaw Sensations[a]	1.2%	0.6%	1.6%	2.3%
Neurological				
Head/Face Sensations[a]	0.8%	1.4%	2.4%	2.4%
Dizziness	1.2%	1.6%	1.5%	1.2%
Headache	0.7%	1.4%	0.9%	0.8%
Migraine	2.6%	3.2%	2.4%	1.8%
Gastrointestinal				
Nausea	10.4%	14.3%	9.6%	8.3%
Vomiting	7.6%	11.1%	9.6%	6.8%
Ear, Nose and Throat				
Sensitivity to Noise	3.1%	4.4%	2.5%	1.5%
Nasal Signs and Symptoms	1.3%	3.0%	1.6%	1.8%
Infections	0.9%	1.8%	1.3%	0.5%
Upper Respiratory Inflammation	0.5%	1.0%	0.6%	0.7%
Throat and Tonsil Symptoms	0.8%	0.2%	1.0%	0.7%
Non-Site Specific				
Sensations[a] (body region unspecified)	1.8%	2.4%	2.7%	2.4%
Malaise/Fatigue	1.3%	1.8%	1.3%	0.8%
Descriptions of Odor or Taste	1.8%	15.3%	20.2%	20.8%

[a] The term "sensations" encompasses adverse events described as pain and discomfort, pressure, heaviness, constriction, tightness, heat/burning or cold sensation, paresthesia, hypoesthesia, numbness, and strange sensations.
[b] Includes patients receiving up to 3 doses of 20 mg.

IMITREX is generally well tolerated. Most of the events were transient in nature and resolved within 45 minutes of subcutaneous administration and within 2 hours of oral or intranasal administration.

Of the 3630 patients treated with IMITREX Nasal Spray in clinical trials, there was one report of a coronary vasospasm related to IMITREX administration.

Other Events Observed During Clinical Trials: Minor disturbances of liver function tests have occasionally been observed with sumatriptan treatment. There is no evidence that clinically significant abnormalities occurred more frequently with sumatriptan than with placebo.

Dyspnea has commonly been observed following sumatriptan treatment.

Post-Market Adverse Drug Reactions: The following section enumerates potentially important adverse events that have occurred in clinical practice and that have been reported spontaneously to various surveillance systems. The events enumerated represent reports arising from both domestic and nondomestic use of sumatriptan. These events do not include those already listed in the Adverse Reactions section above. Because the reports cite events reported spontaneously from worldwide postmarketing experience, the frequency of such events and the role of sumatriptan in their causation cannot be reliably determined.

Cardiac Disorders: bradycardia, tachycardia, palpitations, cardiac arrhythmias, transient ischaemic ECG changes, coronary artery vasospasm, angina, myocardial infarction (see Contraindications and Warnings and Precautions).

Ophthalmologic Disorders: Patients treated with IMITREX rarely exhibit visual disorders like flickering and diplopia. Additionally, cases of reduced vision have been observed. Very rarely, both transient and permanent losses of vision have occurred. These occurrences have included reports of retinal vascular occlusion, ocular venous thrombosis, vasospasm of the eye and ischemic optic neuropathy. Visual disorders may also occur during a migraine attack itself.

Gastrointestinal Disorders: colonic ischemia (see Warnings and Precautions, Cardiovascular, Other Vasospasm Related Events).

Immune System Disorders: hypersensitivity reactions ranging from cutaneous hypersensitivity to anaphylaxis (see Warnings and Precautions, Immune).

Nervous System Disorders: Seizures, although some have occurred in patients with either a history of seizures or concurrent conditions predisposing to seizures there are also reports in patients where no such predisposing factors are apparent (see Warnings and Precautions, Neurologic).

There have been very rare reports of dystonia and related extrapyramidal disorders, such as choreoathetoid movement, akathisia, parkinsonism and akinesia following both subcutaneous and oral treatments of IMITREX. Patients with previous history of drug related dystonia and patients taking medications recognised to be associated with movement disorders such as SSRIs, may be at higher risk.

Nystagmus, scotoma.

Vascular Disorders: hypotension, Raynaud's phenomenon, peripheral vascular ischemia (see Contraindications and Warnings and Precautions, Cardiovascular, Increase in Blood Pressure and Other Vasospasm Related Events).

DRUG INTERACTIONS: Drug-Drug Interactions: Single dose pharmacokinetic drug interaction studies have not shown evidence of interactions with propranolol, flunarizine, pizotifen or alcohol. Multiple dose interaction studies have not been performed. The pharmacokinetics of sumatriptan nasal spray were unaltered when preceded by a single clinical dose of the nasal decongestant xylometazoline (Otrivin).

Ergot-Containing Drugs: Ergot-containing drugs have been reported to cause prolonged vasospastic reactions. Because there is a theoretical basis for these effects being additive, ergot-containing or ergot-type medications (like dihydroergotamine or methysergide) are contraindicated within 24 hours of IMITREX DF or IMITREX administration (see Contraindications).

MAO Inhibitors: In studies conducted in a limited number of patients, MAO inhibitors reduce sumatriptan clearance, significantly increasing systemic exposure. Therefore, the use of IMITREX DF or IMITREX in patients receiving MAO inhibitors is contraindicated (see Contraindications and Action and Clinical Pharmacology).

Selective Serotonin Reuptake Inhibitors (SSRIs)/Serotonin Norepinephrine Reuptake Inhibitors (SNRIs): Cases of life-threatening serotonin syndrome have been reported during combined use of selective serotonin reuptake inhibitors (SSRIs) or serotonin norepinephrine reuptake inhibitors (SNRIs) and triptans (see Warnings and Precautions).

Other 5-HT$_1$ agonists: The administration of IMITREX DF or IMITREX with other 5-HT$_1$ agonists has not been evaluated in migraine patients. As an increased risk of coronary vasospasm is a theoretical possibility with co-administration of 5-HT$_1$ agonists, use of these drugs within 24 hours of each other is contraindicated.

Drug-Laboratory Test Interactions: IMITREX DF or IMITREX are not known to interfere with commonly employed clinical laboratory tests.

DOSAGE AND ADMINISTRATION: Dosing Considerations: IMITREX DF and IMITREX are indicated for the acute treatment of migraine headache with or without aura. Sumatriptan should not be used prophylactically. Sumatriptan may be given orally, subcutaneously or as a nasal spray. The safety of treating an average of more than four headaches in a 30 day period has not been established.

In selecting the appropriate formulation for individual patients, consideration should be given to the patient's preference for formulation and the patient's requirement for rapid onset of relief. Significant relief begins about 10-15 minutes following subcutaneous injection, 15 minutes following intranasal administration and 30 minutes following oral administration.

In addition to relieving the pain of migraine, sumatriptan (all formulations) has also been shown to be effective in relieving associated symptoms of migraine (nausea, vomiting, phonophobia, photophobia). Sumatriptan is equally effective when administered at any stage of a migraine attack. Long term (12-24 months) clinical studies with maximum recommended doses of sumatriptan indicate that there is no evidence of the development of tachyphylaxis, or medication-induced (rebound) headache.

The safety and efficacy of IMITREX DF or IMITREX in children has not been established and its use in this age group is not recommended. (See Warnings and Precautions.)

Recommended Dose and Dosage Adjustment: Tablets: The minimal effective single adult dose of IMITREX DF Tablets is 25† mg. The maximum recommended single dose is 100 mg.

The optimal dose is a single 50 mg tablet. However, depending on individual patient's needs and response to treatment, some patients may require 100 mg.

Clinical trials have shown that approximately 50-75% of patients have headache relief within two hours after oral dosing with 100 mg, and that a further 15-25% have headache relief by 4 hours. Comparator studies have shown similar efficacy rates with the 50 mg and 100 mg tablets.

If the migraine headache returns, or if a patient has a partial response to the initial dose, the dose may be repeated after 2 hours. Not more than 200 mg should be taken in any 24 hour period.

If a patient does not respond to the first dose of IMITREX DF Tablets, a second dose should not be taken for the same attack, as it is unlikely to be of clinical benefit. IMITREX DF may be taken to treat subsequent migraine attacks.

Hepatic Impairment: In patients with mild or moderate hepatic impairment, plasma sumatriptan concentrations up to two times those seen in healthy subjects have been observed (see Warnings and Precautions). Sumatriptan should not be administered to patients with severe hepatic impairment (see Contraindications).

Injection: IMITREX Injection should be injected subcutaneously (on the outside of the thigh or in the upper arm) using an autoinjector.

The recommended adult dose of sumatriptan is a single 6 mg subcutaneous injection. Clinical trials have shown that approximately 70-72% of patients have headache relief within one hour after a single subcutaneous injection. This number increases to 82% by 2 hours.

If the migraine headache returns, or if a patient has a partial response to the initial dose, the dose may be repeated after 1 hour. Not more than 12 mg (two 6 mg injections) should be taken in any 24 hour period.

If a patient does not respond to the first dose of IMITREX Injection, a second dose should not be taken for the same attack, as it is unlikely to be of clinical benefit. IMITREX may be taken for subsequent attacks.

Administration during migraine aura prior to other symptoms occurring may not prevent the development of a headache.

Nasal Spray: The minimal effective single adult dose of sumatriptan nasal spray is 5 mg. The maximum recommended single dose is 20 mg.

If the migraine headache returns, or if a patient has a partial response to the initial dose, the dose may be repeated after 2 hours. Not more than 40 mg should be taken in any 24 hour period.

Optimal rates of headache relief were seen with the 20 mg dose. Single doses above 20 mg should not be used due to limited safety data and lack of increased efficacy relative to the 20 mg single dose. Within the range of 5-20 mg, an increase in dose was not associated with any significant increase in the incidence or severity of adverse events other than taste disturbance (see Adverse Reactions).

Administration: Tablets: The tablet should be swallowed whole with water, not crushed, chewed or split.

Injection: Patients should be advised to read the patient instruction leaflet regarding the safe disposal of syringes and needles.

Nasal Spray: The nasal spray should be administered into one nostril **only**. The device is a ready to use single dose unit and must **not be** primed before administration. Patients should be advised to read the patient instruction leaflet regarding the use of the nasal spray device before administration.

† 25 mg tablets are not available in Canada.

OVERDOSAGE:

There have been some reports of overdosage with IMITREX. Patients have received single injections of up to 12 mg subcutaneously without significant adverse effects. Doses up to 16 mg subcutaneously and up to 400 mg orally were not associated with side effects other than those mentioned. The highest dose of IMITREX Nasal Spray administered without significant adverse effects was 20 mg given three times daily for 4 days.

If overdosage with sumatriptan occurs, the patient should be monitored and standard supportive treatment applied as required. Toxicokinetic data are not available.

The effect of haemodialysis or peritoneal dialysis on the serum concentration of sumatriptan is unknown.

For management of a suspected drug overdose, CPhA recommends that you contact your **regional Poison Control Centre**. See the *CPS* Directory section for a list of Poison Control Centres.

ACTION AND CLINICAL PHARMACOLOGY: Mechanism of Action: IMITREX DF and IMITREX have been shown to be effective in relieving migraine headache. Sumatriptan is an agonist for a vascular 5-hydroxytryptamine$_{1D}$ (5-HT$_{1D}$) receptor subtype (a member of the 5-HT$_1$ family), and has only weak affinity for 5-HT$_{1A}$ receptors and no significant activity (as measured using standard radioligand binding assays) or pharmacological activity at 5-HT$_2$, 5-HT$_3$, 5-HT$_4$, 5-HT$_{5A}$, or 5-HT$_7$ receptor subtypes, or at alpha$_1$-, alpha$_2$-, or beta-adrenergic; dopamine$_1$ or dopamine$_2$; muscarinic; or benzodiazepine receptors.

The therapeutic activity of IMITREX DF and IMITREX in migraine is generally attributed to its agonist activity at 5-HT$_{1B}$/5-HT$_{1D}$ receptors. Two current theories have been proposed to explain the efficacy of 5-HT$_1$ receptor agonists in migraine. One theory suggests that activation of 5-HT$_1$ receptors located on intracranial blood vessels, including those on the arteriovenous anastomoses, leads to vasoconstriction, which is believed to be correlated with the relief of migraine headache. The other hypothesis suggests that activation of 5-HT$_1$ receptors on perivascular fibres of the trigeminal system results in the inhibition of pro-inflammatory neuropeptide release. These theories are not mutually exclusive.

Experimental data from animal studies shows that sumatriptan also activates 5-HT$_1$ receptors on peripheral terminals of the trigeminal nerve which innervates cranial blood vessels. This causes the inhibition of neuropeptide release. It is thought that such an action may contribute to the anti-migraine action of sumatriptan in humans.

Cardiovascular Effects: In vitro studies in human isolated epicardial coronary arteries suggest that the predominant contractile effect of 5-HT is mediated via 5-HT$_2$ receptors. However, 5-HT$_1$ receptors also contribute to some degree to the contractile effect seen. Transient increases in systolic and diastolic blood pressure (up to 20 mmHg) of rapid onset (within minutes), have occurred after intravenous administration of up to 64 µg/kg (3.2 mg for 50 kg subject) to healthy volunteers. These changes were not dose related and returned to normal within 10-15 minutes. Following oral administration of 200 mg or intranasal administration of 40 mg, however, mean peak increases in blood pressure were smaller and of slower onset than after intravenous or subcutaneous administration.

Pharmacodynamics: Significant relief begins about 10-15 minutes following subcutaneous injection, 15 minutes following intranasal administration and 30 minutes following oral administration.

Pharmacokinetics: Pharmacokinetic parameters following subcutaneous, oral or intranasal administration are shown in Table 5.

Inter-patient and intra-patient variability was noted in most pharmacokinetic parameters assessed.

Table 5: IMITREX/IMITREX DF

Summary of Pharmacokinetic Parameters

Parameter	Subcutaneous	Oral	Intranasal
Bioavailability	96%	14%	16%
C_{max} (ng/mL)	6 mg: 72 ng/mL	100 mg: 50–60 ng/mL 25 mg: 18 ng/mL	5 mg: 4.7 ng/mL 10 mg: 8.5 ng/mL 20 mg: 14.4 ng/mL
T_{max}	6 mg: 15 min	100 mg: 0.5–5 h[a]	1–1.5 h
$T_{1/2}$	2 h (1.7–2.3 h)	2 h (1.9–2.2 h)	2 h (1.3–5.4 h)
Protein Binding	14–21%		
Volume of Distribution	170 L		
Total Plasma Clearance	1160 mL/min		
Renal Plasma Clearance	260 mL/min		

[a] 70% to 80% of C_{max} values were attained within 30–45 minutes of dosing.

Absorption/Metabolism: Sumatriptan is rapidly absorbed after oral, subcutaneous and intranasal administration. The low oral and intranasal bioavailability is primarily due to metabolism (hepatic and pre-systemic) and partly due to incomplete absorption. The oral absorption of sumatriptan is not significantly affected either during migraine attacks or by food.

In vitro studies with human microsomes suggest that sumatriptan is metabolized by monoamine oxidase (MAO), predominantly the A isoenzyme. In studies conducted in a limited number of patients, MAO inhibitors reduce sumatriptan clearance, significantly increasing systemic exposure.

Excretion: Non-renal clearance of sumatriptan accounts for about 80% of the total clearance. The major metabolite, the indole acetic acid analogue of sumatriptan is mainly excreted in the urine where it is present as a free acid (35%) and the glucuronide conjugate (11%). It has no known 5-HT$_1$ or 5-HT$_2$ activity. Minor metabolites have not been identified.

Special Populations and Conditions: Geriatrics: No differences have been observed between the pharmacokinetic parameters in healthy elderly volunteers compared with younger volunteers (less than 65 years old).

STORAGE AND STABILITY: IMITREX DF Tablets should be stored between 15 and 30°C.

IMITREX Injection and Nasal Spray should be stored between 2 to 30°C and protected from light.

INFORMATION FOR THE PATIENT: Published in e-CPS, available by subscription at www.e-cps.ca.

DOSAGE FORMS, COMPOSITION AND PACKAGING: IMITREX: Injection: Each prefilled syringe contains: sumatriptan (base) 6 mg as the succinate salt; total volume=0.5 mL. Syringes are placed in a tamper-evident carrying/disposal case. Two prefilled syringes plus an Imitrex Statdose Pen autoinjector are packed in an Imitrex Statdose System autoinjector kit. Refill pack of 2 prefilled syringes in a carton. Also available to physicians or hospitals in a single dose vial (6 mg; total volume=0.5 mL). Carton of 5.

Nasal Spray: 5 mg: Each unit dose spray contains: sumatriptan (base) as the hemisulfate salt 5 mg in an aqueous buffered solution. Nonmedicinal ingredients: anhydrous dibasic sodium phosphate, monobasic potassium phosphate, purified water, sodium hydroxide and sulfuric acid. Boxes of 6 nasal spray devices (3×2 devices).

20 mg: Each unit dose spray contains: sumatriptan (base) as the hemisulfate salt 20 mg in an aqueous buffered solution. Nonmedicinal ingredients: anhydrous dibasic sodium phosphate, monobasic potassium phosphate, purified water, sodium hydroxide and sulfuric acid. Boxes of 6 nasal spray devices (3×2 devices).

IMITREX DF: 50 mg: Each white, film-coated tablet contains: sumatriptan (base) 50 mg as the succinate salt. Nonmedicinal ingredients: croscarmellose sodium, dibasic calcium phosphate anhydrous, magnesium stearate, methylhydroxypropyl cellulose, microcrystalline cellulose, sodium bicarbonate, titanium dioxide and triacetin. Gluten- and tartrazine-free. Blister packs of 6.

100 mg: Each pink, film-coated tablet contains: sumatriptan (base) 100 mg as the succinate salt. Nonmedicinal ingredients: croscarmellose sodium, dibasic calcium phosphate anhydrous, iron oxide red, magnesium stearate, methylhydroxypropyl cellulose, microcrystalline cellulose, sodium bicarbonate, titanium dioxide and triacetin. Gluten- and tartrazine-free. Blister packs of 6.

(Shown in Product Identification Section)

ImmuCyst®

Bacillus Calmette-Guérin (BCG), substrain Connaught

Antineoplastic

sanofi pasteur

Date of Revision: June 2010

SUMMARY PRODUCT INFORMATION:

Route of Administration	Dosage Form/ Strength	Clinically Relevant Nonmedicinal Ingredients
Intravesical instillation	Powder for suspension: 81 mg (dry weight) equivalent to 10.5±8.7×10[8] colony forming units (CFU)	Monosodium glutamate For a complete listing see Dosage Forms, Composition and Packaging.

DESCRIPTION: ImmuCyst [Bacillus Calmette-Guérin (BCG), substrain Connaught] is a freeze-dried preparation made from the Connaught substrain of Bacillus Calmette-Guérin, which is an attenuated strain of *M. bovis* for treatment of non-muscle invasive bladder cancer (Ta/T1 papillary tumours and CIS).

The BCG organisms are viable upon reconstitution. The reconstituted product contains 10.5±8.7×10[8] colony-forming units (CFU) per instillation dose.

INDICATIONS AND CLINICAL USE: ImmuCyst is indicated for intravesical use in the treatment of primary or recurrent carcinoma in situ (CIS) of the urinary bladder, for prophylaxis of recurrence of CIS of the urinary bladder and for prophylaxis following transurethral resection (TUR) of primary or recurrent stage Ta and/or T1 papillary tumours, or any combination thereof, regardless of antecedent intravesical treatment.

ImmuCyst is not indicated as an immunizing agent for the prevention of tuberculosis.

CONTRAINDICATIONS:

- Known systemic hypersensitivity reaction to any component (see Description and Warnings and Precautions) of ImmuCyst or after previous administration of the medicinal product or a medicinal product containing the same substances.
- Active tuberculosis: Active tuberculosis should be ruled out before starting treatment with ImmuCyst.
- Current symptoms or previous history of systemic BCG reaction. (See Warnings and Precautions.)
- Concurrent febrile illness, urinary tract infection, or gross hematuria. Treatment with ImmuCyst should be postponed until their resolution. (See Warnings and Precautions, Serious and Severe Adverse Events Related Precautions.)
- Congenital or acquired immune deficiencies, whether due to concurrent disease (e.g., AIDS, leukemia, and lymphoma), or immunosuppressive therapy (e.g., corticosteroids cancer therapy [cytotoxic drugs, radiation]) (see Drug Interactions, Drug-Drug Interactions) because of the risk of disseminated BCG infection.
- A minimum of 14 days should elapse before ImmuCyst is administered following biopsy, TUR or traumatic catheterization.

WARNINGS AND PRECAUTIONS:

Serious Warnings and Precautions

Systemic BCG Reactions: A systemic BCG reaction, which may be fatal, is a systemic granulomatous illness, which may occur (although rarely) subsequent to exposure to BCG.

Because it is usually difficult to isolate BCG organisms from affected organs, it is often unclear to what extent such a reaction is caused by an infectious process versus an inflammatory hypersensitivity reaction, hence the term "systemic BCG reaction".

Based on past clinical experience with intravesical BCG, "systemic BCG reaction" may be defined as the presence of any of the following signs, if no other etiologies for such signs are detectable: fever ≥39.5°C for 12 hours; fever ≥38.5°C for 48 hours; pneumonitis; hepatitis; other organ dysfunction outside of the genitourinary tract with granulomatous inflammation on biopsy; or the classical signs of sepsis, including circulatory collapse, acute respiratory distress and disseminated intravascular coagulation. (See Adverse Reactions.)

Although rare, a systemic BCG reaction is much more likely to occur if ImmuCyst is administered within 14 days of biopsy, TUR or traumatic bladder catheterization (associated with hematuria).

General: For intravesical instillation only. Do not inject subcutaneously intradermally or intravenously.

Advice for Patients: Fever, chills, malaise, flu-like symptoms, increased fatigue or an increase in urinary symptoms, (such as burning or pain on urination) can occur. However, patients should be advised to notify their physicians if any of these symptoms last more than 48 hours or increase in severity. Patients should also notify their physicians if they experience any of the following: an increase in urinary symptoms (such as urgency, frequency of urination, blood in urine), joint pain, eye complaints (such as pain, irritation or redness), cough, skin rash, jaundice, nausea or vomiting.

Because ImmuCyst contains live mycobacteria, excreted urine may also contain live bacteria. Patients should be advised on appropriate infection control procedures to protect family and close contacts from infection. Patients living with or in close quarters to persons who are immunocompromised (on chemotherapy, etc.) should exercise special caution to avoid inadvertently transmitting BCG infection to such susceptible persons. ImmuCyst is retained in the bladder for as long as possible up to 2 hours and then voided. To avoid transmission of BCG to others, for 6 hours after treatment patients should void while seated to avoid splashing of urine. Urine voided during this time should be disinfected with an equal volume of household bleach for 15 minutes before flushing or disposal. Unless medically contraindicated, patients should be instructed to increase fluid intake to "flush" the bladder for several hours following treatment with ImmuCyst. Patients may experience burning with the first void after treatment.

Handling Precautions: Handle as infectious. ImmuCyst contains live attenuated mycobacteria and should be prepared and handled using aseptic technique. (See Dosage And Administration, Reconstitution of Freeze-Dried Product.) BCG infections have been reported in health-care workers preparing BCG for administration.

Nosocomial infections have been reported in immunosuppressed patients receiving parenteral drugs, which were prepared in areas in which BCG was prepared.

Carcinogenesis and Mutagenesis: Mutagenesis and carcinogenesis studies have not been conducted with ImmuCyst in animals or in humans. Results from clinical trials do not indicate any increased potential for mutagenesis or carcinogenesis although that was not specifically monitored.

Cardiovascular: The risk of ectopic BCG infections has not been determined but is considered to be very small. BCG infection of aneurysms, arterial grafts and cardiac devices can also occur. The benefits of BCG therapy must be carefully weighed against the possibility of ectopic BCG infection in patients with arterial aneurysms or prosthetic devices of any kind.

Genitourinary: Some male genitourinary tract infections (orchitis/epididymitis) have been refractory to multiple drug antimycobacterial therapy and required orchiectomy.

If a bacterial urinary tract infection (UTI) occurs during the course of ImmuCyst treatment, ImmuCyst instillation should be withheld until complete resolution of the bacterial UTI, since the combination of a UTI and BCG-induced cystitis may lead to more severe adverse effects on the genitourinary tract; moreover, because BCG bacilli are sensitive to a wide variety of antibiotics; antimicrobial administration may diminish the efficacy of ImmuCyst.

Hypersensitivity: Acute allergic reaction has been very rarely reported following intradermal injection of BCG vaccine for the prevention of tuberculosis and therefore should be taken into consideration when administering ImmuCyst.

The stopper of the vial for this product contains natural rubber latex, which may cause allergic reactions.

Immune: For patients with a condition that may in the future require mandatory immunosuppression (e.g., awaiting organ transplant, myasthenia gravis) the decision to treat with ImmuCyst should be considered carefully.

Treatments using immunosuppressants and/or radiation interfere with the immune response to ImmuCyst and increase the risk of disseminated BCG infection. Because of the risk of BCG infection, ImmuCyst should not be used in immunosuppressed patients or persons with congenital or acquired immune deficiencies, whether due to concurrent disease (e.g., AIDS, leukemia, lymphoma), cancer therapy (e.g., cytotoxic drugs, radiation), or immunosuppressive therapy (e.g., corticosteroids).

Intravesical treatment with ImmuCyst may induce a positive response to purified protein derivative (PPD). (See Drug Interactions.) Determination of a patient's reactivity to PPD should be conducted before administration of ImmuCyst.

ImmuCyst should not be handled by persons with an immunologic deficiency.

Peri-Operative Considerations: A minimum of 14 days should elapse before ImmuCyst is administered following biopsy, TUR or traumatic catheterization. There should be no evidence of hematuria prior to instillation of ImmuCyst.

Sensitivity/Resistance: ImmuCyst is not sensitive to pyrazinamide.

Serious and Severe Adverse Events Related Precautions: To prevent serious infections, avoid trauma and/or introduction of contaminants to the urinary tract, a minimum of 14 days should elapse before ImmuCyst is administered following traumatic catheterization. (See Contraindications.) The treatment schedule should subsequently be resumed as if no interruption in treatment had occurred.

Patients should be monitored for the presence of symptoms and signs of toxicity after each intravesical treatment. If a patient develops persistent fever or experiences an acute febrile illness consistent with BCG infection, BCG instillations should be permanently discontinued, the patient immediately evaluated and treated for BCG infection and an infectious diseases consultation sought. (See Contraindications.) As standard therapy for BCG infection, treatment with two or more antimycobacterial agents must be initiated promptly while diagnostic evaluation, including cultures, is conducted. Use of single antibiotic therapy is not recommended. Negative cultures do not necessarily rule out infection.

Special Populations: ImmuCyst is not recommended for prophylactic treatment following TUR of stage TaG1 papillary tumours unless they are judged to be at high risk of tumour recurrence.

In patients with small bladder capacity, increased risk of bladder contracture should be considered in decisions to treat with ImmuCyst.

Patients undergoing antimicrobial therapy for other infections should be evaluated to assess whether the therapy might diminish the efficacy of ImmuCyst. (See Drug Interactions, Drug-Drug Interactions.)

Pregnant Women: Animal reproduction studies have not been conducted with ImmuCyst. It is also not known whether ImmuCyst can cause fetal harm when administered to a pregnant woman or can affect reproduction capacity. ImmuCyst should be given to a pregnant woman only if clearly needed. Women should be advised not to become pregnant while on therapy.

Nursing Women: It is not known whether ImmuCyst can be excreted in human milk. Because many medicinal products are excreted in human milk and because of the potential for serious adverse reactions from ImmuCyst in nursing infants, it is advisable to discontinue breastfeeding if the mother's condition requires treatment with ImmuCyst.

Pediatrics: Safety and effectiveness of therapy with ImmuCyst in pediatric patients have not been established. Therefore, ImmuCyst should not be used in pediatric patients.

ADVERSE REACTIONS: Adverse event information is derived from clinical trials and worldwide post-marketing experience.

Administration of ImmuCyst causes an inflammatory response in the bladder and can provoke signs and symptoms of cystitis. (See Table 1 and Table 2.) Such reactions may to some degree be taken as evidence that BCG is evoking the desired response, but careful patient monitoring is required.

Symptoms of bladder irritability are reported in approximately 50% of patients receiving ImmuCyst and typically begin a few hours after instillation and last 6-48 hours. The symptoms are usually seen following the third instillation and tend to increase in severity after each administration. The mechanism of action of the irritative side effects has not been studied, but is most consistent with an immunological mechanism. There is no evidence that dose reduction or antituberculous drug therapy can prevent or lessen the irritative symptoms of ImmuCyst.

Clinical Trial Adverse Drug Reactions: Because clinical trials are conducted under very specific conditions the adverse drug reaction rates observed in the clinical trials may not reflect the rates observed in practice and should not be compared to the rates in the clinical trials of another drug. Adverse drug reaction information from clinical trials is useful for identifying drug-related adverse events and for approximating rules.

Description of Data Sources: The adverse reactions which occurred among recipients of ImmuCyst during clinical trials SWOG 8216 and SWOG 8507 (see Action and Clinical Pharmacology) are listed in Table 1 and Table 2.

Data are categorized by Medical Dictionary for Regulatory Activities (MedDRA) system organ class and by decreasing frequency.

Table 1: ImmuCyst

SWOG Study 8216—Adverse Reactions (n=112)

Adverse Reaction	Percent of Patients	
	Overall Induction Plus Maintenance	**(Grade ≥3) (Total of 11 Instillations)**
Infections and Infestations		
Cystitis	29.5%	(0.0%)
Urinary tract infection	17.9%	(0.0%)
Pulmonary infection	2.7%	(0.0%)
Systemic infection	2.7%	(1.8%)
Infection	0.9%	(0.9%)
Blood and Lymphatic System Disorders		
Anemia	20.5%	(0.0%)
Leukopenia	5.4%	(0.0%)
Coagulopathy/thrombocytopenia	0.9%	(0.0%)
Metabolism and Nutrition Disorders		
Anorexia	10.7%	(0.0%)
Nervous System Disorders		
Headache	1.8%	(0.0%)
Dizziness	0.9%	(0.0%)
Cardiac Disorders		
Cardiac (unclassified)	2.7%	(0.0%)
Gastrointestinal Disorders		
Nausea/vomiting	16.1%	(0.0%)
Diarrhea	6.3%	(0.0%)
Abdominal pain	2.7%	(0.0%)
Constipation	0.9	(0.0%)
Hepatobiliary Disorders		
Liver involvement	2.7%	(0.0%)
Skin and Subcutaneous Tissue Disorders		

(cont'd)

Table 1: ImmuCyst *(cont'd)*

SWOG Study 8216—Adverse Reactions (n=112)

Adverse Reaction	Percent of Patients: Overall Induction Plus Maintenance	Percent of Patients: (Grade ≥3) (Total of 11 Instillations)
Skin rash	1.8%	(0.0%)
Musculoskeletal and Connective Tissue and Bone Disorders		
Arthralgia/myalgia/arthritis	7.1%	(0.9%)
Flank pain	0.9%	0.0%
Renal and Urinary Disorders		
Dysuria	51.8%	(3.6%)
Urinary frequency	40.2%	(1.8%)
Hematuria	39.3%	(7.1%)
Urinary urgency	17.9%	(0.9%)
Renal toxicity (NOS)	9.8%	(1.8%)
Urinary incontinence	6.3%	(0.0%)
Bladder cramps/pain	6.3%	(0.0%)
Contracted bladder	5.4%	(0.9%)
Tissue in urine	0.9%	(0.0%)
Ureteral obstruction	0.9%	(0.0%)
Reproductive System and Breast Disorders		
Genital pain	9.8%	(0.0%)
General Disorders and Administration Site Conditions		
Malaise	40.2%	(1.8%)
Fever	38.4%	(2.7%)
Chills	33.9%	(2.7%)
Fatigue	0.9%	(0.0%)

Table 2: ImmuCyst

SWOG Study 8507—Adverse Reactions

Adverse Reaction	Induction (n=587/587) 6 Instillations: Overall	Induction: (Grade ≥3)	Induction + Maintenance (n=247/587) 6+21 Instillations: Overall	Induction + Maintenance: (Grade ≥3)
Infections and Infestations				
Urinary tract infection	1.0%	(0.0%)	4.5%	(0.4%)
Systemic infection	0.9%	(0.5%)	0.4%	(0.4%)
Pulmonary infection	0.5%	(0.2%)	NR[a]	NR
Infection	0.3%	(0.0%)	NR	NR
Cystitis	0.2%	(0.0%)	2.0%	(0.4%)
Blood and Lymphatic Disorders				
Anemia	0.7%	(0.0%)	NR	NR
Leukopenia	0.3%	(0.0%)	NR	NR
Coagulopathy/thrombocytopenia	0.2%	(0.2%)	NR	NR
Metabolism and Nutrition Disorders				
Anorexia	4.6%	(0.3%)	7.7%	(0.4%)
Nervous System Disorders				
Headache	0.3%	(0.0%)	0.4%	(0.0%)
Dizziness	0.2%	(0.0%)	NR	NR
Cardiac Disorders				
Cardiac (unclassified)	0.3%	(0.0%)	1.2%	(0.0%)
Gastrointestinal Disorders				

(cont'd)

Table 2: ImmuCyst *(cont'd)*

SWOG Study 8507—Adverse Reactions

Adverse Reaction	Induction (n=587/587) 6 Instillations: Overall	Induction: (Grade ≥3)	Induction + Maintenance (n=247/587) 6+21 Instillations: Overall	Induction + Maintenance: (Grade ≥3)
Nausea/vomiting	2.6%	(0.3%)	4.9%	(0.8%)
Diarrhea	0.9%	(0.0%)	1.2%	(0.4%)
Abdominal pain	0.3%	(0.0%)	NR	NR
Constipation	NR	NR	0.8%	(0.0%)
Mucositis/ulcers/stomatitis	0.2%	(0.0%)	NR	NR
Hepatobiliary Disorders				
Liver involvement	0.3%	(0.2%)	2.0%	(0.0%)
Granulomatous hepatitis	0.2%	(0.2%)	NR	NR
Skin and Subcutaneous Tissue Disorders				
Skin rash	0.7%	(0.3%)	1.2%	(0.0%)
Hypersensitivity reaction skin	NR	NR	0.4%	(0.4%)
Skin abscess	NR	NR	0.4%	(0.0%)
Musculoskeletal and Connective Tissue Disorders				
Arthralgia/myalgia/arthritis	0.3%	(0.0%)	1.2%	(0.4%)
Renal and Urinary Disorders				
Dysuria	26.4%	(1.7%)	45.8%	(8.9%)
Hematuria	18.6%	(3.6%)	28.3%	(7.3%)
Urinary frequency	14.1%	(1.7%)	34.0%	(7.3%)
Urinary urgency	3.2%	(0.3%)	12.2%	(2.8%)
Bladder cramps/pain	1.4%	(0.3%)	3.6%	(1.2%)
Urinary incontinence	0.9%	(0.3%)	2.0%	(0.8%)
Renal toxicity	0.9%	(0.0%)	0.8%	(0.0%)
Contracted bladder	0.5%	(0.2%)	3.6%	(2.0%)
Ureteral obstruction	0.2%	(0.2%)	NR	NR
Tissue in urine	NR	NR	0.8%	(0.0%)
Reproductive System and Breast Disorders				
Genital pain	0.3%	(0.0%)	NR	NR
General Disorders and Administration Site Conditions				
Fever	17.2%	(0.3%)	31.12%	(2.0%)
Malaise	16.7%	(0.7%)	24.7%	(2.0%)
Chills	14.1%	(0.9%)	31.6%	(2.0%)
Fatigue	1.0%	(0.3%)	0.8%	(0.0%)

[a] NR=not reported.

Post-Market Adverse Drug Reactions: The following additional adverse events have been spontaneously reported during the post-marketing use of ImmuCyst worldwide. Because these events were reported voluntarily from a population of uncertain size, it is not always possible to reliably estimate their frequency or establish a causal relationship to product exposure. Decisions to include these events in labeling were based on one or more of the following factors: 1) severity of the event, 2) frequency of reporting, or 3) strength of causal connection to ImmuCyst.

Data are categorized by MedDRA system organ class.

Infections and Infestations: BCG Infection (rare): BCG is capable of dissemination when administered by the intravesical route. Serious infections, including sepsis with associated mortality, have been reported. BCG infections have also been reported in eye, lung, liver, bone, bone marrow, kidney, regional lymph nodes, peritoneum, genitourinary tract (orchitis/epididymitis) and prostate (e.g., granulomatous prostatitis).

BCG infection of aneurysms and prosthetic devices (including arterial grafts, cardiac devices and artificial joints) has also been reported.

Joint symptoms (arthritis, arthralgia), ocular symptoms (including conjunctivitis, uveitis, iritis, keratitis, granulomatous choreoretinitis), urinary symptoms (including urethritis), skin rash, alone or in combination (Reiter's syndrome), have been reported following administration of ImmuCyst. For the reports of Reiter's syndrome, the risk seems to be more elevated among patients who are positive for HLA-B27.

Renal abscess (very rare).

Respiratory, Thoracic and Mediastinal Disorders: pneumonia, interstitial lung disease.

Skin and Subcutaneous Tissue Disorders: erythema nodosum.

Renal and Urinary Disorders: renal failure, pyelonephritis, nephritis (including tubulointerstitial nephritis, interstitial nephritis and glomerulonephritis).

urinary retention (including bladder tamponade and feeling of residual urine).

General Disorders and Administration Site Conditions: flu like symptoms (rare).

Investigations (Laboratory Tests): abnormal/increased blood creatinine or blood urea nitrogen (BUN).

Physicians, nurses and pharmacists should report any adverse reaction related to the administration of the product to the appropriate health authorities in accordance with local requirements and to the Global Pharmacovigilance Department, Sanofi Pasteur Limited, 1755 Steeles Avenue West, Toronto, ON, M2R 3T4 Canada. 1-888-621-1146 (phone) or 416-667-2435 (fax). The report should include details of the treatment history with ImmuCyst, relevant medical history, the symptoms and signs of the adverse reaction, the treatment administered for the reaction and the response to such treatment.

DRUG INTERACTIONS:

> **Serious Drug Interactions**
> **Immunosuppressive Treatments:** Treatment combinations using immunosuppressants and/or radiation interfere with the immune response to ImmuCyst and increase the risk of disseminated BCG infection. (See Warnings and Precautions.)

Drug-Drug Interactions: Intravesical treatment with ImmuCyst may induce a positive response to PPD, which may complicate future interpretations of skin test reactions to PPD when used to diagnose suspected mycobacterial infections. Determination of a patient's reactivity to PPD should be conducted before administration of ImmuCyst.
Antibacterial Drugs: Antimicrobial therapy for other infections may interfere with the effectiveness of ImmuCyst. Patients undergoing antimicrobial therapy should be evaluated to assess whether the therapy might diminish the efficacy of ImmuCyst.
Antituberculosis Drugs: Antituberculosis drugs should not be used prophylactically to prevent the local, irritative side effects of ImmuCyst. There are no data to suggest that the acute, local urinary tract symptoms common with intravesical BCG are due to mycobacterial infection.

ImmuCyst is not sensitive to pyrazinamide.

DOSAGE AND ADMINISTRATION: Recommended Dose: One dose of ImmuCyst consists of the intravesical instillation of 81 mg BCG.

Intravesical treatment of the urinary bladder should begin a minimum of 14 days after biopsy or TUR (see Contraindications and Warnings and Precautions) and consists of induction and maintenance therapy.

- The induction therapy schedule consists of one intravesical instillation of ImmuCyst each week for 6 weeks for a total of 6 doses.
- Based on clinical studies performed with ImmuCyst, maintenance therapy following induction is highly recommended. After a 6-week pause, one intravesical dose should be given each week for 1 to 3 weeks. Then one dose should be given each week for 1 to 3 weeks at 6, 12, 18, 24, 30 and 36 months following the initiation of induction treatment.

Reconstitution of Freeze-Dried Product: For the reconstitution and further dilution of one dose of ImmuCyst, 50 mL sterile, preservative-free saline is required.

The preparation of ImmuCyst should be done using **aseptic technique**. A separate area for the preparation of the ImmuCyst suspension is recommended in order to avoid cross contamination. The person responsible for mixing the agent should wear gloves, eye protection, a mask and gown to avoid inhalation of BCG organisms and inadvertent exposure of broken skin to BCG organisms.

When handling and reconstituting ImmuCyst, care should be taken so as to avoid needle stick injuries.

ImmuCyst should not be handled by persons with an immunologic deficiency. (See Warnings and Precautions.)

Do not remove the rubber stopper from the vial.

Prepare the surface of the ImmuCyst and diluent vials (if provided) using a suitable antiseptic.

Presentation with Diluent: Using a 5 mL sterile syringe and needle, draw into the syringe a volume of air equal to the volume of diluent in the vial. Pierce the center of the rubber stopper in the vial containing diluent with the sterile needle of the syringe, invert the vial and slowly inject into it the air contained in the syringe. Keeping the point of the needle immersed in the diluent, withdraw into the syringe 3 mL of diluent for the 81 mg vial presentation. Then, holding the syringe-plunger steady, withdraw the needle from the vial.
Presentation without Diluent: Using a 5 mL sterile syringe and needle, draw up 3 mL of sterile preservative-free saline solution.
For Both Presentations: Using the same syringe and needle, pierce the rubber stopper in the vial of freeze-dried material with the needle. Hold the vial of freeze-dried material upright and pull the plunger of the syringe back to create a mild vacuum in the vial. Release the plunger and allow the vacuum to pull the saline from the syringe into the vial of freeze-dried material. After all the saline has passed into the freeze-dried material, remove the needle and syringe.

Shake the vial gently until a fine, even suspension results. Avoid foaming since this will prevent withdrawal of the proper dose. Withdraw the entire contents of the reconstituted material from the vial into the same 5 mL syringe. Return the vial to an upright position before removing the syringe from the vial.

Further dilute the reconstituted material from the vial (1 dose) in sterile, preservative-free saline to a final volume of 50 mL for intravesical instillation.

Any reconstituted product which exhibits flocculation or clumping that cannot be dispersed with gentle shaking should not be used.

Administration: For intravesical instillation only. Do not inject subcutaneously or intravenously.

This dose is prepared by reconstituting 1 vial containing 81 mg freeze-dried BCG with 3 mL of diluent or with 3 mL of sterile, preservative-free saline. The reconstituted BCG is further diluted in sterile, preservative-free saline, for a total of 50 mL instillation volume. (See Warnings and Precautions and Dosage and Administration, Reconstitution of Freeze-Dried Product.)

A urethral catheter is inserted into the bladder under **aseptic conditions**, the bladder is drained and then the 50 mL suspension of ImmuCyst is instilled slowly by gravity, following which the catheter is withdrawn.

The patient retains the suspension for as long as possible up to two hours. The patient should lie prone for the first 15 minutes following instillation. Thereafter, the patient is allowed to be up. At two hours after the instillation, all patients should void in a seated position for hygienic safety reasons. (See Warnings and Precautions and Special Handling Instructions.) Unless medically contraindicated, patients should be instructed to increase fluid intake in order to flush the bladder in the hours following BCG treatment.

OVERDOSAGE:
Not documented.

> For management of a suspected drug overdose, CPhA recommends that you contact your **regional Poison Control Centre**. See the *CPS* Directory section for a list of Poison Control Centres.

ACTION AND CLINICAL PHARMACOLOGY: Pharmacodynamics: When administered intravesically as a cancer therapy, BCG promotes a local acute inflammatory and sub-acute granulomatous reaction with macrophage and leukocyte infiltration in the urothelium and lamina propria of the urinary bladder. The local inflammatory effects are associated with an elimination or reduction of non-muscle invasive cancerous tumours of the urinary bladder (Ta/T1 papillary tumours and CIS). The exact mechanism of action is unknown, but the anti-tumour effect appears to be T-lymphocyte dependent.
Pharmacokinetics: Because ImmuCyst contains live mycobacteria, excreted urine may also contain live bacteria. (See Warnings and Precautions and Special Handling Instructions.)

STORAGE AND STABILITY: ImmuCyst should be stored at 2 to 8°C (i.e., in a refrigerator). It should not be used after the expiration date marked on the vial, otherwise it may be inactive.

At no time should the freeze-dried ImmuCyst be exposed to direct or indirect sunlight. Exposure to artificial light should also be kept to a minimum.
Reconstituted Product: Once reconstituted, the product should be used immediately.

Reconstituted product should not be exposed to direct or indirect sunlight. Exposure to artificial light should also be kept to a minimum.

If there is an unavoidable delay between reconstitution and administration, this delay should not exceed 2 hours at a temperature between 2 to 25°C.

Any reconstituted product, which exhibits flocculation or clumping that cannot be dispersed with gentle shaking, should not be used.

SPECIAL HANDLING INSTRUCTIONS: Instructions for Disposal: Unused product, packaging and all equipment and materials used for instillation of the product (e.g., syringes, catheters) should be placed immediately in a container for biohazardous materials and disposed of according to local requirements applicable to biohazardous materials.

Urine voided during the 6-hour period following ImmuCyst instillation should be disinfected with an equal volume of 5% hypochlorite solution (undiluted household bleach) and allowed to stand for 15 minutes before flushing. (See Warnings and Precautions.)

INFORMATION FOR THE PATIENT: Published in e-CPS, available by subscription at www.e-cps.ca.

DOSAGE FORMS, COMPOSITION AND PACKAGING: ImmuCyst is supplied as a sterile lyophilized white powder in a vial containing 81 mg. If provided, the diluent is a sterile clear colourless solution supplied in a vial containing 3 mL.
Each vial contains: Bacillus Calmette-Guérin (BCG), substrain Connaught 81 mg and monosodium glutamate 150 mg (5% w/v). The diluent if provided consists of sodium chloride 25.5 mg (0.85% w/v), disodium hydrogen phosphate 7.5 mg (0.25% w/v), sodium dihydrogen phosphate 1.7 mg (0.06% w/v), polysorbate 80 0.75 mg (0.025% w/v), water for injection up to 3 mL. No preservative added. Packages of either one 81 mg vial BCG with one 3 mL vial diluent or one 81 mg vial of BCG.

ImmuCyst is supplied in an amber Type 1 glass vial and the diluent (if provided) is supplied in a clear Type 1 glass vial. The stopper for both vials contains natural latex rubber.

Immunocal®
protein isolate
Glutathione Precursor

Immunotec

PHARMACOLOGY: IMMUNOCAL is a natural source of the glutathione precursor cysteine for the maintenance of a strong immune system. It is fat-free and contains less then 1% lactose and has a high protein biological value (>110 BV) providing all essential amino acids.

The systemic availability of oral glutathione is negligible; the vast majority of it must be manufactured intracellularly from precursors. Glutathione is a tripeptide made intracellularly from its constituent amino acids L-glutamate, L-cysteine and glycine. The sulfhydryl (thiol) group (SH) of cysteine serves as a proton donor and is responsible for the biological activity of glutathione. Provision of this amino acid is the rate-limiting factor in glutathione synthesis by the cells since bioavailable cysteine is relatively rare in foodstuffs. Furthermore, cysteine if ingested as the free amino acid L-cysteine, has toxic potential and is spontaneously catabolized in the gastrointestinal tract and blood plasma. Toxicity is avoided when cysteine is integrated into larger proteins such as serum albumin, alpha lactalbumin and lactoferrin.

IMMUNOCAL is a bovine whey protein isolate specially prepared to provide a rich source of bioavailable cysteine. Following digestion, the cysteine remains as the stable form cystine (2 molecules of cysteine linked by a disulfide bond) and glutamylcystine. After absorption, these dipeptides travel safely in the blood stream and readily enter the cells to release free cysteine for intracellular glutathione synthesis. IMMUNOCAL is a cysteine delivery system.

The disulphide bond in cystine is pepsin and trypsin resistant but may be split by heat, low pH or mechanical stress, releasing free cysteine. When subject to heat or shearing forces (inherent in most extraction processes), the fragile disulfide bonds within the peptides are broken and the bioavailability of cysteine is greatly diminished.
Glutathione has multiple functions:

1. It is the major endogenous antioxidant produced by the cells, participating directly in the neutralization of free radicals and reactive oxygen compounds, as well as the maintenance of exogenous antioxidants such as vitamins C and E in their reduced (active) forms.
2. Through direct conjugation, it detoxifies many xenobiotics (foreign compounds) and carcinogens, both organic and inorganic such as heavy metals, aromatic hydrocarbons, nitrosamines, benzopirines and others including pharmacological agents such as acetaminophen.
3. It is essential for the immune system to exert its full potential, e.g. (1) modulating antigen presentation to lymphocytes, thereby influencing cytokine production and the type of response (cellular or humoral) that develops, (2) enhancing proliferation of lymphocytes thereby increasing magnitude of response, (3) enhancing killing activity of cytotoxic T cells and NK cells, and (4) regulating apoptosis, thereby maintaining control of the immune response.
4. It plays a fundamental role in numerous metabolic and biochemical reactions such as DNA synthesis and repair, protein synthesis, prostaglandin synthesis, amino acid transport and enzyme activation. Many systems in the body are adversely affected by low glutathione levels, including the immune system, the nervous system, the gastrointestinal system and the cardiovascular-pulmonary system.

INDICATIONS: Glutathione augmentation is a strategy developed to address states of glutathione deficiency, high oxidative stress, immune deficiency, and xenobiotic overload in which glutathione plays a part in the detoxification of the xenobiotic in question. Many clinical pathologies are associated with glutathione deficiency and oxidative stress and are elaborated upon in numerous medical references. Low glutathione is also strongly implicated in wasting and negative nitrogen balance seen in muscle wasting.

CONTRAINDICATIONS: In individuals who develop or have known hypersensitivity to specific milk proteins (this does not include lactose intolerance).

WARNINGS: Patients undergoing immunosuppressive therapy should discuss the use of this product with their health care practitioner.

Heating or adding IMMUNOCAL to a hot liquid or use of a high-speed blender to reconstitute it will significantly decrease the effectiveness of the product.

PRECAUTIONS: Each pouch of IMMUNOCAL provides 9 g of protein. Patients on a protein-restricted diet need to take this into account when calculating their daily protein load. Although a bovine milk derivative, IMMUNOCAL is well tolerated by lactose-intolerant individuals. IMMUNOCAL is contraindicated in individuals who develop or have known hypersensitivity to specific milk proteins (this does not include lactose intolerance).

Individuals with the autosomal-recessive metabolic disorder cystinuria, are at higher risk of developing cysteine nephrolithiasis (1-2% of renal calculi).
Pregnancy: No adverse effects have been reported. A health care practitioner should be consulted prior to use if the patient is pregnant or has reason to believe she is.
Lactation: No adverse effects have been reported. A health care practitioner should be consulted prior to use if the patient breast feeds.
Geriatrics: Glutathione levels drop with age. Dosage recommendations may rise with increasing age.

ADVERSE EFFECTS: IMMUNOCAL is a natural source of protein classified as a Natural Health Product and has not been statistically assessed for adverse effects. Gastrointestinal bloating and cramps are possible if the product is not sufficiently rehydrated. Transient urticarial-like skin rash has been reported in rare individuals undergoing severe detoxification reaction. Skin rash abates when the intake is stopped or reduced.

OVERDOSE:

Symptoms and Treatment: There have been no reports of toxicity from overdosing on IMMUNOCAL. Glutathione is a tightly regulated intracellular constituent and is limited in its production by negative feedback inhibition of its own synthesis through the enzyme gamma-glutamylcysteine synthetase.

> For management of a suspected drug overdose, CPhA recommends that you contact your **regional Poison Control Centre**. See the *CPS* Directory section for a list of Poison Control Centres.

DOSAGE: As a natural source of the glutathione cysteine precursor for the maintenance of a strong immune system, 10 g per day (one pouch) is recommended. As a natural source of the glutathione precursor cysteine for the maintenance of a strong immune system, 20 g per day is recommended. 30-40 g per day has been used in clinical trials without ill effects.

IMMUNOCAL is best administered on an empty stomach or with a light meal. Concomitant intake of another high protein load may adversely affect absorption.

INFORMATION FOR THE PATIENT: Published in e-CPS, available by subscription at www.e-cps.ca.

SUPPLIED: Each individually-sealed foil pouch contains: 10 g of powder, 9 g of which is protein. The other is represented by naturally occurring ingredients including ash, trace minerals and trace amounts of vitamins. Boxes of 30 pouches.

IMMUNOCAL is a dehydrated powdered protein isolate. It must be appropriately rehydrated before use. Ideally, it should be consumed immediately after mixing. Should the product be premixed for later consumption, it should be refrigerated and consumed within a short period after mixing. Do not heat or use a hot liquid to rehydrate the product or use a high-speed blender for reconstitution. These methods will decrease the effect of the product. Proper mixing is imperative. Consult instructions included in packaging. Store in a cool dry environment. Avoid excessive heat. Refrigeration is not necessary.

Imodium® Advanced

loperamide HCl—simethicone

Oral Antidiarrheal—Oral Antiflatulent

McNeil Consumer Healthcare

Date of Revision: October 17, 2008

PHARMACOLOGY: Diarrhea may be defined as a failure or imbalance of one or a combination of activities in the gut which include secretion, absorption and motility. Loperamide hydrochloride has been shown to act on all of these functions via cholinergic, non-cholinergic, opiate and non-opiate receptor-mediated mechanisms. In this way, loperamide HCl effectively reduces fecal output and frequency, improves stool consistency and relieves symptoms of abdominal cramping and fecal incontinence.

Pharmacodynamics: Loperamide binds to the opiate receptor in the gut wall. Consequently, it inhibits the release of acetylcholine and prostaglandins, thereby reducing propulsive peristalsis, increasing intestinal transit time and enhancing resorption of water and electrolytes. Loperamide does not change the physiological flora. Loperamide increases the tone of the anal sphincter, thereby reducing incontinence and urgency. Loperamide does not act centrally. Loperamide has a high affinity for the gut wall and is extensively metabolized on first-pass through the liver. Therefore, loperamide hardly reaches the systemic circulation.

Simethicone is an inert surface-active agent with anti-foaming properties which relieves symptoms associated with diarrhea, particularly flatulence, abdominal discomfort, bloating and cramping.

Pharmacokinetics: Absorption: Loperamide is easily absorbed from the gut, but it is almost completely extracted by the liver, where it is metabolized, conjugated and excreted via the bile. Simethicone is not absorbed.

Distribution: Studies on distribution in rats show a high affinity for the gut wall with a preference for binding to receptors of the longitudinal muscle layer.

Metabolism: Elimination mainly occurs by oxidative N-demethylation, which is the main metabolic pathway for loperamide.

Excretion: Excretion of the unchanged loperamide and the metabolites mainly occurs through the feces. The half-life of loperamide in man is about 11 hours with a range of 9-14 hours.

Diarrhea is often associated with gas-related abdominal discomfort. Simethicone (poly-dimethylsiloxane) acts as a defoaming agent in the stomach and intestines, by changing the surface tension of gas bubbles, thus enabling them to coalesce and be eliminated more easily.

The combination of loperamide hydrochloride and simethicone has been shown in clinical trials to be overall more effective than either of its active components in controlling the symptoms of both diarrhea and gas-related discomfort.

Only very small amounts (0.3%) of the administered dose of loperamide are absorbed from the G.I. tract. Plasma concentrations of unchanged drug remained below 1.5 ng/mL after oral intake of four Loperamide HCl/Simethicone Chewable Tablets by 24 healthy adult volunteers. Peak loperamide levels were reached at 6.6 hours following ingestion, with an apparent elimination half-life of about 22 hours. There is no evidence that simethicone is absorbed from the G.I. tract. It is thought to be physiologically inert and devoid of toxicity.

Comparative Bioavailability: A single dose [4×(2 mg loperamide/125 mg simethicone)], open-label, randomized, two-treatment crossover study comparing the bioavailability of loperamide from IMODIUM Advanced Caplets and IMODIUM Advanced Chewable Tablets was conducted in 28 healthy male and female volunteers under fasting conditions. Results from the study are presented in Table 1.

Table 1: IMODIUM Advanced

Summary Table of the Comparative Bioavailability Data

LOPERAMIDE 4×(2 mg loperamide HCl/125 mg simethicone) From Measured Data Geometric Mean Arithmetic Mean (CV%)				
Parameter	Test IMODIUM Advanced Caplets[a]	Reference IMODIUM Advanced Chewable Tablets[a]	% RATIO of Geometric Means	90% Confidence Interval
AUC_T (ng·h/mL)	29.3 32.4 (51)	27.4 30.0 (49)	106.9	102.1–113.3
AUC_I (ng·h/mL)	33.6 37.1 (52)	31.4 34.6 (52)	107.0	102.0–113.0
C_{max} (ng/mL)	1.70 1.94 (62)	1.58 1.74 (53)	107.6%	101.9–115.2
T_{max}[b] (h)	5.7 (14)	5.9 (16)	—	—
$T_{½}$[b] (h)	16.3 (27)	16.2 (20)	—	—

[a] Manufactured by McNeil Consumer Healthcare.
[b] Expressed as the arithmetic mean (CV%) only.

INDICATIONS: Loperamide hydrochloride/Simethicone is indicated as an adjunct to rehydration therapy for the symptomatic control of acute, nonspecific diarrhea associated with gas-related abdominal discomfort, such as distention, bloating, flatulence, abdominal pain and cramping.

Treatment of diarrhea with Loperamide hydrochloride/Simethicone is only symptomatic. Whenever an underlying etiology can be determined, specific treatment should be given when appropriate (or when indicated).

CONTRAINDICATIONS: Loperamide hydrochloride/Simethicone is contraindicated for use in children under 2 years of age.

Loperamide hydrochloride/Simethicone is contraindicated in patients with known hypersensitivity to loperamide, simethicone, any of the excipients of the drug and in those in whom constipation must be avoided.

Loperamide hydrochloride/Simethicone should not be used in the case of acute dysentery that is characterized by blood in stools and elevated temperature. Fluid and electrolyte depletion may occur in patients who have diarrhea. The use of Loperamide hydrochloride/Simethicone does not preclude the administration of appropriate fluid and electrolyte therapy.

Loperamide hydrochloride/Simethicone should not be used in patients with bacterial enterocolitis caused by invasive organisms including Salmonella, Shigella, and Campylobacter.

Loperamide hydrochloride/Simethicone must not be used in patients with acute ulcerative colitis or pseudomembranous colitis associated with broad-spectrum antibiotics. In such patients, agents which inhibit intestinal motility or delay intestinal transit time have increased the possible risk of significant sequelae including ileus, megacolon and toxic megacolon. Loperamide hydrochloride/Simethicone therapy should be discontinued promptly if abdominal distention occurs or if untoward symptoms develop. In general, Loperamide hydrochloride/Simethicone should not be used when the inhibition of peristalsis is to be avoided.

WARNINGS: The use of Loperamide hydrochloride/Simethicone is not recommended for children under 12 years of age except on the advice of a physician (see Dosage).

Loperamide hydrochloride/Simethicone should be used with special caution in young children and those with compromised blood brain barrier (eg, meningitis) because of the greater variability of response in these groups. Dehydration, particularly in young children, may further influence the variability of response to Loperamide hydrochloride/Simethicone.

In patients with (severe) diarrhea, especially in children, fluid and electrolyte depletion may occur. In such cases administration of appropriate fluid and electrolyte replacement should be considered. Loperamide hydrochloride/Simethicone should not be given to children under 6 years of age without medical prescription and supervision.

Non-clinical data have shown that loperamide is a P-glycoprotein substrate. Concomitant administration of loperamide (16 mg single dose) with quinidine, or ritonavir, which are both P-glycoprotein inhibitors, resulted in a 2 to 3-fold increase in loperamide plasma levels. The clinical relevance of this pharmacokinetic interaction with P-glycoprotein inhibitors, when loperamide is given at recommended dosages (2 mg, up to 8 mg maximum daily dose), is unknown.

In case of accidental ingestion of Loperamide hydrochloride/Simethicone by children, see Overdose.

Tiredness, dizziness, or drowsiness may occur in the setting of diarrheal syndromes treated with loperamide. Therefore, it is advisable to use caution when driving a car or operating machinery.

PRECAUTIONS: *Pregnancy:* Safe use of Loperamide hydrochloride/Simethicone during pregnancy has not been established. Reproduction studies performed with loperamide hydrochloride in the rat and the rabbit revealed no evidence of impaired fertility or harm to the fetus at dosage levels up to 30-fold the therapeutic dose for man. Therefore, Loperamide hydrochloride/Simethicone should be used in pregnant women only when, in the opinion of the physician, the potential benefits outweigh the potential risks.

Although there are no indications that loperamide or simethicone possess teratogenic or embryotoxic properties, the anticipated therapeutic benefits should be weighed against potential hazards before Loperamide hydrochloride/Simethicone is given during pregnancy, especially during the first trimester.

Lactation: Small amounts of loperamide may appear in human breast milk. Therefore, Loperamide hydrochloride/Simethicone is not recommended during breast-feeding.

Dependence Liability: Physical dependence to loperamide hydrochloride in humans has not been observed. However, studies in morphine-dependent monkeys demonstrated that loperamide hydrochloride at doses above those recommended for humans prevented signs of morphine withdrawal. However, in humans, the naloxone challenge pupil test, which when positive indicates opiate-like effects was negative, when performed after a single high dose, or after more than two years of therapeutic use of loperamide hydrochloride. There is no evidence of any dependence potential for simethicone.

Patients with hepatic dysfunction should be monitored for signs of CNS toxicity due to the extensive first pass metabolism of loperamide in the liver. IMODIUM Advanced should be used under medical supervision in patients with severe hepatic dysfunction.

If clinical improvement is not observed within 48 hours, the administration of Loperamide hydrochloride/Simethicone should be discontinued and patients should be advised to consult their physician.

Patients with AIDS treated with Loperamide hydrochloride/Simethicone for diarrhea should have therapy stopped at the earliest signs of abdominal distension. There have been isolated reports of toxic megacolon in AIDS patients with infectious colitis from both viral and bacterial pathogens treated with loperamide hydrochloride.

Since the majority of loperamide is metabolized, and metabolites or the unchanged drug is excreted in the feces, dose adjustments in patients with a kidney disorder are not required.

ADVERSE EFFECTS: The standard for defining frequency terms will be based on the Council for International Organizations of Medical Science (CIOMS) convention. Specifically: Very common (>1/10). Common (>1/100, <1/10). Uncommon (>1/ 1000, <1/100). Rare (>1/10 000, <1/1000). Very rare (<1/10 000), including isolated reports.

With use of loperamide hydrochloride, occasional hypersensitivity reactions have been reported, such as skin rash and urticaria, and extremely rare cases of anaphylactic shock and bullous eruption including Toxic Epidermal Necrolysis. In the majority of these cases, the patients were on other medications which may have caused or contributed to the events.

The adverse effects reported in adults during clinical trials with Loperamide hydrochloride/Simethicone Chewable Tablets were generally of a minor and self-limiting nature and infrequent: nausea, altered taste (<2%); headache, chills, dry mouth, cough, skin rash (<1%); constipation (<1%) and/or abdominal distension have also been reported. In some very rare cases, particularly in which the treatment information had not been respected, these latter effects have been associated with ileus. Urinary retention has been reported rarely.

Clinical Trial Adverse Drug Reactions: The frequency provided is a reflection of adverse experiences in clinical trials and does not represent true incidence or frequency as seen with epidemiologic studies.

1) Common Adverse events in patients with acute diarrhea.

The following adverse events with an incidence of 1.0% or greater or classified as "common", which were more frequently reported in patients on loperamide/simethicone than on placebo, are presented in the Table 2.

Table 2: IMODIUM Advanced

Listing of Common Adverse Events in Patients with Acute Diarrhea with an Incidence of 1.0% or Greater as Measured in Clinical Trials

	Loperamide 2 mg + Simethicone 125 mg	Loperamide 2 mg	Simethicone 125 mg	Placebo
No. of treated patients	462	456	462	456
Gastrointestinal Disorders %				
Nausea	1.7%	0.4%	0.4%	0.4%
Nervous System Disorders %				
Dysgeusia	1.9%	4.2%	0.0%	0.2%

The adverse event with an incidence of 1.0% or greater or classified as "common", which was more frequently reported in patients on placebo than on loperamide/simethicone, was: dizziness.

Post-Market Adverse Drug Reactions: Loperamide/Simethicone is a combination product containing loperamide hydrochloride. Therefore, adverse experiences considered significant for loperamide hydrochloride will also be included in this section due to the theoretical expectation of a similar adverse event profile even in the absence of actual reports for Loperamide/Simethicone.

Adverse events which may be causally related to the administration of Loperamide/Simethicone that have come to light as a result of reports received in relation to administration of the marketed product are provided in this section. Because these reactions are reported voluntarily from a population of uncertain size, it is not always possible to reliably estimate their frequency or establish a causal relationship to drug exposure.

Immune System Disorders: Allergic reactions and in some cases severe hypersensitivity reactions including anaphylactic shock and anaphylactoid reactions have been reported for loperamide hydrochloride.

Nervous System Disorders: Dizziness, loss of consciousness and depressed level of consciousness have been reported for loperamide hydrochloride.

Gastrointestinal Disorders: abdominal pain, nausea, constipation, flatulence, vomiting and dyspepsia. Abdominal distension, ileus and megacolon including toxic megacolon have been reported for loperamide hydrochloride (see Precautions).

Renal and Urinary Disorders: Urinary retention has been reported for loperamide hydrochloride.

Psychiatric System Disorders: drowsiness.

Skin and Subcutaneous Tissue Disorders: rash, urticaria and pruritus.

Angioedema, and bullous eruptions including Stevens-Johnson syndrome, erythema multiforme, and toxic epidermal necrolysis have been reported for loperamide hydrochloride.

Special Senses: dysgeusia.

A number of the adverse events reported during the clinical investigations and post-marketing experience with loperamide are frequent symptoms of the underlying diarrheal syndrome (abdominal pain/discomfort, nausea, vomiting, dry mouth, tiredness, drowsiness, dizziness, constipation, and flatulence). These symptoms are often difficult to distinguish from undesirable drug effects.

OVERDOSE:

Symptoms: In case of overdosage (including relative overdosage due to hepatic dysfunction), central nervous system depression (stupor, coordination, abnormality, somnolence, miosis, muscular hypertonia, respiratory depression), urinary retention and paralytic ileus may occur. Children may be more sensitive to CNS effects than adults.

In clinical trials with loperamide hydrochloride, an adult who took three 20 mg doses within a 24-hour period was nauseated after the second dose and vomited after the third dose. In studies designed to examine the potential for side effects, intentional ingestion of up to 60 mg of loperamide hydrochloride in a single dose to healthy subjects resulted in no significant adverse effects.

Treatment: Clinical trials have demonstrated that a slurry of activated charcoal administered promptly after ingestion of loperamide hydrochloride can reduce the amount of drug which is absorbed into the systemic circulation by as much as ninefold. If vomiting occurs spontaneously upon ingestion, a slurry of 100 gms of activated charcoal should be administered orally as soon as fluids can be retained.

If vomiting has not occurred, gastric lavage should be performed followed by administration of 100 gms of the activated charcoal slurry through the gastric tube. In the event of overdosage, patients should be monitored for signs of CNS depression for at least 48 hours. If symptoms of overdose occur, naloxone can be given as an antidote. If responsive to naloxone, vital signs must be monitored carefully for recurrence of symptoms of drug overdose for at least 48 hours after the last dose of naloxone.

In view of the prolonged action of loperamide and the short duration (one to three hours) of naloxone, the patient must be monitored closely and treated repeatedly with naloxone as indicated. Since relatively little drug is excreted in the urine, forced diuresis is not expected to be effective for overdosage with Loperamide hydrochloride/Simethicone.

For management of a suspected drug overdose, CPhA recommends that you contact your **regional Poison Control Centre**. See the *CPS* Directory section for a list of Poison Control Centres.

DOSAGE: Adults and Children 12 Years of Age and Older: Chew 2 IMODIUM Advanced Chewable Tablets or swallow 2 IMODIUM Advanced Caplets after the first loose bowel movement and one tablet or caplet after each subsequent loose bowel movement, up to a maximum of 4 tablets or caplets a day for no more than 2 days.

Children 6-11 Years of Age: Chew 1 IMODIUM Advanced Chewable Tablet or swallow 1 IMODIUM Advanced Caplet after the first loose bowel movement and 1/2 tablet or caplet after each subsequent loose bowel movement, up to a maximum 3 tablets or caplets (for ages 9-11 years) or maximum 2 tablets or caplets (for ages 6-8 years) per day, for no longer than 2 days.

Drink plenty of clear fluids to help prevent dehydration which may accompany diarrhea. Take only on an empty stomach (1 hour before or 2 hours after a meal).

Geriatrics (>65 years of age): No dose adjustments are required for the elderly.

Renal Impairment: No dosage adjustment necessary in renal impairment.

Hepatic Impairment: Although no pharmacokinetic data are available in patients with hepatic impairment, IMODIUM Advanced should be used with caution in such patients because of reduced first pass metabolism.

INFORMATION FOR THE PATIENT: Published in e-CPS, available by subscription at www.e-cps.ca.

SUPPLIED: Caplets: Each white caplet with a vanilla odour, debossed with "IMO" on one side and scored and debossed with "2" and "125" on the other side, contains: loperamide HCl 2 mg and simethicone 125 mg. Nonmedicinal ingredients: acesulfame potassium, croscarmellose sodium, dibasic calcium phosphate, flavour, maltodextrin, microcrystalline cellulose, propylene glycol and stearic acid. Energy: 0.42 kJ (0.1 kcal). Sodium: 0.04 mmol (1.05 mg). Bisulfite-, gluten-, lactose- and tartrazine-free. Blister packs of 20. Bottles of 42. Store at controlled room temperature (15 to 30°C).

Chewable Tablets: Each green, round, scored, flat-faced chewable tablet, engraved "IMODIUM" on one side and scored and engraved "2" on top and "125" on the bottom on the other side, contains: loperamide HCl 2 mg and simethicone 125 mg. Nonmedicinal ingredients: basic polymethacrylates, cellulose acetate, cornstarch, D&C Yellow No. 10, dextrates, FD&C Blue No. 1 aluminum lake, microcrystalline cellulose, N&A vanilla mint flavour, sodium saccharin, sorbitol, stearic acid, sucrose and tribasic calcium phosphate. Energy: 16.55 kJ (3.96 kcal). Sodium: 0.002 mmol (0.05 mg). Bisulfite-, gluten-, lactose- and tartrazine-free. Blister packs of 5 and 20. Store at controlled room temperature (15 to 30°C).

Imodium® Caplets
loperamide HCl
Oral Antidiarrheal

McNeil Consumer Healthcare

Imodium® Quick-Dissolve
loperamide HCl
Oral Antidiarrheal

McNeil Consumer Healthcare

Imodium® Oral Solution
loperamide HCl
Oral Antidiarrheal

McNeil Consumer Healthcare

Date of Preparation: January 18, 2007
Date of Revision: November 13, 2008

SUMMARY PRODUCT INFORMATION:

Route of Administration	Dosage Form/ Strength	Clinically Relevant Nonmedicinal Ingredients
Oral	Caplet/2 mg Quick-Dissolve Tablet/2 mg Oral Solution 2 mg/15 mL	None For a complete listing see Dosage Forms, Composition and Packaging.

INDICATIONS AND CLINICAL USE: IMODIUM (loperamide hydrochloride) is indicated:

- as an adjunct to rehydration therapy for the symptomatic control of acute non-specific diarrhea
- for chronic diarrhea associated with inflammatory bowel disease
- for reducing the volume of discharge for ileostomies, colostomies and other intestinal resections

Treatment of diarrhea with IMODIUM is only symptomatic. Whenever an underlying etiology can be determined, specific treatment should be given when appropriate (or when indicated).

In acute diarrhea, if clinical improvement is not observed within 48 hours, the administration of IMODIUM should be discontinued and patients should be advised to consult their physician.

Geriatrics (>65 years of age): No dose adjustments are required for the elderly.

Pediatrics (2 to 12 years of age): Loperamide should be used in children only on the advice of a physician. IMODIUM caplets and Quick-Dissolve tablets are not suited for children under 6 years of age.

Children under 2 years of age: The use of IMODIUM in children under 2 years is contraindicated.

Renal Impairment: No dosage adjustment necessary in renal impairment.

Hepatic Impairment: Although no pharmacokinetic data are available in patients with hepatic impairment, IMODIUM should be used with caution in such patients because of reduced first pass metabolism.

CONTRAINDICATIONS:

- Patients who are hypersensitive to this drug or to any ingredient in the formulation or component of the container. For a complete listing, see Dosage Forms, Composition and Packaging.
- IMODIUM is contraindicated in those in whom constipation must be avoided.
- IMODIUM should not be used in the following cases:
  - in patients with acute dysentery, which is characterized by blood in stools and elevated temperature,
  - in patients with acute ulcerative colitis,
  - in patients with bacterial enterocolitis caused by invasive organisms including Salmonella, Shigella, and Campylobacter,
  - in patients with pseudomembranous colitis associated with the use of broad-spectrum antibiotics.
  - In patients who the inhibition of peristalsis is to be avoided. In such patients, agents which inhibit intestinal motility or delay intestinal transit time have increased the possible risk of significant sequelae including ileus, megacolon and toxic megacolon.
  - Must be discontinued promptly if abdominal distension occurs or if other untoward symptoms develop.

WARNINGS AND PRECAUTIONS: General: Since treatment of diarrhea with IMODIUM is only symptomatic, diarrhea should be treated causally, whenever causal treatment is available. Fluid and electrolyte depletion may occur in patients who have diarrhea. The use of IMODIUM does not preclude the administration of appropriate fluid and electrolyte therapy.

IMODIUM should be kept out of the reach of children. IMODIUM caplets and Quick-Dissolve tablets are not suited for children under 6 years of age. Due to the particular ease with which IMODIUM Quick-Dissolve tablets may be swallowed, special care should be taken when storing this product. In case of accidental ingestion of IMODIUM by children see Overdosage.

Tiredness, dizziness, or drowsiness may occur in the setting of diarrheal syndromes treated with IMODIUM. Therefore, it is advisable to use caution when driving a car or operating machinery.

Dependence/Tolerance: Physical dependence to IMODIUM in humans has not been observed. However, studies in morphine-dependent monkeys demonstrated that loperamide hydrochloride at doses above those recommended for humans prevented signs of morphine withdrawal. However, in humans, the naloxone challenge pupil test, which when positive indicated opiate-like effects, performed after a single high dose, or after more than two years of therapeutic use of IMODIUM, was negative.

Hepatic/Biliary/Pancreatic: Patients with hepatic dysfunction should be monitored for signs of CNS toxicity due to the extensive first pass metabolism of loperamide in the liver.

Immune: Patients with AIDS treated with IMODIUM for diarrhea should have therapy stopped at the earliest signs of abdominal distension. There have been isolated reports of toxic megacolon in AIDS patients with infectious colitis from both viral and bacterial pathogens treated with loperamide hydrochloride.

Neurologic: IMODIUM should be used with special caution in young children and those with compromised blood brain barrier (e.g., meningitis) because of the greater variability of response in these groups. Dehydration, particularly in young children, may further influence the variability of response to IMODIUM.

Renal: Since the majority of the drug is metabolized, and metabolites or the unchanged drug is excreted in the feces, dose adjustments in patients with a kidney disorder are not required.

Special Populations: Pregnant Women: Safe use of IMODIUM during pregnancy has not been established. Reproduction studies performed in the rat and the rabbit revealed no evidence of impaired fertility or harm to the fetus at dosage levels up to 30-fold, the therapeutic dose for man. Therefore, IMODIUM should be used in pregnant women only when, in the opinion of the physician, the potential benefits outweigh the potential risks.

Although there are no indications that loperamide hydrochloride possesses teratogenic or embryotoxic properties, the anticipated therapeutic benefits should be weighed against potential hazards before IMODIUM is given during pregnancy, especially during the first trimester.

The extent of exposure in pregnancy during clinical trials has not been established.

Nursing Women: Small amounts of loperamide may appear in human breast milk. Therefore, IMODIUM is not recommended during breast-feeding.

Pediatrics (<12 years of age): The use of IMODIUM is not recommended for children under 12 years of age except on the advice of a physician (see Dosage and Administration). IMODIUM should be used with special caution in young children because of greater variability of response in this group. Dehydration, particularly in young children, may further influence the variability of response to IMODIUM.

In patients with diarrhea, especially in children, fluid and electrolyte depletion may occur. In such cases administration of appropriate fluid and electrolyte replacement therapy is the most important measure. IMODIUM should not be given to children under 6 years of age without medical prescription and supervision.

The use of the IMODIUM caplet or Quick-Dissolve tablet is not suitable for children under 6 years of age.

The use of IMODIUM is contraindicated for children under 2 years of age.

Geriatrics (>65 years of age): No dose adjustment is required for the elderly.

ADVERSE REACTIONS: The standard for defining frequency terms will be based on the Council for International Organizations of Medical Science (CIOMS) convention. Specifically: Very common (>1/10). Common (>1/100, <1/10). Uncommon (>1/1000, <1/100). Rare (>1/10 000, <1/1000). Very rare (<1/10 000), including isolated reports.

Adverse Drug Reaction Overview: The adverse effects reported in adults during clinical trials are difficult to distinguish from symptoms associated with the diarrheal syndrome. In adults, they were generally of a minor and self-limiting nature e.g., abdominal pain or discomfort; drowsiness or dizziness; tiredness; dry mouth; nausea and vomiting. Hypersensitivity reactions, such as skin rash and urticaria, and extremely rare cases of anaphylactic shock and bullous eruption including Toxic Epidermal Necrolysis, have also been reported. In the majority of these cases, the patients were on other medications which may have caused or contributed to the events. Constipation and/or abdominal distension have also been reported. In some very rare cases, particularly in which the treatment information had not been respected, these effects have been associated with ileus. Urinary retention has been reported rarely. Opiate-like effects (CNS) have been observed in young children (under 3 years of age). No adverse experiences were reported after prolonged use of loperamide.

With the IMODIUM Quick-Dissolve tablet formulation, some subjects have complained about a burning or prickling sensation on the tongue immediately following its use.

Clinical Trial Adverse Drug Reactions: Because clinical trials are conducted under very specific conditions the adverse reaction rates observed in the clinical trials may not reflect the rates observed in practice and should not be compared to the rates in the clinical trials of another drug. Adverse drug reaction information from clinical trials is useful for identifying drug-related adverse events and for approximating rates.

The frequency provided is a reflection of adverse experiences in clinical trials and does not represent true incidence or frequency as seen with epidemiologic studies.

1) Common Adverse events in patients with acute diarrhea: The following adverse events with an incidence of 1.0% or greater or classified as "common", which were more frequently reported in patients on loperamide hydrochloride than on placebo, are presented in Table 1.

Table 1: IMODIUM

Listing of Common Adverse Events in Patients with Acute Diarrhea with an Incidence of 1.0% or Greater as Measured in Clinical Trials

	Acute Diarrhea	
	Loperamide Hydrochloride	**Placebo**
No. of Treated Patients	231	236
Gastrointestinal Disorders %		
Constipation	2.6%	0.8%

The adverse events with an incidence of 1.0% or greater or classified as "common", which were more frequently reported in patients on placebo than on loperamide hydrochloride, were: dry mouth, flatulence, abdominal cramp and colic.

2) Common Adverse events in patients with chronic diarrhea: The adverse events with an incidence of 1.0% or greater or classified as "common", which were more frequently reported in patients on loperamide hydrochloride than on placebo, are presented in Table 2.

Table 2: IMODIUM

Listing of Common Adverse Events in Patients with Chronic Diarrhea with an Incidence of 1.0% or Greater as Measured in Clinical Trials

	Chronic Diarrhea	
	Loperamide Hydrochloride	**Placebo**
No. of Treated Patients	285	277
Gastrointestinal Disorders %		
Constipation	5.3%	0.0%
Nervous System Disorders %		

(cont'd)

Table 2: IMODIUM *(cont'd)*

Listing of Common Adverse Events in Patients with Chronic Diarrhea with an Incidence of 1.0% or Greater as Measured in Clinical Trials

	Chronic Diarrhea	
	Loperamide Hydrochloride	**Placebo**
Dizziness	1.4%	0.7%

The adverse events with an incidence of 1.0% or greater or classified as "common", which were more frequently reported in patients on placebo than on loperamide hydrochloride were: nausea, vomiting, headache, meteorism, abdominal pain, abdominal cramp and colic.

3) Common Adverse events from seventy-six controlled and uncontrolled studies in patients with acute or chronic diarrhea: The following adverse events with an incidence of 1.0% or greater or classified as "common" in patients from all studies are given in Table 3.

Table 3: IMODIUM

Listing of Common Adverse Events in Patients with Acute and Chronic Diarrhea with an Incidence of 1.0% or Greater as Measured in Clinical Trials

	Acute Diarrhea	Chronic Diarrhea	All Studies[a]
No. of Treated Patients	1913	1371	3740
Gastrointestinal Disorders %			
Nausea	0.7%	3.2%	1.8%
Constipation	1.6%	1.9%	1.7%
Abdominal cramps	0.5%	3.0%	1.4%

[a] All patients in all studies, including those in which it was not specified if the adverse events occurred in patients with acute or chronic diarrhea.

Post-Market Adverse Drug Reactions: Adverse events which may be causally related to the administration of IMODIUM that have come to light as a result of reports received in relation to administration of the marketed product are provided in this section. Because these reactions are reported voluntarily from a population of uncertain size, it is not always possible to reliably estimate their frequency or establish a causal relationship to drug exposure.

Immune System Disorders: Allergic reactions and in some cases severe hypersensitivity reactions including anaphylactic shock and anaphylactoid reactions have been reported with the use of loperamide hydrochloride.

Nervous System Disorders: dizziness, loss of consciousness and depressed level of consciousness.

Gastrointestinal Disorders: abdominal pain, ileus, abdominal distension, nausea, constipation, vomiting, megacolon including toxic megacolon (see Warnings and Precautions), flatulence, and dyspepsia.

Renal and Urinary Disorders: urinary retention.

Psychiatric System Disorders: drowsiness.

Skin and Subcutaneous Tissue Disorders: rash, urticaria and pruritus, angioedema, and bullous eruptions including Stevens-Johnson syndrome, erythema multiforme, and toxic epidermal necrolysis have been reported with use of loperamide hydrochloride.

A number of the adverse events reported during the clinical investigations and post-marketing experience with loperamide are frequent symptoms of the underlying diarrheal syndrome (abdominal pain/discomfort, nausea, vomiting, dry mouth, tiredness, drowsiness, dizziness, constipation, and flatulence). These symptoms are often difficult to distinguish from undesirable drug effects.

DRUG INTERACTIONS: Drug-Drug Interactions: Non-clinical data have shown that loperamide is a P-glycoprotein substrate. Concomitant administration of loperamide (16 mg single dose) with quinidine, or ritonavir, which are both P-glycoprotein inhibitors, resulted in a 2 to 3-fold increase in loperamide plasma levels. The clinical relevance of this pharmacokinetic interaction with P-glycoprotein inhibitors, when loperamide is given at recommended dosages (2 mg, up to 16 mg maximum daily dose), is unknown.

No drug interactions have been reported. However, it is expected that drugs with similar pharmacological properties may potentiate the effect of IMODIUM and that drugs that accelerate gastrointestinal transit may decrease its effect.

Drug-Food Interactions: Interactions with food have not been established.

Drug-Herb Interactions: Interactions with herbal products have not been established.

Drug-Laboratory Test Interactions: Interactions with laboratory tests have not been established.

DOSAGE AND ADMINISTRATION: Recommended Dose and Dosage Adjustment: IMODIUM Quick-Dissolve is a fast-dissolving tablet which can be taken without fluid. The tablet disintegrates within seconds on the surface of the tongue and is then swallowed with the saliva.

Dose for the oral solution should be administered with the attached measuring cup only.

Adults and Children 12 Years of Age and Older: IMODIUM Caplets, IMODIUM Quick-Dissolve Tablets and IMODIUM Oral Solution: Acute Diarrhea: The initial dose of IMODIUM (loperamide hydrochloride) is 2 caplets or 2 Quick-Dissolve Tablets or 30 mL Oral Solution (4 mg) followed by 1 caplet or 1 Quick-Dissolve Tablet or 15 mL Oral Solution (2 mg) after every subsequent loose stool. Clinical studies indicate that diarrheal control may be achieved after the initial dose in 50% of patients. Daily dosage should not exceed 8 caplets or Quick-Dissolve Tablets or 120 mL Oral Solution (16 mg).

Chronic Diarrhea: The recommended initial dosage of IMODIUM is 4 mg (2 caplets or 2 Quick-Dissolve Tablets or 30 mL Oral Solution) followed by 2 mg (1 caplet or 1 Quick-Dissolve Tablet or 15 mL Oral Solution) after each unformed stool until diarrhea is controlled; thereafter, the dosage of IMODIUM should be reduced to meet individual requirements. When the optimal daily dosage has thus been established, this amount can be administered as a single dose daily or in divided doses. The average daily maintenance dosage used in clinical trial has been 4-8 mg.

The maximum dose for chronic diarrhea is 8 caplets or 8 Quick-Dissolve Tablets or 120 mL Oral Solution (16 mg) daily. If improvement is not observed after treatment with 16 mg per day for 10 days, symptoms are unlikely to be controlled by further administration.

Children (6 to 12 years): IMODIUM Caplets and IMODIUM Quick-Dissolve Tablets: The use of IMODIUM caplets and Quick-Dissolve tablets is not suitable for children under 6 years of age. IMODIUM Oral Solution is intended for use in adults and children 12 years of age and older only.

Acute or Chronic Diarrhea: Loperamide should be used in children only on the advice of a physician. For children up to but not including 12 years of age, the following schedule will usually fulfil initial dosage requirements: see Table 4.

Table 4: IMODIUM

Recommended First-Day Dosage Schedule

Six to eight years: (20 to 30 kg)	2 mg b.i.d. (4 mg daily dose)
Eight to twelve years: (greater than 30 kg)	2 mg t.i.d. (6 mg daily dose)

Following the first treatment day, it is recommended that subsequent IMODIUM doses (1 mg/10 kg body weight) be administered only after a loose stool and not exceed the maximum daily dose.

Duration of Treatment: IMODIUM may be administered for prolonged periods of time. Blood, urine, liver and kidney function, ECG and ophthalmological examinations have revealed no significant abnormalities after several years of administration. No tolerance to the antidiarrheal effect has been observed. Naloxone pupil challenge studies in patients with chronic diarrhea who have received IMODIUM orally for prolonged periods indicate a lack of CNS effects.

OVERDOSAGE:

Symptoms: In case of overdose (including relative overdose due to hepatic dysfunction), central nervous system depression (stupor, coordination abnormality, somnolence, miosis, muscular hypertonia, respiratory depression), urinary retention and ileus may occur. Children may be more sensitive to CNS effects than adults.

In clinical trials, an adult who took three 20 mg doses within a 24-hour period was nauseated after the second dose and vomited after the third dose. In studies designed to examine the potential for side effects, intentional ingestion of up to 60 mg of loperamide hydrochloride in a single dose to healthy subjects resulted in no significant adverse effects.

Treatment: Treatment is symptomatic and supportive. Appropriate standard methods of gastrointestinal decontamination may be employed. Activated charcoal administered in appropriate dosages, promptly after ingestion of loperamide hydrochloride can reduce the amount of drug which is absorbed into the systemic circulation by as much as nine fold.

In the event of overdosage, patients should be monitored for signs of CNS depression for at least 48 hours. If symptoms of overdose occur, naloxone can be given as an antidote. Since the duration of action of IMODIUM is longer than that of naloxone (1 to 3 hours), repeated treatment with naloxone might be indicated. If responsive to naloxone, vital signs must be monitored carefully for recurrence of symptoms of drug overdose for at least 48 hours after the last dose of naloxone.

Since relatively little drug is excreted in the urine, forced diuresis is not expected to be effective for IMODIUM overdosage.

Physicians without experience in managing loperamide overdose should seek consultation with a Regional Poison Control Centre.

> For management of a suspected drug overdose, CPhA recommends that you contact your **regional Poison Control Centre**. See the *CPS* Directory section for a list of Poison Control Centres.

ACTION AND CLINICAL PHARMACOLOGY: Mechanism of Action: Diarrhea may be defined as a failure or imbalance of one or a combination of activities in the gut which include secretion, absorption and motility. IMODIUM (loperamide hydrochloride) has been shown to act on all of these functions via cholinergic, non-cholinergic, opiate and non-opiate receptor-mediated mechanisms. In this way, IMODIUM effectively reduces fecal output and frequency, improves stool consistency and relieves symptoms of abdominal cramping and fecal incontinence.

Pharmacodynamics: Loperamide binds to the opiate receptor in the gut wall. Consequently, it inhibits the release of acetylcholine and prostaglandins, thereby reducing propulsive peristalsis, and increasing intestinal transit time. Loperamide increases the tone of the anal sphincter, thereby reducing incontinence and urgency.

Due to its high affinity for the gut wall and its high first-pass metabolism, loperamide hardly reaches the systemic circulation.

Pharmacokinetics: Absorption: Loperamide is easily absorbed from the gut, but it is almost completely extracted by the liver, where it is metabolized, conjugated and excreted via the bile.

Distribution: Studies on distribution in rats show a high affinity for the gut wall with a preference for binding to receptors of the longitudinal muscle layer.

Metabolism: Elimination mainly occurs by oxidative N-demethylation, which is the main metabolic pathway for loperamide.

Excretion: Excretion of the unchanged loperamide and the metabolites mainly occurs through the feces. The half-life of loperamide in man is about 11 hours with a range of 9-14 hours.

STORAGE AND STABILITY: IMODIUM caplets and Oral Solution should be stored at room temperature (15-30°C). Protect from light.

Store IMODIUM Quick-Dissolve tablets at room temperature (15-30°C) and protect from moisture.

SPECIAL HANDLING INSTRUCTIONS: Keep out of reach of children.

INFORMATION FOR THE PATIENT: Published in e-CPS, available by subscription at www.e-cps.ca.

DOSAGE FORMS, COMPOSITION AND PACKAGING: IMODIUM Caplets: Each light green, capsule-shaped tablet, embossed with "Imodium A-D" on one side and "2 mg" on the other side, contains: loperamide HCl 2 mg. Nonmedicinal ingredients: cellulose, colloidal silicon dioxide, D&C yellow No. 10, dibasic calcium phosphate, FD&C blue No. 1 and magnesium stearate. Blister packs of 6, 12, 24 and 42 caplets.

IMODIUM Quick-Dissolve Tablets: Each white, circular tablet contains: loperamide HCl 2 mg. Nonmedicinal ingredients: aspartame, flavour, gelatin, mannitol and sodium bicarbonate. Blister strips of 10 tablets, packages containing one (10 tablets) or two (20 tablets) blister strips. **IMODIUM Quick-Dissolve tablets should not be pushed through the blister, as this would damage them.** To take the tablets out of the blister, pull up the edge of the foil, tear the foil completely off, press out and then remove the tablet.

IMODIUM Oral Solution: Each 15 mL of opaque green liquid with a mint odour contains: loperamide HCl 2 mg. Nonmedicinal ingredients: carboxymethylcellulose sodium, cellulose, citric acid, D&C yellow no. 10, dimethyl siloxane, FD&C blue no. 1, flavour, glycerin, methylcellulose, propylene glycol, purified water, simethicone, sodium benzoate, sorbic acid, sucralose, titanium dioxide and xanthan gum. Plastic bottles of 120, 240 and 360 mL.

IMOGAM® Rabies Pasteurized

rabies immune globulin, pasteurized (human)

Immunotherapeutic Agent (Passive Immunization)

sanofi pasteur

Date of Revision: November 2005

PHARMACOLOGY: Infection with rabies virus characteristically produces an acute illness with rapidly progressive CNS manifestations, including anxiety, dysphagia, and convulsions, and almost invariably progresses to death. Some patients may present with paralysis.

Rabies virus is classified in the Rhabdovirus family.

Rabies virus can infect any mammal. In North America, it occurs mainly in certain wildlife species and is spread by them to domestic livestock and pets. In recent years, most reported wildlife infections in British Columbia have been in bats; in Alberta, Saskatchewan and Manitoba in skunks; in Ontario and Quebec in foxes and skunks; and in the Northwest Territories in foxes. Rabies has been reported sporadically from New Brunswick and Nova Scotia and recently outbreaks in foxes have been reported in Labrador. Bat rabies is found in all regions across Canada and in most of the larger islands as far north as bats are found. Although domestic dogs and cats account for less than 10% of reported animal rabies, bites of these species account for the vast majority of suspected rabies exposures in humans and thus the majority of courses of antirabies postexposure treatment.

Airborne transmission has been reported in the laboratory and in bat-infected caves. Transmission has also occurred by transplantation of corneas from patients dying of undiagnosed rabies. Person-to-person transmission by bite has not been documented, although the virus has been isolated from the saliva of patients.

The incubation period in humans ranges from 5 days to more than 1 year; 2 months is the average. Recently, incubation periods of many years have been confirmed by antigenic typing of strains.

Rabies virus is usually transmitted by the bite of a rabid animal but can occasionally penetrate abraded skin contaminated with the saliva of infected animals. Progress of the virus after exposure is believed to follow a neural pathway and the time between exposure and clinical rabies is a function of the proximity of the bite (or abrasion) to the CNS and the dose of virus injected. The incubation period is usually 2 to 6 weeks but can be longer. After severe bites to the face, neck or arms, it may be as short as 10 days. After initiation of the vaccine series (human diploid cell origin), it takes approximately 1 week for development of immunity to rabies; therefore, the value of immediate passive immunization with rabies antibodies in the form of Rabies Immune Globulin (Human) cannot be overemphasized.

Since reporting began in 1925, 21 persons have died of rabies in Canada. Even though disease may not develop in everyone bitten by a rabid animal, a decision on the management of a person who may have been exposed to rabies virus must be made rapidly and judiciously since delay in starting postexposure prophylaxis reduces its effectiveness. Since it is not possible to distinguish between those in whom rabies will or will not develop if untreated and since the infection is almost always fatal, it is essential that all persons exposed to proved or suspected rabid animals be given postexposure prophylaxis. Between 1000 and 1500 persons in Canada receive postexposure treatment each year because of exposure to rabid or suspected rabid animals.

Among recent human cases in the U.S., infections with bat rabies virus strains have predominated, the problem being failure to recognize the small wound inflicted by a biting bat and thus omission of postexposure prophylaxis.

Rabies antibody provides passive protection when given immediately to individuals exposed to rabies virus. Rabies Immune Globulin (human) of adequate potency was used in conjunction with Rabies Vaccine of duck embryo origin. When a globulin dose of 20 IU/kg of rabies antibody was given simultaneously with the first dose of vaccine, levels of passive rabies antibody were detected 24 hours after injection in all individuals. There was minimal or no interference with the immune response to the initial and subsequent doses of vaccine, including booster doses.

Studies of IMOGAM Rabies Pasteurized, [Rabies Immune Globulin, Pasteurized (Human)] administered with the first of 5 doses of Inactivated Human Rabies Vaccine Mérieux confirmed that passive immunization with 20 IU/kg of Rabies Immune Globulin (Human) provides maximum circulating antibody with minimum interference with the active immunization.

A recent study indicates that the neutralizing antibody levels following administration of IMOGAM Rabies Pasteurized, with and without Rabies Vaccine (HDCV) are not significantly different from that observed following IMOGAM RABIES (not heat treated) administered in the same manner.

A double-blind trial was conducted in 64 healthy veterinary student volunteers randomized into 4 parallel groups of 16 each, to compare the safety and antibody levels achieved following i.m. injection of IMOGAM Rabies Pasteurized and IMOGAM RABIES, (non heat-treated). Each immune globulin was administered on day 0, either alone or in combination with the human diploid cell Rabies Vaccine (IMOVAX RABIES) using the standard postexposure prophylactic schedule of day 0, 3, 7, 14 and 28.

The dosage corresponded to the postexposure recommended dose of 20 IU/kg of rabies immune globulin and was administered in 3, equally divided i.m. injections of under 5 mL in either gluteus. Serum rabies antibody levels were assessed before treatment and on days 3, 7, 14, 28, 35, and 42 by the Rabies Fluorescent Focus Inhibition Test (RFFIT).

Serum antibody levels were similar in the IMOGAM Rabies Pasteurized and IMOGAM RABIES groups. By day 3, 60% of each group had detectable antibody titers of ≥0.05 IU/mL. By day 14, the geometric mean titres (with 95% confidence interval) were 19 IU/mL (11 to 38) in the IMOGAM Rabies Pasteurized + vaccine group and 31 IU/mL (20 to 48) in the IMOGAM RABIES + vaccine group. These differences were not statistically different.

Both IMOGAM Rabies Pasteurized and IMOGAM RABIES were safe and without serious adverse events or allergic reactions.

INDICATIONS: For individuals suspected of exposure to rabies, with one exception: persons who have been previously immunized with Human Diploid Cell Rabies Vaccine, (HDCV) in a pre- or postexposure treatment series receive only vaccine.

Persons previously vaccinated with a vaccine other than HDCV in whom adequate antibody levels have not been demonstrated should receive full postexposure prophylaxis with HDCV and RIG.

If indicated, IMOGAM Rabies Pasteurized should be administered as promptly as possible after exposure. If initiation of treatment is delayed for any reason, IMOGAM Rabies Pasteurized should still be given, regardless of the interval between exposure and treatment. Since vaccine-induced antibody begins to appear within 1 week, there is no value in administering rabies immune globulin more than 8 days after the first dose of a rabies vaccine course.

Recommendations for passive and/or active immunization after exposure to an animal suspected of having rabies have been outlined by the WHO and by the Canadian National Advisory Committee on Immunization (NACI).

Postexposure Immunization: A decision on the management of a person who has been exposed to the risk of rabies infection must be made rapidly and judiciously since delay in starting a course of vaccine reduces its effectiveness, and the disease once established is almost always fatal.

Rabies prophylaxis must be considered in every incident where potential exposure to rabies virus has occurred. The following factors should be taken into consideration.

Species of Animal: The animals in Canada most often proven rabid are foxes, skunks, cattle, dogs, cats and bats. The distribution of animal rabies and the species involved vary considerably across Canada so it is important to consult the local medical officer of health or government veterinarian. Human exposures to livestock are usually confined to salivary contamination, with the exception of horses and swine in which biting incidents have been reported. Risk of infection following exposure to rabid cattle is low, and only about 30 cases have ever been recorded. Squirrels, hamsters, guinea pigs, gerbils, chipmunks, rats, mice, other rodents or rabbits and hares are rarely found to be infected with rabies and are not known to cause human rabies in Canada and the U.S. Postexposure prophylaxis should be considered if the animal's behavior was highly unusual.

Incident: Each incident requires full investigation including an assessment of the risk of rabies in the animal species involved and the behavior of the particular animal. An **unprovoked** attack is more apt to indicate that the animal is rabid. Nevertheless, rabid cats and dogs may become uncharacteristically quiet. Bites inflicted on a person attempting to feed or handle an apparently healthy animal should generally be regarded as **provoked**.

Type of Exposure: Rabies is transmitted when the virus is inoculated into tissues, most commonly when virus in saliva is introduced into tissues by bites. Transmission can also occur when cuts or wounds of skin or mucous membranes are contaminated with virus in saliva or infected tissues. Rarely, transmission has been recorded when virus was inhaled, or infected corneal grafts were transplanted into patients. Thus, 2 broad categories of exposure are recognized as warranting postexposure prophylaxis:

Bite: any penetration of skin by teeth. Bites inflicted by most animals are readily apparent. However, bites inflicted by bats to a sleeping person may not be felt, and these animals' needle-like teeth may leave no visible bite marks. Hence, when persons are sleeping unattended in a room where a bat is present and they cannot reasonably exclude the possibility of a bite, postexposure prophylaxis should be initiated.

Non-bite: includes contamination of scratches, abrasions or cuts of skin or mucous membranes by saliva or other potentially infectious material, such as the brain tissue of a rabid animal. Petting a rabid animal or handling its blood, urine or feces is not considered to be exposure nor is being sprayed by a skunk. Such incidents do not warrant postexposure prophylaxis.

Postexposure prophylaxis is warranted and recommended in rare instances of non-bite exposure, such as inhalation of aerosolized virus by spelunkers exploring caves inhabited by infected bats or by laboratory technicians homogenizing tissues infected with rabies virus; however, the efficacy of prophylaxis after such exposures is unknown. Stringent guidelines concerning the suitability of tissue donors have eliminated the probability that rabies virus will be transmitted iatrogenically.

Non-bite (and bite) exposures incurred in the course of caring for humans with rabies could theoretically transmit the infection. No case of rabies acquired in this way has been documented, but postexposure prophylaxis should be considered for exposed individuals.

Because some bat bites may be less severe, and therefore more difficult to recognize, than bites inflicted by larger mammalian carnivores, rabies postexposure treatment should be considered for any physical contact with bats when bite or mucous membrane contact cannot be excluded.

Vaccination Status of Biting Animal: A small number of vaccinated animals have developed rabies. Therefore, symptoms suggesting rabies, even in a vaccinated animal, must be carefully evaluated. The vaccination history in itself should not influence the need for postexposure treatment nor the need to sacrifice the animal for assessment.

The following recommendations are intended as a guide for the management of persons following possible exposure to rabies and may need to be modified in accordance with the specific circumstances of the exposure to rabies.

Local Treatment of Wounds: **Immediate washing and flushing with soap and water, detergent, or water alone is imperative and is probably the most effective procedure in the prevention of rabies.** Suturing the wound should be avoided if possible. Tetanus prophylaxis and antibacterial drugs should be given as required.

Immunizing Agents: There are 2 types of immunizing products: Vaccines, which contain inactivated virus and induce an active immune response beginning in 7 to 10 days and persisting for at least a year; Rabies Immune Globulin (RIG), which provides rapid protection that persists for only a short period of time (half-life about 21 days).

Vaccine and immune globulin should be used concurrently for optimum postexposure prophylaxis against rabies, except in persons previously vaccinated with HDCV.

Postexposure Treatment Guide: The following recommendations are only a guide (see Table 1). They should be applied in conjunction with knowledge of the animal species involved, circumstances of the bite or other exposure, vaccination status of the animal, and presence of rabies in the region. Local and provincial public health officials should be consulted if questions arise about the need for rabies prophylaxis.

Table 1: IMOGAM Rabies Pasteurized

Postexposure Treatment Guide

Animal Species	Condition of Animal at Time of Exposure	Management of Exposed Person
Dog or cat	Healthy and available for 10 days' observation.	1. Local treatment of wound. 2. At first sign of rabies in animal, give RIG (local and intramuscular) and start HDCV.
	Rabid or suspected rabid.[a] Unknown or escaped.	1. Local treatment of wound. 2. RIG (local and intramuscular) and HDCV.
Skunk, bat, fox, coyote, raccoon and other carnivores. Includes bat found in room when a person was sleeping unattended.	Regard as rabid unless geographic area is known to be rabies-free.[a]	1. Local treatment of wound. 2. RIG (local and intramuscular) and HDCV.
Livestock, rodents or lagomorphs (hares and rabbits)	Consider individually. Consult appropriate public health and Food Inspection Agency officials. Bites of squirrels, chipmunks, rats, mice, hamsters, gerbils, other rodents, rabbits and hares may rarely warrant post-exposure rabies prophylaxis if the behavior of the biting animal was highly unusual.	

[a] If possible, the animal should be humanely killed and the brain tested for rabies as soon as possible; holding for observation is not recommended. Discontinue vaccine if fluorescent antibody test of animal brain is negative.

Legend: RIG=(human) rabies immune globulin. HDCV=human diploid cell vaccine.

CONTRAINDICATIONS: IMOGAM Rabies Pasteurized, [Rabies Immune Globulin, Pasteurized (Human)] should not be administered in repeated doses once vaccine treatment has been initiated. Repeating the dose may interfere with maximum active immunity expected from the vaccine.

WARNINGS: IMOGAM Rabies Pasteurized, [Rabies Immune Globulin, Pasteurized (Human)] is made from human plasma. Products made from human plasma may contain infectious agents, such as viruses, that can cause disease. The risk that such products will transmit an infectious agent has been reduced by screening plasma donors for prior exposure to certain viruses, by testing for the presence of certain current virus infections, and by inactivating and/or removing certain viruses. An alcohol fractionation procedure used to purify the immunoglobulin component removes and/or inactivates both enveloped and nonenveloped viruses. An added heat treatment process (60°C, 10 hours) further inactivates both enveloped and nonenveloped viruses (see Supplied). Despite these measures, it is still theoretically possible that known or unknown infectious agents may be present. All infections thought by a physician possibly to have been transmitted by this product should be reported by the physician or other health care provider to the Medical Director, Sanofi Pasteur Limited, 1755 Steeles Avenue West, Toronto, Ontario, Canada, M2R 3T4. The physician should discuss the risks and benefits of this product with the patient. This should include information that cases of rabies have been attributed to omission of passive immunization in persons who have received rabies vaccine.

IMOGAM Rabies Pasteurized should be given with caution to patients with a history of prior systemic allergic reactions following the administration of human immune globulin preparations.

Persons with specific IgA deficiency have increased potential for developing antibodies to IgA and could have anaphylactic reactions to subsequent administration of blood products containing IgA.

PRECAUTIONS: General: There is no contraindication to the use of rabies vaccine or rabies immune globulin if indicated following exposure to a proven rabid animal. Hypersensitive individuals should be vaccinated only under strict medical supervision.

Infiltration of wounds in some anatomical sites (finger tips) must be carried out with care in order to avoid increased pressure in the tissue compartment (compartment syndrome).

The possibility of allergic reactions in individuals sensitive to components of the product should be evaluated. Epinephrine HCl solution (1:1000) and other appropriate agents should be available for immediate use in case an anaphylactic or acute hypersensitivity reaction occurs. Health care providers should be familiar with current recommendations for the initial management of anaphylaxis in nonhospital settings, including proper airway management.

Before administration of any product, all appropriate precautions should be taken to prevent adverse reactions. This includes a review of the patient's history with respect to possible hypersensitivity to the product or similar product, determination of previous immunization history, and the presence of any contraindications, current health status, and a current knowledge of the literature concerning the use of the product under consideration.

Special care should be taken to ensure that the product is not injected into a blood vessel.

Under no circumstances should RIG vaccine be administered in the same syringe or at the same site as Rabies Vaccine.

A separate sterile needle and syringe, or a sterile disposable unit, must be used for each individual patient to prevent the transmission of infectious agents. There have been case reports of transmission of HIV and hepatitis by failure to scrupulously observe sterile technique.

Needles should not be recapped and should be disposed of properly.

Before administration of IMOGAM Rabies Pasteurized, [Rabies Immune Globulin, Pasteurized (Human)], health care personnel should inform the patient, parent or guardian of the benefits and risks of immunization, and also inquire about the recent health status of the patient to be injected.

IMOGAM Rabies Pasteurized should not be administered i.v because of the potential for serious reactions. Injection should be made i.m. and care should be taken to draw back on the plunger of the syringe before injection in order to be certain that the needle is not in a blood vessel. Although systemic reactions to immunoglobulin preparations are rare, epinephrine (1:1000) should be available for treatment of acute anaphylactoid reactions. As with all preparations given i.m., bleeding complications may be encountered in patients with bleeding disorders.

Drug Interactions: Live virus vaccine such as measles vaccine should not be given for 4 months following IMOGAM Rabies Pasteurized administration because antibodies in the globulin preparation may interfere with the immune response to the vaccination. Interference may also occur if the administration of IMOGAM Rabies Pasteurized becomes necessary within a short time after the administration of a live viral vaccine, and if the time interval between the two is very short (less than 14 days), vaccination may have to be repeated.

Pregnancy: Pregnancy is not a contraindication to rabies postexposure therapy. Based on limited data, there have been no fetal abnormalities associated with rabies vaccination. Clinical experience with other immunoglobulin preparations suggests that there are no known adverse effects on the fetus from immune globulin, but there are no reported studies indicating whether or not such adverse effects occur. Specifically animal reproduction studies have not been conducted with IMOGAM Rabies Pasteurized. It is also not known whether IMOGAM Rabies Pasteurized can cause fetal harm when administered to a pregnant woman or can affect reproductive capacity. IMOGAM Rabies Pasteurized should be given to a pregnant woman only if clearly needed.

ADVERSE EFFECTS: In a recent clinical trial involving 16 volunteers in each of 4 treatment groups, 2 subjects reported severe headaches, 1 in the IMOGAM Rabies Pasteurized, [Rabies Immune Globulin, Pasteurized (Human)] + placebo group and 1 in the IMOGAM Rabies and the IMOVAX Rabies group. One third of the volunteers reported moderately systemic reactions (headache and malaise). These were equally distributed among the 4 treatment groups with no significant differences between the groups.

Local or mild systemic adverse reactions to the globulin are infrequent and may be treated symptomatically.

Local tenderness, soreness or stiffness of the muscles may occur at the injection site and may persist for several hours after injection. Urticaria and angioedema may occur. Anaphylactic reactions although rare, have been reported following injection of human immune globulin preparations. Fever, skin reactions or chills have been reported following human rabies immunoglobulins. Rare cases of nausea, vomiting, hypotension, tachycardia and allergic-type reactions have been reported. In very rare cases, anaphylactic shock has been observed.

Physicians, nurses, and pharmacists should report any adverse occurrences temporally related to the administration of the product in accordance with local requirements and to the Global Pharmacovigilance Department, Sanofi Pasteur Limited, 1755 Steeles Avenue West, Toronto, Ontario, Canada, M2R 3T4.

DOSAGE: Parenteral biological products should be inspected visually for extraneous particulate matter and/or discoloration before administration. If these conditions exist, the product should not be administered.

IMOGAM Rabies Pasteurized, [Rabies Immune Globulin, Pasteurized (Human)] should be used in conjunction with rabies human diploid cell vaccine (HDCV). The recommended dose of IMOGAM Rabies Pasteurized is 20 IU/kg (0.133 mL/kg) of body weight at the time of administration of the first vaccine dose. This formula is applicable to all age groups, including children. If anatomically feasible, the full dose of RIG should be thoroughly infiltrated in the area around and into the wounds. Any remaining volume should be injected i.m. at a site distant from vaccine administration.

IMOGAM Rabies Pasteurized should never be administered in the same syringe or into the same anatomical site as the vaccine. HDCV is never to be administered in the gluteal region. Because IMOGAM Rabies Pasteurized may partially suppress active production of antibody, no more than the recommended dose should be given.

The dose of 20 IU/kg body weight is the same for children and adults. The dose of IMOGAM Rabies Pasteurized, especially following multiple wounds, may be diluted 2-to 3-fold in a solution of 0.9% sodium chloride in order to provide the full amount of human rabies immunoglobulin required for good infiltration of sites at risk of rabies.

Do not heat by placing in warm water or incubator.

When administering a dose from a rubber-stoppered vial, do not remove either the rubber stopper or the metal seal holding it in place. Aseptic technique must be used for withdrawal of each dose (see Precautions).

Before injection, the skin over the site to be injected should be cleansed with a suitable germicide.

After insertion of the needle, aspirate to ensure that the needle has not entered a blood vessel.

Do not inject i.v.

Each person who is immunized should be given a permanent personal immunization record. In addition, it is essential that the physician or nurse record the immunization history in the permanent medical record of each patient. This permanent office record should contain the name of the product, date given, dose, manufacturer and lot number.

SUPPLIED: IMOGAM Rabies Pasteurized, [Rabies Immune Globulin, Pasteurized (Human)] is a sterile solution of antirabies immunoglobulin (10 to 18% protein) for i.m. administration. It is prepared by cold alcohol fractionation from pooled venous plasma of individuals immunized with Rabies Vaccine prepared from human diploid cells (HDCV). The product is stabilized with 0.3 M glycine. The globulin solution has a pH of 6.8±0.4 adjusted with sodium hydroxide or hydrochloric acid. No preservatives are added.

IMOGAM Rabies Pasteurized is a colorless to light opalescent liquid.

A heat-treatment process step (58 to 60°C, 10 hours) to inactivate viruses has been added to further reduce risk of blood-borne viral transmission. The inactivation and removal of model and laboratory strains of enveloped and nonenveloped viruses during the manufacturing and heat treatment processes for IMOGAM Rabies Pasteurized has been validated by spiking experiments. Human immunodeficiency virus, type 1 (HIV-1) and type 2 (HIV-2) were selected as relevant viruses for plasma derived products. Bovine viral diarrhea virus and Sindbis virus were chosen to model hepatitis C virus. Porcine pseudorabies virus was selected to model hepatitis B virus and herpes virus. Avian reovirus was used to model nonenveloped RNA viruses and for its relative resistance to inactivation by chemical and physical methods. Finally, porcine parvovirus was selected to model human parvovirus B19 and its notable resistance to inactivation by heat treatment.

Removal and/or inactivation of the studied enveloped and nonenveloped model viruses was demonstrated at the precipitation III stage of manufacturing. In addition, inactivation was demonstrated to occur during the 10-hour (58 to 60°C) heat treatment process for the studied enveloped and nonenveloped viruses.

The product is standardized against a standard Rabies Immune Globulin of known potency in IU for rabies antibody. Each vial is formulated to contain at least 150 IU/mL. Each mL contains: human proteins 100 to 180 mg containing (IgG-class) human rabies immunoglobulins with a minimum titre of 150 IU*/mL. Nonmedicinal ingredients: glycine 22.5 mg, sodium chloride 1 mg and water for injection up to 1 mL. Vials of 2 mL–300 IU (150 IU/mL) which is sufficient for a child weighing 15 kg; and 10 mL–1500 IU (150 IU/mL) which is sufficient for an adult weighing 75 kg.

Store at refrigerator temperature (2 to 8°C). **Do not freeze.** Product which has been exposed to freezing should not be used. IMOGAM Rabies Pasteurized contains no preservatives and unused portions must be discarded immediately. Do not use after expiration date.

* Titre determined by the Rapid Fluorescent Focus Inhibition Test (RFFIT) technique.

Imovane® Ⓟ

zopiclone

Hypnotic—Sedative

sanofi-aventis

Date of Revision: October 2, 2009

PHARMACOLOGY: IMOVANE (zopiclone), a cyclopyrrolone derivative, is a short-acting hypnotic agent. IMOVANE belongs to a novel chemical class, which is structurally unrelated to existing hypnotics. However, the pharmacological profile of IMOVANE is similar to that of the benzodiazepines.

IMOVANE pharmacological properties are: hypnotic, sedative, anxiolytic, anti-convulsant, muscle-relaxant. These effects are related to a specific agonist action at central receptors belonging to the GABAa macromolecular complex, modulating the opening of the chloride ion channel.

In sleep laboratory studies of one to 21-day duration in man, zopiclone reduced sleep latency, increased the duration of sleep and decreased the number of nocturnal awakenings. Zopiclone delayed the onset of REM sleep but did not reduce consistently the total duration of REM periods. The duration of stage 1 sleep was shortened, and the time spent in stage 2 sleep increased. In most studies, stage 3 and 4 sleep tended to be increased, but no change and actual decreases have also been observed. The effect of zopiclone on stage 3 and 4 sleep differs from that of the benzodiazepines, which suppress slow wave sleep. The clinical significance of this finding is not known.

With hypnotic drugs, the duration of hypnotic effect and the profile of unwanted effects may be influenced by the alpha (distribution) ($t_{½}α$) and beta (elimination) ($t_{½}β$) half-lives of the administered drug and any active metabolites formed. When half-lives are long, the drug or metabolite may accumulate during periods of nightly administration and be associated with impairments of cognitive and motor performance during waking hours. If half-lives are short, the drug and metabolites will be cleared before the next dose is ingested, and carry-over effects related to sedation or CNS depression should be minimal or absent. If the drug has a very short elimination half-life, it is possible that a relative deficiency (i.e., in relation to the receptor site) may occur at some point in the interval between each night's use. This sequence of events may account for two clinical findings reported to occur after several weeks of nightly use of rapidly eliminated benzodiazepines or benzodiazepine-like hypnotics: 1) increased wakefulness during the last third of the night and 2) the appearance of increased day-time anxiety (see Warnings).

During nightly use and for an extended period, pharmacodynamic tolerance or adaptation to some effects of benzodiazepines or benzodiazepine-like hypnotics may develop. However in two sleep laboratory studies involving 17 patients, there was an absence of tolerance with zopiclone for treatment periods of more than 4 weeks.

Rebound Insomnia: Some manifestations of rebound insomnia have been reported both in sleep laboratory and clinical studies following the withdrawal of zopiclone (see Precautions).

Zopiclone treatment was associated with dose-related residual effects (see Precautions).

Pharmacokinetics: Absorption: Zopiclone is rapidly and well absorbed. Bioavailability is more than 75%, indicating the absence of a significant first-pass effect. After the administration of 3.75 and 7.5 mg doses, peak plasma concentrations of 30 and 60 ng/mL, respectively were reached in less than 2 hours. Absorption was similar in males and females.

Repeated daily administration of a 7.5 mg oral dose for 14 days did not change the pharmacokinetic characteristics of zopiclone and did not lead to accumulation.

Distribution: Zopiclone is rapidly distributed from the vascular compartment (distribution half-life [$t_{½}α$]: 1.2 hours) while the elimination half-life is approximately 5 hours (range: 3.8 to 6.5 hours). Plasma protein binding is low (approximately 45% in the 25-100 ng/mL concentration range) and non saturable. The risk of drug interaction arising from displacement of bound drug is low. The distribution volume is 91.8-104.6 liters.

Metabolism: Zopiclone is extensively metabolized by three major pathways; only about 4 to 5% of the drug is excreted unchanged in the urine.

An in vitro study indicates that cytochrome P450 (CYP) 3A4 is the major isoenzyme involved in the metabolism of zopiclone to both metabolites, and that CYP2C8 is also involved with N-desmethyl zopiclone formation.

The principal metabolites are the N-oxide derivative (~12%), which has weak pharmacological activity in animals, and the N-desmethyl metabolite (~16%), which is pharmacologically inactive.

Their apparent half-lives evaluated from the urinary data are approximately 4.5 and 7.4 hours, respectively. Both metabolites are excreted renally.

Other metabolites resulting from oxidative decarboxylation are partly eliminated via the lung as carbon dioxide. In animals, zopiclone did not induce hepatic microsomal enzymes.

Excretion: Excretion studies, using C^{14}-zopiclone have shown that more than 90% of the administered dose was excreted over a period of 5 days, 75% being eliminated in the urine and 16% in the feces.

The low renal clearance of unchanged zopiclone (mean 8.4 mL/min) compared with that of plasma (232 mL/min) indicates that zopiclone clearance is mainly metabolic.

Special Patient Population: Elderly Subjects: The absolute bioavailability of zopiclone was increased (94% vs 77% in young subjects) and the elimination half-life prolonged (~7 hours). Accumulation has not been observed on repeated dosing.

Patients with Hepatic Insufficiency: Elimination half-life was substantially prolonged (11.9 hours) and time to peak plasma levels delayed (3.5 hours). Consequently, lower doses are recommended (see Dosage).

In cirrhotic patients, the plasma clearance of IMOVANE is reduced by approximately 40% in relation with the decrease of the demethylation process. Therefore, dosage will have to be modified in these patients.

Patients with Mild to Moderate Renal Insufficiency: The pharmacokinetics of zopiclone were not affected. In renal insufficiency, no accumulation of zopiclone or of its metabolites has been detected after prolonged administration.

IMOVANE is removed by hemodialysis; however, hemodialysis is of no value in treating overdose due to the large volume of distribution of IMOVANE (see also Overdose, Symptoms, and Treatment). Hemodialysis did not appear to increase the plasma clearance of the drug.

Lactating Women: Zopiclone was present in the milk, its concentration paralleled plasma levels but was about 50% lower (see Precautions, Lactation).

INDICATIONS: Sleep disturbance may be the presenting manifestation of a physical and/or psychiatric disorder. Consequently, a decision to initiate symptomatic treatment of insomnia should only be made after the patient has been carefully evaluated.

IMOVANE (zopiclone) is indicated for the short-term treatment and symptomatic relief of insomnia characterized by difficulty in falling asleep, frequent nocturnal awakenings and/or early morning awakenings.

Treatment with IMOVANE should usually not exceed 7-10 consecutive days. Use for more than 2-3 consecutive weeks requires complete re-evaluation of the patient. Prescriptions for IMOVANE should be written for short-term use (7-10 days) and it should not be prescribed in quantities exceeding a 1-month supply.

The use of hypnotics should be restricted for insomnia where disturbed sleep results in impaired daytime functioning.

CONTRAINDICATIONS: IMOVANE is contraindicated in patients with known hypersensitivity to the drug or any component or its formulation, in patients with myasthenia gravis and severe hepatic insufficiency and in those with severe impairment of respiratory function, e.g., significant sleep apnea syndrome.

WARNINGS: General: Benzodiazepine and benzodiazepine-like compounds should be used with extreme caution in patients with a history of substance or alcohol abuse.

Because some of the adverse effects of IMOVANE may be dose related, the smallest possible effective dose should be prescribed, especially for elderly patients. Inappropriate, heavy sedation in the elderly, may result in accidental events/falls.

The cause of insomnia should be identified wherever possible and the underlying factors treated before a hypnotic is prescribed. The failure of insomnia to remit after 7-10 days of treatment may indicate the presence of a primary psychiatric and/or medical illness or the presence of sleep state misperception.

Worsening of insomnia or the emergence of new abnormalities of thinking or behaviour may be the consequence of an unrecognized psychiatric or physical disorder. These have also been reported to occur in association with the use of drugs that act at the benzodiazepine receptors.

IMOVANE should be used with caution in patients who in the past manifested paradoxical reactions to alcohol and/or sedative medications.

Lactose is a nonmedicinal ingredient in IMOVANE 5 mg. Patients with rare hereditary diseases of galactose intolerance (galactosemia or glucose-galactose malabsorption) should not take IMOVANE 5 mg. IMOVANE 7.5 mg does not contain lactose.

Pregnancy: Benzodiazepines may cause fetal damage when administered during pregnancy. During the first trimester of pregnancy, several studies have suggested an increased risk of congenital malformations associated with the use of benzodiazepines.

Insufficient data are available on zopiclone to assess its safety during human pregnancy. Thus, the use of IMOVANE during pregnancy is not recommended. If IMOVANE is prescribed to a woman of child-bearing potential, the patient should be warned of the potential risk to a fetus and advised to consult her physician regarding the discontinuation of the drug if she intends to become pregnant or suspects that she is pregnant.

During the last weeks of pregnancy or during labor, ingestion of therapeutic doses of benzodiazepine hypnotic drugs has resulted in neonatal CNS depression due to transplacental distribution. Similar effects can be expected to occur with zopiclone, due to its pharmacological effects. If IMOVANE is used during the last three months of pregnancy or during labour, effects on the neonate, such as hypothermia, hypotonia, and respiratory depression can be expected.

A child born to a mother who is on benzodiazepines or benzodiazepine-like agents may be at risk for withdrawal symptoms from the drug during the postnatal period.

Amnesia: Anterograde amnesia of varying severity has been reported following therapeutic doses of benzodiazepines or benzodiazepine-like agents. The event is rare with IMOVANE. Anterograde amnesia may occur, especially when sleep is interrupted or when retiring to bed is delayed after the intake of the tablet. Anterograde amnesia is a dose-related phenomenon and elderly subjects may be at particular risk.

Cases of transient global amnesia and "traveller's amnesia" have also been reported in association with benzodiazepines, the latter in individuals who have taken the drug, often in the middle of the night, to induce sleep while travelling. Transient global amnesia and traveller's amnesia are unpredictable and not necessarily dose-related phenomena.

To reduce the possibility of anterograde amnesia, patients should ensure that they take the tablet strictly when retiring for the night. Patients should be warned not to take IMOVANE under circumstances in which a full night's sleep and clearance of the drug from the body are not possible before they need again to resume full activity.

Abnormal Thinking and Behavioural Changes: Abnormal thinking and other behavioural changes have been reported to occur in association with the use of benzodiazepines and benzodiazepine-like agents including IMOVANE, although rarely (see Adverse Effects). Some of the changes may be characterized by decreased inhibition, e.g., aggression or extroversion that seems excessive, similar to that seen with alcohol and other CNS depressants (e.g., sedative/hypnotics). Particular caution is warranted in patients with a history of violent behaviour and a history of unusual reactions to sedatives including alcohol and the benzodiazepines or benzodiazepine-like agents. Psychotic behavioural changes that have been reported include abnormal behaviour, irritability, hallucinations, anger, nightmare and depersonalization. Abnormal behaviours associated with the use of benzodiazepines or benzodiazepine-like agents have been reported more with chronic use and/or high doses but they may occur during the acute, maintenance or withdrawal phases of treatment.

It can rarely be determined with certainty whether a particular instance of abnormal behaviours listed above is drug induced, spontaneous in origin, or a result of an underlying psychiatric disorder. Nevertheless, the emergence of any new behavioural sign or symptom of concern requires careful and immediate evaluation. Should these occur, use of the product should be discontinued. These reactions are more likely to occur in the elderly.

Cognitive Function: The benzodiazepines and benzodiazepine-like agents affect mental efficiency, e.g., concentration, attention and vigilance. The risk of confusion is greater in the elderly and in patients with cerebral impairment.

Anxiety, Restlessness: An increase in daytime anxiety and/or restlessness have been observed during treatment with IMOVANE. This may be a manifestation of interdose withdrawal, due to the short elimination half-life of the drug.

Depression: Caution should be exercised if IMOVANE is prescribed to patients with signs and symptoms of depression that could be intensified by hypnotic drugs. The potential for self-harm (e.g., intentional overdose) is high in patients with depression and thus, the least amount of drug that is feasible should be available to them at any one time.

As with other hypnotics, IMOVANE does not constitute a treatment of depression and may even mask its symptoms.

Complex Sleep-related Behaviours: Complex sleep-related behaviours such as "sleep-driving" (i.e., driving while not fully awake after ingestion of a sedative-hypnotic, with amnesia for the event) have been reported in patients who have taken IMOVANE. Other potentially dangerous behaviours have been reported in patients who got out of bed after taking a sedative-hypnotic and were not fully awake, including preparing and eating food, making phone calls, leaving the house, etc. As with "sleep-driving", patients usually do not remember these events. The use of alcohol and other CNS-depressants with IMOVANE appears to increase the risk of such behaviours, as does the use of IMOVANE at doses exceeding the maximum recommended dose. IMOVANE **is not to be taken with alcohol**. Caution is needed with concomitant use of other CNS depressants drugs. Due to the risk to the patient and the community, discontinuation of IMOVANE should be strongly considered for patients who report any such complex sleep-related behaviours.

Severe Anaphylactic and Anaphylactoid Reactions: Rare cases of angioedema involving the tongue, glottis or larynx have been reported in patients after taking the first or subsequent doses of sedative-hypnotics, including IMOVANE. Some patients have had additional symptoms such as dyspnea, throat closing or nausea and vomiting that suggest anaphylaxis. Some patients have required medical therapy in the emergency department. If angioedema involves the throat, glottis or larynx, airway obstruction may occur and be fatal. Patients who develop angioedema after treatment with IMOVANE should not be rechallenged with the drug.

PRECAUTIONS: Drug Abuse, Dependence and Withdrawal: Use of sedative/hypnotics agents like IMOVANE may lead to the development of physical and psychological dependence or abuse. The risk of dependence or abuse is increased with the dose and duration of treatment, if used with alcohol or other psychotropics, in patients with a history of alcoholism and/or drug abuse or in patients with marked personality disorders. Interdose daytime anxiety and rebound anxiety may increase the risk of dependency in IMOVANE treated patients.

Once physical dependence has developed, abrupt termination of treatment will be accompanied by withdrawal symptoms.

Withdrawal symptoms, similar in character to those noted with barbiturates and alcohol (convulsions, tremor, abdominal and muscle cramps, vomiting, sweating, dysphoria, perceptual disturbances and insomnia) have occurred following abrupt discontinuation of benzodiazepines and benzodiazepine-like agents, including IMOVANE. The more severe symptoms are usually associated with higher dosages and longer usage, although patients given therapeutic dosages for as few as 1-2 weeks can also have withdrawal symptoms including daytime anxiety between nightly doses.

Consequently, abrupt discontinuation should be avoided and a gradual dosage tapering schedule is recommended in any patient taking the drug for more than a few weeks. The recommendation for tapering is particularly important in patients with a history of seizures (see Adverse Effects).

As with all hypnotics, repeat prescriptions should be limited to those who are under medical supervision.

It may be useful to inform the patient when treatment is started that it will be of limited duration and to explain precisely how the dosage will be progressively decreased.

Rebound Insomnia: A transient syndrome whereby the symptoms that led to treatment with a benzodiazepine or benzodiazepine-like agent recur in an enhanced form, may occur on withdrawal of hypnotic treatment. It may be accompanied by other reactions including mood changes, anxiety and restlessness.

Since the risk of such phenomena is greater after abrupt discontinuation of IMOVANE, especially after prolonged treatment, it is, therefore recommended to decrease the dosage gradually and to advise the patient accordingly (see Adverse Effects). It is important that the patient should be aware of the possibility of rebound phenomena, thereby minimizing anxiety over such symptoms should they occur while the medicinal product is being discontinued.

Tolerance: Some loss of efficacy of other hypnotics may develop after repeated use. However, there was an absence of tolerance with IMOVANE for treatment periods of up to 4 weeks.

Patients with Specific Conditions: IMOVANE should be given with caution to patients with impaired hepatic or renal function, or chronic pulmonary insufficiency. Dosage adjustments are recommended (see Dosage). Respiratory depression has been reported in patients with compromised respiratory function.

IMOVANE is contraindicated in patients with myasthenia gravis and severe hepatic insufficiency and in those with severe impairment of respiratory function, e.g., significant sleep apnea syndrome (see Contraindications).

Patients Requiring Mental Alertness/Driving: Because of IMOVANE pharmacological properties and CNS depressant effect, IMOVANE may adversely affect the ability to drive or use machines. Patients receiving the drug should be cautioned against engaging in hazardous occupations requiring complete mental alertness such as operating machinery or driving a motor vehicle. For the same reason, patients should be warned against the concomitant ingestion of IMOVANE and alcohol or CNS depressant drugs (see Drug Interactions).

Pregnancy: The use of IMOVANE during pregnancy is not recommended (see Warnings).

Lactation: IMOVANE is excreted in human milk, and its concentration may reach 50% of the plasma levels. Insufficient data are available on IMOVANE to assess its safety during lactation. Therefore, the administration of IMOVANE to nursing mothers is not recommended.

Children (<18 years of age): The safety and effectiveness of IMOVANE in children and young adults below the age of 18 have not been established.

Geriatrics (≥65 years of age): Elderly patients are especially susceptible to dose-related adverse effects, such as drowsiness, dizziness, or impaired coordination. Inappropriate, heavy sedation may result in accidental events/fall. Therefore, the lowest possible dose should be used in these subjects (see Dosage, Geriatrics (≥65 years of age)). Anterograde amnesia is a dose-related phenomenon and elderly subjects may be at particular risk.

Drug Interactions: The risk of drug interaction arising from displacement of bound drug is low.

Alcohol: Concomitant intake with alcohol is not recommended (see Warnings, Complex Sleep-related Behaviours). IMOVANE may produce additive CNS depressant effects when co-administered with alcohol.

CNS Depressants: IMOVANE may produce additive CNS depressant effects when co-administered with sedative antihistamines, anticonvulsants, narcotic analgesics, anesthetics, or psychotropic medications such as antipsychotics (neuroleptics), hypnotics, anxiolytics/sedatives, and antidepressant agents which themselves can produce CNS depression. In the case of narcotic analgesics, enhancement of euphoria may also occur leading to an increase in psychological dependence.

Drugs Affecting Cytochrome P450 Enzymes: Since IMOVANE is metabolized by the cytochrome P450 (CYP) 3A4 isoenzyme (see Pharmacology, Pharmacokinetics, Metabolism), plasma levels of IMOVANE may be increased when co-administered with CYP3A4 inhibitors, such as erythromycin, clarithromycin, ketoconazole, itraconazole, and ritonavir. A dose reduction for IMOVANE may be required when it is co-administered with CYP3A4 inhibitors. Conversely, plasma levels of IMOVANE may be decreased when co-administered with CYP3A4 inducers, such as rifampicin or rifampin, carbamazepine, phenobarbital, phenytoin, and St. John's wort. A dose increase for IMOVANE may be required when it is co-administered with CYP3A4 inducers.

The effect of erythromycin on the pharmacokinetics of IMOVANE has been studied in 10 healthy subjects. The AUC of IMOVANE is increased by 80% in presence of erythromycin. The hypnotic effect of IMOVANE may be enhanced when administered with erythromycin.

ADVERSE EFFECTS: The most common adverse reaction seen with IMOVANE is taste alteration (bitter taste). Severe drowsiness and/or impaired coordination are signs of drug intolerance or excessive doses.

The following adverse events were observed in patients receiving IMOVANE. In the absence of an established cause-effect relationship those adverse reactions that were observed more frequently with IMOVANE than with a placebo are in italic.

Central Nervous System: *somnolence, dizziness, confusion, anterograde amnesia* or *memory impairment, feeling of drunkenness, euphoria,* nightmares, agitation, *anxiety* or *nervousness,* hostility, *depression,* decreased libido, *coordination abnormality,* headache, *hypotonia,* tremor, muscle spasms, paresthesia, *speech disorder.*

Hallucinations, aggressiveness, irritability, anger, inappropriate behaviors possibly associated with amnesia, sleep walking (see Warnings, Complex Sleep-related Behaviours), have been reported rarely.

Cardiovascular: palpitations.

Digestive: *bitter taste, dry mouth, coated tongue, bad breath,* nausea, vomiting, *dyspepsia,* diarrhea, *constipation, anorexia* or *increased appetite.*

General Disorders and Administration Site Conditions: *asthenia,* chills.

Respiratory: dyspnea.

Special Senses: amblyopia.

Dermatologic: rash, spots on skin, sweating, pruritus. Rashes and pruritus may be a sign of drug hypersensitivity; discontinue if this occurs.

Angioedema and/or anaphylactic reactions have been reported very rarely.

Metabolic and Nutritional: weight loss.

Musculoskeletal: limb heaviness.

Laboratory Tests: There have been sporadic reports of abnormal laboratory test values. Mild to moderate increases in serum transaminase and/or alkaline phosphatase have been reported very rarely.

Geriatrics: Geriatric patients tended to have a higher incidence of palpitations, vomiting, anorexia, sialorrhea, confusion, agitation, anxiety, tremor and sweating than younger patients. Anterograde amnesia is a dose-related phenomenon and elderly subjects may be at particular risk.

Withdrawal syndrome has been reported upon discontinuation of IMOVANE (see Precautions, Drug Abuse, Dependence and Withdrawal). Withdrawal symptoms vary and may include rebound insomnia, anxiety, tremor, sweating, agitation, confusion, headache, palpitations, tachycardia, delirium, nightmares, hallucinations, and irritability. In very rare cases, seizures may occur.

OVERDOSE:

Symptoms: Overdose is usually manifested by varying degrees of central nervous system depression ranging from drowsiness to coma according to the quantity ingested. In mild cases, symptoms include drowsiness, confusion, and lethargy; in more severe cases, symptoms may include ataxia, hypotonia, hypotension, respiratory depression, and coma. Overdose should not be life threatening unless combined with other CNS depressants, including alcohol. Other risk factors, such as the presence of concomitant illness and the debilitated state of the patient, may contribute to the severity of symptoms and very rarely can result in fatal outcome.

In voluntary or accidental cases of IMOVANE overdosage involving doses up to 340 mg, the principal effects reported were prolonged sleep, drowsiness, lethargy and ataxia.

Treatment: Symptomatic and supportive treatment in adequate clinical environment is recommended, attention should be paid to respiratory and cardiovascular functions. Gastric lavage or activated charcoal is only useful when performed soon after ingestion. Hemodialysis is of no value due to the large volume of distribution of IMOVANE. Flumazenil may be a useful antidote; however, flumazenil administration may contribute to the appearance of neurological symptoms (convulsions).

Poison Control Center:

As with the management of all overdosage, the possibility of multiple drug ingestion should be considered. The physician may wish to consider contacting a poison control center for up-to-date information on the management of hypnotic drug product overdosage.

For management of a suspected drug overdose, CPhA recommends that you contact your **regional Poison Control Centre.** See the *CPS* Directory section for a list of Poison Control Centres.

DOSAGE: Treatment with IMOVANE should usually not exceed 7-10 consecutive days. Use for more than 2-3 consecutive weeks requires complete re-evaluation of the patient.

The product should be taken just before retiring for the night.

Adults: The usual adult dose is 5 mg to 7.5 mg. The 7.5 mg dose should not be exceeded (see Precautions).

Geriatrics (≥65 years of age): In the elderly and/or debilitated patient an initial dose of 3.75 mg (one-half of a 7.5 mg tablet) at bedtime is recommended. The dose may be increased to 5 mg or 7.5 mg if the starting dose does not offer adequate therapeutic effect.

Patients with Impaired Liver Function or Chronic Respiratory Insufficiency: The recommended dose is 3.75 mg (one-half of a 7.5 mg tablet) depending on acceptability and efficacy. Up to 7.5 mg may be used with caution in appropriate cases.

IMOVANE is contraindicated in patients with severe hepatic insufficiency and in those with severe impairment of respiratory function, e.g., significant sleep apnea syndrome (see Contraindications).

Patients with Renal Insufficiency: Although no accumulation of IMOVANE or of its metabolites has been detected in cases of renal insufficiency, it is recommended that patients with impaired renal function should start treatment with 3.75 mg (one-half of a 7.5 mg tablet).

Children (<18 years of age): IMOVANE is not indicated for patients under 18 years of age.

INFORMATION FOR THE PATIENT: Published in e-CPS, available by subscription at www.e-cps.ca.

SUPPLIED: 5 mg: Each round, white tablet, marked IMOVANE 5 on one side and the logo rPr on the other, contains: zopiclone 5 mg. Nonmedicinal ingredients: corn starch, dicalcium phosphate, lactose, magnesium stearate and sodium carboxymethyl starch; coating: hydroxypropyl methylcellulose and titanium dioxide. White high-density polyethylene bottles of 100. Store in a dry place, at room temperature (15-30°C). Protect from light. Keep in a safe place out of reach of children.

7.5 mg: Each oval, scored, blue tablet, marked IMOVANE on one side and the logo rPr on each side of the score on the other side, contains: zopiclone 7.5 mg. The 7.5 mg tablet can be broken into two equal parts of 3.75 mg. Nonmedicinal ingredients: calcium phosphate dihydrate dibasic, croscarmellose sodium, magnesium stearate and microcrystalline cellulose; coating: carnauba wax, FD&C Blue #1, Opadry II White and polyethylene glycol. White high-density polyethylene bottles of 100 and 500. Store in a dry place, at room temperature (15-30°C). Protect from light. Keep in a safe place out of reach of children.

(Shown in Product Identification Section)

IMOVAX® Polio

poliomyelitis vaccine, inactivated (Vero cell origin)

Active Immunizing Agent

sanofi pasteur

Date of Revision: October 2007

SUMMARY PRODUCT INFORMATION:

Route of Administration	Dosage Form/ Strength	Clinically Relevant Nonmedicinal Ingredients
Subcutaneous injection	Solution for injection Each 0.5 mL dose is formulated to contain: purified inactivated poliomyelitis vaccine: Type 1 (Mahoney) Type 2 (MEF1) Type 3 (Saukett)	2-phenoxyethanol, formaldehyde, residual calf serum protein, neomycin, streptomycin and polymyxin B, Medium 199 Hanks (without phenol red)

DESCRIPTION: IMOVAX Polio [Inactivated Poliomyelitis Vaccine (Vero Cell Origin)] is a sterile suspension of three types of inactivated poliomyelitis vaccine: type 1 (Mahoney), type 2 (MEF1) and type 3 (Saukett). This vaccine is prepared from types 1, 2 and 3 of poliovirus cultured on Vero cells, purified and then inactivated by formaldehyde.

INDICATIONS AND CLINICAL USE: IMOVAX Polio is indicated for active immunization against poliomyelitis caused by poliovirus types 1, 2 and 3 from 2 months of age in infants, children and adults both for primary immunization and for boosters. (See Dosage and Administration.)

Infants, Children and Adolescents: It is recommended that all infants, unimmunized children and adolescents not previously immunized be vaccinated routinely against paralytic poliomyelitis.

Children Incompletely Immunized: Children of all ages should have their immunization status reviewed and be considered for supplemental immunization.

Adults: All adults at risk of exposure to poliovirus should have their immunization status reviewed. For those who are unvaccinated, who have a history of incomplete immunization, or for whom immunization is uncertain, a primary series of IMOVAX Polio is recommended. (See Dosage and Administration, Adults.) The following categories of persons are at increased risk of exposure to poliovirus:

- travellers to areas of countries where poliomyelitis is still transmitted or may be a risk;
- laboratory workers handling specimens that may contain polioviruses;
- health-care workers in close contact with persons who may be excreting wild or vaccine strains of polioviruses;
- unimmunized parents or child-care workers who will be caring for children or unimmunized adults who may be in contact with children in countries where OPV is used, or in rare instances in which infants receive OPV in a country in which inactivated poliomyelitis vaccine (IPV) is normally used;
- members of communities or specific population groups with disease caused by wild poliovirus.

IMOVAX Polio can be used for completing immunization series in cases of previous clinical poliomyelitis (usually due to only a single poliovirus type) or incomplete immunization with OPV.

Pediatrics: Safety and efficacy of IMOVAX Polio have been shown in children 6 weeks of age and older.

CONTRAINDICATIONS: Immunization with IMOVAX Polio should be deferred in the presence of any acute illness, including febrile illness, to avoid superimposing adverse effects from the vaccine on the underlying illness or mistakenly identifying a manifestation of the underlying illness as a complication of vaccine use. A minor illness such as mild upper respiratory infection is not reason to defer immunization.

Allergy to any component of IMOVAX Polio, or its container, or an anaphylactic or other allergic reaction to a previous dose of IMOVAX Polio is a contraindication to vaccination. For a complete listing, see Dosage Forms, Composition and Packaging.

WARNINGS AND PRECAUTIONS: General: As with any vaccine, immunization with IMOVAX Polio may not protect 100% of susceptible persons.

Aseptic technique must be used. Use a separate sterile needle and syringe, or a sterile disposable unit, for each individual dose to prevent disease transmission.

IMOVAX Polio should not be administered into the buttocks due to the varying amount of fatty tissue in this region, nor by the intradermal route, since these methods of administration may induce a weaker immune response.

Do not inject into a blood vessel.

IPV should not be used for control of outbreaks of poliomyelitis if OPV is available.

Before administration, take all appropriate precautions to prevent adverse reactions. This includes a review of the patient's history concerning possible hypersensitivity to the vaccine or similar vaccine, previous immunization history, the presence of any contraindications to immunization and current health status.

Before administration of IMOVAX Polio, health-care providers should inform the patient, parent or guardian of the benefits and risks of immunization, inquire about the recent health status of the patient and comply with any local requirements regarding information to be provided to the patient before immunization and the importance of completing the immunization series.

It is important that the patient, parent or guardian be questioned concerning any symptoms and/or signs of an adverse reaction after a previous dose of vaccine. (See Contraindications and Adverse Reactions.)

Immune: As with all other products, Epinephrine Hydrochloride Solution (1:1000) and other appropriate agents should be available for immediate use in case an anaphylactic or acute hypersensitivity reaction occurs. Health-care providers should be familiar with current recommendations for the initial management of anaphylaxis in non-hospital settings, including proper airway management. For instructions on recognition and treatment of anaphylactic reactions, see the current edition of the Canadian Immunization Guide or visit the Health Canada website.

As each dose may contain undetectable traces of neomycin, streptomycin and polymyxin B, which are used during vaccine production, caution should be exercised when the vaccine is administered to subjects with hypersensitivity to these antibiotics (and other antibiotics of the same classes).

Immunocompromised persons (whether from disease or treatment) may not obtain the expected immune response. If possible, consideration should be given to delaying vaccination until after the completion of any immunosuppressive treatment. Nevertheless, vaccination of subjects with chronic immunodeficiency such as HIV infection is recommended even if the antibody response might be limited.

Special Populations: Pregnant Women: There are limited data on the use of this vaccine in pregnant woman. Animal studies are insufficient with respect to effects on pregnancy and embryo/fetal development, parturition and postnatal development. No clinical trials with inactivated poliomyelitis vaccine have been conducted on pregnant women. Although there is no convincing evidence documenting adverse effects of inactivated poliomyelitis vaccine on the pregnant woman or the developing fetus, it is prudent on theoretical grounds to avoid vaccinating pregnant woman.

The National Advisory Committee on Immunization (NACI) states that IPV is not contraindicated in pregnancy, but its administration should be delayed until after the first trimester, if possible, to minimize any theoretical risk. If risk of exposure is imminent, IPV should be given and is always the vaccine of choice except for outbreak control.

Nursing Women: It is not known whether IMOVAX Polio is excreted in human milk. Because many drugs are excreted in human milk, caution should be exercised when IMOVAX Polio is administered to a nursing woman.

The National Advisory Committee on Immunization states that inactivated polio vaccine may safely be given to lactating mothers who have not previously been immunized or are travelling to an endemic area.

ADVERSE REACTIONS: Adverse Drug Reaction Overview: Local reactions are usually mild and transient in nature. Systemic adverse reactions reported in infants receiving IPV concomitantly at separate sites or combined with DPT-containing (Diphtheria Tetanus Pertussis) vaccines have been similar to those associated with administration of DPT-containing vaccines alone.

Clinical Trial Adverse Drug Reactions: Because clinical trials are conducted under very specific conditions the adverse reaction rates observed in the clinical trials may not reflect the rates observed in practice and should not be compared to the rates in the clinical trials of another drug. Adverse drug reaction information from clinical trials is useful for identifying drug-related adverse events and for approximating rates.

The local reactogenicity of IMOVAX Polio was evaluated in two multicentre randomized clinical trials involving a total of 395 patients and local reactions were uncommonly to very commonly reported:

- injection site redness: in 0.7% to 2.4% of subjects in each trial
- injection site pain: 0.7% to 34%
- injection site mass: 0.4%

In a multicentre randomized Phase III study involving 205 children, fever >38.1°C was commonly to very commonly observed (in 10% of children after the first dose, in 18% of children after the second dose, in 7% of children after the third dose).

In an other multicentre randomized Phase III study involving 324 children, it was concluded that IMOVAX Polio combined or associated with DPT vaccine was as well-tolerated as DPT vaccine administered alone.

Post-Market Adverse Drug Reactions: These frequencies are based on spontaneous reporting rates and have been calculated using number of reports and estimated number of vaccinated patients.

IMOVAX Polio is rarely administered alone according to the childhood immunization schedules.

Whatever the adverse event reported during the post-marketing experience, its frequency remained very rare (<0.01%).

The most frequently reported adverse events are local reactions and fever (respectively around 20% and 10% of adverse events reported).

Blood and Lymphatic System Disorders: Very rare (<0.01%): lymphadenopathy.

General Disorders and Administration Site Conditions: Very rare (<0.01%): injection site reactions such as injection site edema, injection site pain, injection site rash or injection site mass within 48 hours following the vaccination and lasting one or two days; transient mild fever (pyrexia) within 24 to 48 hours following the vaccination.

Immune System Disorders: Very rare (<0.01%): Type I hypersensitivity reaction to one component of the vaccine such as allergic reaction, anaphylactic reaction or anaphylactic shock.

Musculo-skeletal and Connective Tissue Disorders: Very rare (<0.01%): mild and transitory arthralgia and myalgia within a few days after the vaccination.

Nervous System Disorders: Very rare (<0.01%): short-lasting convulsions, febrile convulsions, within a few days following the vaccination; headache; transient and mild paraesthesia (mainly of limbs) within two weeks after the vaccination.

Psychiatric Disorders: Very rare (<0.01%): within the first hours or days following the vaccination and shortly resolving: agitation, somnolence, irritability.

Skin and Subcutaneous Tissue Disorders: Very rare (<0.01%): rash, urticaria.

Nervous System: Although no causal relationship between IMOVAX Polio and Guillain-Barré syndrome (GBS) has been established, GBS has been temporally related to administration of another inactivated poliovirus vaccine.

An extensive review by the (US) Institute of Medicine of adverse events associated with vaccination suggested that no serious adverse events have been associated with IPV. Although no causal relationship has been established, deaths have occurred in temporal association after vaccination of infants with IPV.

Health professionals should report any adverse occurrences temporally related to the administration of the product in accordance with local requirements and to the Global Pharmacovigilance Department, Sanofi Pasteur Limited, 1755 Steeles Avenue West, Toronto, ON, M2R 3T4, Canada. 1-888-621-1146 (phone) or 416-667-2435 (fax).

DRUG INTERACTIONS: There are no known interactions of IMOVAX Polio with drugs or foods.

Administering the most widely used live and inactivated vaccines during the same patient visit has produced seroconversion rates and rates of adverse reactions similar to those observed when the vaccines are administered separately. Simultaneous administration using separate syringes at separate sites is suggested, particularly when there is concern that an individual may not return for subsequent vaccination.

The first two doses of IMOVAX Polio may be administered at separate sites using separate syringes concomitantly with DPT, acellular pertussis, *H. influenzae* type b (Hib), and hepatitis B vaccines. From historical data on the antibody responses to diphtheria, tetanus, whole-cell or acellular pertussis, Hib, or hepatitis B vaccines used concomitantly or in combination with IMOVAX Polio, no interferences have been observed on the immunological end points accepted for clinical protection.

IMOVAX Polio may be administered simultaneously with other parenteral vaccines at separate sites with separate syringes.

Except in the case of immunosuppressive therapy (see Warnings and Precautions, Immune), no significant clinical interaction with other treatments or biological products has been documented.

IMOVAX Polio should not be mixed in the same syringe with other parenterals.

DOSAGE AND ADMINISTRATION: Children: Primary Immunization: A primary series of IMOVAX Polio consists of three 0.5 mL doses administered subcutaneously. The interval between the first two doses should be at least four weeks, but preferably eight weeks. The third dose should follow at least six months but preferably 12 months later. The primary schedule is usually integrated with combination infant vaccines against diphtheria, tetanus, pertussis and *H. influenzae* type b, beginning at 2 months of age.

Alternatively, three doses of 0.5 mL may be administered at intervals of 8 weeks, followed by a fourth dose of 0.5 mL approximately 12 months after the third dose.

Although it is recommended that immunization be started at 2 months of age, if for any reason it is delayed, the same schedule may be used.

Booster Doses: All children who received a primary series of IMOVAX Polio, or a combination of IPV and OPV, should be given a booster dose at age 4-6 years, unless the last dose of the primary series was administered on or after the fourth birthday. An additional booster dose should be given at age 14-16 years unless OPV was used exclusively during the primary series. Whether there is a need to administer additional doses routinely is unknown at this time.

A final total of at least four doses are necessary to complete a series of primary and booster doses. Children and adolescents with a previously incomplete series of IPV should receive sufficient additional doses to reach this number.

For children who began their polio immunization series in a country where OPV is used, immunization may be completed using IPV; there is no need to re-start the series. Conversely, children who have been started on an immunization series with IPV and who move to an area where OPV is used may receive the necessary doses of OPV to complete their series.

Adults: For unimmunized adults at increased risk, primary immunization with IPV is recommended as two doses given at an interval of 4 to 8 weeks with a further dose 6 months to 1 year later. Additional considerations are as follows:

Travellers who will be departing within 4 weeks should receive a single dose of IPV and the remaining doses later, at the recommended intervals.

Unimmunized parents/child-care workers: in those rare instances in which infants receive OPV, there is a very small risk of OPV-associated paralysis to unimmunized parents or to other household contacts. It will generally not be practical for such persons to be fully protected with IPV before the infant is immunized; their risk may be reduced if they are given one dose of IPV at the same time as the first dose is given to the infant. Arrangements should be made for the adults to complete their basic course of immunization.

Incompletely immunized adults at increased risk (see Indications, Adults) who have previously received less than a full primary course of IPV or OPV should receive the remaining dose(s) of poliovirus vaccine as IPV, regardless of the interval since the last dose.

Adults and adolescents who are at greater risk of exposure to poliovirus than the general population (see above) may be given a single dose of IPV if more than 10 years have elapsed since the last dose of their **complete** IPV and/or OPV vaccination series.

Missed Dose: Time intervals between doses longer than those recommended for routine primary immunization do not necessitate additional doses as long as a final total of four doses is reached.

If a dose is missed, it can be given at any time.

Administration: Inspect for extraneous particulate matter and/or discolouration before use. If these conditions exist, the product should not be administered.

For information on vaccine administration see the current edition of the Canadian Immunization Guide or visit the Health Canada website.

Shake the pre-filled syringe well to uniformly distribute the solution before administration.

Administer IMOVAX Polio subcutaneously. In infants and small children, the mid-lateral aspect of the thigh is the preferred site; in older children and adults in the deltoid or triceps area.

Do not inject intravenously.

Needles should not be recapped and should be disposed of properly.

Give the patient a permanent personal immunization record. In addition, it is essential that the physician or nurse record the immunization history in the permanent medical record of each patient. This permanent office record should contain the name of the vaccine, date given, dose, manufacturer and lot number.

Overdosage:

> For management of a suspected drug overdose, CPhA recommends that you contact your **regional Poison Control Centre**. See the *CPS* Directory section for a list of Poison Control Centres.

Not documented.

ACTION AND CLINICAL PHARMACOLOGY: Mechanism of Action: IMOVAX Polio induces the production of neutralizing antibodies against each type of virus which are related to protective efficacy.

Pharmacodynamics: IMOVAX Polio is a highly purified, inactivated poliovirus vaccine produced by microcarrier culture. These methods allow for the production of vaccine that induces antibody responses in most children after administering only two doses.

Studies in developed and developing countries with a similar inactivated poliovirus vaccine produced by the same technology have shown that a direct relationship exists between the antigenic content of the vaccine and the frequency of seroconversion, antibody titre and immunologic memory.

Inactivated poliovirus vaccine (IPV) reduces fecal and pharyngeal excretion of poliovirus. Field studies in the US and Europe have demonstrated herd immunity in populations immunized with IPV.

Duration of Effect: Immunity following injectable poliovirus vaccines has been shown to persist for 4 or more years after a primary series.

STORAGE AND STABILITY: Store at 2 to 8°C. **Do not freeze.** Discard product if exposed to freezing.

Do not use after expiration date.

SPECIAL HANDLING INSTRUCTIONS: The vaccine should be clear and colourless: do not use the vaccine if it has a cloudy appearance.

INFORMATION FOR THE PATIENT: Published in e-CPS, available by subscription at www.e-cps.ca.

DOSAGE FORMS, COMPOSITION AND PACKAGING: Each dose of 0.5 mL of purified inactivated poliomyelitis vaccine contains: type 1 (Mahoney) 40 D antigen units, type 2 (MEF1) 8 D antigen units, type 3 (Saukett) 32 D antigen units; 2-phenoxyethanol ≤1.0%, formaldehyde ≤0.02%, residual calf serum protein <1 ppm, trace amounts of neomycin, streptomycin and polymyxin B, Medium 199 Hanks (without phenol red) up to 0.5 mL. Syringes of 0.5 mL, packages 1 and packages of 10. The stopper of the syringe for this product does not contain latex (natural rubber).

IMOVAX® Rabies

rabies vaccine inactivated (DCO)

Active Immunizing Agent

sanofi pasteur

Date of Revision: March 2006

SUMMARY PRODUCT INFORMATION:

Route of Administration	Dosage Form/ Strength	Clinically Relevant Nonmedicinal Ingredients (per 1 mL)
Intramuscular injection	Powder and Diluent for Suspension for Injection Each 1 mL dose is formulated to contain: ≥2.5 IU Rabies virus (WISTAR Rabies PM/WI 38 1503-3M Strain)	Human albumin, neomycin **Diluent:** sterile water for injection

DESCRIPTION: IMOVAX Rabies [Rabies Vaccine Inactivated (DCO)] produced by Sanofi Pasteur SA is a sterile, stable, freeze-dried suspension of rabies virus prepared from WISTAR Rabies PM/WI 38 1503-3M strain. The virus is harvested from infected MRC-5 human diploid cells, concentrated by ultrafiltration and inactivated by beta-propiolactone. The vaccine contains no preservative.

INDICATIONS AND CLINICAL USE: IMOVAX Rabies [Rabies Vaccine Inactivated (DCO)] is indicated for the active immunization of individuals of all age groups to prevent disease caused by the rabies virus. It is indicated for both pre-exposure immunization (both primary series and booster doses) and post-exposure immunization.

Pre-Exposure Immunization: Primary Immunization: Pre-exposure rabies immunization is an elective procedure and should be offered to persons at potentially high risk of contact with rabid animals, e.g., certain laboratory workers, veterinarians, animal control and wildlife workers, spelunkers, and hunters and trappers in high-risk areas such as the Far North.

Pre-exposure immunization should be considered for travellers intending to live or work in areas where rabies is enzootic and where rabies control programs for domestic animals are inadequate, or where adequate and safe post-exposure facilities are unavailable. This includes: persons with frequent risk of rabies exposure; children in rabies enzootic areas who are too young to understand the need to avoid animals or to report an animal bite; persons in rabies enzootic areas where there is limited access to tissue culture vaccines and/or immune globulin or where ready transportation to an appropriate health-care facility cannot be assured.

Pre-exposure vaccination does not eliminate the need for prompt prophylaxis following an exposure but it eliminates the need for Rabies Immune Globulin (RIG) except in immunocompromised persons. Any exposed person should receive appropriate wound treatment (see Management of Persons After Possible Exposure to Rabies) and a vaccine post-exposure treatment regimen. (See Dosage and Administration, Dosing Considerations.)

Booster Doses: Persons with continuing high risk of exposure such as veterinarians, should have their serum tested for rabies antibodies every 2 years; others working with live rabies virus in laboratories or vaccine-production facilities and who are at risk of inapparent exposure should be tested every 6 months. Those with inadequate titres should be given a booster dose of IMOVAX

Rabies. Persons previously immunized with other vaccines should be given sufficient doses of IMOVAX Rabies to produce an adequate antibody response. The Canadian national rabies reference laboratory considers an acceptable antibody response to be a titre of ≥0.5 IU/mL by the Rapid Fluorescent-Focus Inhibition Test (RFFIT).

Post-Exposure Management: Because it is not possible to determine which exposed individuals will develop rabies if untreated and because the infection is almost always fatal, it is essential that everyone exposed to animals with proven or suspected rabies be given post-exposure prophylaxis. The essential components of rabies post-exposure prophylaxis are local treatment of wounds and vaccination, and, in most cases RIG.

A decision on the management of a person who may have been exposed to the rabies virus must be made rapidly and judiciously since delays in starting a post-exposure prophylaxis reduce its effectiveness, and the disease, once established, is almost always fatal. Post-exposure prophylaxis should be started as soon as possible after exposure and should be offered to exposed individuals regardless of the elapsed interval. When notification of an exposure is delayed, prophylaxis may be started as late as 6 or more months after exposure.

Rabies prophylaxis must be considered in every incident where potential exposure to rabies virus has occurred. In evaluating each case, local public health officials should be consulted. For further information on the factors to be considered in evaluating exposure consult the current edition of the Canadian Immunization Guide.

Bite: any penetration of the skin by teeth. Bites inflicted by most animals are readily apparent. However, bites inflicted by bats to a sleeping person may not be felt, and may leave no visible bite marks. Hence, when persons are sleeping unattended in a room where a bat is found or when the possibility of a bite cannot be reasonably excluded post-exposure prophylaxis should be initiated.

Non-Bite: including contamination of scratches, abrasions or cuts of the skin or mucous membranes by saliva or other potentially infectious material, such as the brain tissue of a rabid animal. Post-exposure prophylaxis is warranted and recommended in rare instances of non-bite exposure, such as inhalation of aerosolized virus by spelunkers exploring caves inhabited by infected bats or by laboratory technicians homogenizing tissues infected with rabies virus; however, the efficacy of prophylaxis after such exposures is unknown.

Exposures incurred in the course of caring for humans with rabies could theoretically transmit the infection. No case of rabies acquired in this way has been documented, but post-exposure prophylaxis should be considered for exposed individuals.

Management of Persons After Possible Exposure to Rabies: Table 1 outlines the recommendations for the management of persons after possible exposure to rabies. These recommendations are intended as a guide and may need to be modified in accordance with the specific circumstances of the exposure.

Immediate washing and flushing with soap and water and a virucidal agent is imperative and is probably the most effective procedure in the prevention of rabies. Suturing the wound should be avoided if possible. Tetanus prophylaxis and antibacterial drugs should be given as required.

Table 1: IMOVAX Rabies

Post-Exposure Prophylaxis for Persons Not Previously Immunized Against Rabies

Animal Species	Condition of Animal at Time of Exposure	Management of Exposed Person
Dog or cat	Healthy and available for 10 days' observation.	1. Local treatment of wound. 2. At first sign of rabies in animal, give RIG (local +/− intramuscular) and start IMOVAX Rabies
	Rabid or suspected to be rabid. Unknown or escaped.	1. Local treatment of wound 2. RIG (local +/− intramuscular) and IMOVAX Rabies
Skunk, bat, fox, coyote, raccoon and other carnivores. Includes bat found in room when a person was sleeping unattended.	Regard as rabid unless geographic area is known to be rabies-free.	1. Local treatment of wound. 2. RIG (local +/− intramuscular) and IMOVAX Rabies
Livestock, rodents or lagomorphs (hares and rabbits)	Consider individually. Consult appropriate public health and food inspection or agricultural officials. Bites of squirrels, chipmunks, rats, mice, hamsters, gerbils, other rodents, rabbits and hares may warrant post-exposure rabies prophylaxis if the behaviour of the biting animal was highly unusual.	

Legend: RIG=(human) rabies immune globulin.

The course of vaccine may be discontinued after consultation with pubic health/infectious disease experts if the direct fluorescent antibody test of the brain of an animal killed at the time of attack proves to be negative. However, if suspicion of rabies in the animal remains high even in the presence of a negative test, the immunization series should be continued.

Geriatrics: Evidence from experience suggests that rabies vaccine is efficacious in the geriatric population.

Pediatrics: Safety and effectiveness in children have been established. The indications for infants and children are the same as for adults.

CONTRAINDICATIONS: There are no definite contraindications to the use of IMOVAX Rabies [Rabies Vaccine Inactivated (DCO)] in the post-exposure situation; however, care should be taken if the vaccine is to be administered to persons who are hypersensitive to rabies vaccine or to any ingredient in the formulation or component of the container. For a complete listing, see Dosage Forms, Composition and Packaging. Local public health should be consulted if questions arise about the need for post-exposure treatment and expert opinion should be sought in the management of these individuals.

Pre-exposure prophylaxis should not be administered to persons who are hypersensitive to this vaccine or to any ingredient in the formulation or component of the container. For a complete listing, see Dosage Forms, Composition and Packaging. Persons who are at high-risk of contracting rabies disease and who have a hypersensitivity to the vaccine or one of its components may be referred for an evaluation by an allergist.

WARNINGS AND PRECAUTIONS: General: As with any vaccine, immunization with IMOVAX Rabies [Rabies Vaccine Inactivated (DCO)] may not protect 100% of individuals.

Pre-exposure immunization with IMOVAX Rabies should be deferred in the presence of any acute illness, including febrile illness.

Local and/or mild systemic reactions may occur after vaccine injection but these are usually transient and do not contraindicate continuing immunization.

Interchanging IMOVAX Rabies with other rabies vaccines during a pre- or post-exposure series is not recommended because of a lack of data on the safety and efficacy of such a regimen. The immunization series should, whenever possible, be completed with the same product. When this is not feasible, the series may be completed with another WHO-approved cell-culture vaccine.

Although no post-exposure vaccine failures have occurred in Canada or the US since cell culture vaccines have been routinely used, failures have occurred abroad when some deviation was made from the recommended post-exposure treatment protocol or when less than the currently recommended amount of antirabies sera was administered. Specifically, subjects who contracted rabies after post-exposure prophylaxis did not have their wounds cleansed with soap and water, did not receive their rabies vaccine injections in the deltoid area (i.e., vaccine was administered in the gluteal area), or where the wound site was not properly infiltrated with RIG. (See Dosage and Administration.)

This is a single dose of vaccine. In both pre-exposure and post-exposure immunization, the full 1.0 mL dose should be given intramuscularly. (See Dosage and Administration.)

In adults and children the vaccine should be injected into the deltoid muscle. In infants and small children the mid-lateral aspect of the thigh may be preferable. There have been reports of possible vaccine failure when the vaccine has been administered in the gluteal area.

This vaccine must not be used subcutaneously or intradermally. Special care should be taken to ensure that the product is not injected into a blood vessel.

A separate, sterile syringe and needle, or a sterile disposable unit, must be used for each individual patient to prevent the transmission of infectious agents. There have been case reports of transmission of HIV and hepatitis by failure to scrupulously observe sterile technique.

Before administration of IMOVAX Rabies, take all appropriate precautions to prevent adverse reactions. This includes a review of the patient's history concerning possible hypersensitivity to the vaccine or similar vaccine, previous immunization history, the presence of any contraindications to immunization and current health status. The health-care provider should inform the patient, parent or guardian of the benefits and risks of immunization, inquire about the recent health status of the patient and comply with any local requirements with respect to information to be provided to the patient before immunization and the importance of completing the immunization series.

This product contains albumin, a derivative of human blood. Based on effective donor screening and product manufacturing processes, it carries an extremely remote risk for transmission of viral diseases. A theoretical risk for transmission of variant Creutzfeldt-Jakob disease (vCJD) is also considered extremely remote. No cases of transmission of viral diseases or vCJD have ever been attributed to albumin.

Hematologic: Intramuscular injections should be given with care in persons with coagulation disorders or on anticoagulant therapy because intramuscular injection can cause injection site hematoma.

Immune: As with other products, Epinephrine Hydrochloride Solution (1:1000) and other appropriate agents should be available for immediate use in case an anaphylactic or acute hypersensitivity reaction occurs. Health-care providers should be familiar with current recommendations for the initial management of anaphylaxis in non-hospital settings, including proper airway management. For instructions on recognition and treatment of anaphylactic reactions, see the current edition of the Canadian Immunization Guide or visit the Health Canada website.

The possibility of allergic reactions in individuals sensitive to components of the vaccine should be evaluated.

Since the vaccine contains traces of neomycin and phenol red, the possibility of allergic reactions in individuals sensitive to these substances should be borne in mind.

Corticosteroids, immunosuppressive agents, and immunosuppressive illnesses can interfere with the development of active immunity after vaccination. Immunosuppressive agents should not be administered during post-exposure therapy unless essential for the treatment of other conditions. When rabies post-exposure prophylaxis is administered to persons receiving steroids or other immunosuppressive therapy, or who are immunosuppressed, it is important that a serum sample be tested for rabies antibody to ensure that an acceptable antibody response has developed. For immunodeficient individuals, this test can be performed 2 to 4 weeks after the vaccination. Pre-exposure prophylaxis should be administered to such persons with the awareness that the immune response may be inadequate. Antibody titre determination is also advisable after pre-exposure immunization in these populations.

Failures to seroconvert after the third dose should be managed in consultation with appropriate public health officials.

In the case of pre-exposure immunization, a significant increase has been noted in "immune complex-like" reactions in persons receiving booster doses of IMOVAX Rabies. (See Adverse Reactions.)

Special Populations: Pregnant Women: The safety of rabies vaccines in pregnancy has not been established. IMOVAX Rabies has not been studied in animal teratogenicity studies. It is also not known whether IMOVAX Rabies can cause fetal harm when administered to a pregnant woman or can affect reproductive capacity. IMOVAX Rabies should be given to a pregnant woman only if clearly needed.

Pre-Exposure: In the absence of sufficient human data, postponement of pre-exposure vaccination is recommended. If there is a substantial risk of exposure to rabies, pre-exposure prophylaxis may be indicated during pregnancy.

Post-Exposure: Because of the potential consequences of inadequately treated rabies exposure, and because there is no indication that fetal abnormalities have been associated with rabies vaccination, pregnancy is not considered a contraindication to post-exposure prophylaxis.

Nursing Women: It is not known whether this vaccine is excreted in human milk. Caution must be exercised when pre-exposure vaccine is administered to a nursing mother. The US Advisory Committee on Immunization Practices (ACIP) states that inactivated vaccines administered to a lactating woman do not affect the safety of breast-feeding for mothers or infants.

Monitoring and Laboratory Tests: Post-immunization antibody titre determination may be advisable for those anticipating frequent exposure or whose immune response may be reduced by illness, medication or advanced age.

ADVERSE REACTIONS: Clinical Trial Adverse Drug Reactions: Because clinical trials are conducted under very specific conditions, the adverse reaction rates observed in the clinical trials may not reflect the rates observed in practice and should not be compared to the rates in the clinical trials of another drug. Adverse drug reaction information from clinical trials is useful for identifying drug-related adverse events and for approximating rates.

IMOVAX Rabies [Rabies Vaccine Inactivated (DCO)] has been studied in recent randomized controlled trials in both children (N=199) using pre-exposure schedule (3 doses, I.M. plus booster at 1 year) and adults (N=124) using the post exposure schedule (5 doses, I.M.). The most frequent adverse events were injection site pain and headache. (See Table 2.)

Table 2: IMOVAX Rabies

Adverse Reactions Information (Clinical Trials)

Body System	Frequency	Adverse Reactions (Clinical Trials, N=323)
Blood and Lymphatic System Disorders	Common (>1%, <10%)	Adenopathy
Immune System Disorders	Common (>1%, <10%)	Allergic reaction such as urticaria, rash, dyspnea, wheezing
Nervous System Disorders	Very Common (>1/10)	Headache
	Common (>1%, <10%)	Dizziness
Gastrointestinal Disorders	Very Common (>1/10)	Nausea
	Common (>1%, <10%)	Abdominal pain, vomiting, diarrhea
Musculoskeletal and Connective Tissue Disorders	Very Common (>1/10)	Myalgia
	Common (>1%, <10%)	Arthralgia
General Disorders and Administration-Site Condition	Very Common (>1/10)	Injection site pain, erythema, induration, malaise, injection site hematoma
	Common (>1%, <10%)	Injections site pruritus, fever, chills

Post-Market Adverse Drug Reactions: Based on spontaneous reporting, the following additional adverse events have been reported very rarely (>1/10 000) during the post marketing surveillance of IMOVAX Rabies. Their frequencies have been estimated using number of reports and estimated number of patients. However, exact incidence cannot be precisely calculated. (See Table 3.)

Two cases of neurologic illness resembling Guillain-Barré syndrome, a transient neuroparalytic illness, that resolved without sequelae in 12 weeks and a focal subacute central nervous system disorder temporally associated with HDCV, have been reported.

DRUG INTERACTIONS: Corticosteroids and other immunosuppressive agents can interfere with the development of active immunity (See Warnings and Precautions, Immune).

Under no circumstances should rabies vaccine be administered in the same syringe or at the same site as rabies immune globulin.

If any other vaccines are administered during the same visit, they must be given at separate sites and with separate syringes. IMOVAX Rabies [Rabies Vaccine Inactivated (DCO)] must not be mixed in the same syringe with other parenterals.

Table 3: IMOVAX Rabies
Adverse Reactions Information (Post-Marketing)

Body System	Adverse Reactions (Only Observed in Post-Approval Use)
Immune System Disorders	Pruritus, oedema Anaphylactic reactions, Serum sickness type reaction[a]
Nervous System Disorders	Paraesthesia, neuropathy[b]
General Disorders and Administration-Site Condition	Asthenia

[a] Allergic reactions occurred less frequently among persons receiving primary vaccination. These reactions have been associated with the presence of betapropiolactone-altered human albumin in the HDCV.
[b] The use of corticosteroids to treat life-threatening neuroparalytic reactions carries the risk of inhibiting the development of active immunity to rabies. It is especially important in these cases that the serum of the patient be tested for rabies antibodies.

DOSAGE AND ADMINISTRATION: Recommendations for passive and/or active vaccination after exposure to an animal suspected of having rabies have been outlined by the WHO and by the National Advisory Committee on Immunization.

IMOVAX Rabies [Rabies Vaccine Inactivated (DCO)] is indicated for 3-dose pre-exposure and 5-dose post-exposure series in combination with rabies immune globulin for individuals suspected of exposure to rabies, with one exception: persons who have been previously vaccinated with IMOVAX Rabies Vaccine in a pre-exposure or post-exposure treatment series should receive only vaccine.

Needles should not be recapped and should be disposed of properly.

Pre-Exposure Dosage: Primary Vaccination: Three doses of IMOVAX Rabies are required. One dose of 1.0 mL is to be given intramuscularly on each of days 0, 7 and 21.

Booster Doses: The booster dose of 1.0 mL of vaccine should be administered intramuscularly.

Post-Exposure Immunization of Previously Unimmunized Individuals: A series of five doses of 1.0 mL of IMOVAX Rabies should be given. The first 1.0 mL dose on day 0 as soon as possible after exposure, and one 1.0 mL dose on each of days 3, 7, 14 and 28 after the first dose. An appropriate dose of RIG should also be given on day 0 as described below.

RIG: The recommended dose of human RIG is 20 IU/kg body weight. This formula is applicable to all age groups, including children. If anatomically feasible, the full dose of RIG should be thoroughly infiltrated in the area around and into the wounds. When more than one wound exists, each should be locally infiltrated with a portion of the RIG. See RIG package insert for precise information on the administration of RIG. Since vaccine-induced antibody begins to appear within 1 week, there is no value in administering RIG more than 8 days after initiating an approved vaccine course.

IMOVAX Rabies and immune globulin should be used concurrently for optimum post-exposure prophylaxis against rabies, except in certain previously immunized persons, as indicated below.

Post-Exposure Prophylaxis of Previously Immunized Individuals: Post-exposure prophylaxis for persons who have previously received rabies vaccine differs according to which preparation of vaccine was received.

A. Two doses of 1.0 mL of IMOVAX Rabies, one injected immediately and the other 3 days later, without RIG, are recommended for exposed individuals with the following rabies immunization history:
   i. Completion of an approved course of pre- or post-exposure prophylaxis with HDCV, a WHO approved cell-culture rabies vaccine or PCEC (Purified Chick Embryo Culture):
   ii. Completion of immunization with other types of rabies vaccine or with IMOVAX Rabies according to unapproved schedules so long as neutralizing rabies antibody has been demonstrated in serum.

B. A complete course of IMOVAX Rabies plus RIG is recommended for those who may have received rabies vaccines but do not fulfill the criteria listed in A. A serum sample may be collected before vaccine is given, and if antibody is demonstrated the course may be discontinued, provided at least two doses of IMOVAX Rabies have been administered.

Serologic Testing and Booster Doses: Healthy persons immunized with an appropriate regimen will develop rabies antibodies, and therefore routine post-immunization antibody determinations are not recommended. Neutralizing antibodies develop 7-14 days after immunization and persist for at least 2 years.

Post-immunization antibody titre determination may be advisable for those anticipating frequent exposure or whose immune response may be reduced by illness, medication or advanced age. Persons with continuing high risk of exposure, such as veterinarians, should have their serum tested for rabies antibodies every 2 years; others working with live rabies virus in laboratories or vaccine-production facilities and who are at risk of inapparent exposure should be tested every 6 months.

Those with inadequate titres should be given a booster dose of IMOVAX Rabies. Persons previously immunized with other vaccines should be given sufficient doses of IMOVAX Rabies to produce an adequate antibody response.

Missed Dose: It is very important to complete the series of rabies vaccinations on time. Cases of rabies have been reported when the approved schedule was not followed.

Administration: Administer the vaccine **intramuscularly**. For adults and children, the vaccine should always be administered in the deltoid area. In infants and small children, the anterolateral aspect of the thigh is also acceptable. The gluteal area should never be used for injections because administration of rabies vaccine in this area results in lower neutralizing antibody titres. For information on vaccine administration see the current edition of the Canadian Immunization Guide or visit the Health Canada website.

Under no circumstances should vaccine be administered in the same syringe or at the same site as RIG.

Reconstitution: Parenteral Products:

Vial Size	Volume of Diluent to be Added to Vial	Approximate Available Volume	Nominal Concentration per mL
3 mL	1 mL	1 mL	≥2.5 IU

Before administration parenteral drug products should be checked visually for any deviation from normal appearance including container integrity. The syringe and its package should also be inspected prior to use for evidence of leakage, or a faulty tip seal. If evidence of such defects is observed, the syringe should not be used.

The reconstituted vaccine should be used immediately.

After use, any remaining vaccine and container must be disposed of safely, according to biohazardous waste guidelines.

Package with Two Needles: Attach the plunger and reconstitution needle to the syringe and reconstitute the freeze-dried vaccine by introducing the diluent provided into the vial of powder. Gently swirl the contents until completely dissolved. Withdraw the suspension from the vial into the syringe. Remove the reconstitution needle and replace it with an appropriate needle for intramuscular injection.

Package with Attached Needle: Reconstitute the freeze-dried vaccine in its vial with the diluent supplied in the syringe. Gently swirl the contents until completely dissolved.

OVERDOSAGE:
Not documented.

> For management of a suspected drug overdose, CPhA recommends that you contact your **regional Poison Control Centre**. See the *CPS* Directory section for a list of Poison Control Centres.

ACTION AND CLINICAL PHARMACOLOGY: Mechanism of Action: Human diploid cell rabies vaccine (HDCV) together with RIG and local treatment are highly effective in preventing rabies in exposed individuals. No post-exposure HDCV failures have occurred in Canada or the United States. The most important immune response to rabies vaccines is antibodies to the G protein of the viral envelope. Pre-exposure vaccination with potent rabies vaccines leads to the development of virus-neutralizing antibodies (VNAs). Vaccination also induces production of cytotoxic T cells, which have been shown to protect vaccinated mice in the absence of neutralizing antibodies.

STORAGE AND STABILITY: Store at 2 to 8°C.

Do not freeze. Product which has been exposed to freezing should not be used.

SPECIAL HANDLING INSTRUCTIONS: The vaccine should be used immediately after reconstitution. If the vaccine is not administered promptly, discard contents.

Do not use the vaccine after the expiration date.

INFORMATION FOR THE PATIENT: Published in e-CPS, available by subscription at www.e-cps.ca.

DOSAGE FORMS, COMPOSITION AND PACKAGING: Single dose vials of lyophilized vaccine with 1 mL of diluent (sterile water for injection) contained in a disposable syringe with two needles (1 × 25G × 16 mm and 1 × 25G × 25 mm) or single dose vials of lyophilized vaccine with 1 mL of diluent (sterile water for injection) contained in a disposable syringe with an attached needle. The vial stoppers for the vial and plunger stoppers and needle shields for the syringes supplied with this product do not contain dry natural latex rubber.

Each 1 mL dose contains: rabies virus (WISTAR Rabies PM/WI 38 1503-3M Strain) ≥2.5 IU, human albumin <100 mg, neomycin <150 µg, phenol red 20 µg, diluent (sterile water for injection).

The powder is homogenous and pinkish beige to orangey yellow. The diluent is a clear colourless liquid. After reconstitution, IMOVAX Rabies is a clear or slightly opalescent red to purplish red suspension.

Imunovir® Ⓟ
inosine pranobex
Subacute Sclerosing Panencephalitis Therapy

Helix Biopharma

PHARMACOLOGY: Mechanism(s) that might explain the results of the clinical studies employing inosine pranobex have not been completely elucidated. However, possible antiviral and immunomodulating properties of this drug may be involved.

Serum uric acid concentration rose with increasing inosine pranobex doses. Hyperuricemic levels (greater than 7.5 mg%) were seen at doses equal to or exceeding 3 g/day. At doses of 4 g/day, about 60% of the subjects had serum uric acid levels in excess of 7 mg%; 30% of the subjects exceeded 7.5 mg%. Urinary uric acid excretion was also elevated after inosine pranobex administration. The time for urine normalization was usually longer than that required for normalization of serum uric acid level. In 1 case, uricosuria was found to last more than 9 days, and another case was reported in which 3 weeks were required to restore uric acid excretion to normal level.

Inosine pranobex is composed of inosine and the p-acetamidobenzoic acid salt of N, N-dimethylamido-2-propanol. The principal metabolite (about 80%) of p-acetamidobenzoic acid is O-acylglucuronide and the principal metabolite of N, N-dimethylamine-2-propanol is N, N-dimethylamino- 2-propanol-N-oxide. Virtually 100% of the metabolites was recovered in urine within 8 through 24 hours postadministration period. Each of the components of inosine pranobex is rapidly metabolized, the inosine and p-acetamidobenzoic acid more extensively than N, N-dimethylamino-2-propanol.

INDICATIONS: May be beneficial in retarding neurological deterioration and prolonging life in patients with slowly progressive subacute sclerosing panencephalitis (SSPE). Inosine pranobex is not indicated for any condition other than SSPE.

CONTRAINDICATIONS: None for SSPE patients.

WARNINGS: Because the purine (inosine) moiety of inosine pranobex is rapidly catabolized to uric acid, resulting in elevations of serum and uric acid, it should be used with care in patients with a history of gout, urolithiasis, nephrolithiasis, or renal dysfunction. Uricosuric agents may be administered to patients with severely elevated serum uric acid levels.

PRECAUTIONS: *Pregnancy:* Specific studies on the effects of inosine pranobex on animal reproduction have been performed and were negative. However, well-controlled trials concerning fetal risk and impairment of fertility in humans are not available. Therefore, care should be taken in the use of inosine pranobex by pregnant women and women of childbearing age, and the risks involved should be assessed.

ADVERSE EFFECTS: Imunovir tablets may cause unwanted side effects but these are infrequent and are usually of a mild and brief nature. The most consistent side effect is increased uric acid levels in the blood and urine, which return to pre-treatment levels after the dosing is finished. Infrequent side effects can include upset stomach, itching or rashes, headaches, dizziness, joint aches or feeling tired. Rare side effects can include diarrhea or constipation, increased urine volume, insomnia or feeling nervous or "on edge."

OVERDOSE:

Treatment: Toxic effects from an overdose of inosine pranobex have not been observed. Since the drug is rapidly metabolized, reduction in dosage or withdrawal from treatment with symptomatic general management of signs and symptoms would generally suffice should any untoward reaction occur. Similar management would apply to an accidental overdose.

> For management of a suspected drug overdose, CPhA recommends that you contact your **regional Poison Control Centre**. See the *CPS* Directory section for a list of Poison Control Centres.

DOSAGE: Adults and Children: The recommended dosage is 50 mg/kg/day, up to a maximum of 3 g/day, administered orally in 3 to 4 equally divided doses during waking hours.

SUPPLIED: Each white, oblong tablet, engraved D N on one side and with a breakline on the reverse contains inosine pranobex 500 mg. Nonmedicinal ingredients: magnesium stearate, mannitol, microcrystalline cellulose, povidone and wheat starch. Tartrazine free. Cartons of 100 tablets packed as 5 blister strips of 20 tablets. Store at room temperature.

Imuran® Injection Ⓟ
azathioprine sodium
Immunosuppressive Agent

Triton Pharma

Imuran® Tablets Ⓟ
azathioprine
Immunosuppressive Agent

Triton Pharma

Date of Revision: November 4, 2009

SUMMARY PRODUCT INFORMATION:

Route of Administration	Dosage Form/ Strength	Clinically Relevant Nonmedicinal Ingredients
Oral	Tablet 50 mg	For a complete listing see Dosage Forms, Composition and Packaging.
Injection	Solution 50 mg	

INDICATIONS AND CLINICAL USE: Renal Homotransplantation: IMURAN (azathioprine) is indicated as an adjunct for the prevention of rejection in renal homotransplantation.

Rheumatoid Arthritis: IMURAN is indicated only in adult patients meeting criteria for classic or definite rheumatoid arthritis as specified by the American Rheumatism Association. IMURAN should be restricted to patients with severe, active and erosive disease not responsive to conventional management including rest, acetylsalicylic acid or other non-steroidal drugs, or with disease-modifying antirheumatic drugs (DMARD's).

Geriatrics (>65 years of age): No data are available.

Pediatrics (<18 years of age): No data are available.

CONTRAINDICATIONS:

- IMURAN (azathioprine) should not be given to patients who have shown hypersensitivity to the drug.

WARNINGS AND PRECAUTIONS:

- **IMURAN is mutagenic and carcinogenic and may increase the patients' risk of neoplasia, in particular lymphoma and skin cancer (see Carcinogenesis and Mutagenesis).**
- **Severe leukopenia and/or thrombocytopenia may occur in patients on IMURAN (see Hematologic).**
- **Increased susceptibility to infection (see Warnings and Precautions).**
- **IMURAN can cause fetal harm when administered to a pregnant woman (see Special Populations, Pregnant Women).**
- **Transplantation: Only physicians experienced in immunosuppressive therapy and management of organ transplant should prescribe Imuran (Azathioprine). Patients receiving the drug should be managed in facilities equipped and staffed with adequate laboratory and supportive medical resources. The physician responsible for maintenance therapy should have complete information requisite for the follow-up of the patient.**
- **Rheumatiod Arthritis: Careful monitoring of Imuran treated patients is mandatory. Imuran should only be prescribed for rheumatoid arthritis by physicians experienced with the use of immunosuppressants.**

General: The dosage that will be tolerated or effective will vary from patient to patient. Therefore, careful management is necessary to obtain the optimum therapeutic effect and to reduce toxicity. Caution must be exercised to observe early signs of depression of the bone marrow which may result in leukopenia and eventually thrombocytopenia and bleeding. Since this drug may have a delayed action, it is important to withdraw the medication temporarily at the first sign of an abnormally large fall in the white cell count or of abnormal depression of the bone marrow. It must be kept in mind that patients with impaired renal function may have slower elimination of the drug and a greater cumulative effect. Lower dose if there is impaired renal function. It is recommended that the drug be withheld if there is evidence of toxic hepatitis or biliary stasis.

A persistent negative nitrogen balance has been observed in some patients on continuous azathioprine dosage; if this should occur, the dose should be reduced as this has been found to correct the situation.

The combined use of IMURAN with DMARD's have not been studied for either added benefit or unexpected adverse effects. The use of IMURAN with these agents cannot be recommended.

Carcinogenesis and Mutagenesis: Patients with rheumatoid arthritis previously treated with alkylating agents (cyclophosphamide, chlorambucil, melphalan or others) may have a prohibitive risk of neoplasia if treated with IMURAN.

IMURAN is mutagenic in animals and humans, carcinogenic in animals, and may increase the patient's risk of neoplasia. Patients receiving immunosupressive drugs, particularly transplant patients receiving aggressive therapy, are known to have an increased risk of developing non-Hodgkin's lymphomas and other malignancies, notably skin cancers (melanoma and non-melanoma), sarcomas (Kaposi's and non-Kaposi's), uterine cervical cancer in situ, and reticulum cell or lymphomatous tumors. The risk appears to be related to the intensity and duration of immunosuppression rather than to the use of any specific agent. It has been reported that reduction or discontinuation of immunosuppression may be associated with partial or complete regression of non-Hodgkin's lymphomas and Kaposi's sarcomas. The degree of immunosuppression is determined not only by the immunosuppressive regimen, but also by a number of other patient factors. The number of immunosuppressive agents may not necessarily increase the risk of lymphomas. However, patients who receive multiple immunosuppressive agents may be at risk for over-immunosuppression; therefore, immunosuppressive drug therapy should be maintained at the lowest effective levels. As is usual for patients with increased risk for skin cancer, exposure to sunlight and UV light should be limited, and patients should wear protective clothing and use a sunscreen with a high protection factor. Information is available on the spontaneous neoplasia risk in rheumatoid arthritis, and on neoplasia following immunosuppressive therapy of other auto-immune diseases. It has not been possible to define the precise risk of neoplasia due to IMURAN. The increased risk of developing non-Hodgkin's lymphomas in immunosuppressed rheumatoid arthritis patients compared with the general population appears to be related at least in part to the disease itself. However, acute myelogenous leukemia as well as solid tumors have been reported in patients with rheumatoid arthritis who have received azathioprine. Data on neoplasia in patients receiving IMURAN can be found under Adverse Reactions.

Gastrointestinal: A gastrointestinal hypersensitivity reaction characterized by severe nausea and vomiting has been reported. These symptoms may also be accompanied by diarrhea, rash, fever, malaise, myalgias, elevations in liver enzymes, vasculitis, hepatic dysfunction, cholestatis and occasionally, hypotension. Symptoms of gastrointestinal toxicity may often develop within the first several weeks of IMURAN therapy and are reversible upon discontinuation of the drug. The reaction can recur within hours after rechallenge with a single dose of IMURAN.

Hematologic: Severe leukopenia and/or thrombocytopenia may occur in patients on IMURAN (azathioprine). Macrocytic anemia and severe bone marrow depression may also occur. Hematologic toxicities are dose related and may be more severe in renal transplant patients whose homograft is undergoing rejection. It is suggested that patients on IMURAN have complete blood counts, including platelet counts, weekly during the first month, twice monthly for the second and third months of treatment, then monthly or more frequently if dosage alterations or other therapy changes are necessary. Delayed hematologic suppression may occur. Prompt reduction in dosage or temporary withdrawal of the drug may be necessary if there is a rapid fall in, or persistently low leukocyte count or other evidence of bone marrow depression. Leukopenia does not correlate with therapeutic effect; therefore, the dose should not be increased intentionally to lower the white blood cell count.

There are individuals with an inherited deficiency of the enzyme thiopurine methyl-transferase (TPMT) who may be unusually sensitive to the myelosuppressive effect of azathioprine and prone to developing rapid bone marrow depression following the initiation of treatment with IMURAN (azathioprine). This problem could be exacerbated by coadministration with drugs that inhibit TPMT, such as olsalazine, mesalazine or sulphasalazine. Also a possible association between decreased TPMT activity and secondary leukemias and myelodysplasia has been reported in individuals receiving 6-mercaptopurine (the active metabolite of azathioprine) in combination with other cytotoxics. Some laboratories offer testing for TPMT deficiency, although these tests have not been shown to identify all patients at risk of severe toxicity. Therefore close monitoring of blood counts is still necessary.

Immune: Patients receiving IMURAN alone or in combination with other immunosuppressants, particularly corticosteroids, have shown increased susceptibility to infections (e.g. fungal, viral and bacterial), including severe or atypical infection with varicella, herpes zoster and other infections agents (see Adverse Reactions). Fungal, viral, bacterial and protozoal infections may be fatal and should be treated vigorously. Reduction of azathioprine dosage and/or use of other drugs should be considered. Infection with varicella zoster virus (VZV; chickenpox and herpes zoster) may become severe during the administration of immunosuppressants. Caution should be exercised especially with respect to the following:

Before starting the administration of immunosuppressants, the prescriber should check to see if the patient has a history of VZV. Serologic testing may be useful in determining previous exposure. Patients who have no history of exposure should avoid contact with individuals with chickenpox or herpes zoster. If the patient is exposed to VZV, special care must be taken to avoid patients developing chickenpox or herpes zoster, and passive immunisation with varicella-zoster immunoglobulin (VZIG) may be considered.

If the patient is infected with VZV, appropriate measures should be taken, which may include antiviral therapy and supportive care.

Sexual Function/Reproduction: IMURAN has been reported to cause temporary depression in spermatogenesis and reduction in sperm viability and sperm count in mice at doses 10 times the human therapeutic dose; a reduced percentage of fertile matings occurred when animals received 5 mg/kg.

Special Populations: Pregnant Women: There are no adequate and well-controlled studies in pregnant women therefore IMURAN should not be given to patients who are pregnant or likely to become pregnant in the near future without careful assessment of risk versus benefit.

IMURAN can cause fetal harm when administered to a pregnant woman.

IMURAN should not be given during pregnancy or in patients of reproductive potential without careful weighing of risk versus benefit. Use of IMURAN in pregnant patients should be avoided whenever possible. If this drug is used during pregnancy or if the patient becomes pregnant while taking this drug, the patient should be apprised of the potential hazard to the fetus. Women of childbearing age should be advised to avoid becoming pregnant.

There have been reports of premature birth and low birth weight following maternal exposure to azathioprine, particularly in combination with corticosteroids. There have also been reports of spontaneous abortion following either maternal or paternal exposure. IMURAN is teratogenic in rabbits and mice when given in doses equivalent to the human dose (5 mg/kg daily). Abnormalities included skeletal malformations and visceral anomalies.

Leukopenia and/or thrombocytopenia have been reported in a proportion of neonates whose mothers took azathioprine throughout their pregnancies. Extra care in hematological monitoring is advised during pregnancy.

Limited immunologic and other abnormalities have occurred in a few infants born of renal allograft recipients on IMURAN. In a detailed case report, documented lymphopenia, diminished IgG and IgM levels, CMV infection, and a decreased thymic shadow were noted in an infant born to a mother receiving 150 mg azathioprine and 30 mg prednisone daily throughout pregnancy. At 10 weeks most features were normalized. Pancytopenia and severe immune deficiency has been reported in a preterm infant whose mother received 125 mg azathioprine and 12.5 mg prednisone daily. There have been two published reports of abnormal physical findings. In one study an infant born with preaxial polydactyly whose mother received azathioprine 200 mg daily and prednisone 20 mg every other day during pregnancy. The second study described an infant with a large myelomeningocele in the upper lumbar region, bilateral dislocated hips, and bilateral talipes equinovarus. The father was on long-term azathioprine therapy.

Nursing Women: The use of IMURAN in nursing mothers is not recommended. Azathioprine or its metabolites are transferred at low levels, both transplacentally and in breast milk. Because of the potential for tumorigenicity shown for azathioprine, a decision should be made on whether to discontinue nursing or discontinue the drug, taking into account the importance of the drug to the mother.

Pediatrics (<18 years of age): Safety and efficacy of azathioprine in children have not been established.

IMURAN should not be used to treat children with rheumatoid arthritis.

Geriatrics (>65 years of age): Safety and efficacy of azathioprine in geriatrics have not been established.

ADVERSE REACTIONS: Adverse Drug Reaction Overview: The principal and potentially serious toxic effects of IMURAN (azathioprine) are hematologic and gastrointestinal. The risks of secondary infection and neoplasia are also significant (see Warnings and Precautions). The frequency and severity of adverse reactions depend on the dose and duration of IMURAN as well as on the patient's underlying disease or concomitant therapies. The incidence of hematologic toxicities and neoplasia encountered in groups of renal homograft recipients is significantly higher than that in studies employing IMURAN for rheumatoid arthritis.

Clinical Trial Adverse Drug Reactions: Because clinical trials are conducted under very specific conditions the adverse reaction rates observed in the clinical trials may not reflect the rates observed in practice and should not be compared to the rates in the clinical trials of another drug. Adverse drug reaction information from clinical trials is useful for identifying drug-related adverse events and for approximating rates.

The relative incidences in clinical studies are summarized below:

Toxicity	Renal Homograft %	Rheumatoid Arthritis %
Leukopenia Any Degree	>50	28
$<2500/mm^3$	16	5.3
Infections	20	<1
Neoplasia		[a]
Lymphoma	0.5	
Others	2.8	

[a] Data on the rate and risk of neoplasia among persons with rheumatoid arthritis treated with azathioprine are limited. The incidence of lymphoproliferative disease in patients with RA appears to be significantly higher than that in the general population. In one completed study, the rate of lymphoproliferative disease in RA patients receiving higher than recommended doses of azathioprine (5 mg/kg/day) was 1.8 cases per 1000 patient years of follow-up, compared with 0.8 cases per 1000 patient years of follow-up in those not receiving azathioprine. However, the proportion of the increased risk attributable to the azathioprine dosage or to other therapies (i.e., alkylating agents) received by patients treated with azathioprine cannot be determined.

Hematologic: Leukopenia and/or thrombocytopenia and rarely as agranulocytosis, pancytopenia and aplastic anemia are dose dependent and may occur late in the course of IMURAN therapy. Dose reduction or temporary withdrawal allows reversal of these toxicities. These adverse events occur particularly in patients predisposed to myelotoxicity, such as those with TPMT deficiency (see Warnings and Precautions) and renal or hepatic insufficiency and in patients failing to reduce the dose of IMURAN when receiving concurrent allopurinol therapy (see Warnings and Precautions). Infection may occur as a secondary manifestation of bone marrow suppression or leukopenia, but the incidence of infection is 30 to 60 times greater in renal homotransplantation than in rheumatoid arthritis. Macrocytic anemia and/or bleeding have been reported in patients on IMURAN.

Gastrointestinal: Nausea and vomiting may occur within the first few months of IMURAN therapy, and occurred in approximately 12% of 676 rheumatoid arthritis patients. The frequency of gastric disturbance can often be reduced by administration of the drug in divided doses and/or after meals. However, in some patients, nausea and vomiting may be severe and may be accompanied by symptoms such as diarrhea, fever, malaise, vasculitis, hepatic dysfunction, cholestatis and myalgias (see Warnings and Precautions). Vomiting with abdominal pain may occur rarely with a hypersensitivity pancreatitis.

Infections and Infestations: Infections (i.e. viral, fungal and bacterial) occur very commonly in transplant patients receiving azathioprine in combination with other immunosuppressants and uncommonly in other patient populations (see Warnings and Precautions).

Hepatic: Hepatotoxicity manifested by elevation of serum alkaline phosphatase, bilirubin and/or serum transaminases is known to occur with thiopurines including IMURAN and PURINETHOL (6-mercaptopurine). This toxic hepatitis with biliary stasis is known to occur in homograft recipients. Hepatotoxicity has been uncommon in rheumatoid arthritis patients on IMURAN (less than 1%). Hepatotoxicity following transplantation most often occurs within 6 months of transplantation and is generally reversible after interruption of IMURAN. Rare but life-threatening hepatic damage associated with chronic administration of azathioprine has been described primarily in transplant patients and in one patient receiving IMURAN for panuveitis. Histological findings include sinusoidal dilation, peliosis hepatis, veno-occlusive disease and nodular regenerative hyperplasia. Periodic measurement of serum transaminases, alkaline phosphatase, and bilirubin is indicated for early detection of hepatotoxicity. If hepatic veno-occlusive disease is clinically suspected, IMURAN should be permanently withdrawn. In some cases withdrawal of azathioprine has resulted in either a temporary or permanent improvement in liver histology and symptoms.

Less Common Clinical Trial Adverse Drug Reactions (<1%): Additional side effects of low frequency have been reported. These include skin rashes, alopecia, fever, arthralgias, diarrhea, steatorrhea, negative nitrogen balance, and reversible interstitial pneumonitis.

There have been rare reports of neoplasms including non-Hodgkins lymphomas, skin cancers (melanoma and non-melanoma), sarcomas (Kaposi's and non-Kaposi's), uterine cervical cancer in situ, acute myeloid leukaemia and myelodysplasia (some in association with chromosomal abnormalities).

Post-Market Adverse Drug Reactions: Stevens-Johnson syndrome and toxic epidermal necrolysis have been reported very rarely in post-marketing surveillance.

DRUG INTERACTIONS: Overview: Drug-Drug Interactions: Allopurinol: The principal pathway for detoxification of IMURAN is inhibited by allopurinol. In patients receiving IMURAN, the concomitant administration of ZYLOPRIM (allopurinol) will require a reduction in dose to approximately 1/3 to 1/4 of the usual dose of IMURAN. Subsequent adjustment of doses of IMURAN should be made on the basis of therapeutic response and any toxic effects. Other agents affecting myelopoesis: Drugs which may affect leukocyte production, including co-trimoxazole, may lead to exaggerated leukopenia, especially in renal transplant recipients.

Angiotensin Converting Enzyme Inhibitors: The use of angiotensin converting enzyme inhibitors to control hypertension in patients on azathioprine has been reported to induce anemia and severe leukopenia.

Warfarin: IMURAN may inhibit the anticoagulant effect of warfarin.

Non-Depolarizing Muscle Relaxants: There is clinical evidence that IMURAN antagonizes the effect of non-depolarizing muscle relaxants such as curare, d-tubocurarine and pancuronium. Experimental data confirm that azathioprine reverses the neuromuscular blockade caused by d-tubocurarine, and show that azathioprine potentiates the neuromuscular blockade caused by succinylcholine.

As there is in vitro evidence that aminosalicylate derivatives (e.g. olsalazine, mesalazine or sulphasalazine) inhibit the TPMT enzyme, they should be administered with caution to patients receiving concurrent azathioprine therapy (see Warnings and Precautions).

DOSAGE AND ADMINISTRATION: Recommended Dose and Dosage Adjustment: Renal Homotransplantation: The dose of IMURAN (azathioprine) required to prevent rejection and minimize toxicity will vary with individual patients; this necessitates careful management. The initial dose is usually 3-5 mg/kg daily, beginning at the time of transplant. IMURAN is usually given as a single daily dose on the day of, and in a minority of cases one to three days before, transplantation. IMURAN is often initiated with the intravenous administration of the sodium salt, with subsequent use of tablets (at the same dose level) after the post-operative period. Intravenous administration of the sodium salt is indicated only in patients unable to tolerate oral medications. Dose reduction to maintenance levels of 1-3 mg/kg daily is usually possible. The dose of IMURAN should not be increased to toxic levels because of threatened rejection. Discontinuation may be necessary for severe hematologic or other toxicity, even if rejection of the homograft may be a consequence of drug withdrawal.

Rheumatoid Arthritis: IMURAN is usually given on a daily basis. The initial dose should be approximately 1.0 mg/kg (50-100 mg) given as a single dose or on a twice daily schedule. The dose may be increased, beginning at six to eight weeks and thereafter by steps at four-week intervals, if there are no serious toxicities and if initial response is unsatisfactory. Dose increments should be 0.5 mg/kg daily, up to a maximum dose of 2.5 mg/kg/day. Therapeutic response occurs after several weeks of treatment, usually six to eight; an adequate trial should be a minimum of 12 weeks. Patients not improved after twelve weeks can be considered refractory. IMURAN may be continued long-term in patients with clinical response, but patients should be monitored carefully, and gradual dosage reduction should be attempted to reduce risk of toxicities. Maintenance therapy should be at the lowest effective dose, and the dose given can be lowered, with decremental changes of 0.5 mg/kg or approximately 25 mg daily every four weeks, while other therapy is kept constant. The optimum duration of maintenance IMURAN has not been determined. IMURAN can be discontinued abruptly, but delayed effects are possible.

Rest, physiotherapy and salicylates should be continued while IMURAN is given, but it may be possible to reduce the dose of corticosteroids in patients on IMURAN.

Use in Renal Dysfunction: Relatively oliguric patients, especially those with tubular necrosis in the immediate post-cadaveric transplant period, may have delayed clearance of IMURAN or its metabolites, or be particularly sensitive to this drug, and are usually given lower doses.

Parenteral Administration: For intravenous use only. A 50 mg vial should be reconstituted with 5 to 15 mL Sterile Water for Injection, however to obtain a nominal concentration of 10 mg/mL, 5 mL of Sterile Water for Injection should be used. Once the Sterile Water for Injection has been added, swirl until a clear solution results. This solution has a pH of approximately 10-12. No antimicrobial preservative is included. Therefore reconstitution and dilution must be carried out under full aseptic conditions, preferably immediately before use. Any unused solution should be discarded. Further dilution into sterile saline is usually made for infusion; the final volume depends on time for the infusion, usually 30-60 minutes but as short as five minutes and as long as eight hours for the daily dose.

Reconstitution: Parenteral Products:

Vial Size	Volume of Diluent to be Added to Vial	Approximate Available Volume	Nominal Concentration per mL
50 mg	5 mL	5 mL	10 mg/mL

Shake until complete dissolution.

No antimicrobial preservative is included. Therefore reconstitution and dilution must be carried out under full aseptic conditions, preferably immediately before use. Any unused solution should be discarded.

Intravenous Infusion: Further dilution into sterile saline is usually made for infusion. The final volume depends on the time for the infusion, usually 30-60 minutes, but as short as five minutes and as long as eight hours for the daily dose.

As with all parenteral drug products, intravenous admixtures should be inspected visually for clarity, particulate matter, precipitate, discolouration and leakage prior to administration whenever solution and container permit. Solutions showing haziness, particulate matter, precipitate, discolouration or leakage should not be used. Discard unused portion.

OVERDOSAGE:
Initial symptoms are nausea and vomiting; and symptoms appearing later are leukopenia, thrombocytopenia, hepatic necrosis and anorexia.

For the treatment of overdosage, administer gastric lavage and fluids; blood transfusions may be needed due to suppression of the proliferation of granulocytes.

About 30% of IMURAN (azathioprine) is bound to serum proteins, but approximately 45% is removed during an 8-hour hemodialysis. A single case has been reported of a renal transplant patient who ingested a single dose of 7500 mg IMURAN. The immediate toxic reactions were nausea, vomiting, and diarrhea, followed by mild leukopenia and mild abnormalities in liver function. The white blood cell count, AST, and bilirubin returned to normal 6 days after the overdose.

> For management of a suspected drug overdose, CPhA recommends that you contact your **regional Poison Control Centre**. See the *CPS* Directory section for a list of Poison Control Centres.

ACTION AND CLINICAL PHARMACOLOGY: Mechanism of Action: Homograft Survival: Although the use of azathioprine for inhibition of renal homograft rejection is well established, the mechanism(s) for this action are somewhat obscure. The drug suppresses hypersensitivities of the cell-mediated type and causes variable alterations in antibody production. Suppression of T-cell effects, including ablation of T-cell suppression, is dependent on the temporal relationship to antigenic stimulus or engraftment. This agent has little effect on established graft rejections or secondary responses.

Alterations in specific immune responses or immunologic functions in transplant recipients are difficult to relate specifically to immunosuppression by azathioprine. These patients have subnormal responses to vaccines, low numbers of T-cells, and abnormal phagocytosis by peripheral blood cells, but their mitogenic responses, serum immunoglobulins and secondary antibody responses are usually normal.

Immunoinflammatory Response: Azathioprine suppresses disease manifestations as well as underlying pathology in animal models of auto-immune disease. For example, the severity of adjuvant arthritis is reduced by azathioprine.

The mechanisms whereby azathioprine affects auto-immune diseases are not known. Azathioprine is immunosuppressive, delayed hypersensitivity and cellular cytotoxicity tests being suppressed to a greater degree than are antibody responses. In the rat model of adjuvant arthritis, azathioprine has been shown to inhibit the lymph node hyperplasia which precedes the onset of the signs of the disease. Both the immunosuppressive and therapeutic effects in animal models are dose-related. Azathioprine is considered a slow-acting drug and effects may persist after the drug has been discontinued.

Pharmacodynamics: In view of the observations by Schwartz et al. that mercaptopurine suppressed the antibody response in rabbits injected with bovine serum albumin, the effects of azathioprine on the formation of antibodies were investigated. In the suppression of the formation of antibodies in mice to sheep red cells, as determined by hemagglutinin titers, azathioprine was found to be superior to mercaptopurine. Whereas mercaptopurine was active only at its maximum tolerated dose of 75 mg/kg, azathioprine was active at 25 mg/kg and was tolerated in doses up to 60 mg/kg for the dosage schedule employed (intraperitoneal injection for 4 successive days beginning at the time of the antigenic stimulus). The anti-immune effects of azathioprine are not due entirely to the mercaptopurine derived therefrom by splitting in vivo.

Another line of evidence which suggests that part of the activity of azathioprine may be due to its reaction with sulfhydryl compounds is the potentiation of its anti-immune effect by the simultaneous administration of MYLERAN (busulfan). (Busulfan is also known to react with sulfhydryl groups in tissues.) Thus the combination of azathioprine (10 mg/kg) and busulfan (30 mg/kg) produced a marked suppression of the antibody response, whereas the minimum effective dose of azathioprine alone is 25 mg/kg, and busulfan alone is inactive at its maximum tolerated dose of 40 mg/kg. The combination of mercaptopurine (25 mg/kg) and busulfan (25 mg/kg) is inactive.

Pharmacokinetics: Metabolism: Azathioprine is well absorbed following oral administration. Maximum serum radioactivity occurs at one to two hours after oral 35S-azathioprine and decays with a half-life of five hours. This is not an estimate of the half-life of azathioprine itself but is the decay rate for all 35S-containing metabolites of the drug. Because of extensive metabolism, only a fraction of the radioactivity is present as azathioprine. Usual doses produce blood levels of azathioprine, and of mercaptopurine derived from it, which are low (<1 μg/mL). Blood levels are of little predictive value for therapy since the magnitude and duration of clinical effects correlate with thiopurine nucleotide levels in tissues rather than with plasma drug levels. Azathioprine and mercaptopurine are moderately bound to serum proteins (30%) and are partially dialyzable.

Azathioprine is cleaved in vivo to mercaptopurine. Both compounds are rapidly eliminated from blood and are oxidized or methylated in erythrocytes and liver; no azathioprine or mercaptopurine is detectable in urine after eight hours. Conversion to inactive 6-thiouric acid by xanthine oxidase is an important degradative pathway, and the inhibition of this pathway in patients receiving ZYLOPRIM (allopurinol) is the basis for the azathioprine dosage reduction required in these patients (see Drug Interactions). Proportions of metabolites are different in individual patients, and this presumably accounts for variable magnitude and duration of drug effects. Renal clearance is probably not important in predicting biological effectiveness or toxicities, although dose reduction is practiced in patients with poor renal function.

STORAGE AND STABILITY: IMURAN Tablets should be stored in a dry place between 15 and 25°C, protected from light.

IMURAN for Injection should be stored between 15 and 25°C and protected from light. Single dose vials. Discard unused portion.

SPECIAL HANDLING INSTRUCTIONS: Tablets and intact vials should be returned to the manufacturer for destruction. Proper precautions should be taken in packaging these materials for transport.

All materials which have come in contact with cytotoxic drugs should be segregated and incinerated at 1000°C or more. Sealed containers may explode.

Personnel regularly involved in the preparation and handling of cytotoxic agents should have bi-annual blood examinations.

INFORMATION FOR THE PATIENT: Published in e-CPS, available by subscription at www.e-cps.ca.

DOSAGE FORMS, COMPOSITION AND PACKAGING: Injection: Each vial contains: the equivalent of azathioprine 50 mg as the sodium salt, and sodium hydroxide to adjust pH. Single dose vials of 17 mL.

Tablets: Each yellow to off-white, overlapping circle (dumbbell) shape tablet, imprinted IMURAN 50 on one side and with converging scored lines on the other, contains: azathioprine 50 mg. Nonmedicinal ingredients: lactose, magnesium stearate, potato starch, povidone and stearic acid. Bottles of 100.

(Shown in Product Identification Section)

Indapamide ℞

CPhA Monograph

see *Thiazide Diuretics*

Inderal®-LA ℞

propranolol HCl

Beta-adrenergic Receptor Blocking Agent

Pfizer

Date of Preparation: July 18, 1968
Date of Revision: October 31, 2006

PHARMACOLOGY: Propranolol is a non-selective beta-adrenergic receptor blocking drug. It has no other autonomic nervous system activity. Propranolol is a competitive antagonist which specifically competes with beta-adrenergic receptor stimulating agents for available beta-receptor sites. When access to beta-adrenergic receptor sites is blocked by propranolol, the chronotropic, inotropic, and vasodilator responses to beta-adrenergic stimulation are decreased proportionately.

Beta-adrenergic blockade is useful in some clinical conditions in which sympathetic activity is excessive or inappropriate, and therefore, detrimental to the patient. Sympathetic stimulation is however, vital in some situations (e.g. in patients with AV block or with a severely damaged heart) and should be preserved. The basic objective of beta-adrenergic blockade is to decrease adverse sympathetic stimulation but not to the degree that impairs necessary sympathetic support. Beta-blockade may result in bronchial constriction by interfering with endogenously or exogenously induced bronchodilation (see Contraindications and Warnings).

The mechanism of the antihypertensive effects of propranolol has not been established. Among the factors that may be involved are decreased cardiac output, inhibition of renin release by the kidneys, and diminution of tonic sympathetic nerve outflow from vasomotor centers in the brain. It has been suggested, but not established, that propranolol may achieve a better antihypertensive effect in patients with normal or elevated plasma renin activity (PRA) than those with low PRA.

Propranolol may reduce the oxygen requirement of the heart at any level of effort by blocking catecholamine induced increases in the heart rate, systolic blood pressure, and the velocity and extent of myocardial contraction. On the other hand, propranolol may increase oxygen requirements by increasing left ventricular fiber length, end diastolic pressure, and systolic ejection period. When the net effect is beneficial in anginal patients, it manifests itself during exercise or stress by delaying the onset of pain and reducing the incidence and severity of anginal attacks.

Propranolol exerts antiarrhythmic effects in concentrations producing beta-adrenergic blockade, which appears to be its principal antiarrhythmic mechanism of action. Beta-adrenergic blockade is of unique importance in the management of arrhythmias caused by increased levels of circulating catecholamines or enhanced sensitivity of the heart to catecholamines (arrhythmias associated with pheochromocytoma, thyrotoxicosis, exercise).

Mechanisms of the antimigraine and antitremor effects of propranolol have not been established. The antimigraine effect may be due to inhibition of vasodilatation or arteriolar spasms over the cortex. Beta-adrenergic receptors have been demonstrated in the pial vessels of the brain. The antitremor effects may be exerted through both peripheral and central sites of action. The mechanism by which propranolol reduces the incidence of cardiovascular mortality in post-myocardial infarct patients is unknown.

Inderal-LA is a special formulation of propranolol HCl consisting of capsules filled with spheroids of the active drug that have a sustained-release coating.

Pharmacokinetics: Propranolol from Inderal-LA capsules is almost completely absorbed from the gastrointestinal tract. A large part of the absorbed drug is lost from the systemic circulation due to first-pass metabolism in the liver. The first-pass metabolism is saturable. Steady-state plasma propranolol concentrations from Inderal-LA are proportional to the dose over the range of 60 to 160 mg/day although there is considerable intersubject variation. In healthy volunteers steady state was achieved after 2 or 3 days administration of Inderal-LA.

Peak blood levels following administration of Inderal-LA capsules occur at about 6 hours and the apparent plasma half-life has been reported to be between 10 and 12 hours i.e. 2 to 3 times that of the conventional tablet formulation.

When measured at steady state over a 24-hour period the areas under the propranolol plasma concentration-time curve (AUCs) for the LA-capsules are approximately 60 to 65% of the AUCs for a comparable divided daily dose of propranolol tablets. The lower AUCs for the Inderal-LA capsules are due to greater hepatic metabolism of propranolol because of slower absorption. Over a 24-hour period, blood levels are fairly constant for about 12 hours, then decline exponentially.

INDICATIONS: Inderal-LA (propranolol hydrochloride) extended release capsules are indicated for maintenance therapy in the treatment of hypertension and prophylaxis of angina pectoris.

As for Inderal, the combination of Inderal-LA with thiazide-like diuretics and/or peripheral vasodilators has been shown to be compatible and generally more effective than Inderal-LA alone. Experience with most commonly used antihypertensive agents has not suggested evidence of incompatibility.

Treatment must always be initiated and individual titration of dosage carried out using the conventional tablets. The long-acting formulation may be used for maintenance provided the dosage requirement is suitable.

Inderal-LA is not indicated for the emergency treatment of hypertensive crises.

CONTRAINDICATIONS: Bronchospasm, including bronchial asthma; allergic rhinitis during the pollen season; sinus bradycardia and greater than first degree block; cardiogenic shock; right ventricular failure secondary to pulmonary hypertension; congestive heart failure (see Warnings) unless the failure is secondary to a tachyarrhythmia treatable with propranolol.

WARNINGS: Cardiac Failure: Sympathetic stimulation is a vital component supporting circulatory function in congestive heart failure; therefore, inhibition by means of beta-adrenergic blockade is a potential hazard as it may further depress myocardial contractility and precipitate cardiac failure. Propranolol acts selectively without completely abolishing the inotropic action of digitalis on the heart muscle (i.e., that of supporting the strength of myocardial contractions). In patients already receiving digitalis, the positive inotropic action of digitalis may be reduced by propranolol's negative inotropic effect. The effects of propranolol and digitalis are additive in depressing AV conduction.

Patients Without a History of Cardiac Failure: Continued depression of the myocardium over a period of time can, in some patients, lead to cardiac failure. In rare instances, this has been observed during propranolol therapy. Therefore, at the first sign or symptom of impending cardiac failure, patients should be fully digitalized and/or given a diuretic, and the response observed closely: a) if cardiac failure continues, despite adequate digitalization and diuretic therapy, propranolol should be withdrawn immediately; b) if tachyarrhythmia is being controlled, patients should be maintained on combined therapy and closely followed until threat of cardiac failure is over.

Abrupt Cessation of Therapy in Angina Pectoris: Severe exacerbation of angina and the occurrence of myocardial infarction have been reported in some patients with angina pectoris following abrupt discontinuation of propranolol therapy. Therefore, when discontinuation of propranolol is planned in patients with angina pectoris, the dosage should be gradually reduced over a period of about 2 weeks and the patient should be carefully observed. For patients receiving propranolol tablets, the same frequency of administration should be maintained. For patients on Inderal-LA, discontinuation can be achieved by substituting Inderal-LA 60, 80, 120 and 160 mg by the equivalent dosage of conventional propranolol tablets spread throughout the day, and then gradually reducing the dose. In situations of greater urgency, propranolol dosage should be reduced stepwise, in 4 days under close observation. If angina markedly worsens, or acute coronary insufficiency develops, it is recommended that treatment with propranolol be reinstituted promptly, at least temporarily. In addition, patients with angina pectoris should be warned against abrupt discontinuation of propranolol.

Oculomucocutaneous Syndrome: Various skin rashes and conjunctival xerosis have been reported in patients treated with beta-blockers including propranolol. A severe oculomucocutaneous syndrome, whose signs include conjunctivitis sicca and psoriasiform rashes, otitis, and sclerosing serositis has occurred with the long-term use of one beta-adrenergic blocking agent. This syndrome has not been observed with propranolol, however, physicians should be alert to the possibility of such reactions and discontinue treatment if they occur.

Patients with Thyrotoxicosis: Possible deleterious effects from long-term use of propranolol have not yet been adequately appraised. Special consideration should be given to propranolol's potential for aggravating congestive heart failure. Propranolol may mask the clinical signs of developing or continuing hyperthyroidism or its complications, and give a false impression of improvement. Therefore, abrupt withdrawal of propranolol may be followed by an exacerbation of symptoms of hyperthyroidism, including thyroid storm. This may be another instance where propranolol should be withdrawn slowly by reducing dosage. Propranolol does not distort thyroid function tests.

Patients with Wolff-Parkinson-White Syndrome: Propranolol should be used with caution since several cases have been reported in which, after propranolol treatment, the tachycardia was replaced by a severe bradycardia requiring a demand pacemaker. In one patient, this occurred after an initial dose of 5 mg of propranolol.

Patients Undergoing Elective or Emergency Surgery: The management of patients with angina, being treated with beta-blockers and undergoing elective or emergency surgery, is controversial because beta-adrenergic receptor blockade impairs the ability of the heart to respond to beta-adrenergically mediated reflex stimuli, but abrupt discontinuation of therapy with propranolol may be followed by severe complications (see Warnings). Some patients receiving beta-adrenergic blocking agents have been subject to protracted severe hypotension during anesthesia. Difficulty in restarting and maintaining the heartbeat has also been reported.

For these reasons, in patients with angina undergoing elective surgery, propranolol should be withdrawn gradually (see Warnings). According to available evidence, all clinical and physiologic effects of beta-blockade are no longer present 48 hours after cessation of medication.

In emergency surgery, since propranolol is a competitive inhibitor of beta-adrenergic receptor agonists, its effects may be reversed, if necessary, by sufficient doses of such agonists as isoproterenol or dobutamine.

Anesthesia with agents which maintain cardiac contractility by virtue of their effect on catecholamine release (e.g. ether) should be avoided in patients on propranolol therapy.

Patients Prone to Nonallergic Bronchospasm (e.g., chronic bronchitis, emphysema, bronchiectasis): Propranolol should be administered with caution since it may block bronchodilation produced by endogenous and exogenous catecholamine stimulation of beta-adrenergic receptors.

Patients with Diabetes and in Those Subject to Hypoglycemia: Because of its beta-adrenergic blocking activity, propranolol may block premonitory signs and symptoms (pulse rate and pressure changes) of acute hypoglycemia. This is especially important to keep in mind in patients with labile diabetes. Hypoglycemic attacks may be accompanied by a precipitous elevation of blood pressure. Acute increases in blood pressure have occurred after insulin-induced hypoglycemia in subjects on propranolol.

Hypersensitivity reactions, including anaphylactic/anaphylactoid reactions, have been associated with the administration of propranolol (see Adverse Effects).

Skin Reactions: Cutaneous reactions, including Stevens-Johnson Syndrome, toxic epidermal necrolysis, exfoliative dermatitis, erythema multiforme, and urticaria, have been reported with use of propranolol (see Adverse Effects).

Pregnancy: Pregnancy and Fetal Injury: Propranolol can cause fetal harm when administered to a pregnant woman. The safe use of propranolol in pregnancy has not been established. Use of any drug in pregnancy or in women of childbearing potential requires that the possible risk to mother and/or fetus be weighed against the expected therapeutic benefit. Post-marketing case reports including perinatal complications, such as small placentas, intrauterine growth retardation and congenital abnormalities have been reported in neonates where the mother took propranolol during pregnancy. Some infants born to mothers treated with propranolol were reported to have hypoglycemia, bradycardia and/or respiratory depression. Adequate facilities for monitoring such infants at birth should be available. Propranolol should be used in pregnancy only if the potential benefit justifies the potential risk to the fetus.

Lactation: Propranolol is excreted in human milk. Caution should be exercised when propranolol is administered to a nursing woman.

Children: While experience with propranolol in children under 12 is limited, the indications for this drug is recommended occur infrequently in childhood. Although reports fail to indicate that children respond in a manner different from the adult, physicians are advised to undertake treatment with caution.

PRECAUTIONS: There may be increased difficulty in treating an allergic type reaction in patients on beta-blockers. In these patients, the reaction may be more severe due to pharmacological effects of beta-blockers and problems with fluid changes. Epinephrine should be administered with caution since it may not have its usual effects in the treatment of anaphylaxis. On the one hand, larger doses of epinephrine may be needed to overcome the bronchospasm, while on the other, these doses can be associated with excessive alpha adrenergic stimulation with consequent hypertension, reflex bradycardia and heart-block and possible potentiation of bronchospasm. Alternatives to the use of large doses of epinephrine include vigorous supportive care such as fluids, and the use of beta agonists including parenteral salbutamol or isoproterenol to overcome bronchospasm, and norepinephrine to overcome hypotension.

Some slowing of heart due to unopposed vagal activity is usual in patients receiving propranolol; however, occasionally severe bradycardia occurs and may lead to vertigo, syncopal attacks or orthostatic hypotension. Patients, especially those with limited cardiac reserve should be monitored for signs of excessive bradycardia. Should the patient become symptomatic the dose of propranolol should be decreased or, if necessary, the drug should be discontinued. If it is essential to correct the bradycardia i.v. atropine or isoproterenol should be considered.

It has been reported that administration of propranolol to control cardiac arrhythmias in acute myocardial infarction has caused marked reduction in cardiac output. Therefore, the doses of propranolol should be kept to the minimum in patients with severe myocardial infarction. Caution should be exercised when administering propranolol in such situations, especially when a large portion of the myocardium has been damaged due to coronary occlusion since adequate sympathetic drive should be preserved to maintain ventricular function. Prior administration of other antiarrhythmic cardiac depressant drugs, such as procainamide or quinidine may potentiate the cardiac depressant activity of propranolol. Prior digitalization may be indicated and atropine should be at hand to control bradycardia.

The combination of propranolol with a thiazide like diuretic and/or peripheral vasodilator produces a greater fall in blood pressure than either drug alone. This occurs regardless of which drug is administered first. The same degree of blood pressure control can be achieved by lower than usual dosages of each drug. Therefore, when using such combined therapy, careful monitoring of the dosages is required until the patient is stabilized.

Patients receiving catecholamine depleting drugs such as reserpine or guanethidine should be closely observed if propranolol is administered concomitantly. The added catecholamine blocking action of this drug may produce an excessive reduction of the resting sympathetic nervous activity.

In patients on long-term treatment with propranolol, laboratory determinations should be made at regular intervals. The drug should be used with caution in patients with impaired renal and hepatic functions.

ADVERSE EFFECTS: The most serious adverse effects that may be encountered with propranolol are congestive heart failure and bronchospasm (see Contraindications, Warnings and Precautions).

Gastrointestinal disturbances (anorexia, nausea, vomiting, diarrhea, abdominal pain) are the most common adverse effects reported. Other less frequently reported adverse effects are: (in descending order) cold extremities and exacerbation of Raynaud's phenomenon; congestive heart failure; sleep disturbances including vivid dreams; dizziness, fatigue and bronchospasm.

The following adverse reactions have also been reported with the use of propranolol. Hypersensitivity reactions, including anaphylactic/anaphylactoid reactions, Stevens-Johnson Syndrome, toxic epidermal necrolysis, exfoliative dermatitis, erythema multiforme and urticaria.

Reported adverse effects, according to organ systems are recorded below.

Cardiovascular: congestive heart failure (see Warnings); secondary effects of decreased cardiac output which could include: syncope, vertigo, lightheadedness, decreased renal perfusion and rarely, postural hypotension; intensification of AV block and hypotension; severe bradycardia; claudication and cold extremities, Raynaud's phenomenon; dyspnea; palpitations; precordial pain.

Central Nervous System: dizziness, lethargy, weakness, drowsiness, headache, insomnia, fatigue, anorexia, anxiety, mental depression, poor concentration, reversible amnesia and catatonia, vivid dreams with or without insomnia, hallucinations, paresthesia, incoordination.

Gastrointestinal: nausea, vomiting, epigastric distress, anorexia, bloating, mild diarrhea, constipation.

Respiratory: bronchospasm; laryngospasm and respiratory distress (see Contraindications and Warnings).

Dermatologic: A few cases of erythematous rashes and increase of facial acneiform lesions have been reported; urticaria; exfoliative psoriasiform eruption, Stevens-Johnson syndrome, toxic epidermal necrolysis, exfoliative dermatitis and erythema multiforme.

Others: reduction or loss of libido; reversible alopecia and rarely: diminution and loss of hearing; tinnitus; visual disturbances; diminished vision, conjunctivitis; thrombocytopenic purpura; pharyngitis and agranulocytosis, fever combined with aching and sore throat; flushing of the face.

Allergic: hypersensitivity reactions, including anaphylactic/anaphylactoid reactions.

Clinical Laboratory Test Findings: Elevated blood urea levels in patients with severe heart disease, elevated serum transaminase, alkaline phosphatase, and lactate dehydrogenase have been reported.

OVERDOSE:

Symptoms: Several reports in the published literature describe cases in which propranolol was used as a suicide agent. In most cases, other agents, e.g., alcohol, have also been involved. One patient who died was thought to have ingested 3600 mg of propranolol. Survival of patients taking higher single doses has, however, also been reported. The common signs to be expected in overdosage are bradycardia, hypotension, bronchospasm, or acute cardiac failure.

Treatment: If overdosage occurs, in all cases therapy with propranolol should be discontinued and the patient observed closely. In addition the following therapeutic measures are suggested:

Bradycardia: Administer atropine incrementally in 600 µg (0.6 mg) doses. If there is no response to vagal blockade, administer isoproterenol cautiously.

Cardiac Failure: Digitalization and diuretics.

Hypotension: Vasopressors, e.g., epinephrine or levarterenol. (There is evidence that epinephrine is the drug of choice.)

Bronchospasm: Administer isoproterenol and aminophylline.

For management of a suspected drug overdose, CPhA recommends that you contact your **regional Poison Control Centre**. See the *CPS* Directory section for a list of Poison Control Centres.

DOSAGE: Inderal-LA Extended-Release Capsules are intended for maintenance therapy in those patients requiring doses within the range of 60 to 320 mg/day. Initiation of treatment and individual titration of dosage should be carried out using the conventional tablets. Inderal-LA may be preferred for maintenance because of the convenience of once-daily dosage. Patients with angina or hypertension on a maintenance regimen within the range of 60 to 320 mg/day regular tablets taken in divided doses may be changed to the appropriate number of Inderal-LA capsules taken once daily in the morning or evening.

However, Inderal-LA should not be considered a simple mg-for-mg substitute for conventional propranolol tablets and blood levels achieved are lower than those of 2 to 4 times daily dosing with the same dose. When changing to Inderal-LA from conventional propranolol tablets, a possible need for retitration upwards should be considered, especially to maintain effectiveness at the end of the dosing interval. In most clinical settings, however, such as hypertension or angina where there is little correlation between plasma levels and clinical effect, Inderal-LA has been shown to be therapeutically equivalent to the same mg dose of conventional propranolol as assessed by 24-hour effects on blood pressure, and on 24-hour exercise responses of heart rate, systolic pressure, and rate pressure product. Inderal-LA can provide effective beta blockade for 24-hour periods.

When propranolol is combined with another antihypertensive agent which is already being administered, therapy should be initiated with conventional propranolol tablets following usual dosage recommendations. Once adequate blood pressure control has been obtained, Inderal-LA capsules may be used for maintenance provided the dosage requirement is suitable.

In the treatment of hypertension, if required, further reduction of blood pressure may be attained by the addition of diuretic and/or peripheral vasodilator. Addition of another antihypertensive agent should, however, be gradual, beginning with 50% of the usual recommended starting dose, to avoid excessive reduction of blood pressure.

SUPPLIED: 60 mg: Each white/light blue, extended-release capsule, identified by 3 narrow bands, 1 wide band, and INDERAL-LA 60, contains: propranolol HCl 60 mg. Nonmedicinal ingredients: ethylcellulose, hydroxypropyl methylcellulose and microcrystalline cellulose; empty capsule: FD&C Blue No. 1, FD&C Red No. 3, gelatin, silicon dioxide, sodium lauryl sulfate and titanium dioxide. Energy: 0.84 kJ (0.2 kcal). Alcohol-, gluten-, lactose-, sodium-, sugar-, sulfites- and tartrazine-free. Bottles of 100.

80 mg: Each light blue, extended-release capsule, identified by 3 narrow bands, 1 wide band, and INDERAL-LA 80, contains: propranolol HCl 80 mg. Nonmedicinal ingredients: ethylcellulose, hydroxypropyl methylcellulose and microcrystalline cellulose; empty capsule: FD&C Blue No. 1, FD&C Red No. 3, gelatin, silicon dioxide, sodium lauryl sulfate and titanium dioxide. Alcohol-, gluten-, lactose-, sodium-, sugar-, sulfites- and tartrazine-free. Energy: 0.84 kJ (0.2 kcal). Bottles 100.

120 mg: Each light blue/dark blue, extended-release capsule, identified by 3 narrow bands, 1 wide band and INDERAL-LA 120, contains: propranolol HCl 120 mg. Nonmedicinal ingredients: ethylcellulose, hydroxypropyl methylcellulose and microcrystalline cellulose; empty capsule: FD&C Blue No. 1, FD&C Red No. 3, gelatin, silicon dioxide, sodium lauryl sulfate and titanium dioxide. Energy: 0.84 kJ (0.2 kcal). Alcohol-, gluten-, lactose-, sodium-, sugar-, sulfites- and tartrazine-free. Bottles of 100.

160 mg: Each dark blue, extended-release capsule, identified by 3 narrow bands, 1 wide band, and INDERAL-LA 160, contains: propranolol HCl 160 mg. Nonmedicinal ingredients: ethylcellulose, hydroxypropyl methylcellulose and microcrystalline cellulose; empty capsule: FD&C Blue No. 1, gelatin and titanium dioxide. Energy: 1.26 kJ (0.3 kcal). Alcohol-, gluten-, lactose-, sodium-, sugar-, sulfites- and tartrazine-free. Bottles of 100 and 500.

(Shown in Product Identification Section)

Indomethacin Pr

Nonsteroidal Anti-inflammatory Agent

CPhA Monograph

Date of Preparation: November 2004

Date of Revision: August 2009

This monograph has been compiled by CPhA and reviewed by experts. It may contain information different from that found in Health Canada-approved Product Monographs. The reader is referred to the *CPS* Editorial Policy for more information.

SUMMARY PRODUCT INFORMATION:

Route of Administration	Dosage Form	Strength
Oral	Capsule	25 mg, 50 mg
Rectal	Suppository	50 mg, 100 mg

Intravenous indomethacin, which is used to facilitate closure of a patent ductus arteriosus in premature infants, is not discussed in this monograph (please refer to the Indocid P.D.A. product monograph).

INDICATIONS AND CLINICAL USE: Because of the potential for adverse effects indomethacin should not be used as a simple analgesic or antipyretic.

Indomethacin, orally and rectally, has been effective in active stages of the following:

- Moderate to severe rheumatoid arthritis, including acute flares of chronic disease
- Moderate to severe ankylosing spondylitis
- Moderate to severe osteoarthritis
- Acute painful shoulder (bursitis and/or tendonitis)
- Acute gouty arthritis

Oral indomethacin and some other nonsteroidal anti-inflammatory drugs (NSAIDs) appear to be equally efficacious in treating acute gout, based on small randomized trials.

Indomethacin has also been used in other conditions including Reiter's syndrome (reactive arthritis), acute renal colic and dysmenorrhea.

NSAIDs do not prevent disease progression and will only decrease inflammation (and thus relieve symptoms) for as long as the patient continues to take the drug.

Geriatrics: Use with caution in geriatric individuals 65 years or older since increasing age may be associated with increased risk of adverse events. See Warnings and Precautions.

Pediatrics: Indomethacin ordinarily should not be prescribed for children 14 years of age and under. See Warnings and Precautions. However, intravenous indomethacin has been used to facilitate closure of a patent ductus arteriosus in premature infants.

CONTRAINDICATIONS:

- Hypersensitivity to the drug or to any ingredient in the formulation or component of indomethacin capsules or suppositories.
- Known or suspected hypersensitivity to other nonsteroidal anti-inflammatory drugs. The potential for cross-reactivity between different nonsteroidal anti-inflammatory drugs must be kept in mind.
- Active peptic, duodenal or gastric ulcer, a history of recurrent ulceration, or active inflammatory disease of the gastrointestinal tract.
- Indomethacin should not be used perioperatively in coronary artery bypass graft (CABG) surgery. The risk of myocardial infarction and stroke may be increased in this setting.
- Cerebrovascular bleeding or other bleeding disorder.
- Indomethacin should not be used in patients with the complete or partial syndrome of ASA-intolerance (rhinosinusitis, urticaria/angioedema, nasal polyps, asthma) in whom asthma, anaphylaxis, urticaria/angioedema, rhinitis or other allergic manifestations are precipitated by ASA or other nonsteroidal anti-inflammatory drugs. As well, patients with the above conditions are at risk even if they have taken NSAIDs in the past without adverse events.
- Significant hepatic impairment or active liver disease.
- Severely impaired or deteriorating renal function (creatinine clearance <30 mL/min). Individuals with a lesser degree of renal impairment are at risk of deterioration of their renal function when prescribed indomethacin, and must be monitored.
- Severe uncontrolled heart failure.
- Third trimester of pregnancy. Indomethacin use late in pregnancy may prolong parturition and increases the risk of premature closing of the ductus arteriosus.
- Indomethacin should not be used in the presence of known hyperkalemia (see Warnings and Precautions, Fluid and Electrolyte Balance).
- Indomethacin is not recommended for use with other NSAIDs, including ASA, because of the lack of evidence of any additive therapeutic benefits and the potential for increased adverse events. Concurrent use with ketorolac is contraindicated.
- Indomethacin suppositories are contraindicated in patients with a history of proctitis or recent rectal bleeding.

WARNINGS AND PRECAUTIONS:

> **Serious Warnings and Precautions**
> - Indomethacin is associated with an increased risk of cardiovascular thrombotic events such as stroke, myocardial infarction (MI) and new onset or worsening of pre-existing hypertension.
> - Indomethacin may increase the risk of serious gastrointestinal (GI) events such as ulceration, bleeding and perforation as well as GI irritation. These events may occur without prior symptoms.

General: The lowest possible effective dose for the individual patient should be prescribed, for the shortest possible duration. Increasing the dose, particularly over 200 mg per day, increases the risk of adverse effects, without corresponding increase in clinical benefits.

Aseptic Meningitis: In occasional cases, with some nonsteroidal anti-inflammatory drugs, the symptoms of aseptic meningitis (stiff neck, severe headache, nausea and vomiting, fever or clouding of consciousness) have been observed. Patients with autoimmune disorders (e.g., systemic lupus erythematosus, mixed connective tissue diseases) seem to be predisposed. Health care providers must be vigilant in monitoring for this potential adverse effect.

Infection: In common with other NSAIDs, indomethacin may suppress fever.

Cardiovascular: Use of indomethacin has been associated with an increased risk of serious cardiovascular adverse effects (myocardial infarction, stroke, thrombotic events). Patients with pre-existing cardiovascular disease or cardiovascular risk factors and those with a longer duration of therapy may be at higher risk. Use caution when prescribing indomethacin to patients with ischemic heart disease, cerebrovascular disease and/or heart failure, as well as to patients with risk factors for cardiovascular, cerebrovascular or renal disease (e.g., hypertension, dyslipidemias, diabetes, heart failure (NYHA I), coronary or peripheral artery disease, transient ischemic attacks, smoking, ClCr <60 mL/min).

The use of indomethacin can promote sodium retention which may exacerbate hypertension and/or heart failure. Some patients with pre-existing hypertension may develop worsening of blood pressure control when placed on indomethacin, and regular monitoring of blood pressure is essential.

Dermatologic: Serious skin reactions (e.g., Stevens-Johnson syndrome, toxic epidermal necrolysis, exfoliative dermatitis, erythema multiforme) have been associated with the use of some NSAIDs; however, causality is not clear. Patients who experience a skin rash while on indomethacin should be advised to contact their physician for assessment and advice, as these reactions are potentially life threatening but may be reversible if the causative agent is discontinued and appropriate treatment instituted.

Ear/Nose/Throat: Ototoxicity including tinnitus and hearing loss has been reported with all nonsteroidal anti-inflammatory drugs. The incidence of ototoxicity appears to be greater for ASA compared to indomethacin.

Fluid and Electrolyte Balance: Fluid retention and edema have been observed in patients treated with indomethacin. Therefore the possibility of precipitating heart failure in elderly patients or those with compromised cardiac function should be borne in mind. Indomethacin should be used with caution in patients with heart failure, hypertension or other conditions predisposing to fluid retention. Patients who are at risk for fluid retention should weigh themselves at regular intervals to assist in monitoring for fluid accumulation. With indomethacin use there is the potential risk for hyperkalemia, particularly in patients with diabetes mellitus or renal dysfunction or in patients receiving concomitant therapy with potassium supplements, angiotensin-II receptor antagonists, beta-blockers, angiotensin-converting enzyme inhibitors or potassium-sparing diuretics. It is essential that patients at risk be monitored on a routine basis for hyperkalemia. Hyponatremia has also been reported in elderly patients.

Gastrointestinal: Gastrointestinal toxicity and symptoms are possible with both the oral and rectal use of indomethacin.

Serious gastrointestinal toxicity, such as ulceration, perforation, obstruction and gastrointestinal bleeding, sometimes severe and potentially fatal, can occur at any time, with or without symptoms in patients treated with NSAIDs, including indomethacin.

Gastrointestinal symptoms such as dyspepsia are common, usually developing early in therapy. Dyspepsia does not necessarily correlate with mucosal damage. Health care providers should remain alert for ulceration and bleeding in patients treated with NSAIDs, even in the absence of gastrointestinal symptoms.

In patients observed in clinical trials of such drugs, symptomatic upper gastrointestinal ulcers, gross bleeding or perforation appear to occur in approximately 1% of patients treated for 3 to 6 months and in about 2 to 4% of patients treated for 1 year. The risk continues beyond 1 year. The incidence of these complications is related to dose, past history of known ulcer disease, concurrent use of more than one NSAID and advanced age (see Special Populations).

Indomethacin should be given under close medical supervision to patients with a history of ulcer of the upper gastrointestinal tract or inflammatory disease of the gastrointestinal tract such as ulcerative colitis or Crohn's disease. In these cases the health care provider must weigh the benefits of treatment against the potential adverse effects.

Patients should be informed of the signs and symptoms of serious toxicity and instructed to contact a health care provider immediately if they experience persistent dyspepsia or other signs or symptoms suggestive of gastrointestinal bleeding or ulceration. If ulceration is suspected or confirmed, or if gastrointestinal bleeding occurs, discontinue indomethacin immediately, institute appropriate therapy and monitor the patient closely.

Because serious gastrointestinal tract ulceration and bleeding can occur without warning symptoms, health care providers should follow chronically treated patients and watch for signs and symptoms of ulceration and bleeding and should inform patients of the importance of this follow-up.

The major risk factors are a prior history of serious gastrointestinal events and advancing age. Other possible risk factors include *H. pylori* infection, excessive ethanol intake, smoking, concurrent use of more than one NSAID, high doses of NSAID, and concomitant use of oral corticosteroids, anticoagulants, antiplatelet agents (including ASA) or selective serotonin reuptake inhibitors (SSRIs). Consider concomitant cytoprotective therapy (using a proton pump inhibitor, misoprostol or twice the standard dose of an H_2 receptor antagonist such as famotidine or ranitidine) in patients with one or more risk factors for serious gastrointestinal events.

Hematologic: In patients with coagulopathies, in those receiving anticoagulants and in those at risk for blood dyscrasias indomethacin should be used with caution because hematologic side effects may be more likely to occur. See Adverse Reactions, Hematologic.

Hepatic/Biliary/Pancreatic: As with other NSAIDs, borderline elevations of one or more liver enzyme tests (AST, ALT, ALP) may occur in up to 15% of patients. These abnormalities may progress, remain unchanged, and/or be transient with continued therapy.

Fatal hepatitis has been reported in children with juvenile rheumatoid arthritis treated with indomethacin.

Patients with symptoms and/or signs suggesting liver dysfunction, or in whom an abnormal liver test has occurred should be evaluated for evidence of a more serious hepatic reaction while on therapy with indomethacin. Severe hepatic reactions including jaundice and cases of fatal hepatitis have been reported with nonsteroidal anti-inflammatory drugs.

Although such reactions are rare, if abnormal liver tests persist or worsen, if clinical signs and symptoms consistent with liver disease develop (e.g., jaundice) or if systemic manifestations occur (e.g., eosinophilia, rash) indomethacin should be discontinued. In the presence of liver disease, indomethacin should be used with extreme caution.

Immune: Cross-sensitivity: Patients sensitive to any nonsteroidal anti-inflammatory drugs, including acetylsalicylic acid may be sensitive to indomethacin. ASA-intolerance: As with nonsteroidal anti-inflammatory drugs in general, some patients may experience urticaria upon exposure to indomethacin. Patients with partial or complete syndrome of ASA-intolerance should not be given indomethacin (see Contraindications).

Ophthalmologic: Blurred and/or diminished vision have been reported with the use of NSAIDs and may be early symptoms of adverse ocular effects of indomethacin. Corneal deposits and retinal disturbances have been reported in patients receiving chronic indomethacin therapy. Blurred vision warrants evaluation by an ophthalmologist. Generally the symptoms are reversible when indomethacin is stopped. If long-term therapy with indomethacin is warranted, consider routine evaluation by an ophthalmologist since some patients will have no symptoms.

Perioperative Considerations: As with other NSAIDs, indomethacin is a reversible inhibitor of platelet aggregation. The drug should be discontinued 4 to 7 days before surgery to reduce the risk of bleeding. Consider discontinuing indomethacin 2 weeks before surgery where bleeding could be catastrophic, such as with neurosurgery. Indomethacin is contraindicated in the perioperative treatment of pain in coronary artery bypass graft (CABG) surgery (see Contraindications).

Psychiatric: A relationship between indomethacin and the development of psychosis, aggressive behavior and cognitive dysfunction is especially evident in patients of advanced age. Patients do not necessarily have a history of previous psychiatric disturbances or cognitive impairment. Withdrawal of the drug and appropriate therapy usually reverses these symptoms.

Renal: Acute renal failure which is usually reversible has been reported with the use of indomethacin. In many cases onset of renal failure occurs within 2 days to 2 weeks of initiating therapy. Renal failure has occurred in the absence of pre-existing impairment. Patients at greatest risk are those with renal and hepatic impairment, heart failure, diabetes mellitus, hypovolemia, advanced age, concurrent use of other nephrotoxic drugs or pyelonephritis. Renal dysfunction with indomethacin is likely related to inhibition of prostaglandin synthesis and renin-induced vasoconstriction.

As with other NSAIDs, indomethacin has been associated with hyperkalemia (see Fluid and Electrolyte Balance).

Respiratory: ASA-induced asthma is an uncommon but very important indication of ASA and NSAID sensitivity. It occurs more frequently in patients with asthma who have nasal polyps.

Sensitivity/Resistance: Patients sensitive to any one of the NSAIDs may be sensitive to any of the other drugs of this class.

Special Populations: Pregnant Women: As with all NSAIDs, the use of indomethacin in pregnancy should be weighed against the risks and should not be used unless considered essential. The drug is generally considered safe for short periods of time in the second trimester of pregnancy. Long term use (>48 hours) and third trimester use are contraindicated.

Nursing Women: Indomethacin is excreted in breast milk likely in very small amounts. It is considered compatible with breastfeeding.

Pediatrics (birth to 16 years old): Indomethacin should not be used in children under the age of two years except as intravenous indomethacin to facilitate closure of a patent ductus arteriosus in premature infants (see Indocid P.D.A. monograph). Effectiveness of indomethacin in children has not been established. Indomethacin should not be prescribed for children 14 years of age and younger unless toxicity or lack of efficacy associated with other drugs warrants the risk. The lowest effective dose should be used. Limited clinical information suggests the adverse effects experienced by children receiving indomethacin are similar to those in adults. Fatal hepatitis has been reported in children with juvenile rheumatoid arthritis treated with indomethacin. Experience with indomethacin in children >2 years of age is limited to the capsule formulation.

Geriatrics: Elderly, frail or debilitated patients are most susceptible to the adverse effects associated with nonsteroidal anti-inflammatory drugs; the incidence of these adverse effects increases with the dose and duration of treatment. In addition these patients are at increased risk of lower esophageal ulceration and bleeding. Most reports of fatal gastrointestinal events are in this population, especially those with pre-existing cardiovascular disease.

Monitoring and Laboratory Tests: With chronic use of indomethacin, consider obtaining a baseline hemoglobin, serum creatinine, serum potassium and sodium, complete blood count, fecal occult blood test and liver function tests before or within a month of initiating therapy. Repeat these tests periodically during therapy or if toxicities are suspected. High-risk (e.g., older than 65 years; pediatric patients; history of peptic ulcer disease; prolonged use of high-dose indomethacin; concurrent use of potentially nephrotoxic drugs, corticosteroids, antiplatelets, anticoagulants or drugs affecting serum potassium) may require monitoring every 3 months. If long-term therapy with indomethacin is warranted, consider routine evaluation by an ophthalmologist.

Counsel patients to inform their health care providers immediately of symptoms of serious adverse events associated with indomethacin therapy such as gastrointestinal ulceration and bleeding, changes in vision, symptoms of heart or renal failure, bruising and nongastrointestinal bleeding, hypersensitivity and severe headache.

ADVERSE REACTIONS: More Common Adverse Drug Reactions (>1%): The most common adverse reactions encountered with nonsteroidal anti-inflammatory drugs are gastrointestinal, of which gastric or duodenal ulcer, with or without bleeding, is the most severe. Fatalities have occurred, particularly in the elderly. The more common adverse reactions for indomethacin capsules are listed in Table 1.

It is likely similar rates of adverse events will be seen with the use of rectal indomethacin. In addition rectal irritation and tenesmus have been reported with the use of indomethacin suppositories.

Table 1: Indomethacin

More Common Adverse Drug Reactions (>1%)

Gastrointestinal	Nausea (3–9%) Vomiting (3–9%) Dyspepsia (3–9%) Abdominal pain (1–3%) Constipation (1–3%) Diarrhea (2%)
CNS	Headache (11.7%) Dizziness (3–9%) Vertigo (1–3%) Somnolence (1–3%) Depression (1–3%)
Special Senses	Tinnitus (1–3%)

Less Common Adverse Drug Reactions: Cardiovascular: Hypertension, hypotension and heart failure have been reported.

CNS: Anxiety, fatigue, paresthesia, insomnia, psychotic disturbances, mental confusion, light-headedness, syncope, peripheral neuropathy and seizures have all been reported.

Dermatologic: Rarely, rash, urticaria, pruritus, alopecia, Stevens-Johnson syndrome, toxic epidermal necrolysis, purpura, psoriasis and petechiae have been reported with NSAID use.

Endocrine and Metabolism: Isolated cases of male sexual dysfunction have been reported.

Gastrointestinal: Peptic ulcer, gastrointestinal bleeding and perforation, anorexia and gastritis.

Genitourinary: Some NSAIDs are associated with persistent urinary symptoms (bladder pain, dysuria, urinary frequency), hematuria, interstitial nephritis or cystitis. The initiation of these symptoms may occur at any time after the initiation of therapy with a nonsteroidal anti-inflammatory drug. Should urinary symptoms occur, in the absence of an alternative explanation, stop treatment with indomethacin to ascertain if symptoms disappear. This should be done before urological investigations or treatments are considered.

Hematologic: Leukopenia, coagulopathy, and rarely aplastic anemia have reported with the use of indomethacin, especially following chronic ingestion with therapeutic doses. Bone marrow suppression, agranulocytosis and hemolytic anemia have also been reported. Indomethacin as a nonsteroidal anti-inflammatory drug can inhibit platelet aggregation within 2 hours of taking the drug. The mechanism of this response is related to the inhibition of prostaglandin synthetase.

Hepatic/Biliary/Pancreatic: Hepatitis, jaundice and liver function test abnormalities have been reported.

Hypersensitivity: Acute anaphylaxis, acute respiratory distress, angioedema and fever have been reported in patients using NSAIDs.

Neurologic: Indomethacin may cause drowsiness. Therefore patients should be cautioned against engaging in activities requiring mental alertness and motor coordination such as driving or operating machinery.

There have been rare reports of peripheral neuropathy; symptoms disappeared when the drug was discontinued. Pseudotumor cerebri and seizures have been reported rarely with indomethacin use.

Renal: Proteinuria and nephrotic syndrome have been reported.
Miscellaneous: Edema, hyperkalemia and hypo/hyperglycemia, blurred vision, retinal/macular disturbances. Aseptic meningitis has been reported rarely with NSAID use.

DRUG INTERACTIONS: Overview: Because indomethacin is a nonsteroidal anti-inflammatory drug most of the potentially serious drug interactions are related to increasing the risks of serious gastrointestinal adverse effects, hyperkalemia, renal dysfunction and coagulopathies. Most of the drug interactions are potentially pharmacodynamic in nature, rather than pharmacokinetic. (See Table 2.)

Indomethacin is a strong inhibitor as well as a substrate of CYP 2C9; there is a theoretical potential for interaction with other drugs significantly metabolized by this enzyme.
Drug-Drug Interactions: See Table 2.
Drug-Herb Interactions: Feverfew: In theory, concomitant use of feverfew and indomethacin may predispose patients to more adverse effects of nonsteroidal anti-inflammatory agents (e.g., gastropathy, renal dysfunction and increased risk of bleeding). Concurrent use should be avoided. Probable mechanism is additive prostaglandin and thromboxane inhibition.

Table 2: Indomethacin

Drug-Drug Interactions

Interacting Drug	Effect	Clinical Comment
ACE Inhibitors	Indomethacin may diminish the antihypertensive effects of ACEIs. Combination use of ACEIs, diuretics and indomethacin may increase the risk for acute renal failure and hyperkalemia.	Monitor blood pressure, renal function and serum potassium.
Alcohol	There may be an increased risk of GI side effects (including ulceration or GI bleeding) if alcohol is ingested with NSAIDs.	
Anticoagulants	Numerous studies have shown that the concomitant use of NSAIDs and anticoagulants increases the risk of serious gastrointestinal adverse events, such as bleeding and ulceration.	Concurrent use of indomethacin and warfarin requires close monitoring of the INR; increased bleeding may occur in spite of such monitoring.
Corticosteroids	Concomitant use of corticosteroids and NSAIDs can increase the risk of serious gastrointestinal adverse events, such as ulceration and bleeding. Elderly patients are at greater risk.	Avoid concurrent administration. If deemed necessary, monitor closely for signs and symptoms of gastrointestinal toxicity. Cytoprotection with a proton pump inhibitor or misoprostol is advised [*Am J Gastroenterol* 2009;104(3):728-38].
Cyclosporine	Concomitant administration of indomethacin and cyclosporine may increase the nephrotoxic effects of cyclosporine. This interaction may be related to inhibition of the synthesis of the renal prostaglandin, prostacyclin.	Use concomitantly with caution and monitor renal function and cyclosporine levels.
Diflunisal	The administration of diflunisal to normal volunteers receiving indomethacin decreased the renal clearance and significantly increased the plasma levels of indomethacin. Further, the combined use of indomethacin and diflunisal has been associated with fatal GI hemorrhage.	Avoid concurrent use.
Digoxin	Possible increased digoxin levels.	Use with caution and monitor digoxin levels.
Diuretics	Clinical studies as well as post-marketing surveillance have shown that NSAIDs can reduce the clinical effects of diuretics. (See also potassium-sparing diuretics.) The combination of diuretics, ACEIs and indomethacin may increase the risk for acute renal failure and hyperkalemia.	Use concomitantly with caution and monitor effectiveness, renal function and serum potassium.
Lithium	Indomethacin can increase serum lithium concentrations.	Monitor lithium levels when starting or stopping indomethacin and during chronic indomethacin therapy.
Methotrexate	NSAIDs have been reported to decrease the tubular secretion of methotrexate and potentiate the toxicity.	Avoid the concomitant use of high dose methotrexate; in the case of low dose weekly methotrexate use the combination with caution and monitor for signs and symptoms of toxicity.
NSAIDs	The use of indomethacin in addition to any other NSAID (including topical preparations) is not recommended because of the absence of any evidence demonstrating additive effects and the potential for additive adverse events. Also, some NSAIDs may interfere with the antiplatelet effects of low dose ASA, possibly by competing with ASA for access to the active site of cyclooxygenase-1. The concurrent use of 2 NSAIDs increases the risk of serious gastrointestinal adverse events, such as bleeding and ulceration.	Avoid concurrent use of indomethacin with other NSAIDs, including ASA if possible. Concomitant use of ketorolac and indomethacin is contraindicated.
Potassium supplements, potassium-sparing diuretics, drospirenone	Potential for hyperkalemia, especially in patients with renal dysfunction.	Monitor serum potassium especially in susceptible individuals and with chronic use.
Quinolones	The concomitant use of quinolones and NSAIDs may increase the risk of CNS stimulation and seizure activity.	Use with caution, especially in susceptible individuals.
SSRIs	SSRIs increase the risk of gastrointestinal bleeding and this effect can be potentiated by concomitant use of NSAIDs. The mechanism is likely related to additive effects on platelet inhibition.	Monitor patients for increased signs of bleeding.

Garlic: Caution is advised with the concomitant use of indomethacin and garlic because of the increased risk of bleeding. The probable mechanism involves potentiation of antiplatelet aggregation.
Ginkgo: Avoid the concomitant use of indomethacin and ginkgo because of the increased risk of bleeding. The probable mechanism is potentiation of antiplatelet aggregation. If both agents must be used together monitor bleeding time and signs and symptoms of bleeding.

Use caution with concomitant use of indomethacin and other natural health products with anticoagulant or antiplatelet properties.
Drug-Laboratory Interactions: Nonsteroidal anti-inflammatory drugs may cause gastrointestinal bleeding, which may produce positive fecal hemoccult test results in some individuals and therefore interfere with screening for colorectal cancer. When screening for occult fecal blood loss, nonsteroidal anti-inflammatory drugs may need to be withheld for 2 to 4 days prior to testing, as a positive fecal hemoccult test may be attributable to nonsteroidal anti-inflammatory drug therapy.

Indomethacin decreases platelet aggregation and prolongs bleeding time. The effect of indomethacin on bleeding time should be taken into account when the test is performed.

Indomethacin may cause a false negative dexamethasone suppression test in patients with depression.

DOSAGE AND ADMINISTRATION: Dosing Considerations:

- Use the lowest effective dose, for the shortest duration necessary to control symptoms.
- Indomethacin should always be administered with food or immediately after meals.
- Administration with antacids or H_2 receptor antagonists (cimetidine, famotidine, ranitidine) may help with the gastrointestinal intolerance associated with indomethacin, but will not prevent serious gastrointestinal adverse events. Consider concomitant cytoprotective therapy (using a proton pump inhibitor, misoprostol or twice the standard dose of an H_2 receptor antagonist) in patients with one or more risk factors for serious gastrointestinal events.
- Adverse events with indomethacin appear to be dose related in most patients; every effort should be made to determine the smallest effective dose for individual patients.

Recommended Dose and Dosage Adjustment: See Table 3.

Based on pharmacokinetic data, the total amount of drug absorbed from the rectal suppository is expected to be similar to that from the capsule. Clinical trials suggest the amount of indomethacin absorbed from the suppository is between 80 and 90%. It is suggested that the total daily dose of indomethacin administered rectally not exceed 200 mg. In patients who have persistent night pain or morning stiffness, up to 100 mg of the total daily dose may be given at bedtime either orally or rectally to help with symptoms.
Dose in Geriatric Patients: The initial dose should be one-half the usual adult dose. The maintenance dose should be reduced by 25% in elderly patients because pharmacokinetic studies indicate decreased clearance and increased half-life in such patients.
Dose in Pediatric Patients: See Table 4.
Dose in Adult or Pediatric Patients with Renal Impairment: No dosage adjustment is required for patients with renal dysfunction or failure. While there is not a significant prolongation of the drug's half-life, as with any NSAID, indomethacin should be used with caution in patients with renal dysfunction.
Dosage in Dialysis: Dosage supplementation is not necessary following hemodialysis, continuous ambulatory peritoneal dialysis or continuous arteriovenous hemodialysis.
Hepatic Impairment: Indomethacin should be avoided in patients with significant hepatic impairment.
Missed Dose: Patients should be instructed to take a missed dose as soon as they remember, and not to double the dose or exceed their daily recommended dose.
Administration: Indomethacin capsules should be swallowed whole, not crushed or chewed. Indomethacin should be administered with food or meals.

Table 3: Indomethacin

Indomethacin Dose in Adult Patients

Indication	Route	Initial Dose	Usual Dose	Maximum Dose	Duration of Treatment	Detailed Information
Acute gouty arthritis	Oral	50 mg three times daily	50 mg three times daily	200 mg daily	Until pain is tolerable	The dose should then be rapidly reduced to complete cessation of the drug. Tenderness and heat usually subside in 24 to 48 hours and swelling gradually disappears in 3 to 6 days.
• Moderate to severe rheumatoid arthritis, including acute flares of chronic disease • Moderate to severe ankylosing spondylitis • Moderate to severe osteoarthritis	Oral	25 mg two or three times daily	If initial dose is tolerated, increase dose by 25 or 50 mg by weekly intervals. Titrate only if required and until satisfactory response is obtained.	200 mg daily	As required	Indomethacin should be stopped if severe adverse events occur. After acute phase of the disease is under control, an attempt to reduce the daily dose should be made until the patient is receiving the lowest possible effective dose.
Acute painful shoulder (bursitis and/or tendonitis)	Oral	25 to 50 mg three times daily	25 to 50 mg three times daily	200 mg daily	The usual course of therapy is 7 to 14 days	The drug should be discontinued after the signs and symptoms of inflammation have been controlled for several days.

Table 4: Indomethacin

Indomethacin Dose in Pediatric Patients

Indication	Route	Initial Dose	Usual Dose	Maximum Dose	Duration of Treatment	Detailed Information
Juvenile rheumatoid arthritis	Oral	1–2 mg/kg/day in divided doses	Between 2 and 4 mg/kg/day or lowest effective dose	4 mg/kg/day or 150 mg to 200 mg daily (whichever is less)	As required	Indomethacin should be stopped if severe adverse events occur. After acute phase of the disease is controlled, an attempt to reduce the daily dose should be made until the patient is receiving the lowest possible effective dose.

OVERDOSAGE:

For management of a suspected drug overdose, CPhA recommends that you contact your **regional Poison Control Centre**. See the *CPS* Directory section for a list of Poison Control Centres.

ACTION AND CLINICAL PHARMACOLOGY: Mechanism of Action: Indomethacin is a nonsteroidal anti-inflammatory drug with analgesic and antipyretic properties, but exhibits these effects without altering the course of the underlying disease. It is a reversible inhibitor of the enzymes cyclooxygenase-1 and 2, thus decreasing the formation of prostaglandin precursors. This inhibition occurs in vitro and, in the concentrations reached during therapy, also has an in vivo effect.

Pharmacokinetics: Absorption: Indomethacin is readily absorbed orally. Peak plasma concentrations of about 1 and 2 μg/mL are attained about 2 hours following single doses of 25 mg or 50 mg. After 4 hours, 99% of an orally administered dose has been absorbed.

Distribution: At therapeutic plasma concentrations, about 99% of indomethacin is bound to plasma protein. The drug crosses the blood-brain barrier and the placenta, and is excreted in breast milk. Indomethacin and its conjugates undergo enterohepatic circulation.

Metabolism: Indomethacin is metabolized in the liver and exists in the plasma as the parent drug as well as the unconjugated forms of the desmethyl, desbenzoyl and desmethyl-desbenzoyl metabolites.

Excretion: Indomethacin is eliminated via renal and biliary excretion; about 60% of an oral dose is recovered in the urine (as drug and metabolites) and 33% in the feces. Its mean half-life is estimated to be about 4.5 hours. With doses of 25 or 50 mg TID, steady state drug plasma concentrations are on average about 1.4 times those following the first dose.

Infanrix hexa™

combined diphtheria and tetanus toxoids, acellular pertussis, hepatitis B (recombinant), inactivated poliomyelitis and adsorbed conjugated H. influenzae type b vaccine

Active Immunizing Agent

GlaxoSmithKline

Date of Revision: July 18, 2008

SUMMARY PRODUCT INFORMATION:

Route of Administration	Dosage Form/ Strength	Clinically Relevant Nonmedicinal Ingredients
Intramuscular injection	Sterile suspension for injection/25 limit of flocculation (Lf) [30 International Units (IU)] diphtheria toxoid; 10 Lf (40 IU) tetanus toxoid; 25 μg pertussis toxoid (PT); 25 μg filamentous haemagglutinin (FHA); 8 μg pertactin; 10 μg hepatitis B surface antigen (HBsAg); 40 D-antigen units (DU) of type 1 poliovirus, 8 DU type 2 poliovirus, and 32 DU type 3 poliovirus; 10 μg of adsorbed purified capsular polysaccharide of *H. influenzae* type b (Hib) (PRP) covalently bound to 20-40 μg of tetanus toxoid per 0.5 mL dose	Lactose, sodium chloride, aluminum adjuvant (as aluminum salts), water for injection, residual formaldehyde, polysorbate 20 and 80 (Tween 20 and 80), M199, potassium chloride, disodium phosphate, monopotassium phosphate, glycine, neomycin sulphate, and polymyxin B sulphate

DESCRIPTION: INFANRIX hexa (combined diphtheria and tetanus toxoids, acellular pertussis, hepatitis B (recombinant), inactivated poliomyelitis, and adsorbed conjugated *H. influenzae* type b vaccine) contains diphtheria toxoid, tetanus toxoid, three purified pertussis antigens [pertussis toxoid (PT), filamentous haemagglutinin (FHA) and pertactin (69 kiloDalton outer membrane protein)], hepatitis B virus surface antigen recombinant, adsorbed onto aluminum salts, purified, inactivated poliovirus types 1, 2 and 3, *H. influenzae* type b polysaccharide conjugated to tetanus toxoid.

INDICATIONS AND CLINICAL USE: Pediatrics: Primary Immunization: INFANRIX hexa (combined diphtheria and tetanus toxoids, acellular pertussis, hepatitis B (recombinant), inactivated poliomyelitis, and adsorbed conjugated *H. influenzae* type b vaccine) is indicated for:

- active primary immunization against diphtheria, tetanus, pertussis, hepatitis B, poliomyelitis, and disease caused by *H. influenzae* type b in infants and children 6 weeks to 2 years.

INFANRIX hexa will not prevent hepatitis caused by other agents, such as hepatitis A, C and E viruses, or other pathogens known to infect the liver. As hepatitis D (caused by the delta virus) does not occur in the absence of hepatitis B infection, it can be expected that hepatitis D will also be prevented by INFANRIX hexa vaccination.

Where a dose of hepatitis B vaccine is given at birth, INFANRIX hexa can be used for the second dose from the age of six weeks. If a second dose of hepatitis B vaccine is required before this age, monovalent Hepatitis B vaccine should be used.

INFANRIX hexa has not been evaluated in the Canadian Native Population.

Booster Vaccination: The administration of the booster dose should be given at 18 months as stated in the Canadian Immunization Guide.

INFANRIX hexa can be used for the booster dose provided that the infant has received a full primary vaccination course of each of the antigens contained in INFANRIX hexa, regardless of whether these were administered as monovalent or combination vaccines.

Other combinations of antigens have been studied in clinical trials following primary vaccination with INFANRIX hexa and may be used for a booster dose, these include diptheria, tetanus, acellular pertussis (DTPa) and DTPa/Hib.

CONTRAINDICATIONS: INFANRIX hexa (combined diphtheria and tetanus toxoids, acellular pertussis, hepatitis B (recombinant), inactivated poliomyelitis, and adsorbed conjugated *H. influenzae* type b vaccine):

- should not be administered to subjects with known hypersensitivity to any component of this vaccine (see Dosage Forms, Composition and Packaging) or to subjects having shown signs of hypersensitivity after a previous dose of this vaccine or any injection containing diphtheria, tetanus, pertussis, hepatitis B, poliovirus or *H. influenzae* type b (see Warnings and Precautions, General for information on treatment of immediate allergic reactions).
- should be used with caution in subjects with known hypersensitivity to the antibiotics neomycin and polymyxin, as INFANRIX hexa contains traces of these antibiotics.
- is contraindicated for use after an immediate anaphylactic reaction temporally associated with a previous dose of this vaccine or any injection containing diphtheria, tetanus, pertussis, hepatitis B, poliovirus, or *H. influenzae* type b. Because of the uncertainty as to which component of the vaccine might be responsible, no further vaccination with any of these components should be given. Alternatively, because of the importance of tetanus vaccination, such individuals may be referred to an allergist for evaluation.
- should not be administered to persons 7 years of age or older because diphtheria toxoid may cause severe but transient local and febrile reactions in children and adults, the frequency increasing with age, the dose of toxoid and the number of doses given.
- is contraindicated if the infant has experienced an encephalopathy of unknown etiology, occurring within 7 days following previous vaccination with a pertussis containing vaccine. In these circumstances, pertussis vaccination should be discontinued and the vaccination should be continued with diphtheria-tetanus, Hepatitis B, polio, and Hib vaccines.

Immunization should be deferred during the course of a moderate or severe acute febrile illness or acute infection (see Warnings and Precautions). The presence of a minor infection, however is not a contraindication.

Elective immunization of individuals over 6 months should be deferred during an outbreak of poliomyelitis.

WARNINGS AND PRECAUTIONS: General: INFANRIX hexa (combined diphtheria and tetanus toxoids, acellular pertussis, hepatitis B (recombinant), inactivated poliomyelitis, and adsorbed conjugated *H. influenzae* type b vaccine) should under no circumstances be administered intravascularly or intradermally.

As for all diphtheria, tetanus and pertussis vaccines, each injection should be given deep intramuscularly and each injection of the immunization series should be made at a different site.

As with other injectable vaccines, epinephrine injection (1:1000) and other appropriate agents used for the control of immediate allergic reactions must be immediately available should an acute anaphylactic reaction occur. For this reason, the vaccinee should remain under medical supervision for 30 minutes after immunization.

It is good clinical practice that vaccination should be preceded by a review of the medical history (especially with regard to previous vaccination and possible occurrence of undesirable events) and a clinical examination.

INFANRIX hexa will not prevent disease caused by pathogens other than *C. diphtheria*, *C. tetani*, *B. pertussis*, hepatitis B virus, poliovirus or *H. influenzae* type b .

As with any other vaccine, a protective immune response may not be elicited in all vaccinees for all component antigens in the vaccine. This product is not recommended for treatment of actual infections.

Where passive protection is required, Tetanus Immune Globulin and/or Diphtheria Antitoxin may also be administered at separate sites. Because of the substantial risks of complications from pertussis disease, completion of a primary series of vaccine early in life is strongly recommended.

If any of the following events occur in temporal relation to administration of whole-cell DTP or acellular DTP vaccine, the decision to give subsequent doses of vaccine containing the pertussis component should be carefully considered:

- Temperature of >40.5°C within 48 hours of vaccination not due to another identifiable cause.
- Collapse or shock-like state (hypotonic-hyporesponsive episode) within 48 hours of vaccination.
- Persistent, inconsolable crying lasting >3 hours, occurring within 48 hours of vaccination.
- Convulsions with or without fever occurring within 3 days of vaccination.

There may be circumstances, such as high incidence of pertussis, in which the potential benefits outweigh possible risks, particularly since these events have not been proven to cause permanent sequelae.

The Hib component of the vaccine does not protect against diseases due to capsular serotypes other than type b of *H. influenzae* or against meningitis caused by other organisms. Excretion of capsular polysaccharide antigen in the urine has been described following administration of Hib vaccines, and therefore antigen detection may not have a diagnostic value in suspected Hib disease within 1-2 weeks of vaccination. Other tests should be performed in order to confirm Hib infection during this period.

Hematologic: INFANRIX hexa should be administered with caution to subjects with thrombocytopenia or a bleeding disorder since bleeding may occur following intramuscular administration to these subjects.

Immune: Hepatitis B has a long incubation period. Hepatitis B vaccination may not prevent hepatitis B infection in individuals who had an unrecognized hepatitis B infection at the time of vaccine administration.

INFANRIX hexa is not contraindicated for use in individuals with HIV infection. The expected immunological response may not be obtained after vaccination of immunosuppressed patients.

Immunosuppressive therapies, including irradiation, antimetabolites, alkylating agents, cytotoxic drugs and corticosteroids (used in greater than physiologic doses), may reduce the immune response to vaccines (see Drug Interactions).

Hepatitis B: Infants born of HBsAg-positive mothers should receive hepatitis B immune globulin (HBIG) and Hepatitis B vaccine at birth and should complete the Hepatitis B vaccination series given according to a particular schedule. Infants born of mothers of unknown HBsAg status should receive Hepatitis B vaccine at birth and should complete the Hepatitis B vaccination series given according to a particular schedule (see Manufacturer's package insert for Hepatitis B vaccine).

The subsequent administration of INFANRIX hexa for completion of the Hepatitis B vaccination series in infants who were born of HBsAg-positive mothers and received HBIG, or infants born of mothers of unknown status has not been studied.

Neurologic: Experience with INFANRIX (DTPa) and other INFANRIX-based combinations has not revealed any cases of encephalopathy or permanent neurologic damage causally linked to vaccination. While acute encephalopathy and permanent neurologic damage have not been reported to be causally linked nor in a temporal association with administration of INFANRIX hexa data is limited at this time.

In children with progressive neurological disorders, including infantile spasms, uncontrolled epilepsy or progressive encephalopathy, it is better to defer pertussis (Pa or Pw) immunization until the condition is corrected or stable. However, the decision to give pertussis vaccine must be made on an individual basis after careful consideration of the risks and benefits.

A history of convulsions or other central nervous system disorders in parents or siblings is not a contraindication for INFANRIX hexa, an acellular DTP vaccine. Vaccinees with a history of febrile convulsions should be closely followed up as such adverse events may occur within 2 to 3 days post vaccination.

Studies suggest that when given whole-cell DTP vaccine, infants and children with a history of convulsions in first-degree family members (i.e., siblings and parents) have a 2.4-fold increased risk for neurologic events compared to those without such histories.

Respiratory: Although a moderate or severe illness with or without fever is a reason to defer vaccination, minor illnesses such as mild upper respiratory infections with or without low-grade fever are not a contraindication.

Special Populations: Pregnant Women: As INFANRIX hexa is not intended for use in adults, adequate human data on use during pregnancy and adequate animal reproduction studies are not available.

Nursing Women: As INFANRIX hexa is not intended for use in adults, adequate human data on use during lactation and adequate animal reproduction studies are not available.

Pediatrics: Limited data in 169 premature infants indicate that INFANRIX hexa can be given to premature children. However, a lower immune response may be observed and the level of clinical protection remains unknown. The potential risk of apnea and the need for respiratory monitoring for 48-72h should be considered when administering the primary immunization series to very premature infants (born ≤28 weeks of gestation) and particularly for those with a previous history of respiratory immaturity. As the benefit of vaccination is high in this group of infants, vaccination should not be withheld or delayed. Safety and effectiveness of INFANRIX hexa have not been established in infants below the age of 6 weeks and children over 2 years of age.

ADVERSE REACTIONS: Adverse Drug Reaction Overview: INFANRIX hexa (combined diphtheria and tetanus toxoids, acellular pertussis, hepatitis B (recombinant), inactivated poliomyelitis, and adsorbed conjugated *H. influenzae* type b vaccine) is generally well tolerated.

Clinical Trial Adverse Drug Reactions: Because clinical trials are conducted under very specific conditions the adverse reaction rates observed in the clinical trials may not reflect the rates observed in practice and should not be compared to the rates in the clinical trials of another drug. Adverse drug reaction information from clinical trials is useful for identifying drug-related adverse events and for approximating rates.

During a study conducted in the United States, a total of 785 documented doses of study vaccines were given to 267 subjects included in the According To Protocol (ATP) reactogenicity analysis. Solicited and unsolicited symptoms occurring during the 8-day follow-up period after vaccination were reported. Most reported solicited local symptoms and solicited general symptoms were mild to moderate in intensity. There were no statistically significant differences between the two groups in the incidence of soreness, redness or swelling at the injection site (regardless of side/site/dose) or fever. The percentage of subjects per group experiencing symptoms (both solicited and unsolicited) during the 8 days after vaccination is outlined in Table 1.

Table 1: INFANRIX hexa

Percentage of U.S. Infants with Local or Systemic Reactions within 8 Days of Primary Vaccination with either INFANRIX hexa or Commercially Available INFANRIX, ENGERIX-B, and OPV Administered Simultaneously with Hib at Separate Sites (Per subject analysis)

Event	INFANRIX hexa (N=134)	INFANRIX, ENGERIX-B, Hib vaccine, OPV (N=133)
Local	%	%
Pain, any	42.54	52.63
Pain, severe	1.49	2.26
Redness, any	48.51	47.37
Redness, >20 mm	2.24	3.01
Swelling, any	35.82	40.6
Swelling, >20 mm	3.73	4.51
Systemic	%	%
Temperature		
≥38°C	55.97	51.88
>39.5°C	0.75	2.26
Diarrhea, any	35.82	33.08
Grade 3	0.75	2.26
Eating/drinking less than usual, any	49.25	57.14
Grade 3	2.24	2.26
Irritability/fussiness, any	82.84	86.47
Grade 3	6.72	6.02
Sleeping less than usual, any	50.75	56.39
Grade 3	2.24	3.76
Sleeping more than usual, any	62.69	67.67
Grade 3	3.73	1.5
Unusual crying for more than one hour, any	42.54	41.35
Grade 3	3.73	2.26
Vomiting, any	25.37	20.3
Grade 3	0.75	0.75

Legend: N=number of infants.

The safety profile presented below is based on data from more than 16 000 subjects.

As has been observed for DTPa and DTPa-containing combinations, an increase in local reactogenicity and fever was reported after booster vaccination with INFANRIX hexa with respect to the primary course.

Frequencies per dose as defined by CIOMS: Very common: ≥10%: appetite lost, irritability, crying abnormal, restlessness, pain, redness, local swelling at the injection site (≤50 mm), fever ≥38°C, and fatigue.

Common: ≥1% and <10%: nervousness, vomiting, diarrhea, local swelling at the injection site (>50 mm)*, fever >39.5°C, pruritus† and injection site reactions, including induration.

Uncommon: ≥0.1% and <1%: upper respiratory tract infection, somnolence, cough† and diffuse swelling of the injected limb, sometimes involving the adjacent joint*.

Rare: ≥0.01% and <0.1%: bronchitis and rash.

Very rare: < 0.01%: convulsions (with or without fever), dermatitis, bronchospasm, and urticaria†.

Local reactions after immunization usually consist of swelling or induration, tenderness, and redness or erythema at the injection site. More severe local reactions occasionally occur, such as inflammatory cellulitis without bacterial infection after DTP-containing vaccines.

Post-Market Adverse Drug Reactions: Over 12 million doses of INFANRIX hexa have been distributed overall for primary and booster vaccinations. Extremely rare cases of Sudden Unexpected Death (SUD) in close temporal association to vaccination with INFANRIX hexa have been reported in the first year of life. However, a causal relationship has not been established. The observed number of SUD cases following INFANRIX hexa is below the number of cases expected to occur by chance.

Blood and Lymphatic System Disorders: lymphadenopathy, thrombocytopenia.

Immune System Disorders: allergic reactions (including anaphylactic and anaphylactoid reactions).

Nervous System Disorders: collapse or shock-like state (hypotonic-hyporesponsiveness episode).

Respiratory, Thoracic and Mediastinal Disorders: apnea† [see Warnings and Precautions for apnea in very premature infants (≤28 weeks of gestation)].

Skin and Subcutaneous Tissue Disorders: angioneurotic oedema†.

General Disorders and Administration Site Conditions: extensive swelling reactions, swelling of the entire injected limb*, vesicles at the injection site.

Experience with Hepatitis B Vaccine: Paralysis, neuropathy, Guillain-Barré syndrome, encephalopathy, encephalitis and meningitis have been reported extremely rarely during post-marketing surveillance following vaccination with ENGERIX-B (Hepatitis B vaccine, GlaxoSmithKline) in infants <2 years old. The causal relationship to the vaccine has not been established.

DRUG INTERACTIONS: Overview: INFANRIX hexa (combined diphtheria and tetanus toxoids, acellular pertussis, hepatitis B (recombinant), inactivated poliomyelitis, and adsorbed conjugated *H. influenzae* type b vaccine) should not be mixed with any other vaccine in the same syringe or vial.

Drug-Drug Interactions: Tetanus immune globulin or diphtheria antitoxin, if used, should be given at a separate site, with a separate needle and syringe.

Anticoagulants: As with other intramuscular injections, INFANRIX hexa should not be given to infants or children on anticoagulant therapy unless the potential benefit clearly outweighs the risk of administration (see Warnings and Precautions).

* Children primed with acellular pertussis vaccines are more likely to experience swelling reactions after booster administration in comparison with children primed with whole cell vaccines. These reactions resolve over an average of 4 days.

† Observed with other GSK DTPa-containing vaccines.

Immunosuppressive Therapies: Immunosuppressive therapies, including irradiation, antimetabolites, alkylating agents, cytotoxic drugs and corticosteroids (used in greater than physiologic doses), may reduce the immune response to vaccines. Although no specific data are available from studies with INFANRIX hexa under these conditions, if immunosuppressive therapy will be discontinued shortly, it would be reasonable to defer immunization until the patient has been off therapy for 3 months; otherwise, the patient should be vaccinated while still on therapy. If INFANRIX hexa is administered to a person receiving immunosuppressive therapy, or a recent injection of immune globulin, an adequate immunologic response may not be obtained.

Measles-Mumps-Rubella Vaccine: There are insufficient data with regard to the efficacy and safety of simultaneous administration of INFANRIX hexa and Measles-Mumps-Rubella vaccine to allow any recommendation to be made.

Pneumococcal 7-Valent Conjugate Vaccine: Data on concomitant administration of INFANRIX hexa with Prevnar (pneumococcal 7-valent conjugate vaccine; Wyeth Pharmaceuticals) have shown no clinically relevant interference in the antibody response to each of the individual antigens in INFANRIX hexa when given as a 3 dose primary vaccination and as a 4th dose booster vaccination.

However, a higher incidence of fever (including >39.5°C) was reported in infants receiving INFANRIX hexa and Prevnar compared to infants receiving the hexavalent vaccine alone. The incidence of fever following administration of the two vaccines in the primary series was lower than that observed after the booster vaccination. Antipyretic treatment should be initiated according to local treatment guidelines.

Drug-Food Interactions: Interactions with food have not been established.

Drug-Herb Interactions: Interactions with herbal products have not been established.

Drug-Laboratory Test Interactions: Interactions with laboratory tests have not been established.

DOSAGE AND ADMINISTRATION:

The use of reduced volume (fractional doses) is not recommended. The effect of such practices on the frequency of serious adverse events and on protection against disease has not been determined.

Pre-term infants should be vaccinated according to their chronological age from birth.

INFANRIX hexa (combined diphtheria and tetanus toxoids, acellular pertussis, hepatitis B (recombinant), inactivated poliomyelitis, and adsorbed conjugated *H. influenzae* type b vaccine) has not been evaluated in the Canadian Native Population.

Recommended Dose and Dosage Adjustment: Primary Immunization: The primary immunization course for infants born of HBsAg-negative mothers is 3 doses of INFANRIX hexa 0.5 mL, given intramuscularly, at 2, 4, 6 months of age. INFANRIX hexa should not be administered to any infant before the age of 6 weeks.

Children Previously Vaccinated with One or More Doses of Hepatitis B Vaccine: Children who receive one dose of Hepatitis B vaccine at or shortly after birth may be administered a 3 dose series of INFANRIX hexa vaccine starting as early as 6 weeks of age. There is no data to support the use of a 3 dose series of INFANRIX hexa in infants who have previously received more than one dose of Hepatitis B vaccine. INFANRIX hexa may be administered to infants otherwise scheduled to receive concurrent INFANRIX (diphtheria, tetanus and acellular pertussis vaccine) and Hepatitis B vaccine and in whom vaccination against poliovirus is also desired.

Booster Immunization: The administration of the booster dose should be given at 18 months as stated in the Canadian Immunization Guide.

Missed Dose: Interruption of the recommended schedule with a delay between doses should not interfere with the final immunity achieved with INFANRIX hexa. There is no need to start the series over again regardless of the time elapsed between doses.

Additional Dosing Information: If any recommended dose of pertussis vaccine cannot be given, diphtheria and tetanus toxoids (DT) for pediatric use should be given as needed to complete the series.

For persons 7 years of age or older, Tetanus and Diphtheria Toxoids (Td) for adult use should be given for routine booster immunization against tetanus and diphtheria.

Administration: Preparation for Administration: The vaccine is reconstituted by adding the entire contents of the syringe (PEDIARIX) to the vial containing the Hib pellet.

Do not remove the white back-stop from the syringe. Prior to administration, ensure that the plunger rod is firmly attached to the rubber stopper by turning the plunger clockwise until slight resistance is felt. **Do not** over tighten. Remove syringe LUER Tip-cap and needle cap. Attach needle by pressing and twisting in a clockwise rotation until secured to the syringe.

Upon storage, a white deposit and clear supernatant may be observed. This does not constitute a sign of deterioration. Shake the syringe well before use. The vaccine is ready to use without dilution. Parenteral drug products should be inspected visually for particulate matter or discoloration prior to administration. With thorough agitation, DTPa-HBV-IPV (combined diphtheria and tetanus toxoids, acellular pertussis, hepatitis B (recombinant) and inactivated poliomyelitis vaccine, tradename PEDIARIX) is a homogeneous white turbid suspension. Discard if it appears otherwise. The vaccine is reconstituted by adding the entire contents of the syringe (PEDIARIX) to the vial containing the Hib pellet. After the addition of the PEDIARIX vaccine to the pellet, the mixture should be well shaken until the pellet is completely dissolved. The vaccine should not be mixed with other vaccines.

It is good clinical practice to only inject a vaccine when it has reached room temperature. In addition, a vial at room temperature ensures sufficient elasticity of the rubber closure to minimize any coring of rubber particles. To achieve this, the vial should be kept at room temperature (25±3°C) for at least five minutes before connecting the syringe and reconstituting the vaccine.

The reconstituted vaccine presents as a slightly more cloudy suspension than the liquid component alone. This is normal and does not impair the performance of the vaccine. Discard if it appears otherwise.

Since this product is a suspension containing an adjuvant, shake vigorously to obtain a uniform suspension prior to withdrawal from the vial. **Do not use if resuspension does not occur with vigorous shaking.** After removal of the 0.5 mL dose, any vaccine remaining in the vial should be discarded.

INFANRIX hexa should be administered by intramuscular injection. The preferred sites are the anterolateral aspects of the thigh or the deltoid muscle of the upper arm. The vaccine should not be injected in the gluteal area or areas where there may be a major nerve trunk. Before injection, the skin at the injection site should be cleaned and prepared with a suitable germicide. After insertion of the needle, aspirate to ensure that the needle has not entered a blood vessel.

Do not administer this product subcutaneously or intravenously.

Reconstitution: The syringe should be well shaken in order to obtain a homogeneous turbid white suspension.

The vaccine is reconstituted by adding the contents of the syringe to the vial containing the Hib pellet. After the addition of the PEDIARIX vaccine to the pellet, the mixture should be well shaken until the pellet is completely dissolved.

The reconstituted vaccine presents as a slightly more cloudy suspension than the liquid component alone. This is normal and does not impair the performance of the vaccine. In the event of other variation being observed, discard the vaccine.

After reconstitution, the vaccine should be injected promptly. However the vaccine may be kept for up to 8 hours at room temperature (21°C).

OVERDOSAGE:

Insufficient data are available.

> For management of a suspected drug overdose, CPhA recommends that you contact your **regional Poison Control Centre**. See the *CPS* Directory section for a list of Poison Control Centres.

ACTION AND CLINICAL PHARMACOLOGY: Diphtheria: Diphtheria is a serious communicable disease, primarily a localized and generalized intoxication caused by diphtheria toxin, an extracellular protein metabolite of toxigenic strains of *C. diphtheriae*. The disease occurs most frequently in unimmunized or partially immunized individuals. The incidence of diphtheria in Canada has decreased from 9000 cases reported in 1924 to extremely low levels. Only 1 or 2 cases have been reported annually in recent years. The case fatality rate remains 5% to 10%, with the highest death rates in the very young and elderly. If immunization levels are allowed to fall and adults do not receive booster doses, disease re-emergence may appear as demonstrated in the Commonwealth of Independent States (former Soviet Union), where tens of thousands of cases with substantial mortality have been reported. Protection against disease is due to the development of neutralizing antibodies to the diphtheria toxin. Following adequate immunization with diphtheria toxoid, it is thought that protection persists for at least 10 years. Serum antitoxin levels of at least 0.01 antitoxin units per mL are generally regarded as protective.

This significantly reduces both the risk of developing diphtheria and the severity of clinical illness. Immunization with diphtheria toxoid does not, however, eliminate carriage of *C. diphtheriae* in the pharynx, nose or on the skin.

Tetanus: Tetanus is an intoxication manifested primarily by neuromuscular dysfunction caused by a potent exotoxin released by *C. tetani*. Immunization is highly effective, provides long-lasting protection and is recommended for the whole population. Only 1 to 7 with an average of 5 cases of tetanus are now reported annually in Canada, while no deaths have been recorded since 1995. The disease continues to occur almost exclusively among persons who are unvaccinated, inadequately vaccinated or whose vaccination histories are unknown or uncertain.

Spores of *C. tetani* are ubiquitous. Naturally acquired immunity to tetanus toxin does not occur. Thus, universal primary immunization and timed booster doses to maintain adequate tetanus antitoxin levels are necessary to protect all age groups. Protection against disease is due to the development of neutralizing antibodies to the tetanus toxin. Tetanus toxoid is a highly effective antigen and a completed primary series generally induces serum antitoxin levels of at least 0.01 antitoxin units per mL, a level which has been reported to be protective. It is thought that protection persists for at least 10 years.

Pertussis: Pertussis (whooping cough) is a disease of the respiratory tract caused by *B. pertussis*. Pertussis is highly communicable (attack rates in unimmunized household contacts of up to 90% have been reported) and can affect individuals of any age; however, severity is greatest among young infants. Precise epidemiologic data do not exist, since bacteriological confirmation of pertussis can be obtained in less than half of the suspected cases. Most reported illness from *B. pertussis* occurred in infants and young children in whom complications can be severe. Older children, adolescents and adults, in whom classic signs are often absent, may go undiagnosed and may serve as reservoirs of disease. Pertussis epidemics are cyclic and occur every 3 to 4 years. Pertussis has been controlled in Canada through immunization. During the last 40 years, the incidence of pertussis has decreased by >90% although outbreaks continue to occur.

A recent study was conducted in Germany to assess the efficacy of pertussis vaccine after partial and completed primary vaccination series for preventing hospitalizations due to pertussis under field conditions. Data was acquired by a nationwide, hospital based, active surveillance system. After one dose of the vaccine, vaccine effectiveness was as high as 68%, increasing to 91.8% after receipt of the second dose. Vaccine effectiveness of 3 and 4 doses of acellular vaccine were estimated to be 99.8% and 98.6%, respectively.

Antigenic components of *B. pertussis* believed to contribute to protective immunity include: pertussis toxin (PT); filamentous hemagglutinin (FHA); and pertactin. Although the role of these antigens in providing protective immunity in humans is not well understood, clinical trials which evaluated candidate acellular DTP vaccines manufactured by GlaxoSmithKline supported the efficacy of 3 component INFANRIX (DTPa). Recently published data suggests a higher importance of the PT and pertactin components in providing protection against pertussis.

INFANRIX contains 3 pertussis antigens (PT, FHA and pertactin), and has been shown to be effective in preventing World Health Organization (WHO)-defined pertussis as well as clinically milder disease in two published clinical trials when administered as a primary series.

A double-blind, randomized, placebo (DT)-controlled trial conducted in Italy, sponsored by the U.S. National Institutes of Health (NIH), assessed the absolute protective efficacy of INFANRIX when administered at 2, 4 and 6 months of age. A total of 15 601 infants were immunized with 1 of 2 tri-component acellular DTP vaccines (containing inactivated PT, FHA and pertactin), or with a whole-cell DTP vaccine manufactured by Sanofi Pasteur, or with DT vaccine alone. The mean length of follow-up was 17 months, beginning 30 days after the third dose of vaccine. The population used in the primary analysis of vaccine efficacy included 4481 INFANRIX vaccinees, 4348 whole-cell DTP vaccinees and 1470 DT vaccinees. After 3 doses, the protective efficacy of INFANRIX against WHO-defined typical pertussis (21 days or more of paroxysmal cough with infection confirmed by culture and/or serologic testing) was 84% (95% CI: 76% to 89%) while the efficacy of the whole-cell DTP vaccine was 36% (95% CI: 14% to 52%). When the definition of pertussis was expanded to include clinically milder disease with respect to type and duration of cough, with infection confirmed by culture and/or serologic testing, the efficacy of INFANRIX was calculated to be 71% (95% CI: 60% to 78%) against >7 days of any cough and 73% (95% CI: 63% to 80%) against ≥14 days of any cough. A longer follow-up of the Italian trial showed that after 3 doses, the absolute efficacy of INFANRIX against WHO-defined pertussis remained high at 84% among children up to 4 years of age.

A prospective, blinded efficacy trial was also conducted in Germany employing a household contact study design. In preparation for this study, 3 doses of INFANRIX were administered at 3, 4 and 5 months of age to more than 22 000 children living in 6 areas of Germany in a large safety and immunogenicity trial. Infants who did not participate in this trial could have received whole-cell DTP vaccine (manufactured by Chiron Behring, Germany) or DT vaccine. Calculation of vaccine efficacy was based on attack rates of pertussis in household contacts classified by vaccination status. Of the 173 unvaccinated household contacts, 96 developed WHO-defined pertussis (21 days or more of paroxysmal cough with infection confirmed by culture and/or serologic testing), as compared to 7 of 112 contacts vaccinated with INFANRIX and 1 of 75 contacts vaccinated with whole-cell DTP vaccine. The protective efficacy of INFANRIX was calculated to be 89% (95% CI: 77% to 95%), with no indication of waning of immunity up until the time of the booster. The protective efficacy of the whole-cell DTP vaccine was calculated to be 98% (95% CI: 83% to 100%). When the definition of pertussis was expanded to include clinically milder disease, with infection confirmed by culture and/or serologic testing, the efficacy of INFANRIX against ≥7 days of any cough was 67% (95% CI: 52% to 78%) and against ≥7 days of paroxysmal cough was 81% (95% CI: 68% to 89%). The corresponding efficacy rates of INFANRIX against ≥14 days of any cough or paroxysmal cough were 73% (95% CI: 59% to 82%) and 84% (95% CI: 71% to 91%), respectively.

Hepatitis B: Several hepatitis viruses are known to cause a systemic infection resulting in major pathologic changes in the liver (e.g., A, B, C, D, E). Hepatitis B infection can have serious consequences including acute massive hepatic necrosis, chronic active hepatitis and cirrhosis of the liver. It has been estimated that more than 350 million people in the world are persistently infected with hepatitis B virus.

Among infected infants, very few (5-10%) recover completely; the majority (up to 90%) become chronic carriers with the risk of becoming a chronic carrier decreasing with age (children <5 years 25% to 50%, adults 6% to 10%). Those patients who become chronic carriers can infect others and are at increased risk of developing either cirrhosis or primary hepatocellular carcinoma.

Among other factors, infection with hepatitis B may be the single most important factor for development of this carcinoma. Considering the serious consequences of infection, immunization should be considered for all persons.

Mothers infected with hepatitis B virus can infect their infants at, or shortly after, birth if they are carriers of the hepatitis B surface antigen (HBsAg) or develop an active infection during the third trimester of pregnancy. Infected infants usually become chronic carriers. Therefore, screening of pregnant women for hepatitis B is recommended. According to the Canadian Immunization Guide, hepatitis B prevention should include programs for universal immunization of children, pre-exposure vaccination of high-risk groups, universal HBsAg screening of all pregnant women and post-exposure intervention for those exposed to disease, particularly infants born to hepatitis B-infected mothers. There is no specific treatment for acute hepatitis B infection. However, those who develop anti-HBs antibodies after active infection are usually protected against subsequent infection. Antibody titers ≥10 mIU/mL against HBsAg are recognized as conferring protection against hepatitis B. Seroconversion is defined as antibody titers ≥1 mIU/mL.

Poliomyelitis: Poliovirus is an enterovirus that belongs to the picornavirus family. Three serotypes of poliovirus have been identified (types 1, 2 and 3). Poliovirus is highly contagious with the predominant mode of transmission being person-to-person via the fecal-oral route. Infection may be spread indirectly through contact with infectious saliva or feces or by contaminated water or sewage.

Replication of poliovirus in the pharynx and intestine is followed by a viremic phase where involvement of the central nervous system can occur. While poliovirus infections are asymptomatic or cause nonspecific symptoms (low-grade fever, malaise, anorexia and sore throat) in 90% to 95% of individuals, 1% to 2% of infected persons will develop paralytic disease.

Following the introduction of inactivated poliovirus vaccines (IPV) in Canada in 1955, the indigenous disease has been eliminated. Since 1980, 12 paralytic cases have been reported in Canada, 11 of which were determined to be vaccine-associated paralytic poliomyelitis (VAPP), with Oral Polio Vaccine (OPV). The last reported case of VAPP occurred in 1995.

Forty seven studies involving over 19 000 infants and children have been conducted in developed and developing countries with GlaxoSmithKline's enhanced inactivated poliovirus vaccine, as trivalent IPV vaccine or as a part of DTPa-IPV based combinations.

***H. influenzae* Type b:** *H. influenzae* type b (Hib) was the most common cause of bacterial meningitis and a leading cause of other serious invasive infections in young children prior to the introduction of other Hib vaccines. About 55% to 65% of affected children had meningitis while the remainder had epiglottitis, bacteremia, cellulitis, pneumonia or septic arthritis. The case fatality rate of meningitis is about 5%. Severe neurologic sequelae occur in 10% to 15% of survivors and deafness in 15% to 20% (severe in 3% to 7%).

Before the introduction of Hib conjugate vaccines in Canada in 1988, there were approximately 2000 cases of Hib disease annually. Since then the overall incidence has fallen by more than 99%. The majority of cases occur now in children too old to have received primary vaccination. In 1998, only 15 cases were reported in children <5 years of age.

STORAGE AND STABILITY: Store INFANRIX hexa (combined diphtheria and tetanus toxoids, acellular pertussis, hepatitis B (recombinant), inactivated poliomyelitis, and adsorbed conjugated *H. influenzae* type b vaccine) at 2 to 8°C. Do not use after the expiration date shown on the label. After reconstitution, immediate use is recommended. However, stability of the vaccine has been demonstrated for 8 hours at + 21°C after reconstitution.

Do not freeze. Discard if the vaccine has been frozen.

INFORMATION FOR THE PATIENT: Published in e-CPS, available by subscription at www.e-cps.ca.

DOSAGE FORMS, COMPOSITION AND PACKAGING: Syringe and Vial: Each 0.5 mL dose is formulated to contain 25 Lf (30 IU) diphtheria toxoid, 10 Lf (40 IU) tetanus toxoid, 25 µg PT, 25 µg FHA, 8 µg pertactin, 10 µg HBsAg, 40 D-antigen Units (DU) of type 1 poliovirus, 8 DU type 2 poliovirus, 32 DU type 3 poliovirus, and 10 µg of adsorbed purified capsular polysaccharide of Hib (PRP) covalently bound to 20-40 µg of tetanus toxoid.

Each 0.5 mL dose also contains 12.6 mg lactose, 4.5 mg sodium chloride and 0.7 mg aluminum adjuvants (as aluminum salts), water for injection. The vaccine contains residual formaldehyde, polysorbate 20 and 80 (Tween 20 and 80), M199 (as stabilizer), potassium chloride and disodium phosphate, monopotassium phosphate, glycine, neomycin sulphate, polymyxin B sulphate from the manufacturing process. The procedures used to manufacture the antigen result in a product that contains ≤5% yeast protein.

H. influenzae type b vaccine is supplied as a pellet in a 3 mL vial (Type I glass) with stopper (butyl). PEDIARIX (combined diphtheria and tetanus toxoids, acellular pertussis, hepatitis B (recombinant) and inactivated poliomyelitis vaccine) is supplied as a turbid suspension in a pre-filled syringe (Type I glass) (0.5 mL) with plunger stoppers (butyl). Kit in pack sizes of 10 with or without needles.

Infantol®

multiple vitamins

Dietary Supplement

Church & Dwight

SUPPLIED: Each 5 mL of yellow, opaque, viscous, citrus flavored, water miscible liquid contains: vitamin A 1600 IU (as palmitate), vitamin B_1 1.25 mg, riboflavin 2 mg (as riboflavin 5-phosphate sodium), ascorbic acid 80 mg, vitamin D 400 IU, niacinamide 10 mg and vitamin B_6 1.2 mg. Nonmedicinal ingredients: corn oil, flavors, glycerin, methylparaben, polysorbate, propylparaben, simethicone, sodium cyclamate, sorbitol, tocopherol and xanthan gum. Hydrochloric acid and sodium hydroxide to adjust the pH. pH: 3.9 to 4.1. Energy: 24.3 kJ (5.8 kcal)/5 mL. Sodium: <1 mmol (7 mg). Bottles of 350 mL.

Influvac®

influenza vaccine, surface antigen, inactivated

Active Immunizing Agent for the Prevention of Influenza

Abbott Products

Date of Preparation: July 15, 2005
Date of Revision: July 5, 2010

SUMMARY PRODUCT INFORMATION:

Route of Administration	Dosage Form/ Strength	Clinically Relevant Nonmedicinal Ingredients
Intramuscular injection or deep subcutaneous injection	0.5 mL pre-filled syringe containing neuraminidase and 15 µg hemagglutinin per virus strain in a suspension	None For a complete listing see Dosage Forms, Composition and Packaging.

DESCRIPTION: INFLUVAC (influenza vaccine, surface antigen, inactivated) is a trivalent subunit influenza vaccine. Each 0.5 mL dose contains neuraminidase and 15 µg of hemagglutinin antigen for each virus strain present in the vaccine. The composition is adapted annually according to WHO and the National Advisory Committee on Immunization (NACI). The virus strains used in the vaccine for 2010/2011 are: an A/California/7/2009 (H_1N_1)-like virus, an A/Perth/16/2009 (H_3N_2)-like virus, a B/Brisbane/60/2008-like virus.

INFLUVAC is a clear to slightly opalescent liquid. INFLUVAC is thimerosal-free, mercury-free, and contains no preservative.

INDICATIONS AND CLINICAL USE: INFLUVAC (influenza vaccine, surface antigen, inactivated) is indicated for the prevention of influenza infection caused by the specific strains contained in the vaccine, in adults of 18-years of age and older.

The National Advisory Committee on Immunization (NACI) recommends annual vaccination for individuals in the following categories:

People at High Risk of Influenza-related Complications:

- Healthy children aged 6 to 23 months are at increased risk of influenza-associated hospitalization compared with healthy older children and young adults.
- Adults and children with chronic cardiac or pulmonary disorders (including bronchopulmonary dysplasia, cystic fibrosis, and asthma) severe enough to require medical follow-up or hospital care.
- People of any age who are residents of nursing homes or chronic care facilities.
- People 65 years of age and over.
- Adults and children with chronic conditions such as diabetes mellitus and other metabolic diseases, cancer, immunodeficiency, immunosuppression (due to underlying disease and/or therapy), renal disease, anemia, and hemoglobinopathy. Although some immunosuppressed individuals may have a suboptimal immune response, influenza vaccination is safe and can induce protective antibody levels in a substantial proportion of adults and children, including transplant recipients, those with proliferative diseases of the hematopoietic and lymphatic systems, and HIV-infected patients.
- Children and adolescents (aged 6 months to 18 years) with conditions treated for long periods with acetylsalicylic acid (ASA).
- People at high risk of influenza complications who are embarking on travel to destinations where influenza is likely to be circulating.

People Capable of Transmitting Influenza to Those at High Risk of Influenza-related Complications: People who could transmit influenza to those at high risk should receive annual vaccination, regardless of whether the high-risk person(s) has been immunized:

- Health care providers who work in facilities and community settings, such as physicians, nurses, and emergency response workers.
- Health care and other service providers who have contact with residents of continuing care facilities or residences.
- Those who provide home care for persons in high-risk groups.
- Those who provide services within closed or relatively closed settings to persons at high risk (e.g. crew on ships).
- Household contacts (adults and children) of people at high risk of influenza complications. This includes household contacts of children <6 months of age, who are at high risk of complications from influenza but for whom there is no currently licensed vaccine, and of children aged 6 to 23 months whether or not they have been immunized. Pregnant women should be immunized in their third trimester if they are expected to deliver during influenza season, as they will become household contacts of their newborn (unless adoption occurs).
- Those providing regular child care to children aged 0 to 23 months, whether in or out of the home.
- **People who provide essential community services.** Vaccination for these individuals should be encouraged in order to minimize the disruption of routine activities in epidemics. Employers and their employees should consider yearly influenza immunization for healthy working adults, as this has been shown to decrease work absenteeism due to respiratory and other illnesses.
- **People in direct contact with poultry infected with avian influenza during culling operations.** The relevant individuals include those performing the cull as well as others (such as supervising veterinarians and inspectors) who may be directly exposed to the avian virus.

  Those persons who would be expected by reason of their employment to come into direct contact with infected poultry during culling operations in the event of potential avian influenza outbreaks should be immunized with TIV on a yearly basis prior to the human influenza season. Those who are immunized with TIV just before exposure to avian influenza will not produce protective antibodies against the human vaccine strains for approximately 10 to 14 days. Antiviral prophylaxis should be used as an adjunct to TIV immunization in order to prevent infection with either avian or human influenza during the culling operation. Advice should be sought from the local medical health officer regarding the use of TIV and influenza antiviral prophylaxis in the control of avian influenza outbreaks. This is a theoretical concern. For further information, please refer to NACI guidelines.
- **Healthy persons aged 2 to 64 years. Individuals in this age group should be encouraged to receive the vaccine, even if they are not in one of the aforementioned priority groups.**
- **Pregnant and breast-feeding women who are characterized by any of the conditions listed under "Recommended Recipients".** This includes pregnant and breast-feeding women who have chronic conditions that put them at high risk of complications from influenza, as well as those who are close contacts of high-risk individuals. (Refer to Warnings and Precautions, Special Populations, Pregnant Women.)

Pharmacodynamic Properties: Seroprotection is generally obtained within 2 to 3 weeks. The duration of post-vaccinal immunity to homologous strains or to strains closely related to the vaccine strains varies but is usually 6 to 12 months.
Geriatrics (>65 years of age): Studies on healthy elderly showed that INFLUVAC is well tolerated.
Pediatrics (6 months to 4 years of age): A clinical trial in high-risk children with chronic respiratory or congenital heart disease aged 6 months to 4 years showed that the vaccine was well tolerated and induced an immunogenic response against all three hemagglutinin antigens.

CONTRAINDICATIONS: The influenza virus for INFLUVAC (influenza vaccine, surface antigen, inactivated) is propagated in chicken eggs; therefore, this vaccine should not be administered to anyone with a history of hypersensitivity (allergy) and especially anaphylactic reactions to eggs or egg products.

Allergic reactions are extremely rare and are usually attributable to extreme sensitivity to certain components of the vaccine, probably to trace amounts of residual egg protein.

INFLUVAC should not be given to people who have a hypersensitivity to the active substances, to any of the excipients and to residues of eggs, chicken protein (such as ovalbumin), formaldehyde, cetyltrimethylammonium bromide, polysorbate 80, or gentamicin. For a complete listing, see Dosage Forms, Composition and Packaging.

Allergic or anaphylactic reactions to a previous dose of influenza vaccine are contraindications for vaccination.

Immunization with INFLUVAC should be deferred in the presence of any acute illness, including acute or unstable neurologic illness, febrile illness, or active infection.

A minor febrile illness such as mild upper respiratory infection is not usually reason to defer immunization.

WARNINGS AND PRECAUTIONS: General: If INFLUVAC (influenza vaccine, surface antigen, inactivated) is used in persons receiving immunosuppressive therapy, including corticosteroid therapy, the expected immunological response may be diminished. Antibody response in patients with endogenous or iatrogenic immunosuppression may be insufficient.

As with all injectable vaccines, appropriate medical treatment and supervision should always be readily available in case of a rare anaphylactic event following the administration of the vaccine.

INFLUVAC should not be administered into the buttocks due to varying amounts of fatty tissue in this region, nor by the intradermal route, since these methods of administration may induce a weaker response.

INFLUVAC must not be administered intravascularly.

Sterile epinephrine HCl solution (1:1000) and other appropriate agents should be made available for immediate use in case of anaphylactic reaction or acute hypersensitivity to the vaccine occurs. Health care providers should be familiar with current recommendations for the initial management of anaphylaxis in non-hospital settings, including proper airway management. Before administration of any vaccine, all appropriate precautions should be taken to prevent adverse reactions. This includes a review of the patient's history with respect to possible hypersensitivity to the vaccine or similar vaccine, determination of previous immunization history, and the presence of any contraindications to immunization, current health status, and a current knowledge of the literature concerning the use of the vaccine under consideration.

Intramuscular injections should be given with care in persons suffering from coagulation disorders or on anticoagulant therapy because of risk of hemorrhage.

Pneumonococcal vaccine and influenza vaccine can be given at the same visit but at different sites with separate sterile needles and syringes without an increase in side effects. Whereas influenza vaccine is given annually, pneumonococcal vaccine should be given only once to adults. It should be noted that the adverse reactions may be intensified.

Influenza virus undergoes significant antigenic changes from time to time, so different vaccines are made every year. INFLUVAC, as now constituted, is not effective against all possible strains of influenza virus. Protection is limited to those strains of virus from which the vaccine is prepared or against closely-related strains.

The use of fractional doses in an attempt to reduce the severity of adverse reactions cannot be recommended because there is insufficient evidence on the safety or efficacy of such smaller doses.

As with any vaccine, immunization with INFLUVAC may not protect 100% of susceptible individuals.
Hematologic: See Adverse Reactions.
Neurologic: See Adverse Reactions.
Sensitivity/Resistance: See Adverse Reactions.
Special Populations: Pregnant Women: Limited data from vaccinations in pregnant women do not indicate that adverse fetal and maternal outcomes were attributable to the vaccine. The use of this vaccine may be considered from the second trimester of pregnancy. For pregnant women with medical conditions that increase their risk of complications from influenza, administration of the vaccine is recommended, irrespective of their stage of pregnancy (see Indications and Clinical Use).
Nursing Women: Evidence indicates that influenza vaccine is safe for pregnant women at all stages of pregnancy and for breast-feeding mothers.
Geriatrics (>65 years of age): INFLUVAC is indicated in people 65 years of age and over (see Indications and Clinical Use).
Monitoring and Laboratory Tests: Following influenza vaccination, false positive results in serology tests using the ELISA method to detect antibodies against HIV1, Hepatitis C and especially HTLV1 have been observed. The Western Blot technique disproves the results. The transient false positive reactions could be due to the IgM response by the vaccine.

ADVERSE REACTIONS: Adverse Drug Reaction Overview: Vaccination with INFLUVAC (influenza vaccine, surface antigen, inactivated) cannot cause influenza because the vaccine does not contain live virus.
Local reactions include: redness, swelling, itching, warmth, pain on contact, continuous pain, restriction in arm movement, induration and blue spots. The most frequent local reaction is soreness at the injection site lasting up to 2 days in adults but rarely interferes with normal activities. Prophylactic acetaminophen may decrease the frequency of pain at the injection site.
Systemic reactions: fever, increased sweating, headache, malaise, insomnia, shivering, myalgia, arthralgia, and fatigue. The most frequent systemic reaction is headache.

Allergic responses to influenza vaccine, in rare cases could lead to anaphylactic shocks, are probably a consequence of hypersensitivity to some vaccine component, most likely residual egg protein, which is present in minute quantities.

Neurological disorders with influenza vaccination include neuritis, encephalomyelitis, convulsions and paresthesia.

Rare cases of systemic vasculitis have been reported in persons after influenza vaccination, but a causal relation has not been assess.

Guillain-Barré Syndrome (GBS) occurred in adults in association with the 1976 swine influenza vaccine, and evidence favours the existence of a causal relation between the vaccine and GBS during that season. In an extensive review of studies since 1976, the United States Institute of Medicine concluded that the evidence is inadequate to accept or reject a causal relation between GBS in adults and influenza vaccines administered after the swine influenza vaccine program in 1976.

In Canada the background incidence of GBS was estimated at just over 20 cases per million population in a study done in Ontario and Quebec. A variety of infectious agents, such as *C. jejuni*, have been associated with GBS. It is not known whether influenza virus infection itself is associated with GBS. Neither is it known whether influenza vaccination is causally associated with increased risk of recurrent GBS in persons with a previous history of GBS. Avoiding subsequent influenza vaccination of persons known to have developed GBS within 6 to 8 weeks of a previous influenza vaccination appears prudent at this time. In the past 11 years, for INFLUVAC, 40 cases of Guillain-Barré Syndrome (GBS) and one case of possible GBS, classified as ascending neuron paralysis (flaccid paralysis) were reported. The reporting rate of GBS associated with INFLUVAC is concluded to remain within the expected background incidence. Influenza vaccine is not known to predispose to Reye's Syndrome.

Oculorespiratory Syndrome (ORS) has been reported sporadically in Canada, US and Europe following influenza immunization. Starting in the 2000/2001 season, ORS is defined as the onset of bilateral red eyes and/or respiratory symptoms (cough, wheeze, chest tightness, difficulty breathing, difficulty swallowing, hoarseness or sore throat) and/or facial swelling occurring within 24 hours of influenza immunization. The pathophysiologic mechanism underlying ORS remains unknown.

After the 2000-2001 influenza season, fewer ORS cases have been reported to Health Canada. One case of ORS has been seen with the vaccination with INFLUVAC but a causal relation has not been assessed.

Please refer to the Canadian Immunization Guide for further details about administration of vaccine and management of adverse events.

Physicians, nurses and pharmacists should report any immediate adverse reactions arising from any vaccination, or following shortly thereafter, in accordance with local requirements and to the manufacturer: Drug Safety, Abbott Products Inc., 60 Columbia Way, Suite 207, Markham, Ontario L3R 0C9 Canada. Telephone: 1-800-268-4276.
Clinical Trial Adverse Drug Reactions: A total of 1856 patients have been given INFLUVAC with thimerosal or INFLUVAC thimerosal-free in clinical trials. The safety of INFLUVAC was assessed in the following clinical trials: annual strain composition update requirement, including at least 50 adults aged 18- 60 years and at least 50 elderly subjects aged 60 years or older, conducted during the period of 1993 to 2002 using INFLUVAC with thimerosal; a study comparing INFLUVAC thimerosal-free and INFLUVAC with thimerosal; a study with INFLUVAC thimerosal-free; and a study of 52 high-risk children (6 months to 4 years) vaccinated with INFLUVAC with thimerosal.

Safety evaluation (i.e. local and systemic reactogenicity) is performed during the first 3 days following vaccination. Data on reactogenicity can be found in Table 1, Table 2 and Table 3.

Table 1: INFLUVAC
Local and Systemic Reactions During Three Days After Vaccination with INFLUVAC, Containing Thimerosal

Total N=1596	Adults N[a] (aged 18–59 years) % (n/N)	Elderly N=540 (aged 60 years and over) % (n)
Local Reactions		
Redness	12.5 (132/1052)	9.4 (51)
Swelling	10.4 (109/1053)	6.1 (33)
Itching	6.3 (66/1052)	4.4 (24)
Warmth	11.2 (118/1054)	5.9 (32)
Pain on contact	42.6 (449/1055)	9.1 (49)
Continuous pain	8.2 (86/1053)	2.6 (14)
Restriction in arm movement	10.3 (109/1054)	2.2 (12)
Induration	10.2 (107/1048)	6.5 (35)
Blue spots	2.6 (27 /1052)	2.6 (14)
Systemic Reactions		
Fever	4.3 (45/1053)	1.5 (8)
Increased sweating	5.0 (53/1053)	3.7 (20)
Headache	12.9 (136/1052)	8.3 (45)
Malaise	6.0 (63/1053)	4.3 (23)
Insomnia	4.6 (48/1052)	4.8 (26)
Shivering	2.1 (22/1052)	1.9 (10)

[a] Number of subjects with non-missing data.
Legend: %=n/N (number of cases/Number of subjects with non-missing data).

Table 2: INFLUVAC
Local and Systemic Reactions During Three Days After Vaccination with INFLUVAC Without Thimerosal (n=197)

Total N=197	Adults N=144 (aged 18–59 years) % (n)	Elderly N=53 (aged 60 years and over) % (n)
Local Reactions		
Redness	17.4 (25)	3.8 (2)
Swelling	11.8 (17)	3.8 (2)
Itching	3.5 (5)	7.5 (4)
Warmth	7.6 (11)	5.7 (3)
Pain on contact	41.7 (60)	5.7 (3)
Continuous pain	3.5 (5)	1.9 (1)
Restriction in arm movement	13.2 (19)	3.8 (2)
Induration	16.7 (24)	1.9 (1)
Blue spots	4.2 (6)	3.8 (2)
Systemic Reactions		
Increased sweating	3.5 (5)	3.8 (2)
Headache	11.8 (17)	1.9 (1)
Malaise	2.8 (4)	3.8 (2)
Insomnia	3.5 (5)	3.8 (2)
Shivering	2.1 (3)	0.0 (0)

Table 3: INFLUVAC
Local and Systemic Reactions During Three Days After Vaccination in Children with INFLUVAC Containing Thimerosal

Total N=52	Children (aged 6 months to 4 years) % (n)
Local Reactions	
Redness	11.5 (6)
Swelling	3.8 (2)
Itching	0.0 (0)
Warmth	0.0 (0)

(cont'd)

Table 3: INFLUVAC *(cont'd)*

Local and Systemic Reactions During Three Days After Vaccination in Children with INFLUVAC Containing Thimerosal

Total N=52	Children (aged 6 months to 4 years) % (n)
Pain on contact	0.0 (0)
Continuous pain	0.0 (0)
Restriction in arm movement	0.0 (0)
Induration	7.7 (4)
Blue spots	5.8 (3)
Systemic Reactions	
Fever	26.9 (14)
Increased sweating	11.5 (6)
Malaise	11.5 (6)
Insomnia	25.0 (13)
Loss of appetite	15.2 (8)
Increased crying	15.2 (8)
Increased irritability	25.0 (13)

Data from annual update studies with INFLUVAC containing thimerosal show local and systemic reactions occurred most frequently during the first day after vaccination (40.7% and 13.3%, respectively). During the second and third day after vaccination, local reaction rates declined to 25.4% and 10.3%, respectively. Systemic reaction rates declined to 9.2% and 6.5%.

Data from clinical studies with INFLUVAC thimerosal-free show local reactions occurred most frequently the first day after vaccination (37.1%) and declined during the second and third day to 30.5 % and 14.7% respectively. As for the systemic reactions, few participants to the study reported systemic reactions, and the numbers reported remained stable during the first three days (8.6%, 7.6% and 5.1% respectively).

As summarized in Table 4, both local and systemic reactions for both formulations are comparable. The most frequent local reaction was pain on contact (31% and 32% for the thimerosal- containing and thimerosal-free vaccine, respectively), and the most frequent systemic reaction was headache (11% and 9% for the thimerosal-containing and thimerosal-free vaccine, respectively).

Table 4: INFLUVAC

Comparison of Reactogenicity on Thimerosal-free vs Thimerosal-containing INFLUVAC

Measure	Thimerosal-free INFLUVAC n=197 % (n)	Thimerosal-containing INFLUVAC n=1692 % (n)
Pain on contact at vaccination site	32% (63)	31% (52)
Headache	9% (18)	11% (19)
Any local symptom	45% (89)	45% (76)
Any systemic symptom	14% (28)	19% (32)
Moderate or severe inconvenience	0% (0)	3% (51)

A clinical study in high-risk children with chronic respiratory or congenital heart disease aged 6 months to 4 years with thimerosal-containing INFLUVAC showed that following either of the two vaccinations, the incidence of any local (23%) and any systemic reactions (48%) in this particular group was considered comparable with those reported in healthy adults.

These children received two separate vaccinations and had the added parameters of loss of appetite, increased crying and irritability. All reactions were recorded in the questionnaire by the parent/guardian (instead of direct reporting).

The reactions recorded were relatively minor in nature and were resolved within a few days.

Post-Market Adverse Drug Reactions: Since the 1992 season, over 130.5 million doses of INFLUVAC have been administered. A total of 878 adverse event reports, including 421 serious reports, associated with the use of INFLUVAC have been reported.

These reports include all adverse events reported from the market, health authorities, all published cases, serious adverse event from clinical studies and spontaneous reports, irrespective of any causality assessment.

In adults/elderly the most frequently (45 or more) reported symptoms listed in the adverse reaction reports for the production years 1992 to 2002 were 'injection and infusion site reactions' (102), 'febrile disorders' (92), 'asthenic conditions' (67), 'joint related signs and symptoms' (65), 'nausea and vomiting symptoms' (56), 'headaches NEC' (48), 'general signs and symptoms NEC (46). All of these reactions are considered to be in line with the information in the INFLUVAC global labeling.

From post-marketing surveillance additionally, the following adverse events have been reported:

- Uncommon (>1/1000 and <1/100): generalised skin reactions including pruritus, urticaria or non-specific rash.
- Rare (>1/10 000 and <1/1000): neuralgia, paraesthesia, transient thrombocytopenia. Allergic reactions, in rare cases leading to shock, have been reported.
- Very rare (<1/10 000): vasculitis with transient renal involvement. Neurological disorders, such as encephalomyelitis, neuritis and Guillain-Barré syndrome.

Other adverse reactions reported during post-marketing surveillance include transient lymphadenopathy, febrile convulsions and angioedema.

DRUG INTERACTIONS: Overview: No interaction between INFLUVAC (influenza vaccine, surface antigen, inactivated) and other vaccines or medication are known.

Drug-Drug Interactions: INFLUVAC may be given at the same time as other vaccines. Immunization should be carried out on separate limbs. It should be noted that the adverse reactions may be intensified.

The immunological response may be diminished if the patient is undergoing immunosuppressant treatment.

Theophylline: In the literature, some studies and case reports have suggested a possible interaction between influenza vaccine and the use of theophylline. However, literature reviews on the subject have not scientifically substantiated these interactions. Based on the available evidence, the fact that most countries do not issue a warning regarding a possible interaction seems justified.

Anticoagulants: In the literature, some studies and case reports have suggested a possible interaction between influenza vaccine and the use of anticoagulants such as warfarin. However, literature reviews on the subject have not scientifically substantiated these interactions. Based on the available evidence, the fact that most countries do not issue a warning regarding a possible interaction seems justified.

Drug-Food Interactions: Not known.

Drug-Herb Interactions: Not known.

Drug-Laboratory Test Interactions: Following influenza vaccination, false positive results in serology tests using the ELISA method to detect antibodies against HIV1, Hepatitis C and especially HTLV1 have been observed. The Western Blot technique disproves the results. The transient false positive reactions could be due to the IgM response by the vaccine.

Drug-Lifestyle Interactions: INFLUVAC is unlikely to produce an effect on the ability to drive and use machines.

DOSAGE AND ADMINISTRATION: Recommended Dose and Dosage Adjustment: The recommended dose of INFLUVAC for adults above 18 years is 0.5 mL.

Administration: Parenteral biological products should be inspected visually for extraneous particulate matter and/or discolouration before administration. If these conditions exist, the product should not be administered.

For information on vaccine administration, see the current Canadian Immunization Guide and the Health Canada Website.

The patient should be given a permanent personal immunization record. In addition, it is essential that the physician or nurse record the immunization history in the permanent medical record of each patient. Thus the permanent office record should contain the name of the vaccine, date given, dose, manufacturer and lot number.

INFLUVAC should be administered by intramuscular or deep subcutaneous injection.

INFLUVAC is a colourless clear liquid, in pre-filled single-dose syringes.

INFLUVAC should be allowed to reach room temperature before use. Shake the pre-filled syringe well to uniformly distribute the suspension before administration.

Remove the needle protection, and bleed the syringe of air while holding the needle pointing vertically upward by pressing the plunger in slowly.

Do not administer intravascularly.

Needles should not be recapped, and the syringe should be disposed of properly.

Reconstitution: INFLUVAC comes as 0.5 mL suspension ready for injection.

OVERDOSAGE:

Overdosage is unlikely to have any untoward effect.

For management of a suspected drug overdose, contact your regional Poison Control Centre. See the *CPS* Directory section for a list of Poison Control Centres.

ACTION AND CLINICAL PHARMACOLOGY: Mechanism of Action: INFLUVAC (influenza vaccine, surface antigen, inactivated) is an egg-grown, inactivated influenza virus subunit, trivalent vaccine based on isolated surface antigens of A and B strains of myxovirus influenza. The inoculation of antigen prepared from inactivated influenza virus stimulates the production of specific antibodies. Protection is afforded only against those strains of virus from which the vaccine is prepared or closely related strains.

Influenza A viruses are classified into subtypes on the basis of 2 surface antigens: hemagglutinin (H) and neuraminidase (N). Three subtypes of hemagglutinin (H1, H2, H3) and 2 subtypes of neuraminidase (N1, N2) are recognized among influenza A viruses that have caused widespread human disease. Immunity to these antigens, especially to the hemagglutinin, reduces the likelihood of infection and lessens the severity of disease if infection occurs. Infection with a virus of one subtype confers little or no protection against viruses of other subtypes. Antigenic variation over time within a subtype may be so marked that infection or vaccination with one strain may not induce immunity to distantly related strains of the same subtype. Although influenza B viruses have shown more antigenic stability than influenza A viruses, antigenic variation does occur. For these reasons, major epidemics of respiratory disease caused by variants of influenza still occur. The antigenic characteristics of current and emerging influenza virus strains provide the basis for selecting the virus strains included in each year's vaccine.

Each year's influenza vaccine contains 3 virus strains representing the influenza viruses that are likely to be circulating in Canada on the basis of the recommendation from the World Health Organization for the northern hemisphere.

Pharmacodynamics: Protective antibody levels are generally obtained within 2 to 3 weeks after vaccination.

Pharmacokinetics: As this is a vaccine product, pharmacokinetic studies are not applicable.

Duration of Effect: Protective antibody titres generally last for at least 6 months and may last up to one year or longer. New influenza vaccines are produced each year according to the WHO recommended composition. Patients vaccinated a short time before the start of the expected influenza activity (November in the Northern Hemisphere) may therefore be expected to be protected for influenza infections or its complications during the whole influenza season (November to April).

Serological data over a 52-week period since vaccination in healthy adult subjects aged 18 to 60 years showed a substantial decrease in antibody titres, as is to be expected for Influenza vaccines. Still the 52-week GMT values are markedly elevated as compared to the prevaccination values. The observed decline in GMT values over a one year period was approximately 50-70% for both strains. The sustained levels of protective antibody titres are in line with the expectation of protection during an influenza season up to 6 months after vaccination.

STORAGE AND STABILITY: INFLUVAC (influenza vaccine, surface antigen, inactivated) should be stored at 2 to 8°C (in a refrigerator). Do not freeze. Protect from light.

Do not use vaccine after expiration date as stated on the label.

SPECIAL HANDLING INSTRUCTIONS: INFLUVAC (influenza vaccine, surface antigen, inactivated) should be allowed to reach room temperature before use. Shake well before use. For administration of a 0.25 mL dose from a syringe, push the front side of the plunger exactly to the edge of the hub (the knurled polypropylene ring); a reproducible volume of vaccine remains in the syringe, suitable for administration.

INFORMATION FOR THE PATIENT: Published in e-CPS, available by subscription at www.e-cps.ca.

DOSAGE FORMS, COMPOSITION AND PACKAGING: INFLUVAC (influenza vaccine, surface antigen, inactivated) comes in a 0.5 mL suspension for injection in pre-filled syringes (glass, type I) in the following format: single pack—syringe is packed in a tamper evident carton box; ten pack—syringes are packed in a tamper evident carton box for 10 syringes.

For the 2010/2011 season, each dose of INFLUVAC contains: neuraminidase and 15 µg of hemagglutinin of the following virus strains: A/California/7/2009 (H_1N_1): derived strain used reass. virus NYMC X-181; A/Perth/16/2009 (H_3N_2): like strain used reass. virus NYMC X-187 derived from A/Victoria/210/2009; B/Brisbane/60/2008.

Nonmedicinal ingredients: potassium chloride, potassium dihydrogen phosphate, disodium phosphate dihydrate, sodium chloride, calcium chloride dihydrate, magnesium chloride hexahydrate and water for injections. INFLUVAC also contains trace amounts of eggs, chicken protein, formaldehyde, cetyltrimethylammonium bromide, polysorbate 80 and gentamicin. INFLUVAC is thimerosal-free, mercury-free, and contains no preservative.

(Shown in Product Identification Section)

Infufer® Ⓟ

iron dextran

Hematinic—Iron Supplement

Sandoz

PHARMACOLOGY: After intramuscular injection, iron dextran is absorbed from the injection site into the capillaries and the lymphatic system. Circulating iron dextran is dissociated by the reticuloendothelial system. The ferric iron is transported by transferrin and incorporated into hemoglobin and storage sites. Only traces of unmetabolized iron dextran are excreted in urine, bile, or feces. The drug is negligibly removed by hemodialysis. Most of the intramuscular injection of iron dextran is absorbed within 72 hours, with the remainder absorbed over three to four weeks.

The half-life of i.v. administered [^{59}Fe] iron dextran to iron deficient subjects has ranged from 5 hours to more than 20 hours; however, these values do not represent loss of iron from the body, and accumulation of iron to potentially toxic levels should be avoided.

Iron status following INFUFER (Iron Dextran Injection USP) administration by intravenous infusion was assessed in eight chronic hemodialysis patients (3 female, 5 male; mean age 54±9.9 years) not receiving parenteral iron or recombinant human erythropoietin therapy within the previous 8 weeks. INFUFER was administered in doses of 100 mg diluted in 100 mL of NaCl 0.9%, during the last hour of successive dialysis sessions (usually 2 to 3 sessions per week) until the total dose was attained (mean total dose of 950±220 mg). An initial test dose of 25 mg was administered over 5 minutes, the patient observed for 15 minutes for anaphylaxis, and the remaining 75 mg dose administered over 1 hour. INFUFER increased the iron status in these chronic hemodialysis patients. Plasma ferritin and transferrin saturation values increased significantly at the first time point assessed. Plasma ferritin values remained elevated for at least 4 weeks post-completion of dosing, while transferrin saturation values remained elevated only during the INFUFER administration period. Hemoglobin (Hb) and hematocrit tended to increase, with levels 4 weeks post-completion of dosing significantly higher than the time at which half the INFUFER dose had been administered. The greater increase in Hb was observed in patients with a baseline ferritin of <100 µg/L compared to ferritin values of >100 µg/L. Therefore, the presence of both a transferrin saturation <20% and plasma ferritin <100 µg/L may improve the identification of hemodialysis patients who will often respond to parenteral iron with an increase in Hb.

Iron status following INFUFER administration by intravenous infusion was assessed in fourteen r-HuEPO (recombinant human erythropoietin)-treated hemodialysis patients who completed the study (3 female, 11 male; mean age 59±5.2 years; mean r-HuEPO dose per week 11 429±2142 Units) not receiving parenteral iron therapy within the previous 12 months. INFUFER was administered in doses of 100 mg diluted in 100 mL NaCl 0.9%, during the last half-hour of hemodialysis. Doses were given once a week for ten consecutive weeks, for a total dose of 1000 mg. An initial test dose of 25 mg was administered and the patient observed for one hour for anaphylaxis. INFUFER had a significant impact on the ferritin levels, which is reflective of the patient's iron stores. Significant increases in serum iron and transferrin saturation were observed, with a peak at 8 weeks following initiation of iron dextran therapy. These changes did not translate into an increase in hemoglobin levels.

For patients concurrently taking r-HuEPO, twenty percent of those enrolled (5/25) experienced an adverse reaction to iron dextran. Hypertension was observed in 2 patients (one 3 hours following the test dose, the other during the second dose at week 2). In addition, 1 patient had an anaphylactic response to the test dose. Finally, in the 5 patients who experienced adverse reactions, the following were observed: dizziness, headache, faintness, unconsciousness, distress, palpitations, increased heart rate and blood flow, hypotension, chest pain, flushing, cyanosis, diarrhea, limb cramps, shortness of breath, urticaria and itching.

INDICATIONS: INFUFER (Iron Dextran Injection USP) is indicated for treatment of patients with documented iron deficiency in whom oral administration is unsatisfactory or impossible. It may be administered by intramuscular injection, or by intravenous infusion. **Intravenous infusion must be confined to the hospital treatment of patients for whom the intramuscular route or other forms of therapy are inappropriate or are not available.**

CONTRAINDICATIONS: Hypersensitivity to the product. All anemias not associated with iron deficiency.

INFUFER is not to be used during the acute phase of infectious kidney disease, not to be given intravenously to patients with a history of asthma and not to be administered concomitantly with oral iron preparations.

WARNINGS: The parenteral use of complexes of iron and carbohydrates has resulted in anaphylactic-type reactions. Deaths associated with such administration have been reported. Therefore, INFUFER should be used only in those patients in whom the indications have been clearly established and laboratory investigations confirm an iron deficient state not amenable to oral iron therapy.

Large i.v. doses, such as those used with total dose infusions (TDIs) have been associated with an increased incidence of adverse effects. The adverse effects frequently are delayed (1 to 2 days) and include one or more of the following symptoms: arthralgia, backache, chills, dizziness, moderate to high fever, headache, malaise, myalgia, nausea and vomiting. The onset is usually 24 to 48 hours after administration and symptoms generally subside within 3 to 4 days. Similar symptoms reported following intramuscular injection usually subside within 3 to 7 days. The estimate of risk/benefit should take into consideration the potential for a delayed reaction.

Iron dextran injection should be used with extreme care in patients with serious impairment of liver function.

Iron dextran injection should not be used during the acute phase of infectious kidney disease.

Adverse reactions experienced following administration of iron dextran injection may exacerbate cardiovascular complications in patients with preexisting cardiovascular disease.

Animal studies have shown a risk of carcinogenesis associated with the intramuscular injection of iron-carbohydrate complexes. Sarcomas were produced when large doses were given to rodents, or when small doses were injected repeatedly into the same site in rodents and rabbits.

The long latent period between the injection of a potential carcinogen and the appearance of a tumour makes it impossible to measure accurately the risk in man. There have, however, been several reports in the literature describing tumours at the injection site in humans who had previously received intramuscular injections of iron-dextran.

PRECAUTIONS: Unwarranted therapy with parenteral iron will cause excess storage of iron with the consequent possibility of exogenous hemosiderosis. Such iron overload is particularly apt to occur in patients with hemoglobinopathies and other refractory anemias that might be erroneously diagnosed as iron deficiency anemias.

Iron dextran injection should be used with caution in individuals with histories of significant allergies and/or asthma.

Anaphylaxis and other hypersensitivity reactions have been reported after uneventful test doses as well as therapeutic doses of iron dextran injection. Therefore, administration of subsequent test doses during therapy should be considered (see Dosage).

Epinephrine should be immediately available in the event of acute hypersensitivity reactions. The usual dose of epinephrine is 0.5 mL of a 1:1000 solution, by subcutaneous or intramuscular injection. Patients using beta-blocking agents may not respond adequately to epinephrine, and they may require isoproterenol or similar beta-agonist agents.

Patients with rheumatoid arthritis may have an acute exacerbation of joint pain and swelling following the administration of iron dextran injection.

There have been published reports, from New Zealand, associating the use of intramuscular iron dextran in neonates with an increased incidence of gram-negative sepsis, primarily due to *E. coli*.

Information to Be Provided to the Patient: Patients should be advised of the potential adverse reactions associated with the use of iron dextran injection (see Adverse Effects).

Drug/Laboratory Test Interactions: Large doses of iron dextran (5 mL or more) have been reported to give a brown colour to serum from a blood sample drawn 4 hours after administration. Iron dextran injection may cause falsely elevated values of serum bilirubin and falsely decreased values of serum calcium.

Serum iron determinations by colorimetric assays may not be meaningful for three weeks following the administration of iron dextran.

Serum ferritin peaks approximately 7 to 9 days after an intravenous dose and slowly returns to baseline after about 3 weeks.

Examination of the bone marrow for iron stores may not be meaningful for prolonged periods following therapy with iron dextran injection because residual iron dextran may remain in the reticuloendothelial cells.

Bone scans involving 99m Tc-diphosphonate have been reported to show a dense, crescentic area of activity in the buttocks, following the contour of the iliac crest, 1 to 6 days after intramuscular injections of iron dextran.

Bone scans with 99m Tc-labeled bone seeking agents, in the presence of high serum ferritin levels or following iron dextran infusions, have been reported to show reduction of bony uptake, marked renal activity and increased blood pool and soft tissue accumulation.

Pregnancy: Iron dextran has been shown to be teratogenic and embryocidal in non-anemic mice, rats, rabbits, dogs and monkeys when given in doses of about 3 times the maximum human dose. No consistent adverse fetal effects were observed in mice, rats, rabbits, dogs, and monkeys at doses of 50 mg iron/kg or less. Fetal and maternal toxicity have been reported in monkeys at a total intravenous dose of 90 mg iron/kg over a 14 day period. Similar effects were observed in mice and rats after administration of a single dose of 125 mg iron/kg. Fetal abnormalities in rats and dogs were observed at doses of 250 mg iron/kg and higher. The animals used in these tests were not iron deficient. There are no adequate and well-controlled studies in pregnant women. **Iron dextran injection should be used in pregnant women only if the potential benefit justifies the potential risk to the fetus.**

Placental Transfer: Various animal studies have demonstrated placental transfer of iron dextran complex, and studies in pregnant humans have demonstrated inconclusive results. It appears that some iron does reach the fetus, but the form in which it crosses the placenta is not clear.

Lactation: Caution should be exercised when INFUFER is administered to a nursing woman. Traces of unmetabolized iron dextran are excreted in human milk.

Children: **Not recommended for use in infants under 4 months of age (see Dosage).**

ADVERSE EFFECTS: Severe/Fatal: Anaphylactic reactions to iron dextran injection, including fatal anaphylaxis, have been reported. Such reactions which occur most often within the first several minutes of administration are generally characterized by the sudden onset of respiratory difficulty and/or cardiovascular collapse.

The incidence of these acute hypersensitivity reactions has been estimated between 0.1 to 0.6% (see Warnings). (See Precautions, pertaining to immediate availability of epinephrine.) Administration must be stopped **immediately** when signs of an anaphylactoid reaction are seen.

Mild/moderate: Delayed reactions may occur (see Warnings). In a surveillance program of 1260 patients treated with Total Dose Infusion of iron dextran injection, the overall reaction rate was 29.8%, with 14.3% immediate reactions occurring on the day of infusion and 17.7% delayed reactions occurring on later days; 2.1% of patients experienced both immediate and delayed reactions. (Severe reactions were recorded in 5.3% of patients.)

Cardiovascular: chest pain, chest tightness, shock, hypotension, hypertension, tachycardia, flushing, arrhythmias. (Flushing and hypotension may occur from too rapid intravenous administration.)

Dermatologic: urticaria, pruritus, purpura, rash.

Gastrointestinal: abdominal pain, nausea, vomiting, diarrhea.

Hematologic/Lymphatic: leukocytosis, lymphadenopathy.

Musculoskeletal/Soft Tissue: arthralgia, arthritis (may represent reactivation in patients with quiescent rheumatoid arthritis [see Precautions]), myalgia; backache; sterile abscess, atrophy/fibrosis (intramuscular injection site); brown skin and/or underlying tissue discoloration (staining), soreness or pain at or near intramuscular injection sites; cellulitis; swelling; inflammation; local phlebitis at or near intravenous injection site.

Neurologic: convulsions, seizures, syncope, headache, weakness, unresponsiveness, paresthesia, febrile episodes, chills, dizziness, disorientation, numbness.

Respiratory: respiratory arrest, dyspnea, bronchospasm.

Urologic: hematuria.

Delayed Reactions: arthralgia, backache, chills, dizziness, fever, headache, malaise, myalgia, nausea, vomiting (see Warnings).

Miscellaneous: febrile episodes, sweating, shivering, chills, malaise, altered taste.

OVERDOSE:

Symptoms: Overdosage with iron dextran injection is unlikely to produce acute adverse reactions. Excessive doses beyond the requirements for restoration of hemoglobin and replenishment of iron stores, may lead to hemosiderosis. Periodic monitoring of serum ferritin levels may be helpful in recognizing adverse accumulation of iron in concurrent medical conditions such as chronic renal failure, Hodgkin's disease, and rheumatoid arthritis.

For management of a suspected drug overdose, CPhA recommends that you contact your **regional Poison Control Centre**. See the *CPS* Directory section for a list of Poison Control Centres.

DOSAGE: Oral iron should be discontinued prior to administration of INFUFER (Iron Dextran Injection USP).

Dosage is calculated specifically for each patient dependent upon body weight, age, sex and degree of anemia, using a dosage table or some suitable formula. It is preferred that INFUFER be given by the intramuscular route, unless there are valid reasons for intravenous administration. The intravenous infusion of INFUFER should be restricted to hospital usage only.

Dosage Determinations in Patients with Iron Deficiency Anemia: Periodic hematologic determination of hemoglobin and hematocrit should be used as a guide for monitoring hematological response. As iron storage may lag behind the appearance of normal blood morphology, other tests, such as serum iron, total iron binding capacity (TIBC), serum ferritin and percent saturation of transferrin, may be needed for detecting and monitoring the iron deficient state of the patient.

Reticulocyte count should increase within a few days of iron dextran administration.

Serum ferritin levels may not correlate with body iron stores in patients on chronic renal dialysis who are also receiving iron dextran complex.

Although there are significant variations in body build and weight distribution among males and females, Table 1 and the accompanying formula represent a convenient means for estimating the total iron required. This total iron requirement reflects the amount of iron needed to restore hemoglobin concentration to normal or near normal levels plus an additional allowance to provide adequate replenishment of iron stores in most individuals with moderately or severely reduced levels of hemoglobin. It should be remembered that iron deficiency anemia will not appear until essentially all iron stores have been depleted. Thus, therapy should aim at not only the restoration of hemoglobin but also the replenishment of iron stores.

Factors contributing to the formula include:

$$\frac{\text{mg blood iron}}{\text{lb body weight}} = \frac{\text{mL blood}}{\text{lb body weight}} \times \frac{\text{g hemoglobin}}{\text{mL blood}} \times \frac{\text{mg iron}}{\text{g hemoglobin}}$$

a) Blood volume=65 mL/kg of body weight. b) Normal hemoglobin (males and females) over 15 kg (33 lbs)=14.8 g/100 mL, 15 kg (33 lbs) or less=12 g/100 mL. c) Iron content of hemoglobin=0.34%. d) Hemoglobin deficit. e) Weight.

Based on the above factors, individuals with normal hemoglobin levels will have approximately 33 mg of blood iron/kg of body weight (15 mg/lb).

Note: The formula and accompanying table (Table 1) are applicable for dosage determinations only in patients with iron deficiency anemia; they are not to be used for dosage determinations in patients requiring iron replacement for blood loss.

Table 1: INFUFER

Total INFUFER Requirement For Hemoglobin Restoration and Iron Stores Replacement

Patient Lean Body Weight		**mL Requirement of INFUFER Based on Observed Hemoglobin of**							
kg	**lb**	**3 g/dL**	**4 g/dL**	**5 g/dL**	**6 g/dL**	**7 g/dL**	**8 g/dL**	**9 g/dL**	**10 g/dL**
5	11	3	3	3	3	2	2	2	2
10	22	7	6	6	5	5	4	4	3
15	33	10	9	9	8	7	7	6	5
20	44	16	15	14	13	12	11	10	9
25	55	20	18	17	16	15	14	13	12
30	66	23	22	21	19	18	17	15	14
35	77	27	26	24	23	21	20	18	17
40	88	31	29	28	26	24	22	21	19
45	99	35	33	31	29	27	25	23	21
50	110	39	37	35	32	30	28	26	24
55	121	43	41	38	36	33	31	28	26
60	132	47	44	42	39	36	34	31	28
65	143	51	48	45	42	39	36	34	31
70	154	55	52	49	45	42	39	36	33
75	165	59	55	52	49	45	42	39	35
80	176	63	59	55	52	48	45	41	38
85	187	66	63	59	55	51	48	44	40
90	198	70	66	62	58	54	50	46	42
95	209	74	70	66	62	57	53	49	45
100	220	78	74	69	65	60	56	52	47
105	231	82	77	73	68	63	59	54	50
110	242	86	81	76	71	67	62	57	52
115	253	90	85	80	75	70	64	59	54

(cont'd)

Table 1: INFUFER *(cont'd)*

Total INFUFER Requirement For Hemoglobin Restoration and Iron Stores Replacement

Patient Lean Body Weight		mL Requirement of INFUFER Based on Observed Hemoglobin of							
kg	lb	3 g/dL	4 g/dL	5 g/dL	6 g/dL	7 g/dL	8 g/dL	9 g/dL	10 g/dL
120	264	94	88	83	78	73	67	62	57

Table values were calculated based on a normal adult hemoglobin of 14.8 g/dL for body weights greater than 15 kg (33 lbs) and a hemoglobin of 12 g/dL for body weights less than or equal to 15 kg (33 lbs).

The total amount of INFUFER in mL required to treat the anemia and replenish iron stores may be approximated as follows:
For Adults and Children Over 15 kg (33 lbs): see Table 1.

Alternatively, the total dose may be calculated as follows:
Dose (mL)=0.0442 (Desired Hb-Observed Hb)×LBW+(0.26×LBW)
Based on: Desired Hb=the target Hb in g/dL. Observed Hb=the patient's current hemoglobin in g/dL. LBW=Lean body weight in kg. A patient's lean body weight (or actual body weight if less than lean body weight) should be utilized when determining dosage. To convert the patient's weight from pounds to kg: patient's weight in pounds/2.2=weight in kg. For males: LBW=50 kg+2.3 kg for each inch of patient's height over 5 feet. For females: LBW=45.5 kg+2.3 kg for each inch of patient's height over 5 feet.
Children 5 to 15 kg (11 to 33 lbs): see Table 1. Iron dextran should not normally be given in the first 4 months of life (see Precautions, Children).

Alternatively, the total dose may be calculated as follows:
Dose (mL)=0.0442 (Desired Hb-Observed Hb)×W+(0.26×W)
Based on: Desired Hb=the target Hb in g/dL. (Normal Hb for children 15 kg or less is 12 g/dL.) Observed Hb=the patient's current Hb in g/dL. W=Weight in kg. To convert the patient's weight from pounds to kg: Patient's weight in pounds/2.2=weight in kg.
Iron Replacement for Blood Loss: Some individuals sustain blood losses on an intermittent or repetitive basis. Such blood losses may occur periodically in patients with hemorrhagic diatheses (familial telangiectasia, hemophilia, gastrointestinal bleeding) and on a repetitive basis from procedures such as renal hemodialysis.

Iron therapy in these patients should be directed toward replacement of the equivalent amount of iron represented in the lost blood. **The Table 1 and formula presented under iron deficiency anemia are not applicable for simple iron replacement values.**

Quantitative estimates of the individual's periodic blood loss and hematocrit during the bleeding episode provide a convenient method for the calculation of the required iron dose.

The formula shown below is based on the approximation that 1 mL of normocytic, normochromic red cells contains 1 mg of elemental iron:
Replacement iron (in mg)=Blood loss (in mL)×hematocrit.
Example: Blood loss of 500 mL with 20% hematocrit.
Replacement iron=500×0.20=100 mg.

$$\text{INFUFER dose} = \frac{100\text{ mg}}{50\text{ mg/mL}} = 2\text{ mL}$$

Administration: The total amount of INFUFER (Iron Dextran Injection USP) required for the treatment of iron deficiency anemia or iron replacement for blood loss is determined from the table or appropriate formula (see Dosage).
Intramuscular Injection: **Prior to receiving their first therapeutic dose, all patients should be given an intramuscular test dose of 0.5 mL gradually.** The test dose should be administered in the same recommended test site and by the same technique as described in the last paragraph of this section. Although anaphylactic reactions known to occur following iron dextran administration are usually evident within a few minutes or sooner, it is recommended that at least an hour or longer elapse before the remainder of the initial therapeutic dose is given.

If no adverse reactions are observed, INFUFER can be given according to the following schedule until the calculated total amount required has been reached. Each day's dose should ordinarily not exceed 0.5 mL (25 mg of iron) for infants under 5 kg (11 lbs); 1 mL (50 mg of iron) for children under 10 kg (22 lbs); and 2 mL (100 mg of iron) for other patients. It is recommended that these be **given as a graded series of injections starting with a test dose of 0.5 mL (25 mg elemental iron)**, 1 mL, then 2 mL, while the patient is observed carefully for adverse reactions. The injections should be administered gradually. If the patient is moderately active, injections may be given daily into alternate buttocks. In inactive or bedridden patients, the frequency of injections should be reduced to once or twice weekly.

Deep intramuscular injection in the upper outer quadrant of the buttock, using a Z-track technique (with displacement of the skin laterally prior to injection) insures absorption and will help to avoid staining of the skin. A 5 cm needle is recommended for the adult of average size.

The intramuscular route of administration is to be used unless there are valid reasons for intravenous administration.
Intravenous Infusion: **Prior to receiving their first therapeutic dose, all patients should be given a test dose of 0.5 mL (equivalent to 25 mg elemental iron) by intravenous infusion administered slowly over at least 5 minutes at a rate of not more than 5 drops/minute.** If the test dose is well tolerated, the rate of infusion may be increased **progressively** to 45 to 60 drops/minute (3 to 4 mL/minute).

Anaphylactoid reactions are usually evident within a few minutes. **If at any time during the intravenous administration, any signs of a hypersensitivity reaction or intolerance are detected, administration must be stopped immediately.** Resuscitative equipment should be available, and the reactions treated with 0.5 mL of aqueous epinephrine 1:1000 given s.c. with general supportive measures, followed by either oral or parenteral antihistamines and/or corticosteroids (see Precautions).

INFUFER may be administered in large volumes via the Total Dose Infusion technique for the hospital treatment of patients for whom the i.m. route or other forms of therapy are inappropriate or are not available.

The intravenous route should not be used for patients with a history of asthma. If the intravenous route is judged necessary for patients with a history of allergy, effective antihistamine cover should be given before administration of the iron dextran.
Total Dose Infusion (TDI) Technique: The total amount of calculated INFUFER required is added aseptically immediately before use to the required volume, usually 500 mL of sterile 0.9% Sodium Chloride Injection or 5% Dextrose Injection solution. The use of 5% Dextrose Injection solution has been associated with a higher incidence of local pain and phlebitis.

A test dose of 25 mg of elemental iron should be administered slowly over 5 minutes at an infusion rate not exceeding 5 drops per minute. If no hypersensitivity reaction occurs following an observation period of at least 1 hour, the remainder of the dose may be infused over one to three hours, or as much as six to eight hours at an infusion rate of 3-4 mL/minute. The vein should then be flushed with about 10 mL of 0.9% Sodium Chloride Injection. Patients should be observed closely during the infusion and for at least 1 hour after it is completed.

The intramuscular route of administration is to be used unless there are valid reasons for intravenous administration.
Preparation of Infusion Solutions: See Table 2. For IV infusion with dilution, INFUFER may be diluted in 0.9% Sodium Chloride Injection or 5% Dextrose Injection. The diluted preparations are chemically stable for 24 hours at room temperature. Discard unused portion.

Solutions of INFUFER in 5% Dextrose Injection solution must not be autoclaved, because precipitation may occur. Other agents should not be added to iron dextran infusions, nor should INFUFER be added to blood for transfusion.

Iron dextran has been reported to be incompatible with oxytetracycline and with sulfadiazine sodium in i.v. infusion.
Note: Do not mix INFUFER with other medications or add to parenteral nutrition solutions for i.v. infusion.
Infusion Following Hemodialysis Procedure: Chronic hemodialysis patients who develop anemia may be administered INFUFER in 100 mg doses diluted in 100 mL of 0.9% Sodium Chloride Injection during the last hour of successive dialysis sessions until the total dose is attained. A test dose of 25 mg of elemental iron should be administered slowly over 5 minutes, and the patient monitored for adverse reactions over a 1-hour period before continuing with the initial infusion, as described previously.
Stability of Infusion Preparations: For IV infusion with dilution, INFUFER may be diluted in 0.9% Sodium Chloride Injection or 5% Dextrose Injection solution. The diluted preparations are chemically stable for 24 hours at room temperature. Discard unused portion.

Solutions of INFUFER in 5% Dextrose Injection solution must not be autoclaved, because precipitation may occur. Other agents should not be added to iron dextran infusions, nor should INFUFER be added to blood for transfusion.

As with all parenteral products, intravenous admixtures should be inspected visually for clarity, particulate matter, precipitation, discolouration and leakage prior to administration whenever solution and container permit.

Table 2: INFUFER

Preparation of Infusion Solutions

	Amount of INFUFER	Amount of Diluent[a]
Total Dose Infusion (TDI)	Total Calculated Dose	500 mL
Infusion Following Hemodialysis	2 mL (100 mg iron)	100 mL

[a] Diluent may be sterile 0.9% Sodium Chloride Injection or 5% Dextrose Injection solution. Note that 5% Dextrose Injection solution has been associated with a higher incidence of local pain and phlebitis.

SUPPLIED: Each mL of injection contains: elemental iron 50 mg as an iron dextran complex and sodium chloride 0.9% in water for injection. Sodium hydroxide and/or hydrochloric acid may be used to adjust pH. Preservative-free. Single use, clear vials of 2 mL, boxes of 10. Single use, clear vials of 5 mL, boxes of 5. Store between 15 and 25°C. Do not freeze. Discard unused portion.

The reader is invited to consult CPhA's monograph **ACE Inhibitors**.

Inhibace® Pr

cilazapril monohydrate

Angiotensin Converting Enzyme Inhibitor

Roche

SUPPLIED: 2.5 mg: Each pinkish-brown, oval-shaped, single-scored, biconvex, film-coated tablet, imprinted CIL 2.5, contains: cilazapril 2.5 mg as cilazapril monohydrate. Nonmedicinal ingredients: cornstarch, hydroxypropyl methylcellulose, iron oxide, lactose monohydrate, sodium stearyl fumarate, talc and titanium dioxide. Bottles of 100. Store 15 to 30°C. Keep container tightly closed.
5 mg: Each reddish-brown, oval-shaped, single-scored, biconvex tablet, imprinted CIL 5, contains: cilazapril 5 mg as cilazapril monohydrate. Nonmedicinal ingredients: cornstarch, hydroxypropyl methylcellulose, iron oxide, lactose monohydrate, sodium stearyl fumarate, talc and titanium dioxide. Bottles of 100. Store 15 to 30°C. Keep container tightly closed.

The reader is invited to consult CPhA's monograph **ACE Inhibitors**.

Inhibace® Plus Pr

cilazapril monohydrate—hydrochlorothiazide

Angiotensin Converting Enzyme Inhibitor—Diuretic

Roche

SUPPLIED: Each pale red, oval-shaped, single-scored, bixonvex, film-coated tablet, imprinted CIL + on the top half and 5 + 12.5 on the bottom half of one side, contains: cilazapril 5 mg (as cilazapril monohydrate) and hydrochlorothiazide 12.5 mg. Nonmedicinal ingredients: cornstarch, hydroxypropyl methylcellulose, lactose, red iron oxide, sodium stearyl fumarate, talc and titanium dioxide. Blister packages of 28. Store 15 to 30°C. Keep container tightly closed.

The reader is invited to consult CPhA's monograph **Heparins, Low Molecular Weight**.

Innohep® Pr

tinzaparin sodium

Anticoagulant—Antithrombotic

LEO Pharma

PHARMACOLOGY: Tinzaparin is a low molecular weight heparin (LMWH), produced by enzymatic depolymerization of unfractionated heparin from porcine intestinal mucosa. It is a heterogeneous mixture of sulfated polysaccharide glycosaminoglycan chains. The mass-average molecular weight mass ranges between 5500 and 7500 daltons. The mass percentage of chains lower than 2000 is not more than 10%. The mass percentage of chains between 2000 and 8000 ranges between 60 and 72%. The mass percentage of chains above 8000 ranges between 22 and 36%. Tinzaparin is composed of molecules with and without a specially characterized pentasaccharide, which is the specific site for high affinity binding to the plasma protein antithrombin III (AT III). This binding to AT III leads to an accelerated inhibition of factor Xa. This results in the antithrombotic effect of tinzaparin, although other mechanisms may also be involved since it potentiates the inhibition of several activated coagulation factors.

Tinzaparin is an antithrombotic agent with higher anti-Xa activity (70 to 120 IU/mg) than anti-IIa activity (approximately 55 IU/mg). The ratio of anti-Xa to anti-IIa activity for tinzaparin is 2.0±0.5, whereas it is 1 for unfractionated heparin.
Pharmacokinetics: The bioavailability following subcutaneous injection is about 90% when measured as anti-Xa activity versus 67% for anti-IIa activity. The absorption half-life of anti-Xa activity is 200 minutes and that of anti-IIa activity is 257 minutes. Peak plasma anti-Xa activity occurs at approximately 4-6 hours. Detectable anti-Xa activity persists for 24 hours after injection, despite elimination half-lives of anti-Xa activity of 82 minutes and anti-IIa of 71 minutes. No evidence of accumulation was found when tinzaparin was administered once daily for five days at a dose of 175 anti-Xa IU/kg. The volume of distribution of anti-Xa activity is 4 L and that of anti-IIa activity is 10.9 L. The effect of tinzaparin on APTT values is inconsistent and generally only shows a dose-dependent effect at doses above 5000 anti-Xa IU.

Neither tinzaparin nor heparin doses can be measured directly in the bloodstream. Their effects on clotting are a function of the dose. Unfractionated heparin is usually measured by prolongation of APTT, although plasma anti-Xa can also be determined. Tinzaparin only causes APTT prolongation at higher doses. In the therapeutic range, the effects of tinzaparin on the plasma anti-Xa activity can be measured as an indication of serum tinzaparin levels. However, clinical trials have not demonstrated a linear correlation between anti-Xa activity and antithrombotic effect. Prophylactic doses of 75 IU/kg of tinzaparin by s.c. administration resulted in peak anti-Xa activity of 0.31 to 0.42 IU/mL in patients whereas the mean ratio of peak APTT (as compared to baseline) was 1.13 to 1.35. Treatment doses of 175 anti-Xa IU/kg resulted in peak anti-Xa activity of approximately 0.4 to 1.8 IU/mL and a mean peak APTT ratio of 1.71 to 2.63. APTT values associated with either the prophylaxis or treatment dose of tinzaparin returned to baseline within 20 to 28 hours after administration. APTT values associated with LMWHs heparin are variable and are not predictive of clinical efficacy or safety.

The primary route of tinzaparin elimination is by the kidney. The half-life for anti-Xa activity for LMWHs is prolonged in patients with impaired renal function relative to people with normal function. The effect of renal impairment on tinzaparin anti-Xa activity has not been fully studied (see Warnings, Precautions, Renal Impairment, and Dosage, Use in Patients with Renal Impairment).
INDICATIONS: For the prevention of postoperative venous thromboembolism in patients undergoing orthopedic surgery and in patients undergoing general surgery who are at high risk of developing postoperative venous thromboembolism (see Precautions, Selection of General Surgery Patients).

Tinzaparin is indicated for the treatment of deep vein thrombosis and/or pulmonary embolism.

Tinzaparin is indicated for the prevention of clotting in indwelling i.v. lines for hemodialysis and extracorporeal circulation in patients without high bleeding risk.

CONTRAINDICATIONS: Hypersensitivity to tinzaparin; or any of its constituents, including benzyl alcohol (when using multi-dose vials) (see Warnings, Pregnancy), or sodium bisulphite (see Warnings); or to other low molecular weight heparins and/or heparin. The multi-dose vials of tinzaparin contain 10 mg/mL benzyl alcohol as preservative and must not be given to children <2 years old, premature infants and neonates, due to the risk of developing gasping syndrome. History of confirmed or suspected immunologically-mediated heparin-induced thrombocytopenia (delayed-onset severe thrombocytopenia), or in patients in whom an in vitro platelet-aggregation test in the presence of tinzaparin is positive. Acute or subacute septic endocarditis. Generalized hemorrhage tendency and other conditions/diseases involving an increased risk of hemorrhage (e.g. severe liver insufficiency, women with abortus imminens). Hemophilia or major blood clotting disorders. Acute cerebral insults or hemorrhagic cerebrovascular accidents (except if there are systemic emboli). Active bleeding from a local lesion such as an acute ulcer (e.g., gastric or duodenal) or ulcerating carcinoma. Uncontrolled severe hypertension. Diabetic or hemorrhagic retinopathy. Injury or surgery involving the CNS, eyes or ears. Spinal/epidural anaesthesia is contraindicated where high (i.e. non-prophylactic) dosages of tinzaparin (175 IU/kg once daily) are required, due to an increased risk of bleeding.

WARNINGS: Tinzaparin must not be administered by intramuscular injection due to risk of hematoma.

Tinzaparin cannot be used interchangeably (unit for unit) with unfractionated heparin or other LMWHs.

Determination of peak anti-Xa activity in plasma at 4-6 hours post-dosing is the only method available for monitoring tinzaparin levels. Routine clotting assays are not suitable for monitoring tinzaparin anticoagulant activity. APTT prolongation is not a suitable test for monitoring the LMWHs.

Measurement of peak anti-Xa levels should be considered in patients at higher risk of bleeding and receiving tinzaparin such as the elderly, patients with renal impairment or the extremes of body weight, during pregnancy, or for children. At treatment doses, peak anti-Xa levels should generally be maintained at no more than 1.5 IU/mL in these patients (see Pharmacology, and Precautions, Patient Monitoring).

Tinzaparin should be used with caution in patients with hepatic insufficiency, renal insufficiency or a history of gastrointestinal ulceration.

The half-life for anti-Xa activity in patients with severe renal impairment being treated with LMWH is much longer compared to those with normal kidney function, and has not been fully studied for tinzaparin (see Pharmacology, Precautions, Renal Impairment, and Dosage, Use in Patients with Renal Impairment). Dosage reduction should be considered in patients with severe renal impairment.

Sodium bisulfite, which may cause allergic reactions including anaphylactic symptoms and life-threatening or less severe asthmatic episodes in certain susceptible people, is present in tinzaparin multi-dose vials (10 000 and 20 000 anti-Xa IU/mL) and tinzaparin 20 000 anti-Xa IU/mL unit dose graduated syringes (10 000 IU/syringe, 14 000 IU/syringe and 18 000 IU/syringe). The overall prevalence of sulfite sensitivity in the general population is unknown. Sulfite sensitivity is seen more frequently in asthmatics than in nonasthmatic people. However, tinzaparin 10 000 anti-Xa IU/mL unit dose syringes (3500 IU/syringe and 4500 IU/syringe) do not contain sodium bisulfite.

Tinzaparin should not be used for the treatment of pulmonary embolism in patients with severe hemodynamic instability.

Hemorrhage: Bleeding may occur in conjunction with unfractionated heparin or LMWH use. As with other anticoagulants, tinzaparin should be used with extreme caution in patients at increased risk of hemorrhage. Bleeding can occur at any site during therapy with tinzaparin. An unexpected drop in hematocrit or blood pressure should lead to a search for a bleeding site (see Adverse Effects, Bleeding).

Metabolic: All unfractionated heparins/LMWHs can suppress adrenal secretion of aldosterone, leading to hyperkalaemia, particularly in partients with diabetes mellitus, chronic renal failure, pre-existing metabolic acidosis, raised plasma potassium or taking potassium sparing drugs. The risk of hyperkalaemia appears to increase with duration of therapy but is usually reversible. Plasma potassium should be measured in patients at risk before starting tinzaparin therapy and monitored regularly thereafter especially if treatment is prolonged beyond 7 days.

Spinal/Epidural Hematomas: There have been cases of intraspinal hematomas with the concurrent use of LMWH and spinal/epidural anesthesia resulting in long-term or permanent paralysis. The risk of these events may be higher with the use of postoperative indwelling epidural catheters or by the concomitant use of drugs affecting hemostasis: NSAIDs, platelet inhibitors, or other drugs affecting coagulation. The risk also appears to be increased by traumatic or repeated epidural or spinal procedure. **Tinzaparin should only be used concurrently with spinal/epidural anaesthesia when the therapeutic benefits to the patient outweigh the possible risks** (also, see Contraindications). When used concurrently, no spinal invasion should be performed for 12 hours following the dose of LMWH and the next dose should be held until at least 2 hours after the anesthesia procedure. The same rules apply to the withdrawal or manipulation of the catheter. Careful vigilance for neurological signs is recommended, with rapid diagnosis and treatment; if such signs occur (see Adverse Effects).

Thrombocytopenia: Thrombocytopenia of any degree should be monitored closely. Heparin-induced thrombocytopenia can occur with the administration of tinzaparin. Its incidence is unknown at present.

Thrombocytosis: As with other LMWHs, the administration of tinzaparin in some patients undergoing surgical procedures (especially orthopaedic) or having a concomitant inflammatory process has coincided with an asymptomatic increase in platelet count. If an increase in platelet count occurs, tinzaparin should be stopped, the benefit of continuing therapy for that patient should be re-evaluated against the risk. Drugs affecting platelet function or the coagulation system should in general not be given concomitantly with tinzaparin.

Patients with Prosthetic Heart Valves: Cases of prosthetic valve thrombosis have been reported in patients who received low molecular weight heparins for thromboprophylaxis. Some of these patients were pregnant women in whom thrombosis led to maternal and/or fetal deaths. Pregnant women are at higher risk of thromboembolism (see Warnings, Pregnancy).

Pregnancy: The 2 mL multi-dose vials of tinzaparin (10 000 anti-Xa IU/mL and 20 000 anti-Xa IU/mL) contain 20 mg of benzyl alcohol as a preservative (10 mg of benzyl alcohol per mL). Cases of fatal "Gasping Syndrome" have been reported in the literature, which occurred in premature infants and neonates when large amounts (99-404 mg/kg/day) of benzyl alcohol have been administered. Manifestations of the disease include: metabolic acidosis, respiratory distress, gasping respirations, central nervous system dysfunction, convulsions, intracranial hemorrhages, hypoactivity, hypotonia, cardiovascular collapse and death. Therefore the multi-dose vials of tinzaparin preserved with benzyl alcohol must not be used in children <2 years old, newborn and preterm babies (see Contraindications). Because benzyl alcohol may cross the placenta, tinzaparin preserved with benzyl alcohol should not be used in pregnant women. Prefilled syringes of tinzaparin do not contain benzyl alcohol.

The use of tinzaparin in women with abortus imminens is contraindicated (see Contraindications).

Teratogenic effects: As with other low molecular weight heparins, tinzaparin should not be used in pregnant women unless the therapeutic benefits to the patients outweigh the possible risks. There have been reports of congenital anomalies in infants born to women who received LMWH during pregnancy, including cerebral anomalies, limb anomalies, hypospadias, peripheral vascular malformation, fibrotic dysplasia and cardiac defects. A causal relationship has not been established nor has the incidence been shown to be higher than in the general population.

Non-teratogenic effects: There have been post-marketing reports of fetal death when pregnant women received LMWH. Causality for these cases has not been established. Pregnant women receiving anticoagulants, including tinzaparin, are at increased risk for bleeding. Hemorrhage can occur at any site and may lead to death of mother and/or fetus. Pregnant women receiving tinzaparin should be carefully monitored. Pregnant women and women of child-bearing potential should be informed of the potential hazard to the fetus and the mother if tinzaparin is administered during pregnancy.

There are also post-marketing reports of prosthetic valve thrombosis in pregnant women with prosthetic heart valves while receiving low molecular weight heparins for thromboprophylaxis. These events led to maternal death or surgical interventions.

Pregnant women with prosthetic heart valves appear to be at exceedingly high risk of thromboembolism. An incidence of thromboembolism approaching 30% has been reported in these patients, in some cases even with apparent adequate anticoagulation at treatment doses of low molecular weight heparins or unfractionated heparin. Any attempt to anticoagulate such patients should normally only be undertaken by medical practitioners with documented expertise and experience in this clinical area.

Lactation: It is not known whether tinzaparin is excreted in human breast milk. Because many drugs are excreted in human milk, caution should be exercised when tinzaparin is administered to nursing women.

Children: The safety and effectiveness of tinzaparin in children has not been established.

PRECAUTIONS: Tinzaparin cannot be used interchangeably (unit for unit) with unfractionated heparin or other LMWHs as they differ in their manufacturing process, molecular weight distribution, anti-Xa and anti-IIA activities, units and dosages. Special attention and compliance with instructions for use of each specific product is required during any change in treatment.

Due to the increased risk of bleeding, concomitant medications should not be given by intramuscular injection and care should be taken when giving lumbar puncture and similar procedures.

Drug Interactions: Tinzaparin should be used with caution in patients receiving oral anticoagulants, NSAIDs, platelet inhibitors and thrombolytic agents because of increased risk of bleeding.

Patient Monitoring: Tinzaparin has only a moderate prolonging effect on clotting time assays such as APTT or thrombin time. For laboratory monitoring of tinzaparin plasma anti-Xa levels are recommended. Clinically meaningful prolongation of APTT during hemodialysis or treatment of acute deep vein thrombophlebitis with tinzaparin should only be used as an indication of overdosage.

Tinzaparin is administered subcutaneously and therefore the individual patient's anti-Xa activity level will not remain within the range that would be expected with unfractionated heparin by continuous intravenous infusion throughout the entire dosing interval. In clinical studies the median peak plasma anti-Xa levels achieved approximately 4 hours after subcutaneous administration of 3500 IU, 75 IU/kg or 175 IU/kg were 0.15, 0.34 and 0.70 anti-Xa IU/mL respectively. Clinical studies demonstrate no relevant accumulation after repeated once daily subcutaneous administration of tinzaparin. Tinzaparin should be administered as directed (see Dosage).

As with all anti-thrombotic agents, there is a risk of systemic bleeding with tinzaparin. Care should be taken with tinzaparin use in high dose treatment of newly operated patients. In the event of excessive blood loss from the surgical wound, the first injection of tinzaparin should be deferred until the bleeding has stopped.

After treatment is initiated, patients should be carefully monitored for bleeding complications. This may be done by regular physical examination of the patients, close observation of the surgical drain and periodic measurements of haemoglobin and anti-Xa determinations.

With normal prophylactic doses, tinzaparin does not modify global clotting tests of activated partial thromboplastin time (APTT), prothrombin time (PT) and thrombin clotting time (TT). Therefore, treatment cannot be monitored with these tests.

At higher doses, increases in APTT and ACT (activated clotting time) may occur. Increases in APTT and ACT are not linearly correlated with increasing tinzaparin antithrombotic activity and therefore are unsuitable and unreliable for monitoring tinzaparin activity.

In the case of minor bleeding, the drug should be postponed or withdrawn. When serious bleeding requires reversal of tinzaparin, protamine sulphate (1% solution) by slow infusion will largely neutralize tinzaparin (see Overdose, Treatment). The effect of protamine sulphate should be monitored by the APTT.

Platelets: Platelet counts should be determined prior to the start of treatment with tinzaparin and, subsequently, twice weekly for the duration of treatment.

Caution is recommended when administering tinzaparin to patients with congenital or drug-induced thrombocytopenia or platelet defects.

During tinzaparin administration, special caution is necessary in rapidly developing thrombocytopenia and severe thrombocytopenia <100 000/mcL). A positive or indeterminate result obtained from in vitro tests for antiplatelet antibody in the presence of tinzaparin or other LMWHs and/or heparin would contraindicate tinzaparin.

Renal Impairment: Patients with impaired renal function should be carefully monitored because the half-life for anti-Xa activity after administration of LMWH may be prolonged in this patient population (see Warnings, and Dosage, Use in Patients with Renal Impairment).

Selection of General Surgery Patients: General surgery patients, who have one or more of the following risk factors, are at high risk of developing postoperative venous thromboembolism: previous venous thromboembolism; varicose veins; obesity; heart failure; malignancy; previous long bone fracture of lower limb; bed rest more than 5 days prior to surgery; predicted duration of surgery more than 30 minutes; age 60 years or above.

Geriatrics: Elderly patients receiving LMWHs are at increased risk of bleeding. Careful attention to dosing and concomitant medications, especially anti-platelet preparations, is advised. Close monitoring of elderly patients with low body weight (eg. <45 kg) and those predisposed to decreased renal function is recommended.

Dosing in Patients with Extreme Body Weight: Safety and efficacy of low molecular weight heparins in high weight (eg. >120 kg) and low weight (eg. <45 kg) patients has not been fully determined. Individualized clinical and laboratory monitoring is recommended in these patients.

Laboratory Testing: Since tinzaparin use may be associated with a rise in hepatic transaminases, this observation should be considered when liver function tests are assessed (see Adverse Effects, Liver).

ADVERSE EFFECTS: Bleeding: As with any antithrombotic treatment, hemorrhagic manifestations can occur. Injection site hematomas are a common side effect with tinzaparin, occurring at a frequency of 5% or less with lower (prophylaxis) doses to 10% or more with higher (treatment) doses.

The incidence of major hemorrhagic complications during tinzaparin treatment has been low and generally did not differ from that observed with unfractionated heparin. In clinical trials, the definition of major bleeding included bleeding accompanied by ≥2 g/dL decrease in haemoglobin, requiring transfusion of two or more units of blood products, or bleeding which was intracranial, retroperitoneal, or into a major prosthetic joint. Results from pivotal clinical trials for each indication are provided in Table 1.

Table 1: Innohep

Major Bleeding Events in Clinical Trials for Treatment of Acute DVT and/or PE, DVT Prophylaxis, and Hemodialysis[a]

Indication	Treatment Group	
	Innohep N=213 %	**Heparin N=219 %**
Treatment of Acute DVT with or without PE	0.5[b]	5.0[b]
	Innohep N=304 %	**Heparin N=308 %**
Treatment of PE	1.0[c]	1.6[c]
	Innohep[d] N=715 %	**Warfarin[d] N=721 %**
Prevention of Postoperative DVT in Orthopaedic Surgery	2.8[e]	1.2[e]
	Innohep[f] N=73 %	**Dalteparin[f] N=76 %**
Haemodialysis	1.4	1.3

[a] Bleeding accompanied by ≥2 gram/dL decline in hemoglobin, requiring transfusion of 2 or more units of blood products, or bleeding which was intracranial, retroperitoneal, or into a major prosthetic joint.

[b] Innohep 175 IU/kg once daily SC. Unfractionated heparin initial IV bolus of 5,000 IU followed by continuous IV Infusion adjusted to an aPTT of 1.5 to 2.5 followed by continuous IV infusion adjusted to an aPTT of 2.0 to 3.0 In all groups treatment continued for approximately 6 to 8 days, and all patients received oral anticoagulant treatment commencing in the first 2 to 3 days (p<0.01).

[c] Innohep 175 IU/kg once daily SC. Unfractionated heparin initial IV bolus of 50 IU/kg followed by continuous IV infusion adjusted to an aPTT of 2.0 to 3.0 In all groups treatment continued for approximately 6 to 8 days, and all patients received oral anticoagulant treatment commencing in the first 2 to 3 days.

[d] Innohep 75 IU/kg once daily SC starting 18-24 hours post-surgery. Warfarin starting at 10 mg on the evening post-surgery and dose adjusted to maintain an INR of 2.0 to 3.0. In all groups treatment continued until 14 days post-surgery or until hospital discharge if this occurred earlier.

[e] The 95% CI on the difference in major bleeding event rates (−1.6%) was −3.0%, −0.1%.

[f] Bolus dose into arterial side of dialyzer immediately prior to start of dialysis. Innohep 4500 IU for dialyses ≤4 hours or 6,700 IU for dialyses >4 hours. Dalteparin 5,000 IU for dialyses ≤4 hours or 35 IU/kg plus 12 IU/kg/hour for dialyses >4 hours.

Patients taking tinzaparin are at risk for major bleeding complications when the plasma anti-Xa levels approach 2.0 IU/mL. Other risk factors associated with bleeding on therapy with heparins include a serious concurrent illness, chronic heavy alcohol consumption, use of platelet inhibiting drugs, renal failure, age and possibly, the female gender. Petechiae or easy bruising may precede frank hemorrhage. Bleeding may range from minor local hematoma or major hemorrhage. The early signs of bleeding may include epistaxis, hematuria, or melena. Bleeding may occur at any site and may be difficult to detect, such as retroperitoneal bleeding. Bleeding may also occur from surgical sites. Major hemorrhage, including retroperitoneal or intracranial bleeding, has been reported in association with tinzaparin use, in some cases leading to fatality.

There have been cases of intra-spinal hematomas with the concurrent use of LMWH and spinal/epidural anaesthesia resulting in long term or permanent paralysis (incidence: 1:45 000) (see Warnings).

Skeletal Effects: Use of LMWH over extended periods has been reported to be associated with development of osteopenia.

Liver: A significant but transient increase of the liver transaminases (AST and ALT) has been observed with tinzaparin. This is a consistent finding with all members of the LMWH class, as well as with unfractionated heparin. However, no consistent irreversible liver damage has been observed. Normalization of transaminase levels can be expected within 2 to 4 weeks of the last dose of tinzaparin. The mechanism associated with the increased levels of liver transaminases has not been elucidated.

Transaminase increases occurred after more than three days of tinzaparin treatment in clinical studies. The increase is dose-dependent and has been observed at doses as low as 50 anti-Xa IU/kg once daily. In one study, at a dose of 150 anti-Xa IU/kg twice daily, all subjects showed increased plasma levels of AST and ALT from a mean of 17.8 to 128.5 U/L and 19.3 to 257.0 U/L respectively. These elevations correspond to a seven to twelve-fold increase as compared to the post-study evaluation performed within seven days of study completion.

Hypersensitivity: Thrombocytopenia, skin rash, allergic reactions and skin necrosis are rare, and occur with all LMWHs. Hypersensitivity reactions, including angioedema and anaphylactoid reactions, have been observed rarely with unfractionated heparin and low molecular weight heparins. Tinzaparin should be discontinued in patients showing local or systemic allergic responses.

Heparin-induced Thrombocytopenia: Severe immunologically-mediated thrombocytopenia has been observed rarely with tinzaparin use, resulting in arterial and/or venous thrombosis or thromboembolism (see Warnings, Thrombocytopenia and Precautions, Platelets).

Other: Rare cases of priapism have been reported.

Adverse Events: Adverse events with tinzaparin or heparin reported at a frequency of ≥1% in clinical trials with patients undergoing treatment for proximal DVT and/or PE, are provided in Table 2.

Table 2: Innohep

Adverse Events Occurring in ≥1% in Treatment of Acute Deep Vein Thrombosis and/or PE

Adverse Event	Treatment Group[a] Innohep N=519 n (%)	Heparin N=524 n (%)
Urinary Tract Infection	19 (3.7%)	18 (3.4%)
Chest Pain	12 (2.3%)	8 (1.5%)
Epistaxis	10 (1.9%)	7 (1.3%)
Headache	9 (1.7%)	9 (1.7%)
Nausea	9 (1.7%)	10 (1.9%)
Hemorrhage NOS	8 (1.5%)	23 (4.4%)
Back Pain	8 (1.5%)	2 (0.4%)
Fever	8 (1.5%)	11 (2.1%)
Pain	8 (1.5%)	7 (1.3%)
Constipation	7 (1.3%)	9 (1.7%)
Rash	6 (1.2%)	8 (1.5%)
Dyspnea	6 (1.2%)	9 (1.7%)
Vomiting	5 (1.0%)	8 (1.5%)
Hematuria	5 (1.0%)	6 (1.1%)
Abdominal Pain	4 (0.8%)	6 (1.1%)
Diarrhea	3 (0.6%)	7 (1.3%)
Anemia	0	7 (1.3%)

a Innohep 175 IU/kg once daily SC. Unfractionated heparin initial IV bolus of 5,000 IU followed by continuous IV infusion adjusted to an aPTT of 1.5 to 2.5 or initial IV bolus of 50 IU/kg followed by continuous IV infusion adjusted to an aPTT of 2.0 to 3.0. In all groups treatment continued for approximately 6 to 8 days, and all patients received oral anticoagulant treatment commencing in the first 2 to 3 days.

Legend: NOS=not otherwise specified.

Other Adverse Events in Completed or Ongoing Trials: Other serious adverse events reported at a frequency greater than or equal to 1% in 4000 patients who received tinzaparin in completed or ongoing clinical trials are provided in Table 3.

Table 3: Innohep *(cont'd)*

Serious Adverse Events Associated with Innohep in Clinical Trials

Category	Serious Adverse Event
Bleeding-related	Anorectal bleeding Cerebral/intracranial bleeding Epistaxis Gastrointestinal hemorrhage Hemarthrosis Hematemesis Hematuria Hemopericardium Hemorrhage NOS Injection site bleeding Melena Purpura Retroperitoneal/intra-abdominal bleeding Vaginal hemorrhage Wound hematoma
Organ dysfunction	Angina pectoris Cardiac arrhythmia Dependent edema Myocardial infarction/coronary thrombosis Thromboembolism
Fetal/neonatal	Congenital anomaly Fetal death Fetal distress
Cutaneous	Bullous eruption Erythematous rash Maculopapular rash Skin necrosis
Hematologic	Granulocytopenia Thrombocytopenia
Allergic reactions	Allergic reaction
Injection site reaction	Cellulitis
Neoplastic	Neoplasm

OVERDOSE:

Symptoms: Accidental overdosage following administration of tinzaparin may lead to hemorrhagic complications.

Treatment: Tinzaparin should be immediately discontinued, at least temporarily, in cases of significant excess dosage. In more serious cases, protamine should be administered.

The anticoagulant effect of tinzaparin is inhibited by protamine. This effect may be largely neutralized by slow intravenous injection of protamine sulphate. Each mg of protamine sulphate neutralizes approximately 100 anti-Xa IU of tinzaparin sodium. A second infusion of 0.5 mg protamine per 100 anti-Xa IU of tinzaparin may be administered if the APTT measured 2 to 4 hours after the first infusion remains prolonged. However, even with higher doses of protamine, the APTT may remain prolonged to a greater extent than usually seen with unfractionated heparin. Anti-factor Xa activity is never completely neutralized (maximum about 60-65%).

Particular care should be taken to avoid overdosage with protamine sulphate. Administration of protamine sulphate can cause severe hypotensive and anaphylactoid reactions. Because fatal reactions, often resembling anaphylaxis, have been reported with protamine sulphate, it should be given only when resuscitation equipment and treatment of anaphylactic shock are readily available.

For management of a suspected drug overdose, CPhA recommends that you contact your **regional Poison Control Centre**. See the *CPS* Directory section for a list of Poison Control Centres.

DOSAGE: Tinzaparin is administered by subcutaneous injection, or systemically in the setting of hemodialysis. It must **not** be administered by intramuscular injection (see Warnings).

Prevention of Postoperative Venous Thromboembolism in Orthopaedic Surgery: Hip Surgery: Tinzaparin 50 anti-Xa IU/kg b.w. given by subcutaneous injection two hours before surgery, followed by 50 anti-Xa IU/kg b.w. once daily for 7-10 days. Or, tinzaparin 75 anti-Xa IU/kg b.w. given post-operatively by subcutaneous injection once daily for 7-10 days.

Knee Surgery: Tinzaparin 75 anti-Xa IU/kg b.w. given post-operatively by subcutaneous injection once daily for 7-10 days.

For convenience, the following prefilled syringes are available for dosing by body weight: See Table 4.

Table 4: Innohep

Availability of Prefilled Syringes for Dosing by Body Weight

Dose per syringe	Preoperative 50 anti-Xa IU/kg Body weight	Postoperative 75 anti-Xa IU/kg Body weight
3500 anti-Xa IU	60–80 kg	35–55 kg
4500 anti-Xa IU	80–100 kg	50–70 kg

Patients outside of these weight ranges should be dosed on an individual basis.

Prevention of Postoperative Venous Thromboembolism in General Surgery: Tinzaparin 3500 anti-Xa IU (available in a prefilled syringe) given by s.c. injection 2 hours before surgery followed by 3500 anti-Xa IU once daily for 7 to 10 days.

Treatment of Deep Vein Thrombosis, with or without Pulmonary Embolism or, Treatment of Pulmonary Embolism: The recommended dosage is 175 anti-Xa IU/kg body weight given s.c. once daily at the same time every day. Although trials for DVT treatment did not include a maximum daily dose, few patients were included who exceeded 105 kg. Therefore, the recommended maximum daily dose for tinzaparin is 18 000 anti-Xa IU/day. In clinical trials, plasma anti-Xa levels were typically in the range of <0.3 anti-Xa IU/mL before injection and <1.8 anti-Xa IU/mL approximately 5 hours after injection as determined by a functional anti-Xa assay.

Concomitant treatment with oral anticoagulants (vitamin K antagonists) is usually started immediately. Treatment with tinzaparin should be continued until therapeutic oral anticoagulant effect has been achieved (INR 2.0 to 3.0), usually within 5 days. The average duration of tinzaparin administration is 7 days.

Use in Patients with Renal Impairment: All patients with renal impairment treated with low molecular weight heparins should be monitored carefully.

Administration of LMWHs to patients with renal impairment has been shown to result in prolongation of anti-Xa activity, especially in those with severe renal impairment (creatinine clearance <30 mL/min), leading to increased risk of bleeding. The effect of renal impairment on tinzaparin anti-Xa activity has not been fully studied. Consideration of dosage adjustment in patients with severe renal impairment should be undertaken.

Anticoagulation of Extracorporeal Circulation and Hemodialysis: All patients participating in clinical trials were stable, chronic renal failure patients. The following dosage recommendations are for that patient population, in patients with lower risk of hemorrhage.

Optimization of dosage is required for each individual patient (different clotting stimuli are produced by different dialysis circuits and membranes, and there is inter-patient variability).

The recommended starting dose is tinzaparin 4500 anti-Xa IU administered as a bolus dose into the arterial side of the dialyzer (or intravenously) at the beginning of the dialysis for a session lasting 4 hours or less in patients with no risk of hemorrhage. This dose normally produces plasma anti-Xa levels in the range of 0.5-1.0 IU anti-Xa/mL. Dosage modifications should consider the outcome of the previous dialysis and should be made by increasing or decreasing the dose in steps of 500 anti-Xa IU until a satisfactory dose is obtained.

A larger starting dose may be given for dialysis sessions lasting longer than 4 hours. Doses in subsequent dialysis sessions should be adjusted as required.

In patients with a risk of hemorrhage, dialysis sessions may be carried out using halved doses. An additional smaller dose may be given during dialysis for sessions lasting longer than 4 hours. The dose in subsequent dialysis sessions should be adjusted as necessary to achieve plasma levels within the range of 0.2-0.4 IU anti-Xa/mL.

No anticoagulant should be added to the dialyzer circuit when using this regimen.

INFORMATION FOR THE PATIENT: Published in e-CPS, available by subscription at www.e-cps.ca.

SUPPLIED: Syringes: 10 000 anti-Xa IU/mL: Each mL of sterile solution contains: tinzaparin sodium 10 000 anti-Xa IU. Nonmedicinal ingredients: sodium acetate·$3H_2O$, sodium hydroxide* and water for injection. pH range of the final solution is 5.0 to 7.5. Preservative-free. Unit dose safety syringes (27 gauge, ½ inch needle) of 0.25 mL (2500 anti-Xa IU), 0.35 mL (3500 anti-Xa IU) and 0.45 mL (4500 anti-Xa IU). All syringes except the 2500 anti-Xa IU/mL format are available as safety syringes.

20 000 anti-Xa IU/mL: Each mL of sterile solution contains: tinzaparin sodium 20 000 anti-Xa IU. Nonmedicinal ingredients: sodium metabisulfite, sodium hydroxide* and water for injection. pH range of the final solution is 5.0 to 7.5. Preservative-free. Unit dose graduated safety syringes (27 gauge, ½ inch needle) of 0.5 mL (10 000 anti-Xa IU), 0.7 mL (14 000 anti-Xa IU) and 0.9 mL (18 000 anti-Xa IU).

Multi-dose Vials: 10 000 anti-Xa IU/mL: Each mL of sterile solution contains: tinzaparin sodium 10 000 anti-Xa IU. Nonmedicinal ingredients: benzyl alcohol, sodium hydroxide*, sodium metabisulfite and water for injection. pH range of the final solution is 5.0 to 7.5. Multi-dose preserved vials of 2 mL (total of 20 000 anti-Xa IU per vial).

20 000 anti-Xa IU/mL: Each mL of sterile solution contains: tinzaparin sodium 20 000 anti-Xa IU. Nonmedicinal ingredients: benzyl alcohol, sodium hydroxide*, sodium metabisulfite and water for injection. pH range of the final solution is 5.0 to 7.5. Multi-dose preserved vials of 2 mL (total of 40 000 anti-Xa IU per vial).

Store at 15 to 25°C. Innohep multi-use vials for injection are not affected significantly chemically, physically or microbiologically following multiple puncture (7 times) over a 28 day period when stored at 25°C±2°C. All Innohep syringes and vials are latex-free.

* Quantity sufficient for pH adjustment.

Inspra™ Ⓟ

eplerenone

Aldosterone Antagonist

Pfizer

Date of Preparation: February 25, 2009

SUMMARY PRODUCT INFORMATION:

Route of Administration	Dosage Form/ Strength	All Nonmedicinal Ingredients
Oral	Tablets 25 mg, 50 mg	Croscarmellose sodium, hypromellose, lactose, magnesium stearate, microcrystalline cellulose, polyethylene glycol, polysorbate 80, sodium lauryl sulfate, talc, titanium dioxide, iron oxide yellow, and iron oxide red

INDICATIONS AND CLINICAL USE: INSPRA (eplerenone) is indicated as an adjunct to standard therapy, to reduce the risk of mortality following myocardial infarction, in clinically stable patients who have evidence of heart failure and left ventricular systolic dysfunction (ejection fraction ≤40%).

Serum potassium level should be measured before starting INSPRA therapy and INSPRA should not be administered if initial serum potassium is >5.0 mmol/L.

CONTRAINDICATIONS: INSPRA (eplerenone) is contraindicated in all patients with the following:

- hypersensitivity to INSPRA or any component of this medication (for a complete listing of the INSPRA components, see Dosage Forms, Composition and Packaging);
- patients with clinically significant hyperkalemia;
- severe hepatic impairment (Child-Pugh Class C);
- serum potassium >5.0 mmol/L at initiation;
- moderate to severe renal impairment [creatinine clearance <50 mL/min];
- serum creatinine >221 µmol/L;
- concomitant use with potassium-sparing diuretics, potassium supplements or strong CYP3A4 inhibitors such as ketoconazole, itraconazole, nefazodone, telithromycin, clarithromycin, ritonavir, and nelfinavir (see Drug Interactions and Dosage and Administration).

WARNINGS AND PRECAUTIONS: Hyperkalemia: The principal risk of INSPRA (eplerenone) is hyperkalemia. Hyperkalemia, if not recognized in a timely manner, can cause serious, sometimes fatal, arrhythmias. All patients prescribed INSPRA must have their serum potassium level measured before initiating INSPRA therapy, within one week after the first dose, and measured periodically thereafter (see Dosage and Administration).

Hyperkalemia can be minimized by appropriate patient selection, avoidance of certain concomitant treatments, thoroughly informing the patient and periodic monitoring until the effect of INSPRA has been established.

For patient selection and medications which should not be prescribed concomitantly with INSPRA or prescribed with caution, see Contraindications, Drug Interactions; and Adverse Reactions.

INSPRA should not be administered to patients with initial serum potassium >5.0 mmol/L, serum creatinine >221 µmol/L and/or creatinine clearance <50 mL/min. The incidence of hyperkalemia increases with declining renal function (see Adverse Reactions, Table 3).

Diabetic patients with heart failure (HF) post myocardial infarction (MI), especially those with proteinuria, should also be treated with caution. The subset of patients in EPHESUS with both diabetes and proteinuria on the baseline urinalysis had increased rates of hyperkalemia (see Adverse Reactions, Other Abnormal Hematologic and Clinical Chemistry Findings, Potassium).

Impaired Hepatic Function: In 16 subjects with mild-to-moderate hepatic impairment (Child-Pugh Class B) who received 400 mg of INSPRA, no elevations of serum potassium above 5.5 mmol/L were observed. C_{max} was not significantly changed but AUC was increased by 42% and INSPRA clearance 30% lower compared to matched controls. The dose recommended is 8 times smaller and, therefore, no dose adjustment is necessary in patients with **mild to moderate** hepatic impairment.

The use of INSPRA in patients with severe hepatic impairment has not been evaluated and therefore, INSPRA is not recommended in these patients (see Dosage and Administration and Action and Clinical Pharmacology, Special Populations and Conditions).

Impaired Renal Function: See Contraindications; Warnings and Precautions, Hyperkalemia and Adverse Reactions.

Carcinogenesis and Mutagenesis: Preclinical studies on safety pharmacology, genotoxicity, carcinogenic potential and toxicity to reproduction revealed no special hazard for humans.

In repeat dose toxicity studies, prostate atrophy was observed in rats and dogs at exposure levels several-fold above clinical exposure levels. The prostatic changes were not associated with adverse functional consequences. The clinical relevance of these findings is unknown.

Studies in rats and rabbits showed no teratogenic effects, although decreased body weight in maternal rabbits and increased rabbit fetal resorptions and post-implantation loss were observed at the highest administered dosage.

Special Populations: Pregnant Women: Pregnancy: There are no INSPRA studies in pregnant women. Eplerenone did not impair fertility and was not teratogenic in animals but the risk to the fetus of pregnant women is not known. Therefore, INSPRA should be used during pregnancy only if the potential benefit to the mother justifies the potential risk to the fetus.

Nursing Women: It has not been determined if INSPRA is present in human breast milk, however it was present in rat breast milk at a milk to plasma ratio of 0.85. Because many drugs are excreted in human milk and because of the unknown potential for adverse effects on the nursing infant, a decision should be made whether to discontinue nursing or discontinue the drug, taking into account the importance of the drug to the mother.

Pediatrics: The safety and effectiveness of INSPRA have not been established in pediatric patients and INSPRA is not recommended in this patient population.

Geriatrics: There were 1641 (46%) patients treated with INSPRA in EPHESUS who were 65 and over, while 616 (18.6%) were 75 and over. Patients greater than 75 years did not appear to benefit from the use of INSPRA. No differences in overall incidence of adverse events were observed between elderly and younger patients. However, due at least in part, to age-related decreases in creatinine clearance, the incidence of laboratory-documented hyperkalemia was increased in patients 65 and older (see Hyperkalemia).

ADVERSE REACTIONS: In the eplerenone post-acute myocardial infarction heart failure efficacy and survival study (EPHESUS), safety was evaluated in 3307 patients treated with INSPRA and 3301 placebo-treated patients. Patients were followed for an average of 16 months. Vital status was confirmed for 99.7% of patients. The overall incidence of adverse events reported with INSPRA was similar to placebo (summarized in Table 1).

The most serious adverse events in EPHESUS were endpoint events (e.g., death, cardiac failure) and these were significantly more frequent in the placebo treatment group. Serious adverse events that were significantly associated with eplerenone treatment included dehydration, arterial leg thrombosis, increased creatinine, and pyelonephritis; the incidence of these was low (≤0.5%).

Headache was the most frequent adverse reaction among eplerenone subjects in single- and multiple-dose trials. Adverse events that occurred more frequently in patients treated with INSPRA than placebo were hyperkalemia (summarized in Table 3). Eplerenone-treated patients also experienced more postural hypotension (0.7% vs 0.3% on placebo). Other adverse events more frequent during eplerenone treatment were increased blood urea nitrogen (BUN), increased creatinine, hypothyroidism, gastroesophageal reflux, pancreatitis, ketosis, arterial leg thrombosis, sepsis, and varicose veins. Hypokalemia (<3.5 mmol/L) occurred less frequently in patients treated with INSPRA (8.4% vs 13.1%).

Elevation of serum potassium led to appropriate dose adjustments of eplerenone (see Table 7, Dose adjustment). Permanent discontinuations of eplerenone treatment due to hyperkalemia were infrequent (0.7% eplerenone vs 0.3% placebo); no eplerenone patient died from hyperkalemia. Sepsis led to permanent discontinuation of study medication in 2 eplerenone patients. No patients permanently discontinued study medication due to postural hypotension.

Adverse events experienced by >2.0% of patients in either treatment group or with a statistically significant difference between treatment groups are presented in Table 1.

Table 1: INSPRA

Analysis of Treatment-Emergent Adverse Events[a] in EPHESUS (Treated Patients)

Body System Adverse Event	INSPRA 25–50 mg QD N=3307	Placebo N=3301	p-value[b]
Any event	2608 (78.9%)	2623 (79.5%)	
Autonomic Nervous System Disorders			
Hypotension	119 (3.6%)	109 (3.3%)	—
Hypotension Postural	24 (0.7%)	11 (0.3%)	0.040
Syncope	71 (2.1%)	58 (1.8%)	—
Body as a Whole—General Disorders			
Asthenia	89 (2.7%)	68 (2.1%)	—
Back Pain	91 (2.8%)	95 (2.9%)	—
Chest Pain Non-Cardiac	213 (6.4%)	206 (6.2%)	—
Edema Peripheral	87 (2.6%)	110 (3.3%)	—
Fatigue	95 (2.9%)	91 (2.8%)	—
Fever	67 (2.0%)	65 (2.0%)	—
Injury-Accidental	50 (1.5%)	69 (2.1%)	—
Peripheral Pain	62 (1.9%)	68 (2.1%)	—
Sudden Death	116 (3.5%)	177 (5.4%)	<0.001
Cardiovascular Disorders, General			
Cardiac Failure	376 (11.4%)	460 (13.9%)	0.002
Cardiac Failure Left	153 (4.6%)	194 (5.9%)	0.024
Unstable Angina	305 (9.2%)	315 (9.5%)	—
Central and Peripheral Nervous System Disorders			
Convulsions	2 (<0.1%)	9 (0.3%)	0.038
Dizziness	214 (6.5%)	197 (6.0%)	—
Headache	126 (3.8%)	119 (3.6%)	—
Endocrine Disorders			
Hypothyroidism	15 (0.5%)	5 (0.2%)	0.041
Gastrointestinal System Disorders			
Abdominal Pain	97 (2.9%)	103 (3.1%)	—
Constipation	98 (3.0%)	92 (2.8%)	—
Diarrhea	115 (3.5%)	113 (3.4%)	—
Dyspepsia	129 (3.9%)	120 (3.6%)	—
Gastroesophageal Reflux	17 (0.5%)	6 (0.2%)	0.034
Nausea	139 (4.2%)	133 (4.0%)	—
Pancreatitis	18 (0.5%)	5 (0.2%)	0.010
Tooth Disorder	12 (0.4%)	28 (0.8%)	0.011
Vomiting	76 (2.3%)	59 (1.8%)	—
Heart Rate and Rhythm Disorders			
Arrhythmia Ventricular	73 (2.2%)	73 (2.2%)	—
Fibrillation Atrial	150 (4.5%)	161 (4.9%)	—
Tachycardia Ventricular	70 (2.1%)	63 (1.9%)	—

(cont'd)

Table 1: INSPRA *(cont'd)*

Analysis of Treatment-Emergent Adverse Events[a] in EPHESUS (Treated Patients)

Body System Adverse Event	INSPRA 25–50 mg QD N=3307	Placebo N=3301	p-value[b]
Metabolic and Nutritional Disorders			
Hypercholesterolemia	102 (3.1%)	119 (3.6%)	—
Hyperglycemia	67 (2.0%)	79 (2.4%)	—
Hyperkalemia	113 (3.4%)	66 (2.0%)	<0.001
Hyperuricemia	87 (2.6%)	111 (3.4%)	—
Hypoglycemia	20 (0.6%)	35 (1.1%)	0.043
Hypokalemia	15 (0.5%)	49 (1.5%)	<0.001
Ketosis	9 (0.3%)	1 (<0.1%)	0.021
Musculoskeletal System Disorders			
Arthralgia	71 (2.1%)	89 (2.7%)	—
Myo Endo Pericardial and Valve Disorders			
Angina Pectoris	459 (13.9%)	415 (12.6%)	—
Coronary Artery Disorder	100 (3.0%)	91 (2.8%)	—
Myocardial Infarction	267 (8.1%)	270 (8.2%)	—
Platelet, Bleeding and Clotting Disorders			
Thrombosis Arterial Leg	13 (0.4%)	3 (<0.1%)	0.021
Psychiatric Disorders			
Confusion	6 (0.2%)	16 (0.5%)	0.034
Depression	48 (1.5%)	66 (2.0%)	—
Insomnia	88 (2.7%)	105 (3.2%)	—
Red Blood Cell Disorders			
Anemia	115 (3.5%)	98 (3.0%)	—
Resistance Mechanism Disorders			
Sepsis	18 (0.5%)	5 (0.2%)	0.010
Respiratory System Disorders			
Bronchitis	111 (3.4%)	137 (4.2%)	—
Coughing	167 (5.0%)	207 (6.3%)	0.033
Dyspnea	243 (7.3%)	307 (9.3%)	0.004
Pneumonia	92 (2.8%)	123 (3.7%)	0.032
Upper Respiratory Tract Infection	156 (4.7%)	171 (5.2%)	—
Urinary System Disorders			
BUN Increased	52 (1.6%)	32 (1.0%)	0.036
Creatinine Increase	81 (2.4%)	51 (1.5%)	0.011
Hematuria	70 (2.1%)	55 (1.7%)	—
Renal Function Abnormal	96 (2.9%)	79 (2.4%)	—
Renal Pain	2 (<0.1%)	9 (0.3%)	0.038
Urinary Tract Infection	111 (3.4%)	113 (3.4%)	—
Vascular Disorders			
Cerebrovascular Disorder	103 (3.1%)	101 (3.1%)	—
Vein Varicose	10 (0.3%)	1 (<0.1%)	0.012

[a] A treatment-emergent adverse event is defined as any event not present prior to the initiation of treatment or any event already present that worsens in either intensity or frequency following exposure to the treatment.
[b] From Fisher's exact test. A dash indicates no statistically significant difference between treatment groups (p>0.05).
Data include any events with ≥2.0% incidence in either group or with a significant difference between groups (p≤0.05).

Table 2: INSPRA

Summary of Elevated Serum Potassium in Treated Patients in EPHESUS

Serum Potassium mmol/L	INSPRA 25–50 mg N=3251	Placebo N=3237
>5.5	15.6%	11.2 %
≥6.0	5.5%	3.9%

(cont'd)

Table 2: INSPRA *(cont'd)*

Summary of Elevated Serum Potassium in Treated Patients in EPHESUS

Serum Potassium mmol/L	INSPRA 25–50 mg N=3251	Placebo N=3237
>5.5 at least 2 consecutive measurements	3.0%	1.7%

The higher risk of hyperkalemia in patients with renal impairment and, proteinuria and history of diabetes mellitus are shown in Table 3 and Table 4 respectively.

Table 3: INSPRA

Rates of Hyperkalemia (>5.5 mmol/L) in EPHESUS by Baseline Creatinine Clearance[a]

Baseline Creatinine Clearance	INSPRA	Placebo
≤30 mL/min	31.5%	22.6%
31–50 mL/min	24.1%	12.7%
51–70 mL/min	16.9%	13.1%
>70 mL/min	10.8%	8.7%

[a] Estimated using the Cockroft-Gault formula.

Table 4: INSPRA

Rates of Hyperkalemia (>5.5 mmol/L) in EPHESUS by Proteinuria and History of Diabetes[a]

	INSPRA	Placebo
Proteinuria, no Diabetes	16%	11%
Diabetes, no Proteinuria	18%	13%
Proteinuria and Diabetes	26%	16%

[a] Diabetes assessed as positive medical history at baseline; proteinuria assessed by positive dipstick urinalysis at baseline.

Other Abnormal Hematologic and Clinical Chemistry Findings: Creatinine: Increases of more than 44 µmol/L were reported in 6.5% of patients administered INSPRA and in 4.9% of placebo-treated patients.
Blood Urea Nitrogen: In EPHESUS, a mean increase of 0.17 mmol/L in blood urea nitrogen (BUN) was reported in patients treated with INSPRA and a mean 0.31 mmol/L decrease for placebo-treated patients. BUN increased in 1.6% and 1.0% of subjects, respectively.
Sex Related-Hormone Adverse Events: The incidences of sex hormone-related adverse events are shown in Table 5.

Table 5: INSPRA

Rates of Sex Hormone-Related Adverse Events in EPHESUS

	Rates in Males		Rates in Females
	Gynecomastia	Mastodynia	Abnormal Vaginal Bleeding
INSPRA	0.4%	0.1%	0.4%
Placebo	0.5%	0.1%	0.4%

Adverse Events: Adverse events reported below are those with suspected relationship to treatment and in excess of placebo, taken from EPHESUS. Adverse events are listed by body system and absolute frequency. Frequencies are defined as common (>1% to ≤10%) or uncommon (>0.1% to ≤1%).
Blood and Lymphatic System Disorders: Uncommon: eosinophilia.
Metabolism and Nutrition Disorders: Common: hyperkalemia. Uncommon: dehydration, hypercholesterolemia, hypertriglyceridemia, hyponatremia.
Psychiatric Disorders: Uncommon: insomnia.
Nervous System Disorders: Common: dizziness. Uncommon: headache.
Cardiac Disorders: Uncommon: atrial fibrillation, myocardial infarction, cardiac failure left.
Vascular Disorders: Common: hypotension. Uncommon: postural hypotension.
Respiratory, Thoracic and Mediastinal Disorders: Uncommon: pharyngitis.
Gastrointestinal Disorders: Common: diarrhea, nausea. Uncommon: flatulence, vomiting.
Skin and Subcutaneous Tissue Disorders: Uncommon: pruritus, sweating increased.
Musculoskeletal and Connective Tissue Disorders: Uncommon: back pain, leg cramp.
Renal and Urinary Disorders: Common: renal function abnormal.
General Disorders and Administration Site Conditions: Uncommon: asthenia, malaise.
Investigations: Uncommon: BUN increase, creatinine increase.
Post-Market Adverse Drug Reactions: In post-marketing experience, the following additional undesirable effects have been reported:
Skin and Subcutaneous Tissue Disorders: angioneurotic edema, rash.
DRUG INTERACTIONS: Overview: Inhibitors of CYP3A4: INSPRA (eplerenone) metabolism is predominantly mediated via CYP3A4 and therefore, INSPRA should not be used with drugs described as strong inhibitors of CYP3A4 in their labeling (see Contraindications and Dosage and Administration).

Caution should be used in patients treated with **moderate** 3A4 inhibitors; dosing should not exceed 25 mg QD.
Inducers of CYP3A4: St. John's Wort was found to decrease exposure and to increase clearance of INSPRA significantly indicating that concomitant use of strong inducers of CYP3A4 such as phenobarbital, phenytoin, rifampicin, carbamazepine should be avoided.
ACE Inhibitors and Angiotensin II Receptor Antagonists: In EPHESUS, 3020 (91%) patients receiving INSPRA 25 to 50 mg also received ACE inhibitors or angiotensin II receptor antagonists (ACEI/ARB). Rates of patients with maximum potassium levels >5.5 mmol/L were similar regardless of the use of ACEI/ARB. However, as ACEI/ARB can also increase serum potassium levels in some patients, concomitant use with INSPRA dictates that greater caution should be exercised.
Lithium: A drug interaction study of INSPRA with lithium has not been conducted. Lithium toxicity has been reported in patients receiving lithium concomitantly with diuretics and ACE inhibitors. Serum lithium levels should be monitored frequently if INSPRA is administered concomitantly with lithium, as excretion may be altered as a result of modifications in sodium balance induced by the aldosterone antagonist. Lithium has also been reported to increase plasma renin activity and aldosterone levels.
Nonsteroidal Anti-Inflammatory Drugs (NSAIDs): A drug interaction study of INSPRA with an NSAID has not been conducted. The administration of potassium-sparing antihypertensives drugs with NSAIDs has been shown to reduce the antihypertensive effect in some patients and result in severe hyperkalemia in patients with impaired renal function. Therefore, when INSPRA and NSAIDs or COX-2 Inhibitors are used concomitantly, blood pressure, renal function and serum potassium should be closely monitored.
Herbal Preparations and Salt Substitutes: The full consequence of using INSPRA in patients taking herbal preparations and/or salt substitutes has not been established, and caution should be exercised. Theoretically, patients who are taking herbal preparations that affect blood pressure or contain high levels of potassium may be at risk of hypotension/hypertension or hyperkalemia

(see Warnings and Precautions). Clinicians should consider discontinuing the herbal preparation or salt substitute or closely monitoring patients using such a combination. Such preparations may include (but not limited to): dandelion, potassium iodine, laminaria, morinda, oleander, phosphate salts and potassium preparations, cat's claw, cod liver oil, and licorice.

Drug-Drug Interactions: Drug-drug interaction studies were conducted with a 100 mg dose of INSPRA and the outcomes are summarized in Table 6.

Table 6: INSPRA

Established or Potential Drug-Drug Interactions

Proper Name	Ref	Effect	Clinical Comment
Digoxin	CT	No clinically significant interactions	Systemic Exposure (AUC) to digoxin increases by 16% (90% CI: 4–30%) when co-administered with INSPRA. Caution is warranted when digoxin is dosed near the upper limit of the therapeutic range.
Warfarin	CT	No clinically significant interactions	
CYP3A4 substrates (e.g. midazolam, cisapride)	T and CT	No clinically significant interactions	
Potent CYP3A4 inhibitors (e.g. ketoconazole, itraconazole, ritonavir, nelfinavir, clarithromycin, telithromycin, nefazodone)	T and CT	Significant increases in eplerenone AUC	Concomitant use is contraindicated (see Contraindications).
Mild to Moderate CYP3A4 inhibitors (erythromycin, saquinavir, amiodarone, diltiazem, verapamil, fluconazole)	T and CT	Significant increases in eplerenone AUC	Eplerenone dosing should not exceed 25 mg when mild to moderate inhibitors of CYP3A4 are co-administered (see Dosage and Administration).
Potent CYP3A4 Inducers (e.g. carbamazepine, phenytoin, Phenobarbital, St John's Wort, rifampicin)	T and CT	Decreases eplerenone AUC	Due to the risk. of decreased eplerenone efficacy, concomitant use of strong CYP3A4 inducers with INSPRA is not recommended.
Aluminum and magnesium-containing antacids	CT	No significant changes in eplerenone pharmacokinetics	

Legend: CT=clinical trial; T=theoretical.

Drug-Food Interactions: INSPRA may be administered with or without food.

DOSAGE AND ADMINISTRATION: Recommended Dose and Dosage Adjustment: Serum potassium should be measured before initiating INSPRA (eplerenone) therapy and within the first week after the first dose or after increasing the dose. Serum potassium should be measured periodically thereafter.

INSPRA should not be administered to patients with initial serum potassium >5.0 mmol/L, serum creatinine >221 µmol/L and/or creatinine clearance <50 mL/min.

Efforts should be made to decrease the dietary potassium intake. Patients should be asked about their use of potassium containing salt substitutes and dietary supplements. Factors, such as patient characteristics, serum potassium levels and concomitant medications, may indicate that additional monitoring of serum potassium is appropriate (see Warnings and Precautions, Hyperkalemia; Adverse Reactions, and Drug Interactions). In EPHESUS, the majority of hyperkalemia was observed within the first 3 months after randomization.

INSPRA therapy should be initiated within 3-14 days after acute myocardial infarction.

Treatment should be initiated at 25 mg once daily and titrated to the target dose of 50 mg once daily preferably within 4 weeks as tolerated by the patient. The maximum daily dose is 50 mg daily. INSPRA may be administered with or without food.

Patients who develop hyperkalemia (>5.5 mmol/L) may still benefit from INSPRA with proper dose adjustment. The dose should be adjusted based on the serum potassium level and the dose adjustment table shown in Table 7.

Table 7: INSPRA

Dose Adjustment in Heart Failure Post MI

Serum Potassium (mmol/L)	Action	Dose Adjustment
<5.0	Increase	25 mg QOD to 25 mg QD 25 mg QD to 50 mg QD
5.0–5.4	Maintain	No adjustment
5.5–5.9	Decrease	50 mg QD to 25 mg QD 25 mg QD to 25 mg QOD 25 mg QOD to withhold
≥6.0	Withhold	

Legend: QOD: every other day; QD: every day.

Following withholding INSPRA due to serum potassium ≥6.0 mmol/L and the return of potassium levels within acceptable limits, INSPRA can be restarted at a **test** dose of 25 mg every other day. There are no conclusive data to demonstrate that 25 mg every other day is effective. After a test period of one week on 25 mg every other day, serum potassium levels should be measured. If potassium levels return within acceptable limits, the dose can be increased to 25 mg every day and serum potassium should be measured after one week. It could then be determined if INSPRA therapy should be continued or stopped.

INSPRA dosing should not exceed 25 mg when mild to moderate inhibitors of CYP3A4 are co-administered (see Drug Interactions).

Hepatic Impairment: Mild-to-Moderate Hepatic Impairment: No initial dosage adjustment is necessary. Severe Hepatic Impairment (see Contraindications and Warnings and Precautions).

Renal Impairment: Mild Renal Impairment: No initial dosage adjustment is necessary. Moderate-to-Severe Renal Impairment (see Contraindications and Warnings and Precautions).

OVERDOSAGE:

No cases of human overdosage with INSPRA (eplerenone) have been reported. Lethality was not observed in mice, rats, or dogs after single oral doses that provided C_{max} exposures at least 25 times higher than in humans receiving eplerenone 100 mg/day. Dogs showed emesis, salivation, and tremors at a C_{max} 41 times the human therapeutic C_{max}, progressing to sedation and convulsions at higher exposures.

The most likely manifestation of human overdosage would be anticipated to be hypotension and/or hyperkalemia. Eplerenone cannot be removed by hemodialysis. Eplerenone has been shown to bind extensively to charcoal. If symptomatic hypotension should occur, supportive treatment should be instituted. If hyperkalemia develops, standard treatment should be initiated.

For management of a suspected drug overdose, CPhA recommends that you contact your **regional Poison Control Centre**. See the *CPS* Directory section for a list of Poison Control Centres.

ACTION AND CLINICAL PHARMACOLOGY: Mechanism of Action: Eplerenone binds to the mineralocorticoid receptor and blocks the binding of aldosterone, a component of the renin-angiotensin-aldosterone-system (RAAS). Aldosterone synthesis, which occurs primarily in the adrenal gland, is modulated by multiple factors, including angiotensin II and non-RAAS mediators, such as adrenocorticotropic hormone (ACTH) and potassium. Aldosterone binds to mineralocorticoid receptors in both epithelial (e.g., kidney) and nonepithelial (e.g., heart, blood vessels, and brain) tissues, and increases blood pressure through induction of sodium reabsorption and possibly other mechanisms through both genomic and non-genomic effects.

Pharmacodynamics: Eplerenone has been shown to produce sustained increases in plasma renin and serum aldosterone, consistent with inhibition of the negative regulatory feedback of aldosterone on renin secretion. The resulting increased plasma renin activity and aldosterone circulating levels do not overcome the effects of eplerenone.

Eplerenone selectively binds to recombinant human mineralocorticoid receptors relative to its binding to recombinant human glucocorticoid, progesterone and androgen receptors.

In dose-ranging studies of chronic heart failure (NYHA classification II-IV), the addition of eplerenone to standard therapy resulted in expected dose-dependent increases in aldosterone. Similarly, in a cardiorenal substudy of EPHESUS, therapy with eplerenone led to a significant increase in aldosterone. These results are consistent with blockade of the mineralocorticoid receptor in these populations.

No consistent effects of eplerenone on heart rate, QRS duration, or PR or QT interval were observed in 147 normal subjects evaluated for electrocardiographic changes during pharmacokinetic studies.

Pharmacokinetics: General: Eplerenone is cleared predominantly by cytochrome P450 (CYP) 3A4 metabolism, with an elimination half-life of 4 to 6 hours. Steady state is reached within 2 days. Absorption is not affected by food. Inhibitors of CYP3A4 increase blood levels of eplerenone.

Absorption and Distribution: Mean peak plasma concentrations of eplerenone are reached approximately 1.5 hours following oral administration. The absolute bioavailability of eplerenone is 69% following administration of a 100 mg oral tablet. Both peak plasma levels (C_{max}) and area under the curve (AUC) are dose proportional for doses of 25 to 100 mg and less than proportional at doses above 100 mg.

The plasma protein binding of eplerenone is about 50% and it is primarily bound to alpha 1-acid glycoproteins. The apparent volume of distribution at steady state ranged from 43 to 90 L. Eplerenone does not preferentially bind to red blood cells.

Metabolism and Excretion: Eplerenone metabolism is primarily mediated via CYP3A4. No active metabolites of eplerenone have been identified in human plasma.

Less than 5% of an eplerenone dose is recovered as unchanged drug in the urine and feces. Following a single oral dose of radiolabeled drug, approximately 32% of the dose was excreted in the feces and approximately 67% was excreted in the urine. The elimination half-life of eplerenone is approximately 4 to 6 hours. The apparent plasma clearance is approximately 10 L/hr.

Special Populations and Conditions: Age, Gender, and Race: The pharmacokinetics of eplerenone at a dose of 100 mg once daily has been investigated in the elderly (≥65 years), in males and females, and in blacks. The pharmacokinetics of eplerenone did not differ significantly between males and females. At steady state, elderly subjects had increases in C_{max} (22%) and AUC (45%) compared with younger subjects (18 to 45 years). At steady state, C_{max} was 19% lower and AUC was 26% lower in blacks (see Warnings and Precautions, Geriatrics and Dosage and Administration).

Renal Insufficiency: The pharmacokinetics of eplerenone was evaluated in patients with varying degrees of renal insufficiency and in patients undergoing hemodialysis. Compared with control subjects, steady-state AUC and C_{max} were increased by 38% and 24%, respectively, in patients with severe renal impairment and were decreased by 26% and 3%, respectively, in patients undergoing hemodialysis. No correlation was observed between plasma clearance of eplerenone and creatinine clearance. Eplerenone is not removed by hemodialysis (see Warnings and Precautions, Hyperkalemia).

Hepatic Insufficiency: The pharmacokinetics of eplerenone 400 mg has been investigated in patients with moderate (Child-Pugh Class B) hepatic impairment and compared with normal subjects. Steady-state C_{max} and AUC of eplerenone were increased by 3.6% and 42%, respectively (see Dosage and Administration).

Heart Failure: The pharmacokinetics of eplerenone 50 mg was evaluated in 8 patients with heart failure (NYHA classification II-IV) and 8 matched (gender, age, weight) healthy controls. Compared with the controls, steady state AUC and C_{max} in patients with stable heart failure were 38% and 30% higher, respectively.

Drug-Drug Interactions: (See Drug Interactions.)

Drug-drug interaction studies were conducted with a 100 mg dose of eplerenone.

Eplerenone is metabolized primarily by CYP3A4. A potent inhibitor of CYP3A4 (ketoconazole) caused increased exposure of 5.4 fold; while less potent CYP3A4 inhibitors (erythromycin, saquinavir, verapamil, and fluconazole) resulted in increases ranging from 2.0-2.9 fold. Grapefruit juice caused only a small increase (about 25%) in exposure (see Drug Interactions).

Eplerenone is not an inhibitor of CYP1A2, CYP3A4, CYP2C19, CYP2C9, or CYP2D6. Eplerenone did not inhibit the metabolism of amiodarone, amlodipine, astemizole, chlorzoxazone, cisapride, dexamethasone, dextromethorphan, diclofenac, 17α-ethinyl estradiol, fluoxetine, losartan, lovastatin, mephobarbital, methylphenidate, methylprednisolone, metoprolol, midazolam, nifedipine, phenacetin, phenytoin, simvastatin, tolbutamide, triazolam, verapamil, and warfarin in vitro. Eplerenone is not a substrate or an inhibitor of P-Glycoprotein at clinically relevant doses.

No clinically significant drug-drug pharmacokinetic interactions were observed when eplerenone was administered with cisapride, cyclosporine, digoxin, glyburide, midazolam, oral contraceptives (norethindrone/ethinyl estradiol), simvastatin, or warfarin. St. Johns Wort (a CYP3A4 inducer) caused a small (about 30%) decrease in eplerenone AUC.

No significant changes in eplerenone pharmacokinetics were observed when eplerenone was administered with aluminum and magnesium-containing antacids.

STORAGE AND STABILITY: Store at controlled room temperature (15-30°C)

SPECIAL HANDLING INSTRUCTIONS: Not applicable.

INFORMATION FOR THE PATIENT: Published in e-CPS, available by subscription at www.e-cps.ca.

DOSAGE FORMS, COMPOSITION AND PACKAGING: 25 mg: Each yellow, diamond, biconvex film-coated tablet, debossed with Pfizer on one side and NSR over 25 on the other, contains: eplerenone 25 mg. Nonmedicinal ingredients: croscarmellose sodium, hypromellose, iron oxide red, iron oxide yellow, lactose, magnesium stearate, microcrystalline cellulose, polyethylene glycol, polysorbate 80, sodium lauryl sulfate, talc and titanium dioxide. Blister packs of 30.

50 mg: Each yellow, diamond, biconvex film-coated tablet, debossed with Pfizer on one side and NSR over 50 on the other, contains: eplerenone 50 mg. Nonmedicinal ingredients: croscarmellose sodium, hypromellose, iron oxide red, iron oxide yellow, lactose, magnesium stearate, microcrystalline cellulose, polyethylene glycol, polysorbate 80, sodium lauryl sulfate, talc and titanium dioxide. Blister packs of 30.

Intanza™

influenza vaccine (split virion, inactivated)

Active Immunization Against Influenza

sanofi pasteur

Date of Preparation: May 2010

SUMMARY PRODUCT INFORMATION:

Route of Administration	Dosage Form/ Strength	Clinically Relevant Nonmedicinal Ingredients
Intradermal injection	Suspension for injection. Each 0.1 mL dose is formulated to contain: 9 µg of influenza virus haemagglutinin antigens (HA) of each strain listed in the Description section.	Manufacturing process residuals: neomycin, formaldehyde, ovalbumin and Triton X-100 may be present in trace amounts. For a complete listing see Dosage Forms, Composition and Packaging.

DESCRIPTION: INTANZA [Influenza Vaccine (Split Virion, Inactivated)] is a sterile, colourless and opalescent suspension containing 3 strains of influenza virus cultivated on embryonated eggs, concentrated, purified by zonal centrifugation in a sucrose gradient, split by Triton X-100, inactivated by formaldehyde, concentrated and then diluted in phosphate buffered saline solution. The type of viral antigens contained in INTANZA conform to the current requirements of the World Health Organization (WHO). The strains for the 2010-2011 season are: A/California/7/2009 (H1N1)-like strain, A/Perth/16/2009 (H3N2)-like strain and B/Brisbane/60/2008.

INDICATIONS AND CLINICAL USE: INTANZA is indicated for active immunization against influenza caused by the specific strains of influenza virus contained in the vaccine in adults from 18 years of age and over. The vaccine is provided in two different strengths with specific indications:

- 9 µg/strain/0.1 mL in adults from 18 to 59 years of age, and
- 15 µg/strain/0.1 mL in individuals 60 years of age and over.

Although the current influenza vaccine can contain one or more of the antigens administered in previous years, annual vaccination using the current vaccine is necessary because immunity declines in the year following vaccination.

NACI encourages annual influenza vaccination for all Canadians who have no contraindications.

Vaccine should be offered up to and even after influenza virus activity is documented in a community.

Geriatrics: INTANZA 15 µg is indicated in persons 60 years of age and over.

Pediatrics: INTANZA is not indicated for persons less than 18 years of age.

CONTRAINDICATIONS: Hypersensitivity: INTANZA should not be administered to anyone with a history of severe allergic reaction to any component of the vaccine (see Dosage Forms, Composition and Packaging) or after previous administration of the vaccine or a vaccine containing the same components or constituents.

WARNINGS AND PRECAUTIONS: General: Before administration of INTANZA, health-care providers should inform the recipient of the benefits and risks of immunization, inquire about the recent health status of the recipient, review the recipient's history concerning possible hypersensitivity to the vaccine or similar vaccine, previous immunization history, the presence of any contra-indications to immunization and comply with any local requirements with respect to information to be provided to the recipient before immunization.

As with any vaccine, INTANZA may not protect 100% of vaccinated individuals.

Influenza virus is remarkably unpredictable in that significant antigenic changes may occur from time to time. It is known that INTANZA as now constituted is not effective against all possible strains of influenza virus. Protection is limited to those strains of virus from which the vaccine is prepared or against closely related strains.

Febrile or Acute Disease: Vaccination should be postponed in case of febrile or acute disease.

Immune: As with all products, epinephrine hydrochloride solution (1:1000) and other appropriate agents should be available for immediate use in case an anaphylactic or acute hypersensitivity reaction occurs. Health-care providers should be familiar with current recommendations for the initial management of anaphylaxis in non-hospital settings including proper airway management. For instructions on recognition and treatment of anaphylactic reactions see the current edition of the Canadian Immunization Guide or visit the Health Canada website.

Immunocompromised persons (whether from disease or treatment) may not obtain the expected immune response.

As each dose may contain traces of formaldehyde, Triton X-100 and undetectable traces of neomycin, which are used during vaccine production, caution should be exercised when the vaccine is administered to subjects with hypersensitivity to any of these substances. (See Contraindications.)

Neurologic: Immunization should be delayed in a patient with an active neurologic disorder, but should be considered when the disease process has been stabilized.

Guillain-Barré syndrome (GBS) has been reported after influenza vaccination. However, it is not known whether influenza vaccination specifically might increase the risk for recurrence of GBS. Therefore, NACI and ACIP state it is prudent to avoid vaccinating persons who are known to have experienced GBS within 6 to 8 weeks after a previous influenza vaccination.

Special Populations: Pregnant Women: For INTANZA, no clinical data on pregnant women are available.

In general, data from intramuscular influenza vaccinations in pregnant women do not indicate adverse fetal and maternal outcomes attributable to the vaccine. One animal study with INTANZA did not indicate direct or indirect harmful effects with respect to pregnancy, embryonic/fetal development, parturition or postnatal development.

INTANZA should be given to pregnant women following an assessment of the risks and benefits in the person to be vaccinated.

NACI states that influenza vaccination is recommended for all pregnant women.

Nursing Women: It is not known whether INTANZA is excreted in human milk. Caution must be exercised when INTANZA is administered to a nursing mother.

For INTANZA, no clinical data on nursing women are available.

NACI states that influenza vaccination is considered safe for breastfeeding women.

Pediatrics: INTANZA is not indicated for persons less than 18 years of age.

ADVERSE REACTIONS: Adverse Drug Reaction Overview: Adverse event information is derived from clinical trials and world-wide post-marketing experience with intramuscular influenza vaccines of similar composition.

Because INTANZA does not contain infectious viral particles, it cannot cause influenza. Respiratory disease after vaccination represents coincidental illness unrelated to influenza vaccination.

Clinical Trial Adverse Drug Reactions: Because clinical trials are conducted under widely varying conditions, adverse reaction rates observed in the clinical trials of a vaccine cannot be directly compared to rates in the clinical trials of another vaccine and may not reflect rates observed in practice. The adverse reaction information from clinical trials does, however, provide a basis for identifying the adverse events that appear to be related to vaccine use and for approximating rates of those events.

The safety of INTANZA was evaluated in four open-label randomized clinical trials. In these trials, 2384 adults 18 to 59 years of age received a single 9 µg dose of INTANZA, and 2974 adults 60 years of age and over received a single 15 µg dose of INTANZA. Table 1 presents the frequency of solicited adverse reactions reported in these clinical trials within 7 days of vaccination.

The most common reactions occurring after vaccine administration were injection site reactions. Since the immune response is activated close to the surface of the skin, as expected, apparent injection site reactions after intradermal administration were more frequent than after the control intramuscular (IM) influenza vaccine. The systemic safety profile observed after INTANZA was similar to the control IM influenza vaccine.

In both age groups, the most frequently reported reactions were injection site erythema, swelling and induration and the most frequently reported systemic reactions were headache, myalgia and malaise. Most reactions were mild in intensity, with the exception of severe injection site erythema, which was reported in 13.5% and 17%, respectively, in adults 18 to 59 years of age and adults 60 years of age and over. Most reactions resolved spontaneously within 1 to 3 days after onset. In some cases local redness lasted up to 7 days.

Data from clinical studies of INTANZA indicated that yearly repeated administration of intradermal influenza vaccination or alternating intramuscular and intradermal influenza vaccination did not alter the frequency or severity of adverse events.

Table 1: INTANZA

Frequency (%) of Solicited Reactions Observed in Clinical Trials in Adults Within 7 Days Following a Single Dose of Either INTANZA 9 µg or INTANZA 15 µg

Solicited Reactions	INTANZA 9 µg 18 to 59 Years of Age N=2384	INTANZA 15 µg ≥60 Years of Age N=2974
Injection Site Reactions		
Erythema	85.0	71.9
Swelling	62.7	39.0
Induration	61.5	40.9
Pruritus	42.7	29.2
Pain	41.9	22.2
Ecchymosis	8.3	4.3

(cont'd)

Table 1: INTANZA *(cont'd)*

Frequency (%) of Solicited Reactions Observed in Clinical Trials in Adults Within 7 Days Following a Single Dose of Either INTANZA 9 µg or INTANZA 15 µg

Solicited Reactions	INTANZA 9 µg 18 to 59 Years of Age N=2384	INTANZA 15 µg ≥60 Years of Age N=2974
Systemic Reactions		
Headache	30.2	13.7
Myalgia	22.6	10.8
Malaise	17.3	9.0
Shivering	8.7	4.1
Fever (≥38.0°C)	3.8	2.4

In addition, arthralgia, asthenia (including fatigue), increased sweating, paresthesia, rash, erythema and pruritus, were reported as unsolicited adverse reactions by up to 0.6% of participants in both age groups, including isolated reports. Six cases (0.2%) of lymphadenopathy were reported in clinical trials of INTANZA in adults 18 to 59 years of age, as non-serious unsolicited adverse events, within 21 days after vaccine administration. One case of neuritis (brachial radiculitis) was reported as a serious adverse reaction 15 days following vaccination, among adults ≥60 years of age receiving INTANZA 15 µg.

Data from Post-Marketing Experience: There currently is no data from post-marketing experience with INTANZA. However, the following additional systemic adverse events have been spontaneously reported during the post-marketing use of VAXIGRIP, a trivalent inactivated influenza vaccine containing the same antigens as INTANZA and administered intramuscularly. Because these events are reported voluntarily from a population of uncertain size, it is not possible to reliably estimate their frequency or establish a causal relationship to vaccine exposure.

Blood and Lymphatic System Disorders: transient thrombocytopenia, lymphadenopathy.

Immune System Disorders: allergic reactions: urticaria, dyspnea, angioneurotic edema, anaphylaxis including shock.

Nervous System Disorders: Guillain-Barré syndrome (GBS), neuritis, neuralgia, convulsions, encephalomyelitis.

Vascular Disorders: vasculitis, such as Henoch-Schonlein purpura, with transient renal involvement in certain cases.

Additional Adverse Reactions: Neurological disorders temporally associated with influenza vaccination such as encephalopathy (with or without permanent neurological—motor and/or sensory—deficit and/or intellectual impairment), optic neuritis, facial paralysis, labyrinthitis and brachial plexus neuropathy have been reported. However, no cause and effect relationship has been established.

Physicians, nurses and pharmacists should report any adverse occurrences temporally related to the administration of the product in accordance with local requirements and to the Global Pharmacovigilance Department, Sanofi Pasteur Limited, 1755 Steeles Avenue West, Toronto, ON, M2R 3T4, Canada. 1-888-621-1146 (phone) or 416-667-2435 (fax).

DRUG INTERACTIONS: Concomitant Vaccine Administration: No studies have been conducted regarding the concomitant administration of INTANZA and other vaccines.

According to NACI, inactivated vaccines usually do not interfere with the immune response to other inactivated or live vaccines and influenza vaccine may be given at the same time as other vaccines, provided different sites and administration devices are used.

Vaccine-Drug Interactions: Immunosuppressive treatments may interfere with the development of the expected immune response. (See Warnings and Precautions.)

DOSAGE AND ADMINISTRATION: Recommended Dose and Dosage Adjustment: Annual influenza vaccination consists of 1 dose of INTANZA.

Table 2: INTANZA

Recommended Influenza Vaccine Dosage, by Age

Age Group	Dose
18 to 59 years	0.1 mL—9 µg/strain
60 years and over	0.1 mL—15 µg/strain

Administration: Inspect for extraneous particulate matter and/or discolouration before use. If these conditions exist, the product should not be administered.

The vaccine should be at ambient temperature before being administered. This may be safely accomplished by holding the pre-filled micro-injection system in one's hand.

Do not shake the vaccine before use.

INTANZA is supplied in a micro-injection system for intradermal injection consisting of a pre-filled syringe with a micro-needle (1.5 mm) and a needle shielding system. The needle shielding system is designed to cover the micro-needle after use.

Administer the vaccine **intradermally**. The preferred site is in the region of the deltoid.

Clinical data suggests that re-vaccination is not required if there is liquid observed at the injection site after vaccine administration. A wheal is not required for successful vaccination.

Aseptic technique must be used.

Give the patient a permanent personal immunization record. In addition, it is essential that the physician or nurse record the immunization history in the permanent medical record of each patient. This permanent office record should contain the name of the vaccine, date given, dose, manufacturer and lot number.

1. **Remove Needle Cap**
   Remove the needle cap from the micro-injection system. **Do not shake the vaccine or attempt to remove the air bubble.**
2. **Hold Micro-Injection System Between Thumb and Middle Finger**
   Hold the system by placing the thumb and middle finger only on the finger pads, the index finger remains free. **Do not place fingers on the windows.**
3. **Insert Needle Rapidly Perpendicular to the Skin**
   Insert the needle perpendicular to the skin, in the region of the deltoid, in a short, quick movement.
4. **Inject Using the Index Finger**
   Once the micro-needle has been inserted, maintain a light pressure on the surface of the skin and inject using the index finger to push on the plunger. Do not aspirate.
5. **Activate Needle Shield by Pushing Firmly on Plunger**
   Remove the needle from the skin.
   Direct the needle away from you and others.
   With the same hand, push very firmly with the thumb on the plunger to activate the needle shield.
   You hear a click and a shield comes out to cover the needle.
   Immediately dispose of the system in the nearest sharps collector.

OVERDOSAGE:
Not applicable.

For management of a suspected drug overdose, contact your regional Poison Control Centre. See the *CPS Directory* section for a list of Poison Control Centres.

ACTION AND CLINICAL PHARMACOLOGY: Mechanism of Action: The following information is a summary of intradermal immune stimulation, and of the mechanism of action of influenza vaccines in general derived from published scientific and clinical research, and has not been generated specifically with INTANZA.

Antigens administered into the dermis are rapidly captured by the dendritic cells present in high density in the skin. In addition, the dermis contains a high density of lymphatic vessels and blood vessels, favouring rapid cellular and fluid exchanges and allowing direct access to the immune system. Following migration to the draining lymph node, the dendritic cells, potent stimulators and modulators of the immune response, present the captured antigens to T cells, leading to T and B cell activation/expansion, thereby resulting in the induction of a sustained antigen-specific humoral and cellular immunity.

Immunity to the surface antigens, especially to the haemagglutinin, reduces the likelihood of infection and lessens the severity of disease if infection occurs. Each year's influenza vaccine contains three virus strains (usually two type A and one type B) representing the influenza viruses that are believed likely to circulate in the coming winter. The antigenic characteristics of current and emerging influenza virus strains provide the basis for selecting the strains included in each year's vaccine.

Protection is afforded only against those strains of virus from which the vaccine is prepared, or closely related strains. Immune response against one influenza virus type or subtype confers limited or no protection against another. Furthermore, immune response to one antigenic variant of influenza virus might not protect against a new antigenic variant of the same type or subtype. Frequent development of antigenic variants through antigenic drift is the virologic basis for seasonal epidemics and the reason for the usual incorporation of one or more new strains in each year's influenza vaccine.

Pharmacodynamics: Seroprotection is expected within 2 to 3 weeks following influenza vaccination.

Haemagglutination inhibiting serum antibody titres are considered appropriate surrogates of protection. Comparative evaluation of the humoral immune response was the primary objective in all clinical trials with INTANZA. The humoral immune response was assessed through the measurement of Geometric Mean Titres of HI antibodies, as well as through the evaluation of seroconversion rates, GMT increases and seroprotection rates. In clinical trials in adults 18 to 59 years of age INTANZA 9 µg elicited at least as high an immune response as the control IM influenza vaccine for each of the vaccine strains tested. INTANZA 15 µg in adults 60 years and over was demonstrated to elicit a statistically significant increase in humoral immune response when compared to the control IM influenza vaccine for each of the vaccine strains tested.

Specific sub-analyses conducted in the pivotal clinical trials of INTANZA in both dosages (9 µg and 15 µg) demonstrated that the absence of a wheal at the injection site or the presence of risk factors for severe influenza disease did not affect the seroprotection afforded by INTANZA vaccination. Participants with co-morbidity factors or with low pre-vaccination titres showed an even more pronounced increase in immune response compared to the control IM influenza vaccination. Similar sub-analyses also suggest that the presence of liquid at the injection site after vaccine administration (due to the superficial nature of the injection) does not impact the immune response to INTANZA.

Pharmacokinetics: No pharmacokinetic studies have been performed.

Duration of Effect: Annual vaccination against influenza is recommended.

Results from serology follow-up of adults 18 to 59 years of age immunized with INTANZA 9 µg in a clinical study demonstrated that seroprotection rates and GMTs above pre-vaccination levels persisted up to 12 months following vaccination. The magnitude of the immune response observed within 21 days post-vaccination with INTANZA 15 µg in adults 60 years of age and over suggests that a similar duration of protection can be expected in this age group.

STORAGE AND STABILITY: Store at 2 to 8°C. **Do not freeze.** Discard product if exposed to freezing.

Do not use after expiration date.

INFORMATION FOR THE PATIENT: Published in e-CPS, available by subscription at www.e-cps.ca.

DOSAGE FORMS, COMPOSITION AND PACKAGING: Each 0.1 mL dose of sterile, colourless, opalescent suspension is formulated to contain: 9 µg per strain of haemagglutinin (HA) of split influenza virus, inactivated, of A/California/7/2009 (H1N1)-like strain, A/Perth/16/2009 (H3N2)-like strain and B/Brisbane/60/2008. Buffer solution (up to 0.1 mL) containing: sodium chloride 0.8 mg, potassium chloride 0.02 mg, disodium phosphate dihydrate 0.115 mg, potassium dihydrogen phosphate 0.02 mg. Manufacturing process residuals: neomycin, formaldehyde, ovalbumin and Triton X-100 may be present in trace amounts. Single-dose pre-filled syringes with micro-injection systems equipped with a needle shield to be activated post-administration. The syringes are made of Ph. Eur. Type I glass. The container closure system for INTANZA does not contain latex (natural rubber). Packages of: 1×0.1 mL pre-filled Micro-Injection System, 10×0.1 mL pre-filled Micro-Injection Systems. Not all pack sizes may be marketed. Vaccine Information Service: 1-888-621-1146 or 416-667-2779. Business Hours: 8 a.m. to 5 p.m. Eastern Time, Monday to Friday.

Full product monograph available on request or visit us at www.sanofipasteur.ca

Integrilin® ℞

eptifibatide

Platelet Aggregation Inhibitor

Schering-Plough

Date of Revision: December 19, 2008

PHARMACOLOGY: General: Eptifibatide reversibly inhibits platelet aggregation by preventing the binding of fibrinogen, von Willebrand factor and other adhesive ligands to glycoprotein IIb/IIIa (GP IIb/IIIa). When administered intravenously, eptifibatide inhibits ex vivo platelet aggregation in a dose- and concentration-dependent manner. Platelet aggregation inhibition is reversible following cessation of eptifibatide; this is thought to result from dissociation of eptifibatide from the platelet receptor.

Pharmacodynamics: Eptifibatide inhibits platelet aggregation induced by adenosine diphosphate (ADP) and other agonists in a dose- and concentration-dependent manner. The effect of eptifibatide is observed immediately after administration of a 180 µg/kg intravenous bolus. When followed by a 2 µg/kg/min continuous infusion, this regimen produces a >80% inhibition of 20 µM ADP-induced ex vivo platelet aggregation, (at physiologic calcium concentrations) in more than 80% of patients, after more than 8 hours of infusion. Platelet inhibition was reversed, with a >50% return of platelet function towards baseline 4 hours after discontinuation of an infusion of 2 µg/kg/min.

The eptifibatide dosing regimen used in the ESPRIT study was similar to that used in the PURSUIT study (a 180 µg/kg bolus followed by a 2 µg/kg/min infusion), but added a second 180 µg/kg bolus ten minutes after the first bolus to avoid a transient decrease in platelet aggregation inhibition before reaching steady-state with the continuous 2 µg/kg/min infusion. This dosing regimen is recommended in order to maintain platelet aggregation inhibition above 80% in the early time points when percutaneous coronary intervention (PCI) is performed (see Pharmacokinetics).

Administration of eptifibatide by intravenous bolus and infusion to healthy male subjects causes up to a 5-fold increase in bleeding time, which is reversible upon discontinuation of the infusion with bleeding times returning toward baseline within 4 to 6 hours. When administered alone, eptifibatide has no measurable effect on prothrombin time (PT) or activated partial thromboplastin time (aPTT) (see also Precautions, Drug Interactions).

There were no important differences between age groups on the inhibition by eptifibatide of adenosine diphosphate-induced platelet aggregation. Differences among ethnic groups have not been assessed.

Pharmacokinetics: The pharmacokinetics of eptifibatide are linear and dose-proportional for bolus doses ranging from 90 to 250 µg/kg and infusion rates from 0.5 to 3 µg/kg/min. The administration of a single bolus followed by an infusion produces an early peak level, followed by a small decline until steady state plasma concentrations are achieved (within 4-6 hours). In situations in which continuous inhibition is critical during the first 1-2 hours, e.g., when PCI is performed, this decline can be prevented by administering a second 180 µg/kg bolus ten minutes after the first. Plasma elimination half-life is approximately 2.5 hours. The extent of eptifibatide binding to human plasma protein is about 25%. In patients with unstable angina/non-ST-segment elevation myocardial infarction (UA/NSTEMI), plasma clearance is 55 mL/kg/h and the volume of distribution is approximately 185 mL/kg. In healthy subjects, renal clearance accounts for approximately 50% of total body clearance, with the majority of the drug excreted in the urine as eptifibatide, deamidated eptifibatide, and other more polar metabolites. No major metabolites have been detected in human plasma. Total drug clearance is decreased by approximately 50% and steady-state plasma eptifibatide concentrations are doubled in patients with moderate renal impairment (creatinine clearance of ≥30-<50 mL/min, using the Cockcroft-Gault equation) (see Dosage for the Cockcroft-Gault equation).

Clinical studies have included 2418 patients with serum creatinine between 1 and 2 mg/dL (for the 180 µg/kg bolus followed by a 2 µg/kg/min infusion) and 7 patients with serum creatinine between 2 and 4 mg/dL (for the 135 µg/kg bolus and the 0.5 µg/kg/min infusion), without dose adjustment. An additional 8 patients with serum creatinine between 2 and 4 mg/dL were enrolled in the ESPRIT study and received an intravenous bolus of 180 µg/kg, immediately followed by a continuous infusion of 1 µg/kg/min and a second 180 µg/kg bolus administered ten minutes after the first.

Special Populations: Patients in clinical studies were older than the subjects in clinical pharmacology studies, and they had lower total body clearance and higher eptifibatide plasma levels. However, clinical studies were conducted in patients with UA/NSTEMI ranging in age from 20 to 94 years, without dose adjustment for age. Limited data are available for patients over 75 years of age weighing less than 50 kg. Men and women showed no important differences in the pharmacokinetics of eptifibatide.

INDICATIONS: INTEGRILIN (eptifibatide injection) is indicated for the treatment of patients presenting with symptoms of unstable angina (UA)/non-ST-segment elevation myocardial infarction (NSTEMI), including those patients who may subsequently undergo percutaneous coronary intervention (PCI) as well as those who will be managed medically.

INTEGRILIN is indicated for the treatment of patients undergoing PCI including those undergoing intracoronary stenting.

INTEGRILIN is intended for use with ASA and heparin.

CONTRAINDICATIONS: Treatment with eptifibatide is contraindicated in patients with: A history of bleeding diathesis, or evidence of active abnormal bleeding within the previous 30 days. Thrombocytopenia (<100 000 cells/mm³). Prothrombin time >1.2 times control, or International Normalized Ration (INR) ≥2.0. Severe hypertension (systolic blood pressure >200 mmHg or diastolic blood pressure >110 mmHg) not adequately controlled on antihypertensive therapy. Major surgery within the preceding 6 weeks. History of stroke within 30 days or any history of hemorrhagic stroke. Known history of intracranial disease (neoplasm, arteriovenous malformation, aneurysm). Current or planned administration of another parenteral GP IIb-IIIa inhibitor. Severe renal impairment (creatinine clearance <30 mL/min) or dependency on renal dialysis. Known hypersensitivity to any component of the product. Clinically significant liver disease.

WARNINGS: Bleeding: Bleeding is the most common complication encountered during INTEGRILIN therapy. Administration of INTEGRILIN is associated with an increase in major and minor bleeding, as classified by the Thrombolysis in Myocardial Infarction Study group (TIMI) criteria (see Adverse Effects). Most major bleeding associated with INTEGRILIN has been at the arterial access site for cardiac catheterization or from the gastrointestinal or genitourinary tract.

All potential bleeding sites (e.g., catheter insertion sites, arterial, venous or needle puncture sites; cutdown sites; gastrointestinal, genitourinary and retroperitoneal sites) should be observed carefully.

In patients undergoing PCI, patients receiving INTEGRILIN experienced an increase in major bleeding compared to those receiving placebo without a significant increase in transfusion requirement. Special care should be employed to minimize the risk of bleeding among these patients (see Precautions). **If bleeding cannot be controlled with pressure, infusion of INTEGRILIN and any concomitant heparin should be stopped immediately.**

Clinical data suggest that the risk of major and minor bleeding due to INTEGRILIN therapy may be increased in patients weighing less than 70 kg.

Platelet Count <100 000/mm³: Because it is an inhibitor of platelet aggregation, caution should be exercised when administering eptifibatide to patients with a platelet count <100 000/mm³; there has been no clinical experience with eptifibatide initiated in patients with a platelet count <100 000/mm³.

PRECAUTIONS: Bleeding: Coronary artery bypass grafting (CABG): Treatment with INTEGRILIN is not associated with an increase in bleeding in association with CABG. INTEGRILIN infusion should be discontinued prior to undergoing CABG.

Percutaneous coronary intervention—Care of the femoral artery access site: Treatment with INTEGRILIN is associated with an increase in major and minor bleeding particularly at the site of arterial access for femoral sheath placement. In patients undergoing PCI, INTEGRILIN infusion should be continued for up to 18-24 hours post-procedure or until hospital discharge, whichever comes first. Heparin use is discouraged after the PCI procedure. The femoral artery sheath may be removed during treatment with INTEGRILIN. It is recommended that heparin be discontinued 3-4 hours prior to sheath removal and a decline in aPTT to <45 seconds or activated clotting time (ACT) to <150 seconds be documented. Heparin and INTEGRILIN should be discontinued and sheath hemostasis should be achieved at least 2-4 hours before hospital discharge.

Maintaining Target aPTT and ACT: The aPTT should be maintained between 50 and 70 seconds unless PCI is to be performed. For angioplasty done during the PURSUIT study, a target ACT of 300 to 350 seconds was stipulated. Patients receiving an INTEGRILIN 180 µg/kg bolus followed by a 2 µg/kg/min infusion experienced an increased incidence of bleeding relative to placebo, primarily at the femoral access site. The ESPRIT study stipulated a target ACT of 200 to 300 seconds during intracoronary stenting. Patients receiving an INTEGRILIN 180 µg/kg bolus followed by a 2 µg/kg/min infusion and a second 180 µg/kg bolus ten minutes after the first (mean ACT 284 seconds) experienced an increased incidence of bleeding relative to placebo (mean ACT 276 seconds), primarily at the femoral artery access site. At these lower ACTs, bleeding was less than previously reported with eptifibatide in the PURSUIT and IMPACT II studies. Moreover, there was little increase in transfusion requirements.

PRIDE was a randomized, placebo-controlled, multi-center trial conducted in 126 patients with coronary artery disease undergoing angioplasty, prior to the PURSUIT study. The pharmacodynamics of three dosing regimens of INTEGRILIN were assessed. All infusions were continued for 24 hours post-angioplasty. The incidence of bleeding events in patients receiving INTEGRILIN as a 180 µg/kg bolus and 2 µg/kg/min infusion and heparin targeted at an ACT of 200-250 was similar to that seen in patients receiving placebo and heparin targeted at an ACT of 300-350 seconds. The study was not powered to assess clinical efficacy.

The aPTT or ACT should be checked prior to arterial sheath removal. The sheath should not be removed unless the aPTT is <45 seconds or the ACT is <150 seconds.

Table 1 displays the risk of major bleeding according to the maximum aPTT attained within 72 hours in the PURSUIT study.

Table 1: INTEGRILIN

Major Bleeding by Maximal aPTT within 72 Hours in the PURSUIT Study

Maximum aPTT (seconds)	Placebo n (%)	Eptifibatide 180 µg/kg Bolus, 2 µg/kg/min Infusion n (%)
<50	44/721 (6.1%)	44/743 (5.9%)
50–70 (recommended)	92/908 (10.1%)	99/883 (11.2%)
>70	281/2786 (10.1%)	345/2811 (12.3%)

Care of puncture sites: Arterial and venous punctures, intramuscular injections, and the use of urinary catheters, nasotracheal intubation, nasogastric tubes, and automatic blood pressure cuffs should be minimized. When obtaining intravenous access, non-compressible sites (e.g., subclavian or jugular veins) should be avoided. Document and monitor vascular puncture sites. Consider using saline or heparin locks for blood drawing. Remove dressings gently.

Laboratory Monitoring: Before infusion of INTEGRILIN, the following tests should be conducted: platelet count, hematocrit or hemoglobin, serum creatinine and PT/aPTT. In patients undergoing PCI, the ACT should also be measured in patients who have already received heparin. During and following INTEGRILIN treatment, platelet counts and extent of heparin anticoagulation, as assessed by ACT, should be monitored closely. Platelet counts should be monitored 2 to 4 hours following administration of the INTEGRILIN bolus, and at 24 hours post-infusion termination or prior to patient discharge, whichever occurs first.

Thrombocytopenia: If a patient experiences a platelet decrease (<100 000/mm³), additional platelet counts should be determined (see Adverse Effects, Table 9, Table 10 and Table 11). If thrombocytopenia is confirmed, INTEGRILIN and heparin should be discontinued immediately and the condition appropriately monitored and treated.

From post market experience, acute thrombocytopenia has been reported. Upon discontinuation of INTEGRILIN, acute thrombocytopenia has been reported to be reversible. The rapid reversibility of the pharmacologic action is due to the short plasma half-life of INTEGRILIN (approximately 2.5 hours) and the rapid disassociation of INTEGRILIN from the platelet receptor GP IIb/IIIa.

Prolongation of Bleeding Time: Administration of INTEGRILIN by intravenous bolus and infusion causes up to a 5-fold increase in bleeding time. This increase is reversible upon discontinuation of the infusion with bleeding times returning towards baseline within 4 to 6 hours. When administered alone, INTEGRILIN has no measurable effect on prothrombin time (PT) or activated partial thromboplastin time (aPTT).

Renal Impairment: Renal and non-renal clearance of eptifibatide account for approximately 50% each. Total drug clearance is decreased by approximately 50% and steady-state plasma eptifibatide concentrations are doubled in patients with moderate renal impairment (creatinine clearance of ≥30-<50 mL/min, using Cockcroft-Gault equation) (see Dosage for the Cockcroft-Gault equation). Therefore, the infusion dose should be reduced to 1.0 µg/kg/min in such patients.

No clinical data are available for patients dependent on renal dialysis. In vitro studies have indicated that eptifibatide may be cleared from plasma by dialysis.

Pregnancy: Reproduction and teratology studies have been performed by continuous intravenous infusion of eptifibatide in pregnant rats at total daily doses of up to 72 mg/kg/day (24 times the recommended maximum daily human dose of 3 mg/kg/day) and pregnant rabbits at total daily doses of up to 36 mg/kg/day (12 times the recommended maximum daily human dose). These studies revealed no evidence of impaired fertility or harm to the fetus due to eptifibatide. Eptifibatide has been shown to cross the placenta in pregnant rats. There are, however, no adequate and well-controlled studies in pregnant women with eptifibatide. Because animal reproduction studies are not always predictive of human response, this drug should be used during pregnancy only if clearly needed.

Lactation: It is not known whether eptifibatide is excreted in human milk. Therefore, nursing should be discontinued during the period of drug administration.

Children: Safety and effectiveness of eptifibatide in children have not been established.

Geriatrics: Table 2 and Table 3 show bleeding events and transfusions for patients ≥65 years old and ≥75 years old, respectively, in the PURSUIT study. The incidence of bleeding complications was higher in the elderly in both placebo and eptifibatide groups, and the incremental risk of eptifibatide-associated bleeding was greater in older patients. No dose adjustment was made in the elderly population, but patients over 75 years of age had to weigh at least 50 kg to be enrolled in the PURSUIT study; no such limitation was stipulated in the ESPRIT study (see Adverse Effects).

Table 2: INTEGRILIN

Bleeding Events and Transfusions within 30 Days of Randomization for Patients ≥65 Years Old PURSUIT Study

	Placebo	Eptifibatide 180 µg/kg Bolus, 2 µg/kg/min Infusion
	n (%) of Patients	
Major Bleeding[a,c]	230/2220 (10.4%)	269/2209 (12.2%)
Minor Bleeding[a,c]	190/2220 (8.6%)	358/2209 (16.2%)
Bleeding requiring transfusions[b]	307/2270 (13.5%)	375/2237 (16.8%)

[a] For major and minor bleeding, patients are counted only once according to the most severe classification.
[b] Includes transfusions of any type: whole blood, packed red blood cells, fresh frozen plasma, cryoprecipitate, platelets, and autotransfusion during the initial hospitalization.
[c] Incidence in patients with sufficient clinical information to determine bleeding status.

Table 3: INTEGRILIN

Bleeding Events and Transfusions within 30 Days of Randomization for Patients ≥75 Years Old PURSUIT Study

	Placebo	Eptifibatide 180 µg/kg Bolus, 2 µg/kg/min Infusion
	n (%) of Patients	
Major Bleeding[a,c]	53/655 (8.1%)	78/663 (11.8%)
Minor Bleeding[a,c]	56/655 (8.5%)	130/663 (19.6%)
Bleeding requiring transfusions[b]	81/672 (12.1%)	121/673 (18.0%)

[a] For major and minor bleeding, patients are counted only once according to the most severe classification.
[b] Includes transfusions of any type: whole blood, packed red blood cells, fresh frozen plasma, cryoprecipitate, platelets, and autotransfusion during the initial hospitalization.
[c] Incidence in patients with sufficient clinical information to determine bleeding status.

Drug Interactions: INTEGRILIN has been studied concomitantly with heparin and ASA. The use of INTEGRILIN, in combination with heparin and ASA, has been associated with an increase in bleeding compared to heparin and ASA alone. Because eptifibatide inhibits platelet aggregation, caution should be employed when it is used with other medications that affect hemostasis, including **thrombolytics, oral anticoagulants, non-steroidal anti-inflammatory drugs, dipyridamole, ticlopidine and clopidogrel**. To avoid potentially additive pharmacological effects, concomitant treatment with **other inhibitors of platelet receptor GP IIb/IIIa** should be avoided.

In the ESPRIT study, clopidogrel or, in a few cases, ticlopidine were used routinely starting the day of intracoronary stenting.

Bleeding events were more frequent in patients receiving concurrent heparin while undergoing PCI when ACT exceeded 350 seconds (see Precautions).

Thrombolytics: Limited data are available on the use of INTEGRILIN with thrombolytic agents. In a 180 patient study with the accelerated alteplase regimen, the coadministration of INTEGRILIN up to 180 µg/kg and 0.75 µg/kg/min did not increase the incidence of major bleeding or transfusions compared to patients receiving alteplase alone. In another 181 patient study with streptokinase (1.5 million units over 60 minutes), the coadministration of increasing INTEGRILIN doses was well tolerated up to an infusion rate of 1.3 and 2 µg/kg/min, where there was an increased incidence of bleeding and transfusions.

Based on the limited data on the use of INTEGRILIN in patients receiving thrombolytic agents, the bleeding risk due to combination with thrombolytic therapy cannot be estimated. Therefore, the concomitant treatment with thrombolytic agents should be used judiciously after the risk and benefit are carefully assessed for individual patients by the physician.

Lastly, experience in 40 patients who received a combination of full dose INTEGRILIN (180 µg/kg and 2 µg/kg/min) and full dose thrombolytic therapy revealed a 25% incidence of major bleeding events.

Pharmacokinetic and Pharmacodynamic Interaction with Enoxaparin: The use of enoxaparin dosed as a 1 mg/kg subcutaneous injection every 12 hours in place of unfractionated heparin did not alter the pharmacokinetics of eptifibatide or the level of platelet aggregation inhibition.

ADVERSE EFFECTS: A total of 16 782 patients were treated in the Phase III clinical trials (PURSUIT, IMPACT II and ESPRIT). These 16 782 patients had a mean age of 62 years (range 20 to 94). Eighty-nine percent of the patients were Caucasian, with the remainder being predominantly Black (5%) and Hispanic (5%). Sixty-eight percent were men. Because of the different regimens used in PURSUIT, IMPACT II and ESPRIT, data from the 3 studies were not pooled.

Bleeding: The results of bleeding events and transfusions in the PURSUIT study during infusion and within 30 days are displayed in Table 4, and Table 5 respectively. The results of bleeding events and transfusions in the IMPACT II and ESPRIT studies are displayed in Table 6 and Table 7, respectively.

Bleeding was classified as major or minor by the criteria of the TIMI study group. Major bleeding events were defined as either an intracranial hemorrhage or other bleeding that led to a decrease in hemoglobin greater than 5 g/dL. Minor bleeding events included spontaneous gross hematuria, spontaneous hematemesis, observed blood loss with a hemoglobin decrease of more than 3 g/dL or more than 4 g/dL in the absence of an observed bleeding site. In patients who received transfusions, the corresponding loss in hemoglobin was estimated through an adaptation of the method of Landefeld et al.

Table 4: INTEGRILIN

Bleeding Events and Transfusions during Infusion PURSUIT Study

	Placebo	Eptifibatide 180 µg/kg Bolus, 2 µg/kg/min Infusion
	n (%) of Patients	
Major Bleeding[a,c]	59/4577 (1.3%)	96/4604 (2.1%)
Minor Bleeding[a,c]	89/4577 (1.9%)	186/4604 (4.0%)
Bleeding requiring transfusions[b]	19/4696 (0.4%)	34/4679 (0.7%)

(cont'd)

Table 4: INTEGRILIN *(cont'd)*

[a] For major and minor bleeding, patients are counted only once according to the most severe classification.
[b] Includes transfusions of any type: whole blood, packed red blood cells, fresh frozen plasma, cryoprecipitate, platelets, and autotransfusion during the initial hospitalization.
[c] Incidence in patients with sufficient clinical information to determine bleeding status.

Table 5: INTEGRILIN

Bleeding Events and Transfusions within 30 Days PURSUIT Study

	Placebo	Eptifibatide 180 µg/kg Bolus, 2 µg/kg/min Infusion
	n (%) of Patients	
Major Bleeding[a,c]	425/4577 (9.3%)	498/4604 (10.8%)
Minor Bleeding[a,c]	347/4577 (7.6%)	604/4604 (13.1%)
Bleeding requiring transfusions[b]	490/4696 (10.4%)	601/4679 (12.8%)

[a] For major and minor bleeding, patients are counted only once according to the most severe classification.
[b] Includes transfusions of any type: whole blood, packed red blood cells, fresh frozen plasma, cryoprecipitate, platelets, and autotransfusion during the initial hospitalization.
[c] Incidence in patients with sufficient clinical information to determine bleeding status.

Table 6: INTEGRILIN

Bleeding Events and Transfusions within 30 Days IMPACT II Study

	Placebo n (%)	Eptifibatide 135 µg/kg Bolus, 0.5 µg/kg/min Infusion n (%)	Eptifibatide 135 µg/kg Bolus, 0.75 µg/kg/min Infusion (%)
Patients	1285	1300	1286
Major bleeding[a]	55 (4.5%)	55 (4.4%)	58 (4.7%)
Minor bleeding[a]	115 (9.3%)	146 (11.7%)	177 (14.2%)
Bleeding requiring transfusions[b]	66 (5.1%)	71 (5.5%)	74 (5.8%)

[a] For major and minor bleeding, patients are counted only once according to the most severe classification.
[b] Includes transfusions of whole blood, packed red blood cells, fresh frozen plasma, cryoprecipitate, platelets, and autotransfusion during the initial hospitalization.

Note: Denominator is based on patients for whom data are available.

Table 7: INTEGRILIN

Bleeding Events and Transfusions within 48 Hours[a] ESPRIT Study

	Placebo n (%)	Eptifibatide 180 µg/kg Bolus, 2 µg/kg/min Infusion, 180 µg/kg Bolus 10 min After First n (%)
Patients	1024	1040
Major Bleeding[b]	4 (0.4%)	13 (1.3%)
Minor Bleeding[b]	18 (2.0%)	29 (3.0%)
Bleeding requiring transfusions[c]	11 (1.1%)	16 (1.5%)
Unresolved[d]	102	68

[a] Or discharge, whichever occurred first.
[b] For major and minor bleeding, patients are counted only once according to the most severe classification.
[c] Includes transfusions of any type: whole blood, packed red blood cells, fresh frozen plasma, cryoprecipitate, platelets, and autotransfusion during the initial hospitalization.
[d] Number of patients in who TIMI grade could not be ascertained; these patients are excluded from the denominator in the computation of percents.

In the PURSUIT study, treatment with INTEGRILIN resulted in an incremental risk of major bleeding (increase of 1.5%) and a higher incidence of transfusion (increase of 2.4%) than occurred with placebo. There was also an increase in minor bleeding events in patients treated with eptifibatide (increase of 5.5%) compared to placebo.

In the PURSUIT study, the greatest increase in major bleeding in eptifibatide-treated patients compared to placebo was associated with bleeding at the femoral artery access site (2.8% vs 1.3%). Oropharyngeal (primarily gingival), genitourinary, gastrointestinal, and retroperitoneal bleeding were also seen more commonly in eptifibatide-treated patients compared to placebo.

Among patients experiencing a major bleed in the IMPACT II study, an increase in bleeding on eptifibatide versus placebo was observed only for the femoral artery access site (3.2% vs 2.8%).

The majority of major bleeding events in the ESPRIT study occurred at the vascular access site (1 and 8 patients, or 0.1% and 0.8% in the placebo and eptifibatide groups, respectively). Bleeding at "other" locations occurred in 0.2% and 0.4% of patients, respectively, while the number was even lower at the remaining sites (such as genitourinary, gastrointestinal, and retroperitoneal bleeding).

Table 8 displays the incidence of TIMI major bleeding according to the cardiac procedures carried out in the PURSUIT study. The most common bleeding complications were associated with cardiac revascularization procedures (CABG-related or femoral artery access site bleeding).

A corresponding table for ESPRIT is not presented as every patient underwent PTCA in the ESPRIT study and only 11 patients underwent CABG.

Patients undergoing CABG accounted for most instances of major bleeding in both treatment groups. Patients undergoing coronary angioplasty accounted for most of the increased incidence of major bleeding among patients treated with INTEGRILIN compared to placebo.

Table 8: INTEGRILIN

Major Bleeding by Procedures in the PURSUIT Study[a]

Abnormalities	Placebo n (%)	Eptifibatide 180 µg/kg Bolus, 2 µg/kg/min Infusion n (%)
Patients	4577	4604
Overall Incidence of Major Bleeding	425 (9.3%)	498 (10.8%)
Breakdown by Procedure:		
CABG	375 (8.2%)	377 (8.2%)
Angioplasty without CABG	27 (0.6%)	64 (1.4%)
Angiography without Angioplasty or CABG	11 (0.2%)	29 (0.6%)
Medical Therapy Only	12 (0.3%)	12 (0.3%)

[a] Data through hospital discharge, including patients undergoing CABG.

In the PURSUIT and ESPRIT studies, the risk of major bleeding with INTEGRILIN increased inversely with patient weight. This relationship was most apparent for patients weighing less than 70 kg.

Bleeding adverse events resulting in discontinuation of study drug were more frequent among patients receiving INTEGRILIN than placebo (4.6% versus 0.9% in ESPRIT, 8% versus 1% in PURSUIT, and 3.5% versus 1.9% in IMPACT II).

Intracranial Hemorrhage And Stroke: Intracranial hemorrhage was rare in the PURSUIT, IMPACT II and ESPRIT clinical studies. In the PURSUIT study, only 3 patients in the placebo group and 5 patients in the group treated with INTEGRILIN 180 µg/kg bolus followed by a continuous infusion of 2 µg/kg/min experienced hemorrhagic stroke. The overall incidence of stroke was 0.7% in patients receiving INTEGRILIN 180 µg/kg bolus followed by a continuous infusion of 2 µg/kg/min and 0.8% in placebo patients.

Investigator's assessment of all strokes within 6 months of randomization was 1.3% in patients receiving eptifibatide 180 µg/kg bolus followed by a continuous infusion of 2 µg/kg/min, and 1.5% in placebo patients, in the PURSUIT study.

In the IMPACT II study, intracranial hemorrhage was experienced by 1 patient treated with eptifibatide 135 µg/kg bolus followed by a continuous infusion of 0.5 µg/kg/min, 2 patients treated with eptifibatide 135/0.75 and 2 patients in the placebo group. The overall incidence of stroke was 0.5% in patients receiving 135 µg/kg bolus followed by a continuous infusion of 0.5 µg/kg/min eptifibatide, 0.7% in patients receiving eptifibatide 135 µg/kg bolus followed by a continuous infusion of 0.75 µg/kg/min and 0.7% in the placebo group.

In the ESPRIT study, there were 3 hemorrhagic strokes, 1 in the placebo group and 2 in the eptifibatide (180 µg/kg bolus, followed by a continuous infusion of 2 µg/kg/min, and a 180 µg/kg bolus 10 minutes after the first) group. In addition, there was 1 case of cerebral infarction in the eptifibatide group. Both patients who experienced a hemorrhagic stroke while receiving eptifibatide had received >10 000 units of heparin.

Thrombocytopenia: In the PURSUIT and IMPACT II studies, the incidence of thrombocytopenia (<100 000/mm^3 or >50% reduction from baseline) (see Table 9 and Table 10) and the incidence of platelet transfusions were similar between patients treated with INTEGRILIN and placebo. In the ESPRIT study, the incidence was 0.6% in the placebo group and 1.2% in the eptifibatide group (see Table 11).

Table 9: INTEGRILIN

Incidence of Marked Abnormalities in Platelets Postbaseline for Patients Treated with Placebo or INTEGRILIN[a] **PURSUIT Study**

Abnormalities	Placebo	Eptifibatide 180 µg/kg Bolus, 2 µg/kg/min Infusion
Platelet Count		
<100 000/mm^3	225/4587 (5%)	226/4599 (5%)
≥50% Decrease from Baseline[b]	231/4516 (5%)	250/4544 (5%)
<50 000/mm^3	19/4587 (<1%)	26/4599 (1%)
<20 000/mm^3	2/4587 (<1%)	9/4599 (<1%)

[a] Data through hospital discharge, including patients undergoing CABG.
[b] Requires a baseline value and at least one post-baseline value. All other computations requires only a post-baseline value.

Table 10: INTEGRILIN

Incidence of Marked Abnormalities in Platelets Postbaseline for Patients Treated with Placebo or INTEGRILIN IMPACT II Study

Abnormalities	Placebo	Eptifibatide 135 µg/kg Bolus, 0.5 µg/kg/min Infusion	Eptifibatide 135 µg/kg Bolus, 0.75 µg/kg/min Infusion
Platelet Count			
<100 000/mm^3	31/1285 (2.4%)	34/1300 (2.6%)	36/1286 (2.8%)
≥50% Decrease from Baseline	39/1285 (3.0%)	29/1300 (2.2%)	33/1286 (2.6%)
<50 000/mm^3	8/1285 (0.6%)	2/1300 (0.2%)	5/1286 (0.4%)

Note: Percentage based on total population.

Allergic Reactions: The incidence of anaphylaxis in large randomized studies ranged from 0% to 0.16% for INTEGRILIN and from 0% to 0.15% for placebo. The number of patients who discontinued drug due to allergic reactions in these studies ranged from 0.04% to 0.2% for INTEGRILIN and from 0% to 0.1% for placebo. The potential for the development of antibodies to INTEGRILIN has been studied in 433 subjects, 21 of whom received a second INTEGRILIN administration after 28 days. No antibodies against INTEGRILIN were detected in blood samples collected at baseline and 30 days after drug administration.

Other Adverse Reactions: Table 12 displays serious adverse events other than bleeding from the PURSUIT study which occurred in greater than or equal to 1% of treated patients in the INTEGRILIN or placebo group within 30 days of treatment initiation.

In the ESPRIT study, the incidence of serious non-bleeding adverse events was similar in patients receiving placebo or eptifibatide (6% and 7%, respectively). In the IMPACT II study, serious non-bleeding events that occurred in greater than 1% of patients were uncommon and similar in incidence between placebo- and eptifibatide-treated patients.

There were no significant increases in serious non-bleeding events with INTEGRILIN relative to placebo. Serious non-bleeding adverse events were generally of a cardiovascular etiology and are expected in a patient population presenting with UA/NSTEMI.

Table 11: INTEGRILIN

Incidence of Marked Abnormalities in Platelets Postbaseline for Patients Treated with Placebo or INTEGRILIN[a] **ESPRIT Study**

Abnormalities	Placebo n (%)	Eptifibatide 180 µg/kg Bolus, 2 µg/kg/min Infusion, 180 µg/kg Bolus 10 Minutes After First n (%)
Platelet Count		
<100 000/mm^3	4/1024 (0.4%)	9/1040 (0.9%)
<100 000/mm^3 or ≥50% Decrease from Baseline	6/1024 (0.6%)	12/1040 (1.2%)
>50% Decrease from Baseline[b]	2/1024 (0.2%)	9/1040 (0.9%)
≥20 000 to <50 000/mm^3	0/1024 (0%)	0/1040 (0%)
<20 000/mm^3	0/1024 (0%)	2/1040 (0.2%)

[a] Data within 48 hours of treatment with INTEGRILIN or Placebo.
[b] Requires a baseline value and at least one post-baseline value. All other computations requires only a post-baseline value.

Table 12: INTEGRILIN

Serious Nonbleeding Adverse Events among Treated Patients in the PURSUIT Study

	Placebo (n=4696)	Eptifibatide 180 µg/kg Bolus, 2 µg/kg/min Infusion (n=4679)
Any Serious Nonbleeding Adverse Event	**877 (19%)**	**890 (19%)**
Cardiovascular System		
Atrial Fibrillation	301 (6%)	294 (6%)
Hypotension	290 (6%)	324 (7%)
Congestive Heart Failure	257 (5%)	240 (5%)
Cardiac Arrest	127 (3%)	109 (2%)
Shock	117 (2%)	120 (3%)
Phlebitis	69 (1%)	64 (1%)
Atrioventricular Block	61 (1%)	70 (1%)
Ventricular Fibrillation	65 (1%)	59 (1%)
Ventricular Tachycardia	54 (1%)	51 (1%)
Hemic/Lymphatic System		
Thrombocytopenia	3 (<1%)	11 (<1%)
Nervous System		
Cerebral Ischemia	24 (1%)	18 (<1%)

In the PURSUIT, IMPACT II and ESPRIT trials, discontinuation of study drug due to adverse events other than bleeding was uncommon, with no single event occurring at >0.5% of the study population, except for "cardiovascular" in the IMPACT II study and "other" in the ESPRIT study. In the PURSUIT study, the non-bleeding adverse events (>0.1%) leading to discontinuation occurred in the eptifibatide and placebo groups in the following body systems: cardiovascular system (0.3% and 0.3%), digestive system (0.1% and 0.1%), hemic/lymphatic system (0.1% and 0.1%), nervous system (0.3% and 0.4%), urogenital system (0.1% and 0.1%) and whole body system (0.2% and 0.2%).

In the IMPACT II study, non-bleeding adverse events leading to discontinuation occurred in the 135/0.5 eptifibatide and placebo groups in the following body systems with an incidence of >0.1%: whole body (0.3% and 0.1%), cardiovascular system (1.4% and 1.4%), digestive system (0.2% and 0%), hemic/lymphatic system (0.2% and 0%), nervous system (0.3% and 0.2%), and respiratory system (0.1% and 0.1%).

In the ESPRIT study, the following non-bleeding adverse events leading to discontinuation occurred in the eptifibatide and placebo groups with an incidence of >0.1%: "other adverse events" (1.2% and 1.1%).

Postmarketing Experience: The following adverse events have been reported in post-marketing experience, primarily with eptifibatide in combination with heparin and aspirin: cerebral, gastrointestinal and pulmonary hemorrhage. Fatal bleeding events have been reported. Acute profound thrombocytopenia has been reported.

OVERDOSE:

Symptoms: Potentially, an overdose of INTEGRILIN (eptifibatide) could result in bleeding. Because of its short half-life and rapid clearance, the activity of INTEGRILIN may be halted readily by discontinuing the infusion. INTEGRILIN can also be dialyzed. In certain cases, treatment of overdose may require transfusion.

There was no indication of severe adverse events associated with administration of accidental large bolus doses, rapid infusion reported as overdose, or large cumulative doses.

There has been only limited experience with overdosage of eptifibatide. There were 9 patients in the PURSUIT study, 8 patients in the IMPACT II study and no patient in the ESPRIT study who received bolus doses and/or infusion doses more than double those called for in the protocols. In the PURSUIT study, there was no excessive bleeding in any of these patients, although one patient undergoing CABG was reported as having had a moderate bleed. None of these patients experienced an intracranial bleed or other major bleeding.

Treatment: See Symptoms.

For management of a suspected drug overdose, CPhA recommends that you contact your **regional Poison Control Centre**. See the *CPS* Directory section for a list of Poison Control Centres.

DOSAGE: INTEGRILIN solution for injection must always be given as an intravenous bolus followed by the INTEGRILIN solution for infusion.

Unstable Angina/Non-ST-Segment Elevation Myocardial Infarction: The recommended adult dosage of INTEGRILIN in patients with UA/NSTEMI is an intravenous bolus of 180 µg/kg (as soon as possible following diagnosis), followed immediately by a continuous infusion of 2 µg/kg/min until hospital discharge or initiation of CABG surgery, up to 72 hours. If a patient undergoes PCI, INTEGRILIN infusion should be continued until hospital discharge or for up to 18-24 hours after the procedure, whichever comes first, allowing for 96 hours of therapy.

Patients weighing more than 121 kg should receive a maximum bolus of 22.6 mg (11.3 mL of the 2 mg/mL injection) followed by a maximum infusion rate of 15 mg (20 mL of the 0.75 mg/mL injection) per hour.

The recommended adult dosage of eptifibatide in patients with moderate renal impairment (creatinine clearance of ≥30-<50 mL/min, using the Cockcroft-Gault* equation) is an intravenous bolus of 180 µg/kg as soon as possible following diagnosis, immediately followed by a continuous infusion of 1.0 µg/kg/min. Patients weighing more than 121 kg should receive a maximum bolus of 22.6 mg (11.3 mL of the 2 mg/mL injection) followed by a maximum infusion rate of 7.5 mg (10 mL of the 0.75 mg/mL injection) per hour.

Percutaneous Coronary Intervention (PCI): The recommended adult dosage of INTEGRILIN is an intravenous bolus of 180 µg/kg administered immediately before the initiation of PCI followed by a continuous infusion of 2 µg/kg/min and a second 180 µg/kg bolus 10 minutes after the first bolus. Infusion should be continued until hospital discharge or for up to 18-24 hours, whichever comes first. A minimum of 12 hours of infusion is recommended. Patients weighing more than 121 kg should receive a maximum of 22.6 mg (11.3 mL of the 2 mg/mL injection) per bolus followed by a maximum infusion rate of 15 mg (20 mL of the 0.75 mg/mL injection) per hour.

The recommended adult dose of eptifibatide in patients with moderate renal impairment (creatinine clearance of ≥30-<50 mL/min, using the Cockcroft-Gault* equation), is an intravenous bolus of 180 µg/kg administered immediately before the initiation of the procedure, followed by a second 180 µg/kg bolus administered 10 minutes after the first bolus injection. Simultaneously with the first bolus dose, a continuous infusion of 1.0 µg/kg/min should be started. Continue the infusion until hospital discharge or up to a maximum of 18-24 hours post PCI. A minimum of 12 hours of infusion is recommended. For severe renal impairment see Contraindications.

Patients weighing more than 121 kg should receive a maximum bolus of 22.6 mg (11.3 mL of the 2 mg/mL injection) followed by a maximum infusion rate of 7.5 mg (10 mL of the 0.75 mg/mL injection) per hour.

In patients who undergo coronary artery bypass graft surgery, eptifibatide infusion should be discontinued prior to surgery.

*Using the Cockcroft-Gault equation, with actual body weight, creatinine clearance in mL/min is calculated as:

$$\text{Males} = \frac{(140\text{-age in years})\times(\text{body weight in kg})}{72\times(\text{serum creatinine in mg/dL})}$$

$$\text{Females} = \frac{(140\text{-age in years})\times(\text{body weight in kg})\times(0.85)}{72\times(\text{serum creatinine in mg/dL})}$$

Heparin and ASA Dosing Recommendations: In the PURSUIT, IMPACT II and ESPRIT trials, most patients received concomitant ASA and heparin.

Unstable Angina/Non-ST-Segment Elevation Myocardial infarction ASA: 160-325 mg, given orally, initially and daily thereafter.

Heparin: Target aPTT 50 to 70 seconds during medical management: if weight ≥70 kg, 5000 U bolus followed by infusion of 1000 U/h; if weight <70 kg, 60 U/kg bolus followed by infusion of 12 U/kg/h.

Target ACT 200 to 300 seconds during PCI: If heparin is initiated prior to PCI, additional boluses during PCI to maintain an ACT target of 200-300 seconds. Heparin infusion after the PCI is discouraged.

Percutaneous coronary intervention ASA: 160-325 mg po 1-24 hours prior to PCI and daily thereafter.

Heparin: Target ACT 200 to 300 seconds: 60 U/kg bolus initially in patients not treated with heparin within 6 hours prior to PCI. Additional boluses during PCI to maintain ACT within target. Heparin infusion after the PCI is strongly discouraged.

Patients requiring thrombolytic therapy should have eptifibatide infusions stopped (see Precautions, Thrombolytics).

Instructions for Administration: Like other parenteral drug products, INTEGRILIN solutions should be inspected visually for particulate matter and discoloration prior to administration, whenever solution and container permit.

INTEGRILIN may be administered in the same intravenous line as alteplase, atropine, dobutamine, heparin, lidocaine, meperidine, metoprolol, midazolam, morphine, nitroglycerin, or verapamil. INTEGRILIN should not be administered through the same intravenous line as furosemide.

INTEGRILIN may be administered in the same IV line with 0.9% NaCl or 0.9% NaCl/5% dextrose. With either vehicle, the infusion may also contain up to 60 mEq/L of potassium chloride. No incompatibilities have been observed with intravenous administration sets. No compatibility studies have been performed with PVC bags. INTEGRILIN is for direct infusion and is piggy backed onto an existing intravenous line and should be administered undiluted directly from the vial.

The bolus dose(s) of INTEGRILIN should be withdrawn from the 10 mL vial into a syringe. The bolus dose(s) should be administered by IV push.

Immediately following the bolus dose administration, a continuous infusion of INTEGRILIN should be initiated. Using an intravenous infusion pump, INTEGRILIN should be administered undiluted directly from the 100 mL vial. The 100 mL vial should be spiked with a vented infusion set. Care should be taken to center the spike within the circle on the stopper top.

INTEGRILIN is to be administered by volume according to patient weight. Patients should receive INTEGRILIN according to Table 13.

Table 13: INTEGRILIN

INTEGRILIN Dosing Chart by Weight

Patient Weight (kg)	Bolus Volume (from 2 mg/mL vial) 180 µg/kg	Infusion Volume (from 0.75 mg/mL 100 mL vial)	
		2 µg/kg/min Clcr≥50 mL/min	1 µg/kg/min Clcr<50 mL/min
37–41	3.4 mL	6 mL/h	3 mL/h
42–46	4 mL	7 mL/h	3.5 mL/h
47–53	4.5 mL	8 mL/h	4 mL/h
54–59	5 mL	9 mL/h	4.5 mL/h
60–65	5.6 mL	10 mL/h	5 mL/h
66–71	6.2 mL	11 mL/h	5.5 mL/h
72–78	6.8 mL	12 mL/h	6 mL/h
79–84	7.3 mL	13 mL/h	6.5 mL/h
85–90	7.9 mL	14 mL/h	7 mL/h
91–96	8.5 mL	15 mL/h	7.5 mL/h
97–103	9 mL	16 mL/h	8 mL/h
104–109	9.5 mL	17 mL/h	8.5 mL/h
110–115	10.2 mL	18 mL/h	9 mL/h
116–121	10.7 mL	19 mL/h	9.5 mL/h
>121	11.3 mL	20 mL/h	10 mL/h

Compatibility: INTEGRILIN may be administered in the same IV line with the following IV solutions: 0.9% NaCl, 0.9% NaCl and 5% dextrose and with IV solutions containing up to 60 mEq potassium chloride per liter. No incompatibilities have been observed with intravenous administration sets. No compatibility studies have been performed with PVC bags. Physical and chemical compatibility testing indicate that INTEGRILIN may be administered through an intravenous line with alteplase, atropine, dobutamine, heparin, lidocaine, meperidine, metoprolol, midazolam, morphine, nitroglycerin, or verapamil.

INTEGRILIN should not be administered through an intravenous line with furosemide.

SUPPLIED: 2 mg/mL: Each mL of clear, colorless, sterile, nonpyrogenic solution for i.v. use contains: eptifibatide 2 mg in a 25 mM citric acid buffer, pH 5.0 to 5.5. Nonmedicinal ingredients: citric acid monohydrate, sodium hydroxide (for adjusting pH) and water for injection. Single use vials for bolus injection of 10 mL (20 mg).

0.75 mg/mL: Each mL of clear, colorless, sterile, nonpyrogenic solution for i.v. use contains: eptifibatide 0.75 mg in a 25 mM citric acid buffer, pH 5.0 to 5.5. Nonmedicinal ingredients: citric acid monohydrate, sodium hydroxide (for adjusting pH) and water for injection. Single use vials for intravenous infusion of 100 mL (75 mg).

Store refrigerated at 2 to 8°C. Vials may be transferred to controlled room temperature storage (25°C with excursions permitted between 15 to 30°C) protected from light, for a period not to exceed 2 months. Upon transfer, vials must be marked with a "**Discard By**" date (2 months from the transfer date) which may not exceed the labeled expiration date.

Intelence™ Ⓟ

etravirine

Human Immunodeficiency Virus (HIV) Non-nucleoside Reverse Transcriptase inhibitor

Janssen-Ortho

Date of Preparation: March 27, 2008
Date of Revision: January 8, 2010

SUMMARY PRODUCT INFORMATION:

Route of Administration	Dosage Form/ Strength	Clinically Relevant Nonmedicinal Ingredients
Oral	Tablet, 100 mg	Lactose monohydrate For a complete listing see Dosage Forms, Composition and Packaging.

INDICATIONS AND CLINICAL USE: INTELENCE (etravirine), in combination with other antiretroviral agents, is indicated for the treatment of human immunodeficiency virus type 1 (HIV-1) infection in treatment-experienced adult patients who have failed prior therapy and have HIV-1 strains resistant to multiple antiretroviral agents, including NNRTIs.

This indication is based on safety and efficacy data at 24 weeks from two Phase 3, double-blinded, placebo-controlled trials in treatment-experienced patients who had a least one NNRTI resistance-associated mutation and multiple primary protease inhibitor mutations.

The following points should be considered when initiating therapy with INTELENCE:

- Do not use INTELENCE with only N[t]RTIs in the setting of previous NNRTI failure. This is based on an analysis of an exploratory Phase 2 clinical trial in patients who had experienced virologic failure on an NNRTI- and N[t]RTI-containing regimen.
- The use of other active antiretroviral agents with INTELENCE is associated with an increased likelihood of treatment response.
- Treatment history and, when available, resistance testing, should guide the use of INTELENCE.

Geriatrics (>65 years of age): Clinical studies of INTELENCE did not include sufficient numbers of subjects aged 65 and over to determine whether they respond differently from younger subjects. In general, caution should be exercised when administering INTELENCE in elderly patients, reflecting the greater frequency of decreased hepatic, renal or cardiac function, concomitant disease or other drug therapy (see Warnings and Precautions, Dosage and Administration, and Action and Clinical Pharmacology).

Pediatrics (<18 years of age): Safety and effectiveness of INTELENCE in pediatric patients have not been established. Treatment with INTELENCE is not recommended in children and adolescents (see Warnings and Precautions, Dosage and Administration, and Action and Clinical Pharmacology).

CONTRAINDICATIONS: INTELENCE (etravirine) is contraindicated in patients who are hypersensitive to etravirine or to any ingredient in the formulation or component of the container. For a complete listing, see Dosage Forms, Composition and Packaging.

WARNINGS AND PRECAUTIONS: Skin: Severe, potentially life-threatening, and fatal skin reactions have been reported in patients taking INTELENCE (etravirine). These include cases of Stevens-Johnson Syndrome, toxic epidermal necrolysis and erythema multiforme. Hypersensitivity reactions have also been reported and were characterized by rash, constitutional findings, and infrequently organ dysfunction, including hepatic failure.

Discontinue INTELENCE immediately if signs or symptoms of severe skin reactions or hypersensitivity reactions develop (including, but not limited to, severe rash or rash accompanied by fever, general malaise, fatigue, muscle or joint aches, blisters, oral lesions, conjunctivitis, facial edema, hepatitis, eosinophilia). Clinical status including liver transaminases should be monitored and appropriate therapy initiated. Delay in stopping INTELENCE treatment after the onset of severe rash may result in a life-threatening reaction.

In Phase III clinical trials, Grade 3 and 4 rashes were reported in 1.3% of subjects receiving INTELENCE compared to 0.2% of placebo subjects. A total of 2% of HIV-1-infected patients receiving INTELENCE discontinued from Phase III trials due to rash. Rash occurred most commonly during the first 6 weeks of therapy (see Adverse Reactions, Skin Rash).

General: Patients with hereditary problems of lactose intolerance should not take this medicine.

Carcinogenesis and Mutagenesis: Long-term carcinogenicity studies of etravirine have not been completed.

Etravirine tested negative in the in vitro Ames reverse mutation assay, in vitro chromosomal aberration assay in human lymphocyte, and in vitro clastogenicity mouse lymphoma assay, tested in the presence and absence of the metabolic activation system. Etravirine did not induce chromosomal damage in the in vivo micronucleus test in mice.

Endocrine and Metabolism: Fat Redistribution: Redistribution/accumulation of body fat, including central obesity, dorsocervical fat enlargement (buffalo hump), peripheral wasting, facial wasting, breast enlargement, and "cushingoid appearance" have been observed in patients receiving antiretroviral therapy. The mechanism and long-term consequences of these events are currently unknown. A causal relationship has not been established.

Hepatic/Biliary/Pancreatic: Hepatic Impairment: No dose adjustment is required in patients with mild or moderate hepatic impairment. The pharmacokinetics of INTELENCE have not been studied in patients with severe hepatic impairment (see Action and Clinical Pharmacology, Special Populations and Conditions, Hepatic Insufficiency and Dosage and Administration, Recommended Dosage and Dosage Adjustment, Hepatic Impairment).

Pancreatitis: Pancreatitis has been reported infrequently (<1%) during clinical trials with INTELENCE. In the placebo-controlled Phase III DUET-1 and DUET-2 trials, the rate of clinical pancreatitis was similar in patients receiving INTELENCE 4/599 (0.7%) and placebo 2/604 (0.3%). Pancreatitis has been reported in one healthy volunteer (1/1093, 0.09%).

In the DUET trials asymptomatic grade 3 or 4 increases in serum amylase levels were observed in a similar number of patients treated with INTELENCE (7.5%) and placebo (7.9%) (see Adverse Reactions, Laboratory Abnormalities). Grade 3 or 4 elevated lipase levels were reported in 2.7% patients receiving INTELENCE compared to 1.7% of patients receiving placebo.

Immune: Immune Reconstitution: Immune reconstitution syndrome has been reported in patients treated with combination antiretroviral therapy, including INTELENCE. During the initial phase of treatment, patients responding to antiretroviral therapy may develop an inflammatory response to indolent or residual opportunistic infections (such as MAC, CMV, PCP and TB), which may necessitate further evaluation and treatment.

Renal: Renal Impairment: Since the renal clearance of etravirine is minimal (<1.2%), a decrease in total body clearance is not expected in patients with renal impairment. No special precautions or dose adjustments are required in patients with renal impairment. As etravirine is highly bound to plasma proteins, it is unlikely that it will be significantly removed by haemodialysis or peritoneal dialysis (see Dosage and Administration and Action and Clinical Pharmacology, Special Populations and Conditions, Renal Insufficiency).

Special Populations: Pregnant Women: There are no adequate and well-controlled studies with etravirine in pregnant women. Studies in animals have not shown evidence of developmental toxicity or effect on reproductive function and fertility.

INTELENCE should be used during pregnancy only if the potential benefit justifies the potential risk.

Antiretroviral Pregnancy Registry: To monitor maternal-fetal outcomes of pregnant women exposed to INTELENCE, an Antiretroviral Pregnancy Registry has been established. Physicians are encouraged to register patients by calling 1-800-258-4263.

Nursing Women: There were indirect indications of the presence of etravirine in the milk of lactating rats. It is not yet known if etravirine is excreted in human milk and whether there is potential for adverse events in nursing infants. Because of both the potential for HIV transmission and the potential for adverse events in nursing infants, mothers should be instructed not to breast-feed if they are receiving INTELENCE.

Pediatrics (<18 years of age): The safety and effectiveness of INTELENCE in pediatric patients have not been established.

Geriatrics (>65 years of age): There were insufficient numbers of subjects aged 65 and over in the clinical studies to determine whether they respond differently from younger subjects. In general, caution should be exercised when administering INTELENCE in elderly patients, reflecting the greater frequency of decreased hepatic, renal or cardiac function, concomitant disease or other drug therapy.

ADVERSE REACTIONS: Adverse Drug Reaction Overview: The safety assessment is based on all data from 1203 patients in the ongoing Phase III placebo-controlled trials in antiretroviral treatment-experienced HIV-1-infected adult patients [DUET-1 (TMC125-C206) and DUET-2 (TMC125-C216)], 599 of whom received INTELENCE (etravirine), 200 mg b.i.d. In these pooled trials, the median exposure for subjects in the INTELENCE arm and placebo arm was 30.0 and 29.1 weeks, respectively.

In the pooled DUET trials, 92.5% of both INTELENCE-treated subjects and placebo-treated subjects experienced adverse events. The most commonly (>10%) reported adverse events of all intensities and regardless of causality that occurred at a higher rate in INTELENCE-treated subjects as compared to placebo-treated subjects were rash (any type) in 17.0% and 9.4%, and nausea 13.9% and 11.1% of INTELENCE-treated subjects and placebo-treated subjects, respectively.

In total, 71.0% and 66.9% of the subjects experienced adverse drug reactions (ADRs; i.e. adverse events considered related to INTELENCE) with INTELENCE and placebo, respectively. The majority of the ADRs reported during treatment with INTELENCE were grade 1 to 2 in severity. Grade 3 or 4 ADRs were reported in 16.9% and 12.7% of the INTELENCE- and placebo-treated subjects. ADRs were reported as SAEs in 5.0% and 6.5% of subjects treated with INTELENCE and placebo, respectively. ADRs that led to permanent discontinuation of the investigational medication were reported in 4.5% of the INTELENCE-treated subjects and in 2.2% of the placebo-treated subjects. The most commonly reported ADRs with INTELENCE identified from the pooled DUET trials were rash (any type), reported by 17.0% of INTELENCE-treated subjects and by 9.4% of placebo-treated subjects, diarrhea (15.0% and 20.4%), and nausea (13.9% and 11.1%).

Clinical Trial Adverse Drug Reactions: Because clinical trials are conducted under very specific conditions the adverse reaction rates observed in the clinical trials may not reflect the rates observed in practice and should not be compared to the rates in the clinical trials of another drug. Adverse drug reaction information from clinical trials is useful for identifying drug-related adverse events and for approximating rates.

ADRs of moderate intensity or greater (≥Grade 2) and reported in ≥1% of subjects treated with INTELENCE (200 mg b.i.d.) in the DUET-1 and DUET-2 trials are presented in Table 1. Laboratory abnormalities considered ADRs are included in Table 3.

Table 1: INTELENCE

Treatment-Emergent Adverse Reactions[a] of at Least Moderate Intensity (Grades 2-4) in ≥1% of Adult Subjects in the INTELENCE Treatment Groups

System Organ Class, Preferred Term, %	DUET-1 and DUET-2 Trials INTELENCE+BR N=599	Placebo+BR N=604
Blood and Lymphatic System Disorders		
Anemia	3.5	3.6
Thrombocytopenia	1.3	1.3
Gastrointestinal Disorders		
Diarrhea	5.2	9.6
Nausea	4.7	3.5
Abdominal pain	3.0	2.5
Vomiting	2.3	2.0
Gastroesophageal reflux disease	1.5	1.0
Flatulence	1.0	1.0
Gastritis	1.0	0.7
General Disorders and Administration Site Conditions		
Fatigue	3.3	4.0
Metabolism and Nutrition Disorders		
Hypertriglyceridemia	4.7	3.0
Hypercholesterolemia	3.5	2.2
Hyperlipidemia	1.5	0.7
Hyperglycemia	1.2	0.5
Diabetes mellitus	1.0	0.2
Dyslipidemia	1.0	0.3

(cont'd)

Table 1: INTELENCE *(cont'd)*

Treatment-Emergent Adverse Reactions[a] of at Least Moderate Intensity (Grades 2-4) in ≥1% of Adult Subjects in the INTELENCE Treatment Groups

System Organ Class, Preferred Term, %	DUET-1 and DUET-2 Trials INTELENCE+BR N=599	Placebo+BR N=604
Nervous System Disorders		
Peripheral neuropathy	2.8	1.8
Headache	2.7	4.1
Psychiatric Disorders		
Insomnia	1.8	2.2
Anxiety	1.2	1.7
Renal and Urinary Disorders		
Renal failure	1.5	1.5
Skin and Subcutaneous Tissue Disorders		
Rash	9.0	3.1
Vascular Disorders		
Hypertension	2.8	2.2

[a] Includes adverse reactions at least possibly, probably, or very likely related to the drug.
Legend: N=total number of subjects per treatment group; BR=background regimen.

Skin Rash: The most frequently reported adverse drug reaction of at least Grade 2 in severity in the Phase III studies was rash (9.0%). Stevens-Johnson Syndrome, severe hypersensitivity reaction, and erythema multiforme were reported in <0.1% of subjects during clinical development with INTELENCE. A total of 2% of HIV-1-infected subjects receiving INTELENCE discontinued from Phase III trials due to rash. In general, rash was mild to moderate, macular to maculopapular or erythematous, occurred primarily in the second week of therapy and was infrequent after Week 4. Rash generally resolved within 1-2 weeks on continued therapy. In Phase III studies, the incidence of rash was higher in women compared to men in the INTELENCE arm. Patients with a history of NNRTI-related rash did not appear to be at increased risk for the development of INTELENCE-related rash compared to patients without a history of NNRTI-related. See Table 2 for a summary of rash events.

Table 2: INTELENCE

Rash (Any Type)

Rash Summary, n (%)	Placebo N=604	Pooled DUET Trials N=599
Rash (any type)	**57 (9.4)**	**102 (17.0)**
Grade 1	40 (6.6)	56 (9.3)
Grade 2	19 (3.1)	47 (7.8)
Grade 3	0	8 (1.3)
Onset in days, median	45	12
Duration in days, median	17	11
Leading to permanent stop	**0**	**13 (2.2)**
Vesicular Rash	**1 (0.2)**	**0**

Legend: N=number of subjects; n=number of subjects with observations.

Less Common Clinical Trial Adverse Drug Reactions (<1%): Treatment-emergent adverse drug reactions in the DUET-1 and DUET-2 trials (n=599) occurring in less than 1% of patients receiving INTELENCE (200 mg b.i.d.), and of at least moderate intensity (≥Grade 2) are listed below by body system:

Cardiac Disorders: angina pectoris, atrial fibrillation, myocardial infarction.
Ear and Labyrinth Disorders: vertigo.
Eye Disorders: blurred vision.
Gastrointestinal Disorders: abdominal distension, constipation, dry mouth, hematemesis, pancreatitis, retching, stomatitis.
General Disorders and Administration Site Conditions: sluggishness.
Hepatobiliary Disorders: cytolytic hepatitis, hepatic steatosis, hepatitis, hepatomegaly.
Immune System Disorders: drug hypersensitivity, immune reconstitution syndrome.
Metabolism and Nutrition Disorders: anorexia.
Nervous System Disorders: convulsion, hypoesthesia, syncope, amnesia, hypersomnia, paraesthesia, somnolence, tremor.
Psychiatric Disorders: abnormal dreams, confusional state, disorientation, nervousness, nightmares, sleep disorders.
Reproductive System and Breast Disorders: gynecomastia.
Respiratory, Thoracic and Mediastinal Disorders: bronchospasm, exertional dyspnea.
Skin and Subcutaneous Tissue Disorders: dry skin, hyperhidrosis, lipohypertrophy, night sweats, prurigo, swelling face.

Additional ADRs observed in other trials occurring in less than 1% of patients receiving INTELENCE (200 mg b.i.d.), and of at least moderate intensity (≥Grade 2) are listed below by body system:

Metabolism and Nutrition Disorders: acquired lipodystrophy.
Nervous System Disorders: haemorrhagic stroke.
Skin and Subcutaneous Tissue Disorders: angioneurotic edema, erythema multiforme, Stevens-Johnson Syndrome, toxic epidermal necrolysis.

Abnormal Hematologic and Clinical Chemistry Findings: Laboratory Abnormalities: Treatment-emergent clinical laboratory abnormalities (Grade 3 or 4) observed in patients and reported in greater than or equal to 2% of INTELENCE-treated subjects are presented in Table 3. All other grade 3 or 4 abnormal laboratory parameters were observed in less than 2% of the INTELENCE-treated subjects.

Patients Co-infected with Hepatitis B and/or Hepatitis C Virus: In the pooled analysis for DUET-1 and DUET-2, the safety profile in co-infected subjects (n=140) was generally comparable between subjects receiving INTELENCE and subjects receiving placebo. There was a higher incidence of hepatic and biliary system disorders in co-infected subjects treated with INTELENCE (6.9% of 72 subjects) compared to co-infected subjects in the placebo group (1.5% of 68 subjects). No specific pattern or type of event was observed.

Table 3: INTELENCE

Treatment Emergent Grade 3 to 4 Laboratory Abnormalities Reported in ≥2% of Subjects

	Pooled DUET-1 and DUET-2 Trials	
Laboratory Parameter Preferred Term, n (%)	**INTELENCE+BR N=599**	**Placebo+BR N=604**
General Biochemistry		
Pancreatic amylase	44 (7.5)	48 (7.9)
Grade 3	37 (6.3)	42 (7.0)
Grade 4	7 (1.2)	6 (1.0)
Lipase	**16 (2.7)**	**10 (1.7)**
Grade 3	10 (1.7)	7 (1.2)
Grade 4	6 (1.0)	3 (0.5)
Hematology Differential Counts		
Neutrophils	**22 (3.7)**	**38 (6.3)**
Grade 3	16 (2.7)	21 (3.5)
Grade 4	6 (1.0)	17 (2.8)
Lipids and Glucose		
Total cholesterol	**34 (5.8)**	**25 (4.1)**
Grade 3	34 (5.8)	25 (4.1)
Low density lipoprotein	**30 (5.2)**	**32 (5.4)**
Grade 3	30 (5.2)	32 (5.4)
Elevated glucose levels	**15 (2.5)**	**12 (2.0)**
Grade 3	15 (2.5)	11 (1.8)
Grade 4	0 (0)	1 (0.2)
Triglycerides	**41 (7.0)**	**26 (4.3)**
Grade 3	24 (4.1)	18 (3.0)
Grade 4	17 (2.9)	8 (1.3)
Hepatic Parameters		
Alanine amino transferase	**15 (2.5)**	**10 (1.7)**
Grade 3	11 (1.9)	8 (1.3)
Grade 4	4 (0.7)	2 (0.3)
Aspartate amino transferase	**15 (2.5)**	**10 (1.7)**
Grade 3	12 (2.0)	8 (1.3)
Grade 4	3 (0.5)	2 (0.3)

Among co-infected subjects: Grade 3 or 4 elevations in AST developed in 5.7% of subjects in the INTELENCE arm compared to 4.4% of subjects in the placebo arm; Grade 3 or 4 elevations in ALT developed in 7.1% of subjects in the INTELENCE arm compared to 5.9% of subjects in the placebo arm; Grade 3 or 4 elevations in bilirubin developed in 5.7% of subjects in the INTELENCE arm compared to 1.5% of subjects in the placebo arm.

Post-Market Adverse Drug Reactions: Fatal cases of toxic epidermal necrolysis have been reported. Severe hypersensitivity including cases of hepatic failure have been reported (see Warnings and Precautions).

DRUG INTERACTIONS: Overview: Etravirine is a substrate of CYP3A4, CYP2C9 and CYP2C19. Therefore, co-administration of INTELENCE (etravirine) with drugs that induce or inhibit CYP3A4, CYP2C9 and CYP2C19 may alter the therapeutic effect or adverse reaction profile of INTELENCE.

Etravirine is an inducer of CYP3A4, and an inhibitor of CYP2C9 and CYP2C19. Therefore, co-administration of drugs that are substrates of CYP3A4, CYP2C9 and CYP2C19 with INTELENCE may alter the therapeutic effect or adverse reaction profile of the co-administered drug(s).

Drug-Drug Interactions: Drugs that are not recommended for co-administration with INTELENCE are included in Table 4. These recommendations are based on either drug interaction studies or predicted interactions due to the expected magnitude of interaction and potential for serious events or loss of efficacy.

Table 4: INTELENCE

Drugs That Should Not Be Co-administered with INTELENCE

Concomitant Drug Class: Drug Name	Clinical Comment
HIV-Antiviral Agents: Non-Nucleoside Reverse Transcriptase Inhibitors (NNRTIs)	
efavirenz nevirapine delavirdine	Combining two NNRTIs has not been shown to be beneficial. Concomitant use of INTELENCE with efavirenz or nevirapine may cause a decrease in the plasma concentrations of etravirine and loss of therapeutic effect of INTELENCE. INTELENCE and other NNRTIs should not be co-administered. Combining two NNRTIs has not been shown to be beneficial. INTELENCE and delavirdine should not be co-administered.
HIV-Antiviral Agents: Protease Inhibitors (PIs)—Unboosted (i.e., without co-administration of low-dose ritonavir)	

(cont'd)

Table 4: INTELENCE *(cont'd)*

Drugs That Should Not Be Co-administered with INTELENCE

Concomitant Drug Class: Drug Name	Clinical Comment
ritonavir	Concomitant use of INTELENCE with full-dose ritonavir (600 mg b.i.d.) may cause a significant decrease in the plasma concentration of etravirine. This may result in loss of therapeutic effect of INTELENCE. It is not recommended to co-administer full-dose ritonavir (600 mg b.i.d.) with INTELENCE.
atazanavir nelfinavir indinavir	Concomitant use of INTELENCE without co-administration of low-dose ritonavir may cause a significant alteration in the plasma concentrations of the PI. INTELENCE should not be co-administered with PIs without low-dose ritonavir.
HIV-Antiviral Agents: Protease Inhibitors (PIs)—Boosted (with co-administration of low-dose ritonavir)	
atazanavir/ritonavir	Concomitant use of INTELENCE with atazanivir/ritonavir may cause a significant decrease in atazanavir C_{min} by about 38%. INTELENCE and atazanavir/ritonavir should not be co-administered.
fosamprenavir/ritonavir	An increase of 69% for amprenavir exposure was observed when fosamprenavir/ritonavir was co-administered in the presence of etravirine. Appropriate doses of the combination of INTELENCE and fosamprenavir/ritonavir have not been established. INTELENCE and fosamprenavir/ritonavir should not be co-administered.
tipranavir/ritonavir	Concomitant use of INTELENCE with tipranavir/low-dose ritonavir may cause a significant decrease in the plasma concentration of etravirine and loss of therapeutic effect of INTELENCE. Tipranavir/low-dose ritonavir and INTELENCE should not be co-administered.
Anticonvulsants: carbamazepine, phenobarbital, phenytoin	Carbamazepine, phenobarbital and phenytoin are inducers of CYP450 enzymes. INTELENCE should not be used in combination with carbamazepine, phenobarbital, or phenytoin as co-administration may cause significant decreases in etravirine plasma concentrations and loss of therapeutic effect of INTELENCE.
Antimycobacterials: rifampin	Rifampin is a potent inducer of CYP450 enzymes. INTELENCE should not be used in combination with rifampin as co-administration may cause significant decreases in etravirine plasma concentrations and loss of therapeutic effect of INTELENCE.
Herbal Products: St. John's wort (Hypericum perforatum)	INTELENCE should not be used concomitantly with products containing St. John's wort because co-administration may cause significant decreases in etravirine plasma concentrations and loss of therapeutic effect of INTELENCE.

Established and other potentially significant drug interactions with INTELENCE are included in Table 5. These recommendations are based on either drug interaction studies or predicated interactions due to the expected magnitude of interaction and potential for serious events or loss of efficacy.

Drug interaction studies were performed with etravirine and other drugs likely to be co-administered and some drugs commonly used as probes for pharmacokinetic interactions. The effects of co-administration of etravirine on the AUC, C_{max}, and C_{min} values are summarized in Table 6 and Table 7. Different formulations and/or doses were used which led to similar exposures and, therefore, interactions relevant for one formulation are relevant for the other.

Drug-Food Interactions: The systemic exposure (AUC) to etravirine was decreased by about 50% when INTELENCE was administered under fasting conditions, as compared to when INTELENCE was administered following a meal. Therefore, INTELENCE should always be taken following a meal. The caloric and fat content of the meal is irrelevant.

Drug-Herb Interactions: Concomitant use of INTELENCE and St. John's wort (Hypericum perforatum), or products containing St. John's wort, is not recommended. Co-administration of etravirine with St. John's wort may cause significant decreases in etravirine plasma concentrations, which may result in loss of therapeutic effect of INTELENCE (see Drug-Drug Interactions, Table 4).

Interactions with other herbal products have not been established.

Drug-Laboratory Test Interactions: Interactions with laboratory tests have not been established.

Table 5: INTELENCE

Established and Other Potentially Significant Drug Interactions: Alterations in Dose or Regimen May Be Recommended Based on Drug Interaction Trials or Predicted Interaction

Concomitant Drug Class: Drug Name	Effect on Concentration of Etravirine or Concomitant Drug	Clinical Comment
HIV-Antiviral Agents: Nucleoside or Nucleotide Reverse Transcriptase Inhibitors (NRTIs/N[t]RTIs)		
didanosine[a]	↔ etravirine ↔ didanosine	The combination of INTELENCE and didanosine can be used without dose adjustments. As didanosine is administered on an empty stomach, didanosine should be administered one hour before or two hours after INTELENCE (which should be administered following a meal).
tenofovir disoproxil fumarate[a]	↓ etravirine ↔ tenofovir	The combination of INTELENCE and tenofovir disoproxil fumarate can be used without dose adjustments.
Other NRTIs: Based on the primarily renal elimination route for other NRTIs (e.g., abacavir, emtricitabine, lamivudine, stavudine, and zidovudine), no drug interactions are expected between these drugs and INTELENCE.		
HIV-Antiviral Agents: Protease Inhibitors (PIs)—Boosted (with co-administration of low-dose ritonavir)		
darunavir/ritonavir[a]	↓ etravirine ↔ darunavir	The mean systemic exposure (AUC) of etravirine was reduced by 37% when INTELENCE was co-administered with darunavir/ritonavir. However, the combination of darunavir/ritonavir and etravirine was used safely and effectively in the Phase 3 trials, therefore, INTELENCE and darunavir/ritonavir can be co-administered without any dose adjustments.

(cont'd)

Table 5: INTELENCE *(cont'd)*

Established and Other Potentially Significant Drug Interactions: Alterations in Dose or Regimen May Be Recommended Based on Drug Interaction Trials or Predicted Interaction

Concomitant Drug Class: Drug Name	Effect on Concentration of Etravirine or Concomitant Drug	Clinical Comment
lopinavir/ritonavir (soft gel capsule)[a]	↑ etravirine ↓ lopinavir	The mean systemic exposure (AUC) of etravirine after co-administration of INTELENCE with lopinavir/ritonavir is anticipated to be about 85% higher than the mean AUC of etravirine observed in the Phase 3 trials[b]. The amount of safety data at these increased etravirine exposures is limited, therefore, INTELENCE and lopinavir/ritonavir should be co-administered with caution.
Lopinavir/ritonavir (tablet)[a]	↔ lopinavir ↓ etravirine	The mean systemic exposure (AUC) of etravirine was reduced by approximately 35% after co-administration with lopinavir/ritonavir. This reduction is similar to the reduction in the mean systemic exposure of etravirine in the presence of darunavir/ritonavir observed in Phase 3 trials, therefore INTELENCE can be co-administered with the tablet formulation of lopinavir/ritonavir without dose adjustments.
saquinavir/ritonavir[a]	↓ etravirine ↔ saquinavir	The mean systemic exposure (AUC) of etravirine was reduced by about 33% after co-administration of INTELENCE and saquinavir/ritonavir. The reduction in the mean systemic exposures of etravirine in the presence of saquinavir/ritonavir is similar to the reduction in mean systemic exposures of etravirine in the presence of darunavir/ritonavir, therefore, INTELENCE and saquinavir/ritonavir can be co-administered without any dose adjustments.
HIV-Antiviral Agents: Dual Boosted Protease Inhibitors		
lopinavir/saquinavir/ritonavir[a]	↔ etravirine ↓ lopinavir ↓ saquinavir	The combination of INTELENCE and lopinavir/saquinavir/ritonavir can be used without dose adjustments.
HIV-Antiviral Agents: Fusion Inhibitors		
enfuvirtide	↔ etravirine ↔ enfuvirtide	No interaction is expected for either INTELENCE or enfuvirtide when co-administered.
HIV-Antiviral Agents: Integrase Strand Transfer Inhibitors		
raltegravir[a]	↔ etravirine ↓ raltegravir	The combination of INTELENCE and raltegravir can be used without dose adjustments.
Other Agents		
Antiarrhythmics: amiodarone, bepridil, disopyramide, flecainide, lidocaine (systemic), mexiletine, propafenone, quinidine	↓ antiarrhythmics	Concentrations of these antiarrhythmics may be decreased when co-administered with INTELENCE. Caution is warranted and therapeutic concentration monitoring, if available, is recommended for antiarrhythmics when co-administered with INTELENCE.
Anticoagulants: Warfarin	↑ warfarin	Warfarin concentrations may be affected when co-administered with INTELENCE. Co-administration of INTELENCE and warfarin is anticipated to cause an increase in warfarin exposures, while etravirine exposures are not expected to change. It is recommended that the international normalized ratio (INR) be monitored when warfarin is combined with INTELENCE.
Anti-infectives: azithromycin	↔ etravirine ↔ azithromycin	Based on the renal elimination pathway of azithromycin, no drug interactions are expected between azithromycin and INTELENCE.
Clarithromycin[a]	↑ etravirine ↓ clarithromycin ↑ 14-OH-clarithromycin	Clarithromycin exposure was decreased by etravirine; however, concentrations of the active metabolite, 14-hydroxy-clarithromycin, were increased. Because 14-hydroxy-clarithromycin has reduced activity against Mycobacterium avium complex (MAC), overall activity against this pathogen may be altered; therefore, alternatives to clarithromycin, such as azithromycin, should be considered for the treatment of MAC.
Antifungals: fluconazole	↔ fluconazole ↑ etravirine ↑ voriconazole	The plasma concentrations of INTELENCE are increased when co-administered with fluconazole (a potent inhibitor of CYP2C9) or with voriconazole, (a substrate and inhibitor of CYP3A4, CYP2C9 and CYP2C19). The mean systemic exposure (AUC) of etravirine after co-administration of INTELENCE with fluconazole or voriconazole in the absence of a boosted HIV protease inhibitor is anticipated to be about 194% and 114% higher, respectively, as compared to the mean AUC of etravirine observed in Phase III trials[b]. There is limited safety data on these increased etravirine exposures. Therefore INTELENCE and either fluconazole or voriconazole should be co-administered with caution. Dose adjustments for voriconazole may be necessary depending on other co-administered drugs.

(cont'd)

Table 5: INTELENCE *(cont'd)*

Established and Other Potentially Significant Drug Interactions: Alterations in Dose or Regimen May Be Recommended Based on Drug Interaction Trials or Predicted Interaction

Concomitant Drug Class: Drug Name	Effect on Concentration of Etravirine or Concomitant Drug	Clinical Comment
itraconazole posaconazole ketoconazole	↑ etravirine ↓ itraconazole ↔ posaconazole ↓ ketoconazole	Posaconazole is a potent inhibitor of CYP3A4 and may increase plasma concentrations of etravirine. Itraconazole and ketoconazole are potent inhibitors as well as substrates of CYP3A4. Concomitant systemic use of itraconazole or ketoconazole and INTELENCE may increase plasma concentrations of etravirine. Simultaneously, plasma concentrations of itraconazole or ketoconazole may be decreased by INTELENCE. Dose adjustments for itraconazole or ketoconazole may be necessary depending on other co-administered drugs.
Antimycobacterials: rifabutin[a]	↓ etravirine ↓ rifabutin ↓ 25-O- desacetylrifabutin	The combination of INTELENCE and rifabutin should be used with caution due to the risk of decrease in etravirine and rifabutin exposures. If INTELENCE is co-administered with darunavir/ritonavir, saquinavir/ritonavir or the tablet formulation of lopinavir/ritonavir, then rifabutin should not be co-administered due to the potential for significant reductions in etravirine exposure.
Antivirals: ribavirin	↔ etravirine ↔ ribavirin	Based on the renal elimination pathway of ribavirin, no drug interactions are expected between ribavirin and INTELENCE.
Benzodiazepines: diazepam	↑ diazepam	Concomitant use of INTELENCE with diazepam may increase plasma concentrations of diazepam. A decrease in diazepam dose may be needed.
Corticosteroids: dexamethasone (systemic)	↓ etravirine	Systemic dexamethasone induces CYP3A4 and can decrease etravirine plasma concentrations. This may result in loss of therapeutic effect of INTELENCE. Systemic dexamethasone should be used with caution or alternatives should be considered, particularly for long-term use.
Estrogen-based Contraceptives: ethinylestradiol[a] norethindrone[a]	↔ etravirine ↑ ethinylestradiol ↔ norethindrone	The combination of estrogen-and/or progesterone-based contraceptives and INTELENCE can be used without dose adjustment.
HMG-CoA Reductase Inhibitors: atorvastatin[a]	↔ etravirine ↓ atorvastatin ↑ 2-OH-atorvastatin	Atorvastatin plasma concentrations are decreased 37% and plasma concentrations of the active metabolite, 2-hydroxy-atorvastatin, are increased by 27% when combined with INTELENCE. Dose adjustment of atorvastatin may be necessary to tailor the clinical response when combined with INTELENCE.
fluvastatin, lovastatin, pravastatin, rosuvastatin, simvastatin	↔ etravirine ↑ fluvastatin, ↓ lovastatin, ↔ pravastatin, ↔ rosuvastatin, ↓ simvastatin	No interaction between pravastatin and INTELENCE is expected. Lovastatin, rosuvastatin, and simvastatin are CYP3A4 substrates and co-administration with INTELENCE may result in lower plasma concentrations of the HMG-CoA reductase inhibitor. Fluvastatin and rosuvastatin are metabolized by CYP2C9. Co-administration of fluvastatin with INTELENCE may result in higher plasma concentrations of the HMG-CoA reductase inhibitor. Dose adjustments for fluvastatin may be necessary. No interaction between rosuvastatin and INTELENCE is expected.
H_2-Receptor Antagonists: ranitidine[a]	↓ etravirine	INTELENCE can be co-administered with H_2-receptor antagonists without dose adjustments.
Immunosuppressants: cyclosporine, sirolimus, tacrolimus	↓ cyclosporine ↓ sirolimus ↓ tacrolimus	Co-administration with systemic immunosuppressants should be done with caution because plasma concentrations of cyclosporine, sirolimus, or tacrolimus may be affected when co-administered with INTELENCE.
Narcotic Analgesics: methadone[a]	↔ etravirine ↔ R(−) methadone ↔ S(+) methadone	INTELENCE and methadone may be co-administered without dose adjustments, however, clinical monitoring for withdrawal symptoms is recommended as methadone maintenance therapy may need to be adjusted in some patients.
Phosphodiesterase Type 5 (PDE-5) Inhibitors: sildenafil[a], vardenafil, tadalafil	↓ sildenafil ↓ N-desmethyl-sildenafil	Sildenafil plasma concentrations are decreased by 57% and plasma concentrations of the active metabolite, N-desmethyl-sildenafil, are decreased by 41% when combined with INTELENCE. Concomitant use of PDE-5 inhibitors with INTELENCE may require dose adjustment of the PDE-5 inhibitor to attain the desired clinical effect.
Proton Pump Inhibitors: omeprazole[a]	↑ etravirine	INTELENCE can be co-administered with proton pump inhibitors without dose adjustments.
Selective Serotonin Reuptake Inhibitors (SSRIs): paroxetine[a]	↔ etravirine ↔ paroxetine	INTELENCE can be co-administered with paroxetine without dose adjustments.

a The interaction between INTELENCE and the drug was evaluated in a clinical trial. All other drug interactions shown are predicted.
b The expected increase in systemic exposure of etravirine when co-administered with either lopinavir/ritonavir tablet (~85%), fluconazole (~194%) or voriconazole (~114%) is theoretical and is based on comparisons of etravirine exposures from drug-drug interaction studies to those in the pivotal Phase III trials (in which darunavir/ritonavir was co-administered as part of the background regimen).
Legend: ↑=increases; ↓=decreases, ↔=no change.

Table 6: INTELENCE
Drug Interactions: Pharmacokinetic Parameters for Etravirine in the Presence of Co-administered Drugs[a]

Co-administered Drug	Dose/Schedule of Co-administered Drug	N	PK	Mean Ratio of Etravirine Pharmacokinetic Parameters 90% CI; No Effect=1.00		
				C_{max}	AUC	C_{min}
Co-Administration with Protease Inhibitors (PIs)						
Atazanavir	400 mg q.d.	14	↑	1.47 (1.36–1.59)	1.50 (1.41–1.59)	1.58 (1.46–1.70)
Atazanavir/Ritonavir	300/100 mg q.d.	14	↑	1.30 (1.17–1.44)	1.30 (1.18–1.44)	1.26 (1.12–1.42)
Darunavir/Ritonavir	600/100 mg b.i.d.	14	↓	0.68 (0.57–0.82)	0.63 (0.54–0.73)	0.51 (0.44–0.61)
Fosamprenavir/Ritonavir	700/100 mg b.i.d.	8	↔	N.A.	N.A.	N.A.
Lopinavir/ritonavir (soft gel capsule)	400/100 mg b.i.d.	13	↑	1.15 (0.94–1.41)	1.17 (0.96–1.43)	1.23 (0.98–1.53)
Lopinavir/ritonavir (tablet)	400/100 mg b.i.d.	16	↓	0.70 (0.64–0.78)	0.65 (0.59–0.71)	0.55 (0.49–0.62)
Ritonavir	100 mg single dose	18	↔	1.00 (0.89–1.12)	1.03 (0.91–1.17)	N.A.
Ritonavir	600 mg b.i.d.	11	↓	0.68 (0.55–0.85)	0.54 (0.41–0.73)	N.A.
Saquinavir/ritonavir	1000/100 mg b.i.d.	14	↓	0.63 (0.53–0.75)	0.67 (0.56–0.80)	0.71 (0.58–0.87)
Tipranavir/Ritonavir	500/200 mg b.i.d.	19	↓	0.29 (0.22–0.40)	0.24 (0.18–0.33)	0.18 (0.13–0.25)
Co-Administration with Dual Boosted Protease Inhibitors (PIs)						
Lopinavir/Saquinavir/ritonavir	400 mg/800–1000 mg/100 mg b.i.d.	11	↔	N.A.	N.A.	N.A.
Co-Administration with Nucleoside Reverse Transcriptase Inhibitors (NRTIs)						
Didanosine	400 mg q.d.	15	↔	1.16 (1.02–1.32)	1.11 (0.99–1.25)	1.05 (0.93–1.18)
Tenofovir disoproxil fumarate	300 mg q.d.	23	↓	0.81 (0.75–0.88)	0.81 (0.75–0.88)	0.82 (0.73–0.91)
Co-Administration with Fusion Inhibitors						
Enfuvirtide	90 mg b.i.d.	261	↔[b]	N.A.	N.A.	N.A.
Co-Administration with Integrase Strand Transfer Inhibitors						
Raltegravir	400 mg b.i.d.	19	↔	1.04 (0.97–1.12)	1.10 (1.03–1.16)	1.17 (1.10–1.26)
Co-Administration with Other Drugs						
Atorvastatin	40 mg q.d.	16	↔	0.97 (0.93–1.02)	1.02 (0.97–1.07)	1.10 (1.02–1.19)
Clarithromycin	500 mg b.i.d.	15	↑	1.46 (1.38–1.56)	1.42 (1.34–1.50)	1.46 (1.36–1.58)
Ethinylestradiol/norethindrone	0.035 mg q.d./1 mg q.d.	16	↔	N.A.	N.A.	N.A.
Fluconazole	200 mg q.a.m.	16	↑	1.75 (1.60–1.91)	1.86 (1.73–2.00)	2.09 (1.90–2.31)
Methadone	Individual dose regimen ranging from 60 to 130 mg/day	16	↔	N.A.	N.A.	N.A.
Omeprazole	40 mg q.d.	18	↑	1.17 (0.96–1.43)	1.41 (1.22–1.62)	N.A.
Paroxetine	20 mg q.d.	16	↔	1.05 (0.96–1.15)	1.01 (0.93–1.10)	1.07 (0.98–1.17)
Ranitidine	150 mg b.i.d.	18	↓	0.94 (0.75–1.17)	0.86 (0.76–0.97)	N.A.
Rifabutin	300 mg q.d.	12	↓	0.63 (0.53–0.74)	0.63 (0.54–0.74)	0.65 (0.56–0.74)
Voriconazole	200 mg b.i.d.	16	↑	1.26 (1.16–1.38)	1.36 (1.25–1.47)	1.52 (1.41–1.64)

[a] In drug-drug interaction studies, different formulations and/or doses of INTELENCE were used which led to similar exposures, and, therefore, interactions relevant for one formulation are relevant for the other.
[b] Based on population pharmacokinetic analysis.
Legend: CI=Confidence Interval; N=maximum number of subjects with data; N.A.=not available; ↑=increases; ↓=decreases; ↔=no change; q.d.=once daily; b.i.d.=twice daily; q.a.m.=once daily in the morning.

DOSAGE AND ADMINISTRATION: Dosing Considerations:

- INTELENCE must always be given in combination other antiretroviral medicinal products.
- It is recommended that the dosage of INTELENCE be taken following a meal. The type of food does not affect the exposure to etravirine.

Recommended Dose and Dosage Adjustment: Adults: The recommended oral dose of INTELENCE tablets is 200 mg (two 100 mg tablets) taken twice daily (b.i.d.) following a meal (see Action and Clinical Pharmacology, Pharmacokinetics).

Geriatric Patients: In general, caution should be exercised in the administration of INTELENCE in elderly patients, reflecting the greater frequency of decreased hepatic, renal or cardiac function, concomitant disease or other drug therapy. (see Indications and Clinical Use, Warnings and Precautions and Action and Clinical Pharmacology).

Pediatric Patients: The safety and efficacy of INTELENCE in pediatric patients have not yet been established. Treatment with INTELENCE is not recommended in children and adolescents (see Indications and Clinical Use, Warnings and Precautions and Action and Clinical Pharmacology).

Hepatic Impairment: No dose adjustment is required in patients with mild or moderate hepatic impairment. The pharmacokinetics of INTELENCE has not been studied in patients with severe hepatic impairment (see Warnings and Precautions, Hepatic/Biliary/Pancreatic, and Action and Clinical Pharmacology, Special Populations and Conditions, Hepatic Insufficiency).

Renal Impairment: No dose adjustment is required in patients with renal impairment (see Warnings and Precautions, Renal and Action and Clinical Pharmacology, Pharmacokinetics).

Missed Dose: If the patient misses a dose of INTELENCE within 6 hours of the time it is usually taken, the patient should be told to take INTELENCE following a meal as soon as possible, and then take the next dose of INTELENCE at the regularly scheduled time.

If a patient misses a dose of INTELENCE by more than 6 hours of the time it is usually taken, the patient should be told not to take the missed dose and simply resume the usual dosing schedule.

Table 7: INTELENCE

Drug Interactions: Pharmacokinetic Parameters for Co-administered Drugs in the Presence of Etravirine[a]

Co-administered Drug	Dose/Schedule of Co-administered Drug	N	PK	Mean Ratio of Co-administered Drug Pharmacokinetic Parameters 90% CI; No effect=1.00		
				C_{max}	AUC	C_{min}
Co-Administration with Protease Inhibitors (PIs)						
Atazanavir	400 mg q.d.	14	↓	0.97 (0.73–1.29)	0.83 (0.63–1.09)	0.53 (0.38–0.73)
Atazanavir/ritonavir	300/100 mg q.d.	13	↓	0.97 (0.89–1.05)	0.86 (0.79–0.93)	0.62 (0.55–0.71)
Darunavir/ritonavir	600/100 mg b.i.d.	15	↔	1.11 (1.01–1.22)	1.15 (1.05–1.26)	1.02 (0.90–1.17)
Fosamprenavir/ritonavir	700/100 mg b.i.d.	8	↑	1.62 (1.47–1.79)	1.69 (1.53–1.86)	1.77 (1.39–2.25)
Lopinavir/ritonavir (soft gel capsule)	400/100 b.i.d.	14	↓	0.85 (0.62–1.05)	0.80 (0.49–1.07)	0.92 (0.15–1.68)
Lopinavir/ritonavir (tablet)	400/100 b.i.d.	16	↔	0.89 (0.82–0.96)	0.87 (0.83–0.92)	0.80 (0.73–0.88)
Lopinavir/saquinavir/ritonavir	400 mg b.i.d./800–1000 mg b.i.d./100 mg b.i.d.	11 11	↓ LPV ↓ SQV	0.84 (0.74–0.95) 0.85 (0.61–1.19)	0.82 (0.70–0.96) 0.87 (0.62–1.21)	0.76 (0.54–1.08) 0.87 (0.60–1.28)
Saquinavir/ritonavir	1000/100 mg b.i.d.	15	↔	1.00 (0.70–1.42)	0.95 (0.64–1.42)	0.80 (0.46–1.38)
Tipranavir/ritonavir	500/200 mg b.i.d.	19	↑	1.14 (1.02–1.27)	1.18 (1.03–1.36)	1.24 (0.96–1.59)
Co-Administration with Nucleoside Reverse Transcriptase Inhibitors (NRTIs)						
Didanosine	400 mg q.d.	14	↔	0.91 (0.58–1.42)	0.99 (0.79–1.25)	N.A.
Tenofovir disoproxil fumarate	300 mg q.d.	19	↔	1.15 (1.04–1.27)	1.15 (1.09–1.21)	1.19 (1.13–1.26)
Co-Administration with Integrase Strand Transfer Inhibitors						
Raltegravir	400 mg b.i.d.	19	↓	0.89 (0.68–1.15)	0.90 (0.68–1.18)	0.66 (0.34–1.26)
Co-Administration with Other Drugs						
Atorvastatin	40 mg q.d.	16	↓	1.04 (0.84–1.30)	0.63 (0.58–0.68)	N.A.
2-hydroxy-atorvastatin		16	↑	1.76 (1.60–1.94)	1.27 (1.19–1.36)	N.A.
Clarithromycin	500 mg b.i.d.	15	↓	0.66 (0.57–0.77)	0.61 (0.53–0.69)	0.47 (0.38–0.57)
14-hydroxy-clarithromycin		15	↑	1.33 (1.13–1.56)	1.21 (1.05–1.39)	1.05 (0.90–1.22)
Ethinyl estradiol	0.035 mg q.d.	16	↑	1.33 (1.21–1.46)	1.22 (1.13–1.31)	1.09 (1.01–1.18)
Norethindrone	1 mg q.d.	16	↔	1.05 (0.98–1.12)	0.95 (0.90–0.99)	0.78 (0.68–0.90)
Fluconazole	200 mg q.a.m.	15	↔	0.92 (0.85–1.00)	0.94 (0.88–1.01)	0.91 (0.84–0.98)
R(−) methadone	Individual dose regimen ranging from 60 to 130 mg/day	16	↔	1.02 (0.96–1.09)	1.06 (0.99–1.13)	1.10 (1.02–1.19)
S(+) methadone		16	↔	0.89 (0.83–0.97)	0.89 (0.82–0.96)	0.89 (0.81–0.98)
Paroxetine	20 mg q.d.	16	↔	1.06 (0.95–1.20)	1.03 (0.90–1.18)	0.87 (0.75–1.02)
Rifabutin	300 mg q.d.	12	↓	0.90 (0.78–1.03)	0.83 (0.75–0.94)	0.76 (0.66–0.87)
25-O-desacetylrifabutin	300 mg q.d.	12	↓	0.85 (0.72–1.00)	0.83 (0.74–0.92)	0.78 (0.70–0.87)
Sildenafil	50 mg single dose	15	↓	0.55 (0.40–0.75)	0.43 (0.36–0.51)	N.A.

(cont'd)

Table 7: INTELENCE *(cont'd)*

Drug Interactions: Pharmacokinetic Parameters for Co-administered Drugs in the Presence of Etravirine[a]

Co-administered Drug	Dose/Schedule of Co-administered Drug	N	PK	Mean Ratio of Co-administered Drug Pharmacokinetic Parameters 90% CI; No effect=1.00		
				C_{max}	AUC	C_{min}
N-desmethyl-sildenafil		15	↓	0.75 (0.59–0.96)	0.59 (0.52–0.68)	N.A.
Voriconazole	200 mg b.i.d.	14	↑	0.95 (0.75–1.21)	1.14 (0.88–1.47)	1.23 (0.87–1.75)

[a] In drug-drug interaction studies, different formulations and/or doses of INTELENCE were used which led to similar exposures, and, therefore, interactions relevant for one formulation are relevant for the other.
Legend: CI=Confidence Interval; N=number of subjects with data; N.A.=not available; ↑=increases; ↓=decreases; ↔=no change; q.d.=once daily; b.i.d.=twice daily; q.a.m.=once daily in the morning.

OVERDOSAGE:
There is no specific antidote for overdose with INTELENCE. Treatment of overdose with INTELENCE consists of general supportive measures including monitoring of vital signs and observation of the clinical status of the patient. Administration of activated charcoal may be used to aid in removal of unabsorbed active substance. Since etravirine is highly protein bound, dialysis is unlikely to be beneficial in significant removal of the active substance.

For management of a suspected drug overdose, contact your **regional Poison Control Centre**. See the *CPS* Directory section for a list of Poison Control Centres.

ACTION AND CLINICAL PHARMACOLOGY: Mechanism of Action: Etravirine is a non-nucleoside reverse transcriptase inhibitor (NNRTI) of human immunodeficiency virus type 1 (HIV-1). Etravirine binds directly to reverse transcriptase (RT) and blocks the RNA-dependent and DNA-dependent DNA polymerase activities by causing a disruption of the enzyme's catalytic site. Etravirine can bind in at least 2 conformationally distinct modes. Within a given binding mode, torsional flexibility of etravirine permits access to numerous conformational variants, while the compact design of etravirine permits significant repositioning and reorientation (translation and rotation) within the pocket. Etravirine does not inhibit the human DNA polymerases α, β, and γ.

Decreases in plasma viral load were typically observed as early as 1-2 days after the start of INTELENCE administration in monotherapy trials.

Resistance: Development of resistance against etravirine in vitro typically required multiple NNRTI-resistance associated mutations (RAMs) of which the following were observed most frequently: L100I, E138K, E138G, V179I, Y181C and M230I.

In the Phase 3 trials, DUET 1 and DUET 2, mutations that developed most commonly in subjects with virologic failure to the INTELENCE-containing regimen were V179F, V179I, Y181C and Y181I, generally within a background of other NNRTI RAMs.

Cross-Resistance: Limited cross-resistance between etravirine and efavirenz was observed in vitro in 3 of the 65 site directed HIV-1 mutant strains containing an NNRTI resistance associated mutation. Cross-resistance to delavirdine, efavirenz and/or nevirapine is expected after virologic failure with an etravirine-containing regimen for the virologic failure isolates. Therefore, the treatment of patients with delavirdine, efavirenz or nevirapine following virologic failure of an etravirine-containing regimen is not recommended.

Pharmacokinetics: The pharmacokinetic properties of etravirine have been evaluated in adult healthy subjects and in adult treatment-experienced HIV-1-infected patients. Exposure to etravirine was slightly lower in HIV-1-infected patients than in healthy subjects. See Table 8.

Table 8: INTELENCE

Population Pharmacokinetic Estimates of Etravirine 200 mg b.i.d. in HIV-1-Infected Subjects[a] **(Integrated Data from Phase III DUET Trials at Week 24)**

Parameter	Etravirine 200 mg b.i.d. N=574
AUC_{12h} (ng·h/mL)	
Geometric Mean ± Standard Deviation	4531.53±4543.69
Median (Interquartile Range)	4450.7 (3091.3–6315.0)
C_{0h} (ng/mL)	
Geometric Mean±Standard Deviation	296.74±377.52
Median (Interquartile Range)	298.8 (188.5–462.3)

[a] PK values are about 30% higher in healthy volunteers.
All HIV-infected subjects enrolled in Phase 3 clinical trials received darunavir/ritonavir 600/100 mg b.i.d. as part of their background regimen. Therefore, the pharmacokinetic parameter estimates in Table 8 account for reductions in the pharmacokinetic parameters of etravirine due to co-administration of INTELENCE with darunavir/ritonavir.

When INTELENCE was administered for 8 days to healthy volunteers, the increase in exposure to etravirine was generally dose proportional between total daily doses of 200 and 400 mg, and the total exposure to etravirine was similar irrespective of whether the total daily dose was administered in a once-daily or twice-daily regimen.

Absorption: An intravenous formulation of etravirine is unavailable: thus, the absolute bioavailability of INTELENCE is unknown. After oral administration with food, the maximum plasma concentration of etravirine is generally achieved within 4 hours.

In healthy subjects, the absorption of etravirine is not affected by co-administration of oral ranitidine or omeprazole, drugs that are known to increase gastric pH.

Effect of Food on Absorption: The exposure to etravirine is similar when taken after a standard normal caloric meal (561 kcal) or high-fat high caloric meal (1160 kcal). When compared to administration following a standard normal caloric meal, exposures decreased when etravirine was taken before a standard normal caloric meal (17%), following a croissant (20%), or fasted (51%). Therefore, to achieve optimal exposure, INTELENCE should be taken following a meal.

Distribution: Etravirine is about 99.9% bound to plasma proteins, primarily to albumin (99.6%) and α_1-acid glycoprotein (94.48%-97.66%) in vitro.

In rats, the highest concentrations of radiolabeled etravirine and its metabolites were measured in the gastrointestinal tract, liver and adrenal gland and the lowest levels were associated with blood, plasma, brain, lung and bone. There was no evidence of undue retention or accumulation. The elimination of radioactivity was complete in rats within 96 hours of etravirine oral administration.

In pregnant rats, there was distribution of radiolabeled etravirine and its metabolites to the placenta, vagina, uterus, mammary glands and fetus. Total radioactivity levels in placenta and fetus were about twice the levels observed in maternal blood.

Metabolism: In vitro experiments with human liver microsomes (HLMs) indicate that etravirine primarily undergoes oxidative metabolism by CYP3A4, CYP2C9 and CYP2C19 enzymes. The major metabolites, formed by methyl hydroxylation of the dimethylbenzonitrile moiety, were at least 90% less active than etravirine against wild-type HIV in cell culture.

Etravirine is not a substrate for P-glycoprotein in in vitro studies. Etravirine is an inhibitor of P-glycoprotein in vitro with a 50% inhibitory concentration (IC_{50}) value of 10 500 ng/mL for the probe paclitaxel. This value is approximately 20-fold higher than the average maximum plasma concentration observed in HIV-1 infected patients and is unlikely to have a clinically relevant impact. The extent of first-pass metabolism of etravirine has not been evaluated due to the absence of a suitable intravenous formulation. Etravirine has no pharmacologically active metabolites in the presence of NNRTI-resistant strains of HIV. No dose-dependent changes in metabolism have been observed for etravirine over the daily dose range of 200-400 mg.

Excretion: After administration of a radiolabelled ^{14}C-etravirine dose in human subjects, 93.7% and 1.2% of the administered dose of ^{14}C-etravirine could be retrieved in feces and urine, respectively. Unchanged etravirine accounted for 81.2% to 86.4% of the administered dose in feces. Unchanged etravirine was not detected in urine. The terminal elimination half-life of etravirine was approximately 30-40 hours.

Effects on Electrocardiogram: In a randomized, double-blind, active- and placebo-controlled crossover study, 41 healthy male and female volunteers were administered INTELENCE 200 mg b.i.d., INTELENCE 400 mg q.d., placebo and moxifloxacin 400 mg. After 8 days of dosing, etravirine did not prolong the QT interval. The placebo-adjusted mean maximum increases in QTcF from baseline after 200 mg b.i.d. and 400 mg q.d. of etravirine were 0.1 msec and –0.2 msec, respectively, and 10.1 msec for moxifloxacin 400 mg q.d. No subject in any group had an increase in QTcF of ≥60 msec. No subject experienced an interval exceeding the potentially clinically relevant threshold of 500 msec.

Special Populations and Conditions: Pediatrics: The pharmacokinetics of etravirine in paediatric patients are under investigation. There are insufficient data at this time to recommend a dose.

Geriatrics: Population pharmacokinetic analysis in HIV-infected subjects showed that etravirine pharmacokinetics are not considerably different in the age range (18 to 77 years) evaluated (see Warnings and Precautions, Special Populations, Geriatrics (>65 years of age)).

Gender: A limited number of women were included in studies.

Race: Population pharmacokinetic analysis of etravirine in HIV-infected patients indicated that race had no apparent effect on the exposure to etravirine.

Hepatic Insufficiency: Hepatic Impairment: Etravirine is primarily metabolized and eliminated by the liver. In a study comparing 8 patients with mild hepatic impairment to 8 matched controls and 8 patients with moderate hepatic impairment to 8 matched controls, the multiple dose pharmacokinetic disposition of etravirine was not altered in patients with mild to moderate hepatic impairment. No dosing adjustment is required in patients with mild or moderate hepatic impairment. INTELENCE has not been studied in patients with severe hepatic impairment (see Warnings and Precautions, and Dosage and Administration).

Hepatitis B or Hepatitis C Virus Co-infection: Population pharmacokinetic analysis of the DUET-1 and DUET-2 trials showed reduced clearance for INTELENCE in HIV-1-infected subjects with hepatitis B and/or C virus co-infection. Based upon the safety profile, no dose adjustment is necessary in patients co-infected with hepatitis B and/or C virus.

Renal Insufficiency: The pharmacokinetics of etravirine have not been studied in patients with renal insufficiency. Results from a mass balance study with radioactive ^{14}C-etravirine showed that <1.2% of the administered dose of etravirine is excreted in the urine. No unchanged drug was detected in urine so the impact of renal impairment on etravirine elimination is expected to be minimal. As etravirine is highly bound to plasma proteins, it is unlikely that it will be significantly removed by hemodialysis or peritoneal dialysis (see Warnings and Precautions, Renal and Dosage and Administration, Recommended Dose and Dosage Adjustment, Renal Impairment).

STORAGE AND STABILITY: Store INTELENCE tablets between 15-30°C. Store in the original bottle. Keep the bottle tightly closed in order to protect from moisture. Do not remove the desiccant pouches.

INFORMATION FOR THE PATIENT: Published in e-CPS, available by subscription at www.e-cps.ca.

DOSAGE FORMS, COMPOSITION AND PACKAGING: Each white to off-white oval tablet, debossed with "T125" on one side and "100" on the other side, contains: etravirine 100 mg. Nonmedicinal ingredients: colloidal silicon dioxide, croscarmellose sodium, hypromellose, lactose monohydrate, magnesium stearate and microcrystalline cellulose. Bottles of 120 containing 3 desiccant pouches.

(Shown in Product Identification Section)

Intron A® Ⓟ

interferon alfa-2b

Biological Response Modifier

Schering-Plough

Date of Revision: July 28, 2010

SUMMARY PRODUCT INFORMATION:

Route of Administration	Dosage Form/ Strength	Clinically Relevant Nonmedicinal Ingredients
Subcutaneous; Intramuscular; Intralesional; and Intravenous	Lyophilized Powder with diluent 10 million IU interferon alfa-2b/vial 18 million IU interferon alfa-2b/vial	For a complete listing see Dosage Forms, Composition and Packaging.
Subcutaneous; Intramuscular; and Intravenous	Ready-to-Use Solution (Albumin (human) free) 10 million IU interferon alfa-2b/vial (10 million IU/mL) 18 million IU interferon alfa-2b/vial (6 million IU/mL) 25 million IU interferon alfa-2b/vial (10 million IU/mL)	For a complete listing see Dosage Forms, Composition and Packaging.
Subcutaneous	Solution for Injection (Albumin (human) free), Multi-Dose Pen 18 million IU interferon alfa-2b/pen (15 million IU/mL) 30 million IU interferon alfa-2b/pen (25 million IU/mL) 60 million IU interferon alfa-2b/pen (50 million IU/mL)	For a complete listing see Dosage Forms, Composition and Packaging.

DESCRIPTION: INTRON A (interferon alfa-2b) is a water-soluble protein produced by recombinant DNA techniques. It is obtained from a clone of *E. coli*, which has a genetically engineered plasmid hybridized with an interferon alfa-2b gene from human leukocytes.

INDICATIONS AND CLINICAL USE:

- **Chronic Hepatitis C**
  INTRON A is indicated for the treatment of chronic hepatitis C in patients 18 years or older with compensated liver disease who have a history of blood or blood product exposure and/or are Hepatitis C Virus (HCV) antibody positive. Studies in these patients demonstrated that INTRON A can produce normalization of serum alanine aminotransferase (ALT), clearance of serum HCV RNA and improvement in liver histology.
- **Chronic Active Hepatitis B**

INTRON A is indicated for the treatment of chronic active hepatitis B in patients 18 years of age or older with compensated liver disease and who have evidence of viral replication. Patients must be serum hepatitis B surface antigen (HBsAg) positive for at least 6 months and have Hepatitis B Virus (HBV) replication, as demonstrated by positive serum HBeAg, with elevated serum ALT.

Studies in these patients demonstrated that INTRON A therapy can produce virologic remission of this disease (loss of serum HBeAg and HBV-DNA), and normalization of serum aminotransferases. INTRON A therapy resulted in the loss of serum HBsAg in some responding patients.

INTRON A is not indicated for the treatment of patients who are chronic carriers of hepatitis B surface antigen (HBsAg) but lack evidence of viral replication (serum HBeAg negative).

- **Chronic Myelogenous Leukemia**

  INTRON A is indicated for the treatment of patients with chronic myelogenous leukemia (CML). Studies have demonstrated a greater likelihood of response to INTRON A therapy in patients who are in the chronic phase of the disease.

  Thrombocytosis associated with CML: Thrombocytosis is frequently associated with CML. During the clinical experience accumulated to date, approximately one-quarter (26%) of the patients diagnosed with CML had concomitant thrombocytosis, with a baseline platelet count of greater than 500×10^9/L. Platelet control was achieved in all patients within two months of treatment. At no time were monthly platelet counts $<80 \times 10^9$/L.
- **Multiple Myeloma**

  INTRON A maintenance is a therapeutic option for multiple myeloma patients who achieved objective remission on induction therapy (i.e., melphalan and prednisone). In the relatively older patient population, the potential interferon-mediated benefit of prolonged remission duration must be weighed against the toxicity associated with interferon therapy. The approach to these patients should be individualised.
- **Non-Hodgkin's Lymphoma**

  INTRON A is indicated as adjuvant treatment of high tumor burden follicular lymphoma (Stage 3 or 4) in combination with appropriate chemotherapy, such as a CHOP-like regimen.
- **Malignant Melanoma**

  INTRON A is indicated as adjuvant to surgical treatment in patients 18 years of age or older with malignant melanoma who are free of disease but at high risk for systemic recurrence, within 56 days of surgery.
- **AIDS-Related Kaposi's Sarcoma**

  INTRON A is indicated for the treatment of select patients, above 18 years of age with AIDS-Related Kaposi's Sarcoma. Studies have demonstrated a greater likelihood of response to INTRON A therapy in patients who are without systemic symptoms, who have limited lymphadenopathy and who have a relatively intact immune system.
- **Hairy Cell Leukemia**

  INTRON A is indicated for the treatment of patients with hairy cell leukemia either following or replacing splenectomy.
- **Basal Cell Carcinoma**

  INTRON A, administered intralesionally, should be considered as an alternative treatment for patients with primary superficial and noduloulcerative basal cell carcinoma, where surgery or radiation are considered inappropriate. The basal cell lesion should be subtyped prior to initiation of treatment since no data exist for the use of INTRON A in the following conditions: 1) recurrent basal cell carcinoma; 2) genetic or nevoid basal cell carcinoma; 3) basal cell carcinoma with evidence of deep tissue involvement; 4) morphealike basal cell carcinoma.
- **Condylomata Acuminata**

  INTRON A is indicated for intralesional treatment of selected patients with condylomata acuminata involving external surfaces of the genital and perianal areas.

  In selecting patients for INTRON A treatment, the physician should consider the nature of the patient's lesion and the patient's past treatment history, in addition to the patient's ability to comply with the treatment regimen. INTRON A therapy offers an additional approach to treatment in condylomata and is particularly useful for those patients who do not respond satisfactorily to other treatment modalities (e.g., podophyllin resin, surgery, cryotherapy, chemotherapy, and laser therapy), or whose lesions are more readily treatable by INTRON A than by other treatments.

CONTRAINDICATIONS:

- Patients who are hypersensitive to this drug, to any ingredient in the formulation or component of the container or to any interferon. For a complete listing, see Dosage Forms, Composition and Packaging.
- Patients with severe renal dysfunction (creatinine clearance <50 mL/min) must not be treated with INTRON A injection when used in combination with ribavirin.
- Patients with autoimmune hepatitis.
- Patients with a decompensated liver disease.

WARNINGS AND PRECAUTIONS:

Serious Warnings and Precautions

Alpha interferons, including INTRON A, cause or aggravate fatal or life-threatening neuropsychiatric, autoimmune, ischemic, and infectious disorders. Patients should be monitored closely with periodic clinical and laboratory evaluations. Patients with persistently severe or worsening signs or symptoms of these conditions should be withdrawn from therapy. In many cases, but not all cases, these disorders resolve after stopping interferon therapy.

General: When INTRON A Products are administered in combination with ribavirin in patients with chronic hepatitis C, please also refer to ribavirin product information. When INTRON A is administered in combination with ribavirin, subjects with impaired renal function and/or those over the age of 50 should be more carefully monitored with respect to the development of anemia.

Variations in dosage, routes of administration, and adverse reactions exist among different brands of interferon. Therefore, do not use different brands of interferon in any single treatment regimen.

Because of the fever and other "flu-like" symptoms associated with INTRON A administration, it should be used cautiously in patients with debilitating medical conditions, such as those with a history of cardiovascular (CVS) disease (e.g., unstable angina, uncontrolled congestive heart failure), pulmonary disease (e.g., chronic obstructive pulmonary disease), or diabetes mellitus prone to ketoacidosis.

Cardiovascular: Cardiovascular: Chest pain, hypertension, cardiac arrhythmia, cardiac ischemia, and myocardial infarction have been reported in patients with and without a history of cardiac disorder or abnormality in association with the use of alpha interferon therapies including INTRON A. INTRON A should not be administered to patients with a history of severe pre-existing cardiac disease including unstable or uncontrolled cardiac disease in the previous 6 months. Patients with a history of cardiac disease (e.g., congestive heart failure, myocardial infarction and/or previous or current arrhythmic disorders) or with AIDS-Related Kaposi's Sarcoma, who require INTRON A therapy, should be closely monitored (see Monitoring and Laboratory Tests). Those patients who have pre-existing cardiac abnormalities and/or are in advanced stages of cancer, should have electrocardiograms taken prior to and during the course of treatment. Cardiac arrhythmias (primarily supraventricular) occurred rarely and appeared to be correlated with pre-existing conditions and prior therapy with cardiotoxic agents. These adverse experiences usually respond to conventional therapy but may require dose modification or discontinuation of INTRON A therapy.

Transient reversible cardiomyopathy was reported in approximately 2% of the AIDS-Related Kaposi's Sarcoma patients treated with INTRON A. Cardiomyopathy has also been reported in Acquired Immune Deficiency Syndrome (AIDS) patients not receiving INTRON A therapy. Baseline chest X-rays are suggested and should be repeated if clinically indicated.

Hydration: Adequate hydration must be maintained in patients undergoing INTRON A therapy since hypotension related to fluid depletion has been seen in some patients during therapy and up to two days post-therapy. Fluid replacement may be necessary.

Cerebrovascular Disorders: Ischemic and hemorrhagic cerebrovascular events have been observed in patients treated with interferon alfa-based therapies, including INTRON A. Events occurred in patients with few or no reported risk factors for stroke, including patients less than 45 years of age. Because these are spontaneous reports, estimates of frequency cannot be made and a causal relationship between interferon alfa-based therapies and these events is difficult to establish.

Dental and Periodontal Disorders: Dental and periodontal disorders have been reported in patients receiving ribavirin and interferon combination therapy. In addition, dry mouth could have a damaging effect on teeth and mucous membranes of the mouth during long-term treatment with the combination of ribavirin and INTRON A. Patients should brush their teeth thoroughly twice daily and have regular dental examinations. In addition some patients may experience vomiting. If this reaction occurs, they should be advised to rinse out their mouth thoroughly afterwards.

Endocrine and Metabolism: Hypertriglyceridemia: Hypertriglyceridemia and aggravation of hypertriglyceridemia, sometimes severe, have been observed with INTRON A. Monitoring of lipid levels is, therefore, recommended.

Thyroid Changes: Infrequently, patients treated with alpha interferons, including INTRON A have developed thyroid abnormalities, either hypothyroidism or hyperthyroidism. After discontinuation of therapy, thyroid dysfunction may or may not be reversed. Determine thyroid stimulating hormone (TSH) levels if, during the course of therapy, a patient develops symptoms consistent with possible thyroid dysfunction. In the presence of thyroid dysfunction, INTRON A treatment may be initiated or continued only if TSH levels can be maintained in the normal range by medication.

Diabetes Mellitus and Hyperglycemia: As with other alpha interferons, diabetes mellitus and hyperglycemia have been observed in patients treated with INTRON A. Symptomatic patients should have their blood glucose measured and followed-up accordingly. Patients with diabetes mellitus may require adjustment of their anti-diabetic regimen (see Adverse Reactions).

Gastrointestinal: Colitis: As seen with other interferons, colitis, sometimes serious, have been observed within 12 weeks of starting INTRON A therapy. INTRON A should be discontinued immediately if symptoms of colitis develop (typical manifestations include abdominal pain, bloody diarrhea and fever). The colitis usually resolves within 1 to 3 weeks of discontinuation of alpha interferon.

Hepatic/Biliary/Pancreatic: Liver Function—Chronic Hepatitis C and Chronic Active Hepatitis B: Patients with decompensated liver disease (including prolongation of coagulation markers or other markers of hepatic function), autoimmune hepatitis, a history of autoimmune disease or immune suppressed transplant recipients should not be treated with INTRON A. There are reports of worsening liver disease, including jaundice, hepatic encephalopathy, hepatic failure and death following INTRON A therapy in patients with decompensated liver disease.

Patients with chronic hepatitis B with evidence of decreasing hepatic synthetic function, such as decreasing albumin levels or prolongation of prothrombin time, who nevertheless meet the criteria for therapy, may be at increased risk of clinical decompensation if a flare of aminotransferases occurs. In considering these patients for INTRON A therapy, the potential risks must be evaluated against the potential benefits of treatment.

Hepatic Function: Hepatotoxicity resulting in fatality has been observed rarely in INTRON A treated patients. Any patient developing liver function abnormalities or hepatopathy during treatment should be monitored closely and if appropriate, treatment should be discontinued.

Pancreatitis: Pancreatitis, sometimes life-threatening, has occurred in patients treated with alpha interferons including INTRON A. INTRON A therapy should be suspended if symptoms or signs of pancreatitis are observed. INTRON A should be discontinued in patients diagnosed with pancreatitis.

Immune: AIDS-Related Kaposi's Sarcoma: INTRON A should not be used for patients with rapidly progressive visceral disease. Patients receiving concomitant zidovudine (AZT) have had a higher incidence of neutropenia than that expected with AZT alone. Careful monitoring of the WBC counts is indicated in all patients who are myelosuppressed and in all patients receiving other myelosuppressive medications. The effects of INTRON A when administered in association with drugs used in the treatment of AIDS-Related disease are unknown.

Autoimmune Disease: The development of different auto-antibodies has been reported during treatment with alpha interferons including INTRON A. Clinical manifestations of autoimmune disease during interferon therapy including INTRON A, may occur more frequently in patients predisposed to the development of autoimmune disorders.

Transplantation: The safety and efficacy of INTRON A treatment have not been established for patients with liver or other organ transplants. Preliminary data indicates that interferon alpha, including INTRON A therapy may be associated with an increased rate of kidney graft rejection. Liver graft rejection has also been reported but a causal association with interferon alpha or INTRON A has not been established.

Fever: While fever may be associated with interferon therapy, other causes of persistent fever should be ruled out. Caution should also be observed in patients with coagulation disorders (e.g., thrombophlebitis, pulmonary embolism) or severe myelosuppression.

Neurologic: Effects on Ability to Drive and Use Machines: Patients who develop fatigue, somnolence or confusion during treatment with INTRON A therapy are cautioned to avoid driving or operating machinery.

Ophthalmologic: Ocular Changes: As with other alpha interferons, ophthalmologic disorders, including retinopathies (including macular edema), retinal hemorrhages, cotton wool spots, retinal artery or vein obstruction, serous retinal detachment, loss of visual acuity or visual field, optic neuritis and papilledema have been reported in rare instances after treatment with INTRON A (see Adverse Reactions). All patients should have a baseline eye examination. Any patient complaining of ocular symptoms, including loss of visual acuity or visual field must have a prompt and complete eye examination. Because these ocular events may occur in conjunction with other disease states, periodic visual examinations during INTRON A therapy are recommended in patients with disorders that may be associated with retinopathy, such as diabetes mellitus or hypertension. Discontinuation of INTRON A should be considered in patients who develop new or worsening ophthalmological disorders.

Psychiatric: Psychiatric and Central Nervous System (CNS): Patients with Existence of or History of Severe Psychiatric Conditions: Patients with a pre-existing psychiatric condition or a history of severe psychiatric disorder should not be treated with INTRON A. If treatment with INTRON A is judged necessary in adult patients with existence or history of severe psychiatric conditions, this should only be initiated after having ensured appropriate individualized diagnostic and therapeutic management of the psychiatric condition. Patients should be monitored and therapy discontinued for any patient developing severe depression and suicidal behaviour, and psychosis including hallucinations and aggressive behaviour during treatment.

If severe neuropsychiatric effects, particularly depression, are observed, INTRON A therapy should be discontinued. CNS effects manifested by depression, confusion and other alterations of mental status have been observed in some INTRON A-treated patients; suicidal ideation, attempted suicide and aggressive behavior sometimes directed towards others have been observed rarely. These adverse effects have occurred in patients treated with recommended doses as well as in patients treated with higher INTRON A doses. More significant obtundation and coma have been observed in some patients, usually elderly, treated at higher doses. While these effects are generally reversible upon discontinuation of therapy, in a few patients full resolution took up to three weeks. Very rarely, seizures have occurred with high doses of INTRON A. If patients develop psychiatric problems or CNS problems, including clinical depression, it is recommended that the patients be carefully monitored by the prescribing physician during treatment and in the 6 month-follow-up period, due to the potential seriousness of these undesirable effects. Consideration should be given to discontinue therapy, if psychiatric intervention and/or dose reduction is unsuccessful in controlling psychiatric symptoms. If psychiatric symptoms persist or worsen, or suicidal ideation or aggressive behavior towards others is identified, it is recommended that treatment with INTRON A be discontinued and the patient followed, with psychiatric intervention as appropriate.

Renal: Renal Function: Patients with severe renal dysfunction (creatinine clearance <50 mL/min) should be monitored closely during treatment with INTRON A. Increases in serum creatinine levels have been observed in patients with renal insufficiency treated with interferons, including INTRON A. Patients with impairment of renal function should be closely monitored for signs and symptoms of toxicity, including increases in serum creatinine, and careful adjustments of doses are required.

Respiratory: Pulmonary Changes: As with other alpha interferons, pulmonary infiltrates, pneumonitis, pulmonary hypertension, and pneumonia, occasionally resulting in fatality, have been observed rarely in INTRON A treated patients. The etiology has not been defined. Any patient developing fever, cough, dyspnea or other respiratory symptoms must have a chest X-ray taken. If the chest X-ray shows pulmonary infiltrates or there is evidence of pulmonary function impairment, the patient should be monitored closely, and, if appropriate, interferon-alpha treatment should be discontinued. While this has been reported more often in patients with chronic hepatitis C treated with interferon-alpha, it has also been reported in patients with oncologic diseases treated with interferon-alpha. Prompt discontinuation of interferon alpha administration and supportive treatment (including treatment with corticosteroids) appear to be associated with resolution of pulmonary events. Moreover, these symptoms have been reported more frequently when Shosaikoto (Xiao-Chai-Hu-Tang), a Chinese herbal medication, has been administered concomitantly with interferon-alpha.

Sensitivity/Resistance: Acute Hypersensitivity: Acute serious hypersensitivity reactions (e.g., urticaria, angioedema, bronchoconstriction, anaphylaxis) to INTRON A have been observed rarely during INTRON A therapy. If such a reaction develops, the drug should be discontinued and appropriate medical therapy instituted immediately. Transient rashes do not necessitate interruption of treatment.

INTRON A Ready-to-Use Solution (Albumin (human) free) and Solution for Injection (Albumin (human) free) Multi-Dose Pen contain m-cresol as preservative; some patients may experience allergic reaction to this ingredient.

Sexual Function/Reproduction: INTRON A has been shown to have abortifacient effects in Macaca mulatta (rhesus monkeys) at 90 and 180 times the intramuscular (IM) or subcutaneous (SC) dose of 2 million IU/m^2. Although abortion was observed in all dose groups (7.5 million, 15 million, and 30 million IU/kg), it was only statistically significant versus control at the mid- and high-dose groups (corresponding to 90 and 180 times the IM or SC dose of 2 million IU/m^2). High doses of other forms of interferons alpha and beta are known to produce dose-related anovulatory and abortifacient effects in rhesus monkeys. There are no adequate and well controlled studies on the use of INTRON A in pregnant women. INTRON A should be used during pregnancy only if the potential benefit justifies the potential risk to the fetus.

Effect on Fertility: Interferons, including INTRON A may impair fertility. In studies of interferon use in non-human primates, menstrual cycle abnormalities have been observed. Decreased serum estradiol and progesterone concentrations have been reported in women treated with human leukocyte interferon. Therefore, fertile women should not receive INTRON A unless they are using effective contraception during the treatment period. The effects of INTRON A on male fertility have not been studied. Therefore, a possible effect on male fertility should be considered.

Skin: Psoriatic Disease and Sarcoidosis: Use of alpha interferons including INTRON A, has been associated with exacerbating pre-existing psoriatic disease and sarcoidosis. Use of INTRON A in patients with psoriasis or sarcoidosis is recommended only if the potential benefit justifies the potential risk.

Immunological Effects: A number of immune-mediated dermatological reactions associated with the use of alpha interferons have been reported ranging from erythema multiforme to more severe but very rare occurrences of Stevens-Johnson Syndrome and toxic epidermal necrolysis.

Special Populations: Pregnant Women: There are no adequate and well controlled studies on the use of INTRON A in pregnant women. INTRON A should be used during pregnancy only if the potential benefit justifies the potential risk to the fetus.

Nursing Women: It is not known whether INTRON A is excreted in human milk. However, studies in mice have shown that mouse interferons are excreted into the milk, and because of the potential for serious adverse reactions from INTRON A in nursing infants, a decision to use or discontinue the drug should be based on a benefit to risk assessment.

Pediatrics: Safety and effectiveness of INTRON A have not been established in patients below the age of 18 years.

Monitoring and Laboratory Tests: Laboratory Tests: In addition to those tests normally required for monitoring patients, the following laboratory tests are recommended for all patients on INTRON A therapy prior to beginning treatment and then periodically thereafter:

- Standard hematologic tests: including hemoglobin, complete and differential white blood cell (WBC) counts and platelet count.
- Blood chemistries: including electrolytes, calcium, liver enzyme tests, serum creatinine and thyroid function.

The hematologic parameters of the patients should be followed closely as part of the treatment because a certain degree of myelodepression, including very rare incidences of aplastic anemia and pancytopenia, has been detected in some patients under treatment with INTRON A.

Mild to moderate leukopenia and elevated serum liver enzyme (AST) levels have been reported with intralesional administration of INTRON A; therefore, the monitoring of these laboratory parameters should be considered.

For specific laboratory testing recommendations on chronic hepatitis C and chronic active hepatitis B, see Dosage and Administration.

ADVERSE REACTIONS: Adverse Drug Reaction Overview: The most common adverse reactions were "flu-like" symptoms.

Adverse Drug Reactions: Systemic administration: The most commonly reported adverse effects were fever, fatigue, headache and myalgia ("flu-like" symptoms). Fever and fatigue were reversible within 72 hours of interruption or cessation of treatment and were dose related. While fever may be related to the "flu-like" symptoms commonly reported in patients treated with interferons, other causes of persistent fever should be excluded.

Common adverse effects include rigors/chills, anorexia and nausea. Less common adverse effects include vomiting, diarrhea, arthralgia, asthenia, somnolence, dizziness, dry mouth, alopecia, "flu-like" symptoms (unspecified), back pain, musculoskeletal pain, depression, suicidal ideation, suicide attempts, suicide, malaise, pain, increased sweating, taste alteration, irritability, insomnia, confusion, impaired concentration and hypotension.

Rarely reported adverse reactions include abdominal pain, right upper quadrant (RUQ) pain, rash (e.g., erythematous and maculopapular), nervousness, injection site disorders, paresthesia, viral infection, herpes simplex, dry skin, erythema, pruritus, conjunctivitis, eye pain, abnormal/blurred vision, lacrimal gland disorder, anxiety, emotional lability, psychosis including hallucinations, aggressive behavior sometimes directed towards others, agitation, epistaxis, migraine, nasal congestion, sinusitis, rhinitis, coughing, pharyngitis, resistance mechanism disorders (e.g., altered resistance to infection; these effects rarely have been life-threatening or fatal), respiratory disorders, pulmonary infiltrates, pneumonitis and pneumonia, seizures, impaired consciousness, weight decrease, facial edema, dyspnea, dyspepsia, chest pain, tachycardia, hypertension, increased appetite, decreased libido, menstrual disorders (e.g., amenorrhea, menorrhagia), hypoesthesia, taste perversion, glossitis, stomatitis, loose stool, constipation, gingival bleeding, leg cramps, peripheral ischemia, neuropathy, polyneuropathy, peripheral neuropathy, rhabdomyolysis (sometimes serious), hearing disorder, vertigo, hyperuricemia, and renal insufficiency. Hyperthyroidism or hypothyroidism have also been observed rarely. Hepatotoxicity, including fatality, has been observed rarely. (See Warnings and Precautions.)

Retinal hemorrhages, retinopathies (including macular edema), cotton-wool spots, and retinal artery or vein obstruction; loss of visual acuity or visual field, optic neuritis, and papilledema have been observed rarely in patients treated with interferon alpha, including INTRON A (see Warnings and Precautions).

Very rarely following the marketing of INTRON A, cases of nephrotic syndrome, renal failure, aggravated diabetes mellitus, diabetes mellitus, hyperglycemia, colitis, pancreatitis, hypertriglyceridemia, hearing disorders, cardiac ischemia, myocardial infarction, erythema multiforme, Stevens-Johnson syndrome, and toxic epidermal necrolysis and injection site necrosis have been reported.

CVS adverse reactions, particularly arrhythmia, appeared to be correlated mostly with pre-existing CVS disease and prior cardiotoxic therapy. Transient reversible cardiomyopathy has been reported rarely in patients without prior evidence of cardiac disease. Very rarely reported adverse reactions include pancreatitis, cardiac ischemia and myocardial infarction.

When INTRON A is used with hydroxyurea, the occurrence of cutaneous vasculitides may be increased.

Very rarely INTRON A used alone or in combination with ribavirin may be associated with aplastic anemia or pure red cell aplasia.

Very rarely sarcoidosis or exacerbation of sarcoidosis has been reported.

Clinically significant laboratory abnormalities, most frequently occurring at doses greater than 10 million IU (MIU) daily, include reduction in granulocyte and WBC counts; decreases in hemoglobin level and platelet count; increases in alkaline phosphatase, lactate dehydrogenase (LDH), serum creatinine, serum urea nitrogen, and TSH levels. Moderate and usually reversible reduction in all three blood elements—white blood cells, red blood cells and platelets, have been reported. Increase in serum ALT/AST levels have been noted as an abnormality in some non-hepatitis subjects and also in some patients with chronic hepatitis B coincident with clearance of viral DNAp.

There were no new or unusual toxicities associated with the use of INTRON A for the treatment of malignant melanoma. The most commonly reported adverse reactions were gastrointestinal events, hematologic events, hepatic toxicity, neurologic toxicity, vomiting, chills, fatigue, fever and myalgia. In the surgical adjuvant trial involving 280 patients, 100% of patients treated with INTRON A experienced at least one adverse event compared to 43% for the observation patients. Severe adverse events occurred in 78% of INTRON A treated patients versus 6% of observation patients. 65% of patients had at least one dose modification due to toxicity. 24% of patients discontinued INTRON A treatment due to adverse events.

The following adverse reactions were reported to be possibly or probably treatment-related in the trial involving 143 INTRON A treated patients. The most commonly reported adverse reactions were fatigue, fever, myalgia, anorexia, nausea, headache and chills. Less common adverse reactions were depression, diarrhea, alopecia, taste alteration, dizziness, rash, pain (unspecified), dyspnea, paresthesia, influenza-like symptoms, confusion, bleeding, coughing, increased sweating, arthralgia, malaise and insomnia.

Intralesional Administration: Most reported adverse reactions were mild to moderate, transient and rapidly reversible. The incidence of reported adverse reactions in the patients treated for condylomata acuminata appears to increase in proportion to the number of lesions treated and consequently, is dose related.

The most common adverse reactions were "flu-like" symptoms, (rigors/chills fever, headache, myalgia and malaise). Other commonly reported side effects included nausea, fatigue, dizziness, arthralgia, back pain and injection site reactions (burning, itching, pain and injection site bleeding). In patients treated for condylomata acuminata injection site reactions appeared to be due to manipulation of the lesion rather than the INTRON A therapy.

Rarely reported side effects include diarrhea, somnolence, depression, pain, dyspepsia, increased sweating, unspecified "flu-like" symptoms, confusion, weakness, vomiting, flushing, leg cramps, asthenia, taste perversion, dermatitis and pruritus.

Low WBC counts, elevated serum liver enzyme (AST) levels and low platelet counts have been reported in some patients with intralesional administration of INTRON A. Most of these laboratory findings were transient, rapidly reversible and mild to moderate in severity.

Reported adverse reactions and abnormal laboratory test values observed in patients who were re-treated for condylomata acuminata with INTRON A were qualitatively and quantitatively similar to those reported above.

The following adverse events have been reported very rarely after administration of INTRON A: Blood Disorders: hemolytic anemia, granulocytopenia, leukopenia, increased gamma globulins, coagulation disorder.

Body as a Whole: dehydration, hypercalcemia, cachexia, peripheral edema, lymphadenopathy, periorbital edema, malignant hyperpyrexia, transplant rejection, acidosis, ascites.

CVS: palpitations, postural hypotension, chest pain, chest pain substernal, bradycardia, cardiac failure, cardiomyopathy, atrial fibrillation, arrhythmia, extrasystole, angina pectoris, thrombophlebitis, peripheral ischemia.

Central and Peripheral Nervous System: amnesia, stupor, convulsions, hypertonia, hyperesthesia, hot flashes, migraine, encephalopathy, tremor, coma, extrapyramidal disorder, paresis, speech disorder, dysphonia, syncope, tinnitus, vertigo, abnormal coordination, ataxia, aphasia, CNS dysfunction, abnormal gait, hyperkinesia, dystonia, paralysis, hyperparesthesia.

Endocrine System: gynecomastia, virilism, aggravation of diabetes mellitus, hyperglycemia, adrenal hypercorticism.

Gastrointestinal System: eructation, stomatitis, stomatitis ulcerative, constipation, tenesmus, ileus, thirst, melena, increased saliva, esophagitis, rectal bleeding after stool, dysphagia, gastrointestinal hemorrhage, gastric ulcer, gingivitis, gum hyperplasia, rectal hemorrhage, oral leukoplakia, gastrointestinal mucosal discoloration, abdominal distention, flatulence, tongue discoloration, glossitis, taste loss, discolored feces.

Liver and Biliary System: abnormal hepatic function tests, bilirubinemia, jaundice, RUQ pain, hepatosplenomegaly, splenomegaly, hepatic encephalopathy.

Musculoskeletal System: bone pain, muscle weakness, arthritis, arthrosis, myopathy.

Psychiatric Disorders: agitation, emotional lability, personality disorder, abnormal thinking, abnormal dreaming, sleep disorder, dysphonia, flushing, hypokinesia, suicide attempt, paroniria, apathy, aggravated depression, neurosis, aggressive reaction, feeling of ebriety, psychosis including hallucination, dementia, paranoid reactions.

Reproduction System: impotence, leukorrhea, menorrhagia, uterine bleeding, vaginal hemorrhage, amenorrhea.

Resistance Mechanism Disorders: (i.e., altered resistance to infection): stye, conjunctivitis, viral and fungal infections, moniliasis, sepsis.

Respiratory System: hypoxia, stridor, nasal congestion, pneumonia, sinusitis, rhinitis, rhinorrhea, bronchospasm, cyanosis, wheezing, pleural pain, sneezing, nonproductive coughing, pulmonary embolism, pulmonary edema, laryngitis, cold.

Skin and Appendages: urticaria, acne, nail disorders, hypertrichosis, purpura, peripheral ischemia, furunculosis, non-herpetic cold sores, epidermal necrolysis, lacrimal gland disorder, cyanosis of the hand, photosensitivity, skin discoloration, chloasma, abnormal hair texture, increased hair growth, skin depigmentation, dermatitis lichenoides, melanosis, vitiligo, dry skin, dermatitis, erythema, maculopapular rash, pustular rash, clammy skin, injection site reaction.

Urinary System: micturition disorder, nocturia, polyuria, hematuria, micturition frequency, cystitis, oliguria, nephrosis, urinary incontinence, hyperuricemia.

Visual and Auditory Disorders: photophobia, blurred vision, abnormal vision, diplopia, dry eyes, oculomotor nerve paralysis, retinal disorder, retinal hemorrhage, night blindness, twitching, earache, deafness, hyperacusis.

Post-Market Adverse Drug Reactions: A wide variety of autoimmune and immune-mediated disorders have been reported with alpha interferons including idiopathic thrombocytopenic purpura, thrombotic thrombocytopenic purpura, rheumatoid arthritis, systemic lupus erythematosus, vasculitis, and Vogt-Koyanagi-Harada syndrome.

Cases of acute hypersensitivity reactions, including anaphylaxis, urticaria, and angioedema have been reported.

Asthenic conditions (including asthenia, malaise and fatigue), homicidal ideation, dehydration, palpitations, psoriasis, fungal infection, bacterial infection (including sepsis), and serous retinal detachment have been reported.

DRUG INTERACTIONS: Drug-Drug Interactions: Administration of INTRON A in combination with other chemotherapeutic agents may lead to increased risk of toxicity (severity and duration), which may be life-threatening or fatal as a result of the concomitantly administered drug. The most commonly reported potentially life-threatening or fatal adverse events include mucositis, diarrhea, neutropenia, renal impairment, and electrolyte disturbance. Because of the risk of increased toxicity, careful adjustments of doses are required for INTRON A and for the concomitant chemotherapeutic agents.

An increased risk of developing peripheral neuropathy cannot be ruled out for treatments combining telbivudine with any alfa (standard or pegylated types) and beta interferon products. This risk might occur when the drug is used with interferon products other than pegylated interferon alfa-2a. Development of peripheral neuropathy was reported in a small clinical trial in Hepatitis B investigating the use of both 600 mg daily of telbivudine and 180 micrograms once weekly by subcutaneous administration of pegylated interferon alfa-2a. The safety and efficacy of telbivudine in combination with interferon alfa-2b has not been established in patients with Hepatitis B; therefore, telbivudine in combination with alpha interferons is not recommended.

Concomitant Therapy: Acetaminophen (paracetamol) has been used successfully to alleviate the symptoms of fever and headache, which can occur with INTRON A therapy. The recommended acetaminophen dosage is 500 mg to 1 g given 30 minutes before administration of INTRON A. The maximum dosage of acetaminophen to be given is 1 g four times daily. In order to properly assess the source of fever, adjunctive acetaminophen should be limited to a maximum of 5 consecutive days unless otherwise specified by the prescribing physician.

Narcotics, hypnotics or sedatives should be administered with caution concomitantly with INTRON A Injection.

A synergistic adverse effect on the WBC count may occur when INTRON A is administered concomitantly with AZT. Patients receiving the two agents concomitantly have had a dose-dependent higher incidence of neutropenia than expected when AZT is administered alone.

Interactions between INTRON A and other drugs have not been fully evaluated. Caution should be exercised when administering INTRON A in combination with other potentially myelosuppressive agents.

Drug-Food Interactions: Interactions with food have not been established.

Drug-Herb Interactions: As with other alpha interferons, pulmonary infiltrates, pneumonitis and pneumonia, occasionally resulting in fatality, have been observed rarely in INTRON A treated patients. These symptoms have been reported more frequently when Shosaikoto (Xiao-Chai-Hu-Tang), a Chinese herbal medication, has been administered concomitantly with interferon-alpha.

Drug-Laboratory Test Interactions: Interactions with laboratory tests have not been established.

DOSAGE AND ADMINISTRATION: Dosing Considerations: INTRON A may be administered using either sterilized glass or plastic disposable syringes or the INTRON A Multi-Dose Pen.

In general, the dosage may be adjusted according to the patient's tolerance to the medication. If severe adverse reactions develop, the dosage should be modified (50% reduction) or therapy should be temporarily discontinued until the adverse reactions abate. If persistent or recurrent intolerance develops following adequate dosage adjustment, or if the disease progresses rapidly, treatment with INTRON A should be discontinued.

For maintenance dosage regimens administered subcutaneously or intramuscularly, the patient may self administer the dose at the discretion of the physician.

Laboratory Tests: Standard hematologic tests and blood chemistries (complete blood count and differential, platelet count, electrolytes, liver enzymes, including serum ALT, serum bilirubin, and albumin, serum protein, and serum creatinine) should be conducted in all patients prior to and periodically during treatment with INTRON A. TSH levels must be within normal limits prior to initiation of INTRON A therapy. Any patient developing symptoms consistent with possible thyroid dysfunction during INTRON A therapy should have an evaluation of thyroid function.

In patients treated for hepatitis, the recommended testing schedule is at weeks 1, 2, 4, 8, 12, 16, and every other month, thereafter, throughout treatment. If ALT flares (≥2 times baseline) during INTRON A therapy, INTRON A may be continued unless signs or symptoms of liver failure are observed. During ALT flare, liver function tests for prothrombin time, ALT, alkaline phosphatase, albumin and bilirubin levels should be performed at two-week intervals.

Recommended Dose and Dosage Adjustment: Chronic Hepatitis C: The recommended dosage of INTRON A is 3 MIU administered subcutaneously or intramuscularly three times per week (every other day) for up to 18 months. Most patients who respond demonstrate improvement in serum ALT levels within 12 weeks. Some patients who fail to respond to 3 MIU may benefit from higher doses of up to 10 MIU three times per week (every other day).

Current clinical experience in patients who remain on INTRON A for 12-18 months indicates that a higher proportion of patients demonstrated a sustained response after longer durations of therapy than those who discontinued therapy after six months.

Patients who relapse following INTRON A therapy may be retreated with the same dosage regimen to which they had previously responded.

Patients should be tested for the presence of antibody to HCV and other causes of chronic hepatitis, including autoimmune hepatitis should be excluded. Prior to initiation of INTRON A therapy, the physician should establish that the patient has compensated liver disease with no evidence of hepatic failure. Serum bilirubin, serum albumin, and serum creatinine should be within normal limits.

Prior to initiation of INTRON A therapy, CBC and platelet counts should be evaluated in order to establish baselines for monitoring potential toxicity. During treatment with INTRON A, these tests should be repeated at weeks 1 and 2, and monthly thereafter.

ALT levels should be evaluated after 2, 4, 12 and 24 weeks of therapy to assess response to treatment.

TSH must be within normal limits upon initiation of INTRON A treatment. Patients with pre-existing thyroid abnormalities may be treated if TSH levels can be maintained in the normal range by medication.

Chronic Active Hepatitis B: The recommended dosage of INTRON A is 30 to 35 MIU per week, administered subcutaneously or intramuscularly either as 5 MIU daily or 10 MIU three times per week (every other day), for 16 weeks.

Prior to initiation of INTRON A therapy, a liver biopsy may be useful in establishing a diagnosis of chronic hepatitis. The physician should establish that the patient has compensated liver disease. The following patient entrance criteria for compensated liver disease were used in the clinical studies:

• No history of hepatic encephalopathy, variceal bleeding, ascites, or other clinical signs of decompensation	
• Bilirubin	Normal
• Albumin	Stable and within normal limits
• Prothrombin time	<3 seconds prolonged
• WBC	≥4000/mm³
• Platelets	≥100 000/mm³

Patients with other causes of chronic hepatitis should be excluded. CBC and platelet counts should be evaluated prior to initiation of INTRON A therapy in order to establish baselines for monitoring potential toxicity. These tests should be repeated at treatment weeks 1, 2, 4 and monthly thereafter. Liver function tests, including serum ALT, albumin and bilirubin, should be evaluated after 1, 2, 4, 8, 12, and 16 weeks of therapy. HBeAg, HBsAg, and ALT should be evaluated at the end of therapy, as well as at 3 and 6 months posttherapy, since patients may become virologic responders during the 6 month period following the end of treatment.

For patients with decreases in granulocyte or platelet counts, the following guidelines for dose modifications were used in the clinical trials: See Table 1.

Table 1: INTRON A

Laboratory Values for Dose Modification

Dose	Granulocytes	Platelets
Reduce 50%	<750/mm³	<50 000/mm³
Interrupt	<500/mm³	<30 000/mm³

INTRON A therapy was resumed at 50% or increased to 100% of the initial dose when granulocytes and/or platelets increased above the appropriate values.

A transient increase in ALT ≥2 times baseline value (flare) can occur during INTRON A therapy for chronic active hepatitis B. In clinical trials, this flare generally occurred 8 to 12 weeks after initiation of therapy and was more frequent in responders (63%, 24/38) than in nonresponders (27%, 13/48). However, coincident elevation in bilirubin ≥3 mg/dL occurred infrequently (2%, 2/85). When ALT flare occurs, in general INTRON A therapy should be continued unless signs and symptoms of liver failure are observed. During ALT flare, clinical symptomatology and liver function tests including ALT, albumin and bilirubin, should be monitored at approximately 2 week intervals.

Chronic Myelogenous Leukemia: The recommended dosage of INTRON A is 4 to 5 MIU/m² administered daily subcutaneously. Dosages as little as 0.5 MIU/m² or as high as 10 MIU/m² may be necessary to achieve or maintain control of the WBC count. When the WBC count is controlled, the dosage may be administered three times per week (every other day). The dosage may be adjusted according to the patient's tolerance to the medication.

Treatment should be initiated as early as possible after diagnosis, and continued until complete hematological response is achieved or for a maximum of 18 months. Responding patients generally show a hematologic response within two to three months of treatment. These patients should continue to be treated until a complete hematologic response is obtained, as defined by a WBC count of 3 to 4×10⁹/L. All patients with a complete hematological response should further continue treatment in order to achieve a cytogenetic response which in some patients may not occur until two years after treatment initiation.

In patients, who at the time of initiation of therapy with INTRON A, present with extremely high WBC counts leading to possible life-threatening complications, consideration should be given to concomitant interventions such as leukapheresis in order to quickly lower the WBC count. Once the immediate risk to the patient has been reduced, INTRON A therapy should be initiated.

Thrombocytosis Associated with CML: The recommended dosage for the control of thrombocytosis in CML is the same as that recommended above for the treatment of CML. Dose adjustments made for the control of the WBC counts should also be appropriate to control platelet counts.

Multiple Myeloma: In patients who are in the plateau phase following induction chemotherapy, INTRON A may be administered as monotherapy, subcutaneously, at a dose of 3 MIU/m², three times a week (every other day).

Treatment should continue unless clear disease progression or severe intolerance occurs.

Non-Hodgkin's Lymphoma: When used adjunctively with chemotherapy, the recommended dosage of INTRON A is 5 MIU three times a week on alternate days administered subcutaneously for a duration of 18 months.

The standard chemotherapeutic treatment for patients with high tumor burden follicular lymphomas is the administration of a combination chemotherapy regimen. Most of these regimens are related to the well-known CHOP [cyclophosphamide, doxorubicin, vincristine, and prednisone] regimen such as the CHVP regimen of doxorubicin, cyclophosphamide, teniposide and prednisolone.

At diagnosis, most follicular lymphoma patients have a disseminated disease, stage III or stage IV. Despite this advanced disease, many patients have an indolent course and survive several years after diagnosis. A wait and watch approach may be appropriate for these patients, especially if their tumor burden is low. Treatment is frequently initiated without delay for patients with high-tumor burden such as bulky lymphadenopathy, major organ obstruction or compression syndromes, malignant effusions, bone marrow failure, or rapidly enlarging tumors.

Malignant Melanoma: The recommended INTRON A treatment regimen includes an induction treatment of 5 consecutive days per week for 4 weeks as an intravenous (IV) infusion at a dose of 20 MIU/m², followed by a maintenance treatment of 3 times per week for 48 weeks as a SC injection, at a dose of 10 MIU/m². Therapy should be administered for a total of one year unless the disease progresses.

Induction therapy is administered as a 20 minute IV infusion of INTRON A in 100 mL of normal saline.

If severe adverse reactions develop during INTRON A treatment, particularly if granulocytes decrease to <500/mL or ALT/AST rises to >5×upper limit of normal, treatment should be temporarily discontinued until the adverse reaction abates. INTRON A treatment should be restarted at 50% of the previous dose. If intolerance persists after dose adjustment or if granulocytes decrease to <250/mL or ALT/AST rises to >10×upper limit of normal, INTRON A therapy should be discontinued. In the clinical trial, patients were able to maintain clinical benefit in conjunction with appropriate dose modifications.

For patients treated for malignant melanoma, liver function and WBC and differential counts should be monitored weekly during the induction phase of therapy and monthly during the maintenance phase of therapy.

AIDS-Related Kaposi's Sarcoma: The recommended dosage of INTRON A is 30 MIU/m² three times a week (every other day) administered subcutaneously or intramuscularly.

When patients initiate therapy at 30 MIU/m² three times per week, the average dose tolerated at the end of 12 weeks of therapy is approximately 75% of the weekly dose and 50% of the weekly dose at the end of 24 weeks of therapy.

Lesion measurements and blood counts should be performed prior to initiation of therapy and should be monitored periodically during treatment to determine whether response to treatment or disease stabilization has occurred.

When disease stabilization or a response to treatment occurs, treatment should continue until there is no further evidence of tumor or until discontinuation is required by evidence of a severe opportunistic infection or adverse effect.

Hairy Cell Leukemia: The recommended dosage of INTRON A is 2 MIU/m² administered subcutaneously three times a week (every other day).

Prior to initiation of therapy, tests should be performed to quantitate peripheral blood hemoglobin, platelets, granulocytes and hairy cells and bone marrow hairy cells. These parameters should be monitored periodically during treatment to determine whether response to treatment has occurred. The normalization of one or more hematologic variables usually begins within 2 months of initiation of therapy. Improvement in all three hematologic variables (granulocyte count, platelet count and hemoglobin level) may require 6 months or more of therapy.

If a patient does not respond within 6 months, treatment should be discontinued. If a response to treatment does occur, treatment usually should be continued until no further improvement is observed and the laboratory parameters have been stable for about 3 months. It is not known whether continued treatment after that point is beneficial.

Basal Cell Carcinoma: The lesion to be injected should be cleaned first with a sterile alcohol pad. The intralesional injection should be made into the base and substance of the lesion using a fine needle (30 gauge) and a 1 mL syringe. Care should be taken not to go too deeply beneath the lesion. SC injection should be avoided. For lesions with an initial area below two cm², inject 0.15 mL of reconstituted solution containing 1.5 MIU INTRON A (see Reconstitution) into the lesion three times a week on alternate days, for three weeks. The cumulative dose administered per lesion should be 13.5 MIU. As many as three lesions can be treated at one time.

Large superficial and noduloulcerative basal cell lesions (lesions with an area between two and ten cm²) should be treated three times a week (every other day) for three weeks with 0.5 MIU/cm² of the lesion's initial size (the minimum dose being 1.5 MIU and the maximum dose being 5.0 MIU). Only one large lesion should be treated at a time.

The improvement in clinical status (appearance, size, erythema, etc) of the treated lesion is a reliable predictor of biopsy-proven cures. Therefore, the clinical status should be monitored periodically after treatment end. Improvement in disease signs usually begins at approximately eight weeks after treatment initiation. If no clinical improvement on the lesion is observed after eight to twelve weeks, excision should be re-considered.

Condylomata Acuminata: Inject 1 MIU of INTRON A (0.1 mL of reconstituted INTRON A solution) into each lesion three times per week on alternate days, for 3 weeks. Only the 10 MIU vial of INTRON A when reconstituted with 1 mL of designated diluent results in an isotonic solution at the desired concentration of 1 MIU per 0.1 mL. The injection should be administered intralesionally using a Tuberculin or similar syringe and a 25-30 gauge needle. The needle should be directed at the center of the base of the wart and at an angle almost parallel to the plane of the skin (approximating that in the commonly used PPD test). This will deliver the interferon to the dermal core of the lesion, infiltrating the lesion and causing a small wheal. Care should be taken not to go beneath the lesion too deeply; SC injection should be avoided, since this area is below the base of the lesion. Do not inject too superficially since this will result in possible leakage, infiltrating only the keratinized layer, and not the dermal core. As many as 5 lesions can be treated at one time. To reduce side effects, INTRON A injections may be administered in the evening, when possible. Additionally, acetaminophen may be administered at the time of injection to alleviate some of the potential side effects.

The maximum response usually occurs 4 to 8 weeks after initiation of the first treatment course. If results at 12 to 16 weeks after the initial treatment course has concluded are not satisfactory, a second course of treatment using the above dosage schedule may be instituted providing that clinical symptoms and signs, or changes in laboratory parameters (liver function tests, WBC and platelets) do not preclude such a course of action.

Patients with six to ten condylomata may receive a second (sequential) course of treatment at the above dosage schedule, to treat up to five additional condylomata per course of treatment. Patients with greater than ten condylomata may receive additional sequences depending on how large a number of condylomata are present.

Administration: INTRON A Lyophilized Powder: INTRON A lyophilized powder should be reconstituted with 1 mL of the accompanying sterile water for injection, as diluent. If the patient is not allergic to benzyl alcohol and if it is preferred by the physician, bacteriostatic water for injection (preserved with benzyl alcohol, 0.9%) may be used.

The reconstituted solution is clear and colorless to light yellow in color. The reconstituted material, as for all parenteral drug products, should be inspected visually for particulate matter and discoloration prior to administration.

For SC or IM Administration: Following reconstitution, the appropriate dose should be withdrawn with a sterile syringe and injected slowly subcutaneously or intramuscularly.

For Intralesional Administration: An isotonic solution of INTRON A is recommended for the treatment of basal cell carcinoma. Only the 10 MIU vial of INTRON A when reconstituted with 1 mL of designated diluent results in an isotonic solution at the desired concentration of 1 MIU per 0.1 mL. Reconstitution of other vial sizes to prepare the dilution required for intralesional use will result in a hypertonic solution.

For IV Administration: Following reconstitution, the calculated amount of interferon for the appropriate dose should be withdrawn from the vial(s), added to 100 mL of Sterile Normal Saline solution, and administered over 20 minutes. The final concentration of INTRON A must not be less than 0.1 MIU/mL. **No other drug can be infused concomitantly with INTRON A.**

Compatibility with Other IV Fluids: In addition to IV normal saline solution, INTRON A Lyophilized Powder, at final concentrations of 0.05 to one MIU per mL is stable and compatible in the following mixtures for up to 24 hours at refrigerated or at room temperature in glass bottles:

Ringers Injection	Lactate Ringers Injection
Amino Acid Injections	5% Sodium Bicarbonate Injection

INTRON A Ready-to-Use Solution: Note: All vials containing INTRON A Ready-to-Use Solution are provided with an overfill designed to take into consideration loss of solution in the needle/needle hub, thereby accommodating the appropriate prescribed dose to be withdrawn from the vial for injection.

For SC or IM Administration: INTRON A Ready-to-Use Solution (Albumin (human) free) may be injected directly after withdrawal of the appropriate doses from the vial with a sterile syringe.

For IV Infusion: The infusion of INTRON A Ready-to-use Solution (Albumin (human) free) should be prepared immediately prior to use. Any size vial may be used to measure the required dose; however, the final concentration of interferon in normal saline must not be less than 0.3 MIU/mL. The appropriate dose should then be withdrawn from the vial(s), added to 50 mL of sterile normal saline solution in a PVC bag or glass bottle for intravenous use and administered over 20 minutes. The admixture is stable for at least 24 hours when stored between 2°C and 25°C. **No other drug can be infused concomitantly with INTRON A Ready-to-Use Solution (albumin (human) free).**

As with all parenteral drug products, INTRON A Injectable Solution should be inspected visually prior to administration. INTRON A Injectable Solution is clear and colorless.

Compatibility with IV Administration Sets: The following IV drip sets can be considered compatible with the admixture containing INTRON A Ready-to-Use-Solution (Albumin (human) free):

IV Administration Set	Product Code	Manufacturer
Venoset 78 Primary IV Set	1881	Abbott
Solution Administration Set	2C0001s	Travenol
Basic Solution Set w/5 µm filter	2c5455s	Baxter
IV Set	v1400	McGaw

INTRON A Solution for Injection (Albumin (human) free), Multi-Dose Pen: INTRON A Solution for Injection (Albumin (human) free), Multi-Dose Pen contains a pre-filled multi-dose cartridge for SC administration. It is designed to deliver fixed doses as required using a simple dial mechanism.

The needles provided in the packaging will be used for the INTRON A Pen only. A new needle is to be used each time the pen delivers a dose. Each INTRON A Pen is for an individual patient's use only.

The Multi-Dose Pen should be at room temperature (15-25°C) before administering each dose. The pen should be removed from the refrigerator approximately 30 minutes before administration to allow the injectable solution to reach room temperature (15-25°C). After each use, the needle should be discarded safely and the pen must be returned to the refrigerator immediately (see Storage and Stability).

Table 2: INTRON A

Dosing Chart for INTRON A Multi-dose Pen

Clicks	Strength (MIU)		
	18 MIU PEN	30 MIU PEN	60 MIU PEN
1	0.3 MIU	0.5 MIU	1 MIU
2	0.6	1.0	2
3	0.9	1.5	3
4	1.2	2.0	4

(cont'd)

Table 2: INTRON A *(cont'd)*

Dosing Chart for INTRON A Multi-dose Pen

Clicks	Strength (MIU) 18 MIU PEN	30 MIU PEN	60 MIU PEN
5 (1 full turn)	**1.5**	**2.5**	**5**
6	1.8	3.0	6
7	2.1	3.5	7
8	2.4	4.0	8
9	2.7	4.5	9
10 (2 full turns)	**3.0**	**5.0**	**10**
11	3.3	5.5	11
12	3.6	6.0	12
13	3.9	6.5	13
14	4.2	7.0	14
15 (3 full turns)	**4.5**	**7.5**	**15**
16	4.8	8.0	16
17	5.1	8.5	17
18	5.4	9.0	18
19	5.7	9.5	19
20 (4 full turns – maximum)	**6.0**	**10.0**	**20**

Each Pen contains 1.5 mL of interferon alfa-2b solution: 1.2 mL for therapeutic use and 0.3 mL of extra solution added to clear air from the needle before injection.

As with all parenteral drug products, INTRON A Injectable Solution should be inspected visually prior to administration. INTRON A Injectable Solution is clear and colorless.

OVERDOSAGE:

Symptoms and Treatment of Overdosage: Distinction between the therapeutic dose of INTRON A and overdose has not been clearly defined. Symptoms of overdose may include amplification of the adverse effects, notably "flu-like" symptoms, leukopenia or thrombocytopenia and increased serum liver enzyme levels. The severity of the adverse reactions can be ameliorated by adjusting the dose level and schedule, or in some cases termination of INTRON A therapy. CVS side effects such as hypotension and arrhythmia may require supportive therapy.

As for any pharmacologically active compound, symptomatic treatment with frequent monitoring of vital signs and close observation of the patient are indicated.

> For management of a suspected drug overdose, contact your regional Poison Control Centre. See the *CPS* Directory section for a list of Poison Control Centres.

ACTION AND CLINICAL PHARMACOLOGY: Mechanism of Action: INTRON A has exhibited antiproliferative effects in preclinical studies employing both cell culture systems and human tumor xenografts in animals, and has demonstrated significant immunomodulatory activity in vitro. INTRON A also inhibits viral replication in vitro and in vivo.

Interferons exert their cellular activities by binding to specific membrane receptors on the cell surface. The results of several studies suggest that, once bound to the cell membrane, interferon initiates a complex sequence of intracellular events that include the induction of certain enzymes. It is thought that this process, at least in part, is responsible for the various cellular responses to interferon, including inhibition of virus replication in virus-infected cells, suppression of cell proliferation and such immunomodulation activities as enhancement of the phagocytic activity of macrophages and augmentation of the specific cytotoxicity of lymphocytes for target cells. All of these activities possibly contribute to interferon's therapeutic effects.

Pharmacodynamics: Interferons exert their cellular activities by binding to specific membrane receptors on the cell surface. Preliminary studies to characterize these membrane receptors and to determine the subsequent fate of the human interferon-receptor complex have been carried out using ^{125}I-labelled alfa-2b interferon. Human interferon receptors, as isolated from human lymphoblastoid (Daudi) cells, appear to be highly asymmetric and hydrophobic membrane proteins. They exhibit selectivity for human but not murine interferons, suggesting species specificity. Studies with other interferons have demonstrated species specificity.

Alfa-2 interferon has exhibited antiproliferative effects in preclinical studies employing both cell culture systems and human tumor xenografts in animals, and has demonstrated significant immunomodulatory activity in vitro.

The antiproliferative activity of alfa-2b interferon was evaluated in vitro using mouse and human leukemia cell lines, and human osteosarcoma, melanoma, and normal amnion cells. The antiproliferative effect of alfa-2b interferon was most pronounced against human osteosarcoma cells and the human lymphocytic leukemia cell line RPMI-8402. Growth of both cell lines was inhibited 80 to 100% by alfa-2b interferon. No activity was seen in mouse leukemia cells, which again suggests species specificity.

The immunomodulating activity of alfa-2b interferon was demonstrated in vitro by its augmentation of the spontaneous "natural killer" activity of human lymphocytes, its enhancement of the tumoricidal activity of human monocytes against human tumor cells and its induction of Class 1 histocompatibility antigens on the surface of a number of cells. These effects appear to be dose dependent.

In a study using human hepatoblastoma cell line, HB 611, the in vitro antiviral activity of alpha interferon was demonstrated by its inhibition of hepatitis B virus (HBV) replication.

Mixed results were obtained in the in vivo studies of antitumor activity of alfa-2b interferon. Intraperitoneal administration of alfa-2b interferon (0.1 to 1 MIU for 9 days) had no effect on the growth of human tumor xenografts in athymic mice or on murine leukemia cells implanted in BDF1 mice. Alfa-2b interferon injected intralesionally (0.2 or 0.8 MIU once daily for 7 days), however, delayed the development and reduced the volume of human osteosarcoma implants in athymic mice. The effect was dose related. Additionally, SC administration of alfa-2b interferon at a dose of 0.2 million units/day inhibited the growth of implanted human breast tumor xenografts in athymic mice by about 50% after 23 days.

A human tumor stem cell assay was used to study the effects of recombinant interferon alfa-2b in combination with doxorubicin. Study results indicated that a schedule dependent synergistic effect was exhibited when doxorubicin and recombinant interferon alfa-2b were combined in the cell lines tested. Antagonistic effects or cell growth enhancement over control levels were not observed.

Preliminary studies with isolated and perfused rabbit kidneys have shown that the kidney may be the main site of interferon alpha catabolism.

Pharmacokinetics: The pharmacokinetics of INTRON A were studied in 12 healthy male volunteers following single doses of 5 MIU/m^2 administered intramuscularly, subcutaneously and as a 30 minute IV infusion in a cross-over design. Interferon concentrations were determined using a radioimmunoassay (RIA) with a detection limit equal to 10 IU/mL. The mean serum interferon concentrations following IM and SC injections were comparable. The maximum serum concentrations obtained via these routes were approximately 18 to 116 IU/mL and occurred 3 to 12 hours after administration. The elimination half-lives of interferon following both IM and SC injections were approximately two to three hours. Serum levels were below the detection limit 16 hours post-injection. After IV administration, serum interferon levels peaked (135 to 273 IU/mL) by the end of the infusion, then declined at a slightly more rapid rate than after SC or IM drug administration, becoming undetectable four hours after the infusion. The elimination half-life was approximately two hours. Urine levels of interferon following a single dose (5 MIU/m^2) were below the detection limit following each of the three routes of administration.

In another study, the pharmacokinetics of INTRON A were studied in 12 healthy male volunteers following single 10 MIU doses administered subcutaneously, intramuscularly and as a 30 minute IV infusion. The mean serum level profiles of interferon following SC and IM injections were comparable. The maximum serum levels obtained at six to eight hours after injection were approximately 150-180 IU/mL. The elimination half-lives of interferon following both SC and IM injections were approximately six to seven hours. Serum levels were below the detection limit of 25 IU/mL, 24 hours after the injections. Serum levels of interferon after IV administration peaked (546 IU/mL) by the end of the infusion, then declined rapidly with time, becoming undetectable four hours after the infusion. Urine levels of interferon were below the detection limit following each of the three routes of administration.

There are no pharmacokinetic data available for the intralesional route of administration.

Serum Anti-Interferon Neutralizing Antibodies: Interferon neutralizing factor assays were performed on serum samples of patients who received INTRON A in Schering-Plough monitored clinical trials. The clinical incidence of neutralizing activity developing in cancer patients treated systemically is approximately 3%, and in chronic hepatitis patients is 6.2% with no loss of response due to the low titers.

Serum interferon neutralizing activity was detected in approximately 1% of patients who received INTRON A intralesionally for condylomata acuminata. The detectable titres are low in almost all cases and have not been regularly associated with loss of response or any other autoimmune phenomenon. No development of neutralizing antibodies has been demonstrated in patients who received INTRON A intralesionally in the treatment of basal cell carcinoma or in patients who received INTRON A intravesically in the treatment of bladder cancer.

Serum anti-interferon neutralizing antibodies were detected in 15% (9/58) of the patients who received INTRON A for chronic hepatitis C at 3 MIU three times per week for 6 months and were tested for antibody activity. The titers detected were low in all patients and had no discernible effect on the course of disease or the response to interferon treatment.

Serum anti-interferon neutralizing antibodies were detected in 7% (6/85) of the patients who received INTRON A therapy for chronic hepatitis B at 5 MIU daily for 4 months and in 3% (1/38) of patients treated at 10 MIU, three times per week. The titers were low and did not appear to affect efficacy. The significance of the appearance of serum neutralizing activity is not known.

STORAGE AND STABILITY: Stability and Storage Recommendations: Store lyophilized powder, Ready-to-Use Solution, and Multi-Dose Pen between 2-8°C. INTRON A should not be frozen. Do not use past expiry date on labels.

INTRON A Lyophilized Powder: Before reconstitution, INTRON A should be stored in the refrigerator between 2 and 8°C. For the purpose of transport and/or to facilitate ambulatory use, the non-reconstituted product can be kept at room temperature (up to 25°C) for a period up to four weeks before use. If the product is not reconstituted during the four-week period, it cannot be put back in the refrigerator for a new storage period and should be discarded.

Reconstituted Lyophilized INTRON A Diluted with Bacteriostatic Water for Injection USP (preserved with benzyl alcohol, 0.9%): If stored between 2 to 8°C, use within 30 days.

If stored between 15 to 30°C, use within 14 days.

Discard any unused portion.

Reconstituted Lyophilized INTRON A Diluted with Sterile Water for Injection USP—Supplied with INTRON A: After reconstitution with Sterile Water for Injection, the product is to be used immediately. Since no preservative is present, it is recommended that administration of the solution occur as soon as possible and within 3 hours of reconstitution. For reconstitution under controlled and validated aseptic conditions such as a hospital pharmacy, the chemical and physical in-use stability for the reconstituted solution has been demonstrated 24 hours at 2-8°C. Discard any unused portion.

INTRON A Ready-to-Use-Solution (Albumin (human) free): 10 MIU vials: After first use, any unused solution is stable for 7 days maximum when refrigerated at 2-8°C.

18 and 25 MIU vials: After first use, the solution is stable four weeks maximum when refrigerated at 2-8°C. Any solution remaining after four weeks must be discarded.

For the purpose of transport and/or to facilitate ambulatory use, the solution can be kept at room temperature (up to 25°C) for a period up to seven days before use. INTRON A Ready-to-Use Solution (Albumin (human) free) can be put back in the refrigerator at any time during this seven-day period. If the product is not used during the seven-day period, it cannot be put back in the refrigerator for a new storage period and should be discarded.

INTRON A Solution for Injection (Albumin (human) free), Multi-Dose Pen: Refrigerate at 2-8°C. Each pen is intended for a maximum four-week use period and then must be discarded. A new needle must be used for each dose. After each use, the needle should be discarded safely, and the pen must be returned to the refrigerator immediately. In case the product is left inadvertently at room temperature (15-25°C), a maximum total of 48 hours (two days) of exposure at room temperature (15-25°C) is permitted over the four-week use period.

No other drug can be infused concomitantly with INTRON A.

INFORMATION FOR THE PATIENT: Published in e-CPS, available by subscription at www.e-cps.ca.

DOSAGE FORMS, COMPOSITION AND PACKAGING: Lyophilized Powder with Diluent: Each vial contains: 10 or 18 MIU of interferon alfa-2b, aminoacetic acid, sodium phosphate dibasic anhydrous, sodium phosphate monobasic monohydrate and human albumin. Each vial of lyophilized powder is packaged with 1 vial of diluent containing 1 mL sterile water for injection.

Ready-to-Use Solution (Albumin [human] free): Each vial contains: 18 MIU of interferon alfa-2b, in which each mL contains 6 MIU of interferon alfa-2b; or 10 or 25 MIU of interferon alfa-2b, in which each mL contains 10 MIU of interferon alfa-2b. Nonmedicinal ingredients: edetate disodium, m-cresol, polysorbate 80, sodium chloride, sodium phosphate dibasic anhydrous, sodium phosphate monobasic monohydrate and water for injection.

Solution for Injection (Albumin [human] free), Multi-dose Pen: Each glass carpoule contains: 18 MIU (15 MIU/mL), 30 MIU (25 MIU/mL) or 60 MIU (50 MIU/mL) of interferon alfa-2b. Nonmedicinal ingredients: edetate disodium, m-cresol, polysorbate 80, sodium chloride, sodium phosphate dibasic anhydrous, sodium phosphate monobasic monohydrate and water for injection. Each pre-filled pen is packaged with 12 Novofine 30G 8 mm needles and alcohol swabs.

Invanz® Ⓟ

ertapenem sodium

Antibiotic

Merck Frosst

Date of Revision: July 21, 2010

SUMMARY PRODUCT INFORMATION:

Route of Administration	Dosage Form/ Strength	Clinically Relevant Nonmedicinal Ingredients
Intravenous Intramuscular	1 g ertapenem/vial	Sodium bicarbonate and sodium hydroxide This is a complete listing of nonmedicinal ingredients.

INDICATIONS AND CLINICAL USE: Treatment : INVANZ (ertapenem sodium) is indicated for the treatment of patients with the following moderate to severe infections caused by susceptible strains of the designated microorganisms (see Dosage and Administration).

Complicated intra-abdominal infections due to *E. coli*, *C. clostridioforme*, *E. lentum*, Peptostreptococcus species, *B. fragilis*, *B. distasonis*, *B. ovatus*, *B. uniformis*, or *B. thetaiotaomicron*.

Complicated skin and skin-structure infections due to *S. aureus* (methicillin-susceptible strain only), *S. pyogenes*, *E. coli* and Peptostreptococcus species, as well as, diabetic foot infections due to *S. aureus* (methicillin-susceptible strain only) and Peptostreptococcus species. INVANZ has not been studied in diabetic foot infections with concomitant osteomyelitis or severe ischemia.

Community-acquired pneumonia due to *S. pneumoniae* (penicillin-susceptible strain only), *H. influenzae* (β-lactamase negative strain only), or *M. catarrhalis*.

Complicated urinary tract infections including pyelonephritis due to *E. coli*, *K. pneumoniae* or *P. mirabilis*.

Acute pelvic infections including postpartum endomyometritis, septic abortion and post-surgical gynecologic infections due to *S. agalactiae*, *E. coli*, Peptostreptococcus species, *B. fragilis*, *P. asaccharolytica*, or Prevotella species.

Appropriate specimens for bacteriological examination should be obtained in order to isolate and identify the causative organisms and to determine their susceptibility to ertapenem. Initial therapy with INVANZ may be instituted empirically for the treatment of bacterial infections, including mixed infections, while awaiting the results of these tests. Once these results become available, antimicrobial therapy should be adjusted accordingly.

Prevention: INVANZ is indicated in adults for the prophylaxis of surgical site infection following elective colorectal surgery.

CONTRAINDICATIONS: INVANZ (ertapenem sodium) is contraindicated in patients with known hypersensitivity to any component of this product or to other drugs in the same class or in patients who have demonstrated anaphylactic reactions to beta-lactams. For a complete listing of components, see Dosage Forms, Composition and Packaging.

Due to the use of lidocaine HCl as a diluent, INVANZ administered intramuscularly is contraindicated in patients with a known hypersensitivity to local anesthetics of the amide type and in patients with severe shock or heart block (refer to the Product Monograph for lidocaine HCl).

WARNINGS AND PRECAUTIONS:

Serious Warnings and Precautions

Serious and occasionally fatal hypersensitivity (anaphylactic) and other serious skin reactions have been reported in patients receiving therapy with beta-lactams, including INVANZ (see Warnings and Precautions, Immune and Adverse Reactions, Post-Market Adverse Drug Reactions).

Seizures and other CNS (Central Nervous System) adverse experiences have been reported during treatment with INVANZ. These experiences have occurred most commonly in patients with CNS disorders (e.g., brain lesions or history of seizures) and/or compromised renal function (see Warnings and Precautions, Neurologic, Renal and Adverse Reactions).

Case reports in the literature have shown that co-administration of carbapenems, including ertapenem, to patients receiving valproic acid or divalproex sodium results in a reduction in serum valproic acid concentrations. The valproic acid concentrations may drop below the therapeutic range as a result of this interaction, therefore increasing the risk of breakthrough seizures. In some cases of co-administration of ertapenem with valproic acid, breakthrough seizures have occurred. Increasing the dose of valproic acid or divalproex sodium may not be sufficient to overcome this interaction. The concomitant use of ertapenem and valproic acid/divalproex sodium is generally not recommended. Anti-bacterials other than carbapenems should be considered to treat infections in patients whose seizures are well controlled on valproic acid or divalproex sodium. If administration of INVANZ is necessary, supplemental anticonvulsant therapy should be considered (see Drug Interactions).

General: As with other antibiotics, prolonged use of INVANZ may result in overgrowth of non-susceptible organisms. Repeated evaluation of the patient's condition is essential. If superinfection occurs during therapy, appropriate measures should be taken.

Caution should be taken when administering INVANZ intramuscularly to avoid inadvertent injection into a blood vessel (see Dosage and Administration, Administration).

Lidocaine HCl is the diluent for intramuscular administration of INVANZ. Refer to the Product Monograph for lidocaine HCl for additional precautions.

Gastrointestinal: *C. difficile*-associated disease: *C. difficile*-associated disease (CDAD) has been reported with use of many antibacterial agents, including ertapenem. CDAD may range in severity from mild diarrhea to fatal colitis. It is important to consider this diagnosis in patients who present with diarrhea, or symptoms of colitis, pseudomembranous colitis, toxic megacolon, or perforation of colon subsequent to the administration of any antibacterial agent. CDAD has been reported to occur over 2 months after the administration of antibacterial agents.

Treatment with antibacterial agents may alter the normal flora of the colon and may permit overgrowth of *C. difficile*. *C. difficile* produces toxins A and B, which contribute to the development of CDAD. CDAD may cause significant morbidity and mortality. CDAD can be refractory to antimicrobial therapy.

If the diagnosis of CDAD is suspected or confirmed, appropriate therapeutic measures should be initiated. Mild cases of CDAD usually respond to discontinuation of antibacterial agents not directed against *C. difficile*. In moderate to severe cases, consideration should be given to management with fluids and electrolytes, protein supplementation, and treatment with an antibacterial agent clinically effective against *C. difficile*. Surgical evaluation should be instituted as clinically indicated; as surgical intervention may be required in certain severe cases (see Adverse Reactions).

Hepatic/Biliary/Pancreatic: The pharmacokinetics of ertapenem in patients with hepatic insufficiency have not been established. Of the total number of patients in clinical studies, 37 patients receiving ertapenem 1 g daily and 36 patients receiving comparator drugs were considered to have Child-Pugh Class A, B or C liver impairment. The incidence of adverse experiences in patients with hepatic impairment was similar between the ertapenem group and the comparator groups.

Immune: Hypersensitivity: Serious and occasionally fatal hypersensitivity (anaphylactic) and other serious skin reactions have been reported in patients receiving beta-lactam antibiotics, including INVANZ. Hypersensitivity (anaphylactic) reactions are more likely to occur in individuals with a history of sensitivity to multiple allergens. There have been reports of individuals with a history of penicillin hypersensitivity who have experienced severe hypersensitivity reactions when treated with another beta-lactam. Cross-reactivities between beta-lactam antibiotics have been clearly documented. Before initiating therapy with INVANZ (ertapenem sodium), careful inquiry should be made concerning previous hypersensitivity reactions to penicillins, cephalosporins, other beta-lactams and other allergens. If an allergic reaction to INVANZ occurs, discontinue the drug immediately. Serious anaphylactic reactions require immediate emergency treatment with epinephrine, oxygen, intravenous steroids, and airway management, including intubation. Other therapy may also be administered as indicated (see Contraindications and Adverse Reactions, Post-Market Adverse Drug Reactions).

Neurologic: During clinical investigations in adult patients treated with INVANZ (1 g once a day), seizures, irrespective of drug relationship, occurred in 0.5% of patients during study therapy plus 14-day follow-up period (see Adverse Reactions). These experiences have occurred most commonly in patients with CNS disorders (e.g., brain lesions or history of seizures and/or compromised renal function. Close adherence to the recommended dosage regimen is urged, especially in patients with known factors that predispose to convulsive activity. Anticonvulsant therapy should be continued in patients with known seizure disorders. If focal tremors, myoclonus, or seizures occur, patients should be evaluated neurologically, placed on anticonvulsant therapy if not already instituted, and the dosage of INVANZ re-examined to determine whether it should be decreased or the antibiotic discontinued (see Adverse Reactions).

Renal: Dosage adjustment of INVANZ is recommended in patients with reduced renal function (see Dosage and Administration). A supplementary dose may be recommended in patients following hemodialysis (see Dosage and Administration, Patients on Hemodialysis).

Special Populations: Pregnant Women: There are no adequate and well-controlled studies in pregnant women. INVANZ should be used during pregnancy only if the potential benefit justifies the potential risk to the mother and fetus.

Nursing Women: Ertapenem is excreted in human milk. INVANZ should be administered to nursing mothers only when the potential benefit outweighs the potential risk (see Action and Clinical Pharmacology, Pharmacokinetics).

Pediatrics (<18 years of age): Safety and effectiveness of INVANZ in pediatric patients 3 months to 17 years of age are supported by evidence from adequate and well-controlled studies in adults, pharmacokinetic data in pediatric patients, and additional data from comparator-controlled studies in pediatric patients 3 months to 17 years of age with the following infections (see Indications and Clinical Use).

- Complicated Intra-Abdominal Infections
- Complicated Skin and Skin Structure Infections
- Community Acquired Pneumonia
- Complicated Urinary Tract Infections
- Acute Pelvic Infections

INVANZ is not recommended in infants under 3 months of age as no data are available. INVANZ is not recommended in the treatment of meningitis in the pediatric population due to lack of sufficient CSF penetration.

Geriatrics (≥65 years of age): In clinical studies, the efficacy and safety of INVANZ in the elderly ≥65 years) was comparable to that seen in younger patients (<65 years).

This drug is known to be substantially excreted by the kidney, and the risk of toxic reactions to this drug may be greater in patients with impaired renal function. Because elderly patients are more likely to have decreased renal function, care should be taken in dose selection, and it may be useful to monitor renal function (see Dosage and Administration).

Monitoring and Laboratory Tests: While INVANZ possesses toxicity similar to the beta-lactam group of antibiotics, periodic assessment of organ system function, including renal, hepatic, and hematopoietic, is advisable during prolonged therapy.

ADVERSE REACTIONS: Adverse Drug Reaction Overview: Adult Patients: The total number of patients treated with ertapenem in clinical studies was over 1900 of which over 1850 received a 1 g dose of INVANZ (ertapenem sodium). Most adverse experiences reported in these clinical studies were described as mild to moderate in severity. Drug-related adverse experiences were reported in approximately 20% of patients treated with ertapenem. Ertapenem was discontinued due to adverse experiences thought to be drug-related in 1.3% of patients.

Pediatric Patients: The total number of pediatric patients treated with ertapenem in clinical studies was 384. The overall safety profile is comparable to that in adult patients. In clinical trials, the most common drug-related clinical adverse experiences reported during parenteral therapy were diarrhea (5.5%), infusion site pain (5.5%) and infusion site erythema (2.6%).

Clinical Trial Adverse Drug Reactions: Because clinical trials are conducted under very specific conditions the adverse reaction rates observed in the clinical trials may not reflect the rates observed in practice and should not be compared to the rates in the clinical trials of another drug. Adverse drug reaction information from clinical trials is useful for identifying drug-related adverse events and for approximating rates.

Adult Patients: Table 1 shows the incidence of drug-related adverse experiences reported during parenteral therapy.

Table 1: INVANZ

Incidence (%) of Drug-Related Adverse Experiences[a] Reported During Parenteral Therapy in ≥1.0% of Adult Patients Treated with INVANZ in Clinical Studies

Adverse Events	INVANZ 1 g daily (N=1866)	Piperacillin/Tazobactam 3.375 g q6h (N=775)	Ceftriaxone 1 or 2 g daily (N=912)
Nervous System Disorders			
Headache	2.1	1.0	2.2
Vascular Disorders			
Phlebitis/thrombophlebitis	1.3	1.3	1.4
Gastrointestinal Disorders			
Diarrhea	4.3	6.6	3.7
Nausea	2.9	3.2	2.6
Vomiting	1.0	1.5	0.9
General Disorders and Administration Site Conditions			
Infused vein complication	3.9	5.5	4.3

[a] Determined by the investigator to be possibly, probably, or definitely drug-related.

In clinical studies, seizure was reported during parenteral therapy in 0.2% of patients treated with ertapenem, 0.3% of patients treated with piperacillin/tazobactam and 0% of patients treated with ceftriaxone.

Less Common Clinical Trial Adverse Drug Reactions (<1%): Table 2 lists the less common drug-related adverse experiences that were reported during parenteral therapy with INVANZ within each body system.

Table 2: INVANZ

Less Common Clinical Trial Adverse Drug Reactions (<1%) in Adult Patients

System Organ Class	Uncommon Clinical Trial Adverse Drug Reactions (≥0.1% but <1.0%) Ertapenem (N=1866)	Rare Clinical Trial Adverse Drug Reactions (<0.1%) Ertapenem (N=1866)
Infections and Infestations	Oral candidiasis	Cellulitis, dermatomycosis, fungal infection, herpes simplex, postoperative wound infection, urinary tract infection
Blood and Lymphatic System Disorders		Eosinophilia, neutropenia, thrombocytopenia
Immune System Disorders		Allergy
Metabolism and Nutrition Disorders	Anorexia	Hypoglycemia
Psychiatric Disorders		Agitation, anxiety, depression, hallucinations, syncope
Nervous System Disorders	Confusion, dizziness, insomnia, somnolence, seizures	Restless leg syndrome, grand mal seizure, parasthesia, tremor
Cardiac Disorders		Arrhythmia, tachycardia
Vascular Disorders	Hypotension	Flushing, hot flashes, vasculitis
Respiratory, Thoracic and Mediastinal Disorders	Dyspnea	Nasal congestion, cough, epistaxis, pharyngeal discomfort, pneumonia, rales/rhonchi, wheezing
Gastrointestinal Disorders	Acid regurgitation, constipation, *C. difficile*-associated diarrhea, dry mouth, dyspepsia	Colitis, dysphagia, tongue edema, flatulence, gastritis, gastric ulcer, fecal incontinence, mouth ulcer, pelvic peritonitis
Hepatobiliary Disorders		Cholecystitis, jaundice, liver disorder
Skin and Subcutaneous Tissue Disorders	Erythema, pruritus	Dermatitis, desquamation
Musculoskeletal and Connective Tissue Disorders		Muscle cramps, elbow pain, shoulder pain
Renal and Urinary Disorders		Acute renal insufficiency, renal insufficiency
Pregnancy, Puerperium and Perinatal Conditions		Abortion

(cont'd)

Table 2: INVANZ *(cont'd)*

Less Common Clinical Trial Adverse Drug Reactions (<1%) in Adult Patients

System Organ Class	Uncommon Clinical Trial Adverse Drug Reactions (≥0.1% but <1.0%) Ertapenem (N=1866)	Rare Clinical Trial Adverse Drug Reactions (<0.1%) Ertapenem (N=1866)
Reproductive System And Breast Disorders	Vaginal pruritus	Genital bleeding, vaginal dryness
General Disorders and Administration Site Conditions	Asthenia/fatigue, edema/swelling, fever, pain, abdominal pain, chest pain, extravasation, candidiasis, taste perversion	Chills, cold extremities, facial edema, injection site induration, injection site stinging, malaise, thirst, warm sensation
Investigations		Increased blood pressure
Injury, Poisoning and Procedural Complications		Drug overdose

Pediatric Patients: Table 3 shows the incidence of drug-related adverse experiences reported during parenteral therapy.

Table 3: INVANZ

Incidence (%) of Drug-Related Adverse Experiences[a] Reported During Parenteral Therapy in ≥1.0% of Pediatric Patients Treated with INVANZ in Clinical Studies

Adverse Events	INVANZ (N=384)	Ceftriaxone (N=100)	Ticarcillin/Clavulanate (N=24)
Gastrointestinal Disorders			
Diarrhea	5.5	10.0	4.2
Vomiting	1.6	2.0	0.0
Skin and Subcutaneous Tissue Disorders			
Rash	1.3	1.0	4.2
General Disorders and Administration Site Conditions			
Infusion site erythema	2.6	2.0	0.0
Infusion site pain	5.5	1.0	12.5
Infusion site phlebitis	1.8	3.0	0.0
Infusion site swelling	1.0	0.0	0.0

[a] Determined by the investigator to be possibly, probably, or definitely drug-related.

In the pediatric clinical studies, the majority of the patients had parenteral therapy followed by a switch to an appropriate oral antimicrobial. During the entire treatment period and a 14 day posttreatment follow-up period, drug-related adverse experiences reported with an incidence of ≥1.0% in patients treated with INVANZ were no different than those listed in Table 3.

Less Common Clinical Trial Adverse Drug Reactions (<1%): Additional drug-related adverse experiences that were reported during parenteral therapy with INVANZ with an incidence of >0.2% but <1% in pediatric studies within each body system are listed below in Table 4.

Table 4: INVANZ

Less Common Clinical Trial Adverse Drug Reactions (>0.2% but <1%) in Pediatric Patients

System Organ Class	Ertapenem (N=384)
Infections and Infestations	Oral candidiasis
Metabolism and Nutritional	Decreased appetite
Nervous System	Headache
Vascular Disorders	Hot flash, hypertension, phlebitis
Respiratory, Thoracic and Mediastinal Disorders	Wheezing
Gastrointestinal	Abdominal pain, enteritis, flatulence, loose stools, nausea, toothache
Skin and Subcutaneous Tissue Disorders	Dermatitis diaper, erythema, petechiae, pruritus, rash erythematous, rash macular
Reproductive System and Breast Disorders	Genital rash
General Disorders and Administration Site Conditions	Chest pain, hypothermia, infusion site burning, infusion site induration, infusion site oedema, infusion site pruritus, infusion site reaction, infusion site warmth, injection site bruising, injection site erythema

Laboratory Test Findings: Adult Patients: Table 5 shows the most frequently observed drug-related laboratory abnormalities during parenteral therapy in patients receiving INVANZ.

Other drug-related laboratory abnormalities that were reported during parenteral therapy in >0.1% but <1.0% of patients treated with INVANZ in clinical studies included the following:

Chemistry: increases in direct serum bilirubin, total serum bilirubin, indirect serum bilirubin, BUN, serum creatinine, serum glucose.

Hematology: increases in eosinophils, PTT, monocytes; decreases in segmented neutrophils, white blood cells, hematocrit, hemoglobin and platelet count.

Urinalysis: increases in urine bacteria, urine epithelial cells, urine red blood cells.

In the majority of clinical studies, parenteral therapy was followed by a switch to an appropriate oral antimicrobial. During the entire treatment period and a 14-day post-treatment follow-up period, drug-related laboratory abnormalities in patients treated with INVANZ were no different than those listed in Table 5.

Pediatric Patients: Table 6 shows the most frequently observed drug-related laboratory abnormality during parenteral therapy in patients receiving INVANZ.

Table 5: INVANZ

Incidence[a] (%) of Specific Drug-Related Laboratory Adverse Experiences Reported During Parenteral Therapy in ≥1.0% of Adult Patients Treated with INVANZ in Clinical Studies

Laboratory Adverse Experiences	INVANZ 1 g daily n[b]=1766	Piperacillin/Tazobactam 3.375 g q6h n[b]=750	Ceftriaxone 1 or 2 g daily n[b]=870
Chemistry			
ALT ↑	5.5	4.4	4.9
AST ↑	4.8	4.5	4.2
Alkaline Phosphatase ↑	2.9	3.9	1.4
Hematology			
Platelet Count ↑	2.0	3.9	0.4

[a] Number of patients with laboratory adverse experiences/Number of patients with the laboratory test; where at least 1516 patients had the test.
[b] Number of patients with one or more laboratory tests.

Table 6: INVANZ

Incidence[a] (%) of Specific Drug-Related Laboratory Adverse Experiences Reported During Parenteral Therapy in ≥1.0% of Pediatric Patients Treated with INVANZ in Clinical Studies

Laboratory Adverse Experiences	INVANZ N[b]=384	Ceftriaxone N[b]=100	Ticarcillin/Clavulanate N[b]=24
Chemistry			
ALT ↑	1.9	0.0	4.3
AST ↑	1.9	0.0	4.3
Hematology			
Neutrophil Count ↓	2.5	1.1	0.0

[a] Number of patients with laboratory adverse experiences/Number of patients with the laboratory test; where at least 300 patients had the test.
[b] Number of patients with one or more laboratory tests.

Additional drug-related laboratory adverse experiences that were reported during parenteral therapy in >0.5% but <1.0% of pediatric patients treated with INVANZ in clinical studies include: increase in eosinophils.

Prevention: In a clinical study for the prophylaxis of surgical site infections following elective colorectal surgery in which 476 adult patients received a 1 g dose of ertapenem and 476 adult patients received a 2 g dose of cefotetan prior to surgery, the following additional (i.e., in addition to Adverse Experiences listed in Table 1) drug-related adverse experience was reported with an incidence of ≥1.0% (common): wound infection (1.7% for patients treated with ertapenem and 2.1% for patients treated with cefotetan).

The following additional (i.e., in addition to Adverse Experiences listed in Table 2) drug-related adverse experiences were reported with an incidence of <1.0% (uncommon) as listed below:

Cardiac Disorders: sinus bradycardia.

Infections and Infestations: cellulitis, clostridial infection, Clostridium colitis, postoperative infection.

Injury and Poisoning: wound complication.

Skin and Subcutaneous Tissue Disorders: erythematous rash, urticaria.

The following additional (i.e., in addition to adverse experiences listed in the Laboratory Test Findings) drug related laboratory adverse experiences were reported with an incidence of <1.0% (uncommon): increases in white blood cells and prothrombin time (PT).

Patients with Renal Insufficiency: There are limited data in adults patients with renal insufficiency from the study of prophylaxis of surgical site infection following elective colorectal surgery. In a clinical study in which 476 treated patients received a 1 g dose of ertapenem 1 hour prior to surgery, the AE profile observed in five patients with creatinine clearance ≤30 mL/min./1.73 m² is consistent with their underlying renal condition and/or having just undergone major elective colorectal surgery.

Post-Market Adverse Drug Reactions: The following post-marketing adverse experiences have been reported:

Immune System: anaphylaxis including anaphylactoid reactions.

Nervous System Disorders: dyskinesia, myoclonus, tremor.

Psychiatric Disorders: altered mental status (e.g., aggression, agitation, confusion/confusional state, delirium, disorientation, mental status changes), hallucinations.

Skin and Subcutaneous Tissue Disorders: urticaria, Drug Rash with Eosinophilia and Systemic Symptoms (DRESS syndrome).

DRUG INTERACTIONS: Overview: In vitro studies indicate that ertapenem does not inhibit P-glycoprotein-mediated transport of digoxin or vinblastine and that ertapenem is not a substrate for P-glycoprotein-mediated transport. In vitro studies in human liver microsomes indicate that ertapenem does not inhibit metabolism mediated by any of the following six cytochrome P450 (CYP) isoforms: 1A2, 2C9, 2C19, 2D6, 2E1 and 3A4. Drug interactions caused by inhibition of P-glycoprotein-mediated drug clearance or CYP-mediated drug clearance with the listed isoforms are unlikely (see Action and Clinical Pharmacology, Pharmacokinetics). In vitro studies indicate that ertapenem, over its therapeutic concentration range, has little effect on the unbound fraction of warfarin in human plasma.

Drug-Drug Interactions: Probenecid: When ertapenem is administered with probenecid (500 mg of probenecid every 6 hours), probenecid competes for active tubular secretion and reduces the renal excretion of ertapenem. This leads to small but statistically significant increases in the elimination half-life (19%, mean half-life with probenecid is 4.8 hours and mean half-life without probenecid is 4.0 hours) and in the extent of systemic exposure (25%, mean $AUC_{0-\infty}$ of total ertapenem with probenecid is 767.6 μg·hr/mL and mean $AUC_{0-\infty}$ of total ertapenem without probenecid is 616.2 μg·hr/mL). The coadministration of ertapenem with probenecid is not recommended, unless clinically necessary, due to the small effect on half-life. No dosage adjustment is recommended when patients receive probenecid concomitantly with ertapenem.

Valproic Acid: Case reports in the literature have shown that co-administration of carbapenems, including ertapenem, to patients receiving valproic acid or divalproex sodium results in a reduction of serum valproic acid concentrations. The valproic acid concentrations may drop below the therapeutic range as a result of this interaction, therefore increasing the risk of breakthrough seizures. In some cases of co-administration of ertapenem with valproic acid, breakthrough seizures have occurred. The mechanism of this interaction is unknown, (see Warnings and Precautions).

DOSAGE AND ADMINISTRATION: Treatment: Recommended Dose and Dosage Adjustment: The recommended dose of INVANZ (ertapenem sodium) in patients 13 years of age and older is 1 gram (g) given once a day. The recommended dose of INVANZ in patients 3 months to 12 years of age is 15 mg/kg twice daily (not to exceed 1 g/day).

Table 7 presents treatment guidelines for INVANZ.

Table 7: INVANZ

Daily Treatment Guidelines for Adult and Pediatric Patients with Normal Renal Function[a]

Infection[b]	Patients 13 Years of Age and Older	Patients 3 Months to 12 Years of Age	Recommended Duration of Total Antimicrobial Treatment
Complicated Intra-abdominal Infections	1 g daily	15 mg/kg/dose to a maximum of 500 mg twice daily[d]	5 to 14 days
Complicated Skin and Skin-Structure Infections	1 g daily	15 mg/kg/dose to a maximum of 500 mg twice daily[d]	7 to 14 days
Diabetic Foot Infections	1 g daily (patients ≥18 years old only)	not applicable	5 to 28 days[c]
Community-Acquired Pneumonia	1 g daily	15 mg/kg/dose to a maximum of 500 mg twice daily[d]	10 to 14 days[c]
Complicated Urinary Tract Infections including pyelonephritis	1 g daily	15 mg/kg/dose to a maximum of 500 mg twice daily[d]	10 to 14 days[c]
Acute Pelvic Infections including postpartum endomyometritis, septic abortion and post-surgical gynecologic infections	1 g daily	15 mg/kg/dose to a maximum of 500 mg twice daily[d]	3 to 10 days

[a] Defined as creatinine clearance >90 mL/min/1.73 m².
[b] Due to the designated pathogens (see Indications and Clinical Use).
[c] Duration includes a possible switch to an appropriate oral therapy once clinical improvement has been demonstrated.
[d] Not to exceed 1 g/day.

Special Populations: Patients with Renal Insufficiency: INVANZ may be used for the treatment of infections in adult patients with renal insufficiency. In patients whose creatinine clearance is >30 mL/min/1.73 m² (SI=>0.5 mL/s/1.73 m²), no dosage adjustment is necessary. Adult patients with advanced renal insufficiency (creatinine clearance ≤30 mL/min/1.73 m² (SI=≤0.5 mL/s/1.73 m²)), and end-stage renal insufficiency on hemodialysis (creatinine clearance ≤10 mL/min/1.73 m² (SI=≤0.17 mL/s/1.73 m²)) **should receive 500 mg daily**. There are no data in pediatric patients with renal insufficiency. This recommended dosage reduction is based on pharmacokinetic modeling of data collected from a clinical safety and pharmacokinetic study in adult patients with varying degrees of renal insufficiency (including those with creatinine clearance <30 mL/min/1.73 m² (SI=<0.5 mL/s/1.73 m²)) receiving a single 1 g IV dose of ertapenem (see Action and Clinical Pharmacology, Renal Insufficiency). The efficacy of the recommended adjusted dose (500 mg) for adult patients with advanced or end-stage renal insufficiency has not been established.

Patients on Hemodialysis: When adult patients on hemodialysis are given the recommended daily dose of 500 mg of INVANZ within 6 hours prior to hemodialysis, a supplementary dose of 150 mg is recommended following the hemodialysis session. If INVANZ is given at least 6 hours prior to hemodialysis, no supplementary dose is recommended. There are no data in patients undergoing peritoneal dialysis or hemofiltration. There are no data in pediatric patients on hemodialysis.

When only the serum creatinine is available, the following formula* may be used to estimate creatinine clearance (mL/min). The serum creatinine should represent a steady state of renal function.

$$\text{Males} = \frac{(\text{weight in kg}) \times (140 - \text{age in years})}{(72) \times \text{serum creatinine (mg/100 mL)}}$$

$$\text{Females} = (0.85) \times (\text{value calculated for males})$$

When using the International System of units (SI), the estimated creatinine clearance (mL/s) can be calculated as follows:

$$\text{Males} = \frac{(\text{weight in kg}) \times (140 - \text{age in years}) \times 1.4736}{(72) \times \text{serum creatinine } (\mu\text{mol/L})}$$

$$\text{Females} = (0.85) \times (\text{value calculated for males})$$

Patients with Hepatic Impairment: No dosage adjustment recommendation can be made in patients with impaired hepatic function (see Action and Clinical Pharmacology, Special Populations and Conditions and Warnings and Precautions, Hepatic/Biliary/Pancreatic).

Age/Gender: No dosage adjustment is recommended based on age **(13 years of age and older)** or gender. Dosing adjustment is needed based on age 3 months to 12 years of age (see Action and Clinical Pharmacology, Special Populations and Conditions and Warnings and Precautions, Pediatrics (<18 years of age)).

Prevention: Table 8 presents prophylaxis guidelines for INVANZ.

Table 8: INVANZ

Prophylaxis Guidelines for Adults

Indication	Daily Dose (IV) Adults	Recommended Duration of Total Antimicrobial Treatment
Prophylaxis of surgical site infection following elective colorectal surgery[a]	1 g	Single intravenous dose given 1 hour prior to the surgical incision

[a] Limited data are available in patients with advanced renal insufficiency (creatinine clearance ≤30 mL/min/1.73 m² [SI=≤0.5 mL/s/1.73 m²]). (See Adverse Reactions, Prevention, Patients with Renal Insufficiency.)

Missed Dose: The injection schedule will be set by the physician, who will monitor the response and condition to determine what treatment is needed.

Administration: INVANZ may be administered by intravenous infusion or intramuscular injection. When administered intravenously, INVANZ should be infused over a period of 30 minutes.

Intramuscular administration of INVANZ may be used as an alternative to intravenous administration in the treatment of those infections for which intramuscular therapy is appropriate.

Reconstitution: Patients 13 Years of Age and Older: Preparation for Intravenous Administration: Do not mix or co-infuse INVANZ with other medications.

Do not use diluents containing dextrose (α D-glucose).

INVANZ must be reconstituted and then diluted prior to administration.

1. Reconstitute the contents of a 1 g vial of INVANZ with 10 mL Water for Injection, 0.9% Sodium Chloride Injection or Bacteriostatic Water for Injection to yield a reconstituted solution of approximately 100 mg/mL. Shake well to dissolve.
2. To withdraw a 1 gram dose, immediately withdraw 9.8 mL of the reconstituted vial and transfer to 50 mL of 0.9% Sodium Chloride Injection.
3. The reconstituted IV solution should be used within 6 hours after preparation.

Preparation for Intramuscular Administration: INVANZ must be reconstituted prior to administration.

1. Reconstitute the contents of a 1 g vial of INVANZ with 3.2 mL of 1.0% lidocaine HCl injection† **(without epinephrine)** to yield a reconstituted solution of approximately 280 mg/mL. Shake vial thoroughly to form solution. To withdraw a 1 gram dose, the contents of the reconstituted vial should be withdrawn as completely as possible.
2. Immediately withdraw the contents of the vial and administer by deep intramuscular injection into a large muscle mass (such as the gluteal muscles or lateral part of the thigh).
3. The reconstituted IM solution should be used within 1 hour after preparation. **Note: The reconstituted solution should not be administered intravenously.**

Pediatric Patients 3 Months to 12 Years of Age: Preparation for Intravenous Administration: Do not mix or co-infuse INVANZ with other medications.

Do not use diluents containing dextrose (α D-glucose).

INVANZ must be reconstituted and then diluted prior to administration.

1. Reconstitute the contents of a 1 g vial of INVANZ with 10 mL Water for Injection, 0.9% Sodium Chloride Injection or Bacteriostatic Water for Injection to yield a reconstituted solution of approximately 100 mg/mL. Shake well to dissolve.
2. Immediately withdraw a volume equal to 15 mg/kg of body weight (not to exceed 500 mg per dose) and dilute in 0.9% Sodium Chloride Injection to a final concentration of 20 mg/mL or less (not to exceed 1 g/day).
3. The reconstituted IV solution should be used within 6 hours after preparation. Discard unused portion of the vial.

Preparation for Intramuscular Administration: INVANZ must be reconstituted prior to administration.

1. Reconstitute the contents of a 1 g vial of INVANZ with 3.2 mL of 1.0% lidocaine HCl injection† **(without epinephrine)** to yield a reconstituted solution of approximately 280 mg/mL. Shake vial thoroughly to form solution.
2. Immediately withdraw a volume equal to 15 mg/kg of body weight (not to exceed 500 mg per dose and 1 g/day) and administer by deep intramuscular injection into a large muscle mass (such as the gluteal muscles or lateral part of the thigh).
3. The reconstituted IM solution should be used within 1 hour after preparation. **Note: The reconstituted solution should not be administered intravenously. Discard unused portion of the vial.**

Parenteral drug products should be inspected visually for particulate matter and discoloration prior to use, whenever solution and container permit. As with all parenteral drug products, intravenous admixtures should be inspected visually for clarity, particulate matter, precipitate, discoloration and leakage prior to administration, whenever solution and container permit. Solutions showing haziness, particulate matter, precipitate, discoloration or leakage should not be used. Discard unused portion. Solutions of INVANZ range from colorless to pale yellow. Variations of color within this range do not affect the potency of the product.

The vials are for single use only. Unused portions should be discarded.

OVERDOSAGE:

No specific information is available on the treatment of overdosage with INVANZ (ertapenem sodium). Intentional overdosing of INVANZ is unlikely. Intravenous administration of INVANZ at a 3 g daily dose for 8 days to healthy adult volunteers did not result in significant toxicity. In clinical studies in adults, inadvertent administration of up to 3 g in a day did not result in clinically important adverse experiences. In pediatric clinical studies, a single IV dose of 40 mg/kg up to a maximum of 2 g did not result in toxicity.

In the event of an overdose, INVANZ should be discontinued and general supportive treatment given until renal elimination takes place.

INVANZ can be removed by hemodialysis; however, no information is available on the use of hemodialysis to treat overdosage.

For management of a suspected drug overdose, contact your regional Poison Control Centre. See the *CPS* Directory section for a list of Poison Control Centres.

ACTION AND CLINICAL PHARMACOLOGY: Mechanism of Action: INVANZ (ertapenem sodium) is a sterile, synthetic, parenteral, 1-β methyl-carbapenem that is structurally related to beta-lactam antibiotics, such as penicillins and cephalosporins, with in vitro activity against a range of gram-positive and gram-negative aerobic and anaerobic bacteria.

The bactericidal activity of ertapenem results from the inhibition of cell wall synthesis and is mediated through ertapenem binding to penicillin binding proteins (PBPs). In *E. coli*, it has strong affinity toward PBPs 1a, 1b, 2, 3, 4 and 5 with preference for PBPs 2 and 3.

Ertapenem is stable against hydrolysis by a variety of beta-lactamases, including penicillinases, and cephalosporinases and extended spectrum beta-lactamases. Ertapenem is hydrolyzed by metallo-beta-lactamases.

Pharmacokinetics: Overall, ertapenem pharmacokinetics were approximately linear. The plasma concentration of total ertapenem declines in a poly-exponential fashion following single 30-minute intravenous infusion. Area under the plasma concentration curve (AUC) of ertapenem increased slightly less than dose-proportionally based on total ertapenem concentrations over the 0.5 to 2 g dose range and that the AUC increased slightly greater than dose proportionally based on unbound ertapenem concentrations over the 0.5 to 2 g dose range. The slight deviations from strict dose proportionality are thought to be due to concentration-dependent plasma protein binding at the proposed therapeutic dose. The departure from dose-proportionality is very slight and, given the apparent wide therapeutic index of ertapenem, is not considered clinically relevant. The apparent volume of distribution of ertapenem at steady state is approximately 8.2 liters. The major metabolite of ertapenem is the bacteriologically inactive ring-opened derivative formed predominantly by the kidney by hydrolysis of the beta-lactam ring. Ertapenem is eliminated primarily by the kidneys. Plasma radioactivity consists predominantly (94%) of ertapenem. The mean plasma half-life of ertapenem in healthy young adults and patients 13 to 17 years of age is approximately 4 hours and approximately 2.5 hours in pediatric patients 3 months to 12 years of age. The mean bioavailability of 1 g IM dose is approximately 92%. There is no accumulation of ertapenem following multiple IV doses ranging from 0.5 to 2 g daily or IM doses of 1 g daily.

Average plasma concentrations (μg/mL) and mean $AUC_{0-\infty}$ of total ertapenem following a single 30-minute IV infusion of a 1 or 2 g dose and IM administration of a single 1 g dose in healthy young adults are presented in Table 9.

Table 9: INVANZ

Plasma Concentrations and Mean $AUC_{0-\infty}$ of Total Ertapenem After Single Dose Administration in Healthy Young Adults

Route/ Dose	Average Plasma Concentrations (μg/mL) 0.5 hr	1 hr	2 hr	4 hr	6 hr	8 hr	12 hr	18 hr	24 hr	$AUC_{0-\infty}$ (μg·h/mL)
IV 1 g[a]	155	115	83	48	31	20	9	3	1	572
IV 2 g[a]	283	202	145	86	58	36	16	5	2	1011
IM 1 g	33	53	67	57	40	27	13	4	2	555

[a] IV doses were infused at a constant rate over 30 minutes.

Mean $AUC_{0-\infty}$ values (μg·hr/mL) of unbound ertapenem for intravenous doses of 1 g and 2 g are 33.2 and 76.6, respectively.

Average plasma concentrations (μg/mL) of ertapenem in pediatric patients are presented in Table 10.

Absorption: Ertapenem, reconstituted with 1% lidocaine HCl injection, USP (in saline without epinephrine), is well absorbed following IM administration at the recommended dose of 1 g. The mean bioavailability is approximately 92%. Following 1 g daily IM administration, mean peak plasma concentrations (mean C_{max}=70.6 μg/mL) are reached in approximately 2 hours (mean T_{max}=2.2 hours) [see Table 9].

Distribution: Ertapenem is highly bound to human plasma proteins. In healthy young adults, the proportion of protein binding of ertapenem decreases as plasma concentrations of total ertapenem increase, from approximately 95% bound at an approximate plasma concentration of <100 micrograms (μg)/mL to approximately 85% protein bound at an approximate plasma concentration of 300 μg/mL.

The apparent volume of distribution (V_{dss}) of ertapenem in adults at steady state is approximately 8.2 liters (0.12 liter/kg), approximately 0.2 liter/kg in pediatric patients 3 months to 12 years of age and approximately 0.16 liter/kg in pediatric patients 13 to 17 years of age.

* Cockcroft and Gault equation: Cockcroft DW, Gault MH. Prediction of creatinine clearance from serum creatinine. Nephron. 1976.

† Refer to the prescribing information for lidocaine HCl.

Concentrations of ertapenem achieved in skin blister fluid at each sampling point on the third day of 1 g once daily IV doses are presented in Table 11. The ratio of AUC_{0-24} of total ertapenem in skin blister fluid to AUC_{0-24} of total ertapenem in plasma is 0.61.

Table 10: INVANZ

Plasma Concentrations of Ertapenem in Pediatric Patients After Single IV[a] Dose Administration

Age Group (Dose)	Average Plasma Concentrations (µg/mL) 0.5 hr	1 hr	2 hr	4 hr	6 hr	8 hr	12 hr	24 hr
3 to 23 months								
(15 mg/kg)[b]	103.8	57.3	43.6	23.7	13.5	8.2	2.5	—
(20 mg/kg)[b]	126.8	87.6	58.7	28.4	—	12.0	3.4	0.4
(40 mg/kg)[c]	199.1	144.1	95.7	58.0	—	20.2	7.7	0.6
2 to 12 years								
(15 mg/kg)[b]	113.2	63.9	42.1	21.9	12.8	7.6	3.0	—
(20 mg/kg)[b]	147.6	97.6	63.2	34.5	—	12.3	4.9	0.5
(40 mg/kg)[c]	241.7	152.7	96.3	55.6	—	18.8	7.2	0.6
13 to 17 years								
(20 mg/kg)[b]	170.4	98.3	67.8	40.4	—	16.0	7.0	1.1
(1 g)[d]	155.9	110.9	74.8	—	24.0	—	6.2	—
(40 mg/kg)[c]	255	188.7	127.9	76.2	—	31.0	15.3	2.1

[a] IV doses were infused at a constant rate over 30 minutes.
[b] Up to a maximum dose of 1 g/day.
[c] Up to a maximum dose of 2 g/day.
[d] Based on three patients receiving 1 g ertapenem who volunteered for pharmacokinetic assessment in one of the two safety and efficacy studies.

Table 11: INVANZ

Concentrations (µg/mL) of Total Ertapenem in Adult Skin Blister Fluid at Each Sampling Point on the Third Day of 1 g Once Daily IV Doses

0.5 hr	1 hr	2 hr	4 hr	8 hr	12 hr	24 hr
7	12	17	24	24	21	8

The concentration of ertapenem in breast milk of 5 lactating women was measured at random time points daily for 5 consecutive days following the last 1 g dose of a 3- to 6-day, once daily intravenous therapy. The measured concentration of ertapenem in breast milk on the last day of therapy (5 to 14 days postpartum) in all 5 women was <0.38 µg/mL; peak concentrations were not assessed. By Day 5 after discontinuation of therapy, the level of ertapenem was undetectable in the breast milk of 4 women and was detected at trace levels (<0.13 µg/mL) in 1 woman.

In vitro studies indicate that ertapenem does not inhibit P-glycoprotein-mediated transport of digoxin or vinblastine and that ertapenem is not a substrate for P-glycoprotein-mediated transport (see Drug Interactions).

Metabolism: In healthy young adults, after IV infusion of radiolabeled 1 g ertapenem, the plasma radioactivity consists predominantly (94%) of ertapenem. The major metabolite of ertapenem is the bacteriologically inactive ring-opened derivative formed predominantly by the kidney by hydrolysis of the beta-lactam ring. This metabolite is found in urine (approximately 37% of the administered dose).

In vitro studies in human liver microsomes indicate that ertapenem does not inhibit metabolism mediated by any of the six major cytochrome P450 (CYP) isoforms: 1A2, 2C9, 2C19, 2D6, 2E1 and 3A4 (see Drug Interactions). In vitro studies in human liver microsomes indicate that ertapenem is a poor substrate of cytochrome P450 (CYP) isoforms.

Coadministration of cilastatin (renal dehydropeptidase-1 inhibitor) significantly reduced the plasma clearance of ertapenem and increased the urinary excretion of ertapenem in rats and mice consistent with the view that dehydropeptidase-1 catalyzed the metabolism of ertapenem.

Excretion: Ertapenem is eliminated primarily by the kidneys. The mean plasma half-life in healthy young adults and patients 13 to 17 years of age is approximately 4 hours and approximately 2.5 hours in pediatric patients 3 months to 12 years of age.

Following administration of a 1 g radiolabeled IV dose of ertapenem to healthy young adults, approximately 80% is recovered in urine and 10% in feces. Of the 80% recovered in urine, approximately 38% is excreted as unchanged drug and approximately 37% as the bacteriologically inactive ring-opened metabolite.

In healthy young adults given a 1 g IV dose, average concentrations of ertapenem in urine exceed 984 µg/mL during the period 0 to 2 hours postdose and exceed 52 µg/mL during the period 12 to 24 hours postdose.

Special Populations and Conditions: Pediatrics: Plasma concentrations of ertapenem are comparable in pediatric patients 13 to 17 years of age and adults following a 1 g once daily IV dose.

Following the 20 mg/kg dose (up to a maximum dose of 1 g), the pharmacokinetic parameter values in patients 13 to 17 years of age were generally comparable to those in healthy young adults. Three out of six patients 13 to 17 years of age received less than a 1 g dose. To provide an estimate of the pharmacokinetic data if all patients in this age group were to receive a 1 g dose, the pharmacokinetic data were calculated adjusting for a 1 g dose, assuming linearity. A comparison of results shows that a 1 g once daily dose of ertapenem achieves a pharmacokinetic profile in patients 13 to 17 years of age comparable to that of adults. The ratios (13 to 17 years/Adults) for AUC, the end of infusion concentration and the concentration at the midpoint of the dosing interval were 0.99, 1.20, and 0.84 respectively.

Plasma concentrations at the midpoint of the dosing interval following a single 15 mg/kg IV dose of ertapenem in patients 3 months to 12 years of age are comparable to plasma concentrations at the midpoint of the dosing interval following a 1 g once daily IV dose in adults (see Action and Clinical Pharmacology, Pharmacokinetics, Distribution). The plasma clearance (mL/min/kg) of ertapenem in patients 3 months to 12 years of age is approximately 2-fold higher as compared to that in adults. At the 15 mg/kg dose, the AUC value (doubled to model a twice daily dosing regimen, i.e., 30 mg/kg/day exposure) in patients 3 months to 12 years of age was comparable to the AUC value in young healthy adults receiving a 1g IV dose of ertapenem.

Geriatrics: Plasma concentrations (AUC) following a 1 g and 2 g IV dose of ertapenem are slightly higher (approximately 39% and 22% for total ertapenem, respectively, and approximately 71% and 65% for unbound ertapenem, respectively) in elderly adults (≥65 years) relative to young adults (<65 years). These differences could be attributed partly to age-related changes in renal function. No dosage adjustment is necessary for elderly patients with normal (for their age) renal function.

Gender: The plasma concentration profiles of ertapenem are comparable in healthy men and women when body weight differences are taken into consideration. No dosage adjustment is recommended based on gender.

Hepatic Insufficiency: The pharmacokinetics of ertapenem in patients with hepatic insufficiency have not been established. In vitro studies indicate that ertapenem is metabolically stable in human liver microsomes. Following administration of a 1 g radiolabeled IV dose of ertapenem to healthy young adults, only 10% of ^{14}C-ertapenem was recovered in feces (see Action and Clinical Pharmacology, Pharmacokinetics, Metabolism and Excretion). Due to the limited extent of hepatic metabolism of ertapenem, its pharmacokinetics are not expected to be affected by hepatic impairment. No dosage adjustment recommendations can be made in patients with hepatic impairment.

Renal Insufficiency: Single 1 g IV doses of ertapenem were administered to 26 adult subjects with varying degrees of renal impairment, AUC was similar in patients with mild renal insufficiency (Cl_{cr} 60-90 mL/min/1.73 m² (when using International System of Units (SI), SI=1.0-1.5 mL/s/1.73 m²)) compared with healthy subjects (ages 25 to 82 years). AUC was increased in patients with moderate renal insufficiency (Cl_{cr} 31-59 mL/min/1.73 m² (SI=0.52-0.98 mL/s/1.73 m²)) approximately 1.5-fold compared with healthy subjects. AUC was increased in patients with advanced renal insufficiency (Cl_{cr} 5-30 mL/min/1.73 m² (SI=0.08-0.50 mL/s/1.73 m²)) approximately 2.6-fold compared with healthy subjects. AUC was increased in patients with end-stage renal insufficiency (Cl_{cr} <10 mL/min/1.73 m² (SI=<0.17 mL/s/1.73 m²)) approximately 2.9-fold compared with healthy subjects. There are no data in pediatric patients with renal insufficiency.

A dosage adjustment (500 mg once daily) is recommended for adult patients with advanced or end-stage renal insufficiency (see Dosage and Administration). The recommended dosage reduction is based on pharmacokinetic modeling of data collected from the clinical safety and pharmacokinetic study in patients with varying degrees of renal insufficiency (including those with creatinine clearance <30 mL/min/1.73 m² (SI=<0.5 mL/s/1.73 m²)) receiving a single 1 g IV dose of ertapenem. Pharmacokinetic modeling was used to determine a dosing regimen, which would provide equivalent drug exposure for which clinical efficacy has been demonstrated.

Following a single 1 g IV dose in 5 patients with end-stage renal insufficiency given immediately prior to a 4-hour hemodialysis session, approximately 30% of the dose was recovered in the dialysate. When patients on hemodialysis are given the recommended daily dose of 500 mg of INVANZ (ertapenem sodium) within 6 hours prior to hemodialysis, a supplementary dose of 150 mg is recommended following the hemodialysis session (see Dosage and Administration).

Table 12 displays the mean plasma AUCs and the geometric mean AUC ratios (RI/Pooled Control) for total and unbound ertapenem in adult patients with varying degrees of renal insufficiency (RI).

Table 12: INVANZ

Mean Plasma AUCs and Geometric Mean Ratios (GMR) for Total and Unbound Ertapenem Following a 1 g Intravenous Dose of Ertapenem in Adult Patients with Varying Degrees of Renal Insufficiency (RI) Versus the Pooled Control Group

Pharmacokinetic Parameter	Pooled Control[a]	Mild RI[b]	Moderate RI[b]	Advanced RI[b]	End-Stage RI[b]
Total Drug					
$AUC_{0-\infty}$ (µg·h/mL)	665.9	712.2	1016.5	1719.9	1941.5
GMR[c]	—	1.1	1.5	2.6	2.9
Unbound Drug					
$AUC_{0-\infty}$ (µg·h/mL)	42.5	44.2	76.1	144.6	252.7
GMR	—	1.0	1.8	3.4	6.0

[a] Pooled Control: Healthy young adult and healthy elderly subjects.
[b] Mild RI=Cl_{cr} 60-90 mL/min/1.73 m²; Moderate RI=Cl_{cr} 31-59 mL/min/1.73 m²; Advanced RI=Cl_{cr} 5-30 mL/min/1.73 m²; End-Stage RI=Cl_{cr} <10 mL/min/1.73 m².
[c] GMR=Geometric Mean Ratio of RI/Pooled Control.

STORAGE AND STABILITY: Before Reconstitution: Store lyophilized powder between 15 and 25°C.
Reconstituted and Infusion Solutions: The reconstituted solution, immediately diluted in 0.9% Sodium Chloride Injection (see Dosage and Administration, Administration), may be stored at room temperature (25°C) and used within 6 hours or stored for 24 hours under refrigeration (5°C) and used within 4 hours after removal from refrigeration. Solutions of INVANZ (ertapenem sodium) should not be frozen (see Dosage and Administration, Reconstitution).

INFORMATION FOR THE PATIENT: Published in e-CPS, available by subscription at www.e-cps.ca.

DOSAGE FORMS, COMPOSITION AND PACKAGING: Each vial of sterile lyophilized powder contains: ertapenem 1 g as free acid for intravenous infusion or for intramuscular injection. Nonmedicinal ingredients: sodium bicarbonate and sodium hydroxide to adjust pH to 7.5. The sodium content is approximately 137 mg (approximately 6.0 mEq). Single dose glass vials.

Invega™ Ⓟ
paliperidone
Antipsychotic

Janssen-Ortho

Date of Preparation: September 26, 2007
Date of Revision: July 23, 2009

SUMMARY PRODUCT INFORMATION:

Route of Administration	Dosage Form/ Strength	Clinically Relevant Nonmedicinal Ingredients
Oral	Extended-release tablets/ 3 mg, 6 mg, and 9 mg	Lactose For a complete listing see Dosage Forms, Composition and Packaging.

INDICATIONS AND CLINICAL USE: INVEGA (paliperidone) is indicated for the treatment of schizophrenia. In controlled clinical trials, INVEGA was found to improve the symptoms of schizophrenia, including positive and negative symptoms.
Geriatrics (>65 years of age): See Warnings and Precautions, Serious Warnings and Precautions Box and Special Populations.
Pediatrics (<18 years of age): The safety and efficacy of INVEGA in children under the age of 18 have not been established.

CONTRAINDICATIONS: INVEGA is contraindicated in patients who are hypersensitive to paliperidone, risperidone, or to any ingredient in the formulation or component of the container. For a complete listing, see Dosage Forms, Composition and Packaging.

WARNINGS AND PRECAUTIONS:

Serious Warnings and Precautions
Increased Mortality in Elderly Patients with Dementia: Elderly patients with dementia treated with atypical antipsychotic drugs are at an increased risk of death compared to placebo. Analyses of thirteen placebo-controlled trials with various atypical antipsychotics (modal duration of 10 weeks) in these patients showed a mean 1.6-fold increase in the death rate in the drug-treated patients. Although the causes of death were varied, most of the deaths appeared to be either cardiovascular (e.g., heart failure, sudden death) or infectious (e.g., pneumonia) in nature (see Warnings and Precautions, Special Populations, Use in Geriatric Patients with Dementia).

General: QT Prolongation: Paliperidone causes a modest increase in the corrected QT (QTc) interval. The use of paliperidone should be avoided in combination with other drugs that are known to prolong QTc including Class 1A (e.g., quinidine, procainamide) or Class III (e.g., amiodarone, sotalol) antiarrhythmic medications, antipsychotic medications (e.g., chlorpromazine, thioridazine), antibiotics (e.g., gatifloxacin, moxifloxacin), or any other class of medications known to prolong the QTc interval. Paliperidone should also be avoided in patients with congenital long QT syndrome and in patients with a history of cardiac arrhythmias.

Certain circumstances may increase the risk of the occurrence of torsades de pointes and/or sudden death in association with the use of drugs that prolong the QTc interval, including (1) bradycardia; (2) hypokalemia or hypomagnesemia; (3) concomitant use of other drugs that prolong the QTc interval; and (4) presence of congenital prolongation of the QT interval.

QT Prolongation Study R076477-SCH-1009: The effects of paliperidone on the QT interval were evaluated in a double-blind, active-controlled (moxifloxacin 400 mg single dose), multicenter QT study in adults with schizophrenia and schizoaffective disorder. Serial ECG assessments were scheduled at multiple days and multiple timepoints during the day. Least square mean changes from baseline in QTcLD were calculated at each scheduled ECG assessment timepoint and day.

In study R076477-SCH-1009 (n=141), the 8 mg dose of immediate-release oral paliperidone (n=44) showed a maximal (least square) mean change from baseline in QTcLD of 10.9 msec (90% CI:8.24; 13.62) and was noted on day 8 at 1.5 hours post dose. The mean steady-state peak plasma concentration for this 8 mg dose of paliperidone immediate-release was more than twice the exposure observed with the maximum recommended 12 mg dose of INVEGA ($C_{max\ ss}$=113 and 45 ng/mL, respectively, when administered with a standard breakfast). In this same study, a 4 mg dose of the immediate-release oral formulation of paliperidone ($C_{max\ ss}$=35 ng/mL) showed a maximal (least square) mean change from baseline in QTcLD of 9.3 msec (90% CI: 6.56; 11.98) and was noted on day 2 at 1.5 hours post-dose. None of the subjects had a change exceeding 60 msec or a QTcLD exceeding 500 msec at any time during this study.

Also, in this study, a 400 mg dose of moxifloxacin (n=58) showed a maximal least square mean change from baseline in QTcLD of 6.1 msec (90% CI: 3.64; 8.53) and was noted on day 8 at 3 hours post-dose. Placebo (n=58) showed a maximal least square mean change from baseline in QTcLD of 3.5 msec (90% CI: 1.05; 5.95) and was noted on day 2 at 30 minutes post-dose.

Concomitant Use of INVEGA with Oral Risperidone: Since paliperidone (9-hydroxy-risperidone) is the major active metabolite of risperidone, concomitant use of INVEGA with oral risperidone is not recommended since the combination of the two will lead to additive paliperidone exposure.

Body Temperature Regulation: Disruption of the body's ability to reduce core body temperature has been attributed to antipsychotic agents. Appropriate care is advised when prescribing INVEGA to patients who will be experiencing conditions which may contribute to an elevation in core body temperature, e.g., exercising strenuously, exposure to extreme heat, receiving concomitant medication with anticholinergic activity, or being subject to dehydration.

Cardiovascular: Orthostatic Hypotension: Paliperidone may induce orthostatic hypotension in some patients based on its alpha-blocking activity. Based on pooled data from the three placebo-controlled, 6-week, fixed-dose trials with INVEGA (3, 6, 9 and 12 mg), orthostatic hypotension was reported by 2.5% of subjects treated with INVEGA compared with 0.8% of subjects treated with placebo.

INVEGA should be used with caution in patients with known cardiovascular disease (e.g., heart failure, myocardial infarction or ischemia, conduction abnormalities), cerebrovascular disease or conditions that predispose the patient to hypotension such as dehydration and hypovolemia. Special care should be taken to avoid hypotension in patients with a history of cerebrovascular insufficiency or ischemic heart disease, and in patients taking medications to lower blood pressure.

Endocrine and Metabolism: Hyperglycemia: Hyperglycemia, in some cases extreme and associated with ketoacidosis or hyperosmolar coma or death, has been reported in patients treated with all atypical antipsychotics. These cases were, for the most part, seen in post-marketing clinical use and epidemiologic studies, and not in clinical trials.

In clinical trials, there have been few reports of glucose-related adverse events (e.g., hyperglycemia) in subjects treated with INVEGA.

Assessment of the relationship between atypical antipsychotic use and glucose abnormalities is complicated by the possibility of an increased background risk of diabetes mellitus in patients with schizophrenia and the increasing incidence of diabetes mellitus in the general population. Given these confounders, the relationship between atypical antipsychotic use and hyperglycemia-related adverse events is not completely understood. However, epidemiological studies, which did not include INVEGA, suggest an increased risk of treatment-emergent hyperglycemia-related adverse events in patients treated with the atypical antipsychotics. Because INVEGA was not marketed at the time these studies were performed, it is not known if INVEGA is associated with this increased risk. Precise risk estimates for hyperglycemia-related adverse events in patients treated with atypical antipsychotics are not available.

Any patient treated with atypical antipsychotics should be monitored for symptoms of hyperglycemia including polydipsia, polyuria, polyphagia, and weakness. Patients who develop symptoms of hyperglycemia during treatment with atypical antipsychotics should undergo fasting blood glucose testing. In some cases, hyperglycemia has resolved when the atypical antipsychotic was discontinued; however, some patients required continuation of antidiabetic treatment despite discontinuation of the suspect drug. Patients with risk factors for diabetes mellitus (e.g., obesity, family history of diabetes) who are starting treatment with atypical antipsychotics should undergo fasting blood glucose testing at the beginning of treatment and periodically during treatment. Patients with an established diagnosis of diabetes mellitus who are started on atypical antipsychotics should be monitored regularly for worsening of glucose control.

Hyperprolactinemia: As with other atypical antipsychotics that antagonize dopamine D_2 receptors, paliperidone elevates prolactin levels and the elevation persists during chronic administration. Paliperidone has a prolactin-elevating effect similar to that seen with risperidone.

Tissue culture experiments indicate that approximately one-third of human breast cancers are prolactin dependent in vitro, a factor of potential importance if the prescription of these drugs is considered in a patient with previously detected breast cancer. Although disturbances such as galactorrhea, amenorrhea, gynecomastia, and impotence have been reported with prolactin-elevating compounds, the clinical significance of elevated serum prolactin levels is unknown for most patients. As is common with dopamine D_2 antagonists, prolonged administration of risperidone in rodent carcinogenicity studies resulted in an increase in the incidence of pituitary gland, mammary gland, and endocrine pancreas hyperplasia and/or tumours. However, neither clinical studies nor epidemiologic studies conducted to date have shown an association between chronic administration of this class of drugs and tumorigenesis in humans; the available evidence is considered too limited to be conclusive at this time. The carcinogenic potential of paliperidone, an active metabolite of risperidone, was assessed based on studies with risperidone conducted in mice and rats.

In the three placebo-controlled, 6-week, fixed-dose trials with INVEGA (3, 6, 9, and 12 mg), the proportion of subjects who experienced potentially prolactin-related adverse events was similar for the placebo (1%) and INVEGA (1-2%) groups.

Gastrointestinal: Potential for Gastrointestinal Obstruction: Because the INVEGA tablet is nondeformable and does not appreciably change in shape in the GI tract, INVEGA should not be administered to patients with pre-existing severe gastrointestinal narrowing (pathologic or iatrogenic, for example: esophageal motility disorders, small bowel inflammatory disease, "short gut" syndrome due to adhesions or decreased transit time, past history of peritonitis, cystic fibrosis, chronic intestinal pseudo-obstruction, or Meckel's diverticulum) or in patients with dysphagia or significant difficulty in swallowing tablets. There have been rare reports of obstructive symptoms in patients with known strictures in association with the ingestion of drugs in non-deformable controlled-release formulations. Due to the controlled-release design of the tablet, INVEGA should only be used in patients who are able to swallow the tablet whole (see Dosage and Administration, Dosing Considerations).

Antiemetic Effect: An antiemetic effect was observed in preclinical studies with paliperidone. This effect, if it occurs in humans, may mask the signs and symptoms of overdosage with certain drugs or of conditions such as intestinal obstruction, Reye's syndrome, and brain tumour.

Genitourinary: Priapism: Drugs with alpha-adrenergic blocking effects have been reported to induce priapism. Priapism has been reported with INVEGA during post-marketing surveillance (see Adverse Reactions, Post-Market Adverse Drug Reactions).

Hepatic/Biliary/Pancreatic: Paliperidone is not extensively metabolized in the liver. In a study in subjects with moderate hepatic impairment (Child-Pugh class B), the plasma concentrations of unbound paliperidone were similar to those of healthy subjects. No dose adjustment is required in patients with mild to moderate hepatic impairment. The effect of severe hepatic impairment is unknown.

Neurologic: Neuroleptic Malignant Syndrome (NMS): Neuroleptic malignant syndrome is a potentially fatal symptom complex that has been reported in association with antipsychotic drugs, including paliperidone.

Clinical manifestations of NMS are hyperthermia, muscle rigidity, altered mental status (including catatonic signs) and evidence of autonomic instability (irregular blood pressure, tachycardia, cardiac arrhythmias, and diaphoresis). Additional signs may include elevated creatine phosphokinase, myoglobinuria (rhabdomyolysis), and acute renal failure.

In arriving at a diagnosis, it is important to identify cases in which the clinical presentation includes both serious medical illness (e.g., pneumonia, systemic infection, etc.) and untreated or inadequately treated extrapyramidal signs and symptoms. Other important considerations in the differential diagnosis include central anticholinergic toxicity, heat stroke, drug fever, and primary central nervous system pathology.

The management of NMS should include: (1) immediate discontinuation of antipsychotic drugs including INVEGA, and other drugs not essential to concurrent therapy; (2) intensive symptomatic treatment and medical monitoring; and (3) treatment of any concomitant serious medical problems for which specific treatments are available. There is no general agreement about specific pharmacological treatment regimens for uncomplicated NMS.

If a patient requires antipsychotic drug treatment after recovery from NMS, the potential reintroduction of drug therapy should be carefully considered. The patient should be carefully monitored, since recurrence of NMS has been reported.

Tardive Dyskinesia (TD): A syndrome of potentially irreversible, involuntary, dyskinetic movements may develop in patients treated with antipsychotic drugs. Although TD appears to be most prevalent in the elderly, especially elderly females, it is impossible to predict at the onset of treatment which patients are likely to develop TD. It has been suggested that the occurrence of parkinsonian side effects is a predictor for the development of TD.

The risk of developing TD and the likelihood that it will become irreversible are believed to increase as the duration of treatment and the total cumulative dose of antipsychotic drugs administered to the patient increase. However, the syndrome can develop, although much less commonly, after relatively brief treatment periods at low doses. There is no known treatment for established cases of TD. The syndrome may remit, partially or completely, if antipsychotic treatment is withdrawn. However, antipsychotic treatment itself may suppress the signs and symptoms of TD, thereby masking the underlying process. The effect of symptom suppression upon the long-term course of TD is unknown.

In view of these considerations, INVEGA should be prescribed in a manner that is most likely to minimize the risk of TD. As with any antipsychotic, INVEGA should generally be reserved for patients who appear to be obtaining substantial benefit from the drug. In such patients, the smallest dose and the shortest duration of treatment should be sought. The need for continued treatment should be reassessed periodically.

If signs and symptoms of TD develop during treatment with INVEGA, withdrawal of the drug should be considered. However, some patients may require treatment with INVEGA despite the presence of the syndrome.

Potential Effect on Cognitive and Motor Performance: Somnolence, sedation and blurred vision were reported in subjects treated with INVEGA (see Adverse Reactions). Antipsychotics, including INVEGA, have the potential to impair judgment, thinking, or motor skills. Patients should be cautioned about performing activities requiring mental alertness, such as operating hazardous machinery or operating a motor vehicle, until they are reasonably certain that paliperidone therapy does not adversely affect them.

Seizures: Antipsychotic drugs are known to lower the seizure threshold. During premarketing clinical trials (the three placebo-controlled, 6-week, fixed-dose studies and a study conducted in elderly schizophrenic subjects), the number of reports of seizures was similar between subjects treated with INVEGA (3, 6, 9, 12 mg, 0.22%) and subjects treated with placebo (0.25%). As with other antipsychotic drugs, INVEGA should be used cautiously in patients with a history of seizures or other conditions that potentially lower the seizure threshold.

Parkinson's Disease and Dementia with Lewy Bodies: Physicians should weigh the risks versus the benefits when prescribing antipsychotic drugs, including INVEGA, to patients with Parkinson's disease or dementia with Lewy bodies (DLB) since both groups may be at increased risk of neuroleptic malignant syndrome as well as having an increased sensitivity to antipsychotic medications. Manifestation of this increased sensitivity can include confusion, obtundation, postural instability with frequent falls, in addition to extrapyramidal symptoms.

Psychiatric: Suicide: The possibility of suicide or attempted suicide is inherent in psychosis, and thus, close supervision and appropriate clinical management of high-risk patients should accompany drug therapy.

Renal: The dose should be reduced in patients with moderate to severe renal impairment (see Dosage and Administration). The disposition of paliperidone was studied in subjects with varying degrees of renal function. Elimination of paliperidone decreased with decreasing creatinine clearance. Total clearance of paliperidone was reduced in subjects with impaired renal function by 32% in mild (CrCl=50 to <80 mL/min), 64% in moderate (CrCl=30 to <50 mL/min), and 71% in severe (CrCl=10 to <30 mL/min) renal impairment. The mean terminal elimination half-life of paliperidone was 24, 40, and 51 hours in subjects with mild, moderate, and severe renal impairment, respectively, compared with 23 hours in subjects with normal renal function (CrCl ≥80 mL/min). INVEGA has not been studied in subjects with creatinine clearance <10 mL/min.

Special Populations: Pregnant Women: The safety of INVEGA during pregnancy has not been established. No teratogenic effect was noted in any animal study. Laboratory animals treated with a high dose of paliperidone showed a slight increase in fetal deaths. This high dose was toxic to the mothers. The offspring were not affected at exposures 20- to 34-fold the maximum human exposure. INVEGA should only be used if the benefits outweigh the risks. The effect of INVEGA on labour and delivery in humans is unknown.

Use of antipsychotic drugs during the last trimester of pregnancy has been associated with reversible extrapyramidal symptoms in the neonate.

Nursing Women: In animal studies with paliperidone and in human studies with risperidone, paliperidone was excreted in the milk. Patients should be advised not to breast-feed an infant if they are taking INVEGA.

Pediatrics (<18 years of age): The safety and efficacy of INVEGA in children under the age of 18 years have not been established.

Geriatrics (>65 years of age): The number of patients 65 years of age or older exposed to INVEGA during a placebo-controlled clinical trial in elderly subjects receiving flexible doses (3-12 mg/day) was limited (n=76). In general, the types and frequencies of adverse events reported in these subjects in this study were similar to those reported in the younger population of adult subjects studied in three placebo-controlled, 6-week, fixed-dose trials. Based on the limited data and consistent with general clinical practice, a greater sensitivity of older individuals to adverse events, including cardiac events, cannot be ruled out.

Because elderly subjects may have diminished renal function, dose adjustments may be required according to their renal function status (see Renal and Dosage and Administration).

Use in Geriatric Patients with Dementia: Overall Mortality: In a meta-analysis of 13 controlled clinical trials, elderly patients with dementia treated with other atypical antipsychotic drugs had an increased risk of mortality compared to placebo. INVEGA is not indicated for the treatment of elderly patients with dementia.

Cerebrovascular Adverse Events (CVAEs) in Elderly Patients With Dementia: In placebo-controlled trials in elderly patients with dementia treated with some atypical antipsychotic drugs, including risperidone and olanzapine, there was a higher incidence of cerebrovascular adverse events (cerebrovascular accidents and transient ischemic attacks) including fatalities compared to placebo. INVEGA is not indicated for the treatment of elderly patients with dementia.

Dysphagia: Esophageal dysmotility and aspiration have been associated with antipsychotic drug use. Aspiration pneumonia is a common cause of morbidity and mortality in patients with advanced Alzheimer's dementia. INVEGA and other antipsychotic drugs should be used cautiously in patients at risk for aspiration pneumonia.

ADVERSE REACTIONS: Clinical Trial Adverse Drug Reactions: Because clinical trials are conducted under very specific conditions the adverse reaction rates observed in the clinical trials may not reflect the rates observed in practice and should not be compared to the rates in the clinical trials of another drug. Adverse drug reaction information from clinical trials is useful for identifying drug-related adverse events and for approximating rates.

Short-Term, Placebo-Controlled, Fixed-Dose Studies: The information presented in this section was derived from pooled data from three placebo-controlled, 6-week, fixed-dose studies conducted in non-elderly (mean age 38 years) patients with schizophrenia. The doses studied among these three trials included 3, 6, 9, 12, and 15 mg/day. Body systems and adverse event/adverse drug reaction (ADR) terms are based on the MedDRA dictionary.

Adverse Events Associated with Discontinuation of Treatment: Overall, there was no difference in the incidence of discontinuation due to adverse events between patients who received INVEGA (5%) and placebo-treated patients (5%). The types of adverse events that led to discontinuation were similar between patients treated with INVEGA and placebo-treated patients, except for Nervous System Disorders (2% and 0%, respectively) and Gastrointestinal Disorders (1% and 0%, respectively) which were of greater incidence among patients treated with INVEGA than placebo-treated patients, and Psychiatric Disorders which were of greater incidence among placebo-treated patients than patients treated with INVEGA (3% and 1%, respectively).

Commonly Observed Adverse Drug Reactions: Table 1 enumerates all treatment-emergent adverse events, regardless of causality, reported at an incidence of ≥1% of patients treated with INVEGA in these studies, and for which the incidence in patients treated with INVEGA was greater than the incidence in patients treated with placebo.

The most frequently reported ADRs, reported by ≥2% of patients treated with INVEGA, included: headache (13.2%; placebo 11.8%), tachycardia (6.6%; placebo 2.8%), akathisia (6.5%; placebo 3.9%), sinus tachycardia (5.5%; placebo 4.2%), extrapyramidal disorder (5.4%; placebo 2.3%), somnolence (4.9%; placebo 3.4%), dizziness (4.8%; placebo 3.9%), sedation (4.2%; placebo 3.7%), tremor (3.4%; placebo 3.4%), hypertonia (2.8%; placebo 1.1%), dystonia (2.6%; placebo 0.6%), orthostatic hypotension (2.5%; placebo 0.8%), and dry mouth (2.4%; placebo 0.6%).

Dose-Related Adverse Reactions: Based on the pooled data from the three placebo-controlled, 6-week, fixed-dose studies, among the adverse reactions that occurred with a greater than 2% incidence in the subjects treated with INVEGA, the incidences of the following adverse reactions increased with dose: somnolence, orthostatic hypotension, akathisia, dystonia, extrapyramidal disorder, hypertonia, Parkinsonism, and salivary hypersecretion. For most of these, the increased incidence was seen primarily at the 12 mg dose, and, in some cases, the 9 mg dose.

Elderly: The number of patients 65 years of age or older exposed to INVEGA during a placebo-controlled clinical trial in elderly subjects receiving flexible doses (3-12 mg/day) was limited (n=76). In general, the types and frequencies of adverse events reported in these subjects in this study were similar to those reported in the younger population of adult subjects studied in three placebo-controlled, 6-week, fixed-dose trials. Based on the limited data and consistent with general clinical practice, a greater sensitivity of older individuals to adverse events, including cardiac events, cannot be ruled out.

Extrapyramidal Symptoms (EPS): Pooled data from the three placebo-controlled, 6-week, fixed-dose studies provided information regarding treatment-emergent EPS. Several methods were used to measure EPS: (1) the Simpson-Angus global score, (2) the Barnes Akathisia Rating Scale global clinical rating score, (3) use of anticholinergic medications to treat emergent EPS, and (4) incidence of spontaneous reports of EPS. For the Simpson-Angus Scale, spontaneous EPS reports and use of anticholinergic medications, there was a dose-related increase observed for the 9 mg and 12 mg doses. There was no difference observed between placebo and INVEGA 3 mg and 6 mg doses for any of these EPS measures. See Table 2 and Table 3.

Table 1: INVEGA

Treatment-Emergent Adverse Events, Regardless of Causality, Reported by ≥1% of Patients with Schizophrenia in Any INVEGA Group and Which Occurred at Greater Incidence Than in the Placebo Group in the Three Placebo-Controlled, 6-Week, Double-Blind, Fixed-Dose Clinical Trials. (Safety Analysis Set)

Body System or Organ Class Dictionary-derived Term	Placebo (N=355) %	INVEGA 3 mg (N=127) %	INVEGA 6 mg (N=235) %	INVEGA 9 mg (N=246) %	INVEGA 12 mg (N=242) %
Cardiac Disorders					
Atrioventricular block first degree	1	2	0	2	1
Bradycardia	1	0	1	1	2
Bundle branch block	2	3	1	3	<1
Palpitations	0	2	1	0	1
Sinus arrhythmia	0	2	1	1	<1
Sinus tachycardia	4	9	4	4	7
Tachycardia	3	2	7	7	7
Eye Disorders					
Dry eye	0	2	0	<1	<1
Oculogyration	0	0	0	2	0
Vision blurred	1	1	<1	0	2
Gastrointestinal Disorders					
Abdominal pain	1	0	2	1	1
Abdominal pain upper	1	1	3	2	2
Diarrhea	2	1	1	1	2
Dry mouth	1	2	3	1	3
Dyspepsia	4	2	3	2	5
Nausea	5	6	4	4	4
Salivary hypersecretion	<1	0	<1	1	4
Stomach discomfort	<1	2	1	<1	1
Toothache	1	2	2	2	2
Vomiting	5	2	3	4	5
General Disorders and Administration Site Conditions					
Asthenia	1	2	<1	2	2
Fatigue	1	2	1	2	2
Pyrexia	1	1	<1	2	2
Infections and Infestations					
Bronchitis	<1	0	1	<1	1
Nasopharyngitis	3	3	2	2	2
Rhinitis	<1	0	1	0	<1
Upper respiratory tract infection	1	1	1	1	1
Viral infection	<1	0	<1	1	1
Injury, Poisoning and Procedural Complications					
Fall	<1	0	1	0	0
Investigations					
Alanine aminotransferase increased	1	1	2	1	1
Blood creatine phosphokinase increased	1	1	2	0	<1
Blood insulin increased	1	2	1	1	<1
Blood pressure increased	1	2	<1	<1	1
Blood triglycerides increased	<1	2	<1	0	0
Electrocardiogram QT corrected interval prolonged	3	3	4	3	5
Electrocardiogram T wave abnormal	1	2	1	2	1

(cont'd)

Table 1: INVEGA *(cont'd)*

Treatment-Emergent Adverse Events, Regardless of Causality, Reported by ≥1% of Patients with Schizophrenia in Any INVEGA Group and Which Occurred at Greater Incidence Than in the Placebo Group in the Three Placebo-Controlled, 6-Week, Double-Blind, Fixed-Dose Clinical Trials. (Safety Analysis Set)

Body System or Organ Class Dictionary-derived Term	Placebo (N=355) %	INVEGA 3 mg (N=127) %	INVEGA 6 mg (N=235) %	INVEGA 9 mg (N=246) %	INVEGA 12 mg (N=242) %
Electrocardiogram T wave inversion	1	0	<1	1	1
Electrocardiogram abnormal	0	0	0	2	1
Heart rate increased	1	3	1	<1	1
Insulin C-peptide increased	1	2	1	1	0
Weight decreased	1	2	0	0	0
Weight increased	1	1	0	2	2
Metabolism and Nutrition Disorders					
Decreased appetite	0	2	<1	<1	1
Increased appetite	<1	2	0	1	1
Musculoskeletal and Connective Tissue Disorders					
Arthralgia	1	0	2	1	0
Back pain	1	1	1	1	2
Muscle rigidity	0	1	0	1	<1
Neck pain	<1	0	0	0	1
Pain in extremity	1	0	1	0	2
Shoulder pain	0	1	1	1	1
Nervous System Disorders					
Akathisia	4	4	3	8	10
Dizziness	4	6	5	4	5
Dyskinesia	1	0	<1	<1	2
Dystonia	1	1	1	4	4
Extrapyramidal disorder	2	5	2	7	7
Headache	12	11	12	14	14
Hypertonia	1	2	1	4	3
Parkinsonism	0	0	<1	2	1
Sedation	4	1	5	3	6
Somnolence	3	5	3	7	5
Syncope	<1	1	1	1	<1
Tremor	3	3	3	4	3
Psychiatric Disorders					
Aggression	1	2	<1	1	1
Anxiety	8	9	7	6	5
Depression	<1	0	1	<1	<1
Nightmare	0	0	<1	1	<1
Suicidal ideation	1	2	1	<1	<1
Respiratory, Thoracic and Mediastinal Disorders					
Cough	1	3	2	3	2
Nasal congestion	1	1	1	1	1
Skin and Subcutaneous Tissue Disorders					
Pruritus	1	0	1	1	0
Vascular Disorders					
Hypotension	<1	2	<1	1	1
Orthostatic hypotension	1	2	1	2	4

Table 2: INVEGA
Results of Extrapyramidal Symptoms (EPS) Studies

EPS Group	Percentage of Patients				
		INVEGA			
	Placebo (N=355)	3 mg once daily (N=127)	6 mg once daily (N=235)	9 mg once daily (N=246)	12 mg once daily (N=242)
Parkinsonism[a]	9	11	3	15	14
Akathisia[b]	6	6	4	7	9
Use of anticholinergic medications[c]	10	10	9	22	22

[a] For Parkinsonism, percent of patients with Simpson-Angus global score >0.3 (Global score defined as total sum of items score divided by the number of items).
[b] For Akathisia, percent of patients with Barnes Akathisia Rating Scale global score ≥2.
[c] Percent of patients who received anticholinergic medications to treat emergent EPS.

Table 3: INVEGA
Results of Extrapyramidal Symptoms (EPS) Studies

EPS Group	Percentage of Patients				
		INVEGA			
	Placebo (N=355)	3 mg once daily (N=127)	6 mg once daily (N=235)	9 mg once daily (N=246)	12 mg once daily (N=242)
Overall percentage of patients with EPS-related AE	11.0	12.6	10.2	25.2	26.0
Dyskinesia	3.4	4.7	2.6	7.7	8.7
Dystonia	1.1	0.8	1.3	5.3	4.5
Hyperkinesia	3.9	3.9	3.0	8.1	9.9
Parkinsonism	2.3	3.1	2.6	7.3	6.2
Tremor	3.4	3.1	2.6	4.5	3.3

Dyskinesia group includes: Dyskinesia, Extrapyramidal disorder, Muscle twitching, Tardive dyskinesia.
Dystonia group includes: Dystonia, Muscle spasms, Oculogyration, Trismus.
Hyperkinesia group includes: Akathisia, Hyperkinesia.
Parkinsonism group includes: Bradykinesia, Cogwheel rigidity, Drooling, Hypertonia, Hypokinesia, Muscle rigidity, Musculoskeletal stiffness, Parkinsonism.
Tremor group includes: Tremor.

Weight Gain: In the pooled data from the three placebo-controlled, 6-week, fixed-dose studies, the proportions of patients meeting a weight gain criterion of ≥7% of body weight were compared, revealing a similar incidence of weight gain for INVEGA 3 mg and 6 mg (7% and 6%, respectively) compared with placebo (5%), and a higher incidence of weight gain for INVEGA 9 mg and 12 mg (9% and 9%, respectively).

ECG Changes: In the pooled data from the three placebo-controlled, 6-week, fixed-dose studies, between-group comparisons revealed no clinically important differences between INVEGA and placebo in the incidence of ECG parameters outside clinically important limits, with the exception of heart rate. Compared with placebo (23%), a higher percentage of subjects treated with INVEGA (36% , 3, 6, 9, 12 mg) had heart rate values ≥100 bpm.

Abnormal Hematologic and Clinical Chemistry Findings: In the pooled data from the three placebo-controlled, 6-week, fixed-dose studies, a between-group comparison revealed no medically important differences between INVEGA and placebo in the proportions of subjects experiencing potentially clinically significant changes in routine serum chemistry, hematology, or urinalysis parameters. Similarly, there were no differences between INVEGA and placebo in the incidence of discontinuations due to changes in hematology, urinalysis, or serum chemistry, including mean changes from baseline in fasting glucose, insulin, c-peptide, triglyceride, HDL, LDL, and total cholesterol measurements. However, INVEGA was associated with increases in serum prolactin (see Warnings and Precautions, Endocrine and Metabolism). Maximum mean increases of serum prolactin concentrations were generally observed on Day 15 of treatment (first post-baseline measurement), and remained above baseline levels at study endpoint. The incidence of potentially prolactin-related adverse events was small and similar to that for placebo.

Clinical Trial Adverse Drug Reactions in Short-Term, Placebo-Controlled, Fixed-Dose Studies: The following ADRs, where a causal relationship is suspected between the drug and the reported event, were reported in patients treated with INVEGA (n=850) in the three placebo-controlled, 6-week, double-blind, fixed-dose clinical trials in patients with schizophrenia. The following terms and frequencies were applied: very common (≥10%), common (frequent) (≥1% to <10%), uncommon (infrequent) (≥0.1% to <1%), rare (≥0.01% to <0.1%), and very rare (<0.01%). The majority of ADRs were mild to moderate in severity.

Cardiac Disorders: common: atrioventricular block first degree, bradycardia, sinus tachycardia, tachycardia, bundle branch block; uncommon: palpitations, sinus arrhythmia.

Eye Disorders: uncommon: oculogyration.

Gastrointestinal Disorders: common: abdominal pain upper, dry mouth, salivary hypersecretion, vomiting.

General Disorders: common: asthenia, fatigue; uncommon: edema.

Immune System Disorders: uncommon: anaphylactic reaction.

Investigations: common: weight increased; uncommon: electrocardiogram abnormal.

Metabolism and Nutrition Disorders: uncommon: increased appetite.

Musculoskeletal and Connective Tissue Disorders: uncommon: muscle rigidity.

Nervous System Disorders: very common: headache; common: akathisia, dizziness, dystonia, extrapyramidal disorder, hypertonia, Parkinsonism, sedation, somnolence, tremor; uncommon: dizziness postural, dyskinesia, grand mal convulsion, syncope.

Psychiatric Disorders: uncommon: nightmare.

Reproductive System and Breast Disorders: uncommon: amenorrhea, breast discharge, erectile dysfunction, galactorrhea, gynecomastia, menstruation irregular.

Vascular Disorders: common: orthostatic hypotension; uncommon: hypotension, ischemia.

Adverse Drug Reactions in a Long-term, Placebo-Controlled Study : The safety of INVEGA was also evaluated in a longer-term trial in adults with schizophrenia. In general, the types, frequencies, and severities of ADRs reported during the initial 14-week open-label phase of this study were comparable to those reported in the 6-week, placebo-controlled, fixed-dose studies. The ADRs reported during the longer-term double-blind phase of this study were similar in type and severity to those observed in the initial 14-week open-label phase, but occurred at generally lower frequencies.

Post-Market Adverse Drug Reactions: Adverse events first identified as ADRs during postmarketing experience with INVEGA are included in Table 4. The frequencies are provided according to the following convention: very common ≥1/10, common ≥1/100 to <1/10, uncommon ≥1/1000 to <1/100, rare ≥1/10 000 to <1/1000, very rare <1/10 000, including isolated reports.

Table 4: INVEGA
Adverse Drug Reactions Identified During Postmarketing Experience with INVEGA by Frequency Category Estimated from Spontaneous Reporting Rates

Reproductive System and Breast Disorders	
Very rare	Priapism

Safety Information Reported with Risperidone: Paliperidone is the major active metabolite of risperidone. The release profile and pharmacokinetic characteristics of INVEGA are considerably different than those observed with oral immediate-release risperidone formulations (see Action and Clinical Pharmacology), however, the receptor binding profile of paliperidone is very similar to that of the parent compound. Safety information reported with risperidone in clinical trials and postmarketing experience that may be relevant to INVEGA can be found in local labelling for risperidone.

DRUG INTERACTIONS: Drug-Drug Interactions: Caution is advised when prescribing INVEGA with drugs known to prolong the QT interval.

Potential for INVEGA to Affect Other Drugs: Paliperidone is not expected to cause clinically important pharmacokinetic interactions with drugs that are metabolized by cytochrome P-450 isozymes. In vitro studies in human liver microsomes showed that paliperidone does not substantially inhibit the metabolism of drugs metabolized by cytochrome P450 isozymes, including CYP1A2, CYP2A6, CYP2C8/9/10, CYP2D6, CYP2E1, CYP3A4, and CYP3A5. Therefore, paliperidone is not expected to inhibit clearance of drugs that are metabolized by these metabolic pathways in a clinically relevant manner. Paliperidone is also not expected to have enzyme-inducing properties.

A population pharmacokinetic analysis to evaluate the influence of predicted CYP2D6 phenotype on exposure indicated that no adjustment in the paliperidone dose on the basis of predicted phenotype is warranted.

Paliperidone is a weak inhibitor of P-glycoprotein (P-gp) at high concentrations. No in vivo data are available and the clinical relevance of this with respect to P-gp mediated transport of other drugs is unknown.

Given the primary CNS effects of paliperidone (see Adverse Reactions), INVEGA should be used with caution in combination with other centrally acting drugs and alcohol. Paliperidone may antagonize the effect of levodopa and other dopamine agonists.

Because of its potential for inducing orthostatic hypotension (see Warnings and Precautions, Cardiovascular), an additive effect may be observed when INVEGA is administered with other therapeutic agents that have this potential.

Potential for Other Drugs to Affect INVEGA: Paliperidone is not a substrate of CYP1A2, CYP2A6, CYP2C9, CYP2C19, and CYP3A5. This suggests that an interaction with inhibitors or inducers of these isozymes is unlikely.

While in vitro studies indicate that CYP2D6 and CYP3A4 may be minimally involved in paliperidone metabolism, there are no indications in vitro nor in vivo that these isozymes play a significant role in the metabolism of paliperidone (see Action and Clinical Pharmacology, Pharmacokinetics).

In an interaction study in healthy subjects in which INVEGA was administered concomitantly with paroxetine, a potent CYP2D6 inhibitor, no clinically relevant effects on the pharmacokinetics of paliperidone were observed.

Carbamazepine and Other Potent CYP3A4 Inducers: Co-administration of INVEGA once daily with carbamazepine 200 mg twice daily caused a decrease of approximately 37% in the mean steady-state Cmax and AUC of paliperidone. As is typical of CYP3A4 inducers, carbamazepine is also a P-glycoprotein (P-gp) inducer. Although in-vitro studies have shown that paliperidone is a substrate of both P-gp and CYP3A4, the relative contributions of P-gp and CYP3A4 to changes in the pharmacokinetic parameters are unclear.

On initiation of carbmazepine, the dose of INVEGA should be re-evaluated and increased if necessary. Conversely, on discontinuation of carbamazepine, the dose of INVEGA should be re-evaluated and decreased if necessary. Until more data are available, these recommendation should be extended to other potent CYP3A4 inducers and/or P-glycoprotein upregulators.

Paliperidone, a cation under physiological pH, is primarily excreted unchanged by the kidneys, approximately half via filtration and half via active secretion. Concomitant administration of trimethoprim, a drug known to inhibit active renal cation drug transport, did not influence the pharmacokinetics of paliperidone.

Concomitant Use of INVEGA with Risperidone: Since paliperidone (9-hydroxy-risperidone) is the major active metabolite of risperidone, concomitant use of INVEGA with oral risperidone is not recommended since the combination of the two will lead to additive paliperidone exposure.

Drug-Food Interactions: Following administration of a single 12 mg paliperidone extended-release tablet to healthy ambulatory subjects with a standard high-fat/high-caloric meal, the mean C_{max} and AUC values of paliperidone increased by 60% and 54%, respectively, compared with administration under fasting conditions. Although the presence or absence of food at the time of administration of INVEGA may increase or decrease exposure to paliperidone, these changes are not considered clinically relevant. Clinical trials establishing the safety and efficacy of INVEGA were carried out in subjects without regard to the timing of meals.

Drug-Herb Interactions: Interactions with herbal products have not been established.

Drug-Laboratory Test Interactions: Interactions with laboratory tests have not been established.

Drug-Lifestyle Interactions: Smoking: No dosage adjustment is recommended based on smoking status. Based on in vitro studies utilizing human liver enzymes, paliperidone is not a substrate for CYP1A2; smoking should, therefore, not have an effect on the pharmacokinetics of paliperidone. Consistent with these in vitro results, population pharmacokinetic evaluation has not revealed any differences between smokers and non-smokers.

DOSAGE AND ADMINISTRATION: Dosing Considerations:

- Since paliperidone (9-hydroxy-risperidone) is the major active metabolite of risperidone, concomitant use of INVEGA with oral risperidone is not recommended since the combination of the two will lead to additive paliperidone exposure.
- INVEGA should be administered orally once daily, preferably in the morning, without regard to meals. Clinical trials establishing the safety and efficacy of INVEGA were carried out in patients without regard to food intake. INVEGA must be swallowed whole with the aid of liquids, and must not be chewed, divided, or crushed. The medication is contained within a nonabsorbable shell designed to release the drug at a controlled rate. The tablet shell, along with insoluble core components, is eliminated from the body; patients should not be concerned if they occasionally notice something that looks like a tablet in their stool.

Recommended Dose and Dosage Adjustment: Adult: The recommended starting and target dose of INVEGA is 6 mg once daily. No initial dose titration is required. However, in some cases a lower dose of 3 mg/day may be sufficient.

In clinical trials a dose range of 3 to 12 mg/day was studied and while efficacy was observed across all doses, there was a dose-related increase in adverse effects (see Adverse Reactions).

Dose adjustments should be made after clinical reassessment and generally should occur at intervals of more than 5 days. When dose adjustments are indicated, small increments/decrements of 3 mg/day are recommended, up to a maximum of 12 mg/day.

Patients with Hepatic Impairment : No dose adjustment is required in patients with mild to moderate hepatic impairment. INVEGA has not been studied in patients with severe hepatic impairment.

Patients with Renal Impairment: For patients with mild renal impairment (creatinine clearance=50 to <80 mL/min), the maximum recommended initial dose is 3 mg once daily. The dose may be increased to a maximum of 6 mg once daily based on clinical response and tolerability.

For patients with moderate to severe renal impairment (creatinine clearance=10 to <50 mL/min), the recommended initial dose of INVEGA is 1.5 mg once daily which may then be increased to 3 mg once daily after clinical reassessment.

As INVEGA has not been studied in patients with creatinine clearance <10 mL/min, use is not recommended in such patients.

Elderly: Dosing recommendations for elderly patients with normal renal function (≥80 mL/min) are the same as for adults with normal renal function. However, because elderly patients may have diminished renal function, dose adjustments may be required according to their renal function status (see Patients with Renal Impairment).

Pediatrics: Safety and effectiveness of INVEGA in patients <18 years of age have not been studied.

Other Special Populations: No dose adjustment for INVEGA is recommended based on gender, race, or smoking status.

OVERDOSAGE:

Symptoms: In general, expected signs and symptoms are those resulting from an exaggeration of paliperidone's known pharmacological effects, i.e., drowsiness and sedation, tachycardia and hypotension, QT prolongation, and extrapyramidal symptoms. In the case of acute overdosage, the possibility of multiple drug involvement should be considered.

Treatment: Consideration should be given to the extended-release nature of the product when assessing treatment needs and recovery. There is no specific antidote to paliperidone. General supportive measures should be employed. Establish and maintain a clear airway and ensure adequate oxygenation and ventilation. Cardiovascular monitoring should commence immediately and should include continuous electrocardiographic monitoring for possible arrhythmias. Hypotension and circulatory collapse should be treated with appropriate measures such as intravenous fluid and/or sympathomimetic agents. Gastric lavage (after intubation if the patient is unconscious) and administration of activated charcoal together with a laxative should be considered. In case of severe extrapyramidal symptoms, anticholinergic agents should be administered. Close supervision and monitoring should continue until the patient recovers.

> For management of a suspected drug overdose, CPhA recommends that you contact your **regional Poison Control Centre**. See the *CPS* Directory section for a list of Poison Control Centres.

ACTION AND CLINICAL PHARMACOLOGY: Mechanism of Action: Paliperidone is a centrally active dopamine D_2 antagonist with predominant serotonergic 5-HT_{2A} antagonistic activity. Paliperidone is also active as an antagonist at α_1 and α_2 adrenergic receptors and H_1 histaminergic receptors. Paliperidone has no affinity for cholinergic muscarinic or β_1- and β_2-adrenergic receptors. The pharmacological activity of the (+)- and (−)-paliperidone enantiomers is qualitatively and quantitatively similar.

The mechanism of action of paliperidone, as with other drugs having efficacy in schizophrenia, is unknown. However, it has been proposed that the drug's therapeutic activity in schizophrenia is mediated through a combination of dopamine Type 2 (D_2) and serotonin Type 2 (5HT_{2A}) receptor antagonism. Antagonism at receptors other than D_2 and 5HT_{2A} may explain some of the other effects of paliperidone.

Pharmacodynamics: Formulation Characteristics : The controlled rate of release of paliperidone from the extended-release technology results in a pharmacokinetic profile with a slower rate of absorption than an immediate-release formulation, leading to an ascending plasma concentration profile over 24 hours on Day 1 of dosing. In studies with paliperidone and risperidone, an ascending profile paliperidone formulation concept demonstrated a differential effect on orthostatic hypotension compared to a flat or immediate-release profile. In one study (n=27), paliperidone administered to achieve an ascending profile with a total dose of 4 mg compared to a lower dose (2 mg) of immediate release risperidone resulted in lower incidences of orthostatic hypotension (32% vs. 46%). The extended-release profile showed a lower incidence of orthostatic hypotension and allows for initiation of treatment at an effective dose without titration, as is the typical practice with antipsychotic drugs to address initial orthostatic intolerance.

Pharmacokinetics: Following a single dose, the plasma concentrations of paliperidone steadily rise to reach peak plasma concentration (C_{max}) in approximately 24 hours after dosing. The pharmacokinetics of paliperidone following INVEGA administration are dose-proportional within the available dose range. The terminal elimination half-life of paliperidone, regardless of formulation, is approximately 23 hours.

Steady-state concentrations of paliperidone are attained within 4-5 days of dosing in most subjects. The release characteristics of INVEGA result in minimal peak-trough fluctuations as compared to those observed with immediate-release risperidone. In a study comparing the steady-state pharmacokinetics following once-daily administration of 12 mg paliperidone (administered as extended-release tablets) with 4 mg immediate-release risperidone in schizophrenic subjects, the fluctuation indexes were 38% for paliperidone extended-release compared to 125% for risperidone immediate-release (Figure 1).

Figure 1: INVEGA

Steady-State Concentration Profile Following Administration of 12 mg Paliperidone Administered as Six 2 mg Extended-release Tablets Once Daily for 6 Days (Paliperidone Concentrations are Represented) Compared with Risperidone Immediate-release Administered as 2 mg Once Daily on Day 1 and 4 mg Once Daily On Days 2 to 6 (Paliperidone+Risperidone Concentrations are Represented)

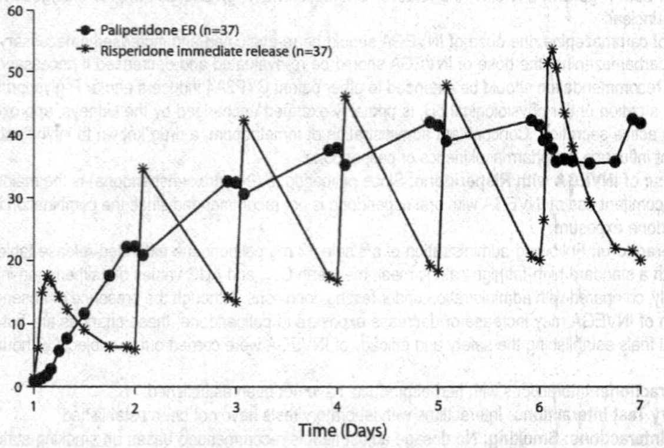

Following administration of INVEGA, the (+) and (−) enantiomers of paliperidone interconvert, reaching an AUC (+) to (−) ratio of approximately 1.6 at steady state.

Absorption: The absolute oral bioavailability of paliperidone from INVEGA (i.e., the extended release formulation) is 28%. It is thought that this is due to a higher fraction of paliperidone being released in the colon, where absorption is lower.

Following administration of a single 12 mg paliperidone extended-release tablet to healthy ambulatory subjects with a standard high-fat/high-caloric meal, the mean C_{max} and AUC values of paliperidone increased by 60% and 54%, respectively, compared with administration under fasting conditions. Although the presence or absence of food at the time of INVEGA administration may increase or decrease exposure to paliperidone, these changes are not considered clinically relevant. Clinical trials establishing the safety and efficacy of INVEGA were carried out in subjects without regard to the timing of meals (see Dosage and Administration).

Distribution: Paliperidone is rapidly distributed. The apparent volume of distribution is 487 L. The plasma protein binding of paliperidone is 74%. It binds primarily to α_1-acid glycoprotein and albumin. In vitro, high therapeutic concentrations of diazepam (3 μg/mL), sulfamethazine (100 μg/mL), warfarin (10 μg/mL), and carbamazepine (10 μg/mL) caused a slight increase in the free fraction of paliperidone at 50 ng/mL. These changes are not expected to be of clinical significance.

Metabolism and Excretion: The following data are based on a human mass balance study using oral solution of ^{14}C-paliperidone, a dosage form which has approximately 100% bioavailability. One week following administration of a single 1 mg dose of oral solution ^{14}C-paliperidone, 59% of the administered dose was excreted unchanged into urine, indicating that paliperidone is not extensively metabolized in the liver. Approximately 80% of the administered radioactivity was recovered in urine and 11% in the feces.

Four metabolic pathways have been identified in vivo, of which each accounted for no more than 6.5% of the administered dose: dealkylation, hydroxylation, dehydrogenation, and benzisoxazole scission. In vitro studies suggested a role for CYP2D6 and CYP3A4 in the metabolism of paliperidone; however, in vivo results indicate that these isozymes play a very limited role in the metabolism of paliperidone. Despite the large variation in the general population with regard to the ability to metabolize CYP2D6 substrates, population pharmacokinetic analyses indicated no discernable difference on the exposure and apparent clearance of paliperidone after administration of INVEGA between extensive metabolizers and poor metabolizers of CYP2D6 substrates. In vitro studies using microsomal preparations of heterologous systems indicate that CYP1A2, CYP2A6, CYP2C9, CYP2C19, and CYP3A5 are not involved in the metabolism of paliperidone. Paliperidone is not expected to have enzyme-inducing properties.

Special Populations and Conditions: Pediatrics: No data available.

Geriatrics: No dosage adjustment is recommended based on age alone. However, because elderly subjects may have diminished renal function, dose adjustments may be required according to their renal function status (see Renal Insufficiency). Data from a pharmacokinetic study in elderly subjects (≥65 years of age, n=26) indicated that the apparent steady-state clearance of paliperidone following INVEGA administration was 20% lower compared to that of adult subjects (18-45 years of age, n=28). However, there was no discernable effect of age in the population pharmacokinetic analysis involving schizophrenia subjects after correction for age-related decreases in CrCl.

Gender: No dosage adjustment is recommended based on gender. The apparent clearance of paliperidone following INVEGA administration is approximately 19% lower in women than men. This difference is largely explained by differences in lean body mass and creatinine clearance between men and women, as a population pharmacokinetics evaluation revealed no evidence of clinically significant gender-related differences in the pharmacokinetics of paliperidone following INVEGA administration after correction for lean body mass and creatinine clearance.

Race: No dosage adjustment is recommended based on race. Population pharmacokinetics analysis revealed no evidence of race-related differences in the pharmacokinetics of paliperidone following INVEGA administration.

Hepatic Insufficiency: Paliperidone is not extensively metabolized in the liver. In a study in subjects with moderate hepatic impairment (Child-Pugh class B), the plasma concentrations of unbound paliperidone were similar to those of healthy subjects. No dose adjustment is required in patients with mild to moderate hepatic impairment. INVEGA has not been studied in patients with severe hepatic impairment.

Renal Insufficiency: The dose should be reduced in patients with mild and moderate to severe renal impairment (see Dosage and Administration). The disposition of paliperidone was studied in subjects with varying degrees of renal function. Elimination of paliperidone decreased with decreasing estimated creatinine clearance. Total clearance of paliperidone was reduced in subjects with impaired renal function by 32% in mild (CrCl=50 to <80 mL/min), 64% in moderate (CrCl=30 to <50 mL/min), and 71% in severe (CrCl=10 to <30 mL/min) renal impairment. The mean terminal elimination half-life of paliperidone was 24, 40, and 51 hours in subjects with mild, moderate, and severe renal impairment, respectively, compared with 23 hours in subjects with normal renal function (CrCl ≥80 mL/min). INVEGA has not been studied in subjects with creatinine clearance <10 mL/min.

Smoking Status: No dosage adjustment is recommended based on smoking status. Based on in vitro studies utilizing human liver enzymes, paliperidone is not a substrate for CYP1A2; smoking should, therefore, not have an effect on the pharmacokinetics of paliperidone. Consistent with these in vitro results, population pharmacokinetic evaluation has not revealed any differences between smokers and non-smokers.

STORAGE AND STABILITY: INVEGA should be stored at 15-30°C. Protect from moisture.

Keep out of the reach of children.

INFORMATION FOR THE PATIENT: Published in e-CPS, available by subscription at www.e-cps.ca.

DOSAGE FORMS, COMPOSITION AND PACKAGING: 3 mg: Each white, extended-release, capsule-shaped tablet, printed with "PAL 3", contains: paliperidone 3 mg. Orifices may or may not be visible. Nonmedicinal ingredients: butylated hydroxytoluene, carnauba wax, cellulose acetate, ferric oxide red, ferric oxide yellow, hydroxyethyl cellulose, hypromellose, iron oxide black, lactose monohydrate, polyethylene oxides, polyethylene glycol, propylene glycol, povidone, sodium chloride, stearic acid, titanium dioxide and triacetin. Bottles of 30.

6 mg: Each beige, extended-release, capsule-shaped tablet, printed with "PAL 6", contains: paliperidone 6 mg. Orifices may or may not be visible. Nonmedicinal ingredients: butylated hydroxytoluene, carnauba wax, cellulose acetate, ferric oxide red, ferric oxide yellow, hydroxyethyl cellulose, hypromellose, iron oxide black, polyethylene oxides, polyethylene glycol, propylene glycol, povidone, sodium chloride, stearic acid and titanium dioxide. Bottles of 30.

9 mg: Each pink, extended-release, capsule-shaped tablet, printed with "PAL 9", contains: paliperidone 9 mg. Orifices may or may not be visible. Nonmedicinal ingredients: butylated hydroxytoluene, carnauba wax, cellulose acetate, ferric oxide red, ferric oxide yellow, hydroxyethyl cellulose, hypromellose, iron oxide black, polyethylene oxides, polyethylene glycol, propylene glycol, povidone, sodium chloride, stearic acid and titanium dioxide. Bottles of 30.

System Components and Performance: INVEGA tablets utilize osmotic pressure to deliver paliperidone from the dosage form at a controlled rate. The system, which resembles a capsule-shaped tablet in appearance, comprises an osmotically active trilayer core surrounded by a subcoat and semipermeable membrane. The trilayer core is composed of two drug layers containing the drug and excipients, and a push layer containing osmotically active components. There are two precision laser-drilled orifices on the drug-layer dome of the tablet. Each strength is identified by a unique colour overcoat and print markings. In an aqueous environment, such as the gastrointestinal tract, the water-dispersible colour overcoat erodes quickly. Water is then imbibed through the semi-permeable, rate-controlling membrane. The membrane controls the rate at which water enters the tablet core, which, in turn, controls drug delivery. The hydrophilic polymers of the core hydrate and swell, creating a gel containing paliperidone that is then pushed out through the tablet orifices. The drug release rate from the system is designed to increase with time over a period of approximately 16 to 22 hours due to the drug-concentration gradient incorporated into the two drug layers of INVEGA. The ascending release rate of INVEGA allows patients to receive a therapeutically effective dose of paliperidone without the need for dose titration. The biologically inert components of the tablet remain intact during gastrointestinal transit and are eliminated in the stool, along with insoluble core components.

(Shown in Product Identification Section)

Invega® Sustenna™ Ⓟ

paliperidone palmitate

Antipsychotic

Janssen-Ortho

Date of Preparation: June 29, 2010
Date of Revision: July 21, 2010

SUMMARY PRODUCT INFORMATION:

Route of Administration	Dosage Form/Strength	Nonmedicinal Ingredients
Intramuscular injection	Prolonged-Release Injectable Suspension/supplied as prefilled syringes containing 50 mg/0.5 mL, 75 mg/0.75 mL, 100 mg/1 mL, and 150 mg/1.5 mL paliperidone as paliperidone palmitate	Citric acid monohydrate, disodium hydrogen phosphate anhydrous, polyethylene glycol 4000, polysorbate 20, sodium dihydrogen phosphate monohydrate, sodium hydroxide, water for injection

INDICATIONS AND CLINICAL USE: INVEGA SUSTENNA (paliperidone palmitate) is indicated for the treatment of schizophrenia. In controlled clinical trials, INVEGA SUSTENNA was found to improve the symptoms of schizophrenia, including positive and negative symptoms.

Geriatrics (>65 years of age): See Warnings and Precautions, Boxed Serious Warnings and Precautions and Special Populations.

Pediatrics (<18 years of age): The safety and efficacy of INVEGA SUSTENNA in children under the age of 18 have not been established.

CONTRAINDICATIONS: INVEGA SUSTENNA is contraindicated in patients who are hypersensitive to paliperidone, risperidone, or to any ingredient in the formulation or component of the container.

WARNINGS AND PRECAUTIONS:

> **Serious Warnings and Precautions**
> **Increased Mortality in Elderly Patients with Dementia**
> **Elderly patients with dementia treated with atypical antipsychotic drugs are at an increased risk of death compared to placebo. Analyses of thirteen placebo-controlled trials with various atypical antipsychotics (modal duration of 10 weeks) in these patients showed a mean 1.6-fold increase in the death rate in the drug-treated patients. Although the causes of death were varied, most of the deaths appeared to be either cardiovascular (e.g., heart failure, sudden death) or infectious (e.g., pneumonia) in nature (see Warnings and Precautions, Special Populations, Use in Geriatric Patients with Dementia).**

General: Administration: Care must be taken to avoid inadvertent injection of INVEGA SUSTENNA into a blood vessel.

QT Prolongation: Paliperidone causes a modest increase in the corrected QT (QTc) interval. The use of paliperidone should be avoided in combination with other drugs that are known to prolong QTc including Class 1A (e.g., quinidine, procainamide) or Class III (e.g., amiodarone, sotalol) antiarrhythmic medications, antipsychotic medications (e.g., chlorpromazine, thioridazine), antibiotics (e.g., gatifloxacin, moxifloxacin), or any other class of medications known to prolong the QTc interval. Paliperidone should also be avoided in patients with congenital long QT syndrome and in patients with a history of cardiac arrhythmias.

Certain circumstances may increase the risk of the occurrence of torsades de pointes and/or sudden death in association with the use of drugs that prolong the QTc interval, including (1) bradycardia; (2) hypokalemia or hypomagnesemia; (3) concomitant use of other drugs that prolong the QTc interval; and (4) presence of congenital prolongation of the QT interval.

QT Prolongation Study R076477-SCH-1009: The effects of oral paliperidone on the QT interval were evaluated in a double-blind, active-controlled (moxifloxacin 400 mg single dose), multicentre QT study in adults with schizophrenia and schizoaffective disorder. Serial ECG assessments were scheduled at multiple days and multiple time points during the day. Least square mean changes from baseline in QTcLD were calculated at each scheduled ECG assessment time point and day.

In study R076477-SCH-1009 (n=141), the 8 mg dose of immediate-release oral paliperidone (n=44) showed a maximal (least square) mean change from baseline in QTcLD of 10.9 msec (90% CI:8.24; 13.62) and was noted on day 8 at 1.5 hours post-dose. The mean steady-state peak plasma concentration for this 8 mg dose of paliperidone immediate release ($C_{max\ ss}$=113 ng/mL) was more than 2-fold the exposure predicted for the maximum recommended 150 mg dose of INVEGA SUSTENNA administered in the deltoid muscle (predicted median $C_{max\ ss}$=50 ng/mL).

In this same study, a 4 mg dose of the immediate-release oral formulation of paliperidone ($C_{max\ ss}$=35 ng/mL) showed a maximal (least square) mean change from baseline in QTcLD of 9.3 msec (90% CI: 6.56; 11.98) and was noted on day 2 at 1.5 hours post-dose. None of the subjects had a change exceeding 60 msec or a QTcLD exceeding 500 msec at any time during this study. Also, in this study, a 400 mg dose of moxifloxacin (n=58) showed a maximal least square mean change from baseline in QTcLD of 6.1 msec (90% CI: 3.64; 8.53) and was noted on day 8 at 3 hours post-dose. Placebo (n=58) showed a maximal least square mean change from baseline in QTcLD of 3.5 msec (90% CI: 1.05; 5.95) and was noted on day 2 at 30 minutes post-dose.

In the four fixed-dose, double-blind, placebo-controlled studies of INVEGA SUSTENNA in which 1293 subjects received active drug, no subject experienced a change in QTcLD exceeding 60 msec and no subject had a QTcLD value of >500 msec at any time point. In the long-term study, in which 849 subjects received INVEGA SUSTENNA, no subject had a QTcLD change >60 msec, and one subject had a QTcLD value of 507 msec (Bazett's QT corrected interval [QTcB] value of 483 msec); this latter subject also had a heart rate of 45 beats per minute.

Concomitant Use of INVEGA SUSTENNA with Risperidone or Oral Paliperidone: Concomitant use of INVEGA SUSTENNA with oral paliperidone or oral or injectable risperidone has not been studied. Since paliperidone (9-hydroxy-risperidone) is the major active metabolite of risperidone, concomitant use of INVEGA SUSTENNA with risperidone or oral paliperidone is not recommended since the combination of any of these medications will lead to additive paliperidone exposure.

Body Temperature Regulation: Disruption of the body's ability to reduce core body temperature has been attributed to antipsychotic agents. Appropriate care is advised when prescribing INVEGA SUSTENNA to patients who will be experiencing conditions which may contribute to an elevation in core body temperature, e.g., exercising strenuously, exposure to extreme heat, receiving concomitant medication with anticholinergic activity, or being subject to dehydration.

Cardiovascular: Orthostatic Hypotension: Paliperidone can induce orthostatic hypotension and syncope in some patients because of its alpha-blocking activity. Syncope was reported in <1% (4/1293) of subjects treated with INVEGA SUSTENNA in the recommended dose range of 25 mg-150 mg in the four fixed-dose, double-blind, placebo-controlled trials compared with 0% (0/510) of subjects treated with placebo. In the long-term study, syncope was not reported as an adverse event in the open-label transition/maintenance phases or the subsequent double-blind phase. However, presyncope was reported as an adverse event in one subject (<1% [1/849]) in the open-label transition/maintenance phase and syncope was reported as an adverse event in one subject (<1%) during the open-label extension phase of the study.

In the four fixed-dose, double-blind, placebo-controlled studies, orthostatic hypotension was reported as an adverse event by <1% (2/1293) of INVEGA SUSTENNA-treated subjects. Further, 2% (29/1293) of INVEGA SUSTENNA-treated subjects in the recommended dose range of 25 mg-150 mg and 2% (11/510) of placebo-treated subjects met predefined criteria for orthostatic hypotension based on vital signs measurements.

In the long-term study, there were no reported adverse events of orthostatic hypotension. No more than 1% of INVEGA SUSTENNA-treated subjects met the predefined criteria for orthostatic hypotension based on vital signs measurements (1% [6/849]) during the open-label transition/maintenance phases, <1% [1/205] during the double-blind phase, and 1% [4/388] during the open-label extension phase) compared with 1% (2/203) of placebo-treated subjects in the double-blind phase.

INVEGA SUSTENNA should be used with caution in patients with known cardiovascular disease (e.g., heart failure, history of myocardial infarction or ischemia, conduction abnormalities), cerebrovascular disease, or conditions that predispose the patient to hypotension (e.g., dehydration, hypovolemia). Special care should be taken to avoid hypotension in patients with a history of cerebrovascular insufficiency or ischemic heart disease, and in patients taking medications to lower blood pressure.

Endocrine and Metabolism: Hyperglycemia: Hyperglycemia, in some cases extreme and associated with ketoacidosis or hyperosmolar coma or death, has been reported in patients treated with all atypical antipsychotics. These cases were, for the most part, seen in post-marketing clinical use and epidemiologic studies, and not in clinical trials.

In clinical trials, there have been few reports of hyperglycemia or diabetes (<3%) in subjects treated with INVEGA SUSTENNA.

Assessment of the relationship between atypical antipsychotic use and glucose abnormalities is complicated by the possibility of an increased background risk of diabetes mellitus in patients with schizophrenia and the increasing incidence of diabetes mellitus in the general population. Given these confounders, the relationship between atypical antipsychotic use and hyperglycemia-related adverse events is not completely understood. However, epidemiological studies, which did not include INVEGA SUSTENNA, suggest an increased risk of treatment-emergent hyperglycemia-related adverse events in patients treated with the atypical antipsychotics. Because INVEGA SUSTENNA was not marketed at the time these studies were performed, it is not known if INVEGA SUSTENNA is associated with this increased risk. Precise risk estimates for hyperglycemia-related adverse events in patients treated with atypical antipsychotics are not available.

Any patient treated with atypical antipsychotics should be monitored for symptoms of hyperglycemia including polydipsia, polyuria, polyphagia, and weakness. Patients who develop symptoms of hyperglycemia during treatment with atypical antipsychotics should undergo fasting blood glucose testing. In some cases, hyperglycemia has resolved when the atypical antipsychotic was discontinued; however, some patients required continuation of anti-diabetic treatment despite discontinuation of the suspect drug. Patients with risk factors for diabetes mellitus (e.g., obesity, family history of diabetes) who are starting treatment with atypical antipsychotics should undergo fasting blood glucose testing at the beginning of treatment and periodically during treatment. Patients with an established diagnosis of diabetes mellitus who are started on atypical antipsychotics should be monitored regularly for worsening of glucose control.

Hyperprolactinemia: As with other atypical antipsychotics that antagonize dopamine D_2 receptors, paliperidone elevates prolactin levels and the elevation persists during chronic administration. Paliperidone has a prolactin-elevating effect similar to that seen with risperidone.

Tissue culture experiments indicate that approximately one-third of human breast cancers are prolactin dependent in vitro, a factor of potential importance if the prescription of these drugs is considered in a patient with previously detected breast cancer. Although disturbances such as galactorrhea, amenorrhea, gynecomastia, and impotence have been reported with prolactin-elevating compounds, the clinical significance of elevated serum prolactin levels is unknown for most patients. As is common with dopamine D_2 antagonists, prolonged administration of risperidone in rodent carcinogenicity studies resulted in an increase in the incidence of pituitary gland, mammary gland, and endocrine pancreas hyperplasia and/or tumours. However, neither clinical studies nor epidemiologic studies conducted to date have shown an association between chronic administration of this class of drugs and tumorigenesis in humans; the available evidence is considered too limited to be conclusive at this time. The carcinogenic potential of paliperidone, an active metabolite of risperidone, was assessed based on studies with risperidone conducted in mice and rats.

In the four fixed-dose, double-blind, placebo-controlled studies with INVEGA SUSTENNA (25 mg-150 mg), the proportion of subjects who experienced potentially prolactin-related adverse events was similar for the placebo (1%) and INVEGA SUSTENNA (1-2%) groups.

Gastrointestinal: Antiemetic Effect: An antiemetic effect was observed in preclinical studies with paliperidone. This effect, if it occurs in humans, may mask the signs and symptoms of overdosage with certain drugs or of conditions such as intestinal obstruction, Reye's syndrome, and brain tumour.

Genitourinary: Priapism: Drugs with alpha-adrenergic blocking effects have been reported to induce priapism. Although no cases of priapism have been reported in clinical trials with INVEGA SUSTENNA, priapism has been reported with oral paliperidone during post-marketing surveillance.

Hepatic/Biliary/Pancreatic: Paliperidone is not extensively metabolized in the liver. In a study with oral paliperidone in subjects with moderate hepatic impairment (Child-Pugh class B), the plasma concentrations of unbound paliperidone were similar to those of healthy subjects. No dose adjustment is required in patients with mild to moderate hepatic impairment. The effect of severe hepatic impairment is unknown.

Neurologic: Neuroleptic Malignant Syndrome (NMS): Neuroleptic malignant syndrome is a potentially fatal symptom complex that has been reported in association with antipsychotic drugs, including paliperidone.

Clinical manifestations of NMS are hyperthermia, muscle rigidity, altered mental status (including catatonic signs) and evidence of autonomic instability (irregular blood pressure, tachycardia, cardiac arrhythmias, and diaphoresis). Additional signs may include elevated creatine phosphokinase, myoglobinuria (rhabdomyolysis), and acute renal failure.

In arriving at a diagnosis, it is important to identify cases in which the clinical presentation includes both serious medical illness (e.g., pneumonia, systemic infection, etc.) and untreated or inadequately treated extrapyramidal signs and symptoms. Other important considerations in the differential diagnosis include central anticholinergic toxicity, heat stroke, drug fever, and primary central nervous system pathology.

The management of NMS should include: (1) immediate discontinuation of antipsychotic drugs including INVEGA SUSTENNA, and other drugs not essential to concurrent therapy; (2) intensive symptomatic treatment and medical monitoring; and (3) treatment of any concomitant serious medical problems for which specific treatments are available. There is no general agreement about specific pharmacological treatment regimens for uncomplicated NMS.

If a patient requires antipsychotic drug treatment after recovery from NMS, the potential reintroduction of drug therapy should be carefully considered. The patient should be carefully monitored, since recurrence of NMS has been reported.

Tardive Dyskinesia (TD): A syndrome of potentially irreversible, involuntary, dyskinetic movements may develop in patients treated with antipsychotic drugs. Although TD appears to be most prevalent in the elderly, especially elderly females, it is impossible to predict at the onset of treatment which patients are likely to develop TD. It has been suggested that the occurrence of parkinsonian side effects is a predictor for the development of TD.

The risk of developing TD and the likelihood that it will become irreversible are believed to increase as the duration of treatment and the total cumulative dose of antipsychotic drugs administered to the patient increase. However, the syndrome can develop, although much less commonly, after relatively brief treatment periods at low doses. There is no known treatment for established cases of TD. The syndrome may remit, partially or completely, if antipsychotic treatment is withdrawn. However, antipsychotic treatment itself may suppress the signs and symptoms of TD, thereby masking the underlying process. The effect of symptom suppression upon the long-term course of TD is unknown.

In view of these considerations, INVEGA SUSTENNA should be prescribed in a manner that is most likely to minimize the risk of TD. As with any antipsychotic, INVEGA SUSTENNA should generally be reserved for patients who appear to be obtaining substantial benefit from the drug. In such patients, the smallest dose and the shortest duration of treatment should be sought. The need for continued treatment should be reassessed periodically.

If signs and symptoms of TD develop during treatment with INVEGA SUSTENNA, withdrawal of the drug should be considered. However, some patients may require treatment with INVEGA SUSTENNA despite the presence of the syndrome.

Potential Effect on Cognitive and Motor Performance: Somnolence, sedation and dizziness were reported as adverse reactions in subjects treated with INVEGA SUSTENNA (see Adverse Reactions). Antipsychotics, including INVEGA SUSTENNA, have the potential to impair judgment, thinking, or motor skills. Patients should be cautioned about performing activities requiring mental alertness, such as operating hazardous machinery or operating a motor vehicle, until they are reasonably certain that paliperidone therapy does not adversely affect them.

Seizures: Antipsychotic drugs are known to lower the seizure threshold. In the four fixed-dose, double-blind, placebo-controlled studies, <1% (1/1293) of subjects treated with INVEGA SUSTENNA in the recommended dose range of 25 mg-150 mg experienced an adverse event of convulsion compared with <1% (1/510) of placebo-treated subjects who experienced an adverse event of grand mal convulsion.

In the long-term study, <1% (3/849) INVEGA SUSTENNA-treated subjects in the open-label transition/maintenance phase reported adverse events of convulsion (2 subjects) or epilepsy (1 subject). In the double-blind phase, <1% (1/205) of INVEGA SUSTENNA-treated subjects reported an adverse event of epilepsy compared with 0% (0/203) of placebo-treated subjects. No cases of epilepsy or convulsion were reported in the open-label extension phase of this study.

As with other antipsychotic drugs, INVEGA SUSTENNA should be used cautiously in patients with a history of seizures or other conditions that potentially lower the seizure threshold.

Parkinson's Disease and Dementia with Lewy Bodies: Physicians should weigh the risks versus the benefits when prescribing antipsychotic drugs, including INVEGA SUSTENNA, to patients with Parkinson's disease or dementia with Lewy bodies (DLB) since both groups may be at increased risk of neuroleptic malignant syndrome as well as having an increased sensitivity to antipsychotic medications. Manifestation of this increased sensitivity can include confusion, obtundation, postural instability with frequent falls, in addition to extrapyramidal symptoms.

Psychiatric: Suicide: The possibility of suicide or attempted suicide is inherent in psychosis, and thus, close supervision and appropriate clinical management of high-risk patients should accompany drug therapy. INVEGA SUSTENNA is to be administered by a health care professional (see Dosage and Administration); therefore, suicide due to an overdose is unlikely.

Renal: INVEGA SUSTENNA has not been systematically studied in patients with renal impairment. Based on a limited number of observations with INVEGA SUSTENNA in subjects with mild renal impairment and pharmacokinetic simulations, the dose of INVEGA SUSTENNA should be reduced in patients with mild renal impairment (see Dosage and Administration). INVEGA SUSTENNA is not recommended in patients with moderate or severe renal impairment.

The disposition of oral paliperidone was studied in subjects with varying degrees of renal function. Elimination of paliperidone decreased with decreasing creatinine clearance. Total clearance of paliperidone was reduced in subjects with impaired renal function by 32% in mild (CrCl=50 to <80 mL/min), 64% in moderate (CrCl=30 to <50 mL/min), and 71% in severe (CrCl=10 to <30 mL/min) renal impairment, corresponding to an average increase in exposure (AUC_{inf}) of 1.5-fold, 2.6-fold, and 4.8-fold, respectively, compared to healthy subjects. The mean terminal elimination half-life of paliperidone was 24, 40, and 51 hours in subjects with mild, moderate, and severe renal impairment, respectively, compared with 23 hours in subjects with normal renal function (CrCl ≥80 mL/min).

Special Populations: Pregnant Women: The safety of intramuscularly-injected paliperidone palmitate or orally-dosed paliperidone for use during human pregnancy has not been established. No teratogenic effect was noted in any animal study. Laboratory animals treated with a high dose of paliperidone showed a slight increase in fetal deaths. Pregnancy parameters were not affected in rats given the intramuscular injection of paliperidone palmitate. The high doses were toxic to the mothers. The offspring were not affected at exposures 20- to 22-fold the maximum human exposure, or intramuscular exposures 6-fold the maximum human exposure. INVEGA SUSTENNA should only be used if the benefits outweigh the risks. The effect of INVEGA SUSTENNA on labour and delivery in humans is unknown.

Use of antipsychotic drugs during the last trimester of pregnancy has been associated with reversible extrapyramidal symptoms in the neonate.

Nursing Women: In animal studies with paliperidone and in human studies with risperidone, paliperidone was excreted in the milk. Patients should be advised not to breast-feed an infant if they are taking INVEGA SUSTENNA.

Pediatrics (<18 years of age): The safety and efficacy of INVEGA SUSTENNA in children under the age of 18 years has not been established.

Geriatrics (>65 years of age): Clinical studies of INVEGA SUSTENNA did not include sufficient numbers of subjects aged 65 and over to determine whether they respond differently from younger subjects. Other reported clinical experience has not identified differences in responses between elderly and younger patients.

This drug is known to be substantially excreted by the kidney and clearance is decreased in patients with renal impairment who should be given reduced doses. Because elderly subjects may have diminished renal function, dose adjustments may be required according to their renal function status (see Renal and Dosage and Administration).

Use in Geriatric Patients with Dementia: Overall Mortality: In a meta-analysis of 13 controlled clinical trials, elderly patients with dementia treated with other atypical antipsychotic drugs had an increased risk of mortality compared to placebo. INVEGA SUSTENNA is not indicated for the treatment of elderly patients with dementia.

Cerebrovascular Adverse Events (CVAEs) in Elderly Patients with Dementia: In placebo controlled trials in elderly patients with dementia treated with some atypical antipsychotic drugs, including risperidone and olanzapine, there was a higher incidence of cerebrovascular adverse events (cerebrovascular accidents and transient ischemic attacks) including fatalities compared to placebo. INVEGA SUSTENNA is not indicated for the treatment of elderly patients with dementia.

Dysphagia: Esophageal dysmotility and aspiration have been associated with antipsychotic drug use. Aspiration pneumonia is a common cause of morbidity and mortality in patients with advanced Alzheimer's dementia. INVEGA SUSTENNA and other antipsychotic drugs should be used cautiously in patients at risk for aspiration pneumonia.

ADVERSE REACTIONS: Clinical Trial Adverse Drug Reactions: Because clinical trials are conducted under very specific conditions the adverse reaction rates observed in the clinical trials may not reflect the rates observed in practice and should not be compared to the rates in the clinical trials of another drug. Adverse drug reaction information from clinical trials is useful for identifying drug-related adverse events and for approximating rates.

The data described in this section are derived from a clinical trial database consisting of a total of 3817 subjects with schizophrenia who received at least one dose of INVEGA SUSTENNA in the recommended dose range of 25 mg to 150 mg and a total of 510 subjects with schizophrenia who received placebo. Among the 3817 INVEGA SUSTENNA-treated subjects, 1293 received INVEGA SUSTENNA in four fixed-dose, double-blind, placebo-controlled trials (one 9-week and three 13-week studies), 849 received INVEGA SUSTENNA in the long-term trial (of whom 205 continued to receive INVEGA SUSTENNA during the double-blind placebo-controlled phase of this study), and 1675 received INVEGA SUSTENNA in five non-placebo controlled trials (three noninferiority active-comparator trials, one long-term open-label pharmacokinetic and safety study, and an injection site [deltoid-gluteal] cross-over trial). One of the 13-week studies included a 150 mg INVEGA SUSTENNA initiation dose followed by treatment with either 25 mg, 100 mg, or 150 mg every 4 weeks.

Adverse events during exposure to study treatment were obtained by general inquiry and recorded by clinical investigators using their own terminology. Consequently, to provide a meaningful estimate of the proportion of individuals experiencing adverse events, events were grouped in standardized categories using MedDRA terminology.

A causal association for INVEGA SUSTENNA often cannot be reliably established in individual cases. Further, because clinical trials are conducted under widely varying conditions, adverse event rates observed in the clinical trials of a drug cannot be directly compared to rates in the clinical trials of another drug and may not reflect the rates observed in clinical practice.

The majority of all adverse events were mild to moderate in severity.

Short-Term, Placebo-Controlled Studies: The most common adverse events (reported by ≥5% in any INVEGA SUSTENNA dose group in the four fixed-dose, double-blind, placebo-controlled trials and at least twice that for placebo) were: injection site reactions, dizziness, extrapyramidal disorder, somnolence and akathisia.

Discontinuations Due to Adverse Events : In the four fixed-dose, double-blind placebo controlled trials, 5.0% of subjects treated with INVEGA SUSTENNA discontinued due to adverse events as compared to 7.8% of subjects treated with placebo. Schizophrenia (1.5%), psychotic disorder (0.5%), suicidal ideation (0.5%), and agitation (0.5%) were the most common adverse events leading to discontinuation in the INVEGA SUSTENNA treatment group. In the overall clinical trial program, one INVEGA SUSTENNA-treated subject also discontinued due to neuroleptic malignant syndrome.

Commonly Observed Adverse Drug Events in Double-Blind, Placebo-Controlled Trials: Table 1 enumerates the adverse events reported in ≥2% of patients treated with INVEGA SUSTENNA in the four fixed-dose, double-blind, placebo-controlled studies.

Table 1: INVEGA SUSTENNA

Adverse Events in ≥2% of INVEGA SUSTENNA-Treated Subjects and Equal or Greater Than Placebo with Schizophrenia in Four Fixed-Dose, Double-Blind, Placebo-Controlled Trials

Body System or Organ Class Preferred Term	Placebo (N=510) %	R092670 25 mg eq. (N=130) %	R092670 50 mg eq. (N=302) %	R092670 100 mg eq. (N=312) %	R092670 150/25 mg eq. (N=160) %	R092670 150/100 mg eq. (N=165) %	R092670 150/150 mg eq. (N=163) %	Total Pali (N=1232) %
Total Percentage of Subjects with Adverse Events	70	75	68	69	63	60	63	67
Infections and Infestations								
Bronchitis	1	2	<1	1	0	1	1	1
Influenza	<1	0	0	<1	2	1	0	<1
Nasopharyngitis	2	0	2	2	4	2	2	2
Upper respiratory tract infection	2	2	2	2	1	2	4	2
Urinary tract infection	1	0	1	<1	1	1	2	1
Metabolism and Nutrition Disorders								
Decreased appetite	1	2	1	1	0	1	1	1
Psychiatric Disorders								
Agitation	7	10	5	9	8	5	4	6
Anxiety	7	8	5	3	5	6	6	5
Depression	1	1	2	1	1	0	1	1
Hallucination, auditory	1	2	2	1	1	1	1	1
Insomnia	15	15	15	13	12	10	13	13
Nightmare	<1	2	0	0	0	0	0	<1
Suicidal ideation	2	0	1	2	2	2	1	1
Tension	1	2	1	1	0	0	0	1
Nervous System Disorders								
Akathisia	3	2	2	3	1	5	6	3
Dizziness	1	6	2	4	1	4	2	3
Dyskinesia	1	1	2	1	0	1	1	1
Extrapyramidal disorder	1	5	2	3	1	0	0	2
Headache	12	11	11	15	11	7	6	11
Hypertonia	<1	1	2	1	0	0	0	1
Somnolence	3	5	7	4	1	5	5	5
Eye Disorders								
Eye swelling	0	2	0	0	0	0	0	<1
Cardiac Disorders								
Conduction disorder	1	0	2	1	0	0	0	1

(cont'd)

Table 1: INVEGA SUSTENNA *(cont'd)*

Adverse Events in ≥2% of INVEGA SUSTENNA-Treated Subjects and Equal or Greater Than Placebo with Schizophrenia in Four Fixed-Dose, Double-Blind, Placebo-Controlled Trials

Body System or Organ Class Preferred Term	Placebo (N=510) %	R092670 25 mg eq. (N=130) %	R092670 50 mg eq. (N=302) %	R092670 100 mg eq. (N=312) %	R092670 150/25 mg eq. (N=160) %	R092670 150/100 mg eq. (N=165) %	R092670 150/150 mg eq. (N=163) %	Total Pali (N=1232) %
Sinus bradycardia	1	0	1	<1	2	0	0	<1
Tachycardia	<1	1	0	1	1	1	2	1
Vascular Disorders								
Hypertension	1	2	1	1	1	1	0	1
Respiratory, Thoracic and Mediastinal Disorders								
Cough	1	2	3	1	0	1	1	1
Dyspnea	1	2	<1	1	1	0	0	1
Oropharyngeal pain	1	1	2	<1	1	1	0	1
Gastrointestinal Disorders								
Abdominal discomfort/abdominal pain upper	2	2	4	4	1	2	4	3
Constipation	5	3	5	5	2	4	1	4
Diarrhea	2	0	3	2	1	2	2	2
Dry mouth	1	3	1	0	1	1	1	1
Gastroesophageal reflux disease	0	2	<1	<1	0	0	0	<1
Nausea	3	4	4	3	2	2	2	3
Toothache	1	1	1	3	1	2	3	2
Vomiting	4	5	4	2	3	2	2	3
Skin and Subcutaneous Tissue Disorders								
Pruritus	1	1	2	1	1	0	1	1
Rash	1	2	1	<1	2	1	2	1
Musculoskeletal and Connective Tissue Disorders								
Back pain	2	2	1	3	1	1	1	1
Musculoskeletal stiffness	1	1	<1	<1	1	1	2	1
Myalgia	1	2	1	<1	1	0	2	1
Pain in extremity	1	0	2	2	2	3	0	2
General Disorders and Administration Site Conditions								
Asthenia	0	2	1	<1	0	1	1	1
Fatigue	1	1	2	2	1	2	1	2
Injection site reactions	2	0	4	6	9	7	10	6
Pain	1	0	2	1	0	1	1	1
Investigations								
Alanine aminotransferase increased	2	0	2	1	1	1	1	1
Aspartate aminotransferase increased	1	0	2	0	1	1	2	1
Blood cholesterol increased	<1	2	1	0	0	0	0	<1

(cont'd)

Table 1: INVEGA SUSTENNA *(cont'd)*

Adverse Events in ≥2% of INVEGA SUSTENNA-Treated Subjects and Equal or Greater Than Placebo with Schizophrenia in Four Fixed-Dose, Double-Blind, Placebo-Controlled Trials

Body System or Organ Class Preferred Term	Placebo (N=510) %	R092670 25 mg eq. (N=130) %	R092670 50 mg eq. (N=302) %	R092670 100 mg eq. (N=312) %	R092670 150/25 mg eq. (N=160) %	R092670 150/100 mg eq. (N=165) %	R092670 150/150 mg eq. (N=163) %	Total Pali (N=1232) %
Electrocardiogram qt prolonged	1	1	1	1	2	2	0	1
Low density lipoprotein increased	<1	2	1	0	0	1	0	<1
Weight increased	1	4	4	1	1	1	2	2
Injury, Poisoning and Procedural Complications								
Skin laceration	<1	2	<1	0	1	0	0	<1

Note: The following preferred terms were combined: "Somnolence" and "Sedation" into "Somnolence"; "Injection site pain", "Injection site pruritus", "Injection site nodule", "Injection site induration", "Administration site pain", "Administration site reaction", "Application site erythema", "Application site swelling", "Injection site bruising", "Injection site discomfort", "Injection site erythema", "Injection site extravasation", "Injection site inflammation", "Injection site irritation", "Injection site mass", "Injection site oedema", "Injection site reaction", "Injection site swelling", "Injection site haematoma", "Injection site joint pain", "Vessel puncture site pain", and "Vessel puncture site reaction" into "Injection site reactions"; and "Abdominal discomfort", "Stomach discomfort" and "Abdominal pain upper" into "Abdominal discomfort/Abdominal pain upper".
Note: The adverse events in the studies were coded using the MedDRA version 12.0.
Note: The cut-off criteria (incidence ≥2% and ≥ placebo) are based on percentages after rounding.

Less Common Clinical Trial Adverse Drug Reactions: The following additional adverse events occurred in <2% of INVEGA SUSTENNA-treated subjects in the above four fixed-dose, double-blind, placebo-controlled trials. In addition, the following also includes adverse events reported in INVEGA SUSTENNA-treated subjects with schizophrenia at any rate who participated in other trials. All events assessed as possible drug-related adverse events are included. In addition, medically/clinically meaningful events particularly those that are likely to be useful to the prescriber or that have pharmacologic plausibility, have been included. Although the events reported occurred during treatment with INVEGA SUSTENNA, they were not necessarily caused by it.

Events are categorized by organ class and listed in order of decreasing frequency according to the following definitions: common ≥1/100 to <1/10, uncommon ≥1/1000 to <1/100, rare ≥1/10 000 to <1/1000, very rare <1/10 000, including isolated reports.

Immune System Disorders: Uncommon: hypersensitivity.
Endocrine Disorders: Uncommon: hyperprolactinemia.
Metabolism and Nutrition Disorders: Uncommon: hyperglycemia, hyperinsulinemia, increased appetite.
Psychiatric Disorders: Uncommon: restlessness.
Nervous System Disorders: Common: tremor. Uncommon: bradykinesia, convulsion, dizziness postural, drooling, dysarthria, dystonia, lethargy, oromandibular dystonia, parkinsonism, psychomotor hyperactivity, syncope, tardive dyskinesia. Rare: cerebrovascular accident, neuroleptic malignant syndrome.
Eye Disorders: Uncommon: oculogyric crisis, vision blurred. Rare: eye movement disorder, eye rolling.
Ear and Labyrinth Disorders: Uncommon: vertigo.
Cardiac Disorders: Uncommon: atrioventricular block first degree, bradycardia, palpitations, bundle branch block, postural orthostatic tachycardia syndrome, sinus tachycardia.
Vascular Disorders: Uncommon: orthostatic hypotension.
Gastrointestinal Disorders: Uncommon: salivary hypersecretion.
Skin and Subcutaneous Tissue Disorders: Uncommon: pruritus generalized, urticaria. Rare: drug eruption.
Musculoskeletal and Connective Tissue Disorders: Uncommon: joint stiffness, muscle rigidity, muscle spasms, muscle tightness, muscle twitching. Rare: nuchal rigidity.
Reproductive System and Breast Disorders: Uncommon: amenorrhea, erectile dysfunction, galactorrhea, gynecomastia, menstrual disorder, menstruation delayed, menstruation irregular, sexual dysfunction. Rare: breast discharge.
Investigations: Common: blood glucose increased, blood triglycerides increased. Uncommon: electrocardiogram abnormal.

In the long-term trial, the nature and frequencies of adverse events during the open-label phases of this study were generally comparable to those observed in the four placebo-controlled fixed-dose studies shown in Table 1. The nature of adverse events reported during the double-blind phase of this study was also generally similar to those observed in the open-label phases.

Dose-Related Adverse Events: Based on the pooled data from the four fixed-dose, double-blind, placebo-controlled trials, among the adverse events that occurred at ≥2% incidence in the subjects treated with INVEGA SUSTENNA, only akathisia and injection site reactions display a clear dose-related trend. Hyperprolactinemia also exhibited a dose relationship, but did not occur at ≥2% incidence in subjects treated with INVEGA SUSTENNA.

Demographics: An examination of population subgroups in the double-blind, placebo-controlled trials did not reveal any evidence of differences in safety on the basis of age, gender, or race alone; however, there were few subjects ≥65 years of age.

Extrapyramidal Symptoms (EPS): Pooled data from the two double-blind, placebo-controlled, 13-week, fixed-dose trials provided information regarding treatment-emergent EPS. Several methods were used to measure EPS: (1) the Simpson-Angus global score (mean change from baseline or score at the end of trial) which broadly evaluates Parkinsonism, (2) the Barnes Akathisia Rating Scale global clinical rating score (mean change from baseline or score at the end of trial) which evaluates akathisia, (3) use of anticholinergic medications to treat emergent EPS, (4) the Abnormal Involuntary Movement Scale scores (mean change from baseline or scores at the end of trial) (Table 2), and (5) incidence of spontaneous reports of EPS (Table 3).

The results across all phases of the long-term trial exhibited comparable findings. In the 9-week, fixed-dose, double-blind, placebo-controlled trial, the proportions of Parkinsonism and akathisia assessed by incidence of rating scales were higher in the INVEGA SUSTENNA 100 mg group (18% and 11%, respectively) than in the INVEGA SUSTENNA 50 mg group (9% and 5%, respectively) and placebo group (7% and 4%, respectively).

In the 13-week study involving 150 mg initiation dosing, the incidence of any treatment-emergent EPS-related adverse events was similar to that of the placebo group (8%), but exhibited a dose-related pattern with 6%, 10%, and 11% in the INVEGA SUSTENNA 150/25 mg, 150/100 mg, and 150/150 mg groups, respectively. Hyperkinesia was the most frequent category of EPS-related adverse events in this study, and was reported at a similar rate between the placebo (4.9%) and INVEGA SUSTENNA 150/100 mg (4.8%) and 150/150 mg (5.5%) groups, but at a lower rate in the 150/25 mg group (1.3%). The percentage of subjects who required use of an anticholinergic medication was low and similar across the placebo and paliperidone palmitate groups (11% to 13%).

Weight Gain: In the 13-week study involving the recommended initiation regimen (i.e., the initial 150 mg and 100 mg deltoid injections), the proportions of subjects with a weight increase from baseline of ≥7% were more common among subjects in the INVEGA SUSTENNA groups than in the placebo group. The proportion of subjects with an abnormal weight increase ≥7% showed a dose-related trend, with a 5% incidence rate in the placebo group compared with rates of 6%, 8%, and 13% in the INVEGA SUSTENNA 25 mg, 100 mg, and 150 mg groups, respectively.

In the two 13-week, fixed-dose, double-blind, placebo-controlled trials (pooled data), the proportions of subjects meeting a weight gain criterion of ≥7% of body weight were 6%, 9%, and 10% in the INVEGA SUSTENNA 25 mg, 50 mg, and 100 mg groups, respectively, compared with 2% in the placebo group. In the 9-week, fixed-dose, double-blind, placebo-controlled trial, 8% and 6% in the INVEGA SUSTENNA 50 mg and 100 mg groups, respectively, met this criterion compared with 4% in the placebo group.

Table 2: INVEGA SUSTENNA

Treatment-Emergent Extrapyramidal Symptoms (EPS) Assessed by Incidence of Rating Scales and Use of Anticholinergic Medication

Scale	Percentage of Subjects			
		INVEGA SUSTENNA		
	Placebo (N=262)	25 mg (N=130)	50 mg (N=223)	100 mg (N=228)
Parkinsonism[a]	9	12	10	6
Akathisia[b]	5	5	6	5
Dyskinesia[c]	3	4	6	4
Use of Anticholinergic Medications[d]	12	10	12	11

[a] For Parkinsonism, percent of subjects with Simpson-Angus Total score >0.3 at endpoint (Total score defined as total sum of items score divided by the number of items).
[b] For Akathisia, percent of subjects with Barnes Akathisia Rating Scale global score ≥2 at endpoint.
[c] For Dyskinesia, percent of subjects with a score ≥3 on any of the first 7 items or a score ≥2 on two or more of any of the first 7 items of the Abnormal Involuntary Movement Scale at endpoint.
[d] Percent of subjects who received anticholinergic medications to treat emergent EPS.

Table 3: INVEGA SUSTENNA

Treatment-Emergent Extrapyramidal Symptoms (EPS)-Related Adverse Events by MedDRA Preferred Term

EPS Group	Percentage of Subjects			
		INVEGA SUSTENNA		
	Placebo (N=262)	25 mg (N=130)	50 mg (N=223)	100 mg (N=228)
Overall percentage of subjects with EPS-related adverse events	10	12	11	11
Parkinsonism	5	6	6	4
Hyperkinesia	2	2	2	4
Tremor	3	2	2	3
Dyskinesia	1	2	3	1
Dystonia	0	1	1	2

Parkinsonism group includes: Extrapyramidal disorder, hypertonia, musculoskeletal stiffness, parkinsonism, drooling, masked facies, muscle tightness, hypokinesia.
Hyperkinesia group includes: Akathisia, restless legs syndrome, restlessness.
Dyskinesia group includes: Dyskinesia, choreoathetosis, muscle twitching, myoclonus, tardive dyskinesia.
Dystonia group includes: Dystonia, muscle spasms.

Table 4: INVEGA SUSTENNA

Treatment-Emergent Extrapyramidal Symptoms (EPS)-Related Adverse Events by MedDRA Preferred Term in a 13-week 150 mg Initiation Dose Study

EPS Group	Percentage of Subjects			
		INVEGA SUSTENNA		
	Placebo (N=164)	150/25 mg[a] (N=160)	150/100 mg[a] (N=165)	150/150 mg[a] (N=163)
Hyperkinesia	4.9	1.3	4.8	5.5
Parkinsonism	1.8	3.1	3.0	4.3
Tremor	2.4	0.6	1.8	1.2
Dyskinesia	0.6	0	1.2	0.8
Dystonia	0.6	1.9	0	0

[a] Initial deltoid injection of 150 mg followed by either 25 mg, 100 mg, or 150 mg every 4 weeks by deltoid or gluteal injection.
Parkinsonism group includes: Extrapyramidal disorder, hypertonia, musculoskeletal stiffness, parkinsonism, drooling, masked facies, muscle tightness, hypokinesia.
Hyperkinesia group includes: Akathisia, restless legs syndrome, restlessness.
Dyskinesia group includes: Dyskinesia, choreoathetosis, muscle twitching, myoclonus, tardive dyskinesia.
Dystonia group includes: Dystonia, muscle spasms.

During the 33-week open-label transition/maintenance period of the long-term trial, 12% of INVEGA SUSTENNA-treated subjects met this criterion; the mean weight change from open-label baseline was +0.7 kg. In the variable length double-blind phase, this criterion (weight gain of ≥7% from double-blind phase to endpoint) was met by 6% of INVEGA SUSTENNA-treated subjects (median duration 171 days [range 1 day-407 days]) compared with 3% of placebo-treated subjects (median duration 105 days [range 8 days-441 days]); the mean weight change from double-blind baseline was +0.5 kg for INVEGA SUSTENNA compared with −1.0 kg for placebo. Similar results were observed in the open-label extension phase of this study.

Abnormal Hematologic and Clinical Chemistry Findings: In the pooled data from the two double-blind, placebo-controlled, 13-week, fixed-dose trials, a between-group comparison revealed no medically important differences between INVEGA SUSTENNA and placebo in the proportions of subjects experiencing potentially clinically significant changes in routine serum chemistry, hematology, or urinalysis parameters. Similarly, there were no differences between INVEGA SUSTENNA and placebo in the incidence of discontinuations due to changes in hematology, urinalysis, or serum chemistry, including mean changes from baseline in fasting glucose, insulin, c-peptide, triglyceride, HDL, LDL, and total cholesterol measurements. However, INVEGA SUSTENNA was associated with increases in serum prolactin (see Warnings and Precautions, Endocrine and Metabolism). Observed increases in serum prolactin concentrations were mostly asymptomatic and infrequently associated with reports of potentially prolactin-related adverse events. The results from the 13-week study involving 150 mg initiation dosing, the 9-week, fixed-dose, double-blind, placebo-controlled trial, and the double-blind phase of the long-term trial exhibited comparable findings.

Pain Assessment and Local Injection Site Reactions: In the 13-week study involving the recommended initiation regimen (i.e., the initial 150 mg and 100 mg deltoid injections, the mean intensity of injection pain reported by subjects using a visual analog scale (0 mm=no pain to 100 mm=unbearably painful) at first injection was 22 and 18 for INVEGA SUSTENNA and placebo groups, respectively. Throughout the rest of the study when injections could be administered in either the gluteal or deltoid site, mean pain scores ranged between 10-15 mm for gluteal injections, and from 15-21 mm for deltoid injections. Thus, pain at the deltoid site tended to be greater, although still usually mild. Investigator ratings of pain were consistent with the subject ratings. Although less frequent, there was also more swelling at the deltoid site as compared to the gluteal site.

Overall, occurrences of pain, induration, redness, or swelling, at injection sites, as assessed by blinded study personnel, were infrequent, generally mild, and tended to decrease over time.

Adverse Events Reported with Oral Paliperidone: The following is a list of additional adverse events that have been reported with oral paliperidone:

Infections and Infestations: rhinitis, viral infection.

Immune System Disorders: anaphylactic reaction.

Psychiatric Disorders: aggression, sleep disorder.

Nervous System Disorders: cogwheel rigidity, grand mal convulsion, parkinsonian gait, transient ischemic attack.

Eye Disorders: dry eye.

Cardiac Disorders: bundle branch block left, sinus arrhythmia.

Vascular Disorders: hypotension, ischemia.

Respiratory, Thoracic and Mediastinal Disorders: nasal congestion, pneumonia aspiration.

Gastrointestinal Disorders: dyspepsia, flatulence, small intestinal obstruction.

Skin and Subcutaneous Tissue Disorders: rash papular.

Musculoskeletal and Connective Tissue Disorders: arthralgia, musculoskeletal pain, neck pain, shoulder pain, torticollis, trismus.

Reproductive System and Breast Disorders: breast engorgement, breast pain, breast tenderness, retrograde ejaculation.

General Disorders and Administration Site Conditions: edema, edema peripheral, pyrexia.

Injury, Poisoning and Procedural Complications: fall.

Investigations: blood creatine phosphokinase increased, blood insulin increased, blood pressure increased, electrocardiogram QT corrected interval prolonged, electrocardiogram T wave abnormal, electrocardiogram T wave inversion, heart rate increased, insulin C-peptide increased, weight decreased.

Post-Market Adverse Drug Reactions: Adverse events first identified as ADRs during postmarketing experience with paliperidone are included in Table 5. In this table, the frequencies are provided according to the following convention: very common ≥1/10, common ≥1/100 to <1/10, uncommon ≥1/1000 to <1/100, rare ≥1/10 000 to <1/1000, very rare <1/10 000, including isolated reports.

In Table 5, ADRs are presented by frequency category based on spontaneous reporting rates.

Table 5: INVEGA SUSTENNA

Adverse Drug Reactions Identified During Post-Marketing Experience with Paliperidone by Frequency Category Estimated from Spontaneous Reporting Rates

Adverse Drug Reactions	
Immune System Disorders	
Rare	Angioedema
Gastrointestinal Disorders	
Very rare	Swollen tongue
Renal and Urinary Disorders	
Very rare	Urinary incontinence
Very rare	Urinary retention
Reproductive System and Breast Disorders	
Very rare	Priapism

Safety Information Reported with Risperidone: Paliperidone is the major active metabolite of risperidone. The release profile and pharmacokinetic characteristics of INVEGA SUSTENNA are considerably different from those observed with oral immediate-release risperidone formulations, as well as those from risperidone long-acting injection (see Action and Clinical Pharmacology); however, the receptor binding profile of paliperidone is very similar to that of the parent compound. Safety information reported with oral risperidone and risperidone long-acting injection in clinical trials and postmarketing experience that may be relevant to INVEGA SUSTENNA can be found in local labelling for risperidone.

DRUG INTERACTIONS: Drug-Drug Interactions: Caution is advised when prescribing INVEGA SUSTENNA with drugs known to prolong the QT interval.

Since paliperidone palmitate is hydrolyzed to paliperidone (see Action and Clinical Pharmacology), results from studies with oral paliperidone should be taken into consideration when assessing drug-drug interaction potential.

Potential for INVEGA SUSTENNA to Affect Other Drugs: Paliperidone is not expected to cause clinically important pharmacokinetic interactions with drugs that are metabolized by cytochrome P-450 isozymes. In vitro studies in human liver microsomes showed that paliperidone does not substantially inhibit the metabolism of drugs metabolized by cytochrome P450 isozymes, including CYP1A2, CYP2A6, CYP2C8/9/10, CYP2D6, CYP2E1, CYP3A4, and CYP3A5. Therefore, paliperidone is not expected to inhibit clearance of drugs that are metabolized by these metabolic pathways in a clinically relevant manner. Paliperidone is also not expected to have enzyme-inducing properties.

A population pharmacokinetic analysis from a study using oral paliperidone extended-release to evaluate the influence of predicted CYP2D6 phenotype on exposure indicated that no adjustment in the paliperidone dose on the basis of predicted phenotype is warranted.

Paliperidone is a weak inhibitor of P-glycoprotein (P-gp) at high concentrations. No in vivo data are available and the clinical relevance of this with respect to P-gp mediated transport of other drugs is unknown.

Given the primary CNS effects of paliperidone (see Adverse Reactions), INVEGA SUSTENNA should be used with caution in combination with other centrally acting drugs and alcohol. Paliperidone may antagonize the effect of levodopa and other dopamine agonists.

Because of its potential for inducing orthostatic hypotension (see Warnings and Precautions, Cardiovascular), an additive effect may be observed when INVEGA SUSTENNA is administered with other therapeutic agents that have this potential.

Potential for Other Drugs to Affect INVEGA SUSTENNA: Paliperidone is not a substrate of CYP1A2, CYP2A6, CYP2C9, CYP2C19, and CYP3A5. This suggests that an interaction with inhibitors or inducers of these isozymes is unlikely.

While in vitro studies indicate that CYP2D6 and CYP3A4 may be minimally involved in paliperidone metabolism, there are no indications in vitro nor in vivo that these isozymes play a significant role in the metabolism of paliperidone (see Action and Clinical Pharmacology, Pharmacokinetics).

In an interaction study in healthy subjects in which oral paliperidone extended-release once daily was administered concomitantly with paroxetine, a potent CYP2D6 inhibitor, no clinically relevant effects on the pharmacokinetics of paliperidone were observed.

Carbamazepine and Other Potent CYP3A4 Inducers: Co-administration of oral paliperidone extended-release once daily with carbamazepine 200 mg twice daily caused a decrease of approximately 37% in the mean steady-state Cmax and AUC of paliperidone. As is typical of CYP3A4 inducers, carbamazepine is also a P-glycoprotein (P-gp) inducer. Although in-vitro studies have shown that paliperidone is a substrate of both P-gp and CYP3A4, the relative contributions of P-gp and CYP3A4 to changes in the pharmacokinetic parameters are unclear.

On initiation of carbamazepine, the dose of INVEGA SUSTENNA should be re-evaluated and increased if necessary. Conversely, on discontinuation of carbamazepine, the dose of INVEGA SUSTENNA should be re-evaluated and decreased if necessary. Until more data are available, these recommendations should be extended to other potent CYP3A4 inducers and/or P-glycoprotein upregulators.

Paliperidone, a cation under physiological pH, is primarily excreted unchanged by the kidneys, approximately half via filtration and half via active secretion. Concomitant administration of trimethoprim, a drug known to inhibit active renal cation drug transport, did not influence the pharmacokinetics of paliperidone.

Concomitant Use of INVEGA SUSTENNA with Risperidone or Oral Paliperidone : Concomitant use of INVEGA SUSTENNA with oral paliperidone or oral or injectable risperidone has not been studied. Since paliperidone (9-hydroxy-risperidone) is the major active metabolite of risperidone, concomitant use of INVEGA SUSTENNA with risperidone or oral paliperidone is not recommended since the combination of any of these medications will lead to additive paliperidone exposure.

Drug-Food Interactions: Interactions with food have not been established.

Drug-Herb Interactions: Interactions with herbal products have not been established.

Drug-Laboratory Test Interactions: Interactions with laboratory tests have not been established.

Drug-Lifestyle Interactions: Smoking: No dosage adjustment is recommended based on smoking status. Based on in vitro studies utilizing human liver enzymes, paliperidone is not a substrate for CYP1A2; smoking should, therefore, not have an effect on the pharmacokinetics of paliperidone. Consistent with these in vitro results, population pharmacokinetic evaluation has not revealed any statistically significant differences between smokers and non-smokers in an analysis performed with oral paliperidone extended-release tablets.

DOSAGE AND ADMINISTRATION: Recommended Dose and Dosage Adjustment: Adult: For patients who have never taken oral paliperidone or oral/injectable risperidone, it is recommended to establish tolerability with oral paliperidone or oral risperidone prior to initiating treatment with INVEGA SUSTENNA.

Recommended **initiation regimen** of INVEGA SUSTENNA is with a dose of 150 mg on treatment day 1 and 100 mg on day 8 (one week later), both administered in the deltoid muscle in order to attain therapeutic concentrations rapidly (see Action and Clinical Pharmacology). Recommendations for switching from other antipsychotics are provided in the section For Patients who are SWITCHING From Other Antipsychotic Agents.

The recommended subsequent monthly maintenance dose is 75 mg; this dose can be higher or lower within the range of 25 to 150 mg based on individual patient tolerability and/or efficacy. Following the initiation regimen, monthly maintenance doses can be administered in either the deltoid or gluteal muscle.

Adjustment of the maintenance dose may be made monthly. When making dose adjustments, the prolonged-release characteristics of INVEGA SUSTENNA should be considered (see Action and Clinical Pharmacology), as the full effect of the dose adjustment may not be evident for several months.

Administration Information: INVEGA SUSTENNA is intended for intramuscular use only. Inject slowly, deep into the muscle. Care should be taken to avoid inadvertent injection into a blood vessel. Each injection should be administered by a health care professional. Administration should be in a single injection. Do not administer the dose in divided injections. Do not administer intravascularly or subcutaneously.

The recommended needle size for administration of INVEGA SUSTENNA into the deltoid muscle is determined by the patient's weight. For those ≥90 kg (≥200 lb), the 1½ inch, 22 gauge needle is recommended. For those <90 kg (<200 lb), the 1-inch, 23 gauge needle is recommended. Deltoid injections should be alternated between the two deltoid muscles.

The recommended needle size for administration of INVEGA SUSTENNA into the gluteal muscle is the 1½-inch, 22 gauge needle. Administration should be made into the upper-outer quadrant of the gluteal area. Gluteal injections should be alternated between the two gluteal muscles.

Concomitant use of INVEGA SUSTENNA with oral paliperidone or oral or injectable risperidone has not been studied. Since paliperidone (9-hydroxyrisperidone) is the major active metabolite of risperidone, concomitant use of INVEGA SUSTENNA with risperidone or oral paliperidone is not recommended since the combination of any of these medications will lead to additive paliperidone exposure.

Missed Dose: Guidance for Avoiding Missed Doses: It is recommended that the second dose of the initiation regimen of INVEGA SUSTENNA be given one week after the first dose. To avoid a missed dose, patients may be given the second dose 2 days before or after the one-week time point. Similarly, the third and subsequent injections after the initiation regimen are recommended to be given monthly. To avoid a missed monthly dose, patients may be given the injection up to 7 days before or after the monthly time point.

Missed Dose (1 Month to 6 Weeks): After administration of the initiation regimen, the recommended injection cycle of INVEGA SUSTENNA is monthly. If less than 6 weeks have elapsed since the last injection, then the previous maintenance dose should be administered as soon as possible, followed by injections at monthly intervals.

Missed Dose (>6 Weeks to 6 Months): If more than 6 weeks have elapsed since the last injection of INVEGA SUSTENNA, the recommendation is as follows:

For patients with previous maintenance doses of 25 to 100 mg:

1. A deltoid injection as soon as possible at the same maintenance dose the patient was previously on,
2. Another deltoid injection (same dose) one week later (day 8),
3. Resumption of the normal monthly cycle of injections in either the deltoid or gluteal muscle of 25 mg to 150 mg.

For patients with previous maintenance dose of 150 mg:

1. A deltoid injection as soon as possible at the 100 mg dose
2. Another deltoid injection one week later (day 8) at the 100 mg dose
3. Resumption of the normal monthly cycle of injections in either the deltoid or gluteal muscle of 25 mg to 150 mg.

Missed Dose (>6 Months): Subsequent to administration of the initiation regimen, if more than 6 months have elapsed since the last injection of INVEGA SUSTENNA, initiate dosing as described for the initial recommended initiation of INVEGA SUSTENNA above.

Patients with Hepatic Impairment: INVEGA SUSTENNA has not been studied in patients with hepatic impairment. Based on a study with oral paliperidone, no dose adjustment is required in patients with mild or moderate hepatic impairment. Paliperidone has not been studied in patients with severe hepatic impairment (see Action and Clinical Pharmacology).

Patients with Renal Impairment: INVEGA SUSTENNA has not been systematically studied in patients with renal impairment (see Action and Clinical Pharmacology). For patients with mild renal impairment (creatinine clearance ≥50 to <80 mL/min), recommended initiation of INVEGA SUSTENNA is with a dose of 100 mg on treatment day 1 and 75 mg one week later, both administered in the deltoid muscle. Thereafter, follow with monthly injections of 50 mg in either the deltoid or gluteal muscle.

INVEGA SUSTENNA is not recommended in patients with moderate or severe renal impairment (creatinine clearance <50 mL/min).

Elderly: In general, recommended dosing for elderly patients with normal renal function (≥80 mL/min) is the same as for younger adults with normal renal function. As elderly patients may have diminished renal function, dose adjustments may be required according to their renal function status (see Patients with Renal Impairment).

Pediatrics: Safety and effectiveness of INVEGA SUSTENNA in patients <18 years of age have not been studied.

Other Special Populations: No dose adjustment for INVEGA SUSTENNA is recommended based on gender, race, or smoking status.

For Patients who are SWITCHING From Other Antipsychotic Agents: There are no systematically collected data to specifically address switching schizophrenic patients from other antipsychotics to INVEGA SUSTENNA, or concerning concomitant administration with other antipsychotics.

Switching from Oral Antipsychotics: For patients who have never taken oral paliperidone or oral/injectable risperidone, tolerability should be established with oral paliperidone or oral risperidone prior to initiating treatment with INVEGA SUSTENNA.

Previous oral antipsychotics can be discontinued at the time of initiation of treatment with INVEGA SUSTENNA. INVEGA SUSTENNA should be started according to the one-week initiation dosing regimen (i.e., the initial 150 mg and 100 mg deltoid injections) as described in Recommended Dose and Dosage Adjustment. Patients previously stabilized on different doses of INVEGA Extended-Release Tablets can attain similar paliperidone steady-state exposure with INVEGA SUSTENNA following administration of the initiation regimen as described in Recommended Dose and Dosage Adjustment and subsequent monthly doses as in Table 6.

Switching from Long-Acting Injectable Antipsychotics: For patients who have never taken oral paliperidone or oral/injectable risperidone, tolerability should be established with oral paliperidone or oral risperidone prior to initiating treatment with INVEGA SUSTENNA.

When switching patients from previous long-acting injectable antipsychotics (including RISPERDAL CONSTA), initiate INVEGA SUSTENNA therapy in place of the next scheduled injection. INVEGA SUSTENNA should then be continued at monthly intervals.

The one-week initiation dosing regimen (i.e., the initial 150 mg and 100 mg deltoid injections) as described at the beginning of the Dosage and Administration is not required.

Patients previously stabilized on different doses of RISPERDAL CONSTA risperidone powder for Injectable Prolonged-Release Suspension can attain similar active drug steady-state exposure during maintenance treatment with INVEGA SUSTENNA monthly doses according to the following: see Table 7.

Table 6: INVEGA SUSTENNA

Doses of INVEGA and INVEGA SUSTENNA Needed to Attain Similar Paliperidone Exposure at Steady-state

Formulation	INVEGA Extended-Release Tablets	INVEGA SUSTENNA Prolonged-Release Suspension
Dosing Frequency	Once Daily	Once every 4 weeks
Dose (mg)	12	150
	6	75
	3	25–50

Table 7: INVEGA SUSTENNA

Doses of RISPERDAL CONSTA and INVEGA SUSTENNA Needed to Attain Similar Paliperidone Exposure at Steady-state

Previous RISPERDAL CONSTA Dose	INVEGA SUSTENNA Dose
25 mg every 2 weeks	50 mg monthly
37.5 mg every 2 weeks	75 mg monthly
50 mg every 2 weeks	100 mg monthly

If INVEGA SUSTENNA is discontinued, its prolonged-release characteristics must be considered. As recommended with other antipsychotic medications, the need for continuing existing extrapyramidal symptoms (EPS) medication should be re-evaluated periodically.

Instructions for Use: The kit contains a prefilled syringe and 2 safety needles (a 1 ½-inch 22 gauge needle and a 1-inch 23 gauge needle) for intramuscular injection.

INVEGA SUSTENNA is for single use only.

Note: The 1 ½-inch 22 gauge needle hub colour appears gray but corresponds to ISO needle hub colour "black".

1. Shake the syringe vigorously for a minimum of 10 seconds to ensure a homogeneous suspension.
2. Select the appropriate needle.
   For DELTOID injection, if the patient weighs <200 lb (<90 kg), use the 1-inch **23** gauge needle (needle with **blue** coloured hub); if the patient weighs ≥200 lb (≥90 kg), use the 1½-inch **22** gauge needle (needle with **gray** coloured hub).
   For GLUTEAL injection, use the 1½-inch **22** gauge needle (needle with **gray** coloured hub).
3. While holding the syringe upright, remove the rubber tip cap with an easy clockwise twisting motion.
4. Peel the safety needle pouch half way open. Grasp the needle sheath using the plastic peel pouch. Attach the safety needle to the luer connection of the syringe with an easy clockwise twisting motion.
5. Pull the needle sheath away from the needle with a straight pull. Do not twist the sheath as the needle may be loosened from the syringe.
6. Bring the syringe with the attached needle in upright position to de-aerate. De-aerate the syringe by moving the plunger rod carefully forward.
7. Inject the entire contents intramuscularly into the selected deltoid or gluteal muscle of the patient. **Do not administer intravascularly or subcutaneously.**
8. After the injection is complete, use either thumb or finger of one hand or a flat surface to activate the needle protection system. The needle protection system is fully activated when a 'click' is heard. Discard the syringe with needle appropriately.

OVERDOSAGE:

Because INVEGA SUSTENNA is to be administered by health care professionals, the potential for overdosage by patients is low.

Symptoms: In general, expected signs and symptoms are those resulting from an exaggeration of paliperidone's known pharmacological effects, i.e., drowsiness and sedation, tachycardia and hypotension, QT prolongation, and extrapyramidal symptoms. Torsades de pointes and ventricular fibrillation have been reported in a patient in the setting of overdose with oral paliperidone. In the case of acute overdosage, the possibility of multiple drug involvement should be considered.

Treatment: Consideration should be given to the prolonged-release nature of INVEGA SUSTENNA and the long apparent half-life of paliperidone when assessing treatment needs and recovery. There is no specific antidote to paliperidone. General supportive measures should be employed. Establish and maintain a clear airway and ensure adequate oxygenation and ventilation. Cardiovascular monitoring should commence immediately and should include continuous electrocardiographic monitoring for possible arrhythmias. Hypotension and circulatory collapse should be treated with appropriate measures such as intravenous fluids and/or sympathomimetic agents. In case of severe extrapyramidal symptoms, anticholinergic agents should be administered. Close supervision and monitoring should continue until the patient recovers.

For management of a suspected drug overdose, contact your regional Poison Control Centre. See the *CPS Directory* section for a list of Poison Control Centres.

ACTION AND CLINICAL PHARMACOLOGY: Mechanism of Action: Paliperidone palmitate is hydrolyzed to paliperidone (see Pharmacokinetics). The mechanism of action of paliperidone, as with other drugs having efficacy in schizophrenia, is unknown. However, it has been proposed that the drug's therapeutic activity in schizophrenia is mediated through a combination of dopamine Type 2 (D_2) and serotonin Type 2 ($5HT_{2A}$) receptor antagonism. Antagonism at receptors other than D_2 and $5HT_{2A}$ may explain some of the other effects of paliperidone.

Pharmacodynamics: Paliperidone is a centrally active dopamine D_2 antagonist with predominant serotonergic $5\text{-}HT_{2A}$ antagonistic activity. Paliperidone is also active as an antagonist at α_1 and α_2 adrenergic receptors and H_1 histaminergic receptors. Paliperidone has no affinity for cholinergic muscarinic or β_1- and β_2-adrenergic receptors. The pharmacological activity of the (+)- and (−)- paliperidone enantiomers is qualitatively and quantitatively similar.

Pharmacokinetics: Absorption and Distribution: Due to its extremely low water solubility, paliperidone palmitate dissolves slowly after intramuscular injection before being hydrolyzed to paliperidone and absorbed into the systemic circulation. Following a single intramuscular dose, the plasma concentrations of paliperidone gradually rise to reach maximum plasma concentrations at a median t_{max} of 13 days. The release of the drug starts as early as day 1 and lasts for as long as 126 days.

Following intramuscular injection of single doses (25 mg-150 mg) in the deltoid muscle, on average, a 28% higher C_{max} was observed compared with injection in the gluteal muscle. The two initial deltoid intramuscular injections of 150 mg on day 1 and 100 mg on day 8 help attain therapeutic concentrations rapidly.

This dosing regimen and the release profile of INVEGA SUSTENNA results in rapid attainment of sustained therapeutic concentrations similar to the steady state concentrations obtained by monthly dosing at 75 mg. At lower or higher monthly doses of INVEGA SUSTENNA, plasma concentrations gradually decrease or increase respectively until steady state for the lower or higher doses is achieved; see Figure 1.

The AUC of paliperidone following INVEGA SUSTENNA administration was dose proportional over a 25 mg-150 mg dose range, and less than dose proportional for C_{max} for doses exceeding 50 mg. The mean steady state peak: trough ratio for an INVEGA SUSTENNA dose of 100 mg was 1.8 following gluteal administration and 2.2 following deltoid administration. The median apparent half-life of paliperidone following INVEGA SUSTENNA administration increased over the dose range of 25 mg-150 mg from 25-49 days.

Following administration of paliperidone palmitate the (+) and (−) enantiomers of paliperidone interconvert, reaching an AUC (+) to (−) ratio of approximately 1.6-1.8.

Based on a population analysis, the apparent volume of distribution of paliperidone is 391 L. The plasma protein binding of racemic paliperidone is 74%.

Metabolism and Excretion: The following data are based on a human mass balance study using oral solution of ^{14}C-paliperidone which has approximately 100% bioavailability. One week following administration of a single 1 mg dose of oral solution ^{14}C-paliperidone, 59% of the dose was excreted unchanged into urine, indicating that paliperidone is not extensively metabolized in the liver. Approximately 80% of the administered radioactivity was recovered in urine and 11% in the feces.

Figure 1: INVEGA SUSTENNA

Population PK Simulations of Plasma Paliperidone Concentrations with a Range of Maintenance Doses. The Solid Line and the Shaded Area Represent the Median and the 90% Prediction Interval Based on the Population PK Simulation

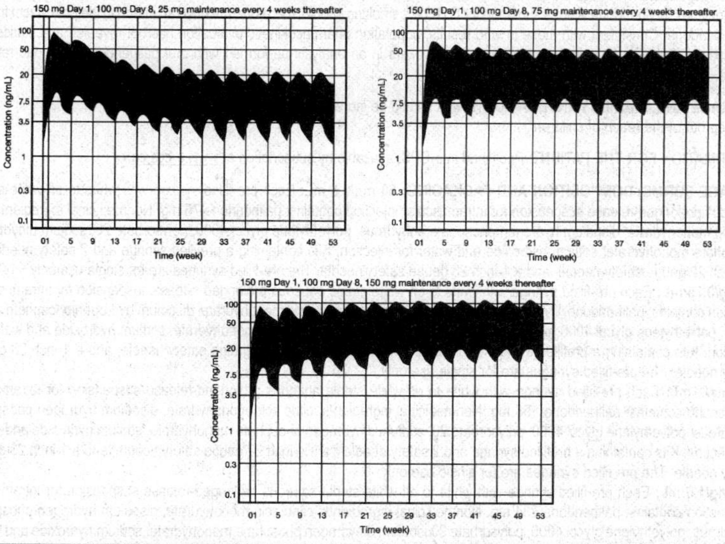

Four metabolic pathways have been identified in vivo, none of which accounted for more than 6.5% of the dose: dealkylation, hydroxylation, dehydrogenation, and benzisoxazole scission. Although in vitro studies suggested a role for CYP2D6 and CYP3A4 in the metabolism of paliperidone, there is no evidence in vivo that these isozymes play a significant role in the metabolism of paliperidone. Population pharmacokinetics analyses indicated no discernable difference on the apparent clearance of paliperidone after administration of oral paliperidone between extensive metabolizers and poor metabolizers of CYP2D6 substrates. In vitro studies in human liver microsomes showed that paliperidone does not substantially inhibit the metabolism of medicines metabolized by cytochrome P450 isozymes, including CYP1A2, CYP2A6, CYP2C8/9/10, CYP2D6, CYP2E1, CYP3A4, and CYP3A5.

In vitro studies have shown that paliperidone is a P-gp substrate and a weak inhibitor of P-gp at high concentrations. No in vivo data are available and the clinical relevance is unknown.

Long-Acting Paliperidone Palmitate Injection versus Oral Extended-Release Paliperidone: INVEGA SUSTENNA is designed to deliver paliperidone over a monthly period while extended-release oral paliperidone is administered on a daily basis. Figure 2 presents the median pharmacokinetic profiles for paliperidone for 5 weeks following INVEGA SUSTENNA administration using the recommended initiation regimen compared to the administration of an oral extended-release tablet (6 mg or 12 mg). The initiation regimen for INVEGA SUSTENNA (150 mg/100 mg in the deltoid muscle on Day 1/Day 8) was designed to rapidly attain steady-state paliperidone concentrations when initiating therapy without the use of oral supplementation.

Figure 2: INVEGA SUSTENNA

Median Plasma Concentration-time Profiles Following Median Pharmacokinetic Profiles for Paliperidone for 5 Weeks Following INVEGA SUSTENNA Administration Using the Recommended Initiation Regimen (initiating with paliperidone palmitate equivalent to paliperidone 150 mg/100 mg in the deltoid muscle on Day 1/Day 8) Compared to the Daily Administration of an Oral Extended-release Tablet (6 mg or 12 mg)

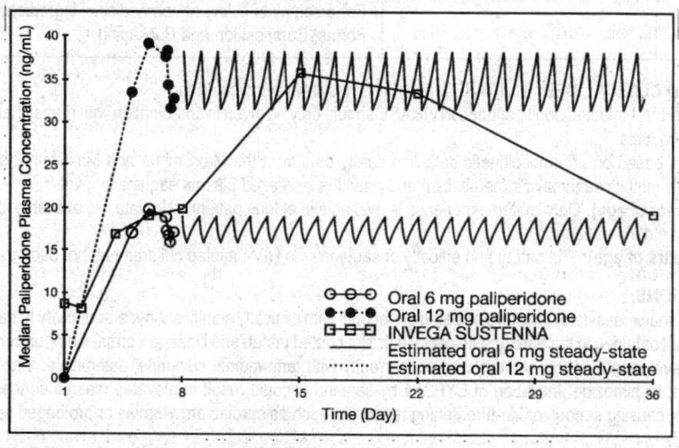

In general, overall initiation plasma levels with INVEGA SUSTENNA were within the exposure range observed with 6-12 mg extended-release oral paliperidone. The use of the INVEGA SUSTENNA initiation regimen allowed patients to stay in this exposure window of 6-12 mg extended-release oral paliperidone even on trough pre-dose days (Day 8 and Day 36). The intersubject variability for paliperidone pharmacokinetics following delivery from INVEGA SUSTENNA was lower relative to the variability determined from extended release oral paliperidone tablets. Because of the difference in median pharmacokinetic profiles between the two products, caution should be exercised when making a direct comparison of their pharmacokinetic properties.

Special Populations and Conditions: Pediatrics: No data available.

Geriatrics: No dosage adjustment is recommended based on age alone. However, dose adjustment may be required because of age-related decreases in creatinine clearance (see Action and Clinical Pharmacology,Renal Insufficiency and Dosage and Administration).

Gender: No clinically significant differences were observed between men and women.

Race: Population pharmacokinetics analysis of data from studies with oral paliperidone revealed no evidence of race-related differences in the pharmacokinetics of paliperidone following INVEGA SUSTENNA administration.

Hepatic Insufficiency: Paliperidone is not extensively metabolized in the liver. Although INVEGA SUSTENNA was not studied in patients with hepatic impairment, no dose adjustment is required in patients with mild or moderate hepatic impairment. In a study in subjects with moderate hepatic impairment (Child-Pugh class B), the plasma concentrations of unbound paliperidone were similar to those of healthy subjects. No dose adjustment is required in patients with mild to moderate hepatic impairment. Paliperidone has not been studied in patients with severe hepatic impairment.

Renal Insufficiency: INVEGA SUSTENNA has not been systematically studied in patients with renal impairment. Based on a limited number of observations with INVEGA SUSTENNA in subjects with mild renal impairment and pharmacokinetic simulations, the dose of INVEGA SUSTENNA should be reduced in patients with mild renal impairment; INVEGA SUSTENNA is not recommended for use in patients with moderate or severe renal impairment (see Dosage and Administration).

The disposition of a single oral dose 3 mg of paliperidone extended-release tablet was studied in subjects with varying degrees of renal function. Elimination of paliperidone decreased with decreasing estimated creatinine clearance. Total clearance of paliperidone was reduced in subjects with impaired renal function by 32% on average in mild (CrCl=50 to <80 mL/min), 64% in moderate (CrCl=30 to <50 mL/min), and 71% in severe (CrCl=10 to <30 mL/min) renal impairment, corresponding to an average increase in exposure (AUC_{inf}) of 1.5, 2.6, and 4.8 fold, respectively, compared to healthy subjects. The mean terminal elimination half-life of paliperidone was 24, 40, and 51 hours in subjects with mild, moderate, and severe renal impairment, respectively, compared with 23 hours in subjects with normal renal function (CrCl ≥80 mL/min). Paliperidone has not been studied in subjects with creatinine clearance <10 mL/min.

Smoking Status: No dosage adjustment is recommended based on smoking status. Based on in vitro studies utilizing human liver enzymes, paliperidone is not a substrate for CYP1A2; smoking should, therefore, not have an effect on the pharmacokinetics of paliperidone. Consistent with these in vitro results, population pharmacokinetic evaluation has not revealed any statistically significant differences between smokers and non-smokers in an analysis performed with oral paliperidone extended-release tablets.

STORAGE AND STABILITY: INVEGA SUSTENNA should be stored at room temperature (15-30°C).

Keep out of the reach of children.

INFORMATION FOR THE PATIENT: Published in e-CPS, available by subscription at www.e-cps.ca.

DOSAGE FORMS, COMPOSITION AND PACKAGING: 50 mg/0.5 mL: Each pre-filled syringe with white to off-white sterile aqueous prolonged-release suspension for intramuscular injection contains: paliperidone 78 mg. Nonmedicinal ingredients: citric acid monohydrate, disodium hydrogen phosphate anhydrous, polyethylene glycol 4000, polysorbate 20, sodium dihydrogen phosphate monohydrate, sodium hydroxide and water for injection. Kits containing a prefilled syringe and 2 safety needles, a 1½-inch 22 gauge safety needle, and a 1-inch 23 gauge safety needle. The pre-filled syringes are for single use only.

75 mg/0.75 mL: Each pre-filled syringe with white to off-white sterile aqueous prolonged-release suspension for intramuscular injection contains: paliperidone 117 mg. Nonmedicinal ingredients: citric acid monohydrate, disodium hydrogen phosphate anhydrous, polyethylene glycol 4000, polysorbate 20, sodium dihydrogen phosphate monohydrate, sodium hydroxide and water for injection. Kits containing a prefilled syringe and 2 safety needles, a 1½-inch 22 gauge safety needle, and a 1-inch 23 gauge safety needle. The pre-filled syringes are for single use only.

100 mg/1 mL: Each pre-filled syringe with white to off-white sterile aqueous prolonged-release suspension for intramuscular injection contains: paliperidone 156 mg. Nonmedicinal ingredients: citric acid monohydrate, disodium hydrogen phosphate anhydrous, polyethylene glycol 4000, polysorbate 20, sodium dihydrogen phosphate monohydrate, sodium hydroxide and water for injection. Kits containing a prefilled syringe and 2 safety needles, a 1½-inch 22 gauge safety needle, and a 1-inch 23 gauge safety needle. The pre-filled syringes are for single use only.

150 mg/1.5 mL: Each pre-filled syringe with white to off-white sterile aqueous prolonged-release suspension for intramuscular injection contains: paliperidone 234 mg. Nonmedicinal ingredients: citric acid monohydrate, disodium hydrogen phosphate anhydrous, polyethylene glycol 4000, polysorbate 20, sodium dihydrogen phosphate monohydrate, sodium hydroxide and water for injection. Kits containing a prefilled syringe and 2 safety needles, a 1½-inch 22 gauge safety needle, and a 1-inch 23 gauge safety needle. The pre-filled syringes are for single use only.

(Shown in Product Identification Section)

Invirase® Ⓟ

saquinavir mesylate

HIV Protease Inhibitor—Antiretroviral Agent

Roche

Date of Revision: March 22, 2010

SUMMARY PRODUCT INFORMATION:

Route of Administration	Dosage Form/ Strength	Clinically Relevant Nonmedicinal Ingredients
Oral	200 mg hard gelatin capsule	Lactose (see Warnings and Precautions) For a complete listing of nonmedicinal ingredients see Dosage Forms, Composition and Packaging.
Oral	500 mg film coated tablet	Lactose (see Warnings and Precautions) For a complete listing of nonmedicinal ingredients see Dosage Forms, Composition and Packaging.

INDICATIONS AND CLINICAL USE: INVIRASE (saquinavir mesylate) is indicated for:

- The treatment of HIV-1 infected adult patients. INVIRASE should only be given in combination with ritonavir and other antiretroviral medicinal products.

This indication is based on pharmacokinetic data and safety data from the MaxCmin 1 and MaxCmin 2 studies. Low dose ritonavir significantly inhibits saquinavir's metabolism and provides increased plasma saquinavir levels.

Geriatrics (>65 years of age): Only limited experience is available in elderly patients. No data are available to establish a dose recommendation in elderly patients.

Pediatrics (<16 years of age): The safety and efficacy of saquinavir in HIV-infected children has not been established.

CONTRAINDICATIONS:

- INVIRASE (saquinavir mesylate) is contraindicated in patients with clinically significant hypersensitivity to saquinavir or to any other component contained in the hard gelatin capsule or film coated tablet (see Dosage Forms, Composition and Packaging).
- INVIRASE/ritonavir should not be administered concurrently with terfenadine, cisapride, astemizole, triazolam, midazolam, ergot derivatives, or pimozide. Inhibition of CYP3A4 by saquinavir could result in elevated plasma concentrations of these drugs, potentially causing serious or life-threatening reactions, such as cardiac arrhythmias or prolonged sedation (see Drug Interactions).
- INVIRASE/ritonavir should not be used in patients already taking medications known to cause QT interval prolongation, such as Class IA (e.g., quinidine, procainamide) or Class III (e.g., amiodarone, sotalol) antiarrhythmic drugs or in patients with a history of QT interval prolongation.
- INVIRASE/ritonavir is contraindicated in patients with severe hepatic impairment (see Warnings and Precautions, Hepatic/Biliary/Pancreatic).
- INVIRASE/ritonavir should not be given together with rifampin, due to the risk of severe hepatocellular toxicity if the three drugs are taken together (see Drug Interactions).

INVIRASE/ritonavir should not be administered concurrently with drugs listed in Table 1 (also see Drug Interactions, Table 3).

Table 1: INVIRASE

Drugs that are Contraindicated with INVIRASE/ritonavir

Drug Class	Drugs within Class that are Contraindicated with INVIRASE/ritonavir
Antiarrhythmics	Amiodarone, bepridil, flecainide, procainamide, propafenone, quinidine, sotalol
Antihistamines	Astemizole[a], terfenadine[a]
Antimycobacterial Agents	Rifampin
Ergot Derivatives	Dihydroergotamine, ergonovine, ergotamine, methylergonovine
GI Motility Agents	Cisapride[a]
Neuroleptics	Pimozide
Sedative/Hypnotics	Triazolam, midazolam

[a] No longer marketed in Canada.

Because ritonavir is coadministered with INVIRASE, prescribers should refer to the prescribing information for ritonavir for additional contraindicated drugs.

WARNINGS AND PRECAUTIONS:

Serious Warnings and Precautions
- INVIRASE (saquinavir mesylate) should only be administered with low dose ritonavir (see Indications and Clinical Use)
- Serious or life-threatening drug-drug interactions (see Contraindications and Drug Interactions)
- INVIRASE/ritonavir is contraindicated in patients with severe hepatic impairment (see Hepatic/Biliary/Pancreatic)

General: INVIRASE should only be used if it is combined with ritonavir.

When INVIRASE is prescribed in combination with other antiretroviral therapies, physicians should refer to the appropriate Product Monographs for safety and prescribing information.

If a serious or severe toxicity occurs during treatment with INVIRASE, treatment with the drug should be interrupted until the etiology of the event is identified or the toxicity resolves. At that time, resumption of treatment with full dose may be considered.

Lactose Intolerance: Each capsule contains lactose (anhydrous) 63.3 mg and each film-coated tablet contains lactose (monohydrate) 38.5 mg. Patients with rare hereditary problems of galactose intolerance, the Lapp lactase deficiency or glucose-galactose malabsorption (autosomal recessive disorder) should not take this medicine.

Body as a Whole: Fat Redistribution: Redistribution/accumulation of body fat including central obesity, dorsocervical fat enlargement (buffalo hump), peripheral wasting, facial wasting, breast enlargement, and "Cushingoid appearance" have been observed in patients receiving antiretroviral therapy. The mechanism and long-term consequences of these events are currently unknown. A causal relationship has not been established.

Carcinogenesis and Mutagenesis: No human data is available.

Cardiovascular: Cardiac Conduction Abnormalities: Dose-dependent prolongations of QT and PR intervals were observed in healthy volunteers receiving ritonavir-boosted INVIRASE. PR interval prolongation of >200 msec (1st degree AV-Block) was observed in 40% of subjects receiving a therapeutic dose of INVIRASE/ritonavir (1000/100 mg bid) and 47% of subjects receiving a supratherapeutic dose of INVIRASE/ritonavir (1500/100 mg bid) on Day 3 compared with 3 % of subjects in the active control (moxifloxacin) arm and 5% in the placebo group. Maximum mean QT prolongations (QTcS: study-specific QTc interval correction) of 18.9 msec, 30.2 msec and 12.2 msec were observed in the 1000/100 mg, 1500/100 mg and moxifloxacin (positive control) groups respectively. The majority of subjects (89% and 80% in the therapeutic dose and supratherapeutic dose groups, respectively) had a QTcS of <450 msec and none had a QTcS interval of >500 msec. (See Action and Clinical Pharmacology, Special Populations and Conditions, Effects on Electrocardiogram.)

Ritonavir-boosted INVIRASE should not be used in patients already taking medications known to cause QT interval prolongation, such as Class IA (e.g. quinidine, procainamide) or Class III (e.g. amiodarone, sotalol) antiarrhythmic drugs, or in patients with a history of QT interval prolongation. Caution should be taken when administering ritonavir-boosted INVIRASE with any medication which can significantly increase either the QT or PR interval. Caution is also warranted when administering ritonavir-boosted INVIRASE to patients with a known history of QT prolongation or medical conditions predisposing to QT prolongation (e.g. electrolyte disturbances) and/or patients with pre-existing conduction system disease (e.g. first-degree AV block or second- or third degree AV block).

Hyperlipidemia: Elevated cholesterol and/or triglyceride levels have been observed in some patients taking saquinavir in combination with ritonavir. Cholesterol and triglyceride levels should be monitored prior to initiating combination therapy with INVIRASE/ritonavir, and at periodic intervals while on such therapy. In these patients, lipid disorders should be managed as clinically appropriate.

Endocrine and Metabolism: Diabetes Mellitus and Hyperglycemia: New onset diabetes mellitus, exacerbation of pre-existing diabetes mellitus and hyperglycemia have been reported during post-marketing surveillance in HIV-infected patients receiving protease inhibitor therapy. Some patients required either initiation or dose adjustments of insulin or oral hypoglycemic agents for treatment of these events. In some cases diabetic ketoacidosis has occurred. In those patients who discontinued protease inhibitor therapy, hyperglycemia persisted in some cases. Because these events have been reported voluntarily during clinical practice, estimates of frequency cannot be made and a causal relationship between protease inhibitor therapy and these events has not been established.

Hematologic: Hemophiliac Patients: There have been reports of increased bleeding including spontaneous skin hematomas and hemarthrosis in patients with Hemophilia Type A and Type B treated with protease inhibitors. In some patients, additional Factor VIII was given. In more than half of the reported cases, treatment with protease inhibitors was continued or re-introduced. There is no proven relationship between protease inhibitors and such bleeding, however, the frequency of bleeding episodes should be closely monitored in patients on saquinavir.

Hepatic/Biliary/Pancreatic: Patients with Hepatic Impairment: In cases of mild impairment no initial dose adjustment is necessary at the recommended dose. The use of INVIRASE (alone or in combination with ritonavir) in patients with moderate hepatic impairment has not been studied. In the absence of such studies, caution should be exercised, as increases in saquinavir levels and/or increases in liver enzymes may occur. In patients with underlying hepatitis B or C, cirrhosis, chronic alcoholism and/or other underlying liver abnormalities there have been reports of worsening liver disease and development of portal hypertension after starting saquinavir. Associated symptoms include jaundice, ascites, edema and, in some cases esophageal varices. Several of these patients died. A causal relationship between saquinavir therapy and development of portal hypertension has not been established. Increased monitoring for signs and symptoms of liver toxicity should be considered. INVIRASE/ritonavir is contraindicated in patients with severe hepatic impairment (see Contraindications).

Pancreatitis: Elevated cholesterol and/or triglyceride levels have been observed in some patients taking saquinavir in combination with ritonavir. Marked elevation in triglyceride levels is a risk factor for development of pancreatitis (see Warnings and Precautions, Cardiac Disorders).

Immune: Immune Reconstitution Syndrome: Immune reconstitution syndrome has been reported in patients treated with combination antiretroviral therapy, including INVIRASE. During the initial phase of combination antiretroviral treatment, patients whose immune system responds may develop an inflammatory response to indolent or residual opportunistic infections (such as *M. avium* infection, cytomegalovirus, *P. jiroveci* pneumonia (PCP), or tuberculosis), which may necessitate further evaluation and treatment.

Renal: Patients with Renal Impairment: Renal clearance is only a minor elimination pathway, the principal route of metabolism and excretion for saquinavir is via the liver. Therefore, no initial dose adjustment is necessary for patients with renal impairment. However, patients with severe renal impairment have not been studied and caution should be exercised when prescribing saquinavir in this population.

Resistance/Cross-Resistance: Varying degrees of cross-resistance among protease inhibitors have been observed. Continued administration of INVIRASE therapy following loss of viral suppression may increase the likelihood of cross-resistance to other protease inhibitors (see also Action and Clinical Pharmacology, Resistance).

Special Populations: Pregnant Women: Reproduction studies with saquinavir in rats have shown no embryotoxicity or teratogenicity at plasma exposures (AUC values) up to 5 times those achieved with human use (1800 mg/day), or in rabbits at dose levels up to 24 times the recommended human dose. There are however, no adequate or well controlled studies of INVIRASE in pregnant women. Because animal reproduction studies are not always predictive of human response, INVIRASE should be used during pregnancy only if the potential benefits are considered to outweigh the potential risks to the fetus.

Antiretroviral Pregnancy Registry: To monitor maternal-fetal outcomes of pregnant women exposed to INVIRASE and other antiretroviral drugs, an Antiretroviral Pregnancy Registry has been established. Physicians are encouraged to register patients by calling 1-800-258-4263.

Nursing Women: It is not known whether saquinavir is excreted in human milk. **Because many drugs are excreted in human milk, it is advisable to caution mothers against breast feeding while taking INVIRASE.** Animal studies indicate that administration of saquinavir to rats through the lactation period at plasma concentrations (AUC values) up to 5 times those achieved with the human-dose (1800 mg/day) had no effect on the survival, growth or development of offspring to weaning. However, the potential for adverse reactions to saquinavir in nursing infants cannot be assessed. **Current medical practice advises against breast-feeding by HIV-infected women, due to the possibility of post-natal transmission.**

Pediatrics (<16 years of age): The safety and efficacy of saquinavir in HIV-infected children has not been established. The safety and efficacy of saquinavir when coadministered with ritonavir to pediatric patients is under investigation.

Geriatrics (>65 years of age): Only limited experience is available in elderly patients. No data are available to establish a dose recommendation in elderly patients.

Monitoring and Laboratory Tests: Clinical chemistry tests, viral load and CD_4 count should be performed prior to initiating therapy and at appropriate intervals thereafter. Elevated nonfasting triglyceride levels have been observed in patients in saquinavir trials. Triglyceride levels should be periodically monitored during therapy. Increases in cholesterol have also been observed and should be monitored. For comprehensive information concerning laboratory test alterations associated with the use of other antiretroviral therapies, physicians should refer to the complete product information for these drugs.

ADVERSE REACTIONS: Clinical Trial Adverse Drug Reactions: Because clinical trials are conducted under very specific conditions the adverse reaction rates observed in the clinical trials may not reflect the rates observed in practice and should not be compared to the rates in the clinical trials of another drug. Adverse drug reaction information from clinical trials is useful for identifying drug-related adverse events and for approximating rates.

The most frequently reported adverse events with at least a possible relationship to saquinavir in combination with low dose ritonavir (i.e. adverse reactions) were nausea, diarrhea, fatigue, vomiting, flatulence, and abdominal pain.

Concomitant Therapy with Ritonavir Adverse Reactions: There have been no large controlled clinical trials with INVIRASE in combination with low dose ritonavir. The safety database is therefore based on trials with saquinavir soft gel capsules in combination with low dose ritonavir. The limited data available are from two studies where the safety of saquinavir soft capsule (1000 mg twice daily) used in combination with low dose ritonavir (100 mg twice daily) for at least 48 weeks was studied in 311 patients. Adverse reactions in these pivotal studies are summarized in Table 2, which also includes marked laboratory abnormalities that have been observed with the saquinavir soft capsule in combination with ritonavir (at 48 weeks).

Table 2: INVIRASE

Clinical Adverse Events Considered at Least Possibly Related to Saquinavir Soft Gel Capsules and of Moderate, Severe or Life-Threatening Intensity, Occurring in ≥1% of Patients in MaxCmin 1 and MaxCmin 2

	MaxCmin 1 (N=148) No. (%)	MaxCmin 2 (N=163) No. (%)
All Body Systems		
Patients having at least one adverse event	56 (38)	63 (39)
Blood and Lymphatic System Disorders		
Anemia	3 (2)	2 (1)
Congenital, Familial and Genetic Disorders		
Lipodystrophy congenital	6 (4)	5 (3)
Gastrointestinal Disorders		
Nausea	11 (7)	11 (7)
Diarrhea	8 (5)	13 (8)
Vomiting	6 (4)	4 (3)
Abdominal pain upper	—	6 (4)
Abdominal pain	4 (3)	4 (3)
Flatulence	4 (3)	—
Dyspepsia	—	2 (1)
General Disorders and Administration Site Conditions		
Fatigue	7 (5)	3 (2)
Asthenia	2 (1)	2 (1)
Fat tissue increased	—	2 (1)
Immune System Disorders		
Hypersensitivity	2 (1)	—
Investigations		
Alanine aminotransferase increased	4 (3)	3 (2)
Aspartate aminotransferase increased	3 (2)	2 (1)
Blood triglycerides	2 (1)	
Blood triglycerides increased	2 (1)	4 (3)
Weight decreased	2 (1)	—
Metabolism and Nutrition Disorders		
Anorexia	2 (1)	—
Diabetes mellitus	2 (1)	—
Hypertriglyceridemia	—	2 (1)
Nervous System Disorders		
Headache	—	4 (3)
Dizziness (excl. vertigo)	—	2 (1)
Peripheral neuropathy	2 (1)	—
Skin and Subcutaneous Tissue Disorders		
Dry skin	2 (1)	—
Pruritus	2 (1)	—
Rash	2 (1)	—

The clinical trial database for INVIRASE consists of >6000 patients, with over 100 patients followed for >2 years. Limited experience is available from three single-dose studies investigating the pharmacokinetics of the INVIRASE 500 mg film coated tablet compared to the INVIRASE 200 mg capsule in healthy volunteers (n=140). In two of these studies saquinavir was boosted with ritonavir; in the other study, saquinavir was administered as single drug. The INVIRASE tablet and the capsule formulations were similarly tolerated. The most common adverse events were gastrointestinal disorders (such as diarrhea). Since bioequivalence was demonstrated, no difference in safety profile is expected between the two formulations of INVIRASE.

Less Common Clinical Trial Adverse Drug Reactions: Additionally, the following adverse experiences of any intensity, at least remotely related to saquinavir, reported in clinical trials using INVIRASE or saquinavir soft gel capsules with or without ritonavir, and not mentioned in Table 2 are provided for completeness and are listed below by body system:

Blood and Lymphatic System Disorders: hemolytic anemia, neutropenia, thrombocytopenia, bleeding dermal, leucopenia, microhemorrhages, pancytopenia, splenomegaly, lymphadenopathy.

Cardiac Disorders: hypertension, cyanosis, heart murmur, heart valve disorder, hypotension, syncope.

Gastrointestinal Disorders: ascites, intestinal obstruction, constipation, eructation, stomatitis, discoloured feces, glossitis, frequent bowel movements, gastralgia, gastritis, gastrointestinal inflammation, pancreatitis, pancreatitis leading to death, tooth disorder, cheilitis, colic abdominal, dysphagia, esophagitis, feces bloodstained, gingivitis, hemorrhage rectum, hemorrhoids, infectious diarrhea, melena, pain pelvic, painful defecation, parotid disorder, salivary glands disorder, stomach upset, toothache, abdominal distention.

General Disorders and Administration Site Conditions: mucosal ulceration, fever, wasting syndrome, allergic reaction, chest pain, shivering, edema, intoxication, parasites external, retrosternal pain and drug fever; abdominal pain.

Hepatobiliary Disorders: jaundice, portal hypertension, and exacerbation of chronic liver disease with Grade 4 elevated liver function test, hepatomegaly, hepatosplenomegaly, hyperbilirubinemia, liver enzyme disorder.

Infections and Infestations: staphylococcal infection, abscess, angina tonsillaris, candidiasis, cellulitis, herpes simplex, herpes zoster, infection bacterial, infection mycotic, influenza, moniliasis.

Investigations: blood glucose increased, and blood glucose decreased, increased alkaline phosphatase, increased creatinine phosphokinase, increased gamma GT, raised amylase, raised LDH, TSH increase, hyperglycemia, hypercalcemia, hyperkalemia, hypernatremia, hyperphosphatemia, hypocalcemia, hypokalemia, hyponatremia, hypophosphatemia; hyperbilirubinemia.

Metabolism and Nutrition Disorders: appetite decreased, weight increase, dehydration, appetite increased.

Musculoskeletal and Connective Tissue Disorder: muscular weakness, polyarthritis, stiffness, arthralgia, arthritis, back pain, cramps leg, cramps muscle, musculoskeletal disorders, tissue changes, trauma, myalgia and musculoskeletal pain.

Neoplasms Benign, Malignant and Unspecified (including cysts and polyps): skin papilloma, acute myeloid leukaemia, tumor.

Nervous System Disorders: hypoaesthesia, coordination abnormal, intracranial hemorrhage, ataxia, confusion, dry mouth, convulsions, dysesthesia, tremor, dysarthria, heart rate disorder, hyperesthesia, hyperreflexia, hyporeflexia, light-headed feeling, myelopolyradiculoneuritis, numbness face, pain facial, paresis, poliomyelitis, prickly sensation, progressive multifocal leukoencephalopathy, spasms, unconsciousness, and extremity numbness.

Psychiatric Disorders: confusional state, suicide attempt, insomnia, euphoria, anxiety, reduced intellectual ability, irritability, agitation, hallucination, somnolence, depression, amnesia, anxiety attack, dreaming excessive, lethargy, libido disorder, overdose effect, psychic disorder, psychosis, speech disorder.

Renal and Urinary Disorders: micturition disorder, renal calculus, urinary tract bleeding, urinary tract infection.

Reproductive System Disorders: impotence, prostate enlarged, vaginal discharge.

Respiratory, Thoracic and Mediastinal Disorders: pharyngitis, dyspnea, laryngitis, rhinitis, bronchitis, cough, epistaxis, hemoptysis, pneumonia, pulmonary disease, respiratory disorder, sinusitis, upper respiratory tract infection.

Skin and Subcutaneous Tissue Disorders: Stevens-Johnson syndrome, dermatitis bullous, drug eruption, severe cutaneous reaction associated with increased liver function tests, sweating increased, hot flushes, skin pigment changes, acne, dermatitis, folliculitis, alopecia, and polyarthritis, chalazion, dermatitis seborrheic, eczema, erythema, furunculosis, hair changes, nail disorder, night sweats, photosensitivity reaction, rash maculopapular, skin disorder, skin nodule, skin ulceration, urticaria, verruca.

Special Senses: visual disturbances, taste alteration, xerophthalmia, blepharitis, earache, ear pressure, eye irritation, hearing decreased, otitis, tinnitus, dry eye syndrome.

Vascular Disorders: vasoconstriction and vein distended.

Post-Market Adverse Drug Reactions: Serious and non-serious adverse events from post-marketing spontaneous reports (where saquinavir was taken as the sole protease inhibitor or in combination with ritonavir), for which a causal relationship to saquinavir cannot be excluded are listed below. As these data come from the spontaneous reporting system, the frequency of adverse reactions is unknown.

- Immune System Disorders: allergic reactions and hypersensitivity.
- Metabolism and Nutrition Disorders:
  - diabetes mellitus or hyperglycemia sometimes associated with ketoacidosis (see Warnings and Precautions, Endocrine and Metabolism, Diabetes Mellitus and Hyperglycemia).
  - Lipodystrophy: Combination antiretroviral therapy has been associated with redistribution of body fat (lipodystrophy) in HIV infected patients including the loss of peripheral and facial subcutaneous fat, increased intra-abdominal and visceral fat, breast hypertrophy and dorsicervical fat accumulation (buffalo hump) (see Warnings and Precautions, Body as a Whole, Fat Redistribution).
  - Combination antiretroviral therapy has been associated with metabolic abnormalities such as hypertriglyceridemia, hypercholesterolemia, insulin resistance, hyperglycemia and hyperlactatemia (see Warnings and Precautions).
- Nervous System Disorders: somnolence, convulsions.
- Vascular Disorders:
  - thrombophlebitis.
  - There have been reports of increased bleeding, including spontaneous skin hematomas and hemarthroses, in hemophilic patients type A and B treated with protease inhibitors (see Warnings and Precautions, Hematologic, Hemophiliac Patients).
- Hepatobiliary Disorders: isolated elevation of transaminases and hepatitis.

Additional adverse events that have been observed during the postmarketing period are similar to those seen in clinical trials with INVIRASE and saquinavir soft gel capsules alone or in combination with ritonavir.

DRUG INTERACTIONS:

Serious Drug Interactions

- INVIRASE (saquinavir mesylate) should not be administered concurrently with some antiarrythmics, antihistamines, ergot derivatives, antimycobacterial agents, GI motility agents, neuroleptics, sedatives or hypnotics. For a listing of drugs within each of the above drug classes see Contraindications.
- INVIRASE/ritonavir should not be used in patients already taking medications known to cause QT interval prolongation, such as Class IA (e.g., quinidine, procainamide) or Class III (e.g., amiodarone, sotalol) antiarrhythmic drugs or in patients with a history of QT interval prolongation
- Caution is warranted when coadministering INVIRASE with HMG-CoA reductase inhibitors as there is an increased risk of mypopathy and rhabdomyolysis (see Table 3 and Table 4).
- In some cases, coadministration of saquinavir and ritonavir has led to severe adverse events, mainly diabetic ketoacidosis and liver disorders, especially with pre-existing liver disease (see Table 4).
- Unless saquinavir is coadministered with ritonavir, saquinavir should not be used with either rifabutin or efavirenz as the concurrent use results in reduced saquinavir concentrations (see Table 3).
- Concomitant use of fluticasone propionate and INVIRASE/ritonavir may increase plasma concentrations of fluticasone propionate, resulting in significantly reduced serum cortisol concentrations. Coadministration of fluticasone propionate and INVIRASE/ritonavir is not recommended unless the potential benefit to the patient outweighs the risk of systemic corticosteroid side effects (see Table 3 and Table 4).
- Concurrent use of INVIRASE and St. John's Wort or products containing St. John's Wort is not recommended (see Drug-Herb Interactions).
- Garlic capsules should not be used if taking saquinavir without ritonavir (see Drug-Herb Interactions).
- When coadministering INVIRASE with any agent having a narrow therapeutic margin, such as anticoagulants, anticonvulsants, and antiarrhythmics, special attention is warranted (see Table 3 and Table 4).
- Coadministration of sildenafil or tadalafil with INVIRASE/ritonavir is expected to substantially increase the concentrations of sildenafil or tadalafil, and may result in associated adverse events such as hypotension, visual changes and priapism. Vardenafil should not be coadministered with INVIRASE/ritonavir (see Table 4).
- Caution should be exercised when INVIRASE and digoxin are coadministered; the serum concentration of digoxin should be monitored and the dose of digoxin may need to be reduced (see Table 4).

Overview: Several drug interaction studies have been completed with both INVIRASE and saquinavir soft gel capsules. Observations from drug interaction studies with saquinavir soft gel capsules may not be predictive for INVIRASE. Because ritonavir is coadministered, prescribers should refer to the prescribing information for ritonavir regarding drug interactions associated with this drug.

The metabolism of saquinavir is mediated by cytochrome P450, with the specific isoenzyme CYP3A4 responsible for 90% of the hepatic metabolism. Additionally, saquinavir is a substrate for P-Glycoprotein (Pgp). Therefore, drugs that affect CYP3A4 and/or Pgp, may modify the pharmacokinetics of saquinavir. Similarly, saquinavir might also modify the pharmacokinetics of other drugs that are substrates for CYP3A4 or Pgp.

Drugs that are Mainly Metabolized by CYP3A4: Compounds that are substrates of CYP3A4 (e.g. alfentanyl, alprazolam, amiodarone, calcium channel blockers, clindamycin, carbamazepine, cyclosporine, dapsone, disopyramide, fentanyl, nefazodone, pimozide, quinidine, quinine, tacrolimus, warfarin) may have elevated plasma concentrations when coadministered with INVIRASE; therefore, these combinations should be used with caution and patients should be monitored for toxicities associated with such drugs.

Since INVIRASE is coadministered with ritonavir, the ritonavir product monograph should be reviewed for additional drugs that should not be coadministered.

Substrates of P-gp: Concomitant use of INVIRASE with drugs that are substrates of P-gp may lead to elevated plasma concentrations of the concomitant drugs. Monitoring for toxicity is therefore recommended. Compounds that are substrates of P-gp include cyclosporine, paclitaxel, and vinblastine.

Inducers of CYP3A4: Coadministration with compounds that are potent inducers of CYP3A4 (e.g., phenobarbital, phenytoin, dexamethasone, carbamazepine) may result in decreased plasma levels of saquinavir.

Ritonavir-Boosted INVIRASE and Rifampin: In a study investigating the drug-drug interaction of rifampin 600 mg/day daily and INVIRASE 1000 mg/ritonavir 100 mg twice daily (ritonavir-boosted INVIRASE) involving 28 healthy volunteers, 11 of 17 healthy volunteers (65%) exposed concomitantly to rifampin and ritonavir-boosted INVIRASE developed severe hepatocellular toxicity presented as increased hepatic transaminases. In some subjects, transaminases increased up to >20-fold the upper limit of normal and were associated with gastrointestinal symptoms including abdominal pain, gastritis, nausea, and vomiting. Following discontinuation of all three drugs, clinical symptoms abated and the increased hepatic transaminases normalized (see Contraindications).

Drug-Drug Interactions: Drugs that are contraindicated or not recommended for coadministration with saquinavir are included in Table 3. Drugs with established and other potentially significant drug interactions are included in Table 4. These recommendations are based on either drug interaction studies or predicted interactions due to the expected magnitude of interaction and potential for serious events or loss of efficacy.

Table 3: INVIRASE

Drugs that are Contraindicated or not Recommended for Coadministration with INVIRASE/ritonavir

Drug Class: Specific Drugs	Clinical Comment
Antiarrhythmics: Amiodarone, bepridil, flecainide, procainamide, propafenone, quinidine, sotalol	**Contraindicated** due to potential for serious and/or life threatening reactions.
Antihistamines: Astemizole[a], terfenadine[a]	**Contraindicated** due to potential for serious and/or life-threatening cardiac arrhythmias.
Antimycobacterial: Rifabutin	**Warning:** Saquinavir should not be given without ritonavir to patients taking rifabutin as coadministration results in significantly reduced plasma concentrations of saquinavir and may lead to loss of virologic response.
Rifampin	**Contraindicated:** Rifampin should not be administered in patients taking INVIRASE/ritonavir as part of an ART regimen due to risk of hepatocellular toxicity.
Corticosteroid (nasal use): Fluticasone	**Warning:** Systemic corticosteroid effects including Cushing's syndrome and adrenal suppression have been reported during postmarketing use in patients receiving ritonavir and inhaled or intranasally administered fluticasone propionate. Therefore, coadministration of fluticasone propionate and INVIRASE/ritonavir is not recommended unless the potential benefit to the patient outweighs the risk of systemic corticosteroid side effects (see Table 4).
Ergot Derivatives: Dihydroergotamine, ergonovine, ergotamine, methylergonovine	**Contraindicated** due to potential for serious and life-threatening reactions such as acute ergot toxicity characterized by peripheral vasospasm and ischemia of the extremities and other tissues.
Garlic Capsules	No data are available for the coadministration of INVIRASE/ritonavir and garlic capsules. **Warning:** Garlic capsules should not be used when taking saquinavir without ritonavir due to the risk of decreased saquinavir plasma concentrations (see Drug-Herb Interactions).
GI Motility Agent: Cisapride[a]	**Contraindicated** due to potential for serious and/or life-threatening reactions such as cardiac arrhythmias.
Herbal Products: St. John's Wort (hypericum perforatum)	Not recommended due to risk of decreased plasma concentrations of saquinavir which may lead to loss of virologic response and possible resistance to saquinavir or to the class of protease inhibitors (see Drug-Herb Interactions).
HMG-CoA Reductase Inhibitors: Lovastatin, simvastatin	Not recommended due to potential for serious reactions such as risk of myopathy including rhabdomyolysis.
Neuroleptic: Pimozide	**Contraindicated** due to potential for serious and/or life-threatening reactions such as cardiac arrhythmias.
Non-Nucleoside Reverse Transcriptase Inhibitor: Efavirenz	**Warning:** Saquinavir should not be given without ritonavir to patients taking efavirenz as coadministration results in significantly reduced plasma concentrations of saquinavir and may lead to loss of virologic response.
Sedatives/Hypnotics: Triazolam, midazolam	**Contraindicated** due to potential for serious and/or life-threatening reactions such as prolonged or increased sedation or respiratory depression.

[a] No longer marketed in Canada.

Since INVIRASE is coadministered with ritonavir, the ritonavir product monograph should be reviewed for additional drugs that should not be coadministered.

Drug-Food Interactions: Coadministration of 600 mg of saquinavir soft gel capsules and quadruple strength grapefruit juice as a single administration in healthy volunteers resulted in a 54% increase in exposure to saquinavir.

Drug-Herb Interactions: Garlic Capsules: Garlic capsules should not be used when taking saquinavir without ritonavir due to the risk of decreased saquinavir plasma concentrations. No data are available for the coadministration of INVIRASE/ritonavir and garlic capsules.

St. John's Wort (hypericum perforatum): Concomitant use of INVIRASE and St John's Wort or products containing St. John's Wort is not recommended due to risk of decreased plasma concentrations of saquinavir which may lead to loss of virologic response and possible resistance to saquinavir or to the class of protease inhibitors.

DOSAGE AND ADMINISTRATION:

Dosing Considerations: INVIRASE (saquinavir mesylate) should only be used in combination with ritonavir, because it significantly inhibits saquinavir's metabolism to provide increased plasma saquinavir levels.

Recommended Dose and Dosage Adjustment: For adults or adolescents over the age of 16 years unable to take INVIRASE 500 mg film-coated tablets, INVIRASE should be given in the form of 200 mg capsules.

Adults and Adolescents Over the Age of 16 Years: INVIRASE should only be used in combination with ritonavir. The recommended dosage regimen is INVIRASE 1000 mg (5×200 mg capsules or 2×500 mg tablets) two times daily with ritonavir 100 mg two times daily, in combination with other antiretroviral agents. Ritonavir should be taken at the same time as INVIRASE, and within 2 hours after a meal.

Concomitant Therapy: INVIRASE with Lopinavir/Ritonavir: When administered with lopinavir/ritonavir 400/100 mg bid, the appropriate dose of INVIRASE is 1000 mg bid (with no additional ritonavir).

Dose Adjustments for Combination Therapy with INVIRASE: For serious toxicities that may be associated with saquinavir, the drug should be interrupted. INVIRASE at doses less than 1000 mg with 100 mg ritonavir bid are not recommended since lower doses have not shown antiviral activity. For recipients of combination therapy with INVIRASE and ritonavir, dose adjustments may be necessary. These adjustments should be based on the known toxicity profile of the individual agent and the pharmacokinetic interaction between saquinavir and the coadministered drug (see Drug Interactions). Physicians should refer to the Product Monographs of these drugs for comprehensive dose adjustment recommendations and drug-associated adverse reactions.

Missed Dose: The missed dose should be taken as soon as it is remembered, then the regular dosing schedule should be continued. Two doses should not be taken at the same time.

Administration: Ritonavir should be taken at the same time as INVIRASE, and within 2 hours after a meal. INVIRASE capsules and tablets should be swallowed unchewed, with water or some other non-alcoholic drink. You should avoid excessive consumption of alcohol during your treatment with INVIRASE.

Table 4: INVIRASE

Established and Other Potentially Significant Drug Interactions: Alteration in Dose or Regimen May Be Recommended Based on Drug Interaction Studies or Predicted Interaction (Information in the table applies to INVIRASE/ritonavir)

Concomitant Drug Class: Drug Name	Effect on Concentration of Saquinavir or Concomitant Drug	Clinical Comment
HIV-Antiviral Agents		
Fusion Inhibitor: Enfuvirtide	Saquinavir soft gel capsules/ritonavir ↔ Enfuvirtide	No clinically significant interaction was noted from a study in 12 HIV patients who received enfuvirtide concomitantly with saquinavir soft gel capsules/ritonavir 1000/100 mg bid. No dose adjustments are required.
Non-Nucleoside Reverse Transcriptase Inhibitor: Delavirdine	↑ Saquinavir Effect on delavirdine not well established INVIRASE/ritonavir Interaction not evaluated	The safety and efficacy of this combination have not been established. In a small, preliminary study, hepatocellular enzyme elevations occurred in 13% of subjects during the first several weeks of treatment with the delavirdine and saquinavir combination (6% Grade 3 or 4). Hepatocellular changes should be monitored frequently if this combination is prescribed.
Non-Nucleoside Reverse Transcriptase Inhibitor: Efavirenz	INVIRASE/ritonavir ↔ Saquinavir ↔ Efavirenz	Saquinavir should not be given without ritonavir to patients taking efavirenz. In the studies performed in HIV patients no clinically significant alterations of either saquinavir or efavirenz concentrations were noted.
Non-Nucleoside Reverse Transcriptase Inhibitor: Nevirapine	Unboosted saquinavir ↓ 24% Saquinavir ↔ Nevirapine INVIRASE/ritonavir Interaction not evaluated	This decrease is not thought to be clinically significant and no dose adjustments of saquinavir or nevirapine are recommended. The safety and efficacy of the combination of nevirapine and INVIRASE/ritonavir have not been established.
Protease Inhibitor: Atazanavir	INVIRASE/ritonavir ↑ Saquinavir ↑ Ritonavir ↔ Atazanavir	The safety and efficacy for this combination have not been established. Saquinavir HC/ritonavir/atazanavir coadministered once daily at 1600/100/300 mg in HIV-infected patients resulted in increased exposure to saquinavir and ritonavir. Hyperbilirubinemia was the most common and most severe adverse event.
Protease Inhibitor: Indinavir	↑ Saquinavir Effect on indinavir not well established INVIRASE/ritonavir Interaction not evaluated	The safety and efficacy of the combination of indinavir and INVIRASE/ritonavir have not been established.
Protease Inhibitor: Lopinavir/ritonavir (coformulated capsule)	↔ Saquinavir ↔ Lopinavir ↓ Ritonavir	Evidence from several clinical trials indicates that saquinavir concentrations achieved with the saquinavir and lopinavir/ritonavir combination are similar to those achieved following saquinavir/ritonavir 1000/100 mg. The recommended dose for this combination is saquinavir 1000 mg plus lopinavir/ritonavir 400/100 mg bid.
Protease Inhibitor: Nelfinavir	Saquinavir Nelfinavir	Ritonavir-boosted INVIRASE combined with nelfinavir administered to 24 HIV-infected patients for a short treatment duration of 7 days was tolerated. However, concomitant administration of nelfinavir and saquinavir soft gel capsules resulted in a moderate increase in the incidence of diarrhea. The concentration of nelfinavir M8 metabolite was increased, in the presence of ritonavir-boosted saquinavir but did not alter the safety profile of nelfinavir.

(cont'd)

Table 4: INVIRASE *(cont'd)*

Established and Other Potentially Significant Drug Interactions: Alteration in Dose or Regimen May Be Recommended Based on Drug Interaction Studies or Predicted Interaction (Information in the table applies to INVIRASE/ritonavir)

Concomitant Drug Class: Drug Name	Effect on Concentration of Saquinavir or Concomitant Drug	Clinical Comment
Protease Inhibitor: Ritonavir	↑ Saquinavir ↔ Ritonavir	The recommended dose regimen when ritonavir is given to increase saquinavir concentrations is 1000 mg saquinavir plus ritonavir 100 mg twice daily. In some cases, coadministration of SQV and RTV has led to severe adverse events, mainly diabetic ketoacidosis and liver disorders, especially in patients with pre-existing liver disease. When used in combination therapy, doses greater than 400 mg BID of either ritonavir or saquinavir were associated with an increase in adverse events. Therefore, combination therapy should be used with caution.
Protease Inhibitor: Tipranavir/ritonavir	↓ Saquinavir	Combining saquinavir with tipranavir/ritonavir is not recommended.
Other Agents		
Antiarrhythmics: Lidocaine (systemic)	↑ Antiarrhythmics	Caution is warranted and therapeutic concentration monitoring, if available, is recommended for antiarrhythmics given with INVIRASE/ritonavir.
Anticoagulant: Warfarin		Concentrations of warfarin may be affected. It is recommended that INR (international normalized ratio) be monitored.
Anticonvulsants: Carbamazepine, phenobarbital, phenytoin	↓ Saquinavir Effects on anticonvulsants are not well established INVIRASE/ritonavir Interaction not evaluated	Use with caution, saquinavir may be less effective due to decreased saquinavir plasma concentrations in patients taking these agents concomitantly.
Antidepressant: Trazodone	↑ Trazodone	Concomitant use of trazodone and INVIRASE/ritonavir may increase plasma concentrations of trazodone. Adverse events of nausea, dizziness, hypotension and syncope have been observed following coadministration of trazodone and ritonavir. If trazodone is used with a CYP3A4 inhibitor such as INVIRASE/ritonavir, the combination should be used with caution and lower dose of trazodone should be considered.
Antidepressants (tricyclic): Amitriptyline, imipramine	↑ Tricyclics	Therapeutic concentration monitoring is recommended for tricyclic antidepressants when coadministered with INVIRASE/ritonavir.
Antifungal: Ketoconazole	↑ Ketoconazole ↔ INVIRASE/ritonavir	No dose adjustment for either saquinavir or ritonavir is required when coadministered with ≤200 mg ketoconazole. High doses of ketoconazole (>200 mg/day) are not recommended.
Itraconazole	INVIRASE/ritonavir Interaction not evaluated	The safety and efficacy of the combination of itraconazole and INVIRASE/ritonavir have not been established.
Anti-infective: Clarithromycin	↑ Saquinavir ↑ Clarithromycin INVIRASE/ritonavir Interaction not evaluated	No dose adjustment is required when the two drugs are coadministered for a limited time at the doses studied (clarithromycin 500 mg bid and saquinavir soft gel capsules 1200 mg tid for 7 days). For patients with renal impairment, the following dosage adjustments should be considered: • For patients with CL_{CR} 30 to 60 mL/min the dose of clarithromycin should be reduced by 50%. • For patients with CL_{CR} <30 mL/min the dose of clarithromycin should be decreased by 75%. No dose adjustment for patients with normal renal function is necessary.
Erythromycin	↑ Saquinavir INVIRASE/ritonavir Interaction not evaluated	When saquinavir is administered without ritonavir, no dose adjustment is required when the two drugs are coadministered.
Antimycobacterial: Rifabutin	↓ Saquinavir/↔ ritonavir ↑ Rifabutin	INVIRASE should not be given as the sole protease inhibitor to patients. No dose adjustment of saquinavir/ritonavir 1000/100 mg bid is required if ritonavir-boosted Invirase is administered in combination with rifabutin. Dose adjustment of rifabutin (150 mg every 4 days) is recommended when used in combination with ritonavir-boosted Invirase. Monitoring of neutropenia and the liver enzyme levels is recommended for patients receiving rifabutin (150 mg every 4 days) and ritonavir-boosted Invirase (1000/100 mg bid) treatment. Based on extrapolation from the existing data, twice weekly dosing of rifabutin (e.g. Monday, Thursday) is not recommended with ritonavir-boosted Invirase (1000/100 mg bid) as this would lead to pharmacokinetic exposure of rifabutin active moiety approximating that achieved at 300 mg qd regimen which may lead to a higher incidence or severity of rifabutin associated adverse events.
Benzodiazepines: Alprazolam, clorazepate, diazepam, flurazepam	↑ Benzodiazepines	Clinical significance is unknown; however, a decrease in benzodiazepine dose may be needed.

(cont'd)

Table 4: INVIRASE *(cont'd)*

Established and Other Potentially Significant Drug Interactions: Alteration in Dose or Regimen May Be Recommended Based on Drug Interaction Studies or Predicted Interaction (Information in the table applies to INVIRASE/ritonavir)

Concomitant Drug Class: Drug Name	Effect on Concentration of Saquinavir or Concomitant Drug	Clinical Comment
Calcium Channel Blockers: Diltiazem, felodipine, nifedipine, nicardipine, nimodipine, verapamil, amlodipine, isradipine	↑ Calcium channel blockers	Caution is warranted and clinical monitoring of patients is recommended.
Corticosteroid: Dexamethasone	↓ Saquinavir INVIRASE/ritonavir Interaction not evaluated	Use with caution, saquinavir may be less effective due to decreased saquinavir plasma concentrations in patients taking these agents concomitantly.
Corticosteroid (nasal use): Fluticasone	INVIRASE/ritonavir ↑ Fluticasone	Ritonavir significantly increases plasma fluticasone propionate exposures, resulting in significantly decreased serum cortisol concentrations. Concomitant use of INVIRASE/ritonavir and fluticasone propionate is expected to produce the same effects. Systemic corticosteroid effects including Cushing's syndrome and adrenal suppression have been reported during postmarketing use in patients receiving ritonavir and inhaled or intranasally administered fluticasone propionate. Therefore, coadministration of fluticasone propionate and INVIRASE/ritonavir is not recommended unless the potential benefit to the patient outweighs the risk of systemic corticosteroid side effects.
Digitalis Glycosides: Digoxin	↑ Digoxin	Concomitant use of INVIRASE/ritonavir with digoxin results in a significant increase in serum concentrations of digoxin. Caution should be exercised when INVIRASE/ritonavir and digoxin are coadministered; the serum concentration of digoxin should be monitored and the dose of digoxin may need to be reduced.
Histamine H_2-Receptor Antagonist: Ranitidine	↑ Saquinavir INVIRASE/ritonavir Interaction not evaluated	The increase is not thought to be clinically relevant. The safety and efficacy of the combination of ranitidine and INVIRASE/ritonavir have not been established.
HMG-CoA Reductase Inhibitors: Simvastatin, lovastatin, atorvastatin, rosuvastatin	↑ HMG-CoA reductase inhibitors	The combination of INVIRASE/ritonavir with simvastatin, lovastatin and rosuvastatin should be avoided. Use lowest possible dose of atorvastatin and with careful monitoring or consider other HMG-CoA reductase inhibitors such as pravastatin, fluvastatin.
Immunosuppressants: Cyclosporine, tacrolimus, rapamycin	↑ Immunosuppressants	Therapeutic concentration monitoring is recommended for immunosuppressant agents when coadministered with INVIRASE/ritonavir.
Narcotic Analgesic: Methadone	↓ Methadone	No dose adjustment is recommended when INVIRASE/ritonavir is combined with methadone.
Oral Contraceptives: Ethinyl estradiol	↓ Ethinyl estradiol	Alternative or additional contraceptive measures should be used when estrogen-based oral contraceptives and INVIRASE/ritonavir are coadministered.
PDE5 Inhibitor (phosphodiesterase type 5 inhibitors): Sildenafil, vardenafil, tadalafil	↔ Saquinavir ↑ Sildenafil ↑ Vardenafil ↑ Tadalafil	Sildenafil may be used with caution at reduced doses of 25 mg every 48 hours, or tadalafil may be used with caution at reduced doses of 10 mg every 72 hours with increased monitoring for adverse events including hypotension, visual changes and priapism. Vardenafil should not be used with INVIRASE/ritonavir.
Proton Pump Inhibitors: Omeprazole	↑ Saquinavir ↔ Ritonavir	No data are available on the concomitant administration of Invirase/ritonavir and other proton pump inhibitors. If omeprazole or other proton pump inhibitors are taken concomitantly with INVIRASE/ritonavir, caution is advised and monitoring for potential saquinavir toxicities is recommended, particularly gastrointestinal symptoms, increased triglycerides, and deep vein thrombosis.

OVERDOSAGE:
There is limited experience of overdose with saquinavir.

Whereas acute or chronic overdose of saquinavir alone did not result in major complications, in combination with other protease inhibitors, overdose symptoms and signs such as general weakness, fatigue, diarrhea, nausea, vomiting, hair loss, dry mouth, hyponatremia, weight loss and orthostatic hypotension have been observed.

There is no specific antidote for overdose with saquinavir. Treatment of overdose with saquinavir, should consist of general supportive measures, including monitoring of vital signs and ECG, and observations of the patient's clinical status. If warranted, patients should be treated with activated charcoal. Since saquinavir is highly protein bound, dialysis is unlikely to be beneficial in significant removal of the active substance.

> For management of a suspected drug overdose, contact your regional Poison Control Centre. See the *CPS* Directory section for a list of Poison Control Centres.

ACTION AND CLINICAL PHARMACOLOGY: Mechanism of Action: Saquinavir is a selective and reversible inhibitor of HIV protease, an essential viral enzyme which is required for specific cleavage of viral gag and gag-pol polyproteins and ultimately, for the release of mature, infectious virus.

Antiviral activity in vitro: Saquinavir demonstrates antiviral activity against a panel of laboratory strains and clinical isolates of HIV-1 with typical EC_{50} and EC_{90} values in the range 1-10 nM and 5-50 nM. In the presence of 50% human serum or alpha-1 glycoprotein (1 mg/mL), the antiviral activity of saquinavir decreases by an average factor of 25-fold and 14-fold, respectively. There is no apparent difference in the antiviral activity of saquinavir between subtype B and non-B clades whereas EC_{50} values are in the range of 0.3-2.4 nM with clinical isolates of HIV-2.

Resistance: In vitro Resistance: In vitro selection of resistance from wild-type HIV-1 virus: The most commonly reported mutations, G48V and L90M, were observed to develop during in vitro passage of HIV-1 wild-type virus in the presence of increasing concentrations of saquinavir. Recombinant virus harboring the G48V and L90M mutations exhibited 7.9-fold and 3.3-fold reductions in viral susceptibility to saquinavir, respectively. Protease mutations such as M36I, I54V, K57R, and L63V developed less frequently in the presence of saquinavir.

In vivo Resistance: Treatment Naïve Patients: Four studies have investigated ritonavir-boosted saquinavir regimens in ART naïve patients [(saquinavir/ritonavir 1600 mg/100 mg qd (n=349); 1000 mg/100 mg bid (n=92)]. Baseline resistance analyses were conducted on 26 patients experiencing virological rebound. Data from two patients was excluded either because PI mutations were present at baseline or a signature protease mutation (D30N) associated with another PI subsequently developed. Virus from two patients (2/24) developed protease mutations (M36I and M46i/m, respectively). These mutations are not typically associated with saquinavir resistance. No specific saquinavir-associated protease mutations were observed to develop following virological failure.

Treatment Experienced Patients: Baseline and on-therapy genotype was evaluated for 22 previously PI-experienced patients who experienced virological failure after receiving a ritonavir-boosted saquinavir regimen (MaxCmin 1 and 2 studies; 1000/100 mg bid, n=171). Virus from eight patients (8/22; 36%) developed additional protease mutations following virological failure. The relative incidence of each mutation was: I84V (n=4, 18%); F53L, A71V or G73S (n=2, 9%); L10V, M46I, I54V, V82A or L90M (n=1, 4.5%).

Pharmacokinetics: The pharmacokinetic properties of saquinavir have been evaluated in healthy volunteers and in HIV-infected patients after single and multiple oral doses of 25, 75, 200 and 600 mg TID; and in healthy volunteers after intravenous infusion doses of 12 mg administered over 1 hour, and 6, 36 and 72 mg administered over 3 hours.

Absorption: Absorption and absolute bioavailability are improved when the drug is taken after a meal. Similarly, the presence of food increases the time required to achieve maximum concentration.

The extent of absorption (as reflected by AUC) after a 600 mg oral dose in fasting healthy volunteers was substantially increased (from 24 ng· h/mL to 161 ng· h/mL) when given following a heavy breakfast (48 g protein, 60 g carbohydrate, 57 g fat; 1006 kcal). The presence of food also increased the time taken to achieve maximum concentration from 2.4 hours to 3.8 hours, and substantially increased the mean maximum plasma concentrations (C_{max}) from 3.0 ng/mL to 35.5 ng/mL. The effect of food has been shown to be present for up to 2 hours. Therefore, INVIRASE (saquinavir mesylate) should be taken within 2 hours after a meal. Gastric pH has been shown not to play a major role in this increased bioavailability which is associated with food.

Additionally, exposure to saquinavir was doubled ($AUC_{(0-12)}$ increased from 183.2 ng· h/mL to 374.4 ng· h/mL) when INVIRASE was coadministered with "double-strength" grapefruit juice; and increased by 30% ($AUC_{(0-12)}$ from 183.2 ng· h/mL to 238.1 ng· h/mL) when taken with normal strength grapefruit juice in a single dose study.

HIV-infected patients administered saquinavir 600 mg TID, with the instructions to take their doses after a meal or substantial snack, had AUC and C_{max} which were about twice those observed in healthy volunteers receiving the same treatment regimen (AUC=757.2 vs 359.0 ng· h/mL; C_{max}=253.3 vs 90.39 ng/mL).

Following administration of a 600 mg (3×200 mg) oral dose to 8 healthy volunteers in the presence of food (heavy breakfast, as defined above), the mean absolute bioavailability is 4% (range: 1% to 9%). This low bioavailability is thought to be due to a combination of incomplete absorption (30%) and extensive first pass metabolism.

After single and multiple oral doses as capsules (25 to 600 mg TID) in the presence of food, the increase in exposure (50-fold) was greater than directly proportional to the increase in dose (24-fold). Accumulation following multiple dosing (600 mg TID) in HIV-infected patients is modest: AUC was increased 150% at steady state compared to single doses.

No food effect data are available for INVIRASE in combination with ritonavir. Saquinavir exposure was similar when saquinavir soft gel capsules plus ritonavir (1000 mg/100 mg bid) were administered following a high-fat (45 g fat) or moderate-fat (20 g fat) breakfast.

Table 5: INVIRASE

Pharmacokinetic Parameters of Saquinavir at Steady-State After Administration of Different Regimens in HIV-Infected Patients. Arithmetic Mean ± Standard Deviation

Dosing Regimen	N	AUCτ (ng· h/mL)	AUC_{24h} (ng· h/mL)	C_{min} (ng/mL)
INVIRASE 600 mg tid	10	866±533	2598	75±62
Saquinavir soft gel capsules 1200 mg tid	31	7249±6174	21747	216±182
INVIRASE 400 mg bid + ritonavir 400 mg bid	7	16 000±8000	32 000	480±360
INVIRASE 1000 mg bid + ritonavir 100 mg bid	24	19 513±14 424	39 026	571±580
Saquinavir soft gel capsules 1000 mg bid + ritonavir 100 mg bid	24	23 852±15 580	47 704	605±551

τ is the dosing interval (ie, 8h if tid and 12h if bid).

Distribution: The mean steady-state volume of distribution following intravenous administration of a 12 mg dose of saquinavir is 700 L (CV 39%), indicating extensive partitioning into tissues. Saquinavir shows a high degree of protein binding (~98%), which is independent of concentration over the range 15-700 ng/mL.

In two patients treated with saquinavir (600 mg TID), cerebrospinal fluid concentrations were negligible when compared to concentrations from matching plasma samples.

Metabolism: Greater than 96% of a radiolabelled I.V. dose appears in the feces within 48 hours, indicating extensive hepatic clearance. Hepatic metabolism is P450-mediated, of which >90% is the work of one isozyme (CYP3A4). The metabolic profile of saquinavir has been investigated in bile, plasma and microsomes in rats and in microsomes from other species, including man. Saquinavir is rapidly metabolized to a range of mono- and di-hydroxylated inactive compounds. Following intravenous administration, 66% of circulating saquinavir is present as unchanged drug and the remainder as metabolites, suggesting that saquinavir undergoes extensive first-pass metabolism.

Excretion: Renal excretion is a very minor route of elimination for saquinavir (<4%). Systemic clearance is rapid, 80 L/h, which is close to hepatic plasma flow. Systemic clearance was constant after intravenous doses of 6, 36 and 72 mg infused over 3 hours. The mean residence time of the drug was found to be 7 hours.

In a mass balance study using ^{14}C-saquinavir (n=8), 88% and 1% of the orally administered radioactivity was recovered in feces and urine, respectively, within 4 days of dosing. In an additional four subjects administered 10.5 mg ^{14}C-saquinavir intravenously, 81% and 3% of the intravenously administered radioactivity was recovered in the feces and urine, respectively, within 4 days of dosing. In mass-balance studies, 13% of circulating saquinavir in plasma was present as unchanged drug after oral administration and the remainder present as metabolites.

Special Populations and Conditions: Pediatrics: The pharmacokinetics of saquinavir when administered as INVIRASE have not been sufficiently investigated in pediatric patients.

Geriatrics: The pharmacokinetics of saquinavir when administered as INVIRASE have not been sufficiently investigated in patients >65 years of age.

Gender: A gender difference was observed, with females showing a higher saquinavir exposure than males (mean AUC increase of 56%, mean C_{max} increase of 26%), in the bioequivalence study comparing INVIRASE 500 mg film coated tablets to the INVIRASE 200 mg capsules in combination with ritonavir. There was no evidence that age and body weight explained the gender difference in this study. A clinically significant difference in safety and efficacy between men and women has not been reported with the 1000 mg INVIRASE/100 mg ritonavir b.i.d. dosage regimen.

Race: The influence of race on the pharmacokinetics of INVIRASE has not been determined.

Hepatic Insufficiency: In cases of mild impairment no initial dosage adjustment is necessary at the recommended dose. The use of INVIRASE (alone or in combination with ritonavir) in patients with moderate hepatic impairment has not been studied. In the absence of such studies, caution should be exercised, as increases in saquinavir levels and/or increases in liver enzymes may occur. In patients with underlying hepatitis B or C, cirrhosis, chronic alcoholism and/or other underlying liver abnormalities there have been reports of worsening liver disease and development of portal hypertension after starting saquinavir. Associated symptoms include jaundice, ascites, edema and, in some cases esophageal varices. Several of these patients died. A causal relationship between saquinavir therapy and development of portal hypertension has not been established. Increased monitoring for signs and symptoms of liver toxicity should be considered (see Contraindications).

Renal Insufficiency: Renal clearance is only a minor elimination pathway, the principal route of metabolism and excretion for saquinavir is via the liver. Therefore, no initial dose adjustment is necessary for patients with renal impairment. However, patients with severe renal impairment have not been studied and caution should be exercised when prescribing saquinavir in this population.

Effects on Electrocardiogram: The effect of 1000/100 mg bid (therapeutic dose) and 1500/100 mg bid (supra-therapeutic dose) of INVIRASE/ritonavir on the QT interval was evaluated over 20 hours on Day 3 of dosing in a 4-way crossover, double-blind, placebo- and active-controlled (moxifloxacin 400 mg) study in healthy male and female volunteers aged 18 to 55 years old (N=59) (see Table 6). The Day 3 timepoint was chosen since the pharmacokinetic exposure was maximum on that day in a previous 14-day multiple dose pharmacokinetic study.

Table 6: INVIRASE

Maximum Mean of ddQTcS[a] (msec) on Day 3 for Therapeutic Dose of INVIRASE/ritonavir, Supra-Therapeutic Dose of INVIRASE/ritonavir and Active Control Moxifloxacin in Healthy Volunteers

Treatment	Post-Dose Time Point	Maximum Mean ddQTcS (msec)	Standard Error	Upper 95%-CI of ddQTcS (msec)
INVIRASE/ritonavir 1000/100 mg bid	12 hours	18.86	1.91	22.01
INVIRASE/ritonavir 1500/100 mg bid	20 hours	30.22	1.91	33.36
Moxifloxacin[b]	4 hours	12.18	1.93	15.36

[a] Derived difference of pre-dose baseline corrected QTcS between active treatment and placebo arms.
[b] 400 mg was administered only on Day 3.
Note: QTcS in this study was $QT/RR^{0.319}$ for males and $QT/RR^{0.337}$ for females, which are similar to Fridericia's correction ($QTcF=QT/RR^{0.333}$).

In this study, PR interval prolongation of >200 msec was also observed in 40% and 47% of subjects receiving INVIRASE/ritonavir 1000/100 mg bid and 1500/100 mg bid, respectively, on Day 3 compared to three (3)% of subjects in the active control moxifloxacin arm and 5% in the placebo arm. The maximum mean PR interval changes relative to the pre-dose baseline value were 25 msec and 34 msec in the two ritonavir-boosted INVIRASE treatment groups, 1000/100 mg bid and 1500/100 mg bid, respectively and remained relatively unchanged in the placebo and moxifloxacin arms (see Warnings and Precautions, Cardiovascular, Cardiac Conduction Abnormalities).

Maximum mean QT prolongations (QTcS; study-specific QTc interval correction) of 18.9 msec, 30.2 msec. and 12.2 msec were observed in the 1000/100 mg, 1500/100 mg, and moxifloxacin (positive control) groups, respectively. The majority of subjects (89% and 80% in the therapeutic dose and supra-therapeutic dose groups, respectively) had a QTcS of <450 msec and none had a QTc interval of >500 msec (see Warnings and Precautions, Cardiovascular, Cardiac Conduction Abnormalities).

STORAGE AND STABILITY: INVIRASE (saquinavir mesylate) tablets and capsules should be kept in a tightly closed container and stored between 15 and 30°C.

INFORMATION FOR THE PATIENT: Published in e-CPS, available by subscription at www.e-cps.ca.

DOSAGE FORMS, COMPOSITION AND PACKAGING: Capsules: Each hard gelatin, light brown and green capsule, imprinted with "Roche" and "0245" on opaque shells, contains: saquinavir 200 mg, present as saquinavir mesylate. Nonmedicinal ingredients: lactose, magnesium stearate, microcrystalline cellulose, povidone, sodium starch glycolate and talc; capsule shell: gelatin, indigotine, iron oxide and titanium dioxide. Glass or plastic (HDPE) bottles of 270.

Tablets: Each light orange to greyish- or brownish-orange, oval cylindrical, biconvex film-coated tablet with "ROCHE" and "SQV 500" imprinted on the tablet face, contains saquinavir 500 mg, present as saquinavir mesylate. Nonmedicinal ingredients: croscarmellose sodium, lactose, magnesium stearate, microcrystalline cellulose and povidone K30; film-coat: hypromellose, iron oxide red, iron oxide yellow, talc, titanium dioxide and triacetin. Plastic (HDPE) bottles of 120.

(Shown in Product Identification Section)

Iopidine® 1% ℞

apraclonidine HCl

Controls Postsurgical Intraocular Pressure

Alcon

Iopidine® 0.5% ℞

apraclonidine HCl

Glaucoma Therapy

Alcon

SUPPLIED: Iopidine 1%: Each mL of sterile, isotonic, aqueous solution contains: apraclonidine HCl 1.15% equivalent to apraclonidine base 1% with benzalkonium chloride 0.01% as preservative. Nonmedicinal ingredients: hydrochloric acid and/or sodium hydroxide (to adjust pH), purified water, sodium acetate and sodium chloride. Plastic ophthalmic dispensers of 0.1 mL. Pouches of 2. These dispensers are enclosed in a foil overwrap as an added barrier to evaporation.

Iopidine 0.5%: Each mL of sterile, isotonic, aqueous solution contains: apraclonidine HCl 0.575% equivalent to apraclonidine base 0.5% with benzalkonium chloride 0.01% as preservative. Nonmedicinal ingredients: hydrochloric acid and/or sodium hydroxide (to adjust pH), purified water, sodium acetate and sodium chloride. Plastic Drop-Tainer dispensers of 5 mL.

Store between 2 and 30°C. Do not freeze. Protect from light.

Ipecac Syrup

Emetic

CPhA Monograph

Date of Revision: October 2006

This monograph has been compiled by CPhA and reviewed by experts. It may contain information different from that found in Health Canada-approved Product Monographs. The reader is referred to the *CPS* Editorial Policy for more information.

PHARMACOLOGY: Ipecac syrup is prepared from powdered ipecac which is derived from the dried roots and rhizomes of Cepha acuminata or Cepha ipecacuanha. Its pharmacologic action is attributed to its major alkaloids, emetine and cephaline. Ipecac syrup should not be confused with ipecac fluidextract which is 14 times more potent. Ipecac induces vomiting by both gastric irritation and central stimulation of the chemoreceptor trigger zone.

Approximately 95% of patients vomit within 15 to 30 minutes of administration of a therapeutic dose and vomiting usually persists for 30 minutes to 2 hours.

INDICATIONS: Ipecac is no longer recommended in the management of poisoned patients.

For management of a suspected poisoning, CPhA recommends that you contact your **regional Poison Control Centre**. See the *CPS* Directory section for a list of Poison Control Centres.

WARNINGS: Ipecac fluidextract is 14 times more potent than ipecac syrup and has been associated with serious toxicity and fatalities.

ADVERSE EFFECTS: Administration of ipecac syrup and the resulting vomiting may induce seizures in patients who have ingested CNS stimulants. The use of ipecac may occasionally result in protracted or prolonged vomiting, diarrhea and lethargy. Less frequently, patients may experience irritability, hyperactivity, fever or diaphoresis. Rare but serious adverse effects include Mallory-Weiss tears, pneumomediastinum and aspiration pneumonia.

Toxicity may occur in patients with eating disorders who chronically consume large amounts of ipecac syrup. Myopathy, with manifestations of muscle weakness and pain, hyporeflexia, tenderness and stiffness, has been the major presenting adverse effect. Cardiotoxicity, including hypotension, chest pain, arrhythmias or cardiac failure, may be serious and life-threatening.

Protracted vomiting produced by the chronic ingestion of ipecac syrup may cause metabolic abnormalities, dental abnormalities, eosophagitis, gastric reflux, Mallory-Weiss syndrome, parotid gland enlargement and aspiration pneumonitis.

OVERDOSE:

Symptoms: Cases of severe toxicity from ipecac have usually involved ingestion of the fluidextract in volumes appropriate only for the syrup.

Ipecac contains a cardiotoxin that can cause edema and necrosis of the heart muscle in high doses. Other symptoms may include nausea, bloody stools, abdominal cramps and pain, hypotension, dyspnea, shock, seizures and coma.

Treatment: Management of acute overdose generally involves symptomatic and supportive care.

> For management of a suspected ipecac overdose, CPhA recommends that you contact your **regional Poison Control Centre**. See the *CPS* Directory section for a list of Poison Control Centres.

Iressa® Ⓟ

gefitinib

Epidermal Growth Factor Receptor (EGFR) Tyrosine Kinase Inhibitor

AstraZeneca

Date of Revision: December 18, 2009

SUMMARY PRODUCT INFORMATION:

Route of Administration	Dosage Form/ Strength	Clinically Relevant Nonmedicinal Ingredients
Oral	Tablet, 250 mg gefitinib	Lactose monohydrate, microcrystalline cellulose, croscarmellose sodium, povidone, sodium lauryl sulfate, magnesium stearate, hypromellose, macrogol 300, titanium dioxide, yellow iron oxide, red iron oxide

INDICATIONS AND CLINICAL USE: IRESSA (gefitinib) is indicated for the first line treatment of patients with locally advanced (not amenable to curative therapy) or metastatic non-small cell lung cancer (NSCLC) who have activating mutations of the EGFR-TK (see Warnings and Precautions, Monitoring and Laboratory Tests).

Geriatrics (≥65 years of age): No differences in safety or efficacy were observed between younger and older patients (see Warnings and Precautions, Special Populations and Conditions).

Pediatrics (≤16 years of age): IRESSA is not indicated for use in paediatric patients, as safety and effectiveness have not been established (see Warnings and Precautions, Special Populations and Conditions).

CONTRAINDICATIONS: Patients who are hypersensitive to gefitinib or to any ingredient in the formulation or component of the container. For a complete listing, see Dosage Forms, Composition and Packaging.

WARNINGS AND PRECAUTIONS:

> **Serious Warnings and Precautions**
> - IRESSA (gefitinib) should be administered under the supervision of a qualified health professional who is experienced in the treatment and management of patients with cancer.
> - IRESSA should not be used in patients with EGFR mutation negative tumours (see Warnings and Precautions, Monitoring and Laboratory Tests);
> - IRESSA has not been studied in patients with severe renal impairment (see Action and Clinical Pharmacology, Special Populations and Conditions).

Effects on Ability to Drive and Use Machinery: IRESSA is not expected to impair a patient's ability to drive or use machines. However, some patients may occasionally feel weak. If this happens, patients should not drive or operate machinery.

Cardiovascular: No thorough QT/QTc study was performed to rule out the effect of IRESSA on QT prolongation. Routine ECG assessments during clinical trials did not identify any concerns regarding QT prolongation.

Carcinogenesis and Mutagenesis: Pre-clinical studies have identified a statistically significant increase in hepatocellular adenomas in rats and mice and in mesenteric lymph node hemangiosarcomas in rats. The clinical relevance of these findings is unknown.

Drug Interactions: Drugs that cause significant sustained elevation in gastric pH may reduce plasma concentrations of IRESSA and therefore may reduce efficacy (see Drug Interactions).

CYP3A4: IRESSA is primarily metabolized by CYP3A4.

Substances that are inducers of CYP3A4 activity may increase metabolism and decrease gefitinib plasma concentrations. Therefore, co-medication with CYP3A4 inducers (e.g., phenytoin, carbamazepine, rifampicin, barbiturates, or St. John's Wort) may potentially reduce efficacy (see Drug Interactions).

Substances that are inhibitors of CYP3A4 activity (e.g. ketoconazole, macrolides, grapefruit juice) may decrease metabolism and increase gefitinib plasma concentrations. This may be clinically relevant and caution is advised as adverse experiences are related to dose and exposure (see Drug Interactions).

CYP2D6: In vitro studies demonstrate gefitinib has potential to inhibit CYP2D6. In a clinical trial in cancer patients, gefitinib was co-administered with metoprolol (a CYP2D6 substrate). This resulted in a 35% increase in metoprolol exposure. Such an increase might potentially be relevant for CYP2D6 substrates with narrow therapeutic index. When the use of CYP2D6 substrates are considered in combination with gefitinib, a dose modification of the CYP2D6 substrate should be considered, especially for products with a narrow therapeutic window (see Drug Interactions).

Gastrointestinal: Diarrhea, Dehydration and Renal Dysfunction: IRESSA use is very commonly associated with diarrhea, nausea, vomiting, stomatitis, and anorexia. Patients should be advised to seek medical advice promptly in the event of developing severe or persistent diarrhoea, nausea, vomiting or anorexia. These symptoms should be managed as clinically indicated. as any subsequent dehydration may lead to renal dysfunction if left untreated (see Dosage and Administration, Recommended Dose and Dosage Adjustment).

Hematologic: International Normalised Ratio (INR) elevations and/or bleeding events have been reported in some patients taking warfarin. Patients taking warfarin should be monitored regularly for changes in Prothrombin Time (PT) or INR (see Drug Interactions).

Two Phase II trials using the combination IRESSA/vinorelbine have been discontinued due to a high incidence of CTC grade 3 and 4 neutropenia. When used in combination, IRESSA aggravated the neutropenic effect of vinorelbine.

Cerebrovascular events have been reported in clinical studies of IRESSA. A relationship with IRESSA has not been established.

Haemorrhage: Throughout the IRESSA lung cancer clinical trials, the incidence of haemoptysis/pulmonary haemorrhage reported on the IRESSA arm has consistently been higher than that reported on the comparator arm (e.g. on IPASS 3.5% vs. 3.1%, IRESSA vs. carboplatin/paclitaxel. Pooled incidence: IRESSA 5.3% vs. placebo 4.4%; IRESSA 5.0% vs. docetaxel 3.5%; IRESSA 3.7% vs. other chemotherapy 2.8%; overall pooled IRESSA incidence: 4.8%). This may in part be explained by the longer duration of treatment on the IRESSA arm.

Epistaxis and haematuria are commonly associated with IRESSA therapy (4.3%).

Hepatic/Biliary/Pancreatic: Hepatotoxicity: Liver function test abnormalities (including increases in alanine aminotransferase, aspartate aminotransferase, bilirubin) have been observed, rarely presenting as hepatitis. Although a causal relationship has not been established, isolated cases of hepatic failure and fulminant hepatitis, including fatalities, have been reported with IRESSA use. Therefore, periodic liver function testing is recommended. IRESSA should be used cautiously in the presence of mild to moderate changes in liver function. Discontinuation should be considered if changes are severe.

Ophthalmologic: Conjunctivitis, blepharitis, and dry eye are commonly seen in patients treated with IRESSA (6.7%) and are generally mild in nature (CTC grade 1). Corneal erosion occurs uncommonly (0.3%), is reversible and sometimes is associated with aberrant eyelash growth. The safety of wearing contact lenses during IRESSA therapy has not been adequately studied.

Patients should be advised to seek medical advice promptly in the event of developing any eye symptoms (see Adverse Reactions).

These symptoms should be managed as clinically indicated (see Dosage and Administration, Recommended Dose and Dosage Adjustment).

Renal: There have been reports of renal failure secondary to dehydration due to diarrhea, nausea, vomiting and/or anorexia, or associated with pre-renal factors such as concurrent infections or concomitant medications including chemotherapy. In more severe or persistent cases of diarrhea, or cases leading to dehydration, particularly in patients with known risk factors (e.g. renal disease, concurrent vomiting, concomitant medications that impair ability to tolerate dehydration such as NSAIDs and diuretics), IRESSA therapy should be interrupted and appropriate measures taken to intensively rehydrate the patient.

In addition, urea, creatinine and electrolytes should be monitored in patients at high risk of dehydration.

Respiratory: Interstitial Lung Disease (ILD), which may be acute in onset, has been observed in patients receiving IRESSA at an overall incidence of about 1%, and approximately 1/3 of the cases have been fatal (see Adverse Reactions, Interstitial Lung Disease (ILD)).

If patients present with worsening of respiratory symptoms such as dyspnoea, cough and fever, IRESSA should be interrupted and prompt investigation initiated. If ILD is confirmed, IRESSA should be discontinued and the patient treated appropriately.

The incidence of ILD-type events was 5.8% in patients receiving IRESSA in a post-marketing surveillance study in Japan (3350 patients) (see Adverse Reactions, Interstitial Lung Disease (ILD)). In a Japanese Pharmacoepidemiological case-control study (see Adverse Reactions, Interstitial Lung Disease (ILD)) in 3159 patients with NSCLC who were followed up for 12 weeks when receiving IRESSA or chemotherapy, the cumulative incidence of ILD (unadjusted for imbalances in patient characteristics) at 12 weeks' follow-up was 4.0% in patients receiving IRESSA and 2.1% in those receiving chemotherapy. The adjusted odds ratio (OR) of developing ILD was 3.2 (95% confidence interval (CI) 1.9 to 5.4) for IRESSA versus chemotherapy. This trial identified the following risk factors for developing ILD (irrespective of whether the patient received IRESSA or chemotherapy): smoking, poor performance status (PS ≥2), CT scan evidence of reduced normal lung (≤50%), recent diagnosis of NSCLC (<6 months), pre-existing ILD, increasing age (≥55 years old) and concurrent cardiac disease. Risk of mortality among patients who developed ILD on both treatments was higher in patients with the following risk factors: smoking, CT scan evidence of reduced normal lung (≤50%), pre-existing ILD, increasing age (≥65 years old), and extensive areas adherent to pleura (≥50%).

Skin: Rash is very common with IRESSA use (57.9%), mainly mild to moderate (CTC grade 1 or 2). Toxic epidermal necrolysis, Stevens-Johnson syndrome and erythema multiforme occur rarely (0.04%), and some cases have been fatal (see Dosage and Administration, Recommended Dose and Dosage Adjustment). Preclinical work in guinea pigs indicates that IRESSA may be a potential skin (contact) sensitiser. Results of an in vitro phototoxicity study demonstrated that IRESSA may have phototoxicity potential.

Special Populations: Pregnant Women: There are no adequate and well-controlled studies in pregnant women using IRESSA. Women of childbearing potential must be advised to avoid becoming pregnant. If IRESSA is used during pregnancy or if the patient becomes pregnant while receiving this drug, she should be apprised of the potential hazard to the fetus or potential risk for loss of the pregnancy. IRESSA may cause fetal harm when administered to a pregnant woman.

Nursing Women: It is not known whether IRESSA is excreted in human milk, however this is documented to occur in pre-clinical testing. Because many drugs are excreted in human milk and because of the potential for serious adverse reactions in nursing infants, women should be advised against breast-feeding while receiving IRESSA therapy.

Pediatrics (≤16 years of age): In a Phase I/II trial of IRESSA and radiation in paediatric patients, newly diagnosed with brain stem glioma or incompletely resected supratentorial malignant glioma, 4 cases (1 fatal) of CNS haemorrhages have been reported in 45 patients enrolled. A further case of CNS haemorrhage has been reported in a child with an ependymoma from a trial with IRESSA alone. An increased risk of cerebral haemorrhage in adult patients with NSCLC receiving IRESSA has not been established. IRESSA is not indicated for use in paediatric patients, as safety and effectiveness have not been established.

Geriatrics (≥65 years of age): Of the total number of patients participating in the INTEREST and ISEL trials, 37% were aged 65 or older. No differences in IRESSA safety or efficacy effect relative to the comparator were observed between younger and older patients.

Hepatic Impairment: Patients with moderate to severe hepatic impairment (Child Pugh B or C) due to cirrhosis have increased plasma concentrations of gefitinib (see Action and Clinical Pharmacology and Dosage and Administration). An average 3.1-fold increase in exposure to gefitinib in patients with moderate and severe hepatic impairment was observed in a phase I hepatic impairment study. None of the patients had cancer, all had cirrhosis and some had hepatitis. This increase in exposure may be of clinical relevance since adverse experiences are related to dose and exposure to gefitinib.

In the pivotal trial IPASS, patients with alanine aminotransferase (ALT) or aspartate aminotransferase (AST) levels greater than 2.5 times upper limit of normal (ULN) with no demonstrable liver metastases or greater than 5 times ULN in the presence of liver metastases were excluded due to potential hepatic concerns associated with the carboplatin/paclitaxel doublet. Consequently, the IPASS study does not contribute any data in this patient population.

CYP2D6 Poor Metabolisers: In a clinical trial of healthy volunteers, CYP2D6 poor metabolisers achieved a 2-fold higher mean exposure to gefitinib than in extensive metabolisers. The higher average gefitinib exposures achieved by individuals with no active CYP2D6 may be clinically relevant since adverse experiences are related to dose and exposure.

Monitoring and Laboratory Tests: Assessment of EGFR Mutation Status: EGFR mutation status must be known prior to starting IRESSA therapy because only patients with an activating mutation of EGFR TK should be treated with IRESSA (see Indications and Clinical Use). When assessing the EGFR mutation status of a patient, it is important that a well-validated and robust methodology is chosen to minimize the possibility of false negative or false positive determinations.

Clinical characteristics of never smoker, adenocarcinoma histology, and female gender have been shown to be independent predictors of positive EGFR mutation status for both non-Asian and Asian patients. Asian patients also have a higher incidence of EGFR mutation positive tumours (approximately 40% positive rate) than non-Asian patients (approximately 10% positive rate). These clinical characteristics should not be used to guide treatment choice, however they may be helpful in guiding mutation testing. A patient must be defined as EGFR mutation positive before starting IRESSA therapy.

Hematology and Chemistry Assessment: Electrolytes, BUN, creatinine, liver function tests (alanine aminotransferase, aspartate aminotransferase, bilirubin) should be performed at baseline and periodically during IRESSA therapy.

Patients taking warfarin should be monitored regularly for changes in Prothrombin Time (PT) or INR (see Drug Interactions).

Other: IRESSA contains lactose. This should be considered when assessing the benefit:risk ratio of IRESSA use in patients with rare hereditary problems of galactose intolerance, Lapp lactase deficiency or glucose-galactose malabsorption.

ADVERSE REACTIONS: Adverse Drug Reaction Overview: Adverse drug reactions (ADR) found to be associated with treatment with IRESSA are shown in Table 1. The most common adverse drug reactions reported at the recommended 250 mg daily dose, occurring in more than 20% of patients, are diarrhoea, sometimes associated with dehydration and mainly mild or moderate in nature (CTC grade 1 or 2) and less commonly, severe (CTC grade 3 or 4); and skin reactions (including rash, acne, dry skin and pruritus) (Table 1). Approximately 10% of patients had a severe ADR (Common Toxicity Criteria, (CTC) grade 3 or 4). Approximately 3% of patients stopped therapy due to an ADR. The onsets of these ADRs usually occurred within the first month of therapy and were generally mild and non-cumulative as well as reversible.

ADRs have been assigned to the frequency categories in Table 1 based on the incidence of comparable adverse event reports in a pooled dataset from the ISEL, INTEREST and IPASS phase III clinical trials (2462 IRESSA-treated patients). In assigning these frequencies no account was taken of the frequency of reports within the comparative treatment groups or whether the investigator considered it to be related to study medication. The frequency of ADRs relating to abnormal laboratory values is based on patients with a change in baseline of 2 or more CTC grades in the relevant laboratory parameters.

Clinical Trial Adverse Drug Reactions: IPASS STUDY (D791A00007): In IPASS, the most commonly reported adverse events for patients treated with IRESSA (gefitinib) were diarrhoea and skin reactions (including rashes/acnes, dry skin and pruritus). Overall, for IRESSA-treated patients with an EGFR mutation positive status, the profile of the most common adverse events was similar to that reported in the overall population and consistent with the known safety profile of IRESSA.

IRESSA had a more favourable tolerability profile than carboplatin/paclitaxel doublet chemotherapy, indicated by fewer CTC grade 3, 4 or 5 adverse events (31.6% versus 62.5%), fewer dose modifications due to toxicity (16.1% versus 35.2% [carboplatin]/37.5% [paclitaxel]) and fewer adverse events leading to discontinuation of randomized treatment (6.9% versus 13.6%). In addition, fewer treatment-related adverse events (88.6% versus 96.6%) were reported with IRESSA compared with carboplatin/paclitaxel.

Table 2 summarizes the most commonly reported adverse events observed with IRESSA and carboplatin/paclitaxel therapies in the IPASS trial irrespective of causality.

Formal statistical analyses were performed for ten pre-specified events possibly associated with IRESSA or carboplatin/paclitaxel treatment. This included relevant adverse events of any CTC grade and laboratory parameter values of CTC grade ≥3 (worsenings from baseline only) occurring during the period on randomized treatment (Table 3). Events of rashes/acnes, diarrhoea and CTC Grade ≥3 liver transaminases were reported at a statistically significantly higher incidence in the IRESSA arm. Events of neurotoxicity, and CTC Grade ≥3 haematological toxicity (CTC Grade ≥3 neutropenia, leukopenia, thrombocytopenia, and anaemia) were reported at a statistically significantly higher incidence in the carboplatin/paclitaxel arm. Although nausea and vomiting were included in the group of five events considered possibly associated with gefitinib treatment, the incidence of both was statistically significantly higher in the carboplatin/paclitaxel arm despite premedication.

Interstitial Lung Disease (ILD): In the phase III open-label IPASS trial comparing IRESSA to carboplatin/paclitaxel doublet chemotherapy as first-line treatment in selected patients with advanced NSCLC in Asia, the incidence of ILD-type events was 2.6% on the IRESSA treatment arm versus 1.4% on the carboplatin/paclitaxel treatment arm.

In the INTEREST trial, the incidence of ILD-type events was similar for both treatments (IRESSA 10 patients [1.4%] versus docetaxel 8 patients [1.1%]).

In the ISEL trial, the incidence of ILD-type events in the overall population was similar, and approximately 1% in both treatment arms. The majority of ILD-type events reported were from patients of Oriental ethnicity and the ILD incidence among patients of Oriental ethnicity receiving IRESSA therapy and placebo was similar, approximately 3% and 4%, respectively. One ILD-type event was fatal, and this occurred in a patient receiving placebo.

In a Post-Marketing Surveillance study in Japan (3350 patients) the reported rate of ILD-type events in patients receiving IRESSA was 5.8%.

In a Japanese Pharmacoepidemiological case-control study (see Warnings and Precautions, Respiratory) in patients with NSCLC, the crude cumulative incidence of ILD (unadjusted for imbalances in patient characteristics) at 12 weeks follow-up was 4.0% in patients receiving IRESSA and 2.1% in those receiving chemotherapy and the adjusted odds ratio (OR) of developing ILD was 3.2 (95% confidence interval (CI) 1.9 to 5.4) for IRESSA versus chemotherapy. An increased risk of ILD on IRESSA relative to chemotherapy was seen predominantly during the first 4 weeks of treatment (adjusted OR 3.8; 95% CI 1.9 to 7.7); thereafter the relative risk was lower (adjusted OR 2.5; 95% CI 1.1 to 5.8).

Gastrointestinal Perforation: Isolated cases of gastrointestinal perforation have been reported in patients with underlying risk factors (e.g. concomitant medications such as steroids, NSAIDs, underlying history of GI ulceration, age, smoking, bowel metastases at sites of perforation). However, a causal relationship with IRESSA has not been established.

Post-Market Adverse Drug Reactions: The following safety signals have been raised from post-marketing adverse event reports: ILD, pancreatitis, allergic reactions (including angioedema and urticaria), hepatitis and pyrexia.

Table 1: IRESSA

Adverse Drug Reactions by Frequency and System/Organ (pooled safety data from ISEL, INTEREST and IPASS phase III clinical trials)

Very common (≥10%)	Gastrointestinal Disorders	Diarrhoea (34.9%), mainly mild or moderate in nature (CTC grade 1 or 2) and, less commonly, severe (CTC grade 3 or 4).
		Nausea (17.8%), mainly mild in nature (CTC grade 1).
		Vomiting (13.8%), mainly mild or moderate in nature (CTC grade 1 or 2).
		Stomatitis (11.0%), predominantly mild in nature (CTC grade 1).
	Hepatobiliary Disorders	Elevations in alanine aminotransferase (11.4%), mainly mild to moderate.
	Metabolism and Nutrition Disorders	Anorexia (19.7%), mild or moderate in nature (CTC grade 1 or 2).
	Skin and Subcutaneous Tissue Disorders	Skin reactions (57.9%), mainly a mild or moderate (CTC grade 1 or 2) pustular rash, sometimes itchy with dry skin, on an erythematous base.
	General Disorders and Administration Site Conditions	Asthenia (17.7%), predominantly mild in nature (CTC grade 1).
Common (≥1– <10%)	Gastrointestinal Disorders	Dehydration (1.8%), secondary to diarrhoea, nausea, vomiting or anorexia
		Dry mouth[a] (2.0%), predominantly mild in nature (CTC grade 1)
	Vascular Disorders	Haemorrhage (4.3%), such as epistaxis and haematuria
	Hepatobiliary Disorders	Elevations in aspartate aminotransferase (7.9%), mainly mild to moderate
		Elevations in total bilirubin (2.7%), mainly mild to moderate
	Renal and Urinary Disorders	Asymptomatic laboratory elevations in blood creatinine (1.5%)
		Proteinuria (7.7%)
	Skin and Subcutaneous Tissue Disorders	Nail disorder (7.9%)
		Alopecia (4.7%)
	General Disorders and Administration Site Conditions	Pyrexia (8.7%)
	Eye Disorders	Conjunctivitis, blepharitis, and dry eye[a] (6.7%), mainly mild in nature (CTC grade 1).
	Respiratory, Thoracic and Mediastinal Disorders	Interstitial lung disease (1.3%), often severe (CTC grade 3-4). Fatal outcomes have been reported.
Uncommon (≥0.1–<1%)	Gastrointestinal Disorders	Pancreatitis (0.1%)
	Eye Disorders	Corneal erosion (0.3%), reversible and sometimes in association with aberrant eyelash growth.
	Skin and Subcutaneous Tissue Disorders	Allergic reactions[b] (0.9%), including angioedema and urticaria.

(cont'd)

Table 1: IRESSA *(cont'd)*

Adverse Drug Reactions by Frequency and System/Organ (pooled safety data from ISEL, INTEREST and IPASS phase III clinical trials)

Rare (≥0.01–<0.1%)	Skin and Subcutaneous Tissue Disorders	Toxic epidermal necrolysis, Stevens-Johnson syndrome and erythema multiforme (0.04%).
	Hepatobiliary Disorders	Hepatitis (0.08%)

[a] This event can occur in association with other dry conditions (mainly skin reactions) seen with IRESSA.

[b] The overall incidence of AEs of allergic reaction reported in the pooled analysis of the ISEL, INTEREST and IPASS trials was 1.5% (36 patients). Fourteen of the 36 patients were excluded from the reported frequency as their reports contained evidence of either a non-allergic aetiology or that the allergic reaction was the result of treatment with another medication.

Table 2: IRESSA

Most Common Adverse Events (those occurring in at least 10% of patients in either treatment group) or Adverse Events with a Difference in Incidence of >5% Between Treatment Groups (IPASS; EFS population)

	Number (%) of patients[a]	
System Organ Class and Preferred Term	**IRESSA 250 mg (N=607) Overall[b]**	**Carboplatin/Paclitaxel (N=589) Overall[b]**
Blood and Lymphatic Disorders[c]		
Anaemia	43 (7.1)	150 (25.5)
Neutropenia	15 (2.5)	223 (37.9)
Leukopenia	13 (2.1)	146 (24.8)
Thrombocytopenia	8 (1.3)	71 (12.1)
Gastrointestinal Disorders		
Diarrhoea	283 (46.6)	128 (21.7)
Nausea	101 (16.6)	261 (44.3)
Stomatitis	81 (13.3)	42 (7.1)
Vomiting	78 (12.9)	196 (33.3)
Constipation	73 (12.0)	173 (29.4)
General Disorders and Administration Site Conditions		
Fatigue	87 (14.3)	219 (37.2)
Pyrexia	54 (8.9)	61 (10.4)
Infections and Infestations		
Paronychia	82 (13.5)	0 (0)
Investigations		
ALT increased	64 (10.5)	31 (5.3)
AST increased	53 (8.7)	19 (3.2)
White blood cell count decreased	5 (0.8)	52 (8.8)
Neutrophil count decreased	0 (0)	40 (6.8)
Metabolism and Nutrition Disorders		
Anorexia	117 (19.3)	235 (39.9)
Musculoskeletal and Connective Tissue Disorders		
Myalgia	47 (7.7)	186 (31.6)
Arthralgia	39 (6.4)	113 (19.2)
Nervous System Disorders		
Peripheral sensory neuropathy	23 (3.8)	141 (23.9)
Hypoaesthesia	21 (3.5)	154 (26.1)
Neuropathy peripheral	9 (1.5)	97 (16.5)
Psychiatric Disorders		
Insomnia	88 (14.5)	108 (18.3)
Respiratory, Thoracic and Mediastinal Disorders		
Cough	57 (9.4)	62 (10.5)
Skin and Subcutaneous Tissue Disorders		
Rash	313 (51.6)	120 (20.4)
Dry skin	145 (23.9)	17 (2.9)
Pruritus	107 (17.6)	71 (12.1)

(cont'd)

Table 2: IRESSA *(cont'd)*

Most Common Adverse Events (those occurring in at least 10% of patients in either treatment group) or Adverse Events with a Difference in Incidence of >5% Between Treatment Groups (IPASS; EFS population)

System Organ Class and Preferred Term	Number (%) of patients[a]	
	IRESSA 250 mg (N=607) Overall[b]	Carboplatin/Paclitaxel (N=589) Overall[b]
Alopecia	67 (11.0)	344 (58.4)
Acne	66 (10.9)	4 (0.7)
Dermatitis acneiform	35 (5.8)	2 (0.3)

[a] Percentages are of total patients in each treatment group presented by decreasing order of incidence in the IRESSA group within the System Organ Class. Patients are counted once within any preferred term.
[b] Overall includes all adverse events that occurred whilst receiving first-line treatment or within 28 days after discontinuation.
[c] Clinically significant laboratory findings were only reported as adverse events if a criterion for a serious adverse event was fulfilled: the abnormality caused study treatment to be discontinued, or the investigator insisted the abnormality was to be reported as an adverse event. Therefore, laboratory findings worsening from baseline to CTC grade 3 or 4 should be referred to for the primary assessment of haematological and liver function toxicity.
Legend: ALT: alanine aminotransferase; AST: aspartate aminotransferase; EFS: Evaluable-for-safety; N: Number of patients.

Table 3: IRESSA

Analysis of Specific Safety Events (IPASS; EFS population)

Event[a]	IRESSA 250 mg (N=607)		Carboplatin/Paclitaxel (N=589)		Adjusted p-value[b]
	n	(%)	n	(%)	
Events Possibly Associated with Gefitinib					
Rashes/Acnes	398	(65.6)	132	(22.4)	<0.0001
Diarrhoea	274	(45.1)	128	(21.7)	<0.0001
Nausea	74	(12.2)	260	(44.1	<0.0001
Vomiting	59	(9.7)	193	(32.8)	<0.0001
Elevated liver transaminases (CTC ≥3)[c]	57	(9.4)	6	(1.0)	<0.0001
Events Possibly Associated with Carboplatin/Paclitaxel					
Neurotoxicity	30	(4.9)	411	(69.8)	<0.0001
Neutropenia (CTC ≥3)[c]	4	(0.7)	385	(65.4)	<0.0001
Leukopenia (CTC ≥3)[c]	1	(0.2)	202	(34.3)	<0.0001
Anaemia (CTC ≥3)[c]	11	(1.8)	56	(9.5)	<0.0001
Thrombocytopenia (CTC ≥3)[c]	5	(0.8)	29	(4.9)	0.0001

[a] Data are derived from adverse events occurring on-treatment and during the 28 day follow-up period, and from laboratory data reported on-treatment. Percentages are of total patients in each treatment group presented in decreasing order of incidence in the IRESSA group for events possibly associated with IRESSA, and in decreasing order of incidence in the carboplatin/paclitaxel group for events possibly associated with carboplatin/paclitaxel.
[b] Calculated using the method of Westfall and Young 1993.
[c] Identified from the laboratory data, as abnormal laboratory results were not to be routinely reported as adverse events.
Legend: CTC: Common Terminology Criteria; EFS: Evaluable-for-safety; N: Number of patients.

DRUG INTERACTIONS: Overview: Gefitinib showed no enzyme induction effects in animal studies. Human liver microsome studies demonstrated that in vitro gefitinib was not a potent inhibitor of any human CYP enzyme activities. At the highest concentration studied, it produced approximately 50% inhibition of CYP2D6. In a clinical trial in cancer patients, gefitinib was co-administered with metoprolol (a CYP2D6 substrate). This resulted in a small (35%) increase in exposure to metoprolol, which is not considered to be clinically relevant. However, such an increase has potential clinical relevance for CYP2D6 substrates with a narrow therapeutic index and caution is advised when co-administered with gefitinib.

In vitro studies have shown that the metabolism of gefitinib is predominantly via CYP3A4. Co-administration with rifampicin (a known potent CYP3A4 inducer) in healthy volunteers reduced mean gefitinib AUC by 83% of that without rifampicin. Substances that are inducers of CYP3A4 activity may increase metabolism and decrease gefitinib plasma concentrations. Therefore, co-medication with CYP3A4 inducers (e.g., phenytoin, carbamazepine, rifampicin, barbiturates, or St. John's Wort) may potentially reduce efficacy.

Co-administration with itraconazole (a potent CYP3A4 inhibitor) resulted in an 80% increase in the mean AUC of gefitinib in healthy volunteers. Substances that are inhibitors of CYP3A4 activity (e.g., azole antifungals such as ketoconazole and itraconazole, macrolide antibiotics such as erythromycin and clarithromycin, protease inhibitors, grapefruit juice etc.) may decrease metabolism and increase gefitinib plasma concentrations. This increase may be clinically relevant as adverse experiences are related to dose and exposure. Therefore, caution should be used when administering CYP3A4 inhibitors with IRESSA.

Co-administration of ranitidine (gastric pH above 5) reduced by 47% the mean gefitinib AUC in healthy volunteers. Drugs that cause significant sustained elevation in gastric pH (histamine H_2-receptor antagonists such as ranitidine or cimetidine; proton-pump inhibitors) may reduce plasma concentrations of gefitinib and therefore potentially may reduce efficacy (see Action and Clinical Pharmacology, Metabolism).

International Normalized Ratio (INR) elevations and/or bleeding events have been reported in some patients taking warfarin while on IRESSA therapy. Patients taking warfarin should be monitored regularly for changes in prothrombin time or INR.

Drug-Drug Interactions: See Table 4.

Table 4: IRESSA

Established or Potential Drug-Drug Interactions

Proper Name	Effect	Clinical Comment
Metoprolol	↑ metoprolol exposure by 35%	Observation made in cancer patients.
Rifampicin	↓ mean AUC of gefitinib by 83%	Observation made in healthy volunteers.
Itraconazole	↑ mean AUC of gefitinib by 80%	Observation made in healthy volunteers.
Ranitidine	↓ mean AUC of gefitinib by 47%	Observation made in healthy volunteers using supratherapeutic doses.

(cont'd)

Table 4: IRESSA *(cont'd)*

Drug-Food Interactions: Grapefruit juice and other inhibitors of CYP3A4 may decrease metabolism and increase gefitinib plasma concentrations.

Drug-Herb Interactions: St. John's Wort and other inducers of CYP3A4 may potentially reduce the efficacy of gefitinib.

Drug-Laboratory Test Interactions: Interactions with laboratory tests have not been established.

DOSAGE AND ADMINISTRATION: Recommended Dose and Dosage Adjustment: The recommended daily dose of IRESSA (gefitinib) is one 250 mg tablet with or without food. Higher doses do not produce a better response and lead to increased toxicity.

Dosage Adjustment: No dosage adjustment is required on the basis of patient age, body weight, gender, ethnicity or renal function. However, data are limited in patients with severe renal impairment (creatinine clearance ≤20 mL/min (see Action and Clinical Pharmacology, Special Populations and Conditions) and caution is advised in these patients.

For patients unable to tolerate treatment after a therapy interruption for toxicity, IRESSA should be discontinued and another treatment option should be considered.

Poorly Tolerated Diarrhoea: Patients with poorly tolerated diarrhoea (sometimes associated with dehydration) or skin adverse drug reactions may be successfully managed by providing a brief (up to 14 days) therapy interruption followed by reinstatement of the 250 mg daily dose once toxicity has resolved.

Eye Symptoms: Patients who develop eye symptoms should be evaluated and managed, including interruption of therapy with IRESSA. Reinstatement of the 250 mg/day IRESSA dose should be considered when symptoms and eye changes have resolved.

Respiratory Symptoms: If patients present with acute onset or worsening of respiratory symptoms such as dyspnoea, cough and fever, IRESSA should be interrupted and prompt investigation initiated. If Interstitial Lung Disease (ILD) is confirmed, IRESSA should be discontinued and the patient treated appropriately (see Warnings and Precautions, Respiratory and Adverse Reactions).

Hepatic Impairment: An average 3.1-fold increase in exposure to gefitinib in patients with moderate and severe hepatic impairment due to cirrhosis was observed in a phase I hepatic impairment study (see Warnings and Precautions, Special Populations and Action and Clinical Pharmacology). This increase in exposure may be of clinical relevance since adverse experiences are related to dose and exposure to gefitinib. No dose adjustments are recommended for patients with moderate to severe hepatic impairment (Child Pugh B or C) however, these patients should be closely monitored. No dose adjustments are recommended for patients with elevated aspartate transaminase (AST), alkaline phosphatase or bilirubin due to liver metastases. These patients should be closely monitored for adverse events.

In patients with impaired liver function secondary to liver metastases, gefitinib exposure was similar for patients with moderate hepatic dysfunction compared to normal hepatic function. Data from four patients with severe hepatic dysfunction due to liver metastases suggested that steady state exposures in these patients are also similar to those in patients with normal hepatic function.

In the pivotal trial IPASS, patients with alanine aminotransferase (ALT) or aspartate aminotransferase (AST) levels greater than 2.5 times upper limit of normal (ULN) with no demonstrable liver metastases or greater than 5 times ULN in the presence of liver metastases were excluded due to potential hepatic concerns associated with the carboplatin/paclitaxel doublet. Consequently, the IPASS study does not contribute any data in this patient population.

OVERDOSAGE:

In non-clinical studies, the median lethal oral dose in rats was 2000 mg/kg (approximately 400 times the clinically recommended daily dose in humans on a mg/kg basis). The median lethal oral dose in mice was found to be in excess of 2000 mg/kg.

There is no specific treatment in the event of overdose of IRESSA and possible symptoms of overdose are not established. However, in phase I clinical trials, a limited number of patients were treated with daily doses of up to 1000 mg. An increase in frequency and severity of some adverse reactions was observed, mainly diarrhoea and skin rash. Adverse reactions associated with overdose should be treated symptomatically; in particular, severe diarrhoea should be managed appropriately.

> For management of a suspected drug overdose, contact your regional Poison Control Centre. See the *CPS* Directory section for a list of Poison Control Centres.

ACTION AND CLINICAL PHARMACOLOGY: Mechanism of Action: IRESSA (gefitinib) is an epidermal growth factor receptor (EGFR) tyrosine kinase inhibitor (TKI). EGFR is expressed on the cell surface of many normal cells as well as cancer cells. Increased EGFR signalling can drive tumour growth through the activation of pathways that are crucial to proliferation, invasion, angiogenesis, metastasis and inhibition of cell death.

Mutations in the tyrosine kinase domain of the EGFR gene are only found in tumour cells and increase the dependency of these tumour cells to the intercellular signalling cascades that result in the promotion of tumour cell growth, blocking of apoptosis, increasing the production of angiogenic factors and facilitating the processes of metastasis.

In patients whose tumour contains an activating mutation of the EGFR-tyrosine kinase (TK), IRESSA binds to the EGFR TK domain with high specificity and affinity, resulting in potent inhibition of the over-active signalling pathways which can lead to tumour shrinkage.

Pharmacokinetics: The pharmacokinetics of gefitinib have been evaluated in healthy volunteers and in cancer patients following both single and multiple dosing.

Absorption: Following single oral administration to volunteers or to cancer patients, absorption was moderately slow and the mean terminal half-life was 30.5 and 41.0 hours, respectively. In volunteers, gefitinib AUC showed up to a 20-fold range at the same dose level and increased proportionally with dose over the dose range 50 to 250 mg. Between 250 and 500 mg, there was a slightly greater than dose proportional increase in exposure but the maximum degree of non-proportionality observed was only 2-fold. In cancer patients, gefitinib AUC increased with dose over the dose range 50 to 700 mg and showed up to an 8-fold range of values within a dose level.

Daily administration of gefitinib to patients resulted in a 2-to 8-fold accumulation with steady state plasma concentrations achieved within 7-10 days. At steady state, plasma concentrations were typically maintained within a 2-to 3-fold range across the 24-hour dosing interval. Population pharmacokinetic data from Trial 0016 showed a mean steady state trough concentration following a 250 mg oral dose of 264 ng/mL (95% CI: 92.2 to 755 ng/mL) with inter-and intra-patient variability of 54 and 21%, respectively.

Mean oral bioavailability of gefitinib was approximately 60% in both healthy volunteers and cancer patients, indicating that it was well absorbed. C_{max} was typically achieved within 3 to 7 hours after dosing in both groups. Relative bioavailability of gefitinib in volunteers was not altered by food to an extent likely to be of clinical significance. In a trial in healthy volunteers where gastric pH was maintained above pH 5 by co-administration of high doses of ranitidine with sodium bicarbonate, relative bioavailability was reduced by 47%.

Distribution: Mean volume of distribution at steady state of gefitinib is 1600 L in volunteers and 1400 L in cancer patients indicating extensive distribution into tissue. At clinically relevant concentrations of gefitinib, binding (in vitro) to human plasma proteins is approximately 90% with the binding proteins involved being serum albumin and α1-acid glycoprotein.

Metabolism: In vitro data indicate that CYP3A4 is the major P450 isozyme involved in the oxidative metabolism of gefitinib. Three sites of biotransformation have been identified in the metabolism of gefitinib: metabolism of the N-propylmorpholino-group, demethylation of the methoxy substituent on the quinazoline, and oxidative defluorination of the halogenated phenyl group. Five metabolites have been fully identified in faecal extracts and the major component was O-desmethyl gefitinib, although this only accounted for 14% of the dose.

In human plasma, 8 metabolites were fully identified. The major metabolite identified was O-desmethyl gefitinib, which was14-fold less potent than gefitinib at inhibiting EGFR-stimulated cell growth and had no inhibitory effect on tumour cell growth in mice. It is therefore considered unlikely that it contributes to the clinical activity of gefitinib.

The production of O-desmethyl gefitinib has also been shown, in vitro, to be via CYP2D6. The role of CYP2D6 in the metabolic clearance of gefitinib has been evaluated in a clinical trial in healthy volunteers genotyped for CYP2D6 status. In poor metabolisers (devoid of CYP2D6) no measurable levels of O-desmethyl gefitinib were produced. The range of gefitinib exposures achieved in both the extensive and the poor metaboliser groups were wide and overlapping but the mean exposure to gefitinib was 2-fold higher in the poor metaboliser group. The higher average exposures that could be achieved by individuals with no active CYP2D6 may be clinically relevant since adverse experiences are related to dose and exposure.

Excretion: Gefitinib total plasma clearance is approximately 500 mL/min. Excretion is predominantly via the faeces with renal elimination of drug and metabolites accounting for less than 4% of the administered dose.

Special Populations and Conditions: Pediatrics: There are no pharmacokinetic data in paediatric patients.

Hepatic Impairment: In a phase I open-label study of single dose gefitinib 250 mg in patients with mild, moderate or severe hepatic impairment due to cirrhosis (according to Child-Pugh classification), there was an increase in exposure in all groups compared with healthy controls. An average 3.1-fold increase in exposure to gefitinib in patients with moderate and severe hepatic impairment was observed. None of the patients had cancer, all had cirrhosis and some had hepatitis. This increase in exposure may be of clinical relevance since adverse experiences are related to dose and exposure to gefitinib (see Warnings and Precautions, Special Populations).

Gefitinib has been evaluated in a clinical trial conducted in 41 patients with solid tumours and normal hepatic function or, moderate or severe hepatic dysfunction due to liver metastases. It was shown that following daily dosing of IRESSA 250 mg, time to steady state, total plasma clearance and steady state exposure (C_{maxss}, AUC_{24ss}) were similar for the groups with normal and moderately impaired hepatic function. Data from 4 patients with severe hepatic dysfunction due to liver metastases suggested that steady state exposures in these patients are also similar to those in patients with normal hepatic function.

Renal Insufficiency: No clinical studies were conducted with IRESSA in patients with severely compromised renal function. Gefitinib and its metabolites are not significantly excreted via the kidney (<4%). A limited number of patients with moderate renal insufficiency (calculated creatinine clearance of 30-50 mL/min) participated in the clinical trials. Based on the data from these studies, no safety concerns were raised regarding the use of IRESSA in patients with mild or moderate renal impairment in comparison to patients with normal renal function at baseline. Due to the small number of patients, there is insufficient data to evaluate the safety profile of IRESSA in patients with severe renal impairment.

STORAGE AND STABILITY: IRESSA (gefitinib) should be stored at room temperature, 15 to 30°C.

INFORMATION FOR THE PATIENT: Published in e-CPS, available by subscription at www.e-cps.ca.

DOSAGE FORMS, COMPOSITION AND PACKAGING: Each brown, round, biconvex, film-coated tablet, impressed with "IRESSA 250" on one side and plain on the other, contains: gefitinib 250 mg. Nonmedicinal ingredients: croscarmellose sodium, hypromellose, lactose monohydrate, macrogol 300, magnesium stearate, microcrystalline cellulose, povidone, red iron oxide, sodium lauryl sulfate, titanium dioxide and yellow iron oxide. Blister packs of 30.

(Shown in Product Identification Section)

Irinotecan Hydrochloride Trihydrate for Injection Ⓟ

irinotecan HCl trihydrate

Antineoplastic

Hospira

SUPPLIED: Each mL of sterile, clear, colourless to pale yellow solution contains: irinotecan HCl trihydrate 20 mg. Nonmedicinal ingredients: lactic acid, sorbitol and water for injection. May contain sodium hydroxide or hydrochloric acid as pH adjusters. Single use amber glass ONCO-TAIN vials of 2, 5 and 25 mL (single packs).

Irinotecan Hydrochloride Trihydrate Injection Ⓟ

irinotecan HCl trihydrate

Antineoplastic

Sandoz

SUPPLIED: Each mL of sterile, pale yellow, clear, aqueous solution contains: irinotecan hydrochloride trihydrate 20 mg. Nonmedicinal ingredients: lactic acid, sorbitol and water for injection. Sodium hydroxide may be used to adjust the pH to 3.0-3.8. Boxes of 1×2 mL (in a 2 mL single use vial). Boxes of 1×5 mL (in a 5 mL single use vial). Boxes of 1×25 mL (in a 50 mL single use vial). Store between 15 and 30°C. Do not refrigerate. Protect from light and freezing.

Iron Salts: Oral

ferrous fumarate

ferrous gluconate

ferrous sulfate

Anemia Therapy

CPhA Monograph

Date of Revision: October 2006

This monograph has been compiled by CPhA and reviewed by experts. It may contain information different from that found in Health Canada-approved Product Monographs. The reader is referred to the *CPS* Editorial Policy for more information.

PHARMACOLOGY: Iron is an important component of a number of enzymes necessary for energy transfer. It is also present in hemoglobin and myoglobin and is important in the metabolism of catecholamines and the functioning of neutrophils.

Administration of iron preparations corrects erythropoietic abnormalities which are due to deficiency of iron. Iron does not stimulate erythropoiesis nor does it correct hemoglobin disturbances not caused by iron deficiency. In fact, it may cause iron storage disease or iron toxicity when used in these conditions.

Administration of iron relieves other symptoms of iron deficiency such as soreness of the tongue, dysphagia, dystrophy of the nails and skin, and fissuring of the angles of the lips.

Pharmacokinetics: Absorption of iron is influenced by many factors including the form in which it is administered, the dose, the status of the patient's iron stores, the degree of erythropoiesis, and the patient's diet and drug therapy. Absorption is increased by iron deficiency, the fasting state and the concurrent administration of Vitamin C (see Precautions: Drug Interactions). In addition, inorganic iron appears to be absorbed better than iron from dietary sources, and heme iron, found in meat, fish and poultry, is absorbed better than non-heme dietary iron. Ferrous salts are absorbed up to three times better than ferric salts. Ferrous iron passes through gastrointestinal mucosal cells directly into the blood and is immediately bound to transferrin which transports iron to the bone marrow where it is incorporated into hemoglobin. Maximal absorption takes place in the duodenum and proximal jejunum; therefore, iron may not be as well absorbed from slow-release and delayed-release preparations which may bypass the site of optimal absorption.

The body has no physiological route for the excretion of excess iron. Most of the iron liberated by destruction of hemoglobin is conserved and reused. Normal daily excretion of iron from cell desquamation varies from 0.5 to 2 mg. The average monthly loss of iron in normal menstruation is 12 to 30 mg.

Frequent blood donors, pregnant women, burn victims, individuals on hemodialysis, or with intestinal diseases (celiac, sprue, inflammatory bowel disease) and premature infants may require prophylactic therapy.

The Canadian Paediatric Society recommends that term infants who are not breast-fed receive iron-fortified formula from birth, and states that term breast-fed infants do not require supplemental iron until after 6 months of age.

INDICATIONS: Prevention and treatment of iron deficiency anemias.

CONTRAINDICATIONS: Hemosiderosis, hemochromatosis. Iron compounds are also contraindicated in the treatment of anemia due to conditions other than iron deficiency. Administration of iron to premature infants with vitamin E deficiency may precipitate red cell hemolysis. Therefore, correction of vitamin E deficiency (usually with parenteral vitamin E) should precede iron administration.

Because of the risk of iron overload, oral and parenteral iron therapy should not be used concomitantly (see Adverse Effects).

PRECAUTIONS: Prolonged administration of iron (i.e., for longer than 6 months) should be avoided except in patients with continued bleeding, malabsorption syndromes that benefit from additional iron therapy or repeated pregnancies.

Orally administered iron salts may not be well absorbed in patients with steatorrhea and those who have had a partial gastrectomy.

Liquid iron preparations may stain the teeth with continued use. Stains may be prevented to a large extent by taking the dose through a straw, first mixing it with water or fruit juice, and by following the dose with a drink of plain water or juice. Brushing the teeth with sodium bicarbonate or hydrogen peroxide 3% will usually remove existing stains.

Because iron overload may increase susceptibility to certain bacterial infections (e.g., *Y. enterocolitica*), some clinicians recommend that iron not be administered to HIV-positive individuals without documented iron-deficiency anemia.

Drug Interactions: Iron may decrease the absorption of the following drugs: bisphosphonates, tetracycline, penicillamine, quinolone antibiotics, levodopa, methyldopa and levothyroxine. These drugs should be administered at least 2 hours before or after the administration of oral iron. Patients should be monitored for inadequate clinical response and switched to alternative therapy if necessary.

Concomitant administration of iron and chloramphenicol may impair the hematologic response to iron.

Concurrent administration of more than 200 mg of vitamin C per 30 mg iron increases absorption of iron from the gastrointestinal tract by approximately 10%.

Concomitant administration of antacids (containing aluminum and magnesium salts or sodium bicarbonate or calcium carbonate) or cholestyramine may impair the absorption of iron.

Drug-Laboratory Test Interactions: Because iron preparations can color the feces black, large amounts may interfere with the guaiac test for occult blood in stool.

Pregnancy: No adverse effects have been reported with intake of normal daily requirements.

Lactation: At therapeutic doses, the amount of iron excreted in breast milk is not sufficient to affect the infant.

Children: Deaths have occurred in children following ingestion of as little as 400 mg of elemental iron. Patients should be warned about the extreme danger to children of accidental iron poisoning.

ADVERSE EFFECTS: Oral iron preparations may cause nausea, vomiting, dyspepsia, constipation, diarrhea or dark stools. These effects are generally dose-related and, with the exception of dark stools, usually subside with continued therapy. The incidence of adverse effects during therapy with a particular salt is a function of the total amount of elemental iron delivered by the daily dose. To minimize gastrointestinal side effects, it may be helpful to take oral iron doses with or after meals, or to initiate therapy at lower doses and gradually increase to the therapeutic dose.

Hemosiderosis may occur secondary to long-term administration of large amounts of iron. This is more likely in patients receiving both oral and parenteral forms of iron, in patients with conditions that may be erroneously diagnosed as iron-deficiency anemia, and in patients receiving large amounts of parenteral iron.

Liquid iron preparations may stain teeth (see Precautions).

OVERDOSE:

Iron can be extremely toxic in overdose.

Iron poisoning is uncommon in adults, but is one of the leading causes of pediatric poisoning deaths. Systemic toxicity following ingestion of greater than 60 mg/kg of elemental iron is likely. Lower doses (i.e., 10 to 40 mg/kg of elemental iron) usually cause gastrointestinal symptoms without significant systemic toxicity.

Symptoms: Initial signs and symptoms of clinically significant iron overdose are gastrointestinal (epigastric pain, nausea, vomiting, and diarrhea). Melena and hematemesis may result in hemodynamic instability. The complete absence of gastrointestinal symptoms during the first 6 hours after ingestion of iron suggests that the dose is nontoxic. A transient period of apparent recovery may occur between 6 and 24 hours after a clinically significant ingestion. The gastrointestinal symptoms may resolve but the patient will continue to appear unwell. Tachycardia and metabolic acidosis may be evident. During this period, toxicity may be ongoing so it is important to continue active management of the patient. In severe overdose, patients may go into shock within a few hours of the ingestion until up to 24 hours or more after the ingestion. Hypotension, circulatory collapse, metabolic acidosis, coagulopathy, coma, convulsions and death may occur. Hepatic failure may occur several days after a large ingestion due to oxidative damage to hepatocytes. Intestinal scarring and obstruction are complications that may occur several weeks after a large ingestion as the gastrointestinal lesions heal.

Serum Iron Studies:

Iron poisoning is a clinical diagnosis and practitioners should not rely solely on toxicological tests as a guide to the potential severity of an overdose. Serum iron levels are useful, but may not correlate well with systemic toxicity. Serum iron levels generally peak 2 to 6 hours after ingestion, although this may not be true for delayed-release formulations. Serum iron concentrations of 50 µmol/L to >90 µmol/L (300 to >500 µg/dL) are generally indicative of significant gastrointestinal toxicity and possible systemic toxicity. Higher levels suggest the possibility of more severe poisoning. Significant morbidity and mortality is associated with serum iron levels >179 µmol/L (>1000 µg/dL). An apparently low serum iron level does not rule out the possibility of significant toxicity. Patients in the later stages of poisoning may have normal or declining serum iron levels. Moreover, deferoxamine can falsely lower serum iron levels unless atomic absorption is used to quantify serum iron concentrations. Total iron binding capacity (TIBC) is not useful in determining the severity of iron poisoning.

Treatment: After initial assessment and stabilization of the patient, iv access should be established, volume repletion begun and appropriate lab tests ordered (hemoglobin, hematocrit, serum iron concentration, serum electrolytes, BUN and creatinine, blood gases and anion gap determination). Liver function tests and coagulation studies may also be helpful. Vital signs should be closely monitored. Iron is radiopaque and abdominal x-ray may reveal the presence of intact tablets in the gastrointestinal tract. This is not true of liquid preparations or multivitamins. Absence of tablets on the x-ray does not rule out a significant ingestion.

Gastric lavage should not be routinely performed, but may be considered on the advice of a Poison Control Centre in unusual cases. Iron is not bound by activated charcoal. Whole bowel irrigation (WBI) is generally regarded as the method of choice for decontaminating the gut. A nasogastric tube is often necessary to facilitate administration of polyethylene glycol solution. The usual dose of polyethylene glycol solution is 250 to 500 mL/h in children and 2 L/h in adults. Beginning with a lower rate and increase as tolerated. An antiemetic such as metoclopramide may be used to treat nausea and vomiting.

Fluid and electrolyte balance should be carefully maintained. Hypotension may require the use of vasopressors. Metabolic acidosis should be treated by correcting hypovolemia and hypoperfusion.

Deferoxamine is a specific antidote for iron poisoning. Deferoxamine forms a complex with ferric iron that is excreted by the kidneys. Oral administration of deferoxamine is not recommended as this may increase absorption of iron from the gastrointestinal tract. Indications for deferoxamine include metabolic acidosis, repetitive vomiting, toxic appearance, lethargy, hypotension or signs of shock. Deferoxamine should also be administered to patients with serum iron levels >90 µmol/L (>500 µg/dL).

Deferoxamine should be administered as an iv infusion, starting slowly and gradually increasing to a dose of 15 mg/kg/h to minimize hypotension, which is common. The manufacturer recommends a maximum dose of 6 g. The deferoxamine-iron complex will usually cause the patient's urine to turn pink. A baseline urine sample may be collected for comparison with samples collected after treatment has begun. The endpoint of deferoxamine therapy is not well defined, but many authors recommend it be discontinued when the patient appears clinically well, the anion-gap acidosis has resolved, and the urine is no longer discoloured. Some experts recommend continuing deferoxamine beyond 24 hours at a lower dose if there are continuing signs of toxicity.

Hemodialysis is not effective in removing iron from the body. However, patients who develop renal failure during deferoxamine therapy may benefit, because hemodialysis can remove the deferoxamine-iron complex.

For management of a suspected drug overdose, CPhA recommends that you contact your **regional Poison Control Centre**. See the *CPS* Directory section for a list of Poison Control Centres.

DOSAGE: In preventing iron deficiency, adequate dietary intake is preferred over supplementation whenever possible. Food sources include red meat, poultry, organ meat (e.g., liver), spinach, dried fruits, whole grains, nuts, beans and clams. Iron from animal sources is better absorbed than that from plant sources.

The recommended daily intake of iron to prevent deficiency is 0.3 mg in infants less than 4 months and 6 to 8 mg in older infants and children. Adolescents and adults should receive 8 to 13 mg daily. An additional 5 mg/day is recommended in the second trimester of pregnancy with an additional 10 mg/day in the third trimester. Additional iron is not usually required during the first trimester or lactation.

Calculation of dosage for iron preparations should always be based on the amount of elemental iron to be administered. Commonly used oral iron salts and their elemental iron content are listed in Table 1.

Table 1: Iron Salts: Oral
Comparison of Elemental Iron Content

Iron Salt	% of Elemental Iron
Ferrous Fumarate	33
Ferrous Gluconate	11.6
Ferrous Sulfate	20
Ferrous Sulfate, anhydrous	30

For iron deficient adults, 50 to 100 mg of elemental iron given orally 3 times daily is usually adequate. Absorption is optimal in the fasting state. To lessen gastrointestinal intolerance, lower doses may be administered initially, and the medication may be given with or after meals. After 4 or 5 days the dose may be gradually increased. After the hemoglobin level returns to normal, oral therapy should be continued for 3 to 6 months to replenish stores.

Premature infants who are not receiving iron-fortified formula should receive 2 to 4 mg elemental iron/kg/day divided BID or as a single daily dose to a maximum of 15 mg/day. Iron supplementation should begin at the age of 8 weeks and continue until the age of 1 year.

For infants and children with severe iron-deficiency anemia, 4 to 6 mg elemental iron/kg/day in 3 divided doses is given. Infants and children with mild to moderate iron-deficiency anemia should receive 3 mg elemental iron/kg/day divided BID or as a single daily dose. Infants and children who require prophylaxis against iron-deficiency anemia should receive 0.5 to 2 mg elemental iron/kg/day (maximum 15 mg/day).

Isentress® ℞

raltegravir potassium

Human Immunodeficiency Virus Integrase Strand Transfer Inhibitor

Merck Frosst

Date of Revision: April 30, 2010

SUMMARY PRODUCT INFORMATION:

Route of Administration	Dosage Form/ Strength	Clinically Relevant Nonmedicinal Ingredients
Oral	Film coated tablets 400 mg raltegravir (as raltegravir potassium)	Lactose For a complete listing see Dosage Forms, Composition and Packaging.

INDICATIONS AND CLINICAL USE: ISENTRESS (raltegravir) is indicated in combination with other antiretroviral agents for the treatment of human immunodeficiency virus (HIV-1) infection in adult patients.

This indication is based on the evidence of efficacy of ISENTRESS from the analysis of 48-week data from 3 ongoing, randomized, double-blind, placebo-controlled trials, BENCHMRK 1 and BENCHMRK 2 (Protocols 018 and 019), in antiretroviral treatment-experienced HIV-1 infected adult patients and the analysis of 48-week data from an ongoing, randomized, double-blind, active-control trial, STARTMRK (Protocol 021). These efficacy results were supported by the 48-week analysis of a randomized, double-blind, controlled, dose-ranging trial, Protocol 005, in antiretroviral treatment-experienced HIV-1 infected adult patients and 96-week analysis of a randomized, double-blind, controlled, dose-ranging trial, Protocol 004, in antiretroviral treatment-naïve HIV-1 infected adult patients.

CONTRAINDICATIONS: ISENTRESS is contraindicated in patients who are hypersensitive to any component of this medicine. For a complete listing of components, see Dosage Forms, Composition and Packaging.

WARNINGS AND PRECAUTIONS: General: Caution should be used when coadministering ISENTRESS with strong inducers of uridine diphosphate glucuronosyltransferase (UGT) 1A1 (e.g., rifampin) due to reduced plasma concentrations of raltegravir (see Drug Interactions).

Immune: During the initial phase of treatment, patients responding to antiretroviral therapy may develop an inflammatory response to indolent or residual opportunistic infections (such as *M. avium* complex, cytomegalovirus, *P. jeroveci* pneumonia, and tuberculosis, or reactivation of varicella zoster virus), which may necessitate further evaluation and treatment.

Musculoskeletal: Grade 2-4 creatine kinase laboratory abnormalities were observed in patients treated with raltegravir (see Adverse Reactions). Cases of myopathy and rhabdomyolysis have been reported with raltegravir. A relationship to raltegravir is not clear in a majority of these cases; however there have been isolated post-market reports of myopathy and rhabdomyolysis either with an association to raltegravir or where a relationship to raltegravir could not be ruled out. Use with caution in patients at increased risk of myopathy or rhabdomyolysis, such as patients receiving concomitant medications known to cause these conditions.

Special Populations: Pregnant Women: Developmental toxicity studies were performed in rabbits (at doses up to 1000 mg/kg/day) and rats (at doses up to 600 mg/kg/day). The highest doses in these studies produced systemic exposures in these species approximately 3-to 4-fold above the exposure at the recommended human dose. No treatment related external, visceral, or skeletal changes were observed in rabbits. Treatment-related increases over controls in the incidence of supernumerary ribs were seen in rats at 600 mg/kg/day (exposures 4.4- fold above the exposure at the recommended human dose). In both rabbits and rats, no treatment related effects on embryonic/fetal survival or fetal weights were observed.

In rats, at a maternal dose of 600 mg/kg/day, mean drug concentrations in fetal plasma were approximately 1.5- to 2.5-fold greater than in maternal plasma at 1 hour and 24 hours postdose, respectively. In rabbits, at a maternal dose of 1000 mg/kg/day, mean drug concentrations in fetal plasma were approximately 2% of the mean maternal concentration at both 1 and 24 hours postdose. Toxicokinetic studies demonstrated placental transfer of drug in both species.

There are no adequate and well-controlled studies in pregnant women; therefore, the safety of ISENTRESS in pregnant women is not known. ISENTRESS, like other antiretroviral agents, is not recommended for use in pregnancy.

Antiretroviral Pregnancy Registry: To monitor maternal-fetal outcomes of pregnant patients exposed to ISENTRESS, an Antiretroviral Pregnancy Registry has been established. Physicians are encouraged to register patients by calling 1-800-567-2594.

Nursing Women: It is not known whether raltegravir is secreted in human milk. However, raltegravir is secreted in the milk of lactating rats. In rats, at a maternal dose of 600 mg/kg/day, mean drug concentrations in milk were approximately 3-fold greater than in maternal plasma. Breast-feeding is not recommended while taking ISENTRESS. In addition, it is recommended that HIV-infected mothers not breast-feed their infants to avoid risking postnatal transmission of HIV.

Pediatrics (<16 years of age): Safety and effectiveness in pediatric patients less than 16 years of age have not been established.

Geriatrics (≥65 years of age): Clinical studies of ISENTRESS did not include sufficient numbers of patients aged 65 and over to determine whether they respond differently from younger patients. In general, dose selection for an elderly patient should be cautious, reflecting the greater frequency of decreased hepatic, renal, or cardiac function, and of concomitant disease or other drug therapy.

ADVERSE REACTIONS: Clinical Trial Adverse Drug Reactions: Because clinical trials are conducted under very specific conditions the adverse reaction rates observed in the clinical trials may not reflect the rates observed in practice and should not be compared to the rates in the clinical trials of another drug. Adverse drug reaction information from clinical trials is useful for identifying drug-related adverse events and for approximating rates.

Treatment-Experienced Adverse Experiences: The safety assessment of ISENTRESS in treatment-experienced patients is based on the pooled safety data from the randomized clinical studies, P005, P018 and P019, reported using the recommended dose of ISENTRESS 400 mg twice daily in combination with optimized background therapy (OBT) in 507 patients, in comparison to 282 patients taking placebo in combination with OBT. During double-blind treatment, the total follow-up was 702.8 patient-years in the group receiving ISENTRESS 400 mg b.i.d. and 257.1 patient-years in the group receiving placebo.

For patients in the group receiving ISENTRESS 400 mg twice daily + OBT (mean follow-up 72.3 weeks) and the comparator group placebo + OBT (mean follow-up 47.6 weeks) in the pooled analysis for studies P005, P018 and P019, the most commonly reported adverse experiences (>10% in either group), of all intensities and regardless of causality were: diarrhea in 20.3% and 21.3%, nausea in 12.2% and 15.6%, headache in 10.8% and 12.8%, fatigue in 10.5% and 5.7%, upper respiratory tract infection in 10.3% and 7.8%, pyrexia in 7.7% and 11.7% of patients, respectively.

The following clinical adverse experiences below are regardless of causality and were considered by investigators to be of mild, moderate or severe intensity.

Clinical adverse events of mild, moderate or severe intensity occurring in ≥2% of treatment-experienced adult patients in either treatment group are presented in Table 1.

Less Common Clinical Trial Adverse Drug Reactions (<2%): Drug-related adverse experiences occurring in less than 2% of treatment-experienced patients (n=507) receiving ISENTRESS + OBT and of moderate to severe intensity are listed below by system organ class:

General Disorders and Administration Site Conditions: asthenia, fatigue, pyrexia, chest discomfort, chills, feeling hot, irritability, drug intolerance, face edema, fat necrosis.

Blood and Lymphatic System Disorders: anaemia, macrocytic anaemia, neutropenia.

Cardiac Disorders: myocardial infarction, palpitations, ventricular extrasystoles.

Ear and Labyrinth Disorders: vertigo.

Eye Disorders: visual disturbance.

Gastrointestinal Disorders: abdominal pain, vomiting, abdominal distension, upper abdominal pain, constipation, gastrointestinal pain, abdominal discomfort, dyspepsia, flatulence, gastritis, glossitis, gastroesophageal reflux disease, dry mouth.

Hepatobiliary Disorders: hepatitis, hepatomegaly, hyperbilirubinemia.

Immune System Disorders: drug hypersensitivity, hypersensitivity.

Infections and Infestations: cellulitis, herpes simplex, genital herpes.

Injury, Poisoning and Procedural Complications: drug toxicity, compression fracture.

Investigations: weight decreased, weight increased.

Table 1: ISENTRESS

Percentage of Patients with Adverse Experience of All Intensities and Regardless of Causality Occurring in ≥2% of Treatment-Experienced Adult Patients in Either Treatment Group

	Randomized Studies P005, P018 and P019			
	ISENTRESS 400 mg b.i.d.+OBT (N=507)		Placebo+OBT (N=282)	
System Organ Class, Preferred Term, %	n	(%)	n	(%)
Patients with One or More Adverse Experiences	463	(91.3)	248	(87.9)
Patients with No Adverse Experience	44	(8.7)	34	(12.1)
Blood and Lymphatic System Disorders	48	(9.5)	26	(9.2)
Anaemia	15	(3.0)	12	(4.3)
Lymphadenopathy	23	(4.5)	9	(3.2)
Cardiac Disorders	26	(5.1)	11	(3.9)
Ear and Labyrinth Disorders	15	(3.0)	6	(2.1)
Eye Disorders	36	(7.1)	16	(5.7)
Conjunctivitis	14	(2.8)	1	(0.4)
Gastrointestinal Disorders	242	(47.7)	141	(50.0)
Abdominal Distension	16	(3.2)	9	(3.2)
Abdominal Pain	31	(6.1)	14	(5.0)
Abdominal Pain Upper	20	(3.9)	10	(3.5)
Constipation	17	(3.4)	1	(0.4)
Diarrhea	103	(20.3)	60	(21.3)
Dyspepsia	11	(2.2)	6	(2.1)
Flatulence	19	(3.7)	10	(3.5)
Gastritis	8	(1.6)	7	(2.5)
Haemorrhoids	8	(1.6)	6	(2.1)
Nausea	62	(12.2)	44	(15.6)
Toothache	5	(1.0)	6	(2.1)
Vomiting	40	(7.9)	26	(9.2)
General Disorders and Administration Site Conditions	195	(38.5)	100	(35.5)
Asthenia	17	(3.4)	12	(4.3)
Chest Pain	11	(2.2)	5	(1.8)
Fatigue	53	(10.5)	16	(5.7)
Oedema Peripheral	11	(2.2)	7	(2.5)
Pyrexia	39	(7.7)	33	(11.7)

(cont'd)

Table 1: ISENTRESS *(cont'd)*

Percentage of Patients with Adverse Experience of All Intensities and Regardless of Causality Occurring in ≥2% of Treatment-Experienced Adult Patients in Either Treatment Group

	Randomized Studies P005, P018 and P019			
	ISENTRESS 400 mg b.i.d.+OBT (N=507)		Placebo+OBT (N=282)	
System Organ Class, Preferred Term, %	n	(%)	n	(%)
Hepatobiliary Disorders	20	(3.9)	9	(3.2)
Immune System Disorders	15	(3.0)	7	(2.5)
Infections and Infestations	316	(62.3)	163	(57.8)
Anogenital Warts	18	(3.6)	2	(0.7)
Bronchitis	39	(7.7)	19	(6.7)
Cellulitis	13	(2.6)	4	(1.4)
Folliculitis	12	(2.4)	3	(1.1)
Gastroenteritis	21	(4.1)	6	(2.1)
Genital Herpes	10	(2.0)	6	(2.1)
Herpes Simplex	12	(2.4)	5	(1.8)
Herpes Zoster	29	(5.7)	4	(1.4)
Influenza	30	(5.9)	10	(3.5)
Nasopharyngitis	48	(9.5)	16	(5.7)
Oesophageal Candidiasis	4	(0.8)	6	(2.1)
Onychomycosis	6	(1.2)	6	(2.1)
Oral Candidiasis	8	(1.6)	22	(7.8)
Oral Herpes	10	(2.0)	3	(1.1)
Pharyngitis	13	(2.6)	4	(1.4)
Pneumonia	22	(4.3)	12	(4.3)
Respiratory Tract Infection	16	(3.2)	3	(1.1)
Sinusitis	24	(4.7)	9	(3.2)
Upper Respiratory Tract Infection	52	(10.3)	22	(7.8)
Urinary Tract Infection	11	(2.2)	8	(2.8)
Injury, Poisoning and Procedural Complications	67	(13.2)	28	(9.9)
Investigations	27	(5.3)	21	(7.4)
Weight Decreased	11	(2.2)	9	(3.2)
Metabolism and Nutrition Disorders	69	(13.6)	31	(11.0)
Anorexia	13	(2.6)	8	(2.8)
Decreased Appetite	10	(2.0)	4	(1.4)
Musculoskeletal and Connective Tissue Disorders	123	(24.3)	48	(17.0)
Arthralgia	26	(5.1)	9	(3.2)
Back Pain	23	(4.5)	10	(3.5)
Muscle Spasms	10	(2.0)	7	(2.5)
Musculoskeletal Pain	10	(2.0)	1	(0.4)
Myalgia	13	(2.6)	8	(2.8)
Pain in Extremity	26	(5.1)	9	(3.2)
Neoplasms Benign, Malignant and Unspecified (Incl Cysts and Polyps)	48	(9.5)	16	(5.7)
Skin Papilloma	22	(4.3)	9	(3.2)
Nervous System Disorders	141	(27.8)	75	(26.6)

(cont'd)

Table 1: ISENTRESS *(cont'd)*

Percentage of Patients with Adverse Experience of All Intensities and Regardless of Causality Occurring in ≥2% of Treatment-Experienced Adult Patients in Either Treatment Group

	Randomized Studies P005, P018 and P019			
	ISENTRESS 400 mg b.i.d.+OBT (N=507)		Placebo+OBT (N=282)	
System Organ Class, Preferred Term, %	n	(%)	n	(%)
Dizziness	25	(4.9)	6	(2.1)
Headache	55	(10.8)	36	(12.8)
Neuropathy	5	(1.0)	7	(2.5)
Neuropathy Peripheral	10	(2.0)	6	(2.1)
Psychiatric Disorders	72	(14.2)	45	(16.0)
Anxiety	13	(2.6)	10	(3.5)
Depression	16	(3.2)	12	(4.3)
Insomnia	29	(5.7)	13	(4.6)
Renal and Urinary Disorders	41	(8.1)	19	(6.7)
Dysuria	4	(0.8)	6	(2.1)
Reproductive System And Breast Disorders	45	(8.9)	12	(4.3)
Erectile Dysfunction	11	(2.2)	1	(0.4)
Respiratory, Thoracic and Mediastinal Disorders	80	(15.8)	46	(16.3)
Cough	28	(5.5)	12	(4.3)
Pharyngolaryngeal Pain	14	(2.8)	13	(4.6)
Sinus Congestion	4	(0.8)	6	(2.1)
Skin and Subcutaneous Tissue Disorders	160	(31.6)	71	(25.2)
Eczema	4	(0.8)	8	(2.8)
Lipodystrophy Acquired	14	(2.8)	5	(1.8)
Night Sweats	16	(3.2)	8	(2.8)
Pruritus	16	(3.2)	9	(3.2)
Rash	34	(6.7)	9	(3.2)
Skin Lesion	10	(2.0)	0	(0.0)
Vascular Disorders	43	(8.5)	15	(5.3)
Hypertension	29	(5.7)	6	(2.1)

Metabolism and Nutrition Disorders: diabetes mellitus, central obesity, dyslipidemia, hyperlactacidemia, hyperlipidemia, hypertriglyceridemia, increased appetite, decreased appetite, lipomatosis.
Musculoskeletal and Connective Tissue Disorders: arthralgia, myalgia, pain in extremity, back pain, muscle spasms, musculoskeletal pain, myositis, muscle atrophy, amyotrophy, osteoporosis.
Nervous System Disorders: dizziness, neuropathy peripheral, allodynia, neuropathy, paraesthesia, polyneuropathy, somnolence, tension headache, tremor, peripheral sensory neuropathy.
Psychiatric Disorders: depression, insomnia, abnormal dreams, anxiety.
Renal and Urinary Disorders: nephropathy toxic, nephrotic syndrome, nephritis, nephritis interstitial, nephrolithiasis, nocturia, pollakiuria, renal failure, renal failure acute, renal failure chronic, renal impairment, renal tubular necrosis.
Reproductive System and Breast Disorders: erectile dysfunction, gynecomastia.
Respiratory, Thoracic and Mediastinal Disorders: epistaxis.
Skin and Subcutaneous Tissue Disorders: rash, hyperhidrosis, acneiform dermatitis, erythema, fat atrophy, lipoatrophy, lipohypertrophy, night sweats, macular rash, maculo-papular rash, pruritic rash, xeroderma, prurigo, facial wasting.
Discontinuations: In the pooled analyses for studies P005, P018 and P019, the rates of discontinuation of therapy due to adverse experiences were 2.6% in patients receiving ISENTRESS + OBT and 3.2% in patients receiving placebo + OBT.
Abnormal Hematologic and Clinical Chemistry Findings: The percentages of treatment experienced adult patients receiving either ISENTRESS 400 mg twice daily or placebo (both with OBT) in P005, P018 and P019 with selected Grades 2 to 4 laboratory abnormalities that represent a worsening from baseline are presented in Table 2.
Treatment-Naïve Adverse Experiences: The following safety assessment of ISENTRESS in treatment-naïve patients is based on the randomized double-blind active controlled study of treatment-naïve patients, STARTMRK (Protocol 021) with ISENTRESS 400 mg twice daily in combination with a fixed dose of emtricitabine 200 mg (+) tenofovir 245 mg, (N=281) versus efavirenz (EFV) 600 mg at bedtime in combination with emtricitabine (+) tenofovir (N=282). During double-blind treatment, the total follow-up for patients receiving ISENTRESS 400 mg twice daily + emtricitabine (+) tenofovir was 392 patient-years and 371 patient-years for patients receiving efavirenz 600 mg at bedtime + emtricitabine (+) tenofovir.

Numbers (%) of patients with adverse experiences and with drug-related adverse experiences in the group receiving ISENTRESS, were less frequent than in the group receiving efavirenz based on the nominal p-values (0.05 and <0.001 respectively).

The most commonly reported adverse experiences (>10% in either group), of all intensities and regardless of causality in patients treated with ISENTRESS + emtricitabine (+) tenofovir versus the patients treated with efavirenz + emtricitabine (+) tenofovir, were: diarrhea in 14.9% and 21.6%, nausea in 14.2% and 12.1%, headache in 21.7% and 24.1%, fatigue in 6.0% and 11.0%, influenza in 6.4% and 11.3%, nasopharyngitis in 14.2% and 11.7%, upper respiratory tract infection in 13.2% and 13.1%, dizziness in 8.5% and 36.9%, abnormal dreams in 7.5% and 13.1%, insomnia in 11.0% and 10.3%, cough in 11.0% and 8.5%, pyrexia in 10.3% and 9.6% and rash in 5.0% and 11.7% of patients, respectively.

The following clinical adverse experiences below are regardless of causality and were considered by investigators to be of mild, moderate or severe intensity.

Table 2: ISENTRESS

Selected Laboratory Abnormalities Reported in Treatment-Experienced Patients (≥2%)

Laboratory Parameter Preferred Term	Limit	Grade	Randomized Studies P005, P018 and P019: ISENTRESS 400 mg b.i.d. (N=507) (%)	Randomized Studies P005, P018 and P019: Placebo (N=282) (%)
Hematology Laboratory Test				
Absolute Neutrophil Count (10^9/L)	0.75–0.999	Grade 2	(3.7)	(7.1)
	0.50–0.749	Grade 3	(2.8)	(2.8)
Hemoglobin (mmol/L)	1.16–1.31	Grade 2	(1.0)	(2.5)
Platelet Count (10^9/L)	50–99.999	Grade 2	(4.1)	(5.7)
Blood Chemistry Test				
Fasting (non-random) Serum LDL-C (mmol/L)	4.13–4.90	Grade 2	(11.6)	(6.7)
	≥4.91	Grade 3	(6.2)	(4.7)
Fasting (non-random) Serum Cholesterol (mmol/L)	6.20–7.77	Grade 2	(19.6)	(15.6)
	>7.77	Grade 3	(9.7)	(5.1)
Fasting (non-random) Serum Triglyceride (mmol/L)	5.65–8.48	Grade 2	(7.3)	(9.8)
	8.49–13.56	Grade 3	(5.9)	(2.9)
	>13.56	Grade 4	(3.4)	(2.2)
Fasting (non-random) Serum Glucose Test (mmol/L)	6.95–13.88	Grade 2	(12.0)	(7.5)
Total Serum Bilirubin	1.6–2.5×ULN	Grade 2	(6.3)	(6.4)
	2.6–5.0×ULN	Grade 3	(3.6)	(3.5)
Serum Creatinine	1.4–1.8×ULN	Grade 2	(3.6)	(2.5)
Serum Aspartate Aminotransferase	2.6–5.0×ULN	Grade 2	(10.3)	(6.7)
	5.1–10.0×ULN	Grade 3	(3.7)	(2.5)
Serum Alanine Aminotransferase	2.6–5.0×ULN	Grade 2	(9.3)	(7.8)
	5.1–10.0×ULN	Grade 3	(3.6)	(1.8)
Serum Alkaline Phosphatase	2.6–5.0×ULN	Grade 2	(2.4)	(0.4)
Serum Pancreatic Amylase Test	2.1–5.0×ULN	Grade 3	(4.3)	(2.5)
Serum Lipase Test	1.6–3.0×ULN	Grade 2	(4.1)	(3.2)
Serum Creatine Kinase	6.0–9.9×ULN	Grade 2	(2.8)	(1.8)
	10.0–19.9×ULN	Grade 3	(3.7)	(2.8)
	≥20.0×ULN	Grade 4	(3.0)	(0.7)

Legend: ULN=Upper limit of normal range.

Clinical adverse events of mild, moderate or severe intensity occurring in ≥2% of treatment-naïve adult patients in either treatment group are presented in Table 3.

Less Common Clinical Trial Adverse Drug Reactions (<2%): Drug-related adverse reactions occurring in less than 2% of treatment-naïve patients (n=281) receiving ISENTRESS + emtricitabine (+) tenofovir and of moderate to severe intensity are listed below by system organ class:

Blood and Lymphatic System Disorders: lymph node pain, neutropenia, anemia.
Ear and Labyrinth Disorders: tinnitus, vertigo.
Gastrointestinal Disorders: diarrhea, abdominal pain, vomiting, abdominal pain upper.
General Disorders and Administration Site Conditions: fatigue, asthenia.
Immune System Disorders: immune reconstitution syndrome.
Infections and Infestations: herpes zoster, gastroenteritis, folliculitis.
Metabolism and Nutrition Disorders: anorexia, decreased appetite.
Musculoskeletal and Connective Tissue Disorders: arthritis, myalgia, muscle spasms, neck pain.
Nervous System Disorders: dizziness, hypersomnia, somnolence, memory impairment, aphasia, disturbance in attention, tremor.
Psychiatric Disorders: abnormal dreams, nightmare, anxiety, mental disorder, confusional state, stuttering.
Reproductive System and Breast Disorders: erectile dysfunction.
Renal and Urinary Disorders: nephrolithiasis.
Skin and Subcutaneous Tissue Disorders: acne, alopecia, skin lesion.

Discontinuations: In the study P021, the rate of discontinuation of therapy due to adverse reactions was 3.2% in patients receiving ISENTRESS + emtricitabine (+) tenofovir and 6.4% in patients receiving efavirenz + emtricitabine (+) tenofovir.

Serious Events: Drug Related: The following serious drug-related adverse reactions were reported in the clinical study, P021: anemia, nausea, immune reconstitution syndrome, accidental overdose, mental disorder, aphasia, disturbance in attention, dizziness, headache, tremor, stuttering.

Table 3: ISENTRESS

Percentage of Patients with Adverse Experience of All Intensities and Regardless of Causality Occurring in (≥2%) of Treatment-Naïve Adult Patients in Either Treatment Group

System Organ Class, Preferred Term, %	ISENTRESS 400 mg b.i.d (N=281) n	ISENTRESS 400 mg b.i.d (N=281) (%)	Efavirenz 600 mg q.h.s. (N=282) n	Efavirenz 600 mg q.h.s. (N=282) (%)
	Randomized Study Protocol 021			
Patients With One Or More Adverse Experiences	259	(99.2)	271	(96.1)
Patients With No Adverse Experience	22	(7.8)	11	(3.9)
Blood and Lymphatic System Disorders	16	(5.7)	6	(2.1)
Lymphadenopathy	7	(2.5)	4	(1.4)
Cardiac Disorders	13	(4.6)	10	(3.5)
Ear And Labyrinth Disorders	17	(6.0)	21	(7.4)
Vertigo	5	(1.8)	12	(4.3)
Eye Disorders	12	(4.3)	25	(8.9)
Conjunctivitis	6	(2.1)	8	(2.8)
Gastrointestinal Disorders	127	(45.2)	140	(49.6)
Abdominal Distension	4	(1.4)	6	(2.1)
Abdominal Pain	17	(6.0)	16	(5.7)
Abdominal Pain Upper	5	(1.8)	8	(2.8)
Diarrhoea	42	(14.9)	61	(21.6)
Dyspepsia	17	(6.0)	10	(3.5)
Flatulence	10	(3.6)	16	(5.7)
Gastritis	7	(2.5)	5	(1.8)
Gastrooesophageal Reflux Disease	7	(2.5)	3	(1.1)
Nausea	40	(14.2)	34	(12.1)
Vomiting	19	(6.8)	24	(8.5)
General Disorders and Administration Site Conditions	66	(23.5)	95	(33.7)
Asthenia	12	(4.3)	11	(3.9)
Chest Pain	4	(1.4)	7	(2.5)
Chills	5	(1.8)	7	(2.5)
Fatigue	17	(6.0)	33	(11.7)
Oedema Peripheral	2	(0.7)	6	(2.1)
Pain	10	(3.6)	5	(1.8)
Pyrexia	29	(10.3)	27	(9.6)
Hepatobiliary Disorders	6	(2.1)	1	(0.4)
Immune System Disorders	10	(3.6)	6	(2.1)
Infections And Infestations	180	(64.1)	191	(67.7)
Body Tinea	3	(1.1)	6	(2.1)
Bronchitis	13	(4.6)	21	(7.4)
Folliculitis	6	(2.1)	5	(1.8)
Gastroenteritis	7	(2.5)	12	(4.3)
Genital Herpes	9	(3.2)	10	(3.5)
Herpes Simplex	4	(1.4)	8	(2.8)
Herpes Zoster	11	(3.9)	11	(3.9)
Influenza	18	(6.4)	32	(11.3)

(cont'd)

Table 3: ISENTRESS *(cont'd)*

Percentage of Patients with Adverse Experience of All Intensities and Regardless of Causality Occurring in (≥2%) of Treatment-Naïve Adult Patients in Either Treatment Group

	Randomized Study Protocol 021			
	ISENTRESS 400 mg b.i.d (N=281)		Efavirenz 600 mg q.h.s. (N=282)	
System Organ Class, Preferred Term, %	n	(%)	n	(%)
Nasopharyngitis	40	(14.2)	33	(11.7)
Onychomycosis	3	(1.1)	6	(2.1)
Oral Candidiasis	6	(2.1)	3	(1.1)
Oral Herpes	4	(1.4)	6	(2.1)
Pharyngitis	13	(4.6)	18	(6.4)
Pneumonia	6	(2.1)	6	(2.1)
Rhinitis	2	(0.7)	6	(2.1)
Sinusitis	13	(4.6)	15	(5.3)
Syphilis	5	(1.8)	8	(2.8)
Upper Respiratory Tract Infection	37	(13.2)	37	(13.1)
Urinary Tract Infection	1	(0.4)	6	(2.1)
Injury, Poisoning And Procedural Complications	30	(10.7)	28	(9.9)
Investigations	7	(2.5)	17	(6.0)
Weight Decreased	2	(0.7)	6	(2.1)
Metabolism And Nutrition Disorders	23	(8.2)	28	(9.9)
Anorexia	9	(3.2)	11	(3.9)
Musculoskeletal And Connective Tissue Disorders	60	(21.4)	65	(23.0)
Arthralgia	19	(6.8)	15	(5.3)
Back Pain	15	(5.3)	17	(6.0)
Muscle Spasms	1	(0.4)	6	(2.1)
Musculoskeletal Pain	2	(0.7)	6	(2.1)
Myalgia	7	(2.5)	11	(3.9)
Neck Pain	6	(2.1)	2	(0.7)
Pain in Extremity	7	(2.5)	5	(1.8)
Neoplasms Benign, Malignant And Unspecified (Incl Cysts And Polyps)	8	(2.8)	15	(5.3)
Kaposi's Sarcoma AIDS Related	1	(0.4)	6	(2.1)
Skin Papilloma	5	(1.8)	6	(2.1)
Nervous System Disorders	97	(34.5)	167	(59.2)
Dizziness	24	(8.5)	104	(36.9)
Headache	61	(21.7)	68	(24.1)
Migraine	6	(2.1)	1	(0.4)
Paraesthesia	6	(2.1)	6	(2.1)
Somnolence	3	(1.1)	22	(7.8)
Psychiatric Disorders	76	(27.0)	101	(35.8)
Abnormal Dreams	21	(7.5)	37	(13.1)
Anxiety	11	(3.9)	12	(4.3)
Depression	12	(4.3)	17	(6.0)
Insomnia	31	(11.0)	29	(10.3)

(cont'd)

Table 3: ISENTRESS *(cont'd)*

Percentage of Patients with Adverse Experience of All Intensities and Regardless of Causality Occurring in (≥2%) of Treatment-Naïve Adult Patients in Either Treatment Group

	Randomized Study Protocol 021			
	ISENTRESS 400 mg b.i.d (N=281)		Efavirenz 600 mg q.h.s. (N=282)	
System Organ Class, Preferred Term, %	n	(%)	n	(%)
Nightmare	7	(2.5)	14	(5.0)
Renal And Urinary Disorders	11	(3.9)	11	(3.9)
Reproductive System And Breast Disorders	15	(5.3)	24	(8.5)
Respiratory, Thoracic And Mediastinal Disorders	76	(27.0)	62	(22.0)
Cough	31	(11.0)	24	(8.5)
Nasal Congestion	10	(3.6)	6	(2.1)
Pharyngolaryngeal Pain	17	(6.0)	10	(3.5)
Productive Cough	6	(2.1)	3	(1.1)
Rhinorrhoea	5	(1.8)	8	(2.8)
Sinus Congestion	4	(1.4)	6	(2.1)
Skin And Subcutaneous Tissue Disorders	75	(26.7)	108	(38.3)
Acne	10	(3.6)	5	(1.8)
Dermatitis	7	(2.5)	8	(2.8)
Dermatitis Allergic	1	(0.4)	6	(2.1)
Night Sweats	9	(3.2)	1	(0.4)
Pruritus	9	(3.2)	11	(3.9)
Rash	15	(5.3)	33	(11.7)
Rash Maculo-Papular	2	(0.7)	9	(3.2)
Rash Papular	4	(1.4)	6	(2.1)
Skin Lesion	7	(2.5)	3	(1.1)
Vascular Disorders	15	(5.3)	15	(5.3)
Hypertension	11	(3.9)	8	(2.8)

CNS Events: In treatment naïve patients (P021) central nervous system (CNS) adverse reactions, as measured by proportion of patients with 1 or more CNS symptoms (described below) were reported significantly less frequently in the group receiving ISENTRESS + emtricitabine (+) tenofovir as compared with the group receiving efavirenz + emtricitabine (+) tenofovir, p <0.001 and <0.001 for cumulative events through Weeks 8 and 48, respectively. In the group receiving ISENTRESS, the percentage of patients with 1 or more CNS symptoms was 20.3% compared to 52.1% in the group receiving efavirenz by Week 8, and 26.0% compared to 58.5% by Week 48. CNS adverse reactions for this analysis were dizziness, insomnia, concentration impaired, somnolence, depression, nightmare, confusional state, suicidal ideation, nervous system disorder, psychotic disorder, abnormal dreams, suicide attempt, acute psychosis, delirium, depressed level of consciousness, hallucination, auditory hallucination, completed suicide and major depression.

Abnormal Hematologic and Clinical Chemistry Findings: The percentages of treatment-naïve adult patients receiving either ISENTRESS 400 mg twice daily or efavirenz (both with emtricitabine (+) tenofovir) in P021 with selected Grades 2 to 4 laboratory abnormalities that represent a worsening from baseline are presented in Table 4.

Table 4: ISENTRESS

Selected Laboratory Abnormalities Reported in Treatment-Naïve Patients (≥2%)

			Randomized Study P021	
Laboratory Parameter Preferred Term	**Limit**	**Grade**	**ISENTRESS 400 mg b.i.d. (N=281) (%)**	**Efavirenz 600 mg q.h.s. (N=282) (%)**
Hematology Laboratory Test				
Absolute neutrophil count (10^9/L)	0.75–0.999	Grade 2	(3.2)	(3.5)
Blood Chemistry Test				
Fasting (non-random) serum LDL-C (mmol/L)	4.13–4.90	Grade 2	(6.4)	(10.7)
	≥4.91	Grade 3	(1.1)	(3.9)

(cont'd)

Table 4: ISENTRESS *(cont'd)*

Selected Laboratory Abnormalities Reported in Treatment-Naïve Patients (≥2%)

Laboratory Parameter Preferred Term	Limit	Grade	Randomized Study P021: ISENTRESS 400 mg b.i.d. (N=281) (%)	Randomized Study P021: Efavirenz 600 mg q.h.s. (N=282) (%)
Fasting (non-random) serum cholesterol (mmol/L)	6.20–7.77	Grade 2	(7.5)	(16.0)
	>7.77	Grade 3	(0.0)	(3.2)
Fasting (non-random) serum triglyceride (mmol/L)	5.65–8.48	Grade 2	(0.4)	(3.2)
Fasting (non-random) serum glucose test (mmol/L)	6.95–13.88	Grade 2	(2.8)	(3.5)
Total serum bilirubin	1.6–2.5×ULN	Grade 2	(3.6)	(0.4)
Serum aspartate aminotransferase	2.6–5.0×ULN	Grade 2	(3.9)	(5.7)
Serum alanine aminotransferase	2.6–5.0×ULN	Grade 2	(6.0)	(7.1)
Serum alkaline phosphatase (IU(alk phos)/L)	2.6–5.0×ULN	Grade 2	(1.4)	(2.8)

Legend: ULN=Upper limit of normal range.

Through 48 weeks of therapy, ISENTRESS demonstrated minimal effects on serum lipids with small increases in total and LDL cholesterol and a decrease in serum triglycerides. The group treated with efavirenz had a significantly higher mean change from baseline in total cholesterol, triglycerides, non-HDL-C, and LDL-C. Modest increases in HDL were observed in both groups, significantly higher for efavirenz.

Long Term Treatment-Naïve Data: The safety profile of ISENTRESS in a 96-week phase II dose-ranging double-blind study of treatment-naïve patients (P004) with ISENTRESS plus tenofovir (TDF) and lamivudine (3TC) (N=160) versus efavirenz (EFV) plus TDF and 3TC (N=38) was consistent with the phase III treatment naïve data (P021), with the exception of the following drug related adverse experiences of moderate to severe intensity reported in one or more patients with ISENTRESS in P004: oral lichen planus, depression, renal impairment, lichen planus and hypertension. In this study patients randomized to ISENTRESS received doses ranging from 100 mg to 600 mg twice daily for the first 48 weeks and subsequently all received 400 mg twice daily.

Selected Adverse Experiences: Additional Neoplasms, Benign, Malignant and Unspecified: Cancers were observed in treatment-experienced patients who initiated ISENTRESS or placebo, both with OBT and in treatment-naïve patients who initiated ISENTRESS or efavirenz, both with emtricitabine (+) tenofovir; several were recurrent. The types and rates of specific cancers were those expected in a highly immunodeficient population (many had CD4+ cell counts below 50 cells/mm³ and most had prior AIDS diagnoses). The risk of developing cancer in these studies was similar in the group receiving ISENTRESS and the group receiving the comparator.

Patients with Co-existing Conditions: Additional Musculoskeletal and Connective Tissue Disorders: Grade 2-4 creatine kinase laboratory abnormalities were observed in patients treated with ISENTRESS (see Table 2). Myopathy and rhabdomyolysis have been reported; however, the relationship of ISENTRESS to these events is not known. Use with caution in patients at increased risk of myopathy or rhabdomyolysis, such as patients receiving concomitant medications known to cause these conditions.

Patients Co-infected with Hepatitis B and/or Hepatitis C Virus: In Phase III studies, treatment-experienced patients (N=113/699 or 16.2%) and treatment-naïve patients (N=42/563 or 7.5%) with chronic (but not acute) active hepatitis B and/or hepatitis C co-infection were permitted to enroll provided that baseline liver function tests did not exceed 5 times the upper limit of normal (ULN). In general the safety profile of ISENTRESS in patients with hepatitis B and/or hepatitis C virus co-infection was similar to that in patients without hepatitis B and/or hepatitis C virus co-infection, although the rates of AST and ALT abnormalities were somewhat higher in the subgroup with hepatitis B and/or hepatitis C virus co-infection for both treatment groups. In treatment-experienced patients, Grade 2 or higher laboratory abnormalities that represent a worsening from baseline of AST, ALT or total bilirubin occurred in 26%, 27% and 12%, respectively, of co-infected patients treated with ISENTRESS as compared to 9%, 8% and 7% of all other patients treated with ISENTRESS. In treatment-naïve patients (P021), Grade 2 or higher laboratory abnormalities that represent a worsening from baseline of AST, ALT or total bilirubin occurred in 20%, 25% and 15%, respectively, of co-infected patients treated with ISENTRESS as compared to 5%, 7% and 3% of all other patients treated with ISENTRESS.

Post-Market Adverse Drug Reactions: The following additional adverse experiences have been reported in post-marketed experience without regard to causality:

Blood and Lymphatic System Disorders: thrombocytopenia.

Musculoskeletal and Connective Tissue Disorders: rhabdomyolysisp.

Psychiatric Disorders: depression (particularly in patients with a pre-existing history of psychiatric illness), including suicidal ideation and behaviors.

Skin and Subcutaneous Tissue Disorders: Stevens-Johnson syndrome.

DRUG INTERACTIONS: Overview: Raltegravir is not a substrate of cytochrome P450 (CYP) enzymes and does not inhibit (IC_{50}>100 μM) CYP1A2, CYP2B6, CYP2C8, CYP2C9, CYP2C19, CYP2D6 or CYP3A in vitro. Moreover, in vitro, raltegravir did not induce CYP3A4. A midazolam drug interaction study confirmed the low propensity of raltegravir to alter the pharmacokinetics of agents metabolized by CYP3A4 in vivo by demonstrating a lack of meaningful effect of raltegravir on the pharmacokinetics of midazolam, a sensitive CYP3A4 substrate.

Similarly, raltegravir is not an inhibitor (IC_{50}>50 μM) of the UDP-glucuronosyltransferases (UGT) tested (UGT1A1, UGT2B7), and raltegravir does not inhibit P-glycoprotein-mediated transport. Based on these data, ISENTRESS is not expected to affect the pharmacokinetics of drugs that are substrates of these enzymes or P-glycoprotein (e.g., protease inhibitors, NNRTIs, methadone, opioid analgesics, statins, azole antifungals, proton pump inhibitors and anti-erectile dysfunction agents).

Based on in vivo and in vitro studies, raltegravir is eliminated mainly by metabolism via a UGT1A1-mediated glucuronidation pathway.

Coadministration of ISENTRESS with drugs that are potent inducers of UGT1A1, such as rifampin (an inducer of numerous drug metabolizing enzymes), reduces plasma concentrations of ISENTRESS. Caution should be used when coadministering ISENTRESS with rifampin or other strong inducers of UGT1A1. (See Warnings and Precautions.) The impact of other potent inducers of drug metabolizing enzymes, such as phenytoin and phenobarbital, on UGT1A1 is unknown. Other less potent inducers (e.g., efavirenz, nevirapine, rifabutin, glucocorticoids, St. John's wort, pioglitazone) may be used with the recommended dose of ISENTRESS.

Coadministration of ISENTRESS with drugs that are known to be potent UGT1A1 inhibitors (e.g., atazanavir; see Table 5) increases plasma levels of ISENTRESS. However, the degree of increase is modest and combination therapy with these inhibitors was well tolerated in the clinical studies such that no dose adjustment is required.

Drug-Drug Interactions: Effect of Raltegravir on the Pharmacokinetics of Other Agents: In drug interaction studies, raltegravir did not have a clinically meaningful effect on the pharmacokinetics of the following: hormonal contraceptive, tenofovir, midazolam and lamivudine. In a multiple-dose drug interaction study, ethinyl estradiol and norelgestromin AUC values were 98% and 114%, respectively, when coadministered with raltegravir as compared to when administered without raltegravir. In a multiple-dose drug interaction study, tenofovir AUC and trough concentrations when coadministered with raltegravir were 90% and 87% of values obtained with tenofovir monotherapy. In another drug interaction study, midazolam AUC from coadministration was 92% of the value obtained with midazolam alone. In a Phase II study, lamivudine pharmacokinetics were similar in patients receiving combinations with raltegravir versus with efavirenz.

Effect of Other Agents on the Pharmacokinetics of Raltegravir: In drug interaction studies, atazanavir, efavirenz, ritonavir, tenofovir, and tipranavir/ritonavir did not have a clinically meaningful effect on the pharmacokinetics of raltegravir. Rifampin, which is a strong inducer of drug metabolizing enzymes, caused a decrease in trough levels of raltegravir. Drug interactions are further described in Table 5.

DOSAGE AND ADMINISTRATION:

Recommended Dose and Dosage Adjustment: For the treatment of adult patients with HIV-1 infection the dosage of ISENTRESS is 400 mg administered orally, twice daily with or without food. ISENTRESS is to be given in a combination regimen with other antiretroviral agents.

Hepatic/Biliary/Pancreatic: There were no clinically important pharmacokinetic differences between patients with moderate hepatic insufficiency and healthy subjects. No dosage adjustment is necessary for patients with mild to moderate hepatic insufficiency. The effect of severe hepatic insufficiency on the pharmacokinetics of raltegravir has not been studied.

Renal: There were no clinically important pharmacokinetic differences between patients with severe renal insufficiency and healthy subjects. No dosage adjustment is necessary.

OVERDOSAGE:

Activated charcoal may be administered to aid in the removal of unabsorbed drug. The extent to which ISENTRESS may be107 dialyzable is unknown.

No specific information is available on the treatment of overdosage with ISENTRESS. Doses as high as 1600 mg single dose and 800 mg b.i.d. multiple doses were studied in Phase I without evidence of toxicity. Occasional doses of 1800 mg per day were taken in Phase II/III studies without evidence of toxicity. Based upon available data, raltegravir appears to be well tolerated at doses up to 800 mg b.i.d. and when administered with drugs that increase exposure by 50-70% (such as tenofovir and atazanavir).

Table 5: ISENTRESS

Effect of Other Agents on the Pharmacokinetics of Raltegravir

Coadministered Drug	Coadministered Drug Dose/Schedule	Raltegravir Dose/ Schedule	Clinical Comment	Ratio (90% Confidence Interval) of Raltegravir Pharmacokinetic Parameters with/without Coadministered Drug; No Effect=1.00: n	C_{max}	AUC	C_{min}
Protease Inhibitors:							
atazanavir	400 mg daily	100 mg single dose	No dosage adjustment required	10	1.53 (1.11, 2.12)	1.72 (1.47, 2.02)	1.95 (1.30, 2.92)
atazanavir/ritonavir	300 mg/100 mg daily	400 mg twice daily	No dosage adjustment required	10	1.24 (0.87, 1.77)	1.41 (1.12, 1.78)	1.77 (1.39, 2.25)
ritonavir	100 mg twice daily	400 mg single dose	No dosage adjustment required	10	0.76 (0.55, 1.04)	0.84 (0.70, 1.01)	0.99 (0.70, 1.40)
tenofovir	300 mg daily	400 mg twice daily	No dosage adjustment required	9	1.64 (1.16, 2.32)	1.49 (1.15, 1.94)	1.03 (0.73, 1,45)
tipranavir/ritonavir	500 mg/200 mg twice daily	400 mg twice daily	No dosage adjustment required	15 (14 for C_{min})	0.82 (0.46, 1.46)	0.76 (0.49, 1.19)	0.45 (0.31, 0.66)
Non-Nucleoside Reverse Transcriptase Inhibitor: efavirenz	600 mg daily	400 mg single dose	No dosage adjustment required	9	0.64 (0.41, 0.98)	0.64 (0.52, 0.80)	0.79 (0.49, 1.28)
Antibacterial: rifampin	600 mg daily	400 mg single dose	Use with caution (see Warnings and Precautions).	9	0.62 (0.37, 1.04)	0.60 (0.39, 0.91)	0.39 (0.30, 0.51)
rifampin	600 mg daily	800 mg twice daily		14	1.62[a] (1.12, 2.33)	1.27[a] (0.94, 1.71)	0.47[a] (0.36, 0.61)

[a] Compared to 400 mg twice daily administered alone.

For management of a suspected drug overdose, contact your regional Poison Control Centre. See the *CPS* Directory section for a list of Poison Control Centres.

ACTION AND CLINICAL PHARMACOLOGY: Mechanism of Action: ISENTRESS contains raltegravir, a human immunodeficiency virus integrase strand transfer inhibitor. Raltegravir inhibits the catalytic activity of HIV integrase, an HIV-encoded enzyme that is required for viral replication. Inhibition of integrase prevents the covalent insertion, or integration, of the HIV genome into the host cell genome during the early phase of infection. HIV genomes that fail to integrate cannot direct the production of new infectious viral particles, so inhibiting integration prevents propagation of the viral infection. Raltegravir did not significantly inhibit human phosphoryltransferases including DNA polymerases α, β, and γ.

Pharmacodynamics: Microbiology: Raltegravir at concentrations of 31±20 nM resulted in 95% inhibition (IC_{95}) of viral spread (relative to an untreated virus-infected culture) in human T-lymphoid cell cultures infected with the cell-line adapted HIV-1 variant H9IIIB. In addition, raltegravir at concentrations of 6 to 50 nM resulted in 95% inhibition of viral spread in cultures of mitogen-activated human peripheral blood mononuclear cells infected with diverse, primary clinical isolates of HIV-1, including isolates from 5 non-B subtypes, and isolates resistant to reverse transcriptase inhibitors and protease inhibitors. In a single-cycle infection assay, raltegravir inhibited infection of 23 HIV isolates representing 5 non-B subtypes and 5 circulating recombinant forms with IC50 values ranging from 5 to 12 nM. Raltegravir also inhibited replication of an HIV-2 isolate when tested in CEM×174 cells (IC_{95}=6 nM). Additive to synergistic antiretroviral activity was observed when human T-lymphoid cells infected with the H9IIIB variant of HIV-1 were incubated with raltegravir in combination with nucleoside analog reverse transcriptase inhibitors (zidovudine, zalcitabine, stavudine, abacavir, tenofovir, didanosine, or lamivudine); non-nucleoside reverse transcriptase inhibitors (efavirenz, nevirapine, or delavirdine); protease inhibitors (indinavir, saquinavir, ritonavir, amprenavir, lopinavir, nelfinavir, or atazanavir); or the entry inhibitor enfuvirtide.

Drug Resistance: The mutations observed in HIV-1 integrase that contributed to raltegravir resistance (evolved either in vitro or in patients treated with raltegravir) generally included a substitution at either Q148 (changed to H, K, or R) or N155 (changed to H) plus one or more additional mutations (e.g., L74I/M, E92Q, E138A/K, G140A/S, or V151I). Amino acid substitution at Y143C/H/R is another pathway to raltegravir resistance.

Recombinant viruses containing a single primary mutation (Q148H, K or R, or N155H) displayed decreased replication capacity and reduced susceptibility to raltegravir in vitro. Secondary mutations further decreased susceptibility to raltegravir and sometimes acted as compensatory mutations for viral replication capacity.

Cardiac Electrophysiology: In a randomized, placebo-controlled, crossover study, 31 healthy subjects were administered a single oral supratherapeutic dose of raltegravir 1600 mg and placebo. There was no effect on the QTc interval. Peak raltegravir plasma concentrations were approximately 4-fold higher than the peak concentrations following a 400-mg dose.

Pharmacokinetics:

Table 6: ISENTRESS

Comparison of Raltegravir Plasma Pharmacokinetics in Healthy Adult Male and Female Subjects Administered Multiple Oral Doses of 400 mg Twice Daily Raltegravir in the Fasted State and After a Specified Meal

	AUC_{0-12h} (μM·h)[a]	C_{max} (μM)[a]	C_{12h} (nM)[a]	T_{max} (h)[b]
Fasted	10.0	2.71	110	3.0
Low-Fat Meal	5.38	1.31	94	3.0
Moderate-Fat Meal	11.3	2.85	182	4.0
High-Fat Meal	21.2	5.32	453	4.0

[a] Geometric mean.
[b] Median.

Absorption: Raltegravir is rapidly absorbed with a T_{max} of approximately 3 hours postdose in the fasted state. Raltegravir AUC and C_{max} increase dose proportionally over the dose range 100 mg to 1600 mg. Raltegravir C_{12h} increases dose proportionally over the dose range of 100 mg to 800 mg and increases slightly less than dose proportionally over the dose range 100 mg to 1600 mg. With twice-daily dosing, pharmacokinetic steady state is achieved rapidly, within approximately the first 2 days of dosing. There is little to no accumulation in AUC and C_{max} and evidence of slight accumulation in C_{12h}. The absolute bioavailability of raltegravir has not been established.

In patients on 400 mg twice daily monotherapy, raltegravir drug exposures were characterized by a geometric mean AUC_{0-12h} of 14.3 μM·h and C_{12h} of 142 nM.

Effect of Food on Oral Absorption: ISENTRESS may be administered with or without food. Raltegravir was administered without regard to food in the pivotal safety and efficacy studies in HIV-infected patients. The effect of consumption of low-, moderate- and high-fat meals on steady-state raltegravir pharmacokinetics was assessed in healthy volunteers. Administration of multiple doses of raltegravir following a moderate-fat meal did not affect raltegravir AUC to a clinically meaningful degree with an increase of 13% relative to fasting. Raltegravir $C_{12\,hr}$ was 66% higher and C_{max} was 5% higher following a moderate-fat meal compared to fasting. Administration of raltegravir following a high-fat meal increased AUC and C_{max} by approximately 2-fold and increased $C_{12\,hr}$ by 4.1-fold. Administration of raltegravir following a low-fat meal decreased AUC and C_{max} by 46% and 52%, respectively; $C_{12\,hr}$ was essentially unchanged. Food appears to increase pharmacokinetic variability relative to fasting.

Distribution: Raltegravir is approximately 83% bound to human plasma protein over the concentration range of 2 to 10 μM.

Metabolism and Excretion: The apparent terminal half-life of raltegravir is approximately 9 hours, with a shorter α-phase half-life (~1 hour) accounting for much of the AUC. Following administration of an oral dose of radiolabeled raltegravir, approximately 51 and 32% of the dose was excreted in feces and urine, respectively. In feces, only raltegravir was present, most of which is likely derived from hydrolysis of raltegravir-glucuronide secreted in bile as observed in preclinical species. Two components, namely raltegravir and raltegravir-glucuronide, were detected in urine and accounted for approximately 9 and 23% of the dose, respectively. The major circulating entity was raltegravir and represented approximately 70% of the total radioactivity; the remaining radioactivity in plasma was accounted for by raltegravir-glucuronide. Studies using isoform-selective chemical inhibitors and cDNA-expressed UGT show that UGT1A1 is the main enzyme responsible for the formation of raltegravir-glucuronide. Thus, the data indicate that the major mechanism of clearance of raltegravir in humans is UGT1A1-mediated glucuronidation.

Special Populations and Conditions: Pediatrics: The pharmacokinetics of raltegravir in pediatric patients has not been established.

Geriatrics: The effect of age on the pharmacokinetics of raltegravir was evaluated in the composite analysis and the population pharmacokinetic (PK) analysis. There was no clinically meaningful effect of age on raltegravir pharmacokinetics. No dosage adjustment is necessary.

Gender: A study of the pharmacokinetics of raltegravir was performed in young healthy males and females. Additionally, the effect of gender was evaluated in a composite analysis of pharmacokinetic data from 103 healthy subjects and 28 HIV patients receiving raltegravir monotherapy with fasted administration. The effect of gender was also evaluated in a population PK analysis of concentration data from 80 healthy subjects and HIV patients receiving raltegravir alone or in combination with other drugs and in fasted and fed conditions. There were no clinically important pharmacokinetic differences due to gender. No dosage adjustment is necessary.

Race: The effect of race on the pharmacokinetics of raltegravir was evaluated in the composite analysis. There was no clinically meaningful effect of race on raltegravir pharmacokinetics. No dosage adjustment is necessary.

Body Mass Index (BMI): The composite analysis assessed the effect of BMI on the pharmacokinetics of raltegravir. There was no clinically meaningful effect of BMI on raltegravir pharmacokinetics. Additionally, no clinically meaningful effect of body weight on raltegravir pharmacokinetics was identified in the population PK analysis. No dosage adjustment is necessary.

Hepatic Insufficiency: Raltegravir is eliminated primarily by glucuronidation in the liver. A study of the pharmacokinetics of raltegravir was performed in patients with moderate hepatic insufficiency. Additionally, hepatic insufficiency was evaluated in the composite pharmacokinetic analysis. There were no clinically important pharmacokinetic differences between patients with moderate hepatic insufficiency and healthy subjects. No dosage adjustment is necessary for patients with mild to moderate hepatic insufficiency. The effect of severe hepatic insufficiency on the pharmacokinetics of raltegravir has not been studied.

Renal Insufficiency: Renal clearance of unchanged drug is a minor pathway of elimination. A study of the pharmacokinetics of raltegravir was performed in patients with severe renal insufficiency. Additionally, renal insufficiency was evaluated in the composite pharmacokinetic analysis. There were no clinically important pharmacokinetic differences between patients with severe renal insufficiency and healthy subjects. No dosage adjustment is necessary. Because the extent to which ISENTRESS may be dialyzable is unknown, dosing before a dialysis session should be avoided.

Genetic Polymorphism: There is no evidence that common UGT1A1 polymorphisms alter raltegravir pharmacokinetics to a clinically meaningful extent. In a comparison of 30 subjects with *28/*28 genotype (associated with reduced activity of UGT1A1) to 27 subjects with wild-type genotype, the geometric mean ratio (90% CI) of AUC was 1.41 (0.96, 2.09).

STORAGE AND STABILITY: Store at room temperature (15-30°C).

INFORMATION FOR THE PATIENT: Published in e-CPS, available by subscription at www.e-cps.ca.

DOSAGE FORMS, COMPOSITION AND PACKAGING: Each pink, oval-shaped, film-coated tablet with 227 on one side, contains: 434.4 mg of raltegravir potassium (as salt), equivalent to 400 mg of raltegravir (free phenol). Nonmedicinal ingredients: calcium phosphate dibasic anhydrous, hypromellose 2208, lactose monohydrate, magnesium stearate, microcrystalline cellulose, poloxamer 407 (contains 0.01% butylated hydroxytoluene as antioxidant) and sodium stearyl fumarate; film coating contains: black iron oxide and red iron oxide, polyethylene glycol 3350, polyvinyl alcohol, talc and titanium dioxide. Unit-of-use bottles of 60.

(Shown in Product Identification Section)

Isoflurane, USP ℞

isoflurane

Inhalation Anesthetic

Abbott

SUPPLIED: Isoflurane contains no additives. Amber-colored bottles of 100 and 250 mL. Store between 15 to 25°C.

Isoniazid ℞

Antimycobacterial

CPhA Monograph

Date of Revision: March 2008

This monograph has been compiled by CPhA and reviewed by experts. It may contain information different from that found in Health Canada-approved Product Monographs. The reader is referred to the *CPS* Editorial Policy for more information.

SUMMARY PRODUCT INFORMATION:

Drug	Route of Administration	Dosage Form	Strength
Isoniazid	Oral	Syrup	10 mg/mL
		Tablet	100 mg, 300 mg
	IV[a]	Solution	100 mg/mL (10 mL vial)
Rifampin/Isoniazid/ Pyrazinamide	Oral	Tablet	120 mg/50 mg/300 mg

[a] Available through Health Canada's Special Access Programme.

INDICATIONS AND CLINICAL USE: Isoniazid, a first-line drug in the treatment of respiratory and nonrespiratory tuberculosis, is used in a regimen with other antituberculosis drugs. Isoniazid is used as monotherapy in the treatment of latent tuberculosis infection [*Canadian tuberculosis standards*. 6th ed. http://www.phac-aspc.gc.ca/tbpc-latb/pubs/pdf/tbstand07_e.pdf].

CONTRAINDICATIONS: Patients who develop severe hypersensitivity reactions to isoniazid, including isoniazid-induced hepatitis, drug fever, chills and arthritis; acute liver disease of any etiology.

WARNINGS AND PRECAUTIONS: Warnings: Severe and sometimes fatal hepatitis associated with isoniazid therapy may occur and may develop even after months of treatment. Baseline serum aminotransferases should be performed prior to initiation of isoniazid therapy. Serum AST levels become elevated in about 10 to 20% of patients, usually during the first few months of therapy, but this can occur at any time. Usually enzyme levels return to normal despite continuance of isoniazid treatment, but in some cases progressive liver dysfunction occurs. Estimated rate of clinical hepatitis in patients given isoniazid alone is approximately 0.6% [American Thoracic Society/Centers for Disease Control and Prevention/Infectious Diseases Society of America: treatment of tuberculosis. *Am J Respir Crit Care Med* 2003;167(4):603-62]. Clinical hepatitis is rare before age 20, and occurs in approximately 0.2% of 20- to 34-year-olds, 1.5% of 35- to 49-year-olds and 2% of 50- to 64-year olds with isoniazid monotherapy. The risk of developing clinical hepatitis is increased with pre-existing liver disease, previous exposure to hepatitis C, concurrent use of other hepatotoxic medications and excessive or chronic use of alcohol. Instruct patients to report immediately any symptoms of hepatitis, such as fatigue, weakness, malaise, anorexia, nausea or vomiting, dark urine or yellowing of the skin.

Routine monitoring of serum liver enzymes is not necessary except for patients with pre-existing liver disease, concomitant hepatotoxic drugs, history of alcohol abuse or prior INH hepatitis, or patients who are 35 years and older, pregnant or who are within 3 months postpartum. Serum aminotransferases should be measured monthly and when symptoms occur. Review signs and symptoms of liver disease, such as nausea, anorexia, dark urine or scleral icterus, with patients on isoniazid therapy. If AST exceeds 5 times the upper limit of normal or if symptoms of liver damage occur, an alternative agent should be used since continued use of isoniazid in these patients may cause fatal hepatitis. If isoniazid must be reinstituted, this should be done only after symptoms and laboratory abnormalities have cleared. Therapy should be reinitiated in very small and gradually increasing doses, and withdrawn immediately if there is any indication of recurrent liver involvement.

Precautions: Isoniazid may cause mild or severe hepatic dysfunction (see Warnings).

Hypersensitivity reactions, including rash, fever, lymphadenopathy or vasculitis have occurred rarely and usually develop within 3 to 7 weeks of starting therapy. If these signs or symptoms occur, isoniazid should be discontinued and reinstituted very gradually, if necessary, after the reaction resolves.

Optic neuritis is a rare complication. Periodic ophthalmoscopic examinations during isoniazid therapy are recommended when visual symptoms occur.

It is believed that isoniazid competes with pyridoxyl phosphate for the enzyme apotryptophanase which may lead to symptoms of pyridoxine (vitamin B_6) deficiency. Pyridoxine administration can prevent and reverse peripheral neuropathy complicating isoniazid use. Prophylactic pyridoxine administration (25 mg/day) should probably be given routinely to individuals predisposed to developing peripheral neuropathies secondary to isoniazid therapy (e.g., patients who are malnourished, pregnant, suffer from alcoholism, with diabetes, or are HIV-infected, or patients receiving higher doses of isoniazid).

Special Populations: Pregnant Women: Although safe use of isoniazid during pregnancy has not been definitely established, isoniazid has been used to treat clinical tuberculosis in pregnant women. The Canadian Thoracic Society, the American Thoracic Society (ATS), the US Centers for Disease Control and Prevention (CDC) and the Infectious Diseases Society of America (IDSA) consider isoniazid to be safe for use in pregnancy, but the risk of hepatitis may be increased in the peripartum. Prophylactic pyridoxine supplementation at a dose of 25 mg daily is recommended.

The Canadian Thoracic Society does not recommend the use of isoniazid as treatment of latent tuberculosis infection during pregnancy, assuming active tuberculosis disease has been or other high risk medical conditions such as HIV infection have been excluded; however, treatment with isoniazid for latent tuberculosis infection may be reconsidered after delivery [*Canadian tuberculosis standards*. 6th ed. http://www.phac-aspc.gc.ca/tbpc-latb/pubs/pdf/tbstand07_e.pdf].

Nursing Women: No adverse effects have been reported, but there is a potential risk of peripheral neuritis or hepatic damage. Breastfed infants should be carefully observed for evidence of adverse effects. Isoniazid is considered compatible with breastfeeding according to the American Academy of Pediatrics.

ADVERSE REACTIONS: Toxic effects are usually encountered only with higher doses of isoniazid, and their incidence is reportedly higher in slow inactivators. The incidence of adverse effects at a dose of 10 mg/kg has been reported to be approximately 15%.

Gastrointestinal: nausea, vomiting, epigastric distress. Liquid preparations of isoniazid containing sorbitol may be associated with diarrhea.

Hematologic: agranulocytosis, hemolytic, sideroblastic or aplastic anemia; thrombocytopenia; eosinophilia.

Hepatic: elevated serum aminotransferases (ALT, AST) and bilirubin concentrations (in 10 to 20% of patients), hepatitis with or without jaundice. Isoniazid-associated hepatotoxicity (sometimes severe and/or fatal) is generally considered to be an unpredictable hypersensitivity reaction (see Warnings). Risk of isoniazid accumulation and isoniazid-induced hepatitis may be increased in the presence of hepatic disease. Isoniazid may be used in patients with stable disease. Monitor serum aminotransferases and signs and symptoms of clinical hepatitis frequently, if isoniazid is used. Consult an expert.

Hypersensitivity (rare): fever, skin eruptions (morbilliform, maculopapular, purpuric, or exfoliative), Stevens-Johnson syndrome, lymphadenopathy, vasculitis, hemolytic anemia, neutropenia. Hypersensitivity reactions usually occur in the first 3 to 7 weeks of therapy (see Precautions).

Metabolic and Endocrine: pyridoxine deficiency, pellagra, hyperglycemia, metabolic acidosis, gynecomastia.

Nervous System: Peripheral neuropathy is dose related and is most common in persons with nutritional deficiency, diabetes, HIV infection, renal failure, alcoholism and also pregnant and breastfeeding women. Recommend pyridoxine supplementation, 25 mg/day, for prevention of peripheral neuropathy.

Convulsions, toxic encephalopathy, optic neuritis and atrophy, and toxic psychosis may occur rarely. Other CNS effects include dysarthria, irritability, seizures, dysphoria or inability to concentrate.

Miscellaneous: rheumatic syndrome and systemic lupus erythematosus-like syndrome.

Approximately 20% of patients treated with isoniazid develop anti-nuclear antibodies. Approximately <1% develop clinical lupus erythematosus; discontinue isoniazid [American Thoracic Society/Centers for Disease Control and Prevention/Infectious Diseases Society of America: treatment of tuberculosis.*Am J Respir Crit Care Med* 2003;167(4):603-62].

Monitor for signs and symptoms of immune reconstitution inflammatory syndrome (fever, malaise, local reactions in organs) during tuberculosis therapy after initiation of antiretroviral therapy in patients co-infected with HIV. [*Canadian tuberculosis standards.* 6th ed. http://www.phac-aspc.gc.ca/tbpc-latb/pubs/pdf/tbstand07_e.pdf].

DRUG INTERACTIONS: Because the chemotherapy of tuberculosis involves the use of at least 2 drugs, the possible adverse reactions of each drug should be borne in mind as well as the potential for drug interactions.

Isoniazid is an inhibitor of cytochrome P450 isoenzymes CYP1A2, CYP2C19 (major) and CYP3A4 (major) and can decrease the metabolism of substrates of these isoenzymes, possibly increasing their serum concentrations and potential toxicity. Isoniazid can also induce CYP2E1. "Tyramine poisoning" is rare but has been reported to occur after ingestion of foods and beverages with high monoamine content. Isoniazid may inhibit plasma monoamine oxidase and diamine oxidase. If flushing occurs, instruct patients to avoid foods and drinks, e.g., certain cheeses (e.g., Swiss), wine.

Alcohol: Concomitant use increases risk of isoniazid-induced hepatotoxicity. Isoniazid metabolism may be increased. Avoid combination.

Aluminum hydroxide gel: Decreases gastrointestinal absorption of isoniazid. Administer isoniazid at least 1 hour before the antacid.

Carbamazepine: Concomitant administration with isoniazid may increase serum carbamazepine concentrations. Monitor serum carbamazepine concentrations and adjust carbamazepine dose if necessary. Monitor for signs and symptoms of carbamazepine toxicity, e.g., ataxia, nausea, vomiting.

Cycloserine: Monitor for CNS side effects such as dizziness or drowsiness when isoniazid and cycloserine are used in combination.

Phenytoin: Concomitant administration with isoniazid may increase serum phenytoin concentrations. Monitor serum phenytoin concentrations and adjust phenytoin dose if necessary. Monitor for signs and symptoms of phenytoin toxicity, e.g., ataxia, nausea, vomiting, nystagmus.

Rifampin: Hepatotoxicity has been reported to occur more frequently when rifampin and isoniazid are given concurrently. The incidence may be higher in slow isoniazid inactivators, those receiving high doses of isoniazid or those with pre-existing liver disease. Monitor for signs and symptoms of hepatitis, e.g., fatigue, weakness, malaise, anorexia.

Theophyllines: Isoniazid inhibits theophylline metabolism. Monitor for signs and symptoms of theophylline toxicity, e.g., nausea, vomiting, diarrhea, arrhythmia, hypotension.

Warfarin: Isoniazid may inhibit the hepatic metabolism of warfarin. Monitor for increases in INR when isoniazid and warfarin are used in combination.

DOSAGE AND ADMINISTRATION: Absorption after oral administration is optimal if taken on an empty stomach but it may be taken with food if gastrointestinal irritation occurs. Once-weekly isoniazid should not be used in treating HIV-infected individuals with active TB disease.

Treatment of Active Tuberculosis Disease: Treatment consists of 2 phases: (1) intensive phase, where medications are given daily to kill rapidly dividing populations of *M. tuberculosis* and to prevent drug resistance and (2) continuation phase, which targets less metabolically active and intermittently dividing organisms. During the continuation phase, medications may be given daily or 2 or 3 times weekly. The duration of each phase varies depending on the other drugs used.

When intermittent (2 or 3 times weekly) regimens are used, drug administration should be directly observed.

In conjunction with other antituberculosis agents, the adult dose is 300 mg daily. When intermittent therapy regimens are used, the adult dose of isoniazid is 900 mg twice weekly or 600 mg three times weekly [*Canadian tuberculosis standards.* 6th ed. http://www.phac-aspc.gc.ca/tbpc-latb/pubs/pdf/tbstand07_e.pdf].

Children: 10 to 15 mg/kg once daily (maximum 300 mg once daily). Intermittent therapy in children: 20 to 30 mg/kg twice weekly (maximum 900 mg per dose).

Treatment of Latent Tuberculosis Infection: Isoniazid is used as monotherapy for treatment of latent tuberculosis infection, for a period of 9 months. Adults: 5 mg/kg once daily (maximum 300 mg once daily) for 9 months. Children: 10 to 15 mg/kg once daily (maximum 300 mg once daily) for 9 months.

For high-risk individuals who are likely to be noncompliant and whose isoniazid treatment needs to be directly observed, a dose of 15 mg/kg twice weekly (maximum 900 mg per dose), may be considered as an alternative to daily therapy. The comparable pediatric dose is 20 to 30 mg/kg (maximum 900 mg per dose), twice weekly.

Renal Impairment: No dose adjustment is necessary.

OVERDOSAGE:

Signs and Symptoms: Toxicity is unlikely to appear more than six hours after a single acute ingestion. Early signs of acute isoniazid toxicity may include dizziness, vomiting, slurred speech and tachycardia. However, seizures may be the first symptom to appear. These may be preceded by hyperreflexia or areflexia. Seizures, coma and severe anion gap acidosis with a high serum lactate concentration are the three primary manifestations of acute isoniazid toxicity. Seizures may occur following a single dose of 20 mg/kg, and appear invariably with ingestions greater than 35 to 40 mg/kg. When acidosis is present, serum pH is generally in the range of 6.80 to 7.30. Coma may be prolonged for 24 to 36 hours and may persist even after seizure activity and acidosis are controlled. Other signs of acute isoniazid overdose include hyperglycemia, glycosuria, and ketonuria, renal failure, hypotension and hyperpyrexia.

Recommended Management: General management of isoniazid overdose includes supportive care with focus on supporting patient's cardiovascular status, protecting the airway, abolishing seizure activity and correcting metabolic acidosis. A single dose of activated charcoal should be considered at a dose of 1 g/kg. Pyridoxine iv should be administered to prevent neurotoxic effects. Dose of pyridoxine should be equal to the amount of isoniazid ingested. If the amount of isoniazid ingested is unknown, pyridoxine can be given empirically, in a dose of 5 g in adults or 70 mg/kg (maximum dose 5 g) in children, at a rate of 1 g every 2-3 minutes. If seizures are not terminated with this dose, doses may be repeated. The nasogastric route may be used to administer crushed tablets if iv pyridoxine is not available. Diazepam iv with addition of phenobarbital or propofol may be used in addition to pyridoxine to treat convulsions. Isoniazid may be removed by hemodialysis and/or peritoneal dialysis (isoniazid clearance is slower).

For management of a suspected drug overdose, CPhA recommends that you contact your **regional Poison Control Centre**. See the *CPS* Directory section for a list of Poison Control Centres.

ACTION AND CLINICAL PHARMACOLOGY: Isoniazid (INH) is a bactericidal agent active against organisms of the genus Mycobacterium, specifically *M. tuberculosis, M. bovis* and *M. kansasii*. It is a highly specific agent, ineffective against other microorganisms. The exact mechanism of action is unknown but the drug is firmly bound to actively growing, sensitive, tubercle bacilli and does not affect these organisms when they are in the metabolic resting state.

When used alone in the treatment of tuberculosis, resistant strains emerge very rapidly; when combined with other antituberculosis agents the emergence of resistant strains may be delayed or prevented. When isoniazid is used alone in the prophylaxis of tuberculosis, the development of resistance does not appear to be a major problem.

Pharmacokinetics: Following oral administration, isoniazid is rapidly and almost completely absorbed, and peak blood levels are reached in about 1 to 2 hours. Oral bioavailability is reduced when isoniazid is administered with food. It diffuses readily into all body fluids (including cerebrospinal, pleural, and ascitic), tissues, organs, and excreta (saliva, sputum and feces). Isoniazid cerebrospinal fluid concentrations are similar to plasma concentrations. The drug also passes through the placental barrier and into milk in concentrations comparable to those in the maternal plasma. Isoniazid is <10% bound to plasma proteins.

Isoniazid is metabolized by the liver mainly by acetylation and dehydrazination. The N-acetylhydrazine metabolite is believed to be responsible for the hepatotoxic effects seen in patients treated with isoniazid. The rate of acetylation is genetically determined. Approximately 50 to 60% of blacks and Caucasians are slow inactivators; 80% of native Alaskans and Asians are rapid inactivators. The half-life in fast acetylators is 1 to 2 hours while in slow acetylators it is 2 to 5 hours. Elimination is largely independent of renal function, however, the half-life may be prolonged in liver disease. The rate of acetylation has not been shown to significantly alter the effectiveness of isoniazid. However, slow acetylation may lead to higher blood concentrations during chronic administration of the drug, with an increased risk of toxicity. Isoniazid and its metabolites are excreted in the urine with 75 to 96% of the dose excreted in 24 hours. Small amounts are also excreted in saliva, sputum and feces. Isoniazid is removed by hemodialysis and peritoneal dialysis.

Isoproterenol HCl Injection USP ℞

isoproterenol HCl

Sympathomimetic

Sandoz

SUPPLIED: Each mL of sterile aqueous solution contains: isoproterenol hydrochloride 0.2 mg. Nonmedicinal ingredients: hydrochloric acid to adjust pH, lactic acid, sodium chloride for isotonicity, sodium lactate, sodium metabisulfite (as preservative) and water for injection. Ampoules of 1 and 5 mL, boxes of 10. Do not use solution if it is pinkish or darker than slightly yellow in colour or contains a precipitate. Store between 15 and 30°C. Protect from light. Discard unused portion.

The reader is invited to consult CPhA's monograph **Calcium Channel Blockers**.

Isoptin® SR ℞

verapamil HCl

Antihypertensive

Abbott

SUPPLIED: 120 mg: Each off-white, biconvex, round, film-coated tablet, with SR 120 embossed on one side, KNOLL on the other side, contains: verapamil HCl 120 mg. Nonmedicinal ingredients: hydroxypropyl methylcellulose, magnesium stearate, microcrystalline cellulose, polyethylene glycol, povidone, sodium alginate, talc, titanium dioxide and wax. Bottles of 100.

180 mg: Each light-pink, football-shaped, film-coated tablet with KNOLL on one side and SR, scored, 180 on the other, contains: verapamil HCl 180 mg. Nonmedicinal ingredients: hydroxypropyl methylcellulose, magnesium stearate, microcrystalline cellulose, polyethylene glycol, povidone, red iron oxide (hydrated ferric oxide), sodium alginate, talc, titanium dioxide and wax. Bottles of 100.

240 mg: Each light-green, scored, capsule-shaped, film-coated tablet, with 2 triangles embossed on one side, contains: verapamil HCl 240 mg. Nonmedicinal ingredients: hydroxypropyl methylcellulose, indigotine lake, magnesium stearate, microcrystalline cellulose, polyethylene glycol, povidone, quinoline yellow lake, sodium alginate, talc, titanium dioxide and wax. Bottles of 100 and 500.

(Shown in Product Identification Section)

Isopto® Atropine ℞

atropine sulfate

Mydriatic—Cycloplegic—Anticholinergic

Alcon

SUPPLIED: A sterile, buffered ophthalmic solution with 1% atropine sulfate. Preserved with benzalkonium chloride. Nonmedicinal ingredients: boric acid, hydrochloric acid, 0.5% hydroxylpropyl methylcellulose, purified water and sodium hydroxide. Drop-Tainer dispensers of 5 mL.

Isopto® Carbachol ℞

carbachol

Miotic—Cholinergic

Alcon

SUPPLIED: A sterile, buffered, isotonic solution with carbachol 1.5% or 3%. Preserved with benzalkonium chloride. Nonmedicinal ingredients: boric acid, hydrochloric acid, 1% hydroxypropyl methylcellulose, purified water, sodium borate, sodium chloride and sodium hydroxide. Drop-Tainer dispensers of 15 mL.

Isopto® Carpine ℞

pilocarpine HCl

Miotic—Cholinergic

Alcon

SUPPLIED: A sterile, buffered solution of pilocarpine HCl 1%, 2% or 4%. Preserved with benzalkonium chloride. Nonmedicinal ingredients: boric acid, citric acid, hydrochloric acid, 0.5% hydroxypropyl methylcellulose, purified water, sodium chloride, sodium citrate and sodium hydroxide. Drop-Tainer dispensers of 15 mL.

Isopto® Homatropine
homatropine HBr
Mydriatic—Cycloplegic—Anticholinergic

Alcon

SUPPLIED: A sterile, buffered solution of homatropine HBr 2% or 5%. Preservative: benzalkonium chloride (in 2%); benzethonium chloride (in 5%). Nonmedicinal ingredients: 0.5% hydroxypropyl methylcellulose, hydrochloric acid and/or sodium hydroxide, polysorbate 80, purified water and sodium chloride. Drop-Tainer dispensers of 15 mL.

Isosorbide Dinitrate

CPhA Monograph

see *Nitrates*

Isosorbide Mononitrate

CPhA Monograph

see *Nitrates*

Isotamine® Ⓟ
isoniazid
Tuberculosis Therapy

Valeant

PHARMACOLOGY: Isoniazid may be bacteriostatic or bactericidal in action, depending on the concentration of the drug attained at the site of infection and the susceptibility of the infecting organism. The exact mechanism of action of isoniazid has not been fully elucidated, but several mechanisms including interference with metabolism of bacterial proteins, nucleic acids, carbohydrates, and lipids have been proposed. One of the principal actions of the drug appears to be inhibition of mycolic acid synthesis in susceptible bacteria which results in loss of acid-fastness and disruption of the bacterial cell wall. Isoniazid is active against susceptible bacteria only when they are undergoing cell division. Susceptible bacteria may undergo 1 or 2 divisions before multiplication is arrested.

Spectrum: Isoniazid is a highly specific agent and is active only against organisms of the genus Mycobacterium. Isoniazid is active in vitro and in vivo against *M. tuberculosis*, *M. bovis*, and some strains of *M. kansasii*. In vitro, the minimum inhibitory concentration (MIC) for most susceptible mycobacteria is 0.02 to 0.2 µg/mL in Lowenstein-Jensen media.

Resistance: Natural and acquired resistance to isoniazid have been demonstrated in vitro and in vivo in strains of *M. tuberculosis*. In vitro, resistance to isoniazid develops in a stepwise manner. The mechanism of resistance may be related to failure of the drug to penetrate or be taken up by the resistant bacteria. Resistant strains of initially susceptible bacteria develop rapidly if isoniazid is used alone in the treatment of clinical tuberculosis; however, development of resistance does not appear to be a major problem when the drug is used alone in preventive therapy. When isoniazid is combined with other antituberculosis agents in the treatment of clinical tuberculosis, emergence of resistant strains may be delayed or prevented. There is no evidence of cross-resistance between isoniazid and other antituberculosis agents currently available.

Pharmacokinetics: Absorption: Isoniazid is readily absorbed from the gastrointestinal tract. When given with food, the extent of absorption and peak plasma concentrations of the drug may be reduced. Following oral application of the drug, peak plasma concentrations are attained within 1 to 2 hours. Plasma concentrations of the drug in rapid isoniazid inactivators are 20 to 50% of those in slow isoniazid inactivators.

Distribution: Isoniazid is distributed into all body tissues and fluids (including cerebrospinal fluid, pleural and ascitic fluids, skin, sputum, saliva, lungs, muscle, and caseous tissue). The drug concentrations found in the cerebrospinal fluid are reported to be 90 to 100% of concurrent plasma concentrations. Isoniazid is not substantially bound to plasma proteins (0 to 10%). Isoniazid readily crosses the placenta. Isoniazid is distributed into milk in concentrations approximately equal to maternal concentrations.

Biotransformation: Biotransformation of isoniazid occurs mainly in the liver. Isoniazid is acetylated by N-acetyl transferase to N-acetylisoniazid; it is biotransformed to isonicotinic acid and monoacetylhydrazine. Monoacetylhydrazine is associated with hepatotoxicity via formation of a reactive intermediate metabolite when N-hydroxylated by the cytochrome P-450 mixed oxidase system. The rate of acetylation is genetically determined; slow acetylators are characterized by a relative lack of hepatic N-acetyl transferase.

Half-life: Adults, including elderly patients: Fast acetylators: 0.5 to 1.6 hours. Slow acetylators: 2 to 5 hours. Acute and chronic liver disease: may be prolonged to 6.7 h vs 3.2 h in controls. Children (age 1.5 to 15 years): 2.3 to 4.9 hours. Neonates 7.8 and 19.8 hours found in 2 newborns who received isoniazid transplacentally. The long half-life may be due to the limited acetylation capacity of neonates.

Peak Serum Concentrations: 3 to 7 µg/mL after a single 300 mg oral dose.

Time to Peak Serum Concentrations: 1 to 2 hours.

Elimination: The plasma half-life of isoniazid in patients with normal renal and hepatic function ranges from 1 to 4 hours, depending on the rate of metabolism. In patients with severely impaired renal or hepatic function, the plasma half-life may be prolonged.

The rate of isoniazid acetylation does not appear to alter efficacy when the drug is administered daily or 2 or 3 times weekly; however, a relationship between rapid inactivation and poor therapeutic response has been noted in once-weekly intermittent regimens.

In adults with normal renal function, approximately 75 to 96% of a 5 mg/kg oral dose of isoniazid is excreted in urine within 24 hours as unchanged drug and metabolites. Small amounts of the drug are also excreted in saliva, sputum and feces. Isoniazid is removed by hemodialysis or peritoneal dialysis.

INDICATIONS: Treatment of Mycobacterial Infections: Isoniazid is used in conjunction with at least 1 other antituberculosis agent in the treatment of clinical tuberculosis. Isoniazid is also used in conjunction with other antituberculosis agents in the treatment of diseases caused by other mycobacteria.

Prevention of Tuberculosis: Household members and other close contacts of individuals with recently diagnosed clinical tuberculosis. Individuals with a significant reaction to the standard Mantoux tuberculin skin test and with findings on chest radiograph consistent with nonprogressive tuberculosis in whom there are neither positive bacteriologic findings nor a history of adequate chemotherapy. Newly infected individuals with a tuberculin skin test conversion within the last 2 years.

Individuals with a significant reaction to the standard Mantoux tuberculin skin test in special clinical situations, including those who are receiving prolonged corticosteroid or immunosuppressive therapy, have hematologic and reticuloendothelial diseases such as leukemia or Hodgkin's disease, or have diabetes mellitus, end-stage renal disease or silicosis. Individuals with clinical situations associated with substantial, rapid weight loss or chronic undernutrition, including intestinal bypass surgery for obesity, the postgastrectomy state, chronic peptic ulcer disease or malabsorption syndromes, or carcinomas of the oropharynx and upper gastrointestinal tract that prevent adequate nutrition, should also receive isoniazid preventive therapy if they have a significant reaction to the standard Mantoux tuberculin skin test.

Individuals with known or suspected human immunodeficiency virus infection.

Other individuals with a significant reaction to the standard Mantoux tuberculin skin test. Preventive therapy is indicated for individuals with a significant reaction who are younger than 35 years of age, even when none of the risk factors listed above is present.

CONTRAINDICATIONS: In patients with chronic or acute liver disease or a history of previous isoniazid-associated hepatic injury, and should be discontinued if serum aminotransferase concentrations are more than 3 times higher than the upper limit of the normal range.

Isoniazid is also contraindicated in patients with a history of severe adverse reactions to the drug, including severe hypersensitivity reactions or drug fever, chills, and arthritis.

WARNINGS: No data supplied by the manufacturer.

PRECAUTIONS: Liver function tests should be performed periodically in patients receiving isoniazid. In addition, patients should be questioned monthly for signs and symptoms of liver disease and should be instructed to report to their physician any of the prodromal symptoms of hepatitis (e.g., fatigue, weakness, malaise, nausea, vomiting, anorexia).

Isoniazid should be used with caution in daily users of alcohol and patients with chronic liver disease or severe renal impairment. Minor dosage adjustments may be necessary in patients with severe renal impairment.

Periodic ophthalmologic examinations should be performed in patients who develop visual symptoms while receiving the drug.

When isoniazid is used in patients who are malnourished or predisposed to neuropathy (e.g., diabetes, alcoholics), pyridoxine should generally be administered concomitantly.

Drug Interactions: The following drug interactions and/or related problems have been reported:

Note: Combinations containing any of the following medications, depending on the amount present, may also interact with this medication.

Acetaminophen: potential of increased hepatotoxicity and, possibly, nephrotoxicity.

Adrenocorticoids, glucocorticoids: increased hepatic metabolism and/or excretion of isoniazid, leading to decreased plasma concentrations and effectiveness of isoniazid, especially in rapid acetylators.

Alcohol: Concurrent daily intake of alcohol may result in increased incidence of isoniazid-induced hepatotoxicity and increased metabolism of isoniazid.

Alfentanil: Chronic preoperative or perioperative use of isoniazid, a hepatic enzyme inhibitor, may decrease the plasma clearance and prolong the duration of action of alfentanil.

Antacids: Antacids may delay and decrease absorption and serum concentrations of orally administered isoniazid.

Anticoagulants: may result in increased anticoagulant effect because of the inhibition of enzymatic metabolism of anticoagulants.

Benzodiazepines: Isoniazid may decrease the hepatic metabolism of benzodiazepines.

Carbamazepine: Serum carbamazepine levels and toxicity may be increased by isoniazid.

Cheese (Swiss, Cheshire) or Fish (tuna, skipjack Sardinella): redness or itching of skin, hot feeling, rapid or pounding heartbeat, sweating, chills or clammy feeling, headache, lightheadedness due to the inhibition of plasma monoamine oxidase and diamine oxidase by isoniazid.

Cycloserine: Increased incidence of CNS effects such as dizziness or drowsiness may occur.

ADVERSE EFFECTS: Nervous System Effects: Peripheral neuritis, usually preceded by paresthesia of the feet and hands, is the most common adverse effect of isoniazid and occurs most frequently in malnourished patients and those predisposed to neuritis (e.g., alcoholics, diabetics). Rarely, other nervous system side effects have also occurred including: seizures, toxic encephalopathy, muscle twitching, ataxia, stupor, tinnitus, euphoria, memory impairment, separation of ideas and reality, loss of self-control, dizziness, and toxic psychosis. Neurotoxic effects may be prevented or relieved by the administration of 10 to 50 mg of pyridoxine HCl daily during isoniazid therapy. In addition, optic neuritis and atrophy have been reported with isoniazid.

Hepatic Effects: Mild hepatic dysfunction (mild and transient increases in serum AST, ALT and bilirubin concentrations has occurred in approximately 10 to 20% of patients receiving isoniazid, usually during the first 4 to 6 months of therapy. In most cases, enzyme concentrations return to pretreatment values despite continuation of isoniazid, but progressive liver dysfunction, bilirubinuria, jaundice, and severe and sometimes fatal hepatitis have occurred rarely. If symptoms of hepatitis or signs suggestive of hepatic damage occur during isoniazid therapy, the drug should be discontinued promptly.

Sensitivity Reactions: Hypersensitivity reactions include fever, skin eruptions (morbilliform, maculopapular, purpuric, exfoliative), lymphadenopathy, vasculitis and, rarely, hypotension, usually 3 to 7 weeks following initiation of therapy. At the first sign of hypersensitivity reaction, all drugs should be discontinued. If isoniazid is reinstituted, the drug should be restarted in small and gradually increasing doses only after symptoms have cleared. If there is any indication of recurrence of hypersensitivity, isoniazid should be discontinued immediately.

Hematologic Effects: Adverse hematologic effects include agranulocytosis, eosinophilia, thrombocytopenia, methemoglobinemia, and hemolytic, sideroblastic, or aplastic anemia.

Other Adverse Effects: nausea, vomiting, epigastric distress, dryness of the mouth, pyridoxine deficiency, pellagra, hyperglycemia, metabolic acidosis, and urinary retention and gynecomastia in males. A systemic lupus erythematosus-like syndrome and a rheumatic syndrome with arthralgia have also occurred.

OVERDOSE:

Symptoms: Symptoms of overdosage usually occur within 30 minutes to 3 hours following ingestion of the drug. Overdosage of isoniazid has produced nausea, vomiting, dizziness, slurred speech, blurred vision, and visual hallucinations, including bright colors and strange designs. After marked overdosage, respiratory distress and CNS depression, progressing rapidly from stupor to coma, severe intractable seizures, metabolic acidosis, acetonuria, and hyperglycemia have occurred. If untreated or treated inadequately, isoniazid overdosage may be fatal. Isoniazid-induced seizures are thought to be associated with decreased g-aminobutyric acid (GABA) concentrations in the CNS, possibly resulting from inhibition by isoniazid of brain pyridoxal-5-phosphate activity.

Treatment: In the management of isoniazid overdosage, an airway should be secured and adequate respiratory exchange established immediately. Seizures may be controlled with i.v. administration of diazepam or short-acting barbiturates and a dosage of pyridoxine HCl equal to the amount of isoniazid ingested. Generally, 1 to 4 g of pyridoxine HCl is given i.v. followed by 1 g i.m. every 30 minutes until the entire dose has been given. If seizures are controlled and overdosage is recent, within the last 2 to 3 hours, the stomach should be emptied by gastric lavage. Blood gases, serum electrolytes, glucose, and BUN determinations should be performed. Blood should be typed and crossmatched in case hemodialysis is required. I.V. administration of sodium bicarbonate should be considered to control metabolic acidosis and repeated as needed; dosage should be adjusted on the basis of laboratory test results. Pyridoxine has also had a beneficial effect in correcting acidosis in some patients, possibly by controlling seizures and resulting lactic acidosis. Pyridoxine has been effective in treating isoniazid-induced seizures as well as other mental status changes associated with isoniazid overdosage. In several patients who remained comatose following initial treatment of seizures with diazepam and pyridoxine, administration of an additional 3 to 5 g dose of pyridoxine HCl after 36 to 42 hours of coma resulted in complete awakening within 30 minutes. The fact that administration of high doses of pyridoxine can result in adverse neurologic effects should be considered whenever the drug is used in the treatment of isoniazid-induced seizures and/or coma.

Forced osmotic diuresis should be initiated as soon as possible following isoniazid overdosage to increase renal clearance of the drug and should be continued several hours after clinical improvement to ensure complete clearance of the drug and prevent relapse. Fluid intake and output should be monitored. In severe cases, hemodialysis or, if hemodialysis is not available, peritoneal dialysis should be used in conjunction with forced diuresis. In addition, measures should be taken to protect against hypoxia, hypotension, and aspiration pneumonia.

> For management of a suspected drug overdose, CPhA recommends that you contact your **regional Poison Control Centre**. See the *CPS* Directory section for a list of Poison Control Centres.

DOSAGE: Isoniazid is usually administered orally. The drug may be given by i.m. injection when oral therapy is impossible. Oral and i.m. dosages of isoniazid are identical.

Treatment of Tuberculosis: In the treatment of clinical tuberculosis and other mycobacterial diseases, isoniazid should not be given alone. Therapy should be continued long enough to prevent relapse.

The usual adult dosage of isoniazid for the treatment of tuberculosis is 5 to 10 mg/kg body weight once daily up to a maximum of 300 mg daily.

Children and infants tolerate larger doses of isoniazid than do adults and may be given 10 to 20 mg/kg of body weight once daily, depending on the severity of the disease. The maximum dosage for children is 300 to 500 mg daily.

When isoniazid is used in combination with rifampin in children, limiting isoniazid dosage to 10 mg/kg and rifampin dosage to 15 mg/kg daily may minimize the risk of hepatotoxicity. When isoniazid is used in combination with other antituberculosis drugs and the drugs are administered twice weekly, the usual adult dosage is 15 mg/kg (up to 900 mg) twice weekly and the usual dosage for children is 20 to 40 mg/kg (up to 900 mg) twice weekly.

Prevention of Tuberculosis: For tuberculosis preventive therapy, isoniazid usually is given alone. Preventive therapy generally should be continued for 6 to 12 months. The **usual adult dosage** of isoniazid for preventive therapy is 300 mg once daily.

Children and infants receive for preventive therapy isoniazid in a dosage of 10 to 15 mg/kg (up to 300 mg) once daily.

SUPPLIED: Syrup: Each mL of strawberry-flavored syrup contains: isoniazid, USP 10 mg. Nonmedicinal ingredients: citric acid, glycerin, methylparaben, propylparaben, sodium citrate and flavor. Bottles of 500 mL.

When a dose less than or not a multiple of 5 mL is prescribed, the syrup may be diluted with water.

Syrup must not be used as diluent as isoniazid is unstable in the presence of sugars. When stored in filled unopened containers at a temperature not exceeding 25°C, the syrup is expected to retain its potency for 1 year. When dispensed, each container should be filled and the contents should represent not more than 1 month's supply.

Tablets: Each white, scored, compressed tablet, imprinted ICN I22, contains: isoniazid, USP 300 mg. Nonmedicinal ingredients: colloidal silicon dioxide, magnesium stearate and microcrystalline cellulose. Bottles of 100 and 1000. Store in well-closed, light-resistant containers at controlled room temperature (15 to 30°C).

Ixiaro®

Japanese encephalitis vaccine (inactivated, adsorbed)

Encephalitis Vaccine

Novartis Pharmaceuticals

Date of Preparation: September 15, 2009

SUMMARY PRODUCT INFORMATION:

Route of Administration	Dosage Form/ Strength	Clinically Relevant Nonmedicinal Ingredients
Intramuscular	0.5 mL suspension for injection containing 6 µg Protein and having a potency ≤460 ng ED_{50}	**Adjuvant:** Aluminium hydroxide **Phosphate Buffered Saline:** Sodium chloride, potassium dihydrogen phosphate, disodium hydrogen phosphate, water for injection For a complete listing see Dosage Forms, Composition and Packaging.

DESCRIPTION: IXIARO Japanese Encephalitis Virus, purified inactivated vaccine is a sterile, ready to use suspension for intramuscular use.

The vaccine is prepared by propagating Japanese encephalitis virus strain (SA_{14}-14-2) in Vero cells. The virus suspension is treated with protamine sulphate to remove contaminating DNA and proteins. The purified virus is then inactivated by treatment with formaldehyde, adjusted to a specified protein concentration and formulated by addition of aluminium hydroxide adjuvant. No preservatives or antibiotics are added to the formulation.

Each dose of vaccine contains 6 µg of purified, inactivated JE virus preparation and 0.1% aluminium hydroxide, hydrated corresponding to 0.25 mg Al/dose. The potency of the vaccine is measured as minimum amount of vaccine required to seroconvert 50 % of mice.

INDICATIONS AND CLINICAL USE: IXIARO is indicated for active immunization against Japanese encephalitis for persons 18 years of age and older.

IXIARO should be considered for use in individuals at risk of exposure through travel or in the course of their occupation.

Geriatrics (>65 years of age): Special studies in the geriatric population were not performed; however, IXIARO has been administered to 120 subjects ≥65 years of age. No overall differences in safety and efficacy were observed between these subjects.

Pediatrics (<18 years of age): IXIARO is not recommended for use in persons below 18 years of age due to limited data on safety and efficacy in this population.

CONTRAINDICATIONS:

- Patients who are hypersensitive to this drug or to any ingredient in the formulation or component of the container. For a complete listing, see Dosage Forms, Composition and Packaging.
- Individuals who show hypersensitivity reactions after receiving the first dose of the vaccine should not be given the second dose.
- As with other vaccines, vaccination with IXIARO must be postponed in persons with acute severe febrile conditions.

WARNINGS AND PRECAUTIONS: As with any other vaccine, vaccination with IXIARO may not result in protection in all cases. IXIARO will not protect against encephalitis caused by other micro-organisms.

> **Serious Warnings and Precautions**
>
> As with all injectable vaccines, appropriate medical treatment and supervision should always be available to treat rare cases of anaphylactic reactions following the administration of the vaccine.
> - IXIARO should under no circumstances be administered intravascularly.
> - Like other intramuscular injections, this vaccine should not be administered intramuscularly to persons with thrombocytopenia, haemophilia or other bleeding disorders.

Special Populations: Pregnant Women: It is not known whether IXIARO can cause harm to the foetus or the pregnant woman. The potential risk for humans is unknown.

IXIARO should be given to a pregnant woman only if the benefit outweighs the risks to mother and fetus.

Nursing Women: It is not known whether IXIARO is excreted in human milk. Therefore, caution should be exercised when IXIARO is administered to a nursing woman.

IXIARO should be given to a nursing woman only if the benefit outweighs the risks to mother and child.

Pediatrics (<18 years of age): IXIARO is not recommended for use in persons below 18 years of age due to a lack of data on safety and efficacy in this population.

Geriatrics (>65 years of age): Special studies in the geriatric population were not performed; however, IXIARO has been administered to 120 subjects ≥65 years of age. No overall differences in safety and efficacy were observed between these subjects.

Immunosuppressed Individuals: In patients receiving immunosuppressive therapy or patients with immunodeficiency an adequate immune response may be diminished.

Monitoring and Laboratory Tests: Not applicable.

ADVERSE REACTIONS: Adverse Drug Reaction Overview: Clinical Trial Adverse Drug Reactions: Because clinical trials are conducted under very specific conditions the adverse reaction rates observed in the clinical trials may not reflect the rates observed in practice and should not be compared to the rates in the clinical trials of another drug. Adverse drug reaction information from clinical trials is useful for identifying drug-related adverse events and for approximating rates.

Data sources: Pooled 6-month Safety Analysis which is a pooled analysis of Phase 3 studies. The treatment groups consisted of IXIARO, placebo, active comparator (JE-VAX) and another typical traveler's vaccine (HAVRIX). Healthy adults 18 years of age and older were included.

Non-study population: pregnant and nursing women, persons younger than 18 years, persons with any underlying disease.

Possibly or Probably Related Treatment-Emergent Adverse Events from Clinical Trials: The percentage of subjects with probably or possibly related TEAEs was similar for IXIARO and placebo during the 6 months after first vaccination (Table 1). This table displays all TEAEs in ≥1.0% of subjects.

Table 1: IXIARO

Possibly or Probably Related Treatment-Emergent Adverse Events, Occurring in ≥1% of Subjects Who Received IXIARO: Pooled 6-Month Safety Analysis

System Organ Class and Preferred Term	IXIARO N=3558		JE-VAX N=435		HAVRIX N=65		Placebo N=657	
	n	(%)	n	(%)	n	(%)	n	(%)
Nervous System Disorders								
Headache	684	19.2	79	18.2	6	9.2	132	20.1
General Disorders and Administration Site Conditions								

(cont'd)

Table 1: IXIARO *(cont'd)*

Possibly or Probably Related Treatment-Emergent Adverse Events, Occurring in ≥1% of Subjects Who Received IXIARO: Pooled 6-Month Safety Analysis

System Organ Class and Preferred Term	IXIARO N=3558		JE-VAX N=435		HAVRIX N=65		Placebo N=657	
	n	(%)	n	(%)	n	(%)	n	(%)
Fatigue	339	9.5	35	8.0	1	1.5	65	9.9
Influenza like illness	313	8.8	30	6.9	1	1.5	57	8.7
Pyrexia	76	2.1	10	2.3	0	0	15	2.3
Injection site pain[a]	1191	33.7	118	27.6	41	64.1	234	35.9
Injection site tenderness[b]	1080	34.2	153	35.8	35	54.7	212	32.5
Injection site erythema[a]	322	9.1	116	27.2	8	12.5	48	7.4
Injection site hardening[a]	282	8.0	74	17.3	15	23.4	48	7.4
Injection site swelling[a]	169	4.8	67	15.7	5	7.8	30	4.6
Injection site itching[a]	121	3.4	88	20.6	6	9.4	29	4.4
Musculoskeletal and Connective Tissue Disorders								
Myalgia	478	13.4	52	12.0	1	1.5	94	14.3
Gastrointestinal Disorders								
Nausea	162	4.6	26	6.0	0	0	37	5.6
Skin and Subcutaneous Tissue Disorders								
Rash	35	1.0	5	1.1	0	0	4	0.6

[a] For injection site pain, erythema, hardening, swelling and itching, subject number in the IXIARO group was 3532, in the JE-VAX group 427, in the HAVRIX group 64 and in the Placebo group 652.

[b] For injection site tenderness, subject number in the IXIARO group was 3158, in the JE-VAX group 427, in the HAVRIX group 64 and in the Placebo group 652.

Less Common Clinical Trial Adverse Drug Reactions (<1%) :

Table 2: IXIARO

Possibly or Probably Related Treatment-Emergent Adverse Events, Occurring in <1% of Subjects: Pooled 6-Month Safety Analysis

System Organ Class and Preferred Term	IC51 N=3558		JE-VAX N=435		HAVRIX N=65		Placebo N=657	
	n	(%)	n	(%)	n	(%)	n	(%)
Nervous System Disorders								
Dizziness	13	0.4	2	0.5	0	0	4	0.6
Migraine	11	0.3	1	0.2	0	0	0	0
Paraesthesia	2	0.1	0	0	0	0	1	0.2
General Disorders and Administration Site Conditions								
Injection site haemorrhage	12	0.3	0	0	1	1.5	0	0
Injection site bruising	7	0.2	3	0.7	0	0	1	0.2
Chills	5	0.1	0	0	0	0	3	0.5
Malaise	4	0.1	0	0	0	0	0	0
Oedema peripheral	1	0.0	0	0	0	0	0	0
Musculoskeletal and Connective Tissue Disorders								
Pain in extremity	3	0.1	1	0.2	0	0	2	0.3
Arthralgia	1	0.0	0	0	0	0	0	0
Gastrointestinal Disorders								
Vomiting	21	0.6	2	0.5	0	0	7	1.1
Diarrhea	19	0.5	3	0.7	0	0	4	0.6
Abdominal pain	4	0.1	0	0	0	0	1	0.2
Skin and Subcutaneous Tissue Disorders								
Pruritus	3	0.1	1	0.2	0	0	1	0.2

(cont'd)

Table 2: IXIARO *(cont'd)*

Possibly or Probably Related Treatment-Emergent Adverse Events, Occurring in <1% of Subjects: Pooled 6-Month Safety Analysis

System Organ Class and Preferred Term	IC51 N=3558		JE-VAX N=435		HAVRIX N=65		Placebo N=657	
	n	(%)	n	(%)	n	(%)	n	(%)
Erythema	2	0.1	1	0.2	0	0	0	0
Respiratory, Thoracic and Mediastinal Disorders								
Dyspnea	2	0.1	0	0	0	0	0	0
Investigations								
Hepatic enzyme increased	8	0.2	0	0	1	1.5	0	0
Blood and Lymphatic System Disorders								
Lymphadenitis	2	0.1	0	0	0	0	0	0
Thrombocytopenia	1	0.0	0	0	0	0	1	0.2
Ear and Labyrinth Disorders								
Vertigo	12	0.3	0	0	0	0	1	0.2
Cardiac Disorders								
Palpitations	2	0.1	0	0	0	0	0	0
Tachycardia	2	0.1	0	0	0	0	0	0

Serious Adverse Events: Summary of Serious Adverse Events reported in Clinical Trials: 72 serious adverse events were reported in 3945 subjects who received Ixiaro in completed clinical trials. Causality was assessed by investigator as not related or unlikely related in the SAEs summarized below (see list and Table 3).

Gastro-intestinal events (10 events; abdominal pain (2 events), acute abdomen, appendicitis (2 events), cholecystitis, diverticulitis, rectal hemorrhage, gastrointestinal infection, reflux oesophagitis); infections (11 events; abscess soft tissue (2 events), erysipelas, herpes zoster, peritonsillar abscess, pneumonia, pyelonephritis, respiratory tract infection, appendiceal abscess, tubo-ovarian abscess, tonsillitis); cancer (8 events; cancer of colon, pancreas, breast (2 events), lung, ovary, prostate, chondroma); accidents and surgical procedures (19 events); vascular or cardiac events (4 events; chest pain (2 events), intracranial aneurysm, myocardial infarction); genitourinary events (9 events; cervix disorder, ectopic pregnancy, nephrolithiasis, ovarian cyst ruptured (2 events), ovarian torsion, renal colic, urinary incontinence, vaginal cyst) and others (8 events; drug toxicity, musculoskeletal pain (2 events), bone marrow donation, retinal detachment, stillbirth, mediastinal mass, convulsion).

The following medically relevant serious adverse events were reported: See Table 3.

Table 3: IXIARO

Medically Relevant Serious Adverse Events Reported in Clinical Trials

Event	Interval to vaccination	Outcome	Causality Assessment by Investigator	Comment
CSF cell count increased[a]	40 days	No symptoms by time of last follow up	Unlikely related	Cause not established
Dermatomyositis	12 days	Ongoing by time of last follow up	Unlikely related	Pre-existing condition

[a] 2 events in 1 subject; initial symptom: ocular fixation difficulties.

In addition, two serious adverse events assessed as possibly related where reported. See Table 4.

Table 4: IXIARO

Serious Adverse Events Assessed as Possibly or Probably Related to Vaccination in or as Follow-up to Clinical Trials Completed and Ongoing to Date

Event	Interval to Vaccination	Outcome	Causality Assessment by Investigator
Syndactyly[a]	8.5 months[b]	not recovered	possibly related
Hypertension	12 days	recovered	possibly related

[a] Syndactyly of 2nd and 3rd toes, in infant of vaccinated subject.

[b] Delivery 8.5 months after vaccination. Estimated interval between last menstrual period and last IXIARO vaccination was 5 weeks.

Abnormal Hematologic and Clinical Chemistry Findings: There were no safety concerns with regard to haematological parameters, clinical chemistry or urinalysis across studies.

Uncommon: increased hepatic enzymes.

Post-Market Adverse Drug Reactions: The following adverse drug reactions have been reported from post marketing use: feeling hot, headache, injection site induration, mild encephalitis (see Table 5), neuritis (see Table 5 and summary information below), rash and pruritic rash, urticaria, vertigo, and vomiting. In all cases where outcome information was provided (8 of 12) patient had recovered or was recovering.

Table 5: IXIARO

Important Post-Market Drug Reactions

Most Important ADR (PT)	Interval to Vaccination	Further ADRs (PT)	Outcome (most important ADR)
Neuritis	Several hours	mononeuritis, paresis, neuralgia, arthralgia, myalgia, sensory disturbance, CSF cell count increased, paraesthesia, muscular weakness	recovering
Encephalitis	One day	headache, neck pain, diarrhea, pain in extremity, performance status decreased, pyrexia	recovered in 3 days

Neuritis: A 24 year old female experienced severe myalgia and arthralgia of both shoulder joints nine hours after vaccination; later paraesthesia and paresis of extremities occurred. She was hospitalized and diagnosed with neuritis; cerebral NMR was normal. By time of hospital discharge after two weeks she was recovering. Causality assessment by reporter: Unlikely as to vaccine, given the short interval between vaccination and event onset. Possible triggering by aluminum adjuvant was assumed.

DRUG INTERACTIONS: Overview: Not applicable.

Use with Other Vaccines: Concomitant administration of IXIARO with inactivated hepatitis A vaccine has been evaluated in one clinical study. There was no interference with the immune response to JEV and HAV vaccines, respectively. Concomitant administration of IXIARO and hepatitis A vaccine was shown to be non-inferior to single vaccinations with regard to geometric mean titres (GMT) of anti-JEV neutralizing antibody and HAV antibody, and for seroconversion rates.

There were no statistically significant higher rates in systemic or injection-site adverse reactions among subjects who received concomitant vaccination with IXIARO and hepatitis A vaccine compared with those who received IXIARO or hepatitis A vaccine alone.

The most frequently reported symptom on the day of the first vaccination in all three groups was injection site pain in 59.0% of subjects receiving IXIARO + HAVRIX, in 48.4% of subjects receiving IXIARO + placebo and in 48.4% of subjects receiving HAVRIX + placebo. The second frequent symptom was tenderness in 45.9%, 43.8% and 42.2% of subjects, respectively.

If co-administration with another vaccine is indicated, immunisation should be carried out on separate limbs.

Drug-Drug Interactions: Interactions with other drugs have not been established.

Drug-Food Interactions: Interactions with food have not been established.

Drug-Herb Interactions: Interactions with herbal products have not been established.

Drug-Laboratory Test Interactions: Interactions with laboratory tests have not been established.

Drug-Lifestyle Interactions: No studies on the effect of IXIARO on the ability to drive or use machines have been performed.

DOSAGE AND ADMINISTRATION: Dosing Considerations: Not applicable.

Recommended Dose and Dosage Adjustment: The primary vaccination series consists of two doses of 0.5 mL each according to the following schedule: First dose at Day 0. Second dose: 28 days after first dose.

A seroconversion rate of 29.4% has been observed 10 days after the first vaccination, and 97.3% one week after the second vaccination. Hence the primary immunization should be completed at least one week prior to potential exposure to Japanese encephalitis virus (JEV).

Missed Dose: If complete vaccination course of two injections is not finished full protection against the disease might not be achieved.

There is limited data from one trial that the second injection can be given up to 11 months after the first one. Seroconversion rate was 99.0% (99/100; GMT 504.3 [95% CI: 367.3, 692.3]) at 1 month after the second vaccination at Month 11 and was 88.5% (85/96; GMT 121.0 [95% CI: 87.4, 167.6]) by Month 24.

Booster Dose: There is limited data on the effect of a booster dose after completed primary immunization in subjects whose neutralizing antibody titre had dropped below the threshold for seroconversion (PRNT50≥1:10). In the per-protocol population, 16 subjects received a booster dose 11 months after the first dose, leading to a SCR of 100% [95%CI 80.6, 100.0] and a GMT of 676.2 [95%CI 365.0, 1252.5]. An additional 24 subjects received a booster dose 23 months after the first dose, resulting in a SCR of 100% [95%CI 86.2, 100.0] and a GMT of 2496.1 [95%CI 1407.5, 4426.7].

Administration: The vaccine should be administered by intramuscular injection into the deltoid muscle. It should never be injected intravascularly.

Exceptionally, IXIARO may also be administered subcutaneously to patients with thrombocytopenia or bleeding disorders since bleeding may occur following an intramuscular administration. Subcutaneous administration could lead to a suboptimal response to the vaccine. However, it should be noted that there are no clinical efficacy data to support administration by the subcutaneous route.

Each pre-filled syringe is for single use only and should not be used for more than one individual. Inject the entire contents of the syringe.

In the absence of compatibility studies, this vaccine must not be mixed with other medicinal products.

OVERDOSAGE:

No case of overdose has been reported.

> For management of a suspected drug overdose, CPhA recommends that you contact your **regional Poison Control Centre**. See the *CPS* Directory section for a list of Poison Control Centres.

ACTION AND CLINICAL PHARMACOLOGY: Disease Burden: Japanese Encephalitis is the one of the most common viral encephalitis with over 50 000 cases reported worldwide annually, although the figure could be much higher due to the lack of proper surveillance systems in many Asian countries where the virus is endemic. JEV is a mosquito-borne flavivirus; humans are an accidental host and are not considered reservoirs for virus transmission. The majority of infections in humans are asymptomatic, and overt encephalitis occurs in only one out of every 50 to 1000 individuals infected. JE disease has an associated mortality rate of 30-40%, and 50% of affected patients are left with permanent neuropsychiatric sequelae. Hence, although the relative mortality rate in a healthy population might be very low, due to the permanent neurological sequelae, the public health burden for the society is much higher.

Visitors to areas where JE is endemic or epidemic are at higher risk of being infected with JE compared to the local population. Incidence rates for JE disease in non-immunized Western troops have been observed to reach up to 2 per 10 000 individuals per week. Sporadic cases of JE disease in travellers from Europe and North America are reported every year.

Mechanism of Action: Studies in animals have shown that the vaccine triggers the immune system to produce antibodies against Japanese encephalitis virus that are most often protective. Challenge studies were performed in mice that were treated with human IXIARO antisera. These studies showed that almost all mice that had a Plaque Reduction Neutralization Test titre of at least 1:10 were protected from a lethal Japanese encephalitis virus challenge. These studies suggest that protection is mediated by antibodies raised against the vaccine.

Duration of Effect: Long-term immunogenicity to IXIARO was assessed in a subset of 181 subjects (ITT or intent to treat population). Immunogenicity data covering a period of 24 months after the first vaccination were as follows: See Table 6 and Table 7.

Table 6: IXIARO

Seroconversion Rates (SCR) and Geometric Mean Titres (GMT) at Month 2, 6, 12 and 24 After Vaccination with IXIARO (ITT population)—Results From a Pivotal Long-term Immunogenicity Study

Month		SCR ITT Population		GMT ITT Population	
		N=181 % (n)	95% Confidence Interval	N=181	95% Confidence Interval
2	Seroconverted	98.9 (179)	[96.1, 99.7]	310.8	[268.8, 359.4]
	Not seroconverted	0.6 (1)			
	Missing	0.6 (1)			
6	Seroconverted	95.0 (172)	[90.8, 97.4]	83.5	[70.9, 98.4]
	Not seroconverted	5.0 (9)			
12	Seroconverted	83.4 (151)	[77.3, 88.1]	41.2	[34.4, 49.3]
	Not seroconverted	16.6 (30)			

(cont'd)

Table 6: IXIARO *(cont'd)*

Seroconversion Rates (SCR) and Geometric Mean Titres (GMT) at Month 2, 6, 12 and 24 After Vaccination with IXIARO (ITT population)—Results From a Pivotal Long-term Immunogenicity Study

		SCR ITT Population		GMT ITT Population	
Month		**N=181 % (n)**	**95% Confidence Interval**	**N=181**	**95% Confidence Interval**
24	Seroconverted	81.8 (148)	[75.5, 86.7]	44.3	[36.7, 53.4]
	Not seroconverted	18.2 (33)			

The observed decline in GMT is as expected and compares well with data from other inactivated JE vaccines.

Table 7: IXIARO

Seroconversion Rates (SCR) and Geometric Mean Titres (GMT) at Month 2 and 6 After Vaccination with JE-VAX (ITT3 population)

		SCR ITT3 Population		GMT ITT3 Population	
Month		**N=82 % (n)**	**95% Confidence Interval**	**N=82 % (n)**	**95% Confidence Interval**
2	Seroconverted	80.0 (97.6)	[91.5, 99.3]	99.5	[76.9, 128.6]
	Not seroconverted	2 (2.4)			
	Missing	0 (0)			
6	Seroconverted	61 (74.4)	[64.0, 82.6]	34.1	[25.1, 46.4]
	Not seroconverted	21 (25.6)			

In another open-label, follow-up Phase 3 study, the persistence of immunogenicity up to 24 months after primary vaccination was assessed. The primary endpoint was the SCR at 24 months after the primary vaccination. A total of 118 subjects who had received the standard schedule of IXIARO were included in the follow-up study. SCRs and GMTs at Month 24 are summarized in Table 8 for the ITT population.

Table 8: IXIARO

Seroconversion Tates (SCR) and Geometric Mean Titres (GMT) at Month 6, 12 and 24 After Vaccination with IXIARO (ITT population)—Results From a Supportive Long Term Persistence Study

		SCR		GMT	
Month		**% (n/N)**	**95% Confidence Interval**	**GMT (n)**	**95% Confidence Interval**
6	Seroconverted	82.8 (96/116)	[74.9, 88.6]	46.6 (116)	[38.7, 56.1]
12	Seroconverted	58.3 (67/115)	[49.1, 66.9]	18.0 (115)	[15.5, 20.8]
24	Seroconverted	48.3 (56/116)	[39.4, 57.3]	16.2 (113)	[13.8, 19.0]

The full duration of protection for IXIARO is currently unknown and one study is ongoing to determine the duration of protection up to 5 years after vaccination. Generally, for inactivated JE vaccines, duration of protection has been derived from the percentage of subjects achieving a neutralizing antibody titre of at least 1:10, determined in a PRNT assay. This is also the cut-off used to determine seroconversion in all clinical studies with IXIARO, and has also been recognized by the WHO.

STORAGE AND STABILITY: Store in a refrigerator (2-8°C). Do not freeze.

Store in the original package to protect from light.

Do not use after the expiry date shown on the label.

SPECIAL HANDLING INSTRUCTIONS: Do not use if the blister foil is not intact or packaging is damaged. Upon storage, a fine white deposit with a clear colorless supernatant can be observed. Do not use if the product appears discolored (i.e. off-white) or if the syringe is damaged. The pre-filled syringe is ready to use. If a needle is not provided, use a sterile needle. Shake before use. Thorough agitation immediately before administration is necessary to maintain suspension of the vaccine. The full recommended dose of the vaccine should be used.

Prior to agitation, IXIARO may appear as a clear liquid with a white precipitate. After thorough agitation, it forms a white, cloudy liquid/suspension. The vaccine should be visually inspected for particulate matter and discoloration prior to administration. Discard the product if particulates are present or if it appears discolored or if the syringe appears to be physically damaged.

Any unused product or waste material should be disposed of in accordance with local requirements.

INFORMATION FOR THE PATIENT: Published in e-CPS, available by subscription at www.e-cps.ca.

DOSAGE FORMS, COMPOSITION AND PACKAGING: A single dose (0.5 mL of sterile suspension) contains: 6 µg (protein content) of inactivated Japanese encephalitis virus (attenuated strain SA14-14-2 produced in Vero cells) adsorbed on aluminum hydroxide, hydrated (0.25 mg Al/dose). Pre-filled syringes (Type I glass) of 0.5 mL with a plunger stopper (halobutyl elastomer). Pack size of 1 syringe with or without a separate needle.

J

Janumet™ Ⓟ

sitagliptin phosphate—metformin HCl

Oral Antihyperglycemic Agent—DPP-4 Inhibitor—Incretin Enhancer

Merck Frosst

Date of Preparation: September 23, 2009

SUMMARY PRODUCT INFORMATION:

Route of Administration	Dosage Form/ Strength	Clinically Relevant Nonmedicinal Ingredients
Oral	Tablet 50 mg/500 mg, 50 mg/850 mg, 50 mg/1000 mg	For a complete listing see Dosage Forms, Composition and Packaging.

INDICATIONS AND CLINICAL USE: JANUMET(sitagliptin/metformin) is indicated as an adjunct to diet and exercise to improve glycemic control in adult patients with type 2 diabetes mellitus inadequately controlled on metformin or in patients already being treated with the combination of sitagliptin and metformin.

Geriatrics (≥65 years of age): Because sitagliptin and metformin are substantially excreted by the kidney and because aging can be associated with reduced renal function, JANUMET should be used with caution as age increases. Care should be taken in dose selection and should be based on careful and regular monitoring of renal function (see Warnings and Precautions, Special Populations, Geriatrics (≥65 years of age)).

Pediatrics (<18 years of age): Safety and effectiveness of JANUMET in pediatric patients have not been established. Therefore, JANUMET should not be used in this population.

CONTRAINDICATIONS:

- Unstable and/or insulin-dependent (Type I) diabetes mellitus.
- Acute or chronic metabolic acidosis, including diabetic ketoacidosis, with or without coma, history of ketoacidosis with or without coma. Diabetic ketoacidosis should be treated with insulin.
- In patients with a history of lactic acidosis, irrespective of precipitating factors.
- In the presence of renal impairment or when renal function is not known, and also in patients with serum creatine levels above the upper limit of normal range. Renal disease or renal dysfunction, e.g., as suggested by serum creatinine levels ≥136 μmol/L [males], ≥124 μmol/L [females], or abnormal creatinine clearance (<60 mL/min), which may also result from conditions such as cardiovascular collapse (shock), acute myocardial infarction, and septicemia (see Warnings and Precautions).
- In excessive alcohol intake, acute or chronic.
- In patients suffering from severe hepatic dysfunction, since severe hepatic dysfunction has been associated with some cases of lactic acidosis, JANUMET should generally be avoided in patients with clinical or laboratory evidence of hepatic disease.
- In cases of cardiovascular collapse and in disease states associated with hypoxemia such as cardiorespiratory insufficiency, which are often associated with hyperlactacidemia.
- During stress conditions, such as severe infections, trauma or surgery and the recovery phase thereafter.
- In patients suffering from severe dehydration.
- Known hypersensitivity to sitagliptin, metformin or to any ingredient in the formulation (see Warnings and Precautions, Hypersensitivity Reactions and Adverse Reactions, Post-Market Adverse Drug Reactions). For a complete listing, see Dosage Forms, Composition and Packaging.
- During pregnancy and breastfeeding.

JANUMET should be temporarily discontinued in patients undergoing radiologic studies involving intravascular administration of iodinated contrast materials, because the use of such products may result in acute alteration of renal function (see Warnings and Precautions, General).

WARNINGS AND PRECAUTIONS:

> **Serious Warnings and Precautions**
> - Lactic acidosis is a rare, but serious, metabolic complication that can occur due to metformin accumulation during treatment with JANUMET (see Endocrine and Metabolism, Lactic Acidosis).
> - Patients should be cautioned against excessive alcohol intake, either acute or chronic, when taking JANUMET, since alcohol intake potentiates the effect of metformin on lactate metabolism (see Endocrine and Metabolism, Lactic Acidosis).

General: JANUMET should not be used in patients with type 1 diabetes or for the treatment of diabetic ketoacidosis.

Patient Selection and Follow-Up: Careful selection of patients is important. It is imperative that there be rigid attention to diet and careful adjustment of dosage. Regular thorough follow-up examinations are necessary.

If vomiting occurs, withdraw drug temporarily, exclude lactic acidosis, then resume dosage cautiously (see Adverse Reactions).

Particular attention should be paid to short range and long range complications which are peculiar to diabetes. Periodic cardiovascular, ophthalmic, hematological, hepatic and renal assessments are advisable.

Use of JANUMET must be considered as treatment in addition to proper dietary regimen and not as a substitute for diet.

Care should be taken to ensure that JANUMET is not given when a contraindication exists.

If during JANUMET therapy the patient develops acute intercurrent disease such as: clinically significant hepatic dysfunction, cardiovascular collapse, congestive heart failure, acute myocardial infarction, or other conditions complicated by hypoxemia, the drug should be discontinued.

Hypersensitivity Reactions: There have been post-marketing reports of serious hypersensitivity reactions in patients treated with sitagliptin, one of the components of JANUMET. These reactions include anaphylaxis, angioedema, and exfoliative skin conditions including Stevens-Johnson syndrome. Onset of these reactions occurred within the first 3 months after initiation of treatment with sitagliptin, with some reports occurring after the first dose. If a hypersensitivity reaction is suspected, discontinue JANUMET, assess for other potential causes for the event, and institute alternative treatment for diabetes (see Contraindications and Adverse Reactions, Post-Market Adverse Drug Reactions).

Cardiovascular: Sitagliptin: Congestive Heart Failure: A limited number of patients with congestive heart failure participated in clinical studies of sitagliptin. In studies of sitagliptin in combination with metformin, patients with congestive heart failure requiring pharmacological therapy or NYHA Class III or IV congestive heart failure were excluded. Patients with Classes I and II were included in small number. Use in this population is not recommended.

Metformin: Hypoxic States: Cardiovascular collapse (shock) from whatever cause, acute congestive heart failure, acute myocardial infarction and other conditions characterized by hypoxemia have been associated with lactic acidosis and may also cause prerenal azotemia. When such events occur in patients on JANUMET therapy, the drug should be promptly discontinued.

Endocrine and Metabolism: Metformin : Lactic Acidosis: Lactic acidosis is a rare, but serious, metabolic complication that can occur due to metformin accumulation during treatment with JANUMET; when it occurs, it is fatal in approximately 50% of cases. Lactic acidosis may also occur in association with a number of pathophysiologic conditions, including diabetes mellitus, and whenever there is significant tissue hypoperfusion and hypoxemia. Lactic acidosis is characterized by elevated blood lactate levels (>5 mmol/L), decreased blood pH, electrolyte disturbances with an increased anion gap, and an increased lactate/pyruvate ratio. When metformin is implicated as the cause of lactic acidosis, metformin plasma levels >5 μg/mL are generally found.

The reported incidence of lactic acidosis in patients receiving metformin hydrochloride is very low (approximately 0.03 cases/1000 patient-years, with approximately 0.015 fatal cases/1000 patient-years). Reported cases have occurred primarily in diabetic patients with significant renal insufficiency, including both intrinsic renal disease and renal hypoperfusion, often in the setting of multiple concomitant medical/surgical problems and multiple concomitant medications. Patients with congestive heart failure requiring pharmacologic management, in particular those with unstable or acute congestive heart failure who are at risk of hypoperfusion and hypoxemia, are at increased risk of lactic acidosis. In particular, treatment of the elderly should be accompanied by careful monitoring of renal function. Metformin treatment should not be initiated in patients ≥80 years of age unless measurement of creatinine clearance demonstrates that renal function is not reduced, as these patients are more susceptible to developing lactic acidosis. The risk of lactic acidosis increases with the degree of renal dysfunction and the patient's age. The risk of lactic acidosis may, therefore, be significantly decreased by regular monitoring of renal function in patients taking metformin and by use of the minimum effective dose of metformin.

In addition, metformin should be promptly withheld in the presence of any condition associated with hypoxemia, dehydration, or sepsis. Because impaired hepatic function may significantly limit the ability to clear lactate, metformin should generally be avoided in patients with clinical or laboratory evidence of hepatic disease.

Patients should be cautioned against excessive alcohol intake, either acute or chronic, when taking metformin, since alcohol potentiates the effects of metformin hydrochloride on lactate metabolism. In addition, metformin should be temporarily discontinued prior to any intravascular radiocontrast study and for any surgical procedure.

The onset of lactic acidosis often is subtle, and accompanied only by nonspecific symptoms such as malaise, myalgias, respiratory distress, increasing somnolence, and nonspecific abdominal distress. There may be associated hypothermia, hypotension, and resistant bradyarrhythmias with more marked acidosis. The patient and the patient's physician must be aware of the possible importance of such symptoms and the patient should be instructed to notify the physician immediately if they occur. Metformin should be withdrawn until the situation is clarified. Serum electrolytes, ketones, blood glucose, and if indicated, blood pH, lactate levels, and even blood metformin levels may be useful. Once a patient is stabilized on any dose level of metformin, gastrointestinal symptoms, which are common during initiation of therapy, are unlikely to be drug related. Later occurrence of gastrointestinal symptoms could be due to lactic acidosis or other serious disease.

Levels of fasting venous plasma lactate above the upper limit of normal but less than 5 mmol/L in patients taking metformin do not necessarily indicate impending lactic acidosis and may be explainable by other mechanisms, such as poorly controlled diabetes or obesity, vigorous physical activity, or technical problems in sample handling.

Lactic acidosis should be suspected in any diabetic patient with metabolic acidosis lacking evidence of ketoacidosis (ketonuria and ketonemia).

Lactic acidosis is a medical emergency that must be treated in a hospital setting. In a patient with lactic acidosis who is taking metformin, the drug should be discontinued immediately and general supportive measures promptly instituted. Because metformin hydrochloride is dialyzable (with a clearance of up to 170 mL/min under good hemodynamic conditions), prompt hemodialysis is recommended to correct the acidosis and remove the accumulated metformin. Such management often results in prompt reversal of symptoms and recovery (see Contraindications and Warnings and Precautions, Cardiovascular, Hepatic/Biliary/Pancreatic).

Physicians should instruct their patients to recognize the symptoms which could be a signal of the onset of lactic acidosis. If acidosis of any kind develops, JANUMET should be discontinued immediately.

Change in Clinical Status of Previously Controlled Diabetes Patients: A diabetic patient previously well controlled on JANUMET who develops laboratory abnormalities or clinical illness (especially vague and poorly defined illness) should be evaluated promptly for evidence of ketoacidosis or lactic acidosis. Evaluation should include serum electrolytes and ketones, blood glucose and, if indicated, blood pH, lactate, pyruvate and metformin levels. If acidosis of either form occurs, JANUMET must be stopped immediately and appropriate corrective measures initiated.

Loss of Control of Blood Glucose: When a patient stabilized on any diabetic regimen is exposed to stress such as fever, trauma, infection, or surgery, a temporary loss of glycemic control may occur. At such times, it may be necessary to withhold JANUMET and temporarily administer insulin. JANUMET may be reinstituted after the acute episode is resolved.

The effectiveness of oral antidiabetic drugs in lowering blood glucose to a targeted level decreases in many patients over a period of time. This phenomenon, which may be due to progression of the underlying disease or to diminished responsiveness to the drug, is known as secondary failure, to distinguish it from primary failure in which the drug is ineffective during initial therapy.

Should secondary failure occur with JANUMET, therapeutic alternatives should be considered.

Vitamin B_{12} Levels: Impairment of vitamin B_{12} absorption has been reported in some patients. Therefore, measurements of serum vitamin B_{12} are advisable at least every one to two years in patients on long-term treatment with JANUMET.

A decrease to subnormal levels of previously normal serum Vitamin B_{12} levels, without clinical manifestations, is observed in approximately 7% of patients receiving metformin in controlled clinical trials of 29 weeks duration. Such decrease, possibly due to interference with B_{12} absorption from the B_{12}-intrinsic factor complex, is, however, very rarely associated with anemia and appears to be rapidly reversible with discontinuation of metformin or Vitamin B_{12} supplementation. Measurement of hematologic parameters on an annual basis is advised in patients on JANUMET and any apparent abnormalities should be appropriately investigated and managed (see Warnings and Precautions, Monitoring and Laboratory Tests). Certain individuals (those with inadequate Vitamin B_{12} or calcium intake or absorption) appear to be predisposed to developing subnormal Vitamin B_{12} levels.

Hypoglycemia: Hypoglycemia does not occur in patients receiving metformin alone under usual circumstances of use, but could occur when caloric intake is deficient, when strenuous exercise is not compensated by caloric supplementation, or during concomitant use with other glucose-lowering agents (such as sulfonylureas and insulin) or ethanol. Elderly, debilitated, or malnourished patients, and those with adrenal or pituitary insufficiency or alcohol intoxication are particularly susceptible to hypoglycemic effects. Hypoglycemia may be difficult to recognize in the elderly, and in people who are taking β-adrenergic blocking drugs.

The patients should be warned about driving a vehicle or operating machinery under these conditions where risk of hypoglycemia is present.

Hepatic/Biliary/Pancreatic: Sitagliptin: There are limited clinical experiences in patients with moderate hepatic insufficiency and no clinical experience in patients with severe hepatic insufficiency. Use in patients with severe hepatic insufficiency is not recommended (see Action and Clinical Pharmacology, Pharmacokinetics).

Metformin: Since impaired hepatic function has been associated with some cases of lactic acidosis, JANUMET should generally be avoided in patients with clinical or laboratory evidence of hepatic disease.

Peri-Operative Considerations: Metformin: JANUMET therapy should be temporarily suspended for any surgical procedure (except minor procedures not associated with restricted intake of food and fluids). JANUMET should be discontinued 2 days before surgical intervention and should not be restarted until the patient's oral intake has resumed and renal function has been evaluated as normal.

Alcohol Intake: Alcohol is known to potentiate the effect of metformin on lactate metabolism. Patients, therefore, should be warned against excessive alcohol intake, acute or chronic, while receiving JANUMET.

Renal: Sitagliptin: Clinical study experience with sitagliptin in patients with moderate or severe renal insufficiency including those with ESRD is limited. Use in these patients is not recommended (see Action and Clinical Pharmacology, Special Populations and Conditions, Renal Insufficiency).

Metformin: Metformin is known to be substantially excreted by the kidney, and the risk of metformin accumulation and lactic acidosis increases with the degree of impairment of renal function. Thus, patients with serum creatinine levels above the upper limit of the normal range for their age should not receive JANUMET. In patients with advanced age, JANUMET should be carefully titrated to establish the minimum dose for adequate glycemic effect, because aging is associated with reduced renal function. In elderly patients, renal function should be monitored regularly.

Before initiation of JANUMET therapy and every 6 months while on JANUMET therapy, renal function should be assessed and verified as being within normal range.

In patients in whom development of renal dysfunction is anticipated, renal function should be assessed more frequently and JANUMET discontinued if evidence of renal impairment is present.

Special caution should be exercised in situations where renal function may become impaired, for example when initiating antihypertensive therapy or diuretic therapy and when starting therapy with an NSAID.

Use of Concomitant Medications That May Affect Renal Function or Metformin Disposition: Concomitant medication(s) that may affect renal function or result in significant hemodynamic change or may interfere with the disposition of metformin, such as cationic drugs that are eliminated by renal tubular secretion (see Drug-Drug Interactions), should be used with caution.

Radiologic Studies Involving the Use of Intravascular Iodinated Contrast Materials (for example, intravenous urogram, intravenous cholangiography, angiography, and computed tomography (CT) scans with intravascular contrast materials): Intravascular contrast studies with iodinated materials can lead to acute alteration of renal function and have been associated with lactic acidosis in patients receiving metformin (see Contraindications). Therefore, in patients in whom any such study is planned, JANUMET should be temporarily discontinued at the time of or prior to the procedure, and withheld for 48 hours subsequent to the procedure and reinstituted only after renal function has been re-evaluated and found to be normal.

Special Populations: Pregnant Women: There are no adequate and well-controlled studies in pregnant women with JANUMET or its individual components; therefore, the safety of JANUMET in pregnant women is not known. JANUMET is not recommended for use in pregnancy.

Because recent information suggests that abnormal blood glucose levels during pregnancy are associated with a higher incidence of congenital abnormalities, there is a consensus among experts that insulin be used during pregnancy to maintain blood glucose levels as close to normal as possible.

Nursing Women: No studies in lactating animals have been conducted with the combined components of JANUMET. In studies performed with the individual components, both sitagliptin and metformin are secreted in the milk of lactating rats. It is not known whether sitagliptin and/or metformin are excreted in human milk. Therefore, JANUMET should not be used by a woman who is nursing.

Pediatrics (<18 years of age): Safety and effectiveness of JANUMET in pediatric patients have not been established. Therefore, JANUMET should not be used in this population.

Geriatrics (≥65 years of age): Sitagliptin and Metformin: Because sitagliptin and metformin are substantially excreted by the kidney and because aging can be associated with reduced renal function, JANUMET should be used with caution as age increases. Care should be taken in dose selection and should be based on careful and regular monitoring of renal function (see Warnings and Precautions, Renal; Dosage and Administration, Geriatrics).

Sitagliptin: In clinical studies, no overall differences in safety or effectiveness were observed between subjects 65 years and over and younger subjects. While this and other reported clinical experience have not identified differences in responses between the geriatric and younger patients, greater sensitivity of some older individuals cannot be ruled out.

Metformin: Controlled clinical studies of metformin did not include sufficient numbers of elderly patients to determine whether they respond differently from younger patients, although other reported clinical experience has not identified differences in responses between the elderly and younger patients. Metformin is known to be substantially excreted by the kidney and because the risk of serious adverse reactions to the drug is greater in patients with impaired renal function, metformin should only be used in patients with normal renal function (see Contraindications). Because aging is associated with reduced renal function, metformin should be used with caution as age increases. Care should be taken in dose selection and should be based on careful and regular monitoring of renal function.

Monitoring and Laboratory Tests: Response to all diabetic therapies should be monitored by periodic measurements of blood glucose and HbA_{1c} levels, with a goal of decreasing these levels towards the normal range. HbA_{1c} is especially useful for evaluating long-term glycemic control.

Initial and periodic monitoring of hematologic parameters (e.g., hemoglobin/hematocrit and red blood cell indices) and renal function (serum creatinine) should be performed, at least on an annual basis. While megaloblastic anemia has rarely been seen with metformin therapy, if this is suspected, Vitamine B_{12} deficiency should be excluded.

Monitoring of Renal Function: Metformin and sitagliptin are known to be substantially excreted by the kidney. The risk of metformin accumulation and lactic acidosis increases with the degree of impairment of renal function. Thus, patients with serum creatinine levels above the upper limit of normal for their age should not receive JANUMET. In patients with advanced age, JANUMET should be carefully titrated to establish the minimum dose for adequate glycemic effect, because aging can be associated with reduced renal function. In elderly patients, particularly those ≥80 years of age, renal function should be monitored regularly.

Before initiation of therapy with JANUMET and at least annually thereafter, renal function should be assessed and verified as normal. In patients in whom development of renal dysfunction is anticipated, renal function should be assessed more frequently and JANUMET discontinued if evidence of renal impairment is present.

ADVERSE REACTIONS: Adverse Drug Reaction Overview: Sitagliptin: Sitagliptin was generally well tolerated in controlled clinical studies as a combination therapy with metformin, with the overall incidence of side effects similar to that reported with placebo.

The incidences of serious adverse experiences and discontinuation of therapy due to clinical adverse experiences were generally similar to placebo. The most frequent adverse reaction in trials of sitagliptin as add-on combination therapy with metformin (reported regardless of causality, and more common with sitagliptin than other treatments) was nasopharyngitis.

Metformin: The adverse events most commonly associated with metformin (sitagliptin/metformin) are diarrhea, nausea, and upset stomach. Lactic acidosis is a rare, but serious side effect. Lactic acidosis is fatal in approximately 50% of cases.

Lactic Acidosis: very rare (<1/10 000 and isolated reports) (see Warnings and Precautions and Overdosage).

Gastrointestinal Reactions: very common (>1/10). Gastrointestinal symptoms (diarrhea, nausea, vomiting, abdominal bloating, flatulence, and anorexia) are the most common reactions to metformin and are approximately 30% more frequent in patients on metformin monotherapy than in placebo-treated patients, particularly during initiation of metformin therapy. These symptoms are generally transient and resolve spontaneously during continued treatment. Occasionally, temporary dose reduction may be useful.

Because gastrointestinal symptoms during therapy initiation appear to be dose-related, they may be decreased by gradual dose escalation and by having patients take metformin (metformin HCl) with meals (see Dosage and Administration).

Because significant diarrhea and/or vomiting can cause dehydration and prerenal azotemia, metformin should be temporarily discontinued, under such circumstances.

For patients who have been stabilized on metformin, nonspecific gastrointestinal symptoms should not be attributed to therapy unless intercurrent illness or lactic acidosis have been excluded.

Special Senses: common (≥1/100). During initiation of metformin therapy complaints of taste disturbance are common, i.e. metallic taste.

Dermatologic Reactions: very rare (<1/10 000 and isolated reports). The incidence of rash/dermatitis in controlled clinical trials was comparable to placebo for metformin monotherapy and to sulfonylurea for metformin/sulfonylurea therapy. Reports of skin reactions such as erythema, pruritus, and urticaria are very rare.

Hematologic: During controlled clinical trials of 29 weeks duration, approximately 9% of patients on metformin monotherapy and 6% of patients on metformin/sulfonylurea therapy developed asymptomatic subnormal serum vitamin B_{12} levels; serum folic acid levels did not decrease significantly. However, only five cases of megaloblastic anemia have been reported with metformin administration (none during U.S. clinical studies) and no increased incidence of neuropathy has been observed (see Warnings and Precautions, Endocrine and Metabolism).

Decrease of vitamin B_{12} absorption with decrease of serum levels during long-term use of metformin is rare (≥1/10 000 and <1/1000). Consideration of such aetiology is recommended if a patient presents with megaloblastic anemia.

Hepatic: very rare (<1/10 000 and isolated reports). Liver function tests abnormalities or hepatitis resolving upon metformin discontinuation has been documented in isolated reports.

Clinical Trial Adverse Drug Reactions: Because clinical trials are conducted under very specific conditions the adverse reaction rates observed in the clinical trials may not reflect the rates observed in practice and should not be compared to the rates in the clinical trials of another drug. Adverse drug reaction information from clinical trials is useful for identifying drug-related adverse events and for approximating rates.

In a 24-week placebo-controlled clinical study of patients receiving sitagliptin (100 mg daily) as add-on combination therapy with metformin, the incidence of adverse reactions, reported regardless of causality assessment, in ≥1% of patients are shown in Table 1.

Table 1: JANUMET

Adverse Reactions ≥1% in Any Treatment Group (regardless of causality) Reported in Patients in a 24-Week Placebo-Controlled, Double-Blind Clinical Trial of Sitagliptin in Add-On Combination Use with Metformin

Body System/Organ Class Adverse Event	Number of Patients (%) Sitagliptin 100 mg + Metformin n=464	 Placebo + Metformin n=237
Ear and Labyrinth Disorders		
Vertigo	5 (1.1)	4 (1.7)
Eye Disorders		
Vision Blurred	1 (0.2)	3 (1.3)
Gastrointestinal Disorders		
Abdominal Pain	2 (0.4)	6 (2.5)
Abdominal Pain Upper	6 (1.3)	2 (0.8)
Constipation	5 (1.1)	1 (0.4)
Diarrhea	11 (2.4)	6 (2.5)
Nausea	6 (1.3)	2 (0.8)
Vomiting	5 (1.1)	2 (0.8)
General Disorders and Administration Site Conditions		
Fatigue	2 (0.4)	4 (1.7)
Edema Peripheral	4 (0.9)	3 (1.3)
Infections and Infestations		
Bronchitis	12 (2.6)	6 (2.5)
Bronchitis Acute	2 (0.4)	3 (1.3)
Gastroenteritis	4 (0.9)	5 (2.1)
Influenza	19 (4.1)	12 (5.1)
Nasopharyngitis	19 (4.1)	7 (3.0)
Pharyngitis	6 (1.3)	1 (0.4)
Pneumonia	5 (1.1)	0 (0.0)
Sinusitis	7 (1.5)	2 (0.8)
Tooth Infection	5 (1.1)	2 (0.8)
Upper Respiratory Tract Infection	34 (7.3)	22 (9.3)
Urinary Tract Infection	9 (1.9)	2 (0.8)
Injury, Poisoning and Procedural Complications		
Contusion	5 (1.1)	1 (0.4)
Investigations		
Blood Glucose Increased	3 (0.6)	6 (2.5)
Metabolism and Nutrition Disorders		
Hyperglycemia	2 (0.4)	7 (3.0)
Hypoglycemia	6 (1.3)	5 (2.1)
Musculoskeletal and Connective Tissue Disorders		
Arthralgia	14 (3.0)	1 (0.4)
Back Pain	15 (3.2)	6 (2.5)
Muscle Spasm	1 (0.2)	3 (1.3)
Myalgia	1 (0.2)	3 (1.3)
Pain in Extremity	5 (1.1)	4 (1.7)
Shoulder Pain	3 (0.6)	3 (1.3)
Nervous System Disorders		
Dizziness	7 (1.5)	2 (0.8)
Headache	12 (2.6)	7 (3.0)
Sciatica	1 (0.2)	3 (1.3)
Sinus Headache	0 (0.0)	3 (1.3)
Psychiatric Disorders		
Insomnia	5 (1.1)	3 (1.3)
Renal and Urinary Disorders		
Nephrolithiasis	3 (0.6)	3 (1.3)

(cont'd)

Table 1: JANUMET *(cont'd)*

Adverse Reactions ≥1% in Any Treatment Group (regardless of causality) Reported in Patients in a 24-Week Placebo-Controlled, Double-Blind Clinical Trial of Sitagliptin in Add-On Combination Use with Metformin

Body System/Organ Class Adverse Event	Number of Patients (%)	
	Sitagliptin 100 mg + Metformin n=464	Placebo + Metformin n=237
Respiratory, Thoracic and Mediastinal Disorders		
Cough	14 (3.0)	4 (1.7)
Vascular Disorders		
Hypertension	7 (1.5)	6 (2.5)

In a pre-specified analysis, the incidence of hypoglycemia in patients treated with sitagliptin plus metformin (1.3%) was similar to patients treated with placebo and metformin (2.1%). The incidence of selected gastrointestinal adverse experiences in patients treated with sitagliptin and metformin was also similar to placebo and metformin.

In pooled studies of up to one year duration which compared sitagliptin added to metformin or a sulfonylurea agent (glipizide) added to metformin, adverse reactions, reported regardless of causality assessment, in ≥1% of patients are shown in Table 2.

Table 2: JANUMET

Adverse Reactions ≥1% in Any Treatment Group (regardless of causality) Reported in Patients From Double-Blind Clinical Trials of Sitapliptin in Add-On Combination Use with Metformin in Studies up to One Year Compared to a Sulfonylurea Agent (glipizide)

Body System/Organ Class Adverse Event	Number of Patients (%)	
	Sitagliptin 100 mg + Metformin n=979	Glipizide + Metformin n=748
Gastrointestinal Disorders		
Abdominal Pain	10 (1.0)	6 (0.8)
Abdominal Pain Upper	13 (1.3)	7 (0.9)
Constipation	17 (1.7)	13 (1.7)
Diarrhea	42 (4.3)	36 (4.8)
Dyspepsia	14 (1.4)	12 (1.6)
Nausea	19 (1.9)	16 (2.1)
Toothache	2 (0.2)	13 (1.7)
Vomiting	11 (1.1)	9 (1.2)
General Disorders and Administration Site Conditions		
Fatigue	20 (2.0)	8 (1.1)
Non-Cardiac Chest Pain	10 (1.0)	6 (0.8)
Edema Peripheral	16 (1.6)	14 (1.9)
Infections and Infestations		
Bronchitis	27 (2.8)	22 (2.9)
Cellulitis	7 (0.7)	10 (1.3)
Gastroenteritis	19 (1.9)	13 (1.7)
Gastroenteritis Viral	8 (0.8)	9 (1.2)
Herpes Zoster	4 (0.4)	8 (1.1)
Influenza	35 (3.6)	32 (4.3)
Nasopharyngitis	75 (7.7)	49 (6.6)
Sinusitis	20 (2.0)	12 (1.6)
Upper Respiratory Tract Infection	78 (8.0)	70 (9.4)
Urinary Tract Infection	41 (4.2)	21 (2.8)
Investigations		
Blood Glucose Decreased	5 (0.5)	16 (2.1)
Blood Glucose Increased	13 (1.3)	5 (0.7)
Weight Increased	1 (0.1)	8 (1.1)
Metabolism and Nutrition Disorders		
Hyperglycemia	10 (1.0)	6 (0.8)
Hypoglycemia	32 (3.3)	217 (29.0)
Musculoskeletal and Connective Tissue Disorders		
Arthralgia	34 (3.5)	29 (3.9)

(cont'd)

Table 2: JANUMET *(cont'd)*

Adverse Reactions ≥1% in Any Treatment Group (regardless of causality) Reported in Patients From Double-Blind Clinical Trials of Sitapliptin in Add-On Combination Use with Metformin in Studies up to One Year Compared to a Sulfonylurea Agent (glipizide)

Body System/Organ Class Adverse Event	Number of Patients (%)	
	Sitagliptin 100 mg + Metformin n=979	Glipizide + Metformin n=748
Back Pain	39 (4.0)	32 (4.3)
Muscle Spasms	9 (0.9)	8 (1.1)
Neck Pain	4 (0.4)	8 (1.1)
Osteoarthritis	18 (1.8)	5 (0.7)
Pain in Extremity	23 (2.3)	9 (1.2)
Shoulder Pain	7 (0.7)	14 (1.9)
Nervous System Disorders		
Dizziness	26 (2.7)	14 (1.9)
Headache	34 (3.5)	31 (4.1)
Hypoaesthesia	3 (0.3)	11 (1.5)
Psychiatric Disorders		
Anxiety	13 (1.3)	7 (0.9)
Depression	10 (1.0)	7 (0.9)
Insomnia	12 (1.2)	11 (1.5)
Reproductive System and Breast Disorders		
Erectile Dysfunction	6 (0.6)	8 (1.1)
Respiratory, Thoracic and Mediastinal Disorders		
Cough	19 (1.9)	23 (3.1)
Pharyngolaryngeal Pain	10 (1.0)	9 (1.2)
Sinus Congestion	5 (0.5)	8 (1.1)
Eczema	4 (0.4)	12 (1.6)
Vascular Disorders		
Hypertension	33 (3.4)	29 (3.9)

Less Common Clinical Trial Adverse Drug Reactions ≥0.1% and <1% (drug-related and greater than placebo): Cardiac Disorders: bundle branch block.
Gastrointestinal Disorders: abdominal discomfort, abdominal pain upper, diarrhea, dyspepsia, flatulence, reflux esophagitis disease, retching.
General Disorders and Administration Site Conditions: face edema, malaise, peripheral edema, pain.
Hepatobiliary Disorders: hepatic steatosis.
Infections and Infestations: gastric ulcer helicobacter, helicobacter gastritis, upper respiratory tract infection.
Investigations: blood glucose decreased.
Metabolism and Nutrition Disorders: decreased appetite, hypoglycemia.
Musculoskeletal and Connective Tissue Disorders: muscle tightness.
Nervous System Disorders: migraine, neuropathy peripheral, parosmia, somnolence.
Reproductive System and Breast Disorders: dysmenorrhea, erectile dysfunction.
Respiratory, Thoracic and Mediastinal Disorders: cough.
Skin and Subcutaneous Tissue Disorders: exanthem, rash, urticaria.
Vascular Disorders: orthostatic hypotension.

Nausea was the only drug-related adverse reaction reported by the investigator that occurred with an incidence ≥1% in patients receiving sitagliptin (1.1%) and greater than in patients receiving placebo (0.4%).

Abnormal Hematologic and Clinical Chemistry Findings: Sitagliptin: The incidence of laboratory adverse experiences was similar in patients treated with sitagliptin 100 mg compared to patients treated with placebo. In most clinical studies, a slight decrease in alkaline phosphatase and small increases in uric acid and white blood cell count (due to an increase in neutrophils) were observed. In active comparator studies versus a sulfonylurea agent (glipizide) similar changes were seen in alkaline phosphatase and uric acid.

Mean Change from Baseline (standard error)

Study	Treatment Group	Alkaline Phosphatase (IU/L)	Uric Acid (mg/dL)	WBC (cell/µL)
Placebo-Controlled	Sitagliptin	−3.1 (0.4)	0.17 (0.04)	346.0 (64.3)
	Placebo	−1.3 (0.7)	0.05 (0.06)	142.4 (98.8)
Active-Controlled	Sitagliptin	−5.7 (0.5)	0.21 (0.05)	207.8 (67.4)
	Glipizide	−3.4 (0.5)	0.20 (0.05)	86.0 (62.5)

Metformin: In controlled clinical trials of metformin of 29 weeks duration, a decrease to subnormal levels of previously normal serum Vitamin B_{12} levels, without clinical manifestations, was observed in approximately 7% of patients. Such decrease, possibly due to interference with B_{12} absorption from the B_{12}-intrinsic factor complex, is, however, very rarely associated with anemia and appears to be rapidly reversible with discontinuation of metformin or Vitamin B_{12} supplementation (see Warnings and Precautions).

Post-Market Adverse Drug Reactions: The following additional adverse reactions have been identified during post-marketing use of JANUMET or sitagliptin, one of the components of JANUMET. Because these reactions are reported voluntarily from a population of uncertain size, it is generally not possible to reliably estimate their frequency or establish a causal relationship to drug exposure.

Hypersensitivity reactions include anaphylaxis, angioedema, rash, urticaria, cutaneous vasculitis and exfoliative skin conditions, including Stevens-Johnson syndrome (see Contraindications and Warnings and Precautions, Hypersensitivity Reactions); pancreatitis.

DRUG INTERACTIONS: Overview: Sitagliptin and Metformin: Co-administration of multiple doses of sitagliptin (50 mg) and metformin (1000 mg) given twice daily did not meaningfully alter the pharmacokinetics of either sitagliptin or metformin in patients with type 2 diabetes.

Pharmacokinetic drug interaction studies with JANUMET have not been performed; however, such studies have been conducted with the individual components of JANUMET (sitagliptin and metformin).

Sitagliptin: Sitagliptin is not an inhibitor of CYP isozymes CYP3A4, 2C8, 2C9, 2D6, 1A2, 2C19 or 2B6, and is not an inducer of CYP3A4. Sitagliptin is a p-glycoprotein substrate, but does not inhibit p-glycoprotein mediated transport of digoxin. Based on these results, sitagliptin is considered unlikely to cause interactions with other drugs that utilize these pathways.

Sitagliptin is not extensively bound to plasma proteins. Therefore, the propensity of sitagliptin to be involved in clinically meaningful drug-drug interactions mediated by plasma protein binding displacement is very low.

Metformin: The simultaneous administration JANUMET and a sulfonylurea could produce a hypoglycemic reaction, especially if they are given in patients already receiving other drugs which, themselves, can potentiate the effect of sulfonylureas. These drugs can be: long-acting sulfonamides, tubercolostatics, phenylbutazone, clofibrate, monoamine oxidase inhibitors, salicylates, probenecid and propanolol.

In healthy volunteers, the pharmacokinetics of propranolol and ibuprofen were not affected by metformin when co-administered in single-dose interaction studies. Metformin is negligibly bound to plasma proteins and is therefore, less likely to interact with highly protein-bound drugs such as salicylates, sulfonamides, chloramphenicol and probenecid.

Drug-Drug Interactions: Sitagliptin: In clinical studies, as described below, sitagliptin did not meaningfully alter the pharmacokinetics of metformin, glyburide, simvastatin, rosiglitazone, warfarin, or oral contraceptives, providing in vivo evidence of a low propensity for causing drug interactions with substrates of CYP3A4, CYP2C8, CYP2C9, and organic cationic transporter (OCT).

Metformin: Co-administration of multiple twice-daily doses of sitagliptin with metformin, an OCT substrate, did not meaningfully alter the pharmacokinetics of metformin or sitagliptin in patients with type 2 diabetes. Therefore, sitagliptin is not an inhibitor of OCT-mediated transport.

Sulfonylureas: Single-dose pharmacokinetics of glyburide, a CYP2C9 substrate, were not meaningfully altered in subjects receiving multiple doses of sitagliptin. Clinically meaningful interactions would not be expected with other sulfonylureas (e.g., glipizide, tolbutamide, and glimepiride) which, like glyburide, are primarily eliminated by CYP2C9. The effect of sulfonylureas on the pharmacokinetics of sitagliptin was not assessed.

Simvastatin: Single-dose pharmacokinetics of simvastatin, a CYP3A4 substrate, were not meaningfully altered in subjects receiving multiple daily doses of sitagliptin. Therefore, sitagliptin is not an inhibitor of CYP3A4-mediated metabolism.

Thiazolidinediones: Single-dose pharmacokinetics of rosiglitazone were not meaningfully altered in subjects receiving multiple daily doses of sitagliptin. Therefore, sitagliptin is not an inhibitor of CYP2C8-mediated metabolism. Clinically meaningful interactions with pioglitazone are not expected because pioglitazone predominantly undergoes CYP2C8- or CYP3A4-mediated metabolism. The effect of thiazolidinediones on the pharmacokinetics of sitagliptin was not assessed.

Warfarin: Multiple daily doses of sitagliptin did not meaningfully alter the pharmacokinetics, as assessed by measurement of S(−) or R(+) warfarin enantiomers, or pharmacodynamics (as assessed by measurement of prothrombin INR) of a single dose of warfarin. Since S(−) warfarin is primarily metabolized by CYP2C9, these data also support the conclusion that sitagliptin is not a CYP2C9 inhibitor.

Oral Contraceptives: Co-administration with sitagliptin did not meaningfully alter the steady-state pharmacokinetics of norethindrone or ethinyl estradiol.

Digoxin: Sitagliptin had a minimal effect on the pharmacokinetics of digoxin. Following administration of 0.25 mg digoxin concomitantly with 100 mg of sitagliptin daily for 10 days, the plasma AUC of digoxin was increased by 11%, and the plasma C_{max} by 18%. These increases are not considered likely to be clinically meaningful. No dosage adjustment of digoxin or JANUMET is recommended.

Cyclosporine: A study was conducted to assess the effect of cyclosporine, a potent inhibitor of p-glycoprotein, on the pharmacokinetics of sitagliptin. Coadministration of a single 100-mg oral dose of sitagliptin and a single 600 mg oral dose of cyclosporine increased the AUC and C_{max} of sitagliptin by approximately 29% and 68%, respectively. These modest changes in sitagliptin pharmacokinetics were not considered to be clinically meaningful. The renal clearance of sitagliptin was also not meaningfully altered. Therefore, meaningful interactions would not be expected with other p-glycoprotein inhibitors. No dosage adjustment for JANUMET is recommended when co-administered with cyclosporine or other p-glycoprotein inhibitors (e.g., ketoconazole).

Metformin: Glyburide: In a single-dose interaction study in type 2 diabetes patients, co-administration of metformin and glyburide did not result in any changes in either metformin pharmacokinetics or pharmacodynamics. Decreases in glyburide AUC and C_{max} were observed, but were highly variable. The single-dose nature of this study and the lack of correlation between glyburide blood levels and pharmacodynamic effects make the clinical significance of this interaction uncertain.

Furosemide: A single-dose, metformin-furosemide drug interaction study in healthy subjects demonstrated that pharmacokinetic parameters of both compounds were affected by co-administration. Furosemide increased the metformin plasma and blood C_{max} by 22% and blood AUC by 15%, without any significant change in metformin renal clearance. When administered with metformin, the C_{max} and AUC of furosemide were 31% and 12% smaller, respectively, than when administered alone, and the terminal half-life was decreased by 32%, without any significant change in furosemide renal clearance. No information is available about the interaction of metformin and furosemide when co-administered chronically.

Nifedipine: A single-dose, metformin-nifedipine drug interaction study in normal healthy volunteers demonstrated that co-administration of nifedipine increased plasma metformin C_{max} and AUC by 20% and 9%, respectively, and increased the amount excreted in the urine. T_{max} and half-life were unaffected. Nifedipine appears to enhance the absorption of metformin. Metformin had minimal effects on nifedipine.

Cationic Drugs: Cationic drugs (e.g., amiloride, digoxin, morphine, procainamide, quinidine, quinine, ranitidine, triamterene, trimethoprim, or vancomycin) that are eliminated by renal tubular secretion theoretically have the potential for interaction with metformin by competing for common renal tubular transport systems. Such interaction between metformin and oral cimetidine has been observed in normal healthy volunteers in both single- and multiple-dose metformin-cimetidine drug interaction studies, with a 60% increase in peak metformin plasma and whole blood concentrations and a 40% increase in plasma and whole blood metformin AUC. There was no change in elimination half-life in the single-dose study. Metformin had no effect on cimetidine pharmacokinetics. Although such interactions remain theoretical (except for cimetidine), careful patient monitoring and dose adjustment of JANUMET and/or the interfering drug is recommended in patients who are taking cationic medications that are excreted via the proximal renal tubular secretory system.

Other: Certain drugs tend to produce hyperglycemia and may lead to loss of glycemic control. These drugs include the thiazides and other diuretics, corticosteroids, phenothiazines, thyroid products, estrogens, estrogen plus progestogen, oral contraceptives, phenytoin, nicotinic acid, sympathomimetics, calcium channel blocking drugs, isoniazid and beta-2-agonists. ACE-inhibitors may decrease the blood glucose levels. When such drugs are administered to a patient receiving JANUMET the patient should be closely observed to maintain adequate glycemic control.

Elimination rate of the anticoagulant phenprocoumon has been reported to be increased by 20% when used concurrently with metformin. Therefore, patients receiving phenprocoumon or other antivitamin K anticoagulants should be monitored carefully when both types of drugs are used simultaneously. In such cases, an important increase of prothrombin time may occur upon cessation of JANUMET therapy, with an increased risk of hemorrhage.

Drug-Food Interactions: There are no known interactions with food.

Drug-Herb Interactions: Interactions with herbal products have not been established.

Drug-Laboratory Test Interactions: Intravascular contrast studies with iodinated materials can lead to acute alteration of renal function and have been associated with lactic acidosis in patients receiving metformin (see Contraindications and Warnings and Precautions).

Drug-Lifestyle Interactions: Sitagliptin and Metformin: No studies of the effects of JANUMET on the ability to drive and use machines have been performed. JANUMET is not expected to affect the ability to drive and use machines under usual circumstances. However, patients should be warned about driving a vehicle or operating machinery under conditions where a risk of hypoglycemia is present (see Warnings and Precautions, Endocrine and Metabolism, Metformin).

Metformin: Patients should be cautioned against excessive alcohol intake, either acute or chronic, when taking JANUMET, since alcohol intake potentiates the effect of metformin on lactate metabolism (see Contraindications).

DOSAGE AND ADMINISTRATION: Dosing Considerations: Over a period of time, patients may become progressively less responsive to therapy with oral hypoglycemic agents because of deterioration of their diabetic state. Patients should therefore be monitored with regular clinical and laboratory evaluations, including blood glucose and glycosylated hemoglobin (A1C) determinations, to determine the minimum effective dosage and to detect primary failure or secondary failure (see Warnings and Precautions).

In patients in whom the maximum dose fails to lower the blood glucose adequately, therapeutic alternatives should be considered.

The dosage of antihyperglycemic therapy with JANUMET should be individualized on the basis of the patient's current regimen, effectiveness, and tolerability while not exceeding the maximum recommended daily dose of 100 mg sitagliptin and 2000 mg metformin.

JANUMET should generally be given twice daily with meals, with gradual dose escalation, to reduce the gastrointestinal (GI) side effects due to metformin.

Recommended Dose and Dosage Adjustment: The starting dose of JANUMET should be based on the patient's current regimen. JANUMET should be given twice daily with meals. The following doses are available:
50 mg sitagliptin/500 mg metformin hydrochloride;
50 mg sitagliptin/850 mg metformin hydrochloride;
50 mg sitagliptin/1000 mg metformin hydrochloride.

No studies have been performed specifically examining the safety and efficacy of JANUMET in patients previously treated with other oral antihyperglycemic agents and switched to JANUMET. Any change in therapy of type 2 diabetes should be undertaken with care and appropriate monitoring as changes in glycemic control can occur.

Patients Inadequately Controlled on Metformin Monotherapy: For patients inadequately controlled on metformin alone, the usual starting dose of JANUMET should provide sitagliptin dosed as 50 mg twice daily (100 mg total daily dose) plus the dose of metformin already being taken.

Patients Switching from Co-Administration of Sitagliptin and Metformin: For patients switching from sitagliptin co-administrated with metformin, JANUMET may be initiated at the dose of sitagliptin and metformin already being taken.

Patients with Renal Insufficiency: JANUMET should not be used in patients with renal failure or renal dysfunction e.g., serum creatinine levels ≥136 µmol/L [males], ≥124 µmol/L [females] or abnormal creatinine clearance (see Contraindications and Warnings and Precautions).

Patients with Hepatic Insufficiency: Use of JANUMET in patients with severe hepatic insufficiency is not recommended (see Contraindications and Warnings and Precautions).

Geriatrics: As metformin and sitagliptin are excreted by the kidney, JANUMET should be used with caution as age increases. Monitoring of renal function is necessary to aid in prevention of metformin-associated lactic acidosis, particularly in the elderly (see Warnings and Precautions, Endocrine and Metabolism, Lactic Acidosis and Action and Clinical Pharmacology, Special Populations and Conditions, Geriatrics).

Pediatrics: There are no data available on the use of JANUMET in patients younger than 18 years of age. Therefore, use of JANUMET in pediatric patients is not recommended.

Missed Dose: If a dose of JANUMET is missed, it should be taken as soon as the patient remembers. If he/she does not remember until it is time for the next dose, the missed dose should be skipped and returned to the regular schedule. Two doses of JANUMET should not be taken at the same time.

OVERDOSAGE:

Sitagliptin: During controlled clinical trials in healthy subjects, single doses of up to 800 mg sitagliptin were generally well tolerated. Minimal increases in QTc, not considered to be clinically relevant, were observed in one study at a dose of 800 mg sitagliptin (see Action and Clinical Pharmacology, Pharmacodynamics). There is no experience with doses above 800 mg in humans. In phase I multiple-dose studies, there were no dose-related clinical adverse reactions observed with sitagliptin with doses of up to 600 mg per day for 10 days and 400 mg per day for periods of up to 28 days.

In the event of an overdose, it is reasonable to employ the usual supportive measures, e.g., remove unabsorbed material from the gastrointestinal tract, employ clinical monitoring (including obtaining an electrocardiogram), and institute supportive therapy if required.

Sitagliptin is modestly dialyzable. In clinical studies, approximately 13.5% of the dose was removed over a 3- to 4-hour hemodialysis session. Prolonged hemodialysis may be considered if clinically appropriate. It is not known if sitagliptin is dialyzable by peritoneal dialysis.

Metformin: Available information concerning treatment of a massive overdosage of metformin hydrochloride is very limited. It would be expected that adverse reactions of a more intense character including epigastric discomfort, nausea and vomiting followed by diarrhea, drowsiness, weakness, dizziness, malaise and headache might be seen. Should those symptoms persist, lactic acidosis should be excluded. The drug should be discontinued and proper supportive therapy instituted.

Overdose of metformin hydrochloride has occurred, including ingestion of amounts greater than 50 grams. Hypoglycemia was reported in approximately 10% of cases, but no causal association with metformin hydrochloride has been established. Lactic acidosis has been reported in approximately 32% of metformin overdose cases (see Warnings and Precautions, Endocrine and Metabolism, Lactic Acidosis). Metformin is dialyzable with a clearance of up to 170 mL/min under good hemodynamic conditions. Therefore, hemodialysis may be useful for removal of accumulated drug from patients in whom metformin overdosage is suspected.

For management of a suspected drug overdose, contact your **regional Poison Control Centre**. See the *CPS* Directory section for a list of Poison Control Centres.

ACTION AND CLINICAL PHARMACOLOGY: Mechanism of Action: JANUMET: JANUMET combines two antihyperglycemic agents with complementary mechanisms of action to improve glycemic control in patients with type 2 diabetes: sitagliptin phosphate, a dipeptidyl peptidase 4 (DPP-4) inhibitor, and metformin hydrochloride, a member of the biguanide class. JANUMET targets three core defects of type 2 diabetes which are: decreased insulin synthesis and release, increased hepatic glucose production and decreased insulin sensitivity.

Sitagliptin: Sitagliptin is an orally-active, potent, and highly selective inhibitor of the dipeptidyl peptidase 4 (DPP-4) enzyme for the treatment of type 2 diabetes. The DPP-4 inhibitors are a class of agents that act as incretin enhancer.

Incretin hormones, including glucagon-like peptide-1 (GLP-1) and glucose-dependent insulinotropic polypeptide (GIP), are released by the intestine throughout the day, and levels are increased in response to a meal. The incretins are part of an endogenous system involved in the physiologic regulation of glucose homeostasis. When blood glucose concentrations are normal or elevated, GLP-1 and GIP increase insulin synthesis and release from pancreatic beta cells by intracellular signaling pathways involving cyclic AMP. Orally administered glucose provokes a higher insulin response than that of intravenously administered glucose by raising circulating incretin levels (the incretin effect). In patients with type 2 diabetes, the incretin effect is diminished. Progressive beta-cell failure is a feature characterizing the pathogenesis of type 2 diabetes. Treatment with GLP-1 or with DPP-4 inhibitors in animal models of type 2 diabetes has been demonstrated to improve beta cell responsiveness to glucose and stimulate insulin biosynthesis and release. With higher insulin levels, tissue glucose uptake is enhanced.

In addition, GLP-1 lowers glucagon secretion from pancreatic alpha cells. Decreased glucagon concentrations, along with higher insulin levels, lead to reduced hepatic glucose production, resulting in a decrease in blood glucose levels. The effects of GLP-1 and GIP are glucose dependent such that when blood glucose concentrations are low, stimulation of insulin release and suppression of glucagon secretion by GLP-1 are not observed. For both GLP-1 and GIP, stimulation of insulin release is enhanced as glucose rises above normal concentrations. Further, GLP-1 does not impair the normal glucagon response to hypoglycemia.

The activity of GLP-1 and GIP is limited by the DPP-4 enzyme, which rapidly hydrolyzes the incretin hormones to produce inactive products. Sitagliptin prevents the hydrolysis of incretin hormones by DPP-4, thereby increasing plasma concentrations of the active forms of GLP-1 and GIP. By enhancing active incretin levels, sitagliptin increases insulin release and decreases glucagon levels in a glucose-dependent manner.

In patients with type 2 diabetes with hyperglycemia, these changes in insulin and glucagon levels lead to lower hemoglobin A_{1c} (HbA_{1c}) and lower fasting and postprandial glucose concentrations. The glucose-dependent mechanism of sitagliptin is distinct from the mechanism of sulfonylureas, which increase insulin secretion even when glucose levels are low, which can lead to hypoglycemia in patients with type 2 diabetes and in normal subjects. Sitagliptin is a potent and highly selective inhibitor of the enzyme DPP-4, and does not inhibit the closely-related enzymes DPP-8 or DPP-9 at therapeutic concentrations. Inhibition of DPP-8 or DPP-9, but not DPP-4, is associated with toxicity in preclinical animal models and alteration of immune function in vitro.

Metformin: Metformin is an antihyperglycemic agent, which improves glucose tolerance in patients with type 2 diabetes, lowering both basal and postprandial plasma glucose. Metformin is a biguanide derivative producing an antihyperglycemic effect which is observed in diabetic patients or in diabetic animals. Its pharmacologic mechanisms of action are different from other classes of oral antihyperglycemic agents. Metformin may decrease hepatic glucose production, decrease intestinal absorption of glucose, and improve insulin sensitivity by increasing peripheral glucose uptake and utilization. Unlike sulfonylureas, metformin does not produce hypoglycemia in either patients with type 2 diabetes or normal subjects (except in special circumstances, see Warnings and Precautions, Hypoglycemia) and does not cause hyperinsulinemia. With metformin therapy, insulin secretion remains unchanged while fasting insulin levels and day-long plasma insulin response may actually decrease.

Pharmacodynamics: Sitagliptin: In patients with type 2 diabetes, administration of single oral doses of sitagliptin leads to inhibition of DPP-4 enzyme activity for a 24-hour period, resulting in a 2- to 3-fold increase in circulating levels of active GLP-1 and GIP, increased plasma levels of insulin and C-peptide, decreased glucagon concentrations, reduced fasting glucose, and reduced glucose excursion following an oral glucose load or a meal. After a single dose, effects on plasma glucose were observed within 2-3 hours.

In a study of patients with type 2 diabetes inadequately controlled on metformin monotherapy (N=26), glucose levels monitored throughout the day were significantly lower (p<0.001) in patients who received sitagliptin 100 mg per day (50 mg twice daily) in combination with metformin compared with patients who received placebo with metformin (see Figure 1).

Figure 1: JANUMET

24-Hour Plasma Glucose Profile After 4-Week Treatment with Sitagliptin 50 mg BID with Metformin or Placebo with Metformin

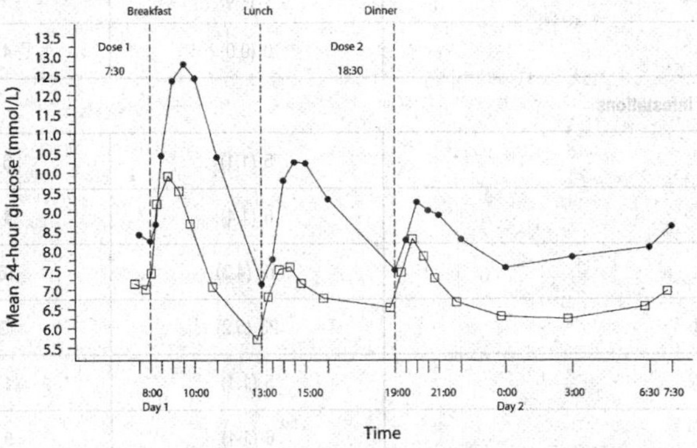

Sitagliptin and Metformin Co-Administration: In a two-day study in healthy subjects, sitagliptin alone increased active GLP-1 concentrations, whereas metformin alone increased active and total GLP-1 concentrations to similar extents. Co-administration of sitagliptin and metformin has an additive effect on active GLP-1 concentrations. Sitagliptin, but not metformin, increased active GIP concentrations. It is unclear what these findings mean for changes in glycemic control in patient with type 2 diabetes.

In studies with healthy subjects, sitagliptin did not lower blood glucose or cause hypoglycemia, suggesting that the insulinotropic and glucagon suppressive actions of the drug are glucose dependent.

Cardiac Electrophysiology: In a randomized, placebo-controlled crossover study, 79 healthy subjects were administered a single oral dose of sitagliptin 100 mg, sitagliptin 800 mg (8 times the recommended dose), and placebo. At the recommended dose of 100 mg, there was no effect on the QTc interval obtained at the peak plasma concentration, or at any other time during the study. Following the 800-mg dose, the maximum increase in the placebo-corrected mean change in QTc from baseline at 3 hours postdose was 8.0 msec. This small increase was not considered to be clinically significant. At the 800-mg dose, peak sitagliptin plasma concentrations were approximately 11-time higher than the peak concentrations following a 100-mg dose.

In patients with type 2 diabetes administered sitagliptin 100 mg (N=81) or sitagliptin 200 mg (N=63) daily, there were no meaningful changes in QTc interval based on ECG data obtained at the time of expected peak plasma concentration.

Pharmacokinetics: In a bioequivalence study of JANUMET 50/500 and 50/1000 (mg/mg sitagliptin/metformin hydrochloride), both the sitagliptin component and the metformin component were bioequivalent to co-administered 50 mg sitagliptin phosphate (JANUVIA) tablet and metformin hydrochloride tablets 500 and 1000 mg, respectively under fasted conditions in healthy subjects.

Because bioequivalence is demonstrated at the lowest and highest combination tablet dose strengths available, bioequivalence is conferred to the (sitagliptin/metformin) 50 mg/850 mg fixed dose combination (FDC) tablet.

Table 3: JANUMET

Geometric Mean Pharmacokinetic Parameters for Sitagliptin and Metformin Following Single Dose of JANUMET or Co-Administration of Corresponding Doses of Sitagliptin and Metformin as Individual Tablets to Healthy Subjects Under Fasted Conditions

		Sitagliptin			
Treatment	Subject Number	$AUC_{0-\infty}$ (µM·hr)	C_{max} (nM)	T_{max}[a] (hr)	$t_{½}$[b] (hr)
A	24	4.09	415	2.5	12.3
B	24	4.01	414	2.75	12.6
C	24	4.05	423	2.5	13.1
D	24	3.94	397	2.5	13.7
		Metformin			
Treatment	Subject Number	$AUC_{0-\infty}$ (µM·hr)	C_{max} (nM)	T_{max}[a] (hr)	$t_{½}$[b] (hr)
A	24	7.26	1180	2.5	9.79
B	24	7.25	1180	2.75	11.6
C	24	11.9	1850	2.5	13.6
D	24	11.9	1870	2	13.9

[a] Median.
[b] Harmonic mean.
Treatment A=sitagliptin 50 mg + metformin hydrochloride 500 mg.
Treatment B=JANUMET sitagliptin (50 mg)/metformin hydrochloride (500 mg).
Treatment C=sitagliptin 50 mg + metformin hydrochloride 1000 mg.
Treatment D=JANUMET sitagliptin (50 mg)/metformin hydrochloride (1000 mg).

When administered in the fed state (following a standard high-fat breakfast), the metformin component of JANUMET was bioequivalent to metformin taken together with sitagliptin as individual tablets.

Absorption: Sitagliptin: The absolute bioavailability of sitagliptin is approximately 87%. Since co-administration of a high-fat meal with sitagliptin had no effect on the pharmacokinetics, sitagliptin may be administered with or without food.

Metformin: The absolute bioavailability of a metformin hydrochloride 500 mg tablet given under fasting conditions is approximately 50-60%. Studies using single oral doses of metformin hydrochloride tablets 500 mg to 1500 mg, and 850 mg to 2550 mg, indicate that there is a lack of dose proportionality with increasing doses, which is due to decreased absorption rather than an alteration in elimination. Food decreases the extent of and slightly delays the absorption of metformin, as shown by approximately a 40% lower mean peak plasma concentration (C_{max}), a 25% lower area under the plasma concentration versus time curve (AUC), and a 35-minute prolongation of time to peak plasma concentration (T_{max}) following administration of a single 850-mg tablet of metformin with food, compared to the same tablet strength administered fasting. The clinical relevance of these decreases is unknown.

Distribution: Sitagliptin: The mean volume of distribution at steady state following a single 100-mg intravenous dose of sitagliptin to healthy subjects is approximately 198 L. The fraction of sitagliptin reversibly bound to plasma proteins is low (38%).

Metformin: The apparent volume of distribution (V/F) of metformin following single oral doses of metformin hydrochloride tablets 850 mg averaged 654±358 L. Metformin is negligibly bound to plasma proteins, in contrast to sulfonylureas, which are more than 90% protein bound. Metformin partitions into erythrocytes, most likely as a function of time. At usual clinical doses and dosing schedules of metformin hydrochloride tablets, steady state plasma concentrations of metformin are reached within 24-48 hours and are generally <1 µg/mL. During controlled clinical trials of metformin, maximum metformin plasma levels did not exceed 5 µg/mL, even at maximum doses.

Metabolism: Sitagliptin: Sitagliptin is primarily eliminated unchanged in urine, and metabolism is a minor pathway. Approximately 79% of sitagliptin is excreted unchanged in the urine.

Following a [^{14}C] sitagliptin oral dose, approximately 16% of the radioactivity was excreted as metabolites of sitagliptin. Six metabolites were detected at trace levels and are not expected to contribute to the plasma DPP-4 inhibitory activity of sitagliptin. In vitro studies indicated that the primary enzyme responsible for the limited metabolism of sitagliptin was CYP3A4, with contribution from CYP2C8.

Metformin: Intravenous single-dose studies in normal subjects demonstrate that metformin is excreted unchanged in the urine and does not undergo hepatic metabolism (no metabolites have been identified in humans) nor biliary excretion.

Excretion: Sitagliptin: Following administration of an oral [^{14}C] sitagliptin dose to healthy subjects, approximately 100% of the administered radioactivity was eliminated in feces (13%) or urine (87%) within one week of dosing. The apparent terminal $t_{½}$ following a 100-mg oral dose of sitagliptin was approximately 12.4 hours and renal clearance was approximately 350 mL/min.

Elimination of sitagliptin occurs primarily via renal excretion and involves active tubular secretion. Sitagliptin is a substrate for human organic anion transporter-3 (hOAT-3), which may be involved in the renal elimination of sitagliptin. The clinical relevance of hOAT-3 in sitagliptin transport has not been established. Sitagliptin is also a substrate of p-glycoprotein, which may also be involved in mediating the renal elimination of sitagliptin. However, cyclosporine, a p-glycoprotein inhibitor, did not reduce the renal clearance of sitagliptin.

Metformin: Renal clearance is approximately 3.5 times greater than creatinine clearance, which indicates that tubular secretion is the major route of metformin elimination. Following oral administration, approximately 90% of the absorbed drug is eliminated via the renal route within the first 24 hours, with a plasma elimination half-life of approximately 6.2 hours. In blood, the elimination half-life is approximately 17.6 hours, suggesting that the erythrocyte mass may be a compartment of distribution.

Special Populations and Conditions: Pediatrics: No studies with JANUMET have been performed in pediatric patients.

Geriatrics: Sitagliptin: No dosage adjustment is required based on age. Age did not have a clinically meaningful impact on the pharmacokinetics of sitagliptin based on a population pharmacokinetic analysis of Phase I and Phase II data. Elderly subjects (65 to 80 years) had approximately 19% higher plasma concentrations of sitagliptin compared to younger subjects.

Metformin: Limited data from controlled pharmacokinetic studies of metformin in healthy elderly subjects suggest that total plasma clearance of metformin is decreased, the half life is prolonged, and C_{max} is increased, compared to healthy young subjects. From these data, it appears that the change in metformin pharmacokinetics with aging is primarily accounted for by a change in renal function (see Warnings and Precautions, Special Populations, Geriatrics (≥65 years of age)).

JANUMET treatment should not be initiated in patients ≥80 years of age unless measurement of creatinine clearance demonstrates that renal function is not reduced (see Warnings and Precautions, Endocrine and Metabolism, Lactic Acidosis).

Gender: No dosage adjustment is necessary based on gender.

Sitagliptin: Gender had no clinically meaningful effect on the pharmacokinetics of sitagliptin based on a composite analysis of Phase I pharmacokinetic data and on a population pharmacokinetic analysis of Phase I and Phase II data.

Metformin: Metformin pharmacokinetic parameters did not differ significantly between normal subjects and patients with type 2 diabetes when analyzed according to gender. Similarly, in controlled clinical studies in patients with type 2 diabetes, the antihyperglycemic effect of metformin was comparable in males and females.

Race: No dosage adjustment is necessary based on race.

Sitagliptin: Race had no clinically meaningful effect on the pharmacokinetics of sitagliptin based on a composite analysis of Phase I pharmacokinetic data and on a population pharmacokinetic analysis of Phase I and Phase II data, including subjects of white, Hispanic, black and Asian racial groups.

Metformin: No studies of metformin pharmacokinetic parameters according to race have been performed. In controlled clinical studies of metformin in patients with type 2 diabetes, the antihyperglycemic effect was comparable in whites (n=249), blacks (n=51), and Hispanics (n=24).

Hepatic Insufficiency: Sitagliptin: In patients with moderate hepatic insufficiency (Child-Pugh score 7 to 9), mean AUC and C_{max} of sitagliptin increased approximately 21% (90% CI: 1%, 46%) and 13% (90% CI: -9%, 42%), respectively, compared to healthy matched controls following administration of a single 100 mg dose of sitagliptin.

Metformin: No pharmacokinetic studies of metformin have been conducted in patients with hepatic insufficiency.

Renal Insufficiency: JANUMET should not be used in patients with renal insufficiency (see Contraindications).

Sitagliptin: An approximately 2-fold increase in the plasma AUC of sitagliptin was observed in patients with moderate renal insufficiency, and an approximately 4-fold increase was observed in patients with severe renal insufficiency and in patients with ESRD on hemodialysis, as compared to normal healthy control subjects.

Metformin: In patients with decreased renal function (based on measured creatinine clearance (<60 mL/min), the plasma and blood half-lifes of metformin are prolonged and the renal clearance is decreased in proportion to the decrease in creatinine clearance.

STORAGE AND STABILITY: The product should be stored at 15-30°C.

INFORMATION FOR THE PATIENT: Published in e-CPS, available by subscription at www.e-cps.ca.

DOSAGE FORMS, COMPOSITION AND PACKAGING: 50 mg/500 mg: Each light pink, capsule-shaped, film-coated tablet with "575" debossed on one side, contains: sitagliptin phosphate monohydrate 64.25 mg and metformin hydrochloride equivalent to sitagliptin 50 mg as free base and metformin hydrochloride 500 mg. Nonmedicinal ingredients: microcrystalline cellulose, polyvinylpyrrolidone, sodium lauryl sulfate and sodium stearyl fumarate; film coating: black iron oxide, polyvinyl alcohol, polyethylene glycol, red iron oxide, talc and titanium dioxide. Bottles of 60.

50 mg/850 mg: Each pink, capsule-shaped, film-coated tablet with "515" debossed on one side, contains: sitagliptin phosphate monohydrate 64.25 mg and metformin hydrochloride equivalent to sitagliptin 50 mg as free base and metformin hydrochloride 850 mg. Nonmedicinal ingredients: microcrystalline cellulose, polyvinylpyrrolidone, sodium lauryl sulfate and sodium stearyl fumarate; film coating: black iron oxide, polyvinyl alcohol, polyethylene glycol, red iron oxide, talc and titanium dioxide. Bottles of 60.

50 mg/1000 mg: Each red, capsule-shaped, film-coated tablet with "577" debossed on one side, contains: sitagliptin phosphate monohydrate 64.25 mg and metformin hydrochloride equivalent to sitagliptin 50 mg as free base and metformin hydrochloride 1000 mg. Nonmedicinal ingredients: microcrystalline cellulose, polyvinylpyrrolidone, sodium lauryl sulfate and sodium stearyl fumarate; film coating: black iron oxide, polyvinyl alcohol, polyethylene glycol, red iron oxide, talc and titanium dioxide. Bottles of 60.

(Shown in Product Identification Section)

Januvia® Ⓟ

sitagliptin phosphate

Oral Antihyperglycemic Agent—DPP-4 Inhibitor—Incretin Enhancer

Merck Frosst

Date of Revision: June 2, 2010

SUMMARY PRODUCT INFORMATION:

Route of Administration	Dosage Form/ Strength	Clinically Relevant Nonmedicinal Ingredients
Oral	Tablet 100 mg	For a complete listing see Dosage Forms, Composition and Packaging.

INDICATIONS AND CLINICAL USE: Monotherapy: JANUVIA (sitagliptin) is indicated as an adjunct to diet and exercise to improve glycemic control in adult patients with type 2 diabetes mellitus and for whom metformin is inappropriate due to contraindications or intolerance.

Combination with Metformin: JANUVIA is indicated in combination with metformin in adult patients with type 2 diabetes mellitus to improve glycemic control when diet and exercise, plus metformin do not provide adequate glycemic control.

Combination with Metformin and a Sulfonylurea: JANUVIA is indicated in combination with metformin and a sulfonylurea in adult patients with type 2 diabetes mellitus to improve glycemic control when diet and exercise, and dual therapy with these agents, do not provide adequate glycemic control.

Geriatrics (≥65 years of age): No dosage adjustment is required based on age however, greater sensitivity of some older individuals cannot be ruled out (see Warnings and Precautions, Dosage and Administration and Action and Clinical Pharmacology).

Pediatrics (<18 years of age): Safety and effectiveness of JANUVIA in pediatric patients have not been established. Therefore, JANUVIA should not be used in this population.

CONTRAINDICATIONS: Patients who are hypersensitive to this drug or to any ingredient in the formulation (see Warnings and Precautions, Hypersensitivity Reactions and Adverse Reactions, Post-Market Adverse Drug Reactions). For a complete listing, see Dosage Forms, Composition and Packaging.

WARNINGS AND PRECAUTIONS: General: JANUVIA should not be used in patients with type 1 diabetes or for the treatment of diabetic ketoacidosis.

The use of JANUVIA in combination with insulin has not been adequately studied. Use of JANUVIA in combination with insulin is not indicated.

Pancreatitis: There have been reports of acute pancreatitis, including fatal and non-fatal hemorrhagic or necrotizing pancreatitis, in patients taking JANUVIA. After initiation of JANUVIA, patients should be observed carefully for signs and symptoms of pancreatitis. If pancreatitis is suspected, JANUVIA should promptly be discontinued and appropriate management should be initiated. Risk factors for pancreatitis include a history of: pancreatitis, gallstones, alcoholism, or hypertriglyceridemia.

Hypoglycemia: When JANUVIA was used in combination with metformin and a sulfonylurea the incidence of hypoglycemia was increased over that of placebo in combination with metformin and a sulfonylurea (see Adverse Reactions). To reduce the risk of hypoglycemia associated with this indication, a lower dose of sulfonylurea may be considered (see Dosage and Administration).

Hypersensitivity Reactions: There have been post-marketing reports of serious hypersensitivity reactions in patients treated with JANUVIA. These reactions include anaphylaxis, angioedema, and exfoliative skin conditions including Stevens-Johnson syndrome. Onset of these reactions occurred within the first 3 months after initiation of treatment with JANUVIA, with some reports occurring after the first dose. If a hypersensitivity reaction is suspected, discontinue JANUVIA, assess for other potential causes for the event, and institute alternative treatment for diabetes (see Contraindications and Adverse Reactions, Post-Market Adverse Drug Reactions).

Special Populations: Pregnant Women: There are no adequate and well-controlled studies in pregnant women; therefore, the safety of JANUVIA in pregnant women is not known. JANUVIA is not recommended for use in pregnancy.

Nursing Women: Sitagliptin is secreted in the milk of lactating rats. It is not known whether sitagliptin is secreted in human milk. Therefore, JANUVIA should not be used by a woman who is nursing.

Pediatrics (<18 years of age): Safety and effectiveness of JANUVIA in pediatric patients have not been established. Therefore, JANUVIA should not be used in this population.

Geriatrics (≥65 years of age): In clinical studies, no overall differences in safety or effectiveness were observed between subjects 65 years and over and younger subjects. While this and other reported clinical experience have not identified differences in responses between the geriatric and younger patients, greater sensitivity of some older individuals cannot be ruled out.

This drug is known to be substantially excreted by the kidney. Renal function should be assessed prior to initiating dosing and periodically thereafter in geriatric patients because they are more likely to have decreased renal function (see Dosage and Administration and Action and Clinical Pharmacology).

Cardiovascular—Patients with Congestive Heart Failure: A limited number of patients with congestive heart failure participated in clinical studies of sitagliptin. In studies of sitagliptin in combination with metformin, patients with congestive heart failure requiring pharmacological therapy or NYHA Class III or IV congestive heart failure were excluded. Patients with Classes I and II were included in small number. Use in this population is not recommended.

Hepatic Insufficiency: There are limited clinical experiences in patients with moderate hepatic insufficiency and no clinical experience in patients with severe hepatic insufficiency. Use in patients with severe hepatic insufficiency is not recommended (see Action and Clinical Pharmacology).

Renal Insufficiency: Clinical study experience with JANUVIA in patients with moderate or severe renal insufficiency including those with ESRD is limited. Use in these patients is not recommended (see Action and Clinical Pharmacology).

Monitoring and Laboratory Tests: Response to all diabetic therapies should be monitored by periodic measurements of blood glucose and HbA_{1c} levels, with a goal of decreasing these levels towards the normal range. HbA_{1c} is especially useful for evaluating long-term glycemic control. Sitagliptin is substantially excreted by the kidney. Renal function should be assessed prior to initiating dosing and periodically thereafter.

ADVERSE REACTIONS: Adverse Drug Reaction Overview: JANUVIA was generally well tolerated in controlled clinical studies as monotherapy and as part of combination therapy with metformin, with the overall incidence of side effects similar to that reported with placebo or combination therapy with metformin and a sulfonylurea.

The incidences of serious adverse reactions and discontinuation of therapy due to clinical adverse reactions were generally similar to placebo. The most frequent adverse reaction in trials of JANUVIA as monotherapy (placebo-controlled) and as add-on combination therapy with metformin (reported regardless of causality, and more common with JANUVIA than other treatments) was nasopharyngitis. The most frequent adverse events with JANUVIA as add-on combination therapy with metformin and a sulfonylurea agent was hypoglycemia.

Clinical Trial Adverse Drug Reactions: Because clinical trials are conducted under very specific conditions the adverse reaction rates observed in the clinical trials may not reflect the rates observed in practice and should not be compared to the rates in the clinical trials of another drug. Adverse drug reaction information from clinical trials is useful for identifying drug-related adverse events and for approximating rates.

Monotherapy: Two placebo-controlled monotherapy studies, one of 18- and one of 24-week duration, included patients treated with JANUVIA 100 mg once daily and patients given placebo. Adverse events, reported regardless of causality assessment, in ≥1% of patients in these two studies pooled are shown in Table 1.

Table 1: JANUVIA

Adverse Events ≥1% in Any Treatment Group (regardless of causality) Reported in Patients Treated with JANUVIA 100 mg or Placebo in Pooled 18 and 24-Week Placebo-Controlled, Double-Blind Clinical Trials of JANUVIA as Monotherapy

Body System/Organ Class Adverse Event	Number of Patients (%) Sitagliptin 100 mg n=443	 Placebo n=363
Eye Disorders		
Conjunctivitis	3 (0.7)	4 (1.1)
Gastrointestinal Disorders		
Abdominal pain	5 (1.1)	6 (1.7)
Constipation	13 (2.9)	5 (1.4)
Diarrhea	19 (4.3)	10 (2.8)
Gastritis	2 (0.5)	4 (1.1)
Nausea	7 (1.6)	3 (0.8)
Vomiting	3 (0.7)	4 (1.1)
General Disorders and Administration Site Conditions		
Fatigue	5 (1.1)	9 (2.5)
Edema peripheral	7 (1.6)	4 (1.1)
Pain	0 (0.0)	4 (1.1)
Infections and Infestations		
Bronchitis	5 (1.1)	6 (1.7)
Gastroenteritis	6 (1.4)	4 (1.1)
Influenza	19 (4.3)	16 (4.4)
Nasopharyngitis	23 (5.2)	12 (3.3)
Pharyngitis	5 (1.1)	1 (0.3)
Sinusitis	6 (1.4)	9 (2.5)
Upper respiratory tract infection	29 (6.5)	24 (6.6)
Urinary tract infection	8 (1.8)	9 (2.5)
Viral infection	2 (0.5)	4 (1.1)
Viral upper respiratory tract infection	5 (1.1)	1 (0.3)
Injury, Poisoning and Procedural Complications		
Limb injury	3 (0.7)	4 (1.1)
Investigations		
Blood glucose increased	7 (1.6)	13 (3.6)
Metabolism and Nutrition Disorders		
Hyperglycemia	5 (1.1)	7 (1.9)
Hypoglycemia	5 (1.1)	2 (0.6)
Musculoskeletal and Connective Tissue Disorders		
Arthralgia	4 (0.9)	9 (2.5)
Back pain	14 (3.2)	12 (3.3)
Muscle spasm	6 (1.4)	4 (1.1)
Myalgia	6 (1.4)	4 (1.1)
Neck pain	1 (0.2)	4 (1.1)
Osteoarthritis	5 (1.1)	1 (0.3)
Pain in extremity	7 (1.6)	6 (1.7)
Nervous System Disorders		
Dizziness	7 (1.6)	8 (2.2)
Headache	18 (4.1)	14 (3.9)
Paresthesia	4 (0.9)	4 (1.1)
Psychiatric Disorders		
Anxiety	3 (0.7)	4 (1.1)
Insomnia	4 (0.9)	6 (1.7)
Respiratory, Thoracic and Mediastinal Disorders		
Cough	8 (1.8)	10 (2.8)
Vascular Disorders		
Hypertension	8 (1.8)	7 (1.9)

In a 24-week study which compared sitagliptin and metformin, adverse events, reported regardless of causality assessment, in ≥1% of patients are shown in Table 2.

Table 2: JANUVIA

Adverse Events ≥1% in Any Treatment Group (regardless of causality) Reported in Patients in 24-Week Active-Controlled, Double-Blind Clinical Trial of JANUVIA as Monotherapy

Body System/Organ Class Adverse Event	Number of Patients (%) Sitagliptin 100 mg n=528	 Metformin n=522
Gastrointestinal Disorders		
Abdominal pain	4 (0.8)	6 (1.1)
Abdominal pain upper	5 (0.9)	12 (2.3)
Constipation	9 (1.7)	5 (1.0)
Diarrhea	19 (3.6)	57 (10.9)
Dyspepsia	1 (0.2)	7 (1.3)
Gastritis	6 (1.1)	11 (2.1)
Nausea	6 (1.1)	16 (3.1)
Vomiting	2 (0.4)	7 (1.3)
General Disorders and Administration Site Conditions		
Fatigue	6 (1.1)	6 (1.1)
Infections and Infestations		
Bronchitis	4 (0.8)	7 (1.3)
Influenza	12 (2.3)	11 (2.1)
Nasopharyngitis	10 (1.9)	17 (3.3)
Upper respiratory tract infection	5 (0.9)	11 (2.1)
Urinary tract infection	3 (0.6)	13 (2.5)
Metabolism and Nutrition Disorders		
Hypoglycemia	9 (1.7)	18 (3.4)
Musculoskeletal and Connective Tissue Disorders		
Back pain	9 (1.7)	9 (1.7)
Pain in extremity	7 (1.3)	2 (0.4)
Nervous System Disorders		
Dizziness	9 (1.7)	5 (1.0)
Headache	17 (3.2)	17 (3.3)
Respiratory, Thoracic and Mediastinal Disorders		
Cough	1 (0.2)	8 (1.5)
Vascular Disorders		
Hypertension	12 (2.3)	4 (0.8)

Combination Therapy—Sitagliptin Add-On to Metformin: In a 24-week placebo-controlled clinical study of patients receiving sitagliptin (100 mg daily) as add-on combination therapy with metformin the incidence of adverse events reported regardless of causality assessment, in ≥1% of patients are shown in Table 3.

Table 3: JANUVIA

Adverse Events ≥1% in Any Treatment Group (regardless of causality) Reported in Patients in a 24-Week Placebo-Controlled, Double-Blind Clinical Trial of JANUVIA in Add-On Combination Use with Metformin

Body System/Organ Class Adverse Event	Number of Patients (%) Sitagliptin 100 mg + Metformin n=464	 Placebo + Metformin n=237
Ear and Labyrinth Disorders		
Vertigo	5 (1.1)	4 (1.7)
Eye Disorders		
Vision blurred	1 (0.2)	3 (1.3)
Gastrointestinal Disorders		
Abdominal pain	2 (0.4)	6 (2.5)
Abdominal pain upper	6 (1.3)	2 (0.8)
Constipation	5 (1.1)	1 (0.4)
Diarrhea	11 (2.4)	6 (2.5)
Nausea	6 (1.3)	2 (0.8)
Vomiting	5 (1.1)	2 (0.8)
General Disorders and Administration Site Conditions		
Fatigue	2 (0.4)	4 (1.7)
Edema peripheral	4 (0.9)	3 (1.3)
Infections and Infestations		
Bronchitis	12 (2.6)	6 (2.5)
Bronchitis acute	2 (0.4)	3 (1.3)
Gastroenteritis	4 (0.9)	5 (2.1)
Influenza	19 (4.1)	12 (5.1)
Nasopharyngitis	19 (4.1)	7 (3.0)
Pharyngitis	6 (1.3)	1 (0.4)
Pneumonia	5 (1.1)	0 (0.0)
Sinusitis	7 (1.5)	2 (0.8)
Tooth infection	5 (1.1)	2 (0.8)
Upper respiratory tract infection	34 (7.3)	22 (9.3)
Urinary tract infection	9 (1.9)	2 (0.8)
Injury, Poisoning and Procedural Complications		
Contusion	5 (1.1)	1 (0.4)
Investigations		
Blood glucose increased	3 (0.6)	6 (2.5)
Metabolism and Nutrition Disorders		
Hyperglycemia	2 (0.4)	7 (3.0)
Hypoglycemia	6 (1.3)	5 (2.1)
Musculoskeletal and Connective Tissue Disorders		
Arthralgia	14 (3.0)	1 (0.4)
Back pain	15 (3.2)	6 (2.5)
Muscle spasm	1 (0.2)	3 (1.3)
Myalgia	1 (0.2)	3 (1.3)
Pain in extremity	5 (1.1)	4 (1.7)
Shoulder pain	3 (0.6)	3 (1.3)
Nervous System Disorders		
Dizziness	7 (1.5)	2 (0.8)
Headache	12 (2.6)	7 (3.0)
Sciatica	1 (0.2)	3 (1.3)
Sinus headache	0 (0.0)	3 (1.3)
Psychiatric Disorders		
Insomnia	5 (1.1)	3 (1.3)
Renal and Urinary Disorders		
Nephrolithiasis	3 (0.6)	3 (1.3)
Respiratory, Thoracic and Mediastinal Disorders		
Cough	14 (3.0)	4 (1.7)
Vascular Disorders		
Hypertension	7 (1.5)	6 (2.5)

In pooled studies of up to one year duration which compared sitagliptin added to metformin or a sulfonylurea agent (glipizide) added to metformin, adverse events, reported regardless of causality assessment, in ≥1% of patients are shown in Table 4.

Table 4: JANUVIA

Adverse Events ≥1% in Any Treatment Group (regardless of causality) Reported in Patients From Double-Blind Clinical Trials of JANUVIA in Add-On Combination Use with Metformin in Studies Up to One Year Compared to a Sulfonylurea Agent (glipizide)

Body System/Organ Class Adverse Event	Number of Patients (%)	
	Sitagliptin 100 mg + Metformin n=979	Glipizide + Metformin n=748
Gastrointestinal Disorders		
Abdominal pain	10 (1.0)	6 (0.8)
Abdominal pain upper	13 (1.3)	7 (0.9)
Constipation	17 (1.7)	13 (1.7)
Diarrhea	42 (4.3)	36 (4.8)
Dyspepsia	14 (1.4)	12 (1.6)
Nausea	19 (1.9)	16 (2.1)
Toothache	2 (0.2)	13 (1.7)
Vomiting	11 (1.1)	9 (1.2)
General Disorders and Administration Site Conditions		
Fatigue	20 (2.0)	8 (1.1)
Non-cardiac chest pain	10 (1.0)	6 (0.8)
Edema peripheral	16 (1.6)	14 (1.9)
Infections and Infestations		
Bronchitis	27 (2.8)	22 (2.9)
Cellulitis	7 (0.7)	10 (1.3)
Gastroenteritis	19 (1.9)	13 (1.7)
Gastroenteritis viral	8 (0.8)	9 (1.2)
Herpes zoster	4 (0.4)	8 (1.1)
Influenza	35 (3.6)	32 (4.3)
Nasopharyngitis	75 (7.7)	49 (6.6)
Sinusitis	20 (2.0)	12 (1.6)
Upper respiratory tract infection	78 (8.0)	70 (9.4)
Urinary tract infection	41 (4.2)	21 (2.8)
Investigations		
Blood glucose decreased	5 (0.5)	16 (2.1)
Blood glucose increased	13 (1.3)	5 (0.7)
Weight increased	1 (0.1)	8 (1.1)
Metabolism and Nutrition Disorders		
Hyperglycemia	10 (1.0)	6 (0.8)
Hypoglycemia	32 (3.3)	217 (29.0)
Musculoskeletal and Connective Tissue Disorders		
Arthralgia	34 (3.5)	29 (3.9)
Back pain	39 (4.0)	32 (4.3)
Muscle spasms	9 (0.9)	8 (1.1)
Neck pain	4 (0.4)	8 (1.1)
Osteoarthritis	18 (1.8)	5 (0.7)
Pain in extremity	23 (2.3)	9 (1.2)
Shoulder pain	7 (0.7)	14 (1.9)
Nervous System Disorders		
Dizziness	26 (2.7)	14 (1.9)
Headache	34 (3.5)	31 (4.1)
Hypoaesthesia	3 (0.3)	11 (1.5)
Psychiatric Disorders		

(cont'd)

Table 4: JANUVIA *(cont'd)*

Adverse Events ≥1% in Any Treatment Group (regardless of causality) Reported in Patients From Double-Blind Clinical Trials of JANUVIA in Add-On Combination Use with Metformin in Studies Up to One Year Compared to a Sulfonylurea Agent (glipizide)

Body System/Organ Class Adverse Event	Number of Patients (%)	
	Sitagliptin 100 mg + Metformin n=979	Glipizide + Metformin n=748
Anxiety	13 (1.3)	7 (0.9)
Depression	10 (1.0)	7 (0.9)
Insomnia	12 (1.2)	11 (1.5)
Reproductive System and Breast Disorders		
Erectile dysfunction	6 (0.6)	8 (1.1)
Respiratory, Thoracic and Mediastinal Disorders		
Cough	19 (1.9)	23 (3.1)
Pharyngolaryngeal pain	10 (1.0)	9 (1.2)
Sinus congestion	5 (0.5)	8 (1.1)
Eczema	4 (0.4)	12 (1.6)
Vascular Disorders		
Hypertension	33 (3.4)	29 (3.9)

Combination Therapy: Sitagliptin Add-On to Metformin and a Sulfonylurea: In a 24-week placebo-controlled study of JANUVIA 100 mg in combination with metformin and glimepiride (JANUVIA, N=116; placebo, N=113), the incidence of adverse events, reported regardless of causality assessment, in ≥1% of patients are shown in Table 5. The overall incidence of adverse events with JANUVIA was higher than with placebo, in part related to higher incidence of hypoglycemia (see Table 5).

Table 5: JANUVIA

Adverse Events ≥1% in Any Treatment Group (regardless of causality) Reported in Patients in a 24-Week Placebo-Controlled, Double-Blind Clinical Trial of JANUVIA in Add-On Combination Use with Metformin and a Sulfonylurea Agent (glimepiride)

Body System/Organ Class Adverse Event	Number of Patients (%)	
	Sitagliptin 100 mg + Metformin + Glimepiride n=116	Placebo + Metformin + Glimepiride n=113
Ear and Labyrinth Disorders		
Vertigo	2 (1.7)	0 (0.0)
Eye Disorders		
Diabetic retinopathy	0 (0.0)	2 (1.8)
Vision blurred	0 (0.0)	2 (1.8)
Gastrointestinal Disorders		
Abdominal pain upper	2 (1.7)	2 (1.8)
Constipation	4 (3.4)	0 (0.0)
Diarrhea	1 (0.9)	4 (3.5)
Dyspepsia	3 (2.6)	2 (1.8)
Gastritis	0 (0.0)	4 (3.5)
Toothache	2 (1.7)	2 (1.8)
Vomiting	2 (1.7)	1 (0.9)
General Disorders and Administration Site Conditions		
Fatigue	0 (0.0)	3 (2.7)
Non-cardiac chest pain	2 (1.7)	1 (0.9)
Pyrexia	0 (0.0)	2 (1.8)
Hepatobiliary Disorders		
Cholelithiasis	0 (0.0)	2 (1.8)
Infections and Infestations		
Bronchitis	2 (1.7)	2 (1.8)
Gastroenteritis	3 (2.6)	0 (0.0)
Gastroenteritis viral	2 (1.7)	2 (1.8)
Influenza	3 (2.6)	2 (1.8)
Nasopharyngitis	7 (6.0)	9 (8.0)

(cont'd)

Table 5: JANUVIA *(cont'd)*

Adverse Events ≥1% in Any Treatment Group (regardless of causality) Reported in Patients in a 24-Week Placebo-Controlled, Double-Blind Clinical Trial of JANUVIA in Add-On Combination Use with Metformin and a Sulfonylurea Agent (glimepiride)

Body System/Organ Class Adverse Event	Number of Patients (%) Sitagliptin 100 mg + Metformin + Glimepiride n=116	Placebo + Metformin + Glimepiride n=113
Pharyngitis	1 (0.9)	3 (2.7)
Pneumonia	3 (2.6)	0 (0.0)
Rhinitis	2 (1.7)	0 (0.0)
Sinusitis	1 (0.9)	2 (1.8)
Tooth abscess	2 (1.7)	1 (0.9)
Upper respiratory tract infection	8 (6.9)	9 (8.0)
Urinary tract infection	2 (1.7)	1 (0.9)
Injury, Poisoning and Procedural Complications		
Fall	0 (0.0)	3 (2.7)
Polytraumatism	1 (0.9)	2 (1.8)
Investigations		
Blood glucose decreased	0 (0.0)	2 (1.8)
Metabolism and Nutrition Disorders		
Hypoglycemia	19 (16.4)	1 (0.9)
Musculoskeletal and Connective Tissue Disorders		
Arthralgia	5 (4.3)	1 (0.9)
Back pain	1 (0.9)	2 (1.8)
Muscle spasms	2 (1.7)	1 (0.9)
Osteoarthritis	2 (1.7)	0 (0.0)
Pain in extremity	4 (3.4)	1 (0.9)
Shoulder pain	0 (0.0)	2 (1.8)
Nervous System Disorders		
Dizziness	3 (2.6)	1 (0.9)
Headache	8 (6.9)	3 (2.7)
Hypoaesthesia	2 (1.7)	0 (0.0)
Somnolence	0 (0.0)	2 (1.8)
Respiratory, Thoracic and Mediastinal Disorders		
Asthma	2 (1.7)	1 (0.9)
Skin and Subcutaneous Tissue Disorders		
Pruritus	2 (1.7)	1 (0.9)
Rash	2 (1.7)	1 (0.9)
Vascular Disorders		
Hypertension	2 (1.7)	0 (0.0)

Less Common Clinical Trial Adverse Drug Reactions ≥0.1% and <1% (Drug-Related and Greater than Placebo in Pooled Monotherapy and in Individual Placebo-Controlled Studies): Blood and Lymphatic System Disorders: anemia.

Cardiac Disorders: bundle branch block, palpitations.

Gastrointestinal Disorders: abdominal discomfort, abdominal pain upper, abdominal tenderness, constipation, diarrhea, dyspepsia, flatulence, reflux esophagitis disease, frequent bowel movements, gastroesophageal reflux disease, retching, salivary hypersecretion.

General Disorders and Administration Site Conditions: asthenia, face edema, hunger, irritability, malaise, peripheral edema, pain, pyrexia, xerosis.

Hepatobiliary Disorders: hepatic steatosis.

Infections and Infestations: gastric ulcer helicobacter, helicobacter gastritis, oropharyngeal candidiasis, upper respiratory tract infection, urinary tract infection.

Investigations: blood glucose decreased, blood glucose increased, blood pressure decreased, blood pressure increased, hepatic enzyme increased.

Metabolism and Nutrition Disorders: decreased appetite, hypoglycemia.

Musculoskeletal and Connective Tissue Disorders: muscle tightness.

Nervous System Disorders: coordination abnormal, dizziness, headache, migraine, neuropathy peripheral, parosmia, somnolence.

Psychiatric Disorders: anxiety, depression.

Renal and Urinary Disorders: renal disorders.

Reproductive System and Breast Disorders: dysmenorrhea, erectile dysfunction.

Respiratory, Thoracic and Mediastinal Disorders: cough.

Skin and Subcutaneous Tissue Disorders: dry skin, erythema, exanthem, hyperhidrosis, prurigo, pruritus generalized, rash, rash macular, rosacea, urticaria.

Vascular Disorders: orthostatic hypotension.

In two monotherapy studies, diarrhea was the only drug-related adverse reaction reported by the investigator that occurred with an incidence ≥1% in patients receiving JANUVIA 100 mg (1.1%) and greater than in patients receiving placebo (0.3%).

In a combination therapy study with metformin, nausea was the only drug-related adverse reaction reported by the investigator that occurred with an incidence ≥1% in patients receiving JANUVIA (1.1%) and greater than in patients receiving placebo (0.4%).

In a combination therapy study with metformin and a sulfonylurea, hypoglycemia (JANUVIA 13.8%; placebo 0.9%) and constipation (JANUVIA 1.7%; placebo 0.0%) were the only drug-related adverse reactions reported by the investigator that occurred with an incidence ≥1% in patients receiving JANUVIA and greater than in patients receiving placebo and metformin and a sulfonylurea.

Abnormal Hematologic and Clinical Chemistry Findings: The incidence of laboratory adverse experiences was similar in patients treated with JANUVIA 100 mg compared to patients treated with placebo. In most clinical studies, a slight decrease in alkaline phosphatase and small increases in uric acid and white blood cell count (due to an increase in neutrophils) were observed. In active comparator studies versus metformin or versus a sulfonylurea agent (glipizide) similar changes were seen in alkaline phosphatase and uric acid.

Study	Treatment Group	Mean Change From Baseline (standard error) Alkaline Phosphatase (IU/L)	Uric Acid (mg/dL)	WBC (cell/microl)
Placebo-controlled (monotherapy)	Sitagliptin	−5.3 (0.5)	0.26 (0.04)	320.2 (71.7)
	Placebo	−0.8 (0.5)	−0.05 (0.05)	58.6 (80.0)
Active-controlled (monotherapy)	Sitagliptin	−3.9 (0.5)	−0.0 (0.0)	220.4 (77.7)
	Metformin	−4.7 (0.5)	0.1 (0.0)	184.7 (66.6)
Placebo-controlled (add-on to metformin)	Sitagliptin	−3.1 (0.4)	0.17 (0.04)	346.0 (64.3)
	Placebo	−1.3 (0.7)	0.05 (0.06)	142.4 (98.8)
Active-controlled (add-on to metformin)	Sitagliptin	−5.7 (0.5)	0.21 (0.05)	207.8 (67.4)
	Glipizide	−3.4 (0.5)	0.20 (0.05)	86.0 (62.5)

Post-Market Adverse Drug Reactions: The following additional adverse reactions have been identified during post-marketing use of JANUVIA. Because these reactions are reported voluntarily from a population of uncertain size, it is generally not possible to reliably estimate their frequency or establish a causal relationship to drug exposure.

Hypersensitivity reactions include anaphylaxis, angioedema, rash, urticaria, cutaneous vasculitis, and exfoliative skin conditions, including Stevens-Johnson syndrome (see Contraindications and Warnings and Precautions, Hypersensitivity Reactions); acute pancreatitis, including fatal and non-fatal hemorrhagic and necrotizing pancreatitis (see Warnings and Precautions).

DRUG INTERACTIONS: Overview: Sitagliptin is not an inhibitor of CYP isozymes CYP3A4, 2C8, 2C9, 2D6, 1A2, 2C19 or 2B6, and is not an inducer of CYP3A4. Sitagliptin is a p-glycoprotein substrate, but does not inhibit p-glycoprotein mediated transport of digoxin. Based on these results, sitagliptin is considered unlikely to cause interactions with other drugs that utilize these pathways.

Sitagliptin is not extensively bound to plasma proteins. Therefore, the propensity of sitagliptin to be involved in clinically meaningful drug-drug interactions mediated by plasma protein binding displacement is very low.

Drug-Drug Interactions: In clinical studies, as described below, sitagliptin did not meaningfully alter the pharmacokinetics of metformin, glyburide, simvastatin, rosiglitazone, warfarin, or oral contraceptives, providing in vivo evidence of a low propensity for causing drug interactions with substrates of CYP3A4, CYP2C8, CYP2C9, and organic cationic transporter (OCT).

Metformin: Co-administration of multiple twice-daily doses of sitagliptin with metformin, an OCT substrate, did not meaningfully alter the pharmacokinetics of metformin or JANUVIA in patients with type 2 diabetes. Therefore, sitagliptin is not an inhibitor of OCT-mediated transport.

Sulfonylureas: Single-dose pharmacokinetics of glyburide, a CYP2C9 substrate, were not meaningfully altered in subjects receiving multiple doses of sitagliptin. Clinically meaningful interactions would not be expected with other sulfonylureas (e.g., glipizide, tolbutamide, and glimepiride) which, like glyburide, are primarily eliminated by CYP2C9. The effect of sulfonylureas on the pharmacokinetics of sitagliptin was not assessed.

Simvastatin: Single-dose pharmacokinetics of simvastatin, a CYP3A4 substrate, were not meaningfully altered in subjects receiving multiple daily doses of sitagliptin. Therefore, sitagliptin is not an inhibitor of CYP3A4-mediated metabolism.

Thiazolidinediones: Single-dose pharmacokinetics of rosiglitazone were not meaningfully altered in subjects receiving multiple daily doses of sitagliptin. Therefore, sitagliptin is not an inhibitor of CYP2C8-mediated metabolism. Clinically meaningful interactions with pioglitazone are not expected because pioglitazone predominantly undergoes CYP2C8- or CYP3A4-mediated metabolism. The effect of thiazolidinediones on the pharmacokinetics of sitagliptin was not assessed.

Warfarin: Multiple daily doses of sitagliptin did not meaningfully alter the pharmacokinetics, as assessed by measurement of S(−) or R(+) warfarin enantiomers, or pharmacodynamics (as assessed by measurement of prothrombin INR) of a single dose of warfarin. Since S(−) warfarin is primarily metabolized by CYP2C9, these data also support the conclusion that sitagliptin is not a CYP2C9 inhibitor.

Oral Contraceptives: Co-administration with sitagliptin did not meaningfully alter the steady-state pharmacokinetics of norethindrone or ethinyl estradiol.

Digoxin: Sitagliptin had a minimal effect on the pharmacokinetics of digoxin. Following administration of 0.25 mg digoxin concomitantly with 100 mg of JANUVIA daily for 10 days, the plasma AUC of digoxin was increased by 11%, and the plasma C_{max} by 18%. These increases are not considered likely to be clinically meaningful. No dosage adjustment of digoxin or JANUVIA is recommended.

Cyclosporine: A study was conducted to assess the effect of cyclosporine, a potent inhibitor of p-glycoprotein, on the pharmacokinetics of sitagliptin. Co-administration of a single 100 mg oral dose of JANUVIA and a single 600 mg oral dose of cyclosporine increased the AUC and C_{max} of sitagliptin by approximately 29% and 68%, respectively. These modest changes in sitagliptin pharmacokinetics were not considered to be clinically meaningful. The renal clearance of sitagliptin was also not meaningfully altered. Therefore, meaningful interactions would not be expected with other p-glycoprotein inhibitors. No dosage adjustment for JANUVIA is recommended when co-administered with cyclosporine or other p-glycoprotein inhibitors (e.g., ketoconazole).

Drug-Food Interactions: There are no known interactions with food.

Drug-Herb Interactions: Interactions with herbal products have not been established.

Drug-Laboratory Test Interactions: Interactions with laboratory tests have not been established.

Drug-Lifestyle Interactions: No studies of the effects of JANUVIA on the ability to drive and use machines have been performed. However, JANUVIA is not expected to affect the ability to drive and use machines. When JANUVIA is used in combination with metformin and sulfonylurea, patients should be advised to take precautions to avoid hypoglycaemia while driving or using machinery.

DOSAGE AND ADMINISTRATION:

Dosing Considerations: JANUVIA can be taken with or without food.

Recommended Dose and Dosage Adjustment: The recommended dose of JANUVIA is 100 mg once daily.

When JANUVIA is used in combination with metformin and a sulfonylurea, a lower dose of sulfonylurea may be considered to reduce the risk of hypoglycemia (see Warnings and Precautions, Hypoglycemia).

Patients with Renal Insufficiency: Use of sitagliptin in patients with moderate or severe renal insufficiency including those with ESRD is not recommended.

Patients with Hepatic Insufficiency: Use of sitagliptin in patients with severe hepatic insufficiency is not recommended.

Geriatrics: No dosage adjustment is necessary for geriatric patients.

Pediatrics: There are no data available on the use of JANUVIA in patients younger than 18 years of age. Therefore, use of JANUVIA in pediatric patients is not recommended.

Missed Dose: If a dose of JANUVIA is missed, it should be taken as soon as the patient remembers. A double dose of JANUVIA should not be taken on the same day.

OVERDOSAGE:
During controlled clinical trials in healthy subjects, single doses of up to 800 mg JANUVIA were generally well tolerated. Minimal increases in QTc, not considered to be clinically relevant, were observed in one study at a dose of 800 mg JANUVIA (see Action and Clinical Pharmacology). There is no experience with doses above 800 mg in clinical trials.

In the event of an overdose, it is reasonable to employ the usual supportive measures, e.g., remove unabsorbed material from the gastrointestinal tract, employ clinical monitoring (including obtaining an electrocardiogram), and institute supportive therapy if required.

Sitagliptin is modestly dialyzable. In clinical studies, approximately 13.5% of the dose was removed over a 3- to 4-hour hemodialysis session. Prolonged hemodialysis may be considered if clinically appropriate. It is not known if sitagliptin is dialyzable by peritoneal dialysis.

> For management of a suspected drug overdose, contact your regional Poison Control Centre. See the *CPS* Directory section for a list of Poison Control Centres.

ACTION AND CLINICAL PHARMACOLOGY: Mechanism of Action: JANUVIA is an orally-active, potent, and highly selective inhibitor of the dipeptidyl peptidase 4 (DPP-4) enzyme for the treatment of type 2 diabetes. The DPP-4 inhibitors are a novel class of agents that act as incretin enhancers.

Incretin hormones, including glucagon-like peptide-1 (GLP-1) and glucose-dependent insulinotropic polypeptide (GIP), are released by the intestine throughout the day, and levels are increased in response to a meal. The incretins are part of an endogenous system involved in the physiologic regulation of glucose homeostasis. When blood glucose concentrations are normal or elevated, GLP-1 and GIP increase insulin synthesis and release from pancreatic beta cells by intracellular signaling pathways involving cyclic AMP. Progressive beta-cell failure is a feature characterizing the pathogenesis of type 2 diabetes. Treatment with GLP-1 or with DPP-4 inhibitors in animal models of type 2 diabetes has been demonstrated to improve beta cell responsiveness to glucose and stimulate insulin biosynthesis and release. With higher insulin levels, tissue glucose uptake is enhanced.

In addition, GLP-1 lowers glucagon secretion from pancreatic alpha cells. Decreased glucagon concentrations, along with higher insulin levels, lead to reduced hepatic glucose production, resulting in a decrease in blood glucose levels. When blood glucose concentrations are low, stimulation of insulin release and suppression of glucagon secretion by GLP-1 are not observed. GLP-1 does not impair the normal glucagon response to hypoglycemia.

The activity of GLP-1 and GIP is limited by the DPP-4 enzyme, which rapidly hydrolyzes the incretin hormones to produce inactive products. Sitagliptin prevents the hydrolysis of incretin hormones by DPP-4, thereby increasing plasma concentrations of the active forms of GLP-1 and GIP. By enhancing active incretin levels, sitagliptin increases insulin release and decreases glucagon levels in a glucose-dependent manner.

In patients with type 2 diabetes with hyperglycemia, these changes in insulin and glucagon levels lead to lower hemoglobin A_{1c} (HbA_{1c}) and lower fasting and postprandial glucose concentrations Sitagliptin demonstrates selectivity for DPP-4, and does not inhibit the DPP-8 or DPP-9 activity in vitro at concentrations approximating those from therapeutic doses. Inhibition of DPP-8 or DPP-9, but not DPP-4, is associated with toxicity in preclinical animal models and alteration of immune function in vitro.

Pharmacodynamics: In patients with type 2 diabetes, administration of single oral doses of JANUVIA leads to inhibition of DPP-4 enzyme activity for a 24-hour period, resulting in a 2- to 3-fold increase in circulating levels of active GLP-1 and GIP, increased plasma levels of insulin and C-peptide, decreased glucagon concentrations, reduced fasting glucose, and reduced glucose excursion following an oral glucose load or a meal.

In a study of patients with type 2 diabetes inadequately controlled on metformin monotherapy (N=26), glucose levels monitored throughout the day were significantly lower (p<0.001) in patients who received sitagliptin 100 mg per day (50 mg twice daily) in combination with metformin compared with patients who received placebo with metformin (see Figure 1).

Figure 1: JANUVIA

24-Hour Plasma Glucose Profile After 4-Week Treatment with Sitagliptin 50 mg BID with Metformin or Placebo with Metformin

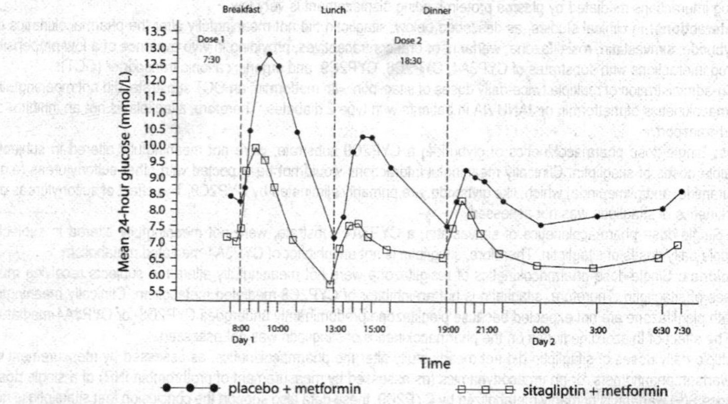

In studies with healthy subjects, JANUVIA did not lower blood glucose or cause hypoglycemia, suggesting that the insulinotropic and glucagon suppressive actions of the drug are glucose dependent.

Cardiac Electrophysiology: In a randomized, placebo-controlled crossover study, 79 healthy subjects were administered a single oral dose of JANUVIA 100 mg, JANUVIA 800 mg (8 times the recommended dose), and placebo. At the recommended dose of 100 mg, there was no effect on the QTc interval obtained at the peak plasma concentration, or at any other time during the study. Following the 800 mg dose, the maximum increase in the placebo-corrected mean change in QTc from baseline at 3 hours postdose was 8.0 msec. This small increase was not considered to be clinically significant. At the 800 mg dose, peak sitagliptin plasma concentrations were approximately 11 times higher than the peak concentrations following a 100 mg dose.

In patients with type 2 diabetes administered JANUVIA 100 mg (N=81) or JANUVIA 200 mg (N=63) daily, there were no meaningful changes in QTc interval based on ECG data obtained at the time of expected peak plasma concentration.

Pharmacokinetics: See Table 6.

Table 6: JANUVIA

Summary of Sitagliptin's Pharmacokinetic Parameters in Healthy Volunteers

	C_{max} nM	$t_{½}$ (h)	$AUC_{0-\infty}$ μM·hr	Renal Clearance mL/min	Volume of Distribution (L)[a]
Single oral dose (100 mg) mean	950	12.4	8.52	350	198

[a] Volume of distribution at steady state following an I.V. dose.

The pharmacokinetics of sitagliptin have been extensively characterized in healthy subjects and patients with type 2 diabetes. After oral administration of a 100 mg dose to healthy subjects, sitagliptin was rapidly absorbed, with peak plasma concentrations (median T_{max}) occurring 1 to 4 hours post-dose. Plasma AUC of sitagliptin increased in a dose-proportional manner. Following a single oral 100 mg dose to healthy volunteers, mean plasma AUC of sitagliptin was 8.52 μM·hr, C_{max} was 950 nM, and apparent terminal half-life ($t_{1/2}$) was 12.4 hours. Plasma AUC of sitagliptin increased approximately 14% following 100 mg doses at steady-state compared to the first dose. The intra-subject and inter-subject coefficients of variation for sitagliptin AUC were small (5.8% and 15.1%). The pharmacokinetics of sitagliptin were generally similar in healthy subjects and in patients with type 2 diabetes.

Absorption: The absolute bioavailability of sitagliptin is approximately 87%. Since coadministration of a high-fat meal with JANUVIA had no effect on the pharmacokinetics, JANUVIA may be administered with or without food.

Distribution: The mean volume of distribution at steady state following a single 100 mg intravenous dose of sitagliptin to healthy subjects is approximately 198 liters. The fraction of sitagliptin reversibly bound to plasma proteins is low (38%).

Metabolism: Sitagliptin is primarily eliminated unchanged in urine, and metabolism is a minor pathway. Approximately 79% of sitagliptin is excreted unchanged in the urine.

Following a [^{14}C] sitagliptin oral dose, approximately 16% of the radioactivity was excreted as metabolites of sitagliptin. Six metabolites were detected at trace levels and are not expected to contribute to the plasma DPP-4 inhibitory activity of sitagliptin. In vitro studies indicated that the primary enzyme responsible for the limited metabolism of sitagliptin was CYP3A4, with contribution from CYP2C8.

Excretion: Following administration of an oral [^{14}C] sitagliptin dose to healthy subjects, approximately 100% of the administered radioactivity was eliminated in feces (13%) or urine (87%) within one week of dosing. The apparent terminal $t_{½}$ following a 100 mg oral dose of sitagliptin was approximately 12.4 hours and renal clearance was approximately 350 mL/min.

Elimination of sitagliptin occurs primarily via renal excretion and involves active tubular secretion. Sitagliptin is a substrate for human organic anion transporter-3 (hOAT-3), which may be involved in the renal elimination of sitagliptin. The clinical relevance of hOAT-3 in sitagliptin transport has not been established. Sitagliptin is also a substrate of p-glycoprotein, which may also be involved in mediating the renal elimination of sitagliptin. However, cyclosporine, a p-glycoprotein inhibitor, did not reduce the renal clearance of sitagliptin.

Special Populations and Conditions: Pediatrics: No studies with JANUVIA have been performed in pediatric patients.

Geriatrics: No dosage adjustment is required based on age. Age did not have a clinically meaningful impact on the pharmacokinetics of sitagliptin based on a population pharmacokinetic analysis of Phase I and Phase II data. Elderly subjects (65 to 80 years) had approximately 19% higher plasma concentrations of sitagliptin compared to younger subjects.

Gender: No dosage adjustment is necessary based on gender. Gender had no clinically meaningful effect on the pharmacokinetics of sitagliptin based on a composite analysis of Phase I pharmacokinetic data and on a population pharmacokinetic analysis of Phase I and Phase II data.

Race: No dosage adjustment is necessary based on race. Race had no clinically meaningful effect on the pharmacokinetics of sitagliptin based on a composite analysis of Phase I pharmacokinetic data and on a population pharmacokinetic analysis of Phase I and Phase II data, including subjects of white, Hispanic, black and Asian racial groups.

Hepatic Insufficiency: In patients with moderate hepatic insufficiency (Child-Pugh score 7 to 9), mean AUC and C_{max} of sitagliptin increased approximately 21% (90% CI: 1%, 46%) and 13% (90% CI: −9%, 42%), respectively, compared to healthy matched controls following administration of a single 100 mg dose of JANUVIA.

Renal Insufficiency: An approximately 2-fold increase in the plasma AUC of sitagliptin was observed in patients with moderate renal insufficiency, and an approximately 4-fold increase was observed in patients with severe renal insufficiency and in patients with ESRD on hemodialysis, as compared to normal healthy control subjects.

STORAGE AND STABILITY: Store at room temperature (15 to 30°C).

INFORMATION FOR THE PATIENT: Published in e-CPS, available by subscription at www.e-cps.ca.

DOSAGE FORMS, COMPOSITION AND PACKAGING: Each beige, round, film-coated tablet with "277" on one side, contains: sitagliptin phosphate monohydrate 128.5 mg which is equivalent to 100 mg of free base. Nonmedicinal ingredients: anhydrous dibasic calcium phosphate (calcium hydrogen phosphate, anhydrous), croscarmellose sodium, magnesium stearate, microcrystalline cellulose and sodium stearyl fumarate; film coating: polyethylene glycol (macrogol), polyvinyl alcohol, red iron oxide, talc, titanium dioxide and yellow iron oxide. Bottles of 30 and 100.

(Shown in Product Identification Section)

Jurnista™ Ⓝ

hydromorphone HCl

Opioid Analgesic

Janssen-Ortho

Date of Preparation: November 17, 2009
Date of Revision: March 8, 2010

SUMMARY PRODUCT INFORMATION:

Route of Administration	Dosage Form/ Strength	All Nonmedicinal Ingredients
Oral	Prolonged-Release Tablet 4 mg, 8 mg, 16 mg and 32 mg	Butyl hydroxytoluene, cellulose acetate, glycerol triacetate, iron oxide black, ferric oxide red (8 mg only), ferric oxide yellow (16 mg and 32 mg only), hypromellose, lactose anhydrous, lactose monohydrate, macrogol, magnesium stearate, polyethylene oxide, povidone, propylene glycol, sodium chloride and titanium dioxide. JURNISTA may contain traces of sodium metabisulfite.

INDICATIONS AND CLINICAL USE: Adults: JURNISTA (hydromorphone hydrochloride) tablets are indicated for the management of moderate to severe chronic pain in adults who require continuous around-the-clock opioid analgesia.

Geriatrics (>65 years of age): The elderly are more prone to central nervous system (CNS) adverse effects, gastrointestinal disturbances and physiological reduction of renal function. Caution is advised during initiation and maintenance treatment, especially if there are concomitant medications (see Dosage and Administration).

Pediatrics (<18 years of age): The use of JURNISTA in children under 18 years of age is not recommended, as dosage requirements for the safe and efficacious use of JURNISTA have not been established for this patient population.

CONTRAINDICATIONS: JURNISTA (hydromorphone hydrochloride) is contraindicated in:

- Patients who are hypersensitive to this drug or to any ingredient in the formulation or component of the container. For a complete listing of excipients, see Dosage Forms, Composition and Packaging.
- Patients who have had surgical procedures and/or underlying disease that may result in narrowing of the gastrointestinal tract, or have "blind loops" of the gastrointestinal tract or gastrointestinal obstruction.
- Patients who have ileus of any type.
- Patients with suspected surgical abdomen (e.g., acute appendicitis or pancreatitis).
- Patients with mild, intermittent or short duration pain that can otherwise be managed.
- The management of acute pain.
- The management of perioperative pain.
- Patients with acute asthma or other obstructive airway, and status asthmaticus.
- Patients with acute respiratory depression, elevated carbon dioxide levels in the blood, and cor pulmonale.
- Patients with acute alcoholism, delirium tremens, and convulsive disorders.
- Patients with severe CNS depression, increased cerebrospinal or intracranial pressure, and head injury.
- Patients taking monoamine oxidase (MAO) inhibitors (or within 14 days of such therapy).
- Women during pregnancy, labour and delivery.

WARNINGS AND PRECAUTIONS: General: JURNISTA (hydromorphone hydrochloride) tablets must be swallowed whole. JURNISTA tablets should never be chewed, divided, or crushed. Taking broken or divided JURNISTA could lead to the uncontrolled release and absorption of a potentially fatal dose of hydromorphone.

Tablet strengths of 16 mg or higher are only for opioid tolerant patients requiring hydromorphone equivalent dosages of 16 mg or higher per day. These doses may lead to severe medical consequences, including fatal respiratory depression, in patients not previously exposed to similar daily doses of opioids at the time of switching to JURNISTA.

JURNISTA is for continuous opioid coverage, given once a day in patients who require treatment for several days or more. Because it may be more time consuming to titrate a patient not routinely taking opioids to adequate analgesia using a controlled-release opioid preparation, it is advisable to have patients titrated to a satisfactory level of pain relief with an immediate-release opioid prior to conversion to the appropriate total daily dose of JURNISTA.

Patients who have received JURNISTA should be closely monitored, especially for signs of respiratory depression, until a stable maintenance dose is reached. Since alcohol increases the sedative effect of opioids, the concomitant use of JURNISTA and alcohol should be avoided.

Gastrointestinal: Potential for Gastrointestinal Obstruction: Because the JURNISTA tablet is non-deformable and does not appreciably change in shape in the gastrointestinal (GI) tract, JURNISTA should not be administered to patients with pre-existing severe GI narrowing (pathologic or iatrogenic, for example: esophageal motility disorders, small bowel inflammatory disease, "short gut" syndrome due to adhesions or decreased transit time, past history of peritonitis, cystic fibrosis, chronic intestinal pseudo-obstruction, or Meckel's diverticulum) or in patients with dysphagia or significant difficulty in swallowing tablets.

There have been very rare reports of obstructive symptoms in patients with known strictures in association with the ingestion of medicinal products in non-deformable controlled-release formulations (see Adverse Reactions).
Constipation: JURNISTA causes a reduction in gastrointestinal motility associated with an increase in smooth muscle tone. Constipation is a frequent side effect reported with opioid treatment. Patients should be advised on measures to prevent constipation and prophylactic laxative use should be considered. Extra caution should be used in patients with chronic constipation.
Gastrointestinal Transition: Clinical conditions or medical products that cause a sudden and significant shortening of gastrointestinal transit time may result in decreased hydromorphone absorption from JURNISTA and may potentially lead to withdrawal symptoms in patients with a physical dependence on opioids. Appropriate coverage with an immediate-release opioid formulation should be considered.

Due to the controlled-release design, JURNISTA tablets should only be used in patients who are able to swallow the tablets whole. The JURNISTA tablet is non-deformable and does not appreciably change in shape in the GI tract. Patients should be advised that the depleted JURNISTA shells are excreted in their stool in the original shape.
Acute Abdominal Conditions: The administration of opioids may obscure the diagnosis or clinical course of acute abdominal conditions. Therefore, it is important to make sure that the patient is not suffering from intestinal occlusion, including ileus, before initiation of treatment.
Abuse and Diversion: JURNISTA tablets are intended for oral use only. Abuse can lead to overdose and even death. This risk is increased when the tablet is crushed, broken, or chewed, and with concurrent consumption of alcohol or other CNS depressants. With abuse by parenteral route, the tablet contents may cause lethal complications.

Patients must be instructed **not** to give JURNISTA to anyone else. Diversion will have serious medical consequences, including death.
Dependence/Tolerance: JURNISTA contains hydromorphone, a strong opioid. Tolerance and physical dependence tend to develop upon repeated administration of hydromorphone, and there is a potential for development of psychological dependence. However, tolerance as well as both physical and psychological dependence, are not by themselves evidence of an addictive disorder or abuse. Iatrogenic addiction following appropriate opioid administration for pain relief is relatively rare.

Physical dependence is a state of adaptation that is manifested by an opioid-specific withdrawal syndrome that can be produced by abrupt cessation, rapid dose reduction, decreasing blood level of the drug, and/or administration of an antagonist. The opioid abstinence or withdrawal syndrome is characterized by some or all of the following: restlessness, lacrimation, rhinorrhea, yawning, perspiration, chills, piloerection, myalgia, mydriasis, irritability, anxiety, backache, joint pain, weakness, abdominal cramps, insomnia, nausea, anorexia, vomiting, diarrhea, or increased blood pressure, respiratory rate, or heart rate. In general, opioids should not be abruptly discontinued (see Dosage and Administration, Cessation of Therapy).

JURNISTA should be used with caution in patients with alcoholism and other drug dependencies, due to the increased frequency of opioid tolerance and psychological dependence observed in these patient populations.

With abuse by parenteral route, the tablet excipients may cause lethal complications.
Cardiovascular: Hypotension: Opioid analgesics, including hydromorphone, may cause severe hypotension in an individual whose ability to maintain blood pressure is compromised because of lower blood volume or concomitant administration of drugs such as phenothiazines or general anesthetics (see Drug Interactions, Drug-Drug Interactions).
Endocrine and Metabolism: JURNISTA should be administered with caution and in reduced dosages in patients with adrenocortical insufficiency, myxedema, and hypothyroidism.
Genitourinary: JURNISTA, like all opioid analgesics, should be administered with caution and in reduced dosages in patients with prostatic hypertrophy or urethral stricture.
Hepatic/Biliary/Pancreatic: Patients with moderate hepatic insufficiency should be started on a reduced JURNISTA dose and be closely monitored. If indicated, great caution and careful monitoring should be exercised for patients with severe hepatic insufficiency (see Dosage and Administration).

Opioids can cause an increase in biliary tract pressure as a result of spasm in the sphincter of Oddi. Caution should, therefore, be exercised in the administration of JURNISTA to patients with inflammatory or obstructive bowel disorders, or acute pancreatitis secondary to biliary tract disease, and in patients about to undergo biliary surgery.
Neurologic: Head Injury and Increased Intracranial Pressure: The respiratory depressant effects of opioids with carbon dioxide retention and secondary elevation of cerebrospinal fluid pressure may be markedly exaggerated in the presence of head injury or raised intracranial pressure. Opioids produce effects that may obscure neurological signs of further increases in intracranial pressure in patients with head injuries. JURNISTA should only be administered under such circumstances when it is considered essential and then with extreme caution, and is contraindicated in patients with increased cerebrospinal or intracranial pressure, and head injury (see Contraindications).
Peri-Operative Considerations: JURNISTA is contraindicated for perioperative pain relief. In the case of planned chordotomy or other pain-relieving operations, patients should not be treated with JURNISTA within 24 hours before or after the operation. Thereafter, if JURNISTA is to be continued after the patient recovers from the postoperative period, a new dosage should be administered in accordance with the changed need for pain relief. The risk of withdrawal in opioid-tolerant patients should be addressed as clinically indicated (see Dosage and Administration, Cessation of Therapy).

The administration of analgesics in the perioperative period should be managed by health care providers with adequate training and experience (e.g., by an anesthesiologist).
Psychomotor Impairment: Hydromorphone may impair mental and/or physical ability required for the performance of potentially hazardous tasks such as driving a car or operating machinery. This is particularly likely at the start of therapy, following an increase in dose or change of preparation. Patients should be advised not to drive a car or operate machinery unless they are tolerant to the effects of JURNISTA.
Renal: Patients with moderate renal insufficiency should be started on a reduced JURNISTA dose and closely monitored during dose titration. In patients with severe renal insufficiency, an increased dosing interval should also be considered and these patients should, in addition, be monitored during maintenance therapy for development of opioid-related adverse reactions (see Dosage and Administration).
Respiratory: Respiratory Depression: Respiratory depression is the most important hazard of opioid preparations. JURNISTA should be used with extreme caution in patients having a substantially decreased respiratory reserve or pre-existing respiratory depression, and in patients with chronic obstructive pulmonary disease, hypoxia, or hypercapnia. Such patients are often less sensitive to the stimulatory effects of carbon dioxide (CO_2) on the respiratory centre and the respiratory depressant effects of hydromorphone may reduce respiratory drive to the point of apnea.

Severe pain antagonizes the respiratory-depressant effects of opioids. However, should pain suddenly subside, these effects may rapidly become manifest. Patients who are scheduled for regional anesthetic procedures or other interruptions of pain transmission pathways should not receive JURNISTA within 24 hours of the procedure. Concomitant administration of hydromorphone with other opioid analgesics is associated with an increased risk of respiratory failure. Therefore, it is important to reduce the dose of hydromorphone when other opioid analgesics are given concomitantly.
Sensitivity/Resistance: Galactose Intolerance: Lactose is a nonmedicinal ingredient in JURNISTA. Patients with rare hereditary diseases of galactose intolerance (galactosemia or glucose-galactose malabsorption) should not take this medicine.
Sulfite Allergy: JURNISTA may contain traces of sodium metabisulfite, a sulfite that may cause allergic-type reactions including anaphylactic symptoms and life-threatening or less severe asthmatic episodes in certain susceptible people. The overall prevalence of sulfite sensitivity in the general population is unknown and probably low. Sulfite sensitivity is seen more frequently in asthmatic than in non-asthmatic people.
Information to Be Provided to the Patient: A patient information sheet is included in the package of JURNISTA tablets dispensed to the patient.

Patients receiving JURNISTA should be given the following instructions by the physician:

1. Patients should be informed that accidental ingestion or use by individuals (including children) other than the patient for whom it was originally prescribed, may lead to severe, even fatal, consequences.
2. Patients should be advised that JURNISTA contains hydromorphone, an opioid pain medicine.
3. Patients should be advised that JURNISTA should only be taken as directed. The dose of JURNISTA should not be adjusted without consulting with a physician or other healthcare professional.
4. JURNISTA should be swallowed whole (not crushed, divided, or chewed) due to a risk of fatal hydromorphone overdose.
5. Patients should not combine JURNISTA with alcohol or other central nervous system depressants (sleep aids, tranquilizers) because dangerous additive effects may occur resulting in serious injury or death.
6. Patients should be advised to consult their physician or pharmacist if other medications are being used or will be used with JURNISTA.
7. Patients should be advised that if they have been receiving treatment with JURNISTA and cessation of therapy is indicated, it may be appropriate to taper the JURNISTA dose, rather than abruptly discontinue it, due to the risk of precipitating withdrawal symptoms.
8. Patients should be advised of the most common adverse reactions that may occur while taking JURNISTA: constipation, nausea, vomiting, somnolence, headache and dizziness.
9. Patients should be advised that JURNISTA may cause drowsiness, dizziness, or lightheadedness and may impair mental and/or physical ability required for the performance of potentially hazardous tasks (e.g., driving, operating machinery). Patients started on JURNISTA or patients whose dose has been adjusted should be advised not to drive a car or operate machinery unless they are tolerant to the effects of JURNISTA.
10. As with other opioids, patients taking JURNISTA should be advised of the potential for constipation; patients should be advised on measures to prevent constipation and prophylactic laxative use should be considered.
11. Patients should be advised that JURNISTA is a potential drug of abuse. They should protect it from theft or misuse.
12. Patients should be advised that JURNISTA should never be given to anyone other than the individual for whom it was prescribed.
13. Patients should be advised that JURNISTA 16 mg or higher is for use only in opioid-tolerant patients.

Special Populations: Pregnant Women: JURNISTA is contraindicated during pregnancy, labour and delivery due to impaired uterine contractility and the risk of neonatal respiratory depression. No clinical data on pregnant women exposed to JURNISTA are available. While studies in rats and rabbits have revealed no teratogenic effects, reproductive toxicity has been observed. Hydromorphone has been shown to cross the placental barrier in experimental animals. The potential teratogenic risk for humans from the use of hydromorphone and other opiates during pregnancy is unknown. Withdrawal symptoms may be observed in the newborn of mothers undergoing chronic opioid treatment (see Contraindications).
Nursing Women: Preclinical studies have shown that hydromorphone can be detected in the milk of lactating rats. Low concentrations of hydromorphone and other opioid analgesics have been detected in human milk in clinical studies. JURNISTA should not be used during breast-feeding.
Pediatrics (<18 years of age): The use of JURNISTA in children under 18 years of age is not recommended, as dosage requirements for the safe and efficacious use of JURNISTA have not been established for this patient population.
Geriatrics (>65 years of age): The elderly are more prone to CNS adverse effects and gastrointestinal disturbances, and physiological reduction of the renal function. Therefore, extra caution should be shown, and the initial dose should be reduced. Concomitant use of other medications, especially tricyclic antidepressants, increases the risk of confusion and constipation. Diseases of the prostate gland and the urinary tract are often seen in the elderly. This contributes to the increased risk of urinary retention.

ADVERSE REACTIONS: Adverse Drug Reaction Overview: The most common adverse reactions related to JURNISTA were opioid-related gastrointestinal events of constipation, nausea, and vomiting, and opioid-related nervous system events of somnolence, headache, and dizziness.

The most serious adverse reaction associated with opioid therapy is respiratory depression. Use of an opioid dose that is higher than the opioid tolerance level of the patient may lead to fatal respiratory depression. Respiratory depression due to overexposure may be more likely in certain subgroups of patients, such as in the elderly, in the debilitated, and in those suffering from conditions accompanied by hypoxia or hypercapnia when even moderate doses may lead to fatal respiratory depression (see Warnings and Precautions).
Clinical Trial Adverse Drug Reactions: Because clinical trials are conducted under very specific conditions the adverse reaction rates observed in the clinical trials may not reflect the rates observed in practice and should not be compared to the rates in the clinical trials of another drug. Adverse drug reaction information from clinical trials is useful for identifying drug-related adverse events and for approximating rates.

The safety of JURNISTA was evaluated from the safety data of 13 studies in chronic pain. The 13 studies were conducted in patients with cancer pain and non-malignant pain, including osteoarthritis (OA) pain, and low back pain. In total, 2335 patients had received JURNISTA for pain treatment.
Placebo-Controlled Studies: The placebo-controlled safety database for JURNISTA contains 268 patients with chronic low back pain, and 981 patients with osteoarthritis pain.
Low Back Pain: The study in chronic low back pain was a 12-week double-blind placebo-controlled, randomized withdrawal study with flexible dosing. A total of 447 patients were enrolled into the open-label titration phase with 268 patients randomized into the double-blind treatment phase. In the open-label phase, patients were converted to and titrated to a stable dose with JURNISTA.

At the beginning of the double-blind phase, patients were randomized (in a 1:1 ratio) to either JURNISTA or the matching placebo dosage, administered daily for up to 12 weeks. Patients who were randomized to placebo received JURNISTA in dosages tapering from their stable Conversion and Titration phase dosage to placebo over a maximum of 14 days.

Overall discontinuation rates during the double-blind phase were 50.7% in JURNISTA-treated patients and 67.2% in placebo-treated patients. There were no occurrences of gastrointestinal obstruction or respiratory depression.

The most common treatment-emergent adverse events (≥2%) reported during the titration phase were constipation, diarrhea, dry mouth, nausea, vomiting, drug withdrawal syndrome, fatigue, oedema peripheral, arthralgia, back pain, dizziness, headache, somnolence, anxiety, insomnia, hyperhidrosis and pruritus. Table 1 summarizes the treatment-emergent adverse events for JURNISTA and placebo-treated patients from the placebo-controlled low back pain study.

Table 1: JURNISTA
Treatment-Emergent Adverse Events Reported in a JURNISTA Chronic Pain Trial in Patients with Low Back Pain (≥1% and more frequent than the placebo group)

	JURNISTA % (n=134)	Placebo % (n=134)
Gastrointestinal Disorders		
Abdominal pain	1.5	0
Constipation	7.5	3.7
Dry mouth	1.5	0
Nausea	9.0	7.5
Toothache	2.2	0
Vomiting	6.0	4.5
General Disorders and Administration Site Conditions		
Irritability	1.5	0
Oedema Peripheral	2.2	0.7
Pyrexia	1.5	0.7
Infections and Infestations		
Bronchitis	1.5	0
Gastroenteritis	1.5	0
Gastroenteritis viral	1.5	0.7
Influenza	3.0	1.5
Sinusitis	4.5	0.7
Upper respiratory tract infection	3.0	2.2

(cont'd)

Table 1: JURNISTA *(cont'd)*

Treatment-Emergent Adverse Events Reported in a JURNISTA Chronic Pain Trial in Patients with Low Back Pain (≥1% and more frequent than the placebo group)

	JURNISTA % (n=134)	Placebo % (n=134)
Urinary tract infections	3.0	1.5
Investigations		
Weight decreased	3.0	2.2
Metabolism and Nutrition Disorders		
Dehydration	1.5	0.7
Musculoskeletal and Connective Tissue Disorders		
Arthralgia	6.0	2.2
Joint Swelling	1.5	0
Muscle Spasms	2.2	0.7
Pain in Extremity	1.5	0.7
Nervous System Disorders		
Dizziness	2.2	1.5
Hypersomnia	1.5	0
Psychiatric Disorders		
Insomnia	5.2	3.7
Respiratory, Thoracic and Mediastinal Disorders		
Nasal Congestion	2.2	1.5
Oropharyngeal Pain	1.5	0
Respiratory Tract Congestion	1.5	0
Rhinorrhoea	1.5	0.7
Vascular Disorders		
Hypotension	1.5	0

Osteoarthritis Pain: In the placebo-controlled study with osteoarthritis pain, both opioid naïve and current opioid users were included. The current opioid users were receiving a daily morphine equivalent dose of <40 mg. All patients were randomly assigned to placebo or a fixed dose of JURNISTA (8 or 16 mg) with no dose adjustments allowed. Overall discontinuation rates were 43.7% (145/332 patients) from placebo treatment, 50.8% (162/319 patients) from the 8 mg treatment, and 61.2% (202/330 patients) from the 16 mg treatment. Adverse events were the predominant reason for discontinuation from active treatment and lack of analgesia was the predominant reason for discontinuation from placebo treatment. Adverse events that led to discontinuation of the active study medication were most frequently the common opioid-related events, constipation, nausea, somnolence, dizziness and headache. No deaths occurred during the study or within 30 days after completion of the study treatments. Table 2 summarizes the treatment-emergent adverse events for JURNISTA and placebo-treated patients from the placebo-controlled study in osteoarthritis pain.

Table 2: JURNISTA

Treatment-Emergent Adverse Events Reported in a JURNISTA Chronic Pain Trial in Patients with Osteoarthritis Pain (≥1% and more frequent than the placebo group)

	JURNISTA % (n=649)	Placebo % (n=332)
Cardiac Disorders		
Palpitations	1.1	0
Ear and Labyrinth Disorders		
Vertigo	1.5	0.6
Gastrointestinal Disorders		
Constipation	44.1	11.7
Nausea	33.3	9.6
Vomiting	10.3	2.1
Dry mouth	5.7	2.7
Dyspepsia	2.2	1.5
Abdominal pain	3.5	1.5
Flatulence	1.5	1.2
General Disorders and Administration Site Conditions		
Fatigue	8.0	2.4

(cont'd)

Table 2: JURNISTA *(cont'd)*

Treatment-Emergent Adverse Events Reported in a JURNISTA Chronic Pain Trial in Patients with Osteoarthritis Pain (≥1% and more frequent than the placebo group)

	JURNISTA % (n=649)	Placebo % (n=332)
Oedema	2.2	1.8
Pyrexia	1.1	0
Infections and Infestations		
Influenza	2.8	2.4
Gastroenteritis viral	2.3	0.9
Urinary tract infections	1.5	0.6
Viral infection	1.5	0.3
Injury, Poisoning and Procedural Complications		
Contusion	1.1	0.9
Investigations		
Weight decreased	1.4	0.3
Metabolism and Nutrition Disorders		
Decreased appetite	2.5	0.6
Anorexia	1.8	0.3
Musculoskeletal and Connective Tissue Disorders		
Arthralgia	2.9	2.1
Nervous System Disorders		
Headache	12.9	11.4
Somnolence	15.7	4.8
Dizziness	12.6	6.0
Lethargy	1.7	0
Paraesthesia	1.1	0.9
Tremor	1.2	0.6
Psychiatric Disorders		
Insomnia	4.8	3.3
Anxiety	2.6	0.9
Depression	1.5	0.3
Irritability	1.1	0.3
Libido decreased	1.2	0
Respiratory, Thoracic and Mediastinal Disorders		
Pharyngolaryngeal pain	1.8	0.6
Dyspnoea	1.4	0.6
Skin and Subcutaneous Tissue Disorders		
Pruritus	11.2	2.4
Hyperhidrosis	2.8	0
Rash	2.0	0.6
Vascular Disorders		
Hot flush	1.1	0

All Clinical Studies: The following treatment-emergent adverse reactions were identified premarketing based on pooling the safety data from the 13 studies. Of the 2335 patients who had received JURNISTA, 420 patients were treated with JURNISTA for at least 6 months, while 141 patients were treated with JURNISTA for more than 12 months.

A total of 64 deaths were reported in the 13 studies during or after JURNISTA treatment. Fifty-eight deaths were attributed to cancer and six were associated with other conditions (cardiac arrest in two patients and sepsis, respiratory failure/dehydration, myocardial infarction, and congestive heart failure, each in one patient). All of the deaths were considered unrelated or unlikely related to drug treatment.

Respiratory depression was reported in one patient with cancer pain. The event, which occurred on day 263 of JURNISTA treatment, was considered mild in intensity and definitely related to drug treatment but did not require cessation of JURNISTA treatment. Six gastrointestinal obstructive events were reported: small intestinal obstruction in two patients; and intestinal obstruction, fecaloma, bezoar, and gastric outlet obstruction, each in one patient. All events occurred in the context of predisposing conditions (i.e., pathologic or iatrogenic gastrointestinal narrowing, Crohn's disease, colon cancer, colon resection, colon tortuosity, previous bowel obstruction, gall bladder surgery, gastric ulcer, vagotomy, antrectomy, pyloroplasty, and chronic constipation with chronic laxative abuse). For the bezoar and fecaloma events, there was no evidence of OROS shells in the impacted material.

The most common treatment-emergent adverse reactions related to JURNISTA were opioid-related gastrointestinal events of constipation, nausea, and vomiting, and opioid-related nervous system events of somnolence, headache, and dizziness. The safety profile for JURNISTA is consistent with those of other strong opioids.

Clinical Trial Treatment-Emergent Adverse Reactions: Following are the treatment-emergent adverse reactions from the 13 JURNISTA studies in patients with chronic pain: See Table 3.

Table 3: JURNISTA
Treatment-Emergent Adverse Reactions

System Organ Class	Treatment-Emergent Adverse Reaction Frequency Very Common (≥10%)	Common (≥1% to <10%)	Uncommon (≥0.1% to 1%)	Rare (≥0.01% to 0. 1%)
Cardiac Disorders		tachycardia	palpitations, extrasystoles	bradycardia
Ear and Labyrinth Disorders		vertigo	tinnitus	
Endocrine Disorders				hypogonadism
Eye Disorders		vision blurred	diplopia, dry eye	miosis
Gastrointestinal Disorders	constipation, nausea, vomiting	diarrhea, abdominal pain, dry mouth, dyspepsia, dysphagia, flatulence	haematochezia, abdominal distension, haemorrhoids, abnormal faeces, intestinal obstruction, diverticulum, eructation, gastrointestinal motility disorder, large intestine perforation	anal fissure, bezoar, duodenitis, ileus, impaired gastric emptying, painful defaecation
General Disorders and Administration Site Conditions	Asthenia	edema, pyrexia, pain, chest discomfort, chills, drug withdrawal syndrome	malaise, feeling abnormal, feeling jittery, difficulty in walking, hangover	feeling drunk, feeling hot and cold, hypothermia
Infections and Infestations			gastroenteritis, diverticulitis	
Injury, Poisoning and Procedural Complications		fall, contusion	overdose	
Investigations		weight decreased	oxygen saturation decreased, blood potassium decreased, hepatic enzyme increased, blood amylase increased	blood testosterone decreased
Metabolism and Nutrition Disorders		anorexia, dehydration	fluid retention, increased appetite, hyperuricaemia	
Musculoskeletal and Connective Tissue Disorders		muscle spasms, back pain, arthralgia, pain in extremity	myalgia	
Nervous System Disorders	somnolence, headache, dizziness	hypoaesthesia paraesthesia, tremor, sedation, memory impairment, disturbance in attention, dysgeusia	dysarthria, syncope, balance disorder, coordination abnormal, depressed level of consciousness, hyperaesthesia, dyskinesia, myoclonus, encephalopathy, cognitive disorder, psychomotor hyperactivity, fits/convulsions	hyperreflexia
Psychiatric Disorders		insomnia, anxiety, depression, confusional state, nervousness, abnormal dreams, restlessness, hallucination, mood altered	libido decreased, panic attack, euphoric mood, listless, paranoia, aggression, crying, suicide ideation	dysphoria
Renal and Urinary Disorders		dysuria, urinary retention	pollakiuria, urinary hesitation, micturition disorder	
Reproductive System and Breast Disorders			erectile dysfunction, sexual dysfunction	
Respiratory, Thoracic and Mediastinal Disorders		dyspnea	rhinorrhoea, hypoxia, respiratory distress, bronchospasm, hyperventilation, sneezing	respiratory depression
Skin and Subcutaneous Tissue Disorders		pruritus, hyperhidrosis, rash	erythema	
Vascular Disorders		flushing, hypertension	hypotension	

DRUG INTERACTIONS: Overview: The low level of protein binding of hydromorphone to human plasma proteins (less than 30%) makes it unlikely to result in protein-displacement drug-drug interactions.

In vitro and in vivo data suggest that hydromorphone in clinical practice has minimal potential to moderate the activity of human hepatic CYP450 activities. Metabolism of hydromorphone is predominantly through conjugation with glucuronic acid as a first-pass effect, with no identified active metabolites and with little potential for drug-drug interactions at the level of metabolizing enzymes.

CNS depressants, such as other opioids, anesthetics, sedatives, hypnotics, barbiturates, phenothiazines, chloral hydrate and glutethimide may enhance the depressant effects of hydromorphone. MAO inhibitors (including procarbazine HCl) should not be taken within two weeks of use. Pyrazolidone antihistamines, beta-blockers and alcohol may also enhance the depressant effects of hydromorphone. When combined therapy is contemplated, the dose of one or both agents should be reduced.

Drug-Drug Interactions: CNS Depressants: CNS depressants, such as other opioids, general anesthetics, sedatives, hypnotics, barbiturates, phenothiazines, other antipsychotics, and glutethimide may enhance the depressant effects of hydromorphone. The concomitant use of central nervous system depressants may cause additive depressant effects and respiratory depression. Additionally, hypotension and profound sedation or coma may occur. Pyrazolidone antihistamines, beta-blockers and alcohol may also enhance the depressant effects of hydromorphone. When this combination therapy is indicated with these drugs, the dose of one or both agents should be reduced.

JURNISTA, like other opioids, may enhance the neuromuscular blocking action of muscle relaxants and may cause an increased degree of respiratory depression.

The concomitant use of alcohol should be avoided. Alcohol increases the sedative effect of hydromorphone.

Monoamine Oxidase Inhibitors: Monoamine oxidase inhibitors (MAOIs) may cause CNS excitation or depression, hypotension or hypertension if co-administered with opioids. JURNISTA is contraindicated in patients taking MAOIs or within 14 days of stopping such treatment. MAO inhibitors (including procarbazine) should not be taken within two weeks of using JURNISTA.

Mixed Agonist-antagonist Opioid Analgesics: The concomitant use of hydromorphone (a pure opioid agonist) with mixed agonist-antagonist opioid analgesics (buprenorphine, nalbuphine, pentazocine) could lead to a reduction of the analgesic effect by competitive blocking of receptors, thus leading to a risk of withdrawal symptoms. Therefore, this combination is not recommended.

Alcohol Interaction Studies: In vitro dissolution studies have demonstrated no dose dumping with JURNISTA in the presence of 4, 20, or 40% alcohol (% v/v) with continuous exposure to alcohol over 24 hours.

The effect of co-administering 240 mL 4-40% alcohol on the pharmacokinetics of hydromorphone from a 16 mg JURNISTA tablet was evaluated in healthy subjects. The maximum concentration of hydromorphone (C_{max}) increased on average between 10 to 31% with the co-administration of alcohol. Median T_{max} values were similar across treatment groups and there were no effects seen in AUC values (see Action and Clinical Pharmacology, Pharmacokinetics).

Co-administration of 240 mL 4%, 20% and 40% alcohol (% v/v) increased C_{max} on average by 17%, 31% and 28% for 4%, 20% and 40% alcohol respectively in the fasting state; C_{max} was less affected in the fed state with increases at 14%, 14% and 10%, respectively. The observed variation in C_{max} is consistent with inter-subject variability associated with the use of immediate-release opioids. Median T_{max} in the presence/absence of alcohol remains between 12-16 hours. No effect was seen on AUC values both in the fed and fasted state. Due to the OROS technology in JURNISTA, the extended-release properties of JURNISTA are maintained in the presence of alcohol. However, concomitant use of alcohol should be avoided (see Warnings and Precautions, General).

Drug-Food Interactions: No effects on the pharmacokinetics of JURNISTA were observed with administration of a high fat meal. JURNISTA can be taken with and without food.

Drug-Herb Interactions: Interactions with herbal products have not been established.

Drug-Laboratory Test Interactions: Interactions with laboratory tests have not been established.

Drug-Lifestyle Interactions: The concomitant use of alcohol should be avoided. Alcohol increases the sedative effect of hydromorphone.

DOSAGE AND ADMINISTRATION: Dosing Considerations:

- Safe and effective administration of JURNISTA to patients with pain depends upon a comprehensive assessment of the patient. The nature of the pain, as well as the patient's medical and analgesic history will affect the selection of the dose. Owing to the varied response to opioids observed between individuals, it is recommended that all patients be started at the lowest possible dose of opioid therapy and titrated to an adequate level of analgesia, balanced against acceptable adverse reactions. The lowest titration increment for JURNISTA is 4 mg.
- **JURNISTA must be swallowed whole. Do not chew, divide, or crush the tablet. Taking broken or crushed tablets could lead to the uncontrolled release and rapid absorption of a potentially fatal dose of hydromorphone.**
- **Tablet strengths of 16 mg and higher are only for opioid-tolerant patients requiring hydromorphone equivalent dosages of 16 mg or higher per day. These doses may lead to severe medical consequences, including fatal respiratory depression, in patients not previously exposed to similar daily doses of opioids.**
- Appropriate prophylaxis for known adverse reactions should be considered. For example, the prescription of antiemetics for nausea and vomiting, and an appropriate regimen of bowel management for constipation (stool softeners, laxatives etc.) should be considered.

Recommended Dose and Dosage Adjustment: The controlled-release nature of the formulation allows JURNISTA to be administered once every 24 hours. JURNISTA tablets should be taken at approximately the same time each day with a glass of water.

JURNISTA tablets can be taken with or without food. JURNISTA should not be taken more than once every 24 hours.

Dose Initiation:

- **Patients Currently Not Routinely Receiving Opioids**

  Because it takes 13-16 hours for JURNISTA to reach its maximum drug release, it is recommended to begin treatment with a conventional immediate-release preparation (e.g. immediate-release morphine or immediate-release hydromorphone). Once the patient achieves a steady balance between pain control and adverse reactions, the patient can be converted to the appropriate total daily dose of JURNISTA.

  The initial dose in patients who are opioid naïve or receiving low intermittent doses of weak opioid analgesics—less than 40 mg daily oral morphine equivalents—should be 4 mg every 24 hours. If the physician, based on clinical judgement, decides that a higher initial dose is warranted, 8 mg every 24 hours should not be exceeded. The dose may be titrated upwards or downwards, if required, in increments of either 4 or 8 mg depending on response and supplementary analgesic requirements.
- **Patients Currently Receiving Opioids Regularly**

  Discontinue all other around-the-clock opioid analgesic medications when JURNISTA therapy is initiated.

  In patients currently taking opioid analgesics, the starting dose of JURNISTA should be based on the prior daily opioid dose, using standard equianalgesic ratios. For opioids other than morphine, first estimate the equivalent total daily dose of morphine, then use Table 4 to determine the equivalent total daily dose of JURNISTA.

Table 4: JURNISTA
Multiplication Factors for Converting the Daily Dose of Prior Opioids to the Daily Dose of JURNISTA[a] (mg/day Prior Opioid×Factor=mg/day JURNISTA)

mg/day of Prior Opioid	Multiplication (factor) to obtain mg/day of JURNISTA
Morphine	0.2
Hydromorphone	1

[a] Conversion factors used in JURNISTA clinical trials.

No fixed conversion ratio is likely to be satisfactory in all patients, due to individual patient and formulation differences. Therefore, conversion to the recommended starting dose of JURNISTA followed by close patient monitoring and titration should be done.

Immediate-release hydromorphone daily dose or converted hydromorphone equivalent doses should be rounded down to the closest dose of JURNISTA available, and given once a day.

JURNISTA may be used with usual doses of non-opioid analgesics and analgesic adjuvants.

Individualization of Dosage and Maintenance of Therapy: After the initiation of therapy with JURNISTA, dose adjustments may be necessary to obtain the patient's best balance between pain relief and opioid-related adverse reactions.

If the pain increases in severity or analgesia is inadequate, a gradual increase in dosage may be required. In order to allow the effects of the dose change to stabilize, the dosage should not be increased more frequently than every two days. As a guideline, dosage increases of 25%-75% of the current daily dose of JURNISTA should be considered for each titration step.

Once patients become stable on a selected once-daily dose of JURNISTA, the dose may be continued for as long as pain relief is necessary. The continued need for around-the-clock opioid therapy and adjustments in therapy should be reassessed periodically as appropriate.

Some patients may require periodic supplemental doses of short-acting analgesic for "breakthrough" pain. The initial individual supplemental analgesia doses should generally not exceed 10% to 25% of the 24-hour JURNISTA dose.

Use in Children and Adolescents: JURNISTA is not recommended for use in children and adolescents below age 18 as dosage requirements for the safe and efficacious use of JURNISTA have not been established for this patient population.

Use in the Elderly: The medical setting of the elderly is often complex. Therefore, treatment with JURNISTA should be initiated cautiously at a reduced initial dose (see Warnings and Precautions, Special Populations).

Renal and Hepatic Impairment: Following single-dose administration of hydromorphone immediate-release tablets, the following results were observed in clinical studies:

- In patients with moderate hepatic insufficiency (scoring 7-9 on Child-Pugh rating scale), both exposure (plasma AUC) and peak plasma concentrations of hydromorphone were approximately 4 times higher compared with healthy controls, and elimination half-life was unaltered.
- In patients with moderate renal insufficiency (creatinine clearance of 40-60 mL/min), exposure (plasma AUC) to hydromorphone was approximately 2 times higher than in those with normal renal function, and elimination half-life was unaltered.
- In patients with severe renal insufficiency (creatinine clearance <30 mL/min), exposure (plasma AUC) to hydromorphone was approximately 4 times greater than in those with normal renal function, and elimination half-life 3 times longer.

Therefore, patients with moderate hepatic or renal insufficiency should be started on a reduced dose and closely monitored during dose titration. In patients with severe renal insufficiency, an increased dosing interval should also be considered and these patients should, in addition, be monitored during maintenance therapy for development of opioid-related adverse reactions.

Cessation of Therapy: In patients who are physically dependent on opioids and receiving daily administration of hydromorphone, abrupt discontinuation of treatment with JURNISTA will result in symptoms of withdrawal syndrome. Therefore, if cessation of therapy with JURNISTA is indicated in patients, a gradual downward titration in small increments, such as in steps of 50%, every 2 days is recommended until the lowest possible dose is reached, at which time therapy may be safely discontinued. If symptoms of withdrawal appear, tapering should be stopped. The dose should be slightly increased until the signs and symptoms of opioid withdrawal disappear. Tapering should then begin again, but with longer periods of time between each JURNISTA dose reduction, or before converting to an equianalgesic dose of another opioid to continue tapering.

Missed Dose: Patients should be advised not to take extra tablets or a double dose to make up for a missed dose. JURNISTA should be taken once approximately every 24 hours.

Administration: JURNISTA tablets should be swallowed whole with a glass of water, at approximately the same time each day. They should never be chewed, divided, or crushed.

OVERDOSAGE:

Symptoms: Opioid overdose is characterized by respiratory depression, drowsiness which progresses to stupor and coma, musculoskeletal flaccidity, cold skin, contracted pupils and, at times, tachycardia and hypotension. In cases of severe overdose apnea, circulatory collapse, cardiac arrest and death may occur.

Treatment: In the treatment of overdose, primary attention should be given to the re-establishment of adequate respiratory exchange by keeping the airway open and instituting assisted or controlled ventilation. If oral ingestion was recent, gastric contents may be emptied by gastric lavage, as indicated.

Supportive measures (including oxygen and vasopressors) should be used to manage the shock and pulmonary edema, which potentially accompany overdose. Cardiac arrest and arrhythmias may require cardiac massage or defibrillation.

In cases of severe overdose, specific antidotes such as naloxone should be used to manage respiratory depression (see the prescribing information for the specific opioid antagonist for details of proper use). The effect of naloxone is relatively short; therefore, the patient should be carefully monitored until respiration has stabilized. JURNISTA will release hydromorphone for approximately 24 hours. This should be taken into account in determining the treatment. Opioid antagonists should not be given in the absence of clinically significant respiratory depression, or circulatory depression caused by opioids. Opioid antagonists should be administered with caution to patients suspected to be physically dependent on hydromorphone, since rapid reversal of an opioid, including hydromorphone, may precipitate symptoms of withdrawal.

For management of a suspected drug overdose, contact your regional Poison Control Centre. See the *CPS* Directory section for a list of Poison Control Centres.

ACTION AND CLINICAL PHARMACOLOGY: Mechanism of Action: Hydromorphone, a semi-synthetic morphine derivative, is a hydrogenated ketone of morphine. Hydromorphone is principally an agonist of μ-receptors, showing a weak affinity for κ-receptors. Comparing relative binding affinity for μ- and κ-opioid receptors, hydromorphone binds more specifically to μ-receptors than structurally related morphine. Hydromorphone produces diverse pharmacological effects by binding to opioid receptors in the CNS and other tissues.

Pharmacodynamics: As with all opioid analgesics, hydromorphone exerts its principal pharmacological effects on the CNS and smooth muscle, including the gastrointestinal tract. These effects are expressed and modulated by binding to specific opioid receptors. Hydromorphone is principally an agonist of μ-receptors, showing a weak affinity for κ-receptors. Analgesia occurs as a consequence of the binding of hydromorphone to the μ-receptors of the CNS. Although estimates vary (from 2 to 10 times), oral hydromorphone appears to be approximately 5 times as potent (by weight) as morphine. Respiratory depression occurs principally by direct action on the cerebral respiratory control centres. Opioids may cause nausea and vomiting due to direct stimulation of the chemoreceptor for emesis in the posterior area of the medulla.

Pharmacokinetics: Absorption: Following a single oral dose of JURNISTA prolonged-release tablets, plasma concentrations gradually increase over 6 to 8 hours, and thereafter concentrations are sustained for approximately 18 to 24 hours post-dose; the mean T_{max} values were approximately 13 to 16 hours. This demonstrates that hydromorphone is released in a controlled manner consistent with once-daily dosing. The mean absolute bioavailability of hydromorphone from JURNISTA ranged from 22% to 26%.

Steady-state plasma concentrations are approximately twice those observed following the first dose, and steady state is reached by the fourth dose of JURNISTA. No time-dependent change in pharmacokinetics was seen with multiple dosing. At steady state, JURNISTA given once daily maintained hydromorphone plasma concentrations within the same concentration range as the immediate-release tablet given 4 times daily at the same total daily dose, and diminished the periodic fluctuations in plasma levels seen with the immediate-release tablet. The degree of fluctuation in plasma concentration at steady state during a 24-hour period was lower with JURNISTA (83%) as compared to the overall fluctuations of the immediate-release tablet (147%) (see Figure 1). At steady state, hydromorphone AUC for JURNISTA is equivalent to that observed for the immediate-release tablet dosed four times daily.

Figure 1: JURNISTA

Steady-State Plasma Hydromorphone Concentration-Time Curves

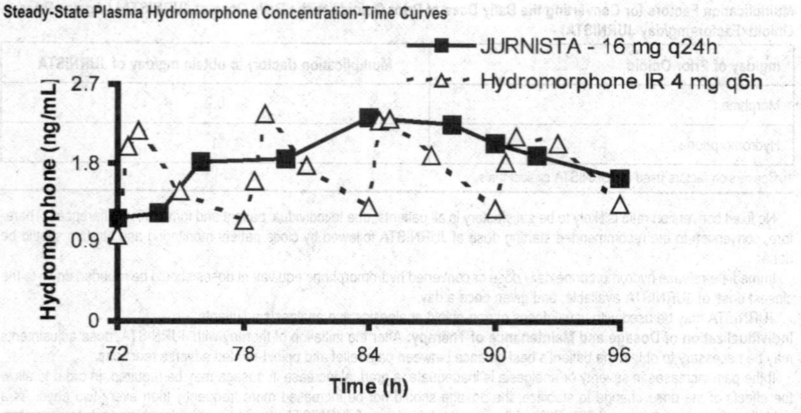

Linear pharmacokinetics has been demonstrated for JURNISTA over the dose range 4 to 64 mg, with a dose-proportional increase in plasma concentrations (C_{max}) and overall exposure ($AUC_{(0-48h)}$ and $AUC_{(0-inf)}$).

Studies with immediate-release hydromorphone indicated that food delayed the rate of absorption of hydromorphone, resulting in a 25% decrease in C_{max} and a 24% increase in AUC. The pharmacokinetics of JURNISTA (single dose 16 mg) was not affected by a high-fat meal. Bioequivalence (AUC and C_{max}) was demonstrated under fast and fed conditions. Therefore, JURNISTA can be administered with or without food.

In a study in patients with chronic pain who had been titrated with JURNISTA to control pain, plasma concentrations began to rise about two hours post-dose, achieving maximal values over a broad and sustained time period, similar to that observed with JURNISTA in healthy subjects. Pharmacokinetic/pharmacodynamic analysis indicated that, in general, rising and falling plasma hydromorphone concentrations correlated with decreasing and increasing pain, respectively.

In a study comparing hydromorphone absorption from JURNISTA taken with no alcohol and taken with 240 mL of 4%, 20% and 40% alcohol, C_{max} increased on average by 17%, 31%, and 28% respectively in the fasting state and was less affected in the fed state with increases of 14%, 14%, and 10%, respectively. Median T_{max} (fasted and fed) with 4%, 20% and 40% alcohol was 12-16 hours and with 0% alcohol was 16 hours. No effect was seen on AUC values both in the fed and fasted state. Concomitant use of alcohol should be avoided. Due to the OROS technology in JURNISTA, the prolonged-release properties of JURNISTA are maintained in the presence of alcohol. For the pharmacodynamic interactions (see Warnings and Precautions, General).

Distribution: The mean extent of binding of hydromorphone to human plasma proteins was determined to be <30% in an in vitro study.

Metabolism: Glucuronidation is the main metabolic pathway and the principal metabolite is the inactive hydromorphone 3-glucuronide, which follows a similar time course to hydromorphone in plasma. Unlike morphine, no active 6-glucuronide metabolite is produced.

First-pass metabolism is rapid and extensive. The elimination half-life for hydromorphone is approximately 2 hours.

Excretion: Following a single dose of [^{14}C]-hydromorphone, hydromorphone and total radiolabelled material disappear from the plasma in approximately 8 hours after dosing, indicating relatively rapid clearance of all drug-related material from the plasma.

Most of the administered hydromorphone dose is excreted as metabolites, with urine as the major route of excretion, accounting for 75% of the administered dose. Approximately 7% and 1% of the dose are excreted as unchanged hydromorphone in urine and feces, respectively.

Special Populations and Conditions: Pediatrics: Very limited data (in published literature) suggest that the pharmacokinetic profile of hydromorphone in children is comparable to that in adults. No clinical studies with JURNISTA have been conducted in children.

Geriatrics: The effect of age on the single-dose pharmacokinetics of immediate-release hydromorphone resulted in a 14% decrease in C_{max} and a modest increase (11%) in AUC in elderly subjects compared to young subjects. No difference in T_{max} was observed. Greater sensitivity of older individuals cannot be excluded. In general, dose selection for an elderly patient should be cautious, usually starting at the low end of the dosing range, reflecting the greater frequency of decreased hepatic, renal, or cardiac function, and of concomitant disease or other drug therapy in this population (see Dosage and Administration).

Gender: Plasma concentrations and pharmacokinetic parameters following administration of JURNISTA are comparable in male and female subjects.

Race: Population pharmacokinetic analysis revealed no evidence of race-related differences in the pharmacokinetics of hydromorphone following JURNISTA administration.

Hepatic Insufficiency: In studies that used single oral dosing with conventional immediate-release hydromorphone tablets, hepatic impairment reduced the first-pass metabolism of hydromorphone such that four-fold increases in plasma levels of hydromorphone were seen in subjects with moderate hepatic dysfunction. See Dosage and Administration for recommendations on dosage.

Renal Insufficiency: Renal impairment affected the pharmacokinetics of hydromorphone and its metabolites hydromorphone 3-glucuronide and hydromorphone 3-sulphate following administration of an immediate-release tablet. The effects of renal impairment on hydromorphone pharmacokinetics were two-fold and four-fold increases in hydromorphone bioavailability in moderate and severe impairment, respectively. There were also substantial changes in hydromorphone 3-glucuronide elimination kinetics for the severe impairment group, although hemodialysis was effective at reducing plasma levels of both hydromorphone and its metabolites. See Dosage and Administration for recommendations on dosage.

STORAGE AND STABILITY: JURNISTA hydromorphone hydrochloride prolonged-release tablets should be stored between 15 and 25°C.

SPECIAL HANDLING INSTRUCTIONS: N/A.

INFORMATION FOR THE PATIENT: Published in e-CPS, available by subscription at www.e-cps.ca.

DOSAGE FORMS, COMPOSITION AND PACKAGING: JURNISTA tablets use the oral osmotic pump (OROS) Push-Pull technology to deliver hydromorphone by a membrane-controlled, osmotically activated process at a constant, controlled rate over 24 hours. All JURNISTA dosage strengths have qualitatively similar formulations, and are designed to deliver proportionately similar amounts of hydromorphone over the 24-hour dosing period.

The JURNISTA tablet is composed of a bilayer tablet core surrounded by a semi-permeable membrane, and coloured and clear overcoating.

4 mg: Each pale beige, round, biconvex, prolonged-release tablet, with 'HM 4' printed in black ink on one side, contains: 4.36 mg and delivers 4 mg hydromorphone HCl, equivalent to 3.56 mg hydromorphone base. Nonmedicinal ingredients: butyl hydroxytoluene, cellulose acetate, ferric oxide red, ferric oxide yellow, hypromellose, iron oxide black, lactose anhydrous, macrogol, magnesium stearate, polyethylene oxide, povidone, propylene glycol, sodium chloride and titanium dioxide. May contain traces of sodium metabisulfite. PVC/Aclar aluminum blisters.

8 mg: Each red, round, biconvex, prolonged-release tablet, with 'HM 8' printed in black ink on one side, contains: 8.72 mg and delivers 8 mg hydromorphone HCl, equivalent to 7.12 mg hydromorphone base. Nonmedicinal ingredients: butyl hydroxytoluene, cellulose acetate, ferric oxide red, glycerol triacetate, hypromellose, iron oxide black, lactose anhydrous, lactose monohydrate, macrogol, magnesium stearate, polyethylene oxide, povidone, propylene glycol, sodium chloride and titanium dioxide. May contain traces of sodium metabisulfite. PVC/Aclar aluminum blisters.

16 mg: Each yellow, round, biconvex, prolonged-release tablet, with 'HM 16' printed in black ink on one side contains: 16.35 mg and delivers 16 mg hydromorphone HCl, equivalent to 14.24 mg of hydromorphone base. Nonmedicinal ingredients: butyl hydroxytoluene, cellulose acetate, ferric oxide yellow, glycerol triacetate, hypromellose, iron oxide black, lactose anhydrous, lactose monohydrate, macrogol, magnesium stearate, polyethylene oxide, povidone, propylene glycol, sodium chloride and titanium dioxide. May contain traces of sodium metabisulfite. PVC/Aclar aluminum blisters.

32 mg: Each white, round, biconvex, prolonged-release tablet, with 'HM 32' printed in black ink on one side contains: prolonged-release tablet contains and delivers 32.00 mg hydromorphone HCl, equivalent to 28.48 mg of hydromorphone base. Nonmedicinal ingredients: butyl hydroxytoluene, cellulose acetate, ferric oxide yellow, glycerol triacetate, hypromellose, iron oxide black, lactose anhydrous, lactose monohydrate, macrogol, magnesium stearate, polyethylene oxide, povidone, propylene glycol, sodium chloride and titanium dioxide. May contain traces of sodium metabisulfite. PVC/Aclar aluminum blisters.

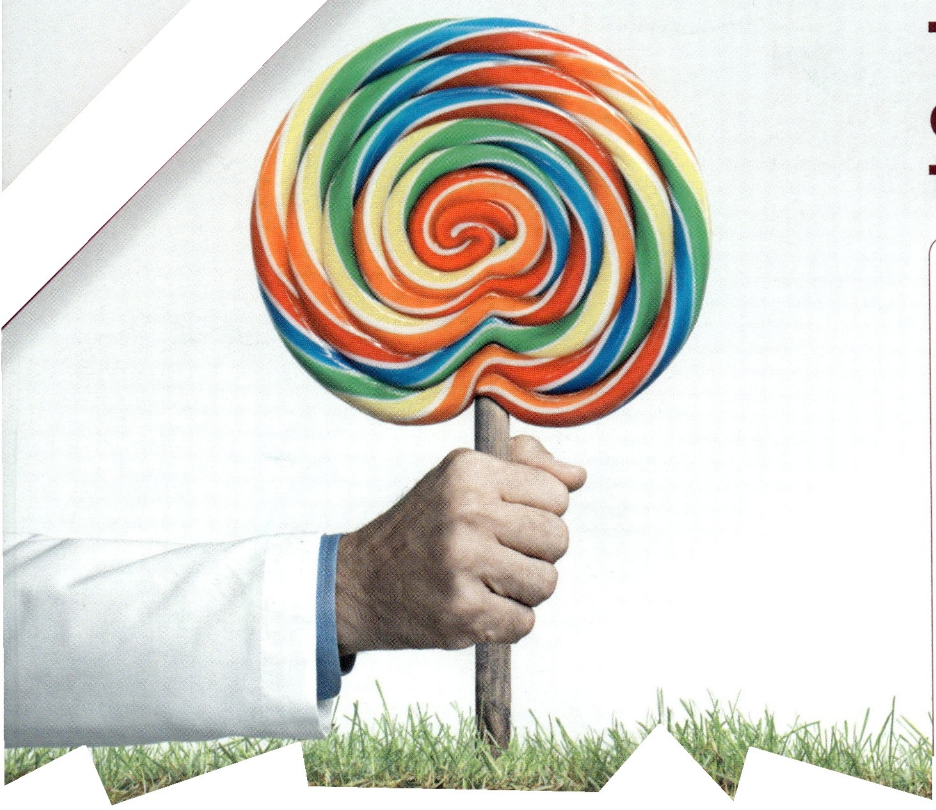

Introducing once-daily Victoza®.

Take a new view of type 2 diabetes treatment.

For treatment of patients who did not achieve adequate glycemic control on metformin, Victoza® + metformin provided:[1, 2]

- Demonstrated **mean reduction in A1C: up to -1.5%*** (p<0.0001 vs. sitagliptin + MET)
  - Victoza® 1.2 mg: -1.2%; Victoza® 1.8 mg: -1.5%; sitagliptin 100 mg: -0.9% (all in combination with MET)
- Demonstrated **mean change in weight: up to -2.8 kg†** (p<0.0001 vs. glimepiride + MET)
  - Victoza® 1.2 mg: -2.6 kg; Victoza® 1.8 mg: -2.8 kg; placebo: -1.5 kg; glimepiride: +1.0 kg (all in combination with MET)

Victoza® was generally well tolerated in clinical trials that included over 4600 patients.[3]

Victoza® (liraglutide) is indicated for once-daily administration for the treatment of adults with type 2 diabetes to improve glycemic control in combination with metformin, when diet and exercise plus maximal tolerated dose of metformin do not achieve adequate glycemic control, or with metformin and a sulfonylurea, when diet and exercise plus dual therapy with metformin and a sulfonylurea do not achieve adequate glycemic control. Victoza® should not be used in type 1 diabetes (formerly known as insulin-dependent diabetes mellitus or IDDM).

Victoza® is contraindicated in patients with a personal or family history of medullary thyroid carcinoma or in patients with Multiple Endocrine Neoplasia syndrome type 2 (MEN 2), in patients who are hypersensitive to liraglutide or to any ingredient in the formulation and in pregnancy or breast-feeding women.

Liraglutide causes dose-dependent and treatment-duration-dependent thyroid C-cell tumours at clinically relevant exposures in both genders of rats and mice. It is unknown whether Victoza® causes thyroid C-cell tumours, including medullary thyroid carcinoma (MTC), in humans, as human relevance could not be ruled out by clinical or nonclinical studies. Victoza® is contraindicated in patients with a personal or family history of MTC and in patients with Multiple Endocrine Neoplasia syndrome type 2 (MEN 2). Based on the findings in rodents, monitoring with serum calcitonin or thyroid ultrasound was performed during clinical trials, but this may have increased the number of unnecessary thyroid surgeries. It is unknown whether monitoring with serum calcitonin or thyroid ultrasound will mitigate human risk of thyroid C-cell tumours. Patients should be counselled regarding the risk and symptoms of thyroid tumours.

Because of limited clinical experience in patients who have cardiac conditions that might be worsened by an increase in heart rate, such as ischemic heart disease and tachyarrhythmia, caution should be observed in these patients. Because of limited clinical experience in patients with pre-existing conduction system abnormalities (e.g., marked first-degree AV block or second- or third-degree AV block) and heart rhythm disturbances (e.g., tachyarrhythmia), caution should be observed in these patients.

Victoza® should not be used in patients with type 1 diabetes mellitus or for the treatment of diabetic ketoacidosis. Victoza® should not be administered intravenously or intramuscularly.

Patients receiving Victoza® in combination with a sulfonylurea may have an increased risk of hypoglycemia. The risk of hypoglycemia can be lowered by reducing the dose of sulfonylurea.

In clinical trials conducted in adult patients with type 2 diabetes, very rare cases of pancreatitis were reported more frequently in the Victoza®-treated group than in the comparator-treated group (2.2 vs. 0.6 cases per 1000 subject-years). In the Victoza®-treated group one fatal case of necrotizing pancreatitis was observed. The causality relationship to Victoza® is unclear.

The most frequently reported adverse events with Victoza® (0.6 to 1.8 mg) treatment were nausea (10.7%-18.6%), diarrhea (8.3%-14.9%), headache (5.4%-12.4%), vomiting (5.4%-7.4%) and dyspepsia (2.1%-7.0%).

Please see Product Monograph for complete recommendations.

References: **1.** Victoza® Product Monograph, Novo Nordisk Canada Inc., 2010. **2.** Pratley R et al. Liraglutide versus sitagliptin for patients with type 2 diabetes who did not have adequate glycaemic control with metformin: a 26-week, randomized, parallel-group, open-label trial. *Lancet.* 2010;375:1447-1456. **3.** Gallwitz B et al. Adding liraglutide to oral antidiabetic drug therapy: onset of treatment effects over time. *Int J Clin Pract.* 2010;64(2):267-276.

*Adapted from Pratley RE et al, 2010.[2] A 26-week, active-comparator, parallel-group, open-label, multicentre trial randomized 665 patients with type 2 diabetes (1:1:1) to once-daily Victoza® (1.2 or 1.8 mg) or once-daily sitagliptin (100 mg) in combination with metformin (≥1500 mg/day). The primary outcome measure was change in A1C. Change in A1C: Victoza® 1.2 mg + MET (-1.2%); Victoza® 1.8 mg + MET (-1.5%); sitagliptin + MET (-0.9%).

†Adapted from Victoza® Product Monograph, 2010.[1] A 26-week, double-blind, double-dummy, placebo- and active-controlled, parallel-group, multicentre trial randomized 1091 patients with type 2 diabetes (2:2:2:1:2) to once-daily Victoza® (0.6, 1.2, or 1.8 mg), to placebo, or to glimepiride (4 mg once-daily) in combination with metformin (1 g bid). Metformin (MET) and glimepiride were gradually titrated up to a maximum dose level. The primary outcome measure was change in weight: Victoza® 1.2 mg + MET (-2.6 kg); Victoza® 1.8 mg + MET (-2.8 kg); glimepiride + MET (+1.0 kg); placebo + MET (-1.5 kg).

NEW

Pr VICTOZA®

liraglutide

novo nordisk®

PAAB

VIC276E/October 2010

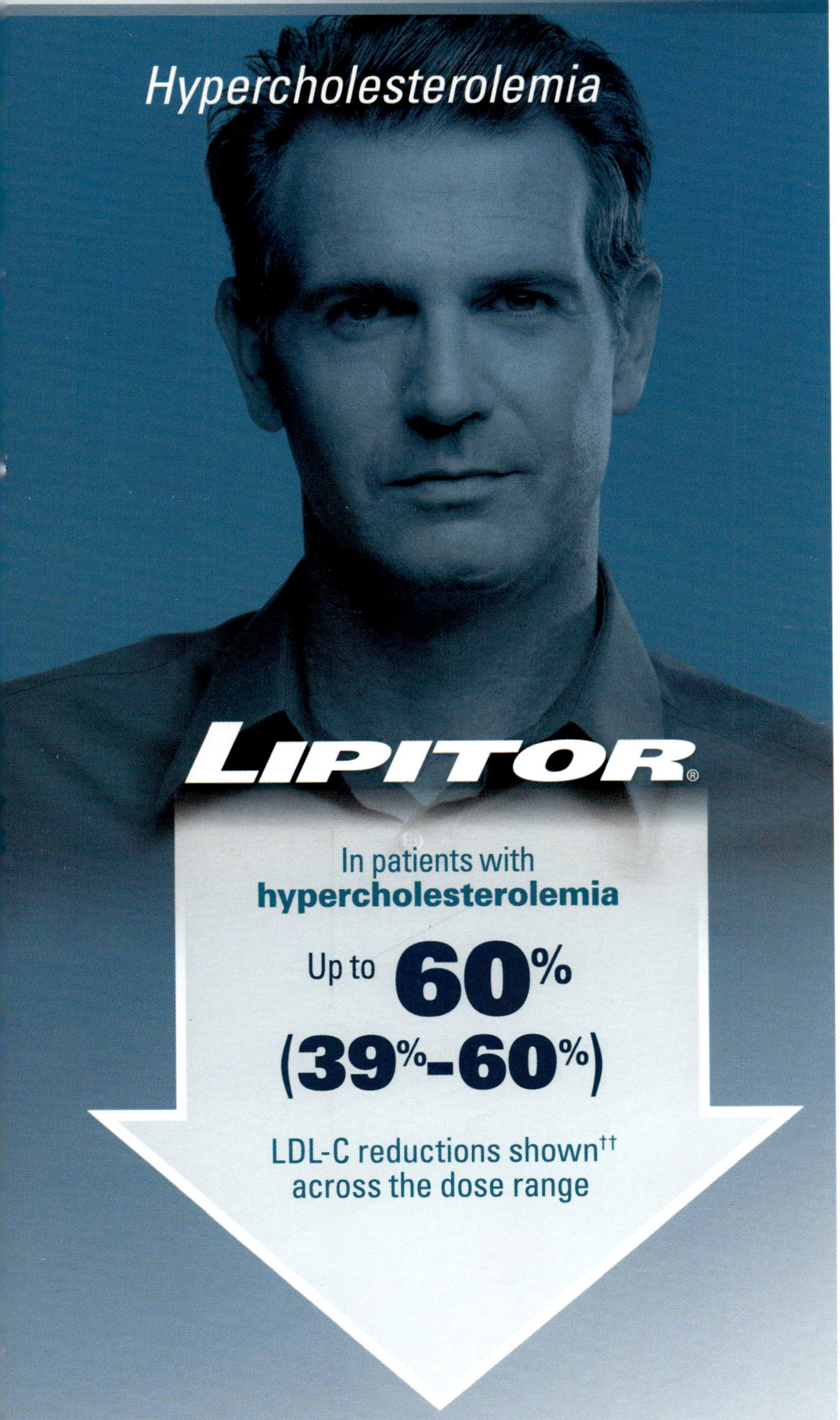

LIPITOR (atorvastatin calcium) is indicated as an adjunct to lifestyle changes, including diet, for the reduction of elevated total cholesterol (total-C), LDL-C, triglycerides (TG), apolipoprotein B (Apo B), the Total-C/HDL-C ratio and for increasing HDL-C in hyperlipidemic and dyslipidemic conditions, when response to diet and other nonpharmacological measures alone has been inadequate, including:

- Primary hypercholesterolemia (Type IIa)
- Combined (mixed) hyperlipidemia (Type IIb), including familial combined hyperlipidemia, regardless of whether cholesterol or triglycerides are the lipid abnormality of concern
- Dysbetalipoproteinemia (Type III)
- Hypertriglyceridemia (Type IV)
- Familial hypercholesterolemia (homozygous and heterozygous). For homozygous familial hypercholesterolemia, LIPITOR should be used as an adjunct to treatments such as LDL apheresis, or as monotherapy if such treatments are not available

An adjunct to diet to reduce total-C, LDL-C, and Apo B levels in boys and postmenarchal girls, 10 to 17 years of age with heterozygous familial hypercholesterolemia, if after an adequate trial of diet therapy the following findings are still present:

a. LDL-C remains ≥4.9 mmol/L (190 mg/dL) or

b. LDL-C remains ≥4.1 mmol/L (160 mg/dL) and:

- there is a positive family history of premature cardiovascular disease or
- two or more other CVD risk factors are present in the pediatric patient

Prior to initiating therapy with LIPITOR, secondary causes should be excluded for elevations in plasma lipid levels (e.g. poorly controlled diabetes mellitus, hypothyroidism, nephrotic syndrome, dysproteinemias, obstructive liver disease, and alcoholism), and a lipid profile performed to measure total cholesterol, LDL-C, HDL-C, and TG.

For patients with TG <4.52 mmol/L (<400 mg/dL), LDL-C can be estimated using the following equation:

LDL-C (mmol/L) = total-C - [(0.37 x (TG) + HDL-C)]

LDL-C (mg/dL) = total-C - [(0.2 x (TG) + HDL-C)]

For patients with TG levels >4.52 mmol/L (>400 mg/dL), this equation is less accurate and LDL-C concentrations should be measured directly or by ultracentrifugation.

Patients with high or very high triglyceride levels, i.e. >2.2 mmol/L (200 mg/dL) or >5.6 mmol/L (500 mg/dL), respectively, may require triglyceride-lowering therapy (fenofibrate, bezafibrate or nicotinic acid) alone or in combination with LIPITOR.

In general, combination therapy with fibrates must be undertaken cautiously and only after risk-benefit analysis (see WARNINGS AND PRECAUTIONS, Muscle Effects, Pharmacokinetic Interactions and DRUG INTERACTIONS).

Elevated serum triglycerides are most often observed in patients with the metabolic syndrome (abdominal obesity, atherogenic dyslipidemia [elevated triglycerides, small dense LDL particles and low HDL-cholesterol], insulin resistance with or without glucose intolerance, raised blood pressure and prothrombic and proinflammatory states).

When drugs are prescribed, attention to therapeutic lifestyle changes (reduced intake of saturated fats and cholesterol, weight reduction, increased physical activity, ingestion of soluble fibres) should always be maintained and reinforced.

Prevention of Cardiovascular Disease

LIPITOR is indicated to reduce the risk of myocardial infarction in adult hypertensive patients without clinically evident coronary heart disease, but with at least three additional risk factors for coronary heart disease such as age >55 years, male sex, smoking, type 2 diabetes, left ventricular hypertrophy, other specified abnormalities on ECG, microalbuminuria or proteinuria, ratio of plasma total cholesterol to HDL-cholesterol >6, or premature family history of coronary heart disease.

LIPITOR is also indicated to reduce the risk of myocardial infarction and stroke in adult patients with type 2 diabetes mellitus and hypertension without clinically evident coronary heart disease, but with other risk factors such as age >55 years, retinopathy, albuminuria or smoking.

LIPITOR is indicated to reduce the risk of myocardial infarction in patients with clinically evident coronary heart disease.

Very rare cases of rhabdomyolysis with acute renal failure secondary to myoglobinuria have been reported with LIPITOR and with other HMG-CoA inhibitors.

Myopathy, defined as muscle pain or muscle weakness in conjunction with increases in creatine kinase (CK) values to greater than ten times the upper limit of normal, should be considered in any patient with diffuse myalgia, muscle tenderness or weakness, and/or marked elevation of CK. Patients should be advised to report promptly any unexplained muscle pain, tenderness or weakness, particularly if accompanied by malaise or fever. Patients who develop any signs or symptoms suggestive of myopathy should have their CK levels measured. LIPITOR therapy should be discontinued if markedly elevated CK levels are measured or myopathy is diagnosed or suspected.

See Prescribing Information for complete warnings, precautions, dosing and administration.

Less than 2% of patients discontinued therapy due to adverse experiences attributable to LIPITOR. Most common adverse effects vs. placebo occurring in patients at an incidence ≥1% were constipation (1% vs. 1%), diarrhea (1% vs. 1%), dyspepsia (1% vs. 2%), flatulence (1% vs. 2%), nausea (1% vs. 0%), headache (1% vs. 2%), pain (1% vs. <1%), myalgia (1% vs. 1%) and asthenia (1% vs. <1%). The adverse events reported in ≥1% of boys and postmenarchal girls (10-17 years of age) were abdominal pain, depression and headache.

LIPITOR is contraindicated: During pregnancy and lactation; active liver disease or unexplained persistent elevations of serum transaminases exceeding 3 times the upper limit of normal; hypersensitivity to any component of this medication.

Lipid levels should be monitored periodically and, if necessary, the dose of LIPITOR adjusted based on desired lipid levels recommended by guidelines. The recommended starting dose of LIPITOR is 10 or 20 mg once daily, depending on patient's LDL-C reduction required. Patients who require a large reduction in LDL-C (more than 45%) may be started at 40 mg once daily. The dosage of LIPITOR should be individualized according to the baseline LDL-C, total-C/HDL-C ratio and/or TG levels to achieve the recommended desired lipid values at the lowest dose needed to achieve the desired LDL-C levels. The pediatric starting dose is 10 mg/day; the maximum recommended dose is 20 mg/day.

Caution should be exercised in patients with severe hypercholesterolemia who are also severely renally impaired, elderly or are concomitantly being administered digoxin or CYP 3A4 inhibitors.

Liver function tests should be performed before the initiation of treatment, and periodically thereafter. Special attention should be paid to patients who develop elevated serum transaminase levels, and in these patients, measurements should be repeated promptly and then performed more frequently.

If increases in alanine aminotransferase (ALT) or aspartate aminotransferase (AST) show evidence of progression, particularly if they rise to greater than 3 times the upper limit of normal and are persistent, the dosage should be reduced or the drug discontinued.

LIPITOR, as well as other HMG-CoA reductase inhibitors, should be used with caution in patients who consume substantial quantities of alcohol and/or have a past history of liver disease.

References: **1.** Colhoun HM *et al.* Primary prevention of cardiovascular disease with atorvastatin in type 2 diabetes in the Collaborative Atorvastatin Diabetes Study (CARDS): multicentre, randomized, placebo-controlled trial. *Lancet* 2004; 364:685-96. **2.** Sever PS *et al.*, for the ASCOT investigators. Prevention of coronary and stroke events with atorvastatin in hypertensive patients who have average or lower-than-average cholesterol concentrations, in the Anglo-Scandinavian Cardiac Outcomes Trial – Lipid Lowering Arm (ASCOT-LLA): a multicentre, randomized, controlled trial. *Lancet* 2003; 361:1149-58. **3.** LIPITOR (atorvastatin calcium) Product Monograph, Pfizer Canada Inc., July 2009.

Pfizer Working together for a healthier world™

Pr LIPITOR®
atorvastatin calcium
tablets

power you can trust™

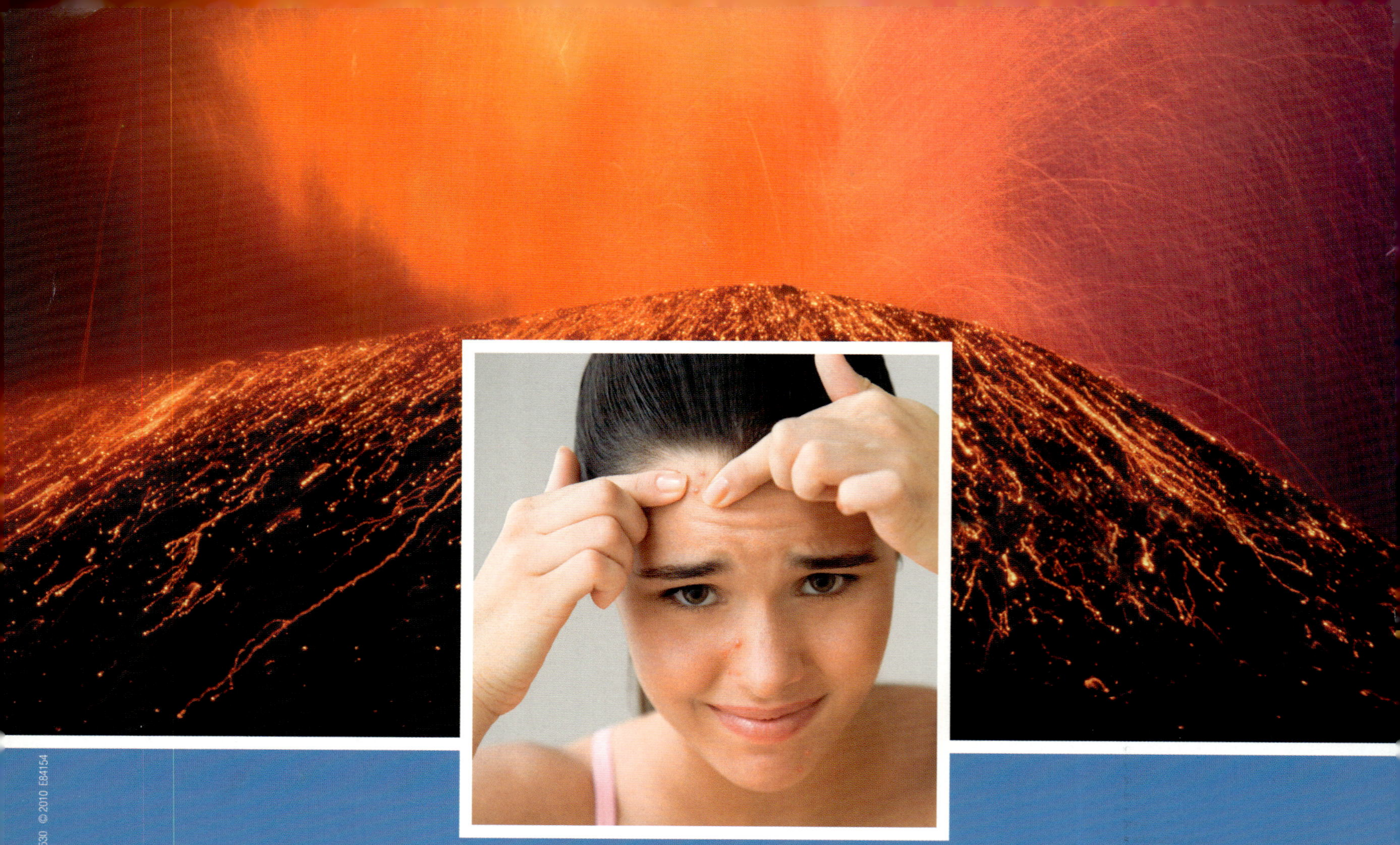

WHICH MAJOR ERUPTION DO YOU THINK SHE'S MOST CONCERNED ABOUT?*

CLINDOXYL® Gel (clindamycin phosphate and benzoyl peroxide) is indicated in the topical treatment of moderate acne vulgaris characterized by the presence of comedones, papules and pustules. CLINDOXYL® Gel is not indicated for the treatment of cystic acne.

Most common side effects in clinical trials were peeling 16.3%, erythema 7.6%, dryness 7.0%, burning 2.3% and pruritus 1.7%.

For external use only. Avoid contact with eyes and mucous membranes. *Clostridium difficile*-associated disease (CDAD) has been reported with the use of topical, oral and parenteral administration of clindamycin. CDAD may range in severity from mild diarrhea to fatal colitis. If the diagnosis of CDAD is suspected or confirmed, appropriate therapeutic measures shoud be initiated. CLINDOXYL® Gel should not be given to pregnant or lactating women. Safety and effectiveness in children under 12 have not been established. Use caution in patients taking neuromuscular blocking agents.

Please refer to the Product Monograph for important information about contra-indications, warnings, precautions, adverse events, dosing and patient selection.

THE #1 TOPICAL ACNE THERAPY DISPENSED IN CANADA[1]

Pr Clindoxyl® once-a-day gel

clindamycin (as phosphate) 1% and benzoyl peroxide 5%, w/w

Help them face their acne

K

K-10®
potassium chloride
Potassium Replacement Therapy

GlaxoSmithKline

INDICATIONS: The prevention and treatment of hypokalemic states which may occur in conjunction with diuretic therapy, digitalis intoxication, corticosteroid therapy, inadequate dietary intake, loss of potassium due to vomiting and diarrhea, hypochloremic alkalosis, diabetic acidosis, and familial periodic paralysis as well as other causes.

CONTRAINDICATIONS: Severe renal impairment, hyperkalemia, untreated Addison's disease, dehydration, heat cramps. Also contraindicated in patients receiving potassium-sparing agents such as aldosterone antagonists and triamterene.

WARNINGS: No data supplied by the manufacturer.

PRECAUTIONS: Potassium must be administered cautiously, since the degree of deficiency or the ideal daily dosage often is not accurately known. Excessive dosage may give rise to potassium intoxication. Frequent checks of the clinical status of the patient and periodic ECG and/or serum potassium levels should be made. This drug should be used with caution in the presence of cardiac disease.

Potassium intoxication may result from overdosage of potassium or from therapeutic dosage in conditions stated under Contraindications.

ADVERSE EFFECTS: Vomiting, diarrhea, nausea, and abdominal discomfort have been reported.

OVERDOSE:

Symptoms: The signs and symptoms of potassium intoxication include paresthesia of the extremities, listlessness, mental confusion, flaccid paralysis, fall in blood pressure, cardiac arrhythmia, and heart block.

Treatment: Hyperkalemia: 1) Dextrose solution. 10 to 25%, containing 10 units of crystalline insulin/20 g dextrose, given i.v. in a dose of 300 to 500 mL/h. 2) Absorption and exchange of potassium using sodium or ammonium cycle cation exchange resin, orally and as retention enema. (Caution: Ammonium compounds should not be used in patients with hepatic cirrhosis.) 3) Hemodialysis and peritoneal dialysis. 4) Eliminate the use of potassium-containing foods or drugs. In case of digitalization, too rapid a lowering of plasma potassium concentration can cause digitalis toxicity.

For management of a suspected drug overdose, CPhA recommends that you contact your **regional Poison Control Centre**. See the *CPS* Directory section for a list of Poison Control Centres.

DOSAGE: Adults: One tablespoonful (15 mL) diluted in a glass of water, tomato or orange juice, twice daily after meals. Deviation from this recommendation may be indicated since no average total daily dose can be defined but must be governed by close observation for clinical effects. In determining dosage, it is well to remember that fruits, vegetables, and their juices contain potassium. Patients should be cautioned to follow directions explicitly in regard to dilution of K-10 to prevent gastrointestinal injury.

SUPPLIED: Each 15 mL contains: potassium chloride 1.5 g (supplying 20 mEq of elemental potassium). Nonmedicinal ingredients: calcium cyclamate, citric acid, glycerin, lemon flavor, orange flavor and sodium benzoate. Bottles of 500 mL.

Kadian® Ⓝ
morphine sulfate
Opioid Analgesic

Abbott

Date of Preparation: November 24, 1995
Date of Revision: December 29, 2006

PHARMACOLOGY: Morphine is an opioid analgesic which exerts an agonist effect at specific, saturable opioid receptors in the CNS and other tissues. Morphine produces diverse pharmacological effects in man including analgesia, suppression of the cough reflex, respiratory depression due to a reduction in the responsiveness of the respiratory centre to carbon dioxide, nausea and emesis through direct stimulation of the chemoreceptor trigger-zone (CTZ), mood changes including euphoria and dysphoria, sedation, mental clouding, alterations in both the endocrine and autonomic nervous systems, and a decrease in gastrointestinal motility leading to constipation.

Pharmacokinetics: Morphine is rapidly absorbed from the gastrointestinal tract, nasal mucosa, and lung after SC and IM injection. When administered orally, it is subject to extensive but variable first pass metabolism, and only about 40% of the administered dose reaches the central compartment.

Once absorbed, morphine is distributed to skeletal muscle, kidneys, liver, intestinal tract, lungs, spleen and brain. It crosses the placental membranes and has been found in breast milk. About 30 to 35% of morphine is reversibly protein bound.

Although, a small fraction of morphine (less than 5%) is demethylated, for all practical purposes, virtually all morphine is converted to glucuronide metabolites including morphine-3-glucuronide and morphine-6-glucuronide. The glucuronide system has very high capacity and is not easily saturated even in disease. Studies in healthy subjects and cancer patients have shown that the glucuronide metabolite to morphine mean molar ratios (based on AUC) are similar following single doses of Kadian and morphine sulfate solution. The morphine to morphine-3-glucuronide to morphine-6-glucuronide mean molar ratios (based on AUC) are approximately 1:26:4, similar to those occurring with morphine sulfate solution.

There has been no evaluation of Kadian in patients with impaired hepatic and renal function. Pharmacokinetic parameters of morphine show considerable inter-subject variation. The average volume of distribution (Vd) is approximately 4 L/kg, and the terminal half-life is 2 to 4 hours.

Following oral administration, the dose normalized extent of absorption (AUC) of morphine from Kadian is similar to that obtained from morphine solutions. However, the rate of absorption of morphine from Kadian is significantly slower.

A single 50 mg oral dose of Kadian in 30 healthy male subjects resulted in a mean peak plasma morphine concentration of 8.1 ng/mL (C_{max}) at 8.5 hours (T_{max}). The extent of absorption was unaffected by food, but the T_{max} was slightly delayed to 10 hours. However, this is not clinically significant. Kadian can be administered with or without food.

When Kadian is given on a fixed dosing regimen, steady state is achieved within about 2 days.

The pharmacokinetic characteristics of Kadian administered once daily for a 7 day period have been investigated in 24 patients with moderate-severe chronic cancer pain requiring opioid analgesia. The mean pharmacokinetic values were calculated from steady-state plasma morphine data and adjusted to a dose of 100 mg (see Table 1).

Table 1: Kadian
Mean Pharmacokinetic Values

Parameter	Mean±S.D.
C_{max} (ng/mL)	37.3±14.0
T_{max} (h)	10.3±3.3
AUC (ng.h/mL)	501±193
C_{min} (ng/mL)	9.9±5.2
T≥0.75 C_{max} (h)	6.0±3.0

Legend: C_{max}=maximum observed plasma morphine concentration; T_{max}=time to reach C_{max}; AUC=area under the plasma concentration time curve; C_{min}=minimum plasma morphine concentration; T≥0.75 C_{max}=time for which the plasma morphine concentration is greater than or equal to 75% of the C_{max}.

Morphine is excreted primarily in the urine as morphine-3-glucuronide and morphine-6-glucuronide. A small amount of the glucuronide metabolites is excreted in the bile, and there is some minor enterohepatic cycling. Seven to 10% of administered morphine is excreted in the feces. Morphine-6-glucuronide has been shown to be pharmacologically active. Because accumulation of this metabolite has been observed in patients with renal disease, caution should be exercised in patients with clinically significant impairment of renal function.

INDICATIONS: For the relief of severe chronic pain requiring the prolonged use of an oral opioid preparation.

CONTRAINDICATIONS: Until further information is available, co-ingestion of Kadian with alcohol is contraindicated. Co-ingestion of Kadian and alcohol can potentially result in rapid increases in opioid plasma concentrations which may be fatal, even in opioid tolerant patients.

In patients with known hypersensitivity to morphine, morphine salts or any of the capsule components, acute or severe bronchial asthma or other obstructive airway disease, respiratory depression, cor pulmonale, biliary colic, gastrointestinal obstruction, particularly paralytic ileus, cardiac arrhythmias, acute alcoholism, delirium tremens, severe CNS depression, convulsive disorder, increased cerebrospinal or intracranial pressure, head injury, brain tumor, suspected surgical abdomen, or concurrent MAO inhibitors or within 14 days of such therapy (see Precautions, Drug Interactions).

WARNINGS: Impaired Respiration: Respiratory depression is the chief hazard of all morphine preparations. Respiratory depression occurs more frequently in elderly and debilitated patients, and in those suffering from conditions accompanied by hypoxia or hypercapnia when even moderate therapeutic doses may significantly decrease pulmonary ventilation.

Morphine should be used with extreme caution in patients with chronic obstructive pulmonary disease or cor pulmonale and in patients having a substantially decreased respiratory reserve, hypoxia, hypercapnia or preexisting respiratory depression. In such patients, even usual therapeutic doses of morphine may increase airway resistance and decrease respiratory drive to the point of apnea. Severe pain antagonizes the respiratory depressant effects of morphine.

Head Injury and Increased Intracranial Pressure: The respiratory depressant effects of morphine with carbon dioxide retention and secondary elevation of cerebrospinal fluid pressure may be markedly exaggerated in the presence of head injury, other intracranial lesions, or a preexisting increase in intracranial pressure. Morphine produces effects which may obscure neurological signs of further increases in pressure in patients with head injuries. Morphine should only be administered under such circumstances when considered essential, and then, with extreme caution.

Hypotensive Effect: Kadian, like all opioid analgesics, may cause severe hypotension in an individual whose ability to maintain blood pressure has already been compromised by a reduced blood volume, or a concurrent administration of drugs such as phenothiazines or general anesthetics (see Precautions, Drug Interactions). Kadian may produce orthostatic hypotension in ambulatory patients.

Kadian, like all opioid analgesics, should be administered with caution to patients in circulatory shock, as vasodilation produced by the drug may further reduce cardiac output and blood pressure.

Gastrointestinal Motility: Kadian should not be given to patients with gastrointestinal obstruction, particularly paralytic ileus, as there is a risk of the product remaining in the stomach for an extended period and the subsequent release of a bolus of morphine when normal gut motility is restored.

As with any other solid dose morphine formulation, diarrhea may reduce Kadian absorption.

Drug Abuse and Dependence: Morphine has a potential for physical and psychological dependence. However, this is not a prime concern in the management of terminally ill patients or patients in severe pain. Abrupt cessation or a sudden reduction in dose after prolonged use may result in withdrawal symptoms. The opioid agonist abstinence syndrome is characterized by some or all of the following symptoms: restlessness, lacrimation, rhinorrhea, yawning, perspiration, gooseflesh, restless sleep or "yen" and mydriasis during the first 24 hours. These symptoms often increase in severity and over the next 72 hours may be accompanied by increasing irritability, anxiety, weakness, twitching and spasms of muscles, kicking movements, severe backache, abdominal and leg pains, abdominal and muscle cramps, hot and cold flashes, insomnia, nausea, anorexia, vomiting, intestinal spasm, diarrhea, coryza and repetitive sneezing, increase in body temperature, blood pressure, respiratory rate and heart rate. Because of excessive loss of fluids through sweating, vomiting and diarrhea, there is usually marked weight loss, dehydration, ketosis, and disturbances in acid base balance. Cardiovascular collapse can occur. Most observable symptoms disappear in 5 to 14 days without treatment; however, there appears to be a phase of secondary or chronic abstinence which may last for 2 to 6 months characterized by insomnia, irritability and muscle aches.

If treatment of physical dependence of patients on Kadian is necessary, detoxification may be achieved by a gradual dosage reduction. Gastrointestinal disturbance or dehydration should be treated appropriately.

Infants born to mothers who are physically dependent on opioid analgesics may also be physically dependent and may exhibit withdrawal symptoms. These infants may have respiratory depression at birth (see Precautions).

Tolerance: Tolerance, in which increasingly large doses are required in order to produce the same degree of analgesia, may develop upon repeated administration of morphine. The dose of Kadian may need to be increased to maintain adequate pain relief (see Dosage).

Pregnancy: Animal reproduction studies have not been performed using morphine. It is not known whether morphine can cause fetal damage when administered throughout pregnancy or if it can affect reproductive capacity in humans. Pregnant patients should be given Kadian only when the benefits clearly outweigh potential risks to the fetus.

PRECAUTIONS: General: Kadian is intended for use in patients who require more than several days of continuous treatment with a potent opioid analgesic.

As with any potent opioid, it is critical to adjust the dosing regimen of Kadian for each patient individually, taking into account the patient's prior analgesic treatment experience. Although, it is clearly impossible to enumerate every consideration that is important to the selection of the initial dose of Kadian, attention should be given to the points listed under Dosage.

Cordotomy: Patients who are scheduled for cordotomy or other interruption of pain transmission pathways should not receive Kadian within 24 hours of the procedure.

Special Risk Groups: Kadian should be administered with caution, and in reduced dosages in elderly or debilitated patients; patients with severe renal or hepatic insufficiency or impaired pulmonary function; patients with Addison's disease; myxedema; hypothyroidism; prostatic hypertrophy or urethral stricture.

Caution should also be exercised in the administration of Kadian to patients with CNS depression; toxic psychosis; acute alcoholism or delirium tremens; severe kyphoscoliosis; convulsive disorders; about to undergo biliary surgery and patients with acute pancreatitis secondary to biliary tract disease.

Occupational Hazards: Driving and Operating Dangerous Machinery: Morphine may impair the mental and/or physical abilities needed to perform potentially hazardous activities such as driving a car or operating machinery. Patients must be cautioned accordingly. Patients should also be warned about the potential combined effects of morphine with other CNS depressants, including other opioids, phenothiazines, sedatives, sedative/hypnotics and alcohol (see Drug Interactions).

Labor/Delivery: Kadian is not recommended for use in women during and immediately before labor. The effects of opioid analgesics are unpredictable. They may prolong labor by temporarily reducing the strength, duration and frequency of uterine contractions, or conversely they may tend to shorten labor by increasing the rate of cervical dilatation. Infants born to mothers receiving opioid analgesics during labor should be observed closely for signs of respiratory depression. Naloxone HCl should be available for reversal of narcotic-induced respiratory depression.

Lactation: As morphine is excreted in human milk, breast-feeding is not recommended while a patient is receiving Kadian. Withdrawal symptoms have been observed in breast-fed infants when maternal administration of morphine is stopped.

Drug Interactions: CNS Depressants: Morphine should be used with great caution and in reduced dosage in patients concurrently receiving other CNS depressants including sedatives, hypnotics, general anesthetics, phenothiazines, other tranquilizers and alcohol because of the risk of respiratory depression, hypotension and profound sedation or coma. When such combined therapy is contemplated, the dose of one or both agents should be reduced.

Muscle Relaxants: Morphine may enhance the neuromuscular blocking action of skeletal relaxants and produce an increased degree of respiratory depression.

Mixed Agonist/Antagonist Opioid Analgesics: From a theoretical perspective, mixed agonist/antagonist opioid analgesics (e.g., pentazocine and buprenorphine) should **not** be administered to a patient who has received or is receiving a course of therapy with a pure opioid agonist analgesic. In these patients, mixed agonist/antagonist analgesics may reduce the analgesic effect or may precipitate withdrawal symptoms.

MAO Inhibitors: The concurrent use of MAO inhibitors and other opioid drugs such as morphine can cause anxiety, confusion and significant depression of respiration, sometimes leading to coma. Morphine should not be given to patients taking MAO inhibitors or within 14 days of stopping such treatment.

Cimetidine: There is a report of confusion and severe respiratory depression when a hemodialysis patient was administered morphine and cimetidine.

Diuretics: Morphine reduces the efficacy of diuretics by inducing the release of antidiuretic hormone. Morphine may also lead to acute retention of urine by causing spasm of the sphincter of the bladder, particularly in men with prostatism.

ADVERSE EFFECTS: The adverse reactions caused by morphine are essentially the same as those observed with other oral and parenteral opioid analgesics. They include the following major hazards: respiratory depression, apnea and to a lesser degree, circulatory depression, respiratory arrest, shock and cardiac arrest.

Most Common Adverse Effects: constipation, dizziness, dysphoria, euphoria, lightheadedness, nausea, sedation, vomiting, sweating.

Sedation: Most patients receiving morphine will experience initial drowsiness. This usually disappears in 3 to 5 days and is not a cause for concern unless it is excessive, or accompanied with unsteadiness or confusion. Excessive or persistent sedation should be investigated. Factors to be considered should include concurrent sedative medications, the presence of hepatic or renal insufficiency, exacerbated respiratory failure, tolerance to the dose used especially in older patients, disease severity and the patient's general condition. If the dose of Kadian has been reduced and pain is not adequately controlled, the dose may be carefully increased again after a few days.

Dizziness and Unsteadiness: May be associated with morphine-induced postural hypotension, particularly in elderly or debilitated patients. The dosage should be adjusted according to individual needs but, because of reduced clearance, dosage may be lower in patients over 50 years of age.

Nausea and Vomiting: Nausea and vomiting are common after single doses of morphine or as an early undesirable effect of regular opioid therapy. The prescription of a suitable antiemetic should be considered. The frequency of nausea and vomiting usually decreases within a week or so but may persist due to opioid-induced gastric stasis.

Constipation: Most patients suffer from constipation while taking opioids on a chronic basis. Some patients, particularly those who are elderly, debilitated or bedridden may become impacted. Patients must be cautioned accordingly and laxatives, softeners and other appropriate treatments should be initiated at the beginning of opioid therapy.

Other adverse reactions include:

Cardiovascular: flushing of the face, chills, tachycardia, bradycardia, palpitations, faintness, syncope, hypotension and hypertension.

Central Nervous System: euphoria, dysphoria, weakness, insomnia, dizziness, confusional symptoms and occasionally hallucinations, disorientation, headache, tremor, muscle rigidity, agitation, uncoordinated muscle movements, seizures, increased intracranial pressure, hypothermia, paresthesia, dyspnea, alterations in mood (nervousness, apprehension, depression, floating feelings).

Gastrointestinal: dry mouth, anorexia, constipation, laryngospasm, colic, taste alterations and biliary colic.

Genitourinary: urine retention or hesitancy, reduced libido or potency.

Endocrine: A syndrome of inappropriate antidiuretic hormone secretion characterized by hyponatremia secondary to decreased free-water excretion may occur (monitoring of electrolytes may be necessary).

Visual Disturbances: blurred vision, nystagmus, diplopia and miosis.

Dermatologic: pruritus, urticaria, other skin rashes and edema, diaphoresis.

Withdrawal (Abstinence) Syndrome: Chronic use of opioid analgesics may be associated with the development of physical dependence. An abstinence syndrome may be precipitated when opioid administration is suddenly discontinued or opioid antagonists administered.

Withdrawal symptoms that may be observed after discontinuation of opioid use include body aches, diarrhea, piloerection, anorexia, nervousness or restlessness, rhinorrhea, sneezing, tremors or shivering, abdominal colic, nausea, sleep disturbance, unusual increase in sweating and yawning, weakness, tachycardia and unexplained fever. With appropriate dose adjustments and gradual withdrawal these symptoms are usually mild.

OVERDOSE:

Symptoms: Acute overdosage with morphine is manifested by respiratory depression, somnolence progressing to stupor or coma, skeletal muscle flaccidity, cold and clammy skin, constricted pupils, and sometimes bradycardia and hypotension.

Treatment: Primary attention should be given to the establishment of a patent airway and institution of assisted or controlled ventilation. The pure opioid antagonist, naloxone HCl, is a specific antidote against respiratory depression which results from opioid overdose. Naloxone (usually 0.4 to 2 mg) should be administered IV. However, because its duration of action is relatively short, the patient must be carefully monitored until spontaneous respiration is reliably re-established. Kadian will continue to release and add to the morphine load for periods longer than the action of a single dose of antagonist, and the management of morphine overdosage should be modified accordingly. If the response to naloxone is suboptimal or not sustained, additional naloxone may be administered as needed, or given by continuous IV infusion to maintain alertness and respiratory function. There is no information available about the cumulative dose of naloxone that may be safely administered.

Naloxone should not be administered in the absence of clinically significant respiratory or circulatory depression secondary to morphine overdosage. Naloxone should be administered cautiously to persons who are known or suspected to be physically dependent on Kadian. In such cases, an abrupt or complete reversal of opioid effects may precipitate an acute withdrawal syndrome. The severity of the withdrawal syndrome produced will depend on the degree of physical dependence and the dose of the antagonist administered. If it is necessary to treat serious respiratory depression in the physically dependent patient, the antagonist should be administered with extreme care and by titration with smaller than usual doses of the antagonist.

Supportive measures (including oxygen, vasopressors) should be employed in the management of circulatory shock and pulmonary edema accompanying overdose as indicated. Cardiac arrest or arrhythmias may require cardiac massage or defibrillation.

Gastric contents may need to be emptied as this can be useful in removing unabsorbed drug, particularly when a sustained-release formulation has been taken.

Morphine toxicity may be a result of overdosage but because of the large inter-individual variation in sensitivity to opioids, it is difficult to assess the exact dose of any opioid that is toxic or lethal. The toxic effects of morphine tend to be overshadowed by the presence of pain or tolerance. Patients having chronic morphine therapy have been known to take in excess of 3000 mg/day with no apparent toxic effects being present.

> For management of a suspected drug overdose, CPhA recommends that you contact your **regional Poison Control Centre**. See the *CPS* Directory section for a list of Poison Control Centres.

DOSAGE: See Warnings and Precautions. **Kadian capsules contain sustained-release pellets which should not be chewed or crushed. Taking chewed or crushed Kadian pellets could lead to the rapid release and absorption of a potentially toxic dose of morphine.**

The capsules are to be administered once daily (every 24 hours).

Selection of the initial dose of Kadian should take into account the following: the total daily dose, potency and characteristics of previous opioid analgesics (e.g., pure agonists or mixed agonist/antagonist); the reliability of the relative potency estimate used to calculate the dose of morphine required (potency estimates vary with the route of administration); the degree of opioid tolerance; the patient's general condition and medical status; and type and severity of pain.

Individual dosing requirements vary considerably based on each patient's size, weight, severity of pain, and medical and analgesic history.

Patients over the age of 50 tend to require much lower doses of morphine than do younger patients. In elderly and debilitated patients and those with impaired respiratory function or significantly decreased renal function, the initial dose should be one half of the usual recommended dose.

For patients who have difficulty swallowing, Kadian capsules may be opened and the sustained-release pellets may be administered in the following way: the pellets may be sprinkled onto a small amount of soft foods (such as yogurt, apple sauce or jam). This should be taken within 30 minutes of sprinkling. The pellets must not be chewed or crushed, and the mouth should be rinsed to ensure that all pellets have been swallowed.

The use of opioid analgesics for the relief of chronic pain, including cancer pain, should be only part of a complete approach to pain control which should include other types of treatment or drug therapy, nondrug measures and psychosocial support.

If signs of excessive opioid effects are observed early in the dosing interval, the next dose should be reduced. If this adjustment leads to inadequate analgesia, that is, breakthrough pain occurs, a supplemental dose of a short acting analgesic may be given. If breakthrough pain repeatedly occurs at the end of a dose interval, it is generally an indication for dosage increase, not more frequent administration. However, where judged necessary, Kadian may be administered more frequently than every 24 hours. The dosing interval should not be reduced below every 12 hours. As experience is gained, adjustments can be made to obtain an appropriate balance between pain relief and opioid side effects.

For essential information on the important details of the management of cancer pain, the reader may wish to consult the following resources: Cancer Pain: A Monograph on the Management of Cancer Pain. Health and Welfare, Canada. Twycross, R.G. and Lack, S.A. Symptom control in far advanced cancer: Pain relief.

Because of the sustained release properties of Kadian, dosage increases should generally be separated by 48 hours.

When properly ingested, no evidence of dose dumping was observed in any of the patients receiving their full daily dose of morphine in the every 24 hours arms of the various steady-state studies.

Use of Kadian as the First Opioid Analgesic: There has been no systematic evaluation of Kadian as an initial opioid analgesic in the management of pain. Because it may be more difficult to titrate a patient using a controlled release morphine, it is ordinarily advisable to begin treatment using an immediate release formulation.

For patients currently receiving opioids, the following dosing recommendations should be considered.

Conversion from Immediate Release Oral Morphine Formulations to Kadian: Patients on Immediate Release oral morphine formulations may be converted to Kadian by administering the patient's total daily morphine dose as Kadian capsules on an every 24 hours dosing regimen. Dose is then adjusted as needed.

The first dose of Kadian should be taken with the last dose of any immediate-release opioid medication due to the prolonged T_{max} after administration of Kadian.

Conversion from Sustained-Release Oral Morphine Formulations to Kadian: Patients on sustained-release oral morphine formulations may be converted to Kadian by administering the patient's total daily morphine dose as Kadian capsules on an every 24 hours dosing regimen at the time of the next scheduled dose of morphine.

Conversion from Parenteral Morphine or Other Parenteral or Oral Opioids to Kadian: If Kadian is administered as the initial oral morphine drug product, particular care must be exercised in the conversion process. Because of uncertainty about an inter-subject variation in relative estimates of opioid potency and cross tolerance, initial dosing regimens should be conservative; that is, an underestimation of the 24 hours oral morphine requirements is preferred to an overestimate. To this end, initial individual doses of Kadian should be estimated conservatively.

Estimates of the relative potency of opioids are only approximate and are influenced by route of administration, individual patient differences, and possibly, by an individual's medical condition.

Consequently, it is difficult to recommend any fixed rule for converting a patient to Kadian directly. The following general points should be considered: Parenteral to Oral Morphine Ratio: Estimates of the oral to parenteral potency of morphine vary. Some authorities suggest that a dose of oral morphine only 2 to 3 times the daily parenteral morphine requirement may be sufficient in chronic use settings.

Other Parenteral or Oral Opioids to Oral Morphine: Because there are no data on these types of analgesic substitutions, specific recommendations are not possible. Physicians are advised to refer to published relative potency data, keeping in mind that such ratios are only approximate (see Table 2). In general, it is safer to underestimate the daily dose of Kadian required and rely upon ad hoc supplementation to deal with inadequate analgesia.

Conversion from Kadian to Other Controlled-Release Oral Morphine Formulations: Kadian is not bioequivalent to other controlled-release morphine preparations. Conversion from Kadian to the same daily dose of other controlled-release morphine preparations may lead to an initial change in the clinical status of the patient and close observation is recommended.

Conversion from Kadian to Parenteral Opioids: When converting a patient from Kadian to parenteral opioids, it is best to assume that the parenteral to oral potency is high. **Note that this is the converse of the strategy used when the direction of conversion is from the parenteral to oral formulations. In both cases however, the aim is to estimate the new dose conservatively.** For example, to estimate the required 24-hour dose of morphine for IM use, one could employ a conversion of 1 mg of morphine IM for every 6 mg of morphine as Kadian. Therefore, the IM 24-hour dose would have to be divided by 6 and administered every 4 hours. This approach is recommended because it is least likely to cause overdose. However, for chronic dosing, clinical experience indicates that this ratio is 2-3:1 and individual titration is recommended (i.e., 20 to 30 mg of oral or rectal morphine is equivalent to 10 mg of parenteral morphine).

Table 2: Kadian

Opioid Analgesics: Approximate Analgesic Equivalences[a]

Drug	Equivalent Dose (mg)[b] (compared to morphine 10 mg IM)		Duration of Action (hours)
	Parenteral	Oral	
Strong Opioid Agonists			
Morphine (single dose)	10	60[c]	3–4
Morphine (chronic dose)	10	20–30[c]	3–4
Hydromorphone	1.5–2	6–7.5	2–4
Anileridine	25	75	2–3
Levorphanol	2	4	4–8
Meperidine[d]	75	300	1–3
Oxymorphone	1.5	5 (rectal)	3–4
Methadone[e]	—	—	—
Heroin	5-8	10–15	3–4
Weak Opioid Agonists			
Codeine	120	200	3–4
Oxycodone	5–10	10–15[f]	2–4
Propoxyphene	50	100	2–4
Mixed Agonist-Antagonists[g]			
Pentazocine[d]	60	180	3–4
Nalbuphine	10	—	3–6

(cont'd)

Table 2: Kadian *(cont'd)*

Opioid Analgesics: Approximate Analgesic Equivalences[a]

Drug	Equivalent Dose (mg)[b] (compared to morphine 10 mg IM)		Duration of Action (hours)
	Parenteral	Oral	
Butorphanol	2	—	3–4

[a] References:
Cancer Pain: A Monograph on the Management of Cancer Pain, Health and Welfare Canada 1984.
Foley K.M., New Engl J. Med 313:84-95,1985.
Aronoff, G.M. and Evans, W.O., In: Evaluation and Treatment of Chronic Pain, 2nd Ed., G.M. Aronoff (Ed.), Williams and Wilkins, Baltimore, pp.359-368,1992.
Cherny, N.I. and Portenoy, R.K., In: Textbook of Pain, 3rd Ed., P.D. Wall and R. Melzack (Eds.), Churchill Livingstone, London, pp.1437-1467,1994.
[b] Most of this data was derived from single-dose, acute pain studies and should be considered an approximation for selection of doses when treating chronic pain.
[c] For acute pain, the oral or rectal dose of morphine is 6 times the injectable dose. However, for chronic dosing, clinical experience indicates that this ratio is 2-3:1 (i.e., 20-30 mg of oral or rectal morphine is equivalent to 10 mg of parenteral morphine).
[d] These drugs are not recommended for the management of chronic pain.
[e] Extremely variable equianalgesic dose. Patients should undergo individualized titration starting at an equivalent to 1/10 of the morphine dose.
[f] In combination with acetaminophen or ASA. For acute pain, single entity oral oxycodone is twice as potent as oral morphine.
[g] Mixed agonist-antagonists can precipitate withdrawal in patients on pure opioid agonists.

Opioid analgesic agents do not effectively relieve dysesthetic pain, post-herpetic neuralgia, stabbing pains, activity-related pain, and some forms of headache. This does not mean that patients with advanced cancer suffering these types of pain should not be given an adequate trial of opioid analgesics. However, such patients may need to be referred early on for other types of pain therapy. Pain without nociception is usually not opioid-responsive.

Dose Titration: Dose titration is the key to success with morphine therapy. Proper optimization of doses scaled to the relief of the individual's pain should aim at the regular administration of the lowest dose of morphine which will maintain the patient free of pain at all times. Dose adjustments should be based on the patient's clinical response. Higher doses may be justified in some patients to cover periods of physical activity.

Because of the sustained release properties of Kadian, dosage adjustments should generally be separated by 48 hours. If dose increments turn out to be required, they should be proportionately greater at lower dose levels (in terms of percentage of the previous dose), than when adjusting a higher dose.

Adjustment or Reduction of Dosage: During the first 2 or 3 days of effective pain relief, the patient may exhibit drowsiness or sleep for prolonged periods. This can be misinterpreted as the effect of excessive analgesic dosing rather than the first sign of relief in a pain-exhausted patient. The dose, therefore, should be maintained for at least 3 days before reduction, provided that the sedation is not excessive or associated with unsteadiness and symptoms of confusion, and that respiratory activity and other vital signs are adequate. If excessive sedation persists, the reason(s) for such an effect must be sought. Some of these are concomitant sedative medications, hepatic or renal failure, exacerbated respiratory failure, higher doses than tolerated by an older patient, or an illness which is more severe than previously recognized. If it is necessary to reduce the dose, it can be carefully increased again after 2 or 4 days if it is obvious that the pain is not being well-controlled.

Following successful relief of severe pain, periodic attempts to reduce the opioid dose should be made. Smaller doses or complete discontinuation of the opioid analgesic may become feasible due to a change in the patient's condition or improved mental state.

Children: The use of Kadian in children has not been evaluated.

Geriatrics: Kadian should be administered with caution and in reduced dosages in elderly patients.

INFORMATION FOR THE PATIENT: Published in e-CPS, available by subscription at www.e-cps.ca.

SUPPLIED: 10 mg: Each size 4 capsule, clear cap imprinted with K10 and clear body imprinted with 1 black band, contains: morphine sulfate 10 mg as creamy-white to light tan polymer-coated sustained-release pellets. Nonmedicinal ingredients: diethyl phthalate, ethylcellulose, gelatin, hypromellose, maize starch, methacrylic acid copolymer, polyethylene glycol, sucrose and talc; black ink: ammonium hydroxide, black iron oxide, potassium hydroxide, propylene glycol and shellac. Gluten-free. Bottles of 100. Store between 15 and 25°C. Protect from light and moisture.

20 mg: Each size 4 capsule, clear cap imprinted with K20 and clear body imprinted with 2 black bands, contains: morphine sulfate 20 mg as creamy-white to light tan polymer-coated sustained-release pellets. Nonmedicinal ingredients: diethyl phthalate, ethylcellulose, gelatin, hypromellose, maize starch, methacrylic acid copolymer, polyethylene glycol, sucrose and talc; black ink: ammonium hydroxide, black iron oxide, potassium hydroxide, propylene glycol and shellac. Gluten-free. Bottles of 100. Store between 15 and 25°C. Protect from light and moisture.

50 mg: Each size 2 capsule, clear cap imprinted with K50 and clear body imprinted with 3 black bands, contains: morphine sulfate 50 mg as creamy-white to light tan polymer-coated sustained-release pellets. Nonmedicinal ingredients: diethyl phthalate, ethylcellulose, gelatin, hypromellose, maize starch, methacrylic acid copolymer, polyethylene glycol, sucrose and talc; black ink: ammonium hydroxide, black iron oxide, potassium hydroxide, propylene glycol and shellac. Gluten-free. Bottles of 100. Store between 15 and 25°C. Protect from light and moisture.

100 mg: Each size 0 capsule, clear cap imprinted with K100 and clear body imprinted with 4 black bands, contains: morphine sulfate 100 mg as creamy-white to light tan polymer-coated sustained-release pellets. Nonmedicinal ingredients: diethyl phthalate, ethylcellulose, gelatin, hypromellose, maize starch, methacrylic acid copolymer, polyethylene glycol, sucrose and talc; black ink: ammonium hydroxide, black iron oxide, potassium hydroxide, propylene glycol and shellac. Gluten-free. Bottles of 50. Store between 15 and 25°C. Protect from light and moisture.

Kaletra® Ⓟ

lopinavir—ritonavir

Human Immunodeficiency Virus (HIV) Protease Inhibitor

Abbott

Date of Preparation: March 9, 2001
Date of Revision: August 9, 2010

SUMMARY PRODUCT INFORMATION:

Route of Administration	Dosage Form/ Strength	Clinically Relevant Nonmedicinal Ingredients
Oral	Film-coated tablets/100 mg/25 mg, 200 mg/50 mg	Sorbitan monolaurate
	Oral solution/80/20 mg/mL	Alcohol, fructose, polyoxyl 40 hydrogenated castor oil and propylene glycol For a complete listing of nonmedicinal ingredients, see Dosage Forms, Composition and Packaging.

DESCRIPTION: KALETRA (lopinavir/ritonavir) is a co-formulation of lopinavir and ritonavir. Lopinavir is an inhibitor of the Human Immunodeficiency Virus (HIV) protease. As co-formulated in KALETRA, ritonavir inhibits the CYP3A-mediated metabolism of lopinavir, thereby providing increased plasma levels of lopinavir.

INDICATIONS AND CLINICAL USE: KALETRA (lopinavir/ritonavir) is indicated in combination with other antiretroviral agents when therapy is warranted for:

- treatment of HIV-1 infection

This indication is based on analyses of plasma HIV RNA levels and CD_4 cell counts in controlled KALETRA studies of 48 weeks duration, and in smaller uncontrolled KALETRA dose-ranging studies of 144 to 360 weeks duration. At present, there are no results from controlled trials evaluating the effect of KALETRA on clinical progression of HIV disease. A limited number of patients between 6 months and 2 years of age have been studied. No data are available on patients less than 6 months of age.

There are insufficient data to support the use of once daily administration of KALETRA for adult patients with three or more protease-inhibitor associated mutations (see Action and Clinical Pharmacology).

Pediatrics (6 months to 18 years of age): The safety and pharmacokinetic profiles of KALETRA in pediatric patients below the age of 6 months have not been established. In HIV-infected patients age 6 months to 12 years, the adverse event profile seen during a clinical trial was similar to that for adult patients. The evaluation of the antiviral activity of KALETRA in pediatric patients in clinical trials is ongoing. KALETRA should not be administered once daily to pediatric patients less than 18 years of age.

Geriatrics (≥65 years of age): Clinical studies of KALETRA did not include sufficient numbers of subjects aged 65 and over to determine whether they respond differently from younger subjects. In general, appropriate caution should be exercised in the administration and monitoring of KALETRA in elderly patients reflecting the greater frequency of decreased hepatic, renal, or cardiac function, and of concomitant disease or other drug therapy.

CONTRAINDICATIONS:

- KALETRA (lopinavir/ritonavir) is contraindicated in patients with known hypersensitivity to any of its ingredients, including ritonavir. For a complete listing, see Dosage Forms, Composition and Packaging.
- Co-administration of KALETRA is contraindicated with drugs that are highly dependent on CYP3A (cytochrome P450 3A) for clearance and for which elevated plasma levels may result in serious and/or life-threatening events. These drugs are listed in Table 1.
- Co-administration of KALETRA is contraindicated with potent CYP3A inducers where significantly reduced lopinavir plasma concentrations may be associated with the potential for loss of virologic response and possible resistance and cross-resistance. These drugs are listed in Table 1.

Table 1: KALETRA

Drugs That Are Contraindicated with KALETRA

Drug Class	Drugs Within Class That Are Contraindicated with KALETRA	Clinical Comment
Antihistamines	astemizole[a], terfenadine[a]	**Contraindicated** due to potential for serious and/or life-threatening reactions such as cardiac arrhythmias.
Antimycobacterial	rifampin	**Contraindicated** due to potential loss of virologic response and possible resistance to KALETRA or to the class of protease inhibitors or other co-administered antiretroviral agents.
Ergot Derivatives	dihydroergotamine, ergonovine, ergotamine, methylergonovine	**Contraindicated** due to potential for serious and/or life-threatening reactions such as acute ergot toxicity characterized by peripheral vasospasm and ischemia of the extremities and other tissues.
Gastrointestinal (GI) Motility Agent	cisapride[a]	**Contraindicated** due to potential for serious and/or life-threatening reactions such as cardiac arrhythmias.
Herbal Products	St. John's Wort (Hypericum perforatum)	**Contraindicated** due to potential loss of virologic response and possible resistance to KALETRA or to the class of protease inhibitors. See also (Drug Interactions, Drug-Herb Interactions).
HMG-CoA Reductase Inhibitors	lovastatin, simvastatin	**Contraindicated** due to potential for serious reactions such as risk of myopathy including rhabdomyolysis. See also (Warnings and Precautions and Drug Interactions, see Boxed Serious Drug Interactions).
Long Acting Beta-Adrenoceptor Agonist	salmeterol	**Contraindicated** due to the potential increased risk of cardiovascular adverse events associated with salmeterol.
Neuroleptic	pimozide	**Contraindicated** due to potential for serious and/or life-threatening reactions such as cardiac arrhythmias.
PDE5 Inhibitors	sildenafil (Revatio; only when used for the treatment of pulmonary arterial hypertension [PAH]), vardenafil	**Contraindicated** due to potential increase in PDE5 inhibitor associated adverse reactions including hypotension, syncope, visual changes and prolonged erection. See Drug Interactions, Drug-Drug Interactions, Table 7 for administration of sildenafil in patients with erectile dysfunction.
Sedatives/Hypnotics	midazolam, triazolam	**Contraindicated** due to potential for serious and/or life-threatening reactions such as prolonged or increased sedation or respiratory depression.

[a] Product not marketed in Canada.

WARNINGS AND PRECAUTIONS:

> **Serious Warnings and Precautions**
> Pancreatitis should be considered if clinical symptoms (nausea, vomiting, abdominal pain) or abnormalities in laboratory values (such as increased serum lipase or amylase values) suggestive of pancreatitis should occur. Patients who exhibit these signs or symptoms should be evaluated and KALETRA and/or other antiretroviral therapy should be suspended as clinically appropriate (see Warnings and Precautions, Hepatic/Biliary/Pancreatic).

General: Lopinavir/ritonavir is an inhibitor of CYP3A and may increase plasma concentrations of agents that are primarily metabolized by CYP3A. Agents that are extensively metabolized by CYP3A and have high first pass metabolism appear to be the most susceptible to large increases in the area under the plasma concentration-time curve (AUC) (>3-fold) when co-administered with KALETRA. Thus, co-administration of KALETRA with drugs highly dependent on CYP3A for clearance and for which elevated plasma concentrations are associated with serious and/or life-threatening events is contraindicated. Co-administration with other CYP3A substrates may require a dose adjustment or additional monitoring. Additionally, KALETRA induces glucuronidation. (See Contraindications, Table 1 and Drug Interactions, Drug-Drug Interactions, Table 7.)

The presence of fructose in KALETRA oral solution may be unsuitable in Hereditary Fructose Intolerance. (See Dosage Forms, Composition and Packaging.)

The presence of high level alcohol in KALETRA oral solution is potentially harmful for those suffering from liver disease, alcoholism, epilepsy, brain injury or disease, as well as for pregnant women and children. It may modify or increase the effects of the other medicines. (See Dosage Forms, Composition and Packaging.)

Patients taking KALETRA oral solution, particularly those with renal impairment or with decreased ability to metabolize propylene glycol (e.g. those of Asian origin), should be monitored for adverse reactions potentially related to propylene glycol toxicity (i.e. seizures, stupor, tachycardia, hyperosmolarity, lactic acidosis, renal toxicity, haemolysis).

Cardiovascular: PR Interval Prolongation: In a Phase 1 study in healthy volunteers, mean change from baseline in PR interval of 11.6 to 31.2 msec was noted in subjects receiving KALETRA on Study Day 3 when exposures were up to 3-fold higher than observed with recommended once daily or twice daily KALETRA doses at steady state. Maximum PR interval was 286 msec and no second- or third-degree heart block was observed.

There have been post-marketing reports of asymptomatic prolongation of the PR interval in some patients receiving combination antiretroviral therapy containing lopinavir/ritonavir. Reports of second- or third-degree atrioventricular block in patients with underlying structural heart disease and pre-existing conduction system abnormalities or in patients receiving drugs known to prolong the PR interval (such as verapamil, calcium blockers, beta-adrenergic blockers, digoxin and atazanavir) have been reported in patients receiving KALETRA. KALETRA should be used with caution in such patients, particularly with those drugs metabolized by CYP3A. (See Action and Clinical Pharmacology, Pharmacodynamics, Effects on the Electrocardiogram.)

Postmarketing cases of QT interval prolongation and torsade de pointes have been reported although causality of KALETRA could not be established. Avoid use in patients with congenital long QT syndrome, those with hypokalemia, and with other drugs that prolong QT interval.

Diabetes Mellitus/Hyperglycemia: New onset diabetes mellitus, exacerbation of pre-existing diabetes mellitus, and hyperglycemia have been reported during post-marketing surveillance in HIV-1 infected patients receiving protease inhibitor (PI) therapy. Some patients required either initiation or dose adjustments of insulin or oral hypoglycemic agents for treatment of these events. In some cases, diabetic ketoacidosis has occurred. In those patients who discontinued PI therapy, hyperglycemia persisted in some cases. Because these events have been reported voluntarily during clinical practice, estimates of frequency cannot be made and a causal relationship between PI therapy and these events has not been established.

Fat Redistribution: Redistribution/accumulation of body fat including central obesity, dorsocervical fat enlargement (buffalo hump), peripheral wasting, facial wasting, breast enlargement, and "cushingoid appearance" have been observed in patients receiving antiretroviral therapy. The mechanism and long-term consequences of these events are currently unknown. A causal relationship has not been established.

Hematologic: There have been reports of increased bleeding, including spontaneous skin hematomas and hemarthrosis, in patients with hemophilia type A and B treated with protease inhibitors (PIs). In some patients additional factor VIII was given. In more than half of the reported cases, treatment with PIs was continued or reintroduced. A causal relationship between PI therapy and these events has not been established; however, the frequency of bleeding episodes should be closely monitored in patients on KALETRA.

Hepatic/Biliary/Pancreatic: Hepatic: KALETRA is principally metabolized by the liver; therefore, caution should be exercised when administering this drug to patients with hepatic impairment. KALETRA has not been studied in patients with severe hepatic impairment. Pharmacokinetic data suggests increases in lopinavir plasma concentrations of approximately 30% as well as decreases in plasma protein binding in HIV and hepatitis C virus (HCV) co-infected patients with mild to moderate hepatic impairment (see Action and Clinical Pharmacology, Pharmacokinetics). Patients with underlying hepatitis B or C or marked elevations in transaminases prior to treatment may be at increased risk for developing or worsening of transaminases elevations or hepatic decompensation with use of KALETRA. There have been post-marketing reports of hepatic dysfunction, including some fatalities. These have generally occurred in patients with advanced HIV disease taking multiple concomitant medications in the setting of underlying chronic hepatitis or cirrhosis. A causal relationship with KALETRA therapy has not been established. Increased aspartate transaminase (AST) and alanine transaminase (ALT) monitoring should be considered in these patients, especially during the first several months of KALETRA treatment.

Pancreatic: Pancreatitis has been observed in patients receiving KALETRA therapy, including those who developed marked triglyceride elevations. In some cases, fatalities have been observed. Although a causal relationship to KALETRA has not been established, marked triglyceride elevation is a risk factor for development of pancreatitis (see Warnings and Precautions, Monitoring and Laboratory Tests, Lipid Elevations). Patients with advanced HIV disease may be at increased risk of elevated triglycerides and pancreatitis, and patients with a history of pancreatitis may be at increased risk for recurrence during KALETRA therapy.

Immune: Immune Reconstitution: Immune reconstitution syndrome has been reported in patients treated with combination antiretroviral therapy, including KALETRA. During the initial phase of treatment, patients responding to antiretroviral therapy may develop an inflammatory response to indolent or residual opportunistic infections [such as *M. avium*-complex (MAC), cytomegalovirus (CMV), *P. jiroveci pneumonia* (PCP), and tuberculosis (TB)], which may necessitate further evaluation and treatment.

Sensitivity/Resistance: Resistance/Cross-Resistance: Various degrees of cross-resistance among protease inhibitors have been observed. The effect of KALETRA therapy on the efficacy of subsequently-administered PIs is under investigation. HIV 1 isolates with reduced susceptibility to lopinavir have been selected in vitro. The presence of ritonavir does not appear to influence the selection of lopinavir-resistant viruses in vitro. The selection of resistance to KALETRA therapy in antiretroviral treatment-naïve patients has not yet been characterized in vivo (see Action and Clinical Pharmacology, Resistance and Cross-resistance).

Special Populations: Pregnant Women: There are no adequate and well-controlled studies in pregnant women. KALETRA should be used during pregnancy only if the potential benefit justifies the potential risk to the fetus. No treatment-related malformations were observed when lopinavir in combination with ritonavir was administered to pregnant rats or rabbits. Embryonic and fetal developmental toxicities occurred in rats at a maternally toxic dose.

Antiretroviral Pregnancy Registry: To monitor maternal-fetal outcomes of pregnant women exposed to KALETRA, an Antiretroviral Pregnancy Registry has been established. Physicians are encouraged to register patients by calling 1-800-258-4263.

Nursing Women: HIV-infected mothers should not breast-feed their infants to avoid risking postnatal transmission of HIV. Studies in rats have demonstrated that lopinavir is secreted in milk. It is not known whether lopinavir is secreted in human milk. Because of both the potential for HIV transmission and the potential for serious adverse reactions in nursing infants, mothers should be instructed **not to breast-feed if they are receiving KALETRA.**

Pediatrics (6 months to 18 years of age): For a brief discussion, see Indications and Clinical Use.

Geriatrics (≥65 years of age): For a brief discussion, see Indications and Clinical Use.

Monitoring and Laboratory Tests: Lipid Elevations: Treatment with KALETRA has resulted in large increases in the concentration of total cholesterol and triglycerides. (See Adverse Reactions, Abnormal Hematologic and Clinical Chemistry Findings, Table 4 and Table 5.) Triglyceride and cholesterol testing should be performed prior to initiating KALETRA therapy and at periodic intervals during therapy. Lipid disorders should be managed as clinically appropriate. See Table 7 for additional information on potential drug interactions with KALETRA and HMG-CoA reductase inhibitors.

ADVERSE REACTIONS: Clinical Trial Adverse Drug Reactions: Because clinical trials are conducted under very specific conditions the adverse reaction rates observed in the clinical trials may not reflect the rates observed in practice and should not be compared to the rates in the clinical trials of another drug. Adverse drug reaction information from clinical trials is useful for identifying drug-related adverse events and for approximating rates.

Adverse Drug Reaction Overview: Treatment-Emergent Adverse Events: Adults: KALETRA (lopinavir/ritonavir) has been studied in 2154 patients as combination therapy in Phase 1/2 and Phase 3 clinical trials. The most common adverse event associated with KALETRA therapy was diarrhea, which was generally of mild to moderate severity, nausea, abdominal pain, asthenia, vomiting, headache, and dyspepsia. The incidence of diarrhea was greater for KALETRA capsule once daily compared to KALETRA capsule twice daily in Study III (see Table 2).

Drug-related clinical adverse events of moderate or severe intensity in ≥2% of patients treated with combination therapy including KALETRA for up to 48 weeks (Phase 3) and for up to 360 weeks (Phase 1/2) are presented in Table 2. For other information regarding observed or potentially serious adverse events, see Warnings and Precautions.

Percentages of patients with selected treatment-emergent adverse events of moderate or severe intensity reported in ≥2% of adult (PI)-experienced patients are listed in Table 3. The incidence of diarrhea during 48 weeks of therapy was similar for KALETRA tablets dosed once daily compared to KALETRA tablets dosed twice daily in Study XI.

Pediatrics: KALETRA has been studied in 100 pediatric patients 6 months to 12 years of age. The adverse event profile seen during a clinical trial was similar to that for adult patients.

Dysgeusia (22%), vomiting (21%), and diarrhea (12%) were the most common adverse reactions of any severity and of probable, possible or unknown relationship to KALETRA oral solution in pediatric patients treated with combination therapy for up to 48 weeks in Study VI. A total of eight subjects experienced adverse events of moderate to severe intensity and of possible, probable, or unknown relationship to KALETRA. The adverse events meeting these criteria and reported for the eight subjects include: allergic reaction (characterized by fever, rash, and jaundice), fever, viral infection, constipation, hepatomegaly, pancreatitis, vomiting, serum glutamic pyruvic transaminase (ALT) increased, dry skin, rash, and dysgeusia. Rash was the only event of those listed that occurred in two or more subjects (n=3).

Less Common Clinical Trial Adverse Drug Reactions (<2%): Treatment-emergent adverse events occurring in less than 2% of adult patients receiving KALETRA in all Phase 2/3 clinical trials and considered at least possibly related or of unknown relationship to treatment with KALETRA and of at least moderate intensity are listed below by system organ class.

Table 2: KALETRA

Percentage of Patients with Selected Treatment-Emergent[a] Adverse Events of Moderate or Severe Intensity Reported in ≥2% of Adult Antiretroviral-Naïve Patients

	Study I (48 Weeks)			Study III (48 Weeks)	Study II (360 Weeks)	Study XI (48 Weeks)	
	KALETRA Capsules 400/100 mg b.i.d.+d4T+3TC (N=326)	Nelfinavir 750 mg t.i.d.+d4T+3TC (N=327)	KALETRA Capsules 800/200 mg Daily+TDF+FTC (N=115)	KALETRA Capsules 400/100 mg b.i.d.+TDF+FTC (N=75)	KALETRA Capsules b.i.d.[b]+d4T+3TC (N=100)	KALETRA Tablets[c] 800/200mg daily+TDF+FTC (N=333)	KALETRA Tablets[c] 400/100mg b.i.d.+TDF+FTC (N=331)
Endocrine Disorders							
Hypogonadism Male	0%	0%	0%	0%	2%	0%	0%
Gastrointestinal Disorders							
Diarrhea	16%	17%	16%	5%	28%	17%	15%
Nausea	7%	5%	9%	8%	16%	7%	5%
Vomiting	2%	2%	3%	4%	6%	3%	4%
Abdominal Pain	4%	3%	3%	3%	11%	1%	1%
Dyspepsia	2%	<1%	0%	1%	6%	0%	0%
Flatulence	2%	1%	2%	1%	4%	1%	1%
Abdominal Distension	<1%	1%	1%	0%	4%	<1%	<1%
Abnormal Feces	0%	<1%	0%	0%	8%	0%	0%
General Disorders and Administration Site Conditions							
Asthenia	4%	3%	0%	0%	9%	<1%	<1%
Pain	1%	0%	0%	0%	3%	0%	0%
Infections and Infestations							
Bronchitis	0%	0%	0%	0%	2%	0%	<1%
Investigations							
Weight Decreased	1%	<1%	0%	0%	2%	0%	<1%
Metabolism and Nutrition Disorders							
Anorexia	1%	<1%	1%	1%	2%	<1%	1%

(cont'd)

Table 2: KALETRA *(cont'd)*

Percentage of Patients with Selected Treatment-Emergent[a] Adverse Events of Moderate or Severe Intensity Reported in ≥2% of Adult Antiretroviral-Naïve Patients

	Study I (48 Weeks)		Study III (48 Weeks)		Study II (360 Weeks)	Study XI (48 Weeks)	
	KALETRA Capsules 400/100 mg b.i.d.+d4T+3TC (N=326)	Nelfinavir 750 mg t.i.d.+d4T+3TC (N=327)	KALETRA Capsules 800/200 mg Daily+TDF+FTC (N=115)	KALETRA Capsules 400/100 mg b.i.d.+TDF+FTC (N=75)	KALETRA Capsules b.i.d.[b]+d4T+3TC (N=100)	KALETRA Tablets[c] 800/200mg daily+TDF+FTC (N=333)	KALETRA Tablets[c] 400/100mg b.i.d.+TDF+FTC (N=331)
Musculoskeletal and Connective Tissue Disorders							
Myalgia	1%	1%	0%	0%	2%	0%	0%
Nervous System Disorders							
Headache	2%	2%	3%	3%	6%	2%	1%
Paresthesia	1%	1%	0%	0%	2%	0%	0%
Psychiatric Disorders							
Insomnia	2%	1%	0%	0%	3%	1%	0%
Depression	1%	2%	1%	0%	0%	0%	0%
Libido Decreased	<1%	<1%	0%	1%	2%	0%	<1%
Reproductive System and Breast Disorders							
Amenorrhea	0%	0%	5%	0%	0%	0%	0%
Skin and Subcutaneous Tissue Disorders							
Lipodystrophy Acquired	1%	1%	0%	0%	12%	0%	0%
Rash	1%	2%	1%	0%	5%	<1%	1%
Vascular Disorders							
Vasodilatation	0%	0%	0%	0%	3%	0%	0%

[a] Includes adverse events of possible or probable relationship to study drug.
[b] Includes adverse event data from dose group I (200/100 mg twice daily [N=16] and 400/100 mg twice daily only [N=16]) and dose group II (400/100 mg b.i.d. [N=35] and 400/200 mg twice daily [N=33]). Within dosing groups, moderate to severe nausea of probable/possible relationship to KALETRA occurred at a higher rate in the 400/200 mg dose arm compared to the 400/100 mg dose arm in group II.
[c] In the first 8 weeks of the study, 166 and 165 of the patients received KALETRA capsule once daily and twice daily, respectively. After that period, all patients received KALETRA tablet.
Legend: b.i.d.=twice daily; t.i.d.=three times daily; d4T=stavudine; 3TC=lamivudine; FTC=emtricitabine; TDF=tenofovir DF.

Table 3: KALETRA

Percentage of Patients with Selected Treatment-Emergent[a] Adverse Events of Moderate or Severe Intensity Reported in ≥2% of Adult Protease Inhibitor-Experienced Patients

	Study IV (48 Weeks)		Study VII[b] and Study V[c] (84 to 144 Weeks)	Study XII (48 Weeks)	
	KALETRA Capsules 400/100 mg b.i.d.+ NVP+NRTIs (N=148)	Investigator-Selected PI(s)+ NVP+NRTIs (N=140)	KALETRA Capsules b.i.d.+ NNRTI+NRTIs (N=127)	KALETRA Tablets 800/200 mg daily+NRTIs (N=300)	KALETRA Tablets 400/100 mg b.i.d.+NRTIs (N=299)
Gastrointestinal Disorders					
Diarrhea	7%	9%	23%	14%	11%
Nausea	7%	16%	5%	3%	7%
Vomiting	4%	12%	2%	2%	3%
Abdominal Pain	2%	2%	4%	2%	<1%
Abdominal Pain Upper	N/A	N/A	N/A	1%	2%
Flatulence	1%	2%	2%	1%	1%
Dysphagia	2%	1%	0%	0%	0%
Abnormal Feces	0%	0%	2%	0%	0%
General Disorders and Administration Site Conditions					
Asthenia	3%	6%	9%	<1%	<1%
Pyrexia	2%	1%	2%	0%	<1%
Pain	0%	0%	4%	0%	0%
Chills	2%	0%	0%	0%	0%
Investigations					
Weight Decreased	0%	1%	3%	<1%	<1%
Metabolism and Nutrition Disorders					
Anorexia	1%	3%	0%	0%	1%
Nervous System Disorders					
Headache	2%	3%	2%	<1%	0%
Paresthesia	0%	1%	2%	0%	0%
Psychiatric Disorders					
Depression	1%	2%	3%	<1%	0%
Insomnia	0%	2%	2%	0%	<1%
Skin and Subcutaneous Tissue Disorders					
Lipodystrophy Acquired	1%	1%	6%	1%	1%
Rash	2%	1%	2%	0%	0%
Vascular Disorders					
Hypertention	0%	0%	2%	0%	0%

[a] Includes adverse events of possible or probable relationship to study drug.
[b] Includes adverse event data from patients receiving 400/100 mg twice daily (n=29) or 533/133 mg twice daily (n=28) for 84 weeks. Patients received KALETRA in combination with NRTIs and efavirenz.
Average of Studies VII and V; both studies have subjects dosed with KALETRA + NNRTI + NRTIs.
[c] Includes adverse event data from patients receiving 400/100 mg twice daily (n=36) or 400/200 mg twice daily (n=34) for 144 weeks. Patients received KALETRA in combination with NRTIs and nevirapine.
Average of Studies VII and V; both studies have subjects dosed with KALETRA + NNRTI + NRTIs.
Legend: b.i.d.=twice daily; NNRTI=non-nucleoside reverse transciptase inhibitor; NRTI=nucleoside reverse transciptase inhibitor; NVP=nevirapine; PI=protease inhibitor; N/A=not applicable.

(cont'd)

Blood and Lymphatic System Disorders: anemia, leucopenia, lymphadenopathy, neutropenia, and splenomegaly.
Cardiac Disorders: angina pectoris, atrial fibrillation, atrioventricular block, hypertension, myocardial infarction, palpitations, and tricuspid valve incompetence.
Ear and Labyrinth Disorders: hyperacusis, tinnitus, and vertigo.
Endocrine Disorders: Cushing's syndrome, and hypothyroidism.
Eye Disorders: eye disorder and visual disturbance.
Gastrointestinal Disorders: abdominal discomfort, abdominal pain lower, constipation, duodenitis, dry mouth, enteritis, enterocolitis, enterocolitis hemorrhagic, eructation, esophagitis, fecal incontinence, gastric disorder, gastric ulcer, gastritis, gastroesophageal reflux disease, hemorrhoids, mouth ulceration, pancreatitis, periodontitis, rectal hemorrhage, stomach discomfort, and stomatitis.
General Disorders and Administration Site Conditions: chest pain, cyst, drug interaction, edema, edema peripheral, face edema, fatigue, hypertrophy, and malaise.
Hepatobiliary Disorders: cholangitis, cholecystitis, cytolytic hepatitis, hepatic steatosis, hepatitis, hepatomegaly, jaundice, and liver tenderness.
Immune System Disorders: drug hypersensitivity, hypersensitivity, and immune reconstitution syndrome.
Infection and Infestations: bacterial infection, bronchopneumonia, cellulitis, folliculitis, furuncle, gastroenteritis, influenza, otitis media, perineal abscess, pharyngitis, rhinitis, sialoadenitis, sinusitis, and viral infections.
Investigations: drug level increased, glucose tolerance decreased, and weight increased.
Metabolism and Nutrition Disorders: decreased appetite, dehydration, diabetes mellitus, dislipidaemia, hypovitaminosis, increased appetite, lactic acidosis, lipomatosis, and obesity.
Musculoskeletal and Connective Tissue Disorders: arthralgia, arthropathy, back pain, muscular weakness, osteoarthritis, osteonecrosis, and pain in extremity.
Neoplasms Benign, Malignant and Unspecified (incl. Cysts and Polyps): benign neoplasm of skin, lipoma, and neoplasm.
Nervous System Disorders: ageusia, amnesia, ataxia, balance disorder, cerebral infarction, convulsion, dizziness, dysgeusia, dyskinesia, encephalopathy, extrapyramidal disorder, facial palsy, hypertonia, migraine, neuropathy, neuropathy peripheral, somnolence, and tremor.
Psychiatric Disorders: abnormal dreams, affect lability, agitation, anxiety, apathy, confusional state, disorientation, mood swings, nervousness, and thinking abnormal.
Renal and Urinary Disorders: hematuria, nephritis, nephrolithiasis, renal disorder, urine abnormality, and urine odor abnormal.
Reproductive System and Breast Disorders: breast enlargement, ejaculation disorder, erectile dysfunction, gynecomastia, and menorrhagia.
Respiratory, Thoracic and Mediastinal Disorders: asthma, cough, dyspnea, and pulmonary edema.
Skin and Subcutaneous Tissue Disorders: acne, alopecia, dermatitis acneiform, dermatitis allergic, dermatitis exfoliative, dry skin, eczema, hyperhidrosis, idiopathic capillaritis, nail disorder, pruritus, rash generalized, rash maculo-papular, seborrhea, skin discoloration, skin hypertrophy, skin striae, skin ulcer, and swelling face.
Vascular Disorders: deep vein thrombophlebitis, deep vein thrombosis, orthostatic hypotension, thrombophlebitis, varicose vein, and vasculitis.
Abnormal Hematologic and Clinical Chemistry Findings: The percentages of adult antiretroviral-naïve and PI-experienced patients treated with combination therapy including KALETRA with Grade 3-4 laboratory abnormalities are presented in Table 4 and Table 5.

Table 4: KALETRA

Grade 3-4 Laboratory Abnormalities Reported in ≥2% of Adult Antiretroviral-Naïve Patients

		Study I (48 Weeks)		Study III (48 Weeks)		Study II (360 Weeks)	Study XI (48 Weeks)	
Variable	**Limit**	**KALETRA Capsules 400/100 mg b.i.d.+d4T+3TC (N=326)**	**Nelfinavir 750 mg t.i.d.+d4T+3TC (N=327)**	**KALETRA Capsules 800/200 mg Daily+TDF+FTC (N=115)**	**KALETRA Capsules 400/100 mg b.i.d.+TDF+FTC (N=75)**	**KALETRA Capsules b.i.d.[a]+d4T+3TC (N=100)**	**KALETRA Tablets[b] 800/200mg daily+TDF+FTC (N=333)**	**KALETRA Tablets[b] 400/100mg b.i.d.+TDF+FTC (N=331)**
Chemistry	**High**							
Glucose	>13.8 mmol/L	2%	2%	3%	1%	4%	0%	<1%
Uric Acid	>0.71 mmol/L	2%	2%	0%	3%	5%	<1%	1%
AST[c]	>5×ULN	2%	4%	5%	3%	10%	1%	2%
ALT[c]	>5×ULN	4%	4%	4%	3%	11%	1%	1%
GGT	>5×ULN	N/A	N/A	N/A	N/A	10%	N/A	N/A
Total Cholesterol	>7.77 mmol/L	9%	5%	3%	3%	27%	4%	3%
Triglycerides	>8.25 mmol/L	9%	1%	5%	4%	29%	3%	6%
Amylase	>2×ULN	3%	2%	7%	5%	4%	N/A	N/A
Lipase	>2×ULN	N/A	N/A	N/A	N/A	N/A	3%	5%
Chemistry	**Low**							
Calculated Creatinine Clearance[d]	<50 mL/min	N/A	N/A	N/A	N/A	N/A	2%	2%
Hematology	**Low**							
Neutrophils	0.75×10^9/L	1%	3%	5%	1%	5%	2%	1%

a Includes adverse event data from dose group I (200/100 mg twice daily [N=16] and 400/100 mg twice daily only [N=16]) and dose group II (400/100 mg b.i.d. [N=35] and 400/200 mg twice daily [N=33]). Within dosing groups, moderate to severe nausea of probable/possible relationship to KALETRA occurred at a higher rate in the 400/200 mg dose arm compared to the 400/100 mg dose arm in group II.
b In the first 8 weeks of the study, 166 and 165 of the patients received KALETRA capsule once daily and twice daily, respectively. After that period, all patients received KALETRA tablet.
c Criterion for Study XI was >5×ULN (AST/ALT).
d The Cockcroft-Gault formula was used to calculate creatinine clearance.
Legend: b.i.d.=twice daily; t.i.d.=three times daily; d4T=stavudine; 3TC=lamivudine; FTC=emtricitabine; TDF=tenofovir DF; ULN=upper limit of the normal range; N/A=Not Applicable; ALT=alanine aminotransferase; AST=aspartate aminotransferase; GGT=gamma-glutamyl transpeptidase.

Table 5: KALETRA

Grade 3-4 Laboratory Abnormalities Reported in ≥2% of Adult Protease Inhibitor-Experienced Patients

		Study IV (48 Weeks)		Studies VII[a] and V[b] (84 to 144 Weeks)	Study XII (48 Weeks)	
Variable	**Limit**	**KALETRA Capsules 400/100 mg b.i.d.+NVP+NRTIs (N=148)**	**Investigator-selected PI(s)+NVP+NRTIs (N=140)**	**KALETRA Capsules b.i.d.+NNRTI +NRTIs (N=127)**	**KALETRA Tablets 800/200 mg daily+NRTIs (N=300)**	**KALETRA Tablets 400/100 mg b.i.d.+NRTIs (N=299)**
Chemistry	**High**					
Glucose	>13.8 mmol/L	1%	2%	5%	2%	2%
Total Bilirubin	>59.5 micromol/L	1%	3%	1%	1%	1%
AST[c]	>5×ULN	5%	11%	8%	3%	2%
ALT[c]	>5×ULN	6%	13%	10%	2%	2%
GGT	>5×ULN	N/A	N/A	29%	N/A	N/A
Total Cholesterol	>7.77 mmol/L	20%	21%	39%	6%	7%

(cont'd)

Table 5: KALETRA *(cont'd)*

Grade 3-4 Laboratory Abnormalities Reported in ≥2% of Adult Protease Inhibitor-Experienced Patients

		Study IV (48 Weeks)		Studies VII[a] and V[b] (84 to 144 Weeks)	Study XII (48 Weeks)	
Variable	**Limit**	**KALETRA Capsules 400/100 mg b.i.d.+NVP+NRTIs (N=148)**	**Investigator-selected PI(s)+NVP+NRTIs (N=140)**	**KALETRA Capsules b.i.d.+NNRTI +NRTIs (N=127)**	**KALETRA Tablets 800/200 mg daily+NRTIs (N=300)**	**KALETRA Tablets 400/100 mg b.i.d.+NRTIs (N=299)**
Triglycerides	>8.25 mmol/L	25%	21%	36%	5%	6%
Amylase	>2×ULN	4%	8%	8%	4%	4%
Lipase	>2×ULN	N/A	N/A	N/A	4%	1%
Creatinine Phosphokinase	>4×ULN	N/A	N/A	N/A	4%	5%
Chemistry	**Low**					
Calculated Creatinine Clearance[d]	<50 mL/min	N/A	N/A	N/A	3%	3%
Inorganic Phosphorous	< 0.48 mmol/L	1%	0%	2%	1%	<1%
Hematology	**Low**					
Neutrophils	0.75×10^9/L	1%	2%	4%	3%	4%
Hemoglobin	<80 g/L	1%	1%	1%	1%	2%

[a] Includes clinical laboratory data from patients receiving 400/100 mg capsules twice daily (n=29) or 533/133 mg capsules twice daily (n=28) for 84 weeks. Patients received KALETRA capsules in combination with NRTIs and efavirenz.
[b] Includes clinical laboratory data from patients receiving 400/100 mg capsules twice daily (n=36) or 400/200 mg capsules twice daily (n=34) for 144 weeks. Patients received KALETRA capsules in combination with NRTIs and nevirapine.
[c] Criterion for Study XII was >5×ULN (AST/ALT).
[d] The Cockcroft-Gault formula was used to calculate creatinine clearance.
Legend: b.i.d.=twice daily; NRTI=nucleoside reverse transciptase inhibitor; NNRTI =non-nucleoside reverse transciptase inhibitor; NVP=nevirapine; PI=protease inhibitor; ULN=upper limit of the normal range; N/A=Not Applicable; ALT=alanine aminotransferase; AST=aspartate aminotransferase; GGT=gamma-glutamyl transpeptidase.

The percentages of pediatric patients treated with combination therapy including KALETRA with Grade 3-4 laboratory abnormalities are presented in Table 6.

Post-Market Adverse Drug Reactions: Hepatitis has been reported in patients on KALETRA therapy.

New onset diabetes mellitus, exacerbation of pre-existing diabetes mellitus, and hyperglycemia has been reported during post-marketing surveillance in HIV-infected patients receiving PI therapy. Some patients required either initiation or dose adjustments of insulin or oral hypoglycemic agents for treatment of these events.

Toxic epidermal necrolysis, Stevens-Johnson Syndrome and erythema multiforme have been reported.

Bradyarrhythmia has been reported.

DRUG INTERACTIONS:

Serious Drug Interactions

- **Analgesics** (fentanyl): Careful monitoring of therapeutic and adverse effects (including respiratory depression) is recommended when KALETRA is co-administered with fentanyl, including extended-release, transdermal or transmucosal preparations.
- **Antihistamines** (astemizole*, terfenadine*): **Contraindicated** due to potential for serious and/or life-threatening reactions such as cardiac arrhythmias.
- **Antimycobacterial** (rifampin): **Contraindicated** due to potential loss of virologic response and possible resistance to KALETRA (lopinavir/ritonavir) or to the class of protease inhibitors or other co-administered antiretroviral agents. KALETRA should not be co-administered with rifampin.
- **Ergot Derivatives** (dihydroergotamine, ergonovine, ergotamine, methylergonovine): **Contraindicated** due to potential for serious and/or life-threatening reactions such as acute ergot toxicity characterized by peripheral vasospasm and ischemia of the extremities and other tissues.
- **GI (Gastrointestinal) Motility Agent** (cisapride*): **Contraindicated** due to potential for serious and/or life-threatening reactions such as cardiac arrhythmias.
- **Herbal Products** (St. John's Wort): **Contraindicated** due to potential loss of virologic response and possible resistance to KALETRA or to the class of protease inhibitors.
- **HMG-CoA Reductase Inhibitors** (lovastatin, simvastatin): **Contraindicated** due to potential for serious reactions such as risk of myopathy including rhabdomyolysis. KALETRA should not be co-administered with these drugs.
- **Long Acting Beta-Adrenoceptor Agonist** (salmeterol): **Contraindicated** due to the potential increased risk of cardiovascular adverse events associated with salmeterol.
- **Neuroleptic** (pimozide): **Contraindicated** due to the potential for serious and/or life-threatening reactions such as cardiac arrhythmias.
- **PDE5 Inhibitors** (sildenafil [only when used for the treatment of pulmonary arterial hypertension], vardenafil): **Contraindicated** due to potential increase in PDE5 inhibitor associated adverse reactions including hypotension, syncope, visual changes and prolonged erection.
- **Sedatives/Hypnotics** (midazolam, triazolam): **Contraindicated** due to potential for serious and/or life-threatening reactions such as prolonged or increased sedation or respiratory depression.

Overview: No drug interaction studies were performed with the once daily regimen of KALETRA (lopinavir/ritonavir).

KALETRA is an inhibitor of CYP3A (cytochrome P450 3A) both in vitro and in vivo. Co-administration of KALETRA and drugs primarily metabolized by CYP3A (e.g., dihydropyridine calcium channel blockers, HMG-CoA reductase inhibitors, immunosuppressants and PDE5 inhibitors) may result in increased plasma concentrations of the other drugs that could increase or prolong their therapeutic and adverse effects. (See Drug Interactions, Drug-Drug Interactions, Table 7.) Agents that are extensively metabolized by CYP3A and have high first pass metabolism appear to be the most susceptible to large increases in AUC (>3-fold) when co-administered with KALETRA.

KALETRA does not inhibit CYP2D6, CYP2C9, CYP2C19, CYP2E1, CYP2B6 or CYP1A2 at clinically relevant concentrations.

KALETRA has been shown in vivo to induce its own metabolism and to increase the biotransformation of some drugs metabolized by cytochrome P450 enzymes and by glucuronidation

KALETRA is metabolized by CYP3A. Co-administration of KALETRA and drugs that induce CYP3A may decrease lopinavir plasma concentrations and reduce its therapeutic effect. (See Drug Interactions, Drug-Drug Interactions, Table 7.) Co-administration of KALETRA and other drugs that inhibit CYP3A may increase lopinavir plasma concentrations.

Drug interaction studies were performed with KALETRA and other drugs likely to be co-administered and some drugs commonly used as probes for pharmacokinetic interactions. Table 7 presents established and other potentially significant drug interactions with lopinavir. The effects of other drugs on ritonavir are not shown since they generally correlate with those observed with lopinavir (if lopinavir concentrations are decreased, ritonavir concentrations are decreased). For information regarding clinical recommendations, see Drug Interactions, Drug-Drug Interactions, Table 7.

* Product not marketed in Canada.

Table 6: KALETRA

Grade 3-4 Laboratory Abnormalities Reported in ≥2% Pediatric Patients

Variable	**Limit**	**KALETRA Oral Solution b.i.d.[a]+NRTIs (n=100)**
Chemistry	**High**	
Sodium	>149 mmol/L	3%
Total Bilirubin	>2.9×ULN	4%
AST	>180 U/L	8%
ALT	>215 U/L	7%
Total Cholesterol	>7.77 mmol/L	4%
Amylase	>2.5×ULN	6%
Chemistry	**Low**	
Sodium	<130 mmol/L	3%
Calcium	<1.75 mmol/dL	2%
Hematology	**Low**	
Hemoglobin	<70 g/L	2%
Platelet Count	$<50 \times 10^9$/L	4%
Neutrophils	$<0.40 \times 10^9$/L	2%

[a] Includes clinical laboratory data from the 230/57.5 mg/m² (n=49) and 300/75 mg/m² (n=51) dose arms.
Legend: b.i.d.=twice daily; NRTI=nucleoside reverse transcriptase inhibitor; ULN=upper limit of the normal range; ALT=alanine aminotransferase; AST=aspartate aminotransferase.

Drug-Drug Interactions: Possible Dose Adjustments Based on Drug-Drug Interactions:

Other Drugs: Drugs with No Observed or Predicted Interactions with KALETRA: Drug interaction studies reveal no clinically significant interaction between KALETRA and desipramine (CYP2D6 probe), pravastatin, stavudine, lamivudine, omeprazole or ranitidine.

Based on known metabolic profiles, clinically significant drug interactions are not expected between KALETRA and fluvastatin, dapsone, trimethoprim/sulfamethoxazole, azithromycin, erythromycin or fluconazole.

Flecainide and Propafenone: Based on results of a desipramine interaction study, KALETRA does not inhibit CYP2D6-mediated metabolism at clinically relevant concentrations. However, caution should be used when co-administering either flecainide or propafenone with KALETRA.

Drug-Herb Interactions: St. John's Wort (Hypericum perforatum): Concomitant use of KALETRA and St. John's Wort (Hypericum perforatum), or products containing St. John's Wort, is contraindictated (see Contraindications, Table 1). Co-administration of protease inhibitors, including KALETRA, with St. John's Wort is expected to substantially decrease protease inhibitor concentrations and may result in sub-optimal levels of lopinavir and lead to loss of virologic response and possible resistance to lopinavir or to the class of protease inhibitors.

Table 7: KALETRA

Established and Other Potentially Significant Drug Interactions: Alteration in Dose or Regimen May Be Recommended Based on Drug Interaction Studies or Predicted Interaction

Concomitant Drug Class: Drug Name	Effect on Concentration of Lopinavir or Concomitant Drug	Clinical Comment
HIV-Antiviral Agents		
Non-nucleoside Reverse Transcriptase Inhibitors: efavirenz, nevirapine	↓ lopinavir ↔ efavirenz ↔ nevirapine	A dose increase of KALETRA tablets to 500/125 mg twice daily (given as two 200/50 mg tablets and one 100/25 mg tablet) when used in combination with efavirenz resulted in similar lopinavir plasma concentrations compared to KALETRA tablets 400/100 mg twice daily without efavirenz. See Dosage and Administration. A dose increase of KALETRA oral solution to 533/133 mg (6.5 mL) twice daily taken with food may be considered when used in combination with efavirenz or nevirapine in patients where reduced susceptibility to lopinavir is clinically suspected (by treatment history or laboratory evidence). KALETRA should not be administered once daily in combination with efavirenz or nevirapine (see Dosage and Administration). **Note:** Efavirenz and nevirapine induce the activity of CYP3A and thus have the potential to decrease plasma concentrations of other protease inhibitors when used in combination with KALETRA. The effect of KALETRA on both efavirenz and nevirapine was assessed in healthy volunteers. Although no significant interaction was apparent, due to study discontinuations, both studies had limited power to detect changes in efavirenz and nevirapine pharmacokinetics in the presence of KALETRA.
Non-nucleoside Reverse Transcriptase Inhibitor: delavirdine	↑ lopinavir	The safety and efficacy of this combination have not been established.
Nucleoside Reverse Transcriptase Inhibitor: didanosine		KALETRA tablets can be administered simultaneously with didanosine without food. For KALETRA oral solution, it is recommended that didanosine be administered on an empty stomach; therefore, didanosine should be given one hour before or two hours after KALETRA oral solution (given with food).
Nucleoside Reverse Transcriptase Inhibitor: tenofovir	↑ tenofovir ↔ lopinavir	KALETRA increases tenofovir concentrations. The mechanism of this interaction is unknown. Patients receiving KALETRA and tenofovir should be monitored for tenofovir-associated adverse events.
Nucleoside Reverse Transcriptase Inhibitor: abacavir, zidovudine	↓ abacavir ↓ zidovudine	KALETRA induces glucuronidation; therefore, KALETRA has the potential to reduce zidovudine and abacavir plasma concentrations. The clinical significance of this potential interaction is unknown.
HIV Protease Inhibitor: amprenavir[a]	↑ amprenavir (amprenavir 750 mg b.i.d. + KALETRA produces ↑ AUC, similar C_{max}, ↑ C_{min} relative to amprenavir 1200 mg b.i.d) ↓ lopinavir	KALETRA at a dose of 400/100 mg, when co-administered with amprenavir, is not recommended. Safety and efficacy of increased doses of KALETRA in combination with amprenavir have not been established. KALETRA should not be administered once daily in combination with amprenavir. Amprenavir induces the activity of CYP3A and thus has the potential to decrease plasma concentrations of other protease inhibitors when used in combination with KALETRA (see Dosage and Administration).
HIV Protease Inhibitors: fosamprenavir	↓ amprenavir ↓ lopinavir	An increased rate of adverse events has been observed with the co-administration of the medications. The safety and efficacy of this combination have not been established.
fosamprenavir/ritonavir	↓ amprenavir ↑ lopinavir	The concomitant use of fosamprenavir/ritonavir and lopinavir/ritonavir is not recommended because of significant pharmacokinetic interactions. KALETRA should not be administered once daily in combination with fosamprenavir (see Dosage and Administration).
HIV Protease Inhibitors: indinavir	↑ indinavir (indinavir 600 mg b.i.d. + KALETRA produces similar AUC, ↓ C_{max}, ↑ C_{min} relative to indinavir 800 mg t.i.d.) ↔ lopinavir	Decrease indinavir dose to 600 mg twice daily when co-administered with KALETRA 400/100 mg twice daily. KALETRA tablets once daily has not been studied in combination with indinavir.
HIV Protease Inhibitors: nelfinavir	↑ nelfinavir (nelfinavir 1000 mg b.i.d. + KALETRA produces similar AUC, similar C_{max}, ↑ C_{min} relative to nelfinavir 1250 mg b.i.d.) ↑ M8 metabolite of nelfinavir ↓ lopinavir	A dose increase of KALETRA to 533/133 mg (6.5 mL of oral solution) or 500/125 mg (given as two 200/50 mg tablets and one 100/25 mg tablet) twice daily may be considered in patients where reduced susceptibility to lopinavir is clinically suspected (by treatment history or laboratory evidence). The safety and efficacy of this combination have not been established. KALETRA should not be administered once daily in combination with nelfinavir. Nelfinavir induces the activity of CYP3A and thus has the potential to decrease plasma concentrations of other protease inhibitors when used in combination with KALETRA (see Dosage and Administration).
HIV Protease Inhibitors: saquinavir	↑ saquinavir (saquinavir 800 mg b.i.d. + KALETRA produces ↑ AUC, ↑ C_{max}, ↑ C_{min} relative to saquinavir 1200 mg t.i.d.) ↔ lopinavir	Saquinavir 1000 mg twice daily may be considered when co-administered with KALETRA 400/100 mg twice daily. KALETRA tablets once daily has not been studied in combination with saquinavir.
HIV Protease Inhibitors: ritonavir	↑ lopinavir	The safety and efficacy of this combination have not been established.
HIV Protease Inhibitors: tipranavir/ritonavir	tipranavir/ritonavir + KALETRA produces ↓ AUC and ↓ C_{min} of lopinavir	The concomitant administration of KALETRA and tipranavir co-administered with low-dose ritonavir is not recommended. Tipranavir (500 mg twice daily) with ritonavir (200 mg twice daily), co-administered with lopinavir/ritonavir (400/100 mg twice daily), resulted in a 55 and 70% reduction in lopinavir AUC and C_{min}, respectively.
Other Agents		
Analgesic: fentanyl	↑ fentanyl	The CYP3A inhibitor activity of KALETRA is expected to increase the plasma concentrations of fentanyl. Careful monitoring of therapeutic and adverse effects (including respiratory depression) is recommended when KALETRA is co-administered with fentanyl, including extended-release, transdermal or transmucosal preparations.
Antiarrhythmics: amiodarone, bepridil[a], lidocaine (systemic), and quinidine	↑ antiarrhythmics	Caution is warranted and therapeutic concentration monitoring is recommended for antiarrhythmics when co-administered with KALETRA, if available.
Anticancer Agents: dasatinib, nilotinib, vinblastine, vincristine	↑ anticancer agents	Potentially life-threatening adverse events associated with these anticancer agents have occurred as a result of having their serum concentrations increased when co-administered with KALETRA. Concomitant administration of KALETRA and nilotinib or dasatinib should be avoided where possible. Where co-administration is unavoidable, refer to the drug's prescribing information for dosing instructions and relevant warnings and precautions.
Anticoagulant: warfarin		Concentrations of warfarin may be affected. It is recommended that INR (International Normalized Ratio) be monitored.
Anticonvulsants: carbamazepine, phenobarbital, phenytoin	↓ lopinavir ↓ phenytoin	Use with caution. KALETRA may be less effective due to decreased lopinavir plasma concentrations in patients taking these agents concomitantly. KALETRA should not be administered once daily in combination with carbamazepine, phenobarbital, or phenytoin. In addition, co-administration of phenytoin and lopinavir/ritonavir resulted in moderate decreases in steady-state phenytoin concentrations. Phenytoin levels should be monitored when co-administering with lopinavir/ritonavir.
Antidepressants: bupropion,	↓ bupropion ↓ hydroxybupropion ↔ lopinavir	Concurrent administration of bupropion with lopinavir/ ritonavir will decrease plasma levels of both bupropion and its active metabolite (hydroxybupropion).
trazodone	↑ trazodone	Adverse events of nausea, dizziness, hypotension and syncope have been observed. If trazodone is used with a CYP3A4 inhibitor such as KALETRA, the combination should be used with caution and a lower dose of trazodone should be considered.

(cont'd)

Table 7: KALETRA *(cont'd)*

Established and Other Potentially Significant Drug Interactions: Alteration in Dose or Regimen May Be Recommended Based on Drug Interaction Studies or Predicted Interaction

Concomitant Drug Class: Drug Name	Effect on Concentration of Lopinavir or Concomitant Drug	Clinical Comment
Anti-infective: clarithromycin	↑ clarithromycin	For patients with renal impairment, the following dosage adjustments should be considered: • For patients with CL_{CR} 30 to 60 mL/min the dose of clarithromycin should be reduced by 50%. • For patients with CL_{CR} <30 mL/min the dose of clarithromycin should be decreased by 75%. No dose adjustment for patients with normal renal function is necessary.
Antifungals: itraconazole, ketoconazole, voriconazole	↑ itraconazole ↑ ketoconazole ↔ lopinavir ↓ voriconazole	High doses of ketoconazole or itraconazole (>200 mg/day) are not recommended. Careful monitoring for adverse events and cautious use of ketoconazole or itraconazole is warranted at doses >200 mg/day when administered with KALETRA. Administration of a single 200 mg dose of ketoconazole did not increase the C_{max}, AUC or C_{min} of lopinavir during KALETRA 400/100 mg twice daily administration. However, it is possible that with multiple administration or higher doses of ketoconazole, lopinavir concentrations could be moderately increased. A study has shown that co-administration of ritonavir 100 mg every 12 hours decreased voriconazole steady-state AUC by an average of 39%; therefore, co-administration of lopinavir/ritonavir and voriconazole should be avoided, unless an assessment of the benefit/risk to the patient justifies the use of voriconazole.
Antimycobacterial: rifabutin,	↑ rifabutin and rifabutin metabolite ↔ lopinavir	Co-administration of KALETRA with rifabutin substantially increases concentration of rifabutin and its active metabolite by >5-fold which may result in an increase in rifabutin-associated adverse events, including fever, neutropenia and uveitis. Dosage reduction of rifabutin by at least 75% of the usual dose of 300 mg/day is recommended (i.e., a maximum dose of 150 mg every other day or three times per week). Increased monitoring for adverse events is warranted in patients receiving the combination. Further dosage reduction of rifabutin may be necessary.
rifampin	↓ lopinavir	Due to the large reductions in lopinavir plasma concentrations observed in a study evaluating the combination of rifampin 600 mg once a day with KALETRA 400/100 mg twice daily, KALETRA should not be co-administered with rifampin as it may significantly decrease lopinavir's therapeutic effect. Results from studies using higher doses of lopinavir/ ritonavir co-administered with rifampin indicated higher incidences of liver and gastrointestinal toxicity.
Antiparasitic: atovaquone	↓ atovaquone	Clinical significance is unknown; however, increase in atovaquone doses may be needed.
Calcium Channel Blockers, Dihydropyridine: e.g., felodipine, nicardipine[a], nifedipine	↑ dihydropyridine calcium channel blockers	Caution is warranted and clinical monitoring of patients is recommended.
Cardiotonic Glycoside: digoxin	↑ digoxin	Co-administration of ritonavir (300 mg every 12 hours) and digoxin resulted in significantly increased digoxin levels. Caution should be exercised when co-administering KALETRA with digoxin, with appropriate monitoring of serum digoxin levels.
Corticosteroid: dexamethasone,	↓ lopinavir	Use with caution. KALETRA may be less effective due to decreased lopinavir plasma concentrations in patients taking these agents concomitantly.
Fluticasone propionate	↑ fluticasone propionate	Concomitant use of ritonavir and fluticasone propionate can significantly increase fluticasone propionate plasma concentrations and reduce serum cortisol concentrations. Systemic corticosteroid effects including Cushing's syndrome and adrenal suppression have been reported when ritonavir has been co-administered with inhaled or intranasally administered fluticasone propionate. Use with caution. Consider alternatives to fluticasone propionate, particularly for long-term use.
Disulfiram/metronidazole		KALETRA oral solution contains alcohol which can produce disulfiram-like reactions when co-administered with disulfiram or other drugs that produce this reaction (e.g., metronidazole).
Erectile Dysfunction Agents—PDE5 inhibitors: sildenafil, tadalafil, vardenafil	↑ sildenafil ↑ tadalafil ↑ vardenafil lopinavir (study not done)	Particular caution should be used when prescribing sildenafil or tadalafil for the treatment of erectile dysfunction in patients receiving KALETRA. Co-administration of KALETRA with these drugs is expected to substantially increase their concentrations and may result in increase in associated adverse events such as hypotension, syncope, visual changes, and prolonged erection. Sildenafil may be used with caution at reduced doses of 25 mg every 48 hours with increased monitoring for adverse events. Concomitant use of sildenafil with KALETRA is contraindicated in pulmonary arterial hypertension (PAH) patients (see Contraindications, Table 1). Tadalafil may be used with caution at reduced doses of 10 mg every 72 hours with increased monitoring for adverse events. Combination of vardenafil with KALETRA is contraindicated (see Contraindications, Table 1).
HMG-CoA Reductase Inhibitors: atorvastatin, rosuvastatin, pravastatin	↑ atorvastatin ↔ lopinavir ↑ rosuvastatin ↔ lopinavir ↑ pravastatin ↔ lopinavir	HMG-CoA reductase inhibitors (statins) may interact with protease inhibitors and increase the risk of myopathy including rhabdomyolysis. The long-term safety when co-administering HMG-CoA reductase inhibitors with KALETRA has not been established. Concomitant use of protease inhibitors with lovastatin or simvastatin is contraindicated (see Contraindications). Other HMG-CoA reductase inhibitors (statins) may also interact with protease inhibitors. This warning is based on clinical reports and on indirect evidence from studies on the cytochrome P450 CYP3A4 metabolism pathway. Use lowest possible dose of atorvastatin or rosuvastatin with careful monitoring. Consider other HMG-CoA reductase inhibitors such as pravastatin or fluvastatin in combination with KALETRA lopinavir/ritonavir. Note that an approximate 30% increase in pravastatin concentrations was observed and careful monitoring is warranted.
Immunosuppressants: cyclosporine, rapamycin, tacrolimus	↑ immunosuppressants	Therapeutic concentration monitoring is recommended for immunosuppressant agents when co-administered with KALETRA.
Narcotic Analgesic: methadone	↓ methadone	Dosage of methadone may need to be increased when co-administered with KALETRA.
Oral or Patch Contraceptive: ethinyl estradiol, norethindrone	↓ ethinyl estradiol ↓ norethindrone	Alternative or additional contraceptive measures should be used when estrogen-progesterone-based oral or patch contraceptives and KALETRA are co-administered.

[a] Product not marketed in Canada.
Legend: b.i.d.=twice daily; t.i.d.=three times a day.

DOSAGE AND ADMINISTRATION: **Dosing Considerations:**

- Do not use once daily administration of KALETRA (lopinavir/ritonavir) in:
  - combination with efavirenz, nevirapine or nelfinavir
  - combination with carbamazepine, phenobarbital or phenytoin
  - pediatric patients
- Concomitant therapy may affect the dose of KALETRA (see Dosage and Administration, Recommended Dose and Dosage Adjustment, Adults, Concomitant Therapy) and (Dosage and Administration, Recommended Dose and Dosage Adjustment, Pediatric Patients, Concomitant Therapy).
- For children 6 months to 18 years of age, the pediatric dose based on body weight or body surface area calculations.

Recommended Dose and Dosage Adjustment:

- KALETRA tablets may be taken with or without food.
- KALETRA oral solution must be taken with food.
- KALETRA tablets should be swallowed whole and not chewed, broken, or crushed.

The recommended oral dose of KALETRA is as follows (please also refer to Indications and Clinical Use and Adverse Reactions):

Adults: Twice Daily Administration:

- KALETRA tablets 400/100 mg (given as two 200/50 mg tablets) twice daily.
- KALETRA oral solution 400/100 mg (given as 5 mL) twice daily.

Once Daily Administration:

- KALETRA tablets 800/200 mg (given as four 200/50 mg tablets) once daily in patients with less than three protease-inhibitor associated mutations.
- KALETRA oral solution 800/200 mg (given as 10 mL) once daily in patients with less than three protease-inhibitor associated mutations.

There are insufficient data to support the use of once daily administration of KALETRA for adult patients with three or more protease-inhibitor associated mutations (see Action and Clinical Pharmacology).

Concomitant Therapy: Omeprazole and Ranitidine:

- KALETRA can be used in combination with acid-reducing agents (omeprazole and ranitidine) with no dose adjustment.

Efavirenz, Nevirapine, Amprenavir or Nelfinavir:

- A dose increase of KALETRA tablets to 500/125 mg twice daily (given as two 200/50 mg tablets and one 100/25 mg tablet) should be considered when used in combination with efavirenz, nevirapine, amprenavir or nelfinavir in treatment experienced patients where reduced susceptibility to lopinavir is clinically suspected (by treatment history or laboratory evidence). See Drug Interactions, Table 7.
- A dose increase of KALETRA oral solution to 533/133 mg (given as 6.5 mL oral solution) twice daily may be considered when used in combination with efavirenz, nevirapine, amprenavir or nelfinavir in the treatment of experienced patients where reduced susceptibility to lopinavir is clinically suspected (by treatment history or laboratory evidence). See Drug Interactions, Table 7).

Increasing the dose of KALETRA tablets to 600/150 mg (given as three 200/50 mg tablets) twice daily when co-administered with efavirenz significantly increased the lopinavir plasma concentrations approximately 35%, and ritonavir concentrations approximately 56 to 92%, compared to KALETRA tablets 400/100 mg (given as two 200/50 mg tablets) twice daily without efavirenz (see Drug Interactions, Table 7). The clinical significance in terms of safety and efficacy is not known.

KALETRA tablets and oral solution should not be administered as a once daily regimen in combination with efavirenz, nevirapine or nelfinavir.

Pediatric Patients: Pediatric Patients (6 months to 18 years): KALETRA tablets and oral solution should not be administered once daily in pediatric patients less than 18 years of age.

In children 6 months to 18 years of age, the recommended dosage of KALETRA should be calculated based on body weight (kg) or body surface area (BSA—m^2) and should not exceed the recommended adult dose.

Healthcare professionals should pay special attention to the accurate calculation of the dose of KALETRA, transcription of the medication orders, dispensing information and dosing instructions to minimize the risk for medication errors, overdose (see Overdosage) and underdose. Prescribers should calculate the appropriate dose based on body weight or body surface area (BSA) recommendations in Table 8, Table 9, Table 10, Table 11, Table 12 and Table 13 for each individual child and depending on concomitant therapy.

Before prescribing KALETRA 100/25 mg tablets, children should be assessed for the ability to swallow intact tablets. If a child is unable to reliably swallow a KALETRA tablet, the KALETRA oral solution formulation should be prescribed. The dose of the oral solution should be administered using a calibrated oral dosing syringe.

Table 8: KALETRA

Pediatric Dosing Guidelines Based on BSA for KALETRA Oral Solution[a]—Without Concomitant Efavirenz, Nevirapine, Nelfinavir or Amprenavir

Body Surface Area (m²)[b]	Twice Daily Dose (230/57.5 mg/m²)
0.25	0.7 mL (57.5/14.4 mg)
0.5	1.4 mL (115/28.8 mg)
0.75	2.2 mL (172.5/43.1 mg)
1.0	2.9 mL (230/57.5 mg)
1.25	3.6 mL (287.5/71.9 mg)
1.5	4.3 mL (345/86.3 mg)
1.75	5 mL (400/100 mg)

a KALETRA oral solution should be taken with food.

b

$$BSA\ (m^2) = \sqrt{\frac{Height\ (cm) \times Weight\ (kg)}{3600}}$$

Table 9: KALETRA

Pediatric Dosing Guidelines Based on BSA for KALETRA 100/25 mg Tablets[a]—Without Concomitant Efavirenz, Nevirapine, Nelfinavir or Amprenavir

Body Surface Area (m²)[b]	Recommended Number of 100/25 mg Tablets Twice-Daily
0.4 to <0.6	Tablets are not recommended. Use oral solution
≥0.6 to <0.9	2 tablets (200/50 mg)
≥0.9 to <1.4	3 tablets (300/75 mg)
≥1.4	4 tablets (400/100 mg)

a KALETRA tablets may be taken with or without food.

b

$$BSA\ (m^2) = \sqrt{\frac{Height\ (cm) \times Weight\ (kg)}{3600}}$$

Table 10: KALETRA

Pediatric Dosing Guidelines Based on Weight for KALETRA Oral Solution and 100/25 mg Tablets—Without Concomitant Efavirenz, Nevirapine, Nelfinavir or Amprenavir

Weight (kg)	Twice Daily Dose (mg/kg)[a]	Volume of Oral Solution Twice Daily (80 mg lopinavir/20 mg ritonavir per mL)[b]	Number of 100/25 mg Tablets Twice Daily[c]
7 to <15 kg	**12 mg/kg**		
7 to 10 kg		1.25 mL	Tablets are not recommended. Use oral solution.
>10 to <15 kg		1.75 mL	
15 to 40 kg	**10 mg/kg**		
15 to 20 kg		2.25 mL	2
>20 to 25 kg		2.75 mL	2
>25 to 30 kg		3.50 mL	3
>30 to 35 kg		4.00 mL	3
>35 to 40 kg		4.75 mL	4 (or two 200/50 mg tablets)
>40 kg	See adult dosage recommendation.		

a Dosing based on the lopinavir component of KALETRA oral solution (80 mg/20 mg per mL).
b KALETRA oral solution should be taken with food.
c KALETRA Tablets may be taken with or without food.

Concomitant Therapy: Efavirenz, nevirapine, amprenavir or nelfinavir: A dose increase of KALETRA oral solution to 300/75 mg/m² twice daily taken with food, should be considered when used in combination with efavirenz, nevirapine, amprenavir, or nelfinavir in the treatment of experienced children 6 months to 18 years of age in which reduced susceptibility to lopinavir is clinically suspected (by treatment history or laboratory evidence). Children >45 kg in weight should receive the adult dose (see Table 13). Table 11 and Table 12 contain dosing guidelines for KALETRA oral solution and KALETRA 100/25 mg tablets based on body surface area, respectively, and Table 13 contains dosing guidelines for KALETRA oral solution or the KALETRA 100/25 mg tablets based on body weight, when used in combination with efavirenz, nevirapine, amprenavir, or nelfinavir in children (see Drug Interactions and (Table 7).

Missed Dose: If a dose of this medication has been missed, it should be taken as soon as possible. However, if it is almost time for the next dose, skip the missed dose and go back to the regular dosing schedule. Do not double doses.

Table 11: KALETRA

Pediatric Dosing Guidelines Based on BSA for KALETRA Oral Solution[a]—with Concomitant Efavirenz, Nevirapine, Nelfinavir or Amprenavir

Body Surface Area (m²)[b]	Twice Daily Dose (300/75 mg/m²)
0.25	0.9 mL (75/18.8 mg)
0.5	1.9 mL (150/37.5 mg)
0.75	2.8 mL (225/56.3 mg)
1.0	3.8 mL (300/75 mg)
1.25	4.7 mL (375/93.8 mg)
1.5	5.6 mL (450/112.5 mg)
1.75	6.5 mL (525/131.3 mg)

a KALETRA oral solution should be taken with food.

b

$$BSA\ (m^2) = \sqrt{\frac{Height\ (cm) \times Weight\ (kg)}{3600}}$$

Table 12: KALETRA

Pediatric Dosing Guidelines Based on BSA for KALETRA 100/25 mg Tablets[a]—with Concomitant Efavirenz, Nevirapine, Nelfinavir or Amprenavir

Body Surface Area (m²)[b]	Recommended Number of 100/25 mg Tablets Twice-Daily
0.4 to <0.6	Tablets are not recommended. Use oral solution.
≥0.6 to <0.8	2 tablet (200/50 mg)
≥0.8 to <1.2	3 tablets (300/75 mg)
≥1.2 to <1.4	4 tablets (400/100 mg)
≥1.4	5 tablets (500/125 mg)

a KALETRA tablets may be taken with or without food.

b

$$BSA\ (m^2) = \sqrt{\frac{Height\ (cm) \times Weight\ (kg)}{3600}}$$

Table 13: KALETRA

Pediatric Dosing Guidelines Based on Weight for KALETRA Oral Solution and 100/25 mg Tablets—with Concomitant Efavirenz, Nevirapine, Nelfinavir or Amprenavir

Weight (kg)	Twice Daily Dose (mg/kg)[a]	Volume of Oral Solution Twice daily (80 mg lopinavir/20 mg ritonavir per mL)[b]	Number of 100/25 mg Tablets Twice Daily[c]
7 to <15 kg	**13 mg/kg**		
7 to 10 kg		1.50 mL	Tablets are not recommended. Use oral solution.
>10 to <15 kg		2.00 mL	
15 to 45 kg	**11 mg/kg**		
15 to 20 kg		2.50 mL	2
>20 to 25 kg		3.25 mL	3
>25 to 30 kg		4.00 mL	3
>30 to 35 kg		4.50 mL	4 (or two 200/50 mg tablets)
>35 to 45 kg		5.00 mL	4 (or two 200/50 mg tablets)
>45 kg		6.5 mL	5 (or two 200/50 mg tablets and one 100/25 mg tablet)

a Dosing based on the lopinavir component of KALETRA oral solution (80 mg/20 mg per mL).
b KALETRA oral solution should be taken with food.
c KALETRA tablets may be taken with or without food.

OVERDOSAGE:

Overdoses with KALETRA (lopinavir/ritonavir) oral solution have been reported. One of these reports described fatal cardiogenic shock in a 2.1 kg infant who received a single dose of 6.5 mL of KALETRA oral solution nine days prior. However, a causal relationship between the overdose and the outcome could not be established. Healthcare professionals should be aware that KALETRA oral solution is highly concentrated and therefore, should pay special attention to accurate calculation of the dose of KALETRA, transcription of the medication order, dispensing information and dosing instructions to minimize the risk for medication errors and overdose. This is especially important for infants and young children.

KALETRA (lopinavir/ritonavir) oral solution contains 42.4% alcohol (v/v). Accidental ingestion of the product by a young child could result in significant alcohol-related toxicity and could approach the potential lethal dose of alcohol.

- There is no specific antidote for overdose with KALETRA.
- Treatment of overdose with KALETRA should consist of general supportive measures including monitoring of vital signs and observation of the clinical status of the patient.
- Administration of activated charcoal should be used to aid in removal of unabsorbed drug.
- Human experience of acute overdosage with KALETRA is limited.
- Since KALETRA is highly protein bound, dialysis is unlikely to be beneficial.

For management of a suspected drug overdose, contact your regional Poison Control Centre. See the *CPS Directory* section for a list of Poison Control Centres.

ACTION AND CLINICAL PHARMACOLOGY: Mechanism of Action: Lopinavir, an inhibitor of the HIV protease, prevents cleavage of the Gag-Pol polyprotein, resulting in the production of immature, non-infectious viral particles. Ritonavir inhibits the metabolism of lopinavir, thereby increasing the plasma levels of lopinavir. The antiviral activity of KALETRA (lopinavir/ritonavir) is due to lopinavir.

Antiviral Activity In Vitro: The in vitro antiviral activity of lopinavir against laboratory HIV strains and clinical HIV isolates was evaluated in acutely infected lymphoblastic cell lines and peripheral blood lymphocytes, respectively. In the absence of human serum, the mean 50% effective concentration (EC_{50}) of lopinavir against five different HIV-1 laboratory strains ranged from 10 to 27 nM (0.006 to 0.017 µg/mL, 1 µg/mL=1.6 microM) and ranged from 4 to 11 nM (0.003 to 0.007 µg/mL) against several HIV-1 subtype B clinical isolates (n=6). In the presence of 50% human serum, the mean EC_{50} of lopinavir against these five laboratory strains ranged from 65 to 289 nM (0.04 to 0.18 µg/mL), representing a 7- to 11-fold attenuation.

Resistance: The selection of resistance to KALETRA therapy in antiretroviral treatment-naïve patients has not yet been characterized. In a Phase 3 study of 653 antiretroviral treatment naïve patients (Study I), plasma viral isolates from each patient on treatment with plasma HIV >400 copies/mL at Week 24, 32, 40 and/or 48 were analysed. No evidence of resistance to KALETRA was observed in 37 evaluable KALETRA-treated patients (0%). Evidence of genotypic resistance to nelfinavir, defined as the presence of D30N and/or L90M mutation in HIV protease, was observed in 25/76 (33%) of evaluable nelfinavir-treated patients. The selection of resistance to KALETRA in antiretroviral-naïve pediatric patients (Study VI) appears to be consistent with that seen in adult patients (Study I).

There are insufficient data at this time to identify lopinavir-associated mutational patterns in isolates from patients on KALETRA therapy. However, in Phase 2 studies of 227 antiretroviral treatment naïve and PI-experienced patients, isolates from 4 of 23 patients with quantifiable (>400 copies/mL) viral RNA following treatment with KALETRA for 12 to 100 weeks displayed significantly reduced susceptibility to lopinavir compared to the corresponding baseline viral isolates. Three of these patients had previously received treatment with a single protease inhibitor (nelfinavir, indinavir, or saquinavir) and one patient had received treatment with multiple protease inhibitors (indinavir, saquinavir and ritonavir). All four of these patients had at least four mutations associated with PI resistance immediately prior to KALETRA therapy. Following viral rebound, isolates from these patients all contained additional mutations, some of which were recognized to be associated with PI resistance.

Cross-resistance: Preclinical Studies: Varying degrees of cross-resistance have been observed among HIV protease inhibitors. Little information is available on the cross-resistance of viruses that developed decreased susceptibility to lopinavir during KALETRA therapy.

The in vitro activity of lopinavir against clinical isolates from patients previously treated with a single PI was determined. Isolates that displayed >4-fold reduced susceptibility to nelfinavir (n=13) and saquinavir (n=4), displayed <4-fold reduced susceptibility to lopinavir. Isolates with >4-fold reduced susceptibility to indinavir (n=16) and ritonavir (n=3) displayed a mean of 5.7 to 8.3-fold reduced susceptibility to lopinavir, respectively. Isolates from patients previously treated with two or more PIs showed greater reductions in susceptibility to lopinavir, as described in the Clinical Studies section that follows.

Clinical Studies—Antiviral Activity of KALETRA in Patients with Previous Protease Inhibitor (PI) Therapy: The clinical relevance of reduced in vitro susceptibility to lopinavir has been examined by assessing the virologic response to KALETRA therapy, with respect to baseline viral genotype and phenotype, in 56 NNRTI-naïve patients with HIV RNA >1000 copies/mL despite previous therapy with at least two PIs selected from nelfinavir, indinavir, saquinavir and ritonavir (Study VII). In this study, patients were initially randomized to receive one of two doses of KALETRA in combination with efavirenz and nucleoside reverse transcriptase inhibitors (NRTIs). The EC_{50} of lopinavir against the 56 baseline viral isolates ranged from 0.5- to 96-fold higher than the EC_{50} against wild type HIV. Fifty-five percent (31/56) of these baseline isolates displayed a >4-fold reduced susceptibility to lopinavir with a mean reduction in lopinavir susceptibility of 27.9-fold.

Table 14 shows the 48-week virologic response (HIV RNA <400 and <50 copies) according to susceptibility and number of genotypic mutations at baseline in 50 evaluable patients enrolled in the Study VII described above. Because this was a select patient population and the sample size was small, the data depicted in Table 14 do not constitute definitive clinical susceptibility breakpoints. Additional data are needed to determine clinically significant breakpoints for KALETRA.

Table 14: KALETRA

HIV RNA Response at Week 48 by Baseline KALETRA Susceptibility and by Number of Protease Inhibitor-Associated Mutations[a]—Study VII

Lopinavir Susceptibility[b] at Baseline	HIV RNA <400 copies/mL (%)	HIV RNA <50 copies/mL (%)
<10 fold	25/27 (93)	22/27 (81)
>10 and <40 fold	11/15 (73)	9/15 (60)
≥40 fold	2/8 (25)	2/8 (25)
Number of Protease Inhibitor Mutations at Baseline		
Up to 5	21/23 (91)[c]	19/23 (83)
>5	17/27 (63)	14/27 (52)

[a] Lopinavir susceptibility was determined by recombinant phenotypic technology performed by Virologic; genotype also performed by Virologic.
[b] Fold change in susceptibility from wild type.
[c] Thirteen of the 23 patient isolates contained PI mutations at positions 82, 84, and/or 90.

After 48 weeks of treatment with KALETRA, efavirenz and NRTIs, plasma HIV RNA ≤400 copies/mL was observed in 93% (25/27), 73% (11/15), and 25% (2/8) of patients with <10-fold, 10- to 40-fold, and ≥40-fold reduced susceptibility to lopinavir at baseline, respectively.

There are insufficient data at this time to identify lopinavir-associated mutational patterns in isolates from patients on KALETRA therapy. Further studies are needed to assess the association between specific mutational patterns and virologic response rates.

Genotypic Correlates of Reduced Virologic Response in Antiretroviral-Experienced Patients Initiating a KALETRA-Based Combination Regimen: Virologic response to KALETRA has been shown to be affected by the presence of three or more of the following amino acid substitutions in protease at baseline: L10F/I/R/V, K20M/N/R, L24I, L33F, M36I, I47V, G48V, I54L/T/V, V82A/C/F/S/T, and I84V. Table 15 shows the 48 week virologic response (HIV RNA <400 copies/ mL) according to the number of the above PI resistance mutations at baseline in Studies IV, V and VII.

Table 15: KALETRA

Virologic Response (HIV RNA <400 copies/mL) at Week 48 by Baseline KALETRA Susceptibility and by Number of Protease Substitutions Associated with Reduced Response to KALETRA[a]

Number of PI Mutations at Baseline[a]	Study IV Single PI-Experienced[b], NNRTI-Naive n=130	Study V Single PI-Experienced[c], NNRTI-Naive n=56	Study VII Multiple PI-Experienced[d], NNRTI-Naive n=50
0–2	76/103 (74%)	34/45 (76%)	19/20 (95%)
3–5	13/26 (50%)	8/11 (73%)	18/26 (69%)
6 or more	0/1 (0%)	n/a	1/4 (25%)

[a] Substitutions considered in the analysis included L10F/I/R/V, K20M/N/R, L24I, L33F, M36I, I47V, G48V, I54L/T/V, V82A/C/F/S/T, and I84V.
[b] 43% indinavir, 42% nelfinavir, 10% ritonavir, 15% saquinavir.
[c] 41% indinavir, 38% nelfinavir, 4% ritonavir, 16% saquinavir.
[d] 86% indinavir, 54% nelfinavir, 80% ritonavir, 70% saquinavir.
Legend: NNRTI=Non-nucleoside reverse transciptase inhibitor; PI=protease inhibitor; N/A=not applicable.

Table 16 shows the 48-week virologic response (HIV-1 RNA <50 copies/mL) in Study XII according to the number of protease-inhibitor associated mutations resistance mutations listed in Table 15 present at baseline. There are insufficient data to support once daily administration of KALETRA for adult patients with three or more protease-inhibitor associated mutations.

Table 16: KALETRA

Virologic Response (HIV RNA <50 copies/mL) at Week 48 by Baseline Number of Protease Substitutions Associated with Reduced Response to KALETRA[a]

Number of PI Mutations at Baseline[a]	Study XII (Treatment-Experienced[b]) KALETRA Once Daily+NRTIs (n=268)	Study XII (Treatment-Experienced[c]) KALETRA Twice Daily+NRTIs (n=264)
0 to 2	167/255 (65%)	154/250 (62%)
3 to 5	4/13 (31%)	8/14 (57%)
6 or more	N/A	N/A

[a] Substitutions considered in the analysis included L10F/I/R/V, K20M/N/R, L24I, L33F, M36I, I47V, G48V, I54L/T/V, V82A/C/F/S/T, and I84V.
[b] 88% NNRTI-experienced, 47% PI-experienced (24% nelfinavir, 19% indinavir, 13% atazanavir).
[c] 81% NNRTI-experienced, 46% PI-experienced (20% nelfinavir, 17% indinavir, 13% atazanavir).
Legend: NRTI=Nucleoside/Nucleotide reverse transcriptase inhibitor; PI=protease inhibitor; N/A=not applicable.

Pharmacodynamics: Viral Effects: Lopinavir is virologically ten-fold more active than ritonavir, with an EC_{50} of 0.07 µg/mL against $HIV\text{-}1_{IIIB}$ activity in MT_4 cells in a medium containing 50% human serum and 10% calf serum. The protein binding corrected EC_{50} against wild-type HIV for ritonavir under the same conditions is 0.9 µg/mL. Against ritonavir-resistant HIV, lopinavir displays potency similar to that observed by ritonavir against wild-type HIV. In the Phase 2 and Phase 3 trials, lopinavir has been tested in HIV PI-naïve subjects, as well as HIV-infected subjects with single PI experience who have developed various degrees of genotypic and phenotypic resistance to PIs and to NRTIs. Pharmacokinetic/pharmacodynamic modelling of the antiviral effect of lopinavir in these studies has shown little relationship between exposure and virologic outcome. In a study that evaluated subjects who were multiple PI-experienced, the C_{trough} to EC_{50} (of the pretreatment HIV viral isolate) ratio was determined to be an important factor for durable virologic suppression with lopinavir/ritonavir.

The incidence of diarrhea showed increased rates with increased dose within individual studies; however, no statistically significant dose group differences were observed. Also, no apparent difference was observed in the incidence of diarrhea between the antiretroviral-naïve and experienced groups. The incidence of nausea was higher for treatment-naïve subjects who received the KALETRA capsule 400/200 mg dose than subjects who received the 400/100 mg dose. In addition, across-study comparisons suggested that naïve subjects receiving a KALETRA capsule 400/200 mg dose tended to have higher incidence rates of nausea compared to experienced subjects receiving the same dose.

Effects on the Electrocardiogram: QTcF interval was evaluated in a randomized, placebo and active (moxifloxacin 400 mg once daily) controlled crossover study in 39 healthy adults, with 10 measurements over 12 hours on Day 3. The maximum mean (95% upper confidence bound) differences in QTcF from placebo were 3.6 (6.3) msec and 13.1 (15.8) msec for the 400/100 mg twice daily and supratherapeutic 800/200 mg twice daily KALETRA regimen, respectively. The two regimens resulted in exposures on Day 3 which were approximately 1.5 and 3-fold higher than those observed with recommended once daily or twice daily KALETRA doses at steady state. No subject experienced an increase in QTcF of >60 msec from baseline or a QTcF interval exceeding the potentially clinically relevant threshold of 500 msec.

Mean change from baseline in PR interval of 11.6 to 31.2 msec was also noted in subjects receiving KALETRA tablets in the same study on Day 3. Maximum PR interval was 286 msec and no second- or third-degree heart block was observed (see Warnings and Precautions).

Pharmacokinetics: The pharmacokinetic properties of lopinavir co-administered with ritonavir have been evaluated in healthy adult volunteers and in HIV-infected patients; no substantial differences were observed between the two groups. Lopinavir is essentially completely metabolized by CYP3A. Ritonavir inhibits the metabolism of lopinavir, thereby increasing the plasma levels of lopinavir. Across studies, administration of KALETRA capsules 400/100 mg twice daily yields mean steady-state lopinavir plasma concentrations 15- to 20-fold higher than those of ritonavir in HIV infected patients. The plasma levels of ritonavir are less than 7% of those obtained after the ritonavir dose of 600 mg twice daily. The in vitro antiviral EC_{50} of lopinavir is approximately 10-fold lower than that of ritonavir. Therefore, the antiviral activity of KALETRA is due to lopinavir.

At steady state, KALETRA capsules 400/100 mg twice daily taken without meal restrictions produced a mean±SD (standard deviation) lopinavir C_{max} of 9.6±4.4 µg/mL, occurring approximately 4 hours after administration. The mean steady-state trough concentration prior to the morning dose was 5.5±4.0 µg/mL. Lopinavir AUC over a 12-hour dosing interval averaged 82.8±44.5 µg·h/mL. Administration of a single 400/100 mg dose of KALETRA capsules with a moderate-fat meal (500 to 682 Kcal, 23 to 25% calories from fat) was associated with a mean increase of 48 and 23% in lopinavir AUC and C_{max}, respectively, relative to fasting. To enhance bioavailability and minimize pharmacokinetic variability, KALETRA capsules should be taken with food.

Lopinavir is approximately 98 to 99% bound to plasma proteins. Lopinavir is extensively metabolized by the hepatic cytochrome P450 system, almost exclusively by the CYP3A isozyme. Ritonavir is a potent CYP3A inhibitor which inhibits the metabolism of lopinavir, and therefore increases plasma levels of lopinavir. A [^{14}C]-lopinavir study in humans showed that 89% of the plasma radioactivity after a single 400/100 mg KALETRA capsule dose was due to parent drug. After multiple dosing, less than 3% of the lopinavir dose is excreted unchanged in the urine. The half-life ($t_{½}$) of lopinavir over a 12-hour dosing interval averaged 5 to 6 hours, and the apparent oral clearance (CL/F) of lopinavir is 6 to 7 L/h.

Absorption: In a pharmacokinetic study in HIV-positive subjects (n=19), multiple dosing with 400/100 mg KALETRA capsules twice daily with food for 3 weeks produced a mean±SD lopinavir C_{max} of 9.8±3.7 µg/mL (95% CI: 8.0 to 11.6 µg/mL), occurring approximately 4 hours after administration. The mean steady-state trough concentration prior to the morning dose was 7.1±2.9 µg/mL (95% CI: 5.7 to 8.5 µg/mL) and minimum concentration within a dosing interval was 5.5±2.7 µg/mL (95% CI: 4.2 to 6.8 µg/mL). Lopinavir AUC over a 12-hour dosing interval averaged 92.6±36.7 µg·h/mL (95% CI: 74.9 to 110.3 µg·h/mL). The absolute bioavailability of lopinavir co-formulated with ritonavir in humans has not been established. Under nonfasting conditions (500 Kcal, 25% from fat), lopinavir concentrations were similar following administration of KALETRA co-formulated capsules and oral solution. When administered under fasting conditions, both the mean AUC and C_{max} of lopinavir were 22% lower for the KALETRA oral solution relative to the capsule formulation.

The relative bioavailability of KALETRA 200/50 mg tablets compared to KALETRA capsules was assessed in two Phase 1, single-center, open-label, randomized, cross-over studies (Studies VIII and IX) in 111 healthy adults under fed conditions (moderate-fat meal, 490 to 560 Kcal, 20 to 30% of calories from fat) as a single 400/100 mg dose. Plasma concentrations of lopinavir and ritonavir after administration of two 200/50 mg KALETRA tablets are similar to three 133.3/33.3 mg KALETRA capsules under fed conditions with less pharmacokinetic variability. Following a moderate-fat meal, relative to the KALETRA capsule, administration of KALETRA 200/50 mg tablets increased lopinavir AUC_t and C_{max} by 18 and 24%, respectively, and increased ritonavir AUC_t and C_{max} by 20 and 35%, respectively.

In a Phase 1, single-center, open-label, randomized, cross-over study (Study VIII) in 63 healthy adults (46 males, 17 females), no clinically significant changes in C_{max} and AUC were observed following the administration of a single 400/100 mg dose of KALETRA 200/50 mg tablets under fasting conditions or following a moderate-fat meal (558 Kcal, 24.1% from fat) or a high-fat meal (998 Kcal, 51.3% from fat) relative to the KALETRA capsule dose following a moderate-fat meal. Relative to the KALETRA capsule dose following a moderate-fat meal, administration of KALETRA 200/50 mg tablets under fasting conditions increased lopinavir C_{max} by 10% with no change in AUC_t, and increased ritonavir AUC_t and C_{max} by 10 and 33%, respectively. Relative to the KALETRA capsule dose following a moderate-fat meal, administration of KALETRA 200/50 mg tablets following a moderate-fat meal increased lopinavir AUC_t and C_{max} by 27 and 30%, respectively, and increased ritonavir AUC_t and C_{max} by 27 and 40%, respectively. Relative to the KALETRA capsule dose following a moderate-fat meal, administration of KALETRA 200/50 mg tablets following a high-fat meal showed no change in lopinavir AUC_t and C_{max}, and increased ritonavir AUC_t and C_{max} each by 15%.

In a Phase 1, single-center, open-label, randomized, cross-over study (Study IX) in 48 healthy adults (34 males, 14 females) following a moderate-fat meal (492 Kcal, 22.9% from fat) and a single 400/100 mg dose, the relative bioavailability of KALETRA 200/50 mg tablets from two production lots compared to KALETRA capsules was increased for lopinavir AUC_t and C_{max} by 10 to 13% and 17 to 23%, respectively and increased for ritonavir AUC_t and C_{max} by 15% and 29 to 38%, respectively.

In a Phase 3, multicenter, open-label, randomized study (Study XI) in 664 HIV-1 infected adult subjects (502 males, 144 females) , following multiple-dose administration of KALETRA in a parallel group comparison of Week 2 data (n=18 for twice daily and n=17 for once daily), lopinavir concentrations are approximately 14 to 25% higher following twice daily administration of the tablet compared to the capsule and 19 to 38% higher following once daily administration of the tablet compared to the capsule. Ritonavir plasma levels were similarly increased 25 to 54% following twice daily and once daily dosing of the KALETRA tablet compared to the capsule. In a within-subject analysis comparing the tablet at Week 10 to the capsule at Week 2 (n=18 for twice daily and n=16 for once daily), lopinavir and ritonavir plasma levels did not appear to be clinically significantly increased. The maximum average changes following twice daily and once daily dosing were 4 and 16%, respectively, for lopinavir and 10 and 18%, respectively, for ritonavir.

The relative bioavailability of KALETRA 100/25 mg tablets compared to KALETRA 200/50 mg tablets was assessed in a Phase 1, single-center, open-label, randomized, cross-over study (Study X) in 44 healthy adults (35 males, 9 females) under fasting conditions as a single 400/100 mg dose. Plasma concentrations of lopinavir and ritonavir after administration of four 100/25 mg KALETRA tablets are similar to two 200/50 mg KALETRA tablets under fasting conditions.

Effects of Food on Oral Absorption: KALETRA Tablets: The relative bioavailability of KALETRA 200/50 mg tablets under fasting conditions was compared to KALETRA 200/50 mg tablets following meals in a Phase 1, single-center, open-label, randomized, cross-over study (Study VIII) in 63 healthy adults as a 400/100 mg dose. No clinically significant changes in C_{max} and AUC were observed following administration of KALETRA 200/50 mg tablets under fed conditions compared to fasted conditions. Relative to fasting, administration of KALETRA 200/50 mg tablets with a moderate-fat meal (558 Kcal, 24.1% calories from fat) increased lopinavir AUC_t and C_{max} by 26.9 and 17.6%, respectively, and ritonavir AUC_t and C_{max} by 15.6 and 4.9%, respectively. Relative to fasting, administration of KALETRA 200/50 mg tablets with a high fat meal (998 Kcal, 51.3% from fat) increased lopinavir AUC_t by 18.7% but not C_{max}, and ritonavir AUC_t and C_{max} were increased 24.7 and 10.3%, respectively. The average lopinavir T_{max} for the 200/50 mg tablet under fasting conditions, following a moderate-fat meal and following a high-fat meal were 3.6, 4.0 and 5.4 hours, respectively. The average ritonavir T_{max} for the 200/50 mg tablet under fasting conditions, following a moderate-fat meal and following a high-fat meal were 3.4, 4.0 and 5.4 hours, respectively. The lopinavir terminal phase half-lives were similar for all regimens and ranged, on average, from 2.6 to 2.7 hours. The ritonavir terminal phase half-lives were similar for all regimens and ranged, on average, from 4.2 to 4.7 hours. Additional details regarding the pharmacokinetics of the KALETRA capsule and 200/50 mg tablet formulations under various meal conditions may be found in Action and Clinical Pharmacology, Pharmacokinetics, Absorption. KALETRA tablets may therefore be taken with or without food.

KALETRA Oral Solution: Relative to fasting, KALETRA oral solution dosed with a moderate-fat meal (500 to 683 Kcal, 23 to 25% calories from fat) in healthy adults was associated with increases in lopinavir AUC and C_{max} of 80 and 54%, respectively. Relative to fasting, administration of KALETRA oral solution with a high-fat meal (872 Kcal, 56% from fat) increased lopinavir AUC and C_{max} by 130 and 56%, respectively. To enhance bioavailability and minimize pharmacokinetic variability, KALETRA oral solution should be taken with food.

Distribution: At steady-state, lopinavir is approximately 98 to 99% bound to plasma proteins. Lopinavir binds to both alpha-1-acid glycoprotein (AAG) and albumin; however, it has a higher affinity for AAG. At steady state, lopinavir protein binding remains constant over the range of observed concentrations after 400/100 mg KALETRA twice daily, and is similar between healthy volunteers and HIV-positive patients.

After a single dose of [^{14}C]lopinavir/ritonavir (10/5 mg/kg) in rats the radioactivity was distributed well throughout the body. With the exception of the adrenal gland, thyroid gland, liver and gastrointestinal tract, at 4 hours the tissue to plasma ratios of the remaining tissues were less than one. The highest concentrations were found in the liver and the lowest concentrations in the brain. The brain concentrations were approximately equal to the free concentrations in the plasma (approximately 2%). Concentrations in the lymphatic system were 6 to 61% of those in the plasma.

Metabolism: In vitro experiments with human hepatic microsomes indicate that lopinavir primarily undergoes oxidative metabolism. Lopinavir is extensively metabolized by the hepatic cytochrome P450 system, almost exclusively by the CYP3A isozyme. Ritonavir is a potent CYP3A inhibitor, which inhibits the metabolism of lopinavir, and therefore increases plasma levels of lopinavir. A [^{14}C]-lopinavir study in humans showed that 89% of the plasma radioactivity after a single 400/100 mg KALETRA dose was due to parent drug. At least 13 lopinavir oxidative metabolites have been identified in man. Ritonavir has been shown to induce metabolic enzymes, resulting in the induction of its own metabolism. Pre-dose lopinavir concentrations decline with time during multiple dosing, stabilizing after approximately 10 to 16 days.

Excretion: Following a 400/100 mg [^{14}C]-lopinavir/ritonavir dose, approximately 10.4±2.3% and 82.6±2.5% of an administered dose of [^{14}C]-lopinavir can be accounted for in urine and feces, respectively, after 8 days. Unchanged lopinavir accounted for approximately 2.2 and 19.8% of the administered dose in urine and feces, respectively. After multiple dosing, less than 3% of the lopinavir dose is excreted unchanged in the urine. The apparent oral clearance (CL/F) of lopinavir is 5.98±5.75 L/hr (mean ± SD, n=19).

Once Daily Dosing: The pharmacokinetics of once daily KALETRA have been evaluated in HIV-infected subjects naïve to antiretroviral treatment. KALETRA capsules 800/200 mg was administered in combination with emtricitabine 200 mg and tenofovir DF 300 mg as part of a once daily regimen. Multiple dosing of 800/200 mg KALETRA capsules once a day for 4 weeks with food (n=24) produced a mean±SD lopinavir C_{max} of 11.8±3.7 µg/mL, occurring approximately 6 hours after administration. The mean steady-state lopinavir trough concentration prior to the morning dose was 3.2±2.1 µg/mL and minimum concentration within a dosing interval was 1.7±1.6 µg/mL. Lopinavir AUC over a 24-hour dosing interval averaged 154.1±61.4 µg·h/mL.

Special Populations and Conditions: Pediatrics: The pharmacokinetics of KALETRA oral solution 300/75 mg/m^2 twice daily and 230/57.5 mg/m^2 twice daily have been studied in a total of 53 pediatric patients, ranging in age from 6 months to 12 years. The 230/57.5 mg/m^2 twice daily regimen without nevirapine and the 300/75 mg/m^2 twice daily regimen with nevirapine provided lopinavir plasma concentrations similar to those obtained in adult patients receiving the 400/100 mg twice daily regimen (without nevirapine). KALETRA once daily has not been evaluated in pediatric patients.

The following describes the KALETRA-nevirapine interaction. The nevirapine regimen was 7 mg/kg twice daily (6 months to 8 years) or 4 mg/kg twice daily (>8 years). The lopinavir mean steady-state AUC, C_{max}, and C_{min} were 72.6±31.1, 8.2±2.9 and 3.4±2.1 µg/mL respectively, after KALETRA 230/57.5 mg/m^2 twice daily without nevirapine (n=12), and were 85.8±36.9, 10.0±3.3 and 3.6±3.5 µg/mL respectively, after 300/75 mg/m^2 twice daily with nevirapine (n=12).

Geriatrics: Lopinavir pharmacokinetics has not been studied in elderly patients.

Gender: No gender-related pharmacokinetic differences have been observed in adult patients. Population pharmacokinetic analysis of lopinavir in HIV-infected subjects indicated that gender had no apparent effect on the exposure to lopinavir.

Race: No clinically important pharmacokinetic differences due to race have been identified. Population pharmacokinetic analysis of lopinavir in HIV-infected subjects indicated that race had no apparent effect on the exposure to lopinavir.

Hepatic Insufficiency: Lopinavir is principally metabolized and eliminated by the liver. Multiple dosing of KALETRA capsules 400/100 mg twice daily to HIV and HCV co-infected patients with mild to moderate hepatic impairment (n=12) resulted in a 30% increase in lopinavir AUC and 20% increase in C_{max} compared to HIV-infected subjects with normal hepatic function (n=12). Additionally, the plasma protein binding of lopinavir was lower in both mild and moderate hepatic impairment compared to controls (99.09 vs. 99.31% respectively). Caution should be exercised when administering KALETRA to subjects with hepatic impairment. KALETRA has not been studied in patients with severe hepatic impairment (see Warnings and Precautions, Hepatic/Biliary/Pancreatic).

Renal Insufficiency: Lopinavir pharmacokinetics have not been studied in patients with renal insufficiency; however, since less than 3% of the dose of lopinavir is eliminated unchanged in the urine, a decrease in total body clearance is not expected in patients with renal insufficiency. Population pharmacokinetic analysis of lopinavir in HIV-infected subjects indicated that subjects with mild renal impairment (CL_{CR} between 50 to 80 mL/min, n=79) had no apparent effect on the exposure to lopinavir.

STORAGE AND STABILITY: KALETRA Film-coated Tablets: Store KALETRA film-coated tablets between 15 to 25°C. It is recommended that the product be stored and dispensed in the original container.

KALETRA Oral Solution: Store KALETRA oral solution between 2 to 8°C until dispensed. Avoid exposure to excessive heat. Keep cap tightly closed. Product must be stored and dispensed in the original container. Refrigeration of KALETRA oral solution by the patient is not required if used within 42 days and stored below 25°C.

INFORMATION FOR THE PATIENT: Published in e-CPS, available by subscription at www.e-cps.ca.

DOSAGE FORMS, COMPOSITION AND PACKAGING: Film-Coated Tablets: 100 mg/25 mg: Each pale yellow, film-coated tablet, embossed with the Abbott logo and the Abbo-Code KC, contains: lopinavir 100 mg and ritonavir 25 mg. Nonmedicinal ingredients: colloidal silicon dioxide, copovidone, sodium stearyl fumarate and sorbitan monolaurate; film-coating: polyethylene glycol 3350, polyvinyl alcohol, talc, titanium dioxide and yellow ferric oxide E172. Bottles of 60.

200 mg/50 mg: Each yellow, film-coated tablet, embossed with the Abbott logo and the Abbo-Code KA, contains: lopinavir 200 mg and ritonavir 50 mg. Nonmedicinal ingredients: colloidal silicon dioxide, copovidone, sodium stearyl fumarate and sorbitan monolaurate; film-coating: colloidal silicon dioxide, hydroxypropyl cellulose, hypromellose, polyethylene glycol 400, polyethylene glycol 3350, polysorbate 80, talc, yellow ferric oxide E172 and titanium dioxide. Bottles of 120.

Oral Solution: Each mL of light yellow to orange-colored liquid contains: lopinavir 80 mg and ritonavir 20 mg. Nonmedicinal ingredients: acesulfame potassium, alcohol, artificial cotton candy flavor, citric acid, glycerin, high fructose corn syrup, Magnasweet-110 flavor, menthol, natural and artificial vanilla flavor, peppermint oil, polyoxyl 40 hydrogenated castor oil, povidone, propylene glycol, saccharin sodium, sodium chloride, sodium citrate and water. Alcohol: 42.4% (v/v). Amber-colored multiple-dose bottles of 160 mL, packaged with a marked dosing cup.

Kaopectate®

attapulgite

Antidiarrheal

Paladin

SUPPLIED: Children's: Each 15 mL of cherry-flavored oral suspension contains: activated attapulgite 600 mg. Nonmedicinal ingredients: FD&C Red No. 40, flavor, glucono-delta-lactone, magnesium aluminum silicate, methylparaben, purified water, sorbic acid, sucrose, titanium dioxide and xanthan gum. Energy: 28.7 kJ (7.1 kcal)/15 mL. Sodium: <1 mmol (4.88 mg)/15 mL. Gluten-, lactose- and tartrazine-free. Bottles of 180 mL. Protect from freezing.

Extra Strength: Each 15 mL of peppermint-flavored oral suspension contains: activated attapulgite 750 mg. Nonmedicinal ingredients: flavor, glucono-delta-lactone, magnesium aluminum silicate, methylparaben, purified water, sorbic acid, sucrose, titanium dioxide and xanthan gum. Energy: 29.7 kJ (7.1 kcal)/15 mL. Sodium: <1 mmol (4.88 mg)/15 mL. Gluten-, lactose- and tartrazine-free. Bottles of 250 and 350 mL. Protect from freezing.

Regular Strength: Each 15 mL of vanilla-flavored oral suspension contains: activated attapulgite 600 mg. Nonmedicinal ingredients: flavor, glucono-delta-lactone, magnesium aluminum silicate, methylparaben, purified water, sorbic acid, sucrose, titanium dioxide and xanthan gum. Energy: 29.7 kJ (7.1 kcal)/15 mL. Sodium: <1 mmol (2.2 mg)/15 mL. Gluten-, lactose- and tartrazine-free. Bottles of 250 and 350 mL. Protect from freezing.

Kayexalate® ℞

sodium polystyrene sulfonate

Cation-Exchange Resin

sanofi-aventis

SUPPLIED: Light brown, to brown, finely powdered sodium polystyrene sulfonate, a cation-exchange resin prepared in the sodium phase with an in vivo exchange capacity of approximately 1 mmol (in vitro approximately 3.1 mmol) of potassium/g. Sodium: 4.1 mmol (100 mg)/g. Gluten-, lactose-, starch-, sucrose- and tartrazine-free. Jars of 454 g.

K-Dur®

potassium chloride

Potassium Supplement

Schering-Plough

PHARMACOLOGY: Potassium ion is the principal intracellular cation of most body tissues. Potassium ions participate in a number of essential physiological processes including the maintenance of intracellular tonicity, the transmission of nerve impulses, the contraction of cardiac, skeletal and smooth muscle and the maintenance of normal renal function. Potassium depletion may occur whenever the rate of potassium loss exceeds the rate of potassium intake. Such depletion usually develops slowly as a consequence of prolonged therapy with oral diuretics, primary or secondary hyperaldosternism, diabetic ketoacidosis, severe diarrhea, or inadequate replacement of potassium in patients on prolonged parenteral nutrition. Potassium depletion due to these causes is usually accompanied by a concomitant deficiency of chloride and is manifested by hypokalemia and metabolic alkalosis.

K-DUR tablets contain microcrystalloids which disperse upon disintegration of the tablet. The microcrystalloids are formulated to provide a controlled release of potassium chloride. The dispersibility of the microcrystalloids and the controlled release of ions from them are intended to minimize the possibility of high local concentrations of potassium within the gastrointestinal tract.

INDICATIONS: For the treatment of patients with hypokalemia with or without metabolic alkalosis in the treatment of digitalis intoxication, and for the treatment of patients with hypokalemic familial periodic paralysis.

For the prevention of potassium depletion when the dietary intake is inadequate in the following conditions: patients receiving digitalis and diuretics for congestive heart failure, selected patients with hypertension on long-term diuretic therapy, hepatic cirrhosis with ascites, states of aldosterone excess with normal renal function, potassium-losing nephropathy, and with certain diarrheal states.

CONTRAINDICATIONS: Potassium supplements are contraindicated in patients with hyperkalemia since a further increase in potassium concentration in such patients can produce cardiac arrest. Hyperkalemia may complicate any of the following conditions: acute and chronic renal failure, extensive tissue breakdown as in severe burns, adrenal insufficiency, or the administration of a potassium-sparing diuretic (e.g. spironolactone, triamterene), or other drugs causing hyperkalemia such as captopril and enalapril.

Slow release potassium chloride preparations have produced esophageal ulceration in certain cardiac patients with esophageal compression due to enlarged left atrium. The administration of these preparations is contraindicated in such patients as well as in patients with dysphagia.

All solid dosage forms of potassium supplements are contraindicated in any patients in whom there is cause for arrest or delay in tablet passage through the gastrointestinal tract. In these instances, potassium supplementation should be with a liquid preparation.

WARNINGS: Hyperkalemia: In patients with impaired mechanisms for excreting potassium, the administration of potassium salts can produce hyperkalemia and cardiac arrest. This occurs most commonly in patients given potassium by the i.v. route but may also occur in patients given potassium orally. Potentially fatal hyperkalemia can develop rapidly and be asymptomatic. The use of potassium salts in patients with chronic renal disease, or any other condition which impairs potassium excretion, requires particularly careful monitoring of the serum potassium concentration and appropriate dosage adjustment. Hyperkalemia has the potential to promote quinidine toxicity.

Hypokalemia: Hypokalemia should not be treated by the concomitant administration of potassium salts and a potassium-sparing diuretic (e.g. spironolactone, triamterene) or other drugs causing hyperkalemia such as captopril or enalapril since the simultaneous administration of these agents can produce severe hyperkalemia. Hypokalemia in patients with metabolic acidosis should be treated with an alkalinizing potassium salt such as potassium acetate, potassium bicarbonate or potassium citrate.

Gastrointestinal Lesions: Potassium chloride tablets have produced stenotic and/or ulcerative lesions of the small bowel and deaths, in addition to upper gastrointestinal bleeding. These lesions are caused by a high localized concentration of potassium ions in the region of a rapidly dissolving tablet, which injures the bowel wall and thereby produces obstruction, hemorrhage or perforation.

The frequency of gastrointestinal lesions with K-DUR tablet is, at present, unknown. K-DUR tablet should be discontinued immediately and the possibility of bowel obstruction or perforation considered if severe vomiting, abdominal pain, distention, or gastrointestinal bleeding occurs. All oral potassium preparations should be prescribed with particular caution in patients with a history of peptic ulcer.

PRECAUTIONS: The treatment of potassium depletion, particularly in the presence of cardiac disease, renal disease, or acidosis, requires careful attention to acid-base balance and appropriate monitoring of the serum electrolytes, the ECG and the clinical status of the patient.

Potassium supplements should be used with caution in diseases associated with heart block since increased serum potassium may increase the degree of block.

Since anticholinergic agents have the potential to slow gastrointestinal motility, caution should be exercised when prescribing solid oral potassium preparations to patients concurrently receiving anticholinergic agents.

Pregnancy: Because of gastrointestinal hypomotility associated with pregnancy, solid oral potassium supplements should be given to pregnant women only if clearly needed.

Lactation: See Pregnancy.

ADVERSE EFFECTS: The most common adverse reactions to oral potassium salts are nausea, vomiting, abdominal discomfort and diarrhea. These symptoms are due to irritation of the gastrointestinal tract and are best avoided by increasing fluid intake when possible, taking the dose with meals or reducing the dose. Intestinal bleeding, ulceration, perforation and obstruction have been reported in patients treated with solid dosage forms of potassium salts and may occur with K-DUR (see Contraindications and Warnings).

One of the most severe adverse effects is hyperkalemia (see Contraindications, Warnings and Overdose). Skin rash has been reported rarely with potassium preparations.

OVERDOSE:

Overdosage from therapeutic doses of solid oral potassium salts in persons with normal excretory mechanism rarely occurs; however, if excretory mechanisms are impaired, potentially fatal hyperkalemia may occur. Acute (accidental or intentional) overdosages of solid oral potassium salts have resulted in severe and/or fatal hyperkalemia.

Symptoms: Overdosage with potassium is characterized chiefly by cardiovascular, neuromuscular and gastrointestinal disturbances.

Cardiovascular: ECG changes, hypotension and shock, bundle-branch block, ventricular arrhythmias, ventricular fibrillation leading possibly to cardiac arrest.

Neuromuscular: paresthesia, areflexia, convulsions, flaccid paralysis of striated muscle leading possibly to respiratory paralysis.

Gastrointestinal: nausea, vomiting, diarrhea and abdominal cramps.

Hyperkalemia: It is important to recognize that hyperkalemia is usually asymptomatic and may be manifested only by an increased serum potassium concentration and characteristic ECG changes which include increased amplitude and peaking of the T-wave, and flattening or absence of the P-wave. As hyperkalemia worsens prolongation of the P-R interval, widening of the QRS complex with S-T segment depression and arrhythmias may develop.

Widening of the QRS complex is one of the most ominous signs and indicates the need for aggressive treatment.

Treatment: The plasma concentration and ECG must be monitored in every case of potassium overdosage, as well as serum electrolytes, BUN, glucose and arterial blood gases.

ECG signs of hyperkalemia (tall peaked T-waves, P-R prolongation, disappearance of P-waves, QRS widening, heart block) are indications for immediate treatment.

In severe hyperkalemia (plasma potassium exceeded 8 mEq/L or ECG abnormalities include absence of P-wave, presence of widened QRS complex or ventricular arrhythmia): administer i.v. 300 to 500 mL/hour of 10% dextrose solution containing 10-20 units of insulin/1000 mL. Correct acidosis, if present, with i.v. sodium bicarbonate (44 to 132 mEq/L of glucose solution). Administer 10 to 30 mL of 10% calcium gluconate i.v. over 1 to 5 minutes under continuous ECG monitoring.

Administer cation exchange resin by high retention enema. 30 to 50 g sodium polystyrene sulfonate suspended in 100 mL warm aqueous sorbital solution should be kept in the sigmoid colon for several hours, if possible. The colon is then irrigated with non-sodium containing solution to remove the resin. Repeated enemas can be administered, or the resin given repeatedly by mouth to maintain a physiologic potassium concentration.

Hemodialysis or peritoneal dialysis may be of use, particularly in patients with renal failure.

In moderately severe hyperkalemia (plasma potassium between 6.5 and 8 mmol/L (mEq/L) or ECG peaking of T-wave): administer i.v. 300 to 500 mL/hour of 10% dextrose solution containing 10-20 units of insulin/1000 mL. Correct acidosis, if present, with i.v. sodium bicarbonate (44 to 132 mEq/L of glucose solution). Correct hyponatremia and hypovolemia, if present.

Once the patient's cardiac state has been stabilized, in the case of a recent **acute** ingestion of K-DUR, consideration should be given to the standard measures to remove any unabsorbed drug in the stomach, such as adsorption by activated charcoal administered as a slurry with water or administration of gastric lavage. When overdosage is the result of **chronic** therapeutic ingestion, the drug should be discontinued immediately as well as potassium containing foods and medications and also potassium sparing diuretics.

For management of a suspected drug overdose, CPhA recommends that you contact your **regional Poison Control Centre**. See the *CPS* Directory section for a list of Poison Control Centres.

DOSAGE: The usual dietary intake of potassium by the average adult is 40 to 80 mmol (mEq) (3000 to 6000 mg)/day.

Potassium depletion sufficient to cause hypokalemia usually requires the loss of 200 or more mmol (mEq) (15 000 mg) of potassium from the total body store.

Dosage must be adjusted to the individual needs of each patient but is typically in the range of 20 mmol (mEq) (1500 mg)/day for the prevention of hypokalemia to 40-100 mmol (mEq) (3000-7500 mg)/day or more for the treatment of potassium depletion (see Table 1).

Table 1: K-DUR
Dosage

K-DUR Tablets	For Prevention	For Treatment
20 mmol (mEq) (1500 mg)	1 tablet/day 20 mmol (mEq) (1500 mg)	2 to 5 tablets/day 40 to 100 mmol (mEq) (3000 to 7500 mg)

If more than one (1) K-DUR 20 mmol (mEq) (1500 mg) tablet is prescribed/day, the total daily dosage should be divided into 2 or more separate doses.

Tablets should be taken with a glass of water or other liquid.

Patients having difficulty swallowing whole tablets may try one of the following alternate methods of administration. Break the tablet in half, and take each half separately with a glass of water; or prepare an aqueous suspension as follows: Place the whole tablet in approximately one-half glass of water (115 mL). Allow 2 to 3 minutes for the tablet to disintegrate. Stir for about half a minute after the tablet has disintegrated. Drink the entire contents of the glass immediately. Add another small quantity of water, stir and drink immediately. Aqueous suspensions of K-DUR tablets that are not taken immediately should be discarded. The use of other liquids for suspending the tablets is not recommended.

SUPPLIED: Each sustained-release, capsule-shaped, white to off-white mottled tablets imprinted "K-DUR 20" on one side and scored on the other, contains: potassium chloride USP 20 mmol (mEq) (1500 mg). Nonmedicinal ingredients: crospovidone, ethylcellulose, hydroxypropylcellulose, magensium stearate, and microcrystalline cellulose. Bottles of 100. Keep tightly closed. Store at controlled room temperature 15 to 30°C.

(Shown in Product Identification Section)

Kenalog®-10 Injection Ⓟ

triamcinolone acetonide

Corticosteroid

Bristol-Myers Squibb

Date of Revision: July 19, 2010

Note: KENALOG-10 INJECTION is triamcinolone acetonide, a synthetic glucocorticoid corticosteroid with marked anti-inflammatory action, in a sterile aqueous suspension suitable for intradermal, intra-articular, and intra bursal injection and for injection into tendon sheaths. **This formulation is not for intravenous, intramuscular, intraocular, epidural or intrathecal injection.**

PHARMACOLOGY: Naturally occurring glucocorticoids (e.g., hydrocortisone), which also have salt-retaining properties, are used as replacement therapy in adrenocortical deficiency states. Synthetic analogs such as triamcinolone are primarily used for their potent anti-inflammatory effects in disorders of many organ systems.

Glucocorticoids cause profound and varied metabolic effects. In addition, they modify the body's immune responses to diverse stimuli.

INDICATIONS: Intra-Articular: For intra-articular or intrabursal administration, and for injections into tendon sheaths, as adjunctive therapy for short-term administration in the following conditions: synovitis of osteoarthritis, rheumatoid arthritis, acute and subacute bursitis, acute gouty arthritis, epicondylitis, acute nonspecific tenosynovitis, and post-traumatic osteoarthritis.

Intradermal: Intralesional administration is indicated for the treatment of keloids, discoid lupus erythematosus, necrobiosis lipoidica diabeticorum, alopecia areata, and localized hypertrophic, infiltrated, inflammatory lesions of: lichen planus, psoriatic plaques, granuloma annulare, and lichen simplex chronicus (neurodermatitis).

CONTRAINDICATIONS: Corticosteroids are generally contraindicated in patients with systemic infections. KENALOG-10 is also contraindicated in patients with a sensitivity to the medicinal or nonmedicinal ingredients.

The preparation should not be injected into infected areas.

WARNINGS: Because KENALOG-10 is a suspension, it should **not** be administered i.v.

Epidural and intrathecal administration of this product should not be used. Reports of serious medical events have been associated with epidural and intrathecal routes of administration.

KENALOG-10 is a long-acting preparation, and is **not** suitable for use in acute situations.

Prolonged use of corticosteroids may produce posterior subcapsular cataracts or glaucoma with possible damage to the optic nerve. Prolonged use may also enhance the likelihood of secondary ocular infections.

Average and large doses of hydrocortisone or cortisone can cause elevation of blood pressure, salt and water retention, and increased excretion of potassium. These effects are less likely to occur with the synthetic derivatives except when they are used in large doses; dietary salt restriction and potassium supplementation may be necessary (see Precautions). All corticosteroids increase calcium excretion, which may be associated with osteoporosis or aggravate preexisting osteoporosis.

Corticosteroids may mask some signs of infection, and new infections may appear during their use. There may be decreased resistance and inability to localize infection when corticosteroids are used. In addition, patients who are on immunosuppressant drugs including corticosteroids are more susceptible to infections than those not taking these drugs. Moreover, chickenpox and measles can have a more serious or even fatal course in patients on corticosteroids. In such children, or adults receiving corticosteroids who have not had these diseases, particular care should be taken to avoid exposure. If exposed, therapy with varicella zoster immune globulin (VZIG) or pooled i.v. immunoglobulin (IVIG), as appropriate, may be indicated. If chickenpox or herpes zoster develops, treatment with antiviral agents may be considered. Similarly, corticosteroids should be used with great caution in patients with Strongyloides (threadworm) infestation because corticosteroid-induced immunosuppression may lead to Strongyloides hyperinfection and dissemination with widespread larval migration, often accompanied by severe enterocolitis and potentially fatal Gram-negative septicemia.

Patients should not be vaccinated or immunized while on corticosteroid therapy, especially on high doses, because of a lack of antibody response predisposing to medical complications, particularly neurological ones.

The use of triamcinolone in patients with active tuberculosis should be restricted to those cases of fulminating or disseminated tuberculosis in which the corticosteroid is used for the management of the disease in conjunction with an appropriate antituberculous regimen. Chemoprophylaxis should be used in patients with latent tuberculosis or tuberculin reactivity who are taking corticosteroids.

Rare instances of anaphylactoid reactions have occurred in patients receiving parenteral corticosteroid therapy. Appropriate precautionary measures should be taken prior to administration, especially when the patient has a history of allergy to any drug.

Adequate studies to demonstrate the safety of KENALOG-10 use by intraturbinal, subconjunctival, sub-tenons, retrobulbar and intraocular (intravitreal) injections have not been performed.

Endophthalmitis, eye inflammation, increased intraocular pressure and visual disturbances including vision loss have been reported with intravitreal administration. Several instances of blindness have been reported following injection of corticosteroid suspensions into the nasal turbinates and intralesional injection about the head. Administration of KENALOG-10 (Triamcinolone Acetonide Injectable Suspension) by any of these routes is not recommended.

This product contains benzyl alcohol as a preservative. Benzyl alcohol has been associated with serious adverse events and death, particularly in pediatric patients. The "gasping syndrome" has been associated with benzyl alcohol. Although normal therapeutic doses of this product deliver amounts of benzyl alcohol that are substantially lower than those reported in association with the "gasping syndrome", the minimum amount of benzyl alcohol at which toxicity may occur is not known. Premature and low-birth-weight infants, as well as patients receiving high dosages, may be more likely to develop toxicity.

Pregnancy: Many corticosteroids have been shown to be teratogenic in laboratory animals at low doses. Since adequate human reproduction studies have not been performed with corticosteroids, the use of these drugs in pregnancy, nursing mothers, or women of childbearing potential requires that the possible benefits of the drug be weighed against the potential hazards to the mother and the embryo, fetus, or breast-fed infant. Other systemic corticosteroids have been shown to appear in breast milk and to slightly elevate (by 1%) the risk of cleft palate in human fetuses. Infants born to mothers who have received substantial doses of corticosteroids during pregnancy should be carefully observed for signs of adrenal suppression.

Lactation: See Pregnancy.

Children: Because corticosteroids can suppress growth, the development of infants and children on prolonged corticosteroid therapy should be carefully observed. Caution should be used in the event of exposure to chickenpox, measles or other communicable diseases. Children should not be vaccinated or immunized while on corticosteroid therapy (see Warnings). Corticosteroids may also affect endogenous steroid production.

Exposure to excessive amounts of benzyl alcohol has been associated with toxicity (hypotension, metabolic acidosis), particularly in neonates, and an increased incidence of kernicterus, particularly in small preterm infants. There have been rare reports of deaths, primarily in preterm infants, associated with exposure to excessive amounts of benzyl alcohol (see Warnings).

PRECAUTIONS: Drug induced adrenocortical insufficiency may occur with corticosteroids and persist for months after discontinuation of therapy; therefore, in any situation of stress such as trauma, surgery or severe illness occurring during that period, hormone therapy should be reinstituted. Since mineralocorticoid secretion may be impaired, salt and/or a mineralocorticoid should be administered concurrently.

There is an enhanced corticosteroid effect in patients with hypothyroidism and in those with cirrhosis.

Corticosteroids should be used cautiously in patients with ocular herpes simplex because of possible corneal perforation.

Psychiatric disturbances may appear when corticosteroids are used. These can include insomnia, depression (sometimes severe), euphoria, mood swings, psychotic symptoms and personality changes. Pre-existing emotional instability or psychosis may also be aggravated by corticosteroids. The use of antidepressant drugs does not relieve and may exacerbate adrenocorticoid-induced mental disturbances.

Corticosteroids should be used with caution in the following conditions: Nonspecific ulcerative colitis (if there is a probability of perforation, abscess, or other pyogenic infection); diverticulitis; recent intestinal anastomoses; active or latent peptic ulcer; renal insufficiency; acute glomerulonephritis; chronic nephritis; hypertension; congestive heart failure; thrombophlebitis; thromboembolism; osteoporosis; exanthema; Cushing's syndrome; diabetes mellitus; convulsive disorders; metastatic carcinoma; myasthenia gravis.

Although therapy with KENALOG-10 may ameliorate symptoms of inflammation, it does not obviate the need to treat the cause.

Intra-articular injection of a corticosteroid may produce systemic as well as local effects. The inadvertent injection of the suspension into the soft tissues surrounding a joint may lead to the occurrence of systemic effects and is the most common cause of failure to achieve the desired local results.

Following intra-articular steroid therapy, patients should be specifically warned to avoid overuse of joints in which symptomatic benefit has been obtained. Otherwise an increase in joint deterioration can occur.

Overdistention of the joint capsule and deposition of steroid along the needle track should be avoided in intra-articular injection, since this may lead to s.c. atrophy.

Corticosteroids should not be injected into unstable joints. Repeated intra-articular injection may in some cases itself result in instability of the joint. In selected cases, particularly where repeated injections are given, x-ray follow-up is suggested.

An increase in joint discomfort has seldom occurred. A marked increase in pain accompanied by local swelling, further restriction of joint motion, fever, and malaise are suggestive of a septic arthritis. If these complications should appear, and the diagnosis of septic arthritis is confirmed, administration of triamcinolone should be stopped, and antimicrobial therapy should be instituted immediately and continued for 7 to 10 days after all evidence of infection has disappeared. Appropriate examination of any joint fluid present is necessary to exclude a septic process. Injection of a steroid into a previously infected joint should therefore be avoided. Repeated injection into inflamed tendons has been followed by tendon rupture. Therefore, it should also be avoided.

Like other potent corticosteroids, triamcinolone should be used under close clinical supervision. Triamcinolone can cause elevation of blood pressure, salt and water retention, and increased potassium and calcium excretion necessitating dietary salt restriction and potassium supplementation. Edema may occur in the presence of renal disease with a fixed or decreased glomerular filtration rate.

During prolonged therapy, **an adequate protein intake is essential** to counteract the tendency to gradual weight loss sometimes associated with negative nitrogen balance, wasting and weakness of skeletal muscles.

Menstrual irregularities may also occur with corticosteroid treatment.

In peptic ulcer, recurrence may be asymptomatic until perforation or hemorrhage occurs. Long-term adrenocortical therapy may itself produce hyperacidity or peptic ulcer. Therefore, antiulcer therapy is recommended.

Continued supervision of the patient after termination of triamcinolone therapy is essential, since there may be a sudden reappearance of severe manifestations of the disease for which the patient was treated.

Patients should be advised to inform subsequent physicians of the prior use of corticosteroids.

Geriatrics: The common adverse effects of systemic corticosteroids such as osteoporosis or hypertension may be associated with more serious consequences in old age. Close clinical supervision is recommended.

Occupational Hazards: The effects of corticosteroid therapy on the ability to drive or operate machinery have not been studied.
Drug Interactions: Amphotericin B injection and Potassium-Depleting Agents: Patients should be observed for hypokalemia.
Anticholinesterases: Effects of the anticholinesterase agent may be antagonized.
Anticoagulants, Oral: Corticosteroids may potentiate or decrease anticoagulant action. Patients receiving oral anticoagulants and corticosteroids should therefore be closely monitored.
Antidiabetics: Corticosteroids may increase blood glucose; diabetic control should be monitored, especially when corticosteroids are initiated, discontinued, or changed in dosage.
Antitubercular Drugs: Isoniazid serum concentrations may be decreased.
Cyclosporine: Monitor for evidence of increased toxicity of cyclosporine when the two are used concurrently.
Digitalis Glycosides: Coadministration may enhance the possibility of digitalis toxicity.
Estrogens, Including Oral Contraceptives: Corticosteroid half-life and concentration may be increased and clearance decreased.
Hepatic Enzyme Inducers (e.g., barbiturates, phenytoin, carbamazepine, rifampin): There may be increased metabolic clearance of KENALOG-10 injection. Patients should be carefully observed for possible diminished effect of steroid, and the dosage of KENALOG-10 injection should be adjusted accordingly.
Human Growth Hormone (e.g., somatrem): The growth-promotion effect of somatrem may be inhibited.
Ketoconazole: Corticosteroid clearance may be decreased, resulting in increased effects.
Nondepolarizing Muscle Relaxants: Corticosteroids may decrease or enhance the neuromuscular blocking action.
Nonsteroidal Anti-inflammatory Agents (NSAIDs): Corticosteroids may increase the incidence and/or severity of gastrointestinal bleeding and ulceration associated with NSAIDS. Also, corticosteroids can reduce serum salicylate levels and therefore decrease their effectiveness. Conversely, discontinuing corticosteroids during high-dose salicylate therapy may result in salicylate toxicity. ASA should be used cautiously in conjunction with corticosteroids in patients with hypoprothrombinemia.
Thyroid Drugs: Metabolic clearance of adrenocorticoids is decreased in hypothyroid patients and increased in hyperthyroid patients. Changes in thyroid status of the patient may necessitate adjustment in adrenocorticoid dosage.
Vaccines: Neurological complications and lack of antibody response may occur when patients taking corticosteroids are vaccinated (see Warnings).
Laboratory Test Interactions: Corticosteroids may affect the nitroblue tetrazolium test for bacterial infection, producing false-negative results.

ADVERSE EFFECTS: Undesirable reactions following intra-articular administration of the preparation have included postinjection flare, transient pain, irritation at the injection site, sterile abscesses, hyper- or hypopigmentation, Charcot-like arthropathy, and occasional increase in joint discomfort; following intradermal administration, rare instances of blindness associated with intralesional therapy around the face and head, transient local discomfort, sterile abscesses, hyper- or hypopigmentation, cutaneous and s.c. atrophy (which usually disappears, unless the basic disease process is itself atrophic) have occurred.

Since systemic absorption may occasionally occur with intra-articular or other local administration, patients should be watched closely for the following adverse reactions which may be associated with any corticosteroid therapy:
General: anaphylactoid reactions; aggravation or masking of infections.
Cardiovascular: hypertension, syncope, congestive heart failure, arrhythmias, necrotizing angiitis, thromboembolism, thrombophlebitis.
Fluid and Electrolyte Disturbances: sodium retention, fluid retention associated with hypertension or congestive heart failure, potassium loss which may lead to cardiac arrhythmias or ECG changes, and hypokalemic alkalosis.
Musculoskeletal: muscle weakness, fatigue, steroid myopathy, loss of muscle mass, osteoporosis, vertebral compression fractures, delayed healing of fractures, aseptic necrosis of femoral and humeral heads, pathologic fractures of long bones, and spontaneous fractures.
Gastrointestinal: peptic ulcer with possible subsequent perforation and hemorrhage, pancreatitis, abdominal distention, ulcerative esophagitis.
Dermatologic: impaired wound healing, thin fragile skin, petechiae and ecchymoses, facial erythema, increased sweating, purpura, striae, hirsutism, acneiform eruptions, lupus erythematosus-like lesions, hives, rash, suppressed reactions to skin tests.
Neuropsychiatric: convulsions, increased intracranial pressure with papilledema (pseudotumor cerebri) usually after treatment, vertigo, headache, insomnia, neuritis, parasthesias, and aggravation of pre-existing psychiatric conditions, depression (sometimes severe), euphoria, mood swings, psychotic symptoms and personality changes.
Endocrine: menstrual irregularities; development of the cushingoid state; suppression of growth in children; secondary adrenocortical and pituitary unresponsiveness, particularly in times of stress (e.g., trauma, surgery, or illness); decreased carbohydrate tolerance; manifestations of latent diabetes mellitus; and increased requirements for insulin or oral hypoglycemic agents in diabetics.
Ophthalmic: posterior subcapsular cataracts, increased intra-ocular pressure, glaucoma, and exophthalmos, corneal perforation.
Metabolic: hyperglycemia, glycosuria, and negative nitrogen balance due to protein catabolism.

OVERDOSE:

Symptoms: Chronic: The symptoms of glucocorticoid overdose may include confusion, anxiety, depression, gastrointestinal cramping or bleeding, ecchymosis, moon face and hypertension. After long-term use, rapid withdrawal can result in acute adrenal insufficiency (which also may occur in times of stress); Cushingoid changes can result from continued use of large doses.

Treatment: Acute: There is no specific treatment for overdose, but supportive therapy should be instituted and, if gastrointestinal bleeding occurs, it should be treated as peptic ulcer.

> For management of a suspected drug overdose, CPhA recommends that you contact your **regional Poison Control Centre**. See the *CPS* Directory section for a list of Poison Control Centres.

DOSAGE: This preparation contains benzyl alcohol. Not for use in newborn or premature infants (see Warnings, Children).
Intra-articular or intrabursal and tendon sheaths: The initial dose of KENALOG-10 for intra-articular or intrabursal administration and for injection into tendon sheaths may vary from 2.5 to 5 mg (0.25 to 0.5 mL) for smaller joints and from 5 to 15 mg (0.5 to 1.5 mL) for larger joints, depending on the specific disease entity being treated. Single injections into several joints, up to a total of 20 mg (2 mL) or more, have been given without incident.
Intradermal: The initial dose of triamcinolone will vary depending upon the specific disease entity being treated but should be limited to 1 mg (0.1 mL) per injection site, since larger volumes are more likely to produce cutaneous atrophy.
Multiple sites separated by 1 cm or more may be injected, keeping in mind that the greater the total volume employed the more corticosteroid becomes available for systemic absorption and systemic effects. Such injections may be repeated, if necessary, at weekly or less frequent intervals.
Localization of Dose: The lower dosages in the initial dosage range of triamcinolone may produce the desired effect when the corticosteroid is administered to provide a localized concentration. The site and volume of the injection should be carefully considered when triamcinolone is administered for this purpose.
General: The initial dosage should be maintained or adjusted until a satisfactory response is noted. If after a reasonable period of time there is a lack of satisfactory clinical response, KENALOG-10 should be gradually discontinued and the patient transferred to other appropriate therapy.
Dosage requirements are variable and must be individualized on the basis of the disease under treatment and the response of the patient. Dosage adjustments may be necessary in accordance with changes in clinical status.
Administration: **Strict aseptic technique is mandatory.** The vial should be shaken before use to ensure a uniform suspension. Prior to withdrawal, the suspension should be inspected for clumping or granular appearance (agglomeration). An agglomerated product results from exposure to freezing temperatures and should not be used. After withdrawal, inject without delay to prevent settling in the syringe. Careful technique should be employed to avoid the possibility of entering a blood vessel or introducing infection.
Injection Technique: For treatment of joints, the usual intra-articular injection techniques should be followed. If an excessive amount of synovial fluid is present in the joint, some, but not all, should be aspirated to aid in the relief of pain and to prevent undue dilution of the steroid.

With intra-articular or intrabursal administration, and with injection of KENALOG-10 into tendon sheaths or ganglia, prior use of a local anesthetic may often be desirable. Care should be taken with this kind of injection, particularly in the deltoid region, to avoid injecting the suspension into the tissues surrounding the site, since this may lead to tissue atrophy.

For treatment of ganglia, KENALOG-10 injection is injected directly into the cyst cavity.

In treating acute tenosynovitis, care should be taken to ensure that the injection of KENALOG-10 is made into the tendon sheath rather than the tendon substance. Epicondylitis may be treated by infiltrating the preparation into the area of greatest tenderness.

Intralesional: For treatment of dermal lesions, KENALOG-10 should be injected directly into the lesion, i.e., intradermally or s.c. For accuracy of dosage measurement and ease of administration, it is preferable to employ a tuberculin syringe and a small bore needle (23 to 25 gauge). Ethyl chloride spray may be used to alleviate the discomfort of the injection.
Safety in Handling: Due to the high potency of this drug and its potential for absorption through the skin, persons who handle KENALOG-10 should avoid skin and eye contact, as well as inhalation of airborne drug.

SUPPLIED: Each mL of sterile, aqueous suspension contains: triamcinolone acetonide 10 mg. Nonmedicinal ingredients: benzyl alcohol, carboxymethylcellulose sodium, hydrochloric acid, polysorbate, sodium chloride, sodium hydroxide and water. pH between 5.0 and 7.5. At the time of manufacture, the air in the container is replaced by nitrogen. Vials of 5 mL. Store at controlled room temperature (15 to 30°C), avoid freezing and protect from light.

Kenalog®-40 Injection Ⓟ

triamcinolone acetonide
Corticosteroid

Bristol-Myers Squibb

Date of Revision: July 19, 2010

Note: KENALOG-40 INJECTION (triamcinolone acetonide) is a synthetic glucocorticoid corticosteroid with marked anti-inflammatory action, in a sterile aqueous suspension suitable for intramuscular, intra-articular and intrabursal injection. **This formulation is not suitable for intravenous, intradermal, intraocular, epidural or intrathecal injection.**

PHARMACOLOGY: Naturally occurring glucocorticoids (e.g., hydrocortisone), which also have salt-retaining properties, are used as replacement therapy in adrenocortical deficiency states. Synthetic analogs such as triamcinolone are primarily used for their potent anti-inflammatory effects in disorders of many organ systems.

Glucocorticoids cause profound and varied metabolic effects. In addition, they modify the body's immune responses to diverse stimuli.

KENALOG-40 has an extended duration of effect which may be permanent, or sustained over a period of several weeks. Studies indicate that following a single i.m. dose of 60 to 100 mg of triamcinolone acetonide, adrenal suppression occurs within 24 to 48 hours and then gradually returns to normal, usually in 30 to 40 days. This finding correlates closely with the extended duration of therapeutic action achieved with the drug.

INDICATIONS: I.M.: The i.m. administration is indicated for systemic corticosteroid therapy in such conditions as dermatoses, or generalized rheumatoid arthritis and other connective tissue disorders. It is also indicated for allergic diseases; however, for acute allergic reactions, epinephrine is the drug of choice, steroid therapy being adjunctive.

I.M. administration is particularly valuable in such conditions when oral corticosteroid therapy is not feasible. Triamcinolone is not an agent of choice in the treatment of adrenocortical insufficiency or the salt-losing form of the adrenogenital syndrome.
Intra-Articular: For intra-articular or intrabursal administration, and for injections into tendon sheaths, as adjunctive therapy for short-term administration in the following conditions: synovitis of osteoarthritis; rheumatoid arthritis; acute and subacute bursitis; acute gouty arthritis; epicondylitis; acute nonspecific tenosynovitis; and post-traumatic osteoarthritis.

CONTRAINDICATIONS: Corticosteroids are contraindicated in patients with systemic infections. I.M. corticosteroid preparations are contraindicated for idiopathic thrombocytopenic purpura. KENALOG-40 is also contraindicated in patients with a sensitivity to the medicinal or non-medicinal ingredients.

WARNINGS: Because KENALOG-40 is a suspension, it should **not** be administered i.v.. The s.c. route of administration must not be used, due to the possibility of local atrophy.

Epidural and intrathecal administration of this product should not be used. Reports of serious medical events have been associated with epidural and intrathecal routes of administration.

Adequate studies to demonstrate the safety of KENALOG-40 use by intraturbinal, subconjunctival, sub-tenons, retrobulbar injection and intraocular (intravitreal) have not been performed. Endophthalmitis, eye inflammation, increased intraocular pressure and visual disturbances including vision loss have been reported with intravitreal administration. Several instances of blindness have been reported following injection of corticosteroid suspensions into the nasal turbinates and intralesional injection about the head. Administration of KENALOG-40 (Triamcinolone Acetonide Injectable Suspension) by any of these routes is not recommended.

KENALOG-40 is a long-acting preparation and is not suitable for use in acute situations. To avoid drug-induced adrenal insufficiency, supportive dosage may be required in times of stress (such as trauma, surgery or severe illness) both during treatment with KENALOG-40 and for a year afterwards.

Prolonged use of corticosteroids may produce posterior subcapsular cataracts or glaucoma, with possible damage to the optic nerve. Prolonged use may also enhance the likelihood of secondary ocular infections.

Average and large doses of hydrocortisone or cortisone can cause elevation of blood pressure, salt and water retention, and increased excretion of potassium. These effects are less likely to occur with the synthetic derivatives except when they are used in large doses; dietary salt restriction and potassium supplementation may be necessary (see Precautions). All corticosteroids increase calcium excretion, which may be associated with or aggravate preexisting osteoporosis.

Corticosteroids may mask some signs of infection, and new infections may appear during their use. There may be decreased resistance and inability to localize infection when corticosteroids are used. In addition, patients who are on immunosuppressant drugs including corticosteroids are more susceptible to infections than those not taking these drugs. Moreover, chickenpox and measles can have a more serious or even fatal course in patients on corticosteroids. In such children, or adults receiving corticosteroids who have not had these diseases, particular care should be taken to avoid exposure. If exposed, therapy with varicella zoster immune globulin (VZIG) or pooled i.v. immunoglobulin (IVIG), as appropriate, may be indicated. If chickenpox or herpes zoster develops, treatment with antiviral agents may be considered. Similarly, corticosteroids should be used with great caution in patients with Strongyloides (threadworm) infestation because corticosteroid-induced immunosuppression may lead to Strongyloides hyperinfection and dissemination with widespread larval migration, often accompanied by severe enterocolitis and potentially fatal Gram-negative septicemia.

Patients should not be vaccinated or immunized while on corticosteroid therapy, especially on high doses, because of a lack of antibody response predisposing to medical complications, particularly neurological ones.

The use of triamcinolone in patients with active tuberculosis should be restricted to those cases of fulminating or disseminated tuberculosis in which the corticosteroid is used for the management of the disease in conjunction with an appropriate antituberculous regimen. Chemoprophylaxis should be used in patients with latent tuberculosis or tuberculin reactivity who are taking corticosteroids.

Rare instances of anaphylactoid reactions have occurred in patients receiving parenteral corticosteroid therapy. Appropriate precautionary measures should be taken prior to administration, especially when the patient has a history of allergy to any drug.

Unless a **deep** i.m. injection is given, local atrophy is likely to occur. (For recommendations on injection techniques, see Dosage.) Due to the significantly higher incidence of local atrophy when the material is injected into the deltoid area, this injection site should be avoided in favor of the gluteal area.

This product contains benzyl alcohol as a preservative. Benzyl alcohol has been associated with serious adverse events and death, particularly in pediatric patients. The "gasping syndrome" has been associated with benzyl alcohol. Although normal therapeutic doses of this product deliver amounts of benzyl alcohol that are substantially lower than those reported in association with the "gasping syndrome", the minimum amount of benzyl alcohol at which toxicity may occur is not known. Premature and low-birth-weight infants, as well as patients receiving high dosages, may be more likely to develop toxicity.
Pregnancy: Many corticosteroids have been shown to be teratogenic in laboratory animals at low doses. Since adequate human reproduction studies have not been performed with corticosteroids, the use of these drugs in pregnancy, nursing mothers, or women of child-bearing potential requires that the possible benefits of the drug be weighed against the potential hazards to the mother and the embryo, fetus, or breast-fed infant. Other systemic corticosteroids have been shown to appear in breast milk and to slightly elevate (by 1%) the risk of cleft palate in human fetuses. Infants born to mothers who have received substantial doses of corticosteroids during pregnancy should be carefully observed for signs of adrenal suppression.
Lactation: See Pregnancy.
Children: This preparation is not recommended for children under 6 years of age. Because corticosteroids can suppress growth, the development of children on prolonged corticosteroid therapy should be carefully observed. Caution should be used in the event of exposure to chickenpox, measles or other communicable diseases. Children should not be vaccinated or immunized while on corticosteroid therapy (see Warnings). Corticosteroids may also affect endogenous steroid production.

Exposure to excessive amounts of benzyl alcohol has been associated with toxicity (hypotension, metabolic acidosis), particularly in neonates, and an increased incidence of kernicterus, particularly in small preterm infants. There have been rare reports of deaths, primarily in preterm infants, associated with exposure to excessive amounts of benzyl alcohol (see Warnings).

PRECAUTIONS: Drug induced adrenocortical insufficiency may occur with corticosteroids and persist for months after discontinuation of therapy; therefore, in any situation of stress (such as trauma, surgery or severe illness) occurring during that period, hormone therapy should be reinstituted. Since mineralocorticoid secretion may be impaired, salt and/or a mineralocorticoid should be administered concurrently.

There is an enhanced corticosteroid effect in patients with hypothyroidism and in those with cirrhosis.

Corticosteroids should be used cautiously in patients with ocular herpes simplex because of possible corneal perforation.

Psychiatric disturbances may appear when corticosteroids are used. These can include insomnia, depression (sometimes severe), euphoria, mood swings, psychotic symptoms and personality changes. Pre-existing emotional instability or psychosis may also be aggravated by corticosteroids. The use of antidepressant drugs does not relieve and may exacerbate adrenocorticoid-induced mental disturbances.

Corticosteroids should be used with caution in the following conditions: nonspecific ulcerative colitis (if there is a probability of perforation, abscess, or other pyogenic infection); diverticulitis; recent intestinal anastomoses; active or latent peptic ulcer; renal insufficiency; acute glomerulonephritis; chronic nephritis; hypertension; congestive heart failure; thrombophlebitis; thromboembolism; osteoporosis; exanthema; Cushing's syndrome; diabetes mellitus; convulsive disorders; metastatic carcinoma; myasthenia gravis.

Although therapy with KENALOG-40 may ameliorate symptoms of inflammation, it does not obviate the need to treat the cause.

Intra-articular injection of a corticosteroid may produce systemic as well as local effects. The inadvertent injection of the suspension into the soft tissues surrounding a joint may also lead to the occurrence of systemic effects, and is the most common cause of failure to achieve the desired local results.

Following intra-articular steroid therapy, patients should be specifically warned to avoid overuse of joints in which symptomatic benefit has been obtained. Otherwise an increase in joint deterioration can occur.

Overdistention of the joint capsule and deposition of steroid along the needle track should be avoided in intra-articular injection, since this may lead to s.c. atrophy.

Corticosteroids should not be injected into unstable joints. Repeated intra-articular injection may in some cases itself result in instability of the joint. In selected cases, particularly where repeated injections are given, x-ray follow-up is suggested.

An increase in joint discomfort has seldom occurred. A marked increase is pain accompanied by local swelling, further restriction of joint motion, fever, and malaise are suggestive of a septic arthritis. If these complications should appear, and the diagnosis of septic arthritis is confirmed, administration of triamcinolone should be stopped, and antimicrobial therapy should be instituted immediately and continued for 7 to 10 days after all evidence of infection has disappeared. Appropriate examination of any joint fluid present is necessary to exclude a septic process. Injection of a steroid into a previously infected joint should therefore be avoided. Repeated injection into inflamed tendons has been followed by tendon rupture. Therefore, it should also be avoided.

Like other potent corticosteroids, triamcinolone should be used under close clinical supervision. Triamcinolone can cause elevation of blood pressure, salt and water retention, and increased potassium and calcium excretion necessitating dietary salt restriction and potassium supplementation. Edema may occur in the presence of renal disease with a fixed or decreased glomerular filtration rate.

During prolonged therapy, **an adequate protein intake is essential** to counteract the tendency to gradual weight loss sometimes associated with negative nitrogen balance, wasting and weakness of skeletal muscles.

Menstrual irregularities may also occur with corticosteroid treatment.

In peptic ulcer, recurrence may be asymptomatic until perforation or hemorrhage occurs. Long-term adrenocortical therapy may itself produce hyperacidity or peptic ulcer. Therefore, antiulcer therapy is recommended.

Continued supervision of the patient after termination of triamcinolone therapy is essential, since there may be a sudden reappearance of severe manifestations of the disease for which the patient was treated.

Patients should be advised to inform subsequent physicians of the prior use of corticosteroids.

Geriatrics: The common adverse effects of systemic corticosteroids such as osteoporosis or hypertension may be associated with more serious consequences in old age. Close clinical supervision is recommended.

Occupational Hazards: The effects of corticosteroid therapy on the ability to drive or operate machinery have not been studied.

Drug Interactions: Amphotericin B Injection and Potassium-Depleting Agents: Patients should be observed for hypokalemia.

Anticholinesterases: Effects of the anticholinesterase agent may be antagonized.

Anticoagulants, Oral: Corticosteroids may potentiate or decrease anticoagulant action. Patients receiving oral anticoagulants and corticosteroids should therefore be closely monitored.

Antidiabetics: Corticosteroids may increase blood glucose; diabetic control should be monitored, especially when corticosteroids are initiated, discontinued, or changed in dosage.

Antitubercular Drugs: Isoniazid serum concentrations may be decreased.

Cyclosporine: Increased activity of both cyclosporine and corticosteroids may occur when the two are used concurrently.

Digitalis Glycosides: Coadministration may enhance the possibility of digitalis toxicity.

Estrogens, Including Oral Contraceptives: Corticosteroid half-life and concentration may be increased and clearance decreased.

Hepatic Enzyme Inducers (e.g., barbiturates, phenytoin, carbamazepine, rifampin): There may be increased metabolic clearance of KENALOG-40 injection. Patients should be carefully observed for possible diminished effect of steroid, and the dosage of KENALOG-40 injection should be adjusted accordingly.

Human Growth Hormone (e.g., somatrem): The growth-promoting effect of somatrem may be inhibited.

Ketoconazole: Corticosteroid clearance may be decreased, resulting in increased effects.

Nondepolarizing Muscle Relaxants: Corticosteroids may decrease or enhance the neuromuscular blocking action.

Nonsteroidal Anti-inflammatory Agents (NSAIDs): Corticosteroids may increase the incidence and/or severity of gastrointestinal bleeding and ulceration associated with NSAIDS. Also, corticosteroids can reduce serum salicylate levels and therefore decrease their effectiveness. Conversely, discontinuing corticosteroids during high-dose salicylate therapy may result in salicylate toxicity. ASA should be used cautiously in conjunction with corticosteroids in patients with hypoprothrombinemia.

Thyroid Drugs: Metabolic clearance of adrenocorticoids is decreased in hypothyroid patients and increased in hyperthyroid patients. Changes in thyroid status of the patient may necessitate adjustment in adrenocorticoid dosage.

Vaccines: Neurological complications and lack of antibody response may occur when patients taking corticosteroids are vaccinated (see Warnings).

Laboratory Test Interactions: Corticosteroids may affect the nitroblue tetrazolium test for bacterial infection, producing false-negative results.

ADVERSE EFFECTS: General: Following administration by any route, anaphylactoid reactions; aggravation or masking of infections.

Cardiovascular: hypertension, syncope, congestive heart failure, arrhythmias, necrotizing angiitis, thromboembolism, thrombophlebitis.

Fluid and Electrolyte Disturbances: sodium retention, fluid retention associated with hypertension or congestive heart failure, potassium loss which may lead to cardiac arrhythmias or ECG changes, hypokalemic alkalosis.

Musculoskeletal: muscle weakness, fatigue, myopathy, loss of muscle mass, osteoporosis, vertebral compression fractures, delayed healing of fractures, aseptic necrosis of femoral and humeral heads, pathologic fractures of long bones, spontaneous fractures.

Gastrointestinal: peptic ulcer with possible subsequent perforation and hemorrhage, pancreatitis, abdominal distention, ulcerative esophagitis.

Dermatologic: impaired wound healing, thin fragile skin, petechiae and ecchymoses, facial erythema, increased sweating, purpura, striae, hirsutism, acneiform eruptions, lupus erythematosus-like lesions, hives, rash, suppressed reactions to skin tests.

Neuropsychiatric: convulsions, increased intracranial pressure with papilledema (pseudotumor cerebri) usually after treatment, vertigo, headache, insomnia, neuritis, parasthesias, aggravation of pre-existing psychiatric conditions, depression (sometimes severe), euphoria, mood swings, psychotic symptoms and personality changes.

Endocrine: menstrual irregularities; development of the cushingoid state; suppression of growth in children; secondary adrenocortical and pituitary unresponsiveness, particularly in times of stress (e.g., trauma, surgery, or illness); decreased carbohydrate tolerance; manifestations of latent diabetes mellitus; and increased requirements for insulin or oral hypoglycemic agents in diabetics.

Ophthalmic: posterior subcapsular cataracts, increased intra-ocular pressure, glaucoma, and exophthalmos, corneal perforation.

Metabolic: hyperglycemia, glycosuria, and negative nitrogen balance due to protein catabolism.

Following I.M. Administration: Severe pain has been reported following i.m. administration. Sterile abscesses, cutaneous and s.c. atrophy, hyperpigmentation, hypopigmentaion and Charcot-like arthropathy have also occurred.

Intra-Articular Administration: Undesirable reactions have included postinjection flare, transient irritation at the injection site, sterile abscesses, cutaneous and subcutaneous atrophy, hyper-or hypopigmentation, Charcot-like arthropathy and occasional increase in joint discomfort (see Precautions).

OVERDOSE:

Symptoms: Chronic: The symptoms of glucocorticoid overdose may include confusion, anxiety, depression, gastrointestinal cramping or bleeding, ecchymosis, moon face and hypertension. After long-term use, rapid withdrawal can result in acute adrenal insufficiency (which also may occur in times of stress); Cushingoid changes can result from continued use of large doses.

Treatment: Acute: There is no specific treatment for acute overdose, but supportive therapy should be instituted and, if gastrointestinal bleeding occurs, it should be managed.

For management of a suspected drug overdose, CPhA recommends that you contact your **regional Poison Control Centre**. See the *CPS* Directory section for a list of Poison Control Centres.

DOSAGE: General: This preparation contains benzyl alcohol. Not for use in newborn or premature infants (see Children).

The initial dose of KENALOG-40 may vary from 2.5 to 60 mg/day depending on the specific disease entity being treated (see below). In less severe conditions, lower doses generally suffice, while in other patients, higher initial doses may be required. Usually the parenteral dosage range is one-third to one-half the oral dose, given every 12 hours. In life-threatening situations, administration of higher dosages may be justified.

The initial dosage should be maintained or adjusted until a satisfactory response is noted. If after a reasonable period of time there is a lack of satisfactory clinical response, KENALOG-40 should be gradually discontinued and the patient transferred to other appropriate therapy.

Dosage requirements are variable and must be individualized on the basis of the disease under treatment and the response of the patient. The lowest possible dose of corticosteroid should be used to control the condition being treated. After a favorable response is noted, the proper maintenance dosage should be determined by decreasing the initial drug dosage in small decrements at appropriate time intervals down to the lowest dosage which will maintain the desired clinical response. Constant monitoring of drug dosage is necessary. Dose adjustments may be necessary in accordance with changes in clinical status. Patient exposure to stressful situations not directly related to the disease may necessitate increasing the dosage. After long-term therapy, it is recommended that KENALOG-40 be withdrawn gradually.

Systemic: Adults and children over 12 years of age: The suggested initial dose is 60 mg (1.5 mL), **injected deeply into the gluteal muscle**. Atrophy of s.c. fat may occur if the injection is not properly given. Dosage is usually adjusted within the range of 40 to 80 mg, depending upon patient response and duration of relief. However, some patients may be well controlled on doses as low as 20 mg or less.

Hay Fever or Pollen Asthma: Patients with hay fever or pollen asthma who are not responding to pollen administration and other conventional therapy may obtain a remission of symptoms lasting throughout the pollen season after a single injection of 40 to 100 mg (1 to 2.5 mL).

Children 6 to 12 years: The suggested initial dose is 40 mg (1 mL), although dosage depends more on the severity of symptoms than on age or weight. There is insufficient clinical experience with KENALOG-40 to recommend its use in children under 6 years of age.

Local: Intra-articular or intrabursal administration and for injection into tendon sheaths: A single local injection of triamcinolone is frequently sufficient, but several injections may be needed for adequate relief of symptoms.

Initial Dose: 2.5 to 5 mg (0.063 to 0.125 mL) for smaller joints and from 5 to 15 mg (0.125 to 0.375 mL) for larger joints, depending on the specific disease entity being treated. For adults, doses up to 10 mg (0.25 mL) for smaller areas and up to 40 mg (1 mL) for larger areas have usually been sufficient. Single injections into several joints, up to a total of 80 mg (2 mL), have been given without undue reactions.

Administration: General: **Strict aseptic technique is mandatory.** The vial should be shaken before use to ensure a uniform suspension. Prior to withdrawal, the suspension should be inspected for clumping or granular appearance (agglomeration). An agglomerated product results from exposure to freezing temperatures and should not be used. After withdrawal, KENALOG-40 should be injected without delay to prevent settling in the syringe. Careful technique should be employed to avoid the possibility of entering a blood vessel or introducing infection.

Systemic: For systemic therapy, injection should be made **deeply into the gluteal muscle** (see Warnings). For adults, a minimum needle length of 4 cm is recommended. In obese patients, a longer needle may be required. Use alternative sites for subsequent injections.

Local: For treatment of joints, usual intra-articular injection techniques should be followed. If an excessive amount of synovial fluid is present in the joint, some, but not all, should be aspirated to aid in the relief of pain and to prevent undue dilution of the steroid.

With intra-articular or intrabursal administration, and with injection into tendon sheaths, prior use of a local anesthetic may often be desirable. Care should be taken with this kind of injection, particularly in the deltoid region, and with injection into tendon sheaths to avoid injecting the suspension into the tissues surrounding the site, since this may lead to tissue atrophy.

In treating acute nonspecific tenosynovitis, care should be taken to ensure that the injection of the corticosteroid is made into the tendon sheath rather than the tendon substance. Epicondylitis may be treated by infiltrating the preparation into the area of greatest tenderness.

Safety in Handling: Due to the high potency of this drug and its potential for absorption through the skin, persons who handle KENALOG-40 should avoid skin and eye contact, as well as inhalation of airborne drug.

SUPPLIED: Each mL of sterile, aqueous suspension contains: triamcinolone acetonide 40 mg. Nonmedicinal ingredients: benzyl alcohol, carboxymethylcellulose sodium, hydrochloric acid, polysorbate, sodium chloride, sodium hydroxide and water. pH is between 5.0 and 7.5. At the time of manufacture, the air in the container is replaced by nitrogen. Vials of 1 and 5 mL. Store at controlled room temperature (15 to 30°C), avoid freezing and protect from light.

Keppra® P
levetiracetam
Antiepileptic

UCB

Date of Revision: September 20, 2010

PHARMACOLOGY: Mechanism of Action: Levetiracetam is a drug of the pyrrolidine class chemically unrelated to existing antiepileptic drugs (AEDs). As with other drugs in this class, the mechanism of action of levetiracetam in man is not known.

Pharmacokinetics: Summary: Single- and multiple-dose pharmacokinetics of levetiracetam have included healthy volunteers, adult and pediatric patients with epilepsy, elderly subjects, and subjects with renal and hepatic impairment. Results of these studies indicate that levetiracetam is rapidly and almost completely absorbed after oral administration. The pharmacokinetic profile is linear with low intra- and inter-subject variability. There is no modification of the clearance after repeated administration. Food does not affect the extent of absorption of levetiracetam, although the rate is decreased. Levetiracetam is not protein-bound (<10% bound) and its volume of distribution is close to the volume of intracellular and extracellular water. Sixty-six percent (66%) of the dose is renally excreted unchanged. The major metabolic pathway of levetiracetam (24% of the dose) is an enzymatic hydrolysis of the acetamide group. It is not liver cytochrome P450 dependent. The metabolites have no known pharmacodynamic activity and are renally excreted. Plasma half-life of levetiracetam across studies is 6-8 hours. Plasma half-life is increased in subjects with renal impairment, and in the elderly primarily due to impaired renal clearance.

Based on its pharmacokinetic characteristics, levetiracetam is unlikely to produce or to be subject to metabolic interactions.

The pharmacokinetic profile is comparable in healthy volunteers and in patients with epilepsy.

Due to its complete and linear absorption, plasma levels can be predicted from the oral dose of levetiracetam expressed as mg/kg body weight. Therefore, there is no need for plasma level monitoring of levetiracetam.

Human Pharmacology: Pharmacokinetics: The pharmacokinetics of levetiracetam have been characterized in single-and multiple-dose PK studies, with doses up to 5000 mg; these studies included healthy volunteers (N=98), patients with epilepsy (N=58 adult patients and N=24 pediatric patients), elderly subjects (N=16) and subjects with renal and hepatic impairment (N=36 and 16, respectively).

Absorption and Distribution: Levetiracetam is rapidly and almost completely absorbed after oral administration. The oral bioavailability of levetiracetam tablets is 100%. Plasma peak concentrations (C_{max}) are achieved at 1.3 hours after dosing. The extent of absorption is independent of both dose and the presence of food, but the latter delays T_{max} by 1.5 hours and decreases C_{max} by 20%. The pharmacokinetics of levetiracetam are linear over the dose range of 500-5000 mg. Steady-state is achieved after two days of a twice daily administration schedule. Mean peak concentrations (C_{max}) are 31 and 43 µg/mL, respectively, following a single 1000 mg dose, and a repeated 1000 mg twice daily dose.

Neither levetiracetam nor its primary metabolite is significantly bound to plasma proteins (<10%). The volume of distribution of levetiracetam is approximately 0.5 to 0.7 L/kg, a value that is close to the total body water volume. No tissue distribution data for humans are available.

Metabolism: Levetiracetam is not extensively metabolized in humans. The major metabolic pathway is the enzymatic hydrolysis of the acetamide group, which produces the pharmacologically inactive carboxylic acid metabolite, ucb L057 (24% of dose). The production of this metabolite is not dependent on any liver cytochrome P450 isoenzymes and is mediated by serine esterase(s) in various tissues, including blood cells. Two minor metabolites were identified as the product of hydroxylation of the 2-oxo-pyrrolidine ring (2% of dose) and opening of the 2-oxo-pyrrolidine ring in position 5 (1% of dose). There is no evidence for enantiomeric interconversion of levetiracetam or its major metabolite.

Elimination: Levetiracetam plasma half-life in adults is 7±1 hours and was unaffected by dose, route of administration or repeated administration. Levetiracetam is eliminated from the systemic circulation by renal excretion as unchanged drug, which represents 66% of administered dose. The total body clearance is 0.96 mL/min/kg and the renal clearance is 0.6 mL/min/kg. Approximately 93% of the dose was excreted within 48 hours. The mechanism of excretion is glomerular filtration with subsequent partial tubular reabsorption. The primary metabolite, ucb L057, is excreted by glomerular filtration and active tubular secretion with a renal clearance of 4 mL/min/kg. Levetiracetam elimination is correlated to creatinine clearance and clearance is thus reduced in patients with impaired renal function (see Precautions and Dosage).

Special Populations: Elderly: Pharmacokinetics of levetiracetam were evaluated in 16 elderly patients, ranging in age from 61-88 years, with 11 of the 16 patients aged 75 years of age or over with creatinine clearance ranging from 30 to 74 mL/min. Following oral administration of 500 mg bid for 10 days, total body clearance decreased by 38% and the half-life was increased about 40% (10 to 11 hours) when compared to healthy adults. This is most likely due to the decrease in renal function in these subjects.

Pediatrics (6 to 12 years): Pharmacokinetics of levetiracetam were evaluated in 24 pediatric patients (age 6-12 years) after a single dose. The apparent clearance of levetiracetam adjusted to body weight was approximately 40% higher than in epileptic adults.

Gender: Levetiracetam C_{max} and AUC were 20% higher in women (N=11) compared to men (N=12). However, clearances adjusted for body weight were comparable.

Race: Formal pharmacokinetic studies of the effects of race have not been conducted. Because levetiracetam is primarily renally excreted and there are no known important racial differences in creatinine clearance, significant pharmacokinetic differences due to race are not expected.

Renal Impairment: Single dose pharmacokinetics were performed in 20 subjects with renal impairment (N=7 mild/CL_{cr} of 50-79 mL/min; N=8 moderate/CL_{cr} of 30-49 mL/min; N=5 severe/CL_{cr} <30 mL/min), and N=11 matching healthy volunteers. Clearance of levetiracetam is correlated with creatinine clearance and levetiracetam pharmacokinetics following repeat administration were well predicted from single dose data. The apparent body clearance of the parent drug levetiracetam is reduced in patients with impaired renal function by approximately 40% in the mild group, 50% in the moderate group, and 60% in the severe renal impairment group. For the primary metabolite ucb L057, the decrease in clearance values from baseline was greater than that seen for the parent drug in all subject groups.

In anuric (end stage renal disease) patients, the apparent body clearance was approximately 30% compared to that of normal subjects. Approximately 50% of the pool of levetiracetam in the body is removed during a standard 4-hour hemodialysis procedure.

Dosage should be reduced in patients with impaired renal function receiving levetiracetam, and supplemental doses should be given to patients after dialysis (see Precautions and Dosage).

Hepatic Impairment: A single-dose pharmacokinetic study was performed in 16 subjects with hepatic impairment (N=5 mild/Child-Pugh Grade A; N=6 moderate/Grade B; N=5 severe/Grade C vs 5 healthy controls). For the mild and moderate subgroups neither mean nor individual pharmacokinetic values were clinically different from those of controls. In patients with severe hepatic impairment, mean apparent body clearance was 50% that of normal subjects, with decreased renal clearance accounting for most of the decrease. Therefore a 50% reduction of the daily maintenance dose is recommended when the creatinine clearance is <60 mL/min (see Precautions and Dosage).

Clinical Efficacy: The efficacy of Keppra as adjunctive therapy (added to other antiepileptic drugs) in adults was established in three multicenter, randomized, double-blind, placebo-controlled clinical studies in a total of 904 adult patients who had a history of partial onset seizures with or without secondary generalization.

General Methodology: Patient Population: Patients in these three studies had refractory partial onset seizures for a minimum of 1 (or 2) year(s) prior to enrollment. They had previously taken a minimum number of classical AEDs (either one or two), and at the time of the study were taking a stable dose regimen of at least one AED. During the baseline period, it was required that patients experienced a minimum of 12 partial onset seizures over 12 weeks (Study N132) or 4 partial onset seizures during each 4-week period (Study N051) or 2 partial onset seizures per 4-week period (Study N138).

Dosing Schedules: After a prospective baseline period of approximately 12 weeks, patients were randomized to placebo, or levetiracetam 1000 mg, 2000 mg or 3000 mg/day (depending on the study), given as twice daily doses. In all trials, there was a 2 or 4 week titration period, followed by a 12-14 week maintenance period.

Measures of Efficacy: The primary measure of efficacy was a between group comparison of the percent reduction in weekly partial seizure frequency relative to placebo over the entire randomized treatment period (titration+maintenance). Secondary efficacy parameters include the 50% and 100% responder rate in partial onset seizure frequency over the entire randomized treatment period. Efficacy results are based on the ITT population with the exception of a few patients lacking evaluable seizure frequency data.

The above trial description applies to all three studies below. Thus for each trial, only primary distinguishing information is stated below.

Study N132: Study N132 was a parallel-group study conducted in the United States comparing placebo, Keppra 1000 mg/day, and Keppra 3000 mg/day in 95, 98, and 101 randomized patients, respectively. The efficacy for Study N132 is displayed in Table 1.

Table 1: Keppra

Median Percent Reduction from Baseline in Weekly Frequency of Partial Onset Seizures in Study N132

	AEDs+ Placebo	AEDs+Keppra 1000 mg/day	AEDs+Keppra 3000 mg/day
N	95	97	101
Median Baseline Seizure Frequency	1.77	2.53	2.08
Percent Reduction in Partial Seizure Frequency from Baseline	6.9%	36.9%[a]	38.1%[a]

[a] p<0.001 versus placebo.

Study N051: Study N051 was a crossover study conducted in Europe comparing placebo, Keppra 1000 mg/day, and Keppra 2000 mg/day in 112, 106, and 106 randomized patients, respectively.

The first period of the study (Period A) was designed to be analyzed as a parallel-group study. The efficacy results for Period A are displayed in Table 2.

Study N138: Study N138 was a parallel-group study conducted in Europe comparing placebo and Keppra 3000 mg/day in 105 and 181 randomized patients, respectively. Table 3 displays the efficacy results for Study N138.

Responder Rates: Each patient is categorized according to their efficacy data: percent reduction from baseline in weekly frequency of partial onset seizures, calculated over the entire randomized treatment period. The percentage of patients who remained on Keppra for at least 21 days and achieved ≥50% reduction, or a 100% reduction (seizure free) within each of the three pivotal studies is presented in Table 4.

INDICATIONS: Adults: Keppra (levetiracetam) is indicated as adjunctive therapy in the management of patients with epilepsy who are not satisfactorily controlled by conventional therapy.

CONTRAINDICATIONS: This product should not be administered to patients who have previously exhibited hypersensitivity to levetiracetam or any of the inactive ingredients in Keppra tablets.

Table 2: Keppra

Median Percent Reduction from Baseline in Weekly Frequency of Partial Onset Seizures in Study N051 Period A

	AEDs+ Placebo	AEDs+Keppra 1000 mg/day	AEDs+Keppra 2000 mg/day
N	111	106	105
Median Baseline Seizure Frequency	2.46	2.82	2.59
Percent Reduction in Partial Seizure Frequency from Baseline	1.1%	20.7%[a]	24.4%[a]

[a] p<0.001 versus placebo.

Table 3: Keppra

Median Percent Reduction from Baseline in Weekly Frequency of Partial Onset Seizures in Study N138

	AEDs+ Placebo	AEDs+Keppra 3000 mg/day
N	104	180
Median Baseline Seizure Frequency	1.78	1.67
Percent Reduction in Partial Seizure Frequency from Baseline	7.3%	36.8%[a]

[a] p<0.001 versus placebo.

Table 4: Keppra

Partial Onset Responder Rate over the Entire Treatment Period by Randomized Dose

Percent Reduction	AEDs+ Placebo	AEDs+ Keppra 1000 mg/day	AEDs+Keppra 2000 mg/day	AEDs+Keppra 3000 mg/day
Study N132				
N	95	97	—	101
≥50%	7%	36%	—	40%
Seizure free (100%)	0%	3%	—	6%
Study N051				
N	111	106	105	—
≥50%	6%	21%	34%	—
Seizure free (100%)	1%	2%	3%	—
Study N138				
N	104	—	—	180
≥50%	14%	—	—	39%
Seizure free (100%)	0%	—	—	7%

WARNINGS: Central Nervous System Adverse Events: Keppra (levetiracetam) use is associated with the occurrence of central nervous system (CNS) adverse events; the most significant of these can be classified into the following categories: 1) somnolence and fatigue, 2) behavioral/psychiatric symptoms and 3) coordination difficulties.

There was no clear dose response relationship for any of the three categories of CNS adverse events, within the recommended dose range of up to 3000 mg/day. Somnolence/asthenia and coordination difficulties occurred most frequently within the first four weeks of treatment and usually resolved while patients remained on treatment. In the case of behavioral/psychiatric symptoms (including such adverse events as aggression, agitation, anger, anxiety, emotional lability, hostility, irritability), approximately half of the patients reported these events within the first four weeks, with the remaining events occurring throughout the duration of the trials.

See also Precautions, Central Nervous System Adverse Events.

Withdrawal of Anti-epileptic Drugs: As with all antiepileptic drugs, Keppra should be withdrawn gradually to minimize the potential of increased seizure frequency.

Suicidal Ideation and Behavior: Suicidal ideation and behavior have been reported in patients treated with antiepileptic agents in several indications.

All patients treated with antiepileptic drugs, irrespective of indication, should be monitored for signs of suicidal ideation and behavior and appropriate treatment should be considered. Patients (and caregivers of patients) should be advised to seek medical advice should signs of suicidal ideation or behavior emerge.

An FDA meta-analysis of randomized placebo controlled trials, in which antiepileptic drugs were used for various indications, has shown a small increased risk of suicidal ideation and behavior in patients treated with these drugs. The mechanism of this risk is not known.

There were 43 892 patients in the placebo controlled clinical trials that were included in the meta-analysis. Approximately 75% of patients in these clinical trials were treated for indications other than epilepsy and, for the majority of non-epilepsy indications the treatment (antiepileptic drug or placebo) was administered as monotherapy. Patients with epilepsy represented approximately 25% of the total number of patients treated in the placebo controlled clinical trials and, for the majority of epilepsy patients, treatment (antiepileptic drug or placebo) was administered as adjunct to other antiepileptic agents (i.e., patients in both treatment arms were being treated with one or more antiepileptic drug). Therefore, the small increased risk of suicidal ideation and behavior from the meta-analysis (0.43% for patients on antiepileptic drugs compared to 0.24% for patients on placebo) is based largely on patients that received monotherapy treatment (antiepileptic drug or placebo) for non-epilepsy indications. The study design does not allow an estimation of the risk of suicidal ideation and behavior for patients with epilepsy that are taking antiepileptic drugs, due both to this population being the minority in the study, and the drug-placebo comparison in this population being confounded by the presence of adjunct antiepileptic drug treatment in both arms.

Serious Dermatological Reactions: Serious dermatological reactions, including Stevens-Johnson syndrome (SJS) and toxic epidermal necrolysis (TEN), have been reported in both children and adults in association with Keppra use. The median time of onset for reported cases was 12 days. Such serious skin reactions may be life-threatening, and some patients have required hospitalization with very rare reports of fatal outcome. Recurrence of the serious skin reactions following re-challenge with Keppra has been reported.

The reporting rate of TEN and SJS associated with Keppra use, which is generally accepted to be an underestimate due to underreporting, is 9 cases/million patient years. This exceeds the background incidence rate estimates for these serious skin reactions in the general population; background estimates range between 0.5 to 6 cases per million-person years. Therefore, if a patient develops a skin reaction while taking Keppra, consideration should be given to discontinuing Keppra and prescribing another antiepileptic medication.

PRECAUTIONS: General: Hematological Abnormalities: Minor but statistically significant decreases compared to placebo were seen in total mean RBC count, mean hemoglobin, and mean hematocrit in Keppra-treated patients in controlled trials. For hemoglobin values, the percentage of Keppra or placebo treated patients with possibly clinically significant abnormalities were less than 0.5% each. For hematocrit values, a total of 5.1% of Keppra-treated versus 3.2% of placebo patients had at least one possibly significant decrease in hematocrit (≤37% in males and 32% in females).

For white blood cells (WBC), 2.9% of treated versus 2.3% of placebo patients had at least one possibly clinically significant decrease in WBC count (≤2.8×10^9/L), while 2.6% of treated vs 1.7% of placebo patients had at least one possibly significant decrease in neutrophil count (≤1.0×10^9/L). Of the Keppra-treated patients with a low neutrophil count, all but one rose towards or reached baseline with continued treatment. No patient was discontinued secondary to low neutrophil counts.

Central Nervous System Adverse Events: (See Warnings.)

Keppra (levetiracetam) use is associated with the occurrence of central nervous system (CNS) adverse events; the most significant of these can be classified into the following categories: 1) somnolence and fatigue, 2) behavioral/psychiatric symptoms and 3) coordination difficulties.

The following CNS adverse events were observed in controlled clinical trials (see Table 5).

Table 5: Keppra

Total Combined Incidence Rate for Each of the Three Categories of CNS Adverse Events in Placebo-Controlled Add-On Clinical Trials

Category of CNS Adverse Event	Keppra[a]+AED therapy (N=672)	Placebo+AED therapy (N=351)
Somnolence and Fatigue		
Somnolence	15%	10%
Asthenia	14%	10%
Behavioral/Psychiatric Symptoms		
Nonpsychotic[b]	14%	6%
Psychotic[c]	1%	0%
Coordination Difficulties[d]	3%	2%

[a] Reflects Keppra doses of 1000 mg, 2000 mg, 3000 mg, and 4000 mg per day.

[b] "Non-psychotic behavioral/psychiatric symptoms" encompasses the following terms: agitation, antisocial reaction, anxiety, apathy, depersonalization, depression, emotional lability, euphoria, hostility, nervousness, neurosis, personality disorder and suicide attempt.

[c] "Psychotic behavioral/psychiatric symptoms" encompasses the following terms: hallucinations, paranoid reaction, psychosis and psychotic depression.

[d] "Coordination difficulties" encompasses the following terms: ataxia, abnormal gait, incoordination.

See Adverse Effects, Table 6 for incidence rate of individual AEs contained within the categories.

Behavioral/psychiatric symptoms (including agitation, emotional lability, hostility, anxiety etc.) have been reported approximately equally in patients with and without a psychiatric history.

There was no clear dose response relationship for any of the three categories of CNS adverse events, within the recommended dose range of up to 3000 mg/day. In a controlled study including a dose of 4000 mg, administered without titration, the incidence rate of somnolence during the first four weeks of treatment for patients receiving the high dose was 42%, compared to 21% for patients receiving 2000 mg/day.

Occupational Hazards: No studies on the effects on the ability to drive and use machines have been performed. Due to possible different individual sensitivity, some patients might experience somnolence or other central nervous system related symptoms, at the beginning of treatment or following a dose increase. Therefore, caution is recommended in those patients when performing skilled tasks, e.g. driving vehicles or operating machinery.

Special Populations: Patients with Renal Impairment: Renal excretion of unchanged drug accounts for approximately 66% of administered levetiracetam dose. Consistent with this, pharmacokinetic studies in renally-impaired patients indicate that apparent clearance is significantly reduced in subjects with renal impairment (see Pharmacology, Special Populations).

In patients with renal impairment Keppra dosage should be appropriately reduced. Patients with end stage renal disease, i.e. those undergoing dialysis should be given supplemental doses after dialysis (see Dosage).

Pregnancy: There are no adequate and well-controlled studies on the use of Keppra in pregnant women. Levetiracetam and/or its metabolites cross the placental barrier in animal species and in humans.

In reproductive toxicity studies in rats and rabbits, levetiracetam induced developmental toxicity at exposure levels similar to or greater than the human exposure. There was evidence of increased skeletal variations/minor anomalies, retarded growth, embryonic death, and increased pup mortality. In the rat, fetal abnormalities occurred in the absence of overt maternal toxicity. The systemic exposure at the observed no effect level in the rabbit was about 4 to 5 times the human exposure. The potential risk for humans is unknown. Keppra should not be used during pregnancy unless potential benefits to mother and fetus are considered to outweigh potential risks to both. Discontinuation of antiepileptic treatments may result in disease worsening, which can be harmful to the mother and the fetus.

As with other antiepileptic drugs, physiological changes during pregnancy may affect levetiracetam concentration. There have been reports of decreased levetiracetam concentration during pregnancy. This decrease is more pronounced during the third trimester (up to 60% of baseline concentration before pregnancy). It is recommended that clinical response should be monitored carefully in women receiving Keppra treatment during pregnancy, and determination of changes in plasma concentrations should be considered to ensure that adequate seizure control is maintained throughout pregnancy. In the event that medication is increased during pregnancy, the dose may need to be adjusted postpartum.

UCB AED Pregnancy Registry: UCB, Inc. has established the UCB AED Pregnancy Registry to advance scientific knowledge about safety and outcomes associated with pregnant women being treated with all UCB antiepileptic drugs including Keppra. Physicians should encourage patients to register before fetal outcome is known (e.g., ultrasound, results of amniocentesis, etc.). To ensure broad program access and reach, either a healthcare provider or the patient can initiate enrollment in the UCB AED Pregnancy Registry by calling 1-888-537-7734 (toll free). Patients may also enroll in the North American Antiepileptic Drug Pregnancy Registry by calling 1-888-233-2334 (toll free).

Lactation: Levetiracetam is excreted in breast milk. Therefore, there is a potential for serious adverse reactions from Keppra in nursing infants. A decision should be made whether to discontinue nursing or discontinue the drug, taking into account the importance of the drug to the mother, and the as-yet uncharacterized risks to the infant.

Children: Safety and efficacy in patients below the age of 18 have not been established.

Geriatrics: Renal function can be decreased in the elderly and levetiracetam is known to be substantially excreted by the kidney, the risk of adverse reactions to the drug may be greater in patients with impaired renal function. A pharmacokinetic study in 16 elderly subjects (age 61-88 years) showed a decrease in clearance by about 40% with oral administration of both single dose and 10 days of multiple twice-daily dosing. This decrease is most likely due to the expected decrease in renal function in these elderly subjects. Care should therefore be taken in dose selection for elderly patients, and it may be useful to monitor renal function.

There were insufficient numbers of elderly patients in controlled trials of epilepsy to adequately assess the efficacy or safety of Keppra in these patients. Nine of 672 patients treated with Keppra were 65 or over.

Drug Interactions: In Vitro Studies on Metabolic Interaction Potential: In vitro, levetiracetam and its primary metabolite have been shown not to inhibit the major human liver cytochrome P450 isoforms (CYP3A4, 2A6, 2C8/9/10, 2C19, 2D6, 2E1 and 1A2), glucuronyl transferase (paracetamol UGT i.e. UGT1A6, ethinyl estradiol UGT i.e. UGT1A1 and p-nitrophenol UGT i.e. UGT [pl6.2]) and epoxide hydrolase activities. In addition, levetiracetam does not affect the in vitro glucuronidation of valproic acid. In human hepatocytes in culture, levetiracetam did not cause enzyme induction.

Levetiracetam circulates largely unbound (<10% bound) to plasma proteins; therefore clinically significant interactions with other drugs through competition for protein binding sites are unlikely.

Thus in vitro data, in combination with the pharmacokinetic characteristics of the drug, indicate that Keppra is unlikely to produce, or be subject to, pharmacokinetic interactions.

Clinical Pharmacokinetic Data: Other Antiepileptic Drugs (AEDs): Potential drug interactions between Keppra and other AEDs (phenytoin, carbamazepine, valproic acid, phenobarbital, lamotrigine, gabapentin and primidone) were assessed by evaluating the serum concentrations of levetiracetam and these AEDs during placebocontrolled clinical studies. These data suggest that levetiracetam may not significantly influence the plasma concentrations of these other AEDs, and that the other AEDs may not significantly influence the plasma concentrations of levetiracetam.

For two of these AEDs-phenytoin and valproate- formal pharmacokinetic interaction studies with Keppra were performed. Keppra was co-administered with either phenytoin or valproate at doses of 3000 mg/day and 1000 mg/day respectively. No clinically significant interactions were observed.

Other Drug Interactions: No data on the influence of antacids on the absorption of levetiracetam is available.

No data on the interaction of levetiracetam with alcohol is available.

Oral Contraceptives: A pharmacokinetic clinical interaction study has been performed in healthy subjects between the oral contraceptive containing 0.03 mg ethinyl estradiol and 0.15 mg levonorgesterol, and the lowest therapeutic dose of Keppra (500 mg bid). No clinically significant pharmacokinetic interactions were observed.

However, pharmacokinetic interaction studies using Keppra as adjunctive therapy and covering the recommended dosage range, have not been conducted. Therefore, physicians should advise their female patients to be alert to any irregular vaginal bleeding or spotting, and to immediately report to them any occurrences.

Digoxin: Keppra (1000 mg bid) did not influence the pharmacokinetics and pharmacodynamics (ECG) of digoxin given as a 0.25 mg dose every day. Coadministration of digoxin did not influence the pharmacokinetics of levetiracetam.

Warfarin: Keppra (1000 mg bid) did not influence the pharmacokinetics of R and S warfarin (2.5 mg, 5 mg, or 7.5 mg daily). Prothrombin time was not affected by levetiracetam. Coadministration of warfarin did not affect the pharmacokinetics of levetiracetam.

Probenecid: Probenecid, a renal tubular secretion blocking agent, administered at a dose of 500 mg four times a day, did not change the pharmacokinetics of levetiracetam (1000 mg bid). C^{ss}_{max} of the metabolite, ucb L057, was approximately doubled in the presence of probenecid and the renal clearance of the metabolite ucb L057 was decreased by 60%; this alteration is likely related to competitive inhibition of tubular secretion of ucb L057. The effect of Keppra on probenecid was not studied.

ADVERSE EFFECTS: Commonly Observed: In well-controlled clinical studies, the most frequently reported adverse events associated with the use of Keppra in combination with other AEDs, not seen at an equivalent frequency among placebo-treated patients, were somnolence, asthenia, dizziness and infection. Of the most frequently reported adverse events, asthenia, somnolence and dizziness appeared to occur predominantly during the first four weeks of treatment with Keppra.

Incidence of AEs in Controlled Clinical Trials: See Table 6.

Table 6: Keppra

Incidence (%) of Treatment-Emergent Adverse Events In Placebo-Controlled, Add-on Studies By Body System. (Adverse Events Occurred in at Least 1% Of Keppra-treated Patients and Occurred More Frequently than Placebo-treated Patients) (Studies N051, N052, N132 and N138)

Body System/Adverse Event	Keppra+AED therapy (N=672) %	Placebo+AED therapy (N=351) %
Body as a Whole		
Asthenia	14	10
Infection[a]	13	7
Digestive System		
Tooth Disorders	2	1
Hemic and Lymphatic System		
Ecchymosis	2	1
Nervous System		
Amnesia	2	0
Anxiety	2	1
Ataxia	3	1
Depression	4	2
Dizziness	9	4
Emotional Lability	2	0
Hostility	2	1
Nervousness	4	2
Personality Disorders	1	0
Somnolence	15	10
Thinking Abnormal	2	1
Vertigo	3	1
Respiratory System		
Pharyngitis	6	4
Rhinitis	4	3
Sinusitis	2	1

[a] In levetiracetam-treated patients, the majority of "Infection" events (93%) were coded to reported terms of "common cold" or "infection upper respiratory".

Other events reported by 1% or more of patients treated with Keppra but as or more frequent in the placebo group were: abdominal pain, accidental injury, amblyopia, anorexia, back pain, bronchitis, chest pain, confusion, constipation, convulsion, cough increased, diarrhea, diplopia, drug level increased, dysmenorrhea, dyspepsia, fever, flu syndrome, fungal infection, gastroenteritis, gingivitis, grand mal convulsion, headache, insomnia, nausea, otitis media, pain, paresthesia, rash, tremor, urinary tract infection, vomiting and weight gain.

Additional Events Observed in Placebo Controlled Trials: Lack of Dose-Related Incidence of Adverse Events within Therapeutic Range: Based on the data from the controlled clinical trials, there was no evidence of dose relationship within the recommended dose range of 1000 to 3000 mg/day.

Discontinuation or Dose Reduction in Well-Controlled Clinical Studies: In well-controlled clinical studies, 14.3% of patients receiving Keppra and 11.7% receiving placebo either discontinued or had a dose reduction as a result of an adverse event. Table 7 lists the most common (>1%) adverse events that resulted in discontinuation or dose reduction.

Table 7: Keppra

Adverse Events That Most Commonly Resulted in Discontinuation or Dose Reduction in Placebo-controlled Studies in Patients with Epilepsy

	Keppra (N=672)	Placebo (N=351)
Asthenia	9 (1.3%)	3 (0.9%)
Headache	8 (1.2%)	2 (0.6%)
Convulsion	16 (2.4%)	10 (2.8%)
Dizziness	11 (1.6%)	0
Somnolence	31 (4.6%)	6 (1.7%)
Rash	0	5 (1.4%)

The overall adverse experience profile of Keppra was similar between females and males. There are insufficient data to support a statement regarding the distribution of adverse experience reports by age and race.

The following adverse events were seen in well-controlled studies of Keppra for indications in epilepsy other than those approved in this labeling: balance disorder, disturbance in attention, eczema, hyperkinesia, memory impairment, myalgia, nasopharyngitis, pruritus, mood swings, and vision blurred, aggression, agitation, depression, and irritability.

Post-marketing Experience: In post-marketing experience, nervous system and psychiatric disorders have most frequently been reported. In addition to adverse reactions during clinical studies, and listed above, the following adverse reactions have been reported in post-marketing experience. Data are insufficient to support an estimate of their incidence in the population to be treated.

Blood and Lymphatic Disorders: leukopenia, neutropenia, pancytopenia (with bone marrow suppression identified in some of these cases), thrombocytopenia.

Nervous System Disorders: paraesthesia.

Metabolism and Nutrition Disorders: weight loss.

Hepatic/Biliary/Pancreatic: abnormal liver function test, hepatitis, hepatic failure, pancreatitis (see Hepatic Failure).

Psychiatric: abnormal behavior, anger, anxiety, confusion, hallucination, psychotic disorders (see Warnings, Central Nervous System Adverse Events), suicidal behavior (including completed suicide) (see Warnings, Suicidal Ideation and Behavior).

Skin and Subcutaneous Tissue Disorders: toxic epidermal necrolysis, Stevens-Johnson syndrome, erythema multiforme (see Warnings, Serious Dermatological Reactions), alopecia: in several alopecia cases, recovery was observed when levetiracetam was discontinued.

Hepatic Failure: Reports of increases in liver function tests in patients taking Keppra, with and without other medications, have been received. Reports of hepatitis and hepatic failure in patients taking Keppra, with and without other medications, have been received.

OVERDOSE:

Symptoms: The highest reported Keppra overdose is approximately 10 times the therapeutic dose. In the majority of overdose cases, multiple drugs were involved. Somnolence, agitation, aggression, depressed level of consciousness, respiratory depression, and coma were observed with Keppra overdoses. The minimal lethal oral dose in rodents is at least 233 times the maximum clinically studied dose.

Treatment: There is no antidote for overdose with Keppra; treatment is symptomatic and may include hemodialysis. If indicated, elimination of unabsorbed drug should be attempted by emesis or gastric lavage; usual precautions should be observed to maintain airway. General supportive care of the patient is indicated including monitoring of vital signs and observation of the clinical status of the patient.

Standard hemodialysis procedures result in significant removal of levetiracetam (approximately 50% in 4 hours) and should be considered in cases of overdose. Although hemodialysis has not been performed in the few known cases of overdose, it may be indicated by the patient's clinical state or in patients with significant renal impairment.

For management of a suspected drug overdose, CPhA recommends that you contact your **regional Poison Control Centre**. See the *CPS* Directory section for a list of Poison Control Centres.

DOSAGE: General: Renal excretion of unchanged drug accounts for approximately 66% of administered levetiracetam dose. Consistent with this, reduced doses are recommended for patients with renal impairment.

Keppra is given orally with or without food.

Adults: Treatment should be initiated at a dose of 1000 mg/day, given as twice daily dosing (500 mg bid). Depending on clinical response and tolerability, the daily dose may be increased every two weeks by increments of 1000 mg, to a maximum recommended daily dose of 3000 mg.

In clinical trials, daily doses of 1000 mg, 2000 mg, and 3000 mg, given as twice a day dosing, were shown to be effective. Although there was a tendency toward greater response rate with higher dose, a consistent statistically significant increase in response with increased dose has not been shown. There are limited safety data from controlled clinical trials at doses higher than 3000 mg/day (approximately 40 patients), therefore these doses are not recommended.

Patients with Impaired Renal Function: Keppra dosage should be reduced in patients with impaired renal function (see Table 8). Patients with end stage renal disease should receive supplemental doses following dialysis. To use this dosing table, an estimate of the patient's creatinine clearance is needed.

CL_{cr} in mL/min may be estimated from serum creatinine (mg/dL) determination using the following formula:

$$CL_{cr} = \frac{[140\text{-age (years)}]\times\text{weight (kg)}}{72\times\text{serum creatinine (mg/dL)}} \quad (\times 0.85 \text{ for female patients})$$

Then CL_{cr} is adjusted for body surface area (BSA) as follows:

$$\underset{(\text{mL/min/1.73 m}^2)}{CL_{cr}} = \frac{Cl_{cr}\ (\text{mL/min})}{\text{BSA subject (m}^2)} \times 1.73$$

Table 8: Keppra

Dosing Adjustment for Patients with Impaired Renal Function

Group	Creatinine Clearance (mL/min/1.73 m²)	Dosage and Frequency
Normal	≥80	500 to 1500 mg twice daily
Mild	50–79	500 to 1000 mg twice daily
Moderate	30–49	250 to 750 mg twice daily
Severe[a]	<30	250 to 500 mg twice daily
End-stage renal disease patients undergoing dialysis[b]	—	500 to 1000 mg once daily

[a] Or according to best clinical judgement.

[b] Following dialysis, a 250 to 500 mg supplemental dose is recommended.

Patients with Impaired Hepatic Function: No dose adjustment is needed in patients with mild to moderate hepatic impairment. In patients with severe hepatic impairment, the creatinine clearance may underestimate the renal insufficiency. Therefore a 50% reduction of the daily maintenance dose is recommended when the creatinine clearance is <60 mL/min/1.73 m².

Geriatrics: Dose selection and titration should proceed cautiously in elderly patients, as renal function decreases with age.

INFORMATION FOR THE PATIENT: Published in e-CPS, available by subscription at www.e-cps.ca.

SUPPLIED: 250 mg: Each blue, oblong-shaped, film-coated tablet, scored, debossed with "ucb 250" on one side, contains: levetiracetam 250 mg. Nonmedicinal ingredients: colloidal anhydrous silica, FD&C blue #2/indigo carmine aluminum lake, magnesium stearate, polyethylene glycol 3350, polyethylene glycol 6000, polyvinyl alcohol, sodium croscarmellose, talc and titanium dioxide. Bottles of 120. Store between 15-30°C.

500 mg: Each yellow, oblong-shaped, film-coated tablet, scored, debossed with "ucb 500" on one side, contains: levetiracetam 500 mg. Nonmedicinal ingredients: colloidal anhydrous silica, iron oxide yellow, magnesium stearate, polyethylene glycol 3350, polyethylene glycol 6000, polyvinyl alcohol, sodium croscarmellose, talc and titanium dioxide. Bottles of 120. Store between 15-30°C.

750 mg: Each orange, oblong-shaped, film-coated tablet, scored, debossed with "ucb 750" on one side, contains: levetiracetam 750 mg. Nonmedicinal ingredients: colloidal anhydrous silica, FD&C yellow #6/sunset yellow FCF aluminum lake, iron oxide red, magnesium stearate, polyethylene glycol 3350, polyethylene glycol 6000, polyvinyl alcohol, sodium croscarmellose, talc and titanium dioxide. Bottles of 120. Store between 15-30°C.

(Shown in Product Identification Section)

Ketamine Hydrochloride Injection USP Ⓝ

ketamine HCl

General Anesthetic

Sandoz

SUPPLIED: 10 mg/mL: Each mL contains: ketamine (as hydrochloride) 10 mg, sodium chloride, benzethonium chloride 0.01% (as preservative), sodium hydroxide and/or hydrochloric acid to adjust pH and water for injection. Multidose vials of 20 mL, boxes of 1. Multidose vials of 2 mL, boxes of 10. Store between 15 and 30°C. Protect from light and heat. Discard 28 days after initial use.

50 mg/mL: Each mL contains: ketamine (as hydrochloride) 50 mg, benzethonium chloride 0.01% (as preservative), sodium hydroxide and/or hydrochloric acid to adjust pH and water for injection. Multidose vials of 10 mL, boxes of 1. Multidose vials of 2 mL, boxes of 10. Store between 15 and 30°C. Protect from light and heat. Discard 28 days after initial use.

Ketek® Pr

telithromycin

Antibacterial

sanofi-aventis

Date of Revision: July 10, 2009

SUMMARY PRODUCT INFORMATION:

Route of Administration	Dosage Form/ Strength	Clinically Relevant Nonmedicinal Ingredients
Oral	Reduced size tablet 400 mg	New formulation without lactose and corn starch For a complete listing see Dosage Forms, Composition and Packaging.

INDICATIONS AND CLINICAL USE: When prescribing telithromycin, consideration should be given to guidance on the appropriate use of antibacterial agents, and the local prevalence of resistance.

KETEK (telithromycin) tablets are indicated for the treatment of community-acquired pneumonia (of mild to moderate severity) due to *S. pneumoniae*, including multi-drug resistant strains (MDRSP)*, *H. influenzae*, *M. catarrhalis*, *C. (Chlamydia) pneumoniae*, *L. pneumophila*, *M. pneumoniae*, *S. aureus*, in patients 18 years old and older.

To reduce the development of drug-resistant bacteria and maintain the effectiveness of KETEK and other antibacterial drugs, KETEK should be used only to treat infections that are proven or strongly suspected to be caused by susceptible bacteria. When culture and susceptibility information are available, they should be considered in selecting or modifying antibacterial therapy. In the absence of such data, local epidemiology and susceptibility patterns may contribute to the empiric selection of therapy.

CONTRAINDICATIONS:

- **KETEK (telithromycin) is contraindicated in patients with myasthenia gravis.** Exacerbations of myasthenia gravis have been reported in patients and sometimes occurred within a few hours of the first dose of telithromycin. Reports have included death and life-threatening acute respiratory failure with a rapid onset and progression.
- KETEK is contraindicated in patients with a previous history of hepatitis and/or jaundice associated with the use of KETEK tablets, or any macrolide antibiotic.
- KETEK is contraindicated in patients who are hypersensitive to telithromycin, any ingredient in the formulation, or to any macrolide antibiotic. For a complete listing, see Dosage Forms, Composition and Packaging.
- Concomitant administration of KETEK with any of the following drugs is contraindicated: cisapride†, pimozide, astemizole†, terfenadine† and ergot alkaloids.

WARNINGS AND PRECAUTIONS: General: Telithromycin is a strong inhibitor of CYP3A4 and a mild inhibitor of CYP2D6. Thus it is reasonable to expect that the concomitant administration of KETEK and drugs primarily metabolized by these enzymes (i.e. CYP3A4 substrates) may result in increased plasma concentration levels of those drugs that could increase or prolong their therapeutic effect and/or increase adverse reactions. Caution should be exercised during concomitant administration of KETEK and other drugs that are CYP3A4 substrates, especially those drugs with low bioavailability.

Telithromycin is primarily metabolized by cytochrome P450 3A4 (CYP3A4) and to a lesser extent by cytochrome P450 1A (CYP1A). Concomitant administration of CYP3A4 inducers is likely to result in subtherapeutic levels of telithromycin and loss of effect. Concomitant administration of potent CYP3A4 inhibitors may lead to increases in plasma levels of telithromycin (see Drug Interactions, Drug-Drug Interactions).

* MDRSP: Multi-drug resistant *S. pneumoniae* are isolates resistant to two or more of the following antibiotics: penicillin (penicillin-resistant *S. pneumoniae* or PRSP), macrolides (erythromycin/macrolide-resistant *S. pneumoniae* or ERSP/MRSP), 2nd generation cephalosporins (e.g., cefuroxime), tetracyclines and trimethoprim-sulfamethoxazole.

† No longer marketed in Canada.

Cardiovascular: KETEK has the potential to prolong the QTc interval of the electrocardiogram in some patients as observed with some macrolides. QTc interval prolongation may lead to an increased risk for ventricular arrhythmias, including Torsades de Pointes (TdP). Thus, KETEK should be avoided in patients with congenital prolongation of the QTc interval, history of long QT syndrome, and in patients with ongoing proarrythmic conditions such as uncorrected hypokalemia or hypomagnesaemia, clinically significant bradycardia (<50 bpm) and in patients receiving Class IA (e.g. quinidine and procainamide) or Class III (e.g. amiodarone, sotalol) antiarrhythmic agents.

KETEK should be avoided in patients who experienced a confirmed cardiogenic syncope, ventricular tachyarrhythmia or TdP while taking a medicinal product with QT-prolonging potential, such as a macrolide or quinolone antibiotic, or other non-antibiotic suspected of prolonging the QT interval.

In clinical trials the effect on QTc interval was small (mean approximately 1 millisecond). There were no reports of TdP or other serious ventricular arrhythmias or related syncope in the clinical program and no subgroups at risk were identified.

In clinical trials no increased cardiovascular morbidity or mortality attributable to the QTc interval prolongation occurred with KETEK treatment in 4780 patients, including 204 patients having a prolonged QTc interval at baseline.

Cases of torsades de pointes have been reported in post-marketing experience with KETEK.

Statins: The risk of myopathy and rhabdomyolysis may be increased with high statin plasma levels. Therefore, concomitant administration of telithromycin with statins primarily metabolized by CYP3A4 should be avoided.

Gastrointestinal: *C. difficile*-associated disease (CDAD): *C. difficile*-associated disease (CDAD) has been reported with use of many antibacterial agents, including KETEK. CDAD may range in severity from mild diarrhea to fatal colitis. It is important to consider this diagnosis in patients who present with diarrhea or symptoms of colitis, pseudomembranous colitis, toxic megacolon, or perforation of the colon subsequent to the administration of any antibacterial agent. CDAD has been reported to occur over 2 months after the administration of antibacterial agents.

Treatment with antibacterial agents may alter the normal flora of the colon and may permit overgrowth of *C. difficile*. *C. difficile* produces toxins A and B, which contribute to the development of CDAD. CDAD may cause significant morbidity and mortality. CDAD can be refractory to antimicrobial therapy.

If the diagnosis of CDAD is suspected or confirmed, appropriate therapeutic measures should be initiated. Mild cases of CDAD usually respond to discontinuation of antibacterial agents not directed against *C. difficile*. In moderate to severe cases, consideration should be given to management with fluids and electrolytes, protein supplementation, and treatment with an antibacterial agent clinically effective against *C. difficile*. Surgical evaluation should be instituted as clinically indicated since surgical intervention may be required in certain severe cases (see Adverse Reactions).

Hepatic/Biliary/Pancreatic: Hepatotoxicity: Acute hepatic failure and severe liver injury, in some cases fatal have been reported in patients treated with KETEK. These hepatic reactions included fulminant hepatitis and hepatic necrosis leading to liver transplant, and were observed during or immediately after treatment with KETEK. Liver injury progressed rapidly and occurred after administration of only a few doses of KETEK (see Adverse Reactions).

In addition, less severe hepatic dysfunction associated with increased liver enzymes, hepatitis and in some cases jaundice was reported with the use of KETEK. These events associated with less severe forms of liver toxicity were reversible.

Physicians and patients should monitor for the appearance of signs or symptoms of hepatitis, such as fatigue, malaise, anorexia, nausea, jaundice, bilirubinuria, acholic stools, liver tenderness, hepatomegaly or pruritus. Patients with signs or symptoms of hepatitis must be advised to discontinue KETEK and immediately seek medical evaluation, which should include liver function tests (see Adverse Reactions). If clinical hepatitis or transaminase elevations combined with other systemic symptoms occur, KETEK should be permanently discontinued.

KETEK must not be re-administered to patients with a previous history of hepatitis and/or jaundice associated with the use of KETEK tablets, or any macrolide antibiotic (see Contraindications).

Use in Patients with Hepatic Impairment: No dose adjustment is needed in patients with severe hepatic impairment, unless renal function is severely impaired. Experience in patients with impaired hepatic function is limited; hence, KETEK should be used with caution in these patients (see Dosage and Administration, Dosing Considerations and Action and Clinical Pharmacology, Special Populations and Conditions).

In patients with severely impaired renal and/or hepatic function, concomitant administration of KETEK and strong CYP3A4 inhibitors, such as protease inhibitors or ketoconazole, is not recommended (see Action and Clinical Pharmacology, Special Populations and Conditions).

Immune: Hypersensitivity Reactions: Serious allergic reactions, including anaphylaxis and angioedema have been very rarely reported in patients on KETEK therapy. If an allergic reaction occurs, KETEK should be discontinued and appropriate therapy should be instituted.

Neurologic: Loss of Consciousness: There have been post-marketing adverse event reports of loss of consciousness, including syncope, sometimes associated with vagal syndrome.

Ophthalmologic: Visual Disturbances: KETEK may cause visual disturbances particularly in slowing the ability to accommodate and the ability to release accommodation. Visual disturbances included blurred vision, difficulty focusing, and diplopia. Most events were mild to moderate however, severe cases have been reported (see Adverse Reactions, Less Common Clinical Trial Adverse Drug Reactions, Eye Disorders).

Renal: Use in Patients with Renal Insufficiency: No dose adjustment is needed in patients with mild to moderate renal impairment. In the presence of severe renal impairment (creatinine clearance <30 mL/min), the dose should be reduced to 400 mg once daily (see Dosage and Administration, Dosing Considerations and Action and Clinical Pharmacology, Special Populations and Conditions and Warnings And Precautions, Hepatic/Biliary/Pancreatic, Use in Patients with Hepatic Impairment).

In patients with severely impaired renal and/or hepatic function, concomitant administration of KETEK and strong CYP3A4 inhibitors, such as protease inhibitors or ketoconazole, is not recommended (see Action and Clinical Pharmacology, Special Populations and Conditions).

Special Populations: Pregnant Women: There are no adequate and well-controlled studies in pregnant women.

Studies in animals have shown embryofetal toxicity only at doses inducing maternal toxicity. The effects occurred at doses of 300 mg/kg/day in rats and 60 mg/kg/day in rabbits, which correspond to 18.8 and 3.75 times the recommended human clinical dose, respectively. The potential risk for humans is unknown. KETEK should not be used during pregnancy unless the expected benefit to the mother outweighs any possible risk to the foetus.

Nursing Women: It is not known whether telithromycin is excreted in human milk; however, it is excreted in the milk of lactating animals at concentrations about five times those of maternal plasma. Preweaned rats, exposed indirectly via consumption of milk from dams treated with 200 mg/kg/day for 3 weeks, were not adversely affected, despite data indicating higher drug levels in milk than in plasma. Because animal data are not always predictive of human response, KETEK should not be used during lactation unless the expected benefit to the mother outweighs any possible risk to the baby.

Pediatrics (birth to 18 years old): The safety of KETEK in pediatric populations less than 13 years of age has not been established. A total of 124 subjects aged 13 to 18 years were treated with KETEK in 16 Phase III trials. Efficacy and safety were similar to that observed in older patients.

Geriatrics: In the 16 Phase III clinical trials (n=4780 analysed for safety), KETEK was administered to 694 patients who were 65 years and older, including 231 patients who were 75 years and older.

Efficacy and safety were similar to that observed in younger patients. However, greater sensitivity of older individuals to KETEK or telithromycin cannot be ruled out.

No dosage adjustment is required based on age alone; however, a dosage adjustment is recommended in elderly patients with severe renal impairment (CL_{CR} <30 mL/min) (see Dosage and Administration, Dosing Considerations and Action and Clinical Pharmacology, Special Populations and Conditions, Geriatrics).

Monitoring and Laboratory Tests: There are no reported laboratory test interactions.

Occupational Hazards: Visual Disturbances: KETEK may cause visual disturbances particularly in slowing the ability to accommodate and the ability to release accommodation. Visual disturbances included blurred vision, difficulty focusing, and diplopia. Most events were mild to moderate; however severe cases have been reported. If a patient experiences these events, a healthcare professional should be consulted and consideration may be given to taking KETEK at bedtime (see Adverse Reactions, Less Common Clinical Trial Adverse Drug Reactions, Eye Disorders).

Loss of Consciousness: There have been post-marketing adverse event reports of loss of consciousness, including syncope sometimes associated with vagal syndrome.

Driving a Vehicle or Operating Machinery: Because of potential visual difficulties, loss of consciousness, confusion or hallucination, patients should attempt to minimize activities such as driving a motor vehicle, operating heavy machinery or engaging in other hazardous activities during treatment with KETEK. If patients experience visual disorders, loss of consciousness, confusion or hallucination, while taking KETEK, patients should not drive a motor vehicle, operate heavy machinery or engage in other potentially hazardous activities.

ADVERSE REACTIONS: Adverse Drug Reaction Overview: During clinical trials, some patients experienced adverse reactions inherent to the use of antibacterials. Most of these events were mild to moderate in severity and transient. In all Phase III studies, discontinuation due to a possibly related treatment-emergent adverse event occurred in 2.3% of KETEK (telithromycin) treated patients. Most discontinuations in the KETEK groups were due to treatment-emergent adverse events in the gastrointestinal body system, primarily diarrhea (0.5%), nausea (0.4%), and vomiting (0.5%).

Clinical Trials Adverse Drug Reactions: Because clinical trials are conducted under very specific conditions the adverse reaction rates observed in the clinical trials may not reflect the rates observed in practice and should not be compared to the rates in the clinical trials of another drug. Adverse drug reaction information from clinical trials is useful for identifying drug-related adverse events and for approximating rates.

The safety of KETEK 800 mg once daily was evaluated in a total of 4780 patients (N=2702 in controlled trials) treated for 5 days or for 7 to 10 days. Treatment-emergent adverse reactions judged by investigators to be at least possibly drug related and occurring in ≥1.0 % of all KETEK-treated patients in all Phase III trials are listed in Table 1.

Table 1: KETEK

Possibly-related Treatment-emergent Adverse Events Reported in All Phase III Clinical Trials (percent incidence)

Adverse Event System Organ Class/Preferred Term	KETEK (all studies) n=4780 (% of subjects)	KETEK (controlled studies) n=2702 (% of subjects)	Comparator n=2139 (% of subjects)
Gastrointestinal Disorders			
Diarrhea NOS	8.1	10.0	8.0
Nausea	5.5	7.0	4.1
Vomiting NOS	1.9	2.4	1.4
Loose stools	1.5	2.1	1.4
Abdominal pain NOS	1.0	1.3	0.7
Flatulence	0.9	1.4	0.9
Dyspepsia	0.9	1.4	1.0
Nervous System Disorders			
Dizziness (excl. vertigo)	1.9	2.8	1.5
Headache	1.5	2.0	2.5
Dysgeusia	1.1	1.5	3.6

Legend: NOS=not otherwise specified.

Visual Adverse Events: Table 2 provides the incidence of treatment-emergent visual adverse events, by age and gender, in all controlled Phase III studies.

Table 2: KETEK

Incidence, by Age and Gender, of All Treatment-emergent Visual Adverse Events in All Controlled Phase III Studies

Gender/Age	Phase III Studies Telithromycin	Comparators[a]
Female ≤40	2.05% (14/682)	0.00% (0/534)
Female >40	1.00% (7/703)	0.35% (2/574)
Male ≤40	1.24% (7/563)	0.48% (2/417)
Male >40	0.27% (2/754)	0.33% (2/614)
Total	1.11% (30/2702)	0.28% (6/2139)

[a] Includes all comparators combined.

For Phase III studies, the group with the highest incidence of visual adverse events was females 40 years of age or less, while males over the age of 40 had rates of visual events similar to comparator-treated patients.

In clinical trials, increases in liver enzymes (AST, ALT, ALP) have been reported. The overall frequency of transaminase increases was similar to that seen in comparators. Elevations above 3×ULN were uncommon. Liver enzyme increases were usually asymptomatic and reversible.

Less Common Clinical Trial Adverse Drug Reactions: All Studies: In the controlled studies including the large trial in a usual care setting, additional events, judged by investigators to be at least possibly drug related that occurred in ≥0.1% and <1% of KETEK-treated patients were:

Blood and Lymphatic System Disorders: anemia, eosinophilia, leukopenia, neutropenia, thrombocythaemia.

Cardiac Disorders: bundle branch block, palpitations.

Ear and Labyrinth Disorders: vertigo.

Eye Disorders: Visual adverse events most often included blurred vision, difficulty focusing and diplopia. Most events were mild to moderate however, severe cases have been reported. Some patients discontinued therapy due to these adverse events. Visual adverse events were reported as having occurred after any dose during treatment, but most adverse events occurred after the first or second dose. Visual events lasted several hours and recurred upon subsequent dosing in some patients. For patients who continued treatment, some resolved on therapy while others continued to have symptoms until they completed the full course of treatment. These events have not been associated with signs of ocular abnormality.

Gastrointestinal Disorders: abdominal distension, abdominal pain, abdominal pain (lower), abdominal pain (upper), abdominal tenderness, antibiotic associated colitis, aphthous stomatitis, aptyalism, constipation, dry lips, dry mouth, dyspepsia, eructation, flatulence, frequent bowel movements, gastritis, gastrointestinal disorder, gastrointestinal upset, gastro-oesophageal reflux disease, glossitis, glossodynia, mouth ulceration, pharyngolaryngeal pain, reflux oesophagitis, stomach discomfort, stomatitis, vomiting, watery stools.

General Disorders and Administration Site Conditions: asthenia, fatigue, oedema peripheral.

Hepatobiliary Disorders: cholestasis, hepatitis, hepatocellular damage. Symptomatic hepatic injury, with or without jaundice, was rare and reversible.

Immune System Disorders: drug hypersensitivity, hypersensitivity.

Infections and Infestations: fungal infections NOS (NOS=not otherwise specified), gastroenteritis, oral candidiasis, sinusitis, vaginal candidiasis, vaginitis, vaginosis fungal.

Metabolism and Nutrition Disorders: anorexia, appetite decreased, hypokalemia.

Musculoskeletal and Connective Tissue Disorder: back pain, muscle cramps.
Nervous System Disorders: ageusia, disturbance in attention, dysgeusia, paresthesia, paresthesia oral, somnolence.
Psychiatric Disorders: abnormal dreams, anxiety, insomnia, nervousness, nightmare.
Renal and Urinary Disorder: chromaturia, creatinine renal clearance decreased, polyuria.
Reproductive System and Breast Disorders: dysmenorrhea, vaginal irritation.
Skin and Subcutaneous Tissue Disorders: allergic dermatitis, eczema, pruritus, rash, sweating increased, urticaria.
Vascular Disorders: flushing.
Other Rare Events Included (<0.1%): alkaline phosphatase increased, bradycardia, coagulopathy (coagulation disorder), elevated blood bilirubin, erythema multiforme, face edema, hyperkalemia, hypotension, QT interval prolonged, sinus (atrial) arrhythmia.
Abnormal Hematologic and Clinical Chemistry Findings: Clinically noteworthy changes in clinical chemistry and hematologic variables were assessed for all Phase III studies and their incidence was compared between studies in patients with community-acquired pneumonia (CAP) and non-CAP studies (see Table 3).

Table 3: KETEK
Common Clinically Noteworthy Changes in Clinical Chemistry and Hematologic Variables in Controlled Phase III CAP and Non-CAP Studies

	Clinically Noteworthy Change	CAP Studies (% of subjects)		Non-CAP Studies (% of subjects)	
		KETEK	Comparator	KETEK	Comparator
Clinical Chemistry					
Creatinine clearance ↓	<50 mL/min	4.0	5.7	4.2	4.9
ALT ↑	>3 ULN	2.5	2.8	1.2	1.1
AST ↑	>3 ULN	2.4	2.2	0.6	0.8
Hematology					
Eosinophils ↑	>1000/mm³	1.6	1.5	0.8	1.2
Leucocytes ↓	<3000/mm³	1.1	1.7	0.8	0.2
Neutrophils ↓	<1500/mm³	3.0	4.0	2.0	1.7
Potassium ↑	>5.5 mmol/L	3.6	3.8	1.1	1.1

Legend: ULN=upper limit of normal, using the laboratory normal range.

A higher incidence of clinically noteworthy changes in hepatic analytes was observed in CAP studies, which is due to the severity of the underlying disease. The increase in hepatic analytes was more common in subjects with elevated levels at baseline. Similarly, decreases in creatinine clearance were more commonly seen in subjects with clearances below the extended normal range at study entry. None of these changes are considered clinically significant.
Post-Market Adverse Drug Reactions: The following adverse events have been reported during post-marketing surveillance: exacerbation of myasthenia gravis, severe allergic reactions including anaphylaxis and angioedema, pancreatitis, torsades de pointes, loss of consciousness including syncope, sometimes associated with vagal syndrome (see Contraindications and Warnings and Precautions), confusion, hallucination, anosmia, arthralgia and myalgia.

Severe and in some cases fatal hepatotoxicity, including fulminant hepatitis, hepatic necrosis and hepatic failure have been reported in some patients treated with KETEK. These hepatic reactions were observed during or shortly after treatment. In some of these cases, liver injury progressed rapidly and occurred after administration of only a few doses of KETEK (see Contraindications and Warnings and Precautions). Severe reactions, in some but not all cases, have been associated with serious underlying diseases or concomitant medications. Data from post-marketing reports and clinical trials show that most cases of hepatic dysfunction were mild to moderate.

Spontaneous cases of toxic epidermal necrolysis (TEN) and Stevens-Johnson syndrome (SJS) have been reported; however, a causal association between the administration of KETEK and development of SJS and TEN has not been established.

DRUG INTERACTIONS:

Telithromycin, like certain other macrolides, is primarily metabolized by CYP3A4 and inhibits CYP3A4. The concomitant administration of telithromycin and other drugs mainly metabolized by this enzyme may lead to increased plasma concentrations of the co-administered drugs (see Drug-Drug Interactions).

Overview: Drug-Drug: KETEK (telithromycin) is primarily metabolized by cytochrome P450 3A4 (CYP3A4) and to a lesser extent by cytochrome P450 1A (CYP1A).
Effects of Telithromycin on Other Drugs: In vitro drug interaction studies have demonstrated that telithromycin is a strong inhibitor of CYP3A4 and a mild inhibitor of CYP2D6. Thus it is reasonable to expect that the concomitant administration of KETEK and drugs primarily metabolized by these enzymes (i.e. CYP3A4 substrates) may result in increased plasma concentration levels of those drugs that could increase or prolong their therapeutic effect and/or increase adverse reactions. Caution should be exercised during concomitant administration of KETEK and other drugs that are CYP3A4 substrates, especially those drugs with low bioavailability.

In vivo studies with midazolam, simvastatin and cisapride have demonstrated a potent inhibition of intestinal CYP3A4 and a moderate inhibition of hepatic CYP3A4 by telithromycin. The degree of inhibition with different CYP3A4 substrates is difficult to predict. Hence, patients taking medicinal products that are CYP3A4 substrates and have a narrow therapeutic window, should be clinically monitored while taking KETEK. Concomitant administration of drugs mainly metabolized by this enzyme may lead to increased plasma concentrations, possibly resulting in increased adverse events. Telithromycin is a mild inhibitor of CYP2D6.
Effects of Other Drugs on Telithromycin: Concomitant administration of CYP3A4 inducers (such as rifampin, phenytoin, carbamazepine, phenobarbital, St. John's wort) is likely to result in subtherapeutic levels of telithromycin and loss of effect.

Concomitant administration of potent CYP3A4 inhibitors (such as ritonavir and ketoconazole) may lead to increases in plasma levels of telithromycin.
Drug-Drug Interactions: See Table 4.

No specific drug interaction studies have been performed to evaluate the following potential drug-drug interactions between KETEK and drugs metabolized by cytochrome P450 systems, such as: carbamazepine, cyclosporine, disopyramide, hexobarbital, phenytoin, quinidine, and triazolam. However, drug interactions have been observed with macrolide products. Elevation of serum levels of these drugs may be observed when co-administered with telithromycin.
Drug-Food Interactions: Studies have shown that there is no interaction with food for the regular size tablet‡ and that the reduced-size tablet is bioequivalent to the regular size tablet in the fasted state. KETEK tablets can be taken with or without food.

When KETEK was given with 240 mL of grapefruit juice after an overnight fast to healthy subjects, the pharmacokinetics of telithromycin were not affected.
Drug-Herb Interactions: Interactions with herbal products have not been established (for information on St. John's wort see Warnings and Precautions, General and Drug Interactions, Overview, Drug-Drug).
Drug-Laboratory Test Interactions: There are no reported laboratory test interactions.

‡ Regular size tablet was the previous formulation, no longer available on Canadian market.

Table 4: KETEK
Established or Predicted Drug-Drug Interactions

Proper Name	Ref	Effect	Clinical Comments
CYP3A4 Inhibitors			
Itraconazole	CT	↑ telithromycin plasma conc.	This interaction does not necessitate a dosage adjustment for telithromycin. A multiple-dose interaction study with itraconazole, a CYP3A4 inhibitor, and KETEK showed that maximum plasma concentrations of telithromycin were increased by 22% and AUC by 54% when co-administered with itraconazole.
Ketoconazole	CT	↑ telithromycin plasma conc. ↓ ketoconazole plasma conc.	This interaction does not necessitate a dosage adjustment for telithromycin. A multiple-dose interaction study with ketoconazole, a CYP3A4 inhibitor, and KETEK showed that maximum plasma concentrations of telithromycin were increased by 51% and AUC by 95%. The maximum ketoconazole plasma concentrations and AUC were both decreased by 20% when co-administered with KETEK.
CYP3A4 Inducers			
Rifampin	CT	↓ telithromycin conc.	Concomitant treatment of KETEK with rifampin should be avoided. During concomitant administration of rifampin and telithromycin in repeated doses, C_{max} and AUC of telithromycin were decreased by 79% and 86%, respectively. The induction gradually decreases during 2 weeks after cessation of treatment with rifampin.
CYP3A4 Substrates			
Benzodiazepines	CT	↑ midazolam conc.	Oral or intravenous administration of midazolam concomitant with KETEK is associated with an increase in plasma levels of midazolam. Therefore, dosage of midazolam should be adjusted as necessary and patient should be clinically monitored. Similar precautions should be used with other benzodiazepines, which are metabolized by CYP3A4, for example triazolam and to a lesser extent alprazolam. Concomitant administration of KETEK with intravenous or oral midazolam resulted in 2- and 6-fold increases respectively, in the AUC of midazolam due to inhibition of CYP3A4-dependent metabolism of midazolam. For those benzodiazepines that are not metabolized by CYP3A4 (temazepam, nitrazepam, lorazepam) interaction with KETEK is unlikely.
Cisapride	CT	↑ cisapride plasma conc.	The concomitant administration of KETEK and cisapride is contraindicated (see Contraindications). Steady-state peak plasma concentrations of cisapride (an agent with the potential to increase QT interval) were increased by 95% when co-administered with repeated doses of KETEK, resulting in significant increases in QTc.
Ergotamine or dihydroergotamine	T		Acute ergot toxicity characterized by severe peripheral vasospasm and dyesthesia has been reported when macrolide antibiotics were co-administered with vasoconstrictive ergot alkaloids. Without further data, the co-administration of KETEK and these drugs is contraindicated (see Contraindications).
Pimozide	T	risk of ↑ pimozide plasma conc.	The use of KETEK is contraindicated with pimozide (see Contraindications). Although there are no studies looking at the interaction between KETEK and pimozide (an agent with the potential to increase QT intervals), there is a potential risk of increased pimozide plasma levels by inhibition of CYP3A4 pathways by KETEK as with macrolides.
Statins	CT	↑ simvastatin conc. ↑ simvastatin acid conc.	High levels of simvastatin may increase the risk of myopathy and rhabdomyolysis. Therefore, concomitant administration of telithromycin with simvastatin or other statins primarily metabolized by CYP3A4 should be avoided. If KETEK is prescribed, consideration should be given to either suspending therapy of these statins for the duration of treatment, or to separating the administration of both products by 12 hours. Patients should be carefully monitored to detect any signs or symptoms of myopathy or rhabdomyolysis. When simvastatin was co-administered with telithromycin, there was a 5.3-fold increase in simvastatin C_{max} and an 8.9-fold increase in simvastatin AUC, a 15-fold increase in simvastatin acid C_{max} and a 12-fold increase in simvastatin acid AUC. In another study, when simvastatin and telithromycin were administered 12 hours apart, there was a 3.4-fold increase in simvastatin C_{max}, a 3.8-fold increase in simvastatin AUC, a 3.2-fold increase in the active metabolite C_{max} and a 4.3-fold increase in the active metabolite AUC. These levels are approximately one-half of the levels reported when simvastatin and telithromycin were administered concomitantly. Simvastatin levels were increased due to CYP3A4 inhibition by telithromycin.

(cont'd)

Table 4: KETEK *(cont'd)*

Established or Predicted Drug-Drug Interactions

Proper Name	Ref	Effect	Clinical Comments
	T T T	↑ lovastatin and atorvastatin conc. ↑ pravastatin conc. ↑ rosuvastatin conc.	Similarly, an interaction may be expected with lovastatin and to a lesser extent atorvastatin. Although pravastatin is not metabolized by CYPs, hepatic cell OATP1 transporters play an important role in its elimination from the body. In vitro OATP1 transporter inhibition has been demonstrated for macrolides and telithromycin. Telithromycin slightly inhibits the in vitro transporter uptake of pravastatin. The in vivo relevance of this in vitro finding has not been established for telithromycin. Fluvastatin is essentially metabolized by CYP2C9 rather than CYP3A4, and in vitro transporter inhibition was shown not to be significantly increase fluvastatin exposure in patients. Therefore, no drug interaction is expected with this product. Rosuvastatin is mainly excreted unchanged (only 10% is metabolized by CYP2C9). Although it is known to be a substrate of OATP1B1 in vitro, alternate transporting proteins are thought to be involved. Given the current available information, the relevance of these findings for drug-drug interaction with telithromycin has not been established.
CYP2D6 Substrates			
Paroxetine	CT		There was no pharmacokinetic effect on paroxetine, when KETEK was co-administered.
Metoprolol	CT	↑ metoprolol conc.	When metoprolol was co-administered with KETEK, there was an increase of approximately 38% on the C_{max} and AUC of metoprolol, however, there was no effect on the elimination half-life of metoprolol. Telithromycin exposure is not modified with concomitant single-dose administration of metoprolol. In patients with heart failure, the increased exposure to metoprolol, a CYP2D6 substrate, may be of clinical importance. Therefore, co-administration of KETEK and metoprolol in patients with heart failure should be considered with caution.
CYP1A2 Substrates			
Theophylline	CT		There was no clinically relevant pharmacokinetic effect on theophylline when KETEK was co-administered. However, the administration of both drugs should be separated by one hour in order to decrease the likelihood of gastrointestinal side effects.
Other Drug Interactions			
Digoxin	CT	↑ digoxin plasma conc.	Monitoring of digoxin side effects or serum levels should be considered during concomitant administration of digoxin and KETEK. KETEK has been shown to increase the plasma concentrations of digoxin. The plasma peak and trough levels were increased by 73% and 21%, respectively, in healthy volunteers. There were no significant changes in ECG parameters and no signs of digoxin toxicity were observed. However, pharmacokinetic interactions in healthy volunteers have been observed after co-administration of KETEK tablets with digoxin.
Sotalol	CT	↓ sotalol conc.	KETEK has been shown to decrease the C_{max} of sotalol by 34% and to decrease the AUC of sotalol by 20% due to decreased absorption.
Warfarin	C, CT		During concomitant administration of telithromycin and warfarin, INR should be closely monitored, and if necessary, the oral anticoagulant dosage should be adjusted as appropriate. There are reports of increased anticoagulant effects when telithromycin and warfarin are used concurrently. However, there were no pharmacodynamic or pharmacokinetic effects on racemic warfarin in healthy subjects.
Oral Contraceptives	CT		Based on a pharmacokinetic/pharmacodynamic interaction study, KETEK did not interfere with the antiovulatory effect of oral contraceptives containing ethinyl estradiol and levonorgestrel.
Ranitidine, antacids	CT		There was no clinically relevant pharmacokinetic interaction of ranitidine or antacids containing aluminium and magnesium hydroxide on KETEK.

Legend: C=case study; CT=clinical trial; T=theoretical.

DOSAGE AND ADMINISTRATION:

Dosing Considerations: KETEK (telithromycin) tablets can be administered with or without food (see Drug Interactions, Drug-Food Interactions).

Consideration may be given to taking telithromycin at bedtime, to reduce the potential impact of visual disturbances and loss of consciousness (see Warnings and Precautions, Occupational Hazards).

Impaired Renal Function: No dosage adjustment for KETEK is necessary in patients with mild to moderate renal impairment. In the presence of severe renal impairment (creatinine clearance <30 mL/min), the dose should be reduced to 400 mg once daily. For hemodialysis patients, on dialysis days, KETEK 800 mg should be given after each dialysis session (see also Warnings and Precautions, Renal and Action and Clinical Pharmacology, Special Populations and Conditions).

Impaired Hepatic Function: No dosage adjustment is required in patients with mild, moderate, or severe hepatic impairment, unless renal function is severely impaired in which case the dose of KETEK should be reduced to 400 mg once daily. Experience in patients with impaired hepatic function is limited; hence, KETEK should be used with caution in these patients (see also Warnings and Precautions, Hepatic/Biliary/Pancreatic and Action and Clinical Pharmacology, Special Populations and Conditions).

Recommended Dose and Dosage Adjustment: See Table 5.

Missed Dose: If a dose is missed, it should be taken as soon as possible. However, if it is almost time for the next dose, no additional dose should be taken and the regular dosing schedule should be resumed. No more than one dose of KETEK (2 tablets) should be taken in a 24-hour period.

OVERDOSAGE:

Administration of activated charcoal may be considered.

The patient should be carefully observed (e.g. ECG, electrolytes) and given symptomatic and supportive treatment. Adequate hydration should be maintained. The effectiveness of hemodialysis in an overdose situation with KETEK is unknown.

Post-market reports indicate that an overdose with KETEK (telithromycin) may produce gastrointestinal symptoms, such as nausea, vomiting and diarrhea.

In animal studies, telithromycin had low acute toxicity with an LD_{50} value in the range of 1500-2000 mg/kg in the mouse and a minimum lethal dose of greater than 2000 mg/kg in the rat. No clinical signs were observed in rats; in mice, hypotonia was seen at 1500 mg/kg and above, with tremors prior to death.

For management of a suspected drug overdose, contact your **regional Poison Control Centre**. See the *CPS* Directory section for a list of Poison Control Centres.

ACTION AND CLINICAL PHARMACOLOGY: Mechanism of Action: KETEK (telithromycin) is a novel antimicrobial that belongs to a new chemical family, the ketolides. Ketolides are recent additions to the macrolide-lincosamide streptogramin (MLS) class. Telithromycin exerts its antimicrobial effects by inhibiting bacterial protein synthesis. This occurs not only by directly blocking translation of the bacterial 23S ribosomal RNA but also by inhibiting the assembly of new bacterial ribosomes.

Telithromycin blocks protein synthesis by binding to two sites on the 50S ribosomal subunit: domain II and V of the 23S rRNA. The affinity of telithromycin for the 23S rRNA has been measured to be 10 times greater than that of erythromycin A in erythromycin-susceptible strains and 25 times greater in macrolide-resistant strains. The difference in binding strength can be attributed to the C11-12 carbamate side chain. It allows telithromycin to maintain binding at domain II, even in the presence of resistance that alters the domain V binding site.

Table 5: KETEK

Recommended Dose and Dosage Adjustment

Infection	Daily Dose and Route of Administration	Frequency of Administration	Duration of Treatment
Community-acquired pneumonia—Adults 18 years and older	800 mg oral (2×400 mg tablets)	once daily	7 to 10 days

Pharmacokinetics: Telithromycin displays non-linear kinetics over a wide dose range.

The mean pharmacokinetic characteristics of telithromycin after administration of single and multiple (7 days) once-daily 800 mg doses to healthy adult subjects are shown in Table 6.

Table 6: KETEK

Summary of Telithromycin's Pharmacokinetic Parameters in Healthy Adult Subjects (single and multiple [7 days] once-daily 800 mg doses)

	C_{max} (µg/mL)	T_{max} (h)[a]	$t_{½}$ (h)	AUC_{0-24} (µg·h/mL)	$C_{24}h$ (µg/mL)
Single Oral Dose, mean (n=18)	1.9	1	7.16	8.25	0.03
Multiple Oral Doses, mean (n=18)	2.27	1	9.81	12.5	0.07

[a] Median values.

Legend: C_{max}=maximum plasma concentration; T_{max}=time to C_{max}; AUC=area under concentration vs. time curve; $t_{½}$=terminal plasma half-life; C_{24h}=plasma concentration at 24 hours postdose.

In a patient population, mean peak and trough plasma concentrations were 2.9 µg/mL (±1.55), (n=219) and 0.2 µg/mL (±0.22) (n=204) respectively, after 3 to 5 days of KETEK 800 mg once daily.

Absorption: Following oral administration, telithromycin reached maximal concentration at about 1 hour (0.5 to 4 hours). It has an absolute bioavailability of approximately 57% in both young and elderly subjects after a single dose of 800 mg (undergoes first-pass metabolism).

The rate and extent of absorption of the regular-size tablet‡ are unaffected by food intake. Under fasting conditions in adult healthy volunteers the "reduced-size" tablet was found to be equivalent to the "regular-sized" tablet, and thus KETEK tablets can be given without regard to food.

In fasting healthy adult subjects, peak plasma telithromycin concentrations of approximately 2 µg/mL are attained within a median of 1 hour after an 800 mg oral dose.

Steady-state plasma concentrations are reached within 2 to 3 days of once-daily dosing with telithromycin 800 mg and are approximately 1.5 times the single-dose concentration after 7 days of dosing.

Comparative Bioavailability Study: In a 2-way crossover comparative bioavailability study, the reformulated 400 mg reduced-size tablet vs the 400 mg regular size tablet of telithromycin, after a single oral dose of 2×400 mg telithromycin under fasting conditions in adult healthy volunteers, was found to be bioequivalent with the regular size telithromycin tablets.

Table 7: KETEK

Summary Table of the Comparative Bioavailability Data for Telithromycin

	Telithromycin (2×400 mg) From Measured Data Geometric Mean Arithmetic Mean (CV %)			
Parameter	Test[a]	Reference[b]	% Ratio of Geometric Means	Confidence Interval (90%)
AUC_T (ng·h/mL)	6136 6723 (48)	6807 7359 (42)	90.1	84.1; 96.6
AUC_I (ng·h/mL)	6492 7030 (46)	7023 7558 (41)	92.4	86.7; 98.6
C_{MAX} (ng/mL)	1067 1161 (43)	1188 1276 (39)	89.8	82.1; 98.3
T_{MAX}(h)	— 2.5	— 3		
$t_{½}$ (h)	7.87 8.10 (25)	7.36 7.51 (21)		

[a] Telithromycin 400 mg regular-size tablets, Quintiles, Kansas City. (Identical to the telithromycin regular-size tablets no longer available on the Canadian market.)

[b] Telithromycin 400 mg reduced size tablets, Quintiles, Kansas City. (Identical to the telithromycin regular-size tablets currently available on the Canadian market.)

Distribution: Over a clinically relevant concentration range, total in vitro protein binding is approximately 60% to 70% and is primarily due to human serum albumin. Protein binding is not modified in elderly subjects and in patients with hepatic impairment.

Telithromycin is widely distributed throughout the body and the distribution is similar between young and elderly subjects. Rapid distribution of telithromycin into tissues results in significantly higher telithromycin concentrations in most target tissues than in plasma.

Metabolism: Telithromycin is primarily metabolized by the liver.

After oral administration, two-thirds of the dose is eliminated as metabolites and one third unchanged. The main circulating compound in plasma is telithromycin. Its main circulating metabolite represented 12.6% of the AUC of telithromycin and has little antimicrobial activity compared with the parent medicinal product. Three other plasma metabolites were detected in plasma, urine and faeces, each representing 3% or less of the AUC of telithromycin. It is estimated that approximately 50% of telithromycin's metabolism is mediated by cytochrome P450 (3A4) and the remaining 50% is cytochrome P450 independent.

Excretion: Prior to entering the systemic circulation, 33% of the dose of telithromycin undergoes metabolism by a first-pass effect and 57% reaches the systemic circulation. The unchanged dose reaching the systemic circulation is eliminated by multiple pathways as follows: 7% of the dose is excreted unchanged in faeces by biliary and/or intestinal secretion; 13% is excreted unchanged in urine by renal excretion; and 37% is metabolized by the liver.

The main elimination half-life of telithromycin is 2-3 hours and the terminal elimination half-life is about 10 hours at a dose of 800 mg once daily.

Special Populations and Conditions: Pediatrics: The pharmacokinetics of telithromycin in pediatric populations, 12 years of age and under, have not been studied. In clinical trials, population pharmacokinetic analysis, including limited data (n=18) obtained in pediatric patients 13 to 17 years of age, showed that telithromycin concentrations in this age group were similar to the concentrations in patients 18 to 60 years of age (n=1329).

Geriatrics: In patients with respiratory infections, aged greater than 65 years (n=20), plasma telithromycin C_{max} and AUC were increased 30% and 40%, respectively, compared to patients less than 65 years of age (n=142). In subjects aged 65 to 92 years (n=14), plasma telithromycin C_{max} and AUC were increased 100% and 120%, respectively, compared to healthy adults aged 19 to 29 (n=12) after once daily dosing of 800 mg for 10 days. There was no statistically significant change in the elimination half-life.

No dosage adjustment is required based on age alone; however, a dosage adjustment is recommended in elderly patients with severe renal impairment (CL_{CR} <30 mL/min) (see Warnings and Precautions, Renal and Dosage and Administration, Dosing Considerations).

Gender: In 18 healthy young volunteers (20 to 34 years of age) and in 14 healthy elderly volunteers (65 to 92 years of age) given single and multiple doses of 800 mg KETEK, there was no statistical difference between males and females in mean AUC, C_{max} and elimination half-life.

Hepatic Insufficiency: In a single-dose study (800 mg) in 12 patients and a multiple-dose study (800 mg) in 13 patients with mild to severe hepatic insufficiency (Child Pugh Class A, B and C), the C_{max}, AUC and $t_{½}$ of telithromycin were similar compared to those obtained in age- and sex-matched healthy subjects. In both studies, an increase in renal elimination was observed in hepatically impaired patients indicating that this pathway may compensate for some of the decrease in metabolic clearance.

No dosage adjustment is necessary in patients with mild, moderate, or severe hepatic impairment, unless renal function is severely impaired. Experience in patients with impaired hepatic function is limited; hence, KETEK should be used with caution in these patients (see Warnings and Precautions, Hepatic/Biliary/Pancreatic and Dosage and Administration, Dosing Considerations).

Renal Insufficiency: In 20 patients with mild to severe renal impairment, increases in C_{max} and AUC values ranged from 37 to 38% and 41 to 52%, respectively, compared to normal healthy subjects.

In the presence of severe renal impairment (creatinine clearance <30 mL/min), the dose should be reduced to 400 mg once daily (see Dosage and Administration, Dosing Considerations).

In a single-dose study in patients with end-stage renal failure on hemodialysis (n=10), the mean C_{max} and AUC values were similar to normal healthy subjects when telithromycin was administered 2 hours post-dialysis (see Warnings and Precautions, Renal and Dosage and Administration, Dosing Considerations).

Multiple Insufficiency: The effects of impairment of multiple elimination pathways were studied in 12 subjects ≥60 years of age, with diminished renal function (CL_{CR}=24 to 80 mL/min) and given ketoconazole to block the CYP3A4 pathway. In this study, when severe renal insufficiency (CL_{CR} <30 mL/min) and concomitant impairment of hepatic metabolism were present, telithromycin exposure was at the highest end of values observed in Phase III clinical studies. In the presence of severe renal impairment (CL_{CR} <30 mL/min), with or without coexisting hepatic impairment, a reduced dosage of KETEK is recommended (see Warnings and Precautions, Renal, Hepatic/Biliary/Pancreatic and Dosage and Administration, Dosing Considerations).

STORAGE AND STABILITY: Store at room temperature between 15-30°C. Protect from exposure to heat and light and keep in a safe place out of the reach of children.

INFORMATION FOR THE PATIENT: Published in e-CPS, available by subscription at www.e-cps.ca.

DOSAGE FORMS, COMPOSITION AND PACKAGING: Reduced size tablets (new formulation without lactose and corn starch): Each light-orange, oval, film-coated tablet (approx. 8.7×13.9 mm), imprinted "H3647" on one side and "400" on the other side, contains: telithromycinin 400 mg. Nonmedicinal ingredients: croscarmellose sodium, magnesium stearate, microcrystalline cellulose and povidone; coating: hydroxypropyl methylcellulose, polyethylene glycol, red ferric oxide, talc, titanium dioxide and yellow ferric oxide. Bottles of 60.

(Shown in Product Identification Section)

Ketoconazole, Oral ℞
Antifungal

CPhA Monograph

Date of Preparation: November 2003
Date of Revision: October 2006

This monograph has been compiled by CPhA and reviewed by experts. It may contain information different from that found in Health Canada-approved Product Monographs. The reader is referred to the *CPS* Editorial Policy for more information.

SUMMARY PRODUCT INFORMATION:

Route of Administration	Dosage Form	Product Strength
Oral	Tablet	200 mg

INDICATIONS AND CLINICAL USE: Health Canada-approved indications include:

- treatment of serious or life-threatening systemic fungal infections in normal, predisposed or immunocompromised patients where alternate therapy is considered inappropriate or has been unsuccessful: systemic candidiasis, chronic mucocutaneous candidiasis, coccidioidomycosis and paracoccidioidomycosis, histoplasmosis and chromomycosis
- treatment of severe recalcitrant dermatophytoses unresponsive to other forms of therapy

Due to poor penetration into the CNS, ketoconazole is not recommended for the treatment of fungal infections of the CNS.

Uses Not Approved in Canada: Ketoconazole has been used in the treatment of prostatic carcinoma, Cushing's syndrome, hirsutism, hypercalcemia in patients with sarcoidosis and tuberculosis-associated hypercalcemia.

CONTRAINDICATIONS: Contraindicated in patients with known hypersensitivity to ketoconazole. Cross-sensitivity with other azole antifungals is possible. Also contraindicated in patients with hepatic dysfunction and women of childbearing potential, unless effective forms of contraception are employed.

WARNINGS AND PRECAUTIONS: Endocrine and Metabolism: Ketoconazole may inhibit the synthesis of cortisol and testosterone, especially in patients on high doses of the drug. It is recommended that the daily dose of ketoconazole not exceed 400 mg.

Hepatic/Biliary/Pancreatic: Hepatotoxicity has occurred rarely during ketoconazole therapy. The risk is higher for women over 50, patients with a history of hepatic disease or alcohol abuse and patients on prolonged ketoconazole therapy (>2 weeks) or concurrently taking other hepatotoxic drugs. It is recommended to perform liver function tests prior to treatment, after 2 weeks and periodically during treatment (monthly or more frequently). Patients should report any signs and symptoms of liver dysfunction (i.e., unusual fatigue, fever, anorexia, nasuea, vomiting, jaundice, dark urine, pale stool). Mild transient increases in transaminases or alkaline phosphatase may occur; however, ketoconazole should be discontinued if liver function tests increase substantially or are persistently elevated.

Special Populations: Pregnant Women: There are no adequate studies using ketoconazole in pregnant women; however there have been reports of limb defects in newborns exposed to ketoconazole in the first trimester. Ketoconazole is teratogenic in rats at a dose of 80 mg/kg (10 times the recommended human dose). Oral ketoconazole should only be used in pregnant women when the benefits outweigh the risks.

Nursing Women: Ketoconazole is excreted in breast milk. Ketoconazole is generally considered compatible with breast-feeding.

Pediatrics: Ketoconazole should only be used in children when the benefits outweigh the risks. Careful hepatic and hematologic monitoring is indicated. Ketoconazole is not recommended in children less than 2 years of age.

Geriatrics: No information is available on the relationship of age to the effects of ketoconazole in geriatric patients.

Monitoring and Laboratory Tests: Monitor liver function tests (GGT, alkaline phosphatase, AST, ALT and bilirubin) prior to treatment, after 2 weeks and periodically during treatment (monthly or more frequently), particularly in patients at high risk of liver dysfunction (see Warnings and Precautions, Hepatic/Biliary/Pancreatic).

DRUG INTERACTIONS: See Table 1 and Table 2.

Table 1: Ketoconazole, Oral

Drug-Drug Interactions

Interacting Drug	Source of Data	Effect	Clinical Comment
Alfentanil	T	↓ hepatic metabolism of alfentanil	Monitor for increased opioid side effects, including increased or prolonged respiratory depression
Aminoglycosides	T	May ↓aminoglycoside peak serum concentration	Monitor aminoglycoside levels. Consider an alternative antifungal to ketoconazole
Antacids	CT	↓absorption of ketoconazole due to ↑ gastric pH	Avoid antacids for 2 hours before or after taking ketoconazole
Benzodiazepines	CT	May inhibit hepatic metabolism of benzodiazepine via CYP3A4	Monitor for increased sedation and other adverse effects - Use alternative benzodiazepine (not metabolized by 3A4) such as lorazepam and temazepam
Buspirone	T	↓ metabolism of buspirone	Monitor patient for increased sedation. Alternative to buspirone: lorazepam, temazepam
Busulfan	T	Unknown mechanism of action leads to small ↑ in busulfan plasma concentration	Low to no clinical significance; monitor patient for busulfan toxicity (e.g. hepatic veno-occlusive disease, hepatotoxicity, bone marrow hypoplasia)
Calcium Channel Blockers	CT	↑ plasma concentration of the calcium channel blocker metabolized by CYP3A4 (e.g. dihydropyridines, verapamil)	Monitor for orthostatic hypotension, increased heart rate (with dihydropyridines)
Carbamazepine	CT	↓ metabolism of carbamazepine and possibility of ↑ metabolism of ketoconazole	Monitor for increased carbamazepine levels and possible toxicity if both drugs administered
Cyclosporine	C, CT	↓ metabolism of cyclosporine	Monitor cyclosporine levels
Didanosine	CT	↑ gastric pH caused by didanosine buffers (magnesium hydroxide) ↓ absorption of ketoconazole	Administer ketoconazole at least 2 hours before didanosine. Use an enteric coated didanosine tablet
Domperidone	C, CT	Approximate three-fold increase in domperidone plasma levels resulting in possible QT prolongation	Avoid use of this combination
Donepezil	CT	↓ metabolism of donepezil	Monitor for increased donezepril adverse effects including nausea, vomiting and abdominal pain
H_2-receptor antagonists	CT	↓ GI absorption of ketoconazole due to↑ gastric pH	Administer ketoconazole at least 2 hours before H_2-receptor antagonists and monitor for ↓ antifungal efficacy
Loratidine	CT	↓ metabolism of loratadine and its active metabolite	Monitor for increased effects of loratadine
Methadone	T	↑ plasma concentration of methadone	Use an alternative opioid; codeine and morphine are not metabolized by CYP 3A4; monitor for ↑ narcotic effects
Methylprednisolone	CT	May ↓ metabolism of methylprednisolone, leading to enhanced suppression of cortisol secretion	Methylprednisolone may need to be adjusted
Protease Inhibitors	C, CT	May ↑ plasma levels of protease inhibitors	Dose of protease inhibitors may need to be adjusted; consider an alternate antifungal
Proton Pump Inhibitors	C	↓ GI absorption of ketoconazole due to↑ gastric pH	Monitor for ↓ antifungal activity; avoid combination if possible
Rifampin	C	↑ metabolism of ketoconazole and ↓ levels of rifampin	Separate doses by 12 h. Monitor for therapeutic failure of both drugs
Sirolimus	CT	↓ metabolism of sirolimus	Avoid concurrent administration; monitor for symptoms of sirolimus toxicity, e.g. hyperlipidemia, bone marrow depression

(cont'd)

Table 1: Ketoconazole, Oral *(cont'd)*

Drug-Drug Interactions

Interacting Drug	Source of Data	Effect	Clinical Comment
Sucralfate	CT	↓ levels of ketoconazole	Administer ketoconazole at least 2 hours before sucralfate and monitor for ↓ antifungal efficacy
Tacrolimus	CT	Inhibition of CYP 3A4 and p-glycoprotein may lead to↑ levels of tacrolimus	Monitor tacrolimus levels
Tolbutamide	T	↓ metabolism of tolbutamide	Monitor blood glucose concentrations
Trazodone	T	↓ metabolism of trazodone	A lower dose of trazodone may be considered. Monitor patient for adverse effects such as nausea, hypotension and syncope.
Vincristine	T	↑ levels of vincristine and risk of neurotoxicity	Monitor patient for neurotoxicity
Warfarin	C	Probably decreased warfarin metabolism	Monitor PT and INR if ketoconazole initiated, discontinued, or with dosage change

Legend:
C=case study; CT=clinical trial; T=theoretical

Table 2: Ketoconazole, Oral

Drug-Food Interactions

Interacting Food	Reference	Effect	Clinical Comment
Alcohol	C	Disulfiram-like reaction seen rarely	Counsel patient to decrease alcohol intake; advise patient to monitor for flushing, nausea, headache
Grapefruit Juice	T	Possible ↓ absorption or ↑ metabolism of ketoconazole.	Counsel patient to avoid grapefruit and grapefruit juice during period of ketoconazole therapy

Legend:
C=case study; CT=clinical trial; T=theoretical

ACTION AND CLINICAL PHARMACOLOGY: The exact mechanism of action of ketoconazole is unknown. It is believed that ketoconazole exerts its antifungal effects by inhibiting the synthesis of ergosterol in fungal and yeast cells, resulting in increased permeability of the cell walls and cell membranes.
Pharmacokinetics: See Table 3.

Table 3: Ketoconazole, Oral

Summary of Pharmacokinetic Parameters

	C_{max}	$t_{1/2}$ (h)	Clearance	Volume of Distribution
Single dose mean	3.4 ± 0.3 mg/L	8.7 ± 0.2		0.36 ± 0.1 L/kg
Long-term therapy (steady state)		3.3 ± 1.0	0.5 ± 0.25 L/h/kg	2.4 ± 1.6 L/kg

Absorption: 75% of an oral dose is absorbed. Absorption is dependent on gastric acidity.
Distribution: Distributed into bile, saliva, cerumen, synovial fluid, and sebum. CSF penetration is erratic and considered minimal. Ketoconazole is 84% to 99% bound to plasma proteins.
Metabolism: Ketoconazole is partially metabolized in the liver via liver enzymes CYP3A4 to several inactive metabolites. Ketoconazole inhibits CYP1A2, CYP2C9 and is a potent inhibitor of CYP3A4.
Excretion: Ketoconazole and its metabolites are primarily eliminated by excretion into the feces (57%) and urine (13%).

ADVERSE REACTIONS: More Common Adverse Reactions: Dermatologic: Pruritus (1.5%).
Gastrointestinal: Dyspepsia (3%), nausea and vomiting (3%), abdominal pain (3%).
Less Common Adverse Drug Reactions: CNS: Headache, dizziness, somnolence, tremors, nervousness, paresthesias.
Dermatologic: Alopecia, purpura, rash, dermatitis.
Endocrine and Metabolism: Gynecomastia, dose-dependent increase in testosterone serum levels, decrease in basal and ACTH-induced cortisol levels, increased serum levels of 17-OH progesterone and decreased urinary levels of 17-ketosteroids, hypoparathyroidism, oligospermia and azoospermia, impotence, loss of libido, menstrual irregularities.
Gastrointestinal: Diarrhea, GI hemorrhage.
Hematologic: Thrombocytopenia, eosinophilia, decreased hematocrit, anemia, leukopenia, neutropenia.
Hepatic/Biliary/Pancreatic: Idiosyncratic hepatocellular dysfunction, transient increases in liver enzymes (ALT, alkaline phosphatase, AST and serum bilirubin).
Immune: Anaphylaxis after first dose (rare), hypersensitivity reactions including urticaria.
Ophthalmologic: Corneal deposits, cataract enlargement.
Psychiatric: Suicidal tendencies and severe depression (rare).
Respiratory: Dypsnea.
Miscellaneous: Fever and chills, photophobia, arthralgia, sensation of detachment (at 800 mg/day).

DOSAGE AND ADMINISTRATION: **Adults:** See Table 4.
Pediatrics: Infants and Children (other than neonates): 3.3 to 6.6 mg/kg/day orally once daily.
Doses of 5 to 10 mg/kg/day given as a single daily dose or divided every 12 hours have also been used.
Renal Impairment: Dose reduction is not required in patients with renal failure.
Hepatic Impairment: It is recommended to adjust the dose of ketoconazole in patients with severe hepatic impairment.
Missed Dose: A missed dose should be taken as soon as the patient remembers. If it is almost time for the next dose, the missed dose should not be taken and the patient should return to the regular dosage schedule.
Administration: Oral: This drug should be taken daily with meals.

Table 4: Ketoconazole, Oral

Dose in Adult Patients

Indication	Route	Usual Dose	Maximum Dose	Duration of Treatment	Response Time[a]
Dermatomycoses				4–8 weeks	4 weeks
Hair or Scalp Mycoses				4–8 weeks	4 weeks
Pityriasis Versicolor				3–6 weeks[b]	3 weeks
Oral Thrush				1–2 weeks	1 week
Chronic Mucocutaneous Candidiasis	Oral	200 mg daily	400 mg daily	6–12 months	4 months
Systemic Candidiasis				2–4 weeks	4 weeks
Paracoccidioidomycosis				2–4 months	2 months
Coccidioidomycosis				>6 months	6 months
Histoplasmosis				2–4 months	2 months
Chromomycosis				>6 months	6 months

[a] If there is no response during this period, increasing the dosage may improve response depending on sensitivity of the organism.
[b] 5 days is usually effective for most cases. A longer duration of treatment is reserved for resistant cases.

OVERDOSAGE:

For management of a suspected drug overdose, CPhA recommends that you contact your **regional Poison Control Centre**. See the *CPS* Directory section for a list of Poison Control Centres.

Ketoderm® Ⓟ
ketoconazole
Topical Antifungal

TaroPharma

SUPPLIED: Each g of white, odorless cream contains: ketoconazole 20 mg (2%). Nonmedicinal ingredients: butylated hydroxyanisole (BHA), isopropyl myristate, polysorbate 60, polysorbate 80, propylene glycol, sorbitan monostearate, stearyl and cetyl alcohols and water. Tubes of 30 g. Store at room temperature, between 15 and 25°C. Keep from freezing.

Ketorolac Ⓟ
NSAID Analgesic

CPhA Monograph

Date of Preparation: August 2006
Date of Revision: October 2009

This monograph has been compiled by CPhA and reviewed by experts. It may contain information different from that found in Health Canada-approved Product Monographs. The reader is referred to the *CPS* Editorial Policy for more information.

SUMMARY PRODUCT INFORMATION:

Route of Administration	Dosage Form	Strength
Oral	Tablet	10 mg
Parenteral (im)	Ampoule	10 mg/mL, 30 mg/mL

INDICATIONS AND CLINICAL USE: Ketorolac is indicated for the short-term management of moderate to acute pain, as follows:
Oral: For the short-term management (no greater than 5 days for post-surgical patients or 7 days for patients with musculoskeletal pain) of moderate to moderately severe acute pain, including post-surgical pain (such as general orthopedic and dental surgery), acute musculoskeletal trauma pain and postpartum uterine cramping pain.
IM: For the short-term management (no greater than 2 days) of moderate to severe acute pain, including pain following major abdominal, orthopedic and gynecologic procedures. Combined use of im and oral therapy should not exceed 5 days.
IV: The iv route is not approved by Health Canada; however its use is supported in the medical literature and in clinical practice. See Dosage and Administration.
The drug is not indicated for use in minor or chronic painful conditions.

CONTRAINDICATIONS:
- Hypersensitivity to ketorolac tromethamine or to any ingredient in the formulation.
- Hypersensitivity to other NSAIDs or ASA.
- Complete or partial nasal polyps, those with asthma, anaphylaxis, urticaria, rhinitis or other allergic symptoms.
- Active peptic ulcer, a history of recurrent ulceration or active gastrointestinal inflammatory disease.
- History of or active gastrointestinal bleeding or perforation.
- Significant hepatic impairment or active liver disease.
- Renal impairment (serum creatinine >442 µmol/L) or those at risk for renal failure. Those with lesser degrees of renal impairment (serum creatinine 170 to 442 µmol/L) are at risk of deteriorating renal function when taking an NSAID.
- Concurrent use with other NSAIDs.
- Immediately before any major surgery or intraoperatively.
- Perioperatively in coronary artery bypass graft (CABG) surgery; other nonsteroidal anti-inflammatory drugs (NSAIDs) studied in this setting showed an increased incidence of cardiovascular thromboembolic events, deep surgical infections and sternal wound complications.
- Coagulation disorders, cerebrovascular bleeding or postoperative patients with high risk of bleeding.
- Epidural or intrathecal administration.
- Concomitant use of ketorolac and probenecid or pentoxifylline.
- During labour and delivery. Ketorolac may have adverse effects on fetal circulation and may increase the risk of uterine hemorrhage due to inhibition of uterine contractions.

WARNINGS AND PRECAUTIONS:

> **Serious Warnings and Precautions**
> - Long-term use of ketorolac is not recommended (see Dosage and Administration).
> - The most serious risks associated with ketorolac use are gastrointestinal, including: bleeding, peptic ulceration, perforation and gastrointestinal bleeding, which can occur at any time, with or without warning symptoms. Elderly patients are more susceptible to serious adverse effects.

General: Long-term use of ketorolac is not recommended as the incidence of side effects increases with duration of treatment.

Hypovolemia should be corrected before starting therapy with ketorolac.

Cardiovascular: Data have shown an increased risk of cardiovascular adverse events (myocardial infarction, stroke, thrombotic events) associated with some NSAIDs (both selective and nonselective inhibitors of cyclooxygenase-2). Short-term use, especially at low dosages, does not appear to be associated with an increased risk of serious cardiovascular events except immediately following coronary artery bypass graft [CABG] surgery.

NSAID use may lead to new hypertension or may worsen pre-existing hypertension. Use with caution in patients with heart failure or hypertension since fluid retention may occur.

Endocrine and Metabolism: With NSAID treatment there is a potential risk of hyperkalemia, particularly in patients with conditions such as diabetes mellitus or renal failure, elderly patients or in patients receiving concomitant therapy with β-adrenergic blockers, angiotensin converting enzyme inhibitors, angiotensin receptor blockers, potassium supplements or potassium-sparing diuretics.

Gastrointestinal: Ketorolac should be given under close medical supervision to those susceptible to gastrointestinal tract irritation, particularly those with a history of peptic ulcer, diverticulosis, ulcerative colitis and Crohn's disease. Discontinue ketorolac if ulceration is suspected or confirmed.

Genitourinary: Some NSAIDs can cause persistent urinary symptoms (dysuria, urinary frequency) or hematuria. Should these symptoms occur, treatment with ketorolac must be stopped immediately.

Hematologic: Ketorolac may inhibit platelet adhesion and aggregation and prolong bleeding time (generally by approximately three minutes from baseline values). Ketorolac has a transient effect on platelet function, and aggregation usually returns to normal within 24 to 48 hours after discontinuation. Ketorolac does not affect prothrombin time or partial thromboplastin time. Platelet count may be affected by ketorolac.

Hepatic/Biliary/Pancreatic: Use caution in patients with impaired hepatic function or a history of liver disease. Patients with abnormal liver function tests or signs and symptoms suggesting hepatic dysfunction should be monitored carefully while on ketorolac. Discontinue the drug if liver dysfunction progresses. Increases in serum transaminases (ALT, AST) may occur in patients taking ketorolac.

Immune: Severe anaphylactic reactions have been reported in patients receiving ketorolac. Such reactions may occur in patients with known hypersensitivity to ASA or other NSAIDs including ketorolac; however these reactions also have been reported in patients without a history of hypersensitivity. Asthmatic patients may be at particular risk for severe hypersensitivity reactions.

Neurologic: Drowsiness, dizziness, vertigo, insomnia or depression have been reported. Patients should use caution engaging in activities that require alertness.

Ophthalmologic: Blurred and/or diminished vision have been reported. If these symptoms develop, therapy should be discontinued and an ophthalmologic examination performed.

Perioperative Considerations: Postoperative hematomas and other symptoms of wound bleeding have been reported with perioperative use of im ketorolac. Physicians should be aware of the potential risk of bleeding in cases where hemostasis is critical such as resection of the prostate, tonsillectomy or cosmetic surgery.

Renal: The following renal abnormalities have been associated with ketorolac: acute renal failure, nephrotic syndrome, interstitial nephritis, and renal papillary necrosis. See Table 6 (Dose in Adult Patients with Renal Impairment). Elevations of creatinine and blood urea nitrogen have occurred.

Special Populations: Pregnant Women: Although it is unknown whether ketorolac crosses the human placenta, the molecular weight is small enough that passage should be expected. A positive association has been reported between NSAIDs and spontaneous abortions. Because human data are not available, ketorolac should only be used in the first and second trimesters of pregnancy if necessary. The administration of ketorolac is not recommended during the third trimester of pregnancy.

Ketorolac is contraindicated in labor and delivery because it may inhibit prostaglandin synthesis which may affect the fetal circulation and inhibit uterine contractions, increasing the risk of uterine hemorrhage. Also, ketorolac should not be used during the third trimester, labor or delivery because of the possibility of premature closure of the ductus arteriosus.

Nursing Women: Ketorolac is excreted into breast milk in small quantities. Although the manufacturer does not recommend the administration of ketorolac during lactation, the American Academy of Pediatrics considers ketorolac compatible with breast-feeding.

Pediatrics: The manufacturer does not recommend the use of ketorolac in children under the age of 16 years in Canada. However, there is evidence for the use of single doses of ketorolac injection (iv or im) for children over 2 years of age (see Dosage and Administration); there is limited data to support administration of more than one parenteral dose in pediatric patients. The drug should not be used in children <2 years of age. Use of the oral formulation is not recommended in children as it has no advantages over other available oral NSAIDs.

Geriatrics: Patients older than 65 years, frail or debilitated patients are more susceptible to adverse reactions from NSAIDs. The incidence may increase with dose and duration of treatment. Older patients are also at risk of lower esophageal ulceration and gastrointestinal bleeding. CNS effects may include confusion. Elderly patients are at increased risk of reduced renal function so caution is required. The lower end of the dosing range should be used in geriatric patients and the total daily dose should not exceed 60 mg.

ADVERSE REACTIONS: More Common Adverse Drug Reactions: See Table 1.

Table 1: Ketorolac

More Common Adverse Drug Reactions (≥1%)

Body System	Effect
Cardiovascular	Edema, hypertension
CNS	Oral: somnolence, insomnia, nervousness, headache, dizziness IM: somnolence, headache, sweating, dizziness
Dermatologic	Urticaria Sweating (usually with im only)
Gastrointestinal	Oral: nausea, vomiting, feeling of fullness, diarrhea, dyspepsia, gastrointestinal pain, constipation, peptic ulcers, flatulence IM: nausea, vomiting
Body as a Whole	Oral: fever, edema IM: injection site pain, vasodilatation

Less Common Adverse Drug Reactions (<1%): Cardiovascular: Oral: vasodilatation, palpitation, hypertension, substernal chest pain.

IM: hypertension, chest pain, tachycardia, hemorrhage, palpitation, pulmonary embolus, syncope, ventricular tachycardia, pallor, flushing.

Central Nervous System: Oral: abnormal dreams, anxiety, dry mouth, hyperkinesias, paresthesia, increased sweating, euphoria, hallucinations, migraine.

IM: insomnia, increased dry mouth, abnormal dreams, anxiety, depression, paresthesia, nervousness, paranoid reaction, speech disorder, euphoria, increased libido, excessive thirst, inability to concentrate, stimulation.

Dermatologic: Oral: rash, urticaria, pruritus, burning sensation.

IM: injection site reactions, pruritus, rash, subcutaneous hematoma.

Ear/Nose/Throat: Oral: ear pain.

IM: tinnitus, taste perversion, deafness.

Endocrine and Metabolism: Oral: edema, weight gain, elevated alkaline phosphatase, elevated BUN, excessive thirst, generalized edema, hyperuricemia.

IM: edema, hypokalemia, hypovolemia.

Gastrointestinal: Oral: anorexia, flatulence, vomiting, stomatitis, gastritis, gastrointestinal disorder, sore throat, duodenal ulcer, gastrointestinal hemorrhage, increased appetite, melena, rectal bleeding.

IM: flatulence, anorexia, constipation, diarrhea, dyspepsia, gastrointestinal fullness, gastrointestinal hemorrhage, gastrointestinal pain, melena, sore throat, rectal bleeding, stomatitis.

Genitourinary: Oral: dysuria, hematuria, increased urinary frequency, oliguria, polyuria.

IM: dysuria, urinary retention, oliguria, increased urinary frequency, vaginitis.

Hematologic: Oral: anemia, purpura.

IM: anemia, coagulation disorder, purpura.

Hepatic/Biliary/Pancreatic: increase in liver enzymes.

Ophthalmologic: Oral: blurred vision, lacrimation disorder, abnormal vision.

IM: blurred vision, diplopia, retinal hemorrhage.

Respiratory: Oral: increased cough, rhinitis, dry nose, dyspnea, asthma, epistaxis.

IM: asthma, increased cough, dyspnea, epistaxis, hiccup, rhinitis.

DRUG INTERACTIONS:

> **Serious Drug Interactions**
> - Pentoxifylline: concurrent administration is contraindicated due to increased tendency to bleeding.
> - Probenecid: probenecid decreases clearance and increases half-life of ketorolac by two-fold; concurrent administration is contraindicated.

Drug-Drug Interactions: See Table 2.

Table 2: Ketorolac

Drug-Drug Interactions

Interacting Drug	Effect	Clinical Comment
ACE inhibitors	May increase risk of renal impairment especially in volume-depleted patients. NSAIDs may diminish the antihypertensive effects of ACE inhibitors.	Avoid concurrent use.
Alcohol	There may be increased risk of GI side effects (bleeding) when alcohol is ingested with NSAIDs.	Avoid concurrent use.
Anticoagulants and thrombolytic agents	Concomitant use of NSAIDs and warfarin/heparin is associated with a higher risk of GI bleeding compared with use of either agent alone (synergistic effect). Prostaglandins play an important role in hemostasis, and NSAIDs affect platelet function.	Avoid concurrent use. However, if concurrent therapy is required, close monitoring to be certain that no change in anticoagulant dosage is necessary.
Anticonvulsants (e.g., phenytoin, carbamazepine)	Seizures have been reported rarely in patients receiving concomitant therapy. There may be a reduced therapeutic effect of the anticonvulsant.	Monitor appropriately.
Corticosteroids	Increased risk of GI side effects such as ulceration and bleeding	Avoid concurrent use.
Furosemide and diuretics	Ketorolac reduces the diuretic response to furosemide by about 20% in normovolemic individuals. This effect may be related to inhibition of renal prostaglandin synthesis.	Avoid concurrent use.
Lithium	Some NSAIDs have been reported to inhibit renal lithium clearance leading to potential lithium toxicity.	This potential reaction has not been studied with ketorolac. Avoid concurrent use.
Methotrexate	Concomitant administration has been reported to reduce the renal clearance of methotrexate with some NSAIDs; severe, sometimes fatal toxicity has occurred.	Avoid high-dose methotrexate. For low-dose methotrexate monitor renal function and for signs of methotrexate toxicity; reduced dose may be necessary.
NSAIDs including ASA	See Contraindications.	Contraindicated due to risk of additive adverse effects.
Pentoxifylline	Increased tendency to bleeding with concomitant use. See Serious Drug Interactions.	Concurrent administration is contraindicated.
Potassium supplements/ potassium-sparing diuretics	Potential for hyperkalemia, especially in patients with renal dysfunction.	Monitor serum potassium especially in susceptible individuals.
Probenecid	Probenecid decreases clearance and increases half-life of ketorolac by two-fold. See Serious Drug Interactions.	Concurrent administration is contraindicated.
Protein-bound drugs	Ketorolac is highly protein bound to human plasma protein (mean 99.2%). It could theoretically displace other protein-bound drugs significantly.	Therapeutic concentrations of digoxin, warfarin, acetaminophen, phenytoin, tolbutamide, ibuprofen, naproxen and piroxicam did not alter ketorolac protein binding.
Psychoactive drugs (e.g., fluoxetine, thiothixene, alprazolam)	Hallucinations have been reported in patients receiving concomitant therapy.	Monitor appropriately.
Selective serotonin reuptake inhibitors	SSRIs increase the risk of gastrointestinal bleeding and this effect can be potentiated by concomitant use of NSAIDs.	Monitor patients for increased signs of bleeding.

Table 3: Ketorolac
Dose in Adult Patients

Indication	Route	Initial Dose	Dose Titration	Usual Dose	Maximum Dose	Duration of Therapy	Clinical Comment
Acute post-surgical pain	Oral	10 mg	Q4–6H PRN	10 mg	40 mg/24 hours	Max. 5 days	Use lowest possible dose for shortest duration of therapy. For adults weighing less than 50 kg, use geriatric dosing (Table 4).
Acute musculoskeletal pain	Oral	10 mg	Q4–6H PRN	10 mg	40 mg/24 hours	Max. 7 days	Use lowest possible dose for shortest duration of therapy.
Moderate to severe acute pain	IM	10–30 mg	Q4–6H PRN	10–30 mg	120 mg/24 hours	Max. 2 days	Administration of continuous multiple im doses not extensively studied. Risk of toxicity appears to increase with longer use at recommended doses. In adults weighing <50 kg, use geriatric dosing (Table 4).
Moderate to severe acute pain	IV	30 mg	Q6H PRN	30 mg	120 mg/24 hours	Max. 2 days	The iv route is not approved by Health Canada; however its use is supported in the medical literature and in clinical practice. In adults weighing <50 kg, use geriatric dosing (Table 4).

Table 4: Ketorolac
Dose in Geriatric Patients and Adults Weighing Less Than 50 kg

Indication	Route	Initial Dose	Dose Titration	Usual Dose	Maximum Dose	Duration of Therapy	Clinical Comment
Acute post-surgical pain	IM	10 mg	Q4–6H PRN	10–15 mg	60 mg/24 hours	Not to exceed 2 days.	The lower end of the dosage range is recommended.
Moderate to severe acute pain	IV	10 mg	Q6H PRN	10–15 mg	60 mg/24 hours	Not to exceed 2 days.	The lower end of the dosage range is recommended. The iv route is not approved by Health Canada; however its use is supported in the medical literature and in clinical practice.

Table 5: Ketorolac
Dose in Pediatric Patients

Indication	Route	Age/Weight	Initial Dose	Dose Titration	Maximum Dose	Duration of Therapy	Clinical Comment
Acute post-surgical pain	IM/IV	2 to 16 years	IM: 1 mg/kg/dose IV: 0.5 mg/kg/dose	IM: Single dose only IV: IV doses have been given Q6H PRN (maximum duration of 2 days)	IM: 30 mg dose IV: Patients <16 years: 15 mg dose Patients ≥16 years: 30 mg dose	Data available for single doses. If multiple doses are used maximum duration of iv ketorolac is 2 days.	IV administration is not approved by Health Canada although it is supported in the literature and is used in practice. Not for use in tonsillectomy patients due to increased risk of bleeding.

Drug-Herb Interactions: Feverfew: In theory, concomitant use of feverfew and ketorolac may predispose patients to more adverse effects of NSAIDs (e.g., gastropathy, renal dysfunction, increased risk of bleeding). Concurrent use should be avoided. Probable mechanism is additive prostaglandin and thromboxane inhibition.
Garlic: Caution is advised with the concomitant use of garlic and ketorolac because of the increased risk of bleeding. The probable mechanism involves potentiation of platelet aggregation.
Ginkgo: Avoid concomitant use of ginkgo and ketorolac because of the increased risk of bleeding. The probable mechanism is potentiation of platelet aggregation. If both agents must be used together monitor bleeding time and signs and symptoms of bleeding.
Caution is advised with concomitant use of ketorolac and any herb that exhibits anticoagulant or antiplatelet properties.

DOSAGE AND ADMINISTRATION: Dosing Considerations:
- Adjust dosage depending on patient response. Supplement with low-dose opioids if required for pain control.
- In pediatrics, the oral formulation of ketorolac is not considered to have advantages over other available oral NSAIDs.

Recommended Dose and Dosage Adjustment: Adults: See Table 3.
For adults weighing less than 50 kg, use geriatric dosing (see Table 4).
Geriatrics: See Table 4.
Pediatrics: See Table 5.
Renal Impairment: See Table 6.

Table 6: Ketorolac
Dose in Adult Patients with Renal Impairment

Route	Creatinine Clearance (mL/min)	Dosage Adjustment
Oral/IM	>50	None
Oral/IM	10–50	Total daily dose should be reduced by 50%. Do not exceed a total daily dose of 60 mg.
Oral/IM	<10	Do not use in patients with advanced renal impairment.

Dialysis: Dosage in dialysis has not been determined. Dialysis does not significantly clear ketorolac from blood.
Hepatic Impairment: Dosage in hepatic impairment has not been determined.
Conversion from Parenteral to Oral therapy: Replace ketorolac im by an oral analgesic as soon as possible. When ketorolac tablets are used as a follow-on therapy to parenteral ketorolac, the total combined daily dose of ketorolac (oral + parenteral) should not exceed 120 mg in younger adult patients or 60 mg in elderly patients on the day the change of formulation is made. Subsequently, oral dosing should not exceed the recommended daily maximum of 40 mg. The total daily duration of combined oral and im treatment should not exceed 5 days.
Administration: Oral: Administration with food or milk may decrease GI upset.
IM: Administer slowly via deep im injection.
IV: IV doses must be given over no less than 15 seconds.

OVERDOSAGE:

> For management of a suspected drug overdose, CPhA recommends that you contact your **regional Poison Control Centre**. See the *CPS* Directory section for a list of Poison Control Centres.

ACTION AND CLINICAL PHARMACOLOGY: Mechanism of Action: Ketorolac tromethamine is a nonsteroidal anti-inflammatory drug (NSAID) exhibiting anti-inflammatory, analgesic and antipyretic effects. Ketorolac inhibits the synthesis of prostaglandins through inhibition of cyclo-oxygenase (COX-1 and COX-2) isoenzymes.
Pharmacokinetics: Adults: Absorption: Ketorolac is rapidly and completely absorbed following both oral and im administration.
Oral: Peak plasma concentrations occur at an average of 44 minutes after a single 10 mg dose. The rate of absorption, but not the extent, is decreased by food. Onset of analgesia occurs 30 to 60 minutes after oral dosing.
IM: Peak plasma concentrations of ketorolac occur an average of 50 minutes after a single 30 mg dose. Analgesic onset occurs within 10 minutes of im dosing.

Distribution: Ketorolac is more than 99% bound to plasma proteins.
Metabolism: Ketorolac is metabolized mainly by glucuronidation. It is mostly metabolized to inactive compounds.
Excretion: In adults the terminal elimination half-life is 4 to 6 hours. In elderly individuals, it is 5 to 8 hours. The elimination half-life is prolonged in renal impairment.
Oral and IM: Ketorolac and its metabolites are mainly excreted in the urine (91.4%) while the remainder is excreted in the feces (6.1%).
STORAGE AND STABILITY: Ketorolac Tablets: Store at room temperature with protection from light.
Ketorolac IM: Store at room temperature with protection from light.

Ketorolac Tromethamine Injection USP Ⓟ
ketorolac tromethamine
NSAID—Analgesic

Sandoz

SUPPLIED: Each mL of clear, slightly yellow, sterile solution contains: ketorolac tromethamine 30 mg. Nonmedicinal ingredients: ethyl alcohol 10% (w/v), sodium chloride for tonicity, sodium hydroxide and/or hydrochloric acid to adjust pH and water for injection. Multidose vials of 1 and 10 mL, boxes of 10. Store between 15 and 30°C. Protect from light. Discard 28 days after initial use.

Kivexa® Ⓟ
abacavir sulfate—lamivudine
Antiretroviral Agent

ViiV Healthcare ULC

Date of Revision: April 23, 2010

SUMMARY PRODUCT INFORMATION:

Route of Administration	Dosage Form/ Strength	Clinically Relevant Nonmedicinal Ingredients
Oral	Tablet/600 mg abacavir (as abacavir sulfate) and 300 mg lamivudine	None For a complete listing see Dosage Forms, Composition and Packaging.

INDICATIONS AND CLINICAL USE: KIVEXA (abacavir sulfate/lamivudine) is indicated in antiretroviral combination therapy for the treatment of Human Immunodeficiency Virus (HIV) infection in adults.
In one controlled study (CNA30021), more patients taking abacavir 600 mg once daily had severe hypersensitivity reactions than patients taking abacavir 300 mg twice daily. (See Warnings and Precautions, Adverse Reactions and Dosage and Administration.)
KIVEXA is one of multiple products containing abacavir. Before starting KIVEXA, review medical history for prior exposure to any abacavir containing product, in order to avoid reintroduction in a patient with a history of hypersensitivity to abacavir.
CONTRAINDICATIONS: KIVEXA (abacavir sulfate/lamivudine) is contraindicated in:
- patients who are hypersensitive to this drug or to any ingredient in the formulation or component of the container. For a complete listing, see Dosage Forms, Composition and Packaging.
- patients with known hypersensitivity to abacavir or lamivudine, or to any of the excipients.
- patients with hepatic impairment (see Warnings and Precautions).

Following a hypersensitivity reaction to abacavir, **never** restart KIVEXA or any other abacavir containing product. Fatal rechallenge reactions have been associated with re-administration of abacavir to patients with a prior history of a hypersensitivity reaction to abacavir (see Warnings and Precautions).

WARNINGS AND PRECAUTIONS:

Serious Warnings and Precautions

- **Fatal Hypersensitivity Reactions:** Fatal hypersensitivity reactions have been associated with therapy with abacavir sulphate and other abacavir containing products. Therapy with KIVEXA (abacavir sulfate/lamivudine) should be discontinued in patients developing signs or symptoms of hypersensitivity in 2 or more of the following groups: 1) fever, 2) rash, 3) gastrointestinal (including nausea, vomiting, diarrhea or abdominal pain, 4) constitutional (including generalized malaise, fatigue or achiness, 5) respiratory (including pharyngitis, dyspnea, cough and abnormal chest x-ray findings, predominantly infiltrates, which can be localized). (See Warnings and Precautions, Hypersensitivity Reactions to Abacavir.) To minimize the risk of a life threatening hypersensitivity reaction, KIVEXA should be permanently discontinued if hypersensitivity cannot be ruled out, even when other diagnoses are possible (acute onset of respiratory diseases, gastroenteritis or reactions to other medications).
  The symptoms of a hypersensitivity reaction can occur at any time during treatment with abacavir, but usually occur within the fist six weeks of therapy. **KIVEXA or any other medicinal product containing abacavir (e.g. ZIAGEN, TRIZIVIR) must never be restarted following a hypersensitivity reaction, as more severe symptoms will recur within hours and may include life threatening hypotension and death.** Severe or fatal hypersensitivity reactions can occur within hours after KIVEXA re-introduction in patients who have no identified history or undiagnosed symptoms of hypersensitivity during their initial period of use of KIVEXA.
  Patients who carry the HLA-B*5701 allele are at a significant increased risk for experiencing a hypersensitivity reaction to abacavir. Prior to initiating therapy with abacavir, it is recommended that screening for HLA-B*5701 status be undertaken. Screening is also recommended prior to re-initiation of abacavir in patients of unknown HLA-B*5701 status who have previously tolerated abacavir. Use of abacavir in patients known to carry the HLA-B*5701 allele is not recommended.
  Cases of abacavir hypersensitivity have occurred in patients who are HLA-B*5701 negative. The clinical diagnosis of suspected hypersensitivity to abacavir remains the basis for clinical decision making in all patients. Therefore, it is important to permanently discontinue abacavir and not rechallenge with abacavir if hypersensitivity cannot be ruled out, regardless of the presence or absence of the HLA-B*5701 allele due to the potential for a severe or even fatal reaction (see Warnings and Precautions, Hypersensitivity Reactions to Abacavir, Risk Factors: HLA-B*5701 Allele).
- **Lactic Acidosis and Severe Hepatomegaly with Steatosis:** Lactic acidosis and severe hepatomegaly with steatosis, including fatal cases, have been reported with the use of nucleoside analogues alone or in combination, including KIVEXA and other antiretrovirals. A majority of these cases have been in women. Obesity and prolonged nucleoside exposure may be risk factors. However, cases have also been reported in patients with no known risk factors. Treatment with KIVEXA should be suspended in any patient who develops clinical or laboratory findings suggestive of lactic acidosis or pronounced hepatotoxicity (which may include hepatomegaly and steatosis even in the absence of marked transaminase elevations) (see Warnings and Precautions, Hepatic/Biliary/Pancreatic).
- **Post-Treatment Exacerbation of Hepatitis:** It is recommended that all patients with HIV be tested for the presence of chronic hepatitis B virus (HBV) before initiating antiretroviral therapy. KIVEXA is not indicated for the treatment of chronic HBV infection and the safety and efficacy of KIVEXA have not been established in patients coinfected with HBV and HIV. Exacerbations of hepatitis B have been reported in patients after the discontinuation of antiretroviral therapy. Patients coinfected with HIV and HBV should be closely monitored with both clinical and laboratory follow-up for at least several months after stopping treatment with KIVEXA (see Adverse Reactions, Post-Market Adverse Drug Reactions).
- **Pancreatitis:** Pancreatitis has been observed in some patients receiving abacavir and lamivudine. However it is not clear whether these cases were due to drug treatment or to the underlying HIV disease. Pancreatitis must be considered whenever a patient develops abdominal pain, nausea, vomiting or elevated biochemical markers. Discontinue use of KIVEXA until diagnosis of pancreatitis is excluded (see Adverse Reactions, Post-Market Adverse Drug Reactions).
- **Pancreatitis in Pediatric Patients:** In pediatric patients with a history of prior antiretroviral nucleoside exposure, a history of pancreatitis, or other significant risk factors for the development of pancreatitis, lamivudine containing products should be used with caution. Treatment with lamivudine containing products should be stopped immediately if clinical signs, symptoms, or laboratory abnormalities suggestive of pancreatitis occur (see Adverse Reactions, Post-Market Adverse Drug Reactions).

General: KIVEXA (abacavir sulfate/lamivudine) is a fixed-dose combination of abacavir sulfate and lamivudine. KIVEXA should not be administered concomitantly with either abacavir or lamivudine.

Hypersensitivity Reactions to Abacavir: Serious and sometimes fatal hypersensitivity reactions have been associated with therapy with abacavir sulfate, one of the two active ingredients of KIVEXA. Patients who carry the HLA-B*5701 allele are at a significantly increased risk for experiencing a hypersensitivity reaction to abacavir. Other less common signs or symptoms of hypersensitivity include fever, skin rash, fatigue, myolysis, edema, paresthesia, anaphylaxis, liver failure, renal failure, hypotension, adult respiratory distress syndrome, respiratory failure, and death have occurred in association with hypersensitivity reactions, gastrointestinal symptoms such as nausea, vomiting, diarrhea or abdominal pain, and respiratory signs and symptoms such as pharyngitis, dyspnea, cough and abnormal chest x-ray findings predominantly infiltrates, which can be localized.

Physical findings associated with hypersensitivity to abacavir in some patients include lymphadenopathy, mucous membrane lesions (conjunctivitis and mouth ulcerations), and rash. The rash usually appears maculopapular or urticarial, but may be variable in appearance. There have been reports of erythema multiforme. Hypersensitivity reactions have occurred without rash.

Laboratory abnormalities associated with hypersensitivity to abacavir in some patients include elevated liver function tests, elevated creatine phosphokinase, elevated creatinine, and lymphopenia.

The diagnosis of a hypersensitivity reaction should be carefully considered for patients presenting with symptoms of acute onset respiratory diseases, even if alternative respiratory diagnoses (pneumonia, bronchitis, pharyngitis or flu-like illness) are possible. KIVEXA or any other medicinal product containing abacavir (ZIAGEN, TRIZIVIR), **must never** be restarted following a hypersensitivity reaction, as more severe symptoms will recur within hours and may include life threatening hypotension and death.

To avoid a delay in diagnosis and minimize the risk of a life threatening hypersensitivity reaction, KIVEXA should be permanently discontinued if hypersensitivity cannot be ruled out, even when other diagnoses are possible (respiratory diseases, flu-like illness, gastroenteritis or reactions to other medications). KIVEXA, or any other medicinal product containing abacavir (ZIAGEN, TRIZIVIR), should not be re-started even if a recurrence of symptoms occurs following rechallenge with alternative medication(s).

Severe or fatal hypersensitivity reactions can occur within hours after KIVEXA re-introduction in patients who have no identified history or unrecognized symptoms of hypersensitivity during their initial period of use of KIVEXA.

Regardless of a patient's HLA-B*5701 status, if therapy with KIVEXA or any other medicinal product containing abacavir (ZIAGEN, TRIZIVIR) has been discontinued and restarting therapy is under consideration, the reason for discontinuation should be evaluated to ensure that the patient did not have symptoms of a hypersensitivity reaction. **If a hypersensitivity reaction cannot be ruled out, KIVEXA or any other medicinal product containing abacavir (e.g. ZIAGEN, TRIVIZIR) should not be restarted.**

If symptoms consistent with hypersensitivity are not identified, reintroduction can be undertaken with continued monitoring for symptoms of a hypersensitivity reaction. Make patients aware that a hypersensitivity reaction can occur with reintroduction of KIVEXA or any other abacavir containing product and that reintroduction of KIVEXA or introduction of any other abacavir containing product needs to be undertaken only if medical care can be readily accessed by the patient or others.

Overall, in clinical trials conducted before the introduction of screening for the HLA-B*5701 allele, hypersensitivity reactions have been reported in approximately 8% of 2670 patients (n=206) in 9 clinical trials (range: 2% to 9%) with enrolment from November 1999 to February 2002. Data on time to onset and symptoms of suspected hypersensitivity in the nine studies were collected on a detailed data collection module. This reaction is characterized by the appearance of symptoms indicating multi-organ/body-system involvement. Symptoms can occur at any time during therapy however, they usually appear within the first 6 weeks (median time to onset is 11 days) of initiation of treatment with abacavir (see Adverse Reactions).

In a controlled study (CNA30021), more patients taking abacavir 600 mg once daily had severe hypersensitivity reactions than patients taking abacavir 300 mg twice daily (see Warnings and Precautions and Dosage and Administration). In this study, 4 patients (11%) receiving abacavir 600 mg once daily experienced hypotension with a hypersensitivity reaction compared with 0 patients receiving abacavir 300 mg twice daily.

A warning card with information for the patient about this hypersensitivity reaction is included in the KIVEXA pack (see Information for the Patient: Warning Card).

Risk Factors: HLA-B*5701 Allele: Studies have shown that carriage of the HLA-B*5701 allele is associated with a significantly increased risk of a hypersensitivity reaction to abacavir. CNA106030 (PREDICT-1), a randomized, double blind study, evaluated the clinical utility of prospective HLA-B*5701 screening on the incidence of abacavir hypersensitivity reaction in abacavir-naïve HIV-1 infected adults (n=1650). In this study, use of pre-therapy screening for the HLA-B*5701 allele and exclusion of subjects with this allele reduced the incidence of clinically suspected abacavir hypersensitivity reactions from 7.8% (66/847) to 3.4% (27/803) (p<0.0001). Based on this study, it is estimated that 61% of patients with the HLA-B*5701 allele will develop a clinically suspected hypersensitivity reaction during the course of abacavir treatment compared with 4% of patients who do not have the HLA-B*5701 allele.

Figure 1: KIVEXA

Hypersensitivity Related Symptoms Reported with Greater Than or Equal to 10 Percent Frequency in Clinical Trials (n=206 Patients)

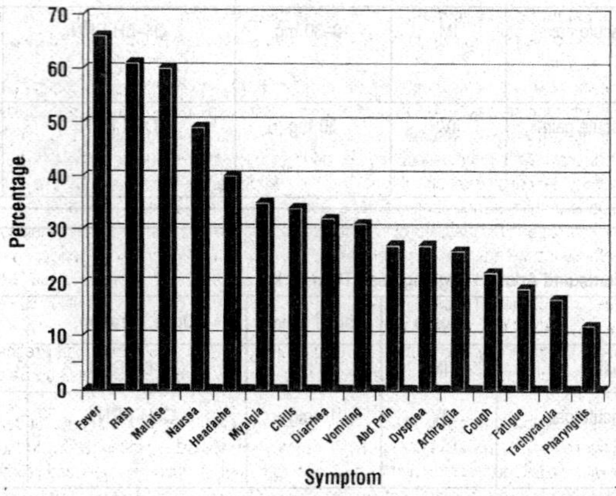

Screening for carriage of the HLA-B*5701 allele is recommended prior to initiating treatment with abacavir. Screening is also recommended prior to re-initiating abacavir in patients of unknown HLA-B*5701 status who have previously tolerated abacavir. For HLA-B*5701-positive patients, initiating or re-initiating treatment with an abacavir containing regimen is not recommended and should be considered only with close medical supervision and under exceptional circumstances where potential benefit outweighs the risk.

Skin patch testing is used as a research tool and should not be used to aid in the clinical diagnosis of abacavir hypersensitivity.

In any patient treated with abacavir, the clinical diagnosis of a hypersensitivity reaction must remain the basis of clinical decision making. Even in the absence of the HLA- B*5701 allele, it is important to permanently discontinue abacavir and not rechallenge with abacavir if a hypersensitivity reaction cannot be ruled out on clinical grounds, due to the potential for a severe or even fatal reaction.

Carcinogenesis and Mutagenesis: Abacavir induced chromosomal aberrations both in the presence and absence of metabolic activation in an in vitro cytogenetic study in human lymphocytes. Abacavir was mutagenic in the absence of metabolic activation, although it was not mutagenic in the presence of metabolic activation in an L5178Y mouse lymphoma assay. At systemic exposures approximately nine times higher than those in humans at the therapeutic dose, abacavir was clastogenic in males and not clastogenic in females in an in vivo mouse bone marrow micronucleus assay.

Abacavir was not mutagenic in bacterial mutagenicity assays in the presence and absence of metabolic activation.

Carcinogenicity studies with orally administered abacavir in mice and rats showed an increase in the incidence of malignant and non-malignant tumours. Malignant tumours occurred in the preputial gland of males and the clitoral gland of females of both species, and in the liver, urinary bladder, lymph nodes and subcutis of female rats.

The majority of these tumours occurred at the highest abacavir dose of 330 mg/kg/day in mice and 600 mg/kg/day in rats. These dose levels were equivalent to 24 to 33 times the expected systemic exposure in humans.

Cardiovascular: The results of a prospective, observational, epidemiological study designed to investigate the rate of myocardial infarction in patients on combination antiretroviral therapy (N=33 347) suggest that current or recent use (within the past 6 months) of abacavir may be associated with a potential increased risk of myocardial infarction. This elevated risk does not appear to increase further over time, and no excess risk was present in patients who had stopped taking abacavir more than 6 months previously. The relative risk of myocardial infarction was estimated to be 1.9 (95% CI 1.47-2.45). The absolute myocardial infarction rate was 6.1/1000 patient years of exposure for those recently exposed to abacavir compared to an absolute myocardial infarction rate of 2.6/1000 patient years of exposure for those not recently exposed. In addition, the absolute myocardial infarction rate ranged from 3.4 to 3.7/1000 patient years of exposure for patients recently exposed to other NRTIs (i.e. zidovudine, stavudine and lamivudine).

In a pooled analysis of GSK sponsored clinical trials (N=9639), no increased risk of myocardial infarction was observed with abacavir use. At this time, though the available data do not allow a definitive conclusion regarding the association between the use of abacavir and an increased risk of myocardial infarction, it is recommended that physicians discuss the potential benefits and risks of abacavir with their patients.

As a precaution, the underlying risk of coronary heart disease should be considered when prescribing antiretroviral therapies, including abacavir, and action taken to minimize all modifiable risk factors (e.g. hypertension, hyperlipidemia, diabetes mellitus and smoking).

Endocrine and Metabolism: Fat Redistribution: Redistribution/accumulation of body fat, including central obesity, dorsocervical fat enlargement ("buffalo hump"), peripheral wasting, facial wasting, breast enlargement, and "cushingoid appearance" have been observed in patients receiving antiretroviral therapy.

The mechanism and long term consequences of these events are currently unknown. A causal relationship has not been established.

Hematologic: Very rare occurrences of pure red cell aplasia have been reported with lamivudine use. Discontinuation of lamivudine has resulted in normalization of hematologic parameters in patients with suspected lamivudine induced pure red cell aplasia.

Hepatic/Biliary/Pancreatic: Lactic Acidosis/Severe Hepatomegaly with Steatosis: Lactic acidosis and severe hepatomegaly with steatosis, including fatal cases, have been reported with the use of antiretroviral nucleoside analogues alone or in combination, including abacavir and lamivudine, in the treatment of HIV infection. A majority of these cases have been in women. Clinical features which may be indicative of the development of lactic acidosis include generalized weakness, anorexia and sudden unexplained weight loss, gastrointestinal symptoms and respiratory symptoms (dyspnea and tachypnea).

Obesity and prolonged nucleoside exposure may be risk factors. Particular caution should be exercised when administering KIVEXA to any patient, and particularly to those with known risk factors for liver disease. Treatment with KIVEXA should be suspended in any patient who develops clinical or laboratory findings suggestive of lactic acidosis or hepatotoxicity, which may include hepatomegaly and steatosis even in the absence of marked transaminase elevations.

Use with Interferon and Ribavirin Based Regimens: In vitro studies have shown ribavirin can reduce the phosphorylation of pyrimidine nucleoside analogues such as lamivudine, a component of KIVEXA. Although no evidence of a pharmacokinetic or pharmacodynamic interaction (e.g. loss of HIV/HCV virologic suppression) was seen when ribavirin was coadministered with lamivudine in HIV/HCV coinfected patients (see Drug Interactions), hepatic decompensation (some fatal) has occurred in HIV/HCV coinfected patients receiving combination antiretroviral therapy for HIV and interferon alfa with or without ribavirin. Patients receiving interferon alfa with or without ribavirin and KIVEXA should be closely monitored for treatment associated toxicities, especially hepatic decompensation. Discontinuation of KIVEXA should be considered as medically appropriate. Dose reduction or discontinuation of interferon alfa, ribavirin, or both should also be considered if worsening clinical toxicities are observed, including hepatic decompensation.

Patients with Impaired Hepatic Function: Abacavir is contraindicated in patients with moderate to severe hepatic impairment and dose reduction is required in patients with mild hepatic impairment. Because KIVEXA is a fixed dose combination and cannot be dose adjusted, KIVEXA is contraindicated for patients with hepatic impairment.

Abacavir is metabolised primarily by the liver. The pharmacokinetics of abacavir have been studied inpatients with mild hepatic impairment (Child-Pugh score 5-6) who had confirmed cirrhosis.

The results showed that there was a mean increase of 1.89 fold in the abacavir AUC, and 1.58 fold in the half life of abacavir. The AUCs of the metabolites were not modified by the liver disease. However, the rates of formation and elimination of these were decreased. Dosage reduction of abacavir is therefore required in patients with mild hepatic impairment. The pharmacokinetics of abacavir have not been studied in patients with moderate or severe hepatic impairment.

Data obtained in patients with moderate to severe hepatic impairment show that lamivudine pharmacokinetics are not significantly affected by hepatic dysfunction.

Patients Coinfected with Hepatitis B Virus: Clinical study and marketed use of lamivudine have shown that some patients with chronic hepatitis B virus (HBV) disease may experience clinical or laboratory evidence of recurrent hepatitis upon discontinuation of lamivudine, which may have more severe consequences in patients with decompensated liver disease. If abacavir/lamivudine is discontinued in patients coinfected with hepatitis B virus, periodic monitoring of both liver function tests and markers of HBV replication should be considered.

Immune: Immune Reconstitution Syndrome: During the initial phase of treatment, patients responding to antiretroviral therapy may develop an inflammatory response to indolent or residual opportunistic infections (such as MAC, CMV, PCP and TB), which may necessitate further evaluation and treatment.

Renal: Patients with Impaired Renal Function: Lamivudine requires dose adjustment in the presence of renal insufficiency. Because KIVEXA is a fixed dose combination and cannot be dose adjusted, it is not recommended for use in patients with creatine clearance <50 mL/min.

Respiratory: Severe respiratory symptoms, some indicative of adult respiratory distress syndrome (ARDS), occur in a small proportion of hypersensitivity reaction cases. ARDS or respiratory failure appears more likely to occur in a rechallenge situation.

Special Populations: Pregnant Women: The safe use of abacavir sulfate/lamivudine in human pregnancy has not been established. Lamivudine and abacavir have been associated with findings in animal reproductive studies. Therefore, administration of KIVEXA in pregnancy should be considered only if the benefit to the mother outweighs the possible risk to the fetus.

There have been reports of mild, transient elevations in serum lactate levels, which may be due to mitochondrial dysfunction, in neonates and infants exposed in utero or peri-partum to nucleoside reverse transcriptase inhibitors (NRTIs). The clinical relevance of transient elevations in serum lactate is unknown. There have also been very rare reports of developmental delay, seizures and other neurological disease. However, a causal relationship between these events and NRTI exposure in utero or peri-partum has not been established. These findings do not affect current recommendations to use antiretroviral therapy in pregnant women to prevent vertical transmission of HIV.

To monitor maternal-fetal outcomes of pregnant women exposed to KIVEXA, an Antiretroviral Pregnancy Registry has been established. Physicians are encouraged to register patients by calling ViiV Healthcare ULC's Drug Safety Department (1-877-393-8448).

Nursing Women: It is recommended that HIV infected women do not breast-feed their infants, under any circumstances, in order to avoid transmission of HIV. Lamivudine is excreted in human milk at similar concentrations to those found in serum. It is expected that abacavir will also be secreted into human milk, although this has not been confirmed. It is therefore recommended that mothers do not breast-feed while receiving treatment with KIVEXA.

Pediatrics (<18 years of age): The safety and effectiveness of KIVEXA has not been studied in patients <18 years of age. Physicians should refer to the individual product information for lamivudine and abacavir.

Geriatrics (>65 years of age): KIVEXA should not be used in patients over 65 years of age. Physicians should refer to the individual product information for lamivudine and abacavir (see Use of KIVEXA in Patients with Comorbid Conditions and in the Elderly).

Use of KIVEXA in Patients with Comorbid Conditions and in the Elderly: KIVEXA should not be used in patients over 65 years of age, or in patients with comorbid conditions such as hepatic or renal failure, as this dosing regimen has not been studied in this population. The use of KIVEXA has not been studied in elderly patients or patients with comorbid conditions.

Therapy Experienced Patients: In clinical trials, patients with prolonged prior nucleoside reverse transcriptase inhibitor (NRTI) exposure or who had HIV-1 isolates that contained multiple mutations conferring resistance to NRTIs had limited response to abacavir. The potential for cross resistance between abacavir and other NRTIs should be considered when choosing new therapeutic regimens in therapy experienced patients.

ADVERSE REACTIONS: Adverse Drug Reaction Overview: KIVEXA (abacavir sulfate/lamivudine) contains abacavir and lamivudine; therefore the adverse events associated with these may be expected. For many of the adverse events listed it is unclear whether they are related to the active substance, the wide range of other medicinal products used in the management of HIV infection, or whether they are a result of the underlying disease process.

Clinical Trial Adverse Drug Reactions: Because clinical trials are conducted under very specific conditions the adverse reaction rates observed in the clinical trials may not reflect the rates observed in practice and should not be compared to the rates in the clinical trials of another drug. Adverse drug reaction information from clinical trials is useful for identifying drug-related adverse events and for approximating rates.

Hypersensitivity to Abacavir: Overall, in clinical trials conducted before the introduction of screening for the HLA-B*5701 allele, hypersensitivity to abacavir was reported in 8% of patients in 9 clinical trials (range: 2 to 9%). This reaction is characterized by the appearance of symptoms indicating multi-organ/body system involvement.

Product containing abacavir **must not** be restarted following a hypersensitivity reaction because more severe symptoms will recur within hours and may include life threatening hypotension and death. Patients developing signs or symptoms of hypersensitivity should discontinue treatment as soon as a hypersensitivity reaction is first suspected, and must seek medical evaluation immediately. To avoid a delay in diagnosis and minimize the risk of a life threatening hypersensitivity reaction, KIVEXA should be permanently discontinued if hypersensitivity cannot be ruled out, even when other diagnoses are possible (e.g. respiratory diseases, flu-like illness, gastroenteritis or reactions to other medications). KIVEXA, or any other medicinal product containing abacavir, should not be restarted even if a recurrence of symptoms occurs following rechallenge with alternative medication(s).

Severe or fatal hypersensitivity reactions can occur within hours after KIVEXA re-introduction in patients who have no identified history or unrecognized symptoms of hypersensitivity during their initial period of use of KIVEXA (see Warnings and Precautions).

Almost all patients developing hypersensitivity reactions will have fever and/or rash (usually maculopapular or urticarial) as part of the syndrome, however reactions have occurred without rash or fever.

Symptoms can occur at any time while being treated with abacavir, but usually appear within the first six weeks of initiation of treatment (median time to onset 11 days).

The signs and symptoms of this hypersensitivity reaction are listed below. Those reported **in at least 10% of patients** with a hypersensitivity reaction are in bold text.

Gastrointestinal Tract: abdominal pain, diarrhea, mouth ulceration, **nausea, vomiting**.
Hematological: lymphopenia.
Liver/Pancreas: elevated liver function tests, hepatic failure.
Miscellaneous: anaphylaxis, conjunctivitis, edema, **fatigue, fever**, hypotension, lymphadenopathy, **malaise**.
Musculoskeletal: arthralgia, elevated creatine phosphokinase, **myalgia**, rarely myolysis.
Neurological/Psychiatry: headache, paresthesia.
Respiratory Tract: adult respiratory distress syndrome, **cough, dyspnea**, respiratory failure, sore throat.
Skin: rash (usually maculopapular or urticarial).
Urology: elevated creatinine, renal failure.

Some patients with hypersensitivity were initially thought to have respiratory disease (e.g. pneumonia, bronchitis, or pharyngitis), a flu-like illness, gastroenteritis or reactions to other medications. This delay in diagnosis of hypersensitivity resulted in abacavir being continued or re-introduced, leading to a more severe hypersensitivity reaction or death. Therefore, the diagnosis of hypersensitivity reaction should be carefully considered for patients presenting with symptoms of these diseases. If a hypersensitivity reaction cannot be ruled out, KIVEXA, or any other medicinal product containing abacavir (e.g. ZIAGEN, TRIZIVIR), should not be restarted.

The symptoms related to this hypersensitivity reaction worsen with continued therapy, and usually resolve upon discontinuation of abacavir.

Restarting abacavir following a hypersensitivity reaction results in a prompt return of symptoms within hours. This recurrence of the hypersensitivity reaction may be more severe than on initial presentation, and may include life threatening hypotension and death. Regardless of their HLA-B*5701 status, patients who develop this hypersensitivity reaction must discontinue KIVEXA and must never be rechallenged with KIVEXA, or any other medicinal product containing abacavir (e.g. ZIAGEN, TRIZIVIR).

There have been infrequent reports of hypersensitivity reactions following re-introduction of abacavir, where the interruption was preceded by a single key symptom of hypersensitivity (i.e. rash, fever, malaise/fatigue, gastrointestinal or a respiratory symptom).

On very rare occasions, hypersensitivity reactions have been reported in patients who have restarted therapy, and who had no preceding symptoms of a hypersensitivity reaction.

The adverse events for abacavir or lamivudine are listed in Table 1 by body system and absolute frequency. Frequencies are defined as very common (>1/10), common (>1/100, <1/10), uncommon (>1/1000, <1/100), rare (>1/10 000, <1/1000), and very rare (<1/10 000).

Many of the adverse events listed occur commonly (i.e. nausea, vomiting, diarrhea, fever, lethargy, and rash) in patients with abacavir hypersensitivity. Therefore, patients with any of these symptoms should be carefully evaluated for the presence of this hypersensitivity reaction. If KIVEXA has been discontinued in patients due to their experiencing any one of these symptoms and a decision is made to restart abacavir, this must be done only under direct medical supervision (see Warnings and Precautions).

Table 1: KIVEXA

Adverse Events Observed During Clinical Trials

Body System	Abacavir	Lamivudine
Blood and Lymphatic Systems Disorders		Uncommon: neutropenia, anemia, thrombocytopenia
Immune System Disorders	Common: drug hypersensitivity	
Metabolism and Nutrition Disorders	Common: anorexia, hyperlactatemia Rare: lactic acidosis (see Warnings and Precautions)	
Nervous System Disorders	Common: headache	Common: headache
Gastrointestinal Disorders	Common: nausea, vomiting, diarrhea Rare: pancreatitis has been reported, but a causal relationship to abacavir treatment is uncertain	Common: nausea, vomiting, upper abdominal pain, diarrhea
Hepatobiliary Disorders		Uncommon: transient rises in liver enzymes (AST, ALT)
Skin and Subcutaneous Tissue Disorders	Common: rash (without systemic symptoms) Very rare: erythema multiforme, SJS and TEN	Common: rash
General Disorders and Administration Site Conditions	Common: fever, lethargy, fatigue	Common: fatigue, malaise, fever

In study CNA30021, treatment emergent clinical adverse reactions (rated by the investigator as at least moderate) with a ≥5% frequency during therapy with abacavir 600 mg once daily and efavirenz 600 mg once daily were similar. For hypersensitivity reactions, patients receiving abacavir once daily showed a rate of 9% in comparison to a rate of 7% for patients receiving abacavir twice daily. However, patients receiving abacavir 600 mg once daily experienced a significantly higher incidence of severe drug hypersensitivity reactions and severe diarrhea compared to patients who received abacavir 300 mg twice daily. Five percent (5%) of patients receiving abacavir 600 mg once daily had severe drug hypersensitivity reactions compared to 2% of patients receiving abacavir 300 mg twice daily. Two percent (2%) of patients receiving abacavir 600 mg once daily had severe diarrhea while none of the patients receiving abacavir 300 mg twice daily had this event.

Pancreatitis, which has been fatal in some cases, has been observed in antiretroviral nucleoside experienced pediatric patients receiving 3TC alone or in combination with other antiretroviral agents. In an open label, dose escalation study (NUCA2002), 14 patients (14%) developed pancreatitis while receiving monotherapy with 3TC. Three of these patients died of complications of pancreatitis. In a second open label study (NUCA2005), 12 patients (18%) developed pancreatitis. In study ACTG300, pancreatitis was not observed in 236 patients randomized to 3TC plus RETROVIR (AZT). Pancreatitis was observed in one patient in this study who received open label 3TC in combination with RETROVIR (AZT) and ritonavir following discontinuation of didanosine monotherapy.

Post-Market Adverse Drug Reactions: In addition to the adverse events included from clinical trial data, the following adverse events listed below have been identified during post-approval use of abacavir and lamivudine.

These events have been chosen for inclusion due to either their seriousness, frequency of reporting, potential causal connection to abacavir and lamivudine, or a combination of these factors. Because they are reported voluntarily from a population of unknown size, estimates of frequency cannot be made.

Body as a Whole: anaphylaxis, redistribution/accumulation of body fat, weakness.
Digestive: stomatitis.
Endocrine/Metabolic: hepatic steatosis, hyperglycemia, hyperlactatemia, lactic acidosis.
Hematological: pure red cell aplasia.
Hemic and Lymphatic: anemia, lymphadenophathy, splenomegaly.
Hepatic: hepatic steatosis, lactic acidosis.
Musculoskeletal: muscle disorders including rarely rhabdomyolosis, arthralgia.
Nervous: paresthesia, peripheral neuropathy.
Other: alopecia.
Skin: pruritus, rash, urticaria. Suspected Stevens-Johnson syndrome (SJS) and toxic epidermal necrolysis (TEN) have been reported in patients receiving abacavir, primarily in combination with medications known to be associated with SJS and TEN, respectively. Because of the overlap of the clinical signs and symptoms between hypersensitivity to abacavir, SJS and TEN and the possibility of multiple drug sensitivities in some patients, abacavir should be discontinued and not restarted in such cases. There have been reports of erythema multiforme with abacavir use.

DRUG INTERACTIONS: Overview: As KIVEXA (abacavir sulfate/lamivudine) contains abacavir and lamivudine, any interactions that have been identified with these agents individually may occur with KIVEXA. Clinical studies have shown that there are no clinically significant interactions between abacavir and lamivudine. Abacavir and lamivudine are not significantly metabolized by cytochrome P450 enzymes (such as CYP 3A4, CYP 2C9 or CYP 2D6) nor do they inhibit or induce this enzyme system. Therefore, there is little potential for interactions with antiretroviral protease inhibitors, non-nucleosides and other medicinal products metabolized by major P450 enzymes.

The likelihood of metabolic interactions with lamivudine is low due to limited metabolism and plasma protein binding, and almost complete renal clearance. Lamivudine is predominantly eliminated by active organic cationic secretion. The possibility of interactions with other medicinal products administered concurrently should be considered, particularly when the main route of elimination is renal.

Drug-Drug Interactions: The drugs listed in Table 2 and Table 3 are based on either drug interaction case reports or studies, or potential interactions due to the expected magnitude and seriousness of the interaction (i.e. those identified as contraindicated).

Table 2: KIVEXA

Interactions Relevant to Abacavir

Proper Name	Effect	Clinical Comment
Ethanol	In men, the metabolism of abacavir sulfate is altered by concomitant ethanol resulting in an increase in AUC of abacavir of about 41%.	The clinical significance of this is unknown. In men, abacavir sulfate has no effect on the metabolism of ethanol. This interaction has not been studied in women.
Methadone	In a pharmacokinetic study, coadministration of 600 mg abacavir twice daily with methadone showed a 35% reduction in abacavir C_{max} and a one hour delay in t_{max}, but AUC was unchanged.	The changes in abacavir pharmacokinetics are not considered clinically relevant. In this study, abacavir increased the mean methadone systemic clearance by 22%. This change is not considered clinically relevant for the majority of patients, however occasionally methadone dose retitration may be required.
Retinoids		Retinoid compounds, such as isotretinoin, are eliminated via alcohol dehydrogenase. Interaction with abacavir is possible but has not been studied.

(cont'd)

Table 2: KIVEXA *(cont'd)*

Interactions Relevant to Abacavir

Proper Name	Effect	Clinical Comment
Ribavirin	In vitro data indicate ribavirin reduces phosphorylation of lamivudine, stavudine, and zidovudine.	No pharmacokinetic (e.g. plasma concentrations or intracellular triphosphorylated active metabolite concentrations) or pharmacodynamic (e.g. loss of HIV/HCV virologic suppression) interaction was observed when ribavirin and lamivudine (n=18), stavudine (n=10), or zidovudine (n=6) were coadministered as part of a multi drug regimen to HIV/HCV coinfected patients (see Warnings and Precautions, Hepatic/Biliary/Pancreatic).

Table 3: KIVEXA

Interactions Relevant to Lamivudine

Proper Name	Effect	Clinical Comment
Trimethoprim	Administration of trimethoprim/sulphamethoxazole 160 mg/800 mg (co-trimoxazole) causes a 40% increase in lamivudine exposure because of the trimethoprim component.	Unless the patient has renal impairment, no dosage adjustment of lamivudine is necessary (see Dosage and Administration). Lamivudine has no effect on the pharmacokinetics of trimethoprim or sulphamethoxazole. The effect of coadministration of lamivudine with higher doses of co-trimoxazole used for the treatment of *P. carinii* pneumonia and toxoplasmosis has not been studied.
Zalcitabine	Lamivudine may inhibit the intracellular phosphorylation of zalcitabine when the two medicinal products are used concurrently.	KIVEXA is not recommended to be used in combination with zalcitabine.

Drug-Food Interactions: Interactions with food have not been established.
Drug-Herb Interactions: Interactions with herbs have not been established.
Drug-Laboratory Test Interactions: Interactions with laboratory tests have not been established.

DOSAGE AND ADMINISTRATION: Dosing Considerations: Therapy should be initiated by a physician experienced in the management of HIV infection.

A patient information leaflet and warning card that provide information about recognition of hypersensitivity reactions should be dispensed with each new prescription and refill.

KIVEXA (abacavir sulfate/lamivudine) can be taken with or without food.

Recommended Dose and Dosage Adjustment: Because KIVEXA is a fixed dose tablet it should not be prescribed for patients requiring dosage adjustments, such as those who weigh less than 40 kg, those with creatinine clearance <50 mL/min, those with hepatic impairment or those experiencing dose limiting adverse events. Separate preparations of abacavir (ZIAGEN) or lamivudine (3TC) should be administered in cases where discontinuation or dose adjustment is indicated. In these cases the physician should refer to the individual product information for these medicinal products.

Adults (≥18 years): The recommended dose of KIVEXA is one tablet once daily. The use of abacavir 600 mg once daily may be associated with a higher incidence of severe hypersensitivity reactions.

Children: Physicians should refer to the individual product information for lamivudine and abacavir. The safety and effectiveness of KIVEXA have not been studied in patients less than 18 years of age (see Warnings and Precautions).

Elderly: The use of KIVEXA has not been studied in elderly patients or patients with comorbid conditions (see Warnings and Precautions).

Missed Dose: It is important to take KIVEXA as prescribed to ensure the patient gets maximum benefit. If the patient forgets to take a dose, they should take it as soon as they remember, and then continue as before. Patients must not take more than one tablet to make up for forgotten individual doses.

OVERDOSAGE:
There is no known antidote for KIVEXA (abacavir sulfate/lamivudine). If overdosage occurs, the patient should be monitored, and standard supportive treatment applied as required. Although no data are available, administration of activated charcoal may be used to aid in the removal of unabsorbed drug. It is not known whether abacavir can be removed by peritoneal dialysis or hemodialysis. Because a negligible amount of lamivudine was removed via (4 hour) hemodialysis, continuous ambulatory peritoneal dialysis, and automated peritoneal dialysis, it is not known if continuous hemodialysis would provide clinical benefit in a lamivudine overdose event.

Limited data are available on the consequences of ingestion of acute overdoses in humans. No fatalities occurred, and the patients recovered.

Single doses up to 1200 mg and daily doses up to 1800 mg of abacavir sulfate have been administered to patients in clinical studies. No unexpected adverse reactions were reported. The effects of higher doses are not known. No specific signs or symptoms have been identified following such overdose.

One case of acute overdose in an adult ingesting 6 g of 3TC was reported; there were no clinical signs or symptoms noted and hematologic tests remained normal. One other adult patient in error ingested lamivudine 1200 mg per day plus zidovudine 1200 mg per day for approximately 2 weeks; he had a Grade 3 decrease in absolute neutrophil count that resolved upon reduction of doses of lamivudine and zidovudine. Two cases of pediatric overdose were reported in ACTG300. One case was a single dose of 7 mg/kg of 3TC; the second case involved the use of 5 mg/kg of 3TC twice daily for 30 days. There were no clinical signs or symptoms noted in either case.

In Phase I studies, lamivudine was administered at doses up to 20 mg/kg per day (i.e. approximately five times the usual recommended dose in adults) without serious consequences.

> For management of a suspected drug overdose, contact your regional Poison Control Centre. See the *CPS* Directory section for a list of Poison Control Centres.

ACTION AND CLINICAL PHARMACOLOGY: Mechanism of Action: KIVEXA (abacavir sulfate/lamivudine) is a fixed dose combination of two nucleoside analogues (abacavir and lamivudine). Abacavir and lamivudine are nucleoside reverse transcriptase inhibitors (NRTIs), and are potent, selective inhibitors of HIV-1 and HIV-2. Both abacavir and lamivudine are metabolized sequentially by intracellular kinases to the respective triphosphate (TP), which are the active moieties. Lamivudine-TP and carbovir-TP (the active triphosphate form of abacavir) are substrates for and competitive inhibitors of HIV reverse transcriptase (RT). Inhibition of RT is via viral DNA chain termination after nucleoside analogue. Carbovir and lamivudine triphosphates show significantly less affinity for host cell DNA polymerases.

In a study of 20 HIV-infected patients receiving abacavir 300 mg twice daily, with only one 300 mg dose taken prior to the 24 h sampling period, the geometric mean terminal carbovir-TP intracellular half-life at steady-state was 20.6 h, compared to the geometric mean abacavir plasma half-life in this study of 2.6 h.

The steady state pharmacokinetic properties of abacavir 600 mg once daily was compared to abacavir 300 mg twice daily in a crossover study in 27 HIV-infected patients. Intracellular carbovir triphosphate exposures in peripheral blood mononuclear cells were higher for abacavir 600 mg once daily with respect to $AUC_{24,ss}$ (32 %, higher), $C_{max\ 24,ss}$ (99% higher) and trough values (18% higher), compared to the 300 mg twice daily regimen.

For patients receiving lamivudine 300 mg once daily, the terminal intracellular half-life of lamivudine-TP was prolonged to 16 to 19 h, compared to the plasma lamivudine half-life of 5 to 7 h.

The steady state pharmacokinetic properties of lamivudine 300 mg once daily for 7 days compared to lamivudine 150 mg twice daily for 7 days were assessed in a crossover study in 60 healthy volunteers. Intracellular lamivudine triphosphate exposures in peripheral blood mononuclear cells were similar with respect to $AUC_{24,ss}$ and $C_{max\ 24,ss}$; however, trough values were lower compared to the 150 mg twice daily regimen. Inter subject variability was greater for intracellular lamivudine triphosphate concentrations versus lamivudine plasma trough concentrations. These data support the use of lamivudine 300 mg and abacavir 600 mg once daily for the treatment of HIV-infected patients. Additionally, the efficacy and safety of this combination given once daily has been demonstrated in a pivotal clinical study.

STORAGE AND STABILITY: Stability and Storage Recommendations: Store KIVEXA (abacavir sulfate/lamivudine) tablets between 15 to 30°C.

INFORMATION FOR THE PATIENT: Published in e-CPS, available by subscription at www.e-cps.ca.

DOSAGE FORMS, COMPOSITION AND PACKAGING: Each orange, film coated, modified capsule shaped tablet, debossed with GS FC2 on one side and the other side plain, contains: abacavir 600 mg as abacavir sulfate and lamivudine 300 mg. Nonmedicinal ingredients: FD&C Yellow #6 Aluminum Lake, hypromellose, magnesium stearate, microcrystalline cellulose, polyethylene glycol 400, polysorbate 80, sodium starch glycolate and titanium dioxide. Blisters of 30.

(Shown in Product Identification Section)

Klean-Prep®
polyethylene glycol—electrolytes
Laxative

Helix Biopharma

PHARMACOLOGY: Klean-Prep is a balanced electrolyte solution containing polyethylene glycol 3350, sodium sulfate, potassium chloride, sodium chloride and sodium bicarbonate. The solution prepared as recommended is iso-osmotic. It has been found that very little net absorption or secretion of electrolytes from the bowel occurs with this mixture. The sodium sulfate inhibits net sodium absorption, and the other electrolytes prevent net absorption or secretion of other ions, so that the patient can ingest large volumes of the solution to effect bowel cleansing without significant changes in water and electrolyte balance.

It is known that sodium is actively absorbed (against an electrochemical gradient) by the intestinal mucosa when the accompanying anion is chloride. However, sodium absorption is markedly reduced when sulfate is substituted for chloride. Total gut perfusion with this product is, thus, not associated with significant sodium and water absorption. The solution is useful in cleansing the colon of patients who are about to undergo gastrointestinal examinations (barium x-rays, colonoscopy, etc.) or surgical procedures requiring a clean colon.

Fordtran and his colleagues have recommended that oral ingestion of 1.2 to 1.8 L/hour until 4 L have been consumed, would result in satisfactory cleansing of the colon. Orally administered Klean-Prep induces diarrhea, which rapidly cleanses the bowel, usually within 3 to 4 hours. Polyethylene glycol 3350 acts as an osmotic agent and the electrolyte concentration results in virtually no net absorption or secretion of ions. Large volumes may be administered without significant changes in water or electrolyte balance.

INDICATIONS: For cleansing of the bowel prior to colonoscopy, barium enema x-ray examination or surgical procedures requiring a clean colon.

CONTRAINDICATIONS: In patients with gastrointestinal obstruction, gastric retention, bowel perforation, severe colitis or toxic megacolon.

WARNINGS: No additional ingredients, flavorings, etc. should be added to the solution before administration.

PRECAUTIONS: Patients with impaired gag reflex or a stuporous or unconscious state or who are otherwise prone to regurgitation or aspiration, should be observed during the administration of Klean-Prep, especially if it is given via nasogastric tube. If gastrointestinal obstruction or perforation is suspected, appropriate studies should be performed to rule out these contraindications before administering Klean-Prep.

Pregnancy: Animal reproduction studies have not been conducted with Klean-Prep. It is also not known whether Klean-Prep can cause fetal harm when it is administered to a pregnant woman or whether it can affect reproductive capacity. Klean-Prep should be given to a pregnant woman only if clearly needed.

Children: Safety and effectiveness in children have not been established.

Long-term studies have not been done on animals to determine carcinogenic potential or effects on reproduction.

ADVERSE EFFECTS: Klean-Prep administration is associated with a low incidence of side effects, primarily nausea, abdominal fullness and bloating and occasional cramps and vomiting. These side effects are transient and usually subside rapidly.

OVERDOSE:
No data supplied by the manufacturer.

> For management of a suspected drug overdose, CPhA recommends that you contact your **regional Poison Control Centre**. See the *CPS* Directory section for a list of Poison Control Centres.

DOSAGE: The recommended dose for adults is 4 L of solution prior to gastrointestinal examination or procedures. The usual procedure is to have the patient drink 250 mL every 10 minutes until the 4 L is consumed or the rectal effluent is clear. Rapid drinking of each portion is preferred rather than drinking small amounts continuously. The first bowel movement should occur approximately 1 hour after the start of administration. Patient acceptance may be improved by chilling the solution before administration (but not serving with ice). If the patient is unable or unwilling to drink the solution, it may be administered via nasogastric tube.

Various regimens have been used. Ideally, the patient should fast approximately 3 to 4 hours prior to Klean-Prep ingestion, but in no case should solid foods be given for at least 2 hours before the solution is administered. One method is to schedule patients for examination at mid-morning, allowing the patient 3 hours for drinking and 1 hour waiting period to completed bowel evacuation. Another method is to administer Klean-Prep on the evening before the examination, particularly if the patient is to have a barium enema. No food except clear liquids are permitted after Klean-Prep administration and prior to examination.

SUPPLIED: Each sachet of powder for oral administration as a solution following reconstitution contains: polyethylene glycol 3350, 59 g; sodium sulfate 5.68 g; sodium bicarbonate 1.68 g; sodium chloride 1.46 g and potassium chloride 0.74 g. Also contains natural vanilla flavor and aspartame.

When made up to a 1 L volume with water, the solution contains: polyethylene glycol 3350, 17.6 mmol/L; sodium 125 mmol/L; sulfate 40 mmol/L; chloride 35 mmol/L; bicarbonate 20 mmol/L and potassium 10 mmol/L.

Four sachets of 1 L in a clear, graduated 1 L container for reconstitution. Makes 4 L of solution. Store in a dry place at room temperature. When reconstituted, keep solution refrigerated. Use reconstituted solution within 72 hours. Discard unused portion.

K-Lyte®
potassium citrate
Potassium Supplement

WellSpring

INDICATIONS: Oral potassium supplement for the therapy or prophylaxis of potassium deficiency. Especially useful for routine use with thiazide diuretics or corticosteroid hormones to replace excessive potassium losses.

CONTRAINDICATIONS: In ventricular fibrillation, hyperkalemia of any etiology, in association with Addison's disease, salt losing adrenal hyperplasia, in extensive tissue breakdown as in severe burns, acute dehydration and heat cramps. Renal impairment with oliguria or azotemia. Increased sensitivity to potassium administration, e.g., in congenital paramyotonia or adynamia episodica hereditaria.

WARNINGS: In patients with impaired mechanisms for excreting potassium, e.g. chronic renal disease, administration of potassium salts can produce hyperkalemia and cardiac arrest. This occurs most commonly in patients given i.v. potassium but may also occur in patients given oral potassium. Potentially fatal hyperkalemia can develop rapidly and be asymptomatic. Careful monitoring of the serum potassium concentration and appropriate dosage adjustment is recommended.

Caution is advised with concomitant administration of potassium and potassium sparing diuretics e.g., spironolactone or triamterene, since hyperkalemia may develop. Hypokalemia in patients with metabolic acidosis should be treated with an alkalinizing potassium salt such as the acetate, bicarbonate, gluconate or citrate.

In patients on a low salt diet particularly, hypokalemic hypochloremic alkalosis is a possibility that may require chloride as well as potassium supplementation.

PRECAUTIONS: The treatment of potassium depletion, particularly in the presence of cardiac disease, renal disease or acidosis, requires careful attention to acid base balance and appropriate monitoring of serum electrolytes, the ECG and the patient's clinical status.

Use potassium with caution in diseases associated with heart block since increased serum potassium may increase the degree of block.

ADVERSE EFFECTS: Nausea, vomiting and diarrhea have been reported. These symptoms are due to irritation of the gastrointestinal tract and are best avoided by dissolving each dose completely in the stated amount of water, increasing fluid intake when possible, taking the dose with meals or reducing dose.

OVERDOSE:

Symptoms: In patients under normal conditions of exertion, concentrations of potassium in the blood of greater than 4 mmol (mEq)/L, and in the urine of greater than 2.0 g/24 hours, may indicate hyperkalemia.

Paresthesia of the extremities, listlessness, mental confusion, weakness, paralysis, hypotension, cardiac arrhythmias, heart block and cardiac arrest may occur. ECG changes include increased amplitude and peaking of the T waves, depression of the ST segment, reduction in the amplitude of the R wave, widening of the QRS complex, prolongation of the PR interval and a decrease in the amplitude and ultimately disappearance of the P wave. Widening of the QRS complex is one of the most ominous signs and indicates the need for aggressive treatment.

Frequently hyperkalemia is asymptomatic and may be manifested only by increased serum potassium concentration and characteristic electrocardiographic changes as above.

Treatment:

1. Eliminate foods and medications containing potassium, and discontinue potassium sparing diuretics.
2. I.V. administration of 300 to 500 mL/hour of 10% dextrose solution containing 10 to 20 units of crystalline insulin/1000 mL.
3. Correct acidosis, if present, with i.v. sodium bicarbonate.
4. Use exchange resins, hemodialysis or peritoneal dialysis.
5. In the presence of life threatening cardiac arrhythmias, to antagonize the cardiac toxicity, administer i.v. 10 to 50 mL calcium gluconate 10% over 1 to 5 mins. Continuous ECG monitoring is mandatory.

In treating hyperkalemia in digitalized patients, too rapid a lowering of the serum potassium concentration can produce digitalis toxicity.

For management of a suspected drug overdose, CPhA recommends that you contact your regional Poison Control Centre. See the *CPS* Directory section for a list of Poison Control Centres.

DOSAGE: In general a daily dose exceeding 60 mmol (mEq) should not be required.

Adults: Completely dissolve 1 K-Lyte tablet in 85 to 115 mL of cold or ice water and administer 2 to 4 times daily, depending upon the patient's requirements.

Note: K-Lyte should be taken with meals and sipped slowly over a 5 to 10 minute period.

The usual dietary intake of potassium is 40 to 80 mmol (mEq)/day. Potassium depletion sufficient to cause hypokalemia usually requires the loss of 200 or more mmol (mEq) of potassium from the total body store.

If given concomitantly in chronic diuretic therapy, administer on alternating days.

Prevention of hypokalemia: supplementally, approximately 20 to 40 mmol (mEq)/day.

Treatment of depletion: 40 to a maximum of 100 mmol (mEq) daily.

SUPPLIED: Each effervescent, orange flavored and colored tablet, when dissolved in water, contains: potassium citrate 2.5 g or elemental potassium 25 mmol (mEq). Boxes of 30 individually foil wrapped tablets.

Koffex DM

dextromethorphan HBr

Antitussive

Rougier Pharma

SUPPLIED: Syrup: Each 5 mL of red, cherry-flavored syrup contains: dextromethorphan HBr 15 mg. Nonmedicinal ingredients: artificial coloring and flavoring, citric acid, potassium sorbate, propylene glycol, purified water, sodium benzoate and sucrose. Energy: 51 kJ (12 kcal)/5 mL. Alcohol-, gluten-, lactose-, parabens-, sulfite- and tartrazine-free. Bottles of 250 mL and 2 L.

Syrup (sucrose-free): Each 5 mL of orange, melon-flavored syrup contains: dextromethorphan HBr 15 mg. Nonmedicinal ingredients: artificial flavoring, citric acid, FD&C Yellow #6, potassium sorbate, propylene glycol, purified water, sodium benzoate and sorbitol. Energy: 29.8 kJ (7 kcal)/5 mL. Alcohol-, gluten-, lactose-, parabens-, sucrose-, sulfite- and tartrazine-free. Bottles of 2 L.

Kogenate® FS Supplied with BIO-SET Needle-less Reconstitution Set

antihemophilic factor (recombinant)

Coagulation Factor

Bayer

Date of Revision: January 27, 2010

SUMMARY PRODUCT INFORMATION:

Route of Administration	Dosage Form/ Strength	Clinically Relevant Nonmedicinal Ingredients
Intravenous	Lyophilized powder for injection 250, 500, 1000, 2000, 3000 IU/vial	Sucrose, glycine, histidine, calcium chloride, sodium, chloride, polysorbate 80 For a complete listing see Dosage Forms, Composition and Packaging.

DESCRIPTION: KOGENATE FS (Antihemophilic Factor [Recombinant]) is a sterile purified, non-pyrogenic, dried product, which has been manufactured by recombinant DNA technology.

KOGENATE FS supplied with BIO-SET Needle-less Reconstitution Set is a self-contained system provided with a prefilled syringe containing diluent for reconstitution.

INDICATIONS AND CLINICAL USE: KOGENATE FS (Antihemophilic Factor [Recombinant]) is indicated for the treatment of classical hemophilia (hemophilia A), in which there is a demonstrated deficiency of activity of the plasma clotting factor, factor VIII (FVIII). KOGENATE FS provides a means of temporarily replacing the missing clotting factor in order to correct or prevent bleeding episodes, or in order to perform emergency or elective surgery in hemophiliacs.

When used as a regular prophylactic treatment, KOGENATE FS is also indicated to prevent the occurrence of spontaneous hemorrhagic episodes and to prevent joint damage in children with no pre-existing joint damage.

Because KOGENATE FS showed comparable biological activity to other FVIII preparations, it should be used in the same manner as KOGENATE (Antihemophilic Factor [Recombinant]). This includes treatment of bleeding in certain patients with inhibitors to FVIII. In clinical studies of KOGENATE, some patients who developed inhibitors on study continued to manifest a clinical response when inhibitor titers were less than 10 Bethesda Units (B.U.) per mL. When an inhibitor is present, the dosage requirement for FVIII is variable. The dosage can be determined only by clinical response and by monitoring of circulating FVIII levels after treatment (see Dosage and Administration).

KOGENATE FS does not contain von Willebrand Factor and therefore, is not indicated for the treatment of von Willebrand disease.

Geriatrics (>65 years of age): Clinical studies with KOGENATE FS did not include sufficient numbers of patients aged 65 and over to be able to determine whether they respond differently from younger patients. However, clinical experience with KOGENATE and other FVIII products has not identified differences between the elderly and younger patients. As with any patient receiving KOGENATE FS, dose selection for an elderly patient should be individualized.

Pediatrics (<18 years of age): KOGENATE FS is appropriate for use in pediatric patients. Safety and efficacy studies have been performed in two studies (n=60) in less than 4 year old previously untreated and minimally treated pediatric patients.

CONTRAINDICATIONS:

- Patients who are hypersensitive to this drug or to any ingredient in the formulation or component of the container. For a complete listing, see Dosage Forms, Composition and Packaging.
- Known hypersensitivity to mouse or hamster protein.

WARNINGS AND PRECAUTIONS:

Serious Warnings and Precautions

The development of circulating neutralizing antibodies to FVIII may occur during the treatment of patients with hemophilia A (see Warnings and Precautions, Immune).

General: KOGENATE FS (Antihemophilic Factor [Recombinant]) is intended for the treatment of bleeding disorders arising from a deficiency in FVIII. This deficiency should be proven prior to administering KOGENATE FS.

Reconstitution, product administration, and handling of the administration set and needles must be done with caution. Percutaneous puncture with a needle contaminated with blood can transmit infectious viruses including HIV (AIDS) and hepatitis. Obtain immediate medical attention if injury occurs. Place needles in a sharps container after single use. Discard all equipment, including any reconstituted KOGENATE FS product in an appropriate container.

Immune: The development of circulating neutralizing antibodies to FVIII may occur during the treatment of patients with hemophilia A. Inhibitor formation is especially common in young children with severe hemophilia during their first years of treatment or in patients of any age who have received little previous treatment with FVIII. Nonetheless, inhibitor formation may occur at any time in the treatment of a patient with hemophilia A. Patients treated with any rFVIII preparation, including rFVIII-FS, should be carefully monitored for the development of antibodies to rFVIII by appropriate clinical observation and laboratory tests, according to the recommendation of the patient's hemophilia treatment center. In a clinical study about the use of continuous infusion in surgeries, heparin was used to prevent thrombophlebitis at the infusion site, as with any other long-term intravenous infusions.

Among patients treated with antihemophilic factor products, cases of hypotension, urticaria, and chest tightness in association with hypersensitivity reactions have been reported in the literature. Very rare cases of allergic and anaphylactic reactions have been reported with the predecessor product KOGENATE (Antihemophilic Factor [Recombinant]), particularly in very young patients or patients who have previously reacted to other FVIII products (see Adverse Reactions, Post-Market Adverse Drug Reactions). Serious anaphylactic reactions require immediate emergency treatment with resuscitative measures such as the administration of epinephrine and oxygen.

In clinical studies, KOGENATE FS has been used in the treatment of bleeding episodes in 37 previously untreated patients (PUPs) and 23 minimally treated pediatric patients ([MTP], defined as having equal to or less than 4 exposure days). Bleeding episodes were treated effectively with 1 or 2 infusions of rFVIII-FS. Overall, 9 out of 60 (15%) patients developed inhibitors. This included 5 out of 37 (14%) PUPs and 4 out of 23 (17%) MTPs treated with KOGENATE FS; overall 6 out of 60 (10%) with a titer above 10 BU and 3 out of 60 (5%) with a titer below 10 BU. The median number of exposure days at the time of inhibitor detection in these patients was 9 days (range: 3-18 days).

The median number of exposure days in the clinical studies was 114 (range: 4-478). Four of the five patients, who had not achieved 20 exposure days at the end of the study, ultimately achieved more than 20 exposure days in poststudy follow-up and 1 of them developed a low titer inhibitor. The fifth patient was lost to follow-up.

Formation of Antibodies to Mouse and Hamster Protein: Assays to detect seroconversion to mouse and hamster protein were conducted on all patients in clinical studies. None of the patients developed specific antibodies to these proteins following study enrollment and no animal protein associated serious allergic reactions have been observed with rFVIII-FS infusions. Although no such reactions were observed, patients should be made aware of the possibility of a hypersensitivity reaction to mouse and/or hamster protein and alerted to the early signs of such a reaction (eg, hives, localized or generalized urticaria, wheezing, and hypotension). Patients should be advised to discontinue use of the product and contact their physician if such symptoms occur.

Special Populations: Pregnant Women: Animal reproduction studies have not been conducted with KOGENATE FS. It is also not known whether KOGENATE FS can cause fetal harm when administered to a pregnant woman or whether it affects reproduction capacity. KOGENATE FS should not be used during pregnancy unless the benefits clearly outweigh any potential risks. As the disease almost exclusively affects males, no females have been included in clinical studies.

Nursing Women: KOGENATE FS should not be used during lactation unless the benefits clearly outweigh any potential risks.

Geriatrics (>65 years of age): Clinical studies with KOGENATE FS did not include sufficient numbers of patients aged 65 and over to be able to determine whether they respond differently from younger patients. However, clinical experience with KOGENATE and other FVIII products has not identified differences between the elderly and younger patients. As with any patient receiving KOGENATE FS, dose selection for an elderly patient should be individualized.

Pediatrics (<18 years of age): KOGENATE FS is appropriate for use in pediatric patients. Safety and efficacy studies have been performed in two studies (n=60) in less than 4 year old previously untreated and minimally treated pediatric patients.

According to a published study, children in comparison to adults present higher FVIII clearance values and thus lower recovery of FVIII, which may be explained by differences in pharmacokinetics. This information should be taken into account when dosing or following FVIII levels in such a population (see Dosage and Administration, Dosing Considerations).

Monitoring and Laboratory Tests: The clinical effect of KOGENATE FS is the most important element in evaluating the effectiveness of treatment. It may be necessary to administer more KOGENATE FS than would be estimated in order to attain satisfactory clinical results. If the calculated dose fails to attain the expected FVIII levels or if bleeding is not controlled after administration of the calculated dosage, the presence of a circulating inhibitor in the patient should be suspected. Its presence should be substantiated and the inhibitor level quantitated by appropriate laboratory tests. When an inhibitor is present, the dosage requirement for rFVIII-FS is extremely variable and the dosage can be determined only by the clinical response.

ADVERSE REACTIONS: Adverse Drug Reaction Overview: During the clinical studies conducted in previously treated patients ([PTPs], defined as having more than 100 exposure days), 451 adverse events were reported in the course of 24 936 infusions (1.8%). Only 24 events in 13 patients were considered to be at least remotely related to rFVIII-FS administration (0.1%, relative to the number of infusions). In clinical studies with 73 PTPs, one patient had a pre-existing inhibitor. In the other 72 patients, followed over four years, no de novo inhibitors were observed.

Table 1: KOGENATE FS

Adverse Events in PTPs With an Established Relationship to KOGENATE FS, FVIII Products, or Parenterally Administered Proteins

System Organ Class Adverse Event	Number of Patients with AE (%) (Total Number of Patients=73)	AE per Infusion (%) (Total Number of Infusions=24 936)
General Disorders and Administration Site Conditions		
Infusion site reactions	3 (4.1)	0.01
Skin and Subcutaneous Tissue Disorders		
Rash, Pruritus	6 (8.2)	0.02

In clinical studies with previously untreated patients (PUPs) and minimally treated (MTPs) pediatric patients, 726 adverse events were reported in the course of 9389 infusions (7.7%). These included the expected complication of inhibitor development in 9 patients (see Warnings and Precautions, Immune).

Table 2: KOGENATE FS

Adverse Events in PUPs/MTPs With an Established Relationship to KOGENATE FS, FVIII Products, or Parenterally Administered Proteins

System Organ Class Adverse Event	Number of Patients with AE (%) (Total number of patients=61)	AE per Infusion (%) (Total number of infusions=9389)
Blood and Lymphatic System Disorders		
Factor VIII inhibition	9 (15)[a]	N/A
General Disorders and Administration Site Conditions		
Infusion site reactions	4 (6.6)	0.04
Skin and Subcutaneous Tissues Disorders		
Rash, Pruritus	10 (16.4)	0.01

[a] Denominator for de novo inhibitors is N=60 since one patient had a preexisting inhibitor.

Post-Market Adverse Drug Reactions: The following adverse reactions have been identified during postapproval use of KOGENATE FS. Because these reactions are reported voluntarily from a population of uncertain size, it is not always possible to reliably estimate their frequency or establish a causal relationship to drug exposure.

Among patients treated with KOGENATE FS, rare cases of serious allergic/hypersensitivity reactions (which may include facial swelling, flushing, hives, blood pressure decrease, nausea, rash, restlessness, shortness of breath, tachycardia, tightness of the chest, tingling, urticaria, and vomiting,) have been reported, particularly in very young patients or patients who had previously reacted to other FVIII concentrates.

In extensive post-registration studies with KOGENATE FS involving more than 1000 patients, the following was observed: less than 0.2% PTPs developed de novo inhibitors. In a subset defined as having less than 20 exposure days at study entry, less than 11% developed de novo inhibitors. See Table 3.

Table 3: KOGENATE FS

Post-Market Adverse Drug Reactions

System Organ Class	Adverse Event
Blood and Lymphatic System Disorders	FVIII inhibition
Skin and Subcutaneous Tissue Disorders[a]	Pruritus, urticaria, rash
General Disorders and Administration Site Conditions[a]	Infusion site reaction Pyrexia
Immune System Disorders	Anaphylactic reaction, other hypersensitivity signs and symptoms

[a] One patient may have reported more than one event.

Since the launch of KOGENATE/KOGENATE FS, no confirmed cases of viral transmission have been reported.

DRUG INTERACTIONS: Drug-Drug Interactions: KOGENATE FS is a recombinant version of FVIII, a physiological human protein. Besides the known interactions of FVIII with other coagulation proteins, no other interactions with other drugs have been established.

Drug-Food Interactions: Interactions with food have not been established.

Drug-Herb Interactions: Interactions with herbal preparations have not been established.

Drug-Laboratory Test Interactions: There are no known laboratory interactions.

DOSAGE AND ADMINISTRATION: Dosing Considerations: Each bottle of KOGENATE FS (Antihemophilic Factor [Recombinant]) has the rFVIII-FS potency in international units stated on the label based on the one-stage assay methodology. The reconstituted product must be administered intravenously by direct syringe injection. The product must be administered within 3 hours after reconstitution. It is recommended to use the administration set provided to minimize losses of product due to adsorption and volume retention. KOGENATE FS should not be mixed with other medicinal products or infusion solutions.

According to a published study, children in comparison to adults present higher FVIII clearance values and thus lower recovery of FVIII which may be explained by differences in pharmacokinetics. This information should be taken into account when dosing or following FVIII levels in such a population.

Recommended Dose and Dosage Adjustment: The dosages described below are presented as general guidance. It should be emphasized that the dosage of KOGENATE FS required for hemostasis must be individualized according to the needs of the patient, the severity of the deficiency, the severity of the hemorrhage, the presence of inhibitors and the FVIII level desired. It is often critical to follow the course of therapy with FVIII level assays.

The clinical effect of KOGENATE FS is the most important element in evaluating the effectiveness of treatment. It may be necessary to administer more KOGENATE FS than would be estimated in order to attain satisfactory clinical results.

It has been shown in a clinical study performed in 14 adults with severe hemophilia A (≤1% FVIII:C) undergoing a major surgery that KOGENATE FS can be used for continuous infusion in surgeries (pre- and postoperative). In this study, heparin was used to prevent thrombophlebitis at the infusion site, as with any other long-term intravenous infusions. For the calculation of the initial infusion rate, clearance can be obtained by performing a presurgery decay curve, or by starting from an average population value (3.0-3.5 mL/h/kg) and then adjusting accordingly.

Infusion rate (in IU/kg/h)=Clearance (in mL/h/kg)×desired factor VIII level (in IU/mL).

Continuous infusion, clinical, and in vitro stability has been demonstrated using ambulatory pumps with a polyvinyl chloride (PVC) reservoir. KOGENATE FS contains low levels of polysorbate-80 as an excipient, which is known to increase the rate of di-(2-ethylhexyl) phthalate (DEHP) extraction from PVC materials. This should be considered for a continuous infusion administration (see Reconstitution, For Continuous Infusion).

If the calculated dose fails to attain the expected FVIII levels or if bleeding is not controlled after administration of the calculated dosage, the presence of a circulating inhibitor in the patient should be suspected. Its presence should be substantiated and the inhibitor level quantitated by appropriate laboratory tests. When an inhibitor is present, the dosage requirement for rFVIII-FS is extremely variable and the dosage can be determined only by the clinical response.

Some patients with low titer inhibitors (<10 B.U.) can be successfully treated with rFVIII-FS without a resultant anamnestic rise in inhibitor titer. Factor VIII levels and clinical response to treatment must be assessed to ensure adequate response. Use of alternative treatment products, such as Factor IX Complex products, Antihemophilic Factor (Porcine), recombinant Factor VIIa or Activated Procoagulant Protein may be necessary for patients with anamnestic responses to FVIII treatment and/or high titer inhibitors.

Calculation of Dosage: The in vivo percent increase in FVIII level can be estimated by multiplying the dose of rFVIII-FS per kilogram of body weight (IU/kg) by 2%. This method of calculation is based on clinical findings by Abildgaard et al and is illustrated in the following examples.

Equation 1—Calculation of KOGENATE FS Dosage (Expected % FVIII Increase):

$$\text{Expected \% FVIII increase} = \frac{\text{\# units administered} \times 2\%/\text{IU/kg}}{\text{body weight (kg)}}$$

$$\text{Example for a 70 kg adult:} \quad \frac{1400\ \text{IU} \times 2\%/\text{IU/kg}}{70\ \text{kg}} = 40\%$$

Equation 2—Calculation of KOGENATE FS Dosage (Dosage Required):

$$\text{Dosage required (IU)} = \frac{\text{body weight (kg)} \times \text{desired \% FVIII increase}}{2\%/\text{IU/kg}}$$

$$\text{Example for a 15 kg child:} \quad \frac{15\ \text{kg} \times 100\%}{2\ \%/\text{IU/kg}} = 750\ \text{IU required}$$

The dosage necessary to achieve hemostasis depends upon the type and severity of the bleeding episode, according to the following general guidelines (see Table 4).

Table 4: KOGENATE FS

Dosage Necessary to Achieve Hemostasis

Hemorrhagic Event	Therapeutically Necessary Plasma Level of FVIII Activity	Dosage Necessary to Maintain the Therapeutic Plasma Level
Minor Hemorrhage (superficial, early hemorrhages, hemorrhages into joints)	20–40%	10–20 IU per kg Repeat dose if evidence of further bleeding.
Moderate to Major Hemorrhage (hemorrhages into muscles, hemorrhages into the oral cavity, definite hemarthroses, known trauma)	30–60%	15–30 IU per kg Repeat one dose at 12–24 hours if needed.
Surgery (minor surgical procedures)		
Major to Life-Threatening Hemorrhage (intracranial, intra-abdominal or intra thoracic hemorrhages, gastrointestinal bleeding, central nervous system bleeding, bleeding in the retro pharyngeal or retro peritoneal spaces or iliopsoas sheath)	80–100%	Initial dose 40–50 IU per kg Repeat dose 20–25 IU per kg every 8–12 hours.
Fractures		
Head Trauma		
Surgery (major surgical procedures)	~100%	a) By bolus infusions Preoperative dose 50 IU/kg. Verify ~100% activity prior to surgery. Repeat as necessary after 6 to 12 hours initially and for 10 to 14 days until healing is complete. b) By continuous infusion Raise factor VIII activity presurgery with an initial bolus infusion and immediately follow with continuous infusion (in IU/h/kg) adjusting according to patient's daily clearance and desired factor VIII levels for at least 7 days.

Prophylaxis: FVIII products may also be administered on a regular schedule for prophylaxis of bleeding, as reported by Nilsson et al. In children, the recommended dose for a regular prophylaxis schedule is 25 IU/kg of body weight every other day.

Immune Tolerance: FVIII products have been administered to patients on a high dose schedule in order to induce immune tolerance to FVIII, which resulted in disappearance of the inhibitor activity. There is currently no consensus among treaters to the optimal treatment schedule.

Administration: KOGENATE FS (Antihemophilic Factor [Recombinant]) supplied with BIO-SET Needle-less Reconstitution Set is a self-contained system that prevents needlestick injuries during reconstitution (see Warnings and Precautions, General).

Rate of Administration: Data from clinical trials, including patients between 0-68 years old, shows that the entire dose is administered in a median of 5 minutes. The rate of administration, however, should be adapted to the response of each patient.

KOGENATE FS can be infused by continuous infusion. The infusion rate should be calculated based on the clearance and the desired FVIII level. In a clinical study performed in 14 adults with severe hemophilia A (≤1% FVIII:C) who underwent a major surgery, the range of infusion rates for KOGENATE FS was 0.2 to 3.6 mL/h. Example: For a 75 kg patient with a clearance of 3 mL/h/kg, the initial infusion rate would be 3 IU/h/kg to achieve a FVIII level of 100%. For calculation of mL/h, multiply infusion rate in IU/h/kg by kg bw/concentration of solution (IU/mL).

Table 5: KOGENATE FS

Calculation of Infusion Rate Based on Clearance and the Desired FVIII Level

Clearance: 3 mL/h/kg	Desired Plasma FVIII Level	Infusion Rate, IU/h/kg	Infusion Rate for 75 kg Patient, mL/h		
			Concentrations of rFVIII Solution		
			100 IU/mL	200 IU/mL	400 IU/mL
	100% (1 IU/mL)	3.0	2.25	1.125	0.56
	60% (0.6 IU/mL)	1.8	1.35	0.68	0.34
	40% (0.4 IU/mL)	1.2	0.9	0.45	0.225

Higher infusion rates may be required in conditions with accelerated clearance during major bleeds and extensive tissue damage during surgical interventions. Subsequent infusion rates should be calculated based on the actual FVIII levels and recalculated clearance for each day post surgery based on the equation: clearance=infusion rate/actual FVIII level.

Reconstitution: Parenteral Products: KOGENATE FS powder should only be reconstituted with the supplied diluent (2.5 or 5.0 mL Sterile Water for Injection) using the supplied sterile transfer device. Reconstitution and dilution should be performed in accordance with good practices rules, particularly with attention to asepsis. Always work on a clean surface and wash your hands before performing the following procedures:

1. Warm the unopened diluent (as needed) and the product to room temperature not to exceed 37°C.
2. Remove the cap from the concentrate. Take out the diluent prefilled syringe and remove the tip cap.
3. Connect the diluent prefilled syringe to the product vial by gently screwing on to the BIO-SET connection.
4. Place the vial on a rigid, non-skid surface and hold it firmly with one hand. With the other hand, strongly press down the fingerplate near the syringe tip using your thumb and index finger until the fingerplate meets the top edge of the BIO-SET. This confirms that the system is activated.

5. Grasp the plunger rod by the top plate and remove from protective packaging. **Avoid touching the sides and threads of the plunger rod.** Immediately screw plunger rod into the syringe rubber stopper.
6. Inject the diluent into the product by pushing down the plunger rod slowly.
7. Swirl gently until completely dissolved without creating excessive foaming.
8. Parenteral drug products should be inspected visually for particulate matter and discoloration prior to administration, whenever solution and container permit.
9. Invert vial/syringe and transfer the solution into syringe that was used to deliver the diluent. Ensure that the entire contents of the reconstituted KOGENATE FS vial are drawn into the syringe.
10. Unscrew the filled syringe to disconnect it from the empty concentrate vial.

For Bolus Injection:

11. Attach the filled syringe to the administration set (made with microbore tubing) provided and immediately inject intravenously. **Note:** Firmly grasp one or both wings of the administration set to perform venipuncture; do not use the post-use needle shield for this purpose. Use of other administration sets without microbore tubing may result in a larger retention of the solution within the administration set.
12. After infusion, lock post-use needle shield in place using one of the following methods:
    a. One-hand technique: Hold tubing in hand and advance needle shield with thumb and index finger until locked over needle tip.
    b. Two-hand technique: Hold wing stationary and slide needle shield forward with other hand until locked over needle tip.
13. If the same patient is to receive more than one bottle, the diluent syringe provided should be used to reconstitute the powder in the product vials as described above. The reconstituted solutions should then be combined in a larger plastic syringe (not provided) and administered as usual.

Table 6: KOGENATE FS

Reconstitution of Parenteral Products

Vial Size	Volume of Diluent to be Added to Vial	Approximate Available Volume	Nominal Concentration per mL
250 IU	2.5 mL	2.5 mL	100 IU/ mL
500 IU	2.5 mL	2.5 mL	200 IU/mL
1000 IU	2.5 mL	2.5 mL	400 IU/mL
2000 IU	5.0 mL	5.0 mL	400 IU/mL
3000 IU	5.0 mL	5.0 mL	600 IU/mL

For Continuous Infusion: Reconstitute KOGENATE FS according to Steps 1-10 above. Continuous infusion of KOGENATE FS must employ an infusion pump that can provide continuous delivery, deal with low volumes and low infusion speeds. Technical instructions of the pump manufacturer, including the devices to be used, should be followed. The reservoir of the pump should be filled under aseptic conditions and the reservoir and tubing should be changed at least every 24 hours. During in vitro studies, reconstituted product for continuous infusion was shown to be stable for 24 hours at temperatures up to 30°C. This should be kept in mind if the continuous infusion is not intended to be started immediately after reconstitution. In a clinical study performed in 14 adults with severe hemophilia A (≤1% FVIII:C) undergoing a major surgery, a minute amount of heparin was added to the infusion solution (final concentration of 5 U/mL) in order to prevent local thrombophlebitis at the site of the infusion. Refer to Table 5 for infusion rates.

Note: KOGENATE FS reconstituted with 2.5 or 5.0 mL Sterile Water for Injection should not be further diluted for continuous infusion.

OVERDOSAGE:

No symptoms of overdose have been reported.

For management of a suspected drug overdose, CPhA recommends that you contact your **regional Poison Control Centre**. See the *CPS* Directory section for a list of Poison Control Centres.

ACTION AND CLINICAL PHARMACOLOGY: Mechanism of Action: See Indications and Clinical Use.

Pharmacodynamics: The activated partial thromboplastin time (aPTT) is prolonged in people with hemophilia. Determination of aPTT is a conventional in vitro assay for biological activity of factor VIII. Treatment with KOGENATE FS normalizes the aPTT over the effective dosing period.

Pharmacokinetics: Initial pharmacokinetic studies were conducted in 35 patients, with severe hemophilia A.

Absorption: Not applicable. KOGENATE FS is administered directly into the blood stream by IV injection.

Distribution: No specific distribution studies have been performed, **however** after administration of KOGENATE FS (Antihemophilic Factor [Recombinant]), peak factor VIII activity decreases by a two-phase exponential decay. This is similar to that of plasma-derived factor VIII. KOGENATE FS binds to its natural protein carrier vWF and is mostly confined into the vascular space.

Metabolism: KOGENATE FS is metabolized as it produces its biological activity during the activation of the coagulation cascade.

Excretion: After administration of KOGENATE FS (Antihemophilic Factor [Recombinant]), peak factor VIII activity decreased by a two-phase exponential decay with a mean terminal half-life of about 15 hours. This is similar to that of plasma-derived factor VIII which has a mean terminal half-life of approximately 13 hours. The half-life data for rFVIII-FS were unchanged after 24 weeks of exclusive treatment, indicating continued efficacy and no evidence of FVIII inhibition.

Duration of Effect: The duration of effect is variable and dependent on the individual patient, the severity of the bleed and the clinical situation.

STORAGE AND STABILITY: KOGENATE FS (Antihemophilic Factor [Recombinant]) should be stored under refrigeration (2-8°C). Do not use beyond the expiration date indicated on the bottle. Storage of lyophilized powder at room temperature (up to 25°C) for 3 months, such as in home storage situations, may be done. If the product is stored outside the refrigerator, please add the date removed from refrigeration and note a new expiry date on the carton and vial. The new expiry date should be 3 months from the date product is removed from the refrigerator, or the previously stamped expiry date, whichever is shorter. Once product is removed from refrigeration, it cannot be returned to the refrigerator. Freezing must be avoided. Protect from extreme exposure to light and store the lyophilized powder in the carton prior to use.

After reconstitution, the product should be used immediately (within 3 hours) for direct syringe injection. For continuous infusion, stability has been demonstrated for 24 hours at 30°C.

SPECIAL HANDLING INSTRUCTIONS: Not applicable.

INFORMATION FOR THE PATIENT: Published in e-CPS, available by subscription at www.e-cps.ca.

DOSAGE FORMS, COMPOSITION AND PACKAGING: KOGENATE FS (Antihemophilic Factor [Recombinant]) is supplied in the following single use bottles and with a BIO-SET Needle-less Reconstitution Set. A prefilled diluent syringe containing Sterile Water for Injection, EP for reconstitution, a sterile administration set, two alcohol swabs, one sterile bandage, and one sterile cotton pad are also provided (see Table 7).

Table 7: KOGENATE FS

Vial Sizes

Product Code	Approximate Factor VIII Activity	Diluent
08950035	250 IU	2.5 mL
08950043	500 IU	2.5 mL
08950051	1000 IU	2.5 mL
80185600	2000 IU	5.0 mL
80959096	3000 IU	5.0 mL

(cont'd)

Table 7: KOGENATE FS *(cont'd)*

Each vial of KOGENATE FS contains the labelled amount of rFVIII in international units (IU). One IU, as defined by the World Health Organization standard for blood coagulation FVIII, human, is approximately equal to the level of FVIII activity found in 1 mL of fresh pooled human plasma. The final product, when reconstituted as directed, contains the following nonmedicinal ingredients: calcium chloride, chloride, glycine, histidine, polysorbate 80, sodium and sucrose (0.9-1.3%/250 IU, 500 IU, 1000 IU Vial Size; 0.9-1.2%/2000 IU, 3000 IU Vial Size). The product contains no preservative. KOGENATE FS must be administered by the intravenous route.

Kwellada-P® Creme Rinse

permethrin

Topical Pediculicide—Ovicide

GlaxoSmithKline Consumer Healthcare

PHARMACOLOGY: Permethrin, a synthetic pyrethroid, has a broad spectrum of insecticidal activity combined with high potency when applied topically to insects, including head lice, Pediculus capitis.

Like other pyrethroids, permethrin is a sodium channel toxin. In susceptible nerve cells small amounts of permethrin cause a change in the kinetics of the sodium channel. Although the activation of the sodium current is unaffected, the rate of inactivation of the current is greatly slowed. This tail current, even at low doses, is adequate to cause repetitive activity. One normal action potential, in the presence of permethrin, leads to a series of abnormal action potentials. Consequently, there is repetitive firing of the neuron.

Studies, both in vitro and in vivo, have demonstrated that permethrin is active against both the adults and eggs of head lice. In clinical trials 1% permethrin was found to be an efficacious treatment for head lice. After 1 treatment, over 98% of patients were free of head lice at 7 days and over 93% of patients were free of lice at 14 days, indicating that permethrin continues to exert activity after treatment. In the same study, fewer than 2% of patients had viable eggs 7 days after a single application of 1% permethrin creme rinse and at 14 days less than 4% of patients had viable eggs.

INDICATIONS: For the treatment of Pediculus capitis, including adults, nymphs and eggs. One application is usually adequate to eradicate the infestation of head lice. Should reinfestation occur, or the first application not completely eradicate the head lice, a second treatment should be administered 7 days after the initial treatment.

CONTRAINDICATIONS: Patients with a known sensitivity or reaction to permethrin, any synthetic pyrethroid or pyrethrins, or to chrysanthemums.

WARNINGS: Should be discontinued if hypersensitivity occurs.

PRECAUTIONS: General: If permethrin creme rinse comes in contact with the eyes it can cause irritation. If this occurs, the eyes should be rinsed. During a head lice infestation the scalp and surrounding skin are often irritated resulting in erythema, edema and frequently pruritus. These symptoms can be exacerbated after treatment.

Children: Permethrin creme rinse is safe and efficacious in children over 2 years of age. The safety and efficacy of permethrin has not been established in children under the age of 2 years.

Pregnancy: Safety has not been established during controlled clinical trials for use in pregnant women. Permethrin creme rinse should be used when the expected benefits outweigh the potential risks.

Lactation: Because it is not known whether permethrin is excreted during lactation, consideration should be given to discontinuing nursing during treatment with permethrin creme rinse or withholding treatment if it is not possible to discontinue nursing.

ADVERSE EFFECTS: Clinical trials have indicated that adverse reactions are reported infrequently. Adverse reactions which do occur are usually mild and resolve rapidly. They are local in nature.

In clinical trials pruritus was the most frequently reported adverse event with fewer than 3% of patients reporting it. The next most frequently reported adverse event was burning and stinging followed by erythema, which was reported by less than 1% of patients.

OVERDOSE:

Symptoms: There has been no incidence of ingestion of permethrin creme rinse.

Treatment: If permethrin creme rinse is ingested, gastric lavage can be initiated.

For management of a suspected drug overdose, CPhA recommends that you contact your **regional Poison Control Centre**. See the *CPS* Directory section for a list of Poison Control Centres.

DOSAGE: After the hair has been shampooed, rinsed and towelled dry, apply enough creme rinse to saturate the hair and scalp, between 25 to 50 mL. Leave on for 10 minutes. The creme rinse should then be thoroughly rinsed off with water and the hair towelled dry. Nits can be combed out with the comb provided, if desired.

One treatment is usually adequate to eliminate the head lice.

Kwellada-P should be shaken before use.

INFORMATION FOR THE PATIENT: Published in e-CPS, available by subscription at www.e-cps.ca.

SUPPLIED: Each mL of creme rinse liquid contains: permethrin 1% w/w cis/trans ratio of 25:75. Nonmedicinal ingredients: carbomer 980, isopropyl alcohol, lauryl alcohol, polyoxyethylene 4 lauryl ether, polyquarternium-24, propylene glycol, purified water, stearalkonium chloride and trolamine. Plastic bottles of 50 and 200 mL. Store between 15 and 30°C.

Kwellada-P® Lotion

permethrin

Topical Scabicide

GlaxoSmithKline Consumer Healthcare

PHARMACOLOGY: Permethrin, a synthetic pyrethroid, has a broad spectrum of insecticidal activity combined with high potency when applied topically to insects.

Like other pyrethroids, permethrin is a sodium channel toxin. In susceptible nerve cells small amounts of permethrin cause a change in the kinetics of the sodium channel. Although the activation of the sodium current in unaffected, the rate of inactivation of the current is greatly slowed. This tail current, even at low doses, is adequate to cause repetitive activity. One normal action potential, in the presence of permethrin, leads to a series of abnormal action potentials. Consequently, there is a repetitive firing of the neuron.

Clinical studies have demonstrated that permethrin is active against (*S. scabiei*), scabies. In clinical trials 5% permethrin was found to be an effective treatment for scabies. After one application of 5% permethrin lotion 93% of patients were cured at 28 days. At the interim assessment at 14 days 37% were already cured and 61% were improving.

Only a very minimal amount of permethrin is absorbed when applied topically. In a bioavailability study it was determined that <0.032% of a topically applied dose of 5% permethrin lotion was absorbed.

INDICATIONS: For the treatment of scabies (*S. scabiei*). One application is usually adequate to eradicate the infestation of scabies. If new lesions appear or live scabies mites are seen, a second treatment can occur 7 to 10 days after the initial treatment.

CONTRAINDICATIONS: Patients with a known sensitivity or reaction to permethrin, any synthetic pyrethroid or pyrethrins or to chrysanthemums.

WARNINGS: Permethrin should be discontinued if hypersensitivity occurs.

PRECAUTIONS: General: If permethrin lotion comes in contact with the eyes it can cause irritation. If this occurs, the eyes should be rinsed. During a scabies infestation the skin is often irritated resulting in erythema, edema and pruritus. These symptoms can be temporarily exacerbated after treatment, with pruritus often persisting for several weeks after treatment.

Children: Permethrin lotion is efficacious in children over 2 months of age. The safety and efficacy of permethrin has not been established in children under the age of 2 months.

Pregnancy: Safety has not been established during controlled clinical trials for use in pregnant women. Permethrin should be used when the expected benefits outweigh the potential risks.

Lactation: Because it is not known whether permethrin is excreted during lactation, consideration should be given to discontinuing nursing during treatment with permethrin lotion or withholding treatment if it is not possible to discontinue nursing.

ADVERSE EFFECTS: Clinical trials have indicated that adverse reactions are reported infrequently. Adverse reactions which do occur are usually mild and resolve rapidly. They are local in nature.

In clinical trials burning, stinging and tingling were the most frequently reported adverse events with fewer than 1% of patients reporting them. The next most frequently reported event was pruritus followed by erythema which was reported by less than 0.02% of patients. Pruritus is not considered to be an adverse reaction to permethrin because pruritus characteristically remains for several weeks after successful treatment. The itching gradually subsides with the natural loss of the upper layer of skin.

OVERDOSE:

Symptoms: There has been no incidence of ingestion of permethrin lotion.

Treatment: If permethrin lotion is accidently ingested, vomiting can be induced.

For management of a suspected drug overdose, CPhA recommends that you contact your **regional Poison Control Centre**. See the *CPS* Directory section for a list of Poison Control Centres.

DOSAGE: Prior to application the skin should be clean, dry and cool. A hot bath should not be taken prior to treatment. The lotion should be thoroughly massaged into the skin from the neck to the soles of the feet, paying particular attention to the areas between fingers and toes, under the fingernails and toenails, wrists, armpits, genital area and buttocks. Permethrin lotion disappears when rubbed gently into the skin; therefore, it is not necessary for the patient to apply the medication until it remains detectable on the skin. If the hands are washed with soap and water during the treatment period, permethrin lotion should be reapplied.

The patient should put on clean clothes and leave the lotion in place for 12 to 14 hours. The lotion should then be thoroughly washed off during a shower or bath. Patients should again change into clean clothes.

One treatment is usually adequate to eliminate the scabies. However, if live scabies mites are present or new skin lesions appear a second application can be given 7 to 10 days later.

Permethrin should be shaken before use.

INFORMATION FOR THE PATIENT: Published in e-CPS, available by subscription at www.e-cps.ca.

SUPPLIED: Each mL of lotion contains: permethrin 5% (w/w) cis-trans. Nonmedicinal ingredients: carbomer 980, edetate disodium, imidurea, methylparaben, polysorbate 20, propylene glycol, propylparaben, purified water, sorbitan monolaurate and sodium hydroxide. Plastic bottles of 50 and 200 mL. Store between 15 and 30°C.

Kytril® Ⓟ

granisetron HCl

Antiemetic

Roche

Date of Preparation: February 7, 2001
Date of Revision: October 29, 2009

SUMMARY PRODUCT INFORMATION:

Route of Administration	Dosage Form/Strength	Nonmedicinal Ingredients
Oral	Tablets, 1 mg and 2 mg	Hydroxypropyl methylcellulose, lactose, magnesium stearate, microcrystalline cellulose, sodium starch glycollate and Opadry YS-1-18027-A (hypromellose, titanium dioxide, macrogol 400, and polysorbate 80). **Contains lactose.**
I.V. injection	1 mL and 4 mL vials, 1 mg/mL injection	Sodium chloride, benzyl alcohol, citric acid monohydrate, water for injection and hydrochloric acid and/or sodium hydroxide for pH adjustment. **Contains benzyl alcohol.**

INDICATIONS AND CLINICAL USE: KYTRIL (granisetron hydrochloride) is indicated for:

Adults:

- The prevention of nausea and vomiting associated with emetogenic cancer chemotherapy, including high dose cisplatin;
- The prevention of nausea and vomiting associated with radiation, including total body irradiation and fractionated abdominal radiation;
- The prevention and treatment of postoperative nausea and vomiting. As with other antiemetics, routine prophylaxis is not recommended in patients in whom there is little expectation that nausea and/or vomiting will occur postoperatively. In patients where nausea and/or vomiting must be avoided during the postoperative period, KYTRIL Injection is recommended even where the incidence of postoperative nausea and/or vomiting is low.

Geriatrics (>65 years of age): Chemotherapy-induced and Radiation-induced Nausea and Vomiting : Safety and efficacy of KYTRIL appear to be similar to that observed in younger adults (see Warnings and Precautions and Dosage and Administration).

Post-Operative Nausea and Vomiting: Clinical experience in the use of KYTRIL in the prevention and treatment of post-operative nausea and vomiting is limited and it is not indicated for use in this population (see Warnings and Precautions and Dosage and Administration).

Pediatrics: Safety and efficacy of KYTRIL has not been adequately studied in children or adolescents under 18 years of age and it is not indicated for use in this population (see Warnings and Precautions and Dosage and Administration).

CONTRAINDICATIONS:

- KYTRIL (granisetron hydrochloride) is contraindicated in patients with a known hypersensitivity to the drug or to any component of its formulations.

WARNINGS AND PRECAUTIONS: Carcinogenesis and Mutagenesis: KYTRIL (granisetron hydrochloride) has been associated with an increased occurrence of hepatocellular tumours in carcinogenicity studies performed in rodents at doses in excess of the recommended human dose. Although the clinical significance of these findings has not been determined, the use of this drug should be restricted to the treatment of nausea and vomiting in patients undergoing emetogenic cancer chemotherapy. The recommended dosage of KYTRIL should not be exceeded.

Granisetron was administered to rats in the diet in a 24 month carcinogenicity study. The incidence of hepatocellular carcinomas and adenomas was significantly increased in male rats treated at doses of 5 mg/kg/day and in rats of both sexes treated with 25 mg/kg/day. No increase in the rate of occurrence of liver tumours was observed in the 1 mg/kg/day treatment group (100 times the recommended human dose given intravenously).

In another 24 month carcinogenicity study, mice were administered granisetron in the diet at doses of 1, 5, and 50 mg/kg/day. There was a statistically significant increase in the incidence of hepatocellular carcinomas in males and hepatocellular adenomas in females dosed with 50 mg/kg/day. No statistically significant increase in liver tumours was observed in mice at a dose of 5 mg/kg/day (500 times the recommended human dose given intravenously).

Cardiovascular: As for other 5-HT_3 antagonists, cases of ECG modifications including QT prolongation have been reported with KYTRIL. These ECG changes with KYTRIL were minor and generally not of clinical significance, specifically with no evidence of proarrhythmia. However, in patients with pre-existing arrhythmias or cardiac conduction disorders, this might lead to clinical consequences. Therefore, caution should be exercised in patients with cardiac co-morbidities, on cardio-toxic chemotherapy and/or with concomitant electrolyte abnormalities. See also Drug Interactions and Adverse Reactions, Post-Market Adverse Drug Reactions.

Gastrointestinal: KYTRIL is not a drug that stimulates gastric or intestinal peristalsis. It should not be used instead of nasogastric suction. The use of KYTRIL in patients following abdominal surgery or in patients with chemotherapy-induced nausea and vomiting may mask a progressive ileus and/or gastric distention. Patients with signs of sub-acute intestinal obstruction should be monitored following administration of KYTRIL.

Sensitivity/Resistance: Hypersensitivity reactions may occur in patients who have exhibited hypersensitivity to other selective 5-HT_3 receptor antagonists.

Special Populations: Pregnant Women: The use of KYTRIL in pregnant women has not been studied and is not recommended. Reproduction studies performed in pregnant rats given granisetron at intravenous dosages up to 9 mg/kg/day and pregnant rabbits at intravenous dosage up to 3 mg/kg/day revealed no evidence of impaired fertility or harm to the fetus due to granisetron.

Nursing Women: It is not known whether granisetron is excreted in human milk. Nursing is not recommended during treatment with KYTRIL.

Pediatrics: The safety and efficacy of KYTRIL has not been adequately studied in children or adolescents under 18 years of age (see Indications and Clinical Use and Dosage and Administration).

Geriatrics (> 65 years of age): During clinical trials, 713 patients 65 years of age or older received intravenous KYTRIL and of 325 patients 65 years of age or older who received oral KYTRIL, 298 were 65 to 74 years of age and 27 were 75 years of age or older. The efficacy and safety of KYTRIL did not appear to be age dependent (see Indications and Clinical Use and Dosage and Administration).

During postoperative nausea and vomiting clinical trials, 168 patients 65 years of age or older, of which 47 were 75 years of age or older, received KYTRIL Injection. Clinical studies of KYTRIL Injection did not include sufficient numbers of subjects aged 65 years and over to determine whether they respond differently from younger subjects. Other reported clinical experience has not identified differences in responses between the elderly and younger patients (see Indications and Clinical Use and Dosage and Administration).

Information to Be Provided to the Patient: Effect on Ability to Drive and Use Machinery: In healthy subjects, no clinically relevant effects on resting EEG or on the performance of psychometric tests were observed after i.v. KYTRIL at any dose tested (up to 200 µg/kg). There are no data on the effect of KYTRIL on the ability to drive. As there have been occasional reports of somnolence in clinical studies, patients should be advised to avoid driving a car or operating hazardous machinery until they are reasonably certain that the drug treatment does not affect them adversely.

ADVERSE REACTIONS: Because clinical trials are conducted under very specific conditions the adverse reaction rates observed in the clinical trials may not reflect the rates observed in practice and should not be compared to the rates in the clinical trials of another drug. Adverse drug reaction information from clinical trials is useful for identifying drug-related adverse events and for approximating rates.

Adverse Drug Reaction Overview: The most common adverse events reported by patients receiving intravenous or oral KYTRIL in single-day chemotherapy trials are: headache, asthenia, somnolence, diarrhea, constipation, and abdominal pain (see Table 1 for the percentages of patients with these events). The only two common adverse experiences recognized to be causally related to KYTRIL are constipation and headache.

As for other 5-HT_3 antagonists, cases of ECG modifications including QT prolongation have been reported with KYTRIL. These ECG changes with KYTRIL were minor and generally not of clinical significance, specifically with no evidence of proarrhythmia (see Warnings and Precautions, Cardiovascular, Drug Interactions, and Adverse Reactions, Post-Market Adverse Drug Reactions).

Clinical Trial Adverse Drug Reactions: Chemotherapy-induced Nausea and Vomiting: Intravenous KYTRIL was given as a single dose. Oral KYTRIL was given either as a single dose or divided dose for 1, 7, or 14 days. Patients received cancer chemotherapy which consisted primarily of cisplatin or cyclophosphamide regimens. During the 24-hour period following intravenous administration of KYTRIL, I.V. fluids were also given. Adverse events were recorded over seven days when KYTRIL was given on a single day and up to 28 days when KYTRIL was administered for 7 or 14 days. In the absence of a placebo group, the relationship of observed adverse events to treatment with KYTRIL is difficult to judge.

Table 1 gives the frequencies of the six adverse events most commonly reported by patients receiving intravenous or oral KYTRIL in single-day chemotherapy trials. This table does not include those events that are commonly associated with chemotherapy or the underlying malignant disease.

Table 1: KYTRIL

Principal Adverse Events in Clinical Trials of Single-Day Chemotherapy

	Percentage of Patients with Event Intravenous KYTRIL (10–40 µg/kg) (n=1519)	Percentage of Patients with Event Oral KYTRIL (1.0 mg b.i.d. or 2.0 mg u.i.d.) (n=1322)
Headache	14%	22%
Asthenia	5%	15%
Somnolence	4%	2%
Diarrhea	5%	8%
Constipation	4%	17%
Abdominal Pain	3%	6%

The only two common adverse experiences recognized to be causally related to KYTRIL are constipation and headache. As with other drugs of this class, rare cases of hypersensitivity reactions, sometimes severe (e.g. anaphylaxis, shortness of breath, hypotension, urticaria) have been reported.

Radiation-induced Nausea and Vomiting: In controlled clinical trials, the adverse events reported by patients receiving KYTRIL Tablets and concurrent radiation were similar to those reported by patients receiving KYTRIL Tablets prior to chemotherapy. The most frequently reported adverse events were diarrhea (25.6%), asthenia (22.0%) and constipation (15.5%). Headache (7.7%), however, was less prevalent in this patient population. Table 2 lists the adverse experiences (>5%) in patients who received KYTRIL Tablets or placebo.

Table 2: KYTRIL

Principal Adverse Events in Clinical Trials- RINV

	Percentage of Patients with Event Oral KYTRIL 1.0 mg b.i.d. (n=134)	Percentage of Patients with Event Placebo (n=128)
Diarrhea	28%	34%
Asthenia	25%	20%
Constipation	19%	5%
Abdominal Pain	11%	9%
Nausea (after 20 radiation fractions)	11%	9%

(cont'd)

Table 2: KYTRIL *(cont'd)*

Principal Adverse Events in Clinical Trials- RINV

	Percentage of Patients with Event Oral KYTRIL 1.0 mg b.i.d. (n=134)	Percentage of Patients with Event Placebo (n=128)
Decreased appetite	10%	7%
Pain	8%	4%
Headache	5%	11%

Postoperative Nausea and Vomiting: The adverse events listed in Table 3 were reported in ≥ 2% of adults receiving KYTRIL Injection 1 mg during controlled clinical trials.

Table 3: ZYTRIL

Adverse Events ≥2%

	Percent of Patients with Event	
	KYTRIL Injection 1 mg (n=267)	Placebo (n=266)
Pain	10.1	8.3
Constipation	9.4	12.0
Anemia	9.4	10.2
Headache	8.6	7.1
Fever	7.9	4.5
Abdominal Pain	6	6.0
Hepatic Enzymes Increased	5.6	4.1
Insomnia	4.9	6.0
Bradycardia	4.5	5.3
Dizziness	4.1	3.4
Leukocytosis	3.7	4.1
Anxiety	3.4	3.8
Hypotension	3.4	3.8
Diarrhea	3.4	1.1
Flatulence	3	3
Infection	3	2.3
Dyspepsia	3	1.9
Hypertension	2.6	4.1
Urinary Tract Infection	2.6	3.4
Oliguria	2.2	1.5
Coughing	2.2	1.1

In a clinical study conducted in Japan, the types of adverse events differed notably from those reported in Table 3. The adverse events in the Japanese study that occurred in ≥ 2% of patients and were more frequent with KYTRIL 1 mg than with placebo were: fever (56 to 50%), sputum increased (2.7 to 1.7%), and dermatitis (2.7 to 0%).

Less Common Clinical Trial Adverse Drug Reactions: Chemotherapy-induced Nausea and Vomiting: The safety profile of KYTRIL has been evaluated in 3269 patients receiving intravenous KYTRIL (2 to 160 µg/kg) and 2600 patients receiving oral KYTRIL (0.25-20 mg) in single-day and multiple-day clinical trials with emetogenic cancer therapies. In the listings which follow, a COSTART-based dictionary terminology has been used to classify reported adverse experiences. The frequencies presented, therefore, represent the proportion of the patients who experienced an event of the type cited on at least one occasion while receiving KYTRIL.

Experiences are further classified within body system categories and enumerated in order of decreasing frequency using the following definitions: **frequent** experiences are defined as: those occurring on one or more occasion in at least 1/100 patients; **infrequent** adverse experiences as: those occurring in less than 1/100 but at least 1/1000 patients; **rare** experiences as: those occurring in less than 1/1000 patients.

Many adverse experiences are observed in cancer chemotherapy patients. All adverse experiences are included except those for which the drug cause was remote, those reported in terms so general as to be uninformative and those already listed in Table 1.

Body as a Whole: Frequent: abdominal pain.
Infrequent: abdomen enlarged, chills, fever, malaise.
Rare: allergic reaction, chest pain.
Cardiovascular System: Infrequent: hypertension, hypotension, migraine, syncope, vasodilatation.
Rare: arrhythmia, bradycardia, palpitation, postural hypotension, tachycardia, ventricular arrhythmia, angina pectoris, and atrial fibrillation.
Gastrointestinal System: Frequent: decreased appetite.
Infrequent: dry mouth, dyspepsia, flatulence, jaundice, liver function tests abnormal [Elevation of AST and ALT (>2 times the upper limit of normal)], nausea.
Rare: gastrointestinal haemorrhage, hepatic coma, ileus, liver damage, melena, vomiting.
Hemic and Lymphatic System: Rare: coagulation time increased, eosinophilia, leukopenia, anemia, thrombocytopenia.
Metabolic and Nutritional: Infrequent: hypokalemia.
Rare: bilirubinemia, edema, hyperphosphatemia, hyponatremia.
Nervous System: Infrequent: agitation, anxiety, dizziness, drugged feeling, insomnia, nervousness, paresthesia, tremor.
Rare: coma, depersonalisation, grand mal convulsion, vertigo.
Respiratory System: Infrequent: dyspnea, hiccup.
Rare: epistaxis, rhinitis, sinusitis.
Skin and Appendages: Infrequent: pruritus, rash, sweating.
Rare: photosensitivity.
Special Searches: Rare: puncture site pain.
Special Senses: Infrequent: taste perversion.
Rare: abnormal vision.
Urogenital System: Infrequent: dysuria.
Rare: urinary incontinence.

Post-Market Adverse Drug Reactions: The post-marketing safety experience in over 4 million patients is consistent with the clinical trial safety information.

Cases of cardiac arrest, ventricular fibrillation, ventricular tachycardia, ECG QT prolonged, sudden death and syncope were reported rarely in post-marketing experience. Some reports showed temporal association with granisetron, most of them also presenting confounding factors such as concomitant medications, medical history, and/or known risk factors. The relationship to granisetron cannot be established or excluded, either as an effect of the drug alone or in combination with other factors (see Warnings and Precautions, Cardiovascular, and Drug Interactions).

DRUG INTERACTIONS: Overview: No pharmacodynamic interaction was found between single 160 µg/kg i.v. doses of granisetron and single oral doses of 2.5 mg lorazepam or 3 mg haloperidol. Pharmacokinetic interactions with these drugs were not investigated.

The pharmacokinetic characteristics of a single 40 µg/kg i.v. dose of granisetron were not significantly different whether it was administered alone or following 8 days of treatment with the hepatic enzyme inhibitor, cimetidine (200 mg q.i.d.).

Granisetron does not induce or inhibit the cytochrome P450 drug metabolizing enzyme system.

As for other 5-HT_3 antagonists, cases of ECG modifications including QT prolongation have been reported with KYTRIL. These ECG changes with KYTRIL were minor and generally not of clinical significance, specifically with no evidence of proarrhythmia. However, in patients concurrently treated with drugs known to prolong QT interval and/or are arrhythmogenic, this may lead to clinical consequences

DOSAGE AND ADMINISTRATION: Recommended Dose and Dosage Adjustment: Emetogenic Chemotherapy:
Adults: Injection: The recommended dosage of KYTRIL is 10 µg/kg infused intravenously over 5 minutes, beginning within 30 minutes before initiation of chemotherapy only on the day(s) when chemotherapy is given (see Reconstitution for dilution instructions).
Oral: The recommended dosage of oral KYTRIL is 2 mg on the day of chemotherapy. This may be administered either as a single dose (2×1 mg or 1×2 mg) one hour before chemotherapy or as a divided dose of 1 mg one hour before chemotherapy followed by a second 1 mg dose 12 hours post-chemotherapy. The need for additional doses beyond 24 hours post-chemotherapy has not been investigated.
Geriatrics: Available clinical data suggest that dosage reductions may not be necessary in this patient population (see Indications and Clinical Use and Warnings and Precautions).
Pediatrics: See Indications and Clinical Use and Warnings and Precautions.
Renally Impaired Patients: Available clinical data suggest that dosage reductions may not be necessary in this patient population.
Hepatically Impaired Patients: The clearance of KYTRIL is reduced by half in patients with hepatic impairment. The dose response of KYTRIL in patients with hepatic impairment has not been determined.
Radiation (either Total Irradiation or Fractionated Abdominal Radiation): Adults: Oral: The recommended adult dosage of oral KYTRIL is 2 mg once daily. 2×1 mg or 1×2 mg tablets are taken one hour before radiation.
Geriatrics: Available clinical data suggest that dosage reductions may not be necessary in this patient population (see Indications and Clinical Use and Warnings and Precautions).
Pediatrics: See Indications and Clinical Use and Warnings and Precautions.
Prevention and Treatment of Postoperative Nausea and Vomiting : Adults: Injection: The recommended dosage for prevention of postoperative nausea and vomiting is 1 mg of KYTRIL, undiluted, administered intravenously over 30 seconds, before induction of anesthesia or immediately before reversal of anesthesia.

The recommended dosage for the treatment of nausea and/or vomiting after surgery is 1 mg of KYTRIL, undiluted, administered intravenously over 30 seconds.
Geriatrics: Clinical experience in the use of KYTRIL in the prevention and treatment of post-operative nausea and vomiting is limited and it is not indicated for use in this population (see Indications and Clinical Use and Warnings and Precautions).
Pediatrics: See Indications and Clinical Use and Warnings and Precautions.
Reconstitution: Diluted Solutions: Infusion Preparation: To prepare granisetron hydrochloride injection for i.v. infusion, aseptically transfer the appropriate amount of granisetron hydrochloride injection to the desired volume of any of the following solutions: 0.9% sodium chloride, 0.18% sodium chloride and 4% dextrose, 5% dextrose, Hartmann's solution, sodium lactate, mannitol (see Storage and Stability).

OVERDOSAGE:
There is no specific antidote for KYTRIL (granisetron hydrochloride) overdosage. In the case of overdosage, symptomatic treatment should be given. Overdose has been reported with both the intravenous and oral formulations. Overdosage of up to 38.5 mg of granisetron hydrochloride injection has been reported without symptoms or with the occurrence of a slight headache.

For management of a suspected drug overdose, contact your regional Poison Control Centre. See the *CPS* Directory section for a list of Poison Control Centres.

ACTION AND CLINICAL PHARMACOLOGY: Mechanism of Action: KYTRIL (granisetron hydrochloride) is a selective antagonist of 5 hydroxytryptamine (5 HT_3) receptors. Following exposure to emetogenic cancer chemotherapy, mucosal enterochromaffin cells release serotonin which stimulates 5 HT_3 receptors located peripherally on vagal nerve terminals and centrally in the nucleus tractus solitarus. The antiemetic effect of granisetron appears to involve antagonism of the serotonin-induced stimulation of vagal afferent activity.

Radioligand binding studies have demonstrated that KYTRIL has negligible affinity for other 5 HT receptors or for dopamine D_2 receptor binding sites.
Pharmacodynamics: In healthy subjects, KYTRIL produced no consistent or clinically significant changes in pulse rate, blood pressure or ECG. There was no evidence of an effect on psychomotor performance at intravenous doses of up to 200 µg/kg i.v. KYTRIL did not affect the plasma levels of prolactin or aldosterone at single intravenous doses of up to 300 µg/kg or after repeat intravenous doses of 40 µg/kg for 5.5 days.

Following single and multiple oral doses, KYTRIL slowed colonic transit in normal volunteers.
Pharmacokinetics: Chemotherapy-Induced Nausea and Vomiting: Injection: In adult cancer patients undergoing chemotherapy and in healthy volunteers, infusion of a single 40 µg/kg dose of KYTRIL produced the following mean pharmacokinetic data presented in Table 4.

Table 4: KYTRIL

Pharmacokinetic Parameters in Adult Cancer Patients Undergoing Chemotherapy and in Volunteers, Following a Single Intravenous 40 µg/kg Dose of KYTRIL (granisetron hydrochloride) Injection

	Peak Plasma Concentration (ng/mL)	Terminal Phase Plasma Half-Life (h)	AUC (ng·h/mL)	Total Clearance (L/h)
Cancer Patients (N=14)				
Mean	63.8[a]	8.95[a]	167[a]	25.8[a]
Range	18.0 to 176	0.90 to 31.1	26.0 to 294	8.92 to 95.2

(cont'd)

Table 4: KYTRIL *(cont'd)*

Pharmacokinetic Parameters in Adult Cancer Patients Undergoing Chemotherapy and in Volunteers, Following a Single Intravenous 40 µg/kg Dose of KYTRIL (granisetron hydrochloride) Injection

	Peak Plasma Concentration (ng/mL)	Terminal Phase Plasma Half-Life (h)	AUC (ng·h/mL)	Total Clearance (L/h)
Young Adult Volunteers 21 to 42 years (N=20)				
Mean	64.3[b]	4.91[b]	89.7[b]	51.8[b]
Range	11.2 to 182	0.88 to 15.2	15.6 to 201	11.3 to 176
Elderly Volunteers 65 to 81 years (N=20)				
Mean	57.0[b]	7.69[b]	115[b]	27.1[b]
Range	14.6 to 153	2.65 to 17.7	37.7 to 240	10.9 to 58.4

[a] 5 minute infusion.
[b] 3 minute infusion.

Oral: In healthy volunteers and adult cancer patients undergoing chemotherapy, administration of oral KYTRIL produced the following mean pharmacokinetic data presented: See Table 5.

Table 5: KYTRIL

Pharmacokinetic Parameters (Mean [range]) in Adult Cancer Patients Undergoing Chemotherapy and in Volunteers Following Oral KYTRIL (granisetron hydrochloride)

	Peak Plasma Concentration (ng/mL)	Terminal Plasma Half-Life (h)	Area Under Curve (ng·h/mL)	Total Clearance (L/h)
Cancer Patients				
1.0 mg, b.i.d., 7 days (n=24)	8.19 [1.97 to 18.4]	N.D.[a]	54.2 [10.2 to 126]	34.1 [7.94 to 98.0]
Volunteers single dose (n=25)				
1.0 mg	4.10 [0.58 to 7.37]	8.74 [2.40 to 19.9]	43.7 [2.85 to 142]	53.3 [7.04 to 351]
2.5 mg	9.44 [1.68 to 19.5]	7.24 [2.54 to 17.0]	105 [7.75 to 319]	67.2 [7.84 to 323]

[a] Not determined after oral administration.

Distribution: KYTRIL is extensively distributed between plasma and red blood cells with a mean volume of distribution of approximately 3 L/kg. Plasma protein binding is approximately 65%.

Metabolism: The clearance of granisetron occurs predominantly through hepatic metabolism. Biotransformation pathways involve N-demethylation and aromatic ring oxidation followed by conjugation.

Excretion: In normal volunteers, the urinary excretion of unchanged KYTRIL averages 12% of the administered dose over a period of 48 hours, while the remainder of the dose is excreted as metabolites, 47% in the urine and 34% in the feces. The metabolism of granisetron involves N-demethylation and aromatic ring oxidation followed by conjugation.

Postoperative Nausea and Vomiting: Injection: In adult patients (age range, 18 to 64 years) recovering from elective surgery and receiving general anesthesia, mean pharmacokinetic data obtained from a single 1 mg dose of KYTRIL administered intravenously over 30 seconds are shown in Table 6.

Table 6: KYTRIL

Pharmacokinetic Parameters in 16 Adult Surgical Patients Following a Single Intravenous 1 mg Dose of KYTRIL (granisetron hydrochloride) Injection

	Peak Plasma Concentration (ng/mL)	Terminal Plasma Half-Life (h)	Area Under Curve (ng·h/mL)	Total Clearance (L/h)
Mean	75.5	8.63	72.2	19.1
Range	16.8–187	1.77–17.73	21.0–137	7.30–47.6

The pharmacokinetics of granisetron in patients undergoing surgery were similar to those seen in cancer patients undergoing chemotherapy.

Special Populations and Conditions: Pediatrics: The safety and efficacy of KYTRIL has not been adequately studied in children or adolescents under 18 years of age.

Geriatrics: In geriatric (mean age 71 yrs) subjects after single intravenous doses of 40 µg/kg, pharmacokinetic parameters were within the range found for young subjects (mean age 29 yrs). Although the elimination half-life was prolonged and the total plasma clearance reduced in the geriatric relative to the young subject group, no significant differences were determined between the two groups with regard to maximum plasma concentration or area under the plasma concentration time curve values (see Table 4).

Gender and Race: There were too few male and Black patients to adequately assess differences in effect in either population.

Hepatic Insufficiency: A pharmacokinetic study in patients with hepatic impairment due to neoplastic liver involvement showed that total clearance was approximately halved and mean area under the plasma concentration time curve (AUC) values were approximately doubled compared to patients without hepatic impairment.

Renal Insufficiency: Although renal clearance was decreased in subjects with severe renal impairment (N=11) relative to normal volunteers (N=12), total plasma clearance was numerically higher in this renally impaired group (43 L/h) than in the normal volunteers (32 L/h). Mean area under the plasma concentration time curve values were similar for the two subject groups.

Cancer Patients: Following intravenous administration, mean terminal elimination half-life values are approximately twice as long in cancer patients as they are in healthy adult volunteers, while clearance values are decreased by approximately 50% (see Table 4). Available data do not allow a formal comparison of elimination half-life or clearance between volunteers and cancer patients receiving oral KYTRIL.

STORAGE AND STABILITY: Vials should be stored between 15-30°C. Protect from light. Once the vial is penetrated, its contents should be used within 30 days. Discard unused portion.

Store tablets at controlled room temperature (15-30°C).

KYTRIL has been shown to be stable for at least 24 hours in the following solutions: 0.9% sodium chloride, 0.18% sodium chloride and 4% dextrose, 5% dextrose, Hartmann's solution, sodium lactate, mannitol when stored at ambient temperature in normal indoor illumination (natural daylight supplemented by fluorescent light). As with all parenteral drug products, intravenous admixtures should be inspected visually for clarity, particulate matter, precipitate, discoloration and leakage prior to administration, whenever solution and container permit. Appropriate precautions should be taken to maintain the sterility of the infusion solution once prepared.

Pharmaceutical Precautions: As a general precaution, KYTRIL should not be mixed in solution with other drugs.

INFORMATION FOR THE PATIENT: Published in e-CPS, available by subscription at www.e-cps.ca.

DOSAGE FORMS, COMPOSITION AND PACKAGING: Injection: Each mL contains: granisetron HCl 1 mg, sodium chloride 0.9%, benzyl alcohol 1.0%, citric acid monohydrate 0.2%, water for injection and hydrochloric acid and/or sodium hydroxide for pH adjustment. Clear glass multi-use vials of 1 and 4 mL, boxes of 1.

Tablets: 1 mg: Each white, triangular, biconvex, film-coated tablet, debossed with "K1" on one face, contains: granisetron hydrochloride equivalent to granisetron 1 mg. Nonmedicinal ingredients: hydroxypropyl methylcellulose, lactose, magnesium stearate, microcrystalline cellulose, sodium starch glycolate and Opadry YS-1-18027-A (hypromellose, titanium dioxide, macrogol 400, and polysorbate 80). Blister cards of 2 and 10.

2 mg: Each white, triangular, biconvex, film-coated tablet, debossed with "K2" on one face, contains: granisetron hydrochloride equivalent to granisetron 2 mg. Nonmedicinal ingredients: hydroxypropyl methylcellulose, lactose, magnesium stearate, microcrystalline cellulose, sodium starch glycolate and Opadry YS-1-18027-A (hypromellose, titanium dioxide, macrogol 400, and polysorbate 80). Blister cards of 1 and 5.

L

Labetalol Hydrochloride Injection USP

labetalol HCl

Antihypertensive

Sandoz

SUPPLIED: Each mL contains: labetalol hydrochloride 5 mg. Nonmedicinal ingredients: dextrose anhydrous, disodium edetate, methylparaben, propylparaben, anhydrous citric acid and/or sodium hydroxide to adjust pH and water for injection. Multidose amber vials of 20 mL, boxes of 1. Store between 15 and 30°C. Protect from light.

Lacrisert®

hydroxypropyl cellulose

Ophthalmic Insert

Aton Pharma

Date of Preparation: June 10, 1980
Date of Revision: February 2006

PHARMACOLOGY: Lacrisert (hydroxypropyl cellulose ocular system, USP) ophthalmic insert is a rod-shaped, water soluble, ophthalmic preparation made of hydroxypropyl cellulose, 5 mg. Lacrisert contains no preservatives or other ingredients. It is about 1.27 mm in diameter by about 3.5 mm long.

Lacrisert acts to stabilize and thicken the precorneal tear film and prolong the tear film breakup time which is usually accelerated in patients with dry eye states. Lacrisert also acts to lubricate and protect the eye. Lacrisert usually reduces the signs and symptoms resulting from moderate to severe dry eye syndromes, such as conjunctival hyperemia, corneal and conjunctival staining with rose bengal, exudation, tearing, itching, burning, foreign body sensation, smarting, photophobia, dryness and blurred vision. Progressive visual deterioration which occurs in some patients may be retarded, halted, or sometimes reversed.

In four crossover studies the 5 mg Lacrisert administered once a day during the waking hours was compared to artificial tears used four or more times daily. Prolongation of tear film breakup time was statistically significant in two of the four studies and lessening of foreign body sensation, burning, tearing, itching, soreness, and dryness in the majority of patients during treatment with inserts as compared to artificial tears. Improvement, as measured by lessening of symptoms, by rose bengal staining, slit lamp examination of the cornea and conjunctiva, was greater in most patients with moderate to severe symptoms during treatment with Lacrisert. Patient comfort was usually better with Lacrisert than with artificial tears solution, and most patients preferred Lacrisert.

In most patients treated with Lacrisert for over one year, improvement was observed as evidenced by lessening of symptoms generally associated with keratoconjunctivitis sicca such as burning, tearing, foreign body sensation, itching, photophobia and blurred vision.

In healty volunteers, a thickened precorneal tear film was usually observed through the slit lamp while Lacrisert was present in the conjunctival sac.

INDICATIONS: Lacrisert (hydroxypropyl cellulose ocular system, USP) ophthalmic insert is indicated in patients with moderate to severe dry eye syndromes, including keratoconjunctivitis sicca. Lacrisert is indicated in patients who remain symptomatic after an adequate trial of therapy with artificial tear solutions.

Lacrisert is also indicated for patients with: Exposure keratitis, Decreased corneal sensitivity.

CONTRAINDICATIONS: Hypersensitivity to hydroxypropyl cellulose.

PRECAUTIONS: Instructions for inserting and removing Lacrisert (hydroxypropyl cellulose ocular system, USP) ophthalmic insert should be carefully followed. If improperly placed in the inferior cul-de-sac, Lacrisert may result in corneal abrasion.

Because this product may produce transient blurring of vision, patients should be instructed to exercise caution when operating hazardous machinery or driving a motor vehicle.

The safety and efficacy of Lacrisert has not been evaluated in patients with the following conditions: ocular infections or history of infection, eye region surgery or history of ocular trauma, contact lenses use, history of dendritic keratitis, intraocular diseases, severe cicatricial changes in the conjunctiva, significant corneal or conjunctival structural changes, acute ocular disease unrelated to keratoconjunctivitis sicca (KCS), and patients with evidence of recent ocular or adnexal surgery.

Pediatrics: Safety and efficacy in pediatric patients have not been established.

ADVERSE EFFECTS: The following adverse reactions have been reported in patients treated with Lacrisert (hydroxypropyl cellulose ocular system, USP), but were in most instances mild and transient: transient blurring of vision (see Precautions), ocular discomfort or irritation, matting or stickiness of eyelashes, photophobia, hypersensitivity, edema of the eyelids, hyperemia, tearing, foreign body sensation.

OVERDOSE:

> For management of a suspected drug overdose, CPhA recommends that you contact your regional Poison Control Centre. See the *CPS* Directory section for a list of Poison Control Centres.

DOSAGE: One Lacrisert (hydroxypropyl cellulose ocular system, USP) ophthalmic insert in each eye once daily is usually sufficient to relieve the symptoms associated with moderate to severe dry eye syndromes. Individual patients may require more flexibility in the use of Lacrisert, some patients may require twice daily use for optimal results.

In some patients, the concomitant administration of a replacement tear solution at the time of insertion may be of benefit to assist in the dissolution of the insert and removal of debris. Saline drops may be used with Lacrisert in cases with severe dry eyes to assist in the dissolution of the insert and removal of debris. Clinical experience with Lacrisert indicates that in some patients several weeks may be required before satisfactory improvement of symptoms is achieved.

Lacrisert is inserted into the inferior cul-de-sac of the eye beneath the base of the tarsus, not in apposition to the cornea.

NOTE: Occasionally Lacrisert is inadvertently expelled from the eye, especially in patients with shallow conjunctival fornices or when the eye is rubbed. The patient should be cautioned against rubbing the eye(s) containing Lacrisert, especially upon awakening, so as to not dislodge or expel the insert. If required, another Lacrisert ophthalmic insert may be inserted. If experience indicates that transient blurred vision develops in an individual patient, the patient may want to remove Lacrisert a few hours after insertion to avoid this. Another Lacrisert ophthalmic insert may be inserted if needed. Box of 60. Conserve below 30°C.

Expulsion of undissolved inserts one to several hours after application may occur in patients with Schirmer tests of 0 mm.

If Lacrisert causes worsening of symptoms, the patient should be instructed to inspect the conjunctival sac to make certain Lacrisert is in the proper location, deep in the inferior cul-de-sac of the eye, beneath the base of the tarsus. If these symptoms persist, Lacrisert should be removed and the patient should contact the physician.

INFORMATION FOR THE PATIENT: Published in e-CPS, available by subscription at www.e-cps.ca.

SUPPLIED: A rod-shaped (about 1.27mm in diameter by about 3.5 mm long), watersoluble, ophthalmic preparation made of hydroxypropyl cellulose, 5 mg. It contains no preservatives or other ingredients. Packages of 60 units, together with illustrated instructions and a special applicator for removing Lacrisert from the unit dose blister and inserting it into the eye. A spare applicator is included in each package. Store below 30°C.

Illustrated instructions are included in each package, but initially patients must be instructed in the correct method of insertion. While in the ophthalmologist's office, the patient should read the instructions, then practice insertions and removal of Lacrisert until proficiency is achieved.

Lactaid®

lactase

Lactose Digestant

McNeil Consumer Healthcare

PHARMACOLOGY: Converts the disaccharide lactose via hydrolysis into its monosaccharide components, glucose and galactose.

Tablets: In vivo activity has been demonstrated with drug administration at time of milk consumption and at time of consumption of other lactose containing solid and liquid foods.

Drops: Fifteen drops will hydrolyze nearly all of the lactose in 1 L of milk at refrigerator temperature (6°C) in 24 hours. 1 L of any type of milk will contain approximately 50 g lactose prior to lactose hydrolysis.

INDICATIONS: Lactase insufficiency either suspected because of gastrointestinal disturbances (bloating, flatulence, diarrhea) after consumption of milk or milk products or identified by a lactose tolerance test, or a breath hydrogen test after lactose challenge.

PRECAUTIONS: Lactase deficient diabetics should be made aware that milk sugar (lactose) which was previously indigestible by them will now be metabolized and provide calories which must be accounted for in their diet (e.g., 50 g of lactose will yield 25 g of glucose and 25 g of galactose sugar each of which may be converted to energy by metabolism).

Galactosemics may not have milk in any form, lactase enzyme modified or not.

Drug Interactions: No drug interactions reported.

ADVERSE EFFECTS: The most frequently reported adverse effects to the tablets are gastrointestinal in nature, sometimes mimicking the symptoms of lactose intolerance. No reactions of any kind were observed from the liquid drops. Total reactions were estimated at under 0.1% of users.

OVERDOSE:

Overdose has not been reported with this drug.

> For management of a suspected drug overdose, CPhA recommends that you contact your **regional Poison Control Centre**. See the *CPS* Directory section for a list of Poison Control Centres.

DOSAGE: Drops: Add up 15 drops to each L of milk to convert nearly all of the lactose.

Tablets Regular Strength: 3 tablets to be taken **just before** eating a meal or food that contains lactose. The tablet can either be swallowed or chewed.

Extra Strength: 2 tablets to be taken **just before** eating a meal or food that contains lactose. The tablets can either be swallowed or chewed.

Fast Act Caplets: 1 caplet to be taken **just before** eating a meal or food that contains lactose. The caplet must be swallowed whole.

Fast Act Chewable Tablets: 1 tablet to be taken **just before** eating a meal or food that contains lactose. The tablets must be chewed.

Dosage requirements may vary substantially between individuals and between situations.

SUPPLIED: Drops: Each mL of solution contains: lactase (β-D-galactosidase derived from Kluyveromyces lactis yeast). Nonmedicinal ingredients: glycerin and water. Dropper bottles of 15.5 mL. Sufficient to treat 75 L respectively, with doses of 5 drops/L. Treats 25 L with doses of 15 drops/L.

Tablets: Regular Strength: Each white, capsule-shaped tablet, engraved "Lactaid" on one side, contains: at least 3000 FCC lactase units of β-D-galactosidase from *Aspergillus oryzae*. Nonmedicinal ingredients: cellulose, magnesium stearate and mannitol. Packages of 100.

Extra Strength: Each white, capsule-shaped tablet, engraved "Lactaid ES" on one side, contains: at least 4500 FCC lactase units of β-D-galactosidase from *Aspergillus oryzae*. Nonmedicinal ingredients: cellulose, magnesium stearate and mannitol. Packages of 40 and 80.

Fast Act Caplets: Each white to off-white caplet, engraved "Lactaid" on one side, contains: at least 9000 FCC lactase units of β-D-galactosidase from *Aspergillus oryzae*. Nonmedicinal ingredients: colloidal silicon dioxide, croscarmellose sodium, crospovidone, magnesium stearate and microcrystalline cellulose. Packages of 40.

Fast Act Chewable Tablets: Each white to off-white, round, bevel-edged chewable tablet with lemon-vanilla flavor and odour, engraved "Lactaid" on one side contains: at least 9000 FCC lactase units of β-D-galactosidase from *Aspergillus oryzae*. Nonmedicinal ingredients: citric acid, croscarmellose sodium, crospovidone, flavor, magnesium stearate, mannitol, microcrystalline cellulose and sucralose. Phenylketonurics: Contains phenylalanine (aspartame). Packages of 40.

Lactulose

Laxative

CPhA Monograph

Date of Preparation: November 2004
Date of Revision: June 2009

> This monograph has been compiled by CPhA and reviewed by experts. It may contain information different from that found in Health Canada-approved Product Monographs. The reader is referred to the *CPS* Editorial Policy for more information.

SUMMARY PRODUCT INFORMATION:

Route of Administration	Dosage Form	Product Strength
Oral	Solution	667 mg/mL

INDICATIONS AND CLINICAL USE: Lactulose is indicated for:

- Relief of constipation in chronically constipated patients.

Lactulose, an osmotic laxative, may be used in patients in palliative care to manage constipation in combination with a stimulant [*Palliat Med* 2008;22(7):796-807]. Constipation in patients in palliative care may be caused by organic (e.g., pharmacologic agents such as vinca alkaloids, opioid analgesics or oral iron; metabolic disturbances such as dehydration or hypercalcemia; neurologic disorders such as spinal cord involvement; structural abnormalities such as pelvic tumour mass) and/or functional factors (e.g., diet including poor appetite, low fibre intake; environmental factors such as lack of privacy; advanced age).

Other Clinical Uses:

- Prevention and treatment of portal-systemic encephalopathy (PSE), also known as hepatic encephalopathy, including the stages of hepatic pre-coma and coma.

According to controlled studies, lactulose solution therapy reduces blood ammonia levels by 25 to 50% which is, in general, paralleled by an improvement in the patient's mental state and by an improvement in EEG patterns. According to a Cochrane review insufficient data exist on the effects of lactulose in patients with hepatic encephalopathy and lactulose may be less effective than antibiotics in improving this condition [*Cochrane Database Syst Rev* 2004;(2):CD003044]. Patients on lactulose therapy may experience an increase in their protein tolerance level. Lactulose has been given over 2 years in controlled studies for the treatment of chronic PSE. Compared to placebo, lactulose has no significant effect on mortality [*BMJ* 2004;328(7447):1046].

The American College of Gastroenterology hepatic encephalopathy guidelines recommend that lactulose be administered via enema or nasogastric tube in deep encephalopathy. Oral lactulose should be optimally dosed and administered every hour until stool evacuation appears. For cirrhotic patients with chronic encephalopathy, administer lactulose at a dose that results in two or three soft bowel movements per day [*Am J Gastroenterol* 2001;96(7):1968-76]. Compared with placebo, lactulose has been shown to prevent recurrence of hepatic encephalopathy in patients with cirrhosis who had recovered from a previous episode [*Gastroenterology* 2009 Jun 6. Epub ahead of print]. Lactulose 30 to 60 mL divided in 2 or 3 doses was titrated to produce 2 to 3 stools per day.

Geriatrics: Following a barium meal examination, the drug has been used to induce bowel evacuation in geriatric patients with colonic retention of barium and severe constipation.

Pediatrics: Information is limited on the use of lactulose for prevention and treatment of PSE in young children and adolescents. The drug has been used in the treatment of chronic constipation in children; however, the manufacturers state that safety and efficacy of lactulose for the treatment of chronic constipation in children have not been established.

CONTRAINDICATIONS:

- Patients who are hypersensitive to lactulose or to any ingredient in the formulation.
- Patients who require a low galactose diet. Lactulose solution contains galactose at a concentration of less than 107 mg/mL.

WARNINGS AND PRECAUTIONS: General: Slower absorption of medication from the intestine due to acidification. Ideally, do not take within 2 hours of other medications.

Dependence/Tolerance/Withdrawal: Lactulose should not be taken for more than 1 week unless ordered by a physician. Overuse or extended use may cause dependence for bowel function.

Gastrointestinal: Lactulose should not be used in the presence of abdominal pain, nausea, fever or vomiting.

Special Populations: Patients with Diabetes: Lactulose is not absorbed systemically. Lactulose solution contains less than 80 mg/mL of lactose so may be used with caution in patients with diabetes.

Pregnant Women: Pregnancy Category B_M. Animal studies have not revealed significant adverse effects. According to the American College of Gastroenterology, lactulose may be considered if constipation is refractory to dietary fibre or stimulant laxatives [www.gi.org/physicians/pdfs/PregnancyMonograph.pdf]. However, the use of lactulose by women who are pregnant or may become pregnant requires that the potential benefits be weighed against the potential risks.

Nursing Women: It is not known if lactulose is distributed into breast milk. Use lactulose with caution in nursing women.

Pediatrics (birth to 16 years old): According to the manufacturer, safety and effectiveness in pediatric patients have not been established.

ADVERSE REACTIONS: Adverse Drug Reaction Overview: Initial dosing may produce flatulence and abdominal cramps, which are usually transient. Nausea is more common with higher doses. Excessive dosage can lead to diarrhea. Reduce the dose immediately if initial lactulose dose causes diarrhea. If diarrhea persists, discontinue lactulose.

DRUG INTERACTIONS: Overview:

Table 1: Lactulose

Drug-Drug Interactions

Interacting Drug	Effect	Clinical Comment
Antacids	Concurrent administration of nonabsorbable antacids with lactulose may inhibit the desired lactulose-induced drop in colonic pH.	Concurrent administration may result in a possible lack of desired treatment effect which should be considered before such drugs are given concomitantly with lactulose.
Anti-infective agents	Theoretically, the elimination of certain colonic bacteria by anti-infective agents may interfere with the desired degradation of lactulose and thus prevent the acidification of colonic contents.	The status of the lactulose-treated patient should be closely monitored in the event of concomitant oral anti-infective therapy.
Laxatives	The loose stools resulting from their use may falsely suggest that adequate lactulose dosage has been achieved.	Other laxatives should not be used, especially during the initial phase of therapy for PSE.

DOSAGE AND ADMINISTRATION: Recommended Dose and Dosage Adjustment:

Table 2: Lactulose

Dose in Adult Patients

Indication	Usual Dose	Detailed Information
Chronic constipation	15–30 mL daily to BID, maximum 60 mL daily	May require 24 to 48 hours to restore normal bowel movements.
Portal-systemic encephalopathy or hepatic encephalopathy	Acute encephalopathy: 45 mL Q1H until evacuation occurs, then titrate to produce 2 to 3 loose bowel movements per day. Usual dose: 15 to 45 mL Q8-12H.	Chronic encephalopathy may not require hourly dosing [*Am J Gastroenterol* 2001;96(7):1968-76]. Aim is to produce 2 to 3 loose bowel movements per day. Consider decreasing the dose if >2 to 3 bowel movements per day. Discontinue if severe diarrhea.

Table 3: Lactulose

Dose in Geriatric Patients

Indication	Usual Dose
Colonic retention of barium and severe constipation	5–10 mL BID for 1–4 weeks

Table 4: Lactulose

Dose in Pediatric Patients

Indication	Oral Dose	Detailed Information
Chronic constipation	Infants and older children: Initial dose: 5 to 10 mL once daily May double daily dose until stool is produced	Do not exceed recommended adult dose. Onset of action: 24 to 48 hours.
Portal-systemic encephalopathy or hepatic encephalopathy	Infants <1 year: 2.5 mL twice daily Older Children and Adolescents: Adjust dose every 1–2 days as necessary to produce 2–3 soft stools daily. Total daily dose: 10 to 30 mL TID	If the initial dose of lactulose produces diarrhea, reduce dose immediately; if diarrhea persists, discontinue lactulose. Monitor electrolytes especially sodium and potassium.

Administration: Oral: Lactulose is usually administered orally. The sweet taste of lactulose solution, which may be unpleasant to some patients, can be minimized by diluting the solution with water, fruit juice, or milk or administering it in food such as desserts.

Rectal: Lactulose may also be administered rectally to adults with PSE during stages of hepatic pre-coma or coma when the possibility of aspiration exists, or if endoscopic or intubation procedures interfere with oral administration.

When lactulose is used rectally in the treatment of PSE to reverse hepatic coma in adults, 200 g is diluted in 700 mL of water or 0.9% sodium chloride solution; the diluted solution is administered rectally via a rectal balloon catheter and retained for 30 to 60 minutes. Lactulose retention enemas may be administered every 4 to 6 hours; if the enema is retained for less than 30 minutes, it may be repeated immediately. In some patients, reversal of hepatic coma may occur within 2 hours of the first enema. Before discontinuance of lactulose retention enemas, recommended oral dosages of the drug should be started. Cleansing enemas containing soapsuds or other alkaline agents should not be used concomitantly with lactulose enemas.

OVERDOSAGE:

For management of a suspected drug overdose, CPhA recommends that you contact your **regional Poison Control Centre**. See the *CPS* Directory section for a list of Poison Control Centres.

ACTION AND CLINICAL PHARMACOLOGY: Lactulose is a synthetic nonabsorbable disaccharide analog of lactose. Lactulose improves stool frequency and consistency [*Am J Gastroenterol* 2005;100(Suppl 1):S1-4]. In the colon, lactulose is broken down by Lactobacillus and Bacteroides to lactic acid, formic acid and acetic acid by the action of colonic bacteria. The resulting increase in osmotic pressure and acidification of portions of the colonic contents are believed to be responsible for the increase in stool volume and frequency observed during lactulose administration. In hepatic encephalopathy, free ammonia is transformed into ammonium ions in the acidic environment in the colon, which is consequently trapped in the colon.

Pharmacokinetics: Absorption: Lactulose is poorly absorbed from the GI tract and no enzyme capable of hydrolysis of this disaccharide is present in human GI tissue. As a result, oral doses of lactulose reach the colon virtually unchanged.

Excretion: Urinary excretion has been determined to be 3% or less and is essentially complete within 24 hours.

Lamictal® Ⓟ

lamotrigine

Antiepileptic

GlaxoSmithKline

Date of Revision: July 3, 2009

Do not exceed the recommended initial dose and subsequent dose escalations of LAMICTAL. More rapid initial titration has been associated with an increased incidence of serious dermatological reactions (see Warnings).

PHARMACOLOGY: LAMICTAL (lamotrigine) is a drug of the phenyltriazine class chemically unrelated to existing antiepileptic drugs (AEDs).

Lamotrigine is thought to act at voltage-sensitive sodium channels to stabilize neuronal membranes and inhibit the release of excitatory amino acid neurotransmitters (e.g., glutamate, aspartate) that are thought to play a role in the generation and spread of epileptic seizures.

Clinical Trials: In adult placebo controlled clinical studies, LAMICTAL has been shown to be effective in reducing seizure frequency and the number of days with seizures, when added to existing antiepileptic drug therapy in adult patients with partial seizures, with or without generalized tonic-clonic seizures, that are not satisfactorily controlled.

The effectiveness of lamotrigine adjunctive therapy has also been shown in pediatric and adult patients with Lennox-Gastaut syndrome. A significant reduction in major motor seizures, drop attacks, and tonic-clonic seizures was seen following lamotrigine treatment compared with placebo-treated patients. Improvements in cognitive skills (speech, nonverbal communication, alertness, attention, intellectual capacity), behavior, and fine coordination have been seen with lamotrigine treatment in these patients.

Studies have also been conducted using lamotrigine monotherapy in adult patients (n=443) newly diagnosed with epilepsy (partial seizures, with or without secondary generalization or primary generalized tonic clonic). Results have shown comparable efficacy (time to first seizure, seizure frequency, percentage of patients seizure-free) with fewer side effects than currently approved therapies.

Clinical trials have also demonstrated that adult patients (any seizure type) can be converted to lamotrigine monotherapy from polytherapy, with significant numbers of patients maintaining or improving seizure control. Efficacy was maintained during long-term treatment (up to 152 weeks).

A 24-week monotherapy trial was conducted in elderly newly diagnosed patients (102 patients received lamotrigine and 48 received carbamazepine). The findings indicate comparable efficacy and demonstrate that lamotrigine was well tolerated in the elderly. However, the small and unbalanced number of patients in the study precludes any firm conclusions on the relative safety of the two drugs.

Pharmacokinetics: Adults: LAMICTAL is rapidly and completely absorbed following oral administration, reaching peak plasma concentrations 1.4 to 4.8 hours (T_{max}) post-dosing. When administered with food, the rate of absorption is slightly reduced, but the extent remains unchanged. Following single LAMICTAL doses of 50 to 400 mg, peak plasma concentration (C_{max}=0.6 to 4.6 μg/mL) and the area under the plasma concentration-versus-time curve (AUC=29.9 to 211 h·μg/mL) increase linearly with dose. The time-to-peak concentration, elimination half-life ($t_{1/2}$) and volume of distribution (Vd/F) are independent of dose. The $t_{1/2}$ averages 33 hours after single doses and Vd/F ranges from 0.9 to 1.4 L/kg. Following repeated dosing in healthy volunteers for 14 days, the $t_{1/2}$ decreased by an average of 26% (mean steady state $t_{1/2}$ of 26.4 hours) and plasma clearance increased by an average of 33%. In a single-dose study where healthy volunteers were administered both oral and i.v. doses of lamotrigine, the absolute bioavailability of oral lamotrigine was 98%.

Lamotrigine is approximately 55% bound to human plasma proteins. This binding is unaffected by therapeutic concentrations of phenytoin, phenobarbital or valproic acid. Lamotrigine does not displace other antiepileptic drugs (carbamazepine, phenytoin, phenobarbital) from protein binding sites.

Lamotrigine is metabolized predominantly in the liver by glucuronic acid conjugation. The major metabolite is an inactive 2-N-glucuronide conjugate that can be hydrolyzed by β-glucuronidase. Approximately 70% of an oral LAMICTAL dose is recovered in urine as this metabolite.

Pediatrics: Lamotrigine was rapidly absorbed in children, with a T_{max} ranging from 1 to 6 hours. The mean Vd/F of lamotrigine in children aged 5 to 11 years (1.3 to 1.4 L/kg) was similar to that seen in adults (0.9 to 1.4 L/kg) but was larger in younger children (1.8 to 2.3 L/kg). As with adults, the elimination of lamotrigine in pediatric patients was similarly affected by concomitant AEDs. While the CL/F was higher and $t_{1/2}$ was shorter in younger children than in older children, the mean CL/F was higher and mean $t_{1/2}$ was shorter in both pediatric groups than in adults. Population analysis results showed that the estimated apparent plasma clearances in patients aged 13 to 18 years were similar to those found in adult patients.

Geriatrics (≥65 years): Results of a population pharmacokinetic analysis, based on individual trials in which both adult (n=138) and elderly (n=13) patients with epilepsy were enrolled, indicated that the clearance of lamotrigine in elderly patients did not change to a clinically relevant extent. After single doses, apparent clearance was lower in the elderly by 12% (31 mL/min at age 70 vs 35 mL/min at age 20). After 48 weeks of treatment, the difference in clearance was 10% (37 mL/min at age 70 vs 41 mL/min at age 20). In addition, the pharmacokinetics of lamotrigine were studied in 12 healthy elderly volunteers who each received a single oral dose of 150 mg. The mean clearance in the elderly (0.39 mL/min) lies within the range of mean clearance values (0.31 to 0.65 mL/min) obtained in 9 studies with non-elderly adults after single doses of 30 to 450 mg (see also Dosage and Adverse Effects).

Renal Impairment: The pharmacokinetics of a single oral dose of LAMICTAL (100 mg) were evaluated in 12 individuals with chronic renal failure (with mean creatinine clearance of 13 mL/min) who were not receiving other antiepileptic drugs. In this study, the elimination half-life of unchanged lamotrigine was prolonged (by an average of 63%) relative to individuals with normal renal function (see Precautions, Renal Failure and Dosage).

Hemodialysis: In 6 hemodialysis patients, the elimination half-life of unchanged lamotrigine was doubled off dialysis, and reduced by 50% on dialysis, relative to individuals with normal renal function.

Hepatic Impairment: A single-dose pharmacokinetic study was performed in 24 subjects with hepatic impairment (n=12 mild/Grade A; n=5 moderate/Grade B and n=7 severe/Grade C) versus 12 healthy controls. For the moderate and severe subgroups, the mean values for AUC and plasma half-life were increased approximately 2-fold and 3-fold respectively over control values, with clearance decreased proportionately. For the mild group, while mean values were not statistically different from those of controls, a subgroup of 1- to 4 subjects (dependent on pharmacokinetic parameter examined) showed abnormal individual values which were in the range of the moderately impaired subjects (see also Dosage and Precautions).

Gilbert's Syndrome: Gilbert's syndrome (idiopathic unconjugated hyperbilirubinemia) does not appear to affect the pharmacokinetic profile of lamotrigine.

Concomitant Antiepileptic Drugs: In patients with epilepsy, concomitant administration of LAMICTAL with enzyme-inducing AEDs (phenytoin, carbamazepine, primidone or phenobarbital) decreases the mean lamotrigine $t_{1/2}$ to 13 hours. Concomitant administration of LAMICTAL with valproic acid significantly increases $t_{1/2}$ and decreases the clearance of lamotrigine, whereas concomitant administration of LAMICTAL with valproic acid plus enzyme-inducing AEDs can prolong $t_{1/2}$ up to approximately 27 hours. The key lamotrigine parameters for adult patients and healthy volunteers are summarized in Table 1, and for pediatric patients in Table 2.

Table 1: LAMICTAL

Mean Pharmacokinetic Parameters in Adult Patients with Epilepsy or Healthy Volunteers

		Healthy Young Volunteers		Patients with Epilepsy			
	LAMICTAL Adminis-tered	LAMICTAL	LAMICTAL+ Valproic Acid[b]	LAMICTAL+ Enzyme-Inducing AEDs	LAMICTAL+ Valproic Acid	LAMICTAL+ Valproic Acid + Enzyme-Inducing AEDs
T_{max} (h)	Single Dose	2.2 (0.25–12.0)[a]	1.8 (1.0–4.0)	2.3 (0.5–5.0)	4.8 (1.8–8.4)	3.8 (1.0–10.0)
	Multiple Dose	1.7 (0.5–4.0)	1.9 (0.5–3.5)	2.0 (0.75–5.93)	ND	ND
$t_{1/2}$ (h)	Single Dose	32.8 (14.0–103.0)	48.3 (31.5–88.6)	14.4 (6.4–30.4)	58.8 (30.5–88.8)	27.2 (11.2–51.6)
	Multiple Dose	25.4 (11.6–61.6)	70.3 (41.9–113.5)	12.6 (7.5–23.1)	ND	ND
Plasma Clearance (mL/min/kg)	Single Dose	0.44 (0.12–1.10)	0.30 (0.14–0.42)	1.10 (0.51–2.22)	0.28 (0.16–0.40)	0.53 (0.27–1.04)
	Multiple Dose	0.58 (0.24–1.15)	0.18 (0.12–0.33)	1.21 (0.66–1.82)	ND	ND

[a] Range of individual values across studies.
[b] Valproic acid administered chronically (Multiple Dose Study) or for 2 days (Single Dose Study).
Legend: ND=not done.

Table 2: LAMICTAL

Mean Pharmacokinetic Parameters in Pediatric Patients with Epilepsy

Pediatric Study Population	Number of Subjects	T_{max} (h)	$t_{1/2}$ (h)	CL/F (mL/min/kg)
Ages 10 months to 5.3 years				
Patients taking EIAEDs	10	3.0 (1.0–5.9)	7.7 (5.7–11.4)	3.62 (2.44–5.28)
Patients taking AEDs with no known effect on drug-metabolizing enzymes	7	5.2 (2.9–6.1)	19.0 (12.9–27.1)	1.2 (0.75–2.42)
Patients taking VPA only	8	2.9 (1.0–6.0)	44.9 (29.5–52.5)	0.47 (0.23–0.77)
Ages 5 to 11 years				
Patients taking EIAEDs	7	1.6 (1.0–3.0)	7.0 (3.8–9.8)	2.54 (1.35–5.58)
Patients taking EIAEDs plus VPA	8	3.3 (1.0–6.4)	19.1 (7.0–31.2)	0.89 (0.39–1.93)
Patients taking VPA only[b]	3	4.5 (3.0–6.0)	55.4 (24.3–73.7)	0.31 (0.20–0.54)
Ages 13 to 18 years				
Patients taking EIAEDs	11	[a]	[a]	1.3
Patients taking EIAEDs plus VPA	8	[a]	[a]	0.5
Patients taking VPA only	4	[a]	[a]	0.3

[a] Parameter not estimated.
[b] Two subjects were included in the calculation for mean t_{max}.
Legend: EIAEDs=enzyme inducing antiepileptic drugs; VPA=valproic acid.

Oxcarbazepine did not affect the apparent clearance of lamotrigine (see Precautions, Drug Interactions).

Other Drug Interactions: Chronic administration of acetaminophen was shown to slightly decrease the t½ and increase the clearance of a single dose of lamotrigine. Oral contraceptives and rifampin have also been shown to increase the apparent clearance of lamotrigine (see Precautions, Drug Interactions). Co-administration of olanzapine did not have a clinically relevant effect on LAMICTAL pharmacokinetics (see Precautions, Drug Interactions).

INDICATIONS: LAMICTAL (lamotrigine) is indicated: as adjunctive therapy for the management of adult patients with epilepsy who are not satisfactorily controlled by conventional therapy; for use as monotherapy in adults following withdrawal of concomitant antiepileptic drugs; as adjunctive therapy for the management of the seizures associated with Lennox-Gastaut syndrome in pediatric and adult patients.

CONTRAINDICATIONS: LAMICTAL (lamotrigine) is contraindicated in patients with known hypersensitivity to lamotrigine or to any components of the formulation.

WARNINGS: Serious rashes associated with hospitalization have occurred with the use of LAMICTAL (lamotrigine). The incidence of these rashes in clinical trials was 1% (1/100) in pediatric patients (age <16 years) and 0.3% (3/1000) in adults. The incidence of serious rash reported as Stevens-Johnson syndrome (SJS) in clinical trials was 0.5% (1/200) in pediatric patients and 0.1% (1/1000) in adults. In worldwide postmarketing experience, rare cases of toxic epidermal necrolysis and/or death associated with rash have been reported, but their numbers are too few to permit a precise estimate of the rate.

Serious Rash Associated with Rapid Titration: A higher incidence of serious dermatologic events (see Precautions, Skin-related Events, Table 3 and Table 4; see also Dosage) has been associated with more rapid initial titration (exceeding the recommended initial dose or exceeding the recommended dose escalation), and use of concomitant valproic acid.

Rash Associated with a History of Rash to Other Antiepileptic Drugs: In two studies (n=767 and n=988), the frequency of rash with lamotrigine treatment was approximately 3-4 times higher in patients with a history of allergy or rash to other antiepileptics, compared to those without such history.

Nearly all cases of rash associated with LAMICTAL have occurred within 2 to 8 weeks of treatment initiation. However, isolated cases have been reported after prolonged treatment (e.g., 6 months). Accordingly, duration of therapy cannot be relied upon as a means to predict the potential risk signalled by the first appearance of a rash.

Although benign rashes also occur with LAMICTAL, it is not possible to predict reliably which rashes will prove to be life-threatening. Accordingly, all patients who develop rash should be promptly evaluated and LAMICTAL withdrawn immediately, unless the rash is clearly not drug-related.

Hypersensitivity Reactions: Rash has also been reported as part of a hypersensitivity syndrome associated with a variable pattern of systemic symptoms including fever, lymphadenopathy, facial edema and abnormalities of the blood and liver (see Adverse Effects). The syndrome shows a wide spectrum of clinical severity and may rarely lead to disseminated intravascular coagulation (DIC) and multiorgan failure. It is important to note that early manifestations of hypersensitivity (e.g., fever, lymphadenopathy) may be present even though rash is not evident. If such signs and symptoms are present, the patient should be evaluated immediately and LAMICTAL discontinued if an alternative etiology cannot be established.

Prior to initiation of treatment with LAMICTAL, the patient should be instructed that a rash or other signs or symptoms of hypersensitivity (e.g., fever, lymphadenopathy) may herald a serious medical event and that the patient should report any such occurrence to a physician immediately.

Hormonal Contraceptives: Patients taking LAMICTAL should be advised not to start or stop their oral contraceptives without consulting their physician. Significant adjustments in the maintenance dose of LAMICTAL may be required in some patients (see Precautions, Drug Interactions, Oral Contraceptives and Dosage, Women and Oral Contraceptives).

Suicide Risk: Symptoms of depression and/or bipolar disorder may occur in patients with epilepsy, and there is evidence that patients with epilepsy and bipolar disorder have an elevated risk for suicidality.

Twenty-five to 50% of patients with bipolar disorder attempt suicide at least once, and may experience worsening of their depressive symptoms and/or the emergence of suicidal ideation and behaviours (suicidality) whether or not they are taking medications for bipolar disorder, including lamotrigine.

The incidence of suicidal ideation and behaviour was evaluated in a pooled analysis of placebo-controlled clinical trials with lamotrigine involving a total of 6467 patients from a number of indications, including studies in epilepsy and bipolar disorder.

In the subset of bipolar disorder trials, the rate of events was numerically, but not statistically significantly, greater for lamotrigine (29/1212 [2.4%]) compared with placebo (19/1054 [1.8%]). In a pooled analysis of psychiatric indications, events were more common in the first month of treatment, in patients taking lamotrigine. Behavioural events were more common in males.

In the subset of epilepsy trials, there were no statistically significant differences in the rate of events between lamotrigine and placebo; the number of events of suicidal ideation and behaviour was too low (6/1073 [0.6%] on lamotrigine and 2/805 [0.3%] on placebo) to allow a meaningful comparison of these rates.

PRECAUTIONS: Drug Discontinuation: Abrupt discontinuation of any antiepileptic drug (AED) in a responsive patient with epilepsy may provoke rebound seizures. In general, withdrawal of an AED should be gradual, to minimize this risk. Unless safety concerns (i.e., rash) require a more rapid withdrawal, the dose of LAMICTAL (lamotrigine) should be tapered over a period of at least 2 weeks (see Dosage).

Occupational Hazards: Patients with uncontrolled epilepsy should not drive or handle potentially dangerous machinery. During clinical trials, common adverse effects included dizziness, ataxia, drowsiness, diplopia and blurred vision. Patients should be advised to refrain from activities requiring mental alertness or physical coordination until they are sure that LAMICTAL does not affect them adversely.

Skin-related Events: In adult controlled studies of adjunctive lamotrigine therapy, the incidence of rash (usually maculopapular and/or erythematous) in patients receiving LAMICTAL was 10%, compared with 5% in placebo patients. The rash usually occurred within the first 6 weeks of therapy and resolved during continued administration of LAMICTAL. LAMICTAL was discontinued because of rash in 1.1% of adult patients in controlled studies and 3.8% of all patients in all studies. The rate of rash-related withdrawal in clinical studies was higher with more rapid initial titration dosing, and in patients receiving concomitant valproic acid (VPA), particularly in the absence of enzyme-inducing AEDs. (See Table 3 and Table 4; see also Warnings and Dosage).

Table 3: LAMICTAL

Effect of Concomitant AEDs on Rash Associated with LAMICTAL in All Adult Controlled and Uncontrolled Clinical Trials Regardless of Dosing Escalation Scheme

AED Group	Total Patient Number	All Rashes	Withdrawal Due to Rash	Hospitalization in Association with Rash
Enzyme-inducing AEDs[a]	1788	9.2%	1.8%	0.1%
Enzyme-inducing AEDs[a] + VPA	318	8.8%	3.5%	0.9%
VPA ± Non-enzyme-inducing AEDs[b]	159	20.8%	11.9%	2.5%
Non-enzyme-inducing AEDs[b]	27	18.5%	0.0%	0.0%

[a] Enzyme-inducing AEDs include carbamazepine, phenobarbital, phenytoin and primidone.
[b] Non-enzyme-inducing AEDs include clonazepam, clobazam, ethosuximide, methsuximide, vigabatrin and gabapentin.

Table 4: LAMICTAL

Effect of the Initial Daily Dose[a] of LAMICTAL in the Presence of Concomitant AEDs on the Incidence of Rash Leading to Withdrawal of Treatment in Adult Add-on Clinical Trials

AED Group	Enzyme-inducing AEDs[b]		Enzyme-inducing AEDs[b] + VPA		VPA ± Non-enzyme-inducing AEDs[c]	
LAMICTAL Average Daily Dose (mg)	Total Patient Number	Percentage of Patients Withdrawn	Total Patient Number	Percentage of Patients Withdrawn	Total Patient Number	Percentage of Patients Withdrawn
12.5	9	0.0	10	0.0	51	7.8
25	3	0.0	7	0.0	58	12.1
50	182	1.1	111	0.9	35	5.7
100	993	1.4	179	4.5	15	40.0

(cont'd)

Table 4: LAMICTAL *(cont'd)*

Effect of the Initial Daily Dose[a] of LAMICTAL in the Presence of Concomitant AEDs on the Incidence of Rash Leading to Withdrawal of Treatment in Adult Add-on Clinical Trials

AED Group	Enzyme-inducing AEDs[b]		Enzyme-inducing AEDs[b] + VPA		VPA ± Non-enzyme-inducing AEDs[c]	
LAMICTAL Average Daily Dose (mg)	Total Patient Number	Percentage of Patients Withdrawn	Total Patient Number	Percentage of Patients Withdrawn	Total Patient Number	Percentage of Patients Withdrawn
≥125	601	2.8	11	18.2	0	0.0

a Average daily dose in week 1.
b Enzyme-inducing AEDs include carbamazepine, phenobarbital, phenytoin and primidone.
c Non-enzyme-inducing AEDs include clonazepam, clobazam, ethosuximide, methsuximide, vigabatrin and gabapentin.

Increased incidence of rash-related withdrawal was seen when initial doses were higher and titration more rapid than recommended under Dosage.

Patients with a History of Allergy or Rash to Other Antiepileptic Drugs: Caution is also required when treating patients with a history of allergy or rash to other antiepileptic drugs, as it was found in two studies (n=767 and n=988) on the frequency of rash after treatment with lamotrigine that the rate of rash was approximately three to four times higher in patients with such a history, than those without.

Restarting LAMICTAL Therapy: It is recommended that LAMICTAL not be restarted in patients who discontinued due to rash associated with prior treatment with LAMICTAL unless the potential benefits clearly outweigh the risks. If the decision is made to restart a patient who has discontinued LAMICTAL for any reason, the need to restart with the initial dosing recommendations should be assessed. The greater the interval of time since the previous dose, the greater consideration should be given to restarting with the initial dosing recommendations. If a patient has discontinued LAMICTAL for a period of more than 5 half-lives, it is recommended that initial dosing recommendations and guidelines be followed. The half-life of LAMICTAL is affected by other concomitant medications (see Pharmacology, Pharmacokinetics and Dosage).

Drug Interactions: Antiepileptic Drugs (AEDs): Lamotrigine does not affect the plasma concentrations of concomitantly administered enzyme-inducing AEDs. Antiepileptic drugs that induce hepatic drug-metabolizing enzymes (phenytoin, carbamazepine, phenobarbital, primidone) increase the plasma clearance and reduce the elimination half-life of lamotrigine (see Pharmacology).

Valproic acid reduces the plasma clearance and prolongs the elimination half-life of lamotrigine (see Pharmacology). When LAMICTAL was administered to 18 healthy volunteers already receiving valproic acid, a modest decrease (25% on average) in the trough steady-state valproic acid plasma concentrations was observed over a 3-week period, followed by stabilization. However, the addition of LAMICTAL did not affect the plasma concentration of valproic acid in patients receiving enzyme-inducing AEDs in combination with valproic acid (see Precautions, Skin-related Events).

The AUC and C_{max} of oxcarbazepine and its active 10-monohydroxy oxcarbazepine metabolite were not significantly different following the addition of oxcarbazepine (600 mg twice daily) to LAMICTAL (200 mg once daily) in healthy male volunteers (n=13) compared to healthy male volunteers receiving oxcarbazepine alone (n=13). Limited clinical data suggest a higher incidence of headache, dizziness, nausea, and somnolence with co-administration of LAMICTAL and oxcarbazepine compared to LAMICTAL alone or oxcarbazepine alone.

The net effects of co-administration of LAMICTAL with phenytoin, carbamazepine, oxcarbazepine, or valproic acid are summarized in Table 5.

Table 5: LAMICTAL

Summary of AED Interactions with LAMICTAL

AED	AED Plasma Concentration with Adjunctive Lamotrigine[a]	Lamotrigine Plasma Concentration with Adjunctive AEDs[b]
Phenytoin (PHT)	No significant effect	↓ 50%
Carbamazepine (CBZ)	No significant effect	↓ 40%
CBZ epoxide[c]	Conflicting data	
Oxcarbazepine	No significant effect	No significant effect
10-monohydroxy oxcarbazepine metabolite	No significant effect	Not evaluated
Valproic Acid (VPA)	Decreased	↑ 200%
VPA+PHT and/or CBZ	Not evaluated	No significant effect

a From adjunctive clinical trials and volunteer studies.
b Net effects were estimated by comparing the mean clearance values obtained in adjunctive clinical trials and volunteer studies.
c Not administered, but an active metabolite of carbamazepine.

Oral Contraceptives: Effect of Oral Contraceptives on LAMICTAL: In a study in 16 female volunteers, an oral contraceptive preparation containing 30 µg ethinylestradiol and 150 µg levonorgestrel increased the apparent clearance of lamotrigine (300 mg/day) by approximately 2-fold with a mean decrease in AUC of 52% and in C_{max} of 39%. In this study, trough serum lamotrigine concentrations gradually increased and were approximately 2-fold higher on average at the end of the week of the inactive preparation compared to trough lamotrigine concentrations at the end of the active hormone cycle.

Gradual transient increases in lamotrigine levels will occur during the week of no active hormone preparation (pill-free week) for women not also taking a drug that increases the clearance of lamotrigine (carbamazepine, phenytoin, phenobarbital, primidone, or rifampin). The increase in lamotrigine levels will be greater if the dose of LAMICTAL is increased in the few days before or during the pill-free week.

Dosage adjustments may be necessary for women receiving oral contraceptive preparations (see Dosage, Women and Oral Contraceptives).

Effect of LAMICTAL on Oral Contraceptives: Co-administration of LAMICTAL: (300 mg/day) in 16 female volunteers did not affect the pharmacokinetics of the ethinylestradiol component of an oral contraceptive preparation containing 30 µg ethinylestradiol and 150 µg levonorgestrel. There was a mean decrease in the AUC and C_{max} of the levonorgestrel component of 19% and 12%, respectively. Measurement of serum progesterone indicated that there was no hormonal evidence of ovulation in any of the 16 volunteers, although measurement of serum FSH, LH, and estradiol indicated that there was some loss of suppression of the hypothalamic-pituitary-ovarian axis.

The effects of doses of LAMICTAL other than 300 mg/day have not been studied.

The clinical significance of the observed hormonal changes on ovulatory activity is unknown. However, the possibility of decreased contraceptive efficacy in some patients cannot be excluded. Therefore, patients should be instructed to promptly report changes in their menstrual pattern (e.g., break-through bleeding).

Interactions with Other Hormonal Contraceptives or Hormone Replacement Therapy: The effect of other hormonal contraceptive preparations or hormone replacement therapy on the pharmacokinetics of lamotrigine has not been evaluated, although the effect may be similar to oral contraceptive preparations. Therefore, as for oral contraceptives, dosage adjustments may be necessary (see Dosage, Women and Oral Contraceptives).

Olanzapine: The AUC and C_{max} of lamotrigine was reduced on average by 24% and 20%, respectively, following the addition of olanzapine (15 mg once daily) to LAMICTAL (200 mg once daily) in healthy male volunteers (n=16) compared to healthy male volunteers receiving LAMICTAL alone (n=12). This reduction in lamotrigine plasma concentrations is not expected to be clinically relevant.

Risperidone: Following the co-administration of 2 mg risperidone with lamotrigine (up to 400 mg daily), 12 out of the 14 healthy adult volunteers reported somnolence compared to 1 out of 20 when risperidone was given alone, and 0 out of 20 when lamotrigine was administered alone.

Rifampin: In a study in 10 male volunteers, rifampin (600 mg/day for 5 days) significantly increased the apparent clearance of a single 25 mg dose of lamotrigine by approximately 2-fold (AUC decreased by approximately 40%). For patients taking rifampin with LAMICTAL, follow the titration schedule for concomitant enzyme-inducing AEDs (without VPA) (see Dosage, Table 9).

Lopinavir/Ritonavir: In a study in healthy volunteers, lopinavir/ritonavir approximately halved the plasma concentrations of lamotrigine. At least 14 out of 22 healthy adult volunteers reported diarrhea and 5 out of 22 subjects reported rash following the addition of lopinavir/ ritonavir (400 mg/100 mg b.i.d.) to lamotrigine (up to 200 mg b.i.d.), compared to 1 out of 24 reporting diarrhea or rash, when lamotrigine was administered alone (up to 100 mg b.i.d.). Diarrhea is a common adverse event reported for lopinavir/ritonavir. The titration of lamotrigine in this study was rapid, which is a known risk factor for the development of a rash. The rashes necessitated the discontinuation of the medications. One subject also discontinued the medications due to elevated AST and ALT levels. Caution is advised for the co-administration of lopinavir/ritonavir with lamotrigine. In patients receiving concomitant therapy with lopinavir/ritonavir, the treatment regimen recommended for concomitant enzyme-inducing AEDs (without VPA) should be used (see Dosage and Administration, Table 9).

Drugs Depressing Cardiac Conduction: See Patients with Special Diseases and Conditions and Cardiac Conduction Abnormalities.

Drug/Laboratory Test Interactions: LAMICTAL has not been associated with any assay interferences in clinical laboratory tests.

Children: Safety and efficacy in patients below the age of 16 years, other than those with Lennox-Gastaut Syndrome, have not been established.

Geriatrics: As the pharmacokinetics in this age group do not differ significantly from a non-elderly adult population, no dosage adjustment from the recommended adult schedule is required (see also Dosage, Adverse Effects and Pharmacology).

Pregnancy: Studies in mice, rats and rabbits given lamotrigine orally or i.v. revealed no evidence of teratogenicity; however, maternal and secondary fetal toxicity were observed. Studies in rats and rabbits indicate that lamotrigine crosses the placenta; placental and fetal levels of lamotrigine were low and comparable to levels in maternal plasma.

Clinical trial data indicate that lamotrigine has no effect on blood folate concentrations in adults; however, its effects during human fetal development are unknown.

Postmarketing data from six prospective pregnancy registries have documented outcomes in approximately 4000 women exposed to lamotrigine monotherapy during the first trimester of pregnancy. Two registries have reported an increase in the risk of isolated oral cleft (isolated) malformations with exposure to lamotrigine in the first trimester, over both the study reference population and reported background rates from the literature.

The North American Anti-Epileptic Drug Registry reported rates of: 7.3/1000 for lamotrigine exposures in the registry with n=684 vs 0.70/1000 for the reference population and 0.50-2.16/1000 for the background rates.

The Swedish Medical Birth Register reported rates of 9.9/1000 for lamotrigine exposures in the registry with n=403 vs 2.0/1000 for the registry reference population and 0.50-2.16/1000 for the background rates. In the remaining registries with approximately 3000 women, 4 cases of isolated oral cleft malformation were found (1.3/1000 vs 0.50-2.16/1000 for the background rates).

EUROCAT: The European Network of Congenital Anomaly and Twin Registries (EUROCAT) is a network of 40 registries across 20 European countries. The results of a case control design using the EUROCAT dataset demonstrated that the risk of development of oral clefts in the newborn infants was similar to other defects following exposure to lamotrigine in the first trimester. Within the EUROCAT network, rates of exposure to lamotrigine in the first trimester of pregnancy were similar among 4571 non chromosomal, isolated oral cleft cases and 80 052 non chromosomal, non oral cleft defect controls.

The data on use of lamotrigine in polytherapy combinations are insufficient to assess whether the risk of malformation associated with other agents is affected by concomitant lamotrigine use.

As with other medicines, LAMICTAL should only be used during pregnancy if the expected benefits outweigh the potential risks.

Physiological changes during pregnancy may affect lamotrigine levels and/or therapeutic effect. There have been reports of decreased lamotrigine levels during pregnancy. Appropriate clinical management of pregnant women during lamotrigine therapy should be ensured.

To facilitate monitoring fetal outcomes of pregnant women exposed to lamotrigine, physicians are encouraged to register patients, before fetal outcome (e.g., ultrasound, results of amniocentesis, birth, etc.) is known, in the Lamotrigine Drug Pregnancy Registry by calling 1-800-336-2176 (toll free).

Labour and Delivery: The effect of LAMICTAL on labour and delivery in humans is unknown.

Lactation: There is limited information on the use of LAMICTAL in lactation. Preliminary data indicate that lamotrigine passes into human milk in concentrations usually of the order 40 to 60% of the serum concentration. In a small number of infants known to have been breast-fed, the serum concentrations of lamotrigine reached levels at which pharmacological effects may occur. Because of the potential for adverse reactions from LAMICTAL in nursing infants, breast-feeding while taking this medication is not recommended.

Patients with Special Diseases and Conditions: Clinical experience with LAMICTAL in patients with concomitant illness is limited. Caution is advised when using LAMICTAL in patients with diseases or conditions that could affect the metabolism or elimination of the drug.

Renal Failure: A study in individuals with chronic renal failure (not receiving other AEDs) indicated that the elimination half-life of unchanged lamotrigine is prolonged relative to individuals with normal renal function (see Pharmacology). Use of LAMICTAL in patients with severe renal impairment should proceed with caution.

Hepatic Impairment: Results from a single-dose pharmacokinetic study indicate that the apparent clearance of lamotrigine decreased in subjects with Grades A, B or C hepatic impairment. A reduced dosage should be used for all hepatically impaired patients, and lamotrigine should be administered with caution particularly in those patients with severe hepatic impairment (see also Dosage and Pharmacology).

Cardiac Conduction Abnormalities: One placebo-controlled trial that compared ECGs at baseline and during treatment demonstrated a mild prolongation of the PR interval associated with LAMICTAL administration. The prolongation was statistically significant but clinically insignificant. Patients with significant cardiovascular disease or electrocardiographic abnormalities were, however, systematically excluded from clinical trials. Thus, LAMICTAL should be used with caution in patients with cardiac conduction abnormalities, and in patients taking concomitant medications which depress AV conduction.

Dependence Liability: No evidence of abuse potential has been associated with LAMICTAL, nor is there evidence of psychological or physical dependence in humans.

Laboratory Tests: The relationship between clinical efficacy and plasma concentrations has not been clearly established. Based on the possible pharmacokinetic interactions between LAMICTAL and other drugs including AEDs, monitoring of the plasma levels of LAMICTAL and concomitant drugs may be indicated, particularly during dosage adjustments. In general, clinical judgment should be exercised regarding monitoring of plasma levels of LAMICTAL and other drugs and whether or not dosage adjustments are necessary.

ADVERSE EFFECTS: Rarely, serious skin rashes, including Stevens-Johnson syndrome and toxic epidermal necrolysis (Lyell's syndrome) have been reported. Although the majority recover following drug withdrawal, some patients experience irreversible scarring and there have been rare cases of associated death (see Warnings).

Adverse experiences in patients receiving LAMICTAL (lamotrigine) were generally mild, occurred within the first 2 weeks of therapy, and resolved without discontinuation of the drug.

Commonly Observed: The most commonly observed adverse experiences associated with the use of adjunctive therapy with LAMICTAL (incidence of at least 10%) were dizziness, headache, diplopia, somnolence, ataxia, nausea and asthenia.

Dizziness, diplopia, ataxia and blurred vision were dose-related and occurred more commonly in patients receiving carbamazepine in combination with LAMICTAL than in patients receiving other enzyme-inducing AEDs with LAMICTAL. Reduction of the daily dose and/or alteration of the timing of doses of concomitant antiepileptic drugs and/or LAMICTAL may reduce or eliminate these symptoms. Clinical data suggest a higher incidence of rash in patients who are receiving concomitant valproic acid, or non-inducing AEDs (see Warnings and Precautions, Skin-related Events, Table 3).

Adverse Events Associated with Discontinuation of Treatment: Across all adult add-on studies, the most common adverse experiences associated with discontinuation of LAMICTAL were rash, dizziness, headache, ataxia, nausea, diplopia, somnolence, seizure exacerbation, asthenia and blurred vision. In controlled clinical trials, 6.9% of the 711 patients receiving LAMICTAL discontinued therapy due to an adverse experience, versus 2.9% of the 419 patients receiving placebo. Of 3501 patients and volunteers who received LAMICTAL in premarketing clinical studies, 358 (10.2%) discontinued therapy due to an adverse experience.

Serious Adverse Events Associated with Discontinuation of Treatment: Discontinuation due to an adverse experience classified as serious occurred in 2.3% of adult patients and volunteers who received lamotrigine in the premarketing studies. Rash accounted for almost half of the discontinuations due to serious adverse experiences. More rapid initial titration dosing of lamotrigine, and concomitant use of valproic acid were associated with higher incidences of rash-related withdrawal in clinical studies (see Warnings and Precautions, Skin-related Events, Table 4).

Adult Controlled Add-on Clinical Studies: Table 6 enumerates adverse experiences that occurred with an incidence of 2% or greater among refractory patients with epilepsy treated with LAMICTAL.

Other Events Observed During Clinical Studies: During clinical testing, multiple doses of LAMICTAL were administered to 3501 patients and volunteers. The conditions and duration of exposure to LAMICTAL during these clinical studies varied greatly. Studies included monotherapy and pediatric trials. A substantial proportion of the exposure was gained in open, uncontrolled clinical studies. Adverse experiences associated with exposure to lamotrigine were recorded by clinical investigators using terminology of their own choosing. Consequently, it is not possible to provide a meaningful estimate of the proportion of individuals experiencing adverse events without first grouping similar types of adverse experiences into a smaller number of standardized event categories.

Since the adverse experiences reported occurred during treatment with LAMICTAL in combination with other antiepileptic drugs, they were not necessarily caused by LAMICTAL.

The following adverse events have been reported on one or more occasions by at least 1% of patients and volunteers exposed to LAMICTAL: anorexia, weight gain, amnesia, concentration disturbance, confusion, emotional lability, nervousness, nystagmus, paresthesia, thinking abnormality and vertigo. (All types of events are included except those already listed in Table 6.)

Adult Monotherapy Clinical Studies: Withdrawals due to adverse events were reported in 42 (9.5%) of newly diagnosed patients treated with LAMICTAL monotherapy. The most common adverse experiences associated with discontinuation of LAMICTAL were rash (6.1%), asthenia (1.1%), headache (1.1%), nausea (0.7%) and vomiting (0.7%).

Elderly Monotherapy Clinical Studies: A study with elderly newly diagnosed epilepsy patients yielded rates of adverse events which were generally similar to those reported in adults (see Table 6). The rate of withdrawal due to adverse events was 21.6%, with rash (3%), nausea (3%) and coordination abnormalities (3%) representing the most common events associated with withdrawal, followed by somnolence (2%), depression (2%), accidental injury (2%) and malaise (2%) (see also Dosage and Pharmacology).

Adjunctive Therapy in Lennox-Gastaut Syndrome: In 169 adult and pediatric patients with Lennox-Gastaut syndrome, 3.8% of patients on lamotrigine and 7.8% of patients on placebo discontinued treatment due to adverse experiences. The most commonly reported adverse experiences that led to discontinuation were rash for patients treated with LAMICTAL and deterioration of seizure control for patients treated with placebo. Fever and infection occurred at least 10% more frequently in patients ≤12 years of age than in patients >12 years of age on LAMICTAL. Rash occurred at least 10% more frequently in female patients than male patients on LAMICTAL. Table 7 lists adverse events that occurred in at least 1% of 79 adult and pediatric patients who received LAMICTAL up to 15 mg/kg/day or a maximum of 400 mg/day.

Table 6: LAMICTAL

Percentage of Treatment-emergent Adverse Experiences in Adult Placebo or Comparator-controlled Clinical Studies[a]

	Adults (Adjunctive Therapy)[b]		Elderly (Monotherapy)[c]
Total Number of Patients	**LAMICTAL (and other AEDs) (n=711)**	**Placebo (and other AEDs) (n=419)**	**LAMICTAL (n=102)**
Body System/Adverse Experience[d]			
Body as a Whole			
Headache	29.1	19.1	8.8
Accidental Injury	9.1	8.6	8.8
Asthenia	8.6	8.8	4.9
Flu Syndrome	7.0	5.5	4.9
Pain	6.2	2.9	5.9
Back Pain	5.8	6.2	3.9
Fever	5.5	3.6	0.9
Abdominal Pain	5.2	3.6	3.9
Infection	4.4	4.1	5.9
Neck Pain	2.4	1.2	0
Malaise	2.3	1.9	4.9
Seizure Exacerbation	2.3	0.5	n/a
Cardiovascular			
Chest Pain	n/a	n/a	2.9
Syncope	n/a	n/a	2.9
Cerebrovascular Accident	n/a	n/a	3.9
Digestive			
Nausea	18.6	9.5	8.8
Vomiting	9.4	4.3	8.8
Diarrhea	6.3	4.1	6.9
Dyspepsia	5.3	2.1	5.9
Constipation	4.1	3.1	8.9
Tooth Disorder	3.2	1.7	0
Musculoskeletal			
Myalgia	2.8	3.1	0.9
Arthralgia	2.0	0.2	2.9
Nervous			
Dizziness	38.4	13.4	9.8
Ataxia	21.7	5.5	0
Somnolence	14.2	6.9	11.8
Incoordination	6.0	2.1	12.7
Insomnia	5.6	1.9	3.9
Tremor	4.4	1.4	0.9
Depression	4.2	2.6	4.9
Anxiety	3.8	2.6	0.9
Convulsion	3.2	1.2	1.9
Irritability	3.0	1.9	0
Speech Disorder	2.5	0.2	0.9
Memory Decreased	2.4	1.9	n/a
Memory Decreased (memory rating question)	n/a	n/a	19.6
Respiratory			
Rhinitis	13.6	9.3	0.9
Pharyngitis	9.8	8.8	1.9
Cough Increased	7.5	5.7	2.9
Respiratory Disorder	5.3	5.5	0.9
Asthma	n/a	n/a	3.0
Skin and Appendages			
Rash	10.0	5.0	8.8
Pruritus	3.1	1.7	5.9
Herpes Zoster	n/a	n/a	3.0
Eczema	n/a	n/a	2.0
Ulcer Skin	n/a	n/a	2.0
Special Senses			
Diplopia	27.6	6.7	0
Blurred Vision	15.5	4.5	0
Vision Abnormality	3.4	1.0	0
Urogenital			
Female Patients	**(n=365)**	**(n=207)**	**(n=47)**
Dysmenorrhea	6.6	6.3	n/a
Menstrual Disorder	5.2	5.8	n/a
Vaginitis	4.1	0.5	0

[a] Patients from the studies summarized in the first 2 columns were receiving 1 to 3 concomitant enzyme-inducing antiepileptic drugs in addition to LAMICTAL or placebo. Patients from the single study summarized in the last column were compared to n=48 patients receiving carbamazepine. Patients may have reported multiple adverse experiences during the study or at discontinuation. Thus, patients may be included in more than one category.

[b] Studies 05, 06, 16 (US) &16, 21, 35 & 37 (UK).

[c] Study 105-124-C93.

[d] All adverse experiences reported by at least 2% of patients treated with either LAMICTAL add-on or monotherapy are included.

Table 7: LAMICTAL

Treatment-emergent Adverse Experience Incidence in Placebo-controlled Add-on Trial in Adult and Pediatric Patients with Lennox-Gastaut Syndrome[a]

Body System/ Adverse Experience	Percent of Patients Receiving LAMICTAL (n=79)	Percent of Patients Receiving Placebo (n=90)
Body as a Whole		
Infection	13	8
Accidental Injury	9	7
Flu Syndrome	5	0
Asthenia	3	1
Abdominal Pain	3	

(cont'd)

Table 7: LAMICTAL *(cont'd)*

Treatment-emergent Adverse Experience Incidence in Placebo-controlled Add-on Trial in Adult and Pediatric Patients with Lennox-Gastaut Syndrome[a]

Body System/ Adverse Experience	Percent of Patients Receiving LAMICTAL (n=79)	Percent of Patients Receiving Placebo (n=90)
Back Pain	1	0
Edema of the Face	1	0
Lab test Abnormal	1	0
Pain	1	0
Cardiovascular		
Hemorrhage	3	0
Digestive		
Vomiting	9	7
Constipation	5	2
Diarrhea	4	2
Nausea	4	1
Anorexia	3	1
Stomatitis Aphtha	1	0
Tooth Disorder	1	0
Endocrine		
Cushing's Syndrome	1	0
Hypothyroidism	1	0
Hemic and Lymphatic		
Lymphadenopathy (enlarged cervical nodes)	1	0
Nervous System		
Ataxia	4	1
Convulsions	4	1
Tremor	3	0
Agitation	1	0
Coordination	1	0
Dizziness	1	0
Emotional Lability	1	0
Nervousness	1	0
Vertigo	1	0
Respiratory		
Pharyngitis	14	10
Bronchitis	9	7
Pneumonia	3	0
Dyspnea	1	0
Skin		
Rash	9	7
Eczema	4	0
Nail Disorder	1	0
Special Senses		
Blepharitis	1	0
Conjunctivitis	1	0
Keratitis	1	0
Ear Pain	1	0
Eye Pain	1	0
Urogenital		
Urinary Tract Infection	3	0

(cont'd)

Table 7: LAMICTAL *(cont'd)*

Treatment-emergent Adverse Experience Incidence in Placebo-controlled Add-on Trial in Adult and Pediatric Patients with Lennox-Gastaut Syndrome[a]

Body System/ Adverse Experience	Percent of Patients Receiving LAMICTAL (n=79)	Percent of Patients Receiving Placebo (n=90)
Balanitis	2	0
Penis Disorder	2	0

[a] The most frequently reported adverse reactions in children ≤12 years of age in both treatment groups were pharyngitis, fever and infection.

Postmarketing and Other Experience: In addition to the adverse experiences reported during clinical testing of LAMICTAL, the following adverse experiences have been reported in patients receiving marketed LAMICTAL and from worldwide noncontrolled investigational use. These adverse experiences have not been listed above, and data are insufficient to support an estimate of their incidence or to establish causation.

Blood and Lymphatic: There have been reports of hematological abnormalities which may or may not be associated with hypersensitivity syndrome. These have included disseminated intravascular coagulation, hemolytic anemia, neutropenia, leukopenia, pancytopenia, anemia, thrombocytopenia, red cell aplasia, and very rarely agranulocytosis and aplastic anemia.

There have been reported cases of lymphadenopathy in the absence of hypersensitivity reactions, in patients with or without previous history, and taking LAMICTAL alone or in combination with other medications (including other AEDs). Discontinuation of LAMICTAL or, in some cases, dose reduction resolved the reaction.

Gastrointestinal: esophagitis.

Hepatobiliary Tract and Pancreas: pancreatitis. Elevations of liver function tests and rare reports of hepatic dysfunction, including hepatic failure, have been reported. Hepatic dysfunction usually occurs in association with hypersensitivity reactions but isolated cases have been reported without overt signs of hypersensitivity.

Immunologic: lupus-like reaction, vasculitis.

Lower Respiratory: apnea.

Musculoskeletal: Rhabdomyolysis has been observed in patients experiencing hypersensitivity reactions.

Neurology: hallucinations. Exacerbation of parkinsonian symptoms in patients with pre-existing Parkinson's disease and isolated reports of extrapyramidal effects and choreoathetosis in patients without this underlying condition. Movement disorders such as tics and unsteadiness have also been reported.

There have been very rare reports of aseptic meningitis in patients taking LAMICTAL alone or in combination with other AEDs. In some cases, discontinuation of LAMICTAL resolved this reaction.

Non-site Specific: hypersensitivity reaction, multiorgan failure, progressive immunosuppression.

OVERDOSE:

Symptoms: Adults: Acute ingestion of doses in excess of 20 times the maximum therapeutic dose has been reported. In general, overdose has resulted in symptoms including nystagmus, ataxia, impaired consciousness and coma.

However, there has been one fatality reported, a 22 year-old female who intentionally ingested 15 g of LAMICTAL. The patient experienced acute clonic seizures and heart failure, then became asystolic and was resuscitated, but she died 2 days later.

Children: Among patients ≤16 years of age, the two highest known single doses of LAMICTAL have been 3000 mg by a 14 year-old female and approximately 1000 mg by a 4 year-old male. The 14 year-old female was taking marketed LAMICTAL; after the dose, she lost consciousness and was admitted to the hospital for supportive therapy, where she recovered fully (time to recovery not reported). The 4 year-old male was drowsy and agitated when found, and his condition worsened to coma level II after hospitalization. He was given supportive therapy and his condition improved rapidly, with full recovery in 3 days.

Treatment: There are no specific antidotes for LAMICTAL. Following a suspected overdose, hospitalization of the patient is advised. General supportive care is indicated, including frequent monitoring of vital signs and close observation of the patient. If indicated, emesis should be induced or gastric lavage should be performed. It is uncertain whether hemodialysis is an effective means of removing lamotrigine from the blood. In 6 renal failure patients, about 20% of the amount of lamotrigine in the body was removed during 4 hours of hemodialysis.

For management of a suspected drug overdose, CPhA recommends that you contact your **regional Poison Control Centre**. See the *CPS* Directory section for a list of Poison Control Centres.

DOSAGE: Potential for Serious Dermatological Reactions: **Do not exceed the recommended initial dose and subsequent dose escalations of LAMICTAL. More rapid initial titration has been associated with an increased incidence of serious dermatological reactions (see Warnings), as has concomitant use of valproic acid, particularly in the absence of enzyme-inducing AEDs (see Warnings and Precautions). Patients with a history of rash or allergy to other AEDs are more at risk for LAMICTAL-associated rash than those without such history (see Warnings and Precautions).**

General: LAMICTAL (lamotrigine) is intended for oral administration and may be taken with or without food. LAMICTAL should be added to the patient's current antiepileptic therapy.

Valproic acid more than doubles the elimination half-life of lamotrigine and reduces the plasma clearance by 50%; conversely, hepatic enzyme-inducing drugs such as carbamazepine, phenytoin, phenobarbital, and primidone reduce the elimination half-life of lamotrigine by 50% and double the plasma clearance (see Pharmacology). These clinically important interactions require dosage schedules of LAMICTAL as summarized in Table 8, Table 9, Table 10 and Table 11.

LAMICTAL does not alter plasma concentrations of concomitantly administered enzyme-inducing AEDs, and therefore, they do not usually require dose adjustment to maintain therapeutic plasma concentrations. For patients receiving LAMICTAL in combination with other AEDs, an evaluation of all AEDs in the regimen should be considered if a change in seizure control or an appearance or worsening of adverse experiences is observed. If there is a need to discontinue therapy with LAMICTAL, a step-wise reduction of dose over at least 2 weeks (approximately 50% per week) is recommended unless safety concerns (i.e., rash) require a more rapid withdrawal (see Warnings and Precautions).

The relationship of plasma concentration to clinical response has not been established for LAMICTAL. Dosing of LAMICTAL should be based on therapeutic response. In controlled clinical studies, doses of LAMICTAL that were efficacious generally produced steady-state trough plasma lamotrigine concentrations of 1 to 4 µg/mL in patients receiving one or more concomitant AEDs. Doses of LAMICTAL producing this plasma concentration range were well tolerated. As with any antiepileptic drug, the oral dose of LAMICTAL should be adjusted to the needs of the individual patient, taking into consideration the concomitant AED therapy the patient is receiving.

Women and Oral Contraceptives: Starting LAMICTAL in Women Taking Oral Contraceptives: Although oral contraceptives have been shown to increase the clearance of lamotrigine (see Precautions, Drug Interactions), no adjustments to the recommended dose escalation guidelines for LAMICTAL should be necessary solely based on the use of oral contraceptives. Therefore, dose escalation should follow the recommended guidelines based on whether LAMICTAL is added to valproate, whether LAMICTAL is added to carbamazepine, phenytoin, phenobarbital, primidone, or rifampin, or whether LAMICTAL is added in the absence of valproate, carbamazepine, phenytoin, phenobarbital, primidone, or rifampin.

Adjustments to the Maintenance Dose of LAMICTAL: Taking or Starting Oral Contraceptives: For women not taking carbamazepine, phenytoin, phenobarbital, primidone, or rifampin, the maintenance dose of LAMICTAL may need to be increased, by as much as 2-fold over the recommended target maintenance dose, according to clinical response (see Precautions, Drug Interactions). For women taking LAMICTAL in addition to carbamazepine, phenytoin, phenobarbital, primidone, or rifampin, no adjustment should be necessary.

Stopping Oral Contraceptives: For women not taking carbamazepine, phenytoin, phenobarbital, primidone, or rifampin, the maintenance dose of LAMICTAL may need to be to be decreased by as much as 50% of the maintenance dose with concurrent oral contraceptives, according to clinical response (see Precautions, Drug Interactions). For women taking LAMICTAL in addition to carbamazepine, phenytoin, phenobarbital, primidone or rifampin, no adjustment should be necessary.

Women and Other Hormonal Contraceptive Preparations or Hormone Replacement Therapy: Although the effect of other hormonal contraceptive preparations or hormone replacement therapy on the pharmacokinetics of lamotrigine has not been evaluated, the effect may be similar to oral contraceptives (see Precautions, Drug Interactions). Therefore, similar adjustments to the dosage of LAMICTAL may be needed, based on clinical response.

Restarting LAMICTAL Therapy: It is recommended that LAMICTAL not be restarted in patients who discontinued due to rash associated with prior treatment with LAMICTAL, unless the potential benefits clearly outweigh the risks. If the decision is made to restart a patient who has discontinued LAMICTAL for any reason, the need to restart with the initial dosing recommendations should be assessed. The greater the interval of time since the previous dose, the greater consideration should be given to restarting with the initial dosing recommendations. If a patient has discontinued LAMICTAL for a period of more than 5 half-lives, it is recommended that initial dosing recommendations and guidelines be followed. The half-life of LAMICTAL is affected by other concomitant medications (see Pharmacology, Pharmacokinetics).

Adults and Children Over 12 Years of Age: **Do not exceed the recommended initial dose and subsequent dose escalations of LAMICTAL. More rapid initial titration has been associated with an increased incidence of serious dermatological reactions (see Warnings).** For patients taking AEDs whose pharmacokinetic interactions with LAMICTAL are currently unknown, follow the titration schedule for concomitant VPA and non-enzyme-inducing AEDs.

Table 8: LAMICTAL

LAMICTAL Added to VPA with Enzyme-inducing AEDs[a] in Patients Over 12 Years of Age

		For Information[b] Patients Taking Valproic Acid Only or VPA and Non-enzyme-inducing AEDs
Weeks 1+2	25 mg once a day	25 mg every other day
Weeks 3+4	25 mg twice a day	25 mg once a day
Usual Maintenance	To achieve maintenance, doses may be increased by 25–50 mg every 1 to 2 weeks. Usual dose is between 50–100 mg twice a day	To achieve maintenance, doses may be increased by 25–50 mg every 1 to 2 weeks. Usual dose is between 50–100 mg twice a day

a Enzyme-inducing AEDs include carbamazepine, phenobarbital, phenytoin, and primidone.
b Column reflects dosage recommendations in the United Kingdom and is provided for information.

Table 9: LAMICTAL

LAMICTAL Added to Enzyme-inducing AEDs[a] (without VPA) and Selected Other Drugs[b] in Patients Over 12 Years of Age

Weeks 1+2	50 mg once a day
Weeks 3+4	50 mg twice a day
Usual Maintenance	To achieve maintenance, doses may be increased by 100 mg every 1 to 2 weeks. Usual dose is between 150–250 mg twice a day

a Enzyme-inducing AEDs include carbamazepine, phenobarbital, phenytoin, and primidone.
b Rifampin, lopinavir/ritonavir.

There have been no controlled studies to establish the effectiveness or optimal dosing regimen of add-on LAMICTAL therapy in patients receiving only non-enzyme-inducing AEDs or valproic acid. However, available data from open clinical trials indicate that the addition of LAMICTAL under these conditions is associated with a higher incidence of serious rash or rash-related withdrawal, even at an initial titration dose of 12.5 mg daily (see Precautions, Skin-related Events, Table 3 and Table 4; see also Warnings). The potential medical benefits of addition of LAMICTAL under these conditions must be weighed against the increased risk of serious rash. If use of LAMICTAL under these conditions is considered clinically indicated, titration should proceed with extreme caution, especially during the first 6 weeks of treatment.

Withdrawal of Concomitant AEDs in Adults: Concomitant AEDs may be decreased over a 5-week period, by approximately 20% of the original dose every week. However, a slower taper may be used if clinically indicated. During this period, the dose of LAMICTAL administered will be dependent upon the effect of the drug being withdrawn on the pharmacokinetics of lamotrigine, together with the overall clinical response of the patient. The withdrawal of enzyme inducing AEDs (i.e., phenytoin, phenobarbital, primidone, and carbamazepine) will result in an approximate doubling of the $t_{1/2}$ of lamotrigine. Under these conditions, it may be necessary to reduce the dose of LAMICTAL. In contrast, the withdrawal of enzyme-inhibiting AEDs (i.e., valproic acid) will result in a decrease in the $t_{1/2}$ of lamotrigine and may require an increase in the dose of LAMICTAL.

Children: **Do not exceed the recommended initial dose and subsequent dose escalations of LAMICTAL. More rapid initial titration has been associated with an increased incidence of serious dermatological reactions (see Warnings). Safety and efficacy in patients below the age of 16 years, other than those with Lennox-Gastaut Syndrome, have not been established.**

The starting doses and dose escalations listed below are different than those used in clinical trials; however, the maintenance doses are the same as those used in clinical trials. Smaller starting doses and slower dose escalations than those used in clinical trials are recommended because of concern that the risk of serious rash may be greater with higher initial doses and more rapid dose escalation. Consequently, it may take several weeks to months to achieve an individualized maintenance dose.

The smallest available strength of LAMICTAL Chewable/Dispersible Tablets is 2 mg. Only whole tablets should be administered (scoreline on the 5 mg tablet is not intended for tablet splitting). Recommended doses have been determined based on the individual tablet strengths which most closely approximates, but does **not** exceed, the target dose calculated on the basis of patient weight. In patients on concomitant VPA, LAMICTAL should not be administered if the calculated daily dose is less than 1 mg (e.g., patients weighing less than 9 kg). If the initial calculated daily dose of LAMICTAL is 1 to 2 mg or 2.5 to 5 mg, then 2 or 5 mg respectively of LAMICTAL should be taken on alternate days for the first 2 weeks.

For patients taking AEDs whose pharmacokinetic interactions with LAMICTAL are currently unknown, follow the titration schedule for concomitant VPA.

Table 10: LAMICTAL

Pediatric Dosing with LAMICTAL for Patients Receiving Valproic Acid with or Without Enzyme-inducing AEDs[a]

Weight Range	Weeks 1+2 0.15 mg/kg once a day	Weeks 3+4 0.3 mg/kg once a day	Weeks 5 and Onwards to Usual Maintenance Dose[b] To achieve maintenance, doses may be increased by 0.3 mg/kg every 1–2 weeks, to a maximum of 200 mg/day. Usual dose is between 1–5 mg/kg once a day[c]
<9 kg	Do not take LAMICTAL since there is insufficient experience in children weighing less than 9 kg.		
9–13 kg	2 mg every other day	2 mg/day	Increase dose by no more than 2 mg/day every 1–2 weeks
14–16 kg	2 mg/day	4 mg/day	Increase dose by no more than 4 mg/day every 1–2 weeks
17–33 kg	5 mg every other day	5 mg/day	Increase dose by no more than 5 mg/day every 1–2 weeks
34–49 kg	5 mg/day	10 mg/day	Increase dose by no more than 10 mg/day every 1–2 weeks
≥50 kg[d]	5 mg/day	15 mg/day	Increase dose by no more than 15 mg/day every 1–2 weeks

a Enzyme-inducing AEDs include carbamazepine, phenobarbital, phenytoin, and primidone.
b It may take several weeks to months to achieve an individualized maintenance dose.
c Can be given as 2 divided doses.
d Insufficient data are available to be able to support the mg/kg dosing in patients weighing more than 50 kg.

Table 11: LAMICTAL

Pediatric Dosing with LAMICTAL for Patients Receiving Enzyme-inducing AEDs[a,b,c] Without Valproic Acid

Weight Range	Weeks 1+2 0.3 mg/kg twice a day	Weeks 3+4 0.6 mg/kg twice a day	Weeks 5 and Onwards to Usual Maintenance Dose[d] To achieve maintenance, doses may be increased by 1.2 mg/kg every 1–2 weeks, to a maximum of 400 mg/day. Usual dose is between 2.5–7.5 mg/kg twice a day
<9 kg	Do not take LAMICTAL since there is insufficient experience in children weighing less than 9 kg.		
9–12 kg	5 mg/day	10 mg/day	Increase dose by no more than 10 mg/day every 1–2 weeks
13–16 kg	5 mg/day	15 mg/day	Increase dose by no more than 15 mg/day every 1–2 weeks
17–20 kg	10 mg/day	20 mg/day	Increase dose by no more than 20 mg/day every 1–2 weeks
21–24 kg	10 mg/day	25 mg/day	Increase dose by no more than 25 mg/day every 1–2 weeks
25–29 kg	15 mg/day	30 mg/day	Increase dose by no more than 30 mg/day every 1–2 weeks
30–33 kg	15 mg/day	35 mg/day	Increase dose by no more than 35 mg/day every 1–2 weeks
34–37 kg	20 mg/day	40 mg/day	Increase dose by no more than 40 mg/day every 1–2 weeks
38–41 kg	20 mg/day	45 mg/day	Increase dose by no more than 45 mg/day every 1–2 weeks
42–45 kg	25 mg/day	50 mg/day	Increase dose by no more than 50 mg/day every 1–2 weeks
46–49 kg	25 mg/day	55 mg/day	Increase dose by no more than 55 mg/day every 1–2 weeks
50–54 kg	30 mg/day	60 mg/day	Increase dose by no more than 60 mg/day every 1–2 weeks
55–58 kg	30 mg/day	65 mg/day	Increase dose by no more than 65 mg/day every 1–2 weeks
≥59 kg[e]	35 mg/day	70 mg/day	Increase dose by no more than 70 mg/day every 1–2 weeks

a Enzyme-inducing AEDs include carbamazepine, phenobarbital, phenytoin, and primidone.
b Can be given as two divided doses.
c Total daily dose can be divided.
d It may take several weeks to months to achieve an individualized maintenance dose.
e Insufficient data are available to be able to support the mg/kg dosing in patients weighing more than 59 kg.

Geriatrics (≥65 years of age): No dosage adjustment from the recommended adult schedule is required. The pharmacokinetics of lamotrigine in this age group do not differ significantly from a non-elderly population (see also Pharmacology and Adverse Effects).

Patients with Impaired Renal Function: The elimination half-life of lamotrigine is prolonged in patients with impaired renal function (see Pharmacology). Caution should be exercised in dose selection for patients with impaired renal function.

Patients with Impaired Hepatic Function: Mild and Moderate Hepatic-impaired Patients: It is recommended that initial, escalation and maintenance doses be reduced by approximately 50% in patients with either mild or moderate (Child-Pugh Grade A or B) hepatic impairment; dosage schedules based on pharmacokinetic data are summarized in Table 12. Maintenance doses may be adjusted according to clinical response and tolerance (see also Pharmacology and Precautions).

Severe Hepatic-impaired Patients: Caution should be exercised with severe hepatic-impaired patients with epilepsy, as there is no clinical experience with LAMICTAL in this group. It is recommended that initial, escalation and maintenance doses be reduced by approximately 75% in severe (Child-Pugh Grade C) hepatic impairment; dosage schedules based on pharmacokinetic data are summarized in Table 13. Maintenance doses may be adjusted according to clinical response and tolerance (see also Pharmacology and Precautions).

Table 12: LAMICTAL

Dosing for Mild (Child-Pugh Grade A) and Moderate (Child-Pugh Grade B) Hepatic-impaired Adult Patients (based on pharmacokinetic data from 12 mild and 5 moderate hepatic-impaired subjects given a single 100 mg dose)

	Weeks 1+2	Weeks 3+4[c]	Week 5 and Onwards to Usual Maintenance Dose[b]
LAMICTAL + EI AEDS[a]	25 mg/day	50 mg/day	To achieve maintenance, doses may be increased by 50 mg every 1 to 2 weeks.
LAMICTAL + EI AEDS + VPA	10 mg/day	20 mg/day	To achieve maintenance, doses may be increased by 10–20 mg every 1 to 2 weeks.
LAMICTAL + VPA[d] (± non-EI AEDS)	5 mg/day	10 mg/day	To achieve maintenance, doses may be increased by 10–20 mg every 1 to 2 weeks.

a Enzyme-inducing AEDs (EI AEDS) include carbamazepine, phenobarbital, phenytoin, and primidone.
b It may take several weeks to months to achieve an individualized maintenance dose.
c Can be given as 2 divided doses.
d Based on dosage recommendations from the United Kingdom.

Administration of LAMICTAL Chewable/Dispersible Tablets: LAMICTAL Chewable/Dispersible Tablets may be swallowed whole, chewed, or dispersed in water or diluted fruit juice. The scoreline on the 5 mg tablet is not intended for tablet splitting. If the tablets are chewed, consume a small amount of water or diluted fruit juice to aid in swallowing. To disperse the tablets, add the tablets to a small amount of liquid (1 teaspoon, or enough to cover the medication). Approximately 1 minute later, when the tablets are completely dispersed, swirl the solution and consume the entire quantity immediately. No attempt should be made to administer partial quantities of the dispersed tablets.

Table 13: LAMICTAL

Dosing for Severe (Child-Pugh Grade C) Hepatic-impaired Adult Patients (based on pharmacokinetic data from 7 severe hepatic-impaired subjects given a single 100 mg dose)

	Weeks 1+2	Weeks 3+4[c]	Week 5 and Onwards to Usual Maintenance Dose[b]
LAMICTAL + EI AEDS[a]	10 mg/day	20 mg/day	To achieve maintenance, doses may be increased by 20 mg every 1 to 2 weeks.
LAMICTAL + EI AEDS + VPA	5 mg/day	10 mg/day	To achieve maintenance, doses may be increased by 5–10 mg every 1 to 2 weeks.

(cont'd)

Table 13: LAMICTAL *(cont'd)*

Dosing for Severe (Child-Pugh Grade C) Hepatic-impaired Adult Patients (based on pharmacokinetic data from 7 severe hepatic-impaired subjects given a single 100 mg dose)

	Weeks 1+2	Weeks 3+4[c]	Week 5 and Onwards to Usual Maintenance Dose[b]
LAMICTAL + VPA[d] (± non-EI AEDS)	5 mg every other day	5 mg/day	To achieve maintenance, doses may be increased by 5–10 mg every 1 to 2 weeks.

[a] Enzyme-inducing AEDs (EI AEDS) include carbamazepine, phenobarbital, phenytoin, and primidone.
[b] It may take several weeks to months to achieve an individualized maintenance dose.
[c] Can be given as 2 divided doses.
[d] Based on dosage recommendations from the United Kingdom.

INFORMATION FOR THE PATIENT: Published in e-CPS, available by subscription at www.e-cps.ca.

SUPPLIED: Chewable/Dispersible Tablets: 2 mg: Each white, round tablet, engraved "LTG" over "2", contains: lamotrigine 2 mg. Nonmedicinal ingredients: aluminum magnesium silicate, blackcurrant flavor, calcium carbonate, hydroxypropylcellulose, magnesium stearate, povidone, saccharin sodium and sodium starch glycolate. Bottles of 30. Store at controlled room temperature (15 to 30°C) in a dry place and protect from light.

5 mg: Each white to off-white, elongated and biconvex tablet, engraved "GS CL2" on one side and "5" on the other (initiation dose only), contains: lamotrigine 5 mg. Nonmedicinal ingredients: aluminum magnesium silicate, blackcurrant flavor, calcium carbonate, hydroxypropylcellulose, magnesium stearate, povidone, saccharin sodium and sodium starch glycolate. Blisters of 28. Store at controlled room temperature (15 to 30°C) in a dry place and protect from light.

Tablets: 25 mg: Each white, scored, shield-shaped tablet, engraved with "LAMICTAL" and "25", contains: lamotrigine 25 mg. Nonmedicinal ingredients: cellulose, lactose, magnesium stearate, povidone and sodium starch glycolate. Bottles of 100. Store at controlled room temperature (15 to 30°C) in a dry place and protect from light.

100 mg: Each peach, scored, shield-shaped tablet, engraved with "LAMICTAL" and "100", contains: lamotrigine 100 mg. Nonmedicinal ingredients: cellulose, lactose, magnesium stearate, povidone, sunset yellow FCF lake and sodium starch glycolate. Bottles of 100. Store at controlled room temperature (15 to 30°C) in a dry place and protect from light.

150 mg: Each cream, scored, shield-shaped tablet, engraved with "LAMICTAL" and "150", contains: lamotrigine 150 mg. Nonmedicinal ingredients: cellulose, ferric oxide (yellow), lactose, magnesium stearate, povidone and sodium starch glycolate. Bottles of 60. Store at controlled room temperature (15 to 30°C) in a dry place and protect from light.

(Shown in Product Identification Section)

Lamisil® Pr
terbinafine HCl
Antifungal

Novartis Pharmaceuticals

Date of Preparation: April 28, 1993
Date of Revision: March 2, 2010

SUMMARY PRODUCT INFORMATION:

Route of Administration	Dosage Form/ Strength	Clinically Relevant Nonmedicinal Ingredients
Oral	Tablets 250 mg terbinafine (as terbinafine hydrochloride)	Carboxymethyl starch For a complete listing see Dosage Forms, Composition and Packaging.
Topical	Topical cream 1% terbinafine hydrochloride 10 mg/g	For a complete listing see Dosage Forms, Composition and Packaging.
	Topical spray solution 1% terbinafine hydrochloride 10 mg/g	

INDICATIONS AND CLINICAL USE: LAMISIL (terbinafine) is indicated in the treatment of fungal infections of the skin and nails caused by dermatophytes such as Trichophyton (e.g. *T. rubrum, T. mentagrophytes, T. verrucosum, T. violaceum*), *M. canis, E. floccosum* and yeasts of the genus Candida (eg. *C. albicans*), as well as *M. furfur*.

Oral LAMISIL: Oral LAMISIL is indicated in the treatment of onychomycosis (fungal infection of the nail) caused by dermatophyte fungi.

Prior to initiating treatment with LAMISIL Tablets, appropriate nail or skin specimens should be obtained for laboratory testing (KOH preparation, fungal culture, or nail biopsy) in order to confirm the diagnosis of onychomycosis or dermatomycosis.

Oral LAMISIL may be considered for the treatment of severe tineal skin infections (tinea corporis, tinea cruris and tinea pedis) which have been unresponsive to topical treatment.

Note: Oral LAMISIL is not effective in pityriasis versicolor.

Topical LAMISIL: Cream: LAMISIL cream is indicated in the treatment of fungal infections of the skin caused by dermatophytes such as trichophyton, as well as yeast infections of the skin, principally those caused by the genus Candida (e.g. *C. albicans*).

LAMISIL cream is also indicated in the treatment of pityriasis (tinea) versicolor due to *M. furfur*.

Spray: LAMISIL spray is indicated in the treatment of fungal infections of the skin caused by dermatophytes such as trichophyton.

LAMISIL spray is also indicated in the treatment of pityriasis (tinea) versicolor due to *M. furfur*.

Note: Topical LAMISIL is not effective in onychomycosis.

CONTRAINDICATIONS: LAMISIL (terbinafine) is contraindicated in patients with a known hypersensitivity to terbinafine or to any of the excipients of LAMISIL (see Dosage Forms, Composition and Packaging).

WARNINGS AND PRECAUTIONS: Oral LAMISIL:

Serious Warnings and Precautions

Rare cases of liver failure, some leading to death or liver transplant, have occurred with the use of LAMISIL (terbinafine) tablets for the treatment of onychomycosis and dermatomycosis in individuals with and without pre-existing liver disease.

In the majority of liver cases reported in association with LAMISIL use, the patients had serious underlying systemic conditions and an uncertain causal association with LAMISIL. The severity of hepatic events and/or their outcome may be worse in patients with active or chronic liver disease. Treatment with LAMISIL tablets should be discontinued if biochemical or clinical evidence of liver injury develops.

Hepatic/Biliary/Pancreatic: LAMISIL (terbinafine) tablets are not recommended for patients with chronic or active liver disease. Before prescribing LAMISIL tablets, pre-existing liver disease should be assessed. Hepatotoxicity may occur in patients with and without pre-existing liver disease. Pre-treatment serum transaminase (ALT and AST) tests are advised for all patients before taking LAMISIL tablets. Patients prescribed LAMISIL tablets should be warned to report immediately to their physician any symptoms of persistent nausea, anorexia, fatigue, vomiting, right upper abdominal pain or jaundice, dark urine or pale stools. Patients with these symptoms should discontinue taking oral terbinafine, and the patient's liver function should be immediately evaluated.

Renal: The pharmacokinetics of LAMISIL have been investigated in patients with renal impairment (creatinine clearance ≤50 mL/min); based on this study the use of LAMISIL in renally impaired patients is not recommended (see Action and Clinical Pharmacology, Pharmacokinetics).

Endocrine and Metabolism: In vitro and in vivo studies have shown that terbinafine inhibits the CYP2D6 metabolism. Therefore, patients receiving concomitant treatment with drugs predominantly metabolised by this enzyme, e.g. certain members of the following drug classes, tricyclic antidepressants (TCAs), β-blockers, selective serotonine reuptake inhibitors (SSRIs), antiarrhythmics class 1A, 1B and 1C and monoamine oxidase inhibitors (MAO-Is) Type B, should be followed up, if the coadministered drug has a narrow therapeutic window (see Drug Interactions).

Skin: Serious skin reactions (e.g. Stevens-Johnson syndrome, toxic epidermal necrolysis) have been very rarely reported in patients taking LAMISIL tablets. If progressive skin rash occurs, treatment with LAMISIL tablets should be discontinued.

Ophthalmologic: Changes in the ocular lens and retina have been reported following the use of LAMISIL tablets in controlled trials. The changes noted were non-specific and the significance of these changes is unknown.

Immune: Transient decreases in absolute lymphocyte counts (ALC) have been observed in controlled clinical trials. The clinical significance of this observation is unknown. However, in patients with known or suspected immunodeficiency, physicians should consider monitoring complete blood counts in individuals using LAMISIL therapy for greater than six weeks.

Lupus Erythematosus: During post-marketing experience, precipitation and exacerbation of cutaneous and systemic lupus erythematosus have been reported infrequently in patients taking LAMISIL. LAMISIL therapy should be discontinued in patients with clinical signs and symptoms suggestive of lupus erythematosus.

Hematologic: Very rare cases of blood dyscrasias (neutropenia, agranulocytosis, thrombocytopenia, pancytopenia) have been reported in patients treated with LAMISIL tablets. Aetiology of any blood dyscrasias that occur in patients treated with LAMISIL tablets should be evaluated and consideration should be given for a possible change in medication regimen, including discontinuation of treatment with LAMISIL tablets.

Carcinogenesis and Mutagenesis: An increase in liver tumours was observed in male rats at the highest dose level (69 mg/kg) during a life-time (123 weeks) carcinogenicity study. The changes included increased enzyme activity, peroxisome proliferation and altered triglyceride metabolism. The changes have been shown to be species specific since they were not seen in mice or monkeys.

Topical LAMISIL: LAMISIL cream and spray are for external use only. Contact with the eyes should be avoided. LAMISIL spray should not be used on the face.

In the case of accidental ocular contact, the eyes should be rinsed thoroughly with running water and patients should consult a physician if any symptoms persist. In case of accidental inhalation, patients should be advised to consult a physician if any symptoms develop and persist.

LAMISIL spray should be used with caution in patients with lesions where alcohol could be irritating.

Special Populations: Pregnant Women: Animal fetal toxicity and fertility studies did not reveal any teratogenic or embryofetotoxic potential of terbinafine. However, there is only very limited clinical experience with LAMISIL (terbinafine) in pregnant women; therefore, unless the potential benefits outweigh any potential risks, oral LAMISIL or LAMISIL cream should not be used during pregnancy.

Nursing Women: Terbinafine is excreted in breast milk; therefore mothers receiving oral treatment with LAMISIL should not breast-feed. However, with LAMISIL cream and spray treatment, the small amounts absorbed through the skin are unlikely to affect the infant. Nursing mothers should **not** apply LAMISIL topical formulations to the breast. In addition, infants must not come into contact with any treated skin area, including the breasts.

Pediatrics: The safety and efficacy of LAMISIL have not been established in pediatric patients.

LAMISIL should be kept out of the reach of children.

Geriatrics: Plasma concentrations and drug half-life appear to be slightly higher in elderly patients than in the general population. In addition, the incidence of all adverse events in a Post Marketing Surveillance study appeared to be slightly higher in the elderly at normal adult doses; however, the overall rate of adverse events possibly or probably related to terbinafine did not appear to be different compared to the general population. When prescribing tablets for patients in this age group, the possibility of pre-existing impairment of liver or kidney function should be considered (see Action and Clinical Pharmacology, Pharmacokinetics, Oral LAMISIL).

Occupational Hazards: Effects on Ability to Drive and Use Machines: No studies on the effects of LAMISIL tablets treatment on the ability to drive and use machines have been performed. Patients who experience dizziness as an undesirable effect should avoid driving vehicles or using machines.

ADVERSE REACTIONS: Adverse Drug Reaction Overview: Because clinical trials are conducted under very specific conditions, the adverse reaction rates observed in the clinical trials may not reflect the rates observed in practice and should not be compared to the rates in the clinical trials of another drug. Adverse drug reaction information from clinical trials is useful for identifying drug-related adverse events and for approximating rates.

Frequency estimate: very common ≥10%, common ≥1% to <10%, uncommon ≥0.1% to <1%, rare ≥0.01% to <0.1%, very rare <0.01% (includes isolated reports).

LAMISIL Tablets: In general LAMISIL (terbinafine) is well tolerated. Side effects are usually mild to moderate in severity and transient.

Clinical Trial Adverse Drug Reactions: In clinical trials submitted for purposes of marketing approval in Canada adverse events occurred in 10.4% of patients receiving the recommended oral dose. Of these, 5% were mild to moderate gastrointestinal events (feeling of fullness, loss of appetite, dyspepsia, nausea, mild abdominal pain, diarrhoea), 3% were non-serious forms of skin reactions (rash, urticaria) and the remainder were for musculoskeletal reactions (arthralgia, myalgia) and other nonspecific events such as malaise or tiredness.

Table 1 illustrates some of these results.

Table 1: LAMISIL Tablets

Adverse Effects

Organ System Adverse Event	LAMISIL 250 mg (n=998)	(%)
Skin (overall)	27	2.7
Erythema or rash	9	0.9
Urticaria	5	0.5
Eczema	1	0.1
Pruritus	4	0.4
Other	8	0.8
GI (overall)	52	5.2
Diarrhea and/or cramps	10	1.0
Nausea and/or vomiting	11	1.1
Fullness	5	0.5
Sickness	1	0.1
Gastrointestinal irritation, dyspepsia, gastritis	22	2.2
Other	3	0.3
CNS (overall)	12	1.2
Headache	9	0.9

(cont'd)

Table 1: **LAMISIL Tablets** *(cont'd)*

Adverse Effects

Organ System Adverse Event	LAMISIL 250 mg (n=998)	(%)
Concentration	2	0.2
Other	1	0.1
Other (overall)	11	1.1
Tiredness, fatigue	3	0.3
Pain (back, knee, legs, feet, kidney)	1	0.1
Change of taste or dry mouth	1	0.1
Other	6	0.6
Laboratory Adverse Changes (overall)	2	0.2
Hypoglycemia	1	0.1
Elevated liver enzymes	1	0.1
Total	104	10.4

Less Common Clinical Trial Adverse Drug Reactions (<1%): Adverse events not frequently observed include the following:
Uncommon: Taste disturbances, including taste loss, which usually recover within several weeks after discontinuation of the drug were reported. Isolated cases of prolonged taste disturbances have been reported. A decrease of food intake leading to significant weight loss was observed in very few severe cases.
Rare: Idiosyncratic and symptomatic hepatobiliary reactions (2/3 primarily cholestatic in nature and the remainder involving hepatocytic damage or both) have been reported in association with LAMISIL treatment, including very rare cases of serious liver failure (some leading to liver transplant or death). Unspecific prodromal symptoms (nausea, anorexia, fatigue, general malaise) have been reported. Liver enzyme increases have been noted in asymptomatic patients as well as in patients with more specific symptoms of hepatic dysfunction (jaundice, upper abdominal right quadrant pain, pruritus, pale stools, dark urine) (see Warnings and Precautions).

The frequency of reported apparent hepatic dysfunctions has varied. An analysis of 7 key placebo-controlled trials (262 placebo vs 1624 LAMISIL patients) suggested increases of 1.4% vs 3.4% in liver function test indicators (APase, AST, ALT, g-GT, bilirubin >2× above upper normal). In a European post-marketing study in 25 884 patients, asymptomatic liver enzyme increases were reported in 0.17% of patients treated. The reporting frequency for symptomatic liver disorder possibly related to LAMISIL was 1:13 000. The relative risk of acute liver injury in this group was considered to be 4.2 times the background incidence.

In the less controlled circumstances of spontaneous worldwide reporting, the development of clinically significant signs and symptoms of hepatobiliary dysfunction for which no other cause was apparent, and in which LAMISIL was considered the possible causative agent, was calculated to be approximately 1:37 000 treated patients. The reporting frequency overall for hepatobiliary events including elevations in liver enzymes was 1:15 000. Very rare cases of liver failure, some fatal, have been associated with LAMISIL treatment and the incidence rate is about 1:1 000 000 exposed patients.

Hepatobiliary dysfunction (primarily cholestatic in nature), very rare cases of serious liver failure (some with a fatal outcome, or requiring liver transplant). In the majority of liver failure cases the patients had serious underlying systemic conditions and a causal association with the intake of LAMISIL was uncertain.

Oral terbinafine has been rarely associated with systemic allergic reactions including urticaria, angioedema, arthralgia, arthritis and serum-sickness like reactions.
Very Rare: Serious skin reactions (e.g. Stevens Johnson Syndrome, Toxic Epidermal Necrolysis and Erythema Multiforme), acute generalized exanthematous pustulosis psoriasiform eruptions or exacerbation of psoriasis (if progressive skin rash occurs, LAMISIL treatment should be discontinued). Anaphylactic reactions (including angioedema) have been reported. Precipitation or exacerbation of cutaneous and systemic lupus erythematosus have been reported.

Hair loss has been reported, however, a causal relationship has not been established.

Hematologic disorders such as neutropenia, agranulocytosis, pancytopenia and thrombocytopenia have been reported (very rare). Very rare cases of thrombotic thrombocytopenic purpura (TTP) have been reported. The mechanism of TPP induction and the role of LAMISIL have not been elucidated.

Isolated cases of photosensitivity have been reported in association with LAMISIL.

LAMISIL Cream and Spray: Redness, itching, stinging may occur at the site of application; however, treatment rarely has to be discontinued for this reason. These minor symptoms must be distinguished from allergic reactions (e.g. pruritus, bullous eruptions, hives, widespread rash and/or redness, urticaria, angioedema, or positive rechallenge) which are rare but require discontinuation of the drug. In clinical trials, adverse reactions were recorded in 33 of the 1757 (1.8%) patients who received LAMISIL cream, and in 39 of the 898 (4.3%) patients who received LAMISIL spray.

Post-Market Adverse Drug Reactions: During post-marketing experience with LAMISIL tablets, precipitation and exacerbation of cutaneous and systemic lupus erythematosus have been reported infrequently in patients taking LAMISIL. LAMISIL therapy should be discontinued in patients with clinical signs and symptoms suggestive of lupus erythematosus.

The following adverse events were also reported: dizziness, anemia, CPK elevations, rhabdomyolysis, pancytopenia, paraesthesia and hypoaesthesia.

DRUG INTERACTIONS: Overview: Tablets: Many categories of drugs are known to inhibit or induce drug metabolism by cytochrome P450 (CYP) enzymes located in the liver and intestine. Coadministration of such drugs may impact metabolic elimination of drugs, and in some cases, bioavailability may be either increased or decreased and accordingly, possibly necessitate dosage adjustments.

Drug-Drug Interactions: Effects of Other Medicinal Products on Terbinafine: The following medicinal products may increase the effect or plasma concentration of terbinafine: Cimetidine decreased the clearance of terbinafine by 33%.

The following medicinal products may decrease the effect or plasma concentration of terbinafine: Rifampicin increased the clearance of terbinafine by 100%.

Effect of Terbinafine on Other Medicinal Products: According to the results from studies undertaken in vitro and in healthy volunteers, terbinafine shows negligible potential for inhibiting or enhancing the clearance of most drugs that are metabolised via the cytochrome P450 system (e.g. terfenadine, triazolam, tolbutamide or oral contraceptives) with exception of those metabolised through CYP2D6 (see below).

Terbinafine does not interfere with the clearance of antipyrine or digoxin.

Some cases of menstrual irregularities have been reported in patients taking LAMISIL tablets concomitantly with oral contraceptives, although the incidence of these disorders remains within the background incidence of patients taking oral contraceptives alone.

Terbinafine may increase the effect or plasma concentration of the following medicinal products: Caffeine: Terbinafine decreased the clearance of caffeine administered intravenously by 19%.

Compounds Predominantly Metabolised by CYP2D6: In vitro and in vivo studies have shown that terbinafine inhibits the CYP2D6-mediated metabolism. This finding may be of clinical relevance for compounds predominantly metabolized by CYP2D6, e.g. certain members of the following drug classes: tricyclic antidepressants (TCAs), beta-blockers, selective serotonine reuptake inhibitors (SSRIs), antiarrhythmics (including class 1A, 1B and 1C) and monoamine oxidase inhibitors (MAO-Is) Type B, particularly if they also have a narrow therapeutic window (see Warnings and Precautions).

Terbinafine decreased the clearance of desipramine by 82%.

Terbinafine may decrease the effect or plasma concentration of the following medicinal products: terbinafine increased the clearance of ciclosporin by 15%.

Cream and Spray: No drug interactions are known to date.

DOSAGE AND ADMINISTRATION: Oral: LAMISIL Tablets: Adults: 250 mg once daily.

The duration of treatment varies according to the indication and the severity of infection (see Table 2).

Table 2: **LAMISIL Tablets**

Duration of Treatment

Indication	Duration of Treatment
Onychomycosis (of fingers and toes)[a]	6 weeks to 3 months
Skin infections[b]	
Tinea pedis (interdigital and plantar/moccasin type)	2–6 weeks
Tinea corporis, cruris	2–4 weeks

[a] In patients with fingernail infections or toenail infections other than the big toe, or in younger patients, treatment periods of less than 3 months may be adequate. In patients with infections of the big toenail, treatment for 3 months is usually sufficient, although some patients may require treatment for 6 months or longer. Poor nail outgrowth during the first weeks of treatment may enable identification of those patients in whom longer therapy is required. In onychomycosis the optimal clinical effect is seen some months after mycological cure and cessation of treatment. This is related to the period required for outgrowth of healthy nail tissue.

[b] Complete resolution of the signs and symptoms may not occur until several weeks after mycological cure.

Topical: LAMISIL Cream: LAMISIL cream can be applied once or twice daily depending on the indication. The affected areas should be cleansed and dried thoroughly before application of LAMISIL. The cream should be applied to the affected skin and surrounding area in a thin layer and rubbed in lightly. In the case of intertriginous infections (submammary, interdigital, intergluteal, inguinal) the area to which the cream has been applied may be covered with a gauze strip, especially at night.

The duration and frequency of treatment varies with the indication and is dependent on the severity of the infection (see Table 3).

Table 3: **LAMISIL Cream**

Duration of Treatment

Indication	Duration of Treatment
Tinea pedis	1 week, once a day
Tinea corporis/cruris	1 week, once a day
Cutaneous candidiasis	1–2 weeks, once or twice a day[a]
Pityriasis versicolor	2 weeks, once or twice a day

[a] Two weeks of treatment with LAMISIL cream produced slightly improved efficacy over treatment for one week. The difference in outcome may not be clinically significant.

Many patients treated with shorter durations of therapy (1-2 weeks) continue to improve during the 2-4 weeks after therapy has been completed. As a consequence, patients should not be considered therapeutic failures until they have been observed for a period of 2-4 weeks after cessation of treatment.

Relief of clinical symptoms usually occurs within a few days. Irregular use or premature discontinuation of treatment increases the risk of recurrence. If there are no signs of improvement after two weeks the diagnosis should be verified.

LAMISIL Spray : LAMISIL spray is applied once or twice daily, depending on the indication. The affected areas should be cleansed and dried thoroughly before application of LAMISIL. A sufficient amount of solution should be applied to wet the treatment area(s) thoroughly, and to cover the affected skin and surrounding area (see Warnings and Precautions).

The duration of treatment varies with the indication and is dependent on the severity of the infection (see Table 4).

Table 4: **LAMISIL Spray**

Duration of Treatment

Indication	Duration of Treatment
Tinea pedis	1 week, once a day
Tinea corporis/cruris	1 week, once a day
Pityriasis versicolor	1 week, twice a day

Relief of clinical symptoms usually occurs within a few days. Irregular use or premature discontinuation of treatment increases the risk of recurrence. If there are no signs of improvement after two weeks the diagnosis should be verified.

Dosing Considerations: Special Populations: Liver Impairment: LAMISIL tablets are not recommended for patients with chronic or active liver disease (see Warnings and Precautions).

Renal Impairment: The use of LAMISIL tablets has not been adequately studied in patients with renal impairment and is therefore not recommended in this population (see Warnings and Precautions).

OVERDOSAGE:
A few cases of overdosage with LAMISIL tablets (up to 5 g) have been reported giving rise to headache, nausea, epigastric pain and dizziness. The recommended treatment of overdosage consists of eliminating the drug, primarily by the administration of activated charcoal and giving, symptomatic supportive therapy, if needed.

No case of overdosage has been reported with LAMISIL cream and spray. The low systemic absorption of topical terbinafine renders overdosage extremely unlikely. Accidental ingestion of one 30 g tube of LAMISIL cream or one 30 mL bottle of LAMISIL spray, which contain 300 mg terbinafine hydrochloride, is comparable to one LAMISIL 250 mg tablet. However, should larger amounts of topical LAMISIL be inadvertently ingested, adverse effects similar to those observed with an overdosage of LAMISIL tablets are to be expected (e.g. headache, nausea, epigastric pain and dizziness). The alcohol content of the spray (28.8% v/v) and gel (11.3% v/v) has to be taken into account.

> For management of a suspected drug overdose, CPhA recommends that you contact your **regional Poison Control Centre**. See the *CPS* Directory section for a list of Poison Control Centres.

ACTION AND CLINICAL PHARMACOLOGY: Mechanism of Action: LAMISIL (terbinafine) is an allylamine which has a broad spectrum of antifungal activity. At low concentrations LAMISIL is fungicidal against dermatophytes, molds and certain dimorphic fungi. Its activity against yeasts is fungicidal or fungistatic, depending on the species.

Pharmacodynamics: Terbinafine interferes specifically with fungal sterol biosynthesis at an early step. This leads to a deficiency in ergosterol and to an intracellular accumulation of squalene, resulting in fungal cell death. Terbinafine acts by inhibition of squalene epoxidase in the fungal cell membrane. The enzyme squalene epoxidase is not linked to the cytochrome P450 system.

When given orally, the drug concentrates rapidly in skin, hair and nails at levels associated with fungicidal activity.

Pharmacokinetics: Oral LAMISIL: Absorption: Following oral administration, terbinafine is well absorbed (>70%) and the absolute bioavailability of terbinafine from LAMISIL tablets as a result of first-pass metabolism is approximately 50 %. A single 250 mg dose of LAMISIL tablets resulted in mean peak plasma concentration of 1.3 µg/mL within 1.5 hours after administration. At steady-state, in comparison to a single dose, peak concentration of terbinafine was on average 25% higher and plasma AUC increased by a factor of 2.3. From the increase in plasma AUC an effective half-life of ~30 hours can be calculated. The bioavailability of terbinafine is moderately affected by food (increase in the AUC of less than 20%), (20%) by food, but not sufficiently to require dosing adjustments.

Distribution: LAMISIL binds strongly to plasma proteins (99%) and is lipophilic. LAMISIL is widely distributed in the body including adipose tissue. It rapidly diffuses through the dermis and concentrates in lipophilic stratum corneum. It is also secreted in sebum, thus achieving high concentrations in hair follicles, hair and sebum-rich skin. There is evidence that LAMISIL is distributed in the nail plate within the first few weeks of commencing therapy.

Metabolism and Excretion: Oral LAMISIL is excreted mainly in urine (80%) and in feces (20%). Following absorption terbinafine is metabolised rapidly and extensively by the liver. At least seven cytochrome isoenzymes are involved in its metabolism with major contributions from CYP 2C9, CYP 1A2, CYP 3A4, CYP 2C8 and CYP 2C19. Biotransformation results in metabolites with no antifungal activity which are excreted predominantly through the urine. No clinically relevant age-dependent changes in steady-state plasma concentrations of terbinafine have been observed.

Following a single 250 mg dose in 12 hepatically impaired cirrhotic (alcoholic) patients, total clearance of terbinafine was reduced by about 40%. In a sample of 12 renally impaired patients (median creatinine clearance of 17.6 mL/min), LAMISIL clearance following a single 250 mg dose was halved resulting in the doubling or more of peak plasma concentrations or AUC. Patients at the highest and lowest ends of the renal impairment spectrum were not represented. There was no direct correlation between creatinine clearance and terbinafine clearance in renally impaired patients, the metabolism of the drug having been impaired in these patients due to competition between metabolite and parent drug.

Topical LAMISIL: Less than 5% of the dose is absorbed after topical application to humans; systemic exposure is thus very slight.

In healthy volunteers who were administered the gel formulation once daily for 7 days, terbinafine reached concentrations of 909 ng/mL in the stratum corneum 4 hours after the Day 7 application. The stratum corneum half-life was 27.2 hours.

STORAGE AND STABILITY: Store at temperatures between 15 and 30°C.

SPECIAL HANDLING INSTRUCTIONS: Protect tablets from light.

INFORMATION FOR THE PATIENT: Published in e-CPS, available by subscription at www.e-cps.ca.

DOSAGE FORMS, COMPOSITION AND PACKAGING: Cream: Each g of white, smooth, glossy cream contains: terbinafine HCl 10 mg. Nonmedicinal ingredients: benzyl alcohol, cetyl alcohol, cetyl palmitate, isopropyl myristate, polysorbate 60, purified water, sodium hydroxide, sorbitan monostearate and stearyl alcohol. Tubes of 15 and 30 g.

Spray: Each g of clear solution contains: terbinafine HCl 10 mg. Nonmedicinal ingredients: cetomacrogol 1000, ethanol, propylene glycol and water. Alcohol: 28.8% v/v. Bottles of 30 mL.

Tablets: Each whitish to yellow tinged white, circular, biconvex, with bevelled edges tablet, scored on one side and embossed "LAMISIL 250", contains: terbinafine 250 mg, present as the hydrochloride salt. Nonmedicinal ingredients: cellulose microcrystalline granulate, hypromellose, magnesium stearate, silica colloidal anhydrous and sodium starch glycolate. Bottles of 100 and 500. Blister packs of 28 (14 tablets per blister).

(Shown in Product Identification Section)

Lanoxin® Ⓟ

digoxin

Cardiotonic Glycoside

Pharmascience

Date of Revision: April 7, 2010

SUMMARY PRODUCT INFORMATION:

Route of Administration	Dosage Form/Strength	All Nonmedicinal Ingredients
Oral	Digoxin Oral Solution: 0.05 mg per mL	Alcohol, calcined diatomaceous earth, citric acid, D&C Green No. 5, D&C Yellow No. 10, lime flavour, methylparaben, propylene glycol, sodium phosphate, sucrose and water

INDICATIONS AND CLINICAL USE: LANOXIN (Digoxin Oral Solution, C.S.D.) is indicated for:

Congestive Heart Failure: LANOXIN is indicated for the treatment of mild to moderate heart failure. LANOXIN increases left ventricular ejection fraction and improves heart failure symptoms as evidenced by exercise capacity and heart failure-related hospitalizations and emergency care, while having no effect on mortality. Where possible, digoxin should be used with a diuretic and angiotensin-converting enzyme inhibitor, but an optimal order for starting these three drugs cannot be specified.

Digoxin is usually continued after failure is controlled unless some known precipitating factor is corrected. Studies have shown that withdrawal of digoxin may worsen functional status, exercise capacity, and the left ventricular ejection fraction in patients with heart failure. In patients in whom digoxin may be difficult to regulate, or in whom the risk of toxicity may be great (e.g., patients with unstable renal function or whose potassium levels tend to fluctuate) a cautious withdrawal of digoxin may be considered. If digoxin is discontinued, the patient should be regularly monitored for clinical evidence of recurrent heart failure.

Atrial Fibrillation: LANOXIN is indicated for the control of ventricular response rate in patients with chronic atrial fibrillation.

Geriatrics (>70 years of age): Although appropriate studies on the relationship of age to the effects of digitalis glycosides have not been performed in the geriatric population, the majority of experience with digoxin is in this population. This drug is known to be substantially excreted by the kidneys, and the risk of toxic reactions to this drug may be greater in patients with impaired renal function. Because elderly patients may be more likely to have age-related renal function impairment, which may significantly increase the elimination half-life of digoxin, care should be taken in dose selection, which should be based on renal function, and it may be useful to monitor renal function (see Dosage and Administration).

Pediatrics (<10 years of age): Newborn infants display considerable variability in their tolerance to digoxin. Premature and immature infants are particularly sensitive to the effect of digoxin, and the dosage of the drug must not only be reduced but must be individualized according to their degree of maturity. Digitalization in infants and children must be individualized (see Dosage and Administration).

CONTRAINDICATIONS: Digitalis glycosides are contraindicated in ventricular fibrillation.

In a given patient, an untoward effect requiring permanent discontinuation of other digitalis preparations usually constitutes a contraindication to LANOXIN (Digoxin Oral Solution, C.S.D.). Hypersensitivity to LANOXIN itself is a contraindication to its use. Allergy to digoxin, though rare, does occur. It may not extend to all such preparations, and another digitalis glycoside may be tried with caution.

WARNINGS AND PRECAUTIONS:

Serious Warnings and Precautions
- **Do not take other prescription, non-prescription and herbal medications without advice from your doctor.**

General: Digitalis alone or with other drugs has been used in the treatment of obesity. This use of digoxin or other digitalis glycosides is unwarranted. Moreover, since they may cause potentially fatal arrhythmias or other adverse effects, the use of these drugs solely for the treatment of obesity is dangerous.

Anorexia, nausea, vomiting and arrhythmias may accompany heart failure or may be indications of digitalis intoxication. Clinical evaluation of the cause of the symptoms should be attempted before further digitalis administration. In such circumstances determination of the serum digoxin concentration may be an aid in deciding whether or not digitalis toxicity is likely to be present. If the possibility of digitalis intoxication cannot be excluded, cardiac glycosides should be temporarily withheld, if permitted by the clinical situation.

Patients with renal insufficiency require smaller than usual maintenance doses of LANOXIN (Digoxin Oral Solution, C.S.D.) (see Dosage and Administration).

Heart failure accompanying acute glomerulonephritis requires extreme care in digitalization. Relatively low loading and maintenance doses and concomitant use of antihypertensive drugs may be necessary and careful monitoring is essential. LANOXIN (Digoxin Oral Solution, C.S.D.) should be discontinued as soon as possible, especially if a therapeutic trial does not result in improvement. Patients with severe carditis, such as carditis associated with rheumatic fever or viral myocarditis, are especially sensitive to digoxin-induced disturbances of rhythm.

Newborn infants display considerable variability in their tolerance to digoxin. Premature and immature infants are particularly sensitive and dosage must not only be reduced but must be individualized according to their degree of maturity. Impaired renal function must also be carefully taken into consideration.

Dosage of digoxin must be carefully titrated and differences in the bioavailability of parenteral preparations, oral solution and tablets taken into account when changing patients from one preparation to another.

Carcinogenesis and Mutagenesis: There have been no long-term studies performed in animals to evaluate carcinogenic potential, nor have studies been conducted to assess the mutagenic potential of digoxin or its potential to affect fertility.

Cardiovascular: Use During Electrical Cardioversion: Reduction of digoxin dosage may be desirable prior to electrical cardioversion to avoid induction of ventricular arrhythmias, but the physician must consider the consequences of rapid increase in ventricular response to atrial fibrillation if digoxin is withheld 1 to 2 days prior to cardioversion. If there is a suspicion that digitalis toxicity exists, elective cardioversion should be delayed. If it is not prudent to delay cardioversion, the energy level selected should be minimal at first and carefully increased in an attempt to avoid precipitating ventricular arrhythmias.

Sinus Node Disease and AV Block: Incomplete AV block, especially in patients with Stokes-Adams attacks, may progress to advanced or complete heart block if digoxin is given. Heart failure in these patients can usually be controlled by other measures and by increasing the heart rate. If digitalization is essential, electrical pacing of the ventricles may be indicated. In some patients with sinus node disease (i.e., Sick Sinus Syndrome), digoxin may worsen sinus bradycardia or sinoatrial block. Digoxin is not indicated for the treatment of sinus tachycardia unless it is associated with heart failure.

Accessory AV Pathway (Wolff-Parkinson-White Syndrome): In patients with Wolff-Parkinson-White Syndrome and atrial fibrillation, digoxin can enhance transmission of impulses through the accessory pathway. This effect may result in extremely rapid ventricular rates and even ventricular fibrillation.

Use in Patients with Preserved Left Ventricular Systolic Function: Digoxin may worsen the outflow obstruction in patients with idiopathic hypertrophic subaortic stenosis (IHSS). Unless cardiac failure is severe, it is doubtful whether digoxin should be employed. Patients with chronic constrictive pericarditis may fail to respond to digoxin. In addition, slowing of the heart rate by digoxin in some patients may further decrease cardiac output. Patients with heart failure from amyloid heart disease or constrictive cardiomyopathies respond poorly to treatment with digoxin. Patients with severe carditis, such as carditis associated with rheumatic fever or viral myocarditis, are especially sensitive to digoxin-induced disturbances of rhythm.

Use in Patients with Acute Myocardial Infarction: Digoxin should be used with caution in patients with acute myocardial infarction. The use of inotropic drugs in some patients in this setting may result in undesirable increases in myocardial oxygen demand and ischemia.

Dependence/Tolerance: No drug dependence has been reported with the use of digoxin.

Endocrine and Metabolism: In Patients with Electrolyte Disorders: In patients with hypokalemia, toxicity may occur despite serum digoxin concentrations within the normal range, because potassium depletion sensitizes the myocardium to digoxin. Therefore, it is desirable to maintain normal serum potassium levels in patients being treated with digoxin. Hypokalemia may result from diuretic, amphotericin B or corticosteroid therapy, and from peritoneal or hemodialysis or mechanical suction of gastrointestinal secretions. It may also accompany malnutrition, diarrhea, prolonged vomiting, old age, long-standing heart failure, long-standing wasting diseases and treatment with ion-exchange resins or carbenoxolone. In general, rapid changes in serum potassium or other electrolytes should be avoided, and i.v. treatment with potassium should be reserved for special circumstances as described below (see Overdosage).

Calcium, particularly when administered rapidly by the intravenous route, may produce serious arrhythmias in digitalized patients. Hypercalcemia from any cause predisposes the patient to digitalis toxicity. On the other hand, hypocalcemia can nullify the effects of digoxin in man; thus digoxin may be ineffective until serum calcium is restored to normal. These interactions are related to the fact that calcium affects contractility and excitability of the heart in a manner similar to digoxin.

Hypomagnesemia may predispose to digitalis toxicity. If low magnesium levels are detected in a patient on digoxin, replacement therapy should be instituted.

Use in Thyroid Disorders and Hypermetabolic States: In hypothyroidism the digoxin requirements are reduced. Digoxin responses in patients with compensated thyroid disease are normal. Heart failure and/or atrial arrhythmias resulting from hypermetabolic or hyperdynamic states (e.g., hyperthyroidism, hypoxia, or arteriovenous shunt) are best treated by addressing the underlying condition. Atrial arrhythmias associated with hypermetabolic states are particularly resistant to digoxin treatment. Care must be taken to avoid toxicity if digoxin is used.

Renal: In Patients with Renal Disease: Patients with renal insufficiency require smaller than usual maintenance doses of digoxin (see Dosage and Administration).

If the patient has been given digoxin during the previous week or any other less rapidly excreted drug of the digitalis group during the previous 2 weeks, the dose of digoxin must be reduced accordingly. Digoxin toxicity develops more frequently and lasts longer in patients with renal impairment because of the decreased excretion of digoxin. Therefore, it should be anticipated that dosage requirements will be decreased in patients with moderate to severe renal disease (see Dosage and Administration). Because of impaired renal function and excretion in elderly patients, they frequently require lower than recommended doses. Because of the prolonged half-life, a longer period of time is required to achieve an initial or new steady-state concentration in patients with renal impairment than in patients with normal renal function.

Special Populations: Pregnant Women: Teratogenic Effects: Animal reproduction studies have not been conducted with digoxin. It is also not known whether digoxin can cause fetal harm when administered to a pregnant woman or can affect reproduction capacity, although there have been no reports of teratogenic effects following the use of digoxin in pregnancy since its availability in 1929. Digoxin should be given to pregnant women only if clearly needed.

Nursing Women: Studies have shown that digoxin concentrations in the mother's serum and milk are similar. However, the estimated daily dose to a nursing infant will be far below the usual infant maintenance dose. Therefore, this amount should have no pharmacologic effect upon the infant. Nevertheless, caution should be exercised when digoxin is administered to a nursing woman.

Pediatrics (<10 years of age): Digitalis glycosides are a major cause of poisoning in children. The tolerance of newborn infants to digitalis glycosides is variable, since their renal clearance of the medication is reduced. Premature and immature infants are especially sensitive. Dosage of digoxin should be reduced and individualized according to the infant's degree of maturity, since renal clearance increases as the infant matures. Children older than 1 month of age generally require proportionally larger doses than adults on the basis of body weight or body surface area.

Geriatrics (>70 years of age): Although appropriate studies on the relationship of age to the effects of digitalis glycosides have not been performed in the geriatric population, the majority of experience with digoxin is in this population. Elderly patients may be more likely to have age-related renal function impairment, which may significantly increase the elimination half-life of digoxin. Additionally, elderly patients may have a decreased volume of distribution of digitalis due to decreased muscle mass. These factors may contribute to digitalis toxicity in elderly patients.

Monitoring and Laboratory Tests: Patients receiving LANOXIN (Digoxin Oral Solution, C.S.D.) should have their serum electrolytes and renal function (BUN and/or serum creatinine) assessed periodically; the frequency of assessments will depend on the clinical setting. For discussion of serum digoxin concentrations, see Dosage and Administration.

The use of therapeutic doses of digoxin may cause prolongation of the PR interval and depression of the ST segment on the electrocardiogram. Digoxin may produce false positive ST-T changes on the electrocardiogram during exercise testing. These electrophysiologic effects reflect an expected effect of the drug and are not indicative of toxicity.

ADVERSE REACTIONS: Adverse Drug Reaction Overview: In general, the adverse reactions of digoxin are dose-dependent and occur at doses higher than those needed to achieve a therapeutic effect. Hence, adverse reactions are less common when digoxin is used within the recommended dose range or therapeutic serum concentration range and when there is careful attention to concurrent medications and conditions.

Because some patients may be particularly susceptible to side effects with digoxin, the dosage of the drug should always be selected carefully and adjusted as the clinical condition of the patient warrants. In the past, when high doses of digoxin were used and little attention was paid to clinical status or concurrent medications, adverse reactions to digoxin were more frequent and severe. Cardiac adverse reactions accounted for about one-half, gastrointestinal disturbances for about one-fourth, and CNS and other toxicity for about one-fourth of these adverse reactions. However, available evidence suggests that the incidence and severity of digoxin toxicity has decreased substantially in recent years. In recent controlled clinical trials, in patients with predominantly mild to moderate heart failure, the incidence of adverse experiences was comparable in patients taking digoxin and in those taking placebo. In a large mortality trial, the incidence of hospitalization for suspected digoxin toxicity was 2% in patients taking digoxin compared to 0.9% in patients taking placebo. In this trial, the most common manifestations of digoxin toxicity included gastrointestinal and cardiac disturbances; CNS manifestations were less common.

Clinical Trial Adverse Drug Reactions: Adults: Cardiac: Unifocal or multiform ventricular premature contractions, especially in bigeminal or trigeminal patterns, are the most common arrhythmias associated with digoxin toxicity in adults with heart disease. Persistent bigeminy at rest but not on exercise when the sinus rate increases has traditionally been acceptable in the management of some arrhythmias. Ventricular tachycardia and ventricular fibrillation may result from digitalis toxicity. Atrioventricular (AV) dissociation, accelerated junctional (nodal) rhythm and atrial tachycardia with block are also common arrhythmias caused by digoxin overdosage. Excessive slowing of the pulse is a clinical sign of digoxin overdosage. AV block (Wenckebach) of increasing degree may proceed to complete heart block (including asystole).

Note: The electrocardiogram is fundamental in determining the presence and nature of these cardiac disturbances.

Digoxin may also induce other changes in the ECG (e.g., PR prolongation, ST depression), which represent digoxin effect and may or may not be associated with digitalis toxicity. Cardiac toxicity can also occur at therapeutic doses in patients who have conditions which may alter their sensitivity to digoxin (see Warnings and Precautions).

Gastrointestinal: Anorexia, nausea, vomiting, and less commonly, diarrhea are common early symptoms of overdosage. However, uncontrolled heart failure may also produce such symptoms. Rarely, the use of digoxin has been associated with abdominal pain.

It is inadvisable to rely on nausea as an early warning of excessive digoxin as arrhythmias may occur first.

Central Nervous System: Visual disturbances (blurred or yellow vision), headache, weakness, apathy, psychosis, and mental disturbances (such as anxiety, depression, delirium, and hallucination) can occur.

Other: Gynecomastia is occasionally observed following prolonged use of digoxin. Thrombocytopenia and maculopapular rash and other skin reactions have been rarely observed.

Table 1 summarizes the incidence of those adverse experiences listed above for patients treated with digoxin tablets or placebo from two randomized, double-blind, placebo-controlled withdrawal trials. Patients in these trials were also receiving diuretics with or without angiotensin-converting enzyme inhibitors. These patients had been stable on digoxin, and were randomized to digoxin or placebo. The results shown in Table 1 reflect the experience in patients following dosage titration with the use of serum digoxin concentrations and careful follow-up. These adverse experiences are consistent with results from a large, placebo-controlled mortality trial (DIG trial) wherein over half the patients were not receiving digoxin prior to enrolment.

Table 1: LANOXIN

Adverse Experiences in Two Parallel, Double-blind, Placebo-controlled Withdrawal Trials with Digoxin Tablets (Number of Patients Reporting)

Adverse Experience	Digoxin Patients (n=123) (%)	Placebo Patients (n=125) (%)
Cardiac		
Palpitation	1 (0.8)	4 (3.2)
Ventricular extrasystole	1 (0.8)	1 (0.8)
Tachycardia	2 (1.6)	1 (0.8)
Heart arrest	1 (0.8)	1 (0.8)
Gastrointestinal		
Anorexia	1 (0.8)	4 (3.2)
Nausea	4 (3.3)	2 (1.6)
Vomiting	2 (1.6)	1 (0.8)
Diarrhea	4 (3.3)	1 (0.8)
Abdominal pain	0	6 (4.8)
CNS		
Headache	4 (3.3)	4 (3.2)
Dizziness	6 (4.9)	5 (4.0)
Mental disturbances	5 (4.1)	1 (0.8)
Other		
Rash	2 (1.6)	1 (0.8)
Death	4 (3.3)	3 (2.4)

Less Common Clinical Trial Adverse Drug Reactions (<1%): Gastrointestinal: Rarely, the use of digoxin has been associated with abdominal pain, intestinal ischemia, and hemorrhagic necrosis of the intestines.

Other: Thrombocytopenia and maculopapular rash and other skin reactions have been rarely observed.

Infants and Children: Toxicity differs from the adult in a number of respects. Anorexia, nausea, vomiting, diarrhea and CNS disturbances may be present but are rare as initial symptoms in infants. Cardiac arrhythmias are more reliable signs of toxicity. Digoxin in children may produce any arrhythmia. The most commonly encountered are conduction disturbances or supraventricular tachyarrhythmias, such as atrial tachycardia with or without block and junctional (nodal) tachycardia. Ventricular arrhythmias are less common. Sinus bradycardia may also be a sign of impending digoxin intoxication, especially in infants, even in the absence of first-degree heart block. Any arrhythmia or alteration in cardiac conduction that develops in a child taking digoxin should initially be assumed to be a consequence of digoxin intoxication, until further evaluation proves otherwise.

Post-Market Adverse Drug Reactions: Adverse reactions to digoxin are usually dose dependent and occur at dosages higher than those needed to achieve a therapeutic effect.

DRUG INTERACTIONS: Overview: Digitalis glycosides have a narrow therapeutic range and changes in digoxin pharmacokinetics and/or pharmacodynamics caused by a digoxin-drug interaction can result in toxicity or underdigitalization. The presence of or a change in an underlying disease state also can cause changes in digoxin pharmacokinetics and/or pharmacodynamics and may complicate or contribute to a digoxin-drug interaction. Because a risk of digoxin toxicity exists, and the clinical significance of an interaction may be variable and not necessarily predictable, it is important that the addition or withdrawal of a drug to or from a therapeutic regimen that includes digoxin be carefully evaluated in the context of the patient and the clinical situation.

Potassium-depleting corticosteroids and diuretics may be major contributing factors to digitalis toxicity. Calcium, particularly if administered rapidly by the intravenous route, may produce serious arrhythmias in digitalized patients. Quinidine, verapamil, amiodarone, propafenone, indomethacin, itraconazole, alprazolam, and spironolactone raise the serum digoxin concentration due to a reduction in clearance and/or in volume of distribution of the drug, cause a rise in serum digoxin concentration, with the implication that digitalis intoxication may result. This rise appears to be proportional to the dose.

Certain antibiotics [erythromycin and clarithromycin (and possibly other macrolide antibiotics) and tetracycline] may increase digoxin absorption in patients who inactivate digoxin by bacterial metabolism in the lower intestine, so that digitalis intoxication may result. Recent studies have shown that specific colonic bacteria in the lower gastrointestinal tract convert digoxin to cardioinactive reduction products, thereby reducing its bioavailability. Although inactivation of these bacteria by antibiotics is rapid, the serum digoxin concentration will rise at a rate consistent with the elimination half-life of digoxin. The magnitude of rise in serum digoxin concentrations relates to the extent of bacterial inactivation, and may be as much as 2 fold in some cases.

Propantheline and diphenoxylate, by decreasing gut motility, may increase digoxin absorption. Antacids, kaolin-pectin, sulfasalazine, neomycin, cholestyramine, phenytoin, St. John's wort (Hypericum perforatum) and certain anticancer drugs may interfere with intestinal digoxin absorption, resulting in unexpectedly low serum concentrations. Thyroid administration to a digitalized hypothyroid patient may increase the dose requirement of digoxin. Concomitant use of digoxin and sympathomimetics increases the risk of cardiac arrhythmias because both enhance ectopic pacemaker activity. Succinylcholine may cause a sudden extrusion of potassium from muscle cells and may thereby cause arrhythmias in digitalized patients. Although α-adrenergic blockers or calcium channel blockers and digoxin may be useful in combination to control atrial fibrillation, their additive effects on AV node conduction can result in complete heart block.

Due to the considerable variability of these interactions, digoxin dosage should be carefully individualized when patients receive coadministered medications. Furthermore, caution should be exercised when combining digoxin with any drug that may cause a significant deterioration in renal function, since a decline in glomerular filtration or tubular secretion may impair the excretion of digoxin.

Drug-Drug Interactions: See Table 2.

Drug-Herb Interactions: St. John's wort (Hypericum perforatum) may interfere with intestinal digoxin absorption, resulting in unexpectedly low serum concentrations. Patients are advised to consult with their doctors before taking herbal products.

Drug-Laboratory Test Interactions: The use of therapeutic doses of digoxin may cause prolongation of the PR interval and depression of the ST segment on the electrocardiogram. Digoxin may produce false positive ST-T changes on the electrocardiogram during exercise testing. These electrophysiologic effects reflect an expected effect of the drug and are not indicative of toxicity.

Drug-Lifestyle Interactions: Serum digoxin concentration may decrease acutely during periods of exercise without any associated change in clinical efficacy due to increased binding of digoxin to skeletal muscle.

Table 2: LANOXIN

Established or Potential Drug-Drug Interactions with Digoxin

Interacting Drugs	Ref	Effect	Clinical Comment
Albuterol	USP DI 2004	Concurrent use may decrease serum digoxin concentrations, possibly by redistributing digoxin to other tissues. Albuterol may also decrease serum potassium concentrations, which may increase the risk of digoxin toxicity.	
Alprazolam	USP DI 2004	Concurrent use may increase serum digoxin concentrations, possibly by decreasing the renal clearance of digoxin; although one small study performed in healthy volunteers concluded that alprazolam had no significant effect on digoxin clearance, contradictory evidence has been reported in patients [primarily elderly patients] receiving long-term digoxin therapy.	
Amiodarone	USP DI 2004	Increases in serum digoxin concentrations by as much as 100% have been reported with concurrent use. Although it is thought that amiodarone decreases renal and/or nonrenal clearance and/or the volume of distribution of digoxin, other contributing factors, such as amiodarone-induced displacement of digoxin from tissue binding sites, also may be involved. Amiodarone has a long elimination half-life [15 to 65 days or longer] and digoxin toxicity may not appear until several weeks after the addition of amiodarone or may persist long after discontinuation of amiodarone.	
Antacids or Antidiarrheal adsorbents (e.g., kaolin and pectin) or Sulfasalazine	USP DI 2004	Concurrent use may decrease digoxin bioavailability by decreasing digoxin absorption.	In the case of antidiarrheal adsorbents and sulfasalazine, the digoxin dose may be administered 8 hours before the interacting medication.
Antibiotics, oral, especially Macrolide antibiotics, such as: Clarithromycin or Erythromycin or Tetracycline	USP DI 2004	Concurrent use of some oral antibiotics may increase serum digoxin concentrations in patients who inactivate digoxin in the lower intestine by bacterial metabolism; in these individuals, altering the bowel flora with certain antibiotics may diminish digoxin conversion to inactive metabolites, resulting in increased serum digoxin concentration; the increase in serum digoxin concentration has been as much as twofold in some cases and correlates with the extent of bacterial inactivation. Although there are limited data, this interaction has been reported with oral use of clarithromycin, erythromycin, and tetracycline.	
Anticancer medications (such as bleomycin, cyclophosphamide, cytarabine, doxorubicin, procarbazine, and vincristine) or Radiation therapy	USP DI 2004	Concurrent use may decrease digoxin bioavailability by decreasing digoxin absorption; the reduced absorption that occurs during concurrent use with anticancer medications or radiation therapy may be due to temporary damage to the gastrointestinal mucosa and may continue for several days after treatment. However, digitoxin absorption does not appear to be affected by anticancer agents.	In the case of concurrent use of anticancer medications, a dosage form with greater bioavailability, such as the capsule or solution, may help to minimize decreased bioavailability.
Atorvastatin	USP DI 2004	Concurrent use may increase digoxin serum concentrations; steady-state serum concentration increases of approximately 20% have been reported.	
Beta-adrenergic blocking agents including Atenolol, Carvedilol, Metoprolol and Propranolol	USP DI 2004	Concurrent use with these agents may have additive effects on slowing atrioventricular [AV] nodal conduction; concurrent use with carvedilol in patients with hypertension increased the steady-state area under the plasma concentration—time curve [AUC] and trough concentrations of digoxin by 14% and 16%, respectively.	Plasma digoxin concentrations should be monitored when digoxin is co-administered with beta-adrenergic blocking agents.

(cont'd)

Table 2: LANOXIN *(cont'd)*
Established or Potential Drug-Drug Interactions with Digoxin

Interacting Drugs	Ref	Effect	Clinical Comment
Bran fiber, dietary	USP DI 2004	It is uncertain whether concurrent administration of dietary bran fiber decreases digoxin bioavailability. In one small study, there was presumed to be a decrease in digoxin absorption when concurrent administration of digoxin with 5 grams of fiber resulted in a decrease in urinary excretion of digoxin. Another small study found no change in steady-state serum digoxin concentrations when digoxin was administered 15 to 30 minutes before administration of 11 grams of bran [as a bran muffin], with a second bran muffin administered several hours later.	
Calcium channel blocking agents, especially Bepridil or Diltiazem or Nifedipine or Verapamil	USP DI 2004	Concurrent use with calcium channel blocking agents may have additive effects on AV nodal conduction, which could result in complete heart block; concurrent use also may increase serum digoxin concentrations by reducing digoxin renal clearance, possibly as a result of inhibition of active tubular secretion of digoxin; verapamil may increase serum digoxin concentrations by 30 to 200%; bepridil may increase serum digoxin concentrations by approximately 34%; some studies have reported no interaction with diltiazem while others have reported increases in serum digoxin concentrations of 20 to 60%; contradictory evidence of an interaction also exists for nifedipine, although serum digoxin increases of 15 to 50% have been reported; increases in serum digitoxin concentrations also have been reported with concurrent use of diltiazem and verapamil, although increases were less pronounced than with digoxin use and may be due to a reduction in extrarenal digitoxin clearance.	Serum digitalis concentrations and electrocardiogram [ECG] should be monitored and dosages should be adjusted accordingly.
Cholestyramine or Colestipol	USP DI 2004	Colestipol and cholestyramine may delay and reduce the absorption of digoxin.	Digoxin dose may be administered 8 hours before the interacting medication to minimize the interference with digoxin absorption.
Cyclosporine	USP DI 2004	Concurrent use has resulted in increases in serum digoxin concentrations, possibly as a result of decreased apparent volume of distribution and/or plasma clearance of digoxin.	
Diphenoxylate or Propantheline	USP DI 2004	Concurrent use may increase digoxin bioavailability; diphenoxylate and propantheline increase digoxin absorption by decreasing intestinal motility.	
Diuretics, potassium-depleting (such as bumetanide, ethacrynic acid, furosemide, indapamide, mannitol, or thiazides) or Hypokalemia-causing medications	USP DI 2004	Decreases in serum potassium concentrations that can occur with these medications may increase the risk of digitalis toxicity.	Frequent serum potassium concentration determinations are recommended when these medications are concurrently administered with digoxin.
Flecainide	USP DI 2004	Concurrent use has increased serum digoxin concentrations, on average, by 24%; it also has been speculated that concurrent use may cause a slight additive increase in the PR interval.	
Hepatic enzyme inducers, such as: Barbiturates or Phenytoin or Rifampin	USP DI 2004	Concurrent use may increase the metabolism of digitoxin; serum digitoxin concentrations have been reported to decrease by 50% in patients who received 180 mg of phenobarbital per day for 12 weeks; decreases in serum digoxin concentrations also have been reported with concurrent use of rifampin, although the mechanism for this interaction is not completely understood.	Serum digitalis concentrations should be monitored and dosages adjusted accordingly.
Indomethacin	USP DI 2004	Concurrent use may increase digoxin serum concentrations, possibly by inhibiting the renal elimination of digoxin; two small studies that evaluated the interaction in healthy adult patients did not find a clinically significant interaction. Another small study found a significant increase [about 40% on average] in serum digoxin concentrations in adult heart failure patients treated with digoxin on a long-term basis. A small study in premature infants treated conventionally with indomethacin for patent ductus arteriosus [PDA] found an increase in serum digoxin concentrations of approximately 50% with concurrent use.	

(cont'd)

Table 2: LANOXIN *(cont'd)*
Established or Potential Drug-Drug Interactions with Digoxin

Interacting Drugs	Ref	Effect	Clinical Comment
Itraconazol	USP DI 2004	Concurrent use may increase serum digoxin concentrations, possibly by decreasing renal elimination of digoxin; serum digoxin concentration increases of approximately 50% have been reported.	
Metoclopramide	USP DI 2004	Concurrent use of metoclopramide may decrease digoxin absorption by increasing gastrointestinal motility; serum digoxin concentrations as determined by AUC have been reported to decrease by about 24%.	
Neomycin, oral	USP DI 2004	Concurrent use decreases the rate and extent of absorption of digoxin. In a study in healthy volunteers, the extent of absorption of digoxin was decreased by as much as 51% after single doses of digoxin and neomycin. The absorption of digoxin also was decreased when the antibiotic was given 3 or 6 hours before the digoxin dose. The mechanism of this interaction has not been established.	It is recommended that digoxin be administered at least 8 hours before neomycin.
Omeprazole	USP DI 2004	Concurrent use with digoxin may increase digoxin absorption, possibly by altering gastric acidity; on average, C_{max} and AUC values have been reported to be about 10% higher with concurrent use.	
Propafenone	USP DI 2004	Concurrent use of propafenone with digoxin results in an increase in serum digoxin concentrations ranging from 35 to 85%, which appears to be unrelated to digoxin renal clearance but may be related to a decrease in the volume of distribution and nonrenal clearance of digoxin.	Careful monitoring of digoxin concentrations and dosage reduction of digoxin are recommended when propafenone is initiated.
Quinidine or Quinine	USP DI 2004	Concurrent use with quinidine has resulted in increased digoxin plasma concentrations, possibly due to an initial displacement of digoxin from quinidine binding sites, and a reduction in the renal and nonrenal clearance and volume of distribution of digoxin; the extent of the interaction is proportional to plasma quinidine concentrations and, on average, concurrent use results in 100% increases in serum digoxin concentrations, although increases of over 300% have been reported; concurrent use of quinidine with digitoxin has resulted in increases in serum digitoxin concentrations of 30 to 67%, the smaller increases possibly resulting from impairment of extrarenal clearance of digitoxin by quinidine; increases in serum digoxin concentrations also have been reported with concurrent use of quinine.	Serum digitalis concentrations should be monitored and dosage adjusted as indicated.
Spironolactone	USP DI 2004	Concurrent use with digoxin may increase serum digoxin concentrations, possibly by decreasing digoxin renal and nonrenal clearance and/or digoxin volume of distribution; it has been estimated that digoxin plasma concentrations may increase by one third with concurrent use.	
Succinylcholine	USP DI 2004	Concurrent use may cause a sudden release of potassium from muscle cells, increasing the risk of arrhythmias in digitalized patients.	
Sucralfate	USP DI 2004	Sucralfate was reported to reduce digoxin plasma concentrations by about 19%, presumably by reducing the bioavailability of digoxin.	Sucralfate should not be taken within 2 hours of digoxin.
Sympathomimetics	USP DI 2004	Concurrent use may increase the risk of cardiac arrhythmias.	
Thyroid hormones	USP DI 2004	Patients with thyroid disease may have an altered sensitivity to digitalis: hyperthyroid patients may have a reduced response to digitalis and hypothyroid patients may have an increased risk of digitalis toxicity.	Increase in digitalis dose may be required with the use of thyroid hormones in a hypothyroid patient.

DOSAGE AND ADMINISTRATION: General: Recommended dosages of digoxin may require considerable modification because of individual sensitivity of the patient to the drug, the presence of associated conditions, or the use of concurrent medications.

In selecting the dose of digoxin, several factors must be considered:

1. The body weight of the patient. Doses should be calculated based upon lean (i.e., ideal) body weight.
2. The patient's renal function, preferably evaluated on the basis of estimated creatinine clearance.
3. The patient's age. Infants and children require different doses of digoxin than adults. Also, advanced age may be indicative of diminished renal function even in patients with normal serum creatinine concentration (i.e., below 1.5 mg/dL).
4. Concomitant disease states, concurrent medication or other factors likely to alter the pharmacokinetic or pharmacodynamic profile of digoxin (see Warnings and Precautions).
5. To minimize toxic side effects, the lowest effective dose should be used as the maintenance dose.

Serum Digoxin Concentrations: In general, the dose of digoxin used should be determined on clinical grounds. However, measurement of serum digoxin concentrations can be helpful to the clinician in determining the adequacy of digoxin therapy and in assigning certain probabilities to the likelihood of digoxin intoxication. About two-thirds of adults considered adequately digitalized (without evidence of toxicity) have serum digoxin concentrations ranging from 0.8 to 2.0 ng/mL. However, digoxin may produce clinical benefits even at serum concentrations below this range. About two-thirds of adult patients with clinical toxicity have serum digoxin concentrations greater than 2.0 ng/mL. However, since one-third of patients with clinical toxicity have concentrations less than 2.0 ng/mL, values below 2.0 ng/mL do not rule out the possibility that a certain sign or symptom is related to digoxin therapy. Rarely, there are patients who are unable to tolerate digoxin at serum concentrations below 0.8 ng/mL. Consequently, the serum concentration of digoxin should always be interpreted in the overall clinical context, and an isolated measurement should not be used alone as the basis for increasing or decreasing the dose of the drug.

To allow adequate time for equilibration of digoxin between serum and tissue, sampling of serum concentrations should be done just before the next scheduled dose of the drug. If this is not possible, sampling should be done at least 6 to 8 hours after the last dose, regardless of the route of administration or the formulation used. On a once-daily dosing schedule, the concentration of digoxin will be 10% to 25% lower when sampled at 24 versus 8 hours, depending upon the patient's renal function. On a twice-daily dosing schedule, there will be only minor differences in serum digoxin concentrations whether sampling is done at 8 or 12 hours after a dose.

If a discrepancy exists between the reported serum concentration and the observed clinical response, the clinician should consider the following possibilities:

1. Analytical problems in the assay procedure.
2. Inappropriate serum sampling time.
3. Administration of a digitalis glycoside other than digoxin.
4. Conditions (described in Warnings and Precautions) causing an alteration in the sensitivity of the patient to digoxin.
5. Serum digoxin concentration may decrease acutely during periods of exercise without any associated change in clinical efficacy due to increased binding of digoxin to skeletal muscle.

Heart Failure: Adults: Digitalization may be accomplished by either of two general approaches that vary in dosage and frequency of administration, but reach the same endpoint in terms of total amount of digoxin accumulated in the body.

1. Rapid digitalization may be achieved by administering a loading dose based upon projected peak body digoxin stores, then calculating the maintenance dose as a percentage of the loading dose.
2. More gradual digitalization may be obtained by beginning an appropriate maintenance dose, thus allowing digoxin body stores to accumulate slowly. Steady-state serum digoxin concentrations will be achieved in approximately 5 half-lives of the drug for the individual patient. Depending upon the patient's renal function, this will take between 1 and 3 weeks.

Rapid Digitalization with a Loading Dose: Peak body digoxin stores of 8 to 12 µg/kg should provide therapeutic effect with minimum risk of toxicity in most patients with heart failure and normal sinus rhythm. Because of altered digoxin distribution and elimination, projected peak body stores for patients with renal insufficiency should be conservative (i.e., 6 to 10 µg/kg) [see Warnings and Precautions].

The loading dose should be administered in several portions, with roughly half the total given as the first dose. Additional fractions of this planned total dose may be given at 6- to 8-hour intervals, **with careful assessment of clinical response before each additional dose.**

If the patient's clinical response necessitates a change from the calculated dose of digoxin, then calculation of the maintenance dose should be based upon the amount actually given.

A single initial dose of 500 to 750 µg (0.5 to 0.75 mg) of digoxin tablets usually produces a detectable effect in 0.5 to 2 hours that becomes maximal in 2 to 6 hours. Additional doses of 125 to 375 µg (0.125 to 0.375 mg) may be given cautiously at 6 to 8-hour intervals until clinical evidence of an adequate effect is noted. The usual amount of digoxin tablets that a 70-kg patient requires to achieve 8 to 12 µg/kg peak body stores is 750 to 1250 µg (0.75 to 1.25 mg).

Digoxin injection is frequently used to achieve rapid digitalization, with conversion to digoxin tablets for maintenance therapy. If patients are switched from intravenous to oral digoxin formulations, allowances must be made for differences in bioavailability when calculating maintenance dosages (see Table 5).

Table 3: LANOXIN

Usual Daily Maintenance Dose Requirements of Digoxin Tablets (µg) for Estimated Peak Body Stores of 10 µg/kg

Corrected Ccr (mL/min per 70 kg)[a]	Lean Body Weight kg / lb	50 / 110	60 / 132	70 / 154	80 / 176	90 / 198	100 / 220	Number of Days Before Steady State Achieved[b]
0		62.5[c]	125	125	125	187.5	187.5	22
10		125	125	125	187.5	187.5	187.5	19
20		125	125	187.5	187.5	187.5	250	16
30		125	187.5	187.5	187.5	250	250	14
40		125	187.5	187.5	250	250	250	13
50		187.5	187.5	250	250	250	250	12
60		187.5	187.5	250	250	250	375	11
70		187.5	250	250	250	250	375	10
80		187.5	250	250	250	375	375	9
90		187.5	250	250	250	375	500	8
100		250	250	250	375	375	500	7

[a] Ccr is creatinine clearance, corrected to 70 kg body weight or 1.73 m² body surface area. For adults, if only serum creatinine concentrations (Scr) are available, a Ccr (corrected to 70 kg body weight) may be estimated in men as (140−Age)/Scr. For women, this result should be multiplied by 0.85. Note: This equation cannot be used for estimating creatinine clearance in infants or children.

[b] If no loading dose administered.

[c] 62.5 µg=0.0625 mg.

Example: Based on Table 3, a patient in heart failure with an estimated lean body weight of 70 kg and a Ccr of 60 mL/min, should be given 250 µg (0.25 mg) daily of digoxin tablet, usually taken after the morning meal. If no loading dose is administered, steady-state serum concentration in this patient should be anticipated at approximately 11 days.

Infants and Children: In general, divided daily dosing is recommended for infants and young children (under age 10). In the newborn period, renal clearance of digoxin is diminished and suitable dosage adjustments must be observed. This is especially pronounced in the premature infant. Beyond the immediate newborn period, children generally require proportionally larger doses than adults on the basis of body weight or body surface area. Children over 10 years of age require adult dosages in proportion to their body weight. Some researchers have suggested that infants and young children tolerate slightly higher serum concentrations than do adults.

Daily maintenance doses for each age group are given in Table 4 and should provide therapeutic effect with minimum risk of toxicity in most patients with heart failure and normal sinus rhythm. These recommendations assume the presence of normal renal function:

Table 4: LANOXIN

Daily Maintenance Doses of Digoxin Tablets in Children with Normal Renal Function

Age	Daily Maintenance Dose (µg/kg)
2 to 5 years	10 to 15
5 to 10 years	7 to 10
Over 10 years	3 to 5

Additional Information for LANOXIN Oral Solution: Rapid Digitalization with a Loading Dose: A pediatric digoxin injection can be used to achieve rapid digitalization, with conversion to an oral formulation of digoxin tablets or LANOXIN oral solution for maintenance therapy. If patients are switched from intravenous to oral digoxin formulations, allowances must be made for differences in bioavailability when calculating maintenance dosages (see also Dosing Table 5). Peak digoxin stores of 8 to 12 µg/kg should provide therapeutic effect with minimum risk of toxicity in most patients with heart failure and normal sinus rhythm. Because of altered digoxin distribution and elimination, projected peak body stores for patients with renal insufficiency should be conservative (i.e., 6 to 10 µg/kg [see Warnings and Precautions]).

Digitalizing and daily maintenance doses for each age are given in Table 5 and should provide therapeutic effect with minimum risk of toxicity in most patients with heart failure and normal sinus rhythm. These recommendations assume the presence of normal renal function.

The loading dose should be administered in several portions, with roughly half the total given as the first dose. Additional fractions of this planned total dose may be given at 6- to 8-hour intervals, **with careful assessment of clinical response before each additional dose**. If the patients' clinical response necessitates a change from the calculated loading dose of digoxin, then calculation of the maintenance dose should be based upon the amount actually given.

Table 5: LANOXIN

Usual Digitalizing and Maintenance Dosages for LANOXIN Oral Solution in Children with Normal Renal Function Based on Lean Body Weight

Age	Oral Digitalizing[a] Dose (µg/kg)	IV Digitalizing Dose (µg/kg)	Daily Maintenance Dose[b] (µg/kg)
Premature	20 to 30	15 to 25	20% to 30% of oral [or IV] digitalizing dose[c]
Full-Term	25 to 35	20 to 30	25% to 35% of oral [or IV] digitalizing dose[c]
1 to 24 Months	35 to 60	30 to 50	
2 to 5 Years	30 to 40	25 to 35	
2 to 10 Years	20 to 35	15 to 30	
Over 10 Years	10 to 15	8 to 12	

[a] IV digitalizing doses are 80% of oral digitalizing doses.

[b] Divided daily dosing is recommended for children under 10 years of age.

[c] Projected or actual digitalizing dose providing clinical response.

In children with renal disease, digoxin must be carefully titrated based upon clinical response.

Gradual Digitalization with a Maintenance Dose: More gradual digitalization can also be accomplished by beginning an appropriate maintenance dose. The range of percentages provided in Table 5 can be used in calculating this dose for patients with normal renal function.

It cannot be overemphasized that both the adult and pediatric dosage guidelines provided are based upon average patient response and substantial individual variation can be expected. Accordingly, ultimate dosage selection must be based upon clinical assessment of the patient.

Missed Dose: If a dose is missed patients are advised to take the dose as soon as remembered if within 12 hours of scheduled dose and not taking if remembered later. Patients are advised not to double doses and to consult their doctor if a dose is missed for 2 days or more.

Administration: Digoxin is usually administered orally as a single daily dose. Divided daily dosing is recommended in infants and young children.

OVERDOSAGE:

Adults: Digoxin should be temporarily discontinued until the adverse reaction resolves.

Every effort should also be made to correct factors that may contribute to the adverse reaction (such as electrolyte disturbances or concurrent medications). Once the adverse reaction has resolved, therapy with digoxin may be reinstituted, following a careful reassessment of dose.

Withdrawal of digoxin may be all that is required to treat the adverse reaction. However, when the primary manifestation of digoxin overdosage is a cardiac arrhythmia, additional therapy may be needed.

If the rhythm disturbance is a symptomatic bradyarrhythmia or heart block, consideration should be given to the reversal of toxicity with DIGIBIND [Digoxin Immune Fab (Ovine) (see Massive Digitalis Overdosage), the use of atropine, or the insertion of a temporary cardiac pacemaker. However, asymptomatic bradycardia or heart block related to digoxin may require only temporary withdrawal of the drug and cardiac monitoring of the patient. If the rhythm disturbance is a ventricular arrhythmia, consideration should be given to the correction of electrolyte disorders, particularly if hypokalemia (see Administration of Potassium) or hypomagnesemia is present. DIGIBIND is a specific antidote for digoxin and may be used to reverse potentially life-threatening ventricular arrhythmias due to digoxin overdosage.

Administration of Potassium: Every effort should be made to maintain the serum potassium concentration between 4.0 and 5.5 mmol/L. Potassium is usually administered orally, but when correction of the arrhythmia is urgent and the serum potassium concentration is low, potassium may be administered cautiously by the intravenous route. The electrocardiogram should be monitored for any evidence of potassium toxicity (e.g., peaking of T waves) and to observe the effect on the arrhythmia. Potassium salts may be dangerous in patients who manifest bradycardia or heart block due to digoxin (unless primarily related to supraventricular tachycardia) and in the setting of massive digitalis overdosage (see Massive Digitalis Overdosage).

Massive Digitalis Overdosage: Manifestations of life-threatening toxicity include severe ventricular tachycardia or ventricular fibrillation, or progressive bradyarrhythmias or heart block. The administration of more than 10 mg of digoxin in a previously healthy adult, or more than 4 mg in a previously healthy child or a steady-state serum concentration greater than 10 ng/mL, often results in cardiac arrest.

DIGIBIND should be used to reverse the toxic effect of a massive overdose. The decision to administer DIGIBIND to a patient who has ingested a massive dose of digoxin but who has not yet manifested life-threatening toxicity should depend on the likelihood that the life-threatening toxicity will occur (see above).

Patients with massive digitalis ingestion should receive large doses of activated charcoal to prevent absorption and bind digoxin in the gut during enteroenteric recirculation. Emesis or gastric lavage may be indicated especially if ingestion has occurred within 30 minutes of the patient's presentation at the hospital. Emesis should not be induced in patients who are obtunded. If a patient presents more than 2 hours after ingestion or already has toxic manifestations, it may be unsafe to induce vomiting or attempt passage of a gastric tube, because such manoeuvers may induce an acute vagal episode that can worsen digitalis-related arrhythmias.

Severe digitalis intoxication can cause a massive shift of potassium from inside to outside the cell, leading to life-threatening hyperkalemia. The administration of potassium supplements in the setting of massive intoxication may be hazardous and should be avoided. Hyperkalemia caused by massive digitalis toxicity is best treated with DIGIBIND; initial treatment with glucose and insulin may also be required if hyperkalemia itself is acutely life-threatening.

For management of a suspected drug overdose, contact your regional Poison Control Centre. See the *CPS* Directory section for a list of Poison Control Centres.

ACTION AND CLINICAL PHARMACOLOGY: Mechanism of Action: The influence of digitalis glycosides on the myocardium is dose related, and involves both direct action on cardiac muscle and the specialized conduction system, and indirect actions on cardiovascular system mediated by the autonomic nervous system. The indirect actions mediated by the autonomic nervous system involve a vagomimetic action, which is responsible for the effects of digitalis on the sinoatrial (SA) and atrioventricular (AV) nodes; and also a baroreceptor sensitization which results in increased carotid sinus nerve activity and enhanced sympathetic withdrawal for any given increment in mean arterial pressure. The pharmacologic consequences of these direct and indirect effects are: an increase in the force and velocity of myocardial systolic contraction (positive inotropic action); a slowing of heart rate (negative chronotropic effect); and decreased conduction velocity through the AV node. In higher doses, digitalis increases sympathetic outflow from the CNS to both cardiac and peripheral sympathetic nerves. This increase in sympathetic activity may be an important factor in digitalis cardiac toxicity. Most of the extracardiac manifestations of digitalis toxicity are also mediated by the CNS.

Pharmacodynamics: Digoxin produces hemodynamic improvement in patients with heart failure. Short- and long-term therapy with the drug increases cardiac output and lowers pulmonary artery pressure, pulmonary capillary wedge pressure, and systemic vascular resistance. These hemodynamic effects are accompanied by an increase in the left ventricular ejection fraction and a decrease in end-systolic and end-diastolic dimensions.

The times to onset of pharmacologic effect and to peak effect of preparations of digoxin tablets are shown in Table 6.

Table 6: LANOXIN

Time to Onset of Effect and Peak Effect for Digoxin Tablets and LANOXIN Products

Product	Time to Onset of Effect[a]	Time to peak Effect[a]
Digoxin Tablets, C.S.D.	0.5 to 2 hours	2 to 6 hours
LANOXIN (Digoxin Oral Solution, C.S.D.)	0.5 to 2 hours	2 to 6 hours

[a] Documented for ventricular response rate in atrial fibrillation, inotropic effect and electrocardiograph changes.

Congestive Heart Failure: Two 12-week, double-blind, placebo-controlled studies enrolled 178 (RADIANCE trial) and 88 (PROVED trial) patients with NYHA class II or III heart failure previously treated with digoxin, a diuretic, and an ACE inhibitor (RADIANCE only) and randomized them to placebo or treatment with digoxin. Both trials demonstrated better preservation of exercise capacity in patients randomized to digoxin. Continued treatment with digoxin reduced the risk of developing worsening heart failure, as evidenced by heart failure-related hospitalizations and emergency care and the need for concomitant heart failure therapy. The larger study also showed treatment-related benefits in NYHA class and patients' global assessment. In the smaller trial, these trended in favour of a treatment benefit.

The Digitalis Investigation Group (DIG) main trial was a multicenter, randomized, double-blind, placebo-controlled mortality study of 6801 patients with heart failure and left ventricular ejection fraction ≤0.45. At randomization, 67% were NYHA class I or II, 71% had heart failure of ischemic etiology, 44% had been receiving digoxin, and most were receiving concomitant ACE inhibitor (94%) and diuretic (82%). Patients were randomized to placebo or digoxin, the dose of which was adjusted for the patient's age, sex, lean body weight, and serum creatinine (see Dosage and Administration), and followed for up to 58 months (median 37 months). The median daily dose prescribed was 0.25 mg. Overall all-cause mortality was 35% with no difference between groups (95% confidence limits for relative risk of 0.91 to 1.07). Digoxin was associated with a 25% reduction in the number of hospitalizations for heart failure, a 28% reduction in the risk of a patient having at least one hospitalization for heart failure, and a 6.5% reduction in total hospitalizations (for any cause).

Use of digoxin was associated with a trend to increase time to all-cause death or hospitalization. The trend was evident in subgroups of patients with mild heart failure as well as more severe disease, as shown in Table 7. Although the effect on all-cause death or hospitalization was not statistically significant, much of the apparent benefit derived from effects on mortality and hospitalization attributed to heart failure. In situations where there is no statistically significant benefit of treatment evident from a trial's primary end point, results pertaining to secondary endpoint should be interpreted cautiously.

Table 7: LANOXIN

Subgroup Analyses of Mortality and Hospitalization During the First Two Years Following Randomization in the DIG Trial with Digoxin Tablets

		Risk of All-Cause Mortality or All-Cause Hospitalization[a]			Risk of HF-related Mortality or HF-related Hospitalization[a]		
	n	Placebo	Digoxin	Relative risk[b]	Placebo	Digoxin	Relative risk[b]
All patients (EF ≤0.45)	6801	604	593	0.94 (0.88–1.00)	294	217	0.69 (0.63–0.76)
NYHA I/II	4571	549	541	0.96 (0.89–1.04)	242	178	0.70 (0.62–0.80)
EF 0.25–0.45	4543	568	571	0.99 (0.91–1.07)	244	190	0.74 (0.66–0.84)
CTR ≤0.55	4455	561	563	0.98 (0.91–1.06)	239	180	0.71 (0.63–0.81)
NYHA III/IV	2224	719	696	0.88 (0.80–0.97)	402	295	0.65 (0.57–0.75)
EF <0.25	2258	677	637	0.84 (0.76–0.93)	394	270	0.61 (0.53–0.71)
CTR >0.55	2346	687	650	0.85 (0.77–0.94)	398	287	0.65 (0.57–0.75)
EF >0.45[c]	987	571	585	1.04 (0.88–1.23)	179	136	0.72 (0.53–0.99)

[a] Number of patients with an event during the first 2 years per 1000 randomized patients.
[b] Relative risk (95% confidence interval).
[c] DIG Ancillary Study.

Chronic Atrial Fibrillation: In patients with chronic atrial fibrillation, digoxin slows rapid ventricular response rate in a linear dose-response fashion from 0.25 to 0.75 mg/day. Digoxin should not be used for the treatment of multifocal atrial tachycardia.

Pharmacokinetics: Absorption: Gastrointestinal absorption of digoxin is a passive process. Absorption of digoxin from tablets is 60 to 80%. Absorption of Digoxin Oral Solution formulation has been demonstrated to be 70% to 85% complete compared to an identical intravenous dose of digoxin (absolute bioavailability). When digoxin oral solution/tablets are taken after meals, the rate of absorption is slowed, but the total amount of digoxin absorbed is usually unchanged. When taken with meals high in bran fibre; however, the amount absorbed from an oral dose may be reduced.

In some patients, orally administered digoxin is converted to cardioinactive reduction products (e.g., dihydrodigoxin) by colonic bacteria in the gut. Data suggest that 1 in 10 patients treated with digoxin tablets will degrade 40% or more of the ingested dose. As a result, certain antibiotics may increase the absorption of digoxin in such patients. Although inactivation of these bacteria by antibiotics is rapid, the serum digoxin concentration will rise at a rate constant with the extent of bacterial interaction and may be as much as two-fold in some cases.

Distribution: Following drug administration, a 6- to 8-hour distribution phase is observed. This is followed by a much more gradual serum concentration decline, which is dependent on digoxin elimination from the body. The peak height and slope of the early portion (absorption/distribution phases) of the serum concentration-time curve are dependent upon the route of administration and the absorption characteristics of the formulation. Clinical evidence indicates that the early high serum concentrations do not reflect the concentration of digoxin at its site of action, but that with chronic use, the steady-state postdistribution serum levels are in equilibrium with tissue levels and correlate with pharmacologic effects. In individual patients, these postdistribution serum concentrations are linearly related to maintenance dosage and may be useful in evaluating therapeutic and toxic effects.

Digoxin is concentrated in tissues and therefore has a large apparent volume of distribution. Digoxin crosses both the blood-brain barrier and the placenta. At delivery, serum digoxin concentration in the newborn is similar to the serum level in the mother. Approximately 20 to 25% of plasma digoxin is bound to protein. Serum digoxin concentrations are not significantly altered by large changes in fat tissue weight, so that its distribution space correlates best with lean (ideal) body weight, not total body weight.

Metabolism: Metabolism occurs partially in the stomach, but also may occur in the liver and, although only about 16% of a dose of digoxin is metabolized, several metabolites of digoxin and their metabolic pathways have been identified. The bis-digitoxoside and mono-digitoxoside metabolites are considered to be cardioactive. Other metabolites, such as digoxigenin, are considered to be less cardioactive than digoxin. In some patients (estimated to be approximately 10% of patients taking digoxin), other cardioinactive metabolites, such as dihydrodigoxin and dihydrodigoxigenin, may result from the metabolism of digoxin by intestinal bacteria. In these individuals, as much as 40% or more of the oral dose of digoxin may be converted to these inactive reduction products. The metabolism of digoxin is not dependent upon the cytochrome P-450 system.

Excretion: Elimination of digoxin follows first-order kinetics (that is, the quantity of digoxin eliminated at any time is proportional to the total body content). Following i.v. administration to normal subjects, 50 to 70% of a digoxin dose is excreted unchanged in the urine. Renal excretion of digoxin is proportional to glomerular filtration rate and is largely independent of urine flow. In subjects with normal renal function, digoxin has a half-life of 1.5 to 2 days.

Special Populations and Conditions: Pediatrics: The tolerance of newborn infants to digitalis glycosides is variable, since their renal clearance of the medication is reduced. Premature and immature infants are especially sensitive. Dosage should be reduced and individualized according to the infant's degree of maturity, since renal clearance increases as the infant matures. Children older than 1 month of age generally require proportionally larger doses than adults on the basis of body weight or body surface area (see Dosage and Administration).

Geriatrics: Elderly patients may be more likely to have age-related renal function impairment, which may significantly increase the elimination half-life of digoxin. Additionally, elderly patients may have a decreased volume of distribution of digitalis due to decreased muscle mass. These factors may contribute to digitalis toxicity in elderly patients.

Gender: Digoxin is primarily removed from the body by renal elimination. Although the digoxin clearance in women is about 10-15% lower than in men, the effect of gender on the pharmacokinetics of digoxin is not expected to be clinically significant when initiating and monitoring digoxin therapy in patients.

Race: Race differences in digoxin pharmacokinetics have not been formally studied. Because digoxin is primarily eliminated as unchanged drug via the kidney and because there are no important differences in creatinine clearance among races, pharmacokinetic differences due to race are not expected.

Hepatic Insufficiency: Plasma digoxin concentration profiles in patients with acute hepatitis generally fell within the range of profiles in a group of healthy subjects.

Renal Insufficiency: The clearance of digoxin can be primarily correlated with renal function as indicated by creatinine clearance. In children with renal disease, digoxin must be carefully titrated based on clinical response.

The half-life of digoxin in anuric patients is prolonged to 4 to 6 days. Digoxin is not effectively removed from the body by dialysis, exchange transfusion or during cardiopulmonary bypass because most of the drug is in the tissue rather than circulating in the blood.

Genetic Polymorphism: The effect of genetic polymorphism on the pharmacokinetics of digoxin was not studied.

STORAGE AND STABILITY: Store between 15 to 30°C in a dry place and protect from light. Avoid exposure to excessive heat.

INFORMATION FOR THE PATIENT: Published in e-CPS, available by subscription at www.e-cps.ca.

DOSAGE FORMS, COMPOSITION AND PACKAGING: Each mL of clear, light-green coloured liquid with a lime odour and taste, contains: digoxin 0.05 mg (50 μg). Nonmedicinal ingredients: alcohol, calcined diatomaceous earth, citric acid, D&C Green No. 5, D&C Yellow No. 10, lime flavour, methylparaben, propylene glycol, sodium phosphate, sucrose and water. Alcohol: 10.0 mL/100 mL. Tartrazine-free. Bottles of 115 mL with calibrated dropper.

Lantus®

insulin glargine (rDNA origin)

Antidiabetic

sanofi-aventis

Date of Revision: June 8, 2010

SUMMARY PRODUCT INFORMATION:

Route of Administration	Dosage Form/ Strength	Clinically Relevant Nonmedicinal Ingredients
Subcutaneous	Solution for injection 100 U/mL	Glycerol 85%, m-cresol, polysorbate 20 (10 mL vial only), zinc, and water for injection Hydrochloric acid and sodium hydroxide for pH adjustment

DESCRIPTION: LANTUS [insulin glargine injection (rDNA origin)] is a recombinant human insulin analogue that is a long-acting, parenteral blood-glucose-lowering agent. LANTUS is produced by recombinant DNA technology utilizing a non-pathogenic laboratory strain of *E. coli* (K12) as the production organism.

Insulin glargine differs from natural human insulin in that the amino acid asparagine at position 21 of the A-chain is replaced by glycine and two arginines are added to the C-terminus of the B-chain.

INDICATIONS AND CLINICAL USE: LANTUS [insulin glargine injection (rDNA origin)] is a novel recombinant human insulin analogue indicated for once-daily subcutaneous administration in the treatment of patients over 17 years of age with Type 1 or Type 2 diabetes mellitus who require basal (long-acting) insulin for the control of hyperglycemia.

LANTUS is also indicated in the treatment of pediatric patients with Type 1 diabetes mellitus who require basal (long-acting) insulin for the control of hyperglycemia.

CONTRAINDICATIONS: LANTUS [insulin glargine injection (rDNA origin)] is contraindicated in patients who are hypersensitive to this drug or to any ingredient in the formulation or component of the container. For a complete listing, see Dosage Forms, Composition and Packaging.

WARNINGS AND PRECAUTIONS: Hypoglycemia is the most common adverse effect of insulin, including LANTUS. As with all insulins, the timing of hypoglycemia may differ among various insulin formulations. Glucose monitoring is recommended for all patients with diabetes.

Any change of insulin should be made cautiously and only under medical supervision. Changes in insulin strength, timing of administration, manufacturer, type (e.g., regular, NPH, or insulin analogs), species (animal, human), or method of manufacture (recombinant DNA versus animal-source insulin) may result in the need for a change in dosage. Concomitant oral antidiabetic treatment may need to be adjusted. As with all insulins, when transferring to LANTUS, the early warnings symptoms of hypoglycemia may be changed, be less pronounced, or absent. The prolonged effect of subcutaneous LANTUS may delay recovery from hypoglycemia.

LANTUS must not be mixed with any other insulin or diluted with any other solution (see Dosage and Administration, Administration). If LANTUS is diluted or mixed, the solution may become cloudy, and the pharmacokinetic/pharmacodynamic profile (e.g., onset of action, time to peak effect) of LANTUS and/or the mixed insulin may be altered in an unpredictable manner. When LANTUS and regular human insulin were mixed immediately before injection in dogs, a delayed onset of action and time to maximum effect for regular human insulin was observed. The total bioavailability of the mixture was also slightly decreased compared to separate injections of LANTUS and regular human insulin. The relevance of these observations in dogs to humans is not known.

General: LANTUS [insulin glargine injection (rDNA origin)] is not intended for intravenous or intramuscular administration. The prolonged duration of activity of insulin glargine is dependent on injection into subcutaneous tissue. Intravenous administration of the usual subcutaneous dose could result in severe hypoglycemia.

Hypoglycemia may occur if the insulin dose is too high in relation to the insulin requirement (see Hypoglycemia). The use of too low insulin dosages or discontinuation of treatment, especially in Type 1 diabetes, may lead to hyperglycemia and diabetic ketoacidosis. Uncorrected hypoglycemic or hyperglycemic reactions can cause loss of consciousness, coma, or death.

Glucose monitoring is recommended for all patients with diabetes.

As with all insulin preparations, the time course of LANTUS action may vary in different individuals or at different times in the same individual and the rate of absorption is dependent on blood supply, temperature, and physical activity.

Insulin may cause sodium retention and edema, particularly if previously poor metabolic control is improved by intensified insulin therapy.

Patients with human insulin antibodies may be hypersensitive to other insulins, with a risk of hypoglycemia and/or cross-reactivity.

Thiazolidinediones (TZDs), alone or in combination with other antidiabetic agents (including insulin), can cause heart failure and edema. The combination of TZD with insulin is not indicated for the treatment of Type 2 Diabetes Mellitus. Please refer to the respective TZD product monograph Warnings and Precautions information when the use of these drugs in combination with any insulin, including LANTUS, is contemplated.

Hepatic/Biliary/Pancreas: Although studies have not been performed in patients with diabetes and hepatic impairment, LANTUS requirements may be diminished due to reduced capacity for gluconeogenesis and reduced insulin metabolism (see Action and Clinical Pharmacology, Special Populations and Conditions).

Hypoglycemia: As with all insulin preparations, hypoglycemic reactions, especially during initiation of therapy, may be associated with the administration of LANTUS. Hypoglycemia is the most common adverse effect of insulins. Early warning symptoms of hypoglycemia may be different, be less pronounced or absent, under certain conditions, as for example, in patients whose glycemic control is markedly improved, in elderly patients, in patients where an autonomic neuropathy is present, in patients whose hypoglycemia is developing gradually, in patients with a long history of diabetes, in patients with psychiatric illness, or in patients receiving concurrent treatment with certain other drugs such as beta-blockers. Hypoglycemia may occur with other substances including alcohol and psychiatric medications, street drugs, birth control pills, injections and patches (see Drug Interactions, Drug-Drug Interactions).

Such situations may result in severe hypoglycemia (and possibly, loss of consciousness) prior to patients' awareness of hypoglycemia.

The time of occurrence of hypoglycemia depends on the action profile of the insulins used and may, therefore, change when the treatment regimen or timing of administration is changed. As with all insulins, additional caution (including intensified blood glucose monitoring) should be exercised in patient populations who are at greater risk for clinically significant sequelae from hypoglycemic episodes.

In a clinical study, symptoms of hypoglycemia or counter regulatory hormone responses were similar after intravenous insulin glargine and regular human insulin both in healthy subjects and adult patients with type 1 diabetes.

Immune: Insulin administration may cause insulin antibodies to form. In clinical studies, antibodies that cross-react with human insulin and insulin glargine were observed in both NPH human insulin and insulin glargine treatment groups with similar percents of increased and decreased titers. There was no correlation in either treatment group between increases or decreases in these antibody titers and changes in either $A1_C$ or total insulin requirements. In theory, the presence of such insulin antibodies may necessitate adjustment of the insulin dose in order to correct a tendency to hyperglycemia or hypoglycemia, but has not been found on review of LANTUS clinical trials and available post-marketing data.

Injection Site and Allergic Reactions: As with any insulin therapy, lipodystrophy may occur at the injection site and delay insulin absorption. Other injection site reactions with insulin therapy include redness, pain, itching, hives, swelling, and inflammation. Continuous rotation of the injection site within a given area may help to reduce or prevent these reactions. Most minor reactions to insulins usually resolve in a few days to a few weeks.

Immediate-type allergic reactions are rare. Such reactions to insulin (including insulin glargine) or the excipients may, for example, be associated with generalized skin reactions, angioedema, bronchospasm, hypotension, or shock and may be life threatening.

Reports of injection site pain were more frequent with LANTUS than NPH human insulin (2.7% insulin glargine versus 0.7% human NPH). The reports of pain at the injection site were usually mild and did not result in discontinuation of therapy. Other possibly related treatment-emergent injection site reactions occurred at similar incidences with both insulin glargine and NPH human insulin.

Intercurrent Conditions: Insulin requirements may be altered during intercurrent conditions such as infection or illness, emotional disturbances, or stress.

Renal: Although studies have not been performed in patients with diabetes and renal impairment, LANTUS requirements may be diminished due to reduced insulin metabolism (see Warnings and Precautions, Special Populations). Careful glucose monitoring and dose adjustments of insulin or insulin analogues including LANTUS may be necessary in patients with renal dysfunction.

Special Populations: Pregnant Women: Teratogenic Effects: There are no well-controlled clinical studies of the use of insulin glargine in pregnant women. Only a limited number of pregnancies were exposed during Post Marketing Surveillance with insulin glargine. As with other insulins, adverse pregnancy outcomes did not indicate any trends suggesting a link to insulin glargine. To date, no other relevant epidemiological data are available. It is essential for patients with diabetes or a history of gestational diabetes to maintain good metabolic control before conception and throughout pregnancy. Insulin requirements may decrease during the first trimester, generally increase during the second and third trimesters, and rapidly decline after delivery. Careful monitoring of glucose control is essential in such patients. Patients with diabetes should be advised to inform their doctor if they are pregnant or are contemplating pregnancy.

Nursing Women: It is unknown whether insulin glargine is excreted in significant amounts in human milk. Many drugs, including human insulin, are excreted in human milk. For this reason, caution should be exercised when LANTUS is administered to a nursing woman. Lactating women may require adjustments in insulin dose and diet.

Pediatrics (>6 years of age): Safety and effectiveness of LANTUS has been established in children over 6 years of age with Type 1 diabetes mellitus (see Action and Clinical Pharmacology, Special Populations and Conditions and Indications and Clinical Use).

Geriatrics (>65 years of age): In controlled clinical studies comparing insulin glargine to NPH human insulin, 593 of 3890 patients with type 1 and type 2 diabetes were 65 years and older. The only difference in safety or effectiveness in this subpopulation compared to the entire study population was an expected higher incidence of cardiovascular events in both insulin glargine and NPH human insulin treated patients.

In elderly patients with diabetes, the initial dosing, dose increments, and maintenance dosage should be conservative to avoid hypoglycemic reactions.

Hypoglycemia may be difficult to recognize in the elderly (see Warnings and Precautions, Hypoglycemia). In the elderly, progressive deterioration of renal function may lead to steady decrease in insulin requirements. Careful glucose monitoring and dose adjustments of insulin or insulin analogues including LANTUS may be necessary (see Warnings and Precautions, Renal).

ADVERSE REACTIONS: Adverse Drug Reaction Overview: Type 1 and Type 2 Diabetes in Adults: The adverse events most commonly associated with LANTUS [insulin glargine injection (rDNA origin)] include the following:

Body as a Whole: allergic reaction (see Warnings and Precautions).

Hypoglycemia: Hypoglycemia, a frequent adverse reaction to insulin therapy, may occur if the insulin dose is too high in relation to the insulin requirement.

As with all insulins, prolonged or severe hypoglycemic attacks, especially if recurrent, may lead to neurological damage, loss of consciousness, coma or death (see Warnings and Precautions).

Skin and Appendages: injection site reaction, lipodystrophy, pruritus, and rash (see Warnings and Precautions).

Other: antibodies formation (see Warnings and Precautions).

Eyes: A marked change in glycemic control may cause temporary visual impairment, due to temporary alteration in the turgidity and refractive index of the lens.

Long-term improved glycemic control decreases the risk of progression of diabetic retinopathy. However, as for all insulin regimens, intensification of insulin therapy with abrupt improvement in glycemic control may be associated with temporary worsening of diabetic retinopathy.

In patients with proliferative retinopathy, particularly if not treated with photocoagulation, severe hypoglycemic episodes may result in transient amaurosis.

Retinopathy was evaluated in the clinical studies by means of retinal adverse events reported and fundus photography. The numbers of retinal adverse events reported for LANTUS and human NPH treatment groups were similar for patients with type 1 and type 2 diabetes. Progression of retinopathy was investigated by fundus photography using a grading protocol derived from the Early Treatment Diabetic Retinopathy Study (ETDRS). In one clinical study involving patients with type 2 diabetes, a difference in the number of subjects with ≥3-step progression in ETDRS scale over a 6-month period was noted by fundus photography (7.5% in LANTUS group versus 2.7% in human NPH treated group). The overall relevance of this isolated finding cannot be determined due to the small number of patients involved, the short follow-up period, and the fact that this finding was not observed in other clinical studies.

Type 1 Diabetes in Children and Adolescents: Adverse events, that occurred in a pediatric controlled trial in at least 1% of patients treated with LANTUS are shown in Table 1.

Study 3003: The most commonly reported event was lipodystrophy, a known consequence of insulin injections. The intensity was mostly mild. Injection site events were assessed as possibly related in 9 (5.2%) LANTUS subjects and 5 (2.9%) human NPH subjects however none of these subjects discontinued due to these events.

Study 3013: extension of Study 3003, uncontrolled long-term follow-up study of 143 patients who were well-controlled on LANTUS from 3003, for 201-1159 days. The most common adverse events were upper respiratory infections, infection, and rhinitis. Note that when comparing safety findings between studies, the difference in length of exposure needs to be kept in mind.

Table 1: LANTUS

Adverse Events by Body System ≥1% Reported in Study 3003. (Percent Incidence)

Adverse Event (diagnosis) Body System/Coded Term	Number (%) of Subjects LANTUS n=174	Human NPH n=175
Body as a Whole		
Infection	24 (13.8)	31 (17.7)
Accidental Injury	5 (2.9)	4 (2.3)
Abdominal Pain	2 (1.1)	2 (1.1)
Allergic Reaction	2 (1.1)	- (-)
Flu Syndrome	- (-)	3 (1.7)
Pain in Extremity	2 (1.1)	- (-)
Digestive System		
Gastroenteritis	8 (4.6)	10 (5.7)
Diarrhea	2 (1.1)	2 (1.1)
Sore Throat	2 (1.1)	- (-)
Endocrine System		
Diabetes Mellitus	1 (0.6)	4 (2.3)
Injection Site Reactions		
Injection Site Mass	8 (4.6)	6 (3.4)
Injection Site Reaction	5 (2.9)	6 (3.4)
Injection Site Hemorrhage	2 (1.1)	2 (1.1)
Metabolic and Nutritional Disorders		
Hypoglycemic Reaction[a]	3 (1.7)	7 (4.0)
Hyperglycemia	1 (0.6)	3 (1.7)
Ketosis	1 (0.6)	5 (2.9)
Lipodystrophy	3 (1.7)	2 (1.1)
Musculoskeletal System		
Bone Fracture (not spontaneous)	3 (1.7)	3 (1.7)
Bone Disorder	2 (1.1)	- (-)
Nervous System		
Headache	6 (3.4)	5 (2.9)
Respiratory System		
Upper Respiratory Infection	24 (13.8)	28 (16.0)
Pharyngitis	13 (7.5)	15 (8.6)
Rhinitis	9 (5.2)	9 (5.1)
Bronchitis	6 (3.4)	7 (4.0)
Sinusitis	5 (2.9)	5 (2.9)
Asthma	1 (0.6)	2 (1.1)
Cough Increased	3 (1.7)	- (-)
Skin and Appendages		
Fungal Dermatitis	1 (0.6)	2 (1.1)
Skin Benign Neoplasm	1 (0.6)	2 (1.1)
Eczema	2 (1.1)	1 (0.6)
Herpes Zoster	2 (1.1)	1 (0.6)
Urticaria	2 (1.1)	- (-)

[a] Non-serious hypoglycemia episodes are reported separately.

Study 4005: controlled, randomized, double-cross-over: 26 subjects (age range 12-20), regimen of LANTUS + lispro vs. human NPH + human regular. Adverse events were equally distributed between the two treatment regimens. The most common adverse events were upper respiratory tract infection and gastroenteritis.

Patients in the pediatric clinical trials of LANTUS were treated with a human NPH-based regimen pre-study, and patients assigned to receive human NPH during the study began study treatment on the same human NPH regimen they had taken pre-study. This may have been a factor in the increased incidence of hypoglycemia seen in LANTUS-treated patients during (but not following) initial titration in these trials, as an increase in hypoglycemia may be expected when switching from one insulin to another and titrating the dose of the new insulin.

Post-Market Adverse Drug Reactions: Other: Medication errors have been reported in which other insulins, particularly short-acting insulins, have been accidentally administered instead of LANTUS.

DRUG INTERACTIONS: A number of substances affect glucose metabolism and may require insulin dose adjustment and particularly close monitoring.

Drug-Drug Interactions: Substances that may increase the blood-glucose-lowering effect and susceptibility to hypoglycemia, for example: oral antidiabetic products, ACE inhibitors, disopyramide, fibrates, fluoxetine, MAO inhibitors, pentoxifylline, propoxyphene, salicylates, somatostatin analog (e.g. octreotide), sulfonamide antibiotics.

Substances that may reduce the blood-glucose-lowering effect, for example: corticosteroids, danazol, diazoxide, diuretics, sympathomimetic agents (e.g., epinephrine, salbutamol, terbutaline), glucagon, isoniazid, phenothiazine derivatives, somatropin, thyroid hormones, estrogens, progestogens (e.g., in oral contraceptives), protease inhibitors and atypical antipsychotic medications (e.g., olanzapine and clozapine).

Beta-blockers, clonidine, lithium salts, and alcohol may either potentiate or weaken the blood-glucose-lowering effect of insulin. Pentamidine may cause hypoglycemia, which may sometimes be followed by hyperglycemia. In addition, under the influence of sympatholytic medicinal products such as beta-blockers, clonidine, guanethidine, and reserpine, the signs of hypoglycemia may be reduced or absent.

Drug-Food Interactions: Interactions with food have not been established.

Drug-Herb Interactions: Interactions with herbal products have not been established.

Drug-Laboratory Test Interactions: Interactions with laboratory tests have not been established.

DOSAGE AND ADMINISTRATION: Dosing Considerations: LANTUS [insulin glargine injection (rDNA origin)] is a novel recombinant human insulin analogue. Its potency is approximately the same as human insulin. It exhibits a glucose-lowering profile with no pronounced peak with a prolonged duration of action that permits once-daily basal dosing. LANTUS is administered subcutaneously once a day. It may be administered at any time during the day as long as it is administered at the same time every day.

The desired blood glucose levels as well as the doses and timing of antidiabetic medications must be determined and adjusted individually.

Dose adjustment may be required, for example, if the patient's timing of administration, weight or lifestyle changes or other circumstances arise that increase susceptibility to hypoglycemia or hyperglycemia (see Warnings and Precautions, Hypoglycemia). The dose may also have to be adjusted during intercurrent illness (see Warnings and Precautions, Intercurrent Conditions). Any change in insulin dose should be made under medical supervision.

The prolonged duration of activity of LANTUS is dependent on injection into subcutaneous space. LANTUS is not intended for intravenous or intramuscular administration. Intravenous administration of the usual subcutaneous dose could result in severe hypoglycemia (see Warnings and Precautions).

In cases of insufficient glucose control or a tendency to hyper- or hypoglycemic episodes, patient's compliance with the prescribed insulin regimen, injections sites and proper injection techniques, the handling of injection devices and all other relevant factors must be reviewed before dose adjustment is considered.

Blood glucose monitoring is recommended for all patients with diabetes.

LANTUS must not be used for the treatment of diabetic ketoacidosis. Intravenous short-acting insulin should be the preferred treatment.

Recommended Dose and Dosage Adjustment: Initiation of LANTUS therapy: In clinical studies with insulin naive patients with type 2 diabetes LANTUS was started at a dose of 10 U once daily, and subsequently adjusted according to the patient's needs.

Changeover to LANTUS: When changing from a treatment regimen with an intermediate or long-acting insulin to a regimen with LANTUS, the amount and timing of short-acting insulin or fast-acting insulin analogue or the dose of any oral antidiabetic drug may need to be adjusted secondary to the risk of hypoglycemia. In clinical studies when patients were transferred from once-daily NPH human insulin or ultralente human insulin to once-daily LANTUS, the initial dose was usually not changed.

However, in studies when patients were transferred from twice-daily NPH human insulin to LANTUS once daily, the initial dose (U) was usually reduced by approximately 20% (compared to total daily IU of NPH human insulin) and then adjusted based on patient response.

A program of close metabolic monitoring under medical supervision is recommended during transfer and in the initial weeks thereafter. The amount and timing of short-acting insulin or fast-acting insulin analogue may need to be adjusted. This is particularly true for patients with acquired antibodies to human insulin needing high-insulin doses and occurs with all insulin analogues. Such patients may experience a greater insulin response to LANTUS.

With improved metabolic control and resulting increase in insulin sensitivity, adjustment of the dose(s) of antidiabetic treatments may become necessary.

Administration: LANTUS is administered by subcutaneous injection. The injection area must not be rubbed.

As with all insulins, injection sites within an injection area (abdomen, thigh or deltoid) must be alternated from one injection to the next. Patients should be rigorous with site rotation secondary to prolonged deposition. In clinical studies, there was no relevant difference in insulin glargine absorption after abdominal, deltoid, or thigh subcutaneous administration. As for all insulins, the rate of absorption, and consequently the onset and duration of action, may be affected by exercise and other variables.

Preparation and Handling: LANTUS is a clear solution, not a suspension.

Parenteral drug products should be inspected visually prior to administration whenever the solution and the container permit. LANTUS must only be used if the solution is clear and colorless with no particles visible. To minimize local irritation at the injection site, it is recommended to allow the insulin to reach room temperature before injection.

Cartridge version only: If the injection pen malfunctions, LANTUS may be drawn from the cartridge into a U 100 syringe and injected. **A new sterile syringe must be used.**

Mixing and Diluting: LANTUS must not be mixed with any other insulin. Mixing can change the time/action profile of LANTUS and cause precipitation.

LANTUS must not be diluted. Diluting can change the time/action profile of LANTUS.

OVERDOSAGE:

Symptoms: An excess of insulin relative to food intake, energy expenditure or both may lead to severe and sometimes prolonged and life-threatening hypoglycemia (see Warnings and Precautions).

Management: Mild episodes of hypoglycemia can usually be treated with oral carbohydrates. Adjustments in drug dosage, meal patterns, or exercise may be needed.

More severe episodes with coma, seizure, or neurologic impairment may be treated with intramuscular/subcutaneous glucagon or concentrated intravenous glucose.

After apparent clinical recovery from hypoglycemia, continued observation and additional carbohydrate intake may be necessary to avoid reoccurrence of hypoglycemia.

> For management of a suspected drug overdose, contact your regional Poison Control Centre. See the *CPS* Directory section for a list of Poison Control Centres.

ACTION AND CLINICAL PHARMACOLOGY: Pharmacodynamics: The primary activity of insulin, including insulin glargine, is regulation of glucose metabolism. Insulin and its analogues lower blood glucose levels by stimulating peripheral glucose uptake, especially by skeletal muscle and fat, and by inhibiting hepatic glucose production. Insulin inhibits lipolysis in the adipocyte, inhibits proteolysis, and enhances protein synthesis.

Insulin glargine is a human insulin analogue designed to have low solubility at neutral pH. At pH 4, as in the LANTUS injection solution, it is completely soluble. After injection into the subcutaneous tissue, the acidic solution is neutralized, leading to formation of microprecipitates from which small amounts of insulin glargine are slowly released, resulting in a relatively constant concentration/time profile over 24 hours with no pronounced peak. This allows once-daily dosing to meet a patient's basal insulin needs.

Insulin glargine and human insulin have been shown to be equipotent in glucose-lowering effect on a molar basis (when administered intravenously at the same doses). In euglycemic clamp studies in healthy subjects or in patients with type 1 diabetes, the onset of action of subcutaneous insulin glargine was slower than NPH human insulin. The effect profile of insulin glargine was relatively constant with no pronounced peak, and the duration of its effect was prolonged compared to NPH human insulin.

Figure 1 shows results from a study in patients with type 1 diabetes conducted for a maximum of 24 hours after the injection. The median time between injection and the end of pharmacological effect was 14.5 hours (range: 9.5 to 19.3 hours) for NPH human insulin, and 24 hours (range: 10.8 to >24.0 hours) (24 hours was the end of the observation period) for insulin glargine.

Pharmacokinetics: Absorption and Bioavailability: After subcutaneous injection of insulin glargine in healthy subjects, and patients with diabetes, the insulin serum concentrations indicated a slower, more prolonged absorption and a relatively constant concentration/time profile over 24 hours with no pronounced peak in comparison to NPH human insulin. Serum insulin concentrations were thus consistent with the time profile of the pharmacodynamic activity of insulin glargine.

Figure 1: LANTUS
Activity Profile in Patients with Type 1 Diabetes

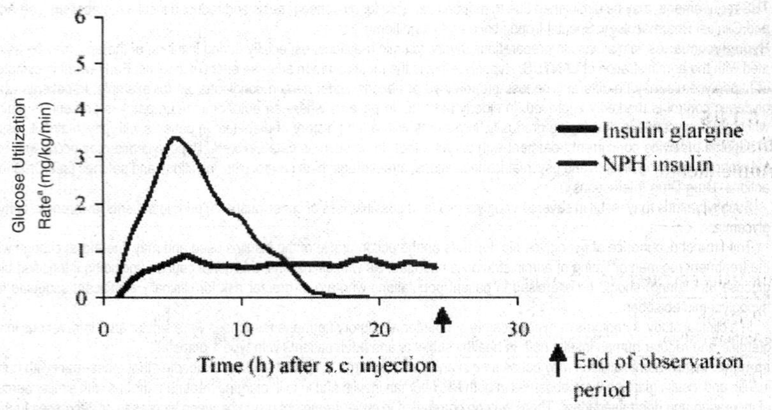

[a] Determined as amount of glucose infused to maintain constant plasma glucose levels (hourly mean values). Indicative of insulin activity. Between-patient variability (CV, coefficient of variation), insulin glargine, 84% and human NPH, 78%.

After subcutaneous injection of 0.3 U/kg insulin glargine in patients with type 1 diabetes, a relatively constant concentration-time profile has been demonstrated. The duration of action after abdominal, deltoid, or thigh subcutaneous administration was similar.

Metabolism: A metabolism study in man indicates that insulin glargine is partly metabolized at the carboxyl terminus of the B chain in the subcutaneous depot to form two active metabolites with similar in vitro activity to insulin, M1 (21^A-Gly-insulin) and M2 (21^A-Gly-des-30^B-Thr-insulin). Unchanged drug and degradation products are also present in the circulation.

Special Populations and Conditions: Age, Race, and Gender: Information on the effect of age, race, and gender on the pharmacokinetics of LANTUS is unavailable. However, in controlled clinical trials in adults (n=3890, Studies 3001, 3002, 3004, 3005, and 3006), and a controlled clinical trial in pediatric patients (n=349, Study 3003) subgroup analyses based on age, race (white, black, Asian/oriental, multiracial and Hispanic) and gender did not show differences in safety and efficacy between insulin glargine and NPH human insulin.

Hepatic Insufficiency: No studies were performed in patients with hepatic insufficiency. However, some studies with human insulin have shown increased circulating levels of insulin in patients with liver failure. Careful glucose monitoring and dose adjustments of insulin or insulin analogues including LANTUS may be necessary in patients with hepatic dysfunction (see Warnings and Precautions, Hepatic/Biliary/Pancreas).

Renal Insufficiency: No studies were performed in patients with renal insufficiency. However, some studies with human insulin have shown increased circulating levels of insulin in patients with renal failure. Careful glucose monitoring and dose adjustments of insulin or insulin analogues including LANTUS may be necessary in patients with renal dysfunction (see Warnings and Precautions, Renal).

Pregnancy: The effect of pregnancy on the pharmacokinetics and pharmacodynamics of LANTUS has not been studied (see Warnings and Precautions, Special Populations).

Obesity: In controlled clinical trials, which included patients with Body Mass Index (BMI) up to and including 49.6 kg/m², subgroup analyses based on BMI did not show any differences in safety and efficacy between insulin glargine and NPH human insulin.

Smoking: Information on the effect of smoking on the pharmacokinetics of LANTUS is unavailable.

Duration of Effect: The longer duration of action (up to 24 hours) of LANTUS is directly related to its slower rate of absorption and supports once-daily subcutaneous administration. The time course of action of insulins including LANTUS may vary between individuals and/or within the same individual. The doses and timing of antidiabetic medications must be determined and adjusted individually, to achieve the desired blood glucose levels.

STORAGE AND STABILITY: Vials: Unopened Vial: Unopened LANTUS vials should be stored in a refrigerator, between 2-8°C. Keep LANTUS away from direct heat and light. LANTUS should not be stored in the freezer and should not be allowed to freeze. If LANTUS freezes or overheats, discard it.

Opened (in use) Vial: The opened vial can be kept refrigerated or unrefrigerated (15-30°C) for up to 28 days away from direct heat and light, as long as the temperature is not greater than 30°C. Opened LANTUS vials, whether or not refrigerated, must be discarded after 28 days even if they contain insulin.

Opened LANTUS vials should not be stored in the freezer and should not be allowed to freeze. If a vial freezes or overheats, discard it.

Cartridges: Unopened Cartridge: Unopened LANTUS cartridges should be stored in a refrigerator, between 2-8°C. Keep LANTUS away from direct heat and light. LANTUS should not be stored in the freezer and should not be allowed to freeze. If LANTUS freezes or overheats, discard it.

Opened (in use) Cartridge: The opened cartridge in use must be kept unrefrigerated (15-30°C) for up to 28 days away from direct heat and light, as long as the temperature is not greater than 30°C. If the cartridge overheats or if there is any remaining insulin after 28 days, discard it. The opened cartridge in use must never be removed from and reinserted into the injection pen.

SoloSTAR: Unopened SoloSTAR: Unopened LANTUS SoloSTAR should be stored in a refrigerator, between 2-8°C. Keep LANTUS away from direct heat and light. LANTUS SoloSTAR should not be stored in the freezer and should not be allowed to freeze. If LANTUS SoloSTAR freezes or overheats, discard it.

Opened (In Use) SoloSTAR: Opened LANTUS SoloSTAR in use must be kept unrefrigerated (15-30°C) for up to 28 days away from direct heat and light, as long as the temperature is not greater than 30°C. If the LANTUS SoloSTAR overheats or if there is any remaining insulin after 28 days, discard it.

Opened LANTUS SoloSTAR should not be stored in the freezer and should not be allowed to freeze. If LANTUS SoloSTAR freezes, discard it.

As with all medications and devices, keep out of reach of children.

SPECIAL HANDLING INSTRUCTIONS: Information to Be Provided to the Patient: LANTUS must only be used if the solution is clear and colorless with no particles visible (see Dosage and Administration, Administration). LANTUS is a clear solution, not a suspension. LANTUS can be confused with other insulin types, since it visually resembles short-acting insulins and its name resembles the "Lente" brand of insulins. It is not necessary to shake or rotate the vial/cartridge/SoloSTAR before use. Patients must be advised that LANTUS must not be mixed with any other insulin or diluted with any other solution (see Warnings and Precautions, General).

Patients should be instructed on self-management procedures including glucose monitoring, proper injection technique, and hypoglycemia and hyperglycemia management. Patients must be instructed on handling of special situations such as intercurrent conditions (illness, stress, or emotional disturbances), an inadequate or skipped insulin dose, inadvertent administration of an increased insulin dose, inadequate food intake or skipped meals. The extent of patient participation in his/her diabetes management is variable and is generally determined by the physician.

Insulin treatment requires constant alertness to the possibility of hyper- and hypoglycemia. Patients and their relatives must know what steps to take if hyperglycemia or hypoglycemia occurs or is suspected, and they must know when to inform a physician.

Patients with diabetes should be advised to inform their doctor if they are pregnant or are contemplating pregnancy.

As with all patients who have diabetes, the ability to concentrate and/or react may be impaired as a result of hypoglycemia or hyperglycemia. Patients should be advised to take precautions to avoid hypoglycemia while driving. This is particularly important in those who have reduced or absent awareness of the warning symptoms of hypoglycemia or have frequent episodes of hypoglycemia. The advisability of driving should be considered in these circumstances.

See also Information for the Patient and refer patients to the LANTUS Information for the Patient circular for LANTUS Vials, LANTUS Cartridge, and LANTUS SoloSTAR for additional information. Refer patients to the User Manual for sanofi-aventis insulin injection pens or injection pens suitable for LANTUS cartridges **as recommended in the information provided by the injection pen manufacturer**, and User Manual for the LANTUS SoloSTAR, for additional information on use of the pens.

INFORMATION FOR THE PATIENT: Published in e-CPS, available by subscription at www.e-cps.ca.

DOSAGE FORMS, COMPOSITION AND PACKAGING: The vials, cartridges and SoloSTAR contain a sterile solution of insulin glargine for use as an injection. LANTUS (insulin glargine injection (rDNA origin)) consists of insulin glargine dissolved in a clear aqueous fluid. Each mL contains: insulin glargine 100 units. Nonmedicinal ingredients: glycerol, m-cresol, polysorbate 20 (10 mL vial only), water for injection and zinc. LANTUS has a pH of approximately 4. The pH is adjusted by addition of aqueous solutions of hydrochloric acid and sodium hydroxide. Vials of 10 mL. Cartridges of 3 mL, packages of 5, for use with sanofi-aventis insulin injection pens or injection pens suitable for LANTUS cartridges as recommended in the information provided by the injection pen manufacturer only. SoloSTAR (pre-filled disposable pen) of 3 mL, package of 5.

Lanvis® Pr
thioguanine
Antileukemic

GlaxoSmithKline

Date of Revision: June 27, 2006

SUMMARY PRODUCT INFORMATION:

Route of Administration	Dosage Form/Strength	Clinically Relevant Nonmedicinal Ingredients
Oral	Tablet/40 mg	gum acacia, lactose, magnesium stearate, potato starch, and stearic acid.

INDICATIONS AND CLINICAL USE:
- LANVIS (thioguanine) is indicated for treatment of acute leukemia.
- LANVIS has also been used in chronic granulocytic (myelocytic, myeloid, myelogenous) leukemia.

CONTRAINDICATIONS:
- Patients who are hypersensitive to this drug or to any ingredient in the formulation or component of the container. For a complete listing, see Summary Product Information, or Dosage Forms, Composition and Packaging. LANVIS (thioguanine) should not be given to patients who experienced a previous hypersensitivity reaction to the drug or any of its components.
- LANVIS should not be used in patients whose disease has demonstrated prior resistance to this drug. In animals and man, there is usually complete cross-resistance between mercaptopurine and thioguanine.

WARNINGS AND PRECAUTIONS: General: LANVIS (thioguanine) is a potent drug and should be used only by physicians experienced with cancer chemotherapeutic drugs. Blood counts should be taken weekly. Discontinue or reduce the dosage immediately at the first sign of abnormal depression of the bone marrow.

Thioguanine is not recommended for maintenance therapy or similar long term continuous treatments due to the high risk of liver toxicity associated with vascular endothelial damage (see Warnings and Precautions, Hepatic/Biliary/Pancreatic).

Carcinogenesis, Mutagenesis and Impairment of Fertility: In view of its action on cellular DNA, thioguanine is potentially mutagenic and carcinogenic, and consideration should be given to the theoretical risk of carcinogenesis when thioguanine is administered (see Warnings and Precautions, Special Populations, Pregnant Women).

Hematologic: The most consistent, dose-related toxicity is bone marrow suppression. This may be manifested by anemia, leukopenia, thrombocytopenia, or any combination of these. Any one of these findings may also reflect progression of the underlying disease. Since thioguanine may have a delayed effect, it is important to withdraw the medication temporarily at the first sign of an abnormally large decrease in any of the formed elements of the blood. Blood counts should be made at least once weekly. Life-threatening infections and bleeding have been observed as consequences of thioguanine-induced granulocytopenia and thrombocytopenia.

It is recommended that evaluation of the hemoglobin concentration or hematocrit, total white blood cell count and differential count, and quantitative platelet count be obtained frequently while the patient is on thioguanine therapy. In cases where the cause of fluctuations in the formed elements in the peripheral blood is obscure, bone marrow examination may be useful for the evaluation of marrow status. The decision to increase, decrease, continue, or discontinue a given dosage of thioguanine must be based not only on the absolute hematologic values, but also upon the rapidity with which changes are occurring. In many instances, particularly during the induction phase of acute leukemia, complete blood counts will need to be done more frequently in order to evaluate the effect of the therapy. The dosage of thioguanine may need to be reduced when this agent is combined with other drugs whose primary toxicity is myelosuppression.

There are individuals with an inherited deficiency of the enzyme thiopurine methyltransferase (TPMT) who may be unusually sensitive to the myelosuppressive effect of thioguanine and prone to developing rapid bone marrow depression following the initiation of treatment with LANVIS. This problem could be exacerbated by coadministration with drugs that inhibit TPMT, such as olsalazine, mesalazine or sulphasalazine. Some laboratories offer testing for TPMT deficiency, although these tests have not been shown to identify all patients at risk of severe toxicity. Therefore, close monitoring of blood counts is still necessary.

Hepatic/Biliary/Pancreatic: Thioguanine is not recommended for maintenance therapy or similar long term continuous treatments due to the high risk of liver toxicity associated with vascular endothelial damage (see Dosage and Administration and Adverse Reactions). This liver toxicity has been observed in a high proportion of children receiving thioguanine as part of maintenance therapy for acute lymphoblastic leukemia and in other conditions associated with continuous use of thioguanine. This liver toxicity is particularly prevalent in males. Liver toxicity usually presents as the clinical syndrome of veno-occlusive disease (hyperbilirubinaemia, tender hepatomegaly, weight gain due to fluid retention and ascites) or with signs of portal hypertension (splenomegaly, thrombocytopenia and oesophageal varices). Histopathological features associated with this toxicity include hepatoportal sclerosis, nodular regenerative hyperplasia, peliosis hepatis and periportal fibrosis.

Thioguanine therapy should be discontinued in patients with evidence of liver toxicity as reversal of signs and symptoms of liver toxicity have been reported upon withdrawal.

Patients must be carefully monitored (see Warnings and Precautions, Monitoring and Laboratory Tests). Early indications of liver toxicity are signs associated with portal hypertension such as thrombocytopenia out of proportion with neutropenia and splenomegaly. Elevations of liver enzymes have also been reported in association with liver toxicity but do not always occur.

A few cases of jaundice have been reported in patients with leukemia who received thioguanine. Among these were two adult male patients and four children with acute myelogenous leukemia, and an adult male with acute lymphocytic leukemia who developed hepatic veno-occlusive disease while receiving chemotherapy for their leukemia. Six patients had received cytarabine prior to treatment with thioguanine, and some were receiving other chemotherapy in addition to thioguanine when they became symptomatic. While hepatic veno-occlusive disease has not been reported in patients treated with thioguanine alone, it is recommended that thioguanine be withheld if there is evidence of toxic hepatitis or biliary stasis, and that appropriate clinical and laboratory investigations be initiated to establish the etiology of the hepatic dysfunction. Deterioration in liver function studies during thioguanine therapy should prompt discontinuation of treatment and a search for an explanation of the hepatotoxicity.

During remission induction particularly, when rapid cell lyis is occurring, adequate precautions should be taken to avoid hyperuricemia and/or hyperuricosuria and the risk of uric acid nephropathy.

Consideration should be given to reducing the dosage in patients with impaired hepatic function.

Immune: Immunisation using a live organism vaccine has the potential to cause infection in immunocompromised hosts. Therefore, immunisation with live organism vaccines (e.g. measles, mumps, etc.) are not recommended.

The effect of thioguanine on the immunocompetence of patients is unknown.

Renal: Consideration should be given to reducing the dosage in patients with impaired renal function.

Sensitivity/Resistance: Since the enzyme hypoxanthine guanine phosphoribosyltransferase is responsible for the conversion of thioguanine to its active metabolite, it is possible that patients deficient in this enzyme, such as those suffering from Lesch-Nyhan syndrome, may be resistant to thioguanine.

Special Populations: Pregnant Women: Thioguanine has been shown to be teratogenic in rats when given in doses 5 times the human dose. When given to the rat on the 4th and 5th days of gestation, 13% of surviving placentas did not contain fetuses, and 19% of offspring were malformed or stunted. The malformations noted included generalized edema, cranial defects, and general skeletal hypoplasia, hydrocephalus, ventral hernia, situs inversus, and incomplete development of the limbs.

There are no adequate and well-controlled studies in pregnant women. Drugs of this type have potential teratogenic activity and the benefits and risks must be weighed before use during pregnancy. If this drug is used during pregnancy, or if the patient becomes pregnant while taking the drug, the patient should be apprised of the hazard to the fetus. Whenever possible, use of the drug should be deferred until after the first trimester of pregnancy.

As with all cytotoxic chemotherapy, adequate contraceptive precautions should be advised when either partner is receiving thioguanine. Women of childbearing potential should be advised to avoid becoming pregnant.

Nursing Women: It is not known whether thioguanine is excreted in human milk. Because of the potential for tumorigenicity shown for thioguanine, a decision should be made whether to discontinue nursing or to discontinue the drug, taking into account the importance of the drug to the mother.

Geriatrics: Clinical studies of thioguanine did not include sufficient numbers of subjects aged 65 and over to determine whether they respond differently from younger subjects. Other reported clinical experience has not identified differences in responses between the elderly and younger patients. In general, dose selection for an elderly patient should be cautious, usually starting at the low end of the dosing range, reflecting the greater frequency of decreased hepatic, renal, or cardiac function, and of concomitant disease or other drug therapy.

Monitoring and Laboratory Tests: It is advisable to monitor liver function tests (serum transaminases, alkaline phosphatase, bilirubin) at weekly intervals when first beginning therapy and at monthly intervals thereafter. It may be advisable to perform liver function tests more frequently in patients with known pre-existing liver disease or in patients who are receiving thioguanine with other hepatotoxic drugs. Patients should be instructed to discontinue thioguanine immediately if clinical jaundice is detected (see Warnings and Precautions, Hepatic/Biliary/Pancreatic).

ADVERSE REACTIONS: Adverse Drug Reaction Overview: Gastrointestinal: Less frequent adverse reactions include nausea, vomiting, anorexia, and stomatitis. Intestinal necrosis and perforation have been reported in patients who received multiple drug chemotherapy including thioguanine. Esophageal varices have been reported in patients receiving continuous busulfan and thioguanine therapy for treatment of chronic myelogenous leukemia (see Drug Interactions).

While on the whole no significant clinical difference between thioguanine and mercaptopurine has been noted with respect to action or side effects, it has been observed that occasionally patients may experience better gastrointestinal tolerance to one or another drug of this type.

Hematologic: The most frequent adverse reaction to thioguanine is myelosuppression. The induction of complete remission of acute myelogenous leukemia usually requires combination chemotherapy in dosages which produce marrow hypoplasia. Since consolidation and maintenance of remission are also affected by multiple drug regimens whose component agents cause myelosuppression, pancytopenia is observed in nearly all patients. Dosages and schedules must be adjusted to prevent life-threatening cytopenias whenever these adverse reactions are observed.

Hyperuricemia frequently occurs in patients receiving thioguanine as a consequence of rapid cell lysis accompanying the antineoplastic effect. Adverse effects can be minimized by increased hydration, urine alkalinization, and the prophylactic administration of a xanthine oxidase inhibitor such as ZYLOPRIM (allopurinol). Unlike PURINETHOL (mercaptopurine) and IMURAN (azathioprine), thioguanine may be continued in the usual dosage when allopurinol is used conjointly to inhibit uric acid formation.

Hepatic: Liver toxicity associated with vascular endothelial damage has been reported when thioguanine is used in maintenance or similar long term continuous therapy which is not recommended (see Dosage and Administration, Warnings and Precautions). This usually presents as the clinical syndrome of hepatic veno-occlusive disease (hyperbilirubinaemia, tender hepatomegaly, weight gain due to fluid retention and ascites) or signs and symptoms of portal hypertension (splenomegaly, thrombocytopenia and oesophageal varices). Elevation of liver transaminases, alkaline phosphatase and gamma glutamyl transferase and jaundice may also occur.

Histopathological features associated with this toxicity include hepatoportal sclerosis, nodular regenerative hyperplasia, peliosis hepatis and periportal fibrosis.

Liver toxicity during short term cyclical therapy presents as veno-occlusive disease. Reversal of signs and symptoms of this liver toxicity has been reported upon withdrawal of short term or long term continuous therapy.

Centrilobular hepatic necrosis has been reported in a few cases; however, the reports are confounded by the use of high doses of thioguanine, other chemotherapeutic agents, oral contraceptives and chronic alcohol abuse.

DRUG INTERACTIONS: Drug-Drug Interactions: See Table 1.

Table 1: LANVIS

Established or Potential Drug-Drug Interactions

Thioguanine	Effect	Clinical comment
Mercaptopurine	Complete cross resistance	Between PURINETHOL (mercaptopurine) and LANVIS.
Busulfan (MYLERAN)	Esophageal varices Liver toxicity	In one study, 12 of approximately 330 patients receiving continuous busulfan and thioguanine therapy for treatment of chronic myelogenous leukemia were found to have esophageal varices associated with abnormal liver function tests. Subsequent liver biopsies were performed in four of these patients, all of which showed evidence of nodular regenerative hyperplasia. Duration of combination therapy prior to the appearance of esophageal varices ranged from 6 to 45 months. With the present analysis of the data, no cases of hepatotoxicity have appeared in the busulfan alone arm of the study.
Aminosalicylate derivatives [(e.g. olsalazine, mesalazine or sulphasalazine)]	Inhibit Thiopurine methyltransferase (TPMT)	Based on in vitro evidence aminosalicylate derivatives should be administered with caution to patients receiving concurrent thioguanine therapy (See Warnings and Precautions).
Live viral vaccines	Potential to cause infection in immunocompromised hosts.	Vaccinations with live organism vaccines are not recommended in immunocompromised individuals (see Warnings and Precautions).

DOSAGE AND ADMINISTRATION: LANVIS (thioguanine) is a potent drug and should be used only by physicians experienced with cancer chemotherapeutic drugs. Blood counts should be taken weekly. Discontinue or reduce the dosage immediately at the first sign of abnormal depression of the bone marrow.

Dosing Considerations: Thioguanine can be used for remission induction and remission consolidation. However, it is not recommended for use during maintenance therapy or similar long term continuous treatments due to the high risk of liver toxicity (see Warnings and Precautions and Adverse Reactions). Unlike mercaptopurine and azathioprine, thioguanine may be continued in the usual dosage when allopurinol is used conjointly to inhibit uric acid formation.

Recommended Dose and Dosage Adjustment: The dosage of thioguanine must be carefully adjusted for each patient to obtain optimum benefit without toxic effects. The usual initial dose is approximately 2 mg/kg body weight/day, orally. If after four weeks on this dosage there is no clinical improvement and no leukocyte depression, the dosage may be cautiously increased to 3 mg/kg/day.

The total daily dose may be given at one time. It is usually calculated to the closest multiple of 20 mg. Although the effect usually occurs slowly over a period of two to four weeks, occasionally there may be a rapid fall in leukocyte count within one or two weeks. This may occur in some adults with acute leukemia and high total leukocyte counts as well as in certain adults with chronic granulocytic leukemia. For this reason it is important to observe such patients closely.

OVERDOSAGE:

Signs and symptoms of overdosage may be immediate, such as nausea, vomiting, malaise, hypertension, and diaphoresis; or delayed, such as myelosuppression and azotemia. It is not known whether thioguanine is dialyzable. Hemodialysis is thought to be of marginal use due to the rapid metabolism of thioguanine into active intracellular derivatives with longer persistence than the parent drug.

There is no known pharmacologic antagonist of thioguanine. The drug should be discontinued immediately if unintended toxicity occurs during treatment. Severe hematologic toxicity may require supportive therapy with platelet transfusions for bleeding, and granulocyte transfusions and antibiotics if sepsis is documented. If a patient is seen immediately following an accidental overdosage of the drug, it may be useful to induce emesis.

For management of a suspected drug overdose, CPhA recommends that you contact your **regional Poison Control Centre**. See the *CPS* Directory section for a list of Poison Control Centres.

ACTION AND CLINICAL PHARMACOLOGY: Mechanism of Action: Thioguanine is a close relative of mercaptopurine and like the latter is an antimetabolite which blocks purine metabolism. Studies by Philips et al. have shown that unlike certain other purine antagonists, thioguanine does not produce substantial pathological changes in the intestinal epithelium of rodents and dogs, in the thoracic organs of rats or in the liver of animals studied. Direct radiation-like damage to lymphoid tissues does not occur. Pathologic changes are virtually limited to bone marrow and consist of neutropenia, reticulopenia, anemia, thrombopenia and prolongation of clotting time. The protracted but reversible aplasia of bone marrow closely resembles the effects of ionizing radiations. In man, thioguanine is extensively converted to 2-amino-6-methyl-mercaptopurine which is much less toxic and less effective than the parent compound. Unlike mercaptopurine and azathioprine, its metabolism is not inhibited by the xanthine oxidase inhibitor, allopurinol.

Thioguanine has multiple metabolic effects and at present it is not possible to designate one major site of action. Its tumor inhibitory properties may be due to one or more of its effects on (a) feedback inhibition of de novo purine synthesis; (b) inhibition of purine nucleotide interconversions; or (c) incorporation into the DNA and the RNA. The net consequence of its actions is a sequential blockade of the synthesis and utilization of the purine nucleotides.

Pharmacodynamics: Thioguanine is incorporated into the DNA and the RNA of human bone marrow cells. Studies with intravenous ^{35}S-6-thioguanine have shown that the amount of thioguanine incorporated into nucleic acids is more than 100 times higher after five daily doses than after a single dose. With the 5-dose schedule, from one-half to virtually all of the guanine in the residual DNA was replaced by thioguanine. Tissue distribution studies of ^{35}S-6-thioguanine in mice showed only traces of radioactivity in the brain after oral administration. Thioguanine concentrations in human cerebrospinal fluid (CSF) have not been measured, but observations on tissue distribution in animals, together with the lack of CNS penetration by the closely related compound, mercaptopurine, suggest that thioguanine does not reach therapeutic concentrations in the CSF.

Thioguanine is extensively metabolized in vivo. There are two principal catabolic routes: methylation to 2-amino-6-methylthiopurine and deamination to 2-hydroxy-6-mercaptopurine, followed by oxidation to 6-thiouric acid. Deamination and subsequent oxidation to thiouric acid occurs only to a small extent. The product of deamination by guanase, 6-thioxanthine is inactive, having negligible antitumor activity. This pathway of thioguanine inactivation is not dependent on the action of xanthine oxidase, and an inhibitor of that enzyme (such as allopurinol) will not block the detoxification of thioguanine even though the inactive 6-thioxanthine is normally further oxidized by xanthine oxidase to thiouric acid before it is eliminated. The product of methylation, 2-amino-6-methylthiopurine, is also substantially less active and less toxic than thioguanine, and its formation is likewise unaffected by the presence of allopurinol. Appreciable amounts of inorganic sulfate are also found in the urine, presumably arising from further metabolism of the methylated derivatives.

Monitoring of plasma levels of thioguanine during therapy is of questionable value. There is technical difficulty in determining plasma concentrations, which are seldom greater than 1 to 2 μg/mL after a therapeutic oral dose. More significantly, thioguanine enters rapidly into the anabolic and catabolic pathways for purines, and the active intracellular metabolites have appreciably longer half-lives than the parent drug. The biochemical effects of a single dose of thioguanine are evident long after the parent drug has disappeared from the plasma. Because of this rapid metabolism of thioguanine to active intracellular derivatives, hemodialysis would not be expected to appreciably reduce toxicity of the drug.

In some animal tumors, resistance to the effect of thioguanine correlates with the loss of HGPRTase activity and the resulting inability to convert thioguanine to thioguanylic acid. However, other resistance mechanisms, such as increased catabolism of TGMP by a nonspecific phosphatase, may be operative. Although not invariable, it is usual to find cross-resistance between thioguanine and its close analogue, PURINETHOL (mercaptopurine).

Pharmacokinetics: Clinical studies have shown that the absorption of an oral dose of thioguanine in man is incomplete and variable, averaging approximately 30% of the administered dose (range: 14% to 46%). Following oral administration of ^{35}S-6-thioguanine, total plasma radioactivity reached a maximum at eight hours and declined slowly thereafter. The parent drug represented only a very small fraction of the total plasma radioactivity at any time, being virtually undetectable throughout the period of measurements.

The oral administration of radiolabeled thioguanine revealed only trace quantities of parent drug in the urine. However, the methylated metabolite, 2-amino-6-methylthiopurine (MTG), appeared very early, rose to a maximum six to eight hours after drug administration, and was still being excreted after 12 to 22 hours. Radiolabeled sulfate appeared somewhat later than MTG but was the principal metabolite after eight hours. Thiouric acid and some unidentified products were found in the urine in small amounts.

Plasma levels decay biexponentially with initial and terminal half-lives of 3 and 5-9 hours respectively.

There are individuals with an inherited deficiency of the enzyme thiopurine methyltransferase (TPMT) who may be unusually sensitive to the myelosuppressive effect of thioguanine. (see Warnings and Precautions, Hematologic).

STORAGE AND STABILITY: LANVIS (thioguanine) tablets should be stored between 15 and 25°C, in a dry place, protected from light.

SPECIAL HANDLING INSTRUCTIONS: Care should be taken when handling or halving the tablets so as not to contaminate hands or to inhale the drug.

Tablets should be returned to the manufacturer for destruction. Proper precautions should be taken in packaging these materials for transport. All materials which have come in contact with cytotoxic drugs should be segregated and incinerated at 1000°C or more.

Personnel regularly involved in the preparation and handling of cytotoxic agents should have bi-annual blood examinations.

INFORMATION FOR THE PATIENT: Published in e-CPS, available by subscription at www.e-cps.ca.

DOSAGE FORMS, COMPOSITION AND PACKAGING: Each pale, greenish-yellow, biconvex tablet, plain on one side and scored on the other side, with "Wellcome" on the upper half and "U3B" on the lower half, contains: thioguanine 40 mg. Nonmedicinal ingredients: gum acacia, lactose, magnesium stearate, potato starch and stearic acid. Bottles of 25.

(Shown in Product Identification Section)

Lariam® Pr

mefloquine HCl

Antimalarial

Roche

SUPPLIED: Each cross-scored (both sides), white, cylindrical, biplane tablet with bevelled edges imprinted ROCHE with hexagon on one side, contains: mefloquine base 250 mg as mefloquine HCl. Nonmedicinal ingredients: ammonium-calcium alginate, cornstarch, crospovidone, lactose, magnesium stearate, microcrystalline cellulose, poloxamer and talc. Blister packs of 8. Store at 15 to 30°C. The tablets are sensitive to moisture and should remain in their blister until consumed.

Lasix® Pr

furosemide

Diuretic

sanofi-aventis

Date of Revision: August 27, 2010

SUMMARY PRODUCT INFORMATION:

Route of Administration	Dosage Form/Strength	Nonmedicinal Ingredients
Oral	Tablet 20 mg, 40 mg	20 mg: Colloidal silicon dioxide, lactose monohydrate, magnesium stearate, starch and talc. 40 mg: Colloidal silicon dioxide, D&C Yellow #10, FD&C Yellow #6, lactose monohydrate, magnesium stearate, starch and talc.
Oral	Solution 10 mg/mL	Alcohol, butylated hydroxyanisol, butylated hydroxytoluene, glycerine, methylparaben, natural orange flavour, polysorbate 80 non-animal, potassium sorbate, purified water, sodium hydroxide and sorbitol.

INDICATIONS AND CLINICAL USE: LASIX (furosemide) is indicated for:

- The treatment of edema associated with congestive heart failure, cirrhosis of the liver and renal disease including, nephrotic syndrome, as well as other edematous states amenable to diuretic therapy.
- Can also be used alone, in the control of mild to moderate hypertension, or in combination with other antihypertensive agents in more severe cases.

Hypertensive patients who cannot be adequately controlled with thiazides will probably also not be adequately controllable with LASIX alone.

Geriatrics (>61 years of age): Use in the geriatric population is associated with differences in safety (see Warnings and Precautions).

Pediatrics: When administered to children, LASIX therapy should be instituted in the hospital, in carefully selected patients, under close observation with frequent monitoring of serum electrolytes. (See Dosage and Administration.)

The available pediatric data does not allow for a recommendation of a specific age range in this population.

CONTRAINDICATIONS: LASIX (furosemide) is contraindicated in:

- Patients who are hypersensitive to furosemide, sulfonamide-derived drugs or to any ingredient in the formulation or component of the container. For a complete listing, see Dosage Forms, Composition and Packaging. Patients allergic to sulfonamides (e.g. sulfonamide antibiotics or sulfonylureas) may show cross-sensitivity to furosemide.
- Patients with complete renal shutdown. If increasing azotemia and oliguria occur during treatment of severe progressive renal disease, the drug should be discontinued.
- Patients with hepatic coma and precoma or in states of electrolyte depletion until the basic condition is improved or corrected. Therapy with LASIX should not be initiated in these patients (see Warnings and Precautions, Hepatic/Biliary/Pancreatic).
- Severe hyponatremia, hypokalemia, hypovolemia, dehydration or hypotension must be regarded as contraindications until serum electrolytes and fluid balance and blood pressure have been restored to normal levels. (See Warnings and Precautions and Adverse Reactions.)
- As furosemide may be capable of displacing bilirubin from albumin at least "in vitro", it should not be administered to jaundiced newborn infants or to infants suffering from diseases (e.g. Rh incompatibility, familial non-hemolytic jaundice, etc.) with the potential of causing hyperbilirubinemia and possibly kernicterus.
- Women must not breast-feed if they are treated with furosemide (see Warnings and Precautions).

WARNINGS AND PRECAUTIONS: General: LASIX (furosemide) is a potent diuretic which if given in excessive amounts can lead to a profound diuresis with water and electrolyte depletion. Therefore, careful medical supervision is required, and dose and dose schedule have to be adjusted to the individual patient's needs (see Dosage and Administration).

All patients receiving LASIX therapy should be observed for signs and symptoms of fluid or electrolyte imbalance, hyponatremia, hypochloremic alkalosis, hypovolemia, hypomagnesemia, or hypocalcemia: dryness of the mouth, thirst, weakness, lethargy, drowsiness, restlessness, muscle pain or cramps, muscular fatigue, hypotension, oligourea, tachycardia, arrhythmia, or gastro-intestinal disturbances such as nausea and vomiting, increases in blood glucose and alteration in glucose tolerance tests.

During long-term therapy a high-potassium diet is recommended. Potassium supplements may be required especially when high doses are used for prolonged periods. Some electrolyte disturbances (e.g. hypokalemia, hypomagnesemia) may increase the toxicity of certain other drugs (e.g. digitalis preparations and drugs inducing QT interval prolongation syndrome. Particular caution with potassium levels is necessary when the patient is on digitalis glycosides, potassium-depleting steroids, or in the case of infants and children. Potassium supplementation, diminution in dose, or discontinuation of LASIX therapy may be required.

Since rigid sodium restriction is conducive to both hyponatremia and hypokalemia, strict restriction in sodium intake is not advisable in patients receiving LASIX therapy.

Urinary outflow must be secured. Patients with urinary outflow require careful monitoring—especially during the initial stages of treatment (see Adverse Reactions, Post-Market Adverse Drug Reactions, Renal and Urinary Disorders).

Concomitant Use with Risperidone: In risperidone placebo-controlled trials in elderly patients with dementia, a higher incidence of mortality was observed in patients treated with furosemide plus risperidone (7.3%; mean age 89 years, range 75-97 years) when compared to patients treated with risperidone alone (3.1%; mean age 84 years, range 70-96 years) or furosemide alone (4.1%; mean age 80 years, range 67-90 years). Concomitant use of risperidone with other diuretics (mainly thiazide diuretics used in low dose) was not associated with similar findings.

No pathophysiological mechanism has been identified to explain this finding, and no consistent pattern for cause of death observed. Nevertheless, caution should be exercised and the risks and benefits of this combination or co-treatment with other potent diuretics should be considered prior to the decision to use. There was no increased incidence of mortality among patients taking other diuretics as concomitant treatment with risperidone. Irrespective of treatment, dehydration was an overall risk factor for mortality (see Contraindications) and should therefore be avoided in elderly patients with dementia.

Carcinogenesis and Mutagenesis: Carcinogenicity: Furosemide in the approximate amount of 200 mg/kg body weight daily was administered to female mice and rats over a 2-year period with their diet. An increased incidence of mammary adenocarcinoma was noted in the mice, but not in the rats. These tumors occurred with a positive trend, and the incidence in the high dose group was increased compared to the control, in addition, the high-dose rate was about five fold over the historical rate. These tumors are considered to be associated with furosemide administration. This dose is considerably greater than the therapeutic dose administered in human patients.

In a carcinogenicity study, rats were administered furosemide in daily doses of 15 and 30 mg/kg body weight. Male rats in the 15 mg/kg-dose category, but not in the 30 mg/kg-dose category, showed a marginal increase in uncommon tumours.

Mutagenicity: In in-vitro tests on bacteria and mammalian cells, both positive and negative results have been obtained. Induction of gene and chromosome mutations, however, has been observed only where furosemide reached cytotoxic concentrations.

Ear/Nose/Throat: Cases of tinnitus and reversible deafness have been reported. There have also been some reports of cases, the majority in children undergoing renal transplantation, in which permanent deafness has occurred. In these latter cases, the onset of deafness was usually insidious and gradually progressive up to 6 months after furosemide therapy. Hearing impairment is more likely to occur in patients with hypoproteinaemia or severely reduced renal function or in patients who are also receiving drugs known to be ototoxic. Since this may lead to irreversible damage, these drugs must only be used with furosemide if there are compelling medical reasons.

Endocrine and Metabolism: Increases in blood glucose and alterations in glucose tolerance tests with abnormalities of the fasting and two-hour postprandial blood sugar levels have been observed. Rare cases of precipitation of diabetes mellitus have been reported.

Asymptomatic hyperuricemia can occur and a gout attack may rarely be precipitated.

Hepatic/Biliary/Pancreatic: It may be advisable to hospitalize patients with hepatic cirrhosis and ascites prior to initiating therapy. Sudden alterations of fluid and electrolyte balance in patients with cirrhosis may precipitate hepatic coma, therefore, strict observation is necessary during the period of diuresis. Supplemental potassium chloride and, if required, an aldosterone antagonist, are helpful in preventing hypokalemia and metabolic alkalosis. (See Contraindications.)

Particularly careful monitoring is necessary in patients with hepatorenal syndrome.

Peri-Operative Considerations: Sulfonamide diuretics have been reported to decrease arterial responsiveness to pressor amines and to enhance the effect of tubocurarine. Great caution should be exercised in administering curare or its derivatives to patients undergoing therapy with LASIX and it is advisable to discontinue LASIX for one week prior to any elective surgery.

Special Populations: Pregnant Women: The teratogenic and embryotoxic potential of furosemide in humans is unknown. The drug should not be used in pregnant women or in women of childbearing potential unless in the opinion of the attending physician the benefits to the patient outweigh the possible risk to the fetus.

Reproductive and teratological studies have been performed in mice, rats, rabbits, cats, dogs and monkeys. With the exception of mice and rabbits, no abnormalities attributed to furosemide were detected. Furosemide caused unexplained maternal deaths and abortions in the rabbit at a daily dose of 50 mg/kg (approximately three times the maximum recommended human daily dose of 1000 mg orally) when administered between days 12 to 17 of gestation. In another study in rabbits, a dose of 25 mg/kg caused maternal deaths and abortions. In a third study, none of the pregnant rabbits survived a dose of 100 mg/kg. Data from the above studies indicate fetal lethality which can precede maternal deaths.

The results of a mouse study and one of the three rabbit studies also showed an increased incidence of distention of the renal pelvis and, in some cases, of the ureters in fetuses derived from treated dams as compared to the incidence of fetuses from the control group.

Treatment during pregnancy requires monitoring of fetal growth.

Nursing Women: It should be noted that diuretics may partially inhibit lactation and that LASIX passes into the breast milk. Women must not breast-feed if they are treated with furosemide (see Contraindications).

Pediatrics: LASIX may lower serum calcium levels, and rare cases of tetany have been reported. Accordingly, periodic serum calcium levels should be obtained.

In premature infants LASIX may precipitate nephrocalcinosis/nephrolithiasis. When administered to premature infants with respiratory distress syndrome in the first few weeks of life, diuretic treatment with LASIX may accentuate the risk of a patent ductus arteriosus. (See Warnings and Precautions, Monitoring and Laboratory Tests.)

Caution is required in neonates because of prolonged half-life of furosemide.

Geriatrics (>61 years of age): Excessive diuresis induced by LASIX may result in dehydration and reduction of blood volume, with circulatory collapse and with the possibility of vascular thrombosis and embolism particularly in elderly patients. LASIX may cause electrolyte depletion.

Furosemide binding to albumin may be reduced in elderly patients.

The drug is known to be substantially excreted unchanged by the kidney, and the risk of toxic reactions to this drug may be greater in patients with impaired renal function. Because elderly patients are more likely to have decreased renal functions, care should be taken in dose selection and may be useful to monitor renal function.

In general dose selection for the elderly patients should be cautious, usually starting at the low end of dosage range, reflecting the greater frequency of decreased hepatic, renal or cardiac function, and the concomitant disease or other drug therapy.

Monitoring and Laboratory Tests: Frequent serum electrolyte, creatinine and CO_2 content determinations should be performed during the first few months of therapy and periodically thereafter. It is essential to replace electrolyte losses and to maintain fluid balance so as to avoid any risk of electrolyte depletion (hyponatremia, hypochloremia, hypokalemia, hypomagnesemia or hypocalcemia), hypovolemia, or hypotension.

Checks on urine and blood glucose should be made at regular intervals especially in diabetics and in those suspected of latent diabetes when receiving LASIX. Increases in blood glucose and alterations in glucose tolerance tests with abnormalities of the fasting and two-hour postprandial blood sugar levels have been observed.

Frequent BUN determinations during the first few months of therapy and periodically thereafter, as well as regular observations for possible occurence of blood dyscrasias, liver damage or idiosyncratic reactions are advisable.

Particularly careful monitoring is necessary in:

- patients with hypoproteinaemia. Cautious dose titration is required.
- premature infants. Renal function must be monitored and renal ultrasonography performed.
- patients with hypotension.
- patients who would be at particular risk from a pronounced fall in blood pressure (e.g. patients with significant stenoses of the coronary arteries or of the blood vessels supplying the brain).
- patients with hepatorenal syndrome.
- patients with latent and manifest diabetes mellitus.
- patients with gout.

Occupational Hazards: LASIX may lower the state of patient alertness and/or reactivity particularly at the start of treatment as a result of a reduction in blood pressure and of other adverse reactions (see Adverse Reactions).

ADVERSE REACTIONS: Clinical Trial Adverse Drug Reactions: No data available.

Post-Market Adverse Drug Reactions: Adverse reactions are categorized below by body system.

Blood and Lymphatic System Disorders: Anemia, eosinophilia, leukopenia and thrombocytopenia (with purpura) have occurred, as well as agranulocytosis, aplastic anemia and hemolytic anemia.

Ear and Labyrinth Disorders: Cases of tinnitus and reversible deafness have been reported. There have also been some reports of cases, the majority in children undergoing renal transplantation, in which permanent deafness has occurred. In these latter cases, the onset of deafness is usually insidious and gradually progressive up to 6 months after furosemide therapy. Hearing impairment is more likely to occur in patients with hypoproteinaemia or severely reduced renal function who are also receiving drugs known to be ototoxic.

Vertigo has been reported.

Eye Disorders: Xanthopsia and blurred vision have been reported.

Gastrointestinal Disorders: Acute pancreatitis, oral and gastric burning, diarrhea, nausea, vomiting and constipation have been reported. Rare occurrence of sweet taste has been reported.

Hepatobiliary Disorders: Jaundice (intrahepatic cholestatic jaundice) has been reported.

Immune System Disorders: Hypersensitivity reactions to furosemide also include photosensitivity, paresthesia and fever. Systemic hypersensitivity reactions include vasculitis and necrotizing angiitis.

Severe anaphylactic or anaphylactoid reactions (e.g. with shock) occur rarely.

Investigations: Increase in liver transaminases has been reported.

Transient elevations of BUN have been observed, especially in patients with renal insufficiency.

As with other diuretics, there may be a transient rise in serum creatinine, uric acid (this may lead to gout attack in predisposed patients), cholesterol and triglyceride levels during furosemide treatment.

Metabolism and Nutrition Disorders: Electrolyte depletion has occurred during therapy with LASIX, especially in patients receiving higher doses with a restricted salt intake. Electrolyte depletion manifests itself by adverse reactions attributed to various body systems: weakness, dizziness, drowsiness, polyuria, polydipsia, orthostatic hypotension, lethargy, sweating, bladder spasms, anorexia, vomiting, mental confusion, meteorism, thirst, headache, muscle cramp, muscle weakness, tetany and disorder of cardiac rhythm. (See Warnings and Precautions.)

The development of electrolyte disturbances is influenced by factors such as underlying diseases (e.g. liver cirrhosis, cardiac failure), concomitant medication and nutrition.

Treatment with LASIX has occasionally caused some deterioration of metabolic control in cases of manifest diabetes, or has made latent diabetes manifest.

Metabolic alkalosis may develop in the form of a gradually increasing electrolyte deficit or, e.g. where higher furosemide doses are administered to patients with normal renal function, acute severe electrolyte losses.

Pre-existing metabolic alkalosis (e.g. in decompensated cirrhosis of the liver) may be aggravated.

In extreme cases, hypovolemia may lead to dehydration, circulatory collapse, hemoconcentration and thrombophilia. Thrombophlebitis and emboli have been reported.

Nervous System Disorders: At the commencement of treatment, excessive diuresis may give rise, especially in elderly patients, to a feeling of pressure in the head, dizziness.

Paresthesia has been reported.

Hepatic encephalopathy in patients with hepatocellular insufficiency has been reported.

Renal and Urinary Disorders: Symptoms of obstructed micturition (e.g. in hydronephrosis, prostatic hypertrophy, ureterostenosis) may become manifest or may be aggravated during medication with diuretics. Interstitial nephritis has been reported.

Increased production of urine may provoke or aggravate complaints in patients with an obstruction of urinary outflow. Thus, acute retention of urine with possible secondary complications may occur.

Skin and Subcutaneous Tissue Disorders: Various forms of dermatitis (e.g. dermatitis bullous), including urticaria, erythema multiforme, bullous pemphigoid, Stevens-Johnson syndrome, toxic epidermal necrolysis, exfoliative dermatitis, pruritus and epidermolysis bullosa have occurred. Dermatologic reactions to furosemide also include purpura and rash.

Vascular Disorders: Too vigorous diuresis may induce orthostatic hypotension or acute hypotensive episodes, which may cause signs and symptoms such as impairment of concentration and reactions, lightheadedness or orthostatic intolerance.

DRUG INTERACTIONS: Overview: Sulfonamide diuretics have been reported to decrease arterial responsiveness to pressor amines and to enhance the effect of tubocurarine or curare-type muscle relaxants. (See Warnings and Precautions, Peri-Operative Considerations.)

In case of concomitant abuse of laxatives, the risk of an increased potassium loss should be considered.

Glucocorticoids, carbenoxolone and licorice may also increase potassium loss.

Administration of LASIX to diabetic patients may result in possible decrease of diabetic control. Dosage adjustments of the anti-diabetic agent may be needed.

Hearing impairment is more likely to occur in patients who are also receiving drugs known to be ototoxic (e.g. aminoglycosides antibiotics, ethacrynic acid and cisplatin) (see Warnings and Precautions).

In edematous hypertensive patients being treated with antihypertensive agents, care should be taken to reduce the dose of these drugs when LASIX is administered, since LASIX potentiates their hypotensive effect.

Non-steroidal anti-inflammatory drugs (e.g. indomethacin, acetyl-salicylic acid) may attenuate the effect of LASIX and may cause renal failure in case of pre-existing hypovolemia.

Drug-Drug Interactions: The drug interactions discussed in this section are based on either drug interaction case reports, or studies, or potential interactions due to the expected magnitude and seriousness of the interaction (i.e., those identified as contraindicated). See Table 1.

Table 1: LASIX

Established or Predicted Drug-Drug Interactions

Proper Name	Ref	Effect	Clinical Comments
Anticonvulsants			
Carbamazepine Phenobarbital Phenytoin	T	↓ furosemide diuretic effect	Anticonvulsant drugs (phenytoin, carbamazepine, phenobarbital), which, like furosemide, undergo significant renal tubular secretion, may also attenuate the effect of furosemide.
Antidiabetics			
Antidiabetics	T	↓ antidiabetic drug effect	The effects of antidiabetic drugs may be reduced.
Antihypertensive Agents			
ACE inhibitors	CT	↓ blood pressure and renal function	Especially in combination with ACE inhibitors, a marked hypotension may be seen sometimes progressing to shock. The concomitant administration of LASIX with ACE-inhibitors may lead to deterioration in renal function and, in isolated cases, to acute renal failure. Consideration must be given to interrupting the administration of furosemide temporarily or at least reducing the dose of furosemide for three days before starting treatment with, or increasing the dose of, an ACE inhibitor.
Angiotensin II receptor antagonists	CT	↓ blood pressure and renal function	Especially in combination with angiotensin II receptor antagonists, a marked hypotension may be seen sometimes progressing to shock. The concomitant administration of LASIX with angiotensin II receptor antagonists may lead to deterioration in renal function and, in isolated cases, to acute renal failure. Consideration must be given to interrupting the administration of furosemide temporarily or at least reducing the dose of furosemide for three days before starting treatment with, or increasing the dose of, an angiotensin II receptor antagonist.
Cephalosporins			
Cephalosporins	T	↓ renal function	Impairment of renal function may develop in patients receiving concurrent treatment with furosemide and high doses of certain cephalosporins.
Chloral Hydrate			
Chloral Hydrate	C	—	In isolated cases intravenous administration of furosemide within 24 hours of taking chloral hydrate may lead to flushing, sweating attacks, restlessness, nausea, increase in blood pressure and tachycardia. Use of furosemide concomitantly with chloral hydrate is therefore not recommended.
Chlorothiazides			
Chlorothiazides	T	—	The concurrent use of LASIX with chlorothiazide has been reported to decrease hypercalciuria and to dissolve some calculi.
Cisplatin			
Cisplatin	T	↑ nephrotoxicity ↑ ototoxicity	Nephrotoxicity of cisplatin may be enhanced if furosemide is not given in low doses and with positive fluid balance when used to achieve forced diuresis during cisplatin treatment. There is also a risk of ototoxic effects if cisplatin and furosemide are given concomitantly.
Cyclosporine			
Cyclosporine	CT	—	Concomitant use of cyclosporine A and furosemide is associated with increased risk of gouty arthritis secondary to furosemide-induced hyperuricemia and cyclosporine impairment of renal urate excretion.
Digitalis Glycosides			
Digitalis Glycosides	T	↓ potassium plasma concentration	Some electrolyte disturbances (e.g. hypokalemia, hypomagnesemia) may increase the toxicity of certain other drugs (e.g. digitalis preparations and drugs inducing QT interval prolongation syndrome). Particular caution with potassium levels is necessary when the patient is on digitalis glycosides. Potassium supplementation, diminution in dose, or discontinuation of LASIX therapy may be required (see Warnings and Precautions).

(cont'd)

Table 1: LASIX *(cont'd)*

Established or Predicted Drug-Drug Interactions

Proper Name	Ref	Effect	Clinical Comments
Lithium			
Lithium	T	↑ lithium plasma concentration	Renal clearance of lithium is decreased in patients receiving LASIX, resulting in increased risk of cardiotoxic and neurotoxic effects of lithium. Therefore, it is recommended that lithium levels be carefully monitored in patients receiving this combination.
Methotrexate			
Methotrexate	T	↓ furosemide diuretic effect	Methotrexate, which like furosemide, undergoes significant renal tubular secretion, may also attenuate the effect of furosemide.
Nephrotoxic Drugs			
Nephrotoxic Drugs	T	↑ nephrotoxicity	The harmful effects of nephrotoxic drugs on the kidney may be increased.
Non-Steroidal Anti-Inflammatory Drugs (NSAIDs)			
Indomethacin	CT	↓ furosemide diuretic effect	Clinical studies have shown that the administration of indomethacin can reduce the natriuretic and anti-hypertensive effect of LASIX in some patients. This response has been attributed to inhibition of prostaglandin synthesis by indomethacin. Therefore, when indomethacin is added to the treatment of a patient receiving LASIX, or LASIX is added to the treatment of a patient receiving indomethacin, the patient should be closely observed to determine if the desired effect of LASIX is obtained. Indomethacin blocks the LASIX-induced increase in plasma-renin activity. This fact should be kept in mind when evaluating plasma-renin activity in hypertensive patients.
Potassium-depleting Steroids			
Potassium-depleting Steroids	T	↓ potassium plasma concentration	Some electrolyte disturbances (e.g. hypokalemia, hypomagnesemia) may increase the toxicity of certain other drugs (e.g. digitalis preparations and drugs inducing QT interval prolongation syndrome). Particular caution with potassium levels is necessary when the patient is on potassium-depleting steroids. Potassium supplementation, diminution in dose, or discontinuation of LASIX therapy may be required (see Warnings and Precautions).
Probenecid			
Probenecid	T	↓ furosemide diuretic effect	Probenecid, which like furosemide, undergoes significant renal tubular secretion, may also attenuate the effect of furosemide.
Radiocontrast Agents			
Radiocontrast Agents	CT	↑ radiocontrast nephropathy	Patients who were at high risk for radiocontrast nephropathy treated with furosemide experienced a higher incidence of deterioration in renal function after receiving radiocontrast compared to high-risk patients who received only intravenous hydration prior to receiving radiocontrast.
Risperidone			
Risperidone	CT	—	Caution should be exercised and the risks and benefits of the combination or co-treatment with furosemide or with other potent diuretics should be considered prior to the decision to use. See Warnings and Precautions, regarding increased mortality in elderly patients with dementia concomitantly receiving risperidone.
Salicylates			
Salicylates	T	↑ salicylate toxicity	Patients receiving high doses of salicylates in conjunction with LASIX may experience salicylate toxicity at lower doses because of competition for renal excretory sites.
Sucralfate			
Sucralfate	T	↓ furosemide absorption	Concurrent administration of LASIX and sucralfate should be avoided, as sucralfate reduces the absorption of furosemide from the intestine and hence weakens its effect.
Theophylline			
Theophylline	T	↑ theophylline effect	The effects of theophylline may be increased.

Legend: C=Case Study; CT=Clinical Trial; T=Theoretical.

Interactions with other drugs have not been established.

Drug-Food Interactions: Interactions with food have not been established.

Drug-Herb Interactions: Interactions with herbal product have not been established.

Drug-Laboratory Test Interactions: Interactions with laboratory tests have not been established.

DOSAGE AND ADMINISTRATION: Dosing Considerations: Careful observations for changes in blood pressure must be made when LASIX is used with other antihypertensive drugs, especially during initial therapy. The dosage of other agents must be reduced by at least 50% as soon as LASIX is added to the regimen to prevent excessive drop in blood pressure. As the blood pressure falls under the potentiating effect of LASIX, a further reduction in dosage or even discontinuation of other antihypertensive drugs may be necessary.

Recommended Dose and Dosage Adjustment: Adults (oral): Edema: The usual initial dose of LASIX is 40 to 80 mg. Ordinarily a prompt diuresis ensues and the starting dose can then be maintained or even reduced. If a satisfactory diuresis has not occurred within 6 hours, succeeding doses should be increased by increments of 20 to 40 mg, if necessary. Maximum daily dose: 200 mg. Once the effective single dose has been determined, it may be repeated 1 to 3 times a day.

The mobilization of edema may be most efficiently and safely accomplished by utilizing an intermittent dosage schedule in which LASIX is given for 2 to 4 consecutive days each week. With doses exceeding 120 mg/day, careful clinical and laboratory observations are particularly advisable.

Hypertension: A dosage schedule of 20 to 40 mg twice daily is recommended. Individualized therapy is of great importance. It is further recommended, if 40 mg twice daily does not lead to a clinically satisfactory response, to add other antihypertensive agents, rather than to increase the dose of LASIX.

Pediatrics (oral): LASIX therapy should be instituted in the hospital, in carefully selected patients, under close observation with frequent monitoring of serum electrolytes.

Orally, the initial dose should be in the range of 0.5 to 1 mg/kg body weight.

The total daily dose (given in divided doses of 6 to 12 hours apart) should not exceed 2 mg/kg orally. In the newborn and in premature babies, the daily dose should not exceed 1 mg/kg.

An intermittent dosage schedule should be adopted as soon as possible using the minimum effective dose at the longest possible intervals. Particular caution with regard to potassium levels is always desirable when LASIX is used in infants and children.

OVERDOSAGE:

Symptoms: Dehydration, electrolyte depletion and hypotension may be caused by overdosage or accidental ingestion. In cirrhotic patients, overdosage might precipitate hepatic coma.

The clinical picture in acute or chronic overdose depends primarily on the extent and consequences of electrolyte and fluide loss, e.g. hypovolemia, dehydration, hemoconcentration, cardiac arrhythmias (including A-V block and ventricular fibrillation). Symptoms of these disturbances include severe hypotension (progressing to shock), acute renal failure, thrombosis, delirious states, flaccid paralysis, apathy and confusion.

Treatment: The drug should be discontinued and appropriate corrective treatment applied: replacement of excessive fluid and electrolyte losses; serum electrolytes, carbon dioxide level and blood pressure should be determined frequently. Adequate drainage must be assured in patients with urinary bladder outlet obstruction (such as prostatic hypertrophy).

No specific antidote to furosemide is known. If ingestion has only just taken place, attempts may be made to limit further systemic absorption of the active ingredient by measures such as gastric lavage or those designed to reduce absorption (e.g. activated charcoal).

> For management of a suspected drug overdose, contact your regional Poison Control Centre. See the *CPS* Directory section for a list of Poison Control Centres.

ACTION AND CLINICAL PHARMACOLOGY: Mechanism of Action: Animal experiments using stop-flow and micropuncture techniques have demonstrated that LASIX inhibits sodium reabsorption in the ascending limb of Henle's loop as well as in both proximal and distal tubules. The action of LASIX on the distal tubule is independent of any inhibitory effect on carbonic anhydrase or aldosterone.

LASIX may promote diuresis in cases which have previously proved resistant to other diuretics.

Pharmacodynamics: A continuous infusion of furosemide is more effective than repetitive bolus injections. Moreover, above a certain bolus dose of the drug there is no significant increase in effect.

The effect of furosemide is reduced if there is lowered tubular secretion or intra-tubular albumin binding of the drug.

Pharmacokinetics: Absorption: In man, LASIX is rapidly absorbed from the gastro-intestinal tract. The diuretic effect of furosemide is apparent within one hour following oral administration and the peak effect occurs in the first or second hour. The duration of action is 4-6 hours but may continue up to 8 hours.

Following intravenous administration of the drug, the diuresis occurs within 30 minutes and the duration of action is about 2 hours.

Metabolism: A small fraction is metabolized by cleavage of the side chain.

Excretion: Urinary excretion is accomplished both by glomerular filtration and proximal tubular secretion, together this accounts for roughly only 2/3 of the ingested dose, the remainder being excreted in the feces.

Table 2 summarizes the elimination kinetics of furosemide.

Table 2: LASIX

Summary of Furosemide's Elimination Kinetics

Subjects	Route of Administration	Dose (mg)	Rate of Administration	Biliary Excretion	Max. Serum Concentration	$t_{½}$ (h)
Normal	Oral	40	—	10–15%	<1 µg/mL	4.0
Normal	I.V.	40	Bolus	10–15%	2.5 µg/mL	4.5
Renal insufficiency	I.V.	1000	25 mg/min	60%	53 µg/mL	13.5
Renal insufficiency	I.V.	1000	4 mg/min	—	29 µg/mL	—

Special Populations and Conditions: Pediatrics: Depending on the maturity of the kidney, the elimination of furosemide may be slowed down. The metabolism of the drug is also reduced if the infant's glucuronisation capacity is impaired.

The terminal half-life is below 12 hours in infants with a post-conceptional age of more than 33 weeks.

In infants of 2 months and older, the terminal clearance is the same as in adults.

Geriatrics: The elimination of furosemide is slowed down due to reduced renal function in the elderly.

Gender: Data unavailable.

Race: Data unavailable.

Hepatic Insufficiency: In liver failure, the half-life of furosemide is increased by 30% to 90% mainly due to a larger volume of distribution. Additionally, in this patient group there is a wide variation in all pharmacokinetic parameters.

Renal Insufficiency: In renal failure, the elimination furosemide is slowed down and the half-life prolonged; the terminal half-life may be up to 24 hours in patients with severe renal failure.

In nephrotic syndrome the reduced plasma protein concentration leads to a higher concentration of unbound (free) furosemide. On the other hand, efficacy of furosemide is reduced in these patients due to binding to intratubular albumin and lowered tubular secretion.

Furosemide is poorly dialyzable in patients undergoing haemodialysis, peritoneal dialysis and CAPD.

Genetic Polymorphism: Data unavailable.

STORAGE AND STABILITY: Temperature: Tablets: Store between 15 and 30°C. Protect from light.

Oral solution: Store between 15 and 30°C. Protect from light.

INFORMATION FOR THE PATIENT: Published in e-CPS, available by subscription at www.e-cps.ca.

DOSAGE FORMS, COMPOSITION AND PACKAGING: Oral Solution: Each mL of clear, slightly yellowish solution with an orange odor, contains: furosemide 10 mg. Nonmedicinal ingredients: alcohol, butylated hydroxyanisol, butylated hydroxytoluene, glycerin, methylparaben, natural orange flavor, polysorbate 80 non-animal, potassium sorbate, purified water, sodium hydroxide and sorbitol. Bottles of 120 mL.

Tablets: 20 mg: Each white, round tablet, with one surface debossed "DLF" and the other debossed with the Hoechst logo, contains: furosemide 20 mg. Nonmedicinal ingredients: colloidal silicon dioxide, lactose monohydrate, magnesium stearate, starch and talc. Blister packs of 30 (2×15).

40 mg: Each yellow, round tablet, debossed with the Hoechst logo on one face, and the other face single scored with "LASIX" debossed above score and "40" debossed below score line, contains: furosemide 40 mg. Nonmedicinal ingredients: colloidal silicon dioxide, D&C Yellow #10, FD&C Yellow #6, lactose monohydrate, magnesium stearate, starch and talc. Blister packs of 30 (2×15).

(Shown in Product Identification Section)

Lasix® Special

furosemide

Diuretic

sanofi-aventis

Date of Revision: August 27, 2010

SUMMARY PRODUCT INFORMATION:

Route of Administration	Dosage Form/Strength	Nonmedicinal Ingredients
Oral	Tablet 500 mg	Cellulose, corn starch, colloidal silicon dioxide, D Yellow #10, FD Yellow #6, lactose monohydrate, magnesium stearate, sodium starch glycolate and talc.

INDICATIONS AND CLINICAL USE: LASIX SPECIAL (furosemide 500 mg) is a high-dosage formulation of furosemide and is intended exclusively for patients with severely impaired renal function. LASIX SPECIAL is to be used under strict medical supervision in a hospital setting (see Dosage and Administration).

High doses of LASIX SPECIAL may be used as an adjuvant treatment of oliguria and in the promotion of diuresis in the treatment of edema:

- in selected patients with acute renal failure, e.g. in the postoperative phase and in association with septic infections;
- in selected patients with chronic renal failure with fluid retention, both in the predialysis phase and when dialysis has become unavoidable, especially in the presence of acute pulmonary edema;
- in selected patients with the nephrotic syndrome with severe impairment of renal function, e.g. in chronic glomerular nephritis, lupus erythematosus and Kimmelstiel-Wilson syndrome.

Geriatrics (>61 years of age): Use in the geriatric population is associated with differences in safety (see Warnings and Precautions).

Pediatrics (newborn-15 years): LASIX SPECIAL is not recommended for pediatric use (see Warnings and Precautions, Special Populations, Pediatrics (newborn-15 years)).

CONTRAINDICATIONS: LASIX SPECIAL is contraindicated in:

- Patients who are hypersensitive to furosemide, sulfonamide-derived drugs, or to any ingredient in the formulation or component of the container. For a complete listing, see Dosage Forms, Composition and Packaging. Patients allergic to sulfonamides (e.g. sulfonamide antibiotics or sulfonylureas) may show cross-sensitivity to furosemide.
- Patients with complete renal shutdown and glomerular filtration rate below 5 mL/min.
- **Patients whose glomerular filtration rate is above 20 mL/min. In such cases, it might cause extremely severe water and electrolyte losses.**
- Patients with hepatic cirrhosis, patients with renal failure due to poisoning with nephrotoxic or hepatotoxic substances and patients with renal failure accompanied by hepatic coma and precoma (see Warnings and Precautions and Adverse Reactions).
- Severe hyponatremia, hypokalemia, hypovolemia, dehydration or hypotension must be regarded as contraindications until serum electrolytes and fluid balance and blood pressure have been restored to normal levels (see Warnings and Precautions and Adverse Reactions).
- As furosemide may be capable of displacing bilirubin from albumin at least "in vitro", it should not be administered to jaundiced newborn infants or to infants suffering from diseases (e.g. Rh incompatibility, familial non-hemolytic jaundice, etc.) with the potential of causing hyperbilirubinemia and possibly kernicterus.
- Women must not breast-feed if they are treated with furosemide (see Warnings and Precautions).

WARNINGS AND PRECAUTIONS: General: LASIX SPECIAL is a potent diuretic which if given in excessive amounts can lead to a profound diuresis with water and electrolyte depletion. Therefore, careful medical supervision is required, and dose and dose schedule have to be adjusted to the individual patient's needs (see Dosage and Administration).

All patients receiving LASIX SPECIAL therapy should be observed for signs and symptoms of fluid or electrolyte imbalance, hyponatremia, hypochloremic alkalosis, hypovolemia, hypomagnesemia, or hypocalcemia: dryness of the mouth, thirst, weakness, lethargy, drowsiness, restlessness, muscle pain or cramps, muscular fatigue, hypotension, oligourea, tachycardia, arrhythmia, or gastro-intestinal disturbances such as nausea and vomiting, increases in blood glucose and alteration in glucose tolerance tests.

During long-term therapy a high-potassium diet is recommended. Potassium supplements may be required especially when high doses are used for prolonged periods. Some electrolyte disturbances (e.g. hypokalemia, hypomagnesemia) may increase the toxicity of certain other drugs (e.g. digitalis preparations and drugs inducing QT interval prolongation syndrome). Particular caution with potassium levels is necessary when the patient is on digitalis glycosides or potassium-depleting steroids. Potassium supplementation, diminution in dose, or discontinuation of LASIX SPECIAL therapy may be required.

Since rigid sodium restriction is conducive to both hyponatremia and hypokalemia, strict restriction in sodium intake is not advisable in patients receiving LASIX SPECIAL therapy.

During treatment with LASIX SPECIAL, extreme care must always be taken to adjust dosage to individual requirements.

Since furosemide is a sulfonamide derivative, it should be used with caution in patients with known sulfonamide sensitivity.

Urinary outflow must be secured. Patients with urinary outflow require careful monitoring-especially during the initial stages of treatment (see Adverse Reactions, Post-Market Adverse Drug Reactions, Renal and Urinary Disorders).

Concomitant Use with Risperidone: In risperidone placebo-controlled trials in elderly patients with dementia, a higher incidence of mortality was observed in patients treated with furosemide plus risperidone (7.3%; mean age 89 years, range 75-97 years) when compared to patients treated with risperidone alone (3.1%; mean age 84 years, range 70-96 years) or furosemide alone (4.1%; mean age 80 years, range 67-90 years). Concomitant use of risperidone with other diuretics (mainly thiazide diuretics used in low dose) was not associated with similar findings.

No pathophysiological mechanism has been identified to explain this finding, and no consistent pattern for cause of death observed. Nevertheless, caution should be exercised and the risks and benefits of this combination or co-treatment with other potent diuretics should be considered prior to the decision to use. There was no increased incidence of mortality among patients taking other diuretics as concomitant treatment with risperidone. Irrespective of treatment, dehydration was an overall risk factor for mortality (see Contraindications) and should therefore be avoided in elderly patients with dementia.

Carcinogenesis and Mutagenesis: Carcinogenicity: Furosemide in the approximate amount of 200 mg/kg body weight daily was administered to female mice and rats over a 2-year period with their diet. An increased incidence of mammary adenocarcinoma was noted in the mice, but not in the rats. These tumors occurred with a positive trend, and the incidence in the high dose group was increased compared to the control, in addition, the high-dose rate was about five fold over the historical rate. These tumors are considered to be associated with furosemide administration. This dose is considerably greater than the therapeutic dose administered in human patients.

In a carcinogenicity study, rats were administered furosemide in daily doses of 15 and 30 mg/kg body weight. Male rats in the 15 mg/kg-dose category, but not in the 30 mg/kg-dose category, showed a marginal increase in uncommon tumours.

Mutagenicity: In in-vitro tests on bacteria and mammalian cells, both positive and negative results have been obtained. Induction of gene and chromosome mutations, however, has been observed only where furosemide reached cytotoxic concentrations.

Ear/Nose/Throat: Cases of tinnitus and reversible deafness have been reported. There have also been some reports of cases, the majority in children undergoing renal transplantation, in which permanent deafness has occurred. In these latter cases, the onset of deafness was usually insidious and gradually progressive up to 6 months after furosemide therapy. (The 500 mg furosemide tablet is for adults only.) Hearing impairment is more likely to occur in patients with hypoproteinaemia or severely reduced renal function, or in patients who are also receiving drugs known to be ototoxic. Since this may lead to irreversible damage, these drugs must only be used with furosemide if there are compelling medical reasons.

Endocrine and Metabolism: Increases in blood glucose and alterations in glucose tolerance tests with abnormalities of the fasting and two-hour postprandial blood sugar levels have been observed. Rare cases of precipitation of diabetes mellitus have been reported.

Asymptomatic hyperuricemia can occur and a gout attack may rarely be precipitated.

Peri-Operative Considerations: Sulfonamide diuretics have been reported to decrease arterial responsiveness to pressor amines and to enhance the effect of tubocurarine or curare-type muscle relaxants. Great caution should be exercised in administering curare or its derivatives to patients undergoing therapy with LASIX SPECIAL and it is advisable to discontinue LASIX SPECIAL for one week prior to any elective surgery.

Special Populations: Pregnant Women: The teratogenic and embryotoxic potential of furosemide in humans is unknown. The drug should not be used in pregnant women or in women of childbearing potential unless in the opinion of the attending physician the benefits to the patient outweigh the possible risk to the fetus.

Reproductive and teratological studies have been performed in mice, rats, rabbits, cats, dogs and monkeys. With the exception of mice and rabbits, no abnormalities attributed to furosemide were detected. Furosemide caused unexplained maternal deaths and abortions in the rabbit at a daily dose of 50 mg/kg (approximately three times the maximum recommended human daily dose of 1000 mg orally) when administered between days 12 to 17 of gestation. In another study in rabbits, a dose of 25 mg/kg caused maternal deaths and abortions. In a third study, none of the pregnant rabbits survived a dose of 100 mg/kg. Data from the above studies indicate fetal lethality which can precede maternal deaths.

The results of a mouse study and one of the three rabbit studies also showed an increased incidence of distention of the renal pelvis and, in some cases, of the ureters in fetuses derived from treated dams as compared to the incidence of fetuses from the control group.

Treatment during pregnancy requires monitoring of fetal growth.

Nursing Women: It should be noted that diuretics may partially inhibit lactation and that LASIX SPECIAL passes into the breast milk. Women must not breast-feed during treatment with furosemide (see Contraindications).

Pediatrics (newborn-15 years): LASIX SPECIAL is not recommended for pediatric use.

LASIX SPECIAL may lower serum calcium levels, and rare cases of tetany have been reported.

In premature infants LASIX may precipitate nephrocalcinosis/nephrolithiasis. When administered to premature infants with respiratory distress syndrome in the first few weeks of life, diuretic treatment with LASIX may accentuate the risk of a patent ductus arteriosus.

Geriatrics (>61 years of age): Excessive diuresis induced by LASIX SPECIAL may result in dehydration and reduction of blood volume, with circulatory collapse and with the possibility of vascular thrombosis and embolism particularly in elderly patients. LASIX SPECIAL may cause electrolyte depletion.

Furosemide binding to albumin may be reduced in elderly patients.

The drug is known to be substantially excreted unchanged by the kidney, and the risk of toxic reactions to this drug may be greater in patients with impaired renal function. Because elderly patients are more likely to have decreased renal functions, care should be taken in dose selection and may be useful to monitor renal function.

In general dose selection for the elderly patients should be cautious, usually starting at the low end of dosage range, reflecting the greater frequency of decreased hepatic, renal or cardiac function, and the concomitant disease or other drug therapy.

Monitoring and Laboratory Tests: Frequent serum electrolyte, creatinine and CO_2 content determinations should be performed during the first few months of therapy and periodically thereafter. It is essential to replace electrolyte losses and to maintain fluid balance so as to avoid any risk of electrolyte depletion (hyponatremia, hypochloremia, hypokalemia, hypomagnesemia or hypocalcemia), hypovolemia, or hypotension.

Checks on urine and blood glucose should be made at regular intervals especially in diabetics and in those suspected of latent diabetes when receiving LASIX SPECIAL. Increases in blood glucose and alterations in glucose tolerance tests with abnormalities of the fasting and two-hour postprandial blood sugar levels have been observed.

Frequent BUN determinations during the first few months of therapy and periodically thereafter, as well as regular observations for possible occurence of blood dyscrasias, liver damage or idiosyncratic reactions are advisable.

Particularly careful monitoring is necessary in:

- patients with hypoproteinaemia. Cautious dose titration is required.
- patients with hypotension.
- patients who would be at particular risk from a pronounced fall in blood pressure (e.g. patients with significant stenoses of the coronary arteries or of the blood vessels supplying the brain).
- patients with hepatorenal syndrome.
- patients with latent and manifest diabetes mellitus
- patients with gout

Occupational Hazards: LASIX SPECIAL may lower the state of patient alertness and/or reactivity particularly at the start of treatment as a result of a reduction in blood pressure and of other adverse reactions (see Adverse Reactions).

ADVERSE REACTIONS: Clinical Trial Adverse Drug Reactions: No data available.

Post-Market Adverse Drug Reactions: Adverse reactions are categorized below by body system.

Blood and Lymphatic System Disorders: Anemia, eosinophilia, leukopenia and thrombocytopenia (with purpura) have occurred, as well as agranulocytosis, aplastic anemia and hemolytic anemia.

Ear and Labyrinth Disorders: Cases of tinnitus and reversible deafness have been reported. There have also been some reports of cases, the majority in children undergoing renal transplantation, in which permanent deafness has occurred. In these latter cases, the onset of deafness is usually insidious and gradually progressive up to 6 months after furosemide therapy. Hearing impairment is more likely to occur in patients with hypoproteinaemia or severely reduced renal function who are also receiving drugs known to be ototoxic.

Vertigo has been reported.

Eye Disorders: Xanthopsia and blurred vision have been reported.

Gastrointestinal Disorders: Acute pancreatitis, oral and gastric burning, diarrhea, nausea, vomiting and constipation have been reported. Rare occurrences of sweet taste have been reported.

Hepatobiliary Disorders: Jaundice (intrahepatic cholestatic jaundice) has been reported.

Immune System Disorders: Hypersensitivity reactions to furosemide also include photosensitivity, paresthesia and fever. Systemic hypersensitivity reactions include vasculitis and necrotizing angiitis.

Severe anaphylactic or anaphylactoid reactions (e.g. with shock) occur rarely.

Investigations: Increase in liver transaminases has been reported.

Transient elevations of BUN have been observed, especially in patients with renal insufficiency.

As with other diuretics, there may be a transient rise in serum creatinine, uric acid (this may lead to gout attack in predisposed patients), cholesterol and triglyceride levels during furosemide treatment.

Metabolism and Nutrition Disorders: Electrolyte depletion has occurred during therapy with LASIX SPECIAL, especially in patients receiving higher doses with a restricted salt intake. Electrolyte depletion manifests itself by adverse reactions attributed to various body systems: weakness, dizziness, drowsiness, polyuria, polydipsia, orthostatic hypotension, lethargy, sweating, bladder spasms, anorexia, vomiting, mental confusion, meteorism, thirst, headache, muscle cramp, muscle weakness, tetany and disorder of cardiac rhythm (see Warnings and Precautions).

The development of electrolyte disturbances is influenced by factors such as underlying diseases (e.g. liver cirrhosis, cardiac failure), concomitant medication and nutrition.

Treatment with LASIX SPECIAL has occasionally caused some deterioration of metabolic control in cases of manifest diabetes, or has made latent diabetes manifest.

Metabolic alkalosis may develop in the form of a gradually increasing electrolyte deficit or, e.g. where higher furosemide doses are administered to patients with normal renal function, acute severe electrolyte losses.

Pre-existing metabolic alkalosis (e.g. in decompensated cirrhosis of the liver) may be aggravated.

In extreme cases, hypovolemia may lead to dehydration, circulatory collapse, hemoconcentration and thrombophilia. Thrombophlebitis and emboli have been reported.

Nervous System Disorders: At the commencement of treatment, excessive diuresis may give rise, especially in elderly patients, to a feeling of pressure in the head, dizziness.

Paresthesia has been reported.

Hepatic encephalopathy in patients with hepatocellular insufficiency has been reported.

Renal and Urinary Disorders: Symptoms of obstructed micturition (e.g. in hydronephrosis, prostatic hypertrophy, ureterostenosis) may become manifest or may be aggravated during medication with diuretics.

Interstitial nephritis has been reported.

Increased production of urine may provoke or aggravate complaints in patients with an obstruction of urinary outflow. Thus, acute retention of urine with possible secondary complications may occur.

Skin and Subcutaneous Tissue Disorders: Various forms of dermatitis (e.g. dermatitis bullous), including urticaria, erythema multiforme, bullous pemphigoid, Stevens-Johnson syndrome, toxic epidermal necrolysis, exfoliative dermatitis, pruritus and epidermolysis bullosa have occurred.

Dermatologic reactions to furosemide also include purpura and rash.

Vascular Disorders: Too vigorous diuresis may induce orthostatic hypotension or acute hypotensive episodes, which may cause signs and symptoms such as impairment of concentration and reactions, lightheadedness or orthostatic intolerance.

DRUG INTERACTIONS: Overview: Sulfonamide diuretics have been reported to decrease arterial responsiveness to pressor amines and to enhance the effect of tubocurarine or curare-type muscle relaxants (see Warnings and Precautions, Peri-Operative Considerations).

In case of concomitant abuse of laxatives, the risk of an increased potassium loss should be considered.

Glucocorticoids, carbenoxolone and licorice may also increase potassium loss.

Administration of LASIX SPECIAL to diabetic patients may result in possible decrease of diabetic control. Dosage adjustments of the anti-diabetic agent may be needed.

Hearing impairment is more likely to occur in patients who are also receiving drugs known to be ototoxic (e.g. aminoglycosides antibiotics, ethacrynic acid and cisplatin) (see Warnings and Precautions).

In edematous hypertensive patients being treated with antihypertensive agents, care should be taken to reduce the dose of these drugs when LASIX SPECIAL is administered, since LASIX SPECIAL potentiates their hypotensive effect.

Non-steroidal anti-inflammatory drugs (e.g. indomethacin, acetylsalicylic acid) may attenuate the effect of LASIX SPECIAL and may cause renal failure in case of pre-existing hypovolemia.

Drug-Drug Interactions: The drug interactions discussed in this section are based on either drug interaction case reports, or studies, or potential interactions due to the expected magnitude and seriousness of the interaction (i.e., those identified as contraindicated). See Table 1.

Interactions with other drugs have not been established.

Drug-Food Interactions: Interactions with food have not been established.

Drug-Herb Interactions: Interactions with herbal products have not been established.

Drug-Laboratory Test Interactions: Interactions with laboratory tests have not been established.

Table 1: LASIX SPECIAL

Established or Predicted Drug-Drug Interactions

Proper Name	Ref	Effect	Clinical Comments
Anticonvulsants			
Carbamazepine Phenobarbital Phenytoin	T	↓ furosemide diuretic effect	Anticonvulsant drugs (phenytoin, carbamazepine, phenobarbital), which, like furosemide, undergo significant renal tubular secretion, may also attenuate the effect of furosemide.
Antidiabetics			
Antidiabetics	T	↓ antidiabetic drug effect	The effects of antidiabetic drugs may be reduced.
Antihypertensive Agents			
ACE inhibitors	CT	↓ blood pressure and renal function	Especially in combination with ACE inhibitors, a marked hypotension may be seen sometimes progressing to shock. The concomitant administration of LASIX SPECIAL with ACE-inhibitors may lead to deterioration in renal function and, in isolated cases, to acute renal failure. Consideration must be given to interrupting the administration of furosemide temporarily or at least reducing the dose of furosemide for three days before starting treatment with, or increasing the dose of, an ACE inhibitor.
Angiotensin II receptor antagonists	CT	↓ blood pressure and renal function	Especially in combination with angiotensin II receptor antagonists, a marked hypotension may be seen sometimes progressing to shock. The concomitant administration of LASIX SPECIAL with angiotensin II receptor antagonists may lead to deterioration in renal function and, in isolated cases, to acute renal failure. Consideration must be given to interrupting the administration of furosemide temporarily or at least reducing the dose of furosemide for three days before starting treatment with, or increasing the dose of, an angiotensin II receptor antagonist.
Cephalosporins			
Cephalosporins	T	↓ renal function	Impairment of renal function may develop in patients receiving concurrent treatment with furosemide and high doses of certain cephalosporins.
Chloral Hydrate			
Chloral Hydrate	C	—	In isolated cases intravenous administration of furosemide within 24 hours of taking chloral hydrate may lead to flushing, sweating attacks, restlessness, nausea, increase in blood pressure and tachycardia. Use of furosemide concomitantly with chloral hydrate is therefore not recommended.
Chlorothiazides			
Chlorothiazides	T	—	The concurrent use of LASIX SPECIAL with chlorothiazide has been reported to decrease hypercalciuria and to dissolve some calculi.
Cisplatin			
Cisplatin	T	↑ nephrotoxicity ↑ ototoxicity	Nephrotoxicity of cisplatin may be enhanced if furosemide is not given in low doses and with positive fluid balance when used to achieve forced diuresis during cisplatin treatment. There is also a risk of ototoxic effects if cisplatin and furosemide are given concomitantly.
Cyclosporine			

(cont'd)

Table 1: LASIX SPECIAL *(cont'd)*

Established or Predicted Drug-Drug Interactions

Proper Name	Ref	Effect	Clinical Comments
Cyclosporine	CT	—	Concomitant use of cyclosporine A and furosemide is associated with increased risk of gouty arthritis secondary to furosemide-induced hyperuricemia and cyclosporine impairment of renal urate excretion.
Digitalis Glycosides			
Digitalis Glycosides	T	↓ potassium plasma concentration	Some electrolyte disturbances (e.g. hypokalemia, hypomagnesemia) may increase the toxicity of certain other drugs (e.g. digitalis preparations and drugs inducing QT interval prolongation syndrome). Particular caution with potassium levels is necessary when the patient is on digitalis glycosides. Potassium supplementation, diminution in dose, or discontinuation of LASIX SPECIAL therapy may be required (see Warnings and Precautions).
Lithium			
Lithium	T	↑ lithium plasma concentration	Renal clearance of lithium is decreased in patients receiving LASIX SPECIAL, resulting in increased risk of cardiotoxic and neurotoxic effects of lithium. Therefore, it is recommended that lithium levels be carefully monitored in patients receiving this combination.
Methotrexate			
Methotrexate	T	↓ furosemide diuretic effect	Methotrexate, which like furosemide, undergoes significant renal tubular secretion, may also attenuate the effect of furosemide.
Nephrotoxic Drugs			
Nephrotoxic Drugs	T	↑ nephrotoxicity	The harmful effects of nephrotoxic drugs on the kidney may be increased.
Non-Steroidal Anti-Inflammatory Drugs (NSAIDs)			
Indomethacin	CT	↓ furosemide diuretic effect	Clinical studies have shown that the administration of indomethacin can reduce the natriuretic and anti-hypertensive effect of LASIX SPECIAL in some patients. This response has been attributed to inhibition of prostaglandin synthesis by indomethacin. Therefore, when indomethacin is added to the treatment of a patient receiving LASIX SPECIAL, or LASIX SPECIAL is added to the treatment of a patient receiving indomethacin, the patient should be closely observed to determine if the desired effect of LASIX SPECIAL is obtained. Indomethacin blocks the LASIX SPECIAL-induced increase in plasma-renin activity. This fact should be kept in mind when evaluating plasma-renin activity in hypertensive patients.
Potassium-depleting Steroids			
Potassium-depleting Steroids	T	↓ potassium plasma concentration	Some electrolyte disturbances (e.g. hypokalemia, hypomagnesemia) may increase the toxicity of certain other drugs (e.g. digitalis preparations and drugs inducing QT interval prolongation syndrome). Particular caution with potassium levels is necessary when the patient is on potassium-depleting steroids. Potassium supplementation, diminution in dose, or discontinuation of LASIX SPECIAL therapy may be required (see Warnings and Precautions).
Probenecid			
Probenecid	T	↓ furosemide diuretic effect	Probenecid, which like furosemide, undergoes significant renal tubular secretion, may also attenuate the effect of furosemide.
Radiocontrast Agents			
Radiocontrast Agents	CT	↑ radiocontrast nephropathy	Patients who were at high risk for radiocontrast nephropathy treated with furosemide experienced a higher incidence of deterioration in renal function after receiving radiocontrast compared to high-risk patients who received only intravenous hydration prior to receiving radiocontrast.
Risperidone			
Risperidone	CT	—	Caution should be exercised and the risks and benefits of the combination or co-treatment with furosemide or with other potent diuretics should be considered prior to the decision to use. See Warnings and Precautions, regarding increased mortality in elderly patients with dementia concomitantly receiving risperidone.
Salicylates			
Salicylates	T	↑ salicylate toxicity	Patients receiving high doses of salicylates in conjunction with LASIX SPECIAL may experience salicylate toxicity at lower doses because of competition for renal excretory sites.

(cont'd)

Table 1: LASIX SPECIAL *(cont'd)*

Established or Predicted Drug-Drug Interactions

Proper Name	Ref	Effect	Clinical Comments
Sucralfate			
Sucralfate	T	↓ furosemide absorption	Concurrent administration of LASIX SPECIAL and sucralfate should be avoided, as sucralfate reduces the absorption of furosemide from the intestine and hence weakens its effect.
Theophylline			
Theophylline	T	↑ theophylline effect	The effects of theophylline may be increased.

Legend: C=Case Study; CT=Clinical Trial; T=Theoretical.

DOSAGE AND ADMINISTRATION: Dosing Considerations: LASIX SPECIAL is to be used under strict medical supervision in a hospital setting.

The high-dosage formulation LASIX SPECIAL is intended exclusively for selected patients with severely impaired glomerular filtration (GFR of less than 20 mL/min. but greater than 5 mL/min.), who have not responded to conventional doses of LASIX (see Indications and Clinical Use).

When LASIX SPECIAL is used in high doses careful attention must be paid to the following points:

- **If the patient is in shock, hypovolemia and hypotension must be corrected by appropriate measures before starting therapy.**
- **Any serious abnormalities of serum electrolytes or acid-base balance must be corrected beforehand.**
- **When treating patients with conditions likely to interfere with micturition, such as prostatic hypertrophy or disturbed consciousness, it is absolutely essential to ensure free urinary drainage.**
- **Because of the wide and unpredictable individual variations in responsiveness it is important to adjust dosage and route of administration to individual needs.**
- **Once the desired rise in urinary output has begun, exact balance of water intake and water output must be maintained throughout the course of treatment, so as to avoid hypovolemia or hypotension. Careful electrolyte replacement is also necessary.**

The dosage of high strength LASIX SPECIAL given below is for adults only. The administration of large doses of furosemide in children has been associated with permanent deafness (see Warnings and Precautions).

Recommended Dose and Dosage Adjustment: Oral: Initial Dose: The dose of furosemide which has been found to produce an effective diuresis when given intravenously is used as the initial dose.

For the initial intravenous dose, follow the manufacturer's dosage recommendations for the administration of intravenous furosemide as stated in the appropriate Product Monograph.

Additional Dose: Should the initial dose fail to produce an adequate increase (at least 40-50 mL) in urinary output within 4-6 hours, the dose may be raised by 250 to 500 mg at a time.

For selected patients with advanced chronic renal failure, diuretic therapy may be started with LASIX orally. If conventional doses (80 to 160 mg orally) fail to produce an adequate diuresis, a single dose of 250 mg is given as a starting dose. If a satisfactory diuresis does not ensue within 4-6 hours, the initial dose may be doubled to 500 mg.

The criterion of optimal dosage is a urinary output of at least 2.5 litres per day.

A maximum daily dose of 1000 mg should not be exceeded.

OVERDOSAGE:

Symptoms: Dehydration, electrolyte depletion and hypotension may be caused by overdosage or accidental ingestion. In cirrhotic patients, overdosage might precipitate hepatic coma.

The clinical picture in acute or chronic overdose depends primarily on the extent and consequences of electrolyte and fluid loss, e.g. hypovolemia, dehydration, hemoconcentration, cardiac arrhythmias (including A-V block and ventricular fibrillation). Symptoms of these disturbances include severe hypotension (progressing to shock), acute renal failure, thrombosis, delirious states, flaccid paralysis, apathy and confusion.

Treatment: The drug should be discontinued and appropriate corrective treatment applied: replacement of excessive fluid and electrolyte losses; serum electrolytes, carbon dioxide level and blood pressure should be determined frequently. Adequate drainage must be assured in patients with urinary bladder outlet obstruction (such as prostatic hypertrophy).

No specific antidote to furosemide is known. If ingestion has only just taken place, attempts may be made to limit further systemic absorption of the active ingredient by measures such as gastric lavage or those designed to reduce absorption (e.g. activated charcoal).

For management of a suspected drug overdose, contact your regional Poison Control Centre. See the *CPS* Directory section for a list of Poison Control Centres.

ACTION AND CLINICAL PHARMACOLOGY: Mechanism of Action: Animal experiments using stop-flow and micropuncture techniques have demonstrated that furosemide inhibits sodium reabsorption in the ascending limb of Henle's loop as well as in both proximal and distal tubules. The action of LASIX SPECIAL on the distal tubule is independent of any inhibitory effect on carbonic anhydrase or aldosterone.

Furosemide may promote diuresis in cases which have previously proved resistant to other diuretics.

Pharmacodynamics: A continuous infusion of furosemide is more effective than repetitive bolus injections. Moreover, above a certain bolus dose of the drug there is no significant increase in effect.

The effect of furosemide is reduced if there is lowered tubular secretion or intra-tubular albumin binding of the drug.

Pharmacokinetics: Absorption: In man, LASIX SPECIAL is rapidly absorbed from the gastro-intestinal tract. The diuretic effect of furosemide is apparent within one hour following oral administration and the peak effect occurs in the first or second hour. The duration of action is 4-6 hours but may continue up to 8 hours. Following intravenous administration of the drug, the diuresis occurs within 30 minutes and the duration of action is about 2 hours.

Metabolism: A small fraction is metabolized by cleavage of the side chain.

Excretion: Urinary excretion is accomplished both by glomerular filtration and proximal tubular secretion, together this accounts for roughly only 2/3 of the ingested dose, the remainder being excreted in the feces.

Table 2 summarizes the elimination kinetics of furosemide.

Table 2: LASIX SPECIAL

Summary of Furosemide's Elimination Kinetics

Subjects	Route of Administration	Dose (mg)	Rate of Administration	Biliary Excretion	Max. Serum Concentration	$t_{½}$ (h)
Normal	Oral	40	—	10–15%	<1 μg/mL	4.0
Normal	I.V.	40	Bolus	10–15%	2.5 μg/mL	4.5
Renal insufficiency	I.V.	1000	25 mg/min	60%	53 μg/mL	13.5
Renal insufficiency	I.V.	1000	4 mg/min	—	29 μg/mL	—

Special Populations and Conditions: Pediatrics: Depending on the maturity of the kidney, the elimination of furosemide may be slowed down. The metabolism of the drug is also reduced if the infant's glucuronisation capacity is impaired.

The terminal half-life is below 12 hours in infants with a post-conceptional age of more than 33 weeks.

In infants of 2 months and older, the terminal clearance is the same as in adults.

Geriatrics: The elimination of furosemide is slowed down due to reduced renal function in the elderly.

Gender: Data unavailable.

Race: Data unavailable.

Hepatic Insufficiency: In liver failure, the half-life of furosemide is increased by 30% to 90% mainly due to a larger volume of distribution. Additionally, in this patient group there is a wide variation in all pharmacokinetic parameters.

Renal Insufficiency: In renal failure, the elimination of furosemide is slowed down and the half-life prolonged; the terminal half-life may be up to 24 hours in patients with severe renal failure.

In nephrotic syndrome the reduced plasma protein concentration leads to a higher concentration of unbound (free) furosemide. On the other hand, efficacy of furosemide is reduced in these patients due to binding to intratubular albumin and lowered tubular secretion.

Furosemide is poorly dialyzable in patients undergoing haemodialysis, peritoneal dialysis and CAPD.

Genetic Polymorphism: Data unavailable.

STORAGE AND STABILITY: Temperature: Tablets: Store between 15 and 30°C.

Light: Protect from light.

INFORMATION FOR THE PATIENT: Published in e-CPS, available by subscription at www.e-cps.ca.

DOSAGE FORMS, COMPOSITION AND PACKAGING: Each yellow, round, tablet, double-scored on one side, debossed with the letters "D", "L" and "X" (each in a separate field) on the scored side, the other side debossed with the Hoechst "Tower and Bridge" logo, contains: furosemide 500 mg. Nonmedicinal ingredients: cellulose, corn starch, colloidal silicon dioxide, D&C Yellow #10, FD&C Yellow #6, lactose monohydrate, magnesium stearate, sodium starch glycolate and talc. HDPE bottles of 20.

(Shown in Product Identification Section)

Lax-A-Day™
polyethylene glycol
Laxative

PendoPharm

Date of Preparation: July 24, 2008
Date of Revision: October 27, 2008

SUMMARY PRODUCT INFORMATION:

Route of Administration	Dosage Form/ Strength	Clinically Relevant Nonmedicinal Ingredients
Oral	Powder for oral solution	None. For a complete listing see Dosage Forms, Composition and Packaging.

INDICATIONS AND CLINICAL USE: Adults: LAX-A-DAY (Polyethylene Glycol 3350 Powder for Oral Solution) is indicated for:

- Constipation: LAX-A-DAY is indicated as a laxative for the treatment of occasional constipation (see Dosage and Administration).

CONTRAINDICATIONS: LAX-A-DAY is contraindicated in patients with:

- known or suspected bowel obstruction, and
- known allergies to polyethylene glycol.

WARNINGS AND PRECAUTIONS: General: Patients with symptoms suggestive of bowel obstruction, appendicitis or inflamed bowels (fever, nausea, vomiting, abdominal pain or distention) should consult a doctor to rule out these conditions before initiating LAX-A-DAY therapy.

Overuse or extended use of any laxative may cause dependence for bowel function.

Do not take any type of laxative for more than one (1) week, unless recommended by a physician.

A laxative should not be taken within two (2) hours of another medicine because the desired effect of the other medicine may be reduced.

Patients presenting with complaints of constipation should have a thorough medical history and physical examination to detect associated metabolic, endocrine and neurogenic conditions, and medications. A diagnostic evaluation should include a structural examination of the colon. Patients should be educated about good defecatory and eating habits (such as high fiber diets) and lifestyle changes (adequate dietary fiber and fluid intake, regular exercise) which may produce more regular bowel habits.

LAX-A-DAY should be administered after being dissolved in approximately 250 mL of water, juice, soda, coffee, or tea.

Special Populations: Pregnant Women: Animal reproductive studies have not been performed with Polyethylene Glycol 3350. It is also not known whether Polyethylene Glycol 3350 can cause fetal harm when administered to a pregnant woman, or can affect reproductive capacity. The use of LAX-A-DAY should be avoided in women who are pregnant unless clearly needed and directed by a physician.

Nursing Women: It is unknown if LAX-A-DAY is excreted in human milk. Because many drugs are excreted in human milk, precaution should be exercised. The use of LAX-A-DAY should be avoided in nursing women unless clearly needed and directed by a physician.

Pediatrics (<18 years of age): Safety and effectiveness of LAX-A-DAY in pediatric patients has not been established.

Geriatrics (>65 years of age) : There is no evidence for special considerations when LAX-A-DAY is administered to elderly patients. If diarrhea occurs, LAX-A-DAY should be discontinued.

Monitoring and Laboratory Tests: No clinically significant effects on laboratory tests have been demonstrated.

In one study, CBC, blood chemistry, and urinalysis were performed after the 14-day treatment period. Laboratory data were compared by repeated measures of analysis of variance. A value $p < 0.05$ was considered statistically significant. No statistically or clinically significant differences between placebo and laxative groups were detected for laboratory measurements.

In another study, CBC, blood chemistry, and urinalysis were performed before and after each 10-day treatment period. No clinically significant changes in laboratory measurements were seen.

ADVERSE REACTIONS: Adverse Drug Reaction Overview: Occasionally, LAX-A-DAY may cause nausea, abdominal bloating, cramping, diarrhea and/or gas. High doses may produce diarrhea and excessive stool frequency, particularly in elderly nursing home patients.

On rare occasions, hives and skin rashes have been reported which are suggestive of an allergic reaction. Patients taking other medications containing polyethylene glycol have occasionally developed urticaria suggestive of an allergic reaction.

DRUG INTERACTIONS: No specific drug interactions have been demonstrated.

A laxative should not be taken within two (2) hours of taking another medicine because the desired effect of the other medicine may be reduced.

DOSAGE AND ADMINISTRATION: Recommended Dose and Dosage Adjustment: Adults: The usual dose is 17 grams (about 1 heaping tablespoon) of LAX-A-DAY powder per day (or as directed by physician) to be stirred in a cup (250 mL) of water, juice, soda, coffee, or tea until completely dissolved.

This product should be used for one week or less or as directed by a physician. Treatment for two to four days (48 to 96 hours) may be required to produce a bowel movement.

Each bottle of LAX-A-DAY is supplied with a dosing cup marked to contain 17 grams of laxative powder when filled to the indicated line. Two to 4 days (48 to 96 hours) may be required to produce a bowel movement.

Special Patient Populations: Treatment of Pregnant or Nursing Women: LAX-A-DAY should only be administered to a pregnant or nursing woman on the advice of a physician (see Warnings and Precautions).

Elderly Patients: No dose adjustment is recommended for elderly patients solely on the basis of their age (see Warnings and Precautions).

Pediatrics: LAX-A-DAY is not indicated for use in children under 18 years of age unless recommended by a physician (see Warnings and Precautions).

OVERDOSAGE:
There have been no reports of accidental overdosage. In the event of overdosage, diarrhea would be the expected major event. If an overdose of drug occurred without concomitant ingestion of fluid, dehydration due to diarrhea may result. In the event of overdose, medication should be terminated and free water administered.

> For management of a suspected drug overdose, CPhA recommends that you contact your **regional Poison Control Centre**. See the *CPS* Directory section for a list of Poison Control Centres.

ACTION AND CLINICAL PHARMACOLOGY: Mechanism of Action: Pharmacology: Polyethylene Glycol 3350 is an osmotic agent which causes water to be retained with the stool.

Essentially, complete recovery of Polyethylene Glycol 3350 was shown in normal subjects without constipation. Attempts at recovery of Polyethylene Glycol 3350 in constipated patients resulted in incomplete and highly variable recovery.

An in vitro study showed indirectly that Polyethylene Glycol 3350 was not fermented into hydrogen or methane by the colonic microflora in human feces. Polyethylene Glycol 3350 appears to have no effect on the active absorption or secretion of glucose or electrolytes. There is no evidence of tachyphylaxis.

Pharmacokinetics: Special Populations and Conditions: Pediatrics: The safety and efficacy of LAX-A-DAY for use in children under 18 years of age have not been established. LAX-A-DAY is not indicated for use in children under 18 years of age.

Geriatrics: There is no evidence for special considerations when LAX-A-DAY is administered to elderly patients. In geriatric nursing home patients a higher incidence of diarrhea occurred at the recommended 17 gram dose.

STORAGE AND STABILITY: Store at room temperature (15 to 30°C).

SPECIAL HANDLING INSTRUCTIONS: None.

INFORMATION FOR THE PATIENT: Published in e-CPS, available by subscription at www.e-cps.ca.

DOSAGE FORMS, COMPOSITION AND PACKAGING: LAX-A-DAY is available in powdered form, for oral administration after complete dissolution in water, juice, soda, coffee, or tea. LAX-A-DAY is available in two package sizes, 238 g and 510 g.

The dosing cup with each bottle is marked with a measuring line and should be used to measure a single daily dose of LAX-A-DAY (17 grams, or about 1 heaping tablespoon).

Lectopam® $^{C}_{T}$

bromazepam

Anxiolytic—Sedative

Roche

SUPPLIED: 3 mg: Each pale red in colour, slightly speckled, cylindrical and biplane in shape tablet, single scored on one side, engraved with Roche/3 on the other side contains: bromazepam 3 mg. Nonmedicinal ingredients: iron oxide red, lactose monohydrate, magnesium stearate, microcrystalline cellulose and talc. PVC blister packs. There are 10 tablets per blister card and 10 blister cards per carton, for a total of 100 tablets per unit. Store at 15 to 30°C.

6 mg: Each greenish-grey to greyish-green in colour, slightly speckled, cylindrical and biplane in shape tablet, single scored on one side, engraved with Roche/6 on the other side contains: bromazepam 6 mg. Nonmedicinal ingredients: indigotine aluminum lake, iron oxide yellow, lactose monohydrate, magnesium stearate, microcrystalline cellulose and talc. PVC blister packs. There are 10 tablets per blister card and 10 blister cards per carton, for a total of 100 tablets per unit. Store at 15 to 30°C.

Lederle Leucovorin® Pr

calcium folinate

Folic Acid Derivative

Pfizer

Date of Preparation: October 10, 1995
Date of Revision: January 25, 2008

Since leucovorin may enhance the toxicity of fluorouracil, leucovorin/fluorouracil combination therapy for advanced colorectal cancer should be administered under the supervision of a physician experienced in the use of antimetabolite cancer chemotherapy. Particular care should be taken in the treatment of elderly or debilitated colorectal cancer patients, as these patients may be at increased risk of severe toxicity. Deaths from severe enterocolitis, diarrhea and dehydration have been reported in elderly patients receiving leucovorin and fluorouracil. Concomitant granulocytopenia and fever were present in some but not all of the patients.

PHARMACOLOGY: Lederle LEUCOVORIN (calcium folinate), the calcium salt of folinic acid (citrovorum factor), is a mixture of the diastereoisomers of the 5-formyl derivative of tetrahydrofolic acid. The biologically active component of the mixture is the (-)-L-isomer. It is a metabolite of folic acid and an essential coenzyme for nucleic acid synthesis used in cytotoxic therapy.

Leucovorin is a reduced form of folic acid, which is readily converted to other reduced folic acid derivatives (e.g., tetrahydrofolate).

Because it does not require reduction by dihydrofolate reductase as does folic acid, leucovorin is not affected by blockage of this enzyme by folic acid antagonists (dihydrofolate reductase inhibitors). This allows purine and thymidine synthesis, and thus DNA, RNA and protein synthesis, to occur. Leucovorin may limit methotrexate action on normal cells by competing with methotrexate for the same transport processes into the cell. Leucovorin rescues bone marrow and gastrointestinal cells from methotrexate but has no apparent effect on pre-existing methotrexate nephrotoxicity.

Leucovorin is extensively converted to 5-methyltetrahydrofolate in the intestine prior to absorption. In this form, it is a major component of the total active human serum folate. Oral absorption is saturable at doses above 25 mg.

Leucovorin enhances the cytotoxicity of fluoropyrimidines such as 5-fluorouracil (5-FU) by their metabolites, methylene tetrahydrofolate and fluorodeoxyuridine monophosphate, forming a stable ternary complex with thymidylate synthase, and thereby, decreasing intracellular levels of that enzyme and the product thymidylate. The cell then dies as a result of thymine starvation.

INDICATIONS: To diminish the toxicity and counteract the effect of impaired methotrexate elimination. To treat the megaloblastic anemias due to folate deficiency, as in sprue, nutritional deficiency, megaloblastic anemias of pregnancy and infancy.

CONTRAINDICATIONS: Calcium folinate therapy is contraindicated for the following: Known hypersensitivity to calcium folinate, or to any components of the product formulation; Pernicious anemia or other megaloblastic anemias where Vitamin B_{12} is deficient. A hematologic remission may occur while neurologic manifestations continue to progress.

WARNINGS: Cases of Stevens-Johnson Syndrome (SJS) and Toxic Epidermal Necrolysis (TEN), some fatal, have been reported in patients receiving leucovorin in combination with other agents known to be associated with these disorders. A contributory role of leucovorin in these occurrences of SJS/TEN cannot be excluded.

In the treatment of accidental overdosages of folic acid antagonists, leucovorin should be administered as promptly as possible. As the time interval between the administration of antifolate and leucovorin rescue increases, the effectiveness of leucovorin in counteracting toxicity decreases. Monitoring of the serum methotrexate concentration is essential in determining the optimal dose and duration of therapy. Delayed methotrexate excretion may be caused by a third space fluid accumulation (i.e., ascites, pleural effusion), renal insufficiency, low pH of urine, or inadequate hydration. Under such circumstances, higher doses of leucovorin or prolonged administration may be indicated.

Treatment-related deaths have been sporadically reported in patients treated with leucovorin plus fluorouracil combination therapy regimens. In general, diarrhea or stomatitis/mucositis are the first indications that severe and potentially life-threatening toxicity could develop. Patients who experience these symptoms while receiving any combination therapy regimen incorporating leucovorin plus fluorouracil should be carefully followed and further therapy should be withheld until these symptoms resolve.

Leucovorin enhances the toxicity of fluorouracil. When these drugs are administered concurrently in the palliative therapy of advanced colorectal cancer, the dosage of fluorouracil must be reduced. Although the toxicities observed in patients treated with the combination of leucovorin plus fluorouracil are qualitatively similar to those observed in patients treated with fluorouracil alone, gastrointestinal toxicities (particularly stomatitis and diarrhea) are observed more commonly and may be more severe in patients receiving the combination (see Precautions).

Therapy with leucovorin/fluorouracil must not be initiated or continued in patients who have symptoms of gastrointestinal toxicity of any severity, until those symptoms have resolved. Patients with diarrhea must be monitored with particular care until the diarrhea has resolved, as rapid clinical deterioration leading to death can occur. Elderly or debilitated patients are at greater risk for severe toxicity receiving this therapy.

Seizures and/or syncope have been reported rarely in cancer patients receiving leucovorin, usually in association with fluoropyrimidine administration, and most commonly in those with CNS metastases or other predisposing factors; however, a causal relationship has not been established.

PRECAUTIONS: Calcium folinate treatment may mask pernicious anemia and other megaloblastic anemias resulting from vitamin B_{12} deficiency.

Calcium folinate should only be used with 5-fluorouracil or methotrexate under the direct supervision of a clinician experienced in the use of cancer chemotherapeutic agents.

Many cytotoxic medicinal products—direct or indirect DNA synthesis inhibitors—lead to macrocytosis (hydroxycarbamide, cytarabine, mercaptopurine, thioguanine). Such macrocytosis should not be treated with folinic acid.

In epileptic patients treated with phenobarbital, phenytoin, primidone, and succinimides there is a risk to increase the frequency of seizures due to a decrease of plasma concentrations of anti-epileptic drugs. Clinical monitoring, possibly monitoring of the plasma concentrations and, if necessary, dose adaptation of the anti-epileptic drug during calcium folinate administration and after discontinuation is recommended.

Drug Interactions: **Calcium folinate may diminish the effect of anti-epileptic substances: phenobarbital, primidone, phenytoin and succinimides, and may increase the frequency of seizures (a decrease of plasma levels of enzymatic inductor anticonvulsant drugs may be observed because the hepatic metabolism is increased as folates are one of the cofactors).**

When calcium folinate is given in conjunction with a folic acid antagonist (eg, cotrimoxazole, pyrimethamine) the efficacy of the folic acid antagonist may either be reduced or completely neutralised.

Preliminary animal and human studies have shown that small quantities of systemically administered leucovorin enter the CSF primarily as 5-methyltetrahydrofolate and, in humans, remain 1 to 3 orders of magnitude lower than the usual methotrexate concentrations following intrathecal administration. However, high doses of leucovorin may reduce the efficacy of intrathecally administered methotrexate.

Leucovorin may enhance the toxicity of fluorouracil (see Warnings).

Pregnancy: **Teratogenic Effects: There are no adequate and well-controlled clinical studies conducted in pregnant or breast-feeding women. No formal animal reproductive toxicity studies with calcium folinate have been conducted. There are no indications that folic acid induces harmful effects if administered during pregnancy. During pregnancy, methotrexate should only be administered on strict indications, where the benefits of the drug to the mother should be weighed against possible hazards to the foetus. Should treatment with methotrexate or other folate antagonists take place despite pregnancy or lactation, there are no limitations as to the use of calcium folinate to diminish toxicity or counteract the effects.**

5-fluorouracil use is generally contraindicated during pregnancy and contraindicated during breast-feeding; this applies also to the combined use of calcium folinate with 5-fluorouracil.

Please refer also to the health-care professional label for methotrexate, other folate antagonists and 5-fluorouracil-containing medicinal products.

Lactation: It is not known whether this drug is excreted in human milk. Because many drugs are excreted in human milk, caution should be exercised when leucovorin is administered to a nursing mother.

Children: There are no data available in children.

Laboratory Tests: The following provides general advice for monitoring patients; however, specific monitoring recommendations may vary with local medical practice.

5-FU/calcium folinate therapy: Complete blood count (CBC) with differential and platelets: prior to each treatment; weekly during the first two courses; at time of anticipated white blood cell (WBC) nadir in all courses thereafter.

Electrolytes and liver function tests: prior to each treatment for the first three courses and prior to every other course thereafter.

Methotrexate/calcium folinate therapy: Serum creatinine levels and serum methotrexate levels: at least once daily.

Urine pH: in cases of methotrexate overdose or delayed excretion, monitor as appropriate, to ensure maintenance of pH ≥7.0.

ADVERSE EFFECTS: Allergic sensitization, including anaphylactoid/ anaphylactic reactions (including shock) and urticaria, has been reported following administration of Leucovorin.

In combination regimens, the toxicity profile of 5-FU is enhanced by leucovorin. The most common manifestations are mucositis, stomatitis, leukopenia, and/or diarrhea which may be dose-limiting. In clinical trials with this drug combination, these toxicities were found to be reversible with appropriate modification of 5-FU administration.

LEUCOVORIN: Immune System Disorders: Frequency undetermined: **allergic reactions, urticaria**. Very Rare: **anaphylactoid/anaphylactoid reactions (including shock).**

Nervous System Disorders: Rare: seizures and/or syncope.

General Disorders and Administration Site Conditions: Frequency undetermined: fever.

Cases of Stevens-Johnson Syndrome (SJS) and Toxic Epidermal Necrolysis (TEN), some fatal, have been reported in patients receiving leucovorin in combination with other agents known to be associated with these disorders. A contributory role of leucovorin in these occurrences of SJS/TEN cannot be excluded.

LEUCOVORIN in Combination with 5-FU: **In combination regimens, the toxicity profile of 5-FU is enhanced by Leucovorin (calcium folinate). The most common manifestations are mucositis, stomatitis, leukopenia and/or diarrhea, which may be dose-limiting. In clinical trials with this drug combination, these toxicities were found to be reversible with appropriate modification of 5-FU administration.**

Generally, the safety profile depends on the applied regimen of 5-fluorouracil due to enhancement of the 5-fluorouracil induced toxicities. Additional undesirable effects when used in combination with 5-fluorouracil:

Gastrointestinal Disorders: Very common: **nausea and vomiting, diarrhea**.

Hepatobiliary Disorders: Frequency undetermined: hyperammonemia.

Skin and Subcutaneous Tissue Disorders: Frequency undetermined: **Palmar-Plantar Erythrodysaesthesia**.

General Disorders and Administration Site Conditions: Frequency undetermined: **mucositis, including stomatitis** and chelitis.

Fatalities have occurred as a result of gastrointestinal toxicity (predominantly mucositis and diarrhea) and myelosuppression. In patients with diarrhea, rapid clinical deterioration leading to death can occur.

OVERDOSE:

Symptoms: Folic acid is a water soluble vitamin converted in the body by the action of folate reductase to folinic acid (Leucovorin) which is rapidly eliminated in the urine.

Folic acid has low acute and chronic toxicities in man. **There have been no reported sequelae in patients who have received significantly more calcium folinate than the recommended dosage. However, excessive amounts of Leucovorin (calcium folinate) may nullify the chemotherapeutic effect of folic acid antagonists.** No adverse effects have been noted in adults after the ingestion of 400 mg/day for 5 months or 10 mg/day for 5 years.

Should overdosage of the combination of 5-fluorouracil and calcium folinate occur, the overdosage instructions for 5-FU should be followed.

> For management of a suspected drug overdose, CPhA recommends that you contact your **regional Poison Control Centre**. See the *CPS* Directory section for a list of Poison Control Centres.

DOSAGE: Tablets are administered orally.

Impaired Methotrexate Elimination or Accidental Overdosage: Leucovorin rescue should begin as soon as possible after an inadvertent overdosage and within 24 hours of Methotrexate administration when there is delayed excretion (see Warnings).

There are no fixed guidelines regarding the dose of methotrexate that triggers an automatic subsequent calcium folinate administration, since tolerance to this folate antagonist depends on various factors. The dose of methotrexate varies, nevertheless folinate rescue is necessary when methotrexate is given at doses exceeding 500 mg/m² and has to be considered with doses of 100 mg-500 mg/m².

Calcium folinate rescue treatment should commence approximately 24 hours after the beginning of methotrexate infusion. Dosage regimens vary depending upon the dose of methotrexate administered. In general, calcium folinate should be administered at a dose of 15 mg (approximately 10 mg/m²) every 6 hours for 10 doses, either parenterally by intramuscular injection, bolus intravenous injection, intravenous infusion, or orally using calcium folinate tablets.

If serum creatinine increases after methotrexate therapy or if methotrexate plasma concentrations are above certain threshold (see Table 1), the dose of calcium folinate should be increased according to the plasma methotrexate concentrations, as soon as the risk is recognized. In the presence of gastrointestinal toxicity, nausea, or vomiting, calcium folinate should be administered parenterally. In the case of intravenous administration, no more than 160 mg of calcium folinate should be injected per minute due to the calcium content of the solution. Further, oral administration of doses greater than 25 mg is not recommended since the digestive absorption of calcium folinate is saturable; these doses should be administered parenterally.

In addition to calcium folinate administration, measures to ensure the prompt excretion of methotrexate are an integral part of the calcium folinate rescue treatment. These measures include: a) Maintenance of urine output above 2500 mL/24 h in adults by increased oral or intravenous fluids 12 hours before and for 36 hours after the end of methotrexate infusion. b) Alkalinisation of urine so that the urinary pH is greater than 7.0 before methotrexate infusion. c) Plasma methotrexate concentration and serum creatinine should be measured at least 24, 48, and 72 hours after the initiation of the methotrexate infusion. These measurements must be continued until the plasma methotrexate level is less than 10-7 molar (0.1µM).

Delayed methotrexate excretion may be seen in some patients. This may be caused by a third space accumulation (as seen in ascites or pleural effusion for example), renal insufficiency or inadequate hydration. See Precautions. Under such circumstances, higher doses of calcium folinate and/or prolonged administration may be indicated. Some dosage and administration guidelines are given in Table 1.

Table 1: Lederle LEUCOVORIN

Dosage and Administration Guidelines for Calcium Folinate Rescue

Clinical Situation	Laboratory Findings	Calcium Folinate Dosage and Duration
Normal methotrexate elimination	Serum methotrexate level ≤10 µM at 24 hours after administration, ≤1 µM at 48 hours, and <0.1 µM at 72 hours.	15 mg PO, IM, or IV every 6 hours for 60 hours (10 doses starting at 24 hours after start of methotrexate infusion).
Delayed late methotrexate elimination	Serum methotrexate level remaining >0.1 µM at 72 hours, and >0.1 µM at 96 hours after administration.	Continue 15 mg PO, IM, or IV every 6 hours, until methotrexate level is less than 0.1 µM.
Delayed early methotrexate elimination and/or evidence of acute renal failure	Serum methotrexate level of >10 µM at 24 hours, or >1 µM at 48 hours after administration **or** a 100% or greater increase in serum creatinine level at 24 hours after methotrexate administration.	150 mg IV every 3 hours, until methotrexate level is less than 1 µM; then 15 mg IV every 3 hours until methotrexate level is less than 0.1 µM.

Hydration (3 L/d) and urinary alkalinization with $NaHCO_3$ should be employed concomitantly. The bicarbonate dose should be adjusted to maintain the urine pH at 7.0 or greater.

Megaloblastic Anemia Due to Folic Acid Deficiency: Doses up to 15 mg daily have been suggested.

INFORMATION FOR THE PATIENT: Published in e-CPS, available by subscription at www.e-cps.ca.

SUPPLIED: Each round, light yellow, scored tablet, engraved "LL5" and "U2", contains: leucovorin (as calcium) 5 mg. Nonmedicinal ingredients: lactose, magnesium stearate, microcrystalline cellulose, sodium starch glycolate and starch pregelatinized 1500. Tartrazine-free. Bottles of 24 and 100. Store at 15 to 30°C. Protect from light.

The reader is invited to consult CPhA's monograph **HMG-CoA Reductase Inhibitors**.

Lescol® Ⓟ
fluvastatin sodium
Lipid Metabolism Regulator

Novartis Pharmaceuticals

Lescol® XL Ⓟ
fluvastatin sodium
Lipid Metabolism Regulator

Novartis Pharmaceuticals

Date of Preparation: August 13, 1997
Date of Revision: September 24, 2009

SUMMARY PRODUCT INFORMATION:

Route of Administration	Dosage Form/ Strength	Clinically Relevant Nonmedicinal Ingredients
Oral	LESCOL 20 and 40 mg capsules	Not applicable For a complete listing see Dosage Forms, Composition and Packaging.
Oral	LESCOL XL 80 mg extended release tablets	Not applicable For a complete listing see Dosage Forms, Composition and Packaging.

INDICATIONS AND CLINICAL USE: Therapy with lipid-altering agents should be considered a component of multiple risk factor intervention in those individuals at increased risk for atherosclerotic vascular disease due to hypercholesterolemia. LESCOL/LESCOL XL (fluvastatin sodium) should be used in addition to a diet restricted in saturated fat and cholesterol when the response to diet and other non-pharmacological measures alone has been inadequate.

Hypercholesterolemia and Mixed Hyperlipidemia: Adults: LESCOL/LESCOL XL are indicated as an adjunct to diet (at least equivalent to the Adult Treatment Panel III (ATP III TLC diet)) in the treatment of elevated total cholesterol (Total-C), LDL-C and triglycerides (TG) and Apo B levels in patients with primary hypercholesterolemia and mixed hyperlipidemia (Fredrickson Type IIa and IIb) whose response to dietary restriction of saturated fat and cholesterol and other nonpharmacological measures has not been adequate.

Pediatrics (10-17 years of age): LESCOL/LESCOL XL are indicated as an adjunct to diet for the reduction of elevated total cholesterol (Total-C), LDL-C and Apo B levels in children and adolescents aged 10 years and older with heterozygous familial hypercholesterolemia.

Therapy with lipid-altering agents should be considered only after secondary causes for hyperlipidemia such as poorly controlled diabetes mellitus, hypothyroidism, nephrotic syndrome, dysproteinemias, obstructive liver disease, other medication, or alcoholism, have been excluded. Prior to initiation of fluvastatin sodium, a lipid profile should be performed to measure Total-C, HDL-C and TG. For patients with TG <4.52 mmol/L (<400 mg/dL), LDL-C can be estimated using the following equation:

$$\text{LDL-C (mmol/L)} = \text{Total-C} - \text{HDL-C} - 0.37\ \text{TG}.$$

For TG levels >4.52 mmol/L (>400 mg/dL), this equation is less accurate and LDL-C concentrations should be determined by ultracentrifugation. In many hypertriglyceridemic patients, LDL-C may be low or normal despite elevated Total-C. In such cases, as with other HMG-CoA reductase inhibitors, LESCOL is not indicated.

Since the goal of treatment is to lower LDL-C, LDL-C levels should be used to initiate and assess treatment response. Only if LDL-C levels are not available, should the total-C be used to monitor therapy.

LESCOL/LESCOL XL have not been studied in conditions where the major abnormality is elevation of chylomicrons, VLDL, or IDL (i.e. hyperlipoproteinemia Types I, III, IV, or V).

Secondary Prevention of Cardiovascular Events: In patients with coronary heart diseases who had undergone a percutaneous intervention (PCI) procedures, LESCOL has been shown to delay the occurrence of major adverse cardiac events (MACE), defined as the first occurrence of cardiac death, nonfatal myocardial infarction or re-intervention procedures.

CONTRAINDICATIONS:

- LESCOL/LESCOL XL (fluvastatin sodium) are contraindicated in patients with known hypersensitivity to any component of this medication (see Dosage Forms, Composition and Packaging).
- LESCOL/LESCOL XL are contraindicated in patients with active liver disease or unexplained, persistent clinically relevant elevations in serum transaminases (see Warnings and Precautions, Hepatic/Biliary/Pancreatic).
- As with other drugs of this class, LESCOL/LESCOL XL are contraindicated during pregnancy and in nursing mothers (see Warnings and Precautions, Special Populations, Pregnant Women/Nursing Women). Cholesterol and other products of cholesterol biosynthesis are essential components for fetal development (including synthesis of steroids and cell membranes). LESCOL/LESCOL XL should be administered to women of childbearing age only when such patients are highly unlikely to conceive and have been informed of the possible harm. If the patient becomes pregnant while taking LESCOL/LESCOL XL, the drug should be discontinued immediately and the patient apprised of the potential harm to the fetus. Atherosclerosis being a chronic process, discontinuation of lipid metabolism regulating drugs during pregnancy should have little impact on the outcome of long-term therapy of primary hypercholesterolemia (see Warnings and Precautions, Special Populations, Pregnant Women/Nursing Women).

WARNINGS AND PRECAUTIONS: General: Before instituting therapy with LESCOL/LESCOL XL (fluvastatin sodium), an attempt should be made to control hypercholesterolemia with appropriate diet, exercise, weight reduction in overweight and obese patients, and to treat other underlying medical problems (see Indications and Clinical Use). The patient should be advised to inform subsequent physicians of the prior use of LESCOL/LESCOL XL or any other lipid metabolism regulator.

Muscle Effects: Effects on skeletal muscle such as rare cases of myalgia, myopathy and, very rarely, rhabdomyolysis have been reported in patients treated with LESCOL/LESCOL XL.

Rare cases of rhabdomyolysis with acute renal failure secondary to myoglobinuria have been reported with LESCOL/LESCOL XL and with other HMG-CoA reductase inhibitors.

Myopathy, defined as muscle pain or muscle weakness in conjunction with increases in creatine phosphokinase (CK) values to greater than ten times the upper limit of normal, should be considered in any patient with diffuse myalgias, muscle tenderness or weakness, and/or a marked elevation of CK. Patients should be advised to report promptly any unexplained muscle pain, tenderness or weakness, particularly if associated with malaise or fever. Patients who develop any signs or symptoms suggestive of myopathy should have their CK levels measured. LESCOL/LESCOL XL therapy should be discontinued if markedly elevated CK levels are measured or myopathy is diagnosed or suspected.

Creatine Kinase Measurement: There is no current evidence to require routine monitoring of plasma total creatine kinase levels in asymptomatic patients on statins. If creatine kinase has to be measured it should not be done following strenuous exercise or in the presence of any plausible alternative cause of CK increase as this makes interpretation difficult.

Pre-disposing Factors for Myopathy/Rhabdomyolysis: LESCOL/LESCOL XL, as with other HMG-CoA reductase inhibitors, should be prescribed with caution in patients with pre-disposing factors for myopathy/rhabdomyolysis. Such factors include: personal or family history of hereditary muscular disorders, previous history of muscle toxicity with another HMG-CoA reductase inhibitor, concomitant use of a fibrate or niacin, hypothyroidism, alcohol abuse, excessive physical exercise, age >70 years, renal impairment, hepatic impairment, diabetes with hepatic fatty change, surgery and trauma, frailty, situations where an increase in plasma levels of active ingredient may occur.

In such situations, the risk of treatment should be considered in relation to the possible benefit and clinical monitoring is recommended. If CK levels are significantly elevated at baseline (>5×Upper Levels of Normal [ULN]), levels should be re-measured within 5 to 7 days later to confirm the results. If CK levels are still significantly elevated (>5×ULN) at baseline, treatment should not be started.

LESCOL/LESCOL XL therapy should be temporarily withheld or discontinued in any patient with an acute serious condition suggestive of myopathy or predisposing to the development of rhabdomyolysis (e.g. sepsis, hypotension, major surgery, trauma, severe metabolic endocrine and electrolyte disorders, or uncontrolled seizures).

Whilst on Treatment: If muscular symptoms like pain, weakness or cramps occur in patients receiving fluvastatin, their CK levels should be measured. Treatment should be stopped, if these levels are found to be significantly elevated (>5×ULN).

LESCOL/LESCOL XL withdrawal should be considered if muscular symptoms are severe and cause daily discomfort, even if CK levels are not significantly elevated (i.e. ≤5×ULN).

Should the symptoms resolve and CK levels return to normal, then reintroduction of fluvastatin or another statin may be considered at the lowest dose and under close monitoring.

An increased risk of myopathy has been reported with HMG-CoA reductase inhibitors which are predominantly CYP3A4 substrates when administered concomitantly with other drugs metabolized by the CYP3A4 isoenzymes such as immunosuppressive drugs, including cyclosporine, colchicines, fibrates, macrolide antibiotics, azole antifungal agents, selective serotonine reuptake inhibitors, or niacin at lipid lowering doses.

Since LESCOL/LESCOL XL are predominantly metabolized by the CYP2C9 subclass of the P450 cytochromes and not metabolized to a significant extent by other cytochrome subclasses, including CYP3A4, it is not expected to increase the risks of myopathy when co-administered with other drugs metabolized by the P450 isoenzyme system. The benefits and risks of using HMG-CoA reductase inhibitors concomitantly with immunosuppressive drugs, erythromycin, or other drugs metabolized by the P450 enzyme system, fibrates or lipid-lowering doses of niacin should nevertheless be carefully considered (see Warnings and Precautions, Pharmacokinetic Interactions, and Drug Interactions, Cytochrome P450).

Experience to date with the use of fluvastatin together with cyclosporine consists of 3 pharmacokinetics studies (fluvastatin doses of 20 mg, 40 mg), 17 clinical trials of small-medium size and short-, medium-term duration (fluvastatin doses of 20 mg, 40 mg, 40 mg BID) in renal and heart transplant recipients, and one large prospective placebo-controlled trial in 2,102 renal transplant recipients followed up for 5 to 6 years (fluvastatin doses of 40 mg and 40 mg BID). Published data indicate that the trough concentration of cyclosporine A was not changed (see Drug Interactions, Drug-Drug Interactions, Immunosuppressive Drugs). No correlation between systemic fluvastatin levels and musculoskeletal adverse events or biochemical markers of musculoskeletal damage or renal function impairment have been observed in clinical trials conducted to date. In post-marketing experience, isolated cases of myopathy have been reported when fluvastatin was co-administered with cyclosporine.

Myopathy has not been observed in clinical trials involving small numbers of patients who were treated with LESCOL together with niacin at lipid lowering doses.

The use of fibrates alone or in combination with HMG-CoA reductase inhibitors has been occasionally associated with myopathy. In short-term studies involving a small number of patients, myopathy was not reported during administration of bezafibrate and LESCOL at doses of 40 mg/day and 60 mg/day. To date, the 80 mg/day dose has not been evaluated with bezafibrate.

Interruption of therapy with LESCOL/LESCOL XL should be considered in any patient with an acute serious condition suggestive of myopathy or having a risk factor predisposing to the development of renal failure or rhabdomyolysis, such as severe acute infection, hypotension, major surgery, trauma, severe metabolic, endocrine or electrolyte disorders and uncontrolled seizures.

Pediatric Population: Fluvastatin has only been investigated in children of 9 years and older with heterozygous familial hypercholesterolemia and efficacy and safety have not been studied for treatment periods longer than two years. In these limited uncontrolled studies, there was no detectable effect on growth or sexual maturation in the adolescent boys or on menstrual cycle length in girls. No data are available about the physical, intellectual and sexual maturation for prolonged treatment period.

Adolescent females should be counselled on appropriate contraceptive methods while on fluvastatin therapy (see Contra-indications). No specific drug-drug interaction studies were conducted in the pediatric patient population (see Drug Interactions).

Pharmacokinetic Interactions: The use of HMG-CoA reductase inhibitors has been associated with rhabdomyolysis, which may be more frequent when they are co-administered with drugs that inhibit the same cytochrome P450 isoenzyme system particularly the CYP3A4. The various HMG-CoA reductase inhibitors differ with respect to the P450 isoenzyme involved in their metabolism. LESCOL/LESCOL XL are predominantly metabolized by the CYP2C9 subclass of the P450 cytochromes and therefore is not expected to interact with drugs known to be CYP3A4 substrates, such as immunosuppressants, macrolide antibiotics, selective serotonine reuptake inhibitors, azole antifungal agents, or grapefruit juice. It may interact, however, with CYP2C9 substrates, e.g. nonsteroidal antiinflammatory drugs or oral anticoagulants. These potential interactions may be less clinically relevant due to the overlap between the different CYP2C isoenzymes (see Warnings and Precautions, Muscle Effects and Drug Interactions).

Cardiovascular: Effect on CoQ10 Levels (ubiquinone): A significant decrease in plasma CoQ_{10} levels in patients treated with fluvastatin sodium and other statins has been observed in short-term clinical trials. The clinical significance of a potential long-term statin-induced deficiency of CoQ10 has not yet been established. It has been reported that a decrease in myocardial ubiquinone levels could lead to impaired cardiac function in patients with borderline congestive heart failure.

Endocrine and Metabolism: Homozygous Familial Hypercholesterolemia: LESCOL/LESCOL XL has not been evaluated in patients with rare homozygous familial hypercholesterolemia. Most HMG-CoA reductase inhibitors are less or not effective in this subgroup of hypercholesterolemic patients.

Effect on Lipoprotein(A) [Lp(a)]: In some patients the beneficial effect of lowered total cholesterol and LDL cholesterol levels may be partly blunted by a concomitant increase in the Lp(a) levels. Until further experience is obtained from controlled clinical trials, it is suggested, where feasible, that Lp(a) measurements be carried out in patients placed on therapy with LESCOL/LESCOL XL.

Endocrine and Metabolism: HMG-CoA reductase inhibitors interfere with cholesterol synthesis and as such could theoretically blunt adrenal and/or gonadal steroid production.

Fluvastatin sodium exhibited no effect upon non-stimulated cortisol levels, FSH (males only) or thyroid metabolism as assessed by TSH. Small declines in total testosterone have been noted in treated groups, but no commensurate elevation in LH occurred. However, the effects of HMG-CoA reductase inhibitors on male fertility have not been studied in an adequate number of patients. The effects, if any, on the pituitary-gonadal axis in premenopausal women are unknown.

Patients treated with fluvastatin sodium who develop clinical evidence of endocrine dysfunction should be evaluated appropriately. Caution should be exercised if an HMG-CoA reductase inhibitor or other agent used to lower cholesterol levels is administered to patients receiving other drugs (e.g. ketoconazole, spironolactone, or cimetidine) that may decrease the levels of endogenous steroid hormones.

Hepatic/Biliary/Pancreatic: LESCOL/LESCOL XL, as well as other HMG-CoA reductase inhibitors should be used with caution in patients who consume substantial quantities of alcohol and/or have a past history of liver disease.

Active liver disease or unexplained transaminase elevations are contraindications to the use of LESCOL/LESCOL XL; if such condition develops during therapy, the drug should be discontinued.

Biochemical abnormalities of liver function have been associated with HMG-CoA reductase inhibitors and other lipid-lowering agents.

Overall, 25 of 2373 patients (1.1%) treated with LESCOL capsules in worldwide controlled clinical trials developed marked persistent elevations (to more than 3 times the upper limit of normal) in transaminase levels requiring discontinuation of treatment in 14 (0.6%) patients. The incidence of such elevations varied from 0.9% at 20 mg/day to 1.9 % at 80 mg/day.

In all clinical trials (controlled and uncontrolled) with LESCOL capsules, ranging from 28 to 71.2 weeks of exposure, 33 of 2969 (1.1%) patients had persistent transaminase elevations requiring discontinuation of treatment in 19 (0.6%) patients. In the majority of patients, these abnormal biochemical findings were asymptomatic.

In a retrospective pooled analysis of all placebo-controlled studies of at least 6 weeks and up to 130 weeks with LESCOL capsules, all patients with transaminase elevations >3 times the upper limit of normal were evaluated. A total of 1814 patients received daily either 20 mg, 40 mg or 80 mg (40 mg b.i.d.) fluvastatin sodium.

All patients with persistent (two consecutive occasions) transaminase elevations >3 times the upper limit of normal had abnormal transaminase elevations at either baseline (before initiation of therapy) and/or by 8 weeks after the start of therapy or dose increase.

In a pooled analysis of three 24-week controlled trials in 854 patients, persistent transaminase elevation occurred in 1.9% of patients treated with LESCOL XL 80 mg, and in 13 of 16 patients the abnormality occurred within 12 weeks of initiation of treatment with LESCOL XL 80 mg.

It is recommended that liver function tests be performed at baseline and 8 weeks after initiation of treatment as well as after an increase in the dose. Particular attention should be paid to patients who develop abnormal serum transaminase levels or signs and symptoms of liver disease. In these patients, measurements should be repeated promptly to confirm the finding and then performed more frequently until the abnormality(ies) return to normal.

If the transaminase levels show evidence of progression, particularly if they rise to three times the upper limit of normal and are persistent, the drug should be discontinued.

Immune: Rare cases of hypersensitivity reactions, such as rash, urticaria, eczema and other skin reactions (e.g. dermatitis, bullous exanthema), thrombocytopenia, angioedema, face edema, vasculitis and lupus erythematosus syndrome have been reported during post-marketing experience with LESCOL capsules. If hypersensitivity is suspected, LESCOL/LESCOL XL should be discontinued. Patients should be advised to report to their doctors promptly any signs of hypersensitivity such as rash, angioedema, urticaria, photosensitivity, polyarthralgia, fever and malaise.

Ophthalmologic: Current data from long-term clinical trials do not indicate an adverse effect of LESCOL/LESCOL XL on the human lens.

Renal: Because fluvastatin sodium does not undergo significant renal excretion modification of dosage should not be necessary in patients with mild to moderate renal impairment (creatinine clearance >30 mL/min).

As there is no experience with LESCOL/LESCOL XL in patients with severe renal insufficiency (creatinine >260 µmol/L, i.e. creatinine clearance <30 mL/min), its use cannot be recommended in this patient population.

Special Populations: Pregnant Women: LESCOL/LESCOL XL are contraindicated during pregnancy (see Contraindications). Data on the use of LESCOL/LESCOL XL in pregnant women is limited. A few reports have been received of congenital anomalies in infants whose mothers were treated during a critical period of pregnancy with other HMG-CoA reductase inhibitors. During the clinical program, a total of 5 women who were receiving LESCOL capsules became pregnant and were discontinued from the studies. Of these 5 women, 3 gave birth to healthy babies, one experienced an ectopic pregnancy which was attributed to a severely scarred Fallopian tube and one spontaneously aborted.

Atherosclerosis is a chronic process and discontinuation of lipid metabolism regulators during pregnancy should have little impact on the outcome of long-term therapy of primary hypercholesterolemia. Cholesterol and other products of cholesterol biosynthesis are essential components for fetal development (including synthesis of steroids and cell membranes). Since HMG-CoA reductase inhibitors decrease cholesterol synthesis and possibly the synthesis of other biologically active substances derived from cholesterol, they may cause fetal harm when administered to pregnant women.

LESCOL/LESCOL XL should be administered to women of childbearing age only when such patients are highly unlikely to conceive and have been informed of the potential hazards. If the patient becomes pregnant while taking this class of drug, therapy should be discontinued and the patient apprised of the potential hazard to the fetus (see Contraindications).

Nursing Women: It is not known whether fluvastatin sodium is excreted in human milk. Because many drugs are excreted in human milk and because of the potential for serious adverse reactions in nursing infants from fluvastatin sodium, women receiving LESCOL/LESCOL XL should not breast-feed (see Contraindications).

Pediatrics (10-17 years of age): (See Warnings and Precautions, General, Pediatric Population.)

Geriatrics: The effect of age on the pharmacokinetics of immediate release fluvastatin sodium capsules was evaluated. Results indicate that for the general patient population plasma concentrations of fluvastatin sodium do not vary either as a function of age or gender (see Actions and Clinical Pharmacology, Pharmacokinetics). Elderly patients may be more susceptible to myopathy (see Warnings and Precautions, Muscle Effects, Pre-disposing Factors for Myopathy/Rhabdomyolysis).

ADVERSE REACTIONS: Clinical Trial Adverse Drug Reactions: Because clinical trials are conducted under very specific conditions the adverse reaction rates observed in the clinical trials may not reflect the rates observed in practice and should not be compared to the rates in the clinical trials of another drug. Adverse drug reaction information from clinical trials is useful for identifying drug-related adverse events and for approximating rates.

In all clinical studies (controlled and uncontrolled) with LESCOL capsules, 1% (32/2969) of LESCOL patients were discontinued due to adverse experiences attributed to study drug (mean exposure of approximately 16 months ranging in duration from one to more than 36 months). This results, in controlled studies, in an exposure adjusted incidence of 0.8 % per patient year in fluvastatin patients compared to an incidence of 1.1% in placebo patients. Adverse events were usually mild and transient.

In controlled phase IIb and phase III clinical studies, 3.9% (51/1318) of patients treated with LESCOL XL 80 mg discontinued due to adverse events (causality not determined).

Clinical adverse reactions of positive or uncertain relationship to study medication occurring at a frequency ≥1% in controlled clinical trials with LESCOL capsules and LESCOL XL tablets are shown in Table 1.

Other adverse events occurring more than 1% in controlled clinical trials include: heartburn, tooth disorder, pharyngitis, sinusitis, coughing, and accidental trauma.

Clinical studies have shown that adverse events observed with LESCOL XL 80 mg used once daily are similar in frequency, nature, and severity to those reported with a 40 mg capsule administered once or twice daily.

Pediatric Population: In two open-label, uncontrolled studies, patients aged 9 years and older were treated for 2 years with LESCOL and LESCOL XL. The most common adverse events observed with an occurrence of 80% were influenza and infections. No data are available about the physical, intellectual and sexual maturation for prolonged treatment period (see Action and Clinical Pharmacology, Pediatrics (10-17 years of age)).

Less Common Clinical Trial Adverse Drug Reactions (<1%): Other clinical adverse reactions of positive or uncertain relationship to study medication occurring in 0.5% to 1.0% of patients receiving 20-80 mg LESCOL capsules monotherapy in controlled clinical trials (N=2326) are listed below:

Gastrointestinal: vomiting, gastritis.

Musculoskeletal: arthritis.

Central Nervous System: conjunctivitis, paresthesia.

Respiratory: rhinitis.

Integumentary: pruritus.

Miscellaneous: leg pain, influenza-like symptoms, allergy.

Table 1: LESCOL/LESCOL XL

Adverse Events of Positive or Uncertain Relationship to Study Medication Occurring ≥1% in Controlled Clinical Trials with LESCOL

	LESCOL[a]			Placebo[a]	LESCOL XL[b]
Adverse Event	**20 mg OD (N=1425) %**	**40 mg OD (N=1136) %**	**40 mg BID (N=369) %**	**(N=960) %**	**80 mg OD N=1318 %**
Gastrointestinal					
Dyspepsia	4.7	4.8	7.3	2.3	1.4
Constipation	2.8	1.8	2.4	2.5	0.8
Abdominal Pain	2.7	2.1	3.8	2.0	0.9
Flatulence	2.5	1.9	1.6	2.2	0.8
Diarrhea	2.5	1.5	1.6	2.1	1.5
Nausea	2.0	1.6	0.8	1.4	1.4
Eructation	1.4	0.6	0.5	1.1	0.0
Musculoskeletal					
Myalgia	1.7	1.8	2.7	2.3	1.5
Arthralgia	1.4	1.4	1.4	1.5	0.2
Back Pain	1.0	0.8	1.1	1.6	0.4
Central Nervous System					
Dizziness	0.9	1.1	0.5	1.8	0.5
Abnormal Vision	1.0	0.9	1.1	1.4	0.0
Psychiatric					
Insomnia	1.9	1.3	0.3	0.9	0.2
Respiratory					
Upper Respiratory Infection	1.1	0.9	2.4	1.9	0.2
Integumentary					
Rash	1.5	0.8	1.9	1.6	0.2
Miscellaneous					
Headache	3.8	2.7	1.9	3.0	0.9
Fatigue	1.8	1.5	0.5	1.8	0.6
Chest Pain	0.3	0.9	1.4	0.5	0.2

[a] Controlled trials with LESCOL capsules (20 and 40 mg daily and 40 mg twice daily).
[b] Controlled trials with LESCOL XL 80 mg tablets.

Post-Market Adverse Drug Reactions: The following adverse events have also been reported during post-marketing experience with LESCOL/LESCOL XL, regardless of causality assessment.

Hypersensitivity Reactions: Rare cases of hypersensitivity reactions, such as rash, urticaria, eczema, and other skin reactions (e.g. dermatitis, bullous exanthema), thrombocytopenia, angioedema, face edema, vasculitis, and lupus erythematosus syndrome have been reported during post-marketing experience.

An apparent hypersensitivity syndrome has also been reported rarely with other HMG-CoA reductase inhibitors and has included one or more of the following features: anaphylaxis, angioedema, lupus erythematous-like syndrome, polymyalgia rheumatica, vasculitis, purpura, thrombocytopenia, leukopenia, hemolytic anemia, positive antinuclear antibody (ANA), erythrocytes sedimentation rate (ESR) increase, arthritis, arthralgia, urticaria, asthenia, photosensitivity, fever, chills, flushing, malaise, dyspnea, toxic epidermal necrolysis, erythema multiforme, including Stevens-Johnson syndrome.

Very rare cases of anaphylactic reaction have been reported with LESCOL/LESCOL XL.

Skeletal: Rarely: muscle tenderness, muscle weakness and myopathy. Very rarely: myositis, rhabdomyolysis (see Warnings and Precautions, Muscle Effects).

Central and Peripheral Nervous System: Very rarely: dysesthesia and hypoesthesia, also know to be associated with the underlying hyperlipidemic disorder.

Gastrointestinal: Very rarely: pancreatitis.

Liver: Very rarely: hepatitis.

The following effects have been reported with drugs of this class:

Skeletal: myopathy, rhabdomyolysis (see Warnings and Precautions, Muscle Effects), muscle cramping/pain.

Neurological: paresthesia, peripheral neuropathy, psychiatric disturbances/anxiety.

Gastrointestinal: hepatitis, cholestatic jaundice, anorexia, vomiting. Very rarely: acute pancreatitis.

Skin: alopecia.

Miscellaneous: asthenia, sweating, hot flushes, gynecomastia.

DRUG INTERACTIONS: Overview: Pharmacokinetic and pharmacodynamic studies conducted with drugs in healthy subjects may not detect the possibility of potential drug interactions in some patients due to differences in underlying disease(s), age or renal function (see Warnings and Precautions, Renal; Special Populations, Geriatrics; and Drug Interactions, Patients with Severe Hypercholesterolemia).

Concomitant Therapy with Other Lipid Metabolism Regulators: Information on combination drug therapy from controlled studies is limited. Based on post-marketing surveillance, gemfibrozil, fenofibrate, other fibrates and lipid lowering doses of niacin (nicotinic acid) may increase the risk of myopathy when given concomitantly with HMG-CoA reductase inhibitors, probably because they can produce myopathy when given alone (see Warnings and Precautions, Muscle Effects). Therefore, combined drug therapy should be approached with caution.

Drug-Drug Interactions: No specific drug-drug interaction studies were conducted in the pediatric patient population.

A drug interactive effect (pharmacokinetic and/or clinical) has been shown for the following drugs in combination with fluvastatin sodium:

Cholestyramine: The cholesterol-lowering effects of LESCOL/LESCOL XL and the bile acid sequestrant, cholestyramine, are additive.

Administration of immediate release fluvastatin sodium concomitantly 2 to 4 hours after cholestyramine, results in fluvastatin decreases of more than 50% for the fluvastatin AUC and 50-80% for the fluvastatin C_{max}. However, administration of immediate release fluvastatin sodium 4 hours after cholestyramine resulted in a clinically significant additive effect in reducing Total-C and LDL-C compared with that achieved with either component drug.

Gemfibrozil/Fenofibrate/Niacin: Myopathy, including rhabdomyolysis, has occurred in patients who were receiving co-administration of HMG-CoA reductase inhibitors with fibric acid derivatives and niacin (in lipid lowering doses), particularly in subjects with pre-existing renal insufficiency (see Warnings and Precautions, Muscle Effects). LESCOL capsules have been safely administered concomitantly with nicotinic acid, gemfibrozil and bezafibrate in clinical studies.

In short-term studies involving a small number of patients, myopathy was not reported during administration of bezafibrate and LESCOL capsules at doses of 40 mg/day and 60 mg/day. To date, the 80 mg/day dose has not been evaluated with bezafibrate. An additional interaction study between 20 mg o.d. fluvastatin and 200 mg t.d.s. bezafibrate showed that mean AUC and C_{max} values of fluvastatin were increased on average by about 50-60%. No effect was seen on bezafibrate pharmacokinetics. This combination should be used with caution, however, due to the increased risk of developing myopathy and/or rhabdomyolysis when HMG-CoA reductase inhibitors including fluvastatin have been combined with fibrates. Any patient complaining of myalgia should be carefully evaluated.

Cimetidine/Ranitidine/Omeprazole: Concomitant administration of LESCOL capsules with cimetidine, ranitidine and omeprazole results in a significant increase in the fluvastatin C_{max} (43%, 70% and 50%, respectively) and AUC (24 to 33%), with an 18 to 23% decrease in apparent oral plasma clearance (Cl/F).

Digoxin: In a crossover study involving 18 patients chronically receiving digoxin, concomitant administration of a single 40 mg dose of LESCOL capsule had no effect on digoxin AUC and small but clinically insignificant increases in the digoxin C_{max} and urinary clearance were noted.

Rifampicin: Administration of LESCOL capsules to subjects pre-treated with rifampicin results in significant reduction in C_{max} (59%) and AUC (51%) of fluvastatin, with a large increase (95%) in plasma clearance.

Antipyrine: Administration of fluvastatin sodium does not influence the metabolism and excretion of antipyrine, either by induction or inhibition.

Cardiovascular Agents: Concomitant administration of propranolol has no effect on the bioavailability of fluvastatin sodium. No clinically significant pharmacokinetic interactions occur when fluvastatin is concomitantly administered with losartan or amlodipine, although mild to moderate adverse events were reported upon concomitant administration of fluvastatin and amlodipine (see Adverse Reactions).

Warfarin and Other Coumarin Derivatives: In vitro protein binding studies demonstrated no interaction at therapeutic concentrations. In a drug interaction study, the concomitant use of LESCOL capsules and warfarin did not alter the plasma levels and prothrombin times compared to warfarin alone. However, isolated incidences of bleeding episodes and/or increased prothrombin times have been reported very rarely in patients on fluvastatin receiving concomitant warfarin or other coumarin derivatives. It is recommended that prothrombin times are monitored when fluvastatin treatment is initiated, discontinued, or the dosage changed in patients receiving warfarin or other coumarin derivatives.

Cytochrome P450: Fluvastatin is predominantly metabolized by the hepatic microsomal CYP2C9 subclass of the P450 cytochromes. It is not metabolized to a significant extent by other cytochrome subclasses, including CYP3A4. The clearance of drugs which are also CYP2C9 substrates may decrease when co-administered with fluvastatin. However, for those CYP2C9-metabolized drugs which have been studied directly, including diclofenac, tolbutamide, and warfarin, the effect on clearance is small and no clinically significant drug interactions of fluvastatin with other CYP2C9 substrates have been demonstrated. Caution should nevertheless be exercised with concomitant use of drugs metabolized by the CYP2C9 subclass of the P450 cytochromes such as phenytoin, oral anticoagulants (e.g. warfarin), oral hypoglycemic agents (e.g. tolbutamide, chlorpropamide) and nonsteroidal anti-inflammatory drugs (e.g. diclofenac) (see Warnings and Precautions, Muscle Effects).

Since LESCOL/LESCOL XL are predominantly metabolized by the CYP2C9 subclass of the P450 cytochromes and not metabolized to a significant extent by other cytochrome subclasses, including CYP3A4, it is not expected to increase the risks of drug interactions when combined with drugs or common agents such as grapefruit juice that inhibit this enzyme (immunosuppressants, azole-type antifungal agents, macrolide antibiotics or antidepressants) (see Warnings and Precautions, Pharmacokinetic Interactions and Muscle Effects).

Itraconazole and Erythromycin: Concomitant administration of fluvastatin with the potent cytochrome P450 (CYP) 3A4 inhibitors itraconazole and erythromycin has minimal effects on the bioavailability of fluvastatin. Given the minimal involvement of this enzyme in the metabolism of fluvastatin, it is expected that other CYP3A4 inhibitors (e.g. ketoconazole, cyclosporin) are unlikely to affect the bioavailability of fluvastatin (see Warnings and Precautions, Muscle Effects).

Fluconazole: Administration of fluvastatin to healthy volunteers pre-treated with fluconazole (CYP2C9 inhibitor) resulted in a significant increase in the exposure, elimination half-life and peak concentration of fluvastatin by about 84%, 80% and 44%, respectively. Although there was no clinical evidence that the safety profile of fluvastatin was altered in patients pre-treated with fluconazole for 4 days, caution should be exercised when fluvastatin is administered concomitantly with fluconazole.

Oral Antidiabetic Agents: For patients receiving oral sulfonylureas (glibenclamide [glyburide], tolbutamide) for the treatment of non-insulin-dependent (type 2) diabetes mellitus (NIDDM), addition of fluvastatin does not lead to clinically significant changes in glycemic control.

In glyburide-treated NIDDM patients (n=32), administration of fluvastatin (40 mg twice daily for 14 days) increased the mean C_{max}, AUC, and $t_{1/2}$ of glyburide approximately 50%, 69% and 121%, respectively. Glyburide (5 to 20 mg daily) increased the mean C_{max} and AUC of fluvastatin by 44% and 51%, respectively. In this study there were no changes in glucose, insulin and C-peptide levels. However, patients on concomitant therapy with glyburide (glibenclamide) and fluvastatin should continue to be monitored appropriately when their fluvastatin dose is increased to 80 mg per day.

Phenytoin: The overall magnitude of the changes in phenytoin pharmacokinetics during co-administration with fluvastatin are relatively small and not clinically significant. Thus, routine monitoring of phenytoin plasma levels is sufficient during co-administration with fluvastatin. The minimal effect of phenytoin on fluvastatin pharmacokinetics indicates that dosage adjustment of fluvastatin is not warranted when co-administered with phenytoin.

Colchicines: Myotoxicity, including muscle pain and weakness and rhabdomyolysis, has been reported anecdotally with concomitant administration of fluvastatin and colchicine during acute exacerbation of gouty arthritis.

Patients with Severe Hypercholesterolemia: Higher dosages (80 mg/day) required for some patients with severe hypercholesterolemia are associated with increased plasma levels of fluvastatin. Caution should be exercised in such patients who are also significantly renally impaired, elderly, or are also concomitantly being administered digoxin, or CYP 450 inhibitors (see Warnings and Precautions, Pharmacokinetic Interactions, and Muscle Effects; and Drug Interactions).

Although specific interaction studies were not performed with all drugs listed below, in clinical studies, LESCOL capsules was used concomitantly with angiotensin converting enzyme (ACE) inhibitors, beta blockers, calcium channel blockers, oral sulphonylureas, antacids, diuretics and nonsteroidal anti-inflammatory drugs (NSAIDs) without evidence to date of clinically significant interactions.

Immunosuppressive Drugs: In a pharmacokinetic study conducted in 19 stable renal transplant patients receiving cyclosporine A concomitantly with fluvastatin 20 mg/day, the AUC for fluvastatin was increased by 1.9 times. Similarly, in a pharmacokinetic study conducted in 19 stable renal transplant patients on stable cyclosporine A regimen who received fluvastatin extended release 80 mg/day for 1 week, both the AUC and C_{max} for fluvastatin were increased by two fold as compared with data from historical controls treated with the same fluvastatin regimen. The trough concentration of cyclosporine A was not changed. In heart transplant patients treated with fluvastatin 40 mg/day and cyclosporine A for four weeks, AUC for fluvastatin was increased 3.5 times and 3.1 times in patients than in the age-matched healthy controls on study days 1 and 28, respectively. In post-marketing experience, isolated cases of myopathy have been reported when fluvastatin was co-administered with cyclosporine (see Warnings and Precautions, Muscle Effects).

Drug-Food Interactions: There were no apparent differences in the lipid-lowering effects of fluvastatin when administered with the evening meal or four (4) hours after the evening meal (see Actions and Clinical Pharmacology, Pharmacokinetics, Absorption). Based on the lack of interaction of fluvastatin with other CYP3A4 substrates, fluvastatin is not expected to interact with grapefruit juice.

Drug-Laboratory Test Interactions: The HMG-CoA reductase inhibitors may cause elevation of transaminase levels (see Warnings and Precautions). Marked elevations of CK levels to more than 5×ULN developed in a very small number (0.3-1.0%) of patients on fluvastatin sodium. In the differential diagnosis of chest pain in a patient on LESCOL/LESCOL XL, cardiac and noncardiac fractions of these enzymes should be determined.

DOSAGE AND ADMINISTRATION: **Dosing Considerations:** Patients should be placed on a standard cholesterol-lowering diet (at least equivalent to the Adult Treatment Panel III [ATP III TLC diet]) before receiving LESCOL/LESCOL XL, and should continue on this diet during treatment with LESCOL/LESCOL XL. If appropriate, a program of weight control and physical exercise should be implemented.

Prior to initiating therapy with LESCOL/LESCOL XL, secondary causes for elevations in plasma lipid levels should be excluded. A lipid profile should also be performed.

Cholesterol levels should be monitored periodically and consideration should be given to reducing the dosage of LESCOL capsule or LESCOL XL tablet if cholesterol levels fall below the desired range.

Recommended Dose and Dosage Adjustment: Adults: Hypercholesterolemia and Mixed Hyperlipidemia: For patients requiring LDL-C reduction of less than 25%, a starting dose of 20 mg LESCOL capsule taken once daily is recommended.

For patients requiring LDL-C reduction of at least 25%, the recommended starting dose is 40 mg daily of LESCOL capsule taken once daily. If necessary, the dosage of fluvastatin may then be increased to 80 mg of LESCOL XL tablet, taken once daily at any time, or alternatively, 80 mg of LESCOL capsule, taken in divided doses of 40 mg twice daily.

LESCOL capsules may be taken consistently with or without food, in the evening or at bedtime. LESCOL capsules must be swallowed whole with a glass of water.

A single dose of LESCOL XL tablets can be administered at any time of the day with or without food. LESCOL XL tablets must be swallowed whole with a glass of water.

Since maximal reduction in LDL-C is seen within 4 weeks of administration of a given dose of LESCOL capsule or LESCOL XL tablet, periodic lipid level determination should be performed with dosage adjusted to a maximum of 80 mg of fluvastatin daily, according to patient response.

Pediatric Population: Prior to initiating treatment with LESCOL/LESCOL XL, the patient should be placed on a standard cholesterol-lowering diet for 6 months. Dietary therapy should be continued during treatment.

The recommended starting dose is 20 mg daily of LESCOL capsule taken once daily.

If the patients did not achieve the desired LDL-C level, the dosage of fluvastatin may then be increased in a step-wise fashion at approximately 6-week intervals to a maximum daily dose of 80 mg. The patient may take 80 mg of LESCOL XL tablet, once daily at any time of the day, or alternatively, 80 mg of LESCOL capsule, in divided doses of 40 mg twice daily.

Starting doses should be individualized according to baseline LDL-C levels and the recommended goal of therapy to be accomplished.

The use of fluvastatin in combination with nicotinic acid, cholestyramine, or fibrate in children and adolescents has not been investigated.

Severe Hypercholesterolemia: In patients with severe hypercholesterolemia, higher dosages (up to 80 mg/day) may be required (see Warnings and Precautions, Pharmacokinetic Interactions and Muscle Effects and Drug Interactions). The maximum recommended daily dosage is 80 mg/day.

Secondary Prevention of Cardiovascular Events (see Hypercholesterolemia and Mixed Hyperlipidemia): During the LESCOL Intervention Prevention Study (LIPS), patients were initiated on fluvastatin treatment at 40 mg twice a day with no titration from a lower dose level. This daily dose was proven to be as well tolerated as placebo.

Therefore, in patients with coronary heart disease who have undergone a percutaneous intervention procedure, the appropriate dose of LESCOL is 40 mg twice a day.

Concomitant Therapy: See Drug Interactions

Dosage in Patients with Renal Impairment: See Warnings and Precautions, Renal.

Dosage in Patients with Hepatic Impairment: See Contraindications and Warnings and Precautions, Hepatic/Biliary/Pancreatic.

Use in the Elderly: See Warnings and Precautions, Geriatrics.

Use in Children: See Warnings and Precautions, Pediatrics (10-17 years of age).

The dosage of LESCOL/LESCOL XL should be individualized according to baseline LDL-C, total-C/HDL-C ratio and/or TG levels to achieve the desired lipid values at the lowest possible dose. Lipid levels should be monitored periodically and, if necessary, the dose of LESCOL/LESCOL XL adjusted accordingly.

OVERDOSAGE:

The maximum single oral dose of LESCOL (fluvastatin sodium) capsules received by healthy volunteers was 80 mg. No clinically significant adverse experiences were seen at this dose.

The maximum dose administered with an extended release formulation was 640 mg for two weeks. This dose was not well tolerated and produced a variety of GI complaints and an increase in transaminase values (i.e., ALT and AST).

There has been a single report of two children, one 2 year old and the other 3 years of age, either of whom may have possibly ingested fluvastatin sodium. The maximum amount of fluvastatin sodium ingested was 80 mg (4×20 mg capsules). Vomiting was induced by ipecac in both children and no capsules were noted in their emesis. Neither child experienced any adverse symptoms and both recovered from the incident without problems.

Should an overdose occur, treatment should be symptomatic and supporting measures should be undertaken as required. The dialysability of LESCOL/LESCOL XL and its metabolites in man is not known at present.

For management of a suspected drug overdose, CPhA recommends that you contact your regional Poison Control Centre. See the *CPS* Directory section for a list of Poison Control Centres.

ACTION AND CLINICAL PHARMACOLOGY: LESCOL (fluvastatin sodium) is a fully synthetic HMG-CoA reductase inhibitor and is hydrophilic. Fluvastatin sodium is a racemate of two erythro enantiomers of which one exerts the pharmacological activity.

Mechanism of Action: Fluvastatin sodium is a competitive inhibitor of HMG-CoA reductase, which is responsible for the conversion of 3-hydroxy-3-methylglutaryl-coenzyme A (HMG-CoA) to mevalonate, a precursor of sterols, including cholesterol. Fluvastatin exerts its main effect in the liver and is mainly a racemate of the two erythro enantiomers of which the 3R,5S enantiomer exerts the pharmacological activity. The inhibition of cholesterol biosynthesis reduces the cholesterol in hepatic cells, which stimulates the synthesis of LDL receptors and thereby increases the uptake of LDL particles. The ultimate result of these mechanisms is a reduction of the plasma total cholesterol (Total-C) and low density lipoprotein cholesterol (LDL-C) concentrations.

Epidemiologic and clinical studies have associated the risk of coronary artery disease (CAD) with elevated levels of Total-C, LDL-C and decreased levels of HDL-C. These abnormalities of lipoprotein metabolism are considered as major contributors to the development of the disease. Other factors, e.g. interactions between lipids/lipoproteins and endothelium, platelets and macrophages, have also been incriminated in the development of human atherosclerosis and of its complications. Effective treatment of hypercholesterolemia/dyslipidemia in long-term clinical trials has consistently been associated with a reduced risk of CAD.

Pharmacodynamics: A variety of clinical studies has demonstrated that elevated levels of total cholesterol (total-C), low density lipoprotein cholesterol (LDL-C) and apolipoprotein B (a membrane transport complex for LDL-C) promote human atherosclerosis. Similarly, decreased levels of high density lipoprotein cholesterol (HDL-C) and its transport complex, apolipoprotein A, are associated with the development of atherosclerosis. Epidemiological investigations have established that cardiovascular morbidity and mortality vary directly with the level of total-C and LDL-C and inversely with the level of HDL-C. In multicentre clinical trials, those pharmacologic and/or non-pharmacologic interventions that simultaneously lowered LDL-C and increased HDL-C reduced the rate of cardiovascular events (both fatal and non-fatal myocardial infarctions) in high risk males or in males and females with established coronary artery disease.

LESCOL/LESCOL XL reduces total-C, LDL-C, apo-B, and TG, and marginally increases HDL-C in patients with hypercholesterolemia and mixed dyslipidemia. Therapeutic response is well established within 2 weeks, and maximum response is achieved within 4 weeks from treatment initiation and maintained during chronic therapy.

Pharmacokinetics:

Table 2: LESCOL/LESCOL XL

Summary of LESCOL/LESCOL XL's Pharmacokinetic Parameters in Single-Dose and Steady-State Studies

	C_{max} (ng/mL) mean±SD (range)	$t_{1/2}$ (h) mean±SD (range)	$AUC_{0-\infty}$ (ng·h/mL) mean±SD (range)	Clearance (L/h) mean±SD (range)	T_{max} (h) mean±SD (range)
Capsules					
20 mg single dose (n=17)	166±106 (48.9-517)	2.5±1.7 (0.5-6.6)	207±65 (111-288)	107±38.1 (69.5-181)	0.9±0.4 (0.5-2.0)
20 mg twice daily (n=17)	200±86 (71.8-366)	2.8±1.7 (0.9-6.0)	275±111 (91.6-467)	87.8±45 (42.8-218)	1.2±0.9 (0.5-4.0)

(cont'd)

Table 2: LESCOL/LESCOL XL *(cont'd)*

Summary of LESCOL/LESCOL XL's Pharmacokinetic Parameters in Single-Dose and Steady-State Studies

	C_{max} (ng/mL) mean±SD (range)	$t_{½}$ (h) mean±SD (range)	$AUC_{0-\infty}$ (ng·h/mL) mean±SD (range)	Clearance (L/h) mean±SD (range)	T_{max} (h) mean±SD (range)
40 mg single dose (n=16)	273±189 (72.8-812)	2.7±1.3 (0.8-5.9)	456±259 (207-1221)	108±44.7 (32.8-193)	1.2±0.7 (0.75-3.0)
40 mg twice daily (n=16)	432±236 (119-990)	2.7±1.3 (0.7-5.0)	697±275 (359-1559)	64.2±21.1 (25.7-111)	1.2±0.6 (0.5-2.5)
Extended-release 80 mg tablets					
80 mg single dose, fasting (n=24)	126±53 (37-242)	—	579±341 (144-1760)	—	3.2±2.6 (1-12)
80 mg single dose, fed-state high fat meal (n=24)	183±163 (21-733)	—	861±632 (199-3132)	—	6 (2-24)
80 mg once daily fasting 7 day steady-state (n=11)	102±42 (43.9-181)	—	630±326 (247-1406)	—	2.6±0.91 (1.5-4)

Absorption: LESCOL is absorbed rapidly and completely following oral administration of the capsule, with peak concentrations reached in less than 1 hour. Following administration of a 10 mg dose, the absolute bioavailability is 24% (range 9%-50%). Administration with food reduces the rate but not the extent of absorption. At steady-state, administration of fluvastatin with the evening meal results in a two-fold decrease in C_{max} and more than two fold increase in T_{max} as compared to administration 4 hours after the evening meal. No significant differences in extent of absorption or in the lipid-lowering effects were observed between the two administrations. After single or multiple doses above 20 mg, fluvastatin exhibits saturable first-pass metabolism resulting in higher-than-expected plasma fluvastatin concentrations.

Fluvastatin has two optical enantiomers, an active 3R,5S and an inactive 3S,5R form. In vivo studies showed that stereo-selective hepatic binding of the active form occurs during the first pass resulting in a difference in the peak levels of the two enantiomers, with the active to inactive peak concentration ratio being about 0.7. The approximate ratio of the active to inactive approaches unity after the peak is seen and thereafter the two enantiomers decline with the same half-life. After an intravenous administration, bypassing the first-pass metabolism, the ratios of the enantiomers in plasma were similar throughout the concentration time profiles.

Fluvastatin administered as LESCOL XL 80 mg tablets reaches peak concentration in approximately 3 hours under either: fasting conditions; or immediately after a low-fat meal; or 2.5 hours after a low fat meal. The mean relative bioavailability of the XL tablet is approximately 29% (range: 9%-66%) compared to that of the LESCOL immediate release capsule administered under fasting conditions. Administration of a high fat meal delayed the absorption (T_{max}: 6 hours) and increased the bioavailability of the XL tablet by approximately 50%. Once LESCOL XL begins to be absorbed, fluvastatin concentrations rise rapidly. The maximum concentration seen after a high fat meal is much less than the peak concentration following a single dose or twice-daily dose of the 40 mg LESCOL capsule. Overall variability in the pharmacokinetics of LESCOL XL is large (42%-64% CV for C_{max} and AUC), and especially so after a high fat meal (63%-89% for C_{max} and AUC). Intrasubject variability in the pharmacokinetics of LESCOL XL under fasting conditions (about 25% for C_{max} and AUC) tends to be much smaller as compared to the overall variability. Multiple peaks in plasma fluvastatin concentrations have been observed after LESCOL XL administration.

Distribution: Fluvastatin is 98% bound to plasma proteins. The mean volume of distribution (VDss) is estimated at 0.35 L/kg. The parent drug is targeted to the liver and no active metabolites are present systemically. At therapeutic concentrations, the protein binding of fluvastatin is not affected by warfarin, salicylic acid and glyburide.

Metabolism: Fluvastatin is metabolized in the liver, primarily via hydroxylation of the indole ring at the 5 and 6-positions. N-dealkylation and beta-oxidation of the side-chain also occurs. The hydroxy metabolites have some pharmacologic activity, but do not circulate in the blood. Both enantiomers of fluvastatin are metabolized in a similar manner.

In vitro studies demonstrated that fluvastatin undergoes oxidative metabolism, predominantly via 2C9 isozyme systems (75%). Other isozymes that contribute to fluvastatin metabolism are 2C8 (~5%) and 3A4 (~20%) (see Drug Interactions).

Excretion: Fluvastatin is primarily (about 90%) eliminated in the feces as metabolites, with less than 2% present as unchanged drug. Urinary recovery is about 5%. After a radiolabeled dose of fluvastatin, the clearance was 0.8 L/h/kg. Following multiple oral doses of radiolabeled compound, there was no accumulation of fluvastatin; however, there was a 2.3 fold accumulation of total radioactivity.

Steady-state plasma concentrations show no evidence of accumulation of fluvastatin following immediate release capsule administration of up to 80 mg daily, as evidenced by a beta-elimination half-life of less than 3 hours. However, under conditions of maximum rate of absorption (i.e., fasting) systemic exposure to fluvastatin is increased 33% to 53% compared to a single 20 mg or 40 mg dose of the immediate release capsule. Following once daily administration of the 80 mg LESCOL XL tablet for 7 days, systemic exposure to fluvastatin is increased (20%-30%) compared to a single dose of the 80 mg LESCOL XL tablet. Terminal half-life of LESCOL XL was about 9 hours as a result of the slow release formulation.

Special Populations and Conditions: Pediatrics (10-17 years of age): Pharmacokinetic data in the pediatric population are not available.

STORAGE AND STABILITY: LESCOL capsules: Store between 15 and 30°C in a tight container. Protect from light and humidity. LESCOL XL tablets: Store between 15 and 30°C.

SPECIAL HANDLING INSTRUCTIONS: Not applicable.

INFORMATION FOR THE PATIENT: Published in e-CPS, available by subscription at www.e-cps.ca.

DOSAGE FORMS, COMPOSITION AND PACKAGING: Capsules: 20 mg: Each strong reddish brown opaque cap and pale yellow opaque body capsule, "XU 20MG" printed in red ink on the body, contains: fluvastatin 20 mg (from fluvastatin sodium 21.06 mg). Nonmedicinal ingredients: calcium carbonate, magnesium stearate, microcrystalline cellulose, pregelatinized starch, sodium bicarbonate and talc; capsule shell and printing ink: benzyl alcohol, butyl paraben, carboxymethyl cellulose sodium, edetate calcium disodium, gelatin, iron oxide red, iron oxide yellow, methyl paraben, propyl paraben, sodium laurel sulphate, sodium propionate and titanium dioxide. Bottles of 100.

40 mg: Each strong reddish brown opaque cap and orange yellow opaque body capsule, "XU 40MG" printed in red ink on the body contains: fluvastatin 40 mg (from fluvastatin sodium 42.12 mg). Nonmedicinal ingredients: calcium carbonate, magnesium stearate, microcrystalline cellulose, pregelatinized starch, sodium bicarbonate and talc; capsule shell and printing ink: benzyl alcohol, butyl paraben, carboxymethyl cellulose sodium, edetate calcium disodium, gelatin, iron oxide red, iron oxide yellow, methyl paraben, propyl paraben, sodium laurel sulphate, sodium propionate and titanium dioxide. Bottles of 100.

Extended Release Tablets: Each yellow, round, slightly biconvex film-coated, extended-release tablet with beveled edges debossed with "LESCOL XL" on one side and "80" on the other, contains: fluvastatin 80 mg (from 84.24 mg fluvastatin sodium). Nonmedicinal ingredients: hydroxypropyl cellulose, hydroxypropyl methylcellulose, iron oxide yellow, magnesium stearate, microcrystalline cellulose, polyethylene glycol 8000, potassium bicarbonate, povidone and titanium dioxide. Blister packs of 28.

(Shown in Product Identification Section)

Letrozole ℞

letrozole

Nonsteroidal Aromatase Inhibitor—Inhibitor of Estrogen Biosynthesis—Antitumour Agent

Cobalt

SUPPLIED: Each yellow, round, biconvex film-coated tablet, plain on both sides, contains: letrozole 2.5 mg. Nonmedicinal ingredients: cellulose compounds (microcrystalline cellulose and hypromellose), colloidal anhydrous silica, iron oxide yellow, lactose monohydrate, magnesium stearate, maize starch, polyethylene glycol, sodium starch glycolate, talc and titanium dioxide. Blister packages of 30. Protect from heat and moisture (store at 15 to 30°C).

Letrozole Tablets USP ℞

letrozole

Nonsteroidal Aromatase Inhibitor—Inhibitor of Estrogen Biosynthesis—Antitumor Agent

Accord Healthcare

SUPPLIED: Each yellow, round, biconvex film-coated tablet, embossed with "LT" on one side and plain on the other side, contains: letrozole 2.5 mg. Nonmedicinal ingredients: cellulose compounds (microcrystalline cellulose and hypromellose), colloidal anhydrous silica, iron oxide yellow, lactose monohydrate, magnesium stearate, maize starch, polyethylene glycol, sodium starch glycolate, talc and titanium dioxide. Blister packages of 30. Protect from heat and moisture (store at 15 to 30°C). Keep out of reach and sight of children and pets.

Leucovorin Calcium Injection USP ℞

calcium folinate

Folic Acid Derivative

Hospira

SUPPLIED: Each mL of sterile aqueous isotonic solution contains: leucovorin 10 mg (as the calcium salt). Nonmedicinal ingredients: 8.5 mg sodium chloride. May contain hydrochloric acid or sodium hydroxide as pH adjusters. Contains no preservative. Single use vials of 5 mL. Discard unused portion. Pharmacy bulk vials of 50 mL, cartons of 1. Store between 2 and 8°C. Protect from light.

Leukeran® ℞

chlorambucil

Antineoplastic

GlaxoSmithKline

Date of Revision: October 29, 2008

Caution: LEUKERAN (chlorambucil) is a potent drug product and should be used only by physicians experienced with cancer chemotherapeutic drugs. Blood counts should be taken once or twice weekly. Discontinue or reduce the dosage upon evidence of abnormal depression of the bone marrow (see Contraindications, Warnings and Precautions).

PHARMACOLOGY: LEUKERAN (chlorambucil) is an aromatic nitrogen mustard derivative which acts as a bifunctional alkylating agent. Alkylation takes place through the formation of a highly reactive ethylenimonium radical. A probable mode of action involves cross-linkage of the ethylenimonium derivative between 2 strands of helical DNA and subsequent interference with replication.

After oral administration of carbon-14 labelled chlorambucil, maximum plasma radioactivity occurs between 40 and 70 minutes later. Studies have shown that chlorambucil disappears from the plasma with a mean terminal phase half-life of 1.5 hours and that its urinary excretion is low. A high level of urinary radioactivity after oral or i.v. administration of carbon-14 labelled chlorambucil indicates that the drug is well absorbed after oral dosage.

Chlorambucil and its metabolites are extensively bound to plasma and tissue proteins. In vitro, chlorambucil is 99% bound to plasma proteins, specifically albumin. Cerebrospinal fluid levels of chlorambucil have not been determined. Evidence of human teratogenicity suggests that the drug crosses the placenta.

Chlorambucil is extensively metabolized in the liver, primarily to phenylacetic acid mustard which has antineoplastic activity. Chlorambucil and its major metabolite spontaneously degrade in vivo, forming monohydroxy and dihydroxy derivatives. After a single dose of radiolabelled chlorambucil (carbon-14), approximately 15 to 60% of the radioactivity appears in the urine after 24 hours. Less than 1% of the urinary radioactivity is in the form of chlorambucil or phenylacetic acid mustard. In summary, the pharmacokinetic data suggest that oral chlorambucil undergoes rapid gastrointestinal absorption and plasma clearance and that it is almost completely metabolized, having extremely low urinary excretion.

INDICATIONS: LEUKERAN (chlorambucil) is indicated as monotherapy in the treatment of chronic lymphocytic leukemia. It is also indicated as monotherapy or in combination with other agents in non-Hodgkin's lymphomas including follicular lymphoma, indolent lymphoma, MALT-lymphoma, mantle-cell lymphoma; Waldenstrom's macroglobulinemia and Hodgkin's disease. It is not curative but produces remissions.

CONTRAINDICATIONS: LEUKERAN (chlorambucil) should not be administered to patients who are resistant to the drug or who have developed hypersensitivity to it. There may be cross-hypersensitivity (skin rash) between chlorambucil and other alkylating agents.

Chlorambucil should not be used within 4 weeks of a full course of radiation or chemotherapy.

WARNINGS: LEUKERAN (chlorambucil), a derivative of nitrogen mustard, is a potent drug. It is for use only under the direction of physicians experienced in the administration of cancer chemotherapeutic drugs.

Rare instances of skin rash progressing to erythema multiforme, toxic epidermal necrolysis, or Stevens-Johnson syndrome have been reported. Chlorambucil should be discontinued promptly in patients who develop skin reactions.

Pregnancy: The use of chlorambucil should be avoided whenever possible during pregnancy. However, when cytotoxic drugs are used in pregnancy, the possible teratogenic effect on the fetus should be kept in mind. It is therefore advisable to delay treatment with these drugs as long as possible and certainly until after the first 3 months of pregnancy. In any individual case, the potential hazard to the fetus must be balanced against the expected benefit to the mother.

Lactation: Mothers receiving LEUKERAN should not breast-feed.

Vaccination: Immunisation using a live organism vaccine has a potential to cause infection in immunocompromised hosts. Therefore, immunisations with live organism vaccines are not recommended.

PRECAUTIONS: General: Since LEUKERAN (chlorambucil) is capable of producing irreversible bone marrow depression, blood counts should be monitored once or twice weekly in patients under treatment.

At therapeutic dosage, LEUKERAN depresses lymphocytes and has less effect on neutrophil and platelet counts and on hemoglobin levels. Discontinuation of LEUKERAN is not necessary at the first sign of a fall in neutrophils, but it must be remembered that the fall may continue for 10 days or more after the last dose.

When lymphocytic infiltration of the bone marrow is present, or the bone marrow is hypoplastic, the daily dose should not exceed 0.1 mg/kg body weight.

Patients with nephrotic syndrome, patients prescribed high pulse dose regimens and patients with a history of seizure disorder, should be closely monitored following administration of chlorambucil, as they may have an increased risk of seizures. As with any potentially epileptogenic drug, caution should be exercised when administering chlorambucil to patients with a history of seizure disorder, head trauma, or receiving other potentially epileptogenic drugs.

Children: The safety and effectiveness in children have not been established.

Patients with Impaired Renal Function: Patients with evidence of impaired renal function should be carefully monitored as they are prone to additional myelosuppression associated with azotemia.

Patients with Impaired Hepatic Function: Consideration should be given to dose reduction in patients with gross hepatic dysfunction.

Carcinogenicity: Acute secondary hematologic malignancies (especially leukemia and myelodysplastic syndrome) have been reported, particularly after long term treatment (see Adverse Effects).

A comparison of patients with ovarian cancer who received alkylating agents with those who did not, showed that the use of alkylating agents including chlorambucil, significantly increased the incidence of acute leukemia.

Acute myelogenous leukemia has been reported in a small proportion of patients receiving chlorambucil as long-term adjuvant therapy for breast cancer.

The leukemogenic risk must be balanced against the potential therapeutic benefit when considering the use of chlorambucil.

Impairment of Fertility, Teratogenic Effects, Mutagenesis: Chlorambucil may cause suppression of ovarian function. Amenorrhea has been reported following chlorambucil therapy.

Azoospermia has been observed as a result of therapy with chlorambucil, although it is estimated that a total dose of at least 400 mg is necessary.

Varying degrees of recovery of spermatogenesis have been reported in patients with lymphoma following treatment with chlorambucil in total doses of 410 to 2600 mg.

As with other cytotoxic agents, LEUKERAN is potentially teratogenic.

As with all cytotoxic chemotherapy, adequate contraceptive precautions should be advised when either partner is receiving chlorambucil.

Chlorambucil has been shown to cause chromatid or chromosome damage in man.

Drug Interactions: Vaccinations with live organism vaccines are not recommended in immunocompromised individuals (see Warnings).

Animal studies indicate that patients who receive phenylbutazone may require a reduction of the standard chlorambucil doses because of the possibility of enhanced chlorambucil toxicity.

ADVERSE EFFECTS: Leucopenia, neutropenia, thrombocytopenia, pancytopenia, anemia or bone marrow suppression is very common. Although bone marrow suppression frequently occurs, it is usually reversible if the chlorambucil is withdrawn early enough. However, irreversible bone marrow failure has been reported.

Acute secondary hematologic malignancies (especially leukemia and myelodysplastic syndrome) are common, particularly after long term treatment.

Gastrointestinal disturbances such as nausea and vomiting, diarrhea and oral ulceration occur infrequently. Other side effects may be encountered, but usually only when the therapeutic dosage has been exceeded.

Severe interstitial pulmonary fibrosis has occasionally been reported in patients with chronic lymphocytic leukemia on long-term chlorambucil therapy. Pulmonary fibrosis may be reversible on withdrawal of chlorambucil.

Allergic reactions to LEUKERAN (chlorambucil) such as urticaria and angioneurotic edema have been rarely reported following initial or subsequent dosing. Skin hypersensitivity (including rare reports of skin rash progressing to erythema multiforme, toxic epidermal necrolysis, and Stevens-Johnson syndrome) has been reported (see Warnings).

Other reported adverse reactions include hepatotoxicity and jaundice, drug fever, peripheral neuropathy, interstitial pneumonia, sterile cystitis, infertility, leukemia, and secondary malignancies (see Precautions).

Seizures have occurred in children with nephrotic syndrome treated with chlorambucil. Rare, focal and/or generalized seizures have been reported to occur in children and adults receiving therapeutic daily doses or high pulse dosing regimens of chlorambucil. Patients with a history of seizure disorder may be particularly susceptible (see Precautions).

Movement disorders including tremor, twitching and myoclonia in the absence of convulsions have also been reported.

OVERDOSE:

Symptoms: Reversible pancytopenia was the main finding of inadvertent overdose of chlorambucil. Neurological toxicity ranging from agitated behavior and ataxia to multiple grand mal seizures has also occurred.

Treatment: As there is no known antidote, the blood picture should be closely monitored and general supportive measures should be instituted together with appropriate blood transfusion, if necessary. Chlorambucil is not dialyzable. The physician should consider contacting a poison centre for additional information on the treatment of any overdose.

> For management of a suspected drug overdose, CPhA recommends that you contact your **regional Poison Control Centre**. See the *CPS* Directory section for a list of Poison Control Centres.

DOSAGE: Chronic Lymphocytic Leukemia: Treatment with LEUKERAN (chlorambucil) is usually started after the patient has developed symptoms or when there is evidence of impaired bone marrow function (but not marrow failure) as indicated by the peripheral blood count.

Initially, LEUKERAN is given at the dose of 0.15 mg/kg/day until the total leukocyte count is formed to 10 000/µL. Treatment may be resumed 4 weeks after the end of the first course and continued at a dosage of 0.1 mg/kg/day.

In a proportion of patients, usually after about 2 years of treatment, the blood leukocyte count is reduced to the normal range, enlarged spleen and lymph nodes become impalpable and the proportion of lymphocytes in the bone marrow is reduced to less than 20%.

Patients with evidence of bone marrow failure should first be treated with prednisolone and evidence of marrow regeneration should be obtained before commencing treatment with LEUKERAN.

Non-Hodgkin's Lymphoma: Used as a single agent, the usual dosage is 0.1 to 0.2 mg/kg/day for 4 to 8 weeks initially. Maintenance therapy is then given, either by a reduced daily dosage or intermittent courses of treatment.

LEUKERAN is useful in the management of patients with advanced lymphocytic lymphoma and those who have relapsed after radiotherapy.

There is no significant difference in the overall response rate obtained with chlorambucil as a single agent and combination chemotherapy in patients with advanced non-Hodgkin's lymphocytic lymphoma.

Hodgkin's Disease: Used as a single agent in the palliative treatment of advanced disease, a typical dosage is 0.2 mg/kg/day for 4 to 8 weeks. LEUKERAN is usually included in combination therapy and a number of regimes have been used. LEUKERAN may also be used as an alternative to nitrogen mustard with a reduction in toxicity but similar therapy results.

Special Instructions: Tablets should be returned to the manufacturer for destruction. Proper precautions should be taken in packaging those materials for transport.

All materials which have come in contact with cytotoxic drugs should be segregated and incinerated at 1000°C or more. Sealed containers may explode.

Personnel regularly involved in the preparation and handling of cytotoxic agents should have bi-annual blood examinations. Provided the outer coating is intact, there is no risk to handling. LEUKERAN Tablets should not be divided.

INFORMATION FOR THE PATIENT: Published in e-CPS, available by subscription at www.e-cps.ca.

SUPPLIED: Each brown, film-coated, round, biconvex tablet, engraved "GX EG3" on one face and "L" on the other face, contains: chlorambucil 2 mg. Nonmedicinal ingredients: anhydrous lactose, colloidal silicon dioxide, microcrystalline cellulose and stearic acid; tablet coating: hydroxypropylmethylcellulose, macrogol, synthetic red iron oxide, synthetic yellow iron oxide and titanium dioxide. Bottles of 25. Store in a refrigerator, between 2 and 8°C.

(Shown in Product Identification Section)

Leustatin® Ⓟ

cladribine

Antineoplastic—Chemotherapeutic Agent

Janssen-Ortho

Date of Preparation: March 8, 1996
Date of Revision: July 31, 2006

SUMMARY PRODUCT INFORMATION:

Route of Administration	Dosage Form/Strength	Clinically Relevant Nonmedicinal Ingredients
Intravenous Infusion	Liquid for Injection/1 mg/mL	Not Applicable For a complete listing see Dosage Forms, Composition and Packaging.

LEUSTATIN (cladribine) for Injection will be referenced as LEUSTATIN and/or cladribine throughout the Product Monograph.

INDICATIONS AND CLINICAL USE: LEUSTATIN (cladribine) for Injection is indicated for:

- Treatment of patients with Hairy Cell Leukemia.

LEUSTATIN should be administered under the supervision of a qualified physician experienced in the use of antineoplastic therapy.

Geriatrics (>65 years of age): See Warnings and Precautions, Special Populations.

Pediatrics, adolescents and young adults (<21 years of age): Safety and effectiveness in children have not been established (see Warnings and Precautions, Special Populations).

CONTRAINDICATIONS:

- LEUSTATIN (cladribine) for Injection is contraindicated in those patients who are hypersensitive to this drug or any of its components. (For a complete listing, see Dosage Forms, Composition and Packaging.)

WARNINGS AND PRECAUTIONS:

> **Serious Warnings and Precautions**
>
> LEUSTATIN (cladribine) for Injection should be administered under the supervision of a qualified physician experienced in the use of antineoplastic therapy.
>
> - Suppression of bone marrow function should be anticipated. This is usually reversible and appears to be dose dependent
> - Significant and prolonged lymphopenia has been noted
> - Serious neurological toxicity (including irreversible paraparesis and quadriparesis) has been reported in patients who received LEUSTATIN by continuous infusion at high doses (4 to 9 times the recommended dose for Hairy Cell Leukemia)
> - Neurologic toxicity appears to demonstrate a dose relationship; however, severe neurological toxicity has been reported rarely following treatment with standard cladribine dosing regimens
> - Acute nephrotoxicity has been observed with high doses of LEUSTATIN (4 to 9 times the recommended dose for Hairy Cell Leukemia), especially when given concomitantly with other nephrotoxic agents/therapies

General: LEUSTATIN (cladribine) for Injection is a potent antineoplastic agent with potentially significant toxic side effects. It should be administered only under the supervision of a physician experienced with the use of cancer chemotherapeutic agents. Patients undergoing therapy should be closely observed for signs of hematologic and non-hematologic toxicity. Careful hematologic monitoring (assessment of peripheral blood counts), particularly during the first 4 to 8 weeks post-treatment, is recommended to detect the development of anemia, neutropenia and thrombocytopenia and for early detection of any potential sequelae (e.g., infection or bleeding). Since fever is a frequently observed side effect during the first month on therapy, patients should be kept well hydrated. As with other potent chemotherapeutic agents, monitoring of renal and hepatic function is also recommended, especially in patients with underlying kidney or liver dysfunction (see Warnings and Precautions, Adverse Reactions and Dosage and Administration).

Tumour Lysis Syndrome: Rare cases of Tumour Lysis Syndrome have been reported in patients treated with cladribine with other hematologic malignancies having a high tumour burden.

Administration of LEUSTATIN (cladribine) for Injection: LEUSTATIN must be diluted in designated intravenous solution prior to administration (see Dosage and Administration).

Benzyl alcohol as a Diluent: Benzyl alcohol is a constituent of the recommended diluent for the 7-day infusion solution. Benzyl alcohol has been reported to be associated with a fatal "Gasping Syndrome" in premature infants (see Dosage and Administration).

Carcinogenesis and Mutagenesis: As expected for compounds in this class, the actions of cladribine yield DNA damage.

Hematologic: Bone Marrow Suppression: Severe bone marrow suppression, including neutropenia, anemia and thrombocytopenia, has been commonly observed in patients treated with LEUSTATIN (cladribine) for Injection, especially at high doses. The myelosuppressive effects of LEUSTATIN were most notable during the first month following treatment. Forty-four percent (44%) of patients received transfusions with RBCs and 14% received transfusions with platelets during Month 1. Careful hematologic monitoring (assessment of peripheral blood counts), particularly during the first 4 to 8 weeks post-treatment, is recommended. Most patients in the clinical studies had hematologic impairment as a manifestation of active Hairy Cell Leukemia. Consequently care should be taken to distinguish disease-related bone marrow suppression from that which may result following treatment with LEUSTATIN. (During the first two weeks after treatment initiation, Mean Platelet Count, Absolute Neutrophil Count (ANC), and Hemoglobin concentration declined and subsequently increased with normalization of mean counts by Day 12, Week 5 and Week 8, respectively). Proceed carefully in patients with severe bone marrow impairment of any etiology since further suppression of bone marrow function should be anticipated.

Hepatic/Biliary/Pancreatic: There are inadequate data on dosing of patients with hepatic insufficiency. Therefore, caution is advised when administering LEUSTATIN (cladribine) for Injection to patients with known or suspected hepatic insufficiency.

Immune: Fever: Fever (T≥37.8°C) was associated with the use of LEUSTATIN (cladribine) for Injection in approximately two-thirds of patients (131/196) in the first month of therapy. Virtually all of these patients were treated empirically with parenteral antibiotics. Overall, 47% (93/196) of all patients had fever in the setting of neutropenia (ANC≤1000×10^6/L), including 62 patients (32%) with severe neutropenia (ANC≤500×10^6/L) (see Adverse Reactions, Clinical Trial Adverse Drug Reactions).

Opportunistic infections have occurred in the acute phase of treatment due to the immunosuppression mediated by LEUSTATIN.

Neurologic: Neurotoxicity was observed in patients, undergoing bone marrow transplantation for acute leukemia. High doses (4 to 9 times the recommended dose for Hairy Cell Leukemia), in conjunction with cyclophosphamide and total body irradiation as preparation for bone marrow transplantation, have been associated with severe, irreversible, neurologic toxicity (paraparesis/quadriparesis) and/or acute renal insufficiency. These toxicities occurred in 45% of patients treated for 7-14 days.

Axonal peripheral polyneuropathy was observed in a dose escalation study at the highest dose levels (approximately 4 times the recommended dose for Hairy Cell Leukemia) in patients not receiving cyclophosphamide or total body irradiation. Severe neurological toxicity has been reported rarely following treatment with standard cladribine dosing regimens.

Renal: Acute renal insufficiency has developed in some patients receiving high doses of LEUSTATIN (cladribine) for Injection. In one study, following a one-hour infusion, the recovery of cladribine in the urine over a 24-hour period was between 10-30% of the administered dose. There are inadequate data on dosing of patients with renal insufficiency. Therefore, caution is advised when administering LEUSTATIN Injection to patients with known or suspected renal insufficiency.

High doses (4 to 9 times the recommended dose for Hairy Cell Leukemia), in conjunction with cyclophosphamide and total body irradiation as preparation for bone marrow transplantation, have been associated with severe, irreversible, neurologic toxicity (paraparesis/quadriparesis) and/or acute renal insufficiency. These toxicities occurred in 45% of patients treated for 7-14 days. In patients with Hairy Cell Leukemia treated with the recommended dose (0.09 mg/kg/day for 7 days), no nephrotoxicity has been reported. Deviations from the dosing regimen recommended for Hairy Cell Leukemia are not advised.

Sexual Function/Reproduction: Impairment of Fertility: The effect on human fertility is unknown. When administered intravenously to Cynomolgus monkeys, cladribine has been shown to cause suppression of rapidly generating cells, including testicular cells.

Special Populations: Pregnant Women: Although there is no evidence of teratogenicity due to LEUSTATIN (cladribine) for Injection in humans, other drugs that inhibit DNA synthesis (e.g. methotrexate and aminopterin) have been reported to be teratogenic in humans. LEUSTATIN has been shown to be embryotoxic in mice when given at doses equivalent to the recommended dose. LEUSTATIN should not be given during pregnancy. There are no adequate and well-controlled studies in pregnant women. If LEUSTATIN is used during pregnancy or if the patient becomes pregnant while taking this drug, the patient should be apprised of the potential hazard to the fetus. Women of childbearing age should be advised to avoid becoming pregnant.

Fetotoxicity: Cladribine is teratogenic in mice and rabbits and consequently has the potential to cause fetal harm when administered to a pregnant woman. A significant increase in variations of fetal growth/development (i.e. increases in cervical ribs, irregularly-shaped exoccipital bones, and variations in sternal ossification) was observed in mice receiving 1.5 mg/kg/day (4.5 mg/m^2) and increased resorptions, reduced litter size and increased fetal malformations were observed when mice received 3.0 mg/kg/day (9 mg/m^2). Fetal death and malformations were observed in rabbits that received 3.0 mg/kg/day (33.0 mg/m^2). No fetal effects were seen in mice at 0.5 mg/kg/day (1.5 mg/m^2) or in rabbits at 1.0 mg/kg/day (11.0 mg/m^2).

Nursing Women: It is not known whether this drug is excreted in human milk. LEUSTATIN (cladribine) for Injection should not be given to a nursing mother.

Pediatrics, Adolescents, and Young Adults (1-21 years of age): In a Phase I study involving patients 1-21 years old with relapsed acute leukemia, LEUSTATIN (cladribine) for Injection was given by continuous intravenous infusion in doses ranging from 3 to 10.7 mg/m^2/day for 5 days (one-half to twice the dose recommended in Hairy Cell Leukemia). In this study, the dose-limiting toxicity was severe myelosuppression with profound neutropenia and thrombocytopenia. At the highest dose (10.7 mg/m^2/day), 3 of 7 patients developed irreversible myelosuppression and fatal systemic bacterial or fungal infections. No unique toxicities were noted in this study (see Indications and Clinical Use).

Geriatrics (>65 years of age): Clinical studies of LEUSTATIN (cladribine) for Injection did not include sufficient numbers of subject's aged 65 and over to determine whether they respond differently from younger subjects. Other reported clinical experience has not identified differences in responses between the elderly and younger patients. In general, dose selection for an elderly patient should be cautious, reflecting the greater frequency of decreased hepatic, renal, or cardiac function, and of concomitant disease or other drug therapy in elderly patients (see Indications and Clinical Use).

Monitoring and Laboratory Tests: During and following treatment, the patient's hematologic profile should be monitored regularly to determine the degree of hematopoietic suppression. In the clinical studies, following reversible declines in all cell counts, the Mean Platelet Count reached 100×10⁹/L by Day 12, the Mean Absolute Neutrophil Count reached 1500×10⁶/L by Week 5 and the Mean Hemoglobin reached 12 g/dL by Week 8. After peripheral counts have normalized, bone marrow aspiration and biopsy should be performed to confirm response to treatment with LEUSTATIN (cladribine) for Injection. Febrile events should be investigated with appropriate laboratory and radiologic studies. Periodic assessment of renal function and hepatic function should be performed as clinically indicated.

ADVERSE REACTIONS: Adverse Drug Reaction Overview: Safety data are based on 196 patients with Hairy Cell Leukemia. The original cohort of 124 patients plus an additional 72 patients enrolled at the same 2 centres after the original enrolment cut-off. Of the 196 patients with Hairy Cell Leukemia entered in the two trials, there were 8 deaths following treatment. Of these, 6 were of infectious etiology, including 3 pneumonias, and 2 occurred in the first month following LEUSTATIN (cladribine) for Injection therapy. Of the 8 deaths, 6 occurred in previously treated patients who were refractory to α-interferon.

In Month 1 of the clinical trials for Hairy Cell Leukemia, severe neutropenia was noted in 70% of patients, fever in 69%, and infection was documented in 28%. Other adverse experiences reported frequently during the first 14 days after initiating treatment included: fatigue (45%), nausea (28%), rash (27%), headache (22%) and injection site reactions (19%). Most of the non-hematologic adverse experiences were mild to moderate in severity.

Clinical Trial Adverse Drug Reactions: Because clinical trials are conducted under very specific conditions the adverse reaction rates observed in the clinical trials may not reflect the rates observed in practice and should not be compared to the rates in the clinical trials of another drug. Adverse drug reaction information from clinical trials is useful for identifying drug-related adverse events and for approximating rates.

Effects of High Doses: In a Phase I investigational study using LEUSTATIN (cladribine) for Injection in high doses (4 to 9 times the recommended dose for Hairy Cell Leukemia) as part of a bone marrow transplant conditioning regimen, which also included high dose cyclophosphamide and total body irradiation, acute nephrotoxicity and delayed onset neurotoxicity were observed.

Thirty-one poor-risk patients with drug-resistant acute leukemia in relapse (29 cases) or non-Hodgkins lymphoma (2 cases) received doses of LEUSTATIN for 7 to 14 days prior to bone marrow transplantation. During LEUSTATIN infusion, 8 patients experienced gastrointestinal symptoms. While the bone marrow was initially cleared of all hematopoietic elements, including tumor cells, leukemia eventually recurred in all treated patients. Within 7 to 13 days after starting treatment with LEUSTATIN, 6 patients (19%) developed manifestations of renal dysfunction (i.e., acidosis, anuria, elevated serum creatinine, etc.) and 5 required dialysis. Several of these patients were also being treated with other medications having known nephrotoxic potential. Renal dysfunction was reversible in 2 of these patients. In the 4 patients whose renal function had not recovered at the time of death, autopsies were performed; in 2 of these, evidence of tubular damage was noted. Eleven patients (35%) experienced delayed onset neurologic toxicity. In the majority, this was characterized by progressive irreversible motor weakness (paraparesis/quadriparesis) of the upper and/or lower extremities, first noted 35 to 84 days after starting high dose therapy with LEUSTATIN. Non-invasive testing (electromyography and nerve conduction studies) was consistent with demyelinating disease.

Axonal peripheral polyneuropathy was observed in a dose escalation study at the highest dose levels (approximately 4 times the recommended dose for Hairy Cell Leukemia) in patients not receiving cyclophosphamide or total body irradiation. Severe neurological toxicity has been reported rarely following treatment with standard cladribine dosing regimens (see Warnings and Precautions, Neurologic and Renal).

Myelosuppression: Myelosuppression was frequently observed during the first month after starting treatment. Neutropenia (ANC<500×10⁶/L) was noted in 70% of patients, compared with 26% in whom it was present initially. Severe anemia (Hemoglobin <8.5 g/dL) developed in 37% of patients, compared with 10% initially, and thrombocytopenia (Platelets <20×10⁹/L) developed in 12% of patients, compared with 4% in whom it was noted initially. During the first month, 54 of 196 patients (28%) exhibited documented evidence of infection: serious infections (e.g. septicemia, pneumonia) were reported in 6% of all patients; the remainder were mild or moderate. Several deaths were attributable to infection and/or complications related to the underlying disease. During the second month, the overall rate of documented infection was 6%; these infections were mild to moderate and no severe systemic infections were seen. After the third month, the monthly incidence of infection was either less than or equal to that of the months immediately preceding LEUSTATIN (cladribine) for Injection therapy.

Infection: Documented infections were noted in fewer than one-third of febrile episodes. Of the 196 patients studied, 19 were noted to have a documented infection in the month prior to treatment. In the month following treatment, there were 54 episodes of documented infection: 23 (42%) were bacterial, 11 (20%) were viral and 11 (20%) were fungal. Seven of 8 documented episodes of herpes zoster occurred during the month following treatment. Fourteen of 16 episodes of documented fungal infections occurred in the first two months following treatment. Virtually all of these patients were treated empirically with antibiotics.

Effects on Lymphocytes: Analysis of lymphocyte subsets indicates that treatment with cladribine is associated with prolonged depression of the CD4 counts and transient suppression of CD8 counts. Prior to treatment, the mean CD4 count was 766/µL. The mean CD4 count nadir, which occurred 4 to 6 months following treatment, was 272/µL. Fifteen months after treatment, mean CD4 counts remained below 500/µL. CD8 counts decreased initially, though increasing counts were observed after 9 months. In a study of 46 patients, the median time to reach a normal absolute CD4+ lymphocyte count was 40 months. Although depletion of these cells may contribute to the risk of opportunistic infection, no direct correlation has been reported between the CD4+ count and the incidence of infection. The clinical significance of the prolonged CD4 lymphopenia is unclear.

Bone Marrow Hypocellularity: Another event of unknown clinical significance includes the observation of prolonged bone marrow hypocellularity. Bone marrow hypocellularity (<35%) was noted after 4 months in 42 of 124 patients (34%) treated in the two pivotal trials. This hypocellularity was noted as late as Day 1010. It is not known whether the hypocellularity is the result of disease-related marrow fibrosis or if it is the result of cladribine toxicity. There was no apparent clinical effect on the peripheral blood counts.

Adverse experiences related to intravenous administration: Injection site reactions (9%; i.e. redness, swelling, pain), Thrombosis (2%), Phlebitis (2%) and a Broken Catheter (1%). These appear to be related to the infusion procedure and/or indwelling catheter, rather than the medication or the vehicle.

Skin: The vast majority of rashes were mild and occurred in patients who were receiving or had recently been treated with other medications (e.g. allopurinol or antibiotics) known to cause rash.

Gastrointestinal: Most episodes of nausea were mild, not accompanied by vomiting, and did not require treatment with antiemetics. In patients requiring antiemetics, nausea was easily controlled, most frequently with chlorpromazine.

Fever: Fever was a frequently observed side effect during the first month on study. During the first month, 11% of patients experienced severe fever (i.e. ≥40°C). Since fever may be accompanied by increased fluid loss, patients should be kept well hydrated during treatment. Since the majority of fevers occurred in neutropenic patients, patients should be closely monitored during the first month of treatment and empiric antibiotics should be initiated as clinically indicated. Although 69% of patients developed fevers, less than 1/3 of febrile events were associated with documented infection. Given the known myelosuppressive effects of LEUSTATIN (cladribine) for Injection, practitioners should carefully evaluate the risks and benefits of administering this drug to patients with active infections (see Warnings and Precautions).

Adverse reactions reported during the first 2 weeks following treatment initiation (regardless of relationship to drug) by ≥5% of patients are listed in Table 1.

From Day 15 to the last follow-up visit, the only events reported by ≥5% of patients were: fatigue (11%), rash (10%), headache (7%), cough (7%), and malaise (5%).

Post-Market Adverse Drug Reactions: The following additional adverse events have been reported since the drug became commercially available. These adverse events have been reported primarily in patients who received multiple courses of LEUSTATIN (cladribine) for Injection.

Hematologic: bone marrow suppression with prolonged pancytopenia, including some reports of aplastic anemia; hemolytic anemia which was reported in patients with lymphoid malignancies, occurring within the first few weeks following treatment; hypereosinophilia. Cases of myelodysplastic syndrome have been reported (0.03%).

Hepatic: reversible, generally mild increases in bilirubin and transaminases.

Nervous system: neurological toxicity; however, severe neurotoxicity has been reported rarely following treatment with standard cladribine dosing regimens.

Respiratory system: pulmonary interstitial infiltrates; in most cases, an infectious etiology was identified.

Skin/subcutaneous: urticaria, hypereosinophilia. In isolated cases Stevens-Johnson and toxic epidermal necrolysis have been reported in patients who were receiving or had recently been treated with other medications (e.g. allopurinol or antibiotics) known to cause these syndromes. For a description of adverse reactions associated with the use of high doses in non-Hairy Cell Leukemia patients see Warnings and Precautions.

Table 1: LEUSTATIN

Adverse Reactions Reported by ≥5% of Patients During the First 2 Weeks Following Treatment Initiation (regardless of relationship to drug)

Body System	Adverse Event
Body as a Whole	Fever, chills, fatigue, asthenia, malaise, trunk pain, diaphoresis
Gastrointestinal System	Nausea, decreased appetite, constipation, vomiting, diarrhea, abdominal pain
Hemic/Lymphatic System	Purpura, petechiae, epistaxis
Nervous System	Headache, dizziness, insomnia
Cardiovascular System	Edema, tachycardia
Respiratory System	Abnormal breath sounds, abnormal chest sounds, cough, shortness of breath
Skin/Subcutaneous Tissue	Rash, injection site reactions, pruritus, pain, erythema
Musculoskeletal System	Myalgia, arthralgia

DRUG INTERACTIONS: Overview: There are no known drug interactions with LEUSTATIN (cladribine) for Injection. Caution should be exercised if LEUSTATIN is administered before, after or in conjunction with other drugs known to cause immunosuppression or myelosuppression (see Warnings and Precautions).

Drug-Drug Interactions: Interactions with other drugs have not been established.

Drug-Food Interactions: Interactions with food have not been established.

Drug-Herb Interactions: Interactions with herbal products have not been established.

Drug-Laboratory Test Interactions: Interactions with laboratory tests have not been established.

DOSAGE AND ADMINISTRATION: Dosing Considerations: High doses of LEUSTATIN (cladribine) for Injection have been associated with:

- Irreversible neurologic toxicity (paraparesis/quadriparesis)
- Acute nephrotoxicity
- Severe bone marrow suppression resulting in neutropenia, anemia and thrombocytopenia

Recommended Dose and Dosage Adjustment: The recommended dose and schedule of LEUSTATIN (cladribine) for Injection for Hairy Cell Leukemia is a single course given by continuous infusion for 7 consecutive days at a dose of 0.09 mg/kg/day. Deviations from this dosage regimen are not advised. If the patient does not respond to the initial course of LEUSTATIN for Hairy Cell Leukemia, it is unlikely that they will benefit from additional courses. Physicians should consider delaying or discontinuing the drug if neurotoxicity or renal toxicity occur (see Warnings and Precautions).

Specific risk factors predisposing to increased toxicity from LEUSTATIN have not been defined. In view of the known toxicities of agents of this class, it would be prudent to proceed carefully in patients with known or suspected renal insufficiency or severe bone marrow impairment of any etiology. Patients should be monitored closely for hematologic or non-hematologic toxicity (see Warnings and Precautions).

Acute renal insufficiency has developed in some patients receiving high doses of LEUSTATIN. In one study, following a one-hour infusion, the recovery of cladribine in the urine over a 24-hour period was between 10-30% of the administered dose. In addition, there are inadequate data on dosing of patients with renal or hepatic insufficiency. Therefore, caution is advised when administering LEUSTATIN to patients with known or suspected renal or hepatic insufficiency (see Warnings and Precautions).

Administration: Reconstitution: Parenteral Products: LEUSTATIN (cladribine) for Injection must be diluted with the designated diluent prior to administration. **Since the drug product does not contain any antimicrobial preservative or bacteriostatic agent, aseptic technique and proper environmental precautions must be observed in preparation of LEUSTATIN solutions.**

Preparation of a Single Daily Dose: Add the calculated dose (0.09 mg/kg or 0.09 mL/kg) of LEUSTATIN (cladribine) for Injection to an infusion bag containing 500 mL of 0.9% Sodium Chloride Injection, USP. Infuse continuously over 24 hours. Repeat daily for a total of 7 consecutive days. **The use of 5% dextrose as a diluent is not recommended because of increased degradation of cladribine.** Admixtures of LEUSTATIN are chemically and physically stable for at least 24 hours at room temperature under normal room fluorescent light in Baxter Viaflex PVC infusion containers. See Table 2.

Table 2: LEUSTATIN

24-Hour Infusion Method

Dose of LEUSTATIN (cladribine) for Injection	Recommended Diluent	Quantity of Diluent
0.09 mg/kg 1 (day)×0.09 mg/kg	0.9% Sodium Chloride Injection	500 mL

Preparation of a 7-Day Infusion: The 7-day infusion solution should only be prepared with Bacteriostatic 0.9% Sodium Chloride Injection, USP (0.9% benzyl alcohol preserved). In order to minimize the risk of microbial contamination, both LEUSTATIN (cladribine) for Injection and the diluent should be passed through a sterile 0.22 µ disposable hydrophilic syringe filter as each solution is being introduced into the infusion reservoir. First add the calculated dose of LEUSTATIN (7 days×0.09 mg/kg) to the infusion reservoir through the sterile filter. Then add a calculated amount of Bacteriostatic 0.9% Sodium Chloride Injection, USP (0.9% benzyl alcohol preserved) also through the filter to bring the total volume of the solution to 100 mL. After completing solution preparation, clamp off the line, disconnect and discard the filter. Aseptically aspirate air bubbles from the reservoir as necessary using the syringe and a dry second sterile filter or a sterile vent filter assembly. Reclamp the line and discard the syringe and filter assembly. Infuse continuously over 7 days. Solutions prepared with Bacteriostatic Sodium Chloride injection for individuals weighing more than 85 kg may have reduced preservative effectiveness due to greater dilution of the benzyl alcohol preservative. Admixtures for the 7-day infusion have demonstrated acceptable chemical and physical stability for at least 7 days in SIMS Deltec Inc. Medication cassettes. See Table 3.

Table 3: LEUSTATIN

7-Day Infusion Method

Dose of LEUSTATIN (cladribine) for Injection	Recommended Diluent	Quantity of Diluent
7 (days)×0.09 mg/kg	Bacteriostatic 0.9% Sodium Chloride Injection, USP (0.9% benzyl alcohol)	q.s. to 100 mL

N.B.: Use sterile 0.22 µ filter when preparing infusion solution.

Since limited compatibility data are available, adherence to the recommended diluents and infusion systems is advised. Solutions containing LEUSTATIN should not be mixed with other intravenous drugs or additives, or infused simultaneously via a common intravenous line, since compatibility testing has not been performed. Preparations containing benzyl alcohol should not be used in neonates (see Warnings and Precautions, Special Populations).

If the same intravenous line is used for sequential infusion of several different drugs, the line should be flushed with a compatible diluent before and after infusion of LEUSTATIN.

Care must be taken to assure the sterility of prepared solutions. Once diluted, solutions of LEUSTATIN should be administered promptly or stored in the refrigerator (2 to 8°C) for no more than 8 hours prior to start of administration. Vials of LEUSTATIN are for single use only. Any unused portion should be discarded in an appropriate manner.

Parenteral drug products should be inspected visually for particulate matter and discoloration prior to administration, whenever solution and container permit. A precipitate may occur during the exposure of LEUSTATIN to low temperatures; it may be resolubilized by allowing the solution to warm naturally to room temperature and by shaking vigorously. **Do not heat or microwave.**

OVERDOSAGE:
There is no known specific antidote to overdosage. Treatment of overdosage consists of discontinuation of LEUSTATIN (cladribine) for Injection, careful observation and appropriate supportive measures. It is not known whether cladribine can be removed from the circulation by any form of dialysis or hemofiltration.

> For management of a suspected drug overdose, CPhA recommends that you contact your **regional Poison Control Centre**. See the *CPS* Directory section for a list of Poison Control Centres.

ACTION AND CLINICAL PHARMACOLOGY: Mechanism of Action: LEUSTATIN (cladribine) for Injection (also commonly known as 2-chloro-2'-deoxy-β-D-adenosine) is a synthetic antineoplastic agent. The selective toxicity of cladribine towards certain normal and malignant lymphocyte and monocyte populations is based on the relative activities of deoxycytidine kinase, and deoxynucleotidase. Like some other deoxypurine nucleosides, cladribine crosses the cell membrane passively. In cells with a high ratio of deoxycytidine kinase to deoxynucleotidase, it is phosphorylated by deoxycytidine kinase to 2-chloro-2'-deoxy-β-D-adenosine monophosphate (2-CdAMP). Since cladribine is resistant to deamination by adenosine deaminase and there is little deoxynucleotidase in lymphocytes and monocytes, 2-CdAMP accumulates intracellularly and is subsequently converted into the active triphosphate deoxynucleotide, 2-chloro-2'-deoxy-β-D-adenosine triphosphate (2-CdATP). It is postulated that cells with high deoxycytidine kinase and low deoxynucleotidase activities will be selectively killed by cladribine as toxic deoxynucleotides accumulate intracellularly.

Cells containing high concentrations of deoxynucleotides are unable to properly repair single-strand DNA breaks. The broken ends of DNA activate the enzyme poly (ADP-ribose) polymerase resulting in NAD and ATP depletion and disruption of cellular metabolism. There is evidence also, that 2-CdATP is incorporated into the DNA of dividing cells, resulting in impairment of DNA synthesis. Thus cladribine can be distinguished from other chemotherapeutic agents affecting purine metabolism in that it is cytotoxic to both actively dividing and quiescent lymphocytes and monocytes, inhibiting both DNA synthesis and repair.

Pharmacokinetics: Absorption: In a clinical investigation, 17 patients with Hairy Cell Leukemia and normal renal function were treated for 7 days with the recommended treatment regimen of LEUSTATIN (cladribine) for Injection (0.09 mg/kg/day) by continuous intravenous infusion. The mean steady-state serum concentration was estimated to be 5.7 ng/mL with a systemic clearance of 663.5 mL/hr/kg. Accumulation of cladribine over the seven day treatment period was not noted.

In a study using two (2) hour infusion of LEUSTATIN at 0.14 mg/kg (8 patients with hematologic malignancies), the mean end-of-infusion plasma cladribine concentration was 48±19 ng/mL. For 5 of the 8 patients with hematologic malignancies, the disappearance of cladribine could be described by either a biphasic or triphasic decline. The mean harmonic terminal half-life for both studies was 5.4 hours, with mean values for clearance and steady-state volume of distribution represented as 978±422 mL/hr/kg and 4.52±2.82 L/kg, respectively. In patients with Hairy Cell Leukemia, there does not appear to be a relationship between serum concentrations and ultimate clinical outcome.

Plasma cladribine concentrations were reported to decline multi-exponentially after intravenous infusions. In one study, thirteen patients with B-cell CLL and low-grade NHL were treated with LEUSTATIN for 5 consecutive days. LEUSTATIN was administered as a 2-hour IV infusion (0.14 mg/kg), SC (0.14 mg/kg), or orally (0.28 mg/kg) with alternate order between patients. Cladribine declined bi-exponentially after the IV administration with α and β half-lives ranging from 0.24 to 2.33 hours (mean±SD=0.70±0.60 hours) and 4.5 to 21.8 hours (mean±SD=9.9±4.6 hours), respectively. The mean±SD C_{max}, clearance, and apparent volume of distribution of cladribine when the 2-hour infusion was administered as the initiate dose were 213±193 nmol/L (n=3), 29.5±8.3 L/h/m² (n=6), and 67.6±28.9 L/m² (n=6), respectively. In another study, twelve patients with lymphoproliferative diseases were treated with LEUSTATIN at a dose of 0.14 mg/kg for 5 consecutive days. LEUSTATIN was administered as a 2-hour IV infusion on Days 1, 3, 4 and 5 and as a 24-hour IV infusion on Day 2. Cladribine declined bi-exponentially after the first IV dose with α and β half-lives ranging from 19 to 58 minutes (mean±SD=35±12 minutes) and 2.8 to 12.1 hours (mean±SD=6.7±2.5 hours), respectively. The mean±SD C_{max} and apparent volume of distribution of cladribine after the first IV dose was 198±87 nmol/L and 9.2±5.4 L/kg, respectively. There was no apparent difference in area under the plasma concentration time curve between the first 2-hour infusion dose and the second 24-hour IV infusion dose, suggesting the disposition of cladribine is independent of infusion rate ranging from 6 to 70 mg/kg/h. The mean half-life of cladribine in leukemic cells has been reported to be 23 hours.

Distribution: Cladribine is bound approximately 20% to plasma proteins and penetrates into cerebrospinal fluid. One report indicates that the CSF concentrations are approximately 25% of those in plasma.

Metabolism: In man, following a 2 hour infusion, the terminal half-life of cladribine has been estimated at ~5.4 hours. Except for limited understanding of the mechanism of cellular toxicity and route of excretion, no other information is available on the metabolism of cladribine in man.

Excretion: An average of 18% of the administered dose has been reported to be excreted in urine of patients with solid tumours during a 5-day continuous intravenous infusion of 3.5-8.1 mg/m²/day of cladribine. Other investigators reported approximately 30% of urinary recovery of cladribine during the first 24 hour post-infusion period during a 5-day 2-hour intravenous infusion of 3.5-10.5 mg/m²/day of cladribine in patients with solid tumours and during 5-day 2-hour intravenous infusion of 6-12 mg/m²/day of cladribine in 10 patients with leukemia or lymphoma. The effect of renal and hepatic impairment on the elimination of cladribine has not been investigated in humans.

STORAGE AND STABILITY: When vials and infusion solutions are stored between 2 to 8°C protected from light, unopened vials of LEUSTATIN (cladribine) for Injection are stable until the expiration date indicated on the package. Freezing does not adversely affect the solution. If freezing occurs, thaw naturally to room temperature. **Do not** heat or microwave. Once thawed, the vial of LEUSTATIN is stable until expiry if refrigerated. **Do not** refreeze. Once diluted, solutions containing LEUSTATIN should be administered promptly or stored in the refrigerator (2 to 8°C) for no more than 8 hours prior to administration.

Store refrigerated 2 to 8°C.

Protect from light during storage.

SPECIAL HANDLING INSTRUCTIONS: The potential hazards associated with cytotoxic agents are well established and proper precautions should be taken when handling, preparing, and administering LEUSTATIN (cladribine) for Injection. The use of disposable gloves and protective garments is recommended. If LEUSTATIN comes in contact with the skin or mucous membranes, wash the involved surface immediately with copious amounts of water. Several guidelines on this subject have been published. Refer to your institution's guidelines for disposal of cytotoxic waste.

LEUSTATIN must be diluted with the designated intravenous solutions prior to administration. **Since the drug product does not contain any antimicrobial preservative or bacteriostatic agent, aseptic technique and proper environmental precautions must be observed in preparation of LEUSTATIN solutions.**

INFORMATION FOR THE PATIENT: Published in e-CPS, available by subscription at www.e-cps.ca.

DOSAGE FORMS, COMPOSITION AND PACKAGING: Each mL of sterile, preservative-free, isotonic solution contains: cladribine 1 mg. Single-use clear flint glass 20 mL vials containing 10 mL (1 mg/mL), boxes of 1.

> The reader is invited to consult CPhA's monograph **Fluoroquinolones**.

Levaquin® Pr
levofloxacin
Antibacterial

Janssen-Ortho

Date of Preparation: November 5, 1997
Date of Revision: May 6, 2010

SUMMARY PRODUCT INFORMATION:

Route of Administration	Dosage Form/ Strength	Clinically Relevant Nonmedicinal Ingredients
Oral	Tablet 250 mg, 500 mg, 750 mg	None For a complete listing see Dosage Forms, Composition and Packaging.
Intravenous Infusion	Injection 5 mg/mL in 5% dextrose	None For a complete listing see Dosage Forms, Composition and Packaging.

INDICATIONS AND CLINICAL USE: LEVAQUIN levofloxacin Tablets and Injection are indicated for the treatment of adults with bacterial infections caused by susceptible strains of the designated microorganisms in the infections listed below.

Note: Since i.v. and oral formulations are interchangeable, i.v. administration is recommended only when it offers a route of administration advantageous to the patient (e.g. patient cannot tolerate oral dosage form).

Upper Respiratory Tract: Acute sinusitis (mild to moderate) due to *S. pneumoniae*, *H. influenzae*, or *M. (Branhamella) catarrhalis*.

Lower Respiratory Tract: Acute bacterial exacerbations of chronic bronchitis (mild to moderate) due to *S. aureus*, *S. pneumoniae*, *H. influenzae*, *H. parainfluenzae*, or *M. (Branhamella) catarrhalis*.

Community-acquired pneumonia (mild, moderate and severe infections) due to *S. aureus*, *S. pneumoniae* (including penicillin-resistant strains), *H. influenzae*, *H. parainfluenzae*, *K. pneumoniae*, *M. (Branhamella) catarrhalis*, *C. pneumoniae*, *L. pneumophila*, or *M. pneumoniae* (see Dosage and Administration).

Nosocomial pneumonia due to methicillin-susceptible *S. aureus*, *P. aeruginosa*, *S. marcescens*, *E. coli*, *K. pneumoniae*, *H. influenzae* or *S. pneumoniae*. Adjunctive therapy should be used as clinically indicated. Where *P. aeruginosa* is a documented or presumptive pathogen, combination therapy with an anti-pseudomonal β-lactam is recommended.

Skin and Skin Structure: Uncomplicated skin and skin structure infections (mild to moderate) due to *S. aureus* or *S. pyogenes*.

Complicated skin and skin structure infections (mild to moderate), excluding burns, due to *E. faecalis*, methicillin-sensitive *S. aureus*, *S. pyogenes*, *P. mirabilis*, or *S. agalactiae*.

Urinary Tract: Complicated urinary tract infections (mild to moderate) due to *E. (Streptococcus) faecalis*, *E. cloacae*, *E. coli*, *K. pneumoniae*, *P. mirabilis*, or *P. aeruginosa* (see Dosage and Administration).

Uncomplicated urinary tract infections (mild to moderate) due to *E. coli*, *K. pneumoniae*, or *S. saprophyticus*.

Acute pyelonephritis (mild to moderate) caused by *E. coli* (see Dosage and Administration).

Chronic bacterial prostatitis due to *E. coli*, *E. faecalis*, or *S. epidermidis*.

Appropriate culture and susceptibility tests should be performed before treatment in order to isolate and identify the organisms causing the infection, and to determine their susceptibility to levofloxacin. Therapy with levofloxacin may be initiated before the results of these tests are known; once results become available, appropriate therapy should be continued.

As with other drugs in this class, some strains of *P. aeruginosa* may develop resistance fairly rapidly during treatment with levofloxacin. Culture and susceptibility testing performed periodically during therapy, will reveal not only the therapeutic effect of the antimicrobial agent, but also the possible emergence of bacterial resistance.

Geriatrics (≥65 years of age): Drug absorption appears to be unaffected by age. Dose adjustment based on age alone is not necessary (see Warnings and Precautions, Special Populations and Action and Clinical Pharmacology).

Pediatrics (<18 years of age) : Safety and effectiveness in children under 18 years of age have not been established (see Warnings and Precautions, Special Populations).

CONTRAINDICATIONS: LEVAQUIN levofloxacin Tablets and Injection are contraindicated in persons with a history of hypersensitivity to levofloxacin, quinolone antimicrobial agents, or any other components of this product. For a complete listing, see the Dosage Forms, Composition and Packaging.

Levofloxacin is also contraindicated in persons with a history of tendinitis or tendon rupture associated with the use of any member of the quinolone group of antimicrobial agents.

WARNINGS AND PRECAUTIONS:

> **Serious Warnings and Precautions**
> - LEVAQUIN (levofloxacin) has been shown to prolong the QT interval of the electrocardiogram in some patients (see Warnings and Precautions, Cardiovascular).
> - Serious hypersensitivity and/or anaphylactic reactions have been reported in patients receiving quinolone therapy, including LEVAQUIN.
> - Seizures may occur with quinolone therapy. LEVAQUIN should be used with caution in patients with known or suspected CNS disorders which may predispose to seizures or lower the seizure threshold (see Warnings and Precautions, Neurologic).
> - LEVAQUIN should not be used in pregnant women unless the potential benefits outweigh the potential risk to the fetus (see Warnings and Precautions, Special Populations).
> - For nursing mothers, a decision should be made to either discontinue nursing or discontinue the administration of LEVAQUIN, taking into account the importance of LEVAQUIN therapy to the mother and the possible risk to the infant (see Warnings and Precautions, Special Populations).
> - LEVAQUIN is not recommended for children under the age of 18 years (see Warnings and Precautions, Special Populations).

General: The oral and intravenous administration of levofloxacin increased the incidence and severity of osteochondrosis in immature rats and dogs. Other quinolones also produce similar erosions in the weight-bearing joints and other signs of arthropathy in immature animals of various species. Consequently, levofloxacin should not be used in pre-pubertal patients.

Although levofloxacin is soluble, adequate hydration of patients receiving LEVAQUIN levofloxacin should be maintained to prevent the formation of a highly concentrated urine. Crystalluria has been observed rarely in patients receiving other quinolones, when associated with high doses and an alkaline urine. Although crystalluria was not observed in clinical trials with levofloxacin, patients are encouraged to remain adequately hydrated.

As with any antimicrobial drug, periodic assessment of organ system functions, including renal, hepatic, and hematopoietic, is advisable during prolonged therapy (see Adverse Reactions).

I.V. Administration: Because rapid or bolus intravenous injection may result in hypotension, **levofloxacin injection should only be administered by slow intravenous infusion over a period of 60 minutes for a 500 mg dose, and 90 minutes for a 750 mg dose** (see Dosage and Administration).

Sexually Transmitted Diseases: Levofloxacin is not indicated for the treatment of syphilis or gonorrhea. Levofloxacin is not effective in the treatment of syphilis. Antimicrobial agents used in high doses for short periods of time to treat gonorrhea may mask or delay the symptoms of incubating syphilis. All patients with gonorrhea should have a serologic test for syphilis at the time of diagnosis. Patients treated with antimicrobial agents with limited or no activity against *T. pallidum* should have a follow-up serologic test for syphilis after 3 months.

Cardiovascular: QT Prolongation: Some quinolones, including levofloxacin, have been associated with prolongation of the QT interval on the electrocardiogram and infrequent cases of arrhythmia. During post-marketing surveillance, very rare cases of torsades de pointes have been reported in patients taking levofloxacin. These reports generally involved patients with concurrent medical conditions or concomitant medications that may have been contributory. The risk of arrhythmias may be reduced by avoiding concurrent use with other drugs that prolong the QT interval including macrolide antibiotics, antipsychotics, tricyclic antidepressants, Class IA (e.g. quinidine, procainamide) or Class III (e.g. amiodarone, sotalol) antiarrhythmic agents, and cisapride. In addition, use of levofloxacin in the presence of risk factors for torsades de pointes such as hypokalemia, significant bradycardia, cardiomyopathy, patients with myocardial ischemia, and patients with congenital prolongation of the QT interval should be avoided.

Endocrine and Metabolism: Disturbances of Blood Glucose: Disturbances of blood glucose, including symptomatic hyper- and hypoglycemia, have been reported with the use of quinolones, including LEVAQUIN. In patients treated with LEVAQUIN, some of these cases were serious. Blood glucose disturbances were usually in diabetic patients receiving concomitant treatment with an oral hypoglycemic agent (e.g. glyburide/glibenclamide) or with insulin. In these patients, careful monitoring of blood glucose is recommended. If a hypoglycemic reaction occurs in a patient being treated with levofloxacin, discontinue levofloxacin immediately and initiate appropriate therapy (see Drug Interactions, and Adverse Reactions). Serious hypoglycaemia and hyperglycemia have also occurred in patients without a history of diabetes.

Gastrointestinal: *C. difficile*-associated disease: *C. difficile*-associated disease (CDAD) has been reported with use of many antibacterial agents, including levofloxacin. CDAD may range in severity from mild diarrhea to fatal colitis. It is important to consider this diagnosis in patients who present with diarrhea or symptoms of colitis, pseudomembranous colitis, toxic megacolon, or perforation of the colon subsequent to the administration of any antibacterial agent. CDAD has been reported to occur over 2 months after the administration of antibacterial agents.

Treatment with antibacterial agents may alter the normal flora of the colon and may permit overgrowth of *C. difficile*. *C. difficile* produces toxins A and B, which contribute to the development of CDAD. CDAD may cause significant morbidity and mortality. CDAD can be refractory to antimicrobial therapy.

If the diagnosis of CDAD is suspected or confirmed, appropriate therapeutic measures should be initiated. Mild cases of CDAD usually respond to discontinuation of antibacterial agents not directed against *C. difficile*. In moderate to severe cases, consideration should be given to management with fluids and electrolytes, protein supplementation, and treatment with an antibacterial agent clinically effective against *C. difficile*. Surgical evaluation should be instituted as clinically indicated since surgical intervention may be required in certain severe cases (see Adverse Reactions).

Hepatic/Biliary/Pancreatic: Very rare post-marketing reports of severe hepatotoxicity (including acute hepatitis and fatal events) have been received for patients treated with levofloxacin. No evidence of serious drug-associated hepatotoxicity was detected in clinical trials of over 7000 patients. Severe hepatotoxicity generally occurred within 14 days of initiation of therapy and most cases occurred within 6 days. Most cases of severe hepatotoxicity were not associated with hypersensitivity. The majority of fatal hepatotoxicity reports occurred in patients 65 years of age or older and most were not associated with hypersensitivity. Levofloxacin should be discontinued immediately if the patient develops signs and symptoms of hepatitis (see Adverse Reactions, Post-Market Adverse Drug Reactions).

Immune: Hypersensitivity: Serious and occasionally fatal hypersensitivity and/or anaphylactic reactions have been reported in patients receiving therapy with quinolones, including levofloxacin. These reactions often occur following the first dose. Some reactions have been accompanied by cardiovascular collapse, hypotension/shock, seizure, loss of consciousness, tingling, angioedema (including tongue, laryngeal, throat or facial edema/swelling), airway obstruction (including bronchospasm, shortness of breath, and acute respiratory distress), dyspnea, urticaria, itching, and other serious skin reactions. Levofloxacin should be discontinued immediately at the first appearance of a skin rash or any other sign of hypersensitivity. Serious acute hypersensitivity reactions may require treatment with epinephrine and other resuscitative measures, including oxygen, intravenous fluids, antihistamines, corticosteroids, pressor, amines and airway management, as clinically indicated (see Adverse Reactions).

Serious and sometimes fatal events, some due to hypersensitivity and some due to uncertain etiology, have rarely been reported in patients receiving therapy with quinolones, including levofloxacin. These events may be severe, and generally occur following the administration of multiple doses. Clinical manifestations may include one or more of the following: fever; rash or severe dermatologic reactions (e.g. toxic epidermal necrolysis, Stevens-Johnson syndrome); vasculitis; arthralgia; myalgia; serum sickness; allergic pneumonitis; interstitial nephritis; acute renal insufficiency or failure; hepatitis, including acute hepatitis; jaundice; acute hepatic necrosis or failure; anemia, including hemolytic and aplastic; thrombocytopenia, including thrombotic thrombocytopenic purpura; leukopenia; agranulocytosis; pancytopenia; and/or other hematologic abnormalities. The administration of levofloxacin should be discontinued immediately, at the first appearance of a skin rash or any other sign of hypersensitivity, and supportive measures instituted (see Adverse Reactions).

Musculoskeletal : Rupture of the shoulder, hand and Achilles tendons that required surgical repair or resulted in prolonged disability have been reported in patients receiving quinolones, including LEVAQUIN. LEVAQUIN should be discontinued if the patient experiences pain, inflammation or rupture of a tendon. Patients should rest and refrain from exercise until the diagnosis of tendinitis or tendon rupture has been confidently excluded. The risk of developing fluoroquinolone-associated tendinitis and tendon rupture is further increased in older patients usually over 60 years of age, in patients taking corticosteroid drugs, and in patients with kidney, heart or lung transplants. Factors, in addition to age and corticosteroid use, that may independently increase the risk of tendon rupture include strenuous physical activity, renal failure, and previous tendon disorders such as rheumatoid arthritis. Tendinitis and tendon rupture have also occurred in patients taking fluoroquinolones who do not have the above risk factors. Tendon rupture can occur during or after completion of therapy; cases occurring up to several months after completion of therapy have been reported. LEVAQUIN should be discontinued if the patient experiences pain, swelling, inflammation or rupture of a tendon. Patients should be advised to rest at the first sign of tendinitis or tendon rupture, and to contact their healthcare provider regarding changing to a non-quinolone antimicrobial drug.

Levofloxacin should not be used in patients with a history of tendon disease/disorder related to previous quinolone treatment (see Contraindications).

Neurologic: CNS and Psychiatric Effects: Convulsions and toxic psychoses have been reported in patients receiving quinolones, including levofloxacin. Quinolones including levofloxacin, may also cause increased intracranial pressure and central nervous system stimulation which may lead to tremors, restlessness, anxiety, lightheadedness, dizziness, confusion and hallucinations, paranoia, depression, nightmares, insomnia and, rarely, suicidal thoughts or acts. These reactions may occur following the first dose. If these reactions occur in patients receiving levofloxacin, the drug should be discontinued and appropriate measures instituted. As with all quinolones, levofloxacin should be used with caution in patients with a known or suspected CNS disorder that may predispose to seizures or lower the seizure threshold (e.g. severe cerebral arteriosclerosis, epilepsy), or in the presence of other risk factors that may predispose to seizures or lower the seizure threshold (e.g. alcohol abuse, certain drug therapies such as NSAIDs and theophylline, renal dysfunction). Levofloxacin should be used with caution in patients with unstable psychiatric illness (see Drug Interactions, and Adverse Reactions).

Rare cases of sensory or sensorimotor axonal polyneuropathy affecting small and/or large axons resulting in paresthesias, hypoesthesias, dysesthesias and weakness have been reported in patients receiving quinolones, including levofloxacin. Levofloxacin should be discontinued if the patient experiences symptoms of neuropathy including pain, burning, tingling, numbness, and/or weakness or other alterations of sensation including light touch, pain, temperature, position sense, and vibratory sensation in order to prevent the development of an irreversible condition.

Renal: Safety and efficacy of levofloxacin in patients with impaired renal function (creatinine clearance ≤80 mL/min) have not been studied. Since levofloxacin is known to be substantially excreted by the kidney, the risk of toxic reactions to this drug may be greater in patients with impaired renal function. The potential effects of levofloxacin associated with possible increased serum/tissue levels in renal impaired patients, such as effect on QTc interval, have not been studied. Adjustment of the dosage regimen may be necessary to avoid the accumulation of levofloxacin due to decreased clearance. Careful clinical observation and appropriate laboratory studies should be performed prior to and during therapy, since elimination of levofloxacin may be reduced. Because elderly patients are more likely to have decreased renal function, care should be taken in dose selection, and it may be useful to monitor renal function. Administer levofloxacin with caution in the presence of renal insufficiency (see Dosage and Administration, Recommended Dose and Dosage Adjustment, Patients with Impaired Renal Function).

Skin: Phototoxicity: Moderate to severe phototoxicity reactions have been observed in patients exposed to direct sunlight or ultraviolet (UV) light while receiving drugs in this class. Excessive exposure to sunlight or UV light should be avoided. However, in clinical trials with levofloxacin, phototoxicity has been observed in less than 0.1% of patients. Therapy should be discontinued if phototoxicity (e.g. skin eruption) occurs.

Special Populations: The safety and efficacy of LEVAQUIN levofloxacin tablets and injection in children, adolescents (under the age of 18 years), pregnant women, and nursing mothers have not been established.

Pregnant Women: There are no adequate and well-controlled studies in pregnant women. Levofloxacin should be used during pregnancy only if the potential benefit justifies the potential risk to the fetus.

Nursing Women: Levofloxacin has not been measured in human milk. Based upon data from ofloxacin, it can be presumed that levofloxacin can be excreted in human milk. Because of the potential for serious adverse reactions from levofloxacin in nursing infants, a decision should be made whether to discontinue nursing or to discontinue the drug, taking into account the importance of the drug to the mother.

Pediatrics (<18 years of age): Levofloxacin is not indicated for the treatment of patients younger than 18 years of age. Quinolones, including levofloxacin, cause arthropathy in juvenile animals of several species. The incidence of protocol-defined musculoskeletal disorders in a prospective long-term surveillance study was higher in children treated for approximately 10 days with levofloxacin than in children treated with non-fluoroquinolone antibiotics for approximately 10 days (see Adverse Reactions).

Geriatrics (≥65 years of age): The pharmacokinetic properties of levofloxacin in younger adults and elderly adults do not differ significantly when creatinine clearance is taken into consideration. However, since the drug is known to be substantially excreted by the kidney, the risk of toxic reactions to this drug may be greater in patients with impaired renal function. Because elderly patients are more likely to have decreased renal function, care should be taken in dose selection. It may also be useful to monitor renal function.

Elderly patients may be more susceptible to drug-associated effects on the QT interval (see Warnings and Precautions, Cardiovascular).

ADVERSE REACTIONS: Adverse Drug Reaction Overview: In North American Phase 3 clinical trials involving 7537 subjects, the incidence of treatment-emergent adverse events in patients treated with LEVAQUIN levofloxacin Tablets and Injection was comparable to comparators. The majority of adverse events were considered to be mild to moderate, with 5.6% of patients considered to have severe adverse events. Among patients receiving multiple-dose therapy, 4.2% discontinued therapy with levofloxacin due to adverse experiences. The incidence of drug-related adverse reactions was 6.7%.

In clinical trials, the most frequently reported adverse drug reaction occurring in >3% of the study population were nausea, headache, diarrhea, insomnia, dizziness and constipation.

Serious and otherwise important adverse drug reactions are discussed in greater detail in other sections (see Warnings and Precautions).

Clinical Trial Adverse Drug Reactions: Because clinical trials are conducted under very specific conditions the adverse reaction rates observed in the clinical trials may not reflect the rates observed in practice and should not be compared to the rates in the clinical trials of another drug. Adverse drug reaction information from clinical trials is useful for identifying drug-related adverse events and for approximating rates.

The data described below reflect exposure to LEVAQUIN levofloxacin in 7537 patients in 29 pooled Phase 3 clinical trials. The population studied had a mean age of 49.6 years (74.2% of the population was <65 years), 50.1% were male, 71.0% were Caucasian, 18.8% were Black. Patients were treated with LEVAQUIN levofloxacin for a wide variety of infectious diseases (see Indications and Clinical Use). Treatment duration was usually 3-14 days, the mean number of days on therapy was 9.6 days and the mean number of doses was 10.2. Patients received LEVAQUIN levofloxacin doses of 750 mg once daily, 250 mg once daily, or 500 mg once or twice daily. The overall incidence, type and distribution of adverse reactions was similar in patients receiving LEVAQUIN levofloxacin doses of 750 mg once daily, 250 mg once daily, and 500 mg once or twice daily.

Adverse reactions (characterized as likely related to drug-therapy) occurring in ≥1% of LEVAQUIN-treated patients are shown in Table 1.

Table 1: LEVAQUIN

Common (≥1%) Adverse Reactions Reported in Clinical Trials with LEVAQUIN

System/Organ Class	Adverse Reaction	% (N=7537)
Infections and Infestations	moniliasis	1
Psychiatric Disorders	insomnia	4[a]
Nervous System Disorders	headache	6
	dizziness	3
Respiratory, Thoracic and Mediastinal Disorders	dyspnea	1
Gastrointestinal Disorders	nausea	7
	diarrhoea	5
	constipation	3
	abdominal pain	2
	vomiting	2
	dyspepsia	2
Skin and Subcutaneous Tissue Disorders	rash	2
	pruritus	1
Reproductive System and Breast Disorders	vaginitis	1[b]
General Disorders and Administration Site Conditions	oedema	1
	injection site reaction	1
	chest pain	1

[a] N=7274.
[b] N=3758 (women).

Less Common Clinical Trial Adverse Drug Reactions (<1%): Less common adverse reactions occurring in 0.1 to <1% of LEVAQUIN-treated patients are shown in Table 2.

Table 2: LEVAQUIN

Less Common (0.1 to 1%) Adverse Reactions Reported in Clinical Trials with LEVAQUIN

System/Organ Class	Adverse Reaction
Infections and Infestations	genital moniliasis
Blood and Lymphatic System Disorders	anaemia, thrombocytopenia, granulocytopoenia
Immune System Disorders	allergic reaction
Metabolism and Nutrition Disorders	hyperglycaemia, hypoglycaemia, hyperkalaemia
Psychiatric Disorders	anxiety, agitation, confusion, depression, hallucination, nightmare[a], sleep disorder[a], anorexia, abnormal dreaming[a]
Nervous System Disorders	tremor, convulsions, parasthaesia, vertigo, hypertonia, hyperkinaesias, abnormal gait, somnolence[a], syncope
Respiratory, Thoracic and Mediastinal Disorders	epistaxis
Cardiac Disorders	cardiac arrest, palpitation, ventricular tachycardia, ventricular arrhythmia
Vascular Disorders	phlebitis
Gastrointestinal Disorders	gastritis, stomatitis, pancreatitis, oesophagitis, gastroenteritis, glossitis, pseudomembraneous/*C. difficile* colitis
Hepatobiliary Disorders	abnormal hepatic function, increased hepatic enzymes, increased alkaline phosphatase

(cont'd)

Table 2: LEVAQUIN *(cont'd)*

Less Common (0.1 to 1%) Adverse Reactions Reported in Clinical Trials with LEVAQUIN

System/Organ Class	Adverse Reaction
Skin and Subcutaneous Tissue Disorders	urticaria
Musculoskeletal and Connective Tissue Disorders	tendonitis, arthralgia, myalgia, skeletal pain
Renal and Urinary Disorders	abnormal renal function, acute renal failure

[a] N=7274.

Rare (<0.1%) adverse reactions from Phase 3 studies include dyspnea and rash maculo-papular.

In clinical trials using multiple-dose therapy, ophthalmologic abnormalities, including cataracts and multiple punctate lenticular opacities, have been noted in patients undergoing treatment with other quinolones. The relationship of the drugs to these events is not presently established.

Crystalluria and cylindruria have been reported with other quinolones.

Abnormal Hematologic and Clinical Chemistry Findings: Laboratory abnormalities seen in >2% of patients receiving multiple doses of levofloxacin: decreased glucose 2.1%.

It is not known whether this abnormality was caused by the drug or the underlying condition being treated.

Pediatric Data : In a group of 1534 pediatric patients (6 months to 16 years of age) treated with levofloxacin for respiratory infections, children 6 months to 5 years of age received 10 mg/kg of levofloxacin twice a day for approximately 10 days and children greater than 5 years of age received 10 mg/kg to a maximum of 500 mg of levofloxacin once a day for approximately 10 days. The adverse reaction profile was similar to that reported in adult patients. Vomiting and diarrhea were reported more frequently in children than reported in adults. However, the frequency of vomiting and diarrhea was similar in levofloxacin-treated and non-fluoroquinolone antibiotic comparator-treated children.

A subset of 1340 of these children treated with levofloxacin for approximately 10 days was enrolled in a prospective, long term, surveillance study to assess the incidence of protocol-defined musculoskeletal disorders (arthralgia, arthritis, tendonopathy, gait abnormality) during 60 days and 1 year following the first dose of levofloxacin.

During the 60-day period following the first dose, the incidence of protocol-defined musculoskeletal disorders was greater in levofloxacin-treated children than in non-fluoroquinolone antibiotic comparator-treated children (2.1% v 0.9%, respectively [p=0.038]). In 22/28 (78%) of these children, reported disorders were characterized as arthralgia. A similar observation was made during the 1-year period, with a greater incidence of protocol-defined musculoskeletal disorders in levofloxacin-treated children than in non-fluoroquinolone antibiotic comparator-treated children (3.4% v 1.8%, respectively [p=0.025]). The majority of these disorders occurring in children treated with levofloxacin were mild and resolved within 7 days. Disorders were moderate in 8 children and mild in 35 (76%) children.

Post-Market Adverse Drug Reactions: Table 3 lists adverse reactions that have been identified during post-approval use of LEVAQUIN levofloxacin. Because these reactions are reported voluntarily from a population of uncertain size, reliably estimating their frequency or establishing a causal relationship to drug exposure is not always possible.

Table 3: LEVAQUIN

Postmarketing Reports of Adverse Drug Reactions

System Organ Class	Adverse Reaction
Blood and Lymphatic System Disorders	pancytopenia, aplastic anemia, leucopenia, hemolytic anemia, eosinophilia, thrombocytopenia including thrombotic thrombocytopenic purpura, agranulocytosis
Immune System Disorders	hypersensitivity reactions, sometimes fatal including: anaphylactic/anaphylactoid reactions, anaphylactic shock, angioneurotic edema, serum sickness
Psychiatric Disorders	psychosis, paranoia, isolated reports of suicide attempt and suicidal ideation
Nervous System Disorders	anosmia, ageusia, parosmia, dysgeusia, peripheral neuropathy, isolated reports of encephalopathy, abnormal EEG, dysphonia, exacerbation of myasthenia gravis, amnesia
Eye Disorders	vision disturbance (including diplopia), visual acuity reduced, vision blurred, scotoma
Ear and Labyrinth Disorders	hypoacusis, tinnitus
Cardiac Disorders	isolated reports of torsade de pointes, electrocardiogram QT prolonged, tachycardia
Vascular Disorders	vasodilation, vasculitis, DIC
Respiratory, Thoracic and Mediastinal Disorders	isolated reports of allergic pneumonitis, interstitial pneumonia, laryngeal edema, apnea
Hepatobiliary Disorders	hepatic failure (including fatal cases), hepatitis, jaundice, hepatic necrosis
Skin and Subcutaneous Tissue Disorders	bullous eruptions to include: Stevens-Johnson Syndrome, toxic epidermal necrolysis, erythema multiforme photosensitivity/phototoxicity reaction, leukocytoclastic vasculitis
Musculoskeletal and Connective Tissue Disorders	tendon rupture, muscle injury (including rupture), rhabdomyolysis, myositis, myalgia
Renal and Urinary Disorders	interstitial nephritis, nephrosis, glomerulonephritis
General Disorders and Administration Site Conditions	multi-organ failure, pyrexia, rash
Investigations	prothrombin time prolonged, international normalized ratio (INR) prolonged, muscle enzymes increased (CPK)

DRUG INTERACTIONS: Overview: Levofloxacin undergoes limited metabolism in humans and is primarily excreted as unchanged drug in the urine. The P450 system is not involved in the levofloxacin metabolism, and is not affected by levofloxacin. Levofloxacin is unlikely to alter the pharmacokinetics of drugs metabolized by these enzymes. Disturbances of blood glucose have been reported in patients treated concomitantly with levofloxacin and an antidiabetic agent. Therefore, careful monitoring of blood glucose is recommended when these agents, including levofloxacin, are co-administered. As with all other quinolones, iron and antacids significantly reduced bioavailability of levofloxacin.

Drug-Drug Interactions: See Table 4.

Table 4: LEVAQUIN

Established or Potential Drug-Drug Interactions

Proper Name	Ref	Effect	Clinical Comment
Antacids, Sucralfate, Metal Cations, Multi-Vitamins	T	**Tablets:** Due to the chelation of levofloxacin by multivalent cations, concurrent administration of LEVAQUIN Tablets with antacids containing calcium, magnesium, or aluminum, as well as sucralfate, metal cations such as iron, multi-vitamin preparations with zinc, or any products containing any of these components may interfere with the gastrointestinal absorption of levofloxacin, resulting in systemic levels considerably lower than desired.	These agents should be taken at least 2 hours before or 2 hours after levofloxacin tablet administration.
	T	**Injection:** There are no data concerning an interaction of intravenous quinolones with oral antacids, sucralfate, multi-vitamins, or metal cations.	Levofloxacin should not be co-administered with any solution containing multivalent cations (e.g. magnesium) through the same intravenous line (see Dosage and Administration, Administration).
Theophylline	CT/T	No significant effect of levofloxacin on the plasma concentrations, AUC, and other disposition parameters for theophylline was detected in a clinical study involving 14 healthy volunteers. Similarly, no apparent effect of theophylline on levofloxacin absorption and disposition was observed. However, concomitant administration of other quinolones with theophylline has resulted in prolonged elimination, elevated serum theophylline levels, and a subsequent increase in the risk of theophylline-related adverse reactions in the patient population	Theophylline levels should be closely monitored, and theophylline dosage adjustments made if appropriate, when levofloxacin is co-administered. Adverse reactions, including seizures, may occur with or without an elevation in serum theophylline level (see Warnings and Precautions).
Warfarin	T	Certain quinolones, including levofloxacin, may enhance the effects of oral anticoagulant warfarin or its derivatives.	When these products are administered concomitantly, prothrombin time, International Normalized Ratio (INR), or other suitable coagulation tests should be monitored closely, especially in the elderly patients.
Cyclosporine	CT	No significant effect of levofloxacin on the peak plasma concentrations, AUC, and other disposition parameters for cyclosporine was detected in a clinical study involving healthy volunteers. However, elevated serum levels of cyclosporine have been reported in the patient population when co-administered with some other quinolones. Levofloxacin C_{max} and k_e were slightly lower, while T_{max} and $t_{½}$ were slightly longer in the presence of cyclosporine, than those observed in other studies without concomitant medication. The differences, however, are not considered to be clinically significant.	No dosage adjustment is required for levofloxacin or cyclosporine when administered concomitantly.
Digoxin	CT	No significant effect of levofloxacin on the peak plasma concentrations, AUC, and, other disposition parameters for digoxin was detected in a clinical study involving healthy volunteers. Levofloxacin absorption and disposition kinetics were similar in the presence or absence of digoxin.	No dosage adjustment for levofloxacin or digoxin is required when administered concomitantly.
Probenecid and Cimetidine	CT	No significant effect of probenecid or cimetidine on the rate and extent of levofloxacin absorption was observed in a clinical study involving healthy volunteers. The AUC and $t_{½}$ of levofloxacin were 27-38% and 30% higher, respectively, while CL/F and Cl_r were 21-35% lower during concomitant treatment with probenecid or cimetidine compared to levofloxacin alone.	Although the differences were statistically significant, the changes were not high enough to warrant dosage adjustment for levofloxacin when probenecid or cimetidine is co-administered.
Non-Steroidal Anti-Inflammatory Drugs (NSAIDs)	T	Although not observed with levofloxacin in clinical trials, some quinolones have been reported to have proconvulsant activity that is exacerbated with concominant use of NSAIDs.	The concomitant administration of a non-steroidal anti-inflammatory drug with a quinolone, including levofloxacin, may increase the risk of CNS stimulation and convulsive seizures (see Warnings and Precautions, Neurologic).
Antidiabetic Agents	C	Disturbances of blood glucose, including hyperglycemia and hypoglycemia, have been reported in patients treated concomitantly with levofloxacin and an antidiabetic agent. Some of these cases were serious.	Careful monitoring of blood glucose is recommended when these agents, including levofloxacin, are co-administered.

(cont'd)

Table 4: LEVAQUIN *(cont'd)*

Established or Potential Drug-Drug Interactions

Proper Name	Ref	Effect	Clinical Comment
Zidovudine	CT	Levofloxacin absorption and disposition in HIV-infected subjects, with or without concomitant zidovudine treatment, were similar. The effect of levofloxacin on zidovudine pharmacokinetics has not been studied.	No dosage adjustment for levofloxacin appears to be required when co-administered with zidovudine.

Legend: C=case study; CT=clinical trial; T=theoretical.

Drug-Food Interactions: LEVAQUIN may be taken with or without food.
Drug-Herb Interactions: Interactions with herbal products have not been established.
Drug-Laboratory Test Interactions: Some quinolones, including levofloxacin, may produce false-positive urine screening results for opiates using commercially available immunoassay kits. Confirmation of positive opiate screens by more specific methods may be necessary.

DOSAGE AND ADMINISTRATION: Dosing Considerations: The dosage of LEVAQUIN levofloxacin Tablets and Injection for patients with normal renal function (i.e. Cl_{Cr} >80 mL/min) is described in the following dosing chart. For patients with altered renal function (i.e. Cl_{Cr} ≤80 mL/min), see the Patients with Impaired Renal Function. The 250 mg and 500 mg doses of LEVAQUIN Injection should be administered by slow infusion over 60 minutes every 24 hours while the 750 mg dose is administered by slow infusion over 90 minutes every 24 hours.
Recommended Dose and Dosage Adjustment: Patients with Normal Renal Function: See Table 5.

Table 5: LEVAQUIN

Dosing Chart—Patients with Normal Renal Function

Infection[a]	Dose	Freq.	Duration[b]
Acute Bacterial Exacerbation of Chronic Bronchitis	500 mg	q24h	7 days
	750 mg	q24h	5 days
Comm.-Acquired Pneumonia	500 mg	q24h	7–14 days (10–14 days for severe infections)
	750 mg[c]	q24h	5 days
Sinusitis	500 mg	q24h	10–14 days
	750 mg[d]	q24h	5 days
Nosocomial Pneumonia	750 mg	q24h	7–14 days
Uncomplicated SSSI	500 mg	q24h	7–10 days
Complicated SSSI	750 mg	q24h	7–14 days
Chronic Bacterial Prostatitis	500 mg	q24h	28 days
Complicated UTI	250 mg	q24h	10 days
	750 mg[e]	q24h	5 days
Acute Pyelonephritis	250 mg	q24h	10 days
	750 mg	q24h	5 days
Uncomplicated UTI	250 mg	q24h	3 days

[a] **Due to the designated pathogens** (see Indications and Clinical Use).
[b] **Total therapy duration.** When appropriate, patients may be converted from LEVAQUIN Injection to an equivalent dose of LEVAQUIN Tablets.
[c] Efficacy of this alternative regimen has only been documented for infections caused by penicillin-susceptible *S. pneumoniae*, *H. influenzae*, *H. parainfluenzae*, *M. pneumoniae*, *C. pneumoniae*, and *L. pneumophila*.
[d] The efficacy of a regimen of 750 mg daily for 5 days has been demonstrated to be non-inferior to a regimen of 500 mg daily for 10 days. The 750 mg daily 5 day regimen has not been compared to a regimen of 500 mg daily for 11-14 days.
[e] The efficacy of this alternative regimen has been documented for infections caused by *E. coli*, *K. pneumoniae*, and *P. mirabilis*. Efficacy against infections caused by *E. faecalis*, *E. cloacae*, or *P. aeruginosa* has not been demonstrated with this regimen.

Patients with Impaired Renal Function: On the basis of the altered levofloxacin disposition pharmacokinetics in subjects with impaired renal function, dose adjustment is recommended for patients with impaired renal function as given below (see Action and Clinical Pharmacology, and Warnings and Precautions, Renal).

Dosing recommendations for renally impaired patients are based on data collected from a clinical safety and pharmacokinetic study in renally impaired patients treated with a single 500 mg oral dose of levofloxacin. There is no clinical experience available in this patient population for the 250 mg dose or 750 mg dose. Pharmacokinetic modeling was used to determine a recommended dosing regimen which would provide equivalent drug exposures for which clinical efficacy has been demonstrated. The potential effects of levofloxacin associated with possible increased serum/tissue levels in renal-impaired patients, such as effect on QTc interval, have not been studied.

Table 6: LEVAQUIN

Dosing Chart—Patients with Impaired Renal Function

Renal Status	Initial Dose	Subsequent Dose
Acute Sinusitis/Acute Bacterial Exacerbation of Chronic Bronchitis/Community Acquired Pneumonia/Uncomplicated SSSI/Chronic Bacterial Prostatitis		
Cl_{Cr} 50–80 mL/min	No dosage adjustment required	
Cl_{Cr} 20–49 mL/min	500 mg	250 mg q24h
Cl_{Cr} 10–19 mL/min	500 mg	250 mg q48h
Hemodialysis	500 mg	250 mg q48h
CAPD	500 mg	250 mg q48h

(cont'd)

Table 6: LEVAQUIN *(cont'd)*

Dosing Chart—Patients with Impaired Renal Function

Renal Status	Initial Dose	Subsequent Dose
Complicated UTI/Acute Pyelonephritis		
Cl_{Cr} ≥20 mL/min	No dosage adjustment required	
Cl_{Cr} 10–19 mL/min	250 mg	250 mg q48h
Complicated SSSI/Nosocomial Pneumonia/Community Acquired Pneumonia/Acute Bacterial Exacerbation of Chronic Bronchitis/Acute Sinusitis/Complicated UTI/Acute Pyelonephritis		
Cl_{Cr} 50–80 mL/min	No dosage adjustment required	
Cl_{Cr} 20–49 mL/min	750 mg	750 mg q48h
Cl_{Cr} 10–19 mL/min	750 mg	500 mg q48h
Hemodialysis	750 mg	500 mg q48h
CAPD	750 mg	500 mg q48h
Uncomplicated UTI	No dosage adjustment required	

Legend: Cl_{Cr}=creatinine clearances. CAPD=chronic ambulatory peritoneal dialysis.

When only the serum creatinine is known, the following formula may be used to estimate creatinine clearance.

Men:

$$\text{Creatinine Clearance (mL/min)} = \frac{\text{Weight (kg)} \times (140-\text{age})}{\text{serum creatinine } (\mu\text{mol/L})} \times 1.2$$

Women: 0.85 × the value calculated for men.

The serum creatinine should represent a steady state of renal function.

Missed Dose: More than the prescribed dose of LEVAQUIN should not be taken, even if a dose is missed.

Administration: Tablets: Levofloxacin can be administered without regard to food. Doses should be administered at least 2 hours before or 2 hours after antacids containing calcium, magnesium, aluminum, sucralfate, metal cations such as iron, multivitamin preparations with zinc, or products containing any of these components.

Injection: Caution: Rapid or bolus intravenous infusion must be avoided. Levofloxacin injection should be infused intravenously, slowly over a period of not less than 60 minutes for a 250 mg or a 500 mg dose, and not less than 90 minutes for a 750 mg dose. LEVAQUIN Injection should only be administered by intravenous infusion. It is not for intramuscular, intrathecal, intraperitoneal, or subcutaneous administration (see Warnings and Precautions).

LEVAQUIN Injection Premix in single-use flexible containers does not require further dilution. Consequently, each 50 mL, 100 mL and 150 mL of PREMIXED solution contains the equivalent of 250 mg, 500 mg and 750 mg of levofloxacin (5 mg/mL), respectively in 5% Dextrose (D_5W).

This parenteral drug product should be inspected visually for clarity, discoloration, particulate matter, precipitate, and leakage prior to administration. Samples containing visible particles should be discarded.

Since the premix flexible containers are for single use only, any unused portion should be discarded.

Since only limited data are available on the compatibility of levofloxacin intravenous injection with other intravenous substances, **additives or other medications should not be added to LEVAQUIN Injection or infused simultaneously through the same intravenous line.** If the same intravenous line is used for sequential infusion of several different drugs, the line should be flushed before and after infusion of LEVAQUIN Injection with an infusion solution compatible with LEVAQUIN Injection and with any other drug(s) administered via this common line.

Instructions for the Use of LEVAQUIN Injection PREMIX in Flexible Containers: To open:
1. Tear outer wrap at the notch and remove solution container.
2. Check the container for minute leaks by squeezing the inner bag firmly. If leaks are found, or if the seal is not intact, discard the solution, as the sterility may be compromised.
3. Do not use if the solution is cloudy or a precipitate is present.
4. Use sterile equipment.
5. **Warning: Do not use flexible containers in series connections.** Such use could result in air embolism due to residual air being drawn from the primary container before administration of the fluid from the secondary container is complete.

Preparation for administration:
1. Close flow control clamp of administration set.
2. Remove cover from port at bottom of container.
3. Insert piercing pin of administration set into port with a twisting motion until the pin is firmly seated.
   Note: See full directions on administration set carton.
4. Suspend container from hanger.
5. Squeeze and release drip chamber to establish proper fluid level in chamber during infusion of LEVAQUIN Injection in PREMIX flexible containers.
6. Open flow control clamp to expel air from set. Close clamp.
7. Regulate rate of administration with flow control clamp.

OVERDOSAGE:
In the event of an acute overdosage, the stomach should be emptied. The patient should be observed, including ECG monitoring (see Action and Clinical Pharmacology, Pharmacodynamics, Studies Measuring Effects on QT and Corrected QT (QTc) Intervals), and appropriate hydration maintained. Treatment should be supportive. Levofloxacin is not efficiently removed by hemodialysis or peritoneal dialysis.

The administration of activated charcoal as soon as possible after oral overdose may prevent excessive increase of systemic levofloxacin exposure.

LEVAQUIN exhibits a low potential for acute toxicity. Mice, rats, dogs and monkeys exhibited the following clinical signs after receiving a single high dose of LEVAQUIN: ataxia, ptosis, decreased locomotor activity, dyspnea, prostration, tremors, and convulsions. Doses in excess of 1500 mg/kg orally and 250 mg/kg IV produced significant mortality in rodents.

For management of a suspected drug overdose, contact your regional Poison Control Centre. See the *CPS* Directory section for a list of Poison Control Centres.

ACTION AND CLINICAL PHARMACOLOGY: Mechanism of Action: LEVAQUIN levofloxacin is a synthetic broad-spectrum antibacterial agent for oral and intravenous administration.

Levofloxacin is the L-isomer of the racemate, ofloxacin, a quinolone antibacterial agent. The antibacterial activity of ofloxacin resides primarily in the L-isomer. The mechanism of action of levofloxacin and other quinolone antibacterials involves inhibition of bacterial topoisomerase II (DNA gyrase) and topoisomerase IV. Topoisomerases are essential in controlling the topological state of DNA, and are vital for DNA replication, transcription, repair and recombination.

Table 7: LEVAQUIN

Summary of Pharmacokinetic Parameters (mean±SD)

Regimen	N	C_{max} (μg/mL)	T_{max} (h)	AUC[k] (μg·h/mL)	CL/F (mL/min)	Vd/F (L)	$t_{1/2}$ (h)	Cl_r (mL/min)
Single Dose								
250 mg p.o.[a]	15	2.8±0.4	1.6±1.0	27.2±3.9	156±20	ND	7.3±0.9	142±21
500 mg p.o.[a,n]	23	5.1±0.8	1.3±0.6	47.9±6.8	178±28	ND	6.3±0.6	103±30
500 mg i.v.[a]	23	6.2±1.0	1.0±0.1	48.3±5.4	175±20	90±11	6.4±0.7	112±25
750 mg p.o.[d]	10	7.1±1.4	1.9±0.7	82.2±14.3	157±28	90±14	7.7±1.3	118±28
750 mg i.v.[c]	4	7.99±1.2[b]	ND	74.4±8.0	170±19	97.0±14.8	7.5±1.9	ND
Multiple Dose								
500 mg q24h p.o.[a]	10	5.7±1.4	1.1±0.4	47.5±6.7[m]	175±25	102±22	7.6±1.6	116±31
500 mg q24h i.v.[a]	10	6.4±0.8	ND	54.6±11.1[m]	158±29	91±12	7.0±0.8	99±28
500 mg or 250 mg q24h i.v. patients with bacterial infections[e]	272	8.7±4.0[j]	ND	72.5±51.2[j,m]	154±72	111±58	ND	ND
750 mg q24h p.o[d]	10	8.6±1.9	1.4±0.5	90.7±17.6	143±29	100±16	8.8±1.5	116±28
750 mg q24h i.v.[c]	4	7.92±0.91[b]	ND	72.5±0.8[m]	172±2	111±12	8.1±2.1	ND
500 mg p.o. Single Dose, Effects of Gender and Age								
Male[f]	12	5.5±1.1	1.2±0.4	54.4±18.9	166±44	89±13	7.5±2.1	126±38
Female[g]	12	7.0±1.6	1.7±0.5	67.7±24.2	136±44	62±16	6.1±0.8	106±40
Young[h]	12	5.5±1.0	1.5±0.6	47.5±9.8	182±35	83±18	6.0±0.9	140±33
Elderly[i]	12	7.0±1.6	1.4±0.5	74.7±23.3	121±33	67±19	7.6±2.0	91±29
500 mg p.o. Single Dose, Patients with Renal Insufficiency								
Cl_{Cr} 50–80 mL/min	3	7.5±1.8	1.5±0.5	95.6±11.8	88±10	ND	9.1±0.9	57±8
Cl_{Cr} 20–49 mL/min	8	7.1±3.1	2.1±1.3	182.1±62.6	51±19	ND	27±10	26±13
Cl_{Cr} <20 mL/min	6	8.2±2.6	1.1±1.0	263.5±72.5	33±8	ND	35±5	13±3
Hemodialysis	4	5.7±1.0	2.8±2.2	ND	ND	ND	76±42	ND
CAPD	4	6.9±2.3	1.4±1.1	ND	ND	ND	51±24	ND
750 mg i.v. Single Dose and Multiple Dose, Patients with Renal Insufficiency								
Single dose—Cl_{Cr} 50–80 mL/min[l]	8	13.3±3.6	ND	128±37	104±25	62.7±15.1	7.5±1.5	ND
Multiple q24h dose—Cl_{Cr} 50–80 mL/min[l]	8	14.3±3.2	ND	145±36	103±20	64.2±16.9	7.8±2.0	ND

[a] Healthy males 18–53 years of age.
[b] 60 min. infusion for 250 mg and 500 mg doses, 90 min. infusion for 750 mg dose.
[c] Healthy male subjects 32–46 years of age.
[d] Healthy male subjects 19–51 years of age.
[e] Including 500 mg q48h for 8 patients with moderate renal impairment (Cl_{Cr} 20–50 mL/min) and infections of the respiratory tract or skin.
[f] Healthy males 22–75 years of age.
[g] Healthy females 18–80 years of age.
[h] Young healthy male and female subjects 18–36 years of age.
[i] Healthy elderly male and female subjects 66–80 years of age.
[j] Dose-normalized values (to 500 mg dose), estimated by population pharmacokinetic modelling.
[k] AUC for 0-∞ reported, unless otherwise specified.
[l] Male and female subjects 34–54 years of age.
[m] $AUC_{0\text{-}24\ h}$.
[n] Absolute bioavailability; F=0.99±0.08 from a 500 mg tablet and F=0.99±0.06 from a 750 mg tablet.
Legend: ND=not determined.

Fluoroquinolones, including levofloxacin, differ in chemical structure and mode of action from other classes of antimicrobial agents, such as β-lactam antibiotics, aminoglycosides, and macrolides. Therefore, microorganisms resistant to these latter classes of antimicrobial agents may be susceptible to fluoroquinolones. For example, β-lactamase production and alterations in penicillin-binding proteins have no effect on levofloxacin activity. Conversely, microorganisms resistant to fluoroquinolones may be susceptible to other classes of antimicrobial agents.

Pharmacodynamics: Studies Measuring Effects on QT and Corrected QT (QTc) Intervals: Two studies have been conducted to assess specifically the effect of levofloxacin on QT and corrected QT (QTc) intervals in healthy adult volunteers. In a dose escalation study (n=48) where the effect on average QTc, after single doses of 500, 1000, and 1500 mg of levofloxacin, was measured between the baseline QTc (calculated as the average QTc measured 24, 20, 16 hours and immediately before treatment) and the average post-dose QTc interval (calculated from measurements taken every half hour for two hours and at 4, 8, 12 and 24 hours after treatment), an effect on the average QTc (Bazett) was −1.84, 1.55 and 6.40 msec, respectively. In a study which compared the effect of 3 antimicrobials (n=48) where the difference was measured between the baseline QTc (calculated as the average QTc measured 24, 20, 16 hours and immediately before treatment) and the average post-dose QTc interval (calculated from measurements taken every half hour for four hours and at 8, 12 and 24 hours after treatment), an effect on the average QTc was an increase of 3.58 msec after the 1000 mg dose of levofloxacin. The mean increase compared to baseline of QTc at C_{max} in these two trials was 7.82 msec and 5.32 msec after a single 1000 mg dose. In these trials, no effect on QT intervals compared to placebo was evident at any of the doses studied. The clinical relevance of the results of these studies is not known.

Pharmacokinetics: The mean (±SD) pharmacokinetic parameters of levofloxacin determined under single and steady-state conditions following oral (p.o.) or intravenous (i.v.) doses of levofloxacin are summarized in Table 7.

Absorption: Oral: Levofloxacin is rapidly and essentially completely absorbed after oral administration. Peak plasma concentrations are usually attained 1 to 2 hours after oral dosing. The absolute bioavailability of a 500 mg tablet and a 750 mg tablet of levofloxacin is approximately 99% in both cases, demonstrating complete oral absorption of levofloxacin. Levofloxacin pharmacokinetics are linear and predictable after single and multiple oral dosing regimens. Steady-state conditions are reached within 48 hours following a 500 mg or 750 mg once-daily dosage regimen. The peak and trough plasma concentrations attained following multiple once-daily oral dosage regimens were approximately 5.7 μg/mL and 0.5 μg/mL after the 500 mg doses, and 8.6 μg/mL and 1.1 μg/mL after the 750 mg doses, respectively.

There was no clinically significant effect of food on the extent of absorption of levofloxacin. Oral administration with food slightly prolongs the time to peak concentration by approximately 1 hour, and slightly decreases the peak concentration by approximately 14%. Therefore, levofloxacin can be administered without regard to food.

I.V.: Following a single intravenous dose of levofloxacin to healthy volunteers, the mean peak plasma concentration attained was 6.2 μg/mL after a 500 mg dose infused over 60 minutes, and 7.99 μg/mL after a 750 mg dose infused over 90 minutes. Levofloxacin pharmacokinetics are linear and predictable after single and multiple i.v. dosing regimens. Steady-state conditions are reached within 48 hours following a 500 mg or 750 mg once-daily dosing regimen. The peak and trough plasma concentrations attained following multiple once-daily i.v. regimens were approximately 6.4 μg/mL and 0.6 μg/mL after the 500 mg doses, and 7.92 μg/mL and 0.85 μg/mL after the 750 mg doses, respectively.

The plasma concentration profile of levofloxacin after i.v. administration is similar and comparable in extent of exposure (AUC) to that observed for levofloxacin tablets when equal doses (mg/mg) are administered. Therefore, the oral and i.v. routes of administration can be considered interchangeable (see Figure 1).

Distribution: The mean volume of distribution of levofloxacin generally ranges from 74 to 112 L after single and multiple 500 mg or 750 mg doses, indicating widespread distribution into body tissues. Levofloxacin reaches its peak levels in skin tissues (11.7 μg/g for a 750 mg dose) and in blister fluid (4.33 μg/g for a 500 mg dose) at approximately 3-4 hours after dosing. The skin tissue biopsy to plasma AUC ratio is approximately 2. The blister fluid to plasma AUC ratio is approximately 1, following multiple once-daily oral administration of 750 mg and 500 mg levofloxacin to healthy subjects, respectively. Levofloxacin also penetrates into lung tissues. Lung tissue concentrations were generally 2- to 5-fold higher than plasma concentrations, and ranged from approximately 2.4 to 11.3 μg/g over a 24-hour period after a single 500 mg oral dose.

Levofloxacin is 24 to 38% bound to serum proteins across all species studied. Levofloxacin binding to serum proteins is independent of the drug concentration.

Metabolism: Levofloxacin is stereochemically stable in plasma and urine, and does not invert metabolically to its enantiomer, D-ofloxacin. Levofloxacin undergoes limited metabolism in humans, and is primarily excreted as unchanged drug (87%) in the urine within 48 hours.

Excretion: The major route of elimination of levofloxacin in humans is as unchanged drug in the urine. The mean terminal plasma elimination half-life of levofloxacin ranges from approximately 6 to 8 hours following single or multiple doses of levofloxacin given orally or intravenously.

Figure 1: LEVAQUIN
Mean Levofloxacin Plasma Concentration:Time Profiles

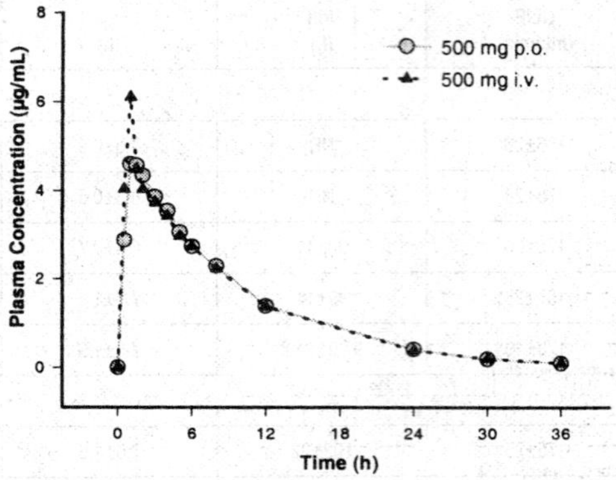

Special Populations and Conditions: Pediatrics: The pharmacokinetics of levofloxacin in pediatric patients have not been studied.

Geriatrics: There are no significant differences in levofloxacin pharmacokinetics between young and elderly subjects when the subjects' differences in creatinine clearance are taken into consideration. Drug absorption appears to be unaffected by age. Levofloxacin dose adjustment based on age alone is not necessary.

Gender: There are no significant differences in levofloxacin pharmacokinetics between male and female subjects when the differences in creatinine clearance are taken into consideration. Dose adjustment based on gender alone is not necessary.

Race: The apparent total body clearance and apparent volume of distribution were not affected by race in a covariate analysis performed on data from 72 subjects.

Hepatic Insufficiency: Pharmacokinetic studies in hepatically impaired patients have not been conducted. Due to the limited extent of levofloxacin metabolism, the pharmacokinetics of levofloxacin are not expected to be affected by hepatic impairment.

Renal Insufficiency: Pharmacokinetic parameters of levofloxacin following oral or intravenous doses of levofloxacin in patients with impaired renal function (creatinine clearance ≤80 mL/min) are presented in Table 7. Clearance of levofloxacin is reduced and plasma elimination half-life is prolonged in this patient population. Dosage adjustment may be required in such patients to avoid accumulation.

A dosage reduction is being recommended depending on the levels of renal insufficiency. Dosing recommendations are based on pharmacokinetic modeling of data collected from a clinical safety and pharmacokinetic study in renally impaired patients treated with a single 500 mg oral dose of levofloxacin (see Warnings and Precautions, Renal, and Dosage and Administration, Recommended Dose and Dosage Adjustment, Patients with Impaired Renal Function).

Neither hemodialysis nor continuous ambulatory peritoneal dialysis (CAPD) is effective in removal of levofloxacin from the body, indicating supplemental doses of levofloxacin are not required following hemodialysis or CAPD.

Bacterial Infection: The pharmacokinetics of levofloxacin in patients with community-acquired bacterial infections are comparable to those observed in healthy subjects.

STORAGE AND STABILITY: Tablets: LEVAQUIN Tablets should be stored at controlled room temperature (15-30°C) in well-closed containers.

Injection: When stored under recommended conditions, LEVAQUIN Injection, as supplied in flexible containers, is stable through the expiration date printed on the label.

LEVAQUIN Injection PREMIX in flexible containers should be stored at 2-25°C; however, brief exposure up to 40°C does not adversely affect the product. Avoid excessive heat and protect from freezing and light. Store with protective overwrap and use immediately once removed from the overwrap.

INFORMATION FOR THE PATIENT: Published in e-CPS, available by subscription at www.e-cps.ca.

DOSAGE FORMS, COMPOSITION AND PACKAGING: Injection: Each mL of sterile, non-pyrogenic, premixed, ready-to-use solution contains: levofloxacin 5 mg in 5% Dextrose (D_5W). pH: 3.8 to 5.8. Solutions of hydrochloric acid and/or sodium hydroxide may have been added to adjust the pH. Preservative-free. The flexible container is fabricated from a specially formulated non-plasticized, thermoplastic copolyester (CR3). The amount of water that can permeate from the container into the overwrap is insufficient to affect the solution significantly. Solutions in contact with the flexible container can leach out certain of the container's chemical components in very small amounts within the expiration period. The suitability of the container material has been confirmed by tests in animals according to USP biological tests for plastic containers. Single-use flexible containers of 100 mL with a fill volume of 50 or 100 mL, 150 mL with a fill volume of 150 mL, cases of 12.

Tablets: 250 mg: Each modified rectangular, film-coated, terra cotta pink tablet, embossed "LEVAQUIN" on one side and "250" on the other, contains: levofloxacin 250 mg. Nonmedicinal ingredients: crospovidone, hydroxypropyl methylcellulose, magnesium stearate, microcrystalline cellulose, polyethylene glycol, polysorbate 80, synthetic red iron oxide and titanium dioxide. Bottles of 50.

500 mg: Each modified rectangular, film-coated, peach tablet, embossed "LEVAQUIN" on one side and "500" on the other, contains: levofloxacin 500 mg. Nonmedicinal ingredients: crospovidone, hydroxypropyl methylcellulose, magnesium stearate, microcrystalline cellulose, polyethylene glycol, polysorbate 80, synthetic red and yellow iron oxides and titanium dioxide. Bottles of 50.

750 mg: Each modified rectangular, film-coated, white tablet, embossed "LEVAQUIN" on one side and "750" on the other, contains: levofloxacin 750 mg. Nonmedicinal ingredients: crospovidone, hydroxypropyl methylcellulose, magnesium stearate, microcrystalline cellulose, polyethylene glycol, polysorbate 80 and titanium dioxide. Bottles of 50.

(Shown in Product Identification Section)

Levemir®
insulin detemir
Antidiabetic

Novo Nordisk

Date of Revision: December 15, 2009

SUMMARY PRODUCT INFORMATION:

Route of Administration	Dosage Form/ Strength	Clinically Relevant Nonmedicinal Ingredients
Subcutaneous	Solution for injection/ 100 U/mL	Disodium phosphate dehydrate, glycerol, metacresol, phenol, sodium chloride, acetate and water for injection. Hydrochloric acid and/or sodium hydroxide may be added to adjust pH.

DESCRIPTION: Levemir (insulin detemir) is a sterile solution of insulin detemir for use as an injection. Insulin detemir is a long-acting basal insulin analogue, with up to 24 hours duration of action, produced by a process that includes expression of recombinant DNA in *S. cerevisiae* followed by chemical modification.

INDICATIONS AND CLINICAL USE: Levemir (insulin detemir) is indicated for:

- the treatment of adult patients with type 1 or type 2 diabetes mellitus who require a long-acting (basal) insulin for the control of hyperglycemia;
- the treatment of pediatric patients with type 1 diabetes mellitus who require a long-acting (basal) insulin for the control of hyperglycemia. The safety and efficacy of Levemir has not been studied in children below the age of 6 years.
- the treatment of type 2 diabetes mellitus in combination with oral anti-diabetic agents (OADs) [metformin or sulfonylureas] in adult patients who are not in adequate metabolic control on OADs alone. For safety reasons, the use of insulin in combination with a thiazolidinedione is not indicated (See Warnings and Precautions).

Levemir is also recommended in combination with short- or rapid-acting meal time insulin.

CONTRAINDICATIONS:

- Patients who are hypersensitive to this drug or to any ingredient in the formulation or component of the container. For a complete listing, see Dosage Forms, Composition and Packaging.

Levemir (insulin detemir) is contraindicated during episodes of hypoglycemia (see Hypoglycemia and Treatment of Overdosage).

WARNINGS AND PRECAUTIONS: General: Hypoglycemia is the most common adverse effect of insulin, including Levemir.

Inadequate dosing or discontinuation of treatment, especially in type 1 diabetes, may lead to hyperglycemia and diabetic ketoacidosis. Usually the first symptoms of hyperglycemia develop gradually over a period of hours or days. They include thirst; increased frequency of urination; nausea; vomiting; drowsiness; flushed dry skin; dry mouth; loss of appetite as well as acetone odour of breath. In type 1 diabetes, untreated hyperglycemic events eventually lead to diabetic ketoacidosis, which is potentially lethal.

Concomitant illness, especially infections and feverish conditions, usually increases the patient's insulin requirement.

Transferring a patient to another type or brand of insulin should be done under medical supervision. Changes in strength, brand (manufacturer), type, origin (animal, human, human insulin analogue) and/or method of manufacture (recombinant DNA versus animal source insulin) may result in the need for a change in dosage. Patients taking Levemir (insulin detemir) may require a change in dosage from that used with their usual insulin. If an adjustment is needed, it may occur with the first dose or during the first few weeks or months.

Levemir should not be administered intravenously as it may result in severe hypoglycemia.

Levemir is not to be used in insulin infusion pumps.

Absorption after intramuscular administration is faster and greater than absorption after subcutaneous administration.

Insulin may cause sodium retention and edema particularly if previously poor metabolic control is improved by intensified insulin therapy.

When using Levemir in combination with oral anti-diabetic agents (OADs) [metformin or sulfonylureas], please refer to the respective product monograph for OADs for their Warnings and Precautions Information.

Thiazolidinediones may induce oedema and/or heart failure with higher rates of heart failure when combined with insulin. Therefore, the combination of Insulin with a thiazolidinedione is not indicated for the treatment of Type 2 Diabetes Mellitus.

Mixture with Other Insulin: Levemir should not be mixed with other insulin for injection.

If Levemir is mixed with other insulin preparations the profile of action of one or both individual components will change. Mixing Levemir with a rapid-acting insulin analogue like NovoRapid (insulin aspart), results in an action profile with a lower and delayed maximum effect compared to separate injections.

Hypoglycemia: As with other insulins, hypoglycemia is the most common adverse effect of insulin therapy, including Levemir.

As with all insulin preparations, hypoglycemic reactions may be associated with the administration of Levemir. Early warning symptoms of hypoglycemia may be different or less pronounced under certain conditions, such as long duration of diabetes, diabetic nerve disease, use of medications such as beta-blockers, or intensified diabetes control.

Hypoglycemia may occur if the insulin dose is too high in relation to the insulin requirement (see Adverse Reactions and Hypoglycemia and Treatment of Overdosage).

Omission of a meal or unplanned strenuous physical exercise may lead to hypoglycemia.

Glucose monitoring is recommended for all patients with diabetes.

Hepatic/Biliary/Pancreas: Hepatic Impairment: As with other insulins, the requirements for Levemir may need to be adjusted in patients with hepatic impairment (see Action and Clinical Pharmacology, Pharmacokinetics).

Immune: Local Allergic Reaction: As with any insulin therapy, injection site reactions may occur and include pain; itching; hives; swelling and inflammation. Continuous rotation of the injection site within a given area may help to reduce or prevent these reactions. Reactions usually resolve in a few days to a few weeks. On rare occasions, injection site reactions may require discontinuation of Levemir.

Systemic Allergic Reactions: Systemic allergic reactions have rarely occurred with insulin treatment. These reactions may be characterized by a generalized rash (with pruritus); shortness of breath; wheezing and a drop in blood pressure. Severe cases of generalized allergy including anaphylactic reaction may be life threatening.

Insulin administration may cause formation of insulin antibodies. A positive correlation was observed in clinical trials between the dose of Levemir (insulin detemir) and the formation of insulin detemir specific antibodies, but this did not appear to affect HbA_{1C}. The long term impact of insulin detemir antibodies on glycemic control is under investigation.

Renal: Renal Impairment: As with other insulins, the requirements for Levemir may need to be adjusted in patients with renal impairment (see Action and Clinical Pharmacology, Pharmacokinetics).

Special Populations: Pregnant Women: There is no clinical experience with Levemir during pregnancy or lactation. Animal reproduction studies have not revealed any differences between Levemir and human insulin regarding embryotoxicity and teratogenicity.

In general, intensified blood glucose control and monitoring of pregnant women with diabetes are recommended throughout pregnancy and when contemplating pregnancy. Insulin requirements usually fall in the first trimester and increase subsequently during the second and third trimester. After delivery, insulin requirements normally return rapidly to pre-pregnancy values.

Nursing Women: It is unknown whether Levemir is excreted in significant amounts in human milk. For this reason, caution should be exercised when Levemir is administered to a nursing mother. Patients with diabetes who are lactating may require adjustments in insulin dose, meal plan or both.

Geriatrics: There was no clinically relevant difference in pharmacokinetics of Levemir between elderly and young subjects.

As with all insulins, in elderly patients and patients with renal or hepatic impairment, glucose monitoring should be intensified and insulin detemir dosage adjusted on an individual basis.

Pediatrics: The pharmacokinetic properties of Levemir were investigated in children (6-12 years) and adolescents (13-17 years) and compared to adults with type 1 diabetes. The pharmacokinetic properties were similar in the three groups. The efficacy and safety of Levemir were demonstrated in children and adolescents aged 6 to 17 years. No evaluated pediatric efficacy and safety data are available to support pediatric dosing advice below the age of 6 years.

Monitoring and Laboratory Tests: As with all insulin therapy, the therapeutic response to Levemir should be monitored by periodic blood glucose tests. Glycosylated hemoglobin should be measured every 3 to 4 months in all patients taking insulin.

Information for Patients: Patients should be informed about the potential advantages and disadvantages of Levemir (insulin detemir) therapy including possible side effects. Patients should also be offered continued education and advice on insulin therapies, delivery device options, life-style management, self-monitoring, complications of insulin therapy, timing of dosage, instruction for use of injection devices and storage of insulin.

To obtain optimal glycemic control, the need for regular blood glucose self-monitoring should be considered when using Levemir.

Female patients should be advised to discuss with their physician if they are pregnant or if they intend to become pregnant.

ADVERSE REACTIONS: Adverse Drug Reaction Overview: The safety profile of Levemir (insulin detemir) observed in clinical trials is similar to the safety profile reported for Novo Nordisk human insulin products.

Adverse drug reactions observed in patients using Levemir are mainly dose-dependent and are due to the pharmacologic effect of insulin. Hypoglycemia is a common undesirable effect. It may occur if the insulin dose is too high in relation to the insulin requirement. From clinical investigations it is known that major hypoglycemia, defined as requirement for third party intervention, occurs in approximately 6% of adult patients treated with Levemir. Severe hypoglycemia may lead to unconsciousness and/or convulsions and may result in temporary or permanent impairment of brain function or even death.

Injection site reactions are seen more frequently during treatment with Levemir, than with human insulin. These reactions include redness, inflammation, bruising, swelling and itching at the injection site. Most of the injection site reactions are minor and of a transitory nature, i.e. they normally disappear during continued treatment in a few days to a few weeks.

Adverse Drug Reactions in Adult and Paediatric Patients: The overall percentage of adult patients treated with Levemir expected to experience adverse drug reactions is estimated to be 12%. In the clinical study in pediatric subjects aged 6 to 17 years; adverse drug reactions were reported for 9.5% of patients treated with Levemir.

Clinical Trial Adverse Drug Reactions: Because clinical trials are conducted under very specific conditions the adverse reaction rates observed in the clinical trials may not reflect the rates observed in practice and should not be compared to the rates in the clinical trials of another drug. Adverse drug reaction information from clinical trials is useful for identifying drug-related adverse events and for approximating rates.

Levemir has been evaluated for safety in 3747 subjects treated for type 1 or type 2 diabetes: 518 in pharmacology trials, 195 in short-term trials and 3034 in the intermediate and long-term trials (including Trials 1385, 1372 and 1379). An additional 862 subjects were exposed to Levemir during three (intermediate and long-term) phase 3 trials in which Levemir was used as an add-on treatment to oral antidiabetic drugs (OADs) in subjects with type 2 diabetes (data summarized below).

In controlled clinical trials, discontinuation due to adverse events occurred in 1.7% of subjects with Levemir and in 1.1% of subjects treated with comparators (mainly NPH insulin).

In controlled clinical trials, adverse drug reactions reported in children and adolescents with type 1 diabetes aged 6-17 years were similar to those observed in adult patients. The overall frequency, however, of major hypoglycemic episodes requiring third party assistance was higher in this age group (16% with Levemir, and 20% with NPH insulin). Only few of these episodes were reported as adverse drug reactions. Serious adverse events reported with Levemir, and NPH insulin in pediatric subjects (irrespective of correlation to trial products) included: gastroenteritis (2.2 vs. 0%), bone fractures (0.9 vs. 0%), ketosis (1.3 vs. 1.9%), accidental injury (0.4 vs. 1.7%) and convulsions (0.9% in both groups).

Serious Adverse Events with Possible or Probable Relationship to Trial Drug: No serious adverse events with possible or probable relation to trial drug were reported with Levemir or NPH insulin in ≥1% of subjects.

The following serious adverse events with possible or probable relationship to trial drug were reported at an incidence of <1% for Levemir and NPH insulin in controlled clinical trials (in more than 1 subject, with higher frequency with Levemir than with NPH insulin):
Metabolic and Nutritional Disorders: hyperglycemia.

Adverse Events Regardless of Relationship to Trial Drug: See Table 1.

Table 1: Levemir

Adverse Events Reported with Levemir and NPH Insulin Occurring in ≥1% of Subjects Regardless of Drug Relationship

System Organ Class	Levemir n=3747 (%)	NPH Insulin n=2084 (%)
Respiratory System Disorders		
Upper Respiratory Tract Infection	16.4	16.3
Pharyngitis	5.2	5.3
Bronchitis	2.4	2.1
Rhinitis	2.2	2.4
Sinusitis	2.0	2.1
Coughing	2.0	1.8
Central and Peripheral Nervous Systems Disorders		
Headache	16.0	14.5
Dizziness	1.8	0.9
Gastro-intestinal System Disorders		
Abdominal Pain	4.2	3.0
Diarrhoea	3.2	4.2
Nausea	3.0	2.6
Gastroenteritis	3.4	3.1
Vomiting	1.9	2.1
Toothache	1.5	1.6
Dyspepsia	1.2	1.8
Body as a Whole—General Disorders		
Influenza-like Symptoms	5.4	5.4
Back Pain	3.3	3.0
Fatigue	1.5	0.9
Fever	1.4	1.2
Pain	1.2	0.9
Musculo-skeletal System Disorders		
Arthralgia	1.9	1.9
Skeletal Pain	1.0	1.3
Myalgia	0.7	1.4
Resistance Mechanism Disorders		
Viral Infection	2.0	2.2
Infection	1.2	1.4
Vision Disorders		
Retinal Disorder	2.4	2.4
Conjunctivitis	0.7	1.1
Secondary Terms		
Accidental Injury	3.0	3.2
Other Events	1.1	0.0
Metabolic and Nutritional Disorders		

(cont'd)

Table 1: Levemir (cont'd)

Adverse Events Reported with Levemir and NPH Insulin Occurring in ≥1% of Subjects Regardless of Drug Relationship

System Organ Class	Levemir n=3747 (%)	NPH Insulin n=2084 (%)
Hypoglycemia	1.4	0.8
Application Site Disorders		
Injection Site Reaction	1.7	0.6
Urinary System Disorders		
Urinary Tract Infection	1.5	1.3
Cardiovascular Disorders, General		
Hypertension	0.8	1.0
Reproductive Disorders, Female		
Dysmenorrhoea	1.1	0.9

Adverse Events in Trials of Levemir in Combination with Oral Antidiabetic Drugs (OADs): Three intermediate and long-term phase 3 trials (NN304-1632, NN304-1373, NN304-1530) were conducted, in which Levemir was used as an add-on treatment to oral antidiabetic drugs (OADs) in subjects with type 2 diabetes. The therapeutic response to Levemir was compared to that of NPH insulin or insulin glargine. A total of 862 subjects with type 2 diabetes were exposed to Levemir during these three studies. The percentage of subjects reporting adverse events with insulin detemir was 56%, NPH insulin was 49% and insulin glargine was 80%. The majority of the adverse events were mild in severity. A total of 3% subjects withdrew due to adverse events: 4% in the Levemir group, 2% in the NPH insulin group and 4% in the insulin glargine group.

The most common adverse events with Levemir were upper respiratory tract infection and headache. For adverse events reported in ≥1% of subjects, the only events reported in higher frequency with Levemir than with comparators were injection site disorders, cystitis and hyperhidrosis.

The only possibly or probably related adverse events that were reported in ≥1% of subjects were: headache (all treatment groups), injection site disorders (insulin detemir and NPH insulin groups) and additionally peripheral edema, hypoglycemia and dizziness in the insulin glargine group.

No severe adverse events were reported in ≥1% of subjects in the Levemir or the NPH insulin groups. In the insulin glargine group, severe adverse events reported in ≥1% of subjects were coronary artery disease, cholelithiasis, hypoglycaemia, cerebrovascular disorder and chest pain.

Less Common Clinical Trial Adverse Drug Reactions (<1%): In addition, the following adverse events were reported at an incidence of <1% for Levemir and NPH insulin in controlled clinical trials (in more than 1 subject, with higher frequency with Levemir than NPH insulin), regardless of drug relationship.

Respiratory System Disorders: pneumonia, laryngitis, asthma, tracheitis, respiratory disorder and pulmonary edema.

Central and Peripheral Nervous Systems Disorders: migraine, tremor, hypertonia, neuralgia, dysphonia, hyperkinesia, hyporeflexia, carpal tunnel syndrome, hyperaesthesia and paralysis.

Gastro-intestinal System Disorders: gastritis, constipation, tooth disorder, gingivitis, gastrointestinal disorder (not otherwise specified), haemorrhoids, dry mouth, colitis, gastroesophageal reflux, tooth caries aggravated, dysphagia, rectum hemorrhage, irritable bowel syndrome and mucositis (not otherwise specified).

Body as a Whole—General Disorders: allergic reaction (anaphylactic shock), potentially allergic reaction, headache, asthenia, hot flushes, syncope, carpal tunnel syndrome, neck rigidity, enlarged abdomen, substernal chest pain, aggravated condition, face edema, mouth edema and sudden death.

Musculo-skeletal System Disorders: arthrosis, bone fracture, tendon disorder, back pain, ischias, osteoporosis, tenosynovitis, torticollis and muscle weakness.

Resistance Mechanism Disorders: abscess, rhinitis, otitis media and parasitic infection.

Vision Disorders: abnormal vision, eye pain, eye infection, eye abnormality, keratitis, corneal ulceration, ocular hemorrhage and retinal hemorrhage.

Skin and Appendages Disorders: skin disorder, pruritus, increased sweating, eczema, skin ulceration, onychomycosis, skin hypertrophy, acne, photosensitivity reaction, dry skin, alopecia, bullous eruption, dermatitis contact, dermatitis, cold clammy skin, lichenoid dermatitis, pilonidal cyst, skin discolouration, otitis externa and verruca.

Secondary Terms: other events, bite food poisoning, medication error, varicella and under assessment.

Metabolic and Nutritional Disorders: hyperglycemia, hypoglycemic coma, hyperlipemia, gout, thirst, weight decrease, aggravated diabetes mellitus, hyperkalaemia, xerophthalmia and diabetic coma.

Application Site Disorders: injection site hematoma, injection site inflammation, cellulitis and needle injury.

Psychiatric Disorders: anxiety, somnolence, confusion, anorexia, emotional lability and thinking abnormally.

Urinary System Disorders: renal pain, albuminuria, hematuria, polyuria, abnormal glomerular renal function and abnormal urine.

Cardiovascular Disorders, General: cardiac failure, edema dependent, heart murmur, weak pulse, aneurysm, left cardiac failure and heart disorder.

Reproductive Disorders, Female: dysmenorrhea, vaginitis, menorrhagia, premenstrual tension, amenorrhoea, breast disorder (not otherwise specified) and mastitis.

Platelet, Bleeding and Clotting Disorders: epistaxis, hematoma and arterial leg thrombosis.

Hearing and Vestibular Disorders: earache, ear disorder (not otherwise specified), motion sickness and vestibular disorder.

Vascular (extracardiac) Disorders: phlebitis, flushing, vascular disorder, leg thrombophlebitis, vein disorder and purpura.

Heart Rate and Rhythm Disorders: palpitation, bradycardia and heart block.

Myo-endo-pericardial and Valve Disorders: angina pectoris, cardiomyopathy and myocardial infarction.

Neoplasm: lipoma, ovarian cyst and lymphoma malignant.

Endocrine Disorders: hypothyroidism and hyperthyroidism and goitre.

Red Blood Cell Disorders: hypochromic anaemia.

Liver and Biliary System Disorders: biliary pain.

White Cell and RES Disorders: lymphadenopathy.

Special Senses Other, Disorders: taste perversion.

Collagen Disorders: rheumatoid arthritis.

Post-Market Adverse Drug Reactions: As of 31 October 2006, Novo Nordisk has received 115 adverse drug reaction reports in pediatric patients. Of these cases, 52 were serious (hereunder 8 unexpected). Most adverse reactions were reported in the following SOCs (System Organ Class): General disorders and administration site conditions, Metabolism and nutrition disorders, Investigations and Skin and subcutaneous tissue disorders (see Table 2). The nature of the events reported is expected in relation to administration of an insulin product. Furthermore, the type of adverse events in pediatric population is similar to that seen in adults. A higher frequency of hypoglycemia was reported in children compared to adults; however this can be explained by underreporting of these events in adults.

In children aged 6-11 years, 39 cases of adverse drug reactions were reported spontaneously, of which 11 were serious (one of them was unlisted). In children aged 12-17 years, 64 cases of adverse drug reactions were reported, of which 35 were serious (four of them were unexpected).

Twelve (12) cases of spontaneously reported adverse drug reactions occurred in children below 6 years of age and were thus recorded in relation to off-label use—three of these cases were serious.

Table 2: Levemir

Distribution of Post-Market Adverse Events in Children and Adults by System Organ Class

SOC (System Organ Class)[a]	General Disorders and Administration Site Conditions (most frequent events—injection site reactions)	Metabolism and Nutrition Disorders (most frequent events—hypoglycemia)	Investigations (most frequent events—blood glucose increased)	Skin and Subcutaneous Tissue Disorders (most frequent events—rash, pruritus and urticaria)
Children (<18 years)	29%	27%	12%	12%
Adults	30%	13%	20%	9%

[a] System Organ Class are coded by use of MedDRA (Medical Dictionary for Regulatory Affairs).

DRUG INTERACTIONS: Overview: As with insulins in general, concomitant use of other drugs may influence insulin requirements.

The following substances may reduce insulin requirements: oral antidiabetic drugs, monoamine oxidase inhibitors (MAOI), non-selective beta-blocking agents, angiotensin converting enzyme (ACE) inhibitors, salicylates, and alcohol.

The following substances may increase insulin requirements: oral contraceptives, thiazides, glucocorticoids, thyroid hormones, beta-sympathomimetics, growth hormone and danazol.

Beta-blocking agents may mask the symptoms of hypoglycemia and delay recovery from hypoglycemia.

Octreotide/lanreotide may both increase and decrease insulin requirement.

Alcohol may intensify and prolong the hypoglycemic effect of insulin.

Drug-Drug Interactions: Interactions with other drugs have not been established.

Drug-Food Interactions: Interactions with food have not been established.

Drug-Herb Interactions: Interactions with herbal products have not been established.

Drug-Laboratory Test Interactions: Interactions with laboratory tests have not been established.

Drug-Lifestyle Interactions: Hypoglycemia may occur as a result of an excess of insulin relative to food intake, energy expenditure, or both. Omission of a meal or unplanned strenuous physical exercise may lead to hypoglycemia. (See Hypoglycemia and Treatment of Overdosage.)

DOSAGE AND ADMINISTRATION: Dosing Considerations: Levemir (insulin detemir) is indicated for the treatment of both adult and pediatric patients with type 1 diabetes mellitus, and adult patients with type 2 diabetes mellitus.

Levemir should be used once daily in combination with:

- Oral antidiabetic drugs (OADs); or
- Short- or rapid-acting meal time insulin.

When Levemir is used as part of a basal-bolus insulin regimen, Levemir has the option of being administered twice daily, depending on patients' needs.

For patients who require twice daily dosing to optimize blood glucose control, the evening dose can be administered either with the evening meal or at bedtime.

Dosage of Levemir is individual and determined, based on the physician's advice, in accordance with the needs of the patient.

Recommended Dose and Dosage Adjustment: New Patients: Patients being initiated on insulin for the first time can be started on Levemir in the same manner as they would be on human insulin.

Type 2 Patients Adding Levemir to OAD: In combination with oral antidiabetic agents, it is recommended to initiate Levemir treatment with once daily administration at a dose of 10 U or 0.1-0.2 U/kg. The dose of Levemir should be titrated on individual patients' needs.

The following titration guideline is recommended based on the average of three self-measured pre-breakfast plasma glucose concentrations: see Table 3.

Table 3: Levemir

Titration Guideline

Average Pre-Breakfast Self-Measured Plasma Glucose (SMPG)	Levemir Dose Adjustment
>10.0 mmol/L	+8
9.1–10.0 mmol/L	+6
8.1–9.0 mmol/L	+4
7.1–8.0 mmol/L	+2
6.1–7.0 mmol/L	+2
4.1–6.0 mmol/L	no change (target)
If one SMPG measurement	
3.1–4.0 mmol/L	–2
<3.1 mmol/L	–4

Transfer Patients: When patients are transferred from other insulin to Levemir, the change should be made as directed by the physician.

Patients transferring to Levemir from intermediate or long-acting insulin may require adjustment of dose and timing of administration to achieve glycemic target.

Close glucose monitoring is recommended during the transition and in the initial weeks thereafter. Concomitant antidiabetic treatment may need to be adjusted (dose and timing of concurrent short-acting insulins or the dose of oral antidiabetic agents, see Warnings and Precautions, General).

Administration: Levemir should not be mixed or diluted with any other insulin for injection (see Warnings and Precautions).

Levemir (insulin detemir) is administered subcutaneously in the abdominal wall, the buttock, the thigh or the upper arm. Injection sites should be rotated within the same region. As with all insulins, the duration of action will vary according to the dose, injection site, blood flow, temperature and level of physical activity.

Parenteral drug products should be inspected visually for particulate matter and discolouration prior to administration, whenever solution and container permit. Levemir should never be used if it has become viscous (thickened) or cloudy; it should only be used if it is clear and colourless. Levemir should not be used after its expiration date.

In patients with diabetes mellitus, optimized metabolic control effectively delays the onset and slows the progression of late diabetic complications. Optimized metabolic control, including glucose monitoring is therefore recommended.

As a precautionary measure, patients should carry a spare syringe and extra insulin in case the insulin delivery device is lost or damaged.

OVERDOSAGE:

Hypoglycemia and Treatment of Overdosage: Hypoglycemia may occur as a result of an excessive dose of insulin relative to food intake, energy expenditure, or both. Omission of a meal or unplanned strenuous physical exercise may lead to hypoglycemia. Symptoms of hypoglycemia may occur suddenly. They may include cold sweat, cool pale skin, fatigue, drowsiness, excessive hunger, vision changes, headache, nausea and palpitation. Severe hypoglycemia may lead to unconsciousness and/or convulsions and may be fatal.

Mild hypoglycemic episodes can be treated by oral administration of glucose or sugary products. It is therefore recommended that patients with diabetes carry sugar-containing products.

Severe hypoglycemic episodes, where the patient has become unconscious, can be treated by glucagon (0.5 to 1 mg) given intramuscularly or subcutaneously by a trained person, or by glucose given intravenously by a medical professional. Glucose must also be given intravenously if the patient does not respond to glucagon within 10 to 15 minutes. Upon regaining consciousness, administration of oral carbohydrates is recommended for the patient in order to prevent a relapse.

> For management of a suspected drug overdose, CPhA recommends that you contact your **regional Poison Control Centre**. See the *CPS* Directory section for a list of Poison Control Centres.

ACTION AND CLINICAL PHARMACOLOGY: Mechanism of Action: Levemir (insulin detemir) is a soluble, long-acting basal insulin analogue with a flat and predictable action profile with a prolonged duration of action. The nocturnal glucose profile is flatter and smoother with Levemir than with NPH insulin. Levemir has improved predictability of action compared to other basal preparations such as NPH (Neutral Protamine Hagedorn) insulin.

The prolonged action of Levemir is mediated by the slower systemic absorption of insulin detemir molecules at the injection site due to strong self-association of the drug molecule and albumin binding via the fatty acid side-chain. More than 98% of insulin detemir in the bloodstream is albumin bound and insulin detemir is distributed more slowly to peripheral target tissues compared to NPH insulin. The absorption kinetics and action profile of Levemir has less intra-patient variability compared to NPH insulin and insulin glargine in our studies.

Pharmacodynamics: Intra-patient variability of Levemir actions was compared to NPH insulin and insulin glargine in a parallel group, randomized, double-blind, clinical pharmacology study of 52 patients Study NN304-1450with type 1 diabetes each receiving 4 doses of assigned treatments. Variability in glucodynamic effects (intra-patient variability in average and maximum glucose infusion rates) from one injection to another, as expressed by the coefficient of variation, was 2- to 2.5-fold less for Levemir than for NPH insulin , (p<0.001) vs. insulin detemir, and 1.6- to 1.8-fold less than for insulin glargine (p<0.001).

The blood glucose lowering effect of Levemir is due to the facilitated uptake of glucose following binding of insulin detemir to receptors on muscle and fat cells and to the simultaneous inhibition of glucose output from the liver.

Figure 1 shows Glucose Infusion Rate results from an isoglycemic clamp study in patients with type 1 diabetes.

Figure 1: Levemir

Activity Profiles for Levemir

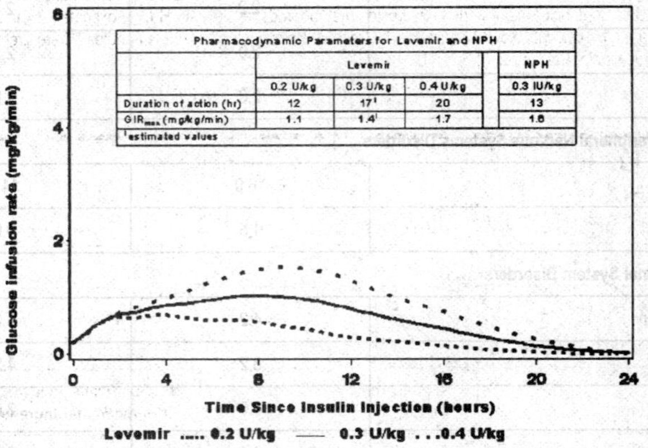

The duration of action is up to 24 hours (see Figure 1), depending on dose, providing an opportunity for once or twice daily administration. If administered twice daily, steady state will occur after 2-3 dose administrations. For doses in the interval of 0.2-0.4 U/kg, Levemir exerts more than 50% of its maximum effect from 3-4 hours and up to approximately 14 hours after dose administration.

Dose proportionality in pharmacodynamic response [maximum effect, duration of action (range: 6-24 hours), total effect] is observed after subcutaneous administration.

The time action profile of Levemir shows significantly less intra-patient variability than other basal insulins. This reduced variability results in a more predictable glycemic response for an individual.

In long-term treatment trials (≥6 months) in patients with type 1 diabetes, fasting plasma glucose was improved with Levemir compared with NPH insulin when given as basal-bolus therapy. Glycemic control, measured as glycosylated hemoglobin (HbA_{1C}) with Levemir is comparable to NPH insulin.

The overall risk of hypoglycemia did not differ between type 1 patients treated with Levemir, NPH or insulin glargine.

The risk of nocturnal hypoglycemia was reduced by 22% for Levemir as compared to NPH.

The risk of severe hypoglycemia was 72% lower (p<0.047) and nocturnal hypoglycaemia was 32% (p<0.046) lower with insulin detemir when compared to insulin glargine, Study NN304-1372.

The risk of hypoglycemia is a major limiting factor in achieving targets for glycemic control in insulin-treated patients with diabetes. Therefore, risk of hypoglycemia is addressed in the context of clinical efficacy.

Our studies in patients with type 2 diabetes treated with basal insulin in combination with oral antidiabetic drugs demonstrated that glycemic control (HbA_{1C}) with Levemir is comparable to NPH and insulin glargine and associated with less weight gain.

In trials with the use of OAD-insulin combination therapy Levemir treatment resulted in a lower risk of minor nocturnal hypoglycemia compared to NPH.

Pharmacokinetics: See Table 4.

Table 4: Levemir

Summary of Insulin Detemir's Pharmacokinetic Parameters in Subjects with Type 1 Diabetes

Single Dose (U/kg)	C_{max} (pmol/L) mean (SD)	T_{max} (min) median (min; max)	$AUC_{0-\infty}$ (pmol·10³-min/L) mean (SD)
0.1	1434 (920)	240 (119; 480)	1232 (1119)
0.2	2896 (1910)	360 (119; 660)	1681 (925)
0.4	4422 (1774)	420 (300; 540)	3709 (1766)
0.8	7278 (2809)	420 (300; 600)	6715 (2665)
1.6	16 535 (9344)	420 (180; 480)	14 235 (6181)

Absorption: In our studies, after subcutaneous injection of Levemir in healthy subjects and in patients with diabetes, intra-subject variation in absorption is lower for Levemir than NPH insulin and insulin glargine. Dose proportionality in serum concentrations was observed after subcutaneous administration.

Maximum serum concentration is reached between 6 and 8 hours after administration.

Bioavailability of insulin detemir is approximately 60%.

Distribution, Metabolism and Excretion: The terminal half-life after subcutaneous administration is determined by the rate of absorption from the subcutaneous tissue. The terminal half-life is between 5 and 7 hours depending on dose.

An apparent volume of distribution for insulin detemir (approximately 0.1 L/kg) indicates that a high fraction of insulin detemir is circulating in the blood.

Degradation of insulin detemir is similar to that of human insulin; all metabolites formed are inactive.

The results of the in vitro and in vivo protein binding studies demonstrate that there is no clinically relevant interaction between insulin detemir and fatty acids or other protein bound drugs.

Special Populations and Conditions: Pediatrics: The pharmacokinetic properties of Levemir were investigated in children (6-12 years) and adolescents (13-17 years) and compared to adults with type 1 diabetes. The pharmacokinetic properties were similar in the three groups. The efficacy and safety of Levemir were demonstrated in children and adolescents aged 6 to 17 years. No pediatric efficacy and safety data are available to support pediatric dosing advice below the age of 6 years.

Geriatrics: There was no clinically relevant difference in pharmacokinetics of Levemir between elderly and young subjects.

Gender: No clinically relevant difference between genders is seen in pharmacokinetic parameters.

Obesity: In controlled clinical trials, which included patients with Body Mass Index (BMI) up to 50 kg/m², subgroup analyses based on BMI did not show any differences in safety and efficacy between Levemir and NPH insulin.

Race: In two trials in healthy Japanese and Caucasian subjects, there were no clinically relevant differences seen in pharmacokinetic parameters.

Hepatic Insufficiency: Individuals with severe hepatic dysfunction, without diabetes, were observed to have lower AUCs as compared to healthy volunteers.

Caution should be taken when making general dosing recommendations for subjects with liver impairment. As with other insulin preparations, titration with Levemir and glucose monitoring should be intensified in patients with liver impairment.

Renal Insufficiency: There was no clinically relevant difference in pharmacokinetics of Levemir between subjects with renal impairment and healthy subjects.

Pregnancy: The effect of pregnancy on the pharmacokinetics and pharmacodynamics of Levemir has not been studied (see Warnings and Precautions, Pregnant Women).

Smoking: The effect of smoking on the pharmacokinetics and pharmacodynamics of Levemir has not been studied.

STORAGE AND STABILITY: Levemir (insulin detemir) should be stored between 2 and 8°C (in a refrigerator) not near a freezing compartment. Do not freeze. In order to protect from light, Levemir Penfill cartridges should be kept in the outer carton.

Levemir Penfill in use or carried as a spare can be kept at temperatures not above 30°C for up to 42 days. Levemir is not to be kept in the refrigerator.

Levemir should not be used after the expiry date printed on the package.

INFORMATION FOR THE PATIENT: Published in e-CPS, available by subscription at www.e-cps.ca.

DOSAGE FORMS, COMPOSITION AND PACKAGING: Each mL of sterile, aqueous, clear, colourless and neutral solution, contains: salt-free anhydrous insulin detemir 100 U (14.2 mg/mL). One unit of Levemir corresponds to one IU of human insulin. Nonmedicinal ingredients: disodium phosphate dihydrate, mannitol, metacresol, phenol, sodium chloride, zinc acetate and water for Injection. Hydrochloric acid and/or sodium hydroxide may be added to adjust pH (approximately 7.4). Levemir Penfill cartridges are designed for use with Novo Nordisk Insulin Delivery Devices and NovoFine needles. There are 100 Units of insulin detemir per mL of insulin. Pack sizes of 5x3 mL.

(Shown in Product Identification Section)

Levitra® Ⓟ

vardenafil HCl

Treatment of Erectile Dysfunction

Bayer

Date of Revision: August 26, 2009

SUMMARY PRODUCT INFORMATION:

Route of Administration	Dosage Form/ Strength	Clinically Relevant Nonmedicinal Ingredients
Oral	Tablets/(equivalent to) vardenafil 5 mg, 10 mg, 20 mg	None For a complete listing see Dosage Forms, Composition and Packaging.

INDICATIONS AND CLINICAL USE: LEVITRA (vardenafil hydrochloride) is indicated for:

- Treatment of erectile dysfunction (difficulties or the inability to achieve or maintain penile erection sufficient for satisfactory sexual performance).

Special Populations: Pregnant Women: LEVITRA is not indicated for use in women. There are no trials of vardenafil in pregnant women.

Nursing Women: See Pregnant Women.

Pediatrics (<18 years of age): LEVITRA is not indicated for use in individuals less than 18 years old.

Geriatrics (≥65 years of age): A starting dose of 5 mg LEVITRA should be considered in patients 65 years and older. On average, elderly males (65 years and over) had a 52% higher vardenafil AUC than younger males (18-45 years); however, this difference was not statistically significant. (See Action and Clinical Pharmacology.)

CONTRAINDICATIONS:

- Patients who are hypersensitive to this drug or to any ingredient in the formulation or component of the container. For a complete listing, see Dosage Forms, Composition and Packaging.
- Consistent with the effects of PDE5 inhibition on the nitric oxide/cyclic guanosine monophosphate pathway, PDE5 inhibitors may potentiate the hypotensive effects of nitrates, and therefore **coadministration of LEVITRA (vardenafil hydrochloride) with nitrates and nitric oxide donors is contraindicated.**

  In a patient prescribed vardenafil hydrochloride, where nitrate administration is deemed medically necessary in a life-threatening situation, at least 24 hours should have elapsed after the last dose of vardenafil hydrochloride before nitrate administration is considered. In such circumstances, nitrates should only be administered under close medical supervision with appropriate hemodynamic monitoring.
- Concomitant use of vardenafil hydrochloride with indinavir, ritonavir, ketoconazole, or itraconazole is contraindicated, as they are potent inhibitors of CYP3A4 (see Warnings and Precautions and Dosage and Administration).

WARNINGS AND PRECAUTIONS: General: The evaluation of erectile dysfunction should include a determination of potential underlying causes, a medical assessment and the identification of appropriate treatment.

Before prescribing LEVITRA (vardenafil hydrochloride), it is important to note the following:

- LEVITRA has not been administered to patients with bleeding disorders or significant active peptic ulceration. Therefore LEVITRA should be administered to these patients after careful benefit-risk assessment. In humans, LEVITRA has no effect on bleeding time alone or with acetylsalicylic acid (ie, ASPIRIN*). In vitro studies with human platelets indicate that LEVITRA does not inhibit platelet aggregation induced by a variety of platelet agonists. A small, concentration-dependent, enhancement of the anti-aggregation effects of a nitric oxide donor, nitroprusside, was observed with supra-therapeutic concentrations of LEVITRA in the presence of platelet agonists. The bleeding time in rats with a combination of heparin and vardenafil was not different from that observed with heparin alone. However, this interaction has not been studied in humans.
- Treatment for erectile dysfunction should generally be used with caution in patients with anatomical deformation of the penis (such as angulation, cavernosal fibrosis or Peyronie's disease) or in patients who have conditions that may predispose them to priapism (such as sickle cell anemia, multiple myeloma, or leukemia).

LEVITRA has not been studied in patients with CNS disease (other than spinal cord injury), hypoactive sexual desire, or in patients who have undergone pelvic surgery (except nerve sparing prostatectomy), pelvic trauma, or radiotherapy.

Postmarketing reports of sudden loss of vision have occurred rarely, in temporal association with the use of PDE5 inhibitors. It is not clear whether these are related directly to the use of PDE5 inhibitors or to other factors. There may be an increased risk to patients who have already experienced Nonarteritic Anterior Ischemic Optic Neuropathy (NAION).

Cardiovascular: Physicians should consider the cardiovascular status of their patients, since there is a degree of cardiac risk associated with sexual activity. In men for whom sexual activity is not recommended because of their underlying cardiovascular status, including uncontrolled hypertension (with BP >140/90 mmHg), any treatment for erectile dysfunction, including LEVITRA, generally should not be used. Physicians are advised to consult the recommendations of the Princeton Consensus Panel (DeBusk et al. Am J Cardiol 2000;86:175-81). The following groups of patients with cardiovascular disease were not included in clinical trials:

- patients with a myocardial infarction or stroke within the last 6 months,
- patients with unstable angina pectoris or acute myocardial ischemia,
- patients with uncontrolled arrhythmias, hypotension (<90/50 mmHg), uncontrolled hypertension (>170/110 mmHg),
- patients with symptomatic postural hypotension in the last six months

LEVITRA has vasodilator properties which may result in mild and transient decreases in blood pressure. Patients with left ventricular outflow obstruction, eg, aortic stenosis and idiopathic hypertrophic subaortic stenosis, can be sensitive to the action of vasodilators, including Type 5 phosphodiesterase inhibitors.

Patients should be stable on alpha-blocker therapy before prescribing LEVITRA.

Patients receiving alpha-blocker therapy should be initiated at the lowest dose of 5 mg LEVITRA.

Congenital and Acquired QT Prolongation: In a study of the effect of LEVITRA on the QT interval in 59 healthy males, therapeutic (10 mg) and supratherapeutic (80 mg) doses of LEVITRA produced minimal increases in QTc interval. (See Action and Clinical Pharmacology.) In a postmarketing study evaluating the effect of combining LEVITRA with another drug of comparable QT effect (400 mg gatifloxacin), it was shown that the drug combination produced an additive QT effect when compared with either drug alone. (See Drug Interactions, Action and Clinical Pharmacology.) These observations should be considered in clinical decisions when prescribing LEVITRA to patients with known history of QT prolongation or patients who are taking medications known to prolong the QT interval. Patients with congenital QT prolongation (long QT syndrome) and those taking Class IA (eg, quinidine, procainamide) or Class III (eg, amiodarone, sotalol) antiarrhythmic medications should avoid using LEVITRA.

Hepatic: No dose adjustment is required in patients with mild hepatic impairment. (See Warnings and Precautions and Action and Clinical Pharmacology.)

In patients with mild hepatic impairment (Child-Pugh A), following a 10 mg dose of LEVITRA, the vardenafil AUC was increased 17% and the maximum concentration (C_{max}) was increased 22%, compared to healthy male volunteers. In patients with moderate impairment (Child-Pugh B), following a 10 mg dose of LEVITRA, the vardenafil AUC was increased 160% and C_{max} was increased 133%, compared to healthy male volunteers.

In patients with moderate hepatic impairment, a 5 mg starting dose of LEVITRA is recommended, which may subsequently be increased to a maximum dose of 10 mg, based on tolerability and efficacy. (See Warnings and Precautions, Dosage and Administration, and Action and Clinical Pharmacology.)

There are no controlled clinical data on the efficacy and safety of LEVITRA in severe hepatic impairment; its use is therefore not recommended until further information is available.

Ophthalmologic: There are no controlled clinical data on the efficacy and safety of LEVITRA in known hereditary degenerative retinal disorders such as retinitis pigmentosa; its use is therefore not recommended until further information is available.

Otologic: Sudden decrease or loss of hearing has been reported in a few postmarketing and clinical trial cases with the use of PDE5 inhibitors, including LEVITRA. These events, which may be accompanied by tinnitus and dizziness, have been reported in temporal association to the intake of PDE5 inhibitors, including LEVITRA. In some of the cases, medical conditions and other factors were reported that may have also played a role in the otologic adverse events. In many cases, medical follow-up information was limited. It is not possible to determine whether these events are related directly to the use of PDE5 inhibitors or to other factors (see Adverse Reactions, Post-Market Adverse Drug Reactions and Information for the Patient). Physicians should advise patients to stop taking LEVITRA and seek prompt medical attention in case of sudden decrease or loss of hearing.

Renal: No dose adjustment is required in patients with renal impairment. In patients with mild, moderate, or severe renal impairment, the pharmacokinetics of LEVITRA were similar to that of control groups with normal renal function. LEVITRA pharmacokinetics have not been evaluated in patients requiring dialysis.

There are no controlled clinical data on the efficacy and safety of LEVITRA in end stage renal disease requiring dialysis; its use is therefore not recommended until further information is available.

Sexual Function/Reproduction: Prolonged erection greater than 4 hours and priapism (painful erections greater than 6 hours in duration) have been reported infrequently with the use of PDE5 inhibitors, including LEVITRA. The incidence of priapism may increase when PDE5 inhibitors are used in combination with intrapenile injections containing vasoactive agents, or other drugs with a known risk of priapism. In the event of an erection that persists longer than 4 hours, the patient should seek immediate medical assistance. If priapism is not treated immediately, penile tissue damage and permanent loss of potency could result. (See Overdosage, Treatment of Priapism.)

The safety and efficacy of combinations of LEVITRA with other agents for the treatment of erectile dysfunction have not been studied. Therefore, the use of such combinations is not recommended.

Information to Be Provided to the Patient: Physicians should discuss with patients the contraindications of LEVITRA with regular and/or intermittent use of organic nitrates. Patients should be advised that concomitant use of LEVITRA and nitrates could cause a sudden drop in blood pressure, dizziness, syncope, heart attack, or stroke.

Physicians should advise patients to stop taking PDE5 inhibitors, including LEVITRA, and seek prompt medical attention in the event of sudden decrease or loss of hearing. These events, which may be accompanied by tinnitus and dizziness, have been reported in temporal association to the intake of PDE5 inhibitors, including LEVITRA. It is not possible to determine whether these events are related directly to the use of PDE5 inhibitors or to other factors. (See Adverse Reactions.)

Physicians should consider the potential cardiac risk of sexual activity in patients with pre-existing cardiovascular disease. Patients who experience symptoms upon initiation of sexual activity should be advised to refrain from further sexual activity and should report the episode to their physician.

Physicians should discuss with patients the appropriate use of LEVITRA and its potential benefits. The patient should be told that sexual stimulation is necessary for an erection if LEVITRA is consumed. Patients should be told that LEVITRA should be taken approximately 25-60 minutes before sexual activity and no more than the recommended dose should be taken. They should be advised to contact their physician for dose adjustment if they are not satisfied with the quality of their erection or if they have an undesirable effect. Patients should be counselled about the importance of notifying their physicians about other medications they have been prescribed, including LEVITRA. Physicians should counsel patients that the concomitant use of PDE5 inhibitors, including LEVITRA with alpha-blockers may lead to symptomatic hypotension in some patients. PDE5 inhibitor therapy should only be initiated if the patient is stable on his alpha-blocker therapy. Patients should be advised that vardenafil may be administered at any time with tamsulosin. With other alpha-blockers, a time separation of dosing should be considered when vardenafil is prescribed concomitantly. In those patients already taking an optimized dose of vardenafil, alpha-blocker therapy should be initiated at the lowest dose. A stepwise increase in alpha-blocker dose may be associated with further lowering of blood pressure in patients taking a PDE5 inhibitor, including vardenafil. Patients should be advised that after stable concomitant therapy is established, vardenafil may be titrated as needed and tolerated. (See Dosage and Administration.)

Physicians should inform patients that erectile disturbances including prolonged erections greater than 4 hours and priapism have been reported with PDE5 inhibitors, including LEVITRA. Patients who experience erections lasting 4 hours or more should be instructed to seek immediate medical assistance. If priapism is not treated immediately, penile tissue damage and permanent loss of potency may result. The incidence of priapism may increase when PDE5 inhibitors, including LEVITRA, are used in combination with intra-penile injections containing vasoactive agents (eg, CAVERJECT).

LEVITRA should be used with caution in patients who have conditions that might predispose them to priapism (such as sickle cell anemia, multiple myeloma, or leukemia), or in patients with anatomical deformation of the penis (such as angulation, cavernosal fibrosis or Peyronie's disease).

Non-arteritic Anterior Ischemic Optic Neuropathy (NAION) has been reported rarely in postmarketing surveillance with PDE5 inhibitors, including vardenafil. Physicians should discuss with their patients the increased risk of NAION before prescribing LEVITRA. If an individual experiences reduction or loss of vision in one or both eyes after the use of LEVITRA, he should immediately report the episode to his physician.

The use of LEVITRA offers no protection against sexually transmitted diseases. Counselling of patients about the protective measures necessary to guard against sexually transmitted diseases, including Human Immunodeficiency Virus (HIV), should be considered.

ADVERSE REACTIONS: Adverse Drug Reaction Overview: LEVITRA (vardenafil hydrochloride) was administered to over 7800 patients (ages 18-89 years) during clinical trials worldwide. Over 625 patients were treated for 6 months and 557 were treated for at least one year. In placebo-controlled clinical trials, the discontinuation rate due to adverse events was low for LEVITRA (3.5% compared to 1.2% for placebo). The most common reasons for discontinuation in the LEVITRA-treated patients were headache (0.9%) and flushing (0.5%). Adverse events with LEVITRA were generally transient, mild to moderate in nature, and decreased with continued dosing.

Clinical Trial Adverse Drug Reactions: Because clinical trials are conducted under very specific conditions, the adverse reaction rates observed in the clinical trials may not reflect the rates observed in practice and should not be compared to the rates in the clinical trials of another drug. Adverse drug reaction information from clinical trials is useful for identifying drug-related adverse events and for approximating rates.

When LEVITRA was taken as recommended, the following adverse events in Table 1 were reported in placebo-controlled clinical trials.

* ASPIRIN is a registered trademark of Bayer AG, used under license by Bayer Inc., Toronto, ON M9W 1G6

Table 1: LEVITRA

Adverse Events Reported by ≥1% of Patients Treated with LEVITRA and More Frequent on Drug than Placebo in All Placebo-controlled Trials of 5 mg, 10 mg, and 20 mg LEVITRA

	LEVITRA (N=3293) (%)	Placebo (N=1861) (%)
Gastrointestinal Disorders		
Dyspepsia	2.5	<0.1
Nausea	1.2	0.3
Nervous System		
Dizziness	1.6	0.3
Headache	10.4	2.0
Respiratory, Thoracic and Mediastinal		
Nasal congestion, (including edema mucosal, rhinitis, rhinorrhea)	4	0.3
Vascular		
Flushing (including hot flush, feeling hot, erythema)	11.3	0.8

Less Common Clinical Trial Adverse Drug Reactions (<1%): The following additional adverse events where a causal relationship is uncertain (but plausible) occurred in <1% of patients receiving LEVITRA in all clinical trials:

Body as a Whole: abdominal pain (including abdominal pain upper), asthenia, back pain, chest pain, face edema, hypersensitivity, influenza (including influenza like illness), laryngeal edema, neck pain, photosensitivity reaction.

Cardiovascular: angina pectoris, hypertension, hypotension, myocardial ischemia, palpitations, postural hypotension, syncope, tachycardia (including heart rate increased).

Gastrointestinal Including Related Investigations: abnormal liver function tests (including hepatic enzyme increased, alanine aminotransferase increased, aspartate aminotransferase increased), diarrhea, dry mouth, dysphagia, esophagitis (including reflux esophagitis), gastritis, gastroesophageal reflux disease, GGTP increased, increased creatinine kinase, nausea, vomiting.

Musculoskeletal: arthralgia, muscle rigidity, myalgia.

Nervous: anxiety, burning sensation, dizziness, feeling abnormal, hypesthesia, insomnia, paresthesia, somnolence, vertigo, seizure, transient global amnesia.

Respiratory, Thoracic and Mediastinal: dyspnea, epistaxis, sinus congestion (including sinus pain).

Skin and Appendages: hyperhidrosis, pruritus, rash, sweating.

Special Senses: amblyopia, chromatopsia (including cyanopsia), conjunctivitis (including eye redness), eye pain (including abnormal sensation in eye), intraocular pressure increased, lacrimation increased, photophobia, sudden decrease or loss of hearing, tinnitus, vision blurred, visual disturbance (including visual brightness).

Urogenital: ejaculation disorder (including premature ejaculation), priapism (including prolonged or painful erections).

Post-Market Adverse Drug Reactions: Myocardial infarction (MI) has been reported in temporal association with the use of LEVITRA and sexual activity, but it is not possible to determine whether MI is related directly to vardenafil, to sexual activity, to the patient's underlying cardiovascular disease, or to a combination of these factors.

From post-marketing experience with drugs of this class, the following serious adverse events have been reported in temporal association with the use of the PDE5 inhibitors: abnormal accommodation, abnormal vision, amnesia, anxiety, cardiovascular hemorrhage, cerebrovascular hemorrhage, decreased vision, hematemesis, hematuria, intraocular hemorrhage, pulmonary hemorrhage, seizure, sudden cardiac death, temporary vision loss, and ventricular arrhythmia.

Cases of sudden decrease or loss of hearing have been reported in temporal association with the use of PDE5 inhibitors including LEVITRA. In some cases, medical conditions and other factors were reported that may have also played a role in the otologic adverse events. In many cases, medical follow-up information was limited. It is not possible to determine whether these reported events are related directly to the use of LEVITRA, to the patient's underlying risk factors for hearing loss, a combination of these factors, or to other factors. (See Warnings and Precautions, Adverse Reactions and Information for the Patient.)

Special Senses: nonarteritic anterior ischemic optic neuropathy, retinal vein occlusion, visual field defect.

DRUG INTERACTIONS: Overview: CYP3A4 Inhibitors: Vardenafil is metabolized predominantly by hepatic enzymes via cytochrome P450 (CYP) isoform 3A4, with some contribution from CYP3A5 and CYP2C isoforms. Therefore, inhibitors of these enzymes may reduce vardenafil clearance. Concomitant use of LEVITRA with indinavir, ritonavir, ketoconazole, and itraconazole is contraindicated, as they are potent inhibitors of CYP3A4. (See Contraindications and Dosage and Administration.)

Antihypertensive Agents: The potential for LEVITRA to augment the hypotensive effects of antihypertensive agents was examined in a clinical pharmacology study and in placebo-controlled clinical trials.

LEVITRA (20 mg), when coadministered with slow-release nifedipine (30 mg or 60 mg once daily to hypertensive patients), did not affect the relative AUC or C_{max} of nifedipine, a drug that is metabolized via CYP3A4. LEVITRA (20 mg) produced mean additional blood pressure reductions of 5.9 mmHg and 5.2 mmHg for supine systolic and diastolic blood pressure, respectively, compared to placebo.

In the placebo-controlled studies of 5, 10, and 20 mg LEVITRA, a total of 41% of patients on placebo and 42% of patients on LEVITRA received at least one antihypertensive medication during their treatment with study medication. Major classes of antihypertensive agents were represented, including: calcium channel blockers (N=353), ACE inhibitors (N=650), beta-blockers (N=346), angiotensin receptor blockers (N=188), and diuretics (N=312). Analysis of these data showed no difference in adverse events, cardiovascular adverse events or discontinuations due to adverse events, in patients taking LEVITRA with or without antihypertensive medications.

Alcohol: The pharmacokinetics of LEVITRA were not influenced by alcohol, and the pharmacokinetics of alcohol were not influenced by coadministration with LEVITRA. No additive effects on blood pressure, heart rate, or bleeding time are seen when LEVITRA (20 mg) is administered with alcohol compared to placebo plus alcohol.

Androgens, Pertinent Anti-androgens: Vardenafil has not been studied in patients using androgen replacement therapy or anti-androgens.

See Table 2.

Table 2: LEVITRA

Established or Potential Drug-Drug Interactions

Proper Name	Ref	Effect	Clinical Comment
Nitrates and nitric oxide donors	CT	Potentiates blood pressure lowering effects of sublingual nitrates taken 1 and 4 hours after a 20 mg dose of LEVITRA in healthy middle-aged subjects. These effects were not observed when 20 mg LEVITRA was taken 24 hours before the NTG.	**Potentiation of the hypotensive effects of nitrates for patients with ischemic heart disease have not been evaluated, and concomitant use of nitrates with LEVITRA is contraindicated.** (See Contraindications.)

(cont'd)

Table 2: LEVITRA *(cont'd)*

Established or Potential Drug-Drug Interactions

Proper Name	Ref	Effect	Clinical Comment
Potent CYP3A4 Inhibitors	CT/T	May decrease vardenafil clearance	Concomitant use of LEVITRA with indinavir, ritonavir, ketoconazole, and itraconazole is contraindicated, as they are potent inhibitors of CYP3A4. (See Contraindications and Dosage and Administration.)
Erythromycin	CT	4-fold increase in vardenafil AUC and a 3-fold increase in C_{max} when 500 mg t.i.d. erythromycin was coadministered with vardenafil (5 mg) to healthy volunteers.	A dose not exceeding 5 mg LEVITRA should be prescribed when used in combination with erythromycin. (See Dosage and Administration.)
Clarithromycin	T	Expected to be similar to that for erythromycin.	A dose not exceeding 5 mg LEVITRA should be prescribed when used in combination with clarithromycin. (See Dosage and Administration.)
Gatifloxacin	CT	An increase in QTcF (Fridericia) was observed when 10 mg vardenafil and 400 mg gatifloxacin were coadministered. The combined effect on QTcF appears to be small (Point Estimate of 4 msec with a 90% Confidence Interval of 1-6 msec) and additive when compared to either drug alone.	The clinical impact of these QT changes is unknown. Patients with congenital QT prolongation (long QT syndrome) and those taking Class IA (eg, quinidine, procainamide) or Class III (eg, amiodarone, sotalol) antiarrhythmic medications should avoid using LEVITRA.
Cimetidine	CT	No effect on AUC and C_{max} of vardenafil 20 mg when coadministered with 400 mg b.i.d. cimetidine in healthy male volunteers.	Cimetidine, a non-specific CYP3A4 inhibitor, has no interaction with vardenafil.
Alpha-adrenergic Receptor-blocking Agents	CT	Consistent with the vasodilatory effects of alpha-blockers and vardenafil, the concomitant use of vardenafil with alpha-blockers may lead to symptomatic hypotension in some patients.	Concomitant treatment should only be initiated if the patient is stable on his alpha-blocker therapy. In these patients, LEVITRA should be initiated at the lowest recommended starting dose of 5 mg. Vardenafil may be administered at any time with tamsulosin; with other alpha-adrenergic blocking agents a time separation of dosing should be considered. In those patients already taking an optimized dose of vardenafil, alpha-blocker therapy should be initiated at the lowest dose. A stepwise increase in alpha-blocker dose may be associated with further lowering of blood pressure in patients taking a PDE5 inhibitor, including vardenafil. Patients should be advised that after stable concomitant therapy is established, vardenafil may be titrated as needed and tolerated. (See Dosage and Administration).
Warfarin	CT	Warfarin, which is metabolized by CYP2C9, did not alter the plasma levels of LEVITRA when coadministered. No effect on pharmacokinetic or pharmacodynamic activity of warfarin (25 mg) when coadministered with LEVITRA (20 mg).	No clinically relevant interactions.
Glyburide	CT	The AUC and C_{max} of glyburide was not altered, by coadministration of LEVITRA (20 mg). No evidence that LEVITRA pharmacokinetics were altered by coadministration of 3.5 mg o.d. glyburide, which is metabolized by CYP3A4.	No clinically relevant interactions.
Digoxin	CT	Digoxin (0.375 mg o.d.) did not alter the plasma levels of LEVITRA when taken in combination. The steady-state pharmacokinetics of digoxin was not altered by the coadministration of LEVITRA (20 mg).	No clinically relevant interactions.
Antacids (magnesium hydroxide/aluminum hydroxide (MAALOX)	CT	A single dose of MAALOX did not affect the AUC or the C_{max} of LEVITRA.	No clinically relevant interactions.
H_2 Antagonists Ranitidine	CT	The AUC and C_{max} of LEVITRA was not affected by coadministration of ranitidine (150 mg b.i.d.).	No clinically relevant interactions.
Acetylsalicylic Acid (ASA) ASPIRIN	CT	LEVITRA (10 and 20 mg) did not potentiate the increase in bleeding time caused by ASPIRIN (two 81 mg tablets o.d.).	No clinically relevant interactions.

(cont'd)

Table 2: LEVITRA *(cont'd)*

Established or Potential Drug-Drug Interactions

Proper Name	Ref	Effect	Clinical Comment
Nifedipine	CT	LEVITRA (20 mg), when coadministered with slow-release nifedipine (30 mg or 60 mg once daily to hypertensive patients), did not affect the relative AUC or C_{max} of nifedipine, a drug that is metabolized via CYP3A4. LEVITRA (20 mg) produced mean additional blood pressure reductions of 5.9 mmHg and 5.2 mmHg for supine systolic and diastolic blood pressure, respectively, compared to placebo.	No clinically relevant interactions.

Legend: C=Case Study; CT=Clinical Trial; T=Theoretical.

Drug-Food Interactions: Grapefruit juice, a weak inhibitor of CYP3A4 gut wall metabolism, may give rise to modest increases in plasma levels of LEVITRA. The combination should be avoided. A high-fat meal may delay t_{max} by one hour. (See Action and Clinical Pharmacology.)

Drug-Herb Interactions: Interactions with herbal products have not been established.

Drug-Laboratory Interactions: Interactions with laboratory tests have not been established.

DOSAGE AND ADMINISTRATION: **Dosing Considerations:** LEVITRA (vardenafil hydrochloride) can be taken with or without food. LEVITRA is not affected by moderate amounts of alcohol (0.5 g/kg body weight; approximately 3.4 fluid ounces of 40% alcohol in a 70 kg person). Sexual stimulation is required to achieve an erection.

Recommended Dose and Dosage Adjustment: The recommended starting dose of LEVITRA is 10 mg, taken orally 25 to 60 minutes before sexual activity. Sexual activity can be initiated as soon as 15 minutes and as long as 8-10 hours after taking LEVITRA. The dose may be increased to a maximum recommended dose of 20 mg or decreased to 5 mg based on efficacy and tolerability. In patients with more severe erectile dysfunction (eg, diabetics) a more rapid titration may be appropriate. The recommended dose frequency is a maximum of once per day (as desired).

Geriatrics: A starting dose of 5 mg LEVITRA should be considered in patients 65 years or older. (See Warnings and Precautions and Action and Clinical Pharmacology.)

Hepatic Insufficiency: No dose adjustment for patients with mild hepatic impairment is required. Vardenafil clearance is reduced in patients with moderate hepatic impairment. **In patients with moderate hepatic impairment, a 5 mg starting dose of LEVITRA is recommended, which may subsequently be increased to a maximum dose of 10 mg, based on tolerability and efficacy.** (See Warnings and Precautions and Action and Clinical Pharmacology.) Vardenafil has not been evaluated in patients with severe hepatic impairment (Child-Pugh C).

Renal Insufficiency: No dose adjustment is required for patients with mild, moderate, or severe renal impairment. Vardenafil has not been evaluated in patients on dialysis.

OVERDOSAGE:

LEVITRA (vardenafil hydrochloride) in single doses up to 80 mg per day was tolerated in healthy male volunteers without producing serious adverse side effects. A 40 mg once daily dose of LEVITRA demonstrated mild adverse events while 40 mg twice daily resulted in cases of severe back pain. No muscle or neurological toxicity was identified.

In cases of overdose, standard supportive measures should be taken as required. Renal dialysis is not expected to accelerate clearance because LEVITRA is highly bound to plasma proteins and is not significantly eliminated in the urine.

Treatment of Priapism: Health professionals should warn patients that there have been rare reports of prolonged erections greater than 4 hours and priapism (painful erections greater than 6 hours in duration) for this class of compounds. In the event that an erection persists longer than 4 hours, the patient should seek immediate medical assistance. If priapism is not treated immediately, penile tissue damage and permanent loss of potency may result.

Detumescence Protocols:

1. Aspirate 40 to 60 mL blood from either left or right corpora using a vacutainer and holder for drawing blood. Patient will often detumesce while blood is being aspirated. Apply ice for 20 minutes post aspiration if erection persists. If the first procedure is unsuccessful, try Procedure 2.
2. Put patient in supine position. Dilute 10 mg phenylephrine into 20 mL distilled water for injection (0.05%). With an insulin syringe, inject 0.1 to 0.2 mL (50-100 µg) into the corpora every 2 to 5 minutes until the detumescence occurs. The occasional patient may experience transient bradycardia and hypertension when given phenylephrine injections; therefore, monitor the patient's blood pressure and pulse every 10 minutes. Patients at risk include those with cardiac arrhythmias and diabetes. Refer to the prescribing information for phenylephrine before use. **Do not give phenylephrine to patients on monoamine oxidase (MAO) inhibitors.** When phenylephrine is used within the first 12 hours of erection, the majority of patients will respond. If Procedure 2 is unsuccessful, try Procedure 3.
3. If the above measures fail to detumesce the patient, a urologist should be consulted as soon as possible, especially if the erection has been present for many hours. If priapism is not treated immediately, penile tissue damage and/or permanent loss of potency may result.

> For management of a suspected drug overdose, contact your **regional Poison Control Centre**. See the *CPS* Directory section for a list of Poison Control Centres.

ACTION AND CLINICAL PHARMACOLOGY: Mechanism of Action: LEVITRA (vardenafil hydrochloride) is a highly selective cyclic GMP-specific phosphodiesterase type 5 (PDE5) inhibitor used for the treatment of male erectile dysfunction/difficulties.

Penile erection is a hemodynamic process initiated by the relaxation of smooth muscle in the corpus cavernosum and its associated arterioles. During sexual stimulation, nitric oxide is released from nerve endings and endothelial cells in the corpus cavernosum. Nitric oxide activates the soluble enzyme guanylate cyclase, resulting in increased synthesis of cyclic guanosine monophosphate (cGMP) in the corpus cavernosum smooth muscle cells. The cGMP in turn triggers smooth muscle relaxation, allowing increased blood flow into the penis and resulting in an erection. The tissue concentration of cGMP is regulated by both the rates of synthesis and degradation via phosphodiesterases (PDEs). The most prominent PDE in the human corpus cavernosum is the cGMP-specific phosphodiesterase type 5 (PDE5); by inhibiting PDE5, the enzyme responsible for cGMP degradation in the corpus cavernosum, vardenafil potently enhances the effect of endogenous nitric oxide, locally released in the corpus cavernosum upon sexual stimulation.

Studies on purified enzyme preparations have shown that vardenafil is a potent and selective inhibitor of human PDE5 with an IC50 (concentration that inhibits 50% of enzyme activity) of 0.7 nM. The inhibitory effect of vardenafil is more potent on PDE5 than on other known phosphodiesterases (>15-fold relative to PDE6 [found in the retina], >130-fold relative to PDE1 [found in the brain, heart, and vascular system], >300-fold relative to PDE11 [found in the testes, penile vasculature, vascular smooth muscle, skeletal muscle, prostate, pituitary], and >1000-fold relative to PDE2, 3, 4, 7, 8, 9, and 10). In vitro, vardenafil causes an elevation of cGMP in the isolated human corpus cavernosum, resulting in muscle relaxation. In the conscious rabbit, vardenafil causes a penile erection that is dependent upon endogenous nitric oxide synthesis and is potentiated by nitric oxide donors.

Pharmacodynamics: Studies of LEVITRA on Erectile Response: In patients with erectile dysfunction, erections considered sufficient for penetration (greater than or equal to 60% rigidity as measured by RIGISCAN device [RigiScan Ambulatory Rigidity and Tumescence Monitor, Dacomed Corp., Minneapolis, USA]) occurred in 64% of men on 20 mg LEVITRA as early as 15 minutes post dosing compared to 52% of men on placebo. The overall erectile response of these subjects treated with LEVITRA became statistically significant compared to placebo at 25 minutes post dosing. In two separate double-blind, placebo-controlled crossover RIGISCAN trials of men with erectile dysfunction of at least 6 months duration, 10 mg and 20 mg LEVITRA significantly improved erections initiated by visual sexual stimulation. Objective measurements of rigidity at the base and tip of the penis (by RIGISCAN) during visual sexual stimulation showed significantly better results at all doses and time points with LEVITRA than with placebo. The mean duration of an erection, in response to visual sexual stimulation, sufficient for penetration was 54 and 67 minutes at the base and 39 and 45 minutes at the tip of the penis for the 10 mg and 20 mg doses of LEVITRA respectively, compared to 31 minutes at the base and 17 minutes at the tip for placebo.

The earliest elapsed time from dosing to attainment of an erection perceived to be sufficient for penetration and resulting in successful completion of intercourse was evaluated in a randomized, double-blind parallel group study in men with ED. The percentage of men reporting successful completion of intercourse after dosing with 10 mg or 20 mg vardenafil was greater than with placebo ($p<0.025$) at all times ≥10 minutes and ≥11 minutes, respectively.

The amount of time from dosing (flexible dose) to attainment of an erection perceived to be sufficient for penetration and resulting in successful intercourse was evaluated in a randomized, double-blind, parallel group study in men with ED. The percentage of men reporting successful completion of intercourse 8 to 10 hours after dosing was greater with vardenafil compared to placebo ($p<0.001$).

Studies of LEVITRA on Blood Pressure and Heart Rate: In a clinical pharmacology study of patients with erectile dysfunction, single doses of 20 mg LEVITRA caused a mean maximum decrease in supine blood pressure of 7 mmHg systolic and 8 mmHg diastolic (compared to placebo), accompanied by a mean maximum increase of heart rate of 4 beats per minute. The maximum decrease in blood pressure occurred between 1 and 4 hours after dosing. Following multiple dosing for 31 days, blood pressure responses were observed on Day 31 that were similar to those observed on Day 1. PDE5 inhibitors, including LEVITRA, may add to the blood pressure lowering effects of antihypertensive agents. (See Drug Interactions.)

Larger effects were recorded among subjects receiving concomitant nitrates. (See Contraindications.)

Studies of LEVITRA on Cardiac Parameters: PDE5 inhibitors, including LEVITRA, have been shown to increase the QT interval. In a study of the effect of vardenafil on the QT interval in 59 healthy males, therapeutic and supratherapeutic doses of vardenafil and another member of the PDE5 inhibitor class produced minimal increases in the QTc interval. This effect on the QT interval is consistent with that observed with other members of the PDE5 inhibitor class. In a postmarketing study evaluating the effect of combining LEVITRA with another drug of comparable QT effect (400 mg gatifloxacin), it was shown that the drug combination produced an additive QT effect when compared with either drug alone. (See Warnings and Precautions, Drug Interactions.)

Studies of LEVITRA on Exercise Performance in Patients with Coronary Artery Disease (CAD): In two independent trials that assessed 10 mg (N=41) and 20 mg (N=39) LEVITRA respectively, LEVITRA did not alter the total treadmill exercise time compared to placebo. The patient population included men aged 40-80 years with stable exercise-induced angina documented by at least one of the following: 1) prior history of MI, CABG, PTCA, or stenting (not within 6 months); 2) positive coronary angiogram showing at least 60% narrowing of the diameter of at least one major coronary artery; or 3) a positive stress echocardiogram or stress nuclear perfusion. The results of the 20 mg study are shown in Table 3.

Table 3: LEVITRA

Effect of 20 mg LEVITRA on Exercise Treadmill Completion Times (Mean in Seconds ± S.D.)

Parameter	20 mg LEVITRA (Mean in Seconds)	Placebo (Mean in Seconds)
Total Treadmill Exercise Time	414±114 (N=36)	411±124 (N=36)
Total Time to Develop Symptoms of Angina Pectoris (first awareness)	354±137 (N=36)	347±143 (N=36)
Total Time to ST-Segment depression (1 mm or greater change from baseline)	364±101 (N=35)	366±105 (N=36)

Studies of LEVITRA on Vision: Single oral doses of phosphodiesterase inhibitors have demonstrated transient dose-related impairment of colour discrimination (blue/green) using the Farnsworth-Munsell 100-hue test and reductions in electroretinogram (ERG) b-wave amplitudes, with peak effects near the time of peak plasma levels. These findings are consistent with the inhibition of PDE6 in rods and cones, which is involved in phototransduction in the retina. The findings were most evident one hour after administration, diminishing but still present 6 hours after administration. In a single dose study in 25 normal males, 40 mg LEVITRA, twice the maximum daily recommended dose, did not alter visual acuity, intraocular pressure, fundoscopic and slit lamp findings.

Studies of LEVITRA on Sperm Characteristics: In healthy male volunteers, there was no effect on sperm motility, morphology, or a variety of other parameters relevant to male reproductive function 1.5 hours after single 20 mg oral doses of LEVITRA were administered.

In a 6-month placebo-controlled study conducted with healthy males or males with erectile dysfunction, aged 25-64 years, daily treatment with 20 mg vardenafil had no effect on sperm concentration, count, motility, or morphology. In addition, vardenafil had no effect on serum levels of testosterone, luteinizing hormone, or follicle-stimulating hormone. The effect of vardenafil on human fertility was not directly evaluated in this study. Although daily treatment with vardenafil 20 mg for six months in this study did not demonstrate significant effects on sperm characteristics, the effect of longer duration of treatment with vardenafil on sperm characteristics is unknown.

Pharmacokinetics: See Table 4.

Table 4: LEVITRA

Summary of Vardenafil Pharmacokinetic Parameters in Healthy Male Volunteers

	C_{max}	$t_{½}$	$AUC_{0-\infty}$	Clearance	Volume of distribution
Single 20 mg dose (mean)	15-17 µg·L/h	4-5 h	70 µg·h/L	56 L/h	208 L

LEVITRA (vardenafil hydrochloride) is rapidly absorbed after oral administration, with a mean absolute bioavailability of about 15%. Its pharmacokinetics approximate dose-proportionality over the recommended dose range (5 mg, 10 mg, and 20 mg). Vardenafil is eliminated predominantly by hepatic metabolism. The elimination half-life is approximately 4-5 hours. Mean vardenafil plasma concentrations measured over 24 hours after the administration of a single oral dose of 20 mg vardenafil to healthy male volunteers are shown in Figure 1.

Figure 1: LEVITRA

Mean Plasma Concentration Curve for 20 mg Vardenafil after Oral Administration

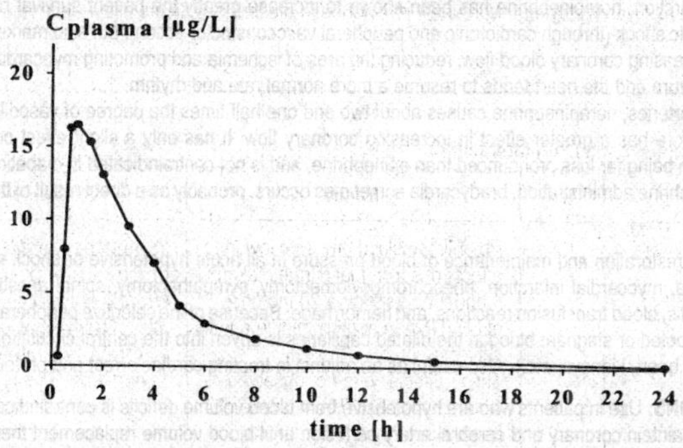

Absorption: Vardenafil is rapidly absorbed, with maximum observed plasma concentrations detected as early as 15 minutes post administration. In the fasted state, maximum plasma concentrations are achieved between 30 to 120 minutes (median 60 minutes) 90% of the time after oral dosing of vardenafil.

When LEVITRA is taken with a typical meal comprised of 30% fat, the rate and extent of absorption of vardenafil are unchanged compared to administration under fasting conditions. Consumption of a high-fat meal caused a reduction in C_{max} of 18-50% without change in AUC (Area Under the Curve); t_{max} was delayed by one hour.

Absorption levels are unchanged with a moderate amount of alcohol.

Distribution: The mean steady-state volume of distribution (V_{ss}) for vardenafil is 208 L, indicating extensive tissue distribution. Vardenafil and its major metabolite, M-1, are highly bound to plasma proteins (about 95% for parent drug and M-1). This protein binding is reversible and independent of total drug concentrations.

Ninety minutes after administration of a single dose of 20 mg LEVITRA, less than 0.0002% of the administered dose is detected in the semen. The concentrations of vardenafil and its primary metabolite in the ejaculate 1.5 hours post dose were 49% and 71%, respectively, of the concentrations in plasma at the same time point.

Metabolism: Vardenafil is eliminated predominantly by hepatic metabolism via cytochrome P450 (CYP) 3A4, with some contribution from the CYP3A5 and CYP2C isoforms. The major circulating metabolite, M-1, results from desethylation at the piperazine moiety of vardenafil. M-1 is subject to further metabolism. The plasma concentration of M-1 is approximately 26% of the parent compound. This metabolite shows a phosphodiesterase selectivity profile similar to that of vardenafil and an in vitro inhibitory potency for PDE5 of 28% compared to vardenafil. Therefore, M-1 accounts for approximately 7% of the total pharmacologic activity.

Excretion: The total body clearance of vardenafil is 56 L/h and the terminal half-life is approximately 4-5 hours. After oral administration, vardenafil is excreted as metabolites predominantly in the feces (approximately 91-95% of administered oral dose) and to a lesser extent in the urine (approximately 2-6% of administered oral dose).

Special Populations and Conditions: Pediatrics (<18 years of age): Vardenafil has not been evaluated in individuals less than 18 years old.

Geriatrics (≥65 years of age): A starting dose of 5 mg LEVITRA should be considered in patients 65 years and older. On average, elderly males (65 years and over) had a 52% higher vardenafil AUC and a 34% higher maximum concentration (C_{max}) than younger males (18-45 years); however, this difference was not statistically significant. (See Warnings and Precautions and Dosage and Administration.)

Hepatic Insufficiency: No dose adjustment is required in patients with mild hepatic impairment. In patients with mild hepatic impairment (Child-Pugh A), the vardenafil AUC was increased 17% and the C_{max} was increased 22%, compared to healthy male volunteers, following a 10 mg vardenafil dose. In patients with moderate impairment (Child-Pugh B), the vardenafil AUC was increased 160% and C_{max} was increased 133%, compared to healthy male volunteers, following a 10 mg vardenafil dose.

In patients with moderate hepatic impairment, a 5 mg starting dose of LEVITRA is recommended, which may subsequently be increased to a maximum dose of 10 mg, based on tolerability and efficacy. (See Warnings and Precautions and Dosage and Administration.) Vardenafil has not been evaluated in patients with severe hepatic impairment (Child-Pugh C).

Renal Insufficiency: No dose adjustment is required in patients with renal impairment. In patients with mild (creatine clearance (Cl_{cr} ≥50-80 mL/min), moderate (Cl_{cr} >30-50 mL/min), or severe (Cl_{cr} ≤30 mL/min) renal impairment, the pharmacokinetics of vardenafil were similar to that of a control group with normal renal function. Vardenafil pharmacokinetics have not been evaluated in patients requiring dialysis.

STORAGE AND STABILITY: Store between 15-30°C. Do not freeze.

INFORMATION FOR THE PATIENT: Published in e-CPS, available by subscription at www.e-cps.ca.

DOSAGE FORMS, COMPOSITION AND PACKAGING: 5 mg: Each orange, film coated, round tablet with embossed "BAYER" cross on one side and "5" on the other side, contains: vardenafil hydrochloride equivalent to 5 mg of vardenafil. Nonmedicinal ingredients: anhydrous colloidal silica, crospovidone, hydroxypropyl methylcellulose, magnesium stearate, microcrystalline cellulose, polyethylene glycol, red ferric oxide, titanium dioxide and yellow ferric oxide. Blister packages of 4.

10 mg: Each orange, film coated, round tablet with embossed "BAYER" cross on one side and "10" on the other side, contains: vardenafil hydrochloride equivalent to 10 mg of vardenafil. Nonmedicinal ingredients: anhydrous colloidal silica, crospovidone, hydroxypropyl methylcellulose, magnesium stearate, microcrystalline cellulose, polyethylene glycol, red ferric oxide, titanium dioxide and yellow ferric oxide. Blister packages of 4.

20 mg: Each orange, film coated, round tablet with embossed "BAYER" cross on one side and "20" on the other side, contains: vardenafil hydrochloride equivalent to 20 mg of vardenafil. Nonmedicinal ingredients: anhydrous colloidal silica, crospovidone, hydroxypropyl methylcellulose, magnesium stearate, microcrystalline cellulose, polyethylene glycol, red ferric oxide, titanium dioxide and yellow ferric oxide. Blister packages of 4.

(Shown in Product Identification Section)

Levofloxacin

CPhA Monograph

see *Fluoroquinolones*

Levophed®

norepinephrine bitartrate

Sympathomimetic

Hospira

PHARMACOLOGY: Norepinephrine functions as a powerful peripheral vasoconstrictor (alpha-adrenergic action) and as a potent inotropic stimulator of the heart and dilator of coronary arteries (beta-adrenergic action). Both of these actions result in an increase in systemic blood pressure and coronary artery blood flow. Cardiac output will vary reflexly in response to systemic hypertension but is usually increased in hypotensive man when the blood pressure is raised to an optimal level. In myocardial infarction accompanied by hypotension, norepinephrine usually increases aortic blood pressure, coronary artery blood flow, and myocardial oxygenation, thereby helping to limit the area of myocardial ischemia and infarction. Venous return is increased and the heart tends to resume a more normal rate and rhythm than in the hypotensive state.

In hypotension that persists after correction of blood volume deficits, norepinephrine helps raise the blood pressure to an optimal level and establish a more adequate circulation.

In myocardial infarction, norepinephrine has been shown to increase greatly the patient survival rate. Norepinephrine not only corrects systemic shock (through cardiotonic and peripheral vasoconstrictor action), but also markedly dilates the coronary arteries, thereby increasing coronary blood flow, reducing the area of ischemia and promoting myocardial oxygenation. There is increased venous return and the heart tends to resume a more normal rate and rhythm.

On the coronary arteries, norepinephrine causes about two and one half times the degree of vasodilatation that epinephrine produces and therefore has a greater effect in increasing coronary flow. It has only a slight effect on sugar metabolism, its hyperglycemic action being far less pronounced than epinephrine, and is not contraindicated in diabetic patients.

Note: With norepinephrine administration, bradycardia sometimes occurs, probably as a direct result of the rise in blood pressure to normal levels.

INDICATIONS: The restoration and maintenance of blood pressure in all acute hypotensive or shock states, which may result from surgery, trauma, myocardial infarction, pheochromocytomectomy, sympathectomy, spinal anesthesia, septicemia, drug reactions, poliomyelitis, blood transfusion reactions, and hemorrhage. Because of the selective peripheral vasoconstrictive action of norepinephrine, pooled or stagnant blood in the dilated capillaries is driven into the central circulation, thus maintaining vital functions (e.g. brain, heart, kidneys, etc.). Also useful as an adjunct in treating cardiac arrest and profound hypotension.

CONTRAINDICATIONS: Use in patients who are hypotensive from blood volume deficits is contraindicated except as an emergency measure to maintain coronary and cerebral artery perfusion until blood volume replacement therapy can be completed. If norepinephrine is continuously administered to maintain blood pressure in the absence of blood volume replacement, the following may occur: severe peripheral and visceral vasoconstriction, decreased renal perfusion and urine output, poor systemic blood flow despite "normal" blood pressure, tissue hypoxia, and lactate acidosis.

Norepinephrine should also not be given to patients with mesenteric or peripheral vascular thrombosis (because of the risk of increasing ischemia and extending the area of infarction) unless, in the opinion of the attending physician, the administration of norepinephrine is necessary as a life-saving procedure.

Cyclopropane and halothane anesthetics increase cardiac autonomic irritability and therefore seem to sensitize the myocardium to the action of i.v. administered epinephrine or levarterenol. Hence, the use of norepinephrine during cyclopropane and halothane anesthesia is generally considered contraindicated because of the risk of producing ventricular tachycardia or fibrillation. The same type of cardiac arrhythmias may result from the use of norepinephrine in patients with profound hypoxia or hypercarbia.

WARNINGS: Norepinephrine should be used with extreme caution in patients receiving MAO inhibitors or antidepressants of the triptyline or imipramine types, because severe, prolonged hypertension may result.

Norepinephrine contains sodium metabisulfite, a sulfite that may cause allergic-type reactions including anaphylactic symptoms and life-threatening or less severe asthmatic episodes in certain susceptible people. The overall prevalence of sulfite sensitivity in the general population is unknown. Sulfite sensitivity is seen more frequently in asthmatic than in nonasthmatic people.

PRECAUTIONS: Avoid Hypertension: Because of the potency of norepinephrine and because of varying response to pressor substances, the possibility always exists that dangerously high blood pressure may be produced with overdoses of this pressor agent. It is desirable, therefore, to record the blood pressure every 2 minutes from the time administration is started until the desired blood pressure is obtained, then every 5 minutes if administration is to be continued. The rate of flow must be watched constantly, and the patient should never be left unattended while receiving norepinephrine. Headache may be a symptom of hypertension due to overdosage.

Site of infusion: Whenever possible, norepinephrine should be given into a large vein, particularly an antecubital vein because, when administered into this vein, the risk of necrosis of the overlying skin from prolonged vasoconstriction is apparently very slight. Some authors have indicated that the femoral vein is also an acceptable route of administration. A catheter tie-in technique should be avoided, if possible, since the obstruction to blood flow around the tubing may cause stasis and increased local concentration of the drug. Occlusive vascular diseases (for example, atherosclerosis, arteriosclerosis, diabetic endarteritis, Buerger's disease) are more likely to occur in the lower than in the upper extremity. Therefore, one should avoid the veins of the leg or dorsum of the hand in elderly patients, or in those suffering from such disorders. Gangrene has been reported in a lower extremity when norepinephrine was given in an ankle vein.

Extravasation: **The infusion site should be checked frequently for free flow.** Care should be taken to avoid extravasation of norepinephrine into the tissues, as local necrosis might ensue due to the vasoconstrictive action of the drug. **Blanching along the course of the infused vein,** sometimes without obvious extravasation, has been attributed to vasa vasorum constriction with increased permeability of the vein wall, permitting some leakage. This also may progress on rare occasions to superficial slough, particularly during infusion into leg veins, in elderly patients or in those suffering from obliterative vascular disease. Hence, if blanching occurs, consideration should be given to the advisability of changing the infusion site at intervals to allow the effects of local vasoconstriction to subside.

Important: Antidote for Extravasation Ischemia: To prevent sloughing and necrosis in areas in which extravasation has taken place, the area should be infiltrated as soon as possible with 10 to 15 mL of saline solution containing from 5 to 10 mg of phentolamine, an adrenergic blocking agent. A syringe with a fine hypodermic needle is used, and the solution is infiltrated liberally throughout the area, which is easily identified by its cold, hard, and pallid appearance. Sympathetic blockage with phentolamine causes immediate and conspicuous local hyperemic changes if the area is infiltrated within 12 hours. Therefore, **phentolamine should be given as soon as possible after the extravasation is noted.**

Some investigators add phentolamine (5 to 10 mg) directly to the infusion flask because it is believed that the drug used in this manner is an effective antidote against sloughing should extravasation occur, whereas the systemic vasopressor activity of the norepinephrine is not impaired.

Two investigators stated that, in the treatment of patients with severe hypotension following **myocardial infarction**, thrombosis in the infused vein and perivenous reactions and necrosis may usually be prevented if 10 mg of heparin are added to each 500 mL of infusion fluid (5% dextrose) containing norepinephrine.

Sympathetic nerve block has also been suggested.

Pregnancy: It is not known whether norepinephrine can cause fetal harm when administered to a pregnant woman or can affect reproduction capacity. It should be given to a pregnant woman only if clearly needed.

Lactation: It is not known whether this drug is excreted in human milk. Because many drugs are excreted in human milk, caution should be exercised when norepinephrine is administered to a nursing woman.

ADVERSE EFFECTS: Body as a Whole: ischemic injury due to potent vasoconstrictor action and tissue hypoxia.

Cardiovascular: bradycardia, probably as a reflex result of a rise in blood pressure, arrhythmias.

Nervous System: anxiety, transient headache.

Respiratory: respiratory difficulty.

Skin and Appendages: extravasation necrosis at injection site.

Prolonged administration of any potent vasopressor may result in plasma volume depletion which should be continuously corrected by appropriate fluid and electrolyte replacement therapy. If plasma volumes are not corrected, hypotension may recur when norepinephrine is discontinued, or blood pressure may be maintained at the risk of severe peripheral and visceral vasoconstriction (e.g., decreased renal perfusion) with diminution in blood flow and tissue perfusion with subsequent tissue hypoxia and lactic acidosis and possible ischemic injury. Gangrene of extremities has been rarely reported.

Overdoses or conventional doses in hypersensitive persons (e.g., hyperthyroid patients) cause severe hypertension with violent headache, photophobia, stabbing retrosternal pain, pallor, intense sweating, and vomiting.

OVERDOSE:

Symptoms: Overdosage with norepinephrine may result in headache, severe hypertension, reflex bradycardia, marked increase in peripheral resistance and decreased cardiac output.

Treatment: In case of accidental overdosage, as evidenced by excessive blood pressure elevation, discontinue the drug until the condition of the patient stabilizes.

> For management of a suspected drug overdose, CPhA recommends that you contact your **regional Poison Control Centre**. See the *CPS* Directory section for a list of Poison Control Centres.

DOSAGE: Restoration of Blood Pressure in Acute Hypotensive States: Blood volume depletion should always be corrected as fully as possible before any vasopressor is administered. When, as an emergency measure, intraaortic pressures must be maintained to prevent cerebral or coronary artery ischemia, norepinephrine can be administered before and concurrently with blood volume replacement.

Diluent: Levophed solution should be administered in 5% Dextrose Solution in Distilled Water or 5% Dextrose in Saline Solution. These fluids containing dextrose are protection against significant loss of potency due to oxidation. Administration in saline solution alone is not recommended. Whole blood or plasma, if indicated to increase blood volume, should be administered separately (for example by use of a Y-tube and individual flasks if given simultaneously).

Average Dosage: Add 4 mL of Levophed solution to 1 000 mL of 5% dextrose solution. Each 1 mL of this dilution contains 4 µg of Levophed base. Give this dilution i.v. Insert a plastic i.v. catheter through a suitable bore needle well advanced centrally into the vein and securely fixed with adhesive tape, avoiding if possible, a catheter tie-in technique as this promotes stasis. A drip bulb is necessary to permit an accurate estimation of the rate of flow in drops per minute. After observing the response to an initial dose of 2 to 3 mL (from 8 to 12 µg of base)/minute, adjust the rate of flow to establish and maintain a low normal blood pressure (usually 80 to 100 mm Hg systolic) sufficient to maintain the circulation to vital organs. In previously hypertensive patients, it is recommended that the blood pressure should be raised no higher than 40 mm Hg below the preexisting systolic pressure. The average maintenance dose ranges from 0.5 to 1 mL/minute (from 2 to 4 µg of base).

High Dosage: Great individual variation occurs in the dose required to attain and maintain an adequate blood pressure. In all cases, dosage of norepinephrine should be titrated according to the response of the patient. Occasionally much larger or even enormous daily doses (as high as 68 mg base or 17 ampuls) may be necessary if the patient remains hypotensive, but occult blood volume depletion should always be suspected and corrected when present. Central venous pressure monitoring is usually helpful in detecting and treating this situation.

Fluid Intake: The degree of dilution depends on clinical fluid volume requirements. If large volumes of fluid (dextrose) are needed at a flow rate that would involve an excessive dose of the pressor agent per unit of time, a more dilute solution than 4 µg/mL should be used. On the other hand, when large volumes of fluid are clinically undesirable, a concentration greater than 4 µg/mL may be used.

Duration of Therapy: The infusion should be continued until adequate blood pressure and tissue perfusion are maintained without therapy. Norepinephrine infusion should be reduced gradually, avoiding abrupt withdrawal. In some of the reported cases of vascular collapse due to acute myocardial infarction, treatment was required for up to 6 days.

Adjunctive Treatment in Cardiac Arrest: Norepinephrine is usually administered i.v. during cardiac resuscitation to restore and maintain an adequate blood pressure after an effective heartbeat and ventilation have been established by other means. (Norepinephrine's powerful beta-adrenergic stimulating action is also thought to increase the strength and effectiveness of systolic contractions once they occur.)
Average Dosage: To maintain systemic blood pressure during the management of cardiac arrest, norepinephrine is used in the same manner as described under Restoration of Blood Pressure in Acute Hypotensive States.

SUPPLIED: Each mL of solution contains: norepinephrine bitartrate equivalent to 1 mg (base). Also contains sodium metabisulfite, sodium chloride, and water for injection. Ampuls of 4 mL, boxes of 10. Caution: Destroy when expired and do not use if the solution is pinkish or darker than slightly yellow or contains a precipitate. Protect from light. Store ampuls inside carton.

Librax® T/C

chlordiazepoxide HCl—clidinium bromide

Anxiolytic—Anticholinergic

Valeant

PHARMACOLOGY: Chlordiazepoxide: Benzodiazepines, such as chlordiazepoxide, act as depressants of the CNS, producing all levels of CNS depression from mild sedation to hypnosis to coma depending on the dose taken.
Clidinium: Anticholinergics, such as clidinium, inhibit the muscarinic actions of acetylcholine on structures innervated by postganglionic cholinergic nerves as well as on smooth muscles that respond to acetylcholine but lack cholinergic innervation. These postganglionic receptor sites are present in the autonomic effector cells of the smooth muscle, cardiac muscle, sinoatrial and atrioventricular nodes, and exocrine glands. Depending on the dose, anticholinergics may reduce the motility and secretory activity of the gastrointestinal system.
Pharmacokinetics: Absorption: Chlordiazepoxide is well absorbed from the gastrointestinal tract within 1 to 2 hours.
Clidinium is poorly and very irregularly absorbed from the gastrointestinal tract.
Protein Binding: Chlordiazepoxide is highly protein bound (96 %).
Biotransformation: Chlordiazepoxide and clidinium are both metabolized in the liver.
Half-life: The biological half-life for chlordiazepoxide is between 5 and 30 hours.
Onset of Action: The action of clidinium starts at about 1 hour after ingestion and lasts for approximately 3 hours.
Elimination: Chlordiazepoxide is eliminated by the kidneys and clidinium by the kidneys and in the feces.

INDICATIONS: As adjunctive therapy in the treatment of peptic ulcer and in the treatment of the irritable bowel syndrome (irritable colon, spastic colon, mucous colitis) and acute enterocolitis, when these are associated with excessive anxiety and tension.

CONTRAINDICATIONS: Cardiovascular instability; history of drug abuse or dependence (chlordiazepoxide may predispose to habituation and dependence); angle-closure, or predisposition to glaucoma (clidinium has a possible mydriatic effect resulting in increased intraocular pressure and may precipitate an acute attack of angle-closure glaucoma); impaired hepatic function (because of decreased metabolism); hiatal hernia with reflux esophagitis (clidinium may aggravate condition); intestinal atony of the elderly or debilitated (may result in obstruction due to clidinium's anticholinergic/antispasmodic effect); intestinal obstruction (may be exacerbated by clidinium); myasthenia gravis (clidinium may aggravate condition because of inhibition of acetylcholine action); prostatic hypertrophy or urinary retention (anticholinergic effects may precipitate or aggravate urinary retention); ulcerative colitis (clidinium may suppress intestinal motility and cause paralytic ileus; also, use may precipitate or aggravate the serious complications of toxic megacolon); sensitivity to chlordiazepoxide and/or clidinium.

WARNINGS: When clidinium is given to patients where the environmental temperature is high, there is risk of a rapid increase in body temperature because of suppression of sweat gland activity.
Risk-benefit should be considered when the following medical problems exist: open-angle glaucoma (clidinium's possible mydriatic effect may cause a slight increase in intraocular pressure; glaucoma therapy may need to be adjusted).
Hypertension (may be aggravated by clidinium).
Hyperthyroidism (characterized by tachycardia, which may be increased by clidinium).
Mental depression (chlordiazepoxide may increase depression).
Psychoses (paradoxical reactions may occur due to chlordiazepoxide).
Severe, chronic obstructive pulmonary disease (anticholinergic effects may cause thickening of secretions and impair expectorations; ventilatory failure may be exacerbated with the use of chlordiazepoxide).
Renal function impairment (decreased excretion may increase risk of side effects).
Xerostomia (prolonged use of clidinium may further reduce limited salivary flow).

PRECAUTIONS: Caution is recommended in debilitated patients since they may show an increased susceptibility to this medication.
Patients who are sensitive to other benzodiazepines or any of the belladonna alkaloids may be sensitive to Librax as well.
Pregnancy: Pregnancy/Reproduction: The use of Librax (anticholinergic and sedative combination) in pregnancy is generally not recommended.
Chlordiazepoxide: Chlordiazepoxide crosses the placenta. It has been reported to increase the risk of congenital malformations when used during the first trimester of pregnancy. Chronic use of chlordiazepoxide during pregnancy may cause physical dependence with resulting withdrawal symptoms in the neonate. Use of chlordiazepoxide just prior to or during labor may cause neonatal flaccidity.
Clidinium: Appropriate studies in humans have not been performed. However, reproduction studies in rats have not shown that clidinium has adverse effects on the fetus.
Lactation: Chlordiazepoxide or its metabolites may be excreted in breast milk; use by nursing mothers may cause sedation in the infant. Clidinium may tend to inhibit lactation.
Children: No information is available on the relationship of age to the effect of chlordiazepoxide and clidinium in pediatric patients. However, it is known that infants and young children are especially susceptible to the toxic effects of atropine-like drugs, such as clidinium, and to the CNS effects of benzodiazepines, such as chlordiazepoxide.
Geriatrics: Geriatric patients may respond to usual doses of chlordiazepoxide and clidinium with excitement, agitation, drowsiness, or confusion.
Geriatric patients are especially susceptible to the anticholinergic side effects, such as constipation, dryness of mouth, and urinary retention (especially in males), of clidinium. If these side effects occur and continue or are severe, medication should be discontinued.
Caution is also recommended when clidinium is given to geriatric patients, because of the danger of precipitating undiagnosed glaucoma.
Memory may become severely impaired in geriatric patients, especially those who already have memory problems, with the continued use of clidinium since this medication blocks the action of acetylcholine, which is responsible for many functions of the brain, including memory function.
Dental: Prolonged use of clidinium may decrease or inhibit salivary flow, thus contributing to the development of caries, periodontal disease, oral candidiasis, and discomfort.

ADVERSE EFFECTS: The following adverse reactions have been reported with the use of Librax:
Hematopoietic: agranulocytosis; granulocytopenia; leukopenia.
CNS: depression (slow heartbeat, shortness of breath, or troubled breathing).
Gastrointestinal: decreased peristalsis—possible paralytic ileus (constipation).
Others: skin rash or hives; increased intraocular pressure (eye pain); jaundice; paradoxical reaction (trouble in sleeping; unusual excitement; nervousness, or irritability); bloated feeling; decreased sweating; dizziness; drowsiness; dryness of mouth; headache; blurred vision; decreased sexual ability; nausea; unusual tiredness or weakness; muscle cramps; stomach cramps; trembling; seizures.

OVERDOSE:

Symptoms: confusion; difficulty in urination; severe drowsiness; severe dryness of mouth, nose, or throat; fast heartbeat; unusual warmth, dryness, and flushing of the skin.

Treatment: The recommended treatment of overdosage includes: emesis or gastric lavage with 4% tannic acid solution; s.c. administration of 5 mg of pilocarpine, repeated as needed, until mouth is moist; norepinephrine bitartrate or metaraminol infusions, to restore blood pressure; caffeine and sodium benzoate, to treat CNS depression; if excitation occurs, barbiturates should not be used since they may exacerbate excitation and/or prolong CNS depression; artificial respiration, if needed, for respiratory depression; symptomatic treatment as necessary.

For management of a suspected drug overdose, CPhA recommends that you contact your **regional Poison Control Centre**. See the *CPS* Directory section for a list of Poison Control Centres.

DOSAGE: General Dosing Information: Dosage should be adjusted to meet the individual requirements of each patient since response varies according to the severity of the condition.
Geriatric and debilitated patients may respond to the usual doses with excitement, agitation, drowsiness, or confusion; lower doses may be required for such patients.
Administration of Librax 30 to 60 minutes before meals is recommended to maximize absorption and, when used for reducing stomach acid formation, to allow its effect to coincide better with any antacid administration following the meal.
Prolonged use of larger than usual therapeutic doses of chlordiazepoxide may result in psychic or physical dependence.
Following prolonged administration, chlordiazepoxide should be withdrawn gradually in order to avoid the possibility of precipitating withdrawal symptoms.
Adults: Usual Oral Dose: 1 or 2 capsules 1 to 4 times a day, 30 to 60 minutes before meals or food, the dosage then being adjusted as needed and tolerated.
Usual Prescribing Limits: up to a total of 8 capsules daily (40 mg of chlordiazepoxide HCl and 20 mg of clidinium bromide).
Children: Usual Oral Dose: Dosage has not been established.
Geriatrics: Usual Oral Dose: Initially no more than 1 capsule 2 times a day, the dosage then being adjusted as needed and tolerated.

SUPPLIED: Each No. 4 hard gelatin capsule with green, opaque cap and body, imprinted LIBRAX (black ink) on the body and cap, contains: chlordiazepoxide HCl, USP 5 mg and clidinium bromide, USP 2.5 mg. Nonmedicinal ingredients: cornstarch, D&C yellow No. 10, FD&C green No. 3, gelatin, lactose (104 mg), talc and titanium dioxide. Energy: 2.1 kJ (0.5 kcal). Gluten-, paraben-, sodium-, sulfite- and tartrazine-free. Bottles of 100 and 500. Store in a well-closed container at controlled room temperature (15 to 30°C).

Lidocaine HCl 0.2%, 0.4% and 0.8% in 5% Dextrose for I.V. Infusion

lidocaine HCl—dextrose

Antiarrhythmic

Baxter

SUPPLIED: Each mL of i.v. infusion contains: lidocaine HCl 0.2%, 0.4%, or 0.8% in 5% dextrose. Viaflex Plus plastic (polyvinyl chloride) containers in the following sizes and concentrations: see Table 1.

Table 1: Lidocaine HCl 0.2%, 0.4% and 0.8% in 5% Dextrose for I.V. Infusion Supplied

Total Volume (mL)	Total Lidocaine HCl Content (mg)	Lidocaine HCl Concentration (mg/mL)
250	1000	4
500	2000	4
250	2000	8

Do not store above 30°C. Protect from freezing.

Lidocaine Parenteral (Antiarrhythmic Agent)

lidocaine HCl

Antiarrhythmic

Hospira

SUPPLIED: Continuous I.V. Infusion: Each mL contains: lidocaine HCl 0.4% in Dextrose 5% for i.v. infusion (lidocaine 0.4% D5W). Nonmedicinal ingredients: hydrochloric acid, sodium hydroxide and water for injection. Plastic bags of 250 and 500 mL.
Single I.V. Injection: Each 5 mL ABBOJECT Disposable Syringe and 25 G, ⅝" or 21 G, 1½" needle contains: lidocaine HCl 2%. Nonmedicinal ingredients: hydrochloric acid, sodium chloride, sodium hydroxide and water for injection. Boxes of 10.
Medication, fluid path and needle are sterile and nonpyrogenic if caps and needle-guard are in place and the package has not been damaged or opened.

Lidodan™ Endotracheal

lidocaine HCl

Topical Anesthetic

Odan

Lidodan™ Ointment

lidocaine

Topical Anesthetic

Odan

Lidodan™ Viscous

lidocaine HCl

Topical Anesthetic

Odan

SUPPLIED: Endotracheal: Each metered dose contains: lidocaine HCl 12 mg (equivalent to 10 mg lidocaine base). Nonmedicinal ingredients: sodium hydroxide and/or hydrochloric acid to adjust pH 5.0 to 7.0 and purified water. Non aerosol spray bottles of 30 mL with a metered dose valve. Single pak: 1 bottle with 1×20 cm stainless steel nozzle. Two pak: 2×30 mL bottles with 2×12 cm disposable plastic nozzles. Three pak: 3×30 mL non aerosol spray bottles.
Banana Flavor: Each metered dose contains: lidocaine HCl 12 mg (equivalent to 10 mg lidocaine base). Nonmedicinal ingredients: banana flavor, sodium hydroxide and/or hydrochloric acid to adjust pH 5.0 to 7.0 and purified water. Non aerosol spray bottles of 60 mL with a metered dose valve. Single pak: 1 bottle with 1×10 cm disposable plastic nozzle.
Stainless Steel Nozzle Pak: 2×20 cm nozzles.
Disposable Plastic Nozzle Pak: 24×12 cm, 50×12 cm, 96×12 cm, 24×20 cm and 96×20 cm nozzles.
Clean stainless steel nozzles may be steam sterilized at 121°C for 15 minutes.
Store between 15 to 30°C. Protect from freezing.
Ointment: Each g contains: lidocaine USP 50 mg (5%) in a water miscible ointment base. Nonmedicinal ingredients: polyethylene glycols and propylene glycol. Tubes of 15 and 30 g. Store between 15 to 30°C.

Viscous: Each mL contains: lidocaine HCl USP 20 mg (2%). Nonmedicinal ingredients: amaranth red #2, cellulose gum, cherry flavor, methylparaben, propylparaben, purified water and sodium cyclamate. Gluten- and tartrazine-free. Unbreakable natural polyethylene bottles of 50 and 100 mL with child-resistant closures. Store between 15 to 30°C.

Limonade Asepta
sodium tartrate
Laxative

Rougier Pharma

SUPPLIED: Each mL of clear, colorless oral solution, with odor of lemon-lime contains: sodium tartrate 56.10 mg (16.84 g per bottle). Nonmedicinal ingredients: artificial and natural flavoring, citric acid, purified water and sodium benzoate. Bottles of 300 mL. Persons on low sodium diets should avoid use of this product. Keep out of reach of children.

Lincocin® Ⓟ
lincomycin HCl monohydrate
Antibiotic

Pfizer

Date of Preparation: September 17, 2003
Date of Revision: April 8, 2008

PHARMACOLOGY: The mode of action of lincomycin is the inhibition of protein synthesis by the inhibition of the binding of aminoacyl sRNA to the messenger ribosome complex at the 50S ribosomal unit.

INDICATIONS: LINCOCIN (lincomycin hydrochloride) is indicated in the treatment of serious infections due to sensitive gram positive organisms (staphylococci, including penicillinase-producing staphylococci, streptococci and pneumococci) when the patient is intolerant of, or the organism resistant to other appropriate antibiotics.

LINCOCIN is indicated in the treatment of osteomyelitis, when the causative organism has been found to be sensitive to this antibiotic.

CONTRAINDICATIONS: As with all drugs, the use of LINCOCIN (lincomycin hydrochloride) is contraindicated in patients previously found to be hypersensitive to the drug or patients who have previously been found hypersensitive to clindamycin (Dalacin C) or to any other component of the product.

LINCOCIN should not be given to persons with known pre-existing monilial infections.

Until further clinical experience is obtained, LINCOCIN is not indicated in the newborn.

WARNINGS: *Clostridium difficile*-associated disease (CDAD) has been reported with use of many antibacterial agents, including LINCOCIN (lincomycin hydrochloride). CDAD may range in severity from mild diarrhoea to fatal colitis. It is important to consider this diagnosis in patients who present with diarrhoea, or symptoms of colitis, pseudomembranous colitis, toxic megacolon, or perforation of colon subsequent to the administration of any antibacterial agent. CDAD has been reported to occur over 2 months after the administration of antibacterial agents.

Treatment with antibacterial agents may alter the normal flora of the colon and may permit overgrowth of *C. difficile*. *C. difficile* produces toxins A and B, which contribute to the development of CDAD. CDAD may cause significant morbidity and mortality. CDAD can be refractory to antimicrobial therapy.

If the diagnosis of CDAD is suspected or confirmed, appropriate therapeutic measures should be initiated. Mild cases of CDAD usually respond to discontinuation of antibacterial agents not directed against *C. difficile*. In moderate to severe cases, consideration should be given to management with fluids and electrolytes, protein supplementation, and treatment with an antibacterial agent clinically effective against *C. difficile*. Surgical evaluation should be instituted as clinically indicated, as surgical intervention may be required in certain severe cases (see Adverse Effects).

LINCOCIN should not be administered undiluted intravenously. All intravenous doses of LINCOCIN should be given by infusion over a period of 30 to 120 minutes. Cases of cardiopulmonary arrest have been reported during the treatment of severe endocarditis when large intravenous doses (over 4 grams) were given rapidly without dilution. These reactions do not occur when the drug is diluted as noted under Dosage.

This product contains benzyl alcohol. Benzyl alcohol has been reported to be associated with a fatal "Gasping Syndrome" in premature infants.

PRECAUTIONS: General: LINCOCIN (lincomycin HCl) should be used with caution in those patients with a history of gastro-intestinal disease, specifically colitis.

LINCOCIN is not indicated for use in the treatment of meningitis as the levels within the cerebral spinal fluid do not reach an adequate concentration to combat this infection.

No serious renal or neurologic abnormalities have been reported to date. No ototoxicity has been demonstrated in any of a large number of patients treated with LINCOCIN.

Pregnancy: No adverse effects on survival of offspring from birth to weaning were seen in studies performed in rates using oral doses of lincomycin up to 1000 mg/kg (7.5 times the maximum human dose of 8 g/day). No teratogenic effects were seen in a study conducted in rats treated with more than 55 times the highest recommended adult human dose of 8 g/day.

In humans, lincomycin crosses the placenta and results in cord serum levels about 25% of the maternal serum levels. No significant accumulation occurs in the amniotic fluid.

Limited experience with 322 women receiving LINCOCIN orally at a dosage of 500 mg four times per day for seven days during pregnancy revealed no ill effect in the mother or the fetus. One hundred and ten of these patients were treated in the first trimester of pregnancy, 105 in the second trimester and 107 in the third trimester. All were suffering from cervicitis and/or vaginitis of bacterial origin in conjunction with their pregnancy.

One hundred and twelve of the children, ages 6½ to 7½ years, from these patients have been examined and compared with a control group of 65 children born at the same time in the same hospital. LINCOCIN treatment did not result in any drug related abnormalities (physical, dental or developmental) when compared with the control group.

Lactation: LINCOCIN has been reported in breast milk at concentrations of 0.5-2.4 µg/mL. However, the use of lincomycin in pregnant and/or breast-feeding women should involve careful consideration of expected benefits and possible risks.

Patients with Special Diseases and Conditions: The serum half-life of LINCOCIN is increased in those patients with impaired renal or hepatic function. Therefore, consideration should be given to reducing the frequency of administration in these patients.

Since adequate data are not yet available in patients with pre-existing endocrine or metabolic diseases, its use in such patients is not recommended at this time unless special clinical circumstances so indicate. Efficacy of LINCOCIN in the prophylactic treatment of rheumatic fever has not been established.

Drug Interactions: In vitro studies have shown antagonistic activity between LINCOCIN and erythromycin; therefore, these agents should not be used concurrently.

Because LINCOCIN has been shown to have neuromuscular blocking properties which may enhance the action of other neuromuscular blocking agents, it should be used with caution in patients receiving such agents.

Laboratory Tests: The use of antibiotics occasionally results in overgrowth of non-susceptible organisms—particularly yeasts. Should superinfections occur, appropriate measures should be taken. No direct relationship of the drug to liver disease has been established. However, it is recommended that all patients receiving treatment for longer than 1 or 2 weeks have liver and kidney function tests performed. If abnormal tests appear, the drug should be discontinued unless, in the opinion of the physician, the drug should be continued for the treatment of a serious infection.

During clinical studies of LINCOCIN in the therapy of infectious disease, a few cases of neutropenia and/or leukopenia were reported. No cases of irreversible toxicity to the hematopoietic system have been reported; however, it is recommended that blood counts be obtained early and repeated periodically during the course of LINCOCIN therapy.

ADVERSE EFFECTS: The following adverse reactions have been reported with the use of LINCOCIN (lincomycin hydrochloride):

Gastrointestinal: nausea, vomiting, esophagitis, colitis, persistent diarrhoea and abdominal distress. *C. difficile*-associated disease has been observed and the syndrome has manifested as a spectrum of symptoms from watery to severe diarrhoea, fever, abdominal cramps and leucocytosis. This may be accompanied by the passage of blood and mucous with resultant peritonitis, shock and toxic megacolon when the offending antibiotic is not discontinued and/or the condition treated) (see Warnings).

Hematopoietic: neutropenia, leukopenia, agranulocytosis, and thrombocytopenic purpura have been reported. There have been rare reports of aplastic anemia and pancytopenia in which lincomycin could not be ruled out as the causative agent.

Hypersensitivity Reactions: Hypersensitivity reactions such as angioneurotic edema, serum sickness and anaphylaxis have been reported, some of these in patients sensitive to penicillin. Rare instances of erythema multiforme, some resembling Stevens-Johnson syndrome, have been associated with LINCOCIN administration.

Skin and Mucous Membranes: Pruritus, skin rashes, urticaria, vaginitis, and rare instances of exfoliative and vesiculobullous dermatitis have been reported.

Liver: Jaundice and abnormal liver function tests (particularly elevation of serum transaminase) have been observed during lincomycin therapy.

Cardiovascular: Instances of hypotension following parenteral administration have been reported, particularly after too rapid administration.

Rare instances of cardiopulmonary arrest have been reported after too rapid i.v. administration (see Dosage).

Local Reactions: Local irritation, pain, induration, and sterile abscess formation have been seen with i.m. injection. Thrombophlebitis has been reported with i.v. injection. These reactions can be minimized by deep i.m. injection and avoidance of indwelling i.v. catheters.

OVERDOSE:

Symptoms: No cases of large overdosage have been reported. It would be expected however that should overdosage occur, gastrointestinal side effects, including abdominal pain, nausea, vomiting and diarrhea, might be seen.

Treatment: Overdosage should be treated with simple gastric lavage. No specific antidote is known.

Hemodialysis or peritoneal dialysis does not effectively remove lincomycin from the blood.

For management of a suspected drug overdose, contact your **regional Poison Control Centre**. See the *CPS* Directory section for a list of Poison Control Centres.

DOSAGE: See Table 1.

Table 1: LINCOCIN

Dosage

	I.M. (Sterile Solution)	I.V. (Sterile Solution)
Adults	600 mg (2 mL) every 24 h	600 mg (2 mL) every 8 to 12[b] hours. Administer as infusion in 250 mL or more of 5% glucose in water or normal saline over a period of 30 to 120 minutes.
Severe Infections	600 mg (2 mL) every 12 h	
Children[a]	10 mg/kg every 24 h	10 to 20 mg/kg/day in 2 or 3 doses at 8 to 12 hour intervals. Administer as infusion diluted as for adults.
Severe Infections	10 mg/kg every 12 h	

[a] Over 1 month of age.
[b] All doses may be increased in more severe infections. Doses as high as 8.4 g/day, for 7 days, in 4 divided doses of 2100 mg in an infusion of 250 mL, of normal saline, over a period of 120 minutes, were well tolerated in normal volunteers.

In β-hemolytic streptococcal infections, continue treatment for at least 10 days to diminish the likelihood of subsequent rheumatic fever or glomerulonephritis.

When therapy with lincomycin is required in individuals with severe impairment of renal function, an appropriate dose is 25% to 30% of that recommended for patients with normally functioning kidneys.

Reconstituted Solutions: LINCOCIN (600 mg/2 mL and 1800 mg/6 mL) was found to be compatible with 500 mL of the following solutions for a period of 24 hours at room temperature: 5% Dextrose in Water, 5% Dextrose in Saline, 10% Dextrose in Water, 10% Dextrose in Saline, Invert sugar 10%, Polysal M with 5% dextrose, Ringer's Solution, Sodium lactate 1/6 molar.

Compatibility was determined by a study which indicated no appreciable change in the pH of the resultant mixture and no loss of potency of the LINCOCIN when diluted as indicated above.

Incompatibilities: When combined with lincomycin in an infusion solution, novobiocin, kanamycin, and phenytoin are each physically incompatible with lincomycin. This list may not be all-inclusive due to the multiple factors influencing drug compatibility data.

SUPPLIED: Each mL of sterile solution contains: lincomycin HCl monohydrate equivalent to lincomycin base 300 mg. Also contains benzyl alcohol and Water for Injection q.s. Vials of 2 mL. Store at room temperature (15- 30°C), protect from light.

Lindane
Pediculicide—Scabicide

CPhA Monograph

Date of Preparation: October 2005
Date of Revision: May 2009

This monograph has been compiled by CPhA and reviewed by experts. It may contain information different from that found in Health Canada-approved Product Monographs. The reader is referred to the *CPS* Editorial Policy for more information.

SUMMARY PRODUCT INFORMATION:

Route of Administration	Dosage Form	Dosage Strength
Topical	Shampoo	1%
Topical	Lotion	1%

INDICATIONS AND CLINICAL USE: Lindane (also known as gamma benzene hexachloride) is indicated in the topical treatment of pediculosis capitis (head lice infestation) caused by *P. humanus* var *capitis* and pediculosis pubis (pubic lice infestation) caused by *P. pubis* in patients who have not responded to or who cannot tolerate other therapies (e.g., permethrin, pyrethrins). It is also used in the topical treatment of scabies caused by *S. scabiei* in patients who have not responded to or who cannot tolerate other therapies (e.g., permethrin 5% cream). Several jurisdictions have banned this agent because of concerns about neurotoxicity and adverse effects on the environment (contamination of waste water). Lindane remains on the Canadian market but is reserved as a second-line agent because of concerns about neurotoxicity and bone marrow suppression following percutaneous absorption. Lindane is not indicated for the treatment of Norwegian scabies (crusted scabies) since the skin breakdown present in this condition poses a risk of increased systemic absorption.

CONTRAINDICATIONS: Patients who are hypersensitive to lindane or to any ingredient in the various formulations.

Lindane is contraindicated in patients with a history of seizures as they may be at increased risk of neurotoxicity.

It is also contraindicated in patients with extensive dermatitis such as atopic dermatitis or psoriasis and in patients with skin rash, skin abrasion, inflammation, or Norwegian (crusted) scabies because of increased systemic absorption.

Using lindane in premature neonates is contraindicated because their skin may be more permeable than full-term neonates; increasing systemic absorption. Furthermore, their liver enzymes may not be sufficiently developed to be able to metabolize the medication.

WARNINGS AND PRECAUTIONS: General: Owing to concerns of bone marrow suppression and neurotoxicity, lindane is considered a second-line therapy only to be used in patients who have not responded to or who cannot tolerate other therapies. See Indications and Clinical Use. Lindane is not effective in preventing lice or scabies. It should be used only if there is a definitive diagnosis. Avoid contact with face, eyes, mucous membranes and urethral meatus. If contact with eyes occurs, flush thoroughly with water.

Hematologic: There has been at least one report of aplastic anemia with prolonged administration of lindane lotion.

Neurologic: Caution must be exercised when using lindane in: infants, children, the elderly, individuals who weigh less than 50 kg, patients with other skin conditions, and patients with a history of head trauma or prior seizure, as they may be at risk of serious neurotoxicity. Lindane should also be used with caution in individuals at risk of seizures such as those: with HIV infection, taking agents that lower the seizure threshold, undergoing abrupt discontinuation of alcohol or sedatives, with excessive alcohol consumption, with severe hepatic disease and with CNS tumors. See Adverse Reactions, Central Nervous System.

Dermatologic: Pruritus caused by sensitivity to the parasites and their products can persist for up to several weeks after successful treatment. In addition scalp itchiness has been reported following topical treatment for scabies and lice. Therefore pruritus may not indicate treatment failure and is not an indication for further treatment. If reinfestation and treatment failure have been ruled out, bothersome post-treatment itching can be relieved with oral antihistamines or topical steroids if needed.

Special Populations: Pregnant Women: There are no published reports of congenital or toxic effects due to lindane use during pregnancy, however, because of the potential toxicity associated with lindane, the Centers for Disease Control and Prevention (CDC) recommends safer alternatives in pregnancy such as permethrin for the treatment of scabies and permethrin or the combination of pyrethrin with piperonyl butoxide for the treatment of lice infestations. Lindane should be avoided when possible in pregnancy and it is advisable for this group of patients to avoid applying lindane on others.

Nursing Women: After topical application, lindane levels in human milk are increased (above the normal baseline level due to persistent environmental contamination) for at least several days. Thus, there may be a risk of toxicity if lindane is ingested via the breast milk by a nursing infant. Topical application of lindane to the chest area of a nursing mother may also result in absorption by the infant via skin to skin contact. Lindane should be avoided in favour of safer alternatives (e.g., permethrins, pyrethrin with piperonyl butoxide) whenever possible. Lindane appears to possess some estrogenic activity, which could suppress lactation.

Geriatrics: Safety and efficacy of lindane have not been specifically studied in geriatric patients. The elderly may be at an increased risk of neurotoxicity. There have been reports of 4 deaths in geriatric patients following application of lindane for the treatment of scabies.

Pediatrics: Since pediatric patients have higher surface area to volume ratio than adults, they may be at an increased risk of greater systemic absorption following topical application of lindane. Caution must be exercised when using lindane in infants, children, and individuals who weigh less than 50 kg as they may be at risk of serious neurotoxicity. Safer alternative therapies should be used whenever possible.

If lindane lotion is used in infants or young children for treatment of scabies, long sleeves, long pants, and gloves or mitts should be worn by the child to prevent accidental ingestion of the drug via thumbsucking or licking.

ADVERSE REACTIONS: Central Nervous System: Dizziness, seizures and death have been associated with lindane ingestion or with prolonged and repeated use of lindane shampoo or lotion. There are rare reports of seizures and death after a single application used according to manufacturer's instructions. CNS effects have been reported more frequently with lindane lotion than shampoo. Also see Warnings and Precautions, Neurologic.

Dermatologic: Alopecia, contact dermatitis, eczematous eruptions, pruritus, urticaria, burning and stinging have been reported following use of lindane shampoo or lotion. Also see Warnings and Precautions, Dermatologic for information on post-treatment itching.

Hematologic: There has been 1 report of severe aplastic anemia and elevated liver function tests in a patient after prolonged application of lindane lotion (twice daily for 3 weeks from neck to knees).

Endocrine and Metabolism: There is evidence to suggest that lindane may possess some estrogenic activity, which could suppress lactation.

Sexual Function/Reproduction: Oral ingestion of lindane in rats (at levels 12 times the estimated human exposure) showed significant reduction in number of spermatids in the testes compared to controls.

Other Adverse Effects: Inhalation of lindane vapours may lead to nausea, vomiting, headache, and irritation of ears, nose and throat.

The following adverse effects have been reported in post-marketing surveillance, however, causality has not been established: cardiac arrythmia, headache, pain, restlessness, nausea, vomiting, hepatitis, paresthesias, hematuria, pulmonary edema.

DRUG INTERACTIONS: Lindane should be used with caution in patients receiving drugs that may lower seizure threshold such as antidepressants, antipsychotics, centrally acting cholinesterase inhibitors, chloroquine, cyclosporine, imipenem, isoniazid, meperidine, methocarbamol, mycophenolate mofetil, penicillins, quinolones, radiographic contrast agents, tacrolimus and theophylline.

Oil may enhance the percutaneous absorption of lindane. Thus it is advisable to avoid oil treatments or oil-based hair preparations immediately before or after applying lindane shampoo. Moreover, lindane lotion should not be applied simultaneously with any other cream, ointment or oil.

DOSAGE AND ADMINISTRATION: Parents or caregivers applying lindane on affected individuals should wear gloves made of nitrile, latex with neoprene, or sheer vinyl. Natural latex gloves should be avoided due to the medication's ability to diffuse through them.

Pediculosis (using Lindane Shampoo):

- **Carefully follow directions on the product label.**
- Wash the hair with regular shampoo (without conditioner) and completely dry it. Wait at least 1 hour after washing and drying hair and then shake the bottle well and apply the lindane shampoo directly to the dry hair until it is thoroughly saturated. Apply the shampoo over a sink to minimize body exposure. The amount of lindane used depends on the length of hair but is usually approximately 30–60 mL.
- Work the shampoo thoroughly into the hair giving special attention to the hairs along the neck and behind the ears: allow it to remain in contact with the hair and scalp for 4 minutes.
- After 4 minutes, add small quantities of warm (not hot) water to the hair until a good lather forms, then rinse the hair immediately with warm water until all the lather is gone. Do not sit the patient in the bathtub to rinse the hair as this could lead to increased skin contact and therefore greater systemic absorption.
- Use a clean towel to dry the hair and a fine-toothed nit comb to remove nits.
- Although retreatment in 7–10 days is recommended with most pediculicides (because of limited ovicidal activity) there has not been a safe interval for reapplication established for lindane. As a result some recommend that lindane not be repeated and that an alternative pediculicide may be appropriate on the advice of the clinician if live lice and nits are detected after 1 week.
- Itching can occur after successful treatment thus continued itching is not necessarily an indication for retreatment with lindane. Also see Warnings and Precautions, Dermatologic for information on post-treatment itching.

Scabies (using Lindane Lotion): All contacts of scabies, even if asymptomatic, require simultaneous treatment (use lindane only if contact has not responded to or cannot tolerate safer alternatives). This includes sexual and close personal or household contacts within the preceding month.

- **Carefully follow directions on the product.**
- During treatment, discontinue use of other topical medications and cosmetics.
- Shake the bottle well.
- Apply a thin layer of lotion uniformly and gently massage into all skin surfaces from chin to toes especially to the creases in the skin, hands, feet (including the soles), between fingers and toes, and underarms and groin. Avoid contact with face, eyes, mucous membranes and urethral meatus. Do not use occlusion.
- Should not be used immediately after bathing since applying to warm wet skin may lead to greater absorption. During treatment, avoid wearing tight fitting or plastic clothing as this may also lead to warmer, moister skin and subsequent increased absorption.
- For adults, remove lotion after 8–12 hours with warm water. Do not leave lotion on skin for longer than 12 hours.
- Lindane is generally not recommended for use in children <6 years of age. If lindane is used in infants, treatment from head to toe (scabies can affect the scalp in this population) is suggested with removal of lotion with warm (not hot) water after 6 hours. Children should be treated from chin to toes with removal with warm water after 6–8 hours. Long sleeves, long pants, and gloves or mitts should be worn by the child during treatment to prevent accidental ingestion of the drug via thumbsucking or licking.
- Do not retreat with lindane. If evidence of infestation persists (e.g., appearance of live mites or new lesions) consult your physician.
- Itching can occur after successful treatment, thus continued itching is not necessarily an indication for retreatment with lindane. Also see Warnings and Precautions, Dermatologic for information on post-treatment itching.

OVERDOSAGE:

For management of a suspected drug overdose, CPhA recommends that you contact your **regional Poison Control Centre**. See the *CPS* Directory section for a list of Poison Control Centres.

ACTION AND CLINICAL PHARMACOLOGY: Lindane, an organochloride insecticide with similar neurotoxic properties as DDT, is absorbed by parasites through their exoskeleton causing overstimulation of their central nervous system resulting in paralysis of the louse and death due to inability to feed. Resistance to lindane as a pediculicide has been well documented. It displays very low ovicidal activity.

Pharmacokinetics: Lindane is rapidly absorbed through the intestine, mucous membranes and the skin. Though it is distributed in all compartments after percutaneous absorption, lindane concentrates mostly in body fat and the skin. It is metabolized by the liver and excreted in the urine and feces.

STORAGE AND STABILITY: Store at 15–30°C.

Linessa® 21 Ⓟ
desogestrel—ethinyl estradiol
Oral Contraceptive

Schering-Plough

Linessa® 28 Ⓟ
desogestrel—ethinyl estradiol
Oral Contraceptive

Schering-Plough

Date of Preparation: December 9, 2005
Date of Revision: February 3, 2010

SUMMARY PRODUCT INFORMATION:

Route of Administration	Dosage Form/Strength	Clinically Relevant Nonmedicinal Ingredients
Oral	Tablets/ desogestrel, ethinyl estradiol 0.100 mg, 0.025 mg 0.125 mg, 0.025 mg 0.150 mg, 0.025 mg	Lactose monohydrate For a complete listing see Dosage Forms, Composition and Packaging.

INDICATIONS AND CLINICAL USE: LINESSA (desogestrel, ethinyl Estradiol tablets) is indicated for:

- prevention of pregnancy

CONTRAINDICATIONS: LINESSA should not be used in women with:

- a history of or actual thrombophlebitis or thromboembolic disorders;
- a history of or actual cerebrovascular disorders;
- a history of or actual myocardial infarction or coronary artery disease;
- valvular heart disease with complications;
- history of or prodromi of a thrombosis (e.g., transient ischaemic attack, angina pectoris);
- active liver disease, or history of or actual benign or malignant liver tumours;
- known or suspected carcinoma of the breast;
- carcinoma of the endometrium or other known or suspected estrogen-dependent neoplasia;
- undiagnosed abnormal vaginal bleeding;
- steroid-dependent jaundice, cholestatic jaundice, history of jaundice of pregnancy;
- any ocular lesion arising from ophthalmic vascular disease, such as partial or complete loss of vision or defect in visual fields;
- known or suspected pregnancy;
- current or history of migraine with focal aura;
- history of actual pancreatitis if associated with severe hypertriglyceridaemia.
- presence of severe or multiple risk factor(s) for arterial or venous or thrombosis:
  - severe hypertension (persistent values of ≥160/100 mmHg)
  - hereditary or acquired predisposition for venous or arterial thrombosis, such as Factor V Leiden mutation and activated protein C (APC-) resistance, antithrombin-III-deficiency, protein C deficiency, protein S deficiency, hyperhomocysteinemia (eg, due to MTHFR C677T, A1298 mutations), prothrombin mutation G20210A, and antiphospholipid-antibodies (anticardiolipin antibodies, lupus anticoagulant)
  - severe dyslipoproteinemia
  - heavy smoking (>15 cigarettes per day) and over age 35
  - diabetes mellitus with vascular involvement
  - major surgery associated with an increased risk of postoperative thromboembolism
  - prolonged immobilization
- hypersensitivity to this product or to any ingredient in the formulation or component of the container. For a complete listing, see Dosage Forms, Composition and Packaging.

WARNINGS AND PRECAUTIONS:

Serious Warnings and Precautions
Cigarette smoking increases the risk of serious adverse effects on the heart and blood vessels. This risk increases with age and becomes significant in oral contraceptive users older than 35 years of age. Women should be counseled not to smoke (see Cardiovascular).

Patients should be counseled that birth control pills **DO NOT PROTECT** against sexually transmitted infections including HIV/AIDS. For protection against STIs, patients should be counseled to use condoms **IN COMBINATION WITH** birth control pills.

General: Discontinue Medication at the Earliest Manifestation of:

A. **Thromboembolic and cardiovascular disorders**, such asthrombophlebitis, pulmonary embolism, cerebrovascular disorders, myocardial ischemia, mesenteric thrombosis, and retinal thrombosis.
B. **Conditions which predispose to venous stasis and to vascular thrombosis** (eg, immobilization after accidents or confinement to bed during long-term illness). Other non-hormonal methods of contraception should be used until regular activities are resumed. For use of oral contraceptives when surgery is contemplated, see Peri-Operative Considerations.
C. **Visual defects- partial or complete**
D. **Papilledema or ophthalmic vascular lesions**
E. **Severe headache of unknown etiology or worsening of pre-existing migraine headache**
F. **Increase in epileptic seizures**

The following information is provided from studies of combination oral contraceptives (COCs).

The use of combination hormonal contraceptives is associated with increased risks of several serious conditions including myocardial infarction, thromboembolism, stroke, hepatic neoplasia and gallbladder disease, although the risk of serious morbidity and mortality is small in healthy women without underlying risk factors. The risk of morbidity and mortality increases significantly if associated with the presence of other risk factors such as hypertension, hyperlipidemias, obesity and diabetes. Other medical conditions which have been associated with adverse circulatory events include systemic lupus erythematosus, hemolytic uremic syndrome, chronic inflammatory bowel disease (Crohn's disease or ulcerative colitis), sickle cell disease, valvular heart disease and atrial fibrillation.

The following conditions have been reported to occur or deteriorate with both pregnancy and COC use, although a direct association with COC's has not been firmly established: porphyria, systemic lupus erythematosus, hemolytic uremic syndrome, Sydenham's chorea, herpes gestationis, and otosclerosis-related hearing loss.

The information contained in this section is principally from studies carried out in women who used combination oral contraceptives with higher formulations of estrogens and progestogens than those in common use today. The effect of long-term use of combination hormonal contraceptives with lower doses of both estrogen and progestogen administered orally remains to be determined.

Carcinogenesis and Mutagenesis: Breast Cancer: Increasing age and a strong family history are the most significant risk factors for the development of breast cancer. Other established risk factors include obesity, nulliparity and late age at first full-term pregnancy. The identified groups of women that may be at increased risk of developing breast cancer before menopause are long-term users of oral contraceptives (more than eight years) and starters at early age. In a few women, the use of oral contraceptives may accelerate the growth of an existing but undiagnosed breast cancer. Since any potential increased risk related to oral contraceptive use is small, there is no reason to change prescribing habits at present.

Women receiving oral contraceptives should be instructed in self-examination of their breasts. Their physicians should be notified whenever any masses are detected. A yearly clinical breast examination is also recommended because, if a breast cancer should develop, estrogen-containing drugs may cause a rapid progression.

Cervical Cancer : The most important risk factor for cervical cancer is persistent human papillomavirus (HPV) infection. Some epidemiological studies have indicated that long-term use of Combination Oral Contraceptives (COCs) may further contribute to this increased risk but there continues to be controversy about the extent to which this finding is attributable to the confounding effects, eg, cervical screening and sexual behavior including use of barrier contraceptives.

Hepatocellular Carcinoma: Hepatocellular carcinoma may be associated with oral contraceptives. The risk appears to increase with duration of hormonal contraceptive use. However, the attributable risk (the excess incidence) of liver cancers in oral contraceptive users is extremely small.

Cardiovascular: Predisposing Factors for Coronary Artery Disease: Cigarette smoking increases the risk of serious cardiovascular side effects and mortality. Birth control pills increase this risk, especially with increasing age. Convincing data are available to support an upper age limit of 35 years for oral contraceptive use in women who smoke.

Other women who are independently at high risk for cardiovascular disease include those with diabetes, hypertension, abnormal lipid profile, or a family history of these. Whether oral contraceptives accentuate this risk is unclear.

In low risk, non-smoking women of any age, the benefits of oral contraceptive use outweigh the possible cardiovascular risks associated with low-dose formulations. Consequently, oral contraceptives may be prescribed for these women up to the age of menopause.

Hypertension: Patients with essential hypertension whose blood pressure is well-controlled may be given hormonal contraceptives but only under close supervision. If a significant elevation of blood pressure in previously normotensive or hypertensive subjects occurs at any time during the administration of the drug, cessation of medication is necessary.

Endocrine and Metabolism: Diabetes: Current low dose oral contraceptives exert minimal impact on glucose metabolism. Diabetic patients, or those with a family history of diabetes, should be observed closely to detect any worsening of carbohydrate metabolism. Patients predisposed to diabetes who can be kept under close supervision may be given oral contraceptives. Young diabetic patients whose disease is of recent origin, well controlled, and not associated with hypertension or other signs of vascular disease, such as ocular fundal changes, should be monitored more frequently while using oral contraceptives.

Lipid and Other Metabolic Effects: A small proportion of women will have adverse lipid changes while on oral contraceptives. Alternative contraception should be used in women with uncontrolled dyslipidemias. (See Contraindications). Elevations of plasma triglycerides may lead to pancreatitis and other complications.

Gastrointestinal: Published epidemiological studies indicate a possible association of COC use and the development of Crohn's disease and ulcerative colitis, although this has not been firmly established.

Genitourinary: Vaginal Bleeding: Persistent irregular vaginal bleeding requires assessment to exclude underlying pathology.

Fibroids: Patients with fibroids (leiomyomata) should be carefully observed. Sudden enlargement, pain, or tenderness require discontinuation of the use of oral contraceptives.

Hematologic: Epidemiological studies have shown that the incidence of venous thromboembolism (VTE) in users of oral contraceptives with low estrogen content (<50 µg ethinyl estradiol) ranges from about 20 to 40 cases per 100 000 women-years, but this risk estimate varies according to the progestogen. This compares with 5 to 10 cases per 100 000 women-years for non-users.

The use of any combined oral contraceptive carries an increased risk of VTE compared with no use. The excess risk of VTE is highest during the first year a woman ever uses a combined oral contraceptive. The increased risk is less than the risk of VTE associated with pregnancy, which is estimated as 60 cases per 100 000 pregnancies. VTE is fatal in 1-2% of cases.

Several epidemiological studies indicate that third generation oral contraceptives, including those containing desogestrel, are associated with a higher risk of venous thromboembolism than certain second generation oral contraceptives. These studies indicate an approximate 2-fold difference in risk, which corresponds to 1-2 cases of venous thromboembolism per 10 000 women-years of use. However, data from additional studies have not shown this difference in risk.

Other Risk Factors for Venous Thromboembolism: Other generalized risk factors for venous thromboembolism include but are not limited to a personal history, a family history (the occurrence of VTE in a direct relative at a relatively early age may indicate genetic predisposition), severe obesity (body mass index >30 kg/m^2) and systemic lupus erythematosus. The risk of VTE also increases with age and smoking. The risk of VTE may be temporarily increased with prolonged immobilization, major surgery, or trauma. Also, patients with varicose veins and leg cast should be closely supervised.

If a hereditary or acquired predisposition for venous thromboembolism is suspected, the woman should be referred to a specialist for advice before deciding on any COC use.

Hepatic/Biliary/Pancreatic: Acute or chronic disturbances of liver function may necessitate the discontinuation of COC use until markers of liver function return to normal.

Jaundice: Patients who have had jaundice should be given oral contraceptives only with great care and under close observation. Oral contraceptive-related cholestasis has been described in women with a history of pregnancy-related cholestasis. Women with a history of cholestasis may have the condition recur with subsequent hormonal contraceptive use.

The development of severe generalized pruritus or icterus requires that the medication be withdrawn until the problem is resolved.

If a patient develops jaundice that proves to be cholestatic in type, the use of oral contraceptives should not be resumed. In patients taking hormonal contraceptives, changes in the composition of the bile may occur and an increased incidence of gallstones has been reported.

Gallbladder Disease: Patients taking oral contraceptives have a greater risk of developing gallbladder disease requiring surgery within the first year of use. The risk may double after four or five years.

Hepatic Nodules: Hepatic nodules (adenoma and focal nodular hyperplasia) have been reported, particularly in long-term users of oral contraceptives. Although these lesions are extremely rare, they have caused fatal intra-abdominal hemorrhage and should be considered in women presenting with an abdominal mass, acute abdominal pain, or evidence of intra-abdominal bleeding.

Immune: Angioedema: Exogenous estrogens may induce or exacerbate symptoms of angioedema, in particular in women with hereditary angioedema.

Neurologic: Migraine and Headache: The onset or exacerbation of migraine or the development of headache of a new pattern that is recurrent, persistent or severe, requires discontinuation of hormonal contraceptives and evaluation of the cause. Women with migraine headaches who take oral contraceptives may be at increased risk of stroke (see Contraindications).

Ophthalmologic: Ocular Disease: Patients who are pregnant or are taking oral contraceptives, may experience corneal edema that may cause visual disturbances and changes in tolerance to contact lenses, especially of the rigid type. Soft contact lenses usually do not cause disturbances. If visual changes or alterations in tolerance to contact lenses occur, temporary or permanent cessation of wear may be advised.

Peri-Operative Considerations: There is an increased risk of thromboembolic complications in oral contraceptive users after major surgery. If feasible, oral contraceptives should be discontinued and an alternative method substituted at least one month prior to **MAJOR** elective surgery. Oral contraceptives should not be resumed until the first menstrual period after hospital discharge following surgery.

Psychiatric: Patients with a history of emotional disturbances, especially the depressive type, may be more prone to have a recurrence of depression while taking oral contraceptives. In cases of a serious recurrence, a trial of an alternate method of contraception should be made, which may help to clarify the possible relationship. Women with premenstrual syndrome (PMS) may have a varied response to oral contraceptives, ranging from symptomatic improvement to worsening of the condition.

Renal: Fluid Retention: Hormonal contraceptives may cause some degree of fluid retention. They should be prescribed with caution, and only with careful monitoring in patients with conditions which might be aggravated by fluid retention.

Sexual Function/Reproduction: Return to Fertility: After discontinuing oral contraceptive therapy, the patient should delay pregnancy until at least one normal spontaneous cycle has occurred in order to date the pregnancy. An alternate contraceptive method should be used during this time.

Amenorrhea: In some women, withdrawal bleeding may not occur during the tablet-free interval. If the COC has been taken according to directions, it is unlikely that the woman is pregnant. However, if the COC has not been taken according to directions prior to the first missed withdrawal bleed, or if two withdrawal bleeds are missed, pregnancy must be ruled out before COC use is continued.

Women having a history of oligomenorrhea, secondary amenorrhea, or irregular cycles may remain anovulatory or become amenorrheic following discontinuation of estrogen-progestin combination therapy.

Amenorrhea, especially if associated with breast secretion that continues for six months or more after withdrawal warrants a careful assessment of hypothalamic-pituitary function.

Reduced Efficacy: The efficacy of COCs may be reduced in the event of missed tablets, gastro-intestinal disturbances or concomitant medication (see Drug Interactions).

Skin: Chloasma may occasionally occur with use of COCs, especially in women with a history of chloasma gravidarum. Women with a tendency to chloasma should avoid exposure to the sun or ultraviolet radiation while taking COCs.

Special Populations: Pregnant Women: Oral contraceptives should not be taken by pregnant women. If pregnancy occurs during treatment with LINESSA, further intake should be stopped. However, if conception accidentally occurs while taking the pill, there is no conclusive evidence that the estrogen and progestin contained in the oral contraceptive will damage the developing child.

Nursing Women: In breastfeeding women, the use of oral contraceptives results in the hormonal components being excreted in breast milk and may reduce its quantity and quality. Published studies have indicated that during lactation, 0.1% of the daily maternal dose of levonorgestrel and 0.02% of the daily maternal dose of ethinyl estradiol could be transferred to the newborn via milk. Adverse effects on the child have been reported, including jaundice and breast enlargement. The nursing mother should be advised not to use oral contraceptives but to use other forms of contraception until she has completely weaned her child.

Pediatrics: The safety and efficacy of LINESSA has not been established in women under the age of 18 years.

Use of this product before menarche is not indicated.

Geriatrics: LINESSA is not indicated for use in postmenopausal women.

Monitoring and Laboratory Tests: Physical Examination and Follow-up: Before oral contraceptives are used, a thorough history and physical examination should be performed, including a blood pressure determination and the family case history carefully noted. In addition, disturbances of the clotting system must be ruled out if any members of the family have suffered from thromboembolic diseases (e.g., deep vein thrombosis, stroke, myocardial infarction) at a young age. Breasts, liver, extremities and pelvic organs should be examined and a Papanicolaou (PAP) smear should be taken if the patient has been sexually active.

The first follow-up visit should be done three months after oral contraceptives are prescribed. Thereafter, examinations should be performed at least once a year or more frequently if indicated. At each annual visit, examination should include those procedures that were done at the initial visit as outlined above or per recommendations of the Canadian Task Force on the Periodic Health Examination.

ADVERSE REACTIONS: Adverse Drug Reaction Overview: An increased risk of the following serious adverse reactions has been associated with the use of oral contraceptives: thrombophlebitis; pulmonary embolism; mesenteric thrombosis; neuro-ocular lesions, e.g., retinal thrombosis; myocardial infarction; cerebral thrombosis; cerebral hemorrhage; hypertension; benign hepatic tumours; gallbladder disease; congenital anomalies.

The following adverse reactions also have been reported in patients receiving oral contraceptives:

Nausea and vomiting, usually the most common adverse reaction, occurs in approximately 10% or less of patients during the first cycle. Other reactions, as a general rule, are seen less frequently or only occasionally, as follows: gastrointestinal symptoms (such as abdominal cramps and bloating); breakthrough bleeding; spotting; change in menstrual flow; dysmenorrhea; amenorrhea during and after treatment; temporary infertility after discontinuance of treatment; edema; chloasma or melasma which may persist; breast changes: tenderness, enlargement, and secretion; change in weight (increase or decrease; endocervical hyperplasias; possible diminution in lactation when given immediately post-partum; cholestatic jaundice; migraine; increase in size of uterine leiomyomata; rash (allergic); mental depression; reduced tolerance to carbohydrates; vaginal candidiasis; premenstrual-like syndrome; intolerance to contact lenses; change in corneal curvature (steepening); cataracts; optic neuritis; retinal thrombosis; changes in libido; chorea; changes in appetite; cystitis-like syndrome; rhinitis; headache; nervousness; dizziness; hirsutism; loss of scalp hair; erythema multiforme; erythema nodosum; hemorrhagic eruption; vaginitis; porphyria; impaired renal function; Raynaud's phenomenon; auditory disturbances; hemolytic uremic syndrome; pancreatitis; abdominal pain; diarrhea; hypersensitivity; vaginal discharge; rash; urticaria.

Clinical Trial Adverse Drug Reactions: Because clinical trials are conducted under very specific conditions the adverse drug reaction rates observed in the clinical trials may not reflect the rates observed in practice and should not be compared to the rates in the clinical trials of another drug. Adverse drug reaction information from clinical trials is useful for identifying drug-related adverse events and for approximating rates.

Two multicentre, 6-cycle, controlled efficacy and safety studies were conducted in 5552 women.

A list of adverse events experienced by >1% of the subjects are listed in Table 1.

Table 1: LINESSA

Incidence of All Adverse Experiences (>1%) (All Subjects Treated Group) to LINESSA

Preferred (WHOART) Term	Incidence During Study	
	n	%
LINESSA (Number of Subjects)	(N=2768)	
Body as a Whole–General		
Influenza-like Symptoms	97	3.5
Back Pain	80	2.9
Allergy	59	2.1
Fatigue	48	1.7
Fever	29	1.0
Central & Peripheral Nervous System		
Headache	420	15.2
Migraine	34	1.2
Gastrointestinal System		
Nausea	225	8.1
Diarrhea	61	2.2
Flatulence	53	1.9
Dyspepsia	46	1.7
Vomiting	43	1.6
Abdominal Pain	33	1.2
Metabolic & Nutritional		
Weight Increase	64	2.3
Musculoskeletal System		
Myalgia	40	1.4
Arthralgia	37	1.3

(cont'd)

Table 1: LINESSA *(cont'd)*

Incidence of All Adverse Experiences (>1%) (All Subjects Treated Group) to LINESSA

Preferred (WHOART) Term	Incidence During Study n	%
Psychiatric		
Emotional Lability	117	4.2
Depression	45	1.6
Insomnia	30	1.1
Nervousness	28	1.0
Reproductive, Female		
Intermenstrual Bleeding	181	6.5
Dysmenorrhea	150	5.4
Breast Pain Female	139	5.0
Moniliasis Genital	132	4.8
Vaginitis	57	2.1
Pelvic Cramping	36	1.3
Resistance Mechanism		
Herpes Simplex	30	1.1
Respiratory System		
Upper Respiratory Tract Infection	328	11.8
Sinusitis	227	8.2
Pharyngitis	134	4.8
Bronchitis	70	2.5
Coughing	50	1.8
Rhinitis	51	1.8
Secondary Terms-Events		
Cervical Smear Test PAP II	51	1.8
Inflicted Injury	47	1.7
Skin & Appendages		
Acne	80	2.9
Rash	35	1.3
Urinary System		
Urinary Tract Infection	112	4.0
Cystitis	30	1.1

Notes: This table contains all adverse events which occurred during treatment, including those deemed to be not related or unlikely related, in addition to those which were deemed to be possibly related, probably related and definitely related. This table contains counts of subjects. Within each treatment group, percentages are based on the number of subjects with an event or without an event divided by the total number of subjects in each demographic subgroup. Adverse experiences that stopped before first dose date or started after last dose date were excluded from this table.

Less Common Clinical Trial Adverse Drug Reactions (<1%): Rare adverse events (<1%) which were observed in clinical trials and deemed to be at least possibly related to LINESSA are as follows:

Body as a Whole-General: chest pain, crying abnormal, hot flushes, leg pain, edema, edema peripheral, pain, rigors, syncope, vertebral disk disorder.

Cardiovascular, General: hypertension.

Central & Peripheral Nervous System: leg Cramps, dizziness, involuntary muscle contractions, tremor.

Gastrointestinal System: constipation, eructation, irritable bowel syndrome.

Hearing & Vestibular: ear disorder, earache, motion sickness.

Liver & Biliary System: bilirubinaemia, cholecystitis, cholelithiasis, increased hepatic enzymes, abnormal hepatic function, AST increased, ALT increased.

Metabolic & Nutritional: hypercholesterolaemia, hyperglycemia, hypertriglyceridemia, LDH increased, generalised edema, edema of the legs, peripheral edema.

Neoplasms: breast fibroadenosis, female breast neoplasm, cervical uterine polyp, ovarian cyst, uterine fibroid.

Platelet Bleeding & Clotting: epistaxis, gingival bleeding, purpura.

Psychiatric: agitation, anorexia, anxiety, increased appetite, impaired concentration, confusion, dyspareunia, decreased libido, neurosis, somnolence, suicide attempt.

Red Blood Cell: anaemia.

Reproductive Female: amenorrhea, breast discharge, breast engorgement, breast enlargement, cervicitis, cervix lesion, non-puerperal lactation, leukorrhea, menorrhagia, menstrual disorder, ovarian pain, female perineal pain, premenstrual tension, uterine contractions, uterine haemorrhage, vaginal bleeding, vaginal discomfort, vaginal haemorrhage, vulva disorder.

Resistance Mechanism: infection, viral infection.

Secondary Terms, Events: ectropion.

Skin & Appendages: alopecia, chloasma, dermatitis, eczema, erythema nodosum, folliculitis, abnormal hair texture, hypertrichosis, melanosis, abnormal pigmentation, pruritus, genital pruritus, skin discolouration, dry skin, increased sweating.

Urinary System: dysuria, haematuria, micturition frequency, abnormal urine.

Vascular: flushing, thrombophlebitis, deep vein disorders.

Vision: photophobia, abnormal vision, xerophthalmia.

White Cell & Reticular Endothelial System: lymphadenopathy.

Post-Market Adverse Drug Reactions: Additional adverse events which have been reported occasionally since the introduction of LINESSA to the market include: peripheral edema, cyst , hypoaesthesia, menorrhagia, metrorrhagia, mood swings, abdominal distention, bleeding tendency, angioneurotic edema, drug exposure during pregnancy, pruritic rash, emotional lability, back pain, pollakiuria, fluid retention, pruritus, frequent bowel movements. These adverse events are compiled from spontaneous reports and are listed regardless of whether or not there was a possible causal relation to LINESSA.

The most serious undesirable effects associated with the use of COCs are listed in Warnings and Precautions. Other side effects that have been reported in users of COCs but for which the association has been neither confirmed nor refuted are found in Table 2.

Table 2: LINESSA

Post Market Adverse Events occurring with Combined Oral Contraceptives

Body system	Common/Uncommon (more than 1/1000)	Rare (less than 1/1000)
Immune system disorders		Hypersensitivity
Metabolism and nutrition disorders	Weight increased, fluid retention	Weight decreased
Nervous system disorders	Headache, migraine, libido decreased, depressed mood, mood altered	Libido increased
Eye disorders		Contact lens intolerance
Gastrointestinal disorders	Nausea, vomiting, abdominal pain, diarrhea	
Skin and subcutaneous tissue disorders	Rash, urticaria	Erythema nodosum, erythema multiforme
Reproductive system and breast disorders	Breast pain, breast tenderness, breast hypertrophy	Vaginal discharge, breast discharge

The most appropriate MedDRA term (version 6.1) to describe a certain adverse reaction is listed. Synonyms or related conditions are not listed, but should be taken into account as well.

DRUG INTERACTIONS: Overview: Interactions between desogestrel/ethinyl estradiol and other drugs have been reported in the literature (see Drug-Drug Interactions). No formal drug-drug interaction studies were conducted with LINESSA.

Drug-Drug Interactions: The concurrent administration of oral contraceptives with other drugs may result in an altered response to either agent (Table 3 and Table 4). Reduced effectiveness of the oral contraceptive, should it occur, is more likely with the low-dose formulations. It is important to ascertain all drugs that a patient is taking, both prescription and non-prescription, before oral contraceptives are prescribed.

Table 3: LINESSA

Drugs Which May Decrease the Efficacy of Oral Contraceptives

Class of Compound	Drug	Proposed Mechanism	Suggested Management
Antacids		Decreased intestinal absorption of progestins.	Dose two hours apart.
Antibiotics	ampicillin cotrimoxazole penicillin	Enterohepatic circulation disturbance, intestinal hurry.	For short course, use additional method or use another drug. For long course, use another method.
	rifampicin	Increased metabolism of progestins. Suspected acceleration of estrogen metabolism.	Use another method.
	chloramphenicol metronidazole neomycin nitrofurantoin sulfonamides tetracyclines	Induction of hepatic microsomal enzymes. Also disturbance of enterohepatic circulation.	For short course, use additional method or use another drug. For long course, use another method.
	troleandomycin	May retard metabolism of oral contraceptives, increasing the risk of cholestatic jaundice.	
Anticonvulsants	carbamazepine ethosuximide felbamate lamotrigine oxcarbazepine phenobarbital phenytoin primidone topiramate	Induction of hepatic microsomal enzymes. Rapid metabolism of estrogen and increased binding of progestin and ethinyl estradiol to SHBG.	Use higher dose oral contraceptives (50 mcg ethinyl estradiol) another drug or another method.
Antifungal	griseofulvin	Stimulation of hepatic metabolism of contraceptive steroids may occur.	Use another method.
Cholesterol Lowering Agents	clofibrate	Reduces elevated serum triglycerides and cholesterol; this reduces oral contraceptive efficacy.	Use another method.
HIV protease inhibitors	ritonavir	Induction of hepatic microsomal enzymes.	Use another drug or another method.
Non-nucleoside reverse transcriptase inhibitors	nevirapine	Induction of hepatic microsomal enzymes.	Use another drug or another method.

(cont'd)

Table 3: LINESSA *(cont'd)*

Drugs Which May Decrease the Efficacy of Oral Contraceptives

Class of Compound	Drug	Proposed Mechanism	Suggested Management
Sedatives and Hypnotics	barbiturates benzodiazepines chloral hydrate glutethimide meprobamate	Induction of hepatic microsomal enzymes.	For short course, use additional method or another drug. For long course use another method or higher dose OCs.
Other Drugs	Analgesics Antihistamines Antimigraine preparations phenylbutazone vitamin E	Reduced oral contraceptive efficacy has been reported. Remains to be confirmed.	

Oral contraceptives may interfere with the metabolism of other drugs. Accordingly, plasma and tissue concentrations may either increase (eg, cyclosporine) or decrease (eg, lamotrigine).

Several of the anti-HIV protease inhibitors (eg, ritonavir) and non-nucleoside reverse transcriptase inhibitors (eg, nevirapine) have been studied with coadministration of oral combination hormonal contraceptives; significant changes (increase and decrease) in the mean AUC of the estrogen and progestin and the potential to affect hepatic metabolism have been noted in some cases. The efficacy and safety of oral contraceptive products may be affected. Healthcare providers should refer to the label of the individual anti-HIV protease inhibitors for further drug-drug interaction information.

Table 4: LINESSA

Modification of Other Drug Action by Oral Contraceptives

Class of Compound	Drug	Modification of Other Drug Action	Suggested Management
Alcohol		Possible increased levels of ethanol or acetaldehyde.	Use with caution.
Alpha-II Adrenoreceptor Agents	clonidine	Sedation effect increased.	Use with caution.
Anticoagulants	All	Oral contraceptives increase clotting factors, decrease efficacy. However oral contraceptives may potentiate action in some patients.	Use another method.
Anticonvulsants	All	Estrogens may increase risk of seizures.	Use another method.
	lamotrigine	Decrease lamotrigine levels, may lead to breakthrough seizures.	Use another method.
Antidiabetic Drugs	Oral hypoglycemics and insulin	Oral contraceptives may impair glucose tolerance and increase blood glucose.	Use low dose estrogen and progestin oral contraceptiveor another method. Monitor blood glucose.
Antihypertensive Agents	guanethidine and methyldopa	Estrogen component causes sodium retention, progestin has no effect.	Use low oral contraceptive estrogen or use another method.
	Beta blockers	Increased drug effect (decreased metabolism).	Adjust dose of drug if necessary. Monitor cardiovascular status.
Antipyretics	acetaminophen	Increased metabolism and renal clearance.	Dose of drug may have to be increased.
	antipyridine	Impaired metabolism.	Decrease dose of drug.
	ASA	Effects of ASA may be decreased by the short-term use of oral contraceptives.	Patients on chronic ASA therapy may require an increase in ASA dosage.
Aminocaproic Acid		Theoretically, a hypercoagulable state may occur because oral contraceptives augment clotting factors.	Avoid concomitant use.
Betamimetic Agents	isoproterenol	Estrogen causes decreased response to these drugs.	Adjust dose of drug as necessary. Discontinuing oral contraceptives can result in excessive drug activity.
Caffeine		The actions of caffeine may be enhanced as oral contraceptives may impair the hepatic metabolism of caffeine.	Use with caution.
Cholesterol-lowering Agents	clofibrate	Their action may be antagonized by oral contraceptives. Oral contraceptives may also increase metabolism of clofibrate.	May need to increase dose of clofibrate.
Corticosteroids	prednisone	Markedly increased serum levels.	Possible need for decrease in dose.

(cont'd)

Table 4: LINESSA *(cont'd)*

Modification of Other Drug Action by Oral Contraceptives

Class of Compound	Drug	Modification of Other Drug Action	Suggested Management
Cyclosporine		May lead to an increase in cyclosporine levels and hepatotoxicity.	Monitor hepatic function. The cyclosporine dose may have to be decreased.
Folic Acid		Oral contraceptives have been reported to impair folate metabolism.	May need to increase dietary intake, or supplement.
Meperedine		Possible increased analgesia and CNS depression due to decreased metabolism of meperidine.	Use combination with caution.
Phenothiazine Tranquilizers	All phenothiazines, reserpine and similar drugs	Estrogen potentiates the hyperprolactinemia effect of these drugs.	Use other drugs or lower dose oral contraceptives. If galactorrhea or hyperprolactinemia occurs, use other method.
Sedatives and Hypnotics	chlordiazepoxide lorazepam oxazepam diazepam	Increased effect (increased metabolism).	Use with caution.
Theophylline	All	Decreased oxidation, leading to possible toxicity.	Use with caution. Monitor theophylline levels.
Tricyclic Antidepressants	clomipramine (possibly others)	Increased side effects; i.e., depression.	Use with caution.
Vitamin B_{12}		oral contraceptives have been reported to reduce serum levels of Vitamin B_{12}.	May need to increase dietary intake, or supplement.

Drug-Food Interactions: Interactions with food have not been established.

Drug-Herb Interactions: Herbal products containing St. John's Wort (hypericum perforatum) may induce hepatic enzymes (cytochrome P450) and p-glycoprotein transporter and may reduce the effectiveness of contraceptive steroids. This may also result in breakthrough bleeding. Physicians and other health care providers should be made aware of the non-prescription products concomitantly used by the patient, including herbal and natural products.

Drug-Laboratory Test Interactions: Laboratory Tests: Results of laboratory tests should be interpreted in the light that the patient is on oral contraceptives. The following laboratory tests are modified.

A. Liver function tests: Aspartate serum transaminase (AST)—variously reported elevations. Alkaline phosphatase and gamma glutamine transaminase (GGT)—slightly elevated.
B. Coagulation tests: Minimal elevation of test values reported for such parameters as prothrombin and Factors VII, VIII, IX and X.
C. Thyroid function tests: Protein binding of thyroxine is increased as indicated by increased total serum thyroxine concentrations and decreased T_3 resin uptake.
D. Lipoproteins: Small changes of unproven clinical significance may occur in lipoprotein cholesterol fractions.
E. Gonadotropins: LH and FSH levels are suppressed by the use of oral contraceptives. Wait two weeks after discontinuing the use of oral contraceptives before measurements are made.
F. Glucose tolerance: Oral glucose tolerance remained unchanged or was slightly decreased.
G. Tissue Specimens: Pathologists should be advised of oral contraceptive therapy when specimens obtained from surgical procedures and Pap smears are submitted for examination.

Drug-Lifestyle Interactions: Non-Contraceptive Benefits of Oral Contraceptives: Several health advantages other than contraception have been reported:

1. Combination oral contraceptives reduce the incidence of cancer of the endometrium and ovaries.
2. Oral contraceptives reduce the likelihood of developing benign breast disease, and as a result, decrease the incidence of breast biopsies.
3. Oral contraceptives reduce the likelihood of development of functional ovarian cysts.
4. Pill-users have less menstrual blood loss and have more regular cycles, thereby reducing the chance of developing iron-deficiency anemia.
5. The use of oral contraceptives may decrease the severity of dysmenorrhea and premenstrual syndrome and may improve acne vulgaris, hirsutism and other androgen-mediated disorders.
6. Oral contraceptives decrease the incidence of acute pelvic inflammatory disease and thereby reduce as well the incidence of ectopic pregnancy.
7. Oral contraceptives have potential beneficial effects on endometriosis.

DOSAGE AND ADMINISTRATION: Patients should be instructed to read the package insert prior to starting LINESSA and any time they are unsure of administration. If they have additional questions they should call their doctor or clinic.

LINESSA tablets are prescribed as a 21-day or 28-day regimen. LINESSA tablets must be taken at approximately the same time every day until the pack is empty. The patient may begin taking LINESSA on Day 1 of her menstrual cycle (i.e. the first day of menstrual flow) or on the first Sunday after her period begins. If the period starts on Sunday, she should start that same day.

Dosage: LINESSA 21 (21-Day Regimen): One coloured tablet is to be taken as follows for 21 consecutive days (three weeks): light yellow for 7 days; orange for 7 days and red for 7 days. Tablets are then discontinued for one week. The patient must not be off the pill for more than seven consecutive days. A new pack will be started on the eighth day. The patient will have a period during the seven days off the pill (the bleeding may be lighter and shorter than their usual period).

LINESSA 28 (28-Day Regimen): Tablets are taken sequentially following the arrows marked on the dispenser. One light yellow tablet is taken daily for 7 days; followed by one orange tablet for 7 days then one red tablet daily for 7 days. On the fourth week the patient will take one "inactive" green pill daily for the next seven consecutive days. A new pack will be started on the eighth day following completion of the green tablets. The patient will have a period during the seven days on the green pill. On this regimen he patient must not go a day without taking a pill.

Management of Missed Tablets: The patient should be instructed to use the following chart if she misses one or more birth control pill (light yellow, orange, or red). She should be told to match the number of pills missed with the appropriate starting time for her dosing regimen.

Missing pills can cause spotting or light bleeding, even if the missed pills are made up. The woman may also feel a little sick to her stomach on the days she takes two pills to make up for missed pills.

If a woman misses pills at any time she could get pregnant. The greatest risks for pregnancy are starting a pack late or missing a pill(s) at the beginning or at the very end of the pack.

The patient should be counseled to always have another kind of birth control (such as condoms and spermicidal foam or gel) to use as a back-up in case they miss pills, and an extra full pack of pills available.

If the patient forgets more that one pill, two months in a row, they should be instructed to talk to their doctor or clinic. The patient may require further counseling about ways to make pill-taking easier or about using another method of birth control.

NOTE to patients on the 28-day regimen (LINESSA 28): If the patient forgets any of the 7 green pills (inactive pills) in Week 4, she should be advised to safely dispose of the pills she missed and then keep taking one pill each day until the pack is empty. A back-up method is not needed.

Administration: It is recommended that LINESSA be taken at the same time each day. The patient should be counseled to associate the pill with some regular activity like eating a meal or going to bed.

The first-time user may wish to use a second method of birth control (e.g. condoms and spermicidal foam or gel) for the first seven days of the first cycle of pill use. This will provide a back-up in case pills are forgotten while they are getting used to taking them.

If spotting, light bleeding or feeling sick to their stomach occurs during the first three months the woman should be counseled to not stop taking the pill. The problem will usually go away. If it does not subside, the patient should consult with her doctor or clinic.

The dosage regimen should not be altered (i.e. the pill should not be stopped) even if the woman does not have sex very often.

Table 5: LINESSA

What to Do if You Miss Pills:

Sunday Start	**Day 1 Start**
Miss 1 pill	**Miss 1 pill**
Take it as soon as you remember, and take the next pill at the usual time. This means that you might take 2 pills in one day.	Take it as soon as you remember, and take the next pill at the usual time. This means that you might take 2 pills in one day.
Miss 2 pills in a row	**Miss 2 pills in a row**
First 2 Weeks: 1. Take 2 pills the day you remember and 2 pills the next day. 2. Then take 1 pill a day until you finish the pack. 3. Use a back-up method of birth control if you have sex in the 7 days after you miss the pills. **Third Week:** 1. Keep taking 1 pill a day until Sunday. 2. On Sunday, safely discard the rest of the pack and start a new pack that day. 3. Use a back-up method of birth control if you have sex in the 7 days after you miss the pills. 4. You may not have a period this month. **If you miss 2 periods in a row, call your doctor or clinic.**	**First 2 Weeks:** 1. Take 2 pills the day you remember and 2 pills the next day. 2. Then take 1 pill a day until you finish the pack. 3. Use a back-up method of birth control if you have sex in the 7 days after you miss the pills. **Third Week:** 1. Safely dispose of the rest of the pill pack and start a new pack that same day. 2. Use a back-up method of birth control if you have sex in the 7 days after you miss the pills. 3. You may not have a period this month. **If you miss 2 periods in a row, call your doctor or clinic.**
Miss 3 or more pills in a row	**Miss 3 or more pills in a row**
Anytime in the Cycle: 1. Keep taking 1 pill a day until Sunday. 2. On Sunday, safely discard the rest of the pack and start a new pack that day. 3. Use a back-up method of birth control if you have sex in the 7 days after you miss the pills. 4. You may not have a period this month. **If you miss 2 periods in a row, call your doctor or clinic.**	**Anytime in the Cycle:** 1. Safely dispose of the rest of the pill pack and start a new pack that same day. 2. Use a back-up method of birth control if you have sex in the 7 days after you miss the pills. 3. You may not have a period this month. **If you miss 2 periods in a row, call your doctor or clinic.**

When receiving any medical treatment, patients should tell their doctor that they are using birth control pills.

Advice in case of vomiting: In case of severe gastro-intestinal disturbance, absorption may not be complete and additional contraceptive measures should be taken. If vomiting occurs within 3-4 hours after tablet-taking, the advice concerning missed tablets (Dosage and Administration, Management of Missed Tablets) is applicable. If the woman does not want to change her normal tablet-taking schedule, she has to take the extra tablet(s) needed from another pack.

Special Notes on Administration: When to start LINESSA: No hormonal contraceptive use in the preceeding cycle: Tablet taking should start on Day 1 of the woman's menstrual cycle or on the first Sunday after her period begins.

Switching from another combination hormonal contraceptive (combined oral contraceptive (COC), vaginal ring, or transdermal patch): The woman should start LINESSA preferably on the day after the last active tablet of her previous COC, but at the latest on the day following the usual tablet-free or inactive tablet of her previous COC. In case a vaginal ring or transdermal patch has been used, the woman should start using LINESSA preferably on the day of removal, but at the latest when the next application would have been due.

Switching from a progestogen-only-method (mini-pill, injection, implant) or from a progestogen-releasing intrauterine system (IUS): The woman may switch from the mini-pill to LINESSA on any day of her cycle. Patients using a progestogen injection should start LINESSA on the day the next injection is due. Patients using an implant or an IUS should start LINESSA on the day it is removed. In all cases, the woman should be advised to use an additional barrier method for the first 7 days of LINESSA use.

Following first-trimester abortion: The woman may start LINESSA immediately. When doing so, she need not take additional contraceptive measures.

Following delivery or second-trimester abortion: Women should be advised to start LINESSA at day 21 to 28 after delivery or second trimester abortion, after consulting with their physician. When starting later, the woman should be advised to additionally use a barrier method for the first 7 days of tablet-taking. However, if intercourse has already occurred, pregnancy should be excluded before the actual start of use or the woman should be advised to wait for her first menstrual period prior to starting LINESSA.

For breastfeeding women see Warnings and Precautions, Nursing Women.

OVERDOSAGE:

Serious ill effects have not been reported following acute ingestion of large doses of oral contraceptives by young children. Overdosage may cause nausea, and withdrawal bleeding may occur in females. There are no antidotes and further treatment should be symptomatic.

For management of a suspected drug overdose, contact your regional Poison Control Centre. See the *CPS* Directory section for a list of Poison Control Centres.

ACTION AND CLINICAL PHARMACOLOGY: Mechanism of Action: Combination oral contraceptives act by the suppression of gonadotropins. The primary mechanism of action is inhibition of ovulation, but other alterations include impaired sperm penetration and "spinnbarkeit" of the cervical mucus, and changes to the endometrium to reduce the likelihood of implantation. Receptor binding studies, as well as studies in animals and humans, have shown etonogestrel, the biologically active metabolite of desogestrel, combines high progestational activity with minimal intrinsic androgenicity. DSG in combination with EE, does not counteract the estrogen-induced increase in SHBG resulting in lower serum levels of free testosterone.

Pharmacodynamics: The contraceptive effect of COCs is based on the interaction of various factors, the most important of which are seen as the inhibition of ovulation and the changes in the cervical secretion.

Desogestrel, the progestogen component of LINESSA, displays low androgenic activity in relation to its progestogenic effects and may increase the HDL/LDL ratio. Like other oral contraceptives, these changes in lipid profile are associated with an increase in triglycerides.

Pharmacokinetics: Absorption: Desogestrel (DSG) is rapidly and almost completely absorbed and converted into etonogestrel, (ENG), its biologically active metabolite. Following oral administration, the relative bioavailability of desogestrel, based on the lowest and highest tablet strengths, 0.100 mg desogestrel/0.025 mg ethinyl estradiol and 0.150 mg desogestrel/0.025 mg ethinyl estradiol, compared to solution, as measured by serum levels of etonogestrel, is approximately 100%. Ethinyl estradiol is rapidly and almost completely absorbed. When the lowest and highest tablet strengths, 0.100 mg desogestrel/0.025 ethinyl estradiol and 0.150 mg desogestrel/0.025 mg ethinyl estradiol, were compared to solution, the relative bioavailability of ethinyl estradiol was 92% and 98% respectively. The effect of food on the bioavailability of LINESSA tablets following oral administration has not been evaluated.

The pharmacokinetics of etonogestrel and ethinyl estradiol following multiple dose administration of LINESSA tablets were determined during the third cycle in 21 subjects. After multiple dosing with LINESSA, plasma concentrations of etonogestrel reached steady-state after four days of treatment during dosing Phases 1 and 3. During dosing Phase 2, steady-state was reached after five days of treatment. The dose-normalized $AUC_{0\text{-}24}$ for etonogestrel was increased approximately 20% from Phase 1 to Phase 2 and approximately 10% from Phase 2 to Phase 3, indicating a possibility of time-dependent kinetics. Time dependency may be explained by a decreased clearance, presumably due to increased binding of etonogestrel to sex hormone-binding globulin (SHBG). SHBG concentrations were shown to be induced by the daily administration of ethinyl estradiol. Steady-state for ethinyl estradiol was reached after four days of dosing in all dosing phases. The pharmacokinetic parameters of etonogestrel and ethinyl estradiol during the third cycle following multiple dose administration of LINESSA tablets are summarized in Table 6.

Table 6: LINESSA

Mean (SD) Pharmacokinetic Parameters of LINESSA Over a 21-Day Dosing Period in the Third Cycle (n=21)

Phase (days)	Dose[H] (mg)	C_{max} (pg/mL)	T_{max} (h)	n-$AUC_{0\text{-}24}$ (pgxh/mL/mg)	CL/F (L/h)
Etonogestrel					
1 (1–7)	0.1	2163.3 (856.4)	1.6 (0.7)	196.0 (75.4)	6.1 (2.3)
2 (8–14)	0.125	3241.5 (1296.5)[a]	1.1 (0.3)[a]	234.4 (85.0)[a]	5.1 (1.9)[a]
3 (15–21)	0.15	3855.7 (1273.1)	1.5 (0.8)	256.6 (104.0)	4.6 (1.6)
Ethinyl Estradiol					
1 (1–7)	0.025	85.4 (51.7)	1.5 (0.8)	26.4 (11.5)	43.5 (15.0)
2 (8–14)	0.025	91.3 (52.2)[a]	1.2 (1.2)[a]	29.0 (15.5)[a]	41.7 (15.5)[a]
3 (15–21)	0.025	90.1 (48.2)	1.2 (0.7)	28.3 (13.2)	42.5 (18.7)

[a] n=20.

Legend: H=Desogestrel; C_{max}=Maximum serum drug concentration; T_{max}=Time at which maximum serum drug concentration occurs; n-$AUC_{0\text{-}24}$=Area under the concentration-vs time curve -0 to 24 hours normalised to 1 µg administered; CL/F=Apparent clearance.

Distribution: Etonogestrel, the active metabolite of desogestrel, was found to be 98% protein bound, primarily to sex hormone-binding globulin (SHBG). Ethinyl estradiol is primarily bound to plasma albumin. Ethinyl estradiol does not bind to SHBG, but induces SHBG synthesis. Desogestrel, in combination with ethinyl estradiol, does not counteract the estrogen-induced increase in SHBG, resulting in lower serum levels of free testosterone.

Metabolism: Desogestrel: Desogestrel is rapidly and completely metabolized by hydroxylation in the intestinal mucosa and on first pass through the liver to etonogestrel. In vitro data suggest an important role for the cytochrome P450 CYP2C9 in the bioactivation of desogestrel. Further metabolism of etonogestrel into 6β-hydroxy, etonogestrel and 6β-13ethyl-dihydroxylated as major metabolites is catalyzed by CYP3A4. Other metabolites (i.e. 3α-OH-desogestrel, 3β-OH-desogestrel, and 3α-OH-5α-H-desogestrel) also have been identified and these metabolites may undergo glucuronide and sulfate conjugation.

Ethinyl estradiol: Ethinyl estradiol is subject to a significant degree of presystemic conjugation (phase II metabolism). Ethinyl estradiol, escaping gut wall conjugation, undergoes phase I metabolism and hepatic conjugation (phase II metabolism). Major phase I metabolites are 2-OH-ethinyl estradiol and 2-methoxy-ethinyl estradiol. Sulfate and glucuronide conjugates of both ethinyl estradiol and phase I metabolites, which are excreted in bile, can undergo enterohepatic circulation.

Excretion: Etonogestrel and ethinyl estradiol are primarily eliminated in urine, bile and feces. At steady state, on Day 21, the elimination half-lives of etonogestrel and ethinyl estradiol are 37.1±14.8 hours and 28.2±10.5 hours, respectively.

Special Populations and Conditions: Race: There is no information to determine the effect of race on the pharmacokinetics of LINESSA (desogestrel/ethinyl estradiol) Tablets.

Hepatic Insufficiency: No formal studies were conducted to evaluate the effect of hepatic disease on the disposition of LINESSA. However, steroid hormones may be poorly metabolized in patients with impaired liver function (see Warnings and Precautions, Hepatic/Biliary/Pancreatic).

Renal Insufficiency: No formal studies were conducted to evaluate the effect of renal disease on the disposition of LINESSA.

STORAGE AND STABILITY: Store between 15-30°C.

Keep in a safe place out of the reach of children and pets.

INFORMATION FOR THE PATIENT: Published in e-CPS, available by subscription at www.e-cps.ca.

DOSAGE FORMS, COMPOSITION AND PACKAGING: LINESSA 21: Each 21-day treatment cycle pack consists of three active dosing phases: 7 light yellow, coated, round tablets, debossed with "TR" above "0" on one side and "Organon*" on the other side containing 0.100 mg desogestrel and 0.025 mg ethinyl estradiol; 7 orange, coated, round tablets, debossed with "TR" above "0" on one side and "Organon*" on the other side, containing 0.125 mg desogestrel and 0.025 mg ethinyl estradiol; and 7 red, coated, round tablets, debossed with "TR" above "0" on one side and "Organon*" on the other side containing 0.150 mg desogestrel and 0.025 mg ethinyl estradiol. Nonmedicinal ingredients: hydroxypropyl methylcellulose, lactose monohydrate, polyethylene glycol, pregelatinized starch, red ferric oxide (in orange and red tablets), stearic acid, talc, titanium dioxide, vitamin E and yellow ferric oxide (in light yellow and orange tablets). 21-day blister cards.

LINESSA 28: Each 28-day treatment cycle pack consists of the same three active dosing phases as the LINESSA 21 pack and also contains 7 green, round tablets, debossed with "KH" above "2" on one side and "Organon*" on the other side, with the following inert ingredients: lactose monohydrate, corn starch, magnesium stearate, hydroxypropyl methylcellulose, polyethylene glycol, titanium dioxide, FD&C Blue No. 2 aluminum lake, yellow ferric oxide and talc. 28-day blister cards.

(Shown in Product Identification Section)

Lioresal® Intrathecal

baclofen

Muscle Relaxant—Antispastic

Novartis Pharmaceuticals

Date of Preparation: September 13, 1994

Date of Revision: July 18, 2006

PHARMACOLOGY: The precise mechanisms of action of baclofen as a muscle relaxant and antispastic agent are not fully understood. Baclofen inhibits both monosynaptic and polysynaptic reflex transmission at the spinal level, possibly by decreasing excitatory neurotransmitter release from primary afferent terminals. Actions at supraspinal sites may also contribute to its clinical effect. Baclofen is an analogue of the inhibitory neurotransmitter gamma-aminobutyric acid (GABA), and may exert its effects by stimulation of the $GABA_B$ receptor subtype.

Baclofen has been shown to have general CNS depressant properties as indicated by the production of sedation with tolerance, somnolence, ataxia and respiratory and cardiovascular depression.

Neuromuscular transmission is not affected by baclofen. Baclofen exerts an antinociceptive effect. In neurological diseases associated with spasm of the skeletal muscles, the clinical effects of baclofen take the form of a beneficial action on reflex muscle contractions and of marked relief from painful spasm, automatism, and clonus.

Intrathecal baclofen, when introduced directly into the spinal subarachnoid space, permits the attainment of effective CSF concentrations with resultant plasma concentrations 100 times lower than those occurring following oral administration.

Clinical Use in Special Patient Populations: Intrathecal baclofen has also been used for the treatment of 21 patients with spinal cord disease and 18 patients with cerebral palsy.

A small number of patients with tetanus (7 patients) have been treated with intrathecal baclofen to reduce hyperreflexia, clonus, and trismus.

The safety and efficacy of intrathecal baclofen in these patient populations have not been systematically evaluated.

Pharmacodynamics: Intrathecal Bolus: The onset of action is generally 0.5 to 1 hour after administration of an intrathecal bolus dose. Peak spasmolytic effect is seen at approximately 4 hours after dosing and effects may last 4 to 8 hours. Onset, peak response, and duration of action may vary with individual patients depending on the dose and severity of symptoms.

Continuous Infusion: The antispastic action is first seen at 6 to 8 hours after initiation of continuous infusion. Maximum efficacy is observed in 24 to 48 hours.

Pharmacokinetics: The pharmacokinetics of cerebrospinal fluid (CSF) clearance of intrathecal baclofen, calculated from intrathecal bolus or continuous infusion studies, approximate CSF turnover, suggesting elimination is by bulk-flow removal of CSF. Direct infusion into the spinal subarachnoid space bypasses absorption processes and allows exposure to the receptor sites in the dorsal horn of the spinal cord.

Intrathecal Bolus: After a bolus lumbar injection of 50 or 100 μg intrathecal baclofen in 7 patients, the average CSF elimination half-life was 1.51 hours over the first 4 hours and the average CSF clearance was approximately 30 mL/h.

After single intrathecal bolus injection/short-term infusion the volume of distribution, calculated from CSF levels, ranges from 22 to 157 mL.

Continuous Infusion: A study, conducted in 10 patients, suggests that the mean CSF clearance for continuous intrathecal infusion of baclofen is approximately 30 mL/h.

Continuous intrathecal infusion daily doses of 50 to 1200 μg result in lumbar CSF concentrations of baclofen as high as 130 to 1240 ng/mL at steady state. According to the half-life measured in the CSF, CSF steady-state concentrations will be reached within 1 to 2 days. Concurrent plasma concentrations of baclofen during intrathecal administration are expected to be low (0 to 5 ng/mL).

Limited pharmacokinetic data suggest that a lumbar-cisternal baclofen concentration gradient of about 4:1 is established during continuous baclofen infusion. This is based upon simultaneous CSF sampling via cisternal and lumbar tap during continuous baclofen infusion at the lumbar level in doses associated with therapeutic efficacy; the interpatient variability was great. This is of clinical importance insofar as spasticity in the lower extremities can be effectively treated with little effect on the upper limbs and with fewer CNS adverse reactions due to effects on the brain centres.

INDICATIONS: For the management of patients with severe spasticity due to spinal cord injury or multiple sclerosis who are unresponsive to oral baclofen or who experience unacceptable side effects at effective oral doses.

Intrathecal baclofen therapy may be considered as an alternative to destructive neurosurgical procedures.

Prior to implantation of a device for chronic intrathecal infusion, patients must demonstrate a positive clinical response to an intrathecal baclofen screening trial (see Dosage).

Intrathecal baclofen has been used in patients with spasticity of cerebral origin, e.g., spasticity following hypoxic encephalopathy, head injury, or stroke; however, clinical experience is limited.

CONTRAINDICATIONS: Known or suspected hypersensitivity to baclofen or to any of the excipients.

The drug should not be administered by the i.v., i.m., s.c. or epidural routes.

WARNINGS: Because of the possibility of potential life-threatening CNS depression, cardiovascular collapse and/or respiratory failure, physicians must be adequately trained in chronic intrathecal infusion therapy.

Specific instructions for programming and/or refilling the implantable pump are given by the pump manufacturers, and must be strictly adhered to. Consult pump manufacturer's literature for information on the appropriate use and care of these devices.

Because of the risks associated with the screening procedure and the adjustment of dosage following pump implantation, these phases must be conducted in a medically supervised and adequately equipped environment (see Dosage).

Resuscitative equipment should be available.

The pump system should not be implanted until the patient's response to bolus intrathecal injection of intrathecal baclofen has been properly evaluated and found to be clinically safe and effective.

Following surgical implantation of the pump, particularly during the initial phase of pump use the patient should be monitored closely until it is certain that the patient's response to the infusion is acceptable and reasonably stable.

On each occasion that the dosing rate of the pump and/or the concentration of intrathecal baclofen in the reservoir is adjusted, close medical monitoring is required until it is certain that the patient's response to the infusion is acceptable and reasonably stable.

It is mandatory that the patient and all those involved in the care of the patient receive adequate information regarding the risks of this mode of treatment. All medical personnel and care givers should be instructed in 1) the signs and symptoms of overdose, 2) procedures to be followed in the event of overdose and 3) proper home care of the pump and insertion site.

Overdose: Signs of overdose may appear suddenly or insidiously (see Overdose: Symptoms and Treatment).

Abrupt Drug Withdrawal:

> Abrupt discontinuation of intrathecal baclofen, regardless of the cause, has resulted in sequelae that include high fever, altered mental status, exaggerated rebound spasticity, and muscle rigidity, that in rare cases has advanced to rhabdomyolysis, multiple organ-system failure and death.
>
> Prevention of abrupt discontinuation of intrathecal baclofen requires careful attention to proper programming and monitoring of the infusion system, refill scheduling and procedures, and pump alarms. Patients and caregivers should be advised of the importance of keeping scheduled refill visits and should be educated on the early symptoms of baclofen withdrawal. Special attention should be given to patients at apparent risk (e.g., spinal cord injuries at T-6 or above, communication difficulties, history of withdrawal symptoms from oral or intrathecal baclofen). Consult the technical manual of the implantable infusion system for additional postimplant clinician and patient information. (See Warnings.)

Abrupt withdrawal of intrathecal baclofen, regardless of the cause, has resulted in sequelae that included high fever, altered mental status, exaggerated rebound spasticity, and muscle rigidity that in rare cases progressed to rhabdomyolysis, multiple organ-system failure, and death. In the first 9 years of postmarketing experience, 27 cases of withdrawal temporally related to the cessation of baclofen therapy were reported; 6 patients died. In most cases, symptoms of withdrawal appeared within hours to a few days following interruption of baclofen therapy. Common reasons for abrupt interruption of intrathecal baclofen therapy included malfunction of the catheter (especially disconnection), low volume in the pump reservoir, and end of pump battery life; human error may have played a causal or contributing role in some cases. Prevention of abrupt discontinuation of intrathecal baclofen requires careful attention to programming and monitoring of the infusion system, refill scheduling and procedures, and pump alarms. Patients and caregivers should be advised of the importance of keeping scheduled refill visits and should be educated on the early symptoms of baclofen withdrawal.

All patients receiving intrathecal baclofen therapy are potentially at risk for withdrawal. Early symptoms of baclofen withdrawal may include return of baseline spasticity, pruritus, hypotension, and paresthesias. Some clinical characteristics of the advanced intrathecal baclofen withdrawal syndrome may resemble autonomic dysreflexia, infection (sepsis), malignant hyperthermia, neuroleptic-malignant syndrome, or other conditions associated with a hypermetabolic state or widespread rhabdomyolysis.

Rapid, accurate diagnosis and treatment in an emergency room or intensive care setting are important in order to prevent the potentially life-threatening CNS and systemic effects of intrathecal baclofen withdrawal. The suggested treatment for intrathecal baclofen withdrawal is the restoration of intrathecal baclofen at or near the same dosage as before therapy was interrupted. However, if restoration of intrathecal delivery is delayed, treatment with GABA-ergic agonist drugs such as oral baclofen, or oral, enteral, or i.v. benzodiazepines may prevent potentially fatal sequelae. Oral baclofen alone should not be relied upon to halt the progression of the effects of intrathecal baclofen withdrawal.

Seizures have been reported during overdose and with withdrawal from baclofen intrathecal as well as in patients maintained on therapeutic doses of baclofen intrathecal.

Therefore, except for serious adverse reactions and overdose related emergencies, the dose should always be reduced slowly when the drug is discontinued (over a period of approximately 1 to 2 weeks).

PRECAUTIONS: Screening: Patients should be infection-free prior to the screening trial with intrathecal baclofen because the presence of a systemic infection may interfere with an assessment of the patient's response to bolus intrathecal baclofen.

Careful monitoring of respiratory and cardiovascular functions is essential during initial test dose administrations (screening phase), especially in patients with cardiopulmonary disease and respiratory muscle weakness as well as those being treated concomitantly with benzodiazepine-type preparations or opiates, who are at higher risk of respiratory depression.

Pump Implantation: Patients should be infection-free prior to pump implantation because the presence of infection may increase the risk of surgical complications. Moreover, a systemic infection may complicate attempts to adjust the dose.

Patient Monitoring: Following surgical implantation of the pump, particularly during the initial phases of pump use, and on each occasion that the dosing rate of the pump and/or the concentration of baclofen in the reservoir is adjusted, the patient should be monitored closely until it is certain that the patient's response to the infusion is acceptable and stable.

Pump Adjustment and Titration: In most patients, it will be necessary to increase the dose gradually over time to maintain effectiveness; a sudden requirement for substantial dose escalation typically indicates a catheter complication (i.e., catheter kink or dislodgment).

Reservoir Filling: Reservoir refilling must be performed by fully trained and qualified personnel following the directions provided by the pump manufacturer. Refill intervals should be carefully calculated to prevent depletion of the reservoir, as this would result in the return of severe spasticity. Depending on individual daily dose requirements and the flow rate of the pump, refill intervals generally vary between 1 and 3 months.

Strict aseptic filling is required to avoid microbial contamination and serious infection. A period of observation appropriate to the clinical situation should follow each refill or manipulation of the drug reservoir.

Extreme caution must be used when filling an implantable pump equipped with an injection port that allows direct access to the intrathecal catheter. Direct injection into the catheter through the access port may cause a life-threatening overdose.

In order to prevent excessive weakness and falling, intrathecal baclofen should be used with caution when spasticity is needed to sustain upright posture and balance in locomotion or whenever spasticity is used to maintain function.

It may be important to maintain some degree of muscle tone and allow occasional spasms to help support circulatory function and possibly prevent the formation of deep vein thrombosis.

An attempt should be made to discontinue concomitant oral antispastic medication to avoid possible overdose or adverse drug interactions, preferably before initiating baclofen infusion, with careful monitoring by the physician. However, abrupt reduction or discontinuation of concomitant antispastics during chronic intrathecal therapy with baclofen should be avoided.

Occupational Hazards: Drowsiness has been reported in some patients on intrathecal baclofen. Patients should be cautioned regarding the operation of automobiles or dangerous machinery, and activities made hazardous by decreased alertness.

Geriatrics: Several patients over the age of 65 years have been treated with intrathecal baclofen during the clinical trials without specific problems. Elderly patients may be more susceptible to the side effects of oral baclofen in the titration stage and this may also apply to intrathecal baclofen. However, as doses are individually titrated there is not likely to be a particular problem in treating elderly patients.

Children: Clinical experience with intrathecal baclofen in patients under 18 years of age is limited and safe use in this age group has not been established.

Pregnancy: Safe use of intrathecal baclofen during pregnancy has not been established. Baclofen crosses the placental barrier. High doses of oral baclofen are associated with an increased incidence of omphaloceles (abdominal hernias) in the fetuses of rats and of ossification defects in those of rats and rabbits. Therefore, the drug should be administered to pregnant patients or women of childbearing potential only when, in the judgment of the physician, the potential benefits outweigh the possible hazards.

Lactation: In mothers taking oral baclofen in therapeutic doses, the active substance passes into the breast milk. It is not known whether detectable levels of drug are present in breast milk of nursing mothers receiving intrathecal baclofen. As a general rule, nursing should be undertaken while a patient is receiving intrathecal baclofen only if the potential benefits outweigh the possible risks to the infant.

Patients with Special Diseases and Conditions: In patients with abnormal CSF flow, the spread of the drug and therefore, the distribution of antispastic activity may be inadequate.

Patients suffering from psychotic disorders, schizophrenia, confusional states, or Parkinson's disease should be treated cautiously with intrathecal baclofen and kept under careful surveillance, because exacerbations of these conditions have been observed with oral baclofen administration.

Special attention should be given to patients known to suffer from epilepsy since seizures have occasionally been reported during overdose with, and withdrawal from, intrathecal baclofen as well as in patients maintained on therapeutic doses of intrathecal baclofen.

Intrathecal baclofen should be used with caution in patients with a history of autonomic dysreflexia. The presence of nociceptive stimuli or abrupt withdrawal of intrathecal baclofen may cause an autonomic dysreflexic episode.

Baclofen should be used with caution in patients with cerebrovascular or respiratory insufficiency, as these conditions may be exacerbated by baclofen.

Interaction of intrathecal baclofen with underlying, non CNS related diseases is unlikely because the systemic availability of the drug after intrathecal administration is substantially lower than after oral administration. Nevertheless, observations after oral baclofen therapy suggest that caution should be exercised in the following situations: history of peptic ulcers, pre-existing sphincter hypertonia, impaired hepatic or renal function.

In rare instances elevated AST, alkaline phosphatase and glucose levels in the serum have been recorded when using oral baclofen.

Drug Interactions: There is inadequate systemic experience with the use of baclofen intrathecal in combination with other medications to predict specific drug-drug interactions. The combined use of morphine and intrathecal baclofen was responsible for hypotension in 1 patient. The potential for this combination to cause dyspnea or other CNS symptoms cannot be excluded.

The coadministration of other intrathecal agents with intrathecal baclofen has not been tested and the safety of these combinations is unknown.

The CNS depressant effects of alcohol and other compounds affecting the CNS may be additive to the effects of intrathecal baclofen.

When using oral baclofen, concurrent treatment with tricyclic antidepressants may potentiate the effect of baclofen, resulting in pronounced muscular hypotonia. Therefore, caution is advised when using intrathecal baclofen in this combination.

Since concomitant treatment with oral baclofen and antihypertensives is likely to increase antihypertensive effects, it is recommended that blood pressure is checked and if necessary, the dosage of antihypertensive medication adjusted accordingly.

Information to Be Provided to the Patient: See Information for the Patient.

ADVERSE EFFECTS: Baclofen has been shown to have general CNS depressant properties, causing sedation, somnolence, and respiratory and cardiovascular depression.

The most commonly reported adverse events with intrathecal baclofen in clinical trials were drowsiness, weakness in the lower extremities, dizziness/lightheadedness and seizures. Adverse events reported during controlled and uncontrolled studies in the United States of America are shown in Table 1.

A causal link between events observed and the administration of baclofen cannot be reliably assessed in many cases, since many of the adverse events reported are known to occur in association with the underlying conditions being treated.

Adverse events associated with the delivery system (e.g., catheter dislocation, pocket infection, meningitis, overdose due to wrong manipulation of the device) are in addition to those listed below.

In a fatal case of a child (causality with baclofen uncertain), inflammatory signs in the posterior horns and signs of arachnoiditis in proximity of the catheter tip were observed. This corresponds to observations in dogs, where chronic inflammatory reactions to the foreign body of the catheter were observed, independently of baclofen concentration.

Table 1: Lioresal Intrathecal

Incidence of Most Frequent Adverse Events in U.S. Clinical Trials

Adverse Event	Number of Patients Reporting Events (%) Screening (N=244)	Titration (N=214)	Maintenance (N=214)
Drowsiness	13 (5.3%)	11 (5.1%)	18 (8.4%)
Weakness, Lower Extremities	1 (0.4%)	11 (5.1%)	15 (7.0%)
Dizziness/Lightheadedness	6 (2.4%)	5 (2.3%)	12 (5.6%)
Seizures	1 (0.4%)	4 (1.9%)	11 (5.1%)
Headache	0 (0%)	3 (1.4%)	9 (4.2%)
Nausea/Vomiting	3 (1.2%)	5 (2.3%)	3 (1.4%)

(cont'd)

Table 1: Lioresal Intrathecal *(cont'd)*

Incidence of Most Frequent Adverse Events in U.S. Clinical Trials

	Number of Patients Reporting Events (%)		
Adverse Event	**Screening (N=244)**	**Titration (N=214)**	**Maintenance (N=214)**
Numbness/Itching/Tingling	2 (0.8%)	1 (0.5%)	8 (3.7%)
Hypotension	3 (1.2%)	0 (0%)	5 (2.3%)
Blurred Vision	0 (0%)	2 (0.9%)	5 (2.3%)
Constipation	0 (0%)	2 (0.9%)	5 (2.3%)
Hypotonia	2 (0.8%)	3 (1.4%)	2 (0.9%)
Slurred Speech	0 (0%)	1 (0.5%)	6 (2.8%)
Coma (Overdose)	0 (0%)	4 (1.9%)	3 (1.4%)
Lethargy	1 (0.4%)	0 (0%)	4 (1.9%)
Weakness, Upper Extremities	1 (0.4%)	0 (0%)	4 (1.9%)
Hypertension	1 (0.4%)	2 (0.9%)	2 (0.9%)
Dyspnea	1 (0.4%)	2 (0.9%)	1 (0.5%)

In addition to the more common adverse events reported above, the following adverse events were observed during clinical trials elsewhere or reported by clinicians using intrathecal baclofen on a humanitarian basis.

Central Nervous System: Occasional: sedation, accommodation disorders/double vision. Rare: respiratory depression, hypothermia, nystagmus, dysphagia, insomnia, somnolence, fatigue, decreased coordination, memory loss, confusion/disorientation, anxiety, depression, suicide ideation and attempt, euphoria, dysphoria, hallucinations, paranoia.

Cardiovascular: Occasional: bradycardia. Rare: deep vein thrombosis, skin flushing, paleness, pulmonary embolism.

Gastrointestinal Tract: Rare: dry mouth, diarrhea, decreased appetite, dehydration, ileus, decreased taste.

Respiratory: Occasional: bradypnea.

Genitourinary: Rare: urinary incontinence, sluggish bladder, bladder spasm, sexual dysfunction.

Skin and Appendages: Rare: urticaria, alopecia, facial edema, diaphoresis.

OVERDOSE:

Special attention must be given to recognizing the signs and symptoms of overdosage at all times, especially during the initial "screening" and "dose titration" phase of treatment and also during reintroduction of intrathecal baclofen after a period of interruption of therapy.

Symptoms: Signs of overdose may appear suddenly or insidiously.

Less sudden and/or less severe forms of overdose may present with signs of drowsiness, lightheadedness, dizziness, somnolence, seizures, loss of consciousness, hypothermia, excessive salivation, nausea and/or vomiting and cephalad progression of hypotonia. Respiratory depression, apnea, and coma result from serious overdosage.

Serious overdose may occur, for example, by inadvertent delivery of catheter contents during catheter patency/position analysis. Errors in programming, excessively rapid dose increases, and concomitant treatment with oral baclofen are other possible causes of overdosage. Possible pump malfunction should also be investigated.

Symptoms of severe intrathecal baclofen overdose (coma) were reported in a sensitive adult patient after receiving a 25 µg intrathecal bolus dose.

Treatment: There is no specific antidote for treating overdoses of intrathecal baclofen, however, the following steps should generally be undertaken. 1) Residual baclofen solution should be removed from the pump as soon as possible. 2) Patients with respiratory depression should be intubated if necessary, until the drug is eliminated.

If lumbar puncture is not contraindicated, consideration should be given in the early stage of the intoxication to withdrawing 30 to 40 mL of CSF to reduce CSF baclofen concentration.

Institute measures to support cardiovascular function.

In the event of convulsions, administer diazepam i.v. with caution.

Anecdotal reports suggest that i.v. physostigmine may reverse central side effects, notably drowsiness and respiratory depression.

Caution in administering physostigmine i.v. is advised, however, because its use has been associated with the induction of seizures, bradycardia, and cardiac conduction disturbances, a test dose of 0.5 mg i.v. is given initially. Give 1 to 2 mg slowly i.v. (over 2 minutes). Patients should be monitored closely during this time. If no clinical changes or cholinergic signs occur within 15 to 30 minutes, an additional 1 to 2 mg may be cautiously administered. Repeat doses of 1 to 2 mg i.v. every 30 minutes up to 2 hours. Physostigmine may not be effective in reversing large overdoses and patients may need to be maintained with respiratory support.

As the CNS effects of physostigmine may wear off rapidly, it is important to monitor the patient continuously.

Physostigmine is the only drug of this class that may be used. Neostigmine should not be used as it does not have any CNS effects.

If symptoms of cholinergic toxicity develop, physostigmine should be discontinued.

For management of a suspected drug overdose, CPhA recommends that you contact your **regional Poison Control Centre**. See the *CPS* Directory section for a list of Poison Control Centres.

DOSAGE: Establishment of the optimum dose schedule requires that each patient undergoes an initial screening phase with intrathecal bolus, followed by a very careful individual dose titration prior to maintenance therapy. This is due to the great variability in the effective individual therapeutic dose.

General: **The first dose should be performed with resuscitative equipment on stand-by.**

Patients must be monitored closely in a fully equipped and staffed environment during the screening phase and dose titration period immediately following implant. Resuscitative equipment should be available for immediate use in case of life-threatening or intolerable adverse reactions. Implantation of pumps should only be performed in experienced centres in order to minimize the risks in the perioperative phase.

Screening Phase: Prior to initiation of chronic infusion of intrathecal baclofen, patients must demonstrate a response to intrathecal baclofen bolus in a screening trial. A test bolus dose of baclofen is usually administered via a lumbar puncture or an intrathecal catheter to elicit a response. For this purpose low concentration ampuls of 0.05 mg/mL are available.

The usual initial test dose is 25 µg or 50 µg and is stepped up by 25 µg increments at least 24 hours apart, until an approximately 4 to 8 hour response is observed; the dose should be given by barbotage over at least 1 minute. If an adverse reaction occurs at a dose of 25 µg, a lower dose, such as 10 µg may be tested.

Patients should demonstrate a positive clinical response in order to be considered responders to treatment. A positive clinical response is characterized by a significant decrease in muscle tone and/or frequency and/or severity of spasms. There is great variability in sensitivity to intrathecal baclofen.

Patients who do not respond to a 100 µg test dose should not be given further increases of dose or be considered for continuous intrathecal infusion. However, in rare instances some patients, particularly those with spasticity of cerebral origin, have received higher test bolus doses.

Dose Titration Phase: After confirmation that the patient is responsive to intrathecal baclofen by means of test bolus doses, intrathecal infusion is established using a suitable delivery system (see Drug delivery devices).

To determine the initial total daily dose of intrathecal baclofen following implant, the screening dose which gave a positive effect should be doubled and administered over a 24 hour period, unless the efficacy of the bolus dose was maintained for more than 12 hours. In this case the starting daily dose should be the screening dose delivered over a 24 hour period. No dose increases should be administered in the first 24 hours.

After the first 24 hours, the dosage should be adjusted slowly on a daily basis to achieve the desired effect, with dosage increments limited to 10 to 30% to avoid possible overdosing. With programmable pumps, the dose should be increased only once every 24 hours. For nonprogrammable pumps with a 76 cm catheter delivering 1 mL/day, intervals of 48 hours are suggested for evaluation of response. If the daily dose has been significantly increased and no clinical effect is achieved, check for proper pump function and catheter patency.

The clinical goal is to maintain muscle tone as close to normal as possible, and to minimize the frequency and severity of spasms without inducing intolerable side effects.

There is limited experience with doses greater than 1000 µg/day.

Maintenance Therapy: The lowest dose giving an adequate response should be used. Most patients require gradual increases in dose over time to maintain optimum response during chronic therapy due to decreased responsiveness to therapy or to progress of the disease.

The daily dose may be gradually increased by 10 to 30% to maintain adequate symptom control by adjusting the dosing rate of the pump and/or the concentration of intrathecal baclofen in the reservoir. The daily dose may also be reduced by 10 to 20% if patients experience side effects. A sudden requirement for substantial dose escalation suggests a catheter complication (i.e., catheter kink or dislodgment) or pump malfunction.

Maintenance dosage for long-term continuous infusion of intrathecal baclofen ranges from 10 to 1200 µg/day, most patients being adequately maintained on 300 to 800 µg/day. The specific concentration that should be used depends upon the total daily dose required as well as the delivery rate of the pump. Please consult pump manufacturer's manual for specific recommendations.

During long-term treatment approximately 10% of patients become refractory to increasing doses. There is not sufficient experience to make firm recommendations for tolerance management; however, in 17 patients, the use of a "drug holiday" by switching for 10 to 14 days to intrathecal preservative-free morphine sulfate has been reported as an effective approach to the management of tolerance. After a few days the sensitivity to baclofen may be restored; treatment should be resumed at the initial continuous infusion dose and followed by a titration phase to avoid overdose accidents. This must be performed in a hospital unit.

Regular clinical review remains a necessity throughout to assess dosage requirements, functioning of the delivery system, and monitoring for possible adverse drug reactions or evidence of infection.

Delivery Regimen: Intrathecal baclofen is most often administered in a continuous infusion mode immediately following implant. After the patient has stabilized with regard to daily dose and functional status, and provided the pump allows it, a more complex mode of delivery may be started to optimize control of spasticity at different times of the day. For example, patients who have increased spasm at night may require a 20% increase in their hourly infusion rate. Changes in flow rate should be programmed to start 2 hours before the time of desired clinical effect.

Drug Delivery Devices: Intrathecal administration of baclofen through an implanted delivery system should only be undertaken by physicians with the necessary knowledge and experience. Specific instructions for programming and/or refilling the implantable pump are given by the pump manufacturers, and must be strictly adhered to. Consult pump manufacturer's literature for information on the appropriate use and care of these devices.

Evidence demonstrating the efficacy of intrathecal baclofen was obtained using the Medtronic SynchroMed Programmable Infusion System. Other pumps proven to be suitable for intrathecal baclofen administration may be used.

The Medtronic SynchroMed Programmable Infusion System, that is an implantable drug delivery system with refillable reservoirs which, after general or local anesthesia, is implanted in a s.c. pocket usually on the abdominal wall. This device is connected to an intrathecal catheter that passes s.c. to the subarachnoid space.

The Medtronic SynchroMed Programmable Infusion System has an 18 mL drug reservoir and may be programmed to different flow rates such as single bolus, periodic boluses, continuous and complex continuous. However, the lithium battery of the pump has a life span of 3 to 4 years and therefore requires replacement.

Intrathecal baclofen proved to be stable in the implanted SynchroMed Programmable Infusion System for 11 weeks.

Details regarding the availability and use of this drug delivery device can be obtained from the manufacturers: Medtronic of Canada Ltd., 6733 Kitimat Road, Mississauga, Ontario, L5N 1W3. 1-800-268-5346; Fax: 1-905-826-6620.

General guidelines regarding the use of all implantable systems are located under Precautions.

Before using other systems, it must be confirmed that the technical specifications, including chemical stability of baclofen in the reservoir fulfil the requirements for safe and effective use of intrathecal baclofen. Please consult pump manufacturer's manual for this information.

Parenteral Products: Instructions for use/handling: Intrathecal baclofen is intended for intrathecal injection and continuous intrathecal infusion as indicated by the delivery specifications of the infusion system.

Each ampul is intended for single use only. Discard any unused portion.

Parenteral drug products should be inspected for particulate matter and discoloration prior to administration whenever solution and container permit.

The concentration to be used depends upon the total daily dose required as well as the delivery rate of the pump. Please consult manufacturer's manual for specific recommendations.

For patients who require concentrations other than 0.05 mg/mL, 0.5 mg/mL or 2 mg/mL, intrathecal baclofen must be diluted, under aseptic conditions, with sterile preservative-free sodium chloride injection and used immediately.

As a rule baclofen ampuls for intrathecal administration should not be mixed with other infusion or injection solutions. Dextrose proved to be incompatible due to a chemical reaction with baclofen.

INFORMATION FOR THE PATIENT: Published in e-CPS, available by subscription at www.e-cps.ca.

SUPPLIED: 0.05 mg/mL: Each mL of clear, colorless solution contains: baclofen 0.05 mg for intrathecal administration. Nonmedicinal ingredients: sodium chloride and water for injection. Ampuls of 1 mL. Cartons of 5.

0.5 mg/mL: Each mL of clear, colorless solution contains: baclofen 0.5 mg for intrathecal administration. Nonmedicinal ingredients: sodium chloride and water for injection. Ampuls of 20 mL. Cartons of 1.

2 mg/mL: Each mL of clear, colorless solution contains: baclofen 2 mg for intrathecal administration. Nonmedicinal ingredients: sodium chloride and water for injection. Ampuls of 5 mL. Cartons of 5.

Protect from heat (store at 15 to 30°C). Do not freeze. Do not heat sterilize. Lioresal Intrathecal must be kept out of the reach and sight of children.

(Shown in Product Identification Section)

Lioresal® Oral Ⓟ

baclofen

Muscle Relaxant—Antispastic

Novartis Pharmaceuticals

Date of Revision: September 2, 2009

PHARMACOLOGY: The precise mechanisms of action of LIORESAL (baclofen) are not fully known. It inhibits both monosynaptic and polysynaptic reflexes at the spinal level, probably by hyperpolarization of afferent terminals, although actions at supraspinal sites may also occur and contribute to its clinical effect. Although LIORESAL is an analog of the putative inhibitory neurotransmitter gamma-aminobutyric acid (GABA), there is no conclusive evidence that actions on GABA systems are involved in the production of its clinical effects.

Peak plasma concentrations of LIORESAL are achieved within 2 hours and the plasma half-life is 2-4 hours.

INDICATIONS: LIORESAL (baclofen) is useful for the alleviation of signs and symptoms of spasticity resulting from multiple sclerosis.

LIORESAL may also be of some value in patients with spinal cord injuries and other spinal cord diseases.

CONTRAINDICATIONS: Hypersensitivity to LIORESAL (baclofen) or to any of the excipients.

WARNINGS: Abrupt Drug Withdrawal: Following abrupt withdrawal of LIORESAL (baclofen), visual and auditory hallucinations, convulsions (status epilepticus), dyskinesia, confusion, psychotic, manic or paranoid states, anxiety with tachycardia and sweating, insomnia, and worsening of spasticity have occurred. Therefore, except for serious adverse reactions, the dose should be reduced slowly when the drug is discontinued (over a period of approximately 1-2 weeks).

For the intrathecal formulation of LIORESAL, it has been reported that clinical characteristics of withdrawal may resemble autonomic dysreflexia, malignant hyperthermia, neuroleptic-malignant syndrome, or other conditions associated with a hypermetabolic state or widespread rhabdomyolysis.

Impaired Renal Function: Because LIORESAL is primarily excreted unchanged through the kidneys, it should be given with caution in patients with renal insufficiency, and generally with a reduced dose. In patients dependent on dialysis, a particularly low dose of LIORESAL should be selected i.e. approximately 5 mg daily.

Unscheduled hemodialysis may be considered a treatment option in cases of severe baclofen toxicity as hemodialysis has been reported to effectively remove baclofen from the body, alleviate clinical symptoms of overdose and shorten the recovery time in these patients.

End Stage Renal Failure: LIORESAL should only be administered to end stage renal failure patients when benefits are considered acceptable, given potential risks. These patients should be closely monitored for prompt diagnosis of early signs and/or symptoms of toxicity (e.g. somnolence, lethargy) (see Overdose, Symptoms and Treatment).

Concomitant Medications that May Impact Renal Function: Particular caution is required when combining LIORESAL to drugs or medicinal products that can significantly impact renal function. Renal function shall be closely monitored and LIORESAL daily dosage adjusted accordingly to prevent baclofen toxicity (see Precautions, Drug Interactions).

Stroke: LIORESAL has not significantly benefited patients with stroke. These patients have also shown poor tolerability to the drug.

Pregnancy: Safe use of LIORESAL during pregnancy or lactation has not been established. Baclofen crosses the placental barrier. High doses are associated with an increased incidence of abdominal hernias in the fetuses of rats and of ossification defects in those of rats and rabbits. Therefore, the drug should be administered to pregnant patients, or women of child-bearing potential only when, in the judgment of the physician, the potential benefits outweigh the possible hazards.

Epilepsy: Extreme caution should be exercised in patients with epilepsy or a history of convulsive disorders. In such patients, the clinical state and electroencephalogram should be monitored at regular intervals during therapy, as deterioration in seizure control and EEG has been reported occasionally in patients taking LIORESAL.

PRECAUTIONS: Children: Safe use of LIORESAL (baclofen) in children under age 12 has not been established and it is, therefore, not recommended for use in children.

Effects on Ability to Drive and Use Machines: LIORESAL may be associated with dizziness, sedation, somnolence and visual disturbance (see Adverse Effects) which may impair the patient's reaction. Patients experiencing these adverse reactions should be advised to refrain from driving or using machines. Patients should also be cautioned that the central nervous system effects of LIORESAL may be additive to those of alcohol and other CNS depressants.

General: LIORESAL should be used with caution where spasticity is utilized to sustain upright posture and balance in locomotion, or whenever spasticity is utilized to obtain increased function.

Caution should also be used in treating the following populations: patients with peptic ulceration (or a history of); elderly patients with cerebrovascular disorders; and patients with respiratory or hepatic failure. **Regarding patients with renal failure, see Warnings, Impaired Renal Function.**

Urinary Disorders: LIORESAL should be used with caution in patients with underlying bladder sphincter hypertonia, since acute retention of urine may occur.

Psychiatric and Nervous System Disorders: Patients with psychiatric disorders such as psychosis, schizophrenia, or confusional states should be treated cautiously with LIORESAL and kept under close surveillance, since exacerbation of these conditions may occur with LIORESAL treatment.

Laboratory Tests: The following laboratory tests have been found to be abnormal in a few patients receiving LIORESAL: AST, alkaline phosphatase and blood sugar (all elevated). Therefore, in patients with liver diseases or diabetes mellitus, appropriate laboratory tests should be performed periodically in order to ensure that no drug-induced changes in these underlying diseases have occurred.

Drug Interactions: The concomitant administration of baclofen and tricyclic antidepressants may potentiate the pharmacological effects of baclofen, resulting in pronounced muscular hypotonia.

The concurrent use of MAO inhibitors and LIORESAL may result in increased CNS-depressant effects; therefore, caution is advised and the dosage of one or both agents should be adjusted accordingly.

Since combined treatment with LIORESAL and antihypertensives is likely to increase the fall in blood pressure, the dosage of antihypertensive medication should be adjusted accordingly.

In patients with Parkinson's disease receiving treatment with baclofen and levodopa plus carbidopa, there have been several reports of mental confusion, hallucinations and agitation.

Isolated cases of increased blood glucose concentrations have been reported with LIORESAL; dosage adjustments of antidiabetic agents (oral and insulin) may therefore be necessary with combined LIORESAL treatment.

Caution should be exercised when administering LIORESAL and magnesium sulfate (or other neuromuscular blocking agents), since a synergistic effect may theoretically occur.

Drugs or medicinal products that can significantly impact renal function may reduce baclofen excretion leading to toxic effects (see Warnings, Impaired Renal Function).

Lactation: LIORESAL is excreted in human milk. As a general rule, nursing should not be undertaken while a patient is on a drug.

ADVERSE EFFECTS: Adverse effects most frequently occur at the start of treatment (e.g. sedation, somnolence), particularly if the dosage is increased too rapidly, if large doses are administered, and in the elderly patient. However, these effects are often transient and can be alleviated or eliminated by decreasing the dosage; they are seldom severe enough to warrant withdrawal of the medication. In elderly patients or those patients with cerebrovascular disorder or a history of psychiatric illness, more serious adverse reactions may occur, such as hallucinations and confusion.

The most common adverse reactions associated with LIORESAL (baclofen) are transient somnolence, sedation, dizziness, weakness and fatigue. Other adverse reactions reported were:

Neuropsychiatric: headache (<10%), insomnia (<10%), muscular weakness, light-headedness, lassitude, exhaustion, tremor, ataxia, respiratory depression, euphoric mood, depression, confusional state, hallucinations, nightmares, myalgia, nystagmus, and, rarely (≥0.01% to <0.1%), excitement, paresthesia, tinnitus, slurred speech, coordination disorder, rigidity, dystonia, blurred vision, strabismus, miosis, mydriasis, diplopia, dysarthria, epileptic seizures, lowered convulsion threshold, and, very rarely (<0.01%), hypothermia.

Cardiovascular: hypotension (<10%), cardiac output decreased, rare instances (≥0.01% to <0.1%) of dyspnea, palpitation, chest pain, syncope.

Gastrointestinal: nausea (approx. 10%), constipation (<10%), gastrointestinal disturbance, retching, vomiting, diarrhea, dry mouth, and, rarely (≥0.01% to <0.1%), anorexia, dysgeusia, abdominal pain, and positive test for occult blood in stool.

Genitourinary: pollakiuria (<10%), enuresis, dysuria, and, rarely (≥0.01% to <0.1%), inability to ejaculate, nocturia, hematuria, urinary retention and erectile dysfunction.

Other: instances of rash, pruritus, ankle edema, hyperhidrosis, weight gain, nasal congestion, accommodation disorders, visual disturbances, and, rarely (≥0.01% to <0.1%), hepatic function abnormal.

Certain patients have shown increased muscle spasticity as a paradoxical reaction to the medication.

Muscular hypotonia of a degree sufficient to make walking or movement difficult may occur, but is usually relieved by readjusting the dosage. For this purpose, the daytime dose may be reduced and the evening dose increased.

Some of the CNS and genitourinary symptoms reported may be related to the underlying disease rather than to drug therapy.

OVERDOSE:

Symptoms: Symptoms of overdosage are predominantly those of central nervous system depression and include drowsiness, impairment of consciousness, respiratory depression, coma, seizures, confusion, hallucinations, agitation, EEG changes (burst suppression pattern and triphasic waves), accommodation disorders, absent pupillary reflexes, muscular hypotonia, myoclonia, hyporeflexia or areflexia, hypotension or hypertension, bradycardia, tachycardia or cardiac arrhythmias, hypothermia, peripheral vasodilatation, nausea, vomiting, diarrhea, increased salivation, elevated LDH, AST, alkaline phosphatase and blood glucose values.

The signs and symptoms may be further aggravated by co-administration of a variety of other agents including alcohol, diazepam, and tricyclic antidepressants.

Treatment: There is no specific antidote. Supportive measures and symptomatic treatment should be given for complications such as hypotension, hypertension, convulsions, gastrointestinal disturbances, and respiratory or cardiovascular depression.

After ingestion of a potentially toxic amount, activated charcoal should be considered, especially during the early period after ingestion. Gastric decontamination (e.g. gastric lavage) should be considered in individual cases, especially in the early period (60 minutes) after ingestion of a potentially life-threatening overdose. Comatose or convulsing patients should be intubated prior to the initiation of gastric decontamination. A high urinary output should be maintained since LIORESAL (baclofen) is excreted mainly by the kidneys. For this purpose, generous quantities of fluid should be administered, possibly together with a diuretic. Hemodialysis (sometimes unscheduled) is indicated in severe poisoning associated with renal failure (see Warnings, Impaired Renal Function). In the event of convulsions, administer diazepam i.v. with caution.

> For management of a suspected drug overdose, contact your regional Poison Control Centre. See the *CPS* Directory section for a list of Poison Control Centres.

DOSAGE: The determination of optimal dosage of LIORESAL (baclofen) requires individual titration. Start therapy at a low dosage and increase gradually until optimum effect is achieved (usually between 40-80 mg daily).

Treatment should be started with a dosage of 15 mg daily, preferably in divided doses.

The following dosage titration schedule is suggested: 5 mg t.i.d. for 3 days; 10 mg t.i.d. for 3 days; 15 mg t.i.d. for 3 days; 20 mg t.i.d. for 3 days.

Thereafter, additional increases may be necessary but the total daily dose should not exceed a maximum of 80 mg daily (20 mg q.i.d.).

The lowest dose compatible with an optimal response is recommended. If benefits are not evident after a reasonable trial period, patients should be slowly withdrawn from the drug (see Warnings).

Impaired Renal Function: Because LIORESAL is primarily excreted unchanged through the kidneys, it should be given with caution in patients with renal insufficiency, and generally with a reduced dose. In patients dependent on dialysis, a particularly low dose of LIORESAL should be selected i.e. approximately 5 mg daily (see Warnings, Impaired Renal Function).

INFORMATION FOR THE PATIENT: Published in e-CPS, available by subscription at www.e-cps.ca.

SUPPLIED: 10 mg: Each white to off-white, oval, flat-faced, bevel-edged tablet, engraved GEIGY on one side and engraved KJ on the other (fully bisected between the K and J), contains: baclofen 10 mg. Nonmedicinal ingredients: cellulose compounds, cornstarch, magnesium stearate and povidone. Energy: 8.6 kJ (2.05 kcal). Alcohol-, bisulfite-, gluten-, lactose-, parabens-, sodium- and tartrazine-free. Bottles of 100. LIORESAL must be kept out of the reach and sight of children.

D.S. 20 mg: Each white to off-white, capsule-shaped tablet, engraved GEIGY on one side and engraved GW on the other (fully bisected between the G and W), contains: baclofen 20 mg. Nonmedicinal ingredients: cellulose compounds, cornstarch, magnesium stearate and povidone. Energy: 1.7 kJ (0.41 kcal). Alcohol-, bisulfite-, gluten-, lactose-, parabens-, sodium- and tartrazine-free. Bottles of 100. LIORESAL must be kept out of the reach and sight of children.

(Shown in Product Identification Section)

Lipidil EZ® Ⓟ

fenofibrate nanocrystals

Lipid Metabolism Regulator

Fournier Pharma

Date of Preparation: July 12, 2005
Date of Revision: October 1, 2007

PHARMACOLOGY: LIPIDIL EZ (fenofibrate) lowers elevated serum lipids by decreasing the low-density lipoprotein (LDL) fraction rich in cholesterol and the very low-density lipoprotein (VLDL) fraction rich in triglycerides. In addition, fenofibrate increases the high-density lipoprotein (HDL) cholesterol fraction.

Fenofibrate appears to have a greater depressant effect on the very low-density lipoproteins (VLDL) than on the low-density lipoproteins (LDL). Therapeutic doses of fenofibrate produce elevations of HDL cholesterol, a reduction in the content of the low-density lipoprotein cholesterol, and a substantial reduction in the triglyceride content of very low-density lipoproteins.

Recent findings suggest that the lipid modulating effects of fenofibrate are mediated by the activation of a specific nuclear receptor called peroxisome proliferator activated receptor alpha (PPARα), which produces: a reduction in apo C-III, and therefore a reduction in the level of dense atherogenic LDL particles; a stimulation of mitochondrial beta-oxidation, and therefore a reduction in triglyceride secretion; a rise in lipoprotein lipase production, and therefore an acceleration of triglyceride rich lipoprotein breakdown; a rise in apo A-I and apo A-II production, and a corresponding rise in HDL.

After oral administration, fenofibrate is rapidly hydrolysed to fenofibric acid, the active metabolite. In man, fenofibric acid is eliminated as the glucuronic acid conjugate and is mainly excreted through the kidney. In man, the elimination half-life of fenofibric acid is about 20-24 hours, a value that is not modified after multiple dosing.

In healthy elderly patients (77 to 87 years of age), the terminal half-life is prolonged, but no dose adjustment is required due to unchanged clearance.

Concomitant Administration with Ezetimibe: Administration of fenofibrate with ezetimibe is effective in improving serum total-C, LDL-C, Apo-B, TG, HDL-C, and non-HDL-C in patients with mixed hyperlipidemia.

Clinical studies have demonstrated that elevated levels of total-C, low density lipoprotein cholesterol (LDL-C) and apolipoprotein B (Apo B; the major protein constituent of LDL), promote atherosclerosis in humans. In addition, decreased levels of high density lipoprotein cholesterol (HDL-C) are associated with the development of atherosclerosis. Epidemiologic studies have established that cardiovascular morbidity and mortality vary directly with the level of total-C and LDL-C and inversely with the level of HDL-C. Like LDL, cholesterol-enriched triglyceride-rich lipoproteins, including very low density lipoproteins (VLDL), intermediate density lipoproteins (IDL), and remnants, can also promote atherosclerosis. **The effects of fenofibrate given with ezetimibe on cardiovascular morbidity and mortality have not been established.**

Pediatrics: Safety and effectiveness have not been established in pediatric patients.

Renal Insufficiency: In patients with severe renal impairment, the rate of clearance of fenofibric acid is greatly reduced, and the compound accumulates during chronic dosage.

In patients having moderate renal impairment (creatinine clearance of 50 to 90 mL per min), the oral clearance and oral volume of distribution of fenofibric acid are increased compared to healthy adults (2.1 L/h and 95 L versus 1.1 L/h and 30 L, respectively). Therefore, the dosage of LIPIDIL EZ should be minimized in patients who have severe renal impairment, while no modification of dosage is required in patients having moderate renal impairment.

Hepatic insufficiency: No pharmacokinetic studies have been conducted in patients having hepatic insufficiency.

No gender-related differences in pharmacokinetics and metabolism have been observed.

Fenofibric acid is extensively bound (>99%) to plasma albumin. This binding is not saturable.

Absorption of a micronized fenofibrate formulation (LIPIDIL Micro 200 mg capsules) is low and variable when administered under fasting conditions and increases when given with food. Fenofibrate, given in a micro-coated formulation (LIPIDIL Supra 160 mg tablets), requires lower doses (160 mg) to achieve equivalent plasma levels to the micronized (200 mg) formulation. Nanocrystallization of fenofibrate allows for further reduction in the dose (LIPIDIL EZ 145 mg tablets), and LIPIDIL EZ may be taken without regard to meals, because of optimized product absorption.

In a single-dose three-way randomized crossover bioavailability study in 72 healthy male and female volunteers, under low fat fed conditions, one 145 mg LIPIDIL EZ or three 48 mg LIPIDIL EZ tablets were compared to one 200 mg micronized capsule (LIPIDIL Micro 200 mg). Each subject received a single oral dose of each formulation with a low fat breakfast (30% fat, approx. 400 Kcal), with a two-week interval between doses. See Table 1 and Table 2.

These data demonstrate that comparable bioavailability was achieved between LIPIDIL EZ, 145 mg or 3×48 mg tablets, and LIPIDIL Micro 200 mg capsules.

In a single-dose two-way randomized crossover bioavailability study in 40 healthy male volunteers, under low fat fed conditions, one 145 mg LIPIDIL EZ tablet was compared to one 160 mg LIPIDIL Supra tablet. Each subject received a single oral dose of each formulation with a low fat breakfast (30% fat, approx. 400 Kcal), with a two-week interval between doses. See Table 3.

These data demonstrate that comparable bioavailability was achieved between, 145 mg LIPIDIL EZ tablets and LIPIDIL Supra 160 mg tablets.

A study to examine the effect of food on the absorption of nanocrystallized fenofibrate was performed as a single-dose three-way randomized cross-over bioavailability study in 45 healthy male and female volunteers. Each subject received a single dose of 145 mg LIPIDIL EZ with either a high fat breakfast [50% fat, approx. 1000 Kcal, High Fat Fed (HFF)], a low fat breakfast [30% fat, approx. 400 Kcal; Low Fat Fed (LFF)] or no breakfast (fasted state), with a two-week interval between study arms. See Table 4 and Table 5.

Table 1: LIPIDIL EZ

Summary Table of the Comparative Bioavailability Data: A Single Dose Study (LIPIDIL EZ 145 mg tablet vs LIPIDIL Micro 200 mg capsule)

Analyte: Fenofibric Acid From Measured and Log Transformed Data Geometric Mean Arithmetic Mean (CV %)				
Parameter	Test: LIPIDIL EZ 145 mg	Reference: LIPIDIL Micro 200 mg	% Ratio of Geometric Means	90% Confidence Interval
AUC_T (µg·h/mL)	148.47 153.5 (27%)	170.49 174.2 (25%)	87.1%	85.2–89.0%
AUC_I (µg·h/mL)	151.69 157.4 (28%)	176.03 180.4 (27%)	86.2%	84.3–88.1%
C_{MAX} (µg/mL)	8.646 8.80 (19%)	8.582 8.87 (26%)	100.8%	96.8–104.9%
T_{MAX}[a] (h)	3.5 (35%)	4.4 (38%)		
$T_{½}$[a] (h)	20.7 (24%)	22.0 (34%)		

[a] Expressed as arithmetic mean (CV%) only.

Table 2: LIPIDIL EZ

Summary Table of the Comparative Bioavailability Data: A Single Dose Study (LIPIDIL EZ 3×48 mg tablet vs LIPIDIL Micro 200 mg capsule)

Analyte: Fenofibric Acid From Measured and Log Transformed Data Geometric Mean Arithmetic Mean (CV %)				
Parameter	Test: LIPIDIL EZ 3×48 mg	Reference: LIPIDIL Micro 200 mg	% Ratio of Geometric Means	90% Confidence Interval
AUC_T (µg·h/mL)	148.29 153.3 (27%)	170.49 174.2 (25%)	87.0%	85.1–88.9%
AUC_I (µg·h/mL)	151.34 157.0 (29%)	176.03 180.4 (27%)	86.0%	84.3–88.1%
C_{MAX} (µg/mL)	8.399 8.54 (19%)	8.582 8.87 (26%)	97.9%	94.0–101.9%
T_{MAX}[a] (h)	3.6 (35%)	4.4 (38%)		
$T_{½}$[a] (h)	20.1 (23%)	22.0 (34%)		

[a] Expressed as arithmetic mean (CV%) only.

Table 3: LIPIDIL EZ

Summary Table of the Comparative Bioavailability Data: A Single Dose Study (LIPIDIL EZ 145 mg tablet vs LIPIDIL Supra 160 mg tablet)

Analyte: Fenofibric Acid From Measured and Log Transformed Data Geometric Mean Arithmetic Mean (CV %)				
Parameter	Test LIPIDIL EZ 145 mg tablet	Reference LIPIDIL Supra 160 mg tablet	% Ratio of Geometric Means	90% Confidence Interval
AUC_T (µg·h/mL)	103.52 107.99 (29%)	103.93 108.96 (29%)	99.6%	96.2–103.1%
AUC_I (µg·h/mL)	105.00 109.53 (29%)	105.80 110.86 (29%)	99.2%	96.0–102.6%
C_{MAX} (µg/mL)	8.02 8.14 (17%)	6.73 6.91 (23%)	119.2%	111.5–127.4%
T_{MAX}[a] (h)	2.88 (42%)	3.72 (31%)		
$T_{½}$[a] (h)	17.15 (20%)	18.74 (20%)		

[a] Expressed as arithmetic mean (CV %) only.

These data demonstrate that LIPIDIL EZ can be administered with or without food, as there was no effect of food on the bioavailability of the nanocrystallized fenofibrate tablets when compared to the bioavailability under the fasted state.

INDICATIONS: LIPIDIL EZ is indicated as an adjunct to diet, at least equivalent to the Adults Treatment Panel III (ATP III) and Therapeutic Lifestyle Changes (TLC diet), and other therapeutic measures when the response to diet and other measures has been inadequate for: Treatment of patients, including patients with type 2 diabetes (non-insulin dependent), with dyslipoproteinemia (hypercholesterolemia, Fredrickson classification Types IIa and IIb mixed hyperlipidemia), to regulate lipid levels by reducing serum triglycerides and LDL cholesterol levels and increasing HDL cholesterol. Treatment of adult patients with very high serum triglyceride levels, Fredrickson classification Type IV and Type V hyperlipidemia, who are at a high risk of sequelae and complications (i.e., pancreatitis) from their hyperlipidemia.

LIPIDIL EZ, administered in combination with ezetimibe, is indicated for the reduction of elevated total-C, LDL-C, Apo B, and non HDL-C in patients with mixed hyperlipidemia.

LIPIDIL EZ alone may not be adequate therapy in some patients with familial combined hyperlipidemia with Type IIb and Type IV hyperlipoproteinemia.

LIPIDIL EZ (fenofibrate) is not indicated for the treatment of Type I hyperlipoproteinemia.

CONTRAINDICATIONS: Hepatic or severe renal dysfunction (creatinine clearance <20 mL per min), including primary biliary cirrhosis. Pre-existing gallbladder disease (see Warnings). Hypersensitivity to fenofibrate, any component of this medication or other drugs of the fibrate class. Should not be taken in patients allergic to peanut or arachis oil or soya lecithin or related products due to the risk of hypersensitivity reactions. The drug should not be used during pregnancy and breast-feeding. Known photoallergy or phototoxic reaction during treatment with fibrates or ketoprofen. When LIPIDIL EZ is to be administered with ezetimibe, the contraindications to ezetimibe should be reviewed before starting concomitant therapy.

Table 4: LIPIDIL EZ

Summary Table of the Comparative Bioavailability Data: A Single Dose Study (LIPIDIL EZ 145 mg tablets high fat fed vs fasted conditions)

Analyte: Fenofibric Acid From Measured and Log Transformed Data Geometric Mean Arithmetic Mean (CV %)				
Parameter	Test: 145 mg high fat fed	Reference: 145 mg fasted	% Ratio of Geometric Means	90% Confidence Interval
AUC_T (µg·h/mL)	123.0 127.9 (27.7%)	116.5 121.6 (28.1%)	105.4%	102.0–109.0%
AUC_I (µg·h/mL)	124.8 129.9 (28.0%)	118.5 123.8 (28.8%)	105.2%	101.8–108.8%
C_{MAX} (µg/mL)	7.82 7.96 (18.5)	7.77 7.94 (20.1%)	100.7%	96.3–105.4%
T_{MAX}[a] (h)	4.27 (45.5%)	2.33 (31.4%)		
$T_{½}$[a] (h)	17.8 (23.3%)	18.9 (24.9%)		

[a] Expressed as arithmetic mean (CV %) only.

Table 5: LIPIDIL EZ

Summary Table of the Comparative Bioavailability Data: A Single Dose Study (LIPIDIL EZ 145 mg tablets low fat fed vs fasted conditions)

Analyte: Fenofibric Acid From Measured and Log Transformed Data Geometric Mean Arithmetic Mean (CV %)				
Parameter	Test: 145 mg low fat fed	Reference: 145 mg fasted	% Ratio of Geometric Means	90% Confidence Interval
AUC_T (µg·h/mL)	118.1 123.2 (28.4%)	116.5 121.6 (28.1%)	101.3%	98.1–104.7%
AUC_I (µg·h/mL)	119.8 125.1 (28.7%)	118.5 123.8 (28.8%)	101.2%	97.8–104.6%
C_{MAX} (µg/mL)	7.84 7.96 (17.9%)	7.77 7.94 (20.1%)	100.9%	96.4–105.5%
T_{MAX}[a] (h)	3.56 (33.1%)	2.33 (31.4%)		
$T_{½}$[a] (h)	18.7 (19.5%)	18.9 (24.9%)		

[a] Expressed as arithmetic mean (CV %) only.

WARNINGS: General: When LIPIDIL EZ is to be administered with ezetimibe, the ezetimibe Product Monograph should be consulted.

Fenofibrate and HMG-CoA Reductase Inhibitors (Statins): **The concomitant administration of fenofibrate and statins should be avoided unless the benefit for further alteration in lipid levels is likely to outweigh the increased risk of this combination.**

The concomitant administration of fenofibrate (equivalent to 145 mg LIPIDIL EZ) with pravastatin (40 mg) once daily for 10 days, in healthy adults, increased the mean C_{max} and AUC values for pravastatin by 36% (range: from a 69% decrease to a 321% increase) and 28% (range: from a 54% decrease to a 128% increase), respectively. Coadministration of fenofibrate with pravastatin also increased the mean C_{max} and AUC of the major metabolites, 3-alpha-hydroxy-isopravastatin by 55% (range: from a 32% decrease to a 314% increase) and 39% (range: from a 24% decrease to a 261% increase), respectively.

The combined use of fibric acid derivatives and HMG-CoA reductase inhibitors has been associated, in the absence of a marked pharmacokinetic action, in numerous case reports, with rhabdomyolysis, markedly elevated creatine kinase (CK) levels and myoglobinuria, leading to a high proportion of cases to acute renal failure.

This combination therapy must not be used in patients with predisposing factors for myopathy (pre-existing myopathy, age >70 years, renal impairment, hepatic impairment, severe infection, surgery and trauma, frailty, hypothyroidism or electrolyte imbalance, personal or family history of hereditary muscular disorders, previous history of muscle toxicity with another HMG-CoA reductase inhibitor, concomitant use of a fibrate, niacin or ezetimibe, alcohol abuse, excessive physical exercise, diabetes with hepatic fatty change situations where an increase in plasma levels of active ingredient may occur).

For information on a specific HMG-CoA reductase inhibitor, consult a respective Product Monograph.

The use of fibrates alone, including LIPIDIL EZ, may occasionally be associated with myositis, myopathy or rhabdomyolysis. Patients receiving LIPIDIL EZ and complaining of muscle pain, tenderness, or weakness should have prompt medical evaluation for myopathy, including serum creatine kinase level determination. If myopathy and or myositis is suspected or diagnosed, LIPIDIL EZ therapy should be stopped.

Liver Function: Abnormal liver function tests have occasionally been observed during fenofibrate administration, including elevations of transaminases, and decreases or, rarely, increases in alkaline phosphatase. From 5 placebo-controlled trials of 2 to 6 months' duration, increases up to >3 times the upper limit of normal occurred in 2.9% (14/477) of patients taking fenofibrate versus 0.5% (2/386) of those treated with placebo. In the DAIS study (3 years duration), increases up to 3 times the upper limit of normal occurred in 1.9% (4/207) of patients taking fenofibrate versus 0% of those treated with placebo (0/211). Follow-up measurements, performed either at the end of treatment or during continued treatment, showed that transaminase values generally returned to normal limits. **Therefore, regular periodic liver function tests (AST, ALT and GGT) in addition to other baseline tests are recommended every 3 months for the first 12 months and at least yearly thereafter. LIPIDIL EZ (fenofibrate) should be discontinued if abnormalities persist and/or AST and ALT levels increase to more than 3 times the upper limit of normal.**

Concomitant Administration with Ezetimibe: When ezetimibe is initiated in a patient already taking LIPIDIL EZ, liver function tests should be considered at initiation of ezetimibe therapy and then as indicated. When ezetimibe is initiated at the same time as LIPIDIL EZ, liver function tests should be performed at initiation of therapy according to the above recommendations (see Adverse Effects).

Cholelithiasis: Fenofibrate may increase cholesterol excretion into the bile, and may lead to cholelithiasis. If cholelithiasis is suspected, gallbladder studies are indicated. LIPIDIL EZ therapy should be discontinued if gallstones are found.

Haematologic Changes: Mild hemoglobin, haematocrit and white blood cell decreases have been observed occasionally in patients following initiation of fenofibrate therapy. However, these levels stabilize during long-term administration. Periodic blood counts are recommended during the first 12 months of fenofibrate administration.

PRECAUTIONS: General: When LIPIDIL EZ is to be administered with ezetimibe, the ezetimibe Product Monograph should also be consulted.

Initial Therapy: Before instituting fenofibrate therapy, laboratory tests should be conducted to ensure that lipid levels are consistently abnormal. Attempts should be made to control serum lipids with appropriate diet, exercise and weight loss in obese patients. Secondary causes of hypercholesterolemia, such as uncontrolled type 2 diabetes mellitus, hypothyroidism, nephrotic syndrome, dysproteinemia, obstructive liver disease, pharmacological treatment and excessive alcohol intake should be adequately treated before fenofibrate therapy is initiated. In patients at high risk, consideration should be given to the control of other risk factors such as smoking, use of preparations containing estrogen and inadequately controlled hypertension.

Long-term Therapy: Because long-term administration of fenofibrate is recommended, the potential risks and benefits should be carefully weighed. Adequate pretreatment laboratory studies should be performed to ensure that patients have elevated serum cholesterol and/or triglycerides or low HDL-cholesterol levels. Response to therapy should be monitored by determination of serum lipid values (e.g. total cholesterol, LDL-C, triglycerides). If a significant serum lipid response is not obtained in three months, LIPIDIL EZ should be discontinued.

Skeletal Muscle: Treatment with drugs of the fibrate class has been associated on rare occasions with myositis or rhabdomyolysis, usually in patients with impaired renal function and in cases of hypoalbuminemia. Myopathy should be considered in any patient with diffuse myalgias, myositis, muscle cramps, tenderness or weakness, and/or marked elevation of creatine phosphokinase levels.

Patients should be advised to promptly report unexplained muscle pain, tenderness or weakness, particularly if accompanied by malaise or fever. CK levels should be assessed in patients reporting these symptoms, and fenofibrate therapy should be discontinued if markedly elevated CK levels (5 times the upper limit of normal) occur or myopathy is diagnosed.

Patient with pre-disposing factors for myopathy may be at an increased risk of developing rhabdomyolysis (see Warnings). For these patients, the putative benefits and risks of fenofibrate therapy should be carefully weighed.

Concomitant Administration with Ezetimibe: Post marketing reports of adverse events have included rare cases of myopathy/rhabdomyolysis occurring in patients taking ezetimibe. Myopathy/rhabdomyolysis should be considered in patients presenting with muscle pain during treatment with ezetimibe and LIPIDIL EZ, and consideration given to discontinuation of the drugs. Most cases of myopathy/rhabdomyolysis resolved when drugs were discontinued.

Reproduction Studies: Standard tests for teratology, fertility and peri- and post-natal effects in animals have shown a relative absence of risk; however, embryo-toxicity has occurred in animals at maternally toxic doses.

Pregnancy: Safety in pregnant women has not been established. Fenofibrate has been shown to be embryocidal in rats when given in doses 7 to 10 times the maximum recommended human dose (MRHD) and in rabbits when given in doses 9 times the MRHD (on the basis of mg/m² surface area). There are no adequate and well-controlled studies in pregnant women. Fenofibrate should not be used during pregnancy (see Contraindications).

Lactation: In the absence of information concerning the presence of fenofibrate in human breast milk, LIPIDIL EZ should not be used by nursing mothers.

Carcinogenicity: In long-term animal toxicity and carcinogenicity studies, fenofibrate has been shown to be tumorigenic for the liver in male rats at 12 times the human dose. At this dose level in male rats there was also an increase in benign Leydig cell tumors. Pancreatic acinar cell tumors were increased in male rats at 9 and 40 times the human dose. However, mice and female rats were unaffected at similar doses. Florid hepato-cellular peroxisome proliferation has been observed following fenofibrate administration to rats. Such changes have not been found in the human liver after up to 3.5 years of fenofibrate administration.

Hepatobiliary Disease: In patients with a past history of jaundice or hepatic disorder, fenofibrate should be used with caution.

Fenofibrate may increase cholesterol excretion into the bile, and may lead to cholelithiasis.

Concomitant Administration with Ezetimibe: The co-administration of ezetimibe with fibrates other than fenofibrate has not been studied. Therefore, co-administration of ezetimibe and fibrates other than fenofibrate is not recommended (see Drug Interactions, and Product Monograph for ezetimibe).

If cholelithiasis is suspected in a patient receiving ezetimibe and LIPIDIL EZ, gallbladder studies are indicated and alternative lipid-lowering therapy should be considered (see Adverse Effects).

Renal Function: In patients with hypoalbuminemia, e.g., nephrotic syndrome, and in patients with renal insufficiency, the dosage of fenofibrate must be reduced and renal function should be monitored regularly (see Precautions, Skeletal Muscle and Dosage). Fenofibrate should not be used in dialysis patients.

Treatment should be interrupted in case of an increase in creatinine level >50% upper limit of normal. It is recommended that creatinine measurement may be considered during the first three months after initiation of treatment.

Pancreatitis: In common with some other fibrates, pancreatitis has been reported in patients taking fenofibrate. This occurrence may represent a failure of efficacy in patients with severe hypertriglyceridemia, a direct drug effect, or a secondary phenomenon mediated through biliary tract stone or sludge formation with obstruction of the common bile duct.

Geriatrics: Fenofibrate is excreted by the kidney. Therefore, the risk of adverse reactions to LIPIDIL EZ may be greater in the elderly patients with impaired renal function. Since elderly patients are more likely to have a decreased renal function, dose should be carefully selected (see Dosage).

Drug Interactions: General: Fenofibrate is highly protein bound (>99%), mainly to albumin. Consideration should be given to the potential for displacement drug interactions with other highly protein-bound drugs.

Statins: No drug-drug interaction studies with fenofibrate and statins have been conducted in patients.

Pharmacokinetic interaction studies conducted with drugs in healthy subjects may not detect the possibility of a potential drug interaction in some patients due to differences in underlying disease and use of concomitant medications (see Warnings.)

Pravastatin: Concomitant administration in 23 healthy adults of fenofibrate (equivalent to 145 mg LIPIDIL EZ)) with pravastatin, 40 mg once daily for 10 days, has been shown to increase the mean C_{max} and AUC values for pravastatin by 36% (range: from a 69% decrease to a 321% increase) and 28% (range: from a 54% decrease to a 128% increase), respectively. Coadministration of fenofibrate with pravastatin also increased the mean C_{max} and AUC of the major metabolite, 3-alpha-hydroxy-iso-pravastatin by 55% (range: from a 32% decrease to a 314% increase) and 39% (range: from a 24% decrease to a 261% increase), respectively.

Atorvastatin: Concomitant administration of fenofibrate (equivalent to 145 mg LIPIDIL EZ) with atorvastatin (20 mg) once daily for 10 days resulted in a 14% decrease in the mean atorvastatin AUC value (range: from a 67% decrease to a 44% increase) in 22 healthy males. There was a 0% change in the atorvastatin mean C_{max} value (range: from a 60% decrease to a 136% increase). No significant pharmacokinetic interaction was observed in the mean fenofibric acid AUC (2.3% decrease, range: from a 39% decrease to a 40 % increase) or in the mean C_{max} (3.8% decrease, range: from a 29% decrease to a 42% increase) when fenofibrate was coadministered with multiple doses of atorvastatin.

Simvastatin: In a 10-day trial, fenofibrate (equivalent to 145 mg LIPIDIL EZ) was taken once daily. On day 10, simvastatin 40 mg was added to the fenofibrate regimen. The mean AUC of simvastatin acid, the main active metabolite, decreased by 42% (range: from a 77% decrease to a 50% increase) in the presence of fenofibrate. Fenofibrate had no impact (0%) on the mean simvastatin acid C_{max} (range: from a 67% decrease to a 92% increase). The mean fenofibric acid C_{min} plasma levels increased by 14% (range: from a 7% decrease to a 48% increase) following the coadministration of simvastatin, indicating that fenofibric acid concentrations are not significantly affected by the addition of a 40 mg dose of simvastatin.

Rosuvastatin: Coadministration of fenofibrate (67 mg three times daily) and rosuvastatin (10 mg once daily) for seven days did not lead to a clinically significant change in the plasma concentrations of either drug.

Ezetimibe: The safety and effectiveness of fenofibrate co-administered with ezetimibe have been evaluated in a clinical study (see Warnings, Precautions and Adverse Effects). Co-administration of ezetimibe with other fibrates has not been studied (see ezetimibe Product Monograph). Co-administration of ezetimibe with fibrates other than fenofibrate is not recommended until use in patients is studied.

In a pharmacokinetic study, concomitant fenofibrate administration increased total ezetimibe concentrations approximately 1.5-fold. This increase is not considered clinically significant.

Oral Anticoagulants: Caution should be exercised when oral anticoagulants are given in conjunction with LIPIDIL EZ (fenofibrate). The dosage of oral anticoagulant should be reduced to maintain the prothrombin time at the desired level to prevent bleeding complications. Careful monitoring of prothrombin time is therefore recommended until it has been definitely determined that the prothrombin level has been stabilized.

Statins and Cyclosporine: Severe myositis and rhabdomyolysis have occurred when a statin or cyclosporine was administered in combination therapy with a fibrate. Therefore, the benefits and risks of using fenofibrate concomitantly with these drugs should be carefully considered.

Some severe cases of reversible renal function impairment have been reported during concomitant administration of fenofibrate and cyclosporine. The renal function of these patients must therefore be closely monitored and treatment with fenofibrate stopped in the case of severe alteration of laboratory parameters.

Bile Acid Sequestrants: When a fibrate is used concurrently with cholestyramine or any other resin, an interval of at least 2 hours should be maintained between the administration of the two drugs, since the absorption of fibrates is impaired by cholestyramine.

Estrogens: Estrogens may lead to a rise in lipid levels. Prescribing fibrates in patients taking estrogens or estrogen-containing contraceptives must be considered clinically on an individual basis.

ADVERSE EFFECTS: In five placebo-controlled clinical trials, conducted in the U.S. and Europe, a total of 477 patients on fenofibrate and 386 patients on placebo were evaluated for adverse effects during 2 to 6 months of treatment.

Adverse events led to the withdrawal of treatment in 5.5% of patients (26/477) treated with fenofibrate, the most common symptoms being abnormal elevation in transaminases, skin reactions and digestive disorders. Of the placebo-treated patients, 2.6% (10/386) were discontinued due to adverse effects.

The most frequently reported adverse events include: gastrointestinal (epigastric distress, flatulence, abdominal pain, nausea, diarrhea, constipation), dermatologic (erythema, pruritus, urticaria), musculoskeletal (muscle pain and weakness, arthralgia), central nervous system (headache, dizziness, insomnia), miscellaneous (decreased libido, hair loss, weight loss).

Adverse events, regardless of their causality, reported in more than 1% of patients are shown in Table 6.

Table 6: LIPIDIL EZ

Number (%) of Patients Reporting Adverse Events

	Fenofibrate N=477	Placebo N=386
Body as a Whole	68 (14.3%)	51 (13.2%)
Abdominal pain	12 (2.5%)	8 (2.1%)
Asthenia	14 (2.9%)	7 (1.8%)
Headache	15 (3.1%)	11 (2.8%)
Cardiovascular System	15 (3.1%)	13 (3.4%)
Digestive System	63 (13.2%)	47 (12.2%)
Diarrhea	10 (2.1%)	13 (3.4%)
Nausea	12 (2.5%)	7 (1.8%)
Constipation	6 (1.3%)	3 (0.8%)
Dyspepsia	5 (1.0%)	6 (1.6%)
Flatulence	10 (2.1%)	10 (2.6%)
Endocrine System	1 (0.2%)	1 (0.3%)
Haemic & Lymphatic System	3 (0.6%)	1 (0.3%)
Metabolic & Nutritional Disorders	18 (3.8%)	14 (3.6%)
ALT increase	12 (2.5%)	4 (1.0%)
AST increase	8 (1.7%)	1 (0.3%)
ALT/AST increase	9 (4.9%)	0
CPK increase	1 (0.2%)	5 (1.3%)
Creatinine increase	8 (1.7%)	1 (0.3%)
Musculoskeletal System	31 (6.5%)	21 (5.4%)
Arthralgia	11 (2.3%)	11 (2.8%)
Myalgia	3 (0.6%)	4 (1.0%)
Nervous System	31 (6.5%)	11 (2.8%)
Dizziness	5 (1.0%)	4 (1.0%)
Respiratory System	34 (7.1%)	25 (6.5%)
Rhinitis	10 (2.1%)	4 (1.0%)
Skin and Appendages	24 (5.0%)	12 (3.1%)
Rash	11 (2.3%)	3 (0.8%)
Pruritus	10 (2.1%)	3 (0.8%)
Special Senses	14 (2.9%)	10 (2.6%)
Urogenital System	14 (2.9%)	9 (2.3%)

Safety was monitored for 3 years during the placebo-controlled DAIS study for both adverse events and laboratory anomalies. Fenofibrate was used safely in type 2 diabetic patients, as the overall incidence and severity of adverse events were comparable in fenofibrate and placebo groups. Table 7 summarizes the incidence of adverse events, by body system, observed in both treatment groups.

Table 7: LIPIDIL EZ

DAIS Study: Incidence of Adverse Events (AEs) by System, Experienced by Type 2 Diabetic Patients During Treatment with Fenofibrate or Placebo (ITT Population)

	Fenofibrate (N=207)		Placebo (N=211)	
Body System	**AEs**	**Patients**	**AEs**	**Patients**
Total # pts. with at least 1 AE	Total AEs: 1710	201 (97.1%)	Total AEs: 1759	202 (95.7%)
Body as a Whole	371 (21.7%)	136 (65.7%)	362 (20.6%)	146 (69.2%)
Cardiovascular	183 (10.7%)	84 (40.6%)	220 (12.5%)	96 (45.5%)
Digestive	196 (11.5%)	86 (41.6%)	194 (11.0%)	87 (41.2%)
Endocrine	11 (0.6%)	10 (4.8%)	19 (1.1%)	11 (5.2%)

(cont'd)

Table 7: LIPIDIL EZ *(cont'd)*

DAIS Study: Incidence of Adverse Events (AEs) by System, Experienced by Type 2 Diabetic Patients During Treatment with Fenofibrate or Placebo (ITT Population)

	Fenofibrate (N=207)		Placebo (N=211)	
Body System	**AEs**	**Patients**	**AEs**	**Patients**
Haemic/Lymphatic	31 (1.8%)	19 (9.2%)	23 (1.3%)	15 (7.1%)
Metabolic/ Nutritional	50 (2.9%)	32 (15.5%)	70 (4.9%)	41 (19.4%)
Musculoskeletal	155 (9.1%)	84 (40.6%)	180 (10.2%)	84 (39.8%)
CNS	103 (6.0%)	59 (28.5%)	98 (5.6%)	58 (27.5%)
Respiratory	301 (17.6%)	108 (52.2%)	279 (15.9%)	105 (49.8%)
Skin/Appendage	107 (6.3%)	58 (28.0%)	107 (6.1%)	48 (22.8%)
Special Senses	73 (4.3%)	44 (21.3%)	90 (5.1%)	50 (23.7%)
Urogenital	118 (6.9%)	55 (26.6%)	103 (5.9%)	46 (21.8%)
Other	11 (0.6%)	9 (4.4%)	14 (0.8%)	11 (5.2%)

In two open, non-controlled clinical studies conducted in Canada and Germany, a total of 375 patients on fenofibrate, microcoated formulation, were evaluated for adverse events. Listed in Table 8 are the adverse events possibly or probably related to fenofibrate, microcoated formulation and reported by more than 0.5% of the patients.

Table 8: LIPIDIL EZ

Number (%) of Patients Reporting Adverse Events Possibly or Probably Related to Fenofibrate

Canadian and German Multicenter Studies (12-week treatment)	
Adverse Events	**Microcoated Fenofibrate (n=375)**
Digestive System	
Gastrointestinal disorder	4 (1.1%)
Nausea	3 (0.8%)
Flatulence	2 (0.5%)
Diarrhea	2 (0.5%)
Liver function tests abnormal	2 (0.5%)
Dyspepsia	2 (0.5%)
Gastritis	2 (0.5%)
Constipation	2 (0.5%)
Body as a Whole	
Abdominal pain	4 (1.1%)
Headache	2 (0.5%)
Asthenia	2 (0.5%)
Lab test abnormal	2 (0.5%)
Metabolic and Nutritional Disorders	
ALT increased (>3×ULN)	3 (0.8%)
AST increased (>3×ULN)	4 (1.1%)
Creatine kinase increased (>5×ULN)	1 (0.3%)
Nervous System	
Dizziness	2 (0.5%)
Libido decreased	2 (0.5%)

Other adverse events include commonly reported cases of vomiting. Uncommonly reported cases of pancreatitis and venous thromboembolism (pulmonary embolism and deep vein thrombosis). Rarely reported cases of alopecia, sexual asthenia, myositis and muscular cramps. Very rarely reported cases of, rhabdomyolysis and interstitial pneumopathies. Episodes of hepatitis have been reported. When symptoms (e.g. jaundice) indicative of hepatitis occur, laboratory tests are to be conducted for verification and fenofibrate discontinued, if applicable (see Warnings). Photosensitivity reactions, development of gallstones and cutaneous hypersensitivity with erythema and vesiculation or nodulation on parts of the skin exposed to sunlight or artificial UV light in individual cases (even after many months of uncomplicated use) have also been reported.

Combination with Ezetimibe: When LIPIDIL EZ is to be administered with ezetimibe, the ezetimibe Product Monograph should also be consulted.

In a clinical study involving 625 patients treated for up to 12 weeks and 576 patients treated for up to 1 year, co-administration of fenofibrate and ezetimibe was well tolerated. This study was not designed to compare treatment groups for infrequent events. Incidence rates (95% CI) for clinically important elevations (>3 ULN, consecutive) in serum transaminases were 4.5% (1.9, 8.8) and 2.7% (1.2, 5.4) for fenofibrate monotherapy and ezetimibe co-administered with fenofibrate, respectively, adjusted for treatment exposure. Corresponding incidence rates for cholecystectomy were 0.6% (0.0, 3.1) and 1.7% (0.6, 0.4) for fenofibrate monotherapy and ezetimibe co-administered with fenofibrate, respectively (see Warnings, Precautions and Drug Interactions). There were no CPK elevations >10×ULN in either treatment group in this study. No cases of myopathy, rhabdomyolysis, or pancreatitis were reported in this 12 weeks study.

Laboratory Tests: In most trials, sporadic and transient increases in aminotransferase levels have been associated with the use of fenofibrate. The reported frequency of AST and ALT elevations was variable; in the clinical studies conducted in Canada and Germany elevations above three times the upper limit of normal were observed in 2.0% of the patients (7/375) treated with fenofibrate, microcoated formulation. In two dose-ranging studies, the incidence of increases in transaminases (>3×ULN) due to fenofibrate therapy appears to be dose related; 0.6% (1/157) (80 mg tablet), 1.9% (3/158) (160 mg tablet) and 4.0% (6/149) (240 mg tablet). Values usually return to normal without interruption of treatment (see Precautions). Reductions in alkaline phosphatase levels have also been observed.

Mild decreases in hemoglobin, haematocrit, and white blood cell counts have been observed occasionally in patients following initiation of fenofibrate therapy but these observations were without clinical significance. However, these levels stabilize during long-term administration. In addition, a decrease in heptoglobin concentration has been observed in some patients with Type IV hyperlipidemia during long-term use of fenofibrate. However, this decrease in heptoglobin was not associated with any other sign of blood dyscrasia and/or haemolysis.

The mean plasma levels of urea and creatinine showed increases, particularly during long-term fenofibrate treatment, most of them remaining within the limits of normal values.

Fenofibrate also has the potential to provoke CK elevations and changes in haematologic parameters, which generally subside when the drug is discontinued (see Precautions). In the clinical studies conducted in Canada and Germany, the reported frequency of CK elevations above five times the upper limit of normal was approximately 0.3% (2/375) of the patients treated with fenofibrate, microcoated formulation (LIPIDIL Supra).

OVERDOSE:

Treatment: While there has been no reported case of overdosage, symptomatic and supportive measures should be taken. Fenofibrate is not dialysable because the main metabolite (fenofibric acid) is highly bound to plasma proteins.

For management of a suspected drug overdose, CPhA recommends that you contact your **regional Poison Control Centre**. See the *CPS* Directory section for a list of Poison Control Centres.

DOSAGE: Patients should be placed on a standard cholesterol-lowering diet (at least equivalent to the Adult Treatment Panel III (ATP III TLC diet)) before receiving LIPIDIL EZ (fenofibrate,), and should continue on this diet during treatment with LIPIDIL EZ. If appropriate, a program of weight control and physical exercise should be implemented.

Prior to initiating therapy with LIPIDIL EZ, secondary causes for elevations in plasma lipid levels should be excluded. A lipid profile should also be performed.

If a significant serum lipid response is not obtained in three months, LIPIDIL EZ should be discontinued.

The usual recommended dose for LIPIDIL EZ in adults, is one 145 mg tablet daily, taken any time with or without food. In the elderly, the initial dose should be limited to 48 mg per day. The dose should be individualized according to patient response and should be adjusted if necessary following repeat lipid determinations.

The maximum recommended daily dose of LIPIDIL EZ is 145 mg.

In patients having impaired renal function, treatment with LIPIDIL EZ should be initiated at a dose of 48 mg per day and increased only after evaluation of the effects on renal function and lipid levels at this dose.

Concomitant Administration with Ezetimibe: The recommended dose of ezetimibe is 10 mg once daily orally in combination with LIPIDIL EZ. LIPIDIL EZ in combination with ezetimibe, may be taken with or without food, preferably at the same time each day.

INFORMATION FOR THE PATIENT: Published in e-CPS, available by subscription at www.e-cps.ca.

SUPPLIED: 48 mg: Each yellow, oblong, film-coated tablet (NanoCrystal Formulation), embossed with the Fournier logo on one side and 48 on the other, contains: fenofibrate 48 mg. Nonmedicinal ingredients: colloidal silicon dioxide, crospovidone, docusate sodium, hypromellose, lactose monohydrate, magnesium stearate, microcrystalline cellulose, sodium lauryl sulfate and sucrose; coating: D&C Blue #2/Indigo carmine FCF Aluminum Lake, D&C yellow #6/sunset yellow FCF Aluminum Lake, D&C Yellow #10 Aluminum Lake, lecithin, polyvinyl alcohol, talc and titanium dioxide. Blister packs of 30. Store at 15-30°C. Protect from light and moisture.

145 mg: Each white, oblong, film-coated tablet (NanoCrystal Formulation), embossed with the Fournier logo on one side and 145 on the other, contains: fenofibrate 145 mg. Nonmedicinal ingredients: colloidal silicon dioxide, crospovidone, docusate sodium, hypromellose, lactose monohydrate, magnesium stearate, microcrystalline cellulose, sodium lauryl sulfate and sucrose; coating: polyvinyl alcohol, soybean lecithin, talc, titanium dioxide and xanthan gum. Blister packs of 30. Store at 15-30°C. Protect from light and moisture.

(Shown in Product Identification Section)

Lipidil Supra® ℞

fenofibrate microcoated

Lipid Metabolism Regulator

Fournier Pharma

Date of Preparation: February 28, 2000
Date of Revision: November 7, 2007

PHARMACOLOGY: LIPIDIL SUPRA (fenofibrate) lowers elevated serum lipids by decreasing the low density lipoprotein (LDL) fraction rich in cholesterol and the very low density lipoprotein (VLDL) fraction rich in triglycerides. In addition, fenofibrate increases the high density lipoprotein (HDL) cholesterol fraction.

Fenofibrate appears to have a greater depressant effect on the very low density lipoproteins (VLDL) than on the low density lipoproteins (LDL). Therapeutic doses of fenofibrate produce elevations of HDL cholesterol, a reduction in the content of the low density lipoproteins cholesterol, and a substantial reduction in the triglyceride content of very low density lipoproteins.

Recent findings suggest that the lipid modulating effects of fenofibrate are mediated by the activation of a specific nuclear receptor called peroxisome proliferator activated receptor alpha (PPARα), which produces: a reduction in apo C-III, and therefore a reduction in the level of dense atherogenic LDL particles, a stimulation of mitochondrial beta-oxidation, and therefore a reduction in triglyceride secretion, a rise in lipoprotein lipase production, and therefore an acceleration of triglyceride rich lipoprotein breakdown and a rise in apo A-I and apo A-II production, and a corresponding rise in HDL.

Pharmacokinetics: After oral administration, fenofibrate is rapidly hydrolyzed to fenofibric acid, the active metabolite. Fenofibrate's absorption is low and variable when the product is administered under fasting conditions.

Fenofibrate's absorption is increased when the compound is given with food. In man it is mainly excreted through the kidney. Half-life is about 20 hours. In patients with severe renal failure, significant accumulation was observed with a large increase in half-life. Therefore, the dose of fenofibrate may need to be reduced, depending on the rate of creatinine clearance.

Limited experience is available in children and adolescents, at the dose of 5 mg/kg/day fenofibrate non-micronized formulation. However, safety and effectiveness have not been established in this sub-population.

INDICATIONS: LIPIDIL SUPRA (fenofibrate, microcoated formulation) is indicated as an adjunct to diet, at least equivalent to the Adults Treatment Panel III (ATP III) and Therapeutic lifestyle changes (TLC diet) and other therapeutic measures when the response to diet and other measures has been inadequate for: Treatment of patients, including patients with type 2 diabetes (non-insulin dependent), with dyslipoproteinemia (hypercholesterolemia, Fredrickson classification Types IIa and IIb mixed hyperlipidemia), to regulate lipid levels by reducing serum triglycerides and LDL cholesterol levels and increasing HDL cholesterol. Treatment of adult patients with very high serum triglyceride levels, Fredrickson classification Type IV and Type V hyperlipidemia, who are at a high risk of sequelae and complications (i.e., pancreatitis) from their hyperlipidemia.

LIPIDIL SUPRA alone may not be adequate therapy in some patients with familial combined hyperlipidemia with Type IIb and Type IV hyperlipoproteinemia.

LIPIDIL SUPRA is not indicated for the treatment of Type I hyperlipoproteinemia.

CONTRAINDICATIONS: Hepatic or severe renal dysfunction (creatinine clearance <20 mL/min), including primary biliary cirrhosis. Pre-existing gallbladder disease (see Warnings). Hypersensitivity to fenofibrate, any component of this medication or other drugs of the fibrate class. Should not be taken in patients allergic to peanut or arachis oil or soya lecithin or related products due to the risk of hypersensitivity reactions. The drug should not be used during pregnancy and breast-feeding. Known photoallergy or phototoxic reaction during treatment with fibrates or ketoprofen.

WARNINGS: Fenofibrate and HMG-CoA Reductase Inhibitors (Statins): **The concomitant administration of fenofibrate and statins should be avoided unless the benefit for further alteration in lipid levels is likely to outweigh the increased risk of this combination.**

The concomitant administration of fenofibrate with Pravastatin (40 mg) once daily for 10 days, in healthy adults, increased the mean Cmax and AUC values for pravastatin by 36% (range: from a 69% decrease to a 321% increase) and 28% (range: from a 54% decrease to a 128% increase), respectively. Co-administration of fenofibrate with Pravastatin also increased the mean Cmax and AUC of the major metabolites, 3-alpha-hydroxy-isopravastatin by 55% (range: from a 32% decrease to a 314% increase) and 39% (range: from a 24% decrease to a 261% increase), respectively.

The combined use of fibric acid derivatives and HMG-CoA reductase inhibitors has been associated, in the absence of a marked pharmacokinetic action, in numerous case reports, with rhabdomyolysis, markedly elevated creatine kinase (CK) levels and myoglobinuria, leading to a high proportion of cases to acute renal failure.

This combination therapy must not be used in patients with predisposing factors for myopathy (pre-existing myopathy, age >70 years, renal impairment, hepatic impairment, severe infection, surgery and trauma, frailty, hypothyroidism or electrolyte imbalance, personal or family history of hereditary muscular disorders, previous history of muscle toxicity with another HMG-CoA reductase inhibitor, concomitant use of a fibrate, niacin or ezetimibe, alcohol abuse, excessive physical exercise, diabetes with hepatic fatty change situations where an increase in plasma levels of active ingredient may occur).

For information on a specific HMG-CoA reductase inhibitor, consult a respective Product Monograph.

The use of fibrates alone, including LIPIDIL SUPRA, may occasionally be associated with myositis, myopathy or rhabdomyolysis. Patients receiving LIPIDIL SUPRA and complaining of muscle pain, tenderness, or weakness should have prompt medical evaluation for myopathy, including serum creatine kinase level determination. If myopathy and or myositis is suspected or diagnosed, LIPIDIL SUPRA therapy should be stopped.

Liver Function: Abnormal liver function tests have been observed occasionally during fenofibrate administration, including elevations of transaminases, and decreases or, rarely, increases in alkaline phosphatase. From 5 placebo-controlled trials of 2 to 6 months' duration, increases up to >3 times the upper limit of normal occurred in 2.9% (14/477) of patients taking fenofibrate versus 0.5% (2/386) of those treated with placebo. In the DAIS study (3 years duration), increases up to 3 times the upper limit of normal occurred in 1.9% (4/207) of patients taking fenofibrate versus 0% of those treated with placebo (0/211). Follow-up measurements, performed either at the end of treatment or during continued treatment, showed that transaminase values generally returned to normal limits. **Therefore, regular periodic liver function tests (AST, ALT and GGT) in addition to other baseline tests are recommended every 3 months for the first 12 months and at least yearly thereafter. LIPIDIL SUPRA (fenofibrate, microcoated formulation) should be terminated if abnormalities persist and/ or AST and ALT levels increase to more than 3 times the upper limit of normal.**

Cholelithiasis: Fenofibrate may increase cholesterol excretion into the bile, and may lead to cholelithiasis. If cholelithiasis is suspected, gallbladder studies are indicated. LIPIDIL SUPRA therapy should be discontinued if gallstones are found.

Hematologic Changes: Mild hemoglobin, hematocrit and white blood cell decreases have been observed occasionally in patients following initiation of fenofibrate therapy. However, these levels stabilize during long-term administration. Periodic blood counts are recommended during the first 12 months of fenofibrate administration.

PRECAUTIONS: Initial Therapy: Before instituting fenofibrate therapy, laboratory tests should be conducted to ensure that lipid levels are consistently abnormal. Attempts should be made to control serum lipids with appropriate diet, exercise and weight loss in obese patients. Secondary causes of hypercholesterolemia, such as uncontrolled type 2 diabetes mellitus, hypothyroidism, nephrotic syndrome, dysproteinemia, obstructive liver disease, pharmacological treatment and excessive alcohol intake should be adequately treated before fenofibrate therapy is initiated. In patients at high risk, consideration should be given to the control of other risk factors such as smoking, use of preparations containing estrogen and inadequately controlled hypertension.

Long-term Therapy: Because long-term administration of fenofibrate is recommended, the potential risks and benefits should be carefully weighed. Adequate pretreatment laboratory studies should be performed to ensure that patients have elevated serum cholesterol and/or triglycerides or low HDL-cholesterol levels. Response to therapy should be monitored by determination of serum lipid values (e.g. total cholesterol, LDL-C, triglycerides). If a significant serum lipidil response is not obtained in 3 months, LIPIDIL SUPRA should be discontinued.

Skeletal Muscle: Treatment with drugs of the fibrate class has been associated on rare occasions with myositis or rhabdomyolysis, usually in patients with impaired renal function and in cases of hypoalbuminaemia. Myopathy should be considered in any patient with diffuse myalgias, myositis, muscle cramps, tenderness or weakness, and/or marked elevation of creatine phosphokinase levels.

Patients should be advised to promptly report unexplained muscle pain, tenderness or weakness, particularly if accompanied by malaise or fever. CK levels should be assessed in patients reporting these symptoms, and fenofibrate therapy should be discontinued if markedly elevated CK levels (5 times the upper limit of normal) occur or myopathy is diagnosed.

Patients with pre-disposing factors for myopathy may be at an increased risk of developing rhabdomyolysis (see Warnings). For these patients, the putative benefits and risks of fenofibrate therapy should be carefully weighed.

Reproduction Studies: Standard tests for teratology, fertility and peri- and post-natal effects in animals have shown a relative absence of risk; however, embryo-toxicity has occurred in animals at maternally toxic doses.

Pregnancy: Safety in pregnant women has not been established. Fenofibrate has been shown to be embryocidal in rats when given in doses 7 to 10 times the maximum recommended human dose (MRHD) and in rabbits when given in doses 9 times the MRHD (on the basis of mg/m^2 surface area). There are no adequate and well-controlled studies in pregnant women. Fenofibrate should not be used during pregnancy (see Contraindications).

Lactation: In the absence of information concerning the presence of fenofibrate in human breast milk, LIPIDIL SUPRA should not be used by nursing mothers.

Carcinogenicity: In long-term animal toxicity and carcinogenicity studies fenofibrate has been shown to be tumorigenic for the liver in male rats at 12 times the human dose. At this dose level in male rats there was also an increase in benign Leydig cell tumors. Pancreatic acinar cell tumors were increased in male rats at 9 and 40 times the human dose. However, mice and female rats were unaffected at similar doses. Florid hepato-cellular peroxisome proliferation has been observed following fenofibrate administration to rats. Such changes have not been found in the human liver after up to 3.5 years of fenofibrate administration.

Hepatobiliary Disease: In patients with a past history of jaundice or hepatic disorder, fenofibrate should be used with caution. Fenofibrate may increase cholesterol excretion into the bile, and may lead to cholelithiasis.

Renal Function: In patients with hypoalbuminemia, e.g., nephrotic syndrome, and in patients with renal insufficiency, the dosage of fibrates must be reduced and renal function should be monitored regularly (see Precautions, Skeletal Muscle and Dosage). Fenofibrate should not be used in dialysis patients.

Treatment should be interrupted in case of an increase in creatinine levels >50% upper limit of normal. It is recommended that creatinine measurement may be considered during the first three months after initiation of treatment.

Pancreatitis: In common with some other fibrates, pancreatitis has been reported in patients taking fenofibrate. This occurrence may represent a failure of efficacy in patients with severe hypertriglyceridemia, a direct drug effect, or a secondary phenomenon mediated through biliary tract stone or sludge formation with obstruction of the common bile duct.

Geriatrics: Fenofibrate is excreted by the kidney. Therefore, the risk of adverse reactions to LIPIDIL SUPRA may be greater in the elderly patients with impaired renal function. Since elderly patients are more likely to have a decreased renal function, dose should be carefully selected (see Dosage).

Drug Interactions: General: Fenofibrate is highly protein bound (>99%), mainly to albumin. Consideration should be given to the potential for displacement drug interactions with other highly protein-bound drugs.

Statins: No drug-drug interaction studies with fenofibrate and statins have been conducted in patients.

Pharmacokinetic interaction studies conducted with drugs in healthy subjects may not detect the possibility of a potential drug interaction in some patients due to differences in underlying disease and use of concomitant medications (see Warnings).

Pravastatin: Concomitant administration in 23 healthy adults of fenofibrate with pravastatin, 40 mg once daily for 10 days, has been shown to increase the mean Cmax and AUC values for pravastatin by 36% (range: from a 69% decrease to a 321% increase) and 28% (range: from a 54% decrease to a 128% increase), respectively. Co-administration of fenofibrate with pravastatin also increased the mean Cmax and AUC of the major metabolite, 3-alpha-hydroxy-iso-pravastatin by 55% (range: from a 32% decrease to a 314% increase) and 39% (range: from a 24% decrease to a 261% increase), respectively.

Atorvastatin: Concomitant administration of fenofibrate with atorvastatin (20 mg) once daily for 10 days resulted in a 14% decrease in the mean atorvastatin AUC value (range: from a 67% decrease to a 44% increase) in 22 healthy males. There was a 0% change in the atorvastatin mean Cmax value (range: from a 60% decrease to a 136% increase). No significant pharmacokinetic interaction was observed in the mean fenofibric acid AUC (2.3% decrease, range: from a 39% decrease to a 40 % increase) or in the mean Cmax (3.8% decrease, range: from a 29% decrease to a 42% increase) when fenofibrate was co-administered with multiple doses of atorvastatin.

Simvastatin: In a 10-day trial, fenofibrate was taken once daily. On day 10, simvastatin 40 mg was added to the fenofibrate regimen. The mean AUC of simvastatin acid, the main active metabolite, decreased by 42% (range: from a 77% decrease to a 50% increase) in the presence of fenofibrate. Fenofibrate had no impact (0%) on the mean simvastatin acid Cmax (range: from a 67% decrease to a 92% increase). The mean fenofibric acid Cmin plasma levels increased by 14% (range: from a 7% decrease to a 48% increase) following the co-administration of simvastatin, indicating that fenofibric acid concentrations are not significantly affected by the addition of a 40 mg dose of simvastatin.

Rosuvastatin: Co-administration of fenofibrate (67 mg three times daily) and rosuvastatin (10 mg once daily) for seven days did not lead to a clinically significant change in the plasma concentrations of either drug.

Ezetimibe: The safety and effectiveness of ezetimibe and fibrate combination therapy have not been established, therefore co-administration is not recommended until use in patients has been studied.

Oral Anticoagulants: Caution should be exercised when oral anticoagulants are given in conjunction with LIPIDIL SUPRA (fenofibrate, microcoated formulation). The dosage of oral anticoagulant should be reduced to maintain the prothrombin time at the desired level to prevent bleeding complications. Careful monitoring of prothrombin time is therefore recommended until it has been definitely determined that the prothrombin level has been stabilized.

Statins and Cyclosporine: Severe myositis and rhabdomyolisis have occurred when a statin or cyclosporine was administered in combination therapy with a fibrate. Therefore, the benefits and risks of using fenofibrate concomitantly with these drugs should be carefully considered.

Some severe cases of reversible renal function impairment have been reported during concomitant administration of fenofibrate and cyclosporin. The renal function of these patients must therefore be closely monitored and the treatment with fenofibrate stopped in the case of severe alteration of laboratory parameters.

Bile Acid Sequestrants: When a fibrate is used concurrently with cholestyramine or any other resin, an interval of at least 2 hours should be maintained between the administration of the two drugs, since the absorption of fibrates is impaired by cholestyramine.

Estrogens: Estrogens may lead to a rise in lipid levels. Prescribing fibrates in patients taking estrogens or estrogen-containing contraceptives must be considered clinically on an individual basis.

ADVERSE EFFECTS: In five placebo-controlled clinical trials, conducted in the U.S. and Europe, a total of 477 patients on fenofibrate and 386 patients on placebo were evaluated for adverse effects during 2 to 6 months of treatment.

Adverse events led to the withdrawal of treatment in 5.5% of patients (26/477) treated with fenofibrate, the most common symptoms being abnormal elevation in transaminases, skin reactions and digestive disorders. Of the placebo-treated patients, 2.6% (10/386) were discontinued due to adverse effects.

The most frequently reported adverse events include: gastrointestinal (epigastric distress, flatulence, abdominal pain, nausea, diarrhea, constipation), dermatologic (erythema, pruritus, urticaria), musculoskeletal (muscle pain and weakness, arthralgia), central nervous system (headache, dizziness, insomnia), miscellaneous (decreased libido, hair loss, weight loss).

Adverse events, regardless of their causality, reported in more than 1% of patients are shown in Table 1.

Table 1: LIPIDIL SUPRA

Number (%) of Patients Reporting Adverse Events

	Fenofibrate N=477	Placebo N=386
Body as a Whole	68 (14.3%)	51 (13.2%)
Abdominal pain	12 (2.5%)	8 (2.1%)
Asthenia	14 (2.9%)	7 (1.8%)
Headache	15 (3.1%)	11 (2.8%)
Cardiovascular System	15 (3.1%)	13 (3.4%)
Digestive System	63 (13.2%)	47 (12.2%)
Diarrhea	10 (2.1%)	13 (3.4%)
Nausea	12 (2.5%)	7 (1.8%)
Constipation	6 (1.3%)	3 (0.8%)
Dyspepsia	5 (1.0%)	6 (1.6%)
Flatulence	10 (2.1%)	10 (2.6%)
Endocrine System	1 (0.2%)	1 (0.3%)
Haemic & Lymphatic System	3 (0.6%)	1 (0.3%)
Metabolic & Nutritional Disorders	18 (3.8%)	14 (3.6%)
ALT increase	12 (2.5%)	4 (1.0%)
AST increase	8 (1.7%)	1 (0.3%)
ALT/AST increase	9 (4.9%)	0
CPK increase	1 (0.2%)	5 (1.3%)
Creatinine increase	8 (1.7%)	1 (0.3%)
Musculoskeletal System	31 (6.5%)	21 (5.4%)
Arthralgia	11 (2.3%)	11 (2.8%)
Myalgia	3 (0.6%)	4 (1.0%)
Nervous System	31 (6.5%)	11 (2.8%)
Dizziness	5 (1.0%)	4 (1.0%)
Respiratory System	34 (7.1%)	25 (6.5%)
Rhinitis	10 (2.1%)	4 (1.0%)
Skin and Appendages	24 (5.0%)	12 (3.1%)
Rash	11 (2.3%)	3 (0.8%)
Pruritus	10 (2.1%)	3 (0.8%)
Special Senses	14 (2.9%)	10 (2.6%)
Urogenital System	14 (2.9%)	9 (2.3%)

Safety was monitored for 3 years during the placebo-controlled DAIS study for both adverse events and laboratory anomalies. Fenofibrate was used safely in type 2 diabetic patients, as the overall incidence and severity of adverse events were comparable in fenofibrate and placebo groups. Table 2 summarizes the incidence of adverse events, by body system, observed in both treatment groups.

Table 2: LIPIDIL SUPRA

DAIS Study: Incidence of Adverse Events (AEs) by System, Experienced by Type 2 Diabetic Patients During Treatment with Fenofibrate or Placebo (ITT Population)

Body System	Fenofibrate (N=207)		Placebo (N=211)	
	AEs	Patients	AEs	Patients
Total # pts. with at least 1 AE	Total AEs: 1710	201 (97.1%)	Total AEs: 1759	202 (95.7%)
Body as a Whole	371 (21.7%)	136 (65.7%)	362 (20.6%)	146 (69.2%)
Cardiovascular	183 (10.7%)	84 (40.6%)	220 (12.5%)	96 (45.5%)
Digestive	196 (11.5%)	86 (41.6%)	194 (11.0%)	87 (41.2%)
Endocrine	11 (0.6%)	10 (4.8%)	19 (1.1%)	11 (5.2%)
Haemic/Lymphatic	31 (1.8%)	19 (9.2%)	23 (1.3%)	15 (7.1%)
Metabolic/ Nutritional	50 (2.9%)	32 (15.5%)	70 (4.9%)	41 (19.4%)
Musculoskeletal	155 (9.1%)	84 (40.6%)	180 (10.2%)	84 (39.8%)
CNS	103 (6.0%)	59 (28.5%)	98 (5.6%)	58 (27.5%)
Respiratory	301 (17.6%)	108 (52.2%)	279 (15.9%)	105 (49.8%)
Skin/Appendage	107 (6.3%)	58 (28.0%)	107 (6.1%)	48 (22.8%)
Special Senses	73 (4.3%)	44 (21.3%)	90 (5.1%)	50 (23.7%)
Urogenital	118 (6.9%)	55 (26.6%)	103 (5.9%)	46 (21.8%)
Other	11 (0.6%)	9 (4.4%)	14 (0.8%)	11 (5.2%)

In two open, non-controlled clinical studies conducted in Canada and Germany, a total of 375 patients on fenofibrate, microcoated formulation, were evaluated for adverse events. Listed in Table 3 are the adverse events possibly or probably related to fenofibrate, microcoated formulation and reported by more than 0.5% of the patients.

Table 3: LIPIDIL SUPRA

Number (%) of Patients Reporting Adverse Events Possibly or Probably Related to Fenofibrate

Adverse Events	Canadian and German Multicenter Studies (12-Week Treatment) Microcoated Fenofibrate (n=375)
Digestive System	
Gastrointestinal disorder	4 (1.1%)
Nausea	3 (0.8%)
Flatulence	2 (0.5%)
Diarrhea	2 (0.5%)
Liver function tests abnormal	2 (0.5%)
Dyspepsia	2 (0.5%)
Gastritis	2 (0.5%)
Constipation	2 (0.5%)
Body as a Whole	
Abdominal pain	4 (1.1%)
Headache	2 (0.5%)
Asthenia	2 (0.5%)
Lab test abnormal	2 (0.5%)
Metabolic and Nutritional Disorders	
ALT increased (>3×ULN)	3 (0.8%)
AST increased (>3×ULN)	4 (1.1%)
Creatine kinase increased (>5×ULN)	1 (0.3%)
Nervous system	
Dizziness	2 (0.5%)
Libido decreased	2 (0.5%)

)ther adverse events include the following: Common: vomiting. Uncommon: pancreatitis, venous thromboembolism (pul-
ary embolism and deep vein thrombosis). Rare: alopecia, sexual asthenia, myositis, muscular cramps. Very rare: rhab-
volysis, interstitial pneumophaties.
isodes of hepatitis have been reported. When symptoms indicative of hepatitis (e.g. jaundice) occur, laboratory tests are
conducted for verification and fenofibrate discontinued, if applicable (see Warnings).
tosensitivity reactions, development of gallstones and cutaneous hypersensitivity with erythema and vesiculation or nodu-
n parts of the skin exposed to sunlight or artificial UV light in individual cases (even after many months of uncomplicated
ve also been reported.

Laboratory Tests: In most trials, sporadic and transient increases in aminotransferase levels have been associated with the use of fenofibrate. The reported frequency of AST and ALT elevations was variable; in the clinical studies conducted in Canada and Germany elevations above three times the upper limit of normal were observed in 2.0% of the patients (7/375) treated with fenofibrate, microcoated formulation. In two dose-ranging studies, the incidence of increases in transaminases (>3×ULN) due to fenofibrate therapy appears to be dose related; 0.6% (1/157) (80 mg tablet), 1.9% (3/158) (160 mg tablet) and 4.0% (6/149) (240 mg tablet). Values usually return to normal without interruption of treatment (see Precautions). Reductions in alkaline phosphatase levels have also been observed.

Mild decreases in hemoglobin, hematocrit, and white blood cell counts have been observed occasionally in patients following initiation of fenofibrate therapy but these observations were without clinical significance. However, these levels stabilize during long-term administration. In addition, a decrease in haptoglobin concentration has been observed in some patients with Type IV hyperlipidemia during long-term use of fenofibrate. However, this decrease in haptoglobin was not associated with any other sign of blood dyscrasia and/or hemolysis.

The mean plasma levels of urea and creatinine showed increases, particularly during long-term fenofibrate treatment, most of them remaining within the limits of normal values.

Fenofibrate also has the potential to provoke CK elevations and changes in hematologic parameters which generally subside when the drug is discontinued (see Warnings). In the clinical studies conducted in Canada and Germany, the reported frequency of CK elevations above five times the upper limit of normal was approximately 0.3% (2/375) of the patients treated with fenofibrate, microcoated formulation.

OVERDOSE:

Treatment: While there has been no reported case of overdosage, symptomatic and supportive measures should be taken. Fenofibrate is not dialysable because the main metabolite (fenofibric acid) is highly bound to plasma proteins.

> For management of a suspected drug overdose, CPhA recommends that you contact your **regional Poison Control Centre**. See the *CPS* Directory section for a list of Poison Control Centres.

DOSAGE: Patients should be placed on a standard cholesterol-lowering diet (at least equivalent to the Adult Treatment Panel III (ATP III TLC diet)) before receiving LIPIDIL SUPRA (fenofibrate), and should continue on this diet during treatment with LIPIDIL SUPRA. If appropriate, a program of weight control and physical exercise should be implemented.

Prior to initiating therapy with LIPIDIL SUPRA, secondary causes for elevations in plasma lipid levels should be excluded. A lipid profile should also be performed.

If a significant serum lipid response is not obtained in three months, LIPIDIL SUPRA should be discontinued.

The usual recommended dose for LIPIDIL SUPRA (fenofibrate, microcoated formulation) in adults is one 160 mg tablet daily taken with the main meal. The maximum recommended total daily dose of LIPIDIL SUPRA is 200 mg (2 tablets of 100 mg).

In patients with renal insufficiency (creatinine clearance between 20 and 100 mL/min), LIPIDIL SUPRA treatment should be initiated at the dose of 100 mg/day and increased only after evaluation of the tolerance and effects on the lipid parameters. LIPIDIL SUPRA should not be used when the creatinine clearance is lower than 20 mL/min.

INFORMATION FOR THE PATIENT: Published in e-CPS, available by subscription at www.e-cps.ca.

SUPPLIED: 100 mg: Each white, oblong, film-coated tablet, embossed with the Fournier logo on one side and 100 on the other, contains: microcoated fenofibrate 100 mg. Nonmedicinal ingredients: colloidal silicon dioxide, crospovidone, lactose monohydrate, microcrystalline cellulose, povidone, sodium lauryl sulfate and sodium stearyl fumarate; tablet coating: polyvinyl alcohol, soybean lecithin, talc, titanium dioxide and xanthan gum. Blister packs of 30.

160 mg: Each white, oblong, film-coated tablet, embossed with the Fournier logo on one side and 160 on the other, contains: microcoated fenofibrate 160 mg. Nonmedicinal ingredients: colloidal silicon dioxide, crospovidone, lactose monohydrate, microcrystalline cellulose, povidone, sodium lauryl sulfate and sodium stearyl fumarate; tablet coating: polyvinyl alcohol, soybean lecithin, talc, titanium dioxide and xanthan gum. Blister packs of 30.

Store at 15 to 30°C. Protect from light and moisture.

(Shown in Product Identification Section)

> The reader is invited to consult CPhA's monograph **HMG-CoA Reductase Inhibitors.**

Lipitor® Pr

atorvastatin calcium

Lipid Metabolism Regulator

Pfizer

Date of Preparation: January 12, 2001
Date of Revision: July 21, 2009

SUMMARY PRODUCT INFORMATION:

Route of Administration	Dosage Form/Strength	Nonmedicinal Ingredients
Oral	Tablets: 10 mg, 20 mg, 40 mg and 80 mg atorvastatin	Calcium carbonate, candelilla wax (10, 20 and 40 mg), croscarmellose sodium, hydroxypropyl cellulose, hydroxypropyl methylcellulose, lactose monohydrate, magnesium stearate, microcrystalline cellulose, polyethylene glycol, polysorbate 80, simethicone emulsion, talc and titanium dioxide

INDICATIONS AND CLINICAL USE: LIPITOR (atorvastatin calcium) is indicated as an adjunct to lifestyle changes, including diet, for the reduction of elevated total cholesterol (total-C), LDL-C, triglycerides (TG), apolipoprotein B (apo B), the Total-C/HDL-D ratio and for increasing HDL-C; in hyperlipidemic and dyslipidemic conditions, when response to diet and other nonpharmacological measures alone has been inadequate, including:

- Primary hypercholesterolemia (Type IIa);
- Combined (mixed) hyperlipidemia (Type IIb), including familial combined hyperlipidemia, regardless of whether cholesterol or triglycerides are the lipid abnormality of concern;
- Dysbetalipoproteinemia (Type III);
- Hypertriglyceridemia (Type IV);
- Familial hypercholesterolemia (homozygous and heterozygous). For homozygous familial hypercholesterolemia, LIPITOR should be used as an adjunct to treatments such as LDL apheresis, or as monotherapy if such treatments are not available.
- An adjunct to diet to reduce total-C, LDL-C, and apo B levels in boys and postmenarchal girls, 10 to 17 years of age with heterozygous familial hypercholesterolemia, if after an adequate trial of diet therapy the following findings are still present:
  a. LDL-C remains ≥4.9 mmol/L (190 mg/dL) or
  b. LDL-C remains ≥4.1 mmol/L (160 mg/dL) and:
    - there is a positive family history of premature cardiovascular disease or
    - two or more other CVD risk factors are present in the pediatric patient

Prior to initiating therapy with LIPITOR, secondary causes should be excluded for elevations in plasma lipid levels (e.g. poorly controlled diabetes mellitus, hypothyroidism, nephrotic syndrome, dysproteinemias, obstructive liver disease, and alcoholism), and a lipid profile performed to measure total cholesterol, LDL-C, HDL-C, and TG. For patients with TG <4.52 mmol/L (<400 mg/dL), LDL-C can be estimated using the following equation:

LDL-C (mmol/L)=total-C - [(0.37×(TG)+HDL-C)]
LDL-C (mg/dL)=total-C - [(0.2×(TG)+HDL-C)]

For patients with TG levels >4.52 mmol/L (>400 mg/dL), this equation is less accurate and LDL-C concentrations should be measured directly or by ultracentrifugation.

Patients with high or very high triglyceride levels, i.e. >2.2 mmol/L (200 mg/dL) or >5.6 mmol/L (500 mg/dL), respectively, may require triglyceride-lowering therapy (fenofibrate, bezafibrate or nicotinic acid) alone or in combination with LIPITOR.

In general, combination therapy with fibrates must be undertaken cautiously and only after risk-benefit analysis (see Warnings and Precautions, Muscle Effects, Pharmacokinetic Interactions and Drug Interactions).

Elevated serum triglycerides are most often observed in patients with the metabolic syndrome (abdominal obesity, atherogenic dyslipidemia [elevated triglycerides, small dense LDL particles and low HDL-cholesterol], insulin resistance with or without glucose intolerance, raised blood pressure and prothrombic and proinflammatory states).

When drugs are prescribed attention to therapeutic lifestyle changes (reduced intake of saturated fats and cholesterol, weight reduction, increased physical activity, ingestion of soluble fibers) should always be maintained and reinforced.

Prevention of Cardiovascular Disease: LIPITOR is indicated to reduce the risk of myocardial infarction in adult hypertensive patients without clinically evident coronary heart disease, but with at least three additional risk factors for coronary heart disease such as age ≥55 years, male sex, smoking, type 2 diabetes, left ventricular hypertrophy, other specified abnormalities on ECG, microalbuminuria or proteinuria, ratio of plasma total cholesterol to HDL-cholesterol ≥6, or premature family history of coronary heart disease.

LIPITOR is also indicated to reduce the risk of myocardial infarction and stroke in adult patients with type 2 diabetes mellitus and hypertension without clinically evident coronary heart disease, but with other risk factors such as age ≥55 years, retinopathy, albuminuria or smoking.

LIPITOR is indicated to reduce the risk of myocardial infarction in patients with clinically evident coronary heart disease.

CONTRAINDICATIONS: Hypersensitivity to any component of this medication (for a complete listing of the components, see Dosage Forms, Composition and Packaging).

Active liver disease or unexplained persistent elevations of serum transaminases exceeding 3 times the upper limit of normal (see Warnings and Precautions).

Pregnancy and Nursing Women: Cholesterol and other products of cholesterol biosynthesis are essential components for fetal development (including synthesis of steroids and cell membranes). LIPITOR should be administered to women of childbearing age only when such patients are highly unlikely to conceive and have been informed of the possible harm. If the patient becomes pregnant while taking LIPITOR, the drug should be discontinued immediately and the patient apprised of the potential harm to the fetus. Atherosclerosis being a chronic process, discontinuation of lipid metabolism regulating drugs during pregnancy should have little impact on the outcome of long-term therapy of primary hypercholesterolemia (see Warnings and Precautions, Pregnant Women, Nursing Women).

WARNINGS AND PRECAUTIONS: General: Before instituting therapy with LIPITOR (atorvastatin calcium), an attempt should be made to control elevated serum lipoprotein levels with appropriate diet, exercise, and weight reduction in overweight patients, and to treat other underlying medical problems (see Indications and Clinical Use). Patients should be advised to inform subsequent physicians of the prior use of LIPITOR or any other lipid-lowering agents.

Pharmacokinetic Interactions: The use of HMG-CoA reductase inhibitors has been associated with severe myopathy, including rhabdomyolysis, which may be more frequent when they are coadministered with drugs that inhibit the cytochrome P-450 enzyme system. Atorvastatin is metabolized by cytochrome P-450 isoform 3A4 and as such may interact with agents that inhibit this enzyme. (See Warnings and Precautions, Muscle Effects and Drug Interactions.)

Muscle Effects: Effects on skeletal muscle such as myalgia, myopathy and very rarely, rhabdomyolysis have been reported in patients treated with LIPITOR.

Very rare cases of rhabdomyolysis with acute renal failure secondary to myoglobinuria, have been reported with LIPITOR and with other HMG-CoA reductase inhibitors.

Myopathy, defined as muscle pain or muscle weakness in conjunction with increases in creatine kinase (CK) values to greater than ten times the upper limit of normal, should be considered in any patient with diffuse myalgia, muscle tenderness or weakness, and/or marked elevation of CK. Patients should be advised to report promptly any unexplained muscle pain, tenderness or weakness, particularly if accompanied by malaise or fever. Patients who develop any signs or symptoms suggestive of myopathy should have their CK levels measured. LIPITOR therapy should be discontinued if markedly elevated CK levels are measured or myopathy is diagnosed or suspected.

Pre-Disposing Factors for Myopathy/Rhabdomyolysis: LIPITOR, as with other HMG-CoA reductase inhibitors, should be prescribed with caution in patients with pre-disposing factors for myopathy/rhabdomyolysis. Such factors include: personal or family history of hereditary muscular disorders; previous history of muscle toxicity with another HMG-CoA reductase inhibitor; concomitant use of a fibrate, or niacin; hypothyroidism; alcohol abuse; excessive physical exercise; age >70 years; renal impairment; hepatic impairment; diabetes with hepatic fatty change; surgery and trauma; frailty; situations where an increase in plasma levels of active ingredient may occur.

The risk of myopathy and rhabdomyolysis during treatment with HMG-CoA reductase inhibitors is increased with concurrent administration of cyclosporin, fibric acid derivatives, erythromycin, clarithromycin, niacin (nicotinic acid), azole antifungals or nefazodone. Therefore, lower starting and maintenance doses of atorvastatin should also be considered when taken concomitantly with the aforementioned drugs. In cases where coadministration of LIPITOR with cyclosporine is necessary, the dose of LIPITOR should not exceed 10 mg (see Drug Interactions, Overview, Drug-Drug Interactions).

LIPITOR therapy should be temporarily withheld or discontinued in any patient with an acute serious condition suggestive of myopathy or having a risk factor predisposing to the development of renal failure secondary to rhabdomyolysis (such as sepsis, severe acute infection, hypotension, major surgery, trauma, severe metabolic, endocrine and electrolyte disorders, and uncontrolled seizures).

LIPITOR therapy should be discontinued if markedly elevated CPK levels occur or myopathy is diagnosed or suspected.

Cardiovascular: Hemorrhagic Stroke in Patients with Recent Stroke or Transient Ischemic Attack (TIA): A post-hoc analysis of a clinical study in 4,731 patients without coronary heart disease (CHD) who had a stroke or TIA within the preceding six months, revealed a higher incidence of hemorrhagic stroke in the atorvastatin 80mg group compared to placebo. Patients with hemorrhagic stroke on entry appeared to be at increased risk for recurrent hemorrhagic stroke. The potential risk of hemorrhagic stroke should be carefully considered before initiating treatment with atorvastatin in patients with recent (1-6 months) stroke or TIA.

Effect on Ubiquinone (CoQ_{10}) Levels: Significant decreases in circulating ubiquinone levels in patients treated with atorvastatin and other statins have been observed. The clinical significance of a potential long-term statin-induced deficiency of ubiquinone has not been established. It has been reported that a decrease in myocardial ubiquinone levels could lead to impaired cardiac function in patients with borderline congestive heart failure.

Endocrine and Metabolism: Endocrine Function: HMG-CoA reductase inhibitors interfere with cholesterol synthesis and as such might theoretically blunt adrenal and/or gonadal steroid production. Clinical studies with atorvastatin and other HMG-CoA reductase inhibitors have suggested that these agents do not reduce plasma cortisol concentration or impair adrenal reserve and do not reduce basal plasma testosterone concentration. However, the effects of HMG-CoA reductase inhibitors on male fertility have not been studied in adequate numbers of patients. The effects, if any, on the pituitary-gonadal axis in premenopausal women are unknown.

Patients treated with atorvastatin who develop clinical evidence of endocrine dysfunction should be evaluated appropriately. Caution should be exercised if an HMG-CoA reductase inhibitor or other agent used to lower cholesterol levels is administered to patients receiving other drugs (e.g. ketoconazole, spironolactone or cimetidine) that may decrease the levels of endogenous steroid hormones.

Effect on Lipoprotein(a): In some patients, the beneficial effect of lowered total cholesterol and LDL-C levels may be partly blunted by a concomitant increase in Lp(a) lipoprotein concentrations. Present knowledge suggests the importance of high Lp(a) levels as an emerging risk factor for coronary heart disease. It is thus desirable to maintain and reinforce lifestyle changes in high risk patients placed on atorvastatin therapy.

Patients with Severe Hypercholesterolemia: Higher drug dosages (80 mg/day) required for some patients with severe hypercholesterolemia (including familial hypercholesterolemia) are associated with increased plasma levels of atorvastatin. **Caution should be exercised in such patients who are also severely renally impaired, elderly, or are concomitantly being administered digoxin or CYP 3A4 inhibitors** (see Warnings and Precautions, Pharmacokinetic Interactions, Muscle Effects; Drug Interactions; Dosage and Administration).

Hepatic/Biliary/Pancreatic: Hepatic Effects: In clinical trials, persistent increases in serum transaminases greater than three times the upper limit of normal occurred in <1% of patients who received LIPITOR. When the dosage of LIPITOR was reduced, or when drug treatment was interrupted or discontinued, serum transaminase levels returned to pretreatment levels. The increases were generally not associated with jaundice or other clinical signs or symptoms. Most patients continued treatment with a reduced dose of LIPITOR without clinical sequelae.

Liver function tests should be performed before the initiation of treatment, and periodically thereafter. Special attention should be paid to patients who develop elevated serum transaminase levels, and in these patients measurements should be repeated promptly and then performed more frequently.

If increases in alanine aminotransferase (ALT) or aspartate aminotransferase (AST) show evidence of progression, particularly if they rise to greater than 3 times the upper limit of normal and are persistent, the dosage should be reduced or the drug discontinued.

LIPITOR, as well as other HMG-CoA reductase inhibitors, should be used with caution in patients who consume substantial quantities of alcohol and/or have a past history of liver disease. Active liver disease or unexplained transaminase elevations are contraindications to the use of LIPITOR; if such a condition should develop during therapy, the drug should be discontinued.

Ophthalmologic: Effect on the Lens: Current long-term data from clinical trials do not indicate an adverse effect of atorvastatin on the human lens.

Renal: Renal Insufficiency: Plasma concentrations and LDL-C lowering efficacy of LIPITOR was shown to be similar in patients with moderate renal insufficiency compared with patients with normal renal function. However, since several cases of rhabdomyolysis have been reported in patients with a history of renal insufficiency of unknown severity, as a precautionary measure and pending further experience in renal disease, the lowest dose (10 mg/day) of LIPITOR should be used in these patients. Similar precautions apply in patients with severe renal insufficiency [creatinine clearance <30 mL/min (<0.5 mL/sec)]; the lowest dosage should be used and implemented cautiously (see Warnings and Precautions, Muscle Effects; Drug Interactions). Refer also to Dosage and Administration.

Sensitivity/Resistance: Hypersensitivity: An apparent hypersensitivity syndrome has been reported with other HMG-CoA reductase inhibitors which has included 1 or more of the following features: anaphylaxis, angioedema, lupus erythematous-like syndrome, polymyalgia rheumatica, vasculitis, purpura, thrombocytopenia, leukopenia, hemolytic anemia, positive ANA, ESR increase, eosinophilia, arthritis, arthralgia, urticaria, asthenia, photosensitivity, fever, chills, flushing, malaise, dyspnea, toxic epidermal necrolysis, erythema multiforme, including Stevens-Johnson syndrome. Although to date hypersensitivity syndrome has not been described as such, LIPITOR should be discontinued if hypersensitivity is suspected.

Special Populations: Pregnant Women: LIPITOR is contraindicated during pregnancy (see Contraindications).

There are no data on the use of LIPITOR during pregnancy. LIPITOR should be administered to women of childbearing age only when such patients are highly unlikely to conceive and have been informed of the potential hazards. If the patient becomes pregnant while taking LIPITOR, the drug should be discontinued and the patient apprised of the potential risk to the fetus.

Nursing Women: In rats, milk concentrations of atorvastatin are similar to those in plasma. It is not known whether this drug is excreted in human milk. Because of the potential for adverse reactions in nursing infants, women taking LIPITOR should not breast-feed (see Contraindications).

Pediatrics: Safety and effectiveness of LIPITOR in patients 10-17 years of age (N=140) with heterozygous familial hypercholesterolemia have been evaluated in a controlled clinical trial of 6 months duration in adolescent boys and postmenarchal girls. Patients treated with LIPITOR had a safety and tolerability profile generally similar to that of placebo. Doses greater than 20 mg have not been studied in this patient population.

Safety and effectiveness of LIPITOR in pediatric patients has not been determined in the prevention of myocardial infarction.

LIPITOR had no effect on growth or sexual maturation in boys and in girls. The effects on menstrual cycle were not assessed [see Adverse Reactions, Pediatrics Patients and Dosage and Administration for Heterozygous Familial Hypercholesterolemia in Pediatric Patients (10-17 years of age)].

Adolescent females should be counselled on appropriate contraceptive methods while on LIPITOR therapy (see Contraindications and Warnings and Precautions, Pregnant Women). LIPITOR has not been studied in controlled clinical trials involving pre-pubertal patients or patients younger than 10 years of age.

Doses of LIPITOR up to 80 mg/day for 1 year have been evaluated in 8 pediatric patients with homozygous familial hypercholesterolemia.

Geriatrics: Treatment experience in adults 70 years or older (N=221) with doses of LIPITOR up to 80 mg/day has demonstrated that the safety and effectiveness of atorvastatin in this population was similar to that of patients <70 years of age. Pharmacokinetic evaluation of atorvastatin in subjects over the age of 65 years indicates an increased AUC. As a precautionary measure, the lowest dose should be administered initially.

Elderly patients may be more susceptible to myopathy (see Warnings and Precautions, Muscle Effects, Pre-Disposing Factors for Myopathy/Rhabdomyolysis).

ADVERSE REACTIONS: Adverse Drug Reaction Overview: LIPITOR is generally well-tolerated. Adverse reactions have usually been mild and transient. In controlled clinical studies (placebo-controlled and active-controlled comparative studies with other lipid lowering agents) involving 2502 patients, <2% of patients were discontinued due to adverse experiences attributable to LIPITOR. Of these 2502 patients, 1721 were treated for at least 6 months and 1253 for 1 year or more.

Adverse experiences occurring at an incidence ≥1% in patients participating in placebo-controlled clinical studies of LIPITOR and reported to be possibly, probably or definitely drug related are shown in Table 1.

Table 1: LIPITOR

Associated Adverse Events Reported in ≥1% of Patients in Placebo-Controlled Clinical Trials

	Placebo % (n=270)	LIPITOR % (n=1122)
Gastrointestinal		
Constipation	1	1
Diarrhea	1	1
Dyspepsia	2	1
Flatulence	2	1
Nausea	0	1
Nervous System		
Headache	2	1
Miscellaneous		
Pain	<1	1
Myalgia	1	1
Asthenia	<1	1

The following additional adverse events were reported in clinical trials; not all events listed below have been associa
a causal relationship to LIPITOR therapy: muscle cramps, myositis, myopathy, paresthesia, peripheral neuropathy, par
hepatitis, cholestatic jaundice, anorexia, vomiting, alopecia, pruritus, rash, impotence, hyperglycemia, and hypoglyce

Heterozygous Familial Hypercholesterolemia in Pediatric Patients (ages 10-17 years): In a 26-week controll
boys and postmenarchal girls (n=187, where 140 patients received LIPITOR), the safety and tolerability profile of
to 20 mg daily was similar to that of placebo. The adverse events reported in ≥1% of patients were as follows: ab
depression and headache (see Warnings and Precautions, Pediatrics).

Laboratory Changes and Adverse Events: The criteria for clinically significant laboratory changes were >3×
normal (ULN) for liver enzymes, and >5×ULN for creatine kinase. A total of 8 unique subjects met one or mor
during the double-blind phase. Hence, the incidence of patients who experienced abnormally high enzymat
and creatine kinase) was >4% (8/187).

Five atorvastatin and one placebo subjects had increases in CK >5×ULN during the double-blind phase
vastatin treated subjects had increases in CK >10×ULN.

There were 2 subjects who had clinically significant increases in ALT.

Abnormal Hematologic and Clinical Chemistry Findings: Laboratory Tests: Increases in serum tr
been noted in clinical trials (see Warnings and Precautions).

Post-Market Adverse Drug Reactions: The following adverse events have also been reported during post-marketing experience with LIPITOR, regardless of causality assessment:
Very Rare Reports: severe myopathy with or without rhabdomyolysis (see Warnings and Precautions, Muscle Effects, Renal Insufficiency and Drug Interactions).
Isolated Reports: Gynecomastia, thrombocytopenia, arthralgia and allergic reactions (including urticaria, angioneurotic edema, anaphylaxis and bullous rashes [including erytheme multiforme, Stevens-Johnson syndrome and toxic epidermal necrolysis]), fatigue, back pain, chest pain, malaise, dizziness, amnesia, peripheral edema, weight gain, abdominal pain, insomnia, hypoesthesia, tinnitus, tendon rupture and dysgeusia.

These may have no causal relationship to atorvastatin.

Ophthalmologic Observations: See Warnings and Precautions.

DRUG INTERACTIONS: Overview: Pharmacokinetic interaction studies conducted with drugs in healthy subjects may not detect the possibility of a potential drug interaction in some patients due to differences in underlying diseases and use of concomitant medications (see also Warnings and Precautions, Renal Insufficiency, Patients with Severe Hypercholesterolemia; Special Populations, Geriatrics).

Concomitant Therapy with Other Lipid Metabolism Regulators: Based on post-marketing surveillance, gemfibrozil, fenofibrate, other fibrates, and lipid-modifying doses of niacin (nicotinic acid) may increase the risk of myopathy when given concomitantly with HMG-CoA reductase inhibitors, probably because they can produce myopathy when given alone (see Warnings and Precautions, Muscle Effects). Therefore, combined drug therapy should be approached with caution; lower starting and maintenance doses of atorvastatin should be considered.

Cytochrome P-450-Mediated Interactions: Atorvastatin is metabolized by the cytochrome P-450 isoenzyme, CYP 3A4. Erythromycin, a CYP 3A4 inhibitor, increased atorvastatin plasma levels by 40%. Coadministration of CYP 3A4 inhibitors, such as grapefruit juice, some macrolide antibiotics (i.e. erythromycin, clarithromycin), immunosuppressants (cyclosporine), azole antifungal agents (i.e. itraconazole, ketoconazole), protease inhibitors, or the antidepressant, nefazodone, may have the potential to increase plasma concentrations of HMG-CoA reductase inhibitors, including LIPITOR. Caution should thus be exercised with concomitant use of these agents and lower starting and maintenance doses of atorvastatin should be considered when taken concomitantly with the aforementioned drugs (see Warnings and Precautions, Pharmacokinetic Interactions, Muscle Effects, Renal Insufficiency and Endocrine Function; Dosage and Administration).

Transporter Inhibitors: Atorvastatin and atorvastatin-metabolites are substrates of the OATP1B1 transporter. Inhibitors of the OATP1B1 (e.g. cyclosporine) can increase the bioavailability of atorvastatin.

Inducers of Cytochrome P450 3A: Concomitant administration of atorvastatin with inducers of cytochrome P450 3A4 (eg efavirenz, rifampin) can lead to variable reductions in plasma concentrations of atorvastatin. Due to the dual interaction mechanism of rifampin, (cytochrome P450 3A4 induction and inhibition of hepatocyte uptake transporter OATP1B1), simultaneous coadministration of atorvastatin with rifampin resulted in a mean increase in C_{max} and AUC of atorvastatin of 12 and 190%, respectively. In contrast, a delayed administration of atorvastatin after administration of rifampin has been associated with a significant reduction (approximately 80%) in atorvastatin plasma concentrations.

Drug-Drug Interactions: The drugs listed in Table 2 are based on either drug interactions studies, case reports, or potential interactions due to the expected magnitude and seriousness of the interaction (i.e., those identified as contraindicated). Interactions with other drugs have not been established.

Drug-Food Interactions: Coadministration of grapefruit juice has the potential to increase plasma concentrations of HMG-CoA reductase inhibitors including LIPITOR. The equivalent of 1.2 litres per day resulted in a 2.5 fold increase in AUC of atorvastatin.

Drug-Herb Interactions: Interactions with herbal products have not been established.

Drug-Laboratory Test Interactions: LIPITOR may elevate serum transaminase and creatine kinase levels (from skeletal muscle). In the differential diagnosis of chest pain in a patient on therapy with LIPITOR, cardiac and noncardiac fractions of these enzymes should be determined.

Table 2: LIPITOR

Established or Potential Drug-Drug Interactions

Proper Name	Effect	Clinical Comment
Bile Acid Sequestrants	**Patients with mild to moderate HC:** ↑ LDL-C reduction (−45%) when LIPITOR 10 mg and colestipol 20 g were coadministered than when either drug was administered alone (−35% for LIPITOR and −22% for colestipol). **Patients with severe HC:** LDL-C reduction was similar (−53%) when LIPITOR 40 mg and colestipol 20 g were coadministered when compared to that with LIPITOR 80 mg alone. ↓ plasma concentration (~26%) when LIPITOR 40 mg plus colestipol 20 g were coadministered compared with LIPITOR 40 mg alone. However, the combination drug therapy was less effective in lowering TG than LIPITOR monotherapy in both types of hypercholesterolemic patients.	When LIPITOR is used concurrently with colestipol or any other resin, an interval of at least 2 hours should be maintained between the two drugs, since the absorption of LIPITOR may be impaired by the resin.
Fibric Acid Derivatives (gemfibrozil, fenofibrate, bezafibrate) and Niacin (nicotinic acid)	↑ in the risk of myopathy during treatment with other drugs in this class, including atorvastatin, with concurrent administration with a fibric acid derivative	Although there is limited experience with the use of LIPITOR given concurrently with fibric acid derivatives and niacin, the benefits and risks of such combined therapy should be carefully considered (see Warnings and Precautions, Muscle Effects).
Coumarin Anticoagulants	No clinically significant effect on prothrombin time	LIPITOR had no clinically significant effect on prothrombin time when administered to patients receiving chronic warfarin therapy.
Digoxin	In healthy subjects, digoxin PK at steady-state were not significantly altered by coadministration of digoxin 0.25 mg and LIPITOR 10 mg daily. ↑ in digoxin steady-state concentrations by ~20% following coadministration of digoxin 0.25 mg and LIPITOR 80 mg daily).	Patients taking digoxin should be monitored appropriately.
Antihypertensive Agents: Amlodipine	In healthy subjects, atorvastatin PK were not altered by the coadministration of LIPITOR 80 mg and amlodipine 10 mg at steady state. No apparent changes in BP or HR.	
Quinapril	Steady-state quinapril dosing of 80 mg QD did not significantly affect the PK profile of atorvastatin tablets 10 mg QD.	

(cont'd)

Table 2: LIPITOR *(cont'd)*

Established or Potential Drug-Drug Interactions

Proper Name	Effect	Clinical Comment
Oral Contraceptives and Hormone Replacement Therapy	↑ plasma concentrations (AUC levels) of norethindone by ~30% and ethinyl estradiol by ~20% following coadministration of LIPITOR with an oral contraceptive containing 1 mg norethindone and 35 µg ethinyl estradiol. In clinical studies, LIPITOR was used concomitantly with estrogen replacement therapy without evidence to date of clinically significant adverse interactions.	These increases should be considered when selecting an oral contraceptive.
Antacids	↓ in plasma concentrations of LIPITOR by ~35% following administration of aluminum and magnesium based antacids, such as Maalox TC Suspension. LDL-C reduction was not altered; TG-lowering effect of LIPITOR may be affected.	
Cimetidine	No effect on plasma concentrations or LDL-C lowering efficacy of LIPITOR ↓ in TG-lowering effect of LIPITOR from 34% to 26%	
Diltiazem Hydrochloride	Steady-state diltiazem increases the exposure, based on AUC_{LASTs}, of a single dose of atorvastatin by approximately 50%.	
Antipyrine	LIPITOR had no effect on the PK of antipyrine	Antipyrine was used as a non-specific model for drugs metabolized by the microsomal hepatic enzyme system (cytochrome P-450 system). Interactions with other drugs metabolized via the same cytochrome isozymes are not expected.
Macrolide Antibiotics (azithromycin, clarithromycin, erythromycin). Clarithromycin and erythromycin are both CYP3A4 inhibitors	In healthy adults, coadministration of LIPITOR (10 mg QD) and azithromycin (500 mg QD) did not significantly alter the plasma concentrations of atorvastatin. ↑ plasma concentration by ~40% with erythromycin (500 mg QID) and ~80% with clarithromycin (500 mg BID) when coadministered with atorvastatin (10 mg QD)	See Warnings and Precautions, Muscle Effects.
Protease Inhibitors (nelfinavir mesylate)	↑ plasma concentrations of atorvastatin when atorvastatin 10 mg QD is coadministered with nelfinavir mesylate 1250 mg BID ↑ AUC by 74% and ↑ C_{max} by 122%	Nelfinavir is a known CYP3A4 inhibitor.
Cyclosporine	Concomitant administration of atorvastatin 10 mg and cyclosporine 5.2 mg/kg/day resulted in a 7.7 fold increase in exposure to atorvastatin.	In cases where coadministration of atorvastatin with cyclosporine is necessary, the dose of atorvastatin should not exceed 10 mg. See Warnings and Precautions, Muscle Effects.
Itraconazole	Concomitant administration of atorvastatin 20–40 mg and itraconazole 200 mg daily resulted in a 2.5-3.3-fold increase in atorvastatin AUC.	

Legend: HC=hypercholesterolemia; TG=triglycerides; PK=pharmacokinetics; BP=blood pressure; HR=heart rate; AUC=Area under the curve.

DOSAGE AND ADMINISTRATION: Patients should be placed on a standard cholesterol-lowering diet before receiving LIPITOR, and should continue on this diet during treatment with LIPITOR. If appropriate, a program of weight control and physical exercise should be implemented.

Prior to initiating therapy with LIPITOR, secondary causes for elevations in plasma lipid levels should be excluded. A lipid profile should also be performed.

Primary Hypercholesterolemia and Combined (Mixed) Dyslipidemia, Including Familial Combined Hyperlipidemia: The recommended starting dose of LIPITOR is 10 or 20 mg once daily, depending on patient's LDL-C reduction required. Patients who require a large reduction in LDL-C (more than 45%) may be started at 40 mg once daily. The dosage range of LIPITOR is 10 to 80 mg once daily. Doses can be given at any time of the day with or without food, and should preferably be given in the evening. A significant therapeutic response is evident within 2 weeks, and the maximum response is usually achieved within 2-4 weeks. The response is maintained during chronic therapy. Adjustments of dosage, if necessary, should be made at intervals of 2 to 4 weeks. The maximum dose is 80 mg/day.

The dosage of LIPITOR should be individualized according the baseline LDL-C, total-C/HDL-C ratio and/or TG levels to achieve the recommended desired lipid values at the lowest dose needed to achieve LDL-C desired level. Lipid levels should be monitored periodically and, if necessary, the dose of LIPITOR adjusted based on desired lipid levels recommended by guidelines.

Severe Dyslipidemias: In patients with severe dyslipidemias, including homozygous and heterozygous familial hypercholesterolemia and dysbetalipoproteinemia (Type III), higher dosages (up to 80 mg/day) may be required (see Warnings and Precautions, Pharmacokinetic Interactions, Muscle Effects; Drug Interactions).

Heterozygous Familial Hypercholesterolemia in Pediatric Patients (10-17 years of age): In this population, the recommended starting dose of LIPITOR is 10 mg/day; the maximum recommended dose is 20 mg/day (doses greater than 20 mg/day have not been studied in this patient population). Doses should be individualized according to the recommended goal of therapy (see Indications and Clinical Use). Adjustments should be made at intervals of 4 weeks or more.

Prevention of Cardiovascular Disease: Clinical trials conducted that evaluated atorvastatin in the primary prevention of myocardial infarction used a dose of 10 mg atorvastatin once daily.

For secondary prevention of myocardial infarction, optimal dosing may range from 10 mg to 80 mg atorvastatin once daily, to be given at the discretion of the prescriber, taking into account the expected benefit and safety considerations relevant to the patient to be treated.

Concomitant Therapy: See Drug Interactions.

Dosage in Patients with Renal Insufficiency: See Warnings and Precautions.

OVERDOSAGE:
There is no specific treatment for atorvastatin overdosage. Should an overdose occur, the patient should be treated symptomatically and supportive measures instituted as required. Due to extensive drug binding to plasma proteins, hemodialysis is not expected to significantly enhance atorvastatin clearance (see Adverse Reactions).

> For management of a suspected drug overdose, contact your regional Poison Control Centre. See the *CPS* Directory section for a list of Poison Control Centres.

ACTION AND CLINICAL PHARMACOLOGY: Mechanism of Action: LIPITOR (atorvastatin calcium) is a synthetic lipid-lowering agent. It is a selective, competitive inhibitor of 3-hydroxy-3-methylglutaryl-coenzyme A (HMG-CoA) reductase. This enzyme catalyzes the conversion of HMG-CoA to mevalonate, which is an early and rate-limiting step in the biosynthesis of cholesterol.

LIPITOR lowers plasma cholesterol and lipoprotein levels by inhibiting HMG-CoA reductase and cholesterol synthesis in the liver and by increasing the number of hepatic Low Density Lipoprotein (LDL) receptors on the cell surface for enhanced uptake and catabolism of Low Density Lipoprotein (LDL).

LIPITOR reduces LDL-Cholesterol (LDL-C) and the number of LDL particles. Lipitor also reduces Very Low Density Lipoprotein-Cholesterol (VLDL-C), serum triglycerides (TG) and Intermediate Density Lipoproteins (IDL), as well as the number of apolipoprotein B (apo B) containing particles, but increases High Density Lipoprotein-Cholesterol (HDL-C). Elevated serum cholesterol due to elevated LDL-C is a major risk factor for the development of cardiovascular disease. Low serum concentration of HDL-C is also an independent risk factor. Elevated plasma TG is also a risk factor for cardiovascular disease, particularly if due to increased IDL, or associated with decreased HDL-C or increased LDL-C.

Epidemiologic, clinical and experimental studies have established that high LDL-C, low HDL-C and high plasma TG promote human atherosclerosis and are risk factors for developing cardiovascular disease. Some studies have also shown that the total (TC):HDL-C ratio (TC:HDL-C) is the best predictor of coronary artery disease. In contrast, increased levels of HDL-C are associated with decreased cardiovascular risk. Drug therapies that reduce levels of LDL-C or decrease TG while simultaneously increasing HDL-C have demonstrated reductions in rates of cardiovascular mortality and morbidity.

Pharmacodynamics: The lowering of total cholesterol, LDL-C and ApoB have been shown to reduce the risk of cardiovascular events and mortality.

LIPITOR (atorvastatin calcium) is a selective, competitive inhibitor of HMG-CoA reductase. In both subjects and in patients with homozygous and heterozygous familial hypercholesterolemia, nonfamilial forms of hypercholesterolemia, mixed dyslipidemia, hypertriglyceridemia, and dysbetalipoproteinemia, LIPITOR has been shown to reduce levels of total cholesterol (total-C), LDL-C, apo B and total TG, and raises HDL-C levels.

Epidemiologic and clinical studies have associated the risk of coronary artery disease (CAD) with elevated levels of total-C, LDL-C and decreased levels of HDL-C. These abnormalities of lipoprotein metabolism are considered as major contributors to the development of the disease. Like LDL, cholesterol-enriched lipoproteins, including VLDL, IDL and remnants can also promote atherosclerosis. Elevated plasma triglycerides are frequently found in a triad with low HDL-C levels and small LDL particles, as well as in association with non-lipid metabolic risk factors for coronary heart disease (metabolic syndrome). Clinical studies have also shown that serum triglycerides can be an independent risk factor for CAD. CAD risk is especially increased if the hypertriglyceridemia is due to increased intermediate density lipoproteins (IDL) or associated with decreased HDL or increased LDL-C. In addition, high TG levels are associated with an increased risk of pancreatitis. Although epidemiological and preliminary clinical evidence link low HDL-C levels and high triglyceride levels with coronary artery disease and atherosclerosis, the independent effect of raising HDL or lowering TG on the risk of coronary and cerebrovascular morbidity and mortality has not been demonstrated in prospective, well-controlled outcome studies. Other factors, e.g. interactions between lipids/lipoproteins and endothelium, platelets and macrophages, have also been incriminated in the development of human atherosclerosis and of its complications. Regardless of the intervention used (lowfat/low-cholesterol diet, partial ileal bypass surgery or pharmacologic therapy), effective treatment of hypercholesterolemia/dyslipidemia has consistently been shown to reduce the risk of CAD.

LIPITOR reduces LDL-C and the number of LDL particles, lowers Very Low Density Lipoprotein-Cholesterol (VLDL-C) and serum triglyceride, reduces the number of apo B containing particles, and also increases HDL-C. LIPITOR is effective in reducing LDL-C in patients with homozygous familial hypercholesterolemia, a condition that rarely responds to any other lipid-lowering medication. In addition to the above effects, LIPITOR reduces IDL-C and apolipoprotein E (apo E) in patients with dysbetalipoproteinemia (Type III).

In patients with type II hyperlipidemia, atorvastatin improved endothelial dysfunction. Atorvastatin significantly improved flow-mediated endothelium-dependent dilatation induced by reactive hyperemia, as assessed by brachial ultrasound ($p<0.01$).

Pharmacokinetics: Absorption: Atorvastatin is rapidly absorbed after oral administration; maximal plasma concentrations occur within 1 to 2 hours. Extent of absorption and plasma atorvastatin concentrations increase in proportion to atorvastatin dose. Atorvastatin tablets are 95-99% bioavailable compared to solutions. The absolute bioavailability (parent drug) of atorvastatin is approximately 12% and the systemic availability of HMG-CoA reductase inhibitory activity is approximately 30%. The low systemic availability is attributed to presystemic clearance in gastrointestinal mucosa and/or first-pass metabolism in the liver. Although food decreases the rate and extent of drug absorption by approximately 25% and 9%, as assessed by C_{max} and AUC respectively, LDL-C reduction and HDL-C elevation are similar when atorvastatin is given with and without food. Plasma atorvastatin concentrations are lower (approximately 30% for C_{max} and AUC) following drug administration in the evening compared with morning dosing. However, LDL-C reduction and HDL-C elevation are the same regardless of the time of drug administration.

Distribution: Mean volume of distribution of atorvastatin is approximately 381 L. Atorvastatin is ≥98% bound to plasma proteins. A blood/plasma ratio of approximately 0.25 indicates poor drug penetration into red blood cells. Based on observations in rats, atorvastatin is likely to be secreted in human milk.

Metabolism: Atorvastatin is extensively metabolized to ortho- and para-hydroxylated derivatives by cytochrome P-450 3A4 (CYP 3A4) and to various beta-oxidation products. In vitro, inhibition of HMG-CoA reductase by ortho- and para-hydroxylated metabolites is equivalent to that of atorvastatin. Approximately 70% of circulating inhibitory activity for HMG-CoA reductase is attributed to active metabolites. In animals, the ortho-hydroxy metabolite undergoes further glucuronidation. Atorvastatin and its metabolites are eliminated by biliary excretion.

Excretion: Atorvastatin is eliminated primarily in bile following hepatic and/or extrahepatic metabolism; however, the drug does not appear to undergo significant enterohepatic recirculation. Mean plasma elimination half-life of atorvastatin in humans is approximately 14 hours, but the half-life for inhibitory activity for HMG-CoA reductase is 20 to 30 hours due to the contribution of longer-lived active metabolites. Less than 2% of a dose of atorvastatin is recovered in urine following oral administration.

Special Populations and Conditions: Pediatrics: Assessment of pharmacokinetic parameters such as C_{max}, AUC and bioavailability of LIPITOR in pediatric patients (>10-<17 years old, postmenarche) was not performed during the 6-month, placebo-controlled trial referred to earlier (see Warnings and Precautions, Pediatrics).

Geriatrics: Plasma concentrations of atorvastatin are higher (approximately 40% for C_{max} and 30% for AUC) in healthy elderly subjects (age 65 years or older) compared with younger individuals. LDL-C reduction, however, is comparable to that seen in younger patient populations.

Gender: Plasma concentrations of atorvastatin in women differ (approximately 20% higher for C_{max} and 10% lower for AUC) from those in men; however, there is no clinically significant difference in LDL-C reduction between men and women.

Race: Plasma concentrations of atorvastatin are similar in black and white subjects.

Hepatic Insufficiency: Plasma concentrations of atorvastatin are markedly increased (approximately 16-fold in C_{max} and 11-fold in AUC) in patients with chronic alcoholic liver disease (Childs-Pugh B).

Renal Insufficiency: Plasma concentrations and LDL-C lowering efficacy of LIPITOR are similar in patients with moderate renal insufficiency compared with patients with normal renal function. However, since several cases of rhabdomyolysis have been reported in patients with a history of renal insufficiency of unknown severity, as a precautionary measure and pending further experience in renal disease, the lowest dose (10 mg/day) of LIPITOR should be used in these patients. Similar precautions apply in patients with severe renal insufficiency [creatinine clearance <30 mL/min (<0.5 mL/sec)]; the lowest dosage should be used and implemented cautiously (see Warnings and Precautions, Muscle Effects; Drug Interactions; Dosage and Administration).

STORAGE AND STABILITY: Store at controlled room temperature 15 to 30°C.

SPECIAL HANDLING INSTRUCTIONS: Not applicable.

INFORMATION FOR THE PATIENT: Published in e-CPS, available by subscription at www.e-cps.ca.

DOSAGE FORMS, COMPOSITION AND PACKAGING: 10 mg: Each white, elliptical, film-coated tablet, coded "10" on one side and "PD 155" on the other, contains: atorvastatin calcium 10 mg. Nonmedicinal ingredients: calcium carbonate, candelilla wax, croscarmellose sodium, hydroxypropyl cellulose, hydroxypropyl methylcellulose, lactose monohydrate, magnesium stearate, microcrystalline cellulose, polyethylene glycol, polysorbate 80, simethicone emulsion, talc and titanium dioxide. Bottles of 90.

20 mg: Each white, elliptical, film-coated tablet, coded "20" on one side and "PD 156" on the other, contains: atorvastatin calcium 20 mg. Nonmedicinal ingredients: calcium carbonate, candelilla wax, croscarmellose sodium, hydroxypropyl cellulose, hydroxypropyl methylcellulose, lactose monohydrate, magnesium stearate, microcrystalline cellulose, polyethylene glycol, polysorbate 80, simethicone emulsion, talc and titanium dioxide. Bottles of 90.

40 mg: Each white, elliptical, film-coated tablet, coded "40" on one side and "PD 157" on the other, contains: atorvastatin calcium 40 mg. Nonmedicinal ingredients: calcium carbonate, candelilla wax, croscarmellose sodium, hydroxypropyl cellulose, hydroxypropyl methylcellulose, lactose monohydrate, magnesium stearate, microcrystalline cellulose, polyethylene glycol, polysorbate 80, simethicone emulsion, talc, and titanium dioxide. Bottles of 90.

80 mg: Each white, elliptical, film-coated tablet, coded "80" on one side and "PD 158" on the other, contains: atorvastatin calcium 80 mg. Nonmedicinal ingredients: calcium carbonate, croscarmellose sodium, hydroxypropyl cellulose, hydroxypropyl methylcellulose, lactose monohydrate, magnesium stearate, microcrystalline cellulose, polyethylene glycol, polysorbate 80, simethicone emulsion, talc and titanium dioxide. Blisters of 30 (3 strips×10).

(Shown in Product Identification Section)

Liquor Carbonis Detergens

coal tar

Antipsoriasis

Odan

SUPPLIED: Each plastic, amber bottle contains: coal tar solution USP 20%. Bottles of 500 mL.

Lisinopril ℞

CPhA Monograph

see *ACE Inhibitors*

Lithium ℞

lithium carbonate
lithium citrate

Antimanic

CPhA Monograph

Date of Revision: November 2007

> This monograph has been compiled by CPhA and reviewed by experts. It may contain information different from that found in Health Canada-approved Product Monographs. The reader is referred to the *CPS* Editorial Policy for more information.

SUMMARY PRODUCT INFORMATION:

Drug	Route of Administration	Dosage Form	Strength
Lithium carbonate	Oral	Immediate-release capsule	150 mg, 300 mg, 600 mg
		Extended-release tablet	300 mg
Lithium citrate	Oral	Syrup	8 mmol/5 mL (approximately equivalent to lithium carbonate 300 mg/5 mL)

PHARMACOLOGY: Lithium is a monovalent cation that competes at cellular sites with other cations in the body. Cations are involved in the synthesis, storage, release and reuptake of neurotransmitters. The pathogenesis of mania appears to be affected by neurotransmitters such as dopamine and norepinephrine. Lithium alters sodium transport in nerve and muscle cells and may reduce concentrations of catecholamine neurotransmitters and inhibit the intracellular formation of cyclic AMP. However, the specific biochemical mechanism of lithium action in the control of mania is unknown.

Unlike other antimanic agents, lithium does not possess general sedative properties.

Pharmacokinetics: Lithium is well absorbed from the gastrointestinal tract with peak plasma concentrations occurring between 1 and 3 hours after administration. Peak plasma concentrations following administration of extended-release preparations are reached in 4 to 12 hours. Steady-state concentrations are reached in 4 days with the onset of antimanic effect usually occurring within 5 to 7 days. Full therapeutic effect may require 10 to 21 days following initiation of therapy. When lithium is used as augmentation therapy in refractory depression, some patients may respond within 48 hours, but most respond in 1 to 2 weeks.

Lithium is widely distributed into most body tissues and crosses the blood-brain barrier. CSF lithium concentrations are approximately half of plasma concentrations. Lithium does not bind to plasma proteins. Elimination half-life is 24 hours and is increased to 36 hours in geriatric patients and 40 to 50 hours in patients with impaired renal function.

Lithium is excreted primarily in the urine with less than 1% eliminated in the feces. Small amounts are also excreted in sweat. Lithium is filtered by the glomeruli with 80% reabsorbed in the tubules. In patients with normal renal function, 50 to 80% of a single dose is excreted in the urine within 24 hours. Renal lithium excretion varies among individuals and dosage must be individualized. Renal clearance is decreased in geriatric patients and increased in younger patients and during pregnancy. Sodium loading or depletion affects renal clearance of the drug. A low salt intake resulting in low tubular concentration of sodium increases lithium reabsorption and may result in toxicity. Polyuria does not increase renal clearance of the drug. Lithium is removed by hemodialysis. The half-life of lithium is shorter in children.

Routine serum drug concentration monitoring is necessary (see Warnings, Precautions and Dosage).

INDICATIONS: Lithium is used In the treatment of acute manic and hypomanic episodes in patients with bipolar disorder, and in the maintenance treatment of bipolar disorder. Lithium has been used as augmentation therapy in patients with refractory depression. Lithium has also been used in the prophylactic management of chronic cluster headache.

CONTRAINDICATIONS: Patients with significant renal or cardiovascular disease, severe debilitation or dehydration or sodium depletion. The risk of lithium toxicity is increased in these patients. If the psychiatric indication is life-threatening and if the patient fails to respond to other measures, lithium treatment may be undertaken at low doses with extreme caution, including dosage adjustments based on daily serum lithium determinations. In such instances, hospitalization is necessary.

WARNINGS: Lithium toxicity is closely related to serum lithium levels and can occur at levels close to the therapeutic range. Facilities for prompt and accurate serum lithium determinations should be available before initiating therapy.

Prevention of chronic toxicity requires careful screening for pre-existing renal and other diseases, establishment of 12-hour post-dose serum lithium levels that are as low as possible yet clinically effective, maintaining control of treatment by monitoring serum lithium levels, exercising clinical and laboratory surveillance over potential side effects or signs of lithium intoxication, exercising maximum control of at-risk patients and insuring that long-term lithium therapy is maintained only when clinical response has been clearly established.

The ability to tolerate lithium is greater during the acute manic phase and decreases when manic symptoms subside (see Dosage).

Renal Function: Chronic lithium therapy is frequently associated with a decrease in renal concentrating capacity with development of thirst, polyuria, weight gain and altered renal function tests and occasionally presents as nephrogenic diabetes insipidus. Such patients should be carefully managed to avoid dehydration with resulting lithium retention and toxicity. Impaired renal function during chronic therapy may be only partially reversible when lithium is discontinued.

Glomerular sclerosis and interstitial fibrosis as well as tubular lesions have been reported in patients on chronic lithium therapy, but a causal relationship has not been established.

During lithium therapy, progressive or sudden changes in renal function, even within the normal range, indicate the need for re-evaluation of treatment, including dosage and frequency of administration, and a reassessment of the risk-benefit ratio of long-term lithium therapy.

Pregnancy: Administration of lithium during pregnancy may result in an increased incidence of cardiac and other anomalies, especially Ebstein's anomaly. Nephrogenic diabetes insipidus, euthyroid goiter and hypoglycemia have also occurred in women treated with lithium during pregnancy. Lithium should not be used during pregnancy or in women of childbearing potential unless it cannot be substituted by other appropriate therapy and if the expected benefits outweigh the possible hazards to the child.

If lithium is used during pregnancy, serum lithium concentrations should be carefully monitored and the dosage adjusted if necessary since renal clearance and distribution of the drug into erythrocytes may be increased during pregnancy. Pregnant women receiving lithium may have subtherapeutic serum lithium concentrations if the dosage is not increased during pregnancy. Immediately postpartum, renal clearance of lithium may decrease to pre-pregnancy levels. To decrease the risk of postpartum lithium intoxication, dosage of the drug should be reduced 1 week prior to parturition or when labor begins.

Lactation: Lithium is excreted into breast milk in concentrations ranging from 30 to 100% of maternal serum levels. Lithium should be used with caution in breast-feeding mothers and if possible, avoided until the infant is several months old. If it is used during lactation, the mother should be educated about signs and symptoms of lithium toxicity and the increased risk posed by dehydration in the infant. Some clinicians recommend monitoring lithium serum concentrations and periodic monitoring of renal and thyroid function in infants exposed to lithium through breast-feeding.

Children: Lithium has a shorter half-life in children.

PRECAUTIONS: Maintain patients on lithium therapy under careful clinical and laboratory control throughout treatment. Serious adverse reactions and lithium intoxication can occur with serum concentrations greater than 1.5 mmol/L (see Geriatrics). Lithium concentration should be measured before the first lithium dose of the day, i.e., 9 to 12 hours after the last dose was administered. Serum lithium concentrations should usually be monitored 3 times weekly, and blood studies and urinalysis conducted weekly, during the initial period of administration and as required thereafter. If lithium levels exceed 1.5 to 2 mmol/L, discontinue the drug and, if appropriate, resume administration at a lower dose after 24 hours.

Changes in sodium intake may significantly alter the renal elimination of lithium. Sodium intake and lithium clearance are directly related (i.e., decreasing sodium intake may lead to decreased clearance of lithium). Patients should be advised to maintain adequate sodium and fluid intake and to avoid substantial changes in either. They should also be cautioned to avoid dehydration and to report prolonged vomiting, diarrhea or fever to their physician.

Prodromal toxic signs such as fatigue, muscular weakness, incoordination, drowsiness, coarse tremors, diarrhea and vomiting provide an early warning of lithium intoxication. The patient and family should be instructed to notify the physician immediately if any of these adverse reactions occur. Signs of toxicity or a rise in lithium concentration after the dosage is stabilized require investigation to determine the cause of drug accumulation.

There is evidence of decreased tolerance to lithium once the acute manic episode begins to resolve. Therefore, when the acute attack subsides, the dosage should be reduced to maintain serum lithium concentrations between 0.6 and 1 mmol/L.

There have been reports of withdrawal symptoms following lithium discontinuation. Gradual discontinuation is recommended unless abrupt withdrawal is necessary because of toxicity.

Periodic review and monitoring of kidney and cardiovascular function is advisable during therapy with lithium. Patients with underlying cardiovascular disease should be observed carefully for signs of arrhythmias. Perform other laboratory tests as indicated by the patient's clinical condition.

Since the formation of nontoxic goiters has been reported during lithium therapy, examine the thyroid gland before treatment and perform appropriate thyroid function tests. Nontoxic goiters reported during prolonged lithium therapy have disappeared following discontinuation of the medication. Treatment with small doses of thyroxine in patients who develop a diffuse nontoxic goiter may stop further growth or lead to shrinkage of the gland.

Geriatrics: Elderly patients appear to be more susceptible to adverse effects and may experience a higher incidence of neurotoxicity at lithium concentrations considered therapeutic for younger adults. Certain groups of elderly patients are particularly vulnerable, including those with neurologic disease, cardiovascular disorders, renal impairment and those over 80 years of age. The recommended therapeutic range for serum lithium concentrations in older patients is ≤ 0.4 to 0.6 mmol/L, not to exceed 1 mmol/L.

Occupational Hazards: Lithium may cause dizziness or decreased mental alertness. Patients should be appropriately cautioned regarding the operation of motor vehicles or hazardous machinery.

Drug Interactions: ACE Inhibitors: Concomitant administration of lithium and ACE inhibitors may increase the risk of lithium toxicity. Frequently monitor lithium levels during concurrent therapy.

Angiotensin II Receptor Blockers: Cases of lithium intoxication have been reported when angiotensin II receptor blockers were added to the therapeutic regimen. Close monitoring for signs of increased lithium serum concentration is recommended if these drugs are used concurrently.

Anticonvulsants: Concurrent use of lithium and carbamazepine or phenytoin might result in an increased risk of CNS toxicity.

Antipsychotics: Both pharmacokinetic interactions and clinical toxicity (e.g., neurotoxicity) have been described with the combined use of these agents. Monitor for altered response to either drug when lithium and an antipsychotic are used in combination, and when either drug is withdrawn.

Calcium Channel Blockers: Concomitant administration of lithium and calcium channel blockers may increase the risk of neurotoxicity.

Cyclooxygenase-2 (COX-2) Inhibitors: In one study in healthy subjects receiving celecoxib and lithium, mean steady-state levels of lithium were increased by 17% compared to subjects receiving lithium alone. Based on this study, some clinicians suggest monitoring patients maintained on lithium for evidence of an interaction if a COX-2 inhibitor is initiated or withdrawn.

Diuretics: Patients stabilized on lithium therapy who receive a thiazide diuretic may require a reduction of lithium dosage to avoid accumulation and toxicity, since there is often a 20 to 40% reduction of renal lithium clearance. Furosemide may increase the risk of lithium toxicity in patients >65 years, especially during the first month of therapy.

Haloperidol: A type of encephalopathy resembling neuroleptic malignant syndrome (characterized by weakness, lethargy, fever, tremulousness and confusion, extrapyramidal symptoms, leukocytosis, elevated BUN and fasting blood sugar) followed by irreversible brain damage has occurred in a few patients treated with both lithium and haloperidol. Patients receiving combined therapy should be monitored closely for early evidence of neurologic toxicity, such as rigidity and/or hyperpyrexia; discontinue treatment if these signs appear.

Iodides: Concomitant administration of lithium and iodides may increase the hypothyroid effects of either of these medications.

Monoamine Oxidase Inhibitors (MAOIs): Two patients died after developing rigidity, hyperthermia and hepatic failure while taking phenelzine, lithium and L-tryptophan. Though L-tryptophan may have contributed to these reactions, some clinicians recommend avoiding the combination of lithium and nonselective MAOIs.

Methyldopa: Concomitant administration of lithium and methyldopa may increase the risk of lithium toxicity.

Metronidazole: Concomitant administration of lithium and metronidazole may cause renal retention of lithium, leading to lithium toxicity. If possible, lithium should be discontinued during therapy with metronidazole.

Neuromuscular Blockers: The action of neuromuscular blockers may be prolonged in patients receiving lithium. A temporary omission of a few doses of lithium can reduce the risks of this interaction.

NSAIDs: Several NSAIDs have been reported to increase steady-state plasma lithium levels substantially. Increased frequency of monitoring plasma lithium levels is recommended during concurrent therapy with NSAIDs.

Serotonergic Drugs: Combined use of lithium and other serotonergic drugs (e.g., SSRIs, sibutramine) may increase the risk of serotonin syndrome.

Sodium Bicarbonate: Concomitant administration of lithium and sodium bicarbonate may enhance lithium excretion. A higher dose of lithium may be required in these patients.

Tetracycline: Concomitant administration of lithium and tetracycline may increase the risk of lithium toxicity.

Theophylline: The administration of aminophylline or theophylline to patients on lithium may require increased lithium doses to maintain the clinical effects of the drug.

Tricyclic Antidepressants: Concurrent use of lithium and tricyclic antidepressants may increase the risk of toxicity (e.g., tremors, ataxia, seizures). Older patients may be particularly susceptible. If the combination is used, some clinicians suggest using the lowest effective dose of each agent and monitoring the patient closely for adverse effects.

ADVERSE EFFECTS: Mild adverse effects may occur even when serum lithium values remain below 1 mmol/L. Most frequent are the initial postabsorptive symptoms believed to be associated with a rapid rise in serum lithium concentrations. They include gastrointestinal discomfort, nausea, vertigo, muscle weakness and a dazed feeling, and frequently disappear after stabilization of therapy. The more common persistent adverse effects include fine tremor of the hands, fatigue, thirst, polyuria and nephrogenic diabetes insipidus.

Mild to moderate toxic reactions may occur at lithium concentrations from 1.5 to 2 mmol/L, and moderate to severe reactions at concentrations above 2 mmol/L (see Precautions, Geriatrics).

Some patients may experience lithium accumulation during initial therapy, which may result in toxic concentrations that require immediate discontinuation of the drug. Some elderly patients with lower renal clearance may experience varying degrees of lithium toxicity, requiring reduction or temporary withdrawal of medication. However, in patients with normal renal clearance, the toxic manifestations typically occur in a predictable sequence related to serum lithium concentrations. The usually transient gastrointestinal symptoms are the earliest side effects to occur. A mild degree of fine tremor of the hands may persist throughout therapy. Thirst and polyuria may be followed by increased drowsiness, ataxia, tinnitus and blurred vision, indicating early intoxication. As intoxication progresses the following manifestations may be encountered: confusion, increasing disorientation, muscle twitches, hyperreflexia, nystagmus, seizures, diarrhea, vomiting, and eventually coma and death.

The following adverse effects have been reported and appear to be related to serum lithium concentrations:

Autonomic Nervous System: blurred vision, dry mouth.

Cardiovascular: arrhythmia, hypotension, ECG changes consisting of flattening or inversion of T-waves, peripheral circulatory failure, cardiac collapse.

Central Nervous System: anesthesia of the skin, slurred speech, blurred vision, blackout spells, headache, seizures, cranial nerve involvement, psychomotor retardation, somnolence, toxic confusional states, restlessness, stupor, coma, acute dystonia, EEG changes.

Dermatologic: dryness and thinning of the hair, leg ulcers, skin rash, pruritus and exacerbation of psoriasis.

Gastrointestinal: anorexia, nausea, vomiting, diarrhea.

Genitourinary: diabetes insipidus (see Warnings), albuminuria, oliguria, polyuria, glycosuria.

Hematologic: anemia, leukopenia, leukocytosis.

Hypersensitivity: allergic vasculitis.

Metabolic: transient hyperglycemia, slight elevation of plasma magnesium, goiter.

Neuromuscular: general muscle weakness, ataxia, tremor, muscle hyperirritability, (fasciculation, twitchings, especially of facial muscles and clonic movements of the limbs), choreoathetotic movement, hyperactive deep tendon reflexes.

Thyroid Abnormalities: euthyroid goiter and/or hypothyroidism (including myxedema) accompanied by lower T_3 and T_4 levels and elevated TSH. Iodine^{131} uptake may be elevated. On average, 5 to 15% of patients on long-term lithium therapy manifest clinical signs or have altered serum hormone levels (see Precautions). Paradoxically, rare cases of hyperthyroidism have been reported.

Miscellaneous: general fatigue, dehydration, weight loss, tendency to sleep, lethargy, transient scotomata, metallic taste, peripheral edema.

Hypercalcemia, associated with lithium-induced hyper-parathyroidism, has also been reported.

OVERDOSE:

Symptoms: Lithium toxicity is closely related to the concentration of lithium in the blood and is usually associated with serum concentrations in excess of 2 mmol/L. Patients chronically on lithium have more severe symptoms for a given serum level than those with no previous lithium load who have ingested a single large dose. Early signs of toxicity which may occur at lower serum concentrations (see Adverse Effects) usually respond to a reduction in dosage. Chronic lithium intoxication has been preceded by the appearance or aggravation of the following symptoms: sluggishness, drowsiness, lethargy, coarse hand tremor or muscle twitches, loss of appetite, vomiting and diarrhea. Occurrence of these symptoms requires immediate cessation of medication and careful clinical reassessment and management.

Symptoms of overdose vary depending on whether the intoxication is acute or chronic. Patients with acute overdose usually have early gastrointestinal symptoms such as nausea, vomiting and diarrhea. These are often absent in patients experiencing chronic toxicity. In all patients with lithium intoxication, the primary problem is neurologic toxicity that may progress from fine tremor to hyperreflexia, fasciculations, muscular irritability, choreoathesis, clonus, agitation, altered mental status, lethargy, seizures and coma. The serum concentration may not correlate with neurologic symptoms due to the delay in lithium distribution from blood to the central nervous system (i.e., serum concentrations may be elevated before neurologic symptoms appear). Cardiac complications such as arrhythmias or significant hypotension are rare. If hypotension does occur it is generally secondary to volume depletion.

Treatment: Early symptoms of chronic lithium toxicity can usually be treated by reduction or cessation of dosage of the drug and resumption of treatment at a lower dose after 24 to 48 hours. Whole bowel irrigation with a balanced polyethylene glycol-electrolyte solution (e.g., PegLyte) may help minimize lithium absorption. Activated charcoal does not adsorb lithium but may be of value if multiple drug ingestion is suspected. Measure serum lithium levels every 4 to 6 hours until the serum lithium level is below 2 mmol/L.

Maintain fluid and electrolyte balance. Maintain urine output and sodium excretion by administering iv sodium chloride. Administration of large amounts of sodium in the absence of sodium depletion has not been shown to be successful in speeding lithium excretion. Sodium bicarbonate, mannitol, loop and thiazide diuretics, carbonic anhydrase inhibitors or phosphodiesterase inhibitors are *not* recommended.

The definitive therapy for lithium intoxication is hemodialysis. Indications for hemodialysis include: potentially toxic exposures in patients with renal failure; neurologic dysfunction including altered mental status; acute ingestion with serum lithium concentration of ≥4.0 mEq/L; acute-on-chronic or chronic overdose with serum lithium concentration ≥2.5 mEq/L; and moderate to severe neurologic toxicity. Patients who may not be able to tolerate sodium repletion should also be considered for early hemodialysis.

Draw serum lithium levels immediately after hemodialysis and again 6 hours later. If either level is high or the patient continues to exhibit signs of neurotoxicity a second course of hemodialysis may be necessary.

Peritoneal dialysis is not indicated in the management of lithium toxicity in patients with normal renal function. It may be used as a temporizing measure in a patient with a functioning peritoneal dialysis catheter until hemodialysis can be started.

> For management of a suspected drug overdose, CPhA recommends that you contact your **regional Poison Control Centre**. See the *CPS* Directory section for a list of Poison Control Centres.

DOSAGE: Screening of patients should include a medical history and physical examination with emphasis on the CNS, urinary, cardiovascular, gastrointestinal and endocrine systems as well as the skin. It should also include: routine 24-hour urine volume, serum creatinine, record of weight and ECG. Electrolytes and TSH should also be measured and for long-term treatment, creatinine clearance and urine concentration tests should also be performed.

Once therapy is initiated, monitoring of the patient should include: mental status, physical examination, weight, 12-hour post-dose serum lithium and a check for lithium side effects and compliance. It should also include serum creatinine every 12 months, plasma thyroid hormone and TSH every 6 to 12 months, particularly in female patients, and serum calcium every 2 years.

Serum lithium levels should be maintained within the therapeutic range, as high as necessary for efficacy and with the patient free of significant adverse effects. Three daily doses should be used initially, at least until the daily dosage is established. Adjustments in dosage may be required to minimize adverse effects. Switching to a different lithium preparation or changing the frequency of dosing may be necessary to address absorption-related adverse effects or concern over possible renal toxicity.

The therapeutic dose for the treatment of acute mania should be based primarily on the patient's clinical condition. It must be individualized according to serum concentrations and clinical response. For manic patients, the dose should be adjusted to obtain serum concentrations between 0.8 and 1.2 mmol/L (measured before the first lithium dose of the day).

In properly screened adult patients, the suggested initial daily dosage for acute mania is 900 to 1800 mg (15 to 20 mg/kg), in 3 divided doses. In view of the large interindividual variability of renal lithium excretion, it is suggested that lithium treatment be started at a dose between 600 and 900 mg/day, reaching a level of 1200 to 1800 mg in divided doses on the second day. Depending on the patient's clinical condition, the initial dosage should be adjusted to produce the desired serum lithium concentration. The weight of the patient should also influence the magnitude of the initial dose.

After the acute manic episode subsides, usually within a week, the dosage should be reduced to achieve serum concentrations between 0.6 and 1 mmol/L, since tolerance to lithium may decrease as severity of mania subsides. The average suggested dosage at this stage is 900 mg/day, in 3 divided doses, with a range usually between 450 and 1200 mg/day. When the manic attack is controlled, maintain lithium administration during the expected duration of the manic phase, since early withdrawal might lead to relapse.

Once patients are stabilized on a maintenance dose and stable therapeutic blood levels are reached, the dosage schedule may be changed to a once daily regimen. The total daily dose, when administered as a single dose, may be approximately 5 to 30% lower than when given in divided doses over the day. It is essential to maintain clinical supervision of the patient and to monitor serum lithium levels both when using the divided daily dosage regimen and when transferring to the once daily administration dosage regimen (see Precautions).

In uncomplicated cases receiving maintenance therapy during remission, serum lithium levels should be monitored at least every 2 months. Blood samples for serum lithium determination should be drawn 12 hours following a dose (e.g., prior to the morning dose). Total reliance must not be placed on serum levels. Adequate patient evaluation requires both clinical assessment and laboratory analysis.

Elderly and debilitated patients and those with significant renal impairment should be prescribed lithium with particular caution (see Precautions, Geriatrics). Starting dose should not exceed 300 mg/day accompanied by frequent serum level monitoring. Serum concentrations of 0.4 to 0.6 mmol/L are usually effective in elderly patients and should not exceed 1 mmol/L.

Children: Lithium has been used in children in initial doses of 15 to 20 mg/kg/day in 3 to 4 divided doses, titrating to a maximum of 60 mg/kg/day based on response and lithium serum levels. If tolerated, maintenance therapy can be given as a once daily dose.

Depression, Augmentation Therapy: 600 to 900 mg/day; target serum level is 0.6 to 1 mmol/L.

Prophylaxis of Chronic Cluster Headache: Adults 300 mg 3 times daily.

Extended-release lithium carbonate tablets should be swallowed whole or broken in half. They should not be chewed or crushed (see product monographs).

Livostin® Eye Drops

levocabastine HCl

Histamine H1-Antagonist

Novartis Pharmaceuticals

Date of Preparation: June 5, 2008
Date of Revision: June 17, 2010

PHARMACOLOGY: Levocabastine is a potent, fast-acting and highly selective histamine H_1-antagonist with a sustained duration of action.

Within 10 to 15 minutes of topical application to the eyes, levocabastine inhibits: itching, redness and chemosis induced by conjunctival provocation with histamine; itching, redness, chemosis, eyelid swelling, and tearing induced by conjunctival provocation with allergens; and itching and redness induced by conjunctival provocation with compound 48/80.

Orally-administered levocabastine provides a dose dependent inhibition of skin reactions to intradermal histamine. After topical application to the eyes, levocabastine did not produce clinically significant systemic antihistamine effects in patients.

Levocabastine eye drops (2 drops/eye 3 times daily), under acute and steady state conditions, are devoid of CNS effects, as evaluated by objective and subjective psychoperformance tests and measures of general CNS activity.

Following topical application to the eyes, the absorption of levocabastine was incomplete and the absolute bioavailability of levocabastine instilled in the eyes could be estimated at approximately 30% in patients with allergic conjunctivitis and up to 60% in healthy volunteers.

INDICATIONS: The symptomatic management of seasonal allergic conjunctivitis.

CONTRAINDICATIONS: In patients with hypersensitivity to any of the ingredients.

WARNINGS: Children: Levocabastine is not recommended for use in children under the age of 12 years except on the advice of a physician. Clinical experience in children under 5 years of age is limited with ocular levocabastine.

PRECAUTIONS: As with all ophthalmic preparations containing benzalkonium chloride, patients are advised not to wear soft (hydrophilic) contact lenses while under treatment with levocabastine eye drops.

Pregnancy: There are no clinical trials on the use of levocabastine eye drops in pregnant or nursing women; therefore, levocabastine eye drops should not be used during pregnancy, except if the potential benefit justifies the potential risk to the fetus.

Lactation: See Pregnancy.

Geriatrics: The safety and efficacy of topical levocabastine have not been established in patients greater than 65 years of age.

ADVERSE EFFECTS: The most frequent side effect encountered with levocabastine eye drops is eye irritation. Most side effects are transient and rarely necessitate discontinuation of therapy. See Table 1.

Post-Market Adverse Drug Reaction: The following events have been reported in association with levocabastine eye drops use in worldwide post-marketing experience: keratitis.

OVERDOSE:

There has been no experience with overdosage of levocabastine eye drops.

Treatment: Treatment should include general supportive measures.

For management of a suspected drug overdose, CPhA recommends that you contact your **regional Poison Control Centre**. See the *CPS* Directory section for a list of Poison Control Centres.

DOSAGE: Adults and children (12 to 65 years old): 1 drop (15 µg/drop) instilled in each eye, 2 times daily. The dose may be increased to 1 drop 3 to 4 times daily.

It is not useful to continue the treatment for more than 3 days if no improvement is seen. There are no clinical studies to support continuous treatment durations of greater than 16 weeks.

As levocabastine eye drops are available as a microsuspension, the bottle should be shaken before each application. Levocabastine eye drops should be used within 1 month of the first opening of the bottle. Patients should be instructed to take appropriate measures to avoid contamination.

Table 1: Livostin Eye Drops

Incidence of the Most Frequent[a] Adverse Experiences in Patients Treated with Livostin Eye Drops or Placebo Eye Drops

Organ System	Incidence (%) Livostin Eye Drops (n=599)	Incidence (%) Placebo Eye Drops (n=215)
Ocular	**19.9**	**18.6**
Eye irritation	16.4	15.8
Dry conjunctiva	<1.0	0.0
The others (blurred vision, eye discharge, eyelid edema, eye pain and abnormal lacrimation) were <1.0% for both the Livostin and placebo group.		
CNS	**6.0**	**9.3**
Headache	3.5	4.2
Somnolence	2.0	5.1
Insomnia	<1.0	0.0
Respiratory System	**4.2**	**5.1**
Coughing	1.0	1.4
Epistaxis	1.0	<1.0
Nasal congestion	<1.0	0.0
Rhinorrhea	<1.0	1.4
The others (nasal irritation, itchy throat, pharyngitis and dyspnea) were <1.0% for both the Livostin and placebo groups.		
Other		
Tiredness	2.0	1.4
Dry mouth	1.0	4.2
Fever	<1.0	0.0
Rash	<1.0	0.0
Generalized pruritus	<1.0	<1.0
Pruritus	<1.0	0.0
Nausea	<1.0	0.0

[a] Reported more than once in the Livostin group.

INFORMATION FOR THE PATIENT: Published in e-CPS, available by subscription at www.e-cps.ca.

SUPPLIED: Each mL of white sterile ophthalmic microsuspension contains: levocabastine HCl equivalent to levocabastine 0.5 mg. Nonmedicinal ingredients: benzalkonium chloride 0.15 mg as preservative, disodium edetate, disodium phosphate, hypromellose, monosodium phosphate, polysorbate 80, propylene glycol and water. pH 6 to 8. Plastic bottles of 10 mL containing 5 mL of microsuspension. Store between 15 and 30°C. Must be kept out of the reach and sight of children.

Livostin® Nasal Spray

levocabastine HCl

Histamine H1-Antagonist

Janssen-Ortho

Date of Preparation: January 25, 1995
Date of Revision: November 27, 2009

PHARMACOLOGY: LIVOSTIN levocabastine hydrochloride is a potent, fast-acting and highly selective histamine H_1-antagonist with a sustained duration of action.

Within 10 minutes of topical application to the nose, levocabastine inhibits sneezing, itchy nose and rhinorrhea induced by nasal provocation with allergens.

Orally administered levocabastine provides a dose-dependent inhibition of skin reactions to intradermal histamine. After repeated topical application to the nose, topical and systemic antihistamine effects contribute to overall clinical outcome. Although systemic effects may contribute to the therapeutic effects of levocabastine nasal spray, this is not accompanied by any sedative effects.

Levocabastine nasal spray (2 sprays/nostril 3 times daily), under acute and steady-state conditions, is devoid of CNS effects, as evaluated by objective and subjective psychoperformance tests and measures of general CNS activity.

Following topical application to the nose, the absorption of levocabastine was incomplete and the absolute bioavailability of levocabastine administered in the nose could be estimated at 60 to 80% in healthy volunteers and in patients with allergic rhinitis.

INDICATIONS: LIVOSTIN levocabastine hydrochloride nasal spray is indicated for the symptomatic treatment of allergic rhinitis (sneezing, itchy nose, runny nose).

CONTRAINDICATIONS: LIVOSTIN levocabastine hydrochloride nasal spray is contraindicated in patients with hypersensitivity to any of the ingredients.

WARNINGS: *Pregnancy:* There are no clinical trials on the use of LIVOSTIN levocabastine hydrochloride nasal spray in pregnant or nursing women; therefore, LIVOSTIN nasal spray should not be used during pregnancy, except if the potential benefit justifies the potential risk to the fetus.

Lactation: LIVOSTIN can be excreted in human milk. Administration of LIVOSTIN nasal spray to women who are breastfeeding should only be considered if the expected benefit to the mother is greater than any possible risk to the child.

Children: Levocabastine nasal spray is not recommended for use in children under the age of 12 years. Clinical experience with nasal levocabastine is absent in children under 5 years of age.

Occupational Hazards: Effects on Driving Ability and Use of Machinery: LIVOSTIN levocabastine hydrochloride nasal spray will generally not cause clinically relevant sedation nor does it impair psychomotor performance as compared with placebo. LIVOSTIN nasal spray, therefore, would not be expected to interfere with the ability to drive a car or operate machinery. Should drowsiness occur, caution is advised.

PRECAUTIONS: Renal: Limited data are available on the use of levocabastine in patients with renal impairment. Caution should be exercised when administering LIVOSTIN levocabastine hydrochloride nasal spray to patients with renal impairment.

Geriatrics: The safety and efficacy of topical levocabastine has not been established in patients older than 65 years of age.

Drug Interactions: Interactions with alcohol or any other drugs were never reported in clinical trials. In specifically designed studies, there was no evidence of potentiation of the effects of either alcohol or diazepam by LIVOSTIN nasal spray used in normal dosages.

ADVERSE EFFECTS: Clinical Trial Adverse Drug Reactions: The most frequent side effect encountered with LIVOSTIN levocabastine hydrochloride nasal spray during clinical trials is nasal irritation. Most side effects are transient and rarely necessitate discontinuation of therapy. Table 1 lists instances of frequent adverse experiences observed during clinical trials.

Post-Market Adverse Drug Reactions: In addition to the side effects identified in clinical trials (see Table 1), the following post-marketing adverse drug reactions have been very rarely reported: hypersensitivity, dyspnoea, bronchospasm, tachycardia, nasal congestion, epistaxis, headache, eyelid edema, fatigue, malaise, and application site reactions including nasal edema and nasal discomfort. In post-marketing experience, allergic reactions have rarely been reported.

OVERDOSE:

Symptoms: There have been no reports of overdosage of LIVOSTIN levocabastine hydrochloride nasal spray. Some sedation after accidental intake of the contents of the bottle cannot be excluded.

Treatment: In the case of accidental ingestion, the patient should be advised to drink plenty of non-alcoholic fluids in order to accelerate the renal elimination of levocabastine hydrochloride. Treatment of overdosage should include general supportive measures.

For management of a suspected drug overdose, contact your **regional Poison Control Centre**. See the *CPS* Directory section for a list of Poison Control Centres.

DOSAGE: Adults and children (12 to 65 years old): the usual dose is 2 sprays (50 µg/spray) of LIVOSTIN levocabastine hydrochloride per nostril, 2 times daily. The dose may be increased to 2 sprays 3 to 4 times daily.

It is not useful to continue the treatment for more than 3 days if no improvement is seen. There are no clinical studies to support continuous treatment durations of greater than 10 weeks.

As LIVOSTIN nasal spray is available as a microsuspension, the bottle should be shaken before each application. Patients should be instructed to clear the nasal passages prior to administering the spray and to inhale through the nose during spraying. Before using the pump delivery system for the first time, the pump reservoir should be filled up by priming until a fine spray is delivered.

Table 1: LIVOSTIN Nasal Spray

Incidence of the Most Frequent[a] Adverse Experiences in Patients Treated With LIVOSTIN or Placebo Nasal Spray

Organ System	Incidence (%) LIVOSTIN Nasal Spray (n=702)	Incidence (%) Placebo Nasal Spray (n=427)
Respiratory System	**10.4**	**9.6**
Nasal irritation	5.4	5.6
Epistaxis	1.0	<1.0
Coughing, throat irritation, respiratory disorder, aggravated nasal obstruction and nasal pruritus were <1.0% in the LIVOSTIN group and not reported in the placebo group. The others (dry nose, rhinorrhea, dyspnea, itchy throat) were <1.0% for both the LIVOSTIN and placebo groups.		
CNS	**7.7**	**7.0**
Somnolence	3.8	3.5
Headache	3.1	3.0
Dizziness	<1.0	<1.0
Ocular	**3.0**	**2.1**
Eye irritation[b]	2.6	1.9
Other		
Dry mouth	3.3	2.6
Tiredness	1.4	<1.0
Facial edema, rash, decreased hearing, pruritus of external ear and taste perversion were <1.0% in the LIVOSTIN group and not reported in the placebo group. The others (abdominal pain, increased appetite, nausea and increased weight) were <1.0% for both the LIVOSTIN and placebo groups.		

[a] Reported more than once in the LIVOSTIN group.
[b] The eye irritation observed in the levocabastine nasal spray group was mostly reported by the patients receiving both the levocabastine nasal spray and eye drops.

INFORMATION FOR THE PATIENT: Published in e-CPS, available by subscription at www.e-cps.ca.

SUPPLIED: Each mL of white microsuspension contains: levocabastine hydrochloride equivalent to levocabastine 0.5 mg. Nonmedicinal ingredients: benzalkonium chloride, disodium edetate, disodium phosphate, hypromellose, monosodium phosphate, polysorbate 80, propylene glycol and water. pH 6 to 8. Plastic bottles of 15 mL containing 15 mL of microsuspension. Store at room temperature (15 to 30°C).

(Shown in Product Identification Section)

Locacorten® Vioform® Cream ℞

flumethasone pivalate—clioquinol

Topical Corticosteroid—Antibacterial—Antifungal

Paladin

SUPPLIED: Each tube of off-white water soluble cream contains: flumethasone pivalate 0.02% and clioquinol 3%. Nonmedicinal ingredients: cetyl alcohol, cetyl palmitate, glycerin, petrolatum, phenoxyethanol, sodium lauryl sulfate, stearyl alcohol and water. Tubes of 30 g. Protect from heat (store between 15 and 30°C) and freezing.

Locacorten® Vioform® Eardrops ℞

flumethasone pivalate—clioquinol

Topical Aural Corticosteroid—Antibacterial—Antifungal

Paladin

SUPPLIED: Each dispenser of clear solution contains: flumethasone pivalate 0.02% and clioquinol 1%. Nonmedicinal ingredients: polyethylene glycol. Parabens- and tartrazine-free. Plastic controlled-drop dispenser of 10 mL, cartons of 1. Protect from heat (store between 15 and 30°C) and light. The eardrops may turn yellow when exposed to air and may cause staining of the skin, nails, hair or fabrics.

Lomotil® Ⓝ

diphenoxylate HCl—atropine sulfate

Antidiarrheal

Pfizer

PHARMACOLOGY: The mode of action of diphenoxylate in the bowel is similar to that of morphine and related drugs. Gastrointestinal propulsion is inhibited through a direct action on the smooth muscle, resulting in a decrease in peristaltic action and a consequent increase in transit time.

INDICATIONS: As an adjunct in the management of diarrhea. Bacterially-induced diarrhea should be treated with appropriate antimicrobial therapy.

CONTRAINDICATIONS: Known hypersensitivity to diphenoxylate or atropine; patients who are jaundiced; the treatment of diarrhea associated with pseudomembranous enterocolitis; diarrhea caused by enterotoxin producing bacteria.

WARNINGS: This medication should be kept out of the reach of children since accidental overdose may cause severe or even fatal respiratory depression. Lomotil is not recommended for use in children under 2 years of age. Dosage recommendations should be strictly adhered to, especially in children.

Pregnancy: The use of Lomotil during pregnancy, lactation or in women of childbearing potential requires that the expected benefits of the drug be weighed against any possible hazard to the mother and child. Effects of diphenoxylate or atropine may be evident in the infants of nursing mothers taking Lomotil (since these compounds are excreted in breast milk).

Lactation: See Pregnancy.

PRECAUTIONS: General: Occupational Hazards: Lomotil may produce drowsiness or dizziness. The patient should be cautioned regarding activities that require mental alertness, such as driving or operating dangerous machinery.

Slowing of intestinal motility by an agent such as Lomotil does not preclude the need for appropriate fluid and electrolyte replacement. Dehydration may further influence the variability of response to Lomotil and may predispose to delayed diphenoxylate intoxication. Drug-induced inhibition of peristalsis may result in fluid retention in the colon which may further aggravate dehydration and electrolyte imbalance. If severe dehydration or electrolyte imbalance is present, withhold Lomotil until appropriate corrective therapy has been initiated.

Children: Lomotil should be used with special caution, since signs of atropinism may occur even with recommended doses, particularly in patients with Down's syndrome. Lomotil should be used with special caution in young children because of their variable response.

Patients with Special Diseases and Conditions: Lomotil should be used with extreme caution in patients with cirrhosis and other hepatic disease and in all patients with abnormal liver function tests, since hepatic coma may be precipitated.

In some patients with acute ulcerative colitis, agents which inhibit intestinal motility or delay intestinal transit time have been reported to induce toxic megacolon. Consequently, patients with acute ulcerative colitis should be carefully observed and Lomotil therapy should be discontinued promptly if abdominal distension occurs or if other untoward symptoms develop.

Dependence Liability: Addiction to (dependency on) Lomotil is theoretically possible at high dosage. Therefore, the recommended dosage should not be exceeded. Because of the structural and pharmacological similarity of diphenoxylate to meperidine and similar drugs with a definite addiction potential, Lomotil should be administered with considerable caution to patients who are receiving addicting drugs, to individuals known to be addiction-prone, or to those whose histories suggest that they may increase the dosage on their own initiative. Because a subtherapeutic dose of atropine has been added to the diphenoxylate, to discourage deliberate overdosage, there should be strict observance of the contraindications and precautions relative to the use of atropine.

Drug Interactions: Lomotil may potentiate the action of barbiturates, tranquilizers and alcohol. Therefore, the patient should be closely observed when these medications are used concomitantly.

Since the chemical structure of diphenoxylate is similar to that of meperidine, the concurrent use of Lomotil with MAO inhibitors may in theory precipitate a hypertensive crisis.

ADVERSE EFFECTS: The most frequently reported adverse effect is nausea. Other symptoms which have been reported at therapeutic doses are:

Nervous System: drowsiness, coma, lethargy, sedation/drowsiness, restlessness, dizziness, insomnia, headache, blurring of vision, depression, euphoria, confusion, paresthesia, malaise.

Respiratory: respiratory depression.

Gastrointestinal: vomiting, anorexia, nausea, abdominal bloating, cramps, paralytic ileus, toxic megacolon, pancreatitis.

Allergy: anaphylaxis, pruritus, skin eruption, giant urticaria, angioneurotic edema.

Atropine effects such as dryness of the skin and mucous membranes, hyperthermia, tachycardia, urinary retention and flushing may also occur, especially in children.

OVERDOSE:

Symptoms: Initial signs may include dryness of the skin and mucous membranes, mydriasis, restlessness, flushing, hyperthermia and tachycardia followed by lethargy or coma, hypotonic reflexes, nystagmus, pinpoint pupils and respiratory depression. Cardiac arrest has occurred in children.

Treatment: Treat all possible Lomotil overdoses as serious and maintain medical observation for at least 48 hours.

Gastric lavage, establishment of a patent airway, and possibly, mechanically-assisted respiration are advised. Undertake gastric lavage with due caution in an unconscious patient, preferably following insertion of a cuffed endotracheal tube. If the patient is not comatose, administration of a slurry of activated charcoal may be indicated.

Narcotic antagonists such as naloxone HCl may be used for the treatment of respiratory depression caused by narcotic drugs or pharmacologically-related compounds, such as Lomotil.

Naloxone HCl Dosage in Adults: Naloxone HCl may be administered to adults at a dose of 0.4 mg i.v. Additional doses of 0.4 mg may be given at 2- or 3-minute intervals until adequate improvement in pulmonary ventilation is demonstrated. Subsequent injections of this drug must be governed by the degree of respiratory depression present and should be titrated accordingly. Since the duration of action of naloxone HCl is short in comparison to that of diphenoxylate, improvement of respiration after its administration may be followed by subsequent respiratory depression. It should be noted that although signs of overdosage and respiratory depression may not be evident with Lomotil after ingestion, respiratory depression may occur 12 to 30 hours later. Consequently, continuous observation is necessary until the effect of diphenoxylate on respiration, which may persist for many hours, has passed. The period of observation should extend over at least 48 hours, preferably under continuous hospital care.

Naloxone HCl Dosage in Children: For known or suspected narcotic overdosage, the initial dosage of naloxone HCl in children is 0.005 to 0.01 mg/kg body weight when given i.v., i.m. or s.c. This dose may be repeated as for adults above. If necessary, naloxone HCl can be diluted with sterile water for injection.

For management of a suspected drug overdose, CPhA recommends that you contact your **regional Poison Control Centre**. See the *CPS* Directory section for a list of Poison Control Centres.

DOSAGE: Adults: The usual initial dose is 5 mg (2 tablets) 3 or 4 times daily (20 mg/24 hours in divided doses is the maximum recommended dosage). An individual maintenance dose can be subsequently determined. Downward adjustment should be made as soon as initial control of symptoms is accomplished. The maintenance dose may be as low as ¼ of the dose required for initial control.

Children: **Not for use in children under 2 years of age (see Warnings and Precautions).**

The recommended initial dosage determined by the child's weight, is as follows: 0.3 to 0.4 mg/kg **daily** in divided doses. For convenience, **approximate** dosage (in children of average weight) may be determined by Table 1.

Table 1: Lomotil

Approximate Dosage in Children of Average Weight

Age	Approximate Body Weight	Total Daily Dose
2 to 5 years	15–20 kg	2.5 mg b.i.d.
6 to 8 years	20–27 kg	2.5 mg t.i.d.
9 to 12 years	27–36 kg	2.5 mg q.i.d.
13 years and above	—	5 mg q.i.d.

As with adult therapy, adjustment of dosage downward should be made as soon as initial control of symptoms is accomplished.

These pediatric schedules are the best approximation of an average dose recommendation which should be adjusted according to the overall nutritional status and degree of dehydration encountered in the child. The recommended doses must not be exceeded.

SUPPLIED: Each round, white tablet, with "SEARLE" debossed on one side and "61" on the other side, contains: diphenoxylate HCl 2.5 mg and atropine sulfate 0.025 mg. Nonmedicinal ingredients: acacia, cornstarch, magnesium stearate, mineral oil, sorbitol, sucrose and talc. Bottles of 250. Store at 15-25°C and protect from light.

(Shown in Product Identification Section)

Loniten® ℞
minoxidil
Antihypertensive

Pfizer

Date of Preparation: September 23, 2003
Date of Revision: April 26, 2010

PHARMACOLOGY: Minoxidil is an orally effective direct acting peripheral vasodilator that reduces elevated systolic and diastolic blood pressure by decreasing peripheral vascular resistance.

Minoxidil does not directly stimulate the heart or electrolyte reabsorption by the kidney. However, because of peripheral dilatation, minoxidil elicits a reflex mediated increase in cardiac output, salt and water retention, and a rise in plasma renin activity. These adverse effects are diminished by the simultaneous administration of a diuretic and a beta-adrenergic blocking agent or other sympathetic nervous system suppressant.

Minoxidil is at least 95% absorbed from the gastrointestinal tract. Plasma levels of the parent drug reach maximum within the first hour and decline rapidly thereafter. The average plasma half-life in man is 4.2 hours. Approximately 90% of the administered drug is metabolized, predominantly by conjugation with glucuronic acid at the N oxide position in the pyrimidine ring but also by conversion to more polar products.

Known metabolites exert much less pharmacologic effect than minoxidil itself, and all are excreted principally in the urine. Minoxidil does not bind to plasma proteins, and its renal clearance corresponds to the glomerular filtration rate. In the absence of functional renal tissue, minoxidil and its metabolites can be removed by hemodialysis, although this does not rapidly reverse its pharmacological effect.

The extent and time-course of blood pressure reduction by minoxidil do not correspond closely to its concentration in plasma. After a single oral dose, blood pressure usually starts to decline within one half hour, and reaches a minimum between 2 and 3 hours and recovers at an arithmetically linear rate of about 30%/day. The total duration of effect is approximately 72 hours. When minoxidil is administered chronically, the time required to achieve maximum effect on blood pressure is inversely related to the size of the dose.

INDICATIONS: Because of the potential for serious adverse effects, minoxidil is indicated only in the treatment of severe hypertension that is symptomatic or associated with target organ damage and is not manageable with maximum therapeutic doses of a diuretic plus two other antihypertensive drugs. At the present time, use in milder degrees of hypertension is not recommended because the benefit—risk relationship in such patients has not been defined.

CONTRAINDICATIONS: Pheochromocytoma because minoxidil may reflexly stimulate secretion of catecholamines from the tumor; pulmonary hypertension associated with mitral stenosis; hypersensitivity to minoxidil or any components of the preparation.

WARNINGS: Salt and water retention; congestive heart failure—concomitant use of an adequate diuretic is required: Minoxidil must usually be administered concomitantly with a diuretic adequate to prevent fluid retention and possible congestive heart failure; a high-ceiling (loop) diuretic is almost always required. Body weight should be monitored closely. If minoxidil is used without a diuretic, retention of several hundred milli-equivalents of salt and corresponding volumes of water can occur within a few days, leading to increased plasma and interstitial fluid volume and local and generalized edema. Diuretic treatment, alone or in combination with restricted salt intake, will usually minimize fluid retention, although reversible edema did develop in approximately 10% of nondialysis patients so treated. Diuretic effectiveness was limited mostly by disease related impaired renal function. The condition of patients with pre-existing congestive heart failure occasionally deteriorated in association with fluid retention, although because of the fall in blood pressure (reduction of afterload), more than twice as many improved than worsened. Rarely, refractory fluid retention may require discontinuation of minoxidil.

Provided that the patient is under close medical supervision, it may be possible to resolve refractory salt retention by discontinuing minoxidil for 1 or 2 days and then resuming treatment in conjunction with vigorous diuretic therapy.

Concomitant treatment to prevent tachycardia is usually required: Minoxidil increases the heart rate. This increase can be partly or entirely prevented by the concomitant administration of a beta-adrenergic blocking drug or other sympathetic nervous system suppressant. Round-the-clock effectiveness of the sympathetic suppressant should be assured. In addition, angina may worsen or appear for the first time during minoxidil treatment, probably because of the increased oxygen demands associated with increased heart rate and cardiac output. This can usually be prevented by sympathetic blockade.

Pericarditis, Pericardial effusion and Tamponade: Although there is no evidence of a causal relationship, there have been multiple reports of pericarditis occurring in association with minoxidil.

Pericardial effusion, occasionally with tamponade, has been observed in about 3% of treated patients not on dialysis, especially those with inadequate or compromised renal function. Although in many cases the pericardial effusion was associated with a connective tissue disease, the uremic syndrome, congestive heart failure or marked fluid retention, there have been instances in which these potential causes of effusion were not present. Patients should be observed closely for any suggestion of a pericardial disorder, and echocardiographic studies should be carried out if suspicion arises. More vigorous diuretic therapy, dialysis, pericardiocentesis or surgery may be required. If the effusion persists, withdrawal of therapy should be considered in light of other means of controlling the hypertension and the patient's clinical status.

Interaction with Guanethidine: Although minoxidil does not itself cause orthostatic hypotension, its administration to patients already receiving guanethidine can result in profound orthostatic effects. If at all possible guanethidine should be discontinued well before minoxidil is begun. Where this is not possible, minoxidil therapy should be started in the hospital and the patient should remain institutionalized until severe orthostatic effects are no longer present or the patient has learned to avoid activities that provoke them.

Hazard of Rapid Control of Blood Pressure: In patients with very severe blood pressure elevation, too rapid control of blood pressure, especially with i.v. agents, can precipitate cerebrovascular accidents and myocardial infarction. Although such events have not been unequivocally associated with minoxidil use, total experience is limited at present.

Any patient with malignant hypertension should have initial treatment with minoxidil carried out in a hospital setting, both to assure that blood pressure is falling and to assure that it is not falling more rapidly than intended.

Cardiac Lesions in Animals: In non-primate animal studies, minoxidil produced several types of myocardial lesions as well as other adverse cardiac effects. These included necrotic and hemorrhagic lesions of the myocardium and papillary muscles and cardiac hypertrophy and dilatation. As greater experience with minoxidil has accumulated, it has become apparent that these cardiac lesions so described in the dog, minipig and other non-primates do not occur in humans. Human autopsy experience has revealed the following: Among 242 autopsies performed on patients who received minoxidil tablets, cardiac pathology was detected in only 8 instances. In every instance, the conclusion has been reached that the human heart lesions were decidedly different in individual elements and constellation of changes from both the atrial and ventricular lesions seen in animals. Among 224 autopsies performed on patients never exposed to minoxidil tablets, the cardiac pathology observed, especially in the right atrium, entirely encompassed the pathologic findings seen in the minoxidil cases. The inference of these observations is that the pathologic findings in hearts of minoxidil treated hypertensive patients were not attributable to minoxidil administration, but rather to disease processes which were common to patients in these two studies.

PRECAUTIONS: Monitor fluid and electrolyte balance and body weight (see Warnings, Salt and Water Retention).

Observe patients for signs and symptoms of pericardial effusions (see Warnings, Pericarditis, Pericardial Effusion and Tamponade).

Abnormal hair growth is a common occurrence (see Adverse Effects). This is especially disturbing to women and children and patients should be thoroughly informed about this effect before therapy with minoxidil is begun.

When using a concomitant sympatholytic to prevent tachycardia, careful attention to adjusting the dosages of the beta-blocker or other sympathetic nervous system suppressant is required for maximum safety and efficacy (see Dosage, Concomitant Therapy).

When using a concomitant diuretic to prevent or treat fluid retention, careful attention to adjusting the dosage of the diuretic is required for maximum safety and efficacy (see Dosage, Concomitant Therapy).

Minoxidil has not been used in patients who have had a myocardial infarction within the preceding month. It is possible that a reduction of arterial pressure with minoxidil might further limit blood flow to the myocardium, although this might be compensated by decreased oxygen demand because of lower blood pressure.

Hypersensitivity to minoxidil, manifested as a skin rash, including rare reports of bullous eruptions and Stevens-Johnson syndrome, has been seen.

Renal failure or dialysis patients may require smaller doses of minoxidil and should have close medical supervision to prevent exacerbation of renal failure or precipitation of cardiac failure.

If minoxidil therapy must be discontinued in a patient who has been treated effectively, the drug should be phased out gradually or replaced with another antihypertensive agent. Careful monitoring of the patient's blood pressure during the treatment adjustment is necessary.

Pregnancy: The safety for use of minoxidil in pregnancy has not been established. Minoxidil has been shown to reduce the conception rate in rats and to show evidence of increased fetal absorption in rabbits when administered at 5 times the human dose. There was no evidence of teratogenic effects in rats and rabbits. Minoxidil should be used during pregnancy only if the potential benefit justifies the potential risk to the fetus.

Lactation: This drug has been reported to be excreted in human milk. As a general rule, nursing should not be undertaken while a patient is on minoxidil.

Children: Use in children has been limited to date particularly in infants. The recommendations under Dosage can be considered only a rough guide and careful titration is essential.

Information to Be Provided to the Patient: The patient should be made fully aware of the importance of continuing all prescribed antihypertensive medications and of the nature of symptoms that would suggest fluid overload (see Information for the Patient).

ADVERSE EFFECTS: Salt and water retention (see Warnings): Temporary edema, developed in 7% of patients who were not edematous at the start of therapy.

Pericarditis, pericardial effusion and tamponade (see Warnings).

Hypertrichosis: Elongation, thickening, and enhanced pigmentation of fine body hair are seen in about 80% of patients. This develops within 3 to 6 weeks after starting therapy. It is usually first noticed on the temples, between the eyebrows, between the hairline and the eyebrows, or in the sideburn area of the upper lateral cheek, later extending to the back, arms, legs, and scalp. Upon discontinuation of minoxidil, new hair growth stops, but 1 to 6 months may be required for restoration to pretreatment appearance. No endocrine abnormalities have been found to explain the abnormal hair growth; thus, it is hypertrichosis without virilism.

ECG Changes: Changes in direction and magnitude of the ECG T waves occur in approximately 60% of patients treated with minoxidil. In rare instances a large negative amplitude of the T wave may encroach upon the ST segment, but the ST segment is not independently altered. These changes usually disappear with continuance of treatment and revert to the pretreatment state if minoxidil is discontinued. No symptoms have been associated with these changes.

Miscellaneous: Breast tenderness, rash (see Precautions) and gastrointestinal intolerance developed in less than 1% of patients.

Altered Laboratory Findings: Effects of hemodilution-hematocrit, hemoglobin, and erythrocyte count usually fall about 7% initially and then recover to pretreatment levels; thrombocytopenia and leukopenia have been rarely reported; alkaline phosphatase increased varyingly without other evidence of liver or bone abnormality; serum creatinine increased an average of 6% and BUN slightly more, but later declined to pretreatment levels.

OVERDOSE:

Symptoms: There have been only a few instances of deliberate or accidental overdosage with minoxidil. When exaggerated hypotension is encountered, it is most likely to occur in association with residual sympathetic nervous system blockade from previous therapy (guanethidine-like effects of alpha-adrenergic blockade).

Treatment: The recommended treatment is i.v. administration of normal saline. Sympathomimetic drugs, such as norepinephrine or epinephrine, should be avoided because of their excessive cardiac stimulating action. Phenylephrine, angiotensin II, vasopressin and dopamine, which reverse the effects of minoxidil, should only be used if inadequate perfusion of a vital organ is evident.

> For management of a suspected drug overdose, CPhA recommends that you contact your **regional Poison Control Centre**. See the *CPS* Directory section for a list of Poison Control Centres.

DOSAGE: Adults and children over 12 years of age: The recommended initial daily dosage of minoxidil is 5 mg given in 2 divided doses. Daily dosage can be increased to 10, 20 and 40 mg/day in divided doses, at 3 day intervals or longer, if required for optimum blood pressure control. The effective dosage range is usually 10 to 40 mg/day. In certain patients, doses up to a maximum of 100 mg/day may be attempted, recognizing the probability of an increase in the incidence and severity of adverse reactions.

Children under 12 years of age: The initial recommended daily dosage is 0.2 mg/kg minoxidil in 2 divided doses. The dosage may be increased by 0.1 to 0.2 mg/kg/day increments, at 3 day intervals or longer, until optimum blood pressure control is achieved. The effective dosage range is usually 0.25 to 1 mg/kg/day. The maximum recommended dose is 50 mg/day.

Frequency of Dosage Adjustment: Dosage must be titrated carefully according to individual response. Intervals between dosage adjustments normally should be at least 3 days since the full response to a given dose is not obtained for at least that amount of time.

Where a more rapid management of hypertension is required, a 5 mg dose can be given every 6 hours if the patient is hospitalized and carefully monitored (see Warnings).

Dose Frequency: The magnitude of within-day fluctuation of arterial pressure during therapy with minoxidil is directly proportional to the extent of pressure reduction. When the targeted blood pressure has been reached, a change from twice daily to once daily dosing with minoxidil may be tried in those patients in whom the diastolic pressure has been reduced less than 30 mmHg. If supine diastolic pressure has been reduced more than 30 mmHg, the twice daily dosage schedule should be maintained.

Concomitant Therapy: Diuretics: To prevent fluid retention and possible congestive heart failure, minoxidil must be used in conjunction with a high ceiling (loop) diuretic in patients relying on renal function for maintaining salt and water balance. Diuretics have been used at the following dosages when starting therapy with minoxidil: hydrochlorothiazide (50 mg twice daily) or other thiazides at equi-effective dosage; chlorthalidone (50 to 100 mg once daily); furosemide (40 mg twice daily).

If excessive salt and water retention results in a weight gain of more than 2 kg, diuretic therapy should be changed to furosemide; if the patient is already taking furosemide, dosage should be increased in accordance with the patient's requirements. Rarely, refractory fluid retention may require discontinuation of minoxidil. Provided that the patient is under close medical supervision, it may be possible to resolve refractory fluid retention by discontinuing minoxidil for 1 or 2 days and then resuming treatment in conjunction with vigorous diuretic therapy.

In dialysis patients also receiving diuretic therapy, use of minoxidil may create the need to raise diuretic dosage or to increase the frequency or duration of dialysis in order to maintain salt and water balance.

Sympathetic Nervous System Suppressants: The preferred agent to achieve sympathetic nervous system suppression is a beta-blocker equivalent to an adult propranolol dosage of 80 to 160 mg/day. Higher doses may be required when patients, pretreated with a beta-blocker, have an increase in heart rate exceeding 20 beats/minute or when simultaneous introduction of minoxidil and a beta-blocker causes an increase in heart rate exceeding 10 beats/minute.

If beta-blockers are contraindicated, methyldopa (250 to 750 mg twice daily) may be used instead. Methyldopa must be given for at least 24 hours before starting therapy with minoxidil because of the delay in the onset of methyldopa's action. Limited clinical experience indicates that clonidine may also be used to prevent tachycardia induced by minoxidil; the usual dosage is 0.1 to 0.2 mg twice daily.

Sympathetic nervous system suppressants may not completely prevent an increase in heart rate due to minoxidil but usually do prevent tachycardia. Typically, patients receiving a beta-blocker prior to initiation of therapy with minoxidil have a bradycardia and can be expected to have an increase in heart rate toward normal when minoxidil is added. When treatment with minoxidil and a beta-blocker or other sympathetic nervous system suppressant are begun simultaneously, their opposing cardiac effects usually nullify each other, leading to little change in heart rate.

INFORMATION FOR THE PATIENT: Published in e-CPS, available by subscription at www.e-cps.ca.

SUPPLIED: 2.5 mg: Each round, white tablet scored and embossed with a "U" and 121 on one side and 2½ on the other contains: minoxidil 2.5 mg. Nonmedicinal ingredients: cornstarch, lactose, magnesium stearate, microcrystalline cellulose and silicon dioxide. Gluten-free. Bottles of 100. Store at controlled room temperature (15 to 30°C).

10 mg: Each round, white tablet scored and embossed with a "U" and 137 on one side and 10 on the other contains: minoxidil 10 mg. Nonmedicinal ingredients: cornstarch, lactose, magnesium stearate, microcrystalline cellulose and silicon dioxide. Gluten-free. Bottles of 100. Store at controlled room temperature (15 to 30°C).

(Shown in Product Identification Section)

Lopid™

gemfibrozil

Antihyperlipidemic

Pfizer

Date of Preparation: January 9, 2001
Date of Revision: January 22, 2010

PHARMACOLOGY: LOPID (gemfibrozil) is a lipid regulating agent which decreases serum triglycerides and total cholesterol, and increases high density lipoprotein cholesterol. The lipid-lowering changes occur primarily in the very low density lipoprotein (VLDL) fraction (S_f20-400) rich in triglycerides and to a lesser extent in the low density lipoprotein (LDL) fraction (S_f0-20) rich in cholesterol. LOPID treatment of patients with elevated triglycerides due to Type IV hyperlipoproteinemia may cause a rise in LDL-cholesterol. In addition, LOPID increases the high density lipoprotein (HDL) cholesterol subfractions, HDL_2 and HDL_3, as well as apolipoproteins AI and AII.

Epidemiological studies have shown that both low HDL-cholesterol and high LDL-cholesterol are independent risk factors for coronary heart disease. Depending on the type of hyperlipidemia, pharmacological intervention with LOPID raises HDL-cholesterol and may lower LDL-cholesterol, and may be associated with reduced morbidity due to coronary heart disease as reported in the Helsinki Heart Study; a 5-year primary prevention Phase IV clinical trial.

The mechanism of action has not been definitely established. In man, LOPID has been shown to inhibit peripheral lipolysis and to decrease the hepatic extraction of free fatty acids, thus reducing hepatic triglyceride production. LOPID also inhibits the synthesis and increases clearance of VLDL carrier apolipoprotein B, leading to a decrease in VLDL.

Animal studies suggest that LOPID may, in addition to elevating HDL cholesterol (HDL-C), reduce incorporation of long-chain fatty acids into newly formed triglycerides, accelerate turnover and removal of cholesterol from the liver, and increase excretion of cholesterol in the feces.

INDICATIONS: LOPID (gemfibrozil) is indicated as an adjunct to diet and other therapeutic measures for:

1. Treatment of adult patients with very high serum triglyceride levels, Fredrickson classification Type IV and V hyperlipidemias, who are at a high risk of sequelae and complications (i.e. pancreatitis) from their hyperlipidemia.
2. Treatment of patients with hypercholesterolemia, Type IIa and IIb mixed dyslipidemias, to regulate lipid levels (reduce serum triglycerides and LDL cholesterol levels and increase HDL cholesterol).

LOPID alone may not be adequate therapy in some patients with familial combined hyperlipidemia with Type IIb and IV hyperlipoproteinemia.

Initial therapy for hyperlipidemia should include a specific diet, weight reduction, and an exercise program; and for patients with diabetes mellitus, a good diabetic control.

CONTRAINDICATIONS:

1. Hepatic or renal dysfunction, including primary biliary cirrhosis.
2. Pre-existing gallbladder disease (see Precautions).
3. Hypersensitivity to LOPID (gemfibrozil) or any of the inert ingredients.
4. The drug should not be used in pregnant or lactating patients.
5. LOPID is not indicated for the treatment of Type I hyperlipoproteinemia.
6. The concomitant use of gemfibrozil with repaglinide is contraindicated (see Precautions, Drug Interactions).

WARNINGS: Muscle Effects: There have been reports of severe myalgia, myositis and rhabdomyolysis accompanied by markedly elevated creatinine kinase when gemfibrozil and HMG CoA reductase inhibitors were used concomitantly (see Precautions, Drug Interactions). When rhabdomyolysis is severe the ensuing myoglobinuria can lead to acute renal failure. Therefore, HMG CoA reductase inhibitors should not be used concomitantly with LOPID.

Myopathy, defined as muscle aching or muscle weakness, associated with increases in plasma creatine phopsphokinase (CPK) values to greater than 10 times the Upper Limit of Normal (ULN), should be considered in any patient with diffuse myalgias, muscle tenderness or weakness, and/or marked elevation of CPK. Patients should be advised to report promptly unexplained muscle pain, tenderness, or weakness, particularly if accompanied by malaise or fever.

The risk of myopathy and rhabdomyolosis during treatment with HGM-CoA reductase inhibitors in combination with fibric acid derivatives is increased.

The benefits and risks of combined therapy should be carefully considered (see Precautions, Drug Interactions).

Rhabdomyolysis with renal dysfunction secondary to myoglobinuria have been reported with HMG-CoA reductase inhibitors. Gemfibrozil therapy should be discontinued if markedly elevated CPK levels occur or myopathy is diagnosed or suspected. Gemfibrozil should be temporarily withheld in any patient experiencing an acute or serious condition suggestive of a myopathy or having a risk factor predisposing to the development of renal failure secondary to rhabdomyolysis, e.g., sepsis; hypotension; major surgery; trauma; severe metabolic, endocrine or electrolyte disorders; or uncontrolled epilepsy.

Clofibrate: LOPID clinically, pharmacologically and chemically shows similarities with clofibrate. Physicians prescribing gemfibrozil should also be familiar with the risks and benefits of clofibrate.

Toxicology Studies: Long-term studies with gemfibrozil have been conducted in rats and mice at one and ten times the human dose. The incidence of benign liver nodules and liver carcinomas was significantly increased in high dose male rats. The incidence of liver carcinomas was increased also in low dose males, but the increase was not statistically significant (p>0.05). In high dose female rats, there was a significant increase in the combined incidence of benign and malignant liver neoplasms. There were no statistically significant differences from controls in the incidence of liver tumors in male and female mice, but the doses tested were lower than those shown to be carcinogenic with other fibrates. Liver and testicular cell tumors were increased in male rats.

Electron microscopy studies have demonstrated a florid hepatic peroxisome proliferation following gemfibrozil administration to male rats. Such changes have not been found in the liver of patients treated with this drug.

Toxicology studies in male rats revealed a dose-related increase of benign Leydig cell tumors. Subcapsular bilateral cataracts occurred in 10% and unilateral in 6.3% of the high dose males.

Cholelithiasis: LOPID may increase cholesterol excretion into the bile raising the potential for gallstone formation leading to cholelithiasis. If cholelithiasis is suspected, gallbladder studies are indicated. LOPID therapy should be discontinued if gallstones are found. Cases of cholelithiasis have been reported with gemfibrozil therapy.

General: Since a reduction of total mortality has not been demonstrated, LOPID should be administered only in those patients described in the Indications section. If a significant serum lipid response is not obtained in 3 months, LOPID should be discontinued.

If LOPID is chosen for treatment, the prescribing physician should discuss the proposed therapy and inform the patient of the expected benefits and potential risks which may be associated with long-term administration (see Precautions).

Children: Safety and efficacy in children have not been established.

Pregnancy: Strict birth control procedures must be exercised by women of childbearing potential. If pregnancy occurs despite birth control procedures, LOPID should be discontinued.

Women who are planning pregnancy should discontinue LOPID several months prior to conception.

Lactation: Because of the potential for tumorigenicity shown for gemfibrozil in rats, a decision should be made whether to discontinue nursing or discontinue the drug, taking into account the importance of the drug to the mother.

PRECAUTIONS: Initial Therapy: Before instituting LOPID (gemfibrozil) therapy, attempts should be made to control serum lipids and lipoproteins with appropriate diet, exercise, weight loss in obese patients, and control of diabetes mellitus.

Long-term Therapy: Because long-term administration of LOPID is recommended, pretreatment clinical chemistry studies should be performed to ensure that the patient has elevated serum lipid or low HDL cholesterol levels. Periodic determinations of serum lipids and lipoproteins should be done during LOPID administration, including measurement of LDL-cholesterol/HDL-cholesterol ratio, particularly in Type IV hyperlipoproteinemic patients.

Impairment of Fertility: Administration of approximately three and ten times the human dose to male rats for 10 weeks resulted in a dose-related decrease of fertility. Subsequent studies demonstrated that this effect was reversed after a drug-free period of about 8 weeks, and it was not transmitted to their offspring.

Hematologic Changes: Mild hemoglobin, hematocrit and white blood cells (WBC) decrease have been observed occasionally following initiation of LOPID therapy. The levels then stabilize during long-term administration. Rarely, severe anemia, leukopenia, thrombocytopenia, eosinophilia and bone marrow hypoplasia have been reported. Therefore, periodic blood count determinations are recommended during the first 12 months of LOPID administration.

Liver Function: Abnormal liver function tests have been observed occasionally during LOPID administration, including elevations of AST, ALT, LDH, alkaline phosphatase, creatine kinase, and bilirubin. These are usually reversible when LOPID is discontinued. Therefore, periodic liver function studies are recommended and LOPID therapy should be terminated if abnormalities persist.

Hepatobiliary Disease: In patients with a past history of jaundice or hepatic disorder, LOPID should be used with caution.

Cardiac Arrhythmias: Although no clinically significant abnormalities occurred that could be attributed to LOPID, the possibility exists that such abnormalities may occur.

Drug Interactions: When LOPID (gemfibrozil) and lovastatin were used concomitantly there have been reports of severe myalgia, myositis and rhabdomyolysis accompanied by markedly elevated CK. When rhabdomyolysis is severe, the ensuing myoglobinuria can lead to acute renal failure. Therefore, lovastatin should not be used concomitantly with LOPID.

Anticoagulants: Caution should be exercised when anticoagulants are given in conjunction with LOPID. The dosage of the anticoagulant should be reduced to maintain the prothrombin time at the desired level to prevent bleeding complications. Frequent prothrombin determinations are advisable until it has been definitely determined that the prothrombin level has stabilized.

Bile Acid-Binding Resins: Reduced bioavailability of LOPID may result when given simultaneously with resin-granule drugs such as colestipol. Administration of the drugs two hours or more apart is recommended.

HMG-CoA Reductase Inhibitors: There have been reports of severe myalgia, myositis and rhabdomyolysis accompanied by markedly elevated creatine kinase (CK) when gemfibrozil and HMG-CoA reductase inhibitors were used concomitantly. When rhabdomyolysis is severe the ensuing myoglobinuria can lead to acute renal failure. Therefore, HMG-CoA reductase inhibitors should not be used concomitantly with LOPID (see Warnings, Muscle Effects).

Repaglinide: Serious cases of hypoglycemia have been reported following the concomitant use of repaglinide and gemfibrozil. This is likely due to inhibition of CYP 2C8 by gemfibrozil as evidenced by decreases in blood glucose that were proportional to the dose of gemfibrozil. In healthy volunteers, the levels of repaglinide were significantly increased when co-administered with gemfibrozil. The averaged area under the curve (AUC) was increased 8-fold (range 6- to 15 fold) and the half-life increased 3 fold. When itraconazole, an inhibitor of CYP 3A4, was also given with gemfibrozil and repaglinide, even greater effects were observed: AUC for repaglinide was increased 19-fold and the half-life increased from 1.3 to 6 hours (see Contraindications).

CYP2C8 inhibition by gemfibrozil can affect the metabolism of several major cardiovascular drugs such as amiodarone, verapamil, warfarin but also other drugs such as tolbutamide.

Gemfibrozil is also known to potently inhibit CYP2C9 activity. Therefore, CYP2C9 inhibition by gemfibrozil can affect the metabolism of several major cardiovascular drugs such as carvedilol and losartan but also other drugs such as phenytoin and diazepam.

ADVERSE EFFECTS: Pre-Marketing Studies: LOPID (gemfibrozil) has been carefully evaluated in over 3,000 patients having received the drug in monitored clinical studies prior to marketing. Symptoms reported during the controlled phase in studies of 805 subjects were considered for safety. The symptoms listed in Table 1 are those which occurred in at least 5 patients and all skin reactions whatever their incidence. The principal symptoms for which incidence was greater with gemfibrozil than with placebo involved the gastrointestinal system. Nausea and vomiting, and abdominal and epigastric pain occurred more often in the gemfibrozil group than in the placebo group. However, the incidence was low: nausea, 4.3% with gemfibrozil versus 3.8% with placebo; vomiting, 2.3% versus 0.8%; abdominal pain, 6.4% versus 4.2%; and epigastric pain, 3.4% versus 1.7%.

Table 1: LOPID

Incidence of Symptoms Reported in Controlled Premarketing Studies

Symptom	Gemfibrozil (n=529) (%)	Placebo (n=236) (%)
Body as a Whole		
Dizziness	2.8	4.2
Chest pain	2.1	1.7
Fatigue	0.9	0.4
Integumentary		
Rash	2.5	1.3
Pruritus	0.8	1.3
Dermatitis	0.6	0.4
Urticaria	0.2	0.0
Musculoskeletal		
Pain in extremities	1.5	1.7
Gastrointestinal		
Abdominal pain	6.4	4.2
Diarrhea	4.9	5.1
Nausea	4.3	3.8
Epigastric pain	3.4	1.7
Vomiting	2.3	0.8
Flatulence	1.5	2.1
Endocrine		
Gout	0.9	0.8
Central Nervous System		
Headache	2.3	4.2
Paresthesia	0.9	0.4
Special Senses		
Blurred vision	1.1	0.8
Number of Patients Withdrawn for Clinical Symptoms	1.3	1.3

Additional adverse reactions that have been reported, where a causal relationship to treatment with gemfibrozil is probable, are:

Hepatobiliary Disorders: cholestatic jaundice.
Gastrointestinal Disorders: pancreatitis.
Nervous System Disorders: dizziness, somnolence, paresthesia, peripheral neuritis, headache.
Psychiatric Disorders: decreased libido, depression.
Eye Disorder: blurred vision.
Reproductive System and Breast Disorders: impotence.

Musculoskeletal and Connective Tissue Disorders: arthralgia, synovitis, myalgia, myopathy, myasthenia, painful extremities, rhabdomyolysis (see Warnings, Drug Interactions).
Skin and Subcutaneous Tissue Disorders: exfoliative dermatitis, rash, dermatitis, pruritus, angioedema, urticaria, photosensitivity.
Respiratory, Thoracic and Mediastinal Disorders: laryngeal edema.
Blood and Lymphatic System Disorders: severe anemia, leukopenia, thrombocytopenia, eosinophilia, bone marrow hypoplasia (see Precautions, Hematologic Changes).

Additional adverse reactions that have been reported included photosensitivity, alopecia, cholecystitis and cholelithiasis (see Warnings).
Post-Marketing Study (Helsinki Heart Study): The long-term safety of LOPID (gemfibrozil) was established in the Helsinki Heart Study, a 5-year primary prevention Phase IV clinical trial. In the double-blind phase of the Helsinki Heart Study, 2046 patients received LOPID for up to 5 years. Table 2 lists the most frequently reported adverse events and includes those occurring in at least 1% of all subjects treated with gemfibrozil. Dyspepsia (19.6% versus 11.9%), abdominal pain (9.8% versus 5.6%), acute appendicitis (1.2% versus 0.6%) and atrial fibrillation (0.7% versus 0.1%) occurred more often in the gemfibrozil group than the placebo group, while all other adverse events were similar in frequency between the two groups.

Table 2: LOPID

Incidence of Adverse Events in Controlled Phase of Helsinki Heart Study

Adverse Event	Gemfibrozil (n=2046) (%)	Placebo (n=2035) (%)
Body as a Whole		
Fatigue	3.8	3.5
Headache	1.2	1.1
Digestive System		
Dyspepsia	19.6	11.9
Abdominal pain	9.8	5.6
Diarrhea	7.2	6.5
Flatulence	5.3	5.2
Nausea and/or vomiting	2.5	2.1
Constipation	1.4	1.3
Acute appendicitis	1.2	0.6
Nervous System		
Vertigo	1.5	1.3
Skin and Appendages		
Eczema	1.9	1.2
Rash	1.7	1.3
Number of Patients Withdrawn Due to Adverse Events	**10.4**	**7.3**

OVERDOSE:

Symptoms: Overdosage has been reported with gemfibrozil. Symptoms reported with overdosage were abdominal cramps, abnormal liver function tests, diarrhea, increased CPK, joint and muscle pain, nausea and vomiting. In one case of accidental overdosage, where a child ingested 9 g of gemfibrozil, non-specific symptoms of nausea and vomiting were reported. The patient fully recovered.

Treatment: Symptomatic supportive measures should be taken should overdosage occur.

For management of a suspected drug overdose, contact your regional Poison Control Centre. See the *CPS* Directory section for a list of Poison Control Centres.

DOSAGE: The recommended dose for adults is 1200 mg administered in two divided doses (two 300 mg capsules or one 600 mg tablet twice a day) 30 minutes before the morning and evening meal. The maximum recommended daily dose is 1500 mg.

SUPPLIED: 300 mg: Each maroon and white hard gelatin capsule printed "LOPID" in grey on body and printed "PD 669" in gray on cap contains: gemfibrozil 300 mg. Nonmedicinal ingredients: Capsule: cornstarch, polysorbate 80. Capsule shell: contains: silicon dioxide, FD&C Blue No. 1, FD&C Red No. 3, gelatin, sodium lauryl sulfate and titanium dioxide. Energy: 3.4 kJ (0.8 kcal). Gluten-, lactose-, paraben-, sodium-, sulfite- and tartrazine-free. Bottles of 100 and 250. Store at controlled room temperature (15 to 30°C).
600 mg: Each white, ellipsoidal, film-coated tablet, imprinted in black ink "Lopid 600 mg" on one side and "Parke-Davis" on the other, contains: gemfibrozil 600 mg. Nonmedicinal ingredients: calcium stearate, candelilla wax, colloidal silicon dioxide, hypromellose, hydroxypropylcellulose, methylparaben, microcrystalline cellulose, Black Fine ink, polyethylene glycol, polysorbate 80, pregelatinized starch, propylparaben and white Opaspray. Energy: 2.0 kJ (0.47 kcal). Gluten-, lactose-, sodium-, sulfite- and tartrazine-free. Bottles of 100 and 250. Store at controlled room temperature (15 to 30°C).

(Shown in Product Identification Section)

Lopresor® Ⓟ

metoprolol tartrate

Beta-adrenergic Receptor Blocking Agent

Novartis Pharmaceuticals

Date of Preparation: June 21, 1977
Date of Revision: October 7, 2008

PHARMACOLOGY: Metoprolol is a β-adrenergic receptor-blocking agent. In vitro and in vivo animal studies have shown that it has a preferential effect on the β_1-adrenoreceptors, chiefly located in cardiac muscle. This preferential effect is not absolute, however, and at higher doses, metoprolol also inhibits β_2-adrenoreceptors, chiefly located in the bronchial and vascular musculature. Metoprolol has no membrane-stabilizing or partial agonism (intrinsic sympathomimetic activities). It is used in the treatment of hypertension, angina pectoris and to reduce mortality in patients with myocardial infarction.

The mechanism of the antihypertensive effect has not been established. Among the factors that may be involved are: a) competitive ability to antagonize catecholamine-induced tachycardia at the β-receptor sites in the heart, thus decreasing heart rate, cardiac contractility and cardiac output; b) inhibition of renin release by the kidneys; c) inhibition of the vasomotor centres.

By blocking catecholamine-induced increases in heart rate, in velocity and extent of myocardial contraction, and in blood pressure, metoprolol reduces the oxygen requirements of the heart at any given level of effort, thus making it useful in the long-term management of angina pectoris. However, in patients with heart failure, β-adrenergic receptor blockade may increase oxygen requirements by increasing left ventricular fiber length and end-diastolic pressure (preload).

The mechanisms involved in reducing mortality in patients with acute myocardial infarction are not fully understood.
Pharmacokinetics: In humans, absorption of metoprolol is rapid and complete. Plasma levels following oral administration, however, approximate 50% of levels following i.v. administration, indicating about 50% first-pass metabolism.

Intersubject plasma levels achieved are highly variable after oral administration, although they show good reproducibility within each individual. Peak plasma concentrations are attained after approximately 1.5 to 2 hours with conventional metoprolol formulations, and after approximately 4 to 5 hours with slow-release formulations. Upon repeated oral administration, the percentage of the dose systemically available is higher than after a single dose and also increases dose dependently. Ingestion with food may raise the systemic availability of an oral dose by approximately 20 to 40%. Only a small fraction of the drug (about 12%) is bound to human serum albumin.

Metoprolol is extensively metabolised by enzymes of the cytochrome P450 system in the liver. The oxidative metabolism of metoprolol is under genetic control with a major contribution of the polymorphic cytochrome P450 isoform 2D6 (CYP2D6). There are marked ethnic differences in the prevalence of the poor metabolizers (PM) phenotype. Approximately 7% of Caucasians and less than 1% Orientals are PMs.

CYP2D6 poor metabolizers exhibit several-fold higher plasma concentrations of metoprolol than extensive metabolizers with normal CYP2D6 activity. However, the cytochrome P450 2D6 dependent metabolism of metoprolol seems to have little or no effect on safety or tolerability of the drug. None of the metabolites of metoprolol contribute significantly to its β-blocking effect.

Elimination is mainly by biotransformation in the liver, and the plasma half-life averages 3.5 hours (range: 1 to 9 hours). The total clearance rate of an intravenous dose is approximately 1L/min and the protein binding rate is approximately 10%. Less than 5% of an oral dose of metoprolol is recovered unchanged in the urine; the rest is excreted by the kidneys as metabolites that appear to have no clinical significance.

The systemic availability and half-life of metoprolol in patients with renal failure do not differ to a clinically significant degree from those in normal subjects; however metabolite excretion is impaired. Since the resulting metabolite accumulation has no effect on the β-blocking effects, no reduction in dosage is usually needed in patients with chronic renal failure.

Liver impairment may increase metoprolol bioavailability and reduce total clearance.
Pharmacodynamics: Significant beta-blocking effect (as measured by reduction of exercise heart rate) occurs within 1 hour after oral administration, and its duration is dose-related. For example, a 50% reduction of the maximum effect after single oral doses of 20, 50, and 100 mg occurred at 3.3, 5.0 and 6.4 hours, respectively, in normal subjects. After repeated oral dosages of 100 mg twice daily, a significant reduction in exercise systolic blood pressure was evident at 12 hours.
Pharmacokinetic and Pharmacodynamic Relationship: Following i.v. administration of metoprolol, the half-life of the distribution phase is approximately 12 minutes; the urinary recovery of unchanged drug is approximately 10%. When the drug was infused over a 10-minute period, in normal volunteers, maximum β-blockade was achieved at approximately 20 minutes. Doses of 5 mg and 15 mg yielded a maximal reduction in exercise-induced heart rate of approximately 10% and 15%, respectively. The effect on exercise heart rate decreased linearly with time at the same rate for both doses, and disappeared at approximately 5 hours and 8 hours for the 5 mg and 15 mg doses, respectively.

Equivalent maximal β-blocking effect is achieved with oral and i.v. doses in the ratio of approximately 2.5:1.

There is a linear relationship between the log of plasma levels and reduction of exercise heart rate. However, antihypertensive activity does not appear to be related to plasma levels. Because of variable plasma levels attained with a given dose and lack of a consistent relationship of antihypertensive activity to dose, selection of proper dosage requires individual titration.

In several studies of patients with acute myocardial infarction, i.v. followed by oral administration of metoprolol caused a reduction in heart rate, systolic blood pressure, and cardiac output. Stroke volume, diastolic blood pressure, and pulmonary artery end diastolic pressure remained unchanged.

The SR formulation produced lower peak metoprolol plasma concentrations than the regular tablets in studies with volunteers. Between 4 to 6 hours both concentration curves were similar. During the 8- to 24-hour period concentrations were higher after the SR tablets.

INDICATIONS: Hypertension: Metoprolol is indicated for mild or moderate hypertension. Usually combined with other antihypertensive agents (thiazide diuretics), it may be tried alone when the physician judges that a beta-blocker rather than a diuretic, should be the initial treatment.

Combining metoprolol with a diuretic or peripheral vasodilator has been found to be compatible and generally more effective than metoprolol alone. Limited experience with other antihypertensive agents has not shown evidence of incompatibility with metoprolol.

Metoprolol is not recommended for the emergency treatment of hypertensive crises.
Angina Pectoris: Metoprolol is indicated for the long-term treatment of angina pectoris due to ischemic heart disease.
Myocardial Infarction: Metoprolol is indicated in the treatment of hemodynamically stable patients with definite or suspected acute myocardial infarction to reduce cardiovascular mortality.

Treatment with i.v. metoprolol can be initiated as soon as the patient's clinical condition allows (see Dosage, Contraindications and Warnings).

Alternatively, in patients with proven myocardial infarction, oral treatment can begin within 3 to 10 days of the acute event (see Dosage). Data are not available as to whether benefit would ensue if the treatment is initiated later.

Clinical trials have shown that patients with unconfirmed myocardial infarction received no benefit from early drug therapy.

CONTRAINDICATIONS: Metoprolol should not be used in the presence of: known hypersensitivity to metoprolol and derivatives, Lopresor components or hypersensitivity to other beta-blockers (cross-sensitivity between beta-blockers can occur); sinus bradycardia; sick sinus syndrome; second and third degree AV block; right ventricular failure secondary to pulmonary hypertension; overt heart failure; cardiogenic shock; severe peripheral arterial circulatory disorders; anesthesia with agents that produce myocardial depression (e.g., ether); untreated pheochromocytoma; the i.v. form is also contraindicated in the presence of asthma and other obstructive respiratory diseases (for oral treatment, see Precautions, Bronchospastic Diseases).
Myocardial Infarction Patients—Additional Contraindications: In patients with a heart rate <45 beats/min; significant heart block greater than first degree (PR interval ≥0.24 s); systolic blood pressure <100 mmHg; or moderate to severe cardiac failure (see Warnings).

WARNINGS: Cardiac Failure: Special caution should be exercised when administering metoprolol to patients with a history of heart failure. Sympathetic stimulation is a vital component supporting circulatory function in congestive heart failure, and inhibition with β-blockade always carries the potential hazard of further depressing myocardial contractility and precipitating cardiac failure. The positive inotropic action of digitalis may be reduced by the negative inotropic effect of metoprolol when the two drugs are used concomitantly. The effects of β-blockers and digitalis are additive in depressing AV conduction. This also applies to combinations with calcium-antagonists of the verapamil type or some antiarrhythmics (see Precautions, Drug Interactions).

In patients without a history of cardiac failure, continued depression of the myocardium over a period of time can, in some cases, lead to cardiac failure and/or hypotension (systolic blood pressure ≤90 mmHg). Therefore, at the first sign or symptom of impending cardiac failure, patients should be fully digitalized and/or given a diuretic and the response observed closely. If cardiac failure continues, despite adequate digitalization and diuretic therapy, metoprolol therapy should be reduced or withdrawn.
Abrupt Cessation of Therapy: Patients with angina should be warned against abrupt discontinuation of metoprolol. There have been reports of severe exacerbation of angina and of myocardial infarction or ventricular arrhythmias in patients with angina pectoris, following abrupt discontinuation of beta-blocker therapy. The last 2 complications may occur with or without preceding exacerbation of angina pectoris. Therefore, when discontinuation of metoprolol is planned in patients with angina pectoris or previous myocardial infarction, the dosage should be reduced gradually over a period of about 2 weeks. The patient should be carefully observed. The same frequency of administration should be maintained. In situations of greater urgency, metoprolol therapy should be discontinued stepwise and with closer observation. If angina markedly worsens or acute coronary insufficiency develops, it is recommended that treatment with metoprolol be reinstituted promptly, at least temporarily.

Patients should be warned against interruption or discontinuation of therapy without the physician's advice. Because coronary artery disease is common and may be unrecognized, it is prudent not to discontinue metoprolol therapy abruptly even in patients treated only for hypertension.
Oculomucocutaneous Syndrome: Various skin rashes and conjunctival xerosis have been reported with β-blockers, including metoprolol. Oculomucocutaneous syndrome, a severe syndrome whose signs include conjunctivitis sicca and psoriasiform rashes, otitis, and sclerosing serositis, has occurred with the chronic use of one β-adrenergic receptor-blocking agent (practolol). This syndrome has not been observed with metoprolol or any other such agent. However, physicians should be alert to the possibility of such reactions and should discontinue treatment in the event they occur.

Severe Sinus Bradycardia: Severe sinus bradycardia may occur after β_1-adrenergic receptor blockade with metoprolol because of unopposed vagal activity. Very rarely a pre-existing AV conduction disorder of moderate degree may become aggravated, possibly leading to AV block. In such cases, dosage should be reduced or gradually withdrawn. Atropine, isoproterenol or dobutamine should be considered in patients with acute myocardial infarction.
Thyrotoxicosis: Although metoprolol has been used successfully for the symptomatic (adjuvant) therapy of thyrotoxicosis, possible deleterious effects from long-term use of metoprolol have not been adequately appraised. Beta-blockade may mask the clinical signs of continuing hyperthyroidism or its complications, and give a false impression of improvement. Therefore, abrupt withdrawal of metoprolol may be followed by an exacerbation of the symptoms of hyperthyroidism, including thyroid storm.
Myocardial Infarction Patients—Additional Warnings: Acute Intervention: During acute intervention in myocardial infarction, i.v. metoprolol should only be used by experienced staff under circumstances where resuscitation and monitoring equipment is available.
Cardiac Failure: Depression of the myocardium with metoprolol may lead to cardiac failure (see Warnings). Special caution should be exercised when administering metoprolol to patients with a history of cardiac failure or those with minimal cardiac reserve. Should failure occur, treatment should be as described in Warnings.
Severe Sinus Bradycardia: Severe sinus bradycardia may occur with the use of metoprolol (see Warnings). Acute myocardial infarction (particularly inferior infarcts) may significantly decrease sinus rate. If the rate falls below 40 beats/min, especially with signs of decreased cardiac output, administer atropine (0.25 to 0.5 mg) i.v. If atropine treatment is unsuccessful, discontinue metoprolol and consider cautious administration of isoproterenol or installation of a cardiac pacemaker.
AV Conduction: Metoprolol slows AV conduction and may produce significant first- (PR interval ≥0.24 s), second-, or third-degree heart block. Acute myocardial infarction may also produce heart block. If heart block occurs, discontinue metoprolol and administer atropine (0.25 to 0.5 mg) i.v. If atropine treatment is unsuccessful, consider cautious administration of isoproterenol or installation of a cardiac pacemaker. Because of their negative effect on atrioventricular conduction, beta-blockers, including metoprolol, should only be given with caution to patients with first degree atrioventricular block.
Hypotension: If hypotension (systolic blood pressure ≤90 mm Hg) occurs, metoprolol should be discontinued, and the hemodynamic status of the patient and the extent of myocardial damage carefully assessed. Invasive monitoring of central venous, pulmonary capillary wedge, and arterial pressures may be required. Appropriate therapy with fluids, positive inotropic agents, balloon counterpulsation, or other treatment modalities should be instituted. If hypotension is associated with sinus bradycardia or AV block, treatment should be directed at reversing these (see above).

PRECAUTIONS: Bronchospastic Diseases: **In general, patients with bronchospastic diseases should not receive β-blockers, including metoprolol.** However, because of its relative β_1-selectivity, metoprolol may be used with caution in patients with asymptomatic bronchospastic disease who do not respond to, or cannot tolerate, other antihypertensive treatment. Since β_1-selectivity is not absolute, a β_2-stimulating agent should be administered concomitantly, and the lowest possible dose of metoprolol should be used. In these circumstances it would be prudent initially to administer metoprolol in smaller doses 3 times daily, instead of larger doses 2 times daily, to avoid the higher plasma levels associated with the longer dosing interval (see Dosage).

Because it is unknown to what extent β_2-stimulating agents may exacerbate myocardial ischemia and the extent of infarction, these agents should not be used prophylactically in patients with proven or suspected acute myocardial infarction. If bronchospasm not related to congestive heart failure occurs, metoprolol should be discontinued. A theophylline derivative or a β_2-agonist may be administered cautiously, depending on the clinical condition of the patient. Both theophylline derivatives and β_2-agonists may produce serious cardiac arrhythmias.
Diabetes and Hypoglycemia: Metoprolol should be administered cautiously to spontaneously hypoglycemic or diabetic patients (especially those with labile diabetes) who are receiving insulin or oral hypoglycemic agents. β-adrenergic receptor blockers, including metoprolol, may mask the premonitory signs and symptoms of acute hypoglycemia.
Liver Function: Metoprolol should be used with caution in patients with impaired liver function. Liver function tests should be performed at regular intervals during long-term treatment (see Pharmacology, Pharmacokinetics).
Allergen Immunotherapy: There may be increased difficulty in treating an allergic type reaction in patients on β-blockers. Whenever possible, β-blockers, including metoprolol, should be avoided in patients who are at risk of anaphylaxis. In these patients, the reaction may be more severe due to pharmacologic effects of the β-blockers and problems with fluid changes. Epinephrine should be administered with caution since it may not have its usual effects in the treatment of anaphylaxis. On the one hand, larger doses of epinephrine may be needed to overcome the bronchospasm, while on the other, these doses can be associated with excessive alpha-adrenergic stimulation with consequent hypertension, reflex bradycardia and heart block and possible potentiation of bronchospasm. Alternatives to the use of large doses of epinephrine include vigorous supportive care such as fluids and the use of β-agonists including parenteral salbutamol or isoproterenol, to overcome bronchospasm and norepinephrine to overcome hypotension.
Patients Undergoing Surgery: It is not advisable to withdraw β-adrenoceptor blocking drugs, including metoprolol, prior to surgery in the majority of patients especially in those with risk of overt or silent coronary heart disease. However, care should be taken to avoid using anesthetic agents that may depress the myocardium. Vagal dominance, if it occurs, may be corrected with atropine (1-2 mg i.v.).

Some patients receiving β-blocking drugs have been subject to protracted severe hypotension during anesthesia. Difficulty in restarting and maintaining the heartbeat has also been reported.

Since metoprolol is a competitive inhibitor of β-adrenoceptor agonists, its effects may be reversed, if necessary, by sufficient doses of such agonists as isoproterenol or dobutamine.
Peripheral Artery Disorders: Metoprolol may aggravate the symptoms of peripheral arterial circulatory disorders, mainly due to its blood pressure lowering effect.
Pheochromocytoma: Where a β-blocker is prescribed for a patient known to be suffering from a pheochromocytoma, an alpha-blocker should be given concomitantly.
Occupational Hazards: Reaction Time: β-blockers may adversely affect the patient's reaction time. Patients should be advised to avoid operating automobiles and machinery or engaging in other tasks requiring alertness until the patient's response to metoprolol therapy has been determined.
Pregnancy: Metoprolol crosses the placental barrier. Since metoprolol has not been studied in human pregnancy, the drug should not be given to pregnant women. The use of any drug in patients of child-bearing potential requires that the anticipated benefit be weighed against the possible hazards.
Lactation: Metoprolol is excreted in breast milk. If drug use is essential, patients should stop nursing.
Children: The safety and efficacy of metoprolol in children have not been established.
Geriatrics: Caution is indicated when using metoprolol in elderly patients. An excessively pronounced decrease in blood pressure or pulse rate may cause the blood supply to vital organs to fall to inadequate levels.
Drug Interactions: Antihypertensives: Metoprolol dosage should be adjusted to the individual requirements of the patient especially when used concomitantly with other antihypertensive agents (see Dosage).

The following medicinal products may increase the effect or plasma concentrations of metoprolol:
Calcium Channel Blockers: As with other β-blockers, metoprolol should not be given together with verapamil type calcium-antagonists. However, in exceptional cases, when the physician considers concomitant use essential, such use should be instituted gradually in a hospital setting under careful supervision. Negative inotropic, dromotropic and chronotropic effects may occur when metoprolol is given together with calcium antagonists. Verapamil and diltiazem reduce metoprolol clearance.
Antiarrhythmic Agents: β-blockers may enhance the negative inotropic and negative dromotropic effect of antiarrhythmic agents such as quinidine and amiodarone.
Nitroglycerin: Nitroglycerin may enhance the hypotensive effect of metoprolol.
Inhalation Anesthetics: β-blockers enhance the cardiodepression produced by certain anesthetics (see Precautions, Patients Undergoing Surgery).
MAO Inhibitors and Adrenergic Neuron-blockers: Closely monitor patients receiving MAO inhibitors or catecholamine-depleting drugs (such as reserpine or guanethidine). The added β-adrenergic-blockade of metoprolol may excessively reduce sympathetic activity. Metoprolol should not be combined with other β-blockers.
Prazosin (selective alpha-1-adrenergic antagonist): The acute postural hypotension that can follow the first dose of prazosin may be increased in patients already taking a beta-blocker.
CYP2D6 inhibitors: Potent inhibitors of this enzyme may increase the plasma concentration of metoprolol. Strong inhibition of CYP2D6 would result in the change of phenotype into poor metabolizer. Caution should therefore be exercised when co-administering potent CYP2D6 inhibitors with metoprolol. Known clinically significant potent inhibitors of CYP2D6 are antidepressants such as fluoxetine, paroxetine or bupropion, antipsychotics such as thioridazine, antiarrhythmics such as quinidine or propafenone, antiretrovirals such as ritonavir, antihistamines such as diphenhydramine, antimalarials such as hydroxychloroquine or quinine, antifungals such as terbinafine and medications for stomach ulcers such as cimetidine or ranitidine.

The following medicinal products may decrease the effect or plasma concentrations of metoprolol:
Digitalis Glycosides: Concurrent use of digitalis glycosides may result in excessive bradycardia and/or increase in atrioventricular conduction time.
α-Adrenergic Stimulants (cold remedies, nasal drops): Exaggerated hypertensive responses can be produced when β-blockers are combined with α-adrenergic agonists.
NSAIDs: Concurrent treatment with indomethacin may decrease the antihypertensive effect of β-blockers.
Hepatic Enzyme-Inducers: Hepatic enzyme-inducing substances may exert an influence on the plasma level of metoprolol. The plasma concentration of metoprolol is lowered by rifampicin.

Effect of metoprolol on other medicinal products:
Clonidine Withdrawal Syndrome: The hypertensive crisis which may follow clonidine withdrawal may be accentuated in the presence of β-blockade. Withdrawing the β-blocker several days before the clonidine may reduce the danger of rebound effects.
Oral Antidiabetics: The dosage of oral antidiabetics may have to be readjusted in patients receiving β-blockers (see Precautions).
Lidocaine: Metoprolol may reduce the clearance of lidocaine.
Alcohol: Metoprolol may modify the pharmacokinetics (decrease the elimination rate) of alcohol.

ADVERSE EFFECTS: The most common adverse events reported are exertional tiredness, gastrointestinal disorders, and disturbances of sleep patterns. The most serious adverse events reported are congestive heart failure, bronchospasm and hypotension.

Reported adverse effects according to organ systems are:
Cardiovascular: secondary effects of decreased cardiac output which include: syncope, vertigo, light-headedness and postural hypotension; second and third degree AV block (see Contraindications); congestive heart failure (see Warnings); severe bradycardia; lengthening of PR interval; sinus arrest; claudication; gangrene in patients with pre-existing severe peripheral circulatory disorders; precordial pain; hot flushes; edema; cold extremities; Raynaud's phenomenon; cardiac arrhythmias; palpitations; chest pains.

In a placebo-controlled study in patients with acute myocardial infarction the incidence of the following cardiovascular reactions were as shown in Table 1.

Table 1: Lopresor
Incidence of Cardiovascular Reactions

	Metoprolol %	Placebo %
Orthostatic hypotension (systolic BP <90 mmHg)	27.4	23.2
Bradycardia (heart rate <40 beats/min)	15.9	6.7
Second- or third-degree heart block	4.7	4.7
First-degree heart block (PR ≥0.24 s)	5.3	1.9
Heart failure	27.5	29.6

Central Nervous System: headache, dizziness, mental depression, light-headedness, vivid dreams/nightmares, vertigo, anxiety, alertness decreased, weakness, fatigue, sedation, somnolence or insomnia, hallucination, paresthesia, personality disorder.
Gastrointestinal: diarrhea, constipation, flatulence, nausea and vomiting, abdominal pain, heartburn, dry mouth, hepatitis.
Respiratory: shortness of breath, bronchospasm, status asthmaticus, exertional dyspnea, wheezing, rhinitis, worsening of psoriasis.
Allergic/Dermatological: (see Warnings): skin rash (exanthema, urticaria, psoriasiform and dystrophic skin lesions), hyperhydrosis, pruritus, photosensitivity.
Ear, Eye, Nose and Throat (EENT): tinnitus, dry and/or eye irritation, conjunctivitis, hearing disorders (e.g. hypoacusis or deafness) when doses exceed those recommended, blurred vision and nonspecific visual disturbances.
Miscellaneous: muscle cramps, exertional tiredness, weight increase, alopecia, decreased libido, Peyronie's disease, arthritis, retroperitoneal fibrosis.
Clinical Laboratory: The following laboratory parameters have been elevated on rare occasions: transaminases, BUN, alkaline phosphatase and bilirubin.
Hematology: Isolated cases of thrombocytopenia and leukopenia.
Post Marketing Experience: The following adverse reactions have been reported during post-approval use of metoprolol: confusional state, an increase in blood triglycerides and a decrease in High Density Lipoprotein (HDL). Because these reports are from a population of uncertain size and are subject to confounding factors, it is not possible to reliably estimate their frequency.

OVERDOSE:
Symptoms: The most common signs to be expected with overdosage of a β-adrenoreceptor agent are hypotension, bradycardia, congestive heart failure, bronchospasm and hypoglycemia. Atrioventricular block, cardiogenic shock and cardiac arrest may develop. In addition, impairment of consciousness (or even coma), nausea, vomiting and cyanosis may occur.

Concomitant ingestion of alcohol, antihypertensives, quinidine, or barbiturates aggravate the signs and symptoms.

The first manifestations of overdosage set in 20 minutes to 2 hours after drug administration.

Treatment: If overdosage occurs, in all cases therapy with metoprolol should be discontinued, the patient hospitalized and observed closely. Remove any drug remaining in the stomach by induction of emesis or gastric lavage. In addition, if required, the following therapeutic measures are suggested.
Bradycardia and Hypotension: Initially 1 to 2 mg of atropine sulfate should be given i.v. If a satisfactory effect is not achieved, norepinephrine or dopamine may be administered after preceding treatment with atropine. (See Precautions concerning the use of epinephrine in β-blocked patients.) In cases of hypoglycemia glucagon (1 to 10 mg) can be administered.
Heart block (second- or third-degree): Isoproterenol or transvenous cardiac pacemaker.

1. Congestive heart failure: Conventional therapy.
2. Bronchospasm: I.V. aminophylline or a β_2-agonist.
3. Hypoglycemia: I.V. glucose.

It should be remembered that metoprolol is a competitive antagonist of isoproterenol and hence large doses of isoproterenol can be expected to reverse many of the effects of excessive doses of metoprolol. However, the complications of excess isoproterenol, e.g. hypotension and tachycardia, should not be overlooked.

For management of a suspected drug overdose, CPhA recommends that you contact your **regional Poison Control Centre**. See the *CPS* Directory section for a list of Poison Control Centres.

DOSAGE: Hypertension: Metoprolol is usually used in conjunction with other antihypertensive agents, particularly a thiazide diuretic, but may be used alone (see Indications).

The dose must always be adjusted to the individual requirements of the patient, in accordance with the following guidelines.

Metoprolol treatment should be initiated with doses of 50 mg b.i.d. If an adequate response is not seen after 1 week, dosage should be increased to 100 mg b.i.d. In some cases the daily dosage may need to be increased by further 100 mg increments at intervals of not less than 2 weeks up to a maximum of 200 mg b.i.d., which should not be exceeded. The usual maintenance dose is within the range of 100 to 200 mg daily.

When metoprolol is combined with another antihypertensive agent which is already being administered, metoprolol should be added initially at a dose of 50 mg b.i.d. After 1 or 2 weeks the daily dosage may be increased if required, in increments of 100 mg, at intervals of not less than 2 weeks, until adequate blood pressure control is obtained.
Angina Pectoris: The recommended dosage range is 100 to 400 mg/day in divided doses. Initiate treatment with 50 mg b.i.d. for the first week. If response is not adequate, the daily dosage should be increased by 100 mg for the next week. The usual maintenance dose is 200 mg/day. The need for further increases should be closely monitored at weekly intervals and the dosage increased in 100 mg increments to a maximum of 400 mg/day in 2 or 3 divided doses. A metoprolol dose of 400 mg/day should not be exceeded.
Slow-release Lopresor SR Tablets: Treatment must always be initiated and individual titration of dosage carried out using the regular tablets. The SR formulation may be preferred for maintenance because of the convenience of once-daily administration. Lopresor SR tablets should be taken in the morning and swallowed whole.

Lopresor SR 100 mg is intended for maintenance dosing in those patients requiring 100 mg metoprolol/day.

Lopresor SR 200 mg is intended for maintenance dosing in those patients requiring doses of 200 mg/day.

Tablet Residue in Feces: After the active substance has diffused out of the insoluble core of the Lopresor SR Tablet, the tablet residue is excreted in a softened form and may be found in the feces.

Myocardial Infarction: **In addition to the usual contraindications: Only patients with suspected acute myocardial infarction who meet the following criteria are suitable for therapy as described below:** systolic blood pressure ≥100 mmHg; heart rate* ≥45 beats/minute; PR interval <0.24 seconds; rales*: <10 cm; adequate peripheral circulation.

Therapy should be discontinued in patients if the heart rate drops below 45 or the systolic blood pressure drops below 100 mmHg.

Early Treatment: During the early phase of definite or suspected acute myocardial infarction, treatment with metoprolol can be initiated as soon as possible after the patient's arrival in the hospital. Such treatment should be initiated in a coronary care or similar unit immediately after the patient's hemodynamic condition has stabilized.

Treatment in this early phase should begin with the i.v. administration of 3 bolus injections of 5 mg each. The injections should be given at approximately 2-minute intervals. During the i.v. administration, blood pressure, heart rate, and ECG should be carefully monitored. If any of the injections are associated with adverse cardiovascular effects, i.v. administration should be stopped immediately and the patient should be observed carefully and appropriate therapy instituted.

In patients who tolerate the full i.v. dose (15 mg), metoprolol tablets, 50 mg every 6 hours, should be initiated 15 minutes after the last i.v. dose and continued for 48 hours. Thereafter, patients should receive a maintenance dosage of 100 mg twice daily (see Late Treatment).

Patients who appear not to tolerate the full i.v. dose should be started on either 25 or 50 mg every 6 hours (depending on the degree of intolerance) 15 minutes after the last i.v. dose or as soon as their clinical condition allows. In patients with severe intolerance, treatment with metoprolol should be discontinued (see Warnings).

Late Treatment (for proven myocardial infarction patients only): Patients with contraindications to treatment during the early phase of myocardial infarction, patients who appear not to tolerate the full early treatment, and patients in whom the physician wishes to delay therapy for any other reason should be started on metoprolol tablets, 100 mg twice daily, as soon as their clinical condition allows. Treatment can begin within 3 to 10 days of the acute event. Therapy should be continued for at least 3 months. Although the efficacy of treatment beyond 6 months has not been conclusively established data from studies with other β-blockers suggest that the treatment should be continued for 1 to 3 years.

Note: Ampuls: Metoprolol ampuls are single dose ampuls intended for i.v. injection. All parenteral drug products should be inspected for particulate matter and discoloration prior to administration whenever solution and container permit. Discard any unused portion or solution with particulate matter or discoloration.

SUPPLIED: Ampuls: Each mL of aqueous, clear, injectable solution contains: metoprolol tartrate 1 mg. Also contains sodium chloride 9 mg. Alcohol-, bisulfite-, gluten-, lactose-, parabens- and tartrazine-free. Ampuls of 5 mL. Cartons of 5. Protect from heat (store between 2 to 30°C) and light.

Slow-release Tablets: 100 mg: Each round, film-coated, orange-brown tablet, embossed GEIGY on one side and KR/100 engraved on the other, contains: metoprolol tartrate 100 mg in a slow-release formulation. Nonmedicinal ingredients: carnauba wax, castor oil compounds, cellulose compounds, iron oxides, magnesium stearate, phosphates polysorbate, talc and titanium dioxide. Energy: 1.05 kJ (0.26 kcal). Alcohol-, bisulfite-, gluten-, lactose-, parabens-, sodium- and tartrazine-free. Bottles of 100 and 250. Protect from heat (store between 2 and 30°C), light and humidity.

200 mg: Each round, film-coated, light yellow tablet, embossed GEIGY on one side and CDC on the other, contains: metoprolol tartrate 200 mg in a slow-release formulation. Nonmedicinal ingredients: carnauba wax, castor oil compounds, cellulose compounds, iron oxides, magnesium stearate, phosphates polysorbate, talc and titanium dioxide. Energy: 1.05 kJ (0.26 kcal). Alcohol-, bisulfite-, gluten-, lactose-, parabens-, sodium- and tartrazine-free. Bottles of 100 and 250. Protect from heat (store between 2 and 30°C), light and humidity.

Tablets: 50 mg: Each light red, film-coated, capsule-shaped tablet embossed 51/51 and scored on one side and embossed GEIGY on the other, contains: metoprolol tartrate 50 mg. Nonmedicinal ingredients: carnauba wax, cellulose compounds, lactose, magnesium stearate, povidone, polyethylene glycol, silicon dioxide, sodium carboxymethyl starch and talc. Energy: 1.05 kJ (0.25 kcal). Sodium: <1 mmol (0.06 mg). Alcohol-, bisulfite-, gluten-, parabens- and tartrazine-free. Bottles of 100 and 500. Protect from heat (store between 2 and 30°C), light and humidity.

100 mg: Each light blue, film-coated, capsule-shaped tablet embossed 71/71 and scored on one side and embossed GEIGY on the other, contains: metoprolol tartrate 100 mg. Nonmedicinal ingredients: carnauba wax, cellulose compounds, lactose, magnesium stearate, povidone, polyethylene glycol, silicon dioxide, sodium carboxymethyl starch and talc. Energy: 1.05 kJ (0.25 kcal). Sodium: <1 mmol (0.12 mg). Alcohol-, bisulfite-, gluten-, parabens- and tartrazine-free. Bottles of 100. Protect from heat (store between 2 and 30°C), light and humidity.

(Shown in Product Identification Section)

* Extreme caution should be exercised when giving i.v. metoprolol to patients with heart rate between 45 and 60 and/or pulmonary rales less than 10 cm.

Loprox® Ⓟ

ciclopirox olamine

Topical Antifungal

sanofi-aventis

Date of Revision: November 6, 2007

PHARMACOLOGY: Ciclopirox is a synthetic broad spectrum antifungal agent that inhibits the growth of pathogenic dermatophytes, yeasts, and *M. furfur*. It exhibits fungicidal activity in vitro against isolates of *T. rubrum*, *T. mentagrophytes*, *E. floccosum*, *M. canis* and *C. albicans*.

The mode of action of ciclopirox olamine was studied mainly in *C. albicans*. It is presumed that ciclopirox mediated growth inhibition or death of fungal cells is primarily caused by in vitro cellular depletion of some essential substrates and/or ions and that such effects are brought about through blockage of their uptake from the medium.

No data on mechanism of action are available for dermatophytes.

Penetration studies in human cadaverous skin with tagged ciclopirox cream 1% showed the presence of 0.8 and 1.6% of the dose in stratum corneum 1.5 to 6 hours after application. The levels in the dermis were still 10 to 15 times above the minimum inhibitory concentrations.

Autoradiographic studies with human cadaverous skin showed that ciclopirox penetrates through the epidermis, hair follicles, into the dermis, hair and the sebaceous gland with a depot or reservoir in the stratum corneum.

Pharmacokinetic studies in males with tagged ciclopirox cream 1% showed an average of 1.3% absorption of the dose. The cream was applied topically under occlusion to the back, with a total penetration time of 6 hours. Excretion occurred via the kidney, with biological half-life of 1.7 hours. Two days after application only 0.01% of the dose applied could be found in the urine.

Draize Human Sensitization Assay, 21-Day Cumulative Irritancy study, Phototoxicity study and Photo-Draize study conducted in a total of 142 healthy male subjects showed no contact sensitization of the delayed hypersensitivity type, no irritation, no phototoxicity and no photo-contact sensitization due to ciclopirox olamine cream 1%. The ingredients of ciclopirox lotion 1% are qualitatively the same as those of ciclopirox cream 1%.

Microbiology: Ciclopirox can be best described as a broad spectrum antimycotic agent with significant antibacterial activity. It is also effective against several protozoa.

INDICATIONS: For the topical treatment of the following dermal infections: tinea pedis, tinea cruris and tinea corporis due to *T. rubrum*, *T. mentagrophytes*, *E. floccosum*, *M. canis*; cutaneous candidiasis (moniliasis) due to *C. albicans*; and tinea (pityriasis) versicolor due to *M. furfur*.

It is not proposed for vaginal application.

CONTRAINDICATIONS: In individuals who have shown hypersensitivity to any of the product components.

WARNINGS: Not for ophthalmic use.

PRECAUTIONS: If a reaction suggesting sensitivity or chemical irritation should occur with the use of ciclopirox, treatment should be discontinued and appropriate therapy instituted.

Pregnancy: Reproduction studies have been performed in the mouse, rat, rabbit and monkey (via various routes of administration) at doses 10 times or greater than the topical human dose. No significant evidence of impaired fertility or harm to the fetus due to the use of ciclopirox has been revealed. However, a higher incidence of systemic absorption of ciclopirox in the rat was noted in the group given 30 mg/kg orally as compared to controls. There are, however, no adequate or well-controlled studies in pregnant women. Because animal reproduction studies are not always predictive of human response, this drug should be used during pregnancy only if clearly needed.

Lactation: It is not known whether this drug is excreted in human milk. Because many drugs are excreted in human milk, caution should be exercised when ciclopirox is administered to nursing women.

Children: Safety and effectiveness in children below the age of 10 years have not been established.

ADVERSE EFFECTS: Ciclopirox is well tolerated with a low incidence of adverse reactions reported in clinical trials. Ciclopirox cream had a 0.4% incidence of adverse reactions in controlled clinical trials. These included pruritus at the site of application, worsening of clinical signs and symptoms and mild to severe burning reported in a few cases.

In a controlled clinical trial with 89 patients using ciclopirox lotion and 89 patients using the vehicle, the incidence of adverse reactions was low. The side effects included pruritus occurring in 3 patients and burning, which occurred in 1 patient.

OVERDOSE:

There have been no clinical reports of acute overdosage with ciclopirox cream or lotion by any route of administration.

From acute toxicity studies of ciclopirox cream 1% in adult rats, oral doses of 36 g/kg produced no evidence of toxic signs.

> For management of a suspected drug overdose, CPhA recommends that you contact your **regional Poison Control Centre**. See the *CPS* Directory section for a list of Poison Control Centres.

DOSAGE: Gently massage into the affected and surrounding skin areas twice daily, in the morning and evening, for a minimum of 4 weeks. Clinical improvement with relief of pruritus and other symptoms usually occurs within the first week of treatment. If a patient shows no clinical improvement after 2 weeks of treatment with ciclopirox the diagnosis should be redetermined. Patients with tinea versicolor usually exhibit clinical and mycological clearing after 2 weeks of treatment.

SUPPLIED: Cream: Each tube contains: ciclopirox olamine 1%. Nonmedicinal ingredients: benzyl alcohol, cetyl alcohol, cocamide DEA, lactic acid, mineral oil, myristyl alcohol, octyldodecanol, polysorbate 60, sorbitan monostearate and stearyl alcohol. Tubes of 45 g.

Lotion: Each bottle contains: ciclopirox olamine USP 1%. Nonmedicinal ingredients: benzyl alcohol, cetyl alcohol, cocamide DEA, lactic acid, mineral oil, myristyl alcohol, octyldodecanol, polysorbate 60, sorbitan monostearate and stearyl alcohol. Bottles of 60 mL.

Store at 15 to 30°C.

Lorazepam Ⓝ

CPhA Monograph

see *Benzodiazepines*

Lorazepam Injection USP Ⓣ

lorazepam

Anxiolytic—Sedative

Sandoz

SUPPLIED: Each mL of sterile solution for injection contains: lorazepam 4 mg. Nonmedicinal ingredients: benzyl alcohol, polyethylene glycol and propylene glycol. Multidose vials of 1 mL, boxes of 10. Store between 2 and 8°C. Do not use if solution is discoloured or contains a precipitate. Discard within 28 days of initial use. Protect from light. Protect from freezing.

Losec 1-2-3 A®

omeprazole magnesium—amoxicillin—clarithromycin

H. pylori Associated Peptic Ulcer Disease

AstraZeneca

Note: Regimen consists of omeprazole magnesium 20 mg, amoxicillin 1000 mg and clarithromycin 500 mg. All twice daily for 7 days. For further details on this triple therapy for treatment of *H. pylori* eradication, consult the Losec product monograph. For additional safety information on amoxicillin and clarithromycin, consult the product monographs.

Losec 1-2-3 M®

omeprazole magnesium—metronidazole—clarithromycin

H. pylori Associated Peptic Ulcer Disease

AstraZeneca

Note: Regimen consists of omeprazole magnesium 20 mg, metronidazole 500 mg and clarithromycin 250 mg. All twice daily for 7 days. For further details on this triple therapy for treatment of *H. pylori* eradication, consult the Losec product monograph. For additional safety information on metronidazole and clarithromycin, consult the product monographs.

Losec® Capsules Ⓟ

omeprazole

H+, K+-ATPase Inhibitor

AstraZeneca

Date of Preparation: October 24, 2000

Date of Revision: June 30, 2010

Note: When used in combination with amoxicillin, clarithromycin or metronidazole, the Product Monographs for those agents must be consulted and followed.

PHARMACOLOGY: LOSEC (omeprazole) inhibits the gastric enzyme H^+,K^+-ATPase (the proton pump) which catalyzes the exchange of H^+ and K^+. It is effective in the inhibition of both basal acid secretion and stimulated acid secretion. The inhibition is dose-dependent. Daily oral doses of omeprazole 20 mg and higher showed a consistent and effective acid control. A mean reduction of 24-hour intragastric acidity of approximately 80% was achieved during repeated dosing of 20 mg daily.

Treatment with LOSEC alone has been shown to suppress, but not eradicate *H. pylori*, a bacterium that is strongly associated with acid peptic disease. Approximately 90 to 100% of patients with duodenal ulcers, and 80% of patients with gastric ulcers, are infected with *H. pylori*. Clinical evidence indicates a synergistic effect between omeprazole and certain antibiotics in achieving eradication of *H. pylori*. Eradication of *H. pylori* is associated with symptom relief, healing of mucosal lesions, decreased rate of duodenal ulcer recurrence and long-term remission of peptic ulcer disease, reducing the need for prolonged antisecretory therapy.

There is no statistically significant change in the bioavailability (AUC, C_{max}) of amoxicillin during concomitant treatment with omeprazole in healthy volunteers.

There is an increase in the bioavailability (AUC) and half-life of omeprazole, and bioavailability (AUC) and C_{max} of clarithromycin, during concomitant administration in healthy volunteers.

There is no statistically significant change in the bioavailability (AUC,C_{max}) of metronidazole during concomitant treatment with omeprazole in healthy volunteers.

LOSEC is absorbed rapidly. After an initial oral dose of LOSEC, approximately 35% of the drug is absorbed from the gastrointestinal tract. Following one week of therapy the percentage absorbed is 43. Neither food nor antacids have any effect on the bioavailability. Peak plasma levels occur within about four hours.

The terminal plasma half-life is about 40 minutes. The antisecretory effect of omeprazole is directly proportional to the AUC; it is not dependent on the plasma concentration at any given time. Omeprazole is 95% bound to plasma proteins.

The 20 mg tablet and the 20 mg capsule are not bioequivalent in terms of plasma omeprazole AUC, C_{max} and t_{max}. LOSEC 20 mg tablets demonstrate, after repeated dosing, increased plasma omeprazole AUC (18%) and maximum concentration (41%) in comparison to omeprazole 20 mg given as capsules.

The omeprazole capsule (as a multiple unit formulation) is usually emptied gradually from the stomach into the intestine. In contrast to the capsule, the tablet (as a single unit formulation) will enter the intestine and dissolve as one unit. Consequently, the absorption and first pass metabolism of the tablet take place only during a very limited period. This may be one of the reasons for the difference observed in the pharmacokinetic variables of the two formulations.

LOSEC 20 mg tablets and LOSEC 20 mg capsules have an equivalent pharmacodynamic effect assessed by the inhibition of stimulated acid secretion and effect on 24-hour intragastric pH.

Omeprazole undergoes first-pass metabolism by the cytochrome P450 2C19 system, mainly in the liver. Following i.v. and oral administration, 80% of the dose is recovered as urinary metabolites. The remaining 20% is excreted in the feces.

INDICATIONS: LOSEC (omeprazole) is indicated in the treatment of conditions where a reduction of gastric acid secretion is required, such as:

- duodenal ulcer;
- gastric ulcer;
- NSAID-associated gastric and duodenal ulcers;
- reflux esophagitis;
- symptomatic gastroesophageal reflux disease (GERD), i.e., heartburn and regurgitation;
- Zollinger-Ellison syndrome (pathological hypersecretory condition);
- eradication of *H. pylori*.

LOSEC, in combination with clarithromycin and either amoxicillin or metronidazole, is indicated for the treatment of patients with peptic ulcer disease associated with *H. pylori* infection. The optimal timing for eradication therapy in patients whose ulcer is not clinically active (i.e., asymptomatic) remains to be determined.

Patients who fail to have their infection eradicated may be considered to have *H. pylori* resistant to the antimicrobials used in the eradication regimen. Therefore, therapy involving alternative effective antimicrobial agents should be considered (if re-treating).

It has been demonstrated that resistance to metronidazole is a negative predictive factor, decreasing the eradication rate of *H. pylori* obtained with triple therapy (omeprazole, metronidazole and clarithromycin) by 10-20%. The addition of omeprazole to metronidazole and clarithromycin appears to reduce the effect of primary resistance and the development of secondary resistance compared to antimicrobials alone. See Table 1 and Table 2.

Table 1: LOSEC Capsules

Results of Studies in Patients with a History of Duodenal Ulcer Who Were *H. pylori*-positive

		Eradication Rate	
	Treatment	**APT or ITT Analysis**	**PP Analysis**
Study 1	omeprazole 20 mg + amoxicillin 1000 mg + clarithromycin 500 mg, all twice daily for one week	96%	98%
	omeprazole 20 mg + metronidazole 400 mg[a] + clarithromycin 250 mg, all twice daily for one week	95%	94%
Study 2	omeprazole 20 mg + amoxicillin 1000 mg + clarithromycin 500 mg, all twice daily for one week	94%	95%
	omeprazole 20 mg + metronidazole 400 mg[a] + clarithromycin 250 mg, all twice daily for one week	87%	91%

[a] 500 mg metronidazole appears to be equivalent to 400 mg with regards to efficacy and safety.

Study 1: Patients included in the APT and PP analyses were assessed for *H. pylori* status by UBT pre- and post-treatment, n=684 (APT analysis).

Study 2: Patients included in the ITT and PP analyses were assessed for *H. pylori* status by UBT and culture pre- and post-treatment, n=514 (ITT analysis).

Table 2: LOSEC Capsules

Results of Studies in Patients With Active Peptic Ulcer Who Were *H. pylori*-positive (ITT analysis)

	Treatment	**Eradication Rate (PP analysis)**	**Ulcer Healing Rate (post-treatment)**	**Rate of Patients in Remission (6 months after cessation of therapy)**
Study 3	omeprazole 20 mg + amoxicillin 1000 mg + clarithromycin 500 mg, all twice daily for one week	78% (87%)	92%	88%
	omeprazole 20 mg + metronidazole 400 mg[a] + clarithromycin 250 mg, all twice daily for one week	85% (92%)	94%	92%
Study 4	omeprazole 20 mg + amoxicillin 1000 mg + clarithromycin 500 mg, all twice daily for one week	79% (83%)	94%	83%
	omeprazole 20 mg + metronidazole 400 mg[a] + clarithromycin 250 mg, all twice daily for one week	86% (93%)	96%	92%

[a] 500 mg metronidazole appears to be equivalent to 400 mg with regards to efficacy and safety.

Study 3: Patients with duodenal ulcer, included in the ITT analysis, were assessed for *H. pylori* status by UBT and histology pre- and post-treatment, n=146 (ITT analysis).

Study 4: Patients with gastric ulcer, included in the ITT analysis, were assessed for *H. pylori* status by UBT and histology pre- and post-treatment, n=145 (ITT analysis).

CONTRAINDICATIONS: Hypersensitivity to omeprazole or any of the components of this medication (see Supplied).

WARNINGS: When gastric ulcer is suspected, the possibility of malignancy should be excluded before therapy with LOSEC (omeprazole) is instituted, as treatment with LOSEC may alleviate symptoms and delay diagnosis.

Concomitant administration with atazanavir, nelfinavir or clopidogrel is not recommended (see Precautions, Drug Interactions).

Pregnancy: The safety of omeprazole in pregnancy has not been established. LOSEC should not be administered to pregnant women unless the expected benefits outweigh the potential risks.

Lactation: It is not known if omeprazole is secreted in human milk. LOSEC should not be given to nursing mothers unless its use is considered essential.

Children: The safety and effectiveness of LOSEC in children has not yet been established.

PRECAUTIONS: Geriatrics: Elderly subjects showed increased bioavailability (36%), reduced total plasma clearance (to 250 mL/min) and prolonged (50%) elimination half-life (to 1.0 hour). The daily dose in elderly patients should, as a rule, not exceed 20 mg (see Dosage).

Patients with Hepatic Insufficiency: Patients with impaired liver function showed a 75% increase in bioavailability, reduced total plasma clearance (to 67 mL/min), and a four-fold prolongation of the elimination half-life (to 2.8 hours). Twenty mg given once daily to these patients for four weeks was well tolerated, with no accumulation of omeprazole or its metabolites. The daily dose in patients with severe liver disease should, as a rule, not exceed 20 mg (see Dosage).

Patients with Renal Insufficiency: The disposition of intact omeprazole is unchanged in patients with impaired renal function and no dose adjustment is needed in these patients (see Dosage).

Carcinogenicity: The rat carcinogenicity study (24 months) revealed a gradual development from gastric ECL-cell hyperplasia to carcinoids at the end of their normal life span during administration with 14-140 mg/kg/day of omeprazole. No metastasis developed. No carcinoids developed during 18 months' high-dose treatment of mice (14-140 mg/kg/day). Similarly, administration of omeprazole up to 28 mg/kg/day in dogs for seven years did not cause any carcinoids.

The gastric carcinoids in rats were related to sustained hypergastrinemia secondary to acid inhibition and not to omeprazole per se. Similar observations have been made after administration of histamine H_2-receptor blockers and also in partially fundectomized rats.

Short- and long-term treatment in a limited number of patients for up to six years has not resulted in any significant pathological changes in gastric oxyntic endocrine cells.

Drug Interactions: The absorption of some drugs might be altered due to decreased intragastric acidity. Thus, it can be predicted that the absorption of ketoconazole and itraconazole will decrease during omeprazole treatment, as it does during treatment with other acid secretion inhibitors or antacids.

Omeprazole is metabolized by the cytochrome P450 system (CYP), mainly in the liver. The pharmacokinetics of the following drugs which are also metabolized through the cytochrome P450 system have been evaluated during concomitant use of omeprazole in humans: aminopyrine, antipyrine, clopidogrel, diazepam, phenytoin, warfarin (or other vitamin K antagonists), theophylline, voriconazole, propranolol, metoprolol, lidocaine, quinidine, ethanol, piroxicam, diclofenac and naproxen.

Aminopyrine and Antipyrine: After 14 days' administration of 60 mg omeprazole once daily, the clearance of aminopyrine was reduced by 19%; the clearance of antipyrine was reduced by 14%. After 14 days' administration of 30 mg once daily, no significant changes in clearance were noted.

Clopidogrel: Clopidogrel is metabolized to its active metabolite in part by CYP2C19. Co-administration of clopidogrel with omeprazole, an inhibitor of CYP2C19, reduces the pharmacological activity of clopidogrel given concomitantly or 12 hours apart. Concomitant use of drugs that inhibit the activity of this enzyme may result in reduced plasma concentrations of the active metabolite of clopidogrel and a reduction in platelet inhibition.

In a crossover clinical study, 72 healthy subjects were administered clopidogrel (300 mg loading dose followed by 75 mg/day) alone and with omeprazole (80 mg at the same time as clopidogrel) for 5 days. The exposure to the active metabolite of clopidogrel was decreased by 46% (Day 1) and 42% (Day 5) when clopidogrel and omeprazole were administered together. Mean inhibition of platelet aggregation (IPA) was diminished by 47% (24 hours) and 30% (Day 5) when clopidogrel and omeprazole were administered together. In another study 72 healthy subjects were given the same doses of clopidogrel and omeprazole but the drugs were administered 12 hours apart; the results were similar indicating that administering clopidogrel and omeprazole at different times does not prevent their interaction.

The pharmacological interaction between clopidogrel and omeprazole is related to partly shared metabolic pathways. Whether such an interaction translates into negative clinical outcomes is uncertain.

Diazepam, Warfarin and Phenytoin (or other vitamin K antagonists): As LOSEC is metabolized through cytochrome P450 2C19, it can alter the metabolism and prolong elimination of diazepam, warfarin (R-warfarin) and phenytoin.

Diazepam: Following repeated dosing with omeprazole 40 mg once daily, the clearance of diazepam was decreased by 54%. The corresponding decrease after omeprazole 20 mg was 26%.

Warfarin (or other vitamin K antagonists): Concomitant administration of omeprazole 20 mg in healthy subjects had no effect on plasma concentrations of the (S)-enantiomer of warfarin, but caused a slight, though statistically significant increase (12%) in the less potent (R)-enantiomer concentrations. A small but statistically significant increase (11%) in the anticoagulant effect of warfarin was also seen. In patients receiving warfarin or other vitamin K antagonists, monitoring of INR (International Normalised Ratio) is recommended and a reduction of the warfarin (or other vitamin K antagonist) dose may be necessary. Concomitant treatment with omeprazole 20 mg daily did not change coagulation time in patients on continuous treatment with warfarin.

Phenytoin: Following three weeks' treatment with omeprazole 20 mg once daily, the steady-state plasma levels of phenytoin in epileptic patients already receiving concomitant phenytoin treatment were not significantly affected. Urinary excretion of phenytoin and its main metabolite were also unchanged.

After single intravenous and oral doses of omeprazole 40 mg in young, healthy volunteers, the clearance of phenytoin was decreased by 15-20%, and half-life was prolonged by 20-30%. Following repeated dosing with omeprazole 40 mg once daily, the elimination half-life of phenytoin was increased by 27%. Thus, there appears to be a dose-dependent inhibition of elimination of phenytoin by omeprazole.

Patients receiving phenytoin and warfarin (or other vitamin K antagonists) should be monitored to determine if it is necessary to adjust the dosage of these drugs when taken concomitantly with omeprazole. Results from a range of interaction studies with LOSEC versus other drugs indicate that omeprazole, 20-40 mg given repeatedly, has no influence on any other clinically relevant isoforms of CYP, as shown by the lack of metabolic interaction with substrates for CYP 1A2 (caffeine, phenacetin, theophylline), CYP 2C9 (S-warfarin), CYP 2D6 (metoprolol, propranolol), CYP 2E1 (ethanol), and CYP 3A (cyclosporin, lidocaine, quinidine, estradiol).

Antiretroviral Drugs: Omeprazole, like other acid-reducing agents, has been reported to interact with some antiretroviral drugs. The clinical importance and the mechanisms behind these interactions are not always known. A change in gastric pH may change the absorption of the antiretroviral drug. Other possible interaction mechanisms are via CYP 2C19.

Reports indicate that omeprazole has a significant impact on atazanavir exposure, decreasing AUC, C_{max} and C_{min}. This interaction is only partially overcome by the addition of ritonavir to the atazanavir treatment regimen. Similarly, decreased serum levels of nelfinavir have also been reported when given together with omeprazole. Concomitant administration of omeprazole with atazanavir and nelfinavir is therefore not recommended. For other antiretroviral drugs, such as saquinavir, elevated serum levels have been reported. There are also some antiretroviral drugs where unchanged serum levels have been reported when given with omeprazole (see Warnings).

Tacrolimus: Although no clinical studies have been undertaken, there is a possibility that the concomitant administration of omeprazole and tacrolimus may increase serum levels of tacrolimus.

Theophylline: No effects on oral or i.v. theophylline kinetics have been observed after repeated once-daily doses of 40 mg omeprazole.

Voriconazole: Concomitant administration of omeprazole and a CYP 2C19 and CYP 3A4 inhibitor, voriconazole, resulted in more than doubling of the omeprazole exposure. However, a dose adjustment of omeprazole is not required.

Propranolol and Metoprolol: No effects on propranolol kinetics were observed in a steady-state trial with 20 mg of omeprazole daily. Similarly, no effects on steady state plasma levels of metoprolol were observed after concomitant treatment with 40 mg omeprazole daily.

Lidocaine: No interaction with a single intravenous dose of lidocaine or its active metabolite, MEGX, was found after one week of pretreatment with LOSEC 40 mg once daily. There were no interactions between omeprazole and lidocaine or MEGX concerning pharmacokinetic variables.

Quinidine: After one week of omeprazole 40 mg once daily, no effect was observed on the kinetics or pharmacodynamics of quinidine.

Ethanol: There was no significant effect on the pharmacokinetics of ethanol after omeprazole 20 mg.

Piroxicam, Diclofenac and Naproxen: There was no significant effect on the steady-state pharmacokinetics of piroxicam, diclofenac, and naproxen following repeated dosing with omeprazole 20 mg in healthy volunteers.

Antacids: No interaction with concomitantly administered antacids has been found.

Food: No interaction with food has been found.

Other Interactions: As demonstrated with other PPIs, prolonged use may impair the absorption of protein-bound Vitamin B_{12} and may contribute to the development of Vitamin B_{12} deficiency.

ADVERSE EFFECTS: Omeprazole is well tolerated. Most adverse reactions have been mild and transient and there has been no consistent relationship with the treatment. Adverse events have been recorded during controlled clinical investigations in 2764 patients exposed to omeprazole or reported from routine use. In a controlled clinical trial comparing omeprazole to placebo, the prevalence of adverse events with omeprazole 40 mg once daily was similar to the placebo group. In short-term, comparative, double-blind studies with histamine H_2-receptor antagonists, there was no significant difference in the prevalence of adverse events between omeprazole and the H_2-receptor antagonists. An extensive evaluation of laboratory variables has not revealed any significant changes during omeprazole treatment which are considered to be clinically important.

The following adverse events (at a rate of more than one percent) have been reported in individuals receiving omeprazole therapy in controlled clinical situations: diarrhea (2.8%); headache (2.6%); flatulence (2.3%); abdominal pain (1.7%); constipation (1.3%); and dizziness/vertigo (1.1%).

The following is a list of adverse events reported in clinical trials or reported from routine use. Events are classified within body system categories. The following definitions of frequencies are used: common: ≥1/100; uncommon: ≥1/1000 and <1/100; and rare: <1/1000.

Central and Peripheral Nervous System: Common: headache. Uncommon: dizziness, paraesthesia, somnolence, insomnia and vertigo. Rare: reversible mental confusion, agitation, aggression, depression and hallucinations, predominantly in severely ill patients.

Endocrine: Rare: gynaecomastia.

Gastrointestinal: Common: diarrhoea, constipation, abdominal pain, nausea/vomiting and flatulence. Rare: dry mouth, stomatitis and gastrointestinal candidiasis.

Hematologic: Rare: leukopenia, thrombocytopenia, agranulocytosis and pancytopenia.

Hepatic: Uncommon: increased liver enzyme levels. Rare: encephalopathy in patients with pre-existing severe liver disease; hepatitis with or without jaundice and hepatic failure.

Musculoskeletal: Rare: arthralgia, muscular weakness and myalgia.

Skin: Uncommon: rash, dermatitis and/or pruritus, and urticaria. Rare: photosensitivity, erythema multiforme, Stevens-Johnson syndrome, toxic epidermal necrolysis (TEN) and alopecia.

Other: Uncommon: malaise, hypersensitive reactions including urticaria. Rare: hypersensitive reactions including angioedema, fever, bronchospasm, interstitial nephritis and anaphylactic shock; increased sweating, peripheral edema, blurred vision, taste disturbances and hyponatraemia.

H. pylori Eradication Combination Therapy: The following adverse events (at a rate of more than 1%) were recorded during controlled clinical trials in 493 patients receiving omeprazole, amoxicillin and clarithromycin: diarrhea (28%), taste disturbances (15%), headache (5%), flatulence (4%), nausea (3%), abdominal pain (2%), ALT increased (1%), epigastric pain (1%), pharyngitis (1%) and glossitis (1%).

The following adverse events (at a rate of more than 1%) were recorded during controlled clinical trials in 494 patients receiving omeprazole, metronidazole and clarithromycin: taste disturbances (14%), diarrhea (13%), headache (6%), ALT increased (6%), flatulence (5%), nausea (5%), AST increased (5%), dyspepsia (3%), dry mouth (2%), dizziness/vertigo (2%), epigastric pain (1%), pharyngitis (1%), eructation (1%) and fatigue (1%).

OVERDOSE:

Symptoms: No information is available on the effects of higher doses in man and specific recommendations for treatment cannot be given. Single oral doses of up to 400 mg of omeprazole have not resulted in any severe symptoms and no specific treatment has been needed. As in all cases where overdosing is suspected, treatment should be supportive and symptomatic. Any unabsorbed material should be removed from the gastrointestinal tract, and the patient should be carefully monitored.

The oral LD_{50} of omeprazole in male and female rats and mice was greater than 4000 mg/kg. In dogs, the only sign of acute toxicity was vomiting which occurred at doses of approximately 600 mg/kg.

When used in combination with antibiotics, the Prescribing Information/Product Monograph for those antibiotics should be consulted.

Treatment: See Symptoms.

> For management of a suspected drug overdose, contact your regional Poison Control Centre. See the *CPS* Directory section for a list of Poison Control Centres.

DOSAGE: Duodenal Ulcer: Acute Therapy: The recommended adult oral dose is 20 mg given once daily. Healing usually occurs within two weeks. For patients not healed after this initial course of therapy, an additional two weeks of treatment is recommended.

Refractory Patients: In patients with duodenal ulcer refractory to other treatment regimens, the recommended adult doses are 20 mg or 40 mg given once daily. Healing is usually achieved within four weeks in such patients.

Maintenance Therapy for Duodenal Ulcer: Over 95% of duodenal ulcer patients are *H. pylori*-positive, and should be treated with eradication therapy, as described below. A small percentage of patients who are *H. pylori*-negative will experience a disease recurrence and will require maintenance treatment with an antisecretory agent. The recommended LOSEC (omeprazole) dose is 10 mg once daily, increased to 20-40 mg once daily, as necessary.

Gastric Ulcer: Acute Therapy: The recommended adult dose is 20 mg given once daily. Healing usually occurs within four weeks. For patients not healed after this initial course of therapy, an additional four weeks of treatment is recommended.

Refractory Patients: In patients with gastric ulcer refractory to other treatment regimens, the recommended dose is 40 mg given once daily. Healing is usually achieved within eight weeks.

Maintenance Therapy for Gastric Ulcer: About 80% of gastric ulcer patients are *H. pylori*-positive, and should be treated with eradication therapy, as described below. A small percentage of patients who are *H. pylori*-negative will experience a disease recurrence and will require maintenance treatment with an antisecretory agent. The recommended LOSEC dose is 20 mg once daily, increased to 40 mg once daily, as necessary.

NSAID-Associated Gastric or Duodenal Ulcers: The issue of whether or not eradication of *H. pylori* in patients with NSAID-associated ulcers might have beneficial preventive effects has not yet been settled.

Acute Therapy: In patients with NSAID-associated gastric or duodenal ulcers, the recommended adult dose is 20 mg given once daily. Symptom resolution is rapid and healing usually occurs within four weeks. For those patients not healed after this initial course of therapy, an additional four weeks of treatment is recommended.

Maintenance Therapy: For the prevention of relapse in patients with NSAID-associated gastric or duodenal ulcers, the recommended adult dose is 20 mg given once daily, for up to six months.

H. pylori-Associated Peptic Ulcer Disease: Omeprazole, Amoxicillin and Clarithromycin Triple Therapy: The recommended dose for eradication of *H. pylori* is LOSEC 20 mg, amoxicillin 1000 mg and clarithromycin 500 mg, all twice daily for seven days. This dosing regimen can be known as Losec 1-2-3 A.

Omeprazole, Metronidazole and Clarithromycin Triple Therapy: The recommended dose for eradication of *H. pylori* is LOSEC 20 mg, metronidazole 500 mg and clarithromycin 250 mg, all twice daily for seven days. This dosing regimen can be known as Losec 1-2-3 M.

To ensure healing and/or symptom control, further treatment with 20 mg LOSEC once daily for up to three weeks is recommended for patients with active duodenal ulcer, and with 20-40 mg LOSEC once daily for up to 12 weeks for patients with active gastric ulcer.

Patient compliance with treatment regimens for the eradication of *H. pylori* has been demonstrated to have a positive effect on eradication outcome. In clinical trials, patients treated with triple-therapy regimens have shown high compliance rates.

Susceptibility testing (MIC values derived from the Agar dilution method) of *H. pylori* to metronidazole and clarithromycin is available for 486 primary isolates from patients with a history of duodenal ulcer in one European study.

Resistance to metronidazole (MIC >8 mg/L) was detected in 131 strains (27%), while nine strains (2%) were resistant to clarithromycin (MIC >1 mg/L). Secondary resistance to metronidazole developed in strains from four patients treated with omeprazole/metronidazole/clarithromyin. Similarly, in those patients treated with omeprazole/metronidazole/clarithromycin or omeprazole/amoxicillin/clarithromycin combinations, secondary resistance to clarithromycin developed in strains from four patients. For amoxicillin, the MIC values at pre- or post-therapy did not indicate any primary, or the development of secondary, resistance of *H. pylori*.

Reflux Esophagitis: Acute Therapy: The recommended adult dose is 20 mg given once daily. In most patients, healing occurs within four weeks. For patients not healed after this initial course of therapy, an additional four weeks of treatment is recommended.

* A working definition of dyspepsia would include the presence of epigastric pain/discomfort, with or without heartburn and regurgitation which may be accompanied by nausea, vomiting, bloating, belching, flatulence, early satiety or postprandial fullness. Symptoms may occur either during the day or throughout the night.

Refractory Patients: For patients with reflux esophagitis refractory to other treatment regimens, the recommended dose is 40 mg given once daily. Healing is usually achieved within eight weeks.

Maintenance Therapy for Reflux Esophagitis: For the long-term management of patients with healed reflux esophagitis, 10 mg omeprazole once daily has been found to be effective in controlled clinical trials of 12 months' duration, and in continuous maintenance treatment in a limited number of patients for a period of up to six years. In the case of recurrence, the dose can be increased to 20-40 mg omeprazole.

Symptomatic Gastroesophageal Reflux Disease (i.e., Heartburn and Regurgitation): The recommended adult dose is 20 mg given once daily. Symptom relief should be rapid. If symptom control is not achieved after four weeks, further investigation is recommended. Since some patients respond adequately to 10 mg given once daily, individual dose adjustment should be considered. For the maintenance of symptom relief in patients with gastroesophageal reflux disease (i.e., heartburn and regurgitation), the recommended adult dose is 10 mg given once daily.

Zollinger-Ellison Syndrome: The dose used in the treatment of Zollinger-Ellison Syndrome will vary with the individual patient.

The recommended initial dose is 60 mg, given once daily. More than 90% of the patients with the severe form of the disease and inadequate response to other therapies have been adequately controlled with doses of 20 mg to 120 mg daily. With doses greater than 80 mg, the dose should be divided and given twice daily. Doses should be adjusted to the individual patient's need and should continue as long as clinically indicated. Doses up to 120 mg t.i.d. have been administered.

Patients with Renal Insufficiency: No dose adjustment is required (see Precautions).

Patients with Hepatic Insufficiency: No dose adjustment is required. The daily dose should not exceed 20 mg (see Precautions).

Geriatrics: No dose adjustment is required. The daily dose should not exceed 20 mg (see Precautions).

The capsules should be swallowed whole with sufficient water.

Stability and Storage Recommendations: LOSEC (omeprazole) capsules are moisture sensitive and are therefore provided in a package suitable for direct distribution to the patient.

Patients should be advised to keep the bottle tightly capped and to store it in a dry place. Store at controlled room temperature (15-30°C), protected from moisture.

INFORMATION FOR THE PATIENT: Published in e-CPS, available by subscription at www.e-cps.ca.

SUPPLIED: 10 mg: Each two-piece hard gelatin delayed release capsule with an opaque pink body and an opaque pink cap, the body printed "10", and the cap A/OS, in black ink, contains: omeprazole 10 mg. Nonmedicinal ingredients: disodium hydrogen phosphate dihydrate, gelatin, hydroxypropyl cellulose, hydroxypropyl methylcellulose, iron oxide, lactose anhydrous, magnesium stearate, mannitol, methacrylic acid copolymer, microcrystalline cellulose, polyethylene glycol, sodium lauryl sulfate and titanium dioxide. High-density polyethylene bottles of 30 with a child-resistant screw cap which contains a desiccant. Dispense in the original container.

20 mg: Each two-piece hard gelatin delayed release capsule with an opaque pink body and an opaque reddish-brown cap, the body printed "20", and the cap A/OM, in black ink, contains: omeprazole 20 mg. Nonmedicinal ingredients: disodium hydrogen phosphate dihydrate, gelatin, hydroxypropyl cellulose, hydroxypropyl methylcellulose, iron oxide, lactose anhydrous, magnesium stearate, mannitol, methacrylic acid copolymer, microcrystalline cellulose, polyethylene glycol, sodium lauryl sulfate and titanium dioxide. High-density polyethylene bottles of 30 with a child-resistant screw cap which contains a desiccant. Dispense in the original container.

(Shown in Product Identification Section)

Losec® Tablets 🄿

omeprazole magnesium

H+, K+-ATPase Inhibitor

AstraZeneca

Date of Preparation: February 3, 2000
Date of Revision: April 30, 2010

Note: When used in combination with amoxicillin, clarithromycin or metronidazole, the product monographs for those agents must be consulted and followed.

PHARMACOLOGY: Omeprazole inhibits the gastric enzyme H^+, K^+-ATPase (the proton pump) which catalyzes the exchange of H^+ and K^+. It is effective in the inhibition of both basal acid secretion and stimulated acid secretion. The inhibition is dose-dependent. Daily oral doses of 20 mg and higher, showed a consistent and effective acid control. Information from clinical trials in patients with duodenal ulcers in remission indicate that omeprazole magnesium 20 mg tablets demonstrate the same inhibition of stimulated acid secretion and similar effect on 24-hour intragastric pH as omeprazole 20 mg capsules. The mean decrease in peak acid output after pentagastrin stimulation was approximately 70%, after 5 days of dosing with omeprazole magnesium 20 mg tablet once daily.

The 20 mg tablet and the 20 mg capsule are not bioequivalent in terms of plasma omeprazole AUC, C_{max} and t_{max}. Omeprazole magnesium 20 mg tablets demonstrate, after repeated dosing, increased plasma omeprazole AUC (18%) and maximum concentration (41%) in comparison to omeprazole 20 mg given as capsules.

The omeprazole capsule (as a multiple unit formulation) is usually emptied gradually from the stomach into the intestine. In contrast to the capsule, the tablet (as a single unit formulation) will enter the intestine and dissolve as one unit. Consequently, the absorption and first pass metabolism of the tablet take place only during a very limited period. This may be one of the reasons for the difference observed in the pharmacokinetic variables of the two formulations.

Omeprazole magnesium tablets are absorbed rapidly. Food has no effect on the bioavailability of the tablet. Peak plasma levels occur on average within 2 hours.

Omeprazole magnesium 20 mg tablets and omeprazole 20 mg capsules have an equivalent effect on the inhibition of stimulated acid secretion and on 24-hour intragastric pH. These data support the conclusion that the 20 mg tablet and capsule can be used with equivalent efficacy in the treatment of conditions where a reduction of gastric acid secretion is required.

The equivalence of two 10 mg omeprazole magnesium tablets to one 20 mg omeprazole magnesium tablet has been demonstrated by a bioequivalence study in healthy volunteers.

The antisecretory effect of omeprazole is directly proportional to the AUC; it is not dependent on the plasma concentration at any given time. Omeprazole is 95% bound to plasma proteins.

Treatment with omeprazole alone has been shown to suppress, but not eradicate *H. pylori*, a bacterium that is strongly associated with acid peptic disease. Approximately 90 to 100% of patients with duodenal ulcers, and 80% of patients with gastric ulcer, are infected with *H. pylori*. Clinical evidence indicates a synergistic effect between omeprazole and certain antibiotics in achieving eradication of *H. pylori*. Eradication of *H. pylori* is associated with symptom relief, healing of mucosal lesions, decreased rate of duodenal ulcer recurrence and long-term remission of peptic ulcer disease, and reducing the need for prolonged anti-secretory therapy.

There is no statistically significant change in the bioavailability (AUC, C_{max}) of amoxicillin during concomitant treatment with omeprazole, in healthy volunteers.

There is an increase in the bioavailability (AUC) and half-life of omeprazole, and bioavailability (AUC) and C_{max} of clarithromycin, during concomitant administration, in healthy volunteers.

There is no statistically significant change in the bioavailability (AUC, C_{max}) of metronidazole during concomitant treatment with omeprazole, in healthy volunteers.

Omeprazole undergoes first-pass metabolism by the cytochrome P450 2C19 system, mainly in the liver. Following i.v. administration and oral administration (capsules) of omeprazole, 80% of the dose is recovered as urinary metabolites. The remaining 20% is excreted in the feces.

INDICATIONS: In the treatment of conditions where a reduction of gastric acid secretion is required, such as: duodenal ulcer; gastric ulcer; NSAID-associated gastric and duodenal ulcers; reflux esophagitis; symptomatic gastroesophageal reflux disease (GERD), i.e., heartburn and regurgitation; dyspepsia*: a complex of symptoms which may be caused by any of the organic diseases listed above, or upon investigation no identifiable organic cause is found (i.e., functional dyspepsia); Zollinger-Ellison syndrome (pathological hypersecretory condition); eradication of *H. pylori*.

Omeprazole, in combination with clarithromycin and either amoxicillin or metronidazole, is indicated for the treatment of patients with peptic ulcer disease associated with *H. pylori* infection. The optimal timing for eradication therapy in patients whose ulcer is not clinically active (i.e., asymptomatic) remains to be determined.

The issue of whether or not eradication of *H. pylori* in patients with NSAID-associated ulcers might have beneficial preventive effects has not yet been settled.

In dyspeptic patients with an *H. pylori* infection, the concurrent gastritis can be healed with appropriate eradication therapy.

CONTRAINDICATIONS: Hypersensitivity to omeprazole or any of the components of this medication (see Supplied).

WARNINGS: In the presence of any alarm symptom (e.g., significant unintentional weight loss, recurrent vomiting, dysphagia, haematemesis or melena) and when gastric ulcer is suspected or present, malignancy should be excluded, as treatment may alleviate symptoms and delay diagnosis.

Concomitant administration with atazanavir, nelfinavir or clopidogrel is not recommended (see Precautions, Drug Interactions).

Pregnancy: The safety in pregnancy has not been established. Omeprazole should not be administered to pregnant women unless the expected benefits outweigh the potential risks.

Lactation: It is not known if omeprazole is secreted in human milk. It should not be given to nursing mothers unless its use is considered essential.

Children: The safety and effectiveness of omeprazole in children have not yet been established.

PRECAUTIONS: Geriatrics: Elderly subjects showed increased bioavailability (36%), reduced total plasma clearance (to 250 mL/min) and prolonged (50%) elimination half-life (to 1.0 hour) (data obtained from studies with i.v. administration of omeprazole and oral administration of omeprazole capsules). The daily dose in elderly patients should, as a rule, not exceed 20 mg (see Dosage).

Hepatic Insufficiency: Patients with impaired liver function showed a 75% increase in bioavailability, reduced total plasma clearance (to 67 mL/min), and a 4-fold prolongation of the elimination half-life (to 2.8 hours) (data obtained from studies with i.v. administration of omeprazole and oral administration of omeprazole capsules). A dose of 20 mg omeprazole capsules given once daily to these patients for 4 weeks was well tolerated, with no accumulation of omeprazole or its metabolites. The daily dose in patients with severe liver disease should, as a rule, not exceed 20 mg (see Dosage).

Renal Insufficiency: The disposition of intact omeprazole is unchanged in patients with impaired renal function and no dose adjustment is needed in these patients (data obtained from studies with i.v. administration of omeprazole and oral administration of omeprazole capsules) (see Dosage).

Information on the bioavailability of the omeprazole magnesium 20 mg tablet in elderly patients, in patients with hepatic insufficiency, and in patients with renal insufficiency, as well as information on drug interactions are not currently available.

Carcinogenicity: The rat carcinogenicity study (24 months) revealed a gradual development from gastric ECL-cell hyperplasia to carcinoids at the end of their normal life span during administration with 14 to 140 mg/kg/day of omeprazole. No metastasis developed. No carcinoids developed during 18 months' high-dose treatment of mice (14 to 140 mg/kg/day). Similarly, administration of omeprazole up to 28 mg/kg/day in dogs for 7 years did not cause any carcinoids.

The gastric carcinoids in rats were related to sustained hypergastrinemia secondary to acid inhibition and not to omeprazole per se. Similar observations have been made after administration of histamine H_2-receptor blockers and also in partially fundectomized rats.

Short-term treatment and long-term treatment with omeprazole capsules in a limited number of patients for up to 6 years have not resulted in any significant pathological changes in gastric oxyntic endocrine cells.

Drug Interactions: The absorption of some drugs might be altered due to the decreased intragastric acidity. Thus, it can be predicted that the absorption of ketoconazole and itraconazole will decrease during omeprazole treatment, as it does during treatment with other acid secretion inhibitors or antacids.

Omeprazole is metabolized by the cytochrome P450 system (CYP), mainly in the liver. The pharmacokinetics of the following drugs, which are also metabolized through the cytochrome P450 system, have been evaluated during concomitant use of omeprazole capsules in humans: aminopyrine, antipyrine, clopidogrel, diazepam, phenytoin, warfarin (or other vitamin K antagonists), theophylline, voriconazole, propranolol, metoprolol, lidocaine, quinidine, ethanol, piroxicam, diclofenac and naproxen.

Aminopyrine and Antipyrine: After 14 days' administration of 60 mg omeprazole once daily, the clearance of aminopyrine was reduced by 19%; the clearance of antipyrine was reduced by 14%. After 14 days' administration of 30 mg once daily, no significant changes in clearance were noted.

Clopidogrel: Clopidogrel is metabolized to its active metabolite in part by CYP2C19. Co-administration of clopidogrel with omeprazole, an inhibitor of CYP2C19, reduces the pharmacological activity of clopidogrel given concomitantly or 12 hours apart. Concomitant use of drugs that inhibit the activity of this enzyme may result in reduced plasma concentrations of the active metabolite of clopidogrel and a reduction in platelet inhibition.

In a crossover clinical study, 72 healthy subjects were administered clopidogrel (300 mg loading dose followed by 75 mg/day) alone and with omeprazole (80 mg at the same time as clopidogrel) for 5 days. The exposure to the active metabolite of clopidogrel was decreased by 46% (Day 1) and 42% (Day 5) when clopidogrel and omeprazole were administered together. Mean inhibition of platelet aggregation (IPA) was diminished by 47% (24 hours) and 30% (Day 5) when clopidogrel and omeprazole were administered together. In another study 72 healthy subjects were given the same doses of clopidogrel and omeprazole but the drugs were administered 12 hours apart; the results were similar indicating that administering clopidogrel and omeprazole at different times does not prevent their interaction.

The pharmacological interaction between clopidogrel and omeprazole is related to partly shared metabolic pathways. Whether such an interaction translates into negative clinical outcomes is uncertain.

Diazepam, Phenytoin and Warfarin (or other vitamin K antagonists): As omeprazole is metabolized through cytochrome P450 2C19, it can alter the metabolism and prolong elimination of diazepam, warfarin (R-warfarin) and phenytoin.

Diazepam: Following repeated dosing with omeprazole 40 mg once daily, the clearance of diazepam was decreased by 54%. The corresponding decrease after omeprazole 20 mg was 26%.

Warfarin (or other vitamin K antagonists): Concomitant administration of omeprazole 20 mg in healthy subjects had no effect on plasma concentrations of the (S)-enantiomer of warfarin, but caused a slight, though statistically significant increase (12%) in the less potent (R)-enantiomer concentrations. A small but statistically significant increase (11%) in the anticoagulant effect of warfarin was also seen. In patients receiving warfarin or other vitamin K antagonists, monitoring of INR (International Normalised Ratio) is recommended and a reduction of the warfarin (or other vitamin K antagonist) dose may be necessary. Concomitant treatment with omeprazole 20 mg daily did not change coagulation time in patients on continuous treatment with warfarin.

Phenytoin: Following 3 weeks' treatment with omeprazole 20 mg once daily, the steady-state plasma levels of phenytoin in epileptic patients already receiving concomitant phenytoin treatment were not significantly affected. Urinary excretion of phenytoin and its main metabolite were also unchanged.

After single i.v. and oral doses of omeprazole capsules 40 mg in young, healthy volunteers, the clearance of phenytoin was decreased by 15 to 20%, and half-life was prolonged by 20 to 30%. Following repeated dosing with omeprazole 40 mg once daily, the elimination half-life of phenytoin was increased by 27%. Thus, there appears to be a dose-dependent inhibition of elimination of phenytoin by omeprazole.

Patients receiving phenytoin and warfarin (or other vitamin K antagonists) should be monitored to determine if it is necessary to adjust the dosage of these drugs when taken concomitantly with omeprazole.

Results from a range of interaction studies with omeprazole versus other drugs indicate that omeprazole, 20 to 40 mg given repeatedly, has no influence on other clinically relevant isoforms of CYP, as shown by the lack of metabolic interaction with substrates for CYP 1A2 (caffeine, phenacetin, theophylline), CYP 2C9 (S-warfarin), CYP 2D6 (metoprolol, propranolol), CYP 2E1 (ethanol), and CYP 3A (cyclosporin, lidocaine, quinidine, estradiol).

Antiretroviral Drugs: Omeprazole, like other acid-reducing agents, has been reported to interact with some antiretroviral drugs. The clinical importance and the mechanisms behind these interactions are not always known. A change in gastric pH may change the absorption of the antiretroviral drug. Other possible interaction mechanisms are via CYP 2C19.

Reports indicate that omeprazole has a significant impact on atazanavir exposure, decreasing AUC, C_{max} and C_{min}. This interaction is only partially overcome by the addition of ritonavir to the atazanavir treatment regimen. Similarly, decreased serum levels of nelfinavir have also been reported when given together with omeprazole. Concomitant administration of omeprazole with atazanavir and nelfinavir is therefore not recommended. For other antiretroviral drugs, such as saquinavir, elevated serum levels have been reported. There are also some antiretroviral drugs where unchanged serum levels have been reported when given with omeprazole (see Warnings).

Tacrolimus: Although no clinical studies have been undertaken, there is a possibility that the concomitant administration of omeprazole and tacrolimus may increase serum levels of tacrolimus.

Theophylline: No effects on oral or i.v. theophylline kinetics have been observed after repeated once daily doses of 40 mg omeprazole.

Voriconazole: Concomitant administration of omeprazole and a CYP 2C19 and CYP 3A4 inhibitor, voriconazole, resulted in more than doubling of the omeprazole exposure. However, a dose adjustment of omeprazole is not required.

Propranolol and Metoprolol: No effects on propranolol kinetics were observed in a steady-state trial with 20 mg of omeprazole daily. Similarly, no effects on steady-state plasma levels of metoprolol were observed after concomitant treatment with 40 mg omeprazole daily.

Lidocaine: No interaction with a single i.v. dose of lidocaine or its active metabolite, MEGX, was found after 1 week's pre-treatment with omeprazole 40 mg once daily. There were no interactions between omeprazole and lidocaine or MEGX concerning pharmacokinetic variables.

Quinidine: After 1 week of omeprazole 40 mg once daily, no effect was observed on the kinetics or pharmacodynamics of quinidine.

Ethanol: There was no significant effect on the pharmacokinetics of ethanol after omeprazole 20 mg.

Piroxicam, Diclofenac and Naproxen: There was no significant effect on the steady-state pharmacokinetics of piroxicam, diclofenac, and naproxen following repeated dosing with omeprazole 20 mg, in healthy volunteers.

Antacids: No interaction with antacids administered concomitantly with omeprazole (given as capsules) has been found.

Food: No interaction with food after repeated dosing of omeprazole tablets has been found.

Other Interactions: As demonstrated with other PPIs, prolonged use may impair the absorption of protein-bound Vitamin B_{12} and may contribute to the development of Vitamin B_{12} deficiency.

ADVERSE EFFECTS: Omeprazole is well tolerated. Most adverse reactions have been mild and transient, and have shown no consistent relationship with treatment. Adverse events have been recorded during controlled clinical investigations in 2764 patients exposed to omeprazole (data taken from controlled clinical studies with omeprazole capsules) or reported from routine use. In a controlled clinical trial comparing omeprazole to placebo, the prevalence of adverse events with omeprazole 40 mg once daily was similar to that with placebo. In short-term comparative double-blind studies with histamine H_2-receptor antagonists, there was no significant difference in the prevalence of adverse events between omeprazole capsules and the H_2-receptor antagonists. An extensive evaluation of laboratory variables has not revealed any significant changes during omeprazole treatment which are considered to be clinically important.

The following adverse events (at a rate of more than 1%) have been reported in individuals receiving omeprazole capsules in controlled clinical situations: diarrhea (2.8%); headache (2.6%); flatulence (2.3%); abdominal pain (1.7%); constipation (1.3%); and dizziness/vertigo (1.1%).

The following is a list of adverse events reported in clinical trials or reported from routine use. Events are classified within body system categories. The following definitions of frequencies are used: common: ≥1/100; uncommon: ≥1/1000 and <1/100; and rare: <1/1000.

Central and Peripheral Nervous System: Common: headache. Uncommon: dizziness, paresthesia, somnolence, insomnia and vertigo. Rare: reversible mental confusion, agitation, aggression, depression and hallucination occurring predominantly in severely ill patients.

Endocrine: Rare: gynaecomastia.

Gastrointestinal: Common: diarrhoea, constipation, abdominal pain, nausea/vomiting and flatulence. Rare: dry mouth, stomatitis and gastrointestinal candidiasis.

Hematologic: Rare: leukopenia, thrombocytopenia, agranulocytosis and pancytopenia.

Hepatic: Uncommon: increased liver enzyme levels. Rare: encephalopathy in patients with pre-existing severe liver disease; hepatitis with or without jaundice and hepatic failure.

Musculoskeletal: Rare: arthralgia, muscular weakness and myalgia.

Skin: Uncommon: rash, dermatitis and/or pruritus, and uticaria. Rare: photosensitivity, erythema multiforme, Stevens-Johnsons syndrome, toxic epidermal necrolysis (TEN) and alopecia.

Other Adverse Events: Uncommon: malaise, hypersensitive reactions including urticaria Rare: hypersensitive reactions including angioedema, fever, bronchospasm and interstitial nephritis and anaphylactic shock; increased sweating, peripheral edema, blurred vision, taste disturbances and hyponatraemia.

H. pylori Eradication Combination Therapy: The following adverse events (at a rate of more than 1%), were recorded during controlled clinical trials in 493 patients receiving omeprazole, amoxicillin and clarithromycin: diarrhea (28%), taste disturbances (15%), headache (5%), flatulence (4%), nausea (3%), abdominal pain (2%), ALT increased (1%), epigastric pain (1%), pharyngitis (1%) and glossitis (1%).

The following adverse events (at a rate of more than 1%) were recorded during controlled clinical trials in 494 patients receiving omeprazole, metronidazole and clarithromycin: taste disturbances (14%), diarrhea (13%), headache (6%), ALT increased (6%), flatulence (5%), nausea (5%), AST increased (5%), dyspepsia (3%), dry mouth (2%), dizziness/vertigo (2%), epigastric pain (1%), pharyngitis (1%), eructation (1%) and fatigue (1%).

Clinical experience with the use of omeprazole magnesium 20 mg tablet is limited. In 2 short-term studies (20 mg tablet once daily for a maximum duration of 7 days) in a limited number of patients with duodenal ulcer in remission, the adverse event profile seen with the omeprazole magnesium 20 mg tablet is similar to that seen with the omeprazole 20 mg capsule.

OVERDOSE:

Symptoms: No information is available on the effects of higher doses in man, and specific recommendations for treatment cannot be given. Single oral doses of up to 400 mg of omeprazole capsules have not resulted in any severe symptoms, and no specific treatment has been needed. As in all cases where overdosing is suspected, treatment should be supportive and symptomatic. Any unabsorbed material should be removed from the gastrointestinal tract, and the patient should be carefully monitored.

The oral LD_{50} of omeprazole in male and female rats and mice was greater than 4000 mg/kg. In dogs, the only sign of acute toxicity was vomiting which occurred at doses of approximately 600 mg/kg.

When used in combination with antibiotics, the prescribing information/product monograph for those antibiotics should be consulted.

Treatment: See Symptoms.

> For management of a suspected drug overdose, contact your regional Poison Control Centre. See the *CPS Directory* section for a list of Poison Control Centres.

DOSAGE: Duodenal Ulcer: Acute Therapy: The recommended adult oral dose is 20 mg given once daily. Healing usually occurs within 2 weeks. For patients not healed after this initial course of therapy, an additional 2 weeks of treatment is recommended.

Refractory Patients: In patients with duodenal ulcer refractory to other treatment regimens, the recommended adult dose is 20 to 40 mg given once daily. Healing is usually achieved within 4 weeks in such patients.

Maintenance Therapy for Duodenal Ulcer: Over 95% of duodenal ulcer patients are *H. pylori*-positive, and should be treated with eradication therapy, as described below. A small percentage of patients who are *H. pylori*-negative will experience a disease recurrence and will require maintenance treatment with an antisecretory agent. The recommended dose is 10 mg once daily, increased to 20 to 40 mg once daily as necessary.

Gastric Ulcer: Acute Therapy: The recommended adult dose is 20 mg given once daily. Healing usually occurs within 4 weeks. For patients not healed after this initial course of therapy, an additional 4 weeks of treatment is recommended.

Refractory Patients: In patients with gastric ulcer refractory to other treatment regimens, the recommended adult dose is 40 mg given once daily. Healing is usually achieved within 8 weeks.

Maintenance Therapy for Gastric Ulcer: About 80% of gastric ulcer patients are *H. pylori*-positive, and should be treated with eradication therapy, as described below. A small percentage of patients who are *H. pylori*-negative will experience a disease recurrence and will require maintenance treatment with an antisecretory agent. The recommended dose is 20 mg once daily, increased to 40 mg once daily as necessary.

Reflux Esophagitis: Acute Therapy: The recommended adult dose is 20 mg given once daily. In most patients, healing occurs within 4 weeks. For patients not healed after this initial course of therapy, an additional 4 weeks of treatment is recommended.

Refractory Patients: For patients with reflux esophagitis refractory to other treatment regimens, the recommended adult dose is 40 mg given once daily. Healing is usually achieved within 8 weeks.

Maintenance Therapy for Reflux Esophagitis: For the long-term management of patients with healed reflux esophagitis, 10 mg omeprazole (given as capsules) once daily has been found to be effective in controlled clinical trials of 12 months' duration, and in continuous maintenance treatment, in a limited number of patients, for a period of up to 6 years. Therefore, the recommended adult dose of omeprazole magnesium tablets for maintenance treatment of patients with healed reflux esophagitis is 10 mg given once daily. In the case of recurrence, the dose can be increased to 20 to 40 mg once daily.

Symptomatic Gastroesophageal Reflux Disease (i.e., Heartburn and Regurgitation): The recommended adult dose is 20 mg given once daily. Symptom relief should be rapid. If symptom control is not achieved after 4 weeks, further investigation is recommended. Since some patients may respond adequately to 10 mg given once daily, individual dose adjustment can be considered. For the maintenance of symptom relief in patients with gastroesophageal reflux disease (i.e., heartburn and regurgitation) the recommended adult dose is 10 mg given once daily.

NSAID-Associated Gastric or Duodenal Ulcers: The issue of whether or not eradication of *H. pylori* in patients with NSAID-associated ulcers might have beneficial preventive effects has not yet been settled.

Acute Therapy: In patients with NSAID-associated gastric or duodenal ulcers, the recommended adult dose is 20 mg given once daily. Symptom resolution is rapid and healing usually occurs within 4 weeks. For those patients not healed after this initial course of therapy, an additional 4 weeks of treatment is recommended.

Maintenance Therapy: For the prevention of relapse in patients with NSAID-associated gastric or duodenal ulcers, the recommended adult dose is 20 mg given once daily, for up to 6 months.

Dyspepsia: Prior to treating patients presenting with dyspeptic symptoms, it should be determined that these symptoms are originating from the upper gastrointestinal tract. Patients presenting with alarm symptoms (see Warnings), and older patients who are at a greater risk of having a serious organic disease, should be investigated prior to the initiation of therapy. If the dyspeptic symptoms are known to be related to a diagnosis of organic disease, the appropriate treatment regimen listed in the sections above should be employed.

If the dyspeptic symptoms are not known to be related to an organic disease, the recommended daily dose of omeprazole magnesium is 20 mg once daily for 4 weeks. If after 2 weeks' treatment the patient does not respond to therapy, or there is an early clinical indication of a lack of efficacy, the patient should be thoroughly investigated in order to rule out organic disease (see Warnings). If there are indications of a clinical response following the initial 2 weeks of treatment, omeprazole magnesium may be continued for an additional 2 weeks. Patients may respond adequately to 10 mg once daily, therefore, individual dose adjustment may be considered.

Epigastric pain/discomfort (with or without heartburn and regurgitation) as predominant symptoms, are likely to respond to acid suppression therapy. In all cases, patients who do not respond to 4 weeks' treatment, or whose symptoms recur shortly after discontinuation of treatment with omeprazole, should be investigated for underlying organic diseases.

H. pylori Associated Peptic Ulcer Disease: Omeprazole, Amoxicillin and Clarithromycin Triple Therapy: The recommended dose for eradication of *H. pylori* is omeprazole magnesium 20 mg, amoxicillin 1000 mg and clarithromycin 500 mg, all twice daily for 7 days. This dosing regimen can be known as Losec 1-2-3 A.

Omeprazole, Metronidazole and Clarithromycin Triple Therapy: The recommended dose for eradication of *H. pylori* is omeprazole magnesium 20 mg, metronidazole 500 mg and clarithromycin 250 mg, all twice daily for 7 days. This dosing regimen can be known as Losec 1-2-3 M.

To ensure healing and/or symptom control, further treatment with 20 mg omeprazole magnesium once daily for up to 3 weeks is recommended for patients with active duodenal ulcer, and with 20 to 40 mg omeprazole magnesium once daily for up to 12 weeks for patients with active gastric ulcer.

Patient compliance with treatment regimens for the eradication of *H. pylori* has been demonstrated to have a positive effect on eradication outcome. In clinical trials, patients treated with triple therapy regimens have shown high compliance rates.

Patients who fail to have their infection eradicated may be considered to have *H. pylori* resistant to the antimicrobials used in the eradication regimen. Therefore, therapy involving alternative effective antimicrobial agents should be considered (if re-treating).

In dyspeptic patients with an *H. pylori* infection, the concurrent gastritis can be healed with appropriate eradication therapy.

Zollinger-Ellison Syndrome: The dose used in the treatment of Zollinger-Ellison syndrome will vary with the individual patient.

The recommended initial dose is 60 mg, given once daily. More than 90% of patients with the severe form of the disease and inadequate response to other therapies have been adequately controlled with doses of 20 to 120 mg omeprazole capsules daily. With doses greater than 80 mg, the dose should be divided and given twice daily. Doses should be adjusted to the individual patient's need and should continue as long as clinically indicated. Doses up to 120 mg omeprazole capsules 3 times daily have been administered.

Renal Insufficiency: No dose adjustment is required (see Precautions).

Hepatic Insufficiency: No dose adjustment is required. The daily dose should not exceed 20 mg (see Precautions).

Geriatrics: No dose adjustment is required. The daily dose should not exceed 20 mg (see Precautions).

The tablets should be swallowed whole with sufficient water.

Storage: Omeprazole magnesium tablets are moisture sensitive and are therefore provided in blister compliance packages suitable for direct distribution to the patient. Store in a dry place at controlled room temperature (15 to 30°C).

INFORMATION FOR THE PATIENT: Published in e-CPS, available by subscription at www.e-cps.ca.

SUPPLIED: 10 mg: Each pink, circular and biconvex delayed release tablet, printed LOSEC/10 on one side, contains: omeprazole magnesium anhydrous 10.3 mg (equivalent to omeprazole 10 mg). Nonmedicinal ingredients: hydroxypropyl methylcellulose, iron oxide, mannitol, methacrylic acid copolymer, microcrystalline cellulose, paraffin, polyethylene glycol, sodium starch glycolate, sodium stearyl fumarate, talc and titanium dioxide. Press-through blister compliance strips in cartons of 30. Dispense in original container.

20 mg: Each red-brown, circular, biconvex delayed release tablet, printed LOSEC/20 on one side, contains: omeprazole magnesium anhydrous 20.6 mg (equivalent to omeprazole 20 mg). Nonmedicinal ingredients: hydroxypropyl methylcellulose, iron oxide, mannitol, methacrylic acid copolymer, microcrystalline cellulose, paraffin, polyethylene glycol, sodium starch glycolate, sodium stearyl fumarate, talc and titanium dioxide. Press-through blister compliance packs in cartons of 30. 10×10 unit dose blister packages. HDPE bottles of 100. Dispense in the original container.

(Shown in Product Identification Section)

Lotemax™ Ⓟ

loteprednol etabonate

Corticosteroid

Bausch & Lomb

Date of Preparation: January 12, 2009

SUMMARY PRODUCT INFORMATION:

Route of Administration	Dosage Form/ Strength	Clinically Relevant Nonmedicinal Ingredients
Ophthalmic	Suspension, 0.5% w/v	Benzalkonium chloride For a complete listing see Dosage Forms, Composition and Packaging.

INDICATIONS AND CLINICAL USE: Lotemax (loteprednol etabonate) Ophthalmic Suspension is indicated for:

- treatment of post-operative inflammation following cataract surgery.

Pediatrics (<18 years of age): Lotemax should not be used in pediatric patients. The safety and efficacy of Lotemax have not been studied in pediatric patients.

Geriatrics: No overall differences in safety or effectiveness have been observed between elderly and younger patients.

CONTRAINDICATIONS:

- Suspected or confirmed infection of the eye: viral diseases of the cornea and conjunctiva including epithelial herpes simplex keratitis (dendritic keratitis), vaccinia, and varicella; untreated ocular infection of the eye; mycobacterial infection of the eye and fungal diseases of ocular structures.
- Hypersensitivity to this drug or any ingredient in the formulation or container, or to other corticosteroids. For a complete listing, see Dosage Forms, Composition and Packaging.

WARNINGS AND PRECAUTIONS: General: For ophthalmic use only.

Lotemax is indicated for short-term treatment only (up to 14 days). The initial prescription and renewal of Lotemax should be made by a physician only after appropriate ophthalmologic examination is performed. If signs and symptoms fail to improve after two days, the patient should be re-evaluated. If Lotemax is used for 10 days or longer, intraocular pressure should be closely monitored. See Ophthalmologic.

The use of steroids after cataract surgery may delay wound healing.

Prolonged use of corticosteroids may result in cataract and/or glaucoma formation. Lotemax should not be used in the presence of glaucoma or elevated intraocular pressure, unless absolutely necessary and close ophthalmologic monitoring is undertaken. Extreme caution should be exercised, and duration of treatment should be kept as short as possible. See Ophthalmologic.

Lotemax should not be used in cases of existing (suspected or confirmed) ocular viral, fungal, or mycobacterial infections. Lotemax may suppress the host response and thus increase the hazard of secondary ocular infections. The use of Lotemax in patients with a history of herpes simplex requires great caution and close monitoring. See Ophthalmologic.

Lotemax contains benzalkonium chloride. See Dosage and Administration.

Lotemax has not been studied in pregnant or nursing women, but has been found to be teratogenic in animals. Lotemax should not be used in pregnant or nursing women unless the benefits to the mother clearly outweigh the risk to the foetus or the nursing child. See Special Populations.

Carcinogenesis and Mutagenesis: Long-term animal studies have not been conducted to evaluate the carcinogenic potential of loteprednol etabonate. Loteprednol etabonate was not genotoxic in vitro in the Ames test, the mouse lymphoma tk assay, or in a chromosome aberration test in human lymphocytes, or in vivo in the single dose mouse micronucleus assay.

Endocrine and Metabolism: Glucocorticoids, mostly when systemic exposure occurs, decrease the hypoglycemic activity of insulin and oral hypoglycemics, so that a change in dose of the antidiabetic drugs may be necessitated. In high doses, glucocorticoids also decrease the response to somatotropin. The usual doses of mineralocorticoids and large doses of some glucocorticoids cause hypokalemia and may exaggerate the hypokalemic effects of thiazides and high-ceiling diuretics. In combination with amphotericin-B, they also may cause hypokalemia. Glucocorticoids appear to enhance the ulcerogenic effects of non-steroidal anti-inflammatory drugs. They decrease the plasma levels of salicylates, and salicylism may occur on discontinuing steroids. Glucocorticoids may increase or decrease the effects of prothrombopenic anticoagulants. Estrogens, phenobarbital, phenytoin and rifampin increase the metabolic clearance of adrenal steroids and hence necessitate dose adjustments. However, given the very low systemic exposure to loteprednol etabonate when using Lotemax as directed, these possible effects are not likely. See Action and Clinical Pharmacology.

Immune: Cortisol and the synthetic analogs of cortisol have the capacity to prevent or suppress the development of the local heat, redness, swelling, and tenderness by which inflammation is recognized. At the microscopic level, they inhibit not only the early phenomena of the inflammatory process (edema, fibrin deposition, capillary dilation, migration of leukocytes into the inflamed area, and phagocytic activity) but also the later manifestations, such as capillary proliferation, fibroblast proliferation, deposition of collagen, and, still later, cicatrisation.

Neurologic: Disturbances and suppression of the Hypothalamic-Pituitary-Adrenal (HPA) axis can occur with systemic exposure to corticosteroids. However, given the very low systemic exposure to loteprednol etabonate when using Lotemax as directed, these possible effects are not likely. See Action and Clinical Pharmacology.

Ophthalmologic: Lotemax should be used as a short-term treatment. If Lotemax is used for 10 days or longer, intraocular pressure should be monitored. The initial prescription and renewal of Lotemax should be made by a physician only after appropriate ophthalmologic examination is performed with the aid of magnification, such as slit lamp biomicroscopy and, where appropriate, fluorescein staining. If signs and symptoms fail to improve after two days, the patient should be re-evaluated.

Prolonged use of corticosteroids may result in glaucoma with damage to the optic nerve, defects in visual acuity and fields of vision, and in posterior subcapsular cataract formation. Lotemax should not be used in the presence of glaucoma or elevated intraocular pressure, unless absolutely necessary and careful and close appropriate ophthalmologic monitoring (including intraocular pressure and lens clarity) is undertaken.

Fungal infections of the cornea are particularly prone to develop coincidentally with long-term local steroid application. Fungus invasion must be considered in any persistent corneal ulceration where a steroid has been used or is in use. Fungal cultures should be taken when appropriate.

Prolonged use of corticosteroids may suppress the host response and thus increase the hazard of secondary ocular infections. In those diseases causing thinning of the cornea or sclera, perforations have been known to occur with the use of topical steroids. In acute purulent conditions of the eye, steroids may mask infection or enhance existing infection.

Use of ocular steroids may prolong the course and may exacerbate the severity of many viral infections of the eye (including herpes simplex). Employment of a corticosteroid medication in the treatment of patients with a history of herpes simplex requires great caution.

Formulations with benzalkonium chloride should be used with caution in soft contact lens wearer. See Dosage and Administration, Administration.

Sexual Function/Reproduction: The effects of Lotemax on sexual function and reproduction have not been studied in humans. Treatment of male and female rats with up to 50 mg/kg/day and 25 mg/kg/day of loteprednol etabonate, respectively, (400 and 200 times the Lotemax clinical dose) prior to and during mating, was clearly harmful to the rats, but did not impair their copulation performance and fertility (i.e., ability of female rats to become pregnant). However, these doses were highly toxic and had major and significant toxic effects on the pregnancies, and the survival and development of the offspring. Maternal toxicity, possible occurrence of abnormalities and growth retardation started at 4 times the Lotemax clinical dose. See Special Populations, Pregnant Women.

Special Populations: Pregnant Women: Lotemax should not be used in pregnant women, unless the benefit to the mother clearly outweighs the risks to the foetus. Studies in pregnant women have not been conducted. However, studies in animals have shown major reproductive and developmental toxicity when administered orally at ~40 times the Lotemax clinical dose. At lower doses (4 times the Lotemax clinical dose), maternal toxicity was demonstrated and, although there were no major teratogenic effects, growth retardation and a possible increase in the occurrence of some abnormalities were noted.

Nursing Women: Lotemax should not be used in lactating women, unless the benefit to the mother clearly outweighs the risks to the nursing infant/child. Studies in lactating women have not been conducted. Systemic steroids appear in human milk and could suppress growth, interfere with endogenous corticosteroid production, or cause other untoward effects.

It is not known whether topical ophthalmic administration of corticosteroids could result in sufficient systemic absorption to produce detectable quantities in human milk.

Pediatrics: Lotemax should not be used in pediatric patients. The safety and efficacy of Lotemax have not been studied in pediatric patients.

Geriatrics: No overall differences in safety or effectiveness have been observed between elderly and younger patients.

Monitoring and Laboratory Tests: If Lotemax is used for 10 days or longer, intraocular pressure should be monitored. See Warnings and Precautions, General.

ADVERSE REACTIONS: Adverse Drug Reaction Overview: Reactions associated with ophthalmic steroids include elevated intraocular pressure, which may be associated with optic nerve damage, visual acuity and field defects, posterior subcapsular cataract formation, secondary ocular infection from pathogens including herpes simplex, and perforation of the globe where there is thinning of the cornea or sclera.

In nineteen clinical trials ranging from 1 to 42 days in length, 1209 patients received various concentrations of loteprednol etabonate in topical ocular drops (0.005%, 0.05%, 0.1%, 0.2%, 0.5%). Adverse events related to loteprednol etabonate (LE) were generally mild to moderate, non-serious and did not interrupt continuation in the studies. The most frequent ocular event reported as related to therapy was increased IOP: 6% (77/1209) in patients receiving loteprednol etabonate, as compared to 3% (25/806) in the placebo treated patients.

With the exception of elevations in IOP, the incidence of events in the LE group was similar to, or less than that of the placebo control groups. Itching was reported as related to therapy in 3% of the loteprednol treated eyes, injection, epiphora, burning/stinging other than at instillation, foreign body sensation, and burning/stinging at instillation were each reported for 2% of eyes. The most frequent non-ocular event reported as related to therapy was headache, reported for 1.2% of the loteprednol treated subjects and 0.6% of the placebo treated subjects.

Clinical Trial Adverse Drug Reactions: Because clinical trials are conducted under very specific conditions the adverse reaction rates observed in the clinical trials may not reflect the rates observed in practice and should not be compared to the rates in the clinical trials of another drug. Adverse drug reaction information from clinical trials is useful for identifying drug-related adverse events and for approximating rates.

Two phase III studies were conducted to assess the safety and efficacy of Lotemax in the treatment of inflammation following cataract surgery with intraocular lens (IOL) implantation. Both studies were randomized, double-masked, placebo controlled, multi-centre parallel group. Patients with a combined anterior chamber rating of cell and flare ≥3 (moderate, scale 0-9) were enrolled in Study A (N=227) and Study B (N=203). Patients with history of intraocular or laser surgery on the eye within the past six months or the presence of any ocular pathology other than the cataract (for example vernal conjunctivitis, glaucoma of any kind, giant papillary conjunctivitis, viral or bacterial conjunctivitis, uveitis, retinopathies) were excluded from the studies. During these studies, 212 patients were exposed to Lotemax.

Incidence of Medical Events in the phase III studies are outlined in Table 1.

Intraocular Pressure: Elevated IOP is associated with the application of topical corticosteroids. IOP was closely monitored in the phase III studies.

In the phase III studies, IOP increases of 6 to 9 mm Hg were seen in 11 subjects in the Lotemax group and in the placebo group (see Table 2). Four patients, 3 Lotemax and 1 placebo, reached an IOP of 22 to 24 mm Hg. One placebo patient reached an IOP of 29 mm Hg.

Adverse Reactions Reported in Other Controlled Randomized Studies: In nineteen clinical trials ranging from 1 to 42 days in length, 1209 patients received various concentrations of loteprednol etabonate in topical ocular drops (0.005%, 0.05%, 0.1%, 0.2%, 0.5%), the most frequent ocular event reported as related to therapy was increased intraocular pressure: 6% (77/1209) in patients receiving loteprednol etabonate, as compared to 3% (25/806) in the placebo population.

Ocular adverse reactions occurring in 5-15% of patients treated with loteprednol etabonate ophthalmic suspension (0.2%-0.5%) in clinical studies included abnormal vision/blurring, burning on instillation, chemosis, discharge, dry eyes, epiphora, foreign body sensation, itching, injection, and photophobia. Other ocular adverse reactions occurring in less than 5% of patients include conjunctivitis, corneal abnormalities, eyelid erythema, keratoconjunctivitis, ocular irritation/pain/discomfort, papillae, and uveitis. Some of these events were similar to the underlying ocular disease being studied.

Table 1: Lotemax

Incidence of Medical Events in the Phase III Studies

	Lotemax N=212		Placebo N=218	
	N	%	N	%
No signs or symptoms	93	44	48	22
Discomfort, eye	28	13	49	22
Epiphora (eye/app)	25	12	49	22
Itching, eye	24	11	33	15
Photophobia	23	11	72	33
Eye pain	18	8	53	24
Dry eyes	13	6	18	8
Injection	11	5	50	23
Cell, anterior chamber	8	4	20	9
Ciliary flush	6	3	17	8
Erythema, eyelids	6	3	17	8
Discharge, eye	5	2	14	6
Edema, corneal	5	2	17	8
Chemosis	2	1	9	4
Flare, anterior chamber	2	1	23	11
Hyphema	1	<1	1	<1

Table 2: Lotemax

Incidence of IOP Increases From Baseline (number of patients and percentages)

	Visit 2 Day 2-6	Visit 3 Day 7-12	Visit 4 Day 13+	Any Visit
Pivotal Study A				
≥10 mm Hg				
Placebo	0 (0%)	0 (0%)	0 (0%)	0 (0%)
LE	2 (2%)	1 (1%)	0 (0%)	3 (3%)[a]
6 to 9 mm Hg				
Placebo	3 (3%)	1 (1%)	1 (1%)	5 (4%)
LE	1 (1%)	5 (5%)	2 (2%)	7 (6%)
Pivotal Study B				
≥10 mm Hg				
Placebo	0 (0%)	1 (1%)	0 (0%)	1 (1%)[b]
LE	0 (0%)	0 (0%)	0 (0%)	0 (0%)
6 to 9 mm Hg				
Placebo	4 (4%)	2 (2%)	2 (3%)	6 (6%)
LE	0 (0%)	3 (3%)	2 (2%)	4 (4%)

[a] One eye developed severe uveitis and increased from 18 mm Hg pre-op to 50 mm Hg at Visit 3.
One eye increased from 7 mm Hg pre-op to 26 mm Hg post-op and to 30 mm Hg by Visit 2.
One eye increased from 8 mm Hg pre-op to 23 mm Hg post-op and to 25 mm Hg by Visit 2.
[b] One eye increased from 19 mm Hg pre-op and 18 mm Hg post-op to 48 mm Hg by Visit 3.

Non-ocular adverse reactions occurred in less than 15% of patients. These include headache, rhinitis and pharyngitis.

In a summary of controlled, randomized studies of individuals treated for 28 days or longer with loteprednol etabonate, the incidence of significant elevation of intraocular pressure (≥10 mm Hg) was 2% (15/901) among patients receiving loteprednol etabonate and 0.5% (3/583) among patients receiving placebo.

Post-Market Adverse Drug Reactions: In over a decade of post-marketing experience, more than 14 million units of Lotemax have been shipped globally. During that time seven (7) adverse event reports that qualified as serious were received. Table 3 summarizes these events.

DRUG INTERACTIONS: Overview: No specific drug interaction studies have been conducted. There are no known drug interactions.

Lotemax contains benzalkonium chloride which interacts with soft contact lens. See Dosage and Administration, Administration.

Drug-drug, drug-food, drug-herb, and drug-laboratory interactions have not been studied.

DOSAGE AND ADMINISTRATION: Recommended Dose and Dosage Adjustment: Apply one to two drops of Lotemax into the conjunctival sac of the operated eye(s) four times daily beginning 24 hours after surgery and continuing throughout the first 2 weeks of the post-operative period.

Missed Dose: If scheduled dose is missed, patient should be advised to wait until the next dose and then continue as before.

Administration: Shake vigorously before using. Lotemax should be stored upright between 15-25°C for up to 28 days after first opening.

The preservative in Lotemax, benzalkonium chloride, may be absorbed by soft contact lenses, and can discolour soft contact lenses. Therefore, Lotemax should not be used while the patient is wearing soft contact lenses. Patients who wear soft contact lenses and whose eyes are not red should wait ten to fifteen minutes after instilling Lotemax before they insert their contact lenses.

Patients should be advised not to wear a contact lens if their eye is red. Lotemax should not be used to treat contact lens related irritation.

Table 3: Lotemax

Lotemax Serious Adverse Events, March 1998-October 2008

Sex	Age	Event
F	84	Atrioventricular block, Atrial fibrillation, Collapse of lung, Drug toxicity, Bradycardia
M	40	Intraocular pressure increased
F	79	Staphylococcal infection, Corneal ulcer
F	28	Transplant rejection, Corneal perforation, Eye injury
F	60	Corneal scar, Corneal ulcer, Corneal infection, Cataract, Visual acuity reduced, Corneal perforation, Uveitis
F	43	Ocular toxicity, Chemical burns of eye, Corneal epithelium defect, Corneal scar
M	UNK	Blood glucose decreased

OVERDOSAGE:
No cases of overdose have been reported.

For management of a suspected accidental oral ingestion or drug overdose, contact your **regional Poison Control Centre**. See the *CPS* Directory section for a list of Poison Control Centres.

ACTION AND CLINICAL PHARMACOLOGY: Mechanism of Action: There is no generally accepted explanation for the mechanism of action of ocular corticosteroids. However, corticosteroids are thought to act by the induction of phospholipase A_2 inhibitory proteins, collectively called lipocortins. It is postulated that these proteins control the biosynthesis of potent mediators of inflammation such as prostaglandins and leukotrienes by inhibiting the release of their common precursor arachidonic acid. Arachidonic acid is released from membrane phospholipids by phospholipase A_2. Corticosteroids are capable of producing a rise in intraocular pressure.

Pharmacodynamics: Corticosteroids inhibit the inflammatory response to a variety of inciting agents and probably delay or slow healing. They inhibit the edema, fibrin deposition, capillary dilation, leukocyte migration, capillary proliferation, fibroblast proliferation, deposition of collagen, and scar formation associated with inflammation.

Pharmacokinetics: Results from a bioavailability study in normal volunteers (8 females, 2 males; age range of 19-44 years) established that plasma levels of loteprednol etabonate and Δ^1 cortienic acid etabonate (PJ 91), its primary, inactive metabolite, were below the limit of quantitation (1 ng/mL) at all sampling times. The results were obtained following the ocular administration of one drop of 0.5% loteprednol etabonate ophthalmic suspension in each eye 8 times daily for 2 days or 4 times daily for 42 days.

STORAGE AND STABILITY: Store upright between 15-25°C. **Do not freeze. Keep out of reach of children.**

SPECIAL HANDLING INSTRUCTIONS: There is no special handling instruction for Lotemax.

INFORMATION FOR THE PATIENT: Published in e-CPS, available by subscription at www.e-cps.ca.

DOSAGE FORMS, COMPOSITION AND PACKAGING: Loteprednol etabonate ophthalmic suspension 0.5% w/v is supplied in a white low density polyethylene plastic bottle with a white controlled drop tip and a pink polypropylene cap in the following sizes: 5 mL in a 7.5 mL bottle, 10 mL in a 10 mL bottle. Nonmedicinal ingredients: benzalkonium chloride, edetate disodium, glycerin, povidone, purified water and tyloxapol. Hydrochloric acid and/or sodium hydroxide may be added to adjust the pH to 5.5-5.6.

(Shown in Product Identification Section)

The reader is invited to consult CPhA's monograph **ACE Inhibitors**.

Lotensin® 🅿

benzepril HCl

Angiotensin Converting Enzyme Inhibitor

Novartis Pharmaceuticals

Date of Preparation: June 7, 1993
Date of Revision: September 24, 2009

PHARMACOLOGY: Benazepril is an angiotensin converting enzyme (ACE) inhibitor which is used in the treatment of hypertension.

Benazepril, after hydrolytic bioactivation to benazeprilat, inhibits angiotensin converting enzyme (ACE), a peptidyl dipeptidase catalyzing the conversion of angiotensin I to the vasoconstrictor angiotensin II. Angiotensin II also stimulates aldosterone secretion by the adrenal cortex, leading to sodium resorption and potassium secretion by the distal renal tubules.

Inhibition of ACE results in a decrease in plasma angiotensin II, leading to decreased vasoconstriction and a small decrease in aldosterone secretion and plasma aldosterone concentrations. Although the decrease in aldosterone is small, it can result in small increases in serum potassium. Slight increases in serum potassium have been observed in some hypertensive patients treated with benazepril alone. Essentially no change in mean serum potassium was seen in patients treated with benazepril and a thiazide diuretic (see Precautions).

Removal of inhibition of renin secretion by angiotensin II leads to increased plasma renin activity (due to removal of negative feedback of renin release).

ACE is identical to kininase II. Thus, benazepril may interfere with degradation of the potent peptide vasodilator, bradykinin. Whether increased levels of bradykinin play a role in the therapeutic effects of benazepril is unknown.

While the mechanism through which benazepril lowers blood pressure is believed to be primarily suppression of the renin-angiotensin-aldosterone system, benazepril has an antihypertensive effect even in patients with low renin hypertension. In particular, benazepril was antihypertensive in all races studied, although it was somewhat less effective in blacks than in non-blacks.

Pharmacokinetics: Following oral administration of benazepril, peak plasma concentrations of benazepril are reached within 0.5 to 1 hour. The extent of absorption is at least 37% as determined by urinary recovery of unchanged drug and its metabolites. Following absorption, benazepril is rapidly hydrolyzed to its active metabolite, benazeprilat. Peak plasma concentrations of benazeprilat are reached 1 to 2 hours after drug intake in the fasting state and 2 to 4 hours after drug intake in the nonfasting state. While the rate of absorption may be slowed by the presence of food in the gastrointestinal tract, the systemic availability of benazeprilat is not affected. Benazeprilat is eliminated predominantly by renal excretion and has an effective accumulation half-life of 10 to 11 hours. The serum protein binding of benazepril is about 97%, and that of benazeprilat about 95%.

Benazepril is almost completely metabolized to benazeprilat, and to the glucuronide conjugates of benazepril and benazeprilat. Only trace amounts of an administered dose of LOTENSIN can be recovered in the urine as unchanged benazepril, while about 20% of the dose is excreted as benazeprilat, 4% as benazepril glucuronide, and 8% as benazeprilat glucuronide. The kinetics of benazepril are approximately dose-proportional within the dosage range (10 to 40 mg).

The disposition of benazepril and benazeprilat in patients with mild to moderate renal insufficiency (creatinine clearance >30 mL/min [0.5 mL/s]) is similar to that in patients with normal renal function. In patients with creatinine clearance <30 mL/min [0.5 mL/s], peak benazeprilat levels and the initial (alpha phase) half-life increase, and time to steady state may be delayed (see Dosage).

In patients with hepatic dysfunction due to cirrhosis, levels of benazeprilat are essentially unaltered. The pharmacokinetics of benazepril and benazeprilat do not appear to be influenced by age.

Pharmacodynamics: Administration of benazepril to patients with mild to moderate essential hypertension results in a reduction of both supine and standing blood pressure usually with little or no orthostatic change. Orthostatic hypotension is infrequent, although it may occur in patients who are salt- and/or volume-depleted (see Warnings).

After administration of a single oral dose, the onset of antihypertensive activity occurs at approximately 1 hour, with maximum reduction of blood pressure achieved by 2 to 4 hours, in most patients. At recommended doses given once daily, antihypertensive effects have persisted for at least 24 hours. In dose-response studies using once daily dosing in mild to moderate essential hypertensive patients, the minimally effective daily dose of benazepril was 10 mg. In studies comparing the same daily dose of benazepril given as a single morning dose or as a twice daily dose, blood pressure reductions at the time of morning trough blood levels were greater with the divided regimen.

During chronic therapy, the maximum reduction in blood pressure with any dose is generally achieved after 1 to 2 weeks. Abrupt withdrawal of benazepril has not been associated with a rapid increase in blood pressure.

When benazepril is given together with thiazide-type diuretics, its blood pressure lowering effect is approximately additive.

Efficacy and safety appear to be the same for elderly (>65 years of age) and younger adult patients given the same daily dosages.

INDICATIONS: In the treatment of mild to moderate essential hypertension. It may be used alone or in association with thiazide diuretics.

In using benazepril, consideration should be given to the risk of angioedema (see Warnings).

Benazepril should normally be used in those patients in whom treatment with a diuretic or a beta-blocker was found ineffective or has been associated with unacceptable adverse effects.

Benazepril can also be tried as an initial agent in those patients in whom use of diuretics and/or beta-blockers is contraindicated or in patients with medical conditions in which these drugs frequently cause serious adverse effects.

The safety and efficacy of benazepril in congestive heart failure and renovascular hypertension have not been established and therefore, its use in these conditions is not recommended.

The safety and efficacy of concurrent use of benazepril with antihypertensive agents other than thiazide diuretics have not been established.

CONTRAINDICATIONS: In patients with known hypersensitivity to this product or any of its components and in patients with a history of angioedema with or without previous treatment with an ACE inhibitor.

WARNINGS:

Serious Warnings and Precautions

When used in pregnancy, angiotensin converting enzyme (ACE) inhibitors can cause injury or even death of the developing fetus. When pregnancy is detected, benazepril should be discontinued as soon as possible.

Anaphylactoid and Related Reactions: Presumably because angiotensin-converting enzyme inhibitors affect the metabolism of eicosanoids and polypeptides, including endogenous bradykinin, patients receiving ACE inhibitors (including benazepril) may experience a variety of adverse reactions, some of them serious.

Angioedema: Angioedema has been reported in patients with ACE inhibitors, including benazepril. Angioedema associated with laryngeal involvement may be fatal. If laryngeal stridor or angioedema of the face, tongue, or glottis occurs, benazepril should be discontinued immediately, the patient treated appropriately in accordance with accepted medical care, and carefully observed until the swelling disappears. In instances where swelling is confined to the face and lips, the condition generally resolves without treatment, although antihistamines may be useful in relieving symptoms. Where there is involvement of tongue, glottis or larynx, likely to cause airway obstruction, appropriate therapy (including, but not limited to 0.3 to 0.5 mL of s.c. epinephrine solution 1:1000) should be administered promptly (see Adverse Effects).

The incidence of angioedema during ACE inhibitor therapy has been reported to be higher in black patients of African origin than in non-black patients.

Patients with a history of angioedema unrelated to ACE inhibitor therapy may be at increased risk of angioedema while receiving an ACE inhibitor (see Contraindications).

Hypotension: Occasionally, orthostatic hypotension has occurred after administration of benazepril usually after the first or second dose or when the dose was increased. It is more likely to occur in patients who are volume depleted by diuretic therapy, dietary salt restriction, dialysis, diarrhea, or vomiting. In patients with ischemic heart disease or cerebrovascular disease, an excessive fall in blood pressure could result in a myocardial infarction or cerebrovascular accident (see Adverse Effects). Because of the potential fall in blood pressure in these patients, therapy with benazepril should be started under close medical supervision. Such patients should be followed closely for the first weeks of treatment and whenever the dose of benazepril is increased. In patients with severe congestive heart failure, with or without associated renal insufficiency, ACE inhibitor therapy may cause excessive hypotension and has been associated with oliguria, and/or progressive azotemia, and rarely, with acute renal failure and/or death.

If hypotension occurs, the patient should be placed in a supine position and, if necessary, receive an i.v. infusion of normal saline. A transient hypotensive response is not a contraindication to further treatment, which usually can be continued without difficulty once the blood pressure has increased after volume expansion. However, lower doses of benazepril and/or reduced concomitant diuretic therapy should be considered.

Neutropenia/Agranulocytosis: Agranulocytosis and bone marrow depression have been caused by ACE inhibitors. Current experience with benazepril shows the incidence to be rare and a causal relationship to the administration of benazepril has not been established. Periodic monitoring of white blood cell counts should be considered, especially in patients with collagen vascular disease and/or renal disease.

Pregnancy: ACE inhibitors can cause fetal and neonatal morbidity and mortality when administered to pregnant women. When pregnancy is detected, benazepril should be discontinued as soon as possible.

The use of ACE inhibitors during the second and third trimesters of pregnancy has been associated with fetal and neonatal injury including hypotension, neonatal skull hypoplasia, anuria, reversible or irreversible renal failure, and death. Oligohydramnios has also been reported, presumably resulting from decreased fetal renal function, associated with fetal limb contractures, craniofacial deformation, and hypoplastic lung development.

Prematurity, and patent ductus arteriosus and other structural cardiac malformations, as well as neurologic malformations, have also been reported following exposure in the first trimester of pregnancy.

Infants with a history of in utero exposure to ACE inhibitors should be closely observed for hypotension, oliguria, and hyperkalemia. If oliguria occurs, attention should be directed toward support of blood pressure and renal perfusion. Exchange transfusion or dialysis may be required as a means of reversing hypotension and/or substituting for impaired renal function; however, limited experience with those procedures has not been associated with significant clinical benefit.

It is not known if benazepril can be removed from the body by hemodialysis.

Animal Data: Dose related maternal toxicity was observed in studies of pregnant rats, mice and rabbits at doses of 250 mg/kg, 150 mg/kg and 1 mg/kg respectively. No embryotoxic or teratogenic effects of benazepril were seen at doses up to 250 mg/kg in rats (300 times the maximum recommended dose in humans), 150 mg/kg in mice (90 times the maximum recommended dose in humans) and 5 mg/kg in rabbits (more than 3 times the maximum recommended dose in humans).

Lactation: The presence of concentrations of ACE inhibitor have been reported in human milk. Use of ACE inhibitors is not recommended during breast-feeding.

PRECAUTIONS: Renal Impairment: As a consequence of inhibiting the renin-angiotensin-aldosterone system, changes in renal function have been seen in susceptible individuals. In patients whose renal function may depend on the activity of the renin-angiotensin-aldosterone system, such as patients with bilateral renal artery stenosis, unilateral renal artery stenosis to a solitary kidney, or severe congestive heart failure, treatment with agents that inhibit this system has been associated with oliguria, progressive azotemia, and rarely, acute renal failure and/or death. In susceptible patients, concomitant diuretic use may further increase risk.

Use of benazepril should include appropriate assessment of renal function.

Anaphylactoid Reactions During Membrane Exposure: Anaphylactoid reactions have been reported in patients dialyzed with high-flux membranes (e.g., polyacrylonitrile [PAN]) and treated concomitantly with an ACE inhibitor. Dialysis should be stopped immediately if symptoms such as nausea, abdominal cramps, burning, angioedema, shortness of breath and severe hypotension occur. Symptoms are not relieved by antihistamines. In these patients consideration should be given to using a different type of dialysis membrane or a different class of antihypertensive agents.

Anaphylactoid Reactions During Desensitization: There have been isolated reports of patients experiencing sustained life threatening anaphylactoid reactions while receiving ACE inhibitors during desensitizing treatment with hymenoptera (bees, wasps) venom. In the same patients, these reactions have been avoided when ACE inhibitors were temporarily withheld for at least 24 hours, but they have reappeared upon inadvertent rechallenge.

Hyperkalemia and Potassium-Sparing Diuretics: Elevated serum potassium (>5.5 mEq/L) was observed in 1.1% of hypertensive patients in clinical trials treated with benazepril alone and in 0.4% treated with benazepril and hydrochlorothiazide. In most cases these were isolated values which resolved despite continued therapy. Hyperkalemia was a cause of discontinuation of therapy in less than 0.1% of hypertensive patients.

Risk factors for the development of hyperkalemia may include renal insufficiency, diabetes mellitus, and the concomitant use of agents to treat hypokalemia (see Drug Interactions).

Valvular Stenosis: There is concern on theoretical grounds that patients with aortic stenosis might be at particular risk of decreased coronary perfusion when treated with vasodilators because they do not develop as much afterload reduction.

Surgery/Anesthesia: ACE inhibitors may augment the hypotensive effects of anesthetics and analgesics. In patients undergoing surgery or during anesthesia with agents that produce hypotension, benazepril will block the angiotensin II formation that could otherwise occur secondary to compensatory renin release. Hypotension that occurs as a result of this mechanism can be corrected by volume expansion.

Patients with Impaired Liver Function: Hepatitis (hepatocellular and/or cholestatic), elevations of liver enzymes and/or serum bilirubin have occurred during therapy with ACE inhibitors in patients with or without pre-existing liver abnormalities. In most cases the changes were reversed on discontinuation of the drug.

Elevations of liver enzymes and/or serum bilirubin have been reported with benazepril (see Adverse Effects). Should the patient receiving benazepril experience any unexplained symptoms particularly during the first weeks or months of treatment, it is recommended that a full set of liver function tests and any other necessary investigations be carried out. Discontinuation of benazepril should be considered when appropriate.

There are no adequate studies in patients with cirrhosis and/or liver dysfunction. Benazepril should be used with particular caution in patients with pre-existing liver abnormalities. In such patients baseline liver function tests should be obtained before administration of the drug and close monitoring of response and metabolic effects should apply.

Cough: A dry, persistent cough, which usually disappears only after withdrawal or lowering of the dose of benazepril has been reported. Such possibility should be considered as part of the differential diagnosis of the cough.

Children: Safety and effectiveness of benazepril in children have not been established; therefore, its use in this age group is not recommended.

Geriatrics: Although clinical experience has not identified differences in response between the elderly (>65 years) and younger patients, greater sensitivity of some older individuals cannot be ruled out.

Drug Interactions: Concomitant Diuretic Therapy: Patients concomitantly taking ACE inhibitors and diuretics, and especially those in whom diuretic therapy was recently instituted, may occasionally experience an excessive reduction of blood pressure after initiation of therapy. The possibility of hypotensive effects after the first dose of benazepril can be minimized by either discontinuing the diuretic or increasing the salt intake prior to initiation of treatment with benazepril. If it is not possible to discontinue the diuretic, the starting dose of benazepril should be reduced and the patient should be closely observed for several hours following initial dose and until blood pressure has stabilized (see Warnings and Dosage).

Agents Causing Renin Release: The antihypertensive effect of benazepril is augmented by antihypertensive agents that cause renin release (e.g., diuretics).

Agents Increasing Serum Potassium: Since benazepril decreases aldosterone production, increases of serum potassium may occur. Potassium sparing diuretics (e.g., spironolactone, triamterene, amiloride, etc.) or potassium supplements should be given only for documented hypokalemia and with caution and frequent monitoring of serum potassium, since they may lead to a significant increase in serum potassium. Salt substitutes which contain potassium should also be used with caution.

Agents Affecting Sympathetic Activity: Agents affecting sympathetic activity (e.g., ganglionic blocking agents or adrenergic neuron blocking agents) may be used with caution. β-adrenergic blocking agents add some further antihypertensive effect to benazepril.

Indomethacin: Indomethacin may diminish the antihypertensive efficacy of concomitantly administered benazepril.

Oral Anticoagulants: Multiple dose interaction studies failed to identify any clinically important effects on the serum concentrations, the degree of protein binding or the anticoagulant effect (measured by prothrombin time) of warfarin and nicoumalone. The bioavailability of benazeprilat was not assessed during the coadministration of benazepril with warfarin or nicoumalone.

Lithium: Increased lithium levels and symptoms of lithium toxicity have been reported in patients receiving ACE inhibitors (including benazepril) during therapy with lithium. These drugs should be coadministered with caution and frequent monitoring of serum lithium levels is recommended. If a diuretic is also used, the risk of lithium toxicity may be increased.

Hydrochlorothiazide, Chlorthalidone and Furosemide: The bioavailability of benazepril was not altered when single doses were administered concomitantly with the diuretics hydrochlorothiazide, chlorthalidone or furosemide.

Acetylsalicylic Acid: No important changes in pharmacokinetic parameters occurred when single doses of benazepril were administered concomitantly with acetylsalicylic acid.

Digoxin: In a single dose interaction study of benazepril with multiple doses of digoxin, no important changes in pharmacokinetic parameters were observed.

Amlodipine/Nifedipine: Benazepril has been used concomitantly with the calcium channel blockers amlodipine and nifedipine, without evidence of clinically important adverse interactions.

Insulin/Oral Anti-Diabetics: ACE inhibitors (including benazepril) may reduce insulin resistance. In isolated cases, such reduction may lead to hypoglycemic reactions in patients treated concomitantly with anti-diabetics. Particularly close blood glucose monitoring is recommended.

Gold: Nitritoid reactions (symptoms include facial flushing, nausea, vomiting and hypotension) have been reported rarely in patients on therapy with injectable gold (sodium aurothiomalate) and concomitant ACE inhibitor therapy.

Other: In separate single or multiple dose pharmacokinetic interaction studies, the bioavailability of benazepril was not altered by coadministration with propranolol, naproxen, atenolol, nifedipine, amlodipine or cimetidine.

Information to Be Provided to the Patient: Note: As with many other drugs, certain advice to patients being treated with benazepril is warranted. This information is intended to aid in the safe and effective use of this medication. It is not a disclosure of all possible adverse experiences or intended effects.

Angioedema: Angioedema, including laryngeal edema, may occur especially following the first dose of benazepril. Patients should be so advised and told to report immediately any signs or symptoms suggesting angioedema, such as swelling of face, extremities, eyes, lips, tongue, difficulty in swallowing or breathing. They should immediately stop taking benazepril and consult with their physician.

Hypotension: Patients should be cautioned to report light-headedness, especially during the first few days of benazepril therapy. If actual syncope occurs, the patient should be told to discontinue the drug and consult with their physician.

All patients should be cautioned that excessive perspiration and dehydration may lead to an excessive fall in blood pressure because of reduction in fluid volume. Other causes of volume depletion such as vomiting or diarrhea may also lead to a fall in blood pressure, patients should be advised to consult with their physician.

Agranulocytosis/Neutropenia: Patients should be told to report promptly to their physician any indication of infection (e.g., sore throat, fever), as this may be a sign of neutropenia.

Impaired Liver Function: Patients should be advised to return to their physician if he/she experiences any symptoms possibly related to liver dysfunction. This would include "viral-like symptoms" in the first weeks to months of therapy (such as fever, malaise, muscle pain, rash or adenopathy which are possible indicators of hypersensitivity reactions), or if abdominal pain, nausea or vomiting, loss of appetite, jaundice, itching or any other unexplained symptoms occur during therapy.

Hyperkalemia: Patients should be told not to use salt substitutes containing potassium without consulting their physician.

Hypoglycemia: Patients treated concomitantly with anti-diabetics should be advise that ACE inhibitors (including benazepril) may reduce insulin resistance. In isolated cases, such reduction may lead to hypoglycemic reactions in these patients. Particularly close blood glucose monitoring is recommended.

Pregnancy: Since the use of benazepril during pregnancy can cause injury and even death of the developing fetus, patients should be advised to report promptly to their physician if they become pregnant.

Lactation: The presence of concentrations of ACE inhibitor have been reported in human milk. Use of ACE inhibitors is not recommended during breast-feeding.

ADVERSE EFFECTS: Benazepril has been evaluated for safety in over 6000 hypertensive patients. Over 400 elderly patients have participated in controlled hypertension trials. Long-term safety has been assessed in more than 700 patients treated for 1 year or more. There was no increase in the incidence of adverse reactions in elderly patients given the same daily dose. The overall frequency of adverse reactions was not related to duration of therapy or total daily dose.

The most severe adverse reactions occurring in clinical trials with benazepril were: angioedema (full clinical syndrome, 1 case; edema of lips or face without the other manifestations of angioedema, 0.5%), hypotension (0.3%), postural hypotension (0.4%) and syncope (0.1%). Hypotension or postural dizziness was a cause for discontinuation of therapy in <0.2% of patients treated with benazepril alone. Myocardial infarction and cerebral vascular accident occurred, possibly secondary to excessive hypotension in high risk patients (see Warnings).

The most frequent clinical adverse reactions in placebo-controlled clinical trials with benazepril monotherapy (N=964) were headache (6.2%), dizziness (3.6%), fatigue (2.4%), somnolence (1.6%), postural dizziness (1.5%), nausea (1.3%) and cough (1.2%). Discontinuation of therapy due to adverse experiences was required in 4% of patients treated with benazepril.

Adverse reactions occurring in 1% or more of the 2004 patients in controlled hypertension trials who were treated with benazepril monotherapy, are listed in Table 1.

Table 1: Lotensin

Adverse Reactions in Controlled Hypertension Trials

Body System	Patients (N=2004) %
Nervous System	
Headache	10.2
Dizziness	4.2
Somnolence	1.1
Vertigo	1.1
Respiratory	
Symptoms of upper respiratory tract infection	5.4
Increased cough	3.4
Flu symptoms	1.2
Gastrointestinal	
Nausea	2.5
Abdominal pain	2.4
Diarrhea	2.0
Dyspepsia	1.2
Musculoskeletal	
Musculoskeletal pain	2.6
Other	
Fatigue	3.6
Rhinitis	2.4
Pharyngitis	1.7
Back pain	1.7
Chest pain	1.2

Clinical adverse reactions occurring in less than 1% of patients treated with benazepril in controlled and uncontrolled clinical trials, and postmarketing experience, are listed below by body system: Incidence less than 1%:

Body as a Whole: asthenia.

Cardiovascular: excessive hypotension, angina pectoris, palpitations, myocardial infarction, cerebrovascular accident, arrhythmia.

Digestive: constipation, gastritis, vomiting, flatulence, melena, abdominal pain, pancreatitis.

Musculoskeletal: arthritis, arthralgia, myalgia.

Nervous: anxiety, depression, hypertonia, insomnia, nervousness, paresthesia, incoordination, decreased libido.

Respiratory: dyspnea, asthma, bronchitis.

Dermatologic: apparent hypersensitivity reactions (manifested by dermatitis, pruritus, or rash), photosensitivity, pemphigus, Stevens-Johnson syndrome and flushing.

Special Senses: tinnitus and taste disorders.

Urogenital: impaired renal function, impotence, pollakiuria.

Hematologic: leucopenia, eosinophilia, hemolytic anemia and thrombocytopenia.

Allergic and Immune Reactions: angioedema, lip edema, face edema.

Liver: hepatitis (predominantly cholestatic), cholestatic jaundice.

Abnormal Laboratory Findings: hyperkalemia (see Precautions).

Creatinine, Blood Urea Nitrogen: Increases in serum creatinine (>150% of baseline) were observed in 2% of patients treated with benazepril alone. Less than 0.1% of these patients developed simultaneous increases in blood urea nitrogen and serum creatinine. Increases are more likely to occur in patients receiving concomitant diuretic therapy than in those on benazepril alone. These increases often reversed on continued therapy.

Neutropenia: Neutrophil counts of less than 1500/mm³ occurred in 2% of patients treated with benazepril alone. No patient was discontinued from a study because of a low neutrophil or white blood cell (WBC) count. No patient developed a persistent neutrophil count <1000/mm³ and no patient developed a serious infection in association with a reduced neutrophil or WBC count. No patient treated with benazepril developed agranulocytosis (see Warnings).

Hemoglobin: Decreases in hemoglobin (a low value and a decrease of 5 g/dL) occurred in only 1 of 2014 patients receiving benazepril alone and in 1 of 1357 patients receiving benazepril plus a diuretic.

Hepatic: Elevations of liver enzymes and/or serum bilirubin have occurred (see Precautions).

Other: Elevations of uric acid and blood glucose have been reported, as have scattered incidents of hyponatremia and proteinuria.

Post-Market Adverse Drug Reactions: The following adverse events of unknown frequency have been reported during post-marketing use of benazepril: small bowel angioedema, anaphylactoid reactions, hyperkalemia, agranulocytosis, neutropenia (see Warnings).

OVERDOSE:

Symptoms: No data are available on overdosage in humans.

The most likely clinical manifestation of overdosage would be symptoms attributable to severe hypotension, for which the usual treatment is i.v. infusion of normal saline solution.

If ingestion is recent, then emesis should be induced. Although the active metabolite, benazeprilat, is only slightly dialyzable, renal dialysis may be useful in overdosed patients with severely impaired renal function.

Treatment: See Symptoms.

For management of a suspected drug overdose, CPhA recommends that you contact your **regional Poison Control Centre**. See the *CPS* Directory section for a list of Poison Control Centres.

DOSAGE: Dosage must be individualized. Initiation of therapy requires consideration of recent antihypertensive drug treatment, the extent of blood pressure elevation and salt restriction. The dosage of other antihypertensive agents being used with benazepril may need to be adjusted.

Monotherapy: The recommended initial dose of benazepril is 10 mg once daily. Dosage should be adjusted according to blood pressure response, generally, at intervals of at least 2 weeks. The usual maintenance dose is 20 mg daily. The maximum daily dose of benazepril is 40 mg.

In some patients treated once daily, the antihypertensive effect may diminish towards the end of the dosing interval. This can be evaluated by measuring blood pressure just prior to dosing to determine whether satisfactory control is being maintained for 24 hours. If it is not, either twice daily administration with the same total daily dose, or an increase in dose should be considered.

If blood pressure is not controlled with benazepril alone, a diuretic may be added. After the addition of a diuretic, it may be possible to reduce the dose of benazepril.

Concomitant Diuretic Therapy: Orthostatic hypotension occasionally may occur following the initial dose of benazepril and is more likely in patients who are currently being treated with a diuretic. The diuretic should, if possible, be discontinued for 2 to 3 days before beginning therapy with benazepril to reduce the likelihood of hypotension (see Warnings). If the diuretic cannot be discontinued, an initial dose of 5 mg benazepril should be used with careful medical supervision for several hours and until blood pressure has stabilized. The dosage of benazepril should subsequently be titrated (as described above) to the optimal response.

Dosage Adjustment in Renal Impairment: The usual dose of benazepril is recommended for patients with a creatinine clearance >30 mL/min [0.5 mL/s]. For patients with severe renal impairment (creatinine clearance of <30 mL/min [0.5 mL/s]), the initial daily dose is 5 mg. Titration must be individualized. The dosage may be titrated upwards to 10 mg/day. For further reductions in blood pressure the addition of a diuretic or another antihypertensive should be considered or alternatively, the dose of benazepril can be increased.

INFORMATION FOR THE PATIENT: Published in e-CPS, available by subscription at www.e-cps.ca.

SUPPLIED: 5 mg: Each light yellow, ovaloid, slightly biconvex, film-coated tablet, one side is imprinted LV, the other CG with a score on both sides, contains: benazepril HCl 5 mg. Nonmedicinal ingredients: cellulose compounds, colloidal silicon dioxide, cornstarch, crospovidone, hydrogenated castor oil, iron oxide, lactose, polyethylene glycol, talc and titanium dioxide. Blister packages of 28. Protect from heat (i.e., store at 15 to 30°C) and humidity.

10 mg: Each dark yellow, ovaloid, slightly biconvex, film-coated tablet, fully bisected on both sides, one side is engraved CG, the other HO, contains: benazepril HCl 10 mg. Nonmedicinal ingredients: cellulose compounds, colloidal silicon dioxide, cornstarch, crospovidone, hydrogenated castor oil, iron oxide, lactose, polyethylene glycol, talc and titanium dioxide. Blister packages of 28. Protect from heat (i.e., store at 15 to 30°C) and humidity.

20 mg: Each light orange, round, slightly biconvex, film-coated tablet, with bevelled edges, contains: benazepril HCl 20 mg. Nonmedicinal ingredients: cellulose compounds, colloidal silicon dioxide, cornstarch, crospovidone, hydrogenated castor oil, iron oxide, lactose, polyethylene glycol, talc and titanium dioxide. Blister packages of 28. Protect from heat (i.e., store at 15 to 30°C) and humidity.

(Shown in Product Identification Section)

Lotriderm® Ⓟ

clotrimazole—betamethasone dipropionate

Topical Antifungal—Corticosteroid

Schering-Plough

PHARMACOLOGY: Betamethasone dipropionate with clotrimazole combines the anti-inflammatory, antipruritic and vasoconstrictive activity of betamethasone dipropionate with the antifungal activity of clotrimazole. The primary action of clotrimazole is against dividing and growing organisms, possibly through reaction with the cell membrane.

INDICATIONS: For the topical treatment of the following fungal dermal infections complicated by inflammatory pruritus: tinea pedis, tinea cruris and tinea corporis due to *T. rubrum*, *T. mentagrophytes*, *E. floccosum*, and *M. canis*.

CONTRAINDICATIONS: In patients who are sensitive to betamethasone dipropionate, clotrimazole, other corticosteroids or imidazoles, or to any one of the components in this preparation.

Topical steroids are contraindicated in untreated bacterial and tubercular infections involving the skin and in certain viral diseases such as herpes simplex, chickenpox and vaccinia.

WARNINGS: Lotriderm should not be used in or near the eyes since this preparation is not formulated for ophthalmic use.

Pregnancy: There are no adequate and well-controlled studies in pregnant women on teratogenic effects of a topically applied combination of clotrimazole and betamethasone dipropionate. Therefore, this cream should be used during pregnancy only if the potential benefit justifies the potential risk to the fetus.

Drugs containing corticosteroids should not be used extensively on pregnant patients in large amounts or for prolonged periods of time.

Lactation: Since it is not known whether the components of Lotriderm cream are excreted in human milk, caution should be exercised when this product is administered to a nursing woman.

PRECAUTIONS: General: Systemic absorption of topical corticosteroids has produced reversible hypothalamic-pituitary-adrenal (HPA) axis suppression, manifestations of Cushing's syndrome, hyperglycemia and glucosuria in some patients.

Systemic absorption of topical corticosteroid agents will be increased with the use of more potent corticosteroid agents, with prolonged usage or if extensive body surface areas are treated. Therefore, patients receiving large doses of potent topical corticosteroids, applied to a large surface area should be evaluated periodically for evidence of HPA axis suppression. If HPA axis suppression occurs, an attempt should be made to withdraw the drug, to reduce the frequency of application, or to substitute with a less potent corticosteroid agent.

Recovery of HPA axis function is generally prompt and complete upon discontinuation of the drug. Infrequently, signs and symptoms of steroid withdrawal may occur, requiring supplemental systemic corticotherapy.

If irritation or hypersensitivity develops with the use of the cream, treatment should be discontinued and appropriate therapy instituted.

Suitable precautions should be taken in using topical corticosteroids in patients with stasis dermatitis and other skin diseases with impaired circulation.

Prolonged use of corticosteroid preparations may produce striae or atrophy of the skin or s.c. tissue. If this occurs, treatment should be discontinued.

Patients should be advised to inform subsequent physicians of the prior use of corticosteroids.

Children: Safety and effectiveness in children below the age of 12 have not been established with Lotriderm cream.

The use of Lotriderm Cream in diaper dermatitis is not recommended.

Pediatric patients may demonstrate greater susceptibility to topical corticosteroid-induced HPA axis suppression and Cushing's syndrome than mature patients because of a greater absorption due to a larger skin surface area to body weight ratio.

Hypothalamic-pituitary-adrenal (HPA) axis suppression, Cushing's syndrome and intracranial hypertension have been reported in children receiving topical corticosteroids. Manifestations of adrenal suppression in children include linear growth retardation, delayed weight gain, low plasma cortisol levels and absence of response to ACTH stimulation. Manifestations of intracranial hypertension include bulging fontanelles, headaches and bilateral papilledema.

Administration of topical dermatologics containing a corticosteroid to children should be limited to the least amount compatible with an effective therapeutic regimen. Chronic corticosteroid therapy may interfere with the growth and development of children.

Laboratory Tests: If there is a lack of response to the cream, appropriate microbiological studies should be repeated to confirm the diagnosis and rule out other pathogens before instituting another course of antimycotic therapy.

The following tests may be helpful in evaluating HPA axis suppression due to the corticosteroid component: urinary free cortisol test and ACTH stimulation test.

ADVERSE EFFECTS: The following adverse reactions have been reported in connection with the use of Lotriderm cream: paresthesia in 5 of 270 patients (1.85%), maculopapular rash, edema, and secondary infection, each in 1 of 270 (0.37%) patients.

Adverse reactions reported with the use of clotrimazole are as follows: erythema, stinging, blistering, peeling, edema, pruritus, urticaria and general irritation of the skin.

The following local adverse reactions are reported infrequently when topical corticosteroids are used as recommended. These reactions are listed in an approximate decreasing order of occurrence: burning, itching, irritation, dryness, folliculitis, hypertrichosis, acneiform eruptions, hypopigmentation, perioral dermatitis, allergic contact dermatitis, maceration of the skin, secondary infection, skin atrophy, striae and miliaria.

OVERDOSE:

No specific antidote is available and treatment should be symptomatic.

Symptoms: Betamethasone Dipropionate: Excessive or prolonged use of topical corticosteroids can suppress pituitary-adrenal function, resulting in secondary adrenal insufficiency, and produce manifestations of hypercorticism, including Cushing's disease. Clotrimazole: Overdosage by topical clotrimazole administration is highly improbable, since application of C^{14} labeled clotrimazole to intact or diseased skin under occlusive dressing for 6 hours did not yield measurable quantities (lower detection limit 0.001 µg/mL) of radioactive material in the sera of human subjects.

Treatment: Appropriate symptomatic treatment of corticosteroid overdosage is indicated. Acute hypercorticoid symptoms are usually reversible. Treat electrolyte imbalance, if necessary. In cases of chronic toxicity, slow withdrawal of corticosteroids is advised.

> For management of a suspected drug overdose, CPhA recommends that you contact your **regional Poison Control Centre**. See the *CPS* Directory section for a list of Poison Control Centres.

DOSAGE: A thin film of cream should be applied to cover completely the affected and surrounding skin areas twice daily, in the morning and at night, for 2 weeks in tinea cruris and tinea corporis and for 4 weeks in tinea pedis. The use of the cream for longer than 4 weeks is not recommended.

Clinical improvement, with relief of erythema and pruritus, usually occurs within 3 to 5 days of treatment. If a patient with tinea cruris and tinea corporis shows no clinical improvement after 1 week of treatment, the diagnosis should be reviewed. In tinea pedis, the treatment should be applied for 2 weeks prior to making that decision. Treatment with Lotriderm should be discontinued if the condition persists after 2 weeks in tinea cruris and tinea corporis and after 4 weeks in tinea pedis. Alternate therapy may then be instituted, if indicated, with an appropriate antifungal preparation.

Lotriderm cream should **not** be used with occlusive dressings.

SUPPLIED: Each g of white to off-white cream contains: clotrimazole USP 10 mg and 0.64 mg betamethasone dipropionate, USP, equivalent to 0.5 mg (0.05%) betamethasone USP, in a hydrophilic emollient cream. Nonmedicinal ingredients: benzyl alcohol, cetostearyl alcohol, mineral oil, phosphoric acid, polyethylene glycol 1000 monocetyl ether, propylene glycol, purified water, sodium phosphate monobasic monohydrate and white petrolatum. Sodium hydroxide to adjust pH. Tubes of 15 and 50 g. Store between 2 and 30°C.

Lovastatin ℞

CPhA Monograph

see *HMG-CoA Reductase Inhibitors*

> The reader is invited to consult CPhA's monograph **Heparins: Low Molecular Weight**.

Lovenox® ℞

enoxaparin sodium

Anticoagulant—Antithrombotic

sanofi-aventis

Lovenox® HP ℞

enoxaparin sodium

Anticoagulant—Antithrombotic

sanofi-aventis

Date of Revision: August 27, 2009

SUMMARY PRODUCT INFORMATION:

Route of Administration	Dosage Form/ Strength	All Nonmedicinal Ingredients
Subcutaneous injection & Intravenous injection	**LOVENOX–100 mg/mL** Pre-filled syringes with protective shield: 30 mg/0.3 mL, 40 mg/0.4 mL, 60 mg/0.6 mL, 80 mg/0.8 mL, 100 mg/1.0 mL	The pre-filled syringe contains water for injection.
	Multiple dose vial: 300 mg/3 mL	The vial contains 1.5% (w/v) benzyl alcohol as a preservative.
	LOVENOX HP–150 mg/mL Pre-filled syringes with protective shield: 120 mg/0.8 mL, 150 mg/1.0 mL	For composition, see Dosage Forms, Composition and Packaging.

INDICATIONS AND CLINICAL USE: LOVENOX (enoxaparin) is indicated for:

- The prophylaxis of thromboembolic disorders (deep vein thrombosis) in patients undergoing:
  - orthopedic surgery of the hip or knee; In addition, LOVENOX is indicated in hospital or after hospital discharge for long-term prevention of venous thromboembolic diseases following hip replacement surgery.
  - high risk abdominal, gynecological, or urological surgeries;
  - colorectal surgery.
- The prophylaxis of deep vein thrombosis (DVT) in medical patients who are at moderate risk of DVT and who are bedridden due to moderate to severe acute cardiac insufficiency (NYHA Class III or IV heart failure), acute respiratory failure revealing or complicating chronic respiratory insufficiency not requiring ventilatory support and acute respiratory infections (excluding septic shock), who require short-term prophylaxis of deep vein thrombosis.

LOVENOX is also indicated for:

- The treatment of deep vein thrombosis, with or without pulmonary embolism.
- The treatment of unstable angina or non-Q-wave myocardial infarction, concurrently with ASA.
- Treatment of acute ST-segment Elevation Myocardial Infarction (STEMI), including patients to be managed medically or with subsequent Percutaneous Coronary Intervention (PCI).

Geriatrics: Evidence from clinical studies and experience suggests that use in the geriatric population is associated with differences in safety and a brief discussion can be found in Warnings and Precautions, under Special Populations, Geriatrics.

In the clinical study for treatment of acute STEMI, with adjustment in dose for patients ≥75 years of age, there was no evidence of difference in efficacy between patients ≥75 years of age (n=1241) and patients less than 75 years of age (n=9015).

Pediatrics: No data is available.

CONTRAINDICATIONS:

- Hypersensitivity to LOVENOX (enoxaparin); or any of its constituents, including benzyl alcohol (when using multiple dose vials) (see Warnings and Precautions, Special Populations, Pregnant Women); or to other low molecular weight heparins and/or heparin.

  For composition, see Dosage Forms, Composition and Packaging.
- History of confirmed or suspected immunologically-mediated heparin-induced thrombocytopenia (delayed-onset severe thrombocytopenia), or in patients in whom an in vitro platelet-aggregation test in the presence of enoxaparin is positive.
- Acute or subacute bacterial endocarditis.
- Active bleeding.
- Major blood clotting disorders.
- Active gastric or duodenal ulcer.
- Hemorrhagic cerebrovascular accident (except if there are systemic emboli).
- Severe uncontrolled hypertension.
- Diabetic or hemorrhagic retinopathy.
- Other conditions or diseases involving an increased risk of hemorrhage.
- Injuries to and operations on the brain, spinal cord, eyes and ears.
- Spinal/epidural anaesthesia is contraindicated where repeated treatment doses of LOVENOX (1 mg/kg every 12 hours or 1.5 mg/kg once daily) are required, due to an increased risk of bleeding.

WARNINGS AND PRECAUTIONS: General: LOVENOX (enoxaparin) must not be administered by the intramuscular route.

LOVENOX cannot be used interchangeably (unit for unit) with unfractionated heparin (UFH) or other low molecular weight heparins (LMWHs) as they differ in their manufacturing process, molecular weight distribution, anti-Xa and anti-IIa activities, units and dosages. Special attention and compliance with instructions for use of each specific product is required during any change in treatment.

Determination of anti-Xa levels in plasma is the only method available for monitoring LOVENOX activity. The effect of LOVENOX on global clotting tests such as aPTT, PT and TT is dose-dependent. At lower doses, used in prophylaxis, LOVENOX does not prolong these tests. At higher doses, aPTT prolongation is observed but treatment cannot be monitored with these tests.

Measurement of peak anti-Xa levels at about 4 hours post-dose should be considered in patients at higher risk of bleeding and receiving LOVENOX, such as the elderly, patients with renal impairment or the extremes of body weight, during pregnancy, or for children. At treatment doses, peak anti-Xa levels should generally be maintained at no more than 1.5 IU/mL in these patients (see Action and Clinical Pharmacology, and Warnings and Precautions, Monitoring and Laboratory Tests).

Selection of General Surgery Patients: Risk factors associated with postoperative venous thromboembolism following general surgery include history of venous thromboembolism, varicose veins, obesity, heart failure, malignancy, previous long bone fracture of a lower limb, bed rest for more than 5 days prior to surgery, predicted duration of surgery of more than 30 minutes, age 60 years or above.

Selection of Orthopedic Surgery Patients: Major orthopedic surgery carried out on the lower extremities is associated with a higher risk of VTE, and a notable percentage of patients will develop a thrombosis if they are not given prophylaxis. Factors shown to predispose patient to VTE following major orthopedic surgery include a history of VTE, current obesity, delayed mobilization advanced age or cancer. Other risk factors that might be clinically important include congestive heart failure, chronic obstructive pulmonary disease (COPD) as well as female gender. High risk period for VTE lasts up to 3 months after hip surgery, therefore thromboprophylaxis should start as soon as possible and continue for up to 28 to 35 days after surgery. (ACCP guidelines 2004.)

Selection of Medical Patients: The risk factors for the development of thrombosis in the individual medical patient are important in determining whether thromboprophylaxis is appropriate. In one clinical trial, LOVENOX 40 mg once daily reduced the risk of the development of deep vein thrombosis (DVT) from 14.9% to 5.5% during the short term risk period in bedridden patients. Careful consideration should be given to the selection of patients. Patients at high risk of developing DVT or other thrombosis (such as patients with a malignant disease, a history of thrombophilia and known deficiency in antithrombin III, protein C or protein S, or APC resistance) are not candidates for therapy with LOVENOX 40 mg once daily because this dose may be inadequate for those patients. Furthermore, LOVENOX should not be given for thromboprophylaxis in medical patients who are bedridden due to infections with septic shock. Medical patients who require short term thromboprophylaxis for the risk of DVT due to severely restricted mobility during acute illness including moderate to severe heart failure, acute respiratory failure revealing or complicating chronic respiratory insufficiency not requiring ventilatory support, and acute respiratory infections may be selected for thromboprophylaxis with LOVENOX 40 mg once daily.

The safety and efficacy of LOVENOX 40 mg once daily following hospital discharge has not been established in the medical patient population. In the clinical trial mentioned above, thromboembolic events were not common following discontinuation of LOVENOX 40 mg at discharge. However, a significant number of patients did require antithrombotic therapy following discharge; specifically 13.63%. During the 3-month period following discharge, less than 1% of events were serious and included deep vein thrombosis, pulmonary embolism and death which is considered to be thromboembolic in origin. Therefore, the physician should consider whether thromboprophylaxis post-discharge would be necessary for the individual patient.

Gastrointestinal: LOVENOX should be used with caution in patients with gastrointestinal ulceration.

Hematologic: Hemorrhage: Bleeding may occur in conjunction with unfractionated heparin or low molecular weight heparin use. As with other anticoagulants, LOVENOX should be used with extreme caution in patients at increased risk of hemorrhage. Bleeding can occur at any site during therapy with LOVENOX. An unexpected drop in hematocrit or blood pressure should lead to a search for a bleeding site (see Adverse Reactions, Bleeding).

Thrombocytopenia: Thrombocytopenia of any degree should be monitored closely. Heparin-induced thrombocytopenia can occur with the administration of LOVENOX. Its incidence is unknown at present.

Platelets: Platelet counts should be determined prior to the commencement of treatment with LOVENOX and, subsequently, twice weekly for the duration of therapy.

Caution is recommended when administering LOVENOX to patients with congenital or drug induced thrombocytopenia, or platelet defects.

Hepatic/Biliary/Pancreatic: LOVENOX should be used with caution in patients with hepatic insufficiency.

Immune: During LOVENOX administration, special caution is necessary in rapidly developing thrombocytopenia and severe thrombocytopenia (<100 000/µL). A positive or indeterminate result obtained from in vitro tests for antiplatelet antibody in the presence of enoxaparin or other low molecular weight heparins and/or heparin would contraindicate LOVENOX.

Peri-Operative Considerations: Spinal/Epidural Hematomas: There have been cases of intra-spinal hematomas with the concurrent use of LOVENOX and spinal/epidural anesthesia resulting in long-term or permanent paralysis. The risk of these events may be higher with the use of post-operative indwelling epidural catheters or by the concomitant use of drugs affecting hemostasis: nonsteroidal anti-inflammatory drugs (NSAIDs), platelet inhibitors, or other drugs affecting coagulation including glycoprotein IIb/IIIa antagonists. The risk is greater with higher LOVENOX dosage regimens (e.g. at 1 mg/kg twice daily or 1.5 mg/kg once daily) than with prophylactic doses. The risk also appears to be increased by traumatic or repeated epidural or spinal procedure. **LOVENOX should only be used concurrently with spinal/epidural anaesthesia when the therapeutic benefits to the patients outweigh the possible risks (also see Contraindications).** When used concurrently, no spinal invasion should be performed for at least 12 hours following the last dose of LOVENOX (higher doses may require longer delays) and that the next dose should be held until at least 2 hours after the anaesthetic procedure. The same rules apply to the withdrawal or manipulation of the catheter. Careful vigilance for neurological signs such as: midline back pain, sensory and motor deficits (numbness or weakness in lower limbs), bowel and/or bladder dysfunction is recommended with rapid diagnosis and treatment, if signs occur (see Adverse Reactions).

Percutaneous Coronary Revascularisation Procedures: To minimize the risk of bleeding following the vascular instrumentation during the treatment of unstable angina, non-Q-wave myocardial infarction, and acute ST-segment elevation myocardial infarction, adhere precisely to the intervals recommended between LOVENOX injection doses. It is important to achieve hemostasis at the puncture site after PCI. In case a closure device is used, the sheath can be removed immediately. If a manual compression method is used, it is recommended to remove the sheath 6 hours after the last IV/SC injection. If the treatment with enoxaparin sodium is to be continued, the next scheduled dose should be given no sooner than 6 to 8 hours after sheath removal. The site of the procedure should be observed for signs of bleeding or hematoma formation. (See Dosage and Administration, Recommended Dose and Dosage Adjustment, Treatment of Unstable Angina or Non-Q-Wave Myocardial Infarction and Treatment of acute ST-Segment Elevation Myocardial Infarction.)

Renal: LOVENOX should be used with caution in patients with renal insufficiency.

LOVENOX dosage should be reduced in patients with severely impaired renal function (see Action and Clinical Pharmacology, Special Populations and Conditions, Renal Insufficiency, and Dosage and Administration, Use in Patients with Renal Impairment).

Patients with impaired renal function should be carefully monitored because half-life for anti-Xa activity after administration of low molecular weight heparin may be prolonged in this patient population (see Dosage and Administration, Use in Patients with Renal Impairment).

In patients with renal impairment, there is an increase in exposure to enoxaparin which increases the risk of bleeding. Since exposure to enoxaparin is significantly increased in patients with severe renal impairment (creatinine clearance <30 mL/min), a dosage adjustment is recommended for both therapeutic and prophylactic dosage ranges (see Action and Clinical Pharmacology, Special Populations and Conditions, Renal Insufficiency, and Dosage and Administration, Use in Patients with Renal Impairment).

Special Populations: Pregnant Women: The multiple dose vial of LOVENOX (300 mg/3 mL) contains benzyl alcohol as a preservative. Benzyl alcohol has been associated with a potentially fatal "Gasping Syndrome" in neonates. Manifestations of the disease included: metabolic acidosis, respiratory distress, gasping respirations, central nervous system dysfunction, convulsions, intracranial hemorrhages, hypoactivity, hypotonia, cardiovascular collapse and death. Because benzyl alcohol may cross the placenta, LOVENOX preserved with benzyl alcohol should not be used in pregnant women.

Teratogenic effects: As with other low molecular weight heparins, LOVENOX should not be used in pregnant women unless the therapeutic benefits to the patients outweigh the possible risks. There have been reports of congenital anomalies in infants born to women who received low molecular weight heparin during pregnancy including cerebral anomalies, limb anomalies, hypospadias, peripheral vascular malformation, fibrotic dysplasia and cardiac defects. A causal relationship has not been established nor has the incidence been shown to be higher than in the general population.

Non-teratogenic effects: There have been post-marketing reports of fetal death when pregnant women received low molecular weight heparins. Causality for these cases has not been established. Pregnant women receiving anticoagulants, including LOVENOX, are at increased risk for bleeding. Hemorrhage can occur at any site and may lead to death of mother and/or fetus. Pregnant women receiving LOVENOX should be carefully monitored. Pregnant women and women of child-bearing potential should be informed of the potential hazard to the fetus and the mother if LOVENOX is administered during pregnancy.

There are also postmarketing reports of prosthetic valve thrombosis in pregnant women with prosthetic heart valves while receiving low molecular weight heparins for thromboprophylaxis. These events led to maternal death or surgical interventions.

Pregnant women with prosthetic heart valves appear to be at exceedingly high risk of thromboembolism. An incidence of thromboembolism approaching 30% has been reported in these patients, in some cases even with apparent adequate anticoagulation at treatment doses of low molecular weight heparins or unfractionated heparin. Any attempt to anticoagulate such patients should normally only be undertaken by medical practitioners with documented expertise and experience in this clinical area.

Patients with Prosthetic Heart Valves: Cases of prosthetic valve thrombosis have been reported in patients who have received low molecular weight heparins for thromboprophylaxis. Some of these patients were pregnant women in whom thrombosis led to maternal and/or fetal deaths. Pregnant women are at higher risk of thromboembolism (see Warnings and Precautions, Pregnant Women).

Nursing Women: It is not known whether LOVENOX is excreted in human milk. Because many drugs are excreted in human milk, caution should be exercised when LOVENOX is administered to nursing women.

Pediatrics: The safety and effectiveness of LOVENOX in children has not been established.

Geriatrics: Elderly patients (especially patients eighty years of age and older) receiving low molecular weight heparins are at increased risk of bleeding. Careful attention to dosing and concomitant medications, especially anti-platelet preparations, is advised. Close monitoring of elderly patients with low body weight (e.g. <45 kg) and those predisposed to decreased renal function is recommended.

For treatment of acute ST-segment Elevation Myocardial Infarction in geriatric patients, the incidence of bleeding complications was higher in patients ≥65 years of age as compared to younger patients (<65 years). Patients ≥75 years of age did not receive a 30-mg IV bolus prior to the normal dosage regimen and had their SC dose adjusted to 0.75 mg/kg every 12 hours. (See Dosage and Administration, Recommended Dose and Dosage Adjustment, Treatment of acute ST-segment Elevation Myocardial Infarction, Geriatrics (≥75 years of age).)

Acute Coronary Disease: When thrombolytic treatment is considered appropriate in patients with unstable angina, non-Q-wave myocardial infarction and acute ST-segment Elevation Myocardial Infarction, the concomitant use of an anticoagulant such as LOVENOX may increase the risk of bleeding.

Medical Patients: LOVENOX at a dose of 40 mg once daily should not be given for thromboprophylaxis other than deep vein thrombosis (DVT) prevention or in medical patients who, in the opinion of the attending physician, would be at a higher risk of thromboembolism (such as patients with a malignant disease, a history of thrombophilia and known deficiency in antithrombin III, protein C or protein S, or APC resistance). Furthermore, LOVENOX should not be given for thromboprophylaxis in medical patients who are bedridden due to infections with septic shock. Patients with severe COPD complicated by right heart failure are candidates for another form of thromboprophylaxis. LOVENOX at a dose of 40 mg once daily has been studied in medical patients who require short term thromboprophylaxis to prevent the development of DVT while they are bedridden (6 to 11 days). If, in the opinion of the attending physician, longer thromboprophylaxis is necessary, then consideration should be given to a thromboprophylactic agent, which has been proven effective.

Patients with Extreme Body Weight: Safety and efficacy of low molecular weight heparins in high weight (e.g. >120 kg) and low weight (e.g. <45 kg) patients has not been fully determined. Individualised clinical and laboratory monitoring is recommended in these patients (see also Action and Clinical Pharmacology, Special Population and Conditions, Low-Weight Patients).

Monitoring and Laboratory Tests: LOVENOX has only a moderate prolonging effect on clotting time assays such as aPTT or thrombin time. For lab monitoring of effect, anti-Xa methods are recommended. Prolongation of aPTT during therapy with LOVENOX to the same extent as with unfractionated heparin should only be used as a criteria of overdose. Dose increases aimed at prolonging aPTT to the same extent as with unfractionated heparin could cause overdose and bleeding.

LOVENOX is administered subcutaneously, and therefore, the individual patient's antifactor Xa activity level will not remain within the range that would be expected with unfractionated heparin by continuous i.v. infusion throughout the entire dosing interval. In patients treated with enoxaparin 1.0 mg/kg twice daily for proximal deep vein thrombosis, mean peak plasma anti-Xa levels were 0.91 IU/mL. In patients given enoxaparin 1.0 mg/kg twice daily for acute treatment of unstable angina, peak anti-Xa activity levels were 1.0-1.1 IU/mL. At steady-state in patients given a 1.5 mg/kg qd regimen for treatment of DVT, mean peak activity was 1.7 IU anti-Xa/mL. The steady-state is practically achieved at the second or the third dose depending on the dosage regimen, once or twice daily, respectively. LOVENOX should be administered as directed (see Dosage and Administration).

As with all anti-thrombotic agents, there is a risk of systemic bleeding with LOVENOX administration. Consequently, therapy should not be started before primary hemostasis has been established and preferably no sooner than 12 hours after surgery, see Dosage and Administration. Care should be taken with LOVENOX use in high dose treatment of newly operated patients.

After treatment is initiated, patients should be carefully monitored for bleeding complications. This may be done by regular physical examination of the patients, close observation of the surgical drain and periodic measurements of hemoglobin, and anti-factor Xa determinations.

With normal prophylactic doses, LOVENOX does not modify global clotting tests of activated partial thromboplastin time (aPTT), prothrombin time (PT) and thrombin clotting time (TT). Therefore, treatment cannot be monitored with these tests.

At higher doses, increases in aPTT (activated partial thromboplastin time) and ACT (activated clotting time) may occur. Increases in aPTT and ACT are not linearly correlated with increasing enoxaparin antithrombotic activity and therefore are unsuitable and unreliable for monitoring enoxaparin activity.

ADVERSE REACTIONS: Adverse Drug Reaction Overview: Bleeding: As with any antithrombotic treatment, hemorrhagic manifestations can occur (also see Adverse Reactions, Local Reactions).

The incidence of major hemorrhagic complications during LOVENOX treatment has been low and generally did not differ from that observed with unfractionated heparin. Patients taking LOVENOX are at risk for major bleeding complications when the plasma anti-factor Xa levels approach 2.0 IU/mL. Other risk factors associated with bleeding on therapy with heparins include a serious concurrent illness, chronic heavy alcohol consumption, use of platelet inhibiting drugs, renal failure, age and possibly, the female gender. Petechiae or easy bruising may precede frank hemorrhage. Bleeding may range from minor local hematoma to major hemorrhage. The early signs of bleeding may include epistaxis, hematuria, or melena. Bleeding may occur at any site and may be difficult to detect; such as retroperitoneal bleeding. Bleeding may also occur from surgical sites.

Major hemorrhage, including retroperitoneal and intracranial bleeding, has been reported in association with LOVENOX use, in some cases leading to fatality.

Local Reactions: Pain and mild local irritation may follow the subcutaneous injection of enoxaparin sodium. Rarely, hard inflammatory nodules have been observed at the injection site. Injection site hematomas are a common side effect with LOVENOX (enoxaparin) occurring at a frequency of 5% or less with lower (prophylaxis) doses to 10% or more with higher (treatment) doses.

Clinical Trial Adverse Drug Reactions: Because clinical trials are conducted under very specific conditions the adverse drug reaction rates observed in the clinical trials may not reflect the rates observed in practice and should not be compared to the rates in the clinical trials of another drug. Adverse drug reaction information from clinical trials is useful for identifying drug-related adverse events and for approximating rates.

The following rates of major bleeding events have been reported during clinical trials with LOVENOX (see Table 1, Table 2, Table 3, Table 4, Table 5,Table 6 and Table 7).

Table 1: LOVENOX

Major Bleeding Episodes Following Abdominal and Colorectal Surgery[a]

Indications	Dosing Regimen: LOVENOX 40 mg qd SC	Dosing Regimen: Heparin 5000 U q8h SC
Abdominal Surgery[b]	n=555 23 (4%)	n=560 16 (3%)
Colorectal Surgery[b]	n=673 28 (4%)	n=674 21 (3%)

[a] Bleeding complications were considered major: (1) if the hemorrhage caused a significant clinical event, or (2) if accompanied by a hemoglobin decrease ≥2 g/dL or transfusion of 2 or more units of blood products. Retroperitoneal, intraocular, and intracranial hemorrhages were always considered major.

[b] LOVENOX 40 mg qd SC initiated two hours prior to surgery and continued for up to 12 days after surgery.

Table 2: LOVENOX

Major Bleeding Episodes Following Hip or Knee Replacement Surgery[a]

Indications	Dosing Regimen: LOVENOX 30 mg q12h SC	Dosing Regimen: Heparin 15 000 U/24h SC
Hip Replacement Surgery[b]	n=786 31 (4%)	n=541 32 (6%)
Knee Replacement Surgery[b]	n=294 3 (1%)	n=225 3 (1%)

[a] Bleeding complications were considered major: (1) if the hemorrhage caused a significant clinical event, or (2) if accompanied by a hemoglobin decrease ≥2 g/dL or transfusion of 2 or more units of blood products. Retroperitoneal and intracranial hemorrhages were always considered major. In the knee replacement surgery trials, intraocular hemorrhages were also considered major hemorrhages.

[b] LOVENOX 30 mg every 12 hours SC initiated 12 to 24 hours after surgery and continued for up to 14 days after surgery.

Note: At no time point were the 40 mg once a day pre-operative and the 30 mg every 12 hours post-operative hip replacement surgery prophylactic regimens compared in clinical trials.

Table 3: LOVENOX

Major Bleeding Episodes Following Hip or Knee Replacement Surgery with Extended Prophylaxis[a]

Indications	Dosing Regimen: Initial Prophylaxis[b]: LOVENOX 30 mg q12h SC	Initial Prophylaxis[b]: LOVENOX 40 mg qd SC	Extended Prophylaxis[c]: LOVENOX 40 mg qd SC	Extended Prophylaxis[c]: Placebo qd SC
Hip Replacement Surgery	n=475 8 (1.7%)	N=288 3 (1.0%)	n=445 0 (0%)	N=431 (0%)
Knee Replacement Surgery[d]	n=493 8 (1.6%)	—	n=217 0 (0%)	N=221 1 (0%)

[a] Bleeding complications were considered major: (1) if the hemorrhage caused a significant clinical event, or (2) if accompanied by a hemoglobin decrease ≥2 g/dL or transfusion of 2 or more units of blood products. Retroperitoneal and intracranial hemorrhages were always considered major.

[b] Initial Prophylaxis hospital phase: In the multicentre study 307, LOVENOX 30 mg q12h SC for 7–10 days, initiated within 12–24 hours postoperatively; in the single-centre study PK537, LOVENOX 40 mg qd SC initiated 12±2 hours before surgery, repeated on the day of the surgery and continued for 9±2 days.

[c] Extended Prophylaxis outpatient phase: In the multicentre study 307, LOVENOX 40 mg qd SC for 18–21 days; in the single-centre studies PK537 and ENX491001, LOVENOX 40 mg qd SC 21±2 days.

[d] Initial Prophylaxis hospital phase: In the multicentre study 307, LOVENOX 30 mg q12h SC for 7–10 days, initiated within 12–24 hours postoperatively; Extended Prophylaxis outpatient phase: In the multicentre study 307.

Table 4: LOVENOX

Major Bleeding Episodes in Medical Patients with Severely Restricted Mobility During Acute Illness[a]

Indications	Dosing Regimen: LOVENOX[b] 40 mg qd SC	Dosing Regimen: Placebo[b]
Medical Patients During Acute Illness[c]	n=360 3 (<1%)	n=362 2 (<1%)

[a] Bleeding complications were considered major: (1) if the hemorrhage caused a significant clinical event, (2) if the hemorrhage caused a decrease in hemoglobin of ≥2 g/dL or transfusion of 2 or more units of blood products. Retroperitoneal and intracranial hemorrhages were always considered major although none were reported during the trial.

[b] The rates represent major bleeding on study medication up to 24 hours after last dose.

[c] Usual duration of treatment 6 to 11 days.

Adverse Reactions in LOVENOX Injection Treated Patients with Acute ST-Segment Elevation Myocardial Infarction: In a clinical trial in patients with acute ST-segment elevation myocardial infarction, the only additional possibly related adverse reaction that occurred at a rate of at least 0.5% in the Lovenox group was thrombocytopenia (1.5%).

Post-Market Adverse Drug Reactions: Skeletal Effects: Use of low molecular weight heparins over extended periods has been reported to be associated with development of osteopenia.

Liver: Transient, asymptomatic elevations of liver transaminases (AST and ALT) to greater than three times the upper limit of normal has been observed in up to 6% of patients taking LOVENOX. This is a consistent finding with all members of the LMWH class, as well as with unfractionated heparin. The mechanism associated with the increased levels of liver transaminases has not been elucidated. No consistent irreversible liver damage has been observed. Transaminase levels returned to normal within 3 to 7 days after discontinuation of enoxaparin.

Table 5: LOVENOX

Major Bleeding Episodes in Unstable Angina and Non-Q-Wave Myocardial Infarction

Indication	Dosing Regimen	
	LOVENOX[a] 1 mg/kg q12h SC	**Heparin[a] aPTT Adjusted i.v. Therapy**
Unstable Angina and Non-Q-Wave MI[b,c]	n=1578 17 (1%)	n=1529 18 (1%)

[a] The rates represent major bleeding on study medication up to 12 hours after last dose with treatment for up to 8 days.
[b] ASA therapy was administered concurrently (100 to 325 mg per day).
[c] Bleeding complications were considered major: (1) if the hemorrhage caused a significant clinical event, or (2) if accompanied by a hemoglobin decrease by ≥3 g/dL or transfusion of 2 or more units of blood products. Intraocular, retroperitoneal, and intracranial hemorrhages were always considered major.

Table 6: LOVENOX

Major Bleeding Episodes in Treatment of Deep Vein Thrombosis with or Without Pulmonary Embolism Treatment[a]

Indication	Dosing Regimen[b]		
	LOVENOX 1.5 mg/kg qd SC	**LOVENOX 1 mg/kg q12h SC**	**Heparin aPTT Adjusted i.v. Therapy**
Treatment of DVT, with or without PE	n=298 5 (2%)	n=559 9 (2%)	n=554 9 (2%)

[a] Bleeding complications were considered major: (1) if the hemorrhage caused a significant clinical event, or (2) if accompanied by a hemoglobin decrease ≥2 g/dL or transfusion of 2 or more units of blood products. Retroperitoneal, intraocular, and intracranial hemorrhages were always considered major.
[b] All patients also received warfarin (dose-adjusted according to PT to achieve an INR of 2.0 to 3.0) commencing within 72 hours of LOVENOX or standard heparin therapy and continuing for up to 90 days. LOVENOX or standard heparin therapy was discontinued after a therapeutic oral anticoagulant effect was achieved in general about 7 days after treatment initiation.

Table 7: LOVENOX

Major Bleeding Episodes in Acute ST-segment Elevation Myocardial Infarction

Indication	Dosing Regimen	
	Lovenox Initial 30-mg IV bolus followed by 1 mg/kg q12h SC[a]	**Heparin aPTT Adjusted IV Therapy**
Acute ST-segment Elevation Myocardial Infarction	n=10 176	n=10 151
Major bleeding (including ICH)	211 (2.1%)	138 (1.4%)
Intracranial hemorrhages (ICH)	84 (0.8%)	66 (0.7%)

[a] Patients ≥75 years of age did not receive a 30-mg IV bolus prior to the normal dosage regimen and had their SC dose adjusted to 0.75 mg/kg every 12 hours.
The rates represent major bleeding (including ICH) up to 30 days.
Bleedings were considered major if the hemorrhage caused a significant clinical event associated with a hemoglobin decrease by ≥5 g/dL. ICH were always considered major.

Hypersensitivity: Thrombocytopenia, skin rash (including bullous eruptions), purpura, allergic reactions and skin necrosis usually occurring at the injection site are rare, and occur with all low molecular weight heparins. Skin necrosis is usually preceded by purpura or erythematous plaques, infiltrated and painful. In case such reaction is observed, treatment with enoxaparin sodium must be discontinued. Hypersensitivity reactions, including angioedema and anaphylactic/anaphylactoid reactions, have been observed rarely with unfractionated heparin and low molecular weight heparins. Very rare cases of hypersensitivity cutaneous vasculitis have been reported. These cases may include leukocytoclastic vasculitis. LOVENOX should be discontinued in patients showing local or systemic allergic responses.

Heparin-Induced Thrombocytopenia: Severe immunologically-mediated thrombocytopenia has been observed rarely with LOVENOX use, resulting in arterial and/or venous thrombosis or thromboembolism (see Warnings and Precautions, Hematologic, Thrombocytopenia, Platelets, Immune). In some cases thrombosis was complicated by organ infarction or limb ischemia.

Hyperkalaemia: Cases of hyperkalaemia have been reported with heparins and Low Molecular Weight Heparins.

DRUG INTERACTIONS: Drug-Drug Interactions: It is recommended that agents which affect hemostasis should be discontinued prior to LOVENOX therapy unless strictly indicated. If the combination is indicated, LOVENOX should be used with careful clinical and laboratory monitoring when appropriate.

LOVENOX should be used with caution in patients receiving oral anticoagulants, platelet inhibitors and thrombolytic agents because of increased risk of bleeding. Aspirin, unless contraindicated, is recommended in patients treated for unstable angina or non-Q-wave myocardial infarction and acute ST-segment Elevation Myocardial Infarction (see Dosage and Administration).

Drug-Laboratory Interactions: Since LOVENOX use may be associated with a rise in hepatic transaminases, this observation should be considered when liver funtion tests are assessed (see Adverse Reactions, Post-market Adverse Drug Reactions, Liver).

DOSAGE AND ADMINISTRATION: **Dosing Considerations: LOVENOX must not be administered by the intramuscular route.**

Subcutaneous Injection: Enoxaparin sodium is administered by subcutaneous injection for the prevention of venous thromboembolic disease, treatment of deep vein thrombosis, treatment of unstable angina and non-Q-wave myocardial infarction and treatment of acute ST-segment Elevation Myocardial Infarction.

For subcutaneous use LOVENOX should not be mixed with other injections or infusions.

IV Bolus Injection: For acute ST-segment Elevation Myocardial Infarction, treatment is to be initiated with a single IV bolus injection immediately followed by a subcutaneous injection.

Recommended Dose and Dosage Adjustment: Prophylaxis in Conjunction with Hip or Knee Surgery: The recommended dose of LOVENOX is 30 mg (3000 IU) every 12 hours administered by subcutaneous injection. Provided that hemostasis has been established, the initial dose should be given 12 to 24 hours after surgery. The usual duration of treatment is from 7 to 14 days.

Treatment should be continued for as long as the risk of DVT persists. Continued therapy with LOVENOX 40 mg once daily for 3 weeks following the initial phase of thromboprophylaxis in hip replacement surgery patients has been proven to be beneficial.

Prophylaxis in Conjunction with Abdominal or Colorectal Surgery: In patients undergoing abdominal surgery who are at risk for thromboembolic complications, the recommended dose of LOVENOX is 40 mg (4000 IU) once daily administered by subcutaneous injection, with the initial dose given 2 hours prior to surgery (see Warnings and Precautions, General, Selection of General Surgery Patients). The usual duration of treatment is from 7 to 10 days for a maximum of 12 days.

Prophylaxis in Medical Patients: In medical patients at risk for deep vein thrombosis due to severely restricted mobility during acute illness (see Warnings and Precautions, General, Selection of Medical Patients), the recommended dose of LOVENOX is 40 mg (4000 IU) once daily by subcutaneous injection. The usual duration of administration is 6 to 11 days.

Treatment of Deep Vein Thrombosis, with or without Pulmonary Embolism: LOVENOX can be administered subcutaneously either as 1.5 mg/kg once daily or as twice daily injections of 1 mg/kg.

The 1.5 mg/kg once daily dose is the equivalent of 150 IU/kg and should be given at the same time every day. The single daily dose should not exceed 18 000 IU. The expected plasma anti-Xa levels during subcutaneous treatment, when enoxaparin is used as the reference standard, would be <0.3 IU anti-Xa/mL before injection and <1.7 IU anti-Xa/mL 3-4 hours post injection. The measurement of plasma anti-Xa circulating activities depends on the experimental conditions of the assay, particularly on the reference standard used.

In patients with complicated thromboembolic disorders (i.e. with increased risk of recurrent VTE such as obese patients, cancer patients or patients with symptomatic PE), a dose of 1 mg/kg administered twice daily is recommended. This is the equivalent of 100 IU/kg. The expected plasma anti-Xa levels during subcutaneous treatment, when enoxaparin is used as the reference standard, would be <0.3 IU anti-Xa/mL before injection and <1.15 IU anti-Xa/mL 3-4 hours post injection.

Oral anticoagulant therapy should be initiated as soon as possible, and LOVENOX should be continued until a therapeutic anticoagulant effect has been achieved (INR: 2 to 3), in general for approximately 7 days.

Treatment of Unstable Angina or Non-Q-Wave Myocardial Infarction: The recommended dose of LOVENOX is 1 mg/kg every 12 hours by subcutaneous injection. This is the equivalent of 100 IU/kg. The maximum dose should not exceed 10 000 IU / 12 hours. The expected plasma anti-Xa levels during subcutaneous treatment would be <0.3 IU anti-Xa/mL before injection and <1.15 IU anti-Xa/mL 3-4 hours after injection. Treatment should continue for a minimum of 2 days until clinical stabilization has been achieved, in general, for up to 8 days. The effect of the short-term treatment was sustained over a one-year period.

Concomitant therapy with ASA (100 to 325 mg once daily) is recommended. (See Warnings and Precautions, Peri-Operative considerations, Percutaneous Coronary Revascularisation Procedures.)

Treatment of acute ST-Segment Elevation Myocardial Infarction: In patients with acute ST-segment elevation myocardial infarction, the recommended dose of LOVENOX injection is a **single IV bolus of 30 mg** plus a 1 mg/kg SC dose followed by 1 mg/kg administered SC every 12 hours (maximum 100 mg for the first two doses only, followed by 1 mg/kg dosing for the remaining doses). For dosage in patients ≥75 years of age, see section below entitled Geriatrics (≥75 years of age). When administered in conjunction with a thombolytic (fibrin specific or non-fibrin specific), LOVENOX injection should be given between 15 minutes before and 30 minutes after the start of fibrinolytic therapy. All patients should receive acetylsalicylic acid (ASA) as soon as they are identified as having STEMI and maintained with 75 to 325 mg once daily unless contraindicated. The recommended duration of LOVENOX injection treatment is 8 days or until hospital discharge, whichever comes first.

For Patients Managed with Percutaneous Coronary Intervention (PCI): If the last LOVENOX SC administration was given less than 8 hours before balloon inflation, no additional dosing is needed. If the last LOVENOX SC administration was given more than 8 hours before balloon inflation, an IV bolus of 0.3 mg/kg of LOVENOX injection should be administered. (See Warnings and Precautions, Peri-Operative considerations, Percutaneous Coronary Revascularisation Procedures.)

Geriatrics (≥75 years of age): For treatment of acute ST-segment Elevation Myocardial Infarction in geriatric patients ≥75 years of age, do not use an initial IV bolus. Initiate dosing with 0.75 mg/kg SC every 12 hours (maximum 75 mg for the first two doses only, followed by 0.75 mg/kg dosing for the remaining doses). No dose adjustment is necessary for other indications in geriatric patients unless kidney function is impaired.

Use in Patients with Renal Impairment: All patients with renal impairment treated with low molecular weight heparins should be monitored carefully.

Exposure to enoxaparin increases with degree of renal impairment. In patients with renal impairment, the increased exposure to enoxaparin has been shown to increase risk of bleeding (see Action and Clinical Pharmacology, Special Populations and Conditions, Renal Insufficiency).

A dosage adjustment is required for patients with severe renal impairment (creatinine clearance <30 mL/min) since enoxaparin exposure is significantly increased in this patient population. The following dosage adjustments are recommended for prophylaxis and treatment in patients with **severe** renal impairment:

- For prophylaxis in conjunction with hip or knee orthopedic surgery, the recommended dosage is **30 mg (3000 IU) once daily**
- For prophylaxis in conjunction with abdominal or colorectal surgery, or for prophylaxis in medical patients at risk of DVT, the recommended dosage is **20 mg (2000 IU) or 30 mg (3000 IU) once daily** based on individual risk/benefit assessment
- For treatment of deep vein thrombosis, with or without pulmonary embolism, the recommended dosage is **1 mg/kg once daily**
- For treatment of unstable angina or non-Q-wave myocardial infarction, the recommended dosage is **1 mg/kg once daily**.
- For treatment of acute ST-segment Elevation Myocardial Infarction, the recommended dosage is **30 mg-single IV bolus plus a 1 mg/kg SC dose followed by 1 mg/kg administered SC once daily.**
- For treatment of acute ST-segment Elevation Myocardial Infarction in geriatric patients ≥75 years of age, the recommended dosage is **1 mg/kg administered SC once daily (no initial bolus)**.

Dosage adjustment may also need to be considered in patients who have renal characteristics close to those of patients with severe renal impairment.

Administration: Subcutaneous Injection Technique: The subcutaneous injection of LOVENOX should be carried out with the patient sitting or lying down in a comfortable position. Inject in the subcutaneous tissue of the anterolateral and posterolateral abdominal girdle, alternatively on the left and right sides. With the thickness of skin held between the operator's thumb and finger, introduce the entire length of the needle vertically into the skin.

Intravenous (Bolus) Injection Technique: LOVENOX should be administered through an intravenous line. LOVENOX should not be mixed or co-administered with other medications. To avoid the possible mixture of LOVENOX with other drugs, the intravenous access chosen should be flushed with a sufficient amount of saline or dextrose solution prior to and following the intravenous bolus administration of LOVENOX to clear the port of drug. LOVENOX may be safely administered with normal saline solution (0.9%) or 5% dextrose in water.

Initial 30-mg Bolus: The initial 30-mg bolus can be administered, using the multiple dose vial or enoxaparin sodium pre-filled syringe. When pre-filled syringes are used, expel the excessive volume if needed, to retain only 30 mg (0.3 mL) in the syringe. The 30-mg dose can then be directly injected into the intravenous line.

Additional Bolus for PCI When Last SC Administration Was Given More Than 8 Hours Before Balloon Inflation: For patients being managed with Percutaneous Coronary Intervention (PCI), an additional IV bolus of 0.3 mg/kg is to be administered if last SC administration was given more than 8 hours before balloon inflation (see Dosage and Administration, Recommended Dose and Dosage Adjustment, For Patients Managed with Percutaneous Coronary Intervention (PCI)).

In order to assure the accuracy of the small volume to be injected, it is recommended to dilute the drug.

For example, to obtain a 3-mg/mL solution, using a 60-mg enoxaparin sodium pre-filled syringe, it is recommended to use a 50-mL infusion bag (i.e. using either normal saline solution (0.9%) or 5% dextrose in water) as follows: Withdraw 30 mL from the infusion bag with a syringe and discard the liquid. Inject the complete contents of the 60-mg enoxaparin sodium pre-filled syringe into the 20 mL remaining in the bag. Gently mix the contents of the bag. Withdraw the required volume of diluted solution with a syringe for administration into the intravenous line.

After dilution is completed, the volume to be injected can be calculated using the following formula [Volume of diluted solution (mL) = Patient weight (kg)×0.1] or using Table 8. The dilution should be prepared immediately before use.

Table 8: LOVENOX

Volume to Be Injected Through Intravenous Line After Dilution Is Completed

Weight [kg]	Required Dose (0.3 mg/kg) [mg]	Volume to Inject When Diluted to a Final Concentration of 3 mg/mL [mL]
45	13.5	4.5
50	15	5
55	16.5	5.5
60	18	6
65	19.5	6.5
70	21	7
75	22.5	7.5

(cont'd)

Table 8: LOVENOX *(cont'd)*

Volume to Be Injected Through Intravenous Line After Dilution Is Completed

Weight [kg]	Required Dose (0.3 mg/kg) [mg]	Volume to Inject When Diluted to a Final Concentration of 3 mg/mL [mL]
80	24	8
85	25.5	8.5
90	27	9
95	28.5	9.5
100	30	10

Care should be taken to ensure use of the correct formulation, either LOVENOX (100 mg/mL concentration) or LOVENOX HP (150 mg/mL concentration), when using these products.

Important: When the LOVENOX dose to be given is equivalent to the full amount of the pre-filled syringe, no attempt should be made to expel air prior to giving the injection. If the graduated syringes (60 mg/0.6 mL, 80 mg/0.8 mL, 100 mg/1.0 mL, 120 mg/0.8 mL, 150 mg/1.0 mL) are used and the dose of LOVENOX has to be adjusted, it is necessary to expel the air bubble and any excess drug solution.

Under normal conditions of use, LOVENOX does not modify global clotting tests of activated partial thromboplastin time (aPTT), prothrombin time (PT) and thrombin clotting time (TT). Therefore treatment can not be monitored with these tests. The plasma levels of the drug can be verified by measuring anti-Xa and anti-IIa activities.

OVERDOSAGE:

Accidental overdosage following administration of LOVENOX (enoxaparin) may lead to hemorrhagic complications. LOVENOX should be immediately discontinued, at least temporarily, in cases of significant excess dosage. In more serious cases, protamine should be administered.

The anticoagulant effect of LOVENOX is inhibited by protamine. This effect may be largely neutralized by slow intravenous injection of protamine sulfate. However, even with higher doses of protamine, the aPTT may remain prolonged to a greater extent than usually seen with unfractionated heparin. Anti-factor Xa activity is never completely neutralized (maximum about 60%).

In the event that prompt reversal of the anticoagulant effects of enoxaparin is required at any time after LOVENOX dosing, Table 9 is provided as a guide for initial use of protamine. Attending physicians confronted with a potential overdosage of enoxaparin should always use their best clinical judgment in determining the appropriate dosing regimen of protamine to be administered.

Table 9: LOVENOX

Neutralization of Enoxaparin by Protamine

	Time Since LOVENOX Dose		
	≤8 hours	>8 hours and ≤12 hours	>12 hours
Protamine dose	1 mg protamine per 1 mg enoxaparin	0.5 mg protamine per 1 mg enoxaparin	may not be required

A second infusion of 0.5 mg protamine per 1 mg LOVENOX may be administered if the aPTT measured 2 to 4 hours after the first infusion remains prolonged.

Particular care should be taken to avoid overdosage with protamine sulfate. Administration of protamine sulfate can cause severe hypotensive and anaphylactoid reactions. Because fatal reactions, often resembling anaphylaxis, have been reported with protamine sulfate, it should be given only when resuscitation equipment and treatment of anaphylactic shock are readily available.

For management of a suspected drug overdose, contact your **regional Poison Control Centre**. See the *CPS* Directory section for a list of Poison Control Centres.

ACTION AND CLINICAL PHARMACOLOGY: Mechanism of Action: LOVENOX (enoxaparin) is a low molecular weight heparin fragment, which is obtained by controlled depolymerization of natural heparin from porcine intestinal mucosa. It possesses antithrombotic action. Enoxaparin is composed of molecules with and without a specially characterized pentasaccharide, the antithrombin binding site, that is essential for high affinity binding to the plasma protein antithrombin (formerly referred to as antithrombin III). With a molecular weight range of 3800-5000 daltons (versus 15 000 daltons for heparin), the enoxaparin molecule is too small to bind simultaneously to thrombin and antithrombin, the primary anticoagulant factor in blood.

The mechanism of action of enoxaparin is antithrombin-dependent. It acts mainly by accelerating the rate of the neutralization of certain activated coagulation factors by antithrombin, but other mechanisms may also be involved. Enoxaparin potentiates preferentially the inhibition of coagulation factors Xa and IIa and only slightly affects other hemostatic mechanisms such as clotting time. The antithrombotic effect of enoxaparin is well correlated to the inhibition of factor Xa.

The ratio of anti-Xa/anti-IIa activity is greater than 4 with enoxaparin (whereas this ratio is equal to 1 with heparin). This dissociation between anti-Xa and anti-IIa activities has been shown in experimental models with an antithrombotic activity comparable to that of heparin while the bleeding effect is reduced. In man, clinical trials have not shown a causal relationship between the ratio of anti-Xa/anti-IIa activity and clinical/pharmacological effect.

LOVENOX cannot be measured directly in the bloodstream. Rather the effect on clotting mechanisms is measured. Heparin dosage is monitored by both prolongation of aPTT and by anti-Xa activity. For enoxaparin, the aPTT may not be significantly prolonged relative to unfractionated heparin at prophylactic doses, and at therapeutic doses aPTT prolongation is not used to measure the therapeutic effect of LOVENOX. Enoxaparin potency is described in international anti-Xa units (e.g., 1 mg of enoxaparin is equivalent to 100 IU of anti-Xa).

Pharmacokinetics: Absorption: The pharmacokinetics of enoxaparin have been studied on the basis of plasma levels of anti-Xa activity. The mean absolute bioavailability of enoxaparin, when given subcutaneously, is about 92% in healthy volunteers.

The mean peak plasma anti-Xa activity is observed 3 to 5 hours after subcutaneous injection. Levels of approximately 0.2, 0.4, 1.0 and 1.3 anti-Xa IU/mL were seen in healthy volunteers, following a single subcutaneous administration of 20 mg, 40 mg, 1 mg/kg and 1.5 mg/kg, respectively.

Enoxaparin pharmacokinetics appear to be linear over the recommended dosage ranges. After repeated subcutaneous administration of the 1 mg/kg twice daily regimen, the steady-state is reached from Day 3 to 4 with mean exposure about 65% higher than after a single dose. Mean peak and trough levels of about 1.2 and 0.52 IU/mL respectively were seen with this regimen.

A 30 mg IV bolus immediately followed by a 1 mg/kg SC every 12 hours provided initial peak anti-Factor Xa levels of 1.16 IU/mL (n=16) and average exposure corresponding to 88% of steady-state levels. Steady state is achieved on the second day of treatment.

Distribution: The volume of distribution of enoxaparin is about 5 liters. Following subcutaneous dosing, the apparent clearance of enoxaparin is approximately 15 mL/min.

Information from a clinical trial with a very small number of volunteers indicates that enoxaparin, as detected by anti-factor Xa activity, does not appear to cross the placental barrier, at least during the second trimester of pregnancy.

Metabolism: Enoxaparin is metabolized in the liver by desulfation and depolymerization.

Excretion: Elimination appears monophasic with a half-life of about 4 hours after a single subcutaneous dose and about 7 hours after repeated dosing, in healthy volunteers.

The main route of elimination is via the kidney. Renal clearance of active fragments represents about 10% of the administered dose and total renal excretion of active and non-active fragments 40% of the dose.

Pharmacokinetic interaction: No pharmacokinetic interaction was observed between enoxaparin and thrombolytics when administered concomitantly.

Special Populations and Conditions: Geriatrics: Based on the results of a population pharmacokinetic analysis, the enoxaparin kinetic profile is not different in elderly subjects compared to younger subjects when renal function is normal. However, since renal function is known to decline with age, elderly patients may show reduced elimination of enoxaparin (see Warnings and Precautions, Renal and Special Populations, Geriatrics).

Low-Weight Patients: When non-weight-adjusted dosing was administered, after a single-subcutaneous 40 mg dose, anti-Xa exposure was observed to be 52% higher in low-weight women (<45 kg) and 27% higher in low-weight men (<57 kg) when compared to normal weight control subjects, which may lead to a higher risk of bleeding (see Warnings and Precautions, Special Populations, Patients with Extreme Body Weight).

Renal Insufficiency: A linear relationship between anti-Xa plasma clearance and creatinine clearance at steady-state has been observed, indicating decreased clearance of enoxaparin in patients with reduced renal function.

Anti-Xa exposure at steady-state, represented by AUC, is increased about 34% in mild renal impairment (creatinine clearance 50-80 mL/min), about 72% in moderate renal impairment (creatinine clearance 30-50 mL/min), and about 95% in severe renal impairment (creatinine clearance <30 mL/min) upon administration of enoxaparin 1.5 mg/kg once daily sc for 4 days. Anti-Xa exposure at steady-state is increased about 33% in mild renal impairment, about 46% in moderate and about 97% in severe renal impairment upon administration of enoxaparin 1 mg/kg bid sc for 4 days. When enoxaparin was administered at a fixed, prophylaxis dose of 40 mg once daily sc for 4 days, the anti-Xa exposure increased by about 20% in mild renal impairment, about 21% in moderate renal impairment, and about 65% in severe renal impairment (see Warnings and Precautions, Renal, and Dosage and Administration, Use in Patients with Renal Impairment).

The half-life for anti-Xa activity in patients with impaired renal function is much longer than for people with normal renal function ($t_{1/2}$=5.12 h in patients with chronic renal failure vs 2.94 h in young healthy volunteers) when enoxaparin was administered intravenously.

STORAGE AND STABILITY: Temperature: Store at room temperature (15-25°C).

Others: Protect from heat.

Do not store the multiple dose vials for more than 28 days after the first use.

INFORMATION FOR THE PATIENT: Published in e-CPS, available by subscription at www.e-cps.ca.

DOSAGE FORMS, COMPOSITION AND PACKAGING: LOVENOX: Multidose Vials: Each multidose vial contains: enoxaparin sodium 300 mg in 3 mL water for injection (concentration 10 mg/0.1 mL) and 1.5% (w/v) benzyl alcohol as a preservative.

Pre-filled Syringes: 30 mg/0.3 mL: Each syringe contains: enoxaparin sodium 30 mg in 0.3 mL water for injection. The solution is preservative-free and intended for use as a single-dose injection. Pre-filled syringes 27 G of 0.3 mL with protective shield, cartons of 10, blisters of 2, each in individual blister pack.

40 mg/0.4 mL: Each syringe contains: enoxaparin sodium 40 mg in 0.4 mL water for injection. The solution is preservative-free and intended for use as a single-dose injection. Pre-filled syringes 27 G of 0.4 mL with protective shield, cartons of 10, blisters of 2, each in individual blister pack.

60 mg/0.6 mL: Each syringe contains: enoxaparin sodium 60 mg in 0.6 mL water for injection. The solution is preservative-free and intended for use as a single-dose injection. Pre-filled syringes 27 G of 0.6 mL with protective shield, cartons of 10, blisters of 2, each in individual blister pack.

80 mg/0.8 mL: Each syringe contains: enoxaparin sodium 80 mg in 0.8 mL water for injection. The solution is preservative-free and intended for use as a single-dose injection. Pre-filled syringes 27 G of 0.8 mL with protective shield, cartons of 10, blisters of 2, each in individual blister pack.

100 mg/1 mL: Each syringe contains: enoxaparin sodium 100 mg in 1 mL water for injection. The solution is preservative-free and intended for use as a single-dose injection. Pre-filled syringes 27 G of 1 mL with protective shield, cartons of 10, blisters of 2, each in individual blister pack.

The 60 mg/0.6 mL, 80 mg/0.8 mL, and the 100 mg/1 mL syringes are imprinted with a graduation scale of 1 mL with major increments of 0.1 mL and minor increments of 0.025 mL.

Each LOVENOX presentation has a solution pH of 5.5 to 7.5 with an approximate anti-factor Xa activity of 100 IU/1 mg of drug (with reference to the WHO First International Low Molecular Weight Heparin Reference Standard).

LOVENOX HP (High Potency): 120 mg/0.8 mL: Each syringe contains: enoxaparin sodium 120 mg in 0.8 mL water for injection. The solution is preservative-free and intended for use as a single-dose injection. Pre-filled syringes 27 G of 0.8 mL with protective shield, cartons of 10, blisters of 2, each in individual blister pack.

150 mg/1 mL: Each syringe contains: enoxaparin sodium 150 mg in 1 mL water for injection. The solution is preservative-free and intended for use as a single-dose injection. Pre-filled syringes 27 G of 1 mL with protective shield, cartons of 10, blisters of 2, each in individual blister pack.

The 120 mg/0.8 mL and 150 mg/1 mL syringes are imprinted with a graduation scale of 1 mL with major increments of 0.1 mL and minor increments of 0.02 mL.

The pH of the syringe and multiple dose solution is 5.5 to 7.5 with an approximate anti-factor Xa activity of 100 IU/1 mg of drug (with reference to the WHO First International Low Molecular Weight Heparin Reference Standard). Nitrogen is used in the headspace to inhibit oxidation.

Loxapac® IM ℞

loxapine HCl

Antipsychotic

Sandoz

SUPPLIED: Each mL contains: loxapine base (as hydrochloride) 50 mg. Nonmedicinal ingredients: hydrochloric acid and/or sodium hydroxide to adjust pH to approximately 6.0, polysorbate 80, propylene glycol and water for injection. Ampules of 1 mL, boxes of 10. Store between 15 and 30°C.

Loxapine ℞

loxapine HCl—loxapine succinate

Antipsychotic

CPhA Monograph

Date of Preparation: October 2010

This monograph has been compiled by CPhA and reviewed by experts. It may contain information different from that found in Health Canada-approved Product Monographs. The reader is referred to the *CPS* Editorial Policy for more information.

SUMMARY PRODUCT INFORMATION:

Drug	Route of Administration	Dosage Form	Strength
Loxapine succinate	Oral	Tablet	2.5 mg, 5 mg, 10 mg, 25 mg, 50 mg
		Liquid	25 mg/mL
Loxapine HCl	Parenteral (IM)	Injection	25 mg/mL, 50 mg/mL

PHARMACOLOGY: Loxapine is a tricyclic dibenzoxazepine antipsychotic of intermediate potency with pharmacologic actions similar to the phenothiazine, butyrophenone and thioxanthene classes of antipsychotics. Loxapine appears to exert its antipsychotic effects by blocking dopamine receptors in the mesolimbic and mesocortical areas of the brain. Blockade of dopamine receptors in the nigrostriatal and tuberoinfundibular tracts is believed to be the mechanism for adverse effects including extrapyramidal symptoms and hyperprolactinemia. Other adverse effects of loxapine arise from its ability to block muscarinic, alpha-adrenergic, histaminic and serotonergic receptors. Muscarinic blockade causes anticholinergic side effects such as dry mouth, blurred vision and urinary retention. Histamine antagonism can cause CNS side effects such as sedation and drowsiness. Blocking of alpha-adrenergic receptors can cause orthostatic hypotension and reflex tachycardia. Serotonin blockade can result in weight gain.

Pharmacokinetics: Loxapine is well absorbed after oral or im administration. Loxapine is distributed mainly to the brain, lungs, heart, liver, pancreas and CSF. It is extensively metabolized in the liver and excreted in the urine and feces. Loxapine and its active and inactive metabolites are eliminated in a biphasic fashion with half-lives of 5 and 19 hours, respectively.

INDICATIONS: Health Canada-approved indications include:
- management of psychotic disorders such as schizophrenia

CONTRAINDICATIONS: Loxapine is contraindicated in:
- comatose patients
- severe CNS depression from any cause (e.g., alcohol, barbiturates, opiates)
- circulatory collapse
- patients with known hypersensitivity to loxapine or any component of the formulation

WARNINGS:

Serious Warnings and Precautions
- Use of antipsychotics such as loxapine has been associated with acute and chronic extrapyramidal reactions including dystonias, akathisia, parkinsonian symptoms, neuroleptic malignant syndrome (NMS) and tardive dyskinesia (TD). NMS can be life-threatening and loxapine should be promptly discontinued if NMS is suspected. TD may not resolve after drug discontinuation. See also Adverse Effects.
- The use of antipsychotic agents in elderly patients has been associated with a dose-related increase in all-cause mortality, with an inverse relationship to duration of use. The risk may be higher with first-generation or "conventional" antipsychotics compared to second-generation or "atypical" agents [*N Engl J Med* 2005;353(22):2335-41; *CMAJ* 2007;176(5):627-32. doi:10.1503/cmaj.061250]. The use of antipsychotics in older patients should be carefully considered, and first-generation agents should be avoided whenever possible.

PRECAUTIONS: Abrupt Withdrawal: Sudden discontinuation of antipsychotics can result in symptoms such as nausea, vomiting, diarrhea, sweating, insomnia and confusion. Psychosis and movement disorders can also be precipitated. Antipsychotics should be discontinued gradually when possible.

Autonomic Nervous System: Because of potential anticholinergic effects, loxapine should be used with caution in patients with angle closure glaucoma or propensity for urinary retention.

CNS: See also Warnings and Adverse Effects. Loxapine can lower the seizure threshold and should be used with extreme caution in patients with seizure disorders or other risk factors for seizures such as acute alcohol withdrawal.

Antipsychotics have antiemetic properties which may mask signs and symptoms of toxic drug overdoses or diseases (e.g., intestinal obstruction, brain tumor).

Cardiovascular: Because it may cause tachycardia and hypotension, loxapine should be used with caution in patients with cardiovascular disease. Hypotension may occur more frequently with parenteral administration. Patients should be supine during injections and remain supine or sitting for 30 minutes afterward.

Endocrine: Patients with hypocalcemia may be more susceptible to dystonic reactions (see Adverse Effects).

Occupational Hazards: Patients should be warned that loxapine may impair their ability to perform hazardous tasks such as driving or operating heavy machinery.

Pregnancy: There are no published reports of outcomes associated with fetal exposure to loxapine. If loxapine is required during pregnancy, use the lowest effective dose for the shortest possible time. Avoid using loxapine near term to minimize the risk of adverse effects in the neonate such as extrapyramidal symptoms or lethargy.

Lactation: Antipsychotics have been detected in breast milk in concentrations of 0.2% to 11%. There have been no reports of adverse outcomes associated with loxapine exposure through breastfeeding. Use with caution in breastfeeding women because of the possible sedative and anticholinergic side effects in the infant.

Children: Children may be more susceptible to the adverse effects of antipsychotics including extrapyramidal effects, sedation and weight gain. If treatment with an antipsychotic is to be initiated, start at the lowest possible dose, titrate slowly, assess the need for the antipsychotic regularly and limit the duration of therapy.

Geriatrics: See Warnings, Serious Warnings and Precautions. If loxapine is used in elderly patients, use reduced dosages; elderly patients are more susceptible to the therapeutic and adverse effects of phenothiazines, particularly postural hypotension, cognitive impairment, extrapyramidal effects and anticholinergic effects such as constipation, urinary retention and blurred vision.

Drug Interactions: Anticholinergic Agents: Concomitant use of loxapine and other drugs with anticholinergic properties may increase the incidence/severity of adverse effects such as dry mouth, blurred vision, constipation, cognitive impairment and urinary retention.

Antiparkinson's Agents: By blocking dopamine transmission, antipsychotics can antagonize the dopaminergic effects of antiparkinsonian agents.

CNS Depressants: The effects of CNS depressants (e.g., alcohol, benzodiazepines, opiates) may be increased with concomitant loxapine use.

Drugs that Prolong the QTc Interval: Use of loxapine in combination with other drugs that prolong the QTc interval (e.g., amiodarone, chlorpromazine, clarithromycin, disopyramide, domperidone, droperidol, erythromycin, indapamide, lithium, moxifloxacin, pimozide, procainamide, quetiapine, quinidine, quinine, tricyclic antidepressants, ziprasidone) may result in additive prolongation of the QTc interval and increased risk of life-threatening arrhythmias such as torsades de pointes.

Lithium: Rarely, concurrent use of lithium with antipsychotic agents has resulted in acute encephalopathic syndrome. If loxapine and lithium are used concurrently, monitor closely for neurotoxic effects.

ADVERSE EFFECTS: Many adverse effects of loxapine are transient, and persistent symptoms usually respond to a dose reduction. More common adverse effects (≥1%) are described in Table 1.

Table 1: Loxapine

More Common Adverse Effects (≥1%)

Body System	Effect	Clinical Comment
Autonomic Nervous System	Anticholinergic effects such as dry mouth, blurred vision, constipation	When feasible, dosage reduction may improve symptoms.
Central Nervous System	Sedation, memory impairment, confusion, delirium	Very common with initial therapy; usually lessens with continued use.
	Acute onset extrapyramidal effects such as parkinsonism, akathisia, dystonic reactions	Use lowest effective dose for shortest possible time and regularly re-evaluate need for continued therapy. Management options include dosage reduction, switching to a 2nd generation antipsychotic, use of medications such as benzodiazepines (akathisia), anticholinergic agents (dystonia, parkinsonism) or beta-blockers (akathisia).
	Late onset movement disorders such as tardive dyskinesia (TD), characterized by rhythmical involuntary movements of the tongue, face, mouth or jaw (e.g., protrusion of the tongue, puffing of the cheeks, puckering of the mouth and chewing movements)	There is no evidence-based drug treatment for this syndrome. Management includes discontinuing the antipsychotic, switching to a 2nd generation agent if necessary. Fine vermicular movements of the tongue may be an early sign of TD and discontinuing the drug when this occurs might prevent full onset of the syndrome.
Cardiovascular	Orthostatic hypotension Tachycardia	To minimize the risk of orthostasis advise patients to maintain good hydration and to rise slowly from sitting or lying down.
Endocrine	Galactorrhea, gynecomastia, amenorrhea, sexual dysfunction, hyperlipidemia	May improve with dosage reduction (if feasible).

(cont'd)

Table 1: Loxapine (cont'd)

Less Common Adverse Effects (<1%): Autonomic: urinary retention, adynamic ileus.

Cardiovascular: tachycardia and ECG abnormalities (e.g., QTc prolongation).

Central Nervous System: Neuroleptic Malignant Syndrome (NMS): This rare but potentially fatal syndrome, characterized by muscle rigidity, fever/hyperthermia, labile blood pressure and fluctuating levels of consciousness, can occur in patients taking loxapine and other antipsychotics. NMS appears to occur more commonly in young males. Dehydration is an additional risk factor. Patients need to be aware of the importance of adequate hydration, particularly in situations involving environmental exposure to extreme heat.

Dermatological: pruritus, rashes, hyperpigmentation, photosensitivity (recommend the use of sunscreen).

Endocrine: amenorrhea, gynecomastia and menstrual irregularity.

Hematologic: Agranulocytosis, thrombocytopenia and leukopenia have rarely occurred.

Hepatic: jaundice.

Ocular: pigmentary retinopathy and lenticular pigmentation.

Miscellaneous: weight gain, weight loss, sexual dysfunction, seizures, neuroleptic malignant syndrome (see Adverse Effects).

OVERDOSAGE:

Symptoms: Symptoms of loxapine overdose are an extension of its pharmacologic actions. The primary symptoms observed are sedation and hypotension. Mild or early intoxication may appear as restlessness and confusion, which may progress to coma. Altered temperature regulation can occur; both hypothermia and hyperthermia have been reported. Neuroleptic malignant syndrome can occur in overdose, though it most often occurs with therapeutic doses. Other symptoms may include anticholinergic manifestations (mydriasis, dry mouth, agitation, urinary retention, decreased bowel sounds), tachycardia, cardiac arrhythmias, seizures and respiratory and/or vasomotor collapse.

Treatment: Patients who have ingested loxapine in overdose may require respiratory and hemodynamic support. This may include intubation, ventilation, boluses of isotonic iv fluids, and inotropic support. Once the patient's airway is adequately protected, 1 dose of activated charcoal (1 g/kg body weight) can be administered up to 120 minutes after oral overdose, to minimize absorption of loxapine. The utility of this intervention decreases with time, and it may not influence clinical outcome. Patients with seizures should be treated with benzodiazepines, or, if necessary, barbiturates. Phenytoin is generally ineffective for toxin-induced seizures. Ventricular arrhythmias are uncommon, and should be treated with boluses of sodium bicarbonate as well as antiarrhythmics such as lidocaine. In the rare patient with torsades de pointes, iv magnesium sulfate and/or an overdrive pacemaker should be used. Acute dystonic reactions may be treated with iv benztropine or diphenhydramine.

For management of a suspected drug overdose, CPhA recommends that you contact your **regional Poison Control Centre**. See the *CPS* Directory section for a list of Poison Control Centres.

DOSAGE: Oral: Loxapine therapy should be initiated at 10 mg twice daily and titrated over a period of 7 to 10 days. An initial dose of 50 mg daily may be given to individuals with severe symptoms. The usual maintenance dose is 60 to 100 mg daily in 2 to 4 divided doses; however, the lowest effective dose should be used. Many patients have been maintained on doses as low as 20 to 60 mg per day.

Parenteral: IM administration may be used to provide symptomatic control in patients with acute agitation or those who are unable to take the drug orally. The usual dose is 12.5 to 50 mg im every 4 to 6 hours or longer, and adjusted according to the patient's response and side effects. Switch to the oral route as soon as practical.

Geriatrics: Avoid in elderly patients when possible; see Warnings, Serious Warnings and Precautions. If used in older patients, initial dose is 5 to 10 mg once or twice daily.

The reader is invited to consult CPhA's monograph **Thiazide Diuretics**.

Lozide® 🄿

indapamide

Diuretic—Antihypertensive

Servier

Date of Preparation: August 4, 1995
Date of Revision: July 9, 2008

PHARMACOLOGY: Indapamide is a diuretic antihypertensive agent. The mechanism whereby indapamide exerts its action in the control of hypertension is not completely elucidated: both renal and extrarenal actions may be involved. The renal site of action is the proximal part of the distal tubule and the ascending part of Henle's loop. Sodium and chloride ions are excreted in approximately equivalent amounts. The increased delivery of sodium to the distal tubular exchange site results in increased potassium excretion and hypokalemia.

Pharmacokinetics: Indapamide is rapidly and completely absorbed after oral administration. Peak blood levels are obtained after 1 to 2 hours. Indapamide is concentrated in the erythrocytes and is 79% bound to plasma proteins and to erythrocytes.

It is taken up by the vascular wall in smooth vascular muscle according to its high lipid solubility. Seventy per cent of a single oral dose is eliminated by the kidneys and 23% by the gastrointestinal tract. Indapamide is metabolized to a marked degree, the unchanged product representing approximately 5% of the total dose found in the urine during the 48 hours following administration. Elimination of indapamide from the plasma is biphasic with half-lives of 14 and 25 hours respectively.

INDICATIONS: The management of essential hypertension. It may be tried as a sole therapeutic agent in the treatment of mild to moderate hypertension. Normally indapamide, as other diuretics, is used as the initial agent in multiple drug regimens.

CONTRAINDICATIONS: Anuria, progressive and severe oliguria, hepatic coma. Known hypersensitivity to indapamide or to other sulfonamide derivatives.

WARNINGS: Electrolyte changes observed with indapamide become severe at doses above 2.5 mg/day. Therefore the maximum daily dose should not exceed this dose.

Hypokalemia may occur at all doses with consequent weakness, cramps, and cardiac dysrhythmias. Hypokalemia is a particular hazard in digitalized patients; dangerous or fatal arrhythmias may be precipitated.

Hypokalemia occurs commonly with diuretics; electrolyte monitoring is essential particularly in patients who would be at increased risk from hypokalemia, such as patients with cardiac arrhythmias or those who are receiving concomitant cardiac glycosides.

Patients with renal insufficiency receiving indapamide should be carefully monitored. If increasing azotemia and oliguria occur during treatment, the diuretic should be discontinued.

Hyperuricemia may occur during administration of indapamide. Rarely gout has been reported. Blood uric acid levels should be monitored, particularly in patients with a history of gout who should continue to receive appropriate treatment.

PRECAUTIONS: Patients receiving indapamide should be carefully observed and serum electrolytes monitored for signs and symptoms of fluid or electrolyte imbalance; namely hyponatremia, hypochloremia and hypokalemia. BUN, uric acid, and glucose levels should also be assessed during therapy. Hypokalemia, an ever present hazard with most diuretics, will be more common in association with concomitant steroid or ACTH therapy and with inadequate electrolyte intake. The serum potassium should be determined at regular intervals and potassium supplementation instituted when indicated (see Warnings).

The signs of electrolyte imbalance are: dryness of the mouth, thirst, weakness, lethargy, drowsiness, restlessness, muscle pains or cramps, muscle fatigue, hypotension, oliguria, gastrointestinal disturbances such as nausea and vomiting, tachycardia and ECG changes.

Special caution should be used in treating patients with severe hepatic disease since diuretics may induce metabolic alkalosis in cases of potassium depletion which may precipitate episodes of hepatic encephalopathy.

Orthostatic hypotension may occur and may be potentiated by alcohol, barbiturates, narcotics or concurrent therapy with other antihypertensives.

When indapamide is given with other nondiuretic antihypertensive agents, the effects on blood pressure are additive.

Sulfonamide derivatives have been reported to exacerbate or activate systemic lupus erythematosus. These possibilities should be kept in mind with the use of indapamide although no case has been reported to date.

Severe dermatological adverse reactions, some accompanied by systemic manifestations, have been rarely reported with the use of indapamide. In the majority of cases, the condition subsided within 14 days following discontinuation of indapamide therapy (see Adverse Effects).

Caution should be observed when administering the drug to patients with severely impaired renal function, since the drug is excreted primarily by the renal route.

Although indapamide exerts minimal effect on glucose metabolism, insulin requirements may be affected in diabetics and hyperglycemia and glycosuria may occur in patients with latent diabetes.

Calcium excretion is decreased by diuretics pharmacologically related to indapamide. After 6 to 8 weeks of indapamide 1.25 mg treatment and in long-term studies of hypertensive patients with higher doses of indapamide, however, serum concentrations of calcium increased only slightly with indapamide. Prolonged treatment with drugs pharmacologically related to indapamide may in rare instances be associated with hypercalcemia and hypophosphatemia secondary to physiologic changes in the parathyroid gland; however, the common complications of hyperparathyroidism, such as renal lithiasis, bone resorption, and peptic ulcer, have not been seen. Treatment should be discontinued before tests for parathyroid function are performed. Like the thiazides, indapamide may decrease serum PBI levels without signs of thyroid disturbance.

The antihypertensive effect of the drug may be enhanced in the patient postsympathectomy.

Pregnancy: Since indapamide has not been studied in human pregnancy, the drug should not be given to pregnant women. The use in patients of childbearing potential requires that the anticipated benefit be weighed against possible hazards.

Lactation: It is unknown whether or not indapamide appears in breast milk. Indapamide should not be administered to nursing mothers. If use of the drug is deemed essential, the patient should stop nursing.

Children: The safety and effectiveness have not been established.

ADVERSE EFFECTS: The safety data presented under this section involves 2 different databases and was obtained at 2 different time periods. For the earliest database (indapamide 2.5 mg), consisting mainly of European studies performed before 1980, adverse events were collected with respect to a possible causal relationship to treatment, whereas for the most recent database (indapamide 1.25 mg), consisting exclusively of North American studies, adverse events were collected irrespective of such a causal relationship. This explains why the overall incidence of adverse events at the 2.5 mg dose appears to be lower than at the 1.25 mg dose (see below).

Most adverse events for both dosages, 1.25 mg and 2.5 mg, have been mild or moderate.

The adverse reactions represent data from clinical studies involving a total of 992 patients given indapamide 2.5 mg: 349 patients from 4 placebo controlled studies treated for 8 to 12 weeks; 356 patients from 6 active controlled studies treated for 6 up to more than 52 weeks; 287 patients from 4 uncontrolled studies treated for 6 up to 40 weeks.

The overall rate of adverse events, with respect to a possible causal relationship to the drug, was 29% and discontinuation of therapy due to adverse events was required in 5.6% of patients.

The most severe and common adverse event is the electrolyte imbalance. Electrolyte changes reported include hypokalemia (14.2%; requiring potassium supplementation 6%; with clinical symptoms 1.2%), hypochloremia (9.4%) and hyponatremia (3.1%).

The other changes observed in laboratory parameters are minor and infrequent: elevation in blood uric acid (8.6%), blood glucose (6.0%), BUN (5.7%) and blood creatinine (3.6%).

The most frequent adverse events (incidence ≥ 1%) reported for patients treated with indapamide 2.5 mg were: headache (3.4%), vertigo (2.2%), dizziness (1.9%), asthenia (1.7%) and muscle cramps (1.2%).

All other adverse events occurred at an incidence of less than 1% and included by body system:

Central Nervous: drowsiness, sleepiness, insomnia, weakness, lethargy and visual disturbance.

Gastrointestinal: nausea, anorexia, dryness of mouth, gastralgia, vomiting, diarrhea and constipation.

Musculoskeletal: joint pain, back pain and weakness of legs.

Cardiovascular: orthostatic hypotension, tachycardia and ECG changes (nonspecific ST-T change, U waves, left ventricular strain).

Urogenital: impotence, modification of libido and polyuria.

Dermatological: rash and pruritus.

Endocrine: gout.

Other: tinnitus, malaise, fainting and sweat.

In placebo-controlled studies involving 306 patients given indapamide 1.25 mg and 319 given placebo for up to 8 weeks, the overall incidence of adverse events, irrespective of causal relationship, was about 50% in both indapamide and placebo groups. In the indapamide 1.25 mg group, 4.2% of patients discontinued treatment because of adverse events.

In these studies, 20% of patients treated with indapamide 1.25 mg had at least 1 potassium value below 3.4 mEq/L.

The most frequently reported adverse events (incidence ≥ 1%) in the indapamide 1.25 mg group were: headache (17%), infection (12%), pain (8%), dizziness (7%), back pain (5%), rhinitis (5%), asthenia (4%), dyspepsia (4%), flu syndrome (3%), hypertonia (3%), sinusitis (3%), chest pain (2%), constipation (2%), cough (2%), diarrhea (2%), edema (2%), nausea (2%), pharyngitis (2%), conjunctivitis (1%), nervousness (1%) and ECG abnormalities (nonspecific ST-T changes (7%), sinus bradycardia (3%), arrhythmia (2%) or tachycardia (2%).

All other clinical adverse events occurred at an incidence of less than 1%. These are the following:

Central Nervous: agitation, amnesia, anxiety, ataxia, coordination abnormality, depression, dream abnormality, hyperesthesia, insomnia, migraine, paresthesia, somnolence, twitching and vertigo.

Gastrointestinal: increased appetite, dry mouth, GI carcinoma, GI disorders, duodenitis, dysphagia, esophagitis, flatulence, gastritis, gastroenteritis, oral moniliasis, proctitis, rectal disorders, rectal hemorrhoids, stomatitis, tooth disorders and vomiting.

Musculoskeletal: arthralgia, arthritis, bone disorders, joint disorders, bone fracture, bone pain, chondrodystrophy, myalgia, myasthenia and myopathy.

Cardiovascular: angina pectoris, bundle branch block, ventricular extrasystoles, atrial fibrillation, atrial flutter, hypertension, postural hypotension, palpitations, syncope, supraventricular tachycardia and vasodilation.

Urogenital: dysmenorrhea, dysuria, impotence, urinary tract infection, nocturia, oliguria, urinary frequency or urgency, renal pain or calculus, prostate disorders and vaginitis.

Respiratory: bronchitis, dyspnea, laryngitis, lung disorder and sputum increase.

Dermatological: acne, application site reaction, exfoliative dermatitis, nail disorder, skin nodule, rash, bullous eruption and sweat.

Metabolic and Nutritional: diabetes mellitus and gout.

Special Senses: amblyopia, ear disorders, ear pain, otitis, photophobia, taste perversion, tinnitus and vision abnormality.

Other: thyroid disorder, ecchymosis, allergic reaction, edema face, fever, hernia, malaise and monilia.

Postmarketing Experience: Among the less common suspected adverse reactions reported, the following, which are not included elsewhere in the product monograph, have been published in the medical literature and/or are classified as serious or potentially serious: Stevens-Johnson syndrome, bullous eruption, photosensitivity with bullae, erythroderma, purpura, epidermal necrolysis, erythema multiforme, angioedema, cataract, acute myopia, optic neuritis, ventricular arrhythmia, torsades de pointe, stroke, acute hypersensitivity reaction leading to interstitial nephritis and renal failure, anemia, agranulocytosis, metabolic alkalosis, hyperosmolar coma, dehydration, hepatitis, pancreatitis, lithium toxicity, rhabdomyolysis, vasculitis, fever.

One case of synergetic effect of clofibrate with indapamide leading to hyponatremia, hypokalemia, hypoosmolarity, nausea and progressive loss of consciousness.

Relationship with the administration of indapamide has not been proved in all cases.

OVERDOSE:

Symptoms: There have been no reports of overdosage. Based on the pharmacological activities of indapamide, overdosage may lead to excessive diuresis with electrolyte depletion. In cirrhotic patients, overdosage might precipitate hepatic coma.

Treatment: There is no specific antidote. Treatment is symptomatic and supportive. Discontinue drug. Induce emesis or perform gastric lavage. Correct dehydration, electrolyte imbalance, hepatic coma and hypotension by established procedures.

For management of a suspected drug overdose, CPhA recommends that you contact your **regional Poison Control Centre**. See the *CPS* Directory section for a list of Poison Control Centres.

DOSAGE: One 1.25 mg tablet/day taken in the morning as a single dose. If the response is not satisfactory after 4 to 8 weeks, the dose may be increased to a maximum of 2.5 mg as a single dose taken in the morning. If the antihypertensive response to indapamide is insufficient, an increase in dosage is not recommended (see Warnings).

Instead a nondiuretic antihypertensive agent should be added to the drug regimen. Alternatively if in the opinion of the physician, an important diuretic effect is desirable for the patient's control, a different diuretic which allows for dose titration could be tried instead of indapamide.

SUPPLIED: 1.25 mg: Each round, orange, film-coated tablet, with S embossed on one side, contains: indapamide hemihydrate 1.25 mg. Nonmedicinal ingredients: glycerol, hydroxypropylmethyl cellulose, lactose monohydrate, macrogol 6000, magnesium stearate, maize starch, microcrystalline cellulose, pregelatinized starch, sunset yellow S aluminium lake, talc and titanium dioxide. Blister-packs of 30 and 100.

2.5 mg: Each pink, sugar-coated tablet contains: indapamide hemihydrate 2.5 mg. Nonmedicinal ingredients: colloidal silica, corn starch, ethylcellulose, FD&C Red No. 3 lake, FD&C Yellow No. 6 lake, glycerol monooleate, lactose, magnesium stearate, polysorbate, povidone, pregelatinized corn starch, sodium benzoate, sodium carboxymethylcellulose, sucrose, talc, titanium dioxide and white beeswax. Blister-packs of 30 and 100.

Store at room temperature (15-30°C).

(Shown in Product Identification Section)

Lucentis® Pr

ranibizumab

Antivascular Endothelial Growth Factor-A (VEGF-A inhibitor) for Age-Related Macular Degeneration—Antineovascularisation Agent

Novartis Pharmaceuticals

Date of Preparation: December 18, 2008
Date of Revision: April 23, 2009

SUMMARY PRODUCT INFORMATION:

Route of Administration	Dosage Form/ Strength	Clinically Relevant Nonmedicinal Ingredients
Intravitreal injection	Sterile solution/10 mg/mL (2.3 mg/0.23 mL/vial)	Not applicable For a complete listing see Dosage Forms, Composition and Packaging.

INDICATIONS AND CLINICAL USE: LUCENTIS (ranibizumab injection) is indicated for the treatment of neovascular (wet) age-related macular degeneration (AMD).

CONTRAINDICATIONS:

- Patients who are hypersensitive to this drug or to any ingredient in the formulation or component of the container. For a complete listing, see Dosage Forms, Composition and Packaging.
- Patients with active or suspected ocular or periocular infections.
- Patients with active intraocular inflammation.

WARNINGS AND PRECAUTIONS: General: Treatment with LUCENTIS (ranibizumab injection) is for intravitreal injection only.

Thromboembolic Events: There is a potential risk of arterial thromboembolic events following intravitreal use of VEGF inhibitors.

In the Phase III studies, the overall frequency of arterial thromboembolic events was similar between ranibizumab and control. A numerically higher stroke rate was observed in patients treated with ranibizumab 0.5 mg compared to ranibizumab 0.3 mg or control, however the differences were not statistically significant. The difference in stroke rates may be greater in patients with known risk factors for stroke, including history of prior stroke or transient ischemic attack. Therefore, these patients should be carefully evaluated by their physicians as to whether LUCENTIS treatment is appropriate and the benefit outweighs the potential risk. (See Adverse Reactions.)

Patients who suffer a thromboembolic event while being treated with LUCENTIS should be carefully evaluated by their physician who will assess if continuation of LUCENTIS treatment is appropriate, i.e., if the benefit to the patient justifies the risk.

Hepatic/Biliary/Pancreatic: LUCENTIS has not been studied in patients with hepatic impairment.

Immune: As with all therapeutic proteins, there is a potential for immunogenicity with LUCENTIS. Patients should be instructed to report if an intraocular inflammation increases in severity, which may be a clinical sign attributable to intraocular antibody formation. There is a theoretical risk of hypersensitivity reactions including anaphylaxis/anaphlactoid reactions or angioedema which may occur with the use of LUCENTIS.

Immunogenicity: The pre-treatment incidence of immunoreactivity to LUCENTIS was 0%-3% across treatment groups. After monthly dosing with LUCENTIS for 12 to 24 months, low titres of antibodies to LUCENTIS were detected in approximately 1%-6% of patients. The immunogenicity data reflect the percentage of patients whose test results were considered positive for antibodies to LUCENTIS in an electrochemiluminescence assay and are highly dependent on the sensitivity and specificity of the assay. The clinical significance of immunoreactivity to LUCENTIS is unclear at this time, although some patients with the highest levels of immunoreactivity were noted to have iritis or vitritis.

Ophthalmologic: Intravitreous injections, including those with LUCENTIS, have been associated with endophthalmitis, intraocular inflammation, rhegmatogenous retinal detachment, retinal tear and iatrogenic traumatic cataract (see Adverse Reactions). Proper aseptic injection techniques must always be used when administering LUCENTIS. In addition, patients should be monitored during the week following the injection to permit early treatment if an infection occurs. Patients should be instructed to report any symptoms suggestive of endophthalmitis or any of the above mentioned events without delay.

Increases in intraocular pressure have been seen within 60 minutes of injection of LUCENTIS (see Adverse Reactions). Both intraocular pressure and the perfusion of the optic nerve head must therefore be monitored and managed appropriately. Monitoring may consist of a check for perfusion of the optic nerve head immediately after the injection and/or tonometry within 30 minutes following the injection.

LUCENTIS has not been studied in patients who have previously received other types of intravitreal injections.

The safety and efficacy of LUCENTIS therapy administered to both eyes concurrently has not been studied.

Renal: Systemic exposure to LUCENTIS may be increased in patients with renal impairment (see Action and Clinical Pharmacology, Special Populations and Conditions). The clinical significance of increased systemic exposure to LUCENTIS is unknown.

Special Populations: Pregnant Women: There are no data from the use of ranibizumab in pregnant women. It is not known whether ranibizumab can cause fetal harm when administered to a pregnant woman or can affect reproduction capacity. LUCENTIS should not be used in pregnancy unless the potential benefit justifies the potential risk to the fetus.

Women of childbearing potential should use effective contraception during treatment.

Nursing Women: It is not known whether LUCENTIS is excreted in human milk. As a precautionary measure, breast-feeding is not recommended during the use of LUCENTIS.

Pediatrics (<18 years of age): LUCENTIS has not been studied in this sub-population.

Geriatrics (≥65 years of age): No dose adjustment is necessary in the elderly.

Effects on Ability to Drive and Use Machines: The Lucentis treatment procedure may induce temporary visual disturbances, which may affect the ability to drive or use machines (see Adverse Reactions). Patients who experience these signs must not drive or use machines until these temporary visual disturbances subside.

ADVERSE REACTIONS: Adverse Drug Reaction Overview: Serious adverse events related to the injection procedure included endophthalmitis, rhegmatogenous retinal detachment, retinal tear and iatrogenic traumatic cataract (see Warnings and Precautions).

Other serious ocular events observed among LUCENTIS-treated patients included intraocular inflammation (with frequency from 3.3% to 11.7%) and increased intraocular pressure (with frequency from 6.6% to 18.8%). (See Warnings and Precautions.)

Clinical Trial Adverse Drug Reactions: Because clinical trials are conducted under very specific conditions the adverse reaction rates observed in the clinical trials may not reflect the rates observed in practice and should not be compared to the rates in the clinical trials of another drug. Adverse drug reaction information from clinical trials is useful for identifying drug-related adverse events and for approximating rates.

A total of 1315 patients constituted the safety population in the three phase III studies, FVF2598g (MARINA), FVF2587g (ANCHOR) and FVF3192g (PIER) with 24 months exposure to LUCENTIS (ranibizumab injection) and four hundred and forty (440) patients were treated with the recommended dose of 0.5 mg.

The common ocular and non-ocular adverse events with suspected relationship to LUCENTIS treatment occurring in ≥1% of patients receiving treatment with LUCENTIS 0.5 mg in at least one of the three controlled phase III studies FVF2598g (MARINA; 2-year data), FVF2587g (ANCHOR; 2-year data) and FVF3192g (PIER; 2-year data) are summarized in Table 1 and Table 2.

The common ocular and non-ocular adverse events, regardless of treatment relationship to LUCENTIS, with a difference in incidence rate of ≥2% between patients receiving treatment with 0.5 mg LUCENTIS and the control group in at least one of the three controlled phase III studies FVF2598g (MARINA; 2-year data), FVF2587g (ANCHOR; 2-year data) and FVF3192g (PIER; 2-year data) are summarized in Table 3.

Table 1: LUCENTIS

Ocular Adverse Reactions in the Study Eye. Studies MARINA (FVF2598g), ANCHOR (FVF2587g) and PIER (FVF3192g) Safety Population. Adverse Events with Incidence Rate ≥1% for LUCENTIS 0.5 mg in at Least One Study

	% of Patients Study MARINA (Dosage q 1 month) 2 Years			% of Patients Study ANCHOR (Dosage q 1 month) 2 Years			% of Patients Study PIER (Dosage q 1 month for first 3 months then q 3 months) 2 Years		
Preferred Term	**Sham (N=236)**	**LUCENTIS 0.3 mg (N=238)**	**LUCENTIS 0.5 mg (N=239)**	**Verteporfin PDT (N=143)**	**LUCENTIS 0.3 mg (N=137)**	**LUCENTIS 0.5 mg (N=140)**	**Sham (N=62)**	**LUCENTIS 0.3 mg (N=59)**	**LUCENTIS 0.5 mg (N=61)**
Cataract	0.0%	0.0%	1.3%	0.0%	0.0%	1.4%	0.0%	0.0%	0.0%
Cataract nuclear	0.0%	0.0%	0.0%	0.0%	0.7%	0.0%	0.0%	0.0%	1.6%
Conjunctival haemorrhage	11.9%	13.4%	18.4%	11.2%	17.5%	11.4%	0.0%	0.0%	1.6%
Conjunctival hyperaemia	2.1%	0.4%	1.7%	2.1%	5.1%	2.1%	0.0%	0.0%	0.0%
Conjunctivitis	1.3%	1.3%	1.3%	0.0%	0.0%	0.0%	0.0%	0.0%	0.0%
Corneal abrasion	2.5%	1.3%	2.5%	0.7%	0.0%	1.4%	0.0%	0.0%	0.0%
Detachment of retinal pigment epithelium	0.4%	0.0%	0.4%	0.0%	0.0%	0.0%	0.0%	0.0%	1.6%
Dry eye	0.8%	0.4%	2.1%	0.7%	0.0%	0.7%	0.0%	0.0%	0.0%
Eye discharge	3.0%	2.9%	0.4%	2.1%	0.7%	1.4%	0.0%	0.0%	0.0%
Eye irritation	11.4%	10.1%	6.7%	5.6%	4.4%	5.7%	0.0%	1.7%	1.6%
Eye pain	23.7%	26.9%	28.9%	18.2%	22.6%	17.9%	0.0%	0.0%	0.0%
Eye pruritus	4.7%	2.9%	4.2%	1.4%	7.3%	2.9%	0.0%	0.0%	0.0%
Eyelid oedema	1.3%	0.8%	1.7%	1.4%	2.2%	1.4%	0.0%	0.0%	0.0%
Eyelid pain	0.4%	0.8%	0.4%	0.7%	0.0%	1.4%	0.0%	0.0%	0.0%
Foreign body sensation in eyes	10.2%	11.8%	11.3%	6.3%	5.1%	7.9%	0.0%	0.0%	0.0%
Hypoaesthesia eye	0.0%	0.0%	0.0%	0.0%	0.0%	0.0%	0.0%	0.0%	1.6%
Incorrect route of drug administration	0.0%	0.0%	0.0%	0.0%	0.7%	0.0%	0.0%	0.0%	1.6%
Injection site haemorrhage	0.8%	0.0%	1.7%	0.7%	2.2%	2.1%	0.0%	0.0%	0.0%
Injection site pain	0.8%	0.8%	1.3%	0.7%	0.7%	0.0%	0.0%	0.0%	0.0%
Intraocular pressure increased	3.8%	18.9%	18.8%	5.6%	17.5%	15.0%	1.6%	5.1%	6.6%
Iridocyclitis	0.4%	0.8%	1.7%	0.0%	0.0%	2.9%	0.0%	1.7%	1.6%
Iritis	3.8%	5.9%	5.4%	0.0%	2.2%	6.4%	1.6%	0.0%	1.6%
Keratopathy	0.0%	0.0%	0.4%	0.0%	0.0%	0.0%	0.0%	0.0%	1.6%
Lacrimation increased	9.3%	11.8%	7.9%	1.4%	5.1%	5.0%	0.0%	0.0%	0.0%
Ocular discomfort	3.0%	5.9%	3.8%	1.4%	2.9%	5.0%	0.0%	0.0%	1.6%
Ocular hyperaemia	7.2%	5.0%	6.3%	4.2%	6.6%	7.9%	0.0%	0.0%	0.0%
Punctate keratitis	0.8%	0.8%	1.3%	0.0%	0.0%	0.7%	0.0%	0.0%	0.0%
Uveitis	0.0%	0.4%	0.8%	0.0%	0.7%	1.4%	0.0%	0.0%	0.0%
Vision blurred	1.7%	6.3%	2.9%	1.4%	5.1%	2.9%	0.0%	0.0%	0.0%
Visual acuity reduced	0.4%	1.7%	2.9%	2.1%	0.7%	0.7%	0.0%	1.7%	0.0%
Visual disturbance	0.4%	3.8%	6.7%	0.7%	2.9%	1.4%	0.0%	0.0%	0.0%
Vitreous detachment	1.3%	4.2%	2.1%	0.0%	2.2%	0.7%	0.0%	0.0%	0.0%
Vitreous disorder	0.0%	1.3%	0.4%	0.0%	1.5%	1.4%	0.0%	0.0%	0.0%
Vitreous floaters	2.1%	18.9%	17.2%	1.4%	9.5%	4.3%	0.0%	1.7%	1.6%
Vitreous haemorrhage	0.0%	2.1%	1.7%	0.7%	2.2%	2.1%	0.0%	0.0%	0.0%
Vitritis	1.3%	5.5%	8.4%	1.4%	3.6%	5.0%	0.0%	0.0%	1.6%
Total intraocular inflammation[a]	5.1%	10.9%	11.7%	1.4%	5.8%	10.7%	1.6%	1.7%	3.3%

[a] Preferred terms summarized: Anterior chamber inflammation, Hypopyon, Iridocyclitis, Iritis, Uveitis and Vitritis.
Multiple occurrences of the same event were counted once in the overall incidence.

Table 2: LUCENTIS

Non-ocular Adverse Reactions. Studies MARINA (FVF2598g), ANCHOR (FVF2587g) and PIER (FVF3192g) Safety Population. Adverse Events with Incidence Rate ≥1% for LUCENTIS 0.5 mg in at Least One Study

	% of Patients Study MARINA (Dosage q 1 month) 2 years			% of Patients Study ANCHOR (Dosage q 1 month) 2 Years			% of Patients Study PIER (Dosage q 1 month for first 3 months then q 3 months) 2 Years		
Preferred Term	**Sham (N=236)**	**LUCENTIS 0.3 mg (N=238)**	**LUCENTIS 0.5 mg (N=239)**	**Verteporfin PDT (N=143)**	**LUCENTIS 0.3 mg (N=137)**	**LUCENTIS 0.5 mg (N=140)**	**Sham (N=62)**	**LUCENTIS 0.3 mg (N=59)**	**LUCENTIS 0.5 mg (N=61)**
Investigations									
Blood creatinine increased	0.0%	0.0%	0.0%	0.0%	0.0%	0.0%	0.0%	0.0%	1.6%
Blood pressure diastolic increased	0.0%	0.0%	0.0%	0.0%	0.0%	0.0%	0.0%	0.0%	1.6%
Blood urea increased	0.0%	0.0%	0.0%	0.0%	0.0%	0.0%	0.0%	0.0%	1.6%
Musculoskeletal and Connective Tissue Disorders									
Pain in extremity	0.0%	0.0%	0.0%	0.7%	0.0%	0.0%	0.0%	0.0%	1.6%
Nervous System Disorders									
Headache	0.4%	0.8%	2.5%	0.0%	0.7%	0.0%	0.0%	0.0%	0.0%

Multiple occurrences of the same event were counted once in the overall incidence.

Table 3: LUCENTIS

Ocular (in the study eye) and Non Ocular Adverse Events with a Difference in Incidence Rate ≥2% Between LUCENTIS 0.5 mg and the Control in at Least One Study. Studies MARINA (FVF2598g), ANCHOR (FVF2587g) and PIER (FVF3192g) Safety Population

	% of Patients Study MARINA (Dosage q 1 month) 2 years			% of Patients Study ANCHOR (Dosage q 1 month) 2 Years			% of Patients Study PIER (Dosage q 1 month for first 3 months then q 3 months) 2 Years		
Preferred Term	**Sham (N=236)**	**LUCENTIS 0.3 mg (N=238)**	**LUCENTIS 0.5 mg (N=239)**	**Verteporfin PDT (N=143)**	**LUCENTIS 0.3 mg (N=137)**	**LUCENTIS 0.5 mg (N=140)**	**Sham (N=62)**	**LUCENTIS 0.3 mg (N=59)**	**LUCENTIS 0.5 mg (N=61)**
Blood and Lymphatic System Disorders									
Anaemia	8.1%	7.1%	7.5%	4.2%	8.8%	8.6%	0.0%	6.8%	8.2%
Cardiac Disorders									
Angina pectoris	1.7%	2.5%	1.3%	0.7%	0.0%	3.6%	0.0%	0.0%	0.0%
Cardiac failure congestive	4.2%	4.2%	2.5%	3.5%	4.4%	4.3%	3.2%	3.4%	6.6%
Sinus bradycardia	0.0%	0.0%	0.0%	0.0%	1.5%	0.0%	0.0%	0.0%	3.3%
Congenital, Familial and Genetic Disorders									
Corneal dystrophy	2.5%	4.2%	2.9%	0.0%	2.9%	2.1%	0.0%	0.0%	0.0%
Ear and Labyrinth Disorders									
Vertigo	1.7%	4.2%	1.7%	7.0%	5.8%	1.4%	1.6%	0.0%	6.6%
Eye Disorders									
Arcus lipoides	0.0%	1.3%	2.1%	0.0%	2.2%	1.4%	0.0%	1.7%	0.0%
Blepharitis	8.9%	10.9%	13.4%	7.0%	10.2%	9.3%	6.5%	6.8%	4.9%
Cataract	6.8%	7.1%	5.4%	7.0%	9.5%	13.6%	1.6%	6.8%	6.6%
Cataract cortical	2.1%	1.3%	4.6%	1.4%	1.5%	1.4%	1.6%	1.7%	3.3%
Cataract nuclear	5.9%	4.2%	3.8%	1.4%	5.1%	5.0%	3.2%	1.7%	8.2%
Conjunctival haemorrhage	66.1%	77.3%	75.7%	50.3%	71.5%	70.0%	29.0%	50.8%	52.5%
Conjunctival hyperaemia	6.8%	2.9%	7.1%	4.2%	11.7%	7.9%	0.0%	1.7%	0.0%
Conjunctivitis	3.0%	3.8%	3.3%	0.0%	2.2%	2.1%	0.0%	3.4%	3.3%
Conjunctivitis allergic	1.7%	2.1%	3.8%	0.7%	0.7%	1.4%	1.6%	0.0%	3.3%
Detachment of retinal pigment epithelium	15.3%	11.3%	9.2%	3.5%	2.2%	4.3%	3.2%	8.5%	16.4%
Dry eye	6.4%	6.7%	10.0%	9.1%	3.6%	14.3%	8.1%	8.5%	4.9%
Eye irritation	19.9%	16.0%	19.2%	6.3%	4.4%	8.6%	4.8%	13.6%	13.1%
Eye pain	33.5%	36.1%	37.2%	23.1%	29.9%	30.0%	12.9%	18.6%	18.0%
Eyelid pain	0.4%	1.3%	1.3%	0.7%	0.0%	2.9%	0.0%	0.0%	1.6%
Foreign body sensation in eyes	14.4%	18.1%	18.8%	12.6%	8.0%	10.0%	6.5%	10.2%	9.8%
Glaucoma	0.4%	1.3%	2.9%	2.1%	1.5%	2.1%	0.0%	1.7%	1.6%
Iridocyclitis	1.3%	0.8%	1.7%	0.0%	0.0%	3.6%	1.6%	1.7%	1.6%

(cont'd)

Table 3: LUCENTIS *(cont'd)*

Ocular (in the study eye) and Non Ocular Adverse Events with a Difference in Incidence Rate ≥2% Between LUCENTIS 0.5 mg and the Control in at Least One Study. Studies MARINA (FVF2598g), ANCHOR (FVF2587g) and PIER (FVF3192g) Safety Population

	% of Patients Study MARINA (Dosage q 1 month) 2 years			% of Patients Study ANCHOR (Dosage q 1 month) 2 Years			% of Patients Study PIER (Dosage q 1 month for first 3 months then q 3 months) 2 Years		
Preferred Term	**Sham (N=236)**	**LUCENTIS 0.3 mg (N=238)**	**LUCENTIS 0.5 mg (N=239)**	**Verteporfin PDT (N=143)**	**LUCENTIS 0.3 mg (N=137)**	**LUCENTIS 0.5 mg (N=140)**	**Sham (N=62)**	**LUCENTIS 0.3 mg (N=59)**	**LUCENTIS 0.5 mg (N=61)**
Iritis	7.6%	8.0%	7.9%	1.4%	5.8%	7.9%	1.6%	1.7%	1.6%
Lacrimation increased	16.1%	17.2%	16.3%	5.6%	10.2%	9.3%	0.0%	6.8%	3.3%
Maculopathy	11.4%	8.4%	9.6%	4.9%	5.1%	7.9%	3.2%	5.1%	8.2%
Ocular discomfort	4.7%	7.6%	7.1%	2.1%	4.4%	6.4%	0.0%	0.0%	8.2%
Ocular hyperaemia	10.2%	10.1%	10.0%	5.6%	7.3%	12.1%	1.6%	8.5%	6.6%
Photophobia	2.5%	3.8%	2.5%	1.4%	0.7%	3.6%	0.0%	1.7%	0.0%
Posterior capsule opacification	5.1%	6.3%	7.9%	2.8%	3.6%	5.0%	0.0%	3.4%	3.3%
Retinal degeneration	6.8%	10.5%	10.0%	4.2%	2.9%	5.7%	3.2%	1.7%	1.6%
Retinal disorder	9.3%	11.3%	12.6%	2.8%	8.0%	6.4%	0.0%	0.0%	1.6%
Uveitis	0.0%	0.4%	0.8%	0.0%	0.7%	2.1%	0.0%	0.0%	0.0%
Visual disturbance	11.4%	13.9%	15.9%	5.6%	10.2%	7.9%	1.6%	3.4%	4.9%
Vitreous detachment	17.8%	21.8%	22.2%	21.7%	17.5%	18.6%	19.4%	10.2%	8.2%
Vitreous disorder	0.0%	2.1%	0.8%	0.0%	1.5%	2.1%	0.0%	1.7%	0.0%
Vitreous floaters	9.7%	31.9%	29.7%	4.9%	19.0%	22.1%	3.2%	11.9%	13.1%
Vitreous haemorrhage	2.5%	3.4%	2.9%	2.1%	3.6%	5.0%	1.6%	0.0%	1.6%
Vitritis	3.4%	7.1%	12.6%	2.1%	6.6%	10.7%	1.6%	1.7%	4.9%
Gastrointestinal Disorders									
Dental caries	0.8%	2.1%	0.8%	0.0%	1.5%	2.1%	1.6%	0.0%	0.0%
Diarrhoea	8.5%	7.6%	4.2%	4.9%	10.2%	5.7%	1.6%	1.7%	4.9%
Dysphagia	0.8%	2.5%	0.8%	0.0%	0.7%	1.4%	0.0%	0.0%	3.3%
Hiatus hernia	2.1%	0.8%	1.3%	0.7%	1.5%	3.6%	0.0%	1.7%	0.0%
Nausea	5.5%	8.8%	8.8%	7.0%	8.0%	10.0%	4.8%	8.5%	3.3%
General Disorders and Administration Site Conditions									
Asthenia	2.5%	1.7%	1.7%	2.1%	4.4%	1.4%	0.0%	3.4%	3.3%
Chest pain	5.5%	4.2%	3.8%	2.1%	5.1%	5.0%	3.2%	6.8%	3.3%
Injection site haemorrhage	1.7%	1.7%	5.0%	2.8%	5.8%	4.3%	0.0%	0.0%	0.0%
Infections and Infestations									
Bronchitis	8.5%	9.7%	10.5%	9.8%	8.0%	12.1%	4.8%	5.1%	6.6%
Diverticulitis	2.1%	3.8%	2.9%	0.7%	1.5%	2.9%	0.0%	3.4%	1.6%
Gastroenteritis viral	2.1%	1.3%	4.2%	0.0%	2.9%	2.9%	0.0%	1.7%	3.3%
Herpes zoster	2.1%	5.5%	4.2%	2.1%	2.9%	0.0%	1.6%	1.7%	4.9%
Influenza	5.1%	9.7%	7.9%	4.2%	5.8%	6.4%	3.2%	3.4%	4.9%
Localized infection	2.5%	2.1%	0.8%	0.0%	0.7%	1.4%	0.0%	0.0%	3.3%
Nasopharyngitis	13.1%	13.4%	15.9%	12.6%	24.8%	16.4%	9.7%	8.5%	6.6%
Sinusitis	5.5%	7.6%	8.4%	10.5%	10.5%	8.6%	4.8%	5.1%	1.6%
Upper respiratory tract infection	9.7%	15.1%	7.5%	6.3%	7.3%	11.4%	4.8%	11.9%	4.9%
Urinary tract infection	7.6%	8.8%	7.1%	10.5%	12.4%	11.4%	8.1%	8.5%	13.1%
Injury, Poisoning and Procedural Complications									
Corneal abrasion	3.4%	2.5%	2.9%	0.7%	2.2%	3.6%	1.6%	1.7%	0.0%
Foot fracture	0.4%	1.3%	0.0%	0.0%	0.7%	2.9%	1.6%	0.0%	0.0%
Procedural pain	1.7%	1.7%	1.3%	2.8%	2.2%	5.7%	1.6%	5.1%	0.0%
Wrist fracture	2.5%	1.7%	0.4%	0.0%	0.7%	2.1%	0.0%	0.0%	0.0%
Investigations									
Blood cholesterol increased	3.8%	0.8%	3.8%	0.7%	0.7%	2.9%	1.6%	3.4%	1.6%

(cont'd)

Table 3: LUCENTIS *(cont'd)*

Ocular (in the study eye) and Non Ocular Adverse Events with a Difference in Incidence Rate ≥2% Between LUCENTIS 0.5 mg and the Control in at Least One Study. Studies MARINA (FVF2598g), ANCHOR (FVF2587g) and PIER (FVF3192g) Safety Population

	% of Patients Study MARINA (Dosage q 1 month) 2 years			% of Patients Study ANCHOR (Dosage q 1 month) 2 Years			% of Patients Study PIER (Dosage q 1 month for first 3 months then q 3 months) 2 Years		
Preferred Term	**Sham (N=236)**	**LUCENTIS 0.3 mg (N=238)**	**LUCENTIS 0.5 mg (N=239)**	**Verteporfin PDT (N=143)**	**LUCENTIS 0.3 mg (N=137)**	**LUCENTIS 0.5 mg (N=140)**	**Sham (N=62)**	**LUCENTIS 0.3 mg (N=59)**	**LUCENTIS 0.5 mg (N=61)**
Blood glucose increased	4.7%	3.4%	3.8%	1.4%	3.6%	4.3%	0.0%	1.7%	1.6%
Intraocular pressure increased	5.9%	23.9%	23.8%	7.7%	22.6%	25.0%	4.8%	23.7%	31.1%
White blood cell count increased	0.0%	0.0%	2.5%	0.0%	0.7%	0.7%	0.0%	0.0%	0.0%
Metabolism and Nutrition Disorders									
Diabetes mellitus	1.3%	2.9%	3.8%	2.8%	4.4%	3.6%	0.0%	5.1%	1.6%
Gout	1.7%	0.8%	2.5%	0.7%	2.9%	2.9%	0.0%	0.0%	3.3%
Hypokalemia	3.0%	1.3%	1.7%	4.2%	4.4%	2.1%	0.0%	0.0%	8.2%
Musculoskeletal and Connective Tissue Disorders									
Arthralgia	8.9%	10.9%	11.3%	9.8%	5.1%	10.7%	1.6%	6.8%	8.2%
Back pain	9.3%	10.1%	9.2%	13.3%	10.2%	4.3%	3.2%	1.7%	6.6%
Exostosis	0.4%	0.4%	0.4%	1.4%	1.5%	1.4%	0.0%	0.0%	3.3%
Musculoskeletal chest pain	0.0%	0.0%	0.0%	0.0%	1.5%	0.7%	0.0%	0.0%	3.3%
Osteoarthritis	4.2%	3.8%	1.7%	0.7%	2.9%	3.6%	9.7%	1.7%	4.9%
Pain in extremity	5.9%	6.3%	5.4%	4.9%	5.1%	5.0%	0.0%	5.1%	3.3%
Nervous System Disorders									
Dementia	1.3%	0.4%	0.4%	0.7%	0.7%	0.7%	0.0%	0.0%	3.3%
Dizziness	9.7%	7.6%	4.6%	4.9%	5.1%	7.9%	1.6%	3.4%	3.3%
Headache	10.2%	16.0%	10.0%	7.0%	12.4%	15.0%	3.2%	1.7%	8.2%
Sciatica	0.8%	1.3%	1.7%	0.7%	2.2%	2.1%	0.0%	1.7%	3.3%
Psychiatric Disorders									
Anxiety	3.0%	4.2%	5.0%	6.3%	7.3%	3.6%	4.8%	0.0%	1.6%
Respiratory, Thoracic and Mediastinal Disorders									
Chronic obstructive pulmonary disease	2.1%	2.1%	4.6%	3.5%	6.6%	7.9%	0.0%	6.8%	0.0%
Cough	7.2%	9.7%	10.5%	8.4%	12.4%	6.4%	3.2%	3.4%	3.3%
Dyspnoea	2.5%	5.0%	2.9%	3.5%	3.6%	5.7%	3.2%	6.8%	1.6%
Sinus congestion	2.5%	2.1%	2.1%	0.0%	1.5%	2.1%	1.6%	1.7%	1.6%
Skin and Subcutaneous Tissue Disorders									
Ecchymosis	0.4%	1.7%	1.7%	0.0%	2.2%	4.3%	0.0%	1.0%	1.6%
Pruritus	2.1%	3.8%	2.5%	0.7%	0.0%	3.6%	1.6%	1.7%	0.0%
Vascular Disorders									
Hypertension	16.1%	17.2%	16.3%	16.1%	9.5%	12.1%	11.3%	10.2%	18.0%

Multiple occurrences of the same event were counted once in the overall incidence.

Table 4: LUCENTIS

Ocular Adverse Events in the Study Eye Regardless of Relationship to Treatment by System Organ Class and Preferred Term (2-year incidence at least 1.0% in ranibizumab 0.5 mg group) in MARINA, ANCHOR, and PIER (pooled data) Safety Population

Preferred Term	**Sham N=298 (%)**	**PDT N=143 (%)**	**Ranibizumab 0.3 mg N=434 (%)**	**Ranibizumab 0.5 mg N=440 (%)**
Congenital, Familial and Genetic Disorders				
Corneal dystrophy	2.0%	0.0%	3.2%	2.3%
Eye Disorders				
Anterior chamber flare	2.0%	0.0%	2.1%	2.0%
Arcus lipoides	0.0%	0.0%	1.6%	1.6%
Blepharitis	8.4%	7.0%	10.1%	10.9%
Cataract	5.7%	7.0%	7.8%	8.2%

(cont'd)

Table 4: LUCENTIS *(cont'd)*

Ocular Adverse Events in the Study Eye Regardless of Relationship to Treatment by System Organ Class and Preferred Term (2-year incidence at least 1.0% in ranibizumab 0.5 mg group) in MARINA, ANCHOR, and PIER (pooled data) Safety Population

Preferred Term	**Sham N=298 (%)**	**PDT N=143 (%)**	**Ranibizumab 0.3 mg N=434 (%)**	**Ranibizumab 0.5 mg N=440 (%)**
Cataract cortical	2.0%	1.4%	1.4%	3.4%
Cataract nuclear	5.4%	1.4%	4.1%	4.8%
Cataract subcapsular	2.3%	0.7%	3.2%	2.7%
Chalazion	0.3%	0.7%	0.7%	1.6%
Choroidal neovascularisation	16.8%	12.6%	2.5%	2.5%
Conjunctival haemorrhage	58.4%	50.3%	71.9%	70.7%

(cont'd)

Table 4: LUCENTIS *(cont'd)*

Ocular Adverse Events in the Study Eye Regardless of Relationship to Treatment by System Organ Class and Preferred Term (2-year incidence at least 1.0% in ranibizumab 0.5 mg group) in MARINA, ANCHOR, and PIER (pooled data) Safety Population

Preferred Term	Sham N=298 (%)	PDT N=143 (%)	Ranibizumab 0.3 mg N=434 (%)	Ranibizumab 0.5 mg N=440 (%)
Conjunctival hyperemia	5.4%	4.2%	5.5%	6.4%
Conjunctivitis	2.3%	0.0%	3.2%	3.0%
Conjunctivitis allergic	1.7%	0.7%	1.4%	3.0%
Detachment of retinal pigment epithelium	12.8%	3.5%	8.1%	8.6%
Diplopia	0.0%	0.7%	0.9%	1.1%
Dry eye	6.7%	9.1%	6.0%	10.7%
Eye discharge	6.7%	3.5%	6.2%	3.0%
Eye haemorrhage	3.4%	0.0%	0.7%	1.1%
Eye irritation	16.8%	6.3%	12.0%	15.0%
Eye pain	29.2%	23.1%	31.8%	32.3%
Eye pruritus	10.4%	8.4%	8.5%	10.2%
Eye swelling	1.3%	1.4%	1.2%	1.4%
Eyelid edema	2.7%	2.8%	2.8%	3.0%
Eyelid pain	0.3%	0.7%	0.7%	1.8%
Foreign body sensation in eyes	12.8%	12.6%	13.8%	14.8%
Glaucoma	0.3%	2.1%	1.4%	2.5%
Iridocyclitis	1.3%	0.0%	0.7%	2.3%
Iritis	6.4%	1.4%	6.5%	7.0%
Lacrimation increased	12.8%	5.6%	13.6%	12.3%
Macular degeneration	62.4%	70.6%	43.3%	42.0%
Macular edema	10.4%	4.9%	3.2%	3.6%
Macular scar	1.7%	2.1%	2.3%	1.8%
Maculopathy	9.7%	4.9%	6.9%	8.9%
Meibomianitis	0.3%	0.0%	0.9%	1.6%
Ocular discomfort	3.7%	2.1%	5.5%	7.0%
Ocular hyperemia	8.4%	5.6%	9.0%	10.2%
Photophobia	2.0%	1.4%	2.5%	2.5%
Photopsia	5.0%	8.4%	4.8%	4.1%
Posterior capsule opacification	4.0%	2.8%	5.1%	6.4%
Punctate keratitis	3.7%	1.4%	3.9%	3.0%
Retinal degeneration	6.0%	4.2%	6.9%	7.5%
Retinal detachment	7.0%	2.1%	3.9%	1.4%
Retinal disorder	7.4%	2.8%	8.8%	9.1%
Retinal exudates	9.7%	4.9%	5.5%	4.8%
Retinal haemorrhage	52.7%	67.8%	25.8%	25.2%
Retinal pigmentation	1.0%	0.0%	1.4%	1.1%
Retinal tear	1.0%	0.0%	0.9%	1.1%
Retinal vascular disorder	2.7%	0.7%	0.5%	1.4%
Subretinal fibrosis	15.1%	22.4%	9.2%	9.5%
Trichiasis	0.7%	0.7%	1.2%	1.6%
Uveitis	0.0%	0.0%	0.5%	1.1%
Vision blurred	7.4%	9.1%	11.5%	6.8%
Visual acuity reduced	17.8%	16.8%	11.3%	8.6%
Visual disturbance	7.4%	4.9%	9.2%	10.5%
Vitreous detachment	17.8%	21.7%	18.9%	19.1%

(cont'd)

Table 4: LUCENTIS *(cont'd)*

Ocular Adverse Events in the Study Eye Regardless of Relationship to Treatment by System Organ Class and Preferred Term (2-year incidence at least 1.0% in ranibizumab 0.5 mg group) in MARINA, ANCHOR, and PIER (pooled data) Safety Population

Preferred Term	Sham N=298 (%)	PDT N=143 (%)	Ranibizumab 0.3 mg N=434 (%)	Ranibizumab 0.5 mg N=440 (%)
Vitreous disorder	0.0%	0.0%	1.8%	1.1%
Vitreous floaters	8.1%	4.9%	25.1%	25.0%
Vitreous haemorrhage	2.3%	2.1%	3.0%	3.4%
Vitritis	3.0%	2.1%	6.2%	10.9%
General Disorders and Administration Site Conditions				
Injection site haemorrhage	1.3%	2.8%	2.8%	4.1%
Immune System Disorders				
Drug hypersensitivity	2.0%	4.2%	1.4%	1.4%
Injury, Poisoning and Procedural Complications				
Corneal abrasion	3.0%	0.7%	2.3%	2.7%
Investigations				
Intraocular pressure increased	5.7%	7.7%	23.5%	25.2%
Skin and Subcutaneous Tissue Disorders				
Cutis laxa	0.7%	0.7%	1.4%	1.1%
Dandruff	0.7%	0.7%	0.7%	1.1%

Table 5: LUCENTIS

Non-ocular Adverse Events Regardless of Relationship to Treatment by System Organ Class and Preferred Term (2-year incidence at least 1.0% in ranibizumab 0.5 mg group) in MARINA, ANCHOR, and PIER (pooled data) Safety Population

Preferred Term	Sham N=298 (%)	PDT N=143 (%)	Ranibizumab 0.3 mg N=434 (%)	Ranibizumab 0.5 mg N=440 (%)
Blood and Lymphatic System Disorders				
Anaemia	6.4%	4.2%	7.6%	8.0%
Cardiac Disorders				
Angina pectoris	1.3%	0.7%	1.4%	1.8%
Atrial fibrillation	4.0%	3.5%	3.2%	4.5%
Bradycardia	0.7%	2.1%	0.9%	1.1%
Cardiac failure congestive	4.0%	3.5%	4.1%	3.6%
Cardiomegaly	1.7%	0.7%	1.2%	1.1%
Coronary artery disease	3.0%	0.7%	2.8%	2.3%
Myocardial infarction	1.7%	1.4%	1.2%	1.6%
Ear and Labyrinth Disorders				
Vertigo	1.7%	7.0%	4.1%	2.3%
Endocrine Disorders				
Hypothyroidism	2.3%	2.1%	1.6%	1.1%
Gastrointestinal Disorders				
Abdominal pain	1.7%	2.1%	2.8%	1.1%
Colonic polyp	1.0%	2.8%	1.6%	1.6%
Constipation	7.0%	5.6%	6.7%	5.2%
Dental caries	1.0%	0.0%	1.6%	1.1%
Diarrhoea	7.0%	4.9%	7.6%	4.8%
Diverticulum	1.3%	0.7%	2.1%	1.6%
Dyspepsia	3.7%	2.8%	2.1%	1.4%
Dysphagia	0.7%	0.0%	1.6%	1.4%
Gastritis	0.7%	0.7%	1.2%	1.6%
Gastroesophageal reflux disease	5.0%	8.4%	6.0%	3.6%

(cont'd)

Table 5: LUCENTIS *(cont'd)*

Non-ocular Adverse Events Regardless of Relationship to Treatment by System Organ Class and Preferred Term (2-year incidence at least 1.0% in ranibizumab 0.5 mg group) in MARINA, ANCHOR, and PIER (pooled data) Safety Population

Preferred Term	Sham N=298 (%)	PDT N=143 (%)	Ranibizumab 0.3 mg N=434 (%)	Ranibizumab 0.5 mg N=440 (%)
Haemorrhoids	2.3%	1.4%	1.8%	1.8%
Hiatus hernia	1.7%	0.7%	1.2%	1.8%
Inguinal hernia	0.3%	0.0%	0.5%	1.1%
Nausea	5.4%	7.0%	8.5%	8.4%
Toothache	2.0%	1.4%	1.4%	1.6%
Vomiting	1.3%	5.6%	4.4%	2.0%
General Disorders and Administration Site Conditions				
Asthenia	1.0%	2.1%	2.8%	1.4%
Chest pain	5.0%	2.1%	4.8%	3.9%
Fatigue	3.4%	4.9%	3.2%	3.2%
Oedema peripheral	5.7%	2.8%	6.7%	3.6%
Pain	1.7%	2.1%	2.1%	2.0%
Pyrexia	1.7%	1.4%	2.5%	2.3%
Hepatobiliary Disorders				
Cholelithiasis	3.0%	0.7%	0.7%	1.1%
Immune System Disorders				
Drug hypersensitivity	2.7%	1.4%	0.9%	2.0%
Hypersensitivity	1.0%	4.2%	2.8%	2.3%
Seasonal allergy	3.4%	7.0%	3.7%	3.9%
Infections and Infestations				
Bronchitis	8.1%	9.8%	9.0%	10.5%
Cellulitis	2.3%	0.7%	2.1%	1.1%
Cystitis	2.0%	2.8%	3.0%	3.0%
Diverticulitis	1.7%	0.7%	3.0%	2.7%
Ear infection	1.3%	2.1%	1.4%	1.4%
Gastroenteritis viral	1.7%	0.0%	1.8%	3.6%
Herpes zoster	2.0%	2.1%	4.1%	3.0%
Influenza	4.7%	4.2%	7.6%	7.0%
Localised infection	2.0%	0.0%	1.4%	1.4%
Lower respiratory tract infection	0.7%	1.4%	1.8%	1.1%
Nasopharyngitis	12.4%	12.6%	16.4%	14.8%
Pneumonia	5.4%	4.2%	6.2%	4.5%
Sinusitis	5.4%	10.5%	8.1%	7.5%
Tooth abscess	1.7%	1.4%	1.2%	1.6%
Tooth infection	1.3%	0.0%	1.6%	1.1%
Upper respiratory tract infection	8.7%	6.3%	12.2%	8.4%
Urinary tract infection	7.7%	10.5%	9.9%	9.3%
Injury, Poisoning and Procedural Complications				
Contusion	7.4%	5.6%	3.9%	4.1%
Excoriation	1.3%	0.7%	1.6%	1.6%
Fall	4.0%	2.1%	3.2%	3.2%
Joint sprain	0.7%	0.0%	1.2%	1.1%
Procedural pain	1.7%	2.8%	2.3%	2.5%
Skin laceration	2.3%	3.5%	3.5%	1.6%
Investigations				

(cont'd)

Table 5: LUCENTIS *(cont'd)*

Non-ocular Adverse Events Regardless of Relationship to Treatment by System Organ Class and Preferred Term (2-year incidence at least 1.0% in ranibizumab 0.5 mg group) in MARINA, ANCHOR, and PIER (pooled data) Safety Population

Preferred Term	Sham N=298 (%)	PDT N=143 (%)	Ranibizumab 0.3 mg N=434 (%)	Ranibizumab 0.5 mg N=440 (%)
Blood cholesterol increased	3.4%	0.7%	1.2%	3.2%
Blood glucose increased	3.7%	1.4%	3.2%	3.6%
Blood pressure increased	6.0%	2.1%	4.6%	5.5%
Blood urea increased	0.3%	0.7%	0.9%	1.1%
Blood uric acid increased	1.3%	0.0%	0.7%	1.8%
White blood cell count increased	0.0%	0.0%	0.2%	1.6%
Metabolism and Nutrition Disorders				
Dehydration	1.0%	3.5%	2.8%	2.3%
Diabetes mellitus	1.0%	2.8%	3.7%	3.4%
Gout	1.3%	0.7%	1.4%	2.7%
Hypercholesterolaemia	4.4%	5.6%	5.3%	5.0%
Hyperlipidaemia	2.0%	2.8%	1.8%	1.6%
Hypokalaemia	2.3%	4.2%	2.1%	2.7%
Musculoskeletal and Connective Tissue Disorders				
Arthralgia	7.4%	9.8%	8.5%	10.7%
Arthritis	7.0%	7.0%	4.6%	5.7%
Back pain	8.1%	13.3%	9.0%	7.3%
Exostosis	0.3%	1.4%	0.7%	1.1%
Joint swelling	2.0%	1.4%	1.8%	1.1%
Muscle spasms	2.3%	2.8%	2.3%	1.6%
Musculoskeletal pain	4.4%	2.8%	2.8%	3.0%
Musculoskeletal stiffness	0.0%	0.7%	0.2%	1.1%
Myalgia	1.3%	2.8%	1.4%	1.6%
Neck pain	1.0%	0.0%	1.2%	2.0%
Osteoarthritis	5.4%	0.7%	3.2%	2.7%
Osteoporosis	2.0%	3.5%	2.8%	3.0%
Pain in extremity	4.7%	4.9%	5.8%	5.0%
Rotator cuff syndrome	1.3%	0.7%	0.9%	1.1%
Neoplasms Benign, Malignant and Unspecified (incl cysts and polyps)				
Basal cell carcinoma	3.7%	2.1%	5.1%	2.3%
Skin cancer	1.0%	0.0%	0.9%	1.1%
Nervous System Disorders				
Balance disorder	0.3%	0.0%	0.2%	1.1%
Carpal tunnel syndrome	0.3%	0.7%	0.9%	1.4%
Cerebrovascular accident	0.7%	0.7%	0.7%	1.1%
Dizziness	8.1%	4.9%	6.2%	5.2%
Headache	8.7%	7.0%	12.4%	11.4%
Nerve compression	1.0%	0.0%	0.5%	1.1%
Sciatica	0.7%	0.7%	1.6%	2.0%
Syncope	3.0%	2.1%	1.4%	2.7%
Transient ischaemic attack	1.3%	2.8%	0.7%	1.8%
Psychiatric Disorders				
Anxiety	3.4%	6.3%	4.6%	4.1%
Depression	6.7%	9.1%	5.5%	5.0%
Insomnia	5.0%	4.2%	4.1%	5.2%

(cont'd)

Table 5: LUCENTIS *(cont'd)*

Non-ocular Adverse Events Regardless of Relationship to Treatment by System Organ Class and Preferred Term (2-year incidence at least 1.0% in ranibizumab 0.5 mg group) in MARINA, ANCHOR, and PIER (pooled data) Safety Population

Preferred Term	Sham N=298 (%)	PDT N=143 (%)	Ranibizumab 0.3 mg N=434 (%)	Ranibizumab 0.5 mg N=440 (%)
Renal and Urinary Disorders				
Renal cyst	1.3%	3.5%	1.4%	1.1%
Renal failure	0.3%	1.4%	1.8%	1.1%
Reproductive System and Breast Disorders				
Benign prostatic hyperplasia	1.3%	2.8%	2.1%	2.3%
Respiratory, Thoracic and Mediastinal Disorders				
Asthma	2.0%	2.8%	2.5%	2.3%
Chronic obstructive pulmonary disease	1.7%	3.5%	4.1%	5.0%
Cough	6.4%	8.4%	9.7%	8.2%
Dyspnoea	2.7%	3.5%	4.8%	3.6%
Emphysema	1.0%	1.4%	1.2%	1.1%
Epistaxis	1.0%	2.8%	1.8%	1.6%
Pharyngolaryngeal pain	0.7%	2.8%	2.3%	1.8%
Rhinorrhoea	1.7%	1.4%	2.3%	1.4%
Sinus congestion	2.3%	0.0%	1.8%	2.0%
Skin and Subcutaneous Tissue Disorders				
Actinic keratosis	3.0%	0.7%	1.8%	1.4%
Dermatitis contact	0.7%	2.1%	0.9%	1.4%
Ecchymosis	0.0%	0.0%	0.7%	1.6%
Pruritus	1.3%	0.7%	2.1%	2.5%
Rash	3.7%	5.6%	2.8%	3.9%
Vascular Disorders				
Haematoma	1.3%	0.0%	1.4%	1.1%
Hypertension	15.1%	16.1%	13.8%	15.2%
Hypotension	2.3%	4.2%	2.3%	1.8%

Arterial thromboembolic events, as defined by the ANTIPLATELET TRIALISTS' COLLABORATION (APTC), including vascular deaths, non-fatal myocardial infarctions, nonfatal ischemic strokes and non-fatal haemorrhagic strokes, have been linked to the systemic availability of highly potent vascular endothelial growth factor (VEGF) inhibitors. When the first-year data from all three phase III studies (MARINA, ANCHOR and PIER) were combined, the overall incidence of arterial thromboembolic events was higher for patients treated with LUCENTIS 0.5 mg (2.5%) compared with control arm (1.1%). When the second year data from all three phase III (MARINA, ANCHOR and PIER) were combined, the overall incidence of arterial thromboembolic events was similar for patients with LUCENTIS 0.5 mg (4.1%) compared with the control arm (3.6%). For (fatal and non-fatal) cerebrovascular accidents (CVAs) the results were not consistent across studies. In the MARINA study, there was a slight numerical imbalance between LUCENTIS 0.5 mg (1.3%) and the control arm (0.4%) during the first year, which was still present at the end of the 2-year treatment period (3.3% for 0.5 mg vs. 1.3% for sham treatment). The CVA incidence rate in the MARINA, ANCHOR study and PIER study are shown in Table 6. Although there was a low annual rate of arterial thromboembolic events observed in the LUCENTIS (a VEGF inhibitor) clinical trials, there was no imbalance between treatment groups (Table 7). There is a potential risk of arterial thromboembolic events following intravitreal use of VEGF inhibitors.

Table 6: LUCENTIS

Cerebrovascular Accident (CVA) Rates (fatal and non-fatal), Safety Populations (2-year cumulative data)

	Control	0.3 mg LUCENTIS	0.5 mg LUCENTIS
MARINA–1 yr	1/236 (0.4%)	1/238 (0.4%)	3/239 (1.3%)
MARINA–2 yr	3/236 (1.3%)	3/238 (1.3%)	8/239 (3.3%)
ANCHOR–1 yr	1/143 (0.7%)	1/137 (0.7%)	1/140 (0.7%)
ANCHOR– 2 yr	2/143 (1.4%)	3/137 (2.2%)[a]	0/140 (0.0%)
PIER–1 yr	0/62 (0.0%)	0/59 (0.0%)	0/61 (0.0%)
PIER–2 yr[b]	0/62 (0.0%) (before crossover) 1/39 (2.6%) (after crossover)	0/59 (0.0%)	0/61 (0.0%)

[a] Includes one serious adverse event of cerebral infarction (Year 1), one adverse event of ischemic stroke (Year 2) and one non-serious adverse event of cerebral ischemia (Year 2).

[b] After the month 12 visit in the study, patients in the sham-injection group could crossover to the LUCENTIS 0.5 mg group for the remainder of the study.

Table 7: LUCENTIS

Arterial Thromboembolic Events (ATE) as Defined by the Antiplatelet Trialists' Collaboration (APTC), Safety Populations (2-year cumulative data)

	Control	0.3 mg LUCENTIS	0.5 mg LUCENTIS
MARINA–1 yr	2/236 (0.8%)	4/238 (1.7%)	5/239 (2.1%)
MARINA–2 yr	9/236 (3.8%)	11/238 (4.6%)	11/239 (4.6%)
ANCHOR–1 yr	3/143 (2.1%)	3/137 (2.2%)	6/140 (4.3%)
ANCHOR–2 yr	6/143 (4.2%)	6/137 (4.4%)	7/140 (5.0%)
PIER–1 yr	0/62 (0.0%)	0/59 (0.0%)	0/61 (0.0%)
PIER–2 yr[a]	1/62 (1.6%) (before crossover) 1/39 (2.6%) (after crossover)	1/59 (1.7%)	0/61 (0.0%)

[a] After the month 12 visit in the study, patients in the sham-injection group could crossover to the LUCENTIS 0.5 mg group for the remainder of the study.

The SAILOR study, FVF 3689g, was a Phase IIIb, Multicenter Study to Evaluate the Safety and Tolerability of Ranibizumab in Naive and Previously Treated Subjects with Choroidal Neovascularization (CNV) Secondary to Age-Related Macular Degeneration (AMD).

In the study, an interim analysis including data from almost 2400 patients (randomized to the two doses of LUCENTIS 0.3 mg and LUCENTIS 0.5 mg in a 1:1 ratio) with an average follow-up period of 230 days was performed. The overall incidence of CVAs (fatal and non-fatal) was found to be 1.1% for LUCENTIS 0.5 mg compared with 0.3% for LUCENTIS 0.3 mg (p=0.021). The rate of deaths from all causes was (1.6% on 0.5 mg vs. 0.6% on 0.3 mg, p=0.029) whereas the differences in the rate of vascular deaths (0.7% on 0.5 mg vs. 0.4% on 0.3 mg) and in the rate of combined APTC events (1.7% on 0.5 mg vs. 1.1% on 0.3 mg) were smaller.

A second interim analysis which was based on an average follow-up time of 335 days showed that the difference in the incidence of CVAs had decreased with increasing exposure to LUCENTIS treatment (1.3% on 0.5 mg vs. 0.6% on 0.3 mg). The same applied to the difference in the overall death rate (2.0% on 0.5 mg vs. 1.3% on 0.3 mg).

Upon final analysis of the incidence in strokes in SAILOR study, there exists a trend towards a higher stroke rate in the 0.5 mg group compared to the 0.3 mg group. The respective 95% CIs for the overall stroke rate were wide (0.3% to 1.3% for the 0.3 mg group vs. 0.7% to 2.0% for the 0.5 mg group). The number of strokes was small for both dose groups, and there is not sufficient evidence to conclude (or rule out) that there is a true difference in stroke rates among the treatment groups. Forty-nine deaths were reported, with 20 deaths in the 0.3-mg group (1.7%) and 29 deaths in the 0.5-mg group (2.4%). Of these, 21 were classified as vascular deaths, 11 in the 0.3-mg group (0.9%) and 10 in the 0.5-mg group (0.8%).

Less Common Clinical Trial Adverse Drug Reactions: The adverse events with suspected relationship to LUCENTIS treatment listed below occurred in patients receiving treatment with LUCENTIS 0.5 mg for up to 2 years in the controlled Phase III studies MARINA (FVF2598g) and ANCHOR (FVF2587g) at an incidence of <1.0%. The safety data described below also includes procedure and potential drug related adverse events in the 379 patients of the combined 0.5 mg treatment groups.

Cardiac Disorders: atrial fibrillation.

Ear and Labyrinth Disorders: ear pain.

Eye Disorders: abnormal sensation in eye, angle closure glaucoma, anterior chamber flare, blepharitis, blindness, cataract subcapsular, conjunctival edema, conjunctivitis allergic, corneal deposits, corneal edema, corneal epithelium defect, corneal striae, dellen, detachment of retinal pigment epithelium, endophthalmitis, episcleritis, erythema of eyelid, eye hemorrhage, eye swelling, eyelid irritation, eyelid ptosis, glaucoma, hyphema, iris adhesions, keratopathy, lenticular pigmentation, macular degeneration, maculopathy, photophobia, photopsia, pigmentary glaucoma, posterior capsule opacification, pupillary reflex impaired, retinal artery occlusion, etinal disorder, retinal scar, retinal tear, scleral hyperemia, subretinal fibrosis, vitreous degeneration, vitreous opacities.

Gastrointestinal Disorders: nausea.

General Disorders and Administration Site Conditions: asthenia, facial pain, injection site irritation, pain.

Infections and Infestations: hypopyon.

Injury, Poisoning and Procedural Complications: cataract traumatic, contusion, eye injury, scratch.

Investigations: intraocular pressure decreased.

Musculoskeletal and Connective Tissue Disorders: pain in jaw.

Nervous System Disorders: dizziness.

Psychiatric Disorders: anticipatory anxiety, anxiety.

Respiratory, Thoracic and Mediastinal Disorders: cough, increased upper airway secretion, rhinorrhea, wheezing.

Skin and Subcutaneous Tissue Disorders: dermatitis allergic, lichenoid ketatosis.

Abnormal Hematologic and Clinical Chemistry Findings: There were no findings to suggest a relationship between LUCENTIS and the development of clinically significant abnormalities.

Post-Market Adverse Drug Reactions: The common ocular and non-ocular adverse drug reactions been reported with an incidence rate of ≥1.0% of the total adverse reactions reported in Phase IV clinical trials and with marketed use of LUCENTIS are summarized in Table 8.

Table 8: LUCENTIS

LUCENTIS Post-market Ocular and Non-ocular Adverse Reactions: Phase IV Studies [SECURE (CRFB002A2402) and EVEREST (CBPD952A2308)], Literature Cases and Spontaneous Reports. Adverse Reactions with Incidence Rate ≥1% of Total Adverse Reactions Reported (n=4074)

Preferred Term	Studies SECURE and EVEREST	Literature Cases	Spontaneous Reports
Eye Disorders			
Visual acuity reduced	5 (0.1%)	31 (0.8%)	226 (5.5%)
Eye pain	2 (0.0%)	0 (0.0%)	182 (4.5%)
Visual impairment	1 (0.0%)	2 (0.0%)	125 (3.1%)
Endophthalmitis	5 (0.1%)	12 (0.3%)	77 (1.9%)
Ocular hyperaemia	0 (0.0%)	0 (0.0%)	93 (2.3%)
Vision blurred	0 (0.0%)	0 (0.0%)	80 (2.0%)
Myodesopsia	0 (0.0%)	0 (0.0%)	57 (1.4%)
Foreign body sensation in eyes	0 (0.0%)	0 (0.0%)	51 (1.2%)
Eye haemorrhage	0 (0.0%)	1 (0.0%)	45 (1.1%)
Lacrimation increased	0 (0.0%)	0 (0.0%)	45 (1.1%)

(cont'd)

Table 8: LUCENTIS (cont'd)

LUCENTIS Post-market Ocular and Non-ocular Adverse Reactions: Phase IV Studies [SECURE (CRFB002A2402) and EVEREST (CBPD952A2308)], Literature Cases and Spontaneous Reports. Adverse Reactions with Incidence Rate ≥1% of Total Adverse Reactions Reported (n=4074)

Preferred Term	Studies SECURE and EVEREST	Literature Cases	Spontaneous Reports
Retinal pigment epithelial tear	0 (0.0%)	11 (0.3%)	34 (0.8%)
Eye irritation	0 (0.0%)	0 (0.0%)	43 (1.1%)
Gastrointestinal Disorders			
Nausea	0 (0.0%)	0 (0.0%)	39 (1.0%)
General Disorders and Administration Site Conditions			
Drug ineffective	0 (0.0%)	3 (0.1%)	82 (2.0%)
Investigations			
Blood pressure increased	0 (0.0%)	0 (0.0%)	50 (1.2%)
Nervous System Disorders			
Cerebrovascular accident	0 (0.0%)	1 (0.0%)	86 (2.1%)
Headache	0 (0.0%)	0 (0.0%)	85 (2.1%)
Dizziness	1 (0.0%)	0 (0.0%)	51 (1.2%)
Skin and Subcutaneous Disorders			
Allergic reactions[a]	1 (0.0%)	1 (0.0%)	71 (1.7%)

[a] Preferred terms summarized: Rash, Erythema, Urticaria, Pruritus and Pruritus generalized.

DRUG INTERACTIONS: Overview: Nine-month data from open-label study (PROTECT) in which the safety of same-day administration of verteporfin PDT and LUCENTIS 0.5 mg was evaluated, showed that the initial combination of treatment was 6.3% (two of 32 patients).
Drug-Food Interactions: Interactions with food have not been established.
Drug-Herb Interactions: Interactions with herbal products have not been established.
Drug-Laboratory Test Interactions: Interactions with laboratory tests have not been established.

DOSAGE AND ADMINISTRATION: Recommended Dose and Dosage Adjustment: Single-use vial for intravitreal use only.

LUCENTIS must be administered by a qualified ophthalmologist experienced in intravitreal injections.

The recommended dose for LUCENTIS (ranibizumab injection) is 0.5 mg (0.05 mL). LUCENTIS 0.5 mg is recommended to be administered by intravitreal injection once a month. Treatment may be reduced to one injection every 3 months after the first three injections if monthly dosing is not feasible. Compared to monthly dosing, dosing every 3 months will lead to an approximate 5-letter (1 line) loss of visual acuity benefit, on average, over the following 9 months. Patients should be evaluated regularly.

Administration: LUCENTIS treatment is initiated with a loading phase of one injection per month for three consecutive months, followed by a maintenance phase in which patients should be monitored for visual acuity on a regular basis. If the patient experiences a loss of greater than 5 letters in visual acuity (Early Treatment Diabetic Retinopathy Study (ETDRS) or one Snellen line equivalent), or clinical or diagnostic evidence of disease activity, LUCENTIS should be administered. The interval between two doses should not be shorter than 1 month.

As with all medicinal products for parenteral use, LUCENTIS should be inspected visually for particulate matter and discoloration prior to administration.

The injection procedure should be carried out under aseptic conditions, which includes the use of surgical hand disinfection, sterile gloves, a sterile drape and a sterile eyelid speculum (or equivalent) and the availability of sterile paracentesis (if required). The patient's medical history for hypersensitivity reactions should be carefully evaluated prior to performing the intravitreal procedure (see Contraindications). The peri-ocular skin, eyelid and ocular surface should be disinfected. Adequate anaesthesia and a broad-spectrum topical microbicide should be administered prior to the injection.

The patient should be instructed to self-administer antimicrobial drops four times daily for 3 days before and after each injection.

To prepare LUCENTIS for intravitreal administration, please adhere to the following instructions:

1. Before withdrawal, the outer part of the rubber stopper of the vial should be disinfected.
2. Assemble the 5 micrometer filter needle (included in LUCENTIS pack) onto the 1 mL syringe (not included in LUCENTIS pack) using aseptic technique. Push the blunt filter needle into the centre of the vial stopper until the needle touches the bottom edge of the vial.
3. Withdraw all the liquid from the vial, keeping the vial in an upright position, slightly inclined to ease complete withdrawal.
4. Ensure that the plunger rod is drawn sufficiently back when emptying the vial in order to completely empty the filter needle.
5. Leave the blunt filter needle in the vial and disconnect the syringe from the blunt filter needle. The filter needle should be discarded after withdrawal of the vial contents and should not be used for the intravitreal injection.
6. Aseptically and firmly assemble the injection needle (not included in LUCENTIS pack) onto the syringe.
7. Carefully remove the cap from the injection needle without disconnecting the injection needle from the syringe.
   Note: Grip at the hub of the injection needle while removing the cap.
8. Carefully expel the air from the syringe and adjust the dose to the 0.05 mL mark on the syringe. The syringe is ready for injection.
   Note: Do not wipe the injection needle. Do not pull back on the plunger.

Any unused product or waste material should be disposed of in accordance with local requirements.

The injection needle should be inserted 3.5 to 4.0 mm posterior to the limbus into the vitreous cavity, avoiding the horizontal meridian and aiming towards the centre of the globe. The injection volume of 0.05 mL is then delivered. The scleral site should be rotated for subsequent injections.

OVERDOSAGE:
Because LUCENTIS (ranibizumab injection) is administered by qualified ophthalmologists experienced in intravitreal injections, the likelihood of an overdose is very low. Cases of accidental overdose have been reported from the clinical studies and post-marketing data. Adverse reactions most frequently associated with these reported cases were intraocular pressure increased and eye pain. If an overdose occurs, intraocular pressure should be monitored and treated, if deemed necessary by the attending physician.

> For management of a suspected drug overdose, CPhA recommends that you contact your **regional Poison Control Centre**. See the *CPS* Directory section for a list of Poison Control Centres.

ACTION AND CLINICAL PHARMACOLOGY: Mechanism of Action: Ranibizumab is a humanised recombinant monoclonal antibody fragment targeted against human vascular endothelial growth factor-A (VEGF-A). Ranibizumab is designed to penetrate all retinal layers. It binds with high affinity to all active VEGF-A isoforms (e.g. $VEGF_{110}$, $VEGF_{121}$ and $VEGF_{165}$), thereby preventing binding of VEGF-A to its receptors VEGFR-1 and VEGFR-2. Binding of VEGF-A to its receptors leads to endothelial cell proliferation and neovascularisation, as well as vascular leakage, all of which are thought to contribute to the progression of the neovascular form of age-related macular degeneration.

Pharmacokinetics: Following monthly intravitreal administration of LUCENTIS (ranibizumab injection) to patients with neovascular AMD, serum concentrations of ranibizumab were generally low. Maximum serum levels (C_{max}), measured after single administration and estimated using population pharmacokinetics (PK) for repeated administration, were generally below the ranibizumab concentration necessary to inhibit the biological activity of VEGF by 50% (11-27 ng/mL, as assessed in an in vitro cellular proliferation assay). Following single administration, C_{max} was dose proportional over the dose range of 0.05 to 1.0 mg/eye. Although the PK data suggest that serum ranibizumab levels remain below the level necessary to inhibit the biological activity of VEGF by 50%, an assessment of additional time points around the C_{max} would be required to confirm that serum ranibizumab levels do not exceed this threshold at any timepoint upon monthly intravitreal injection of 0.5 mg LUCENTIS in humans.

Based on analysis of limited population pharmacokinetics data from patients treated with the 0.5 mg dose, serum ranibizumab C_{max}, attained approximately 1 day after dosing, is predicted to generally range between 0.79 and 2.90 ng/mL, and C_{min} is predicted to generally range between 0.07 and 0.49 ng/mL.

Special Populations and Conditions: Pediatrics: LUCENTIS has not been studied in this sub-population.
Geriatrics: No dose adjustment is required in the elderly.
Gender: No special considerations are needed.
Hepatic Insufficiency: No formal studies have been conducted to examine the pharmacokinetics of LUCENTIS in patients with hepatic impairment.
Renal Insufficiency: No formal studies have been conducted to examine the pharmacokinetics of LUCENTIS in patients with renal impairment. Sixty-eight percent (136 of 200) of patients in a population pharmacokinetic analysis had renal impairment (46.5% mild [50-80 mL/min], 20% moderate [30-50 mL/min], and 1.5% severe [<30 mL/min]). Systemic clearance was slightly lower in patients with mild and moderate renal impairment. Three patients with severe renal impairment had a clearance that was reduced by approximately 42%. The clinical significance of these findings is unknown.

STORAGE AND STABILITY: Store in a refrigerator (2-8°C). **Do not freeze.**
Keep the vial in the outer carton in order to protect from light.
LUCENTIS must be kept out of the reach and sight of children.

SPECIAL HANDLING INSTRUCTIONS: Do not use if particles, discolouration or cloudiness are evident.
Vials are for single use only.
Any unused product or waste material should be disposed of in accordance with local requirements.
In the absence of compatibility studies, this medicinal product must not be mixed with other medicinal products.

INFORMATION FOR THE PATIENT: Published in e-CPS, available by subscription at www.e-cps.ca.

DOSAGE FORMS, COMPOSITION AND PACKAGING: Each mL of sterile, clear, colourless to pale yellow aqueous solution for injection, contains: ranibizumab 10 mg. Nonmedicinal ingredients: α,α-trehalose dihydrate, histidine, histidine hydrochloride monohydrate, polysorbate 20 and water for injections. Preservative-free. Single-use glass vials (colourless type I glass) with chlorobutyl rubber stopper containing 2.3 mg ranibizumab in 0.23 mL solution for injection. One pack contains one 0.23 mL vial and one filter needle for withdrawal of the vial contents.

Lumigan® Ⓟ
bimatoprost
Elevated Intraocular Pressure Therapy

Allergan

Date of Preparation: May 14, 2002
Date of Revision: December 24, 2007

SUMMARY PRODUCT INFORMATION:

Route of Administration	Dosage Form/ Strength	Clinically Relevant Nonmedicinal Ingredients
Ophthalmic	Solution, 0.03%	Benzalkonium chloride 0.05 mg/mL as preservative For a complete listing see Dosage Forms, Composition and Packaging.

INDICATIONS AND CLINICAL USE: LUMIGAN (bimatoprost) ophthalmic solution 0.03% is indicated for:
- the reduction of elevated intraocular pressure in patients with open angle glaucoma or ocular hypertension.

Geriatrics (>65 years of age): No overall clinical differences in safety or effectiveness have been observed between elderly and other adult patients. Use as for adult patients.
Pediatrics (<18 years of age): Not recommended for pediatric use. Safety and effectiveness in pediatric patients have not been established.

CONTRAINDICATIONS:
- Patients who are hypersensitive to this drug or to any ingredient in the formulation or component of the container. For a complete listing, see Dosage Forms, Composition and Packaging.

WARNINGS AND PRECAUTIONS: General: LUMIGAN (bimatoprost) ophthalmic solution 0.03% has been reported to cause changes to pigmented tissue. The changes include increased pigmentation and growth of eyelashes and increased pigmentation of the iris and periorbital tissue (eyelid). The increased pigmentation may be permanent.

LUMIGAN may gradually change eye color, increasing the amount of brown pigment in the iris by increasing the number of melanosomes (pigment granules) in melanocytes. **The long-term effects on the melanocytes and the consequences of potential injury to the melanocytes and/or deposition of pigment granules to other area of the eye are currently unknown.** The change in iris color occurs slowly and may not be noticeable for several months to years. Pigmentation is expected to increase as long as LUMIGAN is administered. In clinical studies, noticeable darkening of the iris has been reported in 1.5% of patients treated for 12 months with LUMIGAN at the proposed dose of one drop once daily in each affected eye (1.1% of patients treated for 6 months).

Patients should be informed of the possibility of iris color change. In addition, patients who are expected to receive treatment in only one eye should be informed about the potential for increased brown pigmentation of the iris, periorbital tissue, and eyelashes in the treated eye and thus, heterochromia between the eyes. They should be advised of the potential for a disparity between the eyes in length, thickness, and/or number of eyelashes.

Typically the brown pigmentation around the pupil is expected to spread concentrically towards the periphery in affected eyes, but the entire iris or parts of it may also become more brownish. Until more information about increased brown pigmentation is available, patients should be examined regularly and, depending on the clinical situation, treatment may be stopped if increased pigmentation ensues. The increase in brown iris pigment is not expected to progress further upon discontinuation of treatment, but the resultant color change may be permanent. Neither nevi nor freckles of the iris are expected to be affected by treatment.

There have been reports of bacterial keratitis associated with the use of multiple-dose containers of topical ophthalmic products. These containers had been inadvertently contaminated by patients who, in most cases, had a concurrent corneal disease or a disruption of the ocular epithelial surface. See Information for the Patient.

Hepatic/Biliary/Pancreatic: LUMIGAN has not been studied in patients with hepatic impairment and should therefore be used with caution in such patients.
Occupational Hazards: Based on the pharmacodynamic profile, bimatoprost is not expected to influence a patient's ability to drive or operate machinery. As with any ocular medication, if transient blurred vision occurs at instillation, the patient should wait until the vision clears before driving or using machinery.
Ophthalmologic: LUMIGAN should be used with caution in patients with active intraocular inflammation (e.g. uveitis).

Macular edema, including cystoid macular edema, has been reported during treatment with LUMIGAN.

LUMIGAN should be used with caution in aphakic patients, in pseudophakic patients with a torn posterior lens capsule, or in patients with known risk factors for macular edema.

LUMIGAN has not been adequately evaluated for the treatment of angle closure, inflammatory or neovascular glaucoma.

The pivotal clinical studies included patients with pseudoexfoliative and pigmentary glaucoma, in numbers proportionate to the population. All of these patients responded positively to LUMIGAN, however given the low absolute numbers of these patients enrolled no statistical significance can be concluded. None of these patients dropped out due to lack of efficacy or adverse experiences.

Contact lenses should be removed prior to instillation of LUMIGAN and may be reinserted 15 minutes following its administration. Patients should be advised that LUMIGAN contains benzalkonium chloride, which may be absorbed by soft contact lenses.

Renal: LUMIGAN has not been studied in patients with renal impairment and should therefore be used with caution in such patients.

Sexual Function/Reproduction: Bimatoprost did not impair fertility in male or female rats at doses of up to 0.6 mg/kg/day (approximately 103 times the human exposure based on blood AUC levels).

Special Populations: Pregnant Women: In embryo/fetal developmental studies in pregnant mice and rats, abortion was observed at oral doses of bimatoprost which were at least 33 or 97 times, respectively, the intended human exposure as measured by area-under-the curve blood levels.

Maternal toxicity, evidenced by reduced gestation length, late resorptions, fetal death, postnatal mortality and reduced pup body weights were observed when female rats received oral doses which were at least 41 times the intended human exposure (based on blood AUC levels). Cohabitation times in the offspring were increased but neurobehavioural functions were not affected.

There are no adequate and well-controlled studies of LUMIGAN administration in pregnant women. Because animal reproductive studies are not always predictive of human response, LUMIGAN should be administered during pregnancy only if the potential benefit justifies the potential risk to the fetus.

There has been no experience of pregnancy during clinical trials.

Nursing Women: It is not known whether bimatoprost is excreted in human milk. Because many drugs are excreted in human milk, caution should be exercised when LUMIGAN is administered to a nursing woman.

ADVERSE REACTIONS: Adverse Drug Reaction Overview: In 12-month multi-center, double-blind, active-controlled clinical studies, most adverse events were ocular, mild to moderate, and not serious. The most frequently reported treatment related adverse event was conjunctival hyperemia (45% of patients treated with bimatoprost QD). Increased iris pigmentation was reported for 1.5 % of patients in the QD group.

Clinical Trial Adverse Drug Reactions: Because clinical trials are conducted under very specific conditions the adverse reaction rates observed in the clinical trials may not reflect the rates observed in practice and should not be compared to the rates in the clinical trials of another drug. Adverse drug reaction information from clinical trials is useful for identifying drug-related adverse events and for approximating rates.

The data presented below are taken from two randomized, multicentre, double-blind, parallelgroup clinical studies, of 12 months duration, which were conducted on 1198 patients with glaucoma or ocular hypertension. Bimatoprost 0.03% solution was administered once or twice daily and compared to timolol 0.5% solution BID in a 2:2:1 ratio. Treatment-related adverse events reported from these studies (combined) are presented in Table 1.

Table 1: LUMIGAN

Percent of Patients in the 12 Month Phase 3 Studies with Treatment-related Adverse Events Reported at an Incidence ≥1%

	Bimatoprost 0.03% QD n=474 (%)	Bimatoprost 0.03% BID n=483 (%)	Timolol 0.05% BID n=241 (%)
Body as a Whole			
Headache	3.4%	3.1%	3.7%
Asthenia	1.3%	1.4%	0.8%
Infection	1.3%	0.6%	0.4%
Cardiovascular			
Hypertension	1.7%	1.9%	0.8%
Central Nervous System			
Dizziness	0.8%	0.5%	1.2%
Depression	0.0%	1.0%	0.4%
Respiratory			
Rhinitis	0.4%	1.9%	0.0%
Skin			
Hirsutism	1.1%	1.4%	0.0%
Special Senses			
Conjunctival hyperemia	44.7%	56.1%	13.3%
Growth of eyelashes	42.6%	53.6%	5.0%
Eye pruritus	14.6%	17.6%	3.3%
Eye dryness	8.0%	11.6%	2.1%
Burning sensation in eye	7.0%	6.6%	10.4%
Blepharal pigmentation	5.5%	11.4%	0.4%
Foreign body sensation	5.5%	9.9%	2.1%
Eye pain	5.1%	9.3%	3.3%
Visual disturbance	5.1%	7.7%	4.6%
Erythema eyelid	3.8%	3.0%	0.8%
Eyelash discoloration	3.2%	5.2%	0.4%
Eye discharge	2.7%	4.1%	0.8%
Irritation eye	2.7%	3.5%	1.2%
Blepharitis	2.5%	2.9%	1.7%
Superficial punctuate keratitis	2.5%	2.3%	2.5%
Photophobia	1.7%	6.8%	0.4%
Allergic conjunctivitis	1.5%	1.4%	0.0%
Epiphora	1.5%	2.7%	2.5%
Iris pigmentation increased	1.5%	1.9%	0.0%
Visual acuity worsened	1.5%	1.4%	0.8%
Asthenopia	1.3%	3.1%	0.4%
Cataract NOS	1.3%	1.2%	2.9%
Conjunctival oedema	1.3%	1.9%	1.2%
Corneal erosion	0.8%	1.0%	1.2%
Stinging sensation eye	0.8%	2.1%	1.7%
Eyelid pruritus	0.2%	4.1%	0.4%

(cont'd)

Table 1: LUMIGAN (cont'd)

Treatment related adverse events resulted in the discontinuation of 5.7% of patients, principally for conjunctival hyperemia (3.4%). Only 1.1% of patients on LUMIGAN QD were discontinued due to lack of efficacy.

Less Common Clinical Trial Adverse Drug Reactions (<1%): Body as a Whole: chest pain.

Cardiovascular: palpitations.

Digestive: liver function tests abnormal, oral dryness, dyspepsia.

Metabolic: peripheral oedema, hypercholesteremia.

Musculoskeletal: arthritis.

Nervous: anxiety, diplopia, somnolence, insomnia, nervousness.

Respiratory: bronchitis, cough increased, pharyngitis, sinusitis, dyspnoea.

Skin: pruritus, rash.

Special Senses: blepharospasm, conjunctiva (NOS), eyelid oedema, chalazion, eye oedema, hordeolum, conjunctival bleb, conjunctival folliculosis, eyelid (NOS), eyelid pain, iritis (ocular inflammation), keratitis, visual field defect, vitreous floaters.

Urogenital: cystitis, urine abnormality.

Post-Market Adverse Drug Reactions: The following serious, unexpected reactions reported during the post-market use of LUMIGAN in clinical practice and in the literature have been chosen for inclusion based on the frequency of reporting, possible causal connection to LUMIGAN, or a combination of these factors: corneal oedema, keratitis, vision blurred.

DRUG INTERACTIONS: Overview: No specific drug interaction studies have been conducted. However, no drug-drug interactions are anticipated in humans since systemic drug concentrations of bimatoprost are extremely low (less than 0.2 ng/mL) following repeated ocular dosing and as metabolism and excretion involves multiple pathways.

Drug-Food Interactions: Interactions with food have not been established.

Drug-Herb Interactions: Interactions with herbal products have not been established.

Drug-Laboratory Test Interactions: Interactions with laboratory tests have not been established.

DOSAGE AND ADMINISTRATION: Recommended Dose and Dosage Adjustment: The recommended dosage is one drop in the affected eye(s) once daily in the evening. The dosage of LUMIGAN (bimatoprost) ophthalmic solution 0.03% should not exceed once daily since it has been shown that more frequent administration may lessen the intraocular pressure lowering effect, and increase the frequency and severity of adverse events.

Missed Dose: Patients should be instructed to apply a single drop as soon as they remember, and then to return to their regular routine.

Administration: If more than one topical ophthalmic drug is being used, the drugs should be administered at least five (5) minutes apart.

Contact lenses should be removed prior to instillation of LUMIGAN and may be reinserted 15 minutes following its administration.

OVERDOSAGE:

No information is available on overdosage in humans. If overdose with LUMIGAN (bimatoprost) ophthalmic solution 0.03% occurs, treatment should be symptomatic.

In oral (by gavage) mouse and rat studies, doses up to 100 mg/kg/day did not produce any toxicity. This dose, expressed as mg/m^2, is at least 70 times higher than the amount of bimatoprost to which a 10 kg child would be exposed were it to accidentally ingest one 7.5 mL bottle of LUMIGAN.

For management of a suspected drug overdose, CPhA recommends that you contact your **regional Poison Control Centre**. See the *CPS* Directory section for a list of Poison Control Centres.

ACTION AND CLINICAL PHARMACOLOGY: Mechanism of Action: LUMIGAN (bimatoprost) is a synthetic prostamide analogue and is structurally related to prostaglandin F2α in that the carboxylic acid group is replaced with an electronically neutral substituent. Its mechanism of action resembles that of prostamide F2α, a naturally occurring substance. LUMIGAN exhibits no meaningful pharmacological activity at known prostaglandin receptors as well as no uterotonic or mitogenic activity. Studies suggest that it lowers IOP by increasing uveoscleral and trabecular meshwork outflow, with no significant effect on aqueous humor inflow. Pharmacodynamic studies in humans demonstrated a significant 30-35% decrease in outflow resistance compared to vehicle treated eyes based on tonographic data and calculated values of apparent outflow resistance. The ocular hypotensive effect does not involve a COX-dependent mechanism.

Pharmacodynamics: The effect of LUMIGAN within the first 12 hours of dosing was evaluated in two studies. When dosed in the morning, bimatoprost began to take effect within 4 hours after initial instillation, and was followed by continued decreases in IOP through 12 hours. The effect of bimatoprost 0.03% ophthalmic solution between 12 and 24 hours post-instillation also was evaluated. Mean IOP at 12 hours post-dosing was 17.7 mm Hg and 16.9 mm Hg 24 hours after the last dose. Based on this information, once-daily evening dosing is recommended so that the time of anticipated maximal efficacy of the drug coincides with the morning hours (08:00 to 11:00 AM) when untreated IOP is usually highest.

Pharmacokinetics: After one drop of 0.03% bimatoprost ophthalmic solution was administered once daily to both eyes of 15 healthy subjects, blood bimatoprost concentrations peaked within 10 minutes after dosing and were below the lower limit of detection (0.025 ng/mL) in most subjects within 1.5 hours after dosing.

Systemic exposure after repeated ocular application is low. Steady state was achieved after one week of once daily dosing with one drop of 0.03% bimatoprost ophthalmic solution to both eyes, with mean C_{max} values of 0.07 and 0.08 ng/mL on day 7 and 14, respectively, and mean AUC_{0-24h} of 0.074 and 0.096 ng·h/mL on day 7 and 14, respectively.

In patients with glaucoma or ocular hypertension, bimatoprost blood concentrations were similar to those observed in normal healthy subjects.

There was no significant systemic drug accumulation over time with the once daily dosing regimen. Mean blood concentration was around 0.08 ng/mL after 12 months of QD or BID dosing. The once daily regimen corresponded to a total exposure of 6.13 mg (one 28 µL drop in each eye once a day for 12 months) or 0.00028 mg/kg/day for a 60-kg individual over 12 months.

Absorption: Bimatoprost is rapidly absorbed across the human cornea and sclera, with scleral penetration being more efficient. Animal studies show that it is well distributed into ocular tissues following ocular administration, where only minimal metabolism occurs in humans.

Distribution: Bimatoprost is moderately distributed into body tissues with a steady-state volume of distribution of 0.67 L/kg. In human blood, bimatoprost resides mainly in the plasma. Approximately 12% of bimatoprost remains unbound in human plasma.

Metabolism: Bimatoprost is the major circulating species in the blood once it reaches the systemic circulation following ocular dosing. Bimatoprost then undergoes oxidation, N-deethylation and glucuronidation to form a diverse variety of metabolites. Studies using human liver microsomes and recombinant human P450 isozymes, identified CYP 3A4 as one of the enzymes involved in the metabolism of bimatoprost in humans. However, since multiple enzymes and pathways are involved in the biotransformation of bimatoprost, no significant drugdrug interactions are anticipated.

Bimatoprost is only minimally metabolized in ocular tissues in humans, and is active in its intact form, without metabolic modification.

Excretion: Following an intravenous dose of radiolabelled bimatoprost (3.12 µg/kg) to six healthy subjects, the maximum blood concentration of unchanged drug was 12.2 ng/mL and decreased rapidly with an elimination half-life of approximately 45 minutes. The total blood clearance of bimatoprost was 1.5 L/h/kg. Up to 67% of the administered dose was excreted in the urine while 25% of the dose was recovered in the feces. Both urinary and fecal routes are important pathways for elimination of the parent compound and its metabolites, following intravenous administration.

Special Populations and Conditions: Geriatrics: Elderly individuals (>65 years) exhibited higher systemic levels but this was not considered to be clinically relevant since bimatoprost had a similar efficacy and safety profile in both the young and elderly that participated in the clinical trials.

STORAGE AND STABILITY: LUMIGAN (bimatoprost) ophthalmic solution 0.03% should be stored in the original container at 2-25°C. Discard unused solution at the end of treatment.

Keep in a safe place out of the reach of children.

INFORMATION FOR THE PATIENT: Published in e-CPS, available by subscription at www.e-cps.ca.

DOSAGE FORMS, COMPOSITION AND PACKAGING: Each mL of clear, isotonic, buffered, preserved, colorless, sterile ophthalmic solution contains: bimatoprost 0.3 mg. Nonmedicinal ingredients: benzalkonium chloride, citric acid monohydrate, purified water, sodium chloride and sodium phosphate dibasic heptahydrate. Sodium hydroxide and/or hydrochloric acid may be added to adjust pH. pH: 7.3±0.5. Osmolality: approximately 290 mOsmol/kg. Opaque plastic ophthalmic dispenser bottles of 2.5, 3, 5 and 7.5 mL.

Lumigan® RC Pr

bimatoprost

Elevated Intraocular Pressure Therapy—Prostamide Analogue

Allergan

Date of Preparation: September 10, 2009

SUMMARY PRODUCT INFORMATION:

Route of Administration	Dosage Form/ Strength	Clinically Relevant Nonmedicinal Ingredients
Ophthalmic	Solution, 0.01%	Benzalkonium chloride 0.2 mg/mL as preservative For a complete listing see Dosage Forms, Composition and Packaging.

INDICATIONS AND CLINICAL USE: LUMIGAN RC (bimatoprost) ophthalmic solution 0.01% is indicated for:

- the reduction of elevated intraocular pressure in patients with open angle glaucoma or ocular hypertension

Geriatrics (>65 years of age): No overall clinical differences in safety or effectiveness have been observed between elderly and other adult patients. Use as for adult patients.

Pediatrics (<18 years of age): Not recommended for pediatric use. Safety and effectiveness in pediatric patients have not been established.

CONTRAINDICATIONS:

- Patients who are hypersensitive to this drug or to any ingredient in the formulation or component of the container. For a complete listing, see Dosage Forms, Composition and Packaging.

WARNINGS AND PRECAUTIONS: General: Bimatoprost ophthalmic solutions have been reported to cause changes to pigmented tissue. The changes include increased pigmentation and growth of eyelashes and increased pigmentation of the iris and periorbital tissue (eyelid). The increased pigmentation may be permanent.

Bimatoprost ophthalmic solution may gradually change eye color, increasing the amount of brown pigment in the iris by increasing the number of melanosomes (pigment granules) in melanocytes. **The long-term effects on the melanocytes and the consequences of potential injury to the melanocytes and/or deposition of pigment granules to other area of the eye are currently unknown.** The change in iris color occurs slowly and may not be noticeable for several months to years. Pigmentation is expected to increase as long as bimatoprost ophthalmic solution is administered. In a 12-month clinical study, iris colour change was reported in 0.5% of patients treated with bimatoprost ophthalmic solution 0.01%. Noticeable darkening of the iris has been reported in 1.5% of patients treated for 12 months with bimatoprost ophthalmic solution 0.03% at the proposed dose of one drop once daily in each affected eye (1.1% of patients treated for 6 months).

Patients should be informed of the possibility of iris color change. In addition, patients who are expected to receive treatment in only one eye should be informed about the potential for increased brown pigmentation of the iris, periorbital tissue, and eyelashes in the treated eye and thus, heterochromia between the eyes. They should be advised of the potential for a disparity between the eyes in length, thickness, and/or number of eyelashes.

Typically the brown pigmentation around the pupil is expected to spread concentrically towards the periphery in affected eyes, but the entire iris or parts of it may also become more brownish. Until more information about increased brown pigmentation is available, patients should be examined regularly and, depending on the clinical situation, treatment may be stopped if increased pigmentation ensues. The increase in brown iris pigment is not expected to progress further upon discontinuation of treatment, but the resultant color change may be permanent. Neither nevi nor freckles of the iris are expected to be affected by treatment.

LUMIGAN RC contains benzalkonium chloride at a concentration of 0.02% (0.2 mg/mL), compared to 0.005% (0.05 mg/mL) in LUMIGAN. Monitoring is required with frequent or prolonged use in dry eye patients or where the cornea is compromised.

LUMIGAN RC has not been studied in patients with severe dry eye, and therefore, should not be used in patients with severe dry eye (see Warnings and Precautions, Ophthalmologic).

LUMIGAN RC contains the preservative benzalkonium chloride which may be absorbed by soft contact lenses (see Warnings and Precautions, Ophthalmologic).

There have been reports of bacterial keratitis associated with the use of multiple-dose containers of topical ophthalmic products. These containers had been inadvertently contaminated by patients who, in most cases, had a concurrent corneal disease or a disruption of the ocular epithelial surface. See Information for the Patient.

Ophthalmologic: LUMIGAN RC should be used with caution in patients with active intraocular inflammation (e.g. uveitis).

Macular edema, including cystoid macular edema, has been reported during treatment with bimatoprost ophthalmic solution 0.03%.

LUMIGAN RC should be used with caution in aphakic patients, in pseudophakic patients with a torn posterior lens capsule, or in patients with known risk factors for macular edema.

LUMIGAN RC has not been adequately evaluated for the treatment of angle closure, inflammatory or neovascular glaucoma.

The pivotal clinical studies included patients with pseudoexfoliative and pigmentary glaucoma, in numbers proportionate to the population. All of these patients responded positively, however given the low absolute numbers of these patients enrolled no statistical significance can be concluded. None of these patients dropped out due to lack of efficacy or adverse experiences.

Contact lenses should be removed prior to instillation of LUMIGAN RC and may be reinserted 15 minutes following its administration. Patients should be advised that LUMIGAN RC contains benzalkonium chloride, which may be absorbed by soft contact lenses.

The benzalkonium chloride concentration in LUMIGAN RC is 0.02% (0.2 mg/mL), compared to 0.005% (0.05 mg/mL) in LUMIGAN. Benzalkonium chloride, which is commonly used as a preservative in ophthalmic products, has been reported to cause punctate keratopathy and/or toxic ulcerative keratopathy. Therefore, monitoring is required with frequent or prolonged use in dry eye patients or where the cornea is compromised.

LUMIGAN RC has not been studied in patients with severe dry eye, and therefore, should not be used in patients with severe dry eye (see Warnings and Precautions).

Hepatic/Biliary/Pancreatic: LUMIGAN RC (bimatoprost) ophthalmic solution 0.01% has not been studied in patients with hepatic impairment and should therefore be used with caution in such patients.

Occupational Hazards: Based on the pharmacodynamic profile, bimatoprost is not expected to influence a patient's ability to drive or operate machinery. As with any ocular medication, if transient blurred vision occurs at instillation, the patient should wait until the vision clears before driving or using machinery.

Renal: LUMIGAN RC has not been studied in patients with renal impairment and should therefore be used with caution in such patients.

Sexual Function/Reproduction: Bimatoprost did not impair fertility in male or female rats at doses of up to 0.6 mg/kg/day (approximately 103 times the human exposure based on blood AUC levels obtained in subjects administered bimatoprost ophthalmic solution 0.03%, one drop/day in both eyes for 14 days).

Special Populations: Pregnant Women: In embryo/fetal developmental studies in pregnant mice and rats, abortion was observed at oral doses of bimatoprost which were at least 33 or 97 times, respectively, the intended human exposure as measured by blood AUC levels obtained in subjects administered bimatoprost ophthalmic solution 0.03%, one drop/day in both eyes for 14 days.

Maternal toxicity, evidenced by reduced gestation length, late resorptions, fetal death, postnatal mortality and reduced pup body weights were observed when female rats received oral doses which were at least 41 times the intended human exposure (based on blood AUC levels obtained in subjects administered bimatoprost ophthalmic solution 0.03%, one drop/day in both eyes for 14 days). Cohabitation times in the offspring were increased but neurobehavioural functions were not affected.

There are no adequate and well-controlled studies of LUMIGAN RC administration in pregnant women. Because animal reproductive studies are not always predictive of human response, LUMIGAN RC should be administered during pregnancy only if the potential benefit justifies the potential risk to the fetus.

There has been no experience of pregnancy during clinical trials.

Nursing Women: It is not known whether bimatoprost is excreted in human milk. Because many drugs are excreted in human milk, caution should be exercised when LUMIGAN RC is administered to a nursing woman.

ADVERSE REACTIONS: Adverse Drug Reaction Overview: In the 12-month multi-centre, double blind, active controlled clinical study with bimatoprost ophthalmic solution 0.01%, most adverse events were ocular, mild, and not serious. The most frequently reported adverse event was conjunctival hyperaemia (31.4% of patients treated).

Clinical Trial Adverse Drug Reactions: Because clinical trials are conducted under very specific conditions the adverse reaction rates observed in the clinical trials may not reflect the rates observed in practice and should not be compared to the rates in the clinical trials of another drug. Adverse drug reaction information from clinical trials is useful for identifying drug-related adverse events and for approximating rates.

The data presented below are taken from a randomized, multicentre, double-blind, parallel-group clinical study, of 12 months duration, which was conducted in 560 patients with glaucoma or ocular hypertension. Bimatoprost 0.01% solution was administered once daily and was compared to bimatoprost 0.03% and bimatoprost 0.0125% ophthalmic solutions administered once daily. Adverse events, regardless of causality, reported from this study are presented in Table 1, for LUMIGAN RC (bimatoprost) ophthalmic solution 0.01% and LUMIGAN (bimatoprost) ophthalmic solution 0.03%.

Table 1: LUMIGAN RC

Number (%) of Patients with Ocular Adverse Events, Regardless of Causality, Reported by >1% of Patients (Study 192024-031)

SOC[b] Preferred Term	LUMIGAN RC N=185	LUMIGAN N=187
All Ocular Events	88 (47.6%)[c]	116 (62.0%)
Eye Disorders		
Conjunctival hyperaemia[a]	58 (31.4%)	73 (39.0%)
Erythema of eyelid[a]	7 (3.8%)	10 (5.3%)
Eye irritation[a]	7 (3.8%)	3 (1.6%)
Growth of eyelashes[a]	7 (3.8%)	6 (3.2%)
Conjunctival haemorrhage	5 (2.7%)	1 (0.5%)
Vision blurred[a]	5 (2.7%)	3 (1.6%)
Punctate keratitis[a]	4 (2.2%)	11 (5.9%)
Cataract	4 (2.2%)	4 (2.1%)
Eye pruritus[a]	4 (2.2%)	10 (5.3%)
Conjunctival oedema[a]	3 (1.6%)	1 (0.5%)
Visual acuity reduced	2 (1.1%)	4 (2.1%)
Eyelids pruritus[a]	2 (1.1%)	1 (0.5%)
Eye pain	2 (1.1%)	2 (1.1%)
Iris hyperpigmentation[a]	1 (0.5%)	2 (1.1%)
Vitreous floaters	2 (1.1%)	1 (0.5%)
Asthenopia[a]	1 (0.5%)	3 (1.6%)
Vitreous detachment	1 (0.5%)	3 (1.6%)
Lacrimation increased	1 (0.5%)	1 (0.5%)
Visual field defect	1 (0.5%)	2 (1.1%)
Foreign body sensation in eyes	0 (0.0%)	5 (2.7%)
Dry eye	0 (0.0%)	3 (1.6%)
Blepharitis	0 (0.0%)	3 (1.6%)
Abnormal sensation in eye	0 (0.0%)	3 (1.6%)
Eye allergy	0 (0.0%)	1 (0.5%)
Maculopathy	0 (0.0%)	2 (1.1%)
Scotoma	0 (0.0%)	2 (1.1%)
Blepharitis allergic	0 (0.0%)	3 (1.6%)

(cont'd)

Table 1: LUMIGAN RC *(cont'd)*

Number (%) of Patients with Ocular Adverse Events, Regardless of Causality, Reported by >1% of Patients (Study 192024-031)

SOC[b] Preferred Term	LUMIGAN RC N=185	LUMIGAN N=187
Corneal erosion	0 (0.0%)[c]	2 (1.1%)
Photophobia	0 (0.0%)[c]	2 (1.1%)
General Disorders & Administration Site Conditions		
Instillation site irritation[a]	2 (1.1%)	1 (0.5%)
Infections & Infestations		
Hordeolum	1 (0.5%)	2 (1.1%)
Investigations		
Intraocular pressure increased	0 (0.0%)	3 (1.6%)
Skin & Subcutaneous Tissue Disorders		
Skin hyperpigmentation[a]	5 (2.7%)	10 (5.3%)
Hypertrichosis[a, d]	3 (1.6%)	3 (1.6%)

[a] Event reported by an investigator as treatment-related for at least one patient for LUMIGAN RC.
[b] Coding based on MedDRA 10.0.
[c] LUMIGAN RC significantly less than LUMIGAN (p≤0.005).
[d] Hypertrichosis **reported as "hair growth around the eye"**.

Compared to LUMIGAN, LUMIGAN RC had significantly fewer adverse events (all causality and treatment-related), and significantly fewer ocular adverse events. Patients experienced less severe macroscopic hyperaemia.

Treatment related adverse events resulted in the discontinuation of 2.2% of patients on bimatoprost ophthalmic solution 0.01%, principally for conjunctival hyperaemia (1.6%). Of the patients treated with bimatoprost ophthalmic solution 0.03%, 6.4% discontinued as a result of a treatment related effect, principally for conjunctival hyperaemia (2.7%).

Non-Ocular Adverse Events: See Table 2.

Table 2: LUMIGAN RC

Number (%) of Patients with Non-ocular Adverse Events, Regardless of Causality, Reported by >1% of Patients treated with LUMIGAN RC (Study 192024-031)

SOC[a] Preferred Term	LUMIGAN RC N=185	LUMIGAN N=187
All non-ocular events	80 (43.2%)	77 (41.2%)
Blood and Lymphatic System Disorders		
Anaemia	3 (1.6%)	1 (0.5%)
Cardiac Disorders		
Cardiac failure congestive	3 (1.6%)	0 (0.0%)
Endocrine Disorders		
Hypothyroidism	4 (2.2%)	1 (0.5%)
Gastrointestinal Disorders		
Gastrooesophageal reflux disease	6 (3.2%)	1 (0.5%)
Nausea[b]	3 (1.6%)	1 (0.5%)
Toothache	2 (1.1%)	0 (0.0%)
General Disorders & Administration Site Conditions		
Peripheral oedema	3 (1.6%)	2 (1.1%)
Chest pain	2 (1.1%)	2 (1.1%)
Infections and Infestations		
Upper respiratory tract infection	6 (3.2%)	3 (1.6%)
Nasopharyngitis	5 (2.7%)	4 (2.1%)
Pharyngitis streptococcal	3 (1.6%)	0 (0.0%)
Influenza	2 (1.1%)	1 (0.5%)
Bronchitis	2 (1.1%)	0 (0.0%)
Urinary tract infection	2 (1.1%)	2 (1.1%)
Injury, Poisoning & Procedural Complications		
Skin laceration	3 (1.6%)	1 (0.5%)
Procedural pain	2 (1.1%)	1 (0.5%)
Fall	2 (1.1%)	2 (1.1%)
Metabolism and Nutrition Disorders		
Hypercholesterolaemia	5 (2.7%)	5 (2.7%)
Diabetes mellitus	5 (2.7%)	2 (1.1%)
Diabetes mellitus non-insulin dependent	3 (1.6%)	1 (0.5%)
Dyslipidaemia	2 (1.1%)	0 (0.0%)
Musculoskeletal and Connective Tissue Disorders		
Muscle spasms	3 (1.6%)	0 (0.0%)
Back pain	2 (1.1%)	6 (3.2%)
Nervous System Disorders		
Dizziness	3 (1.6%)	2 (1.1%)
Headache[b]	3 (1.6%)	3 (1.6%)
Psychiatric Disorders		
Depression	3 (1.6%)	1 (0.5%)
Renal		
Nephrolithiasis	2 (1.1%)	0 (0.0%)
Respiratory, Thoracic and Mediastinal System		
Cough	2 (1.1%)	1 (0.5%)
Asthma	2 (1.1%)	3 (1.6%)
Dyspnoea	2 (1.1%)	1 (0.5%)
Vascular Disorders		
Hypertension	8 (4.3%)	11 (5.9%)

* Event reported by an investigator as treatment-related for LUMIGAN RC.

(cont'd)

Table 2: LUMIGAN RC *(cont'd)*

[a] Coding based on MedDRA versions 10.0.
[b] Event reported by an investigator as treatment-related for at least one patient for LUMIGAN RC.

Less Common Clinical Trial Adverse Drug Reactions (<1%) : The number of patients reporting an adverse event, regardless of causality, was 1 (0.5%) for each of the following adverse events:
Ocular: eyelid oedema*, eyelid pain, cataract nuclear, conjunctival disorder*, eyelid exfoliation, eyelid margin crusting*, keratoconjunctivitis sicca, meibomianitis, chalazion, chemical eye injury, conjunctivitis viral, corneal epithelium defect, corneal thinning, macular degeneration, macular hole, madarosis*, retinal pigment epitheliopathy, trichiasis.
Infections and Infestations: sinusitis, diverticulitis, pneumonia, cellulitis.
Injury, Poisoning & Procedural Complications: contusion.
Musculoskeletal and Connective Tissue Disorders: musculoskeletal pain.
Psychiatric Disorders: anxiety.
Skin: pruritus*, dry skin*.
Safety Data from Other Clinical Trials: In double-blind, active-controlled clinical studies conducted with LUMIGAN (bimatoprost) ophthalmic solution 0.03% once daily, the following treatment related adverse events were reported:
Body as a Whole: Common (≥1% to <10%): headache, asthenia, infection. Uncommon (≥0.1% to <1%): chest pain.
Cardiovascular: Common (≥1% to <10%): hypertension. Uncommon (≥0.1% to <1%): palpitations.
Central Nervous System: Uncommon (≥0.1% to <1%): dizziness, anxiety, diplopia, somnolence, insomnia, nervousness.
Digestive: Uncommon (≥0.1% to <1%): liver function tests abnormal, oral dryness, dyspepsia.
Metabolic: Uncommon (≥0.1% to <1%): peripheral oedema, hypercholesteremia.
Musculoskeletal: Uncommon (≥0.1% to <1%): arthritis.
Respiratory: Uncommon (≥0.1% to <1%): rhinitis, bronchitis, cough increased, pharyngitis, sinusitis, dyspnoea.
Skin: Common (≥1% to <10%): hirsutism. Uncommon (≥0.1% to <1%): pruritus, rash.
Special Senses: Very common (>10%): conjunctival hyperaemia, growth of eyelashes, eye pruritus. Common (≥1% to <10%): eye dryness, burning sensation in eye, blepharal pigmentation, foreign body sensation, eye pain, visual disturbance, erythema eyelid, eyelash discolouration, eye discharge, irritation eye, blepharitis, superficial punctuate keratitis, photophobia, allergic conjunctivitis, epiphora, iris pigmentation increased, visual acuity worsened, asthenopia, cataract NOS, conjunctival oedema. Uncommon (≥0.1% to <1%): corneal erosion, stinging sensation eye, eyelid pruritus, blepharospasm, conjunctiva (NOS), eyelid oedema, chalazion, eye oedema, hordeolum, conjunctival bleb, conjunctival folliculosis, eyelid (NOS), eyelid pain, iritis (ocular inflammation), keratitis, visual field defect, vitreous floaters.
Urogenital: Uncommon (≥0.1% to <1%): cystitis, urine abnormality.
Post-Market Adverse Drug Reactions: No data on post-market adverse drug reactions is available as yet with LUMIGAN RC (bimatoprost ophthalmic solution 0.01%, with benzalkonium chloride 0.2 mg/mL). The following serious, unexpected reports have been received during the post-market use of LUMIGAN (bimatoprost ophthalmic solution 0.03% with benzalkonium chloride 0.05 mg/mL) and have been chosen for inclusion based on the frequency of reporting, possible causal connection to LUMIGAN (bimatoprost ophthalmic solution 0.03% with 0.05 mg/mL), or a combination of these factors: corneal oedema, keratitis, vision blurred.

DRUG INTERACTIONS: Overview: No specific drug interaction studies have been conducted. However, no drug-drug interactions are anticipated in humans since systemic drug concentrations of bimatoprost are extremely low (less than 0.2 ng/mL) following repeated ocular dosing with bimatoprost ophthalmic solution 0.03% and as metabolism and excretion involves multiple pathways.

Drug-drug, drug-food, drug-herb, and drug-laboratory interactions have not been studied.

DOSAGE AND ADMINISTRATION: Recommended Dose and Dosage Adjustment: The recommended dosage is one drop in the affected eye(s) once daily in the evening. The dosage of LUMIGAN RC (bimatoprost) ophthalmic solution 0.01% should not exceed once daily since it has been shown that more frequent administration of bimatoprost ophthalmic solution may lessen the intraocular pressure lowering effect, and increase the frequency and severity of adverse events.
Missed Dose: Patients should be instructed to apply a single drop as soon as they remember, and then to return to their regular routine.
Administration: If more than one topical ophthalmic drug is being used, the drugs should be administered at least five (5) minutes apart.

Contact lenses should be removed prior to instillation of LUMIGAN RC and may be reinserted 15 minutes following its administration.

OVERDOSAGE:
No information is available on overdosage in humans. If overdose with LUMIGAN RC (bimatoprost) ophthalmic solution 0.01% occurs, treatment should be symptomatic.

In oral (by gavage) mouse and rat studies, doses up to 100 mg/kg/day did not produce any toxicity. This dose, expressed as mg/m², is at least 210 times higher than the amount of bimatoprost to which a 10 kg child would be exposed were it to accidentally ingest the contents of one 7.5 mL bottle of LUMIGAN RC.

> For management of a suspected drug overdose, particularly accidental ingestion, contact your **regional Poison Control Centre**. See the *CPS* Directory section for a list of Poison Control Centres.

ACTION AND CLINICAL PHARMACOLOGY: Mechanism of Action: Bimatoprost is a synthetic prostamide analogue and is structurally related to prostaglandin F2α in that the carboxylic acid group is replaced with an electronically neutral substituent. Its mechanism of action resembles that of prostamide F2α, a naturally occurring substance. Bimatoprost exhibits no meaningful pharmacological activity at known prostaglandin receptors as well as no uterotonic or mitogenic activity. Studies suggest that it lowers intraocular pressure (IOP) by increasing uveoscleral and trabecular meshwork outflow, with no significant effect on aqueous humor inflow. Pharmacodynamic studies in humans demonstrated a significant 30-35% decrease in outflow resistance compared to vehicle treated eyes based on tonographic data and calculated values of apparent outflow resistance. The ocular hypotensive effect does not involve a COX-dependent mechanism.

Pharmacodynamics: The effect of bimatoprost ophthalmic solution 0.03% within the first 12 hours of dosing was evaluated in two studies. When dosed in the morning, bimatoprost began to take effect within 4 hours after initial instillation, and was followed by continued decreases in IOP through 12 hours. The effect of bimatoprost 0.03% ophthalmic solution between 12 and 24 hours post-instillation also was evaluated. Mean IOP at 12 hours post-dosing was 17.7 mm Hg and 16.9 mm Hg 24 hours after the last dose. Based on this information, once-daily evening dosing is recommended so that the time of anticipated maximal efficacy of the drug coincides with the morning hours (08:00 to 11:00 AM) when untreated IOP is usually highest.

Pharmacokinetics: After one drop of bimatoprost ophthalmic solution 0.03% was administered once daily to both eyes of 15 healthy subjects, blood bimatoprost concentrations peaked within 10 minutes after dosing and were below the lower limit of detection (0.025 ng/mL) in most subjects within 1.5 hours after dosing.

Systemic exposure after repeated ocular application is low. Steady state was achieved after one week of once daily dosing with one drop of bimatoprost ophthalmic solution 0.03% to both eyes, with mean C_{max} values of 0.07 and 0.08 ng/mL on day 7 and 14, respectively, and mean $AUC_{0\text{-}24h}$ of 0.074 and 0.096 ng·hr/mL on day 7 and 14, respectively.

In patients with glaucoma or ocular hypertension, bimatoprost blood concentrations were similar to those observed in normal healthy subjects.

There was no significant systemic drug accumulation over time with the once daily dosing regimen. Mean blood concentration was around 0.08 ng/mL after 12 months of QD or BID dosing with bimatoprost ophthalmic solution 0.03%. The once daily regimen corresponded to a total exposure of 6.13 mg (one 28 μL drop in each eye once a day for 12 months) or 0.00028 mg/kg/day for a 60-kg individual over 12 months.

Absorption: Bimatoprost is rapidly absorbed across the human cornea and sclera, with scleral penetration being more efficient. Animal studies show that it is well distributed into ocular tissues following ocular administration, where only minimal metabolism occurs in humans.

Distribution: Bimatoprost is moderately distributed into body tissues with a steady-state volume of distribution of 0.67 L/kg. In human blood, bimatoprost resides mainly in the plasma. Approximately 12% of bimatoprost remains unbound in human plasma.

Metabolism: Bimatoprost is the major circulating species in the blood once it reaches the systemic circulation following ocular dosing. Bimatoprost then undergoes oxidation, N-deethylation and glucuronidation to form a diverse variety of metabolites. Studies using human liver microsomes and recombinant human P450 isozymes, identified CYP 3A4 as one of the enzymes involved in the metabolism of bimatoprost in humans. However, since multiple enzymes and pathways are involved in the biotransformation of bimatoprost, no significant drug-drug interactions are anticipated.

Bimatoprost is only minimally metabolized in ocular tissues in humans, and is active in its intact form, without metabolic modification.

Excretion: Following an intravenous dose of radiolabelled bimatoprost (3.12 μg/kg) to six healthy subjects, the maximum blood concentration of unchanged drug was 12.2 ng/mL and decreased rapidly with an elimination half-life of approximately 45 minutes. The total blood clearance of bimatoprost was 1.5 L/hr/kg. Up to 67% of the administered dose was excreted in the urine while 25% of the dose was recovered in the feces. Both urinary and fecal routes are important pathways for elimination of the parent compound and its metabolites, following intravenous administration.

Special Populations and Conditions: Geriatrics: Elderly individuals (>65 years) exhibited higher systemic levels but this was not considered to be clinically relevant since no overall clinical differences in safety or effectiveness have been observed between elderly and other adult patients.

STORAGE AND STABILITY: LUMIGAN RC (bimatoprost) ophthalmic solution 0.01% should be stored in the original container at 2-25°C. Discard unused solution at the end of treatment.

Keep in a safe place out of the reach of children.

INFORMATION FOR THE PATIENT: Published in e-CPS, available by subscription at www.e-cps.ca.

DOSAGE FORMS, COMPOSITION AND PACKAGING: Each mL of clear, isotonic, buffered, preserved, colorless, sterile ophthalmic solution contains: bimatoprost 0.1 mg. Nonmedicinal ingredients: benzalkonium chloride 0.2 mg as preservative, citric acid monohydrate, purified water, sodium chloride and sodium phosphate dibasic heptahydrate. Sodium hydroxide and/or hydrochloric acid may be added to adjust pH. pH: 7.3±0.5. Osmolality: approximately 290 mOsmol/kg. White opaque plastic ophthalmic dispenser bottles of 2.5, 3, 5 and 7.5 mL.

Lupron® Ⓟ
leuprolide acetate
Gonadotropin-releasing Hormone Analog

Abbott

Lupron Depot® 3.75 mg/7.5 mg Ⓟ
leuprolide acetate
Gonadotropin-releasing Hormone Analog

Abbott

Date of Preparation: November 26, 1986
Date of Revision: March 23, 2010

SUMMARY PRODUCT INFORMATION:

Route of Administration	Dosage Form/ Strength	Clinically Relevant Nonmedicinal Ingredients
LUPRON		
Subcutaneous	Multiple-dose vial/5 mg/mL	Acetic acid, benzyl alcohol, sodium chloride, sodium hydroxide For a complete listing see Dosage Forms, Composition and Packaging.
LUPRON DEPOT		
Intramuscular	Pre-filled dual chamber syringe containing sterile lyophilized microspheres/3.75 mg (1-Month SR) and 7.5 mg (1-Month SR).	Carboxymethylcellulose sodium, DL-lactic and glycolic acids copolymer, D-mannitol, gelatin, glacial acetic acid, polysorbate 80 For a complete listing see Dosage Forms, Composition and Packaging.
Definition: SR=slow release.		

INDICATIONS AND CLINICAL USE: LUPRON (leuprolide acetate injection) and LUPRON DEPOT (leuprolide acetate for depot suspension) are indicated for:
- the treatment of children with central precocious puberty.
  Children should be selected using the following criteria:
  1. Clinical diagnosis of CPP (idiopathic or neurogenic) with onset of secondary sexual characteristics earlier than 8 years in females and 9 years in males.
  2. Clinical diagnosis should be confirmed prior to initiation of therapy as follows:
     a. Confirmation of diagnosis by a pubertal response to a GnRH stimulation test. The sensitivity and methodology of this assay must be understood.
     b. Bone age advanced one year beyond the chronological age.
  3. Baseline evaluation should also include:
     a. Height and weight measurements
     b. Sex steroid levels
     c. Adrenal steroid level to exclude congenital adrenal hyperplasia
     d. Beta human chorionic gonadotropin level to rule out a chorionic gonadotropin secreting tumor
     e. Pelvic/adrenal/testicular ultrasound to rule out a steroid secreting tumor
     f. Computerized tomography of the head to rule out intracranial tumor

  LUPRON DEPOT must be administered under the supervision of a physician.

Geriatrics (>65 years of age): Refer to the "Prostatic Cancer" Product Monograph for the efficacy and safety of LUPRON and LUPRON DEPOT in this population.

CONTRAINDICATIONS:
- LUPRON (leuprolide acetate injection) and LUPRON DEPOT (leuprolide acetate for depot suspension) are contraindicated in patients with hypersensitivity to the drug or its components or similar nonapeptides or component of the container. Isolated cases of anaphylaxis have been reported. For a complete listing, see Dosage Forms, Composition and Packaging.
- LUPRON and LUPRON DEPOT are contraindicated in women who are or may become pregnant. The possibility exists that spontaneous abortion may occur if the drug is administered during pregnancy.

  When LUPRON DEPOT was administered on day 6 of pregnancy at test dosages of 0.00024, 0.0024, and 0.024 mg/kg (1/1200 to 1/12 the human pediatric dose) to rabbits, LUPRON DEPOT produced a dose-related increase in major fetal abnormalities. Similar studies in rats failed to demonstrate an increase in fetal malformations. There was increased fetal mortality and decreased fetal weights with the two higher doses of LUPRON DEPOT in rabbits and with the highest dose (0.024 mg/kg) in rats. The effects on fetal mortality are logical consequences of the alterations in hormonal levels brought about by this drug. Therefore, the possibility exists that spontaneous abortion may occur if the drug is administered during pregnancy.

  Patients treated with LUPRON and LUPRON DEPOT should use non hormonal methods of contraception.
- It is not known whether leuprolide acetate is excreted in human milk; therefore, LUPRON and LUPRON DEPOT are contraindicated in patients who are breast-feeding.

WARNINGS AND PRECAUTIONS: General: Postmarketing reports of convulsions have been observed in patients on leuprolide acetate therapy. These included patients in the female and pediatric populations, patients with a history of seizures, epilepsy, cerebrovascular disorders, central nervous system anomalies or tumors, and in patients on concomitant medications that have been associated with convulsions such as bupropion and SSRIs. Convulsions have also been reported in patients in the absence of any of the conditions mentioned above.

Patients with known allergies to benzyl alcohol, a vehicle ingredient of LUPRON, may present symptoms of hypersensitivity, usually local, in the form of erythema and induration at the injection site.

Carcinogenesis and Mutagenesis: Two-year carcinogenicity studies were conducted in rats and mice. In rats, a dose-related increase of benign pituitary hyperplasia and benign adenomas was noted at 24 months when the drug was administered subcutaneously at high daily doses (0.6 to 4 mg/kg). There was a significant but not dose-related increase of pancreatic islet-cell adenomas in females and of testicular interstitial cell adenomas in males (highest incidence in the low dose group). In mice no pituitary abnormalities were observed at a dose as high as 60 mg/kg for two years.

Patients have been treated with leuprolide acetate for up to three years with doses as high as 10 mg/day and for two years with doses as high as 20 mg/day without demonstrable pituitary abnormalities.

Mutagenicity studies have been performed with leuprolide acetate using bacterial and mammalian systems. These studies provided no evidence of a mutagenic potential.

Central Precocious Puberty: During the early phase of therapy, gonadotropins and sex steroids rise above baseline because of the natural stimulatory effect of the drug. An increase in clinical signs and symptoms may therefore be observed.

Non-compliance with the drug regimen or inadequate dosing may result in inadequate control of the pubertal process. The consequences of poor control include the return of pubertal signs such as menses, breast development, and testicular growth. The long-term consequences of inadequate control of gonadal steroid secretion are unknown, but may include a further compromise of adult stature.

Dependence/Tolerance: No drug-dependence has been reported with the use of leuprolide acetate.

Endocrine and Metabolism: Changes in Bone Density: Bone loss can be expected as part of natural aging and can also be anticipated during the hypoandrogenic state caused by long-term use of leuprolide acetate. In patients with significant risk factors for decreased bone mineral content and/or bone mass such as family history of osteoporosis, chronic use of corticosteroids or anticonvulsants or chronic abuse of alcohol or tobacco, leuprolide acetate may pose additional risk. In these patients, risk versus benefit must be weighed carefully before initiation of leuprolide acetate therapy.

Hypogonadism: Long-term administration of leuprolide acetate will cause suppression of pituitary gonadotropins and gonadal hormone production with clinical symptoms of hypogonadism. These changes have been observed to reverse on discontinuation of therapy. However, whether the clinical symptoms of induced hypogonadism will reverse in all patients has not yet been established.

Hepatic/Biliary/Pancreatic: The pharmacokinetics of the drug in patients with hepatic, biliary or pancreatic impairment have not been determined.

Renal: The pharmacokinetics of the drug in patients with renal impairment have not been determined.

Special Populations: Pregnant Women: The paediatric products LUPRON and LUPRON DEPOT described in this Product Monograph are not indicated for use in women. LUPRON DEPOT treatment of women is covered in the LUPRON DEPOT 3.75 mg and 11.25 mg "Endometriosis" Product Monograph.

Nursing Women: It is not known whether leuprolide acetate is excreted in human milk; therefore, LUPRON and LUPRON DEPOT are contraindicated in patients who are breast-feeding. LUPRON DEPOT treatment of women is covered in the LUPRON DEPOT 3.75 mg and 11.25 mg "Endometriosis" Product Monograph.

Geriatrics (>65 years of age): Refer to the "Prostatic Cancer" Product Monograph for the efficacy and safety of LUPRON and LUPRON DEPOT in this population.

Monitoring and Laboratory Tests: Response to LUPRON and LURPON DEPOT should be monitored 1 to 2 months after the start of therapy with a GnRH stimulation test and sex steroid levels. Measurement of bone age for advancement should be done every 6 to 12 months.

Sex steroids may increase or rise above prepubertal levels if the dose is inadequate. See Warnings and Precautions, Endocrine and Metabolism. Once a therapeutic dose has been established, gonadotropin and sex steroid levels will decline to prepubertal levels.

ADVERSE REACTIONS: Adverse Drug Reaction Overview: Potential exacerbation of signs and symptoms during the first few weeks of the treatment is a concern in patients with rapidly advancing central precocious puberty. See Warnings and Precautions.

Clinical Trial Adverse Drug Reactions: Because clinical trials are conducted under very specific conditions the adverse reaction rates observed in the clinical trials may not reflect the rates observed in practice and should not be compared to the rates in the clinical trials of another drug. Adverse drug reaction information from clinical trials is useful for identifying drug-related adverse events and for approximating rates.

In two studies of children with central precocious puberty, in 2% or more of the patients receiving the drug, the following adverse reactions were reported to have a possible or probable relationship to drug as ascribed by the treating physician (see Table 1). Reactions considered not drug related are excluded.

Table 1: LUPRON/LUPRON DEPOT

Adverse Reactions Reported Having a Possible or Probable Relationship to Drug in 2% or More of Patients Receiving the Drug

	Number of Patients N=421 (%)
Body as a Whole	
General pain	12 (3)
Headache	11 (3)
Injection site reaction including abscess[a]	37 (9)
Cardiovascular System	
Vasodilatation	9 (2)
Integumentary System	
Acne/seborrhea	8 (2)
Rash including erythema multiforme	12 (3)
Nervous System	
Emotional lability	19 (5)
Urogenital System	
Vaginitis/vaginal bleeding/vaginal discharge	13 (3)

[a] Most events were mild or moderate in severity.

Less Common Clinical Trial Adverse Drug Reactions (<2%): In these same studies, the following adverse reactions were reported in less than 2% of the patients.

Body as a Whole: aggravation of pre-existing tumor and decreased vision, allergic reaction, body odor, fever, flu syndrome, infection, hypertrophy.

Cardiovascular System: bradycardia, hypertension, peripheral vascular disorder, syncope.

Digestive System: constipation, dyspepsia, dysphagia, gingivitis, increased appetite, nausea/vomiting.

Endocrine System: accelerated sexual maturity, feminization, goiter.

Hemic and Lymphatic System: purpura.

Metabolic and Nutritional Disorders: growth retarded, peripheral edema, weight gain.

Musculoskeletal System: arthralgia, joint disorder, myalgia, myopathy.

Nervous System: depression, hyperkinesia, nervousness, somnolence.

Respiratory System: asthma, epistaxis, pharyngitis, rhinitis, sinusitis.

Integumentary System: alopecia, hair disorder, hirsutism, leukoedema, nail disorder, skin hypertrophy, urticaria.

Urogenital System: cervix disorder/neoplasm, dysmenorrhea, gynecomastia/breast disorders, menstrual disorder, urinary incontinence.

Abnormal Hematologic and Clinical Chemistry Findings: The following laboratory events were reported as adverse reactions: antinuclear antibody present and increased sedimentation rate.

See Drug-Laboratory Test Interactions under Drug Interactions.

Post-Market Adverse Drug Reactions: Isolated cases of anaphylaxis have been reported. Symptoms consistent with an anaphylactoid or asthmatic process have been rarely reported.

Pituitary Apoplexy: During post-marketing surveillance, rare cases of pituitary apoplexy (a clinical syndrome secondary to infarction of the pituitary gland) have been reported after the administration of gonadotropin-releasing hormone agonists. In a majority of these cases, a pituitary adenoma was diagnosed, with a majority of pituitary apoplexy cases occurring within 2 weeks of the first dose, and some within the first hour. In these cases, pituitary apoplexy has presented as sudden headache, vomiting, visual changes, ophthalmoplegia, altered mental status, and sometimes cardiovascular collapse. Immediate medical attention has been required.

During post-marketing surveillance which include other dosage forms, the following adverse events were reported:

Cardiovascular System: hypotension.

Hemic and Lymphatic System: decreased WBC.

Central/Peripheral Nervous System: convulsion, peripheral neuropathy, spinal fracture/paralysis.

Integumentary System: rash, urticaria, photosensitivity reactions.

Musculoskeletal System: tenosynovitis-like symptoms.

Urogenital System: prostate pain.

Miscellaneous: injection site reactions including pain, inflammation, sterile abscess, induration and hematoma.

See the "Prostatic Cancer" and "Endometriosis" LUPRON and LUPRON DEPOT Product Monographs for other reported events.

DRUG INTERACTIONS: Overview: Leuprolide being approximately 46% bound to plasma proteins, and a peptide that is primarily degraded by peptidase and not by cytochrome P-450 enzymes as noted in specific studies, drug interactions would not be expected to occur.

Drug-Drug Interactions: No pharmacokinetic-based drug-drug interaction studies have been conducted.

Drug-Food Interactions: Interactions with food have not been established.

Drug-Herb Interactions: Interactions with herbal products have not been established.

Drug-Laboratory Test Interactions: Administration of LUPRON DEPOT at therapeutic doses results in suppression of the pituitary-gonadal system. Normal function is usually restored within 4 to 12 weeks after treatment is discontinued. Diagnostic tests of pituitary-gonadal function conducted during treatment and within 4 to 8 weeks after discontinuation of LUPRON DEPOT therapy may therefore be misleading.

As expected, leuprolide acetate administration will initially affect selected serum and urine parameters in the first week of treatment: elevation of BUN, creatinine, acid phosphatase, testosterone and dihydrotestosterone can be expected. With chronic administration, these high values will usually return to normal, or drop below baseline in the case of testosterone, dihydrotestosterone and acid phosphatase.

DOSAGE AND ADMINISTRATION: Dosing Considerations:

- LUPRON DEPOT (leuprolide acetate for depot suspension) must be administered under the supervision of a physician.
- LUPRON DEPOT 3.75 mg (1-Month SR) and 7.5 mg (1-Month SR), administered intramuscularly are designed to provide continuous sustained release of leuprolide for 1 month.

Note: As with all parenteral products, inspect container's solution for discoloration and particulate matter before each use.

Use in Central Precocious Puberty: The dose of leuprolide acetate must be individualized for each child. The dose is based on a mg/kg ratio of drug to body weight. Younger children require higher doses on a mg/kg ratio.

For each dosage form, after 1 to 2 months of initiating therapy or changing doses, the child must be monitored with a GnRH stimulation test, sex steroids, and Tanner staging to confirm downregulation. Measurements of bone age for advancement should be monitored every 6 to 12 months. The dose should be titrated upward until no progression of the condition is noted either clinically and/or by laboratory parameters.

The first dose found to result in adequate downregulation can probably be maintained for the duration of therapy in most children. However, there are insufficient data to guide dosage adjustments as patients move into higher weight categories after beginning therapy at very young ages and low dosages. It is recommended that adequate downregulation be verified in such patients whose weight has increased significantly while on therapy.

Discontinuation of leuprolide acetate should be considered before age 11 for females and age 12 for males.

Recommended Dose and Dosage Adjustment: LUPRON: The recommended starting dose is 50 µg/kg/day administered as a **single subcutaneous injection**. If total downregulation is not achieved, the dose should be titrated upward by 10 µg/kg/day to a maximum of 100 µg/kg/day. This dose will be considered the maintenance dose.

LUPRON DEPOT: The recommended starting dose is 0.3 mg/kg/4 weeks (minimum 7.5 mg) administered as a **single intramuscular injection**, after reconstitution with the special diluent. See Dosage and Administration, Administration. The starting dose will be dictated by the child's weight.

Child's Weight	Total Dose
≤25 kg	7.5 mg
>25–≤37.5 kg	11.25 mg
>37.5 kg	15 mg

If total downregulation is not achieved, the dose should be titrated upward in increments of 3.75 mg every 4 weeks to a maximum of 15 mg per month. This dose will be considered the maintenance dose.

Missed Dose: LUPRON: If the patient forgets to take the injection at the usual time, they should take it as soon as they remember, if they remember on the same day. If not, they should not take the missed dose at all; they should wait until it is time for their next dose. The patient should not take two doses at once.

The patient should not stop taking LUPRON simply because they feel better.

LUPRON DEPOT: Regular injections are important. Adherence to 4-week drug administration schedules must be accepted if therapy is to be successful. If a shot is missed or is administered a week late, the child's pubertal development could begin again. See Warnings and Precautions, General and Central Precocious Puberty.

Administration: LUPRON: As with other drugs administered chronically by injection, the injection site should be varied periodically.

As a guide, the usual sites of injection are indicated in Figure 1.

Figure 1: LUPRON

Suggested Rotation of the Injection Site

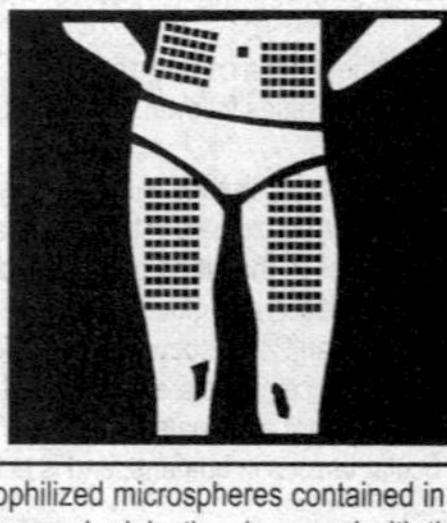

Reconstitution: LUPRON DEPOT: The lyophilized microspheres contained in the front chamber of the prefilled dual-chamber syringe are to be reconstituted prior to intramuscular injection, in accord with the following directions:

For LUPRON DEPOT 3.75 mg (1-Month SR) and 7.5 mg (1-Month SR):

1. The LUPRON DEPOT powder should be visually inspected and the syringe should **not be used** if clumping or caking is evident. A thin layer of powder on the wall of the syringe is considered normal. The diluent should appear clear.
2. To prepare for injection, screw the white plunger into the end stopper until the stopper begins to turn.
3. Remember to tighten the needle by twisting the needle cap clockwise. Do not overtighten.
4. Holding the syringe upright, release the diluent by **slowly pushing** (6 to 8 seconds) the plunger until the first stopper is at the **blue line** in the middle of the barrel.
5. Keep the syringe upright. Gently shake the syringe to thoroughly mix the microspheres (powder) to form a uniform suspension. The suspension will appear milky.
6. If the microspheres adhere to the stopper or caking/clumping is present, tap the syringe against your finger to disperse. **Do not use** if any of the powder has not gone into suspension.
7. Keep the syringe upright. With the opposite hand, remove the needle cap without twisting and advance the plunger to expel the air from the syringe.
8. At the time of reconstitution, inject the entire contents of the syringe intramuscularly. The suspension settles very quickly following reconstitution; therefore, LUPRON DEPOT should be mixed and used immediately.
   Note: Aspirated blood would be visible just below the luer lock connection if a blood vessel is accidentally penetrated. If present, blood can be seen through the transparent LuproLoc safety device.
9. After injection, withdraw the needle. Immediately activate the LuproLoc safety device by pushing the arrow forward with the thumb or finger until the device is fully extended and a **click** is heard or felt.

Although the suspension has been shown to be stable for 24 hours following reconstitution, since the product does not contain a preservative, the suspension should be discarded if not used immediately.

As with other drugs administered by injection, the injection site should be varied periodically.

OVERDOSAGE:

In rats, subcutaneous administration of 250 to 500 times the recommended human pediatric dose, expressed on a per body weight basis resulted in dyspnea, decreased activity, and local irritation at the injection site.

There is no clinical experience with the effects of an acute overdose. Because the acute animal toxicity of the drug is low, adverse effects are not expected. No difference in adverse reactions was observed in patients who received either 1 or 10 mg/day leuprolide acetate for up to three years or 20 mg/day for up to two years.

> For management of a suspected drug overdose, contact your regional Poison Control Centre. See the *CPS* Directory section for a list of Poison Control Centres.

ACTION AND CLINICAL PHARMACOLOGY: Mechanism of Action: Leuprolide acetate is a synthetic nonapeptide analog of naturally-occurring gonadotropin-releasing hormone (GnRH or LHRH). The analog possesses greater potency than the natural hormone. When administered as indicated, leuprolide acetate acts as a potent inhibitor of gonadotropin production. It is chemically unrelated to steroids.

Unlike steroid hormones, leuprolide acetate exerts specific action on the pituitary gonadotrophs and the human reproductive tract.

This specificity reduces the likelihood of secondary adverse effects such as gynecomastia, thromboembolism, edema, liver and gallbladder involvement.

Pharmacodynamics: Human studies indicated that following an initial stimulation of gonadotropins, chronic stimulation with leuprolide acetate results in suppression or "downregulation" of these hormones and consequent suppression of ovarian and testicular steroidogenesis. These effects are reversible on discontinuation of drug therapy.

Central Precocious Puberty: Two chronic studies involving the treatment of children with central precocious puberty (CPP), demonstrated that following the administration of LUPRON (leuprolide acetate) injection and/or LUPRON DEPOT (leuprolide acetate for depot suspension), stimulated and basal gonadotropins are reduced to prepubertal levels. Testosterone and estradiol are reduced to prepubertal levels in males and females, respectively, and a reduction of gonadotropins will allow for normal physical and psychological growth and development. Natural maturation occurs when gonadotropins return to pubertal levels following discontinuation of leuprolide acetate.

The following physiological effects have been noted with the chronic administration of leuprolide acetate in CPP patients.

- **Skeletal Growth:** A measurable increase in body length can be noted since the epiphyseal plates will not close prematurely.
- **Organ Growth:** Reproductive organs will return to a prepubertal state.

- **Menses:** Menses, if present, will cease.

Intramuscular injection of LUPRON DEPOT provides plasma concentrations of leuprolide acetate over a period of one month.

In a study of 22 children with central precocious puberty, doses of LUPRON DEPOT were given every 4 weeks and plasma levels were determined according to weight categories as summarized in Table 2.

Table 2: LUPRON/LUPRON DEPOT

Determination of Leuprolide Plasma Levels According to Weight Categories in Children with Central Precocious Puberty

Patient Weight Range (kg)	Group Weight Average (kg)	Dose (mg)	Trough Plasma Leuprolide Level Mean±SD (ng/mL)[a]
20.2–27.0	22.7	7.5	0.77±0.033
28.4–36.8	32.5	11.25	1.25±1.06
39.3–57.5	44.2	15.0	1.59±0.65

[a] Group average values determined at Week 4 immediately prior to leuprolide injection. Drug levels at 12 and 24 weeks were similar to respective 4 week levels.

Pharmacokinetics: Intramuscular injections of LUPRON DEPOT (leuprolide acetate for depot suspension) 3.75 mg (1-Month SR) and 7.5 mg (1-Month SR) provide effective plasma concentrations of leuprolide acetate over a period of one month.

Leuprolide is not active when given orally.

Absorption: A single dose of LUPRON DEPOT 3.75 mg (1-Month SR) was administered by intramuscular injection to healthy adult female volunteers. The absorption of leuprolide was characterized by an initial increase in plasma concentration, with peak concentration ranging from 4.6 to 10.2 ng/mL at four hours post-dosing. However, intact leuprolide and an inactive metabolite could not be distinguished by the assay used in the study. Following the initial rise, leuprolide concentrations started to plateau within two days after dosing and remained relatively stable for about four to five weeks with plasma concentrations of about 0.30 ng/mL.

Following a single LUPRON DEPOT 7.5 mg (1-Month SR) intramuscular injection to adult patients, the mean peak leuprolide plasma concentration was almost 20 ng/mL at 4 hours and then declined to 0.36 ng/mL at 4 weeks. However, intact leuprolide and an inactive major metabolite could not be distinguished by the assay used in the study. Undetectable leuprolide plasma concentrations have been observed during chronic LUPRON DEPOT 7.5 mg (1-Month SR) administration, but testosterone levels appear to be maintained at castrate levels.

In adults, bioavailability by subcutaneous administration is comparable to that by intravenous administration. Leuprolide acetate has a plasma half-life of 2.9 hours.

Distribution: The mean steady-state volume of distribution of leuprolide following intravenous bolus administration to healthy male volunteers was 27 L. In vitro binding to human plasma proteins ranged from 43 to 49%.

Metabolism: In healthy male volunteers, a 1 mg bolus of leuprolide administered intravenously revealed that the mean systemic clearance was 7.6 L/h, with a terminal elimination half-life of approximately 3 hours based on a two-compartment model.

In rats and dogs, administration of ^{14}C-labelled leuprolide was shown to be metabolized to smaller inactive peptides, pentapeptide (Metabolite I), tripeptides (Metabolites II and III) and dipeptide (Metabolite IV). These fragments may be further catabolized.

The major metabolite (M-I) plasma concentrations measured in 5 prostate cancer patients reached mean maximum concentration 2 to 6 hours after dosing and were approximately 6% of the peak parent drug concentration. One week after dosing, mean plasma M-I concentrations were approximately 20% of leuprolide concentrations.

Excretion: Following administration of LUPRON DEPOT 3.75 mg (1-Month SR) to 3 patients, less than 5% of the dose was recovered as parent and M-I metabolite in the urine.

Special Populations and Conditions: Pediatrics: A pharmacokinetic study of leuprolide acetate in children has not been performed.

Hepatic Insufficiency: The pharmacokinetics of the drug in patients with hepatic impairment have not been determined.

Renal Insufficiency: The pharmacokinetics of the drug in patients with renal impairment have not been determined.

STORAGE AND STABILITY: LUPRON: Store LUPRON (leuprolide acetate injection) 5 mg/mL between 2 and 8°C.

LUPRON DEPOT:

Store LUPRON DEPOT (leuprolide acetate for depot suspension) 3.75 mg (1-Month SR), and 7.5 mg, (1-Month SR) between 15 and 25°C. Protect from freezing.

Although the suspension has been shown to be stable for 24 hours following reconstitution, since the product does not contain a preservative, the suspension should be discarded if not used immediately.

SPECIAL HANDLING INSTRUCTIONS: It is very important to activate the LuproLoc safety device immediately after injection. This is done by pushing the arrow forward with the thumb or finger until the device is fully extended and a **click** is heard or felt. See Dosage and Administration, Administration, Reconstitution.

INFORMATION FOR THE PATIENT: Published in e-CPS, available by subscription at www.e-cps.ca.

DOSAGE FORMS, COMPOSITION AND PACKAGING: LUPRON: Each mL contains: leuprolide acetate 5 mg. Nonmedicinal ingredients: benzyl alcohol, sodium chloride and sterile water for injection USP. The pH may have been adjusted with sodium hydroxide and/or acetic acid. Multiple dose vials of 2.8 mL for subcutaneous use. Supplied as a 14-day kit. Each 14 day Patient Administration Kit contains: 1 vial of Lupron, 28 swabs and 14 syringes and 1 Patient Information/Instructions for Use leaflet.

LUPRON DEPOT: 3.75 mg (1-Month Slow Release): Each prefilled dual-chamber syringe contains: sterile lyophilised microspheres composed of leuprolide acetate incorporated in a biodegradable copolymer of lactic and glycolic acids. The front chamber contains: leuprolide acetate 3.75 mg. Nonmedicinal ingredients: DL-lactic and glycolic acids copolymer, D-mannitol and purified gelatin. The rear chamber of diluent contains: carboxymethylcellulose sodium, D-mannitol, glacial acetic acid USP to control pH, polysorbate 80 and water for injection USP.

7.5 mg (1-Month Slow Release): Each prefilled dual-chamber syringe contains: sterile lyophilised microspheres composed of leuprolide acetate incorporated in a biodegradable copolymer of lactic and glycolic acids. The front chamber contains: leuprolide acetate 7.5 mg. Nonmedicinal ingredients: DL-lactic and glycolic acids copolymer, D-mannitol and purified gelatin. The rear chamber of diluent contains: carboxymethylcellulose sodium, D-mannitol, glacial acetic acid USP to control pH, polysorbate 80 and water for injection USP.

Each kit contains 1 prefilled dual-chamber syringe with 23 G needle, 2 alcohol swabs, Patient Information Leaflet, Special Instructions for Use and Package Insert.

Lupron® Ⓟ

Leuprolide acetate

Gonadotropin-releasing Hormone Analog

Abbott

Lupron Depot® 7.5 mg/22.5 mg/30 mg Ⓟ

Leuprolide acetate

Gonadotropin-releasing Hormone Analog

Abbott

Date of Preparation: March 11, 1999

Date of Revision: March 23, 2010

SUMMARY PRODUCT INFORMATION:

Route of Administration	Dosage Form/ Strength	Clinically Relevant Nonmedicinal Ingredients
LUPRON		
Subcutaneous	Multiple-dose vial/5 mg/mL	Acetic acid, benzyl alcohol, sodium chloride, sodium hydroxide For a complete listing see Dosage Forms, Composition and Packaging.
LUPRON DEPOT		
Intramuscular	Pre-filled dual chamber syringe containing sterile lyophilized microspheres/7.5 mg (1-Month SR)	Carboxymethylcellulose sodium, DL-lactic and glycolic acids copolymer, D-mannitol, gelatin, glacial acetic acid, polysorbate 80
	Pre-filled dual chamber syringe containing sterile lyophilized microspheres/22.5 mg (3-Month SR)	Carboxymethylcellulose sodium, D-mannitol, glacial acetic acid, polylactic acid, polysorbate 80
	Pre-filled dual chamber syringe containing sterile lyophilized microspheres/30.0 mg (4-Month SR)	Carboxymethylcellulose sodium, D-mannitol, glacial acetic acid, polylactic acid, polysorbate 80 For a complete listing see Dosage Forms, Composition and Packaging.
Definition: SR=slow release.		

INDICATIONS AND CLINICAL USE: LUPRON (leuprolide acetate injection) and LUPRON DEPOT (leuprolide acetate for depot suspension) are indicated for:

- the palliative treatment of sex hormone responsive advanced (stage D2) carcinoma of the prostate.

LUPRON DEPOT must be administered under the supervision of a physician.

Geriatrics (>65 years of age): The majority of the patients studied in the clinical trials for LUPRON and LUPRON DEPOT were 65 years and older.

Pediatrics (<18 years of age): LUPRON DEPOT 22.5 mg (3-Month SR) and 30.0 mg (4-Month SR) are not indicated for use in children. LUPRON DEPOT treatment of children is covered in the LUPRON DEPOT 3.75 mg and 7.5 mg "Central Precocious Puberty" Product Monograph.

Women (>18 years of age): LUPRON DEPOT 22.5 mg (3-Month SR) and 30.0 mg (4-Month SR) are not indicated for use in women. LUPRON DEPOT treatment of women is covered in the LUPRON DEPOT 3.75 mg and 11.25 mg "Endometriosis" Product Monograph.

CONTRAINDICATIONS:

- LUPRON (leuprolide acetate injection) and LUPRON DEPOT (leuprolide acetate for depot suspension) are contraindicated in patients with hypersensitivity to the drug or its components or similar nonapeptides or components of the container. Isolated cases of anaphylaxis have been reported. For a complete listing, see Dosage Forms, Composition and Packaging.
- LUPRON and LUPRON DEPOT are contraindicated in women who are or may become pregnant. The possibility exists that spontaneous abortion may occur if the drug is administered during pregnancy.
- It is not known whether leuprolide is excreted in human milk; therefore, LUPRON and LUPRON DEPOT are contraindicated in patients who are breast-feeding.

WARNINGS AND PRECAUTIONS: General: LUPRON (leuprolide acetate injection) and LUPRON DEPOT (leuprolide acetate for depot suspension), like other gonadotropin-releasing hormone (LH-RH) agonists, causes a transient increase in serum concentration of testosterone during the first weeks of treatment. Patients may experience worsening of symptoms or onset of new symptoms, including bone pain, neuropathy, hematuria, or ureteral or bladder outlet obstruction. Cases of spinal cord compression, which may contribute to paralysis with or without fatal complications, have been reported with LH-RH agonists. If spinal cord compression or renal impairment due to ureteral obstruction develops, standard treatment of these complications should be instituted.

Patients with metastatic vertebral lesions and/or with urinary tract obstruction should begin leuprolide acetate therapy under close supervision.

Postmarketing reports of convulsions have been observed in patients on leuprolide acetate therapy. These included patients in the female and pediatric populations, patients with a history of seizures, epilepsy, cerebrovascular disorders, central nervous system anomalies or tumors, and in patients on concomitant medications that have been associated with convulsions such as bupropion and SSRIs. Convulsions have also been reported in patients in the absence of any of the conditions mentioned above.

Patients with known allergies to benzyl alcohol, a vehicle ingredient of LUPRON, may present symptoms of hypersensitivity, usually local, in the form of erythema and induration at the injection site.

Carcinogenesis and Mutagenesis: Two-year carcinogenicity studies were conducted in rats and mice. In rats, a dose-related increase of benign pituitary hyperplasia and benign adenomas was noted at 24 months when the drug was administered subcutaneously at high daily doses (0.6 to 4 mg/kg). There was a significant but not dose-related increase of pancreatic islet-cell adenomas in females and of testicular interstitial cell adenomas in males (highest incidence in the low dose group). In mice, no pituitary abnormalities were observed at a dose as high as 60 mg/kg for two years.

Patients have been treated with leuprolide acetate for up to three years with doses as high as 10 mg/day and for two years with doses as high as 20 mg/day without demonstrable pituitary abnormalities.

Mutagenicity studies have been performed with leuprolide acetate using bacterial and mammalian systems. These studies provided no evidence of a mutagenic potential.

Dependence/Tolerance: No drug-dependence has been reported with the use of leuprolide acetate.

Endocrine and Metabolism: Changes in Bone Density: Bone loss can be expected as part of natural aging and can also be anticipated during the hypoandrogenic state caused by long-term use of leuprolide acetate. In patients with significant risk factors for decreased bone mineral content and/or bone mass such as family history of osteoporosis, chronic use of corticosteroids or anticonvulsants or chronic abuse of alcohol or tobacco, leuprolide acetate may pose additional risk. In these patients, risk versus benefit must be weighed carefully before initiation of leuprolide acetate therapy.

Hypogonadism: Long-term administration of leuprolide acetate will cause suppression of pituitary gonadotropins and gonadal hormone production with clinical symptoms of hypogonadism. These changes have been observed to reverse on discontinuation of therapy. However, whether the clinical symptoms of induced hypogonadism will reverse in all patients has not yet been established.

Hepatic/Biliary/Pancreatic: The pharmacokinetics of the drug in patients with hepatic, biliary or pancreatic impairment have not been determined.

Renal: The pharmacokinetics of the drug in patients with renal impairment have not been determined.

Special Populations: Pregnant Women: LUPRON and LUPRON DEPOT 7.5 mg (1-Month SR), 22.5 mg (3-Month SR) and 30.0 mg (4-Month SR) described in this Product Monograph are not indicated for use in women. LUPRON DEPOT treatment of women is covered in the LUPRON DEPOT 3.75 mg and 11.25 mg "Endometriosis" Product Monograph.

Nursing Women: LUPRON and LUPRON DEPOT 7.5 mg (1-Month SR), 22.5 mg (3-Month SR) and 30.0 mg (4-Month SR) described in this Product Monograph are not indicated for use in women. LUPRON DEPOT treatment of women is covered in the LUPRON DEPOT 3.75 mg and 11.25 mg "Endometriosis" Product Monograph.

Pediatrics (<18 years of age): Safety and effectiveness of LUPRON DEPOT 22.5 mg (3-Month SR) and 30.0 mg (4-Month SR) have not been established in pediatric patients. See "Central Precocious Puberty" Product Monograph for the safety and effectiveness of LUPRON and LUPRON DEPOT in children with central precocious puberty.

Geriatrics (>65 years of age): In prostatic cancer clinical trials for LUPRON and LUPRON DEPOT, the majority of subjects studied were at least 65 years of age. The labelling therefore reflects the pharmacokinetics, efficacy and safety of LUPRON and LUPRON DEPOT in this population.

Monitoring and Laboratory Tests: Response to LUPRON and LUPRON DEPOT should be monitored by measuring serum levels of testosterone, as well as prostate-specific antigen and prostatic acid phosphatase. In the majority of patients, testosterone levels increased above baseline during the first week, declining thereafter to baseline levels or below by the end of the second week. In the LUPRON DEPOT 30.0 mg (4-Month SR) study, castrate levels were reached within two to four weeks, and once achieved, were maintained in most patients (45/49) for as long as the patients received their injections.

The effects of leuprolide acetate on bone lesions may be monitored by bone scans, while its effects on prostatic lesions may be monitored by ultrasonography and/or computed tomography (CT) scan in addition to digital rectal examination.

Intravenous pyelogram, ultrasonography, or CT scan may also be utilized to diagnose or assess the status of obstructive uropathy.

Periodic monitoring of serum testosterone and Prostatic Specific Antigen (PSA) levels is recommended, especially if the anticipated clinical or biochemical response to treatment has not been achieved. It should be noted that results of testosterone determinations are dependent on assay methodology. It is advisable to be aware of the type and precision of the assay methodology to make appropriate clinical and therapeutic decisions.

ADVERSE REACTIONS: Adverse Drug Reaction Overview: In clinical studies, an initial rise in serum testosterone levels usually occurred in non-orchiectomized patients during the first week of treatment.

This occasionally was associated with a worsening of signs and symptoms, usually an increase in bone pain. See Warnings and Precautions. In some cases, temporary renal impairment was accompanied by mental confusion, joint pain, nausea and vomiting. In each case, leuprolide acetate administration was continued and the symptom(s) subsided in one to two weeks.

The potential for exacerbation of signs and symptoms during the first few weeks of treatment is a concern in patients with vertebral metastases and/or in patients with severe obstructive uropathy which, if aggravated, may lead to neurological problems such as temporary weakness and/or paresthesia of the lower limbs or worsening of urinary symptoms, such as hematuria and urinary tract obstruction.

Clinical Trial Adverse Drug Reactions: Because clinical trials are conducted under very specific conditions the adverse reaction rates observed in the clinical trials may not reflect the rates observed in practice and should not be compared to the rates in the clinical trials of another drug. Adverse drug reaction information from clinical trials is useful for identifying drug-related adverse events and for approximating rates.

LUPRON and LUPRON DEPOT 7.5 mg (1-Month SR), 22.5 mg (3-Month SR), 30 mg (4-Month SR): The following possibly or probably related systemic adverse reactions were reported by ≥5% of the patients using LUPRON (leuprolide acetate injection) and LUPRON DEPOT (leuprolide acetate for depot suspension) 7.5 mg, 22.5 mg and 30 mg in clinical studies. Reactions not considered drug related are excluded.

In two clinical studies with LUPRON, hot flashes (49 to 55%), impotence/decrease in libido (3 to 10%), local reactions at injection site/ecchymosis/erythema (4 to 15%), decrease in testicular size/atrophic genitalia (7 to 13%), and itching rash (3%) were reported.

Adverse reactions reported by ≥5% of the patients using LUPRON DEPOT formulations are summarized in Table 1.

Table 1: LUPRON DEPOT

Incidence (%) of Possibly or Probably Related Systemic Adverse Reactions Reported by ≥5% of Patients Treated with LUPRON DEPOT 7.5 mg (1 injection every month), LUPRON DEPOT 22.5 mg (1 injection every 3 months) and LUPRON DEPOT 30 mg (1 injection every 4 months)

Body System	LUPRON DEPOT 7.5 mg (1-Month SR) N=56 (%) Study III	LUPRON DEPOT 22.5 mg (3-Month SR)[a] Non-Orchiectomized N=94 (%) Studies IV and V	LUPRON DEPOT 30 mg (4-Month SR) Non-Orchiectomized N=49 (%) Study VI	LUPRON DEPOT 30 mg (4-Month SR) Orchiectomized N=24 (%) Study VII[b]
Body as a Whole				
Asthenia	3 (5.4)	7 (7.4)	6 (12.2)	1 (4.2)
Flu syndrome			6 (12.2)	0 (0.0)
General pain	4 (7.1)	25 (26.6)	16 (32.7)	1 (4.2)
Headache		6 (6.4)	5 (10.2)	1 (4.2)
Injection site reaction		13 (13.8)	4 (8.2)	9 (37.5)
Cardiovascular System				
Hot flashes/sweats[c]	33 (58.9)	55 (58.5)	23 (46.9)	2 (8.3)
Gastrointestinal System				
Nausea/vomiting	3 (5.4)			
GI disorder		15 (16.0)	5 (10.2)	3 (12.5)
Metabolic and Nutritional Disorders				
Dehydration			4 (8.2)	0 (0.0)
Edema	7 (12.5)		4 (8.2)	5 (20.8)
Musculoskeletal System				
Joint disorder		11 (11.7)	8 (16.3)	1 (4.2)
Myalgia			4 (8.2)	0 (0.0)
Central/Peripheral Nervous Systems				
Dizziness/Vertigo		6 (6.4)	3 (6.1)	2 (8.3)
Insomnia/Sleep disorders		8 (8.5)		
Neuromuscular disorders		9 (9.6)	3 (6.1)	1 (4.2)
Paresthesia			4 (8.2)	1 (4.2)
Respiratory System				
Dyspnea	3 (5.4)			

* Physiologic effects of decreased testosterone.

(cont'd)

Table 1: LUPRON DEPOT *(cont'd)*

Incidence (%) of Possibly or Probably Related Systemic Adverse Reactions Reported by ≥5% of Patients Treated with LUPRON DEPOT 7.5 mg (1 injection every month), LUPRON DEPOT 22.5 mg (1 injection every 3 months) and LUPRON DEPOT 30 mg (1 injection every 4 months)

Body System	LUPRON DEPOT 7.5 mg (1-Month SR) N=56 (%) Study III	LUPRON DEPOT 22.5 mg (3-Month SR)[a] Non-Orchiectomized N=94 (%) Studies IV and V	LUPRON DEPOT 30 mg (4-Month SR) Non-Orchiectomized N=49 (%) Study VI	LUPRON DEPOT 30 mg (4-Month SR) Orchiectomized N=24 (%) Study VII[b]
Respiratory disorders		6 (6.4)	4 (8.2)	1 (4.2)
Skin and Appendages				
Skin reaction		8 (8.5)	6 (12.2)	0 (0.0)
Urogenital System				
Testicular atrophy[c]	3 (5.4)	19 (20.2)		
Impotence[c]	3 (5.4)	0 (0.0)		
Urinary disorders		14 (14.9)	5 (10.2)	4 (16.7)

a The adverse reactions reported for LUPRON DEPOT 22.5 mg (3-Month SR) are based on two clinical trials.
b Study VII was a multicenter, open-label study designed to characterize the pharmacokinetic profile of LUPRON DEPOT 30 mg (4-Month SR) following a single intramuscular injection and to assess the safety of the formulation in prostatic cancer patients.
c Physiological effect of decreased testosterone.

Less Common Clinical Trial Adverse Drug Reactions (<5%): The following possibly or probably related systemic adverse reactions were reported by less than 5% of the patients using LUPRON and LUPRON DEPOT 7.5 mg (1-Month SR), 22.5 mg (3-Month SR) and 30 mg (4-Month SR) in clinical studies. Reactions not considered drug-related are excluded.

LUPRON: Cardiovascular System: cardiac arrhythmias, congestive heart failure, electrocardiogram (ECG) changes/ischemia, high blood pressure, hypotension, myocardial infarction, murmur, phlebitis/thrombosis, pulmonary emboli, transient ischemic attack/stroke.
Central/Peripheral Nervous System: anxiety, blurred vision, dizziness/light-headedness, headache, hearing disorder, lethargy, memory disorder, mood swings, nervousness, numbness, paresthesia, peripheral neuropathy, sleep disorders, spinal fracture/paralysis, syncope/blackouts, taste disorders.
Endocrine System: breast tenderness or pain, gynecomastia, libido increase, thyroid enlargement.
Gastrointestinal System: anorexia, constipation, dysphagia, gastrointestinal bleeding, gastrointestinal disturbance, hepatic dysfunction, peptic ulcer, rectal polyps.
Hemic and Lymphatic Systems: anemia, decreased white blood cell (WBC).
Integumentary System: carcinoma of skin/ear, dry skin, ecchymosis, hair loss, itching, pigmentation, skin lesions.
Musculoskeletal System: ankylosing spondylosis, joint pain, myalgia, pelvic fibrosis, spasms.
Respiratory System: cough, pleural rub, pneumonia, pulmonary fibrosis, pulmonary infiltrate, respiratory disorders, sinus congestion.
Urogenital System: bladder spasms, hematuria, incontinence, penile swelling, prostate pain, urinary obstruction, urinary tract infection.
Miscellaneous: asthenia, depression, fatigue, fever, hypoglycemia, hypoproteinemia, increased blood urea nitrogen (BUN), increased creatinine, infection/inflammation, ophthalmologic disorders, swelling (temporal bone).
LUPRON DEPOT 7.5 mg (1-Month SR): Cardiovascular System: angina, cardiac arrhythmia.
Central/Peripheral Nervous System: insomnia, paresthesia.
Endocrine System: gynecomastia, libido decrease.
Gastrointestinal System: anorexia, diarrhea.
Integumentary System: dermatitis, local skin reactions, hair growth.
Musculoskeletal System: bone pain, myalgia.
Respiratory System: dyspnea, hemoptysis.
Urogenital System: dysuria, frequency/urgency, hematuria, testicular pain.
Miscellaneous: asthenia, diabetes, fever/chills, hard nodule in throat, increased calcium, increased uric acid, serum glutamic oxaloacetic transaminase (AST) (greater than 2 times normal values), weight gain.
LUPRON DEPOT 22.5 mg (3-Month SR): Body as a Whole: enlarged abdomen, fever.
Cardiovascular System: arrhythmia, bradycardia, heart failure, hypertension, hypotension, varicose vein.
Central/Peripheral Nervous System: anxiety, delusions, depression, hypesthesia, libido decrease*, nervousness, paresthesia.
Digestive System: anorexia, duodenal ulcer, increased appetite, thirst/dry mouth.
Hemic and Lymphatic Systems: anemia, lymphedema.
Metabolic and Nutritional Disorders: dehydration, edema.
Respiratory System: epistaxis, pharyngitis, pleural effusion, pneumonia.
Special Senses: abnormal vision, amblyopia, dry eyes, tinnitus.
Urogenital System: gynecomastia, impotence*, penis disorders, testis disorders.
LUPRON DEPOT 22.5 mg (3-Month SR): Body as a Whole: abscess, accidental injury, allergic reaction, cyst, fever, generalized edema, hernia, neck pain, neoplasm.
Cardiovascular System: atrial fibrillation, deep thrombophlebitis, hypertension.
Digestive System: anorexia, eructation, gastrointestinal hemorrhage, gingivitis, gum hemorrhage, hepatomegaly, increased appetite, intestinal obstruction, periodontal abscess.
Hemic and Lymphatic System: lymphadenopathy.
Metabolic and Nutritional Disorders: healing abnormal, hypoxia, weight loss.
Musculoskeletal System: leg cramps, pathological fracture, ptosis.
Nervous System: abnormal thinking, amnesia, confusion, convulsion, dementia, depression, insomnia/sleep disorders, libido decreased†, neuropathy, paralysis.
Respiratory System: asthma, bronchitis, hiccup, lung disorder, sinusitis, voice alteration.
Skin and Appendages: herpes zoster, melanosis.
Urogenital System: bladder carcinoma, epididymitis, impotence†, prostate disorder, testicular atrophy†, urinary incontinence, urinary tract infection.

Abnormal Hematologic and Clinical Chemistry Findings: Abnormalities of certain parameters were observed in hematologic and clinical chemistry determinations were recorded, but relationship to drug is difficult to assess in this population.

The following were recorded in ≥5% of patients in clinical studies with LUPRON DEPOT 7.5 mg (1-Month SR), 22.5 mg (3-Month SR) and 30.0 mg (4-Month SR):

LUPRON DEPOT 7.5 mg (1-Month SR): Lactate dehydrogenase (LDH) (>2 times normal values), alkaline phosphatase (>1.5 times normal values).

LUPRON DEPOT 22.5 mg (3-Month SR): Increased BUN, hyperglycemia, hyperlipidemia [total cholesterol, low-density lipo[illegible] tein (LDL)-cholesterol, triglycerides], hyperphosphatemia, abnormal liver function tests, increased PT, increased PTT. Add[illegible] laboratory abnormalities reported were: decreased platelets, decreased potassium and increased WBC.

LUPRON DEPOT 30 mg (4-Month SR): Abnormalities of certain parameters were observed, but their relationsh[illegible] treatment are difficult to assess in this population. The following were recorded in ≥5% of patients: decreased [illegible] decreased hemoglobin/hematocrit/red blood cell (RBC), hyperlipidemia (total cholesterol, LDL-cholesterol [illegible] decreased high-density lipoprotein(HDL)-cholesterol, eosinophilia, increased glucose, increased liver funct[illegible]

† Physiologic effects of decreased testosterone.

aminotransferase (ALT), aspartate transaminase (AST), gamma-glutamyl transpeptidase (GGTP), lactate dehydrogenase (LDH)], and increased phosphorus. Additional laboratory abnormalities were reported: increased BUN and PT, leukopenia, thrombocytopenia, uricaciduria, urine abnormality.

See Drug-Laboratory Test Interactions under Drug Interactions for more details.

Post-Market Adverse Drug Reactions: Isolated cases of anaphylaxis have been reported. Symptoms consistent with an anaphylactoid or asthmatic process have been rarely reported.

Pituitary Apoplexy: During post-marketing surveillance, rare cases of pituitary apoplexy (a clinical syndrome secondary to infarction of the pituitary gland) have been reported after the administration of gonadotropin-releasing hormone agonists. In a majority of these cases, a pituitary adenoma was diagnosed, with a majority of pituitary apoplexy cases occurring within 2 weeks of the first dose, and some within the first hour. In these cases, pituitary apoplexy has presented as sudden headache, vomiting, visual changes, ophthalmoplegia, altered mental status, and sometimes cardiovascular collapse. Immediate medical attention has been required.

Changes in Bone Density: Decreased bone density has been reported in the medical literature in men who have had orchiectomy or who have been treated with an LH-RH agonist analog. In a clinical trial, 25 men with prostate cancer, 12 of whom had been treated previously with leuprolide acetate for at least six months, underwent bone density studies as a result of pain. The leuprolide acetate-treated group had lower bone density scores than the non-treated control group. From another case report, two additional men, one 64 and the other 70 years, respectively, receiving goserelin acetate, were observed to have collapsed vertebrae thought to be due to decreased bone mineral density. It can be anticipated that long periods of medical castration in men will have effects on bone density.

During post-marketing surveillance, which includes other dosage forms and other patient populations, the following adverse events were reported:

Cardiovascular System: hypotension.
Central/Peripheral Nervous System: convulsion, peripheral neuropathy, spinal fracture/paralysis.
Hemic and Lymphatic System: decreased WBC.
Integumentary System: photosensitivity reactions, rash, urticaria.
Musculoskeletal System: tenosynovitis-like symptoms.
Urogenital System: prostate pain.
Miscellaneous: hematoma, induration, inflammation, injection site reactions including pain, sterile abscess.

See the "Central Precocious Puberty" and "Endometriosis" LUPRON and LUPRON DEPOT Product Monographs for other reported events.

DRUG INTERACTIONS: Overview: Leuprolide being approximately 46% bound to plasma proteins, and a peptide that is primarily degraded by peptidase and not by cytochrome P-450 enzymes as noted in specific studies, drug interactions would not be expected to occur.

Drug-Drug Interactions: No pharmacokinetic-based drug-drug interaction studies have been conducted.
Drug-Food Interactions: Interactions with food have not been established.
Drug-Herb Interactions: Interactions with herbal products have not been established.
Drug-Laboratory Test Interactions: Administration of leuprolide acetate in therapeutic doses results in suppression of the pituitary-gonadal system. Normal function is usually restored within 4 to 12 weeks after treatment is discontinued. Diagnostic tests of pituitary-gonadal function conducted during treatment and within 4 to 8 weeks after discontinuation of LUPRON DEPOT therapy may therefore be misleading.

As expected, leuprolide acetate administration will initially affect selected serum and urine parameters in the first week of treatment: elevation of BUN, creatinine, acid phosphatase, testosterone and dihydrotestosterone can be expected. With chronic administration, these high values will usually return to normal, or drop below baseline in the case of testosterone, dihydrotestosterone and acid phosphatase.

DOSAGE AND ADMINISTRATION: Dosing Considerations:

- LUPRON DEPOT (leuprolide acetate for depot suspension) must be administered under the supervision of a physician.
- LUPRON DEPOT 7.5 mg (1-Month SR), 22.5 mg (3-Month SR) and 30 mg (4-Month SR) administered intramuscularly are designed to provide continuous sustained release of leuprolide for 1, 3, and 4 months, respectively.

Note: As with all parenteral products, inspect container's solution for discoloration and particulate matter before each use.

Recommended Dose and Dosage Adjustment: LUPRON: The recommended dose of LUPRON (leuprolide acetate injection) is 1 mg (0.2 mL), as a **single daily subcutaneous injection**. See Dosage and Administration, Administration and Information for the Patient.

LUPRON DEPOT: The recommended dose of LUPRON DEPOT (1-Month SR) is 7.5 mg administered **monthly as a single intramuscular injection**, after reconstitution with the special diluent. See Dosage and Administration, Administration and Information for the Patient.

The recommended dose of LUPRON DEPOT (3-Month SR) is 22.5 mg administered as a **single intramuscular injection once every three months (12 weeks)**, after reconstitution with the special diluent. See Dosage and Administration, Administration and Information for the Patient. Due to different release characteristics, a fractional dose of this 3-Month depot formulation is not equivalent to the same dose of the monthly formulation and should therefore not be given.

The recommended dose of LUPRON DEPOT (4-Month SR) is 30 mg administered as a **single intramuscular injection once every four months (16 weeks)**, after reconstitution with the special diluent. See Dosage and Administration, Administration and Information for the Patient. Due to different release characteristics, a fractional dose of this 4-Month depot formulation is not equivalent to the same dose of the monthly formulation and should therefore not be given.

Missed Dose: LUPRON: If the patient forgets to take the injection at the usual time, they should take it as soon as they remember, if they remember on the same day. If not, they should not take the missed dose at all; they should wait until it is time for their next dose. The patient should not take two doses at once.

The patient should not stop taking LUPRON simply because they feel better.

LUPRON DEPOT: Maintaining testosterone suppression is important in treating the symptoms of hormone-dependent prostate cancer. Missing an appointment by a few days should not disrupt the benefits of treatment, but keeping a consistent schedule of LUPRON DEPOT injection is an important part of treatment.

Administration: LUPRON: As with other drugs administered chronically by injection, the injection site should be varied periodically.

As a guide, the usual sites of injection are indicated in Figure 1.

Figure 1: LUPRON

Suggested Rotation of the Injection Site

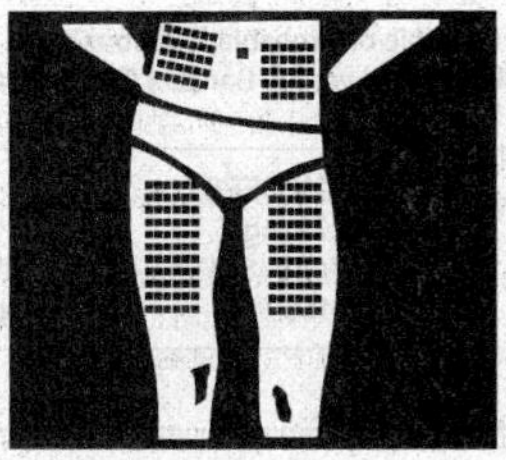

Reconstitution: LUPRON DEPOT: The lyophilized microspheres contained in the front chamber of the prefilled dual-chamber syringe are to be reconstituted prior to intramuscular administration, in accord with the following directions:

Due to different release characteristics, a fractional dose of the 3-month or 4-month depot formulation is not equivalent to the same dose of the monthly formulation and should not be given.

For LUPRON DEPOT 7.5 mg (1-Month SR), 22.5 mg (3-Month SR) and 30 mg (4-Month SR):

1. The LUPRON DEPOT powder should be visually inspected and the syringe should **not be used** if clumping or caking is evident. A thin layer of powder on the wall of the syringe is considered normal. The diluent should appear clear.
2. To prepare for injection, screw the white plunger into the end stopper until the stopper begins to turn.
3. Remember to tighten the needle by twisting the needle cap clockwise. Do not overtighten.
4. Holding the syringe upright, release the diluent by **slowly pushing** (6 to 8 seconds) the plunger until the first stopper is at the **blue line** in the middle of the barrel.
5. Keep the syringe upright. Gently shake the syringe to thoroughly mix the microspheres (powder) to form a uniform suspension. The suspension will appear milky.
6. If the microspheres adhere to the stopper or caking/clumping is present, tap the syringe against your finger to disperse. **Do not use** if any of the powder has not gone into suspension.
7. Keep the syringe upright. With the opposite hand, remove the needle cap without twisting and advance the plunger to expel the air from the syringe.
8. At the time of reconstitution, inject the entire contents of the syringe intramuscularly. The suspension settles very quickly following reconstitution; therefore, LUPRON DEPOT should be mixed and used immediately.
   Note: Aspirated blood would be visible just below the luer lock connection if a blood vessel is accidentally penetrated. If present, blood can be seen through the transparent LuproLoc safety device.
9. After injection, withdraw the needle. Immediately activate the LuproLoc safety device by pushing the arrow forward with the thumb or finger until the device is fully extended and a **click** is heard or felt.

Although the suspension has been shown to be stable for 24 hours following reconstitution, since the product does not contain a preservative, the suspension should be discarded if not used immediately.

As with other drugs administered by injection, the injection site should be varied periodically.

OVERDOSAGE:

There is no clinical experience with the effects of an acute overdose. Because the animal toxicity of the drug is low, adverse effects are not expected. No difference in adverse reactions was observed in patients who received either 1 or 10 mg/day leuprolide acetate for up to three years or 20 mg/day for up to two years.

> For management of a suspected drug overdose, contact your regional Poison Control Centre. See the *CPS* Directory section for a list of Poison Control Centres.

ACTION AND CLINICAL PHARMACOLOGY: Mechanism of Action: Leuprolide acetate is a synthetic nonapeptide analog of naturally-occurring gonadotropin-releasing hormone (GnRH or LHRH). The analog possesses greater potency than the natural hormone. When administered as indicated, leuprolide acetate acts as a potent inhibitor of gonadotropin production. It is chemically unrelated to steroids.

Unlike steroid hormones, leuprolide acetate exerts specific action on the pituitary gonadotrophs and the human reproductive tract.

This specificity reduces the likelihood of secondary adverse effects such as gynecomastia, thromboembolism, edema, liver and gallbladder involvement.

Pharmacodynamics: General: Animal and human studies indicate that, following an initial stimulation, chronic administration of leuprolide acetate results in the inhibition of gonadotropin production. Consequently, ovarian or testicular steroidogenesis is suppressed. The therapeutic effect of leuprolide acetate in the treatment of hormone-dependent tumors, such as in prostatic cancer, results from the reduction in serum gonadotropins and gonadal steroids.

Chronic administration of leuprolide acetate has resulted in inhibition of tumor growth (prostatic tumors in Noble and Dunning male rats, 7-12-dimethylbenz[α]-anthracene (DMBA)-induced mammary tumors in female rats) as well as atrophy of the reproductive organs. An additional mechanism of action, a direct effect on the gonads by downregulation of the gonadotropin receptors, is suggested in some animal studies.

In humans, subcutaneous administration of single daily doses of leuprolide acetate results in an initial increase in circulating levels of luteinizing hormone (LH) and follicle stimulating hormone (FSH), leading to a transient increase in the levels of the gonadal steroids (testosterone and dihydrotestosterone in males and estrone and estradiol in premenopausal females). However, continuous administration results in decreased levels of LH and FSH in all patients. In males, testosterone is reduced to castrate levels. In premenopausal females, estrogens are reduced to post-menopausal levels. These decreases occur within two to four weeks after initiation of treatment, and are maintained as long as treatment continues. Castrate levels of testosterone in prostatic cancer patients have been demonstrated for periods of up to 5 years.

Pharmacokinetics: Intramuscular injections of LUPRON DEPOT (leuprolide acetate for depot suspension) 7.5 mg (1-Month SR), 22.5 mg (3-Month SR), and 30.0 mg (4-Month SR) provide plasma concentrations of leuprolide acetate over a period of one, three, and four months, respectively.

Absorption: Following a single LUPRON DEPOT 7.5 mg (1-Month SR) injection to adult patients, the mean peak leuprolide plasma concentration was almost 20 ng/mL at 4 hours and then declined to 0.36 ng/mL at 4 weeks. However, intact leuprolide and an inactive major metabolite could not be distinguished by the assay used in the study. Undetectable leuprolide plasma concentrations have been observed during chronic LUPRON DEPOT 7.5 mg (1-Month SR) administration, but testosterone levels appear to be maintained at castrate levels.

The pharmacokinetic profile of LUPRON DEPOT 22.5 mg (3-Month SR) was characterized in 23 orchiectomized prostate cancer patients. Following a single injection of the three month formulation of LUPRON DEPOT 22.5 mg (3-Month SR), a mean peak plasma leuprolide concentration of 48.9 ng/mL was observed at 4 hours and then declined to 0.67 ng/mL at 12 weeks. Leuprolide appeared to be released at a constant rate following the onset of steady state level during the third week after dosing, providing steady plasma concentrations through the 12-week dosing interval. Detectable levels of leuprolide were present at all measurement points in all patients during this 12-week period. The initial burst, followed by the rapid decline to a steady-state level, was similar to the release pattern seen with the monthly formulation.

Following a single injection of LUPRON DEPOT 30.0 mg (4-Month SR) in sixteen orchiectomized prostate cancer patients, a mean plasma leuprolide concentration of 59.3 ng/mL was observed at 4 hours and the mean concentration then declined to 0.30 ng/mL at 16 weeks. The mean plasma concentration of leuprolide from weeks 3.5 to 16 was 0.44±0.20 ng/mL (range: 0.20 to 1.06). Leuprolide appeared to be released at a constant rate following the onset of steady-state levels during the fourth week after dosing, providing steady plasma concentrations throughout the 16-week dosing interval. However, intact leuprolide and an inactive major metabolite could not be distinguished by the assay which was employed in the study. The initial burst, followed by the rapid decline to a steady-state level, was similar to the release pattern seen with the other depot formulations.

In adults, bioavailability by subcutaneous administration is comparable to that by intravenous administration. Leuprolide acetate has a plasma half-life of 2.9 hours.

Distribution: The mean steady-state volume of distribution of leuprolide following intravenous bolus administration to healthy male volunteers was 27 L. In vitro binding to human plasma proteins ranged from 43 to 49%.

Metabolism: In healthy male volunteers, a 1 mg bolus of leuprolide acetate administered intravenously revealed that the mean systemic clearance was 7.6 L/h, with a terminal elimination half-life of approximately 3 hours based on a two compartment model.

In rats and dogs, administration of ^{14}C-labelled leuprolide was shown to be metabolized to smaller inactive peptides, pentapeptide (Metabolite I), tripeptides (Metabolites II and III) and dipeptide (Metabolite IV). These fragments may be further catabolized.

The major metabolite (M-I) plasma concentrations measured in 5 prostate cancer patients reached mean maximum concentration 2 to 6 hours after dosing and were approximately 6% of the peak parent drug concentration. One week after dosing, mean plasma M-I concentrations were approximately 20% of leuprolide concentrations.

Excretion: Following administration of LUPRON DEPOT 3.75 mg (1-Month SR) to 3 patients, less than 5% of the dose was recovered as parent and M-I metabolite in the urine.

Special Populations and Conditions: Pediatrics: A pharmacokinetic study of leuprolide acetate in children has not been performed.

Geriatrics: See Warnings and Precautions, Special Populations, Geriatrics (>65 years of age).

Hepatic Insufficiency: The pharmacokinetics of the drug in patients with hepatic impairment have not been determined.

Renal Insufficiency: The pharmacokinetics of the drug in patients with renal impairment have not been determined.

STORAGE AND STABILITY: LUPRON: Store LUPRON (leuprolide acetate injection) 5 mg/mL between 2 and 8°C.

LUPRON DEPOT: Store LUPRON DEPOT (leuprolide acetate for depot suspension) 7.5 mg (1-Month SR), 22.5 mg (3-Month SR), and 30.0 mg (4-Month SR) between 15 and 25°C. Protect from freezing.

Although the suspension has been shown to be stable for 24 hours following reconstitution, since the product does not contain a preservative, the suspension should be discarded if not used immediately.

SPECIAL HANDLING INSTRUCTIONS: It is very important to activate the LuproLoc safety device immediately after injection. This is done by pushing the arrow forward with the thumb or finger until the device is fully extended and a **click** is heard or felt. See Dosage and Administration, Administration, Reconstitution.

INFORMATION FOR THE PATIENT: Published in e-CPS, available by subscription at www.e-cps.ca.

DOSAGE FORMS, COMPOSITION AND PACKAGING: LUPRON: Each mL contains: leuprolide acetate 5 mg. Nonmedicinal ingredients: benzyl alcohol, sodium chloride and sterile water for injection, USP. The pH may have been adjusted with sodium hydroxide and/or acetic acid. Sterile multiple dose vials of 2.8 mL for subcutaneous use supplied as 14-day kit. Each 14-day patient administration kit contains: 1 vial of Lupron, 28 swabs, 14 syringes, and one Patient Information/Instructions for Use leaflet.

LUPRON DEPOT: 7.5 mg (1-Month SR): Each prefilled dual-chamber syringe contains: sterile lyophilized microspheres composed of leuprolide acetate incorporated in a biodegradable copolymer of lactic and glycolic acids. The front chamber contains: leuprolide acetate 7.5 mg. Nonmedicinal ingredients: DL-lactic and glycolic acids copolymer, D-mannitol and purified gelatin. The rear chamber of diluent contains the following nonmedicinal ingredients: carboxymethylcellulose sodium, D-mannitol, glacial acetic acid, USP to control pH, polysorbate 80 and water for injection, USP. When mixed with diluent, the sterile lyophilized microspheres become a suspension, which is intended as an intramuscular injection to be given **once every month**. Supplied in single-dose kits containing 1 prefilled dual-chamber syringe with 23 G needle, 2 alcohol swabs, Patient Information Leaflet, Special Instructions for Use and Package Insert.

During the manufacturing process of LUPRON DEPOT (1-Month SR), acetic acid is lost, leaving the leuprolide peptide.

22.5 mg (3-Month SR): Each prefilled dual-chamber syringe contains: sterile lyophilized microspheres composed of leuprolide acetate incorporated in a biodegradable polymer of polylactic acid. The front chamber contains: leuprolide acetate 22.5 mg. Nonmedicinal ingredients: D-mannitol and polylactic acid. The rear chamber of diluent contains the following nonmedicinal ingredients: carboxymethylcellulose sodium, D-mannitol, glacial acetic acid, USP to control pH, polysorbate 80 and water for injection, USP. When mixed with diluent, the sterile lyophilized microspheres become a suspension, which is intended as an intramuscular injection to be given **once every 3 months**. Supplied in single-dose kits containing 1 prefilled dual-chamber syringe with 23 G needle, 2 alcohol swabs, Patient Information Leaflet, Special Instructions for Use and Package Insert.

During the manufacturing process of LUPRON DEPOT (3-Month SR), acetic acid is lost, leaving the leuprolide peptide.

30 mg (4-Month SR): Each prefilled dual-chamber syringe contains: sterile lyophilized microspheres composed of leuprolide acetate incorporated in a biodegradable polymer of polylactic acid. The front chamber contains: leuprolide acetate 30 mg. Nonmedicinal ingredients: D-mannitol and polylactic acid. The rear chamber of diluent contains following nonmedicinal ingredients: carboxymethylcellulose sodium, D-mannitol, glacial acetic acid, USP to control pH, polysorbate 80 and water for injection, USP. When mixed with diluent, the sterile lyophilized microspheres become a suspension, which is intended as an intramuscular injection to be given **once every 4 months**. Supplied in single-dose kits containing 1 prefilled dual-chamber syringe with 23 G needle, 2 alcohol swabs, Patient Information Leaflet, Special Instructions for Use and Package Insert.

During the manufacturing process of LUPRON DEPOT (4-Month SR), acetic acid is lost, leaving the leuprolide peptide.

Lupron Depot® 3.75 mg/11.25 mg ℞

leuprolide acetate

Gonadotropin-releasing Hormone Analog

Abbott

Date of Preparation: March 11, 1999
Date of Revision: March 23, 2010

SUMMARY PRODUCT INFORMATION:

Route of Administration	Dosage Form/ Strength	Clinically Relevant Nonmedicinal Ingredients
Intramuscular	Prefilled dual chamber syringe containing sterile lyophilized microspheres/3.75 mg (1-month slow release)	Carboxymethylcellulose sodium, DL-lactic and glycolic acids copolymer, D-mannitol, gelatin, glacial acetic acid, polysorbate 80
	Prefilled dual chamber syringe containing sterile lyophilized microspheres/11.25 mg (3-month slow release)	Carboxymethylcellulose sodium, D-mannitol, glacial acetic acid, polylactic acid, polysorbate 80 For a complete listing see Dosage Forms, Composition and Packaging.

INDICATIONS AND CLINICAL USE: Both LUPRON DEPOT (leuprolide acetate for depot suspension) 3.75 mg (1-Month SR) and 11.25 mg (3-Month SR) are indicated for:

- the treatment of endometriosis, including pain relief and reduction of endometriosis lesions, for a period of six months.

LUPRON DEPOT can be used as sole therapy where it may provide symptomatic relief for women close to menopause who do not desire surgery, or as an adjunct to surgery.

Experience with LUPRON DEPOT for the management of endometriosis has been limited to women 18 years of age and older.

LUPRON DEPOT must be administered under the supervision of a physician.

Geriatrics (>65 years of age): LUPRON DEPOT 3.75 mg (1-Month SR) and 11.25 mg (3-Month SR) are not indicated for women over 65 years of age.

Pediatrics (<18 years of age): LUPRON DEPOT 11.25 mg (3-Month SR) is not indicated for pediatric use. LUPRON DEPOT treatment of children is covered in the LUPRON DEPOT 3.75 mg and 7.5 mg, "Central Precocious Puberty" Product Monograph.

CONTRAINDICATIONS:

- LUPRON DEPOT (leuprolide acetate for depot suspension) is contraindicated in patients with hypersensitivity to the drug or its components or similar nonapeptides or components of the container. Isolated cases of anaphylaxis have been reported. For a complete listing, see Dosage Forms, Composition and Packaging.
- LUPRON DEPOT is contraindicated in women who are or may become pregnant. When administered on day 6 of pregnancy at test dosages of 0.00024, 0.0024, and 0.024 mg/kg (1/300 to 1/3 the 3.75 mg LUPRON DEPOT human dose) to rabbits, LUPRON DEPOT produced a dose-related increase in major fetal abnormalities. Similar studies in rats failed to demonstrate an increase in fetal malformations. There was increased fetal mortality and decreased fetal weights with the two higher doses of LUPRON DEPOT in rabbits and with the highest dose (0.024 mg/kg) in rats. The effects on fetal mortality are logical consequences of the alterations in hormonal levels brought about by this drug. Therefore, the possibility exists that spontaneous abortion may occur if the drug is administered during pregnancy.

  Patients treated with LUPRON DEPOT should use nonhormonal methods of contraception.
- LUPRON DEPOT is also contraindicated in patients with undiagnosed abnormal vaginal bleeding.
- It is not known whether leuprolide is excreted in human milk; therefore, LUPRON DEPOT is contraindicated in patients who are breast-feeding.

WARNINGS AND PRECAUTIONS: General: Postmarketing reports of convulsions have been observed in patients on leuprolide acetate therapy. These included patients in the female and pediatric populations, patients with a history of seizures, epilepsy, cerebrovascular disorders, central nervous system anomalies or tumors, and in patients on concomitant medications that have been associated with convulsions such as bupropion and SSRIs. Convulsions have also been reported in patients in the absence of any of the conditions mentioned above.

Isolated cases of short-term worsening of signs and symptoms have been reported during initiation of leuprolide therapy. They are sometimes, but not necessarily, associated with a stimulation of the pituitary gland and an initial increase in the levels of circulating gonadal hormones.

During the early phase of therapy, sex steroids temporarily rise above baseline because of the physiologic effect of the drug. Therefore, an increase in clinical signs and symptoms may be observed during the initial days of therapy, but these will dissipate with continued therapy at adequate doses.

Worsening of the clinical condition may occasionally require discontinuation of therapy and/or surgical intervention.

Before initiating treatment with LUPRON DEPOT (leuprolide acetate for depot suspension), pregnancy must be ruled out (see Warnings and Precautions, Special Populations, Pregnant Women).

Patients on leuprolide therapy should be assessed on a regular basis by their attending physician.

Carcinogenesis and Mutagenesis: Two-year carcinogenicity studies were conducted in rats and mice. In rats, a dose-related increase of benign pituitary hyperplasia and benign adenomas was noted at 24 months when the drug was administered subcutaneously at high daily doses (0.6 to 4 mg/kg). There was a significant but not dose-related increase of pancreatic islet-cell adenomas in females and of testicular interstitial cell adenomas in males (highest incidence in the low dose group). In mice no pituitary abnormalities were observed at a dose as high as 60 mg/kg for two years.

Patients have been treated with leuprolide acetate for up to three years with doses as high as 10 mg/day and for two years with doses as high as 20 mg/day without demonstrable pituitary abnormalities.

Mutagenicity studies have been performed with leuprolide acetate using bacterial and mammalian systems. These studies provided no evidence of a mutagenic potential.

Dependence/Tolerance: No drug-dependence has been reported with the use of leuprolide.

Endocrine and Metabolism: Changes in Bone Density: Since bone loss can be anticipated as part of natural menopause, it may also be expected to occur during the medically induced hypoestrogenic state caused by the long-term use of LUPRON DEPOT. For a period of up to six months, this bone loss should not be important.

In patients with significant risk factors for decreased bone mineral content and/or bone mass such as family history of osteoporosis, chronic use of corticosteroids or anticonvulsants or chronic abuse of alcohol or tobacco, leuprolide may pose additional risk. In these patients, risk versus benefit must be weighed carefully before initiation of leuprolide therapy.

Re-treatment cannot be recommended since safety data for re-treatment are not available. If the symptoms of endometriosis recur after a course of therapy, and further treatment with LUPRON DEPOT is contemplated, it is recommended that bone density be assessed before re-treatment begins to ensure that values are within normal limits.

A controlled study in endometriosis patients showed that vertebral bone density, as measured by dual energy X-ray absorptiometry (DEXA), decreased by an average of 4.1% at six months compared with the pretreatment value.

For those patients who were tested at six or twelve months after discontinuation of therapy, the mean bone density returned to −2.6% of pretreatment.

Earlier studies in endometriosis patients, utilizing quantitative computed tomography (QCT), demonstrated that in the few patients who were retested at six and twelve months, partial to complete recovery of bone density was recorded in the posttreatment period. Use of LUPRON DEPOT for longer than six months or in the presence of other known risk factors for decreased bone mineral content may cause additional bone loss.

The safety of re-treatment as well as treatment beyond 6 months with LUPRON DEPOT has not been established.

Adverse events occurring in clinical studies with LUPRON DEPOT that are associated with hypoestrogenism include hot flashes, headaches, emotional lability, decreased libido, acne, myalgia, reduction in breast size, and vaginal dryness. Estrogen levels returned to normal after treatment was discontinued.

Hepatic/Biliary/Pancreatic: The pharmacokinetics of the drug in patients with hepatic, biliary or pancreatic impairment have not been determined.

Renal: The pharmacokinetics of the drug in patients with renal impairment have not been determined.

Special Populations: Pregnant Women: Safe use of the drug in pregnancy has not been established; therefore, a nonhormonal method of contraception should be used during treatment. Patients should be advised that if they miss or postpone a dose of LUPRON DEPOT, ovulation may occur with the potential for conception. If a patient becomes pregnant during treatment, she should discontinue treatment and consult her physician.

Since menstruation should stop with effective doses of LUPRON DEPOT, the patient should notify her physician if regular menstruation persists. Patients missing successive doses of LUPRON DEPOT may experience breakthrough bleeding.

Before initiating treatment with LUPRON DEPOT, pregnancy must be ruled out.

Nursing Women: It is not known whether leuprolide is excreted in human milk; therefore, LUPRON DEPOT is contraindicated in patients who are breast-feeding.

Pediatrics (<18 years of age): Safety and effectiveness of LUPRON DEPOT 11.25 mg (3-Month SR) have not been established in pediatric patients. Refer to the "Central Precocious Puberty" Product Monograph for the safety and effectiveness of LUPRON DEPOT 3.75 mg (1-Month SR) in children with central precocious puberty.

Geriatrics (>65 years of age): LUPRON DEPOT 3.75 mg (1-Month SR) and 11.25 mg (3-Month SR) have not been studied in women over 65 years of age and are not indicated in this population.

Monitoring and Laboratory Tests: Changes in Laboratory Values During Treatment: Plasma Enzymes: During clinical trials with LUPRON DEPOT, regular laboratory monitoring revealed that AST levels were more than twice the upper limit of normal in only one patient. There was no other clinical or laboratory evidence of abnormal liver function.

Hematology: Slight decreases in hemoglobin and hematocrit values to below normal were noted with receipt of LUPRON DEPOT 11.25 mg (3-Month SR), but none were considered clinically significant.

Lipids: At enrollment, 4% of LUPRON DEPOT 3.75 mg (1-Month SR) patients and 1% of the danazol patients had total cholesterol values above the normal range. These patients also had cholesterol values above the normal range at the end of treatment. Of those patients whose pretreatment cholesterol values were in the normal range, 7% of the LUPRON DEPOT patients and 9% of the danazol patients had posttreatment values above the normal range.

The mean (± SEM) pretreatment values for total cholesterol from all patients were 4.63 (0.08) mmol/L in the LUPRON DEPOT 3.75 mg (1-Month SR) group and 4.54 (0.08) mmol/L in the danazol group. At the end of treatment, the mean values for total cholesterol from all patients were 5.01 mmol/L in the LUPRON DEPOT group and 5.03 mmol/L in the danazol group. These increases from the pretreatment values were statistically significant ($p<0.03$) in both groups.

Triglycerides were increased above the upper limit of normal in 12% of the patients who received LUPRON DEPOT 3.75 mg (1-Month SR) and in 6% of the patients who received danazol.

At the end of treatment, HDL cholesterol fractions decreased below the lower limit of the normal range in 2% of the LUPRON DEPOT 3.75 mg (1-Month SR) patients compared with 54% of those receiving danazol. LDL cholesterol fractions increased above the upper limit of the normal range in 6% of the patients receiving LUPRON DEPOT 3.75 mg (1-Month SR) compared with 23% of those receiving danazol. There was no increase in the LDL/HDL ratio in patients receiving LUPRON DEPOT 3.75 mg (1-Month SR), but there was approximately a two-fold increase in the LDL/HDL ratio in patients receiving danazol. The clinical implication of these changes in this patient population for a restricted therapeutic period is unclear.

Isolated elevations of AST were observed in leuprolide acetate- and danazol-treated patients.

In subjects receiving LUPRON DEPOT 11.25 mg (3-Month SR), triglycerides were slightly elevated (range 142- to 210 mg/dL) in 32% of the subjects who had demonstrated normal baseline values.

Other Changes: In comparative studies, the following changes were seen in approximately 5 to 8% of patients. LUPRON DEPOT was associated with elevations of LDH and phosphorus, and decreases in WBC counts, and danazol therapy was associated with increases in hematocrit, platelet count, and LDH.

ADVERSE REACTIONS: Adverse Drug Reaction Overview: Estradiol levels may increase during the first weeks following the initial injection, but then decline to basal levels. This transient increase in estradiol can be associated with a temporary worsening of signs and symptoms. See Warnings and Precautions.

Clinical Trial Adverse Drug Reactions: Because clinical trials are conducted under very specific conditions the adverse reaction rates observed in the clinical trials may not reflect the rates observed in practice and should not be compared to the rates in the clinical trials of another drug. Adverse drug reaction information from clinical trials is useful for identifying drug-related adverse events and for approximating rates.

LUPRON DEPOT 3.75 mg (1-Month SR): In two controlled clinical trials treating endometriosis, one comparing LUPRON DEPOT 3.75 mg (1-Month SR) with danazol (800 mg/day) and the other with placebo, the following adverse reactions were reported to have a possible or probable relationship to study drugs as ascribed by the treating physician in 5% or more of the patients receiving the drug (Table 1).

Table 1: LUPRON DEPOT 3.75 mg (1-Month SR)

Adverse Reactions Reported Having a Possible or Probable Relationship to Study Drugs in 5% or More of Patients Receiving LUPRON DEPOT 3.75 mg (1-Month SR) versus Danazol (800 mg/day) and LUPRON DEPOT 3.75 mg (1-Month SR) versus Placebo

	LUPRON DEPOT 3.75 mg (1-Month SR) N=166 (%)	Danazol 800 mg/day N=136 (%)	Placebo N=31 (%)
	Number of Reports (%)		
Cardiovascular System			
Edema	12 (7)	17 (13)	1 (3)
Gastrointestinal System			
Nausea/vomiting	21 (13)	17 (13)	1 (3)
Gastrointestinal disturbances[a]	11 (7)	8 (6)	1 (3)

(cont'd)

Table 1: LUPRON DEPOT 3.75 mg (1-Month SR) *(cont'd)*

Adverse Reactions Reported Having a Possible or Probable Relationship to Study Drugs in 5% or More of Patients Receiving LUPRON DEPOT 3.75 mg (1-Month SR) versus Danazol (800 mg/day) and LUPRON DEPOT 3.75 mg (1-Month SR) versus Placebo

	LUPRON DEPOT 3.75 mg (1-Month SR) N=166 (%)	Danazol 800 mg/day N=136 (%)	Placebo N=31 (%)
		Number of Reports (%)	
Endocrine System			
Hot flashes/sweats[a]	139 (84)	77 (57)	9 (29)
Breast changes, tenderness/pain[a]	10 (6)	12 (9)	0 (0)
Decreased libido[a]	19 (11)	6 (4)	0 (0)
Androgen-like effects	22 (13)	44 (32)[b]	1 (3)
virilism	0 (0)	1 (1)	0 (0)
acne	17 (10)	27 (20)	0 (0)
seborrhea	2 (1)	5 (4)	0 (0)
hirsutism	2 (1)	9 (7)	1 (3)
voice alteration	1 (1)	2 (1)	0 (0)
Musculoskeletal System			
Myalgia[a]	1 (1)	7 (5)	0 (0)
Joint disorder[a]	14 (8)	11 (8)	0 (0)
Central/Peripheral Nervous Systems			
Depression/emotional lability[a]	36 (22)	27 (20)	1 (3)
Headaches[a]	53 (32)	30 (22)	2 (6)
Dizziness	19 (11)	4 (3)	0 (0)
Insomnia/sleep disorders[a]	2 (1)	4 (3)	0 (0)
General pain	31 (19)	22 (16)	1 (3)
Neuromuscular disorders[a]	11 (7)	17 (13)	0 (0)
Nervousness[a]	8 (5)	11 (8)	0 (0)
Paresthesias	12 (7)	11 (8)	0 (0)
Integumentary System			
Skin reactions	17 (10)	20 (15)	1 (3)
Urogenital System			
Vaginitis[a]	46 (28)	23 (17)	0 (0)
Miscellaneous			
Asthenia	5 (3)	9 (7)	0 (0)
Weight gain/loss	22 (13)	36 (26)	0 (0)

[a] Physiologic effect of decreased estrogen.
[b] Individual percentages equal 33% due to rounding.
Reactions considered not drug related are excluded.

LUPRON DEPOT 11.25 mg (3-Month SR): In a pharmacokinetic trial involving 20 healthy female subjects receiving LUPRON DEPOT 11.25 mg (3-Month SR), a few adverse events were reported with this formulation that were not reported previously. These included face edema, agitation, laryngitis and ear pain, and are noted in Table 2.

Table 2: LUPRON DEPOT 11.25 mg (3-Month SR)

Adverse Events Reported by 20 Healthy Female Subjects Receiving LUPRON DEPOT 11.25 mg (3-Month SR) in a Pharmacokinetic Trial

	LUPRON DEPOT 11.25 mg (3-Month SR) N=20 (%)
Body as a Whole	
Asthenia	1 (5.0)
Face edema	1 (5.0)
General pain	4 (20.0)
Headache/migraine[a]	16 (80.0)
Cardiovascular System	
Hot flashes/sweats[a]	13 (65.0)

[*] Physiologic effect of decreased estrogen.

(cont'd)

Table 2: LUPRON DEPOT 11.25 mg (3-Month SR) *(cont'd)*

Adverse Events Reported by 20 Healthy Female Subjects Receiving LUPRON DEPOT 11.25 mg (3-Month SR) in a Pharmacokinetic Trial

	LUPRON DEPOT 11.25 mg (3-Month SR) N=20 (%)
Digestive System	
Gastrointestinal disturbance[a]	2 (10.0)
Liver function test abnormal	1 (5.0)
Nausea/vomiting	2 (10.0)
Metabolic and Nutritional Disorders	
Edema	1 (5.0)
Musculoskeletal System	
Myalgia[a]	2 (10.0)
Nervous System	
Agitation	1 (5.0)
Depression/emotional lability[a]	1 (5.0)
Dizziness/vertigo	1 (5.0)
Insomnia/sleep disorders[a]	2 (10.0)
Neuromuscular disorders[a]	1 (5.0)
Respiratory System	
Laryngitis	1 (5.0)
Special Senses	
Ear pain	1 (5.0)
Urogenital System	
Dysmenorrhea	1 (5.0)

[a] Physiologic effect of the drug.

Less Common Clinical Trial Adverse Drug Reactions (<5%): LUPRON DEPOT 3.75 mg (1-Month SR) : The following were reported in less than 5% of patients receiving LUPRON DEPOT:
Body as a Whole: body odor, flu syndrome and injection site reactions.
Cardiovascular System: palpitations, syncope and tachycardia.
Central/Peripheral Nervous Systems: anxiety*, delusions, insomnia/sleep disorders*, memory disorder and personality disorder.
Gastrointestinal System: appetite changes, dry mouth and thirst.
Endocrine System: androgen-like effects.
Hemic and Lymphatic Systems: ecchymosis and lymphadenopathy.
Respiratory System: rhinitis.
Skin and Appendages: alopecia, hair disorder and nail disorder.
Special Senses: conjunctivitis, ophthalmologic disorders* and taste perversion.
Urogenital System: dysuria*, lactation and menstrual disorders.
Abnormal Hematologic and Clinical Chemistry Findings: See Warning and Precautions, Monitoring and Laboratory Tests.
Post-Market Adverse Drug Reactions: Isolated cases of anaphylaxis have been reported. Symptoms consistent with an anaphylactoid or asthmatic process have been rarely reported.

Like other drugs in this class, mood swings, including depression, have been reported as a physiologic effect of decreased sex steroids. There have been very rare reports of suicidal ideation and attempt. Many, but not all, of these patients had a history of depression or other psychiatric illness. Patients should be counselled on the possibility of worsening of depression.

Pituitary Apoplexy: During post-marketing surveillance, rare cases of pituitary apoplexy (a clinical syndrome secondary to infarction of the pituitary gland) have been reported after the administration of gonadotropin-releasing hormone agonists. In a majority of these cases, a pituitary adenoma was diagnosed, with a majority of pituitary apoplexy cases occurring within 2 weeks of the first dose, and some within the first hour. In these cases, pituitary apoplexy has presented as sudden headache, vomiting, visual changes, ophthalmoplegia, altered mental status, and sometimes cardiovascular collapse. Immediate medical attention has been required.

Symptoms consistent with fibromyalgia (e.g., joint and muscle pain, headaches, sleep disorders, gastrointestinal distress, and shortness of breath) have been reported individually and collectively. The relationship of any of these symptoms to leuprolide acetate has not been established.

The following events have been reported during post-marketing surveillance:
Cardiovascular System: hypotension and pulmonary embolism.
Central/Peripheral Nervous Systems: convulsion, peripheral neuropathy and spinal fracture/paralysis.
Gastrointestinal System: hepatic dysfunction.
Hemic and Lymphatic Systems: decreased WBC.
Integumentary System: photosensitivity reactions, rash and urticaria.
Miscellaneous: hematoma, induration, inflammation, injection site reactions including pain and sterile abscess.
Musculoskeletal System: tenosynovitis-like symptoms.
Respiratory System: dyspnea.
Urogenital System: menstrual disorders.

Refer to the "Prostatic Cancer" and "Central Precocious Puberty" LUPRON and LUPRON DEPOT Product Monographs for other reported events.

DRUG INTERACTIONS: Overview: Leuprolide being approximately 46% bound to plasma proteins, and a peptide that is primarily degraded by peptidase and not by cytochrome P-450 enzymes as noted in specific studies, drug interactions would not be expected to occur.
Drug-Drug Interactions: No pharmacokinetic-based drug-drug interaction studies have been conducted.
Drug-Food Interactions: Interactions with food have not been established.
Drug-Herb Interactions: Interactions with herbal products have not been established.
Drug-Laboratory Test Interactions: Administration of LUPRON DEPOT at therapeutic doses results in suppression of the pituitary-gonadal system. Normal function is usually restored within 4 to 12 weeks after the treatment is discontinued. Diagnostic tests of pituitary-gonadal function conducted during the treatment and within 4 to 8 weeks after discontinuation of LUPRON DEPOT therapy may therefore be misleading.

DOSAGE AND ADMINISTRATION: Dosing Considerations: LUPRON DEPOT must be administered under the supervision of a physician.

LUPRON DEPOT 3.75 and 11.25 mg administered intramuscularly is designed to provide continuous sustained release of leuprolide for 1 and 3 months, respectively.

Note: As with all parenteral products, inspect container's solution for discoloration and particulate matter before each use.

Recommended Dose and Dosage Adjustment: LUPRON DEPOT (leuprolide acetate for depot suspension) must be administered under the supervision of a physician. See Table 3.

Table 3: LUPRON DEPOT 3.75 mg (1-Month SR)/11.25 mg (3-Month SR) Dosage

LUPRON DEPOT 3.75 mg (1-Month SR)	LUPRON DEPOT 11.25 mg (3-Month SR)
3.75 mg for 6 months (6 monthly injections)	11.25 mg for 6 months (1 injection every 3 months)

LUPRON DEPOT 3.75 mg (1-Month SR): The recommended dose of LUPRON DEPOT (1-Month SR) is 3.75 mg administered **monthly** as a **single intramuscular injection**, after reconstitution with the special diluent. See Dosage and Administration and Information for the Patient. The treatment course is for six months.

LUPRON DEPOT 11.25 mg (3-Month SR): The recommended dose of LUPRON DEPOT (3-Month SR) is 11.25 mg administered as a **single intramuscular injection once every three months**, after reconstitution with the special diluent. See Dosage and Administration and Information for the Patient.

Due to different release characteristics, a fractional dose of the 3-month depot formulation is not equivalent to the same dose of the monthly formulation and should therefore not be given.

Retreatment cannot be recommended since safety data for re-treatment are not available. If the symptoms of endometriosis recur after a course of therapy, and further treatment with either LUPRON DEPOT 3.75 mg (1-Month SR) or LUPRON DEPOT 11.25 mg (3-Month SR) is contemplated, it is recommended that bone density be assessed before re-treatment begins to ensure that values are within normal limits.

Missed Dose: Missing an appointment by a few days should not disrupt the benefits of treatment, but keeping a consistent schedule of LUPRON DEPOT injections is an important part of treatment.

Reconstitution: Parenteral Products: The lyophilized microspheres contained in the front chamber of the prefilled dual-chamber syringe are to be reconstituted prior to intramuscular injection, in accord with the following directions:

Due to different release characteristics, a fractional dose of the 3-month depot formulation is not equivalent to the same dose of the monthly formulation and should not be given.

For LUPRON DEPOT 3.75 mg (1-Month SR) and 11.25 mg (3-Month SR):

1. The LUPRON DEPOT powder should be visually inspected and the syringe should **not be used** if clumping or caking is evident. A thin layer of powder on the wall of the syringe is considered normal. The diluent should appear clear.
2. To prepare for injection, screw the white plunger into the end stopper until the stopper begins to turn.
3. Remember to tighten the needle by twisting the needle cap clockwise. Do not overtighten.
4. Holding the syringe upright, release the diluent by **slowly pushing** (6- to 8 seconds) the plunger until the first stopper is at the **blue line** in the middle of the barrel.
5. Keep the syringe upright. Gently shake the syringe to thoroughly mix the microspheres (powder) to form a uniform suspension. The suspension will appear milky.
6. If the microspheres adhere to the stopper or caking/clumping is present, tap the syringe against your finger to disperse. **Do not use** if any of the powder has not gone into suspension.
7. Keep the syringe upright. With the opposite hand, remove the needle cap without twisting and advance the plunger to expel the air from the syringe.
8. At the time of reconstitution, inject the entire contents of the syringe intramuscularly. The suspension settles very quickly following reconstitution; therefore, LUPRON DEPOT should be mixed and used immediately.
   Note: Aspirated blood would be visible just below the luer lock connection if a blood vessel is accidentally penetrated. If present, blood can be seen through the transparent LuproLoc safety device.
9. After injection, withdraw the needle. Immediately activate the LuproLoc safety device by pushing the arrow forward with the thumb or finger until the device is fully extended and a CLICK is heard or felt.

Although the suspension has been shown to be stable for 24 hours following reconstitution, since the product does not contain a preservative, the suspension should be discarded if not used immediately.

As with other drugs administered by injection, the injection site should be varied periodically.

OVERDOSAGE:

In rats, subcutaneous administration of 250 to 500 times the recommended human dose, expressed on a per body weight basis, resulted in dyspnea, decreased activity, and local irritation at the injection site. There is no evidence at present that there is a clinical counterpart of this phenomenon.

In early clinical trials using daily subcutaneous leuprolide acetate in patients with prostate cancer, doses as high as 20 mg/day for up to two years caused no adverse effects differing from those observed with the 1 mg/day dose.

For management of a suspected drug overdose, contact your regional Poison Control Centre. See the *CPS* Directory section for a list of Poison Control Centres.

ACTION AND CLINICAL PHARMACOLOGY: Mechanism of Action: Leuprolide is a synthetic nonapeptide analog of naturally-occurring gonadotropin-releasing hormone (GnRH or LHRH). The analog possesses greater potency than the natural hormone. When administered as indicated, leuprolide acts as a potent inhibitor of gonadotropin production. It is chemically unrelated to steroids.

Unlike steroid hormones, leuprolide exerts specific action on the pituitary gonadotrophs and the human reproductive tract.

This specificity reduces the likelihood of secondary adverse effects such as gynecomastia, thromboembolism, edema, liver and gallbladder involvement.

Pharmacodynamics: General: Animal and human studies indicate that, following an initial stimulation, chronic administration of leuprolide acetate results in the inhibition of gonadotropin production. Consequently, ovarian or testicular steroidogenesis is suppressed. The therapeutic effect of leuprolide in the treatment of hormone-dependent tumors, such as in prostatic cancer, results from the reduction in serum gonadotropins and gonadal steroids.

Chronic administration of leuprolide acetate has resulted in inhibition of tumor growth (prostatic tumors in Noble and Dunning male rats, 7-12-dimethylbenz[α]-anthracene(DMBA)-induced mammary tumors in female rats) as well as atrophy of the reproductive organs. An additional mechanism of action, a direct effect on the gonads by down-regulation of the gonadotropin receptors, is suggested in some animal studies.

In humans, subcutaneous administration of single daily doses of leuprolide acetate results in an initial increase in circulating levels of luteinizing hormone (LH) and follicle-stimulating hormone (FSH), leading to a transient increase in the levels of the gonadal steroids (testosterone and dihydrotestosterone in males and estrone and estradiol in pre-menopausal females). However, continuous administration results in decreased levels of LH and FSH in all patients. In males, testosterone is reduced to castrate levels. In pre-menopausal females, estrogens are reduced to post-menopausal levels. These decreases occur within two to four weeks after initiation of treatment, and are maintained as long as treatment continues.

Endometriosis: Endometriosis is a gynecologic disorder wherein endometrial tissue is found to be established in sites outside the endometrial cavity. As definitive diagnosis can only be made during surgery, the true incidence of the disease is unknown.

The etiology of the disease is unclear. An accepted theory of the etiology of endometriosis is the retrograde flow of menstrual fluid with subsequent implantation of viable fragments of endometrium within the pelvic cavity (Sampson's theory). However, this theory does not explain the extra-pelvic sites of endometriosis such as the limbs, thoracic cavity and elsewhere. It has also been suggested that chronic irritation of the peritoneum by menstrual blood may be causative. Another theory is that endometrial tissues are displaced into an implant in new sites during surgery. Genetic and immunologic factors may account for spontaneous endometriosis in a small segment of the population. It is also believed that endometriosis may be caused by lymphatic and hematogenous spread of normal endometrium to distant sites.

Endometriosis may be treated both surgically and medically. Since endometriosis resolves after oophorectomy and menopause, surgical castration may be used to treat the disease. A menopausal state may also be achieved medically. The resultant hypoestrogenic environment results in atrophic changes in both the uterine and ectopic endometrial tissue.

LUPRON DEPOT (leuprolide acetate for depot suspension) achieves a menopausal state by suppression of the pituitary-ovarian axis by inhibiting the output of gonadotropins (FSH and LH) from the pituitary gland.

In female volunteers receiving a single dose of LUPRON DEPOT 3.75 mg (1-Month SR) intramuscularly, an initial burst of leuprolide in plasma was observed. Mean plasma leuprolide levels of approximately 0.23 to 0.34 ng/mL were maintained over a period of four to five weeks, and then slowly tapered off, becoming undetectable eight weeks after injection.

In a pharmacokinetic/pharmacodynamic study of healthy female subjects (N=20), the onset of estradiol suppression was observed for individual subjects between Day 4 and week 4 after dosing. By the third week following the injection, the mean estradiol concentration (8 pg/mL) reached the menopausal range. Throughout the remainder of the dosing period, mean serum estradiol levels ranged from the menopausal to the early follicular range.

LUPRON DEPOT 11.25 mg (3-Month SR) induced amenorrhea in 85% (N=17) of subjects during the initial month and 100% during the second month following the injection. All subjects remained amenorrheic through the remainder of the 12-week dosing interval. Episodes of light bleeding and spotting were reported by a majority of subjects during the first month after the injection and in a few subjects at later time-points. Menses resumed on average 12 weeks (range 2.9 to 20.4 weeks) following the end of the 12-week dosing interval.

LUPRON DEPOT 11.25 mg (3-Month SR) produced similar pharmacodynamic effects in terms of hormonal and menstrual suppression to those achieved with monthly injections of LUPRON DEPOT 3.75 mg (1-Month SR) during the controlled clinical trials for the management of endometriosis. Similar clinical outcome to that with LUPRON DEPOT 3.75 mg (1-Month SR) administered monthly is predicted with LUPRON DEPOT 11.25 mg (3-Month SR) administered every 3 months.

Pharmacokinetics: Intramuscular injections of LUPRON DEPOT 3.75 mg (1-Month SR) and 11.25 mg (3-Month SR) provide effective plasma concentrations of leuprolide acetate over a period of one and three months, respectively.

Leuprolide acetate is not active when given orally.

Absorption: A single dose of LUPRON DEPOT 3.75 mg (1-Month SR) was administered by intramuscular injection to healthy female volunteers. The absorption of leuprolide was characterized by an initial increase in plasma concentration, with peak concentration ranging from 4.6 to 10.2 ng/mL at four hours post-dosing. However, intact leuprolide and an inactive metabolite could not be distinguished by the assay used in the study. Following the initial rise, leuprolide concentrations started to plateau within two days after dosing and remained relatively stable for about four to five weeks with plasma concentrations of about 0.30 ng/mL.

Following a single injection of the three-month formulation of LUPRON DEPOT 11.25 mg (3-Month SR) in female subjects, a mean peak plasma leuprolide concentration of 36.3 ng/mL was observed at 4 hours. Leuprolide appeared to be released at a constant rate following the onset of steady-state levels during the third week after dosing and mean levels then declined gradually to near the lower limit of detection by 12 weeks. The mean (±standard deviation) leuprolide acetate concentration from 3 to 12 weeks was 0.23±0.09 ng/mL. However, intact leuprolide and an inactive major metabolite could not be distinguished by the assay which was employed in the study. The initial burst, followed by the rapid decline to a steady-state level, was similar to the release pattern seen with the monthly formulation.

In adults, bioavailability by subcutaneous administration is comparable to that by intravenous administration. Leuprolide has a plasma half-life of 2.9 hours.

Distribution: The mean steady-state volume of distribution of leuprolide following intravenous bolus administration to healthy male volunteers was 27 L. In vitro binding to human plasma proteins ranged from 43 to 49%.

Metabolism: In healthy male volunteers, a 1 mg bolus of leuprolide administered intravenously revealed that the mean systemic clearance was 7.6 L/h, with a terminal elimination half-life of approximately 3 hours based on a two-compartment model.

In rats and dogs, administration of ^{14}C-labelled leuprolide was shown to be metabolized to smaller inactive peptides, pentapeptide (Metabolite I), tripeptides (Metabolites II and III) and dipeptide (Metabolite IV). These fragments may be further catabolized.

The major metabolite (M-I) plasma concentrations measured in 5 prostate cancer patients reached mean maximum concentration 2 to 6 hours after dosing and were approximately 6% of the peak parent drug concentration. One week after dosing, mean plasma M-I concentrations were approximately 20% of leuprolide concentrations.

Excretion: Following administration of LUPRON DEPOT 3.75 mg (1-Month SR) to 3 patients, less than 5% of the dose was recovered as parent and M-I metabolite in the urine.

Special Populations and Conditions: Pediatrics: A pharmacokinetic study of leuprolide acetate in children has not been performed.

Geriatrics: See Warnings and Precautions, Special Populations, Geriatrics (>65 years of age).

Hepatic Insufficiency: The pharmacokinetics of the drug in patients with hepatic impairment have not been determined.

Renal Insufficiency: The pharmacokinetics of the drug in patients with renal impairment have not been determined.

STORAGE AND STABILITY: Store LUPRON DEPOT (leuprolide acetate for depot suspension) between 15 to 25°C. Protect from freezing.

Although the suspension has been shown to be stable for 24 hours following reconstitution, since the product does not contain a preservative, the suspension should be discarded if not used immediately.

SPECIAL HANDLING INSTRUCTIONS: It is very important to activate the LuproLoc safety device immediately after injection. This is done by pushing the arrow forward with the thumb or finger until the device is fully extended and a CLICK is heard or felt. See Dosage and Administration.

INFORMATION FOR THE PATIENT: Published in e-CPS, available by subscription at www.e-cps.ca.

DOSAGE FORMS, COMPOSITION AND PACKAGING: 3.75 mg (1-Month SR): Each prefilled dual-chamber syringe contains: sterile lyophilized microspheres composed of leuprolide acetate incorporated in a biodegradable copolymer of lactic and glycolic acids. The front chamber contains: leuprolide acetate 3.75 mg. Nonmedicinal ingredients: DL-lactic and glycolic acids copolymer, D-mannitol and purified gelatin. The rear chamber of diluent contains: carboxymethylcellulose sodium, D-mannitol, glacial acetic acid (to control pH), polysorbate 80 and water for injection. When mixed with diluent, the sterile lyophilized microspheres become a suspension, which is intended as an intramuscular injection to be given **once every month**. During the manufacturing process of LUPRON DEPOT (1-Month SR), acetic acid is lost, leaving the leuprolide peptide. Single-dose kits containing one prefilled dual-chamber syringe with 23G needle, two alcohol swabs, Consumer Information leaflet, Special Instructions for Use leaflet, and a Health Professional Information insert.

11.25 mg (3-Month Slow Release): Each prefilled dual-chamber syringe contains: sterile lyophilized microspheres composed of leuprolide acetate incorporated in a biodegradable polymer of polylactic acid. The front chamber contains: leuprolide acetate 11.25 mg. Nonmedicinal ingredients: D-mannitol and polylactic acid. The rear chamber of diluent contains: carboxymethylcellulose sodium, D-mannitol, glacial acetic acid (to control pH), polysorbate 80 and water for injection. When mixed with diluent, the sterile lyophilized microspheres become a suspension, which is intended as an intramuscular injection to be given **once every three months**. During the manufacturing process of LUPRON DEPOT (3-Month SR), acetic acid is lost, leaving the leuprolide peptide. Single-dose kits containing one prefilled dual-chamber syringe with 23G needle, two alcohol swabs, Consumer Information leaflet, Special Instructions for Use leaflet, and a Health Professional Information insert.

Lutrepulse™ Ⓟ
gonadorelin acetate
Ovulatory Agent

Ferring

PHARMACOLOGY: Gonadorelin is a synthetic decapeptide that has the same amino acid sequence as endogenous gonadotropin-releasing hormone (GnRH) synthesized in the human hypothalamus and in various neurons terminating in the hypothalamus. Its pharmacological and toxicological profile is therefore identical to that of endogenous GnRH.

Under physiological conditions, GnRH is released by the hypothalamus in a pulsatile fashion. The primary effect of GnRH is the synthesis and release of luteinizing hormone (LH) in the anterior pituitary gland. GnRH also stimulates the synthesis and release of follicle stimulating hormone (FSH), but this effect is less pronounced. LH and FSH subsequently stimulate the gonads to produce steroids which are instrumental in regulating reproductive hormonal status. Unlike human menopausal gonadotropin (hMG) which supplies pituitary hormones, pulsatile administration of gonadorelin replaces defective hypothalamic secretion of GnRH. Gonadorelin for pulsatile injection approximates the natural hormonal secretory pattern, causing pulsatile release of pituitary gonadotropins. Accordingly, gonadorelin for pulsatile injection is useful in treating conditions of infertility caused by defective GnRH stimulation from the hypothalamus.

The following information summarizes clinical efficacy of gonadorelin administered by pulsatile i.v. or s.c. injection to patients with primary hypothalamic amenorrhea.

In 48 patients with primary hypothalamic amenorrhea (HA) 94% (45/48) patients ovulated and 58% (25/43) patients became pregnant (5 patients did not desire pregnancy).

Treatment was successful even in those patients who failed past attempts at ovulation induction by other methods.

Following i.v. or s.c. injection of GnRH into normal subjects and/or hypogonadotropic patients, plasma GnRH concentrations rapidly declined with initial and terminal half-lives of 2 to 10 min and 10 to 40 min, respectively. In these studies, high clearance values (500 to 1 500 L/day) and low volumes of distribution (9 to 15 L) were calculated. The pharmacokinetics of GnRH in normal subjects and in hypogonadotropic patients were similar. GnRH was rapidly metabolized to various biologically inactive peptide fragments which are readily excreted in urine. Renal failure, but not hepatic disease, prolonged the half-life and reduced the clearance of GnRH.

A comparison of gonadorelin to hCG or hCG + gonadorelin for corpus luteum maintenance revealed the information in Table 1.

Table 1: Lutrepulse

Comparison of Lutrepulse to hCG or hCG+Lutrepulse for Corpus Luteum Maintenance

	hCG		Lutrepulse		hCG+Lutrepulse	
Delivered	43/63	(68%)	19/26	(73%)	19/25	(76%)
Aborted	20/63	(32%)	7/26	(27%)	6/25	(24%)

Gonadorelin alone is therefore able to maintain the corpus luteum during pregnancy.

INDICATIONS: For the induction of ovulation in women with primary hypothalamic amenorrhea.

Differential Diagnosis: Proper diagnosis is critical for successful treatment with gonadorelin. It must be established that hypothalamic amenorrhea or hypogonadism is, in fact, due to a deficiency in quantity or pulsing of endogenous GnRH. The diagnosis of hypothalamic amenorrhea or hypogonadism is based on the exclusion of other causes of the dysfunction, since there is currently no practical technique to directly assess hypothalamic function. Prior to initiation of therapy with gonadorelin the physician should rule out disorders (other than abnormalities of GnRH secretion), that can cause amenorrhea and involve most often general health, reproductive organs, CNS, anterior pituitary, thyroid, adrenals or other endocrine or metabolic disorders.

CONTRAINDICATIONS: Women with any condition that could be exacerbated by pregnancy. For example, pituitary prolactinoma should be considered one such condition. Additionally, any history of sensitivity to gonadorelin or any component of this product is a contraindication.

Patients who have ovarian cysts should not receive gonadorelin.

Gonadorelin is intended to initiate events including the production of reproductive hormones (e.g., estrogens and progesterone). Therefore, any condition that may be worsened by reproductive hormones, such as a hormonally-dependent tumor, is a contraindication to the use of gonadorelin.

WARNINGS: Therapy with gonadorelin should be conducted by physicians familiar with pulsatile GnRH delivery and the clinical ramifications of ovulation induction. While there have been few cases of hyperstimulation (<1%), this possibility must be considered. If hyperstimulation should occur, therapy should be discontinued and spontaneous resolution can be expected. The preservation of the endogenous feedback mechanisms makes severe hyperstimulation (with ascites and pleural effusion) rare. However, the physician should be aware of the possibility and be alert for any evidence of ascites, pleural effusion, hemoconcentration, rupture of a cyst, fluid or electrolyte imbalance, or sepsis.

Multiple pregnancy is a possibility that can be minimized by careful attention to the recommended doses and ultrasonographic monitoring of the ovarian response to therapy. Following a baseline pelvic ultrasound, follow-up studies should be conducted at a minimum on day 7 and day 14 of therapy.

As with any parenteral medication, scrupulous attention to asepsis is important. The infusion area must be monitored as with all indwelling parenteral approaches.

PRECAUTIONS: General: Ovarian hyperstimulation has been reported. This may be related to pulse dosage or concomitant use of other ovulation stimulators. Hyperstimulation may be a greater risk in patients where spontaneous variations in endogenous GnRH secretion occur. Multiple follicle development, multiple pregnancy and spontaneous termination of pregnancy have been reported. Multiple pregnancy can be minimized by appropriate monitoring of follicle formation; nonetheless, the patient and her partner should be advised of the frequency (12%) and potential risks of multiple pregnancy before starting treatment.

Ovarian hyperstimulation, a syndrome of sudden ovarian enlargement, ascites with or without pain, and/or pleural effusion, is rare with pulsatile GnRH therapy. Among 268 patients participating in clinical trials, one case of moderate hyperstimulation has been reported, but this cycle included concomitant use of clomiphene citrate. In contrast, menotropins (hMG) with hCG, have been variously reported to cause some degree of hyperstimulation in up to 50% of conception cycles, and severe hyperstimulation may occur in up to 1.3% of all cycles.

Several cases of allergic reactions to synthetic LHRH have been reported in the published scientific literature. Most of the reports described urticaria following administration of synthetic LHRH although one case described a serious anaphylactic reaction. In cases where it has been investigated, the allergic reactions were associated with anti-LHRH antibodies in the patient's serum. The s.c. route of administration of synthetic LHRH would bear a greater risk of antibody induction compared to i.v. administration. In one study, the incidence of circulating antibodies in patients treated with pulsatile s.c. LHRH was found to be 3%. Some patients who develop antibodies to LHRH may become refractory to treatment.

Gonadorelin should be administered with a suitable pulsatile pump and suitable infusion catheters. The patient should be provided with detailed oral and written instructions regarding infusion pump usage and potential sepsis in order to minimize the frequency of infusion pump malfunction and inflammation, infection, mild phlebitis or hematoma at the catheter site.

Laboratory Tests: Following a diagnosis of primary hypothalamic amenorrhea, initiation of gonadorelin therapy may be monitored by the following: 1) Ovarian ultrasound—baseline, and at least weekly while the patient is on therapy or until ovulation has been documented. 2) Estradiol serum level to assess ovarian response. 3) Mid-luteal phase serum progesterone to confirm ovulation. 4) Recording of basal body temperature. 5) Clinical observation of infusion site at each visit and as needed. 6) Physical examination including pelvic at regularly scheduled visits.

Drug Interactions: None are known. Gonadorelin should not be used concomitantly with other ovulation stimulators.

Drug/Laboratory Test Interactions: None are known.

Carcinogenesis, Mutagenesis, Impairment of Fertility: Since GnRH is a natural substance normally present in humans, long-term studies in animals have not been performed to evaluate carcinogenic potential. Mutagenicity testing was not done.

Pregnancy: Reproductive studies (teratology and embryotoxicity) performed in rats and rabbits have not revealed any evidence of harm to the fetus due to gonadorelin acetate. There was no evidence of teratogenicity when gonadorelin was administered i.v. up to 120 µg/kg/day (>70 times the recommended human dose of 5 µg per pulse) in rats and rabbits.

Studies in pregnant women have shown that gonadorelin does not increase the risk of abnormalities when administered during the first trimester of pregnancy. It appears that the possibility of fetal harm is remote, if the drug is used during pregnancy. In clinical studies, 47 pregnant patients have used gonadorelin during the first trimester of pregnancy (51 pregnancies) and the drug had no apparent adverse effect on the course of pregnancy. Available follow-up reports on infants born to these women revealed no adverse effects or complications that were attributable to gonadorelin. Nevertheless, because the studies in humans cannot rule out the possibility of harm, gonadorelin should be used during pregnancy only for maintenance of the corpus luteum in ovulation induction cycles.

Lactation: It is not known whether this drug is excreted in human milk. There is no indication for use of gonadorelin in a nursing woman.

Children: Not applicable.

ADVERSE EFFECTS: The majority of adverse effects are associated with the parenteral route of administration of the drug and are generally confined to superficial thrombophlebitis and injection site irritation.

Adverse reactions have been reported in approximately 10% of treatment regimens in pivotal clinical trials. Ten of 268 patients interrupted therapy because of an adverse reaction but subsequently resumed treatment. One other subject did not resume treatment.

In clinical studies involving 268 women, one case of moderate ovarian hyperstimulation has been reported. This cycle included concomitant use of clomiphene citrate. This low incidence of hyperstimulation appears to be due to the preservation of normal feedback mechanisms of the pituitary-ovarian axis. Despite the preservation of feedback mechanisms, some incidents of multiple follicle development, multiple pregnancy and spontaneous termination of pregnancy have been reported. In clinical studies involving 142 pregnancies, delivery information was available on 89 pregnancies. Eleven of these gonadorelin-induced pregnancies (12%) were multiple (10 sets of twins, 1 set of triplets).

The following adverse reactions are related to use of an infusion pump: inflammation, infection, mild phlebitis, or hematoma at the catheter site. Additionally, infusion set malfunction and interruption of infusion may occur; this has no known adverse effect other than interruption of therapy.

Anaphylaxis (bronchospasm, tachycardia, flushing, urticaria, induration at injection site) has been reported with the related polypeptide hormone gonadorelin hydrochloride (Factrel). Antibody formation has occurred in approximately 3% of patients treated with Factrel via the s.c. route. In some cases, these appear to be related to a decreased effectiveness of the drug.

Ovarian Cancer: Ovarian cancer has been reported in a very small number of infertile women who have been treated with fertility drugs. A causal relationship between treatment with fertility drugs and ovarian cancer has not been established.

OVERDOSE:

Continuous, non-pulsatile exposure to gonadorelin could temporarily reduce pituitary responsiveness. If the pump should malfunction and deliver the entire contents of the 0.8 mg system, no harmful effects would be expected. Bolus doses as high as 3 000 µg of gonadorelin hydrochloride have not been harmful. Pituitary hyperstimulation and multiple follicle development can be minimized by adhering to recommended doses, and appropriate monitoring of follicle formation (see Precautions).

The LD_{50} values (mg/kg) in the mouse are >400, >3 000, and >4 000 when GnRH is administered i.v., s.c. and orally, respectively. The LD_{50} values (mg/kg) in the rat are >200, >2 000, and >3 000 when GnRH is administered i.v., s.c. and orally, respectively.

Administration of 640 µg/kg in monkeys as a single i.v. bolus resulted in no compound-related effects in clinical observations or gross morphologic evaluations.

For management of a suspected drug overdose, CPhA recommends that you contact your **regional Poison Control Centre**. See the *CPS* Directory section for a list of Poison Control Centres.

DOSAGE: Dosages between 1 and 20 µg have been successfully used in clinical studies. The recommended dose in primary hypothalamic amenorrhea is 5 µg every 90 minutes, administered either s.c. or i.v. This is delivered using the 0.8 mg solution at 50 µL per pulse. Sixty-eight percent of the 5 µg every 90 minutes regimens induced ovulation in patients with primary hypothalamic amenorrhea, when administered i.v.

Some women may require a reduction in the recommended dose of 5 µg should laboratory testing and patient monitoring indicate an inappropriate response. While most primary hypothalamic amenorrhea patients will ovulate during the first cycle of 5 µg therapy, some may be refractory to this dose. The recommended treatment interval before dose adjustment is 21 days. It may be necessary to raise the dose cautiously, and in stepwise fashion if there is no response after 3 treatment intervals. All dose changes should be carefully monitored for inappropriate response.

Table 2 can be used to calculate the dose per pulse when individualizing treatment.

Table 2: Lutrepulse

Calculation of the Dose per Pulse

Vial Size	Volume of Diluent	Volume/pulse	Dose/pulse
0.8 mg	8 mL	25 µL	2.5 µg
0.8 mg	8 mL	50 µL	5 µg

The response to gonadorelin usually occurs within 2 to 3 weeks after therapy initiation. When ovulation occurs, therapy should be continued for another 2 weeks to maintain the corpus luteum. Lutrepulse dose and dosing frequency should remain the same.

Administration: Gonadorelin is to be reconstituted aseptically with 8 mL of the diluent provided (isotonic sterile sodium chloride for injection). The drug product should be reconstituted immediately prior to use and transferred to a plastic reservoir. First withdraw 8 mL of the saline diluent and then inject it onto the lyophile (drug product) cake. The product is shaken for a few seconds to produce a solution which should be clear, colorless, and free of particulate matter. Parenteral drug products should be inspected visually for particulate matter and discoloration prior to administration, whenever solution and container permit. If particulate matter or discoloration are present, the solution should not be used.

The reconstituted solution is administered either i.v. or s.c. using a suitable pulsatile pump. The pump should be set to deliver either 25 or 50 µL of solution, based upon the dose selected, over a pulse period of 1 minute, and at a pulse frequency of 90 minutes. If 50 µL per pulse is used with a pulse frequency of 90 minutes, the 8 mL of solution should last 7 days. If 25 µL per pulse is used with a pulse frequency of 90 minutes, the 8 mL of solution should last 14 days.

SUPPLIED: Each 10 mL vial of lyophilized, sterile powder contains: gonadorelin acetate 0.8 mg (gonadorelin base 0.73 mg) and mannitol 10 mg as a carrier. Packages of 1 vial and a 10 mL vial of sterile, isotonic sodium chloride diluent. The product is stable when stored at room temperature (15 to 30°C) in the unopened package. The reconstituted solution is stable for up to 45 days at 24 to 37°C when stored in vials and reservoir bags, and remains stable and uncontaminated for up to 16 hours in catheter tubing.

Luveris® Ⓟ

lutropin alpha

Gonadotrophin

EMD Canada

Date of Preparation: June 24, 2005
Date of Revision: April 2007

PHARMACOLOGY: Lutropin alpha is a recombinant human luteinizing hormone, r-hLH. r-hLH is a heterodimeric glycoprotein consisting of two non-covalently linked subunits (designated α and β) of 92 and 121 amino acids, respectively. Luteinizing hormone binds on the ovarian theca (and granulosa) cells and testicular Leydig cells, to a receptor shared with human chorionic gonadotropin hormone (hCG). This LH/CG transmembrane receptor is a member of the super-family of G protein-coupled receptors; specifically, it has a large extra-cellular domain. In vitro, the affinity binding of recombinant hLH to the LH/CG receptor on Leydig tumor cells (MA-10) is between that for hCG and that of pituitary hLH, but within the same order of magnitude.

In the ovaries, during the follicular phase, LH stimulates theca cells to secrete androgens, which will be used as the substrate by granulosa cell aromatase enzyme to produce estradiol, supporting FSH-induced follicular development. At mid-cycle, high levels of LH trigger corpus luteum formation and ovulation. After ovulation, LH stimulates progesterone production in the corpus luteum by increasing the conversion of cholesterol to pregnenolone. In the stimulation of follicular development in anovulatory women deficient in LH and FSH, the primary effect resulting from administration of lutropin alpha is an increase in oestradiol secretion by the follicles, the growth of which is stimulated by follitropin alpha.

Following intravenous administration of LUVERIS (lutropin alpha for injection), is rapidly distributed with an initial half-life of approximately one hour and eliminated from the body with a terminal half-life of about 10-12 hours. The steady state volume of distribution is around 10-14 L. When given by intravenous administration, LUVERIS demonstrates linear pharmacokinetics over higher doses (300 to 40 000 IU). However, following administration of the lower dose (75 IU), the concentration range is too small to allow proper quantification of the pharmacokinetic parameters. The disposition of r-hLH is adequately described by a biexponential model. Total clearance is around 2 L/h, and less than 5% of the dose is excreted in the urine. The mean residence time is approximately 5 hours.

Following intramuscular administration, the absolute bioavailability is 0.54; the terminal half-life was found to be longer (mean=16h) after intramuscular injection than after intravenous dosing, indicating that the absorption may be a rate-limiting factor.

Following subcutaneous administration, the absolute bioavailability is 0.56; the terminal half-life is slightly prolonged (mean=21h) compared to i.m. The lutropin alpha pharmacokinetics following single and repeated administration of LUVERIS are comparable and the accumulation ratio of lutropin alpha is minimal. There is no pharmacokinetic interaction with follitropin alpha when administered simultaneously.

INDICATIONS: LUVERIS (lutropin alpha for injection) concomitantly administered with GONAL-F (follitropin alpha for injection) is indicated for stimulation of follicular development in infertile hypogonadotropic hypogonadal women with profound LH deficiency (LH <1.2 IU/L). A definitive effect on pregnancy in this population has not been demonstrated. The safety and effectiveness of concomitant administration of LUVERIS with any other preparation of recombinant human FSH or urinary human FSH is unknown.

CONTRAINDICATIONS: LUVERIS (lutropin alpha for injection) is contraindicated for safety reasons in the presence of:

1. Hypersensitivity to gonadotrophins or to any of the excipients.
2. Ovarian failure.
3. Uncontrolled thyroid or adrenal failure.
4. Active, untreated tumours of the hypothalamus and pituitary gland.
5. Abnormal uterine bleeding of unknown origin.
6. Sex hormone dependent tumours of the reproductive tract and accessory organs.
7. Pregnancy and lactation.

WARNINGS: LUVERIS, (lutropin alpha) should only be used by physicians who are thoroughly familiar with the treatment of hypogonadotrophic hypogonadism (HH) and its management. Possible contraindications for pregnancy should be evaluated. In particular, patients should be evaluated for hypothyroidism, adrenocortical insufficiency, hyperprolactinemia and pituitary or hypothalamic tumours, and appropriate specific treatment instituted.

Patients undergoing stimulation of follicular growth are at an increased risk of developing hyperstimulation in view of possible excessive estrogen response and multiple follicular development.

Overstimulation of the Ovary Following Gonadotropin Therapy: Ovarian Enlargement: Mild to moderate uncomplicated ovarian enlargement which may be accompanied by abdominal distension and/or abdominal pain may occur in patients treated with gonadotropins (such as LUVERIS). These conditions generally regress without treatment within two or three weeks. Careful monitoring of ovarian response can further minimize the risk of overstimulation.

If the ovaries are abnormally enlarged on the last day of therapy with LUVERIS and GONAL-F, hCG should not be administered in this course of therapy. This will reduce the risk of development of Ovarian Hyperstimulation Syndrome.

Ovarian Hyperstimulation Syndrome (OHSS): OHSS is a medical event distinct from uncomplicated ovarian enlargement. Severe OHSS may progress rapidly (within 24 hours to several days) to become a serious medical event. It is characterized by an apparent dramatic increase in vascular permeability which can result in a rapid accumulation of fluid in the peritoneal cavity, thorax, and potentially, the pericardium. The early warning signs of development of OHSS are severe pelvic pain, nausea, vomiting, and weight gain. The following symptomatology has been seen with cases of OHSS: abdominal pain, abdominal distension, gastrointestinal symptoms including nausea, vomiting and diarrhea, severe ovarian enlargement, weight gain, dyspnea, and oliguria. Clinical evaluation may reveal hypovolemia, hemoconcentration, electrolyte imbalances, ascites, hemoperitoneum, pleural effusions, hydrothorax, acute pulmonary distress, and thromboembolic events (see Pulmonary and Vascular Complications). Transient liver function test abnormalities that are suggestive of hepatic dysfunction have been reported in association with Ovarian Hyperstimulation Syndrome (OHSS). These liver function test abnormalities may be accompanied by morphological changes on liver biopsy.

In hypogonadotropic hypogonadal women with profound LH and FSH deficiency from five clinical trials, four cases of OHSS were reported in 4 of 70 (5.7%) patients treated with 75 IU LUVERIS and GONAL-F and one case was reported in 1 of 31 (3.2%) patients treated with GONAL-F alone. Among women treated with any dose of LUVERIS in these studies, five of 96 (5.2%) patients reported 6 cases of OHSS after treatment with LUVERIS and GONAL-F.

OHSS may be more severe and more protracted if pregnancy occurs. OHSS develops rapidly; therefore, patients should be followed for at least two weeks after hCG administration. Most often, OHSS occurs after treatment has been discontinued and reaches its maximum severity at seven to ten days following treatment. Usually, OHSS resolves spontaneously with the onset of menses. If there is evidence that OHSS may be developing prior to hCG administration (see Precautions, Laboratory Tests), hCG must be withheld.

If severe OHSS occurs, treatment with gonadotropins must be stopped and the patient should be hospitalized.

A physician experienced in the management of this syndrome, or who is experienced in the management of fluid and electrolyte imbalances should be consulted.

Multiple Births: Reports of multiple births have been associated with LUVERIS treatment. In patients undergoing induction of ovulation, the incidence of multiple pregnancies and births is increased compared with natural conception. To minimize the risk of multiple pregnancy, ultrasound scans as well as oestradiol measurements are recommended. The patient and her partner should be advised of the potential risk of multiple births before starting treatment.

Pulmonary and Vascular Complications: As with other gonadotropin products, a potential for the occurrence of arterial thromboembolism exists.

PRECAUTIONS: Selection of Patients: Careful attention should be given to diagnose candidates for LUVERIS (lutropin alpha for injection) therapy.

1. Patients should have baseline serum hormone levels of LH <1.2 IU/L and FSH <5 IU/L.
2. Before treatment with gonadotropins is instituted, a thorough gynecologic and endocrinologic evaluation must be performed. This should include an assessment of pelvic anatomy and exclusion of pregnancy.
3. Patients should have a negative progestin challenge test.
4. Patients in later reproductive life have a greater predisposition to endometrial carcinoma as well as a higher incidence of anovulatory disorders. A thorough diagnostic evaluation should always be performed in patients who demonstrate abnormal uterine bleeding or other signs of endometrial abnormalities before starting LUVERIS and follitropin alfa therapy.
5. Evaluation of the partner's fertility potential should be included in the initial evaluation.

Information to Be Provided to the Patient: Prior to therapy with LUVERIS, patients should be informed of the duration of treatment and monitoring of their condition that will be required. The risks of ovarian hyperstimulation syndrome and multiple births (see Warnings) and other possible adverse reactions (see Adverse Effects) should also be discussed.

Laboratory Tests: In most instances, treatment of women with LH and FSH results only in follicular recruitment and development. In the absence of an endogenous LH surge, hCG is given when monitoring of the patient indicates that sufficient follicular development has occurred. This may be estimated by ultrasound alone or in combination with measurement of serum estradiol levels. The combination of both ultrasound and serum estradiol measurement are useful for monitoring the development of follicles, for timing of the ovulatory trigger, as well as for detecting ovarian enlargement and minimizing the risk of the Ovarian Hyperstimulation Syndrome and multiple gestation. It is recommended that the number of growing follicles be confirmed using ultrasonography because serum estrogens do not give an indication of the size or number of follicles.

With the exception of confirmation of pregnancy, the clinical confirmation of ovulation is obtained by direct and indirect indices of progesterone production. The indices most generally used are as follows:

1. A rise in basal body temperature
2. Increase in serum progesterone and
3. Menstruation following a shift in basal body temperature

When used in conjunction with the indices of progesterone production, sonographic visualization of the ovaries will assist in determining if ovulation has occurred. Sonographic evidence of ovulation may include the following:

1. Fluid in the cul-de-sac
2. Ovarian stigmata
3. Collapsed follicle
4. Secretory endometrium

Accurate interpretation of the indices of ovulation require a physician who is experienced in the interpretation of these tests.

Drug Interactions: LUVERIS should only be administered simultaneously or in the same injection with GONAL-F (follitropin alpha for injection). Studies have shown that co-administration of LUVERIS and GONAL-F does not significantly alter the activity, stability, pharmacokinetic or pharmacodynamic properties of either active substance.

Carcinogenesis, Mutagenesis, Impairment of Fertility: Long-term studies to evaluate the carcinogenic potential of LUVERIS in animals have not been performed. In vitro mutagenicity testing of LUVERIS in bacteria and mammalian cell lines, chromosome aberration assay in human lymphocytes and in vivo mouse micronucleus have shown no indication of genetic defects. Impaired fertility has been reported in animals exposed to high doses of lutropin alfa; increased pre- and post-implantation losses were observed in female rats and rabbits given lutropin alfa at doses of 10 IU/kg/day and higher.

Pregnancy: When administered to rats during the late period of pregnancy, doses of 10 IU/kg/day and higher were also shown to affect the postnatal survival and growth of the newborns. There was no evidence of teratogenic effect in either rats or rabbits. LUVERIS is contraindicated in women who are pregnant and may cause fetal harm when administered to a pregnant woman. Reproductive toxicity studies performed in female rats and rabbits showed that lutropin alfa at doses of 10 IU/kg/day and greater caused an increase in pre- and post-implantation losses.

Lactation: It is not known whether LUVERIS is excreted in human milk. Because many drugs are excreted in human milk, the benefits to the mother vs. potential risks to the infant must be weighed before the decision is made to administer LUVERIS to a nursing mother.

Other Age Groups: LUVERIS is not indicated in pediatric or geriatric patients. Safety and effectiveness in these patient populations have not been established.

ADVERSE EFFECTS: Clinical Trials: The safety of LUVERIS was examined in six clinical studies that treated 170 infertile women with hypogonadotropic hypogonadism of whom 152 received LUVERIS and GONAL-F in 283 treatment cycles. Adverse events reported by ≥2% of patients (regardless of causality) treated with any dose of LUVERIS (25, 75, 150, 225 IU) are listed in Table 1.

Table 1: LUVERIS

Adverse Events Reported in ≥2% Patients in All Cycles in All HH Patients in Studies 6253, 6905[a], 7798[b], 8297[c], 21008, and 21415

	0 IU LUVERIS & GONAL-f	75 IU LUVERIS & GONAL-f	All Doses of LUVERIS & GONAL-f
	Patients (n=43) n (%)	Patients (n=118) n (%)	Patients (n=152) n (%)
Patients With Events	20 (46.5)	50 (42.4)	72 (47.4)
Headache	2 (4.7)	12 (10.2)	15 (9.9)
Nausea	0	8 (6.8)	11 (7.2)
Ovarian Hyperstimulation	1 (2.3)	7 (5.9)	9 (5.9)
Breast Pain Female	4 (9.3)	6 (5.1)	9 (5.9)
Abdominal Pain	5 (11.6)	6 (5.1)	13 (8.6)
Ovarian Cyst	4 (9.3)	6 (5.1)	8 (5.3)
Flatulence	3 (7.0)	5 (4.2)	6 (3.9)
Injection Site Reaction	2 (4.7)	4 (3.4)	6 (3.9)
Dysmenorrhoea	1 (2.3)	2 (1.7)	4 (2.6)
Ovarian Disorder	0	2 (1.7)	3 (2.0)
Diarrhoea	1 (2.3)	3 (2.5)	3 (2.0)
Constipation	0	3 (2.5)	3 (2.0)
Pain	3 (7.0)	3 (2.5)	6 (3.9)
Fatigue	0	3 (2.5)	5 (3.3)
Upper Resp Tract Infection	2 (4.7)	1 (0.8)	3 (2.0)

[a] Study 6905 was a randomized, open-label, dose-finding study to assess the efficacy and safety of LUVERIS administered with 150 IU GONAL-F for induction of follicular development in HH women.
[b] Study 7798 was an uncontrolled, multicenter, dose-finding study to assess the efficacy and safety of LUVERIS administered with 150 IU GONAL-F for induction of follicular development in LH and FSH deficient anovulatory women in Germany.
[c] Study 8297 was an uncontrolled, multicenter, dose-finding study to assess the efficacy and safety of LUVERIS administered with 150 IU GONAL-F for induction of follicular development in HH women in Spain.

The following medical events have been reported subsequent to pregnancies resulting from administration of gonadotropins for ovulation induction in controlled clinical studies: spontaneous abortion, ectopic pregnancy, premature labor, postpartum fever, congenital abnormalities.

There is no evidence that use of any gonadotropin drug product for treatment of infertility is associated with an increased risk of congenital malformations.

The following adverse reactions have been previously reported during menotropin therapy: pulmonary and vascular complications (see Warnings); adnexal torsion (as a complication of ovarian enlargement); mild to moderate ovarian enlargement; hemoperitoneum.

There have been infrequent reports of ovarian neoplasms, both benign and malignant, in women who have undergone multiple drug regimens for ovulation induction; however, a causal relationship has not been established.

Post-Marketing Surveillance: Since the introduction of LUVERIS onto the global market in 2000, it is estimated that more than 22 000 patients have been treated. No new unexpected adverse events have been reported during this time. The adverse events collected have been consistent with the safety profile observed during clinical trials and, as a result, there have been no changes made to the core safety information for LUVERIS to date.

OVERDOSE:

Symptoms: In the event of an overdose with LUVERIS, ovarian hyperstimulation syndrome (OHSS) may occur. OHSS is characterized by an apparent dramatic increase in vascular permeability which can result in a rapid accumulation of fluid in the peritoneal cavity, thorax and potentially, the pericardium. The early warning signs of development of OHSS are severe pelvic pain, nausea, vomiting and weight gain.

Treatment: OHSS develops rapidly, therefore, patients should be followed for at least two weeks after hCG administration. If there is evidence that OHSS may be developing prior to hCG administration, hCG must be withheld. If severe OHSS occurs, treatment with gonadotropins must be stopped and the patient should be hospitalised for treatment by an experienced physician (see Warnings for more detailed information on OHSS).

For management of a suspected drug overdose, CPhA recommends that you contact your **regional Poison Control Centre**. See the *CPS* Directory section for a list of Poison Control Centres.

DOSAGE: In LH and FSH deficient women, the objective of LUVERIS (lutropin alpha for injection) therapy in association with GONAL-F (follitropin alpha for injection) is to develop a single mature Graafian follicle from which the oocyte will be liberated after the administration of human Chorionic Gonadotrophin (hCG). LUVERIS should be given as a course of daily injections simultaneously with GONAL-F until adequate follicular development is indicated by ovary ultrasonography and serum estradiol. Since these patients are amenorrhoeic and have low endogenous estrogen secretion, treatment can commence at any time. Treatment duration should not normally exceed 14 days unless signs of follicular development are present.

Treatment should be tailored to the individual patient's response as assessed by measuring (i) follicle size by ultrasound and (ii) estrogen response. The recommended regimen is 75 IU of LUVERIS daily associated with 75-150 IU GONAL-F. The daily dose of LUVERIS should not exceed 75 IU.

To complete follicular development and effect ovulation in the absence of an endogenous LH surge, human chorionic gonadotropin (hCG) should be given one day after the last dose of LUVERIS and GONAL-F. Treatment with hCG should be withheld if the ovaries are abnormally enlarged or if excessive estradiol production has occurred. If the ovaries are abnormally enlarged or abdominal pain occurs, treatment with LUVERIS and GONAL-F should be discontinued and hCG should not be administered, and the patient should be advised not to have intercourse; this may reduce the chances of developing Ovarian Hyperstimulation Syndrome and, should spontaneous ovulation occur, reduce the chances of multiple gestation. A follow-up visit should be conducted in the luteal phase.

Doses administered in subsequent cycles must be individualized for each patient based on her response in the preceding cycle. Doses of GONAL-F greater than 225 IU per day are not routinely recommended. As in the initial cycle, hCG must be given to complete follicular development and induce ovulation. The precautions described above should be followed to minimize the chance of developing Ovarian Hyperstimulation Syndrome.

The couple should be encouraged to have intercourse daily, beginning on the day prior to hCG administration until ovulation becomes apparent in the indices used for the determination of progestational activity.

In light of the indices and parameters mentioned, it should become obvious that, unless a physician is willing to devote considerable time to these patients and be familiar with and conduct the necessary laboratory studies, he/she should not prescribe LUVERIS.

Administration: Dissolve the contents of the vial of LUVERIS in 1 mL Sterile Water for Injection, USP. GONAL-F should be reconstituted and administered as directed in the prescriber labeling for this product. Administer entire contents of the vial SUBCUTANEOUSLY. LUVERIS may be mixed in the same syringe with GONAL-F and the combination given in one injection. For single use. Use immediately after reconstitution. Any unused reconstituted material should be discarded. **Mix gently. Do not shake.**

Parenteral drug products should be inspected visually for particulate matter and discoloration prior to administration.

INFORMATION FOR THE PATIENT: Published in e-CPS, available by subscription at www.e-cps.ca.

SUPPLIED: Each vial of sterile, lyophilized powder contains: 75 IU of r-hLH, 47.75 mg sucrose, 0.1 mg L-methionine, 0.825 mg disodium phosphate dihydrate, 0.052 mg sodium dihydrogen phosphate monohydrate, and 0.05 mg polysorbate 20. Phosphoric acid and/or sodium hydroxide may be used for pH adjustment prior to lyophilization. The diluent provided for reconstitution is Sterile Water for Injections, Ph. Eur./USP. Neutral colourless glass (type I, Ph. Eur) single dose vials of 3 mL. Package combinations of 1 vial 75 IU LUVERIS and solvent (1 mL Sterile Water for Injections, Ph. Eur/USP) or 3 vials 75 IU LUVERIS and solvent (3×1 mL Sterile Water for Injections, Ph. Eur./USP). Lyophilized vials are stable when stored at 2-25°C and protected from light. Do not expose to extreme heat or cold. Do not use the product after the expiry date indicated on the label.

The reader is invited to consult CPhA's monograph **Selective Serotonin Reuptake Inhibitors**.

Luvox®

fluvoxamine maleate

Antidepressant—Antiobsessional

Abbott Products

Date of Preparation: November 13, 1996
Date of Revision: May 28, 2010

PHARMACOLOGY: The antidepressant and antiobsessional actions of LUVOX (fluvoxamine maleate) are believed to be related to its selective inhibition of presynaptic serotonin re-uptake in brain neurones.

There is minimum interference with noradrenergic processes, and, in common with several other specific inhibitors of serotonin uptake, fluvoxamine maleate has very little in vitro affinity for α_1, α_2, β_1, dopamine$_2$, histamine$_1$, serotonin$_1$, serotonin$_2$ or muscarinic receptors.

Pharmacokinetics: In healthy volunteers, fluvoxamine maleate is well absorbed after oral administration. Following a single 100 mg oral dose, peak plasma levels of 31-87 ng/mL were attained 1.5 to 8 hours post-dose. Peak plasma levels and AUC's (0-72 hours) are directly proportionate to dose after single oral doses of 25, 50 and 100 mg. Following single doses, the mean plasma half-life is 15 hours, and slightly longer (17-22 hours), during repeated dosing. Steady-state plasma levels are usually achieved within 10-14 days. The pharmacokinetic profile in the elderly is similar to that in younger patients.

In a dose proportionality study involving fluvoxamine maleate at 100, 200 and 300 mg/day for 10 consecutive days in 30 normal volunteers, steady-state was achieved after about a week of dosing. Maximum plasma concentrations at steady-state occurred within 3-8 hours of dosing and reached concentrations averaging 88, 283 and 546 ng/mL, respectively. Thus, fluvoxamine maleate had nonlinear pharmacokinetics over this dose range, i.e., higher doses of fluvoxamine maleate produced disproportionately higher concentrations than predicted from the lower dose.

Metabolism and Elimination: Fluvoxamine maleate undergoes extensive hepatic transformation, mainly via oxidative demethylation, to at least nine metabolites, which are excreted by the kidney. Ninety-four percent of an oral radioactive dose is recovered in the urine within 48 hours. The two major metabolites showed negligible pharmacological activity. In vitro binding of fluvoxamine maleate to human plasma proteins is about 77% at drug concentrations up to 4000 ng/mL.

INDICATIONS: Depression: LUVOX (fluvoxamine maleate) may be indicated for the symptomatic relief of depressive illness in adults.

The effectiveness of fluvoxamine maleate in long-term use (i.e., for more than 5 to 6 weeks) has not been systematically evaluated in controlled trials. Therefore, the physician who elects to use fluvoxamine maleate for extended periods should periodically re-evaluate the long-term usefulness of the drug for the individual patient.

Obsessive-Compulsive Disorder: LUVOX (fluvoxamine maleate) has been shown to significantly reduce the symptoms of obsessive-compulsive disorder in adults. The obsessions or compulsions must be experienced as intrusive, markedly distressing, time consuming, or interfering significantly with the person's social or occupational functioning.

The efficacy of LUVOX (fluvoxamine maleate) has been studied in double-blind, placebo-controlled clinical trials conducted in obsessive-compulsive outpatients. The usefulness of LUVOX (fluvoxamine maleate) for long-term use (i.e. for more than 10 weeks) has not been systematically evaluated in controlled trials. Therefore, the physician who elects to use LUVOX (fluvoxamine maleate) for extended periods should periodically re-evaluate the long-term usefulness of the drug for the individual patient.

CONTRAINDICATIONS: LUVOX (fluvoxamine maleate) is contraindicated in patients with known hypersensitivity to fluvoxamine maleate or any of the excipients.

Fluvoxamine maleate should not be administered together with tizanidine or monoamine oxidase (MAO) inhibitors, including linezolid, an antibiotic which is a reversible non-selective MAO inhibitor. At least two weeks should elapse after discontinuation of MAO inhibitor therapy before fluvoxamine maleate treatment is initiated. MAO inhibitors should not be introduced within 2 weeks of cessation of therapy with LUVOX (fluvoxamine maleate).

Co-administration of thioridazine, mesoridazine, terfenadine, astemizole, pimozide, or cisapride with LUVOX (fluvoxamine maleate) is contraindicated (see Warnings and Precautions).

WARNINGS: Potential Association with Behavioural and Emotional Changes, Including Self-Harm: **Pediatrics: Placebo-Controlled Clinical Trial Data:**

- **Recent analyses of placebo-controlled clinical trial safety databases from SSRIs and other newer anti-depressants suggests that use of these drugs in patients under the age of 18 may be associated with behavioural and emotional changes, including an increased risk of suicidal ideation and behaviour over that of placebo.**
- **The small denominators in the clinical trial database, as well as the variability in placebo rates, preclude reliable conclusions on the relative safety profiles among these drugs.**

Adults and Pediatrics: Additional Data:

- **There are clinical trial and post-marketing reports with SSRIs and other newer anti-depressants, in both pediatrics and adults, of severe agitation-type adverse events coupled with self-harm or harm to others. The agitation-type events include: akathisia, agitation, disinhibition, emotional lability, hostility, aggression, depersonalization. In some cases, the events occurred within several weeks of starting treatment.**

Rigorous clinical monitoring for suicidal ideation or other indicators of potential for suicidal behaviour is advised in patients of all ages. This includes monitoring for agitation-type emotional and behavioural changes.

Young Adults (ages 18 to 24 years): A recent, FDA meta-analysis of placebo-controlled clinical trials of antidepressant drugs in adult patients with psychiatric disorders showed an increased risk of suicidal behaviour with antidepressants compared to placebo in patients less than 25 years old.

Discontinuation Symptoms: Patients currently taking LUVOX (fluvoxamine maleate) should not be discontinued abruptly, due to risk of discontinuation symptoms. At the time that a medical decision is made to discontinue an SSRI or other newer anti-depressant drug, a gradual reduction in the dose rather an abrupt cessation is recommended.

Potential Interaction with Thioridazine and Mesoridazine: The effect of fluvoxamine (25 mg bid for one week) on thioridazine steady-state concentrations was evaluated in 10 male inpatients with schizophrenia. Concentrations of thioridazine and its two active metabolites, mesoridazine and sulforidazine, increased threefold following co-administration of fluvoxamine.

Thioridazine and mesoridazine administration produces a dose-related prolongation of the QTc interval, which is associated with serious ventricular arrhythmias, such as torsades de pointes-type arrhythmias, and sudden death. It is likely that this experience underestimates the degree of risk that might occur with higher doses of thioridazine. Moreover, the effect of fluvoxamine may even be more pronounced when it is administered at higher doses. Therefore LUVOX (fluvoxamine maleate) and thioridazine or mesoridazine should not be co-administered (see Contraindications) and Precautions).

Potential Interaction with Terfenadine, Astemizole and Cisapride: Terfenadine, astemizole, and cisapride are all metabolized by CYP3A4. Since fluvoxamine maleate is known to inhibit CYP3A4, theoretically, there may be a potential interaction with terfenadine, astemizole, or cisapride. Consequently, it is recommended that fluvoxamine maleate not be used in combination with terfenadine, astemizole, or cisapride (see Contraindications and Precautions, Drug Interactions).

Potential Interaction with Drugs with a Narrow Therapeutic Index: There may be a potential interaction between fluvoxamine maleate and drugs metabolized by CYP3A4 that have a narrow therapeutic index (e.g., carbamazepine, methadone and cyclosporine). Patients administered these combinations should be carefully monitored and, if necessary, dose adjustment of these drugs is recommended (see Precautions, Drug Interactions).

PRECAUTIONS: Discontinuation Symptoms: When discontinuing treatment, patients should be monitored for symptoms which may be associated with discontinuation [e.g., dizziness, abnormal dreams, sensory disturbances (including paresthesias and electric shock sensations), agitation, anxiety, fatigue, confusion, headache, tremor, nausea, vomiting, and sweating or other symptoms which may be of clinical significance (see Adverse Effects)]. A gradual reduction in the dosage over several weeks, rather than abrupt cessation is recommended whenever possible. If intolerable symptoms occur following a decrease in the dose or upon discontinuation of treatment, dose titration should be managed on the basis of the patient's clinical response (see Adverse Effects and Dosage). If fluvoxamine is used until or shortly before giving birth, discontinuation effects in the newborn may occur (see also Precautions, Pregnancy).

Suicide/Suicidal Thoughts or Clinical Worsening: The possibility of a suicide attempt is inherent in depression and may persist until significant remission occurs. Patients with depression may experience worsening of their depressive symptoms and/or the emergence of suicidal ideation and behaviours (suicidality) whether or not they are taking antidepressant medications. Close supervision of high-risk patients should accompany drug therapy and consideration should be given to the possible need for hospitalization. Physicians should encourage patients of all ages to report any new or worsened distressing thoughts or feelings occurring at any time. In order to minimize the opportunity for overdosage, prescriptions for LUVOX (fluvoxamine maleate) should be written for the smallest quantity of drug consistent with good patient management.

Obsessive compulsive disorders can also be associated with an increased risk of suicide-related events.

Patients with a history of suicide-related events or those exhibiting a significant degree of suicidal ideation prior to commencement of treatment are known to be at a greater risk of suicidal thoughts or suicide attempts, and should receive careful monitoring during treatment. Close supervision of patients and in particular those at high risk should accompany drug therapy especially in early treatment and following dose changes. Patients (and caregivers of patients) should be alerted about the need to monitor for any clinical worsening, suicidal behaviour or thoughts and unusual changes in behaviour and to seek medical advice immediately if these symptoms present.

Because of the well established co-morbidity between depression and other psychiatric disorders, the same precautions observed when treating patients with depression should be observed when treating patients with other psychiatric disorders, e.g. obsessive compulsive disorder (see Warnings, Potential Association with Behavioural and Emotional Changes, Including Self-Harm).

Akathisia/Psychomotor Restlessness: The use of fluvoxamine has been associated with the development of akathisia, characterized by a subjectively unpleasant or distressing restlessness and need to move, often accompanied by an inability to sit or stand still. This is most likely to occur within the first few weeks of treatment. In patients who develop these symptoms, increasing the dose may be detrimental and is not recommended.

Seizures: Convulsions have been reported rarely during LUVOX (fluvoxamine maleate) administration. Caution is recommended when the drug is administered to patients with a history of seizures. Fluvoxamine maleate should be avoided in patients with unstable epilepsy and patients with controlled epilepsy should be carefully monitored. Treatment with fluvoxamine maleate should be discontinued if seizures occur or if seizure frequency increases. Seizures have also been reported as a discontinuation symptom (see also Precautions, Discontinuation Symptoms, Adverse Effects, Discontinuation Symptoms, Dosage, Discontinuation of LUVOX Treatment).

Disturbance of Glycemic Control: Glycemic control may be disturbed, especially in the early stages of the treatment. Reported events include hyperglycemia, hypoglycemia, diabetes mellitus and decreased glucose tolerance; these have been reported in both patients with and without pre-existing disturbance of glycemic control. The dosage of anti-diabetic drugs may need to be adjusted.

ECT: Concurrent administration with electroshock therapy should be avoided because of the absence of experience in this area.

Hepatic Enzymes: Treatment with fluvoxamine maleate has been rarely associated with increases in hepatic enzymes, usually accompanied by symptoms. Fluvoxamine maleate administration should be discontinued in such cases.

Combination with Alcohol: Fluvoxamine maleate may potentiate the effects of alcohol and increase the level of psychomotor impairment.

Serotonin Syndrome: On rare occasions, development of a serotonin syndrome or neuroleptic malignant syndrome-like events have been reported in association with treatment of fluvoxamine, particularly when given in combination with other serotonergic and/or neuroleptic drugs. As these syndromes may result in potentially life-threatening conditions, treatment with fluvoxamine maleate should be discontinued and supportive treatment initiated, if characteristic events occur i.e., clusters of symptoms such as hyperthermia, rigidity, myoclonus, autonomic instability with possible rapid fluctuations of vital signs, mental status changes including confusion, irritability, extreme agitation progressing to delirium and coma (see also Precautions, Drug Interactions, Serotonergic Drugs).

Hyponatremia: As with other SSRIs, hyponatremia has been rarely reported, and appeared to be reversible when fluvoxamine maleate was discontinued. Some cases were possibly due to the syndrome of inappropriate antidiuretic hormone secretion. The majority of reports were associated with older patients.

Occupational Hazards: Cognitive and Motor Disturbances: Sedation may occur in some patients. Therefore, patients should be cautioned about participating in activities requiring complete mental alertness, judgement, and physical coordination—such as driving an automobile or performing hazardous tasks—until they are reasonably certain that treatment with LUVOX (fluvoxamine maleate) does not affect them adversely.

Concomitant Illness: LUVOX (fluvoxamine maleate) has not been evaluated or used to any appreciable extent in patients with a recent history of myocardial infarction or unstable heart disease. Patients with these diagnoses were systematically excluded from premarketing clinical studies.

Haemorrhage: SSRIs and serotonin/norepinephrine reuptake inhibitors (SNRIs), including LUVOX (fluvoxamine maleate), may increase the risk of bleeding events. Concomitant use of aspirin, nonsteroidal anti-inflammatory drugs (NSAIDs), warfarin, and other anticoagulants may add to this risk. Case reports and epidemiological studies (case-control and cohort design) have demonstrated an association between use of drugs that interfere with serotonin reuptake and the occurrence of gastrointestinal bleeding. There have been reports of bleeding events ranging from ecchymoses, hematomas, epistaxis, and petechiae to life-threatening haemorrhages, associated with treatment with SSRIs and SNRIs.

Caution is advised in patients taking SSRIs and SNRIs, particularly in concomitant use with drugs known to affect platelet function (e.g. atypical antipsychotics and phenothiazines, most tricyclic antidepressants, anticoagulants, platelet aggregation inhibitors, acetylsalicylic acid and NSAIDs), as well as in patients with a history of bleeding disorders.

Pregnancy: Safe use of fluvoxamine maleate during pregnancy and lactation has not been established. Like other antidepressants, fluvoxamine maleate is excreted via human milk in small quantities. Therefore, it should not be administered to women of childbearing potential or nursing mothers unless, in the opinion of the treating physician, the expected benefits to the patient outweigh the possible hazards to the child or fetus.

Complications Following Late Third Trimester Exposure to SSRIs: Post-marketing reports indicate that some neonates exposed to LUVOX (fluvoxamine maleate), SSRIs (Selective Serotonin Reuptake Inhibitors), or other newer anti-depressants late in the third trimester have developed complications requiring prolonged hospitalization, respiratory support, and tube feeding. Such complications can arise immediately upon delivery. Reported clinical findings have included respiratory distress, cyanosis, apnea, seizures, temperature instability, feeding difficulty, vomiting, hypoglycemia, hypotonia, hypertonia, hyperreflexia, tremor, jitteriness, irritability, and constant crying. These features are consistent with either a direct toxic effect of SSRIs and other newer anti-depressants, or, possibly, a drug discontinuation syndrome. It should be noted that, in some cases, the clinical picture is consistent with serotonin syndrome (see Precautions, Serotonin Syndrome). When treating a pregnant woman with LUVOX (fluvoxamine maleate) the physician should carefully consider the potential risks and benefits of treatment (see Dosage).

Risk of PPHN and Exposure to SSRIs: In one epidemiological case-control study on persistent pulmonary hypertension (PPHN) with n=377 infants with PPHN and n=836 matched control infants, PPHN was six times more common in babies whose mothers took an SSRI antidepressant after the 20th week of pregnancy compared to babies whose mothers did not take an antidepressant. The study was too small to determine relative risks among the specific SSRIs. This information is considered to be preliminary at this time. The absolute risk of PPHN in the general population is reported to be 1-2 per 1000.

Lactation: See Pregnancy.

Children: Safety and efficacy in children under 18 years of age have not been established.

Drug Interactions: LUVOX (fluvoxamine maleate) is contraindicated in combined use with tizanidine, MAO inhibitors, linezolid (an antibiotic which is a reversible non-selective MAO inhibitor), thioridazine, or mesoridazine (see Contraindications and Warnings). Isolated cases of cardiac toxicity have been reported when fluvoxamine was combined with thioridazine (see Contraindications and Warnings).

Cytochrome P450 Enzymes: Fluvoxamine maleate is a potent inhibitor of CYP1A2, and to a lesser extent of CYP2C and CYP3A4. Drugs which are largely metabolised via these isoenzymes are eliminated slower and may have higher plasma concentrations when co-administered with fluvoxamine maleate. This is particularly relevant for drugs with a narrow therapeutic index. Patients should be carefully monitored and, if necessary, dose adjustment of these drugs is recommended.

CYP1A2: An increase in previously stable plasma levels of those tricyclic antidepressants (e.g., clomipramine, imipramine, amitriptyline) and neuroleptics (e.g., clozapine, olanzapine) which are largely metabolized through CYP1A2, has been reported in patients taking fluvoxamine maleate concomitantly. Thus, the combination of these drugs with fluvoxamine is not recommended.

Patients co-administered fluvoxamine maleate and CYP1A2 metabolized drugs with a narrow therapeutic index (such as tacrine, theophylline, methadone, mexiletine, clozapine, warfarin) should be carefully monitored and, if necessary, dose adjustment of these drugs is recommended.

Warfarin plasma concentrations were significantly increased, and prothrombin times prolonged during concurrent administration of fluvoxamine maleate; in interaction studies, a 65% increase in warfarin plasma levels were seen.

As plasma concentrations of propranolol are increased in combination with fluvoxamine maleate, the propranolol dose may need to be lowered; a 5-fold increase in plasma levels of propranolol was seen in interaction studies.

When a single 40 mg dose of tacrine was added to fluvoxamine maleate 100 mg/day administered at steady-state, an associated five and eight fold increase in tacrine C_{max} and AUC, respectively, were observed.

Caffeine plasma levels are likely to be increased during co-administration with fluvoxamine maleate. Thus, patients who consume high quantities of caffeine-containing beverages should lower their intake when fluvoxamine maleate is administered and adverse caffeine effects (like tremor, palpitations, nausea, restlessness, insomnia) are observed.

As plasma concentrations of ropinirole may be increased in combination with fluvoxamine maleate thus increasing the risk of overdose, surveillance and reduction in the dosage of ropinirole during fluvoxamine maleate treatment and after its withdrawal may be required.

CYP2C: Fluvoxamine maleate is also believed to inhibit CYP2C and thus may interact with CYP2C substrates like diazepam. Clearance of both diazepam and its active metabolite N-desmethyldiazepam were reduced with concurrent administration of fluvoxamine maleate.

Patients co-administered fluvoxamine maleate and CYP2C metabolised drugs with a narrow therapeutic index (such as phenytoin) should be carefully monitored and, if necessary, dose adjustment of these drugs is recommended.

CYP3A4: Fluvoxamine maleate is also known to inhibit CYP3A4 and thus may interact with CYP3A4 substrates like diltiazem and alprazolam. A clinically significant interaction is possible with CYP3A4 substrates that have a narrow therapeutic index such as carbamazepine, methadone, and cyclosporine. Such combinations should therefore be administered with caution, and consideration be given to lowering the dose of the concomitant agent. A significantly increased methadone plasma level/dose ratio was seen during concurrent administration of fluvoxamine maleate. When fluvoxamine maleate and alprazolam were co-administered to steady state, plasma concentrations and other pharmacokinetic parameters (AUC, C_{max}, $T_{½}$) of alprazolam were approximately twice those observed when alprazolam was administered alone; clearance was reduced by about 50%. Since terfenadine, astemizole, and cisapride, are metabolized by CYP3A4, theoretically there may be a potential interaction with fluvoxamine maleate that could result in an increased risk for QT prolongation/torsades de pointes. Thus, it is recommended that fluvoxamine maleate not be used in combination with terfenadine, astemizole, or cisapride (see Contraindications).

CYP2D6: CYP2D6 is responsible for the metabolism of substrates such as debrisoquine, sparteine, tricyclic antidepressants (e.g., nortriptyline, amitriptyline, imipramine, and desipramine), phenothiazine neuroleptics (e.g., perphenazine and thioridazine), and Type 1C antiarrhythmics (e.g., propafenone and flecainide). In vitro data suggest that fluvoxamine maleate is a relatively weak inhibitor of CYP2D6, and hence the potential for interactions with compounds metabolized by this isoenzyme is low.

Oxidative Metabolism: The plasma levels of oxidatively metabolised benzodiazepines (e.g., triazolam, midazolam, alprazolam, and diazepam) are likely to be increased when co-administered with fluvoxamine maleate. The dosage of these benzodiazepines should be reduced during co-administration with fluvoxamine.

Glucuronidation: Fluvoxamine maleate does not influence plasma concentrations of digoxin. The clearance of benzodiazepines metabolized by glucuronidation (e.g., lorazepam, oxazepam, temazepam) is unlikely to be affected by fluvoxamine maleate.

Renal Excretion: Fluvoxamine maleate does not influence plasma concentrations of atenolol.

Pharmacodynamic Interactions: CNS Active Drugs: The serotonergic effects of fluvoxamine may be enhanced when used in combination with other serotonergic agents (including triptans, tramodol, SSRIs and St. John's Wort preparations).

St. John's Wort: In common with other SSRIs, pharmacodynamic interactions between fluvoxamine maleate and the herbal remedy St. John's Wort may occur and may result in an increase in undesirable effects.

Lithium, and possibly tryptophan, may enhance the serotonergic effects of fluvoxamine maleate; these combinations should therefore be used with caution. This may, on rare occasions, result in a serotonergic syndrome.

As with other psychotropic drugs patients should be advised to avoid alcohol use while taking fluvoxamine.

Oral Anticoagulants: In patients on oral anticoagulants and fluvoxamine, the risk for haemorrhage may increase and these patients should therefore be closely monitored.

Metabolism of Fluvoxamine: The specific CYP isoenzymes involved in the metabolism of fluvoxamine maleate remains to be identified.

ADVERSE EFFECTS: Commonly Observed: In clinical trials, the most commonly observed adverse events associated with LUVOX (fluvoxamine maleate) administration, and not seen at an equivalent incidence among placebo-treated patients, were gastrointestinal complaints, including nausea (sometimes accompanied by vomiting), constipation, anorexia, diarrhea and dyspepsia; central nervous system complaints, including somnolence, dry mouth, nervousness, insomnia, dizziness, tremor and agitation; and asthenia. Abnormal (mostly delayed) ejaculation was frequently reported by patients with obsessive compulsive disorder, primarily at doses over 150 mg/day.

Adverse Events Leading to Discontinuation of Treatment: Approximately 14% (14.4%) of 34,587 patients who received LUVOX (fluvoxamine maleate) in clinical trials discontinued treatment due to an adverse event. The more common events causing discontinuation from depression trials included nausea and vomiting, insomnia, agitation, headache, abdominal pain, somnolence, dizziness, asthenia and anorexia. The most common events causing discontinuation in patients suffering from obsessive compulsive disorder included insomnia, asthenia and somnolence.

Incidence of Adverse Experiences: Adverse events with an incidence of ≥5% reported in double-blind, placebo-controlled clinical trials in depression and in obsessive-compulsive disorder are presented in Table 1 for each indication.

Table 1: LUVOX

Treatment-Emergent Adverse Experience Incidence (≥5%) in Placebo-Controlled Clinical Trials for Depression and Obsessive-Compulsive Disorder[a]

	Percentage of Patients Reporting Event			
	Depression		OCD	
Body System/Adverse Event	Fluvoxamine (N=222)	Placebo (N=192)	Fluvoxamine (N=160)	Placebo (N=160)
Nervous System				
Somnolence	26.2	9.0	26.9	9.4
Agitation	15.7	8.9	3.8	0
Insomnia	14.4	10.4	31.3	15.0
Dizziness	14.8	13.5	9.4	4.4
Tremor	10.8	4.7	8.1	0.6
Hypokinesia	8.1	3.6	—	—
Hyperkinesia	6.7	8.9	—	—
Depression	4.0	4.2	6.3	4.4
Nervousness	2.2	1.6	15.6	5.0
Anxiety	2.3	2.1	9.4	6.9
Libido Decreased	—	—	7.5	1.9
Thinking Abnormal	—	—	6.9	3.8
Digestive System				
Nausea	36.5	10.9	28.8	6.9
Dry Mouth	25.7	23.9	11.9	3.1
Constipation	18.0	6.8	14.4	8.8
Anorexia	14.9	6.3	5.0	3.1
Diarrhea	5.9	6.3	11.9	8.8
Dyspepsia	3.2	0	13.8	9.4
Body as a Whole				
Headache	21.6	18.7	20.0	23.8
Pain	5.9	3.7	4.4	1.3
Asthenia	4.9	3.2	28.8	9.4
Infection	—	—	11.3	9.4
Abdominal Pain	3.6	3.6	5.6	8.1
Flu Syndrome	—	—	5.0	3.8
Skin				
Sweating Increased	11.2	12.5	6.9	1.9
Respiratory System				
Pharyngitis	—	—	6.3	5.0
Rhinitis	1.3	2.6	5.6	1.9
Special Senses				
Accommodation Abnormal	6.3	6.3	—	—
Taste Perversion	3.2	3.1	5.0	0
Urogenital				
Urinary Frequency	2.2	1.6	5.0	1.3
Abnormal Ejaculation	1.4	0	17.9[b]	0

[a] Dosage titration at study initiation varied between the depression and OCD trials. In depression, fluvoxamine was administered: Day 1, 50 mg; Day 2, 100 mg; Day 3, 150 mg then titrated to response. In OCD, fluvoxamine was administered: Days 1-4, 50 mg; Days 5-8, 100 mg, Days 9-14, 150 mg then titrated to response.

[b] Corrected for gender (males: n=78).

Additional Adverse Events Reported in Clinical Trials: During premarketing and postmarketing studies, multiple doses of LUVOX (fluvoxamine maleate) were administered to approximately 34 587 patients. All events with an incidence of >0.01% are listed, regardless of relation to drug, except those in terms so general as to be uninformative. Events are further classified within body system categories and enumerated in order of decreasing frequency using the following definitions: frequent (occurring on 1 or more occasions in at least 1/100 patients), infrequent (occurring in less than 1/100, but at least 1/1000 patients), or rare (occurring in less than 1/1000 but at least in 1/10 000 patients). Multiple events may have been reported by a single patient. It is important to emphasize that although the events reported did occur during treatment with LUVOX (fluvoxamine maleate), they were not necessarily caused by it.

Nervous: Frequent: agitation, anxiety, dizziness, insomnia, nervousness, somnolence, thinking abnormal, tremor, vertigo. Infrequent: abnormal dreams, abnormal gait, akathisia, amnesia, apathy, ataxia, confusion, depersonalization, depression, drug dependence, emotional lability, euphoria, hallucinations, hostility, hyperkinesia, hypertonia, hypoesthesia, hypokinesia, incoordination, increased salivation, libido decreased, libido increased, manic reaction, neurosis, paraesthesia, psychotic depression, stupor, twitching, vasodilatation. Rare: akinesia, CNS neoplasia, CNS stimulation, coma, convulsion, delirium, delusions, dysarthria, dyskinesia, dystonia, extrapyramidal syndrome, hemiplegia, hyperesthesia, hypotonia, hysteria, myoclonus, neuralgia, neuropathy, paralysis, paranoid reaction, psychosis, reflexes decreased, schizophrenic reaction, screaming syndrome, torticollis, trismus.

Digestive: Frequent: anorexia, constipation, diarrhea, dry mouth, dyspepsia, nausea, vomiting. Infrequent: colitis, dysphagia, eructation, flatulence, gastritis, gastroenteritis, increased appetite, thirst. Rare: biliary pain, esophagitis, fecal incontinence, gastrointestinal carcinoma, gastrointestinal haemorrhage, gingivitis, glossitis, hematemesis, hepatitis, jaundice, liver function tests abnormal, hepatic function abnormal, melena, mouth ulceration, rectal haemorrhage, stomatitis, tenesmus, tongue discoloration, tongue edema, tooth disorder.

Cardiovascular: Frequent: palpitation. Infrequent: angina pectoris, hypertension, hypotension, migraine, postural hypotension, syncope, tachycardia. Rare: arrhythmia, , bradycardia, cerebrovascular accident, extrasystoles, haemorrhage, myocardial infarct, pallor, peripheral vascular disorder, shock.

Body as a Whole: Frequent: abdominal pain, asthenia, headache, malaise. Infrequent: accidental injury, allergic reaction, back pain, chest pain, chills, fever, flu syndrome, infection, neck pain, pain, suicide attempt. Rare: abdomen enlarged, chills and fever, face edema, halitosis, hangover effect, hernia, neck rigidity, overdose, pelvic pain.

Skin: Frequent: sweating increased. Infrequent: cutaneous hypersensitivity reactions (including rash, pruritus, angioedema). Rare: acne, alopecia, dry skin, eczema, furunculosis, herpes simplex, herpes zoster, maculopapular rash, psoriasis, urticaria.

Respiratory: Infrequent: dyspnea, pharyngitis, rhinitis. Rare: asthma, bronchitis, cough increased, epistaxis, hiccup, hyperventilation, laryngismus, laryngitis, pneumonia, sinusitis, voice alteration, yawn.
Special Senses: Infrequent: abnormal vision, amblyopia, hyperacusis. Rare: abnormality of accommodation, blepharitis, conjunctivitis, deafness, diplopia, dry eyes, ear pain, eye pain, lacrimation disorder, mydriasis, parosmia, photophobia, taste loss.
Musculoskeletal: Infrequent: arthralgia, arthrosis, myalgia, myasthenia, tetany. Rare: arthritis, bone pain, leg cramps, pathological fracture, rheumatoid arthritis.
Urogenital: Infrequent: abnormal ejaculation, dysuria, impotence, metrorrhagia, urinary frequency, urinary incontinence. Rare: amenorrhea, anorgasmia, breast pain, cystitis, dysmenorrhea, female lactation, hematuria, kidney pain, leukorrhea, menorrhagia, nocturia, polyuria, prostatic disorder, urinary retention, urinary tract infection, urinary urgency, vaginitis.
Metabolic and Nutritional: Frequent: weight gain. Infrequent: peripheral edema, weight loss. Rare: alcohol intolerance, dehydration, edema, obesity.
Hematic and Lymph Systems: Rare: anemia, cyanosis, ecchymosis, lymphadenopathy, thrombocytopenia.
Hemorrhage: See Precautions.
Adverse Effects Following Discontinuation of Treatment (or dose reduction): There have been reports of adverse reactions upon the discontinuation of LUVOX (fluvoxamine maleate) (particularly when abrupt), including but not limited to the following: dizziness, abnormal dreams, sensory disturbances (including paresthesias and electric shock sensations), agitation, anxiety, fatigue, confusion, headache, tremor, nausea, vomiting and sweating or other symptoms which may be of clinical significance (see Precautions and Dosage).

Patients should be monitored for these or any other symptoms. A gradual reduction in the dosage over several weeks, rather than abrupt cessation is recommended whenever possible. If intolerable symptoms occur following a decrease in the dose or upon discontinuation of treatment, dose titration should be managed on the basis of the patient's clinical response. These events are generally self-limiting. Symptoms associated with discontinuation have been reported for other selective serotonin reuptake inhibitors. Isolated cases of withdrawal symptoms in the newborn child have been described after the use of fluvoxamine maleate at the end of pregnancy (see Precautions and Dosage). Some newborns experience feeding and/or respiratory difficulties, seizures, temperature instability, hypoglycemia, tremor, abnormal muscle tone, jitteriness, and constant crying after third trimester exposure to SSRIs and may require prolonged hospitalization.

Anecdotal spontaneous reports, from the marketplace, but not from clinical trials, have been collected for the following adverse experiences: galactorrhoea, photosensitivity, Stevens-Johnson Syndrome, alopecia, taste perversion, tinnitus, psychomotor restlessness, micturition disorder (including enuresis), drug withdrawal syndrome (including drug withdrawal syndrome neonatal) and haemorrhagic manifestations e.g. ecchymoses, purpura, gastrointestinal bleeding (see Warnings and Precautions). Cases of suicidal ideation and suicidal behaviours have been reported during fluvoxamine therapy or early after treatment discontinuation. Rarely, serotonin syndrome, neuroleptic malignant syndrome-like events, hyponatremia and SIADH have been reported (see Precautions, Serotonin Syndrome; and Precautions, Drug Interactions, CNS Active Drugs).

OVERDOSE:

Symptoms: LUVOX (fluvoxamine maleate) received its first marketing authorization worldwide in 1983 therefore it has been on the market for more than 25 years. In the cumulative post-marketing experience for fluvoxamine, there are over 700 cases in the safety database associated with the adverse drug reaction, overdose (or a similarly-related term). In the majority of these cases, the patients were taking multiple drugs in addition to fluvoxamine. In such cases, it is difficult to differentiate the additive drug effects or drug interactions that may have impacted patient outcome. The smallest estimated dose of fluvoxamine alone associated with a fatal outcome is approximately 1800 mg.

The most common symptoms of overdosage include gastrointestinal complaints (nausea, vomiting, and diarrhoea), somnolence, and dizziness. Cardiac events (tachycardia, bradycardia, hypotension), liver function disturbances, convulsions, and coma have also been reported.

Treatment: There is no specific antidote to fluvoxamine maleate. In situations of overdosage, the stomach should be emptied as soon as possible after tablet ingestion and symptomatic treatment initiated. The repeated use of medicinal charcoal is also recommended. Due to the large distribution volume of fluvoxamine maleate, forced diuresis or dialysis is unlikely to be of benefit.

For management of a suspected drug overdose, contact your regional Poison Control Centre. See the *CPS* Directory section for a list of Poison Control Centres.

DOSAGE: LUVOX (fluvoxamine maleate) is not indicated for use in children under 18 years of age (see Warnings, Potential Association with Behavioural and Emotional Changes, Including Self-Harm).
Depression: Adult Dosage: Treatment should be initiated at the lowest possible dose (50 mg) given once daily at bedtime, and then increased to 100 mg daily at bedtime after a few days, as tolerated. The effective daily dose usually lies between 100 and 200 mg, and should be adjusted gradually according to the individual response of the patient, up to a maximum of 300 mg. Dosage increases should be made in 50 mg increments. Doses above 150 mg should be divided so that a maximum of 150 mg is given in the bedtime dose. Tablets should be swallowed with water and without chewing.
Obsessive-Compulsive Disorder: Adult Dosage: Treatment should be initiated at the lowest possible dose (50 mg) given once daily at bedtime, and then increased to 100 mg daily at bedtime after a few days, as tolerated. The effective daily dose usually lies between 100 mg and 300 mg, and should be adjusted gradually according to the individual response of the patient, up to a maximum of 300 mg. If no improvement is observed within 10 weeks, treatment with LUVOX (fluvoxamine maleate) should be reconsidered. Dosage increases should be made in 50 mg increments. Doses above 150 mg should be divided so that a maximum of 150 mg is given in the bedtime dose. LUVOX (fluvoxamine maleate) should be swallowed with water and without chewing.
Discontinuation of Treatment: Symptoms associated with the discontinuation or dosage reduction of LUVOX (fluvoxamine maleate) have been reported. Patients should be monitored for these and other symptoms when discontinuing treatment or during dosage reduction (see Precautions and Adverse Effects).

A gradual reduction in the dose over several weeks rather than abrupt cessation is recommended whenever possible. If intolerable symptoms occur following a decrease in the dose or upon discontinuation of treatment, dose titration should be managed on the basis of the patient's clinical response (see Precautions and Adverse Effects).
Hepatic or Renal Insufficiency: Patients with hepatic or renal insufficiency should begin treatment with a low dose and be carefully monitored.
Children: The safety and effectiveness of fluvoxamine maleate in children under 18 years of age have not been established (see Warnings, Potential Association with Behavioural and Emotional Changes, Including Self-Harm).
Treatment of Pregnant Women During the Third Trimester: Post-marketing reports indicate that some neonates exposed to LUVOX (fluvoxamine maleate), SSRIs, or other newer anti-depressants late in the third trimester have developed complications requiring prolonged hospitalization, respiratory support, and tube feeding (see Precautions). When treating pregnant women with LUVOX (fluvoxamine maleate) the physician should carefully consider the potential risks and benefits of treatment. The physician may consider tapering LUVOX (fluvoxamine maleate) in the third trimester.
Geriatrics: Since there is limited clinical experience in the geriatric age group, caution is recommended when administering fluvoxamine maleate to elderly patients.

INFORMATION FOR THE PATIENT: Published in e-CPS, available by subscription at www.e-cps.ca.

SUPPLIED: 50 mg: Each film-coated, biconvex, round, scored, white tablet, stamped "291" twice on one side and a stylized "S" on the other, contains: fluvoxamine maleate 50 mg. Nonmedicinal ingredients: colloidal anhydrous silica, hypromellose, maize starch, mannitol, polyethylene glycol 6000, pregelatinized starch, sodium stearyl fumarate, talc and titanium dioxide. Blister packages of 30. Store in a dry place at temperatures between 15-25°C. Protect from light.
100 mg: Each film-coated, biconvex, oval, scored, white tablet, stamped "313" twice on one side and a stylized "S" on the other contains: fluvoxamine maleate 100 mg. Nonmedicinal ingredients: colloidal anhydrous silica, hypromellose, maize starch, mannitol, polyethylene glycol 6000, pregelatinized starch, sodium stearyl fumarate, talc and titanium dioxide. Blister packages of 30. Store in a dry place at temperatures between 15-25°C. Protect from light.

(Shown in Product Identification Section)

Lyderm® Ⓟ
fluocinonide
Topical Corticosteroid

TaroPharma

SUPPLIED: Cream: Each g of cream contains: fluocinonide 0.5 mg (0.05%). Nonmedicinal ingredients: 1, 2, 6-hexanetriol, citric acid, glycerin, polyethylene glycols, propylene glycol and stearyl alcohol. Tubes of 15 and 60 g. Jars of 400 g.
Gel: Each g of gel contains: fluocinonide 0.5 mg (0.05%). Nonmedicinal ingredients: carbomer 940, edetate disodium, propylene glycol, propyl gallate, purified water and sodium hydroxide. Tubes of 15 and 60 g.
Ointment: Each g of ointment contains: fluocinonide 0.5 mg (0.05%). Nonmedicinal ingredients: glyceryl monostearate, propylene carbonate, propylene glycol, white petrolatum and white wax. Tubes of 60 g.
Store at room temperature (15 to 30 °C).

Lyrica® Ⓟ
pregabalin
Analgesic

Pfizer

Date of Revision: June 21, 2010

SUMMARY PRODUCT INFORMATION:

Route of Administration	Dosage Form/Strength	All Nonmedicinal Ingredients
Oral	Capsules, 25 mg, 50 mg, 75 mg, 150 mg, 225 mg, 300 mg	Lactose monohydrate, maize starch, and talc Capsule shells contain gelatin and titanium dioxide. In addition, orange capsule shells contain red iron oxide. White capsule shells contain sodium lauryl sulphate and colloidal silicon dioxide.

INDICATIONS AND CLINICAL USE: Adults: LYRICA (pregabalin) is indicated for the management of neuropathic pain associated with:

- Diabetic peripheral neuropathy and
- Postherpetic neuralgia

LYRICA is indicated for the management of neuropathic pain associated with spinal cord injury.
LYRICA is indicated for the management of pain associated with fibromyalgia.

The efficacy of LYRICA in the management of pain associated with fibromyalgia for up to 6 months was demonstrated in a placebo-controlled trial in patients who had initially responded to LYRICA during a 6-week open-label phase.
Geriatrics (>65 years of age): Pregabalin oral clearance tended to decrease with increasing age. This decrease in pregabalin oral clearance is consistent with age-related decreases in creatinine clearance. Reduction of pregabalin dose may be required in patients who have age related compromised renal function (see Warnings and Precautions, Geriatrics (>65 years of age)).
Pediatrics (<18 years of age): The safety and efficacy of pregabalin in pediatric patients (<18 years of age) have not been established and its use in this patient population is not recommended (see Warnings and Precautions, Pediatrics (<18 years of age)).

CONTRAINDICATIONS: Patients who are hypersensitive to pregabalin or to any ingredient in the formulation or component of the container.

WARNINGS AND PRECAUTIONS: Angioedema: There have been post-marketing reports of angioedema in patients, some without reported previous history/episode(s), during initial/acute and chronic treatment with LYRICA. Specific symptoms included swelling of the face, mouth (tongue, lips, and gums), neck, throat, and larynx/upper airway. There have been reports of life-threatening angioedema with respiratory compromise requiring emergency treatment. Some of these patients did not have reported previous history/episode(s) of angioedema. LYRICA should be immediately discontinued in patients with these symptoms. During the pre-marketing assessment of pregabalin in clinical trials, angioedema was reported as a rare reaction. (See Adverse Reactions, Less Common Clinical Trial Adverse Drug Reactions (<2%) and Post-Marketing Adverse Drug Reactions.)

Caution should be exercised when prescribing LYRICA to patients with previous history/episode(s) of angioedema and related events. In addition, patients who are taking other drugs associated with angioedema (e.g., ACE-inhibitors) may be at increased risk of developing this condition.
Hypersensitivity: There have been postmarketing reports of hypersensitivity reactions (e.g., skin redness, blisters, hives, rash, dyspnea, and wheezing). Pregabalin should be discontinued immediately if such symptoms occur. (See Adverse Reactions, Post-Marketing Adverse Drug Reactions.)
Renal Failure: In both clinical trials of various indications and post-marketing database, there are reports of patients, with or without previous history, experiencing renal failure while receiving pregabalin alone or in combination with other medications. Discontinuation of pregabalin should be considered as it has shown reversibility of this event in some cases. Caution is advised when prescribing pregabalin to the elderly or those with any degree of renal impairment (see Special Populations, Renal, Abrupt or Rapid Discontinuation; Adverse Reactions, Post-Marketing Adverse Drug Reactions; and Dosage and Administration).
Tumorigenic Potential: In standard preclinical in vivo lifetime carcinogenicity studies of pregabalin, a high incidence of hemangiosarcoma was identified in two different strains of mice (see Preclinical Toxicology). The clinical significance of this finding is uncertain. Clinical experience during pregabalin's premarketing development provides no direct means to assess its potential for inducing tumors in humans.

In clinical studies across various patient populations, comprising 6396 patient-years of exposure in 8666 patients ranging in age from 12 to 100 years, new or worsening preexisting tumors were reported in 57 patients. The most common malignant tumor diagnosed was skin carcinoma (17 patients) followed by breast carcinoma (8 patients), prostatic carcinoma (6 patients), carcinoma not otherwise specified (6 patients), and bladder carcinoma (4 patients). Without knowledge of the background incidence and recurrence in similar populations not treated with LYRICA (pregabalin), it is impossible to know whether the incidence seen in these cohorts is or is not affected by treatment.
Ophthalmological Effects: In controlled studies, pregabalin treatment was associated with vision-related adverse events such as blurred vision (amblyopia) [6% pregabalin and 2% placebo] and diplopia (2% pregabalin and 0.5% placebo). Approximately 1% of pregabalin-treated patients discontinued treatment due to vision-related adverse events (primarily blurred vision). Of the patients who did not withdraw, the blurred vision resolved with continued dosing in approximately half of the cases (see Adverse Reactions, Post-Marketing Adverse Drug Reactions).

Prospectively planned ophthalmologic testing, including visual acuity testing, formal visual field testing and dilated funduscopic examination, was performed in over 3600 patients. In these patients, visual acuity was reduced in 7% of patients treated with pregabalin, and 5% of placebo-treated patients. Visual field changes were detected in 13% of pregabalin-treated, and 12% of placebo-treated patients. Funduscopic changes were observed in 2% of pregabalin treated and 2% of placebo-treated patients. At this time, clinical significance of the ophthalmologic findings is unknown.

Patients should be informed that if changes in vision occur, they should notify their physician. If visual disturbance persists, further assessment, including discontinuation of pregabalin, should be considered. More frequent assessments should be considered for patients who are already routinely monitored for ocular conditions.
Peripheral Edema: LYRICA may cause peripheral edema. In controlled peripheral neuropathic pain and fibromyalgia clinical trials, pregabalin treatment caused peripheral edema in 9% of patients compared with 3% of patients in the placebo group. In these studies, 0.7% of pregabalin patients and 0.3% of placebo patients withdrew due to peripheral edema (see Adverse Reactions, Peripheral Edema).

In controlled clinical trials of up to 13 weeks in duration of patients without clinically significant heart or peripheral vascular disease, there was no apparent association between peripheral edema and cardiovascular complications such as hypertension or congestive heart failure. In the same trials, peripheral edema was not associated with laboratory changes suggestive of deterioration in renal or hepatic function.

Higher frequencies of weight gain and peripheral edema were observed in patients taking both LYRICA and a thiazolidinedione antidiabetic agent compared to patients taking either drug alone. The majority of patients using thiazolidinedione antidiabetic agents in the overall safety database were participants in studies of pain associated with diabetic peripheral neuropathy. In this population, peripheral edema was reported in 3% (2/60) of patients who were using thiazolidinedione antidiabetic agents only, 8% (69/859) of patients who were treated with pregabalin only, and 19% (23/120) of patients who were on both pregabalin and thiazolidinedione antidiabetic agents. Similarly, weight gain was reported in 0% (0/60) of patients on thiazolidinediones only; 4% (35/859) of patients on pregabalin only; and 7.5% (9/120) of patients on both drugs.

As the thiazolidinedione class of antidiabetic drugs can cause weight gain and/or fluid retention, possibly exacerbating or leading to heart failure, care should be taken when co-administering LYRICA and these agents.

Congestive Heart Failure: In controlled clinical studies, events of congestive heart failure were reported at an infrequent rate (between 0.1% and 1%; see Adverse Reactions, Less Common Clinical Trial Adverse Drug Reactions (<2%)).

There have been post-marketing reports of congestive heart failure in some patients receiving pregabalin (see Adverse Reactions, Post-Marketing Adverse Drug Reactions). Although this adverse reaction has mostly been observed in elderly cardiovascular compromised patients during pregabalin treatment for a neuropathic pain indication, some cases have occurred in patients without reported edema or previous history of cardiovascular disease. Pregabalin should be used with caution in these patients. Discontinuation of pregabalin may resolve the reaction.

Gastrointestinal: There have been post-marketing reports of events related to reduced lower gastrointestinal tract function (e.g., intestinal obstruction, paralytic ileus, and constipation) in patients, some without reported previous history/episode(s), during initial/acute and chronic treatment with LYRICA, primarily in combination with other medications that have the potential to produce constipation. Some of these events were considered serious and required hospitalization. In a number of instances, patients were taking opioid analgesics including tramadol.

Caution should be exercised when LYRICA and opioid analgesics are used in combination, and measures to prevent constipation may be considered, especially in female patients and elderly as they may be at increased risk of experiencing lower gastrointestinal-related events (see Adverse Reactions, Post-Marketing Adverse Drug Reactions).

Weight Gain: LYRICA may cause weight gain. In pregabalin-controlled peripheral neuropathic pain and fibromyalgia clinical trials with durations of up to 14 weeks, a gain of 7% or more over baseline weight was observed in 8% of pregabalin treated patients and 3% of placebo-treated patients. Few patients treated with pregabalin (0.6%) withdrew from controlled trials due to weight gain (see Adverse Reactions, Weight Gain).

Pregabalin-associated weight gain was related to dose and duration of exposure. Pregabalin-associated weight gain did not appear to be associated with baseline BMI, gender, or age. Weight gain was not limited to patients with edema and was not necessarily due to edema-related events (see Warnings and Precautions, Peripheral Edema).

Although weight gain was not associated with clinically important changes in blood pressure in short-term controlled studies, the long-term cardiovascular effects of pregabalin-associated weight gain are unknown.

Among diabetic patients, pregabalin-treated patients gained an average of 1.6 kg (range: −16 to 16 kg), compared to an average 0.3 kg (range: −10 to 9 kg) weight gain in placebo patients. In a cohort of 333 diabetic patients who received pregabalin for at least 2 years, the average weight gain was 5.2 kg.

In the controlled fibromyalgia clinical trials, 10.7% of pregabalin-treated patients experienced weight gain of 7% or greater compared to 4.9% of placebo-treated patients. Pregabalin-treated patients gained an average of 1.7 kg compared to an average of 0.7 kg weight gain in placebo patients.

While the effects of pregabalin-associated weight gain on glycemic control have not been systematically assessed, in controlled and longer-term open label clinical trials with diabetic patients, pregabalin treatment did not appear to be associated with loss of glycemic control (as measured by HbA_{1C}).

Dizziness and Somnolence: LYRICA may cause dizziness and somnolence. In controlled peripheral neuropathic pain and fibromyalgia studies, pregabalin caused dizziness in 32% of patients compared to 8% in placebo. Somnolence was experienced by 17% and 4% of the patients treated with pregabalin and placebo, respectively. These events begin shortly after the initiation of therapy and generally occur more frequently at higher doses. In these studies, dizziness and somnolence led to withdrawal of 5% (placebo: 0.5%) and 3% (placebo: 0.1%) of the pregabalin-treated patients, respectively. For the remaining patients who experienced these events, dizziness and somnolence persisted until the last dose of pregabalin in 35% and 49% of the patients, respectively (see Adverse Reactions, Table 2 and Table 4, and Table 11 and Post-Marketing Adverse Drug Reactions).

Accordingly, patients should be advised not to drive or operate complex machinery or engage in other hazardous activities until they have gained sufficient experience on pregabalin to gauge whether or not it affects their mental and/or motor performance adversely (see Information for the Patient).

Abrupt or Rapid Discontinuation: Following abrupt or rapid discontinuation of pregabalin, some patients reported symptoms including insomnia, nausea, headache, anxiety, hyperhidrosis, and diarrhea. Pregabalin should be tapered gradually over a minimum of one week rather than discontinued abruptly (see Adverse Reactions, Adverse Events Following Abrupt or Rapid Discontinuation).

Sexual Function/Reproduction: Impairment of Male Fertility: Preclinical Data: In fertility studies in which male rats were orally administered pregabalin (50 to 2500 mg/kg) prior to and during mating with untreated females, a number of adverse reproductive and developmental effects were observed. These included decreased sperm counts and sperm motility, increased sperm abnormalities, reduced fertility, increased preimplantation embryo loss, decreased litter size, decreased fetal body weights, and an increased incidence of fetal abnormalities. Effects on sperm and fertility parameters were reversible in studies of this duration (3-4 months). The no-effect dose for male reproductive toxicity in these studies (100 mg/kg) was associated with a plasma pregabalin exposure (AUC) approximately 3 times human exposure at the maximum recommended dose (MRD) of 600 mg/day.

In addition, adverse effects on reproductive organ (testes, epididymides) histopathology were observed in male rats exposed to pregabalin (500 to 1250 mg/kg) in general toxicology studies of four weeks or greater duration. The no-effect dose for male reproductive organ histopathology in rats (250 mg/kg) was associated with a plasma exposure approximately 8 times human exposure at the MRD.

In a fertility study in which female rats were given pregabalin (500, 1250, or 2500 mg/kg) orally prior to and during mating and early gestation, disrupted estrous cyclicity and an increased number of days to mating were seen at all doses, and embryolethality occurred at the highest dose. The low dose in this study produced a plasma exposure approximately 9 times that in humans receiving the MRD. A no-effect dose for female reproductive toxicity in rats was not established. The clinical significance of female fertility findings in animals is unknown.

Human Data: In a double-blind, placebo-controlled clinical trial to assess the effect of pregabalin on sperm motility, 30 healthy male subjects were exposed to pregabalin 600 mg/day for 3 months (one complete sperm cycle). Pregabalin did not exhibit significant detrimental effects on the reproductive function of healthy male subjects, as measured by semen analysis, when compared with placebo (n=16). However, due to the small sample size and short-term exposure to pregabalin (only one complete sperm cycle), no conclusions can be made regarding possible reproductive effects of pregabalin during long-term exposure. Effects on other male reproductive parameters in humans have not been adequately studied.

Special Populations: Renal: There have been reports of patients, with or without previous history, experiencing renal failure while receiving pregabalin alone or in combination with other medications. Discontinuation of pregabalin showed reversibility of this event in some cases (see Warnings and Precautions; Adverse Reactions, Post-Marketing Adverse Drug Reactions; and Dosage and Administration). Because pregabalin is eliminated primarily by renal excretion, the dose of pregabalin should be adjusted as noted for elderly patients or those with renal impairment (see Action and Clinical Pharmacology and Dosage and Administration).

Adjustment of Dose in Renally-Impaired Patients: In patients with a medical history of significant renal insufficiency, daily dosages should be reduced accordingly (see Table 14 in Dosage and Administration, Dosing Considerations).

Preclinical Data: Pregabalin was not teratogenic in mice, rats, or rabbits. Pregabalin induced fetal toxicity in rats and rabbits at ≥39 times the mean human exposure at the maximum recommended clinical dose of 600 mg/day [$AUC_{(0-24)}$ of 123 μg·h/mL]. In the prenatal-postnatal toxicity study, pregabalin induced offspring developmental toxicity in rats at ≥5 times the maximum recommended human exposure. No developmental effects occurred at 2 times the maximum recommended human exposure.

Human Data: Pregnant Women: There are no adequate and well-controlled studies in pregnant women. Pregabalin should be used during pregnancy only if the potential benefit justifies the potential risk to the fetus.

Labor and Delivery: The effects of pregabalin on labor and delivery in pregnant women are unknown. In the prenatal-postnatal study in rats, pregabalin prolonged gestation and induced dystocia at exposures ≥47 times the mean human exposure [$AUC_{(0-24)}$ of 123 μg·h/mL] at the maximum recommended clinical dose of 600 mg/day.

Nursing Women: It is not known if pregabalin is excreted in human breast milk; however, it is present in the milk of rats. Because of the potential for adverse reactions in nursing infants from pregabalin, a decision should be made whether to discontinue nursing or to discontinue the drug, taking into account the importance of the drug to the mother.

Pediatrics (<18 years of age): The safety and efficacy of pregabalin in pediatric patients (<18 years of age) have not been established.

Geriatrics (>65 years of age): Of the 1831 patients who received pregabalin in neuropathic pain studies, 528 were 65 to 74 years of age, and 452 were 75 years of age or older. No significant differences in efficacy were observed between these patients and younger patients. Pregabalin oral clearance tended to decrease with increasing age. This decrease in pregabalin oral clearance is consistent with age-related decreases in creatinine clearance. Reduction of pregabalin dose may be required in patients who have age-related compromised renal function. In general, the incidence of adverse events did not increase with age.

Creatine Kinase Elevations: Pregabalin treatment was associated with creatine kinase elevations. Mean changes in creatine kinase from baseline to the maximum value were 60 U/L for pregabalin-treated patients and 28 U/L for the placebo patients. In all controlled trials across multiple patient populations, 2% of patients on pregabalin and 1% of placebo patients had a value of creatine kinase at least three times the upper limit of normal. Three pregabalin-treated subjects had events reported as rhabdomyolysis in premarketing clinical trials. The relationship between these myopathy events and pregabalin is not completely understood because the cases had documented factors that may have caused or contributed to these events. Prescribers should instruct patients to promptly report unexplained muscle pain, tenderness, or weakness, particularly if these muscle symptoms are accompanied by malaise or fever. Pregabalin treatment should be discontinued if myopathy is diagnosed or suspected or if markedly elevated creatine kinase levels occur.

Laboratory Changes, Decreased Platelet Count: Pregabalin treatment was associated with a decrease in platelet count. Pregabalin-treated subjects experienced a mean maximal decrease in platelet count of 20×10^3/μL, compared to 11×10^3/μL in placebo patients. In the overall database of controlled trials, 2% of placebo patients and 3% of pregabalin patients experienced a potentially clinically significant decrease in platelets, defined as 20% below baseline value and <150×10^3/μL.

In randomized controlled trials, pregabalin was not associated with an increase in bleeding related adverse events.

ECG Changes, PR Interval Prolongation: Pregabalin treatment was associated with mild PR interval prolongation. In analyses of clinical trial ECG data, the mean PR interval increase was 3-6 msec at pregabalin doses ≥300 mg/day. This mean change difference was not associated with an increased risk of PR increase ≥25% from baseline, an increased percentage of subjects with on-treatment PR >200 msec, or an increased risk of adverse events of second or third degree AV block.

Information to Be Provided to the Patient: Dizziness and Somnolence: Patients should be counseled that LYRICA may cause dizziness, somnolence, blurred vision and other CNS signs and symptoms. Accordingly, they should be advised not to drive, operate complex machinery, or engage in other hazardous activities until they have gained sufficient experience on pregabalin to gauge whether or not it affects their mental, visual, and/or motor performance adversely.

Visual Disturbances: Patients should be counseled that LYRICA may cause visual disturbances. Patients should be informed that if changes in vision occur, they should notify their physician (see Warnings and Precautions, Ophthalmological Effects).

Abrupt or Rapid Discontinuation: Patients should be advised to take LYRICA as prescribed. Abrupt or rapid discontinuation may result in insomnia, nausea, headache, anxiety, hyperhidrosis, or diarrhea.

Edema and Weight Gain: Patients should be counseled that LYRICA may cause edema and weight gain.

Patients should be advised that concomitant treatment with LYRICA and a thiazolidinedione antidiabetic agent may lead to an additive effect on edema and weight gain. For patients with preexisting cardiac conditions, this may increase the risk of heart failure.

Muscle Pain, Tenderness or Weakness: Patients should be instructed to promptly report unexplained muscle pain, tenderness, or weakness, particularly if accompanied by malaise or fever.

Concomitant Treatment with CNS Depressants, Alcohol: Patients who require concomitant treatment with central nervous system depressants such as opiates or benzodiazepines should be informed that they may experience additive CNS side effects, such as somnolence.

In post-marketing experience, there are reports of respiratory failure and coma in patients taking pregabalin alone or in combination with other CNS depressants.

Patients should be told to avoid consuming alcohol while taking LYRICA, as LYRICA may potentiate the impairment of motor skills and sedation of alcohol.

Pregnant Woman: Patients should be instructed to notify their physician if they become pregnant or intend to become pregnant during therapy, and to notify their physician if they are breast-feeding or intend to breast-feed during therapy.

Animal Studies in Male Reproduction: In preclinical studies in rats, pregabalin was associated with an increased risk of male-mediated teratogenicity (see Warnings and Precautions, Sexual Function/Reproduction). The clinical significance of this finding is uncertain; however, men being treated with LYRICA who plan to father a child should be informed of the potential risk of male-mediated teratogenicity.

Skin: Diabetic patients should be instructed to pay particular attention to skin integrity while being treated with LYRICA. Some animals treated with pregabalin developed skin ulcerations, although no increased incidence of skin lesions associated with LYRICA was observed in clinical trials (see Warnings and Precautions, Preclinical Toxicology).

Patients should be informed of the availability of a patient information leaflet, and they should be instructed to read the leaflet prior to taking LYRICA.

Preclinical Toxicology: Carcinogenesis: A dose-dependent increase in the incidence of malignant vascular tumors (hemangiosarcomas) was observed in two strains of mice (B6C3F1 and CD-1) given pregabalin (200, 1000, or 5000 mg/kg) in the diet for two years. Plasma pregabalin exposure (AUC) in mice receiving the lowest dose that increased hemangiosarcomas was approximately equal to the human exposure at the maximum recommended dose (MRD) of 600 mg/day. A no-effect dose for induction of hemangiosarcomas in mice was not established. In an investigative study in female B6C3F1 mice, chronic treatment (24 months) with pregabalin at 1000 mg/kg caused an increased incidence of hemangiosarcoma, consistent with previous studies, but not at 50 or 200 mg/kg. Discontinuation of treatment after 12 months at 1000 mg/kg did not significantly reduce the incidence of hemangiosarcoma at 24 months. Evidence of carcinogenicity was not seen in two studies in Wistar rats following dietary administration of pregabalin for two years at doses (50, 150, or 450 mg/kg in males and 100, 300, or 900 mg/kg in females) that were associated with plasma exposures in males and females up to approximately 14 and 24 times, respectively, human exposure at the MRD. The clinical significance in humans of this finding in mice is unknown.

Mutagenesis: Pregabalin is not genotoxic based on results of a battery of in vitro and in vivo tests. Pregabalin was not mutagenic in bacteria or in mammalian cells in vitro, was not clastogenic in mammalian systems in vitro and in vivo, and did not induce unscheduled DNA synthesis in mouse or rat hepatocytes.

Dermatopathy: Skin lesions ranging from erythema to necrosis were seen in repeated-dose toxicology studies in both rats and monkeys. The etiology of these skin lesions is unknown. At the maximum recommended human dose (MRD) of 600 mg/day, there is a 2-fold safety margin for the dermatological lesions. The more severe dermatopathies involving necrosis were associated with pregabalin exposures (as expressed by plasma AUCs) of approximately 3 to 8 times those achieved in humans given the MRD. No increase in incidence of skin lesions was observed in clinical studies.

Ocular Lesions: Ocular lesions (characterized by retinal atrophy (including loss of photoreceptor cells) and/or corneal inflammation/mineralization) were observed in two lifetime carcinogenicity studies in Wistar rats. These findings were observed at plasma pregabalin exposures (AUC) ≥2 times those achieved in humans given the maximum recommended dose of 600 mg/day. A no-effect dose for ocular lesions was not established. Similar lesions were not observed in lifetime carcinogenicity studies in two strains of mice or in monkeys treated for 1 year. The clinical significance of this finding in rats is unknown.

Monitoring and Laboratory Tests: Routine therapeutic drug monitoring or clinical laboratory testing is not required for patients treated with LYRICA (pregabalin) (see Adverse Reactions).

ADVERSE REACTIONS: Clinical Trial Adverse Drug Reactions: Because clinical trials are conducted under very specific conditions, the adverse reaction rates observed in clinical trials may not reflect the rates observed in practice and should not be compared to the rates in clinical trials of another drug. Adverse drug reaction information from clinical trials is useful for identifying drug-related adverse events and for approximating rates.

In all controlled and uncontrolled trials, during the pre-marketing development of pregabalin, more than 8666 patients have received LYRICA (pregabalin), with 83% of exposure at dosages of 300 mg/day or above and 32% at dosages of 600 mg/day or higher. Approximately 4010 patients had at least 6 months of exposure, 2415 had at least 1 year of exposure, and 939 had at least 2 years of exposure to pregabalin. In controlled trials, 1831 patients with neuropathic pain received pregabalin. In all controlled and uncontrolled studies in fibromyalgia, 3446 patients have received pregabalin doses of 150-600 mg/day. A total of 969 patients had at least 6 months of exposure and 440 patients had at least 1 year exposure to pregabalin. Doses above 600 mg/day have not been studied.

In a controlled study of neuropathic pain due to spinal cord injury, 137 patients were randomized to receive placebo (N=67) or escalating doses (150-600 mg/day) of pregabalin, (N=70). The controlled study was followed by an open-label trial in which 103 patients received pregabalin (150-600 mg/day). The median duration of therapy across the double blind and open-label studies for those subjects treated in the open-label extension was 608 days (range 14-1248). Sixty-nine (67%) subjects received at least 1 year of open-label pregabalin and 31 (30.1%) received at least 2 years of open-label pregabalin.

Most Common Adverse Events in All Pre-marketing Controlled Clinical Studies of Neuropathic Pain: The most commonly observed adverse events (≥5% and twice the rate of that seen in placebo) in pregabalin-treated patients were: dizziness, somnolence, peripheral edema, and dry mouth. Adverse events were usually mild to moderate in intensity.

Discontinuation Due to Adverse Events in Pre-marketing Controlled Clinical Studies: In all pre-marketing controlled studies, the discontinuation rate due to adverse events was 14% for patients receiving pregabalin and 7% for patients receiving placebo. The most common reasons for discontinuation due to adverse events (≥2%) in the pregabalin treatment groups were dizziness and somnolence. Other adverse events that led to withdrawal more frequently in the pregabalin group than the placebo group were ataxia (1%), and asthenia, confusion, headache and nausea (<1% each).

In pre-marketing controlled neuropathic pain studies, the discontinuation rate due to adverse events was 11% for pregabalin and 5% for placebo. The most common reasons for discontinuation due to adverse events (≥2%) in the pregabalin treatment groups were dizziness and somnolence. Other adverse events that led to withdrawal more frequently in the pregabalin group than the placebo group were confusion (1%) and asthenia, peripheral edema and ataxia (<1% each).

Incidence of Adverse Events in Pre-marketing Controlled Clinical Studies of Neuropathic Pain: In summaries of adverse events, investigator's terms for individual adverse events have been grouped into a smaller number of standardized categories using the COSTART IV dictionary. The prescriber should be aware that the percentages in Table 1 through Table 8 cannot be used to predict the frequency of adverse events in the course of usual medical practice where patient characteristics and other factors may differ from those prevailing during clinical studies. Similarly, the cited frequencies cannot be directly compared with figures obtained from other clinical investigations involving different treatments, uses or investigators. An inspection of these frequencies, however, does provide the prescriber with one basis to estimate the relative contribution of drug and non-drug factors to the adverse event incidences in the population studied.

Adverse Events From Pre-marketing Controlled Clinical Studies of Neuropathic Pain: Diabetic Peripheral Neuropathy: Table 1 lists all adverse events, regardless of causality, occurring in ≥2% of patients with neuropathic pain associated with diabetic peripheral neuropathy receiving pregabalin for at least one of the pregabalin groups, and for which the incidence was greater than in the placebo group. A majority of pregabalin-treated patients in these studies had adverse events with a maximum intensity of mild or moderate. In these studies, 979 patients received pregabalin and 459 patients received placebo for up to 13 weeks.

Table 1: LYRICA

Incidence (%) of Treatment-Emergent Adverse Events in Placebo-Controlled Studies in Neuropathic Pain Associated with Diabetic Peripheral Neuropathy (Events in at Least 2% of Patients Receiving Pregabalin and More Frequent Than in Placebo-Treated Patients)

		Pregabalin (mg/day)			
Body System Preferred Term	**Placebo (N=459) %**	**75 (N=77) %**	**150 (N=212) %**	**300 (N=321) %**	**600 (N=369) %**
Body as a Whole					
Infection	6.1	3.9	7.5	8.4	4.6
Asthenia	2.4	3.9	1.9	4.4	7.3
Pain	3.9	5.2	4.2	2.5	4.9
Accidental Injury	2.8	5.2	2.4	2.2	5.7
Back Pain	0.4	0.0	2.4	1.2	1.9
Chest Pain	1.1	3.9	1.4	1.2	1.6
Face Edema	0.4	0.0	0.9	0.9	2.2
Digestive System					
Dry Mouth	1.1	2.6	1.9	4.7	6.5
Constipation	1.5	0.0	2.4	3.7	6.0
Diarrhea	4.8	5.2	2.8	1.9	3.0
Flatulence	1.3	2.6	0	2.2	2.7
Vomiting	1.5	1.3	0.9	2.2	1.1
Hemic and Lymphatic System					
Ecchymosis	0.2	2.6	0.5	0.6	0.3
Metabolic and Nutritional Disorders					
Peripheral Edema	2.4	3.9	6.1	9.3	12.5
Weight Gain	0.4	0.0	4.2	3.7	6.2
Edema	0.0	0.0	1.9	4.0	1.9
Hypoglycemia	1.1	1.3	3.3	1.6	1.1
Nervous System					
Dizziness	4.6	7.8	9.0	23.1	29.0
Somnolence	2.6	3.9	6.1	13.1	16.3
Neuropathy	3.5	9.1	1.9	2.2	5.4
Ataxia	1.3	6.5	0.9	2.2	4.3
Vertigo	1.1	1.3	1.9	2.5	3.5
Confusion	0.7	0.0	1.4	2.2	3.3
Euphoria	0.0	0.0	0.5	3.4	1.6
Thinking Abnormal[a]	0.0	1.3	0.0	0.9	3.0
Abnormal Gait	0.0	1.3	0.0	0.6	2.7
Reflexes Decreased	1.7	3.9	0.5	1.2	1.4
Amnesia	0.2	2.6	0.9	0.0	2.2
Hypesthesia	0.7	2.6	0.0	0.0	0.8
Hyperalgesia	0.2	2.6	0.0	0.0	0.3
Respiratory System					
Dyspnea	0.7	2.6	0.0	1.9	1.9
Skin And Appendages					
Pruritus	1.3	2.6	0.0	0.9	0.0

(cont'd)

Table 1: LYRICA *(cont'd)*

Incidence (%) of Treatment-Emergent Adverse Events in Placebo-Controlled Studies in Neuropathic Pain Associated with Diabetic Peripheral Neuropathy (Events in at Least 2% of Patients Receiving Pregabalin and More Frequent Than in Placebo-Treated Patients)

		Pregabalin (mg/day)			
Body System Preferred Term	**Placebo (N=459) %**	**75 (N=77) %**	**150 (N=212) %**	**300 (N=321) %**	**600 (N=369) %**
Special Senses					
Blurred Vision[b]	1.5	2.6	1.4	2.8	5.7
Conjunctivitis	0.2	2.6	1.4	0.6	0.3

[a] Thinking abnormal primarily consists of events related to difficulty with concentration/attention but also includes events related to cognition and language problems and slow thinking.
[b] Investigator term; summary level term is amblyopia.

Discontinuation in Controlled Clinical Studies of Diabetic Peripheral Neuropathy: Approximately 9% of patients receiving pregabalin and 4% receiving placebo discontinued from controlled diabetic peripheral neuropathy studies due to adverse events. The adverse events most commonly leading to discontinuation are presented in Table 2.

Table 2: LYRICA

Adverse Events Most Frequently (≥2% of patients) Leading to Discontinuation in Placebo-Controlled Studies in Patients with Neuropathic Pain Associated with Diabetic Peripheral Neuropathy

	Number (%) of Patients				
		Pregabalin (mg/day)			
COSTART Preferred Term	**Placebo (N=459)**	**75 (N=77)**	**150 (N=212)**	**300 (N=321)**	**600 (N=369)**
Dizziness	2 (0.4)	0 (0.0)	3 (1.4)	6 (1.9)	21 (5.7)
Somnolence	0 (0.0)	0 (0.0)	0 (0.0)	5 (1.6)	15 (4.1)

Postherpetic Neuralgia: Table 3 lists all adverse events, regardless of causality, occurring in ≥2% of patients with neuropathic pain associated with postherpetic neuralgia receiving pregabalin for at least one of the pregabalin groups, and for which the incidence was greater than in the placebo group. A majority of pregabalin-treated patients in these studies had adverse events with a maximum intensity of mild or moderate. In these studies, 852 patients received pregabalin and 398 patients received placebo for up to 13 weeks.

Table 3: LYRICA

Incidence (%) of Treatment-Emergent Adverse Events in Placebo-Controlled Studies in Neuropathic Pain Associated with Postherpetic Neuralgia (Events in at Least 2% of Patients Receiving Pregabalin and More Frequent Than in Placebo-Treated Patients)

		Pregabalin (mg/day)			
Body System Preferred Term	**Placebo (N=398) %**	**75 (N=84) %**	**150 (N=302) %**	**300 (N=312) %**	**600 (N=154) %**
Body as a Whole					
Infection	3.5	14.3	8.3	6.4	2.6
Headache	5.3	4.8	8.9	4.5	8.4
Pain	3.8	4.8	4.3	5.4	4.5
Asthenia	4	3.6	5	2.6	5.2
Accidental Injury	1.5	3.6	2.6	3.2	5.2
Flu Syndrome	1.3	1.2	1.7	2.2	1.3
Face Edema	0.8	0	1.7	1.3	3.2
Malaise	1	2.4	0.3	0.6	0
Cardiovascular System					
Vasodilatation	1.3	2.4	1	0.6	0
Digestive System					
Dry Mouth	2.8	7.1	7	6.1	14.9
Constipation	2.3	3.6	4.6	5.4	5.2
Diarrhea	4	2.4	4.3	3.5	4.5
Flatulence	1	2.4	1.3	1.6	3.2
Vomiting	0.8	1.2	0.7	2.9	2.6
Metabolic and Nutritional Disorders					
Peripheral Edema	3.5	0	7.9	15.7	16.2
Weight Gain	0.3	1.2	1.7	5.4	6.5
Edema	1.3	0	1	2.2	5.8
Hyperglycemia	0.8	2.4	0.3	0	0

(cont'd)

Table 3: LYRICA *(cont'd)*

Incidence (%) of Treatment-Emergent Adverse Events in Placebo-Controlled Studies in Neuropathic Pain Associated with Postherpetic Neuralgia (Events in at Least 2% of Patients Receiving Pregabalin and More Frequent Than in Placebo-Treated Patients)

Body System Preferred Term	Placebo (N=398) %	Pregabalin (mg/day) 75 (N=84) %	150 (N=302) %	300 (N=312) %	600 (N=154) %
Nervous System					
Dizziness	9.3	10.7	17.9	31.4	37
Somnolence	5.3	8.3	12.3	17.9	24.7
Ataxia	0.5	1.2	2	5.4	9.1
Abnormal Gait	0.5	0	2	3.8	7.8
Confusion	0.3	1.2	2.3	2.9	6.5
Thinking Abnormal[a]	1.5	0	1.7	1.3	5.8
Incoordination	0	2.4	1.7	1.3	2.6
Amnesia	0	0	1	1.3	3.9
Speech Disorder	0	0	0.3	1.3	3.2
Insomnia	1.8	0	0.7	2.2	0
Euphoria	0	2.4	0	1.3	1.3
Nervousness	0.5	0	1	0.3	2.6
Tremor	1.5	1.2	0	1	2.6
Hallucinations	0	0	0.3	0.3	3.2
Hyperesthesia	0.3	2.4	0.3	0	1.3
Respiratory System					
Bronchitis	0.8	0	1.3	1	2.6
Pharyngitis	0.8	0	2.6	0.6	0.6
Rhinitis	1.8	1.2	0.7	0.6	3.2
Skin and Appendages					
Rash	3	2.4	2	2.9	5.2
Special Senses					
Blurred Vision[b]	2.5	1.2	5	5.1	9.1
Diplopia	0	0	1.7	1.9	3.9
Abnormal Vision	0.3	0	1	1.6	5.2
Urogenital System					
Urinary Tract Infection	1.5	0	2.3	1.6	3.2

[a] Thinking abnormal primarily consists of events related to difficulty with concentration/attention but also includes events related to cognition and language problems and slow thinking.
[b] Investigator term; summary level term is amblyopia.

Discontinuation in Controlled Clinical Studies of Postherpetic Neuralgia: Approximately 14% of patients receiving pregabalin and 7% receiving placebo discontinued from controlled postherpetic neuralgia studies due to adverse events. The adverse events most commonly leading to discontinuation are presented in Table 4.

Table 4: LYRICA

Adverse Events Most Frequently (≥2% of patients) Leading to Discontinuation in Placebo-Controlled Studies in Patients with Neuropathic Pain Associated with Postherpetic Neuralgia

COSTART Preferred Term	Number (%) of Patients: Placebo (N=398)	Pregabalin (mg/day) 75 (N=84)	150 (N=302)	300 (N=312)	600 (N=154)
Dizziness	3 (0.8)	0 (0.0)	11 (3.6)	12 (3.8)	12 (7.8)
Somnolence	1 (0.3)	0 (0.0)	6 (2.0)	12 (3.8)	10 (6.5)
Confusion	1 (0.3)	0 (0.0)	2 (0.7)	5 (1.6)	8 (5.2)
Peripheral Edema	1 (0.3)	0 (0.0)	2 (0.7)	5 (1.6)	5 (3.2)
Ataxia	0 (0.0)	0 (0.0)	1 (0.3)	5 (1.6)	4 (2.6)
Abnormal Gait	0 (0.0)	0 (0.0)	0 (0.0)	4 (1.3)	4 (2.6)
Hallucinations	0 (0.0)	0 (0.0)	0 (0.0)	1 (0.3)	4 (2.6)
Dry Mouth	1 (0.3)	0 (0.0)	0 (0.0)	0 (0.0)	4 (2.6)

Incidence of Most Common Dose-Related Treatment-Emergent Adverse Events: Most common dose-related treatment-emergent adverse events are presented in Table 5 (diabetic peripheral neuropathy) and Table 6 (postherpetic neuralgia), and Table 7 (fibromyalgia).

Table 5: LYRICA

Incidence (%) of Most Common Dose-Related Treatment-Emergent Adverse Events in Placebo-Controlled Studies in Neuropathic Pain Associated with Diabetic Peripheral Neuropathy

Adverse Event Preferred Term	Placebo (N=459) %	Pregabalin (mg/day) 75 (N=77) %	150 (N=212) %	300 (N=321) %	600 (N=369) %
Dizziness	4.6	7.8	9	23.1	29
Somnolence	2.6	3.9	6.1	13.1	16.3
Peripheral Edema	2.4	3.9	6.1	9.3	12.5
Asthenia	2.4	3.9	1.9	4.4	7.3
Dry Mouth	1.1	2.6	1.9	4.7	6.5
Weight Gain	0.4	0	4.2	3.7	6.2
Constipation	1.5	0	2.4	3.7	6
Blurred Vision[a]	1.5	2.6	1.4	2.8	5.7

[a] Investigator term; summary level term is amblyopia.

Table 6: LYRICA

Incidence (%) of Most Common Dose-Related Treatment-Emergent Adverse Events in Placebo-Controlled Studies in Neuropathic Pain Associated with Postherpetic Neuralgia

Adverse Event Preferred Term	Placebo (N=398) %	Pregabalin (mg/day) 75 (N=84) %	150 (N=302) %	300 (N=312) %	600 (N=154) %
Dizziness	9.3	10.7	17.9	31.4	37
Somnolence	5.3	8.3	12.3	17.9	24.7
Peripheral Edema	3.5	0	7.9	15.7	16.2
Dry Mouth	2.8	7.1	7	6.1	14.9
Blurred Vision[a]	2.5	1.2	5	5.1	9.1
Ataxia	0.5	1.2	2	5.4	9.1
Weight Gain	0.3	1.2	1.7	5.4	6.5
Abnormal Gait	0.5	0	2	3.8	7.8

[a] Investigator term; summary level term is amblyopia.

Table 7: LYRICA

Incidence (%) of Most Common Dose-Related Treatment-Emergent Adverse Events in Placebo-Controlled Studies in Pain Associated with Fibromyalgia

System Organ Class and Preferred Term (MedDRA version 10.1)	Placebo (N=689) %	Pregabalin (mg/day) 150 (N=132) %	300 (N=685) %	450 (N=687) %	600 (N=564) %
Dizziness	10.4	22.7	32.6	42.5	46.5
Somnolence	4.6	12.9	18.5	19.9	20.7
Weight Increased	2.5	7.6	11.1	10.0	13.7
Peripheral Edema	2.5	5.3	6.7	6.4	10.8
Dry Mouth	1.7	6.8	6.7	9.2	9.4
Constipation	2.8	3.8	5.8	6.8	9.2
Fatigue	5.4	4.5	7.2	8.4	8.2
Balance Disorder	0.1	1.5	3.2	4.9	6.9
Disturbance in Attention	1.3	3.8	4.4	6.4	6.9
Increased Appetite	1.3	3.8	3.4	4.5	5.5
Euphoria	0.9	1.5	4.1	4.8	5.1

Adverse Events From a Controlled Clinical Study in Neuropathic Pain Associated with Spinal Cord Injury: The most commonly observed treatment-related adverse events (≥5% and twice the rate of that seen in placebo) in pregabalin-treated patients were: somnolence, dizziness, asthenia, dry mouth, edema, myasthenia, constipation, thinking abnormal, amblyopia, and amnesia. Adverse events were usually mild to moderate in intensity.

Table 8 lists all adverse events, regardless of causality, occurring in ≥2% of patients receiving pregabalin and for which the incidence was greater than in the placebo group. A majority of pregabalin-treated patients had adverse events with a maximum intensity of mild or moderate. In this study, 70 patients received pregabalin and 67 patients received placebo for up to 12 weeks.

Table 8: LYRICA

Incidence (%) of Treatment-Emergent Adverse Events in a Placebo-Controlled Study in Neuropathic Pain Associated with Spinal Cord Injury (Events in at Least 2% of Patients Receiving Pregabalin and More Frequent Than in Placebo-Treated Patients)

Body System Preferred Term	Placebo N=67 %	Pregabalin (150–600 mg/day) N=70 %
Body as a Whole		
Asthenia	6.0	15.7
Infection	6.0	8.6
Abdomen Enlarged	0.0	4.3
Pain	1.5	4.3
Back Pain	1.5	2.9
Cellulitis	0.0	2.9
Flu Syndrome	1.5	2.9
Neck Pain	1.5	2.9
Cardiovascular System		
Hypotension	0.0	2.9
Digestive System		
Dry mouth	3.0	15.7
Constipation	6.0	12.9
Gastroenteritis	0.0	2.9
Increased Appetite	0.0	2.9
Metabolic and Nutritional Disorders		
Edema	0.0	12.9
Peripheral Edema	6.0	10.0
Weight Gain	0.0	4.3
Musculoskeletal System		
Myasthenia	4.5	8.6
Joint Disorder	0.0	2.9
Nervous System		
Somnolence	9.0	41.4
Dizziness	9.0	24.3
Amnesia	3.0	10.0
Thinking Abnormal[a]	1.5	8.6
Paresthesia	1.5	5.7
Euphoria	0.0	4.3
Speech Disorder	1.5	4.3
Twitching	0.0	4.3
Withdrawal Syndrome	0.0	4.3
Skin and Appendages		
Skin Ulcer	1.5	4.3
Alopecia	0.0	2.9
Vesiculobullous Rash	0.0	2.9
Special Senses		
Blurred Vision[b]	3.0	8.6
Diplopia	1.5	2.9
Tinnitus	0.0	2.9
Urogenital System		
Urinary Incontinence	3.0	5.7

[a] Thinking abnormal primarily consists of events related to difficulty with concentration/attention but also includes events related to cognition and language problems and slow thinking.
[b] Investigator term; summary level term is amblyopia.

Discontinuation in a Controlled Clinical Study in Neuropathic Pain Associated with Spinal Cord Injury: Approximately 21% of patients receiving pregabalin and 13% receiving placebo discontinued due to adverse events. The adverse events most commonly leading to discontinuation are presented in Table 9.

Table 9: LYRICA

Adverse Events Most Frequently (≥2% of patients) Leading to Discontinuation in a Placebo-Controlled Study in Patients with Neuropathic Pain Associated with Spinal Cord Injury

	Number (%) of Patients	
COSTART Preferred Term	Placebo (N=67)	Pregabalin 150–600 mg/day (N=70)
Somnolence	0 (0.0)	4 (5.7)
Edema	0 (0.0)	4 (5.7)
Asthenia	0 (0.0)	3 (4.3)

Overall, the most frequent treatment-related adverse events in the open-label study were related to the nervous system and included: somnolence (18.4%), dizziness (16.5%), and insomnia (10.7%). Other frequent treatment-related adverse events included: asthenia (12.6%), nausea (11.7%), and constipation (10.7%).

Most Common Adverse Events in Controlled Clinical Studies in Fibromyalgia: The most commonly observed treatment-related adverse events (≥5% and twice the rate of that seen in placebo) in pregabalin-treated patients were: dizziness (37.5), somnolence (18.6), weight gain (10.6), dry mouth (7.9), blurred vision (6.7), peripheral edema (6.1), constipation (5.8), and disturbance in attention (5.3). Adverse events were usually mild to moderate in intensity.

Adverse Events from Controlled Clinical Studies in Fibromyalgia: Table 10 lists all adverse events occurring in ≥2% of patients receiving pregabalin and for which the incidence was greater than in the placebo group. A majority of pregabalin-treated patients in these studies had adverse events with mild or moderate intensity. There was a dose-related increase in the incidence of adverse events (see Table 7). Severe adverse events occurred at roughly the same rate in low versus high doses of pregabalin.

Table 10: LYRICA

Incidence (%) of Treatment-Emergent Adverse Events in Controlled Fibromyalgia Studies (in at Least 2% of Pregabalin-Treated Patients and More Frequent Than in Placebo-Treated Patients)

		Pregabalin (mg/day)			
System Organ Class and Preferred Term (MedDRA version 10.1)	Placebo (N=689) %	150 (N=132) %	300 (N=685) %	450 (N=687) %	600 (N=564) %
Ear and Labyrinth Disorders					
Vertigo	0.9	1.5	3.1	3.2	3.5
Eye Disorders					
Blurred Vision[a]	1.0	8.3	5.8	6.4	10.1
Gastrointestinal Disorders					
Dry Mouth	1.7	6.8	6.7	9.2	9.4
Constipation	2.8	3.8	5.8	6.8	9.2
Abdominal Distention	1.5	2.3	2.2	1.9	2.0
Flatulence	1.0	0.8	0.9	2.0	2.3
General Disorders and Administration Site Conditions					
Fatigue	5.4	4.5	7.2	8.4	8.2
Peripheral Edema	2.5	5.3	6.7	6.4	10.8
Feeling Abnormal	0.3	0.8	1.9	1.9	2.0
Feeling Drunk	0	0.8	2.3	1.5	2.1
Infections and Infestations					
Sinusitis	3.0	3.8	3.6	5.2	4.1
Investigations					
Weight Increased	2.5	7.6	11.1	10.9	13.7
Metabolism and Nutritional Disorders					
Increased Appetite	1.3	3.8	3.4	4.5	5.5
Fluid Retention	0.7	1.5	2.2	2.0	2.0
Musculoskeletal and Connective Tissue Disorders					
Arthralgia	2.5	3.8	3.6	3.2	4.6
Muscle Spasm	1.9	2.3	3.4	3.3	3.2
Nervous System Disorders					
Dizziness	10.4	22.7	32.6	42.5	46.5
Somnolence	4.6	12.9	18.5	19.9	20.7
Disturbance in Attention	1.3	3.8	4.4	6.4	6.9
Balance Disorder	0.1	1.5	3.2	4.9	6.9

(cont'd)

Table 10: LYRICA *(cont'd)*

Incidence (%) of Treatment-Emergent Adverse Events in Controlled Fibromyalgia Studies (in at Least 2% of Pregabalin-Treated Patients and More Frequent Than in Placebo-Treated Patients)

System Organ Class and Preferred Term (MedDRA version 10.1)	Placebo (N=689) %	Pregabalin (mg/day) 150 (N=132) %	300 (N=685) %	450 (N=687) %	600 (N=564) %
Memory Impairment	0.6	0.8	2.6	3.5	3.5
Hypoesthesia	0.6	1.5	2.0	2.8	2.3
Tremor	0.6	0	0.6	2.9	3.0
Lethargy	0.4	2.3	1.3	0.7	1.4
Psychiatric Disorders					
Euphoria	0.9	1.5	4.1	4.8	5.1
Anxiety	0.9	1.5	1.9	2.5	1.8
Confusion	0.1	0	2.0	1.9	2.7

[a] Investigator term; summary level term is amblyopia.

Discontinuation Due to Adverse Events in Controlled Clinical Studies in Fibromyalgia: Approximately 20% of patients receiving pregabalin and 11% receiving placebo discontinued due to adverse events. The adverse events most commonly leading to discontinuation were dizziness (6.1%) and somnolence (3.3%) as presented in Table 11. Other events leading to discontinuation in clinical trials of fibromyalgia included weight gain (1.1%), vision blurred (0.8%) and peripheral edema (0.6%). There was a dose-dependent increase in rate of discontinuation due to adverse events.

Table 11: LYRICA

Adverse Events Most Frequently (≥2% of patients) Leading to Discontinuation in Placebo-Controlled Studies in Patients with Pain Associated with Fibromyalgia

System Organ Class and Preferred Term (MedDRA version 10.1)	Number (%) of Patients: Placebo (N=689)	Pregabalin (mg/day) 150 (N=132)	300 (N=675)	450 (N=687)	600 (N=564)
Dizziness	0.4%	1.5%	4.1%	6.6%	9.2%
Somnolence	0.1%	0.8%	2.9%	3.2%	4.6%

Adverse Events Following Abrupt or Rapid Discontinuation: Following abrupt or rapid discontinuation of pregabalin, some patients reported symptoms including insomnia, nausea, headache, anxiety, hyperhidrosis, and diarrhea. Pregabalin should be tapered gradually over a minimum of one week rather than discontinued abruptly (see Warnings and Precautions, Abrupt or Rapid Discontinuation).

Other Events Observed During the Premarketing Evaluation of LYRICA: Following is a list of treatment-emergent adverse events reported during premarketing assessment of LYRICA in clinical trials (over 8600 adult subjects) except those already listed in the previous tables or elsewhere in labeling. In the tabulations that follow, a COSTART based dictionary of terminology has been used to classify reported adverse events. The frequencies presented, therefore, represent the proportion of the over 8600 adult individuals exposed to multiple doses of LYRICA who experienced an event of the type cited on at least 1 occasion while receiving LYRICA. It is important to emphasize that although the events reported occurred during treatment with LYRICA, they were not necessarily caused by it.

Less Common Clinical Trial Adverse Drug Reactions (<2%): Events are further categorized by body system and listed in order of decreasing frequency according to the following definitions: frequent adverse events are those occurring on 1 or more occasions in at least 1/100 patients; infrequent adverse events are those occurring in 1/100 to 1/1000 patients; rare events are those occurring in fewer than 1/1000 patients. See Table 12.

Table 12: LYRICA

Less Common Clinical Trial Adverse Drug Reactions (<2%)

Body System	Adverse Events
Body as a Whole	
Frequent	Flu syndrome, back pain, allergic reaction, fever, generalized edema
Infrequent	Neck pain, neoplasm, cellulitis, cyst, chills, malaise, overdose, moniliasis, hernia, viral infection, photosensitivity reaction, pelvic pain, abdomen enlarged, abscess, neck rigidity, lab test abnormal, drug level increased, carcinoma, sepsis, suicide attempt, reaction unevaluable
Rare	Infection fungal, unexpected benefit, chills and fever, body odor, drug level decreased, halitosis, hangover effect, injection site reaction, hormone level altered, hypothermia, infection bacterial, injection site hemorrhage, intentional overdose, mucous membrane disorder, accidental overdose, adenoma, anaphylactoid reaction, ascites, chest pain substernal, death, sarcoidosis, sudden death, immune system disorder, increased drug effect, injection site pain, Lupus Erythematosus syndrome, medication error, sarcoma, shock, tolerance decreased
Cardiovascular	
Frequent	Hypertension, vasodilatation
Infrequent	Palpitation, migraine, tachycardia, peripheral vascular disorder, electrocardiogram abnormal, cardiovascular disorder, angina pectoris, congestive heart failure, hemorrhage, myocardial infarct, hypotension, postural hypotension, ventricular extrasystoles, atrial fibrillation, coronary artery disorder, bradycardia, cerebrovascular accident, arrhythmia, cerebral ischemia, vascular disorder, sinus bradycardia, myocardial ischemia, bundle branch block, AV block first degree, arteriosclerosis, deep thrombophlebitis, phlebitis, arterial anomaly, heart failure, pulmonary embolus, retinal vascular disorder, varicose vein

(cont'd)

Table 12: LYRICA *(cont'd)*

Less Common Clinical Trial Adverse Drug Reactions (<2%)

Body System	Adverse Events
Rare	Heart arrest, vascular anomaly, occlusion, supraventricular tachycardia, atrial arrhythmia, atrial flutter, cerebral infarct, coronary occlusion, thrombophlebitis, thrombosis, cardiomegaly, extrasystoles, pallor, AV block, AV block second degree, cardiomyopathy, peripheral gangrene, QT interval prolonged, retinal artery occlusion, supraventricular extrasystoles, cerebral hemorrhage, digitalis intoxication, ventricular arrhythmia, aortic stenosis, bigeminy, cerebrovascular disorder, left heart failure, ventricular tachycardia, AV block complete, carotid occlusion, carotid thrombosis, cor pulmonale, embolus lower extremity, endocarditis, heart block, increased capillary fragility, intracranial aneurysm, nodal tachycardia, QT interval shortened, retinal vein thrombosis, ST elevated, T inverted, vascular headache, vasculitis
Digestive System	
Frequent	Nausea, diarrhea, anorexia, gastrointestinal disorder
Infrequent	Gastroenteritis, tooth disorder, periodontal abscess, colitis, gastritis, liver function tests abnormal, increased salivation, thirst, nausea and vomiting, rectal disorder, gingivitis, dysphagia, stomatitis, mouth ulceration, cholelithiasis, rectal hemorrhage, gastrointestinal hemorrhage, glossitis, tooth caries, abnormal stools, cholecystitis, melena, oral moniliasis, esophagitis, tongue disorder, cheilitis, tongue edema
Rare	Eructation, pancreatitis, stomach ulcer, ulcerative stomatitis, esophageal stenosis, fecal incontinence, gum hemorrhage, intestinal obstruction, enteritis, peptic ulcer, enterocolitis, gum hyperplasia, hepatomegaly, liver fatty deposit, tenesmus, biliary pain, fecal impaction, jaundice, periodontitis, ulcerative colitis, aphthous stomatitis, cholestatic jaundice, gastrointestinal carcinoma, hemorrhagic gastritis, hepatitis, liver tenderness, nausea, vomiting and diarrhea, salivary gland enlargement, stomach atony, bloody diarrhea, cardiospasm, duodenal ulcer, gamma glutamyl transpeptidase increased, hematemesis, hepatoma, intestinal perforation, intestinal stenosis, intestinal ulcer, leukoplakia of mouth, necrotizing pancreatitis, pancreas disorder, pseudomembranous colitis, sialadenitis, stomach ulcer hemorrhage, tongue discoloration
Endocrine System	
Infrequent	Diabetes mellitus, hypothyroidism
Rare	Goiter, prolactin increased, thyroid disorder, gonadotropic follicle stim hormone increase, hyperthyroidism, thyroiditis, adrenal insufficiency, parathyroid disorder, thyroid carcinoma, thyroid neoplasia, virilism
Hemic and Lymphatic	
Infrequent	Anemia, leukopenia, thrombocytopenia, lymphadenopathy, hypochromic anemia, leukocytosis, eosinophilia
Rare	Lymphocytosis, petechia, iron deficiency anemia, cyanosis, lymphedema, polycythemia, lymphoma like reaction, megaloblastic anemia, splenomegaly, purpura, thrombocythemia, thrombocytopenic purpura, chronic leukemia, coagulation disorder, erythrocytes abnormal, leukemoid reaction, lymphangitis, macrocytic anemia, neutropenia, pancytopenia, prothrombin decreased, rupture of spleen, sedimentation rate increased
Metabolic and Nutritional	
Infrequent	Hyperglycemia, ALT increased, hypoglycemia, hypokalemia, hypercholesteremia, AST increased, weight loss, hyperlipemia, amylase increased, hyperuricemia, alkaline phosphatase increased, creatinine increased, hyponatremia, gout, dehydration, BUN increased, healing abnormal
Rare	Hypercalcemia, hyperkalemia, hypocalcemia, bilirubinemia, alcohol intolerance, hypoglycemic reaction, ketosis, calcium disorder, hypochloremia, hypomagnesemia, hypoproteinemia, NPN increased, uremia, acidosis, avitaminosis, enzymatic abnormality, gamma globulins increased, hypernatremia, hypophosphatemia, lactic acidosis, obesity
Musculoskeletal System	
Frequent	Arthralgia, myalgia, arthritis, leg cramps, myasthenia
Infrequent	Tendon disorder, arthrosis, joint disorder, bone disorder, tenosynovitis, bursitis, tendinous contracture, osteoporosis, tendon rupture, bone pain
Rare	Rheumatoid arthritis, osteomyelitis, rhabdomyolysis, myopathy, muscle atrophy, myositis, pyogenic arthritis, bone neoplasm, musculoskeletal congenital anomaly, pathological fracture
Nervous System	
Frequent	Insomnia, anxiety, libido decreased, depersonalization, hypertonia, neuropathy
Infrequent	Reflexes decreased, sleep disorder, abnormal dreams, hostility, hallucinations, hyperkinesia, personality disorder, dysarthria, hyperesthesia, hypokinesia, circumoral paresthesia, libido increased, neuralgia, vestibular disorder, aphasia, movement disorder, hyperalgesia, apathy, hypotonia, convulsion, facial paralysis, psychosis
Rare	Drug dependence, neuritis, paranoid reaction, CNS depression, CNS neoplasia, manic reaction, neurosis, extrapyramidal syndrome, meningitis, hemiplegia, reflexes increased, akathisia, delirium, paralysis, withdrawal syndrome, brain edema, CNS stimulation, dyskinesia, encephalopathy, foot drop, grand mal convulsion, hypalgesia, peripheral neuritis, psychotic depression, addiction, arachnoiditis, cerebellar syndrome, cogwheel rigidity, dementia, dystonia, Guillain-Barre syndrome, intracranial hemorrhage, multiple sclerosis, myelitis, schizophrenic reaction, subarachnoid hemorrhage, torticollis
Respiratory System	
Frequent	Sinusitis, rhinitis, dyspnea, cough increased, pneumonia, lung disorder
Infrequent	Asthma, epistaxis, laryngitis, voice alteration, respiratory disorder, sputum increased

(cont'd)

Table 12: LYRICA *(cont'd)*

Less Common Clinical Trial Adverse Drug Reactions (<2%)

Body System	Adverse Events
Rare	Apnea, emphysema, aspiration pneumonia, hyperventilation, lung edema, pleural disorder, atelectasis, hemoptysis, hiccup, hypoxia, laryngismus, lung fibrosis, pleural effusion, lung function decreased, pulmonary hypertension, yawn, bronchiectasis, bronchiolitis, carcinoma of lung, hypoventilation, laryngeal neoplasia, nasal septum disorder, pneumothorax
Skin and Appendages	
Infrequent	Pruritus, sweating, skin disorder, acne, dry skin, alopecia, skin ulcer, herpes simplex, urticaria, nail disorder, eczema, herpes zoster, skin benign neoplasm, fungal dermatitis, maculopapular rash, vesiculobullous rash, skin carcinoma, furunculosis, skin discoloration, skin hypertrophy, psoriasis, seborrhea, hirsutism
Rare	Skin nodule, angioedema, cutaneous moniliasis, skin atrophy, exfoliative dermatitis, pustular rash, ichthyosis, skin melanoma, subcutaneous nodule, sweating decreased, hair disorder, lichenoid dermatitis, melanosis, miliaria, purpuric rash, skin necrosis, Stevens-Johnson Syndrome
Special Sense	
Frequent	Eye disorder, conjunctivitis, otitis media
Infrequent	Retinal disorder, tinnitus, eye pain, cataract specified, dry eyes, taste perversion, ear pain, lacrimation disorder, ear disorder, deafness, eye hemorrhage, photophobia, glaucoma, vitreous disorder, corneal lesion, otitis externa, refraction disorder, blepharitis, retinal edema, taste loss, abnormality of accommodation
Rare	Hyperacusis, keratitis, mydriasis, parosmia, ptosis, retinal hemorrhage, color blindness, retinal depigmentation, retinal detachment, corneal opacity, corneal ulcer, iritis, night blindness, optic atrophy, retinal degeneration, cataract NOS, scleritis, strabismus, anisocoria, blindness, exophthalmos, keratoconjunctivitis, ophthalmoplegia, papilledema
Urogenital System	
Frequent	Anorgasmia
Infrequent	Urinary frequency, urinary incontinence, cystitis, abnormal ejaculation, urination impaired, dysuria, metrorrhagia, hematuria, vaginal moniliasis, prostatic disorder, vaginitis, dysmenorrhea, urinary urgency, kidney calculus, breast pain, menstrual disorder, amenorrhea, menorrhagia, kidney function abnormal, nephritis, urine abnormality, vaginal hemorrhage, urinary retention, urinary tract disorder, leukorrhea, breast neoplasm, menopause, oliguria, polyuria, albuminuria, pyuria
Rare	Breast carcinoma, penis disorder, papanicolau smear suspicious, fibrocystic breast, prostatic carcinoma, uterine fibroids enlarged, acute kidney failure, creatinine clearance decreased, nephrosis, nocturia, polycystic kidney, bladder carcinoma, breast enlargement, cervicitis, cervix disorder, female lactation, glycosuria, gynecomastia, hypomenorrhea, kidney pain, mastitis, pyelonephritis, kidney failure, breast abscess, epididymitis, orchitis, prostate neoplasia, prostatic specific antigen increase, salpingitis, urogenital disorder, urolithiasis, uterine disorder, vulvovaginal disorder, balanitis, bladder calculus, calcium crystalluria, cervix neoplasm, dyspareunia, endometrial carcinoma, endometrial disorder, glomerulitis, hydronephrosis, ovarian cancer, unintended pregnancy, urethral pain, urethritis, urogenital anomaly, urogenital neoplasia, uterine hemorrhage

Comparison of Gender and Race: The overall adverse event profile of pregabalin was similar between women and men. There are insufficient data to support a statement regarding the distribution of adverse experience reports by race.

Peripheral Edema: Incidence of peripheral edema in pre-marketing controlled neuropathic pain studies was 10.4% in the pregabalin group compared with 2.9% in the placebo group. The incidence in the controlled fibromyalgia studies was 7.6% in the pregabalin group compared with 2.5% in the placebo group. In clinical trials, these events of peripheral edema were dose-related, mostly mild to moderate in intensity and rarely led to withdrawal. Peripheral edema was not associated with cardiovascular complications such as hypertension or congestive heart failure and there was no evidence of hemodilution or changes in any laboratory parameters indicative of underlying organ dysfunction (see Warnings and Precautions, Peripheral Edema).

Weight Gain: In the pre-marketing controlled neuropathic pain studies, patients on pregabalin had a higher incidence (5.9%) of weight gain as defined by a ≥7% increase from baseline weight as compared with the placebo group (1.6%). The mean change in the pregabalin group was an increase of 1.5 kg compared with 0.2 kg in the placebo group; few patients (0.1%) withdrew due to weight gain.

The incidence in the controlled fibromyalgia studies was 11.5% in the pregabalin group compared with 2.5% in the placebo group; approximately 1% of pregabalin-treated patients withdrew due to weight gain.

This weight gain was dose-related, and not associated with clinically important changes in blood pressure or cardiovascular adverse events. There was no relationship between baseline body mass index and the incidence of ≥7% weight gain in the controlled trials.

Based on the results of a controlled study of reproductive function in healthy male volunteers, the ≥7% weight gain on pregabalin appeared to be reversible. In this study, there were no reports of peripheral edema (see Warnings and Precautions, Weight Gain).

Abnormal Hematologic and Clinical Chemistry Findings: In all pre-marketing controlled trials, 1.0% of patients on pregabalin and 0.5% of placebo patients had an increase in creatine kinase of >3×upper limit of normal. Renal dysfunction was generally not associated with the elevated creatine kinase in these patients. Mean changes in creatine kinase ranged from 9.6 to 26.3 U/L for pregabalin-treated patients and 4.8 U/L for the placebo patients (see Dosage and Administration, Patients with Impaired Renal Function). Routine therapeutic drug monitoring or clinical laboratory testing is not required for patients treated with LYRICA (see Warnings and Precautions, Creatine Kinase Elevations).

Post-Marketing Adverse Drug Reactions: Since the first global approval of LYRICA on 06 July 2004 through 30 June 2009, there is approximately 6 950 202 patient-years of exposure to LYRICA. Table 13 is based on post-market spontaneous adverse event reports. The percentages shown are calculated by dividing the number of adverse events reported to the company by the estimated number of patient years exposed to LYRICA. Because these adverse reactions are reported spontaneously from a population of uncertain size, it is not possible to reliably estimate their frequency. Furthermore, a causal relationship between LYRICA and the emergence of these events has not been clearly established.

Gastrointestinal: There have been post-marketing events related to reduced lower gastrointestinal tract function e.g., intestinal obstruction, paralytic ileus, and constipation) primarily reported when LYRICA was given in combination with other medications that have the potential to produce constipation, such as opioid analgesics (see Warnings and Precautions, Gastrointestinal).

Urinary and Renal Disorder: renal failure. There have been rare post-marketing reports of patients, with or without previous history, experiencing renal failure while receiving pregabalin alone or in combination with other medications. Discontinuation of pregabalin showed reversibility of this event in some cases. Caution is advised when prescribing pregabalin to the elderly or those with impaired renal function (see Special Populations, Renal; Warnings and Precautions, Renal Failure, and Dosage and Administration).

Cardiovascular: congestive heart failure. These reactions are mostly seen in elderly cardiovascular compromised patients during pregabalin treatment for a neuropathic pain indication (see Warnings and Precautions, Congestive Heart Failure).

Table 13: LYRICA

Post-Market Spontaneous Adverse Event Reports

	Frequency			
Adverse Event	**Common ≥1%**	**Uncommon <1% and ≥0.1%**	**Rare <0.1% and ≥0.01%**	**Very Rare <0.01%**
Cardiovascular				
Congestive Heart Failure[a]				X
Eye Disorders[b]				
Diplopia				X
Vision Blurred				X
Visual Disturbance				X
Psychiatric Disorders				
Confusional State				X
Depression				X
Insomnia				X
Psychotic Disorder[c]				X
Gastrointestinal Disorders				
Diarrhea				X
Dry Mouth				X
Nausea				X
Vomiting				X
Intestinal Obstruction[d]				X
Paralytic Ileus[d]				X
General Disorders and Administration Site Conditions				
Fatigue				X
Feeling Abnormal				X
Pain				X
Immune System Disorders				
Angioedema[e]				X
Hypersensitivity[f]				X
Nervous System Disorders				
Ataxia				X
Coordination Abnormal				X
Dizziness[g]				X
Dysarthria				X
Headache				X
Memory Impairment				X
Paresthesia				X
Somnolence[g]				X
Speech Disorder				X
Tremor				X
Coma				X
Loss of Consciousness				X
Mental Impairment				X
Renal and Urinary Disorders				
Urinary Retention				X
Respiratory, Thoracic and Mediastinal Disorders				
Dyspnea				X
Pulmonary Edema				X
Skin and Subcutaneous Tissue Disorders				

(cont'd)

Table 13: LYRICA *(cont'd)*

Post-Market Spontaneous Adverse Event Reports

Adverse Event	Frequency			
	Common ≥1%	**Uncommon <1% and ≥0.1%**	**Rare <0.1% and ≥0.01%**	**Very Rare <0.01%**
Pruritus				X

[a] These reactions are mostly seen in elderly cardiovascular compromised patients during pregabalin treatment for a neuropathic pain indication (see Warnings and Precautions, Congestive Heart Failure).
[b] There have also been rare reports of accommodation disorder, eyelid edema and eye redness (see Warnings and Precautions, Ophthalmological Effects).
[c] There have been rare reports of psychotic disorders in patients receiving pregabalin.
[d] See below and Warnings and Precautions, Gastrointestinal.
[e] See Warnings and Precautions, Angioedema.
[f] See Warnings and Precautions, Hypersensitivity.
[g] See Warnings and Precautions, Dizziness and Somnolence.

Respiratory, Thoracic and Mediastinal Disorder: pulmonary edema. There have been post-marketing reports of pulmonary edema in patients receiving pregabalin. Although this adverse reaction has mostly been observed in elderly patients with predisposing factors, some cases have occurred in patients with no known previous history or predisposing conditions.
Eye Disorders: diplopia, vision blurred, visual disturbance. There have also been rare reports of accommodation disorder, eyelid edema and eye redness (see Warnings and Precautions, Ophthalmological Effects).
Drug Abuse and Dependence/Liability: In a study of recreational users (N=15) of sedative/hypnotic drugs, including alcohol, a single dose of LYRICA (pregabalin) 450 mg received subjective ratings of "good drug effect", "high", and "liking" to a degree that was similar to a single dose of diazepam 30 mg. In controlled clinical studies in over 5500 patients, 4% of LYRICA-treated patients and 1% of placebo-treated patients overall reported euphoria as an adverse event. However, in clinical trials of diabetic peripheral neuropathy, euphoria was reported as an adverse event by 1.8% of LYRICA-treated patients and 0% of placebo-treated patients, and in clinical trials of postherpetic neuralgia, euphoria was reported as an adverse event by 0.9% of LYRICA-treated patients and 0% of placebo-treated patients. In clinical studies, following abrupt or rapid discontinuation of pregabalin, some patients reported symptoms including insomnia, nausea, headache, anxiety, hyperhidrosis, or diarrhea suggestive of physical dependence (see Warnings and Precautions, Abrupt or Rapid Discontinuation).

Pregabalin is not known to be active at receptor sites associated with drugs of abuse. As with any CNS active drug, physicians should carefully evaluate patients for history of drug abuse and observe them for signs of LYRICA misuse or abuse (e.g., development of tolerance, dose escalation, drug-seeking behaviour).

DRUG INTERACTIONS: Overview: Since pregabalin is predominately excreted unchanged in the urine, undergoes negligible metabolism in humans (<2% of a dose recovered in urine as metabolites), does not inhibit drug metabolism in vitro, and is not bound to plasma proteins, LYRICA (pregabalin) is unlikely to produce, or be subject to, pharmacokinetic interactions.
Pharmacokinetic: In Vitro Studies: In vitro drug metabolism studies revealed that pregabalin at concentrations which were, in general, 10-fold greater than observed in Phase 2/3 clinical trials, does not inhibit human CYP1A2, CYP2A6, CYP2C9, CYP2C19, CYP2D6, CYP2E1, and CYP3A4 enzyme systems.
In Vivo Studies: The drug interaction data described in this section were obtained from studies involving healthy adults, patients with epilepsy, and patients with chronic pain disorders.
Carbamazepine, Valproic Acid, Lamotrigine, Phenytoin, Phenobarbital, and Topiramate: In vitro and in vivo studies showed that LYRICA is unlikely to be involved in significant pharmacokinetic drug interactions. Specifically, there are no clinically significant pharmacokinetic interactions between pregabalin and the following antiepileptic drugs: carbamazepine, valproic acid, lamotrigine, phenytoin, phenobarbital, and topiramate. Important pharmacokinetic interactions would also not be expected to occur between pregabalin and commonly used antiepileptic drugs.
Tiagabine: The results of a population pharmacokinetic analysis indicated that in patients with partial seizures tiagabine had no clinically significant effect on pregabalin clearance.
Gabapentin: The pharmacokinetics of pregabalin and gabapentin were investigated in 12 healthy subjects following concomitant single dose administration of 100 mg pregabalin and 300 mg gabapentin, and in 18 healthy subjects following concomitant multiple dose administration of 200 mg pregabalin q8h and 400 mg gabapentin q8h. Gabapentin pharmacokinetics following single and multiple dose administration were unaltered by pregabalin coadministration. The rate of pregabalin absorption was reduced by approximately 26% (single dose administration) and 18% (multiple dose administration) based on lower C_{max} values; however, the extent of pregabalin absorption was unaffected by gabapentin coadministration.
Oral Contraceptives: Pregabalin coadministration (200 mg TID) had no effect on the steady state pharmacokinetics of norethindrone and ethinyl estradiol (1 mg/35 µg, respectively) in healthy subjects.
Lorazepam: Multiple dose administration of pregabalin (300 mg BID) in healthy subjects had no effect on the rate and extent of lorazepam single dose pharmacokinetics and single dose administration of lorazepam (1 mg) had no clinically significant effect on the steady state pharmacokinetics of pregabalin.
Oxycodone: Multiple dose administration of pregabalin (300 mg BID) in healthy subjects had no effect on the rate and extent of oxycodone single dose pharmacokinetics. Single dose administration of oxycodone (10 mg) had no clinically significant effect on the steady state pharmacokinetics of pregabalin.
Ethanol: Multiple dose administration of pregabalin (300 mg BID) in healthy subjects had no effect on the rate and extent of ethanol single dose pharmacokinetics and single dose administration of ethanol (0.7 g/kg) had no clinically significant effect on the steady state pharmacokinetics of pregabalin.
Diuretics, Oral Hypoglycemics, and Insulin: A population pharmacokinetic analysis in patients with chronic pain showed no clinically significant effect on pregabalin clearance with the concomitant use of diuretics, oral hypoglycemics, and insulin.
Pharmacodynamic: Oxycodone, Lorazepam, Ethanol: Multiple oral doses of pregabalin co-administered with oxycodone, lorazepam, or ethanol did not result in clinically important effects on respiration. Pregabalin may potentiate the effects of ethanol and lorazepam. Pregabalin appears to be additive in the impairment of cognitive and gross motor function caused by oxycodone.

In post-marketing experience, there are reports of respiratory failure and coma in patients taking pregabalin alone or in combination with other CNS depressants.
Thiazolidinedione Antidiabetic Agents: Higher frequencies of weight gain and peripheral edema were observed in patients taking both LYRICA and a thiazolidinedione antidiabetic agent compared to patients taking either drug alone. The majority of patients using thiazolidinedione antidiabetic agents in the overall safety database were participants in studies of pain associated with diabetic peripheral neuropathy.

As the thiazolidinedione class of antidiabetic drugs or LYRICA can cause weight gain and/or fluid retention alone or together, possibly exacerbating or leading to heart failure, caution should be exercised when co-administering LYRICA and these agents (see Warnings and Precautions, Peripheral Edema).
Drug-Food Interactions: The rate of pregabalin absorption is decreased when given with food resulting in a decrease in C_{max} by approximately 25% to 30% and an increase in T_{max} to approximately 3 hours. However, administration of pregabalin with food has no clinically relevant effect on the total amount of pregabalin absorbed. Therefore, pregabalin can be taken with or without food.
Drug-Herb Interactions: LYRICA has no known drug/herb interactions.
Drug-Laboratory Interactions: LYRICA has no known drug/laboratory test interactions.

DOSAGE AND ADMINISTRATION: Dosing Considerations: Patients with Impaired Renal Function: Pregabalin is primarily eliminated from the systemic circulation by renal excretion as unchanged drug. In some elderly patients and those with a medical history of significant renal insufficiency, daily dosages should be reduced accordingly (see Dosage Adjustment Based on Renal Function).

In accordance with current clinical practice, if LYRICA (pregabalin) has to be discontinued, it is recommended this should be done gradually over a minimum of 1 week (see Warnings and Precautions, Abrupt or Rapid Discontinuation).
Adults: Neuropathic Pain Associated with Diabetic Peripheral Neuropathy: The recommended starting dose for LYRICA is 150 mg/day, given in two or three divided doses (75 mg BID or 50 mg TID), with or without food in patients with a creatinine clearance rate of at least 60 mL/min. Efficacy of LYRICA has been demonstrated within the first week. Based on individual patient response and tolerability, the dose may be increased to 150 mg BID (300 mg/day) after one week.

For patients who experience significant and ongoing pain and can tolerate pregabalin 300 mg/day well, maximum daily dose of 600 mg (300 mg twice a day, BID) can be used. However, in clinical trials, LYRICA 600 mg/day did not provide additional significant efficacy and patients treated with this dose experienced markedly higher rates of adverse events and discontinued the trial more frequently (see Adverse Reactions, Table 1 and Table 5). Doses above 600 mg/day have not been studied and are not recommended.
Neuropathic Pain Associated with Postherpetic Neuralgia: The recommended starting dose for LYRICA is 150 mg/day, given in two or three divided doses (75 mg BID or 50 mg TID), with or without food in patients with a creatinine clearance rate of at least 60 mL/min. Efficacy of LYRICA has been demonstrated within the first week. Based on individual patient response and tolerability, the dose may be increased to 150 mg BID (300 mg/day) after one week.

For patients who experience significant and ongoing pain and can tolerate pregabalin 300 mg/day well, maximum daily dose of 600 mg (300 mg twice a day, BID) can be used. However, in clinical trials, LYRICA 600 mg/day did not provide additional significant efficacy and patients treated with this dose experienced markedly higher rates of adverse events and discontinued the trial more frequently (see Adverse Reactions, Table 3 and Table 6). Doses above 600 mg/day have not been studied and are not recommended.
Neuropathic Pain Associated with Spinal Cord Injury: The recommended starting dose for LYRICA is 150 mg/day, given in two divided doses (75 mg BID), with or without food in patients with a creatinine clearance rate of at least 60 mL/min. Efficacy of LYRICA has been demonstrated within the first week. Based on individual patient response and tolerability, the dose may be increased to 150 mg BID (300 mg/day) after one week.

For patients who experience significant and ongoing pain and can tolerate pregabalin 300 mg/day well, a maximum daily dose of 600 mg (300 mg twice a day, BID) may be considered. Doses above 600 mg/day have not been studied and are not recommended.
Pain Associated with Fibromyalgia: The recommended dosage is 300 to 450 mg/day, given in two divided doses. The recommended starting dose for LYRICA is 150 mg/day, given in two divided doses (75 mg BID), with or without food in patients with a creatinine clearance rate of at least 60 mL/min. Based on individual response and tolerability, the dose may be increased to 150 mg BID (300 mg/day) after one week. Patients who do not experience sufficient benefit with 300 mg/day may be further increased to 225 mg BID (450 mg/day). In some patients, efficacy of LYRICA has been demonstrated within the first week.

For patients who experience significant and ongoing pain and can tolerate pregabalin 300 mg/day well, maximum daily dose of 600 mg (300 mg twice a day, BID) can be used. However, in clinical trials of fibromyalgia, LYRICA 600 mg/day did not provide additional significant efficacy and patients treated with this dose experienced significantly higher rates of adverse events and discontinued the trial more frequently (see Adverse Reactions, Table 7 and Table 10). In view of the dose-related adverse events, the decision to treat patients with doses above 450 mg/day should be based on clinical judgment of the treating physician. Doses above 600 mg/day have not been studied and are not recommended.
Dosage Adjustment Based on Renal Function: LYRICA is primarily eliminated by renal excretion. Therefore, the dose should be adjusted for patients with reduced renal function. Pregabalin clearance is directly proportional to creatinine clearance. Therefore, dosing adjustment should be based on creatinine clearance (CL_{Cr}), as indicated in Table 14.

To use this dosing table, an estimate of the patient's creatinine clearance (CL_{Cr}) in mL/min is needed. CL_{Cr} in mL/min may be estimated from serum creatinine (mg/dL) determination using the Cockcroft and Gault equation:

$$CL_{Cr} = \frac{[140\text{-age (years)}] \times \text{weight (kg)}}{72 \times \text{serum creatinine (mg/dL)}} \quad (\times 0.85 \text{ for female patients})$$

Pregabalin is effectively removed from plasma by hemodialysis. Over a 4-hour hemodialysis treatment, plasma pregabalin concentrations are reduced by approximately 50%. For patients receiving hemodialysis, pregabalin daily dose should be adjusted based on renal function. In addition to the daily dose adjustment, a supplemental dose should be given immediately following every 4-hour hemodialysis treatment (see Table 14).

Table 14: LYRICA

Pregabalin Dosage Adjustment Based on Renal Function

Creatinine Clearance (CL_{cr}) (mL/min)	Total Pregabalin Daily Dose (mg/day)[a] Recommended Dose Escalation[c]				Dose Regimen
	Starting Dose	**→ up to**		**Maximum Daily Dose**	
≥60	150	300	450	600	BID or TID
30–60	75	150	225	300	BID or TID
15–30	25–50	75	100–150	150	QD or BID
<15	25	25–50	50–75	75	QD
Supplementary dosage following hemodialysis (mg)[b]					
Patients on the 25 mg QD regimen: take one supplemental dose of 25 mg or 50 mg Patients on the 25-50 mg QD regimen: take one supplemental dose of 50 mg or 75 mg Patients on the 50-75 mg QD regimen: take one supplemental dose of 75 mg or 100 mg Patients on the 75 mg QD regimen: take one supplemental dose of 100 mg or 150 mg					

[a] Total daily dose (mg/day) should be divided as indicated by dose regimen to provide mg/dose.
[b] Supplementary dose is a single additional dose.
[c] Based on individual patient response and tolerability.
Legend: TID=three divided doses; BID=two divided doses; QD=single daily dose.

Geriatrics (>65 years): Pregabalin oral clearance tended to decrease with increasing age. This decrease in pregabalin oral clearance is consistent with age-related decreases in creatinine clearance. Reduction of pregabalin dose may be required in patients who have age-related compromised renal function.
Pediatrics (<18 years of age): The safety and efficacy of pregabalin in pediatric patients (<18 years of age) have not been established and its use in this patient population is not recommended.
Administration: LYRICA is given orally with or without food (see Drug Interactions, Drug-Food Interactions).

OVERDOSAGE:
Signs, Symptoms and Laboratory Findings of Acute Overdosage in Humans: The highest known dose of pregabalin received in the clinical development program in which there was no fatal outcome was 15 000 mg in 1 patient. The types of adverse events experienced by patients who received an overdose were not clinically different from other patients receiving recommended doses of pregabalin.

In post-marketing experience, fatal outcomes in cases in which pregabalin has been taken in combination with other medications have been reported with a pregabalin overdose as low as 800 mg in a day. In none of these cases has pregabalin been established as the cause of death or in pregabalin monotherapy. The lowest fatal dose with pregabalin alone has not yet been identified.

The most commonly reported adverse events observed when pregabalin was taken in overdose (dose range from 800 mg/day up to 11 500 mg as a single dose) included affective disorder, somnolence, confusional state, depression, agitation, and restlessness.
Treatment or Management of Overdose: There is no specific antidote for overdose with pregabalin. If indicated, elimination of unabsorbed drug may be attempted by emesis or gastric lavage; usual precautions should be observed to maintain the airway. General supportive care of the patient is indicated including monitoring of vital signs and observation of the clinical status of the patient. A Certified Poison Control Center should be contacted for up-to-date information on the management of overdose with pregabalin.

Hemodialysis: Standard hemodialysis procedures result in significant clearance of pregabalin (approximately 50% in 4 hours) and should be considered in cases of overdose. Although hemodialysis has not been performed in the few known cases of overdose, it may be indicated by the patient's clinical state or in patients with significant renal impairment.

> For management of a suspected drug overdose, contact your regional Poison Control Centre. See the *CPS* Directory section for a list of Poison Control Centres.

ACTION AND CLINICAL PHARMACOLOGY: Mechanism of Action: LYRICA (pregabalin) binds to the α2-δ subunit of the voltage-gated calcium channels in central nervous system tissues. In vitro, pregabalin reduces calcium influx at nerve terminals, which may inhibit the release of excitatory neurotransmitters such as glutamate. Through this mechanism, LYRICA may modulate nerve impulses involved in the transmission of pain. However, the clinical relevance of these findings in man is unknown.

Pharmacodynamics: LYRICA binds with high affinity to the alpha$_2$-delta protein (a calcium channel subunit) of brain tissues and has analgesic, antiepileptic, and anxiolytic activity. Pregabalin is known chemically as (S)-3-(aminomethyl)-5-methylhexanoic acid.

Although the mechanism of action of pregabalin is unknown, results with genetically modified mice and with compounds structurally-related to pregabalin indicate that selective binding to the alpha$_2$-delta protein is required for analgesic, antiepileptic and anxiolytic action in animal models. In vitro, pregabalin reduces the release of several neurotransmitters, suggesting a modulatory action on calcium channel function.

Pregabalin does not mimic GABA at GABA$_A$ or GABA$_B$ receptors, nor does it augment GABA$_A$ responses like benzodiazepines or barbiturates. In contrast to vascular calcium channel blockers, pregabalin does not alter systemic blood pressure or cardiac function. Various in vitro and in vivo results differentiate pregabalin from GABA uptake inhibitors or GABA transaminase inhibitors. In addition, pregabalin does not block sodium channels, it is not active at opiate receptors, it does not alter cyclooxygenase enzyme activity, it is not a serotonin agonist, it is not a dopamine antagonist, and it is not an inhibitor of dopamine, serotonin or noradrenaline reuptake.

Pregabalin treatment reduces pain-related behavior in neuropathic animal models of diabetes, peripheral nerve damage or chemotherapeutic insult and in a model of musculoskeletal associated pain. Pregabalin given intrathecally prevents pain-related behaviors and reduces pain-related behavior caused by spinally administered agents, suggesting that it acts directly on tissues of the spinal cord or brain.

Pharmacokinetics: All pharmacological actions following pregabalin administration are due to the activity of the parent compound; pregabalin is not appreciably metabolized in humans. Mean steady-state plasma pregabalin concentration-time profiles following 75, 300, and 600 mg/day given in equally divided doses every 8 hours (TID) and 600 mg/day given in equally divided doses every 12 hours (BID) are shown in Table 15. Pregabalin pharmacokinetics are linear over the recommended daily dose range. Inter-subject pharmacokinetic variability for pregabalin is low (<20%).

Table 15: LYRICA

Pregabalin Mean (CV%[a]) Steady-State Pharmacokinetic Parameter Values in Healthy Volunteers

Dose (mg)	Regimen	Daily Dose (mg/day)	N	C_{maxss} (µg/mL)	t_{max} (h)	C_{minss} (µg/mL)	$AUC_{(0-t)}$ (µg·h/mL)	$t_{½}$ (h)	$C_{L/F}$ (mL/min)
25	TID[b]	75	8	1.39	0.9	0.45	6.7	5.9	64.1
				-19.5	-34.2	-25	-18.3	-17.3	-16.1
100	TID	300	6	5.03	0.8	1.94	25.2	6.3	68.9
				-21.3	-31	-33.6	-23	-19.6	-20.9
200	TID	600	11	8.52	0.9	3.28	41.7	6.3	81
				-14.8	-22.2	-29.2	-12.8	-13.6	-11.7
300	BID[c]	600	8	9.07	1.4	2.6	59	6.7	85.1
				-10.5	-57.1	-15.5	-6.4	-16.2	-6.4

[a] Percent coefficient of variation.
[b] Total daily dose given in equally divided doses every 8 hours.
[c] Total daily dose given in equally divided doses every 12 hours.
Legend: C_{maxss}=steady-state peak plasma concentration; t_{max}=time of peak plasma concentration at steady state; C_{minss}=steady-state trough plasma concentration; $AUC_{(0-t)}$=area under the plasma concentration-time curve during one dosing interval at steady state; $t_{½}$=elimination half-life; $C_{L/F}$=oral clearance.

Absorption: Pregabalin is rapidly absorbed when administered in the fasted state, with peak plasma concentrations occurring within 1.5 hours following both single- and multiple-dose administration. Pregabalin oral bioavailability is ≥90% and is independent of dose. C_{max} (Figure 1) and AUC values increase proportionally following single- and multiple-dose administration. Following repeated administration, steady state is achieved within 24 to 48 hours. Multiple dose pharmacokinetics are predictable from single-dose data.

Figure 1: LYRICA

Individual and Mean Steady-State Pregabalin C_{max} Values Following 75, 300 and 600 mg/day Given in Equally Divided Doses TID (q8h) to Healthy Volunteers[a]

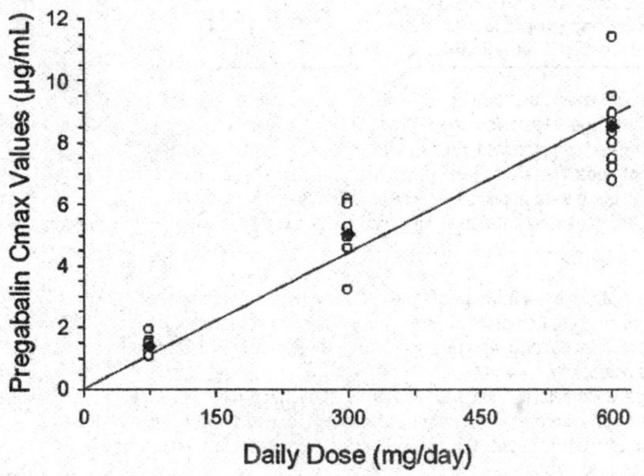

[a] Solid line is the regression line going through the origin; individual (□) and mean (♦) values.

Distribution: In preclinical studies, pregabalin has been shown to readily cross the blood brain barrier in mice, rats, and monkeys. Pregabalin is a substrate for system L transporter which is responsible for the transport of large amino acids across the blood-brain barrier. Pregabalin has been shown to cross the placenta in rats and is present in the milk of lactating rats. In humans, the apparent volume of distribution of pregabalin following oral administration is approximately 0.5 L/kg. Pregabalin is not bound to plasma proteins. At clinically efficacious doses of 150 and 600 mg/day, the average steady-state plasma pregabalin concentrations were approximately 1.5 and 6.0 µg/mL, respectively.

Metabolism: Pregabalin undergoes negligible metabolism in humans. Following a dose of radiolabeled pregabalin, approximately 98% of the radioactivity recovered in the urine was unchanged pregabalin. The N-methylated derivative of pregabalin, the major metabolite of pregabalin found in urine, accounted for 0.9% of the dose. In preclinical studies, pregabalin (S-enantiomer) did not undergo racemization to the R-enantiomer in mice, rats, rabbits, or monkeys.

Excretion: Pregabalin is eliminated from the systemic circulation primarily by renal excretion as unchanged drug. Pregabalin mean $t_{½}$ is 6.3 hours. Pregabalin elimination is proportional to creatinine clearance. Pregabalin clearance is reduced in patients with impaired renal function (see Dosage and Administration).

Special Populations and Conditions: Pregabalin undergoes negligible metabolism, is not bound to plasma proteins, and is eliminated predominately as unchanged drug by renal excretion. Clinically important differences in pregabalin pharmacokinetics due to race and gender have not been observed and are not anticipated.

Pediatrics: Pharmacokinetics of pregabalin have not been studied in paediatric patients.

Geriatrics: Pregabalin oral clearance tended to decrease with increasing age. This decrease in pregabalin oral clearance is consistent with age-related decreases in creatinine clearance. Reduction of pregabalin dose may be required in patients who have age-related compromised renal function (see Warnings and Precautions and Dosage and Administration).

Gender: A population pharmacokinetic analysis of the Phase 2/3 clinical program showed that the relationship between daily dose and pregabalin drug exposure is similar between genders when adjusted for gender-related differences in creatinine clearance.

Race: A population pharmacokinetic analysis of the Phase 2/3 clinical program showed that the relationship between daily dose and pregabalin drug exposure is similar among Caucasians, Blacks, and Hispanics.

Renal Insufficiency: Because renal elimination is the major elimination pathway, dosage reduction in patients with renal dysfunction is necessary. Pregabalin is effectively removed from plasma by hemodialysis. Following a 4-hour hemodialysis treatment, plasma pregabalin concentrations are reduced by approximately 50%. For patients on hemodialysis, dosing must be modified (see Dosage and Administration).

STORAGE AND STABILITY: Store at 15-30°C.

INFORMATION FOR THE PATIENT: Published in e-CPS, available by subscription at www.e-cps.ca.

DOSAGE FORMS, COMPOSITION AND PACKAGING: 25 mg: Each white hard gelatin capsule, printed with black ink "Pfizer" on the cap, "PGN 25" on the body contains: 25 mg pregabalin. Nonmedicinal ingredients: lactose monohydrate, maize starch and talc; capsule shell: colloidal silicon dioxide (manufacturing aid, which may not be present), gelatin, sodium lauryl sulfate and titanium dioxide; black ink: black iron oxide, potassium hydroxide, propylene glycol, shellac and water. HDPE bottles of 60. PVC/aluminum blisters.

50 mg: Each white hard gelatin capsule, printed with black ink "Pfizer" on the cap, "PGN 50" and an ink band on the body contains: 50 mg pregabalin. Nonmedicinal ingredients: lactose monohydrate, maize starch and talc; capsule shell: colloidal silicon dioxide (manufacturing aid, which may not be present), gelatin, sodium lauryl sulfate and titanium dioxide; black ink: black iron oxide, potassium hydroxide, propylene glycol, shellac and water. HDPE bottles of 60. PVC/aluminum blisters.

75 mg: Each white/orange hard gelatin capsule, printed with black ink "Pfizer" on the cap, "PGN 75" on the body contains: 75 mg pregabalin. Nonmedicinal ingredients: lactose monohydrate, maize starch and talc; capsule shell: gelatin and titanium dioxide. In addition, the orange capsule shells contain red iron oxide and the white capsule shells contain sodium lauryl sulfate and colloidal silicon dioxide. Colloidal silicon dioxide is a manufacturing aid, which may not be present. The markings on the capsules are in black ink, which contains shellac, black iron oxide, propylene glycol, potassium hydroxide and water. HDPE bottles of 60. PVC/aluminum blisters.

150 mg: Each white hard gelatin capsule, printed with black ink "Pfizer" on the cap, "PGN 150" on the body contains: 150 mg pregabalin. Nonmedicinal ingredients: lactose monohydrate, maize starch and talc; capsule shell: colloidal silicon dioxide (manufacturing aid, which may not be present), gelatin, sodium lauryl sulfate and titanium dioxide; black ink: black iron oxide, potassium hydroxide, propylene glycol, shellac and water. HDPE bottles of 60. PVC/aluminum blisters.

225 mg: Each white/light orange hard gelatin capsule, printed with black ink "Pfizer" on the cap, "PGN 225" on the body contains: 225 mg pregabalin. Nonmedicinal ingredients: lactose monohydrate, maize starch and talc; capsule shell: gelatin and titanium dioxide. In addition, the orange capsule shells contain red iron oxide and the white capsule shells contain sodium lauryl sulfate and colloidal silicon dioxide. Colloidal silicon dioxide is a manufacturing aid, which may not be present. The markings on the capsules are in black ink, which contains shellac, black iron oxide, propylene glycol, potassium hydroxide and water. HDPE bottles of 60. PVC/aluminum blisters.

300 mg: Each white/orange hard gelatin capsule, printed with black ink "Pfizer" on the cap, "PGN 300" on the body contains: 300 mg pregabalin. Nonmedicinal ingredients: lactose monohydrate, maize starch and talc; capsule shell: gelatin and titanium dioxide. In addition, the orange capsule shells contain red iron oxide and the white capsule shells contain sodium lauryl sulfate and colloidal silicon dioxide. Colloidal silicon dioxide is a manufacturing aid, which may not be present. The markings on the capsules are in black ink, which contains shellac, black iron oxide, propylene glycol, potassium hydroxide and water. HDPE bottles of 60. PVC/aluminum blisters.

(Shown in Product Identification Section)

Lysodren® Pr

mitotane

Antineoplastic

Bristol-Myers Squibb

Date of Preparation: February 25, 1971
Date of Revision: October 26, 2004

PHARMACOLOGY: Mitotane is an adrenal cytotoxic agent, and can cause adrenal inhibition, apparently without cellular destruction. Its biochemical mechanism of action is unknown. Available data suggest that the drug modifies the peripheral metabolism of steroids as well as directly suppressing the adrenal cortex. In man, mitotane administration alters cortisol's extra-adrenal metabolism, leading to a reduction in measurable 17-hydroxy corticosteroids, even though plasma corticosteroid concentrations do not fall. The drug apparently causes increased formation of 6-beta-hydroxy cortisol.

Approximately 40% of oral mitotane is absorbed, and approximately 10% is recovered in the urine as a water soluble metabolite. A small amount is excreted in the bile and the balance is stored in the tissues. When administered parenterally, approximately 25% of the dose is found in the urine as a water soluble metabolite.

Both unchanged drug and a metabolite were measured during and after dosing. The concentrations in patients receiving doses from 5 to 15 g/day varied from 7 to 90 µg/mL of unchanged mitotane and 29 to 54 µg/mL of the metabolite. These studies indicated no relationship between blood concentrations and therapeutic and/or toxic effects.

Following discontinuation of the drug, blood concentrations fell, but persisted for several weeks. In most patients, blood concentrations became undetectable after 6 to 9 weeks. In 1 patient who had received a total of 1 900 g of mitotane, high blood concentrations were found 10 weeks after stopping the drug. Autopsy data have provided evidence that mitotane is found in most body tissues. Fat tissues were the primary storage site. In 1 patient a very large number of tissues were examined and the drug was found in essentially every tissue.

Mitotane appears to be partly converted to a water soluble metabolite. This material has not been characterized, but is only found in the urine and blood of patients receiving mitotane. Examination of bile was made and found to contain no unchanged mitotane. There was metabolite in the bile, and this would indicate that biliary excretion is a significant route of removal of this metabolite from the body.

There is no evidence of a cure as a consequence of mitotane administration. A number of patients have been treated intermittently, treatment being restarted when severe symptoms reappear. Patients often do not respond after the third or fourth such course. Experience accumulated to date suggest that continuous treatment with the maximum possible mitotane dosage would be the best approach.

There was significant reduction in tumor mass following mitotane administration in about 50%, and a significant reduction in elevated steroid excretion in about 80% of the evaluable patients studied to date. Clinical effectiveness can be shown by reduction in tumor mass, reduction in pain, weakness or anorexia, and reduction of steroid symptoms.

INDICATIONS: Mitotane is indicated only in the treatment of inoperable adrenal cortical carcinoma of both functional and nonfunctional type.

CONTRAINDICATIONS: Known hypersensitivity to mitotane.

WARNINGS: Mitotane should be temporarily discontinued immediately following shock or severe trauma since adrenal suppression is its prime action. Exogenous steroids should also be administered in such circumstances since the depressed adrenal may not immediately start to secrete steroids.

Mitotane should be administered with care to patients with liver disease other than metastatic lesion of the adrenal cortex, since the metabolism of mitotane may be interfered with and the drug may accumulate.

All possible tumour tissue should be surgically removed from large metastatic masses before mitotane administration is instituted. This is necessary to minimize the possibility of infarction and hemorrhage in the tumour due to a rapid, positive effect of the drug.

Long-term continuous administration of high doses of mitotane may lead to brain damage and impairment of function. Behavioural and neurological assessments should be made at regular intervals when continuous mitotane treatment exceeds two years.

Pregnancy: Mitotane's safety in pregnancy or lactation has not been established. Treatment of women who are, or who may become pregnant, should be undertaken only after consideration of the benefits versus the possibility of harm to mother and child.

Lactation: See Pregnancy.

PRECAUTIONS: Adrenal insufficiency may develop in patients treated with mitotane, and adrenal steroid replacement should be considered for these patients.

Occupational Hazards: Since sedation, lethargy, vertigo, and other CNS adverse effects can occur, caution ambulatory patients about driving, operating machinery, and other hazardous pursuits requiring mental and physical alertness.

Drug Interactions: Mitotane appears to induce drug metabolizing enzymes in both experimental animals and man. Consequently, the dosage of other drugs given concurrently with mitotane may require adjustment in order to achieve the desired therapeutic effect.

ADVERSE EFFECTS: A very high percentage of patients treated with mitotane have shown at least one type of adverse effect. The main types of adverse reactions consist of the following:

1. Gastrointestinal disturbances, which consisted of anorexia, nausea or vomiting, and in some cases diarrhea, occurred in about 80% of the patients.
2. CNS effects occurred in 40% of the patients and consisted primarily of depression as manifested by lethargy and somnolence (25%), and dizziness or vertigo (15%).
3. Skin toxicity was observed in about 15% of the cases. In some instances, however, this adverse effect subsided while the patients were maintained on the drug.

Infrequently occurring adverse effects involve the eye (visual blurring, diplopia, lens opacity, toxic retinopathy); the genitourinary system (hematuria, hemorrhagic cystitis, albuminuria); cardiovascular system (hypertension, orthostatic hypotension, flushing); and some miscellaneous complaints including generalized aching, hyperpyrexia, and lowered PBI.

OVERDOSE:
No data supplied by the manufacturer.

For management of a suspected drug overdose, CPhA recommends that you contact your **regional Poison Control Centre**. See the *CPS* Directory section for a list of Poison Control Centres.

DOSAGE: Two dosage regimens may be used. The patient may be started on 2-6 g a day, in divided doses q.i.d. or t.i.d. and the dosage increased as quickly as possible to as much drug as can be tolerated, preferably arriving at 8-10 g or more.

or

Start the patient at 9-10 g of mitotane per day in divided doses, either q.i.d. or t.i.d. since most patients will have side effects initially irrespective of starting dosage. If severe side effects appear, the dose should be reduced until the maximum tolerated dose is achieved. If the patient can tolerate higher doses and improved clinical response appears possible, the dose should be increased until adverse reactions interfere.

Experience has shown that the maximum tolerated dose (MTD) will vary from 2 to 16 g/day, but has usually been 8 to 10 g/day. The highest doses used in the studies to date were 18 to 19 g/day.

Treatment should be instituted in the hospital until a stable dosage regimen is achieved.

Treatment should be continued as long as clinical benefits are observed. Maintenance of clinical status or slowing of growth of metastatic lesions can be considered clinical benefits if they can clearly be shown to have occurred.

If no clinical benefits are observed after 3 months at the maximum tolerated dose, the case may be considered a clinical failure. However, 10% of the patients who showed a measurable response required more than 3 months at the MTD.

Early diagnosis and prompt institution of treatment improve the probability of a positive clinical response.

SUPPLIED: Each one-half inch, biconvex, round compressed white tablet, bisected on one side and impressed with "BL" over "L1" on the other side, contains: mitotane 500 mg. Nonmedicinal ingredients: microcrystalline cellulose, polyethylene glycol, silicon dioxide and starch. Bottles of 100.

THE FIRST AND ONLY ANTIARRHYTHMIC DRUG INDICATED TO REDUCE THE RISK OF CV HOSPITALIZATION DUE TO AF IN AF PATIENTS

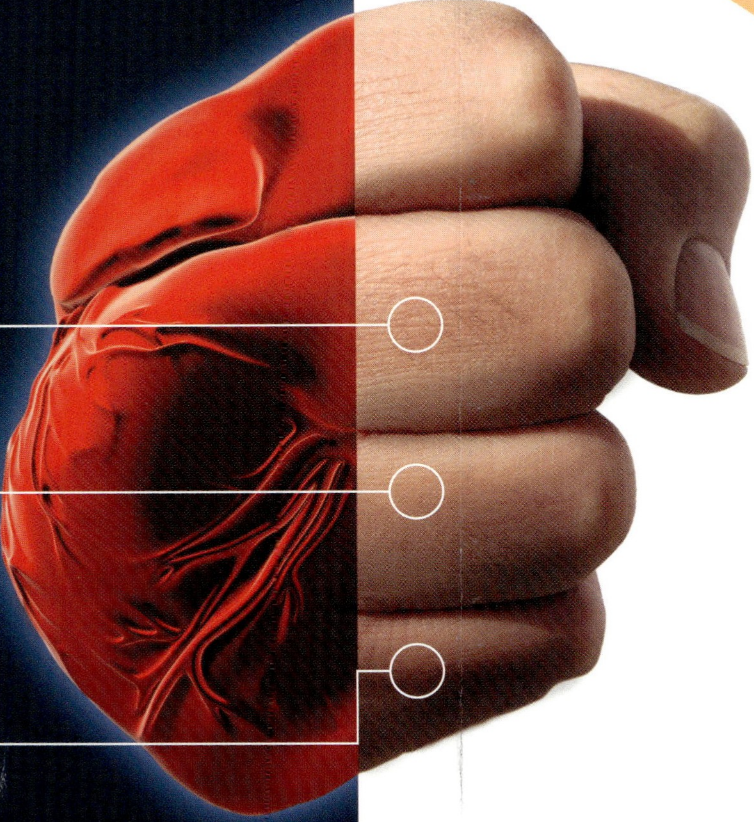

Ⓟ MULTAQ™: Significantly reduced the risk of CV hospitalization (secondary endpoint) 26% RRR

(Incidence of events: 29.3% [*n*=2,301] vs. 36.9% placebo [*n*=2,327]; HR 0.74; 95% CI 0.67 to 0.82; p<0.001)[1,2]*

Generally safe and well-tolerated[1†]

(The most common AEs were diarrhea [9.0%], nausea [4.9%], fatigue [4.3%], abdominal pains [3.5%], and bradycardia [3.3%]. In pooled clinical trials, premature discontinuation due to AEs occurred in 11.8% of MULTAQ™-treated patients [7.7% in the placebo-treated group].)

Easy to dose

(Fixed dose of 400 mg BID)

MULTAQ™ is indicated for the treatment of patients with a history of, or current, atrial fibrillation to reduce the risk of cardiovascular hospitalization due to atrial fibrillation.

In patients with a history of, or current AF, MULTAQ™ significantly reduced the risk of first CV hospitalization or all-cause mortality (primary composite endpoint): 24% RRR (incidence of events: 31.9% vs. 39.4% placebo; HR 0.76; 95% CI 0.69-0.84; p<0.001). With respect to the secondary endpoint of "death from any cause", the difference between the number of deaths in the two treatment groups did not reach statistical significance.[1,2]*

MULTAQ™ is contraindicated in patients with severe congestive heart failure (Stage NYHA IV) and other unstable hemodynamic conditions. It should be used with caution in patients with moderate CHF (Stage NYHA III) and only if the benefits are deemed to outweigh the risks involved. MULTAQ™ is also contraindicated in patients with second- or third-degree AV block or sick sinus syndrome (except when used in conjunction with a functioning pacemaker); bradycardia <50 bpm; QT_c Bazett interval ≥500 msec; severe hepatic impairment; pregnancy; lactation; or a history of hypersensitivity reactions to MULTAQ™ or any of its excipients or component of the container.

MULTAQ™ must not be co-administered with strong CYP 3A4 inhibitors, such as ketoconazole, itraconazole, voriconazole, cyclosporin, telithromycin, clarithromycin, nefazodone, and ritonavir. Co-administration of drugs prolonging the QT interval (such as phenothiazines, bepridil, tricyclic antidepressants certain oral macrolides, and Class I and III antiarrhythmics, which may induce torsades de pointes) is contraindicated because of the potential risk of proarrhythmia.

Treatment with Class I or III antiarrhythmics (such as flecainide, propafenone, quinidine, disopyramide, dofetilide, sotalol, amiodarone) must be stopped before starting MULTAQ™.

The most common adverse reactions observed with MULTAQ™ 400 mg twice daily were diarrhea (9.0%), nausea (4.9%), fatigue (4.3%), abdominal pains (3.5%), bradycardia (3.3%), rashes (including generalized, macular, and maculopapular) (2.7%), asthenia (2.3%), vomiting (2.0%), dyspepsia (1.5%), and pruritus (1.3%).

It is recommended that baseline values of plasma creatinine be established 7 days after initiation of treatment with dronedarone. If the result obtained for the plasma creatinine is above the upper limit of normal as provided by the laboratory, this value should be used as the new reference baseline taking into account that this may be expected with dronedarone, since the drug can affect baseline values. An increase in creatininemia should not necessarily lead to the discontinuation of treatment with dronedarone or discontinuation of treatment with ACE-inhibitors or angiotensin receptor blockers (ARBs). Further laboratory testing is at the discretion of the attending physician.

Consult the MULTAQ™ Product Monograph for information on patient selection, dosing, warnings, and precautions at www.sanofi-aventis.ca.

ACE = angiotensin-converting enzyme; AE = adverse events; AF = atrial fibrillation; AFL = atrial flutter; CHF = congestive heart failure; CI = confidence interval; CV = cardiovascular; HR = hazards ratio; NYHA = New York Heart Association; RRR = relative risk reduction.

Member R&D PAAB

Ⓟ MULTAQ™
dronedarone 400 mg

CDN.DRO.10.08.01E

sanofi aventis
Because health matters

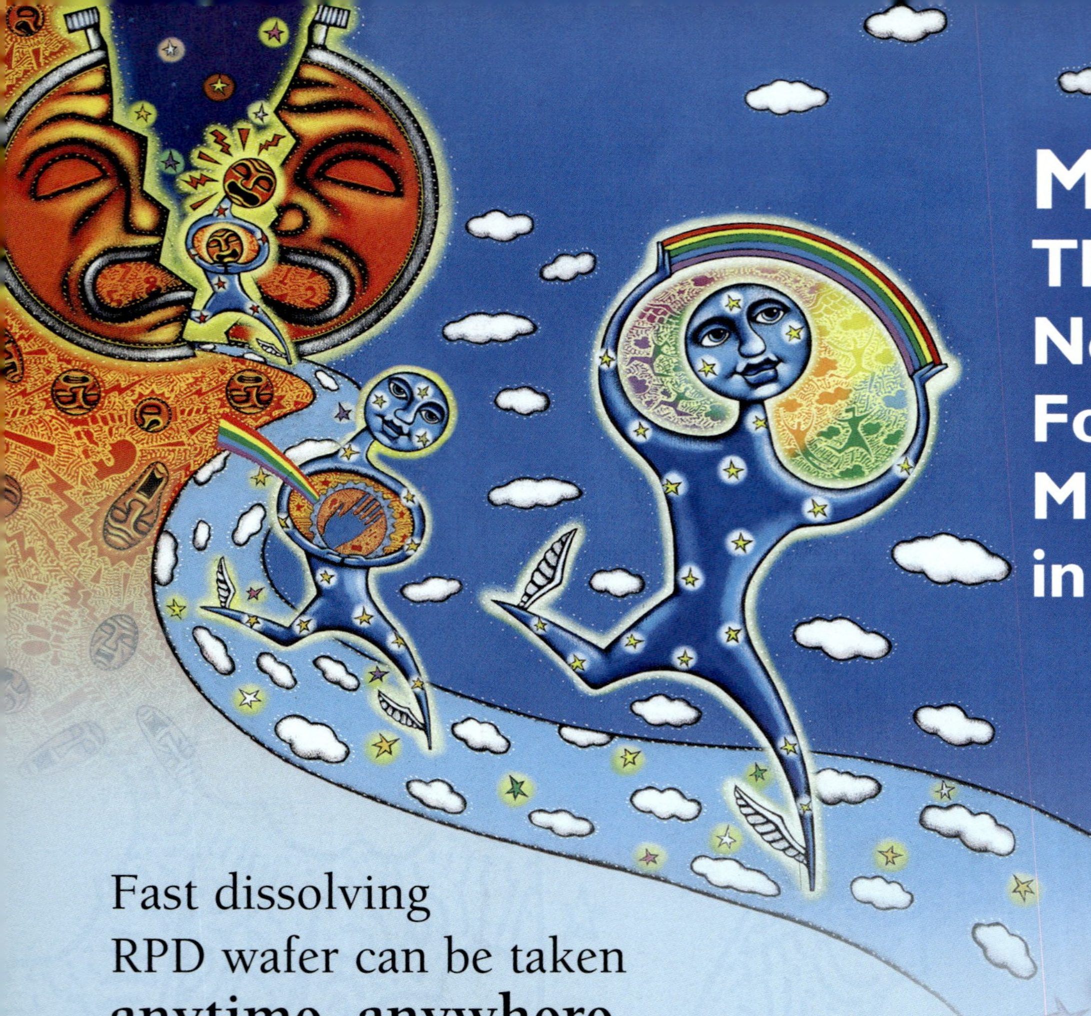

MAXALT RPD®
The #1 Dispensed Non-tablet Formulation Migraine Drug in Canada[1]

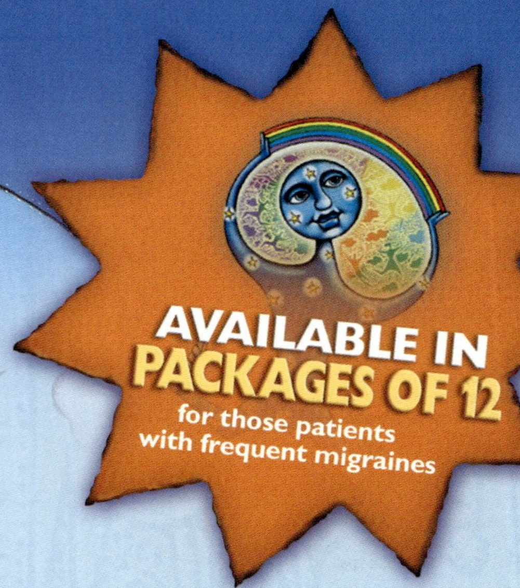

Fast dissolving RPD wafer can be taken **anytime, anywhere** with or without water[2,*]

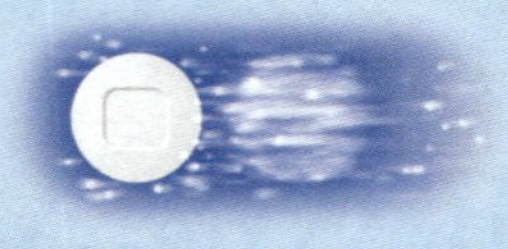

INDICATIONS AND CLINICAL USE

[Pr]MAXALT® (rizatriptan benzoate) is indicated for the acute treatment of migraine attacks with or without aura in adults. MAXALT® is not intended for the prophylactic therapy of migraine or for use in the management of hemiplegic, ophthalmoplegic or basilar migraine. Safety and effectiveness of MAXALT® have not been established for cluster headache, which is present in an older, predominantly male population.

The recommended single adult dose is 5 mg. The maximum recommended single dose is 10 mg. **Redosing:** Doses should be separated by at least 2 hours; no more than a total of 20 mg (Tablets or Wafers) should be taken in any 24-hour period. The safety of treating, on average, more than four headaches in a 30-day period has not been established.

SELECTED IMPORTANT SAFETY INFORMATION

MAXALT® is contraindicated in patients with history, symptoms, or signs of ischemic cardiac, cerebrovascular or peripheral vascular syndromes, valvular heart disease or cardiac arrhythmias (especially tachycardias). In addition, patients with other significant underlying cardiovascular diseases should not receive MAXALT®.

MAXALT® is also contraindicated in patients with uncontrolled or severe hypertension.

MAXALT® is contraindicated in co-administration with monoamine oxidase (MAO) inhibitors within 2 weeks after discontinuation of treatment, and within 24 hours of administration of $5\text{-}HT_1$ agonists or ergot-type medications. For a complete list of contraindications, please consult the Product Monograph.

The most common adverse events during treatment with MAXALT® (rizatriptan benzoate) tablets 10 mg were dizziness (8.9%), somnolence (8.4%), asthenia/fatigue (6.9%), nausea (5.7%) and pain/pressure sensation (chest, 3.1%; neck/throat/jaw, 2.5%; upper limb, 1.8%).

The most common adverse events during treatment with MAXALT RPD® (rizatriptan benzoate) wafers 10 mg were dizziness (8.6%), nausea (7.0%), dry mouth (6.0%), somnolence (5.3%), asthenia/fatigue (3.6%), and pain/pressure sensation (chest, 1.7%; neck/throat/jaw, 2.0%; upper limb, 2.0%).

MAXALT RPD® wafers contain phenylalanine (a component of aspartame).

BEFORE PRESCRIBING, PLEASE CONSULT THE PRODUCT MONOGRAPH FOR WARNINGS, PRECAUTIONS, ADVERSE EVENTS AND IMPORTANT PATIENT SELECTION CRITERIA. PRODUCT MONOGRAPH AVAILABLE FOR DOWNLOAD AT www.merckfrosst.com.

BEFORE PRESCRIBING **MAXALT®/MAXALT RPD®**, PLEASE CONSULT THE ENCLOSED PRESCRIBING INFORMATION.

*The wafer will dissolve rapidly and be swallowed with saliva. No liquid is needed to take the wafer.
RPD=Rapidly dissolving

References:
1. IMS National TRx data ending October 2010.
2. Data on file, Merck Frosst Canada Ltd.: Product Monograph, MAXALT®, 2010.

MERCK
Merck Frosst Canada Ltd., Kirkland, Quebec

PAAB

MXT-08-CDN-34381016-JA-CPS

Maxalt RPD
(rizatriptan benzoate)

M

MabCampath® 🅿

alemtuzumab

Antineoplastic

Genzyme

Date of Preparation: November 30, 2005
Date of Revision: January 27, 2009

SUMMARY PRODUCT INFORMATION:

Route of Administration	Dosage Form/ Strength	Clinically Relevant Nonmedicinal Ingredients
Intravenous injection	Sterile solution 30 mg per 1 mL vial (30 mg/mL)[a]	There are no clinically relevant nonmedicinal ingredients Nonmedicinal ingredients: dibasic sodium phosphate, disodium edetate dihydrate, polysorbate 80, potassium chloride, potassium dihydrogen phosphate and sodium chloride. No preservatives are added.

[a] MabCampath (alemtuzumab) is supplied in single-use clear glass vials containing 30 mg of alemtuzumab in 1 mL of sterile, preservative-free solution. MabCampath is available in boxes of one 30 mg/mL vial (one vial of 30 mg in 1 mL solution) and three 30 mg/mL vials (three vials of 30 mg in 1 mL solution). Note that the three-vial boxes are **not** to be administered as a single dose.

DESCRIPTION: MabCampath (alemtuzumab) is produced in mammalian cell (Chinese hamster ovary) suspension culture in a medium containing neomycin. Neomycin is not detectable in the final product.

INDICATIONS AND CLINICAL USE: MabCampath (alemtuzumab) is indicated for the treatment of patients with previously untreated progressive B-CLL.

The effectiveness of MabCampath as a single agent for the treatment of patients with previously untreated B-CLL is based on progression-free survival (PFS), complete response (CR) and overall response (OR) rates. Currently no data are available that demonstrate an increased overall survival with MabCampath.

MabCampath (alemtuzumab) is also indicated for the treatment of B-CLL patients who have been treated with alkylating agents and who have failed fludarabine therapy.

Physicians should carefully weigh the benefits and risks of treatment with MabCampath, taking into consideration the prognostic characteristics of B-CLL patients such as Rai Stage before initiating treatment.

Geriatrics (>65 years of age): Although no substantial differences in safety and efficacy related to age in B-CLL patients were observed, the number of patients over 65 years of age included in the clinical trials is not sufficient to exclude important differences.

Pediatrics: The safety and efficacy of MabCampath in paediatric patients have not been assessed.

CONTRAINDICATIONS:

- Patients who have active infections.
- Patients with underlying immunodeficiency (e.g., seropositive for HIV).
- Patients who have known Type I hypersensitivity or anaphylactic reactions to MabCampath (alemtuzumab) or to any one of its components.
- Patients with active secondary malignancies.

WARNINGS AND PRECAUTIONS:

Serious Warnings and Precautions

MabCampath (alemtuzumab) should be administered under the supervision of a physician experienced in the use of antineoplastic therapy.

- **Hematologic:** Serious and, in rare instances fatal, pancytopenia/ marrow hypoplasia, autoimmune idiopathic thrombocytopenia, and autoimmune hemolytic anemia have occurred in patients receiving MabCampath therapy. **Single doses of MabCampath greater than 30 mg or cumulative doses greater than 90 mg per week should not be administered because these doses are associated with a higher incidence of pancytopenia.**
- **Infusion Reactions:** MabCampath can result in serious, and in some instances fatal, infusion reactions. Patients should be carefully monitored during infusions and MabCampath withheld for Grade 3 or 4 infusion reactions if indicated. **Gradual escalation to the recommended maintenance dose is required at the initiation of therapy and after interruption of therapy for seven or more days** (see Dosage and Administration).
- **Infections, Opportunistic Infections:** Serious, sometimes fatal bacterial, viral, fungal, and protozoan infections have been reported in patients receiving MabCampath therapy. Prophylaxis directed against *P. jiroveci* pneumonia (PCP) and herpes virus infections has been shown to decrease, but not eliminate, the occurrence of these infections. Anti-viral prophylaxis is strongly recommended.

Warnings and Precautions, including the Serious Warnings and Precautions, apply to all patients (previously untreated and previously treated) who receive MabCampath.

General: Infusion Reactions: MabCampath has been associated with adverse reactions including pyrexia, chills/rigors, nausea, hypotension, urticaria, dyspnea, rash, emesis, and bronchospasm. In clinical trials, the frequency of infusion reactions was highest in the first week of therapy and declined in the second or third weeks of treatment (see Adverse Reactions, Infusion Reactions). Monitor for the signs and symptoms listed above and withhold infusions for Grade 3 or 4 infusion reactions.

The following serious, including fatal, infusion reactions have been identified in post-marketing reports: syncope, pulmonary infiltrates, acute respiratory distress syndrome (ARDS), respiratory arrest, cardiac arrhythmias, myocardial infarction, acute cardiac insufficiency, cardiac arrest, angioedema, and anaphylactoid shock.

MabCampath should be initiated at the recommended dose-escalation scheme (see Dosage and Administration). In order to prevent or decrease the severity of infusion reactions, patients should be premedicated with an oral antihistamine and acetaminophen prior to dosing and monitored closely for infusion reactions. In cases where severe infusion reactions (which may include cytokine release effects) occur, treatment with glucocorticoids, epinephrine and or meperidine can be used (see Dosage and Administration, Recommended Concomitant Medications). For patients who experience an infusion reaction physicians may consider glucocorticoids and/or meperidine as additional premedication for subsequent doses. Careful monitoring of blood pressure and symptoms related to hypotension is recommended especially in patients with ischemic heart disease and in patients on antihypertensive medications. Monitoring and resuscitation facilities should be available. If therapy is interrupted for seven or more days, MabCampath should be reinstituted with gradual dose escalation. For patients with pre-existing cardiac disease, MabCampath should only be administered if the benefits outweigh the risks (see Adverse Reactions and Dosage and Administration).

Hematologic: Prolonged myelosuppression has occurred in patients with leukemia and lymphoma receiving MabCampath. In addition, severe, including fatal, autoimmune anemias and thrombocytopenia were observed in patients receiving MabCampath. Hemolytic anemia, pure red cell aplasia, bone marrow aplasia and hypoplasia were observed in the clinical studies at the recommended dose. Single doses of MabCampath greater than 30 mg or cumulative doses greater than 90 mg per week increase the incidence of pancytopenia.

MabCampath should be discontinued for severe hematologic toxicity (except lymphopenia) or in any patient with evidence of autoimmune hematologic toxicity (see Dosage and Administration, Table 5, Dose Modification and Reinitiation of Therapy for Neutropenia and Thrombocytopenia). Following resolution of transient, non-immune myelosuppression, MabCampath may be reinitiated with caution (see Dosage and Administration). There are no data on the safety of resumption of MabCampath in patients with autoimmune cytopenias or marrow aplasia (see Adverse Reactions).

Tumor Lysis Syndrome: Patients should be well hydrated and, when indicated, allopurinol should be administered for patients with high tumor load, to reduce the risk of tumor lysis syndrome.

Sensitivity/Resistance: Immunosuppression/Opportunistic Infections: MabCampath treatment results in severe and prolonged lymphopenia with a concomitant increased incidence of opportunistic infections (see Adverse Reactions). Prophylaxis against PCP and herpes viruses is recommended upon initiation of therapy and for a minimum of two months following the last dose of MabCampath or until CD4+ counts are ≥200 cells/μL, whichever occurs later (see Dosage and Administration, Recommended Concomitant Medications). Prophylaxis does not eliminate these infections.

A variety of opportunistic infections have been reported in patients receiving MabCampath therapy (see Adverse Reactions, Infections). If a serious infection occurs, MabCampath therapy should be interrupted and may be reinitiated following the resolution of the infection. There have been a significant number of reports of reactivation or new cytomegalovirus (CMV) viremia or infections in patients during clinical studies and in post-marketing reports. Routinely monitor patients for CMV infection during MabCampath treatment and for at least 2 months following completion of treatment. Withhold MabCampath for serious infections and during antiviral treatment for CMV infection or confirmed CMV viremia (e.g. polymerase chain reaction (PCR) positive CMV in 2 consecutive samples obtained 1 week apart) (see Adverse Reactions). Initiate therapeutic ganciclovir (or equivalent) for CMV infection or confirmed CMV viremia (see Dosage and Administration).

Guidelines exist in the published literature for the management of CMV in patients treated with MabCampath (O'Brien, 2006, *Clin Lymphoma*). These guidelines offer a variety of options regarding CMV management and the increased risk of viremia/infection when treated with MabCampath; these options include surveillance, pre-emptive therapy and up front prophylaxis. Although MabCampath therapy was to be withheld during antiviral treatment for CMV in Study 4, these guidelines suggest that MabCampath be held only for those patients with severe infection, who are persistently symptomatic, or both, in order for patients to derive the most benefit from therapy and to avoid unnecessary treatment interruptions.

Because of the potential of transfusion associated Graft versus Host Disease (TAGVHD), it is recommended that patients who have been treated with MabCampath should receive irradiated blood products.

In patients receiving MabCampath as initial therapy, the median time to recovery of CD4+ counts to ≥200 cells/μL occurred by 6 months post-treatment; however at 2 months post-treatment the median was 183 cells/μL. In previously treated patients receiving MabCampath, the median time to recovery of CD4+ counts to ≥200 cells/μL was two months, however, full recovery (to baseline) of CD4+ and CD8+ counts may take more than 12 months (see Boxed Serious Warnings and Precautions and Dosage and Administration).

The potential for an increased risk of infection-related complications may exist following treatment with multiple chemotherapeutic or biological agents.

Immune: Autoimmunity: Autoimmune diseases have been reported, occurring in association with MabCampath treatment, including Graves' disease, hypothyroidism and Goodpasture's syndrome. This may be associated with the severe lymphopenia induced by treatment with MabCampath. Appropriate clinical and laboratory monitoring should be undertaken.

Immunization: Patients who have recently received MabCampath should not be immunized with live viral vaccines, due to their immunosuppression. The safety of immunization with live viral vaccines following MabCampath therapy has not been studied. The ability to generate a primary or anamnestic humoral response to any vaccine following MabCampath therapy has not been studied.

Immunogenicity: As with all therapeutic proteins, there is potential for immunogenicity. Using an ELISA assay, anti-human antibodies were detected in 11 of 133 (8.3%) previously untreated patients. In addition, two patients were weakly positive for neutralizing activity. Limited data suggest that the anti-MabCampath antibodies did not adversely affect tumour response. Four (1.9%) of 211 previously treated patients evaluated for development of an immune response were found to have antibodies to MabCampath.

Cardiovascular: Hypotension, hypertension, bradycardia, atrial fibrillation, cardiac arrest, sinus bradycardia and supraventricular extrasystoles have been observed in patients treated with MabCampath. Assessment and ongoing monitoring of cardiac function (e.g. echocardiography, heart rate and body weight) should be considered in patients previously treated with potentially cardiotoxic agents.

Neurologic: Guillain-Barré syndrome and other neuropathies have been reported in association with MabCampath treatment.

Carcinogenesis and Mutagenesis: No long-term studies in animals have been performed to establish the carcinogenic or mutagenic potential of MabCampath, or to determine its effects on fertility in males or females. Women of childbearing potential and men of reproductive potential should use effective contraceptive methods during treatment and for a minimum of six months following MabCampath therapy.

Sexual Function/Reproduction: Mature sperm are CD52 positive, and MabCampath may cause loss of mature sperm and the possibility of male infertility. Studies have not been carried out to determine the effect or duration of infertility, if any.

Special Populations: Pregnant Women: Animal reproduction studies have not been conducted with MabCampath. It is not known whether MabCampath can affect reproductive capacity or cause fetal harm when administered to a pregnant woman. However, human IgG is known to cross the placental barrier and therefore MabCampath may cross the placental barrier and cause fetal B and T lymphocyte depletion. Males and females of childbearing capacity should use effective contraceptive measures during treatment and for six months following MabCampath therapy. MabCampath should be given to a pregnant woman only if the benefit outweighs the risks to mother and fetus.

Nursing Women: Excretion of MabCampath in human breast milk has not been studied, although it is highly likely that it is excreted in the milk. Because many drugs including human IgG are excreted in human milk, breast-feeding should be discontinued during treatment and for at least 3 months following the last dose of MabCampath.

Pediatrics: The safety and effectiveness of MabCampath in children have not been established.

Geriatrics (>65 years of age): Of 147 previously untreated B-CLL patients treated with MabCampath, 35% were ≥ age 65 and 4% were ≥age 75. Of 149 patients previously treated patients with B-CLL, 44% were ≥65 years of age and 10% were ≥75 years of age. No substantial differences in safety and efficacy related to age in previously untreated or previously treated B-CLL patients were observed; however the size of the database is not sufficient to exclude important differences.

Monitoring and Laboratory Tests: Complete blood counts (CBC) and platelet counts should be obtained at weekly intervals during MabCampath therapy and more frequently if worsening anemia, neutropenia, or thrombocytopenia is observed on therapy. CD4+ counts should be assessed after treatment until recovery to ≥200 cells/μL (see Warnings and Precautions and Adverse Reactions). Recommendations for dose modification and reinitiation of therapy for neutropenia and thrombocytopenia are provided in Table 5 under Dosage and Administration.

ADVERSE REACTIONS: The most common adverse reactions with MabCampath are: infusion reactions (pyrexia, chills, hypotension, urticaria, nausea, rash, tachycardia, dyspnea), cytopenias (neutropenia, lymphopenia, thrombocytopenia, anemia), infections (CMV viremia, CMV infection, other infections), gastrointestinal symptoms (nausea, emesis, abdominal pain), and neurological symptoms (insomnia, anxiety, headache), fatigue and hypertension. The most common serious adverse reactions are cytopenias, infusion reactions, and immunosuppression/ infections (see Warnings and Precautions).

Clinical Trial Adverse Drug Reactions: Because clinical trials are conducted under very specific conditions the adverse reaction rates observed in the clinical trials may not reflect the rates observed in practice and should not be compared to the rates in the clinical trials of another drug. Adverse drug reaction information from clinical trials is useful for identifying drug-related adverse events and for approximating rates.

The data below reflect exposure to MabCampath in 296 patients with CLL of whom 147 were previously untreated and 149 received at least 2 prior chemotherapy regimens. The median duration of exposure was 11.7 weeks for previously untreated patients and 9.0 weeks for previously treated patients.

Infusion Reactions: The pattern of infusion-related reactions reported in previously untreated and previously treated patients was similar; the occurrence of infusion reactions for in all patients was greatest during the initial week of treatment and decreased with subsequent doses of MabCampath.

Antihistamines, acetaminophen, antiemetics, meperidine, and/or glucocorticoids as well as incremental dose escalation were used to prevent or ameliorate infusion-related events (see Warnings and Precautions and Dosage and Administration).

Previously Untreated Patients: Infusion-related reactions including pyrexia, chills, hypotension, urticaria and dyspnea were common in patients treated with MabCampath. Grade 3 and 4 pyrexia and/or chills occurred in approximately 10% of previously untreated patients treated with MabCampath and in none of the patients treated with chlorambucil. All patients were pretreated with antipyretics and antihistamines; additionally, 43% of patients treated with MabCampath received glucocorticoid pre-treatment and 0.7% of patients treated with chlorambucil received glucocorticoid pre-treatment. Premedication with glucocorticoids to prevent infusion reactions would not be expected in patients treated with an antineoplastic agent such as chlorambucil that is administered orally as opposed to an intravenously administered monoclonal antibody such as MabCampath.

Previously Treated Patients: Infusion-related reactions including pyrexia, chills, hypotension, urticaria and dyspnea were common in previously untreated patients treated with MabCampath. Additional infusion-related events reported frequently include nausea, vomiting, rash, fatigue, pruritus, headache and diarrhea. Grade 3 and 4 pyrexia and/or chills were reported in 35% of patients.

Hematologic: Pancytopenia/Marrow Hypoplasia: Previously Untreated Patients: With the exception of one patient who experienced pure red cell aplasia 6 months after completing treatment with MabCampath, there were no reports of pancytopenia or bone marrow aplasia in patients treated with MabCampath or chlorambucil.

Previously Treated Patients: MabCampath therapy was permanently discontinued in 6% of patients due to pancytopenia/marrow hypoplasia; 2% of cases of pancytopenia/ marrow hypoplasia were fatal.

Anemia: Previously Untreated Patients: Grade 3 or 4 anemia was reported in 11% of patients treated with MabCampath with a median time to onset of 31 days and 18% of patients treated with chlorambucil with a median time to onset of 57 days. Sixteen percent of patients treated with MabCampath and 18% of patients treated with chlorambucil received either erythropoiesis stimulating agents, transfusions or both. Autoimmune hemolytic anemia secondary to MabCampath therapy was reported in no patients treated with MabCampath and 1% of patients treated with chlorambucil.

Previously Treated Patients: Grade 3 or 4 anemia was reported in 38% of patients.Sixty seven percent of patients required red blood cell (RBC) transfusions. In addition, the use of erythropoiesis stimulating agents was reported in 20% of patients. Autoimmune hemolytic anemia secondary to MabCampath therapy was reported in 1% of patients. Positive Coombs test without hemolysis was reported in 2% of patients (see Warnings and Precautions, Boxed Serious Warnings and Precautions).

Neutropenia: Previously Untreated Patients: Grade 3 or 4 neutropenia was reported in 41% of patients treated with MabCampath and 25% of patients treated with chlorambucil. The median time to onset of neutropenia was 30 days in the MabCampath arm and 26 days in the chlorambucil arm. Ten percent of patients treated with MabCampath and 4% of patients treated with chlorambucil received granulocyte colony stimulating factors (see Infections).

Previously Treated Patients: Grade 3 or 4 neutropenia was reported in 63% of patients with a median duration of 28 days (range: 2-165 days). Seventeen percent of patients received granulocyte colony stimulating factors (see Infections).

Thrombocytopenia: Previously Untreated Patients: Grade 3 or 4 thrombocytopenia was reported in 12% of patients treated with MabCampath with a median time to onset of 9 days and a median duration of 14 days and in 12% of chlorambucil patients with a median time to onset of 55 days. Three percent of patients treated with MabCampath and 2% of patients treated with chlorambucil required platelet transfusions. Autoimmune thrombocytopenia was not reported in patients treated with MabCampath but was reported in 1% of patients treated with chlorambucil. There were no autoimmune thrombocytopenia fatalities reported in patients treated with either MabCampath or chlorambucil.

Previously Treated Patients: Grade 3 or 4 thrombocytopenia was reported in 50% of patients with a median duration of 21 days (range: 2-165 days). Thirty-eight percent of previously treated patients required platelet transfusions for management of thrombocytopenia. Autoimmune thrombocytopenia was reported in 2% of patients with one fatal case of MabCampath-related autoimmune thrombocytopenia (see Warnings and Precautions, Boxed Serious Warnings and Precautions).

Lymphopenia: Previously Untreated Patients: Severe lymphopenia and a rapid and sustained decrease in lymphocyte subsets occurred in previously untreated patients following administration of MabCampath. The median CD4+ was 0 cell/µL at one month after initiation of therapy, 183 cells/µL at 2 months after discontinuation of therapy and 251 cells/µL at 6 months after discontinuation of therapy. The median CD8+ count was 1.5 cells/µL at 1 month after initiation of therapy, 256 cells/µL at 2 months after discontinuation of therapy and 543 cells/µL at 6 months after discontinuation of therapy.

Previously Treated Patients: Severe lymphopenia and a rapid and sustained decrease in lymphocyte subsets occurred in previously treated patients following administration of MabCampath. The median CD4+ was 2 cells/µL (range 0-564) at 1 month after initiation of therapy, 207 cells/µL (range 0-1876) at 2 months after discontinuation of therapy, 470 cells/µL (range 29-2079) at 6 months after discontinuation of therapy. The median CD8+ count was 2 cells/µL (range 0-1127) at 1 month after initiation of therapy, 251 cells/µL (range 0-3885) at 2 months after discontinuation of therapy, and 578 cells/µL (range 20-2507) at 6 months after discontinuation of therapy. In some previously treated patients treated with MabCampath, CD4+ and CD8+ lymphocyte counts had not returned to baseline levels at longer than 1 year post therapy.

Infections: Previously Untreated Patients: In the study of previously untreated patients, patients treated with MabCampath were tested weekly for CMV using a PCR assay from initiation through completion of therapy, and every 2 weeks for the first 2 months following therapy. CMV infection occurred in 16% (23/147) of patients treated with MabCampath; approximately one-third of these infections were serious or life-threatening however all patients with CMV infection recovered. No events of CMV infection were documented in patients treated with chlorambucil. Approximately 80% of patients treated with MabCampath and 50% of patients treated with chlorambucil experienced at least one infection-related event regardless of relationship to treatment. Infection-related events, excluding CMV, were reported in 46% of patients treated with MabCampath and 50% of chlorambucil treated patients. Infection-related fatalities occurred in 1% of patients treated with MabCampath and 2% of patients treated with chlorambucil. Grade 3 sepsis was reported in 1.4% of patients treated with MabCampath; there were no reports of Grade 4 sepsis. Grade 4 sepsis was reported in 0.7% of chlorambucil treated patients; there were no reports of Grade 3 sepsis. Grade 3-4 febrile neutropenia occurred in 5% of patients treated with MabCampath and 3% of patients treated with chlorambucil.

Previously Treated Patients: In studies of previously treated patients in which routine CMV surveillance was not required, CMV infection was documented in 6% (9/149) of patients; nearly all of these infection-related events were serious or life-threatening. Other infection-related events were reported in approximately 50% of patients. Approximately 55% of patients experienced at least one infection-related event. Infection-related fatalities were reported in 16% of patients. Grade 3 or 4 sepsis and Grade 3 or 4 febrile neutropenia were also reported in 10% of patients.

Cardiac: Previously Untreated Patients: Cardiac dysrhythmias occurred in 15% of patients treated with MabCampath; the majority were tachycardias and were temporally associated with infusion. Dysrhythmias were Grade 3 or 4 in 2% of patients. Cardiac dysrhythmias occurred in 3% of patients treated with chlorambucil; dysrhythmias were Grade 3 or 4 in 2% of patients.

Previously Treated Patients: Cardiac dysrhythmias occurred in 11% of patients treated with MabCampath (Study 1); the majority were tachycardias. Dysrhythmias were Grade 3 or 4 in 2% of patients.

Previously Untreated Patients: Table 1 contains adverse reactions reported in ≥1% of 294 patients randomized (1:1) to receive either MabCampath or chlorambucil as initial therapy for B-CLL. Table 2 contains adverse events regardless of relationship to treatment that were reported in previously untreated patients with ≥2% observed difference in frequency between the MabCampath and chlorambucil treatment groups. Table 3 contains infections observed in two or more previously untreated patients regardless of relationship to treatment with MabCampath or chlorambucil. MabCampath was administered at a dose of 30 mg intravenously three times weekly for up to 12 weeks. The median duration of therapy for patients treated with MabCampath was 11.7 weeks with a median weekly dose of 82 mg (25-75% interquartile range: 69-90 mg). Chlorambucil was administered 40 mg/m² orally every month for up to 12 cycles. The median duration of therapy for patients treated with chlorambucil was 28.3 weeks (7 cycles).

Table 1: MabCampath

Adverse Drug Reactions in ≥1%[a] of the Previously Untreated B-CLL Patient Population (Safety Population) During Treatment or Within 30 Days of Last Study Treatment

	MabCampath (N=147)		Chlorambucil (N=147)	
Preferred Term	**Any Grade (%)**	**Grade 3-4 (%)**	**Any Grade (%)**	**Grade 3-4 (%)**
Body as a Whole—General Disorders				
Pyrexia	64	8	3	0
Chills	50	3	0	0
Fatigue	6	1	5	0
Febrile neutropenia	3	0	2	0

(cont'd)

Table 1: MabCampath *(cont'd)*

Adverse Drug Reactions in ≥1%[a] of the Previously Untreated B-CLL Patient Population (Safety Population) During Treatment or Within 30 Days of Last Study Treatment

	MabCampath (N=147)		Chlorambucil (N=147)	
Preferred Term	**Any Grade (%)**	**Grade 3-4 (%)**	**Any Grade (%)**	**Grade 3-4 (%)**
Anorexia	1	0	3	0
Syncope	1	1	0	0
Cardiovascular Disorders—General				
Hypotension	14	1	0	0
Hypertension	8	3	0	0
Central & Peripheral System Disorders				
Headache	7	1	3	0
Tremor	3	0	1	0
Dizziness	3	1	0	0
Hypoaesthesia	2	0	0	0
Gastrointestinal System Disorders				
Nausea	13	0	35	1
Vomiting	7	0	18	1
Abdominal pain	3	0	1	0
Diarrhoea	1	0	2	0
Dyspepsia	0	0	2	0
Heart Rate & Rhythm Disorders				
Tachycardia	7	0	0	0
Bradycardia	2	1	0	0
Sinus tachycardia	2	0	0	0
Palpitations	0	0	1	0
Metabolic & Nutritional Disorders				
Weight decreased	2	0	0	0
Musculo-skeletal System Disorders				
Asthenia	3	0	1	0
Back pain	2	1	0	0
Bone pain	1	0	1	0
Myalgia	1	0	1	0
Musculoskeletal pain	1	0	1	0
Paraesthesia	1	0	0	0
Platelet, Bleeding & Clotting Disorders				
Thrombocytopenia	5	5	5	4
Petechiae	0	0	1	1
Gingival bleeding	0	0	1	0
Psychiatric Disorders				
Anxiety	1	0	0	0
Red Blood Cell Disorders				
Anaemia	3	2	5	3
Resistance Mechanism Disorders				
Cytomegalovirus viraemia	53	4	6	0
Cytomegalovirus infection	13	4	0	0
Oral candidiasis	1	0	0	0
Respiratory System Disorders				
Dyspnoea	7	2	0	0
Haemoptysis	0	0	1	1

(cont'd)

Table 1: MabCampath *(cont'd)*

Adverse Drug Reactions in ≥1%[a] of the Previously Untreated B-CLL Patient Population (Safety Population) During Treatment or Within 30 Days of Last Study Treatment

Preferred Term	MabCampath (N=147) Any Grade (%)	MabCampath (N=147) Grade 3-4 (%)	Chlorambucil (N=147) Any Grade (%)	Chlorambucil (N=147) Grade 3-4 (%)
Pharyngitis	1	0	3	0
Pneumonia	2	1	1	1
Bronchospasm	2	1	0	0
Bronchitis	1	0	1	1
Bronchopneumonia	1	1	1	1
Skin & Appendages Disorders				
Urticaria	15	2	1	0
Rash	12	1	1	0
Pruritus	3	0	1	0
Erythema	3	0	1	0
Cyanosis	1	0	0	0
Dermatitis allergic	1	0	0	0
Hyperhidrosis	1	0	0	0
White Cell & Reticuloendothelial System Disorders				
Neutropenia	9	7	1	1
Leukopenia	1	1	1	1

[a] ≥1% is defined as 2 or more patients treated with MabCampath or 2 or more patients treated with chlorambucil.

Table 2: MabCampath

Adverse Events Regardless of Relationship in Previously Untreated B-CLL Patients Treated with MabCampath or Chlorambucil with ≥2% Observed Difference Between Treatment Groups

System Organ Class Preferred Term	MabCampath (N=147)	Chlorambucil (N=147)
Application Site Disorders		
Cellulitis	0	4 (2.7%)
Gastrointestinal System Disorders		
Abdominal pain upper	5 (3.4%)	2 (1.4%)
Musculo-skeletal System Disorders		
Muscle spasms	1 (0.7%)	4 (2.7%)
Muscular weakness	3 (2.0%)	0
Psychiatric Disorders		
Insomnia	15 (10.2%)	5 (3.4%)
Resistance Mechanism Disorders		
Candidiasis	6 (4.1%)	2 (1.4%)
Herpes simplex	1 (0.7%)	5 (3.4%)
Viral infection	5 (3.4%)	2 (1.4%)
Respiratory System Disorders		
Upper respiratory tract infection	2 (1.4%)	7 (4.8%)
Pharyngolaryngeal pain	1 (0.7%)	5 (3.4%)
Skin and Appendages Disorders		
Night sweats	2 (1.4%)	7 (4.8%)
Urinary System Disorders		
Urinary tract infection	3 (2.0%)	6 (4.1%)

This table does not include terms already reported in Table 1.

Infection related events regardless of relationship to treatment were reported in 80.3% of previously untreated patients treated with MabCampath and 55.4% of previously untreated patients treated with chlorambucil. Two deaths were reported in previously untreated patients treated with MabCampath neither of which were considered related to treatment. Three deaths were reported in previously untreated patients treated with chlorambucil one of which (Listeria encephalitis) was considered related to treatment. With the exception of one nonfatal case of pneumonia in a MabCampath treated patient and one fatal case in a chlorambucil treated patient, all previously untreated patients who experienced infection-related ADRs recovered.

Table 3: MabCampath

Infections Observed in 2 or More Previously Untreated Patients Regardless of Relationship to Treatment with MabCampath or Chlorambucil

	MabCampath N=147 N (%)	Chlorambucil N=147 N (%)
Bronchitis	11 (7.5%)	7 (4.8%)
Bronchitis acute	2 (1.4%)	4 (2.7%)
Bronchopneumonia	3 (2.0%)	4 (2.7%)
Candidiasis	6 (4.1%)	2 (1.4%)
Cellulitis	0	4 (2.7%)
Cystitis	1 (0.7%)	1 (0.7%)
Cytomegalovirus infection	23 (15.6%)	0
Cytomegalovirus viraemia	82 (55.8%)	12 (8.2%)
Furuncle	0	2 (1.4%)
Herpes simplex	1 (0.7%)	5 (3.4%)
Herpes zoster	3 (2.0%)	4 (2.7%)
Infection	3 (2.0%)	1 (0.7%)
Influenza	0	2 (1.4%)
Laryngopharyngitis	1 (0.7%)	1 (0.7%)
Lobar pneumonia	1 (0.7%)	1 (0.7%)
Nasopharyngitis	2 (1.4%)	4 (2.7%)
Oral candidiasis	3 (2.0%)	0
Pharyngitis	10 (6.8%)	15 (10.2%)
Pneumonia	13 (8.8%)	7 (4.8%)
Rhinitis	7 (4.8%)	8 (5.4%)
Sepsis	2 (1.4%)	2 (1.4%)
Sinusitis	3 (2.0%)	1 (0.7%)
Tonsillitis	1 (0.7%)	3 (2.0%)
Upper respiratory tract infection	2 (1.4%)	7 (4.8%)
Urethritis	1 (0.7%)	1 (0.7%)
Urinary tract infection	3 (2.0%)	6 (4.1%)
Viral infection	5 (3.4%)	2 (1.4%)

In the clinical trial of previously untreated patients, the following ADRs, listed by body system, that are not described in Table 1 were observed in <1% of all patients in the MabCampath arm during the on-treatment period: Application site disorders: infusion site erythema, injection site edema. Body as a whole, general disorders: anaphylactic reaction, hypersensitivity, localized edema, lymphadenopathy, malaise, oral discomfort. Cardiovascular disorders general: angina pectoris, cardiac arrest, myocardial infarction. Central and peripheral nervous system disorders: vertigo. Gastrointestinal system disorders: ileus, mucosal inflammation, stomach discomfort. Heart rate and rhythm disorders: arrhythmia supraventricular, atrial fibrillation, sinus bradycardia, supraventricular extrasystoles. Metabolic and nutritional disorders: hyperglycemia, protein total decreased, tumor lysis syndrome. Musculo-skeletal system disorders: arthralgia, muscle spasms, musculoskeletal chest pain. Platelet, bleeding and clotting disorders: epistaxis. Resistance mechanism disorders: beta hemolytic streptococcal infection, body tinea, candidiasis, genital candidiasis, herpes ophthalmic, sepsis, staphylococcal bacteremia, tuberculosis. Respiratory system disorders: rhinitis, dysphonia, hypoxia, nasopharyngitis, pleural effusion, rhinorrhea. Skin and appendages disorders: dermatitis, rash macular. Urinary system disorders: cystitis, dysuria, urinary tract infection, urine output decreased. Vascular (extracardiac) disorders: flushing, orthostatic hypotension. Vision disorders: conjunctivitis. White cell and reticuloendothelial system disorders: agranulocytosis, lymphopenia.

Previously Treated Patients: Additional safety information was obtained from 3 single arm studies of 149 previously treated patients with CLL administered 30 mg MabCampath intravenously three times weekly for 4 to 12 weeks (median cumulative dose 673 mg [range 2-1106 mg]; median duration of therapy 9.0 weeks). Table 4 lists adverse events including severe or life threatening (National Cancer Institute Common Toxicity Criteria v.2.0 [NCI-CTC] Grade 3 or 4) adverse events reported in ≥1% of the previously treated patients.

Table 4: MabCampath

Adverse Drug Reactions in ≥1% of the Previously-Treated B-CLL Patient Population During Treatment or Within 30 Days of Last Study Treatment (Studies 1, 2 and 3)

Preferred Term	B-CLL Studies In Previously Treated Patients (N=149) Any Grade (%)	B-CLL Studies In Previously Treated Patients (N=149) Grade 3 or 4 (%)
Application Site Disorders		
Cellulitis	1	1
Injection site reaction	1	0
Body as a Whole—General Disorders		

(cont'd)

Table 4: MabCampath *(cont'd)*

Adverse Drug Reactions in ≥1% of the Previously-Treated B-CLL Patient Population During Treatment or Within 30 Days of Last Study Treatment (Studies 1, 2 and 3)

Preferred Term	B-CLL Studies In Previously Treated Patients (N=149) Any Grade (%)	Grade 3 or 4 (%)
Rigors	85	15
Fever	82	14
Fatigue	27	4
Anorexia	13	1
Asthenia	9	0
Pain	7	1
Chest pain	6	1
Malaise	5	0
Temperature changed sensation	5	0
Back pain	5	2
Influenza-like symptoms	5	0
Neutropenic fever	5	1
Edema	1	0
Edema mouth	1	1
Cardiovascular Disorders, General		
Hypotension	30	3
Hypertension	9	1
Central and Peripheric Nervous Systems Disorders		
Headache	18	1
Paresthesia	6	0
Tremor	6	0
Dizziness	5	0
Hypoesthesia	3	0
Vertigo	3	0
Hyperkinesia	1	0
Gastro-intestinal System Disorders		
Nausea	49	2
Vomiting	37	4
Diarrhea	13	1
Abdominal pain	6	2
Stomatitis	5	1
Dyspepsia	4	0
Stomatitis ulcerative	3	0
Constipation	2	0
Mucositis (not otherwise specified)	2	0
Flatulence	1	0
Heart Rate and Rhythm Disorders		
Tachycardia	5	1
Palpitation	1	0
Liver and Biliary System Disorders		
Hepatic function abnormal	1	0
Metabolic and Nutritional Disorders		
Weight decrease	5	0
Dehydration	2	2
Hypocalcemia	2	0

(cont'd)

Table 4: MabCampath *(cont'd)*

Adverse Drug Reactions in ≥1% of the Previously-Treated B-CLL Patient Population During Treatment or Within 30 Days of Last Study Treatment (Studies 1, 2 and 3)

Preferred Term	B-CLL Studies In Previously Treated Patients (N=149) Any Grade (%)	Grade 3 or 4 (%)
Hyponatremia	1	1
Thirst	1	0
Musculo-skeletal System Disorders		
Myalgia	9	0
Skeletal pain	3	1
Arthralgia	1	0
Platelet, Bleeding and Clotting Disorders		
Thrombocytopenia[a]	72	50
Purpura	2	0
Psychiatric Disorders		
Anxiety	3	0
Somnolence	3	0
Confusion	2	1
Depression	2	0
Insomnia	1	0
Red Blood Cell Disorders		
Anemia[a]	77	38
Resistance Mechanism Disorders		
Sepsis	18	13
Herpes simplex	10	1
Moniliasis	10	1
Infection	7	1
Cytomegalovirus infection	6	3
Herpes zoster	5	1
Abscess	3	0
P. jiroveci infection	3	3
Infection bacterial	2	0
Infection viral	1	1
Respiratory System Disorders		
Dyspnea	18	6
Pneumonia	18	13
Bronchitis	9	1
Bronchospasm	6	2
Sinusitis	6	1
Upper resp. tract infection	6	0
Coughing	4	1
Pharyngitis	4	0
Pneumonitis	3	3
Hypoxia	2	1
Hemoptysis	1	0
Pulmonary infiltration	1	1
Rhinitis	1	0
Skin and Appendages Disorders		
Rash	29	3
Urticaria	28	5

(cont'd)

Table 4: MabCampath (cont'd)

Adverse Drug Reactions in ≥1% of the Previously-Treated B-CLL Patient Population During Treatment or Within 30 Days of Last Study Treatment (Studies 1, 2 and 3)

Preferred Term	B-CLL Studies In Previously Treated Patients (N=149) Any Grade (%)	Grade 3 or 4 (%)
Pruritus	21	1
Sweating increased	15	1
Rash erythematous	4	1
Bullous eruption	1	1
Skin disorder	1	0
Special Senses Other, Disorders		
Taste loss	2	1
Urinary System Disorders		
Urinary tract infection	3	0
Hematuria	1	1
Vascular (Extracardiac) Disorders		
Flushing	4	0
Vasospasm	1	0
Vision Disorders		
Conjunctivitis	2	0
Endophthalmitis	1	1
White Cell and Reticuloendothelial System Disorders		
Granulocytopenia[a]	80	63
Pancytopenia	5	3
Leukopenia	1	1
Lymphocytes atypical	1	1

[a] Abnormal laboratory results were included in the table, based on the NCI-CTC toxicity grades for laboratory values. Patients who had toxicity grades shifted from low to high post-baseline were included in the frequency column for Any Grade. Patients who had toxicity grades shifted from low to Grade 3 or higher post-baseline were included in the frequency column for Grade 3 or 4.

During clinical trials in previously treated patients with B-CLL, no additional, clinically significant, adverse drug reactions were recorded at a rate of less than 1% besides those already mentioned in the Product Monograph.

In Study 1, all patients were required to receive anti-herpes and anti-PCP prophylaxis (see Dosage and Administration) and were followed for infections for six months. Forty (43%) of 93 patients experienced 59 infections (one or more infections per patient) related to MabCampath during treatment or within six months of the last dose. Of these, 34 (37%) patients experienced 42 infections that were of Grade 3 or 4 severity; 11 (18%) were fatal. Fifty-five percent of the Grade 3 or 4 infections occurred during treatment or within 30 days of last dose. In addition one or more episodes of febrile neutropenia (ANC ≤500/µL) were reported in 10% of patients.

The following types of infections were reported in Study 1: Grade 3 or 4 sepsis in 12% of patients with one fatality, Grade 3 or 4 pneumonia in 15% with five fatalities, and opportunistic infections in 17% with four fatalities. Candida infections were reported in 5% of patients; CMV infections in 8% (4% of Grade 3 or 4 severity); Aspergillosis in 2% with fatal Aspergillosis in 1%; fatal Mucormycosis in 2%; fatal Cryptococcal pneumonia in 1%; Listeria monocytogenes meningitis in 1%; disseminated Herpes zoster in 1%; Grade 3 Herpes simplex in 2%; and Torulopsis pneumonia in 1%. PCP pneumonia occurred in one (1%) patient who discontinued PCP prophylaxis.

In Studies 2 and 3 in which anti-herpes and anti-PCP prophylaxis was optional, 37 (66%) patients had 47 infections while or after receiving MabCampath therapy. In addition to the opportunistic infections reported above, the following types of related events were observed on these studies: interstitial pneumonitis of unknown etiology and progressive multifocal leukoencephalopathy.

Serious Adverse Events in Clinical Trials: The following serious adverse events were reported in at least one patient treated on studies where MabCampath was used as a single agent (and are not reported in other sections of the Product Monograph) regardless of relationship. These studies were conducted in patients with lymphocytic leukemia and lymphoma (N=892) and in patients with non-malignant diseases (N=152) such as rheumatoid arthritis, solid organ transplant, or multiple sclerosis.

Body as a Whole: allergic reactions, anaphylactoid reaction, ascites, hypovolemia, influenza-like syndrome, mouth edema, neutropenic fever and syncope.

Cardiovascular Disorders: cardiac failure, cyanosis, atrial fibrillation, cardiac arrest, ventricular arrhythmia, ventricular tachycardia, angina pectoris, coronary artery disorder, myocardial infarction and pericarditis.

Additional SAEs observed only in previously untreated patients include: troponin increased, sudden cardiac death, sinus bradycardia, myocardial ischaemia, supraventricular tachycardia and cardiopulmonary failure.

Central and Peripheral Nervous Systems Disorders: abnormal gait, aphasia, coma, grand mal convulsions, paralysis and meningitis.

Additional SAEs observed only in previously untreated patients include: ischemic cerebral infarction, ischemic stroke and depressed level of consciousness.

Endocrine Disorders: hyperthyroidism.

Gastrointestinal System Disorders: duodenal ulcer, esophagitis, gingivitis, gastroenteritis, GI hemorrhage, hematemesis, hemorrhoids, intestinal obstruction, intestinal perforation, melena, paralytic ileus, peptic ulcer, pseudomembranous colitis, colitis, pancreatitis, peritonitis, hyperbilirubinemia, hepatic failure, hepatocellular damage, hypoalbuminemia and biliary pain.

Additional SAEs observed only in previously untreated patients include: hemorrhoidal hemorrhage, gastrointestinal inflammation, gastritis, hepatitis and cholecystitis.

Hearing and Vestibular Disorders: decreased hearing.

Additional SAEs observed only in previously untreated patients include: acute vestibular syndrome.

Metabolic and Nutritional Disorders: acidosis, aggravated diabetes mellitus, dehydration, fluid overload, hyperglycemia, hyperkalemia, hypokalemia, hypoglycemia, hyponatremia, increased alkaline phosphatase and respiratory alkalosis.

Musculoskeletal System Disorders: arthritis or worsening arthritis, arthropathy, bone fracture, myositis, muscle atrophy, muscle weakness, osteomyelitis and polymyositis.

Neoplasms: malignant lymphoma, malignant testicular neoplasm, prostatic cancer, plasma cell dyscrasia, secondary leukemia, squamous cell carcinoma, transformation to aggressive lymphoma and transformation to prolymphocytic leukemia.

Additional SAEs observed only in previously untreated patients include: malignant pleural effusion and tumor lysis syndrome.

Platelet, Bleeding, and Clotting Disorders: coagulation disorder, disseminated intravascular coagulation, hematoma, pulmonary embolism and thrombocythemia.

Additional SAEs observed only in previously untreated patients include: autoimmune thrombocytopenia (onset may be delayed).

Psychiatric Disorders: confusion, hallucinations, nervousness, abnormal thinking and apathy.

White Cell and Reticuloendothelial System Disorders: agranulocytosis, aplasia, decreased haptoglobin, lymphadenopathy and marrow depression.

Additional SAEs observed only in previously untreated patients include: leukopenia.

Red Blood Cell Disorders: hemolysis, hemolytic anemia, splenic infarction and splenomegaly.

Additional SAEs observed only in previously untreated patients include: pure red cell aplasia.

Reproductive System Disorders: cervical dysplasia.

Resistance Mechanism Disorders: abscess, bacterial infection, herpes zoster infection, *P. jiroveci* infection and otitis media.

Additional SAEs observed only in previously untreated patients include: Varicella Zoster Virus infection, other viral infections (not specified), Cytomegalovirus infections and viraemia, tuberculosis, lobar pneumonia, bronchopneumonia, septic shock, candidiasis, enterococcal infection and hypogammaglobulinemia.

Respiratory System Disorders: asthma, bronchitis, chronic obstructive pulmonary disease, hemoptysis, hypoxia, pleural effusion, pleurisy, pneumothorax, pulmonary edema, pulmonary fibrosis, pulmonary infiltration, respiratory depression, respiratory insufficiency, sinusitis, stridor and throat tightness.

Skin and Appendages Disorders: angioedema, bullous eruption, cellulitis and purpuric rash.

Additional SAEs observed only in previously untreated patients include: dermatitis exfoliative and dermatitis allergic.

Special Senses Disorders: taste loss.

Urinary System Disorders: abnormal renal function, acute renal failure, anuria, facial edema, hematuria, toxic nephropathy, ureteric obstruction, urinary retention and urinary tract infection.

Vascular (Extracardiac) Disorders: cerebral hemorrhage, cerebrovascular disorder, deep vein thrombosis, increased capillary fragility, intracranial hemorrhage, phlebitis, subarachnoid hemorrhage and thrombophlebitis.

Vision Disorders: endophthalmitis.

In previously untreated patients, the only related SAEs reported in at least one patient treated with MabCampath were CMV viremia, CMV infection, febrile neutropenia, pneumonia and bronchopneumonia. The only drug related SAEs that were more common in patients treated with MabCampath were CMV events.

Post-Market Adverse Drug Reactions: Additional adverse reactions have been identified during post-marketing use of MabCampath. Because these reactions are reported voluntarily from a population of uncertain size, it is not always possible to reliably estimate their frequency or establish a causal relationship to MabCampath exposure. Decisions to include these reactions in labeling are typically based on one or more of the following factors: (1) seriousness of the reaction, (2) frequency of the reporting, or (3) strength of causal connection to MabCampath.

Cardiovascular: congestive heart failure, cardiomyopathy, decreased ejection fraction (in patients previously treated with potentially cardiotoxic agents).

Fatal Infusion Reactions: see Warnings and Precautions.

Gastrointestinal: GI hemorrhage.

Hepatic: hepatic function abnormality.

Immune Disorders: Goodpasture's syndrome, Graves' disease, aplastic anemia, Guillain-Barré syndrome, chronic inflammatory demyelinating polyradiculoneuropathy, serum sickness, Coombs test [antibody] positive, transfusion associated Graft versus Host Disease. Neurological symptoms associated with previous multiple sclerosis (MS) lesions (these symptoms are reversible, and appear not to occur in patients pre-medicated with high-dose glucocorticoids).

Infections: Epstein-Barr Virus (EBV) including EBV-associated lymphoproliferative disorder, progressive multifocal leukoencephalopathy (PML). Other serious and sometimes fatal viral (e.g., adenovirus, parainfluenza, hepatitis B), bacterial (including tuberculosis and atypical mycobacterioses, nocardiosis), and fungal infections have occurred during post-marketing surveillance.

Metabolic: dehydration, tumour lysis syndrome.

Neurologic: dizziness, optic neuropathy.

Psychiatric: confusion.

Renal: renal function abnormality.

DRUG INTERACTIONS: No formal drug interaction studies have been performed with MabCampath (alemtuzumab). An immune response to MabCampath may interfere with subsequent diagnostic serum tests that utilize antibodies.

DOSAGE AND ADMINISTRATION: All Dosage and Administration recommendations apply to previously untreated and previously treated B-CLL patients.

Dosing Considerations: MabCampath (alemtuzumab) should be administered under the supervision of a physician experienced in the use of antineoplastic therapy.

Recommended Dose and Dosage Adjustment: MabCampath therapy should be initiated at a dose of 3 mg administered as a two hour IV infusion daily (see Adverse Reactions). When the MabCampath 3 mg daily dose is tolerated (e.g., infusion-related toxicities are ≤Grade 2), the daily dose should be escalated to 10 mg and continued until tolerated. When the 10 mg dose is tolerated, the maintenance dose of MabCampath 30 mg may be initiated. The maintenance dose of MabCampath is 30 mg/day administered three times per week on alternate days (i.e., Monday, Wednesday, and Friday) for up to 12 weeks. In most patients, escalation to 30 mg can be accomplished in three to seven days. **Dose escalation to the recommended maintenance dose of 30 mg administered three times per week is required. Single doses of MabCampath greater than 30 mg or cumulative weekly doses of greater than 90 mg should not be administered since higher doses are associated with an increased incidence of pancytopenia** (see Warnings and Precautions, Boxed Serious Warnings and Precautions). MabCampath should be administered intravenously only. The infusion should be administered over a two hour period. **Do not administer as an intravenous push or bolus.**

Recommended Concomitant Medications: Premedication should be given prior to the first dose, at dose escalations, and as clinically indicated. The premedication used in clinical studies was diphenhydramine 50 mg and acetaminophen 500-1000 mg administered 30 minutes prior to MabCampath infusion.

Institute appropriate medical management (e.g., glucocorticoids, epinephrine, meperidine) for infusion reactions as needed. For patients who experience an infusion reaction physicians may consider glucocorticoids and/or meperidine as additional premedication for subsequent doses, as clinically indicated. In the clinical study in previously untreated patients, if grade 3 or 4 infusion-related adverse events were not prevented or ameliorated sufficiently with the protocol-recommended premedications, meperidine 25 mg or hydrocortisone 200 mg IV (or equivalent) given 1 hour prior to MabCampath administration may have been of benefit. Thirty six percent of previously untreated patients treated with MabCampath and 14% of patients treated with chlorambucil received concomitant glucocorticoid therapy (see Adverse Reactions, Clinical Trial Adverse Drug Reactions).

It is strongly recommended that patients should receive anti-infective prophylaxis to minimize the risks of serious opportunistic infections (see Warnings and Precautions, Boxed Serious Warnings and Precautions). Administer trimethoprim/sulfamethoxazole DS twice daily (BID) three times per week (or equivalent) as PCP prophylaxis and famciclovir 250 mg twice a day (BID) or equivalent as herpetic prophylaxis upon initiation of MabCampath therapy. Prophylaxis should be continued for a minimum of two months after completion of MabCampath therapy or until the $CD4^+$ count is ≥200 cells/µL, whichever occurs later.

See Warnings and Precautions, Sensitivity/Resistance, Immunosuppression/Opportunistic Infections for information on cytomegalovirus (CMV) management.

The use of allopurinol and hydration to reduce the risk of tumor lysis syndrome is recommended. In the clinical study in previously untreated patients, allopurinol was administered orally at a dose of 300 mg per day beginning 1 day before MabCampath treatment began and for the next 14 days for the first month. Allopurinol could be administered thereafter as clinically indicated.

Dose Modification and Reinitiation of Therapy: MabCampath therapy should be withheld during serious infection or other serious adverse reactions until the event resolves (see Warnings and Precautions). MabCampath therapy should be discontinued if evidence of autoimmune anemia or autoimmune thrombocytopenia appears. Table 5 includes recommendations for dose modification for severe neutropenia or thrombocytopenia.

There are no dose modifications recommended for lymphopenia.

Administration: Parenteral drug products should be inspected for visible particulate matter and discoloration prior to administration. If particulate matter is present or the solution is discolored, the 30 mg/mL vial should not be used. **Do not shake vial prior to use.** As with all parenteral drug products, aseptic technique should be used during the preparation and administration of MabCampath.

30 mg/1 mL (30 mg/mL) Vial: Withdraw the necessary amount of MabCampath from the 30 mg/mL vial into a syringe calibrated in increments of 0.01 mL for the 3 mg and 10 mg dose and 0.1 mL for the 30 mg dose (see Table 6). Inject into 100 mL sterile 0.9% Sodium Chloride USP or 5% Dextrose in Water USP. **Gently invert the bag to mix the solution.** Discard syringe.

Table 5: MabCampath

Dose Modification for Neutropenia and Thrombocytopenia

Hematologic Values	Dose Modification[a]
Absolute Neutrophil Count (ANC) <250/µL and/or platelet count ≤25 000/µL.	
For first occurrence	Withhold MabCampath therapy. Resume MabCampath therapy at 30 mg when ANC ≥500/µL and platelet count ≥50 000/µL.
For second occurrence	Withhold MabCampath therapy. Resume MabCampath therapy at 10 mg when ANC ≥500/µL and platelet count ≥50 000/µL.
For third occurrence	Discontinue MabCampath therapy.
≥50% decrease from baseline value in patients initiating therapy with a baseline ANC ≤250/µL and/or a baseline platelet count ≤25 000/µL	
For first occurrence	Withhold MabCampath therapy. Resume MabCampath at 30 mg upon return to baseline value(s).
For second occurrence	Withhold MabCampath therapy. Resume MabCampath at 10 mg upon return to baseline value(s).
For third occurrence	Discontinue MabCampath therapy.

[a] If the delay between dosing is ≥7 days, initiate therapy at MabCampath 3 mg and escalate to 10 mg and then to 30 mg as tolerated (see Dosage and Administration).

Table 6: MabCampath

Administration 30 mg/1 mL (30 mg/mL) Vial

Dose	Amount (mL) Withdrawn from 30 mg/mL Vial	Volume of Diluent	Nominal Concentration per mL
Initial: 3 mg	0.1 mL	100 mL	0.03 mg
Initial: 10 mg	0.33 mL	100 mL	0.10 mg
Maintenance: 30 mg	1 mL	100 mL	0.30 mg

The 30 mg/mL vial contains no preservatives and is intended for single use only. Discard vial including any unused portion after withdrawal of dose.

MabCampath contains no antimicrobial preservative. MabCampath should be used within eight hours after dilution. MabCampath solutions may be stored at room temperature (15-30°C) or refrigerated (2-8°C). MabCampath solutions should be protected from light.

Missed Dose: If therapy is interrupted for seven or more days, MabCampath should be reinstituted with gradual dose escalation.

Incompatibilities: No incompatibilities between MabCampath and polyvinylchloride (PVC) bags, PVC or polyethylene-lined PVC administration sets, or low-protein binding filters have been observed. No data are available concerning the incompatibility of MabCampath with other drug substances. Other drug substances should not be added or simultaneously infused through the same intravenous line.

OVERDOSAGE:

Initial doses of intravenous MabCampath (alemtuzumab) of greater than 3 mg are not well-tolerated. One previously treated patient who received 80 mg as an initial dose by IV infusion experienced acute bronchospasm, cough, and shortness of breath, followed by anuria and death. A review of the case suggested that tumor lysis syndrome may have played a role.

Single doses of MabCampath greater than 30 mg or a cumulative weekly dose greater than 90 mg should not be administered as higher doses have been associated with a higher incidence of pancytopenia (see Warnings and Precautions, Boxed Serious Warnings and Precautions and Dosage and Administration). There is no known specific antidote for MabCampath overdosage in previously untreated or previously treated B-CLL patients. Treatment consists of drug discontinuation and supportive therapy.

> For management of a suspected drug overdose, CPhA recommends that you contact your **regional Poison Control Centre**. See the *CPS* Directory section for a list of Poison Control Centres.

ACTION AND CLINICAL PHARMACOLOGY: Mechanism of Action: Alemtuzumab binds to CD52, a non modulating antigen that is present on the surface of essentially all B and T lymphocytes, a majority of monocytes, macrophages, and natural killer (NK) cells, and a subpopulation of granulocytes. Analysis of samples collected from multiple volunteers has not identified CD52 expression on erythrocytes or hematopoetic stem cells. The proposed mechanism of action is antibody-dependent lysis of leukemic cells following cell surface binding. MabCampath-1H Fab binding was observed in lymphoid tissues and the mononuclear phagocyte system. A proportion of bone marrow cells, including some CD34+ cells, express variable levels of CD52. Significant binding was also observed in the skin and male reproductive tract (epididymis, sperm, seminal vesicle). Mature spermatozoa stain for CD52, but neither spermatogenic cells nor immature spermatozoa show evidence of staining.

Pharmacokinetics: MabCampath (alemtuzumab) pharmacokinetics were characterized in a study of 30 previously treated, yet MabCampath-naïve, patients with chronic lymphocytic leukemia (B-CLL) who had failed previous therapy with purine analogs. MabCampath was administered as a two hour intravenous infusion, at the recommended dosing schedule, starting at 3 mg and increasing to 30 mg three times per week for up to 12 weeks. MabCampath pharmacokinetics displayed nonlinear elimination kinetics. After the last 30 mg dose, the mean volume of distribution at steady-state was 0.18 L/kg (range: 0.1 to 0.4 L/kg). Systemic clearance decreased with repeated administration due to decreased receptor-mediated clearance (i.e., loss of CD52 receptors in the periphery). After 12 weeks of dosing, patients exhibited a seven-fold increase in mean AUC. Mean half-life was 11 hours (range: 2 to 32 hours) after the first 30 mg dose and was six days (range: 1 to 14 days) after the last 30 mg dose.

Special Populations and Conditions: Pediatrics: The pharmacokinetics of MabCampath in pediatric patients have not been studied.

Geriatrics: Comparisons of AUC in previously treated B-CLL patients 65 years or older (n=6) versus previously treated B-CLL patients less than 65 years (n=15) suggested that no dose adjustments are necessary for age.

Gender: Comparisons of AUC in previously treated female B-CLL patients (n=4) versus previously treated male B-CLL patients (n=17) suggested that no dose adjustments are necessary for gender.

Hepatic Insufficiency: The effects of hepatic impairment on the pharmacokinetics of MabCampath have not been studied.

Renal Insufficiency: The effects of renal impairment on the pharmacokinetics of MabCampath have not been studied.

STORAGE AND STABILITY: MabCampath (alemtuzumab) should be stored at 2-8°C. Do not freeze. **Discard if 30 mg/mL vial has been frozen.** Protect from direct sunlight.

MabCampath contains no antimicrobial preservative. MabCampath should be used within eight hours after dilution. MabCampath solutions may be stored at room temperature (15-30°C) or refrigerated (2-8°C). MabCampath solutions should be protected from light.

INFORMATION FOR THE PATIENT: Published in e-CPS, available by subscription at www.e-cps.ca.

DOSAGE FORMS, COMPOSITION AND PACKAGING: Each mL of sterile solution contains: alemtuzumab 30 mg. Nonmedicinal ingredients: dibasic sodium phosphate, disodium edetate dihydrate, polysorbate 80, potassium chloride, potassium dihydrogen phosphate and sodium chloride. Preservative-free. Single-use clear glass vials of 1 mL, boxes of 1 and 3. Note that the three-vial boxes are **not** to be administered as a single dose.

MacroBID® Ⓟ

nitrofurantoin monohydrate/macrocrystals

Urinary Tract Antibacterial

Warner Chilcott

Date of Preparation: February 16, 2010

PHARMACOLOGY: Nitrofurantoin is reduced by bacterial flavoproteins to reactive intermediates which inactivate or alter bacterial ribosomal proteins and other macromolecules. As a result of such inactivations, the vital biochemical processes of protein synthesis, aerobic energy metabolism, DNA synthesis, RNA synthesis, and cell wall synthesis are inhibited. The broad-based nature of this mode of action may explain the lack of acquired bacterial resistance to nitrofurantoin, as the necessary multiple and simultaneous mutations of the target macromolecules would likely be lethal to the bacteria.

Each MacroBID capsule contains two forms of nitrofurantoin. Twenty-five percent is macrocrystalline nitrofurantoin, which has slower dissolution and absorption than nitrofurantoin monohydrate. The remaining 75% is nitrofurantoin monohydrate contained in a powder blend which, upon exposure to gastric and intestinal fluids, forms a gel matrix that releases nitrofurantoin over time.

Following a single 100 mg dose, the extent and rate of nitrofurantoin excretion in the urine are similar for 100 mg capsules of MacroBID and 50 or 100 mg capsules of Macrodantin (nitrofurantoin macrocrystals). Nitrofurantoin bioavailability can be increased by as much as 40% when MacroBID is administered with food. Approximately 20-25% of a single dose of MacroBID is recovered in the urine unchanged over 24 hours and drug concentrations inhibitory of bacterial growth are reached or exceeded in the urine. Plasma levels attained with MacroBID usually do not exceed 1 µg/mL and are not considered systemically therapeutic.

INDICATIONS: MacroBID is indicated for the treatment of acute uncomplicated urinary tract infections, e.g. cystitis, when due to susceptible strains of *E. coli*, and *S. saprophyticus*.

MacroBID is not indicated for the treatment of associated renal cortical or perinephric abscesses.

MacroBID is not indicated for therapy of any systemic infections or for use in prostatitis.

CONTRAINDICATIONS: Anuria, oliguria, or significant impairment of renal function (creatinine clearance under 60 mL per minute or clinically significant elevated serum creatinine) are contraindications to therapy with this drug. Treatment of this type of patient carries an increased risk of toxicity because of impaired excretion of the drug. For the same reason, this drug is much less effective under these circumstances.

The drug is contraindicated in pregnant patients during labour and delivery, or when the onset of labour is imminent, and in infants under one month of age because of the possibility of hemolytic anemia in the fetus or the newborn infant due to their immature erythrocyte enzyme systems (glutathione instability).

MacroBID capsule therapy is also contraindicated in those patients with known hypersensitivity to nitrofurantoin.

WARNINGS: Acute, subacute or chronic pulmonary reactions have been observed in patients treated with nitrofurantoin products (see Adverse Effects). If these reactions occur, the drug should be withdrawn and appropriate measures taken. Reports have cited pulmonary reactions as a contributing cause of death.

Chronic pulmonary reactions (diffuse interstitial pneumonitis or pulmonary fibrosis, or both) can develop insidiously. These reactions occur rarely and generally in patients receiving therapy for six months or longer. Close monitoring of the pulmonary condition of patients receiving long-term therapy is warranted and requires that the benefits of therapy be weighed against potential risks (see Adverse Effects).

Hepatic reactions, including hepatitis, hepatic necrosis, cholestatic jaundice and chronic active hepatitis, occur rarely. Fatalities have been reported. The onset of chronic active hepatitis may be insidious, and patients should be monitored periodically for changes in liver function. If hepatitis occurs, the drug should be withdrawn immediately and appropriate measures taken.

Peripheral neuropathy (including optic neuritis) may occur with nitrofurantoin therapy; this may become severe or irreversible. Fatalities have been reported. Predisposing conditions such as renal impairment (creatinine clearance under 60 mL per minute or clinically significant elevated serum creatinine), anemia, diabetes mellitus, electrolyte imbalance, vitamin B deficiency, and debilitating disease may enhance such occurrence. Patients receiving long-term therapy should be monitored periodically for changes in renal function. If numbness or tingling occurs, discontinue use.

Cases of hemolytic anemia of the primaquine-sensitivity type have been induced by nitrofurantoin. The hemolysis appears to be linked to a glucose-6-phosphate dehydrogenase deficiency in the red blood cells of the affected patients. This deficiency is found in 10 percent of Blacks and a small percentage of ethnic groups of Mediterranean and Near-Eastern origin. Any sign of hemolysis is an indication to discontinue the drug. Hemolysis ceases when the drug is withdrawn.

Pseudomonas is the organism most commonly implicated in superinfections in patients with nitrofurantoin preparations.

Carcinogenesis, Mutagenesis and Impairment of Fertility: Nitrofurantoin presented evidence of carcinogenic activity in female B6C3F1 mice as shown by increased incidences of tubular adenomas, benign mixed tumours, and granulosa cell tumours of the ovary. In male F344/N rats, there were increased incidences of uncommon kidney tubular cell neoplasms, osteosarcomas of the bone, and neoplasms of the subcutaneous tissue. In one study involving three subcutaneous injections of 75 mg/kg nitrofurantoin to pregnant female mice, lung papillary adenomas were observed in the F1 generation.

Nitrofurantoin was not carcinogenic when fed to female Holtzman rats for 44.5 weeks or to female Sprague-Dawley rats for 75 weeks. Two chronic rodent bioassays utilizing male and female Sprague-Dawley rats and two chronic bioassays in Swiss mice and BDF1 mice revealed no evidence of carcinogenicity.

Nitrofurantoin has demonstrated mutagenic potential in a variety of laboratory assays conducted in vitro with mammalian and non-mammalian cells exposed to therapeutically attainable and higher concentrations. Point and possibly other types of mutations were observed in bacteria, yeast and fungi. Damage to DNA or inhibition of DNA synthesis were produced in human fibroblasts and lymphocytes, and Chinese hamster ovaries and lung fibroblasts.

In vivo tests on rodents utilizing a wide range of doses demonstrated similar potential. DNA damage to liver, lung, spleen and kidney were observed in rat (alkaline elution test), immature red blood cells (rat micronucleus test) and sperm (H-test in mouse). Some test results were negative such as the sex-linked recessive lethal assay in Drosophila where nitrofurantoin was administered by feeding or injection.

The significance of the carcinogenicity and mutagenicity findings relative to the therapeutic use of nitrofurantoin in humans is unknown. Because of the potential toxicity of nitrofurantoin when used for long-term therapy, the benefits of long-term therapy should be weighed against potential risks (see Dosage).

The administration of high doses of nitrofurantoin to rats causes temporary spermatogenic arrest, which is reversible on discontinuing the drug. Doses of 10 mg/kg/day or greater in healthy human males may, in certain unpredictable instances, produce slight to moderate spermatogenic arrest with a decrease in sperm count.

PRECAUTIONS: *Drug Interactions:* Antacids containing magnesium trisilicate, when administered concomitantly with nitrofurantoin, reduce both the rate and extent of absorption. The mechanism for this interaction probably is adsorption of drug onto the surface of magnesium trisilicate. Nitrofurantoin should not be given along with drugs which may produce impaired renal function. Uricosuric drugs, such as probenecid and sulfinpyrazone, may inhibit renal tubular secretion of nitrofurantoin. The resulting increase in serum levels may increase toxicity and the decreased urinary levels could lessen its efficacy as a urinary tract antibacterial.

Drug/Laboratory Test Interactions: As a result of administration of nitrofurantoin, a false-positive reaction for glucose in the urine may occur. This has been observed with Benedict's and Fehling's solution but not with the glucose enzymatic test.

Antimicrobial Antagonism: Antagonism has been demonstrated in vitro between nitrofurantoin and quinolone antimicrobials. Although the clinical significance of this finding is unknown, concomitant MacroBID and quinolone therapy should be approached with caution.

Pregnancy: Several reproduction studies performed in rabbits and rats with low multiples of human doses and plasma levels revealed no evidence of general reproductive effects, impaired fertility or harm to the fetus. However, in one published study in which pregnant mice were administered 250 mg/kg subcutaneously on three days, growth retardation and a low incidence of malformations were observed. These effects were not observed at 100 mg/kg. In another controlled study in which cultured rat embryos were exposed for 26 hours to concentrations of 48 µg/mL all were malformed. None of those exposed to 60 µg/mL of nitrofurantoin survived.

The relevance of these findings to humans is uncertain. There are, however, no adequate well controlled studies in pregnant women. Though animal reproduction studies are not always predictive of human response, this drug should not be used during pregnancy unless clearly needed.

Labour and Delivery: Nitrofurantoin should not be given to women during labour and delivery, or when the onset of labour is imminent (see Contraindications).

Lactation: Nitrofurantoin has been detected in trace amounts in breast milk. Caution should be exercised when nitrofurantoin is administered to a nursing woman, especially if the infant is known or suspected to have a glucose-6-phosphate dehydrogenase deficiency (see Contraindications).

Children: Nitrofurantoin is contraindicated in infants under one month of age (see Contraindications and Dosage).

ADVERSE EFFECTS: In limited clinical trials, MacroBID 100 mg capsule b.i.d. demonstrated an equivalent side effect profile to Macrodantin 50 mg q.i.d.

In clinical trials of MacroBID the most frequent clinical adverse events that were reported as possibly or probably drug-related were nausea (8%), headache (6%), and flatulence (1.5%).

The following additional clinical adverse events have been reported with the use of nitrofurantoin:

Respiratory: Chronic, subacute or acute pulmonary hypersensitivity reactions may occur with the use of nitrofurantoin (see Warnings). Chronic pulmonary reactions generally occur in patients who have received continuous treatment for 6 months or longer. Malaise, dyspnea on exertion, cough, and altered pulmonary function are common manifestations which can occur insidiously. Radiologic and histologic findings of diffuse interstitial pneumonitis or fibrosis, or both, are also common manifestations of the chronic pulmonary reaction. Fever is rarely prominent. The severity of chronic pulmonary reactions and the degree of their resolution appear to be related to the duration of therapy after the first clinical signs appear. Pulmonary function may be impaired permanently, even after cessation of nitrofurantoin therapy. The risk is greater when pulmonary reactions are not recognized early.

In subacute pulmonary reactions, fever and eosinophilia occur less often than in the acute form. Upon cessation of therapy, recovery may require several months. If the symptoms are not recognized as being drug-related and nitrofurantoin is not stopped, the symptoms may become more severe.

Acute reactions are commonly manifested by fever, chills, cough, chest pain, dyspnea, pulmonary infiltration with consolidation or pleural effusion on x-ray, and eosinophilia. Acute reactions usually occur within the first week of treatment and are reversible with cessation of therapy. Resolution often is dramatic.

Changes in ECG may occur associated with pulmonary reactions.

Collapse and cyanosis have seldom been reported.

Gastrointestinal: diarrhea, dyspepsia, abdominal pain, constipation, emesis, sialadenitis, pancreatitis.

Pseudomembranous colitis, including that due to an overgrowth by *C. difficile*, has been reported rarely with the use of nitrofurantoin.

Hepatic: Hepatic reactions, including hepatitis, cholestatic jaundice, chronic active hepatitis, and hepatic necrosis occur rarely (see Warnings).

Neurologic: peripheral neuropathy including optic neuritis (see Warnings).

Dizziness, drowsiness, amblyopia, asthenia, vertigo, and nystagmus also have been reported with the use of nitrofurantoin.

Benign intracranial hypertension has seldom been reported.

Confusion, depression, euphoria and psychotic reactions have been reported rarely.

Dermatologic: alopecia.

Exfoliative dermatitis and erythema multiforme (including Stevens-Johnson Syndrome) have been reported rarely.

Allergic Reactions: Lupus-like syndrome associated with pulmonary reaction to nitrofurantoin has been reported. Also, angioedema; maculopapular, erythematous or eczematous eruptions; pruritis; urticaria; anaphylaxis; arthralgia; myalgia; drug fever; chills; and malaise have been reported.

Hematologic: Glucose-6-phosphate dehydrogenase deficiency anemia (see Warnings), agranulocytosis, leukopenia, granulocytopenia, hemolytic anemia, thrombocytopenia, megaloblastic anemia, and eosinophilia have occurred. In most cases, these hematologic abnormalities resolved following cessation of therapy. Aplastic anemia has been reported rarely.

Miscellaneous: As with other antimicrobial agents, superinfections with resistant organisms, e.g., Pseudomonas species or Candida species, may occur with the use of nitrofurantoin. Superinfections have been limited to the genitourinary tract.

Increased AST, increased ALT, decreased hemoglobin and increased serum phosphorus.

Nitrofurantoin may cause a rust yellow to brown discolouration of the urine. The clinical significance is unknown.

OVERDOSE:

Symptoms and Treatment: Occasional incidents of acute overdosage of nitrofurantoin have not resulted in any specific symptomatology other than vomiting.

Treatment: In case vomiting does not occur soon after an excessive dose, induction of emesis is recommended. There is no specific antidote for nitrofurantoin but a high fluid intake should be maintained to promote urinary excretion of the drug. It is dialyzable.

For management of a suspected drug overdose, CPhA recommends that you contact your **regional Poison Control Centre**. See the *CPS* Directory section for a list of Poison Control Centres.

DOSAGE: Adults and Children over 12 years: One MacroBID 100 mg capsule twice a day for 7 days (maximum 200 mg/day). MacroBID should be taken every 12 hours with food or milk to minimize gastric upset.

Therapy for acute urinary tract infections should be continued for 7 days or for at least 3 days after sterility of the urine is obtained. Continued infection indicates the need for re-evaluation.

INFORMATION FOR THE PATIENT: Published in e-CPS, available by subscription at www.e-cps.ca.

SUPPLIED: Each opaque, black and yellow, hard shell gelatin capsule, imprinted "Macrobid" on the black portion and "Norwich Eaton" on the yellow portion contains: the equivalent of 100 mg of nitrofurantoin in the form of nitrofurantoin macrocrystals and nitrofurantoin monohydrate. Nonmedicinal ingredients: carbomer 934P, compressible sugar, corn starch, D&C Yellow No. 10, edible gray ink, FD&C Blue No. 1, FD&C Red No. 40, gelatin, lactose, magnesium stearate, povidone, talc and titanium dioxide. Bottles of 100. Store at controlled room temperature (20 to 25°C).

Macugen™ Ⓟ

pegaptanib sodium

Antivascular Endothelium Growth Factor (VEGF165 inhibitor) for Age-Related Macular Degeneration

Pfizer

Date of Preparation: April 25 2005
Date of Revision: July 19, 2006

SUMMARY PRODUCT INFORMATION:

Route of Administration	Dosage Form/Strength	Clinically Relevant Nonmedicinal Ingredients
Intravitreous injection	Sterile solution/0.3 mg	Not applicable For a complete listing see Dosage Forms, Composition and Packaging.

INDICATIONS AND CLINICAL USE: MACUGEN (pegaptanib sodium injection) is indicated for the treatment of subfoveal choroidal neovascularization (CNV) secondary to age-related macular degeneration.

CONTRAINDICATIONS: MACUGEN (pegaptanib sodium injection) is contraindicated in patients with active or suspected ocular or periocular infection or a known hypersensitivity to any component of this preparation. For a complete listing, see Dosage Forms, Composition and Packaging.

WARNINGS AND PRECAUTIONS: General: For ophthalmic use only.

Hepatic and Renal: MACUGEN has not been studied in patients with hepatic impairment or adequately studied in patients with severe renal insufficiency (i.e. creatinine clearances below 20 mL/min). Therefore, clinicians should exercise appropriate clinical judgment before deciding to administer MACUGEN in these patient populations.

Immune: Rare cases of anaphylaxis/anaphylactoid reactions, including angioedema, have been reported in the post-marketing experience following the pegaptanib intravitreal administration procedure. A direct relationship to pegaptanib or any of the various medications administered, as part of the injection preparation procedure or other factors has not been established in these cases (see Dosage and Administration).

Immunogenicity: No anti-pegaptanib sodium IgG antibodies were detected in patients dosed with MACUGEN.

Ophthalmologic: Increased IOP: Transient increases in intraocular pressure (≥35 mmHg) were seen in 9% of MACUGEN treated patients shortly after injection (usually within 30 minutes). Therefore, the perfusion of the optic nerve head and the intraocular pressure should be monitored and appropriately managed (see Dosage and Administration).

Endophthalmitis: Intravitreous injections have been associated with endophthalmitis. Endophthalmitis may occur within one week from injection (for MACUGEN in clinical setting, 0.14 % per injection). Proper aseptic injection technique should always be utilized when administering MACUGEN and patients should be monitored during the week following the injection to permit early treatment, should the infection occur (see Dosage and Administration).

Traumatic cataracts: Most of the events were associated with contact and/or penetration of the lens with the intravitreous injection needle. Thus proper injection techniques should be applied to avoid touching or puncturing the lens.

Information to Be Provided to the Patient: In the days following MACUGEN administration, patients are at risk for the development of endophthalmitis. If the eye becomes red, sensitive to light, painful or develops a change in vision, the patient should seek immediate care with their ophthalmologist. Patients receiving MACUGEN should be advised to have appropriate ophthalmic follow-up examinations.

Special Populations: Pregnant Women: Developmental toxicology studies of pegaptanib sodium have been performed in mice at intravenous doses of 1 to 40 mg/kg/day. Pegaptanib sodium produced no maternal toxicity and no evidence of teratogenicity or fetal mortality. Reduced fetal body weight (5%) and delayed ossification in forepaw phalanges were observed in the 40 mg/kg/day dose group. These findings were within historical controls for this species. In the 40 mg/kg/day group, the maximum pegaptanib sodium plasma concentrations in dams were 20 000 fold greater than those observed in humans (3 mg dose group, 10 times greater than recommended dose). Pegaptanib sodium crosses the placenta in mice. In the 40 mg/kg/day group, pegaptanib sodium concentrations in the amniotic fluid were 0.05% of the maternal plasma levels. The 40 mg/kg regimen represents about 7000 times the recommended human monocular ophthalmic dose of 0.3 mg/eye.

There are no studies in pregnant women with MACUGEN. It is unknown whether pegaptanib sodium can cause fetal harm when administered to a pregnant woman. MACUGEN should be used during pregnancy only if the potential benefit to the mother justifies the potential risk to the fetus.

Nursing Women: It is not known whether MACUGEN is excreted in human milk.

Pediatrics: Safety and effectiveness of MACUGEN in pediatric patients have not been studied.

Geriatrics: Approximately 94% (834/892) of the patients treated with MACUGEN were ≥65 years of age and approximately 62% (553/892) were ≥75 years of age. No difference in treatment effect or systemic exposure was seen with increasing age.

ADVERSE REACTIONS: Adverse Drug Reaction Overview: MACUGEN (pegaptanib sodium injection) was administered to 892 patients in controlled studies for up to one year (total number of injections=7545, mean number of injections/patient=8.5) at doses of 0.3, 1.0 and 3.0 mg. All three doses shared a similar safety profile. In addition, 128 patients continued to receive MACUGEN 0.3 mg for up to 2 years. The safety data described below summarize the experience of 128 patients exposed for up to two years (total number of injections=2078, mean number of injections/patient=15.6) at the recommended dose of 0.3 mg.

Clinical Trial Adverse Drug Reactions: Because clinical trials are conducted under very specific conditions the adverse reaction rates observed in the clinical trials may not reflect the rates observed in practice and should not be compared to the rates in the clinical trials of another drug. Adverse drug reaction information from clinical trials is useful for identifying drug-related adverse events and for approximating rates.

Ocular Adverse Events: The ocular adverse events in the study eye reported to be at least possibly related to study drug or injection procedure in ≥1% of patients in the 0.3 mg MACUGEN group are presented in Table 1.

Table 1: MACUGEN

Incidence (%) of Ocular Adverse Events in Study Eye of ≥1% of Patients Treated with 0.3 mg MACUGEN for up to 2 years—Reported to Be at Least Possibly Related—Cohort of Studies EOP1003 and EOP1004—Safety Population

MedRA Preferred Term	Incidence (%) 0.3 mg MACUGEN N=128	Incidence (%) Sham N=51
Punctate keratitis	48 (38%)	21 (41%)
Vitreous floaters	45 (35 %)	7 (14%)
Eye pain	44 (34%)	15 (29%)
Intraocular pressure increased	34 (27%)	3 (6%)
Vitreous opacities	28 (22 %)	8 (16%)
Anterior chamber inflammation	22 (17%)	2 (4 %)
Corneal oedema	20 (16%)	7 (14%)
Eye irritation	15 (12%)	7 (14%)
Eye redness	15 (12%)	7 (14%)
Abnormal sensation in eye	14 (11%)	7 (14%)
Cataract	14 (11%)	2 (4%)
Conjunctival haemorrhage	14 (11%)	6 (12%)
Eye discharge	14 (11%)	7 (14%)
Visual disturbance NOS	14 (11%)	3 (6%)
Ocular discomfort	12 (9%)	4 (8%)
Vitreous disorder NOS	12 (9%)	0 (0%)
Lacrimation increased	11 (9%)	6 (12%)
Eye pruritus	9 (7%)	6 (12%)
Photophobia	9 (7%)	4 (8%)
Visual acuity reduced	8 (6%)	2 (4%)
Conjunctival hyperaemia	7 (5 %)	3 (6%)
Corneal epithelium disorder	7 (5%)	1 (2%)
Photopsia	7 (5%)	1 (2%)
Vision blurred	7 (5%)	5 (10%)
Conjunctival oedema	6 (5%)	2 (4%)
Vitreous detachment	6 (5%)	2 (4%)

(cont'd)

Table 1: MACUGEN *(cont'd)*

Incidence (%) of Ocular Adverse Events in Study Eye of ≥1% of Patients Treated with 0.3 mg MACUGEN for up to 2 years—Reported to Be at Least Possibly Related—Cohort of Studies EOP1003 and EOP1004—Safety Population

MedRA Preferred Term	Incidence (%) 0.3 mg MACUGEN N=128	Incidence (%) Sham N=51
Conjunctivitis	3 (2%)	0 (0%)
Corneal epithelium defect	3 (2%)	4 (8%)
Dry eye NOS	3 (2%)	5 (10%)
Eyelid oedema	3 (2%)	4 (8%)
Vitreous haemorrhage	3 (2%)	0 (0%)
Deposit eye	2 (2%)	0 (0%)
Eyelid ptosis	2 (2 %)	0 (0%)
Keratitis	2 (2%)	2 (4%)
Mydriasis	2 (2%)	1 (2%)

The ocular adverse events in the study eye that were reported by a single investigator as at least possibly related to study drug or injection procedure in a single patient, (<1% of all patients) in the 0.3 mg MACUGEN group were the following: Anterior uveitis, blepharitis, conjunctivitis allergic, corneal abrasion, corneal deposits, corneal erosion, diplopia, endophthalmitis, eye inflammation NOS, eye swelling, eyelid bleeding, eyelid disorder NOS, eyelid irritation, eyelid margin crusting, eyelids pruritus, keratoconjunctivitis sicca, keratopathy NOS, macular degeneration, ocular icterus, optic nerve cupping, pupillary deformity, pupillary disorder NOS, pupillary reflex impaired, retinal artery occlusion, retinal artery spasm, retinal haemorrhage, retinal scar, retinal telangiectasia.

The following Ocular AEs were reported in the study eye as serious, regardless of causality, among the 892 MACUGEN treated patients in any MACUGEN group during the first year: endophthalmitis (12 cases, 1%), retinal detachment (4 cases, <1%), retinal hemorrhage (3 cases, <1%), cataract (3 cases, <1%), traumatic cataract (3 cases, <1%), vitreous hemorrhage (2 cases, <1%), glaucoma NOS (1 case, <1%), uveitis NOS (1 case, <1%), intraocular pressure increased (1 case, <1%).

No serious ocular adverse events were reported in the study eye during the second year of continuous treatment with 0.3 mg dose of MACUGEN (128 patients).

The ocular adverse events in the study eye that were reported to be not related to the study drug or injection procedure in ≥1% of patients in the 0.3 mg MACUGEN group were the following: Visual acuity reduced, cataract, visual disturbance NOS, punctuate keratitis, blepharitis, retinal haemorrhage, vision blurred, dry eye NOS, eye pain, macular degeneration, conjunctivitis, eye pruritus, vitreous floaters, eye discharge, photopsia, posterior capsule opacification, vitreous opacities, lacrimation increased, abnormal sensation eye, anterior chamber inflammation, corneal dystrophy, eye irritation, intraocular pressure increased, meibomianitis, photophobia, retinal exudates, colour blindness NOS, corneal abrasion, corneal oedema, eyelid oedema, keratitis, keratopathy NOS, ocular discomfort, retinal oedema, and vitreous detachment.

Non-Ocular Adverse Events: In the 128 patients who were treated with 0.3 mg MACUGEN for up to 2 years, the overall safety data were consistent with the Year 1 safety data, and no new safety signals emerged from Year 2.

The non-ocular adverse events reported as at least possibly related to study drug or injection procedure in >1% of patients in the 0.3 mg MACUGEN group were headache and rhinorrhoea.

The non-ocular adverse events reported by a single investigator as at least possibly related to study drug or injection procedure in a single patient (<1% of all patients) in the 0.3 mg MACUGEN group were: tachycardia NOS, vertigo, dyspepsia, vomiting NOS, chest pain, fatigue, tenderness NOS, drug hypersensitivity, corneal abrasion, corneal erosion, periorbital haematoma, back pain, nightmare, dermatitis contact, eczema pruritus, and hypertension NOS.

The following non-ocular serious adverse events were reported in >1% of patients in the 0.3 mg MACUGEN group regardless of causality: angina pectoris, atrial fibrillation, cardiac failure congestive, cerebrovascular accident, chest pain, fall, pneumonia NOS, Prostate cancer NOS, pulmonary embolism, transient ischaemic attack, urinary retention.

The non-ocular serious adverse events reported at an incidence of <1% of patients in the 0.3 mg MACUGEN group (1 patient each) regardless of causality are breast cancer NOS, carotid artery occlusion, carotid artery stenosis, carotid sinus syndrome, cerebrovascular insufficiency, chronic obstructive airways disease exacerbated, confusional state, coronary artery occlusion, depression, dizziness, duodenal stricture, endometrial cancer NOS, fractured pelvis NOS, gastrointestinal candidiasis, haematuria, hip fracture, humerus fracture, hypertension NOS, hypertensive crisis, localised osteoarthritis, lung squamous cell carcinoma stage unspecified, metastases to brain, nephrolithiasis, orthostatic hypotension, Parkinson's disease NOS, post procedural pain, prostatic adenoma, pubic rami fracture, pulmonary oedema NOS, renal cell carcinoma stage unspecified, silent myocardial infarction, tachycardia NOS, and thrombocytopenia.

The non-ocular reported adverse events **reported to be unrelated to the study drug** or injection procedure, in >1% of patients in the 0.3 mg MACUGEN group include: abdominal pain NOS, abrasion NOS, anaemia NOS, angina pectoris, arthralgia, arthritis NOS, arthritis NOS aggravated, asthenia, atrial fibrillation, back pain, balance impaired NOS, basal cell carcinoma, benign prostatic hyperplasia, blood creatinine increased, bone spur, bronchitis NOS, cardiac failure congestive, carotid artery occlusion, cerebrovascular accident, chest pain, constipation, contusion, corneal abrasion, coronary artery disease NOS, cough, depression, cutis laxa, diarrhoea NOS, diabetes mellitus NOS, dizziness, dyspepsia, dyspnoea NOS, emphysema, epistaxis, fall, fatigue, fractured pelvis NOS, fungal infection NOS, gastroenteritis viral NOS, gastrooesophageal reflux disease, haematoma NOS, haematuria, headache, herpes zoster, hypercholesterolaemia, hyperkalaemia, hyperlipidaemia NOS, hypersensitivity NOS, hypertension NOS, hypertension aggravated, hypoacusis, hypokalaemia, hyponatraemia, hypotension NOS, influenza upper respiratory tract infection NOS, insomnia, intraocular pressure increased, lower respiratory tract infection NOS, malaise, muscle cramp, muscle weakness NOS, nasal congestion, nasopharyngitis, nausea, nerve compression, nervousness, oedema peripheral, osteoarthritis NOS, pain in limb, periorbital haematoma, pharyngitis, pitting oedema, pleural effusion chronic obstructive airways disease exacerbated, pneumonia NOS, post procedural pain, pulmonary congestion, pulmonary embolism, pyrexia, prostate cancer NOS, sinusitis NOS, skin carcinoma NOS, skin cysts NOS, skin laceration, skin lesion NOS, tinnitus, transient ischaemic attack, urinary retention, urinary tract infection NOS, vertigo, vomiting NOS, thrombocytopenia, and weight decreased.

Abnormal Hematological and Clinical Chemistry Findings: There were no findings to suggest a relationship between MACUGEN and the development of clinically significant abnormalities.

Post-Market Adverse Drug Reactions: Rare cases of anaphylaxis/anaphylactoid reactions, including angioedema, have been reported in patients following administration of pegaptanib along with various medications administered as part of the injection preparation procedure (see Dosage and Administration and Warnings and Precautions).

Other adverse events reported during post-marketing experience are listed below. It should be noted that the uncontrolled nature of post-marketing surveillance makes it difficult to determine definitively if a reported event was actually caused by MACUGEN, or to reliably assess causation in individual cases. The serious adverse events reported in one or more post-marketing cases with 0.3 mg MACUGEN were: activated partial thromboplastin time prolonged, anaphylactic reaction, angioneurotic oedema, blindness, choroidal detachment, coeliac disease, colonic polyp, death, feeling abnormal, haematochezia, haemoptysis, haemorrhage, haemorrhage intracranial, idiopathic thrombocytopenic purpura, inflammation, injury, intermediate uveitis, iridocyclitis, iritis, loss of consciousness, lung adenocarcinoma, lung disorder, neuritis, non-cardiac chest pain, obstructive airways disorder, pulmonary haemorrhage, pulmonary mass, rash generalized, retinal detachment, retinal neovascularisation, retinal tear, syncope, temporal arteritis, tremor, urticaria, vitritis, white blood cell count decreased.

Non serious adverse events reported in more than one patient included: arthropathy, diarrhoea, drug ineffective, dysphagia, eye disorder, foreign body in eye, heart rate increased, injection site discomfort, injection site pain, myalgia, ocular hyperaemia, pain, scleral disorder, urticaria.

DRUG INTERACTIONS: Overview: Drug interaction studies have not been conducted with MACUGEN. Pegaptanib sodium is metabolized by nucleases and therefore cytochrome P450 mediated drug interactions are unlikely.

A clinical study conducted in patients who received MACUGEN alone (no PDT within 6 weeks of MACUGEN administration) and in combination with PDT (PDT therapy within 6 weeks of MACUGEN administration) revealed no apparent difference in the plasma pharmacokinetics of pegaptanib.

Specific plasma protein drug interaction studies were not conducted. In vitro pharmacodynamic studies however suggest no such interaction.

Drug-Herb Interactions: Interactions with herbal products have not been established.

Drug-Laboratory Test Interactions: Interactions with laboratory tests have not been established.

DOSAGE AND ADMINISTRATION:

Recommended Dose and Dosage Adjustment: MACUGEN (pegaptanib sodium injection) 0.3 mg should be administered once every six weeks by intravitreous injection into the eligible eye. Parenteral drug products should be inspected visually for particulate matter and discoloration prior to administration.

No special dosage modification is required for any of the special populations that have been studied (i.e. gender, elderly).

Administration: Administration of the syringe contents involves attaching the threaded plastic plunger rod to the rubber stopper inside the barrel of the syringe. Do not pull back on the plunger. The syringe end cap is then removed to allow administration of the product.

In clinical trials, to optimize safety the injection procedure was carried out under controlled aseptic conditions, which included the use of sterile gloves, a sterile drape and a sterile eyelid speculum. Adequate anesthesia, antibiotic drops and a povidone-iodine flush (or a suitable alternative) was given prior to the injection. For patients allergic to, or intolerant of, povidone-iodine, the treating physician was allowed to use topical broad-spectrum antibiotic drops for 3 days prior to the procedure. Treating physicians were discouraged from performing a paracentesis prior to the injection. Broad-spectrum antibiotic drops were to be continued for 2 days following the injection.

The patient's medical history for hypersensitivity reactions should be carefully evaluated prior to performing the intravitreal procedure (see Warnings and Precautions).

Following the injection, patients should be monitored for elevation in intraocular pressure and for endophthalmitis. Monitoring may consist of a check for perfusion of the optic nerve head immediately after the injection, tonometry within 30 minutes following the injection, and appropriate follow-up within seven days following the injection. Patients were instructed to report any symptoms suggestive of endophthalmitis without delay, at any time.

The safety and efficacy of MACUGEN therapy administered to both eyes concurrently has not been studied.

OVERDOSAGE:

Overdosage with MACUGEN (pegaptanib sodium injection) has not been reported in clinical trials. The highest dose administered to patients in the clinical studies was 3 mg per eye which represents 10 times the recommended therapeutic dose (0.3 mg). The adverse events at 3 mg dose were similar to those at 0.3 mg or 1 mg. No additional adverse events have been noted but there is decreased efficacy with doses above 1 mg.

> For management of a suspected drug overdose, CPhA recommends that you contact your **regional Poison Control Centre**. See the *CPS* Directory section for a list of Poison Control Centres.

ACTION AND CLINICAL PHARMACOLOGY: Mechanism of Action: MACUGEN (pegaptanib sodium injection) is a selective Vascular Endothelial Growth Factor (VEGF) antagonist. VEGF is a secreted protein that selectively binds and activates its receptors located primarily on the surface of vascular endothelial cells. VEGF induces angiogenesis, vascular permeability and inflammation, all of which are thought to contribute to the progression of the neovascular (wet) form of Age-Related Macular Degeneration (AMD), a leading cause of blindness. VEGF has been implicated in blood retinal barrier breakdown and pathological ocular neovascularization.

Pegaptanib sodium is a pegylated aptamer, a modified oligonucleotide, which adopts a three-dimensional conformation that enables it to bind to extracellular VEGF with high affinity and selectivity. Pegaptanib sodium binds to the major pathological VEGF isoform, extracellular $VEGF_{165}$, with high affinity (Kd=200 pM) and specificity, thereby inhibiting $VEGF_{165}$ binding to its VEGF receptors. In contrast virtually no binding of the nonpegylated aptamer to $VEGF_{121}$ or the VEGF-related proteins VEGF-B, VEGF-C and placental growth factor (PIGF) was detected using in vitro filter binding assays. Pegaptanib sodium does not bind significantly to $VEGF_{121}$. In animal models, $VEGF_{164}$ (the rodent counterpart of human $VEGF_{165}$) was specifically upregulated in disease. The selective inhibition of $VEGF_{164}$ with pegaptanib sodium proved as effective at suppressing pathological neovascularization as pan-VEGF inhibition, however pegaptanib sodium spared the normal vasculature whereas pan-VEGF inhibition did not.

Pharmacokinetics: The pharmacokinetics of MACUGEN have not been well characterized in humans.

Absorption: In animals, pegaptanib sodium is slowly absorbed into the systemic circulation from the eye after intravitreous administration. The rate of absorption from the eye is the rate limiting step in the disposition of pegaptanib sodium in animals and is likely to be in humans. In humans, the average±standard deviation apparent plasma half-life of pegaptanib sodium after a 3 mg (10-times the recommended dose) monocular dose is 10±4 days.

A mean maximum plasma concentration of about 80 ng/mL occurs within 1 to 4 days after a 3 mg (10-times the recommended dose) monocular dose in humans. The mean area under the plasma concentration-time curve (AUC) is about 25 µg·h/mL at this dose. Pegaptanib sodium does not accumulate in the plasma when administered intravitreously every 6 weeks. At doses below 0.5 mg/eye, pegaptanib sodium plasma concentrations do not likely exceed 10 ng/mL.

The absolute bioavailability of pegaptanib sodium (parent drug) after intravitreous administration has not been assessed in humans, but is approximately 70-100% in rabbits, dogs, and monkeys.

In animals that received doses of pegaptanib sodium of up to 0.5 mg/eye to both eyes, plasma concentrations were 0.03% to 0.15% of those in the vitreous humor.

Distribution/Metabolism/Excretion: No study evaluating the potential accumulation in tissues was conducted. Potential accumulation pegaptanib or pegaptanib metabolites in tissues, and in particular the eye, cannot be excluded.

In mice, rats, rabbits, dogs and monkeys, pegaptanib sodium distributes primarily into plasma volume and is not extensively distributed to peripheral tissues after intravenous administration. Twenty-four hours after intravitreous administration of a radiolabeled dose of pegaptanib sodium to both eyes of rabbits, radioactivity was mainly distributed in vitreous fluid, retina and aqueous fluid. After intravitreous and intravenous administrations of radiolabeled pegaptanib sodium to rabbits, the highest concentrations of radioactivity (excluding the eye for the intravitreous dose) were obtained in the kidney. In rabbits, the component nucleotide, 2'-fluorouridine is found in plasma and urine after single radiolabeled pegaptanib sodium intravenous and intravitreous doses. Pegaptanib sodium is metabolized by endo- and exonucleases. In rabbits, pegaptanib sodium is eliminated as parent drug and metabolites primarily in the urine.

Special Populations and Conditions: Geriatrics: Plasma concentrations of pegaptanib sodium were similar among patients 50 to 90 years of age. The number of patients below 60 (n=27; 3.0%) and above 85 (n=72; 8.1%) years old was however limited in the studies.

Gender: Plasma concentrations of pegaptanib sodium in male and female patients are similar.

Hepatic Insufficiency: MACUGEN has not been studied in patients with hepatic impairment (see Warnings and Precautions).

Renal Insufficiency: Renal Insufficiency: Based on a clinical study (EOP1006) with pegaptanib sodium injection 3 mg, a decrease in creatinine clearance from 70 mL/min to 30 mL/min was associated with a 2.3 fold increase in AUC. However, a dosage adjustment for patients treated with the recommended 0.3 mg pegaptanib sodium dose and whose creatinine clearance was ≥30 mL/min is not warranted. The pharmacokinetic data indicates that 0.3 mg dose would not exceed exposure seen with 3 mg which was a well tolerated dose. Patients with severe renal insufficiency (creatinine clearance <20 mL/min) have not been adequately studied (see Warnings and Precautions).

Hemodialysis: MACUGEN has not been studied in patients requiring hemodialysis.

STORAGE AND STABILITY: Store in the refrigerator at 2 to 8°C. Do not freeze.

The MACUGEN syringe should not be removed from the pouch until the patient has been prepared for injection.

SPECIAL HANDLING INSTRUCTIONS: Do not use if particles, discoloration, or cloudiness is evident.

Administration of the syringe contents involves attaching the threaded plastic plunger rod to the rubber stopper inside the barrel of the syringe. Do not pull back on the plunger. The syringe end cap is then removed to allow administration of the product.

Any unused product or waste material should be disposed of in accordance with local requirements.

INFORMATION FOR THE PATIENT: Published in e-CPS, available by subscription at www.e-cps.ca.

DOSAGE FORMS, COMPOSITION AND PACKAGING: Each syringe of sterile, clear, preservative-free solution, contains: pegaptanib sodium 0.3 mg (as the free acid form of the oligonucleotide). Nonmedicinal ingredients: dibasic sodium phosphate heptahydrate, hydrochloric acid, monobasic sodium phosphate monohydrate, sodium chloride, sodium hydroxide and water for injection. Single use glass syringes of 1 mL containing 0.3 mg in a 90 µL deliverable volume. Each syringe is fitted with an attached 27 gauge needle and is contained in an outer package. The accompanying plunger rod and flange are in a separate package.

Magnesium-Odan

magnesium glucoheptonate

Magnesium Supplement

Odan

SUPPLIED: Each mL of red, transparent, raspberry-flavored solution contains: elemental magnesium 5 mg from magnesium gluceptate (magnesium glucoheptonate) 100 mg per mL. Nonmedicinal ingredients: potassium sorbate, purified water, raspberry flavour, sodium benzoate and sucralose. Energy: <21 kJ (<5 kcal)/bottle of 2 L). Bottles of 500 mL and 2 L. Store at room temperature (15 to 30°C).

Magnesium Salts: Oral

magnesium citrate
magnesium glucoheptonate
magnesium hydroxide
magnesium oxide
magnesium sulfate

Osmotic Laxatives—Antacids—Mineral Supplementation

CPhA Monograph

Date of Preparation: November 2008

This monograph has been compiled by CPhA and reviewed by experts. It may contain information different from that found in Health Canada-approved Product Monographs. The reader is referred to the *CPS* Editorial Policy for more information.

SUMMARY PRODUCT INFORMATION:

Magnesium Salt	Route of Administration	Dosage Form	Strength
Magnesium citrate	Oral	Capsule	60 mg, 150 mg, 250 mg, others
		Tablet	50 mg, 200 mg, 250 mg, 300 mg, others
		Liquid	50 mg/mL, 59 mg/mL
		Powder	87.47 mg/2.5 g
Magnesium glucoheptonate	Oral	Capsule	10.24 mg
		Liquid	100 mg/mL
Magnesium hydroxide	Oral	Tablet	50 mg, 300 mg, 385 mg, others
		Liquid	80 mg/mL
Magnesium oxide	Oral	Tablet	252 mg, 835 mg, others
		Capsule	400 mg
		Powder	750 mg/1.25 mL
Magnesium sulfate	Oral	Capsule	59 mg
		Powder	99 g/100 g

INDICATIONS AND CLINICAL USE:

- Magnesium citrate is used in the short-term treatment of constipation and to evacuate the bowel prior to certain surgical and diagnostic procedures.
- Magnesium glucoheptonate is used in the treatment and prevention of hypomagnesemia.
- Magnesium hydroxide is used: for the short term treatment of constipation; for the relief of symptoms of heartburn and acid indigestion; as a dietary supplement.
- Magnesium oxide is used in the treatment and prevention of hypomagnesemia and as a dietary supplement.
- Magnesium sulfate is used orally in the short-term treatment of constipation.

CONTRAINDICATIONS:

- Patients who are hypersensitive to any ingredient in the formulation or component of the container.
- Patients with heart block.
- All laxatives are contraindicated in patients with acute abdominal pain, nausea, vomiting or other symptoms of appendicitis or undiagnosed abdominal pain.
- Patients with serious renal impairment.

WARNINGS AND PRECAUTIONS: Cardiovascular: Hypermagnesemia can cause heart block. Patients with heart block should not consume magnesium supplements.

Endocrine and Metabolism: Repeated administration of osmotic saline laxatives may result in dehydration if not administered with sufficient fluids. Long-term use or overdosage of osmotic saline laxatives can result in serious and potentially life-threatening electrolyte disturbances.

Gastrointestinal: All laxatives are contraindicated in patients with acute abdominal pain, nausea, vomiting or other symptoms of appendicitis or undiagnosed abdominal pain. It is recommended that patients with ileostomies or colostomies avoid use of laxatives. Magnesium antacids or supplements commonly cause a laxative effect. Repeated doses may cause diarrhea which could result in fluid and electrolyte imbalance.

Neurologic: Use with extreme caution in patients with myasthenia gravis or other neuromuscular disease since magnesium has a significant inhibitory effect on acetylcholine release.

Renal: Use cautiously in individuals with reduced kidney function due to an increased risk of hypermagnesemia. Magnesium serum levels should be monitored in renally impaired patients who are receiving magnesium.

Special Populations: Pregnant Women: Magnesium crosses the placenta. Serum levels in the fetus correlate with those in the mother. Intermittent use of magnesium laxatives and antacids (with the exclusion of those products containing sodium bicarbonate or magnesium trisilicate) is considered safe in pregnancy.

Nursing Women: Use of oral magnesium salts is considered compatible with breast-feeding.

Geriatrics: As kidney function declines with age, older individuals may be at increased risk of developing hypermagnesemia following ingestion of oral magnesium salts.

ADVERSE REACTIONS: Adverse Drug Reactions Overview: Orally, magnesium can cause nausea, vomiting and diarrhea. Rarely, larger amounts of magnesium may cause hypermagnesemia, which predominantly occurs in patients with renal insufficiency. Normal serum level for magnesium in adults is 0.8-1 mmol/L and for children is 0.7-0.95 mmol/L. Symptoms of hypermagnesemia include thirst, decreased blood pressure, nausea and vomiting, flushing, muscle weakness, ECG changes, sedation, confusion, loss of tendon reflexes, respiratory paralysis, cardiac arrhythmias, coma, cardiac arrest and death.

DRUG INTERACTIONS: Overview: Magnesium salts are known for their propensity to chelate other drugs present in the GI tract, forming insoluble compounds that can pass through the GI tract without being absorbed. In addition antacid products may alter gastric and urinary pH affecting dissolution, absorption, bioavailability and renal elimination of some drugs. Laxative products potentially decrease transit time of concomitantly administered oral medication and can therefore decrease their absorption. For these reasons, it is generally considered prudent to avoid concurrent administration of magnesium salts with other medications. If oral magnesium salts must be used with other drugs, many interactions can be avoided by taking the magnesium salt 2 hours before or after other drugs.

Drug-Drug Interactions: See Table 1.

Table 1: Magnesium Salts: Oral
Drug-Drug Interactions

Interacting Drug	Effect	Clinical Comment
ACE Inhibitors	Magnesium antacids may ↓ therapeutic effect of these drugs after oral administration (mechanism unknown).	Monitor for changes in effects of these medications when antacids are stopped/started.
Aldesleukin	↓ magnesium serum levels.	Has been reported to cause decreases in magnesium serum levels.
Allopurinol	Magnesium-containing antacids may ↓ therapeutic effect by decreasing its absorption.	Separating the doses of magnesium-containing antacids and allopurinol may attenuate this interaction.
Aluminum Hydroxide	↑ risk of aluminum toxicity in patients with severe renal dysfunction.	Only a concern for magnesium **citrate** (the citrate component is responsible).
Aminoglycosides (e.g., gentamicin)	↓ magnesium serum levels.	These medications have been reported to cause decreases in magnesium serum levels.
	Risk of ↑ neuromuscular blocking effect as these agents possess neuromuscular-blocking activity.	Monitor for ↑ or prolonged neuromuscular blockade in patients with increased serum magnesium or renal impairment.
Amphetamines	Magnesium-containing antacids may ↑ therapeutic/toxic effect of these drugs.	Monitor for changes in effects of these drugs when antacids are started/stopped.
Amphotericin-B	↓ magnesium serum levels.	Has been reported to cause decreases in magnesium serum levels.
Azole Derivative Antifungals (e.g., ketoconazole)	Magnesium-containing antacids may ↓ therapeutic effect of these drugs by decreasing their absorption.	Separating the doses of magnesium-containing antacids and these drugs may attenuate this interaction.
Bisacodyl	↓ therapeutic effect of bisacodyl due to decreased acidity causing bisacodyl to be released prior to reaching the large intestine.	Avoid use of antacids within 1 hour before taking bisacodyl.
Bisphosphonates	Magnesium may ↓ therapeutic effect of these drugs by decreasing their absorption after oral administration.	Separating the doses of magnesium-containing antacids and these drugs may attenuate this interaction.
Calcitriol	↑ risk of hypermagnesemia especially in patients with chronic renal failure.	Choose a non-magnesium containing antacid or phosphate-binding product.
Calcium Channel Blockers	↑ hypotensive effect of calcium channel blockers (higher risk in patients with impaired renal function).	Monitor for hypotension in patients with renal impairment receiving this combination.
	Calcium channel blockers may enhance the adverse/toxic effects of magnesium.	Monitor for adverse/toxic effects of magnesium.
Carboplatin	↓ magnesium serum levels.	Has been reported to cause decreases in magnesium serum levels.
Cefuroxime	Magnesium antacids may ↓ therapeutic effect of this drug after oral administration (mechanism unknown).	Monitor for changes in effects of cefuroxime when antacids are stopped/started.
Cisplatin	↓ magnesium serum levels.	Has been reported to cause decreases in magnesium serum levels.
Corticosteroids	Magnesium antacids may ↓ therapeutic effect of these drugs after oral administration (mechanism unknown).	Monitor for changes in effects of these medications when antacids are stopped/started.
Cyclosporine	Magnesium antacids may ↓ therapeutic effect of cyclosporine after oral administration (mechanism unknown).	Monitor for changes in effects of cyclosporine when antacids are stopped/started.
	Cyclosporine may ↓ magnesium serum levels.	Has been reported to cause decreases in magnesium serum levels.
Dabigatran	Magnesium-containing antacids may ↓ therapeutic effect of dabigatran by decreasing absorption.	In many cases, separating the doses of magnesium-containing antacids and dabigatran may attenuate this interaction.
Dasatinib	Magnesium-containing antacids may ↓ therapeutic effect of dasatinib by decreasing absorption.	In many cases, separating the doses of magnesium-containing antacids and dasatinib may attenuate this interaction.
Delavirdine	Magnesium-containing antacids may ↓ therapeutic effect of delavirdine by decreasing absorption.	In many cases, separating the doses of magnesium-containing antacids and delavirdine may attenuate this interaction.
Diuretics, loop (e.g., furosemide)	↓ magnesium serum levels.	These medications have been reported to cause decreases in magnesium serum levels.

(cont'd)

Table 1: Magnesium Salts: Oral *(cont'd)*

Drug-Drug Interactions

Interacting Drug	Effect	Clinical Comment
Fexofenadine	Magnesium-containing antacids may ↓ therapeutic effect of fexofenadine by decreasing absorption.	In many cases, separating the doses of magnesium-containing antacids and fexofenadine may attenuate this interaction.
Fluoride	Magnesium may ↓ therapeutic effect of fluoride by decreasing absorption after oral administration.	In many cases, separating the doses of magnesium-containing antacids and fluoride may attenuate this interaction.
Iron Salts (except ferric gluconate, iron dextran complex)	Magnesium-containing antacids may ↓ therapeutic effect of these drugs by decreasing absorption.	In many cases, separating the doses of magnesium-containing antacids and these drugs may attenuate this interaction.
Isoniazid	Magnesium-containing antacids may ↓ therapeutic effect of isoniazid by decreasing absorption.	In many cases, separating the doses of magnesium-containing antacids and isoniazid may attenuate this interaction.
Methenamine	↓ therapeutic effect of methenamine due to alkalinization of the urine if magnesium antacids taken in sufficient quantities.	Choose an agent other than methenamine or discontinue antacid.
Mycophenolate	Magnesium may ↓ therapeutic effect of mycophenolate by decreasing absorption after oral administration.	In many cases, separating the doses of magnesium-containing antacids and mycophenolate may attenuate this interaction.
Neuromuscular Blocking Agents (e.g., atracurium, pancuronium, rocuronium)	Risk of ↑ neuromuscular blocking effect as these agents possess neuromuscular-blocking activity.	Monitor for ↑ or prolonged neuromuscular blockade in patients with increased serum magnesium or renal impairment.
Penicillamine	Magnesium antacids may ↓ therapeutic effect of penicillamine after oral administration (mechanism unknown).	Monitor for changes in effects of penicillamine when antacids are stopped/started.
Pentamidine	↓ magnesium serum levels.	Has been reported to cause decreases in magnesium serum levels.
Phenothiazines	Magnesium-containing antacids may ↓ therapeutic effect of these drugs by decreasing their absorption.	Separating the doses of magnesium-containing antacids and these drugs may attenuate this interaction.
Phenytoin	Magnesium-containing antacids may ↓ therapeutic effect of phenytoin by decreasing their absorption.	In many cases, separating the doses of magnesium-containing antacids and phenytoin may attenuate this interaction.
Phosphate Supplements	Magnesium may ↓ therapeutic effect of these drugs by decreasing their absorption after oral administration.	Separating the doses of magnesium-containing antacids and these drugs may attenuate this interaction.
Protease Inhibitors (except darunavir)	Magnesium-containing antacids may ↓ therapeutic effect of these drugs by decreasing their absorption.	In many cases, separating the doses of magnesium-containing antacids and these drugs may attenuate this interaction (for details, refer to monographs of specific agents).
Quinidine	Magnesium-containing antacids may ↑ therapeutic/toxic effect of quinidine.	Monitor for changes in effects of quinidine when antacids are started/stopped.
Quinolone Antibiotics (e.g., ciprofloxacin)	Magnesium may ↓ therapeutic effect of these drugs by decreasing their absorption after oral administration.	Separating the doses of magnesium-containing antacids and these drugs may attenuate this interaction.
Sodium Polystyrene Sulfonate	↑ risk of metabolic alkalosis Oral sodium polystyrene sulfonate may bind magnesium ions, preventing them from neutralizing bicarbonate ions in the small intestine, making more bicarbonate available for systemic absorption.	Interaction can be minimized by: separating the agents by 2 or more hours, giving sodium polystyrene sulfonate rectally or choosing an alternative antacid agent (e.g., H_2-antagonist).
Tacrolimus	↓ magnesium serum levels	Has been reported to cause decreases in magnesium serum levels.
Tetracycline Derivatives	Magnesium may ↓ therapeutic effect of these drugs by decreasing their absorption after oral administration.	Separating the doses of magnesium-containing antacids and these drugs may attenuate this interaction.

Drug-Food Interactions: The acid neutralizing effect of magnesium-containing antacids persists for 20-60 minutes; in the presence of sufficient food this may be prolonged to as long as 3 hours.

Drug-Laboratory Interactions: Some laboratory methods may result in the reporting of falsely elevated calcium serum levels in the presence of **high** magnesium serum levels. Interference with measurement of calcium is not a concern if the magnesium serum level is at or near the normal range. Consultation with the laboratory involved is necessary to confirm whether the methods they use are affected.

DOSAGE AND ADMINISTRATION:

Elemental magnesium content of the various salts can be found in Table 2.

Dosing of magnesium salts in adults can be found in Table 3.

Recommended daily intake of magnesium in adults can be found in Table 4.

Dosing of magnesium salts in pediatrics can be found in Table 5.

Recommended daily intake of magnesium in pediatrics can be found in Table 6.

Administration: Magnesium citrate solution should be chilled prior to administration to increase palatability.

Magnesium hydroxide suspension should be shaken well before swallowing. Magnesium hydroxide tablets should be chewed well before use. In general, liquid suspensions of magnesium hydroxide are faster acting and more effective than tablets.

Magnesium sulfate powder is to be mixed with water according to manufacturer's instructions before administration.

Magnesium glucoheptonate is recommended to be given with meals.

Table 2: Magnesium Salts: Oral

Elemental Magnesium Content

Magnesium Salt	Percentage elemental Mg^{++}	Elemental Mg^{++}/g (mmol)[a]
Magnesium citrate	16	6.7
Magnesium glucoheptonate	5	2.1
Magnesium hydroxide	41.8	17.6
Magnesium oxide	60.5	25.4
Magnesium sulfate	10	4.1

[a] 1 g elemental magnesium = 83 mEq = 42 mmol.

Table 3: Magnesium Salts: Oral

Dose in Adult Patients

Indication	Magnesium Salt	Adult Dose	Clinical Comment
Hypomagnesemia[a]	Magnesium oxide 420 mg tablet	1–2 tablets (420–840 mg) once or twice daily	Diarrhea limits the amount of oral magnesium that can be administered to correct hypomagnesemia. Doses should be titrated according to serum magnesium.
	Magnesium hydroxide 80 mg/mL suspension	7.5–15 mL (600–1200 mg) once or twice daily	
	Magnesium glucoheptonate 100 mg/mL solution	15–30 mL (1500–3000 mg) one to three times daily	
Constipation	Magnesium citrate 15 g/300 mL	75–150 mL (3.75–7.5 g) daily. Follow doses with 250 mL water	Should be used as short-term intermittent therapy, on an as-needed basis, once or twice weekly at most.
	Magnesium hydroxide 80 mg/mL suspension	30–60 mL (2400–4800 mg) once daily or in divided doses	
	Magnesium sulfate	10–30 g (dissolved in 240 mL water or juice) once daily or divided doses	
Bowel Evacuation (prior to medical procedure)	Magnesium citrate 15 g/300 mL	300 mL (15 g) single dose	Drink 250 mL of water each hour for 4–6 h before and 3 h after administration.
Acid Indigestion	Magnesium hydroxide 80 mg/mL suspension	5–15 mL (400–1200 mg) up to four times daily as required	The laxative effect of magnesium hydroxide is often problematic when it is used alone as an antacid on a frequent basis.

[a] Symptoms of hypomagnesemia include weakness, muscle tremor, tetany, increased reflexes, disorientation, convulsions, psychosis, stupor, coma. Drastic reduction in dietary intake of magnesium is needed to induce a negative balance because of extremely effective renal retention and increasing intestinal absorption.

Table 4: Magnesium Salts: Oral

Recommended Daily Intake of Magnesium in Adults

Life Stage Group	Recommended Daily Intake[a,b] (mg elemental Mg^{++})
19–30 y	Male: 400 Female: 310
>31 y	Male: 420 Female: 320
Pregnant	
≤18 y	400
19–30 y	350
31–50 y	360
Lactation	
≤18 y	360
19–30 y	310
31–50 y	320

[a] Hydroxide and oxide salts most commonly used for daily supplementation.

[b] Dietary intake is preferred over supplementation whenever possible. Food sources of magnesium include: green leafy vegetables, nuts, tofu, unprocessed (outer layer not removed) whole grains, legumes (e.g., beans), avocados and bananas.

Table 5: Magnesium Salts: Oral

Dose in Pediatric Patients

Indication	Magnesium Salt	Pediatric Dose	Clinical Comment
Hypomagnesemia[a]	Magnesium oxide 420 mg tablet	20–40 mg/kg/day (elemental Mg^{++}) divided TID	Diarrhea limits the amount of oral magnesium that can be administered to correct hypomagnesemia. Doses should be titrated according to serum magnesium.
	Magnesium hydroxide 80 mg/mL suspension	20–40 mg/kg/day (elemental Mg^{++}) divided TID	
	Magnesium glucoheptonate 100 mg/mL solution	20–40 mg/kg/day (elemental Mg^{++}) divided TID	

(cont'd)

Table 5: Magnesium Salts: Oral *(cont'd)*

Dose in Pediatric Patients

Indication	Magnesium Salt	Pediatric Dose	Clinical Comment
Constipation	Magnesium citrate 15 g/300 mL	On physician's advice only: <6 y: 1–3 mL/kg once daily 6–12 y: 100–150 mL per day >12 y: 150–300 mL per day Follow doses with 250 mL water	Should be used as short-term intermittent therapy, on an as-needed basis, once or twice weekly at most.
	Magnesium hydroxide 80 mg/mL suspension	<2 y: 0.5 ml/kg/dose 2–5 y: 5–15 mL once daily or divided doses 6–11 y: 15–30 mL once daily or divided doses ≥12 y: 30–60 mL once daily or in divided doses	
	Magnesium sulfate	On physician's advice only	
Bowel Evacuation (prior to medical procedure)	Magnesium citrate 15 g/300 mL	4 mL/kg/dose (max 300 mL/dose)	Drink 250 mL of water each hour for 4–6 h before and 3 h after administration.
Acid Indigestion	Magnesium hydroxide 80 mg/mL suspension	<2 y: 0.5 mL/kg/dose 2–5 y: 5–15 mL once daily or divided doses 6–11 y: 15–30 mL once daily or in divided doses ≥12 y: 30–60 mL once daily or in divided doses	The laxative effect of magnesium hydroxide is often problematic when it is used alone as an antacid on a frequent basis.

[a] Symptoms of hypomagnesemia include weakness, muscle tremor, tetany, increased reflexes, disorientation, convulsions, psychosis, stupor, coma. Drastic reduction in dietary intake of magnesium is needed to induce a negative balance because of extremely effective renal retention and increasing intestinal absorption.

Table 6: Magnesium Salts: Oral

Recommended Daily Intake of Magnesium in Pediatric Patients

Age or Gender	Recommended Daily Intake[a,b] (mg elemental Mg^{++})
Infants	
0–6 mo	30
7–12 mo	75
Children	
1–3 y	80
4–8 y	130
Males	
9–13 y	240
14–18 y	410
Females	
9–13 y	240
14–18 y[c]	360

[a] Hydroxide and oxide salts most commonly used for daily supplementation.
[b] Dietary intake is preferred over supplementation whenever possible. Food sources of magnesium include: green leafy vegetables, nuts, tofu, unprocessed (outer layer not removed) whole grains, legumes (e.g., beans), avocados and bananas.
[c] For recommended daily intake in pregnancy or lactation, see Table 4.

OVERDOSAGE:

For management of a suspected drug overdose, CPhA recommends that you contact your **regional Poison Control Centre**. See the *CPS* Directory section for a list of Poison Control Centres.

ACTION AND CLINICAL PHARMACOLOGY: Mechanism of Action: Laxative and Bowel Evacuation: Promotes bowel evacuation by causing osmotic retention of fluid which distends the colon, resulting in increased peristaltic activity. Stimulation of the release of cholecystokinin leading to increased intraluminal fluid and electrolyte accumulation and increased intestinal motility may also play a role.

Antacids: Reacts with hydrochloric acid in the stomach to form magnesium chloride and water, thus neutralizing the gastric acid.

Hypomagnesemia: Magnesium plays an essential role in many cellular reactions. At least 300 enzymes depend on magnesium to function normally. Normal serum level for magnesium in adults is 0.8-1 mmol/L and for children is 0.7-0.95 mmol/L. Although the magnesium serum concentration is the most commonly used test to evaluate magnesium status, it reflects extracellular magnesium and is not a reliable indicator of intracellular depletion. Food sources of magnesium include: green leafy vegetables, nuts, tofu, unprocessed (outer layer not removed) whole grains, legumes (e.g., beans), avocados and bananas. For recommended daily intakes of magnesium in adults and children see Table 4 and Table 6, respectively.

Pharmacokinetics: Adults: Absorption: Approximately 15-30% of orally administered magnesium-containing saline laxatives may be absorbed, likely from the small intestine. These laxatives generally take effect between 0.5 and 6 hours after ingestion.

As an antacid, magnesium hydroxide provides rapid acid-neutralizing effects. Many antacid products combine magnesium hydroxide (which reacts rapidly with hydrochloric acid) with aluminum hydroxide (which reacts more slowly with hydrochloric acid) to try to provide a more sustained acid neutralizing capacity. Another rationale for this combination is that magnesium's tendency to cause diarrhea should offset aluminum's tendency to cause constipation, though in practice this balance is difficult to achieve.

Duration of action for antacids is determined by gastric emptying time. On an empty stomach, acid neutralizing effects last 20-60 minutes, but can be prolonged up to 3 hours in the presence of sufficient food.

Magnesium Replacement: Oral bioavailability of magnesium salts is approximately 35%.

Distribution: Total body magnesium is distributed as follows: bone 60-65%, muscle 27%, other cells 6%, extracellular fluid 1%. Half of plasma magnesium exists as the free ion; a third is bound to albumin and the remainder forms complexes with citrate, phosphate and other anions.

Metabolism: Magnesium levels are efficiently regulated by the kidneys. Magnesium also undergoes efficient enterohepatic circulation.

Excretion: Magnesium is excreted in the urine. Unabsorbed magnesium is excreted in the feces.

STORAGE AND STABILITY: Magnesium citrate solution should be stored at 2-30°C to minimize decomposition and increase palatability. The presence of white precipitate at the bottom of the solution does not alter the potency of the product.

Magnesium hydroxide suspension should be stored below 35°C but prevented from freezing. It should be well shaken before use since separation of water from the suspension occurs on standing.

Magnesium oxide suspension should be stored in a tightly closed container in a dry location.

Magnesium sulfate crystals should be stored in a tightly closed container at 15-30°C.

Magnevist®

gadopentetate dimeglumine

Contrast Enhancement Agent for Magnetic Resonance Imaging (MRI)

Bayer

Date of Revision: September 17, 2009

PHARMACOLOGY: MAGNEVIST (gadopentetate dimeglumine) was developed as a contrast agent for diagnostic use in magnetic resonance imaging (MRI). Gadolinium is a rare earth element. Its ion (Gd^{+++}) has seven unpaired electrons and, therefore, shows paramagnetic properties. Gd^{+++} has a strong effect on the hydrogen-proton spin-lattice relaxation time (T_1), which causes the observed contrast enhancement in MRI scans. By chelation of Gd^{+++} with diethylenetriamine pentaacetic acid (DTPA), a strongly paramagnetic, well-tolerated, stable complex (gadopentetate dimeglumine salt) is obtained.

The free gadolinium ion is unsuitable for clinical use due to high toxicity; however, the metal chelate is metabolically inert. The organic component of the chelate is not measurably metabolized and the metal does not dissociate. After intravenous injection of gadopentetate dimeglumine, the meglumine ion completely dissociates from the gadopentetate. The hydrophilic chelate is distributed only in the extracellular water and does not cross the intact blood-brain barrier. Gadopentetate is excreted unchanged in the urine. It is rapidly eliminated by the kidneys with a clearance identical to that of inulin (no tubular reabsorption).

Pharmacokinetics: The pharmacokinetic profile of intravenously administered gadopentetate dimeglumine in normal subjects conforms to a two-compartment open model with a mean distribution half-life of about 0.2 hours and a mean elimination half-life of about 1.6 hours. Approximately 80% of the dose was excreted in the urine within 6 hours and 93% within 24 hours post injection of a 0.1 mmol/kg dose. Excretion in the faeces amounted to <0.1% over 5 days. There was no detectable biotransformation, dissociation or decomposition of gadopentetate.

MAGNEVIST has no pharmacodynamic effect when administered as indicated with the exception of slightly increased plasma osmolality.

INDICATIONS: MAGNEVIST (gadopentetate dimeglumine), by intravenous injection, is indicated for contrast enhancement during cranial and spinal MRI investigations in adults and children, to detect lesions associated with abnormal vascularity or those thought to alter the blood-brain barrier.

MAGNEVIST is also indicated for use with MRI in adults to provide contrast enhancement and facilitate visualization of lesions with abnormal vascularity within the head (extracranial) and neck.

CONTRAINDICATIONS: MAGNEVIST (gadopentetate dimeglumine) should not be administered to patients who are known or suspected of being hypersensitive to it.

WARNINGS:

Serious Warnings and Precautions

Nephrogenic Systemic Fibrosis: Gadolinium-based contrast agents (GBCAs) increase the risk for Nephrogenic Systemic Fibrosis (NSF) in patients with:

- acute or chronic severe renal insufficiency (glomerular filtration rate <30 mL/min/1.73 m²), or
- acute renal insufficiency of any severity due to the hepato-renal syndrome or in the perioperative liver transplantation period.

In these patients, avoid use of GBCAs unless the diagnostic information is essential and not available with noncontrast enhanced magnetic resonance imaging (MRI). NSF may result in fatal or debilitating systemic fibrosis affecting the skin, muscle, and internal organs. Screen all patients for renal dysfunction by obtaining a history and/or laboratory tests. When administering a GBCA, do not exceed the recommended dose (see Dosage) and allow a sufficient period of time for elimination of the agent from the body prior to any readministration. (See also Warnings, General; Warnings, Renal Impairment; Precautions, Skin; and Adverse Reactions, Postmarket Adverse Drug Reactions.)

General: MRI procedures which involve the use of MAGNEVIST by injection should be carried out by physicians who have the prerequisite training and a thorough knowledge of the particular procedure to be performed.

Nephrogenic Systemic Fibrosis (NSF): Gadolinium-based contrast agents (GBCAs) increase the risk for Nephrogenic Systemic Fibrosis (NSF) in patients with acute or chronic severe renal insufficiency (glomerular filtration rate <30 mL/min/1.73 m²), and in patients with acute renal insufficiency of any severity due to the hepato-renal syndrome, or in the perioperative liver transplantation period. In these patients, avoid use of GBCAs unless the diagnostic information is essential and not available with noncontrast-enhanced magnetic resonance imaging (MRI). For patients receiving hemodialysis, healthcare professionals may consider prompt hemodialysis following GBCA administration in order to enhance the contrast agent's elimination. However, it is unknown if hemodialysis prevents NSF.

Among the factors that may increase the risk for NSF are repeated or higher than recommended doses of a GBCA and the degree of renal function impairment at the time of exposure.

NSF development is considered a potential class-related effect of all GBCAs.

Postmarketing reports have identified the development of NSF following single and multiple administrations of GBCAs. These reports have not always identified a specific agent. Where a specific agent was identified, the most commonly reported agent was gadodiamide (Omniscan), followed by gadopentetate dimeglumine (MAGNEVIST) and gadoversetamide (OptiMARK). NSF has also developed following the sequential administration of gadodiamide with gadobenate dimeglumine (MultiHance) or gadoteridol (ProHance). The number of postmarketing reports is subject to change over time and may not reflect the true proportion of cases associated with any specific GBCA.

The extent of risk for NSF following exposure to any specific GBCA is unknown and may vary among the agents. Published reports are limited and predominantly estimate NSF risks with gadodiamide. In 1 retrospective study of 370 patients with severe renal insufficiency who received gadodiamide, the estimated risk for development of NSF was 4%. The risk, if any, for the development of NSF among patients with mild to moderate renal insufficiency or normal renal function is unknown, and the cautious utilization of the lowest possible dose of GBCA is preferable.

Screen all patients for renal dysfunction by obtaining a history and/or laboratory tests. When administering a GBCA, do not exceed the recommended dose and allow a sufficient period of time for elimination of the agent from the body prior to any readministration. (See Pharmacology and Dosage.)

A skin biopsy is necessary in order to exclude the diagnosis of similarly presenting skin disorders (eg, scleromyxedema). (See Warnings, Serious Warnings and Precautions; Warnings, Renal Impairment; Precautions, Skin; and Adverse Reactions, Postmarket Adverse Drug Reactions.)

Hypersensitivity Reactions: The decision to use MAGNEVIST (gadopentetate dimeglumine) must be made after careful evaluation of the risk-benefit in patients with a history of allergic disposition or bronchial asthma or with any previous reaction to contrast media, since experience shows that these patients suffer more frequently than others from hypersensitivity reactions.

Patients who experience hypersensitivity reactions while taking beta blockers may be resistant to treatment effects of beta agonists.

Patients with cardiovascular disease are more susceptible to serious, even fatal outcomes of severe hypersensitivity reactions.

As with other intravenous contrast agents, MAGNEVIST can be associated with anaphylactic reactions, anaphylactoid/hypersensitivity or other idiosyncratic reactions characterized by cardiovascular, respiratory, or cutaneous manifestations, and ranging from mild to severe reactions including anaphylactic shock. These reactions often occur at least within half an hour of administration. However, in rare cases delayed reactions (hours later or up to several days) may occur (see Adverse Reactions). If such a reaction occurs, stop MAGNEVIST administration and immediately begin appropriate therapy, including resuscitation.

It is important for prompt action in the event of such incidents and to be familiar with the practice of emergency measures. To permit immediate counter-measures to be taken in emergencies, appropriate drugs and instruments (eg, endotracheal tube and ventilator) should be readily available.

As with other contrast-enhanced diagnostic procedures, it is important to closely observe patients with a history of drug reactions, allergy or hypersensitivity disorders, during and up to several hours after MAGNEVIST injection.

Injection Site Reactions: Skin and soft tissue necrosis, thrombosis, fasciitis, and compartment syndrome requiring surgical intervention (eg, compartment release or amputation) have occurred very rarely at the site of contrast injection or the dosed limb. Total volume and rate of MAGNEVIST injection, extravasation of contrast agent, and patient susceptibility might contribute to these reactions. Phlebitis and thrombophlebitis may be observed generally within 24 hours after MAGNEVIST injection and resolve with supportive treatment. Determine the patency and integrity of the intravenous line before administration of MAGNEVIST injection. Assessment of the dosed limb for the development of injection site reactions is recommended.

Sickle Erythrocytes: Deoxygenated sickle cell erythrocytes have been shown in in vitro studies to align perpendicular to a magnetic field which may result in vaso-occlusive complications in vivo. The enhancement of magnetic moment by gadopentetate dimeglumine may possibly potentiate sickle erythrocyte alignment. MAGNEVIST in patients with sickle cell anemia and other hemoglobinopathies has not been studied.

Renal Impairment: In patients with renal insufficiency, acute renal failure requiring dialysis or worsening renal function have occurred, mostly within 48 hours of MAGNEVIST injection. The risk of these events is higher with increasing dose of contrast agent. MAGNEVIST should only be used after careful risk/benefit assessment in these patients, including consideration of possible alternative imaging methods. Use the lowest possible dose and evaluate renal function in patients with renal insufficiency (see Dosage).

- Exposure to GBCAs increases the risk for NSF in patients with:
  - acute or chronic severe renal insufficiency (glomerular filtration rate <30 mL/min/1.73 m^2), or
  - acute renal insufficiency of any severity due to the hepato-renal syndrome or in the perioperative liver transplantation period.
- Screen all patients for renal dysfunction by obtaining a history and/or laboratory tests.
- The risk, if any, for the development of NSF among patients with mild to moderate renal insufficiency or normal renal function is unknown, and the cautious utilization of the lowest possible dose of GBCA is preferable.

(See Warnings, Serious Warnings and Precautions; Precautions, Skin; and Adverse Reactions, Postmarket Adverse Drug Reactions.)

No studies have been conducted in children with severe renal or hepatic dysfunction, clinically unstable or uncontrolled hypertension, or in premature infants.

PRECAUTIONS: General: MAGNEVIST (gadopentetate dimeglumine) is to be administered strictly by intravenous injection. MAGNEVIST will cause tissue irritation and pain if administered extravascularly or if it leaks interstitially.

A sweet taste may be experienced briefly by patients receiving a bolus injection of MAGNEVIST intravenously.

As with any paramagnetic contrast agent, MAGNEVIST might impair the visualization of lesions seen on noncontrast MRI. Therefore, caution should be exercised when MAGNEVIST MRI scans are interpreted without a companion noncontrast MRI scan.

Hemolytic States: Gadopentetate dimeglumine alters red blood cell morphology resulting in transient, slight, extravascular (splenic) hemolysis with increased serum iron and total bilirubin levels. Although this effect was of no clinical significance during clinical trials, caution is advised in patients with hepatic disease and/or hemolytic states.

Convulsive States: While there is no evidence suggesting that MAGNEVIST directly precipitates convulsion, the possibility that it may decrease the convulsive threshold in susceptible patients cannot be ruled out. Patients with seizure disorders or intracranial lesions may be at increased risk of seizure activity, as has been reported rarely in association with MAGNEVIST administration. Precautionary measures should be taken with patients predisposed to seizure, eg, close monitoring and availability of injectable anticonvulsants (see Dosage).

Skin: NSF was first identified in 1997 and has, so far, been observed only in patients with renal disease. This is a systemic disorder with the most prominent and visible effects on the skin. Cutaneous lesions associated with this disorder are caused by excessive fibrosis and are usually symmetrically distributed on the limbs and trunk. Involved skin becomes thickened, which may inhibit flexion and extension of joints and result in severe contractures. The fibrosis associated with NSF can extend beyond dermis and involve subcutaneous tissues, striated muscles, diaphragm, pleura, pericardium, and myocardium. NSF may be fatal. (See Warnings, Serious Warnings and Precautions; Warnings, General; Warnings, Renal Impairment; and Adverse Reactions, Postmarket Adverse Drug Reactions.)

Pediatric: The cautious utilization of the lowest effective dose (0.1 mmol/kg BW) in children is recommended, particularly for neonates and infants, as the pharmacokinetics of MAGNEVIST in neonates and infants with immature renal function have not been studied (see Warnings, Renal Impairment).

Pregnancy: There are no studies on the use of MAGNEVIST in pregnant women. MAGNEVIST should not be used during human pregnancy unless the potential benefit justifies the potential risk to the fetus.

Lactation: Transfer of MAGNEVIST into the milk of lactating mothers can occur. Thus breast feeding should be interrupted for 24 hours post administration of MAGNEVIST and the milk discarded during this period.

Geriatrics: No special precautions are required for elderly patients (see Warnings, Serious Warnings and Precautions).

Interference with Diagnostic Tests: The result of serum iron determination employing methods measuring complex formation (eg, bathophenanthroline) within 24 hours of MAGNEVIST examination may result in inaccurately low values due to the free DPTA in MAGNEVIST.

Information to Be Provided to the Patient: Patients scheduled to receive MAGNEVIST should be instructed to inform their physician if they are pregnant, breast feed, or have a history of renal insufficiency, asthma or allergic respiratory disorders.

Nephrogenic Systemic Fibrosis: There have been postmarket reports of a rare disease called Nephrogenic Systemic Fibrosis (NSF) following gadolinium-based contrast agent (GBCA) use.

NSF is a rare condition which has only been observed so far in patients with severe kidney disease. At present, there is no evidence that other patient groups are at risk of developing the condition. Due to NSF, the skin becomes thickened, coarse, and hard, which sometimes makes bending of the joints difficult. NSF may spread to other organs and even cause death.

Patients with severe kidney disease should avoid the use of MAGNEVIST unless the health care professional believes the possible benefits outweigh the potential risks. Those who have already had an MR imaging procedure and who have any of the following symptoms should seek medical attention as soon as possible:

- Swelling, hardening, and tightening of the skin
- Reddened or darkened patches on the skin
- Burning or itching of the skin
- Yellow spots on the whites of the eyes
- Stiffness in the joints, problems moving or straightening arms, hands, legs, or feet
- Pain deep in the hip bone or ribs
- Weakness of the muscles

Your doctor will monitor your health after administering MAGNEVIST, if you are considered to be at risk for developing NSF.

ADVERSE REACTIONS: General: Most adverse reactions to MAGNEVIST (gadopentetate dimeglumine) develop soon after injection; however, the possibility of delayed reactions cannot be ruled out. The most frequently reported adverse reactions following administration of MAGNEVIST were: see Table 1.

Adverse reactions occurred in 11 of 319 (3.4%) pediatric patients receiving MAGNEVIST in clinical trials (headache, vasodilatation, dizziness, diarrhea, ear pain, tachycardia, fever, edema, seizure, vomiting, nausea, and urticaria). This adverse reaction profile is consistent with the adverse reaction profile observed in adults.

MAGNEVIST will cause tissue irritation and pain if administered extravascularly.

Occupational Hazards: Transient increases or decreases in blood pressure may occur after the administration of MAGNEVIST. These changes are generally of little consequence although 3 clinically significant cases of hypotension have occurred 2 to 6 hours after MAGNEVIST injection. A relationship to the contrast medium could not be determined; however, caution should be exercised by the patient when driving or operating machinery.

Side effects in association with the use of MAGNEVIST are usually mild to moderate and transient in nature. However, serious or severe and life-threatening reactions as well as death have been reported. Postmarketing anaphylactic reactions have been reported, but are very rare. Convulsions were reported in 4 patients with a history of seizures.

Nausea, vomiting, headache, dizziness, a sensation of pain, a general feeling of warmth and injection site warmth or coldness are the most frequently recorded reactions.

Laboratory Changes: Reversible mild elevations over baseline in serum iron, transaminase and total bilirubin were observed in clinical trials. Other disturbances in laboratory values (transient increases in liver function tests) have not been associated with the use of MAGNEVIST. MAGNEVIST does not interfere with serum and plasma calcium measurements determined by colorimetric assays.

Adverse Drug Reaction Profile: The following adverse reactions, listed according to body system, have been reported after administration of MAGNEVIST:

Table 1: MAGNEVIST

Adverse Reactions

Headache	8.7%[a]
in some cases severe	1.3%
Injection Site Discomfort	6.7%
Nausea	3.2%
Localized Pain in Other Parts of the Body (back, ear, eye, teeth)	2.8%
Hypersensitivity-Type Skin and Mucosal Reactions	2.1%
Dizziness	1.5%
Vomiting	1.2%
Paresthesia	1.2%

[a] 42.3% of all cases of headache were considered unrelated to MAGNEVIST administration.

Cardiovascular: hypotension, vasodilatation, pallor, phlebitis, thrombophlebitis, non-specific ECG changes, substernal pain, angina.

Central Nervous System: headache, dizziness, agitation, paresthesia, tinnitus, visual field defect, convulsions, hyperesthesia, burning sensation.

Gastrointestinal: nausea, vomiting, gastrointestinal distress, stomach pain, thirst, increased salivation, taste abnormality, oral soft tissue pain, and paresthesia.

Respiratory System: dry mouth, throat irritation/throat tightness, pharyngolaryngeal pain/pharynx discomfort, rhinorrhea, wheezing, sneezing, laryngismus, cough, dyspnea/apnea.

Cutaneous/Mucous Membranes: rash, sweating, urticaria, pruritus.

Miscellaneous: injection site reactions (coldness, burning, warmth, pain, edema, paresthesia, swelling, irritation, hemorrhage, erythema), teeth pain, pain in extremity, generalized weakness, fever, localized edema, tiredness, anaphylactoid reactions (characterized by cardiovascular, respiratory, and cutaneous symptoms), conjunctivitis.

Laboratory Tests: transient elevation of serum iron and bilirubin levels.

The following other adverse events were reported. A causal relationship has neither been established nor refuted:

Cardiovascular: hypertension, tachycardia, syncope, death related to myocardial infarction or other undetermined causes, clinically relevant transient disturbance in heart rate, disturbance in cardiac rhythm or function and cardiac arrest, circulatory reactions accompanied by peripheral vasodilatation, dyspnea, confusion, cyanosis possibly leading to unconsciousness.

Central Nervous System: diplopia, migraine, anxiety, drowsiness, nystagmus, stupor, confusion; disturbed vision, smell, hearing or speech; tremor, coma.

Gastrointestinal: constipation, diarrhea, anorexia.

Cutaneous/Mucous Membranes: rhinitis, laryngeal/pharyngeal edema, angioedema, flush reaction with vasodilatation, facial edema, erythema, epidermal necrolysis.

Respiratory: transient disturbance in respiratory rate, respiratory distress, respiratory arrest, pulmonary edema.

Renal and Urinary: urinary incontinence, urinary urgency in patients with pre-existing renal impairment, increased serum creatinine and acute renal failure.

Hepato-biliary: transitory changes of liver enzyme levels.

Miscellaneous: localised pain (back, ear, eye), lacrimation, joint pain, chest pain, vasovagal reactions, alterations in body temperature, extravasation, mild warmth, inflammation, and tissue necrosis.

Postmarket Adverse Drug Reactions: Postmarketing reports have identified the development of NSF following single and multiple administrations of GBCAs. These reports have not always identified a specific agent. Where a specific agent was identified, the most commonly reported agent was gadodiamide (Omniscan), followed by gadopentetate dimeglumine (MAGNEVIST) and gadoversetamide (OptiMARK). NSF has also developed following the sequential administration of gadodiamide with gadobenate dimeglumine (MultiHance) or gadoteridol (ProHance). Cases of nephrogenic systemic fibrosis (NSF) have been reported with MAGNEVIST. The number of postmarketing reports is subject to change over time and may not reflect the true proportion of cases associated with any specific GBCA. The extent of risk for NSF following exposure to any specific GBCA is unknown and may vary among the agents. Published reports are limited and predominantly estimate NSF risks with gadodiamide. In 1 retrospective study of 370 patients with severe renal insufficiency who received gadodiamide, the estimated risk for development of NSF was 4%. The risk, if any, for the development of NSF among patients with mild to moderate renal insufficiency or normal renal function is unknown, and the cautious utilization of the lowest possible dose of GBCA is preferable. (See also Warnings, Serious Warnings and Precautions; Warnings, Renal Impairment; Precautions, General; and Precautions, Skin).

In patients with dialysis-dependent renal failure who received MAGNEVIST, delayed and transient inflammatory-like reactions such as fever, chills, and C-reactive protein increase have been commonly observed. These patients had the MRI examination with MAGNEVIST on the day before hemodialysis.

Additional adverse drug reactions from postapproval (spontaneous reporting) data: shock, bronchospasm, laryngospasm, anaphylactoid shock, injection site necrosis, injection site thrombophlebitis, injection site phlebitis, injection site inflammation.

OVERDOSE:

Treatment: In the event of inadvertent overdosage or in the case of severely impaired renal function, MAGNEVIST (gadopentetate dimeglumine) can be removed from the body by extracorporeal hemodialysis. Renal function should be monitored in patients with renal impairment.

> For management of a suspected drug overdose, CPhA recommends that you contact your **regional Poison Control Centre**. See the *CPS* Directory section for a list of Poison Control Centres.

DOSAGE: Special preparation of the patient for examination with MAGNEVIST (gadopentetate dimeglumine) is not required; however, precautionary measures should be taken with patients predisposed to seizure, eg, close monitoring and availability of injectable anticonvulsants (see Precautions). The usual safety rules for MRI (eg, exclusion of ferromagnetic vascular clips) must be observed.

Young children, infants, and neonates may require sedation prior to undergoing an MRI examination, in order to eliminate movement artifacts.

Use the lowest possible dose and evaluate renal function in patients with renal insufficiency. MAGNEVIST should only be used after careful risk/benefit assessment, including consideration of possible alternative imaging methods, in these patients (see Warnings).

The following dosage guidelines apply to adults and children (including neonates and infants):

Recommended Dose: 0.2 mL/kg (0.1 mmol/kg).

Route of Administration: intravenous (into a large vein, if possible).

Rate of Administration: 10 mL/min or as a bolus injection at 10 mL/15 sec.

Maximum Single Dose per Injection: 0.2 mL/kg body weight, to a maximum of 20 mL.

To ensure complete injection of the contrast medium, the injection should be followed by a 5 mL normal saline flush.

If strong clinical suspicion of an intracranial or intraspinal lesion persists, despite a normal MRI scan, the diagnostic yield of the examination may be increased by giving another injection of MAGNEVIST equivalent to the original total dose within 30 minutes and performing MRI again.

MAGNEVIST should not be drawn into the syringe until immediately before use. The rubber stopper should never be pierced more than once. Any unused portion must be discarded upon completion of the procedure.

In the absence of compatibility studies, this medicinal product must not be mixed with other medicinal products.

T_1-weighted scanning sequences are particularly suitable for contrast-enhanced examinations.

MAGNEVIST has been shown to be effective in a wide range of field strengths (0.14 to 1.5 Tesla).

Important Note: The imaging procedure should be completed within **one hour**. Optimal contrast is generally observed in cranial investigations within 27 minutes following injection of MAGNEVIST and in spinal investigations during the early postadministration phase (10-30 minutes).

In neonates and infants, optimal CNS contrast has been observed to persist for several hours after MAGNEVIST administration. (See Precautions, Pediatrics.)

SUPPLIED: Each mL of sterile, clear colorless to slightly yellow aqueous i.v. injection solution, contains: gadopentetic acid dimeglumine salt 469.01 mg (equivalent to 0.5 mmol/mL). Nonmedicinal ingredients: diethylenetriamine pentaacetic acid and meglumine. Osmolality: 1960 mOsm/kg H_2O at 37°C. Single dose vials of 10, 15 and 20 mL packaged in individual cartons. Store at 15 to 30°C and protect from light.

Malarone® ℞
atovaquone—proguanil HCl
Antimalarial

GlaxoSmithKline

Malarone® Pediatric ℞
atovaquone—proguanil HCl
Antimalarial

GlaxoSmithKline

Date of Revision: November 27, 2008

PHARMACOLOGY: The constituents of MALARONE (a fixed combination product with each tablet containing atovaquone and proguanil hydrochloride), interfere with two different pathways involved in the biosynthesis of pyrimidines required for nucleic acid replication. The mechanism of action of atovaquone against *P. falciparum* is via inhibition of mitochondrial electron transport, at the level of the cytochrome bc_1 complex, and collapse of mitochondrial membrane potential. One mechanism of action of proguanil, via its metabolite cycloguanil, is inhibition of dihydrofolate reductase, which disrupts deoxythymidylate synthesis. Proguanil also has antimalarial activity independent of its metabolism to cycloguanil, and proguanil, but not cycloguanil, is able to potentiate the ability of atovaquone to collapse mitochondrial membrane potential in malaria parasites. This latter mechanism may explain the synergy seen when atovaquone and proguanil are used in combination.

Both atovaquone and proguanil are active against the hepatic stages of *P. falciparum* and against asexual blood stage malarial parasites.

Pharmacokinetics: There are no pharmacokinetic interactions between atovaquone and proguanil at the recommended dose. A population pharmacokinetic analysis in adults and children was used to characterize the pharmacokinetics of atovaquone and proguanil. In clinical trials, trough levels of atovaquone, proguanil and cycloguanil in children (weighing 11-40 kg) are within the range observed in adults after adjusting for body weight.

Table 1 summarizes the pharmacokinetic parameters from an atovaquone-proguanil interaction study using dose levels of MALARONE Tablets utilized in the treatment of malaria.

Table 1: MALARONE

Atovaquone, Proguanil and Cycloguanil Geometric Mean Parameters and Point Estimates for MALARONE Tablets (4×250 mg Atovaquone/100 mg Proguanil HCl) versus Atovaquone Tablets (4×250 mg) Alone, and Proguanil HCl Tablets (4×100 mg) Alone in Healthy Adults Following Daily Administration for 3 Days in the Fed State

	Geometric Means			
Parameter	**Combined**	**Alone**	**Combined/Alone ratio×100 (%)**	**90% Confidence Interval (%)**
Atovaquone				
AUC_{0-24} (h·µg/mL)[a]	193	180	108	(100, 116)
$AUC_{0-\infty}$ (h·µg/mL)[b]	510	549	93	(79, 110)
C_{max} (µg/mL)	11.5	10.5	110	(102, 118)
$t_{1/2}$ (h)	59.0	57.1	103	(96, 111)
Proguanil (PG)				
AUC_{0-24} (h·µg/mL)[a]	5.82	6.30	92	(86, 99)
$AUC_{0-\infty}$ (h·µg/mL)[b]	6.00	6.44	93	(84, 103)
C_{max} (µg/mL)	0.509	0.548	93	(87, 99)
$t_{1/2}$ (h)	14.5	13.7	106	(100, 113)
Cycloguanil (CG)				
AUC_{0-24} (h·µg/mL)[a]	1.19	1.30	92	(86, 98)
$AUC_{0-\infty}$ (h·µg/mL)[b]	1.20	1.36	89	(79, 99)
C_{max} (µg/mL)	0.0792	0.0821	97	(92, 101)
$t_{1/2}$ (h)	11.8	11.1	106	(93, 120)
AUC_{CG}/AUC_{PG}[c]	0.21	0.22	94	(86, 103)

[a] AUC_{0-24}: Trapezoidal area under plasma curve from last dose until 24h postdose.
[b] $AUC_{0-\infty}$: Trapezoidal area under plasma curve from last dose until final measured concentration, extrapolated from last concentration to infinity, corrected for concentration predose. At true steady-state, this is equivalent to $AUC_{0-\infty}$ for a single dose.
[c] Ratio of $AUC_{0-\infty}$ for cycloguanil to proguanil.

Absorption: Atovaquone is a highly lipophilic compound with low aqueous solubility. The pharmacokinetics of atovaquone are comparable between healthy subjects and HIV-infected patients. Although there are no absolute bioavailability data for atovaquone in healthy subjects, in HIV-infected patients the absolute bioavailability of a 750 mg single dose of atovaquone tablets taken with food is 21% (90% CI: 17-27%). Dietary fat taken with atovaquone increases the rate and extent of absorption. When taken with a standard breakfast containing 23 g of fat, AUC was increased 2-3 times and C_{max} 5 times compared to the fasting state. Patients should take MALARONE with food or a milky drink (see Dosage).

Proguanil HCl is rapidly and extensively absorbed regardless of food intake.

Distribution: The apparent volume of distribution of atovaquone and proguanil is a function of body weight. Atovaquone is highly protein bound (>99%) but does not displace other highly protein bound drugs in vitro, indicating that significant drug interactions arising from displacement are unlikely. The volume of distribution of atovaquone following oral administration in both adults and children is approximately 8.8 L/kg. Proguanil is 75% protein bound. The volume of distribution of proguanil following oral administration is 42 to 27 L/kg in adults (weighing 41-80 kg) and 42 to 20 L/kg in children (weighing 11-40 kg). In human plasma the binding of atovaquone and proguanil were unaffected by the presence of the other.

Metabolism: There is no evidence that atovaquone is metabolised and there is negligible excretion of atovaquone in urine with the parent drug being predominantly (>90%) eliminated unchanged in feces.

Proguanil HCl is partially metabolised with less than 40% being excreted unchanged in the urine. Proguanil is metabolized to cycloguanil (primarily via CYP2C19) and 4-chlorophenylbiguanide, and these are also excreted unchanged in the urine.

Elimination: The oral clearance of atovaquone and proguanil is a function of body weight. The elimination half-life of atovaquone is about 2-3 days in adults and 1-2 days in children 6 to 12 years of age. The elimination half-lives of proguanil and cycloguanil are about 12-15 hours in both adults and children 6 to 12 years of age. Following oral administration, the clearance of atovaquone in adults and children (weighing 41-80 kg) is approximately 0.16 to 0.05 L/h/kg. In children (weighing 11-40 kg), the clearance is approximately 0.21 to 0.06 L/h/kg. Following oral administration, the clearance of proguanil in adults (weighing 41-80 kg) is 1.6 to 0.85 L/h/kg. In children (weighing 11-40 kg), the oral clearance is approximately 2.2 to 1.0 L/h/kg.

Special Populations: Renal Impairment: There are no studies in children with renal impairment. The effect of renal impairment was evaluated after single-dose oral administration of MALARONE in adults. In patients with mild to moderate renal impairment, oral clearance and/or AUC data for atovaquone, proguanil, and cycloguanil are within the range of values observed in patients with normal renal function. In patients with severe renal impairment (creatinine clearance <30 mL/min), atovaquone C_{max} and AUC are reduced, while the elimination half-lives for proguanil and cycloguanil are prolonged, with corresponding increases in AUC, resulting in the potential for drug accumulation with repeated dosing (see Contraindications and Precautions, Renal Impairment).

Hepatic Impairment: There are no studies in children with hepatic impairment. In a single-dose study, the pharmacokinetics of atovaquone, proguanil, and cycloguanil were compared in 13 adult patients with hepatic impairment (9 mild, 4 moderate, as indicated by the Child-Pugh method) with 13 adult subjects with normal hepatic function. In patients with mild or moderate hepatic impairment there were no marked differences in the rate or extent of systemic exposure to atovaquone (based on C_{max}, T_{max}, and AUC values). There was also no marked difference in the elimination half-life of atovaquone in these patients. There were no marked changes in the C_{max}, T_{max}, and elimination half-life of proguanil in patients with mild or moderate hepatic impairment. However, there was a marked increase (85%) in proguanil AUC in these patients, which is not considered to be clinically relevant due to proguanil's wide therapeutic range. Consistent with the increase in proguanil AUC, there were marked decreases in the systemic exposure to cycloguanil (C_{max} and AUC). This was particularly evident in patients with moderate hepatic impairment, where few measurable cycloguanil concentrations were seen. The decrease in the systemic exposure to cycloguanil is unlikely to be clinically relevant based on evidence from in vitro and clinical data (in more than 100 patients), which indicate that phenotypic status of proguanil metabolism (i.e., low exposure to cycloguanil in poor metabolizers) does not influence the efficacy of MALARONE (see Precautions, Hepatic Impairment).

The pharmacokinetics of MALARONE have not been studied in patients with severe hepatic impairment.

Geriatrics: A single oral dose pharmacokinetic study indicates that no dosage adjustments are needed in the healthy elderly. There is no clinically significant change in the average rate or extent of absorption of atovaquone or proguanil between healthy elderly and young patients. Systemic availability of cycloguanil is higher in the elderly compared to young subjects, but there is no clinically significant change in its elimination half-life. However, since geriatric patients may have reduced renal function, caution should be taken when treating geriatric patients with MALARONE (see Precautions, Geriatrics and Renal Impairment, and Pharmacology, Special Populations, Renal Impairment).

Pediatrics: The pharmacokinetics of atovaquone, proguanil, and cycloguanil were characterized following the daily oral administration of separate tablets of atovaquone and proguanil hydrochloride for 3 consecutive days. The dose was based on body weight. The pharmacokinetics of proguanil and cycloguanil were found to be similar in adult and pediatric patients. However, the elimination half-life of atovaquone was shorter in pediatric patients (1 to 2 days) than in adult patients (2 to 3 days), resulting in a lower C_{max} and AUC in children (i.e., lower systemic exposure to atovaquone in children than in adults). Clinical cure rates, however, were not affected.

Clinical Studies: The prophylaxis indication for adults weighing above 40 kg is based on 3 placebo-controlled studies of 10 to 12 weeks duration conducted in endemic areas with over 700 subjects and 2 active-controlled studies in non-immune travellers which enrolled more than 2000 non-immune travellers to a malaria-endemic country.

The prophylaxis indication for children weighing between 11 and 40 kg is based on 2 placebo-controlled studies of 12 weeks duration conducted in endemic areas with over 500 subjects aged 4 to 15 years, and 2 active-controlled studies in more than 180 non-immune travellers aged 2 to 14 years who visited a malaria-endemic country.

The treatment indication is based on 5 controlled clinical studies conducted in 466 patients (adults and children) receiving concurrent atovaquone and proguanil hydrochloride at the recommended dose (see Dosage). Most of the patients were residents of malaria-endemic areas and may have had previous malaria infections that could have conferred a degree of immunity.

INDICATIONS: Prevention of Malaria: MALARONE (atovaquone and proguanil hydrochloride) is indicated for the prophylaxis of *P. falciparum* malaria including areas where chloroquine resistance has been reported.

Treatment of Malaria: MALARONE (atovaquone and proguanil hydrochloride) is indicated for the treatment of acute, uncomplicated *P. falciparum* malaria when oral treatment is appropriate.

MALARONE has been shown to be effective in areas where *P. falciparum* may be resistant to some other antimalarials.

CONTRAINDICATIONS: MALARONE (atovaquone and proguanil hydrochloride) is contraindicated in individuals with known hypersensitivity to atovaquone or proguanil hydrochloride or any component of the formulation (see Supplied).

MALARONE is contraindicated for **prophylaxis** of *P. falciparum* malaria in patients with severe renal impairment (creatinine clearance <30 mL/min). In patients with severe renal impairment, an alternative to MALARONE should be recommended for **treatment** of *P. falciparum* malaria whenever possible (see Pharmacology, Special Populations, Renal Impairment and Precautions, Renal Impairment).

WARNINGS: Serious hypersensitivity reactions, including angioedema and anaphylaxis, have been reported rarely following the use of MALARONE (atovaquone and proguanil hydrochloride) for treatment and prophylaxis of malaria. These reactions may occur after the administration of the first dose. In this event, MALARONE should be discontinued immediately and supportive medical treatment should be sought.

MALARONE has not been evaluated for the treatment of cerebral malaria or other severe manifestations of complicated malaria including hyperparasitemia, pulmonary oedema or renal failure. Patients with severe malaria are not candidates for oral therapy.

In the event of recrudescent infections due to *P. falciparum*, or failure of chemoprophylaxis, patients should be treated with a different antimalarial.

Absorption of atovaquone may be reduced in patients with diarrhoea or vomiting, but diarrhoea or vomiting was not associated with reduced efficacy in clinical trials of MALARONE for malaria prophylaxis. Persons taking MALARONE for prophylaxis or treatment of malaria should take a repeat dose if they vomit within 1 hour of dosing. In the event of diarrhoea, normal dosing should be continued. As with other antimalarial agents, patients with diarrhoea or vomiting should be reminded to continue to comply with personal protection measures (repellants, bednets).

In patients with acute malaria who present with diarrhoea or vomiting, alternative therapy should be considered. If MALARONE is used to treat malaria in these patients, parasitemia should be closely monitored.

Parasitemia should be closely monitored in patients receiving concurrent tetracycline or metoclopramide (see Precautions, Drug Interactions).

The concomitant administration of MALARONE and rifampin or rifabutin is not recommended (see Precautions, Drug Interactions).

PRECAUTIONS: General: Patients who have a history of epilepsy or psychiatric illness should take MALARONE (atovaquone and proguanil hydrochloride) with caution. During clinical trials, one adult and one child receiving atovaquone/proguanil hydrochloride for the treatment of malaria had seizures; the child successfully continued treatment. Both subjects had a prior history of seizures and the investigators did not consider the events to be exacerbated by treatment with MALARONE. Two adult subjects receiving atovaquone monotherapy experienced psychiatric symptoms. One subject had a history of psychiatric illness and the other a history of drug and alcohol abuse (see Adverse Effects).

Absorption of orally administered atovaquone is significantly reduced when fasting. Therefore alternative therapy with other agents should be considered for patients who are not able to consume food (see Pharmacology, Pharmacokinetics, Absorption).

Parasite relapse occurred commonly when *P. vivax* malaria was treated with MALARONE alone. Travellers with intense exposure to *P. vivax* or *P. ovale*, and those who develop malaria caused by either of these parasites, will require additional treatment with a drug such as primaquine that is active against hypnozoites.

Geriatrics: A single dose pharmacokinetic study indicates that no dosage adjustments are needed in the healthy elderly (see Pharmacology, Special Populations, Geriatrics).

Pregnancy: There are no studies in pregnant women. The safety of atovaquone and proguanil hydrochloride when administered concurrently for use in human pregnancy has not been established. MALARONE should be considered for use in pregnancy only if the expected benefit to the mother justifies the potential risk to the foetus.

Reproductive toxicity studies in animals did not indicate any teratogenic potential at dosages of atovaquone:proguanil hydrochloride of up to 50:20 mg/kg/day in the rat or 100:40 mg/kg/day in the rabbit. In rabbits given atovaquone alone at doses up to 1200 mg/kg/day, an increased incidence of resorptions and decrease in length and weight of fetuses was noted. These effects were likely to be secondary to toxicity of atovaquone in maternal animals. However, animal studies are not always predictive of human response.

The proguanil component of MALARONE acts by inhibiting parasitic dihydrofolate reductase. There are no clinical data indicating that folate supplementation diminishes drug efficacy. For women of childbearing age receiving folate supplements to prevent neural tube birth defects, such supplements may be continued while taking MALARONE.

Lactation: It is not recommended that mothers receiving MALARONE breast-feed their babies. It is not known whether atovaquone is excreted in human milk. Proguanil is excreted in human milk in small quantities. In a rat study, the atovaquone concentrations in milk were 30% of the concurrent atovaquone concentrations in maternal plasma.

The amount of atovaquone or proguanil found in human breast milk would not provide adequate treatment for the infant against malaria.

Children: Treatment of Malaria: MALARONE is not recommended for treatment of acute, uncomplicated *P. falciparum* malaria in children under 3 years of age or who weigh less than 11 kg as safety and effectiveness has not been shown in this group of patients.

Prophylaxis of Malaria: Safety and effectiveness of MALARONE for the prophylaxis of malaria have not been established in children who weigh less than 11 kg (see Pharmacology, Clinical Studies).

Renal Impairment: There are no studies in children with renal impairment (see Pharmacology, Special Populations, Renal Impairment).

A single-dose pharmacokinetic study in adults indicates that no special precautions or dosage adjustments are needed in patients with mild to moderate renal impairment.

MALARONE is not recommended in patients with severe renal impairment (see Pharmacology, Special Populations, Renal Impairment and Contraindications).

Hepatic Impairment: There are no studies in children with hepatic impairment (see Pharmacology, Special Populations, Hepatic Impairment).

A single dose pharmacokinetic study in adults indicates that no dosage adjustments are needed in patients with mild to moderate hepatic impairment. No studies have been conducted in patients with severe hepatic impairment (see Pharmacology, Special Populations, Hepatic Impairment).

Drug Interactions: General: Atovaquone is highly protein bound (>99%) but does not displace other highly protein bound drugs in vitro, indicating that significant drug interactions arising from displacement are unlikely. Proguanil is metabolized primarily by CYP2C19. Potential pharmacokinetic interactions with other substrates or inhibitors of this pathway are unknown.

Use with Anticoagulants: Proguanil may potentiate the anticoagulant effect of warfarin and other coumarin based anticoagulants. The mechanism of this potential drug interaction has not been established. Caution is advised when initiating or withdrawing malaria prophylaxis or treatment with atovaquone-proguanil in patients on continuous treatment with coumarin based anticoagulants.

Use with Rifampin, Rifabutin, Tetracycline or Metoclopramide: Parasitemia should be closely monitored in patients receiving tetracycline or metoclopramide concurrently with MALARONE.

The concomitant administration of MALARONE and rifampin or rifabutin is not recommended.

Concomitant treatment with tetracycline, metoclopramide, rifabutin and rifampicin has been associated with significant decreases in plasma concentrations of atovaquone. Increased clearance of atovaquone when coadministered with tetracycline, leading to 40% lower atovaquone concentrations, has been observed. Concomitant administration of rifampicin or rifabutin is known to reduce atovaquone levels by approximately 50% and 34% respectively.

Use with Indinavir: Concomitant administration of atovaquone and indinavir results in a decrease in the C_{min} of indinavir (23% decrease; 90% CI 8-35%). Caution should be exercised when prescribing atovaquone with indinavir due to the decrease in trough levels of indinavir.

Use with Other Antimalarial Agents: MALARONE should not be administered in combination with other antimalarial drugs. Interactions between MALARONE and other antimalarial drugs have not been studied.

ADVERSE EFFECTS: As MALARONE contains atovaquone and proguanil hydrochloride, the type and severity of adverse reactions associated with each of the compounds may be expected. At the doses employed for the treatment and prophylaxis of malaria, adverse reactions have generally been mild and of limited duration. There has been no evidence of increased toxicity following concurrent administration of the two compounds.

A summary of adverse events associated with the use of MALARONE, atovaquone, or proguanil HCl is provided below.

Blood and Lymphatic: anemia, neutropenia. Pancytopenia in patients with severe renal impairment.

Endocrine and Metabolic: anorexia, hyponatremia.

Gastrointestinal: abdominal pain, nausea, vomiting, diarrhea, gastric intolerance, oral ulceration, stomatitis.

Hepatobiliary Tract and Pancreas: elevated liver enzyme levels and reports of hepatitis, cholestasis, elevated amylase levels. Clinical trial data for MALARONE indicated that abnormalities in liver function tests (elevated bilirubin and transaminases) were reversible and not associated with untoward clinical events.

Immune System/Hypersensitivity: allergic reactions: including rash, urticaria, pruritus, angioedema, isolated reports of anaphylaxis, and vasculitis.

Lower Respiratory: cough.

Neurology: headache, insomnia, dizziness, asthenia.

Non-site Specific: fever.

Skin: rash, hair loss.

Other events seen in clinical trials with MALARONE include:

Body as a Whole: back pain, lethargy.

Cardiovascular: hypotension, palpitations.

Erythropoietic: splenomegaly.

Gastrointestinal: hepatomegaly, constipation, dyspepsia.

Musculoskeletal: myalgia.

Neurology: strange or vivid dreams, visual difficulties, depression, anxiety.

Of the seven severe or treatment-limiting adverse experiences reported in clinical trials with atovaquone and proguanil hydrochloride, three were considered to be treatment related; two were reports of nausea and/or vomiting and one, a report of an anaphylactic reaction (see Warnings). Two subjects, one adult and one 4-year-old child, receiving atovaquone/proguanil hydrochloride for the treatment of malaria had seizures; the child successfully continued treatment. Both subjects had a prior history of seizures and the investigators did not consider the events to be exacerbated by treatment with MALARONE. During clinical trials, two adult subjects receiving atovaquone monotherapy experienced psychiatric symptoms. One subject had a history of psychiatric illness and the other a history of drug and alcohol abuse. Studies of this size and design would only be able to detect adverse events at a rate of 1:150 (95% CI).

Treatment: Table 2 provides a summary of the adverse events considered by investigators to be attributable to study medication and reported in clinical trials for the treatment of malaria with MALARONE Tablets. Abdominal pain, headache, anorexia, nausea, vomiting, diarrhoea, asthenia and abnormal liver function tests were the most commonly reported adverse experiences.

Table 2: MALARONE

Adverse Events Considered by Investigators to be Attributable to Study Medication, Occurring in ≥1% of Adults with Malaria in Completed Phase III Treatment Studies

Adverse Event	MALARONE (n=304)	PYR+S (n=81)	MFQ (n=91)	ADQ (n=71)	C±PYR+S[a] (n=55)
Gastrointestinal					
Abdominal Pain	15% (45)	21% (17)	0%	8% (6)	0%
Vomiting	12% (35)	15% (12)	0%	25% (18)	2% (1)
Nausea	11% (32)	14% (11)	2% (2)	21% (15)	2% (1)
Diarrhoea	8% (25)	11% (9)	0%	7% (5)	2% (1)
Anorexia	5% (15)	5% (4)	1% (1)	13% (9)	2% (1)
Hepatomegaly	2% (6)	6% (5)	0%	0%	0%
Constipation	1% (2)	0%	0%	0%	0%
Dyspepsia	1% (2)	0%	0%	0%	0%
Nervous/Psychiatric					
Headache	8% (25)	31% (25)	1% (1)	7% (5)	0%
Dizziness	3% (8)	11% (9)	0%	11% (8)	2% (1)
Insomnia	1% (3)	4% (3)	0%	25% (18)	0%
Body as a Whole					
Asthenia	7% (20)	16% (13)	0%	3% (2)	0%
Back Pain	1% (2)	4% (3)	0%	0%	0%
Abnormal Liver Function Tests					
ALT	6% (18)	6% (5)	7% (6)	0%	0%
AST	5% (16)	5% (4)	7% (6)	0%	0%
Bilirubin	2% (7)	0%	1% (1)	0%	0%
Cardiovascular					
Hypotension, postural	2% (6)	17% (14)	0%	0%	0%
Palpitations	2% (5)	0%	0%	6% (4)	0%
Cutaneous					
Pruritus	2% (6)	2% (2)	0%	46% (33)	0%
Rash	1% (2)	0%	0%	0%	0%
Musculoskeletal					
Myalgia	3% (8)	6% (5)	0%	4% (3)	0%
Erythropoietic					
Splenomegaly	1% (4)	2% (2)	0%	0%	0%
Respiratory					
Coughing	1% (3)	0%	0%	2% (2)	0%

[a] Data for both comparator groups of chloroquine alone plus pyrimethamine and sulfadoxine.

Legend: PYR=pyrimethamine; S=sulfadoxine; MFQ=mefloquine; ADQ=amodiaquine; C=chloroquine.

A similar profile of clinical adverse events was reported in children with malaria treated with atovaquone and proguanil hydrochloride in phase III trials as occurred in the adult studies.

Prophylaxis: In clinical trials of MALARONE for **prophylaxis** of malaria in adults weighing above 40 kg, the most commonly reported adverse events, independent of attributability, were headache, abdominal pain and diarrhoea, and were reported in a similar proportion of subjects receiving MALARONE Tablets or placebo.

In clinical trials of MALARONE for **prophylaxis** of malaria in children weighing between 11 and 40 kg, residents of malaria-endemic areas, the most commonly reported adverse events, regardless of drug relationship, were abdominal pain, headache, cough, vomiting and fever. Abdominal pain was reported more commonly in the children receiving MALARONE PEDIATRIC Tablets than in the placebo group (21% versus 16%, respectively), whereas fever was reported more commonly in the placebo group than in the group receiving MALARONE PEDIATRIC Tablets (11% versus 5%, respectively). The reported incidence of other events was identical or similar between the two groups.

Table 3 provides a summary of the most common drug-related adverse events reported in clinical trials of MALARONE Tablets for the prophylaxis of malaria in non-immune travellers weighing above 40 kg.

In clinical trials of MALARONE for **prophylaxis** of malaria in travellers to endemic areas, the most commonly (≥5%) reported adverse events, regardless of drug relationship, in children weighing between 11 and 40 kg receiving MALARONE PEDIATRIC Tablets or chloroquine+proguanil were diarrhoea, fever, abdominal pain, nausea, vomiting and headache. Each of these events was reported in a similar or lower percentage of subjects who received MALARONE PEDIATRIC Tablets than who received chloroquine+proguanil.

Table 4 provides a summary of the most common drug-related adverse events reported in clinical trials of MALARONE PEDIATRIC Tablets for the prophylaxis of malaria in non-immune travellers weighing between 11 and 40 kg.

Over a similar duration of exposure, the reported incidence of drug-related adverse events was similar between groups (10% for those receiving MALARONE PEDIATRIC Tablets compared to 9% for those receiving chloroquine+proguanil). During the treatment period, the reported incidence was higher in subjects receiving chloroquine+proguanil than those receiving MALARONE PEDIATRIC Tablets (16% versus 11%, respectively).

Post-Marketing Adverse Reactions: In addition to adverse events reported from clinical trials, the following events have been identified during worldwide post-approval use of MALARONE. Because they are reported voluntarily from a population of unknown size, estimates of frequency cannot be made. These events have been chosen for inclusion due to a combination of their seriousness, frequency of reporting, or potential causal connection to MALARONE.

Skin: cutaneous reactions ranging from rash, photosensitivity, and urticaria to cases of erythema multiforme and Stevens-Johnson syndrome.

Central Nervous System: Cases of seizures and psychotic events (such as hallucinations); however, a causal relationship has not been established.

Hypersensitivity: allergic reactions: including rash, urticaria, pruritus, angioedema and isolated reports of anaphylaxis (see Warnings).

Hepatobiliary Tract and Pancreas: elevated liver enzyme levels and reports of hepatitis, elevated amylase levels.

Table 3: MALARONE

Common Drug-related, Treatment-emergent Adverse Events (≥5%) in Nonimmune Travellers Weighing Above 40 kg (MALARONE Tablets vs Mefloquine and MALARONE Tablets vs Chloroquine/Proguanil)

	MALARONE[a] (n=993)		Mefloquine[b] (n=471)		Chloroquine[c]/ proguanil[d] (n=511)	
Adverse Event	**Active[e] n (%)**	**All[f] n (%)**	**Active[e] n (%)**	**All[f] n (%)**	**Active[e] n (%)**	**All[f] n (%)**
Any Adverse Event	256 (26)	336 (34)	204 (43)	205 (44)	142 (28)	142 (28)
Digestive System	135 (14)	173 (17)	94 (20)	96 (20)	100 (20)	100 (20)
Neuro-psychiatric[g]	117 (12)	165 (17)	139 (30)	139 (30)	53 (10)	54 (11)
Body as a Whole	55 (6)	84 (8)	58 (12)	58 (12)	34 (7)	34 (7)
Skin and Appendages	32 (3)	39 (4)	23 (5)	23 (5)	14 (3)	14 (3)

[a] 1 to 2 days before travel until 7 days after travel.
[b] Weekly from 1 to 3 weeks before travel until 4 weeks after travel.
[c] 1 week before until 4 weeks after travel.
[d] 1 to 2 days before travel until 4 weeks after travel.
[e] Active—includes adverse events that occurred while the active study drug was being administered.
[f] All—includes adverse events that occurred while any study drug (active or placebo) was being administered.
[g] Neuro-psychiatric adverse events include strange or vivid dreams, dizziness, insomnia, visual difficulties, psychiatric depression and anxiety.

OVERDOSE:

Symptoms: There is limited information regarding overdosage from the administration of MALARONE (atovaquone and proguanil hydrochloride). In cases of suspected overdosage symptomatic and supportive therapy should be given as appropriate.

There is no known antidote for atovaquone, and it is currently unknown if atovaquone is dialyzable. The median lethal dose is higher than the maximum oral dose tested in mice and rats (1825 mg/kg/day). Overdoses up to 31 500 mg of atovaquone have been reported. In one such patient who also took an unspecified dose of dapsone, methemoglobinemia occurred. Rash has also been reported after overdose.

Overdoses of proguanil hydrochloride as large as 1500 mg have been followed by complete recovery, and doses as high as 700 mg twice daily have been taken for over 2 weeks without serious toxicity. Adverse events occasionally associated with proguanil hydrochloride doses of 100 to 200 mg/day, such as epigastric discomfort and vomiting, would be likely to occur with overdose. There are also reports of reversible hair loss and scaling of the skin on the palms and/or soles, reversible aphthous ulceration, and hematologic side effects.

Treatment: See Symptoms.

For management of a suspected drug overdose, contact your **regional Poison Control Centre**. See the *CPS* Directory section for a list of Poison Control Centres.

DOSAGE: Each MALARONE (atovaquone and proguanil hydrochloride) Tablet contains 250 mg of atovaquone and 100 mg proguanil hydrochloride.

Each MALARONE PEDIATRIC (atovaquone and proguanil hydrochloride) Tablet contains 62.5 mg atovaquone and 25 mg proguanil hydrochloride.

The daily dose should be taken with food or a milky drink (to ensure maximum absorption) at the same time each day (see Precautions, General). In the event of vomiting within 1 hour of dosing a repeat dose should be taken. Should vomiting continue, alternative therapy should be considered or the patient's parasitemia should be monitored.

MALARONE Tablets (adult strength) and MALARONE PEDIATRIC Tablets should preferably be swallowed whole. Either tablet may be crushed and mixed with condensed milk just prior to administration for children who may have difficulty swallowing tablets.

Prophylaxis: Prophylaxis with MALARONE should start 1 to 2 days before entering a malaria endemic area and any other non-endemic area where prophylaxis for malaria is recommended by international travel Health Authorities (such as PHAC, CDC, WHO, etc.). Prophylaxis should be continued daily throughout the stay and for 7 additional days after leaving the area of concern.

Dosage in Adults: One MALARONE Tablet (adult strength=250 mg atovaquone and 100 mg proguanil hydrochloride) daily.

Dosage in Children (see Precautions, Children and Pharmacology, Special Populations, Children): The dosage for prevention of malaria in children is based upon body weight.

11–20 kg body weight	One MALARONE PEDIATRIC Tablet daily
21–30 kg body weight	Two MALARONE PEDIATRIC Tablets as a single dose daily
31–40 kg body weight	Three MALARONE PEDIATRIC Tablets as a single dose daily
>40 kg body weight	One MALARONE Tablet (adult strength) daily

MALARONE is not recommended for malaria prophylaxis in children weighing less than 11 kg.

Treatment: Dosage in Adults: Four MALARONE Tablets (adult strength) as a single dose for three consecutive days.

Dosage in Children (see Precautions, Children and Pharmacology, Special Populations, Children): The dosage for treatment of acute malaria in children is based upon body weight:

11–20 kg body weight	One MALARONE Tablet (adult strength) daily for three consecutive days
21–30 kg body weight	Two MALARONE Tablets (adult strength) as a single dose for three consecutive days
31–40 kg body weight	Three MALARONE Tablets (adult strength) as a single dose for three consecutive days
>40 kg body weight	Dose as for adults

Special Populations: Patients with Renal Impairment: There are no studies in children with renal impairment. However, pharmacokinetic studies in adults indicate that no dosage adjustments are needed in patients with mild to moderate renal impairment. MALARONE should not be used for malaria **prophylaxis** in patients with severe renal impairment (creatinine clearance <30 mL/min), and alternatives to MALARONE should be recommended for **treatment** of acute *P. falciparum* malaria whenever possible (see Contraindications, Precautions, Renal Impairment, and Pharmacology, Special Populations).

Patients with Hepatic Impairment: There are no studies in children with hepatic impairment. However, a pharmacokinetic study in adults indicates that no dosage adjustments are needed in patients with mild to moderate hepatic impairment. No studies have been conducted in patients with severe hepatic impairment (see Precautions, Hepatic Impairment and Pharmacology, Special Populations).

INFORMATION FOR THE PATIENT: Published in e-CPS, available by subscription at www.e-cps.ca.

SUPPLIED: MALARONE: Each pink, round, biconvex film-coated tablet, branded GX CM3, contains: atovaquone 250 mg and proguanil HCl 100 mg (equivalent to proguanil base 87.4 mg). Nonmedicinal ingredients: low-substituted hydroxypropyl cellulose, magnesium stearate, microcrystalline cellulose, poloxamer 188, povidone K30 and sodium starch glycollate; coating: hypromellose, macrogol 400, polyethylene glycol 8000, red iron oxide and titanium dioxide. Blister packs of 12. Store between 15 and 30°C.

MALARONE PEDIATRIC: Each pink, round, biconvex, film-coated tablet, branded GX CG7, contains: atovaquone 62.5 mg and proguanil HCl 25 mg (equivalent to proguanil base 21.86 mg). Nonmedicinal ingredients: low-substituted hydroxypropyl cellulose, magnesium stearate, microcrystalline cellulose, poloxamer 188, povidone K30 and sodium starch glycollate; coating: hypromellose, macrogol 400, polyethylene glycol 8000, red iron oxide and titanium dioxide. Blister packs of 12. Store between 15 and 30°C. MALARONE PEDIATRIC Tablets are smaller in size than MALARONE Tablets (adult strength).

(Shown in Product Identification Section)

Table 4: MALARONE PEDIATRIC

Most Common[a] Drug-related Adverse Events (>1 subject) in Non-immune Pediatric Travellers Weighing 11-40 kg

	11–20 kg		>20–30 kg		>30–40 kg		Total			
	MALARONE (n=18)		MALARONE (n=45)		MALARONE (n=30)		MALARONE (n=93)		chlor+prog (n=81)	
	T+7	RX	T+7	RX	T+7	RX	T+7	RX	T+7	RX
Adverse Event	n (%)		n (%)		n (%)		n (%)		n (%)	
At Least One Drug-related AE	2 (11)		3 (7)		4 (13)	5 (17)	9 (10)	10 (11)	7 (9)	13 (16)
Digestive System	2 (11)		3 (7)		2 (7)		7 (8)		6 (7)	12 (15)
Diarrhoea	2 (11)		2 (4)		0		4 (4)		2 (2)	3 (4)
Oral Ulceration	0		1 (2)		1 (3)		2 (2)		2 (2)	
Vomiting	1 (6)		0		0		1 (1)		3 (4)	5 (6)
Abdominal Pain	0		0		0		0		3 (4)	7 (9)
Nausea	0		0		0		0		2 (2)	7 (9)
Nervous System	0		1 (2)		2 (7)		3 (3)		1 (1)	
Dreams	0		1 (2)		2 (7)		3 (3)		0	
Skin and Appendages	0		0		2 (7)		2 (2)		1 (1)	
Pruritus	0		0		2 (7)		2 (2)		1 (1)	
Body as a Whole	1 (6)		0		0	2 (7)	1 (1)	3 (3)	1 (1)	
Lethargy	0		0		0	2 (7)	0	2 (2)	0	
Special Senses	0		0		0		0		2 (2)	
Visual Impairment	0		0		0		0		2 (2)	

[a] Most common was defined as reporting in more than one subject in any treatment group.

Legend: prog=proguanil; chlor=chloroquine; T+7=Travel Period+7 days (adverse events starting between start of travel and 7 days post-travel); RX=Treatment Period (MALARONE: 1-2 days before travel until 7 days after travel; Chloroquine: 1 week before travel until 4 weeks after travel; Proguanil: 1-2 days before travel until 4 weeks after travel).

Maltlevol®-12
multiple vitamins
Dietary Supplement

Church & Dwight

SUPPLIED: Each 45 mL (maximum daily dose) contains: vitamin B_{12} 14 µg, vitamin A 6000 IU, vitamin B_1 4.5 mg, riboflavin 3 mg, vitamin B_6 3 mg, niacinamide 30 mg, vitamin D 400 IU, vitamin E 25 IU, iron 33.75 mg as ferric ammonium citrate in a caramel brown, translucent, sweet base of sherry wine. Nonmedicinal ingredients: alcohol, caramel color, citric acid, flavors, methylparaben, polysorbate, propylparaben, purified water, simethicone emulsion, sodium cyclamate, sodium hydrogen phosphate, sorbitol, sucrose and tocopherol. Sodium hydroxide and hydrochloric acid to adjust pH. pH: 4.4 to 4.6. Alcohol: 16%. Energy: 32.76 kJ (7.8 kcal)/5 mL. Sodium: <1 mmol (12 mg)/15 mL. Gluten- and tartrazine-free. Bottles of 350 mL.

Manerix® Ⓟ
moclobemide
Antidepressant

Meda Valeant

Date of Preparation: October 9, 2009

PHARMACOLOGY: MANERIX (moclobemide) is a short-acting, Reversible Inhibitor of Monoamine oxidase type A (RIMA). It is a benzamide derivative which inhibits the deamination of serotonin, noradrenaline and dopamine. This action leads to increased concentrations of these neurotransmitters, which may account for the antidepressant activity of moclobemide.

Monoamine oxidases are currently subclassified into two types, A and B, which differ in their substrate specificity. Moclobemide preferentially inhibits MAO-A; at a 300 mg dose, the inhibition of MAO-A is approximately 80%, while that of MAO-B is approximately 20-30%. The estimated MAO-A inhibition is short-lasting (maximum 24 hours) and reversible.

Pharmacokinetics: Volunteers: General: Following oral administration, MANERIX (moclobemide) is 98% absorbed from the gastrointestinal tract. Due to hepatic first pass effect, absolute bioavailability is approximately 55% after single doses, but 90% after multiple doses. The apparent volume of distribution is approximately 1.2 L/kg, indicating extensive tissue distribution.

MANERIX is extensively metabolized, largely via oxidative reactions on the morpholine moiety of the molecule. While 95% of the administered dose is excreted in the urine, less than 1% of this is in the unchanged form. Active metabolites recovered in vitro or in animal experiments are present only at very low concentrations in the systemic circulation in man. MANERIX is 50% bound to plasma proteins, mainly to albumin. The presence of food reduces the rate, but not the extent of MANERIX absorption.

Single Dose: Following the administration of a 100 mg single oral dose of MANERIX to healthy subjects, peak plasma concentrations ranged from 488 ng/mL to 1450 ng/mL (mean C_{max}: 849 ng/mL) and were reached in 0.5 to 3.5 hours (mean T_{max}: 49 min). The elimination half-life is 1.5 hours. Up to 200 mg, the pharmacokinetics of MANERIX are linear. At higher doses, non-linear pharmacokinetics are observed. In a dose range of 400 mg to 1200 mg, maximum plasma concentrations increased and clearance decreased in a non dose-proportional manner. With increasing doses, the elimination half-life also becomes prolonged.

Multiple Dose: During the second week of a 100 mg t.i.d. dosing regimen in healthy subjects, the steady-state trough concentrations of MANERIX ranged between 114 ng/mL and 517 ng/mL. An increase in the dose to 150 mg t.i.d. resulted in a greater than proportional increase in MANERIX steady-state trough concentrations, namely to concentrations ranging between 346 ng/mL and 1828 ng/mL.

Patients: Hepatic Impairment, Single Dose: In patients with liver cirrhosis, the administration of a single 100 mg dose of MANERIX resulted in approximately a three-fold increase in peak plasma concentrations (C_{max}: 1607 ng/mL), and elimination half-life ($t_{½β}$: 4.0 hr), while clearance decreased about four-fold (Cl 337 mL/min).

Renal Impairment, Single Dose: In patients with renal insufficiency, the administration of a single 100 mg dose of MANERIX did not appreciably alter the pharmacokinetics of the drug, except for an increase in absorption time.

Elderly Patients, Single and Multiple Dose: Following a 100 mg t.i.d. dosing regimen in elderly subjects (65 to 77 years old), C_{max} and AUC values were somewhat higher than in young subjects (21 to 34 years old), namely 1498 versus 950 ng/mL and 5571 versus 3102 ng·h/mL, respectively. Clearance in the elderly was reduced (19.7 versus 32.3 L/h).

Slow Metabolisers: Because MANERIX is partly metabolized by polymorphic isozymes (CYP2C19 and CYP2D6), blood levels of the drug can be affected in patients with genetically or drug-induced poor metabolism. Approximately 2% of the caucasian population and 15% of the asian population can be genetically phenotyped as slow metabolisers with respect to oxidative hepatic metabolism. It was found that the area under the curve (AUC) measurement in slow metaboliser subjects was approximately 1.5 times greater than in extensive metaboliser subjects for the same dose of MANERIX. This increase is within the normal range of variation (up to two-fold) typically seen in patients.

INDICATIONS: Adults: MANERIX (moclobemide) is indicated for the symptomatic relief of depressive illness.

Children <18 years of age: The safety and efficacy of MANERIX has not been established in the pediatric population, therefore its use is not recommended.

CONTRAINDICATIONS: MANERIX (moclobemide) is contraindicated in the following circumstances: In patients with a known hypersensitivity to MANERIX or any component of the product. As with any other exogenous compound the possibility of hypersensitivity reaction should be considered in susceptible patients. Symptoms of hypersensitivity may include rash and edema. In patients in an acute confusional state. Concomitantly with tricyclic antidepressants (see Drug Interactions, Other Antidepressants). In combination with selective serotonin reuptake inhibitors (SSRIs) or conventional monoamine oxidase (MAO) inhibitors (see Drug Interactions, Other Antidepressants). In combination with selegiline (see Drug Interactions). In combination with meperidine. Although there is limited experience with the concomitant use of MANERIX and narcotics, death has occurred in patients receiving a conventional MAO inhibitor and meperidine (pethidine) given concomitantly. Concomitantly with thioridazine (see Precautions and Drug Interactions).

WARNINGS: Potential Association with the Occurrence of Behavioural and Emotional Changes, Including Self-Harm: It is unknown whether increased risk of suicidal ideation and behaviour is associated with the use of older antidepressants (eg MANERIX) in pediatric patients and/or adults. However, recent analyses of placebo-controlled clinical trial safety databases from SSRIs and other newer antidepressants suggest that use of these drugs may be associated with behavioural and emotional changes, including an increased risk of suicidal ideation and behaviour over that of placebo. Thus, rigorous clinical monitoring for suicidal ideation or other indicators of potential for suicidal behaviour is advised in patients of all ages given any antidepressant drug. This includes monitoring for emotional and behavioural changes.

PRECAUTIONS: General: In patients with thyrotoxicosis or pheochromocytoma, conventional MAO-inhibitors may precipitate a hypertensive reaction. Because there are no data available on the use of MANERIX in such patients, caution is advised when prescribing MANERIX to these subjects.

Occupational Hazards: Patients should be cautioned against driving an automobile or performing hazardous tasks until they are certain of the effect that MANERIX has on them.

Pregnancy: Safety of use in pregnancy has not been established. Therefore, MANERIX is not recommended in women who may be pregnant, unless, in the opinion of the physician, the expected benefits to the patient markedly outweigh the possible risk to the fetus.

Lactation: Clinical data suggest that small quantities of MANERIX are excreted in human milk. Therefore, MANERIX is not recommended in nursing mothers unless the anticipated benefits outweigh the potential harm to the infant.

Hepatic Dysfunction: In patients with severe liver dysfunction, the daily dose of MANERIX should be substantially reduced to one third or one half of the standard dose (see Pharmacology, Pharmacokinetics).

Renal Dysfunction: Single dose pharmacokinetic data suggest that no dosage adjustment may be required in patients with impaired renal function (see Pharmacology, Pharmacokinetics). However, multiple dose studies with MANERIX have not been performed in patients with renal dysfunction, therefore, MANERIX should be used with caution in this patient population. In normal volunteers, the absolute bioavailability almost doubles following multiple dosing as compared to a single dose.

Dextromethorphan: Co-administration of MANERIX and dextromethorphan which may be contained in cough and cold medicines is not recommended (see Drug Interactions).

Thioridazine: A study to evaluate the potential of MANERIX to inhibit the cytochrome enzyme P4502D6 (P4502D6) concluded that MANERIX can affect the pharmakokinetics of drugs (such as thioridazine) that are mainly metabolized by P4502D6. Thioridazine administration results in a dose-dependent prolongation of the QTc interval, which may cause serious ventricular arrhythmias including torsades de pointes-type arrhythmias and sudden death. This risk is expected to increase with MANERIX-induced inhibition of thioridazine metabolism (see Contraindications and Drug Interactions).

Drug Interactions: Selegiline: Studies revealed that the combination of moclobemide and selegiline had a supra—additive effect to the tyramine sensitivity. The tyramine sensitive factor was increased with an individual variability. It was expected that the effect of oral tyramine might potentiate this effect to an even greater extent. It was therefore concluded that food containing tyramine should be omitted. Under daily conditions an absolute omission of food with tyramine is almost impossible. Based on the individual variability of the increase in sensitivity it is also not possible to recommend a specific amount which would be still well tolerated. Therefore the combination of moclobemide and selegiline is contraindicated.

Cimetidine: Cimetidine doubles the AUC (area under the plasma concentration-time curve) of MANERIX (moclobemide) and is expected to approximately double MANERIX steady-state concentrations.

In patients receiving MANERIX concomitantly with cimetidine, a 50% reduction in the dosage of MANERIX may be necessary.

Tyramine: During studies conducted at the maximum recommended MANERIX dose of 600 mg/day, the mean dose of tyramine required to produce a 30 mm Hg increase in systolic blood pressure was 148±50 mg (76-200 mg) when MANERIX was administered immediately after tyramine. The threshold dose of tyramine was reduced to 84±23 mg (54-112 mg) when the sequence of administration was reversed so that MANERIX was administered one hour before tyramine. These findings indicate that the potentiation of tyramine may be minimized by administering MANERIX after, instead of prior to, a tyramine-enriched meal. There is limited experience in patients who took MANERIX before meals. Most clinical trial protocols specified that the drug be taken immediately after meals. Therefore, patients should be instructed to take MANERIX immediately after meals.

Treatment with MANERIX does not necessitate special dietary restrictions. In clinical studies it was demonstrated that up to 100 mg tyramine can be safely ingested during treatment with MANERIX 600 mg/day when MANERIX was given after meals. This amount of tyramine, 100 mg, corresponds to 1000 g to 2000 g mild or 200 g strong cheese, or to 70 g Marmite yeast extract.

As a safety measure, patients should be urged to report immediately the abrupt occurrence of any of the following symptoms; occipital headache, palpitations, neck stiffness, tachycardia or bradycardia or other atypical or unusual symptoms not previously experienced.

Other Antidepressants: Concomitant Use: Clinical interaction studies between MANERIX and a tricyclic antidepressant (clomipramine) resulted in severe adverse reactions (see Contraindications). Data involving other tricyclic antidepressants are limited. Therefore, the concomitant use of MANERIX and tricyclic antidepressants is contraindicated.

Clinical data are not available on the concomitant use of MANERIX and selective serotonin reuptake inhibitors, or conventional monoamine oxidase inhibitors. Therefore, until clinical data become available, MANERIX should not be administered in combination with these agents.

Sequential Use: Treatment with a tricyclic antidepressant may be initiated following the discontinuation of MANERIX with a short washout period of no less than two days.

When switching patients from serotonergic antidepressants to a conventional MAO-inhibitor, it is standard practice to allow for a washout period equivalent to at least 4-5 half-lives of the previously administered drug or any active metabolites. This recommendation also applies to MANERIX.

Prozac: An exception is Prozac (fluoxetine); at least five weeks should elapse between its discontinuation and initiation of treatment with MANERIX.

Buspirone: To date, there is no experience regarding the co-administration of MANERIX and buspirone. Therefore, patients should be carefully monitored should concomitant administration be implemented.

Antipsychotics: In depressed patients with schizophrenic or schizoaffective disorder, psychotic symptoms may be exacerbated during treatment with MANERIX. There is little experience regarding the concomitant use of MANERIX and antipsychotic drugs. Therefore, patients should be carefully monitored should concomitant treatment be undertaken.

Thioridazine: A study to evaluate the potential of moclobemide to inhibit the cytochrome enzyme P4502D6 (P4502D6) concluded that moclobemide can affect the pharmakokinetics of drugs (such as thioridazine) that are mainly metabolized by P4502D6. Thioridazine administration results in a dose-dependent prolongation of the QTc interval, which may cause serious ventricular arrhythmias including torsades de pointes-type arrhythmias and sudden death. This risk is expected to increase with moclobemide-induced inhibition of thioridazine metabolism (see Contraindications).

Alcohol: Excessive alcohol consumption should be avoided. Alcohol interaction studies were performed at blood alcohol concentrations of 0.05%. However, no studies were conducted at blood alcohol concentrations recognized as legally intoxicating.

Anesthetic Agents: While specific data on the use of MANERIX in patients undergoing anesthesia are not available, based on its reversible action and short elimination half-life (see Pharmacology) MANERIX should be discontinued no less than two days before the administration of anesthetic agents, especially spinal or local anesthetic agents that contain epinephrine.

In animals, moclobemide has been shown to potentiate the effects of opiates. The combination of moclobemide and meperidine (pethidine) is not recommended (see Contraindications). Other opioid analgesics should be used with extreme caution, if at all, and a dosage adjustment may be necessary for these drugs.

Sympathomimetics: Following multiple oral doses of MANERIX (total dose: 600 mg/day), a phenylephrine-induced increase in systolic blood pressure was potentiated (1.6 times) after intravenous administration. Patients should be advised to avoid the concomitant use of sympathomimetic amines (e.g., amphetamine and ephedrine like compounds contained in many proprietary cold, hay fever or weight-reducing preparations), until further studies have been conducted.

Dextromethorphan: In isolated cases, the co-administration of MANERIX and dextromethorphan resulted in adverse events, including vertigo, tremor, nausea and vomiting. Since cough and cold medicines may contain dextromethorphan, they should not be taken without prior consultation with the physician, such that non-dextromethorphan containing alternatives may be given (see Precautions).

Antihypertensive Agents: Clinical trials with MANERIX have shown inconsistent effects on the blood pressure of hypertensive patients. Therefore, careful monitoring is recommended during initial treatment.

ADVERSE EFFECTS: Table 1 lists the adverse events reported during clinical trials in which 1922 patients were treated with 50-600 mg/day MANERIX (moclobemide) for depressive illness. Limited experience in 60 patients treated with 601 to 750 mg/day of MANERIX suggests that the incidence of adverse reactions may increase at higher doses.

Table 1: MANERIX

Clinical Adverse Events >1%

Organ System	Adverse Event	% Moclobemide (n=1922)	% Placebo (n=271)
Central Nervous System	headache, pressure in head	8.0	11.1
	insomnia, sleep disturbances	7.3	4.8
	dizziness	5.1	8.1
	tremour	5.0	3.0
	increased agitation	4.5	2.6
	restlessness, nervousness	4.1	2.6
	sleepiness, somnolence	3.7	5.5
	tiredness, sedation	3.0	4.1
	increased anxiety, acute anxiety state	2.8	2.2
	weakness or faintness	1.2	1.8

(cont'd)

Table 1: MANERIX *(cont'd)*

Clinical Adverse Events >1%

Organ System	Adverse Event	% Moclobemide (n=1922)	% Placebo (n=271)
Gastrointestinal	nausea	5.2	4.8
	constipation	3.9	3.3
	gastrointestinal pain, epigastric discomfort	2.3	2.6
	sickness	1.9	1.1
	diarrhea	1.8	1.1
	abdominal fullness, abdominal pain	1.6	1.5
	vomiting	1.6	0.4
Cardiovascular	tachycardia, palpitations	3.8	3.3
	hypotension	3.0	0.4
	orthostatic, reactive hypotension	2.3	3.3
Anticholinergic	dry mouth	9.2	10.7
Miscellaneous	sweating	2.4	2.2
	blurred vision	1.8	1.1
	increase/loss of appetite	1.3	1.8

Other clinical adverse events with an incidence of <1% in clinical studies, or reported in post-marketing surveillance, are as follows:

Psychiatric: difficulties falling asleep, nightmares/dreams, hallucinations, memory disturbances, confusion, disorientation, delusions, increased depression, excitation/irritability, hypomanic symptoms, aggressive behaviour, apathy, tension.

Cases of suicidal ideation and suicidal behaviours have been reported during antidepressant therapy or early after treatment discontinuation (see Warnings).

Central and Peripheral Nervous System: migraine, extrapyramidal effects, tinnitus, paresthesia, dysarthria.

Gastrointestinal: heartburn, gastritis, meteorism, indigestion.

Cardiovascular: hypertension, bradycardia, extrasystoles, angina/chest pain, phlebitic symptoms, flushing.

Dermatological/Mucocutaneous: exanthema/rash, allergic skin reaction, itching, gingivitis, stomatitis, dry skin, conjunctivitis, pruritus, urticaria.

Genito-Urinary: disturbances of micturition (dysuria, polyuria, tenesmus) metrorrhagia, prolonged menstruation.

Miscellaneous: general malaise, skeletal/muscular pain, altered taste sensations, hot flushes/cold sensation, photopsia, dyspnea, visual disturbances.

Laboratory Abnormalities: Laboratory examinations were performed in a total of 1401 patients during clinical trials with MANERIX. Reductions were observed in leucocyte, AST and ALT values, however, these reductions were attributed to raised baseline values returning to normal, and were not considered clinically relevant. No other laboratory abnormalities were noted during clinical trials.

In post-market surveillance, there appeared to be a low incidence of raised liver enzymes, without associated clinical sequelae.

OVERDOSE:

Symptoms: Signs and symptoms of overdosage with MANERIX (moclobemide) include nausea, vomiting drowsiness, disorientation, slurred speech, amnesia, reduced reflexes, agitation, hypertension and convulsions. One patient remained stuporous for 36 hours following an overdose with 1550 mg MANERIX. All abnormal laboratory values and vital signs returned to within normal range one to five days after overdosage. No organ toxicity was reported.

Treatment: The treatment of overdosage should consist of general supportive measures. Gastric lavage or induction of emesis, activated charcoal and fluid control may be of benefit.

As with other antidepressants, mixed overdoses of MANERIX with other drugs (e.g. agents active on the CNS), could be life-threatening. Serotonergic syndrome and death have been reported after combined overdose of MANERIX and other antidepressants. Therefore, such patients should be closely monitored so that appropriate care and treatment may be given.

> For management of a suspected drug overdose, CPhA recommends that you contact your **regional Poison Control Centre**. See the *CPS* Directory section for a list of Poison Control Centres.

DOSAGE: Note: MANERIX (moclobemide) should always be taken after meals (see Drug Interactions).

Usual Adult Dosage: The administration of MANERIX should be initiated at 300 mg daily dose (in two divided doses), and increased gradually to a maximum of 600 mg/day if needed, noting carefully the clinical response and any evidence of intolerance. Individual patient response may allow for a reduction of the daily dose. As with other antidepressants, it should be kept in mind that there may be a lag time in therapeutic response. There is no evidence that increasing the dosage rapidly shortens this latent period and may, in fact, increase the incidence of side-effects. Furthermore, because bioavailability of MANERIX has been shown to increase over the first week of dosing (see Pharmacology, Pharmacokinetics), the initial daily dose of 300 mg should not be increased until after this first week of therapy.

Liver Dysfunction: When hepatic metabolism is severely impaired by hepatic disease or inhibited by a drug that affects microsomal mixed function oxidase activity (e.g. cimetidine), the daily dose of MANERIX should be reduced to one-third or one-half of the standard dose.

Renal Dysfunction: Single dose pharmacokinetic data suggest that no dosage adjustment may be required in patients with impaired renal function. However, multiple dose studies with MANERIX have not been performed in patients with renal dysfunction, therefore, MANERIX should be used with caution in this patient population. In normal volunteers, the absolute bioavailability almost doubles following multiple dosing as compared to a single dose.

Geriatrics: No dosage adjustments are necessary in elderly patients.

Cimetidine: Cimetidine doubles the AUC (area under the plasma concentration-time curve) of MANERIX and is expected to approximately double MANERIX steady-state concentrations (see Drug Interactions).

In patients receiving MANERIX concomitantly with cimetidine, a 50% reduction in the dosage of MANERIX may be necessary.

INFORMATION FOR THE PATIENT: Published in e-CPS, available by subscription at www.e-cps.ca.

SUPPLIED: 150 mg: Each pale yellow, single-scored, biconvex, film-coated tablet imprinted ROCHE/150 on one side, single scored on the other, contains: moclobemide 150 mg. Nonmedicinal ingredients: cornstarch, ethylcellulose, iron oxide, lactose, magnesium stearate, methylhydroxypropyl cellulose, polyethylene glycol, povidone, sodium starch glycolate, talc and titanium dioxide. Gluten-, parabens-, sucrose-, sulfites- and tartrazine-free. Bottles of 100. Store at 15 to 30°C.

300 mg: Each white, single scored, biconvex, film-coated tablet imprinted ROCHE/300 on one side and single scored on the other, contains: moclobemide 300 mg. Nonmedicinal ingredients: cornstarch, ethylcellulose, lactose, magnesium stearate, methylhydroxypropyl cellulose, polyethylene glycol, povidone, sodium starch glycolate, talc and titanium dioxide. Bottles of 100. Store at 15 to 30°C.

Mannitol

mannitol

Osmotic Diuretic

Hospira

SUPPLIED: Each mL contains: mannitol 250 mg. Nonmedicinal ingredients: hydrochloric acid, sodium bicarbonate and water for injection. Single dose: Discard unused portion. Fliptop vials of 50 mL, boxes of 25.

MAP Master Amino Acid Pattern® (MAP™)

amino acids

Protein Synthesis Precursor

Functional Nutrients

PHARMACOLOGY: MAP Master Amino Acid Pattern is a source of amino acids to support body protein synthesis (BPS). It is a patented profile of essential amino acids in a highly purified, free, crystalline form. (Canadian Patent No. 2 054 268) After oral ingestion MAP is absorbed without the aid of peptidases through the first 100 cm of functional small intestine. MAP is amphoteric and does not provide any fecal residue.

The results of comparative, double-blind, triple- and quintuple-crossover Net Nitrogen Utilization (NNU) clinical studies have shown that the subjects, while taking MAP as a source of amino acids, achieved a body's 99% NNU. This means that 99% of MAP's constituent amino acids followed the anabolic pathway, thus acting as precursor of body protein synthesis (BPS). During the studies, each subject's body nitrogen balance was maintained in equilibrium by taking MAP as a sole source of amino acids in a dosage of only 400 mg/kg/day (ideal body weight) which provided less than 2 kcal/day (1 g MAP releases 0.04 kcal). The studies have also shown that 1% of MAP's constituent amino acids followed the catabolic pathway, thus releasing only 1% of nitrogen catabolites and energy.

To illustrate: After amino acids are absorbed they can follow either the anabolic pathway or the catabolic pathway (see Figure 1).

Figure 1: MAP Master Amino Acid Pattern

The Anabolic and Catabolic Pathways

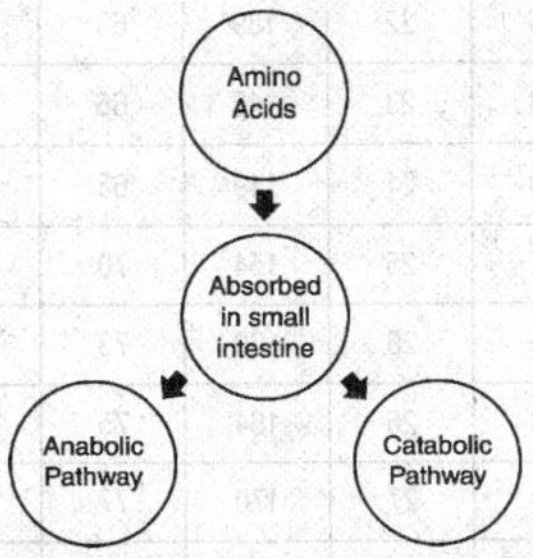

When amino acids follow the anabolic pathway, they act as precursors for body protein synthesis (BPS), thus becoming the body's constituent proteins. Throughout the anabolic pathway, amino acids do not release any nitrogen catabolites or energy (see Figure 2).

Figure 2: MAP Master Amino Acid Pattern

The Anabolic Pathway

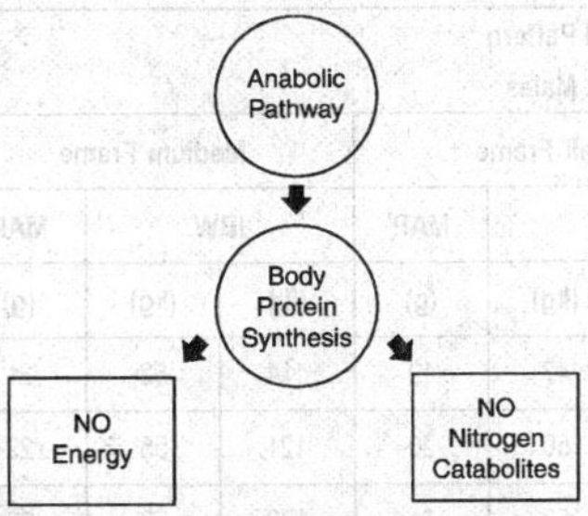

On the other hand, when amino acids follow the catabolic pathway, they act only as a source of energy and not as precursors of body protein synthesis (BPS). Throughout the catabolic pathway, amino acids do release nitrogen catabolites and energy (see Figure 3).

Figure 3: MAP Master Amino Acid Pattern

The Catabolic Pathway

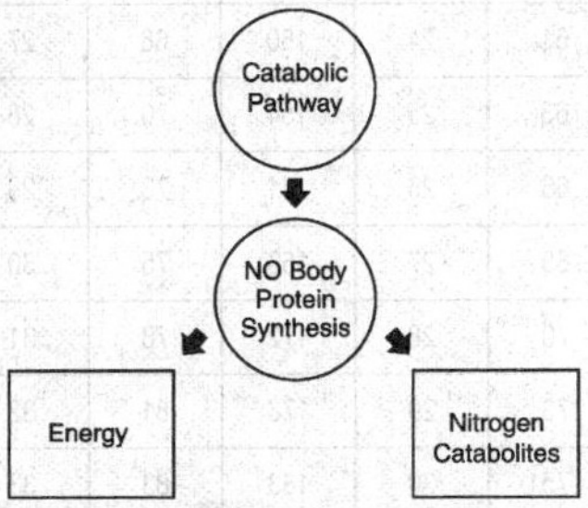

INDICATIONS: MAP is indicated as a source of amino acids to support body protein synthesis.

WARNINGS: Do not use if pregnant or breastfeeding. Consult a health care practitioner prior to use if following a low-protein diet. Caution phenylketonurics: this product contains phenylalanine.

PRECAUTIONS: See Warnings.

ADVERSE EFFECTS: No adverse reactions have been reported.

OVERDOSE:

No adverse reactions have been reported.

> For management of a suspected drug overdose, CPhA recommends that you contact your **regional Poison Control Centre**. See the *CPS* Directory section for a list of Poison Control Centres.

DOSAGE: As a source of amino acids to support body protein synthesis, take 5 to 10 tablets per day preferably with food or as directed by a health care practitioner.

MAP in a dosage of 400 mg/kg/day (ideal body weight) has been shown to be adequate as a sole source of amino acids to maintain the body's nitrogen balance in equilibrium. To calculate the MAP dosage as a sole source of amino acids, see Table 1 and Table 2 or apply the following:

MAP Dosage (g) = Ideal body weight (IBW) kg×0.4 g

Table 1: MAP Master Amino Acid Pattern
IBW and MAP Dosage (g) for Adult Females

Height		Small Frame			Medium Frame			Large Frame		
		IBW		MAP	IBW		MAP	IBW		MAP
(ft)	(cm)	(lb)	(kg)	(g)	(lb)	(kg)	(g)	(lb)	(kg)	(g)
5'	152	92	42	17	103	47	19	114	52	21
5' 1"	155	97	44	17	109	50	20	121	55	22
5' 2"	157	102	46	18	115	52	21	128	58	23
5' 3"	160	106	48	19	119	54	21	132	60	24
5' 4"	163	111	50	20	125	57	23	139	63	25
5' 5"	165	114	52	21	129	59	23	143	65	26
5' 6"	168	120	55	22	135	61	24	150	68	27
5' 7"	170	123	56	22	139	63	25	154	70	28
5' 8"	173	128	58	23	145	66	26	161	73	29
5' 9"	175	132	60	24	149	68	27	165	75	30
5' 10"	178	137	62	25	154	70	28	172	78	31
5' 11"	180	143	65	26	160	73	29	178	81	32
6'	183	146	66	26	164	75	30	183	83	33
6' 1"	185	151	69	27	170	77	31	189	86	34
6' 2"	188	155	70	28	174	79	31	194	88	35
6' 3"	191	160	73	29	180	82	32	200	91	36
6' 4"	193	165	75	30	186	85	33	207	94	37

Table 2: MAP Master Amino Acid Pattern
IBW and MAP Dosage (g) for Adult Males

Height		Small Frame			Medium Frame			Large Frame		
		IBW		MAP	IBW		MAP	IBW		MAP
(ft)	(cm)	(lb)	(kg)	(g)	(lb)	(kg)	(g)	(lb)	(kg)	(g)
5'	152	103	47	19	114	52	21	126	57	23
5' 1"	155	109	50	20	121	55	22	133	62	24
5' 2"	157	115	52	21	128	58	23	140	64	25
5' 3"	160	119	54	21	132	60	24	145	66	26
5' 4"	163	125	57	23	139	63	25	152	69	27
5' 5"	165	129	59	23	143	65	26	157	71	28
5' 6"	168	135	61	24	150	68	27	165	75	30
5' 7"	170	139	63	25	154	70	28	169	77	30
5' 8"	173	145	66	26	161	73	29	177	80	32
5' 9"	175	149	68	27	165	75	30	182	83	33
5' 10"	178	154	70	28	172	78	31	189	86	34
5' 11"	180	160	73	29	178	81	32	196	89	35
6'	183	164	75	30	183	83	33	201	91	36
6' 1"	185	170	77	31	189	86	34	208	95	37
6' 2"	188	174	79	31	194	88	35	213	97	38
6' 3"	191	180	82	32	200	91	36	220	100	40
6' 4"	193	186	85	33	207	94	37	227	103	41
6' 5"	196	190	86	34	211	96	38	232	105	42
6' 6"	198	196	89	35	218	99	39	240	109	43

Tablets can be pulverized and mixed with food or beverage. If administering more than 10 tablets per day, increase dosage gradually. In order to optimize the results, do not take more than 10 tablets of MAP within a two hour period. (If gastrointestinal disorders are present, pulverize tablets.) Consult a health care practitioner for use beyond four weeks.

INFORMATION FOR THE PATIENT: Published in e-CPS, available by subscription at www.e-cps.ca.

SUPPLIED: Tablets of 1000 mg for oral administration. Each tablet contains: L-leucine 189.6 mg, L-lysine HCl 172.4 mg, L-valine 160 mg, L-isoleucine 143.2 mg, L-phenylalanine 124.5 mg, L-threonine 107.3 mg, L-methionine 67.5 mg, L-tryptophan 35.5 mg. Nonmedicinal ingredients: none. Bottles of 120. MAP is also known as SON Formula. Store in a cool dry place.

Maprotiline ℞
Antidepressant

CPhA Monograph

Date of Revision: November 2006

> This monograph has been compiled by CPhA and reviewed by experts. It may contain information different from that found in Health Canada-approved Product Monographs. The reader is referred to the *CPS* Editorial Policy for more information.

SUMMARY PRODUCT INFORMATION:

Route of Administration	Dosage Form	Product Strength
Oral	Tablet	10 mg, 25 mg, 50 mg, 75 mg

INDICATIONS AND CLINICAL USE: Treatment of depressive affective disorders (mood disorders), dysthymic disorder, major depression and anxiety related to depression. Although it has been used for the depressive phase of bipolar disorder, hypomania or mania has occurred in these patients.

When compared to the tricyclic antidepressants (TCAs) (e.g., amitriptyline and imipramine), maprotiline has not shown superior efficacy in the treatment of depression. Maprotiline and paroxetine had similar efficacy in several short-term trials comparing the two agents. However, SSRIs are currently considered first-line treatment for depression because of tolerability and ease of dosing.

Maprotiline is also used in the treatment of neuropathic pain. Amitriptyline is slightly more effective than maprotiline in the treatment of painful diabetic and nondiabetic polyneuropathy.

Pediatrics: Maprotiline is not recommended for use in children since safety and efficacy in children has not been established. There have been cases of sudden death in children treated with maprotiline.

CONTRAINDICATIONS: Maprotiline is contraindicated during the acute recovery period following myocardial infarction and in patients with congestive heart failure.

Because it can lower the seizure threshold, maprotiline should not be given to patients with known or suspected seizure disorders.

Maprotiline is contraindicated in patients with existing liver or kidney damage and in those with a history of blood dyscrasias.

Because of its anticholinergic effects, maprotiline is contraindicated in patients with angle-closure glaucoma. It is contraindicated in patients who have known or suspected hypersensitivity to the drug or its excipients, or have known or suspected hypersensitivity to tricyclic antidepressants belonging to the dibenzazepine group (e.g., imipramine, desipramine, clomipramine). Maprotiline is contraindicated in patients receiving MAOIs or within 14 days before or after treatment with an MAOI (see Table 1).

WARNINGS AND PRECAUTIONS:

> Maprotiline should be used with extreme caution in patients with a history of convulsive disorders, brain damage of varying etiology, those using drugs that may lower the seizure threshold, alcoholism and withdrawal from alcohol and those receiving benzodiazepines that are being tapered rapidly. It appears that the occurrence of seizures is dose-dependent as seizures have usually occurred in patients receiving daily doses of 200 mg or more. To decrease seizure risk patients should be started on low doses with small increases after at least 2 weeks of the same dose.

General: Maprotiline appears to share the toxic potential of tricyclic antidepressants. Concurrent administration of maprotiline and electroconvulsive therapy should only be used by those experienced with this combination.

The potential for attempted suicide must always be considered in depressed patients. It is considered prudent to provide a limited supply of maprotiline to patients thought to be at high risk of suicide.

Maprotiline use in patients with tumors of the adrenal medulla (e.g., pheochromocytoma, neuroblastoma) may provoke a hypertensive crisis.

Cardiovascular: Tricyclic antidepressants and maprotiline may prolong conduction time and produce sinus tachycardia and arrhythmias. The most common ECG changes that occurred in patients using maprotiline were premature ventricular contractions (PVCs), ST-T wave changes, and abnormalities in intraventricular conduction. These changes were rarely associated with significant clinical symptoms.

Myocardial infarct, strokes and cardiac arrest have been reported with tricyclic antidepressants. In patients with cardiovascular disease, especially conduction disorders (e.g., atrioventricular block), other arrhythmias or congestive heart failure, monitor cardiac function and perform ECG examinations during long-term therapy. Gradual dose titration is recommended. Measure patients's lying and standing blood pressure before starting treatment and regularly during treatment as hypotension may occur. Postural hypotension may be controlled by reducing the dosage or administering maprotiline as a single bedtime dose.

Transient cardiac arrhythmias have occurred in rare instances in patients receiving thyroid medications with tricyclic antidepressants.

Dependence/Tolerance/Withdrawal: Abrupt withdrawal of maprotiline may be associated with serious hypotension, dizziness, nausea, vomiting, headache, malaise, sleep disturbance, hyperthermia, irritability, and worsening of the psychiatric condition. Monitor the patient carefully while tapering gradually.

Endocrine and Metabolism: Cases of the syndrome of inappropriate antidiuretic hormone (SIADH) have been reported in patients receiving tricyclic antidepressants.

Gastrointestinal: Because they cause dry mouth, prolonged use of tricyclic antidepressants has been associated with an increased incidence of dental caries. The anticholinergic effects of maprotiline may cause constipation and, rarely, gastrointestinal obstruction.

Genitourinary: The anticholinergic effects of maprotiline cause urinary retention, especially in men with benign prostatic hypertrophy.

Hematologic: Although rare, cases of bone marrow depression with agranulocytosis have been reported. Differential blood cell counts and leukocyte counts are recommended in patients receiving long-term treatment with maprotiline. These blood tests should also be performed in patients receiving maprotiline who present with fever, an influenzal infection or sore throat. Maprotiline should be discontinued in patients with significant neutropenia.

Hepatic/Biliary/Pancreatic: Because isolated cases of obstructive jaundice have been reported, use caution in treating patients with known liver disease. Periodic liver function testing is recommended in these patients.

Neurologic: Seizures have been reported in patients without a history of seizures who were treated with maprotiline at therapeutic doses (see boxed warning above).

Ophthalmologic: Patients with contact lenses may suffer damage to the corneal epithelium as a result of the decreased lacrimation caused by the anticholinergic properties of tricyclic antidepressants. The anticholinergic effects of maprotiline may be harmful in patients with narrow-angle glaucoma.

Perioperative Considerations: Because potential for interaction with general anesthetic is not known, maprotiline use should be tapered prior to elective surgery.

Psychiatric: Agitated patients may become over stimulated when using maprotiline. Reduce dose or discontinue the drug. There have been reports of patients receiving TCAs experiencing activation of latent schizophrenia or aggravation of existing psychotic manifestations in schizophrenia. Individuals with evidence of a bipolar disorder may be at risk of experiencing hypomania or mania.

Skin: Withdraw maprotiline if the patient presents with an allergic skin reaction.

Special Populations: Pregnancy: Safe use of maprotiline in pregnant women has not been established. As a result, maprotiline should not be administered during pregnancy unless the expected benefit to the patient outweighs the potential risk to the fetus. To date there are no published reports of congenital defects, however data from limited surveillance suggest a possible association between oral cleft and first trimester exposure. Neonates whose mothers received tricyclic antidepressants during the third trimester of pregnancy have presented with the following withdrawal symptoms tremors, dyspnea, lethargy, colic, irritability, hypotonia/hypertonia, convulsions, and respiratory depression. If possible, gradually withdraw maprotiline at least 7 weeks before the calculated delivery date.
Lactation: Carefully weigh risk to the infant versus benefit to the mother. Maprotiline passes into breast milk with milk concentrations of 0.2 μg/mL (unchanged maprotiline) after multiple doses. A milk:plasma ratio of approximately 1.5 has been reported after 150 mg per day for three days. It is not known whether the active metabolite is also present in breast milk. Effects of exposure to these small amounts of maprotiline during chronic ingestion is unknown.
Pediatrics: Maprotiline is not recommended for use in children. There have been cases of sudden death in children treated with maprotiline.
Geriatrics: Older individuals generally show a more marked response to maprotiline than younger patients as they are particularly susceptible to anticholinergic, psychiatric, neurological and cardiovascular effects. All older individuals receiving antidepressants should be considered at increased risk of falls and appropriate preventive measures should be taken.

Appropriate measures should be taken to avoid or treat constipation since tricyclic antidepressants have caused paralytic ileus particularly in elderly or hospitalized patients. Older individuals are also at higher risk of urinary retention when taking maprotiline. Especially at night, elderly patients may experience delirious psychosis with the use of tricyclic antidepressants. This symptom disappears within a few days of discontinuing the tricyclic.
Monitoring and Laboratory Tests: Monitor cardiac function and perform ECG examinations during long-term therapy in patients with pre-existing cardiovascular disease. Regularly measure both lying and standing blood pressure in patients susceptible to hypotension.

Differential blood cell counts and leukocyte counts are recommended in patients receiving long-term treatment with maprotiline. These blood tests should also be performed in patients receiving maprotiline who present with fever, a flu-like infection or sore throat.

Periodic liver function testing is recommended in patients with known liver disease.
Occupational Hazards: Especially when starting therapy, maprotiline may produce sedation. Caution patients who may be engaging in activities requiring mental alertness, judgment and physical coordination.
DRUG INTERACTIONS: See Table 1, Table 2 and Table 3.

Table 1: Maprotiline

Serious Drug Interactions
Maprotiline should not be given in conjunction with, or within 14 days before or after treatment with a MAO inhibitor as hypertensive crises, hyperactivity, hyperpyrexia, spasticity, severe convulsions or coma, and death have been reported in patients receiving such combinations. The concomitant treatment with selective, reversible MAO-inhibitors, such as moclobemide, is also contraindicated.

Overview: Since maprotiline is metabolized by the CYP2D6 enzyme system, inhibitors of CYP2D6 may decrease the metabolism of maprotiline.
Drug-Drug Interactions: See Table 2.

Table 2: Maprotiline
Drug-Drug Interactions

Interacting Drug	Effect	Clinical Comment
Anticholinergics	Additive anticholinergic effects (usually minor, but possibility to precipitate adynamic ileus, urinary retention or acute glaucoma) especially in older individuals.	Monitor patient for excessive anticholinergic effects; if necessary, consider using an alternate antidepressant with less anticholinergic activity.
Barbiturates	Barbiturates activate the hepatic enzyme system; may reduce plasma concentrations of maprotiline.	No specific action required, but be alert for evidence of the interaction.
Carbamazepine	Maprotiline may increase plasma concentrations of carbamazepine. Carbamazepine may decrease plasma concentrations of maprotiline through activation of the hepatic enzyme system.	It may be necessary to adjust the dosage of carbamazepine or maprotiline.
Cimetidine	Cimetidine probably inhibits hepatic metabolism of maprotiline.	Use an alternative to cimetidine. Initiate maprotiline at low doses to patients on cimetidine and monitor maprotiline effects in patients initiating/discontinuing or changing doses of cimetidine when stabilized on maprotiline.
CNS Depressants	Increased CNS depression	Use with caution.
Guanethidine (also bethanidine, clonidine, reserpine, alpha-methyldopa)	Maprotiline may antagonize antihypertensive effects.	It has been suggested that if TCAs are used, an alternative antihypertensive should be selected or monitor patient for reduced antihypertensive response.
Lithium	There is some evidence that concurrent use of lithium and TCAs may increase the risk of neurotoxicity, particularly in the elderly.	It has been suggested that reducing the dose of lithium in elderly patients may reduce the risk of neurotoxicity without compromising its clinical effect. Elderly patients should be monitored carefully for signs of neurotoxicity (e.g., tremor, ataxia, seizures) when on combined therapy.
MAOIs, Moclobemide	See Table 1.	
Selective Serotonin Reuptake Inhibitors (e.g., fluoxetine, fluvoxamine)	SSRIs may decrease metabolism of TCAs with corresponding adverse effects.	Avoid this combination or monitor patients for increased maprotiline serum levels or adverse effects; adjust dose as needed (note long half-life of fluoxetine so will dissipate over 2-4 weeks after it is discontinued).
Sympathomimetics	TCAs can enhance the pressor response to norepinephrine and may potentiate the cardiovascular effects (e.g., arrhythmia) of sympathomimetics in general.	Use with caution. Monitor pressor response.

Drug-Herb Interactions: See Table 3.

Table 3: Maprotiline
Drug-Herb Interactions

Interacting Herb	Effect	Clinical Comment
Indian Snakeroot	Indian snakeroot may interact with or potentiate the effects of TCAs.	Unknown clinical significance with maprotiline. Avoid concurrent administration to optimize maprotiline's efficacy.

ACTION AND CLINICAL PHARMACOLOGY: Although the precise mechanism of action of maprotiline is unknown, it is a tetracyclic antidepressant that is pharmacologically similar to the tricyclic antidepressants. It blocks the reuptake of norepinephrine in the brain and peripheral neuronal membranes but does not seem to influence serotonin reuptake. It has stronger antihistaminic activity than amitriptyline and weaker anticholinergic activity. Like the tricyclic antidepressants, maprotiline may cause ECG changes, tachycardia and postural hypotension. It causes sedation, lowers seizure threshold and, at toxic doses, can produce respiratory depression.
Pharmacokinetics: See Table 4.

Table 4: Maprotiline
Pharmacokinetic Parameters in a Healthy Adult Population

$t_{1/2}$ (h)	Clearance	Volume of Distribution
27–58	514 mL/min	16.33 L/kg

Absorption: Maprotiline is slowly but completely absorbed after oral administration. Peak plasma concentrations occur within approximately 8 to 24 hours.
Distribution: Plasma protein binding is 88 to 90%. Antidepressant effects usually occur within 2 to 3 weeks in most patients who respond and may occur within 3 to 7 days.
Metabolism: Maprotiline is metabolized in the liver by hydroxylation and oxidation to form active and inactive metabolites. Maprotiline is metabolized by the CYP2D6 isoenzyme.
Excretion: Maprotiline is excreted primarily in the urine (mostly as glucuronide metabolites) with about 30% excreted in feces. Only 2 to 4% of the dose is excreted unchanged in the urine. Ninety percent of the amount excreted in the urine consists of metabolites, 75% in the form of glucuronides.
Special Populations and Conditions: Geriatrics: Half-life of maprotiline is extended in older individuals (average 66 h).
Hepatic Insufficiency: Maprotiline metabolism may be altered in hepatic function impairment.
Renal Insufficiency: If hepatic function is normal, the half-life and renal excretion of maprotiline are not significantly affected by impaired renal function (creatinine clearance: 24 to 37 mL/min). Urinary excretion of metabolites is reduced. This reduction is normally offset by increased fecal elimination through biliary excretion.
ADVERSE REACTIONS: Adverse Drug Reaction Overview: See Table 5. The most common adverse reactions reported in patients receiving maprotiline are related to its anticholinergic activity. Expected adverse effects are similar to those seen with tricyclic antidepressants. Adverse reactions usually occur at higher dosages. Plasma concentrations may not predict incidence of adverse effects.

Table 5: Maprotiline
More Common Adverse Drug Reactions (1 to >10%)

Body System	Maprotiline (%)
Autonomic	
Delayed micturition, dilation of the urinary tract	>1–10%
Cardiovascular	
Hypotension, particularly orthostatic hypotension with associated dizziness, sinus tachycardia, ECG changes in patients of normal cardiac status (including flattening or inversion of T wave, depressed S-T segments)	>10%
Arrhythmia, disturbances in cardiac conduction (e.g., widening of QRS complex, bundle-branch block), palpitation, syncope	>1–10%
CNS	
Tremors, myoclonus	>10%
Dizziness, headache, nervousness, drowsiness, fatigue, insomnia, anxiety, agitation, decrease in memory	>1–10%
Dermatologic	
Skin rash, urticaria	>1–10%
Endocrine and Metabolism	
Weight gain	>10%
Increased or decreased libido, impotence	>1–10%
Gastrointestinal	
Dry mouth, constipation	>10%
Nausea, vomiting, anorexia, abdominal cramps	>1–10%
Ophthalmologic	
Blurred vision, disturbances of visual accommodation	>10%
Psychiatric	
Confusional states with hallucinations (especially in older individuals and patients suffering from Parkinson's disease), anxiety, agitation, delirium, restlessness, nightmares, hypomania, mania	>1–10%
Miscellaneous	
Perspiration, hot flushes	>10%

Less Common Adverse Drug Reactions: Cardiovascular: Isolated cases (<0.01%) of hypertension, congestive heart failure, myocardial infarction, heart block, asystole, stroke, peripheral vasospastic reactions.

Table 6: Maprotiline

Dose in Adult Patients

Indication	Route	Initial Dose	Titrate	Usual Dose	Maximum Dose	Duration of Treatment	Detailed Information
Depression	Oral	75 mg daily in 2 or 3 divided doses	Maintain initial dose for 2 weeks, then increase gradually in increments of 25 mg (adding to late afternoon or bedtime doses), as needed	75 to 150 mg daily (individualized)	150 mg daily (outpatients) but 200 mg may be required in some of these patients	Medication should be continued for the expected duration of the depressive episode in order to minimize the possibility of relapse following clinical improvement. Maintenance antidepressant therapy is usually recommended for a minimum period of 1 year.	Dosage during maintenance therapy should be kept at the lowest effective level. When maintenance therapy has been established, maprotiline may be administered in a single daily dose at bedtime, if tolerated. However, if the total daily dose exceeds 150 mg, it should be administered in divided doses.
Depression (severely depressed hospitalized patients)	Oral	100 mg daily may be required, in 2 or 3 divided doses	Maintain initial dose for 2 weeks, then increase gradually in increments of 25 mg (adding to late afternoon or bedtime doses), as needed	150 mg daily	225 mg daily (essential to exclude a history of convulsive disorders). Do not exceed 225 mg daily	Medication should be continued for the expected duration of the depressive episode in order to minimize the possibility of relapse following clinical improvement. Maintenance antidepressant therapy is usually recommended for a minimum period of 1 year.	Dosage during maintenance therapy should be kept at the lowest effective level. When maintenance therapy has been established, maprotiline may be administered in a single daily dose at bedtime, if tolerated. However, if the total daily dose exceeds 150 mg, it should be administered in divided doses.

Table 7: Maprotiline

Dose in Geriatric Patients

Indication	Route	Initial Dose	Titrate	Usual Dose	Maximum Dose	Duration of Treatment	Detailed Information
Depression	Oral	10 mg three times daily or 30 mg at bedtime	Very gradual increments, depending on tolerance and response	50 to 75 mg daily	75 mg daily usually adequate	Medication should be continued for the expected duration of the depressive episode in order to minimize the possibility of relapse following clinical improvement. Maintenance antidepressant therapy is usually recommended for a minimum period of 1 year.	In general, lower dosages are recommended for geriatric patients because these individuals usually show a more marked response to maprotiline than patients in younger age groups. Blood pressure and cardiac rhythm should be checked frequently. Dosage during maintenance therapy should be kept at the lowest effective level. When maintenance therapy has been established, maprotiline may be administered in a single daily dose at bedtime, provided such a dosage regimen is well tolerated.

CNS: Rare cases (>0.01-1%) of epileptic seizure; risk of seizures appears to be higher with maprotiline than with the tricyclic antidepressants; isolated cases of tinnitus, incoordination, ataxia, alterations in EEG patterns, extrapyramidal symptoms, myoclonus, speech disorders, weakness, paresthesias.
Dermatologic: Isolated cases of: petechiae, itching, photosensitization. Patients treated with maprotiline should avoid excessive exposure to sunlight.
Ear/Nose/Throat: Isolated cases of nasal congestion.
Endocrine and Metabolism: Isolated cases of gynecomastia (males), breast enlargement and galactorrhea (females), testicular swelling, elevation or depression of blood sugar levels, weight loss, syndrome of inappropriate antidiuretic hormone (SIADH), porphyrinogenicity (in susceptible patients).
Gastrointestinal: Rare cases of diarrhea, elevated transaminases; isolated cases of: paralytic ileus, bitter taste, stomatitis, epigastric distress, black tongue, dysphagia, increased salivation.
Hematologic: Isolated cases of agranulocytosis, eosinophilia, leukopenia, purpura and thrombocytopenia.
Hepatic/Biliary/Pancreatic: Isolated cases of hepatitis with or without jaundice.
Ophthalmologic: Isolated cases of mydriasis, glaucoma.
Psychiatric: Isolated cases of aggressiveness.
Respiratory: Isolated cases of bronchospasm.
Miscellaneous: Isolated cases of alopecia and edema (general or face and tongue), drug fever, systemic anaphylactic/anaphylactoid reactions which may present with hypotension.

DOSAGE AND ADMINISTRATION: See Table 6 and Table 7.

Dosing Considerations: Patients should be kept under medical surveillance during treatment with maprotiline. Individualize dosing. Initiate therapy at the lowest possible dose and increase gradually, watching for adverse reactions. Therapeutic effects usually present after two to three weeks of maprotiline treatment. This lag time to effect is not normally shortened by dosage increases, but incidence of side effects may be increased. Daily dose should not exceed 200 mg to decrease seizure risk. Daily doses may be divided into twice or three-times daily dosing or given as a single evening dose. When discontinuing maprotiline, decrease dose gradually.
Adults: See Table 6.
Geriatrics: See Table 7.
Missed Dose: If the dosing schedule is more than once a day, the patient should take the missed dose as soon as possible unless it is less than 2 hours before the next dose (should not double the dose to make up for the missed one). If the dosing schedule is once at bedtime, don't take the dose in the morning because of sedation.
Administration: Oral: Solid oral dosage forms: 10 mg tablets, 25 mg tablets, 50 mg tablets, 75 mg tablets.
Maprotiline can be taken with or without food.

OVERDOSAGE:

Signs and Symptoms: Because maprotiline shares the pharmacologic properties of tricyclic antidepressants (TCAs), the information in this section pertains to TCAs in general. Note: the incidence of seizures and cardiac arrhythmias and the duration of coma are greater with maprotiline toxicity compared to TCAs.
TCAs are extremely toxic in overdose. Consultation with a Poison Control Centre is recommended. See the *CPS* Directory section for contact numbers.

Cardiac arrhythmias and CNS involvement pose the greatest threat and may occur suddenly even when initial symptoms appear to be mild. The toxic dose is variable but, in general, acute ingestion of 10 to 20 mg/kg may result in serious toxicity and may be lethal. TCA overdose has one of the highest mortality rates of any type of ingestion. Toxicity most commonly begins within two hours of ingestion. The onset of symptoms is frequently precipitous, with patients progressing from a wakeful, interactive state to having severe CNS and cardiac involvement within a matter of minutes.

Peripheral anticholinergic symptoms may include urinary retention, dry mucous membranes, mydriasis, constipation, and occasionally adynamic ileus. Patients may also be hyperpyrexic. CNS signs and symptoms can be highly variable and may range from somnolence to agitation, irritability, confusion, delirium, and hallucinations. In severe cases, patients may display extreme drowsiness, areflexia, respiratory depression, and coma. Patients may occasionally become hypothermic. Seizures are common and may precipitate cardiac toxicity.

Cardiac irregularities are frequent. Sinus tachycardia is common. Its presence is not a reliable predictor of serious toxicity, and its absence does not ensure a benign clinical course. An effect on cardiac conduction similar to that of quinidine may be seen with slowing of conduction, widening of the QRS complex, rightward shift in the axis of the terminal 40 milliseconds of the QRS complex, prolongation of the PR and QT intervals, right bundle branch and AV block, ventricular tachyarrhythmias (including torsades de pointes and fibrillation), and death. Prolongation of the QRS duration to more than 0.1 seconds is generally associated with more severe toxicity. Bradycardia may be seen in severely poisoned patients. Hypotension is common and may be severe, resulting from vasodilation, central and peripheral alpha-adrenergic blockade, and myocardial depression. Metabolic and/or respiratory acidosis may occur secondary to seizures, poor tissue perfusion, respiratory depression or poor gas exchange. In an otherwise healthy young person, prolonged resuscitation may be required.

Recommended Management: All cases of accidental pediatric exposure or adult overdose should be monitored at a health care facility. Asymptomatic cases without ECG abnormalities should be monitored for a minimum of 6 hours. Plasma concentrations of maprotiline are of little use and should not guide management of the patient. In managing overdose, consider the possibility of multiple drug overdose, interactions among drugs and altered pharmacokinetics, including delayed absorption. Protect the patient's airway and support ventilation and perfusion. Closely monitor and maintain the patient's vital signs, ECG, blood gases, serum electrolytes, and acid-base balance. Minimize external stimulation to reduce the risk of seizures.

Consultation with a regional poison centre is advisable in all patients with TCA overdose. Activated charcoal (1 gram per kilogram) may reduce absorption of drug from the gastrointestinal tract, and should be considered in patients who present within 2 hours of ingestion. This can be given through a nasogastric tube if necessary. Although it should not be routinely performed, gastric lavage may be considered in the unusual case where a patient presents within 30 to 60 minutes of a massive TCA overdose, but only on the advice of a Poison Control Centre. If performed, gastric lavage should be followed by administration of activated charcoal. If the patient has a decreased level of consciousness, consideration should be given to placement of an endotracheal tube with cuff inflated before beginning the lavage procedure, to lessen the likelihood of aspiration of gastric contents.

Hypotension should be promptly corrected. If hypotension does not respond to a rapid isotonic fluid bolus and the patient has a widened QRS interval (>0.1 seconds), sodium bicarbonate boluses should be administered at a dose of 1 to 2 mmol/kg (an average adult would typically receive 1 to 3 ampoules of 50 mmol/50 mL). If hypotension still hasn't responded, vasopressors should be employed, with a direct-acting agonist such as norepinephrine being the drug of choice.

Widened QRS intervals (>0.14 seconds) and ventricular arrhythmias should be treated with iv sodium bicarbonate. An iv bolus of 1 to 2 mmol/kg (one or two 50 mmol ampoules) should be administered and repeated if necessary to achieve a serum pH of 7.45 to 7.55. Maintain the pH between 7.45 and 7.55. Do not exceed pH 7.6. Monitor for hypokalemia and fluid overload. Hyperventilation may also be used to maintain alkalemia.

Ventricular arrhythmias refractory to sodium bicarbonate may respond to lidocaine. Quinidine, procainamide and other type IA or IC antiarrhythmics should not be used because they may exacerbate arrhythmias and conduction slowing due to the overdosage. Overdrive pacing should be considered in patients whose arrhythmias are not responsive to drug therapy.

Seizures should be aggressively treated with iv benzodiazepines such as lorazepam or diazepam. If this is unsuccessful, barbiturates and other measures should be employed as for status epilepticus. However, phenytoin is no longer recommended for the treatment of TCA-induced seizures.

Diuresis, hemoperfusion and dialysis are not helpful in TCA overdose.

Flumazenil is contraindicated in any patient with an altered level of consciousness who has or may have taken a TCA or any drug that can cause seizures or arrhythmias, as it may precipitate seizures or even cardiac arrest. This is true even in cases of mixed overdose where the patient is known to have coingested benzodiazepines.

For management of a suspected drug overdose, CPhA recommends that you contact your **regional Poison Control Centre**. See the *CPS* Directory section for a list of Poison Control Centres.

Marcaine
bupivacaine HCl
Local Anesthetic

Hospira

Marcaine Spinal
bupivacaine HCl
Local Anesthetic

Hospira

Marcaine E
bupivacaine HCl—epinephrine
Local Anesthetic

Hospira

Date of Revision: October 15, 2009

SUMMARY PRODUCT INFORMATION:

Route of Administration	Dosage Form/Strength	All Nonmedicinal Ingredients
Parenteral	MARCAINE (bupivacaine hydrochloride) Sterile Solution 2.5 mg/mL, 5 mg/mL and 7.5 mg/mL bupivacaine hydrochloride	Sodium chloride, sodium hydroxide and/or hydrochloric acid and water for injection. Multidose vials contain methylparaben as a preservative.
	MARCAINE E (bupivacaine hydrochloride with epinephrine) Sterile Solution 0.25% with epinephrine 1:200 000 (as barbitrate) 0.50% with epinephrine 1:200 000 (as barbitrate)	Sodium chloride, sodium hydroxide and/or hydrochloric acid, monothioglycerol, ascorbic acid, sodium lactate 60% solution, edetate calcium disodium, sodium metabisulfite and water for injection
	MARCAINE SPINAL (bupivacaine hydrochloride) Sterile Solution 0.75% hyperbaric solution	Dextrose, sodium hydroxide and/or hydrochloric acid and water for injection

INDICATIONS AND CLINICAL USE: Adults (>18 years of age): MARCAINE (bupivacaine hydrochloride), MARCAINE SPINAL (bupivacaine hydrochloride) and MARCAINE E (bupivacaine hydrochloride with epinephrine) are indicated for the production of local or regional anaesthesia and analgesia with the following procedures:

- Local infiltration procedures
- Peripheral nerve blocks
- Retrobulbar blocks
- Caudal, epidural and subarachnoid (spinal) blocks

Standard procedures for local infiltration, minor and major nerve blocks, retrobulbar block or epidural block should be observed.

Geriatrics (>65 years of age): Elderly patients should be given reduced doses commensurate with their age and physical condition.

Pediatrics (<2 years of age): Until further experience is gained in children younger than two years, administration of any presentation of bupivacaine injection in this age group is not recommended.

CONTRAINDICATIONS: MARCAINE (bupivacaine hydrochloride), MARCAINE SPINAL (bupivacaine hydrochloride) and MARCAINE E (bupivacaine hydrochloride with epinephrine) are contraindicated:

- In patients with a hypersensitivity to bupivacaine, or to any local anaesthetic agent of the amide type, or to other components of bupivacaine injections.
- For intravenous regional anaesthesia (Bier Block) since unintentional leakage of bupivacaine over the tourniquet may cause systemic toxic reactions. Cardiac arrest and death have occurred (see Dosage and Administration).
- In obstetric paracervical block anaesthesia. Use of other local anaesthetics in this technique has resulted in foetal bradycardia and death.
- In severe shock and in heart block and when there is inflammation and/or sepsis near the site of the proposed injection.
- MARCAINE parenteral solutions in multidose vials are contraindicated in patients with a known history of hypersensitivity to ester local anesthetics (which are metabolized to para amino benzoic acid (PABA)), methylparaben and propylparaben (antimicrobial preservatives) or to their metabolite, PABA.

MARCAINE E (bupivacaine hydrochloride with epinephrine) is contraindicated in patients with a hypersensitivity to sodium metabisulfite (see Dosage Forms, Composition and Packaging).

MARCAINE parenteral solutions in multidose vials contain methylparaben (antimicrobial preservative) and should not be used for epidural or spinal anesthesia, or for any route of administration that would introduce solution into the cerebrospinal fluid. The safety of these agents has not been established with regard to intrathecal injection, either intentional or accidental. These solutions should not be administered intra-ocularly or retro-ocularly.

Spinal Use: With the exception of serious diseases of the central nervous system or of the lumbar vertebral column, most anesthesiologists consider the following conditions to be only **relative contraindications** to spinal anesthesia. The decision as to whether or not spinal anesthesia should be used for an individual case depends on the physician's appraisal of the advantages, as opposed to the risks, and on his ability to cope with the complications that may arise.

1. Disease of the cerebrospinal system, such as meningitis, spinal fluid block, cranial or spinal hemorrhage, increased intracranial pressure, tumours and syphilis.
2. Shock. This should be treated before any anesthetic is administered. However, in emergency operations, spinal anesthesia may at times be considered the method of choice.
3. Profound anemia, cachexia and when death is imminent.
4. Sepsis with positive blood cultures.
5. High blood pressure. Spinal anesthesia should be well tolerated if particular care is taken to prevent a sudden or appreciable fall in blood pressure.
6. Low blood pressure. The use of suitable pressor agents and methods of controlling the diffusion of the anesthetic should remove the principal objection to spinal anesthesia in patients with low blood pressure.
7. Highly nervous and sensitive persons. Pre-operative medication should overcome this difficulty
8. Visceral perforation, bowel strangulation, acute peritonitis. Some surgeons object to contraction of the gastrointestinal musculature; others, however, consider the associated arrest of peristalsis an advantage. With gastrointestinal hemorrhage, spinal anesthesia should be used with caution or may even be contraindicated.
9. Cardiac decompensation, massive pleural effusion and increased intra-abdominal pressure (e.g. full-term pregnancy, massive ascites, large tumor). High spinal anesthesia should not be used in patients with these conditions unless the Trendelenburg position can be omitted or the intra-abdominal pressure released slowly.

WARNINGS AND PRECAUTIONS: General: Local anaesthetics should only be used by clinicians who are well versed in diagnosis and management of dose-related toxicity and other acute emergencies which may arise from the block to be performed, and then only after ensuring the immediate availability of cardiopulmonary resuscitative equipment, resuscitative drugs, including oxygen, and the personnel resources needed for proper management of toxic reactions and related emergencies (see Adverse Reactions and Overdosage). Delay in proper management of dose-related toxicity, underventilation from any cause and/or altered sensitivity may lead to the development of acidosis, cardiac arrest and, possibly, death.

The highest (0.75%) concentration of isotonic MARCAINE (bupivacaine hydrochloride) injection is not recommended for obstetrical anesthesia. There have been reports of cardiac arrest with difficult resuscitation or death following its use for epidural anesthesia in obstetrical patients. Resuscitation has been difficult or impossible despite apparently adequate preparation and appropriate management. Cardiac arrest has occurred after convulsions resulting from systemic toxicity, probably following unintentional intravascular injection.

An intravenous cannula must be inserted before the local anaesthetic is injected for nerve blocks which may result in hypotension or bradycardia, or where acute systemic toxicity may develop following inadvertent intravascular injection.

The lowest dosage of local anaesthetic that results in effective anaesthesia or analgesia should be used to avoid high plasma levels and serious adverse reactions. Injections should be made slowly or in incremental doses, with frequent aspirations before and during the injection to avoid intravascular injection.

The following precautions apply to all local anesthetics: select needles of proper length and bevel for the technique employed. Inject slowly with frequent aspirations and, if blood is aspirated, relocate the needle. Inadvertent intravascular injection may cause serious complications. Absorption is more rapid when injections are made into highly vascular tissues. In caudal or epidural anesthesia, abandon the method if the subarachnoid space has been entered, as shown by aspiration of spinal fluid. However, a negative aspiration is not 100% reliable.

Injection of repeated doses of bupivacaine may cause a significant increase in blood levels due to accumulation of the drug or its metabolites or slow metabolic degradation. Tolerance to elevated blood levels varies with the physical condition of the patient.

Major peripheral nerve blocks may imply the administration of a large volume of local anaesthetic in areas of high vascularity, often close to large vessels where there is an increased risk of intravascular injection and/or rapid systemic absorption which can lead to high plasma concentrations.

Epinephrine-containing solutions should not be injected into tissues supplied by end arteries, for example, fingers and toes, ears, the nose, and the penis.

Local anaesthetic procedures should be carried out sufficiently away from an inflamed region. Injections should not be performed through inflamed tissue or when there is sepsis at or near the injection site.

Cardiovascular: The decision to use a local anaesthetic containing a vasoconstrictor in patients with peripheral vascular disease will depend on the physician's appraisal of the relative advantages and risks.

There have been reports of cardiac arrest or death during use of bupivacaine for epidural anaesthesia or peripheral nerve blockade. In some instances, resuscitation has been difficult or impossible despite apparently adequate preparation and management.

Ventricular arrhythmia, ventricular fibrillation, sudden cardiovascular collapse and death have been reported when bupivacaine was utilized for local anaesthetic procedures that may have resulted in high systemic concentrations of bupivacaine.

Epidural anaesthesia or analgesia may lead to hypotension and bradycardia. The risk of such effects can be reduced either by preloading the circulation with crystalloidal or colloidal solutions or by injecting a vasopressor such as ephedrine 20-40 mg i.m. Hypotension should be treated promptly, e.g., with ephedrine 5-10 mg intravenously and repeated as necessary. Children should be given ephedrine doses commensurate with their age and weight.

MARCAINE E (bupivacaine hydrochloride with epinephrine) should be used with caution in patients who may have severe or untreated hypertension, ischemic heart disease, cerebral vascular insufficiency, heart block, peripheral vascular disorder and any other pathological condition that might be aggravated by the effects of epinephrine.

Local anaesthetics should be used with caution in patients with impaired cardiovascular function because they may be less able to compensate for functional changes associated with the prolongation of A-V conduction produced by amide-type local anaesthetics.

Patients with partial or complete heart block require special attention since local anaesthetics may depress myocardial conduction. To reduce the risk of potentially serious adverse reactions, attempts should be made to optimize the patient's condition before major blocks are performed. Dosage should be adjusted accordingly.

Central nerve blocks may cause cardiovascular depression, especially in the presence of hypovolemia. Epidural anaesthesia should be used with caution in patients with impaired cardiovascular function.

Endocrine and Metabolism: MARCAINE E (bupivacaine hydrochloride with epinephrine) should be used with caution in patients whose medical history and physical evaluation suggest the existence of poorly controlled hyperthyroidism or advanced diabetes.

Spinal Use: In addition to the above noted precautions, when administering bupivacaine hyperbaric solution for spinal anesthesia, the patient's blood pressure should be carefully monitored. Spinal anesthesia is usually associated with a fall in arterial blood pressure due to sympathetic blockade.

Epidural Use: It is recommended that a test dose be administered initially and the effects monitored before the full dose is given (also see Dosage and Administration). Generally, 2 to 3 mL of 0.50% bupivacaine containing 1:200 000 epinephrine, when clinical conditions permit, should be administered to check that the spinal canal or a blood vessel has not been entered while locating the epidural needle or catheter. In the event of a spinal injection, clinical signs of spinal block would become evident in a few minutes. In the event of intravascular injection, a transient increase in pulse rate and/or systolic blood pressure is usually detectable with a monitor. The other symptoms and signs of "epinephrine response" are less dependable. Concomitantly administered medications may modify these responses. When reinforcing doses are required, the test dose should be used again to check the catheter location. However, an intravascular or subarachnoid injection is still possible even if results of the test dose are negative. Patients on beta-blockers may not manifest changes in heart rate, but blood pressure monitoring can detect an evanescent rise in systolic blood pressure.

During epidural administration, bupivacaine should be administered in incremental doses, with sufficient time between doses to detect toxic manifestations of unintentional intravascular or intrathecal injection. Frequent aspirations for blood or cerebrospinal fluid (where applicable, i.e., when using a "continuous" intermittent catheter technique), should be performed before and during each supplemental injection because plastic tubing in the epidural space can migrate into a blood vessel or through the dura. A negative aspiration, however, does not ensure against an intravascular or intrathecal injection.

Injection in Head and Neck Area: Relatively small doses of local anesthetics injected into the head and neck area, including retrobulbar and stellate ganglion blocks, may produce adverse reactions similar to systemic toxicity seen with unintentional intravascular injections of larger doses. The injection procedures require the utmost care.

Confusion, convulsions, respiratory depression and/or respiratory arrest and cardiovascular stimulation or depression leading to cardiac arrest have been reported. These reactions may be due to intra-arterial injection of the local anesthetic with retrograde flow to the cerebral circulation. They may also be due to puncture of the dural sheath of the optic nerve during retrobulbar block with diffusion of any local anesthetic along the subdural space to the midbrain. Patients receiving these blocks should remain under constant observation and monitoring for their cardiac and pulmonary functions. Resuscitative equipment and personnel for treating adverse reactions should be immediately available. Dosage recommendations should not be exceeded (see Dosage and Administration).

Ophthalmic Surgery: Retrobulbar injections may very occasionally reach the cranial subarachnoid space causing temporary blindness, cardiovascular collapse, apnoea, convulsions, etc. These reactions, which may be due to intra-arterial injection or direct injection into the central nervous system via the sheaths of the optic nerve, must be diagnosed and treated promptly.

Clinicians who perform retrobulbar blocks should be aware that there have been reports of respiratory arrest following local anaesthetic injection. Prior to retrobulbar block, as with all other regional procedures, the immediate availability of equipment, drugs, and personnel to manage respiratory arrest or depression, convulsions, and cardiac stimulation or depression should be assured (see also Warnings and Precautions, Injection in Head and Neck Area). As with other anesthetic procedures, patients should be constantly monitored following ophthalmic blocks for signs of these adverse reactions, which may occur following relatively low total doses. A concentration of 0.75% bupivacaine is indicated for retrobulbar block; however, this concentration is not indicated for any other peripheral nerve block, including the facial nerve, and not indicated for local infiltration, including the conjunctiva.

When 0.75% bupivacaine is used for retrobulbar block, complete corneal anesthesia usually precedes onset of clinically acceptable external ocular muscle akinesia. Therefore, presence of akinesia rather than anesthesia alone should determine readiness of the patient for surgery.

Retrobulbar injections of local anaesthetics carry a low risk of persistent ocular muscle dysfunction. The primary causes include trauma and/or local toxic effects on muscles and/or nerves. The severity of such tissue reactions is related to the degree of trauma, the concentration of the local anaesthetic and the duration of exposure of the tissue to the local anaesthetic. For this reason, as with all local anaesthetics, the lowest effective concentration and dose of local anaesthetic should be used. Vasoconstrictors and other additives may aggravate tissue reactions and should be used only when indicated.

Hepatic/Biliary/Pancreatic: Because amide-type local anaesthetics such as bupivacaine are metabolized by the liver, these drugs should be used cautiously in patients with hepatic disease. Patients with severe hepatic disease, because of their inability to metabolize local anaesthetics normally, are at a greater risk of developing toxic plasma concentrations.

Peri-Operative Considerations: It is essential that aspiration for blood or cerebrospinal fluid be done prior to injecting any local anesthetic, both the original dose and all subsequent doses, to avoid intravascular or subarachnoid injection. During the performance of spinal anesthesia, a free flow of cerebrospinal fluid is indicative of entry into the subarachnoid space. Aspiration should be performed before the anesthetic solution is injected to confirm entry into the subarachnoid space and to avoid intravascular injection. However, a negative aspiration does not ensure against an intravascular or subarachnoid injection.

The safety and effectiveness of local anesthetics depend on proper dosage, correct technique, adequate precautions and readiness for emergencies. Regional or local anesthetic procedures should always be performed in a properly equipped and staffed area.

Resuscitative equipment and resuscitative drugs, including oxygen, should be available for immediate use (see Warnings and Precautions and Adverse Reactions and Overdosage). During major regional nerve blocks, the patients should be in an optimal condition and have i.v. fluids running via an indwelling catheter to assure a functioning intravenous pathway. The clinician responsible should have adequate and appropriate training in the procedure to be performed, should take the necessary precautions to avoid intravascular injection (see Dosage and Administration), and should be familiar with the diagnosis and treatment of side effects, systemic toxicity and other complications (see Adverse Reactions and Overdosage).

Careful and constant monitoring of cardiovascular and respiratory vital signs (adequacy of ventilation) and the patient's state of consciousness should be performed after each local anaesthetic injection. It should be kept in mind at such times that restlessness, anxiety, incoherent speech, lightheadedness, numbness and tingling of the mouth and lips, metallic taste, tinnitus, dizziness, blurred vision, tremors, twitching, depression, or drowsiness may be early warning signs of central nervous system toxicity.

Renal: Local anaesthetics should be used with caution in patients in poor general condition due to severe renal dysfunction although regional anaesthesia is frequently indicated in these patients.

Hypersensitivity: MARCAINE E (bupivacaine hydrochloride with epinephrine) contains sodium metabisulfite, a sulfite that may cause allergic-type reactions including anaphylactic symptoms and life-threatening or less severe asthmatic episodes in certain susceptible people. The overall prevalence of sulfite sensitivity in the general population is unknown and probably low. Sulfite sensitivity is seen more frequently in asthmatic than in nonasthmatic people.

MARCAINE parenteral solutions in multidose vials are contraindicated in patients with known hypersensitivities to local anesthetics of the amide type, to other components in the formulation, parabens and their metabolite para amino benzoic acid (PABA). The use of paraben-containing bupivacaine preparations should also be avoided in patients who are allergic to ester local anesthetics (see Contraindications).

Special Populations: Debilitated and acutely ill patients should be given reduced doses commensurate with their age and physical condition.

Pregnant Women: Decrease pup survival in rats and an embryocidal effect in rabbits have been observed when bupivacaine hydrochloride was administered to these species in doses comparable, respectively, to nine and five times the maximal recommended daily human dose (400 mg).

There are no adequate and well-controlled studies in pregnant women of the effect of bupivacaine on the developing foetus.

Bupivacaine should be used during pregnancy only if the potential benefit justifies the potential risk to the foetus. This does not exclude the use of bupivacaine at term for obstetrical anaesthesia or analgesia.

Labour and Delivery: The highest (0.75%) isotonic concentration is not recommended for obstetrical anesthesia (see Warnings and Precautions). This, however, does not exclude the use of isotonic MARCAINE 0.25% or 0.50% or the spinal use of the hyperbaric MARCAINE 0.75% in dextrose at term for obstetrical anesthesia or analgesia.

Bupivacaine is contraindicated for obstetrical paracervical block anesthesia (see Warnings and Precautions). Local anaesthetics rapidly cross the placenta, and when used for epidural, caudal, or pudendal block anesthesia, can cause varying degrees of maternal, foetal and neonatal toxicity. The incidence and degree of toxicity depend upon the procedure performed, the type and amount of drug used, and the technique of drug administration. Adverse reactions in the parturient, foetus and neonate involve alterations of the central nervous system, peripheral vascular tone and cardiac function.

Maternal hypotension has resulted from regional anaesthesia (see Warnings and Precautions, Cardiovascular). Local anaesthetics produce vasodilation by blocking sympathetic nerves. It is extremely important to avoid aortocaval compression by the gravid uterus during administration of regional block to parturients. Elevating the patient's legs and positioning her on her left side will help prevent decreases in blood pressure. The foetal heart rate also should be monitored continuously, and electronic foetal monitoring is highly advisable.

Epidural anaesthesia may alter the forces of parturition through changes in uterine contractility or maternal expulsive efforts. Epidural anaesthesia has been reported to prolong the second stage of labour by removing the parturient's urge to bear down or by interfering with motor function. The use of MARCAINE 0.25% has been shown to interfere less than the 0.5% solution. Obstetrical anaesthesia may increase the need for forceps assistance.

The addition of epinephrine may potentially decrease uterine blood flow and contractility, especially after inadvertent injection into maternal blood vessels.

Nursing Women: Bupivacaine is excreted in the breast milk, but in such small quantities that there is generally no risk of affecting the infant at therapeutic doses. It is not known whether epinephrine enters breast milk or not, but it is unlikely to affect the breast-fed infant.

Pediatrics: Until further experience is gained in children younger than two years, administration of any presentation of bupivacaine injection in this age group is not recommended.

Until further experience is gained, the following restrictions apply to the use of MARCAINE: (a) isotonic bupivacaine solutions with or without epinephrine are not recommended for spinal use; (b) the 0.75% isotonic solution of bupivacaine with or without epinephrine is not recommended in patients younger than 12 years; (c) MARCAINE SPINAL (bupivacaine hydrochloride 0.75% hyperbaric solution in dextrose) is not recommended for spinal use in patients younger than 18 years.

Geriatrics: Elderly patients should be given reduced doses commensurate with their age and physical condition.

ADVERSE REACTIONS: Reactions to bupivacaine hydrochloride are characteristic of those associated with other local acting anesthetics of the amide type.

Adverse reactions to local anaesthetics are very rare in the absence of overdose or inadvertent intravascular injection. The effects of systemic overdose and unintentional intravascular injections can be serious, but should be distinguished from the physiological effects of the nerve block itself (e.g. a decrease in blood pressure and bradycardia during epidural anaesthesia). Neurological damage, caused directly (e.g. nerve trauma) or indirectly (e.g. epidural abscess) by the needle puncture, is a rare but well recognized consequence of regional, and particularly epidural anaesthesia.

The most commonly encountered acute adverse experiences that demand immediate management are related to the central nervous system and the cardiovascular system. These adverse reactions are generally dose-related and due to high plasma levels which may result from overdosage (see Overdosage), rapid absorption from the injection site, diminished tolerance or from inadvertent intravascular injection. Factors influencing plasma protein binding, e.g. diseases which alter protein synthesis or competition of other drugs for protein binding, may diminish individual tolerances.

In addition to systemic dose-related toxicity, unintentional subarachnoid injection of drug during the intended performance of caudal or lumbar epidural block or nerve blocks near the vertebral column (especially in the head and neck region) may result in underventilation or apnoea ("Total or High Spinal"). Also, hypotension due to loss of sympathetic tone and respiratory paralysis or underventilation due to cephalad extension of the motor level of anaesthesia may occur. This may lead to secondary cardiac arrest if untreated.

Central Nervous System: Restlessness, anxiety, dizziness, tinnitus, blurred vision or tremors may occur, possibly proceeding to convulsions. However, excitement may be transient or absent, with depression being the first manifestation of an adverse reaction. This may quickly be followed by drowsiness merging into unconsciousness and respiratory arrest. Other central nervous system effects may be nausea, vomiting, chills, paraesthesia, numbness of the tongue, hyperacousis, lightheadedness, dysarthria and constriction of the pupils.

Cardiovascular System: High doses or unintentional intravascular injection may lead to high plasma levels and related depression of the myocardium, decreased cardiac output, heart block, hypotension, bradycardia, hypertension, ventricular arrhythmias, including ventricular tachycardia and ventricular fibrillation, and cardiac arrest. Reactions due to systemic absorption may be either slow or rapid in onset. Cardiovascular collapse and cardiac arrest can occur rapidly (see Warnings and Precautions, Cardiovascular and Overdosage).

Allergic: Allergic type reactions are rare (<0.1%) and may occur as a result of sensitivity to local anaesthetics of the amide type. These reactions are characterized by signs such as urticaria, pruritus, erythema, angioneurotic oedema (including laryngeal oedema), tachycardia, sneezing, nausea, vomiting, dizziness, syncope, excessive sweating, elevated temperature, and in the most severe instances, anaphylactic shock.

Neurologic: The incidence of adverse neurologic reactions may be related to the total dose of local anaesthetic administered but is also dependent upon the particular drug used, the route of administration and the physical condition of the patient. Nerve trauma, neuropathy, urinary retention, diplopia and spinal cord dysfunction (e.g., anterior spinal artery syndrome, arachnoiditis, cauda equina syndrome, in rare cases paresis and paraplegia), have been associated with regional anaesthesia. Neurological effects may be related to local anaesthetic techniques, with or without a contribution from the drug.

High or Total Spinal Blockade: In the practice of caudal or lumbar epidural block, occasional unintentional penetration of the subarachnoid space by the catheter may occur, resulting in high or total spinal blockage. Subsequent adverse effects may depend partially on the amount of drug administered subdurally.

Extensive loss of motor and sensory functions, loss of consciousness and cardiovascular and respiratory depression may happen. The cardiovascular depression is caused by extensive sympathetic blockade which may result in profound hypotension and bradycardia, or even cardiac arrest. Respiratory depression is caused by blockade of the innervation of the respiratory muscles, including the diaphragm.

Spinal Use: The most commonly encountered adverse reactions which demand immediate countermeasures are HYPOTENSION due to loss of sympathetic tone and RESPIRATORY PARALYSIS OR UNDERVENTILATION due to cephalad extension of the motor level of anesthesia. These may lead to cardiac arrest if untreated.

In addition, one or several of the following complications or side effects may be observed during or after spinal anesthesia.

Meningitis: With the employment of an aseptic technique, septic meningitis should be practically nonexistent. Some instances of aseptic meningitis, with fever, neck rigidity, and cloudy spinal fluid, have been reported with the use of other spinal anesthetics. In such cases, the course is usually brief and benign, terminating in complete recovery.

However, in a few, permanent paralyses (sometimes terminating fatally) and sensory disturbances have been observed. This type of meningitis has also been observed in rare instances following ordinary diagnostic lumbar puncture.

Palsies: These are rare and affect either the extraocular muscles or the legs and the anal and vesical sphincters (cauda equina syndrome). Paralysis of extraocular muscles usually clears up spontaneously by the third or fourth week.

Clauda equina and lumbosacral cord complications (usually consisting of arachnoiditis and demyelinization) result in loss of impairment of motor and sensory function of the saddle area (bladder, rectum) and one or both legs. The complications have occurred after the use of most, if not all, spinal anesthetics. The loss or impairment of motor function may be permanent or partial recovery may slowly occur. Various explanations for such complications have been advanced, such as hypersensitivity or intolerance to the anesthetic agent with a resultant myelolytic or neurotoxic effect; pooling of relatively high concentrations of anesthetic solution around the cauda equina and spinal cord before diffusion; and accidental injection of irritating antiseptics or detergents (as when syringes and needles are incompletely cleansed or when ampoule storage enters a cracked ampoule). Hence, most anesthesiologists prefer to autoclave ampoules in order to destroy bacteria on the exterior before opening.

Headache: This may largely be prevented by using a small gauge needle to prevent spinal fluid leakage and by placing the patient in the supine position after operation and providing adequate hydration.

Nausea and Vomiting: These may be due to a drop in blood pressure, undue intra-abdominal manipulation or pre-operative medication.

DRUG INTERACTIONS: Drug-Drug Interactions: See Warnings and Precautions concerning solutions containing a vasoconstrictor.

Bupivacaine should be used cautiously in persons with known drug allergies or sensitivities.

Local Anaesthetics: Mixing or the prior or intercurrent use of any other local anesthetic with bupivacaine is not recommended because of insufficient data regarding the interaction and safety of such mixtures. Bupivacaine should be used with caution in patients receiving other amide-type local anaesthetics such as lidocaine, ropivacaine, mepivicaine and prilocaine since the toxic effects are additive.

Antiarrhythmic Drugs: Bupivacaine should also be used with caution with structurally related agents such as the antiarrhythmics, procainamide, disopyramide, tocainide, mexiletine and flecainide.

Class III Antiarrhythmic Drugs: Specific interaction studies with bupivacaine and class III antiarrhythmic drugs (e.g. amiodarone) have not been performed, but caution is advised. Patients being treated with class III antiarrhythmic drugs should be under close surveillance and ECG monitoring since cardiac affects may be additive.

Ergot-Containing Drugs: Bupivacaine with epinephrine or other vasopressors or vasoconstrictors should not be used concomitantly with ergot-type oxytocic drugs, because a severe persistent hypertension may occur and cerebrovascular and cardiac accidents are possible.

Monoamine Oxidase (MAO) Inhibitors: The administration of local anesthetic solutions containing epinephrine or norepinephrine to patients receiving monoamine oxidase inhibitors or tricyclic antidepressants may produce severe, prolonged hypertension. Concurrent use of these agents should generally be avoided. In situations when concurrent therapy is necessary, extreme caution and careful patient monitoring is essential.

Tricyclic Antidepressants (triptyline, imipramine): The administration of local anesthetic solutions containing epinephrine or norepinephrine to patients receiving tricyclic antidepressants may produce severe, prolonged hypertension. Concurrent use of these agents should generally be avoided. In situations when concurrent therapy is necessary, extreme caution and careful patient monitoring is essential.

Neuroleptics (phenothiazines, butyrophenones): Phenothiazines and butyrophenones may reduce or reverse the pressor effect of epinephrine resulting in hypotensive responses and tachycardia.

Sedatives: If sedatives are used to reduce patient apprehension, they should be used in reduced doses, since local anaesthetic agents, like sedatives, are central nervous system depressants which in combination may have an additive effect.

General Anaesthetics—Inhalation Agents (halothane, cyclopropane, trichloroethylene, enflurane and related agents): Dose-related cardiac arrhythmias may occur if preparations containing epinephrine are employed in patients during or immediately following the administration of general anaesthesia with inhalational agents such as halothane, cyclopropane, trichloroethylene, enflurane or other related agents. In deciding whether to use these products concurrently in the same patient, the combined action of both agents upon the myocardium, the concentration and volume of vascoconstrictor used, and the time since injection, when applicable, should be taken into account. Use of chloroprocaine or other local anaesthetics, prior to general anesthesia, may interfere with subsequent use of bupivacaine. Because of this, and because safety of intercurrent use with bupivacaine and other local anaesthetics has not been established, such use is not recommended.

H_2-Antagonists: The H_2-antagonists cimetidine and ranitidine have been shown to reduce the clearance of bupivacaine; ranitidine to a lesser degree than cimetidine. Concomitant administration may increase likelihood of toxicity of bupivacaine. Administration of H_2 blockers prior to epidural anesthesia is inadvisable since toxic levels of local anesthetic may result.

Non-Selective Beta-Blockers: Non-selective beta-blockers such as propranolol enhance the pressor effects of epinephrine, which may lead to severe hypertension and bradycardia.

Drug-Food Interactions: Interactions of bupivacaine with food have not been established.

Drug-Herb Interactions: Interactions of bupivacaine with herbal products have not been established.

Drug-Laboratory Test Interactions: Interactions of bupivacaine with laboratory tests have not been established.

Drug-Lifestyle Interactions: Interactions of bupivacaine with lifestyle have not been established.

DOSAGE AND ADMINISTRATION: Dosing Considerations: General: As with all local anesthetics, the dosage of bupivacaine varies and depends upon the area to be anesthetized, the vascularity of the tissues, the number of neuronal segments to be blocked, the depth of anesthesia and degree of muscle relaxation required, individual tolerance, the technique of anesthesia and the physical condition of the patient. The lowest dosage and concentration needed to provide effective anesthesia should be administered. The rapid injection of a large volume of local anaesthetic solution should be avoided and fractional doses should be used when feasible. In general, complete block of all nerve fibres in large nerves requires the higher concentrations of drug. In smaller nerves, or when a less intense block is required (e.g., in the relief of labour pain), the lower concentrations are indicated. The volume of drug used will affect the extent of spread of anaesthesia.

The use of bupivacaine with epinephrine will prolong the anaesthetic action.

In recommended doses, bupivacaine produces complete sensory block, but the effect on motor function differs among the three concentrations.

- 0.25%, when used for caudal, epidural, or peripheral nerve block, produces incomplete motor block. Should be used for operations in which muscle relaxation is not important, or when another means of providing muscle relaxation is used concurrently. Onset of action may be slower than with the 0.50% or 0.75% solutions.
- 0.50% provides motor blockade for caudal, epidural, or nerve block, but muscle relaxation may be inadequate for operations in which complete muscle relaxation is essential.
- 0.75% produces complete motor block. This concentration is recommended only for epidural block (single dose) in abdominal operations requiring complete muscle relaxation without the aid of other medication, and for retrobulbar anesthesia. It is not recommended for epidural block in obstetrical patients.

Special Populations: Local anaesthetics should be used with caution in patients in poor general condition due to aging or other compromising factors such as advanced liver disease or severe renal dysfunction although regional anaesthesia is frequently indicated in these patients.

Debilitated, elderly patients and acutely ill patients should be given reduced doses commensurate with their age and physical condition.

Recommended Dose and Dosage Adjustment: The duration of anesthesia with bupivacaine is such that, for most procedures, a single dose is sufficient. Maximum dosage limit must be individualized in each case after evaluating the size and physical status of the patient, as well as the usual rate of systemic absorption from a particular injection site. Most experience to date is with single doses of bupivacaine up to 225 mg with epinephrine 1:200 000 and 175 mg without epinephrine; more or less drug may be used depending on individualization of each case. The maximum doses of bupivacaine are considered to apply to a healthy 70 kilogram, young male. However, it is not recommended that they be exceeded in heavier persons.

At present, there is insufficient clinical evidence with multiple dosage or intermittent dose techniques to permit precise recommendations for such procedures to be given. However, limited clinical experience in this area of use indicates that bupivacaine may be repeated in 3 to 6 hours; total daily doses have been up to 400 mg. The duration of anesthetic effect may be prolonged by the addition of a vasoconstricting substance, e.g. epinephrine.

The 0.75% concentration of isotonic MARCAINE (bupivacaine hydrochloride) is not recommended for obstetrical anesthesia or analgesia (see Warnings and Precautions). The 0.50% and 0.25% concentrations of isotonic MARCAINE and the 0.75% hyperbaric solution of MARCAINE in dextrose are recommended at term for obstetrical anesthesia and analgesia.

When prolonged blocks are used, the risks of reaching a toxic plasma concentration or inducing a local neural injury must be considered. The maximum dosage limit must be determined by evaluating the size and physical condition of the patient and considering the usual rate of systemic absorption from a specific injection site. Experience to date indicates that 400 mg administered over 24 hours is well tolerated in average adults. Until further experience is gained, this dose should not be exceeded in 24 hours.

To avoid intravascular injection, aspiration should be repeated prior to and during administration of the main dose, which should be injected slowly or in incremental doses, at a rate of 25-50 mg/min, while closely observing the patient's vital functions and maintaining verbal contact. An inadvertent intravascular injection may be recognized by a temporary increase in heart rate and an accidental intrathecal injection by signs of a spinal block. If toxic symptoms occur, the injection should be stopped immediately.

Adults: Table 1 is presented as a guide to the use of bupivacaine in adults. The doses shown have generally proved satisfactory for the average patient. They may require reduction in relation to age and the physical condition of the patient. The clinician's experience and knowledge of the patient's physical condition are of importance in calculating the required dose.

Table 1: MARCAINE
Dosage Recommendations in Adults

Type of Block	Conc. (%)	Each Dose[a] mL	mg	Onset (min.)	Duration (h) Without Epinephrine	Indication
Local infiltration	0.25 0.5	up to 60[b] up to 30[b]	up to 150[b] up to 150[b]	1–3 1–3	3–4 4–8	Surgical operations and postoperative analgesia.
Epidural	0.5[c]	3–5	15–25			Test dose.
Lumbar epidural	0.25 0.5	6–15 15–30	15–37.5 75–150	2–5 15–30	1–2 2–3	Labour and postoperative pain relief. Surgical operations including Caesarean section.
Thoracic epidural	0.25 0.5	5–15 5–10	12.5–37.5 25–50	10–15 10–15	1.5–2 2–3	Surgical operations.
Caudal epidural	0.25 0.5	20–30 20–30	50–75 100–150	20–30 15–30	1–2 2–3	Pain relief and diagnostic use. Surgical operations and postoperative analgesia.
Intercostal (per nerve)	0.5	2–3	10–15	3–5	4–8	Pain relief for surgery, postoperative and trauma.
Brachial plexus	0.5	30	150	15–30	4–8	Surgical operations.
Sciatic	0.5	10–20	50–100	15–30	4–8	Surgical operations.
Digital[d]	0.25	1–5	2.5–12.5	2–5	3–4	Surgical operations.
Peripheral nerves	0.25 0.5	up to 40[b] up to 30[b]	up to 100[b] up to 150[b]	10–20 5–10	3–5 4–8	Therapeutic (pain relief). Surgical operations.
Sympathetic[e] Stellate block	0.25	5–15	12.5–37.5	20—20	3–6	Ischemic conditions or sympathetic maintained pains e.g., visceral pain conditions such as pancreatitis or cancer, pain of herpes zoster.
Lumbar Paravertebral block	0.25	10–20	25–50	10–20	3–6	
Coeliac Plexus block	0.25	20–40	50–100	10–20	3–6	

[a] For epidural blocks, dose includes test dose.
[b] No more than 400 mg in 24 hours.
[c] With epinephrine 1:200 000 (5 μg/mL).
[d] Without epinephrine.
[e] See Warnings and Precautions.

Children: Until further experience is gained, bupivacaine is not recommended for children younger than two years of age. The following restrictions apply to the use of MARCAINE (bupivacaine hydrochloride), MARCAINE E (bupivacaine hydrochloride with epinephrine) and MARCAINE SPINAL (bupivacaine hydrochloride) for children over two years of age: (a) isotonic bupivacaine solutions with or without epinephrine are not recommended for spinal use; (b) the 0.75% isotonic solution of bupivacaine with or without epinephrine is not recommended in patients younger than 12 years; (c) MARCAINE SPINAL (bupivacaine hydrochloride 0.75% hyperbaric solution in dextrose) is not recommended for spinal use in patients younger than 18 years.

For bolus administration or intermittent injections, unless stated otherwise (see Table 2), a dose of up to 2 mg/kg of bupivacaine or bupivacaine with epinephrine is recommended. The dose administered will depend on the age and body weight of the patient, the site of surgery, and the condition of the patient. The addition of epinephrine will prolong the duration of the block by 50-100%. For the appropriate suggested concentrations and dosage, see Table 2.

Table 2: MARCAINE
Dosage Recommendations in Children (over two years of age) for Bupivacaine with and without Epinephrine—Isotonic Solutions

Type of Block	Conc. (%)	Each Dose mL/kg	Each Dose mg/kg
Local infiltration	0.25 0.5	up to 0.8 up to 0.4	up to 2 up to 2
Caudal epidural[c]			
Lumbosacral	0.25	0.5	1.25[d]
Thoracolumbar	0.25	0.6–1.0	1.5–2.5[d]
Lumbar epidural	0.25 0.5	0.5–1.0 0.3–0.5	1.25–2.5 1.5–2.5
Dorsal (penile)	0.25[a] 0.5[a]	0.1–0.2 0.1–0.2	0.25–0.5 0.5–1.0
Intercostal	0.25[b] 0.5[b]	0.8–1.2 0.4–0.6	2–3 2–3

[a] Without epinephrine.
[b] With epinephrine 1:200 000 (5 μg/mL).
[c] Consider both age and weight for calculation of dosages.
[d] Onset: 20-30 minutes, Duration: 2-6 hours.

Note: The use of bupivacaine with and without epinephrine for anaesthesia and/or analgesia may be supplementary to light general anaesthesia.

Use in Epidural Anaesthesia: When an epidural dose is to be injected, a test dose of a local anaesthetic is recommended (see Warnings and Precautions). MARCAINE E 0.5% (bupivacaine with epinephrine), or 3-5 mL lidocaine (Xylocaine 1-2%) with epinephrine, can be used if a vasoconstrictor is not contraindicated. Verbal contact and repeated monitoring of heart rate and blood pressure should be maintained for five minutes after the test dose. In the absence of signs of subarachnoid or intravascular injection, the main dose may be given.

During epidural administration, bupivacaine should be administered slowly in incremental doses of 3 to 5 mL, with sufficient time between doses to detect toxic manifestations of unintentional intravascular or intrathecal injection.

Solutions in multidose vials contain methylparaben (antimicrobial preservative) and should not be used since their safety has not been established (see Contraindications).

Spinal Use: Bupivacaine for spinal anesthesia is available as a 0.75% hyperbaric solution.

The smallest dose required to produce the desired result should be administered and the dosage should be reduced for elderly and debilitated patients and patients with cardiac and/or liver disease. The use of the hyperbaric solution should permit improved control of the extent of anesthesia since the solution will have a higher specific gravity than spinal fluid.

Bupivacaine in dextrose (0.75% hyperbaric solution) is not recommended in patients younger than 18 years of age.

Table 3: MARCAINE
Recommended Adult Dosage Limits for Spinal Anesthesia

Extent of Anesthesia	Bupivacaine 0.75% Hyperbaric Solution Dosage (mL)	(mg)	Injection Site (lumbar interspace)
Low Spinal and Saddle block for perineal operations	0.8–1.06	6–8	4th
Median Spinal for operations on lower abdomen	1.06–1.6	8–12	3rd or 4th
High Spinal for operations on upper abdomen	1.6–2.0	12–15	2nd, 3rd or 4th

Solutions in multidose vials contain methylparaben (antimicrobial preservative) and should not be used for epidural or spinal anesthesia or for any route of administration that would introduce solution into the cerebrospinal fluid. Local anesthetic solutions containing antimicrobial preservatives solutions should not be administered intra-ocularly or retro-ocularly. These solutions should not be used in doses greater than 15 mL for other types of blockades (see Contraindications).

The extent and degree of spinal anesthesia depend on: the dose of anesthetic (see Table 3), the specific gravity of the anesthetic solution, the volume of solution administered, the force of injection, the level of puncture and the position of the patient during and immediately after injection.

The lateral recumbent position is the customary one for injection; however, when both perineal and abdominal anesthesia are required, the sitting position may be preferred. After preliminary antiseptic preparation of the back, the spinal interspace to be punctured is marked and anesthetized with 1 to 2 mL of 0.25% bupivacaine HCl solution.

Ephedrine (25 mg) may be administered if needed to maintain blood pressure.

After the spinal anesthetic has been administered, the specific gravity of the solution injected determines which position the patient should be placed in, at least for the first 15 to 20 minutes. Continuous sensory tests should be made by gentle strokes with a sharp instrument or by pinching the skin, comparing the sensitivity to that of the inside of the forearm.

Since hypalgesia always precedes anesthesia, it is necessary to determine the line of demarcation between hypalgesia and normal sensation, to avoid extension of anesthesia above the desired segment.

After injection of a 0.75% hyperbaric solution for spinal anesthesia, the patient is immediately placed on his back and the table tilted to a 10 to 20 degree Trendelenburg position in order to allow the solution to flow cephalad.

Under no circumstances should a patient be left in a head-down position longer than one minute from the start of injection without testing the height of anesthesia. The neck is sharply flexed by supporting the head on a double pillow. When hypalgesia is extended to the desired height, the table is promptly brought to the horizontal position and time (about 10 to 20 minutes) allowed for the anesthetic agent to become fixed.

OVERDOSAGE:

Acute systemic toxicity from local anaesthetics is generally related to high plasma levels encountered during therapeutic use of local anaesthetics, or to unintended subarachnoid or intravascular injection, exceptionally rapid absorption from highly vascularized areas or overdosage and originates mainly in the central nervous and the cardiovascular systems (see Adverse Reactions and Warnings and Precautions). Central nervous system reactions are similar for all amide local anaesthetics, while cardiac reactions are more dependent on the drug, both quantitatively and qualitatively.

Symptoms: Accidental intravascular injections of local anaesthetics may cause immediate (within seconds to a few minutes) systemic toxic reactions. In the event of overdose, systemic toxicity appears later (15-60 minutes after injection) due to the slower increase in local anaesthetic blood concentration.

Central nervous system toxicity is a graded response with symptoms and signs of escalating severity. The first symptoms are usually circumoral paresthesia, numbness of the tongue, lightheadedness, hyperacousis, tinnitus and visual disturbances. Dysarthria, muscular twitching or tremors are more serious and precede the onset of generalized convulsions. These signs must not be mistaken for a neurotic behaviour. Unconsciousness and grand mal convulsions may follow which may last from a few seconds to several minutes. Hypoxia and hypercarbia occur rapidly following convulsions due to the increased muscular activity, together with the interference with normal respiration and loss of the airway. In severe cases apnoea may occur. Acidosis, hyperkalaemia, hypocalcaemia and hypoxia increase and extend the toxic effects of local anaesthetics.

Recovery is due to redistribution and subsequent metabolism and excretion of the local anaesthetic drug. Recovery may be rapid unless large amounts of the drug have been administered.

Cardiovascular system toxicity may be seen in severe cases and is generally preceded by signs of toxicity in the central nervous system. In patients under heavy sedation or receiving a general anaesthetic, prodromal CNS symptoms may be absent. Hypotension, bradycardia, arrhythmia and even cardiac arrest may occur as a result of high systemic concentrations of local anaesthetics, but in rare cases cardiac arrest has occurred without prodromal CNS effects.

Cardiovascular toxic reactions are usually related to depression of the conduction system of the heart and myocardium, leading to decreased cardiac output, hypotension, heart block, bradycardia and sometimes ventricular arrhythmias, including ventricular tachycardia, ventricular fibrillation and cardiac arrest.

In children, early signs of local anaesthetic toxicity may be difficult to detect in cases where the block is given during general anaesthesia.

Treatment: The first consideration is prevention, best accomplished by careful and constant monitoring of cardiovascular and respiratory vital signs and the patient's state of consciousness after each local anesthetic injection. At the first sign of change, oxygen should be administered. If signs of acute systemic toxicity appear, injection of the local anaesthetic should be immediately stopped.

The first step in the management of systemic toxic reactions, as well as underventilation or apnea, consists of the immediate establishment and maintenance of a patent airway and assisted or controlled ventilation with 100% oxygen and a delivery system capable of permitting immediate positive airway pressure by mask or endotracheal intubation. This may prevent convulsions if they have not already occurred.

Supportive treatment of the cardiovascular system includes intravenous fluids and, when appropriate, vasopressors (such as epinephrine or ephedrine which enhance myocardial contractility).

If necessary, use drugs to control convulsions. A bolus i.v. injection of a muscle relaxant (e.g., succinylcholine 1 mg/kg bw) will paralyze the patient without depressing the central nervous or cardiovascular systems and facilitate endotracheal intubation, controlled ventilation, and secure optimal oxygenation. An anticonvulsant should be given i.v. if the convulsions do not stop spontaneously in 15-20 seconds. A bolus i.v. dose of diazepam (0.1 mg/kg) or thiopental (1-3 mg/kg) will permit ventilation and counteract central nervous system stimulation, but these drugs also depress central nervous system, respiratory, and cardiac function, add to possible depression, and may result in apnea. Thiopental will control convulsions rapidly, while the action of diazepam will be slower. Prolonged convulsions may jeopardize the patient's ventilation and oxygenation. Intravenous barbiturates, anticonvulsant agents, or muscle relaxants should only be administered by those familiar with their use. For specific techniques and procedures, refer to standard textbooks.

Recent clinical data from patients experiencing local anesthetic-induced convulsions demonstrated rapid development of hypoxia, hypercarbia and acidosis with bupivacaine within a minute of the onset of convulsions. These observations suggest that oxygen consumption and carbon dioxide production are greatly increased during local anesthetic convulsions and emphasize the importance of immediate and effective ventilation with oxygen which may avoid cardiac arrest.

If cardiovascular depression is evident (hypotension, bradycardia), ephedrine 5-10 mg i.v. should be given and may be repeated, if necessary, after 2-3 minutes. Children should be given ephedrine doses commensurate with their age and weight.

Should circulatory arrest occur, immediate cardiopulmonary resuscitation should be instituted. Optimal oxygenation and ventilation and circulatory support as well as treatment of acidosis are of vital importance, since hypoxia and acidosis will increase the systemic toxicity of local anaesthetics. Epinephrine (0.1-0.2 mg intravenous or intracardial injections) should be given as soon as possible and repeated, if necessary. A successful resuscitation may require prolonged efforts.

The supine position is dangerous in pregnant women at term because of aortocaval compression by the gravid uterus. Therefore, during treatment of systemic toxicity, maternal hypotension or foetal bradycardia following regional block, the parturient should be maintained in the left lateral decubitus position if possible, or manual displacement of the uterus off the great vessels should be accomplished. Resuscitation of obstetrical patients may take longer than resuscitation of nonpregnant patients and closed-chest cardiac compression may be ineffective. Rapid delivery of the foetus may improve the response to resuscitative efforts.

If cardiac arrest should occur, a successful outcome may require prolonged resuscitative efforts.

> For management of a suspected drug overdose, contact your regional Poison Control Centre. See the *CPS* Directory section for a list of Poison Control Centres.

ACTION AND CLINICAL PHARMACOLOGY: Bupivacaine is a long-acting, amide-type local anaesthetic with both anaesthetic and analgesic effects. At high doses it produces surgical anaesthesia, while at lower doses it produces sensory block (analgesia) with less pronounced motor block.

Mechanism of Action: Bupivacaine stabilizes the neuronal membrane and prevents both the generation and the conduction of nerve impulses, thereby exerting a local anesthetic action. As with other local anaesthetics, bupivacaine causes a reversible blockade of impulse propagation along nerve fibres by preventing the inward movement of sodium ions through the cell membrane of the nerve fibres. The sodium channel of the nerve membrane is considered a receptor for local anaesthetic molecules.

Onset and Duration of Action: The onset of action is rapid, and anesthesia is long lasting. The duration of action of a local anesthetic is dependent on a number of factors including site of injection, route of administration, concentration and volume (see Dosage and Administration). It has also been noted that there is a period of analgesia that persists after the return of sensation, during which time the need for strong analgesics is reduced. The presence of epinephrine may prolong the duration of action for infiltration and peripheral nerve blocks but has less marked effect on epidural blocks.

MARCAINE 0.5% has a long duration of action of 2-5 hours following a single epidural injection and up to 12 hours after peripheral nerve blocks. The onset of blockade is slower than with lidocaine, especially when anaesthetizing large nerves. When used in low concentrations, i.e., 0.25%, there is less effect on motor nerve fibres and the duration of action is shorter.

Hemodynamics: Bupivacaine, like other local anaesthetics, may also have effects on other excitable membranes e.g. in the brain and myocardium. If excessive amounts of drug reach the systemic circulation rapidly, symptoms and signs of toxicity will appear, emanating mainly from the central nervous and cardiovascular systems.

Central nervous system toxicity (see Overdosage) usually precedes the cardiovascular effects as central nervous system toxicity occurs at lower plasma concentrations. Direct effects of local anaesthetics on the heart include slow conduction, negative inotropism and eventually cardiac arrest.

Indirect cardiovascular effects (hypotension, bradycardia) may occur after epidural administration depending on the extent of the concomitant sympathetic block.

Pharmacokinetics: Absorption: The plasma concentration of local anaesthetics is dependent upon the dose, the route of administration, the patient's hemodynamic/circulatory condition, and the vascularity of the injection site. The addition of epinephrine to bupivacaine may decrease the peak plasma concentration, whereas the time to peak plasma concentration usually is little affected. The effect varies with the type of block, dose and concentration.

Following injection of MARCAINE for caudal, epidural, or peripheral nerve block in man, peak levels of MARCAINE in the blood are reached in 30 to 45 minutes, followed by a gradual decline to insignificant levels during the next three to six hours. Intercostal blocks give the highest peak plasma concentration due to a rapid absorption (maximum plasma concentrations in the order of 1-4 mg/L after a 400 mg dose), while subcutaneous abdominal injections give the lowest plasma concentration. Epidural and major plexus blocks are intermediate. In children, rapid absorption and high plasma concentrations (in the order of 1-1.5 mg/L after a dose of 3 mg/kg) are seen with caudal block.

Bupivacaine shows complete, biphasic absorption from the epidural space with plasma half-lives in the order of seven minutes after initial administration, slowing to six hours over time. The slow absorption is rate-limiting in the elimination of bupivacaine, which explains why the apparent elimination half-life after epidural administration is longer than after intravenous administration.

Distribution: Local anesthetics are bound to plasma proteins in varying degrees. The highly lipophilic agents, such as bupivacaine, are far more highly protein-bound than the more hydrophilic compounds. Bupivacaine is approximately 95% protein-bound in normal adults. Generally, the lower the plasma concentration of drug, the higher the percentage of drug bound to plasma proteins. If plasma protein concentrations are decreased, more of the free drug will be available to exert activity. Bupivacaine is mainly bound to alpha-1-acid glycoprotein.

Bupivacaine readily crosses the placenta and equilibrium in regard to the unbound concentration is rapidly reached. The rate and degree of diffusion is governed by (1) the degree of plasma protein binding, (2) the degree of ionization and (3) the degree of lipid solubility. The degree of plasma protein binding in the foetus is less than in the mother, which results in lower total plasma concentrations in the foetus than in the mother. The free concentration, however, is the same in both mother and foetus.

Fetal/maternal ratios of local anesthetics appear to be inversely related to the degree of plasma protein binding because only the free, unbound drug is available for placental transfer. MARCAINE with a high protein binding capacity (95%) has a low fetal/maternal ratio (0.2 to 0.4).

Bupivacaine has a total plasma clearance of 0.58 L/min a volume of distribution at steady state of 73 L.

An increase in total plasma concentration has been observed during continuous epidural infusion for postoperative pain relief. This is related to a postoperative increase in alpha-1-acid glycoprotein. The unbound, i.e. pharmacologically active, concentration is similar before and after surgery.

Metabolism: Because of its amide structure, bupivacaine is extensively metabolized in the liver predominantly by aromatic hydroxylation to 4-hydroxy-bupivacaine and N-dealkylation to 2,6-pipecoloxylidine (PPX), both mediated by cytochrome P450 3A4. The major metabolite of bupivacaine is pipecoloxylidine, a dealkylated derivative. Patients with hepatic disease may be more susceptible to the potential toxicities of the amide-type local anesthetics.

Excretion: The plasma elimination half-life of MARCAINE in adults is 2.7 hours (range 1.2 to 4.6 hours). In infants, the half-life ranges from 6 to 22 hours, thus it is significantly longer than in adults. Half-life is also prolonged in the elderly. Bupivacaine has an intermediate hepatic extraction ratio of 0.38 after i.v. administration. In children between 1 to 7 years the pharmacokinetics are similar to those in adults.

The kidney is the main excretory organ for most local anesthetics and their metabolites. Urinary excretion is affected by renal perfusion and factors affecting urinary pH.

Clearance of bupivacaine is almost entirely due to liver metabolism and more sensitive to changes in intrinsic hepatic enzyme function than to liver perfusion.

STORAGE AND STABILITY: Store MARCAINE (bupivacaine hydrochloride), MARCAINE SPINAL (bupivacaine hydrochloride) and MARCAINE E (bupivacaine hydrochloride with epinephrine) at 20-25°C. Do not freeze. Protect MARCAINE E (bupivacaine hydrochloride with epinephrine) from light. Do not use if solution is coloured or contains a precipitate.

SPECIAL HANDLING INSTRUCTIONS: Adequate precautions should be taken to avoid prolonged contact between local anaesthetic solutions containing epinephrine (low pH) and metal surfaces (e.g., needles or metal parts of syringes), since dissolved metal ions, particularly copper ions, may cause severe local irritation (swelling, oedema) at the site of injection and accelerate the degradation of epinephrine.

Isotonic Solutions: These solutions are not for spinal anesthesia.

Bupivacaine hydrochloride solutions of MARCAINE that do not contain epinephrine may be autoclaved. Autoclave at 15-pound pressure, 121°C for 15 minutes. Do not use if solution is discoloured or contains a precipitate.

Bupivacaine Hydrochloride with Epinephrine 1:200 000 (as bitartrate): Due to the heat sensitivity of epinephrine, solutions of MARCAINE E (which contain epinephrine) must not be autoclaved and should be protected from light. Do not use if solution is pinkish or darker than slightly yellow or contains a precipitate.

Adequate precautions should be taken to avoid prolonged contact between local anaesthetic solutions containing epinephrine (low pH) and metal surfaces (e.g., needles or metal parts of syringes), since dissolved metal ions, particularly copper ions, may cause severe local irritation (swelling, oedema) at the site of injection and accelerate the degradation of epinephrine.

INFORMATION FOR THE PATIENT: Published in e-CPS, available by subscription at www.e-cps.ca.

DOSAGE FORMS, COMPOSITION AND PACKAGING: The solubility of bupivacaine is limited at pH >6.5. This must be taken into consideration when alkaline solutions, i.e., carbonates, are added since precipitation might occur. In the case of epinephrine-containing solutions, mixing with alkaline solutions may cause rapid degradation of epinephrine.

Isotonic Solutions: 0.25%: Each mL contains: bupivacaine hydrochloride 2.5 mg. Also contains sodium chloride and water for injection. May also contain sodium hydroxide and/or hydrochloric acid (for pH adjustment). Single-dose vials of 10 mL (without preservative), boxes of 5. Single-dose vials of 20 mL (without preservative), boxes of 5. Multiple-dose vials of 50 mL (with methylparaben as preservative), boxes of 1.

0.50%: Each mL contains: bupivacaine hydrochloride 5 mg. Also contains sodium chloride and water for injection. May also contain sodium hydroxide and/or hydrochloric acid (for pH adjustment). Single-dose vials of 10 mL (without preservative), boxes of 5. Single-dose vials of 20 mL (without preservative), boxes of 5. Multiple-dose vials of 50 mL (with methylparaben as preservative), boxes of 1.

0.75%: Each mL contains: bupivacaine hydrochloride 7.5 mg. Also contains sodium chloride and water for injection. May also contain sodium hydroxide and/or hydrochloric acid (for pH adjustment). Single dose vials of 20 mL (without preservative), boxes of 5.

Bupivacaine Hydrochloride with Epinephrine 1:200 000 (as bitartrate): 0.25% with Epinephrine 1:200 000: Each mL contains: bupivacaine hydrochloride 2.5 mg and epinephrine. Single-dose vials of 20 mL (without preservative), boxes of 5.

0.50% with Epinephrine 1:200 000: Each mL contains: bupivacaine hydrochloride 5 mg and epinephrine. Single-dose vials of 20 mL (without preservative), boxes of 5.

These solutions are made isotonic with NaCl and the pH is adjusted with NaOH or HCl. The pH range for solutions without epinephrine is 4.0 to 6.5 and, for solutions with epinephrine, is 3.4 to 4.5. Each mL of solution with epinephrine contains 0.0091 mg epinephrine bitartrate and, as nonmedicinal ingredients, 0.5 mg sodium metabisulfite, 1.25 mg monothioglycerol, and 2 mg ascorbic acid as antioxidants, 1.33 mg sodium lactate buffer and 0.1 mg edetate calcium disodium as stabilizer.

0.75% Hyperbaric Solution for Spinal Use Only: Each mL of solution contains: bupivacaine hydrochloride 7.5 mg and dextrose 82.5 mg in water for injection. The pH is adjusted between 4 and 6.5 with NaOH or HCl. The solution may be autoclaved once at 15 pound pressure, 121°C for 15 minutes. Do not administer any solution which is discolored or contains particulate matter. Single-dose ampoules of 2 mL containing 0.75% hyperbaric solution, boxes of 10.

Marinol® Ⓝ

delta-9-tetrahydrocannabinol

Antiemetic

Abbott Products

Date of Revision: April 14, 2010

SUMMARY PRODUCT INFORMATION:

Route of Administration	Dosage Form/ Strength	Clinically Relevant Nonmedicinal Ingredients
Oral	2.5 mg capsule	Sesame oil
	5 mg capsule	Iron oxide red, iron oxide black, sesame oil
	10 mg capsule	Iron oxide red, iron oxide yellow, sesame oil
For a complete list of nonmedicinal ingredients see Dosage Forms, Composition and Packaging.		

INDICATIONS AND CLINICAL USE: Adults: MARINOL (dronabinol) may be of value in the treatment of:

- AIDS-related anorexia associated with weight loss
- severe nausea and vomiting associated with cancer chemotherapy

MARINOL is a psychotropic agent which may produce physical and psychological dependence and has the potential to be abused. The active component THC is scheduled under the Controlled Drugs and Substances Act and as such cannot be used or prescribed except for its recognized indications.

Long-Term Use of MARINOL: MARINOL has not been systematically evaluated beyond 6 weeks in controlled clinical trials for AIDS-related anorexia associated with weight loss. The physician who elects to use MARINOL for extended periods in this indication should periodically re-evaluate the long-term usefulness of the drug for the individual patient.

Geriatrics (>65 years of age): Evidence from clinical studies and experience indicates that elderly patients are generally more sensitive to the psychoactive effects of drugs and a brief discussion can be found in the appropriate sections (Warnings and Precautions, Special Populations, Geriatrics and Dosage and Administration, Geriatrics).

Pediatrics (<18 years of age): The safety and efficacy of MARINOL have not been established in adolescents or children under 18 years of age, therefore MARINOL should not be used in adolescents or children (see Contraindications).

CONTRAINDICATIONS: MARINOL (dronabinol) is contraindicated in:

- patients with known or suspected allergy to marijuana, other cannabinoids or sesame oil
- patients with significant hepatic or renal impairment
- patients with serious cardiovascular disease, such as ischaemic heart disease, arrhythmias, poorly controlled hypertension or severe heart failure
- patients with a history of schizophrenia or any other psychotic disorder
- children under 18 years of age
- women of child-bearing potential not on a reliable contraceptive or men intending to father a child (see Use in Women of Child-Bearing Potential)
- pregnant or nursing women (see Pregnant Women and Nursing Women)

WARNINGS AND PRECAUTIONS:

> **Serious Warnings and Precautions**
> THC, the active component of MARINOL, can produce physical and psychological dependence and has the potential for being abused.
>
> THC has complex effects on the central nervous system, some of which are called "intoxication type reactions". These can result in changes of mood, decrease in cognitive performances and memory, decrease in ability to control drives and impulses, and alteration of the perception of reality, particularly altered time sense. Fainting episodes have been observed with use of cannabinoids. "Intoxication type reactions" (feeling drunk, disturbance in attention, dizziness, somnolence, disorientation, dissociation, euphoric mood, etc.) appear to be dose-related, increasing in frequency with higher dosages, and subject to great inter-patient variability. They usually remit on reduction of doses, increasing the interval between doses or interruption of the drug. Because of the potential of THC to alter the mental state, MARINOL should be used only as indicated and prescriptions should be limited to the amount necessary for the period between clinic visits.
>
> Drug administration should be discontinued in patients experiencing a psychotic reaction and the patient should be closely observed in an appropriate setting until his/her mental state returns to normal. Patients should be warned not to drive or engage in activities requiring unimpaired judgement and coordination.
>
> Cannabinoids have cardiovascular effects that include tachycardia, and transient changes in blood pressure, including episodes of postural hypotension. Use of MARINOL is not recommended in patients with pre-existing cardiovascular disease, such as ischaemic heart disease, arrhythmias, poorly controlled hypertension or severe heart failure.
>
> Published reports on cannabinoids are equivocal with regard to the effects of THC on seizure threshold. Until further information is available, caution should be used when treating patients with a history of epilepsy or recurrent seizures.

General: The risk/benefit ratio of MARINOL use should be carefully evaluated because of individual variation in response and tolerance to the effects of MARINOL.

The following additional precautions are listed alphabetically.

Cardiovascular: MARINOL is not recommended in patients with cardiac disorders because of occasional hypotension, possible hypertension, syncope, or tachycardia (see Contraindications and Action and Clinical Pharmacology).

Dependence/Tolerance: MARINOL should be used with caution in patients with a history of substance abuse, including alcohol abuse or dependence, because they may be more prone to abuse MARINOL as well. Multiple substance abuse is common and marijuana, which contains the same active compound, is a frequently abused substance.

MARINOL is one of the psychoactive compounds present in cannabis, and is abusable and controlled (Schedule II) under the Controlled Drugs and Substances Act. Both psychological and physiological dependence have been noted in healthy individuals receiving dronabinol, but addiction is uncommon and has only been seen after prolonged high dose administration.

Chronic abuse of cannabis has been associated with decrements in motivation, cognition, judgement, and perception. The etiology of these impairments is unknown, but may be associated with the complex process of addiction rather than an isolated effect of the drug. No such decrements in psychological, social or neurological status have been associated with the administration of MARINOL for therapeutic purposes.

In an open-label study in patients with AIDS who received MARINOL for up to five months, no abuse, diversion or systematic change in personality or social functioning were observed despite the inclusion of a substantial number of patients with a past history of drug abuse.

An abstinence syndrome has been reported after the abrupt discontinuation of dronabinol in volunteers receiving dosages of 210 mg/day for 12 to 16 consecutive days. Within 12 hours after discontinuation, these volunteers manifested symptoms such as irritability, insomnia, and restlessness. By approximately 24 hours post-dronabinol discontinuation, withdrawal symptoms intensified to include "hot flashes", sweating, rhinorrhea, loose stools, hiccoughs and anorexia.

These withdrawal symptoms gradually dissipated over the next 48 hours. Electroencephalographic changes consistent with the effects of drug withdrawal (hyperexcitation) were recorded in patients after abrupt dechallenge. Patients also complained of disturbed sleep for several weeks after discontinuing therapy with high dosages of dronabinol.

Neurologic: Patients receiving treatment with MARINOL should be alerted to the potential for additive central nervous system depression if MARINOL is used concomitantly with alcohol or other CNS depressants such as benzodiazepines and barbiturates.

Patients receiving treatment with MARINOL should be specifically warned not to drive, operate machinery, or engage in any hazardous activity until it is established that they are able to tolerate the drug and to perform such tasks safely.

Psychiatric: MARINOL should not be used in patients with mania, depression, or schizophrenia because MARINOL may exacerbate these illnesses (see Contraindications).

MARINOL should be used with caution, if at all, in patients receiving concomitant therapy with sedatives, hypnotics or other psychoactive drugs because of the potential for additive or synergistic CNS effects.

Patients using MARINOL should be advised of possible changes in mood and other adverse behavioural effects of the drug so as to avoid panic in the event of such manifestations. Patients should remain under the supervision of a responsible adult during initial use of MARINOL and following dosage adjustments.

Use in Women of Child-Bearing Potential: Independent research in laboratory species has found that cannabinoids have been associated with evidence of reproductive toxicity in early gestation and have been found to affect spermatogenesis. Therefore women of child-bearing potential should take reliable contraceptive precautions for the duration of treatment and for three months after discontinuation of therapy. Male patients with a partner of childbearing potential should ensure that reliable contraceptive precautions are maintained for the duration of therapy and for three months after discontinuation of therapy.

Special Populations: Pregnant Women: The safe use of MARINOL during pregnancy has not been established.

Reproduction studies with delta-9-tetrahydrocannabinol have been performed in mice at 15 to 450 mg/m², equivalent to 0.2 to 5 times maximum recommended human dose (MRHD) of 90 mg/m² /day in cancer patients or 1 to 30 times MRHD of 15 mg/m² /day in AIDS patients, and in rats at 74 to 295 mg/m² (equivalent to 0.8 to 3 times MRHD of 90 mg/m² in cancer patients or 5 to 20 times MRHD of 15 mg/m² /day in AIDS patients). These studies have revealed no evidence of teratogenicity due to delta-9-tetrahydrocannabinol. At these dosages in mice and rats, delta-9-tetrahydrocannabinol decreased maternal weight gain and number of viable pups and increased fetal mortality and early resorptions. Such effects were dose dependent and less apparent at lower doses which produced less maternal toxicity. Animal studies have indicated that cannabinoids may have detrimental effects on foetal development. There are no adequate and well-controlled studies in pregnant women. MARINOL is contraindicated in pregnant women. MARINOL should not be used in women who intend to become pregnant.

Nursing Women: There is evidence that delta-9-tetrahydrocannabinol is concentrated in and secreted in human breast milk and is absorbed by the nursing baby. Because the effects on the infant of chronic exposure to MARINOL and its metabolites are unknown, nursing mothers should not use MARINOL (see Contraindications).

Pediatrics: Animal data have indicated that cannabinoids interfere with development of neonatal and adolescent rodents. MARINOL is contraindicated in children under 18 years of age.

Geriatrics: Clinical studies of MARINOL in AIDS and cancer patients did not include the sufficient numbers of subjects aged 65 and over to determine whether they respond differently from younger subjects.

Other reported clinical experience has not identified differences in responses between the elderly and younger patients. In general, dose selection for an elderly patient should be cautious usually starting at the low end of the dosing range, reflecting the greater frequency of decreased hepatic, renal, or cardiac function, increased sensitivity to psychoactive effects and of concomitant disease or other drug therapy.

ADVERSE REACTIONS: Adverse Drug Reaction Overview: The most frequently reported adverse experiences in patients with AIDS during placebocontrolled clinical trials involved the CNS and were reported by 33% of patients receiving MARINOL. About 25% of patients reported a minor CNS adverse event during the first 2 weeks and about 4% reported such an event each week for the next 6 weeks thereafter.

During controlled clinical trials, the most commonly encountered events in anti-emetic studies were drowsiness, dizziness and transient impairment of sensory and perceptual functions; and, in studies in AIDS patients, euphoria, dizziness, somnolence and thinking abnormalities.

A cannabinoid dose-related "high" (easy laughing, elation and heightened awareness) has been reported by patients receiving MARINOL in both the antiemetic (24%) and the lower dose appetite stimulant clinical trials (8%).

Clinical Trial Adverse Drug Reactions: Because clinical trials are conducted under very specific conditions the adverse reaction rates observed in the clinical trials may not reflect the rates observed in practice and should not be compared to the rates in the clinical trials of another drug. Adverse drug reaction information from clinical trials is useful for identifying drug-related adverse events and for approximating rates.

Table 1 lists the adverse reactions experienced by 474 MARINOL-treated patients participating in 11 controlled clinical trials. Studies of AIDS-related weight loss included 157 patients receiving MARINOL at 2.5 mg twice daily and 67 receiving placebo. Studies of different durations were combined by considering the first occurrence of events during the first 28 days. In AIDS patients treated up to 5 months, adverse events related to MARINOL were not related to duration of therapy. Studies of nausea and vomiting related to cancer chemotherapy included 317 patients receiving MARINOL and 68 receiving placebo.

Table 1: MARINOL

Frequency of Adverse Reactions from Clinical Trials in Chemotherapy-related Nausea (N=317) and AIDS-related Anorexia (N=157)

A. Probably Causally Related: Incidence >1%	
Body as a Whole	asthenia
Nervous System	amnesia[b], anxiety/nervousness, ataxia[b], confusion, depersonalization, dizziness[a], euphoria[a], hallucination[b], paranoid reaction[a], somnolence[a], thinking abnormal[a]
Digestive	abdominal pain[a], nausea[a], vomiting
Cardiovascular	palpitations, tachycardia, vasodilation/facial flush
B. Probably Causally Related: Incidence <1%	
Nervous System	depression, nightmares, speech difficulties, tinnitus
Digestive	diarrhea[c], fecal incontinence
Cardiovascular	hypotension[c]
Musculoskeletal	myalgias
Skin/Appendages	flushing[c]
Special Senses	vision difficulties, conjunctivitis[c]
C. Causal Relationship Unknown: Incidence <1% The clinical significance of the association of these events with MARINOL Capsules treatment is unknown, but they are reported as alerting information for the clinician.	
Body as a Whole	chills, headache, malaise
Digestive	anorexia, hepatic enzyme elevation
Respiratory	cough, rhinitis, sinusitis
Skin/Appendages	sweating

(cont'd)

[a] Incidence 3–10%.
[b] Rates generally higher in the antiemetic use.
[c] Incidence 0.3–1%.

Post-Market Adverse Drug Reactions: In addition to those adverse events reported during clinical trials, the following side effects have been identified during post-marketing use of dronabinol. These reactions are reported voluntarily. It is not always possible to reliably estimate the frequency or establish a causal relationship to drug exposure. A frequency of <1% is assumed:
Immune System Disorders: hypersensitivity reactions.
Nervous System Disorders: seizures and seizure like activity.
Skin and Subcutaneous Tissue Disorders: allergic skin reactions (e.g. rash, pruritus).
General Disorders and Administrative Site Reactions: fatigue, dry mouth, drug ineffective.
Injury, Poisoning and Procedural Complications: falls.

DRUG INTERACTIONS:

Serious Drug Interactions
- Care should be taken with sedatives, drugs with sedating effect and hypnotics as coadministration with MARINOL may have an additive effect.
- Alcohol may interact with MARINOL, particularly in affecting coordination, concentration and ability to respond quickly.

Overview: In studies involving patients with AIDS and/or cancer, MARINOL (delta-9- tetrahydrocannabinol) has been co-administered with a variety of medications (e.g. cytotoxic agents, anti-infective agents, sedatives or opioid analgesics) without resulting in any clinically significant drug/drug interactions. Cannabinoids may still interact with other medications through both metabolic and pharmacodynamic mechanisms. Delta-9-tetrahydrocannabinol is highly bound to plasma proteins, and therefore might displace other protein-bound drugs. Although this displacement has not been confirmed in vivo, practitioners should monitor patients for a change in dosage requirements when administering MARINOL to patients receiving other highly protein-bound drugs. Also, the literature contains evidence of drug interactions with smoked marijuana. The potential for drug interactions with MARINOL must be considered.

Drug-Drug Interactions: Published reports of drug/drug interactions involving cannabinoids are summarized in Table 2.

Table 2: MARINOL

Drug Interaction Information on Delta-9-tetrahydrocannabinol

Concomitant Drug	Clinical Effect(s)
Amitriptyline, amoxapine, desipramine, other tricyclic antidepressants	Additive tachycardia, hypertension, drowsiness
Amphetamines, cocaine, other sympathomimetic agents	Additive hypertension, tachycardia, possibly cardiotoxicity
Antipyrine, barbiturates	Decreased clearance of these agents, presumably via competitive inhibition of metabolism
Atropine, scopolamine, antihistamines, other anticholinergic agents	Additive or super-additive tachycardia, drowsiness
Disulfiram	A reversible hypomanic reaction was reported in a 28 year old man who smoked marijuana; confirmed by dechallenge and rechallenge
Fluoxetine	A 21 year old female with depression and bulimia receiving 20 mg/day fluoxetine for 4 weeks became hypomanic after smoking marijuana; symptoms resolved after 4 days
Theophylline	Increased theophylline metabolism reported with smoking of marijuana; effect similar to that following smoking tobacco

DOSAGE AND ADMINISTRATION: Dosing Considerations: The pharmacologic effects of MARINOL (dronabinol) are dose- related and subject to considerable interpatient variability. Therefore, dosage individualization is critical in achieving the maximum benefit of MARINOL treatment.

Recommended Dose and Dosage Adjustment: Adults: AIDS-Related Anorexia Associated with Weight Loss: In the clinical trials, the majority of patients were treated with 5 mg/day MARINOL, although the dosages ranged from 2.5 to 20 mg/day. For an adult:

1. Begin with 2.5 mg before lunch and 2.5 mg before supper. If CNS symptoms (feeling high, dizziness, confusion, somnolence) do occur, they usually resolve in 1 to 3 days with continued dosage.
2. If CNS symptoms are severe or persistent, reduce the dose to 2.5 mg before supper. If symptoms continue to be a problem, taking the single dose in the evening or at bedtime may reduce their severity.
3. When adverse effects are absent or minimal and further therapeutic effect is desired, increase the dose to 2.5 mg before lunch and 5 mg before supper or 5 mg before lunch and 5 mg before supper. Although most patients respond to 2.5 mg twice daily, 10 mg twice daily has been tolerated in about half of the patients in appetite stimulation studies.

Caution should be exercised in escalating the dosage of MARINOL because of the increased frequency of dose-related adverse experiences at higher dosages.

The pharmacologic effects of MARINOL are reversible upon treatment cessation.

Antiemetic in Cancer Chemotherapy-Induced Nausea and Vomiting: Evidence from clinical trials has shown that MARINOL is best administered at an initial dose of 5 mg/m_2, given 1 to 3 hours prior to the administration of chemotherapy, then every 2 to 4 hours after chemotherapy is given, for a total of 4 to 6 doses/day. Should the 5 mg/m_2 dose prove to be ineffective, and in the absence of significant side effects, the dose may be escalated by 2.5 mg/m² increments to a maximum of 15 mg/m² per dose.

Clinical practice experience suggests that a dosage of 5 mg three or four times daily may be adequate for most patients regarding efficacy and tolerability. Dosage may be escalated during a chemotherapy cycle or at subsequent cycles, based upon initial results. Therapy should be initiated at the lowest recommended dosage and titrated to clinical response. Caution should be exercised in escalating the dosage of MARINOL because of the increased frequency of dose related adverse experiences at higher dosages. The pharmacologic effects of MARINOL are reversible upon treatment cessation.

Pediatrics: The safety and efficacy of MARINOL have not been established in adolescents or children under 18 years of age, therefore MARINOL should not be used in adolescents or children.

Geriatrics: Caution is advised in prescribing MARINOL in elderly patients because they are generally more sensitive to the psychoactive effects of drugs. In antiemetic studies, no difference in tolerance or efficacy was apparent in patients >55 years old. In general, dose selection for an elderly patient should be cautious usually starting at the low end of the dosing range, reflecting the greater frequency of decreased hepatic, renal, or cardiac function, increased sensitivity to psychoactive effects and of concomitant disease or other drug therapy.

Missed Dose: If a dose is missed, patients should take it as soon as they remember. However, if it is almost time for the next dose, the missed dose should be skipped and the patient should go back to their regular dosing schedule. The dose should not be doubled.

OVERDOSAGE:

Signs and symptoms following **mild** MARINOL (delta-9-tetrahydrocannabinol) intoxication include drowsiness, euphoria, heightened sensory awareness, altered time perception, reddened conjunctiva, dry mouth and tachycardia; following **moderate** intoxication include memory impairment, depersonalization, mood alteration, urinary retention, and reduced bowel motility; and following **severe** intoxication include decreased motor coordination, lethargy, slurred speech, and postural hypotension. Apprehensive patients may experience panic reactions and seizures may occur in patients with existing seizure disorders.

The estimated lethal human dose of intravenous delta-9-tetrahydrocannabinol is 30 mg/kg (2100 mg/70 kg). Significant CNS symptoms in antiemetic studies followed oral doses of 0.4 mg/kg (28 mg/70 kg) of MARINOL.

Management: A potentially serious oral ingestion, if recent, should be managed with gut decontamination. In unconscious patients with a secure airway, instill activated charcoal (30 to 100 g in adults, 1 to 2 g/kg in infants) via a nasogastric tube. A saline cathartic or sorbitol may be added to the first dose of activated charcoal. Patients experiencing depressive, hallucinatory or psychotic reactions should be placed in a quiet area and offered reassurance. Benzodiazepines (5 to 10 mg diazepam po) may be used for treatment of extreme agitation. Hypotension usually responds to Trendelenburg position and IV fluids. Pressors are rarely required.

> For management of a suspected drug overdose, CPhA recommends that you contact your **regional Poison Control Centre**. See the *CPS* Directory section for a list of Poison Control Centres.

ACTION AND CLINICAL PHARMACOLOGY: Mechanism of Action: MARINOL (dronabinol) is an oral dosage form containing dronabinol which is synthetic delta-9- tetrahydrocannabinol. Delta-9-tetrahydrocannabinol is the main psychotropic component in Cannabis sative (marijuana).

Delta-9-tetrahydrocannabinol is a cannabinoid receptor agonist. There are two known cannabinoid receptors, CB_1 and CB_2. CB_1 receptors are found in large quantities in the cerebral cortex, hippocampus, basal ganglia and cerebellum. Lower amounts are found in the hypothalamus and spinal cord. These locations can be used to predict the pharmacological effects of delta-9-tetrahydrocannabinol. CB_1 receptors are not found in the respiratory centres of the brainstem, CB_2 receptors are found peripherally on immune cells.

Cannabinoids have been shown to stimulate appetite and reduce nausea and vomiting. Specifically, the endocannabinoid anandamide has been shown to stimulate food intake. Delta-9-tetrahydrocannabinol binds to the same cannabinoid receptor, thereby increasing appetite. In addition, delta-9-tetrahydrocannabinol and other cannabinoids have been shown to reduce emesis by binding to CB_1 receptors.

Pharmacodynamics: Dronabinol has been shown to have psychotropic and antiemetic activity. Delta-9- tetrahydrocannabinol can produce changes in mood, decrease in cognitive performance and memory, decrease in ability to control drives and impulses, altered perception of reality, particularly altered time sense, and reversible effects on appetite. These phenomena appear to be dose-related, increasing in frequency with higher dosages, and subject to great interpatient variability.

Animal data has shown that Delta-9-tetrahydrocannabinol has various effects on the central nervous system which are generally reported in the literature including analgesia, reduction of nausea and vomiting in cancer chemotherapy, reduction in intraocular pressure, appetite stimulation in wasting syndromes, relief from muscle spasms and spasticity in multiple sclerosis and decreased intestinal motility. Other effects of Delta-9-tetrahydrocannabinol include changes in cognitive ability and memory, dysphoria and/or euphoria as well as sedation.

Dronabinol induced sympathomimetic activity may result in tachycardia and/or conjunctival injection. Its effects on blood pressure are inconsistent, but occasionally, subjects have experienced orthostatic hypotension and/or syncope upon abrupt standing.

After oral administration, delta-9-tetrahydrocannabinol has an onset of action of approximately 0.5 to 1 hours and peak effect at 2 to 4 hours. Duration of action for psychoactive effects is 4 to 6 hours, but the appetite stimulant effect of delta-9-tetrahydrocannabinol may continue for 24 hours or longer after administration.

Tachyphylaxis and tolerance develop to some of the pharmacologic effects of delta-9-tetrahydrocannabinol and other cannabinoids with chronic use, suggesting an indirect effect on sympathetic neurons. In a study of the pharmacodynamics of chronic delta-9- tetrahydrocannabinol exposure, healthy male volunteers (N=12) received 210 mg/day delta-9- tetrahydrocannabinol, administered orally in divided doses, for 16 days. An initial tachycardia induced by delta-9-tetrahydrocannabinol was replaced successively by normal sinus rhythm and then bradycardia. A decrease in supine blood pressure, made worse by standing, was also observed initially. These volunteers developed tolerance to the cardiovascular and subjective adverse CNS effects of delta-9-tetrahydrocannabinol within 12 days of treatment initiation.

Tachyphylaxis and tolerance do not, however, appear to develop to the appetite stimulant effect of MARINOL. In studies involving patients with Acquired Immune Deficiency Syndrome (AIDS), the appetite stimulant effect of MARINOL has been sustained for up to five months in clinical trials, at dosages ranging from 2.5 mg/day to 20 mg/day.

Pharmacokinetics: The single and multiple dose (twice daily for 10 days) pharmacokinetics of MARINOL and 11-OH-delta-THC, after administration of 2.5, 5 and 10 mg capsules, were assessed in healthy male and female volunteers. Results of this study are presented in Table 3 and Table 4. A slight increase in dose proportionality on mean Cmax and AUC (0-12) of dronabinol was observed with increasing dose over the dose range studied. Limited accumulation (range 1.18 to 2.43) of dronabinol was observed at all doses investigated.

Table 3: MARINOL

Summary of MARINOL's Pharmacokinetic Parameters in Healthy Volunteers

	Arithmetic Mean (SD)				
Dose	**C_{max} (ng/mL)**	**Tmax (h)**	**$t_{½}$ (h)**	**$AUC_{0→∞}$**	**CL/F (L/h)**
Single Dose					
2.5 mg	0.65 (0.304)	2.00 (0.50–4.00)	1.31 (0.659)	2.32 (2.472)	1676.20 (698.7)
5 mg	1.83 (1.429)	1.00 (0.50–3.00)	1.43 (0.490)	3.45 (2.684)	2847.84 (2678.0)
10 mg	6.22 (2.652)	1.50 (0.50–3.00)	4.37 (4.768)	9.67 (3.904)	1254.27 (657.2)
Dose	**C_{max} (ng/mL)**	**Tmax (h)**	**$t_{½}$ (h)**	**$AUC_{0→12}$**	**CL/F (L/h)**
Multiple Dose					
2.5 mg	1.32 (0.617)	1.00 (0.50–4.00)	16.69 (21.723)	2.88 (1.566)	1074.27 (449.9)
5 mg	2.96 (1.807)	2.50 (0.50–4.00)	43.27 (27.986)	6.16 (1.847)	926.15 (444.5)
10 mg	7.88 (4.544)	1.50 (0.50–3.50)	87.04 (22.645)	15.17 (5.516)	754.56 (300.0)

The different strengths of MARINOL are not bioequivalent to each other.

Table 4: MARINOL

Summary of 11-OH-THC's Pharmacokinetic Parameters in Healthy Volunteers

	Arithmetic Mean (SD)			
Dose	**C_{max} (ng/mL)**	**Tmax (h)**	**$t_{½}$ (h)**	**$AUC_{0→∞}$**
Single Dose				
2.5 mg	1.19 (0.763)	3.00 (0.77–4.00)	5.11 (2.719)	4.28 (2.629)
5 mg	2.23 (1.500)	2.00 (1.00–3.00)	6.58 (4.403)	8.03 (4.526)
10 mg	7.51 (5.264)	2.00 (1.00–3.50)	8.51 (1.606)	25.74 (15.156)
Dose	**C_{max} (ng/mL)**	**Tmax (h)**	**$t_{½}$ (h)**	**$AUC_{0→12}$**
Multiple Dose				
2.5 mg	1.65 (0.752)	1.75 (0.50–4.00)	13.65 (9.232)	5.99 (2.459)
5 mg	3.84 (2.322)	2.50 (0.75–4.00)	14.38 (6.428)	12.59 (3.948)
10 mg	7.95 (3.167)	2.00 (0.75–3.50)	23.11 (11.289)	29.50 (9.909)

The different strengths of MARINOL are not bioequivalent to each other.

Absorption and Distribution: Delta-9-tetrahydrocannabinol is almost completely absorbed (90 to 95%) after single oral doses of MARINOL. Due to the combined effects of first pass hepatic metabolism and high lipid solubility, only 10 to 20% of the administered dose reaches the systemic circulation. Delta-9-tetrahydrocannabinol has a large apparent volume of distribution, approximately 10 L/kg, because of its lipid solubility. The plasma protein binding of dronabinol and its metabolites is approximately 97%.

The elimination phase of dronabinol can be described using a two compartment model. Because of its large volume of distribution, dronabinol and its metabolites may be excreted at low levels for prolonged periods of time.

Metabolism: Delta-9-tetrahydrocannabinol undergoes extensive first-pass hepatic metabolism, primarily by microsomal hydroxylation, yielding both active and inactive metabolites. Delta-9- tetrahydrocannabinol and its principal active metabolite, 11-OH-delta-9-THC, are present in approximately equal concentrations in plasma. Concentrations of both parent drug and metabolite peak at approximately 0.5 to 4 hours after oral dosing and decline over several days. Values for clearance average about 0.2 L/kg-h, but are highly variable due to the complexity of cannabinoid distribution.

Excretion: Delta-9-tetrahydrocannabinol and its biotransformation products are excreted in both faeces and urine. Biliary excretion is the major route of elimination with about half of a radio-labelled oral dose being recovered from the faeces within 72 hours as contrasted with 10 to 15 % recovered from urine. Less than 5% of an oral dose is recovered unchanged in the faeces.

Following single dose administration, low levels of dronabinol metabolites have been detected for more than 5 weeks in the urine and faeces.

In a study of MARINOL Capsules involving AIDS patients, urinary cannabinoid/creatinine concentration ratios were studied bi-weekly over a six week period. The urinary cannabinoid/creatinine ratio was closely correlated with dose. No increase in the cannabinoid/creatinine ratio was observed after the first two weeks of treatment, indicating that steady-state cannabinoid levels had been reached. This conclusion is consistent with predictions based on the observed terminal half-life of dronabinol.

Special Populations and Conditions: Pediatrics: The pharmacokinetic profile of MARINOL has not been investigated in pediatric patients.

Geriatrics: The pharmacokinetic profile of MARINOL has not been investigated in geriatric patients.

STORAGE AND STABILITY: MARINOL (delta-9-tetrahydrocannabinol) should be stored at 2 to 8° C, in well sealed HDPE containers.

INFORMATION FOR THE PATIENT: Published in e-CPS, available by subscription at www.e-cps.ca.

DOSAGE FORMS, COMPOSITION AND PACKAGING: 2.5 mg: Each white, soft gelatin capsule, identified "UM", contains: delta-9-tetrahydrocannabinol 2.5 mg. Nonmedicinal ingredients: gelatin, glycerin, methylparaben, propylparaben, sesame oil and titanium dioxide. Bottles of 60.

5 mg: Each brown, soft gelatin capsule, identified "UM", contains: delta-9-tetrahydrocannabinol 5 mg. Nonmedicinal ingredients: iron oxide red, iron oxide black, gelatin, glycerin, sesame oil and titanium dioxide. Bottles of 60.

10 mg: Each orange, soft gelatin capsule, identified "UM", contains: delta-9-tetrahydrocannabinol 10 mg. Nonmedicinal ingredients: iron oxide red, iron oxide yellow, gelatin, glycerin, sesame oil and titanium dioxide. Bottles of 60.

(Shown in Product Identification Section)

Marvelon® ℞

desogestrel—ethinyl estradiol

Oral Contraceptive

Schering-Plough

PHARMACOLOGY: Combination oral contraceptives act by suppression of gonadotropins. Although the primary mechanism of this action is inhibition of ovulation, other alterations include changes in the cervical mucus (which increase the difficulty of sperm entry into the uterus) and the endometrium (which reduce the likelihood of implantation).

Desogestrel, the progestogen component of Marvelon, displays low androgenic activity in relation to its progestogenic effects and may increase the HDL/LDL ratio and apoprotein A-1/B ratio without affecting HDL_2. Like other oral contraceptives, these changes in lipid profile can be associated with an increase in triglycerides.

INDICATIONS: Conception control.

CONTRAINDICATIONS: History of/or actual thrombophlebitis or thromboembolic disorders. History of/or actual cerebrovascular disorders. History of/or actual myocardial infarction or coronary arterial disease. Active liver disease or history of/or actual benign or malignant liver tumors. Known or suspected carcinoma of the breast. Known or suspected estrogen-dependent neoplasia. Undiagnosed abnormal vaginal bleeding. Any ocular lesion arising from ophthalmic vascular disease, such as partial or complete loss of vision or defect in visual fields. When pregnancy is suspected or diagnosed.

WARNINGS: Predisposing Factors for Coronary Artery Disease: Cigarette smoking increases the risk of serious cardiovascular side effects and mortality. Birth control pills increase this risk, especially with increasing age. Convincing data are available to support an upper age limit of 35 years for oral contraceptive use in women who smoke.

Other women who are independently at high risk for cardiovascular disease include those with diabetes, hypertension, abnormal lipid profile, or a family history of these. Whether oral contraceptives accentuate this risk is unclear.

In low-risk, nonsmoking women of any age, the benefits of oral contraceptive use outweigh the possible cardiovascular risks associated with low dose formulations. Consequently, oral contraceptives may be prescribed for these women up to the age of menopause.

> Cigarette smoking increases the risk of serious adverse effects on the heart and blood vessels. This risk increases with age and becomes significant in oral contraceptive users over 35 years of age. Women should be counselled not to smoke.

Epidemiological studies have suggested an association between the use of COCs and an increased risk of venous thrombotic and thromboembolic diseases.

Venous thromboembolism (VTE), manifesting as deep vein thrombosis and/or pulmonary embolism, may occur during the use of all COCs. The approximate incidence of VTE in users of low estrogen dose (<0.05 mg EE) OCs is up to 4 per 10 000 woman years compared to 0.5-3 per 10 000 woman years in non-OC users. The incidence of VTE associated with pregnancy is 6 per 10 000 woman years.

Several epidemiological studies indicate that third generation oral contraceptives, including those containing desogestrel, are associated with a higher risk of venous thromboembolism than certain second generation oral contraceptives. These studies indicate an approximately 2-fold difference in risk, which corresponds to 1-2 cases of venous thromboembolism per 10 000 women-years of use. However, data from additional studies have not shown this difference in risk.

Discontinue medication at the earliest manifestation of:

A. Thromboembolic and cardiovascular disorders such as: thrombophlebitis, pulmonary embolism, cerebrovascular disorders, myocardial ischemia, mesenteric thrombosis and retinal thrombosis.

B. Conditions which predispose to venous stasis and to vascular thrombosis, e.g., immobilization after accidents or confinement to bed during long-term illness. Other nonhormonal methods of contraception should be used until regular activities are resumed. For use of oral contraceptives when surgery is contemplated, see Precautions.

C. Visual defects, partial or complete.

D. Papilledema, or ophthalmic vascular lesions.

E. Severe headache of unknown etiology or worsening of pre-existing migraine headache.

PRECAUTIONS: Physical Examination and Follow-up: Before oral contraceptives are used, a thorough history and physical examination should be performed, including a blood pressure determination. Breasts, liver, extremities and pelvic organs should be examined. A Papanicolaou smear should be taken if the patient has been sexually active.

The first follow-up visit should be done 3 months after oral contraceptives are prescribed. Thereafter, examinations should be performed at least once a year, or more frequently if indicated. At each annual visit, examination should include those procedures that were done at the initial visit as outlined above or per recommendations of the Canadian Task Force on the Periodic Health Examination.

Pregnancy: Oral contraceptives should not be taken by pregnant women. However, if conception accidentally occurs while taking the pill, there is no conclusive evidence that the estrogen and progestin contained in the oral contraceptive will damage the developing child.

Lactation: In breast-feeding women, the use of oral contraceptives results in the hormonal components being excreted in breast milk and may reduce its quantity and quality. If the use of oral contraceptives is initiated after the establishment of lactation, there does not appear to be any effect on the quantity and quality of the milk. There is no evidence that low dose oral contraceptives are harmful to the nursing infant.

Hepatic Function: Patients who have had jaundice including a history of cholestatic jaundice during pregnancy should be given oral contraceptives with great care and under close observation.

The development of severe generalized pruritus or icterus requires that the medication be withdrawn until the problem is resolved.

If the jaundice should prove to be cholestatic in type, the use of oral contraceptives should not be resumed. In patients taking oral contraceptives, changes in the composition of the bile may occur and an increased incidence of gallstones has been reported.

Hepatic nodules (adenoma and focal nodular hyperplasia) have been reported, particularly in long-term users of oral contraceptives. Although these lesions are extremely rare they have caused fatal intra-abdominal hemorrhage and should be considered in women presenting with an abdominal mass, acute abdominal pain or evidence of intra-abdominal bleeding.

Hypertension: Patients with essential hypertension whose blood pressure is well controlled may be given oral contraceptives but only under close supervision. If a significant elevation of blood pressure in previously normotensive or hypertensive subjects occurs at any time during the administration of the drug, cessation of medication is necessary.

Migraine and Headache: The onset or exacerbation of migraine or the development of headache of a new pattern which is recurrent, persistent or severe requires discontinuation of oral contraceptives and evaluation of the cause.

Diabetes: Current low dose oral contraceptives exert minimal impact on glucose metabolism. Diabetic patients, or those with a family history of diabetes, should be observed closely to detect worsening of carbohydrate metabolism. Patients predisposed to diabetes who can be kept under close supervision may be given oral contraceptives. Young diabetic patients whose disease is of recent origin, well-controlled and not associated with hypertension or other signs of vascular disease such as ocular fundal changes should be monitored more frequently while using oral contraceptives.

Ocular Disease: Patients who are pregnant or are taking oral contraceptives may experience corneal edema that may cause visual disturbances and changes in tolerance to contact lenses, especially of the rigid type. Soft contact lenses usually do not cause disturbances. If visual changes or alterations in tolerance to contact lenses occur, temporary or permanent cessation of wear may be advised.

Breasts: Increasing age and a strong family history are the most significant risk factors for the development of breast cancer. Other established risk factors include obesity, nulliparity and late age at first full-term pregnancy. The identified groups of women that may be at increased risk of developing breast cancer before menopause are long-term users of oral contraceptives (more than 8 years) and starters at early age. In a few women, the use of oral contraceptives may accelerate the growth of an existing but undiagnosed breast cancer. Since any potential increased risk related to oral contraceptive use is small, there is no reason to change prescribing habits at present.

Women receiving oral contraceptives should be instructed in self-examination of their breasts. Their physicians should be notified whenever any masses are detected. A yearly clinical breast examination is also recommended because, if a breast cancer should develop, estrogen-containing drugs may cause a rapid progression.

Vaginal Bleeding: Persistent irregular vaginal bleeding requires assessment to exclude underlying pathology.

Fibroids: Patients with fibroids (leiomyomata) should be carefully observed. Sudden enlargement, pain or tenderness requires discontinuation of the use of oral contraceptives.

Emotional Disorders: Patients with a history of emotional disturbances, especially the depressive type, may be more prone to have a recurrence of depression while taking oral contraceptives. In cases of a serious recurrence, a trial of an alternate method of contraception should be made which may help to clarify the possible relationship. Women with premenstrual syndrome (PMS) may have a varied response to oral contraceptives, ranging from symptomatic improvement to worsening of the condition.

Laboratory Tests: Results of laboratory tests should be interpreted in the light that the patient is on oral contraceptives. The following laboratory tests are modified.

A. Liver function tests: Aspartate serum transaminase (AST): variously reported elevations. Alkaline phosphatase and gamma glutamine transaminase (GGT): slightly elevated.

B. Coagulation tests: Minimal elevation of test values reported for such parameters as prothrombin and Factors VII, VIII, IX and X.

C. Thyroid function tests: Protein binding of thyroxine is increased as indicated by increased total serum thyroxine concentrations and decreased T_3 resin uptake.

D. Lipoproteins: Small changes of unproven clinical significance may occur in lipoprotein cholesterol fractions.

E. Gonadotropins: LH and FSH levels are suppressed by the use of oral contraceptives. Wait 2 weeks after discontinuing the use of oral contraceptives before measurements are made.

Tissue Specimens: Pathologists should be advised of oral contraceptive therapy when specimens obtained from surgical procedures and Pap smears are submitted for examination.

Return to Fertility: After discontinuing oral contraceptive therapy, the patient should delay pregnancy until at least 1 normal spontaneous menstrual cycle has occurred in order to date the pregnancy. An alternative contraceptive method should be used during this time.

Amenorrhea: Women having a history of oligomenorrhea, secondary amenorrhea or irregular cycles may remain anovulatory or become amenorrheic following discontinuation of estrogen-progestin combination therapy.

Amenorrhea, especially if associated with breast secretion, that continues for 6 months or more after withdrawal warrants a careful assessment of hypothalamic-pituitary function.

Thromboembolic Complications—Post-surgery: There is an increased risk of post-surgery thromboembolic complications in oral contraceptive users, after major surgery. If feasible, oral contraceptives should be discontinued and an alternative method substituted at least 1 month prior to **major** elective surgery. Oral contraceptives should not be resumed until the first menstrual period after hospital discharge following surgery.

Drug Interactions: The concurrent administration of oral contraceptives with other drugs may result in an altered response to either agent (see Table 1 and Table 2). Reduced effectiveness of the oral contraceptive, should it occur, is more likely with the low-dose formulations. It is important to ascertain all drugs that a patient is taking, both prescription and nonprescription, before oral contraceptives are prescribed.

Table 1: Marvelon

Drugs Which May Decrease the Efficacy of Oral Contraceptives

Class of Compound	Drug	Proposed Mechanism	Suggested Management
Anticonvulsants	Carbamazepine Ethosuximide Phenobarbital Phenytoin Primidone	Induction of hepatic microsomal enzymes: Rapid metabolism of estrogen and increased binding of progestin and ethinyl estradiol to SHBG.	Use higher dose OCs (50 µg ethinyl estradiol), another drug or another method.
Antibiotics	Ampicillin Cotrimoxazole Penicillin	Enterohepatic circulation disturbance, intestinal hurry.	For short course, use additional method or use another drug. For long course, use another method.
	Rifampin	Increased metabolism of progestins. Suspected acceleration of estrogen metabolism.	Use another method.
	Chloramphenicol Metronidazole Neomycin Nitrofurantoin Sulfonamides Tetracyclines	Induction of hepatic microsomal enzymes. Also disturbance of enterohepatic circulation.	For short course, use additional method or use another drug. For long course, use another method.
	Troleandomycin	May retard metabolism of OCs, increasing the risk of cholestatic jaundice.	
Antifungal	Griseofulvin	Stimulation of hepatic metabolism of contraceptive steroids may occur.	Use another method.
Sedatives and Hypnotics	Benzodiazepines Barbiturates Chloral hydrate Glutethimide Meprobamate	Induction of hepatic microsomal enzymes.	For short course, use additional method or another drug. For long course, use another method or higher dose OCs.
Antacids		Decreased intestinal absorption of progestins.	
Other Drugs	Phenylbutazone Antihistamines Analgesics Antimigraine preparations Vitamin E	Reduced OC efficacy has been reported. Remains to be confirmed.	

Table 2: Marvelon

Modification of Other Drug Action by Oral Contraceptives

Class of Compound	Drug	Modification of Other Drug Action	Suggested Management
Alcohol		Possible increased levels of ethanol or acetaldehyde.	Use with caution.
Alpha-II Adrenoreceptor Agents	Clonidine	Sedation effect increased.	Use with caution.
Anticoagulants	All	OCs increase clotting factors, decrease efficacy. However, OCs may potentiate action in some patients.	Use another method.
Anticonvulsants	All	Fluid retention may increase risk of seizures.	Use another method.
Antidiabetic Drugs	Oral hypoglycemics and insulin	OCs may impair glucose tolerance and increase blood glucose.	Use low dose estrogen and progestin OC or another method. Monitor blood glucose.
Antihypertensive Agents	Guanethidine and methyldopa	Estrogen component causes sodium retention, progestin has no effect.	Use low estrogen OC or use another method.
	Beta-blockers	Increased drug effect (decreased metabolism).	Adjust dose of drug if necessary. Monitor cardiovascular status.
Antipyretics	Acetaminophen	Increased renal clearance.	Dose of drug may have to be increased.
	Antipyridine	Impaired metabolism.	Decrease dose of drug.
	ASA	Effects of ASA may be decreased by the short-term use of OCs.	Patients on chronic ASA therapy may require an increase in ASA dosage.
Aminocaproic Acid		Theoretically, a hypercoagulable state may occur because OCs augment clotting factors.	Avoid concomitant use.

(cont'd)

Table 2: Marvelon *(cont'd)*

Modification of Other Drug Action by Oral Contraceptives

Class of Compound	Drug	Modification of Other Drug Action	Suggested Management
Betamimetic Agents	Isoproterenol	Estrogen causes decreased response to these drugs.	Adjust dose of drug as necessary. Discontinuing OCs can result in excessive drug activity.
Caffeine		The actions of caffeine may be enhanced as OCs may impair the hepatic metabolism of caffeine.	Use with caution.
Cholesterol Lowering Agents	Clofibrate	OCs may increase the clearance of clofibrate leading to decreased levels of clofibrate.	Use with caution.
Corticosteroids	Prednisone	Markedly increased serum levels.	Possible need for decrease in dose.
Cyclosporine		May lead to an increase in cyclosporine levels and hepatotoxicity.	Monitor hepatic function. The cyclosporine dose may have to be decreased.
Folic Acid		OCs have been reported to impair folate metabolism.	
Meperedine		Possible increased analgesia and CNS depression due to decreased metabolism of meperidine.	Use combination with caution.
Phenothiazine Tranquilizers	All phenothiazines, reserpine and similar drugs	Estrogen potentiates the hyperprolactinemia effect of these drugs.	Use other drugs or lower dose OCs. If galactorrhea or hyperprolactinemia occurs, use other method.
Sedatives and Hypnotics	Chlordiazepoxide Lorazepam Oxazepam Diazepam	Increased effect (increased metabolism).	Use with caution.
Theophylline	All	Decreased oxidation, leading to possible toxicity.	Use with caution. Monitor theophylline levels.
Tricyclic Antidepressants	Clomipramine (possibly others)	Increased side effects; i.e., depression.	Use with caution.
Vitamin B_{12}		OCs have been reported to reduce serum levels of Vitamin B_{12}.	

Non-contraceptive Benefits of Oral Contraceptives: Several health advantages other than contraception have been reported.

1. Combination oral contraceptives reduce the incidence of cancer of the endometrium and ovaries.
2. Oral contraceptives reduce the likelihood of developing benign breast disease and, as a result, decrease the incidence of breast biopsies.
3. Oral contraceptives reduce the likelihood of development of functional ovarian cysts.
4. Pill-users have less menstrual blood loss and have more regular cycles, thereby reducing the chance of developing iron-deficiency anemia.
5. The use of oral contraceptives may decrease the severity of dysmenorrhea and premenstrual syndrome, and may improve acne vulgaris, hirsutism and other androgen-mediated disorders.
6. Oral contraceptives decrease the incidence of acute pelvic inflammatory disease and, thereby, reduce as well the incidence of ectopic pregnancy.
7. Oral contraceptives have potential beneficial effects on endometriosis.

> Oral contraceptives **do not protect** against sexually transmitted diseases (STDs) including HIV/AIDS. For protection against STDs, it is advisable to use latex condoms **in combination with** oral contraceptives.

ADVERSE EFFECTS: An increased risk of the following serious adverse reactions has been associated with the use of oral contraceptives: thrombophlebitis, pulmonary embolism, mesenteric thrombosis, neuro-ocular lesions, e.g., retinal thrombosis, myocardial infarction, cerebral thrombosis, cerebral hemorrhage, hypertension, benign hepatic tumors, gallbladder disease, congenital anomalies.

The following adverse reactions also have been reported in patients receiving oral contraceptives: Nausea and vomiting, usually the most common adverse reaction, occurs in approximately 10% or less of patients during the first cycle. Other reactions, as a general rule, are seen less frequently or only occasionally, as follows: gastrointestinal symptoms (such as abdominal cramps and bloating), breakthrough bleeding, spotting, change in menstrual flow, dysmenorrhea, amenorrhea during and after treatment, temporary infertility after discontinuance of treatment, edema, chloasma or melasma which may persist, breast changes (tenderness, enlargement and secretion), change in weight (increase or decrease), endocervical hyperplasias, possible diminution in lactation when given immediately postpartum, cholestatic jaundice, migraine, increase in size of uterine leiomyomata, rash (allergic), mental depression, reduced tolerance to carbohydrates, vaginal candidiasis, premenstrual-like syndrome, intolerance to contact lenses, change in corneal curvature (steepening), cataracts, optic neuritis, retinal thrombosis, changes in libido, chorea, changes in appetite, cystitis-like syndrome, rhinitis, headache, nervousness, dizziness, hirsutism, loss of scalp hair, erythema multiforme, erythema nodosum, hemorrhagic eruption, vaginitis, porphyria, impaired renal function, Raynaud's phenomenon, auditory disturbances, hemolytic uremic syndrome, pancreatitis.

OVERDOSE:

Symptoms: Serious ill effects have not been reported following acute ingestion of large doses of oral contraceptives by young children. Overdosage may cause nausea, and withdrawal bleeding may occur in females.

> For management of a suspected drug overdose, CPhA recommends that you contact your **regional Poison Control Centre**. See the *CPS* Directory section for a list of Poison Control Centres.

DOSAGE: **Information for the Patient on How to Take the Birth Control Pill:**

1. **Read these directions:**
   - before you start taking your pills, and
   - any time you are not sure what to do.
2. **Look at your pill pack** to see if it has 21 or 28 pills:
   - 21-Pill Pack: 21 active pills (with hormones) taken daily for 3 weeks, and then take no pills for 1 week

     or
   - 28-Pill Pack: 21 active pills (with hormones) taken daily for 3 weeks, and then 7 "reminder" pills (no hormones) taken daily for 1 week.

Also check the pill pack for instructions on (1) where to start and (2) directions to take pills (see package insert for illustrations).

3. You may wish to use a second method of birth control (e.g., latex condoms and spermicidal foam or gel) for the first 7 days of the first cycle of pill use. This will provide a back-up in case pills are forgotten while you are getting used to taking them.
4. When receiving any medical treatment, be sure to tell your doctor that you are using birth control pills.
5. **Many women have spotting or light bleeding or may feel sick to their stomach during the first 3 months on the pill.** If you do feel sick, do not stop taking the pill. The problem will usually go away. If it does not go away, check with your doctor or clinic.
6. **Missing pills also can cause some spotting or light bleeding,** even if you make up the missed pills. You also could feel a little sick to your stomach on the days you take 2 pills to make up for missed pills.
7. **If you miss pills at any time, you could get pregnant. The greatest risks for pregnancy are:**
   - when you start a pack late, and
   - when you miss pills at the beginning or at the very end of the pack.
8. **Always be sure you have ready:**
   - **another kind of birth control** (such as latex condoms and spermicidal foam or gel) to use as a back-up in case you miss pills, and
   - **an extra, full pack of pills.**
9. **If you have vomiting or diarrhea, or if you take some medicines**, such as antibiotics, your pills may not work as well. Use a back-up method, such as latex condoms and spermicidal foam or gel, until you can check with your doctor or clinic.
10. **If you forget more than 1 pill 2 months in a row,** talk to your doctor or clinic about how to make pill-taking easier or about using another method of birth control.
11. **If your questions are not answered here, call your doctor or clinic.**

When to start the first pack of pills: Be sure to read these instructions:

- before you start taking your pills, and
- any time you are not sure what to do.

Decide with your doctor or clinic what is the best day for you to start taking your first pack of pills. Your pills may be either a 21-day or a 28-day type.

A. 21-Day Combination: With this type of birth control pill, you are 21 days on pills with 7 days off pills. You must not be off the pills for more than 7 days in a row.

1. **The first day of your menstrual period (bleeding) is Day 1 of your cycle.** Your doctor may advise you to start taking the pills on Day 1 or on the first Sunday after your period begins. If your period starts on Sunday, start that same day.
2. Take 1 pill at approximately the same time every day for 21 days; **then take no pills for 7 days.** Start a new pack on the eighth day. You will probably have a period during the 7 days off the pill. (This bleeding may be lighter and shorter than your usual period.)

B. 28-Day Combination: With this type of birth control pill, you take 21 pills which contain hormones and 7 pills which contain no hormones.

1. **The first day of your menstrual period (bleeding) is Day 1 of your cycle.** Your doctor may advise you to start taking the pills on Day 1 or on the first Sunday after your period begins. If your period starts on Sunday, start that same day.

   For Day 1 start: Label the dispenser by selecting the appropriate day label strip that starts with Day 1 of your menstrual period (first day of menstruation is Day 1).

   or

   For Sunday start: Label the dispenser by selecting the day label strip that starts with Sunday.

   Place the day label strip in the space where you see the words "Place Day Label Here". Having the dispenser labelled with the days of the week will help remind you to take your pill every day.
2. Take 1 pill at approximately the same time every day for 28 days. Begin a new pack the next day, **not missing any days on the pills**. Your period should occur during the last 7 days of using that pill pack.

What to do during the month:

1. **Take a pill at approximately the same time every day until the pack is empty.**
   - Try to associate taking your pill with some regular activity like eating a meal or going to bed.
   - Do not skip pills even if you have bleeding between monthly periods or feel sick to your stomach (nausea).
   - Do not skip pills even if you do not have sex very often.
2. **When you finish a pack:**
   - **21 pills: Wait 7 days** to start the next pack. You will have your period during that week.
   - **28 pills:** Start the next pack **on the next day**. Take 1 pill every day. Do not wait any days between packs.

What to do if you miss pills: Table 3 outlines the actions you should take if you miss 1 or more of your birth control pills. Match the number of pills missed with the appropriate starting time for your type of pill pack.

Table 3: Marvelon

What To Do If You Miss Pills

Sunday Start	Day 1 Start
Miss 1 pill	**Miss 1 pill**
Take it as soon as you remember, and take the next pill at the usual time. This means that you might take 2 pills in one day.	Take it as soon as you remember, and take the next pill at the usual time. This means that you might take 2 pills in one day.
Miss 2 pills in a row	**Miss 2 pills in a row**
First two weeks: 1. Take 2 pills the day you remember and 2 pills the next day. 2. Then take 1 pill a day until you finish the pack. 3. Use a back-up method of birth control if you have sex in the 7 days after you miss the pills. **Third Week:** 1. Keep taking 1 pill a day until Sunday. 2. On Sunday, safely discard the rest of the pack and start a new pack that day. 3. Use a back-up method of birth control if you have sex in the 7 days after you miss the pills. 4. You may not have a period this month. **If you miss 2 periods in a row, call your doctor or clinic.**	**First two weeks:** 1. Take 2 pills the day you remember and 2 pills the next day. 2. Then take 1 pill a day until you finish the pack. 3. Use a back-up method of birth control if you have sex in the 7 days after you miss the pills. **Third Week:** 1. Safely dispose of the rest of the pill pack and start a new pack that same day. 2. Use a back-up method of birth control if you have sex in the 7 days after you miss the pills. 3. You may not have a period this month. **If you miss 2 periods in a row, call your doctor or clinic.**
Miss 3 or more pills in a row	**Miss 3 or more pills in a row**
Anytime in the Cycle: 1. Keep taking 1 pill a day until Sunday. 2. On Sunday, safely discard the rest of the pack and start a new pack that day. 3. Use a back-up method of birth control if you have sex in the 7 days after you miss the pills. 4. You may not have a period this month. **If you miss 2 periods in a row, call your doctor or clinic.**	**Anytime in the Cycle:** 1. Safely dispose of the rest of the pill pack and start a new pack that same day. 2. Use a back-up method of birth control if you have sex in the 7 days after you miss the pills. 3. You may not have a period this month. **If you miss 2 periods in a row, call your doctor or clinic.**

Note: 28-Day Pack: If you forget any of the 7 "reminder" pills (without hormones) in Week 4, just safely dispose of the pills you missed. Then keep taking 1 pill each day until the pack is empty. You do not need to use a back-up method.

Always be sure you have on hand:

- a back-up method of birth control (such as latex condoms and spermicidal foam or gel) in case you miss pills, and

• an extra, full pack of pills.

If you forget more than 1 pill 2 months in a row, talk to your doctor or clinic. Talk about ways to make pill-taking easier or about using another method of birth control.

INFORMATION FOR THE PATIENT: Published in e-CPS, available by subscription at www.e-cps.ca.

SUPPLIED: Marvelon 21: Each white, round tablet contains: desogestrel 0.15 mg and ethinyl estradiol 0.03 mg. Nonmedicinal ingredients: colloidal silicon dioxide, hydroxypropyl methylcellulose, lactose, polyethylene glycol, povidone, starch, stearic acid, talc, titanium dioxide and vitamin E. Blister dispensers of 21. Store between 15-30°C.

Marvelon 28: Each white, round tablet contains: desogestrel 0.15 mg and ethinyl estradiol 0.03 mg. Nonmedicinal ingredients: colloidal silicon dioxide, hydroxypropyl methylcellulose, lactose, polyethylene glycol, povidone, starch, stearic acid, talc, titanium dioxide and vitamin E. Each green, round tablet contains the following inactive ingredients: hydroxypropyl methylcellulose, indigotine blue, iron oxide, lactose, magnesium stearate, polyethylene glycol, starch, titanium dioxide and talc. Blister dispensers of 21 white tablets and 7 green tablets. Store between 15-30°C.

(Shown in Product Identification Section)

Matulane® Ⓟ

procarbazine HCl

Antineoplastic

Sigma-Tau

Date of Preparation: November 7, 2006
Date of Revision: April 15, 2008

Matulane (procarbazine hydrochloride) is a potent drug and should only be used by physicians experienced with cancer chemotherapeutic drugs (see Warnings and Precautions). Blood counts as well as renal and hepatic function tests should be performed regularly. Discontinue the drug if abnormal depression of bone marrow or abnormal renal or hepatic function is seen. Capsules should not be opened.

SUMMARY PRODUCT INFORMATION:

Route of Administration	Dosage Form/ Strength	Clinically Relevant Nonmedicinal Ingredients
Oral	50 mg capsule	Not applicable For a complete listing see Dosage Forms, Composition and Packaging.

INDICATIONS AND CLINICAL USE: Matulane (procarbazine hydrochloride) is indicated for use in combination with other anticancer agents for the treatment of Stage III and IV Hodgkin's disease. Matulane is used as part of the MOPP (mechlorethamine, vincristine, procarbazine, prednisone) regimen.

Matulane has also been used successfully alone or in combination with other chemotherapeutic agents to produce regression in a variety of tumour types such as lymphomas and gliomas but data are not yet sufficient to justify specific recommendations.

CONTRAINDICATIONS:

- hypersensitivity to procarbazine or any other component of the product.
- inadequate marrow reserve as demonstrated by bone marrow aspiration. Due consideration of this possible state should be given to each patient who has leukopenia, thrombocytopenia or anemia.

WARNINGS AND PRECAUTIONS:

Matulane (procarbazine hydrochloride) should be prescribed by a qualified health care professional who is experienced with cancer chemotherapy drugs. Clinically significant treatment-related toxicities include:

- **Long-term risk of developing acute leukemia, myelodysplasia, second cancers**
- **Infertility**
- **Neuropathy**
- **MAO (monoamine oxidase) inhibition**

The MOPP regimen is not recommended in treating favourable prognosis CS I-II patients.

General: It is recommended that Matulane (procarbazine hydrochloride) be given only by or under the supervision of a physician experienced in the use of potent antineoplastic drugs. Adequate clinical and laboratory facilities should be available for a proper monitoring of a treatment.

To minimize CNS depression and possible potentiation, barbiturates, antihistamines, narcotics, hypotensive agents or phenothiazines should be used with caution.

Ethyl alcohol should not be used since there may be a disulfiram-like reaction.

Because Matulane exhibits some monoamine oxidase inhibitory activity, sympathomimetic drugs, tricyclic antidepressant drugs (e.g. amitriptyline hydrochloride, imipramine hydrochloride), and other drugs, dietary supplements (e.g. ginseng) and foods known to react with monoamine oxidase inhibitors due to high tyramine content or other physiologic properties should be avoided. High tyramine content is most common in foods that are aged or fermented to increase flavor such as cheeses, yeast or meat extracts, fava or broad bean pods, smoked or pickled meat, poultry, or fish, fermented sausage (bologna, pepperoni, salami, and summer sausage) or other unfresh meat, or dried or overripe fruit.

A further phenomenon of toxicity common to many hydrazine derivatives is hemolysis and the appearance of Heinz-Ehrlich inclusion bodies in erythrocytes.

If radiation or a chemotherapeutic agent known to have marrow-depressant activity has been used, an interval of one month or longer without such therapy is recommended before starting treatment with Matulane. The length of this interval may also be determined by evidence of bone marrow recovery based on successive bone marrow studies.

Prompt cessation of therapy is recommended if any one of the following occurs:

- Central nervous system signs or symptoms such as paresthesias, neuropathies or confusion.
- Leukopenia (white blood count under 4000).
- Thrombocytopenia (platelets under 100 000).
- Hypersensitivity reaction.
- Stomatitis—The first small ulceration or persistent spot soreness around the oral cavity is a signal for cessation of therapy.
- Diarrhea—Frequent bowel movements or watery stools.
- Hemorrhage or bleeding tendencies.

Therapy may be resumed, at the discretion of the physician, after toxic side effects have cleared on clinical evaluation and appropriate laboratory studies.

Carcinogenesis and Mutagenesis: Instances of new nonlymphoid malignancy, including lung cancer and acute myelocytic leukemia, have been reported in patients with Hodgkin's disease treated with procarbazine in combination with other chemotherapy and/or radiation. The risks of secondary lung cancer from treatment appear to be multiplied by tobacco use. The International Agency for Research on Cancer (IARC) considers that there is "sufficient evidence" for the human carcinogenicity of procarbazine hydrochloride when it is given in intensive regimens which include other antineoplastic agents but that there is inadequate evidence of carcinogenicity in humans given procarbazine hydrochloride alone.

The international population-based study Hodgkin Lymphoma patients has demonstrated statistically significant risk of acute myeloid leukemia following Hodgkin lymphoma treatments over a 30-year period [Schonfeld, 2006]. One-year Hodgkin lymphoma survivors (N=35 511) were identified within 14 population-based cancer registries in Nordic countries and North America from January 1, 1970, through December 31, 2001. A total of 217 Hodgkin lymphoma survivors were diagnosed with AML The excess absolute risk of AML declined statistically significantly after 1984 (7.0 to 4.2 and 16.4 to 9.9 in the <35 and ≥35 age groups, respectively, which may be associated with modifications in chemotherapy. Analytical studies with detailed treatment data are required to correlate these decreases with changes in therapy and to better understand the long term risk of AML after Hodgkin's Lymphoma.

The carcinogenicity of procarbazine hydrochloride in animals and mutagenicity in test systems has been reported in a number of studies.

Hematologic: Leukopenia and thrombocytopenia have been reported in patients on Matulane therapy. Platelets and white blood cell counts should be performed prior to each subsequent cycle.

Hepatic/Renal: Undue toxicity may occur if Matulane is used in patients with impairment of renal and/or hepatic function. When appropriate, hospitalization for the initial course of treatment should be considered.

The metabolism of procarbazine is dependent on hepatic transformation and renal elimination. Therefore, dosing modifications may be required in patients with compromised renal or hepatic function.

Sexual Function/Reproduction: Exposure to procarbazine has been reported to be an independent risk factor for acute ovarian failure and acute amenorrhea in females. Azoospermia which can be prolonged resulting in male infertility has been reported to be associated with procarbazine when used in combination with other chemotherapeutic agents.

The standard battery of fertility/reproduction studies in laboratory animals have not been carried out with procarbazine hydrochloride.

Special Populations: Pregnant Women: Procarbazine hydrochloride can cause fetal harm when administered to a pregnant woman. While there are no adequate and well-controlled studies with procarbazine hydrochloride in pregnant women, there are case reports of malformations in the offspring of women who were exposed to procarbazine hydrochloride in combination with other antineoplastic agents during pregnancy. Procarbazine is teratogenic, mutagenic, and carcinogenic. Matulane should be used during pregnancy only if the potential benefit justifies the potential risk to the fetus. If this drug is used during pregnancy, or if the patient becomes pregnant while taking this drug, the patient should be apprised of the potential hazard to the fetus. Women of childbearing potential should be advised to avoid becoming pregnant.

Procarbazine hydrochloride was found to be teratogenic in animal studies. Procarbazine hydrochloride has not been adequately studied in animals for its effects on peri- and postnatal development. However, neurogenic tumours were noted in the offspring in animal studies.

Nursing Women: It is not known whether Matulane is excreted in human milk. Because of the potential for tumorigenicity shown for procarbazine hydrochloride in animal studies, mothers should not nurse while receiving this drug.

Pediatrics: Appropriate prospective controlled studies in the pediatric population have not been performed. Undue toxicity, evidenced by tremors, coma and convulsions, has occurred in a few cases. Dosage, therefore, should be individualized. Very close monitoring is mandatory.

Monitoring and Laboratory Tests: Baseline laboratory data should be obtained prior to initiation of therapy. The hematologic status as indicated by hemoglobin, hematocrit, white blood count (WBC), differential, reticulocytes and platelets should be monitored closely—at least every 3 or 4 days. Bone marrow depression often occurs 2 to 8 weeks after the start of treatment. If leukopenia occurs, hospitalization of the patient may be needed for appropriate treatment to prevent systemic infection.

Hepatic and renal evaluation are indicated prior to beginning therapy. Urinalysis, transaminase, alkaline phosphatase and blood urea nitrogen should be repeated at least weekly.

As part of routine monitoring clinical pulmonary exam, including auscultation, pulmonary toxicity ratings (Cough, SOB) should be performed periodically.

Information to Be Provided to the Patient: Patients should be warned not to drink alcoholic beverages while on Matulane therapy since there may be an Antabuse (disulfiram)-like reaction. They should also be cautioned to avoid foods with known high tyramine content such as wine, yogurt, ripe cheese and bananas. Over-the-counter drug preparations which contain antihistamines or sympathomimetic drugs and tricyclic antidepressants (e.g. amitriptyline HCl, imipramine HCl) should not be used. Patients taking Matulane should also be warned against the use of prescription drugs without the knowledge and consent of their physician. Patients should be advised to discontinue tobacco use.

ADVERSE REACTIONS: In dealing with cancer chemotherapeutic agents, adverse effects are not only common but are to be expected, and actually serve as a guideline to dosage and duration of administration; Matulane (procarbazine hydrochloride) is no exception as to toxicity.

The following adverse reactions include both adverse experiences from clinical trials as well as post-marketing surveillance.

The most serious adverse effects are associated with leukopenia, thrombopenia and a variety of neurological effects (MAO inhibition).

The most commonly reported adverse effects are nausea and vomiting. Leukopenia, anemia and thrombopenia occur frequently.

Other adverse reactions grouped by Body System:

Hematologic: immunosuppression, pancytopenia, eosinophilia, hemolytic anemia, bleeding tendencies such as petechiae, purpura, epistaxis and hemoptysis; thrombosis including pulmonary, deep vein, and mesenteric.

Gastrointestinal: hepatic dysfunction, jaundice, stomatitis, ascites, hematemesis, melena, diarrhea, dysphagia, anorexia, abdominal pain, constipation, dry mouth, pancreatitis.

Neurologic: coma, convulsions, neuropathy, ataxia, paresthesia, nystagmus, diminished reflexes, falling, foot drop, headache, dizziness, unsteadiness, fainting.

Cardiovascular: hypotension, tachycardia, syncope, hypertension, angina, pericarditis, cardiotoxicity, Raynaud-like syndrome.

Ophthalmic: retinal hemorrhage, papilledema, photophobia, diplopia, inability to focus.

Respiratory: pneumonitis, pleural effusion, cough, pneumonia, pulmonary toxicity.

Dermatologic: herpes, dermatitis, pruritus, alopecia, hyperpigmentation, rash, urticaria, flushing, photosensitivity, Lyell syndrome, toxic epidermal necrolysis.

Allergic: generalized allergic reactions.

Genitourinary: hematuria, urinary frequency, nocturia, nephritis.

Musculoskeletal: pain, including myalgia and arthralgia; tremors, osteonecrosis.

Psychiatric: hallucinations, depression, apprehension, nervousness, confusion, nightmares, insomnia.

Endocrine: acute ovarian failure, acute amenorrhea, gynecomastia in prepubertal and early pubertal boys.

Miscellaneous: intercurrent infections, hearing loss, pyrexia, sweating, diaphoresis, lethargy, weakness, fatigue, edema, chills, slurred speech, hoarseness, drowsiness.

Second malignancies (including lung cancer, acute myelocytic leukemia and malignant myelosclerosis) and azoospermia have been reported in patients with Hodgkin's disease treated with procarbazine in combination with other chemotherapy and/or radiation. The risks of secondary lung cancer from treatment appear to be multiplied by tobacco use.

DRUG INTERACTIONS: Matulane (procarbazine hydrochloride) is used in combination with other cytotoxic drugs. Additive toxicity may occur especially with regard to bone marrow/hematologic and gastrointestinal effects (see Warnings and Precautions).

Drug-Drug Interactions: CNS depression and possible potentiation may occur with barbiturates, antihistamines, narcotics, hypotensive agents, phenothiazines, monoamine oxidase (MAO) inhibitors, or catechol-O-methyltransferase (COMT) inhibitors. Matulane can interfere with the absorption of digoxin. The effects of antidiabetics and levodopa may be enhanced by Matulane use. Sensitivity to Matulane can be increased when used with carbamazepine. Concomitant use of these drugs with Matulane should be avoided. Matulane also exhibits monoamine oxidase inhibitory activity. Sympathomimetic drugs and tricyclic antidepressant drugs may interact with Matulane to cause hypertensive reactions (see Warnings and Precautions).

Drug-Food Interactions: Dietary supplements or foods known to react with monoamine oxidase inhibitors due to high tyramine content or other physiologic properties should be avoided (see Warnings and Precautions). Typical reactions include headache, flushed face, palpitations, nausea and vomiting or hypertension.

DOSAGE AND ADMINISTRATION: Matulane (procarbazine hydrochloride) should only be used by physicians experienced with cancer chemotherapeutic drugs.

As part of the MOPP (mechlorethamine, vincristine, and prednisone) and c-MOPP (cyclophosphamide, mechlorethamine, vincristine, and prednisone) regimens Matulane is given orally in a dose of 100 mg/m²/day for 14 days and repeated every 4 weeks.

Upon evidence of hematologic or other toxicity (see Warnings and Precautions), the drug should be discontinued until there has been satisfactory recovery. After toxic side effects have subsided, therapy may then be resumed at the discretion of the physician, based on clinical evaluation and appropriate laboratory studies.

OVERDOSAGE:

The major manifestations of overdosage with Matulane (procarbazine hydrochloride) would be anticipated to be nausea, vomiting, enteritis, diarrhea hypotension, tremors, convulsions and coma. Treatment should consist of either the administration of an emetic or gastric lavage. General supportive measures such as intravenous fluids are advised. Since the major toxicity of procarbazine hydrochloride is hematologic and hepatic, patients should have frequent complete blood counts and liver function tests throughout their period of recovery and for a minimum of two weeks thereafter. Should abnormalities appear in any of these determinations, appropriate measures for correction and stabilization should be immediately undertaken.

For management of a suspected drug overdose, CPhA recommends that you contact your **regional Poison Control Centre**. See the CPS Directory section for a list of Poison Control Centres.

ACTION AND CLINICAL PHARMACOLOGY: Matulane (procarbazine hydrochloride) is one of the methylhydrazine derivatives that has demonstrated an antineoplastic effect against Hodgkin's Disease. The mode of cytotoxic action of Matulane has not yet been clearly defined; however, there is evidence that the drug may act by inhibition of protein, RNA and DNA synthesis. No cross resistance with other chemotherapeutic agents, radiotherapy or steroids has been demonstrated.

Pharmacokinetics: Procarbazine hydrochloride is metabolized primarily in the liver and kidneys. The drug appears to be auto-oxidized to the azo derivative with the release of hydrogen peroxide. The azo derivative isomerizes to the hydrazone, and following hydrolysis splits into a benzylaldehyde derivative and methylhydrazine. The methylhydrazine is further degraded to CO_2 and CH_4 and possibly hydrazine, whereas the aldehyde is oxidized to N-isopropylterephthalamic acid, which is excreted in the urine. Procarbazine hydrochloride is rapidly and completely absorbed. Following oral administration of 30 mg of ^{14}C-labeled procarbazine hydrochloride, maximum peak plasma radioactive concentrations were reached within 60 minutes.

After intravenous injection, the plasma half-life of procarbazine hydrochloride is approximately 10 minutes. Approximately 70% of the radioactivity is excreted in the urine as N-isopropylterephthalamic acid within 24 hours following both oral and intravenous administration of ^{14}C-labeled procarbazine hydrochloride.

Procarbazine hydrochloride crosses the blood-brain barrier and rapidly equilibrates between plasma and cerebrospinal fluid after oral administration.

STORAGE AND STABILITY: Matulane (procarbazine hydrochloride) should be stored at 15-30°C in a tightly closed, light resistant container.

SPECIAL HANDLING INSTRUCTIONS: Procedures for proper handling and disposal of anticancer drugs should be considered. Several guidelines on this subject have been published. Patients and patient caregivers should not open or crush capsules. Do not take Matulane if the capsule is broken. Keep out of reach of children.

INFORMATION FOR THE PATIENT: Published in e-CPS, available by subscription at www.e-cps.ca.

DOSAGE FORMS, COMPOSITION AND PACKAGING: Each No. 2 ivory gelatin capsule contains: procarbazine 50 mg (as procarbazine HCl). Nonmedicinal ingredients: cornstarch, gelatin, mannitol, methylparaben, potassium sorbate, propylparaben, quinoline yellow WS, sunset yellow FCF, talc and titanium dioxide. Plastic bottles of 100.

The reader is invited to consult CPhA's monograph **ACE Inhibitors**.

Mavik® Ⓟ

trandolapril

Angiotensin Converting Enzyme Inhibitor

Abbott

Date of Preparation: May 15, 1997
Date of Revision: December 8, 2008

SUMMARY PRODUCT INFORMATION:

Route of Administration	Dosage Form/ Strength	Clinically Relevant Nonmedicinal Ingredients
Oral	Capsule/0.5 mg, 1 mg, 2 mg and 4 mg	Erythrosine, gelatin, iron oxides and hydroxides, lactose, maize starch, povidone, sodium lauryl sulphate, sodium stearyl fumarate, titanium dioxide

INDICATIONS AND CLINICAL USE: MAVIK (trandolapril) is indicated for:

Essential Hypertension:

- treatment of patients with mild to moderate essential hypertension. It may be used alone or in association with thiazide diuretics.

Trandolapril should normally be used in patients in whom treatment with a diuretic or a beta blocker was found ineffective or has been associated with unacceptable adverse effects.

Trandolapril can also be tried as an initial agent in those patients in whom use of diuretics and/or beta blockers are contraindicated or in patients with medical conditions in which these drugs frequently cause serious adverse effects.

The safety and efficacy of trandolapril in patients with renovascular hypertension has not been established, therefore its use in these conditions is not recommended.

Treatment Following Acute Myocardial Infarction:

- following acute myocardial infarction in clinically stable patients with left ventricular dysfunction, with or without symptoms of heart failure, to improve survival and reduce hospitalizations for heart failure.

Sufficient experience in the treatment of patients with severe heart failure (NYHA Class IV) immediately after myocardial infarction is not yet available.

General: In using trandolapril, consideration should be given to the risk of angioedema (see Warnings and Precautions).

Geriatrics (≥65 years of age): Although clinical experience has not identified differences in response between the elderly (≥65 years) and younger patients (<65 years), greater sensitivity of some older individuals cannot be ruled out (see Action and Clinical Pharmacology, Pharmacodynamics).

Pediatrics (<18 years of age): The safety and effectiveness of trandolapril in children below the age of 18 have not been established. Therefore use in this age group is not recommended.

CONTRAINDICATIONS: MAVIK (trandolapril) is contraindicated in patients who:

- are pregnant or planning to become pregnant.
- are hypersensitive to this drug or to any ingredient in the formulation or component of the container. For a complete listing, see Dosage Forms, Composition and Packaging.
- have a history of angioedema.

WARNINGS AND PRECAUTIONS:

Serious Warnings and Precautions

When used in pregnancy, angiotensin converting enzyme (ACE) inhibitors can cause injury and even death to the developing fetus. When pregnancy is detected or if the patient is planning to become pregnant, MAVIK should be discontinued as soon as possible. See Warnings and Precautions, Special Populations, Pregnant Women.

Cardiovascular: Hypotension: Symptomatic hypotension has occurred after administration of MAVIK (trandolapril), usually after the first or second dose or when the dose was increased. It is more likely to occur in patients who are volume and salt depleted as a result of diuretic therapy, dietary salt restriction, dialysis, diarrhea, or vomiting. In patients with ischemic heart disease or cerebrovascular disease, an excessive fall in blood pressure could result in a myocardial infarction or cerebrovascular accident (see Adverse Reactions). Because of the potential fall in blood pressure in these patients, therapy with trandolapril should be started under close medical supervision. Such patients should be followed closely for the first weeks of treatment and whenever the dose of trandolapril is increased. In patients with severe congestive heart failure, with or without associated renal insufficiency, ACE inhibitor therapy may cause excessive hypotension and has been associated with oliguria, and/or progressive azotemia, and rarely, with acute renal failure and/or death.

If hypotension occurs, the patient should be placed in a supine position and, if necessary, receive an intravenous infusion of 0.9% sodium chloride. A transient hypotensive response is not a contraindication to further doses which can be given, usually without difficulty, once the blood pressure has increased after volume expansion. However, lower doses of trandolapril and/or reduced concomitant diuretic therapy should be considered.

If hypotension develops in patients receiving treatment following acute myocardial infarction, consideration should be given to discontinuation of trandolapril (see Adverse Reactions, Clinical Trial Adverse Drug Reactions, Treatment Following Acute Myocardial Infarction, and Dosage and Administration, Recommended Dose and Dosage Adjustment, Treatment Following Acute Myocardial Infarction).

Aortic Stenosis: There is concern, on theoretical grounds, that patients with aortic stenosis might be at particular risk of decreased coronary perfusion when treated with vasodilators.

Ear/Nose/Throat: As with other ACE inhibitors, dry, persistent cough, which usually disappears only after withdrawal or lowering of the dose of trandolapril, has been reported. Such possibility should be considered as part of the differential diagnosis of cough.

Endocrine and Metabolism: Hyperkalemia and Potassium-Sparing Diuretics: Increases in serum potassium (upper limit of normal range 5.0 mmol/L) were observed in approximately 2.2% of patients in clinical trials treated with trandolapril, in most cases these resolved despite continued therapy. Hyperkalemia was not a cause of discontinuation of therapy in any hypertensive patient. Risk factors for the development of hyperkalemia may include renal insufficiency, diabetes mellitus, and the concomitant use of agents to treat hypokalemia or other drugs associated with increases in serum potassium (see Drug Interactions).

Hematologic: Neutropenia/Agranulocytosis: Agranulocytosis and bone marrow depression have been caused by ACE inhibitors. Current experience with trandolapril shows the incidence to be rare. Periodic monitoring of white blood cell counts should be considered, especially in patients with collagen vascular disease and/or renal disease.

Hepatic/Biliary/Pancreatic: Patients with Impaired Liver Function: Trandolapril should be used with caution in patients with pre-existing liver abnormalities. In such patients, baseline liver function tests should be obtained before administration of the drug and close monitoring of response and metabolic effect should apply.

Hepatitis (hepatocellular and/or cholestatic), elevations of liver enzymes and/or serum bilirubin have occurred during therapy with ACE inhibitors in patients with or without pre-existing liver abnormalities. In most cases the changes were reversed on discontinuation of the drug.

Elevations of liver enzymes and/or serum bilirubin have been reported with trandolapril (see Adverse Reactions). Should the patient receiving trandolapril experience any unexplained symptoms, particularly during the first weeks or months of treatment, it is recommended that a full set of liver function tests and any other necessary investigations be carried out. Discontinuation of trandolapril should be considered when appropriate. (See Action and Clinical Pharmacology, Pharmacokinetics.)

Immune: Angioedema: Angioedema has been reported in patients taking ACE inhibitors, including MAVIK (trandolapril). Angioedema associated with laryngeal involvement may be fatal. If laryngeal stridor or angioedema of the face, tongue, or glottis occurs, trandolapril should be discontinued immediately, the patient treated appropriately in accordance with accepted medical care, and carefully observed until the swelling disappears. In instances where swelling is confined to the face and lips, the condition generally resolves without treatment. Where there is involvement of tongue, glottis, or larynx, likely to cause airway obstruction, appropriate therapy (including, but not limited to 0.3 to 0.5 mL of subcutaneous epinephrine solution 1:1000) should be administered promptly (see Adverse Reactions).

Patients with a history of angioedema unrelated to ACE inhibitor therapy may be at increased risk of angioedema while receiving an ACE inhibitor (see Contraindications).

The incidence of angioedema during ACE inhibition therapy has been reported to be higher in black than in non-black patients.

Intestinal angioedema has also been reported in patients treated with ACE inhibitors. These patients presented with abdominal pain (with or without nausea or vomiting); in some cases there was no prior history of facial angioedema and C-1 esterase levels were normal. The angioedema was diagnosed by procedures including abdominal CT scan or ultrasound, or at surgery, and symptoms resolved after stopping the ACE inhibitor. Intestinal angioedema should be included in the differential diagnosis of patients on ACE inhibitors presenting with abdominal pain.

Anaphylactoid Reactions During Membrane Exposure: Anaphylactoid reactions have been reported in patients dialyzed with high-flux membranes (e.g., polyacrylonitrile [PAN]) and treated concomitantly with an ACE inhibitor. Dialysis should be stopped immediately if symptoms such as nausea, abdominal cramps, burning, angioedema, shortness of breath and severe hypotension occur. Symptoms are not relieved by antihistamines. In these patients consideration should be given to using a different type of dialysis membrane or a different class of antihypertensive agents.

Peri-Operative Considerations: The hypotensive effects of certain inhalation anesthetics may be enhanced by ACE inhibitors. In patients undergoing surgery or anesthesia with agents producing hypotension, trandolapril will block angiotensin II formation secondary to compensatory renin release. If hypotension occurs and is considered to be due to this mechanism, it may be corrected by volume repletion.

Renal: Renal Impairment: As a consequence of inhibiting the renin-angiotensin-aldosterone system, changes in renal function have been seen in susceptible individuals. In patients whose renal function may depend on the activity of the renin-angiotensin-aldosterone system, such as patients with bilateral renal artery stenosis, unilateral renal artery stenosis to a solitary kidney, or severe congestive heart failure, treatment with agents that inhibit this system has been associated with oliguria, progressive azotemia, and rarely, acute renal failure and/or death. In susceptible patients, concomitant diuretic use may further increase risk.

Use of MAVIK (trandolapril) should include appropriate assessment of renal function.

Special Populations: Pregnant Women: ACE inhibitors can cause fetal and neonatal morbidity and mortality when administered to pregnant women. When pregnancy is detected or if the patient is planning to become pregnant, MAVIK should be discontinued as soon as possible.

The use of ACE inhibitors during the second and third trimesters of pregnancy has been associated with fetal and neonatal injury including hypotension, neonatal skull hypoplasia, anuria, reversible or irreversible renal failure, and death. Oligohydramnios has also been reported, presumably resulting from decreased fetal renal function, associated with fetal limb contractures, craniofacial deformation, and hypoplastic lung development.

Prematurity, and patent ductus arteriosus and other structural cardiac malformations, as well as neurologic malformations, have also been reported following ACE inhibitor exposure in the first trimester of pregnancy.

Infants with a history of in utero exposure to ACE inhibitors should be closely observed for hypotension, oliguria, and hyperkalemia. If oliguria occurs, attention should be directed toward support of blood pressure and renal perfusion. Exchange transfusion or dialysis may be required as a means of reversing hypotension and/or substituting for impaired renal function; however, limited experience with those procedures has not been associated with significant clinical benefit.

It is not known if trandolapril or trandolaprilat can be removed from the body by hemodialysis.

Animal Data: Teratology studies in the rat were carried out at doses of 0, 100, 300, or 1000 mg/kg/day. An increased incidence of minor defects (dilation of renal pelvis and ureters) over control values was found at the 1000 mg/kg/day dose series. In fertility studies, where doses of 0, 1, 10 or 100 mg/kg/day were used, the incidence of pelvic cavitation and dilated ureters was increased with the 10 and 100 mg/kg/day dose.

Teratology studies were carried out in the rabbit, both with and without electrolyte supplementation. In two studies without supplementation covering the 0.1 to 0.8 mg/kg dose range, maternal deaths were seen at all doses with a dose-related incidence. These were associated with fetal toxicity and increased fetal loss. No teratological effect was seen. Supplementation with electrolytes allowed doses of 2 to 8 mg/kg to be given: maternal toxicity was again seen, particularly at 8 mg/kg, with weight loss and abortion. No teratological effect was seen.

Two teratology studies were carried out in the cynomolgus monkey (doses of 0, 10, 50 or 250 mg/kg/day and also 5, 25 or 125 mg/kg/day): dosing was on days 20 to 50 of gestation with examination of the fetuses following caesarean section on day 100. Abortions were 3/10, 6/10, 5/11 and 7/10 at respectively 0, 10, 50 or 250 mg/kg/day and 1/10, 4/10, 4/10 and 7/10 at 0, 5, 25 or 125 mg/kg/day. Apart from one animal with a kinked tail in the group receiving 250 mg/kg/day, no other evidence of teratological effects attributable to treatment were observed.

Nursing Women: The presence of concentrations of ACE inhibitor has been reported in human milk. Use of ACE inhibitors is not recommended during breast-feeding. If breast-feeding needs to be continued, alternative measures to control the patient's blood pressure need to be put in place.

Pediatrics (<18 years of age): The safety and effectiveness of trandolapril in children below the age of 18 have not been established. Therefore use in this age group is not recommended.

Geriatrics (≥65 years of age): Although clinical experience has not identified differences in response between the elderly (≥65 years) and younger patients (<65 years), greater sensitivity of some older individuals cannot be ruled out (see Action and Clinical Pharmacology, Pharmacodynamics).

ADVERSE REACTIONS: Clinical Trial Adverse Drug Reactions: Because clinical trials are conducted under very specific conditions the adverse reaction rates observed in the clinical trials may not reflect the rates observed in practice and should not be compared to the rates in the clinical trials of another drug. Adverse drug reaction information from clinical trials is useful for identifying drug-related adverse events and for approximating rates.

Essential Hypertension: The safety experience in double-blind, placebo-controlled and open-label studies includes 2581 patients with mild to moderate essential hypertension who received MAVIK (trandolapril) therapy. Of these, 265 patients were 65 years of age or older. A total of 126 patients prematurely discontinued across the various trials due to adverse events. In long-term open-label trials, 1049 received trandolapril therapy, of which 212 continued treatment for 24 months, 689 for at least 12 months, and 911 for at least 6 months.

Severe adverse reactions occurring in long-term clinical trials (n=1049) with doses of trandolapril ranging from 0.5 mg to 8 mg included cough (3.9%), headache (2.3%), asthenia (2.1%), dizziness (1.7%), palpitations (0.7%), hypotension (0.5%), nausea (0.5%), pruritus (0.5%), and malaise (0.5%).

One serious adverse reaction was judged to be possibly related to trandolapril therapy. This involved a rapid supraventricular arrhythmia with atrial flutter which occurred in a 68 year old male patient with a known history of heart disease.

The adverse reactions (corresponding to possibly, probably or definitely related to treatment) with an incidence ≥1% in all double-blind, placebo-controlled trials and open-label Phase 3 hypertension trials (n=2581) are shown in Table 1.

Table 1: MAVIK

Adverse Reactions by Body System (SOC) Patients Receiving Trandolapril in Phase 3 Hypertension Trials ≥1%

System Organ Class (SOC)	Trandolapril (n=693) %	Placebo (n=194) %
Placebo-Controlled Studies		
Nervous System Disorders		
Headache	2.31	0.5
Gastrointestinal Disorders		
Nausea	1.15	0

System Organ Class (SOC)	Trandolapril (n=1888) %
Active-Controlled and Open-Label Studies	
Nervous System Disorders	
Headache	2.17
Dizziness	1.59
Respiratory, Thoracic and Mediastinal Disorders	
Cough	2.60
General Disorders and Administration Site Conditions	
Asthenia	2.01

Treatment Following Acute Myocardial Infarction: In a survival study in patients with left ventricular dysfunction following myocardial infarction, 876 patients randomized to trandolapril, and 873 to placebo, were treated for an average of two years. A total of 209 patients prematurely discontinued across the various trials due adverse events.

The most serious adverse reactions occurring more frequently with trandolapril than with placebo included dizziness (2.6%) and hypotension (1.5%). The most frequent clinical adverse reactions occurring more frequently with trandolapril than with placebo were cough, dizziness and hypotension.

The adverse reactions (corresponding to possibly, probably or definitely related to treatement) with an incidence ≥1%, occurring in a higher percentage of trandolapril-treated patients than in placebo-treated patients, are presented in Table 2.

Table 2: MAVIK

Adverse Reactions Reported with Trandolapril in Post Myocardial Infarction Patients in the TRACE Study That Occurred at a Frequency ≥1%

System Organ Class (SOC)	Trandolapril (n=876) %	Placebo (n=873) %
Nervous System Disorders		
Dizziness	1.9	1.4
Respiratory, Thoracic and Mediastinal Disorders		
Cough	3.9	0.9
Vascular Disorders		
Hypotension	2.1	0.6

Less Common Clinical Trial Adverse Drug Reactions (<1%): Blood and Lymphatic System Disorders: anaemia, leukopenia, platelet disorder, thrombocytopenia, white blood cell disorder.
Cardiac Disorders: angina pectoris, bradycardia, cardiac failure, myocardial infarction, myocardial ischaemia, palpitations, tachycardia, ventricular tachycardia.
Congenital, Familial and Genetic Disorders: congenital arterial malformation, ichthyosis.
Ear and Labyrinth Disorders: vertigo, tinnitus.
Eye Disorders: abnormal vision, blepharitis, conjunctival oedema, eye disorder, glaucoma*, visual disturbance.
Gastrointestinal Disorders: abdominal pain, constipation, diarrhoea, dry mouth, dyspepsia, esophagitis*, flatulence, gastritis, gastrointestinal disorder, gastrointestinal pain, haematemesis, nausea, vomiting.
General Disorders and Administration Site Conditions: chest pain, fatigue, feeling abnormal, malaise, oedema, oedema peripheral.
Hepatobiliary Disorders: hepatitis, hyperbiliruninaemia.
Immune System Disorders: anaphylactoid reaction*, hypersensitivity.
Infections and Infestations: bronchitis, pharyngitis, upper respiratory tract infection, urinary tract infection.
Injury, Poisoning and Procedural Complications: injury.
Metabolism and Nutritional Disorder: anorexia, enzyme abnormality, gout, hypercholesterolaemia, hyperglycaemia, hyperlipidaemia, hyperuricaemia, hyponatraemia.
Musculoskeletal and Connective Tissue Disorders: arthralgia, back pain, bone pain, muscle spasms, osteoarthritis, pain in extremity.
Nervous System Disorders: cerebrovascular accident, dysgeusia, migraine, migraine without aura, myoclonus, paresthesia, somnolence, syncope, tremor*.
Psychiatric Disorders: agitation, anxiety, apathy, depression, hallucination, insomnia, libido decreased, sleep disorder.
Renal and Urinary Disorders: azotaemia, pollakiuria, polyuria, renal failure.
Reproductive System and Breast Disorders: erectile dysfunction.
Respiratory, Thoracic and Mediastinal Disorders: dyspnoea, epistaxis, pharyngeal inflammation, pharyngolaryngeal pain, productive cough, respiratory disorder, upper respiratory tract congestion, upper respiratory tract inflammation.
Skin and Subcutaneous Tissue Disorders: acne, angioneurotic oedema, dry skin, eczema, hyperhidrosis, pemphigus*, pruritus, psoriasis, rash, skin disorder.
Vascular Disorders: angiopathy, hot flush, hypertension, hypotension, orthostatic hypotension, peripheral vascular disorder, varicose vein.

Rare cases of angioedema affecting the face, extremities, lips, tongue, glottis and/or larynx have been reported in patients treated with ACE inhibitor, including trandolapril.

* These adverse effects represent adverse events; not reactions.

A symptom complex has been reported which may include fever, vasculitis, myalgia, arthralgia/arthritis, a positive anti-nuclear antibody (ANA), elevated erythrocyte sedimentation rate (ESR), eosinophilia and leukocytosis. Rash, photosensitivity or other dermatologic manifestations may also occur.

Rare report of increased appetite has been observed.

Abnormal Hematologic and Clinical Chemistry Findings: Clinical Laboratory Test Findings: Blood creatinine increased, blood alkaline phosphatase increased, blood urea increased, blood lactate dehydrogenase increased, electrocardiogram abnormal, hyperkaelemia, hyperuricaemia, laboratory test abnormal, liver function test abnormal, platelet count decreased, transaminases increased.

Hematologic Findings: Haematocrit decreased, haemoglobin decreased.

Post-Market Adverse Drug Reactions:

System Organ Class	Adverse Event
Blood and Lymphatic System Disorders	Agranulocytosis, pancytopenia
Cardiac Disorders	Arrhythmia, cardiac arrest
Gastrointestinal Disorders	Abdominal pain, ileus, nausea
General Disorders and Administration Site Conditions	Fever
Hepatobiliary Disorders	Jaundice, pancreatitis
Musculoskeletal and Connective Tissue Disorders	Myalgia
Nervous System Disorders	Balance disorder, cerebral haemorrhage, dizziness, syncope, transient ischemic attack
Respiratory, Thoracic and Mediastinal Disorders	Angioedema, bronchospasm (cough, dyspnoea)
Skin and Appendages	Alopecia, leukocytoclastic vasculitis, rash, Stevens-Johnson syndrome, toxic epidermal necrolysis, urticaria

DRUG INTERACTIONS Drug-Drug Interactions: Agents Increasing Serum Potassium: Since trandolapril decreases aldosterone production, elevation of serum potassium may occur. Potassium sparing diuretics such as spironolactone, triamterene or amiloride, or potassium supplements should be given only for documented hypokalemia and with caution and frequent monitoring of serum potassium, since a significant increase in serum potassium could occur.

Salt substitutes which contain potassium should be used with caution.

Agents Causing Renin Release: The antihypertensive effect of trandolapril is augmented by antihypertensive agents that cause renin release (e.g., diuretics).

Alcohol: Alcohol enhances the bioavailability of ACE inhibitors.

Allopurinol, Cytostatic, Immunosuppressive Agents, Systemic Corticosteroids or Procainamide: Concomitant administration with ACE-inhibitors may lead to an increased risk of leukopenia.

Anaphylactoid Reactions During LDL Apheresis: Rarely, patients receiving ACE inhibitors during low density lipoprotein apheresis with dextran sulfate have experienced life-threatening anaphylactoid reactions. These reactions were avoided by temporarily withholding ACE inhibitor therapy prior to each apheresis.

Anaphylactoid Reactions During Desensitization: There have been isolated reports of patients experiencing sustained life-threatening anaphylactoid reactions while receiving ACE inhibitors during desensitization treatment with hymenoptera (bees, wasps) venom. In the same patients, these reactions have been avoided when ACE inhibitors were temporarily withheld for at least 24 hours, but they have reappeared upon inadvertent rechallenge.

Antacids: They decrease the bioavailability of ACE inhibitors (it is recommended to ingest these products separately).

Concomitant Diuretic Therapy: Patients concomitantly taking ACE inhibitors and diuretics, and especially those in whom diuretic therapy was recently instituted, may occasionally experience an excessive reduction of blood pressure after initiation of therapy. The possibility of adverse hypotensive effects after the first dose of trandolapril can be minimized by either discontinuing the diuretic or increasing the salt intake prior to initiation of treatment with trandolapril. If it is not possible to discontinue the diuretic, the starting dose of trandolapril should be reduced and the patient should be closely observed for several hours following the initial dose until blood pressure has stabilized (see Warnings and Precautions and Dosage and Administration).

Digoxin: In one open-label study conducted in 8 healthy male volunteers, in which multiple therapeutic doses of both trandolapril and digoxin were administered, no changes were found in serum levels of trandolapril, trandolaprilat, and digoxin. Pharmacodynamically, the combination had a synergistic effect on left ventricular functions, as evidenced by the improvement in systolic time-intervals.

Lithium: Increased serum lithium levels and symptoms of lithium toxicity have been reported in patients receiving concurrently ACE inhibitors and lithium. Lithium based drugs should be administered with caution, and frequent monitoring of serum lithium levels is recommended. If a diuretic is also used, the risk of lithium toxicity may be further increased.

Nifedipine SR: A study evaluating the potential pharmacokinetic and pharmacodynamic interaction between nifedipine (20 mg) (sustained release) and trandolapril (4 mg) was conducted in 12 healthy male volunteers. After a single dose, no pharmacokinetic or pharmacodynamic interaction was found between the two products.

Non-Steroidal Anti-Inflammatory Agents: The antihypertensive effects of ACE inhibitors may be reduced with concomitant administration of non-steroidal anti-inflammatory agents. As with other ACE inhibitors, the combination of trandolapril with non-steroidal anti-inflammatory agents predisposes to a risk of hyperkalemia particularly in cases of renal failure.

Blood pressure should be monitored more closely when any NSAID is added or discontinued in a patient treated with trandolapril.

Warfarin: In a multi-dose, double-blind, placebo-controlled, pharmacodynamic interaction study with 20 healthy volunteers administered trandolapril (2 mg) and therapeutic doses of warfarin, no clinically significant effects on the anticoagulant properties of warfarin were found.

Drug-Food Interactions: Patients should be told not to use salt substitutes or foods containing potassium without consulting their physician (see Warnings and Precautions). Food does not affect the C_{max} and AUC of trandolapril and trandolaprilat, however food prolongs the T_{max} of trandolaprilat by approximately 2 hours.

Drug-Herb Interactions: Interactions with herbal products have not been evaluated.

Drug-Laboratory Test Interactions: Interactions with laboratory tests have not been evaluated.

Drug-Lifestyle Interactions: Alcohol enhances the bioavailability of ACE inhibitors.

Depending on individual susceptibility, the patients' ability to drive a vehicle or operate machinery may be impaired, especially in the initial stages of treatment.

DOSAGE AND ADMINISTRATION: Dosing Considerations: Essential Hypertension: Dosage of MAVIK (trandolapril) must be individualized. Initiation of therapy requires consideration of recent antihypertensive drug treatment, the extent of blood pressure elevation and salt restriction. The dosage of other antihypertensive agents being used with trandolapril may need to be adjusted.

In some patients treated once daily, the antihypertensive effect may diminish towards the end of the dosing interval. This can be evaluated by measuring blood pressure just prior to dosing to determine whether satisfactory control is being maintained for 24 hours. If it is not an increase in dose should be considered. If blood pressure is not controlled with trandolapril alone, a diuretic may be added.

Diuretic-Treated Patients: Symptomatic hypotension occasionally may occur following the initial dose of trandolapril and is more likely in patients who are currently being treated with a diuretic. The diuretic should, if possible, be discontinued for two to three days before beginning therapy with trandolapril to reduce the likelihood of hypotension (see Warnings and Precautions). If the diuretic cannot be discontinued, an initial dose of 0.5 mg trandolapril should be used with careful medical supervision for several hours and until blood pressure has stabilized. The dosage of trandolapril should subsequently be titrated to the optimal response.

Liver Impairment: A single oral dose of 2 mg of trandolapril was administered to patients with hepatic cirrhosis. Compared to healthy subjects receiving the same dose, C_{max} and AUC values of trandolapril increased by approximately 9 times; C_{max} and AUC of trandolaprilat were nearly doubled. (See Action and Clinical Pharmacology, Pharmacokinetics and Warnings and Precautions, Hepatic/Biliary/Pancreatic, Patients with Impaired Liver Function.)

Recommended Dose and Dosage Adjustment: Monotherapy: Adult: The recommended initial dosage of trandolapril is 1 mg once daily. Dosage should be adjusted according to blood pressure response at intervals of 2 to 4 weeks up to a maximum of 4 mg once daily. The usual maintenance dose is 1 to 2 mg once daily.

Dosage in the Elderly: In elderly patients with normal renal and hepatic function, no dosage adjustment is necessary (see Warnings and Precautions, Special Populations, Geriatrics (≥65 years of age)).

However, as some elderly patients may be particularly susceptible to ACE inhibitors, administration of low initial doses and evaluation of the blood pressure response and of the renal function at the beginning of the treatment is recommended.

Dosage in Renal Impairment: For patients with a creatinine clearance below 30 mL/min/1.73 m², the recommended initial dose is 0.5 mg trandolapril once daily. Dosage may be titrated upward until blood pressure is controlled or to a maximum total daily dose of 1 mg.

In patients with severe renal impairment (creatinine clearance below 10 mL/min/1.73 m²), a daily dosage of 0.5 mg in a single dose should not be exceeded.

Dosage in Liver Impairment: The recommended initial dose is 0.5 mg trandolapril once daily.

Treatment Following Acute Myocardial Infarction: Dosage should be individualized. Initiation of therapy requires consideration of concomitant medication and baseline blood pressure in hemodynamically stable patients.

A starting dose of 1 mg trandolapril once daily should be initiated no earlier than the third day following acute myocardial infarction in patients with left ventricular dysfunction.

After two days at 1 mg once daily, the dose should be increased to 2 mg once daily. For patients who cannot tolerate this dose, the 1 mg once daily dose can be maintained.

After one month, patients tolerating the 2 mg once daily dose should have their dosage increased to 4 mg once daily. Again, for patients who cannot tolerate the 4 mg once daily dose, the 2 mg once daily dose can be maintained.

The dose must be reduced when it is clinically necessary (see Warnings and Precautions, Cardiovascular, Hypotension). If hypotension preventing the patient from standing or walking is observed and is not explained by other factors, the dose must be reduced.

For patients with renal or liver impairment, a starting dose no higher than 0.5 mg once daily should be instituted.

Missed Dose: If the patient forgets to take a capsule, he should take one as soon as he remembers, if he remembers on the same day. If not, he should not take the missed capsule at all. He should wait until it is time to take the next dose. He should never double-up on a dose to make up for the one he has missed.

Administration: Trandolapril may be taken before, during or after meals (see Drug Interactions, Drug-Food Interactions).

OVERDOSAGE:

Limited data are available regarding overdosage of MAVIK (trandolapril) in humans. The most likely clinical manifestation of overdosage of an ACE inhibitor such as trandolapril would be symptoms attributable to severe hypotension, which should normally be treated by intravenous volume expansion with normal saline. It is not known if trandolapril or trandolaprilat can be removed from the body by hemodialysis.

For management of a suspected drug overdose, CPhA recommends that you contact your **regional Poison Control Centre**. See the *CPS* Directory section for a list of Poison Control Centres.

ACTION AND CLINICAL PHARMACOLOGY: Mechanism of Action: MAVIK (trandolapril) is a non-sulphydryl angiotensin converting enzyme (ACE) inhibitor which is used in the treatment of mild to moderate essential hypertension and following acute myocardial infarction in clinically stable patients with left ventricular dysfunction.

Angiotensin-converting enzyme (ACE) is a peptidyl dipeptidase that catalyzes the conversion of angiotensin I to the pharmacologically active substance, angiotensin II, which is a vasopressor agent. In addition, angiotensin II stimulates aldosterone secretion by the adrenal cortex. Inhibition of angiotensin-converting enzyme results in a decreased plasma angiotensin II level. The resulting lack of negative feedback on renal renin secretion leads to an increased plasma renin activity.

Angiotensin-converting enzyme is identical to kininase II. Thus, trandolapril administration may interfere with the degradation of the potent peptide vasodilator bradykinin, which may contribute to the therapeutic activity of trandolapril. Trandolapril is a prodrug, which is hydrolysed to its active diacid form, trandolaprilat, a potent ACE inhibitor.

The antihypertensive effect of trandolapril is due to a reduction in peripheral vascular resistance with little or no change in cardiac output and heart rate. The decrease in blood pressure is not accompanied by water or sodium retention. No modification was found in the urinary excretion of chloride and potassium. Administration of trandolapril to patients with essential hypertension results in reduction of both supine and standing blood pressure.

Pharmacodynamics: Administration of trandolapril to patients with mild to moderate essential hypertension results in a reduction of both supine and standing blood pressure usually with little or no orthostatic change or change in heart rate. Symptomatic postural hypotension is infrequent, although this may occur in patients who are salt- and/or volume-depleted (see Warnings and Precautions).

In mild to moderate hypertensive patients, significant reductions in blood pressure were seen at 2 hours, and peak antihypertensive effects were seen after approximately 8 hours. At the recommended doses, antihypertensive effects are maintained throughout the 24-hour dosing interval in most patients who responded to trandolapril. Abrupt withdrawal of trandolapril has not resulted in rapid increase in blood pressure.

Following single oral therapeutic doses in healthy male volunteers, a rapid onset of ACE inhibition was observed. The peak inhibition was reached between 2 and 4 hours after the initial dose.

The effectiveness of trandolapril appears to be similar in the elderly (over 65 years of age) and younger adult patients given the same daily doses.

The antihypertensive effect of angiotensin converting enzyme inhibitors is generally lower in black patients than in non-blacks.

The antihypertensive effect of trandolapril and thiazide diuretics used concurrently is greater than that seen with either drug used alone.

Pharmacokinetics: Absorption: Following a single oral administration of trandolapril to healthy volunteers, trandolapril was detectable in the plasma 30 minutes later with peak concentrations reached within 1 hour. Trandolaprilat, the active metabolite, reached peak plasma concentrations after approximately 6 hours following trandolapril capsule administration. Plasma concentrations of both trandolapril and trandolaprilat were dose dependent. While food can delay the rate of absorption of trandolapril, there is no clinically significant effect on other pharmacokinetic and pharmacodynamic parameters of trandolaprilat.

Approximately 40 to 60% of an administered oral dose of trandolapril is absorbed.

Distribution: Eighty percent (80%) of the circulating trandolapril and up to 94% of the circulating trandolaprilat are bound to plasma proteins. The protein binding is not saturable for trandolapril but is saturable for trandolaprilat.

Metabolism: Trandolapril undergoes extensive first-pass metabolism in the liver, and this is the reason for its low bioavailability: 7.5% (ranging from 4 to 14%). In the liver it is transformed into its biologically active diacid form, trandolaprilat. Trandolaprilat itself is poorly absorbed after oral administration. Minor metabolic pathways lead to the formation of diketopiperazine derivatives of trandolapril and trandolaprilat. These molecules have no ACE inhibitory activity. Glucuronide conjugated derivatives of trandolapril and trandolaprilat are also produced.

Excretion: With once-daily dosing, a steady-state of trandolaprilat plasma concentrations is reached within 4 days in healthy male and female subjects as well as in patients with chronic renal failure. Similar results were found in young (<65 years) as well as old (≥65 years) male and female patients suffering from mild to moderate essential hypertension. As is the case with several other ACE inhibitors, trandolaprilat has a polyphasic elimination profile with a slow terminal phase, probably the result of binding to ACE and a subsequently slow dissociation from the enzyme. Over the first 16 to 20 hours following oral administration of trandolapril, there is a rapid elimination phase of trandolaprilat. Beyond this time, there is a prolonged terminal elimination phase. The effective half-life ($t_{1/2}$) for accumulation of trandolaprilat has been estimated to be in the range of 16 to 24 hours. The accumulation ratio as measured in hypertensive patients was about 1.5. Trandolapril's elimination half-life ($t_{1/2}$) is on average 0.7 hours.

In healthy male volunteers the excretion, in urine and feces, of trandolapril following an 8 mg single oral dose of ^{14}C-labelled drug is virtually complete after 7 days (99.2±3.4%): eighty-two percent (82%) of the dose was eliminated in 48 hours and 93% of the dose in 72 hours. In this dual route of excretion, urinary and fecal recoveries accounted for 33% and 66% of the total excretion, respectively. Trandolaprilat represents 46% of the urinary and 57% of the fecal excretion. The glucuronide derivatives of trandolapril and trandolaprilat excreted represent each about 13% of total urinary excretion and, 2% and 4% of total fecal excretion. The diketopiperazine of trandolaprilat was 7% of the total urinary excretion. The amounts of trandolapril excreted unchanged and the corresponding diketopiperazine are negligible (<0.5% of the dose).

Renal celarance of trandolaprilat varies depending on dose, as seen in Table 3. Trandolaprilat displays non-linear pharmacokinetics, especially at low doses.

Table 3: MAVIK

Renal Clearance of Trandolaprilat after a Single Oral Administration of Trandolapril to Healthy Subjects

Parameters	0.5 mg	1 mg	2 mg	4 mg
Trandolaprilat $CL_{r0\text{-}96\ h}$ (L/h)	0.15±0.05	1.03±0.18	2.02±0.25	3.93±0.39

Special Populations and Conditions: Pediatrics: Trandolapril pharmacokinetics have not been evaluated in patients less than 18 years of age.

Race: Pharmacokinetic differences have not been evaluated in different races.

Hepatic Insufficiency: In patients with moderate to severe impairment of liver function, plasma trandolapril levels were approximately ten times higher than in healthy subjects. The plasma concentrations of trandolaprilat and the quantities excreted in the urine were also increased, although to a lesser degree. The dose should therefore be reduced in these patients.

In one study, cirrhotic patients who received a single dose of trandolapril 2 mg exhibited a 9-fold increase in trandolapril C_{max} and AUC values. The C_{max} and AUC values of trandolaprilat were about doubled.

Renal Insufficiency: In patients with creatinine clearance ≤30 mL/min/1.73m², the C_{max} and AUC of trandolaprilat were approximately doubled after repeated oral administration, as compared to those of normal subjects.

STORAGE AND STABILITY: Store trandolapril between 15 and 25°C in original container. Trandolapril should not be stored beyond the date indicated on the container.

INFORMATION FOR THE PATIENT: Published in e-CPS, available by subscription at www.e-cps.ca.

DOSAGE FORMS, COMPOSITION AND PACKAGING: 0.5 mg: Each red opaque body and yellow opaque cap, no. 4 gelatin capsule, contains: trandolapril 0.5 mg. Nonmedicinal ingredients: lactose, maize starch, povidone and sodium stearyl fumarate; capsule cap and body: erythrosine, iron oxides and hydroxides, sodium lauryl sulfate and titanium dioxide. HDPE plastic bottles of 100.

1 mg: Each red opaque body and orange opaque cap, no. 4 gelatin capsule, contains: trandolapril 1 mg. Nonmedicinal ingredients: lactose, maize starch, povidone and sodium stearyl fumarate; capsule cap and body: erythrosine, iron oxides and hydroxides, sodium lauryl sulfate and titanium dioxide. HDPE plastic bottles of 100.

2 mg: Each red opaque body and red opaque cap, no. 4 gelatin capsule, contains: trandolapril 2 mg. Nonmedicinal ingredients: lactose, maize starch, povidone and sodium stearyl fumarate; capsule cap and body: erythrosine, iron oxides and hydroxides, sodium lauryl sulfate and titanium dioxide. HDPE plastic bottles of 100.

4 mg: Each red opaque body and brown opaque cap, no. 4 gelatin capsule, contains: trandolapril 4 mg. Nonmedicinal ingredients: lactose, maize starch, povidone and sodium stearyl fumarate; capsule cap and body: erythrosine, iron oxides and hydroxides, sodium lauryl sulfate and titanium dioxide. HDPE plastic bottles of 100.

Maxalt® Pr

rizatriptan benzoate

Migraine Therapy

Merck Frosst

Maxalt RPD® Pr

rizatriptan benzoate

Migraine Therapy

Merck Frosst

Date of Revision: September 17, 2009

SUMMARY PRODUCT INFORMATION:

Route of Administration	Dosage Form/ Strength	Clinically Relevant Nonmedicinal Ingredients
Oral	Tablets 5 mg, 10 mg	Lactose monohydrate For a complete listing see Dosage Forms, Composition and Packaging.
Oral	Wafers 5 mg, 10 mg	For a complete listing see Dosage Forms, Composition and Packaging.

INDICATIONS AND CLINICAL USE: Adults: MAXALT (rizatriptan benzoate) is indicated for:

- acute treatment of migraine attacks with or without aura in adults.

MAXALT is not intended for the prophylactic therapy of migraine or for use in the management of hemiplegic, ophthalmoplegic or basilar migraine (see Contraindications). Safety and effectiveness of MAXALT have not been established for cluster headache, which is present in an older, predominantly male population.

Pediatrics (<18 years of age): The safety and efficacy of MAXALT has not been established in patients under 18 years of age and its use in this age group is not recommended (see Warnings and Precautions).

Geriatrics (>65 years of age): The safety and effectiveness of MAXALT has not been adequately studied in individuals over 65 years of age. Its use in this age group is, therefore, not recommended (see Warnings and Precautions).

CONTRAINDICATIONS: MAXALT is contraindicated in patients with history, symptoms, or signs of ischemic cardiac, cerebrovascular or peripheral vascular syndromes, valvular heart disease or cardiac arrhythmias (especially tachycardias). In addition, patients with other significant underlying cardiovascular diseases (e.g., atherosclerotic disease, congenital heart disease) should not receive MAXALT. Ischemic cardiac syndromes include, but are not restricted to, angina pectoris of any type (e.g., stable angina of effort and vasospastic forms of angina such as the Prinzmetal's variant), all forms of myocardial infarction, and silent myocardial ischemia. Cerebrovascular syndromes include, but are not limited to, strokes of any type as well as transient ischemic attacks (TIAs). Peripheral vascular disease includes, but is not limited to, ischemic bowel disease, or Raynaud's syndrome (see Warnings and Precautions).

Because MAXALT may increase blood pressure, it is contraindicated in patients with uncontrolled or severe hypertension (see Warnings and Precautions).

MAXALT is contraindicated within 24 hours of treatment with another $5\text{-}HT_1$ agonist, or an ergotamine-containing or ergot-type medication like dihydroergotamine or methysergide.

MAXALT is contraindicated in patients with hemiplegic, ophthalmoplegic or basilar migraine.

Concurrent administration of MAO inhibitors or use of rizatriptan within 2 weeks of discontinuation of MAO inhibitor therapy is contraindicated (see Drug Interactions).

Because there are no data available, MAXALT is contraindicated in patients with severe hepatic impairment.

MAXALT is contraindicated in patients who are hypersensitive to rizatriptan or any component of the formulation.

WARNINGS AND PRECAUTIONS: General: MAXALT should only be used where a clear diagnosis of migraine has been established.

For a given attack, if a patient has no response to the first dose of rizatriptan, the diagnosis of migraine should be reconsidered before administration of a second dose.

Psychomotor Effect: Dizziness, somnolence and asthenia/fatigue were experienced by some patients in clinical trials with MAXALT (see Adverse Reactions). Patients should be advised to avoid driving a car or operating hazardous machinery until they are reasonably certain that MAXALT does not adversely affect them.

Cardiovascular: Risk of Myocardial Ischemia and/or Infarction and Other Adverse Cardiac Events: MAXALT has been associated with transient chest and/or neck pain and tightness which may resemble angina pectoris. Following the use of other 5-HT_1 agonists, in rare cases these symptoms have been identified as being the likely result of coronary vasospasm or myocardial ischemia. Rare cases of serious coronary events or arrhythmia have occurred following use of other 5-HT_1 agonists, and may therefore also occur with MAXALT. Because of the potential of this class of compounds (5-$HT_{1B/1D}$ agonists) to cause coronary vasospasm, MAXALT should not be given to patients with documented ischemic or vasospastic coronary artery disease (see Contraindications). It is strongly recommended that MAXALT not be given to patients in whom unrecognized coronary artery disease (CAD) is predicted by the presence of risk factors (e.g., hypertension, hypercholesterolemia, smoker, obesity, diabetes, strong family history of CAD, female with surgical or physiological menopause, or male over 40 years of age) unless a cardiovascular evaluation provides satisfactory clinical evidence that the patient is reasonably free of coronary artery and ischemic myocardial disease or other significant underlying cardiovascular disease. The sensitivity of cardiac diagnostic procedures to detect cardiovascular disease or predisposition to coronary artery vasospasm is unknown. If, during the cardiovascular evaluation, the patient's medical history, electrocardiographic or other investigations reveal findings indicative of, or consistent with, coronary artery vasospasm or myocardial ischemia, MAXALT should not be administered (see Contraindications).

For patients with risk factors predictive of CAD, who are considered to have a satisfactory cardiovascular evaluation, the first dose of rizatriptan should be administered in the setting of a physician's office or similar medically staffed and equipped facility. Because cardiac ischemia can occur in the absence of clinical symptoms, consideration should be given to obtaining on the first occasion of use an electrocardiogram (ECG) during the interval immediately following MAXALT, in these patients with risk factors. However, an absence of drug-induced cardiovascular effects on the occasion of the initial dose does not preclude the possibility of such effects occurring with subsequent administrations.

Intermittent long-term users of MAXALT who have or acquire risk factors predictive of CAD, as described above, should receive periodic interval cardiovascular evaluation as they continue to use MAXALT.

If symptoms consistent with angina occur after the use of MAXALT, ECG evaluation should be carried out to look for ischemic changes.

The systematic approach described above is intended to reduce the likelihood that patients with unrecognized cardiovascular disease will be inadvertently exposed to MAXALT.

Discomfort in the chest, neck, throat and jaw (including pain, pressure, heaviness and tightness) has been reported after administration of rizatriptan. Because drugs in this class may cause coronary artery vasospasm, patients who experience signs or symptoms suggestive of angina following dosing should be evaluated for the presence of CAD or a predisposition to Prinzmetal's variant angina before receiving additional doses of medication, and should be monitored electrocardiographically if dosing is resumed and similar symptoms recur. Similarly, patients who experience other symptoms or signs suggestive of decreased arterial flow, such as ischemic bowel syndrome or Raynaud's syndrome following MAXALT administration should be evaluated for atherosclerosis or predisposition to vasospasm (see Contraindications and Warnings and Precautions).

Cardiac Events and Fatalities Associated with 5-HT_1 Agonists: MAXALT may cause coronary artery vasospasm. Serious adverse cardiac events, including acute myocardial infarction, life-threatening disturbances of cardiac rhythm, and death have been reported within a few hours following the administration of 5-HT_1 agonists. Considering the extent of use of 5-HT_1 agonists in patients with migraine, the incidence of these events is extremely low.

Premarketing Experience with MAXALT: Among the approximately 4200 patients who were treated with at least a single oral dose of either 5 or 10 mg rizatriptan in premarketing clinical trials of MAXALT, electrocardiac adverse experiences were observed in 33 patients. One patient was reported to have chest pain with possible ischemic ECG changes following a single dose of 10 mg.

Postmarketing Experience with MAXALT: Serious cardiovascular events have been reported in association with the use of MAXALT. The uncontrolled nature of postmarketing surveillance, however, makes it impossible to determine definitively the proportion of reported cases that were actually caused by MAXALT or to reliably assess causation in individual cases.

Cerebrovascular Events and Fatalities Associated with 5-HT_1 Agonists: Cerebral hemorrhage, subarachnoid hemorrhage, stroke, and other cerebrovascular events have been reported in patients treated with 5-HT_1 agonists; and some have resulted in fatalities. In a number of cases, it appears possible that the cerebrovascular events were primary, the agonist having been administered in the incorrect belief that the symptoms experienced were a consequence of migraine, when they were not. Before treating migraine headaches with MAXALT in patients not previously diagnosed as migraineurs, and in migraineurs who present with atypical symptoms, care should be taken to exclude other potentially serious neurological conditions. If a patient does not respond to the first dose, the opportunity should be taken to review the diagnosis before a second dose is given. It should be noted that patients with migraine may be at increased risk of certain cerebrovascular events (e.g., stroke, hemorrhage, transient ischemic attack).

Special Cardiovascular Pharmacology Studies with Another 5-HT_1 Agonist: In subjects (n=10) with suspected coronary artery disease undergoing angiography, a 5-HT_1 agonist at a subcutaneous dose of 1.5 mg produced an 8% increase in aortic blood pressure, an 18% increase in pulmonary artery blood pressure, and an 8% increase in systemic vascular resistance. In addition, mild chest pain or tightness was reported by four subjects. Clinically significant increases in blood pressure were experienced by three of the subjects (two of whom also had chest pain/discomfort). Diagnostic angiogram results revealed that 9 subjects had normal coronary arteries and one had insignificant coronary artery disease.

In an additional study with this same drug, migraine patients (n=35) free of cardiovascular disease were subjected to assessments of myocardial perfusion by positron emission tomography while receiving a subcutaneous 1.5 mg dose in the absence of a migraine attack. Reduced coronary vasodilatory reserve (~10%), increased coronary resistance (~20%), and decreased hyperemic myocardial blood flow (~10%) were noted. The relevance of these findings to the use of the recommended oral dose of this 5-HT_1 agonist is not known.

Similar studies have not been done with MAXALT. However, owing to the common pharmacodynamic actions of 5-HT_1 agonists, the possibility of cardiovascular effects of the nature described above should be considered for any agent of this pharmacological class.

Other Vasospasm-Related Events: 5-HT_1 agonists may cause vasospastic reactions other than coronary artery vasospasm. Extensive post-market experience has shown the use of another 5-HT_1 agonist to be associated with rare occurrences of peripheral vascular ischemia and colonic ischemia with abdominal pain and bloody diarrhea.

Increase in Blood Pressure: Significant elevation in blood pressure, including hypertensive crisis, has been reported on rare occasions in patients receiving 5-HT_1 agonists with and without a history of hypertension. In healthy young male and female subjects who received maximal doses of MAXALT (10 mg every 2 hours for 3 doses), slight increases in blood pressure (approximately 2-3 mmHg) were observed. Rizatriptan is contraindicated in patients with uncontrolled or severe hypertension (see Contraindications). In patients with controlled hypertension, MAXALT should be administered with caution, as transient increases in blood pressure and peripheral vascular resistance have been observed in a small portion of patients.

Endocrine and Metabolism: Phenylketonurics: Phenylketonuric patients should be informed that MAXALT RPD Wafers contain phenylalanine (a component of aspartame). Each 5 mg wafer contains 1.05 mg phenylalanine, and each 10 mg wafer contains 2.10 mg phenylalanine.

Hepatic/Biliary/Pancreatic: Rizatriptan should be used with caution in patients with moderate hepatic insufficiency due to an increase in plasma concentrations of approximately 30% (see Action and Clinical Pharmacology, Special Populations and Conditions, and Dosage and Administration). Since there are no data in patients with severe hepatic impairment, rizatriptan is contraindicated in this population (see Contraindications and Dosage and Administration).

Immune: Rare hypersensitivity (anaphylaxis/anaphylactoid) reactions may occur in patients receiving 5-HT_1 agonists such as MAXALT. Such reactions can be life threatening or fatal. In general, hypersensitivity reactions to drugs are more likely to occur in individuals with a history of sensitivity to multiple allergens. Owing to the possibility of cross-reactive hypersensitivity reactions, MAXALT should not be used in patients having a history of hypersensitivity to chemically-related 5-HT_1 receptor agonists.

Neurologic: Care should be taken to exclude other potentially serious neurologic conditions before treating headache in patients not previously diagnosed with migraine or who experience a headache that is atypical for them. There have been rare reports where patients received 5-HT_1 agonists for severe headache that were subsequently shown to have been secondary to an evolving neurological lesion. For newly diagnosed patients or patients presenting with atypical symptoms, the diagnosis of migraine should be reconsidered if no response is seen after the first dose of MAXALT.

Seizures: Caution should be observed if MAXALT is to be used in patients with a history of epilepsy or structural brain lesions which lower the convulsion threshold. There have been very rare reports of seizures following administration of MAXALT in patients with or without risk factors or previous history of seizures (see Adverse Reactions, Post-Marketing Adverse Reactions, Nervous System).

Ophthalmologic: Binding to Melanin-Containing Tissues: The propensity for rizatriptan to bind melanin has not been investigated. Based on its chemical properties, rizatriptan may bind to melanin and accumulate in melanin-rich tissue (e.g., eye) over time. This raises the possibility that rizatriptan could cause toxicity in these tissues after extended use. There were, however, no adverse ophthalmologic changes related to treatment with rizatriptan in the one-year dog toxicity study. Although no systematic monitoring of ophthalmologic function was undertaken in clinical trials, and no specific recommendations for ophthalmologic monitoring are offered, prescribers should be aware of the possibility of long-term ophthalmologic effects.

Renal: Rizatriptan should be used with caution in dialysis patients due to a decrease in the clearance of rizatriptan, resulting in approximately 44% increase in plasma concentrations (see Action and Clinical Pharmacology, Special Populations and Conditions, and Dosage and Administration).

Selective Serotonin Reuptake Inhibitors/Serotonin Norepinephrine Reuptake Inhibitors and Serotonin Syndrome: Cases of life-threatening serotonin syndrome have been reported during combined use of selective serotonin reuptake inhibitors (SSRIs)/serotonin norepinephrine reuptake inhibitors (SNRIs) and triptans. If concomitant treatment with MAXALT and SSRIs (e.g., sertraline, escitalopram oxalate, and fluoxetine) or SNRIs (e.g., venlafaxine, duloxetine) is clinically warranted, careful observation of the patient is advised, particularly during treatment initiation and dose increases. Serotonin syndrome symptoms may include mental status changes (e.g., agitation, hallucinations, coma), autonomic instability (e.g., tachycardia, labile blood pressure, hyperthermia), neuromuscular aberrations (e.g., hyperreflexia, incoordination) and/or gastrointestinal symptoms (e.g., nausea, vomiting, diarrhea) (see Drug Interactions).

Special Populations and Conditions: Pregnant Women: In a reproduction study in rats, birth weights and pre- and post-weaning weight gain were reduced in the offspring of females treated prior to and during mating and throughout gestation and lactation. These effects occurred in the absence of any apparent maternal toxicity (maternal plasma drug exposures were 22 and 337 times, respectively, the exposure in humans receiving the maximum recommended daily dose (MRDD) of 20 mg). The developmental no-effect dose was equivalent to 2.25 times human exposure at the MRDD.

In embryofetal development studies, no teratogenic effects were observed when pregnant rats and rabbits were administered doses at the equivalent of 337 times and 168 times, respectively, the human MRDD, during organogenesis. However, fetal weights were decreased in conjunction with decreased maternal weight gain at these same doses. The developmental no-effect dose in both rats and rabbits was 22 times the human MRDD. Toxicokinetic studies demonstrated placental transfer of drug in both species.

There are no adequate and well-controlled studies in pregnant women; therefore, rizatriptan should be used during pregnancy only if the potential benefit justifies the potential risk to the fetus.

Impairment of Fertility: In a fertility study in rats, altered estrus cyclicity and delays in time to mating were observed in females treated orally with an equivalent of 337 times the maximum recommended daily dose (MRDD) of 20 mg in humans. The no-effect dose was 22 times the MRDD. There was no impairment of fertility or reproductive performance in male rats treated with up to 825 times the MRDD.

Nursing Women: It is not known whether this drug is excreted in human milk. Because many drugs are excreted in human milk, caution should be exercised when MAXALT is administered to women who are breast-feeding. Rizatriptan is extensively excreted in rat milk, at a level of 5-fold or greater than maternal plasma levels.

Pediatrics (<18 years of age): MAXALT is not recommended for use in patients under 18 years of age.

In a randomized placebo-controlled trial of 291 adolescent migraineurs, aged 12-17 years, the efficacy of MAXALT Tablets (5 mg) was not different from that of placebo (see Action and Clinical Pharmacology, Special Populations and Conditions).

Geriatrics (>65 years of age): The safety and effectiveness of MAXALT has not been adequately studied in individuals over 65 years of age. The risk of adverse reactions to this drug may be greater in elderly patients, as they are more likely to have decreased hepatic function, be at higher risk for CAD, and experience blood pressure increases that may be more pronounced. Clinical studies with MAXALT did not include a substantial number of patients over 65 years of age (n=17). Its use in this age group is, therefore, not recommended.

Special Disease Conditions: MAXALT (rizatriptan benzoate) should be administered with caution to patients with diseases that may alter the absorption, metabolism, or excretion of drugs (see Action and Clinical Pharmacology, Special Populations and Conditions).

Monitoring and Laboratory Tests: No specific laboratory tests are recommended for monitoring patients prior to and/or after treatment with MAXALT.

ADVERSE REACTIONS: Adverse Drug Reaction Overview: Serious cardiac events, including some that have been fatal, have occurred following use of 5-HT_1 agonists. These events are extremely rare and most have been reported in patients with risk factors predictive of CAD. Events reported have included coronary artery vasospasm, transient myocardial ischemia, myocardial infarction, ventricular tachycardia, and ventricular fibrillation (see Contraindications and Warnings and Precautions).

Clinical Trial Adverse Drug Reactions: Because clinical trials are conducted under very specific conditions the adverse reaction rates observed in the clinical trials may not reflect the rates observed in practice and should not be compared to the rates in the clinical trials of another drug. Adverse drug reaction information from clinical trials is useful for identifying drug-related adverse events and for approximating rates.

Experience in Controlled Clinical Trials with MAXALT: Typical 5-HT_1 Agonist Adverse Reactions: As with other 5-HT_1 agonists, MAXALT has been associated with sensations of heaviness, pressure, tightness or pain which may be intense. These may occur in any part of the body including the chest, throat, neck, jaw and upper limb.

Acute Safety: Adverse experiences to rizatriptan were assessed in controlled clinical trials that included over 3700 patients who received single or multiple doses of MAXALT Tablets. The most common adverse events during treatment with MAXALT were asthenia/fatigue, somnolence, pain/pressure sensation and dizziness. These events appeared to be dose-related. In long-term extension studies where patients were allowed to treat multiple attacks for up to 1 year, 4% (59 out of 1525 patients) withdrew because of adverse experiences.

Table 1 and Table 2 list the adverse events regardless of drug relationship (incidence ≥1% and greater than placebo) after a single dose of MAXALT Tablets and MAXALT RPD Wafers, respectively. Most of the adverse events appear to be dose-related. The events cited reflect experience gained under closely monitored conditions of clinical trials in a highly selected patient population. In actual clinical practice or in other clinical trials, these frequency estimates may not apply, as the conditions of use, reporting behavior, and the kinds of patients treated may differ.

Table 1: MAXALT

Incidence (≥1% and Greater than Placebo) of Adverse Experiences After a Single Dose of MAXALT Tablets or Placebo (Prior to Subsequent Dose) in Phase III Controlled Clinical Trials[a]

	% of Patients		
	Placebo	**MAXALT 5 mg**	**MAXALT 10 mg**
Number of Patients	627	977	1167
Symptoms of Potentially Cardiac Origin			
Upper Limb Sensations[b]	1.3	1.7	1.8
Chest Sensations[b]	1.0	1.6	3.1
Neck/Throat/Jaw Sensations[b]	0.6	1.4	2.5
Palpitations	0.2	0.9	1.0
Body as a Whole			
Asthenia/Fatigue	2.1	4.2	6.9
Abdominal Pain	1.0	1.7	2.2
Digestive System			
Nausea	3.5	4.1	5.7

(cont'd)

Table 1: MAXALT *(cont'd)*

Incidence (≥1% and Greater than Placebo) of Adverse Experiences After a Single Dose of MAXALT Tablets or Placebo (Prior to Subsequent Dose) in Phase III Controlled Clinical Trials[a]

	% of Patients		
	Placebo	**MAXALT 5 mg**	**MAXALT 10 mg**
Dry Mouth	1.3	2.6	3.0
Vomiting	2.1	1.6	2.3
Nervous System			
Dizziness	4.5	4.2	8.9
Somnolence	3.5	4.2	8.4
Headache	0.8	1.8	2.1
Paresthesia	1.0	1.5	2.9
Tremor	1.0	1.3	0.3
Insomnia	0.3	1.0	0.3
Skin and Skin Appendages			
Flushing	1.0	0.6	1.1

[a] Data from Studies 022, 025, 029 and 030.
[b] The term "sensations" encompasses adverse events described as pain, discomfort, pressure, heaviness, constriction, tightness, heat/burning sensation, paresthesia, numbness, tingling, weakness and strange sensations.

Table 2: MAXALT RPD

Incidence (≥1% and Greater than Placebo) of Adverse Experiences After a Single Dose of MAXALT RPD Wafers or Placebo (Prior to Subsequent Dose) in Phase III Controlled Clinical Trials[a]

	% of Patients		
	Placebo	**MAXALT RPD 5 mg**	**MAXALT RPD 10 mg**
Number of Patients	283	282	302
Symptoms of Potentially Cardiac Origin			
Chest Sensations[b]	0.4	1.4	1.7
Neck/Throat/Jaw Sensations[b]	0.4	1.4	2.0
Tachycardia	1.1	1.4	0.3
Upper Limb Sensations[b]	0.4	0.7	2.0
Palpitations	0.4	0.4	1.0
Body as a Whole			
Asthenia/Fatigue	0.4	2.1	3.6
Digestive System			
Dry Mouth	2.1	6.4	6.0
Nausea	5.7	6.4	7.0
Dyspepsia	0.7	1.1	2.0
Acid Regurgitation	0	1.1	0.7
Salivation Increase	0	0	1.3
Musculoskeletal System			
Regional Heaviness	0	0	1.0
Nervous System			
Dizziness	3.9	6.4	8.6
Somnolence	2.8	4.3	5.3
Headache	0.7	1.8	2.0
Insomnia	0	1.4	0.7
Paresthesia	0.4	1.4	3.0
Hypesthesia	0	1.4	0.7
Mental Acuity Decreased	0	1.1	0.3
Tremor	0.7	1.1	0
Nervousness	0.4	1.1	0.7
Respiratory System			

(cont'd)

Table 2: MAXALT RPD *(cont'd)*

Incidence (≥1% and Greater than Placebo) of Adverse Experiences After a Single Dose of MAXALT RPD Wafers or Placebo (Prior to Subsequent Dose) in Phase III Controlled Clinical Trials[a]

	% of Patients		
	Placebo	**MAXALT RPD 5 mg**	**MAXALT RPD 10 mg**
Pharyngeal Discomfort	0	1.1	0.7
Skin and Skin Appendages			
Sweating	0.7	1.1	1.0
Special Senses			
Taste Perversion	1.1	1.4	2.3
Blurred Vision	0	0.4	1.3

[a] Data from Studies 039 and 049.
[b] The term "sensations" encompasses adverse events described as pain, discomfort, pressure, heaviness, constriction, tightness, heat/burning sensation, paresthesia, numbness, tingling, weakness and strange sensations.

MAXALT was generally well-tolerated. Adverse experiences were typically mild in intensity and were transient. The frequencies of adverse experiences in clinical trials did not increase when up to three doses were taken within 24 hours. The incidences of adverse experiences were not affected by age, gender or use of prophylactic medications. There were insufficient data to assess the impact of race on the incidence of adverse events.

Long-Term Safety: In long-term extension studies, a total of 1854 patients treated 16 150 migraine attacks with MAXALT 5 mg Tablets and 24 043 attacks with MAXALT 10 mg Tablets over a period of up to 1 year. In general, the types of clinical adverse experiences observed in the extension studies were similar to those observed in the acute studies. However, the incidences of most clinical adverse events were approximately 3-fold higher in extension, as expected, based on increased observation time. The most common adverse events per attack (defined as occurring at an incidence of at least 1%) for MAXALT 5 mg and 10 mg, respectively, were as follows: nausea (3%, 4%), dizziness (2%, 2%), somnolence (2%, 4%), asthenia/fatigue (2%, 2%), headache (1%, 2%), vomiting (1%, <1%), chest pain (<1%, 1%) and paresthesia (<1%, 2%). Due to the lack of placebo controls in the extension studies, the role of MAXALT in causation cannot be reliably determined.

Other Events Observed in Association with the Administration of MAXALT: In the section that follows, the frequencies of less commonly reported adverse clinical events are presented. Because the reports include events observed in open studies, the role of MAXALT in their causation cannot be reliably determined. Furthermore, variability associated with adverse event reporting, the terminology used to describe adverse events, etc. limit the value of the quantitative frequency estimates provided. Event frequencies are calculated as the number of patients who used MAXALT 5 mg and 10 mg tablets in Phase II and III studies (n=3716) and reported an event divided by the total number of patients exposed to MAXALT. All reported events are included, except those already listed in the previous table, those too general to be informative, and those not reasonably associated with the use of the drug. Events are further classified within body system categories and enumerated in order of decreasing frequency using the following definitions: frequent adverse events are those defined as those occurring in at least 1/100 patients; infrequent adverse experiences are those occurring in 1/100 to 1/1000 patients; and rare adverse experiences are those occurring in fewer than 1/1000 patients.

Body as a Whole: Frequent were warm sensations, chest pain and chills/cold sensations. Infrequent were heat sensitivity, facial edema, hangover effect, abdominal distention, edema/swelling and malaise. Rare were fever, orthostatic effects, and syncope.

Cardiovascular: Frequent was palpitation. Infrequent were tachycardia, cold extremities, hypertension, arrhythmia, and bradycardia. Rare were angina pectoris and blood pressure increased.

Digestive: Frequent was diarrhea. Infrequent were dyspepsia, thirst, acid regurgitation, dysphagia, constipation, flatulence, and tongue edema. Rare were anorexia, appetite increase, gastritis, paralysis (tongue), eructation and glosodynia.

Metabolic: Infrequent was dehydration.

Musculoskeletal: Infrequent were muscle weakness, stiffness, myalgia, muscle cramp, musculoskeletal pain, and arthralgia.

Neurological/Psychiatric: Frequent were hypesthesia and mental acuity decreased. Infrequent were nervousness, vertigo, insomnia, anxiety, depression, euphoria, disorientation, ataxia, dysarthria, confusion, dream abnormality, gait abnormality, irritability, memory impairment, agitation, hyperesthesia, sleep disorder, speech disorder, migraine and spasm. Rare were dysesthesia, depersonalization, akinesia/bradykinesia, apprehension, hyperkinesia, hypersomnia, and hyporeflexia.

Respiratory: Frequent were dyspnea and pharyngeal discomfort. Infrequent were pharyngitis, irritation (nasal), congestion (nasal), dry throat, upper respiratory infection, yawning, respiratory congestion, dry nose, epistaxis, and sinus disorder. Rare were cough, hiccups, hoarseness, rhinorrhea, sneezing, tachypnea, and pharyngeal edema.

Special Senses: Frequent was taste perversion. Infrequent were blurred vision, tinnitus, dry eyes, burning eye, eye pain, eye irritation, ear pain, and tearing. Rare were hyperacusis, smell perversion, photophobia, photopsia, itching eye, and eye swelling.

Skin and Skin Appendage: Infrequent were sweating, pruritus, rash, and urticaria. Rare were erythema, acne, and photosensitivity.

Urogenital System: Frequent was hot flashes. Infrequent were urinary frequency, polyuria, and menstruation disorder. Rare was dysuria.

The adverse experience profile seen with MAXALT RPD Wafers was similar to that seen with MAXALT Tablets.

Post-Market Adverse Drug Reactions: The following additional adverse reactions have been reported very rarely and most have been reported in patients with risk factors predictive of CAD: Myocardial ischemia or infarction, cerebrovascular accident.

The following adverse reactions have also been reported:

Hypersensitivity: hypersensitivity reaction, anaphylaxis/anaphylactoid reaction, angioedema (e.g., facial edema, tongue swelling, pharyngeal edema), wheezing, urticaria, rash, toxic epidermal necrolysis.

Nervous System: serotonin syndrome.

Seizures: There have been very rare reports of seizures following administration of MAXALT in patients with or without risk factors or previous history of seizures (see Warnings and Precautions).

Musculoskeletal: facial pain.

Special Senses: dysgeusia.

Vascular Disorders: peripheral vascular ischemia.

Drug Abuse and Dependence: Although the abuse potential of MAXALT has not been specifically assessed, no abuse of, tolerance to, withdrawal from, or drug-seeking behavior was observed in patients who received MAXALT in clinical trials or their extensions. The 5-$HT_{1B/1D}$ agonists, as a class, have not been associated with drug abuse.

DRUG INTERACTIONS: Drug-Drug Interactions: Ergot-Containing Drugs: Ergot-containing drugs have been reported to cause prolonged vasospastic reactions. Because there is a theoretical basis that these effects may be additive, use of ergotamine-containing or ergot-type medications (like dihydroergotamine or methysergide) and rizatriptan within 24 hours is contraindicated (see Contraindications).

Monoamine Oxidase Inhibitors: Rizatriptan is principally metabolized via monoamine oxidase, 'A' subtype (MAO-A). In a drug interaction study, when MAXALT 10 mg was administered to subjects (n=12) receiving concomitant therapy with the selective, reversible MAO-A inhibitor, moclobemide 150 mg t.i.d., there were mean increases in rizatriptan AUC and C_{max} of 119% and 41%, respectively; and the AUC of the active N-monodesmethyl metabolite of rizatriptan was increased more than 400%. The interaction would be expected to be greater with irreversible MAO inhibitors. Drug interaction studies were not conducted with selective MAO-B inhibitors. The specificity of MAO-B inhibitors diminishes with higher doses and varies among patients. Therefore, co-administration of rizatriptan in patients taking MAO-A or MAO-B inhibitors is contraindicated (see Contraindications).

Nadolol/Metoprolol: In a drug interactions study, effects of multiple doses of nadolol 80 mg or metoprolol 100 mg every 12 hours on the pharmacokinetics of a single dose of 10 mg rizatriptan were evaluated in healthy subjects (n=12). No pharmacokinetic interactions were observed.

Oral Contraceptives: In a study of concurrent administration of an oral contraceptive during 6 days of administration of MAXALT (10-30 mg/day) in healthy female volunteers (n=18), rizatriptan did not affect plasma concentrations of ethinyl estradiol or norethindrone.

Other 5-HT$_1$ Agonists: The administration of rizatriptan with other 5-HT$_1$ agonists has not been evaluated in migraine patients. Because their vasospastic effects may be additive, co-administration of rizatriptan and other 5-HT$_1$ agonists within 24 hours of each other is contraindicated (see Contraindications).

Propranolol: MAXALT should be used with caution in patients receiving propranolol, since the pharmacokinetic behavior of rizatriptan during co-administration with propranolol may be unpredictable. In a study of concurrent administration of propranolol 240 mg/day and a single dose of rizatriptan 10 mg in healthy subjects (n=11), mean plasma AUC and C_{max} for rizatriptan were increased by 70% and 75%, respectively, during propranolol administration. In one subject, a 4-fold increase in AUC and 5-fold increase in C_{max} was observed. This subject was not distinguishable from the others based on demographic characteristics. The AUC of the active N-monodesmethyl metabolite of rizatriptan was not affected by propranolol. (See Dosage and Administration.)

Selective Serotonin Reuptake Inhibitors/Serotonin Norepinephrine Reuptake Inhibitors and Serotonin Syndrome: Cases of life-threatening serotonin syndrome have been reported in post-marketing experience during combined use of selective serotonin reuptake inhibitors (SSRIs) or serotonin norepinephrine reuptake inhibitors (SNRIs) and triptans. (See Warnings and Precautions.)

In a pharmacokinetic study with paroxetine and rizatriptan, paroxetine had no influence on the plasma levels of rizatriptan.

Drug-Food Interactions: Interactions with food have not been studied. Food has no significant effect on the bioavailability of rizatriptan but delays the time to reach peak concentration by an hour. In clinical trials, MAXALT was administered without regard to food.

Drug-Herb Interactions: Interactions with herbal products have not been studied.

Drug-Laboratory Test Interactions: MAXALT is not known to interfere with commonly employed clinical laboratory tests.

Drug-Lifestyle Interactions: Lifestyle interactions have not been established.

DOSAGE AND ADMINISTRATION:

Dosing Considerations: MAXALT is recommended only for the acute treatment of migraine attacks. MAXALT should not be used prophylactically.

Controlled trials have not established the effectiveness of a second dose if the initial dose is ineffective.

The safety of treating, on average, more than four headaches in a 30-day period has not been established.

Recommended Dose and Dosage Adjustment: Adults: MAXALT Tablets and MAXALT RPD Wafers: The recommended single adult dose is 5 mg. The maximum recommended single dose is 10 mg. There is evidence that the 10 mg dose may provide a greater effect than the 5 mg dose. The choice of dose should therefore be made on an individual basis, weighing the possible benefit of the 10 mg dose with the potential risk for increased adverse events.

For MAXALT RPD Wafers, administration with liquid is not necessary. The wafer is packaged in a blister within an outer aluminum pouch. Patients should be instructed not to remove the blister from the outer pouch until just prior to dosing. The blister pack should then be peeled open with dry hands and the wafer placed on the tongue, where it will dissolve and be swallowed with the saliva.

Redosing: Doses should be separated by at least 2 hours; no more than a total of 20 mg (Tablets or Wafers) should be taken in any 24-hour period.

Patients Receiving Propranolol: A single 5 mg dose of MAXALT should be used. In no instances should the total daily dose exceed 10 mg per day, given in two doses, separated by at least two hours (see Drug Interactions).

Renal Impairment: In hemodialysis patients with severe renal impairment (creatinine clearance <2 mL/min/1.73 m^2), the AUC of rizatriptan was approximately 44% greater than in patients with normal renal function (see Action and Clinical Pharmacology, Special Populations and Conditions). Consequently, if treatment is deemed advisable in these patients, the 5 mg MAXALT Tablet or Wafer should be administered. No more than a total of 10 mg should be taken in any 24-hour period. Repeated dosing in renally impaired patients has not been evaluated.

Hepatic Impairment: MAXALT is contraindicated in patients with severe hepatic impairment (Child-Pugh grade C) due to the absence of safety data. Plasma concentrations of rizatriptan were approximately 30% greater in patients with moderate hepatic insufficiency (see Action and Clinical Pharmacology, Special Populations and Conditions). Consequently, if treatment is deemed advisable in the presence of moderate hepatic impairment, the 5 mg MAXALT Tablet or Wafer should be administered. No more than a total of 10 mg should be taken in any 24-hour period. Repeated dosing in hepatically impaired patients has not been evaluated.

Patients with Hypertension: MAXALT should not be used in patients with uncontrolled or severe hypertension. In patients with mild to moderate controlled hypertension, patients should be treated cautiously at the lowest effective dose.

OVERDOSAGE:

No overdoses of MAXALT (rizatriptan benzoate) were reported during clinical trials.

Rizatriptan 40 mg (administered as either a single dose or as two doses with a 2-hour interdose interval) was generally well tolerated in over 300 patients; dizziness and somnolence were the most common drug-related adverse effects.

In a clinical pharmacology study in which 12 subjects received rizatriptan, at total cumulative doses of 80 mg (given within four hours), two subjects experienced syncope and/or bradycardia. One subject, a female aged 29 years, developed vomiting, bradycardia, and dizziness beginning three hours after receiving a total of 80 mg rizatriptan (administered over two hours); a third degree AV block, responsive to atropine, was observed an hour after the onset of the other symptoms. The second subject, a 25-year-old male, experienced transient dizziness, syncope, incontinence, and a 5-second systolic pause (on ECG monitor) immediately after a painful venipuncture. The venipuncture occurred two hours after the subject had received a total of 80 mg rizatriptan (administered over four hours).

In addition, based on the pharmacology of rizatriptan, hypertension or other more serious cardiovascular symptoms could occur after overdosage. Gastrointestinal decontamination (i.e., gastric lavage followed by activated charcoal) should be considered in patients suspected of an overdose with MAXALT. The elimination half-life of rizatriptan is 2 to 3 hours (see Action and Clinical Pharmacology). Clinical and electrocardiographic monitoring should be continued for at least 12 hours, even if clinical symptoms are not observed.

There is no specific antidote to rizatriptan. In cases of severe intoxication, intensive care procedures are recommended, including establishing and maintaining a patent airway, ensuring adequate oxygenation and ventilation, and monitoring and support of the cardiovascular system.

The effects of hemo- or peritoneal dialysis on serum concentrations of rizatriptan are unknown.

> For management of a suspected drug overdose, CPhA recommends that you contact your **regional Poison Control Centre**. See the *CPS* Directory section for a list of Poison Control Centres.

ACTION AND CLINICAL PHARMACOLOGY: Mechanism of Action: MAXALT is a selective 5-hydroxytryptamine$_{1B/1D}$ (5-HT$_{1B/1D}$) receptor agonist. Rizatriptan binds with high affinity to human cloned 5-HT$_{1B}$ and 5-HT$_{1D}$ receptors. It has weak affinity for other 5-HT$_1$ receptor subtypes (5-HT$_{1A}$, 5-HT$_{1E}$, 5-HT$_{1F}$) and the 5-HT$_7$ receptor, but has no significant activity at 5-HT$_2$, 5-HT$_3$, alpha- and beta-adrenergic, dopaminergic, histaminergic, muscarinic or benzodiazepine receptors.

Current theories on the etiology of migraine headache suggest that symptoms are due to local cranial vasodilatation and/or to the release of vasoactive and pro-inflammatory peptides from sensory nerve endings in an activated trigeminal system. The therapeutic activity of rizatriptan in migraine can most likely be attributed to agonist effects at 5-HT$_{1B/1D}$ receptors on the extracerebral, intracranial blood vessels that become dilated during a migraine attack and on nerve terminals in the trigeminal system. Activation of these receptors results in cranial vessel constriction, inhibition of neuropeptide release and reduced transmission in trigeminal pain pathways.

Pharmacokinetics: Absorption: Rizatriptan is completely absorbed following oral administration. The mean oral absolute bioavailability of the MAXALT Tablet is about 45%, and mean peak plasma concentrations (C_{max}) are reached in approximately 1-1.5 hours (T_{max}). The presence of a migraine headache did not appear to affect the absorption or pharmacokinetics of rizatriptan. Food has no significant effect on the bioavailability of rizatriptan but delays the time to reach peak concentration by an hour. In clinical trials, MAXALT was administered without regard to food. The plasma half-life of rizatriptan in males and females averages 2-3 hours.

When MAXALT 10 mg was administered every 2 hours for three doses on four consecutive days, the plasma concentrations of rizatriptan within each day were approximately 3-fold greater than those seen with a single 10 mg dose and no plasma accumulation of the drug occurred from day to day.

The bioavailability and C_{max} of rizatriptan were similar following administration of MAXALT Tablets and MAXALT RPD Wafers, but the rate of absorption is somewhat slower with MAXALT RPD Wafers, with T_{max} averaging 1.6-2.5 hours. AUC of rizatriptan is approximately 30% higher in females than in males.

Distribution: The mean volume of distribution is approximately 140 liters in male subjects and 110 liters in female subjects. Rizatriptan is minimally bound (14%) to plasma proteins.

Metabolism: The primary route of rizatriptan metabolism is via oxidative deamination by monoamine oxidase-A (MAO-A) to the indole acetic acid metabolite, which is not active at the 5-HT$_{1B/1D}$ receptor. N-monodesmethyl-rizatriptan, a metabolite with activity similar to that of parent compound at the 5-HT$_{1B/1D}$ receptor, is formed to a minor degree. Plasma concentrations of N-monodesmethyl-rizatriptan are approximately 14% of those of parent compound, and it is eliminated at a similar rate. Other minor metabolites, the N-oxide, the 6-hydroxy compound, and the sulfate conjugate of the 6-hydroxy metabolite are not active at the 5-HT$_{1B/1D}$ receptor.

Rizatriptan is not an inhibitor of the activities of human liver cytochrome P450 isoforms 3A4/5, 1A2, 2C9, 2C19, or 2E1; rizatriptan is a competitive inhibitor (Ki=1400 nM) of cytochrome P450 2D6, but only at high, clinically irrelevant concentrations.

Excretion: The total radioactivity of the administered dose recovered over 120 hours in urine and feces was 82% and 12%, respectively, following a single 10 mg oral administration of ^{14}C-rizatriptan. Following oral administration of ^{14}C-rizatriptan, rizatriptan accounted for about 17% of circulating plasma radioactivity. Approximately 14% of an oral dose is excreted in urine as unchanged rizatriptan while 51% is excreted as indole acetic acid metabolite, indicating substantial first pass metabolism.

Pharmacokinetic Parameters of a Single Dose of Rizatriptan in Females (n=12): See Table 3.

Table 3: MAXALT/MAXALT RPD

Pharmacokinetic Parameters of a Single Dose of Rizatriptan in Females (n=12)

	Arithmetic Mean (±SD)			
	MAXALT 5 mg Tablet	**MAXALT RPD 5 mg Wafer**	**MAXALT 10 mg Tablet**	**MAXALT RPD 10 mg Wafer**
$AUC_{(0-\infty)}$ (ng·h/mL)[a]	34.5±13.0	33.2±9.8	73.9±23.4	75.9±24.7
C_{max} (ng/mL)[a]	10.4±3.9	11.1±4.7	21.3±6.9	20.3±7.9
T_{max} (h)	1.0±0.6	1.6±0.8[d]	1.5±0.8	2.5±1.4[d]
$t_{1/2}$ (h)[b]	1.7	1.6	1.7	1.7
Plasma Clearance (mL/min)[c]	1050.5±224.5	1121.2±241.6	1081.6±239.4	1099.3±251.7

a Potency-normalized.
b Harmonic mean.
c Plasma clearance of 1 mg stable, heavy-labeled i.v. dose of rizatriptan given concomitantly with oral dose.
d P<0.05 compared to tablet formulation.

Special Populations and Conditions: Pediatrics: The mean $AUC_{0-\infty}$ and C_{max} of rizatriptan (10 mg orally) were about 12% and 19% higher in adolescents (n=12) as compared to historical data in adults, respectively.

MAXALT is not recommended for use in patients under 18 years of age (see Warnings and Precautions, Pediatrics (<18 years of age)). In a single study in adolescents (n=291), there were no significant differences with respect to headache relief at 2 hours between MAXALT and placebo treated groups.

Geriatrics: Rizatriptan pharmacokinetics in healthy elderly non-migraineur volunteers (age 65-77 years) were similar to those in younger non-migraineur volunteers (age 18-45 years).

Gender: The mean $AUC_{0-\infty}$ and C_{max} of rizatriptan (10 mg orally) were about 30% and 11% higher in females as compared to males, respectively, while T_{max} occurred at approximately the same time.

Race: Pharmacokinetic data revealed no significant differences between African American and Caucasian subjects. The effect of race on the pharmacokinetics of rizatriptan has not been systematically evaluated.

Hepatic Insufficiency: Following oral administration in patients with hepatic impairment caused by mild to moderate alcoholic cirrhosis of the liver, plasma concentrations of rizatriptan were similar in patients with mild hepatic insufficiency compared to a control group of healthy subjects; plasma concentrations of rizatriptan were approximately 30% greater in patients with moderate hepatic insufficiency (see Warnings and Precautions). Since there are no data in patients with severe hepatic impairment (Child-Pugh grade C), rizatriptan is contraindicated in this population (see Contraindications).

Renal Insufficiency: In patients with renal impairment (creatinine clearance 10-60 mL/min/1.73 m^2), the $AUC_{0-\infty}$ of rizatriptan was not significantly different from that in healthy subjects. In hemodialysis patients (creatinine clearance <2 mL/min/1.73 m^2), however, the AUC for rizatriptan was approximately 44% greater than that in patients with normal renal function (see Warnings and Precautions).

STORAGE AND STABILITY: Tablets: Store the tablets at room temperature (15-30°C).

Wafers: Store the wafers at room temperature (15-30°C).

SPECIAL HANDLING INSTRUCTIONS: The patient should be instructed not to remove the blister from the outer aluminum sachet until the patient is ready to consume the wafer inside.

INFORMATION FOR THE PATIENT: Published in e-CPS, available by subscription at www.e-cps.ca.

DOSAGE FORMS, COMPOSITION AND PACKAGING: Tablets: 5 mg: Each pale pink, capsule-shaped compressed tablet, embossed with the code MSD on one side and 266 on the other, contains: rizatriptan 5 mg (corresponding to 7.265 mg of the benzoate salt). Nonmedicinal ingredients: ferric oxide (red), lactose monohydrate, magnesium stearate, microcrystalline cellulose and pregelatinized starch. Blister packages of 6 tablets.

10 mg: Each pale pink, capsule-shaped compressed tablet, embossed with the code MSD 267 on one side and MAXALT on the other, contains: rizatriptan 10 mg (corresponding to 14.53 mg of the benzoate salt). Nonmedicinal ingredients: ferric oxide (red), lactose monohydrate, magnesium stearate, microcrystalline cellulose and pregelatinized starch. Blister packages of 6 and 12 tablets.

Wafers: 5 mg: Each white to off-white, round, rapidly disintegrating tablet, with a flat or slightly irregular surface, debossed with a modified triangle on one side, and with a peppermint flavor, contains: rizatriptan 5 mg (corresponding to 7.265 mg of the benzoate salt). Nonmedicinal ingredients: aspartame, gelatin, glycine, mannitol and peppermint flavor. Individually packaged in blisters inside an aluminum pouch (sachet), blister packages of 6 wafers.

10 mg: Each white to off-white, round, rapidly disintegrating tablet, with a flat or slightly irregular surface, debossed with a modified square on one side, and with a peppermint flavor, contains: rizatriptan 10 mg (corresponding to 14.53 mg of the benzoate salt). Nonmedicinal ingredients: aspartame, gelatin, glycine, mannitol and peppermint flavor. Individually packaged in blisters inside an aluminum pouch (sachet), blister packages of 6 and 12 wafers.

(Shown in Product Identification Section)

Maxidex® 🅿

dexamethasone

Anti-inflammatory

Alcon

SUPPLIED: Ophthalmic Ointment: Each tube of sterile ointment contains: dexamethasone 0.1% in a white petrolatum base. Nonmedicinal ingredients: liquid lanolin, methylparaben and propylparaben. Tubes of 3.5 g.

Ophthalmic Suspension: Each sterile Drop-Tainer dispenser contains: 0.1% dexamethasone. Preserved with benzalkonium chloride. Nonmedicinal ingredients: citric acid, edetate disodium, 0.5% hydroxypropyl methylcellulose, polysorbate 80, purified water, sodium chloride and sodium phosphate. Drop-Tainer dispensers of 5 mL.

Maxipime™ 🅿

cefepime HCl

Antibiotic

Bristol-Myers Squibb

Date of Preparation: May 23, 1995
Date of Revision: September 23, 2008

PHARMACOLOGY: Cefepime is a semi-synthetic broad spectrum cephalosporin antibiotic intended for i.m. or i.v. administration. Cefepime is a bactericidal agent that acts by inhibition of bacterial cell wall synthesis. It has a broad spectrum of activity against a wide range of gram-positive and gram-negative bacteria.

Pharmacokinetics: The average plasma concentrations of cefepime in normal adult males at various times following single 30-minute infusions and single i.m. injections of 500 mg, 1 g and 2 g are summarized in Table 1 and in Figure 1 and Figure 2.

Table 1: Maxipime

Mean Plasma Concentrations of Cefepime (μg/mL)

Cefepime Dose	0.5 h	1 h	2 h	4 h	8 h	12 h
I.V.						
500 mg	38.2	21.6	11.6	5.0	1.4	0.2
1 g	78.7	44.5	24.3	10.5	2.4	0.6
2 g	163.1	85.8	44.8	19.2	3.9	1.1
I.M.						
500 mg	8.2	12.5	12.0	6.9	1.9	0.7
1 g	14.8	25.9	26.3	16.0	4.5	1.4
2 g	36.1	49.9	51.3	31.5	8.7	2.3

Figure 1: Maxipime

Mean Plasma Concentration—Time Profiles After Single Intravenous Infusions Compared to MIC_{90} of Target Pathogens

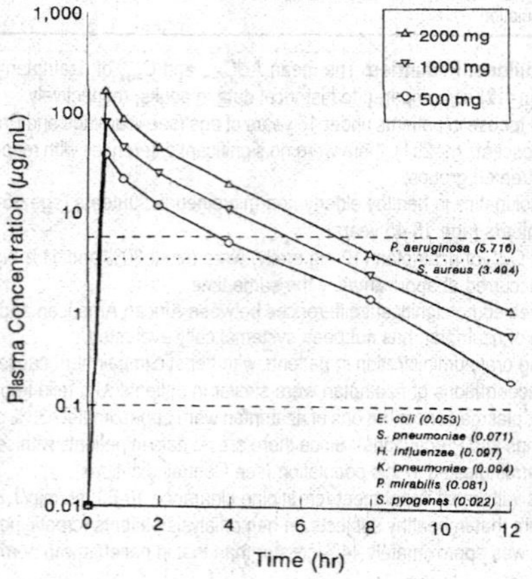

Figure 2: Maxipime

Mean Plasma Concentration—Time Profiles After Single Intramuscular Injections Compared to MIC_{90} of Target Pathogens

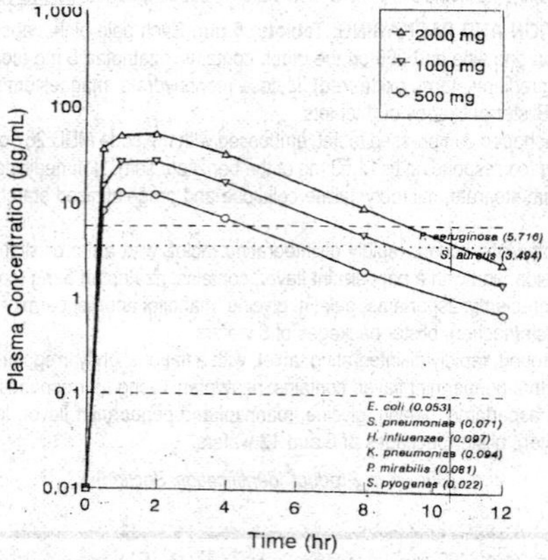

The average elimination half-life of cefepime is approximately 2 hours, and does not vary with respect to dose over the range of 250 mg to 2 g. There was no accumulation in healthy subjects receiving doses up to 2 g i.v. every 8 hours for a period of 9 days. Total body clearance averages 120 mL/minute. The average renal clearance of cefepime is 110 mL/minute, suggesting that the compound is eliminated almost exclusively by renal mechanisms, primarily glomerular filtration.

Urinary recovery of unchanged cefepime represents approximately 85% of dose, resulting in high concentrations of cefepime in the urine. The serum protein binding of cefepime averages 16.4% and is independent of its concentration in the serum. The average steady-state volume of distribution is 18 L.

Following i.m. administration, cefepime is completely absorbed. The pharmacokinetics of cefepime administered i.m. are linear over the range of 500 mg to 2 g and do not vary with respect to treatment duration.

Patients with Renal Impairment: Elimination half-life is prolonged in patients with various degrees of renal insufficiency, with a linear relationship between total body clearance and creatinine clearance. This serves as the basis for dosage adjustment recommendations in this group of patients (see Dosage). The average half-life is 13 hours in patients with severe renal impairment requiring hemodialysis and 19 hours in those requiring continuous ambulatory peritoneal dialysis.

Children: Cefepime pharmacokinetics have been evaluated in pediatric patients following single and multiple 50 mg/kg doses on q8h (n=29) and q12h (n=13) schedules. The mean (±SD) age of the patients was 3.6 (±3.3) years, and ranged from 2.1 months to 11.2 years. Following a single i.v. dose, total body clearance and the steady-state volume of distribution averaged 3.3 (±1.0) mL/min/kg and 0.3 (±0.1) L/kg, respectively. The overall mean elimination half-life was 1.7 (±0.4) hours. The urinary recovery of unchanged cefepime was 60.4 (±30.4)% of the administered dose, and renal clearance was the primary pathway of elimination, averaging 2.0 (±1.1) mL/min/kg. There were no significant differences in the pharmacokinetics of cefepime among pediatric patients of various ages or between male (n=25) and female patients (n=17). There was no evidence of accumulation of cefepime in patients treated for up to 14 days with either regimen. The absolute bioavailability of cefepime after an i.m. dose of 50 mg/kg was 82.3 (±15.6)% in 8 patients. The exposure to cefepime, including minimum plasma concentrations at steady state, following a 50 mg/kg i.v dose in a pediatric patient is comparable to that in adults treated with a 2 g i.v. dose.

INDICATIONS: In the treatment of the following infections when caused by susceptible strains of the designated microorganisms:

Adults: Lower respiratory tract infections: nosocomial and community acquired pneumonia caused by *P. aeruginosa*, *S. aureus* (methicillin-susceptible strains), *S. pneumoniae*, *E. coli* and *H. influenzae*.

Acute exacerbations of chronic bronchitis caused by *S. pneumoniae* and *H. influenzae*.

Uncomplicated and complicated urinary tract infections, including pyelonephritis caused by *P. aeruginosa*, *E. coli*, *K. pneumoniae* and *P. mirabilis*.

Due to the nature of the underlying conditions which usually predispose patients to Pseudomonas infections of the lower respiratory and urinary tracts, a good clinical response accompanied by bacterial eradication may not be achieved despite evidence of in vitro sensitivity.

Skin and skin structure infections caused by *S. aureus* (methicillin-susceptible strains), *S. pyogenes* (Group A streptococci) and *P. aeruginosa*.

Peritonitis due to gangrenous and perforated appendicitis caused by *E. coli*.

Bacterial septicemia caused by *E. coli*, *S. pneumoniae* and *K. pneumoniae*.

Empiric Therapy in Febrile Neutropenic Patients: Cefepime as monotherapy is indicated for empiric treatment of febrile neutropenic patients. In patients at high risk for severe infection (including patients with a history of recent bone marrow transplantation, with hypotension at presentation, with an underlying hematologic malignancy, or with severe or prolonged neutropenia), antimicrobial monotherapy may not be appropriate. Insufficient data exist to support the efficacy of cefepime monotherapy in such patients.

Specimens for bacteriologic culture should be obtained prior to therapy in order to identify the causative organisms and to determine their susceptibilities to cefepime.

Treatment with cefepime may be instituted empirically before results of susceptibility studies are known; however, modification of the antibiotic treatment may be required once these results become available.

In patients who are at risk of infection due to an anaerobic organism, concurrent initial therapy with an antianaerobic agent such as metronidazole or clindamycin is recommended before the causative organism(s) is (are) known. When such concomitant treatment is appropriate, the recommended doses of both antibiotics should be given according to the severity of the infection and the patient's condition.

Children: In pediatric patients for the treatment of infections listed below when caused by susceptible bacteria:

Lower respiratory tract infections: nosocomial and community acquired pneumonia caused by *P. aeruginosa*, *S. aureus* (methicillin-susceptible strains), *S. pneumoniae*, *E. coli*, and *H. influenzae*.

Uncomplicated and complicated urinary tract infections, including pyelonephritis caused by *P. aeruginosa*, *E. coli*, *K. pneumoniae*, and *P. mirabilis*.

Skin and skin structure infections caused by *S. aureus* (methicillin-susceptible strains), *S. pyogenes* (Group A streptococci), and *P. aeruginosa*.

Empiric Therapy in Febrile Neutropenic Patients: Cefepime as monotherapy is indicated for empiric treatment of febrile neutropenic patients. In patients at high risk for severe infection (including patients with a history of recent bone marrow transplantation, with hypotension at presentation, with an underlying hematologic malignancy, or with severe or prolonged neutropenia), antimicrobial monotherapy may not be appropriate. Insufficient data exist to support the efficacy of cefepime monotherapy in such patients.

Specimens for bacteriologic culture should be obtained prior to therapy in order to identify the causative organisms and to determine their susceptibilities to cefepime.

Treatment with cefepime may be instituted empirically before results of susceptibility studies are known; however, modification of the antibiotic treatment may be required once these results become available.

CONTRAINDICATIONS: In patients who have had previous hypersensitivity reactions to cefepime or any component of the formulation or the cephalosporin class of antibiotics, penicillins or other beta-lactam antibiotics (see Supplied).

WARNINGS: Hypersensitivity: Before therapy with cefepime is instituted, careful inquiry should be made to determine whether the patient has had previous immediate hypersensitivity reactions to cefepime, cephalosporins, penicillins or other beta-lactam antibiotics. Antibiotics should be administered with caution to any patient who has demonstrated some form of allergy, particularly to drugs. If an allergic reaction to cefepime occurs, discontinue the drug and institute supportive treatment as appropriate (e.g., maintenance of ventilation, pressor amines, antihistamines, corticosteroids). Serious immediate hypersensitivity reactions may require epinephrine and other supportive therapy.

C. difficile-associated Disease: *C. difficile*-associated disease (CDAD) has been reported with use of many antibacterial agents, including cefepime. CDAD may range in severity from mild diarrhea to fatal colitis. It is important to consider this diagnosis in patients who present with diarrhea, or symptoms of colitis, pseudomembranous colitis, toxic megacolon, or perforation of colon subsequent to the administration of any antibacterial agent. CDAD has been reported to occur over 2 months after the administration of antibacterial agents.

Treatment with antibacterial agents may alter the normal flora of the colon and may permit overgrowth of *C. difficile*. *C. difficile* produces toxins A and B, which contribute to the development of CDAD. CDAD may cause significant morbidity and mortality. CDAD can be refractory to antimicrobial therapy.

If the diagnosis of CDAD is suspected or confirmed, appropriate therapeutic measures should be initiated. Mild cases of CDAD usually respond to discontinuation of antibacterial agents not directed against *C. difficile*. In moderate to severe cases, consideration should be given to management with fluids and electrolytes, protein supplementation, and treatment with an antibacterial agent clinically effective against *C. difficile*. Surgical evaluation should be instituted as clinically indicated, as surgical intervention may be required in certain severe cases (see Adverse Effects).

Renal Impairment: In patients with impaired renal function (creatinine clearance ≤50 mL/min), the dose of cefepime should be adjusted to compensate for the slower rate of renal elimination. Because high and prolonged serum antibiotic concentrations can occur from usual dosages in patients with renal insufficiency or other conditions that may compromise renal function, the maintenance dosage should be reduced when cefepime is administered to such patients. Continued dosage should be determined by degree of renal impairment, severity of infection, and susceptibility of the causative organisms. (See specific recommendations for dosing adjustment in Dosage.) During postmarketing surveillance, serious adverse events have been reported including life-threatening or fatal occurrences of the following: encephalopathy (disturbance of consciousness including confusion, hallucinations, stupor, and coma), myoclonus, seizures (including non convulsive status epilepticus), and/or renal failure (see Adverse Effects, Postmarketing Experience). Most cases occurred in patients with renal impairment who received doses of cefepime that exceeded recommendations in Table 2. In the majority of cases, symptoms of neurotoxicity were reversible and resolved after discontinuation of cefepime and/or after hemodialysis.

PRECAUTIONS: General: As with other antibiotics, prolonged use of cefepime may result in overgrowth of nonsusceptible organisms. Should superinfection occur during therapy, appropriate measures should be taken.

Cefepime should be used with caution in individuals with a history of gastrointestinal disease, particularly colitis.

Many cephalosporins, including cefepime, have been associated with a fall in prothrombin activity. Those at risk include patients with renal or hepatic impairment, or poor nutritional state, as well as patients receiving a protracted course of antimicrobial therapy. Prothrombin time should be monitored in patients at risk, and exogenous vitamin K administered as indicated.

Positive direct Coombs' tests have been reported during treatment with cefepime. In hematologic studies or in transfusion cross-matching procedures when antiglobulin tests are performed on the minor side or in Coombs' testing of newborns whose mothers have received cephalosporin antibiotics before parturition, it should be recognized that a positive Coombs' test may be due to the drug.

Drug Interactions: The combination of cefepime with an aminoglycoside has been shown to be synergistic in vitro. Although there is no evidence that cefepime adversely affects renal function at normal therapeutic doses, the usual precautions, such as the monitoring of renal function, should be applied if drugs with nephrotoxic potential (such as aminoglycosides and potent diuretics) are administered with cefepime.

The administration of cefepime may result in a false-positive reaction for glucose in the urine when using a copper reduction test. It is recommended that glucose tests based on enzymatic glucose oxidase reactions be used.

Pregnancy: There are no adequate and well-controlled studies in pregnant women.

Reproduction studies performed in mice and rats showed no evidence of fetal damage at dose levels equivalent to (mouse) or slightly greater (rat) than the maximum human daily dose when the daily doses are compared to those in man on a mg/m^2 basis. Because animal reproduction studies are not always predictive of human response, this drug should be used during pregnancy only if the potential benefit justifies the potential risk.

Lactation: Cefepime is excreted in human breast milk in very low concentrations. Although less than 0.01% of a 1 g i.v. dose is excreted in milk, caution should be used when cefepime is administered to a nursing woman.

Children: The safety and effectiveness of cefepime in the treatment of uncomplicated and complicated urinary tract infections (including pyelonephritis), uncomplicated skin and skin structure infections, pneumonia (nosocomial and community acquired), and as empiric therapy in febrile neutropenic patients, have been established in the age groups 2 months up to 12 years. Use of cefepime in these age groups is supported by evidence from adequate and well-controlled studies of cefepime in adults with additional pharmacokinetic and safety data from pediatric trials (see Pharmacology and Adverse Effects).

Safety and effectiveness in pediatric patients below the age of 2 months have not been established. However, accumulation of other cephalosporin antibiotics in newborn infants (resulting from prolonged drug half-life in this age group) has been reported.

In those patients in whom meningeal seeding from a distant infection site or in whom meningitis is suspected or documented, an alternate agent with demonstrated clinical efficacy in this setting should be used.

Geriatrics: Healthy elderly male and female volunteers (≥65 years old) who received a single 1 g i.v. dose of cefepime had higher area under the curve (AUC) and lower renal clearance values when compared to younger subjects. However, this appeared to be a function of the decrease in creatinine clearance with increasing age. In patients with age-normalized renal function, a dosage adjustment of cefepime is not necessary. Dosage adjustments are recommended if renal function is compromised.

Of the more than 6400 adults treated with cefepime in clinical studies, 35% were 65 years or older while 16% were 75 years or older. When elderly patients received the usual recommended adult dose, clinical efficacy and safety were comparable to clinical efficacy and safety in nonelderly adult patients unless the patients had renal insufficiency.

Serious adverse events have occurred in elderly patients with renal insufficiency given unadjusted doses of cefepime, including life-threatening or fatal occurrences of the following: encephalopathy (disturbance of consciousness including confusion, hallucinations, stupor and coma), myoclonus, seizures (including nonconvulsive status epilepticus) and/or renal failure (see Warnings and Adverse Effects).

This drug is known to be substantially excreted by the kidney, and the risk of toxic reactions to this drug may be greater in patients with impaired renal function. Because elderly patients are more likely to have decreased renal function, care should be taken in dose selection, and renal function should be monitored (see Warnings and Dosage).

Hepatic Impairment: The pharmacokinetics of cefepime were unaltered in patients with impaired hepatic function who received a single 1 g dose. Therefore, dosage adjustments are not required in patients with hepatic impairment.

Cystic Fibrosis: The pharmacokinetics of cefepime do not change to a clinically significant degree in patients with cystic fibrosis. It is not necessary to alter the dosage of cefepime in this patient population.

ADVERSE EFFECTS: Cefepime is generally well tolerated. In clinical trials (N=5598) the most common adverse events were gastrointestinal symptoms and hypersensitivity reactions. Adverse events considered to be of probable relationship to cefepime are listed below.

Events that occurred at an incidence of >0.1 to 1% (except where noted) were:

Hypersensitivity: rash (1.8%), pruritus, urticaria.

Gastrointestinal: nausea, vomiting, oral moniliasis, diarrhea (1.2%), colitis (including pseudomembranous colitis).

Central Nervous System: headache.

Other: fever, vaginitis, erythema.

Events that occurred between 0.05 to 0.1% were: abdominal pain, constipation, vasodilation, dyspnea, dizziness, paresthesia, genital pruritus, taste perversion, chills, unspecified moniliasis, vaginal moniliasis, urogenital infection and vaginitis.

Events of clinical significance that occurred at an incidence of <0.05% included anaphylaxis and seizures.

At the higher dose of 2 g q8h in **febrile neutropenia**, the incidence of probably related adverse events was higher among 1048 patients who received this dose of cefepime in clinical trials. They consisted of rash (4%), diarrhea (3%), nausea (2%), vomiting (1%), pruritus (1%), fever (1%) and headache (1%).

Local reactions at the site of intravenous infusion occurred in 5.2% of patients; these included phlebitis (2.9%) and inflammation (0.1%). Intramuscular administration of cefepime was very well tolerated with 2.6% of patients experiencing pain or inflammation at the injection site.

Laboratory test abnormalities that developed during clinical trials in patients with normal baseline values were transient. Those that occurred at a frequency between 1 and 2% (unless noted) were: elevations in ALT (3.6%), AST (2.5%), alkaline phosphatase, total bilirubin, anemia, eosinophilia, prolonged prothrombin time and partial thromboplastin time (2.8%); positive Coombs' test without hemolysis (18.7%) also occurred. Additionally, increased phosphorous, decreased phosphorous (2.8%), increased calcium, decreased calcium (which was more common in elderly patients) and increased potassium were observed.

As with some other cephalosporins, transient elevations of blood urea nitrogen and/or serum creatinine and transient thrombocytopenia were observed in 0.5 to 1% of patients. Transient leukopenia and neutropenia were also seen (<0.5%). During postmarketing experience, agranulocytosis has been reported rarely.

Renal insufficiency and hepatic failure have been reported in conjunction with cefepime treatment. However, a causative relationship to cefepime therapy has not been determined (see also Postmarketing Experience).

The following adverse events and altered laboratory tests have been reported for cephalosporin-class antibiotics: Stevens-Johnson syndrome, erythema multiforme, toxic epidermal necrolysis, toxic nephropathy, aplastic anemia, hemolytic anemia, hemorrhage, hepatic dysfunction including cholestasis, false positive test for urinary glucose and pancytopenia.

Pediatric Patients: A similar safety profile has been experienced in infants and children relative to the adult population. No specific concerns have been identified.

Postmarketing Experience: In addition to the events reported during North American clinical trials with cefepime, the following adverse experiences have been reported during worldwide post marketing experience. Because of the uncontrolled nature of spontaneous reports, a causal relationship to cefepime treatment has not been determined.

As with some other drugs in this class, encephalopathy (disturbance of consciousness including confusion, hallucinations, stupor and coma), seizures (including nonconvulsive status epilepticus), myoclonus, and/or renal failure have been reported. Most cases occurred in patients with renal impairment who received doses of cefepime that exceeded recommendations outlined in Dosage. In general, symptoms of neurotoxicity resolved after discontinuation of cefepime and/or after hemodialysis however, some cases included a fatal outcome. Precautions should be taken to adjust daily dosage in patients with renal insufficiency or other conditions that may compromise renal function to reduce antibiotic concentrations that can lead or contribute to these and other serious adverse events, including renal failure.

OVERDOSE:

Symptoms: Accidental overdosing has occurred when large doses were given to patients with impaired renal function (see Warnings). Symptoms of overdose include encephalopathy (disturbance of consciousness including confusion, hallucinations, stupor, and coma), myoclonus, seizures (including nonconvulsive status epilepticus), and neuromuscular excitability.

Treatment: Cefepime is eliminated primarily by the kidneys. In case of severe overdosage, especially in patients with compromised renal function, hemodialysis will aid in the removal of cefepime from the body. Peritoneal dialysis is of no value.

For management of a suspected drug overdose, CPhA recommends that you contact your **regional Poison Control Centre**. See the *CPS* Directory section for a list of Poison Control Centres.

DOSAGE: Can be administered either i.v. or i.m. The dosage and route of administration should be determined according to the susceptibility of the causative organisms, the severity of the infection, and the condition and renal function of the patient. Guidelines for dosage of cefepime in adults with normal renal function are provided in Table 2.

Table 2: Maxipime

Recommended Dosage Schedule for Adults (12 years and older) with Normal Renal Function

Site and Type of Infection	Dose (g)	Route	Frequency	Duration (days)
Mild to moderate urinary tract infection (uncomplicated and complicated), including pyelonephritis	0.5–1	i.v. or i.m.	q12h	7–10
Mild to moderate infections including pneumonia, bronchitis and skin and skin-structure infections	1	i.v. or i.m.	q12h	10
Severe infections including pneumonia, septicemia and complicated intra-abdominal infections	2	i.v.	q12h	10
Empiric therapy in febrile neutropenic patients[a]	2	i.v.	q8h	7[b]

[a] Cefepime has also been used in combination with an aminoglycoside or a glycopeptide in patient populations which excluded high risk patients (see Indications).

[b] Or until resolution of neutropenia.

Pediatric Patients (aged 2 months up to 12 years with normal renal function): Usual Recommended Dosages: Empiric Treatment of Febrile Neutropenia: Patients >2 months of age with body weight ≤40 kg: 50 mg/kg i.v q8h for 7 to 10 days.

Pneumonia, Urinary Tract Infections, Skin and Skin Structure Infections: Patients >2 months of age with body weight ≤40 kg: 50 mg/kg i.v q12h for 10 days.

Experience with the use of cefepime in pediatric patients <2 months of age is limited.

For pediatric patients with body weights >40 kg, adult dosing recommendations apply (see Table 2). Dosage in pediatric patients should not exceed the maximum recommended dosage in adults (2 g q8h). Experience with i.m. administration in pediatric patients is limited.

Infection: The usual duration of therapy is 7 to 10 days; however, more severe infections may require longer treatment.

Impaired Hepatic Function: No adjustment is necessary for patients with impaired hepatic function.

Impaired Renal Function: There is no need to adjust dosage in the elderly unless renal impairment is present. Cefepime is excreted by the kidneys almost exclusively by glomerular filtration. Therefore, in patients with impaired renal function (creatinine clearance ≤50 mL/min), the dose of cefepime should be adjusted to compensate for the slower rate of renal elimination. The recommended initial dose of cefepime in patients with mild to moderate renal impairment should be the same as in patients with normal renal function. An estimate of creatinine clearance should be made to determine the appropriate maintenance dose. The recommended initial dose for patients on hemodialysis and maintenance doses of cefepime in patients with renal insufficiency are presented in Table 3.

Table 3: Maxipime

Maintenance Dosing Schedule in Adult Patients with Renal Impairment

Creatinine Clearance (mL/min)	Recommended Maintenance Schedule: Normal recommended dosing schedules, no adjustments needed		
>50	1 g q12h	2 g q12h	2 g q8h
30–50	1 g q24h	2 g q24h	2 g q12h
11–29	500 mg q24h	1 g q24h	2 g q24h
<11	250 mg q24h	500 mg q24h	1 g q24h
Hemodialysis[a]	500 mg q24h	500 mg q24h	500 mg q24h

[a] Pharmacokinetic modeling indicates that reduced dosing for these patients is necessary. Patients receiving cefepime who are undergoing concomitant hemodialysis should be dosed as follows: 1 gram loading dose on the first day of cefepime therapy and 500 mg per day thereafter. On dialysis days, cefepime should be administered following dialysis. Whenever possible cefepime should be administered at the same time each day.

When only serum creatinine measurement is available, the following formula (proposed by Cockcroft and Gault) may be used to estimate creatinine clearance. The serum creatinine should represent a steady state of renal function:

Males:

$$\text{Creatinine clearance (mL/min)} = \frac{\text{Weight (kg)} \times (140-\text{age})}{72 \times \text{serum creatinine (mg/dL)}}$$

Females: 0.85×value calculated using formula for males.

Pediatric Patients with Impaired Renal Function: Since urinary excretion is the primary route of elimination of cefepime in pediatric patients (see Pharmacology), an adjustment of the dosage of cefepime should also be considered in this population.

A dose of 50 mg/kg in patients aged 2 months up to 12 years is comparable to a dose of 2 g in an adult. As recommended in Table 3, the same increase in interval between doses and/or reduction in dose should be used. When only serum creatinine is available, creatinine clearance may be estimated using either of the following methods (proposed by Schwartz, et al and Dechaux, et al, respectively):

$$\text{Creatinine clearance (mL/min/1.73 m}^2\text{)} = \frac{0.55\times\text{height (cm)}}{\text{serum creatinine (mg/dL)}}$$

or

$$\text{Creatinine clearance (mL/min/1.73 m}^2\text{)} = \frac{0.52\times\text{height (cm)}}{\text{serum creatinine (mg/dL)}} - 3.6$$

Dialysis Patients: In patients undergoing hemodialysis, approximately 68% of the total amount of cefepime present in the body at the start of dialysis will be removed during a 3-hour dialysis period. The recommended initial dose and maintenance schedule for patients on hemodialysis are presented in Table 3.

In patients undergoing continuous ambulatory peritoneal dialysis, cefepime may be administered at the same doses recommended for patients with normal renal function, i.e., 500 mg, 1 g or 2 g (depending on the severity of the infection) at a dosage interval of every 48 hours.

Route of Administration: I.V. Administration: The i.v. route of administration is preferable for patients with severe or life-threatening infections, particularly if the possibility of shock is present.

For direct i.v. injection, the solution reconstituted as recommended (see Dosage, Reconstitution and Compatibility) should be slowly injected directly into the vein over a period of 3 to 5 minutes. Alternatively, the injection can be made into the tubing of an administration set while the patient is receiving a compatible i.v. fluid.

For continuous i.v. infusion, reconstitute the 1 or 2 g vial as recommended (see Dosage, Reconstitution and Compatibility) and add an appropriate quantity of the resulting solution to one of the compatible i.v. fluids in an i.v. administration set. The resulting solution should be administered over a period of approximately 30 minutes.

For intermittent i.v. infusion, a Y-tube administration set can be used with compatible solutions. However, during infusion of a solution containing cefepime, it is desirable to discontinue the other solution.

I.M. Administration: Reconstituted as recommended (see Dosage, Reconstitution and Compatibility) to a final concentration of 280 mg/mL and given by deep i.m. injection into a large muscle mass (such as the upper outer quadrant of the gluteus maximus).

Although cefepime can be constituted with 0.5 or 1% lidocaine HCl, it is usually not required since cefepime causes little or no pain upon i.m. administration.

Reconstitution: I.M. Injection: The following diluents may be used for constituting cefepime for i.m. injection: sterile water for injection, 0.9% sodium chloride injection, 5% dextrose injection, bacteriostatic water for injection with paraben(s), bacteriostatic water for injection with benzyl alcohol, 0.5 or 1% lidocaine HCl (see Table 4).

Table 4: Maxipime

Reconstitution Table—I.M. Injection

Vial Size (g)	Volume of Diluent to be Added (mL)	Approximate Available Volume (mL)	Approximate Cefepime Concentration[a] (mg/mL)
1	2.4	3.6	280

[a] Approximate cefepime concentration includes overages used during manufacturing.

Direct I.V. Injection: Constitute cefepime with 10 mL of sterile water for injection, 5% dextrose injection or 0.9% sodium chloride injection, as directed in Table 5.

Table 5: Maxipime

Reconstitution Table—Direct I.V. Injection

Vial Size (g)	Volume of Diluent to be Added (mL)	Approximate Available Volume (mL)	Approximate Cefepime Concentration[a] (mg/mL)
1	10	11.3	100
2	10	12.5	160

[a] Approximate cefepime concentration includes overages used during manufacturing.

I.V. Infusion: Constitute the 1 g or 2 g vial as recommended and add an appropriate quantity of the resulting solution to one of the compatible i.v. fluids in an i.v. administration set.

At concentrations between 1 and 40 mg/mL, cefepime is compatible with the following i.v. infusion fluids: 0.9% sodium chloride injection, 5% or 10% dextrose injection, M/6 sodium lactate injection, 5% dextrose and 0.9% sodium chloride injection, Lactated Ringers and 5% dextrose injection and Normosol-R and Normosol-M in 5% dextrose injection.

Compatibility: Cefepime, prepared in 0.9% sodium chloride or 5% dextrose injection at a concentration of 4 mg of cefepime/mL, is stable for 72 hours under refrigeration (2 to 8°C) when admixed with: heparin (10 or 50 U/mL), potassium chloride (10 or 40 mEq/mL), theophylline (0.8 mg/mL in 5% dextrose injection).

Cefepime at a concentration of 40 mg/mL in 0.9% sodium chloride solution or 5% dextrose injection was found to be compatible with AMIKIN (amikacin) (6 mg/mL).

Solutions of cefepime, like solutions of most beta-lactam antibiotics, should not be added to solutions of ampicillin, metronidazole, vancomycin, gentamicin, tobramycin sulfate or netilmicin sulfate because of physical or chemical incompatibility. However, if concurrent therapy with cefepime is indicated, each of these antibiotics can be administered separately to the same patient.

As with all parenteral products, i.v. admixtures should be inspected visually for clarity, particulate matter, precipitation, discoloration and leakage prior to administration whenever solution and container permit.

Stability and Storage: Store dry powder at room temperature (15 to 30°C) and protect from light. The dry powder may also be stored in the refrigerator (2 to 8°C), protected from light.

Solutions for i.m. or i.v. use reconstituted as well as diluted as recommended with sterile water for injection, 0.9% sodium chloride injection or 5% dextrose injection are stable for 72 hours when stored under refrigeration (2 to 8°C) and protected from light. Solutions reconstituted as well as diluted with diluents other than those listed above should be used immediately after reconstitution.

Note: Parenteral drugs should be inspected visually for particulate matter before administration, and not used if particulate matter is present.

As with other cephalosporins, the color of Maxipime powder (white to off-white) and constituted solutions (colorless to amber) may darken on storage. The product potency is not adversely affected.

SUPPLIED: Each single use vial of dry powder contains: cefepime HCl equivalent to 1 g and 2 g of cefepime activity. Nonmedicinal ingredients: L-arginine 725 mg per g of cefepime.

Maxitrol® [Pr]

dexamethasone—neomycin sulfate—polymyxin B sulfate

Anti-inflammatory—Antibiotic

Alcon

SUPPLIED: Ophthalmic Ointment: Each g of sterile ointment contains: polymyxin B sulfate 6 000 units, neomycin (as sulfate) 3.5 mg and dexamethasone 1 mg (0.1%) in a white petrolatum base. Nonmedicinal ingredients: anhydrous lanolin, methylparaben and propylparaben. Tubes of 3.5 g.

Ophthalmic Suspension: Each mL contains: dexamethasone 1 mg (0.1%), neomycin (as sulfate) 3.5 mg and polymyxin B sulfate 6 000 units. Preserved with benzalkonium chloride. Nonmedicinal ingredients: hydrochloric acid and/or sodium hydroxide (to adjust pH), 0.5% hydroxypropyl methylcellulose, polysorbate 20, purified water and sodium chloride. Drop-Tainer dispensers of 5 mL.

MED-Letrozole [Pr]

letrozole

Nonsteroidal Aromatase Inhibitor— Inhibitor of Estrogen Biosynthesis— Antitumour Agent

Generic Medical Partners

SUPPLIED: Each yellow, round, film-coated, biconvex tablet, debossed "2.5" on one side and plain on the reverse side contains: letrozole 2.5 mg. Nonmedicinal ingredients: FD&C Yellow #6 aluminium lake, magnesium stearate, polyethylene glycol, polyvinyl alcohol, silicified microcrystalline cellulose, sodium starchglycolatee, talc, titanium dioxide and yellow iron oxide. Blister packages of 30. Protect from heat (store at room temperature 15 to 30°C). Protect from moisture. Keep out of reach and sight of children and pets.

Medrol® [Pr]

methylprednisolone

Glucocorticoid

Pfizer

INDICATIONS: Endocrine Disorders: Primary or secondary adrenocortical insufficiency (hydrocortisone or cortisone is the first choice; synthetic analogs may be used in conjunction with mineralocorticoids where applicable; in infancy mineralocorticoid supplementation is of particular importance). Congenital adrenal hyperplasia. Nonsuppurative thyroiditis. Hypercalcemia associated with cancer.

Nonendocrine Disorders: Rheumatic Disorders: As adjunctive therapy for short-term administration (to tide the patient over an acute episode or exacerbation) in: psoriatic arthritis; rheumatoid arthritis, including juvenile rheumatoid arthritis (selected cases may require low-dose maintenance therapy); ankylosing spondylitis; acute and subacute bursitis; acute nonspecific tenosynovitis; acute gouty arthritis; post-traumatic osteoarthritis; synovitis of osteoarthritis; epicondylitis.

Collagen Diseases: During an exacerbation or as maintenance therapy in selected cases of: systemic lupus erythematosus; systemic dermatomyositis (polymyositis); acute rheumatic carditis; polymyalgia rheumatica; giant cell arteritis.

Dermatologic Diseases: pemphigus; bullous dermatitis herpetiformis; severe erythema multiforme (Stevens-Johnson syndrome); exfoliative dermatitis; mycosis fungoides; severe psoriasis; severe seborrheic dermatitis.

Allergic State: Control of severe or incapacitating allergic conditions intractable to adequate trials of conventional treatment: seasonal or perennial allergic rhinitis; serum sickness; bronchial asthma; drug hypersensitivity reactions; contact dermatitis; atopic dermatitis.

Ophthalmic Diseases: Severe acute and chronic allergic and inflammatory processes involving the eye and its adnexa such as: allergic corneal marginal ulcers; herpes zoster ophthalmicus; anterior segment inflammation; diffuse posterior uveitis and choroiditis; sympathetic ophthalmia; allergic conjunctivitis; keratitis; chorioretinitis; optic neuritis; iritis and iridocyclitis.

Respiratory Diseases: symptomatic sarcoidosis; Löffler's syndrome not manageable by other means; berylliosis; fulminating or disseminated pulmonary tuberculosis when used concurrently with appropriate antituberculous chemotherapy; aspiration pneumonitis.

Hematologic Disorders: idiopathic thrombocytopenic purpura in adults; secondary thrombocytopenia in adults; acquired (autoimmune) hemolytic anemia; erythroblastopenia (RBC anemia); congenital (erythroid) hypoplastic anemia.

Neoplastic Disorders: For palliative management of: leukemias and lymphomas in adults; acute leukemia of childhood.

Edematous States: To induce a diuresis or remission of proteinuria in the nephrotic syndrome, without uremia, of the idiopathic type or that due to lupus erythematosus.

Gastrointestinal Diseases: To tide the patient over a critical period of the disease in: ulcerative colitis; regional enteritis.

Nervous System: acute exacerbations of multiple sclerosis; management of edema associated with brain tumor.

Miscellaneous: Tuberculous meningitis with subarachnoid block or impending block when used concurrently with appropriate antituberculous chemotherapy. Trichinosis with neurologic or myocardial involvement.

Organ Transplantation.

CONTRAINDICATIONS: Systemic fungal infections; known hypersensitivity to methylprenisolone.

WARNINGS: In patients on corticosteroid therapy subjected to unusual stress, increased dosage of rapidly acting corticosteroids before, during, and after the stressful situation is indicated.

Corticosteroids may mask some signs of infection, and new infections may appear during their use. Infections with any pathogen including viral, bacterial, fungal, protozoan or helminthic infections, in any location in the body, may be associated with the use of corticosteroids alone or in combination with other immunosuppressive agents that affect cellular immunity, humoral immunity, or neutrophil function. These infections may be mild, but can be severe and at times fatal. With increasing doses of corticosteroids, the rate of occurrence of infectious complication increases. Do not use intra-articularly, intrabursally, or for intratendonous administration for local effect in the presence of acute infection.

Prolonged use of corticosteroids may produce posterior subcapsular cataracts, glaucoma with possible damage to the optic nerves, and may enhance the establishment of secondary ocular infections due to fungi or viruses. Allergic reactions (e.g., angioedema) may occur.

Average and large doses of hydrocortisone or cortisone can cause elevation of blood pressure, salt and water retention, and increased excretion of potassium. These effects are less likely to occur with the synthetic derivatives except when used in large doses. Dietary salt restriction and potassium supplementation may be necessary. All corticosteroids increase calcium excretion.

Administration of live or live, attenuated vaccines is contraindicated in patients receiving immunosuppressive doses of corticosteroids. Killed or inactivated vaccines may be administered to patients receiving immunosuppressive doses of corticosteroids; however, the response to such vaccines may be diminished. Indicated immunization procedures may be undertaken in patients receiving nonimmunosuppressive doses of corticosteroids.

The use of methylprednisolone in active tuberculosis should be restricted to those cases of fulminating or disseminated tuberculosis in which the corticosteroid is used for the management of the disease in conjunction with an appropriate antituberculosis regimen.

If corticosteroids are indicated in patients with latent tuberculosis reactivity, close observation is necessary as reactivation of the disease may occur. During prolonged corticosteroid therapy, these patients should receive chemoprophylaxis.

There is no universal agreement on whether corticosteroids per se are responsible for peptic ulcers encountered during therapy; however, glucocorticoid therapy may mask the symptoms of peptic ulcer so that perforation or hemorrhage may occur without significant pain.

Osteoporosis is a common but infrequently recognized adverse effect associated with a long-term use of large doses of glucocorticoid.

Growth may be suppressed in children receiving long-term daily, divided dose glucocorticoid therapy and use of such regimen should be restricted to the most urgent indication. Alternate day glucocorticoid therapy usually avoids or minimizes this side effect.

Host defenses are impaired in patients receiving large doses of glucocorticoids and this effect increases susceptibility to fungus infections as well as bacterial and viral infections.

Pregnancy: Some animal studies have shown that corticosteroids, when administered to the mother at high doses, may cause fetal malformations. Adequate human reproductive studies have not been done with corticosteroids. Therefore, the use of this drug in pregnancy, nursing mothers, or women of childbearing potential requires that the benefits of the drug be carefully weighed against the potential risk to the mother and embryo or fetus. Since there is inadequate evidence of safety in human pregnancy, this drug should be used in pregnancy only if clearly needed.

Corticosteroids readily cross the placenta. Infants born of mothers who have received substantial doses of corticosteroids during pregnancy must be carefully observed and evaluated for signs of adrenal insufficiency. There are no known effects of corticosteroids on labor and delivery.

Lactation: Corticosteroids are excreted in breast milk.

PRECAUTIONS: Drug-induced adrenocortical insufficiency may be minimized by gradual reduction of dosage. This type of relative insufficiency may persist for months after discontinuation of therapy; therefore, in any situation of stress occurring during that period, hormone therapy should be reinstituted. Since mineralocorticoid secretion may be impaired, salt and/or mineralocorticoid should be administered concurrently.

There is an enhanced effect of corticosteroids on patients with hypothyroidism and in those with cirrhosis.

Corticosteroids should be used cautiously in patients with ocular herpes simplex because of possible corneal perforation.

The lowest possible dose of corticosteroid should be used to control the condition under treatment, and when reduction in dosage is possible, the reduction should be gradual.

Psychic derangements may appear when corticosteroids are used ranging from euphoria, insomnia, mood swings, personality changes, and severe depression to frank psychotic manifestations. Also, existing emotional instability or psychotic tendencies may be aggravated by corticosteroids.

Corticosteroids should be used with caution in nonspecific ulcerative colitis if there is a probability of impending perforation, abscess or other pyogenic infection; diverticulitis; fresh intestinal anastomoses; active or latent peptic ulcer, renal insufficiency; hypertension; osteoporosis; or myasthenia gravis.

Because complications of treatment with glucocorticoids are dependent on the size of the dose and the duration of treatment, a risk/benefit decision must be made in each individual case as to dose and duration of treatment and as to whether daily or intermittent therapy should be used.

Kaposi's sarcoma has been reported to occur in patients receiving corticosteroid therapy. Discontinuation of corticosteroids may result in clinical remission.

Carcinogenesis, mutagenesis, impairment of fertility: There is no evidence that corticosteroids are carcinogenic, mutagenic, or impair fertility.

Lactation: Corticosteroids are excreted in breast milk.

Drug Interactions: The pharmacokinetic interactions listed below are potentially clinically important. Mutual inhibition of metabolism occurs with concurrent use of cyclosporin and methylprednisolone, therefore, it is possible that adverse events associated with the individual use of either drug may be more apt to occur. Convulsions have been reported with concurrent use of methylprednisolone and cyclosporin. Drugs that induce hepatic enzymes such as phenobarbital, phenytoin and rifampin may increase the clearance of methylprednisolone and may require increase in methylprednisolone dose to achieve desired response. Drugs such as troleandomycin and ketoconazole may inhibit the metabolism of methylprednisolone and thus decrease its clearance. Therefore the dose of methylprednisolone should be titrated to avoid steroid toxicity. Methylprednisolone may increase the clearance of chronic high dose ASA. This could lead to a decrease in salicylate serum levels or increase the risk of salicylate toxicity when methylprednisolone is withdrawn. ASA should be used cautiously in conjunction with corticosteroids in patients suffering from hypoprothrombinemia. The effect of methylprednisolone on oral anticoagulants is variable. There are reports of enhanced as well as diminished effects of anticoagulant when given concurrently with corticosteroids. Therefore coagulation indices should be monitored to maintain the desired anticoagulant effect.

ADVERSE EFFECTS: Note: The following are typical for all systemic corticosteroids. Their inclusion in this list does not necessarily indicate that the specific event has been observed with this particular formulation.

Fluid and electrolyte disturbances: sodium retention; fluid retention; congestive heart failure in susceptible patients; potassium loss, hypokalemic alkalosis; hypertension.
Musculoskeletal: muscle weakness; steroid myopathy; osteoporosis; vertebral compression fractures; aseptic necrosis; pathologic fractures; loss of muscle mass; tendon rupture—particularly of the Achilles tendon.
Gastrointestinal: peptic ulceration with possible perforation and hemorrhage; gastric hemorrhage; pancreatitis; esophagitis; perforation of the bowel.
Dermatologic: impaired wound healing; thin fragile skin; petechiae and ecchymoses; facial erythema; may suppress reactions to skin tests; increased sweating.
Metabolic: negative nitrogen balance due to protein catabolism.
Neurological: increased intracranial pressure; pseudotumor cerebri; psychic derangements; seizures.
Endocrine: menstrual irregularities; development of cushingoid state; suppression of pituitary/adrenal axis; decreased carbohydrate tolerance; manifestations of latent diabetes mellitus; increased requirements for insulin or oral hypoglycemic agents in diabetes; suppression of growth in children.
Ophthalmic: posterior subcapsular cataracts; increased intraocular pressure; exophthalmos; glaucoma.
Immune System: masking of infections; latent infections becoming active; opportunistic infections; hypersensitivity reactions including anaphylaxis; may suppress reactions to skin tests.

Increases in ALT, AST and alkaline phosphatase have been observed following corticosteroid treatment. These changes are usually small, not associated with any clinical syndrome and are reversible upon discontinuation.

OVERDOSE:
No data supplied by the manufacturer.

For management of a suspected drug overdose, CPhA recommends that you contact your **regional Poison Control Centre**. See the *CPS* Directory section for a list of Poison Control Centres.

DOSAGE: The initial dosage of methylprednisolone may vary from 4 to 48 mg of methylprednisolone/day depending on the specific disease entity being treated. In situations of less severity, lower doses will generally suffice while in selected patients higher initial doses may be required. Clinical situations in which high dose therapy may be indicated include multiple sclerosis (200 mg/day), cerebral edema (200 to 1000 mg/day), and organ transplantation (up to 7 mg/kg/day). If after a reasonable period of time there is a lack of satisfactory clinical response, methylprednisolone should be discontinued and the patient transferred to other appropriate therapy. If after long-term therapy the drug is to be stopped, it is recommended that it be withdrawn gradually rather than abruptly.

After a favorable response is noted, the proper maintenance dosage should be determined by decreasing the initial drug dosage in small decrements at appropriate time intervals until the lowest dosage which will maintain an adequate clinical response is reached. It should be kept in mind that constant monitoring is needed in regard to drug dosage. Included in the situations which may make dosage adjustments necessary are changes in clinical status secondary to remissions or exacerbations in the disease process, the patient's individual drug responsiveness, and the effect of patient exposure to stressful situations not directly related to the disease entity under treatment; in this latter situation it may be necessary to increase the dosage of methylprednisolone for a period of time consistent with the patient's condition.

It should be emphasized that dosage requirements are variable and must be individualized on the basis of the disease under treatment and the response of the patient.

ADT Alternate Day Therapy: Alternate day therapy is a corticosteroid dosing regimen in which twice the usual daily dose of corticosteroid is administered every other morning. The purpose of this mode of therapy is to provide a patient requiring long-term, pharmacologic dose treatment with the beneficial effects of corticoids while minimizing certain undesirable effects, including pituitary-adrenal suppression, the cushingoid state, corticoid withdrawal symptoms, and growth suppression in children.

SUPPLIED: 4 mg: Each white, elliptical, cross-scored tablet, engraved "Medrol 4", contains: methylprednisolone 4 mg. Nonmedicinal ingredients: calcium stearate, cornstarch, lactose, mineral oil and sucrose. Gluten-free. Bottles of 100.
16 mg: Each white, elliptical, cross-scored tablet, engraved "Medrol 16", contains: methylprednisolone 16 mg. Nonmedicinal ingredients: calcium stearate, cornstarch, lactose, mineral oil and sucrose. Gluten-free. Bottles of 100.

(Shown in Product Identification Section)

Medrol® Acne Lotion 🅿

methylprednisolone acetate—aluminum chlorhydroxide—sulfur

Acne Therapy

Pfizer

PHARMACOLOGY: Medrol Acne Lotion has an anti-inflammatory action by virtue of its content of methylprednisolone, an astringent and antiperspirant action by virtue of its content of aluminum chlorhydroxide and a keratolytic effect by virtue of its sulfur content. Sulfur has also demonstrated some antibacterial activity at the concentration used.

INDICATIONS: For the control of acne vulgaris in the adolescent and young adult. Also useful in some cases of acne rosacea and seborrheic dermatitis.

CONTRAINDICATIONS: In tuberculosis of the skin and in the presence of skin viral diseases such as herpes simplex, vaccinia and varicella. Also contraindicated in patients known to be sensitive to any ingredients in this lotion.

WARNINGS: *Pregnancy:* Corticosteroids are generally teratogenic in laboratory animals when administered systemically at relatively low dosage levels. The more potent corticosteroids have been shown to be teratogenic after dermal application in laboratory animals. There are no adequate and well-controlled studies in pregnant women on teratogenic effects from topically applied corticosteroids. Therefore, topical corticosteroids should be used during pregnancy only if the potential benefit justifies the potential risk to the fetus. Drugs of this class should not be used extensively on pregnant patients, in large amounts, or for prolonged periods of time.

PRECAUTIONS: General: If irritation develops, topical corticosteroids should be discontinued and appropriate therapy instituted.

In the presence of dermatological infections, the use of an appropriate antifungal or antibacterial agent should be instituted. If a favorable response does not occur promptly, the corticosteroid should be discontinued until the infection has been adequately controlled.

Avoid contact with the eyes. If there are signs of irritation or sensitivity, application should be discontinued. The patient should be advised to inform subsequent physicians of the prior use of corticosteroids.

Systemic absorption of topical corticosteroids has produced reversible hypothalamic-pituitary-adrenal (HPA) axis suppression, manifestations of Cushing's syndrome, hyperglycemia, and glucosuria in some patients. Conditions which augment systemic absorption include the application of the more potent steroids, use over large surface areas, prolonged use, and the addition of occlusive dressings. Therefore, patients receiving a large dose of a potent topical steroid applied to a large surface area or under an occlusive dressing should be evaluated periodically for evidence of HPA axis suppression by using the urinary free cortisol and ACTH stimulation tests. If HPA axis suppression is noted, an attempt should be made to withdraw the drug, to reduce the frequency of application, or to substitute a less potent steroid. Recovery of HPA axis function is generally prompt and complete upon discontinuation of the drug. Infrequently, signs and symptoms of steroid withdrawal may occur, requiring supplemental systemic corticosteroids.

Children: Children may absorb proportionally larger amounts of topical corticosteroids than mature patients because children have a larger skin surface area to body weight ratio. This could lead to greater susceptibility to topical corticosteroid-induced HPA axis suppression and Cushing's syndrome.

HPA axis suppression, Cushing's syndrome, and intracranial hypertension have been reported in children receiving topical corticosteroids. Manifestations of adrenal suppression in children include linear growth retardation, delayed weight gain, low plasma cortisol levels, and absence of response to ACTH stimulation. Manifestations of intracranial hypertension include bulging fontanelles, headaches and bilateral papilledema.

Administration of topical corticosteroids to children should be limited to the least amount compatible with an effective therapeutic regimen. Chronic corticosteroid therapy may interfere with the growth and development of children.

Lactation: It is not known whether topical administration of corticosteroids could result in sufficient systemic absorption to produce detectable quantities in breast milk. Systemically administered corticosteroids are secreted into breast milk in quantities not likely to have a deleterious effect on the infant. Nevertheless, caution should be exercised when topical corticosteroids are administered to a nursing woman.

Laboratory Tests: The following tests may be helpful in evaluating the HPA axis suppression: urinary free cortisol test; ACTH stimulation test.

Information to Be Provided to the Patient: Patients using topical corticosteroids should receive the following information and instructions:

1. This medication is to be used as directed by the physician. It is for external use only. Avoid contact with the eyes.
2. Patients should be advised not to use this medication for any disorder other than for which it was prescribed.
3. The treated skin area should not be bandaged or otherwise covered or wrapped as to be occlusive unless directed by the physician.
4. Patients should report any signs of local adverse reactions especially under occlusive dressing.
5. Parents of pediatric patients should be advised not to use tight-fitting diapers or plastic pants on a child being treated in the diaper area, as these garments may constitute occlusive dressings.

ADVERSE EFFECTS: The following local adverse reactions have been reported with topical corticosteroids, but may occur more frequently with the use of occlusive dressings. These reactions are listed in an approximate decreasing order of occurrence: burning, itching, irritation, dryness, folliculitis, hypertrichosis, acneiform eruptions, hypopigmentation, perioral dermatitis, allergic contact dermatitis, maceration of the skin, secondary infection, skin atrophy, striae, and miliaria.

If excessive dryness of the skin occurs, reduce amount and frequency of application of Medrol Acne Lotion. This effect is more commonly seen in patients with fair complexions or sensitive skin. Localized atrophy or striae have been reported with the use of topical corticosteroids particularly when used in the intertriginous areas. The remote possibility of systemic corticosteroid absorption does exist, particularly if extensive areas are treated or treatment is maintained for prolonged periods. It is estimated that 0.18 mg of methylprednisolone acetate would be absorbed daily if the contents of a 30 mL bottle were used over a period of 7 days.

OVERDOSE:
Treatment: No cases have been reported. Excessive applications should be immediately removed with mild soap and water.

Accidental ingestion has not been reported. Should this occur, vomiting should be induced and appropriate measures taken to treat any irritation of the oral mucosa which might occur. The absorption of a single high dose of methylprednisolone should cause no concern.

For management of a suspected drug overdose, CPhA recommends that you contact your **regional Poison Control Centre**. See the *CPS* Directory section for a list of Poison Control Centres.

DOSAGE: The lotion should be applied to all lesions once or twice a day taking care to avoid contact with the eyes. The skin should be washed with a bland soap prior to each application. The frequency of application will vary from person to person depending on his susceptibility to the drying effect of the lotion. To obtain satisfactory results, dryness of the skin should be produced, but not to the point of flaking or peeling.

In patients with very sensitive skin, application every other day may control acne lesions.

SUPPLIED: Each mL contains: methylprednisolone acetate 2.5 mg, aluminum chlorhydroxide complex 100 mg, sulfur 50 mg. Nonmedicinal ingredients: butylparaben, cetyl palmitate, lexemul AR, methylcellulose, methylparaben, perfume oil, polysorbate 80, polysorbate 85, propylene glycol, polyethylene glycol 400 distearate, and purified water. Gluten-free. Plastic squeeze bottles of 75 mL.

Medroxyprogesterone Acetate Injectable Suspension USP 🅿

medroxyprogesterone acetate

Progestogen

Sandoz

SUPPLIED: Each mL of sterile injectable suspension contains: medroxyprogesterone acetate 150 mg. Nonmedicinal ingredients: hydrochloric acid and/or sodium hydroxide to adjust pH, methylparaben and propylparaben (as preservatives), polyethylene glycol 3350, polysorbate 80, sodium chloride and water for injection. Vials of 1 mL, boxes of 1. Protect from freezing. Store between 15 and 30°C. Shake well before using.

Mefenamic Acid 🅿

Nonsteroidal Anti-inflammatory Agent

CPhA Monograph

Date of Preparation: October 2007

This monograph has been compiled by CPhA and reviewed by experts. It may contain information different from that found in Health Canada-approved Product Monographs. The reader is referred to the *CPS* Editorial Policy for more information.

SUMMARY PRODUCT INFORMATION:

Route of Administration[a]	Dosage Form[a]	Strength[a]
Oral	Capsule	250 mg

[a] For specific product information consult Health Canada's Drug Product Database http://www.hc-sc.gc.ca/dhp-mps/prodpharma/databasdon/index_e.html.

INDICATIONS AND CLINICAL USE: Mefenamic acid is indicated for:

- short-term use (7 days or less) in the relief of mild to moderate pain in conditions such as primary dysmenorrhea, muscular aches and pains, dental pain and headaches.

It has also been used for postoperative pain and pain following insertion of an intrauterine contraceptive device.

Mefenamic acid has been used for fever, especially in children, but should not routinely be used as an antipyretic because of the risk of adverse effects.

Pediatrics: The safety and efficacy of mefenamic acid in children less than 14 years of age has not been established.

CONTRAINDICATIONS:

- Patients who are hypersensitive to mefenamic acid, acetylsalicylic acid (ASA) or other nonsteroidal anti-inflammatory drugs (NSAIDs) or to any ingredient in the formulation or component of the container. Mefenamic acid should not be used in patients with the complete or partial syndrome of ASA-intolerance (rhinosinusitis, urticaria/angioedema, nasal polyps, asthma) in whom asthma, anaphylaxis, urticaria/angioedema, rhinitis or other allergic manifestations are precipitated by ASA or other NSAIDs. As well, patients with the above conditions are at risk even if they have taken NSAIDs in the past without adverse events.
- Patients experiencing perioperative pain associated with coronary artery bypass graft (CABG).
- Mefenamic acid should not be used in patients with pre-existing renal disease.
- It is also contraindicated in patients with active ulceration or chronic inflammation of the GI tract.

WARNINGS AND PRECAUTIONS:

Serious Warnings and Precautions

- NSAIDs, including mefenamic acid, may increase the risk of serious gastrointestinal (GI) events such as ulceration, bleeding and perforation as well as GI irritation. These events may occur without prior symptoms.
- NSAIDs are associated with an increased risk of cardiovascular thrombotic events such as stroke, myocardial infarction (MI) and new onset or worsening of pre-existing hypertension.

Patients considered to be at high risk for either of these types of adverse events should be given an alternate therapy rather than an NSAID. If NSAIDs are used they should be given for the shortest time possible at the lowest effective dose to reduce the risk of GI or cardiovascular events.

General: Patients should be counseled to inform their health care providers immediately of symptoms of serious adverse events associated with mefenamic acid therapy such as GI ulceration and bleeding, changes in vision, symptoms of heart or renal failure, bruising and nongastrointestinal bleeding, hypersensitivity and severe headache. Like other NSAIDs, mefenamic acid may mask fever.

Cardiovascular: See Serious Warnings and Precautions. Pre-existing cardiovascular disease or cardiac risk factors may increase the risk of cardiovascular events in patients taking NSAIDs including mefenamic acid. Individual cardiovascular risk factors must be considered before suggesting any NSAID. Patients should be aware of the signs and symptoms of serious cardiovascular events such as chest pain, weakness, dyspnea and slurred speech.

Use with caution in patients with hypertension, heart failure or fluid retention. Monitor blood pressure.

Dermatologic: Serious adverse events such as toxic epidermal necrolysis (TEN), Stevens-Johnson syndrome (SJS) and exfoliative dermatitis have all been reported in patients treated with NSAIDs. Even patients without prior exposure to NSAIDs may experience anaphylactoid reactions. See Contraindications. Advise patients to consult their clinician if they experience skin rash and/or blisters.

Ear/Nose/Throat: Ototoxicity including tinnitus and hearing loss has been reported with all NSAIDs.

Gastrointestinal: See Serious Warnings and Precautions. Use with caution in elderly or debilitated patients and in those with a history of GI disease such as bleeding or ulcers. NSAIDs should also be used with caution in patients receiving ASA or other antiplatelet agents, anticoagulants, corticosteroids, SSRIs or in those who smoke, consume alcohol or are infected with *H. pylori*.

Mefenamic acid should be given under close medical supervision to patients with a history of ulcer of the upper GI tract or inflammatory disease of the GI tract such as ulcerative colitis or Crohn's disease. In these cases the health care provider must weigh the benefits of treatment against the potential adverse events.

Hematologic: NSAIDs should be used cautiously in anemic patients. Those with coagulopathies, those receiving anticoagulants and those at risk of blood dyscrasias should use mefenamic acid with caution because hematologic side effects may be more likely to occur.

Hepatic/Biliary/Pancreatic: Use mefenamic acid with caution in patients with decreased hepatic function. Monitor patients with abnormal LFT values. As with other NSAIDs, borderline elevations of one or more liver enzyme tests (AST, ALT, ALP) may occur in up to 15% of patients. These abnormalities may progress, remain unchanged, and/or be transient with continued therapy. Probably the most sensitive indicator of NSAID-induced hepatic dysfunction is serum ALT. Discontinue the drug if signs or symptoms of liver disease develop or if the patient presents with systemic manifestations such as rash or eosinophilia.

Immune: Cross-sensitivity: Patients sensitive to any NSAIDs, including ASA may be sensitive to mefenamic acid.

ASA-intolerance: As with nonsteroidal anti-inflammatory drugs in general, some patients may experience urticaria upon exposure to mefenamic acid. Patients with partial or complete syndrome of ASA-intolerance should not be given mefenamic acid (see Contraindications).

Advise patients to consult their clinician and discontinue therapy if skin rash and blisters, fever or other signs of hypersensitivity reaction occur.

Perioperative Considerations: Mefenamic acid should be held for 4 to 7 days prior to surgical procedures since it is a reversible inhibitor of platelet aggregation. Patients are usually encouraged to discontinue NSAIDs two weeks before any surgery where bleeding could be catastrophic e.g., neurosurgery.

Renal: Patients with dehydration or impaired renal function may be at increased risk of experiencing worsening of renal toxicity. Monitor renal function and rehydrate patients before initiating therapy. Mefenamic acid should not be used in patients with advanced renal disease.

Acute renal failure which is usually reversible has been reported with the use of NSAIDs. In many cases onset of renal failure occurs within two days to two weeks of initiating therapy. Renal failure has occurred in the absence of pre-existing impairment. Patients at greatest risk are those with renal and hepatic impairment, heart failure, diabetes mellitus, hypovolemia, advanced age, concurrent use of other nephrotoxic drugs or pyelonephritis. Renal dysfunction with NSAIDs is likely related to inhibition of prostaglandin synthesis and renin-induced vasoconstriction.

Patients with extracellular fluid depletion such as those on diuretics may develop overt renal decompensation as renal prostaglandins may be playing a compensatory role in maintenance of renal perfusion. NSAIDs should also be given cautiously to patients treated with ACE inhibitors or angiotensin II receptor antagonists. These patients should be advised to report any unexpected edema or weight gain to their health care providers.

Respiratory: See Contraindications. Use mefenamic acid with caution in patients with asthma.

Sensitivity/Resistance: Patients sensitive to any one of the nonsteroidal anti-inflammatory drugs may be sensitive to any of the other drugs of this class.

Special Populations: Pregnant Women: Congenital malformations, preterm delivery and low birth weight were not associated with the use of NSAIDs during pregnancy. However, a positive association has been found between the use of NSAIDs and spontaneous abortion. Animal models have revealed that prostaglandin synthesis inhibitors such as NSAIDs can block blastocyste implantation so their use is not recommended in women attempting to conceive.

Avoid in the third trimester of pregnancy as mefenamic acid may cause premature closure of the ductus arteriosus. Persistent pulmonary hypertension of the newborn may also occur when NSAIDs are used close to delivery.

Through their antiprostaglandin effects NSAIDs can prolong gestation, cause excessive uterine bleeding at delivery, impair renal function and cause oligohydramnios.

Nursing Women: There is little experience with the use of mefenamic acid during breastfeeding however it is distributed into milk in small amounts. Because of the risk of potential toxicity, especially when nursing a newborn or preterm infant, some experts recommend that other agents may be preferred if possible. Even other NSAIDs that have been used more widely in breastfeeding women such as ibuprofen are considered by some experts to be safer alternatives. However, if the mother requires mefenamic acid, it is not considered a reason to stop breastfeeding.

Geriatrics: Elderly, frail or debilitated patients are most susceptible to the adverse effects associated with nonsteroidal anti-inflammatory drugs; the incidence of these adverse effects increases with the dose and duration of treatment. In addition these patients are at increased risk of lower esophageal ulceration and bleeding. Most reports of fatal GI events are in this population, especially those with pre-existing cardiovascular disease. Even when using low doses, older individuals are at increased risk of adverse effects of NSAIDs especially CNS effects, renal toxicity and GI ulceration.

ADVERSE REACTIONS: Adverse Drug Reactions Overview: The most common adverse reactions encountered with NSAIDs are gastrointestinal, of which gastric or duodenal ulcer, with or without bleeding, is the most severe. Fatalities have occurred, particularly in the elderly. The more common adverse reactions for mefenamic acid are listed in Table 1.

More Common Adverse Drug Reactions: See Table 1.

Table 1: Mefenamic Acid

More Common Adverse Drug Reactions (≥ 1%)

Body System	Effect
Central nervous system	Headache, dizziness (3–9%), nervousness
Dermatologic	Itching, rash
Endocrine and metabolism	Fluid retention
Gastrointestinal (1–10%)	Abdominal cramps/distress/pain, constipation, diarrhea, dyspepsia, flatulence, gastritis, gastric/duodenal ulcer with bleeding or perforation, heartburn, indigestion, nausea, vomiting
Hematologic	Bleeding (1–10%)
Hepatic/Biliary/Pancreatic	Elevated LFTs (1–10%)
Otic	Tinnitus (1–10%)

Less Common Adverse Drug Reactions (<1%): Cardiovascular: hypertension, heart failure, arrhythmia, tachycardia.

Central Nervous System: confusion, depression, drowsiness, insomnia, hallucinations, aseptic meningitis.

Allergic/Dermatologic: urticaria, Stevens-Johnson syndrome, angioedema, erythema multiforme, toxic epidermal necrolysis.

Ear/Nose/Throat: decreased hearing, epistaxis.

Endocrine and Metabolism: polydipsia, hot flashes.

Gastrointestinal: stomatitis.

Genitourinary: cystitis, polyuria. Renal papillary necrosis and other renal medullary changes have been reported in patients receiving long-term mefenamic acid therapy.

Hematologic: agranulocytosis, anemia, hemolytic anemia, leukopenia, bone marrow suppression, thrombocytopenia.

Hepatic/Biliary/Pancreatic: hepatitis.

Immune: acute anaphylaxis, acute respiratory distress, angioedema and fever have been reported in patients using NSAIDs.

Neurologic: peripheral neuropathy.

Ophthalmologic: blurred vision, toxic amblyopia, conjunctivitis, dry eyes.

Renal: acute renal failure. Some NSAIDs are associated with persistent urinary symptoms (e.g., bladder pain, dysuria, urinary frequency), hematuria, interstitial nephritis or cystitis. The initiation of these symptoms may occur at any time after the initiation of therapy with a nonsteroidal anti-inflammatory drug. Should urinary symptoms occur, in the absence of an alternative explanation, treatment with mefenamic acid should be stopped to ascertain if symptoms disappear. This should be done before urologic investigations or treatments are considered.

Respiratory: dyspnea, allergic rhinitis.

DRUG INTERACTIONS: Overview: Mefenamic acid is an inhibitor of CYP2C9. As such, it may increase the effects of CYP2C9 substrates (e.g., fluoxetine, glipizide, phenytoin). It is also a substrate of CYP2C9.

Drug-Drug Interactions: See Table 2.

Table 2: Mefenamic Acid

Drug-Drug Interactions

Interacting Drug	Effect	Clinical Comment
ACE inhibitors	Mefenamic acid may diminish the antihypertensive effects of ACEIs. Combination of ACEIs, diuretics and mefenamic acid might have an increased risk for acute renal failure and hyperkalemia.	Monitor blood pressure, renal function and serum potassium.
Anticoagulants and antiplatelet medications	Numerous studies have shown that the concomitant use of NSAIDs and anticoagulants increases the risk of serious GI adverse events, such as bleeding and ulceration.	Concurrent use of mefenamic acid and warfarin requires close monitoring of the INR. Even with therapeutic INR monitoring, increased bleeding may occur.
Corticosteroids	Some studies have shown that the concomitant use of corticosteroids and NSAIDs can increase the risk of serious GI adverse events, such as ulceration and bleeding. Elderly patients are at greater risk.	Monitor for signs and symptoms of toxicities.
Cyclosporine	Concomitant administration of mefenamic acid and cyclosporine may increase the nephrotoxic effects of cyclosporine. This interaction may be related to inhibition of the renal prostaglandin, prostacyclin, synthesis.	Use concomitantly with caution and monitor renal function and cyclosporine levels.
Digoxin	Possible increased digoxin levels.	Use with caution and monitor digoxin levels.
Diuretics	Clinical studies as well as post-marketing surveillance have shown that NSAIDs can reduce the clinical effects of diuretics. Potassium-sparing diuretics can increase the risk of hyperkalemia.	Use concomitantly with caution and monitor effectiveness, renal function and serum potassium.
Ethanol	Ethanol used with mefenamic acid may increase the risk of gastric mucosal irritation.	Counsel patients to avoid using ethanol while taking mefenamic acid if possible.
Lithium	Mefenamic acid can increase serum lithium concentrations.	Monitoring lithium levels is advisable when starting or stopping mefenamic acid.
Methotrexate	NSAIDs have been reported to decrease the tubular secretion of methotrexate and potentiate the toxicity.	Avoid the concomitant use of high dose methotrexate; in the case of low dose weekly methotrexate use the combination with caution and monitor for signs and symptoms of toxicity.
NSAIDs	The use of mefenamic acid in addition to any other NSAID is not recommended because of the absence of any evidence demonstrating additive effects and the potential for additive adverse events. Also, some NSAIDs may interfere with the antiplatelet effects of low dose ASA, possibly by competing with ASA for access to the active site of cyclooxygenase-1. The concurrent use of two NSAIDs increases the risk of serious GI adverse events, such as bleeding and ulceration.	Avoid concurrent use of mefenamic acid with other NSAIDs, including ASA if possible.
Potassium supplements/ potassium-sparing diuretics	Potential for hyperkalemia, especially in patients with renal dysfunction.	Monitor serum potassium especially in susceptible individuals.
Quinolones	The concomitant use of quinolones and NSAIDs may increase the risk of CNS stimulation and seizure activity.	Use with caution, especially in susceptible individuals.
SSRIs	SSRIs increase the risk of GI bleeding and this effect can be potentiated by concomitant use of NSAIDs. The mechanism is likely related to additive effects on platelet inhibition.	Monitor patients for increased signs of bleeding.

Drug-Herb Interactions: Many herbal medications have antiplatelet activity that may add to that of mefenamic acid, e.g., dong quai, evening primrose, feverfew, garlic, ginkgo biloba, red clover, ginseng.

Drug-Laboratory Interactions: NSAIDs may cause GI bleeding, which may produce positive fecal hemoccult test results in some individuals and therefore interfere with screening for colorectal cancer. When screening for occult fecal blood loss, nonsteroidal anti-inflammatory drugs may need to be withheld for two to four days prior to testing, as a positive fecal hemoccult test may be attributable to nonsteroidal anti-inflammatory drug therapy.

Mefenamic acid decreases platelet aggregation and may prolong bleeding time. The effect of mefenamic acid on bleeding time should be taken into account when the test is performed.

Use of mefenamic acid may cause a false-positive urinary bilirubin.

DOSAGE AND ADMINISTRATION: **Dosing Considerations:** Safety and efficacy of mefenamic acid in children less than 14 years of age has not been established.

For all indications the lowest effective dose of mefenamic acid should be used for the shortest time necessary in keeping with patient treatment goals.

Mefenamic acid should always be administered with food or immediately after meals. Administration with antacids or H_2-receptor antagonists (e.g., ranitidine) may help with GI intolerance associated with NSAIDs, but will not prevent serious GI adverse events.

Recommended Dose and Dosage Adjustment: Adults: See Table 3.

Table 3: Mefenamic Acid

Dose in Adult Patients

Indication	Route	Initial Dose	Usual Dose	Duration of Treatment	Clinical Comment
Primary dysmenorrhea	Oral	500 mg loading dose	250 mg Q6H	Mefenamic acid should be started immediately at the onset of menses and continued on a regular schedule for 48 to 72 hours.	Mefenamic acid should not be taken prn for primary dysmenorrhea. It is not more effective if started premenstrually.
Pain	Oral	500 mg loading dose	250 mg Q6H prn	1 week	

Dose in Adult Patients with Renal Impairment: No dosage adjustment is required for patients with renal dysfunction or failure. While there does not appear to be a significant prolongation of the drug's half-life, as with any other nonsteroidal anti-inflammatory drug, mefenamic acid should not be used in patients with advanced renal disease.

Dosage in Dialysis: Mefenamic acid does not appear to be dialyzable.

Hepatic Impairment: Use with caution in patients with decreased hepatic function.

Missed Dose: Patients should be instructed to take a missed dose as soon as they remember, and not to double doses or exceed their daily recommended dose.

Administration: Mefenamic acid capsules should be swallowed whole, not crushed or chewed. The drug should be administered with food or meals.

OVERDOSAGE:

For management of a suspected drug overdose, CPhA recommends that you contact your **regional Poison Control Centre**. See the *CPS* Directory section for a list of Poison Control Centres.

ACTION AND CLINICAL PHARMACOLOGY: Mechanism of Action: Mefenamic acid has similar pharmacology to that of other prototypical NSAIDs. The drug inhibits prostaglandin synthesis by decreasing activity of the enzyme cyclooxygenase. It exhibits analgesic, anti-inflammatory and antipyretic activity. The fenemates group of NSAIDs to which mefenamic acid belongs also appear to bind to prostaglandin receptors. This may affect prostaglandins that have already been formed.

Pharmacokinetics: Adults: Absorption: Mefenamic acid is rapidly absorbed from the GI tract. The manufacturer states that there is no evidence of drug accumulation after multiple doses.

Distribution: Mefenamic acid is greater than 90% protein bound. The volume of distribution is 1.06 L/kg.

Metabolism: Mefenamic acid is hepatically metabolized by CYP2C9. The inactive metabolites are 3-hydroxymethyl mefenamic acid and 3-carboxymefenamic acid.

Excretion: The half-life of mefenamic acid is 2 to 3.5 hours. Approximately 50% of a dose is excreted into urine and 20% through the feces.

Mefloquine

Antimalarial

CPhA Monograph

Date of Preparation: May 2006

This monograph has been compiled by CPhA and reviewed by experts. It may contain information different from that found in Health Canada-approved Product Monographs. The reader is referred to the *CPS* Editorial Policy for more information.

SUMMARY PRODUCT INFORMATION:

Route of Administration	Dosage Form	Strength
Oral	Tablet	mefloquine base 250 mg

INDICATIONS AND CLINICAL USE: Mefloquine is indicated for:

- prevention of infection with the malarial parasites *P. falciparum* and *P. vivax*, including chloroquine-resistant strains of *P. falciparum*. Health Canada recommends that mefloquine be used primarily for prophylaxis and not routinely as treatment due to its adverse effect profile.
- treatment of mild to moderate acute malaria caused by susceptible strains of *P. falciparum* including chloroquine-resistant strains and *P. vivax*.

Due to the emergence of mefloquine resistance, mefloquine is not the drug of first choice for malaria chemoprophylaxis in all regions. Up-to-date geographic recommendations for malarial chemoprophylaxis should be consulted before prescribing mefloquine or any other antimalarial.

Patients with life-threatening or overwhelming infections due to *P. falciparum* and those unable to take oral medications should receive intravenous antimalarial agents (e.g., quinine) rather than mefloquine.

CONTRAINDICATIONS:

- Patients who are hypersensitive to mefloquine or to any ingredient in the formulation.
- Patients who are hypersensitive to structurally related compounds (e.g., quinine, quinidine).
- Mefloquine should not be used as prophylaxis for malaria in patients with seizure disorders, generalized anxiety disorders, active depression, recent history of depressive episodes, psychosis or schizophrenia.

WARNINGS AND PRECAUTIONS:

Serious Warnings and Precautions

- Patients with life-threatening or overwhelming infections due to *P. falciparum* should receive intravenous antimalarial agents rather than mefloquine.
- Mefloquine has been associated with seizures. Avoid prophylactic use in patients with a history of seizures.
- Mefloquine is associated with serious psychiatric symptoms including anxiety, depression, suicidal ideation, hallucinations, paranoia and psychosis. For this reason, mefloquine should not be used for prophylaxis of malaria in patients with generalized anxiety disorder, active depression, a recent history of depressive episodes, psychosis or schizophrenia. If psychiatric symptoms emerge during treatment with mefloquine, the drug should be discontinued and an alternative agent used.
- Mefloquine is a myocardial depressant and should be used with caution in patients with abnormal cardiac conduction.
- Concomitant administration of mefloquine with quinine or quinidine has been associated with electrocardiographic abnormalities and increased risk of seizures. For this reason concomitant administration of mefloquine and either quinine or quinidine should be avoided (see Drug Interactions, Drug-Drug Interactions).
- Mefloquine should be avoided during pregnancy unless there is a compelling need to use the drug (see Warnings and Precautions, Special Populations, Pregnant Women).
- Caution is advised when dosing patients with renal or hepatic insufficiency. Elimination of mefloquine may be prolonged, thereby resulting in high plasma mefloquine levels.
- Patients treated with mefloquine in acute *P. vivax* malaria are at high risk of clinical relapse because mefloquine does not eliminate parasites in hepatocytes. To prevent clinical relapse, patients infected with *P. vivax* should subsequently be treated with an 8-aminoquinoline (e.g., primaquine—exclude G-6-PD deficiency prior to use) (see Dosage and Administration)
- Long-term mefloquine use has been associated with ocular lesions in animals. Periodic eye examinations are recommended if mefloquine is used long-term.

Special Populations: Pregnant Women: Pregnancy Category C. Mefloquine readily crosses the placenta. Mefloquine is teratogenic in rats and mice at a dose of 100 mg/kg/day and in rabbits at a dose of 80 mg/kg/day. It has been used to treat *P. falciparum* malaria in pregnant women during the first, second and third trimesters of pregnancy. No increase in the rate of congenital abnormalities and no effects on physical and neurological development up to the age of 12 months have been reported. An increased incidence of stillbirth in women treated with mefloquine cannot be ruled out. Mefloquine is not associated with an increased incidence of teratogenic effects when given after the 1st trimester. If travel to regions where chloroquine-resistant malaria is endemic cannot be avoided, the decision to use mefloquine during pregnancy should be based on whether the expected benefits of therapy justify the potential risk to the exposed fetus. Several studies in pregnant women have revealed no increase in the rate of fetal malformations.

Women of childbearing potential should be warned about the potential teratogenic properties of mefloquine (see Warnings and Precautions) and advised to practise contraception especially during and for 3 months after taking the last dose of mefloquine because of its long half-life. However, in the event that pregnancy occurs during prophylaxis with mefloquine, termination of pregnancy is not automatically indicated. Specialist consultation is recommended.

Nursing Women: Mefloquine is secreted in human breast milk, however, the amount is not considered to be harmful to a nursing infant. WHO considers it to be safe in breastfeeding. Maternal use of mefloquine does not protect the nursing infant from malaria.

Geriatrics: Potentiation of postural hypotension and dizziness may occur with mefloquine use. Caution is advised.

Occupational Hazards: WHO advises against the use of mefloquine chemoprophylaxis in individuals who require a high degree of manual dexterity, coordination and spatial discrimination for their occupations (e.g., pilots). However, a small study in trainee pilots using a flight simulator revealed no significant performance deficit. Some sleep disturbance and decreased concentration were noted.

ADVERSE REACTIONS: More Common Adverse Drug Reactions: See Table 1.

Table 1: Mefloquine

More Common Adverse Drug Reactions (≥1%)

Body System	Effect	Clinical Comment
Central Nervous System	Dizziness (dose-related), headache, light-headedness, vertigo	Usually mild and decreases with continued use
Dermatologic	Maculopapular rash, pruritus	
Gastrointestinal	Dose-related: Abdominal discomfort, nausea and vomiting (~3%) Diarrhea (transient)	Administer with food or in divided doses to minimize side effects. May subside with continued use (see Dosage and Administration).

Less Common Adverse Drug Reactions (<1%): Cardiovascular: A-V block, sinus bradycardia (may occur 4-7 days after mefloquine administration, may last 3-4 days), chest pain (rare), circulatory disturbances (flushing, hypertension, hypotension, syncope), extrasystole, irregular pulse, tachycardia, QTc prolongation.

Central Nervous System (neuropsychiatric): Incidence of serious neuropsychiatry events with prophylactic doses has been documented as 1:10 600. Incidence of seizures and psychosis with treatment doses has been documented as 1:100 to 1:1700.

Abnormal dreams, aggression, agitation and restlessness, anxiety, confusion, depression, emotional problems, fatigue, fever, hallucinations, headache, insomnia, mood changes, panic attacks, seizures, sensory and motor neuropathy (including paresthesias, tremor and ataxia), psychotic or paranoid reactions, suicidal ideation, syncope, tinnitus, vestibular disorders.

Dermatologic: erythema multiforme, exanthema, hair loss, pruritus, sweating, Stevens-Johnson syndrome, urticaria.

Endocrine: hypoglycemia, increased insulin levels, abnormal thyroid function tests.

Gastrointestinal: abdominal pain, loss of appetite.

Hematologic: agranulocytosis, aplastic anemia, hemolytic anemia, leukocytosis, thrombocytopenia.

Musculoskeletal: arthralgia, cramps, muscle weakness, myalgia.

Ophthalmologic: visual disturbances.

DRUG INTERACTIONS:

Serious Drug Interactions

- Administration of the antimalarial agent halofantrine after administration of mefloquine has been associated with prolongation of the QTc interval. Halofantrine should not be administered concomitantly with or consecutive to mefloquine. Data on the administration of mefloquine after halofantrine are not available. Halofantrine is currently not available in Canada.
- Cardiac arrest has been reported in association with concomitant use of propranolol and mefloquine.

Drug-Drug Interactions: See Table 2.

Table 2: Mefloquine

Drug-Drug Interactions

Interacting Drug	Effect	Clinical Comment
Alcohol	Combined use may precipitate neuropsychiatric events. See Less Common Adverse Drug Reactions (<1%).	Avoid concurrent use.

(cont'd)

Table 2: Mefloquine *(cont'd)*

Drug-Drug Interactions

Interacting Drug	Effect	Clinical Comment
Antiepileptics (e.g., carbamazepine)	May decrease plasma concentrations of the epileptic drug. Postulated mechanism is competitive hepatic metabolism.	Monitor blood levels of the antiepileptic before and after mefloquine introduction and adjust dose as necessary. Monitor for decreased therapeutic effects of antiepileptic drug.
Beta-blockers	ECG abnormalities and cardiac arrest	Caution and close monitoring of ECG abnormalities is advised when used in combination. One case report of cardiac arrest in a patient receiving a single prophylactic dose of mefloquine. Avoid concurrent use of propranolol and mefloquine.
Chloroquine, quinine, quinidine	ECG abnormalities and increased risk of convulsions	If these agents are used for initial treatment of acute malaria, introduction of mefloquine should be delayed by at least 12 hours after the last dose.
Drugs that alter cardiac conduction (e.g., beta blockers, calcium channel blockers, antihistamines, tricyclic antidepressants, phenothiazines)	Possible prolongation of QTc interval	There are no conclusive data to establish whether concurrent use will result in cardiac conduction abnormalities. Use with caution.
Ketoconazole	May increase plasma mefloquine concentrations by CYP3A4 inhibition.	Monitor for adverse effects of mefloquine after ketoconazole introduction. May require dose adjustment.
Metoclopramide	May increase plasma concentration of mefloquine. Proposed mechanism is increased rate of mefloquine absorption from the small intestine due to accelerated gastric emptying.	Monitor for adverse effects of mefloquine before and after metoclopramide introduction. May require dose adjustment.
Oral live typhoid vaccine	Possible attenuated effect of the vaccine	Vaccinations with live attenuated bacteria should be completed at least 3 days before the first dose of mefloquine.
Phenothiazines	Increased plasma concentrations of phenothiazines	Monitor for pharmacologic and adverse effects of phenothiazines before and after mefloquine introduction and adjust dose as necessary.
Rifampin	Decreased plasma concentrations of mefloquine secondary to induction of CYP3A4 by rifampin	Avoid concurrent use of rifampin and mefloquine to optimize therapeutic efficacy of mefloquine and prevent risk of resistance.

Drug-Food Interactions: Bioavailability of mefloquine increases by 40% when taken with food.

DOSAGE AND ADMINISTRATION: Recommended Dose and Dosage Adjustment: Adults: See Table 3.
Pediatrics: See Table 4.
Dosage in Dialysis: Neither mefloquine or its major carboxylic metabolite are removed by hemodialysis, thus no dose adjustments are indicated.
Hepatic Impairment: There are no specific recommendations for dose adjustments in patients with hepatic dysfunction. Half-life may be prolonged and plasma levels increased.
Missed Dose: Take as soon as the omission is recognized. Do not take a double dose.

OVERDOSAGE:
Signs and Symptoms: In overdose, the adverse events of mefloquine are more pronounced. The drug has a long half-life so adverse reactions due to overdose may persist for several weeks after administration. Along with neuropsychiatric events reported in cases of mefloquine overdoses, QTc prolongation has also been reported.
Recommended Management: It is recommended that a poison control centre be contacted to obtain expert advice on the management of mefloquine overdose.

General management of mefloquine overdose includes supportive care. Closely observe vital signs especially for hypotension and bradycardia. Monitor cardiac function, i.e. ideally by continuous rhythm monitoring or by serial electrocardiographs. Monitor neuropsychiatric status. For large overdoses of mefloquine, activated charcoal should be considered at a dose of 1 g/kg if it can be administered within 2 hours of ingestion. Mefloquine is not removed by hemodialysis and the drug undergoes enterohepatic recirculation.

> For management of a suspected drug overdose, CPhA recommends that you contact your **regional Poison Control Centre**. See the *CPS* Directory section for a list of Poison Control Centres.

ACTION AND CLINICAL PHARMACOLOGY: Mechanism of Action: Mefloquine is a 4-quinoline-methanol antimalarial agent that is structurally related to quinine and quinidine. The exact mechanism of action of mefloquine is unknown; however, the drug is active against the erythrocytic stages of Plasmodium species, and inactive against the hepatic (exoerythrocytic) stages of the life cycle of these parasites. Mefloquine is active against malarial strains resistant to chloroquine; however, resistance to mefloquine, and cross resistance between mefloquine and halofantrine, and between mefloquine and quinine has been reported.

Data from clinical studies shows that mefloquine blood concentrations of 462, 620 and 915 ng/mL are associated with 90, 95 and 99% prophylactic efficacy.
Pharmacokinetics: See Table 5.
Special Populations: Acute Malaria: Because acute malaria is associated with altered gastrointestinal motility, reduced visceral perfusion and impaired absorption, pharmacokinetics of mefloquine may be altered in patients with acute malaria. Further changes in clearance may occur due to impaired hepatic function and interruption in enterohepatic cycling of mefloquine may result in shorter terminal half-life.
Pediatrics: The pharmacokinetics of mefloquine have been studied in Thai children with uncomplicated *P. falciparum* malaria. In those aged 5 to 12 years, peak plasma concentrations of 3.7 to 3.9 μg/mL were reached in 6.6 to 7.4 hours after a single 20 mg/kg dose of a mefloquine oral suspension. In those aged 6 to 24 months a mean peak plasma concentration of 3.3 μg/mL was achieved 12.8 hours after administration of a 25 mg/kg single dose of a mefloquine oral suspension.
Race: Marked ethnic variation in the plasma concentrations of mefloquine has been reported. After administration of single 500 and 750 mg doses to healthy Asian adults, mean peak concentrations of mefloquine were 1010 and 1401 ng/mL, respectively (see Table 5 for comparison). The reason for the difference between Asian and non-Asian individuals is not known.

Table 3: Mefloquine

Dose in Adult Patients

Indication	Route	Usual Dose	Maximum Dose	Duration of Treatment	Clinical Comment
Prevention of malaria caused by susceptible strains of *P. falciparum* or *P. vivax* and chloroquine-resistant *P. falciparum*	Oral	250 mg base once weekly or Loading dose of 250 mg base once daily for 3 days, then 250 mg base weekly thereafter	250 mg base	Weekly starting one week before travel to a malaria region, weekly during the stay in the region and weekly for four weeks after leaving the region	Administer with a meal and with at least 240 mL of water. Loading dose strategy: steady state levels can be achieved in 4 days rather than 7–9 weeks. It is suggested for last-minute travellers to high-risk chloroquine-resistant areas. Further, loading dose strategies may be used for testing neuropsychiatric side effects prior to departure since they may be related to drug levels. Moreover, to assess neuropsychiatric side effects, the regular weekly dose can be started 3 weeks prior to departure. Though the levels would not have reached steady state after only 3 weeks, the advantage with this regimen is the less prolonged high blood levels if adverse effects are encountered.
Treatment of mild to moderate malaria caused by susceptible strains of *P. falciparum* or *P. vivax* and chloroquine-resistant *P. falciparum*	Oral	Non-immune patients: total therapeutic dose is 20–25 mg/kg; partially immune patients: total therapeutic dose of 15 mg/kg may be used	1500 mg base in non-immune patients; 1000 mg base in partially immune patients	Single dose or if dose is divided, administer 2nd dose 6–8 hours after the 1st dose	**Routine use of mefloquine for treatment of mild to moderate malaria is not recommended in Canada.** Administer with a meal and with at least 240 mL of water. Do not use mefloquine if malaria has resulted from failure of mefloquine prophylaxis. If improvement does not occur within 48 to 72 hours, then mefloquine should not be re-administered. Splitting the dose may decrease the rate of early vomiting and increase oral bioavailability. Patients with acute malaria due to *P. vivax* are at high risk of relapse after treatment with mefloquine because mefloquine does not eliminate the hepatic phase of malaria infection. Prevention of relapse may be achieved by subsequent treatment with primaquine or other 8-aminoquinoline derivative.

Table 4: Mefloquine

Dose in Pediatric Patients

Indication	Route	Usual Dose	Maximum Dose	Duration of Treatment	Clinical Comment
Prevention of malaria caused by susceptible strains of *P. falciparum* or *P. vivax* and chloroquine-resistant *P. falciparum*	Oral	Children aged >3 months and weighing >5 kg: 5 mg/kg body weight once weekly	250 mg base	Weekly starting one week before travel to a malaria region, weekly during the stay in the region and weekly for four weeks after leaving the region	Administer with a meal and with at least 240 mL of water.
		For body weight 5 to <10 kg: 1/8 tablet weekly			
		For body weight 10 to <20 kg: ¼ tablet weekly			
		For body weight 20 to <30 kg: ½ tablet weekly			
		For body weight 30 to <45 kg: ¾ tablet weekly			
		For body weight >45 kg: 1 tablet weekly			
Treatment of mild to moderate malaria caused by susceptible strains of *P. falciparum* or *P. vivax* and chloroquine-resistant *P. falciparum*	Oral	Children aged >3 months and weighing >5 kg: non-immune patients—total therapeutic dose is 20–25 mg/kg; partially immune patients—total therapeutic dose of 15 mg/kg may be used	1500 mg base in non-immune patients; 1000 mg base in partially immune patients	Single dose or if dose is divided, administer 2nd dose 6–8 hours after the 1st dose	**Routine use of mefloquine for treatment of mild to moderate malaria is not recommended in Canada.** If improvement does not occur within 48 to 72 hours then mefloquine should not be re-administered. Administer with a meal and with at least 240 mL of water. Mefloquine has been associated with vomiting in children. If vomiting occurs within 30 minutes of administration, consider re-administration of the full dose; if vomiting occurs between 30 to 60 minutes after administration, consider re-administering an additional one-half dose. If vomiting recurs, consider alternative therapy if improvement does not occur.

Table 5: Mefloquine

Summary of the pharmacokinetic properties of mefloquine after oral administration of a single dose in healthy adult volunteers[a,b]

Oral bioavailability	85%	
Effect of food on oral bioavailability	40% increase in bioavailability Increases rate and extent of absorption	
Absorption half-life	0.4–3.8 hours	
Median time to maximum plasma concentration	17 hours (6 to 24 hours)	
Peak serum concentration following single-dose oral administration	250 mg	286 ng/mL
	500 mg	430 ng/mL
	750 mg	587 ng/mL
	1000 mg	966 ng/mL
Peak and trough serum concentrations at steady state after administration of 250 mg once weekly	peak: 1680 ng/mL trough: 1120 ng/mL	
Time to steady state plasma concentration	8 weeks	
Plasma protein binding (%)	98	
Apparent volume of distribution	20 L/kg	
Erythrocyte: plasma concentration	2:1	
Primary route of elimination	Hepatic metabolism with biliary-fecal excretion of two pharmacologically inactive metabolites	
Mean terminal elimination half-life (range)	21 days (13–33 days)	

[a] Mefloquine is a racemic drug and the pharmacokinetics of the two enantiomers differ. Differences in the pharmacokinetics of (+) and (−) mefloquine contribute to the large interindividual variation in pharmacokinetic parameters.
[b] Interindividual and ethnic variations seen with pharmacokinetic parameters.

Megace® OS ℞

megestrol acetate

Antianorexic—Anticachectic

Bristol-Myers Squibb

Date of Preparation: October 27,1976
Date of Revision: September 22, 1999

PHARMACOLOGY: The precise mechanism of action by which megestrol produces its antianorexic and anticachectic effects is unknown at present. The gain in weight associated with megestrol is associated with increased appetite, an increase in fat and body cell mass.

Pharmacokinetics: In 24* healthy male volunteers (age 19 to 44 years) who received 160 mg of megestrol given as a 40 mg q.i.d. regimen, the oral absorption of Megace appeared to be variable. Peak drug levels for the first 40 mg dose ranged from 10 to 56 ng/mL (mean 27.6 ng/mL) and the times to peak concentrations ranged from 1 to 3 hours (mean 2.2 hours). Plasma elimination half-life ranged from 9.9 to 104.9 hours (mean 34.2 hours). The steady-state plasma concentrations for a 40 mg q.i.d. regimen have not been established.

Plasma steady-state pharmacokinetics of Megace OS were evaluated in 10 adult cachectic male patients (age 26 to 49 years) with acquired immunodeficiency syndrome (AIDS) and an involuntary weight loss greater than 10% of baseline. Patients received a single oral dose of 800 mg/day of megestrol for 21 days. Plasma concentration data obtained on day 21 were evaluated for up to 48 hours past the last dose. A high degree of interpatient variability in rate and extent of absorption was observed. Median peak plasma concentration (C_{max}) of megestrol was 602 ng/mL (range 77 to 1670 ng/mL). Median area under the concentration versus time-curve (AUC) was 7547 ng·h/mL (range 1550 to 27 090 ng·h/mL) and median T_{max} value was 5 h (range 1 to 8 hours).

Steady-state plasma pharmacokinetics of Megace OS were evaluated in 24 asymptomatic HIV seropositive male patients (age 21 to 40 years). Patients received single oral dose of 750 mg of megestrol for 14 days. The mean plasma concentration (C_{max}) of megestrol was 490 ng/mL (range 156 to 1169 ng/mL). The mean area under the concentration vs time curve (AUC) was 6779 ng·h/mL (range 1826 to 14 094 ng·h/mL) and median T_{max} was 3 hours (range 0 to 8 hours).

Estimates of plasma levels of megestrol are dependent on the measurement method used. Plasma levels depend on intestinal and hepatic inactivation of the drug, which may be affected by intestinal tract motility, intestinal bacteria, concomitant antibiotic administration, body weight, diet and hepatic function.

There are no alterations in pharmacokinetic parameters when megestrol (oral suspension) is administered with zidovudine or rifabutin.

Pharmacodynamics: A single oral dose of radioactive megestrol given to 1 male produced a maximum blood level in 1 to 3 hours and gradually fell over a 24-hour period. Megestrol when given orally to women exhibited an average excretion of 86.2% (range 83.1 to 94.7%), fecal excretion accounted for 19.8% (range 7.7 to 30.3%) and urinary excretion for 66.4% (range 56.5 to 78.4%). The biological half-life for doses of 60 to 90 mg was 3.5 days. The half-life of a 160 mg dose was 37.6 hours. The excretion occurred as 3 glucuronide conjugates with hydroxylation occurring at either the 2-α, or the 6-methyl position or at both positions. Other metabolites occur but only account for 5 to 8% of the dose.

Respiratory excretion and fat storage may account for the fraction of an administered dose not found in urine or feces.

INDICATIONS: For the treatment of anorexia, cachexia, or an unexplained significant weight loss in patients with a diagnosis of acquired immunodeficiency syndrome (AIDS).

CONTRAINDICATIONS: In those people who are sensitive to megestrol or any ingredients in the dosage form. Megestrol should not be used as a diagnostic test for pregnancy.

WARNINGS: *Pregnancy:* **The use of progestational agents during the first 4 months of pregnancy is not recommended.**

Progestational agents have been used beginning within the first trimester of pregnancy in an attempt to prevent habitual abortion or treat threatened abortion. There is no adequate evidence that such use is effective and there is evidence of potential harm to the fetus when such drugs are given during the first 4 months of pregnancy. Use of progestational agents, with their uterine-relaxant properties, in patients with fertilized defective ova may cause a delay in spontaneous abortion.

Several reports suggest an association between intrauterine exposure to progestational drugs in the first trimester of pregnancy and genital abnormalities in male and female fetuses. The risk of hypospadias, 5 to 8 per 1000 male births in the general population, may be approximately doubled with exposure to these drugs. There are insufficient data to quantify the risk to exposed female fetuses, however some of these drugs induce mild virilization of the external genitalia of the female fetus.

If the patient is exposed to megestrol during the first 4 months of pregnancy or if she becomes pregnant while taking this drug, she should be apprised of the potential risks to the fetus. Women of childbearing potential should be advised to avoid becoming pregnant.

* Pharmacokinetic data from 1 patient excluded due to unusually high drug levels.

Megestrol oral suspension is not intended for prophylactic use to avoid weight loss.

PRECAUTIONS: General: Therapy with megestrol oral suspension for weight loss should only be instituted after treatable causes of weight loss are sought and addressed. These treatable causes include malignancies, systemic infections, gastrointestinal disorders affecting absorption, endocrine disease and renal or psychiatric disease.

Although the glucocorticoid effects of megestrol oral suspension in HIV-infected individuals have not been evaluated, laboratory evidence of adrenal suppression has been observed rarely in patients shortly after discontinuation of megestrol oral suspension therapy. The significance of these findings has not been fully established. The possibility of adrenal suppression should be considered in all patients taking or withdrawing from chronic megestrol therapy. Replacement stress doses of glucocorticoids may be indicated.

Effects of megestrol oral suspension on HIV viral replication have not been determined.

Use megestrol oral suspension with caution in patients with a history of thrombophlebitis. Close, customary surveillance is indicated as in any patient being treated for recurrent or metastatic cancer. Patients receiving large doses of progestational agents such as megestrol continuously for prolonged periods should be observed closely for possible adrenal cortical suppression.

Children: Safety and effectiveness in pediatric patients have not been established.

Lactation: Because many drugs are excreted in human breast milk and because of the potential for adverse reactions in nursing infants, nursing should be discontinued when receiving megestrol therapy.

HIV Infected Women: Although megestrol has been used extensively in women for the treatment of endometrial and breast cancers, its use in HIV infected women has been limited. All 10 women in clinical trials reported breakthrough bleeding.

Drug Interactions: Possible interactions of megestrol with concomitant medications have not been investigated.

Information to Be Provided to the Patient: Patients should be advised to use megestrol as directed and report any adverse reaction experiences to their physician. Women of childbearing potential should be advised to avoid becoming pregnant and should exercise adequate contraceptive control. If patients become pregnant while taking megestrol, they should promptly notify their physician.

ADVERSE EFFECTS: Weight gain is a frequent side effect of megestrol when it is used in patients with cancer of the breast. This gain has been associated with increased appetite. It is this effect which forms the basis for use of megestrol in patients with anorexia, cachexia or weight loss. Weight gain is associated with an increase in fat and body cell mass.

Untoward reactions that have been reported to occur in patients receiving megestrol include nausea, vomiting, edema, and breakthrough uterine bleeding and occur in approximately 1 to 2% of patients. Gynecomastia and loss of hearing have also been reported. Dyspnea, pain, heart failure, hypertension, hot flashes, mood changes, cushingoid facies, tumor flare (with or without hypercalcemia), hyperglycemia, alopecia, carpal tunnel syndrome, diarrhea, lethargy and rash have also been reported.

Thromboembolic phenomenon including thrombophlebitis and pulmonary embolism (in some cases fatal) have also been reported.

Pituitary adrenal axis abnormalities including glucose intolerance, new onset diabetes, exacerbation of pre-existing diabetes with decreased glucose tolerance and Cushing's syndrome have been reported with the use of megestrol.

In clinical trials of megestrol in patients with acquired immune deficiency syndrome, overall, there was no statistically significant difference between active and placebo treatment in patients reporting at least 1 adverse event. Events reported in ≥5% of these study patients included diarrhea, impotence, rash, flatulence, asthenia and pain. Aside from impotence, all occurred more commonly in patients receiving placebo treatment.

Constipation and urinary frequency also have been reported in patients who received high doses of megestrol in other clinical trials.

OVERDOSE:

Symptoms: Usual safety measures as with the overdose of any medication should be instituted. However, no serious unexpected side effects have resulted from studies involving megestrol administered in dosages as high as 1600 mg/day for 6 months or more.

Treatment: Megestrol has not been tested for dialyzability; however, due to its low solubility, it is postulated that dialysis would not be an effective means of treating overdose.

For management of a suspected drug overdose, CPhA recommends that you contact your **regional Poison Control Centre**. See the *CPS* Directory section for a list of Poison Control Centres.

DOSAGE: For the following indications, at least 2 months of continuous treatment with oral suspension is recommended.

Anorexia, Cachexia, or Significant Weight Loss in Patients with a Diagnosis of Acquired Immunodeficiency Syndrome (AIDS): Usual adult dose: 400 to 800 mg as a single daily dose (10 to 20 mL/day). Ten mL of oral suspension contain 400 mg of megestrol.

Shake container well before use.

Special Instructions: Exposure or overdose at levels approaching recommended dosing levels could result in side effects described above (see Warnings and Adverse Effects). Women at risk of pregnancy should avoid such exposure.

SUPPLIED: Each mL of lemon-lime flavored oral suspension contains: megestrol acetate 40 mg. Nonmedicinal ingredients: anhydrous citric acid, natural and artificial lemon-lime flavor, polyethylene glycol 1450, polysorbate 80, purified water, sodium benzoate, sodium citrate dihydrate, sucrose and xanthan gum. Bottles of 240 mL. Store at room temperature (15 to 30°C). Protect from temperatures above 30°C.

Menactra®

meningococcal (groups A, C, Y and W-135) polysaccharide diphtheria toxoid conjugate vaccine

Active Immunizing Agent for the Prevention of Meningococcal Disease

sanofi pasteur

Date of Revision: September 2008

SUMMARY PRODUCT INFORMATION:

Route of Administration	Dosage Form/ Strength	Clinically Relevant Nonmedicinal Ingredients
Intramuscular Injection	Solution for Injection Each 0.5 mL dose of vaccine is formulated to contain: 4 µg each of meningococcal A, C, Y and W-135 polysaccharides conjugated to a total of approximately 48 µg of a diphtheria toxoid protein carrier. For a complete listing see Dosage Forms, Composition and Packaging.	N/A

DESCRIPTION: Menactra is a sterile, clear to slightly turbid liquid containing *N. meningitidis* serogroups A, C, Y and W-135 capsular polysaccharide antigens individually conjugated to diphtheria toxoid protein. The polysaccharides are covalently linked to diphtheria toxoid and purified by serial diafiltration. The four meningococcal components, present as individual serogroup-specific glycoconjugates, compose the final formulated vaccine.

INDICATIONS AND CLINICAL USE: Menactra is indicated for active immunization for the prevention of invasive meningococcal disease caused by *N. meningitidis* serogroups A, C, Y and W-135 in persons 2 to 55 years of age.

CONTRAINDICATIONS: Known systemic hypersensitivity to any component of Menactra, or its container, or a life-threatening reaction after previous administration of a vaccine containing similar components are contraindications to vaccination. The National Advisory Committee on Immunization (NACI) recommends that such persons may be referred to an allergist for evaluation if immunizations are considered.

Acute Neurological Disorders: Known history of Guillain-Barré syndrome (GBS) is a contraindication to vaccine administration. (See Warnings and Precautions.)

WARNINGS AND PRECAUTIONS: General: Before administration of Menactra, health-care providers should inform the recipient or the parent or guardian of the recipient of the benefits and risks of immunization, inquire about the recent health status of the recipient, review the recipient's history concerning possible hypersensitivity to the vaccine or similar vaccine, previous immunization history, the presence of any contraindications to immunization and comply with any local requirements regarding information to be provided to the recipient/guardian before immunization.

It is extremely important that the recipient, parent or guardian be questioned concerning any signs or symptoms of an adverse reaction after a previous dose of vaccine containing similar components. (See Contraindications and Adverse Reactions.)

As with any vaccine, Menactra may not protect 100% of vaccinated individuals. Very rare cases of meningitis involving a *N. meningitidis* serogroup included in the vaccine have been reported; however, the immune status of the recipients who developed these infections has not been established.

Protection: Menactra can only protect against *N. meningitidis* A, C, Y and W-135 serogroups and will not protect against any other microorganisms.

Menactra is not indicated for the prevention of invasive meningococcal disease caused by serogroup B.

Menactra vaccination is not indicated for immunization against diphtheria.

Menactra is not to be used for treatment of meningococcal infections.

Administration Route Related Precautions: Do not administer Menactra by intravascular injection: ensure that the needle does not penetrate a blood vessel. The subcutaneous routes of administration should not be utilized. There have been reports of subcutaneous use of Menactra, and the safety profile associated with these reports did not differ from that observed with intramuscular use of Menactra. Menactra should not be administered into the buttocks due to the varying amount of fatty tissue in the region since this method of administration may induce a weaker immune response.

Febrile and Acute Disease: The Advisory Committee on Immunization Practices (ACIP) recommends that vaccination should be postponed in cases of acute or febrile disease. However, a disease with low-grade fever should not usually be a reason to postpone vaccination.

Hematologic: Because any intramuscular injection can cause an injection site hematoma in persons with any bleeding disorders, such as hemophilia or thrombocytopenia, or in persons on anticoagulant therapy, intramuscular injections with Menactra should not be administered to such persons unless the potential benefits outweigh the risk of administration. If the decision is made to administer any product by intramuscular injection to such persons, it should be given with caution, with steps taken to avoid the risk of hematoma formation following injection. NACI has published recommendations for the immunization of people with hemophilia and other bleeding disorders.

Immune: The possibility of allergic reactions in persons sensitive to components of the vaccine should be evaluated. Hypersensitivity reactions may occur following the use of Menactra even in persons with no prior history of hypersensitivity to the product components. As vial stoppers contain latex (natural rubber), caution should be exercised when the vaccine is administered to subjects with known hypersensitivity to latex. The syringe presentation of this vaccine contains no latex.

As with all products, epinephrine hydrochloride solution (1:1000) and other appropriate agents should be available for immediate use in case an anaphylactic or acute hypersensitivity reaction occurs. Health-care providers should be familiar with current recommendations for the initial management of anaphylaxis in non-hospital settings, including proper airway management. For instructions on recognition and treatment of anaphylactic reactions, see the current edition of the Canadian Immunization Guide or visit the Health Canada website.

No data are available on the use of Menactra in immunodeficient subjects.

Individuals with functional or anatomical asplenia may produce an immune response to Menactra, however, the degree of protection that would be afforded is unknown.

Immunocompromised persons (whether from disease or treatment) may not achieve the expected immune response. If possible, consideration should be given to delaying vaccination until after the completion of any immunosuppressive treatment. Nevertheless, NACI and ACIP recommend vaccination of persons with chronic immunodeficiency such as HIV infection even if the immune response might be limited.

Neurologic: GBS has been very rarely reported in temporal relationship following administration of Menactra. Based on an evaluation of post-marketing adverse events, a slight increase in the number of GBS reports was observed following administration of Menactra. However, because of the inherent limitations of spontaneous safety reporting, this is not confirmatory of an increased risk and these findings should be viewed with caution. Persons previously diagnosed with GBS should not receive Menactra.

Peri-Operative Considerations: NACI states that if possible, this and other indicated vaccines should be given 10 to 14 days before splenectomy.

Special Populations: Pregnant Women: Animal reproduction studies have not demonstrated a risk with respect to effects on pregnancy and embryo-fetal development, parturition and postnatal development. However, since there are no data on the use of this vaccine in pregnant women, Menactra should be given to a pregnant woman only if clearly needed, such as during an outbreak or prior to necessary travel to an endemic area, and only following an assessment of the risks and benefits.

Nursing Women: It is not known whether the active substances included in the vaccine are excreted in human milk, but antibodies to the polysaccharides have been found to be transferred to the suckling offspring of mice.

Animal studies conducted in mice have not shown any harmful effect on offspring postnatal development caused by maternal antibodies induced by the vaccine. However, the effect on breast-fed infants of the administration of Menactra to their mothers has not been studied. The risks and benefits of vaccination should be assessed before making the decision to immunize a nursing woman.

Geriatrics: Clinical data are available in persons up to the age of 55 years.

Pediatrics: Menactra is not approved for use in children below 2 years of age.

ADVERSE REACTIONS: Clinical Trial Adverse Drug Reactions: Because clinical trials are conducted under widely varying conditions, adverse reaction rates observed in the clinical trials of a vaccine cannot be directly compared to rates in the clinical trials of another vaccine and may not reflect rates observed in practice. The adverse reaction information from clinical trials does, however, provide a basis for identifying the adverse events that appear to be related to vaccine use and for approximating rates of those events.

Children 2 to 10 Years Old: In clinical studies, safety was evaluated within the first 7 days, 28 days and 6 months after vaccination. Menactra was well tolerated among children. The majority of the solicited injection site and systemic reactions reported within 7 days after vaccination were mild, with a mean duration of no more than 3 days for the injection site reactions and less than 4 days for the systemic reactions. The most commonly reported solicited adverse reaction was pain at the injection site (40 to 48% of the participants) (see Table 1).

Study 603-02 was a primary immunogenicity study that also was designed to evaluate the rates of fever post-vaccination. The results show no statistical difference between the treatment groups. Overall the rates of local and systemic reactions were similar. In this study, the rates of severe local and systemic reactions were generally more frequent in Menactra recipients although the study was not statistically powered to detect significant differences for these reactions between the two study groups.

Study MTA-08 was a primary safety study designed to evaluate the rates of severe systemic reactions post-vaccination. The results show no statistical difference between the treatment groups. Rates of local reactions were more frequent in Menactra recipients while the rates of systemic reactions were similar.

Table 1: Menactra

Percentage of Menactra and Menomune-A/C/Y/W-135 Recipients Reporting at Least One Solicited Local and/or Systemic Reaction Within 7 Days, by Reaction Type in Children 2 to 10 Years Old, by Study

	Study 603-02 Menactra N=692		Study 603-02 Menomune-A/C/Y/W-135 N=692		Study MTA08 Menactra N=1704		Study MTA08 Menomune-A/C/Y/W-135 N=1515	
Event	**Any[a]**	**Severe[b]**	**Any**	**Severe**	**Any**	**Severe**	**Any**	**Severe**
Local Reactions								
Pain	48.1	0.7	46.9	0.3	39.7	0.2	30.4	0.0
Redness	29.5	4.3	30.4	0.4	17.9	2.8	9.4	0.0
Induration	22.1	1.0	15.6	0.1	16.1	0.9	5.2	0.0
Swelling	20.5	1.2	14.6	0.3	14.3	1.3	4.9	0.0
Systemic Reactions								
Irritability[c]	35.2	2.7	30.1	0.6	11.0	0.2	12.1	0.4
Drowsiness[c]	26.0	1.6	24.1	1.1	10.4	0.2	10.9	0.3
Anorexia[d]	22.7	1.7	20.3	0.4	8.3	0.3	9.2	0.7
Diarrhea[e]	15.9	1.6	15.7	0.4	12.1	0.2	13.0	0.3
Fever[f]	11.4	0.9	12.0	0.6	5.9	0.2	6.0	0.3
Vomiting[g]	5.9	0.7	7.0	1.1	3.5	0.2	3.1	0.4
Hives[h]	1.2	—	0.4	—	—	—	—	—
Arthralgia[c]	—	—	—	—	7.3	0.1	7.6	0.0
Rash[h]	—	—	—	—	4.1	—	3.5	—
Seizures[h]	—	—	—	—	0.0	—	0.0	—

(cont'd)

Table 1: Menactra *(cont'd)*

[a] Any denotes the proportion of participants reporting any reaction regardless of the severity.
[b] Severe local reaction denotes swelling, redness or induration ≥5 cm in diameter or pain resulting in unwillingness to move the affected arm.
[c] Severe: requiring bed rest.
[d] Severe: skipped ≥3 meals.
[e] Severe: ≥5 episodes.
[f] Severe: ≥39.5°C.
[g] Severe: ≥3 episodes.
[h] These solicited adverse events were reported as present or absent only.

In clinical trial MTA15 conducted in the UK in children 2 to 4 years old, previously immunized with a monovalent meningococcal C conjugate vaccine, Menactra was shown to be well tolerated and had a safety profile comparable to another polysaccharide protein conjugated vaccine [Hib (PRP/T)] used as a control.

Adolescents and Adults (11 to 55 Years Old): Menactra was well tolerated among adolescents and adults. In two clinical trials in adolescents 11-18 years of age (Studies MTA02 and MTA09) and in two clinical studies in adults 18-55 years of age (Studies MTA09 and MTA14), the most commonly reported injection site adverse reactions were pain, induration, redness and swelling. The most common systemic adverse reactions were headache, fatigue and malaise. The majority of injection site and systemic reactions following Menactra were reported as mild in intensity. Except for redness in adults, local reactions were more frequently reported after Menactra than after Menomune-A/C/Y/W-135. The majority of local and systemic reactions following Menactra or Menomune-A/C/Y/W-135 were reported as mild in intensity. No important differences in rates of malaise, diarrhea, anorexia, vomiting, or rash were observed between the vaccine groups (see Table 2).

Table 2: Menactra

Percentage of Menactra and Menomune-A/C/Y/W-135 Subjects from Comparative Trials Reporting at Least One Solicited Local and/or Systemic Reaction within 7 Days, by Reaction Type in Adolescents (11 to 17) and Adults (18 to 55)

	Menactra Adolescents N=2702[a]		Menomune-A/C/Y/W-135 Adolescents N=1411[a]		Menactra Adults N=2824[b]		Menomune-A/C/Y/W-135 Adults N=1613[b]	
Event	**Any[c]**	**Severe[d]**	**Any**	**Severe**	**Any**	**Severe**	**Any**	**Severe**
Local Reactions								
Pain	64.0	0.2	29.4	0	52.2	0.1	33.9	0
Induration	18.0	0.5	6.4	0	16.6	0.6	8.2	0
Redness	11.5	0.4	6.0	0	13.5	0.8	12.9	0
Swelling	12.6	0.6	4.5	0	11.7	0.7	6.1	0
Systemic Reactions								
Headache[e]	37.1	1.1	32.5	0.9	40.7	0.8	39.5	1.0
Fatigue[e]	29.9	1.1	24.6	0.4	34.0	0.7	30.2	0.7
Malaise[e]	21.9	1.1	16.8	0.4	22.9	0.8	21.0	1.1
Arthralgia[e]	17.4	0.4	10.2	0.1	19.5	0.4	15.0	0.2
Diarrhea[f]	11.8	0.3	11.4	0.1	16.6	0.4	14.4	0.4
Anorexia[g]	11.0	0.4	9.1	0.4	11.6	0.3	9.3	0.4
Chills[e]	7.0	0.2	3.5	0.1	8.4	0.3	5.0	0.1
Fever[h]	4.8	0	2.8	0.1	1.2	0	0.5	0
Vomiting[h]	2.0	0.3	1.6	0.3	2.0	0.1	1.4	0.3
Rash[i]	1.6	—	1.5	—	1.4	—	1.2	—

(cont'd)

Table 2: Menactra *(cont'd)*

Percentage of Menactra and Menomune-A/C/Y/W-135 Subjects from Comparative Trials Reporting at Least One Solicited Local and/or Systemic Reaction within 7 Days, by Reaction Type in Adolescents (11 to 17) and Adults (18 to 55)

	Menactra Adolescents N=2702[a]		Menomune-A/C/Y/W-135 Adolescents N=1411[a]		Menactra Adults N=2824[b]		Menomune-A/C/Y/W-135 Adults N=1613[b]	
Event	**Any[c]**	**Severe[d]**	**Any**	**Severe**	**Any**	**Severe**	**Any**	**Severe**
Seizures[j]	0	—	0	—	0	—	0	—

[a] Includes all subjects who provided data from comparative trials 4 and 5.
[b] Includes all subjects who provided data from comparative trials 1 and 2.
[c] Any denotes the proportion of participants reporting any reaction regardless of the severity.
[d] Severe local reaction denotes swelling, redness or induration ≥5 cm in diameter or pain resulting in unwillingness to move the affected arm.
[e] Severe: requiring bed rest.
[f] Severe: ≥5 episodes.
[g] Severe: skipped ≥3 meals.
[h] Severe: ≥3 episodes.
[i] Severe: ≥39.5°C.
[j] These solicited adverse events were reported as present or absent only.

Post-Market Adverse Drug Reactions: The following additional adverse events have been spontaneously reported during the post-marketing use of Menactra. Because these events are reported voluntarily from a population of uncertain size, it is not possible to reliably estimate their frequency or establish a causal relationship to vaccine exposure.
Immune System Disorders: hypersensitivity reactions such as anaphylactic/anaphylactoid reaction, wheezing, difficulty breathing, upper airway swelling, urticaria, erythema, pruritus, hypotension.
Nervous System Disorders: Guillain-Barré syndrome (see Warnings and Precautions), vasovagal syncope, facial palsy, transverse myelitis, acute disseminated encephalomyelitis.
Hematologic Disorders: thrombocytopenia.
Musculoskeletal and Connective Tissue Disorders: myalgia.

Physicians, nurses and pharmacists should report any adverse occurrences temporally associated with the administration of the product in accordance with local requirements and to the Global Pharmacovigilance Department, Sanofi Pasteur Limited, 1755 Steeles Avenue West, Toronto, ON, M2R 3T4 Canada. 1-888-621-1146 (phone) or 416-667-2435 (fax).

DRUG INTERACTIONS: Vaccine Drug Interactions: Immunosuppressive treatments may interfere with the development of the expected immune response. (See Warnings and Precautions.)
Concomitant Vaccine Administration: The concomitant use of Menactra with tetanus and reduced-dose diphtheria vaccine (Td) was evaluated in 11-17 year-old adolescents (N=507). The concomitant administration of the two vaccines to adolescents revealed no apparent increase in reported adverse events or specific safety concern related to the diphtheria toxoid carrier protein content, although the anti-diphtheria response was much higher after concomitant administration of Td with Menactra, compared to the administration of Td followed by Menactra 28 days later. The proportion of participants with a 4-fold rise or more in SBA-BR titre was also higher in subjects who received Menactra and Td concomitantly, than those who were given Td first and Menactra 28 days later. There are currently no data available on the concomitant administration of Menactra with other diphtheria-containing vaccines such as DTaP or Tdap or on intervals considered safe for the administration of diphtheria-containing vaccines before or after Menactra.

The concomitant administration of Menactra and Typhim Vi (*S. typhi* Vi Capsular Polysaccharide Vaccine) was evaluated in 945 adults, 18 to 55 years old. The immune response to the two vaccines was comparable when Menactra and Typhim Vi were given concurrently or separately, 28 days apart.

Vaccines administered simultaneously should be given using separate syringes at separate sites. Menactra should not be mixed in the same syringe with other parenterals.

DOSAGE AND ADMINISTRATION: Recommended Dose and Dosage Adjustment: Menactra should be administered as a single injection of 1 dose (0.5 mL) by the intramuscular route. The preferred site is into the deltoid muscle.

The need for, or timing of, the administration of a booster has not yet been determined.
Administration: Inspect for extraneous particulate matter and/or discolouration before use (see Description). If these conditions exist, the product should not be administered

Shake the vaccine well until a uniform, clear to slightly turbid liquid results. Cleanse the vial stopper with a suitable germicide prior to withdrawing the dose. Do not remove either the stopper or the metal seal holding it in place. Aseptic technique must be used. Use a separate sterile needle and syringe, or a sterile disposable unit for each individual recipient, to prevent disease transmission. Needles should not be recapped and should be disposed of according to biohazard waste guidelines. (See Warnings and Precautions.)

For information on vaccine administration see the current edition of the Canadian Immunization Guide or visit the Health Canada website.

Administer the total volume of 0.5 mL **intramuscularly** (IM). The preferred site of injection is the deltoid muscle.

Give the patient a permanent personal immunization record. In addition, it is essential that the physician or nurse record the immunization history in the permanent medical record of each patient. This permanent office record should contain the name of the vaccine, date given, dose, manufacturer and lot number.

ACTION AND CLINICAL PHARMACOLOGY: Pharmacodynamics: The presence of bactericidal anti-capsular meningococcal antibodies has been associated with protection from invasive meningococcal disease. Menactra induces the production of bactericidal antibodies specific to the capsular polysaccharides of serogroups A,C,Y and W-135. Serum bactericidal antibody (SBA) was established as a serological correlate of protection for group C meningococcal infection in studies in military recruits undertaken in the 1960s. These studies showed that those with naturally acquired SBA titres ≥1:4 measured using human complement (SBA-H) were protected from meningitis caused by *N. meningitidis* serogroup C. An alternative complement source for the SBA is 3 to 4-week-old baby rabbit serum (SBA-BR). While a group C SBA-BR titre ≥1:128 predict protection against meningococcal serogroup C disease it has been shown to underestimate vaccine efficacy; moreover, the cut off ≥1:8 was found to be the most consistent correlate with the observed efficacy of Meningococcal conjugate C vaccine in the UK. A serologic correlate that predicts clinical protection has not been established for serogroups A,Y and W-135.

Menactra was shown to be immunogenic in children >2 years old, adolescents and adults against *N. meningitidis* serogroups A, C, Y and W-135. A group of 2 to 3 year old children (N=92), were followed for 2 to 3 years after a single dose of Menactra. These participants had 1.7 to 5.2 fold higher bactericidal antibody levels than an age matched vaccine naïve control group. A subgroup of these subjects was challenged with a reduced dose of meningococcal polysaccharide vaccine. The bactericidal antibody levels on Day 28 post-challenge were higher in the Menactra-primed subjects (N=46) than the control group (N=26). This antibody response is consistent with immune memory. It is noted, however, that compared to baseline, the fold increase in bactericidal antibody levels after the reduced dose polysaccharide vaccine, was significant in both the Menactra-primed and the control groups.
Duration of Effect: A group of 2 to 3 year old children (N=92) were followed for up to 3 years after a single dose of Menactra. These participants had 1.7 to 5.2 fold higher bactericidal antibody levels than an age-matched vaccine naïve control group. Conjugation of the capsular polysaccharide antigens to the diphtheria protein converts a T-cell independent response to one that is T-cell dependent. However, the duration of protection against invasive meningococcal disease remains unknown.

STORAGE AND STABILITY: Store at 2 to 8°C. **Do not freeze.** Discard product if exposed to freezing.

Do not use after the expiration date.

INFORMATION FOR THE PATIENT: Published in e-CPS, available by subscription at www.e-cps.ca.

DOSAGE FORMS, COMPOSITION AND PACKAGING: Each single dose (0.5 mL) of vaccine is formulated to contain: 4 µg each of meningococcal A, C, Y and W-135 polysaccharides conjugated to a total of approximately 48 µg of a diphtheria toxoid protein carrier; sodium chloride 4.25 mg; sodium phosphate, dibasic, anhydrous qs phosphate 10 mM; sodium phosphate, monobasic qs phosphate 10 mM; Water for Injection qs 0.5 mL. Preservative-free. No adjuvant is added. 1×1 dose syringe, 5×1 dose syringe, 10×1 dose syringe, 1×1 dose vial, 5×1 dose vial. The stopper of the vial presentation of this vaccine contains latex (natural rubber). The syringe presentation of this vaccine contains no latex (natural rubber).
Vaccine Information Service: 1-888-621-1146 or 416-667-2779.

Meningitec®

meningococcal serogroup C conjugate vaccine
Active Immunizing Agent

Pfizer

Date of Preparation: December 12, 2003
Date of Revision: August 22, 2008

PHARMACOLOGY: Meningitec (Meningococcal Serogroup C-CRM_{197} conjugate vaccine) is intended for the prevention of meningitis and/or septicemia caused by *N. meningitidis* serogroup C in infants and older age groups. Meningitec is composed of meningococcal serogroup C oligosaccharides conjugated to a protein carrier, a non-toxic mutant of diphtheria toxin, CRM_{197}. In the final vaccine, aluminum phosphate is used as an adjuvant.

Meningococcal serogroup C infection is a significant public health hazard, causing meningitis and septicemia in all age groups. In Canada, the number of cases of meningococcal disease caused by all serogroups had declined steadily during the period of 1993 to 1999. For example, the incidence was 0.88 cases per 100 000 population in 1997 and 0.57 cases per 100 000 population in 1998. Infants had the highest incidence, with rates of 12.9 and 6.5 cases per 100 000 population in 1997 and 1998, respectively. Most meningococcal disease during that period was caused by serogroups B and C, which were associated with fatality rates of 5.4% and 12.4%, respectively. In 2000, an increase in meningococcal serogroup C disease was noted in Alberta. Since January of 2001, elevated rates of meningococcal serogroup C disease have occurred in Manitoba, Quebec, British Columbia, and Toronto.

Current polysaccharide vaccines have been shown to prevent serogroup C infection in individuals older than 2 years of age for a duration of 3-5 years. Their protective effect is due to their ability to induce bactericidal antibodies specific for the serogroup C capsular polysaccharide. However, their use is limited mainly to cluster control for two important reasons; polysaccharide vaccines are poorly immunogenic and thus ineffective in the young, and secondly, the immune response to polysaccharide vaccines at any age is restricted by the inability of such vaccines to induce immunological memory. Consequently, protection induced by such vaccines is short lived. When polysaccharides are conjugated to protein carrier molecules and used as vaccines their recognition by the immune system changes fundamentally. Such conjugated vaccines generate immunological memory in vaccine recipients of all age groups.

Clinical trials demonstrated that Meningitec is highly immunogenic and induces protective levels of bactericidal antibodies in a significant number of subjects after vaccination (see Table 1). Seven clinical trials were performed to evaluate the appropriate vaccination schedule for subjects of different ages. Data from five trials in infants using a 2-, 3-, 4-month schedule or a 2-, 4-, 6-month schedule demonstrated that 98%-100% of the infants developed serum bactericidal antibody (SBA) titers of at least 1:8 one month after the third dose. A booster dose in the second year of life induced an anamnestic response. Currently, the necessity for a booster dose has not been established.

Data from one trial in toddlers and one trial in adults demonstrated that 91%-100% of the subjects developed SBA titers of at least 1:8 one month after receiving a single dose. The antibody titers following one dose of Meningitec were comparable to those following one dose of licensed unconjugated polysaccharide vaccine in the adult subjects.

To evaluate antibody persistence, blood samples were obtained from infants approximately 1 year after they had been vaccinated on a 2-, 4-, 6-month schedule. Seventy-nine percent (79%) of the infants still had SBA titers of at least 1:8.

Unlike unconjugated polysaccharide vaccines, Meningitec has been shown to induce immunologic memory in infants and toddlers. In two studies, low-dose polysaccharide vaccine was administered 6-12 months after primary vaccination with Meningitec to mimic exposure to natural infection. SBA titers of at least 1:8 were detected in 94% of the infants and 100% of the toddlers. In one of the studies, low-dose polysaccharide vaccine was administered to a second group four years after primary vaccination with Meningitec. SBA titers of at least 1:8 were detected in 95% of the four year old subjects after challenge with low-dose polysaccharide.

Immune tolerance was evaluated in one study in which adult subjects who had been given polysaccharide vaccine 6 months earlier were randomly assigned to receive either Meningitec or a second dose of polysaccharide vaccine. A control group of subjects with no previous exposure to polysaccharide vaccine also received Meningitec. SBA titers of at least 1:8 were detected one month later in 99% of the subjects given Meningitec after polysaccharide vaccine, 93% of the subjects given a second dose of polysaccharide vaccine, and 100% of the control subjects.

Table 1: Meningitec

Immunogenicity 1 Month Following Meningitec by Study Type

Study Number[a]	Vaccination Schedule (Number Vaccinated)	Serum Bactericidal Antibody Titers ≥1:8 1 Month Post-Vaccination (Number Evaluated)[b]
I. Dosing Studies by Age Group		
A. Primary Immunogenicity in Infants After Three Doses		
D110 P2	2, 3, 4 months (58)	98% (53)
D110 P500	2, 3, 4 months (124)	100% (58)
D110 P501	2, 3, 4 months (205)	98% (121)
D110 P502	2, 3, 4 months (117)	98% (50)
D118 P3	2, 4, 6 months (106)	100% (30)
B. Booster Dose in Toddlers After Primary Immunization at 2, 4, 6 Months		
D118 P3	Single dose (64)	100% (49)
C. Immunogenicity of Single Dose in Toddlers (13 months)		
D110 P802	Single dose (75)	91% (75)
D. Immunogenicity of Single Dose in Adults (18–60 years)		
D110 P3	Single dose	
	Group: Meningitec (15)	100% (15)
	Group: PSV[c] (15)	100% (15)
II. Antibody Persistence		

(cont'd)

Table 1: Meningitec *(cont'd)*

Immunogenicity 1 Month Following Meningitec by Study Type

Study Number[a]	Vaccination Schedule (Number Vaccinated)	Serum Bactericidal Antibody Titers ≥1:8 1 Month Post-Vaccination (Number Evaluated)[b]
A. Persistence of Immunogenicity in Infants After Three Doses[d]		
D118 P3	2, 4, 6 months (106)	79% (49)
III. Other Studies		
A. Evidence of Priming by Meningitec in Infants Assessed by PSV Challenge		
D110 P2	Low-dose PSV challenge 1 year after 2, 3, 4 month immunization (17)	94% (17)
D110 P2	Low-dose PSV challenge 4 years after 2, 3, 4 month immunization (22)	95% (22)
B. Evidence of Priming by Meningitec in Toddlers Assessed by PSV Challenge		
D110 P802	Low-dose PSV challenge 6 months after primary immunization (65)	100% (62)
C. Evaluation of Immune Tolerance in Adults (18–25 years)		
D110 P805	Single dose	
	Group: Meningitec after previous PSV (83)	99% (83)
	Group: PSV after previous PSV (85)	93% (85)
	Group: Meningitec no previous PSV (49)	100% (49)

[a] All studies were performed in the United Kingdom, except D118 P3 and D110 P3, which were performed in the United States.
[b] Not all vaccinated subjects were evaluated.
[c] PSV=Polysaccharide vaccine.
[d] For evaluation of antibody persistence, analyses were performed approximately 1 year after primary immunization.

Meningitec was introduced into the UK on November 1, 1999. From March 2000, other meningococcal serogroup C conjugate vaccines were introduced. Reductions in cases of serogroup C disease of between 89% and 94% have been observed in all immunized age groups during 2001/02 when compared to 1998/99, before the meningococcal serogroup C vaccine was introduced. Efficacy estimates have been calculated for all immunized cohorts up to end of December 2001. These are as follows: 89% (95% CI: 69%-96%) for the 3 dose course, 87% (95% CI: 69%-94%) for toddlers vaccinated at 1-2 years, 100% (95% CI: 93%-100%) for pre-schoolers, 95% (95% CI: 87%-97%) for 5-14 year-olds and 94% (95% CI: 79%-99%) for 15-17 year-olds.

INDICATIONS: Meningitec (Meningococcal Serogroup C-CRM$_{197}$ conjugate vaccine) is indicated for the active immunization of children from 2 months of age, adolescents and adults, for the prevention of invasive disease caused by *N. meningitidis* serogroup C.

CONTRAINDICATIONS: Meningitec (Meningococcal Serogroup C-CRM$_{197}$ conjugate vaccine) is contraindicated in patients with a known hypersensitivity to any component of the vaccine, including diphtheria toxoid.

Meningitec is contraindicated in patients who have experienced significant neurologic signs or symptoms, or an allergic or anaphylactoid/anaphylactic reaction following a prior dose of meningococcal serogroup C conjugate vaccine.

WARNINGS: Meningococcal serogroup C conjugate vaccine will only confer protection against serogroup C of *N. meningitidis* and may not protect 100% of persons vaccinated. Invasive serogroup C meningococcal disease has been reported in rare cases in subjects adequately immunized for their age. It will not protect against other serogroups of *N. meningitidis* or other organisms that cause meningitis or septicemia.

As with any intramuscular injection, meningococcal serogroup C conjugate vaccine should be given with caution to individuals with thrombocytopenia or any coagulation disorder or to those receiving anticoagulant therapy.

As with all injectable pediatric vaccines, the potential risk of apnea should be considered when administering the primary immunization series to premature infants. The need for monitoring for at least 48 hours after vaccination should be considered for very premature infants (born ≤30 weeks of gestation).

As the benefit of vaccination is high in this group of infants, vaccination should not be withheld or delayed.

Meningitec should under no circumstances be administered intravenously.

Applies to vial presentation only: The vial stopper contains dry natural rubber that may cause hypersensitivity reactions when handled by or when the product is injected in persons with known or possible latex sensitivity. (See Supplied for packaging components.)

PRECAUTIONS: As with all injectable vaccines, appropriate medical treatment and supervision should always be readily available in case of a rare anaphylatoid/anaphylactic event following the administration of the vaccine. (See Adverse Effects.)

Minor illnesses, such as mild respiratory infection with or without low-grade fever, are not generally contraindications to vaccination. The decision to administer or delay vaccination because of a current or recent febrile illness depends largely on the severity of the symptoms and their etiology. The administration of meningococcal serogroup C conjugate vaccine should be postponed in subjects suffering from acute severe febrile illness.

Meningococcal serogroup C conjugate vaccine may not protect 100% of the individuals receiving the vaccine.

Immunization with this vaccine does not substitute for routine diphtheria vaccination.

Although there is no evidence that the vaccine causes meningococcal C meningitis, symptoms of meningism such as neck pain/stiffness or photophobia have been reported. Clinical alertness to the possibility of coincidental meningitis should therefore be maintained.

Individuals with impaired immune responsiveness whether due to the use of immunosuppressive therapy, a genetic defect, HIV infection, or other causes may have a reduced antibody response to active immunization.

Drug Interactions: Meningococcal serogroup C conjugate vaccine can be administered at the same time as oral polio vaccine, inactivated polio vaccine, hepatitis B vaccine, diphtheria tetanus whole-cell pertussis-Haemophilus influenzae b conjugate vaccine, diphtheria and tetanus toxoids vaccine and acellular pertussis vaccine, diphtheria tetanus vaccine, pneumococcal conjugate vaccine 7-valent, low dose diphtheria and tetanus toxoids vaccine, and measles mumps rubella vaccine, if this fits conveniently in the immunization scheme. There is no data on the concomitant administration of meningococcal serogroup C conjugate vaccine with Varicella vaccine.

Data on concomitant administration of Meningitec with Prevnar (pneumococcal conjugate vaccine 7-valent) have shown no clinically relevant interference in the antibody response to each of the individual antigens when given as primary series vaccinations.

Data for concomitant administration of meningococcal serogroup C conjugate vaccine and DtaP-containing vaccine are derived from a study of concomitant administration of Meningitec with a pediatric combination vaccine (DtaP-HBV-IPV/Hib) and from a study of concomitant administration of Meningitec with DTaP/Hib.

In various studies with different vaccines, concomitant administration of Meningitec with DtaP-containing vaccines has been shown to result in lower SBA GMTs compared to separate administrations. The proportions reaching SBA titres of at least 1:8 or 1:128 are not affected. At present, the potential implications of these observations for the duration of protection are not known.

Different injectable vaccines should be given at separate injection sites.

Table 2 presents data on the immunological response of infants to concomitant vaccines, as measured one month after the third dose of Meningitec or HBV vaccine.

Table 2: Meningitec

Immunogenicity Following Concurrent Administration of Routine Infant Vaccines With Meningitec

Concomitant Vaccine	Immunogenicity	Immunogenicity Results for Concurrently Administered Vaccine Antigens[a]: 1 Month After Third Dose	Booster Dose
Concurrent DTP, mixed before injection with HbOC (Hib) (Study D110 P500)		N=116	Not Done
Hib capsular polysaccharide	GMC[b] (μg/mL) % subjects with ≥1.0 μg/mL	9.8 94%	—
Diphtheria	GMC (IU/mL) % subjects with ≥1.0 μg/mL	1.8 100%	—
Tetanus	GMC (IU/mL) % subjects with ≥1.0 μg/mL	5.8 100%	—
Pertussis toxin	GMC (U/mL) % subjects with ≥2-fold increase in titer	4.2 19%	—
Pertussis FHA[c]	GMC (U/mL) % subjects with ≥2-fold increase in titer	15.4 41%	—
Pertussis fimbriae 2	GMC (U/mL) % subjects with ≥2-fold increase in titer	25.0 87%	—
Concurrent PRP-T (Hib) and DTP (Study D110 P501)		N=81 (Meningitec Lot A)	Not Done
Hib capsular polysaccharide	GMC[b] (μg/mL) % subjects with ≥1.0 μg/mL	1.54 57%	—
		N=85 (Meningitec Lot B)	Not Done
	GMC[b] (μg/mL) % subjects with ≥1.0 μg/mL	1.51 58%	—
Concurrent PRP-T (Hib) (Study D110 P502)		N=92	Not Done
Hib capsular polysaccharide	GMC[b] (μg/mL) % subjects with ≥1.0 μg/m	3.69 84.8%	—
Concurrent DTaP[d] and IPV (Study D118 P8)[e]		N=57[f,g]	Not Done
Pertussis toxin	GMC (U/mL) % subjects with ≥2-fold increase in titer	20.1 80%	—
Pertussis FHA	GMC (U/mL) % subjects with ≥2-fold increase in titer	56.1 69%	—
Pertussis fimbriae 2	GMC (U/mL) % subjects with ≥2-fold increase in titer	4.3 74%	—
Pertussis r69K[h]	GMC (U/mL) % subjects with ≥2-fold increase in titer	63.3 76%	—
Polio Type I	% subjects with titer ≥1:10	75%	—
Polio Type II	% subjects with titer ≥1:10	100%	—
Polio Type III	% subjects with titer ≥1:10	85%	—
Concurrent HBV, OPV and DTP-HbOC administered for primary series; concurrent HbOC (Hib) and DTaP administered for booster dose (Study D118 P7)		N=80[i]	N=25[j]
Hepatitis B	% subjects with ≥10 mIU/mL	100%	Not Done
Polio Type I	% subjects with titer ≥1:10	100%	—
Polio Type II	% subjects with titer ≥1:10	100%	—
Polio Type III	% subjects with titer ≥1:10	100%	—
Diphtheria	GMC IU/mL ≥0.1 IU/mL	Not Done	1.79 100%
Tetanus	GMC IU/mL ≥0.1 IU/mL	—	21.4 100%
Hib capsular polysaccharide	GMC[b] (μg/mL) % subjects with ≥1.0 μg/mL	—	224 96.2%
Pertussis toxoid	GMC (U/mL) % subjects with ≥4-fold increase in titer	—	86.3 64%
Pertussis FHA	GMC (U/mL) % subjects with ≥4-fold increase in titer	—	16.8 64%
Pertussis fimbriae 2	GMC (U/mL) % subjects with ≥4-fold increase in titer	—	13.1 88%
Pertussis r69K[h]	GMC (U/mL) % subjects with ≥4-fold increase in titer	—	86.3 76%
Concurrent DTP-HbOC administered for primary series; concurrent HbOC (Hib) or MMR administered for booster dose (Study D118 P3)		N=95[k]	N=28
Diphtheria	GMC IU/mL ≥0.1 IU/mL	0.69 99.0%	Not Done
Tetanus	GMC IU/mL ≥0.1 IU/mL	4.18 100%	—

(cont'd)

Table 2: Meningitec *(ccnt'd)*

Immunogenicity Following Concurrent Administration of Routine Infant Vaccines With Meningitec

Concomitant Vaccine	Immunogenicity	Immunogenicity Results for Concurrently Administered Vaccine Antigens[a] 1 Month After Third Dose	Booster Dose
Pertussis toxin	GMC (IU/mL) % subjects with ≥4-fold increase in titer	23.01 37.8%	—
Pertussis fimbriae 2	GMC (U/mL) % subjects with ≥4-fold increase in titer	7.51 65.1%	—
Pertussis FHA	GMC (U/mL) % subjects with ≥4-fold increase in titer	9.19 23.3%	—
Pertussis r69K[h]	GMC (U/mL) % subjects with ≥4-fold increase in titer	32.54 59.3%	—
Hib capsular polysaccharide	GMC[b] (μg/mL) % subjects with ≥1.0 μg/mL	5.58 86.5%	21.6 100%
Measles	% subjects seropositive[m]	Not Done	100%
Mumps	% subjects seropositive	—	82%
Rubella	% subjects seropositive	—	89%
Concurrent Diphtheria-tetanus vaccine (DT) in children 3.5 to <6 years of age (Study D110 P801)		Not Done	N=60
Diphtheria	GMC[b] U/mL ≥0.1 IU/mL	—	15.51 100%
Tetanus toxoid	GMC[b] U/mL ≥0.1 IU/mL	—	14.9[n,o] Data Not Available

[a] Results for control groups consisting of the concurrently administered vaccine antigens without Meningitec were not performed in the studies listed below unless otherwise indicated.
[b] GMC=Geometric mean concentration.
[c] FHA=Filamentous hemagglutinin.
[d] Antibody titers were not performed for diphtheria and tetanus.
[e] Results are also available from a separate study where infants received DTaP without concurrent Meningitec. The schedule for DTaP was the same as used in study D118 P8 (see below).

Immunogenicity Results Presented for Pertussis Antigens (n=67) are 1 Month After the Third Dose:		
Pertussis toxin	GMC (U/mL) % subjects with ≥2-fold increase in titer	17.8 83%
Pertussis FHA	GMC (U/mL) % subjects with ≥2-fold increase in titer	46.7 79%
Pertussis fimbriae 2	GMC (U/mL) % subjects with ≥2-fold increase in titer	4.2 75%
Pertussis pertactin r69K	GMC (U/mL) % subjects with ≥2-fold increase in titer	50.9 88%

[f] For ≥2-fold increase in titer, n=38 for fimbriae 2 and r69K, n=39 for pertussis toxin and FHA.
[g] For Polio Types I, II, and III, n=20.
[h] Pertussis r69K=pertactin.
[i] For hepatitis B, n=41.
[j] Booster dose data is also available for a control group where DTaP and HbOC were administered without Meningitec (n=11).
[k] For Pertussis toxin, n=90; for Pertussis fimbriae, n=86; for Pertussis FHA, n=90; for Pertussis pertactin, n=86; for Hib capsular polysaccharide, n=96.
[l] For Hib capsular polysaccharide, n=33.
[m] MMR immunoglobulin G antibodies were measured by an enzyme-linked immunogsorbent assay using Biowhittaker kit and reported as predicted index value, with a value of ≥1 being seropositive.
[n] Results reported in Burrage M, Robinson A, Borrow R, et al. Effect of Vaccination with Carrier Protein on Response to Meningococcal C Conjugate Vaccines and Value of Different Immunoassays as Predictors of Protection. Infection and Immunity. 70(9):4946-54, 2002.
[o] For Tetanus toxoid, n=65.

Pregnancy: Safety during pregnancy has not been established. Meningococcal serogroup C conjugate vaccine is not recommended for use in pregnant women. There is no clinical study data on the use of this vaccine in pregnant women.
Lactation: Safety during lactation has not been established. It is unknown whether vaccine antigens or antibodies are excreted in human milk.
Pediatrics: The safe and effective use of meningococcal serogroup C conjugate vaccine in children below the age of 2 months has not been established.
Geriatrics: Although the vaccine has been studied in adults, studies have not been conducted in adults 65 years or older.
ADVERSE EFFECTS: Adverse Reactions Reported Across All Age Groups Studied: Psychiatric Disorders: Common (≥1% and <10%): irritability.
General Disorders and Administration Site Conditions: Very common (≥10%): injection site erythema; injection site swelling; injection site pain/tenderness. Common (≥1% and <10%): fever ≥38°C.
Additional Reactions Reported in Infants (first year of life) and Toddlers (second year of life): Psychiatric Disorders: Common (≥1% and <10%): crying.
Nervous System Disorders: Very common (≥10%): drowsiness; impaired sleeping.
Gastrointestinal Disorders: Very common (≥10%): vomiting; diarrhea.
Metabolism and Nutrition Disorders: Very common (≥10%): anorexia.
Additional Reactions Reported in Older Age Groups Including Adults (4 to 60 years): Nervous System Disorders: Very Common (≥10%): headache (adults 18 to 60 years). Common (≥1% and <10%): headache (children between 3.5 and 6 years); somnolence.
Musculoskeletal, Connective Tissue and Bone Disorders: Common (≥1% and <10%): myalgia.
Clinical Trials: In all age groups studied, injection site reactions (including redness, swelling and tenderness/pain) were very common. (See Table 3 and Table 6.) Tenderness/pain was the most frequently reported injection site reaction, occurring in approximately 2 of every 10 infants and toddlers and approximately 6 of every 10 older subjects. However, injection site reactions were not usually clinically significant. Redness or swelling of at least 3 cm and tenderness interfering with movement for more than 48 hours was infrequent where studied.

Fever of at least 38.0°C was much more common in infants and toddlers (1 of every 3 or 4 subjects) than in older age groups (1 of every 100 subjects). Temperatures did not usually exceed 39.1°C, particularly in older subjects.
Infants: Table 3 presents the summary of clinical safety data from six studies in infants who received up to three immunizations with Meningitec beginning at the age of 2 months. The reactions listed were the results of specific symptom inquiry by the clinical investigators. Symptoms including crying, irritability, drowsiness, impaired sleeping, anorexia, diarrhea, and vomiting were observed after vaccination, but there was no evidence that these were related to Meningitec rather than to concomitant vaccines, particularly DTP.

Table 3: Meningitec

Summary of All Solicited Local and Systemic Adverse Reactions Within 4 Days Following Any Dose of Meningitec (All Clinical Trials in Infants)

Solicited Adverse Reactions[a]	Incidence (No. with Event/No. Doses Evaluated)	
Injection Site		
Pain (Any) Significant (Interfered With Limb Movement)	20% 5%	(2058/10548) (492/10548)
Redness/Erythema (Any) Significant (≥2.5 cm)	12% 1%	(1263/10724) (126/10724)
Swelling/Induration (Any) Significant (≥2.5 cm)	8% 1%	(849/10720) (148/10720)
Febrile Reactions		
Temperature ≥38.0°C	25%	(2786/10978)
Significant (≥39.1°C)	2%	(192/10978)
Use of Antipyretic Medication	50%	(419/837)
Systemic Reactions		
Increased Crying	70%	(376/537)
Irritability	62%	(6822/11060)
Drowsiness	36%	(4026/11039)
Slept Through Feed	28%	(97/349)
Impaired Sleeping	23%	(2366/10387)
Anorexia	22%	(2423/11049)
Vomiting	14%	(1468/10699)
Diarrhea	10%	(1037/10382)
Unusual High-pitched Cry	2%	(5/299)
Urticaria	<1%	(82/10531)
Blue Skin Tone	<1%	(5/10232)
Convulsions	<1%	(1/10531)
Prolonged Crying	<1%	(98/10709)
Shortness of Breath	<1%	(29/10531)
Twitching	<1%	(10/10232)
Weak/Lethargic/Limp	<1%	(10/10232)

[a] Infants usually received concurrent routine childhood vaccines, including Diphtheria-Tetanus-Pertussis (whole cell) Vaccine (DTP), Diphtheria-Tetanus-Pertussis (acellular) Vaccine (DTaP), Haemophilus b Conjugate Vaccine (Hib), Hepatitis B Vaccine (HBV), Oral Polio Vaccine (OPV), and/or Inactivated Polio Vaccine (IPV). Local reactions were assessed only at the site of Meningitec injection.

In a randomized controlled clinical study performed in the United States (Kaiser Study D118 P8), the profile for Meningitec administered at 2, 4, and 6 months of age with concomitant DTP/HIB (Trivax mixed with HibTITER) or DTaP (Acel-Imune) was similar to that observed in other infant studies. (See Table 4 and Table 5.) The incidence of local reactions was somewhat lower in the Meningitec recipients than in the control Prevnar (7-Valent Pneumococcal Conjugate) vaccine recipients. Pain, redness, and swelling were more common after doses of DTP/Hib than after Meningitec or Prevnar doses, whereas these three local reactions occurred with similar frequencies after doses of DTaP and doses of Meningitec. The most frequently reported systemic reactions were irritability, drowsiness, fever, impaired sleeping, and anorexia, which occurred with similar frequency in Meningitec and Prevnar vaccine recipients.

Table 4: Meningitec

Comparative Local Reactogenicity Profile in Infants Within 4 Days Following Any Dose (Study D118 P8)

Local Reactions[a]	Incidence (No. with Event/No. Doses Evaluated) Meningitec Group		Prevnar Group	
Concurrent DTP/Hib	**Meningitec Site**	**DTP/Hib Site**	**Prevnar Site**	**DTP/Hib Site**
Pain/Tenderness (Any)	20% (1641/8087)	29% (2380/8087)	26% (2146/8153)	33% (2715/8153)
Significant (Interfered with Limb Movement)	5% (424/8087)	7% (595/8087)	8% (628/8153)	10% (792/8153)
Redness (Any)	12% (949/8087)	26% (2065/8087)	14% (1134/8153)	24% (1990/8153)
Significant (≥2.5 cm)	1% (94/8087)	4% (305/8087)	1% (113/8153)	4% (324/8153)
Swelling (Any)	9% (696/8087)	24% (1920/8087	12% (975/8153)	23% (1865/8153)
Significant (≥2.5 cm)	2% (128/8087)	6% (512/8087)	3% (214/8153)	7% (531/8153)
Concurrent DTaP	**Meningitec Site**	**DTaP Site**	**Prevnar Site**	**DTaP Site**

(cont'd)

Table 4: Meningitec *(cont'd)*

Comparative Local Reactogenicity Profile in Infants Within 4 Days Following Any Dose (Study D118 P8)

	Incidence (No. with Event/No. Doses Evaluated)			
Local Reactions[a]	**Meningitec Group**		**Prevnar Group**	
Pain/Tenderness (Any)	16% (242/1557)	16% (251/1557)	18% (288/1641)	9% (149/1641)
Significant (Interfered with Limb Movement)	2% (35/1557)	2% (31/1557)	3% (56/1641)	<1% (10/1641)
Redness (Any)	8% (117/1557)	8% (123/1557)	11% (188/1641)	9% (145/1641)
Significant (≥2.5 cm)	1% (17/1557)	1% (20/1557)	1% (18/1641)	1% (23/1641)
Swelling (Any)	5% (80/1557)	6% (97/1557)	11% (175/1641)	16% (257/1641)
Significant (≥2.5 cm)	<1% (6/1557)	<1% (15/1557)	2% (28/1641)	2% (37/1641)

[a] Local reactions may also have occurred due to concurrent administration of HBV in the same limb as DTP/Hib (Tetramune) or DTaP (Acel-Imune), in some subjects.

Table 5: Meningitec

Comparative Systemic Reactogenicity Profile in Infants Within 4 Days Following Any Dose (Study D118 P8)

	Incidence (No. with Event/No. Doses Evaluated)	
Systemic Reactions[a]	**Meningitec**	**7VPnC**
Irritability	65% (5378/8328)	70% (5862/8382)
Drowsiness	36% (3035/8317)	36% (3046/8363)
Temperature ≥38.0°C	29% (2449/8322)	36% (3019/8370)
Impaired Sleeping	24% (1981/8317)	26% (2163/8363)
Anorexia	23% (1926/8329)	25% (2094/8375)
Vomiting	14% (1171/8332)	17% (1389/8376)
Diarrhea	10% (861/8327)	11% (960/8362)
Temperature ≥39.1°C	2% (171/8322)	3% (260/8344)
Urticaria	<1% (69/8334)	<1% (79/8382)
Prolonged Crying	<1% (42/8263)	<1% (50/8305)
Shortness of Breath	<1% (17/8334)	<1% (14/8382)
Weak/Lethargic/Limp	<1% (9/8334)	<1% (6/8382)
Twitching	<1% (9/8334)	<1% (5/8382)
Blue Skin Tone	<1% (4/8334)	<1% (5/8382)
Convulsions	<1% (1/8334)	<1% (9/8382)
Gray/Ashen Skin Tone	0% (0/8334)	<1% (2/8382)

[a] Systemic reactions may also have occurred due to concurrent administration of routine childhood vaccines, including Diphtheria-Tetanus-Pertussis (whole cell) Vaccine (DTP), Diphtheria-Tetanus-Pertussis (acellular) Vaccine (DTaP), Haemophilus b Conjugate Vaccine (Hib), Hepatitis B Vaccine (HBV), Oral Polio Vaccine (OPV), and/or Inactivated Polio Vaccine (IPV).

Toddlers Through Adults: Table 6 and Table 7 present analysis of local reactions and systemic reactions, respectively, occurring in toddlers and older subjects after one immunization with Meningitec. Data are pooled from seven studies, representing approximately 1100 subjects. The local and febrile reactions listed for both age groups, and the systemic reactions listed for toddlers, were the results of specific symptom inquiry by the clinical investigators. The systemic reactions listed for older subjects were spontaneously reported to the investigators.

The systemic events commonly reported for toddlers (irritability, impaired sleeping, anorexia, drowsiness) were similar to those reported for infants. Commonly reported systemic events in older subjects included headache, drowsiness, myalgia, and vomiting.

Table 6: Meningitec

Summary of Solicited Local and Febrile Reactions Within 4 Days Following One Dose of Meningitec in Toddlers and Older Subjects

	Incidence (No. with Event/No. of Doses Evaluated)	
	13–24 Months	**4–60 Years**
Injection Site		
Pain (Any)	21% (211/991)	63% (123/196)
Significant (Interfered With Limb Movement)	9% (83/919)	7% (1/15)
Redness/Erythema (Any)	9% (94/992)	36% (72/202)
Significant (≥2.5 cm)	1% (6/992)	13% (27/202)
Swelling/Induration (Any)	7% (73/992)	16% (33/202)
Significant (≥2.5 cm)	2% (15/992)	7% (15/202)

(cont'd)

Table 6: Meningitec *(cont'd)*

Summary of Solicited Local and Febrile Reactions Within 4 Days Following One Dose of Meningitec in Toddlers and Older Subjects

	Incidence (No. with Event/No. of Doses Evaluated)	
	13–24 Months	**4–60 Years**
Febrile Reactions		
Temperature ≥38.0°C	30% (337/1136)	1% (3/202)
Significant (≥39.1°C)	4% (41/1136)	0% (0/202)
Use of Antipyretic Medication	41% (26/63)	7% (1/15)

Table 7: Meningitec

Summary of Solicited Systemic Reactions Within 4 Days (Toddlers) and Unsolicited Systemic Reactions Within 4 Weeks (Older Subjects) Following One Dose of Meningitec

	Incidence (No. with Event/No. of Doses Evaluated)	
	13–24 Months	**4–60 Years**[a]
Irritability	55% (635/1165)	2% (5/237)
Impaired Sleeping	25% (270/1100)	None
Anorexia	23% (270/1162)	1% (2/237)
Drowsiness/Somnolence	20% (227/1163)	3% (7/237)
Diarrhea	11% (114/1026)	2% (5/237)
Vomiting	6% (67/1164)	3% (7/237)
Increased Crying	3% (2/73)	None
Urticaria	1% (11/1092)	None
Prolonged Crying	<1% (4/1086)	None
Shortness of Breath/Dyspnea	<1% (1/1092)	1% (2/237)
Twitching	<1% (1/1029)	None
Headache	Not queried	13% (31/237)
Pharyngitis	Not queried	5% (12/237)
Myalgia	Not queried	3% (7/237)
Rhinitis	Not queried	3% (7/237)
Bronchospasm	Not queried	2% (5/237)
Dyspepsia	Not queried	2% (2/237)
Infection Viral	Not queried	2% (5/237)
Otitis Media	Not queried	2% (5/237)
Abdominal Pain	Not queried	1% (2/237)
Infection	Not queried	1% (2/237)
Malaise	Not queried	1% (2/237)
Trauma	Not queried	1% (2/237)
Nausea	Not queried	1% (2/237)
Upper Respiratory Tract Infection	Not queried	1% (2/237)

[a] The rates shown are for unsolicited reactions that occurred in 1% or more of subjects.

Children between the ages of 25 months and 47 months were not included as subjects in clinical trials, and therefore no safety information from clinical trials is available for this age group.

Post-marketing Surveillance (for all age groups): The frequencies given below are based on spontaneous reporting rates for Meningitec in the UK and have been calculated using number of reports received as the numerator and number of doses of Meningitec distributed as the denominator.

Blood and Lymphatic System Disorders: Very rare (<0.01%): lymphadenopathy.

Immune: Very rare (<0.01%): anaphylactic/anaphylactoid reaction including shock; hypersensitivity reactions including bronchospasm, facial edema and angioedema.

Nervous System: Very rare (<0.01%): dizziness; convulsions including febrile convulsions and seizures in patients with pre-existing stable seizure disorder; hypoesthesia and/or paraesthesia; hypotonia.

General Disorders and Administration Site Conditions: Very rare (<0.01%): injection site vesicles; injection site dermatitis; injection site hypersensitivity, including urticaria; injection site induration; injection site inflammation; injection site mass; injection site pruritus.

Musculoskeletal, Connective Tissue and Bone Disorders: Very rare (<0.01%): arthralgia.

Renal and Urinary Disorders: Relapse of nephrotic syndrome has been reported in association with Meningococcal serogroup C conjugate vaccines.

Skin and Subcutaneous Tissue Disorders: Very rare (<0.01%): rash, pruritus, erythema multiforme, Stevens-Johnson syndrome.

Gastrointestinal: Very rare (<0.01%): nausea, abdominal pain.

There have been very rare spontaneous reports of hypotonia (including hypotonic-hyporesponsive episode [HHE]) in temporal association with the administration of meningococcal serogroup C conjugate vaccine. In most cases, meningococcal serogroup C conjugate vaccine was administered concomitantly with other vaccines, the majority of which were pertussis-containing vaccines.

There have been spontaneous reports of very rare petechiae and/or purpura following immunization in the postmarketing experience. Since meningococcal serogroup C conjugate vaccine may not protect against 100% of meningococcal serogroup C disease or disease due to organisms other than *N. meningitidis* serogroup C, individuals who experience petechiae and/or purpura following vaccination should be thoroughly evaluated for the possibility of an infectious or other cause unrelated to vaccination.

As with other pediatric vaccines, there have been spontaneous reports of apnea in temporal association with the administration of meningococcal serogroup C conjugate vaccine. In most cases meningococcal serogroup C conjugate vaccine was administered concomitantly with other vaccines including diphtheria tetanus pertussis vaccine (DTP), inactivated polio vaccine (IPV), oral polio vaccine (OPV), Haemophilus influenzae type b vaccine (Hib), diphtheria tetanus pertussis—Haemophilus influenzae type b vaccine (DTP-Hib), and/or diphtheria tetanus acellular pertussis—hepatitis B vaccine (DTaP-HBV). In addition, in most of the reports existing medical conditions such as history of apnea, infection, prematurity, and/or seizures were present.

OVERDOSE:

There have been reports of overdosage with meningococcal serogroup C conjugate vaccine. Most cases have involved inadvertent revaccination at varying intervals following initial vaccination. Most individuals were asymptomatic. Of the events reported, the majority have also occurred with recommended single doses of meningococcal serogroup C conjugate vaccine.

For management of a suspected drug overdose, CPhA recommends that you contact your **regional Poison Control Centre**. See the *CPS* Directory section for a list of Poison Control Centres.

DOSAGE: The dosage is 0.5 mL given intramuscularly, with care to avoid injection into or near nerves and blood vessels. The vaccine should not be injected in the gluteal area because of the potential risk of injury to the sciatic nerve. The vaccine should not be injected intravenously. Furthermore, the safety and immunogenicity of the intradermal or subcutaneous routes have not been evaluated.

Infants Under the Age of 12 Months: Two doses, each of 0.5 mL, the first dose given not earlier than 2 months and with an interval of at least 2 months between doses.

For Previously Unvaccinated Children Over the Age of 12 Months, Adolescents and Adults: A single dose of 0.5 mL.

Booster Dose: A booster dose should be given after completion of the primary immunization series in infants. The timing of this dose should be in accordance with official recommendations whenever available and preferably at about 12 months of age. The need for further boosters has not yet been established. The need for booster doses in subjects primed with a single dose (i.e. aged 12 months or more when first immunized) has not yet been established.

Method of Administration: Meningitec (Meningococcal Serogroup C-CRM$_{197}$ conjugate vaccine) is a sterile suspension containing an adjuvant. Shake vigorously immediately prior to use to obtain a uniform suspension in the vaccine container. After shaking, the vaccine is a homogeneous, white suspension. The vaccine should not be used if it cannot be resuspended. Parenteral products should be inspected visually for particulate matter and discoloration prior to administration. This product should not be used if particulate matter or discoloration is found.

For the vial presentation, the vaccine is to be administered immediately after being drawn up into a syringe.

The recommended dose is 0.5 mL given intramuscularly. This vaccine should not be injected intradermally, subcutaneously or intravenously since the safety and immunogenicity of these routes have not been evaluated.

The preferred sites are the anterolateral aspect of the thigh in infants or in the deltoid muscle of the upper arm in older children, adolescents and adults. The vaccine should not be injected in the gluteal area or areas where there may be a major nerve trunk and/or blood vessel.

Meningitec should not be mixed with other vaccines or products in the syringe. Separate injection sites should be used if more than one vaccine is being administered.

Before injection, the skin at the injection site should be cleansed and prepared with a suitable germicide. After insertion of the needle, aspirate and wait to see if any blood appears in the syringe, which will help avoid inadvertent injection into a blood vessel. If blood appears, withdraw the needle, discard the syringe and prepare for a new injection at another site.

SUPPLIED: Meningitec (Meningococcal Serogroup C-CRM$_{197}$ conjugate vaccine) is a sterile suspension of the *N. meningitidis* serogroup C oligosaccharide conjugated to *C. diphtheriae* CRM$_{197}$ protein. CRM$_{197}$ is a non-toxic variant of diphtheria toxin isolated from cultures of *C. diphtheriae* strain C7(β197) grown in a casamino acids and yeast-based medium. CRM$_{197}$ is purified through ultra filtration, ammonium sulfate precipitation, and ion-exchange chromatography to high purity.

The liquid suspension contains: *N. meningitidis* serogroup C oligosaccharide 10 µg and diphtheria, CRM$_{197}$ 15 µg. Nonmedicinal ingredients: aluminum phosphate, sodium chloride and Water for Injection. After shaking, the vaccine is a homogenous white suspension. The vaccine does not contain a preservative. Pre-filled syringes(type I glass) with a plunger rod (polypropylene) and a plunger stopper (grey butyl rubber) of 0.5 mL, packages of 10.

Store at 2 to 8°C. Do not freeze. Discard if the vaccine has been frozen. When stored under labelled condition, Meningitec is stable until the expiration date indicated on the container label. Keep out of the reach of children.

Menjugate®

meningococcal group C—CRM197 conjugate vaccine

Active Immunizing Agent

Novartis Pharmaceuticals

Date of Preparation: June 30, 2009

SUMMARY PRODUCT INFORMATION:

Route of Administration	Dosage Form/ Strength	Clinically Relevant Nonmedicinal Ingredients
Intramuscular (IM) Injection	Powder for Suspension for reconstitution with a diluent 10 µg Meningococcal Group C Oligosaccharide conjugated to 12.5 to 25 µg CRM197	Aluminum hydroxide adjuvant For a complete listing see Dosage Forms, Composition and Packaging.

INDICATIONS AND CLINICAL USE: Menjugate (Meningococcal Group C-CRM197 Conjugate Vaccine) is indicated for the active immunization of children from 2 months of age, adolescents and adults, for the prevention of invasive disease caused by *N. meningitidis* serogroup C.

CONTRAINDICATIONS: Menjugate (Meningococcal Group C-CRM197 Conjugate Vaccine) is contraindicated in persons with a known hypersensitivity to any component of the vaccine and in persons who have shown signs of hypersensitivity after previous administration of Menjugate.

As with other vaccines, administration of Menjugate should be postponed in subjects with an acute severe febrile illness.

WARNINGS AND PRECAUTIONS: General: Before the injection of any biological, the health professional responsible for administration should take all precautions known for the prevention of allergic or any other reactions. As with all injectable vaccines, appropriate medical treatment and supervision should always be readily available in case of a rare anaphylactic event following administration of the vaccine.

Prior to administration of any dose of Menjugate (Meningococcal Group C-CRM 197 Conjugate Vaccine), the vaccine recipient (or parent or guardian) should be asked about personal history, family history, and recent health status, including immunization history, current health status and any adverse event associated with previous immunizations.

Menjugate (Meningococcal Group C-CRM197 Conjugate Vaccine) will not protect against meningococcal diseases caused by any of the other types of meningococcal bacteria (A, B, 29-E, H, I, K, L, W-135, X, Y, or Z, including non-typed). Complete protection against meningococcal serogroup C infection cannot be guaranteed.

Although symptoms of meningism such as neck pain/stiffness or photophobia have been reported, there is no evidence that the vaccine causes meningococcal C meningitis. Clinical alertness to the possibility of co-incidental meningitis should therefore be maintained.

Conjugate vaccines containing Cross Reacting Material 197 (CRM197) should not be considered as immunizing agents against diphtheria. No changes in the schedule for administering vaccines containing diphtheria toxoid are recommended.

Any acute infection or febrile illness is reason for delaying the use of Menjugate except when, in the opinion of the physician, withholding the vaccine entails a greater risk. A minor afebrile illness, such as a mild upper respiratory infection, is not usually reason to defer immunization.

The vaccine must not be injected intravenously, subcutaneously or intradermally.

Parents should be informed of the immunization schedule for this vaccine. Precautions such as use of antipyretic measures should be relayed to the parent or guardian, as well as the need to report any adverse event.

The tip cap of the diluent syringe contains 10% Dry Natural Rubber. Although the risk for developing allergic latex reactions is very small, healthcare professionals are encouraged to consider the benefit risk prior to administering this vaccine to patients with known history of hypersensitivity to latex.

Hematologic: Menjugate has not been evaluated in persons with thrombocytopenia or other bleeding disorders. The risk versus benefit for persons at risk of hemorrhage following intramuscular injection must be evaluated.

Immune: In individuals deficient in antibody production, vaccination may not result in an appropriate protective antibody response. While HIV infection is not a contraindication to vaccination, Menjugate has not been specifically evaluated in an immunocompromised population.

Individuals with complement deficiencies and individuals with functional or anatomical asplenia may mount an immune response to meningococcal C conjugate vaccines; however, the degree of protection that would be afforded is unknown.

Special Populations: Pregnant Women: Animal studies have not demonstrated a risk to the fetus following administration of Menjugate. However, since no specific studies in humans have been carried out, caution is advised. The vaccine should not be used during pregnancy unless there is defined risk of meningococcal C disease, in which case the risk-benefit ratio should be evaluated.

Nursing Women: The effect on breast-fed infants of the administration of Menjugate to their mothers has not been studied. The risk-benefit ratio should be examined before making the decision as to whether to immunize during lactation.

Geriatrics (>65 years of age): There are no data in adults aged 65 years and older.

ADVERSE REACTIONS: Clinical Trial Adverse Drug Reactions: Because clinical trials are conducted under very specific conditions the adverse reaction rates observed in the clinical trials may not reflect the rates observed in practice and should not be compared to the rates in the clinical trials of another drug. Adverse drug reaction information from clinical trials is useful for identifying drug-related adverse events and for approximating rates.

In controlled clinical studies performed in all age groups, signs and symptoms were actively monitored and recorded on diary cards following administration of the vaccine.

Of the local solicited symptoms, the most frequently reported were injection-site pain, erythema and swelling, which were normally mild and resolved within 24-72 hours following vaccination.

The general symptoms that have been solicited and reported were predominantly mild and resolved spontaneously. These include headache, malaise, nausea, arthralgia and myalgia in adolescents and adults; and irritability, change in appetite, diarrhea and fever in younger children. These solicited general symptoms were also reported in the control groups and have been reported when Menjugate (Meningococcal Group C-CRM197 Conjugate Vaccine) was administered concomitantly with other vaccines.

In infants and toddlers symptoms including crying, irritability, drowsiness, impaired sleeping, anorexia, diarrhea and vomiting were common after vaccination but there was no evidence that these were related to Menjugate rather than concomitant vaccines, particularly DTP.

Toddlers Through Adults: Table 1 presents an analysis of local and systemic reactions occurring within 7 days after one immunization with Menjugate. Data are pooled from 11 studies, representing approximately 1400 subjects. Most local and systemic reactions occurred by day 1 following immunization. In general, lower percentages of local and systemic reactions were present on days 2 through 6 following the first immunization.

Table 1: Menjugate

Summary of Local and Systemic Post immunization Reactions Within 7 Days Following One Immunization of Menjugate, by Age Group at Enrollment[a]

	Percentage of Subjects		
	Menjugate 1–2 years N=942 (%)	**Menjugate 3–5 years N=198 (%)**	**Menjugate 11–64 years N=269 (%)**
Injection Site			
Pain (Any) Severe	22 <1	25 0	81 2
Temperature (Any) Hot	15 <1	5 1	47 8
Erythema (Any) >50 mm	28 <1	16 0	19 1
Induration (Any) >50 mm	16 <1	7 0	24 1
Systemic			
Change in Eating Habits	16	6	—
Sleepiness	19	9	—
Unusual Crying	4	1	—
Persistent Crying	1	0	—
Irritability	30	10	—
Vomiting	9	5	—
Diarrhea	18	8	—
Rash	9	4	—
Chills	—	—	13
Nausea	—	—	16
Malaise	—	—	25
Myalgia	—	—	29
Arthralgia	—	—	16
Headache	—	—	34
Temperature ≥38°C	9	4	2

(cont'd)

Table 1: Menjugate *(cont'd)*

Summary of Local and Systemic Post immunization Reactions Within 7 Days Following One Immunization of Menjugate, by Age Group at Enrollment[a]

	Percentage of Subjects		
	Menjugate 1–2 years N=942 (%)	**Menjugate 3–5 years N=198 (%)**	**Menjugate 11–64 years N=269 (%)**
Stayed Home Due to Reaction	—	—	7
Analgesic/Antipyretic Medication used	25	9	18

[a] This is a summary of data derived from a meta-analysis of 11 studies conducted in the United States, United Kingdom, Netherlands, and Canada. The recording of systemic reactions varied by age group, not all reactions were collected in all studies.

In clinical studies where subjects received Menjugate or a meningococcal polysaccharide vaccine, the rates of local pain and warmth were significantly lower with Menjugate in toddlers and children 3 to 5 years of age; no differences were seen in the older subjects. In children 3 to 5 years of age, severe pain was seen in 9% of subjects with the polysaccharide vaccine and no subjects with Menjugate. The systemic reactions that were significantly less common in Menjugate subjects were fever, change in eating habits, irritability, and analgesic/antipyretic use in toddlers, and irritability and analgesic/antipyretic use in children 3 to 5 years of age.

In adolescents and adults, the rates of all postimmunization reactions were similar after Menjugate or polysaccharide vaccine administration. The only difference seen in this age group was a tendency for injection-site pain to persist somewhat longer in Menjugate recipients (72 hours) than in polysaccharide vaccine recipients (48 hours). This difference may be due to the aluminum hydroxide adjuvant, which is present in Menjugate but not the polysaccharide vaccine.

Infants: Table 2 presents a summary of clinical safety data from two clinical studies in infants who received up to three immunizations with Menjugate, beginning at the age of two months.

Table 2: Menjugate

Summary of Local and Systemic Post immunization Reactions Within 7 Days Following 1, 2 or 3 Injections of Menjugate

	Percentage of Subjects	
	UK (Multicentre) (N=467)	**Canada (Multicentre) (N=175)**
Age at First Immunization	2 months	2 months
Schedule	3 doses 1 month apart	3 doses 2 months apart
Concomitant Vaccine	DTP, HIB, OPV	DTaP, HIB, IPV (Pentacel)
Local Reactions		
Tenderness	31%	22%
Erythema >25 mm	7%	0%
Induration >25 mm	4%	0%
Systemic Reactions		
Irritability	81%	68%
Sleepiness	69%	54%
Change in eating habits	46%	39%
Diarrhea	43%	28%
Vomiting	34%	19%
Rash	16%	—[a]
Temperature ≥38°C	4%	21%
High-pitched crying	38%	—[a]
Persistent crying	16%	4%

[a] Data not collected.

In a randomized, controlled clinical study performed in infants at three centers in Canada, the profile for Menjugate administered at 2, 4, and 6 months of age with concomitant PENTACEL (DTaP/Hib/IPV) was similar to that observed in earlier infant studies (see Table 3 and Table 4). The frequency of two local adverse events, induration and erythema, was higher in Menjugate recipients than in the control HBV vaccine subjects, however the incidence of these reactions was lower among Menjugate or HBV subjects than following the routine vaccine (DTaP/Hib/IPV) in these same subjects. These differences between the Menjugate and HBV groups may in part be related to the lower dose of aluminum hydroxide in the HBV vaccine relative to the Menjugate vaccine (i.e., 0.5 mg per dose in HBV compared with 1 mg per dose in Menjugate). The most frequently reported systemic reactions were irritability, analgesic/antipyretic medication use, sleepiness and change in eating habits, which were reported with similar frequency in Menjugate and HBV vaccine subjects.

Table 3: Menjugate

Local Reactogenicity Within 7 Days Following Any Immunization, Infant Study—Canada (Multicentre)

	Menjugate Group N=175		HBV Group N=176		P-value MenC vs HBV Droup	
Local Reactions	**Menjugate**	**Pentacel**	**HBV**	**Pentacel**	**Study Vaccine**	**Pentacel**
Tendernes (Any) (Cried when injected leg moved)	38 (22%) 0	53 (30%) 3 (2%)	31 (18%) 0	35 (20%) 0	.33	.025
Erythema (Any) >25 mm	55 (31%) 0	67 (38%) 5 (3%)	33 (19%) 0	63 (36%) 4 (3%)	.006	.63
Induration (Any) >25 mm	42 (24%) 0	65 (37%) 6 (3%)	19 (11%) 1 (1%)	70 (40%) 2 (1%)	.001	.61

Table 4: Menjugate

Systemic Reactogenicity Within 7 Days Following Any Immunization, Infant Study—Canada (Multicentre)

Systemic Reactions	Menjugate Group N=175	HBV Group N=176	P-value
Change in Eating Habits	68 (39%)	63 (36%)	.55
Sleepiness	94 (54%)	98 (56%)	.71
Persistent Crying	7 (4%)	4 (2%)	.35
Irritability	119 (68%)	124 (70%)	.62
Vomiting	34 (19%)	39 (22%)	.53
Diarrhea	49 (28%)	44 (25%)	.52
Rectal Temperature ≥38°C	37 (21%)	47 (27%)	.22
Analgesic/antipyretic Medication Required	96 (55%)	105 (60%)	.36

Less Common Clinical Trial Adverse Drug Reactions (<1%): In clinical trials of Menjugate, approximately 6700 infants through adults were evaluated/monitored for the occurrence of serious adverse experiences (SAEs). There were four SAEs which were considered to be at least possibly related to vaccine. These were one report each of: hypotonia, screaming syndrome, maculopapular rash and agitation, all of which occurred in an open label infant study conducted in the United Kingdom (UK), in which Menjugate was administered concomitantly with DTP, Hib and OPV vaccines. Because these reactions have been reported previously in conjunction with DTP vaccines alone, a causal relationship between these experiences and Menjugate administration cannot be established.

Post-Market Adverse Drug Reactions: The most commonly reported suspected reactions in post marketing surveillance include dizziness, pyrexia, headache, nausea, vomiting and faints.

The frequencies given below are based on spontaneous reporting rates, for this and other Meningococcal C Conjugate vaccines and have been calculated using the number of reports received as the numerator and the total number of doses distributed as the denominator.

Immune System Disorders: Very rare (<0.01%): lymphadenopathy, anaphylaxis, hypersensitivity reactions including bronchospasm, facial edema and angioedema.

Neurologic: Very rare (<0.01%): dizziness, convulsions including febrile convulsions, faints, hypesthesia, paresthesia and hypotonia.

There have been very rare reports of seizures following Menjugate vaccination; individuals have usually recovered rapidly. Some of the reported seizures may have been faints. The reporting rate of seizures was below the background rate of epilepsy in children. In infants seizures were usually associated with fever and were likely to be febrile convulsions.

There have been very rare reports of visual disturbances and photophobia following vaccination with Meningococcal group C conjugate vaccines, usually in conjugation with other neurological symptoms like headache and dizziness.

Skin and Subcutaneous Tissue Disorders: Very rare (<0.01%): rash, urticaria, pruritus, purpura, erythema multiforme and Stevens-Johnson Syndrome.

Gastrointestinal: Very rare (<0.01%): nausea, vomiting and diarrhea.

Musculoskeletal, Connective Tissue and Bone Disorders: Very rare (<0.01%): myalgia and arthralgia.

Renal: Relapse of nephrotic syndrome has been reported in association with Meningococcal group C conjugate vaccines.

DRUG INTERACTIONS: Drug-Drug Interactions: Administration of Menjugate at the same time as IPV, DTP, Hib, DTaP, DT, Td, MMR and HBV vaccines or with OPV does not reduce immunological responses to any of these other antigens. Menjugate should not however, be administered via the same injection as other vaccines. Minor variations in GMT antibody titers were observed between studies; however, the clinical significance, if any, of these observations is not established.

Table 5 presents data on the immunological response of infants to concomitant vaccines, as measured one month after the third dose of Menjugate or HBV vaccine.

Table 5: Menjugate

Response to Routine Infant Concomitant Vaccine (PENTACEL) Antigens Among Menjugate vs HBV Vaccine Recipients Measured at 1 Month After Third Dose. Infant Study—Canada (Multicenter)

Concomitant Vaccine Antigen, Measure of Response		Group		
		MenC	**HBV**	**P-value**
		N=64	**N=61**	
Polio type I	% with antibody titers ≥1:8	97%	95%	.53
Polio type II	% with antibody titers ≥1:8	98%	100%	.32
Polio type III	% with antibody titers ≥1:8	98%	98%	.94
Diphtheria toxin antibody responses	GMT (IU/mL)	4.7	1.9	<.001
	% ≥0.10 IU/mL	100%	100%	1.0
Tetanus antibody response	GMT (IU/mL)	2.4	2.5	.76
	% ≥0.1 IU/mL	100%	100%	1.0
		N=91	**N=89**	
Anti-pertussis with 69K antigen	GMT (EU/mL)	31	36	.29
Anti-pertussis with FHA antigen	GMT (EU/mL)	26	31	.12
Anti-pertussis with PT antigen	GMT (EU/mL)	23	25	.31
		N=148	**N=148**	
PRP-T/Hib antibody responses	GMT (µg/mL)	3.1	3.7	.28
	% ≥1.0 mg/mL	81%	83%	.40

DOSAGE AND ADMINISTRATION: Dosing Considerations: There are no data on the use of different meningococcal group C conjugate vaccines within the primary series or for boosting. Whenever possible, the same vaccine should be used throughout.

Recommended Dose and Dosage Adjustment: Primary Immunization: Infants 2-12 months should receive 3 doses of 0.5 mL each, with an interval of at least 1 month between doses.

Children older than 12 months, adolescents and adults should receive a single dose of 0.5 mL.

Booster Doses: It is recommended that a booster dose should be given after completion of the primary immunization series in infants. The timing of this booster should be in accordance with NACI recommendations. The need for booster doses in subjects primed with a single dose (i.e. aged 12 months or more when first immunized) has not yet been established.

Administration: Do not inject intravenously, subcutaneously or intradermally. Menjugate (Meningococcal Group C-CRM197 Conjugate Vaccine) is to be administered by deep intramuscular injection only, preferably in the anterolateral thigh in infants and in the deltoid region in older children, adolescents and adults.

Care must be taken to ensure the vaccine is not injected into a blood vessel.

Menjugate should not be mixed with other vaccines in the same syringe. Separate injection sites should be used if more than one vaccine is being administered on the same date.

Reconstitution:

Vial Size	Volume of Diluent to be Added to Vial	Approximate Available Volume	Nominal Concentration per mL
3 mL vial containing lyophilised vaccine	0.6 mL	0.5 mL following reconstitution	Meningococcal Group C Oligosaccharide (20 µg) conjugated to CRM197 (25.0 to 50.0 µg)

The following instructions should be adhered to with respect to the reconstitution of lyophilized Menjugate. Use aseptic technique.

Vial of Vaccine Plus Vial of Diluent: Gently agitate the aluminum hydroxide diluent vial. Withdraw 0.6 mL of the suspension and inject it into the Menjugate vial. Gently shake the vial until the cake is dissolved (this will ensure the antigen is bound to the adjuvant). Withdraw 0.5 mL of reconstituted vaccine.

Vial of Vaccine Plus Syringe of Diluent: Gently agitate the syringe containing the aluminum hydroxide diluent. Remove the tip cap from the syringe and attach a suitable needle. Use the whole content of the syringe (0.6 mL of suspension) to reconstitute the Menjugate vial.

Gently shake the reconstituted vial until the vaccine is dissolved (this will ensure the antigen is bound to the adjuvant). Taking care not to withdraw the plunger completely out of the barrel of the syringe, withdraw the full contents of the vial into the syringe. Note that it is normal for a small residual amount of liquid to remain in the vial following withdrawal of the dose. The amount of reconstituted vaccine in the syringe can be compared to the scale in the drawing below, to confirm that a sufficient dose of the vaccine has been withdrawn. See Figure 1.

Figure 1: Menjugate

Recommended Dose (0.5 mL)

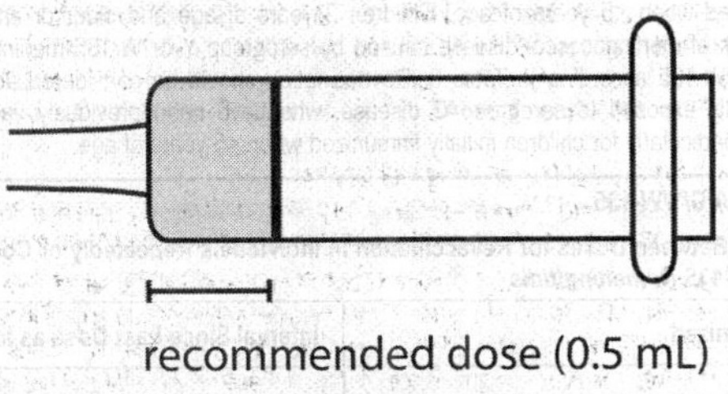

A new needle with a gauge and length suitable for intramuscular injection should be used to administer the product. Ensure that no air bubbles are present in the syringe before injecting the vaccine.

Following reconstitution, Menjugate should be used immediately.

OVERDOSAGE:

There is no experience of overdosage with Menjugate.

> For management of a suspected drug overdose, CPhA recommends that you contact your **regional Poison Control Centre**. See the *CPS* Directory section for a list of Poison Control Centres.

ACTION AND CLINICAL PHARMACOLOGY: Mechanism of Action: Menjugate (Meningococcal Group C-CRM197 Conjugate Vaccine) is intended for the prevention of meningitis and/or septicemia caused by *N. meningitidis* group C in infants and older age groups. Menjugate is composed of meningococcal group C oligosaccharides conjugated to a protein carrier, a non-toxic mutant of diphtheria toxin, CRM197. In the final vaccine, aluminum hydroxide is used as an adjuvant.

As shown in clinical trials, Menjugate is highly immunogenic and induces protective levels of bactericidal antibodies in a significant number of subjects after vaccination.

Compared to licensed unconjugated polysaccharide vaccines, the primary immune response induced by Menjugate is superior in toddlers, children and adolescents, and is comparable in adults.

Additionally, unlike unconjugated polysaccharide vaccines, Menjugate has been shown to induce immunologic memory in infants, toddlers and older children.

No pharmacodynamic or pharmacokinetic studies have been conducted with Menjugate, in accordance with its status as a vaccine. Several immunogenicity studies were conducted in animals, showing that Menjugate induced antibody titers that were dose dependent.

STORAGE AND STABILITY: Primary Storage Condition: Store under refrigeration (+2 to +8°C). Do not freeze. Protect from exposure to light. Stability studies have indicated that the lyophilized product has a shelf life of 36 months. Menjugate vials and the vials or syringes of aluminum hydroxide diluent may have different expiry dates, so health care professionals are advised that the outer carton bears the earlier of the two dates and that this date must be respected. The carton and **all** its contents should be discarded on reaching this outer carton expiry date.

Alternative Storage Condition (Before Reconstitution): Do not store above 25°C. Do not freeze. Protect from exposure to light. The product should be used or discarded within 6 months of the date of removal from the refrigerator (+2 to +8°C) or on reaching the outer carton expiry date (whichever comes first).

INFORMATION FOR THE PATIENT: Published in e-CPS, available by subscription at www.e-cps.ca.

DOSAGE FORMS, COMPOSITION AND PACKAGING: Menjugate is supplied as a 0.5 mL dose, consisting of one vial of vaccine and one vial or syringe of diluent.

The product is provided as a vial of sterile white lyophilised powder (Menjugate) together with a vial or syringe of aluminium hydroxide diluent. The diluent is a sterile white opalescent suspension. Following reconstitution the vaccine is a slightly opaque homogeneous suspension, free from foreign particles.

Each single dose (0.5 mL) of reconstituted vaccine contains: *N. meningitidis* group C (strain C11) oligosaccharide 10 µg conjugated to 12.5 to 25 µg *C. diphtheriae* CRM-197 protein. Nonmedicinal ingredients: disodium phosphate heptahydrate, sodium chloride, sodium dihydrogen phosphate monohydrate, mannitol and Water for Injections. The lyophilized product is to be reconstituted with an adjuvant diluent containing aluminum hydroxide (1 mg/0.5 mL dose). Contains no preservative.

Both the diluent and the lyophilized vaccine are presented in Type I glass vials, with bromobutyl rubber stoppers. The diluent can also be presented in Type I glass syringes with Type I rubber plunger stoppers and tip caps. The tip cap of the diluent syringe contains 10% Dry Natural Rubber. Vial of vaccine plus vial of diluent: pack sizes containing 1 and 5 doses. Vial of vaccine plus syringe of diluent: pack sizes containing 1 dose.

Menomune®-A/C/Y/W-135

meningococcal polysaccharide vaccine, groups A, C, Y and W-135 combined

Active Immunizing Agent

sanofi pasteur

Date of Revision: October 2005

PHARMACOLOGY: *N. meningitidis* causes both endemic and epidemic disease, principally meningitis and meningococcemia. Invasive meningococcal disease is endemic in Canada, and periods of increased activity occur roughly every 10 to 15 years but with no consistent pattern. The incidence of invasive meningococcal disease has varied considerably with different serogroups, age groups, geographic locations and time. Since the last major epidemic of group A meningococcal disease in 1940-1943, the overall incidence has remained at or below 2 per 100 000 population per year. Since 1986, serogroups B and C have been responsible for most of the cases of endemic disease in Canada. The incidence of serogroup C disease has been highest among children <1 year of age (14.8 per 100 000 per year), and has declined with age, except for a smaller peak in the 15 to 19 year age group (2.3 per 100 000 per year). One third of cases occurred in people >20 years. An increasing trend in serogroup Y disease has been observed in the United States during the past decade. In Canada, serogroup Y represented approximately 1-15% of isolates characterized from 1993-2000, however an increased incidence was reported in Ontario in 2001, with serogroup Y disease accounting for 30% of laboratory confirmations during the first 4 months of 2001. Both serogroup A and W-135 (1-12 cases/year) invasive meningococcal disease are reported uncommonly in Canada.

Globally, there are around 1.2 million cases of meningococcal disease annually. Although the disease occurs throughout the world, the most frequent and largest epidemics occur in the African meningitis belt, which includes all or part of 18 sub-Saharan countries. In this area, the majority of outbreaks are caused by *N. meningitidis* serogroup A along with a smaller contribution by serogroup C. More recently, countries in Africa outside of the "meningitis belt" have been affected by epidemic disease as a result of cross-border spread. Since 2000, cases of serogroup W-135 invasive meningococcal disease have been reported in Saudi Arabia and subsequently in various other countries around the world. An epidemiologic association with international travel to Saudi Arabia or close contacts with pilgrims was established in most of these cases. During 2002, a meningitis epidemic associated with W-135 was reported in Burkina Faso, and W-135 has now emerged as an epidemic strain in Africa.

Certain immunodeficiencies result in a marked increase in the risk of meningococcal disease, these may include complement deficiencies (and properdin deficiency), hypogammaglobulinemia, anatomic and functional asplenia (e.g., sickle-cell disease). Individuals with human immunodeficiency virus may also be at increased risk for sporadic meningococcal disease. Persons with cochlear implants have recently been identified as being at greater risk for meningitis.

An elevated risk of meningococcal disease has been observed in the US among freshmen living in dormitories and university students in halls of residence in the UK. Clusters of cases of meningococcal disease in students have been reported in a number of countries and carriage rates increase rapidly amongst freshmen during the first week of the term in the UK. In this age group in Canada, as in other countries, there is an increase of the rate of meningococcal disease infection. In US studies, as much as 83% of cases that occurred in this age group (15-24 years) were potentially vaccine preventable. Infection in this age group was associated with an unusually high case fatality ratio.

Several discoveries affected the future of meningococcal polysaccharide vaccines and demonstrated the significance of anti-capsular antibodies in protection. In the late 1930s, serogroup-specific antigens of meningococcal serogroups A and C were identified as polysaccharides. During the mid 1940s, investigators demonstrated that the protection of mice by anti-serogroup A meningococcal horse serum was directly related to its content of anti-polysaccharide antibodies. Meningococcal polysaccharide vaccines were first demonstrated to be immunogenic in humans by Gotschlich and his co-workers in the 1960s when immunization of US army recruits with serogroup A and C polysaccharides induced protective antibodies. The investigators recorded a significantly reduced acquisition rate of serogroup C carriage among vaccinated recruits compared with unvaccinated persons.

Vaccine Efficacy: The immunogenicity and clinical efficacy of serogroups A and C meningococcal vaccines have been well established. The serogroup A polysaccharide induces antibody in some children as young as 3 months of age, although a response comparable with that among adults is not achieved until 4 or 5 years of age; the serogroup C component is poorly immunogenic in recipients who are less than 18 to 24 months of age. The serogroups A and C vaccines have demonstrated estimated clinical efficacies of 85% to 100% in older children and adults and are useful in controlling epidemics. Serogroups Y and W-135 polysaccharides are safe and immunogenic in adults and in children greater than 2 years of age. Although clinical protection has not been documented, vaccination with these polysaccharides induces bactericidal antibody. The antibody responses to each of the four polysaccharides in the quadrivalent vaccine are serogroup-specific and independent.

Efficacy of serogroup A meningococcal vaccines was demonstrated in the 1970s in Africa and Finland, Egyptian school children aged 6 to 15 years showed 90% or greater protection during the first year after immunization with two different molecular sizes of serogroup A polysaccharide. The higher molecular weight vaccine provided protection for at least three years. In Finland, a randomized controlled mass immunization trial with serogroup A vaccine was conducted in response to a serogroup A epidemic, in children three months to five years of age. Results indicated 90 to 100% protection for three years. In Rwanda, vaccination with bivalent A/C polysaccharide vaccine was performed in response to a serogroup A epidemic. A complete cessation of meningococcal disease was observed within two weeks of vaccination, yet the serogroup A carrier rate remained unchanged.

Efficacy of serogroup C meningococcal vaccines was demonstrated in a field trial involving 20 000 troops in the US Army. Results suggested 90% efficacy under epidemic conditions which existed in basic training centers. In Brazil, 67 300 young children aged 6 to 36 months, were vaccinated with serogroup C polysaccharide in response to a serogroup C epidemic. Results indicated that the vaccine was not effective in children under 24 months of age and only 52% effective in children aged 24 to 36 months. However, studies suggested that the vaccine used in this trial was less immunogenic than other lots of similar vaccine that were used in US children; also, it was shown that the molecular size of the vaccine was smaller than the serogroup C polysaccharide in the present vaccine. Thus, it is quite probable that the current serogroup C polysaccharide vaccine is more effective.

A study performed using 4 lots of MENOMUNE-A/C/Y/W-135 [Meningococcal Polysaccharide Vaccine, Groups A, C, Y and W-135 Combined] in 150 adults showed at least a 4-fold increase in bactericidal antibodies to all groups in greater than 90 percent of the subjects.

A study was conducted in 73 children 2 to 12 years of age. Post-immunization sera were not obtained on four children; seroconversion rates were calculated on 69 paired samples. Seroconversion rates as measured by bactericidal antibody were: Group A-72%, Group C-58%, Group Y-90% and Group W-135-82%. Seroconversion rates as measured by a 2-fold rise in antibody titres based on Solid Phase Radioimmunoassay were: Group A-99%, Group C-99%, Group Y-97% and Group W-135-89%.

Duration of Efficacy: Measurable levels of antibodies against the group A and C polysaccharides decrease markedly during the first 3 years following a single dose of vaccine. This decrease in antibody occurs more rapidly in infants and young children than in adults. Similarly, although vaccine-induced clinical protection probably persists in school children and adults for at least 3 years, the efficacy of the group A vaccine in young children may decrease markedly with the passage of time. In a 3-year study, efficacy declined from greater than 90% to less than 10% among children who were less than 4 years of age at the time of vaccination, whereas among children who were greater than or equal to 4 years of age when vaccinated, efficacy was 67% 3 years later.

In New Zealand, a city-wide vaccine campaign in Auckland was conducted over 6 weeks among children 3 months to 13 years of age. Children 2 to 13 years of age received a single dose of monovalent Group A meningococcal vaccine. Children 3 to 23 months received two doses at least 1 month apart. However, only approximately 26% of the latter group received the recommended second dose. After 2.5 years of active surveillance (1987 to 1989) there were no cases of invasive Group A meningococcal disease in children appropriately vaccinated for age.

INDICATIONS: MENOMUNE-A/C/Y/W-135 [Meningococcal Polysaccharide Vaccine, Groups A, C, Y and W-135 Combined] is indicated for active immunization against invasive meningococcal disease caused by these serogroups. It is recommended for individuals at increased risk of acquiring infection or of having fulminant disease and for the control of outbreaks caused by the serogroups present in the vaccine.

Routine vaccination is recommended for the following high-risk groups: 1) Adults and children >2 years of age with functional or anatomic asplenia, complement, properdin or factor D deficiency. Whenever possible, vaccine should be given at least 10 to 14 days before splenectomy. Children with any of these immunodeficiencies should receive MENOMUNE-A/C/Y/W-135 at 2 years of age. 2) Military recruits and other groups or institutions where there is an increased risk of disease. 3) Research, industrial and clinical laboratory personnel who are routinely exposed to *N. meningitidis* cultures. 4) Persons ≥2 years of age travelling to or living in an area outside of North America in which there is a high incidence of meningococcal disease. When there is risk of exposure to Group A disease because of travel or outbreak, MENOMUNE-A/C/Y/W-135 may be given from 3 months of age (see Table 1). When there is risk of exposure to other vaccine serogroups, MENOMUNE-A/C/Y/W-135 is indicated for persons 2 years of age and older. Pilgrims making the annual Hajj pilgrimage to Mecca should receive a single dose of MENOMUNE-A/C/Y/W-135

>2 weeks before departure. 5) Unimmunized household and intimate social contacts (e.g., kissing, sharing toothbrush) of cases with meningococcal disease known to be caused by serogroup A, C, Y or W-135 meningococci. Clinical health-care workers with significant exposure to infected patients prior to twenty-four hours following commencement of antibiotics. 6) Should be considered for students living in residence or dormitory accommodation. 7) Persons 2 years of age and older who have cochlear implants.

Table 1: MENOMUNE-A/C/Y/W-135

Recommended Doses for Those Exposed or at Risk of Exposure to Serogroup A *N. meningitidis*

Age When First Immunized	Number of Primary Doses
3 to 23 months	Two doses administered 2 to 3 months apart
2 years and older	One dose

Outbreak control: For outbreaks of serogroup C meningococcal disease in adolescents, young adults and adults, one dose of MENOMUNE-A/C/Y/W-135 is recommended.

For the control of outbreaks of serogroup A meningococcal disease, MENOMUNE-A/C/Y/W-135 is recommended as a single dose for children and adults ≥18 months of age. Children 3 to 17 months of age should receive two doses of vaccine given 3 months apart. For the control of outbreaks associated with serogroup Y or W-135 meningococci one dose of MENOMUNE-A/C/Y/W-135 is recommended for persons ≥2 years of age.

For additional information on outbreak control please consult the Health Canada guidelines.

Protective antibody levels may be achieved within 7 to 10 days after vaccination.

MENOMUNE-A/C/Y/W-135 is not indicated for infants and children younger than 2 years of age except as protection of infants 3 months and older against Group A.

For persons remaining at high risk, especially children who were first vaccinated at <4 years of age, revaccination may be indicated (see Dosage).

CONTRAINDICATIONS: General: Immunization with MENOMUNE-A/C/Y/W-135 [Meningococcal Polysaccharide Vaccine, Groups A, C, Y and W-135 Combined] should be deferred in the presence of any acute illness, including febrile illness, to avoid superimposing or potential adverse effects from the vaccine on the underlying illness or mistakenly identifying a manifestation of the underlying illness as a complication of vaccine use. A minor illness such as mild upper respiratory infection is not reason to defer immunization.

Allergy to any component of MENOMUNE-A/C/Y/W-135, the container or an anaphylactic or other allergic reaction to a previous dose of MENOMUNE-A/C/Y/W-135 are contraindications to vaccination (see Supplied).

WARNINGS: This vaccine will not stimulate protection against infections caused by organisms other than Groups A, C, Y and W-135 meningococci.

Immunocompromised persons (whether from disease or treatment) may not obtain the expected immune response. If possible, consideration should be given to delaying vaccination until after the completion of any immunosuppressive treatment.

The stopper of the vial for this product contains dry natural latex rubber. Natural latex rubber has been associated with allergic reactions.

As with any vaccine, immunization with MENOMUNE-A/C/Y/W-135 [Meningococcal Polysaccharide Vaccine, Groups A, C, Y and W-135 Combined] may not protect 100% of susceptible individuals.

PRECAUTIONS: The possibility of allergic reactions in persons sensitive to components of the vaccine should be evaluated. Epinephrine Hydrochloride Solution (1:1000) and other appropriate agents should be available for immediate use in case an anaphylactic or acute hypersensitivity reaction occurs. Health-care providers should be familiar with current recommendations for the initial management of anaphylaxis in non-hospital settings, including proper airway management.

For instructions on recognition and treatment of anaphylactic reactions, see the current edition of the Canadian Immunization Guide or visit the Health Canada website.

Before administration, take all appropriate precautions to prevent adverse reactions. This includes a review of the patient's history concerning possible hypersensitivity to the vaccine or similar vaccine, previous immunization history, the presence of any contraindications to immunization and current health status.

Before administration of MENOMUNE-A/C/Y/W-135 [Meningococcal Polysaccharide Vaccine, Groups A, C, Y and W-135 Combined], health-care providers should inform the patient, parent or guardian of the benefits and risks of immunization, inquire about the recent health status of the patient and comply with any local requirements regarding information to be provided to the patient before immunization as well as the importance of completing the immunization series.

Do not inject into a blood vessel.

Use a separate sterile needle and syringe, or a sterile disposable unit, for each individual dose to prevent disease transmission.

There have been case reports of transmission of HIV and hepatitis by failure to scrupulously observe sterile technique. In particular, the same needle and/or syringe must never be used to re-enter a multidose vial to withdraw vaccine even when it is to be used for inoculation of the same patient. This may lead to contamination of the vial contents and infection of patients who subsequently receive vaccine from the vial.

Pregnancy: Animal reproduction studies have not been conducted with MENOMUNE-A/C/Y/W-135. It is also not known whether MENOMUNE-A/C/Y/W-135 can cause fetal harm when administered to a pregnant woman or can affect reproduction capacity.

MENOMUNE-A/C/Y/W-135 should be given to a pregnant woman only if clearly needed and the expected benefit outweighs any potential risk. Limited data to date have found no evidence of teratogenicity of the polysaccharide quadrivalent meningococcal vaccine when given to pregnant women.

Children: Safety and effectivness of MENOMUNE-A/C/Y/W-135 in children below the age of 2 years have not been established.

Drug Interactions: If any other vaccines are administered during the same visit, they must be given at separate sites and with separate syringes.

MENOMUNE-A/C/Y/W-135 should not be mixed in the same syringe with other parenterals.

ADVERSE EFFECTS: Adverse reactions to meningococcal vaccine are mild and consist principally of pain and redness at the injection site for 1 to 2 days. Pain at the site of injection is the most commonly reported adverse reaction and a transient fever might develop in ≥2% of young children.

The incidence and kinds of reactions reported in adults and children in clinical studies are presented in Table 2. As with the administration of any biological, one should expect possible hypersensitivity reactions.

Table 2: MENOMUNE-A/C/Y/W-135

Systemic or Local Reactions Encountered With Menomune-A/C/Y/W-135 [Meningococcal Polysaccharide Vaccine, Groups A, C, Y and W-135 Combined]

	Systemic Reactions (%)		
	None	Mild	Moderate
Headache	94.7	4.1	1.2
Malaise	97.4	2.6	0
Chills	98.3	1.7	0
Oral Temperature °C	36.7–37.2°C (96.5%)	37.8–38.3°C (3.1%)	38.3°C (0.4%)
	Local Reactions (%)		
	None	**Mild**	**Moderate**
Pain	57.4	17.5	25.1
Tenderness	46.7	24.2	29.1
Diameter of Local Reaction	0	<2 cm	≥2 cm
Erythema	67.5	31.7	0.8
Induration	86.9	8.3	4.8

On very rare occasions, IgA nephropathy has occurred following vaccination with MENOMUNE-A/C/Y/W-135. However, a cause and effect relationship has not been established.

Physicians, nurses and pharmacists should report any adverse occurrences temporally related to the administration of the product in accordance with local requirements and to the Global Pharmacovigilance Department, Sanofi Pasteur Limited, 1755 Steeles Avenue West, Toronto, ON, M2R 3T4, Canada. 1-888-621-1146 (phone) or 416-667-2435 (fax).

DOSAGE: Inspect for extraneous particulate matter and/or discolouration before use. If these conditions exist, the product should not be administered.

For information on vaccine administration, see the current edition of the Canadian Immunization Guide or visit the Health Canada website.

Reconstitution of Freeze-Dried Product and Withdrawal from Stoppered Vial: **Do not remove the stopper from the vial.**

Apply a sterile piece of cotton moistened with a suitable antiseptic to the surface of the stopper of the vial of vaccine and diluent. Withdraw the diluent into a syringe. Holding the plunger of the syringe containing the diluent steady, pierce the center of the stopper in the vial and inject the required volume of sterile diluent into the freeze-dried vaccine. Do not try to force all of the diluent into the vial at once as this will create pressure. It is necessary to gradually allow air to escape into the syringe by intermittently aspirating air from the vial while injecting the diluent into the vial. Do not remove the needle from the stopper until the required volume of diluent has been injected. Shake the vial gently. **Avoid foaming** since this will prevent withdrawal of the proper dose. Withdraw the required dose (0.5 mL) of the reconstituted vaccine into a syringe. Aseptic technique must be used for withdrawal of each dose (see Precautions).

Primary Immunization: The immunizing dose is a single injection of 0.5 mL given subcutaneously.

Primary immunization: for adults and children 2 years of age and older, primary immunization is a single 0.5 mL dose administered subcutaneously. For infants and children 3-23 months of age at risk of Group A infection, primary immunization is two 0.5 mL doses 2-3 months apart.

Where meningococcal group C conjugate vaccine has already been administered and protection against serogroup A, Y or W-135 meningococci is required, a period of 2 weeks should be allowed to elapse before vaccination with MENOMUNE-A/C/Y/W-135 [Meningococcal Polysaccharide Vaccine, Groups A, C, Y and W-135 Combined] if possible.

Revaccination: Revaccination should be considered according to Table 3 for those continuously or repeatedly exposed to serogroup A disease, who have been previously vaccinated with meningococcal polysaccharide vaccine, particularly for children initially immunized when <5 years of age. Children 2 years of age and older or adults with immunodeficiencies resulting in increased risk of meningococcal disease caused by serogroup Y or W-135 meningococci may be revaccinated with MENOMUNE-A/C/Y/W-135 according to Table 3. Revaccination should be considered according to Table 3 for those continuously or repeatedly exposed to serogroup C disease, who have been previously vaccinated with meningococcal polysaccharide vaccine, particularly for children initially immunized when <5 years of age.

Table 3: MENOMUNE-A/C/Y/W-135

Recommended Interval Between Doses for Revaccination in Individuals Repeatedly or Continuously Exposed to Serogroup A, C, Y or W-135 *N. meningitidis*

Age When First Immunized	Interval Since Last Dose as Indication for Repeat Dose
3 to 12 months	6 to 12 months
13 to 23 months	1 to 2 years
2 to 5 years	2 to 3 years
≥6 years	≥5 years

Repeat dosing at 5 year intervals (or sooner in special circumstances) is recommended for individuals at increased risk of fulminant meningococcemia.

Special care should be taken to avoid injecting the vaccine intradermally, intramuscularly, or intravenously since clinical studies have not been done to establish safety and efficacy of the vaccine using these routes of administration.

Needles should not be recapped and should be disposed of properly.

Give the patient a permanent personal immunization record. In addition, it is essential that the physician or nurse record the immunization history in the permanent medical record of each patient. This permanent office record should contain the name of the vaccine, date given, dose, manufacturer and lot number.

SUPPLIED: The vaccine when reconstituted is a clear colourless liquid. Each dose (0.5 mL) contains: *N. meningitidis* group-specific polysaccharide antigens (A, C, Y and W-135) 50 µg, thimerosal (mercury derivative) 1:10 000 (for multidose presentation only), sodium chloride 4.25-4.75 mg, lactose 2.5-5.0 mg, water for injection q.s. Package of 1×1 dose vial of vaccine and 1×0.6 mL vial of diluent. Package of 1×10 dose vial of vaccine and 1×6 mL vial of diluent. The stopper of the vial for this product contains dry natural latex rubber. Store freeze-dried vaccine and reconstituted vaccine, when not in use, at 2 to 8°C. **Do not freeze.** The single dose vial should be used within 24 hours of reconstitution. Discard remainder of 10-dose vials of vaccine within 35 days after reconstitution. Discard product if exposed to freezing. Do not use after expiration date.

Menopur® Ⓟ

menotropins

Gonadotropins for Infertility

Ferring

Date of Preparation: July 7, 2006

SUMMARY PRODUCT INFORMATION:

Route of Administration	Dosage Form/Strength	Clinically Relevant Nonmedicinal Ingredients
Subcutaneous (SC) injection	Lyophilized powder for reconstitution and injection	Lactose monohydrate, polysorbate 20, sodium phosphate buffer (sodium phosphate dibasic, heptahydrate and phosphoric acid)

DESCRIPTION: Menopur (menotropins for injection, USP) is a preparation of gonadotropins, extracted from the urine of postmenopausal women, which has undergone additional steps for purification. Each vial of Menopur contains 75 International Units (IU) of Follicle Stimulating Hormone (FSH) activity and 75 IU of Luteinizing Hormone (LH) activity, plus 21 mg lactose monohydrate and 0.005 mg, polysorbate 20 and sodium phosphate buffer (sodium phosphate dibasic, heptahydrate and phosphoric acid) in a sterile, lyophilized form intended for reconstitution with sterile 0.9% Sodium Chloride Injection, USP.

Menopur is administered by subcutaneous (SC) injection. Human Chorionic Gonadotropin (hCG), a naturally occurring hormone in postmenopausal urine, is present in Menopur and contributes to the overall luteinizing hormone activity.

Both FSH and LH are glycoproteins that are acidic and water soluble.

INDICATIONS AND CLINICAL USE: Menopur (menotropins for injection) is indicated for:

- The development of multiple follicles and pregnancy in the ovulatory patient participating in an ART (Assisted Reproductive Technologies) program.

Selection of Patients:

1. A thorough gynecologic and endocrinologic evaluation, including an assessment of pelvic anatomy, must be performed before treatment with Menopur. Patients with tubal obstruction should receive Menopur only if enrolled in an IVF program.
2. Primary ovarian failure should be excluded by the determination of gonadotropin levels.
3. Careful examination should be made to rule out the presence of an early pregnancy.
4. Patients in late reproductive life have a greater predilection to endometrial carcinoma as well as a higher incidence of anovulatory disorders. A thorough diagnostic evaluation should always be performed in patients who demonstrate abnormal uterine bleeding or other signs of endometrial abnormalities before starting Menopur therapy.
5. Evaluation of the partner's fertility potential should be included in the work-up.

Geriatrics: Menopur is not used in geriatric populations.
Pediatrics: Menopur is not used in pediatric populations.

CONTRAINDICATIONS: Menopur is contraindicated in women who have:

1. A high FSH (Follicle Stimulating Hormone) level indicating primary ovarian failure.
2. Uncontrolled thyroid or adrenal dysfunction.
3. An organic intracranial lesion such as a pituitary tumour.
4. Abnormal vaginal bleeding of undetermined origin.
5. Ovarian cysts or enlargement **not** due to Polycystic Ovarian Syndrome.
6. Prior hypersensitivity to menotropins or Menopur or to any ingredient in the formulation or component of the container. For complete list, see Dosage Forms, Composition and Packaging.
7. Menopur is not indicated in women who are pregnant. There are limited human data on the effects of menotropins when administered during pregnancy.
8. Sex hormone dependent tumours of reproductive tract and accessory organs.

WARNINGS AND PRECAUTIONS: Menopur is a drug that should only be used by physicians who are thoroughly familiar with infertility problems. It is a potent gonadotropic substance, capable of causing mild to severe adverse reactions in women. Gonadotropin therapy requires a certain time commitment by physicians and supportive health professionals, and its use requires the availability of appropriate monitoring facilities (see Warnings and Precautions, Monitoring and Laboratory Tests).

Overstimulation of the Ovary during Menopur Therapy: Ovarian Enlargement: Mild to moderate uncomplicated ovarian enlargement, which may be accompanied by abdominal distension and/or abdominal pain, occurs in approximately 5 to 10% of women treated with menotropins and hCG, and generally regresses without treatment within two or three weeks. The lowest dose consistent with expectation of good results and careful monitoring of ovarian response, can further minimize the risk of overstimulation.

If the ovaries are abnormally enlarged on the last day of Menopur therapy, hCG should not be administered in this course of treatment; this will reduce the chances of development of the Ovarian Hyperstimulation Syndrome (OHSS).

OHSS: OHSS is a medical event distinct from uncomplicated ovarian enlargement. OHSS may progress rapidly to become a serious medical event. It is characterized by an apparent dramatic increase in vascular permeability, which can result in a rapid accumulation of fluid in the peritoneal cavity, thorax, and potentially, the pericardium. The early warning signs of development of OHSS are severe pelvic pain, nausea, vomiting, and weight gain. The following symptomatology has been seen with cases of OHSS: abdominal pain, abdominal distension, gastrointestinal symptoms including nausea, vomiting and diarrhea, severe ovarian enlargement, weight gain, dyspnea, and oliguria. Clinical evaluation may reveal hypovolemia, hemoconcentration, electrolyte imbalances, ascites, hemoperitoneum, pleural effusions, hydrothorax, acute pulmonary distress, and thromboembolic events (see Pulmonary and Vascular Complications). Transient liver function test abnormalities suggestive of hepatic dysfunction, which may be accompanied by morphologic changes on liver biopsy, have been reported in association with the OHSS. In the IVF clinical study, 0399E, OHSS occurred in 7.2% of the 373 Menopur treated women.

Cases of OHSS are more common, more severe and more protracted if pregnancy occurs. OHSS develops rapidly; therefore patients should be followed for at least two weeks after hCG administration. Most often, OHSS occurs after treatment has been discontinued and reaches its maximum at about seven to ten days following treatment. Usually, OHSS resolves spontaneously with the onset of menses. If there is evidence that OHSS may be developing prior to hCG administration (see Monitoring and Laboratory Tests), the hCG should be withheld.

If severe OHSS occurs, treatment must be stopped and the patient should be hospitalized.

A physician experienced in the management of the syndrome, or who is experienced in the management of fluid and electrolyte imbalances, should be consulted.

Pulmonary and Vascular Complications: Serious pulmonary conditions (e.g. atelectasis, acute respiratory distress syndrome) have been reported. In addition, thromboembolic events both in association with, and separate from, the OHSS have been reported following menotropins therapy. Intravascular thrombosis and embolism, which may originate in venous or arterial vessels, can result in reduced blood flow to critical organs or the extremities. Sequelae of such events have included venous thrombophlebitis, pulmonary embolism, pulmonary infarction, cerebral vascular occlusion (stroke), and arterial occlusion resulting in loss of limb. In rare cases, pulmonary complications and/or thromboembolic events have resulted in death.

Multiple Pregnancies: Multiple pregnancies have occurred following treatment with Menopur SC. In the clinical trial of IVF patients in study 0399E, the rates of multiple pregnancies were as follows: Of the 23 continuing pregnancies, fifteen were single and eight were multiple pregnancies. The eight multiple pregnancies included one triplet and seven twin pregnancies. In the IVF study 2002-02 study, the rates of multiple pregnancies were as follows: Of the thirty continuing pregnancies, thirteen were single and sixteen were multiple pregnancies. The multiple pregnancies included two quadruplet, five triplet and ten twin pregnancies.

The patient and her partner should be advised of the potential risk of multiple births before starting treatment.

General: Careful attention should be given to the diagnosis of infertility in the selection of candidates for Menopur therapy (see Indications and Clinical Use, Selection of Patients).

Information to Be Provided to the Patient: Prior to therapy with Menopur, patients should be informed of the duration of treatment and the monitoring of their condition that will be required. Possible adverse reactions (see Adverse Reactions) and the risk of multiple births should also be discussed.

Monitoring and Laboratory Tests: The combination of both estradiol levels and ultrasonography are useful for monitoring the growth and development of follicles, timing of hCG administration, as well as minimizing the risk of the OHSS and multiple gestations.

The clinical confirmation of ovulation is determined by:

a. A rise in basal body temperature;
b. Increase in serum progesterone; and
c. Menstruation following the shift in basal body temperature.

When used in conjunction with indices of progesterone production, sonographic visualization of the ovaries will assist in determining if ovulation has occurred. Sonographic evidence of ovulation may include the following:

a. Fluid in the cul-de-sac;
b. Ovarian stigmata; and
c. Collapsed follicle.

Because of the subjectivity of the various tests for the determination of follicular maturation and ovulation, it cannot be overemphasized that the physician should choose tests with which he/she is thoroughly familiar.

Carcinogenesis and Mutagenesis: Long-term toxicity studies in animals have not been performed to evaluate the carcinogenic potential of menotropins.

Renal and Hepatic Insufficiency: The safety and efficacy of Menopur in renal and hepatic insufficiency have not been studied.

Immune: Local and generalized allergic reactions are known adverse reactions that may be associated with administration of gonadotropin preparations. Two events of anaphylaxis and one event of allergic reaction (hypersensitivity) have been reported from post-market experience.

Special Populations: Pregnant Women: See Contraindications.

Nursing Women: It is not known whether this drug is excreted in human milk. Because many drugs are excreted in human milk, caution should be exercised if menotropins are administered to a nursing woman.

Pediatrics: Menopur is not used in pediatric populations.

Geriatrics: Menopur is not used in geriatric populations.

ADVERSE REACTIONS: Adverse Drug Reaction Overview: Sixty-eight percent (67.7%) of patients treated with Menopur, compared to 75% of patients treated with the precursor compound Repronex, experienced adverse events (AEs). The percentage of patients experiencing AEs following treatment with Menopur is similar to the percentage of patients reporting AEs following treatment with recombinant FSH (Gonal-F).

In general, treatment with Menopur did not appear to increase the incidence or severity of the expected AEs of abdominal pain, cramps, fullness and enlargement, OHSS, nausea and injection site reactions. Furthermore, within each study, Menopur was found to be well-tolerated locally.

In the three studies (0399E, 2000-01 and 2000-02) where pregnancy was a major outcome, there was no difference across treatment groups in the percentage of patients experiencing miscarriage, ectopic pregnancies (all <2%) or elective abortions (all <3%). There also was no notable difference in the percentage of patients with multiple gestations. The number of patients with cycle cancellation due to poor response was small. The most commonly reported serious adverse event was OHSS. The number of patients with OHSS cases considered serious was about 3% in all treatment groups.

No remarkable changes in clinical laboratory parameters or physical examination findings/vital signs were observed with Menopur treatment in any of the studies in which these parameters were assessed.

The percentage of patients experiencing any AEs or expected AEs did not increase as a function of mean total dose of Menopur SC.

Clinical Trial Adverse Drug Reactions: Because clinical trials are conducted under specific conditions the adverse reaction rates observed in the clinical trials may not reflect the rates in practice and should not be compared to the rates in the clinical trials of another drug. Adverse drug reaction information from clinical trials is useful for identifying drug-related AEs and for approximating rates.

The safety of Menopur was examined in 3 clinical studies that enrolled a total of 575 patients receiving Menopur in the IVF and OI studies. All AEs (without regard to causality assessment) occurring at an incidence of >1 % in women treated with Menopur are listed in Table 1.

Table 1: Menopur

Menopur SC and IM in Female Patients Undergoing IVF and OI Adverse Events with Onset on and After GnRH Administration, COSTART Classification (for incidence of 1% or greater)

	IVF[a]		OI[b]	
	N=499		N=76	
Body Systems/Preferred Term	**N**	**%**	**N**	**%**
Body as a Whole				
Abdomen Enlarged	12	2.4	0	0
Abdominal Cramps	30	6	5	6.6
Abdomen Fullness	16	3.2	7	9.2
Abdominal Pain	88	17.6	7	9.2
Back Pain	16	3.2	0	0
Elevated Estradiol	12	2.4	0	0
Fever	7	1.4	0	0
Flu Syndrome	13	2.6	1	1.3
Flushing	12	2.4	0	0
Headache	170	34.1	12	15.8
Injection Site Pain	27	5.4	0	0
Injection Site Reaction	48	9.6	9	11.8
Malaise	14	2.8	2	2.6
Pain	16	3.2	2	2.6
Cardiovascular				
Migraine	12	2.4	0	0
Digestive				
Constipation	8	1.6	0	0
Diarrhea	14	2.8	2	2.6
Hemorrhoids	0	0	1	1.3
Nausea	60	12	6	7.9
Vomiting	21	4.2	2	2.6
Metabolic/Nutritional				
Peripheral Edema	0	0	1	1.3
Musculoskeletal				
Joint Disorder	6	1.2	0	0
Nervous				
Anxiety	1	0.2	1	1.3
Depression	3	0.6	1	1.3
Dizziness	13	2.6	0	0
Emotional Lability	4	0.8	1	1.3
Respiratory				

(cont'd)

Table 1: Menopur *(cont'd)*

Menopur SC and IM in Female Patients Undergoing IVF and OI Adverse Events with Onset on and After GnRH Administration, COSTART Classification (for incidence of 1% or greater)

	IVF[a] N=499		OI[b] N=76	
Body Systems/Preferred Term	**N**	**%**	**N**	**%**
Cough Increased	8	1.6	2	2.6
Nasal Congestion	1	0.2	1	1.3
Pharyngitis	7	1.4	1	1.3
Respiratory Disorder	29	5.8	3	3.9
Rhinorrhea	0	0	1	1.3
Sinusitis	6	1.2	0	0
Strep Throat	0	0	1	1.3
Skin/Appendages				
Puritus	5	1	0	0
Rash	5	1	0	0
Sweating	5	1	0	0
Urogenital				
Abortion	5	1	0	0
Breast Pain	4	0.8	1	1.3
Breast Tenderness	9	1.8	2	2.6
Dysmenorrhea	5	1	0	0
Ectopic Pregnancy	5	1	0	0
Hot Flash	3	0.6	2	2.6
Infection Fungal	5	1	1	1.3
Menstrual Disorder	16	3.2	0	0
OHSS	19	3.8	10	13.2
Ovarian Cyst	7	1.4	0	0
Ovarian Enlargement	0	0	1	1.3
Pelvic Cramps	0	0	3	3.9
Pelvic Discomfort	2	0.4	2	2.6
Persistent Chemical Pregnancy	0	0	1	1.3
Post Retrieval Pain	32	6.4	0	0
Spontaneous Abortion	7	1.4	1	1.3
Urinary Frequency	0	0	1	1.3
Urinary Tract Infection	7	1.4	1	1.3
Uterine Spasm	8	1.6	3	3.9
Vaginal Discharge	5	1	0	0
Vaginal Hemorrhage	15	3	3	3.9
Vaginal Spotting	18	3.6	2	2.6

a Includes IM and SC subjects from Protocol MFK/IVF/0399E and Menopur 2000-02.
b Includes IM and SC subjects from Protocol Menopur 2000-01.

Less Common Clinical Trial Adverse Drug Reactions (<1%) : The following adverse events occurred in <1% of the 575 patients treated with Menopur:

Body as a Whole: ascites, chills and face edema.
Cardiovascular: postural hypotension, palpitation and thrombosis.
Digestive: decreased appetite, duodenitis, flatulence, gastroenteritis, gingivitis, heartburn, increased appetite, rectal pain, tooth disorder and upset stomach.
Hemic/Lympatic: hematoma.
Metabolic/Nutritional: weight gain.
Musculoskeletal: bone pain, leg cramp, muscle pain and twitching.
Nervous: sleeps disorder, thinking abnormal and vertigo.
Respiratory: bronchitis, dyspnea, epistaxis, hyperventilation, pleural effusion and tonsillitis.
Special Senses: ear pain, eye disorder, eye pain and taste perversion.
Urogenital: abnormal breast, cervical polyp, cystitis, hematuria, dysuria, renal pain, ovarian pain, oliguria, urination impaired, uterine disorder, uterine fibroids, uterine hemorrhage, vaginal and genital erythema, and vaginal and genital swelling.

Post-Market Adverse Drug Reactions: Since the first approval of Menopur in 1999, a total number of 73 adverse events have been reported. A total of 41 cases were spontaneously reported, 13 cases from regulatory authorities and 19 cases were serious related cases from clinical trials.

The most frequently reported event was ovarian hyperstimulation syndrome (OHSS), which was reported in 19 cases (2 spontaneously, 1 regulatory report and 16 cases from clinical trials). Two cases of OHSS also included vein thrombosis. OHSS and associated complications, such as thromboembolism, are well-known and related to gonadotropin therapy.

One case of pulmonary embolism without OHSS was reported. According to the literature data, there is a known risk of thromboembolic events without any signs of OHSS related to assisted reproductive technologies.

One case of borderline ovarian cancer was reported. The patient involved was treated with repeated treatment cycles with different gonadotropins and clomiphene citrate, which have been reported as co-suspected drugs. Several epidemiological studies indicated that ovulation induction drugs might be related to borderline ovarian tumors.

Two events of anaphylaxis and one event of allergic reaction (hypersensitivity) have been reported. Allergic reactions, both local and generalized, are known adverse reactions that might be associated following administration of gonadotropin preparations.

A total of 3 cases described injection site reactions, suggesting good local tolerability of Menopur.

DRUG INTERACTIONS: No drug/drug interaction studies have been conducted for Menopur in humans.
Drug Abuse and Dependence: There have been no reports of abuse or dependence with menotropins.

DOSAGE AND ADMINISTRATION: Dosing Considerations: There are great inter-individual variations in response of the ovaries to exogenous gonadotropins. This makes it impossible to set a uniform dosage scheme. The dosage should, therefore, be adjusted individually depending on the ovarian response. Menopur can be given alone or in combination with a gonadotropin-releasing hormone (GnRH) agonist or antagonist. Recommendations about dosage and duration of treatment may change depending on the actual treatment protocols.

To minimize the hazard associated with the occasional abnormal ovarian enlargement which may occur with Menopur therapy, the lowest dose consistent with the expectation of good results should be used. Menopur should be administered subcutaneously until adequate follicular development is indicated by ultrasound alone or in combination with measurement of serum estradiol levels.

Recommended Dose and Dosage Adjustment: Assisted Reproductive: The recommended initial dose of Menopur for patients who have received a GnRH antagonist or GnRH agonist for pituitary suppression is 225 IU. Based on clinical monitoring (including serum estradiol levels and vaginal ultrasound results), subsequent dosing should be adjusted according to individual patient response. Adjustments in dose should not be made more frequently than once every two days and should not exceed 150 IU per adjustment. The maximum daily dose of Menopur given should not exceed 450 IU and dosing beyond 20 days is not recommended.

Once adequate follicular development is evident, hCG (5000-10 000 USP units) should be administered to induce final follicular maturation in preparation for oocyte retrieval. The administration of hCG must be withheld in cases where the ovaries are abnormally enlarged on the last day of therapy. This should reduce the chance of developing OHSS.

Missed Dose: If the patient misses a dose, the patient should be advised to take the missed dose and **not** to double dose.

Administration: Dissolve the contents of one to six vials of Menopur in 1 mL of sterile saline and **administer subcutaneously** immediately. Menopur has been shown to retain its potency and be compatible with Bravelle (urofollitropin for injection, purified) when they are mixed in the same syringe. Any unused reconstituted material should be discarded.

Parenteral drug products should be visually inspected for particulate matter and discoloration prior to administration, whenever solution and container permit.

The lower abdomen (alternating sides) should be used for subcutaneous administration.

OVERDOSAGE:
Aside from possible ovarian hyperstimulation (see Warnings and Precautions), little is known concerning the consequences of acute overdosage with Menopur.

For management of a suspected drug overdose, CPhA recommends that you contact your **regional Poison Control Centre**. See the *CPS* Directory section for a list of Poison Control Centres.

ACTION AND CLINICAL PHARMACOLOGY: Mechanism of Action: Menopur, administered for 7 to 20 days, produces ovarian follicular growth and maturation in women who do not have primary ovarian failure. In order to produce final follicular maturation and ovulation in the absence of an endogenous LH surge, hCG must be administered following Menopur treatment, at a time when patient monitoring indicates sufficient follicular development has occurred.

Pharmacodynamics: Menopur is produced from urine of postmenopausal women. Human Chorionic Gonadotropin (hCG), a naturally occurring hormone in postmenopausal women, is present in Menopur and contributes to the overall luteinizing hormone (LH) activity.

Menopur which contains both FSH and LH activity induces ovarian follicular growth and development as well as gonadal steroid production in women who do not have ovarian failure. FSH is the primary driver of follicular recruitment and growth in early folliculogenesis, while LH is important for ovarian steroidogenesis and is involved in the physiological events leading to development of a competent pre-ovulatory follicle. Follicular growth can be stimulated by FSH in the total absence of LH, but resulting follicles develop abnormally and are associated with low oestradiol levels and inability to luteinize to a normal ovulatory stimulus. In line with the action of LH activity in enhancing steroidogenesis, estradiol levels associated with treatment of Menopur are higher than with recombinant FSH preparations. This should be considered when monitoring patient's response based on estradiol levels.

Pharmacokinetics: Absorption: The SC route of administration trends toward greater bioavailability than the IM route for single and multiple doses of Menopur.

Distribution: Human tissue or organ distribution of FSH and LH has not been studied for Menopur.

Metabolism: Metabolism of FSH and LH has not been studied for Menopur in humans.

Excretion: The elimination half-lives for FSH in the multiple-dose phase were the same at 13 hours for Menopur SC and Menopur IM.

Two open-label, randomized, controlled clinical studies were conducted to assess the pharmacokinetics of Menopur. Study 2003-02 (compared single doses of SC administration of the US and European (EU) formulations of Menopur in 57 pituitary-suppressed, healthy, pre-menopausal females. The study established bioequivalence of the two formulations. Study 2000-03 assessed single and multiple doses of Menopur administered SC and IM in a 3 phase cross-over design in 33 pituitary-suppressed, healthy, pre-menopausal females. The primary pharmacokinetic endpoints were FSH AUC and C_{max} values. The results are summarized in Table 2 and Table 3.

Table 2: Menopur

FSH Pharmacokinetic Parameters (±SD) Following Menopur Administration (Study 2003-02)

PK Parameters	Single Dose (400 IU) SC
C_{max} (mIU/mL)	13.8+3.0
T_{max} (h)	19.6+6.3
$AUC_{0\text{-}120}$ (mIU·h/mL)	1040+215

Table 3: Menopur

FSH Pharmacokinetic Parameters Following Menopur Administration (Study 2000-03)

	Single Dose (225 IU)		Multiple Dose (225 IU×1 day then 150 IU×6 days)	
PK Parameters	**SC**	**IM**	**SC**	**IM**
C_{max} (mIU/mL)	8.5	7.8	15	12.5
T_{max} (h)	17.9	26.8	8	9
AUC (h-mIU/mL)	726.2	656.1	622.7	546.2

Single dose AUC_{120} and multiple dose AUCss.

STORAGE AND STABILITY: Lyophilized powder may be stored refrigerated or at room temperature (15 to 25°C). Protect from light. Use immediately after reconstitution. Discard unused material.

INFORMATION FOR THE PATIENT: Published in e-CPS, available by subscription at www.e-cps.ca.

DOSAGE FORMS, COMPOSITION AND PACKAGING: Menopur (menotropins for injection, USP) is a purified preparation of gonadotropins extracted from the urine of post-menopausal women, which has undergone additional steps of purification. Each sterile vial of lyophilized, white to off-white powder or pellet contains: 75 International Units (IU) FSH activity and 75 IU LH activity, plus 21 mg lactose monohydrate and 0.005 mg polysorbate 20 and sodium phosphate buffer (sodium phosphate dibasic, heptahydrate and phosphoric acid) in a sterile, lyophilized form intended for reconstitution with sterile 0.9% Sodium Chloride Injection, USP. Menopur is administered by subcutaneous (SC) injection. Each vial of Menopur is accompanied by a vial of sterile diluent containing 2 mL of 0.9% Sodium Chloride Injection, USP: 75 IU FSH and 75 IU of LH activity. Boxes of 5 vials+5 vials diluent.

Menveo™

meningococcal (groups A, C, W-135 and Y) oligosaccharide CRM197

Active Immunizing Agent

Novartis Pharmaceuticals

Date of Preparation: May 2010

SUMMARY PRODUCT INFORMATION:

Route of Administration	Dosage Form/ Strength	Clinically Relevant Nonmedicinal Ingredients
Intramuscular Injection	Powder and solution for injection. One dose (0.5 mL of the reconstituted vaccine) contains: Meningococcal group A oligosaccharide 10 µg conjugated to *C. diphtheriae* CRM_{197} protein 16.7 to 33.3 µg. Meningococcal group C oligosaccharide 5 µg conjugated to *C. diphtheriae* CRM_{197} protein 7.1 to 12.5 µg. Meningococcal group W-135 oligosaccharide 5 µg conjugated to *C. diphtheriae* CRM_{197} protein 3.3 to 8.3 µg. Meningococcal group Y oligosaccharide 5 µg conjugated to *C. diphtheriae* CRM_{197} protein 5.6 to 10 µg.	N/A For a complete listing see Dosage Forms, Composition and Packaging.

DESCRIPTION: After reconstitution, Menveo [Meningococcal (Groups A, C, W-135 and Y) Oligosaccharide CRM_{197} Conjugate Vaccine] is a sterile liquid vaccine that contains *N. meningitidis* serogroup A, C, W-135 and Y oligosaccharides conjugated individually to *C. diphtheriae* CRM_{197} protein. The vaccine is to be administered by intramuscular injection. The polysaccharides are produced by bacterial fermentation of N. meningitidis (serogroups A, C, W-135 or Y). MenA, MenW-135 and MenY polysaccharides are purified by several extraction and precipitation steps. MenC polysaccharide is purified by a combination of chromatography and precipitation steps.

The protein carrier (CRM_{197}) is produced by bacterial fermentation and is purified by a series of chromatography and ultrafiltration steps.

The oligosaccharides are prepared for conjugation by hydrolysis, sizing, and reductive amination. After activation, each oligosaccharide is covalently linked to the CRM_{197}. The resulting glycoconjugates are purified to yield the four drug substances, which compose the final vaccine. No preservative or adjuvant is added during manufacturing. The vaccine contains no thimerosal.

The vials in which the vaccine components are contained are composed of Type I glass, USP. The container closures (synthetic rubber stoppers, plunger stopper and tip-cap) are latex-free.

INDICATIONS AND CLINICAL USE: Menveo is indicated for active immunization of adolescents (11 to 18 years of age) and adults (19 to 55 years of age) to prevent invasive disease caused by *N. meningitidis* serogroups A, C, W-135 and Y.

Menveo is not indicated to prevent invasive disease caused by other serogroups of *N. meningitidis* nor to prevent infections caused by other microorganisms. Menveo is not indicated for treatment of meningococcal disease.

CONTRAINDICATIONS: Known hypersensitivity to any component of Menveo, including CRM_{197} or other diphtheria-containing vaccines, or a life-threatening reaction after previous administration of a vaccine containing similar components is a contraindication to vaccine administration. Acute febrile illness of any cause is a contraindication to vaccine administration.

WARNINGS AND PRECAUTIONS: General: Appropriate precautions should be taken before administration of Menveo to minimize the risk of adverse reactions. These precautions include reviewing the subject's immunization and medical history for the presence of any contraindications to immunization, such as possible hypersensitivity to Menveo or similar vaccines (including diphtheria-containing vaccines), and evaluating the patient's current health status.

As a precautionary measure, Epinephrine Hydrochloride Solution (1:1000) and other appropriate agents and equipment must be immediately available in case anaphylactic or serious allergic reactions occur.

As for all vaccines, the date of vaccine administration, the lot number and the manufacturer of the vaccine administered should be recorded in the patient's immunization record.

Menveo should be administered via intramuscular injection (see Dosage and Administration, Dosing Considerations). Care should be taken to avoid injecting Menveo vaccine subcutaneously or intravenously.

An unused sterile syringe and needle should be used for each patient to prevent transmission of blood-borne infectious agents from person to person. Needles should not be recapped and should be disposed of according to guidelines for management of biohazardous waste.

The immune response to Menveo vaccine administered to immunosuppressed persons has not been studied.

Menveo should not be administered to subjects with a known history of Guillain-Barré Syndrome.

Hematologic: Menveo has not been evaluated in persons with thrombocytopenia or bleeding disorders. Because of the risk of hematoma, Menveo should not be administered to persons with any bleeding disorder, such as hemophilia or thrombocytopenia, or to persons receiving anticoagulant therapy, unless the potential benefit outweighs the risk of administration.

NACI has published recommendations for the immunization of people with haemophilia and other bleeding disorders (http://www.phac-aspc.gc.ca/publicat/cig-gci/p03-09-eng.php).

Immune: Immunocompromised patients may have an inadequate response to the vaccination, resulting in lack of protection. The immune response to Menveo vaccine administered to immunosuppressed persons has not been studied.

Special Populations: Pregnant Women: Preclinical Data: Based on reproductive toxicology data in rabbits, Menveo is not predicted to affect pregnancy, parturition, or to increase the risk of embryofetal abnormalities.

Clinical Data: To date no clinical trials have been specifically designed to evaluate the use of Menveo in pregnant or lactating women. There are no data to demonstrate whether or not Menveo affects reproductive capacity or causes fetal harm when administered to a pregnant woman.

Menveo should be given only if the benefits of vaccination clearly outweigh the risks (see Adverse Reactions, Serious Adverse Events).

Nursing Women: Preclinical Data: In a rabbit study, no effects on postnatal development were observed in nursing offspring of vaccinated maternal animals through day 29 of lactation.

Clinical Data: Risk Summary: No studies have been conducted to assess the impact of Menveo on milk production, its presence in breast milk or its effects on the breast-fed child.

Clinical Consideration: There are no specific study data on the effects of vaccination on lactating mothers or their nursing offspring.

Pediatrics (<11 years of age): Safety and immunogenicity of Menveo in children under 11 years old have not been established.

ADVERSE REACTIONS: Adverse Drug Reaction Overview: The incidence and severity of any, local, systemic and other reactions were generally similar in the Menveo groups across all studies and between study groups within the adolescent and adult age groups. The most common local and systemic adverse reactions after Menveo observed in clinical trials were pain at the injection site (41%), headache (30%), myalgia (18%) and nausea (10%).

Clinical Trial Adverse Drug Reactions: Because clinical trials are conducted under very specific conditions the adverse reaction rates observed in the clinical trials may not reflect the rates observed in practice and should not be compared to the rates in the clinical trials of another drug. Adverse drug reaction information from clinical trials is useful for identifying drug-related adverse events and for approximating rates.

The safety of Menveo was evaluated in 5 randomized controlled clinical trials including 6724 participants (from 11 through 55 years of age) who received Menveo and 1966 who received a comparator vaccine (either Menomune, sanofi pasteur or Menactra, sanofi pasteur). Demographic characteristics of subjects who received Menveo were similar to those who received the comparator vaccine

Solicited local and systemic reactions were monitored daily for 7 days after vaccination using a diary card. Participants were monitored for 28 days for unsolicited adverse events which included adverse events requiring a physician visit, Emergency Department visit or which lead to a subject's withdrawal from the study. Unsolicited adverse events were monitored for 6 months after vaccination for medically significant adverse events requiring medical consultation, an Emergency Department visit or that led to a subject's withdrawal with the exclusion of preplanned physician visits, or Emergency Department visits for common acute conditions. Unsolicited adverse event information was obtained either by diary card, telephone interview or home or clinic visit. Serious Adverse Events were collected throughout the duration of the study. Ninety eight percent of participants from the two studies completed the 6-month follow-up evaluation.

Solicited Adverse Reactions: The overall incidence of solicited reactogenic events was similar between subjects that received Menveo and those that received Menactra.

Table 1: Menveo

Overview of Solicited Adverse Reactions among Adults Menveo and Menactra Recipients

Solicited Reaction	Category	Total Menveo N=6185 n (%)	Menactra N=1757 n (%)
Any reaction	Any	3966 (64)	1146 (65)
	Severe	507 (8)	110 (6)
Local	Any	2934 (47)	906 (52)
	Severe[a, b]	225 (4)	54 (3)
Systemic	Any	2740 (44)	725 (41)
	Severe[a, b]	355 (6)	70 (4)
Other[c]	Any[c]	1180 (19)	345 (20)

[a] Most severe across all injections. Any severe=severe local reactions or severe systemic reactions.
[b] Severe local reactions=severe erythema, pain, or induration >50 mm; severe fever=≥39.0°C.
[c] Any other reactions=stayed home; analgesic/antipyretic medication use.
Cell entries are number (percent) of subjects exposed with at least one local, systemic, or other reaction.

Conversely, the rates of systemic and local reactions were somewhat higher with Menveo than with Menomune, and substantially lower than those reported following Tdap.

Table 2: Menveo

Solicited Adverse Reactions among Adolescents Recipients of Menveo and Comparator Vaccines

		11 to 18 Year Age Group							
		V59P6		V59P11		V59P13		V59P18	
Reaction	Category	Menveo N=151 n (%)	Menomune N=209 n (%)	Menveo N=316 n (%)	Tdap N=315 n (%)	Menveo N=1631 n (%)	Menactra N=539 n (%)	Menveo N=541 n (%)	Tdap N=539 n (%)
Any reaction	Any	127 (84)	160 (77)	221 (62)	302 (86)	1044 (64)	379 (70)	373 (69)	443 (82)
	Severe	14 (9)	9 (4)	36 (10)	41 (12)	115 (7)	26 (5)	50 (9)	59 (11)
Local	Any	107 (71)	126 (60)	153 (43)	264 (75)	809 (50)	313 (58)	279 (52)	399 (74)
	Severe	7 (5)	3 (1)	14 (4)	23 (7)	62 (4)	14 (3)	17 (3)	38 (7)
Systemic	Any	85 (56)	102 (49)	171 (48)	202 (57)	710 (44)	234 (43)	274 (51)	309 (57)
	Severe	9 (6)	6 (3)	28 (8)	23 (7)	67 (4)	13 (2)	38 (7)	37 (7)
Other	Any	40 (26)	59 (28)	33 (9)	39 (11)	312 (19)	108 (20)	97 (18)	112 (21)

Of the solicited local reactions, the most common was 'Pain', occurring in 41% and 46% of Menveo and Menactra recipients respectively. Severe pain was uncommon among recipients of both groups. Among systemic reactions, headache was reported most frequently, occurring in 30% and 28% of Menveo and Menactra recipients respectively.

Table 3: Menveo

Summary of Individual Signs of Reactogenicity: Menveo versus Menactra

Reaction	Category	Total Menveo[a] N=6185 n (%)	Menactra N=1757 n (%)
Local Reactions			
Pain	Any	2524 (41)	816 (46)
	Severe	100 (2)	36 (2)
Erythema	Any	926 (15)	231 (13)
	>50 mm	97 (2)	17 (1)
Induration	Any	775 (13)	203 (12)
	>50 mm	86 (1)	15 (1)

(cont'd)

Table 3: Menveo *(cont'd)*

Summary of Individual Signs of Reactogenicity: Menveo versus Menactra

Reaction	Category	Total Menveo[a] N=6185 n (%)	Menactra N=1757 n (%)
Systemic Reactions			
Chills	Any	545 (9)	120 (7)
	Severe	53 (1)	6 (<1)
Nausea	Any	625 (10)	142 (8)
	Severe	47 (1)	9 (1)
Malaise	Any	961 (16)	285 (16)
	Severe	107 (2)	22 (1)
Myalgia	Any	1130 (18)	280 (16)
	Severe	104 (2)	17 (1)
Arthralgia	Any	580 (9)	130 (7)
	Severe	61 (1)	10 (1)
Headache	Any	1881 (30)	491 (28)
	Severe	203 (3)	38 (2)
Rash	Any	160 (3)	42 (2)
Fever	38–38.9°C	125 (2)	27 (2)
	39–39.9°C	30 (<1)	8 (<1)
	≥40°C	6 (<1)	2 (<1)
Other Reactions			
Stayed home	Yes	268 (4)	63 (4)
Analgesic/ antipyretic use	Yes	1066 (17)	326 (19)

[a] This includes subjects who received Menveo alone and subjects who received Menveo with a concomitant vaccine.
[b] Severe was defined as a reaction that prevented an individual's being able to function in their normal daily activities.

Solicited Adverse Reactions in Concomitant Vaccine Studies: In a concomitant vaccination study with Menveo and Tdap + GARDASIL solicited local and systemic reactions were monitored for 7 days after vaccination using a diary card. Unsolicited and serious adverse events were recorded and reported as noted above.

The percentages of subjects reporting each severe systemic reaction to Menveo when administered alone and after Tdap were similar. Subjects in groups receiving either Menveo alone or Menveo concomitant with Tdap and GARDASIL reported similar frequencies of induration and erythema at the Menveo injection site with a slightly lower frequency of injection site pain in the group receiving Menveo alone (45% versus 49% respectively). Pain was the most frequent local reaction reported in both groups. The percentages of subjects reporting systemic reactions after Menveo alone were equal to or lower than those following Menveo with concomitant vaccine administration.

The most commonly reported solicited systemic reactions were headache (36% versus 40%) and malaise (20% versus 24%), myalgia (19% versus 27%) and arthralgia (11% versus 17%) for Menveo alone and Menveo with concomitant vaccine administration, respectively.

Unsolicited Adverse Events: During the first month after vaccination, unsolicited AEs were reported in approximately the same percentage of Menveo and Menactra subjects (17% and 20%, respectively), and only 1% of subjects in each group had unsolicited AEs considered severe. The only unsolicited AE reported in more than 1% of subjects during month 1 postvaccination was headache (2% in each vaccine group). In total, 6% of Menveo subjects and 7% of Menactra subjects reported unsolicited AEs assessed as possibly or probably related to the vaccine within month 1 postvaccination; most of these started within days 1 to 7 postvaccination.

Table 4: Menveo

Unsolicited and Severe Adverse Events Following Menveo or Menactra

Time	Unsolicited Adverse Events (AE)	Total Menveo[a] N or n (%)	Menactra N or n (%)
Month 1	Total exposed: N	6185	1757
	Any AE	1076 (17)	356 (20)
	Any severe AE	59 (1)	16 (1)
	Possibly/probably related AE	357 (6)	128 (7)
	Severe possibly/probably related AE	21 (<1)	5 (<1)
	Any SAE	7 (<1)	4 (<1)
	Possibly/probably related SAE	0	0
	Death	0	0
Months 2 to 6	Total exposed: N	5068	1746
	Any AE	460 (9)	134 (8)
	Any severe AE	42 (1)	14 (1)
	Possibly/probably related AE	3 (<1)	1 (<1)
	Severe possibly/probably related AE	0	0
	Any SAE	31 (1)	10 (1)
	Possibly/probably related SAE	1 (<1)	0
	Death	0	0

[a] This includes subjects who received Menveo alone and subjects who received Menveo with a concomitant vaccine.

Health care professionals should promptly report all clinically significant adverse events after vaccination with Menveo in accordance to the local requirements and to the Global Pharmacovigilance Department Novartis, even if it is not clear that the vaccine caused the event.

To report Suspected Adverse Events, please call Novartis Vaccines at 1-800-363-8883 or Health Canada at 1-866-844-0018.

Serious Adverse Events: The information regarding serious adverse events was derived from 5 randomized, controlled clinical trials. Serious adverse events reported within 6 months of vaccination occurred in 40/6185 (0.6%) of Menveo subjects, 13/1757 (0.7%) of Menactra subjects, and 5/209 (2.4%) of Menomune subjects. During the 6 months following immunization, SAEs reported by more than one subject were as follows: Menveo - appendicitis (3 subjects), road traffic accident (3 subjects), and suicide attempt (5 subjects); Menactra - intervertebral disc protrusion (2 subjects); Menomune - none. Serious adverse events that occurred within 30 days of vaccination were reported by 7 of 6185 (0.1%) subjects in the Menveo group, 4 of 1757 (0.2%) subjects in the Menactra group, and no Menomune subjects. The events that occurred during the first 30 days post immunization with Menveo were: vitello-intestinal duct remnant; Cushing's syndrome; viral hepatitis; pelvic inflammatory disease; intentional multiple drug overdose; simple partial seizure; and suicidal depression. The events that occurred during the first 30 days post immunization with Menactra were: herpes zoster; fall; intervertebral disc protrusion; and angioedema.

To date, no clinical trials have been specifically designed to evaluate the use of Menveo in pregnant or lactating women. Among the 5209 women enrolled in the studies, 43 women were found to be pregnant during the 6-month follow-up period after vaccination. Of these, 37 pregnancies occurred among 4115 Menveo recipients (7 spontaneous abortions, no congenital anomalies). Six pregnancies occurred among 1013 Menactra recipients (no spontaneous abortions, one congenital anomaly (hydrocephalus)). Among the seven subjects with adverse pregnancy outcomes who had received Menveo, the estimated dates of conception were 5 days prior to vaccination (1 subject), 6 to 17 weeks post vaccination (5 subjects), and 6 months post vaccination (1 subject). In the subject who had received Menactra the estimated date of conception was approximately 15 weeks post immunization.

Safety and effectiveness of Menveo have not been established in pregnant women. To enroll in the Novartis Vaccines and Diagnostics Inc. pregnancy registry, please call 1-877-311-8972.

DRUG INTERACTIONS: In general, immunosuppressive therapies, such as irradiation, antimetabolite medications, alkylating agents, cytotoxic drugs, and corticosteroids (used in greater than physiologic doses) may reduce the immune response to vaccines. The immunogenicity of Menveo has not been evaluated in persons receiving such therapies.

Concomitant Vaccine Administration: The immunogenicity and safety of Menveo were evaluated in concomitant use studies with Tdap plus GARDASIL. The non-inferiority of concomitant use of GARDASIL and Tdap with Menveo to Menveo alone has not been established. Co-administration with Tdap and Menveo was associated with a decline in the immune responses to several of the Tdap antigens. However, the clinical relevance of these differences is uncertain. The non-inferiority of sequential administration of Menveo after Tdap to Menveo alone has also not been established. The non-inferiority of HPV alone vs. HPV with Tdap and Menveo has not been established. The concomitant use of Menveo with other licensed vaccines has not been evaluated.

DOSAGE AND ADMINISTRATION: Dosing Considerations: Menveo should be administered as a single 0.5 mL intramuscular injection, preferably into the deltoid muscle (upper arm). Before injection, the skin at the injection site should be cleaned and prepared with a suitable antiseptic. Do not administer Menveo intravenously, subcutaneously or intradermally.

Recommended Dose and Dosage Adjustment: Single dose.

Whether a booster dose of Menveo will be needed has not yet been determined.

Administration: Menveo must be prepared for administration by reconstituting the lyophilized MenA conjugate component with the liquid MenCWY conjugate component. Withdraw the entire contents of the vial of MenCWY solution and inject into the MenA conjugate component vial to reconstitute. Gently shake the reconstituted vial until the vaccine is dissolved. Using a needle of suitable gauge and length for the vaccination, withdraw 0.5 mL of reconstituted product.

1. Withdraw liquid from vial containing **MenCYW-135 liquid conjugate component**
2. Insert MenCYW-135 liquid conjugate component solution into vial containing **MenA lyophilized conjugate component**
3. Gently invert or swirl the vial until the vaccine is dissolved. Administer as a single 0.5 mL intramuscular injection

Please note that it is normal for a small amount of liquid to remain in the vial following withdrawal of the dose. Ensure that no air bubbles are present in the syringe before injecting the vaccine.

Parenteral drug products should be inspected for container integrity, particulate matter and discoloration before administration.

Following reconstitution, the vaccine is a clear, colourless solution, free from visible foreign particles. In the event that any foreign particulate matter and/or variation of physical aspect is observed, discard the vaccine. The reconstituted vaccine should be used immediately. Any unused product or waste material should be disposed in accordance with local requirements for disposal of biohazardous waste.

OVERDOSAGE:

For management of a suspected drug overdose, contact your regional Poison Control Centre. See the *CPS* Directory section for a list of Poison Control Centres.

ACTION AND CLINICAL PHARMACOLOGY: Mechanism of Action: Meningococcal disease is caused by a gram-negative diplococcus, *N. meningitidis*. *N. meningitidis* causes life-threatening disease worldwide. Based on antigenic variations in capsular polysaccharide structure, 13 serogroups of *N. meningitidis* have been identified. Globally, 5 serogroups, A, B, C, W-135 and Y, cause almost all invasive meningococcal infections. Invasive infection by *N. meningitidis* most often manifests as bacteremia and/or meningitis and can also rarely present as arthritis, myocarditis, pericarditis, endophthalmitis, pneumonia or infection at other anatomic sites. Vaccination with Menveo leads to the production of bactericidal antibodies directed against the capsular polysaccharides of serogroups A, C, W-135 and Y.

For epidemiology and further information specific to Canada, please consult Canada Communicable Disease Reports ACS-3 (April 2009) and ACS-4 (June 2009) (http://origin.phac-aspc.gc.ca/publicat/ccdr-rmtc/09vol35/index-eng.php).

Pharmacodynamics: Serum concentrations of complement-mediated bactericidal antibody to *N. meningitidis*, acquired through natural exposure or induced by vaccination, are generally accepted to correlate with protective immunity to meningococcal disease and therefore are used as surrogate markers for vaccine efficacy.

No clinical effectiveness studies have been undertaken with Menveo. The efficacy of Menveo has been inferred from demonstration of immunologic non-inferiority to Menactra among subjects aged 11-55 years. The primary measure of immune response was induction of serogroup-specific anti-capsular antibodies with bactericidal activity. Serum bactericidal activity (SBA) was measured using human serum as the source of exogenous complement (hSBA). The hSBA was the original correlate of protection against meningococcal disease (Goldschneider I., et al, 1969 a, b).

STORAGE AND STABILITY: Store refrigerated, away from the freezer compartment, at 2 to 8°C. Vaccine must be maintained at 2 to 8°C during transport. Do not use Menveo after the expiry date which is stated on the carton. The vaccine consists of one lyophilized vial and one liquid vial. Each of the two components may carry a different expiry date. **All** contents must be discarded on reaching the outer carton expiry date. The reconstituted vaccine should be used immediately, but may be held at or below 25°C for up to 2 hours.

SPECIAL HANDLING INSTRUCTIONS: Do not freeze. Frozen/previously frozen product should not be used. Protect from light.

INFORMATION FOR THE PATIENT: Published in e-CPS, available by subscription at www.e-cps.ca.

DOSAGE FORMS, COMPOSITION AND PACKAGING: Each dose (0.5 mL) of reconstituted vaccine contains: 5 µg each of meningococcal C, W-135 and Y oligosaccharides conjugated and 10 µg of meningococcal A oligosaccharide conjugated to a total of approximately 47 µg of Cross Reactive Material (CRM_{197}) from *C. diphtheriae*. Nonmedicinal ingredients: di-sodium hydrogen phosphate bihydrate, potassium dihydrogen phosphate, sodium chloride, sodium dihydrogen phosphate monohydrate, sucrose and water for injection (WFI). Preservative and adjuvant-free. The vaccine contains no thimerosal and container closures are latex-free. Packs of 5 doses (vial/vial).

Meperidine Ⓝ

CPhA Monograph

see *Opioids*

Meperidine Hydrochloride Injection USP Ⓝ

meperidine HCl

Opioid Analgesic

Sandoz

SUPPLIED: 50 mg/mL: Each mL contains: meperidine hydrochloride 50 mg, sodium hydroxide and/or hydrochloric acid to adjust pH and water for injection. Ampoules of 1 mL, boxes of 10. Store between 15 and 30°C.

75 mg/mL: Each mL contains: meperidine hydrochloride 75 mg, sodium hydroxide and/or hydrochloric acid to adjust pH and water for injection. Ampoules of 1 mL, boxes of 10. Store between 15 and 30°C.

100 mg/mL: Each mL contains: meperidine hydrochloride 100 mg, sodium hydroxide and/or hydrochloric acid to adjust pH and water for injection. Ampoules of 1 mL, boxes of 10. Store between 15 and 30°C.

Mepron® Pr

atovaquone

Antiprotozoal

GlaxoSmithKline

Date of Revision: June 1, 2009

PHARMACOLOGY: Atovaquone is a hydroxy-1,4-naphthoquinone, an analog of ubiquinone, with antipneumocystis activity. The mechanism of action against *P. carinii* has not been fully elucidated.

Pharmacokinetics: The pharmacokinetics of atovaquone have been studied in healthy volunteers, HIV-infected adults with varying stages and manifestations of HIV infection and in immunocompromised children. The half-life of atovaquone is long (2 to 3 days) due to presumed enterohepatic cycling and eventual fecal elimination. There is no evidence that the drug is metabolized in man.

Atovaquone is a highly lipophilic compound with a low aqueous solubility. It is extensively bound to plasma proteins (>99.9%).

The bioavailability of atovaquone is highly dependent on formulation and diet. The atovaquone oral suspension formulation, which has now replaced the atovaquone tablets, has atovaquone particles significantly smaller than those in the tablet formulation, and provides an approximately 2-fold increase in atovaquone bioavailability in the fasting or fed state compared to the tablet formulation studied under the same conditions. The bioavailability of atovaquone suspension can be increased greatly when administered with meals. In healthy volunteers, a standard meal (23 g fat; 610 kcal) increased the bioavailability 2- to 3-fold following 750 mg single doses of atovaquone suspension. The mean area under the atovaquone plasma concentration-time curve (AUC) was increased 2.5-fold and the mean C_{max} was increased 3.4-fold. Fat has been shown to enhance absorption significantly.

In healthy volunteers there is no evidence that the drug is metabolized and there is negligible excretion of atovaquone in the urine, with parent drug being predominantly (>90%) excreted unchanged in feces.

During a multiple-dose study of 4 HIV-seropositive asymptomatic volunteers, the relative oral bioavailability of the tablet formulation decreased at doses above 750 mg once daily with food.

In another multiple-dose escalation study conducted in AIDS patients, lack of dose proportionality was also demonstrated with the tablet formulation; there was, however, a modest increase in concentrations.

INDICATIONS: For the acute oral treatment of mild to moderate *P. carinii* pneumonia (PCP) in patients who are intolerant to trimethoprim-sulfamethoxazole (TMP-SMX).

The efficacy of atovaquone in patients who are failing therapy with TMP-SMX has not been systematically studied (see Warnings).

The indication is based on the results of a comparative pharmacokinetic studies of the oral suspension and tablet formulations and clinical efficacy studies of the tablet formulation which established a relationship between atovaquone plasma concentration and successful treatment. The results of a randomized double-blind trial comparing atovaquone tablets to TMP-SMX in AIDS patients with mild to moderate PCP (defined as an alveolar-arterial oxygen diffusion gradient [$(A\text{-}a)DO_2$] ≤45 mmHg and PaO_2 ≥60 mmHg on room air); and a randomized trial comparing atovaquone tablets and i.v. pentamidine isethionate in patients with mild to moderate PCP intolerant to trimethoprim or sulfa-antimicrobials. These studies are summarized below:

TMP-SMX Comparative Study: This double-blind trial, initiated in 1990, was designed to compare the safety and efficacy of atovaquone tablets to that of TMP-SMX for the treatment of AIDS patients with histologically confirmed PCP. Only patients with mild to moderate PCP were eligible for enrollment.

A total of 408 patients were enrolled into the trial at 37 study centres. Eighty-six patients without histologic confirmation of PCP were excluded from the efficacy analyses. Of the 322 patients with histologically confirmed PCP, 160 were randomized to receive atovaquone tablets and 162 to TMP-SMX.

Study participants randomized to atovaquone treatment were to receive 750 mg atovaquone (three 250 mg tablets) 3 times daily for 21 days and those randomized to trimethoprim-sulfamethoxazole were to receive 320 mg TMP plus 1600 mg SMX 3 times daily for 21 days.

All patients were evaluated for their response to treatment. Each patient was classified as a therapy success or failure. Therapy success was defined as improvement in clinical and respiratory measures persisting at least 4 weeks after cessation of therapy. Therapy failures included lack of response, treatment discontinuation due to an adverse experience, and unevaluable.

There was a significant difference (p=0.03) in mortality rates between the treatment groups. Among the 322 patients with confirmed PCP, 13 of 160 patients treated with atovaquone tablets and 4 of 162 patients receiving TMP-SMX died during the 21-day treatment course or an 8-week follow-up period. In the intent-to-treat analysis for all 408 randomized patients there were 16 deaths in the atovaquone tablets arm and 7 in the TMP-SMX arm (p=0.051).

This difference in mortality between the two treatment groups appeared to be partially due to a disproportionate number of fatal bacterial infections in the atovaquone tablets group. Four of the 13 atovaquone tablets-treated patients died of PCP, while 5 of the 13 died of a combination of bacterial infections and PCP. A correlation between plasma concentrations and death was demonstrated; in general, patients with lower atovaquone plasma concentrations were more likely to die than patients with higher atovaquone plasma concentrations.

Sixty-two percent (62%) of patients on atovaquone tablets and 64% of patients on TMP-SMX were classified as protocol-defined therapy successes. The therapeutic outcomes are presented in Table 1.

The failure rate due to lack of response was significantly larger for patients receiving atovaquone tablets, while the failure rate due to adverse experiences was larger for patients receiving TMP-SMX.

There were no significant differences in the effect of either treatment on additional indicators of response (i.e., arterial blood gas measurements, vital signs, serum LDH levels, clinical symptoms, and chest radiographs).

Pentamidine Comparative Study: This open, randomized trial, initiated in 1991, was designed to compare the safety and efficacy of atovaquone tablets to that of pentamidine for the treatment of histologically confirmed mild or moderate PCP among AIDS patients. Approximately 80% of the patients had a history of, or were currently experiencing, intolerance to trimethoprim or sulfa-antimicrobials.

Patients randomized to atovaquone were to receive 750 mg atovaquone (three 250 mg tablets) 3 times daily for 21 days, and those randomized to pentamidine isethionate were to receive a 3 to 4 mg/kg single i.v. infusion daily for 21 days.

It was anticipated that patients intolerant of TMP-SMX would present in either of 2 ways. They would either have a known intolerance and would represent a primary therapy group, or their intolerance would first become evident during treatment for the current episode of PCP and would represent a study group for salvage therapy.

A total of 135 PCP-positive patients were enrolled: 110 were in the primary therapy group and 25 were in the salvage therapy group.

There was no difference in mortality rates between the treatment groups. Among the 135 patients with confirmed PCP, 10 of 70 patients treated with atovaquone tablets and 9 of 65 patients treated with pentamidine died during the 21-day treatment course or an 8-week follow-up period. Three of the 10 patients treated with atovaquone tablets died of PCP while another 3 patients died with a combination of bacterial infections and PCP. The contribution of PCP in these latter deaths is unclear. One patient died of sepsis, 1 died of lymphoma, 1 died of complications of AIDS and 1 died of refractory pneumothorax. Two of 9 patients treated with pentamidine died of PCP while another 3 patients died with a combination of bacterial infections and PCP. The contribution of PCP in these latter deaths is unclear. One each died of a cerebral mycotic aneurysm and disseminated *C. immitis* and 2 patients died of complications of AIDS. In the intent-to-treat analysis for all randomized patients, there were 11 deaths in the atovaquone tablets arm and 12 deaths in the pentamidine arm. For those patients for whom day 4 atovaquone plasma concentrations are available, 3 of 5 (60%) patients with concentrations <5 µg/mL died during participation in the study. However, only 2 of 21 (9%) patients with day 4 plasma concentrations >5 µg/mL died. The therapeutic outcomes are presented in Table 2.

Table 1: MEPRON

Outcome of Treatment for PCP-positive Patients Enrolled in the TMP-SMX Comparative Study

Outcome of Therapy[a]	Number of Patients (% of Total) MEPRON Tablets (n=160)	TMP-SMX (n=162)	P Value
Therapy Success	99 (62%)	103 (64%)	0.75
Therapy Failure			
Lack of Response	28 (17%)	10 (6%)	<0.01
Adverse Experience	11 (7%)	33 (20%)	<0.01
Unevaluable	22 (14%)	16 (10%)	0.28
Required Alternative PCP Therapy During Study	55 (34%)	55 (34%)	0.95

[a] As defined by the protocol and described in study description above.

Table 2: MEPRON

Outcome of Treatment for PCP-positive Patients Enrolled in the Pentamidine Comparative Study

	Primary Treatment			Salvage Treatment		
Outcome of Therapy	MEPRON Tablets (n=56)	Pentamidine (n=53)	P Value	MEPRON Tablets (n=14)	Pentamidine (n=11)	P Value
Therapy Success	32 (57%)	21 (40%)	0.09	13 (93%)	7 (64%)	0.14
Therapy Failure						
Lack of Response	16 (29%)	9 (17%)	0.18	0	0	
Adverse Experience	2 (3.6%)	19 (36%)	<0.01	0	3 (27%)	0.07
Unevaluable	6 (11%)	4 (8%)	0.75	1 (7%)	1 (9%)	1.00
Required Alternative PCP Therapy During Study	19 (34%)	29 (55%)	0.04	0	4 (36%)	0.03

Data on Chronic Use: Atovaquone oral suspension has not been systematically evaluated as a chronic suppressive agent to prevent the development of PCP in patients at high risk for *P. carinii* disease. In a pilot-dosing study of chronic dosing of atovaquone tablets in AIDS patients, 5 of 31 patients had PCP breakthroughs: one patient at a dose of 750 mg once daily (after 20 days), three patients at 750 mg twice daily (after 14, 70, and 97 days), and one patient at 1500 mg twice daily (after 74 days). The dose used in the acute treatment studies (750 mg 3 times daily) was not studied and, therefore, there are no data on the rate of breakthrough at this dose. Based on these limited observations, no recommendation can be made as to the use of atovaquone oral suspension for prophylaxis.

CONTRAINDICATIONS: In known hypersensitivity to atovaquone or to any of the components of the formulation.

WARNINGS: Clinical experience with atovaquone has been limited to patients with mild to moderate PCP [$(A\text{-}a)DO_2$≤45 mmHg]. Treatment of more severe episodes of PCP has not been systematically studied with this agent.

Also, the efficacy of atovaquone tablets in patients who are failing therapy with TMP-SMX has not been systematically studied and, therefore, cannot be recommended.

Atovaquone has not been evaluated as an agent for PCP prophylaxis.

PRECAUTIONS: General: Absorption of orally administered atovaquone is limited but can be significantly increased when the drug is taken with food. Atovaquone plasma concentrations have been shown to correlate with the likelihood of successful treatment and survival. Therefore, parenteral therapy with other agents should be considered for patients who have difficulty taking atovaquone with food (see Pharmacology).

Gastrointestinal disorders may limit absorption of orally administered drugs. Patients with these disorders also may not achieve plasma concentrations of atovaquone associated with response to therapy in controlled trials. The prescriber must be aware that diarrhea at the start of treatment has been shown to be associated with significantly lower atovaquone plasma levels. These, in turn, are correlated with a higher incidence of therapy failures and a lower survival rate.

Based upon the spectrum of in vitro antimicrobial activity, atovaquone is not effective therapy for concurrent pulmonary conditions such as bacterial, viral or fungal pneumonia or mycobacterial diseases. Clinical deterioration in patients may be due to other pathogens, as well as progressive PCP. All patients with acute PCP should be carefully evaluated for all other possible causes of pulmonary disease and treated with additional agents as appropriate.

Rare cases of hepatitis, elevated liver function tests, and one case of fatal liver failure have been reported in patients treated with atovaquone. A causal relationship between atovaquone use and these events could not be established because of numerous confounding medical conditions and concomitant drug therapies (see Adverse Effects, Post-Marketing Adverse Reactions).

Geriatrics: Atovaquone has not been systematically evaluated in patients greater than 65 years of age. Caution should be exercised when treating elderly patients reflecting the greater frequency of decreased hepatic, renal and cardiac function in this population.

There is no clinically significant change in the average rate or extent of absorption of atovaquone between elderly and young patients. A trend toward an increase in $t_{1/2}$ in elderly subjects after a single dose suggests that atovaquone may accumulate after multiple dosing.

Infants and Young Children: There are no efficacy studies in children. Clinical experience with atovaquone in immunosuppressed pediatric patients is limited to safety data from one pharmacokinetic study (n=11). No children under 4 months of age participated in the Phase I trial.

Pregnancy: There are no adequate and well-controlled studies in pregnant women. Atovaquone should be used during pregnancy only if the potential benefit justifies the potential risk to the fetus.

Lactation: It is not known whether atovaquone is excreted in human milk, and breast-feeding is not recommended. In a rat study, atovaquone concentrations in the milk were 30% of the concurrent atovaquone concentrations in the maternal plasma.

Patients with Hepatic Impairment: In patients with mild to moderate hepatic impairment, there is no clinically significant change in exposure to atovaquone when compared to healthy patients. No data are available in patients with severe hepatic impairment.

Patients with Renal Impairment: In patients with mild to moderate renal impairment, oral clearance and/or AUC data for atovaquone are within the range of values observed in patients with normal renal function. The C_{max} and AUC of total atovaquone (bound+free) are reduced in patients with severe renal impairment. The effect of severe renal impairment on free (unbound) concentrations of atovaquone in plasma is unknown.

Occupational Hazards: Ability to Perform Tasks That Require Judgement, Motor or Cognitive skills: There have been no studies to investigate the effect of atovaquone on driving performance or the ability to operate machinery.

Drug Interactions: As experience is limited, care should be taken when combining other drugs with atovaquone. Atovaquone is highly bound to plasma protein (>99.9%). Therefore, caution should be used when administering atovaquone concurrently with other highly plasma protein bound drugs with narrow therapeutic indices, as competition for binding sites may occur.

The extent of plasma protein binding of atovaquone in human plasma is not affected by the presence of therapeutic concentrations of phenytoin (15 µg/mL). Atovaquone does not affect the pharmacokinetics, metabolism or extent of protein binding of phenytoin in vivo. In vitro there is no plasma protein binding interaction between atovaquone and quinine, phenytoin, warfarin, sulfamethoxazole, indomethacin or diazepam.

The concomitant administration of atovaquone and rifampin or rifabutin is not recommended. Concomitant administration of rifampin or rifabutin is known to reduce atovaquone levels by approximately 50% and 34%, respectively, and could result in subtherapeutic plasma concentrations in some patients.

Concomitant treatment with tetracycline or metoclopramide has been associated with significant decreases in plasma concentrations of atovaquone. Caution should be exercised in prescribing these drugs with atovaquone oral suspension until the potential interaction has been further studied.

In clinical trials of atovaquone oral suspension, small decreases in plasma concentrations of atovaquone (mean <3 µg/mL) were associated with concomitant administration of acetaminophen, benzodiazepines, acyclovir, opiates, cephalosporins, antidiarrheals and laxatives. The causal relationship between the change in plasma concentrations of atovaquone and the administration of these drugs is unknown.

Zidovudine does not appear to affect the pharmacokinetics of atovaquone. However, pharmacokinetic data have shown that atovaquone appears to decrease the rate of metabolism of zidovudine to its glucuronide metabolite (steady-state AUC of zidovudine was increased by 33% and peak plasma concentration of the glucuronide was decreased by 19%). At zidovudine dosages of 500 or 600 mg/day, it would seem unlikely that a 3-week, concomitant course of atovaquone oral suspension for the treatment of acute PCP would result in an increased incidence of adverse reactions attributable to higher plasma concentrations of zidovudine. Extra care should be taken in monitoring patients receiving prolonged atovaquone oral suspension therapy. There are no data available for ddC (zalcitabine).

Didanosine (ddI) does not affect the pharmacokinetics of atovaquone as determined in a prospective multidose drug interaction study of atovaquone and ddI. However, there was a 24% decrease in the AUC for ddI when coadministered with atovaquone which is unlikely to be of clinical significance.

Concomitant administration of atovaquone and indinavir results in a decrease in the C_{min} of indinavir (23% decrease; 90% CI 8 to 35%). Caution should be exercised when prescribing atovaquone with indinavir due to the decrease in trough levels of indinavir.

In clinical trials of atovaquone the following drugs were not associated with a change in steady state plasma concentrations of atovaquone: fluconazole, clotrimazole, ketoconazole, antacids, systemic corticosteroids, nonsteroidal anti-inflammatory drugs, antiemetics (excluding metoclopramide) and H_2-antagonists.

Laboratory Tests: It is not known if atovaquone interferes with clinical laboratory tests or assay results.

Information to Be Provided to the Patient: The importance of taking the prescribed dose of atovaquone oral suspension should be stressed.

Patients should be instructed to take their daily doses with meals, as the presence of food will significantly improve the absorption of the drug.

Patients should be informed that hypersensitivity (allergic) reactions have occurred with this product with symptoms such as hives, swelling of tissues (ie hands, feet, throat), tightening of the throat, and difficulty in breathing. Skin rash, which may blister and look like small targets (central dark spots surrounded by a paler area with a dark ring around the edge [erythema multiforme]) and widespread rash with blisters and peeling skin (particularly occurring around the mouth, nose, eyes and genitals [Stevens-Johnson Syndrome]) are also possible. Other reported events include inflammation of the liver or pancreas, decrease in kidney function, decrease of platelets in the blood, higher than normal level of methemoglobin (metHb) in the blood and deposits in the eye. Patients should contact a doctor, hospital emergency department or regional poison control centre immediately if any of these symptoms occur.

The oral suspension should be shaken gently before use.

ADVERSE EFFECTS: Because many patients who participated in clinical trials with atovaquone tablets had complications of advanced HIV disease, it was often difficult to distinguish adverse events caused by the drug from those caused by underlying medical conditions. There were no life-threatening or fatal adverse experiences caused by atovaquone tablets.

Table 3 summarizes all the clinical adverse experiences reported by ≥5% of the study population during the TMP-SMX comparative study of atovaquone tablets (n=408), regardless of attribution.

Table 3: MEPRON

Treatment-emergent Adverse Experiences in the TMP-SMX Comparative PCP Treatment Study

Treatment-emergent Adverse Experience	Number of Patients with Treatment-emergent Adverse Experience (% of Total)			
	MEPRON Tablets (n=203)		TMP-SMX (n=205)	
Body as a Whole				
Asthenia	17	(8%)	16	(8%)
Fever	28	(14%)	52	(25%)[a]
Headache	33	(16%)	44	(22%)
Gastrointestinal				
Diarrhea	39	(19%)[a]	15	(7%)
Constipation	7	(3%)	35	(17%)[a]
Abdominal Pain	9	(4%)	15	(7%)
Vomiting	29	(14%)	72	(35%)[a]
Nausea	43	(21%)	90	(44%)[a]
Monilia, Oral	11	(5%)	21	(10%)
Nervous				
Dizziness	7	(3%)	17	(8%)[a]
Insomnia	20	(10%)	18	(9%)
Skin				
Rash (including maculopapular)	47	(23%)	69	(34%)[a]
Pruritus	11	(5%)	18	(9%)
No. Patients Discontinuing Therapy due to an Adverse Experience	19	(9%)	50	(24%)[a]
No. Patients Reporting at least one Adverse Experience	127	(63%)	134	(65%)

[a] p<0.05.

Although an equal percentage of patients receiving atovaquone tablets and TMP-SMX reported at least 1 adverse experience, more patients receiving TMP-SMX required discontinuation of therapy due to an adverse event. Nine percent of patients receiving atovaquone tablets were prematurely discontinued from therapy due to an adverse event, versus 24% of patients receiving TMP-SMX. Eight patients receiving atovaquone tablets had therapy discontinued due to development of rash. The majority of cases of rash among patients receiving atovaquone tablets were mild and did not require the discontinuation of dosing. The only other clinical adverse experience which led to premature discontinuation of atovaquone tablets dosing by more than 1 patient was the development of vomiting (n=2). The most common adverse experience requiring discontinuation of dosing in the TMP-SMX group was rash (n=16).

Laboratory test abnormalities reported for ≥5% of the study population during the treatment period are summarized in Table 4. Five patients treated with atovaquone tablets and 15 patients treated with TMP-SMX had therapy prematurely discontinued due to elevations in ALT/AST. In general, patients treated with atovaquone tablets developed fewer abnormalities in measures of hepatocellular function (ALT, AST, alkaline phosphatase) or amylase values than patients treated with TMP-SMX.

Table 4: MEPRON

Treatment-emergent Laboratory Abnormalities

Laboratory Test Abnormality	Number of Patients Developing a Laboratory Test Abnormality % of Total Patients	
	MEPRON Tablets	TMP-SMX
Anemia (Hgb <8.0 g/dL)	6%	7%
Neutropenia (ANC <750 cl/mm³)	3%	9%
Elevated ALT (>5×ULN)	6%	16%
Elevated AST (>5×ULN)	4%	14%
Elevated Alkaline Phosphate (>2.5×ULN)	8%	6%
Elevated Amylase (>1.5×ULN)	7%	12%
Hyponatremia (<0.96×LLN)	7%	26%

Legend: ULN=upper limit of normal range; LLN=lower limit of normal range; ANC=absolute neutrophil count.

Table 5 summarizes the clinical adverse experiences reported by ≥5% of the study population during the comparative trial of atovaquone tablets and i.v. pentamidine (n=144), regardless of attribution. A slightly lower percentage of patients who received atovaquone tablets reported occurrence of adverse events than did those who received pentamidine (63% vs 72%).

However, only 7% of patients discontinued treatment with atovaquone tablets due to adverse events, while 41% of patients who received pentamidine discontinued treatment for this reason (p=<0.001). Of the 5 patients who discontinued therapy with atovaquone tablets, 3 reported rash (4%). Rash was not severe in any patient. No other reason for discontinuation of atovaquone tablets was cited more than once. The most frequently cited reasons for discontinuation of pentamidine therapy were hypoglycemia (8 patients [11%]) and vomiting (6 patients [9%]).

Table 5: MEPRON

Treatment-emergent Adverse Experiences in the Pentamidine Comparative PCP Treatment Study

Treatment-emergent Adverse Experience	Number of Patients with Treatment-emergent Adverse Experience (% of Total)			
	MEPRON Tablets (n=73)		Pentamidine (n=71)	
Body as a Whole				
Asthenia	6	(8%)	10	(14%)
Fever	29	(40%)	18	(25%)
Headache	13	(18%)	20	(28%)
Pain	7	(10%)	7	(10%)
Cardiovascular				
Hypotension	1	(1%)	7	(10%)[a]
Gastrointestinal				
Diarrhea	15	(21%)	22	(31%)

(cont'd)

Table 5: MEPRON *(cont'd)*

Treatment-emergent Adverse Experiences in the Pentamidine Comparative PCP Treatment Study

Treatment-emergent Adverse Experience	Number of Patients with Treatment-emergent Adverse Experience (% of Total)			
	MEPRON Tablets (n=73)		Pentamidine (n=71)	
Dyspepsia	4	(5%)	7	(10%)
Abdominal Pain	7	(10%)	8	(11%)
Vomiting	10	(14%)	12	(17%)
Nausea	16	(22%)	26	(37%)
Monilia, Oral	7	(10%)	2	(3%)
Anorexia	5	(7%)	7	(10%)
Metabolic				
Hypoglycemia	1	(1%)	11	(15%)[a]
Nervous				
Anxiety	5	(7%)	7	(10%)
Dizziness	6	(8%)	10	(14%)
Insomnia	14	(19%)	10	(14%)
Respiratory				
Sinusitis	5	(7%)	4	(6%)
Rhinitis	4	(5%)	5	(7%)
Cough	10	(14%)[a]	1	(1%)
Skin				
Rash	16	(22%)	9	(13%)
Sweat	7	(10%)	2	(3%)
Special Senses				
Taste Perversion	2	(3%)	9	(13%)[a]
No. Patients Discontinuing Therapy due to an Adverse Experience	5	(7%)	29	(41%)[b]
No. Patients Reporting at least one Adverse Experience	46	(63%)	51	(72%)

[a] $p<0.05$.
[b] $p<0.001$.

Laboratory test abnormalities reported in ≥5% of patients in the pentamidine comparative study are presented in Table 6. Laboratory abnormality was reported as the reason for discontinuation of treatment in 2 of 73 patients who received atovaquone tablets. One patient (1%) had elevated creatinine and BUN levels and one patient (1%) had elevated amylase levels. Laboratory abnormalities were the sole or contributing factor in 14 patients who prematurely discontinued pentamidine therapy. In the 71 patients who received pentamidine, laboratory parameters most frequently reported as reasons for discontinuation were hypoglycemia (11%), elevated creatinine levels (6%), and leukopenia (4%).

Table 6: MEPRON

Treatment-emergent Laboratory Test Abnormalities in the Pentamidine Comparative PCP Treatment Study

Laboratory Test Abnormalities	Patients Developing a Laboratory Test Abnormality (% of Total)	
	MEPRON Tablets	Pentamidine
Anemia (Hgb <8.0 g/dL)	4%	9%
Neutropenia (ANC <750 c/mm³)	5%	9%
Hyponatremia (<0.96×LLN)	10%	10%
Hyperkalemia (>1.18×ULN)	0%	5%
Elevated Alkaline Phosphatase (>2.5×ULN)	5%	2%
Hyperglycemia (>1.8×ULN)	9%	13%
Elevated AST (>5×ULN)	0%	5%
Elevated Amylase (>1.5×ULN)	8%	4%
Elevated Creatinine (>1.5×ULN)	0%	7%

Legend: ULN=upper limit of normal range; LLN=lower limit of normal range; ANC: absolute neutrophil count.

Post-Marketing Adverse Reactions: In addition to adverse events reported from clinical trials, the following events have been identified during worldwide post-approval use of atovaquone. Because they are reported voluntarily from a population of unknown size, estimates of frequency cannot be made. These events have been chosen for inclusion due to a combination of their seriousness, frequency of reporting, or potential causal connection to atovaquone.
Blood and Lymphatic System Disorders: methemoglobinemia, thrombocytopenia.
Immune System Disorders: hypersensitivity reactions including angioedema, bronchospasm, throat tightness and urticaria.
Eye Disorders: vortex keratopathy.
Gastrointestinal Disorders: pancreatitis.
Hepatobiliary Disorders: Hepatitis and one case of fatal liver failure have been reported with atovaquone usage.
Skin and Subcutaneous Tissue Disorders: Erythema multiforme and Stevens-Johnson syndrome and skin desquamation have been reported in patients receiving multiple drug therapy including atovaquone.
Renal and Urinary Disorders: acute renal impairment.

OVERDOSE:

Symptoms and Treatment: There is insufficient experience to predict the consequences of or suggest specific management of overdosage from the oral administration of atovaquone oral suspension. If overdosage occurs, the patient should be monitored and standard supportive treatment applied.

For management of a suspected drug overdose, contact your **regional Poison Control Centre**. See the *CPS* Directory section for a list of Poison Control Centres.

DOSAGE: Adults: The recommended oral dose is 750 mg (5 mL) administered with food twice a day (total daily dose 1500 mg) for 21 days.

Failure to administer with food may result in lower plasma concentrations and may limit response to therapy (see Pharmacology and Precautions).

SUPPLIED: Each 5 mL of bright yellow suspension, with a sweet, fruity flavour, contains: atovaquone 750 mg. Nonmedicinal ingredients: benzyl alcohol, flavor (tutti frutti), poloxamer 188, purified water, saccharin sodium and xanthan gum. Bottles of 210 mL with child resistant cap. Store at 15 to 25°C. Keep in tight, light-resistant containers. **Do not freeze.**

(Shown in Product Identification Section)

Merrem® Ⓟr

meropenem

Antibiotic

AstraZeneca

Date of Preparation: June 20, 1996
Date of Revision: February 27, 2007

PHARMACOLOGY: MERREM (meropenem) is a broad spectrum, β-lactamase-resistant, carbapenem antibiotic for parenteral administration.

The bactericidal activity of meropenem results from the inhibition of bacterial cell wall synthesis. Meropenem readily penetrates through the cell wall of most gram-positive and gram-negative bacteria to reach penicillin binding protein (PBP) targets. Its greatest affinity is for PBP 2 of *E. coli*, PBP 2 and 3 of *P. aeruginosa* and 1, 2 and 4 of *S. aureus*.

Meropenem is stable in the presence of all serine β-lactamases (both penicillinases and cephalosporinases) produced by gram-positive and gram-negative bacteria.

Pharmacokinetics: At the end of a 30-minute i.v. infusion of a single dose of meropenem in healthy, male volunteers, mean peak plasma concentrations are approximately 23 µg/mL for the 500 mg dose, 49 µg/mL for the 1 g dose and 115 µg/mL for the 2 g dose.

I.V. bolus injections of a 1 g dose of meropenem over 2 minutes, 3 minutes and 5 minutes were compared in a 3-way crossover trial in healthy male volunteers. This resulted in peak plasma levels of 110, 91 and 94 µg/mL, respectively.

A 5-minute i.v. bolus injection of meropenem in healthy, male volunteers results in mean peak plasma levels of approximately 52 µg/mL for the 500 mg dose and 112 µg/mL for the 1 g dose.

At doses of 500 mg, mean plasma levels of meropenem decline to 1 µg/mL or less, 6 hours after administration.

In subjects with normal renal function, the elimination half-life of meropenem is approximately one hour. Approximately 70% of the administered dose is recovered unchanged in the urine over 12 hours, after which little further urinary excretion is detectable. Urinary concentrations of meropenem in excess of 10 µg/mL are maintained for at least 5 hours at the 500 mg dose. No clinically important accumulation of meropenem in plasma or urine was observed with regimens using 500 mg administered every 8 hours or 1 g administered every 6 hours in volunteers with normal renal function. Plasma protein binding of meropenem is approximately 2%.

There is one metabolite which is microbiologically inactive. In healthy subjects, the AUC for this metabolite was approximately 10% of the AUC for meropenem.

Meropenem penetrates well into most body fluids and tissues. However, it does not penetrate readily into cerebrospinal fluid or aqueous humor in the absence of inflammation at the sites. In children and adults with bacterial meningitis, meropenem concentrations in the cerebrospinal fluid, after intravenous administration of recommended doses, are in excess of those required to inhibit susceptible bacteria.

The pharmacokinetics of MERREM in children over age 2 are essentially similar to those in adults. The elimination half-life for meropenem was approximately 1.5 hours in children of age 3 months to 2 years. The pharmacokinetics for children are linear for doses of 10, 20 and 40 mg/kg and the peak plasma concentrations and AUC values are similar to those seen in healthy adult volunteers after 500 mg, 1 g and 2 g doses, respectively.

Pharmacokinetic studies of MERREM in patients with renal insufficiency have shown that the plasma clearance of meropenem correlates with creatinine clearance. Dosage adjustments are necessary in subjects with renal impairment (see Dosage). A pharmacokinetic study with MERREM in elderly patients with renal insufficiency has shown that a reduction in plasma clearance of meropenem correlates with age-associated reduction in creatinine clearance.

A pharmacokinetic study of MERREM in patients with hepatic impairment has shown no effects of liver disease on the pharmacokinetics of meropenem.

INDICATIONS: For treatment of the following infections when caused by susceptible strains of the designated microorganisms: Lower Respiratory Tract: Community-acquired pneumonia caused by *S. aureus* (β-lactamase-producing and non-β-lactamase-producing), *S. pneumoniae*, *E. coli* and *H. influenzae* (β-lactamase-producing and non-β-lactamase-producing).

Nosocomial pneumonia caused by *S. aureus* (non-β-lactamase-producing), *E. coli*, *H. influenzae* (non-β-lactamase-producing), *K. pneumoniae* and *P. aeruginosa*. As with other antibiotics, caution may be required in critically ill patients with known or suspected *P. aeruginosa* lower respiratory tract infections.

Urinary Tract: Complicated urinary tract infections caused by *E. cloacae*, *E. coli*, *K. pneumoniae*, *P. aeruginosa* and *S. marcescens*.

Intra-abdominal: Complicated intra-abdominal infections caused by *S. milleri*, *S. mitior*, *S. sanguis*, *C. freundii*, *E. cloacae*, *E. coli*, *K. oxytoca*, *K. pneumoniae*, *M. morganii*, *P. aeruginosa*, *B. distasonis*, *B. fragilis*, *B. ovatus*, *B. thetaiotaomicron*, *B. uniformis*, *B. vulgatus*, *C. perfringens*, Clostridium species, *E. lentum*, Fusobacterium species and Peptostreptococcus species.

Clinical trials of MERREM in patients with complicated intra-abdominal infections have demonstrated that the efficacy against *E. faecalis* is 71%.

Gynecologic: Gynecologic infections caused by *E. faecalis*, *S. aureus* (β-lactamase-producing and non-β-lactamase producing), *S. epidermidis* (non-β-lactamase-producing), *E. coli*, Fusobacterium species, *P. bivia*, *P. disiens*, *P. intermedia* and Peptostreptococcus species.

Pelvic inflammatory disease caused by *S. epidermidis* (non-β-lactamase-producing), *S. agalactiae*, *E. coli*, *N. gonorrhoeae* (non-β-lactamase-producing) and *P. bivia*.

Note: MERREM has no activity against *C. trachomatis*. Additional antimicrobial coverage is required if this pathogen is expected.

Uncomplicated Skin and Skin Structure: Uncomplicated skin and skin structure infections caused by *S. aureus* (β-lactamase-producing and non-β-lactamase-producing), *S. agalactiae*, *S. pyogenes* and *E. coli*.

Complicated Skin and Skin Structure: Complicated skin and skin structure infections, except infected burns, due to *S. aureus* (methicillin-susceptible strains), *S. pyogenes*, *S. agalactiae*, *E. faecalis* (excluding vancomycin-resistant isolates), Viridans group streptococci, *E. coli*, *P. aeruginosa*, *P. mirabilis*, *K. pneumoniae*, Peptostreptococcus species, Prevotella species, and *B. fragilis*.

Bacterial Meningitis: Bacterial meningitis caused by *S. pneumoniae*, *H. influenzae* (β-lactamase-producing and non-β-lactamase-producing) and *N. meningitidis*.

Note: There is limited adult efficacy data for MERREM in the treatment of bacterial meningitis. Support for the adult meningitis indication is largely provided by pediatric data.

Bacterial Septicemia: Bacterial septicemia caused by *E. coli*.

Therapy with MERREM may be initiated on the basis of clinical judgement before results of sensitivity testing are available. Continuation of therapy should be re-evaluated on the basis of bacteriological findings and on the patient's clinical condition. Regular sensitivity testing is recommended when treating *P. aeruginosa* infections.

CONTRAINDICATIONS: In patients with known hypersensitivity to any component of this product or in patients who have demonstrated anaphylactic reactions to β-lactam antibiotics.

WARNINGS: Serious and occasionally fatal hypersensitivity (anaphylactic) reactions have been reported in patients receiving therapy with β-lactam antibiotics. These reactions are more likely to occur in individuals with a history of sensitivity to multiple allergens.

There have been reports of individuals with a history of penicillin hypersensitivity who have experienced severe reactions when treated with another β-lactam antibiotic. Before initiating therapy with MERREM (meropenem), careful inquiry should be made concerning previous hypersensitivity reactions to penicillins, cephalosporins, other β-lactam antibiotics, and other allergens. If an allergic reaction to MERREM occurs, discontinue the drug immediately. Anaphylactic reactions require immediate treatment with epinephrine. Oxygen, i.v. steroids, antihistamines and airway management, including intubation, may be required.

Pseudomembranous colitis has been reported with many antibiotics, including MERREM, therefore, it is important to consider this diagnosis in patients who develop diarrhea in association with antibiotic use. This type of colitis may range in severity from mild to life threatening (see Adverse Effects, Post-Marketing Experience).

Treatment with antibacterial agents alters the normal flora of the colon and may permit overgrowth of Clostridia. Studies indicated that a toxin produced by *C. difficile* is one primary cause of antibiotic-associated colitis.

After the diagnosis of pseudomembranous colitis has been established, therapeutic measures should be initiated. Mild cases of pseudomembranous colitis usually respond to drug discontinuation alone. In moderate to severe cases, consideration should be given to management with fluids and electrolytes, protein supplementation and treatment with an antibacterial drug effective against *C. difficile*.

MERREM should not be used to treat infections caused by methicillin resistant staphylococci.

PRECAUTIONS: General: As with other broad-spectrum antibiotics, prolonged use of MERREM (meropenem) may result in overgrowth of nonsusceptible organisms. Repeated evaluation of the patient is essential. If superinfection does occur during therapy, appropriate measures should be taken.

MERREM, like all β-lactam antibiotics, has the potential to cause seizures. Diminished renal function and central nervous system lesions may increase the risk of seizures. When MERREM is indicated in patients with these risk factors, caution is advised.

Convulsions have been observed in a temporal association with use of MERREM, although a causal relationship has not been established.

Use of MERREM may lead to the development of a positive direct or indirect Coombs test.

MERREM may reduce serum valproic acid levels. Subtherapeutic levels of valproic acid may be reached in some patients. Subtherapeutic levels of valproic acid are known to increase patients' pre-disposition to seizure (see Drug Interactions).

Children: The safety and effectiveness of MERREM in the pediatric population 3 months of age and older have been established. MERREM is not recommended for use in infants under the age of 3 months.

The use of MERREM in pediatric patients with bacterial meningitis is supported by evidence from adequate and well controlled studies in the pediatric population. Use of MERREM in pediatric patients for all other indications, as listed in the Indications section, is supported by evidence from adequate and well controlled studies in adults with additional data from pediatric pharmacokinetic studies and controlled clinical trials in pediatric patients (see Dosage, Children).

Note: Inadequate data are available to support the pediatric indications for nosocomial pneumonia, septicemia and complicated skin and skin structure infections.

Pregnancy: There are no adequate and well-controlled studies in pregnant women. Because animal reproduction studies are not always predictive of human response, this drug should be used during pregnancy only if clearly needed. Reproduction studies have been performed in rats and Cynomolgous monkeys at doses up to 1000 mg/kg/day (approximately 16 times the usual human dose of 1 g every 8 hours). These studies revealed no evidence of impaired fertility or harm to the fetus due to meropenem although there were slight changes in fetal body weight at doses of 240 mg/kg/day and above in rats.

Lactation: MERREM is detected in animal breast milk, however, it is not known whether MERREM is excreted in human milk. MERREM should not be given to breast-feeding women unless the potential benefit justifies the potential risk to the baby.

Liver Disease: Patients with pre-existing liver disorders should have their liver function monitored during treatment with MERREM.

Renal Impairment: Dosage adjustment is recommended for patients with renal insufficiency (see Dosage).

Drug Interactions: Probenecid competes with meropenem for active tubular secretion and thus inhibits the renal excretion of meropenem with the effect of increasing the elimination half-life and plasma concentration of MERREM. The coadministration of probenecid with MERREM is neither required nor recommended.

Other than probenecid, no specific drug interaction studies were conducted.

MERREM may reduce serum valproic acid levels. Subtherapeutic levels of valproic acid may be reached in some patients. Subtherapeutic levels of valproic acid are known to increase patients' pre-disposition to seizure (see Precautions, General).

ADVERSE EFFECTS: MERREM (meropenem) is generally well tolerated. Many patients receiving MERREM are severely ill, have multiple background diseases, physiological impairments and receive multiple other drug therapies. In such seriously ill patients, it is difficult to establish the relationship between adverse events and MERREM.

Clinical Trials: The following adverse reaction frequencies were derived from all clinical trials in 3187 patients treated with MERREM administered intravenously.

Local Adverse Reactions: Local adverse clinical reactions that were reported by the investigator as possibly, probably or definitely related to therapy with MERREM were: inflammation at the injection site 1.6%, phlebitis/thrombophlebitis 0.5%, injection site reaction 0.4%, pain at the injection site 0.1% and edema at the injection site 0.1%.

Systemic Adverse Reactions: Systemic adverse clinical reactions that were reported by the investigator as possibly, probably or definitely related to MERREM and occurring in greater than 0.2% of the patients were: diarrhea (2.5%), nausea/vomiting (1.2%), rash (1.1%), pruritus (0.6%), headache (0.5%), urticaria (0.3%), vaginal moniliasis (0.7%), vaginitis (0.3%), oral moniliasis (0.3%) and fever (0.2%).

Additional adverse systemic clinical reactions reported by the investigator as possibly, probably or definitely related to MERREM and occurring in less than 0.2% of the patients are listed below within each body system in order of decreasing frequency.

Body as a Whole: abdominal pain, moniliasis, chills, infection, pain.

Nervous System: agitation, convulsions, dizziness, hallucinations, paresthesias, neuropathy.

Skin and Appendages: sweating.

Special Senses: taste perversion.

Digestive System: constipation.

Metabolic/Nutritional: peripheral edema.

Renal: renal impairment.

Hematological: thrombocytopenia.

Adverse Laboratory Changes: Adverse laboratory changes that were reported by the investigator as possibly, probably or definitely related to MERREM occurring in greater than 0.2% of the patients were as follows:

Hepatic: increased ALT, AST, alkaline phosphatase, LDH and bilirubin.

Hematologic: increased platelets, increased eosinophils, abnormal prothrombin time, abnormal partial thromboplastin time, decreased platelets, decreased WBC, leukopenia and neutropenia (including rare cases of agranulocytosis).

Renal: increased creatinine and increased BUN.

Children: Drug-related diarrhea (5.0%) and increases in platelets (7.0%) appear to occur more frequently in pediatric patients than in adults treated with MERREM.

Post-Marketing Experience: Very rare cases of the following have been reported: pseudomembranous colitis, hypokalemia, hypomagnesemia, severe skin reactions such as erythema multiforme, Stevens-Johnson Syndrome and toxic epidermal necrolysis, thrombocytopenia, and severe hypersensitivity reactions of angioedema and anaphylaxis.

Very rare reports of cholestasis, hepatitis, thrombocytopenia with bleeding and hemolytic anemia have been received. A causal relationship could not be excluded in spite of concomitant medications and/or illnesses.

OVERDOSE:

Symptoms: Intentional overdosing of MERREM (meropenem) is unlikely, although accidental overdosing might occur particularly in patients with reduced renal function. The largest dose of meropenem administered in clinical trials has been 2 g given intravenously every 8 hours to adult patients with normal renal function and 40 mg/kg every 8 hours to children with normal renal function. At these dosages, no adverse pharmacological effects were observed.

Limited post-marketing experience indicates that if adverse events occur following overdosage, they are generally consistent with the adverse event profile described under Adverse Effects.

Treatment: In the event of an overdose, MERREM should be discontinued and general supportive treatment given until renal elimination takes place. MERREM and its metabolite are readily dialyzable and effectively removed by hemodialysis; however, no information is available on the use of hemodialysis to treat overdosage.

The i.v. LD_{50} of meropenem in mice and rats is more than 2500 mg/kg and is approximately 2000 mg/kg in dogs.

For management of a suspected drug overdose, CPhA recommends that you contact your **regional Poison Control Centre**. See the *CPS* Directory section for a list of Poison Control Centres.

DOSAGE: Adults: The usual dose is 500 mg to 1 g by i.v. infusion every 8 hours, depending on type and severity of infection, the known or suspected susceptibility of the pathogens and the condition of the patient (see Table 1). Doses up to 2 g every 8 hours have been used. MERREM (meropenem) should be given by i.v. infusion over approximately 15 to 30 minutes or as an i.v. bolus injection (5 to 20 mL) over approximately 5 minutes.

The recommended dose to be given for adults is shown in Table 1.

Table 1: MERREM

Recommended Dose—Adults

Type of Infection	Dose	Dosage Interval
Complicated urinary tract	500 mg	every 8 hours
Uncomplicated skin and skin structure	500 mg	every 8 hours
Complicated skin and skin structure	500 mg	every 8 hours
Gynecologic and pelvic inflammatory disease	500 mg	every 8 hours
Lower respiratory		
Community-acquired pneumonia	500 mg	every 8 hours
Nosocomial pneumonia	1 g	every 8 hours
Complicated intra-abdominal	1 g	every 8 hours
Meningitis	2 g	every 8 hours
Septicemia	1 g	every 8 hours

Impaired Renal Function: Dosage should be reduced in patients with creatinine clearance less than 51 mL/min (see Table 2).

Table 2: MERREM

Dosage in Impaired Renal Function

Creatinine Clearance (mL/min)	Dose (dependent on type of infection)	Dosing Interval
26–50	recommended dose (500 mg to 2000 mg)	every 12 hours
10–25	one-half recommended dose	every 12 hours
<10	one-half recommended dose	every 24 hours

Meropenem is removed by hemodialysis; if continued treatment with MERREM is necessary, the dose, based on the infection type and severity, should be administered at the completion of the hemodialysis procedure to reinstitute effective treatment.

There are no data on appropriate doses in patients requiring peritoneal dialysis.

Adults with Hepatic Insufficiency: No dosage adjustment is necessary in patients with hepatic dysfunction as long as renal function is normal.

Geriatrics: Dosage adjustment is recommended for the elderly with an estimated or measured creatinine clearance value below 50 mL/min (see Impaired Renal Function).

Children: For infants and children over 3 months of age and weighing up to 50 kg, the recommended dose of MERREM is 10 to 40 mg/kg every 8 hours, depending on type and severity of infection, the known or suspected susceptibility of the pathogens and the condition of the patient (see Table 3). Children weighing over 50 kg require the adult dosage. MERREM should be given as an intravenous infusion over approximately 15 to 30 minutes or as an intravenous bolus injection (5 to 20 mL) over approximately 5 minutes.

Table 3: MERREM

Recommended Dose—Children

Type of Infection	Dose (mg/kg)	Dosing Interval
Complicated urinary tract	10	every 8 hours
Uncomplicated skin and skin structure	10–20	every 8 hours
Community-acquired pneumonia	10–20	every 8 hours
Complicated intra-abdominal	20	every 8 hours
Meningitis	40	every 8 hours

There are no data on appropriate doses for children with renal impairment.

Parenteral Products: Compatibility of MERREM with other drugs has not been established. MERREM should not be mixed with or physically added to solutions containing other drugs.

Freshly prepared solutions of MERREM should be used whenever possible. Solutions of MERREM should not be frozen.

All vials are for single use only. Standard aseptic technique should be employed during constitution and administration.

Parenteral drug products should be inspected visually for particulate matter and discoloration prior to administration, whenever solution and container permit.

I.V. Bolus Administration: Reconstitute injection vials (500 mg/20 mL and 1 g/30 mL) with Sterile Water for Injection (see Table 4). Shake to dissolve and let stand until clear.

MERREM injection vials reconstituted with sterile Water for Injection for bolus administration (up to 50 mg/mL of MERREM) may be stored for up to 2 hours at controlled room temperature 15-25°C or for up to 12 hours at 4°C.

Infusion: Injection vials may be reconstituted, then the resulting solution added to an i.v. container and further diluted with an appropriate infusion fluid (see Table 5).

Stability in Plastic I.V. Bags: Solutions prepared for infusion (MERREM concentrations ranging from 1 to 20 mg/mL) may be stored in plastic i.v. bags with diluents as shown in Table 5. Diluted i.v. infusion solutions should be inspected visually for discoloration, haziness, particulate matter and leakage prior to administration, whenever solution and container permit. Discard unused portion.

Table 4: MERREM
Reconstitution for I.V. Bolus

Vial Size	Amount of Diluent Added (mL)	Approximate Withdrawable Volume (mL)	Approximate Average Concentration (mg/mL)
500 mg/20 mL	10	10	50
1 g/30 mL	20	20	50

Table 5: MERREM
Diluents

Diluent	Number of Hours Stable at Controlled Room Temperature 15 to 25°C	Number of Hours Stable at 4°C
Sodium Chloride 0.9% Injection	4	24
Dextrose 5% Injection	1	4
Dextrose 10% Injection	1	2
Dextrose 5% and Sodium Chloride 0.9% Injection	1	2
Dextrose 5% and Sodium Chloride 0.2% Injection	1	4
Potassium Chloride 0.15% in Dextrose 5% Injection	1	6
Sodium Bicarbonate 0.02% in Dextrose 5% Injection	1	6
Dextrose 5% Injection in Normosol-M	1	8
Dextrose 5% Injection in Ringers Lactate Injection	1	4
Dextrose 2.5% and Sodium Chloride 0.45% Injection	3	12
Mannitol Injection 2.5%	2	16
Ringers Injection	4	24
Ringers Lactate Injection	4	12
Sodium Lactate Injection 1/6 N	2	24
Sodium Bicarbonate 5% Injection	1	4

Stability in Plastic Syringes, Tubing and I.V. Infusion Sets: Solutions of MERREM (MERREM concentrations ranging from 1 to 20 mg/mL) in Water for Injection or Sodium Chloride 0.9% Injection (for up to 4 hours) or in Dextrose 5% Injection (for up to 2 hours) at controlled room temperatures 15 to 25°C are stable in plastic syringes, plastic tubing, drip chambers, and volume control devices of common i.v. infusion sets.

SUPPLIED: 500 mg: Each vial of dry powder contains: meropenem trihydrate equivalent to meropenem anhydrous 500 mg and sodium carbonate equivalent to sodium 45.1 mg. Vials of 20 mL.
1 g: Each vial of dry powder contains: meropenem trihydrate equivalent to meropenem anhydrous 1 g and sodium carbonate equivalent to sodium 90.2 mg. Vials of 30 mL.
Store between 15 and 30°C.

Mersyndol® with Codeine Ⓝ
acetaminophen—codeine phosphate—doxylamine succinate
Analgesic

sanofi-aventis

SUPPLIED: Each round, white, flat-faced, bevelled-edged tablet, with stylized "S" embossed on one side contains: acetaminophen 325 mg, codeine phosphate 8 mg and doxylamine succinate 5 mg. Nonmedicinal ingredients: croscarmellose sodium, magnesium stearate, microcrystalline cellulose, pregelatinized starch, povidone and silicon dioxide. Bisulfites-, gluten-, lactose-, parabens- and tartrazine-free. HDPE bottles of 100. Blister packages of 24.

(Shown in Product Identification Section)

Mesasal® Ⓟ
5-ASA
Lower Gastrointestinal Anti-inflammatory

GlaxoSmithKline

Date of Revision: July 14, 2008

PHARMACOLOGY: 5-Aminosalicylic acid (5-ASA) is considered to be the active component of sulfasalazine. Although its mode of action has not been definitely elucidated, 5-ASA is thought to have a topical anti-inflammatory effect which is produced by inhibition of prostaglandin and/or leukotriene synthesis.

The tablets have an acrylic-based resin coating which is specifically designed to release 5-ASA in the terminal ileum and colon. Urinary recovery studies have shown that 35% of the 5-ASA is absorbed. The absorbed 5-ASA is rapidly acetylated and excreted mainly by the kidney.

Detectable plasma levels of 5-ASA were seen 4 hours after a single oral dose of tablets (2×250 mg). Peak plasma levels of 5-ASA and N-acetyl-5-ASA were 1.2 and 1.9 µg/mL, respectively, and occurred 6.5 to 7 hours post-dosing. Mean steady-state plasma levels of 5-ASA and N-acetyl-5-ASA using a 500 mg 3 times a day dosage schedule are 0.7 and 1.2 µg/mL, respectively.

Except for a delay of 1.5 to 3 hours in time to peak of 5-ASA and N-acetyl-5-ASA plasma levels, Mesasal pharmacokinetics are essentially the same in fasted and fed subjects.

INDICATIONS: The management of acute ulcerative colitis and the prevention of relapse of active ulcerative colitis.

CONTRAINDICATIONS: Hypersensitivity to salicylates; in cases of hemorrhagic diathesis; in patients with existing gastric and duodenal ulcers; in patients with urinary tract obstruction; in children under 2 years of age.

WARNINGS: In cases of kidney or severe liver impairment, caution should be exercised. Interstitial nephritis has been reported following treatment with 5-ASA. Hence, patients with compromised renal function, impaired renal reserve or individuals with an increased risk of developing renal dysfunction due to use of nephrotoxic drugs or other comorbid conditions should be carefully monitored throughout the duration of therapy, and especially during the early months of treatment. Treatment with 5-ASA should be discontinued promptly if renal function significantly deteriorates. Care should be taken to ensure adequate hydration in patients with compromised renal function during exacerbations of inflammatory bowel disease. In view of rare risk of interstitial nephritis associated with 5-ASA treatment, it is recommended that all patients have their renal function monitored (with serum creatinine levels measured) prior to treatment start. Renal function should then be periodically monitored during chronic treatment, based on individual patient history. Treatment with 5-ASA should be discontinued promptly if renal function deteriorates.

Sexual Function/Reproduction: Decreased sperm count and impaired sperm motility, which may affect male fertility, have been reported with mesalazine (5-ASA). This effect may be reversible when treatment is discontinued.

Pregnancy: Adequate human data on use during pregnancy are not available. 5-ASA should not be prescribed during the last weeks of pregnancy or during lactation. In the first 3 months of pregnancy, treatment is recommended only if potential benefits outweigh the possible risks. Adequate human data on use during lactation and adequate animal reproduction studies are not available.

Lactation: See Pregnancy.

Children: There is limited experience with respect to the use of this drug in children; potential benefits should be weighed against possible risks.

PRECAUTIONS: *Drug Interactions:* Caution should be exercised when 5-ASA and sulfonylureas are prescribed concomitantly, since the blood-sugar reducing effect of sulfonylureas may be enhanced. Interactions with coumarins, probenecid, sulfinpyrazone, spironolactone, furosemide and rifampicin cannot be excluded. 5-ASA may delay the excretion of methotrexate.

In long-term therapy, periodic urinalysis should be conducted. Caution should be exercised when therapy is first initiated in patients known to be allergic to sulfasalazine.

There is in vitro evidence that mesalazine (5-ASA) is a weak inhibitor of the azathioprine metabolizing enzyme thiopurine methyltransferase (TPMT). Enhancement of the myelosuppressive effects of azathioprine or 6-mercaptopurine may occur rarely in patients who are treated concomitantly with mesalazine (5-ASA).

ADVERSE EFFECTS: In controlled clinical trials in 395 patients who received 5-ASA, the following adverse reactions were reported: headache (3.0%), nausea (2.0%), abdominal pain (1.5%) and diarrhea (1.5%). Rash (including pruritus and urticaria) has also been reported. Other adverse effects common to salicylates, such as occasional transitory abnormal liver function tests or hypersensitivity reactions, including pulmonary and cardiac changes, may be expected to occur rarely. There have been a few spontaneous reports of pancreatitis, acute and chronic interstitial nephritis and pericarditis associated with 5-ASA therapy. Exacerbation of symptoms of colitis has been reported very rarely. Decreased sperm count, impaired sperm motility, neuropathy, hepatitis and alterations in peripheral blood counts such as leukopenia, neutropenia, thrombocytopenia and aplastic anemia have been rarely reported.

OVERDOSE:

Treatment: There is no specific antidote. Gastric lavage should be employed, followed by promotion of diuresis by the i.v. infusion of an electrolyte solution.

> For management of a suspected drug overdose, contact your **regional Poison Control Centre**. See the *CPS* Directory section for a list of Poison Control Centres.

DOSAGE: During the acute inflammatory stage and in long-term maintenance therapy, 5-ASA must be taken reliably and consistently by the patient in order to ensure therapeutic success.

Although symptomatic relief may be seen as early as 3 to 21 days, therapy should be continued depending on clinical findings.

The following dosage regimens are recommended: Adults: The tablets should be swallowed whole before meals with plenty of fluid.

For the management of acute ulcerative colitis, 1.5 to 3 g daily in divided doses.

For prevention of relapses of acute ulcerative colitis, 1.5 g daily in divided doses.

SUPPLIED: Each oval, red-orange enteric coated tablet contains: 5-aminosalicylic acid 500 mg. Nonmedicinal ingredients: calcium stearate, glycine, iron oxide (red), iron oxide (yellow), methacrylic acid copolymer, microcrystalline cellulose, polyethylene glycol 6000, povidone, silicon dioxide, sodium carbonate, sodium croscarmellose, talc and titanium dioxide. Mesasal tablets are acrylic coated to prevent release of 5-ASA until the tablets reach the terminal ileum and proximal colon. Polyethylene bottles of 100.

(Shown in Product Identification Section)

M-Eslon® Ⓝ
morphine sulfate
Narcotic Analgesic

Ethypharm

Date of Preparation: May 26, 2006

PHARMACOLOGY: Morphine is a narcotic analgesic which exerts an agonist effect at specific, saturable opioid receptors in the CNS and other tissues. In man, morphine produces a variety of effects including analgesia, constipation from decreased gastrointestinal motility, suppression of the cough reflex, respiratory depression from reduced responsiveness of the respiratory centre to CO_2, nausea and vomiting via stimulation of the CTZ, changes in mood including euphoria and dysphoria, sedation, mental clouding, and alterations of the endocrine and autonomic nervous systems.

The psychological effects are of longer duration than that of analgesia. Morphine-induced analgesia is relatively selective in that other sensory modalities (touch, vision, hearing) are not affected. Moderate doses of morphine are effective in relieving clinical (pathological) pain and increasing pain threshold to tolerate pain. The capacity to perceive the sensation of pain may be relatively unaltered. The analgesic effects of morphine are due to its CNS action, i.e., limbic system, hypothalamus, and centrally induced endocrinological effect. At present, the exact mechanism by which the opiates exert their effects remains unknown.

Morphine is readily absorbed from the gastrointestinal tract and after s.c. or i.m. injection. Due to first-pass metabolism in the liver, the effect of an oral dose is less than after parenteral administration. With repeated regular dosing, orally administered morphine is about one-third as potent as when given by i.m. injection. Morphine is primarily excreted in the urine as morphine-3-glucuronide. About 7 to 10% of a dose of morphine is excreted in the feces via the bile.

M-ESLON Capsules (Morphine Sulfate Extended Release Capsules) produce peak morphine levels at steady state in approximately 3 to 4 hours following administration. In human pharmacokinetic studies, they have been shown to have an extended release action, when compared to oral morphine sulfate syrup, as characterized by a flatter peak serum concentration curve which took longer to attain; the elimination half-life was significantly lengthened. Therapeutic levels are maintained over a period of 12 hours.

This product has not been compared to any slow-release morphine preparation on the Canadian market, and therefore is not interchangeable.

INDICATIONS: M-ESLON Capsules (Morphine Sulfate Extended Release Capsules) are indicated for the symptomatic relief of severe pain.

CONTRAINDICATIONS: Until further information is available, co-ingestion of M-ESLON with alcohol is contraindicated. Co-ingestion of M-ESLON and alcohol can potentially result in rapid increases in opioid plasma concentrations, which may be fatal, even in opioid tolerant patients.

M-ESLON Capsules (Morphine Sulfate Extended Release Capsules) should not be given to patients with: hypersensitivity to opiate narcotics; acute asthma or other obstructive airway disease and acute respiratory depression; cor pulmonale; cardiac arrhythmias; acute alcoholism; severe cirrhosis; delirium tremens; severe CNS depression, convulsive disorders; increased cerebrospinal or intracranial pressure; head injury or brain tumor (may cause marked exaggeration of cerebrospinal fluid pressure and mask the clinical course); suspected surgical abdomen; surgical anastomosis (narcotics may cause increase in intraluminal pressure); after surgery of the biliary tract; surgical anastomosis; hypotension; concomitant MAO inhibitors (or within 14 days of such therapy).

WARNINGS: This product has not been compared to any slow-release morphine preparation on the Canadian market, and therefore is not interchangeable.

Drug Dependence: As with other narcotics, tolerance and physical dependence tend to develop upon repeated administration of morphine and there is potential for abuse of the drug and for development of strong psychological dependence. M-ESLON Capsules (Morphine Sulfate Extended Release Capsules) should therefore be prescribed and handled with the high degree of caution appropriate to the use of a drug with strong abuse potential. Drug abuse is not, however, a problem in patients with severe pain in which morphine is appropriately indicated. On the other hand, in the absence of a clear indication for a strong narcotic analgesic, drug-seeking behaviour must be suspected and resisted, particularly in patients with a history of, or propensity for drug abuse. Withdrawal symptoms may occur following abrupt discontinuation of morphine therapy or upon administration of a narcotic antagonist. Therefore, patients on prolonged therapy should be withdrawn gradually from the drug if it is no longer required for pain control.

Severe pain antagonizes the subjective and respiratory depressant actions of morphine. Should pain suddenly subside, these effects may rapidly become manifest. Patients who are scheduled for cordotomy or other interruption of pain transmission pathways should not receive M-ESLON Capsules within 24 hours of the procedure.

Pregnancy: Animals studies indicate that morphine may be teratogenic at high doses in mice, and may cause an increased incidence of abortions and reduced birth weight in rabbits. In humans, it is not known whether morphine can cause fetal harm when administered during pregnancy or can affect reproductive capacity. M-ESLON Capsules should be given to pregnant patients only if clearly needed and when the anticipated benefits outweigh the risks to the fetus and the mother. Infants born to mothers who are physically dependent on narcotics exhibit withdrawal symptoms, such as generalized tremors, hypertonicity, hyperalertness, sleeplessness, excessive crying, vomiting, diarrhea, yawning, and occasional fever.

PRECAUTIONS: General: The respiratory depressant effects of morphine, and the capacity to elevate cerebrospinal fluid pressure, may be greatly increased in the presence of an already elevated intracranial pressure produced by trauma. Also, morphine may produce confusion, miosis, vomiting and other side effects which obscure the clinical course of patients with head injury. In such patients, morphine must be used with extreme caution and only if it is judged to be essential.

Morphine should be used with extreme caution in patients with chronic pulmonary disease; substantially decreased respiratory reserve, preexisting respiratory depression, hypoxia or hypercapnia. Such patients are often less sensitive to the stimulatory effects of carbon dioxide on the respiratory centre and the respiratory depressant effects of morphine may reduce respiratory drive to the point of apnea.

Morphine administration may result in severe hypotension in patients whose ability to maintain adequate blood pressure is compromised by reduced blood volume, or concurrent administration of such drugs as phenothiazines or certain anesthetics.

Morphine may obscure the diagnosis or clinical course of patients with acute abdominal conditions.

Morphine may cause a decrease in systemic vascular resistance in patients with myocardial infarction. A transient fall in systemic arterial pressure may result, leading to severe hypotension. Administered in large doses, morphine may cause severe hypotension even in the supine patient.

Special Risk Groups: Morphine should be administered with caution, and in reduced dosages, to elderly or debilitated patients, to patients with severely reduced hepatic or renal function, and in patients with Addison's disease, hypothyroidism, prostatic hypertrophy or urethral stricture, hypopituitarism, anemia, severe malnutrition, fulminant ulcerative colitis, untreated myxedema.

Labor/delivery : Morphine crosses the placental barrier and its administration during labor can produce respiratory depression in the neonate.

Lactation: Morphine has been detected in human breast milk. Caution should be exercised if morphine is administered to a nursing mother.

Occupational Hazards: Morphine may impair the mental and/or physical abilities needed for certain potentially hazardous activities such as driving a car or operating machinery. Patients should be cautioned accordingly.

Patients should also be cautioned about the combined effects of morphine with other CNS depressants, including other opioids, phenothiazines, sedative/hypnotics and alcohol.

Drug Interactions: Generally, the effects of morphine may be antagonized by acidifying agents and potentiated by alkalinizing agents.

Anticholinergics: The concomitant use of anticholinergics with narcotics, including morphine, may result in an increased risk of severe constipation and urinary retention.

Narcotic Antagonists: Concomitant use of narcotic antagonists may result in reversal of analgesia, and may precipitate withdrawal symptoms in patients who are physically dependent on narcotics.

CNS Depressants: CNS depressants, such as other opioids, alcohol, anesthetics, antihistamines, barbiturates, beta-blockers, chloral hydrate, glutethimide, hypnotics, MAO inhibitors, phenothiazines, pyrazolidone, sedatives, skeletal muscle relaxants and tricyclic antidepressants may enhance the depressant effects of morphine. Concurrent use may result in potentiation of CNS depression and death may occur. If used concurrently with CNS depressants, dosage adjustment may be required.

Amphetamines: Amphetamines potentiate the analgesic effect of morphine.

Oral Anticoagulants: Morphine may increase the anticoagulant activity of coumarin and other anticoagulants.

Alcohol: Until further information is available, co-ingestion of M-ESLON with alcohol is contraindicated. (See Contraindications).

ADVERSE EFFECTS: The major hazards associated with morphine, as with other narcotic analgesics, are respiratory depression and, to a lesser degree, circulatory depression. Respiratory arrest, shock and cardiac arrest have occurred following oral or parenteral use of morphine.

Most Common Adverse Effects Requiring Medical Attention: The most frequently observed side effects of narcotic analgesics such as morphine are sedation, nausea and vomiting, constipation and sweating.

Sedation: Most patients experience initial drowsiness partly for pharmacokinetic reasons and partly because patients often recuperate from prolonged fatigue after the relief of persistent pain. Drowsiness usually clears in 3 to 5 days and is usually not a reason for concern providing that it is not excessive, or associated with unsteadiness or confusional symptoms. If excessive sedation persists the reason for it must be sought. Some of these are: concomitant sedative medications, hepatic or renal failure, exacerbated respiratory failure, higher doses than tolerated in an older patient, or the patient is actually more severely ill than realized. If it is necessary to reduce the dose, it can be carefully increased again after 3 or 4 days if it is obvious that the pain is not being well controlled. Dizziness and unsteadiness may be caused by postural hypotension particularly in elderly or debilitated patients. It can be alleviated if the patient lies down. Because of the slower clearance in patients over 50 years of age, an appropriate dose in this age group may be as low as half or less the usual in the younger age group.

Nausea and Vomiting: Nausea and vomiting occur frequently after single doses of narcotics or as an early unwanted effect of regular narcotic therapy. When instituting prolonged therapy for chronic pain the routine prescription of antiemetic should be considered. Patients taking the equivalent of a single dose of 20 mg or more of morphine every 4 hours (60 mg of M-ESLON Capsules (Morphine Sulfate Extended Release Capsules) every 12 hours) usually require an antiemetic during early therapy. Small doses of prochlorperazine or haloperidol are the most frequently prescribed antiemetics. Nausea and vomiting tend to lessen in a week or so but may persist due to narcotic-induced gastric stasis. In such patients, metoclopramide is often useful.

Constipation: Practically all patients become constipated while taking narcotics on a persistent basis. In some instances, particularly the elderly or bedridden, patients may become impacted. It is essential to caution the patients in this regard and to institute an appropriate regimen of bowel management at the start of prolonged narcotic therapy. Softeners, laxatives and other appropriate measures should be used as required.

CNS: euphoria, dysphoria, weakness, insomnia, dizziness, headache, agitation, tremor, uncoordinated muscle movements, visual disturbances, confusional symptoms and occasionally hallucinations.

Gastrointestinal: dry mouth, anorexia, constipation, cramps, taste alterations and biliary tract spasm.

Genitourinary: urinary retention or hesitance, reduced libido or potency.

Cardiovascular: supraventricular tachycardia, postural hypotension, palpitations, faintness and syncope.

Endocrine: A syndrome of inappropriate antidiuretic hormone secretion characterized by hyponatremia secondary to decreased free-water excretion may be prominent (monitoring of electrolytes may be necessary).

Allergic: pruritus, urticaria, other skin rashes and edema.

Withdrawal (Abstinence) Syndrome: Physical dependence with or without psychological dependence tends to occur on chronic administration. An abstinence syndrome may be precipitated when narcotic administration is discontinued or narcotic antagonists administered. The following withdrawal symptoms may be observed after narcotics are discontinued: body aches, diarrhea, gooseflesh, loss of appetite, nervousness or restlessness, runny nose, sneezing, tremors or shivering, stomach cramps, nausea, trouble with sleeping, unusual increase in sweating and yawning, weakness, tachycardia and unexplained fever. With appropriate medical use of narcotics and gradual withdrawal from the drug, these symptoms are usually mild.

OVERDOSE:

Symptoms: Serious morphine overdosage is characterized by respiratory depression (reduced respiratory rate and/or tidal volume; Cheyne-Stokes respiration; cyanosis), extreme somnolence progressing to stupor or coma, flaccidity of skeletal muscle, cold or clammy skin, and sometimes hypotension and bradycardia. Severe overdosage may result in apnea, circulatory collapse, cardiac arrest and death. Convulsions may occur in young children.

Treatment: Primary attention should be given to the establishment of adequate respiratory exchange through provision of a patent airway and controlled or assisted ventilation. The narcotic antagonist naloxone is a specific antidote against respiratory depression due to overdosage or as a result of unusual sensitivity to morphine. An appropriate dose of this antagonist should therefore be administered, preferably by the i.v. route. The usual initial i.v. adult dose of naloxone is 0.4 mg or higher. Concomitant efforts at respiratory resuscitation should be carried out. Since the duration of action of morphine, particularly extended release formulations, may exceed that of the antagonist, the patient should be under continued surveillance and doses of the antagonist should be repeated as needed to maintain adequate respiration.

An antagonist should not be administered in the absence of clinically significant respiratory or cardiovascular depression. Oxygen, i.v. fluids, vasopressors and other supportive measures should be used as indicated.

Note: In an individual physically dependent on narcotics, the administration of the usual dose of narcotic antagonist will precipitate an acute withdrawal syndrome. The severity of this syndrome will depend on the degree of physical dependence and the dose of antagonist administered. The use of narcotic antagonists in such individuals should be avoided if possible. If a narcotic antagonist must be used to treat serious respiratory depression in the physically dependent patient, the antagonist should be administered with extreme care by using dosage titration, commencing with 10 to 20% of the usual recommended initial dose.

Evacuation of gastric contents may be useful in removing unabsorbed drug, particularly when an extended release formulation has been taken.

For management of a suspected drug overdose, CPhA recommends that you contact your **regional Poison Control Centre.** See the *CPS* Directory section for a list of Poison Control Centres.

DOSAGE: This product has not been compared to any slow-release morphine preparation on the Canadian market, and therefore is not interchangeable.

Administration and dosing of morphine should be individualized bearing in mind the properties of the drug. In addition, the nature and severity of the pain or pains experienced, and the total condition of the patient must be taken into account. Of special importance is other medication given previously or concurrently.

As with other strong narcotic analgesics, use of morphine for the management of persistent pain should be preceded by a thorough assessment of the patient and diagnosis of the specific pain or pains and their causes. Use of narcotics for the relief of chronic pain, including cancer pain, all important as it may be, should be only one part of a comprehensive approach to pain control including other treatment modalities or drug therapy, non-drug measures and psychosocial support.

For essential information on the important details of the management of cancer pain, the reader may wish to consult the following resource: Cancer Pain: A Monograph on the Management of Cancer Pain. Health and Welfare Canada.

The capsules may be opened, and the microgranules given mixed with soft food, liquids or by gastric tube or gastrotomy to dysphagic (e.g. E.N.T. cancer) patients who can benefit from the analgesia obtained from an extended release preparation.

Initial Adult Dose: Individual dosing requirements vary considerably based on each patient's age, weight, severity of pain, and medical and analgesic history.

The most frequent initial dose is 30 mg M-ESLON Capsules (Morphine Sulfate Extended Release Capsules) every 12 hours.

The capsules may be opened, and the microgranules given mixed with soft food, liquids or by gastric tube or gastrotomy to dysphagic (e.g. E.N.T. cancer) patients who can benefit from the analgesia obtained from an extended release preparation.

Patients over the age of 50 tend to require much lower doses of morphine than the younger age group. In elderly and debilitated patients and those with impaired respiratory function or significantly decreased renal function, the initial dose should be one-half the usual recommended dose.

Patients currently receiving other oral morphine immediate release formulations may be transferred to M-ESLON Capsules at the same total daily morphine dosage, equally divided into two 12-hourly M-ESLON doses.

For patients who are receiving an alternate narcotic, the "oral morphine equivalent" of the analgesic presently being used should be determined. Having determined the total daily dosage of the present analgesic, the following equivalence table (Table 1) can be used to calculate the approximate daily oral morphine dosage that should provide equivalent analgesia. This total daily oral morphine dosage should then be equally divided in two 12 hourly M-ESLON doses.

Table 1: M-ESLON

Narcotics: Approximate Analgesic Equivalences[a]

Drug	Equivalent Dose (mg)[b]	
	im	po
Agonists		
Morphine sulfate	10	20–30[c]
Codeine phosphate	120	200
Hydromorphone (Dilaudid)	2	4
Levorphanol (Levo-Dromoran)	2	4
Oxycodone (Percodan, Percocet)		10–15
Anileridine (Leritine)	25	75
Meperidine (pethidine, Demerol)	75	300
Oxymorphone (Numorphan)	1.5	(Supp 5 mg)
Methadone	10	20
Heroin	5–8	10–15
Agonist-Antagonists		
Pentazocine (Talwin)	60	180
Nalbuphine (Nubain)	10	
Butorphanol	2	

[a] Adapted from Cancer Pain: A Monograph on the Management of Cancer Pain, Health & Welfare Canada, 1984.

[b] Most of this data was derived from single-dose, acute pain studies and should be considered a rough approximation for initial selection of doses when treating chronic cancer pain.

[c] The po/im potency ratio of 1/3 to 1/2 for morphine is based on clinical experience in chronic pain.

Dose titration is the key to success with morphine therapy. **Proper optimization of doses scaled to the relief of the individual's pain should aim at the regular administration of the lowest dose of morphine which will maintain the patient free of pain at all times.** Dose adjustments should be based on the patient's clinical response. Higher doses may be justified in some patients to cover periods of physical activity.

Because of the extended release properties of M-ESLON Capsules, dosage adjustments should generally be separated by 48 hours. If dose increments turn out to be required, they should be proportionately greater at the lower dose level (in terms of percentage of previous dose), than when adjusting a higher dose. The usual recommended dose (every 12 hours) increments are 30, 60, 90, 120, 150, 180, 200 mg. Above the 200 mg/dose (400 mg/day) increments should be by 30 to 60 mg/dose.

M-ESLON Capsules (Morphine Sulfate Extended Release Capsules) are designed to allow 12-hourly dosing. If "breakthrough" pain repeatedly occurs at the end of a dose interval, it is generally an indication for a dosage increase, not more frequent administration. However, where judged necessary for optimization of drug effects, the product may be administered every 8 hours. More frequent (than every 8 hours) administration is not recommended.

Adjustment or Reduction of Dosage: During the first 2 or 3 days of effective pain relief, the patient may exhibit drowsiness or sleep for prolonged periods. This can be misinterpreted as the effect of excessive analgesic dosing rather than the first sign of relief in a patient exhausted by pain. The dose, therefore, should be maintained for at least three days before reduction, provided the sedation is not excessive or associated with unsteadiness and confusional symptoms, and respiratory activity and other vital signs are adequate. If excessive sedation persists, the reason(s) for such an effect must be sought. Some of these are: concomitant sedative medications, hepatic or renal failure, exacerbated respiratory failure, higher doses than tolerated by an older patient, or the patient is actually more severely ill than realized. If it is necessary to reduce the dose, it can be carefully increased again after three or four days if it is obvious that the pain is not being well controlled.

Following successful relief of severe pain, periodic attempts to reduce the narcotic dose should be made. Smaller doses or complete discontinuation of the narcotic analgesic may become feasible due to a change in the patient's condition or improved mental state.

Narcotic agents do not relieve effectively dysesthetic pain, post-herpetic neuralgia, stabbing pains, activity-related pain, and some forms of headache. This is not to say that patients with advanced cancer suffering from some of these forms of pain should not be given an adequate trial of opiate analgesics, but it may be necessary to refer such patients at an early time for other forms of pain therapy. Pain without nociception does not respond to narcotics.

INFORMATION FOR THE PATIENT: Published in e-CPS, available by subscription at www.e-cps.ca.

SUPPLIED: 10 mg: Each #4 hard gelatin capsule, printed with the logo "", "M-ESLON" and "10" in black, opaque white cap and body, contains: morphine sulfate 10 mg in the form of extended release microgranules. Nonmedicinal ingredients: cornstarch, dibutyl sebacate, polyoxyethylene glycol, polymeric dispersion of ethylcellulose, sugar and talc; capsule shell: coloring agent, gelatin and sulfur dioxide. Tartrazine-free. Cartons containing blister packs of 20. White, opaque polypropylene bottles of 50, with tamper-evident polyethylene caps. Store at room temperature, and protect from excessive heat.

15 mg: Each #4 hard gelatin capsule, printed with the logo "", "M-ESLON" and "15" in black, opaque yellow cap and transparent natural body, contains: morphine sulfate 15 mg in the form of extended release microgranules. Nonmedicinal ingredients: cornstarch, dibutyl sebacate, polyoxyethylene glycol, polymeric dispersion of ethylcellulose, sugar and talc; capsule shell: coloring agent, gelatin and sulfur dioxide. Tartrazine-free. Cartons containing blister packs of 20. White, opaque polypropylene bottles of 50, with tamper-evident polyethylene caps. Store at room temperature, and protect from excessive heat.

30 mg: Each #4 hard gelatin capsule, printed with the logo "", "M-ESLON" and "30" in black, opaque pink cap and transparent natural body, contains: morphine sulfate 30 mg in the form of extended release microgranules. Nonmedicinal ingredients: cornstarch, dibutyl sebacate, polyoxyethylene glycol, polymeric dispersion of ethylcellulose, sugar and talc; capsule shell: coloring agent, gelatin and sulfur dioxide. Tartrazine-free. Cartons containing blister packs of 20. White, opaque polypropylene bottles of 50, with tamper-evident polyethylene caps. Store at room temperature, and protect from excessive heat.

60 mg: Each #3 hard gelatin capsule, printed with the logo "", "M-ESLON" and "60" in black, opaque orange cap and transparent natural body, contains: morphine sulfate 60 mg in the form of extended release microgranules. Nonmedicinal ingredients: cornstarch, dibutyl sebacate, polyoxyethylene glycol, polymeric dispersion of ethylcellulose, sugar and talc; capsule shell: coloring agent, gelatin and sulfur dioxide. Tartrazine-free. Cartons containing blister packs of 20. White, opaque polypropylene bottles of 50, with tamper-evident polyethylene caps. Store at room temperature, and protect from excessive heat.

100 mg: Each #2 hard gelatin capsule, printed with the logo "", "M-ESLON" and "100" in white, opaque gray cap and transparent natural body, contains: morphine sulfate 100 mg in the form of extended release microgranules. Nonmedicinal ingredients: cornstarch, dibutyl sebacate, polyoxyethylene glycol, polymeric dispersion of ethylcellulose, sugar and talc; capsule shell: coloring agent, gelatin and sulfur dioxide. Tartrazine-free. Cartons containing blister packs of 20. White, opaque polypropylene bottles of 50, with tamper-evident polyethylene caps. Store at room temperature, and protect from excessive heat.

200 mg: Each #0 hard gelatin capsule, printed with the logo "", "M-ESLON" and "200" in white, opaque red cap and transparent natural body, contains: morphine sulfate 200 mg in the form of extended release microgranules. Nonmedicinal ingredients: cornstarch, dibutyl sebacate, polyoxyethylene glycol, polymeric dispersion of ethylcellulose, sugar and talc; capsule shell: coloring agent, gelatin and sulfur dioxide. Tartrazine-free. Cartons containing blister packs of 20. White, opaque polypropylene bottles of 50, with tamper-evident polyethylene caps. Store at room temperature, and protect from excessive heat.

(Shown in Product Identification Section)

Mestinon® ℞
pyridostigmine bromide
Antimyasthenic—Cholinergic

Valeant

Mestinon®-SR ℞
pyridostigmine bromide
Antimyasthenic—Cholinergic

Valeant

PHARMACOLOGY: Pyridostigmine is a cholinergic agent which acts primarily by the inhibition of cholinesterase. It enhances cholinergic action by facilitating the transmission of impulses across neuromuscular junctions. It also has a direct cholinomimetic effect on skeletal muscle and possibly on autonomic ganglion cells and neurons of the CNS. Because of its quaternary ammonium structure, moderate doses of pyridostigmine do not cross the blood-brain barrier to produce CNS effects. Extremely high doses, however, produce CNS stimulation followed by CNS depression, in addition to a depolarizing neuromuscular blockade.

Pyridostigmine is an analog of neostigmine. However, it differs from neostigmine in certain clinically significant respects; for example, pyridostigmine is more effectively absorbed from the alimentary tract than is neostigmine; with equipotent doses, pyridostigmine has a slower onset and longer duration of action, and produces fewer gastrointestinal side effects than neostigmine. After oral administration, Mestinon generally has an onset of action of 20 minutes and a duration of action of approximately 6 hours; as for Mestinon-SR, it has an onset of action of 30 to 60 minutes and a duration of action of 6 to 12 hours.

INDICATIONS: For the symptomatic treatment of myasthenia gravis. In acute myasthenic crises where difficulty in breathing and swallowing is present, the parenteral form should be used. The patient can be transferred to the oral form as soon as it can be tolerated.

CONTRAINDICATIONS: In patients with known hypersensitivity to anticholinesterase agents. Because of the presence of the bromide ion, this product should not be used in patients with a prior history of reaction to bromides. It is also contraindicated in patients with peritonitis or mechanical obstruction of the intestinal or urinary tract.

WARNINGS: Pyridostigmine should be used with caution in patients with epilepsy, bronchial asthma, bradycardia, recent coronary occlusion, vagotonia, hyperthyroidism, cardiac arrhythmias or peptic ulcer. Large oral doses of the drug should be avoided in patients with megacolon or decreased gastrointestinal motility. In these patients, the drug may accumulate and result in toxicity when gastrointestinal motility is restored.

PRECAUTIONS: General: Although failure of patients to show clinical improvement may reflect underdosage, it can also be indicative of overdosage. It is important to differentiate between myasthenic crisis and cholinergic crisis caused by overdosage of pyridostigmine. Both conditions result in extreme muscle weakness but require radically different treatment (see Overdose: Symptoms and Treatment).

Information to Be Provided to the Patient: Complete restoration of muscle strength is rare in myasthenia gravis, and patients should be cautioned not to increase their dose, in an attempt to relieve their symptoms, without consulting their physician. The patient should be encouraged to keep a daily record of his or her condition to assist the physician in determining an optimal therapeutic regimen.

Drug Interactions: Atropine antagonizes the muscarinic effects of pyridostigmine and this interaction may be utilized to counteract the effects of pyridostigmine (see Overdose: Symptoms and Treatment).

Pyridostigmine does not antagonize, and in fact may prolong the phase I block of **depolarizing** muscle relaxants such as succinylcholine or decamethonium.

Certain antibiotics, especially neomycin, streptomycin and kanamycin, have a mild but definite nondepolarizing blocking action which may accentuate neuromuscular block. These antibiotics should be used in the myasthenic patient only where definitely indicated, and then careful adjustment should be made of adjunctive anticholinesterase dosage.

Local and some general anesthetics, antiarrhythmic agents and other drugs that interfere with neuromuscular transmission should be used cautiously, if at all, in patients with myasthenia gravis; the dose of pyridostigmine may have to be increased accordingly.

In severe myasthenia gravis, neostigmine has been used in combination with pyridostigmine to provide the benefits of short and long-term activity; because of the possibility of reduced intestinal motility and increased toxicity, this combination should be used only under strict medical supervision.

Carcinogenesis, Mutagenesis and Impairment of Fertility: Carcinogenicity and mutagenicity studies have not been performed with pyridostigmine.

A fertility and general reproductive performance study was performed in rats at dosages of 15 and 40 mg/kg/day. There were no adverse effects on pregnancy rate, average number of implantation sites, average number of embryos per dam, percent resorptions, duration of gestation, litter size, pup viability or pup growth.

Pregnancy: Teratogenic effects: Pregnancy category B: Reproductive studies have been performed in rats at dosages up to 40 mg/kg/day (2 times the maximum recommended human dose; 4.6 times the average recommended dose). These studies have revealed no evidence of impaired fertility or harm to the fetus due to pyridostigmine. There are, however, no adequate and well controlled studies in pregnant women. However, pyridostigmine, like other cholinesterase inhibitors, contains a quaternary ammonium and, therefore, would be expected to cross the placenta only to a limited extent. Because animal reproductive studies are not always predictive of human response, this drug should be used during pregnancy only if clearly needed.

Nonteratogenic effects: Of newborn infants whose mothers have received anticholinesterase drugs for treatment of myasthenia gravis, 10 to 20% were observed to have transient muscular weakness.

Lactation: It is not known whether pyridostigmine is excreted in human milk. Because many drugs are excreted in human milk, and because of the potential for serious adverse reactions from pyridostigmine in nursing infants, a decision should be made whether to discontinue nursing or to discontinue the drug, taking into account the importance of the drug to the mother.

Children: See Dosage.

ADVERSE EFFECTS: Side effects are generally due to an exaggeration of pharmacological effects of which increased salivation and fasciculation are the most common. Abdominal cramps and diarrhea may also occur.

The following additional adverse reactions have been reported following the use of pyridostigmine:

Respiratory: increased bronchial secretions.
Gastrointestinal: nausea, vomiting, increased peristalsis.
Musculoskeletal: muscle cramps.
Dermatologic: urticaria, rash.
Miscellaneous: miosis, diaphoresis, weakness, allergic reactions.

OVERDOSE:

Symptoms: As is true of all anticholinesterase agents, overdosage of pyridostigmine can cause cholinergic crisis, which is characterized by increasing muscle weakness and which, through involvement of the muscles of respiration, may result in death. Myasthenic crisis, due to an increase in the severity of the disease, is also accompanied by extreme muscle weakness, and thus may be difficult to distinguish from cholinergic crisis on a symptomatic basis. However, such differentiation is extremely important, because increases in the dose of pyridostigmine or other drugs in this class in the presence of cholinergic crisis or of a refractory or "insensitive" state could have grave consequences. The two types of crises may be differentiated by the use of edrophonium chloride as well as by clinical judgment.

Treatment: Treatment of the two conditions differs radically. Whereas the presence of **myasthenic crisis** requires more intensive anticholinesterase therapy, **cholinergic crisis** calls for the prompt **withdrawal** of all drugs of this type. The immediate use of atropine in cholinergic crisis is also recommended. A syringe containing 1 mg of atropine sulfate should be immediately available to be given in aliquots i.v. to counteract severe cholinergic reactions.

Atropine also may be used to abolish or minimize gastrointestinal side effects or other muscarinic reactions; but such use, by masking signs of overdosage, can lead to inadvertent induction of cholinergic crisis.

For management of a suspected drug overdose, CPhA recommends that you contact your **regional Poison Control Centre**. See the *CPS* Directory section for a list of Poison Control Centres.

DOSAGE: The dosage, route and frequency of administration depend on the requirements and clinical response of the patients. The dosage schedule should be adjusted for each patient and changed as the need arises. Dosage requirements in patients with myasthenia gravis may vary from day to day, according to remissions and exacerbations of the disease and the physical and emotional stress suffered by the patient. Larger portions of the label daily dose may be given at times when the patient is more prone to fatigue (afternoon, mealtimes, etc.).

In the initial treatment of myasthenia gravis, oral pyridostigmine should be started at a dosage smaller than that required to produce maximum strength, and daily dosage gradually increased at intervals of 48 hours or more. Changes in oral dosage may take several days to show results. When a further increase in dosage produces no corresponding increase in muscle strength, dosage should be reduced to the previous level so that the patient receives the smallest dose necessary to produce maximum strength.

Note: For information on a diagnostic test for myasthenia gravis, and for the evaluation and stabilization of anticholinesterase therapy, see product monograph on Tensilon.

The immediate effect of a Mestinon-SR 180 mg tablet is about equal to that of a 60 mg conventional tablet; however, the duration of drug action, although varying in individual patients, averages 2½ times that of a 60 mg dose. One to three 180 mg tablets, once or twice daily (180 mg to 1.08 g a day), will usually be sufficient to control symptoms; however, the needs of individual patients may vary markedly from this average. For optimal control, it may be necessary to use conventional tablets or syrup in conjunction with Mestinon-SR therapy. Mestinon-SR tablets are particularly useful for bedtime administration in patients who are very weak upon awakening.

Mestinon and Mestinon-SR tablets should be swallowed whole. Do not crush. However, in certain cases, Mestinon and Mestinon-SR tablets, can be cut in half; but Mestinon-SR tablets should not be crushed or quartered since this would destroy too much of the sustained release matrix.

Due to the slow-release mechanism of the tablet, the matrix may pass through the intestinal system intact. However, it should be noted that the medicinal ingredient has been released through the gastrointestinal tract over an 8 to 12 hour passing time and only the matrix is rejected.

SUPPLIED: Mestinon: Each white, flat compressed tablet, cross-scored on one side and embossed MESTINON 60-V on the other, contains: pyridostigmine bromide 60 mg. Nonmedicinal ingredients: lactose, silicone dioxide and stearic acid. Energy: 4.6 kJ (1.1 kcal). Gluten-, paraben-, sodium-, sulfite- and tartrazine-free. Bottles of 100.

Mestinon-SR: Each capsule-shaped, flattened on 2 sides with a single score on 1 face, light straw colored tablet, embossed MES V 180, contains: pyridostigmine bromide 180 mg. Nonmedicinal ingredients: calcium phosphate, carnauba wax, isopropyl alcohol, magnesium stearate and zein. Energy: 2.3 kJ (0.5 kcal). Gluten-, lactose-, paraben-, sodium-, sulfite- and tartrazine-free. Bottles of 30.

Store in a dry place between 15 and 30°C, in a well-closed container with the desiccant enclosed.

Note: Because of the hygroscopic nature of the Mestinon and Mestinon-SR tablets, mottling may occur. This does not affect their efficacy.

Metadol™ Ⓝ

methadone HCl

Opioid Analgesic

Paladin

Date of Preparation: March 10, 2009

Pursuant to subsection 53(3) of the Narcotic Control Regulations, practitioners seeking to use methadone for the treatment of patients, must first obtain a Federal Ministerial exemption pursuant to section 56 of the Controlled Drugs and Substances Act (CDSA). Such an exemption will effectively allow the named practitioner to administer, prescribe, provide or sell methadone to patients under their professional care for analgesia, subject to certain specified terms and conditions. Exemptions are issued by the Office of Controlled Substances, Healthy Environments and Consumer Safety Branch, Health Canada, directly (see Supplied), or in some provinces, through the College of Physicians and Surgeons.

Pharmacists may supply methadone to a practitioner holding such an exemption.

Warning: MAY BE HABIT FORMING.

PHARMACOLOGY: Methadone hydrochloride is a synthetic opioid analgesic with multiple actions qualitatively similar to those of morphine, the most prominent of which involve the central nervous system and organs composed of smooth muscle. The principal actions of therapeutic value are analgesia and sedation and detoxification or maintenance in opiate addiction. The methadone abstinence syndrome, although qualitatively similar to that of morphine, differs in that the onset is slower, the course is more prolonged, and the symptoms are less severe.

When administered orally, methadone is approximately one-half as potent as when given parenterally. Oral administration results in a delay of the onset, a lowering of the peak, and an increase in the duration of analgesic effect. The steady-state elimination half-life of methadone is approximately 25 hours. Large inter-individual variability in elimination half-life may necessitate 2 to 9 days for steady-state serum levels.

Acutely, methadone has similar effects to other opioids; however, its pharmacological properties are significantly different from other opioid agonists in that it is extremely long-acting (36 to 48 hours) in humans.

After interruption of chronic dosing, if methadone treatment is to be continued, starting doses should be low and patients should be titrated slowly to effect in order to avoid severe toxicity and respiratory depression.

INDICATIONS AND CLINICAL USE: METADOL (Methadone Hydrochloride Tablets, Oral Solution and Concentrate) is indicated for the relief of severe pain. In general, METADOL, as an analgesic, should not be used in opioid naive patients.

CONTRAINDICATIONS: METADOL (Methadone Hydrochloride Tablets, Oral Solution and Concentrate) is contraindicated in individuals with known hypersensitivity to the drug. It is also contraindicated in any situation where opioids are contraindicated such as: patients with respiratory depression (in the absence of resuscitative equipment or in unmonitored settings), and in patients with acute bronchial asthma or hypercarbia.

METADOL should not be given to patients with diarrhea which is associated with pseudomembranous colitis caused by cephalosporins, lincomycins (possibly including topical clindamycin), or penicillins, or to patients having diarrhea caused by poisoning, until toxic material has been eliminated from the gastrointestinal tract.

WARNINGS:

METADOL (Methadone Hydrochloride Tablets, Oral Solution and Concentrate) is for oral administration only. This preparation must not be injected. It is recommended that METADOL tablets, oral solution and concentrate, if dispensed, be packaged in child resistant containers and kept out of the reach of children to prevent accidental ingestion.

Methadone Hydrochloride, a synthetic opioid, is a controlled substance (Classification N) under the Controlled Drugs and Substances Act (CDSA). It is available only through physicians who have received an exemption from the Minister of Health Canada to prescribe methadone pursuant to section 56 of the CDSA. Appropriate security measures should be taken to safeguard stocks of methadone against diversion.

DRUG DEPENDENCE—METHADONE CAN PRODUCE DRUG DEPENDENCE OF THE MORPHINE TYPE AND, THEREFORE, HAS THE POTENTIAL FOR BEING ABUSED. PSYCHOLOGICAL DEPENDENCE, PHYSICAL DEPENDENCE, AND TOLERANCE MAY DEVELOP UPON REPEATED ADMINISTRATION OF METHADONE AND IT SHOULD BE PRESCRIBED AND ADMINISTERED WITH THE SAME DEGREE OF CAUTION APPROPRIATE TO THE USE OF MORPHINE.

Incomplete Cross-Tolerance Between Methadone and Other Opioids: Patients tolerant to other opioids may be incompletely tolerant to methadone. Incomplete cross-tolerance is a particular concern for patients tolerant to other μ-opioid agonists when converting to methadone, making determination of dosing during opioid conversion complex. Deaths have been reported during conversion from chronic, high dose treatment with other opioid agonists. Therefore, it is critical to understand the pharmacokinetics of methadone when converting patients from other opioids (see Dosage and Administration, Table 1 and Table 2, for appropriate conversion schedules). A high degree of "opioid tolerance" does not eliminate the possibility of methadone toxicity.

Interaction with Other Central Nervous System Depressants: Methadone should be used with caution and in reduced dosage in patients who are concurrently receiving other narcotic analgesics, general anaesthetics, phenothiazines, other tranquillizers, sedative hypnotics, tricyclic antidepressants, and other CNS depressants (including alcohol). Respiratory depression, hypotension, and profound sedation or coma may result (see Precautions).

Interactions with Alcohol and Drugs of Abuse: Methadone may be expected to have additive effects when used in conjunction with alcohol, other opioids, or illicit drugs that cause central nervous system depression. Deaths associated with illicit use of methadone have frequently involved concomitant benzodiazepine abuse.

Anxiety: Since methadone, as used by tolerant subjects as a constant maintenance dosage, is not a tranquillizer, patients who are maintained on this drug will react to life problems and stresses with the same symptoms of anxiety as do other individuals. The physician should not confuse such symptoms with those of opioid abstinence and should not attempt to treat anxiety by increasing the dosage of methadone. The action of methadone in maintenance treatment is limited to the control of opioid symptoms and is ineffective for relief of general anxiety.

Head Injury and Increased Intracranial Pressure: The respiratory depressant effects of methadone and its capacity to elevate cerebrospinal fluid pressure may be markedly exaggerated in the presence of head injury, other intracranial lesions or a pre-existing increase in intracranial pressure. Furthermore, opioids produce side effects that may obscure the clinical course of patients with head injuries. In such patients, methadone must be used with caution and only if it is deemed essential.

Asthma and Other Respiratory Conditions: Respiratory depression is the chief hazard from methadone hydrochloride. Respiratory depression is a particular potential problem in elderly or debilitated patients as well as those suffering from conditions accompanied by hypoxia or hypercapnia when even moderate therapeutic doses may dangerously decrease pulmonary ventilation.

Methadone hydrochloride should be administered with extreme caution to patients with conditions accompanied by hypoxia, hypercapnia, or decreased respiratory reserve such as; asthma, chronic obstructive pulmonary disease or cor pulmonale, severe obesity, sleep apnea syndrome, myxedema, kyphoscoliosis, CNS depression or coma. In these patients even usual therapeutic doses of methadone may decrease respiratory drive while simultaneously increasing airway resistance to the pont of apnea. Alternative non-opioid analgesics should be considered, and methadone should be employed only under careful medical supervision at the lowest effective dose.

Hypotensive Effect: The administration of methadone may result in severe hypotension in an individual whose ability to maintain his blood pressure has already been compromised by a depleted blood volume or concurrent administration of such drugs as the phenothiazines or certain anaesthetics.

Analgesia: In general methadone should not be used in opioid naive patients.

Use in Ambulatory Patients: Methadone may impair the mental and/or physical abilities required for the performance of potentially hazardous tasks, such as driving a car or operating machinery. The patient should be cautioned accordingly. Methadone, like other opioids, may produce orthostatic hypotension in ambulatory patients.

Use in Pregnancy/Breastfeeding: Methadone is secreted in saliva, breast milk, amniotic fluid and umbilical cord plasma. The disposition of oral methadone has been studied in approximately 30 pregnant patients in 2nd and 3rd trimesters. Elimination of methadone was significantly changed in pregnancy. Total body clearance of methadone was increased in pregnant patients compared to the same patients postpartum or to non-pregnant opioid-dependent women. The terminal half-life of methadone is decreased during second and third trimesters. The decrease in plasma half-life and increased clearance of methadone resulting in lower methadone trough levels during pregnancy can lead to withdrawal symptoms in some pregnant patients. The dosage may need to be increased or the dosing interval decreased in pregnant patients receiving methadone (see Dosage and Administration).

It is the physician's responsibility to ensure that female patients are fully informed concerning the possible risks to a pregnant woman or her unborn child from the use of methadone. Care of such patients should be under the supervision of a physician experienced in the management of such patients.

Breastfeeding may result in the passage of opioids or other substances into the breast milk. Use of methadone in nursing mothers is not recommended, unless in the opinion of the treating physician, the potential benefits outweigh the possible hazards.

PRECAUTIONS: There is significant risk of respiratory depression if the patient is switched abruptly from other opioids to methadone. Conversion to methadone should be undertaken with caution.

Cardiac Conduction Effects: Laboratory studies, both in vivo and in vitro, have demonstrated that methadone inhibits cardiac potassium channels and prolongs the QT interval. Cases of QT interval prolongation and serious arrhythmia (torsades de pointes) have been observed during treatment with methadone. These cases appear to be more commonly associated with, but not limited to, higher dose treatment (>200 mg/day). Most cases involve patients being treated for pain with large, multiple daily doses of methadone, although cases have been reported in patients receiving doses commonly used for maintenance treatment of opioid addiction.

Methadone should be administered with particular caution to patients already at risk for development of prolonged QT interval (e.g., cardiac hypertrophy, concomitant diuretic use, hypokalemia, hypomagnesemia). Careful monitoring is recommended when using methadone in patients with a history of cardiac conduction abnormalities, those taking medications affecting cardiac conduction, and in other cases where history or physical exam suggest an increased risk of dysrhythmia. QT prolongation has also been reported in patients with no prior cardiac history who have received high doses of methadone. Patients developing QT prolongation while on methadone treatment should be evaluated for the presence of modifiable risk factors, such as concomitant medications with cardiac effects, drugs which might cause electrolyte abnormalities, and drugs which might act as inhibitors of methadone metabolism. For use of methadone to treat pain, the risk of QT prolongation and development of dysrhythmias should be weighed against the benefit of adequate pain management and the availability of alternative therapies.

Methadone treatment for analgesic therapy in patients with acute or chronic pain should only be initiated if the potential analgesic or palliative care benefit of treatment with methadone has been considered to outweigh the risk of QT prolongation that has been reported with high doses of methadone.

The use of methadone in patients already known to have prolonged QT interval has not been systemically studied.

In using methadone an individualized benefit to risk assessment should be carried out and should include evaluation of patient presentation and complete medical history. For patients judged to be at risk, careful monitoring of cardiovascular status, including QT prolongation and dysrhythmias and those described previously should be performed.

Special-Risk Patients: Methadone given on a fixed-dose schedule may have a narrow therapeutic index in certain patient populations, especially when combined with other drugs, and should be reserved for cases where the benefits of opioid analgesia outweigh the known potential risks of cardiac conduction abnormalities, respiratory depression, altered mental states and postural hypotension. METADOL (Methadone Hydrochloride Tablets, Oral Solution and Concentrate) should be given with caution and the initial dose should be reduced in certain patients, such as the elderly or debilitated; those with severe impairment of hepatic or renal function, hypothyroidism, Addison's disease, prostatic hypertrophy, or urethral stricture; patients who are known to be sensitive to central nervous system depressants, such as those with cardiovascular, pulmonary, renal, or hepatic disease; and in patients with comorbid conditions or concomitant medications which may predispose to dysrhythmia.

Acute Abdominal Conditions: The administration of methadone or other narcotics may obscure the diagnosis or clinical course in patients with acute abdominal conditions.

Drug Interactions: Opioid Antagonist, Mixed Agonist/Antagonist, and Partial Agonists Drugs: Patients who are on prolonged methadone therapy may experience withdrawal symptoms when given opioid antagonists or mixed agonist/antagonist drugs. Examples of such agents are naloxone, naltrexone, pentazocine, nalbuphine, butorphanol, and buprenorphine.

Anti-Retroviral Agents: Nevirapine: Based on the known metabolism of methadone, nevirapine may decrease plasma concentrations of methadone by increasing its hepatic metabolism. Opioid withdrawal syndrome has been reported in patients treated with nevirapine and methadone concomitantly. Methadone-maintained patients beginning nevirapine therapy should be monitored for evidence of withdrawal and methadone dose should be adjusted accordingly.

Efavirenz: Coadministration of efavirenz in HIV-infected methadone-maintenance patients has resulted in decreased methadone plasma concentrations associated with signs of opioid withdrawal, and necessitating increases in methadone dose.

Ritonavir and Ritonavir/Lopinavir: Reduced plasma methadone levels have been observed after administration of ritanovir alone or ritanovir/lopinavir combination. Withdrawal symptoms were however, inconsistently observed. Caution is warranted when administering methadone to patients receiving ritonavir-containing regimens in addition to other drugs known to decrease methadone plasma levels.

Zidovudine: Experimental evidence suggests that methadone increases the area under the concentration-time curve (AUC) of zidovudine with possible toxic effects.

Didanosine and Stavudine: Experimental evidence suggests that methadone decreased the AUC and peak levels for didanosine and stavudine, with a more significant decrease for didanosine. Methadone disposition was not substantially altered.

Cytochrome P450 Inducers: The following drug interactions were reported following coadministration of methadone with inducers of cytochrome P450 enzymes.

Rifampin: In patients well-stabilized on methadone, concomitant administration of rifampin resulted in marked reduction in serum methadone levels and concurrent appearance of withdrawal symptoms.

Phenytoin: In a pharmacolinetic study with patients on methadone maintenance therapy, phenytoin administration (250 mg b.i.d. initially for 1 day followed by 300 mg QD for 3-4 days) resulted in ~50% reduction in methadone exposure and concurrently withdrawal symptoms occurred. Upon discontinuation of phenytoin, the incidence of withdrawal symptoms decreased and the methadone exposure increased and was comparable to pre-phenytoin dose scenario.

St. John's Wort, Phenobarbital, Carbamazepine: Administration of methadone along with other CYP3A4 inducers may result in withdrawal symptoms.

Cytochrome P450 Inhibitors: Since the metabolism of methadone is mediated by the CYP3A4 isozyme, coadministration of drugs that inhibit CYP3A4 activity may cause decreased clearance of methadone. The expected clinical results would be increased or prolonged opioid effects. Thus patients coadministered with inhibitors of CYP3A4 such as azole antifungal agents (e.g., ketoconazole), macrolide antibiotics (e.g., erythromycin), while receiving methadone should be carefully monitored and dosage adjustment made if warranted. Some selective serotonin reuptake inhibitors (SSRIs) (i.e. sertraline, fluvoxamine) upon coadministration may increase methadone plasma levels and result in increased opiate effects or toxicity.

Specifically, repeat dose administration of oral voriconazole (400 mg Q12h for 1 day, then 200 mg Q12h for 4 days) increased the C_{max} and AUC_ of pharmacologically active R-methadone by 31% (90% CI: 22%, 40%) and 47% (90% CI: 38%, 57%), respectively, in subjects receiving a methadone maintenance dose (30-100 mg QD). Increased plasma concentrations of methadone have been associated with toxicity including QT prolongation. Frequent monitoring for adverse events and toxicity related to methadone is recommended during coadministration. Dose reduction of methadone may be needed.

Others: Monoamine Oxidase (MAO) Inhibitors: Therapeutic doses of meperidine have precipitated severe reactions in patients concurrently receiving monoamine oxidase inhibitors or those who have received such agents within 14 days. Similar reactions thus far have not been reported with methadone; but if the use of methadone is necessary in such patients, a sensitivity test should be performed in which repeated small incremental doses are administered over the course of several hours while the patient's condition and vital signs are under careful observation.

Protease Inhibitors: **Agenerase**: Coadministration of methadone with Agenerase resulted in a decrease in the C_{max} and AUC of the active methadone enantiomer (R-enantiomer) of 25% and 13% respectively, while the C_{max}, AUC and C_{min} of the inactive methadone enantiomer (S-enantiomer) were decreased by 48%, 40% and 23% respective. When methadone is coadministered with Agenerase, patients should be monitored for methadone underdosing, in particular if low-dose ritonavir is also given. As compared to a nonmatched historical control group, coadministration of methadone and Agenerase resulted in a 30%, 27% and 25% decrease in serum Agenerase AUC, C_{max} and C_{min} respectively. No recommendations can be made regarding adjustment of Agenerase dose when Agenerase is coadministered with methadone.

Viracept: When coadministered with Viracept, changes are reported for total plasma methadone; changes for the individual R-enantiomer and S-enantiomer were similar. Dosage of methadone may need to be increased.

Non-nucleoside Reverse Transcriptase Inhibitors: **Rescriptor**: Dosage of methadone may need to be decreased when coadministered with Rescriptor.

Desipramine: Blood levels of desipramine have increased with concurrent methadone therapy.

Potentially Arrhythmogenic Agents: Extreme caution is necessary when any drug known to have the potential to prolong the QT interval is prescribed in conjunction with methadone. Pharmacodynamic interactions may occur with concomitant use of methadone and potentially arrhythmogenic agents such as class I and III antiarrhythmics, some neuroleptics and tricyclic antidepressants, and calcium channel blockers. Caution should also be exercised when prescribing concomitant drugs capable of inducing electrolyte disturbances that may prolong the QT interval (hypomagnesemia, hypokalemia). These include diuretics, laxatives, and in rare cases mineralocorticoid hormones.

Interactions with Other CNS Depressants: Patients receiving other opioid analgesics, general anesthetics, phenothiazines, other tranquilizers, sedatives, hypnotics, or other CNS depressants (including alcohol) concomitantly with methadone may experience respiratory depression, hypotension, profound sedation, or coma.

Use with Mixed Agonist/Antagonist Opioid Analgesics: Agonist/antagonist analgesics (i.e., pentazocine, nalbuphine, butorphanol, or buprenorphine) should not be administered to patients who have received or are receiving a course of therapy with a pure opioid agonist, such as Methadone Hydrochloride Injection. In this situation, mixed agonist/antagonist analgesics may reduce the analgesic effect of Methadone Hydrochloride Injection and/or may precipitate withdrawal symptoms.

Anxiety: Methadone, used by tolerant patients at a constant maintenance dosage, is not a tranquilizer. Patients who are maintained on this drug will react to life problems and stresses as do other individuals. Anxiety in a patient on methadone should not be confused with narcotic abstinence and should not prompt treatment by increasing the dosage of methadone. The action of methadone in maintenance treatment is limited to the control of symptoms of opioid dependence or pain. Methadone is ineffective for relief of general anxiety.

Acute Pain: Maintenance patients on a stable dose of methadone who experience physical trauma, postoperative pain or other causes of acute pain cannot be expected to derive analgesia from their stable dose of methadone regimens. Such patients should be given analgesics, including opioids, that would be indicated in other patients experiencing similar nociceptive stimulation. Due to the opioid tolerance induced by methadone, when opioids are required for management of acute pain in methadone patients, somewhat higher and/or more frequent doses will often be required than would be the case for other, non-tolerant patients.

Risk of Relapse in Patients on Methadone Maintenance Treatment of Opioid Addiction: Abrupt opioid discontinuation can lead to development of opioid withdrawal symptoms (see Precautions). Presentation of these symptoms has been associated with an increased risk of susceptible patients to relapse to illicit drug use and should be considered when assessing the risks and benefit of methadone use.

Tolerance and Physical Dependence: Tolerance is the need for increasing doses of opioids to maintain a defined effect such as analgesia (in the absence of disease progression or other external factors). Physical dependence is manifested by withdrawal symptoms after abrupt discontinuation of a drug or upon administration of an antagonist . Physical dependence and/or tolerance are not unusual during chronic opioid therapy.

If methadone is abruptly discontinued in a physically dependent patient, an abstinence syndrome may occur. The opioid abstinence or withdrawal syndrome is characterized by some or all of the following: restlessness, lacrimation, rhinorrhea, yawning, perspiration, chills, myalgia, and mydriasis. Other symptoms also may develop, including: irritability, anxiety, backache, joint pain, weakness, abdominal cramps, insomnia, nausea, anorexia, vomiting, diarrhea, or increased blood pressure, respiratory rate, or heart rate.

In general, chronically administered methadone should not be abruptly discontinued.

Special-Risk Patients: Methadone should be given with caution and the initial dose reduced in certain patients, such as the elderly and debilitated and those with severe impairment of hepatic or renal function, hypothyroidism, Addison's disease, prostatic hypertrophy, or urethral stricture. The usual precautions appropriate to the use of parenteral opioids should be observed and the possibility of respiratory depression should always be kept in mind.

Information to Be Provided to the Patient: Methadone, like all opioids, may impair the mental and/or physical abilities required for the performance of potentially hazardous tasks such as driving or operating machinery. The patient should be cautioned accordingly.

Methadone, like other opioids, may produce orthostatic hypotension in ambulatory patients.

Alcohol and other CNS depressants may produce an additive CNS depression, when taken with methadone, and should be avoided.

If a patient taking methadone experiences symptoms suggestive of an arrhythmia (such as palpitations, dizziness, lightheadedness, or syncope), that patient should seek immediate medical attention.

Carcinogenesis, Mutagenesis, Impairment of Fertility: Data from published reports of carcinogenicity studies indicate that there was a significant increase in pituitary adenomas in female B6C2F1 mice consuming 15 mg/kg/day methadone for two years. This dose was approximately 0.6 times a human daily oral dose of 120 mg/day, on a body surface area basis. However, this finding was not seen in mice consuming 60 mg/kg/day (approximately 2.5 times a human daily oral dose of 120 mg/day). Furthermore, in a two-year study of dietary administration of methadone to Fischer 344 rats, there was no clear evidence for treatment related increase in the incidence of neoplasms, at doses as high as 28 mg/kg/day in males and 88 mg/kg/day in females (approximately 2.3 times and 7.1 times, respectively, a human daily oral dose of 120 mg/day) based on body surface area comparison.

In published reports, methadone tested negative in tests for chromosome breakage and disjunction and sex-linked recessive lethal gene mutations in germ cells of Drosophila using feeding and injection procedures. Methadone treatment of male mice increased sex chromosome and autosome univalent chromosomes and translocations in multivalent chromosomes. Methadone tested positive in the *E.coli* DNA repair system and Neurospora crassa and mouse lymphoma forward mutation assays.

Pregnancy: Teratogenic Effects: Pregnancy Category C. There are no controlled studies of methadone use in pregnant women that can be used to establish safety. However, an expert review of published data on experiences with methadone use during pregnancy by TERIS—the Teratogen Information System—concluded that maternal use of methadone during pregnancy as part of a supervised, therapeutic regimen is unlikely to pose a substantial teratogenic risk (quantity and quality of data assessed as "limited to fair"), however, the data are insufficient to state that there is no risk (TERIS, last reviewed October, 2002). Pregnant women involved in methadone maintenance programs have been reported to have significantly improved prenatal care, improved fetal outcomes, and reduced mortality when compared to pregnant women using illicit drugs. Several factors complicate the interpretation of investigations of the children of women who took methadone during pregnancy. These include: the maternal use of illicit drugs, other maternal factors such as nutrition, infection, and psychosocial circumstances, limited information regarding dose and duration of methadone use during pregnancy. In addition, reported studies generally compare the benefit of methadone to the risk of untreated addiction to illicit drugs; the relevance of these findings to pain patients prescribed methadone during pregnancy is unclear.

Methadone has been detected in amniotic fluid and cord plasma at concentrations proportional to maternal plasma and in newborn urine at lower concentrations than corresponding maternal urine.

A retrospective series of 101 pregnant opiate-dependent women who underwent inpatient opiate detoxification with methadone did not demonstrate any increased risk of miscarriage in the 2nd trimester or premature delivery in 3rd trimester.

Several studies have suggested that infants born to narcotic-addicted women treated with methadone during all or part of pregnancy have been found to have decreased fetal growth with reduced birth weight, length, and/or head circumference compared to controls. The growth deficit does not appear to persist into later childhood. However, children born to women treated with methadone during pregnancy have been shown to demonstrate mild but persistent deficits in performance on psychometric and behavioural tests.

Methadone should be used during pregnancy only if the potential benefit justifies the potential risk to the fetus.

Additional information on the potential risks of methadone may be derived from animal data. Methadone does not appear to be teratogenic in the rat or rabbit models. However, following large doses, methadone produced teratogenic effects in the guinea pig, hamster and mouse. One published study found that in hamster fetuses, subcutaneous methadone doses of 31 mg/kg or greater (estimated exposure was approximately 2 times a human daily oral dose of 120 mg/day on a mg/m^2 basis, or equivalent to a human daily intravenous dose of 120 mg/day) on day 8 of gestation produced exencephaly and neurological effects. Some of the reported effects were observed at doses that were maternally toxic. In another study, a single subcutaneous dose of 22-24 mg/kg methadone (estimated exposure was approximately equivalent to a human daily oral dose of 120 mg/day on a mg/m^2 basis; or half a human daily intravenous dose of 120 mg/day) on day 9 of gestation in mice also produced exencephaly in 11% of the embryos. However, no effects were reported in rats and rabbits at oral doses up to 40 mg/kg (estimated exposure was approximately 3 and 6 times, respectively, a human daily oral dose of 120 mg/day on a mg/m^2 basis; or 1.5 and 3 times a human daily intravenous dose of 120 mg/day) during days 6-15 and 6-18, respectively.

Nonteratogenic Effects: Babies born to mothers who have been taking opioids regularly prior to delivery may be physically dependent. Onset of withdrawal symptoms in infants is usually in the first days after birth but may be delayed for two to four weeks. Withdrawal signs in the newborn include irritability and excessive crying, tremors, hyperactive reflexes, increased respiratory rate, increased stools, sneezing, yawning, vomiting, and fever. The intensity of the syndrome does not always correlate with the duration of maternal opioid dose or maternal dose. There is no consensus on the appropriate management of infant withdrawal.

There are conflicting reports on whether the risk of sudden infant death syndrome (SIDS) is increased in infants born to women treated with methadone during pregnancy.

Abnormal fetal nonstress tests (NSTs) have been reported to occur more frequently when the test is performed 1-2 hours after a maintenance dose of methadone in late pregnancy compared to controls. Published animal studies suggest that perinatal exposure to opioids including methadone may alter neuronal development and behaviour in the offspring. Perinatal methadone exposure in rats has been linked to alterations in learning ability, motor activity, thermal regulation, nociception responses and sensitivity to other drugs. Additional animal data demonstrates evidence for neurochemical changes in the brains of methadone-treated offspring, including the cholinergic, dopaminergicn noradrenergic and serotonergic systems.

Clinical Pharmacology for Pregnancy: Pregnant women have significantly lower trough plasma concentrations, increased plasma methadone clearance and shorter half-life than after delivery. Dosage adjustment using higher doses or administering the daily dose in divided doses may be necessary in pregnant women treated with methadone. [See Dosage and Administration].

Labor and Delivery: As with all opioids, administration of methadone to the mother shortly before delivery may result in some degree of respiratory depression in the newborn, especially if higher doses are used. Methadone is not recommended for obstetric analgesia because its long duration of action increases the probability of respiratory depression in the newborn. Narcotics with mixed agonist-antagonist properties should not be used for pain control during labor in patients chronically treated with methadone because they may precipitate acute withdrawal.

Lactation: Methadone is secreted into human milk. There is no information on use of parenteral methadone in breastfeeding, or on the safety of the high doses of methadone typically used in chronic pain treatment. The safety of breastfeeding while taking oral methadone is also controversial. At maternal oral doses of 10-80 mg/day, methadone concentrations from 50 to 570 µg/L in milk have been reported, which, in the majority of samples, were lower than maternal serum drug concentration at steady state. Peak methadone levels in milk occur approximately 4-5 hours after an oral dose. Based on an average milk consumption of 150 mL/kg/day, an infant would consume approximately 17.4 µg/kg/day, which is approximately 2/3% of the oral maternal dose. Methadone has been detected in very low plasma concentrations in some infants whose mothers were taking methadone. Women on high dose methadone maintenance, who are already **breastfeeding , should be counselled to wean breastfeeding gradually in order to prevent neonatal abstinence syndrome**. Methadone-treated mothers considering nursing an opioid-naïve infant should be counselled of the presence of methadone in breast milk.

Because of the potential for serious adverse reactions in nursing infants from methadone, a decision should be made whether to discontinue nursing or to discontinue the drug, taking into account the importance of the drug to the mother.

Pediatric Use: Safety and effectiveness in pediatric patients below the age of 18 years have not been established.

Geriatric Use: Clinical studies of Methadone Hydrochloride Injection did not include sufficient numbers of subjects aged 65 and over to determine whether they respond differently from younger subjects. Other reported clinical experience has not identified differences in responses between the elderly and younger patients. In general, dose selection for an elderly patient should be cautious, usually starting at the low end of the dosing range, reflecting the greater frequency of decreased hepatic, renal, or cardiac function and of concomitant disease or other drug therapy.

Renal Impairment: The use of methadone has not been extensively evaluated in patients with renal insufficiency.

Hepatic Impairment: The use of methadone has not been extensively evaluated in patients with hepatic insufficiency. Methadone is metabolized in the liver and patients with liver impairment may be at risk of accumulating methadone after multiple dosing.

Gender: The use of methadone has not been evaluated for gender specificity.

ADVERSE EFFECTS: Initial Administration: The initial methadone dose should be carefully titrated to the individual. Induction too rapid for the patient's sensitivity is more likely to produce adverse effects.

The major hazards of methadone are respiratory depression and, to a lesser degree, systemic hypotension. Respiratory arrest, shock, cardiac arrest and death have occurred.

The most frequently observed adverse reactions include lightheadedness, dizziness, sedation, nausea, vomiting, and sweating. These effects seem to be more prominent in ambulatory patients and in those who are not suffering severe pain. In such individuals, lower doses of methadone are advisable.

Other adverse reactions that have been reported in patients (including opioid addicts taking methadone for detoxification or maintenance) receiving methadone include the following:

Body as a Whole: asthenia (weakness), edema, headache.

Cardiovascular: arrhythmias, bigeminal rhythms, bradycardia, extrasystoles, tachycardia, torsades de pointes, ventricular fibrillation, ventricular tachycardia. ECG abnormalities, prolonged QT interval, T-wave inversion, cardiomyopathy, flushing, heart failure, hypotension, palpitations, phlebitis, syncope.

Digestive: abdominal pain, anorexia, biliary tract spasm, constipation, dry mouth, glossitis.

Haematologic and Lymphatic: Reversible thrombocytopenia has been described in opioid addicts with chronic hepatitis.

Metabolic and Nutritional: hypokalemia, hypomagnesemia, weight gain.

Nervous: agitation, confusion, seizures, disorientation, dysphoria, euphoria, insomnia.

Respiratory: pulmonary edema.

Skin and Appendages: Intramuscular and Subcutaneous: local tissues reactions (pain, erythema, swelling), particularly with continuous subcutaneous infusion.

Intravenous: pruritus, urticaria, other skin rashes, and rarely, hemorrhagic urticaria.

Special Senses: visual disturbances.

Urogenital: antidiuretic effect, amenorrhea, urinary retention or hesitancy, reduced libido and/or potency.

Maintenance on a Stabilized Dose: During prolonged administration of methadone, there is a gradual, yet progressive disappearance of side effects over a period of several weeks. However, constipation and sweating persist.

Drug Abuse and Dependence: Methadone is a µ-agonist opioid with an abuse liability similar to that of morphine and is a Schedule II controlled substance. Methadone, like morphine and other opioids used for analgesia, has the potential for being abused and is subject to criminal diversion.

Abuse: Drug addiction is characterized by a preoccupation with the procurement, hoarding, and abuse of drugs for nonmedicinal purposes. Drug addiction is treatable, utilizing a multi-disciplinary approach, but relapse is common.

"Drug seeking" behaviour is very common to addicts and drug abusers. Drug seeking tactics include emergency calls or visits near the end of the office hours, refusal to undergo appropriate examination, testing or referral, repeated claims of loss of prescriptions, tampering with prescriptions and reluctance to provide prior medical records or contact information for other treating physician(s). Doctor shopping (visiting multiple prescribers) to obtain additional prescriptions is common among drug abusers and people suffering from untreated addictions.

Physical Dependence and Tolerance: Abuse and addiction are separate and distinct from physical dependence and tolerance. Physicians should be aware that addiction may not be accompanied by concurrent tolerance and symptoms of physical dependence in all addicts. In addition, abuse of opioids can occur in the absence of true addiction and is characterized by misuse for non-medical purposed, often in combination with other psychoactive substances. Methadone Hydrochloride Injection, like other opioids, may be diverted for non-medical use. Careful record-keeping of prescribing information, including quantity, frequency, and renewal requests is strongly advised.

Abuse of Methadone Hydrochloride Injection poses a risk of overdose and death. This risk is increased with concurrent abuse of Methadone Hydrochloride Injection with alcohol and other substances. In addition, parenteral drug abuse is commonly associated with transmission of infectious disease such as hepatitis and HIV.

Proper assessment of the patient, proper prescribing practices, periodic re-evaluation of therapy, and proper dispensing and storage are appropriate measures that help to limit abuse of opioid drugs.

Infants born to mothers physically dependent on opioids may also be physically dependent and may exhibit respiratory difficulties and withdrawal symptoms (See Precautions, Pregnancy and Labor and Delivery).

OVERDOSE:

Symptoms: Serious overdosage of methadone is characterized by respiratory depression (a decrease in respiratory rate and/or tidal volume, Cheyne-Stokes respiration, cyanosis), extreme somnolence progressing to stupor or coma, maximally constricted pupils, skeletal-muscle flaccidity, cold and clammy skin and, sometimes, bradycardia and hypotension. In severe overdosage, particularly by the intravenous route, apnea, circulatory collapse, cardiac arrest, and death may occur.

Treatment: Primary attention should be given to the reestablishment of adequate respiratory exchange through provision of a patent airway and institution of assisted or controlled ventilation. If a non-tolerant person, especially a child, takes a large dose of methadone, effective narcotic antagonists are available to counter-act the potentially lethal respiratory depression. **The physician must remember, however, that methadone is a long-acting depressant (thirty-six to forty-eight hours), whereas the antagonists act for much shorter periods (one to three hours).** The patient must, therefore, be monitored continuously for recurrence of respiratory depression and may need to be treated repeatedly with the narcotic antagonist as needed. If the diagnosis is correct and respiratory depression is due only to overdosage of methadone, the use of respiratory stimulants is not indicated.

Opioid antagonists should not be administered in the absence of clinically significant respiratory or cardiovascular depression. In an individual physically dependent on opioids, the administration of the usual dose of an opioid antagonist may precipitate an acute withdrawal syndrome. The severity of this syndrome will depend on the degree of physical dependence and the dose of the antagonist administered. If antagonists must be used to treat serious respiratory depression in the physically dependent patient, the antagonist should be administered with extreme care and by titration with smaller than usual doses of the antagonist.

Intravenously administered naloxone or nalmefene may be used to reverse signs of intoxication. Because of the relatively short half-life of naloxone as compared with methadone, repeated injections may be required until the status of the patient remains satisfactory. Naloxone may also be administered by continuous intravenous infusion.

Oxygen, intravenous fluids, vasopressors, and other supportive measures should be employed as indicated.

For management of a suspected drug overdose, CPhA recommends that you contact your **regional Poison Control Centre**. See the *CPS* Directory section for a list of Poison Control Centres.

NOTE: IN AN INDIVIDUAL PHYSICALLY DEPENDENT ON OPIOIDS, THE ADMINISTRATION OF THE USUAL DOSE OF OPIOID ANTAGONIST WILL PRECIPITATE AN ACUTE WITHDRAWAL SYNDROME. THE SEVERITY OF THIS SYNDROME WILL DEPEND ON THE DEGREE OF PHYSICAL DEPENDENCE AND THE DOSE OF THE ANTAGONIST ADMINISTERED. THE USE OF AN OPIOID ANTAGONIST IN SUCH A PERSON SHOULD BE AVOIDED IF POSSIBLE. IF IT MUST BE USED TO TREAT SERIOUS RESPIRATORY DEPRESSION IN THE PHYSICALLY DEPENDENT PATIENT, THE ANTAGONIST SHOULD BE ADMINISTERED WITH EXTREME CARE AND BY TITRATION WITH SMALLER THAN USUAL DOSES OF THE ANTAGONIST (10-20% OF THE USUAL RECOMMENDED INITIAL DOSE OF THE ANTAGONIST).

DOSAGE AND ADMINISTRATION: METADOL (Methadone Hydrochloride Tablets, Oral Solution and Concentrate) can only be prescribed by physicians who have received an exemption pursuant to section 56 of the CDSA from the Minister of Health Canada to prescribe methadone (see Supplied). Patients prescribed methadone should be carefully monitored and provided appropriate supportive psychological and social services.

After interruption of chronic dosing, if methadone treatment is to be continued, starting doses should be low and patients should be titrated slowly to effect in order to avoid severe toxicity and respiratory depression.

For Relief of Severe Pain: Dosage should be carefully titrated and adjusted according to the severity of the pain and response of the patient. In general, METADOL, should not be used in opioid naive patients. The usual adult oral dose is 2.5 to 10 mg every 4 hours during the first 3 to 5 days, followed by a fixed dose every 8 to 12 hours depending on the patient's requirements. In geriatric patients the dosage schedule could be given on a once daily basis.

Special Considerations for A Pregnant Patient: Caution shall be taken in the maintenance treatment of pregnant patients. Dosage levels should be kept as low as possible if continued methadone treatment is deemed necessary. It is the physicians responsibility to assure that each female patient be fully informed concerning the possible risks to a pregnant woman or her unborn child from the use of methadone. (See Warnings.)

Special Limitations Treatment of Patients Under Age 18: The safety, effectiveness and dosage regimen of methadone for use in the treatment of adolescents have not been established.

Dispensing Guideline for Opioid Analgesic: Methadone (Oral Solution and Concentrate) must be dispensed in 100 mL of a vehicle that does not easily lend itself to injection.

METADOL (Oral Solution and Concentrate) has been found compatible with 100 mL of the following diluents prepared, where applicable, according to the manufacturer's instructions:

- Grape flavoured Kool-Aid
- Orange flavoured Tang
- Allen's Apple Juice
- Crystal Light Tangerine-Grapefruit flavoured
- Crystal Light Lemonade flavoured

Diluted solutions should be refrigerated (2 to 8°C) and stored for a period not exceeding 7 days in Allen's Apple Juice, and 14 days in all other diluents mentioned above.

Note: For both METADOL Concentrate (10 mg/mL) and METADOL (1 mg/mL) must be mixed with one of the above solutions (diluents) before dispensing.

INFORMATION FOR THE PATIENT: Published in e-CPS, available by subscription at www.e-cps.ca.

SUPPLIED: 1 mg/mL Oral Solution: Each mL of clear unflavoured and colourless liquid contains: methadone hydrochloride USP 1 mg. Nonmedicinal ingredients: citric acid, dextrose, glycerin, methylparaben, polyethylene glycol, purified water, sodium benzoate, sodium cyclamate. Bottles of 100 and 250 mL. Store tightly closed at 15 to 30°C, and protect from light and freezing.

Note: Methadone (Concentrate and Solution) must be dispensed in 100 mL of a vehicle that does not easily lend itself to injection (see Dosage and Administration).

10 mg/mL Oral Concentrate: Each mL of clear unflavoured and colourless liquid contains: methadone hydrochloride 10 mg. Nonmedicinal ingredients: citric acid, dextrose, glycerin, propylene glycol, purified water, sodium benzoate and sodium cyclamate. Bottles of 100 and 250 mL. Store at 15 to 30°C. Keep tightly closed. Protect from light and freezing.

Note: Methadone (Concentrate and Solution) must be dispensed in 100 mL of a vehicle that does not easily lend itself to injection (see Dosage and Administration).

Tablets: 1 mg: Each blue, round, flat-faced beveled-edged tablet, scored and imprinted "1" on one side and "P" logo on the other side, contains: methadone hydrochloride USP 1 mg. Nonmedicinal ingredients: FD&C Blue No.1 Lake, lactose, magnesium stearate and microcrystalline cellulose. Gluten-free. HDPE bottles of 100. Blister packs of 4×25. Store at 15 to 30°C. Keep tightly closed. Protect from light.

5 mg: Each peach, round, beveled-edged tablet, scored and imprinted "5" on one side and "P" logo on the other side, contains: methadone hydrochloride USP 5 mg. Nonmedicinal ingredients: FD&C Yellow No.6 Lake, lactose, magnesium stearate and microcrystalline cellulose. Gluten-free. HDPE bottles of 100. Blister packs of 4×25. Store at 15 to 30°C. Keep tightly closed. Protect from light.

10 mg: Each pale green, round, flat face, beveled-edged tablet, scored and imprinted "10" on one side and "P" logo on the other side, contains: methadone hydrochloride USP 10 mg. Nonmedicinal ingredients: D&C Yellow No.10 Aluminum Lake, FD&C Blue No.1 Lake, lactose, magnesium stearate and microcrystalline cellulose. Gluten-free. HDPE bottles of 100. Blister packs of 4×25. Store at 15 to 30°C. Keep tightly closed. Protect from light.

25 mg: Each white to off-white, biconvex, caplet shaped tablet, scored and imprinted "25" on one side and "P" logo on the other side, contains: methadone hydrochloride USP 25 mg. Nonmedicinal ingredients: lactose, magnesium stearate and microcrystalline cellulose. Gluten-free. HDPE bottles of 100. Blister packs of 4×25. Store at 15 to 30°C. Keep tightly closed. Protect from light.

Physicians who wish to receive an exemption pursuant to section 56 of the CDSA, from the Minister of Health Canada, must contact:

The Office of Controlled Substances
Healthy Environments and Consumer Safety Branch
A/L 3503B
Ottawa, Ontario
K1A 1B9

Pharmacist Compounding Information for Analgesia Preparation Using METADOL Oral Concentrate: To prepare a 100 mL stock solution of various strengths of Methadone, use METADOL concentrate 10 mg/mL and one of the following diluents:

- Grape flavoured Kool-Aid
- Orange flavoured Tang
- Allen's Apple Juice
- Crystal Light Tangerine-Grapefruit flavoured
- Crystal Light Lemonade flavoured

Dilution Chart to Prepare 100 mL of Solution

Concentration of Solution	METADOL (Concentrate)	Diluent
1 mg/mL	10 mL	90 mL
2 mg/mL	20 mL	80 mL
2.5 mg/mL	25 mL	75 mL
5 mg/mL	50 mL	50 mL
7.5 mg/mL	75 mL	25 mL
10 mg/mL	100 mL	0 mL

Note: Solution must be stored under refrigeration, for no longer than 1 week (apple juice) and for no longer than 2 weeks containing any of the other diluents indicated above.

Calculation Table 1 and Table 2 are indicating the individual total quantity of METADOL concentrate and diluent required for the prescribed duration of the treatment of severe pain:

Each 1 mL of these dilutions contains 1 mg of methadone, e.g. 5 mg b.i.d. =>5 mL (prepared solution) b.i.d.

Metadol has been found compatible with the following diluents prepared, where applicable, according to the manufacturer's instructions:

- Grape flavoured Kool-Aid
- Orange flavoured Tang
- Allen's Apple juice
- Crystal Light Tangerine-Grapefruit flavoured
- Crystal Light Lemonade flavoured

Each 1 mL of these dilutions contains 1 mg of methadone, e.g. 5 mg b.i.d. =>5 mL (prepared solution) b.i.d.

Metadol has been found compatible with the following diluents prepared, where applicable, according to the manufacturer's instructions:

- Grape flavoured Kool-Aid
- Orange flavoured Tang
- Crystal Light Tangerine-Grapefruit flavoured
- Crystal Light Lemonade flavoured

Table 1: METADOL

Calculation Table of Different Dilutions for the Quantity Required for 1 WEEK Treatment

	Quantity for 1 Daily Dose Regimen (Once Daily)			Quantity for 2 Times Daily Dose Regimen			Quantity for 3 Times Daily Dose Regimen		
Prescribed Unit Dose	**METADOL 10 mg/mL**	**Diluent**	**Total Quantity of Prepared Solution Per Week**	**METADOL 10 mg/mL**	**Diluent**	**Total Quantity of Prepared Solution Per Week**	**METADOL 10 mg/mL**	**Diluent**	**Total Quantity of Prepared Solution Per Week**
1 mg	0.7 mL	6.3 mL	7 mL	1.4 mL	12.6 mL	14 mL	2.1 mL	18.9 mL	21 mL
2.5 mg	1.75 mL	15.75 mL	17.5 mL	3.5 mL	31.5 mL	35 mL	5.25 mL	47.25 mL	52.5 mL
5 mg	3.5 mL	31.5 mL	35 mL	7 mL	63 mL	70 mL	10.5 mL	94.5 mL	105 mL
7.5 mg	5.25 mL	47.25 mL	52.5 mL	10.5 mL	94.5 mL	105 mL	15.75 mL	141.75 mL	157.5 mL
10 mg	7 mL	63 mL	70 mL	14 mL	126 mL	140 mL	21 mL	189 mL	210 mL

Table 2: METADOL

Calculation Table of Different Dilutions for the Quantity Required for 2 WEEKS Treatment

	Quantity for 1 Daily Dose Regimen (Once Daily)			Quantity for 2 Times Daily Dose Regimen			Quantity for 3 Times Daily Dose Regimen		
Prescribed Unit Dose	**METADOL 10 mg/mL**	**Diluent**	**Total Quantity of Prepared Solution Per Week**	**METADOL 10 mg/mL**	**Diluent**	**Total Quantity of Prepared Solution Per Week**	**METADOL 10 mg/mL**	**Diluent**	**Total Quantity of Prepared Solution Per Week**
1 mg	1.4 mL	12.6 mL	14 mL	2.8 mL	25.2 mL	28 mL	4.2 mL	37.8 mL	42 mL
2.5 mg	3.5 mL	31.5 mL	35 mL	7 mL	63 mL	70 mL	10.5 mL	94.5 mL	105 mL
5 mg	7 mL	63 mL	70 mL	14 mL	126 mL	140 mL	21 mL	189 mL	210 mL
7.5 mg	10.5 mL	94.5 mL	105 mL	21 mL	189 mL	210 mL	31.5 mL	283.5 mL	315 mL
10 mg	14 mL	126 mL	140 mL	28 mL	252 mL	280 mL	42 mL	378 mL	420 mL

Metamucil® Capsules plus Calcium

psyllium husk—calcium carbonate

Dietary Fibre Supplement—Bulk-forming Laxative—Cholesterol-lowering Agent

Procter & Gamble

SUPPLIED: Each capsule contains: psyllium husk (Plantago ovata) 550 mg and calcium (as calcium carbonate) 60 mg. Nonmedicinal ingredients: Blue 1 Lake, caramel colour, crospovidone, gelatin, polysorbate 80, purified water, Red 40 Lake, titanium dioxide and Yellow 6 Lake. Bottles of 75 and 120.

Metamucil® Fibre Therapy Capsules

psyllium husk

Bulk-forming Laxative

Procter & Gamble

SUPPLIED: Each capsule contains: psyllium husk (Plantago ovata) 525 mg. Nonmedicinal ingredients: Blue 1, caramel colour, gelatin, polysorbate 80, Red 40 and Yellow 6. Bottles of 100, 160 and 300.

Metamucil® Fibre Therapy Smooth Texture Pink Lemonade Flavour, Sugar-free

psyllium husk

Bulk-forming Laxative

Procter & Gamble

SUPPLIED: Each g of powder contains: psyllium husk (Plantago ovata) 0.6 g. Nonmedicinal ingredients: acesulfame potassium, aspartame, citric acid, maltodextrin, natural lemon flavour and Red 40. Containers of 429 and 679 g.

Metamucil® Preparations

psyllium hydrophilic mucilloid

Dietary Fibre Supplement—Bulk-forming Laxative—Cholesterol-lowering Agent

Procter & Gamble

PHARMACOLOGY: Metamucil Fibre Therapy is a gel-forming, soluble fibre derived from the seed husks of plants belonging to the genus Plantago. Metamucil has been used for many decades as a bulk-forming laxative for relief of irregularity and as a fibre supplement in individuals who lack sufficient fibre in their diet. Clinical studies have also shown that Metamucil has a hypocholesterolemic effect when taken in conjunction with a low fat diet that is at least equivalent to the AHA Step One diet.

Controlled clinical studies up to 6 months in duration in mild to moderate primary type IIa hypercholesterolemic patients administered 10.2 g/day Metamucil adjunctive to a AHA Step One diet showed significant reductions from baseline in total cholesterol (Tot-C) and low-density lipoprotein (LDL-C) cholesterol in the ranges of 2 to 8% and 5 to 12%, respectively. Consistency across studies, psyllium significantly ($p<0.05$) lowered total cholesterol and LDL cholesterol levels from baseline versus placebo. The percentage change for the psyllium mean versus placebo mean using final week scores ranged from 3 to 7% and 3 to 11% in total and LDL cholesterol, respectively. These studies indicate that adherence to a prudent low-fat diet, supplemented with psyllium significantly lowers total cholesterol and LDL cholesterol levels in patients with mild to moderate primary type IIa hypercholesterolemia. Psyllium had little to no effect on high density lipoprotein cholesterol (HDL-C) and triglyceride levels in patients who were maintained on the AHA Step One diet. As with other lipid-lowering therapies, dietary compliance is an essential element. Monitoring of serum lipid levels by a health care professional at regular intervals is advised so that the therapeutic effect can be determined. Consistent with the Canadian Guidelines on the Detection and Management of Hypercholesterolemia, repeat lipid profiles are recommended 3 to 6 months after initiation of treatment and annually thereafter. Long-term effects of Metamucil therapy for cholesterol reduction beyond 6 months have not been investigated.

A meta-analysis of pivotal efficacy trials, evaluating the hypercholesterolemic effects of 10.2 g total daily psyllium dose for 8 weeks, resulted in significant percent decreases due to psyllium versus placebo in Tot-C −3.8% ($p>0.0001$), LDL-C −5.5% ($p<0.0001$), LDL-C/HDL-C ratio −4.4% ($p=0.002$) and Tot-C/HDL-C ratio −2.5% ($p=0.02$). For each of these variables, a significant ($p<0.05$) decrease from baseline was also detected for the psyllium group but not for the placebo group.

An analysis (psyllium versus placebo) across these controlled clinical studies was conducted to assess the probability of shifting National Cholesterol Education Program (NCEP) risk categories for LDL-C and Total-C. The LDL-C and the Total-C risk categories were measured at baseline and at week 6 to 8 of the treatment phase in each subject involved in the 8 pivotal studies. Table 1 and Figure 1 show the percents of subjects that shifted toward "Decreased Risk," "No Change," and "Increased Risk," for LDL-C. Results of this analysis indicate that the probability of shifting toward a lower risk category was significantly greater in the psyllium group compared to placebo ($p=0.0001$). Thirty-nine percent of the subjects in the psyllium group decreased LDL-C by at least one risk category versus only 23% in the placebo group. Six to eight weeks of psyllium treatment increased the likelihood of shifting to lower risk categories by a factor of 2.33 ($p=0.0001$) compared to placebo. The results for Total-C are similar and are depicted in Table 2 and Figure 2. The risk probabilities in the psyllium group were significantly more concentrated in the lower risk categories than placebo ($p=0.0022$). The percents of subjects with "Decreased Risk" for the psyllium and placebo group were 25% and 15% respectively. Six to eight weeks of psyllium treatment increased the likelihood of lowering Total-C by at least one risk category by a factor of 1.81 ($p=0.0062$) compared to placebo.

Table 1: Metamucil

Distribution Shifts in NCEP Risk at Week 6-8 for LDL-C

	Group			
	Psyllium		Placebo	
Shift in NCEP Risk	n	%	n	%
Decreased Risk	151[a]	39	62[b]	23
No change	198	52	158	58
Increased Risk	34[c]	9	52[c]	19
Total	383		272	

[a] 11 subjects decreased 2 NCEP risk categories.
[b] 6 subjects decreased 2 NCEP risk categories.
[c] 1 subject decreased 2 NCEP risk categories.

Figure 1: Metamucil

Shift in NCEP Risk at Week 6-8 for LDL-C

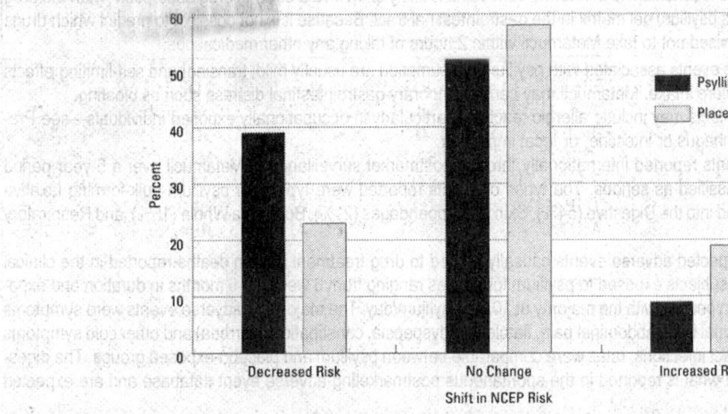

Table 2: Metamucil

Distribution Shifts in NCEP Risk at Week 6-8 for Total-C

	Group			
	Psyllium		Placebo	
Shift in NCEP Risk	n	%	n	%
Decreased Risk	95[a]	25	41[b]	15
No change	250	65	193	71
Increased Risk	39[c]	10	38	14
Total	384		272	

[a] 2 subjects decreased 2 NCEP risk categories.
[b] 1 subject decreased 2 NCEP risk categories.
[c] 1 subject decreased 2 NCEP risk categories.

Figure 2: Metamucil

Shift in NCEP Risk at Week 6-8 for Total-C

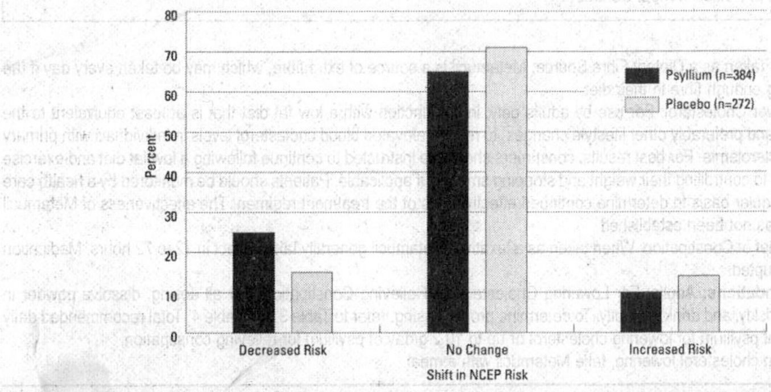

Evidence suggests that psyllium, which acts nonsystemically, exerts its hypocholesterolemic effect at the level of the small intestine and not via absorbed metabolites. It is believed that psyllium increases bile acid excretion by mechanically trapping the bile acids in the digestive tract, thereby producing increased fecal loss of the bile acids. Bile acid synthesis increases, in response to this loss, through increased oxidation of cholesterol, thus depleting the hepatic cholesterol pool. This depletion leads to up-regulation of hepatic LDL receptor activity and the resultant reduction in serum LDL-C concentration.

INDICATIONS: Lowers mild to moderately elevated cholesterol levels when taken with a low fat diet. Gentle relief of irregularity. Dietary fibre supplement. Suitable for daily use by those who lack dietary fibre.

CONTRAINDICATIONS: Nausea, vomiting, fever, abdominal pain or symptoms of an acute abdomen, intestinal obstruction, fecal impaction, undiagnosed rectal bleeding, or dysphagia. Known allergy to any component.

WARNINGS: When used for treatment of constipation, patients should be cautioned that they should not use the product without consulting a doctor if they have noticed a sudden change in bowel habits that persist over a period of 2 weeks. Patients are advised to consult a physician if constipation persists for longer than 1 week, as this may be a sign of a serious medical condition.

Patients are cautioned that taking this product without adequate fluid may cause it to swell and block the throat or esophagus and may cause choking. They should not take the product if they have difficulty in swallowing or have been diagnosed with narrowing of the esophagus. If they experience chest pain, vomiting, or difficulty in swallowing or breathing after taking this product, they are advised to seek immediate medical attention.

Psyllium products may cause allergic reaction in people sensitive to inhaled or ingested psyllium. Keep this and all medications out of the reach of children.

Phenylketonurics: The Smooth Texture, Orange-flavoured, and Berry Burst-flavoured, Sugar-free preparation contains phenylalanine from aspartame.

PRECAUTIONS: Attention Heathcare Professionals: Sensitization to psyllium has occurred in some healthcare professionals chronically exposed to psyllium dust. Therefore, Metamucil Fibre Therapy may cause an allergic reaction in people sensitive to inhaled or ingested psyllium powder. To minimize the potential for allergic reaction, heathcare professionals who frequently dispense powdered psyllium products should follow handling procedures designed to reduce exposure to dust while dispensing, such as spooning the product from the canister rather than pouring. Avoid inhaling the airborne dust while dispensing.

Before instituting therapy with Metamucil, diseases contributing to increased serum cholesterol, such as hypothyroidism, diabetes mellitus, nephrotic syndrome, dysproteinemias, obstructive liver disease and alcoholism, should be ruled out. In addition, the concomitant medications being taken by the patient should be reviewed to determine if they potentially contribute to elevated LDL-C or total cholesterol. It should be verified that an elevated LDL-C is responsible for the high total cholesterol. Patients with primary type IIb hypercholesterolemia or secondary causes of hypercholesterolemia should not be treated with Metamucil. LDL-C and total cholesterol levels should be monitored at regular intervals to ensure that therapeutic effect is being maintained.

Special Populations for Hypercholesterolemia: The safety and effectiveness of Metamucil for cholesterol lowering in children have not been established.

In patients over 65 years, efficacy appears similar to that seen in the population as a whole, with no apparent increase in the frequency of adverse events.

Drug Interactions: Limited information available in the literature, including a single letter to the editor on lithium and one pharmacokinetic study with carbamazepine, suggests that psyllium bulk laxatives may interfere with the absorption of other drugs administered concomitantly. The mechanism is unknown, however, it is likely to involve a delay in drug absorption when the drug is mixed in the hydrated viscous psyllium gel matrix in the gastrointestinal tract. Because it is not possible to predict which drugs are of concern, patients are advised not to take Metamucil within 2 hours of taking any other medications.

ADVERSE EFFECTS: Adverse events associated with psyllium consumption are usually mild, transient and self-limiting effects normally found with increased fibre intake. Metamucil may cause temporary gastrointestinal distress such as bloating.

In rare instances, adverse effects may include allergic reaction (particularly in occupationally exposed individuals—see Precautions), blockage of the esophagus or intestine, or fecal impaction.

The majority of adverse events reported internationally through postmarket surveillance of Metamucil over a 5-year period were nonserious, with <1% classified as serious. The types of events reported were typical for psyllium bulk-forming laxative drugs, with the majority classified into the Digestive (54%), Skin and Appendages (21%), Body as a Whole (15%), and Respiratory (11%) Body Systems.

There were no serious/unexpected adverse events causally related to drug treatment and no deaths reported in the clinical population involving over 1000 subjects exposed to psyllium for studies ranging from 6 weeks to 6 months in duration and exposures from 5.1 to 20.4 g psyllium per day with the majority at 10.2 g psyllium/day. The majority of adverse events were symptoms associated with the gastrointestinal tract (abdominal pain, flatulence, dyspepsia, constipation, diarrhea) and other cold symptoms suggesting upper respiratory tract infections; rates were comparable between psyllium and placebo-exposed groups. The digestive tract events were typical of what is reported in the spontaneous postmarketing adverse event database and are expected side effects of bulk fibre usage.

There were no clinically significant laboratory findings suggesting a safety concern based on results from the clinical program including the clinical laboratory data, hematology, vital signs or vitamin/mineral assessments from the clinical safety data.

There were no special safety concerns found in special populations in the preliminary clinical program including elderly and diabetic populations. Adverse events reported in these groups are comparable to adverse events reported in other clinical subjects. Supportive safety information for psyllium use was found in the literature in diabetics and the elderly, children and subjects with chronic constipation, or with previously resected adenomatous polyps.

OVERDOSE:

Symptoms: Although serious adverse effects are uncommon with Metamucil Fibre Therapy, esophageal and bowel obstruction have occurred in some cases, primarily when insufficient liquid was administered with the dose. Some symptoms that may indicate a serious event include difficulty in breathing (possible allergy or esophageal blockage), difficulty swallowing, chest pain or choking symptoms (possible esophageal obstruction), nausea, vomiting (possible symptoms associated with esophageal or lower intestinal blockage). In some cases, abdominal pain may be indicative of lower intestinal blockage but it is also a side effect associated with the nonserious gas and bloating effects, more commonly associated with fibre intake.

Treatment: Treatment for overdosage is largely symptomatic. Ingestion of additional water is recommended if the patient does not have a history of breathing, swallowing or choking problems. The extra water will help the fibre pass through the system.

If a blockage occurs in the esophagus, generally a probe or scope is used to mechanically break up the blockage under a physician's care. Removal of the blockage through surgery is available as a final option.

For lower intestinal obstructions, an accurate diagnosis of the cause of the blockage is critical. Generally, mechanical removal of the obstruction is the first option, followed by surgery if necessary. Blockages are generally not treated successfully with protein enzymes or enemas.

Bowel movements following an overdose should typically be seen within 72 hours. Follow-up with a physician is essential if this is not the case.

> For management of a suspected drug overdose, contact your regional Poison Control Centre. See the *CPS* Directory section for a list of Poison Control Centres.

DOSAGE: When Taken as a Dietary Fibre Source: Metamucil is a source of extra fibre, which may be taken every day if the patient is not getting enough fibre in their diet.

When Taken to Lower Cholesterol: For use by adults only, in conjunction with a low fat diet that is at least equivalent to the AHA Step One diet and preferably other lifestyle changes, to reduce elevated blood cholesterol levels in individuals with primary type IIa hypercholesterolemia. For best results, consumers should be instructed to continue following a low fat diet and exercise regularly, in addition to controlling their weight and stopping smoking if applicable. Patients should be monitored by a health care professional on a regular basis to determine continued effectiveness of the treatment regimen. The effectiveness of Metamucil beyond 6 months has not been established.

When Taken for Relief of Constipation: When taken as a laxative, Metamucil generally takes effect in 12 to 72 hours. Medication should not be interrupted.

Dosing Recommendations: Adults: For Lowering Cholesterol or Relieving Constipation: For all dosing, dissolve powder in 240 mL liquid, stir briskly, and drink promptly. To determine proper dosing, refer to Table 3 and Table 4. Total recommended daily dose is 10.2 g/day of psyllium for lowering cholesterol or up to 10.2 g/day of psyllium for relieving constipation.

For best results in cholesterol lowering, take Metamucil with a meal.

Table 3: Metamucil

Cholesterol-lowering Dosing Recommendations: Adults

Metamucil Fibre Therapy Product	Adult Dosage[a]	Metamucil g/Dosage	Psyllium g/Dosage	Calories/ Dosage	Frequency of Dosing	Total Daily Dosage (g/psyllium)
Smooth Texture, Unflavoured, sugar-free	Cannister: 3 level teaspoons	5.4 g	3.4 g	20	3 times/day	10.2 g
	4.5 level teaspoons	8.1 g	5.1 g	30	2 times/day	10.2 g
Smooth Texture, Orange Flavoured, sugar-free	Cannister: 3 level teaspoons	5.8 g	3.4 g	20	3 times/day	10.2 g
	Single-dose Packets: 1 packet	5.8 g	3.4 g	20	3 times/day	10.2 g
	4.5 level teaspoons	8.8 g	5.1 g	30	2 times/day	10.2 g
Smooth Texture, Berry Burst Flavoured, sugar-free	Cannister: 3 level teaspoons	5.8 g	3.4 g	20	3 times/day	10.2 g
	Single-dose Packets: 1 packet	5.8 g	3.4 g	20	3 times/day	10.2 g
	4.5 level teaspoons	8.8 g	5.1 g	30	2 times/day	10.2 g
Smooth Texture, Orange Flavour	Cannister: 4 level teaspoons	12.0 g	3.4 g	45	3 times/day	10.2 g
	6 level teaspoons	18.0 g	5.1 g	68	2 times/day	10.2 g
Original Texture, Unflavoured	Cannister: 3 level teaspoons	7.0 g	3.4 g	25	3 times/day	10.2 g
	4.5 level teaspoons	10.5 g	5.1 g	38	2 times/day	10.2 g

(cont'd)

Table 3: Metamucil *(cont'd)*

[a] All doses represent measuring teaspoons.

Table 4: Metamucil

Constipation Dosing Recommendations: Adults

Metamucil Fibre Therapy Product	Adult Dosage[a]	Metamucil g/Dosage	Psyllium g/Dosage	Frequency of Dosing	Total Daily Dosage (g/psyllium)
Smooth Texture, Unflavoured, sugar-free	Cannister: 1 rounded teaspoon	5.4 g	3.4 g	up to 3 times/day	10.2 g
Smooth Texture, Orange Flavoured, sugar-free	Cannister: 1 rounded teaspoon	5.8 g	3.4 g	up to 3 times/day	10.2 g
	Single-dose Packets: 1 packet	5.8 g	3.4 g	up to 3 times/day	10.2 g
Smooth Texture, Berry Burst Flavoured, sugar-free	Cannister: 1 rounded teaspoon	5.8 g	3.4 g	up to 3 times daily	10.2 g
	Single-dose Packets: 1 packet	5.8 g	3.4 g	up to 3 times daily	10.2 g
Smooth Texture, Orange Flavor	Cannister: 1 rounded tablespoon	12.0 g	3.4 g	up to 3 times/day	10.2 g
Original Texture, Unflavoured	Cannister: 1 rounded teaspoon	7.0 g	3.4 g	up to 3 times/day	10.2 g

[a] All doses represent measuring teaspoons.

Children (6 Years of Age and Over): For Constipation: one half the adult dose 1 to 3 times/day, the dose being adjusted for patient size and need (see Table 2. Each dose is taken in 240 mL or more of water or other suitable liquids.

New Users: If patients experience occasional minor bloating, they should reduce the amount of Metamucil that they are taking and gradually increase to the recommended dose.

INFORMATION FOR THE PATIENT: Published in e-CPS, available by subscription at www.e-cps.ca.

SUPPLIED: Original Texture, Unflavoured Powder: Each g of powder contains: psyllium hydrophilic mucilloid 0.5 g. Nonmedicinal ingredients: sucrose. Containers of 336, 504 and 798 g. Store below 30°C. Keep lid tightly closed to protect from humidity.

Smooth Texture, Orange-flavoured: Each g of powder contains: psyllium hydrophilic mucilloid 0.3 g. Nonmedicinal ingredients: citric acid, orange flavour, sucrose and Yellow 6. Containers of 370 and 861 g. Store below 30°C. Keep lid tightly closed to protect from humidity.

Smooth Texture, Orange-flavoured, Sugar-free: Each g of powder contains: psyllium hydrophilic mucilloid 0.6 g. Nonmedicinal ingredients: aspartame, citric acid, maltodextrin, orange flavour and Yellow 6. Containers of 425, 660 and 1044 g. Twin packs of 2×660 g. Boxes of 30 single-dose packets of 5.8 g. Store below 30°C. Keep lid tightly closed to protect from humidity.

Smooth Texture, Berry Burst flavour, Sugar-free: Each g of powder contains: psyllium hydrophilic mucilloid 0.6 g. Nonmedicinal ingredients: aspartame, Blue 1, citric acid, malic acid, maltodextrin, natural and artificial flavour and Red 40. Containers of 425 and 660 g. Twin packs of 2×660 g. Store below 30°C. Keep lid tightly closed to protect from humidity.

Smooth Texture, Unflavoured, Sugar-free: Each g of powder contains: psyllium hydrophilic mucilloid 0.6 g. Nonmedicinal ingredients: citric acid and maltodextrin. Containers of 283 g. Store below 30°C. Keep lid tightly closed to protect from humidity.

Methadone Ⓝ

CPhA Monograph

see *Opioids*

Methazolamide Pr

CPhA Monograph

see *Carbonic Anhydrase Inhibitors: Systemic*

Methenamine

methenamine

methenamine mandelate

Urinary Antibacterial—Antiperspirant

CPhA Monograph

Date of Preparation: October 2008

This monograph has been compiled by CPhA and reviewed by experts. It may contain information different from that found in Health Canada-approved Product Monographs. The reader is referred to the *CPS* Editorial Policy for more information.

SUMMARY PRODUCT INFORMATION:

Drug	Route of Administration	Dosage Form	Strength
Methenamine mandelate	Oral	Tablet	500 mg
Methenamine/sodium bicarbonate/tartaric acid	Oral	Effervescent powder	0.5 g/4.6 g/3.8 g per 10 mL
Methenamine	Topical	Cream	8%

INDICATIONS AND CLINICAL USE: Oral: Methenamine can cause suppression or elimination of bacteriuria, and is therefore used primarily for the prevention rather than treatment of upper and lower urinary tract infections (UTIs). Oral methenamine is approved for the suppression or elimination of bacteriuria associated with pyelonephritis, cystitis and other urinary tract infections. Methenamine is not effective in the treatment of pyelonephritis. It is not used to treat infections outside the urinary tract, because it remains inactive until it is excreted by the kidneys into the urinary tract where formaldehyde is produced and concentrates in the bladder.

Despite many studies in various subgroups of patients, the data on efficacy are not strong largely due to poor quality studies with contradictory results. Compared to placebo, oral methenamine appears effective in preventing either bacteriuria or symptomatic UTIs in young, otherwise healthy people when other antimicrobial agents have not been effective. Oral methenamine has been used for the prevention of recurrent symptomatic UTIs in children when intermittent catheterization techniques used in urinary bladder voiding dysfunction or when other antibiotics have not been effective. Methenamine has been used as short-term prophylaxis (≤7 days) in patients without renal abnormalities, such as women undergoing short-term bladder catheterization, to decrease the incidence of symptomatic UTI; however, effective alternatives such as other oral antibacterial agents should be considered first. Using methenamine in men with chronic bacteriuria resulted in reduced recurrence and fewer acute exacerbations of UTI but superiority to other oral antibacterials has not been demonstrated. Oral methenamine is not effective in preventing UTIs in patients with indwelling bladder catheters as sufficient concentrations of formaldehyde cannot be generated in this clinical setting.

Oral methenamine is not used for the treatment of acute UTIs. Though oral methenamine is approved in patients with neurologic diseases leading to an infected residual urine, in one study, benefit in terms of UTI prevention was not seen in spinal cord–injured patients with neurogenic bladder. Overall, methenamine has not shown to be superior to other antibacterials in the suppression and prevention of urinary tract infections. Oral methenamine should be considered as an alternative to other antibacterial agents in cases of intolerance, allergy, treatment failure or resistance.

Formaldehyde generation from methenamine is dependent on acidic urinary pH; avoid methenamine in patients who are unable to achieve and maintain an acidic urinary pH, e.g., patients with a more alkaline pH (pH >5.5) due to their diet. Using vitamin C or other acidifying agents has not been demonstrated to improve the effectiveness of methenamine, but the effect on urinary pH can be monitored; weigh possible benefits against the unlikely risks associated with these agents. Treatment failures may also be due to urease-producing bacteria in urine such as Proteus and Pseudomonas as methenamine conversion to formaldehyde is prevented by the resulting alkaline urine.

Evidence for the therapeutic use of the effervescent form of methenamine is limited.

Topical: Topical methenamine is indicated for the treatment and prevention of plantar hyperhidrosis and associated malodour, and as adjunct in the treatment of athlete's foot when excessive perspiration contributes to worsening of the condition. Topical methenamine has been shown to be effective in the treatment of palmoplantar hyperhidrosis in adults.

CONTRAINDICATIONS:

- Patients who are hypersensitive to methenamine or any ingredient in the formulation, or to formaldehyde.
- Patients with renal insufficiency (ClCr <50 mL/min).
- Patients with severe hepatic insufficiency.

WARNINGS AND PRECAUTIONS:

Serious Warnings and Precautions

- Avoid methenamine in patients concurrently receiving sulfonamides as there have been reports of insoluble precipitates in acidic urine. Avoid methenamine in patients with a history of gout as they may be at an increased risk of precipitating urate crystals in their urine; also, avoid methenamine in patients at an increased risk of uric acid nephrolithiasis such as those with high serum uric acid levels, low urinary pH and low fractional excretion of urate. Avoid methenamine in patients with severe dehydration and metabolic acidosis.
- Use methenamine with caution in patients with pre-existing hepatic insufficiency as they may be more susceptible to the effects of ammonia and formaldehyde produced in the gastrointestinal tract.
- Prolonged use of methenamine may lead to fungal superinfection or *C. difficile*-associated diarrhea.
- Immediate-type hypersensitivity reactions with methenamine have been reported. If an allergic reaction occurs, discontinue methenamine and institute appropriate therapy.

- Accumulation of formaldehyde in the urinary tract has occurred when methenamine is given for extended periods or at higher than recommended doses, e.g., 8 g daily for three to four weeks, causing bladder irritation and inflammation, dysuria, polyuria, protein and/or blood in the urine. Reducing the dose or acidity of the urine may help alleviate these adverse effects but may limit the clinical effectiveness of methenamine.

Special Populations: Pregnant Women: Pregnancy Category C_M. Use of methenamine during pregnancy has not been adequately studied. It is unknown whether methenamine crosses the placenta. Studies in rats, rabbits and dogs have found little or no evidence of fetal harm. Limited human data does not support a greater incidence of congenital defects relative to the baseline risk. The use of methenamine during pregnancy requires the potential benefits be weighed against the possible risks to the mother and the fetus.

Nursing Women: Methenamine is excreted in small amounts in the breast milk, peaking at 1 hour after ingestion. No adverse effects have been reported in nursing infants. The use of methenamine during nursing requires that potential benefits be weighed against the possible risks to the mother and infant.

Geriatrics: Clinical studies of methenamine did not include significant numbers of subjects over 65 years of age. No differences in toxicity have been observed in older individuals when compared to other age groups. Because of age-related declines in kidney and liver functions, initiate therapy in older individuals at the lower end of the dose range.

Monitoring and Laboratory Tests: Monitor liver enzymes periodically in patients with pre-existing liver insufficiency. Prior to initiation of therapy, perform urinalysis and/or cultures. Monitor for clinical signs and symptoms of a urinary tract infection.

ADVERSE REACTIONS: Adverse Drug Reactions Overview: Methenamine is generally well tolerated by patients. Adverse effects are often mild and reversible. Gastrointestinal adverse effects such as nausea and vomiting, and dermatologic adverse effects such as rash and pruritus are common. Larger doses of methenamine (8 g daily for three to four weeks) are associated with bladder irritation, painful and frequent micturition, albuminuria and gross hematuria, which may be due to higher formaldehyde concentrations in the gastrointestinal and urinary tracts. See Table 1.

Table 1: Methenamine

More Common Adverse Drug Reactions

Body System	Effect	Clinical Comment
Dermatologic	Rash, pruritus	
Gastrointestinal	Nausea, vomiting, diarrhea	Take with food to minimize gastrointestinal upset.
Genitourinary	Dysuria	Decreasing the acidity of urine or the methenamine dose may alleviate or reduce dysuria, but may reduce the effectiveness of methenamine.

Less Common Adverse Drug Reactions: General: generalized edema (rare).
Central Nervous System: headache (rare).
Dermatologic: rash, urticaria, pruritus. **Cream**—Allergic contact dermatitis. Use of methenamine cream, especially in excessive amounts may cause hardening and cracking of the skin which is self-limiting as the top layer of the skin will eventually peel away to reveal a new layer of skin underneath. The use of moisturizing cream or ointment may help retain moisture within the skin.
Gastrointestinal: nausea, vomiting, diarrhea, abdominal cramps, abdominal discomfort, stomatitis, anorexia. There have been instances where these adverse effects have been severe enough to render discontinuation of therapy; however, others have found them to be transient in nature.
Genitourinary: Microscopic and rarely gross hematuria has been reported. Hemorrhagic cystitis with accidental overdose. Reduced urinary flow rates may increase the risk of crystalluria, irritation and inflammation of the urinary tract, where the bladder is most commonly affected. Dysuria, polyuria, albuminuria/proteinuria may occur with prolonged use or taking doses higher than recommended.
Hepatic/Biliary/Pancreatic: Potential to cause increased levels of serum hepatic enzymes, worsening pre-existing hepatic illness with higher methenamine doses due to ammonia production.
Immune: Hypersensitivity reactions have been rarely associated with methenamine therapy. (See Warnings and Precautions.)
Musculoskeletal: muscle cramps (rare).
Neurologic: tinnitus (rare).
Respiratory: dyspnea (rare).
Abnormal Hematologic and Clinical Chemistry Findings: See Table 2.

Table 2: Methenamine

Abnormal Hematologic and Clinical Chemistry Findings

Test	Effect	Clinical Comment
Liver enzymes (e.g., alanine aminotransferase and aspartate aminotransferase)	Reversible increases	Although infrequent, reversible increases in liver enzymes have been observed during therapy, mostly in patients with pre-existing liver dysfunction.
Urinary protein	May be falsely increased	Urinary protein may be falsely elevated by methenamine.
Anion gap	May increase	Seen with mandelate salt.

DRUG INTERACTIONS:

Serious Drug Interactions

- Administration of methenamine to patients who are concurrently receiving a sulfonamide increases the risk of developing crystalluria, potentially leading to renal damage (e.g., renal colic, nephritis, toxic nephrosis).

Overview: Any substance that is capable of changing the pH of the urine can alter the effectiveness of methenamine. Urinary pH is a determining factor in the amount of formaldehyde generated from methenamine. Formaldehyde is responsible for the antibacterial action of methenamine.
Drug-Drug Interactions: See Table 3.

Table 3: Methenamine

Drug-Drug Interactions

Interacting Drug	Effect	Clinical Comment
Antacids (e.g., aluminum hydroxide, calcium carbonate, magnesium hydroxide, sodium bicarbonate)	Antacids, urinary alkalinizers and carbonic anhydrase inhibitors increase urinary pH and as a result, minimize conversion of methenamine to formaldehyde.	Avoid combination. If urine pH cannot be maintained at <5.5 then methenamine should not be used. Alternatively, may use other effective antimicrobials. If used concomitantly, consider administering antacids, urinary alkalizers and carbonic anhydrase inhibitors a few hours after methenamine dosing; however, impact on methenamine effectiveness is unknown. Monitor urinary pH and therapeutic effect of methenamine.
Urinary alkalinizer (e.g., potassium citrate, sodium citrate, sodium acetate)		
Carbonic anhydrase inhibitors (e.g., acetazolamide)		
Sulfonamides	Increased risk of crystalluria due to the low solubility of sulfonamides and metabolites in acidic pH; direct interaction between sulfonamides and formaldehyde to form insoluble precipitates in acidic pH which can result in acute renal failure.	Avoid combination.

Drug-Food Interactions: Intake of alkaline food, e.g., dairy products and most fruits (except citrus fruits, cranberries, prunes, plums) may cause an increase in urinary pH, therefore decreasing the antibacterial effect of methenamine which is optimal at pH <5.5. Patients on methenamine therapy should avoid or limit alkaline foods; separate timing of methenamine administration with regard to alkaline foods by several hours. Clinicians should monitor the effectiveness of methenamine and urinary pH (maintain at <5.5), adding agents to acidify the urine as required. Take methenamine with food to minimize gastrointestinal upset.
Drug-Laboratory Interactions: See Table 4.

DOSAGE AND ADMINISTRATION: Recommended Dose and Dosage Adjustment: Adults: See Table 5 and Table 7.
Geriatrics: No geriatric-specific dosing guidelines have been established. Refer to adult dosing. (See Special Populations, Geriatrics).
Pediatrics: See Table 6.
Dialysis: Do not use in patients on dialysis.
Hepatic Impairment: Avoid in patients with hepatic insufficiency as ammonia is released when methenamine is converted to formaldehyde.

Table 4: Methenamine

Drug-Laboratory Interactions

Test	Effect	Clinical Comment
Urinary catecholamines	Falsely increased levels.	Formaldehyde interferes with the fluorometric procedures used to determine urinary catecholamine levels. Interpret test results with caution if patient on methenamine.
Vanillylmandelic acid (VMA)	Falsely increased levels.	Formaldehyde interferes with the fluorometric procedures used to determine VMA levels. Interpret test results with caution if patient on methenamine.
Urine estriol	Falsely decreased levels.	Formaldehyde reacts with estriol to produce inaccurate results when acid hydrolysis techniques are used. In patients receiving methenamine therapy, enzyme hydrolysis techniques which are not affected by formaldehyde should be used instead.
17-hydroxy-corticosteroid (17-OHCS)	Falsely increased levels.	Formaldehyde interferes with the Porter-Silber method used to determine 17-OHCS levels. Interpret test results with caution if the patient on methenamine.
5-hydroxy-indoleacetic acid (5HIAA)	Falsely decreased levels.	Formaldehyde interferes with colour formation when nitrosonaphthol methods are used to determine 5H1AA levels. Interpret test results with caution if patient on methenamine.

Table 5: Methenamine

Dose in Adult Patients

Indication	Dose	Duration of Therapy	Clinical Comment
Prevention and suppression of recurrent lower urinary tract infections	1 g po QID, maximum 4 g po daily	Methenamine may be used as short-term prophylaxis (≤7 days) in patients without renal abnormalities, such as women undergoing short-term bladder catheterization, to decrease the incidence of symptomatic UTI; however, consider effective alternatives such as other oral antibacterial agents first. Long term use (at least 6 months) has been studied in various populations, with trends toward overall benefit but conflicting results in different studies and with few significant adverse effects.	Used in young, otherwise healthy women when other antibacterial agents have not been effective.
Treatment and prevention of plantar hyperhidrosis and associated malodour	Use topically: apply a thin film to soles, heels, and in between toes daily	Use for 7 consecutive nights, then once or twice weekly thereafter to maintain control for the treatment and prevention of plantar hyperhidrosis and associated malodour.	Following 7 days of therapy, plantar eccrine glands should be suppressed for 1 to 2 months. To maintain control, apply 1-2 times per week **afterwards**. May be used as an adjunct in treating athlete's foot when excessive perspiration contributes to worsening of the condition.
Adjunctive treatment of athlete's foot			

Table 6: Methenamine

Dose in Pediatric Patients

Indication	Dose	Clinical Comment
Prevention of recurrent symptomatic urinary tract infections	5 to 12 years: 500 mg po QID; maximum 2 g po daily <5 years: 250 mg/14 kg po QID; maximum 500 mg QID	Used if intermittent catheterization techniques in children with urinary bladder voiding dysfunction or other antimicrobial agents have not been effective. If patient is unable to swallow, tablets can be split, crushed and dissolved.

Table 7: Methenamine

Dose in Adult Patients with Renal Impairment

Route	Creatinine Clearance	Dosage Adjustment	Clinical Comment
Oral	>50 mL/min	Usual dose	
Oral	≤50 mL/min	Avoid drug	Effective urinary concentrations cannot be achieved.

OVERDOSAGE:

For management of a suspected drug overdose, CPhA recommends that you contact your **regional Poison Control Centre**. See the *CPS* Directory section for a list of Poison Control Centres.

ACTION AND CLINICAL PHARMACOLOGY: Mechanism of Action: Oral methenamine has no systemic antibacterial effects. Methenamine remains inactive until it is excreted by the kidneys into the lower urinary tract. Formaldehyde is produced through hydrolysis of methenamine in acidic urine, and concentrates in the bladder. Urinary pH is an important factor in determining the effectiveness of methenamine due to the amount of formaldehyde liberated. At a pH of 7.4, there is almost no formaldehyde produced; a 6% yield (of the theoretical amount) occurs at a pH of 6 and 20% at a pH of 5. When administered as the mandelate salt, mandelic acid helps to acidify the urine and fosters a bacteriostatic environment by promoting the conversion of methenamine to formaldehyde; a pH of <5 is reached in the stomach, urine and sweat.

Effectiveness of methenamine is influenced not only by the rate of formaldehyde generation but also by the duration of exposure of bacteria to formaldehyde. With methenamine concentrations of 1000 μg/mL, more than 6 h is needed to generate a formaldehyde concentration >25 μg/mL at pH 6.5 and approximately 3 hours at pH 5.85. Approximately 2 hours is needed at this concentration for antibacterial activity. Patients who void frequently or who have their bladders drained frequently may not benefit from methenamine treatment as such actions reduce exposure time of bacteria to formaldehyde and reduce formaldehyde concentrations in the urine.

Almost all bacteria are susceptible to free urine formaldehyde concentration of ≥20 μg/mL. Acquired resistance is deemed unlikely to develop with methenamine; the antibacterial action of methenamine involves non-specific mechanisms and can therefore be used long-term. Formaldehyde is equally effective against Gram-positive and Gram-negative microorganisms, and fungi.

Topical methenamine is hydrolyzed to formaldehyde in sweat. Relief of hyperhidrosis is achieved by decreasing the solubility of protein through a direct interaction between formaldehyde and polypeptides which results in the blockage of affected sweat ducts.

Pharmacokinetics: Adults: Absorption: Methenamine is readily absorbed following oral administration. Approximately 82 to 88% of the administered dose is recovered in the urine of healthy volunteers in a 24-hour period. Approximately 10 to 30% of the methenamine dose is hydrolyzed to ammonia and formaldehyde in the acidic environment of the stomach.

Distribution: The volume of distribution of methenamine is 0.56 L/kg. It is unknown whether methenamine crosses the placenta. Methenamine enters into the breast milk where it achieves concentrations similar to that found in the serum. Mandelic acid also enters breast milk.

Excretion: Methenamine is renally cleared. Approximately 70 to 90% of methenamine is excreted unchanged through glomerular filtration and tubular excretion. The half-life of methenamine is around 4 hours. Bactericidal formaldehyde concentrations in the urine are not achieved until methenamine reaches the bladder.

Methimazole 🅿
Antithyroid Agent

CPhA Monograph

Date of Preparation: October 2006
Date of Revision: November 2007

This monograph has been compiled by CPhA and reviewed by experts. It may contain information different from that found in Health Canada-approved Product Monographs. The reader is referred to the *CPS* Editorial Policy for more information.

SUMMARY PRODUCT INFORMATION:

Route of Administration	Dosage Form	Strength
Oral	Tablet	5 mg, 10 mg

INDICATIONS AND CLINICAL USE: Methimazole is indicated for:

- primary treatment of hyperthyroidism secondary to Graves' disease
- adjunctive therapy to render patients euthyroid prior to thyroidectomy
- management of hyperthyroidism when thyroidectomy is contraindicated or not advisable
- adjunctive therapy to radioactive iodine (RAI) therapy to stabilize thyroid function prior to and potentially after RAI administration until ablative effects of the iodine occur

The treatment of Graves' disease is the only appropriate long-term use of methimazole since this disorder has the potential for spontaneous immunologic remission, i.e., remaining biochemically euthyroid for 1 year after cessation of drug therapy. Female sex, age > 40 years, high thyroid peroxidase antibody positivity, small goiter, mild hyperthyroidism and negative TSH receptor antibody are all factors associated with a higher likelihood of immunologic remission. Antithyroid drug therapy has been shown to achieve sustained remission in 30-40% of cases. Methimazole is not considered a primary treatment for conditions in which spontaneous remissions rarely occur, such as toxic multinodular goiters and solitary autonomous nodules.

Methimazole, 60 to 120 mg/day in divided doses is an alternative to propylthiouracil, 600-1200 mg/day in divided doses, in the management of thyroid storm. Propylthiouracil may be preferred in the management of thyroid storm as it blocks peripheral conversion of thyroxine (T4) to triiodothyronine (T3) by inhibiting 5'-monodeiodinase though the clinical significance of this effect is unknown.

Pediatrics: Methimazole is used in children and adolescents to treat hyperthyroidism, usually in an attempt to delay ablative therapy. If immunologic remission does not occur, surgery or RAI therapy may be considered specifically in older children and adolescents. Maintenance high dose methimazole therapy to achieve euthyroidism may be predictive of no remission.

CONTRAINDICATIONS:

- Patients who are hypersensitive to methimazole or to any ingredient in the formulation or component of the container.

WARNINGS AND PRECAUTIONS:

Serious Warnings and Precautions

- Agranulocytosis (neutrophils < 500/mm³), estimated frequency 0.2 to 0.5%, is the most serious adverse reaction and is probably dose related. It usually occurs in the first 3 months of treatment, though there have been reports of it occurring ≥ 1 year after initiating therapy. Some studies suggest the risk of agranulocytosis is higher in patients > 40 years and those taking doses > 40 mg/day. Patients should be instructed to immediately report any symptoms, such as sore throat or fever, and to discontinue methimazole. Sepsis is suspected if there is rapid onset of fever, chills and prostration. Agranulocytosis is considered a contraindication to further antithyroid therapy because of the cross-reactivity between methimazole and propylthiouracil.
- Cholestatic jaundice has occurred rarely. Patients should be instructed to report symptoms of hepatic dysfunction such as anorexia, pruritus, right upper-quadrant pain. Their presence should prompt evaluation of liver function tests and discontinuation of methimazole.

Special Populations: Pregnant Women: Methimazole readily crosses the placenta. Case reports of aplasia cutis congenita suggest a weak association with methimazole use during gestation. "Methimazole embryopathy," which is characterized by choanal and esophageal atresia, scalp defects, minor facial anomalies and psychomotor delay, is also associated with methimazole use during the first trimester. It is not clear, however, whether the reported congenital abnormalities are associated with in utero exposure to methimazole or to maternal hyperthyroid state. Poorly controlled hyperthyroidism is associated with the following sequelae: spontaneous abortion, premature labor, low birth weight, stillbirth, preeclampsia and heart failure. Good fetal and maternal outcome is dependent on control of maternal hyperthyroidism. If methimazole is to be used in pregnancy, the lowest possible dose should be used to prevent fetal hypothyroidism or goiter. The risk of fetal hypothyroidism or goiter is negligible if the maternal free thyroxine level is maintained at slightly above the upper limit of normal. Methimazole may be discontinued in the last few weeks of pregnancy in some women with Graves' disease because thyroid function diminishes as pregnancy proceeds.

Nursing Women: Methimazole is excreted into breast milk. In a study that involved administration of 2.5 mg of methimazole Q12H, the mean milk: plasma ratio was 16 to 39 μg in the daily milk supply. This is equivalent to 3 mg/day of methimazole in breast milk when extrapolated to the usual daily dose of 20 mg. Methimazole 30 mg/day or less does not appear to pose a major risk to the nursing infant. Closely monitor thyroid function of the infant. Methimazole is considered compatible with breastfeeding by the American Academy of Pediatrics.

ADVERSE REACTIONS: Adverse Drug Reactions Overview: The most serious but rare adverse events include agranulocytosis and cholestatic jaundice. The toxic effects generally resolve upon discontinuation of drug therapy. The most commonly reported reactions include skin rash and gastrointestinal upset. Hypersensitivity reactions can also occur; some resolve with continued therapy, while others may require a short course of corticosteroids.

More Common Adverse Drug Reactions: See Table 1.

Less Common Adverse Drug Reactions (< 1%): Central Nervous System: dizziness, headache.

Dermatologic: urticaria, pruritus, skin pigmentation.

Endocrine and Metabolism: hypothyroidism (due to prolonged therapy), pancreatitis, hypoglycemia.

Gastrointestinal: vomiting, loss of taste (rare), sialadenopathy (rare), neutropenic colitis with cecal perforation.

Hematologic: agranulocytosis (see Warnings and Precautions), granulocytopenia, leukopenia, aplastic anemia, thrombocytopenia.

Hepatic/Biliary/Pancreatic: cholestatic hepatitis (see Warnings and Precautions), immunoallergic hepatitis, jaundice, fulminant hepatitis (rare), hepatic necrosis, encephalopathy (rare).

Immune: lymphadenopathy (rare), anti-neutrophil cytoplasmic antibody (ANCA)-positive vasculitis (rare; discontinue methimazole), lupus-like syndrome.

Neurologic: peripheral neuropathy.

Renal: nephritis.
Abnormal Hematologic and Clinical Chemistry Findings: See Table 2.

Table 1: Methimazole

More Common Adverse Drug Reactions (≥ 1%)

Body System	Effect	Clinical Comment
Musculoskeletal	Arthralgias, polyarthritis	May resolve within 4 weeks of stopping therapy. Arthralgias may be a harbinger of severe transient migratory polyarthritis known as the "antithyroid arthritis syndrome" which may occur within 2 months of starting methimazole.
Dermatologic	Skin rash	Incidence of 3–5%, usually a maculopapular eruption. May also be urticarial or macular. If maculopapular pruritic rash, it may resolve with concomitant antihistamine and/or topical corticosteroid use. Consider switching to propylthiouracil. If rash is urticarial or associated with fever or arthralgias, consider radioiodine therapy as cross-reactivity can be as high as 50%.
Gastrointestinal	Dyspepsia, gastric distress, nausea	Of concern only if persists or becomes bothersome. Dose-dependent; consider dividing the dose.

Table 2: Methimazole

Abnormal Hematologic and Clinical Chemistry Findings

Test	Effect	Clinical Comment
WBC count	Leukopenia	Observed in 10% of patients with untreated hyperthyroidism. Transient, not an indication to discontinue methimazole therapy.
^{123}I, ^{131}I, ^{99m}Tc	↓ uptake	Antithyroid drug should be stopped at least 5 days before the diagnostic test.
ALT, AST, bilirubin, LDH, INR	↑ concentration/time	May indicate an adverse event.

Legend:
WBC=white blood cell; ALT=alanine aminotransferase; AST=aspartate aminotransferase; LDH=lactate dehydrogenase; INR=international normalized ratio.

DRUG INTERACTIONS: Drug-Drug Interactions: See Table 3.

Table 3: Methimazole

Drug-Drug Interactions

Interacting Drug	Effect	Clinical Comment
Warfarin	Increased or decreased warfarin-induced anticoagulation	Hyperthyroidism induces catabolism of clotting factors. Warfarin inhibits synthesis of clotting factors. Concomitant use may enhance warfarin anticoagulant response. Monitor INR and observe for signs of ↑ or ↓ response to warfarin when initiating, discontinuing or changing doses of methimazole. Adjust warfarin dose as necessary.
Digitalis glycosides	↑ serum levels in hyperthyroidism or when euthyroid state is reached with methimazole therapy.	Hyperthyroid patients may not be as sensitive to effects of digoxin as hypothyroid patients. Addition of methimazole may require a reduction in digoxin dose when euthyroid state is reached. Monitor digoxin levels and adjust dose as necessary.
CYP2D6 substrate, e.g., amitriptyline, venlafaxine	Increased plasma concentrations of CYP2D6 substrates	Monitor for potentiation of pharmacologic and adverse effects related to increased levels of CYP2D6 substrates. Adjust dose of CYP2D6 substrates as necessary.
Beta-blockers, e.g., metoprolol, propranolol	↑ clearance of beta-blocker in hyperthyroidism	Addition of methimazole may require a reduction in beta-blocker dose when euthyroid state is reached.

Table 4: Methimazole

Dose in Adult Patients

Indication	Initial Dose	Maintenance Dose	Duration of Therapy	Clinical Comment
Mild hyperthyroidism	15 mg daily	5–15 mg daily	12–18 months of treatment with methimazole is associated with a higher rate of remission compared to 6 months; no additional benefit seen in patients receiving 42 months of therapy.	A latent period of a few days to two weeks may be observed before thyroid hormone stores are depleted and for clinical effect to become evident. Obtain baseline differential white cell count before initiation of therapy. Consider dividing doses (i.e., Q8H) initially to minimize or prevent gastrointestinal adverse effects. Consider dose increase if no improvement in TSH and T4 levels in 4–6 weeks. Monitor thyroid indices monthly until euthyroid state is achieved. The goal is normalizing TSH and tapering the dose of methimazole to 5–15 mg/day. However, it is important to note that the recovery of TSH is slow so initial titration should target normalizing free T3 and free T4 levels. Monitor thyroid indices every 3 months during maintenance therapy. Adjust dose as required to achieve and maintain serum free T3, free T4 and TSH. Inadequate treatment is indicated by elevated free T3. Excessive antithyroid treatment is indicated by elevated TSH.
Moderately severe hyperthyroidism	30–40 mg daily	5–15 mg daily		
Severe hyperthyroidism or large goitres	60 mg daily	5–15 mg daily		

DOSAGE AND ADMINISTRATION: Recommended Dose and Dosage Adjustment: Adults: See Table 4.
Pediatrics: See Table 5.
Hepatic Impairment: The elimination half-life is prolonged in proportion to the degree of impairment. No dose adjustment is needed in patients with liver disease although clearance may be decreased.
Renal Impairment: No dose adjustment needed in renal impairment.
Administration: Methimazole can be taken with or without food. Gastrointestinal side effects may be minimized if taken with food. Consider even spacing the dose throughout the day when given in multidose regimens.

OVERDOSAGE:

For management of a suspected drug overdose, CPhA recommends that you contact your **regional Poison Control Centre**. See the *CPS* Directory section for a list of Poison Control Centres.

ACTION AND CLINICAL PHARMACOLOGY: Mechanism of Action: Methimazole is actively transported into the thyroid gland. It inhibits the formation of thyroid hormones by blocking the incorporation of iodine into tyrosine residues of thyroglobulin. It also inhibits the coupling reaction of these residues to form iodothyronines. Methimazole is believed to interfere with the oxidation of iodide ion and iodotyrosyl groups via inhibition of the peroxidase enzyme. Methimazole does not inactivate stored or circulating T3 and T4 hormones, nor the exogenous thyroxine administered as part of therapy. Unlike propylthiouracil, methimazole does not inhibit the peripheral conversion of T4 to T3.
Pharmacokinetics: Adults: See Table 6.
Absorption: Methimazole is readily absorbed from the gastrointestinal tract with an absolute bioavailability of 93%. The effect of food on absorption is unpredictable.
Distribution: Widely distributed; actively concentrated in the thyroid gland. No significant protein binding is observed.
Metabolism: Rapidly metabolized in the liver by the flavin-containing monooxygenase to sulfenic and sulfinic acids, the latter is converted to N-methylimidazole and sulfite anion upon the reaction with water. Cytochrome P450 metabolism also produces N-methylimidazole. No active metabolites have been found. FMO-mediated metabolism seems to suppress cytochrome P450-catalyzed N-hydroxylation, as well as the content of cytochrome P450 itself.
Excretion: The metabolites and about 11% of unchanged drug are excreted in the urine.

Table 5: Methimazole

Dose in Pediatric Patients

Indication	Initial Dose	Maintenance Dose	Maximum Dose	Clinical Comment
Hyperthyroidism	0.4 mg/kg/day given daily	0.2 mg/kg/day given daily	Maximum 30 mg/24 h	Consider dividing doses (i.e., Q8H) initially to minimize or prevent gastrointestinal adverse effects.

Table 6: Methimazole

Summary of Pharmacokinetic Parameters

C_{max}	Duration of Action	Elimination $t_{½}$	Clearance	Volume of Distribution
0.5–1 h	6–8 h	~ 4–6 h	10 L/h	0.6 L/kg

STORAGE AND STABILITY: Store between 15 and 30°C in a closed, light-resistant container.

Methotrexate Pr

methotrexate sodium

Antimetabolite

Pfizer

SUPPLIED: Each round, yellow, scored tablet, engraved "2.5" and "M1", contains: methotrexate sodium equivalent to methotrexate 2.5 mg. Nonmedicinal ingredients: cornstarch, lactose and magnesium stearate. Dye-free. Bottles of 100.

Methotrexate Injection USP Pr

methotrexate sodium

Antimetabolite—Antirheumatic Agent

Hospira

Date of Revision: July 15, 2009

SUMMARY PRODUCT INFORMATION:

Route of Administration	Dosage Form/ Strength	Clinically Relevant Nonmedicinal Ingredients
Intramuscular, intravenous, intra-arterial, intrathecal	10 mg/mL, 25 mg/mL	Benzyl alcohol as preservative For a complete listing see Dosage Forms, Composition and Packaging.

INDICATIONS AND CLINICAL USE: Two major fields of indication exist for Methotrexate:
- Neoplastic diseases
- Disease Modifying Antirheumatic Drug (DMARD)

Neoplastic Diseases:
- Choriocarcinoma: Methotrexate - as single chemotherapy or in combination with other drugs.
- Intermediate-, or high grade Non-Hodgkin's Lymphoma as part of ProMACE-CytaBOM, ProMACE-MOPP, and Magrath protocols.
- Breast Cancer: as part of CMF (cyclophosphamide-methotrexate-fluorouracil) therapy.
- Acute Lymphoblastic Leukemia (ALL) - as maintenance therapy.
- Head and Neck Cancer - in combination with other chemotherapies.
- Gastric Cancer – palliative combination chemotherapy.
- Metastasis of unknown primary - as palliative combination chemotherapy.
- Osteogenic sarcoma (adjuvant) - high dose Methotrexate with leucovorin rescue (HDMTX-LV).
- Bladder Cancer (advanced) - as part of M-VAC regimen.
- Leptomeningeal spread of malignancies (carcinomatosis/leukemia/lymphoma) as a single chemotherapy or alternating with Ara-C.
- Burkitt's lymphoma.
- Advanced stages of childhood lymphoma (III and IV, St. Jude's Childrens' Research Hospital Staging System).
- Advanced cases of mycosis fungoids (cutaneous T-cell lymphoma).

Disease Modifying Antirheumatic Drug (DMARD): The use of methotrexate as a DMARD in the following diseases where standard therapeutic interventions fail:
- Severe disabling psoriasis/psoriatic arthritis.
- Severe disabling rheumatoid arthritis (RA).

- Severe disabling seronegative arthritides.

In the treatment of psoriasis, methotrexate should be restricted to severe recalcitrant, disabling psoriasis, which is not adequately responsive to other forms of therapy, but only when the diagnosis has been established after dermatologic consultation.

Geriatrics: The clinical pharmacology of methotrexate has not been well studied in older individuals. Due to diminished hepatic and renal function, as well as decreased folate stores in this population, relatively low doses should be considered, and these patients should be closely monitored for early signs of toxicity.

Pediatrics: Safety and effectiveness in pediatric patients have not been established, other than in cancer chemotherapy.

CONTRAINDICATIONS:

- Patients who are hypersensitive to this drug or to any ingredient in the formulation or component of the container. For a complete listing, see Dosage Forms, Composition and Packaging.
- **Pregnancy:** Methotrexate can cause fetal death, embryotoxicity, abortion or teratogenic effects when administered to a pregnant woman. Methotrexate is contraindicated in pregnant patients with psoriasis or rheumatoid arthritis and should be used in the treatment of neoplastic diseases only when the potential benefit outweighs the risk to the fetus.
- Women of childbearing potential should not be started on methotrexate until pregnancy is excluded and should be fully counselled on the serious risk to the fetus should they become pregnant while undergoing treatment. Pregnancy should be avoided if either partner is receiving methotrexate. The optimal time interval between the cessation of methotrexate treatment of either partner and pregnancy has not been clearly established. Published literature recommendations for time intervals vary from 3 months to one year (see Warnings and Precautions).
- Because of the potential for serious adverse reactions in breast fed infants, it is contraindicated in nursing mothers.
- Methotrexate formulations and diluents containing preservatives must not be used for intrathecal or high dose Methotrexate therapy.
- Methotrexate is contraindicated in patients with psoriasis or rheumatoid arthritis in the following situations:
  - Alcoholism, alcoholic liver disease or other chronic liver disease.
  - Overt or laboratory evidence of immunodeficiency syndromes.
  - Pre-existing blood dyscrasias, such as bone marrow hypoplasia, leucopenia, thrombocytopenia or significant anemia.

WARNINGS AND PRECAUTIONS:

Serious Warnings and Precautions

- Methotrexate should be used only by physicians whose knowledge and experience includes the use of antimetabolite therapy (See Indications and Clinical Use).
- Methotrexate injection containing benzyl alcohol must not be used for intrathecal, intraventricular, or high dose therapy (See Dosage and Administration).
- Serious Toxic Reactions (See General).
- Use in pregnancy: Methotrexate has been reported to cause fetal death and/or congenital anomalies (see Special Populations, Pregnant Women). Pregnant patients with psoriasis or rheumatoid arthritis should not receive methotrexate (see Contraindications).

General: Because of the possibility of serious toxic reactions (which can be fatal), Methotrexate should be used only in life-threatening neoplastic diseases, or in patients with psoriasis or rheumatoid arthritis with severe, recalcitrant, disabling disease that is not adequately responsive to other forms of therapy. Deaths have been reported with the use of Methotrexate in the treatment of malignancy, psoriasis and rheumatoid arthritis. Because of the possibility of serious toxic reactions the patient should be informed by the physician of the risks involved and should be under a physician's constant supervision.

The use of methotrexate high dose regimens recommended for osteosarcoma requires meticulous care (see Dosage and Administration). High dosage regimens for other neoplastic diseases are investigational and a therapeutic advantage has not been established.

Methotrexate has the potential for serious toxicity. Toxic effects may be related in frequency and severity to dose or frequency of administration but have been seen at all doses. Because they can occur at any time during therapy, it is necessary to follow patients on methotrexate closely. Most adverse reactions are reversible if detected early. When such reactions do occur, the drug should be reduced in dosage or discontinued and appropriate corrective measures should be taken. If necessary, this could include the use of leucovorin calcium and/or acute, intermittent hemodialysis with a high-flux dialyzer (see Overdosage). If methotrexate therapy is re-instituted, it should be carried out with caution, with adequate consideration of further need for the drug and with increased alertness as to possible recurrence of toxicity.

Methotrexate exits slowly from third space compartments (e.g., pleural effusions or ascites). This results in a prolonged terminal plasma half-life and unexpected toxicity. In patients with significant third space accumulations, it is advisable to evacuate the fluid before treatment and to monitor plasma methotrexate levels.

Unexpectedly severe (sometimes fatal) bone marrow suppression, aplastic anemia and gastrointestinal toxicity have been reported with concomitant administration of methotrexate (usually in high dosage) along with some nonsteroidal anti-inflammatory drugs (NSAIDs) (see Drug Interactions).

Bone marrow and mucosal toxicity of methotrexate depend on: dose and duration of exposure of high levels (>2×10^{-8} mol/L (0.02 micromolar)) of methotrexate. Since the critical time factor has been defined for these organs as being 42 hours in humans, this has the following implications:

- When high doses of Methotrexate are employed (>1 g/m^2), drug levels in serum should be monitored;
- When drug levels exceeding (2×10^{-8} mol/L (0.02 micromolar)) the above for >42 hours may forecast significant toxicity;
- When toxicity can be minimized by appropriate administration of Leucovorin Calcium;
- When high-dose Methotrexate (HDMTX) is employed, it is imperative to alkalinise the urine in order to prevent crystallisation of Methotrexate and its 7-hydroxy metabolite in the urine, which may lead to acute renal failure.

Methotrexate given concomitantly with radiotherapy may increase the risk of soft tissue necrosis and osteonecrosis.

Methotrexate should be used with extreme caution in the presence of debility.

Carcinogenesis and Mutagenesis: Malignant lymphomas, which may regress following withdrawal of methotrexate, may occur in patients receiving low-dose methotrexate and, thus, may not require cytotoxic treatment. Discontinue methotrexate first and, if the lymphoma does not regress, appropriate treatment should be instituted.

Like other cytotoxic drugs, methotrexate may induce "tumour lysis syndrome" in patients with rapidly growing tumours. Appropriate supportive and pharmacologic measures may prevent or alleviate this complication.

No controlled human data exist regarding the risk of neoplasia with methotrexate. Methotrexate has been evaluated in a number of animal studies for carcinogenic potential with inconclusive results. Although there is evidence that methotrexate causes chromosomal damage to animal somatic cells and human bone marrow cells, the clinical significance remains uncertain. Assessment of the carcinogenic potential of methotrexate is complicated by conflicting evidence of an increased risk of certain tumors in rheumatoid arthritis. Benefit should be weighed against this potential risk before using methotrexate alone or in combination with other drugs, especially in children or young adults.

Gastrointestinal: If vomiting, diarrhea, or stomatitis occurs, resulting in dehydration, methotrexate should be discontinued until recovery occurs. Diarrhea and ulcerative stomatitis require interruption of therapy; otherwise, hemorrhagic enteritis and death from intestinal perforation may occur. Methotrexate should be used with extreme caution in the presence of peptic ulcer disease or ulcerative colitis.

Hematologic: Methotrexate should be used with caution in patients with impaired bone marrow function and previous or concomitant wide field radiotherapy. Methotrexate may produce marked bone marrow depression with resultant anemia, aplastic anemia, pancytopenia, leucopenia neutropenia and/or thrombocytopenia. In patients with malignancy and pre-existing hematopoietic impairment, the drug should be used with caution, if at all. In controlled clinical trials in rheumatoid arthritis (n=128), leucopenia (WBC <3000/mm^3) was seen in 2 patients, thrombocytopenia (platelets <1 000 000/mm^3) in 6 patients, and pancytopenia in 2 patients.

In psoriasis and rheumatoid arthritis, Methotrexate should be stopped immediately if there is a significant drop in blood counts. In the treatment of neoplastic diseases, Methotrexate should be continued only if the potential benefit warrants the risk of severe myelosuppression. Patients with profound granulocytopenia and fever should be evaluated immediately and usually require parenteral broad-spectrum antibiotic therapy.

Hepatic/Biliary/Pancreatic: Methotrexate has the potential for acute and chronic hepatotoxicity. Acutely, liver enzyme elevations are frequently seen after Methotrexate administration and are usually not a reason for modification of Methotrexate therapy. Liver enzyme elevations are usually transient and asymptomatic, and also do not appear predictive of subsequent hepatic disease. Persistent liver abnormalities, and/or decrease of serum albumin may be indicators of serious liver toxicity. Chronic toxicity is potentially fatal; it generally has occurred after prolonged use (generally two years or more) and after a total cumulative dose of at least 1.5 grams. Liver biopsy after sustained use often shows histologic changes, and fibrosis and cirrhosis have been reported; these latter lesions may not be preceded by symptoms or abnormal liver function tests in the psoriasis population. Periodic liver biopsies are usually recommended for psoriatic patients who are under long-term treatment. Persistent abnormalities in liver function tests may precede appearance of fibrosis or cirrhosis in the rheumatoid arthritis population. In studies in psoriatic patients, hepatotoxicity appeared to be a function of total cumulative dose and appeared to be enhanced by alcoholism, obesity, diabetes and advanced age. An accurate incidence rate has not been determined; the rate of progression and reversibility of lesions is not known. Special caution is indicated in the presence of pre-existing liver damage or impaired hepatic function.

In psoriasis, liver damage and function tests, including serum albumin and prothrombin time, should be performed several times prior to dosing, but are often normal in the face of developing fibrosis or cirrhosis. These lesions may be detectable only by biopsy.

The usual recommendation is to obtain a liver biopsy: 1) before the start of therapy or shortly after initiation of therapy (4-8 weeks); 2) after a total cumulative dose of 1.5 grams; and 3) after each additional 1.0 to 1.5 grams. Moderate fibrosis or any cirrhosis normally leads to discontinuation of the drug; mild fibrosis normally suggests a repeat biopsy in 6 months. Milder histologic findings such as fatty change and low grade portal inflammation are relatively common pre-therapy. Although these mild changes are usually not a reason to avoid or discontinue methotrexate therapy, the drug should be used with caution.

Clinical experience with liver disease in rheumatoid arthritis is limited, but the same risk factors would be anticipated. Liver function tests are also usually not reliable predictors of histological changes in this population.

In rheumatoid arthritis, advanced age at first use of methotrexate and increasing duration of therapy have been reported as risk factors for hepatotoxicity. Persistent abnormalities in liver function tests may precede appearance of fibrosis or cirrhosis in the rheumatoid population. Liver function tests should be performed at baseline and at 4-8 week intervals in patients receiving methotrexate for rheumatoid arthritis. Pretreatment liver biopsy should be performed for patients with a history of excessive alcohol consumption, persistently abnormal baseline liver function test values, or chronic hepatitis B or C infection. During therapy, liver biopsy should be performed if there are persistent liver function test abnormalities, or there is a decrease in serum albumin below the normal range (in the setting of well controlled rheumatoid arthritis).

If the results of a liver biopsy show mild changes (Roenigk grades I, II, IIIa), methotrexate may be continued and the patient monitored according to the recommendations listed above. Methotrexate should be discontinued in any patient who displays persistently abnormal liver function tests and refuses liver biopsy, or in any patient whose liver biopsy shows moderate to severe changes (Roenigk grade IIIb or IV).

There is a combined reported experience in 217 rheumatoid arthritis patients with liver biopsies both before and during treatment (after a cumulative dose of at least 1500 mg) and in 714 patients with a biopsy only during treatment. There are 64 (7%) cases of fibrosis and 1 (0.1%) case of cirrhosis. Of the 64 cases of fibrosis, 60 were deemed mild. The reticulin stain is more sensitive for early fibrosis and its use may increase these figures. It is unknown whether even longer use will increase these risks.

Immune: Methotrexate should be used with extreme caution in the presence of active infection, and is usually contraindicated in patients with overt or laboratory evidence of immunodeficiency syndromes.

Immunization may be ineffective when given during methotrexate therapy. Immunization with live virus vaccines is generally not recommended. There have been reports of disseminated vaccinia infections after smallpox immunization in patients receiving methotrexate therapy. Hypogammaglobulinemia has been reported rarely.

Information to Be Provided to the Patient: Patients should be informed of the early signs and symptoms of toxicity, of the need to see their physician promptly if they occur, and the need for close follow-up, including periodic laboratory tests to monitor toxicity.

Both the physician and pharmacist should emphasize to the patient that the recommended dose is taken weekly in rheumatoid arthritis and psoriasis, and that mistaken daily use of the recommended dose has led to fatal toxicity.

Patients should be informed of the potential benefit and risk in the use of Methotrexate. The risk of effects on reproduction should be discussed with both male and female patients taking Methotrexate.

Neurologic: There have been reports of leukoencephalopathy following intravenous administration of Methotrexate to patients who have had craniospinal irradiation. Serious neurotoxicity, frequently manifested as generalized or focal seizures, has been reported with unexpectedly increased frequency among pediatric patients with acute lymphoblastic leukemia who were treated with intermediate-dose intravenous Methotrexate (1 g/m^2). Symptomatic patients were commonly noted to have leukoencephalopathy and/or microangiopathic calcifications on diagnostic imaging studies. Chronic leukoencephalopathy has also been reported in patients with osteosarcoma who received repeated doses of high-dose methotrexate with leucovorin rescue even without cranial irradiation. Discontinuation of methotrexate does not always result in complete recovery.

A transient acute neurologic syndrome has been observed in patients treated with high dosage regimens. Manifestations of this neurologic disorder may include behavioural abnormalities, focal sensorimotor signs, including transient blindness and abnormal reflexes. The exact cause is unknown.

After the intrathecal use of Methotrexate, the central nervous system toxicity which may occur can be classified as follows: chemical arachnoiditis manifested by such symptoms as headache, back pain, nuchal rigidity, and fever; paresis, usually transient, manifested by paraplegia associated with involvement with one or more spinal nerve roots; leucoencephalopathy manifested by confusion, irritability, somnolence, ataxia, dementia, and occasionally major convulsions.

Intravenous administration of Methotrexate may also result in acute encephalitis and acute encephalopathy with fatal outcome.

Cases of severe neurological adverse reactions that ranged from headache to paralysis, coma and stroke-like episodes have been reported mostly in juveniles and adolescents given methotrexate in combination with cytarabine.

Renal: Methotrexate therapy in patients with impaired renal function should be undertaken with extreme caution, and at reduced dosages, because renal dysfunction will prolong methotrexate elimination. Methotrexate may cause renal damage that may lead to acute renal failure. High doses of Methotrexate used in the treatment of osteosarcoma may cause renal damage leading to acute renal failure.

Nephrotoxicity is due primarily to the precipitation of methotrexate and 7-hydroxymethotrexate in the renal tubules. Close attention to renal function including adequate hydration, urine alkalization and measurement of serum methotrexate and creatinine levels are essential for safe administration.

Respiratory: Methotrexate-induced lung disease, including acute or chronic interstitial pneumonitis is a potentially dangerous lesion, which may occur at any time during therapy and which has been reported at low doses. It is not always fully reversible and fatalities have been reported. Pulmonary symptoms (especially a dry non-productive cough) or a non-specific pneumonitis occurring during methotrexate therapy may be indicative of a potentially dangerous lesion and require interruption of treatment and careful investigation. Although clinically variable, the typical patient with methotrexate-induced lung disease presents with fever, cough, dyspnea, hypoxemia, and an infiltrate on chest X-ray; infection (including pneumonia) needs to be excluded. This lesion can occur at all dosages.

Pneumonia (in some cases leading to respiratory failure) may occur. Potentially fatal opportunistic infections, especially *P.carinii* pneumonia, may occur with methotrexate therapy. When a patient presents with pulmonary symptoms, the possibility of *P.carinii* should be considered.

Sexual Function/Reproduction: Methotrexate causes embryotoxicity, abortion, and fetal defects in humans. It has also been reported to cause impairment of fertility, oligospermia and menstrual dysfunction in humans, during and for a short period after cessation of therapy.

Skin: Severe, occasionally fatal, dermatologic reactions, including toxic epidermal necrolysis (Lyell's Syndrome), Stevens-Johnson syndrome, exfoliative dermatitis, skin necrosis and erythema multiforme have been reported in children and adults within days of oral methotrexate administration. Reactions were noted after single or multiple, low, intermediate or high doses of methotrexate in patients with neoplastic and non-neoplastic diseases. Recovery has been reported with discontinuation of therapy.

Lesions of psoriasis may be aggravated by concomitant exposure to ultraviolet radiation. Radiation dermatitis and sunburn may be "recalled" by the use of methotrexate.

Special Populations: Pregnant Women: Methotrexate can cause fetal death, embryotoxicity, abortion, or teratogenic effects when administered to a pregnant woman. Methotrexate is contraindicated in pregnant patients with psoriasis or rheumatoid arthritis and should be used in the treatment of neoplastic diseases only when the potential benefit outweighs the risk to the fetus.

Women of childbearing potential should not be started on methotrexate until pregnancy is excluded and should be fully counselled on the serious risk to the fetus should they become pregnant while undergoing treatment. Pregnancy should be avoided if either partner is receiving methotrexate. The optimal time interval between the cessation of methotrexate treatment of either partner and pregnancy has not been clearly established. Published literature recommendations for time intervals vary from 3 months to one year.

Nursing Women: Because of the potential for serious adverse reactions from methotrexate in breast fed infants, Methotrexate is contraindicated in nursing mothers.

Pediatrics: Safety and effectiveness in pediatric patients have not been established, other than in cancer chemotherapy.

Methotrexate injection formulations containing the preservative benzyl alcohol are not recommended for use in neonates (children less than one month of age). There have been reports of fatal 'gasping syndrome' in neonates following the administration of intravenous solutions containing the preservative benzyl alcohol. Symptoms include a striking onset of gasping respiration, hypotension, bradycardia and cardiovascular collapse.

Geriatrics: The clinical pharmacology of methotrexate has not been well studied in older individuals. Due to diminished hepatic and renal function, as well as decreased folate stores in this population, relatively low doses should be considered, and these patients should be closely monitored for early signs of toxicity.

Monitoring and Laboratory Tests: General: Patients undergoing methotrexate therapy should be closely monitored so that toxic effects are detected promptly. Baseline assessment should include a complete blood count (CBC) with differential and platelet counts, hepatic enzymes, renal function tests, and a chest X-ray. During therapy of rheumatoid arthritis and psoriasis, monitoring of these parameters is recommended: hematology at least monthly, and hepatic enzyme levels and renal function every 1 to 2 months. More frequent monitoring is usually indicated during antineoplastic therapy. During initial or changing doses, or during periods of increased risk of elevated methotrexate blood levels (e.g., dehydration), more frequent monitoring may also be indicated.

Liver: Liver biopsies prior to Methotrexate therapy are not indicated routinely. Liver function tests (LFTs) should be determined prior to the initiation of therapy with Methotrexate and they should be monitored regularly throughout therapy. A relationship between abnormal liver function tests and fibrosis or cirrhosis of the liver has not been established. Transient liver function test abnormalities are observed frequently after methotrexate administration and are usually not cause for modification of methotrexate therapy. Persistent liver function test abnormalities just prior to dosing and/or depression of serum albumin may be indicators of serious liver toxicity and require evaluation.

Respiratory: Pulmonary function tests may be useful if methotrexate-induced lung disease is suspected, especially if baseline measurements are available.

Serum Level Monitoring: Serum methotrexate level monitoring can significantly reduce methotrexate toxicity and mortality.

Patients subject to the following conditions are predisposed to developing elevated or prolonged methotrexate levels and benefit from routine monitoring of levels: eg, pleural effusion, ascites, gastrointestinal tract obstruction, previous cisplatin therapy, dehydration, aciduria, impaired renal function.

Some patients may have delayed methotrexate clearance in the absence of these features. It is important that patients be identified within 48 hours since methotrexate toxicity may not be reversible if adequate leucovorin rescue is delayed for more than 42 to 48 hours.

The method of monitoring methotrexate concentrations varies from institution to institution. Monitoring of methotrexate concentrations should include determination of a methotrexate level at 24, 48, or 72 hours, and assessment of the rate of decline in methotrexate concentrations (to determine how long to continue leucovorin rescue).

ADVERSE REACTIONS: Adverse Drug Reaction Overview: In general, the incidence and severity of acute side effects are related to dose, frequency of administration, and the duration of the exposure to significant blood levels of methotrexate to the target organs. The most serious reactions are discussed in Warnings and Precautions. That section should also be consulted when looking for information about adverse reactions with methotrexate.

- Some of the effects mentioned in this section, such as dizziness and fatigue, may affect the ability to drive or operate machinery.
- The most frequently reported adverse reactions include ulcerative stomatitis, leucopenia, nausea, and abdominal distress. Other frequently reported adverse effects are malaise, undue fatigue, chills and fever, dizziness and decreased resistance to infection.

Adverse Drug Reactions by Organ System: Adverse reactions that have been reported with methotrexate are listed below alphabetically by organ system. In the oncology setting, concomitant treatment and the underlying disease make specific attribution of a reaction to methotrexate difficult.

Alimentary System: gingivitis, stomatitis, enteritis, anorexia, nausea, vomiting, diarrhea, hematemesis, melena, gastrointestinal ulceration and bleeding, pancreatitis.

Cardiovascular: pericarditis, pericardial effusion, hypotension, and thromboembolic events (including arterial thrombosis, cerebral thrombosis, deep vein thrombosis, retinal vein thrombosis, thrombophlebitis, and pulmonary embolus).

Central Nervous System: headaches, dizziness, drowsiness, speech impediment including dysarthria and aphasia; hemiparesis, paresis and convulsions have also occurred following administration of methotrexate. Following low doses, there have been occasional reports of transient subtle cognitive dysfunction, mood alteration, or unusual cranial sensations, leucoencephalopathy, or encephalopathy.

Eye Disorders: conjunctivitis, blurred vision, serious visual changes of unknown etiology, and transient blindness/vision loss.

Hematopoietic: Methotrexate can suppress hematopoiesis and cause anemia, leucopenia, and/or thrombocytopenia. Hypogammaglobulinemia has been reported rarely (see Warnings And Precautions, Immune). Lymphadenopathy and lymphoproliferative disorders (including reversible), pancytopenia, neutropenia and agranulocytosis and eosinophilia have also been observed.

Hepatobiliary Disorders: hepatoxocity, acute hepatitis, chronic fibrosis and cirrhosis, decrease in serum albumin, liver enzyme elevations, hepatic failure.

Infection: There have been case reports of sometimes fatal sepsis, sepsis, opportunistic infections, including fatal infections in patients receiving methotrexate therapy for neoplastic and non-neoplastic diseases. *P. carinii* pneumonia was the most common infection. Other reported infections included pneumonia, nocardiosis, histoplasmosis, cryptococcosis, *Herpes zoster*, *H. simplex* hepatitis and disseminated *H. simplex* and cytomegalovirus infection, including cytomegaloviral pneumonia.

Musculoskeletal, Connective Tissue, and Bone Disorders : stress fractures.

Pulmonary System: Respiratory fibrosis, pharyngitis and interstitial pneumonitis deaths have been reported; chronic interstitial obstructive pulmonary disease and alveolitis have occasionally occurred.

Skin: erythematous rashes, pruritus, urticaria, photosensitivity, pigmentary changes, alopecia, ecchymosis, telangiectasia, acne, furunculosis, erythema multiforme, toxic epidermal necrolysis (Lyell's Syndrome), Stevens-Johnson Syndrome, skin necrosis, exfoliative dermatitis, and painful erosion of psoriatic plaques.

Urogenital System: severe nephropathy or renal failure, azotemia, dysuria, cystitis, hematuria; defective oogenesis or spermatogenesis, transient oligospermia, menstrual dysfunction, vaginal discharge and gynecomastia; infertility, abortion, fetal defects, loss of libido/impotence. Proteinuria has also been observed.

Rarer Reactions: Related to or attributed to the use of Methotrexate such as nodulosis, vasculitis, herpes zoster, sepsis, arthralgia/myalgia, diabetes, osteoporosis, sudden death, lymphoma, reversible lymphomas, tumor lysis syndrome, soft tissue necrosis, aplastic anemia, fetal death and osteonecrosis. A few cases of anaphylactoid reactions have been reported.

Malignant lymphomas, which may regress following withdrawal of methotrexate, may occur in patients receiving low-dose methotrexate, and thus may not require cytotoxic treatment. Discontinue methotrexate first and if the lymphoma does not regress, appropriate treatment should be instituted.

Other Adverse Drug Reactions: Adverse Reactions Reported in Rheumatoid Arthritis: Incidence greater than 10%: elevated liver enzymes 15%, nausea/vomiting 10%.

Incidence 1% to 3%: rash/pruritus/dermatitis, alopecia, diarrhea, dizziness, leucopenia and pancytopenia.

Incidence 3% to 10%: stomatitis, thrombocytopenia.

Adverse Reactions in Psoriasis: The adverse reaction rates reported are very similar to those in the rheumatoid arthritis studies. Rarely, painful psoriatic plaque erosions may appear.

Abnormal Hematologic and Clinical Chemistry Findings: Abnormal hematologic and clinical chemistry findings are discussed in Warnings and Precautions, Monitoring and Laboratory Tests.

DRUG INTERACTIONS: Drug-Drug Interactions: The drugs listed below are based on either drug interaction case reports or studies, or potential interactions due to the expected magnitude and seriousness of the interaction (i.e., those identified as contraindicated).

Nonsteroidal Anti-inflammatory Drugs (NSAIDs): Nonsteroidal anti-inflammatory drugs should not be administered prior to or concomitantly with the high doses of Methotrexate used in the treatment of osteosarcoma. Concomitant administration of some NSAIDs with high dose Methotrexate therapy has been reported to elevate and prolong serum Methotrexate levels, resulting in deaths from severe hematologic and gastrointestinal toxicity.

Caution should be used when NSAIDs and salicylates are administered concomitantly with lower doses of methotrexate. These drugs have been reported to reduce the tubular secretion of methotrexate in an animal model, and may enhance its toxicity by increasing methotrexate levels.

In treating rheumatoid arthritis with methotrexate, acetylsalicylic acid (ASA), NSAIDs, and/or low dose steroids may be continued.

The possibility of increased toxicity with concomitant use of NSAIDs including salicylates has not been fully explored. Steroids may be reduced gradually in patients who respond to methotrexate. Combined use of methotrexate with gold, penicillamine, hydroxychloroquine, sulfasalazine, or cytotoxic agents has not been studied and may increase the incidence of adverse effects.

Despite the potential interactions, studies of methotrexate in patients with rheumatoid arthritis have usually included concurrent use of constant dosage regimens of NSAIDs without apparent problems. It should be appreciated however, that the doses used in rheumatoid arthritis (7.5 to 15 mg/week) are somewhat lower than those used in psoriasis and that larger doses could lead to unexpected toxicity.

Leflunomide: Methotrexate in combination with leflunomide may increase the risk of pancytopenia.

Drugs Highly Bound to Plasma Proteins: Methotrexate is partially bound to serum albumin, and toxicity may be increased because of displacement by certain drugs, such as salicylates, phenylbutazone, phenytoin and sulfonamides.

Probenecid: Renal tubular transport is also diminished by probenecid; use of methotrexate with this drug should be carefully monitored.

Nephrotoxic Drugs: In the treatment of patients with osteosarcoma, caution must be exercised if high-dose Methotrexate is administered in combination with a potentially nephrotoxic chemotherapeutic agent (e.g., cisplatin). Methotrexate clearance is decreased by cisplatinum.

Although not documented, other nephrotoxic drugs such as aminoglycosides, amphotericin B and cyclosporin could theoretically increase methotrexate toxicity by decreasing its elimination.

Penicillins and Sulfonamides: Penicillins and sulfonamides may reduce the renal clearance of Methotrexate; hematologic and gastrointestinal toxicity have been observed in combination with Methotrexate.

Oral Antibiotics: Oral antibiotics such as tetracycline, chloramphenicol, and non-absorbable broad spectrum antibiotics, may decrease intestinal absorption of methotrexate or interfere with the enterohepatic circulation by inhibiting bowel flora and suppressing metabolism of the drug by bacteria. For example: neomycin, polymyxin B, nystatin and vancomycin decrease methotrexate absorption, whereas kanamycin increases methotrexate absorption.

Trimethoprim/sulfamethoxazole has been reported rarely to increase bone marrow suppression in patients receiving methotrexate, probably by decreased tubular secretion and/or an additive antifolate effect.

Theophylline: Methotrexate may decrease the clearance of theophylline; theophylline levels should be monitored when used concurrently with methotrexate.

Mercaptopurine: Methotrexate increases the plasma levels of mercaptopurine. Combination of methotrexate and mercaptopurine may therefore require dose adjustment.

Vitamins: Vitamin preparations containing folic acid or its derivatives may decrease responses to systemically administered methotrexate. Preliminary animal and human studies have shown that small quantities of intravenously administered leucovorin enter the cerebrospinal fluid (CSF) primarily as 5-methyl tetrahydrofolate and, in humans, remain 1-3 orders of magnitude lower than the usual methotrexate concentrations following intrathecal administration.

However, high doses of leucovorin may reduce the efficacy of intrathecally administered Methotrexate.

In patients with rheumatoid arthritis or psoriasis, folic acid or folinic acid may reduce methotrexate toxicities such as gastrointestinal symptoms, stomatitis, alopecia and elevated liver enzymes.

Before taking a folate supplement, it is advisable to check B_{12} levels, particularly in adults over the age of 50, since folate administration can mask symptoms of B_{12} deficiency.

Folate deficiency states may increase methotrexate toxicity.

Radiotherapy: Methotrexate given concomitantly with radiotherapy may increase the risk of soft tissue necrosis and osteonecrosis.

Hepatoxins: The potential for increased hepatotoxicity when methotrexate is administered with other hepatotoxic agents has not been evaluated. However, hepatotoxicity has been reported in such cases. Therefore, patients receiving concomitant therapy with methotrexate and other potential hepatotoxic agents (e.g., leflunomide, azathioprine, sulfasalazine, retinoids) should be closely monitored for possible increased risk of hepatotoxicity.

Cytarabine: Methotrexate given concomitantly with cytarabine may increase the risk of severe neurologic adverse events such as headache, paralysis, coma and stroke-like episodes (see Warnings and Precautions, Neurologic).

Drug-Food Interactions: The bioavailability of orally administered methotrexate is reduced by food, particularly milk products.

DOSAGE AND ADMINISTRATION: **Neoplastic Diseases: Dosing Considerations:**

- Parenteral drug products should be inspected visually for particulate matter and discolouration prior to administration, whenever solution and container permit.
- Methotrexate injection may be given by the intramuscular, intravenous, intra-arterial, intrathecal or intraventricular (via Ommaya reservoir into the CNS) routes. The preserved formulation contains benzyl alcohol and must not be used for intrathecal, intraventricular, or high dose therapy.
- Methotrexate may only be administered by physicians experienced in the treatment of neoplasia. The oncologist should consult the current literature for the treatment regimen to be used. Typical dosages reported in the literature for the following malignancies are listed in the following section.

Recommended Dose and Dosage Adjustment: Breast Cancer: The initial doses of CMF will be cyclophosphamide 100 mg/m^2 p.o. days 1 through 14, Methotrexate 40 mg/m^2 IV day 1, 8, and 5 - Fluorouracil 600 mg/m^2 IV day 1, 8. Cycle length will be 28 days ("2 weeks-on, 2 weeks-off"). In patients over 60 years of age, the dosage of Methotrexate will be 30 mg/m^2 IV day 1, 8.

If total bilirubin exceeds 1.5 mg/dL, decrease the dose of Methotrexate only by 50%.

Bladder Cancer: Typical dosage regimens for bladder cancer are the CMV Regimen and the "M-VAC Regimen" which are represented in Table 1 and Table 2.

Table 1: Methotrexate Injection

CMV Regimen[a]

	Days		
Drugs[b]	**1**	**2**	**8**[e]
Cisplatin[c]		100	
Vinblastine	4		4
Methotrexate[d]	30		30

[a] All doses in mg/m^2 with cycles repeated on day 22.
[b] Patients >70 years old receive 80% of all doses; if vomiting persists to day 8, no drug is given.
[c] For each cycle adjust cisplatin to 100% for Ccr >60 mL/min; 50% of dose for Ccr 50-60 mL/min; none for Ccr <50 mL/min.
[d] No drug for a decrease on day 8 of >30 mL/min compared to day 1 or Ccr <50 mL/min or Cr >1.8 mg/dL.
[e] Major dose modifications for both drugs depending on myelosuppression.

Table 2: Methotrexate Injection

M-VAC Regimen[a]

	Days			
Drugs	**1**	**2**	**15**	**22**[c]
Methotrexate	30		30	30
Vinblastine		3	3	3
Doxorubicin		30[b]		
Cisplatin		70		

[a] All doses in mg/m^2 with cycles repeated every 28-32 days.
[b] Patients having prior pelvic irradiation equivalent to >2500 rad in 5 days, reduce the dose of doxorubicin 15 mg/m^2.
[c] No doses given when the WBC <2500 cells/mm^3, platelets >100 000 cells/mm^3, or mucositis present.

Head and Neck Cancer: Methotrexate remains the standard of therapy for patients with recurrent or metastatic disease. It has been given in a wide variety of doses and schedules (a few of which are represented in Table 3).

For palliation of patients with advanced incurable disease and acceptable renal function, it is appropriate to begin oral or intravenous methotrexate with weekly doses of 40-50 mg/m^2 or biweekly doses of 15 to 20 mg/m^2 and escalate the dose in weekly increments until either mild toxicity or therapeutic response is achieved.

Table 3: Methotrexate Injection

Methotrexate Schedule

Methotrexate Schedule[a]
0.8 mg/kg every 4 days IV
25–50 mg every 4 to 7 days
60 mg/m² weekly IV or 40 mg/m² biweekly IV
40–60 mg/m² weekly IV
80 mg/m² for 30 h every 2 wk with escalation to toxicity
40 mg/m² weekly IV
40–200 mg/m² IV on days 1, 4 weekly; Leucovorin on days 2,5
60 mg/m² IV weekly

[a] Excerpt from Devita, et al: CANCER 3rd Ed, p. 496.

Gastric Cancer: A regimen used in a clinical trial in Belgium in patients with resectable gastric cancer follows: methotrexate (1.5 g/m² IV day 1, +5-Fluorouracil (1.5 g/m² IV) + Leucovorin (15 mg/m² orally or IV every 6 hours for 72 hours) + Adriamycin (30 mg/m₂ IV, day 15). The schedule is repeated on day 29 for 6 cycles.

Choriocarcinoma and similar trophoblastic diseases: Methotrexate is administered orally or intramuscularly in doses of 15 to 30 mg daily for a 5 day course. Such courses are usually repeated for 3 to 5 times, as required, with rest periods of one or more weeks interposed between courses, until any manifesting toxic symptoms subside. The effectiveness of therapy is ordinarily evaluated by 24 hour quantitative analysis of urinary chorionic gonadotrophin hormone (beta-HCG), which should return to normal or less than 50 IU/24 hours usually after the third or fourth course, and usually be followed by a complete resolution of measurable lesions in four to six weeks. One to two courses of methotrexate after normalization of beta-HCG is usually recommended. Before each course of the drug, careful clinical assessment is essential. Cyclic combination therapy of methotrexate with other anti tumour drugs has been reported as being useful.

Since hydatiform mole may precede by choriocarcinoma, prophylactic chemotherapy with methotrexate has been recommended.

Chorioadenoma destruens is considered to be an invasive form of hydatiform mole. Methotrexate is administered in these disease states in doses similar to those recommended for choriocarcinoma.

Lymphomas: In Burkitt's tumour, Stages I-II, methotrexate has produced prolonged remissions in some cases. Recommended dosage is 10 to 25 mg/day orally for 4 to 8 days. In Stage III, methotrexate is commonly given concomitantly with other antitumor agents. Treatment in all stages usually consists of several courses of the drug interposed with 7 to 10 day rest periods. Lymphosarcomas in Stage III may respond to combined drug therapy with methotrexate given in doses of 0.625 to 2.5 mg/kg daily.

The treatment of choice for localized histologically aggressive lymphoma is primary combination chemotherapy with or without involved-field radiation therapy. Frequently used regimens for intermediate, or high grade NHL that include methotrexate include groups: the ProMACE/MOPP, ProMACE-CytaBOM, Magrath Protocols. Represented in Table 4 for example, is the ProMACE-CytaBOM Regimen.

Table 4: Methotrexate Injection

ProMACE-CytaBOM Regimen

ProMACE-CytaBOM	Day 1	Day 8	Day 14	Days 15-21
Cyclophosphamide 650 mg/m² IV	x			No therapy
Doxorubicin 25 mg/m² IV	x			
Etoposide 120 mg/m² IV	x			
Cytarabine 300 mg/m² IV		x		
Bleomycin 5 mg/m² IV		x		
Vincristine 1.4 mg/m² IV		x		
Methrotrexate 120 mg/m² IV		x with leucovorin rescue		
Prednisone 60 mg/m² PO	x.....................................	x		
Co-trimoxazole 2 PO bid throughout 6 cycles of therapy				

In early stage childhood non-Hodgkin's lymphoma, methotrexate is used effectively in combination chemotherapy regimens.

Mycosis Fungoides (cutaneous T-cell lymphoma) : Therapy with Methotrexate appears to produce a clinical response, in up to 50% of patients treated, but chemotherapy is not curative. Dosage is usually 2.5 to 10 mg daily by mouth for several weeks or months. Dose levels of drug and adjustment of dose regimen by reduction or cessation of drug are guided by patient response and hematologic monitoring. Methotrexate has also been given intramuscularly in doses of 50 mg once weekly or 25 mg 2 times weekly.

Leukemia: Acute lymphoblastic leukemia (ALL) in children and young adolescents is the most responsive to present day chemotherapy. In young adults and older patients, clinical remission is more difficult to obtain and early relapse is more common.

Methotrexate alone or in combination with steroids was used initially for induction of remission in ALL. More recently, corticosteroid therapy in combination with other antileukemic drugs or in cyclic combinations with methotrexate, has appeared to produce rapid and effective remissions. When used for induction, methotrexate in doses of 3.3 mg/m² in combination with 60 mg/m² of prednisone, given daily, produced remission in 50% of patients treated usually within a period of 4 to 6 weeks. Methotrexate in combination with other agents appears to be the drug of choice for securing maintenance of drug induced remissions. When remission is achieved and supportive care has produced general clinical improvement, maintenance therapy is initiated as follows: Methotrexate is administered 2 times weekly either by mouth or intramuscularly in total weekly doses of 30 mg/m². It has also been given in doses of 2.5 mg/kg intravenously every 14 days. If and when relapse does occur, re-induction of remission can again usually be obtained by repeating the initial induction regimen.

A variety of combination chemotherapy regimens have been used for both induction and maintenance therapy in ALL. The physician should be familiar with recent advances in antileukemic therapy.

Meningeal Leukemia: In the treatment or prophylaxis of meningeal leukemia, Methotrexate must be administered intrathecally.

For intrathecal administration, preservative free Methotrexate is diluted to a concentration of 1 mg/mL in an appropriate sterile, preservative free medium such as 0.9% Sodium Chloride Injection, USP.

The cerebrospinal fluid volume is dependent on age and not on body surface area. The CSF is at 40% of the adult volume at birth and reaches the adult volume in several years.

Intrathecal Methotrexate administration at a dose of 12 mg/m² (maximum 15 mg) has been reported to result in low CSF Methotrexate concentrations and reduced efficacy in children and high concentrations and neurotoxicity in adults.

The following dosage regimen is based on age instead of body surface area:

Age (years)	Dose (mg)
<1	6
1	8
2	10
3 or older	12

In one study in patients under the age of 40, this dosage regimen appeared to result in more consistent CSF Methotrexate concentrations and less neurotoxicity. Another study in children with acute lymphocytic leukemia compared this regimen to a dose of 12 mg/m² (maximum 15 mg), a significant reduction in the rate of CNS relapse was observed in the group whose dose was based on age.

Because the CSF volume and turnover may decrease with age, a dose reduction may be indicated in elderly patients.

For the treatment of meningeal leukemia, intrathecal Methotrexate may be given at intervals of 2 to 5 days. However, administration at intervals of less than 1 week may result in increased subacute toxicity. Methotrexate is administered until the cell count of the cerebrospinal fluid returns to normal. At this point one additional dose is advisable. For prophylaxis against meningeal leukemia, the dosage is the same as for treatment except for the intervals of administration. On this subject, it is advisable for the physician to consult the medical literature.

Untoward side effects may occur with any given intrathecal injection and are commonly neurological in character. Large doses may cause convulsions. Methotrexate given by the intrathecal route appears significantly in the systemic circulation and may cause systemic Methotrexate toxicity. Therefore, systemic antileukemic therapy with the drug should be appropriately adjusted, reduced, or discontinued. Focal leukemic involvement of the central nervous system may not respond to intrathecal chemotherapy and is best treated with radiotherapy.

Leptomeningeal Carcinomatosis: Intrathecal administration of Methotrexate as a single-drug or in combination regimens, is the most common therapy for carcinomatous leptomeningitis.

Treatment is optimally administered through an Ommaya reservoir and is usually started with Methotrexate (10 mg/m²) given twice weekly until the cerebrospinal fluid cytology becomes negative. The treatment regimen is gradually decreased, first to a weekly course, and eventually to a single administration every two months.

Osteosarcoma: An effective adjuvant chemotherapy regimen requires the administration of several cytotoxic chemotherapeutic agents. In addition to high-dose Methotrexate with leucovorin rescue, these agents may include doxorubicin, cisplatin, and the combination of bleomycin, cyclophosphamide and dactinomycin (BCD) in the doses and schedule shown in the table below. The starting dose for high dose Methotrexate treatment is 12 grams/m². If this dose is not sufficient to produce a peak serum Methotrexate concentration of 1000 micromolar (10^{-3} mol/L) at the end of the Methotrexate infusion, the dose may be escalated to 15 grams/m² in subsequent treatments. If the patient is vomiting or is unable to tolerate oral medication, leucovorin is given IV or IM at the same dose and schedule.

Table 5: Methotrexate Injection

Osteosarcoma

Drug[a]	Dose[a]	Treatment Week After Surgery
Methotrexate	12 g/m² IV as 4 hour infusion (starting dose)	4,5,6,7,11,12,15,16,29,30,44,45
Leucovorin	15 mg orally every six hours for 10 doses starting at 24 hours after start of Methotrexate infusion.	4,5,6,7,11,12,15,16,29,30,44,45
Doxorubicin[b] as a single drug	30 mg/m²/day IV×3 days	8,17
Doxorubicin[b] Cisplatin[b]	50 mg/m² IV 100 mg/m² IV	20,23,33,36 20,23,33,36
Bleomycin[b] Cyclophosphamide[b] Dactinomycin[b]	15 units/m² IV × 2 days 600 mg/m² IV × 2 days 0.6 mg/m² IV × 2 days	2,13,26,39,42 2,13,26,39,42 2,13,26,39,42

[a] Link MP, Goorin AM, Miser AW, et al: The effect of adjuvant chemotherapy on relapse-free survival in patients with osteosarcoma of the extremity. N Engl J of Med 1986; 314(No.25):1600-1606.

[b] See each respective package insert for full prescribing information. Dosage modifications may be necessary because of drug-induced toxicity.

When these higher doses of Methotrexate are to be administered, the following safety guidelines should be closely observed.

Guidelines for Methotrexate Therapy with Leucovorin Rescue:

1. Administration of Methotrexate should be delayed until recovery if:
   - The WBC count is less than 1500/microliter
   - The neutrophil count is less than 200/microliter
   - The platelet count is less than 75 000/microliter
   - The serum bilirubin level is greater than 1.2 mg/dL
   - The ALT level is greater than 450 U
   - Mucositis is present, until there is evidence of healing
   - Persistent pleural effusion is present; this should be drained dry prior to infusion.
2. Adequate renal function must be documented.
   a. Serum creatinine must be normal, and creatinine clearance must be greater than 60 mL/min, before initiation of therapy.
   b. Serum creatinine must be measured prior to each subsequent course of therapy. If serum creatinine has increased by 50% or more compared to a prior value, the creatinine clearance must be measured and documented to be greater than 60 mL/min (even if the serum creatinine is still within the normal range).
3. Patients must be well hydrated, and must be treated with sodium bicarbonate for urinary alkalinization.
   a. Administer 1000 mL/m² of intravenous fluid over 6 hours prior to initiation of the Methotrexate infusion. Continue hydration at 125 mL/m² /hr (3 liters/m²/day) during the Methotrexate infusion, and for 2 days after the infusion has been completed.
   b. Alkalinize urine to maintain pH above 7.0 during Methotrexate infusion and leucovorin calcium therapy. This can be accomplished by the administration of sodium bicarbonate orally or by incorporation into a separate intravenous solution.
4. Repeat serum creatinine and serum Methotrexate 24 hours after starting Methotrexate and at least once daily until the Methotrexate level is below 5×10^{-8} mol/L (0.05 micromolar).
5. Table 6 provides guidelines for leucovorin calcium dosage based upon serum Methotrexate levels.
   Patients who experience delayed early Methotrexate elimination are likely to develop non-reversible oliguric renal failure. In addition to appropriate leucovorin therapy, these patients require continuing hydration and urinary alkalinization, and close monitoring of fluid and electrolyte status, until the serum Methotrexate level has fallen to below 0.05 micromolar and the renal failure has resolved. If necessary, acute, intermittent hemodialysis with a high-flux dialyzer may also be beneficial in these patients.
6. Some patients will have abnormalities in Methotrexate elimination, or abnormalities in renal function following Methotrexate administration, which are significant but less severe than the abnormalities described in Table 6. These abnormalities may or may not be associated with significant clinical toxicity. If significant clinical toxicity is observed, leucovorin rescue should be extended for an additional 24 hours (total 14 doses over 84 hours) in subsequent courses of therapy. The possibility that the patient is taking other medications which interact with Methotrexate (e.g., medications which may interfere with Methotrexate binding to serum albumin, or elimination) should always be reconsidered when laboratory abnormalities or clinical toxicities are observed.

Table 6: Methotrexate Injection

Leucovorin Rescue Schedules Following Treatment with Higher Doses of Methotrexate

Clinical Situation	Laboratory Findings	Leucovorin Dosage and Duration
Normal Methotrexate Elimination	Serum Methotrexate level approximately 10 micromolar at 24 hours after administration, 1 micromolar at 48 hours, and less than 0.2 micromolar at 72 hours.	15 mg PO, IM or IV q 6 hours for 60 hours (10 doses starting at 24 hours after start of Methotrexate infusion).
Delayed Late Methotrexate Elimination	Serum Methotrexate level remaining above 0.2 micromolar at 72 hours, and more than 0.05 micromolar at 96 hours after administration.	Continue 15 mg PO, IM or IV q six hours, until Methotrexate level is less than 0.05 micromolar.
Delayed Early Methotrexate Elimination and/or Evidence of Acute Renal Injury	Serum Methotrexate level of 50 micromolar or more at 24 hours, or 5 micromolar or more at 48 hours after administration, OR; a 100% or greater increase in serum creatinine level at 24 hours after Methotrexate administration (e.g., an increase from 0.5 mg/dL to a level of 1 mg/dL or more).	150 mg IV q three hours, until Methotrexate level is less than 1 micromolar; than 15 mg IV q three hours, until Methotrexate level is less than 0.05 micromolar.

Psoriasis and Rheumatoid Arthritis: Dosing Considerations:
- Refer to Neoplastic Diseases, Dosing Considerations
- The patient should be fully informed of the risks involved and should be under constant supervision of the physician (see Warnings and Precautions, Information to Be Provided to the Patient).
- All dosage schedules should be continually tailored to the individual patient. An initial test dose may be given prior to the regular dosing schedule to detect any extreme sensitivity to adverse effects (see Adverse Reactions). Maximal myelosuppression usually occurs in seven to ten days.

Recommended Dose and Dosage Adjustments: Psoriasis: Recommended Starting Dose Schedules
- Weekly single, IM or IV dose schedule: 10 to 25 mg per week until adequate response is achieved.

Dosages in each schedule may be gradually adjusted to achieve optimal clinical response; 30 mg/week should not ordinarily be exceeded.

Once optimal clinical response has been achieved, the dosage schedule should be reduced to the lowest possible amount of drug and to the longest possible rest period. The use of methotrexate may permit the return to conventional topical therapy, which should be encouraged.

Rheumatoid Arthritis: Recommended Starting Dosage Schedules

Therapeutic response usually begins within 3 to 6 weeks and the patient may continue to improve for another 12 weeks or more.

Administration: Dilution: Methotrexate Injection, USP may be diluted with any of the solutions for IV infusion listed below in a concentration range of 0.4 mg/mL to 2 mg/mL. Dilutions should be used within 24 hours if kept at room temperature. Unused solution should be discarded after this time in order to avoid risk of microbial contamination.

Solutions:
- 0.9% Sodium Chloride Injection
- 5% Dextrose Injection
- 4% Dextrose and 0.18% Sodium Chloride Injection
- Ringer's Injection

Since methotrexate is poorly soluble in acid media, use of potassium chloride solution is not advisable.

If a preservative free diluent is used, the solution should be used immediately because of the possibility of microbial growth. It is advisable to protect diluted solutions from light.

Due to the number of brands available, stability data of Methotrexate in plastic syringes and bags are not available.

Unused preservative free products should be discarded due to the possibility of microbial growth.

Dispensing of Pharmacy Bulk Vials: Pharmacy Bulk Vials contain 25 mg/mL Methotrexate (as Methotrexate Sodium) in 20 mL, 40 mL or 100 mL of sterile, **unpreserved**, isotonic solution.

The availability of Pharmacy Bulk Vials is restricted to hospitals with a recognized intravenous admixture program. Methotrexate Injection USP pharmacy bulk vials are packaged in an ONCO-TAIN sleeve to protect from breakage. It is recommended that the vial remains in the carton until time of use. The Methotrexate Injection USP vial should be inspected for damage and visible signs of leaks. If there are signs of breakage or leakage form the vial, do not use. Incinerate the unopened package.

Pharmacy Bulk Vials are intended for multiple dispensing **for intravenous use only** employing a single puncture (see Special Handling Instructions and Disposal of Cytotoxic Drugs).

The Pharmacy Bulk Vial content should be dispensed within eight hours. Any unused solution should be discarded. The diluted solutions prepared from the Pharmacy Bulk vial should be used within 24 hours from the time of the initial puncture of the Pharmacy Bulk Vial, when kept at room temperature.

Pharmacy Bulk Vials contain no preservatives. Care must be taken to minimize the potential for inadvertent introduction of micro organisms during manipulation in the hospital environment.

Incompatibilities: Other drugs should not be mixed with Methotrexate in the same infusion bottle.

Methotrexate has been reported to be incompatible with cytarabine, fluorouracil, and prednisolone sodium phosphate; however, its incompatibility with fluorouracil has been questioned. A mixture of Methotrexate with cytarabine and hydrocortisone sodium succinate in various infusion fluids has been reported to be visually compatible for at least 8 hours at 25°C, although precipitation did not occur on storage for several days.

Contact with acidic solutions should be avoided since Methotrexate is sparingly soluble in acid media and precipitation may occur.

See Warnings and Precautions for clinical incompatibilities.

OVERDOSAGE:

In postmarketing experience, overdose with methotrexate has generally occurred with intrathecal administration, although intravenous and intramuscular overdose have also been reported.

Discontinue or reduce dosage at the first sign of ulceration or bleeding, diarrhea, or marked depression of the hematopoietic system. Leucovorin is indicated to diminish the toxicity and counteract the effect of inadvertently administered overdosages of methotrexate. Leucovorin administration should begin as promptly as possible. As the time interval between methotrexate administration and leucovorin initiation increases, the effectiveness of leucovorin in counteracting toxicity decreases. Monitoring of the serum methotrexate concentration is essential in determining the optimal dose and duration of treatment with leucovorin.

In cases of massive overdosage, hydration and urinary alkalinization may be necessary to prevent the precipitation of methotrexate and/or its metabolites in the renal tubules. Generally, neither standard hemodialysis nor peritoneal dialysis has been shown to improve methotrexate elimination. However, effective clearance of methotrexate has been reported with acute, intermittent hemodialysis using a high-flux dialyzer.

There are published case reports of intravenous carboxypeptidase G2 treatment to hasten clearance of Methotrexate in cases of overdoses.

For management of a suspected drug overdose, contact your regional Poison Control Centre. See the *CPS* Directory section for a list of Poison Control Centres.

ACTION AND CLINICAL PHARMACOLOGY: Mechanism of Action: Methotrexate is a folate antagonist.

Methotrexate inhibits dihydrofolate reductase (DHFR), the enzyme that reduces folic acid to tetrahydrofolic acid. Tetrahydrofolate must be regenerated via the DHFR-catalyzed reaction in order to maintain the intracellular pool of tetrahydrofolate one-carbon derivatives for both thymidylate and purine nucleotide biosynthesis. The inhibition of DHFR by folate antagonists (methotrexate) results in a deficiency in the cellular pools of thymidylate and purines and thus in a decrease in nucleic acid synthesis. Therefore, methotrexate interferes with DNA synthesis, repair, and cellular replication.

Methotrexate is most active against rapidly multiplying cells, because its cytotoxic effects occur primarily during the S phase of the cell cycle. Since cellular proliferation in malignant tissues is greater than in most normal tissues, methotrexate may impair malignant growth without irreversible damage to normal tissues. As a result, actively proliferating tissues, such as malignant cells, bone marrow, fetal cells, buccal and intestinal mucosa, and cells of the urinary bladder, are generally more sensitive to DHFR inhibition effects of methotrexate.

The cytotoxicity of methotrexate results from three important actions: inhibition of DHFR, inhibition of thymidylate synthase, and alteration of the transport of reduced folates. The affinity of DHFR to methotrexate is far greater than its affinity for folic acid or dihydrofolic acid, therefore, large doses of folic acid given simultaneously will not reverse the effects of methotrexate. However, Leucovorin Calcium, a derivative of tetrahydrofolic acid may block the effects of methotrexate if given shortly after the antineoplastic agent. Methotrexate in high doses, followed by leucovorin rescue, is used as a part of the treatment of patients with non-metastatic osteosarcoma.

The original rationale for high dose methotrexate therapy was based on the concept of selective rescue of normal tissues by leucovorin. More recent evidence suggests that high dose methotrexate may also overcome methotrexate resistance caused by impaired active transport, decreased affinity of dihydrofolic acid reductase for methotrexate, increased levels of dihydrofolic acid reductase resulting from gene amplification, or decreased polyglutamination of methotrexate. The actual mechanism of action is unknown.

Methotrexate has immunosuppressive activity. This may be a result of inhibition of lymphocyte multiplication. The mechanisms of action in the management of rheumatoid arthritis of the drug is not known, although suggested mechanisms have included immunosuppressive and/or anti-inflammatory effects.

In psoriasis, the rate of production of epithelial cells in the skin is greatly increased over normal skin. This differential in proliferation rates is the basis for the use of methotrexate to control the psoriatic process.

Pharmacokinetics: Absorption: Orally administered methotrexate is absorbed rapidly in most, but not all patients and reaches peak serum levels in 1 to 4 hours. Methotrexate is generally completely absorbed following parenteral administration, and after intramuscular injection peak serum concentrations occur in 30 to 60 minutes.

Distribution: Methotrexate in serum is approximately 50% protein bound. After intravenous administration, the initial volume of distribution is approximately 0.18 L/kg (18% of body weight) and steady-state volume of distribution is approximately 0.4 to 0.8 L/kg (40% to 80% of body weight). Methotrexate does not penetrate the blood-cerebrospinal fluid barrier in therapeutic amounts when given orally or parenterally.

Metabolism: After absorption, Methotrexate undergoes hepatic and intracellular metabolism to polyglutamated forms which can be converted back to methotrexate by hydrolase enzymes. These polyglutamates act as inhibitors of dihydrofolate reductase and thymidylate syntheses. Small amounts of methotrexate polyglutamates may remain in tissues for extended periods. The retention and prolonged drug action of these active metabolites vary among different cells, tissues and tumours. A small amount of metabolism to 7-hydroxymethotrexate may occur at doses commonly prescribed. The aqueous solubility of 7-hydroxymethotrexate is 3 to 5 fold lower than the parent compound. Methotrexate is partially metabolized by intestinal flora after oral administration.

Excretion: Renal excretion is the primary route of elimination and is dependent upon dosage and route of administration. Excretion of single daily doses occurs through the kidneys in amounts from 80% to 90% within 24 hours. Repeated daily doses result in more sustained serum levels and some retention of methotrexate over each 24-hour period, which may result in accumulation of the drug within the tissues. The liver cells appear to retain certain amounts of the drug for prolonged periods even after a single therapeutic dose. Methotrexate is retained in the presence of impaired renal function and may increase rapidly in the serum and in the tissue cells under such conditions. Methotrexate does not penetrate the blood-cerebrospinal fluid barrier in therapeutic amounts when given orally or parenterally. High concentrations of the drug, when needed, may be attained by direct intrathecal administration.

The terminal half-life reported for methotrexate is approximately 3 to 10 hours for patients receiving treatment for psoriasis, rheumatoid arthritis or low dose antineoplastic therapy (less than 30 mg/m^2). For patients receiving high doses of methotrexate, the terminal half-life is 8 to 15 hours.

Methotrexate clearance rates vary widely and are generally decreased at higher doses.

Special Populations and Conditions: Nursing Women: Methotrexate has been detected in human breast milk and is contraindicated during breast feeding. The highest breast milk to plasma concentration ratio reached was 0.08: 1.

STORAGE AND STABILITY: Keep in a safe place out of the reach of children.

Store Methotrexate Injection, USP vials between 15-25°C. Protect from light.

Multidose vials (50 mg/2 mL and 500 mg/20 mL) Methotrexate with benzyl alcohol) should be stored at 2-8 °C after the vials are punctured for a maximum of four weeks (30 days). Protect from light. Aseptic techniques should be used when handling punctured vials to avoid contamination.

Methotrexate Injection USP vials are packaged in an ONCO-TAIN sleeve to protect form breakage. It is recommended that the vial remains in the carton until time of use. The Methotrexate Injection USP vial should be inspected for damage and visible signs of leaks. If there are signs of breakage or leakage form the vial, do not use. Incinerate the unopened package.

SPECIAL HANDLING INSTRUCTIONS: General: Individuals who have contact with anti-cancer drugs or work in areas where these drugs are used, may be exposed to these agents in air or through direct contact with contaminated objects. Potential health effects may be reduced by adherence to institutional procedures, published guidelines and local regulations for preparation, administration, transportation and disposal of hazardous drugs.

Safe Handling and Disposal: Methotrexate is a potent antineoplastic drug. Good medical practice will minimize exposure of persons involved with frequent handling of this drug as outlined below:

Handling:
1. Methotrexate has no vesicant properties and does not show acute toxicity on topical contact with the skin or mucous membranes. However, persons involved with handling cytotoxic drugs should avoid contact with skin and inhalation of airborne particles.
2. Preparation of antineoplastic solutions should be done in a vertical laminar flow hood (Biological Safety Cabinet - Class II).
3. Personnel preparing Methotrexate solutions should wear PVC gloves, safety glasses and protective clothing such as disposable gowns and masks.
4. Personnel regularly involved in preparation and handling of antineoplastics should have bi-annual blood examinations.

Disposal:
1. Avoid contact with skin and inhalation of airborne particles by use of PVC gloves and disposable gowns and masks.
2. All needles, syringes, vials and other materials for disposal which have come in contact with Methotrexate should be segregated in plastic bags, sealed and marked as hazardous waste. Incinerate at 1000°C or higher. Sealed containers may explode if a tight seal exists.
3. If incineration is not available, rinse all needles, syringes, tubing and other materials for disposal which have come in contact with Methotrexate solutions with water and discard in the sewer system with running water.

Rinse vials with the appropriate quantity of water with the aid of a hypodermic syringe. Withdraw the solution and discard in the sewer system with running water. Dispose of rinsed equipment and vials in a safe manner.

Cleaning: Non-disposable equipment that has come in contact with methotrexate may be rinsed with water and washed thoroughly with soap and water.

Spillage/Contamination: Wear gloves, mask and protective clothing. Place spilled material in an appropriate container (i.e. cardboard for broken glass) and then in a polyethylene bag; absorb remains with gauze pads or towels; wash area with water and absorb with gauze or towels again and place in bag; seal, double bag and mark as a hazardous waste. Dispose of waste by incineration or by other methods approved for hazardous materials. Personnel involved in clean up should wash with soap and water.

INFORMATION FOR THE PATIENT: Published in e-CPS, available by subscription at www.e-cps.ca.

DOSAGE FORMS, COMPOSITION AND PACKAGING: Supplied: 10 mg/mL: Each mL of sterile aqueous isotonic solution contains: methotrexate (as the sodium salt) 10 mg. Nonmedicinal ingredients: sodium chloride 7 mg and sodium hydroxide 2 mg. May contain hydrochloric acid or sodium hydroxide as pH adjusters. Preservative-free. Single use vials of 2 mL, cartons of 5.

25 mg/mL (with preservative): Each mL of sterile aqueous isotonic solution contains: methotrexate (as the sodium salt) 25 mg. Nonmedicinal ingredients: 0.9% v/v benzyl alcohol (as preservative), sodium chloride 2.6 mg. May contain hydrochloric acid or sodium hydroxide as pH adjusters. Single use vials of 2 mL, cartons of 5. Pharmacy bulk vials of 20 mL, cartons of 1.

25 mg/mL (without preservative): Each mL of sterile aqueous isotonic solution contains: methotrexate (as the sodium salt) 25 mg. Nonmedicinal ingredients: sodium chloride 4.9 mg and sodium hydroxide 4.67 mg. May contain hydrochloric acid or sodium hydroxide as pH adjusters. Preservative-free. Single use vials of 2 mL, cartons of 5. Pharmacy bulk vials of 20, 40 and 100 mL, cartons of 1.

Methotrexate Tablets USP ℞

methotrexate sodium

Antimetabolite—Antirheumatic Agent

Hospira

Date of Revision: July 4, 2007

SUMMARY PRODUCT INFORMATION:

Route of Administration	Dosage Form/ Strength	Clinically Relevant Nonmedicinal Ingredients
Oral	Tablet 10 mg	Lactose For a complete listing see Dosage Forms, Composition and Packaging.

INDICATIONS AND CLINICAL USE: Methotrexate Tablets USP is indicated for:

1. Treatment of neoplastic diseases
2. Use as Disease Modifying Antirheumatic Drug (DMARD)

Neoplastic Diseases:

- Choriocarcinoma: methotrexate—as single chemotherapy or in combination with other drugs.
- Intermediate-, or high grade Non Hodgkin's Lymphoma as part of ProMACE-CytaBOM, ProMACE-MOPP, and Magrath protocols.
- Breast cancer: as part of CMF (cyclophosphamide-methotrexate-fluorouracil) therapy.
- Acute Lymphoblastic Leukemia (ALL)—as maintenance therapy.
- Head and neck cancer—in combination with other chemotherapies.
- Gastric cancer—palliative combination chemotherapy.
- Metastasis of unknown primary—as palliative combination chemotherapy.
- Bladder cancer (advanced)—as part of M-VAC regimen.
- Burkitt's lymphoma.
- Advanced stages of childhood lymphoma (III and IV, St. Jude's Childrens' Research Hospital Staging System).
- Advanced cases of mycosis fungoids (cutaneous T-cell lymphoma).

Disease Modifying Antirheumatic Drug (DMARD): The use of methotrexate as a DMARD in the following diseases where standard therapeutic interventions fail:

- severe disabling psoriasis/psoriatic arthritis
- severe disabling rheumatoid arthritis (RA)
- severe disabling seronegative arthritides

In the treatment of psoriasis, methotrexate should be restricted to severe recalcitrant, disabling psoriasis, which is not adequately responsive to other forms of therapy, but only when the diagnosis has been established after dermatologic consultation.

Geriatrics: The clinical pharmacology of methotrexate has not been well studied in older individuals. Due to diminished hepatic and renal function, as well as decreased folate stores in this population, relatively low doses should be considered, and these patients should be closely monitored for early signs of toxicity.

Pediatrics: Safety and effectiveness in pediatric patients have not been established, other than in cancer chemotherapy.

CONTRAINDICATIONS: Patients who are hypersensitive to this drug or to any ingredient in the formulation or component of the container. For a complete listing, see Dosage Forms, Composition and Packaging.

In pregnancy, methotrexate can cause fetal death, embryotoxicity, abortion or teratogenic effects when administered to a pregnant woman. Methotrexate is contraindicated in pregnant patients with psoriasis or rheumatoid arthritis and should be used in the treatment of neoplastic diseases only when the potential benefit outweighs the risk to the fetus.

Women of childbearing potential should not be started on methotrexate until pregnancy is excluded and should be fully counselled on the serious risk to the fetus should they become pregnant while undergoing treatment. Pregnancy should be avoided if either partner is receiving methotrexate. The optimal time interval between the cessation of methotrexate treatment of either partner and pregnancy has not been clearly established. Published literature recommendations for time intervals vary from 3 months to one year (see Warnings and Precautions).

Because of the potential for serious adverse reactions in breast fed infants, it is contraindicated in nursing mothers.

Methotrexate is contraindicated in patients with psoriasis or rheumatoid arthritis in the following situations:

- Alcoholism, alcoholic liver disease or other chronic liver disease.
- Overt or laboratory evidence of immunodeficiency syndromes.
- Pre-existing blood dyscrasias, such as bone marrow hypoplasia, leucopenia, thrombocytopenia or significant anemia.

WARNINGS AND PRECAUTIONS:

> **Serious Warnings and Precautions**
>
> - Because of the possibility of serious toxic reactions (which can be fatal), methotrexate should be used only in life-threatening neoplastic diseases, or in patients with psoriasis or rheumatoid arthritis with severe, recalcitrant, disabling disease that is not adequately responsive to other forms of therapy. Deaths have been reported with the use of methotrexate in the treatment of malignancy, psoriasis and rheumatoid arthritis.
> - Methotrexate should be used only by physicians whose knowledge and experience includes the use of antimetabolite therapy.
> - Because of the possibility of serious toxic reactions, the patient should be informed by the physician of the risks involved and should be under a physician's constant supervision.
> - Use in pregnancy: Methotrexate has been reported to cause fetal death and/or congenital anomalies. Therefore, it is not recommended for the treatment of diseases in women of childbearing potential, unless there is clear medical evidence that the benefits can be expected to outweigh the considered risks. Pregnant patients with psoriasis or rheumatoid arthritis should not receive methotrexate (see Contraindications).

General: Methotrexate has the potential for serious toxicity. Toxic effects may be related in frequency and severity to dose or frequency of administration but have been seen at all doses. Because they can occur at any time during therapy, it is necessary to follow patients on methotrexate closely. Most adverse reactions are reversible if detected early. When such reactions do occur, the drug should be reduced in dosage or discontinued and appropriate corrective measures should be taken. If necessary, this could include the use of leucovorin calcium and/or acute, intermittent hemodialysis with a high-flux dialyzer (see Overdosage). If methotrexate therapy is re-instituted, it should be carried out with caution, with adequate consideration of further need for the drug and with increased alertness as to possible recurrence of toxicity.

Methotrexate exits slowly from third space compartments (e.g., pleural effusions or ascites). This results in a prolonged terminal plasma half-life and unexpected toxicity. In patients with significant third space accumulations, it is advisable to evacuate the fluid before treatment and to monitor plasma methotrexate levels.

Unexpectedly severe (sometimes fatal) bone marrow suppression, aplastic anemia and gastrointestinal toxicity have been reported with concomitant administration of methotrexate (usually in high dosage) along with some nonsteroidal anti-inflammatory drugs (NSAIDs) (see Drug Interactions).

Bone marrow and mucosal toxicity of methotrexate depend on: dose and duration of exposure of high levels (>2×10^{-8} mol/L (0.02 micromolar)) of methotrexate. Since the critical time factor has been defined for these organs as being 42 hours in humans, this has the following implications:

- when drug levels exceeding (2×10^{-8} mol/L (0.02 micromolar)) the above for >42 hours may forecast significant toxicity;
- when toxicity can be minimized by appropriate administration of Leucovorin Calcium;

Methotrexate given concomitantly with radiotherapy may increase the risk of soft tissue necrosis and osteonecrosis.

Methotrexate should be used with extreme caution in the presence of debility.

Carcinogenesis and Mutagenesis: Malignant lymphomas, which may regress following withdrawal of methotrexate, may occur in patients receiving low-dose methotrexate and, thus, may not require cytotoxic treatment. Discontinue methotrexate first and, if the lymphoma does not regress, appropriate treatment should be instituted.

Like other cytotoxic drugs, methotrexate may induce "tumour lysis syndrome" in patients with rapidly growing tumours. Appropriate supportive and pharmacologic measures may prevent or alleviate this complication.

No controlled human data exist regarding the risk of neoplasia with methotrexate. Methotrexate has been evaluated in a number of animal studies for carcinogenic potential with inconclusive results. Although there is evidence that methotrexate causes chromosomal damage to animal somatic cells and human bone marrow cells, the clinical significance remains uncertain. Assessment of the carcinogenic potential of methotrexate is complicated by conflicting evidence of an increased risk of certain tumors in rheumatoid arthritis. Benefit should be weighed against this potential risk before using methotrexate alone or in combination with other drugs, especially in children or young adults.

Gastrointestinal: If vomiting, diarrhea, or stomatitis occurs, resulting in dehydration, methotrexate should be discontinued until recovery occurs. Diarrhea and ulcerative stomatitis require interruption of therapy; otherwise, hemorrhagic enteritis and death from intestinal perforation may occur. Methotrexate should be used with extreme caution in the presence of peptic ulcer disease or ulcerative colitis.

Hematologic: Methotrexate should be used with caution in patients with impaired bone marrow function and previous or concomitant wide field radiotherapy. Methotrexate may produce marked bone marrow depression with resultant anemia, aplastic anemia, pancytopenia, leucopenia neutropenia and/or thrombocytopenia. In patients with malignancy and pre-existing hematopoietic impairment, the drug should be used with caution, if at all. In controlled clinical trials in rheumatoid arthritis (n=128), leucopenia (WBC <3000/mm^3) was seen in 2 patients, thrombocytopenia (platelets <1 000 000/mm^3) in 6 patients, and pancytopenia in 2 patients.

In psoriasis and rheumatoid arthritis, Methotrexate should be stopped immediately if there is a significant drop in blood counts. In the treatment of neoplastic diseases, Methotrexate should be continued only if the potential benefit warrants the risk of severe myelosuppression. Patients with profound granulocytopenia and fever should be evaluated immediately and usually require parenteral broad-spectrum antibiotic therapy.

Hepatic/Biliary/Pancreatic: Methotrexate has the potential for acute and chronic hepatotoxicity. Acutely, liver enzyme elevations are frequently seen after Methotrexate administration and are usually not a reason for modification of Methotrexate therapy. Liver enzyme elevations are usually transient and asymptomatic, and also do not appear predictive of subsequent hepatic disease. Persistent liver abnormalities, and/or decrease of serum albumin may be indicators of serious liver toxicity. Chronic toxicity is potentially fatal; it generally has occurred after prolonged use (generally two years or more) and after a total cumulative dose of at least 1.5 g. Liver biopsy after sustained use often shows histologic changes, and fibrosis and cirrhosis have been reported; these latter lesions may not be preceded by symptoms or abnormal liver function tests in the psoriasis population. Periodic liver biopsies are usually recommended for psoriatic patients who are under long-term treatment. Persistent abnormalities in liver function tests may precede appearance of fibrosis or cirrhosis in the rheumatoid arthritis population. In studies in psoriatic patients, hepatotoxicity appeared to be a function of total cumulative dose and appeared to be enhanced by alcoholism, obesity, diabetes and advanced age. An accurate incidence rate has not been determined; the rate of progression and reversibility of lesions is not known. Special caution is indicated in the presence of pre-existing liver damage or impaired hepatic function.

In psoriasis, liver damage and function tests, including serum albumin and prothrombin time, should be performed several times prior to dosing, but are often normal in the face of developing fibrosis or cirrhosis. These lesions may be detectable only by biopsy.

The usual recommendation is to obtain a liver biopsy: 1) before the start of therapy or shortly after initiation of therapy (4-8 weeks); 2) after a total cumulative dose of 1.5 g; and 3) after each additional 1.0 to 1.5 g. Moderate fibrosis or any cirrhosis normally leads to discontinuation of the drug; mild fibrosis normally suggests a repeat biopsy in 6 months. Milder histologic findings such as fatty change and low grade portal inflammation are relatively common pre-therapy. Although these mild changes are usually not a reason to avoid or discontinue methotrexate therapy, the drug should be used with caution.

Clinical experience with liver disease in rheumatoid arthritis is limited, but the same risk factors would be anticipated. Liver function tests are also usually not reliable predictors of histological changes in this population.

In rheumatoid arthritis, advanced age at first use of methotrexate and increasing duration of therapy have been reported as risk factors for hepatotoxicity. Persistent abnormalities in liver function tests may precede appearance of fibrosis or cirrhosis in the rheumatoid population.

Liver function tests should be performed at baseline and at 4-8 week intervals in patients receiving methotrexate for rheumatoid arthritis. Pretreatment liver biopsy should be performed for patients with a history of excessive alcohol consumption, persistently abnormal baseline liver function test values, or chronic hepatitis B or C infection. During therapy, liver biopsy should be performed if there are persistent liver function test abnormalities, or there is a decrease in serum albumin below the normal range (in the setting of well controlled rheumatoid arthritis).

If the results of a liver biopsy show mild changes (Roenigk grades I, II, IIIa), methotrexate may be continued and the patient monitored according to the recommendations listed above. Methotrexate should be discontinued in any patient who displays persistently abnormal liver function tests and refuses liver biopsy, or in any patient whose liver biopsy shows moderate to severe changes (Roenigk grade IIIb or IV).

There is a combined reported experience in 217 rheumatoid arthritis patients with liver biopsies both before and during treatment (after a cumulative dose of at least 1500 mg) and in 714 patients with a biopsy only during treatment. There are 64 (7%) cases of fibrosis and 1 (0.1%) case of cirrhosis. Of the 64 cases of fibrosis, 60 were deemed mild. The reticulin stain is more sensitive for early fibrosis and its use may increase these figures. It is unknown whether even longer use will increase these risks.

Immune: Methotrexate should be used with extreme caution in the presence of active infection, and is usually contraindicated in patients with overt or laboratory evidence of immunodeficiency syndromes.

Immunization may be ineffective when given during methotrexate therapy. Immunization with live virus vaccines is generally not recommended. There have been reports of disseminated vaccinia infections after smallpox immunization in patients receiving methotrexate therapy. Hypogammaglobulinemia has been reported rarely.

Information to Be Provided to the Patient: Patients should be informed of the early signs and symptoms of toxicity, of the need to see their physician promptly if they occur, and the need for close follow-up, including periodic laboratory tests to monitor toxicity.

Both the physician and pharmacist should emphasize to the patient that the recommended dose is taken weekly in rheumatoid arthritis and psoriasis, and that mistaken daily use of the recommended dose has led to fatal toxicity.

Patients should be informed of the potential benefit and risk in the use of Methotrexate. The risk of effects on reproduction should be discussed with both male and female patients taking Methotrexate.

Neurologic: Chronic leukoencephalopathy has also been reported in patients with osteosarcoma who received repeated doses of high-dose methotrexate with leucovorin rescue even without cranial irradiation. Discontinuation of methotrexate does not always result in complete recovery.

A transient acute neurologic syndrome has been observed in patients treated with high dosage regimens. Manifestations of this neurologic disorder may include behavioural abnormalities, focal sensorimotor signs, including transient blindness and abnormal reflexes. The exact cause is unknown.

Renal: Methotrexate therapy in patients with impaired renal function should be undertaken with extreme caution, and at reduced dosages, because renal dysfunction will prolong methotrexate elimination. Methotrexate may cause renal damage that may lead to acute renal failure. Nephrotoxicity is due primarily to the precipitation of methotrexate and 7-hydroxymethotrexate in the renal tubules. Close attention to renal function including adequate hydration, urine alkalinization and measurement of serum methotrexate and creatinine levels are essential for safe administration.

Respiratory: Methotrexate-induced lung disease, including acute or chronic interstitial pneumonitis is a potentially dangerous lesion, which may occur at any time during therapy and which has been reported at low doses. It is not always fully reversible and fatalities have been reported. Pulmonary symptoms (especially a dry non-productive cough) or a non-specific pneumonitis occurring during methotrexate therapy may be indicative of a potentially dangerous lesion and require interruption of treatment and careful investigation. Although clinically variable, the typical patient with methotrexate-induced lung disease presents with fever, cough, dyspnea, hypoxemia, and an infiltrate on chest X-ray; infection (including pneumonia) needs to be excluded. This lesion can occur at all dosages.

Pneumonia (in some cases leading to respiratory failure) may occur. Potentially fatal opportunistic infections, especially *P. carinii* pneumonia, may occur with methotrexate therapy. When a patient presents with pulmonary symptoms, the possibility of *P. carinii* should be considered.

Sexual Function/Reproduction: Methotrexate causes embryotoxicity, abortion, and fetal defects in humans. It has also been reported to cause impairment of fertility, oligospermia and menstrual dysfunction in humans, during and for a short period after cessation of therapy.

Skin: Severe, occasionally fatal, dermatologic reactions, including toxic epidermal necrolysis (Lyell's Syndrome), Stevens-Johnson syndrome, exfoliative dermatitis, skin necrosis and erythema multiforme have been reported in children and adults within days of oral methotrexate administration. Reactions were noted after single or multiple, low, intermediate or high doses of methotrexate in patients with neoplastic and non-neoplastic diseases. Recovery has been reported with discontinuation of therapy.

Lesions of psoriasis may be aggravated by concomitant exposure to ultraviolet radiation. Radiation dermatitis and sunburn may be "recalled" by the use of methotrexate.

Special Populations: Pregnant Women: Methotrexate can cause fetal death, embryotoxicity, abortion, or teratogenic effects when administered to a pregnant woman. Methotrexate is contraindicated in pregnant patients with psoriasis or rheumatoid arthritis and should be used in the treatment of neoplastic diseases only when the potential benefit outweighs the risk to the fetus.

Women of childbearing potential should not be started on methotrexate until pregnancy is excluded and should be fully counselled on the serious risk to the fetus should they become pregnant while undergoing treatment. Pregnancy should be avoided if either partner is receiving methotrexate. The optimal time interval between the cessation of methotrexate treatment of either partner and pregnancy has not been clearly established. Published literature recommendations for time intervals vary from 3 months to one year.

Nursing Women: Because of the potential for serious adverse reactions from methotrexate in breast fed infants, Methotrexate is contraindicated in nursing mothers.

Pediatrics: Safety and effectiveness in pediatric patients have not been established, other than in cancer chemotherapy.

Geriatrics: The clinical pharmacology of methotrexate has not been well studied in older individuals. Due to diminished hepatic and renal function, as well as decreased folate stores in this population, relatively low doses should be considered, and these patients should be closely monitored for early signs of toxicity.

Monitoring and Laboratory Tests: General: Patients undergoing methotrexate therapy should be closely monitored so that toxic effects are detected promptly. Baseline assessment should include a complete blood count (CBC) with differential and platelet counts, hepatic enzymes, renal function tests, and a chest X-ray. During therapy of rheumatoid arthritis and psoriasis, monitoring of these parameters is recommended: hematology at least monthly, and hepatic enzyme levels and renal function every 1 to 2 months. More frequent monitoring is usually indicated during antineoplastic therapy. During initial or changing doses, or during periods of increased risk of elevated methotrexate blood levels (e.g., dehydration), more frequent monitoring may also be indicated.

Liver: Liver biopsies prior to Methotrexate therapy are not indicated routinely. Liver function tests (LFTs) should be determined prior to the initiation of therapy with Methotrexate and they should be monitored regularly throughout therapy. A relationship between abnormal liver function tests and fibrosis or cirrhosis of the liver has not been established. Transient liver function test abnormalities are observed frequently after methotrexate administration and are usually not cause for modification of methotrexate therapy. Persistent liver function test abnormalities just prior to dosing and/or depression of serum albumin may be indicators of serious liver toxicity and require evaluation.

Respiratory: Pulmonary function tests may be useful if methotrexate-induced lung disease is suspected, especially if baseline measurements are available.

Serum Level Monitoring: Serum methotrexate level monitoring can significantly reduce methotrexate toxicity and mortality.

Patients subject to the following conditions are predisposed to developing elevated or prolonged methotrexate levels and benefit from routine monitoring of levels: eg, pleural effusion, ascites, gastrointestinal tract obstruction, previous cisplatin therapy, dehydration, aciduria, impaired renal function.

Some patients may have delayed methotrexate clearance in the absence of these features. It is important that patients be identified within 48 hours since methotrexate toxicity may not be reversible if adequate leucovorin rescue is delayed for more than 42 to 48 hours.

The method of monitoring methotrexate concentrations varies from institution to institution. Monitoring of methotrexate concentrations should include determination of a methotrexate level at 24, 48, or 72 hours, and assessment of the rate of decline in methotrexate concentrations (to determine how long to continue leucovorin rescue).

ADVERSE REACTIONS: Adverse Drug Reaction Overview: In general, the incidence and severity of acute side effects are related to dose, frequency of administration, and the duration of the exposure to significant blood levels of methotrexate to the target organs. The most serious reactions are discussed in Warnings and Precautions. That section should also be consulted when looking for information about adverse reactions with methotrexate.

- Some of the effects mentioned in this section, such as dizziness and fatigue, may affect the ability to drive or operate machinery.
- The most frequently reported adverse reactions include ulcerative stomatitis, leucopenia, nausea, and abdominal distress. Other frequently reported adverse effects are malaise, undue fatigue, chills and fever, dizziness and decreased resistance to infection.

Adverse Drug Reactions by Organ System: Adverse reactions that have been reported with methotrexate are listed below alphabetically by organ system. In the oncology setting, concomitant treatment and the underlying disease make specific attribution of a reaction to methotrexate difficult.

Alimentary System: gingivitis, stomatitis, enteritis, anorexia, nausea, vomiting, diarrhea, hematemesis, melena, gastrointestinal ulceration and bleeding, pancreatitis.

Cardiovascular: pericarditis, pericardial effusion, hypotension, and thromboembolic events (including arterial thrombosis, cerebral thrombosis, deep vein thrombosis, retinal vein thrombosis, thrombophlebitis, and pulmonary embolus).

Central Nervous System: headaches, dizziness, drowsiness, speech impediment including dysarthria and aphasia; hemiparesis, paresis and convulsions have also occurred following administration of methotrexate. Following low doses, there have been occasional reports of transient subtle cognitive dysfunction, mood alteration, or unusual cranial sensations, leucoencephalopathy, or encephalopathy.

Eye Disorders: conjunctivitis, blurred vision, serious visual changes of unknown etiology, and transient blindness/vision loss.

Hematopoietic: Methotrexate can suppress hematopoiesis and cause anemia, leucopenia, and/or thrombocytopenia. Hypogammaglobulinemia has been reported rarely (see Warnings and Precautions, Immune). Lymphadenopathy and lymphoproliferative disorders (including reversible), pancytopenia, neutropenia and agranulocytosis and eosinophilia have also been observed.

Hepatobiliary Disorders: hepatoxocity, acute hepatitis, chronic fibrosis and cirrhosis, decrease in serum albumin, liver enzyme elevations, hepatic failure.

Infection: There have been case reports of sometimes fatal sepsis, sepsis, opportunistic infections, including fatal infections in patients receiving methotrexate therapy for neoplastic and non-neoplastic diseases. *P. carinii* pneumonia was the most common infection. Other reported infections included pneumonia, nocardiosis, histoplasmosis, cryptococcosis, H. zoster, H. simplex hepatitis and disseminated H. simplex and cytomegaloviral infection, including cytomegaloviral pneumonia.

Musculoskeletal, Connective Tissue, and Bone Disorders: stress fractures.

Pulmonary System: Respiratory fibrosis, pharyngitis and interstitial pneumonitis deaths have been reported; chronic interstitial obstructive pulmonary disease and alveolitis have occasionally occurred.

Skin: erythematous rashes, pruritus, urticaria, photosensitivity, pigmentary changes, alopecia, ecchymosis, telangiectasia, acne, furunculosis, erythema multiforme, toxic epidermal necrolysis (Lyell's Syndrome), Stevens-Johnson Syndrome, skin necrosis, exfoliative dermatitis, and painful erosion of psoriatic plaques.

Urogenital System: severe nephropathy or renal failure, azotemia, dysuria, cystitis, hematuria; defective oogenesis or spermatogenesis, transient oligospermia, menstrual dysfunction, vaginal discharge and gynecomastia; infertility, abortion, fetal defects, loss of libido/impotence. Proteinuria has also been observed.

Rarer Reactions: Related to or attributed to the use of methotrexate such as nodulosis, vasculitis, H. zoster, sepsis, arthralgia/myalgia, diabetes, osteoporosis, sudden death, lymphoma, reversible lymphomas, tumor lysis syndrome, soft tissue necrosis, aplastic anemia, fetal death and osteonecrosis. A few cases of anaphylactoid reactions have been reported.

Malignant lymphomas, which may regress following withdrawal of methotrexate, may occur in patients receiving low-dose methotrexate, and thus may not require cytotoxic treatment. Discontinue methotrexate first and if the lymphoma does not regress, appropriate treatment should be instituted.

Other Adverse Drug Reactions: Adverse Reactions Reported in Rheumatoid Arthritis: Incidence greater than 10%: elevated liver enzymes 15%, nausea/vomiting 10%.

Incidence 3% to 10%: stomatitis, thrombocytopenia.

Incidence 1% to 3%: rash/pruritus/dermatitis, alopecia, diarrhea, dizziness, leucopenia and pancytopenia.

Adverse Reactions in Psoriasis: The adverse reaction rates reported are very similar to those in the rheumatoid arthritis studies. Rarely, painful psoriatic plaque erosions may appear.

Abnormal Hematologic and Clinical Chemistry Findings: Abnormal hematologic and clinical chemistry findings are discussed in Warnings and Precautions, Monitoring and Laboratory Tests.

DRUG INTERACTIONS: Drug-Drug Interactions: The drugs listed below are based on either drug interaction case reports or studies, or potential interactions due to the expected magnitude and seriousness of the interaction (i.e., those identified as contraindicated).

Nonsteroidal Anti-inflammatory Drugs (NSAIDs): Caution should be used when NSAIDs and salicylates are administered concomitantly with lower doses of methotrexate. These drugs have been reported to reduce the tubular secretion of methotrexate in an animal model, and may enhance its toxicity by increasing methotrexate levels.

In treating rheumatoid arthritis with methotrexate, acetylsalicylic acid (ASA), NSAIDs, and/or low dose steroids may be continued.

The possibility of increased toxicity with concomitant use of NSAIDs including salicylates has not been fully explored. Steroids may be reduced gradually in patients who respond to methotrexate. Combined use of methotrexate with gold, penicillamine, hydroxychloroquine, sulfasalazine, or cytotoxic agents has not been studied and may increase the incidence of adverse effects.

Despite the potential interactions, studies of methotrexate in patients with rheumatoid arthritis have usually included concurrent use of constant dosage regimens of NSAIDs without apparent problems. It should be appreciated however, that the doses used in rheumatoid arthritis (7.5 to 15 mg/week) are somewhat lower than those used in psoriasis and that larger doses could lead to unexpected toxicity.

Leflunomide: Methotrexate in combination with leflunomide may increase the risk of pancytopenia.

Drugs Highly Bound to Plasma Proteins: Methotrexate is partially bound to serum albumin, and toxicity may be increased because of displacement by certain drugs, such as salicylates, phenylbutazone, phenytoin and sulfonamides.

Probenecid: Renal tubular transport is also diminished by probenecid; use of methotrexate with this drug should be carefully monitored.

Nephrotoxic Drugs: Although not documented, other nephrotoxic drugs such as aminoglycosides, amphotericin B and cyclosporin could theoretically increase methotrexate toxicity by decreasing its elimination.

Penicillins and Sulfonamides: Penicillins and sulfonamides may reduce the renal clearance of Methotrexate; hematologic and gastrointestinal toxicity have been observed in combination with Methotrexate.

Oral Antibiotics: Oral antibiotics such as tetracycline, chloramphenicol, and non-absorbable broad spectrum antibiotics, may decrease intestinal absorption of methotrexate or interfere with the enterohepatic circulation by inhibiting bowel flora and suppressing metabolism of the drug by bacteria. For example: neomycin, polymyxin B, nystatin and vancomycin decrease methotrexate absorption, whereas kanamycin increases methotrexate absorption.

Trimethoprim/sulfamethoxazole has been reported rarely to increase bone marrow suppression in patients receiving methotrexate, probably by decreased tubular secretion and/or an additive antifolate effect.

Theophylline: Methotrexate may decrease the clearance of theophylline; theophylline levels should be monitored when used concurrently with Methotrexate.

Mercaptopurine: Methotrexate increases the plasma levels of mercaptopurine. Combination of methotrexate and mercaptopurine may therefore require dose adjustment.

Vitamins: Vitamin preparations containing folic acid or its derivatives may decrease responses to systemically administered methotrexate. Preliminary animal and human studies have shown that small quantities of intravenously administered leucovorin enter the cerebrospinal fluid (CSF) primarily as 5-methyl tetrahydrofolate and, in humans, remain 1-3 orders of magnitude lower than the usual methotrexate concentrations following intrathecal administration.

In patients with rheumatoid arthritis or psoriasis, folic acid or folinic acid may reduce methotrexate toxicities such as gastrointestinal symptoms, stomatitis, alopecia and elevated liver enzymes.

Before taking a folate supplement, it is advisable to check B_{12} levels, particularly in adults over the age of 50, since folate administration can mask symptoms of B_{12} deficiency.

Folate deficiency states may increase methotrexate toxicity.

Radiotherapy: Methotrexate given concomitantly with radiotherapy may increase the risk of soft tissue necrosis and osteonecrosis.

Hepatoxins: The potential for increased hepatotoxicity when methotrexate is administered with other hepatotoxic agents has not been evaluated. However, hepatotoxicity has been reported in such cases. Therefore, patients receiving concomitant therapy with methotrexate and other potential hepatotoxic agents (e.g., leflunomide, azathioprine, sulfasalazine, retinoids) should be closely monitored for possible increased risk of hepatotoxicity.

Drug-Food Interactions: The bioavailability of orally administered methotrexate is reduced by food, particularly milk products.

DOSAGE AND ADMINISTRATION: Neoplastic Diseases: Dosing Considerations:

- Oral administration in tablet form is often preferred when low doses are being administered since absorption is rapid and effective serum levels are obtained.
- Methotrexate may only be administered by physicians experienced in the treatment of neoplasia. The oncologist should consult the current literature for the treatment regimen to be used. Typical dosages reported in the literature for the following malignancies are listed in the following section.

Recommended Dose and Dosage Adjustment: Breast Cancer: The initial doses of CMF will be cyclophosphamide 100 mg/m² p.o. days 1 through 14, Methotrexate 40 mg/m² IV day 1, 8, and 5-Fluorouracil 600 mg/m² IV day 1, 8. Cycle length will be 28 days ("2 weeks-on, 2 weeks-off"). In patients over 60 years of age, the dosage of Methotrexate will be 30 mg/m² IV day 1, 8.

If total bilirubin exceeds 1.5 mg/dL, decrease the dose of Methotrexate only by 50%.

Bladder Cancer: Typical dosage regimens for bladder cancer are the CMV Regimen and the "M-VAC Regimen" which are represented in Table 1 and Table 2.

Table 1: Methotrexate Tablets USP

CMV Regimen[a]

	Days		
Drugs[b]	**1**	**2**	**8[e]**
Cisplatin[c]		100	
Vinblastine	4		4
Methotrexate[d]	30		30

[a] All doses in mg/m² with cycles repeated on day 22.
[b] Patients >70 years old receive 80% of all doses; if vomiting persists to day 8, no drug is given.
[c] For each cycle adjust cisplatin to 100% for C_{cr} >60 mL/min; 50% of dose for C_{cr} 50–60 mL/min; none for C_{cr} <50 mL/min.
[d] No drug for a decrease on day 8 of >30 mL/min compared to day 1 or C_{cr} <50 mL/min or C_r >1.8 mg/dL.
[e] Major dose modifications for both drugs depending on myelosuppression.

Table 2: Methotrexate Tablets USP

M-VAC Regimen[a]

	Days			
Drugs	**1**	**2**	**15**	**22[c]**
Methotrexate	30		30	30
Vinblastine		3	3	3
Doxorubicin		30[b]		
Cisplatin		70		

[a] All doses in mg/m² with cycles repeated every 28-32 days.
[b] Patients having prior pelvic irradiation equivalent to >2500 rad in 5 days, reduce the dose of doxorubicin 15 mg/m².
[c] No doses given when the WBC <2500 cells/mm³, platelets >100 000 cells/mm³, or mucositis present.

Head and Neck Cancer: Methotrexate remains the standard of therapy for patients with recurrent or metastatic disease. It has been given in a wide variety of doses and schedules (a few of which are represented in Table 3).

Table 3: Methotrexate Tablets USP

Methotrexate Schedule[a]

0.8 mg/kg every 4 days IV
25–50 mg every 4 to 7 days
60 mg/m² weekly IV or 40 mg/m² biweekly IV
40–60 mg/m² weekly IV
80 mg/m² for 30 h every 2 wk with escalation to toxicity
40 mg/m² weekly IV
40–200 mg/m² IV on days 1, 4 weekly; Leucovorin on days 2,5
60 mg/m² IV weekly

[a] Excerpt from Devita, et al: Cancer 3rd ed., p. 496.

For palliation of patients with advanced incurable disease and acceptable renal function, it is appropriate to begin oral or intravenous methotrexate with weekly doses of 40-50 mg/m² or biweekly doses of 15 to 20 mg/m² and escalate the dose in weekly increments until either mild toxicity or therapeutic response is achieved.

Gastric Cancer: A regimen used in a clinical trial in Belgium in patients with resectable gastric cancer follows: methotrexate (1.5 g/m² IV day 1, + 5-Fluorouracil (1.5 g/m² IV) + Leucovorin (15 mg/m² orally or IV every 6 hours for 72 hours) + Adriamycin (30 mg/m² IV, day 15). The schedule is repeated on day 29 for 6 cycles.

Choriocarcinoma and Similar Trophoblastic Diseases: Methotrexate is administered orally or intramuscularly in doses of 15 to 30 mg daily for a 5 day course. Such courses are usually repeated for 3 to 5 times, as required, with rest periods of one or more weeks interposed between courses, until any manifesting toxic symptoms subside. The effectiveness of therapy is ordinarily evaluated by 24 hour quantitative analysis of urinary chorionic gonadotrophin hormone (beta-HCG), which should return to normal or less than 50 IU/24 hours usually after the third or fourth course, and usually be followed by a complete resolution of measurable lesions in four to six weeks. One to two courses of methotrexate after normalization of beta-HCG is usually recommended. Before each course of the drug, careful clinical assessment is essential. Cyclic combination therapy of methotrexate with other anti tumour drugs has been reported as being useful.

Since hydatiform mole may precede by choriocarcinoma, prophylactic chemotherapy with methotrexate has been recommended.

Chorioadenoma destruens is considered to be an invasive form of hydatiform mole. Methotrexate is administered in these disease states in doses similar to those recommended for choriocarcinoma.

Lymphomas: In Burkitt's tumour, Stages I-II, methotrexate has produced prolonged remissions in some cases. Recommended dosage is 10 to 25 mg/day orally for 4 to 8 days. In Stage III, methotrexate is commonly given concomitantly with other antitumor agents. Treatment in all stages usually consists of several courses of the drug interposed with 7 to 10 day rest periods. Lymphosarcomas in Stage III may respond to combined drug therapy with methotrexate given in doses of 0.625 to 2.5 mg/kg daily.

The treatment of choice for localized histologically aggressive lymphoma is primary combination chemotherapy with or without involved-field radiation therapy. Frequently used regimens for intermediate, or high grade NHL that include methotrexate include groups: the ProMACE/MOPP, ProMACE-CytaBOM, Magrath Protocols. Represented in Table 4 for example, is the ProMACE-CytaBOM Regimen.

Table 4: Methotrexate Tablets USP

ProMACE-CytaBOM Regimen

ProMACE-CytaBOM	Day 1	Day 8	Day 14	Days 15–21
Cyclophosphamide 650 mg/m² IV	x			No therapy
Doxorubicin 25 mg/m² IV	x			
Etoposide 120 mg/m² IV	x			
Cytarabine 300 mg/m² IV		x		
Bleomycin 5 mg/m² IV		x		
Vincristine 1.4 mg/m² IV		x		
Methrotrexate 120 mg/m² IV		x with leucovorin rescue		
Prednisone 60 mg/m² PO	x...................................	x		
Co-trimoxazole 2 PO bid throughout 6 cycles of therapy				

In early stage childhood non-Hodgkin's lymphoma, methotrexate is used effectively in combination chemotherapy regimens.

Mycosis Fungoides (cutaneous T-cell lymphoma): Therapy with methotrexate appears to produce a clinical response, in up to 50% of patients treated, but chemotherapy is not curative. Dosage is usually 2.5 to 10 mg daily by mouth for several weeks or months. Dose levels of drug and adjustment of dose regimen by reduction or cessation of drug are guided by patient response and hematologic monitoring. Methotrexate has also been given intramuscularly in doses of 50 mg once weekly or 25 mg 2 times weekly.

Leukemia: Acute lymphoblastic leukemia (ALL) in children and young adolescents is the most responsive to present day chemotherapy. In young adults and older patients, clinical remission is more difficult to obtain and early relapse is more common.

Methotrexate alone or in combination with steroids was used initially for induction of remission in ALL. More recently, corticosteroid therapy in combination with other antileukemic drugs or in cyclic combinations with methotrexate, has appeared to produce rapid and effective remissions. When used for induction, methotrexate in doses of 3.3 mg/m² in combination with 60 mg/m² of prednisone, given daily, produced remission in 50% of patients treated usually within a period of 4 to 6 weeks. Methotrexate in combination with other agents appears to be the drug of choice for securing maintenance of drug induced remissions. When remission is achieved and supportive care has produced general clinical improvement, maintenance therapy is initiated as follows: Methotrexate is administered 2 times weekly either by mouth or intramuscularly in total weekly doses of 30 mg/m². It has also been given in doses of 2.5 mg/kg intravenously every 14 days. If and when relapse does occur, re-induction of remission can again usually be obtained by repeating the initial induction regimen.

A variety of combination chemotherapy regimens have been used for both induction and maintenance therapy in ALL. The physician should be familiar with recent advances in antileukemic therapy.

Psoriasis and Rheumatoid Arthritis: Dosing Considerations:

- Refer to Neoplastic Diseases, Dosing Considerations.
- The patient should be fully informed of the risks involved and should be under constant supervision of the physician (see Warnings and Precautions, Information to Be Provided to the Patient).
- All dosage schedules should be continually tailored to the individual patient. An initial test dose may be given prior to the regular dosing schedule to detect any extreme sensitivity to adverse effects (see Adverse Reactions). Maximal myelosuppression usually occurs in seven to ten days.

Recommended Dose and Dosage Adjustments: Psoriasis: Recommended Starting Dose Schedules:

- Weekly single oral, IM or IV dose schedule: 10 to 25 mg per week until adequate response is achieved.
- Divided oral dose schedule: 2.5 mg at 12-hour intervals for three doses.

Dosages in each schedule may be gradually adjusted to achieve optimal clinical response; 30 mg/week should not ordinarily be exceeded.

Once optimal clinical response has been achieved, the dosage schedule should be reduced to the lowest possible amount of drug and to the longest possible rest period. The use of methotrexate may permit the return to conventional topical therapy, which should be encouraged.

Rheumatoid Arthritis: Recommended Starting Dosage Schedules:

1. Single oral doses of 7.5 mg once weekly.
2. Divided oral dosages of 2.5 mg at 12 hour intervals for 3 doses given as a course once weekly.

Dosage in each schedule may be adjusted gradually to achieve an optimal response, but not ordinarily to exceed a total weekly dose of 20 mg.

Therapeutic response usually begins within 3 to 6 weeks and the patient may continue to improve for another 12 weeks or more.

Use in Patients with Renal Impairment: See Table 5.

Table 5: Methotrexate Tablets USP

Dose Adjustments in Patients with Renal Insufficiency

Creatinine Clearance (mL/min)	% Standard Dose to Administer
>80	Full Dose
80	75
60	63
50	56
<50	Use alternative therapy

Incompatibilities: See Warnings and Precautions for clinical incompatibilities.

OVERDOSAGE:

In postmarketing experience, overdose with methotrexate has generally occurred with oral and intrathecal administration, although intravenous and intramuscular overdose have also been reported.

Reports of oral overdose indicate accidental daily administration instead of weekly (single or divided doses). Symptoms commonly reported following oral overdose include those symptoms and signs reported at pharmacologic doses, particularly hematologic and gastrointestinal reactions. For example, leukopenia, thrombocytopenia, anemia, pancytopenia, bone marrow suppression, mucositis, stomatitis, oral ulceration, nausea, vomiting, gastrointestinal ulceration, gastrointestinal bleeding. In some cases, no symptoms were reported. There have been reports of death following overdose. In these cases, events such as sepsis or septic shock, renal failure, and aplastic anemia were also reported.

Discontinue or reduce dosage at the first sign of ulceration or bleeding, diarrhea, or marked depression of the hematopoietic system. Leucovorin is indicated to diminish the toxicity and counteract the effect of inadvertently administered overdosages of methotrexate. Leucovorin administration should begin as promptly as possible. As the time interval between methotrexate administration and leucovorin initiation increases, the effectiveness of leucovorin in counteracting toxicity decreases. Monitoring of the serum methotrexate concentration is essential in determining the optimal dose and duration of treatment with leucovorin.

In cases of massive overdosage, hydration and urinary alkalinization may be necessary to prevent the precipitation of methotrexate and/or its metabolites in the renal tubules. Generally, neither standard hemodialysis nor peritoneal dialysis has been shown to improve methotrexate elimination. However, effective clearance of methotrexate has been reported with acute, intermittent hemodialysis using a high-flux dialyzer.

There are published case reports of intravenous carboxypeptidase G2 treatment to hasten clearance of Methotrexate in cases of overdoses.

> For management of a suspected drug overdose, CPhA recommends that you contact your **regional Poison Control Centre**. See the *CPS* Directory section for a list of Poison Control Centres.

ACTION AND CLINICAL PHARMACOLOGY: Mechanism of Action: Methotrexate is a folate antagonist.

Methotrexate inhibits dihydrofolate reductase (DHFR), the enzyme that reduces folic acid to tetrahydrofolic acid. Tetrahydrofolate must be regenerated via the DHFR-catalyzed reaction in order to maintain the intracellular pool of tetrahydrofolate one-carbon derivatives for both thymidylate and purine nucleotide biosynthesis. The inhibition of DHFR by folate antagonists (methotrexate) results in a deficiency in the cellular pools of thymidylate and purines and thus in a decrease in nucleic acid synthesis. Therefore, methotrexate interferes with DNA synthesis, repair, and cellular replication.

Methotrexate is most active against rapidly multiplying cells, because its cytotoxic effects occur primarily during the S phase of the cell cycle. Since cellular proliferation in malignant tissues is greater than in most normal tissues, methotrexate may impair malignant growth without irreversible damage to normal tissues. As a result, actively proliferating tissues, such as malignant cells, bone marrow, fetal cells, buccal and intestinal mucosa, and cells of the urinary bladder, are generally more sensitive to DHFR inhibition effects of methotrexate.

The cytotoxicity of methotrexate results from three important actions: inhibition of DHFR, inhibition of thymidylate synthase, and alteration of the transport of reduced folates. The affinity of DHFR to methotrexate is far greater than its affinity for folic acid or dihydrofolic acid, therefore, large doses of folic acid given simultaneously will not reverse the effects of methotrexate. However, Leucovorin Calcium, a derivative of tetrahydrofolic acid may block the effects of methotrexate if given shortly after the antineoplastic agent.

Methotrexate has immunosuppressive activity. This may be a result of inhibition of lymphocyte multiplication. The mechanisms of action in the management of rheumatoid arthritis of the drug is not known, although suggested mechanisms have included immunosuppressive and/or anti-inflammatory effects.

In psoriasis, the rate of production of epithelial cells in the skin is greatly increased over normal skin. This differential in proliferation rates is the basis for the use of methotrexate to control the psoriatic process.

Pharmacokinetics: Absorption: Orally administered methotrexate is absorbed rapidly in most, but not all patients and reaches peak serum levels in 1 to 4 hours. Methotrexate is generally completely absorbed following parenteral administration, and after intramuscular injection peak serum concentrations occur in 30 to 60 minutes.

Distribution: Methotrexate in serum is approximately 50% protein bound. After intravenous administration, the initial volume of distribution is approximately 0.18 L/kg (18% of body weight) and steady-state volume of distribution is approximately 0.4 to 0.8 L/kg (40% to 80% of body weight). Methotrexate does not penetrate the blood-cerebrospinal fluid barrier in therapeutic amounts when given orally or parenterally.

Metabolism: After absorption, Methotrexate undergoes hepatic and intracellular metabolism to polyglutamated forms which can be converted back to methotrexate by hydrolase enzymes. These polyglutamates act as inhibitors of dihydrofolate reductase and thymidylate syntheses. Small amounts of methotrexate polyglutamates may remain in tissues for extended periods. The retention and prolonged drug action of these active metabolites vary among different cells, tissues and tumours. A small amount of metabolism to 7-hydroxymethotrexate may occur at doses commonly prescribed. The aqueous solubility of 7-hydroxymethotrexate is 3 to 5 fold lower than the parent compound. Methotrexate is partially metabolized by intestinal flora after oral administration.

Excretion: Renal excretion is the primary route of elimination and is dependent upon dosage and route of administration. Excretion of single daily doses occurs through the kidneys in amounts from 80% to 90% within 24 hours. Repeated daily doses result in more sustained serum levels and some retention of methotrexate over each 24-hour period, which may result in accumulation of the drug within the tissues. The liver cells appear to retain certain amounts of the drug for prolonged periods even after a single therapeutic dose. Methotrexate is retained in the presence of impaired renal function and may increase rapidly in the serum and in the tissue cells under such conditions. Methotrexate does not penetrate the blood-cerebrospinal fluid barrier in therapeutic amounts when given orally or parenterally.

The terminal half-life reported for methotrexate is approximately 3 to 10 hours for patients receiving treatment for psoriasis, rheumatoid arthritis or low dose antineoplastic therapy (less than 30 mg/m²).

Methotrexate clearance rates vary widely and are generally decreased at higher doses.

Special Populations and Conditions: Nursing Women: Methotrexate has been detected in human breast milk and is contraindicated during breast feeding. The highest breast milk to plasma concentration ratio reached was 0.08:1.

STORAGE AND STABILITY: Keep in a safe place out of the reach of children.

Store Methotrexate Tablets USP (10 mg) at room temperature, between 15-25°C.

SPECIAL HANDLING INSTRUCTIONS: General: Individuals who have contact with anti-cancer drugs or work in areas where these drugs are used, may be exposed to these agents in air or through direct contact with contaminated objects. Potential health effects may be reduced by adherence to institutional procedures, published guidelines and local regulations for preparation, administration, transportation and disposal of hazardous drugs.

Safe Handling and Disposal: Methotrexate is a potent anti-neoplastic drug. Good medical practice will minimize exposure of persons involved with frequent handling of this drug as outlined below:

Handling:

1. Methotrexate has no vesicant properties and does not show acute toxicity on topical contact with the skin or mucous membranes. However, persons involved with handling cytotoxic drugs should avoid contact with skin and inhalation of airborne particles.
2. Personnel regularly involved in preparation and handling of antineoplastics should have bi-annual blood examinations.

Disposal:

1. Avoid contact with skin and inhalation of airborne particles by use of PVC gloves and disposable gowns and masks.
2. Tablets: Place container and tablets in a plastic bag, seal, and mark as hazardous waste. Incinerate at 1000°C or higher.
3. Tablets: Dissolve tablets in a suitable quantity of normal Sodium Hydroxide (40 g/L of water*) and discard in the sewer system with running water.

Cleaning: Non-disposable equipment that has come in contact with methotrexate may be rinsed with water and washed thoroughly with soap and water.

Spillage/Contamination: Wear gloves, mask and protective clothing. Place spilled material in an appropriate container (i.e. cardboard for broken glass) and then in a polyethylene bag; absorb remains with gauze pads or towels; wash area with water and absorb with gauze or towels again and place in bag; seal, double bag and mark as a hazardous waste. Dispose of waste by incineration or by other methods approved for hazardous materials. Personnel involved in clean up should wash with soap and water.

INFORMATION FOR THE PATIENT: Published in e-CPS, available by subscription at www.e-cps.ca.

DOSAGE FORMS, COMPOSITION AND PACKAGING: Each capsule shaped, yellow, scored tablet, engraved "M 10" contains: methotrexate 10 mg. Nonmedicinal ingredients: lactose monohydrate, magnesium stearate, maize starch, microcrystalline cellulose, polysorbate 80 and starch pregelatinized (Prejel PA 5). Colouring agents- and preservatives-free. Bottles of 100.

Methoxacet

methocarbamol—acetaminophen

Muscle Relaxant—Analgesic

Rougier Pharma

Methoxacet-C⅛ Ⓝ

methocarbamol—acetaminophen—codeine phosphate

Muscle Relaxant—Analgesic

Rougier Pharma

Methoxacet Extra Strength

methocarbamol—acetaminophen

Muscle Relaxant—Analgesic

Rougier Pharma

SUPPLIED: Methoxacet: Each green and white, with a potential presence of green spots on the white part, oblong, film-coated caplet, with one half engraved with "rph" and bisected on the other half, contains: methocarbamol 400 mg and acetaminophen 325 mg. Nonmedicinal ingredients: crospovidone, D&C yellow #10 aluminum lake, FD&C blue #1 aluminum lake, hydroxypropyl methylcellulose, magnesium stearate, maltodextrin, microcrystalline cellulose, polyethylene glycol, povidone, pregelatinized corn starch, sodium croscarmellose, sodium starch glycolate and stearic acid. Blisters of 18. Bottles of 100. Store between 15 and 30°C.

Methoxacet-C⅛: Each oblong caplet, one half is light blue with "rph" engraved, the other is white and bisected and with a potential presence of light blue spots on the white part, contains: methocarbamol 400 mg, acetaminophen 325 mg and codeine phosphate 8 mg. Nonmedicinal ingredients: crospovidone, FD&C blue #1 aluminum lake, magnesium stearate, microcrystalline cellulose, povidone, pregelatinized corn starch, sodium croscarmellose and stearic acid. Blisters of 18. Bottles of 100. Store between 15 and 30°C.

Methoxacet Extra Strength: Each green and white double layer oval film-coated caplet, marked "TEC" on one side and a score line on the other side and with a potential presence of green spots on the white part, contains: methocarbamol 400 mg and acetaminophen 500 mg (which is more than the standard dosage). Nonmedicinal ingredients: crospovidone, D&C yellow #10 aluminum lake, FD&C blue #1 aluminum lake, hydroxypropyl methylcellulose, magnesium stearate, maltodextrin, microcrystalline cellulose, polyethylene glycol, povidone, pregelatinized corn starch, sodium croscarmellose, sodium starch glycolate and stearic acid. Blisters of 18. Bottles of 50. Store between 15 and 30°C.

* Use appropriate safety equipment such as goggles and gloves while working with Sodium Hydroxide, since it can cause severe burns.

Methoxisal

methocarbamol—ASA

Muscle Relaxant—Analgesic

Rougier Pharma

Methoxisal-C⅛ Ⓝ

methocarbamol—ASA—codeine phosphate

Muscle Relaxant—Analgesic

Rougier Pharma

Methoxisal-C¼ Ⓝ

methocarbamol—ASA—codeine phosphate

Muscle Relaxant—Analgesic

Rougier Pharma

Methoxisal-C½ Ⓝ

methocarbamol—ASA—codeine phosphate

Muscle Relaxant—Analgesic

Rougier Pharma

Methoxisal Extra Strength

methocarbamol—ASA

Muscle Relaxant—Analgesic

Rougier Pharma

SUPPLIED: Methoxisal: Each pink and white oblong caplet, with a potential presence of pink spots on the white part, marked "rph" on one side and bisected on the other side, contains: methocarbamol 400 mg and ASA 325 mg. Nonmedicinal ingredients: D&C red #30 aluminum lake, maltodextrin, microcrystalline cellulose, povidone, simethicone, sodium croscarmellose and stearic acid. Blisters of 18. Bottles of 100. Store between 15 and 30°C.

Methoxisal-C⅛: Each yellow and white oblong caplet, with a potential presence of yellow spots on the white part, marked "rph" on one side and bisected on the other side, contains: methocarbamol 400 mg, ASA 325 mg and codeine phosphate 8 mg. Nonmedicinal ingredients: FD&C yellow #6 aluminum lake, D&C yellow #10 aluminum lake, microcrystalline cellulose, povidone, simethicone, sodium croscarmellose and stearic acid. Blisters of 18. Store between 15 and 30°C.

Methoxisal-C¼: Each orange and white oblong caplet, with a potential presence of orange spots on the white part, marked "rph" on one side and bisected on the other side, contains: methocarbamol 400 mg, ASA 325 mg and codeine phosphate 16.2 mg. Nonmedicinal ingredients: D&C red #30 aluminum lake, D&C yellow #10 aluminum lake, microcrystalline cellulose, povidone, simethicone, sodium croscarmellose and stearic acid. Bottles of 100. Store between 15 and 30°C.

Methoxisal-C½: Each peach and white oblong caplet, with a potential presence of peach spots on the white part, marked "rph" on one side and bisected on the other side, contains: methocarbamol 400 mg, ASA 325 mg and codeine phosphate 32.4 mg. Nonmedicinal ingredients: FD&C yellow #6 aluminum lake, microcrystalline cellulose, povidone, simethicone, sodium croscarmellose and stearic acid. Bottles of 100 and 500. Store between 15 and 30°C.

Methoxisal Extra Strength: Each pink and white oblong caplet, with a potential presence of pink spots on the white part, marked "TEC" on one side and bisected on the other side, contains: methocarbamol 400 mg and ASA 500 mg (which is more than the standard dosage). Nonmedicinal ingredients: D&C red #30 aluminum lake, microcrystalline cellulose, povidone, simethicone, sodium croscarmellose and stearic acid. Blisters of 18. Bottles of 50. Store between 15 and 30°C.

Methyldopa Ⓟ

Antihypertensive

CPhA Monograph

Date of Preparation: November 2004
Date of Revision: March 2009

This monograph has been compiled by CPhA and reviewed by experts. It may contain information different from that found in Health Canada-approved Product Monographs. The reader is referred to the *CPS* Editorial Policy for more information.

SUMMARY PRODUCT INFORMATION:

Route of Administration	Dosage Form	Product Strength
Oral	Tablet	125 mg, 250 mg, 500 mg

INDICATIONS AND CLINICAL USE: Methyldopa is indicated for the treatment of hypertension. Methyldopa is one of the drugs of choice for treating hypertension in pregnant women. Methyldopa is not considered a first line agent in the management of hypertension, but may be considered when other agents are ineffective or unsuitable.

CONTRAINDICATIONS:

- Patients who are hypersensitive to this drug or to any ingredient in the formulation
- Active hepatic disease such as acute hepatitis or active cirrhosis
- Previous liver disorder or hemolytic anemia with methyldopa therapy
- Concurrent MAOI therapy

WARNINGS AND PRECAUTIONS: Hematologic: It is recommended to perform a complete blood count and direct Coombs' test prior to and periodically while on methyldopa therapy. Ten to 20% of patients on prolonged methyldopa therapy develop a positive direct Coombs' test, usually 6 to 12 months after starting therapy. Patients with positive Coombs' test should be evaluated for hemolytic anemia. If hemolytic anemia exists, methyldopa must be discontinued and therapy should not be restarted. The anemia should resolve within several weeks after discontinuation of methyldopa. If not, corticosteroid therapy may be indicated. The positive Coombs' test may take weeks to months to return to normal after stopping methyldopa therapy.

Hepatic: Use methyldopa with caution in patients with a history of liver disease. Fever, sometimes associated with eosinophilia or abnormal liver function tests has occurred within 3 weeks of initiating therapy. Jaundice with or without fever has also occurred, usually after 2 to 3 months of therapy. Hepatic necrosis has been reported rarely. It is recommended to check liver function tests prior to and periodically while on methyldopa therapy, especially during the first 6 to 12 weeks or if the patient develops an unexplained fever. Discontinue methyldopa if unexplained fever or jaundice occurs, or if liver function tests are abnormal.

Renal: Lower doses may be required in patients with renal dysfunction. Methyldopa is removed during hemodialysis resulting in loss of blood pressure control. A supplement dose is recommended after hemodialysis (see Dosage and Administration).

Special Populations: Pregnant Women: Methyldopa is the most extensively used antihypertensive in pregnancy and is the initial drug of choice for the treatment of chronic hypertension in pregnant women. Neonates born to women on methyldopa therapy may have decreased systolic blood pressure for the first 2 to 3 days. There have also been reports of tremors. No substantial adverse effects have been detected in long-term follow up of children exposed in utero.

Nursing Women: Methyldopa is excreted in the breast milk. However; the amount is not clinically significant. The American Academy of Pediatrics considers methyldopa to be compatible with breast-feeding.
Pediatrics (birth to 16 years old): There are no well-controlled trials in pediatric patients. Recommended dosages are based on published literature reports of methyldopa therapy in hypertensive pediatric patients (see Dosage and Administration).
Geriatrics: Methyldopa is rarely indicated in the elderly as there are better alternatives for treating hypertension in this age group. If methyldopa is used, start with lower doses since a higher incidence of CNS side effects, postural hypertension and syncope are reported in the elderly.
Monitoring and Laboratory Tests: Obtain a complete blood count, direct Coombs' test and liver function tests prior to initiating therapy and periodically while on therapy (see Warnings and Precautions).
Occupational Hazards: Methyldopa may cause sedation, especially in the first 2 to 3 days of initiating therapy. Advise patients to avoid activities that require mental alertness until they know how methyldopa affects them.

ADVERSE REACTIONS: The most common side effect is transient drowsiness, which occurs in the first 2 to 3 days of initiating therapy, or after a dosage increase.
Cardiovascular: aggravation of angina pectoris, bradycardia (occasional), heart failure, hypertension (rare, following abrupt discontinuation of oral dose), orthostatic hypotension (indicates a need to reduce dosage), prolonged carotid sinus hypersensitivity, sodium and fluid retention (can be controlled with diuretics).
CNS: Common (occurs early in therapy): asthenia, drowsiness, vertigo, weakness, headache. Rare: Bell's palsy, depression, impaired concentration, involuntary choreoathetoid movements (indicates a need to discontinue methyldopa), memory impairment, nightmares, paresthesia, parkinsonism, reversible mild psychosis.
Gastrointestinal: acute pancreatitis, colitis, constipation, diarrhea, distention, dry mouth, flatulence, nausea, sore or black tongue, vomiting.
Hematologic: positive Coombs' test (10–20%), hemolytic anemia (0.1–0.2% of patients who develop a positive Coombs' test), leukopenia (rare, primarily granulocytopenia), immune thrombocytopenia (rare), bone marrow depression, positive lupus and rheumatoid factor tests, hemolysis in patients with glucose-6-phosphate dehydrogenase deficiency.
Hepatic: Rare: abnormal liver function tests, cholestasis, jaundice, hepatitis, hepatic necrosis.
Miscellaneous: nasal congestion (common), decreased libido (frequent), impotence (16%). Rare: amenorrhea, breast enlargement, gynecomastia, hyperprolactinemia, lactation, increased BUN and serum amylase, blurred vision, nocturia.
Immune: drug related fever, myocarditis, pericarditis, lupus-like syndrome.
Skin: eczema, hyperkeratosis, lichenoid eruptions, rash, toxic epidermal necrolysis, ulceration of the soles of the feet, urticaria.
DRUG INTERACTIONS: Drug-Drug Interactions: See Table 1.

Table 1: Methyldopa
Established or Predicted Drug-Drug Interactions

Drug Name	Effect	Clinical Comment
Haloperidol	Methyldopa may increase the effects of haloperidol	Use alternative therapy
Iron	Iron may decrease the extent of methyldopa absorption	Use an alternative antihypertensive or give methyldopa 2 hours before or 6 hours after oral iron. Monitor blood pressure
Levodopa	May increase the effect of both levodopa and methyldopa	Monitor blood pressure and signs of levodopa toxicity. Consider using alternative therapy
Lithium	Methyldopa may increase lithium toxicity	Monitor for lithium toxicity. Consider using an alternative antihypertensive
MAOI	May cause hallucinations, excitation and severe hypertension	MAOIs are contraindicated with methyldopa therapy
Norepinephrine	Methyldopa may prolong the pressor effects of norepinephrine	Monitor for increased blood pressure

Drug-Food Interactions: Methyldopa tablets can be taken with or without food.
Drug-Laboratory Interactions: Methyldopa may cause a positive direct Coombs' test (see Warnings and Precautions). False positive urinary catecholamine testing may occur due to the presence of methyldopa in the urine. Methyldopa may interfere with AST measurement by colorimetry and creatinine using the alkaline picrate method.

DOSAGE AND ADMINISTRATION: Dosing Considerations:
- Tolerance to methyldopa may occur, usually between the second and third month. Increasing the dose or adding a diuretic may help.
- If methyldopa is given with other antihypertensives except for thiazides, the initial dose should be limited to 250 mg BID.

Recommended Dose and Dosage Adjustment:

Table 2: Methyldopa
Dose in Adult Patients

Indication	Route	Initial Dose	Titrate	Usual Dose	Maximum Dose
Hypertension	Oral	250 mg BID or TID	Increase or decrease at intervals of at least 2 days until an adequate response is achieved	500 mg to 2 g daily in 2 to 4 divided doses	3 g daily

Table 3: Methyldopa
Dose in Geriatric Patients

Indication	Route	Initial Dose	Titrate	Maximum Dose
Hypertension	Oral	125 mg daily or BID	Increase by 125 mg every 2 to 3 days as needed	1 g daily

Table 4: Methyldopa
Dose in Pediatric Patients

Indication	Route	Initial Dose	Titrate	Maximum Dose
Hypertension	Oral	10 mg/kg daily in 2 to 4 divided doses	Increase or decrease at intervals of at least 2 days until an adequate response is achieved	65 mg/kg or 3 g daily, whichever is less

Table 5: Methyldopa
Dose in Adult Patients with Renal Impairment

Creatinine Clearance	Dose Adjustment
>50 mL/min	Administer Q8H
10–50 mL/min	Q8–12H
<10 mL/min	Q12–24H

Dosage in Dialysis: It is recommended to give a supplement dose of methyldopa 250 mg following hemodialysis.

OVERDOSAGE:

For management of a suspected drug overdose, CPhA recommends that you contact your **regional Poison Control Centre**. See the *CPS* Directory section for a list of Poison Control Centres.

ACTION AND CLINICAL PHARMACOLOGY: Mechanism of Action: Methyldopa is metabolized to alpha-methylnoradrenaline in the central nervous system. It is thought that this metabolite is responsible for the antihypertensive properties of methyldopa by stimulating α-adrenergic receptors. This stimulation results in a reduction in sympathetic tone and total peripheral resistance. Other properties that may contribute to its therapeutic activity are an ability to reduce plasma renin activity and the inhibition of both central and peripheral norepinephrine and serotonin production .
Pharmacokinetics: Adults: Absorption: The extent of methyldopa absorption following an oral dose is variable, but is approximately 50%. Peak plasma concentrations occur 3 to 6 hours after a dose.
Distribution: There is minimal protein binding of methyldopa. The drug crosses the blood-brain barrier and the placenta and is found in breast milk.
Metabolism: The metabolism of methyldopa is extensive and occurs in the liver and GI tract. The main route is by conjugation to methyldopa mono-O-sulphate. This metabolite may be therapeutically active. Other metabolites have been identified.
Excretion: Methyldopa is primarily excreted in the urine as unchanged drug and as the mono-O-sulphate conjugate. Removal from plasma is biphasic. In patients with normal renal function the first phase plasma half life is 1.8 hours. The half life for the second phase is longer, but undefined. Renal impairment will slow excretion of methyldopa and its metabolites.

Methylprednisolone 🅿

CPhA Monograph

see *Corticosteroids: Systemic*
see *Corticosteroids: Topical*

Methylprednisolone Acetate Injectable Suspension USP 🅿

methylprednisolone acetate
Glucocorticoid

Sandoz

SUPPLIED: 40 mg/mL, multidose formulation: Each mL of sterile aqueous suspension contains: methylprednisolone acetate 40 mg, polyethylene glycol 3350, benzyl alcohol as preservative, polysorbate 80, monobasic sodium phosphate, dibasic sodium phosphate, sodium chloride for tonicity, sodium hydroxide and/or hydrochloric acid to adjust pH and water for injection. Clear multidose vials of 2 mL, boxes of 5. Clear multidose vials of 5 mL, boxes of 5. Discard 28 days after initial use. Shake well before using. Store between 15 and 30°C. Protect from light. Protect from freezing.
80 mg/mL, multidose formulation: Each mL of sterile aqueous suspension contains: methylprednisolone acetate 80 mg, polyethylene glycol 3350, benzyl alcohol as preservative, polysorbate 80, monobasic sodium phosphate, dibasic sodium phosphate, sodium chloride for tonicity, sodium hydroxide and/or hydrochloric acid to adjust pH and water for injection. Clear multidose vials of 5 mL, boxes of 1. Discard 28 days after initial use. Shake well before using. Store between 15 and 30°C. Protect from light. Protect from freezing.
40 mg/mL, preservative-free formulation: Each mL of sterile aqueous suspension contains: methylprednisolone acetate 40 mg, polyethylene glycol 3350, myristyl-gamma-picolinium chloride, sodium chloride for tonicity, sodium hydroxide and/or hydrochloric acid to adjust pH and water for injection. Clear single use vials of 1 mL, boxes of 10. Discard unused portion. Shake well before using. Store between 15 and 30°C. Protect from light. Protect from freezing.
80 mg/mL, preservative-free formulation: Each mL of sterile aqueous suspension contains: methylprednisolone acetate 80 mg, polyethylene glycol 3350, myristyl-gamma-picolinium chloride, sodium chloride for tonicity, sodium hydroxide and/or hydrochloric acid to adjust pH and water for injection. Clear single use vials of 1 mL, boxes of 5. Discard unused portion. Shake well before using. Store between 15 and 30°C. Protect from light. Protect from freezing.

Metoclopramide 🅿

Modifier of Upper Gastrointestinal Motility—Antiemetic

CPhA Monograph

Date of Preparation: November 2003
Date of Revision: July 2009

This monograph has been compiled by CPhA and reviewed by experts. It may contain information different from that found in Health Canada-approved Product Monographs. The reader is referred to the *CPS* Editorial Policy for more information.

SUMMARY PRODUCT INFORMATION:

Route of Administration	Dosage Form	Strength
Intramuscular/Intravenous/Subcutaneous	Liquid	5 mg/mL
Oral	Liquid	1 mg/mL
	Tablet	5 mg, 10 mg

INDICATIONS AND CLINICAL USE: Health Canada-approved indications:
- As an adjunct for the management of delayed gastric emptying associated with subacute and chronic gastritis, or following vagotomy, pyloroplasty and other surgical procedures.
- As an adjunct to facilitate small bowel intubation.
- Diagnostic radiology. Metoclopramide is used as an adjunct to facilitate gastroduodenal evacuation of barium meals and to improve radiological visualization of the gastroduodenal region in patients with gastric atonia, pylorospasm, spasm of the duodenal bulb or with mechanical gastric outlet obstruction. It has also been shown to accelerate small bowel transit of the barium meal and to facilitate fluoroscopy of the terminal ileum.

- Preoperatively, metoclopramide may be useful in reducing narcotic-induced postoperative vomiting.

Uses Not Approved in Canada:

- Prevention of postoperative vomiting. Although indicated for postoperative vomiting prophylaxis, when used in standard clinical doses of 10 mg iv, metoclopramide was shown to be ineffective [*Br J Anaesth* 1999;83(5):761-71]. One study showed that metoclopramide 20 mg was as effective as ondansetron 8 mg when administered at the end of laparoscopic cholecystectomy [*Acta Anaesthesiol Scand* 2002;46(1):109-13]. The 2003 International Anesthesia Research Society Consensus guideline for managing postoperative nausea and vomiting does not recommend metoclopramide for the prevention of postoperative nausea and vomiting due to the lack of evidence of effect, but the decision was not unanimous among panel members [*Acta Anaesthesiol Scand* 2002;46(1):109-13].
- Prevention of nausea and vomiting associated with cancer chemotherapy regimens that contain cisplatin. According to the American Society of Clinical Oncology guideline on the use of antiemetics, the combination of 5-HT_3 serotonin receptor antagonist, dexamethasone and aprepitant is recommended before chemotherapy with cisplatin or other cancer chemotherapeutic agents of high emetic (>90%) risk [*J Clin Oncol* 1999;17(9):2971-94]. To prevent delayed emesis, which occurs ≥24 hours after cancer chemotherapy, a combination of dexamethasone and aprepitant is recommended when using cisplatin or other agents of high emetic risk. High parenteral doses of metoclopramide may be added to the regimen or replace the 5-HT_3 antagonist, in patients who experience nausea and vomiting despite recommended prophylaxis using first-line treatment. Oral metoclopramide is a common component of pre-chemotherapy protocols for low to minimal emetogenic chemotherapies.
- Metoclopramide increases the gastric emptying rate and is considered an alternative to domperidone for the symptomatic treatment of acute and recurrent diabetic gastroparesis. Limited data from randomized trials exist to guide management, however, expert opinion as reflected in the American Gastroenterological Association [*Gastroenterology* 2004;127(5):1592-622] and the American Motility Association [*Neurogastroenterol Motil* 2006;18(4):263-83] guidelines for management of gastroparesis, recommend metoclopramide as one of the treatment modalities. Improvement in nausea occurs early in the course of therapy; relief of vomiting is apparent over the next several weeks, preceding relief of abdominal fullness by about 1 week or more.
- Metoclopramide may be used in pregnant patients experiencing nausea and vomiting despite adequate doses of doxylamine/vitamin B6 combination, dimenhydrinate or promethazine [*Can Fam Physician* 2007;53(12):2109-11].
- According to the American Gastroenterological Association medical position on the management of gastroesophageal reflux disease (GERD), metoclopramide is no longer recommended as monotherapy or as an adjunctive treatment in patients with esophageal or suspected extraesophageal GERD syndromes [*Gastroenterology* 2008;135(4):1383-91].
- For the treatment of persistent hiccoughs, metoclopramide is considered an alternative to chlorpromazine, though it may not be universally effective [*Pharmacotherapy* 1996;16(6):986-95].
- Metoclopramide may be used as primary or adjunctive therapy in headache disorders accompanied by nausea and vomiting. As an antiemetic, it may improve oral absorption of other drugs used to manage the headache.
- Metoclopramide may be used on as-needed basis for prevention of emesis in patients undergoing radiation of minimal emetic risk (<30%) such as breast, head and neck radiation. It is to be continued, prophylactically, for each remaining radiation treatment day [*J Clin Oncol* 2006;24(18):2932-47].
- Patients with anorexia nervosa or bulimia nervosa may have reduced gut motility [*Scand J Gastroenterol* 2003;38(6):573-87], thus, metoclopramide may be used to relieve symptoms of bloating and constipation [*Ann Intern Med* 2001;134(11):1048-59].

CONTRAINDICATIONS:

- Patients who are hypersensitive to metoclopramide or to any ingredient in the formulation.
- Patients with pheochromocytoma; a hypertensive crisis may occur as a result of metoclopramide initiation through the release of catecholamines from the tumor.
- Patients with epilepsy or patients receiving other drugs which are likely to cause extrapyramidal reactions, since frequency and severity of seizures or extrapyramidal reactions may be increased.
- Patients in whom stimulation of gastrointestinal motility may be dangerous such as in those with gastrointestinal hemorrhage, mechanical obstruction or perforation.

WARNINGS AND PRECAUTIONS:

Serious Warnings and Precautions

- Metoclopramide elevates prolactin levels; the elevation persists during chronic administration. Tissue culture experiments indicate that approximately one-third of human breast cancers are prolactin dependent in vitro, a factor of potential importance if metoclopramide therapy is contemplated in a patient with previously detected breast cancer. Although disturbances such as galactorrhea, amenorrhea, gynecomastia and impotence have been reported, the clinical significance of elevated serum prolactin levels is unknown for most patients. An increase in the incidence of mammary neoplasms has been found in rodents after chronic administration of neuroleptic drugs. Neither clinical studies nor epidemiologic studies conducted to date, however, have shown an association between chronic administration of these drugs and mammary tumorigenesis. Evidence is limited and inconclusive.
- In rare instance, tardive dyskinesia may develop early in therapy. Advise and monitor patients for symptoms suggestive of tardive dyskinesia (repetitive, involuntary movements of the body). These symptoms are rarely reversible. If tardive dyskinesia develops, discontinue metoclopramide. Symptoms may lessen or resolve in some patients [www.fda.gov/NewsEvents/Newsroom/PressAnnouncements/2009/ucm149533.htm; www.fda.gov/Safety/MedWatch/SafetyInformation/SafetyAlertsforHumanMedicalProducts/ucm106942.htm].
- Metoclopramide may place increased pressure on suture lines following a gut anastomosis or closure. Metoclopramide should not be used in these patients unless the expected benefits of preventing postoperative nausea and vomiting outweigh the risk of rupture.
- Metoclopramide-induced depression has occurred in patients with or without a prior history of depression. For patients with a prior history of depression, metoclopramide should only be given if the benefits outweigh the risks.
- There may be a risk of cross-sensitivity between metoclopramide and procainamide, because of structural similarities among these drugs.

Cardiovascular: Use caution when administering metoclopramide to patients with hypertension. Metoclopramide iv has been shown to release catecholamines.

Special Populations: Pregnant Women: Pregnancy Category B_M. Metoclopramide has been used for nausea and vomiting related to pregnancy as well as hyperemesis gravidarum. It has been used during all stages of pregnancy. Metoclopramide crosses the placenta. The drug does not appear to be associated with an increased risk of congenital defects or fetal or newborn adverse effects. Exposure to metoclopramide during the first trimester of pregnancy was not associated with significantly increased risks of congenital malformations, low birth weight, preterm delivery or perinatal death [*N Engl J Med* 2009;360(22):2328-39]. Treated pregnant women should be observed for the known adverse effects related to metoclopramide, including more serious neuropsychiatric reactions such as depression and extrapyramidal symptoms.

Nursing Women: Two hours after drug administration, metoclopramide can be found in the breast milk of nursing mothers at concentrations double those found in plasma. In mothers treated with 30 mg daily, total estimated daily dose to the infant is 1 to 45 μg/kg/day which is less than the maximum daily dose of 500 μg/kg recommended in infants. Therefore, with the use of 45 mg daily or less, metoclopramide does not appear to present a risk to breastfed infants. Although no serious adverse effects have been reported in nursing infants, some experts warn that caution should be exercised in using metoclopramide during nursing because of the serious nature of the CNS effects that are possible with the drug. The American Academy of Pediatrics lists metoclopramide as a drug for which the effect on nursing infants is unknown but may be of concern.

Pediatrics: The daily dose should not exceed 0.5 mg/kg, since with higher doses, extrapyramidal symptoms, especially dystonic reactions, frequently occur shortly after therapy is initiated. Neonates may be more susceptible to methemoglobinemia because of their deficiency in NADH methemoglobin reductase.

Geriatrics: Drug-induced parkinsonism may be under-recognized in the elderly. Prolonged dosing appears to increase the likelihood of extrapyramidal effects, especially parkinson-like symptoms. Tardive dyskinesia may develop following drug discontinuation. Prolonged duration of therapy and total cumulative dose may determine risk of developing irreversible tardive dyskinesia.

ADVERSE REACTIONS: Adverse Drug Reactions Overview: Side effects with metoclopramide are generally transient and reversible upon discontinuation of the medication.

More Common Adverse Drug Reactions: Table 1 lists the more common adverse effects of metoclopramide.

Less Common Adverse Drug Reactions: Cardiovascular: Although risk appears low, hypotension, hypertension, supraventricular tachycardia and bradycardia have been reported.

Central Nervous System: A few patients with no previous depressive disorder presented with depression. In some cases, patients exhibited serious symptoms such as suicidal ideation. Persistent generalized anxiety has been reported.

Table 1: Metoclopramide

More Common Adverse Drug Reactions

Body System	Effect	Clinical Comment
Central Nervous System	Drowsiness (dose-related), fatigue and lassitude; insomnia, headache and dizziness; extrapyramidal symptoms, such as motor restlessness (associated with iv administration of high doses of metoclopramide; occurs frequently in children and young adults). Anxiety, restlessness can occur with rapid iv injections.	Drowsiness, fatigue and lassitude occur at the usual recommended dosages. With the higher doses of metoclopramide used to avoid nausea and vomiting related to cancer chemotherapy, dizziness was reported to occur in up to 70% of patients. Extrapyramidal symptoms generally occur within 24 to 48 hours of iv dosing and subside within 24 hours of the drug being discontinued. Most patients respond to treatment with a central anticholinergic (e.g., diphenhydramine and benztropine) or diazepam.
Gastrointestinal	Diarrhea and nausea have been reported.	

The more serious adverse reactions associated with the use of metoclopramide are parkinsonism and/or other extrapyramidal reactions. These often consist of a feeling of restlessness, facial spasms, involuntary movements and in some cases, torticollis, muscular twitching, trismus, oculogyric crisis and opisthotonus. Dystonic reactions resembling tetanus have been reported. Extrapyramidal side effects appear to occur more frequently when the usual recommended dosages are exceeded, but they may be seen with regular therapeutic doses, particularly in children and young adults. Acute dystonia has been reported; it occurs in approximately 0.2% of patients with doses of 30 to 40 mg/day. The incidence increases to 2% in patients over 30 years of age receiving 1 to 2 mg/kg/dose with cancer chemotherapy. Without the prophylactic administration of diphenhydramine accompanying high dose metoclopramide, more than 25% of children and young adults may exhibit dystonic reactions.

Parkinson-like symptoms, which are reversible within 2 to 3 months of discontinuation of metoclopramide, usually occur in the first 6 months of therapy. Use caution if metoclopramide is given to patients with pre-existing Parkinson's disease, as these patients may experience an exacerbation of their symptoms.

Tardive dyskinesia, which in some cases can be irreversible, has been reported after discontinuation of long-term metoclopramide therapy. Therefore, prolonged treatment with metoclopramide should be avoided. Neuroleptic malignant syndrome (NMS) has been reported rarely.

Metoclopramide-induced akathisia and chorea have been reported.

Dermatologic: Metoclopramide-induced delayed non-thrombocytopenic purpuric rash has been reported.

Endocrine and Metabolism: Metoclopramide-induced hyperprolactinemia may cause galactorrhea, menstrual disorders, gynecomastia and impotence. Fluid retention, as a result of stimulation of increased plasma aldosterone concentration, is also possible. Weight gain has been reported.

Gastrointestinal: abdominal pain with rigidity.

Genitourinary: green urine.

Hematologic: Although no causal relationship has been established, agranulocytosis, neutropenia and leukopenia have been reported in patients receiving metoclopramide. Methemoglobinemia has also been reported, especially after overdose in neonates.

Hepatic/Biliary/Pancreatic: Rarely, hepatotoxicity has been reported, with jaundice and increases in liver function tests when metoclopramide was administered with other drugs known to be hepatotoxic.

Immune: Hypersensitivity reactions characterized by rash, urticaria and bronchospasm have been seen occasionally. Anaphylaxis to metoclopramide has been reported.

Abnormal Hematologic and Clinical Chemistry Findings: See Table 2.

Table 2: Metoclopramide

Abnormal Hematologic and Clinical Chemistry Findings

Test	Effect
Alanine aminotransferase, serum	Increased
Aldosterone, plasma	Increased
Alkaline phosphatase, serum	Increased
Aspartate aminotransferase	Increased
Bilirubin, serum	Increased
Cortisol, plasma	Increased
Growth hormone, plasma	Increased
Methemoglobin, blood	Increased
Potassium, serum	Increased
Prolactin, serum	Increased or decreased
Thyroid stimulating hormone	Increased

DRUG INTERACTIONS: Overview: Because metoclopramide increases upper intestinal motility and gastric emptying rate, absorption of concurrently administered drugs may be affected and as a result, the rate of absorption of several orally administered drugs may be affected. Metoclopramide can decrease the extent of absorption of drugs from the stomach (e.g., digoxin). Conversely, absorption from the small bowel may be accelerated (e.g., acetaminophen, tetracyclines, ethanol). Clinical implications of these alterations have not been established.

The effectiveness of metoclopramide as an antiemetic is due to its ability to block dopamine D_2 receptor subtype in the chemoreceptor trigger zone. Other drugs that can block the D_2 receptor are antipsychotics (haloperidol, chlorpromazine) and other antiemetics (prochlorperazine, promethazine); combination of these drugs can result in tardive dyskinesia and other movement disorders.

Drug-Drug Interactions: Drug-drug interactions involving metoclopramide are listed in Table 3.

Table 3: Metoclopramide

Drug-Drug Interactions

Interacting Drug	Effect	Clinical Comment
Anticholinergic agents, e.g., atropine	May antagonize the effects of metoclopramide on gastrointestinal motility.	Avoid combination use.

(cont'd)

Table 3: Metoclopramide *(cont'd)*

Drug-Drug Interactions

Interacting Drug	Effect	Clinical Comment
Antipsychotics, e.g., chlorpromazine, haloperidol, zuclopenthixol	Concurrent use may increase risk of extrapyramidal symptoms.	Monitor for extrapyramidal symptoms (e.g., grinding of teeth, jaw tightness, periauricular pain) if given concurrently. Monitor for tardive dyskinesia.
Atovaquone	May decrease atovaquone plasma concentration.	Clinical significance unknown.
Cimetidine	May decrease cimetidine plasma concentration.	Administer cimetidine at least 2 hours before metoclopramide.
Ciprofloxacin, oral	May accelerate ciprofloxacin absorption resulting in a shorter time to achieve maximum ciprofloxacin plasma concentration; effect on ciprofloxacin bioavailability is unknown.	Clinical significance unknown.
CNS depressants, e.g., alcohol, anxiolytics, opiates, sedatives	Additive effects on sedation may result with concomitant use.	Monitor for excessive sedation. If needed, adjust the dose of the interacting agent.
Cyclosporine	May increase maximum cyclosporine plasma concentrations and bioavailability. Postulated mechanism is increased gastric emptying causing cyclosporine to be absorbed predominantly in the small intestine. Significant differences in oral bioavailability between patients have been noted.	Monitor response and cyclosporine plasma levels; it may be necessary to reduce cyclosporine dose in some patients.
Dantrolene	May increase dantrolene bioavailability.	Avoid combination use.
Digoxin	May decrease time taken to achieve maximum concentration thereby decreasing digoxin absorption.	Monitor digoxin plasma levels before and after metoclopramide introduction. May require dose adjustment.
Ethanol	May increase maximum ethanol plasma concentration. May enhance sedative effects of ethanol. May increase rate of absorption of ethanol by increasing gastrointestinal motility.	Monitor for additive CNS depressive effects, e.g., confusion, drowsiness, respiratory depression and weakness.
Levodopa	May increase bioavailability of levodopa by increasing gastric emptying rate. Metoclopramide may adversely affect control of Parkinson's disease as it is a dopamine antagonist.	Avoid combination use.
Mefloquine	May reduce time to maximum plasma concentration and increase plasma concentration of mefloquine. No significant change in elimination half-life of mefloquine was noted. Proposed mechanism is increased rate of mefloquine absorption from the small intestine due to accelerated gastric emptying.	Monitor for adverse effects of mefloquine before and after metoclopramide introduction. May require adjusting mefloquine dose.
Monoamine oxidase (MAO) inhibitors	Pre-treatment with a MAO inhibitor increased the toxicity of metoclopramide iv in an animal study.	Use with caution in patients with hypertension and those with pheochromocytoma, since metoclopramide releases catecholamines.
Narcotic analgesics	May antagonize the effects of metoclopramide on gastrointestinal motility.	Combination may benefit patients experiencing opioid-induced bowel effects such as slowed gastric emptying or constipation. Monitor for adverse effects and adjust dose accordingly.
Nitrofurantoin	May decrease plasma nitrofurantoin levels. Postulated mechanism is decreased absorption due to increased gastric emptying.	Avoid combination use.
Sertraline	May increase risk of serotonin syndrome and extrapyramidal symptoms when given concurrently.	Based on two case reports. Monitor for extrapyramidal symptoms (e.g., grinding of teeth, jaw tightness, periauricular pain) and serotonin syndrome (e.g., irritability, altered consciousness) if given concurrently.
Succinylcholine	Metoclopramide prolongs neuromuscular blockade induced by succinylcholine. Postulated mechanism is the inhibition of plasma cholinesterase by metoclopramide.	If given concurrently, consider reducing the dose of succinylcholine.
Tacrolimus	May increase tacrolimus plasma levels. Concurrent treatment increases tacrolimus bioavailability by improving delivery of tacrolimus to the small intestine.	Monitor tacrolimus plasma concentrations when administered concurrently with metoclopramide in patients with gastric dysmotility to minimize risk of toxicity.
Venlafaxine	May increase risk of serotonin syndrome and extrapyramidal symptoms when given concurrently.	Based on one case report. Monitor for extrapyramidal symptoms (e.g., grinding of teeth, jaw tightness, periauricular pain) and serotonin syndrome (e.g., irritability, altered consciousness) if given concurrently.

DOSAGE AND ADMINISTRATION: Dosing Considerations: The total adult and pediatric daily dose of metoclopramide should not exceed 0.5 mg/kg/body weight. The exception is when given to patients undergoing chemotherapy. Oral metoclopramide can be given half an hour before meals.

Recommended Dose and Dosage Adjustment: Adults: See Table 4.

Table 4: Metoclopramide

Dose in Adult Patients

Indication	Dose	Duration of Therapy	Clinical Comment
Management of delayed gastric emptying associated with subacute and chronic gastritis, and certain surgical procedures	5 to 10 mg po TID or QID before meals; maximum dose: 0.5 mg/kg/body weight. If require iv: 10 mg im or iv (infused slowly) BID or TID, if necessary.	Duration of treatment depends on response.	Used as adjunct.
Management of small bowel intubation	10 mg iv; infused slowly.	As a single dose.	Used as adjunct. Administer metoclopramide when the tip of the tube reaches the pyloric region.
Diagnostic radiology	20 mg po given 5 to 10 minutes before barium swallow.	As a single dose.	
Reduction of postoperative vomiting induced by narcotics	20 mg po given 2 hours before anesthesia	As a single dose.	
Prevention of postoperative nausea and vomiting (Not an approved use in Canada)	10 mg im given close to termination of surgery; may repeat Q4-6H, if necessary. Larger doses may be needed in high risk patient groups, e.g., general anesthesia ≥2 hours, abdominal or pelvic surgery with visceral manipulation, absence of gastric suction.	As a single dose.	There is evidence that standard clinical doses of 10 mg are ineffective and suboptimal for prevention of postoperative nausea and vomiting. Combining metoclopramide 50 mg with dexamethasone 8 mg given 30 to 60 minutes before the end of surgery was effective in preventing postoperative nausea and vomiting.
Prevention of vomiting associated with cisplatin-containing chemotherapy regimens (Not an approved use in Canada)	For cisplatin doses ≤100 mg/m²: 1 mg/kg of body weight given by iv infusion. For cisplatin doses >100 mg/m²: 2 mg/kg of body weight given by iv infusion		The 2006 update of the American Society of Clinical Oncology guideline for Antiemetics in Oncology recommends the combination of 5-HT_3 serotonin receptor antagonist, dexamethasone and aprepitant for acute emesis. Metoclopramide is no longer used as first-line therapy for cisplatin-induced acute or delayed emesis. High parenteral doses of metoclopramide may be added to the regimen or replace the 5-HT_3 antagonist, in patients who experience nausea and vomiting despite recommended prophylaxis. Administration of metoclopramide is generally by iv infusion over 15 minutes; repeat the dose every 2 hours for two doses, then every 3 hours for three doses.
Prevention of delayed emesis (≥24 hours) in patients receiving chemotherapy (Not an approved use in Canada)	20 to 40 mg BID to QID in conjunction with dexamethasone	3 to 4 days	The 2006 update of the American Society of Clinical Oncology guideline for Antiemetics in Oncology recommends dexamethasone and aprepitant for the prevention of cisplatin-induced delayed emesis.
Management of diabetic gastroparesis (Not an approved use in Canada)	10 mg po TID and HS; given thirty minutes before meals. Dose may be increased to 20 mg QID if 10 mg is inadequate.	Four to twelve weeks	Metoclopramide accelerates gastric emptying. To achieve maximal clinical effects, metoclopramide is given 30 minutes prior to meals. Metoclopramide given at bedtime aids in nocturnal gastric emptying. May switch to im or iv in patients with severe symptoms. Metoclopramide can be given intravenously to patients hospitalized for symptom exacerbations in gastroparesis.
Treatment of nausea and vomiting in pregnancy (Not an approved use in Canada)	5 to 10 mg po/iv every 8 hours	Dependent on patient's symptoms	Metoclopramide may be an option if nausea and vomiting does not respond to doxylamine/vitamin B6, dimenhydrinate and promethazine.
Management of persistent hiccoughs (Not an approved use in Canada)	10 mg iv or im, followed by 10 to 20 mg QID po, has been successful.		Not as effective as chlorpromazine.
Management of nausea and vomiting in headache disorders (Not an approved use in Canada)	10 mg po or iv	As needed	May be used as primary or as adjunctive therapy in headache disorders accompanied by nausea and vomiting. As an antiemetic, metoclopramide may improve oral absorption of other drugs used to manage the headache.

(cont'd)

Table 4: Metoclopramide *(cont'd)*

Dose in Adult Patients

Indication	Dose	Duration of Therapy	Clinical Comment
Prevention of emesis in patients undergoing radiation therapy of minimal emetic risk (<30%) (Not an approved use in Canada)	Pre-radiation therapy: 1 to 2 mg/kg iv		5-HT_3 receptor antagonists are the mainstay of treatment; however, metoclopramide may be used as rescue medication if first-line treatment is ineffective.
Reduced gut motility for patients with anorexia or bulimia nervosa (Not an approved use in Canada)	5 to 20 mg po before meals		Domperidone is preferred as it is associated with a lower incidence of extrapyramidal side effects. By increasing gut motility, metoclopramide may help reduce bloating, early satiety and constipation; it does not impact weight gain.

Pediatrics: See Table 5.

Table 5: Metoclopramide

Dose in Pediatric Patients

Indication	Dose	Duration of Therapy	Clinical Comment
Management of delayed gastric emptying associated with subacute and chronic gastritis, and certain surgical procedures	≤14 y: 2.5 to 5 mg TID before meals; maximum dose: 0.5 mg/kg/body weight.	Duration of treatment depends on response.	Used as adjunct.
Small bowel intubation to facilitate radiographic examination of the upper gastrointestinal tract	<6 y: 0.1 mg/kg iv 6 to 14 y: 2.5 to 5 mg >14 y: 10 mg iv	As a single dose.	Used as adjunct. Administer metoclopramide when the tip of the tube reaches the pyloric region.
Chemotherapy-induced nausea and vomiting (Not an approved use in Canada)	1 to 2 mg/kg/dose every 2 to 4 hours		Administer iv before administration of chemotherapy and every 2 or 3 hours for 3 doses and as required thereafter. Pretreatment with diphenhydramine is recommended to reduce or reverse dystonic reactions.
Management of nausea and vomiting in headache disorders (Not an approved use in Canada)	Oral: 0.1 to 0.2 mg/kg (≤10 mg) IV: 10 mg		
Postoperative nausea and vomiting (Not an approved use in Canada)	≤14 y: 0.1 to 0.2 mg/kg/dose; may repeat Q6-8H PRN >14 y: 10 mg; may repeat Q6-8H PRN		

Renal Impairment: See Table 6 and Table 7.

Table 6: Metoclopramide

Dose in Adult Patients with Renal Impairment

Creatinine Clearance	Dosage Adjustment
>50 mL/min	Usual dose given QID
10–50 mL/min	75% of usual dose
<10 mL/min	50% of usual dose

Table 7: Metoclopramide

Dose in Pediatric Patients with Renal Impairment

Creatinine Clearance	Dosage Adjustment
>30–50 mL/min	75% of usual dose
10–29 mL/min	50% of usual dose
<10 mL/min	25% of usual dose

Dosage in Dialysis: Metoclopramide is not dialyzable and therefore supplemental doses are not necessary.

Hepatic Impairment: Avoid metoclopramide in patients with coexisting hepatic impairment and reduced kidney function. Metoclopramide undergoes minimal hepatic metabolism, except for simple conjugation. Its safe use has been described in patients with advanced liver disease whose renal function was normal.

Administration: Intense feeling of anxiety and restlessness, followed by drowsiness has been associated with rapid iv administration of undiluted metoclopramide injection. These side effects may be averted by injecting slowly, e.g., allowing 1 or 2 minutes to inject 10 mg of metoclopramide. If diluted in a parenteral solution, intravenous metoclopramide should be administered over a period of more than 15 minutes.

OVERDOSAGE:

For management of a suspected drug overdose, CPhA recommends that you contact your **regional Poison Control Centre**. See the *CPS* Directory section for a list of Poison Control Centres.

ACTION AND CLINICAL PHARMACOLOGY: Mechanism of Action: Metoclopramide hydrochloride is a benzamide derivative, structurally related to procainamide. It has dopamine antagonist activity with selective affinity for dopamine D_2-(non-adenylate cyclase linked) receptors (chemoreceptor trigger zone) which contributes to its efficacy as an antiemetic. It has been suggested that the behavioral, motor and neuroendocrine effects of metoclopramide are linked to its antidopaminergic activity. Metoclopramide increases resting pressure in the lower esophageal sphincter and the gastric fundus, and also increases the amplitude of peristaltic movements in the esophagus, gastric antrum and small intestine. These prokinetic actions result in hastened esophageal clearance, accelerated gastric emptying and shortened transit time through the small bowel. The exact mechanism of action is unknown but metoclopramide appears to sensitize tissues to the action of acetylcholine. These effects are blocked by atropine and opioids but not by vagotomy. It does not appear to affect motility in the colon. Metoclopramide has antiemetic properties, which are believed to result from its action on the chemoreceptor trigger zone where the threshold of activity is increased. Stasis related to vomiting is decreased because of accelerated gastric emptying. High-dose metoclopramide may also inhibit serotonin, specifically the 5-HT_3 receptor subtype. Metoclopramide elevates serum prolactin and also causes a transient increase in circulating aldosterone levels. These effects are thought to be due to blockade of dopamine receptors at the pituitary and adrenocortical cellular level. Metabolic clearance of aldosterone is not affected nor is plasma renin activity. During prolonged administration of metoclopramide, plasma aldosterone concentrations are reported to return to pretreatment levels.

Pharmacokinetics: Adults: Absorption: Peak plasma levels occur within minutes following iv administration, and between 45 to 90 minutes after oral administration. Onset of action for im administration is 10 to 15 minutes, for iv administration is 1 to 3 minutes and for oral doses is 30 to 60 minutes. Duration of action is 1 to 2 hours. Oral bioavailability varies from 32 to 97%.

Distribution: There is a first-pass effect after oral administration, and bioavailability varies between 30 and 70%. Metoclopramide is 40% bound to plasma proteins. Volume of distribution is high (approximately 3.5 L/kg in adults).

Metabolism: Metoclopramide is metabolized to sulfate and glucuronide conjugates.

Excretion: The elimination half-life is approximately 3 to 5 hours. About 20% of the drug is eliminated in the urine unchanged, and 30 to 40% is eliminated as the sulfate conjugate. In patients with impaired renal function, the half-life is prolonged and may reach 14 hours or more. Reduced clearance in neonates is also suggested by a prolonged elimination half-life.

Metoclopramide Hydrochloride Injection ℞

metoclopramide HCl

Upper Gastrointestinal Motility Modifier—Antiemetic

Sandoz

SUPPLIED: Each mL contains: metoclopramide hydrochloride 5 mg. Nonmedicinal ingredients: hydrochloric acid and/or sodium hydroxide to adjust pH to 2.5 to 6.5, sodium chloride and water for injection. Preservative-free. Single use amber vials of 2 mL, boxes of 10; of 10 mL, boxes of 5; and of 30 mL, boxes of 1. Store between 15 and 30°C. Protect from light. Discard unused portion.

Metoject® ℞

methotrexate sodium

Antimetabolite—Antirheumatic Agent

Medexus

Date of Preparation: January 8, 2008
Date of Revision: May 6, 2009

SUMMARY PRODUCT INFORMATION:

Route of Administration	Dosage Form/ Strength	Clinically Relevant Nonmedicinal Ingredients
Intramuscular, intravenous, intra-arterial, intrathecal	METOJECT (methotrexate sodium) 10 mg/mL solution for injection is available in single-use pre-filled syringes. METOJECT is available as follows: 1 mL syringe with 0.75 mL solution for injection, equivalent to 7.5 mg methotrexate 1 mL syringe with 1 mL solution for injection, equivalent to 10 mg methotrexate 2.25 mL syringe with 1.5 mL solution for injection, equivalent to 15 mg methotrexate 2.25 mL syringe with 2 mL solution for injection, equivalent to 20 mg methotrexate 3 mL syringe with 2.5 mL solution for injection, equivalent to 25 mg methotrexate	For a complete listing see Dosage Forms, Composition and Packaging.

INDICATIONS AND CLINICAL USE: Two major fields of indication exist for METOJECT (methotrexate sodium):
- Neoplastic diseases
- Disease Modifying Antirheumatic Drug (DMARD)

Neoplastic Diseases:
- Choriocarcinoma: METOJECT—as single chemotherapy or in combination with other drugs.
- Intermediate-, or high grade Non-Hodgkin's Lymphoma as part of ProMACE-CytaBOM, ProMACE-MOPP, and Magrath protocols.
- Breast Cancer: as part of CMF (cyclophosphamide-methotrexate-fluorouracil) therapy.
- Acute Lymphoblastic Leukemia (ALL)—as maintenance therapy.
- Head and Neck Cancer—in combination with other chemotherapies.
- Gastric Cancer—palliative combination chemotherapy.
- Metastasis of unknown primary—as palliative combination chemotherapy.
- Osteogenic sarcoma (adjuvant)—high dose METOJECT with leucovorin rescue (HDMTX-LV).
- Bladder Cancer (advanced)—as part of M-VAC regimen.
- Leptomeningeal spread of malignancies (carcinomatosis/leukemia/lymphoma) as a single chemotherapy or alternating with Ara-C.
- Burkitt's lymphoma.
- Advanced stages of childhood lymphoma (III and IV, St. Jude's Childrens' Research Hospital Staging System).
- Advanced cases of mycosis fungoids (cutaneous T-cell lymphoma).

Disease Modifying Antirheumatic Drug (DMARD): The use of METOJECT as a DMARD in the following diseases where standard therapeutic interventions fail:
- Severe disabling psoriasis/psoriatic arthritis
- Severe disabling rheumatoid arthritis (RA)
- Severe disabling seronegative arthritides

In the treatment of psoriasis, METOJECT should be restricted to severe recalcitrant, disabling psoriasis, which is not adequately responsive to other forms of therapy, but only when the diagnosis has been established after dermatologic consultation.

Geriatrics: The clinical pharmacology of methotrexate has not been well studied in older individuals. Due to diminished hepatic and renal function, as well as decreased folate stores in this population, relatively low doses should be considered, and these patients should be closely monitored for early signs of toxicity.

Pediatrics: Safety and effectiveness in pediatric patients have not been established, other than in cancer chemotherapy.

CONTRAINDICATIONS: Patients who are hypersensitive to this drug or to any ingredient in the formulation or component of the container. For a complete listing, see Dosage Forms, Composition and Packaging.
- Pregnancy: Methotrexate can cause fetal death, embryotoxicity, abortion or teratogenic effects when administered to a pregnant woman. Methotrexate is contraindicated in pregnant patients with psoriasis or rheumatoid arthritis and should be used in the treatment of neoplastic diseases only when the potential benefit outweighs the risk to the fetus.

- Women of childbearing potential should not be started on methotrexate until pregnancy is excluded and should be fully counselled on the serious risk to the fetus should they become pregnant while undergoing treatment. Pregnancy should be avoided if either partner is receiving methotrexate. The optimal time interval between the cessation of methotrexate treatment of either partner and pregnancy has not been clearly established. Published literature recommendations for time intervals vary from 3 months to one year (see Warnings and Precautions).
- Because of the potential for serious adverse reactions in breast fed infants, it is contraindicated in nursing mothers.
- Methotrexate formulations and diluents containing preservatives must not be used for intrathecal or high dose Methotrexate therapy.
- METOJECT (methotrexate sodium) is contraindicated in patients with psoriasis or rheumatoid arthritis in the following situations:
  - Alcoholism, alcoholic liver disease or other chronic liver disease.
  - Overt or laboratory evidence of immunodeficiency syndromes.
  - Pre-existing blood dyscrasias, such as bone marrow hypoplasia, leucopenia, thrombocytopenia or significant anemia.

WARNINGS AND PRECAUTIONS:

Serious Warnings and Precautions
- METOJECT (methotrexate sodium) should be used only by physicians whose knowledge and experience includes the use of antimetabolite therapy (see Indications and Clinical Use).
- Serious Toxic Reactions (see General).
- Use in Pregnancy: Methotrexate has been reported to cause fetal death and/or congenital anomalies (see Special Populations, Pregnant Women). Pregnant patients with psoriasis or rheumatoid arthritis should not receive methotrexate (see Contraindications).

General: Because of the possibility of serious toxic reactions (which can be fatal), METOJECT should be used only in life-threatening neoplastic diseases, or in patients with psoriasis or rheumatoid arthritis with severe, recalcitrant, disabling disease that is not adequately responsive to other forms of therapy. Deaths have been reported with the use of Methotrexate in the treatment of malignancy, psoriasis and rheumatoid arthritis. Because of the possibility of serious toxic reactions the patient should be informed by the physician of the risks involved and should be under a physician's constant supervision.

The use of METOJECT high dose regimens recommended for osteosarcoma requires meticulous care (see Dosage and Administration). High dosage regimens for other neoplastic diseases are investigational and a therapeutic advantage has not been established.

METOJECT has the potential for serious toxicity. Toxic effects may be related in frequency and severity to dose or frequency of administration but have been seen at all doses. Because they can occur at any time during therapy, it is necessary to follow patients on METOJECT closely. Most adverse reactions are reversible if detected early. When such reactions do occur, the drug should be reduced in dosage or discontinued and appropriate corrective measures should be taken. If necessary, this could include the use of leucovorin calcium and/or acute, intermittent hemodialysis with a high-flux dialyzer (see Overdosage). If METOJECT therapy is re-instituted, it should be carried out with caution, with adequate consideration of further need for the drug and with increased alertness as to possible recurrence of toxicity.

Methotrexate exits slowly from third space compartments (e.g., pleural effusions or ascites). This results in a prolonged terminal plasma half-life and unexpected toxicity. In patients with significant third space accumulations, it is advisable to evacuate the fluid before treatment and to monitor plasma methotrexate levels.

Unexpectedly severe (sometimes fatal) bone marrow suppression, aplastic anemia and gastrointestinal toxicity have been reported with concomitant administration of METOJECT (usually in high dosage) along with some non-steroidal anti-inflammatory drugs (NSAIDs) (see Drug Interactions).

Bone marrow and mucosal toxicity of METOJECT depend on: dose and duration of exposure of high levels (>2×10^{-8} mol/L (0.02 micromolar)) of METOJECT. Since the critical time factor has been defined for these organs as being 42 hours in humans, this has the following implications:
- When high doses of METOJECT are employed (>1 g/m^2), drug levels in serum should be monitored;
- When drug levels exceeding (2×10^{-8} mol/L (0.02 micromolar)) the above for >42 hours may forecast significant toxicity;
- When toxicity can be minimized by appropriate administration of Leucovorin Calcium;
- When high-dose METOJECT (HDMTX) is employed, it is imperative to alkalinise the urine in order to prevent crystallisation of METOJECT and its 7-hydroxy metabolite in the urine, which may lead to acute renal failure.

METOJECT given concomitantly with radiotherapy may increase the risk of soft tissue necrosis and osteonecrosis.

METOJECT should be used with extreme caution in the presence of debility.

Carcinogenesis and Mutagenesis: Malignant lymphomas, which may regress following withdrawal of methotrexate, may occur in patients receiving low-dose methotrexate and, thus, may not require cytotoxic treatment. Discontinue methotrexate first and, if the lymphoma does not regress, appropriate treatment should be instituted.

Like other cytotoxic drugs, METOJECT may induce "tumour lysis syndrome" in patients with rapidly growing tumours. Appropriate supportive and pharmacologic measures may prevent or alleviate this complication.

No controlled human data exist regarding the risk of neoplasia with methotrexate. Methotrexate has been evaluated in a number of animal studies for carcinogenic potential with inconclusive results. Although there is evidence that methotrexate causes chromosomal damage to animal somatic cells and human bone marrow cells, the clinical significance remains uncertain. Assessment of the carcinogenic potential of methotrexate is complicated by conflicting evidence of an increased risk of certain tumors in rheumatoid arthritis. Benefit should be weighed against this potential risk before using methotrexate alone or in combination with other drugs, especially in children or young adults.

Gastrointestinal: If vomiting, diarrhea, or stomatitis occurs, resulting in dehydration, METOJECT should be discontinued until recovery occurs. Diarrhea and ulcerative stomatitis require interruption of therapy; otherwise, hemorrhagic enteritis and death from intestinal perforation may occur. METOJECT should be used with extreme caution in the presence of peptic ulcer disease or ulcerative colitis.

Hematologic: METOJECT should be used with caution in patients with impaired bone marrow function and previous or concomitant wide field radiotherapy. METOJECT may produce marked bone marrow depression with resultant anemia, aplastic anemia, pancytopenia, leucopenia neutropenia and/or thrombocytopenia. In patients with malignancy and pre-existing hematopoietic impairment, the drug should be used with caution, if at all. In controlled clinical trials in rheumatoid arthritis (n=128), leucopenia (WBC <3000/mm^3) was seen in 2 patients, thrombocytopenia (platelets <1 000 000/mm^3) in 6 patients, and pancytopenia in 2 patients.

In psoriasis and rheumatoid arthritis, METOJECT should be stopped immediately if there is a significant drop in blood counts. In the treatment of neoplastic diseases, METOJECT should be continued only if the potential benefit warrants the risk of severe myelosuppression. Patients with profound granulocytopenia and fever should be evaluated immediately and usually require parenteral broad-spectrum antibiotic therapy.

Hepatic/Biliary/Pancreatic: METOJECT has the potential for acute and chronic hepatotoxicity. Acutely, liver enzyme elevations are frequently seen after METOJECT administration and are usually not a reason for modification of METOJECT therapy. Liver enzyme elevations are usually transient and asymptomatic, and also do not appear predictive of subsequent hepatic disease. Persistent liver abnormalities, and/or decrease of serum albumin may be indicators of serious liver toxicity. Chronic toxicity is potentially fatal; it generally has occurred after prolonged use (generally two years or more) and after a total cumulative dose of at least 1.5 grams. Liver biopsy after sustained use often shows histologic changes, and fibrosis and cirrhosis have been reported; these latter lesions may not be preceded by symptoms or abnormal liver function tests in the psoriasis population. Periodic liver biopsies are usually recommended for psoriatic patients who are under long-term treatment. Persistent abnormalities in liver function tests may precede appearance of fibrosis or cirrhosis in the rheumatoid arthritis population. In studies in psoriatic patients, hepatotoxicity appeared to be a function of total cumulative dose and appeared to be enhanced by alcoholism, obesity, diabetes and advanced age. An accurate incidence rate has not been determined; the rate of progression and reversibility of lesions is not known. Special caution is indicated in the presence of pre-existing liver damage or impaired hepatic function.

In psoriasis, liver damage and function tests, including serum albumin and prothrombin time, should be performed several times prior to dosing, but are often normal in the face of developing fibrosis or cirrhosis. These lesions may be detectable only by biopsy.

The usual recommendation is to obtain a liver biopsy: 1) before the start of therapy or shortly after initiation of therapy (4-8 weeks); 2) after a total cumulative dose of 1.5 grams; and 3) after each additional 1.0 to 1.5 grams. Moderate fibrosis or any cirrhosis normally leads to discontinuation of the drug; mild fibrosis normally suggests a repeat biopsy in 6 months. Milder histologic findings such as fatty change and low grade portal inflammation are relatively common pre-therapy. Although these mild changes are usually not a reason to avoid or discontinue methotrexate therapy, the drug should be used with caution.

Clinical experience with liver disease in rheumatoid arthritis is limited, but the same risk factors would be anticipated. Liver function tests are also usually not reliable predictors of histological changes in this population.

In rheumatoid arthritis, advanced age at first use of methotrexate and increasing duration of therapy have been reported as risk factors for hepatotoxicity. Persistent abnormalities in liver function tests may precede appearance of fibrosis or cirrhosis in the rheumatoid population. Liver function tests should be performed at baseline and at 4-8 week intervals in patients receiving methotrexate for rheumatoid arthritis. Pretreatment liver biopsy should be performed for patients with a history of excessive alcohol consumption, persistently abnormal baseline liver function test values, or chronic hepatitis B or C infection. During therapy, liver biopsy should be performed if there are persistent liver function test abnormalities, or there is a decrease in serum albumin below the normal range (in the setting of well controlled rheumatoid arthritis).

If the results of a liver biopsy show mild changes (Roenigk grades I, II, IIIa), METOJECT may be continued and the patient monitored according to the recommendations listed above. METOJECT should be discontinued in any patient who displays persistently abnormal liver function tests and refuses liver biopsy, or in any patient whose liver biopsy shows moderate to severe changes (Roenigk grade IIIb or IV).

There is a combined reported experience in 217 rheumatoid arthritis patients with liver biopsies both before and during treatment (after a cumulative dose of at least 1500 mg) and in 714 patients with a biopsy only during treatment. There are 64 (7%) cases of fibrosis and 1 (0.1%) case of cirrhosis. Of the 64 cases of fibrosis, 60 were deemed mild. The reticulin stain is more sensitive for early fibrosis and its use may increase these figures. It is unknown whether even longer use will increase these risks.

Immune: METOJECT should be used with extreme caution in the presence of active infection, and is usually contraindicated in patients with overt or laboratory evidence of immunodeficiency syndromes.

Immunization may be ineffective when given during methotrexate therapy. Immunization with live virus vaccines is generally not recommended. There have been reports of disseminated vaccinia infections after smallpox immunization in patients receiving methotrexate therapy. Hypogammaglobulinemia has been reported rarely.

Information to Be Provided to the Patient: Patients should be informed of the early signs and symptoms of toxicity, of the need to see their physician promptly if they occur, and the need for close follow-up, including periodic laboratory tests to monitor toxicity.

Both the physician and pharmacist should emphasize to the patient that the recommended dose is taken weekly in rheumatoid arthritis and psoriasis, and that mistaken daily use of the recommended dose has led to fatal toxicity.

Patients should be informed of the potential benefit and risk in the use of METOJECT. The risk of effects on reproduction should be discussed with both male and female patients taking METOJECT.

Neurologic: There have been reports of leukoencephalopathy following intravenous administration of METOJECT to patients who have had craniospinal irradiation. Serious neurotoxicity, frequently manifested as generalized or focal seizures, has been reported with unexpectedly increased frequency among pediatric patients with acute lymphoblastic leukemia who were treated with intermediate-dose intravenous METOJECT (1 g/m^2). Symptomatic patients were commonly noted to have leukoencephalopathy and/or microangiopathic calcifications on diagnostic imaging studies. Chronic leukoencephalopathy has also been reported in patients with osteosarcoma who received repeated doses of high-dose METOJECT with leucovorin rescue even without cranial irradiation. Discontinuation of METOJECT does not always result in complete recovery.

A transient acute neurologic syndrome has been observed in patients treated with high dosage regimens. Manifestations of this neurologic disorder may include behavioural abnormalities, focal sensorimotor signs, including transient blindness and abnormal reflexes. The exact cause is unknown.

After the intrathecal use of METOJECT, the central nervous system toxicity which may occur can be classified as follows: chemical arachnoiditis manifested by such symptoms as headache, back pain, nuchal rigidity, and fever; paresis, usually transient, manifested by paraplegia associated with involvement with one or more spinal nerve roots; leucoencephalopathy manifested by confusion, irritability, somnolence, ataxia, dementia, and occasionally major convulsions.

Intravenous administration of METOJECT may also result in acute encephalitis and acute encephalopathy with fatal outcome.

Cases of severe neurological adverse reactions that ranged from headache to paralysis, coma and stroke-like episodes have been reported mostly in juveniles and adolescents given methotrexate in combination with cytarabine.

Renal: METOJECT therapy in patients with impaired renal function should be undertaken with extreme caution, and at reduced dosages, because renal dysfunction will prolong methotrexate elimination. METOJECT may cause renal damage that may lead to acute renal failure. High doses of METOJECT used in the treatment of osteosarcoma may cause renal damage leading to acute renal failure.

Nephrotoxicity is due primarily to the precipitation of methotrexate and 7-hydroxymethotrexate in the renal tubules. Close attention to renal function including adequate hydration, urine alkalization and measurement of serum methotrexate and creatinine levels are essential for safe administration.

Respiratory: Methotrexate-induced lung disease, including acute or chronic interstitial pneumonitis is a potentially dangerous lesion, which may occur at any time during therapy and which has been reported at low doses. It is not always fully reversible and fatalities have been reported. Pulmonary symptoms (especially a dry non-productive cough) or a non-specific pneumonitis occurring during methotrexate therapy may be indicative of a potentially dangerous lesion and require interruption of treatment and careful investigation. Although clinically variable, the typical patient with methotrexate-induced lung disease presents with fever, cough, dyspnea, hypoxemia, and an infiltrate on chest X-ray; infection (including pneumonia) needs to be excluded. This lesion can occur at all dosages.

Pneumonia (in some cases leading to respiratory failure) may occur. Potentially fatal opportunistic infections, especially *P. carinii* pneumonia, may occur with METOJECT therapy. When a patient presents with pulmonary symptoms, the possibility of *P. carinii* should be considered.

Sexual Function/Reproduction: METOJECT causes embryotoxicity, abortion, and fetal defects in humans. It has also been reported to cause impairment of fertility, oligospermia and menstrual dysfunction in humans, during and for a short period after cessation of therapy.

Skin: Severe, occasionally fatal, dermatologic reactions, including toxic epidermal necrolysis (Lyell's Syndrome), Stevens-Johnson syndrome, exfoliative dermatitis, skin necrosis and erythema multiforme have been reported in children and adults within days of oral methotrexate administration. Reactions were noted after single or multiple, low, intermediate or high doses of methotrexate in patients with neoplastic and non-neoplastic diseases. Recovery has been reported with discontinuation of therapy.

Lesions of psoriasis may be aggravated by concomitant exposure to ultraviolet radiation. Radiation dermatitis and sunburn may be "recalled" by the use of methotrexate.

Special Populations: Pregnant Women: METOJECT can cause fetal death, embryotoxicity, abortion, or teratogenic effects when administered to a pregnant woman. METOJECT is contraindicated in pregnant patients with psoriasis or rheumatoid arthritis and should be used in the treatment of neoplastic diseases only when the potential benefit outweighs the risk to the fetus.

Women of childbearing potential should not be started on METOJECT until pregnancy is excluded and should be fully counselled on the serious risk to the fetus should they become pregnant while undergoing treatment. Pregnancy should be avoided if either partner is receiving METOJECT. The optimal time interval between the cessation of METOJECT treatment of either partner and pregnancy has not been clearly established. Published literature recommendations for time intervals vary from 3 months to one year.

Nursing Women: Because of the potential for serious adverse reactions from methotrexate in breast fed infants, METOJECT is contraindicated in nursing mothers.

Pediatrics: Safety and effectiveness in pediatric patients have not been established, other than in cancer chemotherapy.

Geriatrics: The clinical pharmacology of methotrexate has not been well studied in older individuals. Due to diminished hepatic and renal function, as well as decreased folate stores in this population, relatively low doses should be considered, and these patients should be closely monitored for early signs of toxicity.

Monitoring and Laboratory Tests: General: Patients undergoing methotrexate therapy should be closely monitored so that toxic effects are detected promptly. Baseline assessment should include a complete blood count (CBC) with differential and platelet counts, hepatic enzymes, renal function tests, and a chest X-ray. During therapy of rheumatoid arthritis and psoriasis, monitoring of these parameters is recommended: hematology at least monthly, and hepatic enzyme levels and renal function every 1 to 2 months. More frequent monitoring is usually indicated during antineoplastic therapy. During initial or changing doses, or during periods of increased risk of elevated methotrexate blood levels (e.g., dehydration), more frequent monitoring may also be indicated.

Liver: Liver biopsies prior to METOJECT therapy are not indicated routinely. Liver function tests (LFTs) should be determined prior to the initiation of therapy with METOJECT and they should be monitored regularly throughout therapy. A relationship between abnormal liver function tests and fibrosis or cirrhosis of the liver has not been established. Transient liver function test abnormalities are observed frequently after METOJECT administration and are usually not cause for modification of methotrexate therapy. Persistent liver function test abnormalities just prior to dosing and/or depression of serum albumin may be indicators of serious liver toxicity and require evaluation.

Respiratory: Pulmonary function tests may be useful if methotrexate-induced lung disease is suspected, especially if baseline measurements are available.

Serum Level Monitoring: Serum methotrexate level monitoring can significantly reduce methotrexate toxicity and mortality.

Patients subject to the following conditions are predisposed to developing elevated or prolonged methotrexate levels and benefit from routine monitoring of levels: eg, pleural effusion, ascites, gastrointestinal tract obstruction, previous cisplatin therapy, dehydration, aciduria, impaired renal function.

Some patients may have delayed methotrexate clearance in the absence of these features. It is important that patients be identified within 48 hours since methotrexate toxicity may not be reversible if adequate leucovorin rescue is delayed for more than 42 to 48 hours.

The method of monitoring methotrexate concentrations varies from institution to institution. Monitoring of methotrexate concentrations should include determination of a methotrexate level at 24, 48, or 72 hours, and assessment of the rate of decline in methotrexate concentrations (to determine how long to continue leucovorin rescue).

ADVERSE REACTIONS: Adverse Drug Reaction Overview: In general, the incidence and severity of acute side effects are related to dose, frequency of administration, and the duration of the exposure to significant blood levels of methotrexate to the target organs. The most serious reactions are discussed in Warnings and Precautions. That section should also be consulted when looking for information about adverse reactions with methotrexate.

- Some of the effects mentioned in this section, such as dizziness and fatigue, may affect the ability to drive or operate machinery.
- The most frequently reported adverse reactions include ulcerative stomatitis, leucopenia, nausea, and abdominal distress. Other frequently reported adverse effects are malaise, undue fatigue, chills and fever, dizziness and decreased resistance to infection.

Adverse Drug Reactions by Organ System: Adverse reactions that have been reported with methotrexate are listed below alphabetically by organ system. In the oncology setting, concomitant treatment and the underlying disease make specific attribution of a reaction to methotrexate difficult.

Alimentary System: gingivitis, stomatitis, enteritis, anorexia, nausea, vomiting, diarrhea, hematemesis, melena, gastrointestinal ulceration and bleeding, pancreatitis.

Cardiovascular: pericarditis, pericardial effusion, hypotension, and thromboembolic events (including arterial thrombosis, cerebral thrombosis, deep vein thrombosis, retinal vein thrombosis, thrombophlebitis, and pulmonary embolus).

Central Nervous System: headaches, dizziness, drowsiness, speech impediment including dysarthria and aphasia; hemiparesis, paresis and convulsions have also occurred following administration of methotrexate. Following low doses, there have been occasional reports of transient subtle cognitive dysfunction, mood alteration, or unusual cranial sensations, leucoencephalopathy, or encephalopathy.

Eye Disorders: conjuctivitis, blurred vision, serious visual changes of unknown etiology, and transient blindness/vision loss.

Hematopoietic: Methotrexate can suppress hematopoiesis and cause anemia, leucopenia, and/or thrombocytopenia. Hypogammaglobulinemia has been reported rarely (see Warnings and Precautions, Immune). Lymphadenopathy and lymphoproliferative disorders (including reversible), pancytopenia, neutropenia and agranulocytosis and eosinophilia have also been observed.

Hepatobiliary Disorders: hepatotoxicity, acute hepatitis, chronic fibrosis and cirrhosis, decrease in serum albumin, liver enzyme elevations, hepatic failure.

Infection: There have been case reports of sometimes fatal sepsis, sepsis, opportunistic infections, including fatal infections in patients receiving methotrexate therapy for neoplastic and non-neoplastic diseases. *P. carinii* pneumonia was the most common infection. Other reported infections included pneumonia, nocardiosis, histoplasmosis, cryptococcosis, Herpes zoster, H. simplex hepatitis and disseminated H. simplex and cytomegalovirus infection, including cytomegaloviral pneumonia.

Musculoskeletal, Connective Tissue, and Bone Disorders: stress fractures.

Pulmonary System: Respiratory fibrosis, pharyngitis and interstitial pneumonitis deaths have been reported; chronic interstitial obstructive pulmonary disease and alveolitis have occasionally occurred.

Skin: erythematous rashes, pruritus, urticaria, photosensitivity, pigmentary changes, alopecia, ecchymosis, telangiectasia, acne, furunculosis, erythema multiforme, toxic epidermal necrolysis (Lyell's Syndrome), Stevens-Johnson Syndrome, skin necrosis, exfoliative dermatitis, and painful erosion of psoriatic plaques.

Urogenital System: severe nephropathy or renal failure, azotemia, dysuria, cystitis, hematuria; defective oogenesis or spermatogenesis, transient oligospermia, menstrual dysfunction, vaginal discharge and gynecomastia; infertility, abortion, fetal defects, loss of libido/impotence. Proteinuria has also been observed.

Rarer Reactions: Related to or attributed to the use of Methotrexate such as nodulosis, vasculitis, Herpes zoster, sepsis, arthralgia/myalgia, diabetes, osteoporosis, sudden death, lymphoma, reversible lymphomas, tumor lysis syndrome, soft tissue necrosis, aplastic anemia, fetal death and osteonecrosis. A few cases of anaphylactoid reactions have been reported.

Malignant lymphomas, which may regress following withdrawal of methotrexate, may occur in patients receiving low-dose methotrexate, and thus may not require cytotoxic treatment. Discontinue methotrexate first and if the lymphoma does not regress, appropriate treatment should be instituted.

Other Adverse Drug Reactions: Adverse Reactions Reported in Rheumatoid Arthritis: Incidence greater than 10%: elevated liver enzymes 15%, nausea/vomiting 10%.

Incidence 3% to 10%: stomatitis, thrombocytopenia.

Incidence 1% to 3%: rash/pruritus/dermatitis, alopecia, diarrhea, dizziness, leucopenia and pancytopenia.

Adverse Reactions in Psoriasis: The adverse reaction rates reported are very similar to those in the rheumatoid arthritis studies. Rarely, painful psoriatic plaque erosions may appear.

Abnormal Hematologic and Clinical Chemistry Findings: Abnormal hematologic and clinical chemistry findings are discussed in Warnings and Precautions, Monitoring and Laboratory Tests.

DRUG INTERACTIONS: Drug-Drug Interactions: The drugs listed below are based on either drug interaction case reports or studies, or potential interactions due to the expected magnitude and seriousness of the interaction (i.e., those identified as contraindicated).

Nonsteroidal Anti-inflammatory Drugs (NSAIDs): Nonsteroidal anti-inflammatory drugs should not be administered prior to or concomitantly with the high doses of Methotrexate used in the treatment of osteosarcoma. Concomitant administration of some NSAIDs with high dose METOJECT therapy has been reported to elevate and prolong serum methotrexate levels, resulting in deaths from severe hematologic and gastrointestinal toxicity.

Caution should be used when NSAIDs and salicylates are administered concomitantly with lower doses of METOJECT. These drugs have been reported to reduce the tubular secretion of METOJECT in an animal model, and may enhance its toxicity by increasing methotrexate levels.

In treating rheumatoid arthritis with methotrexate, acetyl salicylic acid (ASA), NSAIDs, and/or low dose steroids may be continued.

The possibility of increased toxicity with concomitant use of NSAIDs including salicylates has not been fully explored. Steroids may be reduced gradually in patients who respond to methotrexate. Combined use of methotrexate with gold, penicillamine, hydroxychloroquine, sulfasalazine, or cytotoxic agents has not been studied and may increase the incidence of adverse effects.

Despite the potential interactions, studies of methotrexate in patients with rheumatoid arthritis have usually included concurrent use of constant dosage regimens of NSAIDs without apparent problems. It should be appreciated however, that the doses used in rheumatoid arthritis (7.5 to 15 mg/week) are somewhat lower than those used in psoriasis and that larger doses could lead to unexpected toxicity.

Leflunomide: Methotrexate in combination with leflunomide may increase the risk of pancytopenia.

Drugs Highly Bound to Plasma Proteins: Methotrexate is partially bound to serum albumin, and toxicity may be increased because of displacement by certain drugs, such as salicylates, phenylbutazone, phenytoin and sulfonamides.

Probenecid: Renal tubular transport is also diminished by probenecid; use of METOJECT with this drug should be carefully monitored.

Nephrotoxic Drugs: In the treatment of patients with osteosarcoma, caution must be exercised if high-dose METOJECT is administered in combination with a potentially nephrotoxic chemotherapeutic agent (e.g., cisplatin). METOJECT clearance is decreased by cisplatinum.

Although not documented, other nephrotoxic drugs such as aminoglycosides, Amphotericin B and Cyclosporin could theoretically increase METOJECT toxicity by decreasing its elimination.

Penicillins and Sulfonamides: Penicillins and sulfonamides may reduce the renal clearance of METOJECT; hematologic and gastrointestinal toxicity have been observed in combination with METOJECT.

Oral Antibiotics: Oral antibiotics such as tetracycline, chloramphenicol, and non-absorbable broad spectrum antibiotics, may decrease intestinal absorption of METOJECT or interfere with the enterohepatic circulation by inhibiting bowel flora and suppressing metabolism of the drug by bacteria. For example: Neomycin, Polymyxin B, Nystatin and Vancomycin decrease METOJECT absorption, whereas Kanamycin increases METOJECT absorption.

Trimethoprim/sulfamethoxazole has been reported rarely to increase bone marrow suppression in patients receiving METOJECT, probably by decreased tubular secretion and/or an additive antifolate effect.

Theophylline: METOJECT may decrease the clearance of theophylline; theophylline levels should be monitored when used concurrently with METOJECT.

Mercaptopurine: Methotrexate increases the plasma levels of mercaptopurine. Combination of METOJECT and mercaptopurine may therefore require dose adjustment.

Vitamins: Vitamin preparations containing folic acid or its derivatives may decrease responses to systemically administered METOJECT. Preliminary animal and human studies have shown that small quantities of intravenously administered leucovorin enter the cerebrospinal fluid (CSF) primarily as 5-methyl tetrahydrofolate and, in humans, remain 1-3 orders of magnitude lower than the usual METOJECT concentrations following intrathecal administration. However, high doses of leucovorin may reduce the efficacy of intrathecally administered METOJECT.

In patients with rheumatoid arthritis or psoriasis, folic acid or folinic acid may reduce methotrexate toxicities such as gastrointestinal symptoms, stomatitis, alopecia and elevated liver enzymes.

Before taking a folate supplement, it is advisable to check B_{12} levels, particularly in adults over the age of 50, since folate administration can mask symptoms of B_{12} deficiency.

Folate deficiency states may increase METOJECT toxicity.

Radiotherapy: METOJECT given concomitantly with radiotherapy may increase the risk of soft tissue necrosis and osteonecrosis.

Hepatoxins: The potential for increased hepatotoxicity when METOJECT is administered with other hepatotoxic agents has not been evaluated. However, hepatotoxicity has been reported in such cases. Therefore, patients receiving concomitant therapy with METOJECT and other potential hepatotoxic agents (e.g., leflunomide, azathioprine, sulfasalazine, retinoids) should be closely monitored for possible increased risk of hepatotoxicity.

Cytarabine: METOJECT given concomitantly with cytarabine may increase the risk of severe neurologic adverse events such as headache, paralysis, coma and stroke-like episodes (see Warnings and Precautions, Neurologic).

Drug-Food Interactions: The bioavailability of orally administered methotrexate is reduced by food, particularly milk products.

DOSAGE AND ADMINISTRATION: Neoplastic Diseases: Dosing Considerations:

- Parenteral drug products should be inspected visually for particulate matter and discolouration prior to administration, whenever solution and container permit.
- METOJECT (methotrexate sodium) may be given by the intramuscular, intravenous, intra-arterial, intrathecal or intraventricular (via Ommaya reservoir into the CNS) routes.
- METOJECT may only be administered by physicians experienced in the treatment of neoplasia. The oncologist should consult the current literature for the treatment regimen to be used. Typical dosages reported in the literature for the following malignancies are listed in the following section.

Recommended Dose and Dosage Adjustment: Breast Cancer: The initial doses of CMF will be cyclophosphamide 100 mg/m² p.o. days 1 through 14, METOJECT 40 mg/m² IV day 1, 8, and 5-Fluorouracil 600 mg/m² IV day 1, 8. Cycle length will be 28 days ("2 weeks-on, 2 weeks-off"). In patients over 60 years of age, the dosage of METOJECT will be 30 mg/m² IV day 1, 8.

If total bilirubin exceeds 1.5 mg/dL, decrease the dose of METOJECT only by 50%.

Bladder Cancer: Typical dosage regimens for bladder cancer are the CMV Regimen and the "M-VAC Regimen" which are represented in Table 1 and Table 2.

Table 1: METOJECT

CMV Regimen[a]

	Days		
Drugs[b]	**1**	**2**	**8[e]**
Cisplatin[c]		100	
Vinblastine	4		4
Methotrexate[d]	30		30

[a] All doses in mg/m² with cycles repeated on day 22.
[b] Patients >70 years old receive 80% of all doses; if vomiting persists to day 8, no drug is given.
[c] For each cycle adjust cisplatin to 100% for Ccr >60 mL/min; 50% of dose for Ccr 50–60 mL/min; none for Ccr <50 mL/min.
[d] No drug for a decrease on day 8 of >30 mL/min compared to day 1 or Ccr <50 mL/min or Cr >1.8 mg/dL.
[e] Major dose modifications for both drugs depending on myelosuppression.

Table 2: METOJECT

M-VAC Regimen[a]

	Days			
Drugs	**1**	**2**	**15**	**22[c]**
Methotrexate	30		30	30
Vinblastine		3	3	3
Doxorubicin		30[b]		
Cisplatin		70		

[a] All doses in mg/m² with cycles repeated every 28–32 days.
[b] Patients having prior pelvic irradiation equivalent to >2500 rad in 5 days, reduce the dose of doxorubicin 15 mg/m².
[c] No doses given when the WBC <2500 cells/mm³, platelets >100 000 cells/mm³, or mucositis present.

Head and Neck Cancer: METOJECT remains the standard of therapy for patients with recurrent or metastatic disease. It has been given in a wide variety of doses and schedules (a few of which are represented in Table 3).

Table 3: METOJECT

METOJECT Schedule[a]

0.8 mg/kg every 4 days IV
25–50 mg every 4 to 7 days
60 mg/m² weekly IV or 40 mg/m² biweekly IV
40–60 mg/m² weekly IV
80 mg/m² for 30 h every 2 wk with escalation to toxicity
40 mg/m² weekly IV
40–200 mg/m² IV on days 1, 4 weekly; leucovorin on days 2, 5
60 mg/m² IV weekly

[a] Excerpt from Devita, et al: CANCER 3rd Ed., p. 496.

For palliation of patients with advanced incurable disease and acceptable renal function, it is appropriate to begin oral or intravenous methotrexate with weekly doses of 40-50 mg/m² or biweekly doses of 15 to 20 mg/m² and escalate the dose in weekly increments until either mild toxicity or therapeutic response is achieved.

Gastric Cancer: A regimen used in a clinical trial in Belgium in patients with resectable gastric cancer follows: METOJECT (1.5 g/m² IV day 1, + 5-Fluorouracil (1.5 g/m² IV) + Leucovorin (15 mg/m² orally or IV every 6 hours for 72 hours) + Adriamycin (30 mg/m² IV, day 15). The schedule is repeated on day 29 for 6 cycles.

Choriocarcinoma and Similar Trophoblastic Diseases: METOJECT is administered intramuscularly in doses of 15 to 30 mg daily for a 5 day course. Such courses are usually repeated for 3 to 5 times, as required, with rest periods of one or more weeks interposed between courses, until any manifesting toxic symptoms subside. The effectiveness of therapy is ordinarily evaluated by 24 hour quantitative analysis of urinary chorionic gonadotrophin hormone (beta-HCG), which should return to normal or less than 50 IU/24 hours usually after the third or fourth course, and usually be followed by a complete resolution of measurable lesions in four to six weeks. One to two courses of methotrexate after normalization of beta-HCG is usually recommended. Before each course of the drug, careful clinical assessment is essential. Cyclic combination therapy of METOJECT with other anti tumour drugs has been reported as being useful.

Since hydatiform mole may precede by choriocarcinoma, prophylactic chemotherapy with METOJECT has been recommended.

Chorioadenoma destruens is considered to be an invasive form of hydatiform mole. METOJECT is administered in these disease states in doses similar to those recommended for choriocarcinoma.

Lymphomas: In Burkitt's tumour, Stages I-II, METOJECT has produced prolonged remissions in some cases. Recommended dosage is 10 to 25 mg/day orally for 4 to 8 days. In Stage III, METOJECT is commonly given concomitantly with other antitumor agents. Treatment in all stages usually consists of several courses of the drug interposed with 7 to 10 day rest periods. Lymphosarcomas in Stage III may respond to combined drug therapy with METOJECT given in doses of 0.625 to 2.5 mg/kg daily.

The treatment of choice for localized histologically aggressive lymphoma is primary combination chemotherapy with or without involved-field radiation therapy. Frequently used regimens for intermediate, or high grade NHL that include METOJECT include groups: the ProMACE/MOPP, ProMACE-CytaBOM, Magrath Protocols. Represented in Table 4 for example, is the ProMACE-CytaBOM Regimen.

Table 4: METOJECT
ProMACE-CytaBOM Regimen

ProMACE-CytaBOM	Day 1	Day 8	Day 14	Days 15–21
Cyclophosphamide 650 mg/m² IV	x			No therapy
Doxorubicin 25 mg/m² IV	x			
Etoposide 120 mg/m² IV	x			
Cytarabine 300 mg/m² IV		x		
Bleomycin 5 mg/m² IV		x		
Vincristine 1.4 mg/m² IV		x		
Methotrexate 120 mg/m² IV		x with leucovorin rescue		
Prednisone 60 mg/m² PO	x....................................	x		
Co-trimoxazole 2 PO bid throughout 6 cycles of therapy				

In early stage childhood non-Hodgkin's lymphoma, METOJECT is used effectively in combination chemotherapy regimens.

Mycosis Fungoides (cutaneous T-cell lymphoma): Therapy with METOJECT appears to produce a clinical response, in up to 50% of patients treated, but chemotherapy is not curative. Dosage is usually 2.5 to 10 mg daily by mouth for several weeks or months. Dose levels of drug and adjustment of dose regimen by reduction or cessation of drug are guided by patient response and hematologic monitoring. METOJECT has also been given intramuscularly in doses of 50 mg once weekly or 25 mg 2 times weekly.

Leukemia : Acute lymphoblastic leukemia (ALL) in children and young adolescents is the most responsive to present day chemotherapy. In young adults and older patients, clinical remission is more difficult to obtain and early relapse is more common.

METOJECT alone or in combination with steroids was used initially for induction of remission in ALL. More recently, corticosteroid therapy in combination with other antileukemic drugs or in cyclic combinations with METOJECT, has appeared to produce rapid and effective remissions. When used for induction, METOJECT in doses of 3.3 mg/m² in combination with 60 mg/m² of prednisone, given daily, produced remission in 50% of patients treated usually within a period of 4 to 6 weeks. METOJECT in combination with other agents appears to be the drug of choice for securing maintenance of drug induced remissions. When remission is achieved and supportive care has produced general clinical improvement, maintenance therapy is initiated as follows: METOJECT is administered 2 times weekly either by mouth or intramuscularly in total weekly doses of 30 mg/m². It has also been given in doses of 2.5 mg/kg intravenously every 14 days. If and when relapse does occur, re-induction of remission can again usually be obtained by repeating the initial induction regimen.

A variety of combination chemotherapy regimens have been used for both induction and maintenance therapy in ALL. The physician should be familiar with recent advances in antileukemic therapy.

Meningeal Leukemia: In the treatment or prophylaxis of meningeal leukemia, METOJECT must be administered intrathecally.

For intrathecal administration, preservative free METOJECT is diluted to a concentration of 1 mg/mL in an appropriate sterile, preservative free medium such as 0.9% Sodium Chloride Injection, USP.

The cerebrospinal fluid volume is dependent on age and not on body surface area. The CSF is at 40% of the adult volume at birth and reaches the adult volume in several years.

Intrathecal METOJECT administration at a dose of 12 mg/m² (maximum 15 mg) has been reported to result in low CSF METOJECT concentrations and reduced efficacy in children and high concentrations and neurotoxicity in adults.

The following dosage regimen is based on age instead of body surface area:

Age (years)	Dose (mg)
<1	6
1	8
2	10
3 or older	12

In one study in patients under the age of 40, this dosage regimen appeared to result in more consistent CSF Methotrexate concentrations and less neurotoxicity. Another study in children with acute lymphocytic leukemia compared this regimen to a dose of 12 mg/m² (maximum 15 mg), a significant reduction in the rate of CNS relapse was observed in the group whose dose was based on age.

Because the CSF volume and turnover may decrease with age, a dose reduction may be indicated in elderly patients.

For the treatment of meningeal leukemia, intrathecal METOJECT may be given at intervals of 2 to 5 days. However, administration at intervals of less than 1 week may result in increased subacute toxicity. METOJECT is administered until the cell count of the cerebrospinal fluid returns to normal. At this point one additional dose is advisable. For prophylaxis against meningeal leukemia, the dosage is the same as for treatment except for the intervals of administration. On this subject, it is advisable for the physician to consult the medical literature.

Untoward side effects may occur with any given intrathecal injection and are commonly neurological in character. Large doses may cause convulsions. METOJECT given by the intrathecal route appears significantly in the systemic circulation and may cause systemic METOJECT toxicity. Therefore, systemic antileukemic therapy with the drug should be appropriately adjusted, reduced, or discontinued. Focal leukemic involvement of the central nervous system may not respond to intrathecal chemotherapy and is best treated with radiotherapy.

Leptomeningeal Carcinomatosis: Intrathecal administration of METOJECT as a single-drug or in combination regimens, is the most common therapy for carcinomatous leptomeningitis.

Treatment is optimally administered through an Ommaya reservoir and is usually started with METOJECT (10 mg/m²) given twice weekly until the cerebrospinal fluid cytology becomes negative. The treatment regimen is gradually decreased, first to a weekly course, and eventually to a single administration every two months.

Osteosarcoma: An effective adjuvant chemotherapy regimen requires the administration of several cytotoxic chemotherapeutic agents. In addition to high-dose METOJECT with leucovorin rescue, these agents may include doxorubicin, cisplatin, and the combination of bleomycin, cyclophosphamide and dactinomycin (BCD) in the doses and schedule shown in Table 5. The starting dose for high dose METOJECT treatment is 12 grams/m². If this dose is not sufficient to produce a peak serum METOJECT concentration of 1000 micromolar (10^{-3} mol/L) at the end of the METOJECT infusion, the dose may be escalated to 15 grams/m² in subsequent treatments. If the patient is vomiting or is unable to tolerate oral medication, leucovorin is given IV or IM at the same dose and schedule.

Table 5: METOJECT
Osteosarcoma

Drug[a]	Dose[a]	Treatment Week After Surgery
Methotrexate	12 g/m² IV as 4 hour infusion (starting dose)	4,5,6,7,11,12,15,16,29,30,44,45
Leucovorin	15 mg orally every six hours for 10 doses starting at 24 hours after start of Methotrexate infusion	
Doxorubicin[b] as a single drug	30 mg/m²/day IV×3 days	8,17
Doxorubicin[b]	50 mg/m² IV	20,23,33,36
Cisplatin[b]	100 mg/m² IV	20,23,33,36
Bleomycin[b]	15 units/m² IV × 2 days	2,13,26,39,42
Cyclophosphamide[b]	600 mg/m² IV×2 days	2,13,26,39,42
Dactinomycin[b]	0.6 mg/m² IV×2 days	2,13,26,39,42

[a] Link MP, Goorin AM, Miser AW, et al: The effect of adjuvant chemotherapy on relapse-free survival in patients with osteosarcoma of the extremity. N Engl J of Med 1986;314(No.25):1600-1606.

[b] See each respective package insert for full prescribing information. Dosage modifications may be necessary because of drug-induced toxicity.

When these higher doses of METOJECT are to be administered, the following safety guidelines should be closely observed.

Guidelines for METOJECT Therapy with Leucovorin Rescue:

1. Administration of METOJECT should be delayed until recovery if:
   - The WBC count is less than 1500/microliter
   - The neutrophil count is less than 200/microliter
   - The platelet count is less than 75 000/microliter
   - The serum bilirubin level is greater than 1.2 mg/dL
   - The ALT level is greater than 450 U
   - Mucositis is present, until there is evidence of healing
   - Persistent pleural effusion is present; this should be drained dry prior to infusion.
2. Adequate renal function must be documented.
   a. Serum creatinine must be normal, and creatinine clearance must be greater than 60 mL/min, before initiation of therapy.
   b. Serum creatinine must be measured prior to each subsequent course of therapy. If serum creatinine has increased by 50% or more compared to a prior value, the creatinine clearance must be measured and documented to be greater than 60 mL/min (even if the serum creatinine is still within the normal range).
3. Patients must be well hydrated, and must be treated with sodium bicarbonate for urinary alkalinization.
   a. Administer 1000 mL/m² of intravenous fluid over 6 hours prior to initiation of the METOJECT infusion. Continue hydration at 125 mL/m²/hr (3 liters/m²/day) during the METOJECT infusion, and for 2 days after the infusion has been completed.
   b. Alkalinize urine to maintain pH above 7.0 during METOJECT infusion and leucovorin calcium therapy. This can be accomplished by the administration of sodium bicarbonate orally or by incorporation into a separate intravenous solution.
4. Repeat serum creatinine and serum methotrexate 24 hours after starting METOJECT and at least once daily until the methotrexate level is below 5×10^{-8} mol/L (0.05 micromolar).
5. Table 6 provides guidelines for leucovorin calcium dosage based upon serum METOJECT levels (see Table 6).
   Patients who experience delayed early METOJECT elimination are likely to develop non-reversible oliguric renal failure. In addition to appropriate leucovorin therapy, these patients require continuing hydration and urinary alkalization, and close monitoring of fluid and electrolyte status, until the serum METOJECT level has fallen to below 0.05 micromolar and the renal failure has resolved. If necessary, acute, intermittent hemodialysis with a high-flux dialyzer may also be beneficial in these patients.
6. Some patients will have abnormalities in METOJECT elimination, or abnormalities in renal function following METOJECT administration, which are significant but less severe than the abnormalities described in Table 6. These abnormalities may or may not be associated with significant clinical toxicity. If significant clinical toxicity is observed, leucovorin rescue should be extended for an additional 24 hours (total 14 doses over 84 hours) in subsequent courses of therapy. The possibility that the patient is taking other medications which interact with METOJECT (e.g., medications which may interfere with METOJECT binding to serum albumin, or elimination) should always be reconsidered when laboratory abnormalities or clinical toxicities are observed.

Table 6: METOJECT
Leucovorin Rescue Schedules Following Treatment with Higher Doses of METOJECT

Clinical Situation	Laboratory Findings	Leucovorin Dosage and Duration
Normal Methotrexate Elimination	Serum METOJECT level approximately 10 micromolar at 24 hours after administration, 1 micromolar at 48 hours, and less than 0.2 micromolar at 72 hours.	15 mg PO, IM or IV q 6 hours for 60 hours (10 doses starting at 24 hours after start of METOJECT infusion).
Delayed Late Methotrexate Elimination	Serum METOJECT level remaining above 0.2 micromolar at 72 hours, and more than 0.05 micromolar at 96 hours after administration.	Continue 15 mg PO, IM or IV q six hours, until METOJECT level is less than 0.05 micromolar.

(cont'd)

Table 6: METOJECT *(cont'd)*

Leucovorin Rescue Schedules Following Treatment with Higher Doses of METOJECT

Clinical Situation	Laboratory Findings	Leucovorin Dosage and Duration
Delayed Early Methotrexate Elimination and/or Evidence of Acute Renal Injury	Serum METOJECT level of 50 micromolar or more at 24 hours, or 5 micromolar or more at 48 hours after administration, **or**; a 100% or greater increase in serum creatinine level at 24 hours after METOJECT administration (e.g., an increase from 0.5 mg/dL to a level of 1 mg/dL or more).	150 mg IV q three hours, until METOJECT level is less than 1 micromolar; than 15 mg IV q three hours, until METOJECT level is less than 0.05 micormolar.

Psoriasis and Rheumatoid Arthritis: Dosing Considerations:

- Refer to Neoplastic Diseases, Dosing Considerations.
- The patient should be fully informed of the risks involved and should be under constant supervision of the physician (see Warnings and Precautions, Information to Be Provided to the Patient).
- All dosage schedules should be continually tailored to the individual patient. An initial test dose may be given prior to the regular dosing schedule to detect any extreme sensitivity to adverse effects (see Adverse Reactions). Maximal myelosuppression usually occurs in seven to ten days.

Recommended Dose and Dosage Adjustments: Psoriasis: Recommended Starting Dose Schedules:

- Weekly single, IM or IV dose schedule: 10 to 25 mg per week until adequate response is achieved.

Dosages in each schedule may be gradually adjusted to achieve optimal clinical response; 30 mg/week should not ordinarily be exceeded.

Once optimal clinical response has been achieved, the dosage schedule should be reduced to the lowest possible amount of drug and to the longest possible rest period. The use of METOJECT may permit the return to conventional topical therapy, which should be encouraged.

Rheumatoid Arthritis: Recommended Starting Dosage Schedules: Therapeutic response usually begins within 3 to 6 weeks and the patient may continue to improve for another 12 weeks or more.

Administration: Dilution: METOJECT may be diluted with any of the solutions for IV infusion listed below in a concentration range of 0.4 mg/mL to 2 mg/mL. Dilutions should be used within 24 hours if kept at room temperature. Unused solution should be discarded after this time in order to avoid risk of microbial contamination.

Solutions: 0.9% Sodium Chloride Injection, 5% Dextrose Injection, 4% Dextrose and 0.18% Sodium Chloride Injection, Ringer's Injection.

Since methotrexate is poorly soluble in acid media, use of potassium chloride solution is not advisable.

If a preservative free diluent is used, the solution should be used immediately because of the possibility of microbial growth. It is advisable to protect diluted solutions from light.

Due to the number of brands available, stability data of METOJECT in plastic syringes and bags are not available.

Unused preservative free products should be discarded due to the possibility of microbial growth.

Incompatibilities: Other drugs should not be mixed with METOJECT in the same infusion bottle.

METOJECT has been reported to be incompatible with cytarabine, fluorouracil, and prednisolone sodium phosphate; however, its incompatibility with fluorouracil has been questioned. A mixture of METOJECT with cytarabine and hydrocortisone sodium succinate in various infusion fluids has been reported to be visually compatible for at least 8 hours at 25°C, although precipitation did not occur on storage for several days.

Contact with acidic solutions should be avoided since METOJECT is sparingly soluble in acid media and precipitation may occur.

See Warnings and Precautions for clinical incompatibilities.

OVERDOSAGE:

In post-marketing experience, overdose with methotrexate has generally occurred with intrathecal administration, although intravenous and intramuscular overdose have also been reported.

Discontinue or reduce dosage at the first sign of ulceration or bleeding, diarrhea, or marked depression of the hematopoietic system. Leucovorin is indicated to diminish the toxicity and counteract the effect of inadvertently administered overdosages of methotrexate. Leucovorin administration should begin as promptly as possible. As the time interval between methotrexate administration and leucovorin initiation increases, the effectiveness of leucovorin in counteracting toxicity decreases. Monitoring of the serum methotrexate concentration is essential in determining the optimal dose and duration of treatment with leucovorin.

In cases of massive overdosage, hydration and urinary alkalinization may be necessary to prevent the precipitation of methotrexate and/or its metabolites in the renal tubules. Generally, neither standard hemodialysis nor peritoneal dialysis has been shown to improve methotrexate elimination. However, effective clearance of methotrexate has been reported with acute, intermittent hemodialysis using a high-flux dialyzer.

There are published case reports of intravenous carboxypeptidase G2 treatment to hasten clearance of Methotrexate in cases of overdoses.

> For management of a suspected drug overdose, contact your regional Poison Control Centre. See the *CPS* Directory section for a list of Poison Control Centres.

ACTION AND CLINICAL PHARMACOLOGY: Mechanism of Action: Methotrexate is a folate antagonist.

Methotrexate inhibits dihydrofolate reductase (DHFR), the enzyme that reduces folic acid to tetrahydrofolic acid. Tetrahydrofolate must be regenerated via the DHFR-catalyzed reaction in order to maintain the intracellular pool of tetrahydrofolate one-carbon derivatives for both thymidylate and purine nucleotide biosynthesis. The inhibition of DHFR by folate antagonists (methotrexate) results in a deficiency in the cellular pools of thymidylate and purines and thus in a decrease in nucleic acid synthesis. Therefore, methotrexate interferes with DNA synthesis, repair, and cellular replication.

Methotrexate is most active against rapidly multiplying cells, because its cytotoxic effects occur primarily during the S phase of the cell cycle. Since cellular proliferation in malignant tissues is greater than in most normal tissues, methotrexate may impair malignant growth without irreversible damage to normal tissues. As a result, actively proliferating tissues, such as malignant cells, bone marrow, fetal cells, buccal and intestinal mucosa, and cells of the urinary bladder, are generally more sensitive to DHFR inhibition effects of methotrexate.

The cytotoxicity of methotrexate results from three important actions: inhibition of DHFR, inhibition of thymidylate synthase, and alteration of the transport of reduced folates. The affinity of DHFR to methotrexate is far greater than its affinity for folic acid or dihydrofolic acid, therefore, large doses of folic acid given simultaneously will not reverse the effects of methotrexate. However, Leucovorin Calcium, a derivative of tetrahydrofolic acid may block the effects of methotrexate if given shortly after the antineoplastic agent. Methotrexate in high doses, followed by leucovorin rescue, is used as a part of the treatment of patients with non-metastatic osteosarcoma.

The original rationale for high dose methotrexate therapy was based on the concept of selective rescue of normal tissues by leucovorin. More recent evidence suggests that high dose methotrexate may also overcome methotrexate resistance caused by impaired active transport, decreased affinity of dihydrofolic acid reductase for methotrexate, increased levels of dihydrofolic acid reductase resulting from gene amplification, or decreased polyglutamination of methotrexate. The actual mechanism of action is unknown.

Methotrexate has immunosuppressive activity. This may be a result of inhibition of lymphocyte multiplication. The mechanisms of action in the management of rheumatoid arthritis of the drug is not known, although suggested mechanisms have included immunosuppressive and/or anti-inflammatory effects.

In psoriasis, the rate of production of epithelial cells in the skin is greatly increased over normal skin. This differential in proliferation rates is the basis for the use of methotrexate to control the psoriatic process.

Pharmacokinetics: Absorption: Orally administered methotrexate is absorbed rapidly in most, but not all patients and reaches peak serum levels in 1 to 4 hours. Methotrexate is generally completely absorbed following parenteral administration, and after intramuscular injection peak serum concentrations occur in 30 to 60 minutes.

Distribution: Methotrexate in serum is approximately 50% protein bound. After intravenous administration, the initial volume of distribution is approximately 0.18 L/kg (18% of body weight) and steady-state volume of distribution is approximately 0.4 to 0.8 L/kg (40% to 80% of body weight). Methotrexate does not penetrate the blood-cerebrospinal fluid barrier in therapeutic amounts when given orally or parenterally.

Metabolism: After absorption, Methotrexate undergoes hepatic and intracellular metabolism to polyglutamated forms which can be converted back to methotrexate by hydrolase enzymes. These polyglutamates act as inhibitors of dihydrofolate reductase and thymidylate syntheses. Small amounts of methotrexate polyglutamates may remain in tissues for extended periods. The retention and prolonged drug action of these active metabolites vary among different cells, tissues and tumours. A small amount of metabolism to 7-hydroxymethotrexate may occur at doses commonly prescribed. The aqueous solubility of 7-hydroxymethotrexate is 3 to 5 fold lower than the parent compound. Methotrexate is partially metabolized by intestinal flora after oral administration.

Excretion: Renal excretion is the primary route of elimination and is dependent upon dosage and route of administration. Excretion of single daily doses occurs through the kidneys in amounts from 80% to 90% within 24 hours. Repeated daily doses result in more sustained serum levels and some retention of methotrexate over each 24 hour period, which may result in accumulation of the drug within the tissues. The liver cells appear to retain certain amounts of the drug for prolonged periods even after a single therapeutic dose. Methotrexate is retained in the presence of impaired renal function and may increase rapidly in the serum and in the tissue cells under such conditions. Methotrexate does not penetrate the blood-cerebrospinal fluid barrier in therapeutic amounts when given orally or parenterally. High concentrations of the drug, when needed, may be attained by direct intrathecal administration.

The terminal half-life reported for methotrexate is approximately 3 to 10 hours for patients receiving treatment for psoriasis, rheumatoid arthritis or low dose antineoplastic therapy (less than 30 mg/m²). For patients receiving high doses of methotrexate, the terminal half-life is 8 to 15 hours.

Methotrexate clearance rates vary widely and are generally decreased at higher doses.

Special Populations and Conditions: Nursing Women: Methotrexate has been detected in human breast milk and is contraindicated during breast feeding. The highest breast milk to plasma concentration ratio reached was 0.08:1.

STORAGE AND STABILITY: Keep in a safe place out of the reach of children.

Store METOJECT between 15-25°C. Any unused solution should be discarded. Protect from light.

SPECIAL HANDLING INSTRUCTIONS: General: Individuals who have contact with anti-cancer drugs or work in areas where these drugs are used, may be exposed to these agents in air or through direct contact with contaminated objects. Potential health effects may be reduced by adherence to institutional procedures, published guidelines and local regulations for preparation, administration, transportation and disposal of hazardous drugs.

Safe Handling and Disposal: Methotrexate is a potent anti-neoplastic drug. Good medical practice will minimize exposure of persons involved with frequent handling of this drug as outlined below:

Handling:

1. Methotrexate has no vesicant properties and does not show acute toxicity on topical contact with the skin or mucous membranes. However, persons involved with handling cytotoxic drugs should avoid contact with skin and inhalation of airborne particles.
2. Preparation of antineoplastic solutions should be done in a vertical laminar flow hood (Biological Safety Cabinet—Class II).
3. Personnel preparing Methotrexate solutions should wear PVC gloves, safety glasses and protective clothing such as disposable gowns and masks.
4. Personnel regularly involved in preparation and handling of antineoplastics should have bi-annual blood examinations.

Disposal:

1. Avoid contact with skin and inhalation of airborne particles by use of PVC gloves and disposable gowns and masks.
2. All needles, syringes, vials and other materials for disposal which have come in contact with Methotrexate should be segregated in plastic bags, sealed and marked as hazardous waste. Incinerate at 1000°C or higher. Sealed containers may explode if a tight seal exists.
3. If incineration is not available, rinse all needles, syringes, tubing and other materials for disposal which have come in contact with Methotrexate solutions with water and discard in the sewer system with running water.

Rinse vials with the appropriate quantity of water with the aid of a hypodermic syringe. Withdraw the solution and discard in the sewer system with running water. Dispose of rinsed equipment and vials in a safe manner.

Cleaning: Non-disposable equipment that has come in contact with methotrexate may be rinsed with water and washed thoroughly with soap and water.

Spillage/Contamination: Wear gloves, mask and protective clothing. Place spilled material in an appropriate container (i.e. cardboard for broken glass) and then in a polyethylene bag; absorb remains with gauze pads or towels; wash area with water and absorb with gauze or towels again and place in bag; seal, double bag and mark as a hazardous waste. Dispose of waste by incineration or by other methods approved for hazardous materials. Personnel involved in clean up should wash with soap and water.

INFORMATION FOR THE PATIENT: Published in e-CPS, available by subscription at www.e-cps.ca.

DOSAGE FORMS, COMPOSITION AND PACKAGING: Each mL of solution for injection contains: methotrexate sodium 10 mg. Nonmedicinal ingredients: sodium chloride, sodium hydroxide and water. Syringes of 1 mL with 0.75 mL solution for injection, equivalent to 7.5 mg methotrexate. Syringes of 1 mL with 1 mL solution for injection, equivalent to 10 mg methotrexate. Syringes of 2.25 mL with 1.5 mL solution for injection, equivalent to 15 mg methotrexate. Syringes of 2.25 mL with 2 mL solution for injection, equivalent to 20 mg methotrexate. Syringes of 3 mL with 2.5 mL solution for injection, equivalent to 25 mg methotrexate. Single-use pre-filled syringes, cartons of 1, 5 and 10. Each carton of one syringe will also contain a single needle for use with METOJECT. The sterile hypodermic needle is a Sterican and is for single-use only.

Metolazone ℞

CPhA Monograph

see *Thiazide Diuretics*

Metoprolol Tartrate Injection USP ℞

metoprolol tartrate

Beta-adrenergic Receptor Blocking Agent

Sandoz

SUPPLIED: Each mL contains: metoprolol tartrate 1 mg. Nonmedicinal ingredients: sodium chloride for isotonicity and water for injection. Single use vials of 5 mL, boxes of 5. Store between 2 and 30°C. Protect from light. Protect from freezing. Discard unused portion.

MetroCream® [Rx]
metronidazole
Antirosacea Agent

Galderma

MetroGel® [Rx]
metronidazole
Antirosacea Agent

Galderma

MetroLotion® [Rx]
metronidazole
Antirosacea Agent

Galderma

Date of Revision: July 17, 2007

SUMMARY PRODUCT INFORMATION:

Route of Administration	Dosage Form/ Strength	Clinically Relevant Nonmedicinal Ingredients
Topical	Metronidazole gel USP, 0.75% metronidazole gel Galderma Std, 1 % metronidazole cream, 0.75% metronidazole lotion, 0.75%	Methylparaben, propylparaben, propylene glycol, phenoxyethanol For a complete listing see Dosage Forms, Composition and Packaging.

INDICATIONS AND CLINICAL USE: METROGEL (0.75% and 1%), METROCREAM (0.75%), and METROLOTION (0.75%) (metronidazole topical gel, cream, and lotion) are indicated for:

- topical application in the treatment of inflammatory papules, pustules, and erythema of rosacea. Patients with dry or sensitive skin may prefer using the cream or lotion formulation (i.e., METROCREAM or METROLOTION).

Geriatrics (≥65 years of age): While specific clinical trials in the geriatric population have not been conducted, 66 patients aged 65 years and older treated with METROGEL 1% over 10 weeks showed comparable safety and efficacy as compared to the general study population.

Pediatrics: Safety and effectiveness in pediatrics have not been established.

CONTRAINDICATIONS: METROGEL, METROCREAM, and METROLOTION (metronidazole topical gel, cream, and lotion) are contraindicated:

- in individuals with a history of hypersensitivity to metronidazole, or other ingredients of the formulations. For a complete listing, see Dosage Forms, Composition and Packaging.

WARNINGS AND PRECAUTIONS: General: Because of the minimal absorption of metronidazole, and consequently its insignificant plasma concentration after topical administration, the systemic adverse reactions reported with the oral form of the drug should not be expected with METROGEL, METROCREAM, or METROLOTION (metronidazole topical gel, cream, or lotion).

Physicians should consider the most appropriate formulation (gel, cream, or lotion) for their patients.

Although rosacea is a chronic disease, data on the long-term use of METROGEL, METROCREAM, or METROLOTION in rosacea is not available. In controlled clinical trials, patients were treated for up to12 weeks (see Dosage and Administration).

Carcinogenesis and Mutagenesis: Information from preclinical studies indicates that metronidazole and its principal metabolite are mutagenic in bacteria and that tumours were observed in animal studies after oral administration of metronidazole. The relevance of these findings to the topical use of metronidazole in humans is unknown. The anaerobic or hypoxic conditions that might lead to the production of genotoxic compounds are unlikely to occur in topical use. There is no conclusive evidence after 30 years of clinical use of systemic metronidazole for either a genotoxic or carcinogenic potential.

Hematologic: Metronidazole is a nitroimidazole and should be used with care in patients with evidence of, or history of, blood dyscrasia.

Ophthalmologic: Avoid contact with the eyes. Topical metronidazole has been reported to cause tearing of the eyes. It should not be used in or close to the eye. If contact does occur, flush with water.

Conjunctivitis associated with topical use of metronidazole on the face has been reported.

Sensitivity/Resistance: Exposure to excessive sunlight, including sunlamps and tanning beds, should be avoided when using METROGEL, METROCREAM, or METROLOTION (based on studies in hairless mice treated with intraperitoneal metronidazole).

Skin: If a reaction suggesting local irritation occurs, patients should be directed to use the medication less frequently, discontinue use temporarily, or discontinue use until further instructions.

There were no reports of contact dermatitis attributed to METROGEL and METROCREAM, during clinical trials. However, there have been reports of contact dermatitis/allergic reaction reported during METROLOTION clinical trials and as post marketing adverse reactions (see Adverse Reactions). Physicians should be aware of the possibility of skin sensitivity reactions and of cross-sensitization with other imidazole preparations, such as clotrimazole and tioconazole.

Special Populations: Pregnant Women: There has been no experience to date with the use of METROGEL, METROCREAM, or METROLOTION (metronidazole) in pregnant patients. Metronidazole crosses the placental barrier and enters the fetal circulation rapidly. No fetotoxicity was observed after oral metronidazole in rats or mice. However, because animal reproduction studies are not always predictive of human response, this drug should only be used during pregnancy after careful assessment of the risk/benefit ratio.

Nursing Women: Even though metronidazole blood levels are significantly lower after topical application than after oral administration a decision should be made whether to discontinue nursing or to discontinue the drug, taking into account the importance of the drug to the mother. After oral administration, metronidazole is secreted in breast milk in concentrations similar to those found in the plasma.

ADVERSE REACTIONS: Adverse Drug Reaction Overview: The safety profile of METROGEL (metronidazole topical gel 0.75% and 1%), METROCREAM (metronidazole topical cream 0.75%) and METROLOTION (metronidazole topical lotion 0.75%) has been established in clinical trials. The results of the safety analyses indicate topical application of metronidazole is well tolerated.

Clinical Trial Adverse Drug Reactions: Because clinical trials are conducted under very specific conditions the adverse reaction rates observed in the clinical trials may not reflect the rates observed in practice and should not be compared to the rates in the clinical trials of another drug. Adverse drug reaction information from clinical trials is useful for identifying drug-related adverse events and for approximating rates.

Metronidazole Topical Gel 1%: In a 10-week controlled clinical trial in patients with rosacea, 557 patients used METROGEL (metronidazole gel), 1% and 189 patients used the gel vehicle once daily.

Among the treatment groups, the adverse reactions considered related to treatment were low with comparable frequencies. The majority of the adverse reactions were mild or moderate in severity.

Adverse reactions considered related to once daily treatment with METROGEL 1% were reported at a frequency of <1% and are summarized in Table 1.

Metronidazole Topical Gel 0.75%: The patient safety database included 114 evaluable patients that participated in controlled and uncontrolled METROGEL (metronidazole topical gel) trials. Adverse reactions attributed to the use of METROGEL are summarized in Table 2.

Metronidazole Topical Cream: In controlled clinical trials with METROCREAM (metronidazole topical cream), the patient safety database included 71 evaluable patients. Adverse reactions attributed to the use of METROCREAM are summarized in Table 3.

Metronidazole Topical Lotion: During controlled clinical trials with METROLOTION (metronidazole topical lotion), the patient safety database included 72 evaluable patients. Adverse reactions attributed to the use of METROLOTION are summarized in Table 4.

Table 1: METROGEL

Adverse Reactions Attributed to METROGEL 1% (metronidazole topical gel)[a]

System Organ Class/Adverse Reactions	Incidence (no. of patients)	Severity (no. of patients)	Follow-up Treatment
Skin and Subcutaneous Tissue Disorders			
Dry skin	0.9% (5)	mild (2)	treatment required
		mild	none required
		mild	none required[b]
		moderate	none required[c]
Erythema	0.7% (4)	moderate (3)	none required[b]
		severe	treatment required[b]
Pruritus	0.5% (3)	mild	none required[b]
		moderate	none required[b]
		severe	treatment required[b]
Skin burning sensation	0.2% (1)	mild	none required[c]
Skin irritation	0.2% (1)	severe	treatment required[b]
Rash papular	0.4% (2)	mild	none required
		moderate	none required[b]
Skin desquamation	0.2% (1)	moderate	none required[b]
Skin tightness	0.4% (2)	mild	none required[c]
Facial oedema	0.2% (1)	severe	treatment required[b]
Urticaria	0.2% (1)	moderate	treatment required[b]
Eye Disorders			
Conjunctivitis	0.4% (2)	mild	treatment required
		mild	treatment required[b]
Eye irritation	0.2% (1)	mild	none required
Gastrointestinal Disorders			
Dyspepsia	0.2% (1)	mild	treatment required

[a] MedDRA version 9.0 has been used for coding of adverse reactions.
[b] Drug discontinued.
[c] Therapy interrupted/reduced.

Table 2: METROGEL

Adverse Reactions Attributed to METROGEL 0.75% (metronidazole topical gel)

System Organ Class/Adverse Reactions	Incidence (no. of patients)	Severity	Follow-up Treatment
Skin and Subcutaneous Disorders			
Skin irritation	1.8% (2)	mild	none required
Dry skin	1.8% (2)	mild	none required
Erythema	1.8% (2)	mild	none required
Burning sensation	0.9% (1)	mild	none required
Eye Disorders			
Lacrimation increased	0.9% (1)	mild	none required

Table 3: METROCREAM

Adverse Reactions Attributed to METROCREAM (metronidazole topical cream)

System Organ Class/Adverse Reactions	Incidence (no. of patients)	Severity	Follow-up Treatment
Skin and Subcutaneous Disorders			
Skin discomfort (burning and stinging)	2.8% (2)	moderate	none required
		moderate	drug discontinued
Rosacea	1.4% (1)	mild	drug discontinued
Erythema	1.4% (1)	moderate	drug discontinued
Skin irritation	1.4% (1)	moderate	drug discontinued
Pruritus	1.4% (1)	moderate	none required

Table 4: METROLOTION

Adverse Reactions Attributed to METROLOTION (metronidazole topical lotion)

System Organ Class/Adverse Reactions	Incidence (no. of patients)	Severity	Follow-up Treatment
Skin and Subcutaneous Disorders			
Hypersensitivity	2.8% (2)	moderate	drug discontinued
Dermatitis contact	1.4% (1)	mild	therapy interrupted temporarily
	1.4% (1)	moderate	drug discontinued
Erythema	2.8% (2)	mild	none required
	2.8% (2)	moderate	drug discontinued
Rosacea	1.4% (1)	mild	drug discontinued

Post-Market Adverse Drug Reactions: Since commercialization of METROGEL (0.75%, 1%), METROCREAM and METROLOTION, the following post marketing adverse reactions have been reported.

A causal relationship with topical metronidazole has not been unequivocally established for these adverse drug reactions.

Post Marketing Adverse Drug Reactions by System Organ Class, MedDRA preferred term for METROGEL, METROCREAM and METROLOTION: Blood and Lymphatic Disorders: leucopenia.
Eye Disorders: lacrimation increased.
Gastrointestinal Disorders: dysgeusia, nausea.
General Disorders and Administration: condition aggravated.
Immune System Disorders: hypersensitivity.
Nervous System Disorders: paraesthesia.
Skin and Subcutaneous Tissue Disorders: dermatitis contact, dry skin, erythema, pruritus, rash pustular, dermatitis bullous, skin burning sensation, skin irritation.

DRUG INTERACTIONS: Drug-Drug Interactions: See Table 5.

Table 5: METROCREAM/METROGEL/METROLOTION

Established or Potential Drug-Drug Interactions

Metronidazole	Ref	Effect	Clinical Comment
Coumarin and warfarin	C/CT	Potentiate the anticoagulant effect	Drug interactions are less likely with topical administration but should be kept in mind when metronidazole is prescribed for patients who are receiving anticoagulant treatment. Oral metronidazole has been reported to potentiate the anticoagulant effect of coumarin and warfarin resulting in a prolongation of prothrombin time.
Alcohol	T (topical) C (oral)	Disulfiram-like reaction	Oral metronidazole also interacts with alcohol, producing a disulfiram-like reaction. Although this adverse reaction has not been reported with topical application of metronidazole, a drug interaction of metronidazole-alcohol is a possibility.
Other imidazole preparations such as clotrimazole and tioconazole	T	Skin sensitivity	Physicians should be aware of the possibility of skin sensitivity reactions and of cross-sensitization with other imidazole preparations.

Legend: C=Case Study; CT=Clinical Trial; T=Theoretical.

DOSAGE AND ADMINISTRATION: Recommended Dose and Dosage Adjustment: METROGEL 1%: Apply and rub in a thin film once daily to entire affected area(s).
METROGEL 0.75%, METROCREAM 0.75%, AND METROLOTION 0.75%: Apply and rub in a thin film twice daily, morning and evening, to entire affected areas.

Significant therapeutic results should be noticed within three weeks. Clinical studies have demonstrated continuing improvement through nine weeks of therapy. The dosage required for long-term administration is uncertain (see Warnings and Precautions).

Administration: Areas to be treated should be cleansed before application of METROGEL, METROCREAM, or METROLOTION. The face must be dry before applying medication.

Patients may use cosmetics after application of METROGEL, METROCREAM, or METROLOTION. The medication should have absorbed into the skin ("dry") before the cosmetics are applied.

OVERDOSAGE:
There is no human experience with overdosage of METROGEL, METROCREAM, or METROLOTION (metronidazole topical gel, cream, or lotion). Topically applied metronidazole can be absorbed in sufficient amount to produce systemic effects.

Massive ingestion may produce vomiting and slight disorientation. There is no specific antidote. Ipecac syrup or gastric lavage; then activated charcoal followed by a saline cathartic is suggested. Treatment should include symptomatic and supportive therapy.

> For management of a suspected drug overdose, CPhA recommends that you contact your **regional Poison Control Centre**. See the *CPS* Directory section for a list of Poison Control Centres.

ACTION AND CLINICAL PHARMACOLOGY: Mechanism of Action: METROGEL, METROCREAM, and METROLOTION (metronidazole topical gel, cream, and lotion) preparations are particularly effective against the inflammatory, papulopustular component of rosacea. The mechanisms by which topical metronidazole acts in reducing inflammatory lesions of rosacea are unknown, but may include an anti-bacterial and/or an anti-inflammatory effect.

Pharmacokinetics: Serum metronidazole levels have been shown to be below detection limits (<25 ng/mL) at the majority of time points after administration of topical metronidazole. At the time points that it could be detected, topical metronidazole produced blood levels (C_{max} 40.6 ng/mL) that were approximately 80% less than a similar dose administered orally (C_{max} 212 ng/mL). Therefore, with normal usage, topical metronidazole results in minimal blood levels of metronidazole.

STORAGE AND STABILITY: METROGEL 1% (metronidazole topical gel): Store at room temperature (15 to 30°C).
METROGEL 0.75% and METROCREAM (metronidazole topical gel and cream): Store at 15 to 30°C.
METROLOTION (metronidazole topical lotion): Store at room temperature (15 to 30°C). Protect from freezing.

INFORMATION FOR THE PATIENT: Published in e-CPS, available by subscription at www.e-cps.ca.

DOSAGE FORMS, COMPOSITION AND PACKAGING: METROCREAM: The white, smooth, emollient cream contains: metronidazole 0.75%. Nonmedicinal ingredients: benzyl alcohol, emulsifying wax, glycerin, isopropyl palmitate, lactic acid and/or sodium hydroxide, purified water and sorbitol solution. Aluminum tubes of 60 g.

METROGEL: 0.75%: The clear, colorless gel contains: metronidazole 0.75%. Nonmedicinal ingredients: carbomer 940, edetate disodium, methylparaben, propylene glycol, propylparaben, purified water and sodium hydroxide. Aluminum tubes of 60 g.

1%: The aqueous gel contains: metronidazole 1%. Nonmedicinal ingredients: betadex, edetate disodium, hydroxyethyl cellulose 250 HHX, methylparaben, niacinamide, phenoxyethanol, propylene glycol, propylparaben and purified water. Aluminum tubes of 60 g.

METROLOTION: The fluid, emollient lotion, contains: metronidazole 0.75%. Nonmedicinal ingredients: benzyl alcohol, carbomer 941, cyclomethicone, glycerin, glyceryl stearate, light mineral oil, polyethylene glycol 100 stearate, polyethylene glycol 400, potassium sorbate, purified water, sodium hydroxide and/or lactic acid, stearyl alcohol and steareth-21. Oval plastic bottles of 120 mL.

Metronidazole ℞

Antibacterial—Antiprotozoal

CPhA Monograph

Date of Revision: May 2009

> This monograph has been compiled by CPhA and reviewed by experts. It may contain information different from that found in Health Canada-approved Product Monographs. The reader is referred to the *CPS* Editorial Policy for more information.

SUMMARY PRODUCT INFORMATION:

Drug	Route of Administration	Dosage Form	Strength
Single Entity:			
Metronidazole	Injection	solution	5 mg/mL
	Intravaginal	vaginal cream	10% w/w
	Intravaginal	vaginal gel	7.5 mg/g
	Oral	capsule	500 mg
	Oral	tablet	250 mg
	Oral	tablet—extended release	750 mg
	Topical	cream	1%
	Topical	cream, gel, lotion	0.75%
Combination:			
Metronidazole/nystatin	Intravaginal	vaginal cream, vaginal ovules	metronidazole 500 mg/ nystatin 100 000 units per applicatorful or ovule
Metronidazole/Parsol MCX/Parsol 1789	Topical	cream	metronidazole 1%, parsol MCX 7.5%, parsol 1789 2%

PHARMACOLOGY: Metronidazole, a synthetic nitroimidazole derivative, is amebicidal, trichomonacidal and bactericidal. A chemically reactive, reduced form of metronidazole is thought to be responsible for its pharmacologic activity. The reduced substrate affects anoxic or hypoxic cells causing loss of the helical structure of DNA, strand breakage and impairment of cellular function.

The spectrum of activity of metronidazole includes: anaerobic gram-negative bacilli, including most Bacteroides species, Fusobacterium and Prevotella; anaerobic gram-negative cocci including Veillonellaceae; anaerobic gram-positive bacilli including Clostridium and Eubacterium; anaerobic gram-positive cocci including Peptococcus and Peptostreptococcus. Metronidazole is also active against *Helicobacter pylori*, *Gardnerella vaginalis* and the protozoa *Entamoeba histolytica*, *Trichomonas vaginalis* and *Giardia lamblia*. Metronidazole acts primarily against the trophozoite forms of *E. histolytica* and has limited activity against the encysted forms. Metronidazole is active against *Clostridium difficile*, a common cause of nosocomial diarrhea and nearly all cases of pseudomembranous colitis.

Metronidazole is not active against fungi, viruses and most aerobic and anaerobic gram-positive non-spore-forming bacilli, i.e., Actinomyces, Lactobacillus and Propionibacterium species, including *P. acnes*.

The mechanism by which topical metronidazole reduces inflammatory lesions of rosacea is unknown.

Pharmacokinetics: Following oral administration, metronidazole is well absorbed (>90%) from the gastrointestinal tract. Peak serum levels following an oral dose occur in 1 to 2 hours. Peak metronidazole levels occur at the end of iv infusion.

With normal usage, only trace amounts of metronidazole are found in the serum following topical application of a 0.75% gel. Following vaginal administration of a 5 g dose of a 0.75% gel, systemic absorption is minimal (equivalent to 2% of the mean serum concentration achieved following a single 500 mg oral dose). Peak plasma metronidazole levels were 15.56 µg/mL, 1.86 µg/mL and 1.89 µg/mL after a single 500 mg dose administered orally, as a vaginal cream and as a vaginal insert, respectively [*Obstet Gynecol* 1985;65(6):781-4]. Metronidazole is less than 20% bound to serum proteins and is widely distributed in the body. It reaches all tissues and fluids, with CSF concentrations reaching approximately 43% of serum concentrations. Metronidazole exhibits concentration-dependent killing of susceptible bacteria and is associated with a prolonged post-antibiotic effect. The drug crosses the placenta and is distributed into breast milk. Metronidazole is metabolized in the liver to five metabolites, of which only one is active. The hydroxymetabolite is 30 to 65% active relative to its parent. It is excreted primarily in the urine as metabolites, with approximately 20% of a dose excreted as unchanged drug. The half-life of metronidazole in adults ranges between 6 and 12 hours. Accumulation may occur in patients with severely impaired hepatic function; dose reduction may be indicated. Dose adjustment is generally unnecessary in patients with decreased renal function.

Metronidazole is removed by hemodialysis but is not significantly removed by peritoneal dialysis.

INDICATIONS AND CLINICAL USE: Metronidazole is indicated for:

- Treatment of protozoal infections, i.e., trichomoniasis, giardiasis, intestinal amebiasis, amebic abscesses of the liver

  According to the 2006 Canadian Sexually Transmitted Infections (STI) guidelines (updated January 2008), oral metronidazole is the preferred treatment for patients with trichomoniasis [http://www.phac-aspc.gc.ca/std-mts/sti_2006/pdf/408_Vaginal_Discharge.pdf]
- Treatment of bacterial vaginosis

  According to the 2006 Canadian STI guidelines (updated January 2008), oral/intravaginal metronidazole and intravaginal clindamycin are the preferred treatments in patients with symptomatic bacterial vaginosis [http://www.phac-aspc.gc.ca/std-mts/sti_2006/pdf/408_Vaginal_Discharge.pdf].
- Treatment of serious anaerobic intra-abdominal infections due to susceptible anaerobic bacteria such as *B. fragilis* (and other species of Bacteroides), Clostridium, Fusobacterium, Peptococcus, Peptostreptococcus species

  For mixed aerobic and anaerobic infections, administer appropriate antibiotic(s) for treatment of the aerobic component of the infection (see Warnings). According to the 2003 Guidelines for the Selection of Anti-infective Agents for Complicated Intra-abdominal Infections, metronidazole is used, as an adjunct for the treatment of complicated intra-abdominal infections [*Clin Infect Dis* 2003;37(8):997-1005].
- Treatment of mixed vaginal infection due to *T. vaginalis* and *C. albicans* in combination with nystatin
- Treatment of *H. pylori*-associated peptic ulcer disease

  The American College of Gastroenterology guideline on the management of *H. pylori* infection recommends metronidazole as part of a 3 to 4 drug regimen (except in areas where resistance to metronidazole is exceedingly high). Metronidazole, a proton pump inhibitor (PPI) and clarithromycin comprise a 3-drug regimen. Quadruple therapy includes a PPI or histamine H_2-receptor antagonist, bismuth, tetracycline and metronidazole [*Am J Gastroenterol* 2007;102(8):1808-25].
- Treatment of inflammatory papules, pustules and erythema of rosacea

  Topical metronidazole may be used as initial treatment in mild to moderate rosacea to clear inflammatory lesions. In severe rosacea, it may be used in combination with oral antibiotics.

Other Clinical Uses:

Oral metronidazole is used in the treatment of mild to moderate *C. difficile*-associated diarrhea (CDAD). The major risk factor for CDAD is antimicrobial use. If possible, discontinue offending antimicrobials and provide hydration and electrolyte replacement. Because of its lower cost relative to vancomycin and concern for selection for vancomycin-resistant *E. faecium*, oral metronidazole is considered first-line therapy. Metronidazole iv may be considered for patients where oral therapy is not feasible.

Metronidazole is used in the treatment of periodontal infections. It is also used as an adjunct in acute necrotizing ulcerative gingivitis.

Treatment of anaerobic soft tissue and central nervous system infections. According to the 2005 Practice Guidelines for the Diagnosis and Management of Skin and Soft-Tissue Infections, metronidazole may be used as an adjunct for intestinal or genital tract surgical site infections, animal and human bites, and treatment of necrotizing infections of the skin, fascia and muscle, for its anaerobic activity [*Clin Infect Dis* 2005;41(10):1373-406]. Because of its excellent penetration into the CSF and brain abscess cavities, metronidazole is used as an adjunct for the treatment of brain abscess [*Clin Infect Dis* 1997;25(4):763-79].

Management of diverticulitis includes hydration and broad spectrum antibiotics which include metronidazole [*Dis Colon Rectum* 2006;49(7):939-44].

As an adjunct for the treatment of mixed infections where anaerobes are suspected such as in sepsis and only in aspiration pneumonia in patients with poor dental hygiene or putrid sputum [*N Engl J Med* 2001;344(9):665-71].

According to the American College of Gastroenterology Guidelines on the management of Crohn's disease in adults, metronidazole has been used in patients with mild to moderate active Crohn's disease with ileocolonic or colonic disease who have not responded to sulfasalazine. Metronidazole has not been shown to induce remission. Metronidazole may benefit patients after ileocolonic resections by reducing the likelihood of recurrence when corticosteroids are not effective [*Am J Gastroenterol* 2009;104(2):465-83; *Gastroenterology* 1982;83(3):550-62].

CONTRAINDICATIONS:

- Patients who are hypersensitive to metronidazole, other nitroimidazole derivatives or to any ingredient in the formulation.

The manufacturer states that metronidazole should be used with caution in patients with a history of blood dyscrasias.

WARNINGS: Metronidazole is not active against fungi, viruses and most aerobic and anaerobic gram-positive non-spore-forming bacilli, i.e., Actinomyces, Lactobacillus and Propionibacterium species, including *P. acnes*. In patients with mixed aerobic-anaerobic infections, appropriate concomitant antibiotics active against the aerobic component and anaerobic non-spore-forming gram-positive bacilli should be considered.

Convulsive seizures and peripheral neuropathy, characterized by numbness, tingling, pain, or weakness in the hands or feet, have been reported in patients treated with metronidazole (administered orally or iv). Peripheral neuropathy often occurs in patients receiving large doses and over prolonged periods, e.g., >15 to 20 mg/kg/day for 2 to 4 weeks [*J Child Neurol* 2006;21(5):429-31; *Br Med J* 1977;2(6087):610-1]. If abnormal neurologic symptoms occur, treatment must be discontinued immediately.

Advise patients to avoid consuming alcohol during therapy and 48 h post-treatment. See Table 1 for information on the metronidazole-ethanol interaction.

PRECAUTIONS: When metronidazole is used in the treatment of trichomoniasis, sexual contacts should be treated concurrently regardless of symptomatology. To minimize the risk of reinfection and transmission, patients should be advised to abstain from intercourse or to use a condom during intercourse for the duration of treatment.

When metronidazole is used in the treatment of acute intestinal amebiasis and amebic liver abscess caused by *E. histolytica*, sequential treatment with an intraluminal amebicide (such as iodoquinol or paromomycin) is recommended. Metronidazole is not indicated in cases of asymptomatic amebiasis, as it has limited activity against encysted *E. histolytica*.

Transient eosinophilia and leukopenia have been observed during treatment with metronidazole.

Treatment with metronidazole should be discontinued if ataxia or any other symptom of CNS involvement occurs.

Patients with severe hepatic disease metabolize metronidazole slowly with resultant accumulation of metronidazole and its metabolites in the plasma. Accordingly, for such patients, doses of metronidazole below those usually recommended should be administered and with caution.

<u>*Drug Interactions*</u>: See Table 1.

Table 1: Metronidazole

Drug-Drug Interactions

Interacting Drug	Effect	Clinical Comment
Amprenavir, oral solution	Enhances propylene glycol toxicity; metronidazole inhibits its metabolism	Avoid combination.
Busulfan	Metronidazole may increase busulfan trough serum levels.	Avoid combination. If used concomitantly, monitor for signs and symptoms of busulfan toxicity such as elevated liver enzymes, hemorrhagic cystitis and veno-occlusive disease.
Ethanol	A possible disulfiram-like reaction characterized by flushing, palpitations, tachycardia, nausea and vomiting may occur with concomitant use.	Advise patients to avoid consuming alcohol during therapy and 48 h post-treatment. Advise patients of alcohol content in commercially available medications, e.g., Kaletra oral solution, Septra injection.
Fluorouracil	May increase serum levels of fluorouracil by reducing its clearance.	Monitor for increased adverse effects of fluorouracil such as gastrointestinal and hematological.
Mebendazole	Combination may result in Stevens-Johnson syndrome (SJS) or toxic epidermal necrolysis (TEN).	Avoid concurrent use. If use concomitantly, consider using a lower dose of metronidazole. Monitor for signs and symptoms of SJS/TEN.
Warfarin	Metronidazole may inhibit warfarin metabolism through CYP2C9 inhibition. Potentiation of anticoagulant effect of warfarin resulted in prothrombin time prolongation.	Monitor INR upon addition and discontinuation of metronidazole. Monitor for signs and symptoms of bleeding with concurrent use. Adjust warfarin dose as needed.

Drug-Laboratory Test Interactions: Metronidazole may increase levels of serum amylase and serum lipase, and decrease levels of serum AST, serum LDH, serum cholesterol and platelets.

Pregnant Women: Pregnancy Category B_M. Metronidazole crosses the placental barrier. Oral metronidazole is not recommended during the 1st trimester, although there is no proof of teratogenicity or carcinogenicity in humans. The 2006 Sexually Transmitted Infections guideline recommends the use of oral metronidazole for the treatment of bacterial vaginosis and trichomoniasis in symptomatic women. Evidence suggests that treating bacterial vaginosis in asymptomatic women at high risk of complications of pregnancy (e.g., previous preterm birth) may reduce the risk of preterm delivery. Benefits in treating pregnant women with asymptomatic trichomoniasis has not been demonstrated [http://www.phac-aspc.gc.ca/std-mts/sti-its/pdf/604pregnancy-eng.pdf].

Nursing Women: If a nursing mother is treated with a single 2 g oral dose of metronidazole, an interruption of breastfeeding for 12 to 24 hours is recommended. A brief interruption of breastfeeding for 1 to 2 hours is recommended in breastfeeding women receiving metronidazole iv. Maternal use of topical or vaginal metronidazole during nursing is unlikely to be a concern to the breast-fed baby. There have been no published reports demonstrating untoward effects in breast-fed infants with maternal doses of 250 mg three times daily for 10 days or with the single 2 g oral dose of metronidazole. Although metronidazole is significantly distributed into breast milk, the resulting blood levels in the infant from maternal metronidazole doses is much less than blood levels from therapeutic doses used in infants/children (7.5 to 30 mg/kg/day).

ADVERSE EFFECTS: Cardiovascular: palpitation and chest pain.

Central Nervous System: peripheral neuropathy, convulsive seizures, transient ataxia, dizziness, drowsiness, confusion, insomnia and headache.

Peripheral neuropathies have been reported in a few patients receiving prolonged treatment with large doses of metronidazole. It would appear that the occurrence is not directly related to the daily dosage and that an important predisposing factor is the continuation of oral and/or iv medication for several weeks or months.

Profound neurological deterioration, within 2 hours after metronidazole administration, has been reported. The occurrence is not directly related to the dose.

Dermatologic: rash and pruritus. With topical use: dry skin, skin irritation, stinging or burning of the skin.

Gastrointestinal: diarrhea, nausea, vomiting, unpleasant metallic taste, anorexia, epigastric distress, dyspepsia, constipation, *C. difficile* colitis (rare), dry mouth, glossitis, stomatitis, candidiasis (oral).

Genitourinary: dysuria, proliferation of *C. albicans* in the vagina, vaginal dryness and burning. Darkening of urine has been reported; this is probably due to a metabolite of metronidazole and has no clinical significance. With vaginal administration: burning or increased frequency of urination, vulvitis, burning or irritation of penis of sexual partner.

Hematologic: transient eosinophilia or leukopenia.

Hypersensitivity: Erythematous rash, urticaria, serum sickness-like reactions have been reported rarely.

Local Reactions: Thrombophlebitis has occurred with iv administration.

Metabolic: Gynecomastia has been reported rarely.

OVERDOSE:

For management of a suspected drug overdose, CPhA recommends that you contact your **regional Poison Control Centre**. See the *CPS Directory* section for a list of Poison Control Centres.

DOSAGE: Recommended Dose and Dosage Adjustment:

Table 2: Metronidazole

Dose in Adult Patients

Indication	Dose	Clinical Comment
Trichomoniasis	Oral: 2 g as a single dose or 500 mg BID × 7 days	Routine treatment of male sexual partners is necessary. Intravaginal metronidazole is not effective because the infection usually extends beyond the vagina, e.g., urethra, paraurethral glands, cervix. Can be used in symptomatic pregnant women though not known if treatment will improve pregnancy outcomes such as premature rupture of membranes, preterm birth and low birth weight.
Giardiasis	Oral: 250 mg TID × 5 to 7 days	
Intestinal amebiasis	Oral: 500 to 750 mg TID × 7 to 10 days	Drug of choice as it is quickly absorbed and has good tissue and abscess penetration. Severe cases may require 10 days of treatment. Consider metronidazole IV if patient cannot take oral medications and/or cannot absorb from the small bowel. Treatment should be followed with a course of luminal amebicide as little metronidazole may reach the lumen and eradicate potential intestinal reservoirs [*Mayo Clin Proc* 2008;83(10):1154-9].
Amebic abscesses of the liver	Oral: 500 to 750 mg TID × 7 to 10 days	
Bacterial vaginosis	Preferred: Oral: 500 mg BID × 7 days. Intravaginal gel 0.75%: one applicatorful (5 g) once daily × 5 days. Alternative: Oral: 2 g as a single dose; single dose regimen is associated with higher risk of relapse at 1 month.	Use of metronidazole gel during menses is not recommended. Routine treatment of male sexual partners is not necessary. Pregnancy: Test and treat symptomatic women. Retest 1 month after completion to ensure effective therapy. Treat patients who are asymptomatic for bacterial vaginosis but have a high-risk pregnancy, i.e., history of preterm delivery. Intravaginal antibiotics do not prevent preterm birth and therefore are not recommended.
Bacterial vaginosis, recurrent (≥3 episodes in previous year)	Oral: 500 mg BID × 10 to 14 days. Intravaginal gel: one applicatorful (5 g) once daily, then twice weekly for 4 to 6 months.	
Intra-abdominal infections	Oral: 500 mg every 8 hours (or 7.5 mg/kg every 6 to 8 hours). Max 4 g/24 hours. IV: 500 mg by iv infusion over 30 to 60 minutes, every 8 to 12 hours (or 7.5 mg/kg every 6 to 8 hours). Alternatively, a loading dose of 15 mg/kg iv infusion over 60 minutes can be given followed by a maintenance dose of 7.5 mg/kg every 6 hours. Max 4 g/24 hours.	Duration of therapy depends upon clinical and bacteriological assessment. Treatment for 7 days should be satisfactory for most infections. However, in cases where infection sites cannot be drained or which are liable to endogenous recontamination by anaerobic pathogens, longer duration of treatment may be required.
Mixed vaginal infection (*T. vaginalis* and *C. albicans*)	Use 1 vaginal ovule or 1 applicatorful of the cream once daily × 10 days	A second 10-day course may be given if cure is not achieved. Oral metronidazole can be given if *T. vaginalis* is not completely eliminated.
H. pylori-associated peptic ulcer disease	Oral: 500 mg po BID as part of 3-drug regimen or 250 mg po QID as part of 4-drug regimen used for 7 to 14 days [*Am J Gastroenterol* 2007;102(8):1808-25].	Therapy for 10 to 14 days is associated with better cure rates [*Am J Gastroenterol* 2007;102(8):1808-25]. Local knowledge of antimicrobial resistance may guide therapy; an alternate to metronidazole may be required.
Rosacea	0.75%: Topically applied to affected areas daily or BID for 9 weeks, then as needed. 1%: Topically applied to affected areas daily.	May be used as initial treatment to clear inflammatory lesions in mild to moderate rosacea. In severe rosacea, topical metronidazole can be used in combination with oral antibiotics.
C. difficile-associated diarrhea, mild to moderate	Oral: 250 mg QID or 500 mg TID × 10 to 14 days	For patients where oral therapy is not feasible, consider metronidazole iv 500 mg every 12 hours.
Periodontal infections	Usual oral dose: 250 mg TID × 3 to 5 days; for severe infections, the oral dose is 500 mg BID × 3 to 5 days	As an adjunct in the treatment of acute necrotizing ulcerative gingivitis, the usual oral dose is 250 mg TID for 3 to 5 days or for 7 to 10 days in more severe disease.
Skin and soft tissue infections	500 mg po/iv Q8–12H	As an adjunct in the treatment of intestinal or genital tract surgical site infections, animal and human bites, diabetic foot infections and treatment of necrotizing infections of the skin, fascia and muscle.
Brain abscess	500 mg po/iv Q8H	As an adjunct in a broad spectrum antimicrobial regimen.

(cont'd)

Table 2: Metronidazole *(cont'd)*
Dose in Adult Patients

Indication	Dose	Clinical Comment
Diverticulitis	500 mg po/iv Q8–12H × 5 to 7 days	A component of a broad spectrum antimicrobial regimen [*Dis Colon Rectum* 2006;49(7):939-44].
Sepsis	500 mg iv Q8–12H	Empirically, metronidazole is used as adjunct for the treatment of severe perirectal soft tissue infections or intraperitoneal/gastrointestinal tract infection.
Aspiration pneumonia	500 mg po/iv Q12H	In patients with poor dental hygiene or putrid sputum.
Crohn's disease (see Indications and Clinical Use)	10 to 20 mg/kg po daily divided BID, up to 1 g daily	Benefit seen in patients with ileocolonic or colonic Crohn's disease who did not respond to sulfasalazine. Usually administered over a period of 2 to 4 months.

Dosage in Dialysis: A supplemental full dose should be administered in patients undergoing hemodialysis because both metronidazole and the hydroxy metabolite are removed by dialysis.

Metronidazole 500 mg/100 mL Injection Ⓟ

metronidazole

Antibacterial—Antiprotozoal

Baxter

SUPPLIED: Each mL of sterile, nonpyrogenic solution contains: metronidazole 5 mg in water for injection isotonic with sodium chloride and buffers. Viaflex Plus plastic (polyvinyl chloride) containers of 100 mL. Store at room temperature. Protect from light.

Metronidazole Injection USP Ⓟ

metronidazole

Antibacterial

Hospira

SUPPLIED: Each mL of sterile, nonpyrogenic, isotonic solution, in a single-dose flexible container (PVC) contains: metronidazole 5 mg, sodium chloride for tonicity adjustment with dibasic sodium phosphate anhydrous and citric acid anhydrous as buffers in water for injection. Each 100 mL contains: 14 mEq sodium. Osmolarity: 290 mOsm/L (approx.). pH 5.7 (approx.). Containers of 100 mL. Store between 15 and 25°C. Protect from light.
Incompatibility: Do not mix with sodium lactate 5% w/v injection and dextrose 10% w/v injection.
Reconstitution: Metronidazole injection is a ready to use solution: no dilution or buffering is required.

Metvix™ Ⓟ

methyl aminolevulinate HCl

Antineoplastic Agent

Galderma

Date of Preparation: February 26, 2009

SUMMARY PRODUCT INFORMATION:

Route of Administration	Dosage Form/ Strength	Clinically Relevant Nonmedicinal Ingredients
Topical	Cream/168 mg/g methyl aminolevulinate (as methyl aminolevulinate hydrochloride)	Arachis (peanut) oil, refined almond oil For a complete listing see Dosage Forms, Composition and Packaging.

INDICATIONS AND CLINICAL USE: Metvix cream in combination with 630 nm wavelength red light illumination using the Aktilite CL 128 lamp is indicated for the:
- treatment of thin or non-hyperkeratotic and non-pigmented actinic keratosis on the face and scalp when other therapies are considered less appropriate.
- treatment of primary superficial basal cell carcinoma outside the H-zone of the face (e.g. ears, nose) when other therapies are considered less appropriate. The lesions should have been confirmed previously by biopsy.

This product should be administered in the physician's office by a trained physician only. Care should be taken by the physician when applying Metvix cream to avoid inadvertent skin contact (see Warnings and Precautions).
Geriatrics (>65 years of age): No overall differences in safety and efficacy were observed between patients aged 65 years and older and those who were younger.
Pediatrics: It is not recommended that Metvix cream be used in pediatric patients (see Warnings and Precautions).

CONTRAINDICATIONS:
- Patients who are hypersensitive to this drug or aminolevulinic acid or to any ingredient in the formulation (including peanut and almond oil) or component of the container. For a complete listing, see Dosage Forms, Composition and Packaging.
- Patients with cutaneous photosensitivity/porphyria, or known allergies to porphyrins.
- Patients with morpheaform basal cell carcinoma.

WARNINGS AND PRECAUTIONS:

Serious Warnings and Precautions
- Metvix cream is intended for topical use. Do not apply to the eyes or to mucous membranes.
- This product should be administered by trained physicians only.
- Care should be taken by the physician when applying Metvix cream to avoid inadvertent skin contact (see Sensitivity/Resistance).
- Patients with sBCC treated with Metvix-PDT must have regular follow-up of the treatment site since the efficacy is generally less than with surgery.
- The long-term efficacy of Metvix-PDT with Aktilite CL128 for the treatment of sBCC has not been established. Data from studies performed with a different lamp showed that the sBCC lesion CR at 12 months was similar to that observed with the Aktilite CL128 lamp, but decreased to 29-60% at 60 months post-treatment.

General: Metvix Cream Application: During the time period between the application of Metvix cream and exposure to red light illumination, the treatment site will become photosensitive. After Metvix cream application, patients should avoid exposure of the photosensitive treatment sites to sunlight or bright indoor light (e.g., examination lamps, operating room lamps, tanning beds, or lights at close proximity) during the period prior to red light treatment. Exposure to light may result in a stinging and/or burning sensation and may cause erythema and/or edema of the lesions. Before exposure to sunlight, patients should, therefore, protect treated lesions from the sun by wearing a wide-brimmed hat, protective clothing, or similar covering of light-opaque material. Sunscreens will not protect against photosensitivity reactions caused by visible light. The treated site should be protected from extreme cold with adequate clothing or remaining indoors between application of Metvix cream and photodynamic therapy light treatment.

After illumination of Metvix cream, the area treated should be kept covered and away from light for at least 48 hours.

Because of the potential for skin to become photosensitized, the Metvix cream should be applied by a trained physician to the skin lesion and perilesional skin within 5 mm of the lesion. Redness, swelling, burning and stinging are expected as a result of therapy; however, if these symptoms increase in severity and persist longer than 3 weeks, the patient should contact their doctor.
Photosensitivity and Device Precautions: The patient, operator and other persons present during red light treatment should wear protective goggles that sufficiently screen out red light with wavelengths from 570 to 670 nm.

If for any reason the patient cannot have the red light treatment after application of Metvix cream, the cream should be rinsed off, and the patient should protect the treated area from sunlight, prolonged or intense light for two days. Prolonged exposure for greater than 4 hours to Metvix cream should be avoided.
Carcinogenesis and Mutagenesis: Long-term studies to evaluate the carcinogenic potential of Metvix cream have not been performed.
Hematologic: Metvix cream has not been tested on patients with inherited or acquired coagulation defects.
Hepatic/Biliary/Pancreatic: The results of repeated-dose toxicity studies indicated that the liver was the target organ for high intravenous doses of methyl aminolevulinate in rats, but examination of liver function tests from phase I trials in humans did not reveal any changes that were inconsistent with random variation.
Immune: A study conducted in immunocompromised organ transplant recipients did not identify any safety concern in this population, adverse events being similar to those reported in trials in immunocompetent patients. However, the efficacy of Metvix in immunocompromised patients has not been well established.
Ophthalmologic: Application of Metvix cream to the eyes or to mucous membranes should be avoided.
Sensitivity/Resistance: Contact sensitization (allergenicity) has been observed in 14-52% of subjects previously exposed to Metvix on at least 4 occasions. Care should be taken by the physician applying Metvix cream to avoid inadvertent skin contact. Nitrile gloves should be worn when applying and removing the cream. Vinyl and latex gloves do not provide adequate protection when using this product.

The excipients cetostearyl alcohol and peanut oil may elicit local skin reactions such as contact eczema in rare cases, while methylparaben and propylparaben may sometimes cause allergic reactions.
Sexual Function/Reproduction: The effect of Metvix-PDT on sexual function and reproduction has not been investigated.
Skin: The safety and efficacy of Metvix cream has not been established in patients with porphyria or pigmented or highly infiltrating lesions. Thick (hyperkeratotic) actinic keratosis should not be treated with Metvix cream.

Please see "General" above for precautions regarding photosensitivity reactions.
Special Populations: Pregnant Women: Intravenous methyl aminolevulinate was teratogenic in rabbits at a high dose. It is not known whether Metvix cream can cause fetal harm when administered to a pregnant woman or can affect reproduction capacity.

Treatment with Metvix cream is not recommended during pregnancy. Metvix cream should be given to pregnant women only if the benefit risk ratio is favourable.
Nursing Women: The amount of methyl aminolevulinate secreted into human breast milk following topical administration of Metvix cream is not known. In the absence of clinical studies and because many drugs are excreted in human milk, caution should be exercised when Metvix is administered to a nursing woman.
Pediatrics: Actinic keratosis and basal cell carcinoma are seldom observed under the age of 18 and therefore, there is no experience with the use of Metvix-PDT in this population. Metvix cream is not recommended for use in pediatric patients.
ADVERSE REACTIONS: Adverse Drug Reaction Overview: Adverse drug reactions are categorized as appearing at the treatment site or non-treatment site. The common adverse drug reactions reported in all studies of Metvix-PDT were local phototoxic reactions.
Clinical Trial Adverse Drug Reactions: Actinic Keratosis Studies: A total of 231 subjects, each with 4-10 actinic keratoses were enrolled in 2 double-blind, randomized, vehicle-controlled clinical trials. Subjects were randomized to receive Aktilite PDT with Metvix Cream or Vehicle cream on 2 occasions 1 week apart. Cream was applied for approximately 3 hours under occlusion followed immediately by illumination using the Aktilite CL128 lamp, delivering red light at a dose of 37 J/cm².

Table 1 shows the incidence and severity of adverse drug reactions in these two trials.

Table 1: Metvix
Incidence of Adverse Drug Reactions in ≥1% of Subjects with Actinic Keratoses in Studies 1 and 2 (Safety Population)

	Metvix & Aktilite PDT n=126		Vehicle & Aktilite PDT n=105	
	All Events[a]	Severe	All Events[a]	Severe
Any Treatment Site Adverse Drug Reaction	113 (90%)	28 (22%)	48 (46%)	0 (0%)
Skin burning/pain/discomfort	109 (86%)	25 (20%)	38 (36%)	0 (0%)
Erythema	80 (63%)	7 (6%)	11 (10%)	0 (0%)
Scabbing/crusting/blister/erosions	36 (29%)	2 (2%)	1 (1%)	0 (0%)
Pruritus	28 (22%)	0 (0%)	8 (8%)	0 (0%)
Skin or eyelid edema	23 (18%)	2 (2%)	1 (1%)	0 (0%)
Skin exfoliation	17 (14%)	4 (3%)	3 (3%)	0 (0%)
Skin warm	5 (4%)	0 (0%)	2 (2%)	0 (0%)
Application site discharge	3 (2%)	0 (0%)	0 (0%)	0 (0%)
Skin hemorrhage	2 (2%)	0 (0%)	0 (0%)	0 (0%)
Skin tightness	2 (2%)	0 (0%)	0 (0%)	0 (0%)
Skin hyperpigmentation	2 (2%)	0 (0%)	0 (0%)	0 (0%)
Non Treatment Site Adverse Drug Reaction	13 (10%)	2 (2%)	0 (0%)	0 (0%)
Headache	3 (2%)	1 (1%)	0 (0%)	0 (0%)

[a] Mild, moderate, or severe.

The most common adverse drug reactions were attributable to phototoxicity reactions at the treatment site.
Less Common Clinical Trial Adverse Drug Reactions in Actinic Keratoses Studies (<1%): Eye Disorders: eye pain, lacrimation increased.
Gastrointestinal Disorders: nausea.
General Disorders and Administration Site Conditions: chills.
Injury, Poisoning and Procedural Complications: contusion.
Nervous System Disorders: dizziness.
Skin and Subcutaneous Tissue Disorders: hyperhidrosis.

Superficial Basal Cell Carcinoma Study: A total of 234 subjects were screened and 196 subjects enrolled in the pivotal superficial basal cell carcinoma study. Regarding drug adverse events, there were more events and more subjects in Metvix-PDT group than in surgery group (37% subjects with 65 related adverse events versus 14.6% subjects with 21 related adverse events). Most related adverse events were dermatologic and more frequent in Metvix-PDT group (34% subjects with 61 related dermatologic adverse events versus 7.3% subjects with 8 adverse events). These adverse events are summarised in Table 2.

Table 2: Metvix

Incidence of Adverse Drug Reactions in ≥1% of Subjects in Superficial Basal Cell Carcinoma Study (Safety Population)

		Metvix (N=100)		Surgery (N=96)		
		Mild	**Moderate**	**Mild**	**Moderate**	**Severe**
Any Adverse Event		**26 (26.0%)**	**11 (11%)**	**10 (10.4%)**	**3 (3.1%)**	**1 (1.0%)**
General Disorders and Administration Site Conditions	Pain	1 (1%)	1 (1%)	—	—	1 (1.0%)
Infections and Infestations	**All**	**1 (1%)**	—	**3 (3.1%)**	**1 (1.0%)**	**1 (1.0%)**
	Application site infection	1 (1%)	—	—	—	—
	Wound infection	—	—	3 (3.1%)	1 (1.0%)	1 (1.0%)
Neoplasms Benign, Malignant and Unspecified (incl cysts and polyps)	Basal cell carcinoma	—	1 (1%)	—	—	—
Nervous System Disorders	Headache	1 (1%)	—	—	—	—
Skin and Subcutaneous Tissue Disorders	**All**	**24 (24%)**	**9 (9%)**	**5 (5.2%)**	**1 (1.0%)**	—
	Milia	2 (2%)	—	—	—	—
	Photosensitivity reaction	22 (22%)	9 (9%)	—	—	—
	Skin hyperpigmentation	—	1 (1%)	—	—	—
	Erythema	—	—	3 (3.1%)	—	—
	Keloid scar	—	—	1 (1.0%)	—	—
	Pain of skin	—	—	—	1 (1.0%)	—
	Pruritus	—	—	1 (1.0%)	—	—
	Scar	—	—	1 (1.0%)	—	—
Injury, Poisoning and Procedural Complications	**All**	—	—	**4 (4.2%)**	**1 (1.0%)**	—
	Post procedural pain	—	—	2 (2.1%)	1 (1.0%)	—
	Wound dehiscence	—	—	2 (2.1%)	—	—
Musculoskeletal and Connective Tissue Disorders	Shoulder pain	—	—	1 (1.0%)	—	—
Surgical and Medical Procedures	**All**	—	—	**2 (2.1%)**	—	—
	Skin lesion excision	—	—	1 (1.0%)	—	—
	Suture insertion	—	—	1 (1.0%)	—	—

Related=possibly, probably or definitely related.

The most commonly reported related adverse events were expected: photosensitivity reaction for Metvix-PDT (31% subjects with 57 adverse events), and wound infection for surgery procedure (5.2% subjects with 5 adverse events). Among these subjects, there was 1 subject (1.7%) in surgery group who reported related adverse events of severe intensity. In the Metvix-PDT group, the majority of related adverse events were of mild severity.

Abnormal Hematologic and Clinical Chemistry Findings: No abnormalities attributable to treatment with Metvix-PDT have been observed. The results of repeated-dose toxicity studies indicated that the liver was the target organ for high intravenous doses of methyl aminolevulinate in rats, but examination of liver function tests from phase I trials in humans did not reveal any changes that were inconsistent with random variation.

Adverse Drug Reactions from Other Clinical Trials: In addition, there were reports of parathesia, and, urticaria, rash, skin hypopigmentation, heat rash, and fatigue in Phase III studies in which the illumination was performed with a different lamp (CureLight 01). There were also isolated reports of scar in a dose ranging study performed with CureLight where a relationship to treatment was uncertain.

Post-Market Adverse Drug Reactions: Application site eczema, allergic contact dermatitis and urticaria have been described in post-marketing reports. Most cases were localized to the treatment area and were not severe; some cases of erythema and swelling have been more extensive.

DRUG INTERACTIONS: Overview: There have been no studies of the interaction of Metvix with other drugs, including local anesthetics. It is possible that concomitant use of other known photosensitizing agents might increase photosensitivity reactions when treated with Metvix cream.

The demographic of the treated population is largely elderly patients receiving a variety of concomitant systemic medications, and there is no suggestion of any interaction between Metvix-PDT and these medications.

Drug-Drug Interactions: Interactions with other drugs have not been established.

Drug-Food Interactions: Interactions with food have not been established.

Drug-Herb Interactions: Interactions with herbal products have not been established.

Drug-Laboratory Test Interactions: Interactions with laboratory tests have not been established.

DOSAGE AND ADMINISTRATION:

Dosing Considerations: This product is not intended for application by patients or unqualified medical personnel; therefore, this product is only dispensed to physicians.

Recommended Dose and Dosage Adjustment: Actinic Keratosis: For treatment of thin or non-hyperkeratotic and non-pigmented actinic keratosis lesions on the face and scalp, one treatment session with Metvix-PDT should be performed followed by a second treatment session 7 days later. The treated lesions should be evaluated after 3 months, and up to two additional treatment sessions can be performed if needed. Multiple lesions can be treated in one session. Metvix-PDT is not recommended for treatment of Grade III hyperkeratotic lesions. A maximum of 2 g of Metvix cream per treatment session should be applied.

Superficial Basal Cell Carcinoma (outside the H-zone of the face): One treatment session with Metvix-PDT should be performed with a second treatment session 7 days later. The treated lesions should be evaluated after 3 months, and if needed, two additional treatment sessions 7 days apart should be performed. A maximum of 2 g of Metvix cream per treatment session should be applied.

Missed Dose: If the patient for any reason cannot have the red light treatment within the 3 hour prescribed period after application, the cream should be rinsed off. The patient should be instructed to protect the exposed area from sunlight, and prolonged or intense light for two days.

Administration: One Metvix-PDT session consists of:

1. **Lesion debriding:** Before applying Metvix cream, the surface of the lesions should be prepared with a small dermal curette to remove scales and crusts and to roughen the surface of the lesion. This is to facilitate access of the cream and light to all parts of the lesion.
2. **Application of Metvix cream:** Only nitrile gloves should be worn during this and subsequent steps and universal precautions should be taken. Vinyl and latex gloves do not provide adequate protection when using this product.
   Using a spatula, apply a layer of Metvix cream about 1 mm thick to the lesion and the surrounding 5 mm of normal skin. Multiple lesions may be treated during the same treatment session. Each treatment field should be limited to the size of the light field of the lamp.
3. **Cover the lesion(s):** The area to which the cream has been applied should then be covered with an occlusive, non-absorbent dressing. After cream application, patients should avoid exposure of the treatment sites to sunlight or bright indoor light (e.g., examination lamps, operating room lamps, tanning beds, or lights at close proximity) prior to red light treatment. Exposure to other light sources may result in a stinging and/or burning sensation and may cause erythema and/or edema of the lesions. Patients should protect treated areas from the sun by wearing a wide-brimmed hat, protective clothing or similar covering of light-opaque material. Sunscreens will not protect against photosensitivity reactions caused by visible light. It has not been determined if perspiration can spread the Metvix cream outside the treatment site to the eyes or surrounding skin. The treated site should be protected from extreme cold with adequate clothing or by remaining indoors between the application of Metvix cream and the PDT light treatment.
4. **Wait for 3 hours (at least 2.5 hours, but no more than 4 hours)** (see Warnings and Precautions): Metvix cream should not be applied for longer than the recommended time. If PDT cannot be performed on the patient after the application of Metvix cream, the cream should be rinsed off with saline and gauze and treated areas should be protected from sunlight and prolonged and intense light for 2 days.
5. **Removal of Dressing and Rinse Off Excess Cream:** Following removal of the occlusive dressing, clean the area with saline and gauze. Nitrile gloves should be worn.
6. **Illumination of Metvix Treated Lesion** (see Warnings and Precautions): It is important to ensure that the correct light dose is administered. The light intensity at the lesion surface should not be higher than 200 mW/cm^2. Patient and operator should adhere to safety instructions and precautions provided with the lamp. The patient and operator should wear protective goggles during illumination. The lamp should be carefully positioned so that dosing is accurate and immediately thereafter the lesion should be exposed to red light at 630 nm and a total light dose of 37 J/cm^2.
   Patients should be advised that transient stinging and/or burning at the target lesion sites may occur during the period of light exposure. It is not necessary to protect healthy skin surrounding the lesions during exposure.
   If red light treatment is interrupted or stopped for any reason, it may be restarted. Metvix cream is not intended for use with any device other than the approved lamp: Aktilite CL 128. Use of Metvix cream without subsequent red light illumination is not recommended.

OVERDOSAGE:

Metvix Cream: Metvix cream overdose has not been reported in clinical trials or in post-marketing experience and is not likely to occur in clinical practice due to the nature of the treatment being administered directly by a physician.

No incidences of oral ingestion of Metvix cream have been reported. In the unlikely event that the drug is ingested, monitoring and supportive care is recommended. Methyl aminolevulinate has a low order of single-dose oral and intravenous toxicity in mice and rats; the minimally lethal oral acute dose was more than 2000 mg/kg.

Red Light: There is no information on overdose of red light following Metvix cream application. If red light overexposure and a skin burn occurs, the patient should be treated according to standard practice for the treatment of cutaneous burns.

For management of a suspected drug overdose, CPhA recommends that you contact your **regional Poison Control Centre**. See the *CPS* Directory section for a list of Poison Control Centres.

ACTION AND CLINICAL PHARMACOLOGY: Mechanism of Action: Photosensitization occurs through the metabolic conversion of methyl aminolevulinate (prodrug) to photoactive porphyrins (PAP), which accumulates in the skin lesions where Metvix cream has been applied. When exposed to light of appropriate wavelength and energy, the accumulated photoactive porphyrins produce a photodynamic reaction, resulting in an oxygen dependent cytotoxic process. The absorption of light causes an excited state of the porphyrin molecules, and subsequent spin transfer from photoactive porphyrins to molecular oxygen generates singlet oxygen, which can further react to form superoxide and hydroxyl radicals. Photosensitization of lesions using Metvix cream, plus illumination with Aktilite CL 128 (630 nm wavelength red light) at 37 J/cm^2, is the basis for Metvix photodynamic therapy (PDT).

Pharmacodynamics: See Mechanism of Action.

Pharmacokinetics: Absorption: In vitro dermal absorption of radiolabelled methyl aminolevulinate applied to human cadaver skin has been studied. After 24 hours, the mean cumulative absorption through human skin was 0.26% of the administered dose. A skin depot containing 4.9% of the dose was formed. No corresponding studies in compromised human skin (damage similar to actinic keratosis, BCC, roughened surfaces or without stratum corneum) were performed.

There is no information on the pharmacokinetics of methyl aminolevulinate in human serum due to the instability of the drug in serum.

Metabolism, Distribution and Excretion: The metabolic pathway in humans by which photoactive porphyrins are produced from methyl aminolevulinate is not fully elucidated.

In humans, the levels of photoactive porphyrins in the skin were indirectly determined through a semi-quantitative method measuring the skin fluorescence following methyl aminolevulinate application. A higher degree of accumulation of photoactive porphyrins in lesions compared to normal skin has been demonstrated after topical application of methyl aminolevulinate.

After application of methyl aminolevulinate to the skin of human subjects for 3 hours, a subsequent illumination with a narrow red light spectrum at 630 nm wavelength and a total light dose of 37 J/cm^2 reduced the fluorescence of skin lesions near pre-treatment levels immediately after illumination, but it did not result in complete photobleaching. Thereafter, an increase in fluorescence 2 hours following the illumination was observed. Complete photobleaching was observed 24 hours following the illumination.

Special Populations and Conditions: The pharmacokinetics of methyl aminolevulinate has not been investigated in conditions such as hepatic insufficiency, or renal insufficiency. Any systemic effects are considered to be negligible due to selective accumulation of the compound in lesions compared to normal skin and since systemic absorption is usually minimal after topical administration (see Adverse Reactions).

STORAGE AND STABILITY: Store refrigerated, 2-8°C.

Shelf-life: 18 months.

Use contents within one week after opening. The product should not be used after 24 hours without refrigeration.

SPECIAL HANDLING INSTRUCTIONS: Contact sensitization (allergenicity) has been observed with the use of Metvix cream (see Adverse Reactions). Care should be taken by individuals handling Metvix cream to avoid inadvertent skin contact. Nitrile gloves should be worn when applying and removing the cream. Vinyl and latex gloves do not provide adequate protection from this product.

INFORMATION FOR THE PATIENT: Published in e-CPS, available by subscription at www.e-cps.ca.

DOSAGE FORMS, COMPOSITION AND PACKAGING: Each tube of an oil-in-water emulsion contains: methyl aminolevulinate hydrochloride equivalent to 168 mg/g of methyl aminolevulinate. Nonmedicinal ingredients: arachis (peanut) oil, cetostearyl alcohol, cholesterol, edetate disodium, glycerol, glyceryl monostearate, isopropyl myristate, methylparaben, oleyl alcohol, polyoxyl stearate, propylparaben, purified water, refined almond oil and white soft paraffin. Aluminum tubes of 2 g sealed with an aluminum membrane and a screw cap.

The reader is invited to consult CPhA's monograph **HMG-CoA Reductase Inhibitors**.

Mevacor® ℞
lovastatin
Lipid Metabolism Regulator

Merck Frosst

Date of Revision: December 9, 2008

SUMMARY PRODUCT INFORMATION:

Route of Administration	Dosage Form/ Strength	Clinically Relevant Nonmedicinal Ingredients
Oral	Tablet 20 mg, 40 mg	For a complete listing see Dosage Forms, Composition and Packaging.

INDICATIONS AND CLINICAL USE: Hyperlipidemia: MEVACOR (lovastatin tablets) is indicated as an adjunct to diet, at least equivalent to the American Heart Association (AHA) Step 1 diet, for the reduction of elevated total and Low Density Lipoprotein Cholesterol (LDL-C) levels in patients with primary hypercholesterolemia (Types IIa and IIb), (a disorder of lipid metabolism characterized by elevated serum cholesterol levels in association with normal triglyceride levels (Type IIa) or with increased triglyceride levels [Type IIb]) when the response to diet and other nonpharmacological measures alone has been inadequate.

After establishing that the elevation in plasma lipids represents a primary disorder not due to secondary conditions such as poorly controlled diabetes mellitus, hypothyroidism, the nephrotic syndrome, liver disease, or dysproteinemias, prospective patient should have an elevated LDL-C level as the cause for an elevated total serum cholesterol. This may be particularly relevant for patients with total triglycerides (TG) over 4.52 mmol/L (400 mg/dL) or with markedly elevated High Density Lipoprotein Cholesterol (HDL-C) values, where non-LDL lipoprotein fractions may contribute significantly to total cholesterol levels without apparent increase in cardiovascular risk. In general, LDL-C may be estimated according to the following equations:

LDL-C (mmol/L) = Total cholesterol – [(0.37×triglycerides) + HDL-C]

LDL-C (mg/dL) = Total cholesterol – [(0.16×triglycerides) + HDL-C]

When total triglycerides are greater than 4.52 mmol/L (400 mg/dL) this equation is not applicable. In such patients, LDL-C may be obtained by ultracentrifugation.

Coronary Heart Disease: MEVACOR was also found to slow the progression of coronary atherosclerosis in patients with coronary heart disease as part of a treatment strategy to lower total and LDL-C to the desired levels. In two trials including this type of patient, i.e. in a secondary prevention intervention, MEVACOR monotherapy was shown to slow the progression of coronary atherosclerosis as evaluated by computerized quantitative coronary angiography (QCA). This effect, however, was not accompanied by an improvement in the clinical endpoints (death, fatal/nonfatal myocardial infarction, hospitalization for unstable angina, and coronary revascularization procedure [PTCA and CABG]) within the 2-2½ years' trial period. These trials, however, were not designed to demonstrate a reduction in the risk of coronary morbidity and mortality.

The effect of lovastatin on the progression of atherosclerosis in the coronary arteries has been corroborated by similar findings in carotid vasculature. In the Asymptomatic Carotid Artery Progression Study (ACAPS) which included hyperlipidemic patients with early asymptomatic carotid lesions and without known coronary artery disease, the effect of therapy with lovastatin on carotid atherosclerosis was assessed by B-mode ultrasonography. There was a significant regression of carotid lesions in patients receiving lovastatin alone compared to those receiving placebo alone. The predictive value of changes in the carotid vasculature for stroke has not yet been established. In the lovastatin group there was a significant reduction in the number of patients with major cardiovascular events relative to the placebo group (5 vs 14) and a significant reduction in all-cause mortality (1 vs 8) however, it was not powered to demonstrate a reduction in the risk of coronary morbidity and mortality. This trial should be viewed as supportive and complementary to the others mentioned above.

CONTRAINDICATIONS:

- Patients who are hypersensitive to this drug or to any ingredient in the formulation. For a complete listing, see Dosage Forms, Composition and Packaging.
- Active liver disease or unexplained persistent elevations of serum transaminases.
- Pregnant and nursing women. Cholesterol and other products of cholesterol biosynthesis are essential components for fetal development (including synthesis of steroids and cell membranes). MEVACOR should be administered to women of childbearing age only when such patients are highly unlikely to conceive and have been informed of the possible harm. If the patient becomes pregnant while taking MEVACOR, the drug should be discontinued immediately and the patient appraised of the potential harm to the fetus. Atherosclerosis being a chronic process, discontinuation of lipid metabolism regulating drugs during pregnancy should have little impact on the outcome of long-term therapy of primary hypercholesterolemia (see Warnings and Precautions, Special Populations, Pregnant Women and Nursing Women).

WARNINGS AND PRECAUTIONS: General: Before instituting therapy with MEVACOR, an attempt should be made to control hypercholesterolemia with appropriate diet, exercise, weight reduction in overweight and obese patients, and to treat other underlying medical problems (see Indications and Clinical Use). The patient should be advised to inform subsequent physicians of the prior use of MEVACOR or any other lipid metabolism regulator.

The effects of lovastatin induced changes in lipoprotein levels, including reduction of serum cholesterol, on cardiovascular morbidity or mortality or total mortality has not been established.

Use in Homozygous Familial Hypercholesterolemia (FH): MEVACOR is not effective or is less effective in patients with rare homozygous familial hypercholesterolemia.

Patients with Severe Hypercholesterolemia: Higher dosages (80 mg/day) required for some patients with severe hypercholesterolemia are associated with increased plasma levels of lovastatin.

Caution should be exercised in such patients who are also significantly renally impaired, elderly or are concomitantly administered P-450 inhibitors (see Warnings and Precautions, Myopathy/Rhabdomyolysis and Drug Interactions).

Endocrine and Metabolism: Endocrine Function: HMG-CoA reductase inhibitors interfere with cholesterol synthesis and as such might theoretically blunt adrenal and/or gonadal steroid production. Clinical studies with lovastatin have shown that this agent does not reduce plasma cortisol concentration or impair adrenal reserve, and does not reduce basal plasma testosterone concentration. However, the effects of HMG-CoA reductase inhibitors on male fertility have not been studied in an adequate number of patients. The effects, if any, on the pituitary-gonadal axis in premenopausal women are unknown.

Patients treated with lovastatin who develop clinical evidence of endocrine dysfunction should be evaluated appropriately. Caution should be exercised if an HMG-CoA reductase inhibitor or other agent used to lower cholesterol levels is administered to patients receiving other drugs (e.g. ketoconazole, spironolactone, or cimetidine) that may decrease the levels of endogenous steroid hormones (see Drug Interactions, Cytochrome P-450 Inhibitors (CYP3A4).

Effect on Lipoprotein(a) [Lp(a)]: In some patients the beneficial effect of lowered total cholesterol and LDL-C levels may be partly blunted by a concomitant increase in the Lp(a) levels. Until further experience is obtained from controlled clinical trials, it is suggested, where feasible, that Lp(a) measurements be carried out in patients placed on therapy with MEVACOR.

Effect on CoQ_{10} Levels (ubiquinone): A significant decrease in plasma CoQ_{10} levels in patients treated with MEVACOR and other statins has been observed in short-term clinical trials. The clinical significance of a potential long-term statin-induced deficiency of CoQ_{10} has not yet been established.

Hepatic/Biliary/Pancreatic: In the initial controlled clinical trials performed in 695 patients, marked persistent increases (to more than 3 times the upper limit of normal) in serum transaminases occurred in 1.6% of adult patients who received MEVACOR for at least one year (see Adverse Reactions, Laboratory Tests). When the drug was interrupted or discontinued in these patients, the transaminase levels fell slowly to pretreatment levels. The increases usually appeared 3 to 12 months after the start of therapy with MEVACOR. In most cases they were not associated with jaundice or other clinical signs or symptoms (see Drug Interactions and Adverse Reactions, Post-Market Adverse Drug Reactions).

In the 48-week EXCEL study performed in 8245 patients suffering from moderate hypercholesterolemia, the incidence of marked (more than 3 times the upper limit of normal) increases in serum transaminases on successive testing was 0.1% in patients receiving a placebo and 0.1% at 20 mg/day, 0.9% at 40 mg/day and 1.5% at 80 mg/day in patients administered lovastatin.

It is recommended that liver function tests be performed at baseline and periodically thereafter in all patients. Particular attention should be paid to patients who develop elevated serum transaminase levels and in patients in whom the dose is increased to 40 mg/day or more. In these patients, measurements should be repeated promptly and then performed more frequently.

If the transaminase levels show evidence of progression, particularly if they rise to three times the upper limit of normal and are persistent, the drug should be discontinued.

MEVACOR, as well as other HMG-CoA reductase inhibitors, should be used with caution in patients who consume substantial quantities of alcohol and/or have a past history of liver disease. Active liver disease or unexplained serum transaminase elevations are contraindications to the use of MEVACOR; if such condition develops during therapy, the drug should be discontinued.

Moderate elevations of serum transaminases (less than three times the upper limit of normal) have been reported following therapy with MEVACOR (see Adverse Reactions). These changes were not specific to MEVACOR and were also observed with comparative lipid metabolism regulators. They generally appeared within the first 3 months after initiation of therapy, were often transient and were not accompanied by any other symptoms. They did not necessitate interruption of treatment.

Muscle Effects: Myopathy/Rhabdomyolysis: Effects on skeletal muscle such as myalgia, myopathy and, rarely, rhabdomyolysis have been reported in patients treated with MEVACOR.

Rare cases of rhabdomyolysis with acute renal failure secondary to myoglobinuria, have been reported with MEVACOR and with other HMG-CoA reductase inhibitors.

Myopathy, defined as muscle pain or muscle weakness in conjunction with increases in creatine phosphokinase (CK) values to greater than ten times the upper limit of normal (ULN), should be considered in any patient with diffuse myalgias, muscle tenderness or weakness, and/or a marked elevation of CK. Patients should be advised to report promptly any unexplained muscle pain, tenderness or weakness, particularly if associated with malaise or fever. Patients who develop any signs or symptoms suggestive of myopathy should have their CK levels measured. MEVACOR therapy should be immediately discontinued if markedly elevated CK levels are measured or myopathy is diagnosed or suspected. Myopathy sometimes takes the form of rhabdomyolysis with or without acute renal failure secondary to myoglobinuria, and rare fatalities have occurred. The risk of myopathy is increased with dosage and by high levels of HMG-CoA reductase inhibitory activity in plasma.

Pre-disposing Factors for Myopathy/Rhabdomyolysis: MEVACOR, as with other HMG-CoA reductase inhibitors, should be prescribed with caution in patients with pre-disposing factors for myopathy/rhabdomyolysis. Such factors include: personal or family history of hereditary muscular disorders; previous history of muscle toxicity with another HMG-CoA reductase inhibitor; concomitant use of a fibrate or niacin; hypothyroidism; alcohol abuse; excessive physical exercise; age >70 years; renal impairment; hepatic impairment; diabetes with hepatic fatty change; surgery and trauma; frailty; situations where an increase in plasma levels of active ingredient may occur (see Drug Interactions, Drug-Drug Interactions).

MEVACOR therapy should be temporarily withheld or discontinued in any patient with an acute serious condition suggestive of myopathy or predisposing to the development of rhabdomyolysis (e.g. sepsis, hypotension, major surgery, trauma, severe metabolic endocrine and electrolyte disorders, or uncontrolled seizures).

Myopathy/Rhabdomyolysis Caused by Drug Interactions: Pharmacokinetic Interactions: The use of HMG-CoA reductase inhibitors has been associated with severe myopathy, including rhabdomyolysis, which may be more frequent when they are co-administered with drugs that inhibit the cytochrome P-450 enzyme system. Lovastatin is metabolized by the cytochrome P-450 isoform 3A4 and as such may interact with agents which inhibit this enzyme (see Warnings and Precautions, Myopathy/Rhabdomyolysis and Drug Interactions, Cytochrome P-450 Inhibitors (CYP3A4).

The risk of myopathy/rhabdomyolysis is increased by concomitant use of lovastatin with the following:

- **Potent inhibitors of CYP3A4, e.g., the antifungal azoles itraconazole, and ketoconazole, the antibiotics erythromycin, clarithromycin and telithromycin, the HIV protease inhibitors, or the antidepressant nefazodone, particularly with higher doses of lovastatin** (see Drug Interactions, Cytochrome P-450 Inhibitors (CYP3A4).

Other drugs:

- **Lipid-lowering drugs that can cause myopathy when given alone: Gemfibrozil, other fibrates, or lipid-lowering doses (≥1 g/day) of niacin, particularly with higher doses of lovastatin** (see Drug Interactions, Gemfibrozil and Other Fibrates, Lipid-Lowering Doses (≥1 g/day) of Niacin (nicotinic acid).
- **Cyclosporine or danazol particularly with higher doses of lovastatin** (see Drug Interactions).
- **Amiodarone or verapamil with higher doses of a closely related member of the HMG-CoA reductase inhibitor class** (see Drug Interactions).
- **Fusidic acid (oral or IV):** Patients on fusidic acid (oral or IV) treated concomitantly with lovastatin may have an increased risk of myopathy (see Drug Interactions, Drug-Drug Interactions).

The risk of myopathy/rhabdomyolysis is dose related. In a clinical study Expanded Clinical Evaluation of Lovastatin (EXCEL) in which patients were carefully monitored and some interacting drugs were excluded, there was one case of myopathy among 4933 patients randomized to lovastatin 20-40 mg daily for 48 weeks, and 4 among 1649 patients randomized to 80 mg daily.

Reducing the Risk of Myopathy/Rhabdomyolysis:

1. **General measures: All patients starting therapy with lovastatin, or whose dose of lovastatin is being increased, should be advised of the risk of myopathy and told to report promptly any unexplained muscle pain, tenderness or weakness. Lovastatin therapy should be discontinued immediately if myopathy is diagnosed or suspected.** The presence of these symptoms, and/or a CK level >10 times the upper limit of normal indicates myopathy. In most cases, when patients were promptly discontinued from treatment, muscle symptoms and CK increases resolved. Periodic CK determinations may be considered in patients starting therapy with lovastatin or whose dose is being increased, but there is no assurance that such monitoring will prevent myopathy.

   Many of the patients who have developed rhabdomyolysis on therapy with lovastatin have had complicated medical histories, including renal insufficiency usually as a consequence of long-standing diabetes mellitus. Such patients merit closer monitoring. Therapy with lovastatin should be temporarily stopped a few days prior to elective major surgery and when any major medical or surgical condition supervenes.
2. **Measures to reduce the risk of myopathy/rhabdomyolysis caused by drug interactions** (see Myopathy/Rhabdomyolysis Caused by Drug Interactions): **Use of lovastatin concomitantly with potent CYP3A4 inhibitors (e.g., itraconazole, ketoconazole, erythromycin, clarithromycin, telithromycin, HIV protease inhibitors, or nefazodone) should be avoided.** If treatment with itraconazole, ketoconazole, erythromycin, clarithromycin or telithromycin is unavoidable, therapy with lovastatin should be suspended during the course of treatment. Concomitant use with other medicines labeled as having a potent inhibitory effect on CYP3A4 at therapeutic doses should be avoided unless the benefits of combined therapy outweigh the increased risk.

   The dose of lovastatin should not exceed 20 mg daily in patients receiving concomitant medication with cyclosporine, danazol, gemfibrozil, other fibrates or lipid-lowering doses (≥1 g/day) of niacin. The combined use of lovastatin with gemfibrozil should be avoided unless the benefit of further alteration in lipid levels is likely to outweigh the increased risk of this drug combination. The benefits of the use of lovastatin in patients receiving other fibrates, niacin, cyclosporine, or danazol should be carefully weighed against the risks of these drug combinations. Addition of fibrates or niacin to lovastatin typically provides little additional reduction in LDL-C, but further reductions of TG and further increases in HDL-C may be obtained. Combinations of fibrates or niacin with low doses of lovastatin have been used without myopathy in small, short-term clinical studies with careful monitoring.

   The dose of lovastatin should not exceed 40 mg daily in patients receiving concomitant medication with amiodarone or verapamil. The combined use of lovastatin at doses higher than 40 mg daily with amiodarone or verapamil should be avoided unless the clinical benefit is likely to outweigh the increased risk of myopathy.

   Patients on fusidic acid (oral or IV) and lovastatin should be closely monitored for symptoms and/or signs of myopathy. Temporary suspension of lovastatin treatment may be considered.

Ophthalmologic: Current long-term data from clinical trials do not indicate an adverse effect of lovastatin on the human lens.

Renal: Because MEVACOR does not undergo significant renal excretion, modification of dosage should not be necessary in patients with moderate renal insufficiency.

In patients with severe renal insufficiency (creatinine clearance <0.5 mL/s [30 mL/min]), dosages above 20 mg/day should be carefully considered and, if deemed necessary, implemented cautiously (see Warnings and Precautions, Myopathy/Rhabdomyolysis).

Skin: To date, hypersensitivity syndrome has not been described. In a few instances eosinophilia and skin eruptions appear to be associated with lovastatin treatment. If hypersensitivity is suspected, MEVACOR should be discontinued.

Special Populations: Pregnant Women: MEVACOR is contraindicated during pregnancy.

Safety in pregnant women has not been established. No controlled clinical trials with lovastatin have been conducted in pregnant women. Rare reports of congenital anomalies following intrauterine exposure to HMG-CoA reductase inhibitors have been received. However, in an analysis of approximately 200 prospectively followed pregnancies exposed during the first trimester to MEVACOR or another closely related HMG-CoA reductase inhibitor, the incidence of congenital anomalies was comparable to that seen in the general population. This number of pregnancies was statistically sufficient to exclude a 2.5-fold or greater increase in congenital anomalies over the background incidence.

Atherosclerosis is a chronic process, and ordinarily, discontinuation of lipid-lowering drugs during pregnancy should have little impact on the long-term risk associated with primary hypercholesterolemia. Although there is no evidence that the incidence of congenital anomalies in offspring of patients taking MEVACOR or another closely related HMG-CoA reductase inhibitor differs from that observed in the general population, maternal treatment with MEVACOR may reduce the fetal levels of mevalonate which is a precursor of cholesterol biosynthesis. For these reasons, MEVACOR should not be used in women who are pregnant, trying to become pregnant or suspect they are pregnant. Treatment with MEVACOR should be suspended for the duration of pregnancy or until it has been determined that the woman is not pregnant. (See Contraindications.)

Nursing Women: It is not known whether MEVACOR is excreted in human milk. Because many drugs are excreted in human milk and because of the potential for serious adverse reactions in nursing infants from MEVACOR, women taking MEVACOR should not nurse their infant (see Contraindications).

Pediatrics: Limited experience is available in children. However, safety and effectiveness in children have not been established.

Geriatrics (>60 years of age): In patients over 60 years, efficacy appeared similar to that seen in the population as a whole, with no apparent increase in the frequency of clinical or laboratory adverse findings.

Elderly patients may be more susceptible to myopathy (see Warnings and Precautions, Muscle Effects, Pre-disposing Factors for Myopathy/Rhabdomyolysis).

ADVERSE REACTIONS: Adverse Drug Reaction Overview: MEVACOR was compared to placebo in 8245 patients with hypercholesterolemia (total cholesterol 6.2-7.8 mmol/L) in a randomized, double blind, parallel, 48 week expanded clinical evaluation of lovastatin (EXCEL study). Clinical adverse reactions reported as possible, probably or definitely drug related in any treatment group are shown in Table 1.

Table 1: MEVACOR

Adverse Reactions

	Placebo (n=1663) %	MEVACOR 20 mg q p.m. (n=1642) %	MEVACOR 40 mg q p.m. (n=1645) %	MEVACOR 20 mg b.i.d. (n=1646) %	MEVACOR 40 mg b.i.d. (n=1649) %
Body as a Whole					
Asthenia	1.4	1.7	1.4	1.5	1.2
Gastrointestinal					
Abdominal pain	1.6	2.0	2.0	2.2	2.5
Constipation	1.9	2.0	3.2	3.2	3.5
Diarrhea	2.3	2.6	2.4	2.2	2.6
Dyspepsia	1.9	1.3	1.3	1.0	1.6
Flatulence	4.2	3.7	4.3	3.9	4.5
Nausea	2.5	1.9	2.5	2.2	2.2
Musculoskeletal					
Muscle cramps	0.5	0.6	0.8	1.1	1.0
Myalgia	1.7	2.6	1.8	2.2	3.0
Nervous System/Psychiatric					
Dizziness	0.7	0.7	1.2	0.5	0.5
Headache	2.7	2.6	2.8	2.1	3.2
Skin					
Rash	0.7	0.8	1.0	1.2	1.3
Special Senses					
Blurred vision	0.8	1.1	0.9	0.9	1.2

Other clinical adverse reactions reported as possibly, probably or definitely drug related in 0.5 to 1.0% of patients in any drug treated group are listed below. In all these cases the incidence with drug or placebo was not statistically different.

Body as a Whole: chest pain.

Gastrointestinal: acid regurgitation, dry mouth, vomiting.

Musculoskeletal: leg pain, shoulder pain, arthralgia.

Nervous System/Psychiatric: insomnia, paresthesia.

Skin: alopecia, pruritus.

Special Senses: eye irritation.

No significant difference was found among the different treatment groups including placebo in the incidence of serious clinical adverse experiences including death due to CHD, nonfatal myocardial infarction, cancer, and deaths due to all causes. This study was not designed or powered to evaluate the incidence of these serious clinical adverse experiences. The EXCEL study included a minority of patients at risk of or with coronary artery disease; however, its findings cannot be extrapolated in this respect to other segments of the high-risk population.

Laboratory Tests: Marked persistent increases of serum transaminases have been noted (see Warnings and Precautions, Myopathy/Rhabdomyolysis).

Other liver function test abnormalities including elevated alkaline phosphatase and bilirubin have been reported. In the EXCEL study, 7.3% of the patients on lovastatin had elevations of CK levels of at least twice the normal value on one or more occasions compared to 6.2% on placebo.

The EXCEL study, however, excluded patients with factors known to be associated with an increased risk of myopathy (see Warnings and Precautions, Myopathy/Rhabdomyolysis and Drug Interactions, Drug-Laboratory Test Interactions).

Nervous System: Visual evoked response, nerve conduction measurements and electromyography in over 30 patients showed no evidence of neurotoxic effects of lovastatin.

Effect on the Lens: See Warnings and Precautions.

Post-Market Adverse Drug Reactions: The following adverse events have also been reported during post-marketing experience with MEVACOR, regardless of causality assessment: hepatitis, cholestatic jaundice, vomiting, anorexia, paresthesia, peripheral neuropathy, psychiatric disturbances including anxiety, alopecia, erythema multiforme, including Stevens-Johnson syndrome and toxic epidermal necrolysis.

Gynecomastia has been reported following treatment with other HMG-CoA reductase inhibitors.

An apparent hypersensitivity syndrome has been reported rarely which has included one or more of the following features: anaphylaxis, angioedema, lupus-like syndrome, polymyalgia rheumatica, dermatomyositis, vasculitis, thrombocytopenia, leukopenia, eosinophilia, hemolytic anemia, positive ANA, ESR increase, arthritis, arthralgia, urticaria, asthenia, photosensitivity, fever, flushing, chills, dyspnea and malaise.

DRUG INTERACTIONS: Drug-Drug Interactions: Concomitant Therapy with Other Lipid Metabolism Regulators: Combined drug therapy should be approached with caution as information from controlled studies is limited. Based on post-marketing surveillance, gemfibrozil, other fibrates and lipid lowering doses of niacin (nicotinic acid) may increase the risk of myopathy when given concomitantly with HMG-CoA reductase inhibitors, probably because they can produce myopathy when given alone (see below and Warnings and Precautions, Muscle Effects). Therefore, combined drug therapy should be approached with caution.

Bile Acid Sequestrants: Preliminary evidence suggests that the cholesterol lowering effects of MEVACOR and the bile acid sequestrant, cholestyramine, are additive.

When MEVACOR is used concurrently with cholestyramine or any other resin, an interval of at least two hours should be maintained between the two drugs, since the absorption of MEVACOR may be impaired by the resin.

Gemfibrozil and Other Fibrates, Lipid-Lowering Doses (≥1 g/day) of Niacin (nicotinic acid): These drugs increase the risk of myopathy when given concomitantly with lovastatin, probably because they can produce myopathy when given alone (see Warnings and Precautions, Myopathy/Rhabdomyolysis Caused by Drug Interactions). There is no evidence to suggest that these agents affect the pharmacokinetics of lovastatin.

Myopathy, including rhabdomyolysis, has occurred in patients who were receiving coadministration of MEVACOR with fibric acid derivatives or niacin, particularly in subjects with pre-existing renal insufficiency (see Warnings and Precautions, Myopathy/Rhabdomyolysis Caused by Drug Interactions).

Erythromycin, Clarithromycin and Telithromycin: See Warnings and Precautions, Measures to reduce the risk of myopathy/rhabdomyolysis caused by drug interactions.

Angiotensin-Converting Enzyme Inhibitors: Hyperkalemia associated with myositis (myalgia and elevated CK) has been reported in the case of a single patient with insulin-dependent diabetes mellitus and mild renal insufficiency who received MEVACOR concomitantly with an angiotensin-converting enzyme inhibitor (lisinopril).

Coumarin Anticoagulants: Clinically evident bleeding and/or increased prothrombin time have been reported occasionally in patients taking coumarin anticoagulants concomitantly with lovastatin. It is recommended that in patients taking anticoagulants, prothrombin time be determined before starting lovastatin and frequently enough during early therapy to ensure that no significant alteration of prothrombin time occurs. Once a stable prothrombin time has been documented, prothrombin times can be monitored at intervals usually recommended for patients on coumarin anticoagulants. If the dose of lovastatin is changed, the same procedure should be repeated. Lovastatin therapy has not been associated with bleeding or with changes in prothrombin time in patients not taking anticoagulants.

Cyclosporine or Danazol: The risk of myopathy/rhabdomyolysis is increased by concomitant administration of cyclosporine or danazol particularly with higher doses of lovastatin (see Warnings and Precautions, Myopathy/Rhabdomyolysis).

Digoxin: In patients with hypercholesterolemia, concomitant administration of lovastatin and digoxin had no effect on digoxin plasma concentrations.

Beta-Adrenergic Blocking Drugs: In healthy volunteers, the coadministration of propranolol and lovastatin resulted in a slight decrease of the AUC of lovastatin and its metabolites as well as in a significant decrease of the C_{max} for the lovastatin metabolites.

However there was no clinically relevant interaction reported in patients who have been receiving MEVACOR concomitantly with beta adrenergic blocking agents.

Cytochrome P-450 Inhibitors (CYP3A4): Lovastatin has no CYP3A4 inhibitory activity; therefore, it is not expected to affect the plasma levels of other drugs metabolized by CYP3A4. However, lovastatin itself is a substrate for CYP3A4. Potent inhibitors of CYP3A4 increase the risk of myopathy by increasing the plasma levels of HMG CoA reductase inhibitory activity during lovastatin therapy. These inhibitors include itraconazole, ketoconazole, erythromycin, clarithromycin, telithromycin, HIV protease inhibitors, and nefazodone (see Warnings and Precautions, Myopathy/Rhabdomyolysis Caused by Drug Interactions).

Amiodarone: The risk of myopathy/rhabdomyolysis is increased when amiodarone is used concomitantly with higher doses of a closely related member of the HMG-CoA reductase inhibitor class (see Warnings and Precautions, Myopathy/Rhabdomyolysis Caused by Drug Interactions).

Verapamil: The risk of myopathy/rhabdomyolysis is increased when verapamil is used concomitantly with higher doses of a closely related member of the HMG-CoA reductase inhibitor class (see Warnings and Precautions, Myopathy/Rhabdomyolysis Caused by Drug Interactions).

Fusidic Acid (oral or IV): Patients on fusidic acid (oral or IV) treated concomitantly with lovastatin may have an increased risk of myopathy/rhabdomyolysis (see Warnings and Precautions, Muscle Effects, Other drugs). No clinical data is available regarding drug interaction between fusidic acid and lovastatin.

Other Concomitant Therapy: Although specific interaction studies were not performed, in clinical studies, MEVACOR was used concomitantly with a number of diuretics and nonsteroidal anti inflammatory drugs (NSAIDs), hypoglycemic drugs (chlorpropamide, glipizide, glyburide, insulin), without evidence, to date, of clinically significant adverse interactions.

Drug-Food Interactions: Grapefruit juice contains one or more components that inhibit CYP3A4 and can increase the plasma levels of drugs metabolized by CYP3A4. The effect of typical consumption (one 250 mL glass daily) is minimal (34% increase in active plasma HMG-CoA reductase inhibitory activity as measured by the area under the concentration-time curve) and of no clinical relevance. However, very large quantities (over 1 liter daily) significantly increase the plasma levels of HMG-CoA reductase inhibitory activity during lovastatin therapy and should be avoided (see Warnings and Precautions, Myopathy/Rhabdomyolysis Caused by Drug Interactions).

Drug-Laboratory Test Interactions: Lovastatin may elevate creatine phosphokinase and transaminase levels (see Adverse Reactions, Laboratory Tests). In the differential diagnosis of chest pain in a patient on therapy with MEVACOR, cardiac and non cardiac fractions of these enzymes should be determined.

DOSAGE AND ADMINISTRATION: Dosing Considerations:

- Patients should be placed on a standard cholesterol-lowering diet before receiving MEVACOR and should continue on this diet during treatment with MEVACOR. If appropriate, a program of weight control and physical exercise should be implemented.
- Prior to initiating therapy with MEVACOR, secondary causes for elevations in plasma lipid levels should be excluded. A lipid profile should also be performed.
- **Patients with Hypercholesterolemia:** The usual starting dose is 20 mg/day given as a single dose with the evening meal. Single daily doses given with the evening meal have been shown to be more effective than the same dose given with the morning meal. Adjustments of dosage, if required, should be made at intervals of not less than 4 weeks, to a maximum of 80 mg daily given in single doses or divided doses with the morning and evening meals (see Warnings and Precautions, Myopathy/Rhabdomyolysis and Drug Interactions). Divided doses (i.e., twice daily) tend to be slightly more effective than single daily doses.
- **Patients with Severe Hypercholesterolemia:** In patients with severe hypercholesterolemia, higher doses (80 mg/day) may be required (see Warnings and Precautions, Myopathy/Rhabdomyolysis and Drug Interactions). Cholesterol levels should be monitored periodically and consideration should be given to reducing the dosage of MEVACOR if cholesterol levels fall below the desired range.
- **Patients with Established Coronary Heart Disease:** In the trials involving patients with coronary heart disease and administered MEVACOR with (colestipol) [Familial Atherosclerosis Treatment Study (FATS)] or without concomitant therapy, the dosages used were 20 to 80 mg daily, given in single or divided doses. In the two trials which utilized MEVACOR alone, the dose was reduced if total plasma cholesterol decreased to below 2.85 mmol/L or if LDL-C decreased to below 2.1 mmol/L, respectively.
- **Concomitant Therapy:** (see Drug Interactions, Concomitant Therapy with Other Lipid Metabolism Regulators).

  In patients taking cyclosporine, danazol, gemfibrozil, other fibrates or lipid lowering doses (≥1 g/day) of niacin concomitantly with MEVACOR, the dose of MEVACOR should not exceed 20 mg/day. In patients taking amiodarone or verapamil concomitantly with MEVACOR, the dose of MEVACOR should not exceed 40 mg/day (see Warnings and Precautions, Measures to reduce the risk of myopathy/rhabdomyolysis caused by drug interactions and Drug Interactions).

  The dosage of MEVACOR should be individualized according to baseline LDL-C, total-C/HDL-C ratio and/or TG levels to achieve the recommended desired lipid values at the lowest possible dose and the patient response. Lipid levels should be monitored periodically and, if necessary, the dose of MEVACOR adjusted based on desired lipid levels.

Missed Dose: If a tablet is missed at its usual time, it should be taken as soon as possible. But, if it is too close to the time of the next dose: only the prescribed dose should be taken at the appointed time. **A double dose should not be taken.**

OVERDOSAGE:

Five healthy human volunteers have received up to 200 mg of lovastatin as a single dose without clinically significant adverse experiences. A few cases of accidental overdosage have been reported; no patients had any specific symptoms and all patients recovered without sequelae. The maximum dosage taken was 5-6 g.

In the event of overdosage, treatment should be symptomatic and supportive, liver function should be monitored, and appropriate therapy instituted. Until further experience is obtained, no specific therapy of overdosage can be recommended.

The dialyzability of lovastatin and its metabolites in man is not known.

For management of a suspected drug overdose, CPhA recommends that you contact your **regional Poison Control Centre**. See the *CPS* Directory section for a list of Poison Control Centres.

ACTION AND CLINICAL PHARMACOLOGY: Mechanism of Action: MEVACOR is a cholesterol lowering agent isolated from a strain of *A. terreus*. After oral ingestion, lovastatin, which is an inactive lactone, is hydrolyzed to the corresponding β-hydroxy acid form. This principal metabolite is a specific inhibitor of 3-hydroxy-3-methylglutaryl-coenzyme A (HMG-CoA) reductase.

This enzyme catalyzes the conversion of HMG-CoA to mevalonate, which is an early and rate limiting step in the biosynthesis of cholesterol.

Pharmacodynamics: Lovastatin reduces cholesterol production by the liver and induces some changes in cholesterol transport and disposition in the blood and tissues. The mechanism(s) of this effect is believed to involve both reduction of the synthesis of Low Density Lipoprotein (LDL), and an increase in LDL catabolism as a result of induction of the hepatic LDL receptors.

Pharmacokinetics: Lovastatin has complex pharmacokinetic characteristics.

Metabolism: Lovastatin is metabolized by the microsomal hepatic enzyme system (Cytochrome P-450 isoform 3A4 system). The major active metabolites present in human plasma are the β-hydroxy acid of lovastatin, its 6'-hydroxy, 6'-hydroxymethyl, and 6'-exomethylene derivatives.

STORAGE AND STABILITY: Keep container tightly closed and store at 15-30°C. Protect from light.

INFORMATION FOR THE PATIENT: Published in e-CPS, available by subscription at www.e-cps.ca.

DOSAGE FORMS, COMPOSITION AND PACKAGING: 20 mg: Each light blue-colored, octagon-shaped, flat, bevelled-edge tablet, engraved with MSD 731 on one side and plain on the other side, contains: lovastatin 20 mg. Nonmedicinal ingredients: butylated hydroxyanisole, indigotine on alumina, lactose, magnesium stearate, microcrystalline cellulose and pregelatinized starch. Blister packages of 28.

40 mg: Each green-colored, octagon-shaped, flat, bevelled-edge tablet, engraved with MSD 732 on one side and plain on the other side, contains: lovastatin 40 mg. Nonmedicinal ingredients: butylated hydroxyanisole, indigotine and Quinoline yellow both on alumina substratum, lactose, magnesium stearate, microcrystalline cellulose and pregelatinized starch. Blister packages of 28.

(Shown in Product Identification Section)

Mexiletine

Antiarrhythmic

CPhA Monograph

Date of Preparation: August 2006
Date of Revision: November 2010

This monograph has been compiled by CPhA and reviewed by experts. It may contain information different from that found in Health Canada-approved Product Monographs. The reader is referred to the *CPS* Editorial Policy for more information.

SUMMARY PRODUCT INFORMATION:

Route of Administration	Dosage Form	Strength
Oral	Capsule	100 mg, 200 mg

INDICATIONS AND CLINICAL USE:

No antiarrhythmic drug has been shown to reduce the incidence of sudden death in patients with asymptomatic ventricular arrhythmias. Most antiarrhythmic drugs have the potential to cause dangerous arrhythmias; some have been shown to be associated with an increased incidence of sudden death. In light of the above, physicians should carefully consider the risks and benefits of antiarrhythmic therapy for all patients with ventricular arrhythmias.

Health Canada-approved Indications Include:

- the treatment of documented life-threatening ventricular arrhythmias such as sustained ventricular tachycardia
- the treatment of patients with documented, symptomatic ventricular arrhythmias when the symptoms are of sufficient severity to require treatment

Uses Without Health Canada Approval:

- the management of neuropathic pain of diverse origins

CONTRAINDICATIONS:

- Patients who are hypersensitive to mexiletine as demonstrated by rash, urticaria, or anaphylaxis
- Cardiogenic shock
- Bradycardia
- High degree AV block (in the absence of a pacemaker)

WARNINGS AND PRECAUTIONS: Mortality: The results of the Cardiac Arrhythmia Suppression Trial (CAST) in post-myocardial infarction patients with asymptomatic ventricular arrhythmias showed a significant increase in mortality and in nonfatal cardiac arrest rate in patients treated with certain antiarrhythmic agents compared with a matched placebo group. Whether these results apply to other patient populations, or to other antiarrhythmic agents such as mexiletine, is uncertain, but it is prudent to consider these results when using any antiarrhythmic agent [*N Engl J Med* 1991;324(12):781-8].

Patients with sinus node dysfunction, conduction defects, hypotension or systolic heart failure must be monitored closely when receiving mexiletine.

Patients with poorly compensated liver disease may have impaired clearance of mexiletine and may be more susceptible to adverse events.

Special Populations: Pregnant Women: The safety of mexiletine in pregnancy has not been established. Limited data suggest mexiletine does not present a risk to the fetus. When administered to a pregnant woman near term, detectable serum concentrations were produced in the newborn.

Nursing Women: Mexiletine is excreted in breast milk with a milk: plasma ratio of 1.45. Consider alternatives to breast feeding if administered to a lactating mother.

Monitoring and Laboratory Tests: When used for the treatment of ventricular arrhythmia: ECG.

ADVERSE REACTIONS: Adverse Drug Reactions Overview: Like all antiarrhythmic drugs, mexiletine can give rise to serious life-threatening arrhythmias.

More Common Adverse Drug Reactions: See Table 1.

Table 1: Mexiletine

More Common Adverse Drug Reactions (≥1%)

Body System	Effect	Clinical Comment
Digestive	Gastrointestinal intolerance: heartburn, nausea, vomiting, constipation	Administer with food or after a meal.

Less Common Adverse Drug Reactions (<1%): Cardiovascular: arrhythmias, palpitations, atrial fibrillation, AV block, ventricular arrhythmias, torsades de pointes (polymorphic ventricular tachycardia), systolic heart failure, hypotension.

Dermatologic: erythroderma, flushing, hypersensitivity, rash, Stevens-Johnson syndrome.

Hematologic: agranulocytosis, leucopenia, neutropenia, thrombocytopenia.

Hepatic/Biliary/Pancreatic: elevated liver enzymes, jaundice, hepatic necrosis.

Immune: allergic reactions, lupus-like symptoms.

Neurologic/Central Nervous System: ataxia, dizziness, nystagmus, paresthesia, seizures, tremor.

Ophthalmologic: abnormal vision.

Psychiatric: confusion, hallucination, somnolence, drug-induced psychosis.

Abnormal Hematologic and Clinical Chemistry Findings: See Table 2.

Table 2: Mexiletine

Abnormal Hematologic and Clinical Chemistry Findings

Test	Effect	Clinical Comment
Complete blood count (CBC)	Aplastic anemia, neutropenia, leucopenia thrombocytopenia	Withdraw drug if possible, monitor CBC and provide supportive care as needed.
Liver enzymes	Elevated bilirubin, liver transaminases	Withdraw drug if possible, monitor transaminases.

DRUG INTERACTIONS: Overview: Mexiletine undergoes extensive hepatic metabolism mediated primarily by CYP2D6 and to a lesser extent by CYP1A2. Drugs that alter the function of these enzymes have the potential to alter the pharmacokinetics of mexiletine. Conversely, mexiletine may alter the pharmacokinetics of other drugs metabolized by CYP isozymes.

Concurrent administration of amiodarone did not significantly alter the pharmacokinetics of mexiletine in patients with supraventricular tachyarrhythmias.

Cimetidine did not significantly alter the pharmacokinetics of mexiletine in healthy volunteers.

Drug-Drug Interactions: See Table 3.

Table 3: Mexiletine

Drug-Drug Interactions

Interacting Drug	Effect	Clinical Comment
Caffeine	Mexiletine inhibits the metabolism of caffeine, thereby predisposing patients to symptoms of caffeine excess (nausea, tremor, insomnia). Caffeine does not appreciably alter the pharmacokinetics of mexiletine.	When starting mexiletine, patients should be advised of the potential increase in sensitivity to caffeine.
Cigarette smoking	The $t_{½}$ of mexiletine decreased by 35% and the clearance increased by 32% in volunteers who smoked ≥15 cigarettes per day.	Patients may require larger than usual doses of mexiletine to achieve a therapeutic effect.
Fluvoxamine	Fluvoxamine, an inhibitor of CYP1A2, significantly increased the AUC and C_{max} of mexiletine in healthy volunteers.	If fluvoxamine is added to the regimen of a patient receiving mexiletine, monitor the patient closely for signs of mexiletine excess and titrate the dose downward accordingly.
Opioids	Delay gastric emptying and prolong the time required for absorption of mexiletine from the gastrointestinal tract.	The onset of action of mexiletine may be delayed in patients receiving morphine during the treatment of a myocardial infarction.
Phenytoin	Phenytoin induces metabolism of mexiletine in nonsmoking healthy volunteers resulting in a 55% decrease in AUC and 51% decrease in $t_{½}$ of mexiletine.	Higher doses of mexiletine may be required in patients receiving phenytoin.
Quinidine	In extensive metabolizers of mexiletine, quinidine inhibits CYP2D6 thereby significantly increasing the $t_{½}$ and decreasing clearance of mexiletine. In poor metabolizers, quinidine has no significant effect on mexiletine pharmacokinetics.	The majority of the population are extensive metabolizers and thus susceptible to a significant interaction with quinidine. The dose of mexiletine should therefore be titrated carefully in patients receiving quinidine. Conversely, in patients receiving mexiletine the dose may need to be lowered after the introduction of quinidine.
Rifampin	Rifampin induces metabolism of mexiletine in healthy volunteers resulting in a 39% decrease in AUC and 41% decrease in $t_{½}$ of mexiletine.	Higher doses of mexiletine may be required in patients receiving rifampin.
Theophylline	Mexiletine inhibits CYP1A2-mediated demethylation of theophylline. This results in decreased clearance and increased plasma levels of theophylline and symptoms of theophylline toxicity.	Use the combination of mexiletine and theophylline with caution. Lower dosages of theophylline may be required.
Urinary acidifiers (acetazolamide, ammonium chloride) and alkalinizers (sodium bicarbonate)	Mexiletine is a base. Changes in urinary pH may markedly alter serum concentrations of mexiletine in some patients. Acidification of urine significantly shortens the half-life and increases the fraction of unchanged drug excreted in urine.	Consider the effects of drugs that greatly alter the pH of urine in patients receiving mexiletine (e.g., sodium bicarbonate) and titrate the dose as necessary.

Drug-Food Interactions: As noted in Table 3, mexiletine may increase exposure to caffeine.

DOSAGE AND ADMINISTRATION: Dosing Considerations: The dosage of mexiletine must be individualized based on the therapeutic response and tolerability, both of which are dose-dependent.

When used to treat ventricular arrhythmias it is essential to monitor the ECG (to assess antiarrhythmic effect) and blood pressure closely during the first 24 hours. It is also prudent to monitor the ECG after steady state levels are reached (i.e. after approximately 5 half-lives, see Pharmacokinetics: Adults) initially and after each dose increase.

It is recommended that mexiletine be taken with food.

Recommended Dose and Dosage Adjustment: Adults: See Table 4.

Dosage in Dialysis: The terminal elimination half-life of mexiletine is not increased markedly by renal dysfunction. Thus dosage adjustments are not required in patients with severe renal dysfunction including those receiving dialysis.

Hepatic Impairment: Clearance of mexiletine is significantly impaired in patients with hepatic dysfunction. The terminal elimination half-life is prolonged significantly and plasma concentrations are considerably higher in patients with hepatic cirrhosis compared with control patients with normal liver function. If the drug is used in patients with liver dysfunction (as judged by INR and serum bilirubin concentrations), start with a low initial dose (100 mg) with slow careful titration and monitor the patient closely for signs and symptoms of mexiletine toxicity (cardiovascular, gastrointestinal and neurologic complaints).

Genetic Polymorphism: CYP2D6-mediated hepatic metabolism of mexiletine is affected by a genetic polymorphism (sparteine/debrisoquine polymorphism). Poor metabolizers lack the gene for CYP2D6 and thus do not produce the major hydroxylated metabolite of the drug. The clearance of the drug is prolonged compared with extensive metabolizers of the drug. This is of potential clinical significance particularly with respect to certain drug-drug interactions.

Table 4: Mexiletine

Dose in Adult Patients

Indication	Route	Initial Dose	Dose Titration	Usual Dose	Maximum Dose	Duration of Therapy	Clinical Comment
Ventricular arrhythmia	Oral	400 mg oral loading dose	The first maintenance dose may be given 2 to 6 hours after the loading dose depending on the clinical response.	400–800 mg divided in 2 or 3 equal doses	Some patients may require 1200 mg/day	Varies with severity of the condition and the response of the patient	In the case of ventricular arrhythmia, the therapeutic concentration in serum ranges from 0.5 to 2.0 mg/L [3–11 μmol/L], although the utility of routine serum concentration monitoring is questionable.
Neuropathy (Not an approved use in Canada)	Oral	200 mg once daily	Increase to 200 mg BID then 200 mg TID at 2 day intervals		Not to exceed 1200 mg/day	Varies according to the response	Given that neuropathy is not imminently life-threatening, slow titration of the dose improves tolerability and is preferred.

OVERDOSAGE: The major toxic effects of mexiletine in overdose involve the cardiovascular system and include complete heart block, torsades de pointes and asystole. Seizures may also occur. Administration of activated charcoal may be helpful in preventing absorption of mexiletine from the gastrointestinal tract if given within two hours of overdose.

Management of mexiletine overdose is similar to that for other class Ib antiarrhythmic agents such as lidocaine. Supportive care is the mainstay of therapy. Monitor and manage the hemodynamic status of the patient. Pressors may be required to counteract hypotension. Patients with class Ib antiarrhythmic overdose typically do not respond well to atropine, so dopamine, norepinephrine or isoproterenol may be required to counteract bradyarrhythmias. External pacing may be helpful. Seizures should be treated with benzodiazepines. Cardiopulmonary bypass may be considered in selected cases.

For management of a suspected drug overdose, CPhA recommends that you contact your **Regional Poison Control Centre**. See the *CPS* Directory section for a list of Poison Control Centres.

ACTION AND CLINICAL PHARMACOLOGY: Mechanism of Action: Mexiletine is a class Ib antiarrhythmic agent with local anesthetic and membrane stabilizing properties. The drug is similar in structure and activity to lidocaine, but has a longer terminal elimination half-life, which makes oral administration feasible. The predominant effect on the action potential is mediated through the sodium channel. The drug binds to the sodium channel and impedes sodium influx during phase 0. This slows cardiac conduction. At high tissue concentrations, class Ib agents shorten the duration of the action potential and refractoriness.

Pharmacokinetics: Adults: Absorption: Mexiletine is well absorbed from the gastrointestinal tract with an oral bioavailability of 90%. Maximum plasma concentrations (C_{max}) are achieved in approximately 1.5 to 4 hours after oral administration.

Distribution: The volume of distribution of mexiletine is large (580-707 L in healthy volunteers), is independent of dose and varies greatly between individuals. Approximately 43% of the drug in circulation is bound to albumin and alpha$_1$-acid glycoprotein.

Metabolism: Mexiletine undergoes extensive hepatic metabolism mediated by cytochrome P450 (CYP) isozymes to form a large number of pharmacologically inactive metabolites.

The major metabolites of mexiletine are produced by CYP2D6-mediated hydroxylation. A well described polymorphism in the gene that produces CYP2D6 affects the metabolism of mexiletine. In individuals who lack the gene for CYP2D6 ("poor metabolizers"), mexiletine does not undergo hydroxylation and, thus, there are significant differences in the metabolic profile and in the rate of clearance of the drug in these individuals compared with "extensive metabolizers". The frequency of the poor metabolizer phenotype is variable within any given population, but is generally reported to be <10%.

Mexiletine also undergoes CYP1A2-mediated oxidative metabolism.

The mean terminal elimination half-life has been reported to range from 6.7 to 17.2 hours.

Excretion: Renal excretion is of minor importance in the excretion of mexiletine, although acidification of urine can significantly increase the fraction of drug excreted in urine and decrease the terminal elimination half-life. Under normal physiologic conditions, approximately 5% of an administered dose is recovered unchanged in urine.

Mezavant®

5-ASA

Lower Gastrointestinal Anti-inflammatory

Shire

Date of Revision: August 18, 2010

SUMMARY PRODUCT INFORMATION:

Route of Administration	Dosage Form/ Strength	Clinically Relevant Nonmedicinal Ingredients
Oral	Delayed and extended release tablet 1.2 g	None. For a complete listing see Dosage Forms, Composition and Packaging.

INDICATIONS AND CLINICAL USE: MEZAVANT (mesalamine delayed and extended release tablets) is indicated for:

- Induction of remission (clinical and endoscopic) in patients with active, mild to moderate ulcerative colitis.

Geriatrics (≥65 years of age): Clinical trials of MEZAVANT did not include sufficient numbers of patients aged 65 and over to determine whether they respond differently from younger patients. Other reported clinical experience has not identified differences in responses between the elderly and younger patients. Results of a single dose study on the comparative pharmacokinetic profiles in elderly healthy subjects versus young healthy subjects indicate that systemic exposure to mesalamine increased by up to approximately 2-fold in elderly subjects (>65 years) compared with younger adult subjects (18-35 years) after a 4.8 g single dose of MEZAVANT. Systemic exposures in individual subjects were inversely correlated with renal function as assessed by estimated creatinine clearance. The potential impact on the safe use of MEZAVANT in the elderly population in clinical practice should be considered (see Warnings and Precautions, and Action and Clinical Pharmacology, Pharmacokinetics, Absorption).

Pediatrics (<18 years of age): The safety and effectiveness of mesalamine has not been established in children.

CONTRAINDICATIONS:

- Patients who are hypersensitive to any salicylates (including mesalamine) or to any ingredient in the formulation or component of the container. For a complete listing, see Dosage Forms, Composition and Packaging.

WARNINGS AND PRECAUTIONS: General: The majority of patients who are intolerant or hypersensitive to sulphasalazine can take mesalamine preparations without risk of similar reactions. However, caution should be exercised when treating patients allergic to sulphasalazine.

Mesalamine has been associated with an acute intolerance syndrome that may be difficult to distinguish from a flare of inflammatory bowel disease. Although the exact frequency of occurrence has not been determined, it has occurred in 3% of patients in controlled clinical trials of mesalamine or sulphasalazine. Symptoms include cramping, acute abdominal pain and bloody diarrhoea, sometimes fever, headache and rash. If acute intolerance syndrome is suspected, prompt withdrawal is required.

Patients should be instructed to swallow MEZAVANT tablets whole, taking care not to break the outer coating. The outer coating is designed to remain intact until at least pH 7, normally in the terminal ileum, to protect the active ingredient, mesalamine, and ensure its availability throughout the colon.

Administration of a single dose of MEZAVANT 4.8 g with a high fat meal in healthy volunteers increased systemic exposure of mesalamine compared to results in the fasted state (see Dosage and Administration, Drug-Food Interactions).

Cardiovascular: Mesalamine induced cardiac hypersensitivity reactions (myocarditis and pericarditis) have been reported rarely with MEZAVANT and other mesalamine-containing preparations. Caution should be taken in prescribing this medication to patients with conditions predisposing to the development of myocarditis or pericarditis.

Gastrointestinal: Organic or functional obstruction in the upper gastrointestinal tract may delay onset of action of the product.

Adequate care should be given to patients treated with 5-ASA that have active peptic ulcers.

Acute intolerance syndrome: See General.

Hepatic/Biliary/Pancreatic: No information is available on the use of MEZAVANT in patients with hepatic impairment, and therefore, caution is recommended in these patients.

Renal: Reports of renal impairment, including minimal change in nephrology, and acute or chronic interstitial nephritis have been associated with mesalamine medications and pro-drugs of mesalamine. For any patient with known renal dysfunction, caution should be exercised and MEZAVANT should be used only if the benefits outweigh the risks. It is recommended that all patients have an evaluation of renal function prior to initiation of therapy and periodically while on treatment.

Special Populations: Pregnant Women: There are no adequate and well-controlled studies of mesalamine in pregnant women. Mesalamine is known to cross the placental barrier. MEZAVANT should only be used during pregnancy if the benefits outweigh the risks.

Nursing Women: Low concentrations of mesalamine and higher concentrations of its N-acetyl metabolite have been detected in human breast milk. While there is limited experience of lactating women using mesalamine, caution should be exercised if MEZAVANT is administered to a nursing mother and used only if the benefits outweigh the risks.

Pediatrics (<18 years of age): Safety and effectiveness of MEZAVANT in pediatric patients who are less than 18 years of age have not been established.

Geriatrics (≥65 years of age): Clinical trials of MEZAVANT did not include sufficient numbers of patients aged 65 and over to determine whether they respond differently from younger patients. Other reported clinical experience has not identified differences in responses between the elderly and younger patients. Results of a single dose study on the comparative pharmacokinetic profiles in elderly healthy subjects versus young healthy subjects indicate that systemic exposure to mesalamine increased by up to approximately 2-fold in elderly subjects (>65 years) compared with younger adult subjects (18-35 years) after a 4.8 g single dose of MEZAVANT (see Action and Clinical Pharmacology, Pharmacokinetics, Absorption). Systemic exposures in individual subjects were inversely correlated with renal function as assessed by estimated creatinine clearance. The potential impact on the safe use of MEZAVANT in the elderly population in clinical practice should be considered. In general, dose selection for an elderly patient should be cautious, usually starting at the low end of the dosing range, reflecting the greater frequency of decreased hepatic, renal, or cardiac function, and of concurrent disease or other drug therapy.

ADVERSE REACTIONS: Adverse Drug Reaction Overview: MEZAVANT tablets have been evaluated in 655 ulcerative colitis patients in controlled and open-label studies.

In two 8-week placebo-controlled clinical studies involving 621 (ITT Population) ulcerative colitis patients, 356 received 2.4 g/day or 4.8 g/day MEZAVANT tablets. More adverse events occurred in the placebo group (119) than in each of the MEZAVANT treatment groups (109 in 2.4 g/day, 92 in 4.8 g/day). The most common adverse events with MEZAVANT were headache (4.5%) and flatulence (3.4%). A lower percentage of the 356 MEZAVANT patients discontinued therapy due to adverse events compared to placebo (2.2% vs 7.3%). The most frequent adverse event leading to discontinuation from MEZAVANT therapy was exacerbation of ulcerative colitis (0.8%).

The majority of adverse events in the double blind, placebo-controlled trials were mild or moderate in severity. The percentage of patients with severe adverse events was higher in the placebo treatment group (6.2% in placebo, 1.1% in MEZAVANT 2.4 g/day, 2.2% in MEZAVANT 4.8 g/day). The most common severe adverse events were gastrointestinal disorders which were mainly symptoms associated with ulcerative colitis. Pancreatitis occurred in less than 1% of patients during clinical trials and resulted in discontinuation of therapy with MEZAVANT in patients experiencing this event.

Clinical Trial Adverse Drug Reactions: Because clinical trials are conducted under very specific conditions the adverse reaction rates observed in the clinical trials may not reflect the rates observed in practice and should not be compared to the rates in the clinical trials of another drug. Adverse drug reaction information from clinical trials is useful for identifying drug-related adverse events and for approximating rates.

Overall, the percentage of patients who experienced any adverse event was similar across treatment groups. Treatment related adverse events occurring in MEZAVANT- or placebo-groups at a frequency of at least 1% in two Phase 3, 8-week, double blind, placebo-controlled trials are listed in Table 1.

Table 1: MEZAVANT

Treatment Related Adverse Events in Two Phase 3 Trials Experienced by at Least 1% of the MEZAVANT Group and at a Rate Greater than Placebo

Event[b]	MEZAVANT[a] 2.4 g/day n=177 (%)	MEZAVANT[a] 4.8 g/day n=179 (%)	Placebo[a] n=179 (%)
Nervous System Disorders			
Headache	3	2	0
Gastrointestinal Disorders			
Flatulence	3	2	2
Investigations			
Increased alanine aminotransferase	1	1	0
Skin and Subcutaneous Tissue Disorders			
Pruritus	1	1	0
Alopecia	0	1	0

[a] Percentages are based on the number of patients in the safety population for each treatment group.

[b] Treatment related adverse events for which the placebo rate equals or exceeds the rate for MEZAVANT are nausea, ulcerative colitis, abdominal pain, dizziness, decreased weight (placebo only), and dyspepsia.

The following treatment related adverse events, presented by body system, were reported infrequently (less than 1%) by MEZAVANT-treated ulcerative colitis patients in controlled trials.

Less Common Clinical Trial Adverse Drug Reactions (<1%): Cardiovascular and Vascular Disorders: Uncommon: tachycardia, hypertension, hypotension.

Skin and Subcutaneous Tissue Disorders: Uncommon: acne, rash, urticaria.

Gastrointestinal Disorders: Uncommon: abdominal distension, diarrhoea, pancreatitis, rectal polyp, vomiting.

Investigations: Uncommon: decreased platelet count, elevated total bilirubin.

Musculoskeletal and Connective Tissue Disorders: Uncommon: arthralgia, back pain.

Nervous System Disorders: Uncommon: somnolence, tremor.

Respiratory, Thoracic and Mediastinal Disorders: Uncommon: pharyngolaryngeal pain.

General Disorders and Administrative Site Disorders: Uncommon: asthenia, face oedema, fatigue, pyrexia.

Ear and Labyrinth Disorders: Uncommon: ear pain.

Pooled Safety Analysis: In the pooled safety analysis of patients with ulcerative colitis who participated in the clinical studies, the majority of subjects did not experience treatment emergent adverse events associated with MEZAVANT. Of the events reported, the majority were mild or moderate in severity. The three most frequently reported adverse events within the pooled safety analysis of the ulcerative colitis patient clinical studies were headache, abdominal pain and nausea. Adverse drug reactions observed during clinical trials (pooled safety analysis) are listed in Table 2.

Table 2: MEZAVANT

Adverse Drug Reactions Associated with MEZAVANT from Pooled Safety Analysis

System/Organ Class	Incidence Category	Adverse Drug Reaction
Blood and Lymphatic System Disorders	Uncommon (>0.1% and <1%)	Thrombocytopenia
Ear and Labyrinth Disorders	Uncommon (>0.1% and <1%)	Ear pain
Gastrointestinal Disorders	Common (≥1% and <10%)	Abdominal distension, abdominal pain, diarrhoea, dyspepsia, flatulence, nausea, vomiting
	Uncommon (>0.1% and <1%)	Colitis, pancreatitis, rectal polyp
General Disorders and Administration Site Conditions	Common (≥1% and <10%)	Asthenia, pyrexia
	Uncommon (>0.1% and <1%)	Face oedema, fatigue
Investigations	Common (≥1% and <10%)	Liver-function test abnormal (e.g. ALT, AST, bilirubin)
Musculoskeletal and Connective Tissue Disorders	Common (≥1% and <10%)	Arthralgia associated with myalgia, back pain
Nervous System Disorders	Common (≥1% and <10%)	Headache
	Uncommon (>0.1% and <1%)	Dizziness, somnolence, tremor
Respiratory, Thoracic and Mediastinal Disorders	Uncommon (>0.1% and <1%)	Pharyngolaryngeal pain
Skin and Subcutaneous Tissue Disorders	Common (≥1% and <10%)	Pruritus, rash
	Uncommon (>0.1% and <1%)	Acne, alopecia, urticaria
Cardiovascular and Vascular Disorders	Common (≥1% and <10%)	Hypertension
	Uncommon (>0.1% and <1%)	Hypotension, Tachycardia

Adverse Events Seen with MEZAVANT During Post-Marketing Surveillance: Cardiovascular and Vascular Disorders: myocarditis, pericarditis.

Hepatobiliary Disorders: hepatitis.

Renal Disorders: interstitial nephritis.

Respiratory, Thoracic and Mediastinal Disorders: hypersensitivity pneumonitis (including interstitial pneumonitis, allergic alveolitis, eosinophilic pneumonitis).

Adverse Events Seen with Other Mesalamine Products: Blood and Lymphatic System Disorders: agranulocytosis, aplastic anaemia, leukopenia, neutropenia, pancytopenia.

Nervous System Disorders: neuropathy.

Respiratory, Thoracic and Mediastinal Disorders : bronchospasm.

Hepatobiliary Disorders: cholelithiasis.

Skin and Subcutaneous Tissue Disorders: angioedema.

Musculoskeletal and Connective Tissue Disorders: systemic-lupus erythematosus-like syndrome.

Renal Disorders: nephrotic syndrome.

Abnormal Hematologic and Clinical Chemistry Findings: In the pivotal studies conducted, there has been no notable change from baseline in mean haematology and biochemistry parameters.

DRUG INTERACTIONS: Drug-Drug Interactions: No investigations of interaction between MEZAVANT and other drugs have been performed. However, there have been reports of interactions between products containing mesalamine and other drugs. The concurrent use of mesalamine with known nephrotoxic agents, including non-steroidal anti-inflammatory drugs (NSAIDs) and azathioprine may increase the risk of renal reactions. In patients receiving azathioprine or 6-mercaptopurine, concurrent use of mesalamine can increase the potential for blood disorders, especially leucopenia.

Drug-Food Interactions: Administration of a single dose of MEZAVANT 4.8 g with a high fat meal in healthy volunteers resulted in further delay in absorption and plasma concentrations of mesalamine were detectable 4 hours following dosing. However, high fat meal increased systemic exposure of mesalamine (mean C_{max}: ↑91%; mean AUC: ↑16%) compared to results in the fasted state; consideration should be given to this observation when prescribing to patients expected to consume high-fat meals. However, MEZAVANT was administered with food, part of an unrestricted diet, in the pivotal phase 3 trials.

Drug-Herb Interactions: Interactions with herbal products have not been established.

Drug-Laboratory Test Interactions: Interactions with laboratory tests have not been established.

DOSAGE AND ADMINISTRATION:

Recommended Dose and Dosage Adjustment: MEZAVANT is intended for once daily, oral administration with food. The tablets should be swallowed whole with liquid and should not be crushed or chewed.

The recommended dose for the induction of remission in patients with mild to moderate ulcerative colitis is two to four 1.2 g tablets to be taken once daily for a total daily dose of 2.4 to 4.8 g. No difference in remission rates was noted between doses of 2.4 g/day and 4.8 g/day, but trends in improvement in the sigmoidoscopy score and clinical improvement (reduction in UC-DAI from baseline of ≥3 points) was noted at 4.8 g/day dose versus 2.4 g/day. The studies were not powered to look at differences between MEZAVANT dosing regimens of 2.4 g/day and 4.8 g/day. Similar efficacy was shown when a total daily dose of 2.4 g of MEZAVANT was given as one dose (QD) or when given in two divided doses (BID).

Administration of a single dose of MEZAVANT 4.8 g with a high fat meal in healthy volunteers increased systemic exposure of mesalamine compared to results in the fasted state; consideration should be given to this observation when prescribing to patients expected to consume high-fat meals. However, MEZAVANT was administered with food, part of an unrestricted diet, in the pivotal phase 3 trials. (See Drug Interactions, Drug-Food Interactions and Action and Clinical Pharmacology, Pharmacokinetics.)

Children: The safety and effectiveness of mesalamine has not been established in children. As for tablets needing to be swallowed whole, consideration should be given to the ability to swallow the intact tablet.

Elderly: In general, dose selection for an elderly patient should be cautious, usually starting at the low end of the dosing range, reflecting the greater frequency of decreased hepatic, renal, or cardiac function, and of concurrent disease or other drug therapy.

Missed Dose: If a dose of this medication has been missed, it should be skipped and taken as usual the next day.

OVERDOSAGE:

MEZAVANT is an aminosalicylate, and symptoms of salicylate toxicity may include tinnitus, vertigo, headache, confusion, drowsiness, sweating, hyperventilation, vomiting, and diarrhea. Severe intoxication may lead to disruption of electrolyte balance and blood-pH, hyperthermia, and dehydration.

Conventional therapy for salicylate toxicity may be beneficial in the event of acute overdosage. Fluid and electrolyte imbalance should be corrected by the administration of appropriate intravenous therapy. Adequate renal function should be maintained.

> For management of a suspected drug overdose, contact your regional Poison Control Centre. See the *CPS* Directory section for a list of Poison Control Centres.

ACTION AND CLINICAL PHARMACOLOGY: The MEZAVANT tablet contains a core of mesalamine (5-aminosalicylic acid), 1.2 g, formulated with MMX Multi Matrix System technology. MMX uses a gastro-resistant film of methacrylic acid copolymers, Type A and Type B, which are designed to delay the initial release of mesalamine until exposure to approximately pH 7 and above, normally in the terminal ileum. A consistent and sustained release was observed across the pH range 6.8 to 7.2. The MMX technology also uses a matrix of lipophilic and hydrophilic excipients which facilitate the delayed and extended delivery of effective concentrations of mesalamine through the entire colon with limited systemic absorption.

Mechanism of Action: The mechanism of action of mesalamine is not fully understood, but appears to have a topical anti-inflammatory effect on the colonic epithelial cells.

Mucosal production of arachidonic acid metabolites, both through the cyclooxygenase and lipoxygenase pathways, is increased in patients with chronic inflammatory bowel disease, and it is possible that mesalamine diminishes inflammation by blocking cyclooxygenase and inhibiting prostaglandin production in the colon.

Mesalamine has the potential to inhibit the activation of nuclear factor kappa B (NFκB) and consequently the production of key pro-inflammatory cytokines. More recently, it has been proposed that impairment of PPAR-γ nuclear receptors (γ-form of peroxisome proliferator-activated receptors) may be implicated in ulcerative colitis. PPAR-γ receptor agonists have shown efficacy in ulcerative colitis and evidence has been accumulating that the mechanism of action of mesalamine may be mediated by PPAR-γ receptors.

Pharmacodynamics: The pharmacodynamic actions of mesalamine occur in the colonic/rectal mucosa local to the delivery of drug from MEZAVANT into the lumen. There is information suggesting that severity of colonic inflammation in ulcerative colitis patients treated with mesalamine is inversely correlated with mucosal concentrations of mesalamine. However, plasma concentrations representing systemically absorbed mesalamine are not believed to contribute extensively to efficacy.

Pharmacokinetics: The pharmacokinetic information in this section is based on data from Phase I studies with MEZAVANT and from studies carried out with other formulations of mesalamine.

MEZAVANT contains a 1.2 g core of mesalamine formulated in a multi-matrix system. This system is coated with methacrylic acid copolymers Type A and Type B, which are designed to dissolve at pH 7 and above, facilitating the extended delivery of effective concentrations of mesalamine through the entire colon with limited systemic absorption.

Absorption: The total absorption of mesalamine from MEZAVANT 2.4 g or 4.8 g given once daily for 14 days to healthy volunteers was found to be approximately 21-22% of the administered dose. Steady state was achieved generally by 2 days after dosing.

Gamma-scintigraphy studies have shown that a single dose of MEZAVANT 1.2 g (one tablet) passed rapidly and intact through the upper gastrointestinal tract of fasted healthy volunteers. Scintigraphic images showed a trail of radiolabelled tracer throughout the colon and rectum, indicating that mesalamine had distributed throughout the targeted site of action. Complete disintegration of MEZAVANT and complete release of mesalamine occurred after approximately 17.4 hours. Availability of mesalamine in the colon begins at 6 hours after dosing and continues beyond 24 hours post-dose. Following a single dose of MEZAVANT 4.8 g, detectable levels of mesalamine remain in the plasma for up to 72 hours post dose.

In a single and multiple dose pharmacokinetic study of MEZAVANT 2.4 or 4.8 g was administered once daily with standard meals in 56 healthy volunteers (28 per dose group). Plasma concentrations of mesalamine were detectable after 4 hours and were maximal by 8 hours after the single dose. Accumulation was found to be between 1.7- and 2.4-fold and was independent of dose. This extent of accumulation was only modestly greater (1.1- to 1.4-fold) than predictable from single dose pharmacokinetics.

After a single dose of MEZAVANT, total systemic exposure of 5-ASA appeared to increase slightly more than dose proportionately, with area under the plasma concentration-time curve increasing approximately 2.5-fold for a 2-fold dose increase from 2.4 g to 4.8 g. However there was no evidence of steady state systemic exposure increasing more than proportionately with dose.

In a single dose study, MEZAVANT 1.2 g, 2.4 g and 4.8 g were administered in the fasted state to healthy subjects. Plasma concentrations of mesalamine were detectable after 2 hours and reached a maximum by 9-12 hours on average for the doses studied. The pharmacokinetic parameters are highly variable among subjects (see Table 3). Mesalamine systemic exposure in terms of area under the plasma concentration-time curve (AUC) was slightly more than dose proportional between 1.2 g and 4.8 g MEZAVANT. Maximum plasma concentrations (C_{max}) of mesalamine increased approximately dose proportionately between 1.2 g and 2.4 g and sub-proportionately between 2.4 g and 4.8 g MEZAVANT, with the dose normalized value at 4.8 g representing, on average, 74% of that at 2.4 g based on geometric means.

Table 3: MEZAVANT

Mean (SD) PK Parameters for Mesalamine Following Single Dose Administration of MEZAVANT Under Fasting Conditions

Parameter[a] of Mesalamine	MEZAVANT 1.2 g (N=47)	MEZAVANT 2.4 g (N=48)	MEZAVANT 4.8 g (N=48)
AUC_{0-t} (ng·h/mL)	9039[c] (5054)	20 538 (12 980)	41 434 (26 640)
$AUC_{0-\infty}$ (ng·h/mL)	9578[d] (5214)	21 084 (13 185)	44 775[g] (30 302)
C_{max} (ng/mL)	857 (638)	1595 (1484)	2154 (1140)
T_{max}[b] (h)	9.0[e] (4.0–32.1)	12.0 (4.0–34.1)	12.0 (4.0–34.0)
T_{lag}[b] (h)	2.0[e] (0–8.0)	2.0 (1.0–4.0)	2.0 (1.0–4.0)
$T_{1/2}$ (h) (Terminal Phase)	8.56 (6.38)	7.05[f] (5.54)	7.25[g] (8.32)

a Arithmetic mean of parameter values are presented except for T_{max} and T_{lag}.
b Median (min, max).
c N=43.
d N=27.
e N=46.
f N=33.
g N=36.

Administration of a single dose of MEZAVANT 4.8 g with a high fat meal resulted in further delay in absorption and plasma concentrations of mesalamine were detectable 4 hours following dosing. However, a high fat meal increased systemic exposure of mesalamine (mean C_{max}: ↑91%; mean AUC: ↑16%) compared to results in the fasted state.

In a single-dose pharmacokinetic study of MEZAVANT, 4.8 g was administered in the fasted state to 71 healthy male and female volunteers (28 young (18-35 years); 28 elderly (65-75 years); 15 elderly (>75 years)). Increased age resulted in increased systemic exposure (up to approximately 2-fold, based on AUC_{0-t}, $AUC_{0-\infty}$ and C_{max}) to mesalamine and its metabolite, N-acetyl-5-aminosalicylic acid, but did not affect the percentage of mesalamine absorbed (see Table 4). Increased age resulted in a slower apparent elimination in individual subjects were inversely correlated with renal function as assessed by estimated creatinine clearance.

Distribution: Following dosing of MEZAVANT, the distribution profile of mesalamine is presumed to be the same as that for other mesalamine containing products. Mesalamine has a relatively small volume of distribution of approximately 18 L, confirming minimal extravascular penetration of systemically available drug, which is consistent with the absence of any significant secondary pharmacology. Mesalamine is 43% bound to plasma proteins when in vitro plasma concentrations are 2.5 µg/mL.

Metabolism: The only major metabolite of mesalamine (5-aminosalicylic acid) is N-acetyl-5-aminosalicylic acid, which is pharmacologically inactive. Its formation is brought about by N-acetyltransferase (NAT) activity in the liver and in the cytosol of intestinal mucosal cells, principally by NAT-1. Although this enzyme is known to be subject to genetic polymorphism, NAT-1 genotypes have been shown not to be predictive of mesalamine efficacy or toxicity.

Table 4: MEZAVANT

Mean (SD) PK Parameters for Mesalamine Following Single Dose Administration of MEZAVANT 4.8 g Fasting Conditions to Young and Elderly Subjects

Parameter of 5-ASA	Young Subjects (18–35 yrs) (N=28)	Elderly Subjects (65–75 yrs) (N=28)	Elderly Subjects (>75 yrs) (N=15)
$AUC_{0\text{-}t}$ (ng·h/mL)	51 570 (23 870)	73 001 (42 608)	65 820 (25 283)
$AUC_{0\text{-}\infty}$ (ng·h/mL)	58 057[b] (22 429)	89 612[c] (40 596)	63 067[d] (22 531)
C_{max} (ng/mL)	2243 (1410)	4999 (4381)	4832 (4383)
t_{max}[a] (h)	22.0 (5.98–48.0)	12.5 (4.00–36.0)	16.0 (4.00–26.0)
t_{lag}[a] (h)	2.00 (1.00–6.00)	2.00 (1.00–4.00)	2.00 (2.00–4.00)
$t_{½}$ (h), terminal phase	5.68[b] (2.83)	9.68[c] (7.47)	8.67[d] (5.84)
Renal clearance (L/h)	2.05 (1.33)	2.04 (1.16)	2.13 (1.20)

[a] Median (min-max).
[b] N=15.
[c] N=16.
[d] N=13.
Arithmetic mean (SD) data are presented; N=Number of subjects.

Excretion: Elimination of mesalamine is mainly via the renal route following metabolism to N-acetyl-5-aminosalicylic acid (acetylation). However, there is also limited excretion of the parent drug in urine. Of the approximately 21-22% of the dose absorbed, less than 8% of the dose was excreted unchanged in the urine at steady state, compared with greater than 13% for N-acetyl-5-aminosalicylic acid. The apparent terminal half-lives for mesalamine and its major metabolite, after administration of MEZAVANT 2.4 g and 4.8 g were, on average, 7-9 hours and 8-12 hours, respectively.

Special Populations and Conditions: Pediatrics: No information is available in patients who are less than 18 years of age (see Warnings and Precautions).

Geriatrics: Systemic exposure to mesalamine increased by up to approximately 2-fold in elderly subjects (>65 years) compared with younger adult subjects (18-35 years) after a 4.8 g single dose of MEZAVANT (see Action and Clinical Pharmacology, Pharmacokinetics, Absorption). Systemic exposures in individual subjects were inversely correlated with renal function as assessed by estimated creatinine clearance. The potential impact on the safe use of MEZAVANT in the elderly population in clinical practice should be considered (see Warnings and Precautions).

Gender: No consistent trend on gender effect was observed in the clinical trials.

Race: No pharmacokinetic information is available which examines MEZAVANT in different races.

Hepatic Insufficiency: No information is available for patients with hepatic impairment (see Warnings and Precautions and Adverse Reactions).

Renal Insufficiency: No information is available for patients with mild, moderate and severe renal impairment (see Warnings and Precautions and Adverse Reactions).

Genetic Polymorphism: Mesalamine is principally metabolised by NAT-1. Although this enzyme is known to be subject to genetic polymorphism, NAT-1 genotypes have been shown not to be predictive of mesalamine efficacy or toxicity.

STORAGE AND STABILITY: Store at room temperature 15 to 25°C; excursions permitted to 30°C.

INFORMATION FOR THE PATIENT: Published in e-CPS, available by subscription at www.e-cps.ca.

DOSAGE FORMS, COMPOSITION AND PACKAGING: Each red-brown ellipsoidal, film coated tablet, debossed on one side with S476 contains: mesalamine 1.2 g. Nonmedicinal ingredients: carnauba wax, silica (colloidal hydrated), magnesium stearate, methacrylic acid copolymer types A and B, polyethyleneglycol (macrogol) 6000, red ferric oxide (E172), sodium carboxymethylcellulose (carmellose sodium), sodium starch glycolate (type A), stearic acid, talc, titanium dioxide (E171) and triethylcitrate. Opaque high density polyethylene (HDPE) bottles of 60 and 120 with child-resistant closure.

The MEZAVANT delayed and extended release tablet contains a core of 5-aminosalicylic acid (5-ASA; mesalamine), 1200 mg, formulated with MMX Multi Matrix System technology. MMX uses a gastro-resistant film of methacrylic acid copolymers, Type A and Type B, which are designed to delay the initial release of mesalamine until exposure to approximately pH 7 and above, normally in the terminal ileum. A consistent and sustained release was observed across the pH range 6.8 to 7.2. The MMX technology also uses a matrix of lipophilic and hydrophilic excipients which facilitate the delayed and extended delivery of effective concentrations of mesalamine through the entire colon with limited systemic absorption.

(Shown in Product Identification Section)

Miacalcin® NS Pr

calcitonin salmon

Bone Metabolism Regulator

Novartis Pharmaceuticals

Date of Preparation: August 26, 1999
Date of Revision: February 14, 2008

SUMMARY PRODUCT INFORMATION:

Route of Administration	Dosage Form/ Strength	Clinically Relevant Nonmedicinal Ingredients
Nasal spray	200 IU/actuation	Benzalkonium chloride, hydrochloric acid, sodium chloride and purified water. For a complete listing see Dosage Forms, Composition and Packaging.

INDICATIONS AND CLINICAL USE: MIACALCIN (synthetic calcitonin; salmon) Nasal Spray is indicated for the treatment of postmenopausal osteoporosis in females greater than five years postmenopause with low bone mass relative to healthy premenopausal females. Significant effects on lumbar vertebral bone mineral density , but not on forearm and hip bone mineral density, have been demonstrated.

MIACALCIN Nasal Spray is recommended in conjunction with an adequate calcium (at least 1000 mg elemental calcium per day) and vitamin D (400 IU per day) intake to retard the progressive loss of bone mass.

Geriatrics (>65 years of age): Clinical trials using MIACALCIN NS have included postmenopausal women up to 77 years of age. No unusual adverse events or increased incidence of common adverse events have been noted in patients over 65 years of age.

Pediatrics (<18 years of age): The safety and efficacy of MIACALCIN in children have not been established.

CONTRAINDICATIONS:

- Known hypersensitivity to salmon calcitonin (s-calcitonin) or to any component of the formulation (See Warnings and Precautions and Adverse Reactions).

WARNINGS AND PRECAUTIONS: Immune: Allergic Reactions: Because calcitonin is a polypeptide, the possibility of a systemic allergic reaction exists. There have been rare reports of serious allergic-type reactions, such as bronchospasm, swelling of the tongue or throat, tachycardia, hypotension, collapse and anaphylactic shock in post marketing. The usual provisions should be made for the emergency treatment of such a reaction should it occur. Allergic reactions should be differentiated from generalized flushing and hypotension.

Skin testing should be considered prior to treatment with MIACALCIN NS for patients with suspected sensitivities to calcitonin (see Monitoring and Laboratory Tests).

Ear/Nose/Throat: Nasal Examinations: Nasal adverse events occurred in 17% of patients who received MIACALCIN (synthetic calcitonin; salmon) Nasal Spray and in 14% of patients who received placebo nasal spray in studies in postmenopausal females. Therefore, a nasal examination should be performed prior to start of treatment with nasal calcitonin and at any time nasal complaints occur.

In all postmenopausal patients treated with MIACALCIN Nasal Spray, the most commonly reported nasal adverse events included rhinitis (8.2%), nasal dryness (3.9%), epistaxis (2.4%), and sinusitis (1.6%). In clinical trials in another disorder (Paget's Disease), 2.8% of patients developed nasal ulcerations.

If severe ulceration of the nasal mucosa occurs, as indicated by ulcers greater than 1.5 mm in diameter or penetrating below the mucosa, or those associated with heavy bleeding, MIACALCIN Nasal Spray should be discontinued. Although smaller ulcers often heal without withdrawal of MIACALCIN Nasal Spray, medication should be discontinued temporarily until healing occurs.

Special Populations: Pregnant Women: There are no adequate and well controlled studies in pregnant women with s-calcitonin. MIACALCIN NS is not indicated in pregnancy. Synthetic calcitonin (salmon) has been shown to cause a decrease in fetal birth weights without any fetal abnormalities in rabbits when given by injection in doses 70-278 times the intranasal dose recommended for human use based on body surface area. Since synthetic calcitonin (salmon) does not cross the placental barrier, this may be due to metabolic effects in the pregnant animal.

Nursing Women: It is not known whether this drug is excreted in human milk and should not be administered to nursing mothers. Synthetic calcitonin (salmon) has been shown to inhibit lactation in animals and should not be administered to nursing mothers.

Pediatrics (<18 years of age): The safety and efficacy of MIACALCIN in children have not been established. Its use is not recommended in pediatrics.

Geriatrics (>65 years of age): Clinical trials using MIACALCIN NS have included postmenopausal women up to 77 years of age. No unusual adverse events or increased incidence of common adverse events have been noted in patients over 65 years of age.

Monitoring and Laboratory Tests: Skin testing should be considered prior to treatment with MIACALCIN NS for patients with suspected sensitivities to calcitonin. The following procedure is suggested: Prepare a dilution of 10 IU per mL by withdrawing 0.05 mL of commercially available synthetic calcitonin (salmon) solution for injection in a tuberculin syringe and filling it to 1.0 mL with Dextrose Injection 5%, USP (or Saline Injection, USP). Mix well, discard 0.9 mL and inject intracutaneously 0.1 mL (approximately 1 IU) on the inner aspect of the forearm. Observe the injection site 15 minutes after injection. The appearance of more than mild erythema or wheal constitutes a positive response.

ADVERSE REACTIONS: Adverse Drug Reaction Overview: The most commonly reported adverse events with MIACALCIN (synthetic calcitonin; salmon) Nasal Spray were local effects such as rhinitis, nasal dryness with crusting, non-severe epistaxis and sinusitis.

In normal adults, who have a relatively low rate of bone resorption, the administration of exogenous calcitonin results in only a slight decrease in serum calcium. When bone resorption is more rapid, decreases in serum calcium are more pronounced in response to calcitonin.

Clinical Trial Adverse Drug Reactions: Because clinical trials are conducted under very specific conditions the adverse reaction rates observed in the clinical trials may not reflect the rates observed in practice and should not be compared to the rates in the clinical trials of another drug. Adverse drug reaction information from clinical trials is useful for identifying drug-related adverse events and for approximating rates.

MIACALCIN (synthetic calcitonin; salmon) Nasal Spray has been evaluated for safety in more than 650 patients treated for osteoporosis for up to two years.

Table 1 is based on controlled trials in patients treated with MIACALCIN NS at doses of 50, 100, 200, or 400 IU/day for up to 2 years. The table includes all AEs with an incidence of 1% or greater in the MIACALCIN NS all combined doses treatment group, irrespective of causal relationship to study drug.

In approximately one-half of the patients tested after six months or more of treatment, indications of circulating antibodies to salmon calcitonin were obtained. In most patients the presence of antibodies does not reduce the clinical efficacy of exogenous salmon calcitonin.

Table 1: MIACALCIN NS

Common AEs Occurring in ≥ 1% of Patients Receiving MIACALCIN NS, Combined Doses Treatment Group for up to 2 Years, by Body System (regardless of study drug relationship)

Body System/Adverse Event	MIACALCIN NS (n=697) %	Placebo (n=389) %
Respiratory Thoracic and Mediastinal Disorders		
Rhinitis	8.2	5.4
Nasal Dryness	3.9	3.6
Epistaxis	2.4	2.1
Nasal Crusting	2.2	2.8
Nasal Discomfort	1.6	1.0
Sinusitis	1.6	0.5
Upper Respiratory Tract Infection	1.4	2.3
Nasal Irritation	1.4	1.5
Pharyngitis	1.0	1.0
Gastro-intestinal Disorders		
Abdominal Pain	3.0	1.5
Constipation	1.7	1.8
Nausea	1.7	1.0
Dyspepsia	1.6	0.3
General Disorders		
Influenza Symptoms	1.6	2.6
Fatigue	1.1	0.3
Vascular Disorders		
Hypertension	1.7	0.8
Flushing	4.6	5.1
Nervous System Disorders		

(cont'd)

Table 1: MIACALCIN NS *(cont'd)*

Common AEs Occurring in ≥ 1% of Patients Receiving MIACALCIN NS, Combined Doses Treatment Group for up to 2 Years, by Body System (regardless of study drug relationship)

Body System/Adverse Event	MIACALCIN NS (n=697) %	Placebo (n=389) %
Headache	2.7	2.8
Depression	1.6	1.5
Dizziness	1.6	0.8
Musculoskeletal and Connective Tissue Disorders		
Back Pain	2.9	0.8
Arthralgia	2.0	1.8
Bone Fracture	1.4	1.5
Arthrosis	1.0	1.0
Eye Disorders		
Lacrimation Abnormal	1.0	0.8
Infections and Infestations		
Cystitis	1.1	1.0
Infection	1.4	1.0

MIACALCIN has also been evaluated for safety in more than 900 patients, who were at least 1-year postmenopausal, treated for up to 5 years in the Prevent Recurrence of Osteoporotic Fractures (P.R.O.O.F.) Trial. Similar types of adverse reactions were reported in this study. However, the incidence for adverse reactions in this trial, involving 942 patients exposed to MIACALCIN Nasal Spray and 307 patients exposed to placebo nasal spray, were generally higher than in the 2 year trials due to the longer observation period. In addition, these events were reported with a similar frequency in both the MIACALCIN and placebo groups.

Table 2 includes P.R.O.O.F AEs occuring in ≥1% of patients receiving MIACALCIN NS, assessed as definitely, probably, possibly, or unlikely drug related by the investigators.

Table 2: MIACALCIN NS

P.R.O.O.F: AEs Occurring in ≥1% of Patients Receiving MIACALCIN NS, Regardless of Study Drug Relationship

Body System/Adverse Event	MIACALCIN NS (n=942) %	Placebo (n=307) %
General Disorders and Administration Site Conditions		
Edema (e.g. tongue, extremity, face, generalized)	3.1	2.6
Accidental trauma[a]	1.0	1.3
Asethenia[a]	1.3	1.0
Chest pain[a]	2.9	2.9
Hot flushes[a]	1.3	2.0
Cardiovascular Disorders		
Arrhythmia[a]	1.0	1.6
Gastrointestinal Disorders		
Diarrhea,	1.8	1.0
Dysgeusia	1.3	1.0
Hearing and Vestibular Disorder		
Ear Disorder[a] (e.g. sensation of fullness, stuffiness, blockage)	1.0	1.3
Immune System Disorders		
Allergy	1.6	1.4
Metabolic and Nutritional Disorders		
Hypercalcemia[a]	1.7	1.3
Musculoskeletal Disorders		
Arthropathy[a]	5.5	5.9
Leg pain[a]	2.2	2.3
Pain[a] (e.g. musculoskeletal, general)	4.5	5.5
Nervous System Disorders		
Headache Dysphonia[a] Somnolence[a]	3.9	7.2
Respiratory, Thoracic and Mediastinal Disorders		

(cont'd)

Table 2: MIACALCIN NS *(cont'd)*

P.R.O.O.F: AEs Occurring in ≥1% of Patients Receiving MIACALCIN NS, Regardless of Study Drug Relationship

Body System/Adverse Event	MIACALCIN NS (n=942) %	Placebo (n=307) %
Rhinitis (including nasal edema, nasal congestion, sneezing, allergic rhinitis)	30.6	20.8
Nasal discomfort (e.g. nasal odour, nasal mucosal erythema, mucosal excoriation).	15.8	13.0
Epistaxis	12.6	11.7
Rhinitis ulcerative	3.4	1.6
Abnormal Chest Sounds[a] (e.g. basilar, crepitations, rales)	1.2	1.0
Skin Disorders		
Skin disorder[a] (e.g. fissures,lesions, sores)	1.6	0.7
Dry skin[a]	1.1	0.3
Vascular Disorder		
Purpura	1.3	0.7
Vision Disorders		
Cataract[a]	2.8	1.3
Eye abnormality[a] (dryness, infection, irritation)	1.2	2
Glaucoma[a]	1.0	0.0

[a] Additional adverse reactions that occurred in the P.R.O.O.F. trial not included in the 2 years trial data.

Less Common Clinical Trial Adverse Drug Reactions: Gastrointestinal Disorders: nausea, vomiting. These effects usually subsided spontaneously.

General Disorders and Administration Site Conditions: dizziness, flushing accompanied by a sensation of heat and chills. These effects usually subsided spontaneously.

Genito-urinary Disorders: Uncommonly polyuria. These effects usually subsided spontaneously.

Immune System Disorders: MIACALCIN Nasal Spray may give rise to hypersensitivity reactions such as generalized skin reactions, flushing, edema (facial, extremity and generalized), hypertension and arthralgia. Allergic and anaphylactoid-like reactions and single case of anaphylactic shock have been reported.

Respiratory, Thoracic and Mediastinal Disorders: nasal polyp, nasal septum ulceration, and nasoseptal deviation. Most of the nasal events were mild to moderate in severity and did not prompt discontinuation. MIACALCIN Nasal Spray nasal adverse event rates were 73.5% mild, 24.3% moderate, and 2.2% severe (placebo nasal spray adverse event rates were 69.5% mild, 24.3% moderate, and 6.2% severe).

Abnormal Hematologic and Clinical Chemistry Findings: Antibodies to Salmon Calcitonin: In approximately one-half of the patients tested after six months or more of treatment, indications of circulating antibodies to salmon calcitonin were obtained. In most patients the presence of antibodies does not reduce the clinical efficacy of exogenous salmon calcitonin.

Urine Sediment Abnormalities: Urine sediment abnormalities have not been reported in ambulatory volunteers treated with MIACALCIN Nasal Spray. Coarse granular casts containing renal tubular epithelial cells were reported in the urine of young adult volunteers at bed rest who were given injectable synthetic calcitonin (salmon) in order to determine the effect of MIACALCIN on immobilization osteoporosis. There was no other evidence of renal abnormality and the urine sediment became normal after salmon calcitonin therapy was stopped.

Post-Market Adverse Drug Reactions: rash generalised, pruritus, cough, isolated anaphylactic-type reactions and anaphylactoid reactions including tachycardia, hypotension and collapse. Single case of anaphylactic shock have been reported.

DRUG INTERACTIONS: Drug-Drug Interactions: Concomitant use of calcitonin and lithium may lead to a reduction in plasma lithium concentrations. The dose of lithium may need to be adjusted.

Formal studies designed to evaluate drug interactions with s-calcitonin have not been conducted.

Drug-Food Interactions: The interaction of MIACALCIN NS with food has not been studied.

Drug-Herb Interactions: The interaction of MIACALCIN NS with herbal medications or supplements has not been studied.

Drug-Laboratory Test Interactions: The interaction of MIACALCIN NS with laboratory tests has not been studied.

Drug-Lifestyle Interactions: Effect on ability to drive and use machines: No studies exist on the effects of MIACALCIN NS on ability to drive and use machines. MIACALCIN NS may cause fatigue, dizziness and visual disturbances, which may impair the patient's reactions. Patients must therefore be warned that these effects may occur, in which case they should not drive or use machines.

DOSAGE AND ADMINISTRATION: Dosing Considerations: Pediatrics (<18 years of age): The safety and efficacy of MIACALCIN in children have not been established. Use is therefore not recommended.

Elderly (>65 years of age): Clinical trials using MIACALCIN NS have included postmenopausal women up to 77 years of age.

Recommended Dose and Dosage Adjustment: The recommended dose of MIACALCIN (synthetic calcitonin; salmon) Nasal Spray in postmenopausal women is one spray (200 IU i.e. 0.2 μg) per day administered intranasally, alternating nostrils daily.

Drug effect may be monitored by periodic measurements of lumbar vertebral bone mass to document stabilization of bone mass or increases in bone density.

Missed Dose: Patients who miss one dose of MIACALCIN NS (salmon calcitonin) should not increase the dose of MIACLACIN NS to compensate for the missed dose or doses, but should continue with therapy as soon as possible.

Administration: Instructions on priming of the pump upon first use of the device and nasal introduction of MIACALCIN (synthetic calcitonin; salmon) Nasal Spray should be given to the patient. Instructions for patients are supplied with individual bottles. Patients should be asked to notify their physician if they develop significant nasal irritation.

Patients should be advised of the following:

- Upon, first use only, the pump must be primed. The product should be allowed to reach room temperature before priming.
- After priming and first use, the product should be stored at room temperature in an upright position. Each bottle contains 14 doses.

OVERDOSAGE:

Nausea, vomiting, flushing and dizziness are known to be dose dependent when MIACALCIN is administered parenterally. Such events might therefore also be expected to occur in association with an overdose of MIACALCIN NS. Treatment would be symptomatic. Isolated cases of overdose have been reported but no serious adverse reactions have been associated with high doses.

Single doses of MIACALCIN Nasal Spray up to 1600 IU and doses up to 800 IU per day for three days and chronic administration of doses up to 600 IU per day have been studied without serious adverse effects. A dose of 1000 IU of MIACALCIN (synthetic calcitonin; salmon) injectable solution given subcutaneously may produce nausea and vomiting. A dose of MIACALCIN injectable solution of 32 IU per kg per day for one or two days demonstrated no additional adverse effects.

There have been no reports of hypocalcemic tetany. However, the pharmacologic actions of MIACALCIN Nasal Spray suggest that this could occur in overdose. Therefore, provisions for parenteral administration of calcium should be available for the treatment of overdose.

For management of a suspected drug overdose, CPhA recommends that you contact your **regional Poison Control Centre**. See the *CPS* Directory section for a list of Poison Control Centres.

ACTION AND CLINICAL PHARMACOLOGY: Mechanism of Action: Salmon calcitonin (s-Calcitonin) is a polypeptide hormone secreted by the parafollicular cells of the thyroid gland in mammals and by the ultimobranchial gland of birds and fish. It is of physiological importance in the regulation of calcium metabolism in certain animal species and may also have physiological importance in certain extraskeletal systems (e.g., GI and renal function).

MIACALCIN (synthetic calcitonin; salmon) Nasal Spray (NS) markedly reduces the removal of calcium from bone in conditions with an increased rate of bone resorption such as osteoporosis. Osteoclast activity is inhibited, and osteoblast formation and activity seem to be stimulated. MIACALCIN NS inhibits bone resorption, thus lowering abnormally increased serum calcium. Additionally, at the beginning of treatment it increases the urinary excretion of calcium, phosphorus, and sodium by reducing their tubular re-uptake. Serum calcium, however, is not reduced below the normal range.

Salmon calcitonin acts primarily on bone, but direct renal effects and actions on the gastrointestinal tract are also recognized. Salmon calcitonin appears to have actions essentially identical to calcitonins of mammalian origin, but its potency per mg is greater and it has a longer duration of action. The actions of calcitonin on bone and its role in normal human bone physiology are still incompletely understood.

Single injections of synthetic calcitonin (salmon) result in a marked transient inhibition of the ongoing bone resorptive process. With prolonged use, there is a persistent, smaller decrease in the rate of bone resorption. Histologically this is associated with a decreased number of osteoclasts and an apparent reduction in their resorptive activity. Decreased osteocytic resorption may also be involved.

Because of its chemical nature (a peptide of 32 amino acids), calcitonin may be administered parenterally to achieve maximal absorption. Small percentages of the dose are apparently absorbed when administered by the buccal, oral, topical or inhalation routes; thus far, only the nasal absorption has been well substantiated and demonstrated to show a significant clinical effect.

Pharmacodynamics: All calcitonin structures consist of 32 amino acids in a single chain, with a ring of seven amino-acid residues at the N-terminus, the sequence of which differs from species to species. MIACALCIN (Synthetic Calcitonin; Salmon) Nasal Spray is a synthetic polypeptide of 32 amino acids in the same linear sequence that is found in calcitonin of salmon origin. Due to the greater affinity of salmon calcitonin to receptor binding sites than calcitonins from mammalian species, including the synthetic human calcitonin, MIACALCIN NS is more potent and longer acting. In terms of bioactivity, the potency of MIACALCIN NS was found to be about half that of the drug given by i.m. or s.c. injection.

Osteoporosis is a disease characterized by low bone mass and deterioration of bone tissue architecture leading to enhanced bone fragility and consequent increase in fracture risk. The most common type of osteoporosis occurs in postmenopausal females. Osteoporosis is a result of a disproportionate rate of bone resorption compared to bone formation which disrupts the structural integrity of bone, rendering it more susceptible to fracture. The most common sites of these fractures are the vertebrae, hip, and distal forearm (Colles' fractures). Vertebral fractures occur with the highest frequency and are associated with back pain, spinal deformity and a loss of height.

The primary action of calcitonin is on bone. Studies have shown that calcitonin most consistently affects the osteoclasts. These cells show decreased function, altered morphology and decreased numbers under the influence of calcitonin. Osteocytic osteolysis also appears to be depressed by this hormone. These effects result in the inhibition by calcitonin of bone resorption. Calcitonin may also stimulate osteoblastic bone formation, but decreases in osteoblastic function have also been reported and final conclusions are not yet possible.

Pharmacokinetics: Absorption: The data on bioavailability of MIACALCIN NS obtained by various investigators using different methods show great variability, with a range varying between approximately 3 and 50% relative to intramuscular administration. As is the case with other polypeptide hormones, plasma levels of s-calcitonin are not predictive of the therapeutic response, and hence s-calcitonin activity should be evaluated by biochemical or clinical parameters. MIACALCIN is absorbed rapidly by the nasal mucosa. Maximum plasma concentrations occur within the first hour of administration (median about 10 minutes).

The absolute bioavailability of synthetic calcitonin (salmon) is about 70% after either intramuscular or subcutaneous injection.

Distribution: In the dose range 100-400 IU, area under the plasma concentration curve (AUC) increases roughly in proportion to the dose. However, administration of doses higher than 400 IU does not result in further increases in the AUC for the drug.

The apparent volume of distribution is 0.15-0.3 L/kg, and protein binding amounts to 30 40%.

Metabolism: The patterns of tissue distribution of the hormone seem to differ for the three source species studied thus far and correlate with sites of degradation. Thus, porcine calcitonin tends to accumulate in the liver and kidney and both tissues degrade this form. Human calcitonin shows similar properties except that the kidney is relatively more important for the metabolism of human calcitonin than for porcine calcitonin. In the case of salmon calcitonin, accumulation and degradation seem to occur almost exclusively in the kidney.

Excretion: In the case of salmon calcitonin, accumulation and degradation seem to occur almost exclusively in the kidney. Degradation of all forms of calcitonin occurs by splitting the molecule into smaller fragments which are biologically and immunologically inactive. Very little renal excretion of the intact calcitonin molecule takes place. It appears that salmon calcitonin cannot cross the placental barrier.

For MIACALCIN NS, the half-life of elimination of synthetic calcitonin (salmon) is calculated to be around 20 minutes. There is no accumulation of the drug on repeated admnistration at 10-hour intervals for up to 15 days.

After either intramuscular or subcutaneous injection the elimination half-life is 70 to 90 minutes . Synthetic calcitonin (salmon) and its metabolites are excreted up to 95% by the kidney, the fraction of the parent drug being 2%.

Special Populations and Conditions: Pediatrics: The safety and efficacy of MIACALCIN in children have not been established.

Geriatrics: Clinical trials using MIACALCIN NS have included postmenopausal women up to 77 years of age. No unusual adverse events or increased incidence of common adverse events have been noted in patients over 65 years of age.

STORAGE AND STABILITY: Unopened MIACALCIN Nasal Spray should be stored in the refrigerator between 2 and 8°C and protected from freezing.

After priming, MIACALCIN Nasal Spray should be stored at room temperature (between 15-30°C) and used within 4 weeks. To ensure correct delivery, the bottle should be kept in an upright position.

SPECIAL HANDLING INSTRUCTIONS: To ensure correct delivery, the bottle should be kept in an upright position.

Upon, first use only, the pump must be primed. The product should be allowed to reach room temperature before priming.

Pull up the protective cap, holding the bottle in an upright position, press down the upper part until it clicks. Repeat twice. After the first time the dose counter window shows white and red lines, after the second time white, and after the third time green. It is now ready for use.

After priming and first use, the product should be stored at room temperature in an upright position. Each bottle contains at least 14 doses.

INFORMATION FOR THE PATIENT: Published in e-CPS, available by subscription at www.e-cps.ca.

DOSAGE FORMS, COMPOSITION AND PACKAGING: Spray bottles delivering at least 14 metered doses of 200 IU of synthetic calcitonin (salmon), 1 unit corresponding to about 0.2 µg of synthetic calcitonin (salmon). Nonmedicinal ingredients: benzalkonium chloride, hydrochloric acid, purified water and sodium chloride. Each pack contains 2 bottles of spray solution. The device is composed of a clear, uncolored glass bottle (glass type I) and a spray mechanism containing an integrated, automatic dose-counting mechanism and a built-in mechanical stop.

(Shown in Product Identification Section)

Micardis® Ⓟ

telmisartan

Angiotensin II AT1 Receptor Blocker

Boehringer Ingelheim

Date of Revision: November 24, 2009

SUMMARY PRODUCT INFORMATION:

Route of Administration	Dosage Form/ Strength	All Nonmedicinal Ingredients
Oral	Tablet 40 mg, 80 mg	Sodium hydroxide, meglumine, povidone, sorbitol, and magnesium stearate

INDICATIONS AND CLINICAL USE: Treatment of Essential Hypertension: MICARDIS (telmisartan) is indicated for the treatment of mild to moderate essential hypertension.

MICARDIS may be used alone or in combination with thiazide diuretics.

The concurrent use with angiotensin converting enzyme inhibitors is not recommended.

Risk Reduction of Cardiovascular Morbidity: MICARDIS is indicated to reduce the risk of non-fatal stroke or non-fatal myocardial infarction in patients 55 years or older at high risk of developing major cardiovascular events who cannot tolerate an angiotensin converting enzyme inhibitor (ACEI).

High risk of cardiovascular events includes evidence of coronary artery disease, peripheral arterial disease, stroke, transient ischemic attack, or diabetes mellitus with evidence of end-organ damage. MICARDIS has been used with other required treatment such as other antihypertensives (including ACEI), antiplatelet or statins (see Warnings and Precautions, Drug Interactions).

Geriatrics (>65 years of age): No dosing adjustment is necessary. It should be recognized, however, that greater sensitivity in some older individuals can not be ruled out.

Pediatrics (<18 years of age): MICARDIS is not recommended for use in children below 18 years due to limited data on safety and efficacy.

CONTRAINDICATIONS: MICARDIS (telmisartan) is contraindicated in:

- Patients who are hypersensitive to any components of this product
- Second and third trimesters of pregnancy (see Warnings and Precautions, Special Populations, Pregnant Women)
- Lactation (see Warnings and Precautions, Special Populations, Nursing Women)

Sorbitol: In case of rare hereditary condition of fructose intolerance, the use of MICARDIS is contraindicated. MICARDIS contains 338 mg of sorbitol per maximum recommended daily dose.

WARNINGS AND PRECAUTIONS:

Serious Warnings and Precautions
When used in pregnancy, angiotensin receptor (AT_1) blockers (ARB) can cause injury or even death of the developing fetus. When pregnancy is detected, MICARDIS should be discontinued as soon as possible (see Warnings and Precautions, Special Populations).

Cardiovascular: Valvular Stenosis: There is concern on theoretical grounds that patients with aortic stenosis might be at a particular risk of decreased coronary perfusion, because they do not develop as much afterload reduction.

Hypotension: In patients who are volume-depleted by diuretic therapy, dietary salt restriction, dialysis, diarrhea or vomiting, symptomatic hypotension may occur after initiation of therapy with MICARDIS. Such conditions, especially volume and/or sodium depletion, should be corrected prior to administration of MICARDIS. In these patients, because of the potential fall in blood pressure, therapy should be started under close medical supervision. Similar considerations apply to patients with ischemic heart or cerebrovascular disease, in whom an excessive fall in blood pressure could result in myocardial infarction or cerebrovascular accident.

The use of a dual renin-angiotensin-aldosterone system (RAAS) blockade may lead to increased occurrence of hypotension when given as add-on therapy in patients with controlled blood pressure.

Endocrine and Metabolism: Hyperkalemia: Drugs such as MICARDIS that affect the renin-angiotensin-aldosterone system can cause hyperkalemia. Monitoring of serum potassium in patients at risk is recommended. Based on experience with the use of drugs that affect the renin-angiotensin system, concomitant use with potassium-sparing diuretics, potassium supplements, salt substitutes containing potassium or other medicinal products that may increase the potassium level (heparin, etc.) may lead to a greater risk of an increase in serum potassium.

The use of a dual renin-angiotensin-aldosterone system (RAAS) blockade may lead to increased occurrence of hyperkalemia when given as add-on therapy in patients with controlled blood pressure.

Hepatic/Biliary/Pancreatic: Hepatic Impairment: As the majority of telmisartan is eliminated by biliary excretion, patients with biliary obstructive disorders or hepatic insufficiency have reduced clearance of telmisartan. Three to four fold increases in C_{max} and AUC were observed in patients with liver impairment as compared to healthy subjects. MICARDIS (telmisartan) should be used with caution in these patients (see Dosage and Administration).

Renal: As a consequence of inhibiting the renin-angiotensin-aldosterone system, changes in renal function have been reported in susceptible individuals (such as patients with bilateral renal artery stenosis, unilateral renal artery stenosis to a solitary kidney, or severe congestive heart failure). Dual blockade of the renin-angiotensin-aldosterone system (e.g. concomitant use of an angiotensin II receptor antagonist with an ACE-inhibitor) has been associated with oliguria, progressive azotemia, and rarely, acute renal failure and/or death. Upon treatment with such combination, renal function should be closely monitored.

In patients whose renal function may depend on the activity of the renin-angiotensin-aldosterone system, such as patients with bilateral renal artery stenosis, unilateral renal artery stenosis to a solitary kidney, or severe congestive heart failure, treatment with agents that inhibit this system has been associated with oliguria, progressive azotemia, and rarely acute renal failure and/or death. There is no experience with long term use of MICARDIS (telmisartan) in patients with unilateral or bilateral renal artery stenosis but an effect similar to that seen with ACE inhibitors should be anticipated. In susceptible patients, concomitant diuretic use may further increase the risk. Use of telmisartan should include appropriate assessment of renal function in these types of patients.

There is no experience regarding the administration of MICARDIS (telmisartan) in patients with a recent kidney transplant.

Special Populations: Pregnant Women: Drugs that act directly on the renin-angiotensin-aldosterone system (RAAS) can cause fetal and neonatal morbidity and death when administered to pregnant women. When pregnancy is detected, MICARDIS (telmisartan) should be discontinued as soon as possible.

The use of angiotensin receptor (AT_1) blockers (ARBs) is not recommended during pregnancy. Epidemiological evidence regarding the risk of teratogenicity following exposure to angotensin converting enzyme inhibitors (another class of therapeutic products interfering with the RAAS) during the first trimester of pregnancy has not been conclusive; however a small increase in risk cannot be excluded. Given the current evidence available on the risk with ARB, similar risks may exist for this class of drugs. Patients planning pregnancy should be changed to alternative anti-hypertensive treatments which have an established safety profile for use in pregnancy. When pregnancy is diagnosed, treatment with angiotensin II antagonists should be stopped immediately, and, if appropriate, alternative therapy should be started.

The use of ARBs during the second and third trimesters is known to induce human fetotoxicity (decreased renal function, oligohydramnios, skull ossification retardation) and neonatal toxicity (renal failure, hypotension, hyperkalemia).

Infants with a history of in utero exposure to ARBs should be closely observed for hypotension, oliguria, and hyperkalemia. If oliguria occurs, attention should be directed toward support of blood pressure and renal perfusion. Exchange transfusion may be required as a means of reversing hypotension and/or substituting for disordered renal function; however, limited experience with those procedures has not been associated with significant clinical benefit.

It is not known if telmisartan can be removed from the body by hemodialysis.

Preclinical studies with telmisartan do not indicate teratogenic effect, but have shown fetotoxicity. No teratogenic effects were observed when telmisartan was administered to pregnant rats at oral doses of up to 50 mg/kg/day and to pregnant rabbits at oral doses up to 45 mg/kg/day with saline supplementation. In rabbits, fetotoxicity (total resorptions) associated with maternal toxicity (reduced body weight gain, mortality) was observed at the highest dose level (45 mg/kg/day). In rats, maternally toxic (reduction in body weight gain and food consumption) telmisartan doses of 50 mg/kg/day in late gestation and during lactation were observed to produce adverse effects in rat fetuses and neonates, including reduced viability, low birth weight, delayed maturation, and decreased weight gain. Significant levels of telmisartan were present in rat milk and rat fetuses' blood during late gestation.

Nursing Women: It is not known whether telmisartan is excreted in human milk but significant levels have been found in the milk of lactating rats. Because many drugs are excreted in human milk and because of their potential for affecting the nursing infant adversely, a decision should be made whether to discontinue nursing or discontinue the drug, taking into account the importance of the drug to the mother.

Pediatrics (<18 years of age): MICARDIS is not recommended for use in children below 18 years due to limited data on safety and efficacy.

Geriatrics (>65 years of age): Of the total number of patients receiving MICARDIS (telmisartan) in clinical studies, 551 (18.6%) were 65 to 74 years of age and 130 (4.4%) were 75 years or older. No overall age related differences were seen in the adverse effect profile, but greater sensitivity in some older patients cannot be ruled out.

Monitoring and Laboratory Tests: For specific monitoring and laboratory tests, see Warnings and Precautions (Cardiovascular, Endocrine and Metabolism, Hepatic/Biliary/Pancreatic and Renal) and Drug Interactions.

ADVERSE REACTIONS: Clinical Trial Adverse Drug Reactions: Because clinical trials are conducted under very specific conditions the adverse reaction rates observed in the clinical trials may not reflect the rates observed in practice and should not be compared to the rates in the clinical trials of another drug. Adverse drug reaction information from clinical trials is useful for identifying drug-related adverse events and for approximating rates.

Side effects were reported in clinical trials with telmisartan in the indication hypertension or in patients 50 years or older at high risk of cardiovascular events.

MICARDIS (telmisartan) has been evaluated for safety in 27 clinical trials involving 7968 patients treated for hypertension. Of these 7968 patients, 5788 patients were treated with MICARDIS monotherapy including 1058 patients treated for ≥1 year and 1395 patients treated in placebo-controlled trials.

In 3400 patients, discontinuation of therapy due to adverse events was required in 2.8% of MICARDIS patients and 6.1% of placebo patients. The following potentially serious adverse events have been reported rarely with telmisartan in controlled clinical trials: syncope and hypotension. In placebo-controlled trials, no serious adverse event was reported with a frequency of greater than 0.1% in MICARDIS-treated patients.

The safety profile of MICARDIS in patients treated for risk reduction of cardiovascular morbidity was consistent with that obtained in hypertensive patients. In this program, 11% of patients treated with telmisartan discontinued study medication due to adverse events. The most common adverse events that led to discontinuation were dizziness, hypotension and headache.

The adverse drug reactions listed below have been accumulated from controlled clinical trials in patients treated for hypertension and from post-marketing reports. The listing also takes into account serious adverse events and adverse events leading to discontinuation reported in three clinical long-term studies including 21642 patients treated with telmisartan for prevention of cardiovascular morbidity and mortality for up to six years.

All Clinical Trials: The adverse drug events listed below have been accumulated from 27 clinical trials including 5788 hypertensive patients treated with telmisartan. Adverse events have been ranked under headings of frequency using the following convention: very common (≥1/10); common (≥1/100, <1/10); uncommon (≥1/1000, <1/100); rare (≥1/10 000, <1/1000); very rare (<1/10 000).

Body as a Whole, General: Common: chest pain, influenza-like symptoms, symptoms of infection (e.g. urinary tract infection including cystitis), fatigue, conjunctivitis. Uncommon: hyperhidrosis, asthenia (weakness).

Blood and Lymphatic System: Uncommon: anemia. Rare: thrombocytopenia. Not known: eosinophilia.

Cardiovascular System: Common: edema, palpitation. Uncommon: bradycardia, orthostatic hypotension, hypotension. Rare: tachycardia.

Central and Peripheral Nervous Systems: Very common: headache. Common: dizziness, insomnia. Uncommon: vertigo.

Eye Disorders: Rare: visual disturbance.

Gastrointestinal System: Common: abdominal pain, diarrhoea, dyspepsia, nausea, constipation, gastritis. Uncommon: dry mouth, flatulence, vomiting. Rare: stomach discomfort.

Hepato-biliary Disorders: Rare: hepatic function abnormal/liver disorder.

Immune System: Rare: hypersensitivity. Not known: anaphylactic reaction.

Infections and Infestations: Uncommon: upper respiratory tract infections, urinary tract infections. Not known: sepsis including fatal outcome.

Investigations: Unknown: blood creatinine increased. Rare: blood uric acid increased, hepatic enzymes increased, blood creatinine phosphokinase increased, haemoglobin decreased.

Metabolism and Nutrition Disorders: Uncommon: hyperkalemia.

Musculoskeletal System: Common: arthralgia, muscle spasms (cramps in legs) or pain in extremity (leg pain), myalgia, arthritis, arthrosis. Uncommon: tendon pain (tendonitis like symptoms), back pain.

Nervous System: Uncommon: syncope (faint).

Psychiatric System: Common: anxiety, nervousness. Uncommon: depression.

Renal and Urinary Systems: Uncommon: renal impairment including acute renal failure.

Respiratory System: Common: upper respiratory tract infections including pharyngitis and sinusitis, bronchitis, coughing, dyspnea, rhinitis.

Skin and Appendages System: Common: skin disorders like rash. Uncommon: pruritus. Rare: erythema, drug eruption, angioedema, eczema, toxic skin eruption. Unknown: urticaria.

Hemoglobin: Infrequently, a decrease in hemoglobin has been observed which occurs more often during treatment with telmisartan than with placebo.

Placebo-Controlled Trials: The overall incidence of adverse events reported with MICARDIS (41.4%) was usually comparable to placebo (43.9%) in controlled clinical trials. Adverse events occurring in 1% or more of 1395 hypertensive patients treated with MICARDIS monotherapy in placebo-controlled clinical trials, regardless of drug relationship, include the following (see Table 1).

Table 1: MICARDIS

Adverse Events Occurring in >1% of Hypertensive Patients Treated with MICARDIS Monotherapy

Adverse Event, by System	MICARDIS Total N=1395 %	Placebo N=583 %
Body as a Whole		
Back Pain	2.7	0.9
Chest Pain	1.3	1.2
Fatigue	3.2	3.3
Influenza-Like Symptoms	1.7	1.5
Pain	3.5	4.3
Central and Peripheral Nervous Systems		
Dizziness	3.6	4.6
Headache	8.0	15.6
Somnolence	0.4	1.0
Gastrointestinal System		
Diarrhea	2.6	1.0
Dyspepsia	1.6	1.2
Nausea	1.1	1.4
Vomiting	0.4	1.0
Musculoskeletal System		
Myalgia	1.1	0.7
Respiratory System		
Coughing	1.6	1.7
Pharyngitis	1.1	0.3
Sinusitis	2.2	1.9
Upper Respiratory Tract Infection	6.5	4.6
Heart Rate and Rhythm Disorders		
ECG Abnormal Specific	0.2	1.0
Palpitation	0.6	1.0
Cardiovascular Disorders, General		
Hypertension	1.0	1.7
Oedema Peripheral	1.0	1.2

(cont'd)

Table 1: MICARDIS *(cont'd)*

The incidence of adverse events was not dose-related and did not correlate with the gender, age, or race of patients.

Less Common Clinical Trial Adverse Events (<1%): In addition, the following adverse events, with no established causality, were reported at an incidence <1% in placebo-controlled clinical trials.

Autonomic Nervous System Disorders: sweating increased.

Body as a Whole: abdomen enlarged, allergy, cyst nos, fall, fever, leg pain, rigors, syncope.

Cardiovascular Disorders, General: hypotension, hypotension-postural, leg edema.

Central and Peripheral Nervous Systems Disorders: hypertonia, migraine-aggravated, muscle contraction-involuntary.

Gastrointestinal System Disorders: anorexia, appetite increased, flatulence, gastrointestinal disorder nos, gastroenteritis, gastroesophageal reflux, melena, mouth dry, abdominal pain.

Heart Rate and Rhythm Disorders: arrhythmia, tachycardia.

Metabolic and Nutritional Disorders: diabetes mellitus, hypokalaemia.

Musculoskeletal System Disorders: arthritis, arthritis aggravated, arthrosis, bursitis, fascitis plantar, tendinitis.

Myo Endo Pericardial and Valve Disorders: myocardial infarction.

Psychiatric Disorders: nervousness.

Red Blood Cell Disorders: anemia.

Reproductive Disorders, Female: vaginitis.

Resistance Mechanism Disorders: abscess, infection, bacterial, moniliasis genital, otitis media.

Respiratory System Disorders: bronchospasm, epistaxis, pneumonia, bronchitis.

Skin and Appendage Disorders: rash, skin dry.

Urinary System Disorders: dysuria, hematuria, micturition disorder, urinary tract infection.

Vascular (Extracardiac) Disorders: cerebrovascular disorder, purpura.

Vision Disorders: vision abnormal.

Abnormal Hematologic and Clinical Chemistry Findings: In placebo-controlled clinical trials involving 1041 patients treated with MICARDIS monotherapy, clinically relevant changes in standard laboratory test parameters were rarely associated with administration of MICARDIS.

Creatinine, Blood Urea Nitrogen: Increases in BUN (≥11.2 mg/dL) and creatinine (≥0.5 mg/dL) were observed in 1.5% and 0.6% of MICARDIS-treated patients; the corresponding incidence was 0.3% each for placebo-treated patients. These increases occurred primarily with MICARDIS in combination with hydrochlorothiazide. One telmisartan treated patient discontinued therapy due to increases in creatinine and blood urea nitrogen.

Hemoglobin, Hematocrit: Clinically significant changes in hemoglobin and hematocrit (<10g/dL and <30%, respectively) were rarely observed with MICARDIS treatment and did not differ from rates in placebo-treated patients. No patients discontinued therapy due to anemia.

Serum Uric Acid: An increase in serum uric acid (≥2.7 mg/dL) was reported in 1.7% of patients treated with MICARDIS and in 0.0% of patients treated with placebo. Clinically significant hyperuricemia (>10 mEq/L) was observed in 2.3% of patients with MICARDIS, with 0.4% reported in patients at baseline. Increases in serum uric acid were primarily observed in patients who received MICARDIS in combination with hydrochlorothiazide. No patient was discontinued from treatment due to hyperuricemia.

Liver Function Tests: Clinically significant elevations in AST and ALT (>3 times the upper limit of normal) occurred in 0.1% and 0.5% respectively of patients treated with MICARDIS compared to 0.8% and 1.7% of patients receiving placebo. No telmisartan-treated patients discontinued therapy due to abnormal hepatic function.

Serum Potassium: Marked laboratory changes in serum potassium (≥+/−1.4 mEq/L) occurred rarely and with a lower frequency in MICARDIS-treated patients (0.3%, 0.1%, respectively) than in placebo patients (0.6%, 0.3%, respectively). Clinically significant changes in potassium (that exceeded 3 mEq/L) were found in 0.6% of MICARDIS-treated patients, with 0.5% of these reported at baseline. The corresponding rates for placebo-treated patients were 0.6% and 0.8%.

Cholesterol: In placebo-controlled trials, marked increases in serum cholesterol were reported in a total of 6 telmisartan-treated patients (0.4%) and no placebo patients. Two of these patients were followed over time, in both cases cholesterol values reverted to baseline levels.

Serum elevations in cholesterol were reported as adverse events in 11 of 3445 patients (0.3%) in all clinical trials. There were no reported cases of hypercholesterolemia in telmisartan-treated patients in placebo-controlled trials.

Post-Market Adverse Drug Reactions: Since the introduction of telmisartan in the market, cases of anxiety, dizziness, vision troubled, vertigo, abdominal distension, abdominal pain, retching, hyperhidrosis, arthralgia, myalgia, muscle spasm, back pain, asthenia, pain in extremity, fatigue, chest pain, blood creatinine increased, erythema, pruritus, syncope/faint, insomnia, depression, stomach discomfort, vomiting, hypotension (including orthostatic hypotension), bradycardia, tachycardia, abnormal hepatic function/liver disorder, renal impairment including acute renal failure, hyperkalemia, dyspnoea, anaemia, eosinophilia, thrombocytopenia, and weakness have been reported. The frequency of these effects is unknown. As with other angiotensin II antagonists, rare cases of angioedema, pruritus, rash and urticaria have been reported.

Cases of muscle pain, muscle weakness, myositis and rhabdomyolysis have been reported in patients receiving angiotensin II receptor blockers.

In addition, since the introduction of telmisartan in the market, cases with increased blood creatinine phosphokinase (CPK) have been reported.

DRUG INTERACTIONS: Drug-Drug Interactions: See Table 2.

Table 2: MICARDIS

Established or Potential Drug-Drug Interactions

Telmisartan	Effect	Clinical Comment
Agents increasing serum potassium		Since the telmisartan reduces the production of aldosterone, potassium-sparing diuretics or potassium supplements should be given only for documented hypokalemia and with frequent monitoring of serum potassium. Potassium-containing salt substitutes should also be used with caution. Concomitant thiazide diuretic use may attenuate any effect that telmisartan may have on serum potassium.
Digoxin	When telmisartan was coadministered with digoxin, mean increases in digoxin peak plasma concentration (49%) and in trough concentration (20%) were observed.	It is recommended that digoxin levels be monitored with appropriate dose adjustments when initiating, adjusting or discontinuing MICARDIS, to maintain appropriate plasma digoxin concentrations.

(cont'd)

Table 2: MICARDIS *(cont'd)*

Established or Potential Drug-Drug Interactions

Telmisartan	Effect	Clinical Comment
Diuretics	Patients on diuretics, and especially those in whom diuretic therapy was recently instituted, may occasionally experience an excessive reduction of blood pressure after initiation of therapy with telmisartan.	The possibility of symptomatic hypotension with the use of telmisartan can be minimized by discontinuing the diuretic prior to initiation of treatment and/or lowering the initial dose of telmisartan (see Warnings and Precautions, Cardiovascular, Hypotension and Dosage and Administration). No drug interaction of clinical significance has been identified with thiazide diuretics.
Lithium salts		Reversible increases in serum lithium concentrations and toxicity have been reported during concomitant administration of lithium with angiotensin converting enzyme inhibitors. Rare cases have also been reported with angiotensin II receptor antagonists including MICARDIS. Therefore, serum lithium level monitoring is advisable during concomitant use.
Nonsteroidal Anti-Inflammatory Drugs (NSAIDs)		Combinations of angiotensin-II antagonists (MICARDIS) and NSAIDs (including ASA and COX-2 inhibitors) might have an increased risk for acute renal failure and hyperkalemia. Blood pressure and kidney function should be monitored more closely in this situation, as occasionally there can be a substantial increase in blood pressure. NSAIDs (including ASA and COX-2 inhibitors) and angiotensin-II receptor antagonists exert a synergistic effect on the decrease of glomerular filtration. In patients with pre-existing renal impairment, this may lead to acute renal failure. Monitoring of renal function at the beginning and during the course of the treatment should be recommended. Coadministration of MICARDIS did not result in a clinically significant interaction with ibuprofen.
Ramipril	In one study, the coadministration of telmisartan and ramipril led to an increase of up to 2.5 fold in the AUC_{0-24} and C_{max} of ramipril and ramiprilat.	The clinical relevance of this observation is not known.
Warfarin	MICARDIS (telmisartan) administered for 10 days slightly decreased the mean warfarin trough plasma concentration; this decrease did not result in a change in International Normalized Ratio (INR).	
Other		Coadministration of MICARDIS also did not result in a clinically significant interaction with acetaminophen, amlodipine, glyburide or hydrochlorothiazide.

Drug-Food Interactions: When telmisartan is taken with food, the reduction in the area under the plasma concentration-time curve (AUC) of telmisartan varies from approximately 6% (40 mg) to approximately 19% (160 mg), and the reduction in C_{max} varies from approximately 26% (40 mg) to 56% (160 mg). However, three hours after administration, plasma concentrations are similar whether telmisartan is taken with or without food.

Drug-Herb Interactions: Interactions with herbal products have not been established.

Drug-Laboratory Test Interactions: Interactions with laboratory tests have not been established.

Drug-Lifestyle Interactions: No studies on the effect on the ability to drive and use machines have been performed. However, when driving vehicles or operating machinery it should be taken into account that dizziness or drowsiness may occasionally occur when taking antihypertensive therapy.

DOSAGE AND ADMINISTRATION:

Dosing Considerations: The antihypertensive effect is present within 2 weeks and maximal reduction is generally attained after four weeks. If additional blood pressure reduction is required, a thiazide diuretic may be added.

MICARDIS should be taken consistently with or without food.

Recommended Dose and Dosage Adjustment: Treatment of Essential Hypertension: The recommended dose of MICARDIS (telmisartan) is 80 mg once daily.

No initial dosing adjustment is necessary for elderly patients or for patients with renal impairment, but greater sensitivity in some older individuals cannot be ruled out. Markedly reduced telmisartan plasma levels were observed in patients on hemodialysis.

For patients with hepatic impairment a starting dose of 40 mg is recommended (see Warnings and Precautions, Hepatic/Biliary/Pancreatic).

Risk Reduction of Cardiovascular Morbidity: The recommended dose is 80 mg once daily in patients 55 years or older at high risk for a cardiovascular event. It is not known whether doses lower than 80 mg of MICARDIS are effective in preventing cardiovascular morbidity. It can be administered with other antihypertensive agents except an ACEI.

When initiating telmisartan therapy at this dose, monitoring of blood pressure is recommended, and if appropriate adjustment of medications that lower blood pressure may be necessary.

Missed Dose: MICARDIS should be taken at the same time each day, preferably in the morning. However, if a dose is missed during the day, the next dose should be continued at the usual time. Do not double dose.

OVERDOSAGE:

Limited data are available with regard to overdosage in humans. The most prominent manifestations of overdosage were hypotension and/or tachycardia; bradycardia also occurred. If symptomatic hypotension should occur, supportive treatment should be instituted. Telmisartan is not removed by hemodialysis.

> For management of a suspected drug overdose, contact your **regional Poison Control Centre**. See the *CPS* Directory section for a list of Poison Control Centres.

ACTION AND CLINICAL PHARMACOLOGY: Mechanism of Action: Telmisartan is an orally active angiotensin II AT_1 receptor antagonist. By selectively blocking the binding of angiotensin II to the AT_1 receptors telmisartan blocks the vasoconstrictor and aldosterone secreting effects of angiotensin II. Telmisartan does not exhibit any partial agonist activity at the AT_1 receptors, and has essentially no affinity for the AT_2 receptors. AT_2 receptors have been found in many tissues, but to date they have not been associated with cardiovascular homeostasis. In vitro binding studies indicate that telmisartan has no relevant affinity for other receptors nor does it inhibit human plasma renin.

Telmisartan does not inhibit angiotensin converting enzyme, also known as kininase II, the enzyme that converts angiotensin I to angiotensin II and degrades bradykinin, nor does it affect renin or other hormone receptors or ion channels involved in cardiovascular regulation of blood pressure and sodium homeostasis.

In hypertensive patients blockade of angiotensin II AT_1 receptors results in two to three fold increase in plasma renin and angiotensin II plasma concentrations. Long term effects of increased AT_2 receptor stimulation by angiotensin II are unknown.

Pharmacodynamics: Treatment of Essential Hypertension: In normal volunteers, a dose of telmisartan 80 mg inhibited the pressor response to an intravenous infusion of angiotensin II by about 90% at peak with approximately 40% inhibition persisting for 24 hours.

In hypertensive patients with normal renal function, no clinically significant effects on renal plasma flow, filtration fraction, or glomerular filtration rate were observed. In multiple dose studies in hypertensive patients, telmisartan had no adverse effect on renal function as measured by serum creatinine or blood urea nitrogen.

The antihypertensive effects of telmisartan were demonstrated in six placebo-controlled clinical trials, in a total of 1773 patients, 1031 of whom were treated with MICARDIS (telmisartan). Upon initiation of antihypertensive treatment with telmisartan, blood pressure was reduced after the first dose and there was a gradual increase in the antihypertensive effect during continued treatment for up to 12 weeks, with most of the increase occurring during the first month. Onset of antihypertensive activity occurs within 3 hours after administration of a single oral dose. The antihypertensive effect of once daily administration of telmisartan is maintained for the full 24-hour dose interval. The magnitude of blood pressure reduction from baseline, after placebo subtraction, was on average (SBP/DBP) −11.3/−7.3 mmHg for MICARDIS 40 mg once daily, and −13.7/−8.1 mmHg for MICARDIS 80 mg once daily. Upon abrupt cessation of treatment with MICARDIS, blood pressure gradually returned to baseline values over a period of several days. During long term studies (without placebo control) the effect of telmisartan appeared to be maintained for up to at least one year.

For those patients treated with telmisartan 80 mg once daily who required additional blood pressure reduction, addition of a low dose of hydrochlorothiazide (12.5 mg) resulted in incremental blood pressure reductions of −9.4/−7.0 mmHg.

The antihypertensive effect of once-daily telmisartan (40-80 mg) was similar to that of once-daily amlodipine (5-10 mg), atenolol (50-100 mg), enalapril (5-20 mg) and lisinopril (10-40 mg).

There was essentially no change in heart rate in telmisartan-treated patients in controlled trials.

In clinical trials with post-dose in-clinic monitoring no excessive blood pressure lowering peak effect was observed even after the first dose, and the incidence of symptomatic orthostasis was very low (0.04%). With automated ambulatory blood pressure monitoring, the 24-hour trough-to-peak ratio for telmisartan was determined to be at least 80% for both systolic and diastolic blood pressure.

The antihypertensive effect of telmisartan is not influenced by patient age, weight or body mass index. Blood pressure in hypertensive black patients (usually a low renin population) is significantly reduced by telmisartan (compared to placebo), but less so than in non-black patients.

Pharmacokinetics: Absorption: Following oral administration, telmisartan is well absorbed, with a mean absolute bioavailability of about 50%. Mean peak concentrations of telmisartan are reached in 0.5-1 hour after dosing.

The pharmacokinetic profile is characterized by greater than proportional increases of plasma concentrations (C_{max} and AUC) with increasing doses greater than 40 mg. Telmisartan shows bi-exponential decay kinetics with a terminal elimination half life of approximately 24 hours, and does not accumulate in plasma upon repeated once-daily dosing.

Metabolism: Telmisartan is metabolized by conjugation with glucuronic acid to form an acylglucuronide of telmisartan. This glucuronide is the only metabolite which has been identified in human plasma and urine. Following both oral dosing and intravenous administration of radiolabeled telmisartan, the parent compound represented approximately 85% and the glucuronide approximately 11% of total radioactivity in plasma. No pharmacological activity has been shown for the glucuronide conjugate.

The CYP 450 isoenzymes are not responsible for telmisartan metabolism.

Excretion: Total plasma clearance of telmisartan is >800 mL/min. Half-life and total clearance appear to be independent of dose. Biliary excretion is the main route of elimination of telmisartan and its metabolite. Following intravenous and oral administration of C^{14} labelled telmisartan 0.91% and 0.49% of administered dose were found in the urine as glucuronide, respectively. Most of the oral and intravenous dose, >97%, was excreted in feces as the parent compound.

Women have a lower telmisartan clearance and have a greater systolic blood pressure response at trough than men.

Distribution: Telmisartan is >99.5% bound to plasma protein, mainly albumin and a1-acid glycoprotein. Plasma protein binding is constant over the concentration range achieved with therapeutic doses. The volume of distribution for telmisartan is approximately 500 liters, indicating additional tissue binding sites.

When telmisartan is taken with food, the reduction in the area under the plasma concentration-time curve (AUC) of telmisartan varies from approximately 6% (40 mg) to approximately 19% (160 mg), and the reduction in C_{max} varies from approximately 26% (40 mg) to 56% (160 mg). However, three hours after administration, plasma concentrations are similar whether telmisartan is taken with or without food.

Special Populations and Conditions: Pediatrics: Telmisartan pharmacokinetics have not been investigated in patients <18 years of age.

Geriatrics: The pharmacokinetics of telmisartan do not differ between the elderly and those younger than 65 years (see Dosage and Administration).

Gender: Plasma concentrations of telmisartan are generally 2-3 fold higher in females than in males. No dosage adjustment is necessary.

Hepatic Insufficiency: In patients with hepatic insufficiency, plasma concentrations of telmisartan are increased, and absolute bioavailability approaches 100%. A lower starting dose should be considered (see Warnings and Precautions and Dosage and Administration).

Renal Insufficiency: Renal excretion of telmisartan is negligible. No dosage adjustment is necessary in patients with renal insufficiency. In patients on hemodialysis both C_{max} and AUC of telmisartan were markedly reduced as compared to healthy volunteers. Telmisartan is not removed by hemodialysis (see Warnings and Precautions and Dosage and Administration).

Genetic Polymorphism: No studies were conducted to evaluate the influence of genetic polymorphisms on the pharmacokinetics or pharmacodynamics of telmisartan.

STORAGE AND STABILITY: MICARDIS tablets are hygroscopic and require protection from moisture. Tablets are packaged in blisters and should be stored at room temperature, 15-30°C. Tablets should not be removed from blisters until immediately prior to administration.

INFORMATION FOR THE PATIENT: Published in e-CPS, available by subscription at www.e-cps.ca.

DOSAGE FORMS, COMPOSITION AND PACKAGING: 40 mg: Each white, oblong-shaped, uncoated tablet, marked with the Boehringer Ingelheim logo on one side, and on the other side, with 51H, contains: telmisartan 40 mg. Nonmedicinal ingredients: magnesium stearate, meglumine, povidone, sodium hydroxide and sorbitol. Individually blister sealed in cartons of 28 as 4 cards containing 7 tablets each.

80 mg: Each white, oblong-shaped, uncoated tablet, marked with the Boehringer Ingelheim logo on one side, and on the other side, with 52H, contains: telmisartan 80 mg. Nonmedicinal ingredients: magnesium stearate, meglumine, povidone, sodium hydroxide and sorbitol. Individually blister sealed in cartons of 28 as 4 cards containing 7 tablets each.

(Shown in Product Identification Section)

Micardis® Plus Ⓟ

telmisartan—hydrochlorothiazide

Angiotensin II AT1 Receptor Blocker—Diuretic

Boehringer Ingelheim

Date of Revision: March 2, 2009

SUMMARY PRODUCT INFORMATION:

Route of Administration	Dosage Form/ Strength	All Nonmedicinal Ingredients
Oral	Tablet 80/12.5 mg and 80/25 mg	Iron oxide red (for 80/12.5 mg tablet only), iron oxide yellow (for 80/25 mg tablet only), lactose monohydrate, magnesium stearate, maize starch, meglumine, microcrystalline cellulose, povidone, sodium hydroxide, sodium starch glycolate, and sorbitol

INDICATIONS AND CLINICAL USE: MICARDIS PLUS (80 mg telmisartan/12.5 mg hydrochlorothiazide) is indicated for:

- treatment of mild to moderate essential hypertension in patients in whom combination therapy is considered appropriate.

MICARDIS PLUS (80 mg telmisartan/25 mg hydrochlorothiazide) is indicated for:

- treatment of patients whose blood pressure is not adequately controlled by MICARDIS PLUS 80/12.5 mg or patients who have been previously stabilised on telmisartan and hydrochlorothiazide given separately.

These fixed-dose combinations are not indicated as initial therapy (see Dosage and Administration).

Geriatrics (>65 years of age): No dosage adjustment is necessary. It should be recognized, however, that greater sensitivity in some older individuals can not be ruled out.

Pediatrics (<18 years of age): Safety and efficacy of MICARDIS PLUS have not been established in children and in adolescents up to 18 years.

CONTRAINDICATIONS: MICARDIS PLUS (telmisartan/hydrochlorothiazide) is contraindicated in:
- Patients who are hypersensitive to any component of this product
- Second and third trimesters of pregnancy (see Warnings and Precautions, Special Populations, Pregnant Women)
- Lactation (see Warnings and Precautions, Special Populations, Nursing Women)
- Due to the hydrochlorothiazide component, MICARDIS PLUS is contraindicated in patients with anuria or hypersensitivity to other sulfonamide-related drugs.

Sorbitol: Patients with rare hereditary problems of fructose intolerance should not take this medicine. A recommended daily dose of MICARDIS PLUS tablets contains 338 mg sorbitol. MICARDIS PLUS is therefore unsuitable for patients with rare hereditary fructose intolerance.

Lactose: Patients with rare hereditary problems of galactose intolerance, the Lapp Lactase deficiency or glucose-galactose malabsorption should not take this medication. The maximum recommended daily dose of MICARDIS PLUS contains 112 mg of lactose monohydrate in the dose strength of 80/12.5 mg or 99 mg of lactose monohydrate in the dose strength of 80/25 mg. Patients with rare hereditary conditions of galactose intolerance, e.g. galactosaemia, should not take this medicine.

WARNINGS AND PRECAUTIONS:

Serious Warnings and Precautions
When used in pregnancy, angiotensin receptor (AT_1) blockers (ARB) can cause injury or even death of the developing fetus. When pregnancy is detected, MICARDIS PLUS should be discontinued as soon as possible (see Warnings and Precautions, Special Populations).

Cardiovascular: Hypotension: In patients who are volume-depleted by diuretic therapy, dietary salt restriction, dialysis, diarrhea or vomiting, symptomatic hypotension may occur after initiation of therapy with telmisartan. Such conditions, especially volume and/or sodium depletion, should be corrected prior to administration of telmisartan. In these patients, because of the potential fall in blood pressure, therapy with telmisartan should be initiated under close medical supervision. Similar considerations apply to patients with ischemic heart or cerebrovascular disease, in whom an excessive fall in blood pressure could result in myocardial infarction or cerebrovascular accident.

The use of a dual renin-angiotensin-aldosterone system (RAAS) blockade may lead to increased occurrence of hypotension when given as add-on therapy in patients with controlled blood pressure.

Valvular Stenosis: There is a concern on theoretical grounds that patients with aortic stenosis might be at a particular risk of decreased coronary perfusion, because they do not develop as much afterload reduction.

Endocrine and Metabolism: Electrolyte and Metabolic Imbalances: Telmisartan and Hydrochlorothiazide: In controlled trials using telmisartan (80 mg) and hydrochlorothiazide (12.5 mg) in combination, there were no reports of hyperkalemia. Hypokalemia was reported in 1.4% of patients treated with the combination. No discontinuations due to hypokalemia occurred during treatment. The absence of significant changes in serum potassium levels may be due to the opposing mechanisms of action of telmisartan and hydrochlorothiazide on potassium excretion by the kidney.

The use of a dual renin-angiotensin-aldosterone system (RAAS) blockade may lead to increased occurrence of hyperkalemia when given as add-on therapy in patients with controlled blood pressure.

Hydrochlorothiazide: During thiazide diuretic therapy, periodic determinations of serum electrolytes to detect possible electrolyte imbalances should be performed at appropriate intervals. All patients receiving thiazide therapy should be observed for clinical signs of fluid or electrolyte imbalance, particularly hyponatremia, hypokalemia and hypochloremic alkalosis. Serum and urine electrolyte determinations are particularly important when the patient experiences excessive vomiting or receives parenteral fluids.

Hypokalemia may develop especially with brisk diuresis, when severe cirrhosis is present or after prolonged therapy. Interference with adequate oral electrolyte intake will also contribute to hypokalemia. Hypokalemia may induce cardiac arrhythmia and may also sensitize or exacerbate the response of the heart to the toxic effects of digitalis (e.g. increased ventricular irritability).

Although any chloride deficit is generally mild and usually does not require special treatment except under extraordinary circumstances (as in liver or renal disease), chloride replacement therapy may be required in the treatment of metabolic alkalosis.

Dilutional hyponatremia may occur in edematous patients in hot weather; appropriate therapy is water restriction rather than administration of salt, except in rare instances when the hyponatremia is life-threatening. In actual salt depletion, appropriate replacement is the therapy of choice.

Calcium excretion is decreased by thiazide diuretics which may cause intermittent and slight elevation of serum calcium in the absence of known disorders of calcium metabolism. Marked hypercalcemia may also be evidence of hyperparathyroidism. In the event of significant hypercalcemia, MICARDIS PLUS should be discontinued followed by assessment of parathyroid function.

Thiazide diuretics have been shown to increase the urinary excretion of magnesium, which may result in hypomagnesemia.

Hyperuricemia may occur, and an acute attack of gout may be precipitated in certain patients receiving thiazide therapy.

Insulin requirements in diabetic patients may be altered and latent diabetes mellitus may become manifest during thiazide diuretic therapy.

An increase in cholesterol and triglyceride levels has been associated with thiazide diuretic therapy.

Thiazide may decrease serum PBI levels without signs of thyroid disturbance.

Hepatic/Biliary/Pancreatic: Hepatic Impairment: As the predominant route of elimination of telmisartan is through biliary excretion, patients with cholestasis, biliary obstructive disorders or hepatic insufficiency can be expected to have reduced clearance leading to increased systemic exposure. MICARDIS PLUS should therefore be used with caution in these patients. Dosage reduction should be considered which would necessitate usage of the individual tablet formulations.

MICARDIS PLUS is not recommended for patients with severe hepatic impairment. Thiazides should be used with caution in patients with impaired hepatic function or progressive liver disease, since minor alterations of fluid and electrolyte balance may precipitate hepatic coma (see Dosage and Administration, Patients with Hepatic Impairment).

Immune: Hypersensitivity Reactions: Hypersensitivity reactions to the hydrochlorothiazide component of MICARDIS PLUS may occur in patients with or without a history of allergy or bronchial asthma.

Systemic Lupus Erythematosus: Thiazide diuretics have been reported to cause exacerbation or activation of systemic lupus erythematosus.

Renal: Renal Impairment: As a consequence of inhibiting the renin-angiotensin-aldosterone system, changes in renal function have been reported in susceptible individuals (such as patients with bilateral renal artery stenosis, unilateral renal artery stenosis to a solitary kidney, or severe congestive heart failure). Dual blockade of the renin-angiotensin-aldosterone system (e.g. concomitant use of an angiotensin II receptor antagonist and an ACE-inhibitor) has been associated with oliguria, progressive azotemia, and rarely, acute renal failure and/or death. Upon treatment with such combination, renal function should be closely monitored.

In patients whose renal function may depend on the activity of the renin-angiotensin-aldosterone system such as patients with bilateral renal artery stenosis, unilateral renal artery stenosis to a solitary kidney or severe congestive heart failure, treatment with agents that inhibit this system has been associated with oliguria, progressive azotemia, and rarely, acute renal failure and/or death. In susceptible patients, concomitant diuretic use may further increase risk. Appropriate assessment of renal function should be conducted prior to use of MICARDIS PLUS.

In studies of ACE inhibitors in patients with unilateral or bilateral renal artery stenosis, increases in serum creatinine or blood urea nitrogen were observed. Although there has been no long-term experience with telmisartan in this patient population, an effect similar to that observed with ACE inhibitors should be anticipated.

Due to the hydrochlorothiazide component, MICARDIS PLUS is not recommended in patients with severe renal impairment (creatinine clearance ≤30 mL/min).

Thiazide diuretics should be used with caution in patients with renal impairment.

There is no experience regarding the administration of MICARDIS PLUS in patients with a recent kidney transplant.

Azotemia: Azotemia may be precipitated or increased by the hydrochlorothiazide component of MICARDIS PLUS. Cumulative effects of the drug may develop in patients with impaired renal function since the primary route of excretion is through the urine.

If increasing azotemia and oliguria occur during treatment of severe progressive renal disease, the diuretic should be discontinued.

Special Populations: Pregnant Women: Drugs that act directly on the renin-angiotensin-aldosterone-system (RAAS) can cause fetal and neonatal morbidity and death when administered to pregnant women. When pregnancy is detected, MICARDIS PLUS should be discontinued as soon as possible.

The use of angiotensin receptor (AT_1) blockers (ARBs) is not recommended during pregnancy. Epidemiological evidence regarding the risk of teratogenicity following exposure to angotensin converting enzyme inhibitors (another class of therapeutic products interfering with the RAAS) during the first trimester of pregnancy has not been conclusive; however a small increase in risk cannot be excluded. Given the current evidence available on the risk with ARB, similar risks may exist for this class of drugs. Patients planning pregnancy should be changed to alternative antihypertensive treatments which have an established safety profile for use in pregnancy. When pregnancy is diagnosed, treatment with angiotensin II antagonists should be stopped immediately, and, if appropriate, alternative therapy should be started.

The use of ARBs during the second and third trimesters is known to induce human fetotoxicity (decreased renal function, oligohydramnios, skull ossification retardation) and neonatal toxicity (renal failure, hypotension, hyperkalemia).

Infants with a history of in utero exposure to ARBs should be closely observed for hypotension, oliguria, and hyperkalemia. If oliguria occurs, attention should be directed toward support of blood pressure and renal perfusion. Exchange transfusion may be required as a means of reversing hypotension and/or substituting for disordered renal function; however, limited experience with those procedures has not been associated with significant clinical benefit.

Thiazides cross the placenta and appear in cord blood. The routine use of diuretics in otherwise healthy pregnant women is not recommended and exposes mother and fetus to unnecessary risks, including fetal or neonatal jaundice, thrombocytopenia, and possibly other adverse reactions that have occurred in adults. Diuretics do not prevent development of toxemia of pregnancy and there is no satisfactory evidence that they are useful in the treatment of toxemia.

It is not known if telmisartan can be removed from the body by hemodialysis.

There has been no clinical experience with MICARDIS PLUS (telmisartan/hydrochlorothiazide) in pregnancy.

Preclinical studies with telmisartan do not indicate teratogenic effect, but have shown fetotoxicity.

Nursing Women: MICARDIS PLUS is contraindicated during lactation since it is not known whether telmisartan is excreted in human milk but significant levels have been found in the milk of lactating rats. Animal studies have shown excretion of telmisartan in breast milk. Because many drugs are excreted in human milk and because of their potential for affecting the nursing infant adversely, a decision should be made whether to discontinue nursing or discontinue the drug, taking into account the importance of the drug to the mother. Thiazide diuretics are excreted in human milk at low levels.

Pediatrics (<18 years of age): Safety and effectiveness of MICARDIS PLUS in pediatric patients have not been established.

Geriatrics (>65 years of age): In clinical trials (n=1725) of patients treated with the combination of telmisartan and hydrochlorothiazide, 348 (20.2%) were 65 to 74 years of age and 78 (4.5%) were 75 years of age or older. No overall differences in the safety or efficacy profiles were observed in elderly patients compared with younger patients. It should be recognized however, that greater sensitivity of some older individuals cannot be ruled out.

Monitoring and Laboratory Tests: For specific monitoring and laboratory tests, see Warnings and Precautions (Cardiovascular, Endocrine and Metabolism, Hepatic/Biliary/Pancreatic and Renal) and Drug Interactions.

ADVERSE REACTIONS: Clinical Trial Adverse Drug Reactions: Because clinical trials are conducted under very specific conditions the adverse reaction rates observed in the clinical trials may not reflect the rates observed in practice and should not be compared to the rates in the clinical trials of another drug. Adverse drug reaction information from clinical trials is useful for identifying drug-related adverse events and for approximating rates.

Telmisartan and Hydrochlorothiazide Used in Combination: The overall incidence and pattern of adverse events reported with MICARDIS PLUS (80/25 mg) was comparable with MICARDIS PLUS (80/12.5 mg). A dose-relationship of undesirable effects was not established and they showed no correlation with gender, age or race of the patients.

The combination of telmisartan and hydrochlorothiazide has been evaluated for safety in 1725 patients including 716 treated for over six months and 420 for over one year. In clinical trials with the individual components used in combination, no unexpected adverse events have been observed. Adverse experiences have been limited to those that have been previously reported with telmisartan and hydrochlorothiazide monotherapy. In general, treatment with the combination was well tolerated; most adverse experiences were mild and transient in nature and did not require discontinuation of therapy.

Adverse events at an incidence of 1% or more in patients treated with 80/12.5 mg telmisartan/hydrochlorothiazide combination, irrespective of their causal relationship, are presented in Table 1. This table includes the results of two pivotal studies. One study, a factorial design, compared the use of various doses of telmisartan tablets and hydrochlorothiazide tablets in combination to telmisartan alone, hydrochlorothiazide alone and placebo. The other study compared the fixed dose combination 80/12.5 mg of telmisartan/hydrochlorothiazide to telmisartan 80 mg alone.

Additional adverse reactions reported in clinical trials with telmisartan plus hydrochlorothiazide are listed below according to system organ class:

Autonomic Nervous System: impotence.
Body as a Whole: allergy, leg pain.
Central and Peripheral Nervous Systems: vertigo.
Gastrointestinal System: dyspepsia, gastritis, gastrointestinal disorder.
Metabolic and Nutritional System: hypokalemia, loss of diabetic control, hyperuricemia.
Musculoskeletal System: myalgia, arthralgia, arthrosis.
Psychiatric System: anxiety.
Respiratory System: bronchitis, sinusitis.
Skin and Appendages System: eczema, skin disorder.
Urinary System: urinary tract infection.

In controlled trials with 1017 patients, 0.3% of patients treated with telmisartan (80 mg) and hydrochlorothiazide (12.5 mg) used in combination discontinued due to hypotension.

Adverse events occurred at approximately the same rates in men and women, older and younger patients and black and non-black patients.

Table 1: MICARDIS PLUS
Adverse Events Occurring in ≥1% of Patients Treated with 80/12.5 mg Telmisartan/Hydrochlorothiazide in Pivotal Clinical Trials

	Telmisartan/ HCTZ 80/12.5 mg (n=320) %	Telmisartan 80 mg (n=322) %	HCTZ 12.5 mg (n=75) %	Placebo (n=74) %
Total with Any Adverse Event	39.1	41.3	46.7	41.9
Autonomic Nervous System				
Sweating Increased	1.3	0.3	0	0
Body as a Whole				
Back Pain	1.6	2.5	1.3	0
Fatigue	2.8	2.2	4.0	1.4
Influenza-like Symptoms	1.6	1.2	2.7	1.4
Pain	2.2	2.2	4.0	6.8
Central and Peripheral Nervous Systems				
Dizziness	6.9	3.7	2.7	1.4
Headache	2.5	4.0	13.3	16.2

(cont'd)

Table 1: MICARDIS PLUS *(cont'd)*

Adverse Events Occurring in ≥1% of Patients Treated with 80/12.5 mg Telmisartan/Hydrochlorothiazide in Pivotal Clinical Trials

	Telmisartan/ HCTZ 80/12.5 mg (n=320) %	Telmisartan 80 mg (n=322) %	HCTZ 12.5 mg (n=75) %	Placebo (n=74) %
Gastrointestinal System				
Abdominal Pain	1.6	0.9	0	0
Diarrhea	4.1	1.6	0	0
Nausea	1.6	0.9	1.3	0
Respiratory System				
Pharyngitis	1.6	0.3	0	0
Upper Respiratory Tract Infection	2.5	3.7	9.3	6.8

Note: Telmisartan 80 mg open label treatment is not included in the Telmisartan 80 mg column.
Legend: HCTZ=hydrochlorothiazide.

Abnormal Hematologic and Clinical Chemistry Findings: In controlled trials, clinically relevant changes in standard laboratory test parameters were rarely associated with administration of telmisartan and hydrochlorothiazide in combination. See Table 2.

Table 2: MICARDIS PLUS

Laboratory Parameter Results in Patients Treated with Telmisartan and Hydrochlorothiazide in Combination

Laboratory Parameter	% of Patients Treated with Telmisartan/ Hydrochlorothiazide	Clinical Comment
Increases in Blood Urea Nitrogen (BUN) (≥11.2 mg/dL)	2.8%	No patient discontinued treatment due to an increase in BUN.
Increases in Serum Creatinine (≥0.5 mg/dL)	1.4%	No patient discontinued treatment due to an increase in creatinine.
Decreases in Hemoglobin (≥2 g/dL)	1.2%	Changes in hemoglobin were not considered clinically significant and there were no discontinuations due to anemia.
Decreases in Hematocrit (≥9%)	0.6%	Changes in hematocrit were not considered clinically significant and there were no discontinuations due to anemia.

Liver Function Tests: Occasional elevations of liver enzymes and/or serum bilirubin have occurred. No telmisartan/hydrochlorothiazide treated patients discontinued therapy due to abnormal liver function.
Serum Electrolytes: See Warnings and Precautions.
Telmisartan: Additional side effects were reported in clinical trials with telmisartan in the indication hypertension or in patients 50 years or older at high risk of cardiovascular events.

Telmisartan has been evaluated for safety in 27 clinical trials involving 7968 patients. Of these 7968 patients, 5788 patients were treated with telmisartan monotherapy including 1058 patients treated for ≥1 year and 1395 patients treated in placebo-controlled trials.

The following potentially serious adverse events have been reported rarely with telmisartan in controlled clinical trials: syncope and hypotension. In placebo-controlled trials, no serious adverse event was reported with a frequency of greater than 0.1% in telmisartan-treated patients.

All Clinical Trials: The adverse drug events listed below have been accumulated from 27 clinical trials including 5788 hypertensive patients treated with telmisartan. Adverse events have been ranked under headings of frequency using the following convention: very common (≥1/10); common (≥1/100, <1/10); uncommon (≥1/1000, <1/100); rare (≥1/10 000, <1/1000); very rare (<1/10 000).
Body as a Whole, General: Common: chest pain, influenza-like symptoms, symptoms of infection (e.g. urinary tract infection including cystitis), fatigue, conjunctivitis. Uncommon: hyperhidrosis, asthenia (weakness).
Blood and Lymphatic System: Uncommon: anemia. Rare: thrombocytopenia. Unknown: eosinophilia.
Cardiovascular System: Common: edema, palpitation. Uncommon: bradycardia, orthostatic hypotension, hypotension. Rare: tachycardia.
Central and Peripheral Nervous System: Very common: headache. Common: dizziness, insomnia. Uncommon: vertigo.
Eye Disorders: Rare: visual disturbance.
Gastrointestinal System: Common: abdominal pain, diarrhoea, dyspepsia, nausea, constipation, gastritis. Uncommon: dry mouth, flatulence, vomiting. Rare: stomach discomfort.
Hepato-biliary Disorders: Rare: hepatic function abnormal/liver disorder.
Immune System: Rare: hypersensitivity. Unknown: anaphylactic reaction.
Infections and Infestations: Uncommon: upper respiratory tract infections, urinary tract infections. Not known: sepsis including fatal outcome.
Investigations: Uncommon: blood creatinine increased. Unknown: haemoglobin decreased. Rare: blood uric acid increased, hepatic enzymes increased, blood creatinine phosphokinase increased, haemoglobin decreased.
Metabolism and Nutrition Disorders: Uncommon: hyperkalemia.
Musculoskeletal System: Common: arthralgia, muscle spasms (cramps in legs) or pain in extremity (leg pain), myalgia, arthritis, arthrosis. Uncommon: tendon pain (tendonitis like symptoms), back pain.
Nervous System: Uncommon: syncope (faint).
Psychiatric System: Common: anxiety, nervousness. Uncommon: depression.
Renal and Urinary System: Uncommon: renal impairment including acute renal failure.
Respiratory System: Common: upper respiratory tract infections including pharyngitis and sinusitis, bronchitis, coughing, dyspnea, rhinitis.
Skin and Appendages System: Common: skin disorders like rash. Uncommon: pruritus. Rare: erythema, drug eruption, angioedema, eczema, toxic skin eruption. Unknown: urticaria.
Placebo-Controlled Trials: The overall incidence of adverse events reported with telmisartan (41.4%) was usually comparable to placebo (43.9%) in controlled clinical trials.
Adverse events occurring in 1% or more of 1395 hypertensive patients treated with telmisartan **monotherapy** in placebo-controlled clinical trials, regardless of drug relationship, include the following: see Table 3.

The incidence of adverse events was not dose-related and did not correlate with the gender, age, or race of patients.

Less Common Clinical Trial Adverse Drug Reactions (<1%): In addition, the following adverse events, with no established causality, were reported at an incidence <1% in placebo-controlled clinical trials:
Autonomic Nervous System Disorders: sweating increased.
Body as a Whole: abdomen enlarged, allergy, cyst nos, fall, fever, leg pain, rigors, syncope.
Cardiovascular Disorders, General: hypotension, hypotension-postural, leg edema.
Central and Peripheral Nervous Systems Disorders: hypertonia, migraine-aggravated, muscle contraction-involuntary.

Table 3: MICARDIS PLUS

Adverse Events Occurring in 1% or More of 1395 Patients Treated with Telmisartan Monotherapy

Adverse Event by System	Micardis Total N=1395 %	Placebo N=583 %
Body as a Whole		
Back Pain	2.7	0.9
Chest Pain	1.3	1.2
Fatigue	3.2	3.3
Influenza-like Symptoms	1.7	1.5
Pain	3.5	4.3
Central and Peripheral Nervous Systems		
Dizziness	3.6	4.6
Headache	8.0	15.6
Somnolence	0.4	1.0
Gastrointestinal System		
Diarrhea	2.6	1.0
Dyspepsia	1.6	1.2
Nausea	1.1	1.4
Vomiting	0.4	1.0
Musculoskeletal System		
Myalgia	1.1	0.7
Respiratory System		
Coughing	1.6	1.7
Pharyngitis	1.1	0.3
Sinusitis	2.2	1.9
Upper Respiratory Tract Infection	6.5	4.6
Heart Rate and Rhythm Disorders		
ECG Abnormal Specific	0.2	1.0
Palpitation	0.6	1.0
Cardiovascular Disorders, General		
Hypertension	1.0	1.7
Oedema Peripheral	1.0	1.2

Gastrointestinal System Disorders: anorexia, appetite increased, flatulence, gastrointestinal disorder nos, gastroenteritis, gastroesophageal reflux, melena, mouth dry, abdominal pain.
Heart Rate and Rhythm Disorders: arrhythmia, tachycardia.
Metabolic and Nutritional Disorders: diabetes mellitus, hypokalemia.
Musculoskeletal System Disorders: arthritis, arthritis aggravated, arthrosis, bursitis, fascitis plantar, tendon pain.
Myo Endo Pericardial and Valve Disorders: myocardial infarction.
Psychiatric Disorders: nervousness.
Red Blood Cell Disorders: anemia.
Reproductive Disorders, Female: vaginitis.
Resistance Mechanism Disorders: abscess, infection, bacterial, moniliasis genital, otitis media.
Respiratory System Disorders: bronchospasm, epistaxis, pneumonia, bronchitis.
Skin and Appendage Disorders: rash, skin dry.
Urinary System Disorders: dysuria, hematuria, micturition disorder, urinary tract infection (including cystitis).
Vascular (Extracardiac) Disorders: cerebrovascular disorder, purpura.
Vision Disorders: vision abnormal.

Angioedema has been reported rarely in patients treated with telmisartan.

Abnormal Hematologic and Clinical Chemistry Findings: In placebo-controlled clinical trials involving 1041 patients treated with MICARDIS monotherapy, clinically relevant changes in standard laboratory test parameters were rarely associated with administration of telmisartan. See Table 4.
Hemoglobin, Hemotocrit: Clinically significant changes in hemoglobin and hematocrit (<10 g/dL and <30%, respectively) were rarely observed with telmisartan treatment and did not differ from rates in placebo-treated patients. No patients discontinued therapy due to anemia.
Cholesterol: In placebo-controlled trials, marked increases in serum cholesterol were reported in a total of 6 telmisartan-treated patients (0.4%) and no placebo patients. Two of these patients were followed over time, in both cases cholesterol values reverted to baseline levels.

Serum elevations in cholesterol were reported as adverse events in 11 of 3445 patients (0.3%) in all clinical trials. There were no reported cases of hypercholesterolemia in telmisartan-treated patients in placebo-controlled trials.

Other Clinical Trials: Gastrointestinal: constipation.
Respiratory: rhinitis, dyspnea.
Special senses: conjunctivitis.
Post-Market Adverse Drug Reactions: Telmisartan: Since the introduction of telmisartan in the market, cases of anxiety, dizziness, vision troubled, vertigo, abdominal distension, abdominal pain, retching, hyperhidrosis, arthralgia, myalgia, muscle spasm, back pain, asthenia, pain in extremity, fatigue, chest pain, blood creatinine increased, erythema, pruritus, syncope/faint, insomnia, depression, stomach discomfort, vomiting, hypotension (including orthostatic hypotension), bradycardia, tachycardia, abnormal hepatic function/liver disorder, renal impairment including acute renal failure, hyperkalemia, dyspnoea, anaemia, eosinophilia, thrombocytopenia and weakness have been reported. The frequency of these effects is unknown. As with other angiotensin II antagonists, rare cases of angioedema, pruritus, rash and urticaria have been reported.

Cases of muscle pain, muscle weakness, myositis and rhabdomyolysis have been reported in patients receiving angiotensin II receptor blockers.

In addition, since the introduction of telmisartan in the market, cases with increased blood creatinine phosphokinase (CPK) have been reported.

Hydrochlorothiazide: Adverse experiences that have been reported with hydrochlorothiazide alone without regard to causality are listed below:

Body as a Whole: fever.
Gastrointestinal System: pancreatitis, sialadenitis, gastric irritation, anorexia, nausea, vomiting, diarrhea, constipation.
Hepatobiliary Disorders: jaundice (hepatocellular cholestatic jaundice).
Blood and Lymphatic System: aplastic anemia, agranulocytosis, leukopenia, hemolytic anemia, thrombocytopenia.
Hypersensitivity: purpura.
Respiratory Disorders: respiratory distress including pneumonia and pulmonary edema.
Musculoskeletal: muscle spasm, weakness, cramps in legs.
Central and Peripheral Nervous Systems: dizziness, vertigo, paraesthesia, restlessness, nervousness.
Cardiovascular: orthostatic hypotension.
Heart Rate and Rhythm Disorder: cardiac arrhythmias.
Renal: renal failure, renal dysfunction, interstitial nephritis.
Skin and Subcutaneous Tissue Disorders: rash, urticaria, erythema multiforme including Stevens-Johnson syndrome, exfoliative dermatitis including toxic epidermal necrolysis, photosensitivity reactions, necrotizing angiitis (vasculitis, cutaneous vasculitis), anaphylactic reactions, cutaneous lupus erythematosus-like reactions, reactivation of cutaneous lupus erythematosus.
Eye Disorders: transient blurred vision, xanthopsia.
Laboratory Findings: metabolic: hyperglycaemia, glucosuria, hyperuricaemia.
Other: electrolyte imbalances (including hyponatraemia and hypokalaemia), increases in triglycerides, hypercholesterolemia.

Table 4: MICARDIS PLUS

Laboratory Parameter Results in Placebo-controlled Clinical Trials Involving 1041 Patients Treated with MICARDIS Monotherapy

Laboratory Parameter	% of Placebo Patients	% of Patients Treated with Telmisartan	Clinical Comment
Increases in ALT >3 times the upper limit of normal	1.7%	0.5%	No telmisartan-treated patients discontinued therapy due to abnormal hepatic function.
Increases in AST >3 times the upper limit of normal	0.8%	0.1%	No telmisartan-treated patients discontinued therapy due to abnormal hepatic function.
Increases in Blood Urea Nitrogen (BUN) ≥11.2 mg/dL	0.3%	1.5%	These increases occurred primarily with telmisartan in combination with hydrochlorothiazide. One telmisartan treated patient discontinued therapy due to increases in blood urea nitrogen and creatinine.
Increases in Creatinine ≥0.5 mg/dL	0.3%	0.6%	These increases occurred primarily with telmisartan in combination with hydrochlorothiazide. One telmisartan treated patient discontinued therapy due to increases in blood urea nitrogen and creatinine.
Increases in Serum Potassium ≥1.4 mEq/L	0.6%	0.3%	Clinically significant changes in potassium (that exceeded 3 mEq/L) were found in 0.6% of telmisartan-treated patients, with 0.5% of these reported at baseline. The corresponding rates for placebo-treated patients were 0.6% and 0.8%.
Decreases in Serum Potassium ≥1.4 mEq/L	0.3%	0.1%	Clinically significant changes in potassium (that exceeded 3 mEq/L) were found in 0.6% of telmisartan-treated patients, with 0.5% of these reported at baseline. The corresponding rates for placebo-treated patients were 0.6% and 0.8%.
Increases in Serum Uric Acid ≥2.7 mg/dL	0.0%	1.7%	Clinically significant hyperuricemia (>10 mEq/L) was observed in 2.3% of patients with telmisartan, with 0.4% reported in patients at baseline. Increases in serum uric acid were primarily observed in patients who received telmisartan in combination with hydrochlorothiazide. No patient was discontinued from treatment due to hyperuricemia.

DRUG INTERACTIONS: Overview: Telmisartan: Cytochrome P450: Telmisartan is not metabolized by the cytochrome P450 (CYP) isoenzymes; as such, it is not expected that a pharmacokinetic interaction of telmisartan with drugs which inhibit or induce CYP isozymes will occur.

Hydrochlorothiazide: Cytochrome P450: Hydrochlorothiazide is not metabolized by humans; as such, no pharmacokinetic interaction with agents known to inhibit or induce CYP isozymes or other enzymes systems is expected.

Drug-Drug Interactions: See Table 5 and Table 6.

Table 5: MICARDIS PLUS

Established or Potential Drug-Drug Interactions

Telmisartan	Effect	Clinical comment
Diuretics	Patients on diuretics, and especially those in whom diuretic therapy was recently instituted, may occasionally experience an excessive reduction of blood pressure after initiation of therapy with telmisartan.	The possibility of symptomatic hypotension with the use of telmisartan can be minimized by discontinuing the diuretic prior to initiation of treatment and/or lowering the initial dose of telmisartan (see Warnings and Precautions, Hypotension and Dosage and Administration). No drug interaction of clinical significance has been identified with thiazide diuretics.
Agents increasing serum potassium		Since the telmisartan component of MICARDIS PLUS reduces the production of aldosterone, potassium-sparing diuretics or potassium supplements should be given only for documented hypokalemia and with frequent monitoring of serum potassium. Potassium-containing salt substitutes should also be used with caution. Concomitant thiazide diuretic use may attenuate any effect that telmisartan may have on serum potassium.
Digoxin	When telmisartan was co-administered with digoxin, mean increases in digoxin peak plasma concentration (49%) and in trough concentration (20%) were observed.	It is recommended that digoxin levels be monitored with appropriate dose adjustments when initiating, adjusting or discontinuing MICARDIS PLUS, to maintain appropriate plasma digoxin concentrations.
Lithium Salts	As with other drugs which enhance sodium excretion, lithium clearance may be reduced in the presence of telmisartan.	Lithium generally should not be administered with thiazide diuretics.
Ramipril	In one study, the co-administration of telmisartan and ramipril led to an increase of up to 2.5 fold in the AUC_{0-24} and C_{max} of ramipril and ramiprilat.	The clinical relevance of this observation is not known.
Warfarin	Telmisartan administered for 10 days slightly decreased the mean warfarin trough plasma concentration; this decrease did not result in a change in the International Normalized Ratio (INR).	
Acetaminophen, amlodipine, glibenclamide, hydrochlorothiazide, or ibuprofen		Co-administration of telmisartan did not result in a clinically significant pharmacokinetic interaction.

(cont'd)

Table 6: MICARDIS PLUS

Established or Potential Drug-Drug Interactions

Hydrochlorothiazide	Effect	Clinical comment
Alcohol, barbiturates and narcotics	Potentiation of orthostatic hypotension may occur.	
Anti-diabetic drugs (oral agents and insulin)	Potential for hyperglycemia in patients on thiazides	Dosage adjustment of the antidiabetic drug may be required.
Cholestyramine and colestipol resins	Absorption of hydrochlorothiazide is impaired in the presence of anionic exchange resins. Single doses of either cholestyramine or colestipol resins bind hydrochlorothiazide and reduce its absorption from the gastrointestinal tract by up to 85% and 43% respectively.	
Corticosteroids, ACTH	Intensified electrolyte depletion, particularly hypokalemia may occur.	
Lithium Salts		Lithium should not generally be administered concurrently with diuretics; if lithium must be administered concurrently with MICARDIS PLUS, serum lithium levels should be carefully monitored.
Nonsteroidal Anti-Inflammatory drugs (NSAIDs including ASA and COX-2 inhibitors)	The co-administration of a non-steroidal anti-inflammatory agent can reduce the diuretic, natriuretic, and antihypertensive effects of loop, potassium-sparing and thiazide diuretics. The potential for acute renal insufficiency in patients who are dehydrated may be enhanced.	Patients receiving NSAIDs and MICARDIS PLUS should be adequately hydrated and be monitored for renal function at the beginning of the combined treatment. Monitoring of renal function at the beginning and during the course of the treatment is recommended as well as regular hydration of the patient. Therefore, when MICARDIS PLUS and NSAIDs are used concomitantly, the patient should be observed closely to determine whether the desired effect of the diuretic is obtained.
Pressor amines (e.g. norepinephrine)	Decreased response to pressor amines may occur, but the effect is considered not sufficient to preclude their concurrent use.	
Skeletal muscle relaxants, nondepolarizing (e.g. tubocurarine)	Possible increased responsiveness to the muscle relaxant	
Other antihypertensive drugs	Additive effect or potentiation of antihypertensive effect	
β-adrenergic receptor blocking agents propranolol, metoprolol, sotalol, or acebutolol		No significant pharmacokinetic interactions were noted when these agents were administered concomitantly, separately or in fixed combination.
Spironolactone, indomethacin, allopurinol and phenytoin.		No significant interactions have been noted.

Drug-Food Interactions: Interactions with food have not been established.
Drug-Herb Interactions: Interactions with herbal products have not been established.
Drug-Laboratory Test Interactions: Interactions with laboratory tests have not been established.
Drug-Lifestyle Interactions: Interactions with lifestyle have not been established.

DOSAGE AND ADMINISTRATION: **Dosing Considerations:** MICARDIS PLUS may be substituted in patients who have been stabilized on the individual telmisartan 80 mg and hydrochlorothiazide 12.5 mg components as described below.

MICARDIS PLUS may be administered with or without food, however it should be taken consistently with regard to food intake.

Recommended Dose and Dosage Adjustment: MICARDIS PLUS (telmisartan/hydrochlorothiazide) is not for initial therapy.

A patient whose blood pressure is not adequately controlled with telmisartan monotherapy 80 mg, may be switched to MICARDIS PLUS, (telmisartan 80 mg/hydrochlorothiazide 12.5 mg) once daily.

A patient whose blood pressure is not adequately controlled with MICARDIS PLUS (telmisartan 80 mg/hydrochlorothiazide 12.5 mg), may be switched to MICARDIS PLUS (telmisartan 80 mg/hydrochlorothiazide 25 mg) once daily.

Telmisartan Monotherapy : The recommended dose of telmisartan is 80 mg once daily. The antihypertensive effect is present within 2 weeks and maximal reduction is generally attained after four weeks. If additional blood pressure reduction is required, a thiazide diuretic may be added.

No initial dosing adjustment is necessary for elderly patients or for patients with renal impairment but greater sensitivity in some older individuals cannot be ruled out. Markedly reduced telmisartan plasma levels were observed in patients on hemodialysis.

Diuretic Treated Patients: In patients receiving diuretics, telmisartan therapy should be initiated with caution, since these patients may be volume depleted and thus more likely to experience hypotension following initiation of additional antihypertensive therapy. Whenever possible, all diuretics should be discontinued two to three days prior to the administration of telmisartan to reduce the likelihood of hypotension. (See Warnings and Precautions, Hypotension.) If this is not possible because of the patients's condition, telmisartan should be administered with caution and the blood pressure monitored closely. Thereafter, the dosage should be adjusted according to the individual response of the patient.

Patients with Renal Impairment: The usual regimens of therapy with MICARDIS PLUS may be followed as long as the patient's creatinine clearance is >30 mL/min. In patients with more severe renal impairment, loop diuretics are preferred to thiazides; in this instance, MICARDIS PLUS is not recommended.

Patients with Hepatic Impairment: For patients with hepatic impairment, a starting dose of 40 mg of telmisartan is recommended. MICARDIS PLUS is not recommended for patients with severe hepatic impairment.

Missed Dose: If a dose is missed, patients should not take a double dose; patients should just carry on with the next dose at the usual time.

Administration: MICARDIS PLUS may be administered with or without food, however it should be taken consistently with regard to food intake.

OVERDOSAGE:

Limited information is available for MICARDIS PLUS with regard to overdose in humans. Serum electrolytes and creatinine should be monitored frequently. If hypotension occurs, the patient should be placed in a supine position, with salt and volume replacements given quickly. For the individual components of MICARDIS PLUS, the following information is available:

Telmisartan: Based on limited data, the most prominent manifestations of overdose are hypotension, dizziness and tachycardia; bradycardia also occurred in this setting as a result of parasympathetic (vagal) stimulation. If symptomatic hypotension should occur, supportive treatment should be instituted. Telmisartan is not removed by hemodialysis.

Hydrochlorothiazide: The most common signs and symptoms observed are those caused by electrolyte depletion (hypokalemia, hypochloremia, hyponatremia) and dehydration resulting from excessive diuresis. If digitalis has also been administered, hypokalemia may accentuate cardiac arrhythmias. The degree to which hydrochlorothiazide is removed by hemodialysis has not been established.

For management of a suspected drug overdose, CPhA recommends that you contact your **regional Poison Control Centre**. See the *CPS* Directory section for a list of Poison Control Centres.

ACTION AND CLINICAL PHARMACOLOGY: **Mechanism of Action:** MICARDIS PLUS (telmisartan/hydrochlorothiazide) is a combination of telmisartan, a selective angiotensin II antagonist and hydrochlorothiazide, a thiazide diuretic.

Telmisartan: Telmisartan is an orally active, AT_1 selective angiotensin II receptor antagonist. By selectively blocking the binding of angiotensin II to the AT_1 receptors, telmisartan inhibits the vasoconstrictor and aldosterone-secreting effects of angiotensin II. Telmisartan blocks AT_1 receptors, and has essentially no affinity for the AT_2 receptors. AT_2 receptors have been found in many tissues; to date, they have not been found to be associated with cardiovascular homeostasis.

Telmisartan does not inhibit angiotensin converting enzyme (ACE, also known as kininase II), the enzyme that converts angiotensin I to angiotensin II and degrades bradykinin, nor does it affect renin or other hormone receptors or ion channels involved in cardiovascular regulation of blood pressure and sodium homeostasis.

In hypertensive patients, antagonism of angiotensin II AT_1 receptors results in two to three-fold increases in plasma renin and angiotensin II plasma concentrations. Long term effects of increased AT_2 receptor stimulation by angiotensin II are unknown.

Hydrochlorothiazide: Hydrochlorothiazide is a thiazide diuretic which affects the renal tubular mechanisms of electrolyte reabsorption, directly increasing excretion of sodium and chloride in the distal tubule, thus promoting water excretion. The diuretic action of hydrochlorothiazide reduces plasma volume, with consequent increases in plasma renin activity, increases in aldosterone secretion, increases in urinary potassium loss and decreases in serum potassium. The latter effects of the renin-aldosterone link are mediated by angiotensin II; as such, co-administration of an angiotensin II AT_1 receptor antagonist may prevent the potassium loss associated with thiazide diuretics. The precise mechanism of the antihypertensive effect of thiazides however, is not fully understood.

Pharmacodynamics: Telmisartan: The antihypertensive effects of telmisartan were demonstrated in six placebo-controlled clinical trials, in a total of 1773 patients, 1031 of whom were treated with MICARDIS (telmisartan). Upon initiation of antihypertensive treatment with telmisartan, blood pressure was reduced after the first dose and there was a gradual increase in the antihypertensive effect during continued treatment for up to 12 weeks, with most of the increase occurring during the first month. Onset of antihypertensive activity occurs within 3 hours after administration of a single oral dose. The antihypertensive effect of once daily administration of telmisartan is maintained for the full 24-hour dose interval. The magnitude of blood pressure reduction from baseline, after placebo subtraction, was on average (SBP/DBP) −11.3/−7.3 mmHg for MICARDIS 40 mg once daily, and −13.7/−8.1 mmHg for MICARDIS 80 mg once daily. Upon abrupt cessation of treatment with MICARDIS, blood pressure gradually returned to baseline values over a period of several days. During long term studies (without placebo control) the effect of telmisartan appeared to be maintained for up to at least one year.

For those patients treated with telmisartan 80 mg once daily who required additional blood pressure reduction, addition of a low dose of hydrochlorothiazide (12.5 mg) resulted in incremental blood pressure reductions of −9.4/−7.0 mmHg.

There was essentially no change in heart rate in telmisartan-treated patients in controlled trials.

In clinical trials with post-dose in-clinic monitoring no excessive blood pressure lowering peak effect was observed even after the first dose, and the incidence of symptomatic orthostasis was very low (0.04%).

With automated ambulatory blood pressure monitoring, the 24-hour trough-to-peak ratio for telmisartan was determined to be at least 80% for both systolic and diastolic blood pressure.

The antihypertensive effect of telmisartan is not influenced by patient age, weight or body mass index. Blood pressure in hypertensive black patients is significantly reduced by telmisartan (compared to placebo), but less so than in non-black patients.

In hypertensive patients with normal renal function, no clinically significant effects on renal plasma flow, filtration fraction, or glomerular filtration rate were observed. In multiple dose studies in hypertensive patients, telmisartan had no adverse effect on renal function as measured by serum creatinine or blood urea nitrogen.

Hydrochlorothiazide: After oral administration of hydrochlorothiazide, diuresis begins within 2 hours, peaks in about 4 hours and lasts 6 to 12 hours.

Telmisartan and Hydrochlorothiazide Combination: In a placebo-controlled clinical study, the combination of telmisartan and hydrochlorothiazide resulted in decreases in trough systolic blood pressure (SBP) and diastolic blood pressure (DBP) which were greater than the decreases induced by either agent administered as monotherapy.

In a controlled clinical trial directly comparing MICARDIS PLUS with telmisartan (80 mg) monotherapy, trough SBP and DBP reductions observed with MICARDIS PLUS were significantly greater than with telmisartan alone.

Similarly, in other controlled studies with patients who did not achieve or maintain adequate response with telmisartan monotherapy, the addition of 12.5 mg hydrochlorothiazide to titrated doses of telmisartan further reduced systolic and diastolic pressure.

The antihypertensive effect of telmisartan/hydrochlorothiazide (80 mg/12.5 mg) was independent of age or gender. The overall response to the combination was similar for black and non-black patients.

There was essentially no change in heart rate in patients treated with the combination of telmisartan and hydrochlorothiazide in the placebo-controlled trial.

Pharmacokinetics: There are no pharmacokinetic interactions between telmisartan and hydrochlorothiazide as the pharmacokinetic parameters of the individual components are unchanged by their co-administration as MICARDIS PLUS. The results of a randomized, crossover study demonstrated that the bioavailabilities of telmisartan and hydrochlorothiazide were the same, whether administered as the fixed-dose combination or as the single entity formulations. See Table 7.

Table 7: MICARDIS PLUS

Single Dose Pharmacokinetics in Normotensive Subjects (10 Male and 10 Female Caucasian Subjects, 18 to 45 Years of Age). Given are Arithmetic Means (%CV)

Drug	Therapy	C_{max} (ng/mL)	$t_{½}$ (h)	$AUC_{0-\infty}$ (ng· h/mL)	Clearance (CL/f) (mL/min)	Volume of Distribution (Vz/f) (L)
Telmisartan: monotherapy	A	246 (%CV 69.4)	22.2 (%CV 30)	1439 (%CV 94)	1650 (%CV 62)	2908 (%CV 60)
Telmisartan: combination therapy	B	266 (%CV 103)	24.4 (%CV 33)	1467 (%CV 94)	1565 (%CV 63)	3091 (%CV 63)
Hydrochlorothiazide: combination therapy	A	75.3 (%CV 26)	11.4 (%CV 43)	580.4 (%CV 27)	380 (%CV 23)	363.8 (%CV 43)
Hydrochlorothiazide: monotherapy	B	75.7 (%CV 22)	11.5 (%CV 36)	563.9 (%CV 20)	384 (%CV 20)	380.4 (%CV 40)

Telmisartan: Absorption: Following oral administration, telmisartan is well absorbed with a mean absolute bioavailability of about 50%. Mean peak plasma concentrations (C_{max}) of telmisartan are reached in 0.5-1.0 hour after dosing. The pharmacokinetic profile is characterized by greater than proportional increases in plasma concentrations (C_{max} and AUC) with increasing doses greater than 40 mg. Telmisartan shows bi-exponential decay kinetics with terminal elimination half life of approximately 24 hours, and does not accumulate in plasma upon repeated once daily administration. Food slightly reduces the bioavailability of telmisartan.

Distribution: Telmisartan is extensively bound to plasma proteins (>99.5%) at concentrations achieved at the recommended dosage. The apparent volume of distribution is approximately 500 L, suggesting extensive tissue binding sites.

Metabolism: Telmisartan is metabolized by conjugation to form a pharmacologically inactive acylglucuronide; this is the only metabolite that has been detected in human plasma and urine. Following both oral dosing and intravenous administration of radiolabelled telmisartan, the parent compound represented approximately 85%, and the glucuronide approximately 11% of total radioactivity in plasma. The cytochrome P450 isoenzymes are not involved in the metabolism of telmisartan.

Excretion: Total plasma clearance of telmisartan is >800 mL/min. Biliary excretion is the predominant route of elimination of telmisartan and its metabolite.

Hydrochlorothiazide: Absorption: Following oral administration, peak concentrations of hydrochlorothiazide were reached approximately 2.0 hours after dosing. Based on cumulative renal excretion of hydrochlorothiazide the absolute bioavailability was about 60% to 70%.

Distribution: Hydrochlorothiazide is 40% protein bound in the plasma and its apparent volume of distribution is 2 to 5 L/kg.

Excretion: Hydrochlorothiazide is not metabolized but is eliminated rapidly by the kidney. The plasma-half life has been observed to vary between 5.6 and 14.8 hours when the plasma levels can be followed for up to 24 hours. At least 61 percent of the oral dose is eliminated unchanged within 24 hours. Hydrochlorothiazide crosses the placenta but not the blood-brain barrier and is excreted in breast milk.

Special Populations and Conditions: Telmisartan: Pediatrics: Telmisartan pharmacokinetics have not been investigated in patients <18 years of age.

Geriatrics: The pharmacokinetics of telmisartan does not differ between elderly patients and those younger than 65 years of age.

Gender: Plasma concentrations of telmisartan are generally 2-3 times higher in females than in males administered the same oral dose. In clinical trials however, no significant increases in blood pressure response or in the incidence of orthostatic hypotension were found in women. No dosage adjustment is necessary on the basis of gender.

Hepatic Insufficiency: In patients with hepatic insufficiency, plasma concentrations of telmisartan are increased, and absolute bioavailability approaches 100% (see Warnings and Precautions and Dosage and Administration). Reduction of the dose of telmisartan should be considered which would necessitate usage of the individual tablet formulations.

Renal Insufficiency: Renal excretion of telmisartan is negligible. In patients with mild to moderate renal impairment, (creatinine clearance of 30-80 mL/min), no dosage adjustment is necessary (see Warnings and Precautions, Renal Impairment and Dosage and Administration, Patients with Renal Impairment). Telmisartan is not removed by hemodialysis.

As a consequence of inhibiting the renin-angiotensin-aldosterone system, changes in renal function may be anticipated in susceptible individuals. In patients whose renal function may depend on the activity of the renin-angiotensin-aldosterone system such as patients with bilateral renal artery stenosis, unilateral renal artery stenosis to a solitary kidney or severe congestive heart failure, treatment with agents that inhibit this system has been associated with oliguria, progressive azotemia, and rarely, acute renal failure and/or death. In susceptible patients, concomitant diuretic use may further increase risk. Appropriate assessment of renal function should be conducted prior to use of MICARDIS PLUS.

In studies of ACE inhibitors in patients with unilateral or bilateral renal artery stenosis, increases in serum creatinine or blood urea nitrogen were observed. Although there has been no long-term experience with telmisartan in this patient population, an effect similar to that observed with ACE inhibitors should be anticipated.

Due to the hydrochlorothiazide component, MICARDIS PLUS is not recommended in patients with severe renal impairment (creatinine clearance ≤30 mL/min).

Thiazide diuretics should be used with caution in patients with renal impairment.

There is no experience regarding the administration of MICARDIS PLUS in patients with a recent kidney transplant.

No initial dosing adjustment for telmisartan is necessary for elderly patients or for patients with renal impairment but greater sensitivity in some older individuals cannot be ruled out. Markedly reduced telmisartan plasma levels were observed in patients on hemodialysis.

The usual regimens of therapy with MICARDIS PLUS may be followed as long as the patient's creatinine clearance is >30 mL/min. In patients with more severe renal impairment, loop diuretics are preferred to thiazides; in this instance MICARDIS PLUS is not recommended.

Azotemia: Azotemia may be precipitated or increased by the hydrochlorothiazide component of MICARDIS PLUS. Cumulative effects of the drug may develop in patients with impaired renal function since the primary route of excretion is through the urine.

If increasing azotemia and oliguria occur during treatment of severe progressive renal disease, the diuretic should be discontinued.

Genetic Polymorphism: No studies were conducted to evaluate the influence of genetic polymorphisms on the pharmacokinetics or pharmacodynamics of telmisartan.

STORAGE AND STABILITY: MICARDIS PLUS tablets are packaged in blisters and should be stored at room temperature (15-30°C). MICARDIS PLUS tablets are hygroscopic and require protection from moisture. Tablets should not be removed from blisters until immediately prior to administration.

INFORMATION FOR THE PATIENT: Published in e-CPS, available by subscription at www.e-cps.ca.

DOSAGE FORMS, COMPOSITION AND PACKAGING: 80/12.5 mg: Each bilayered, oblong-shaped, uncoated tablet, the telmisartan layer being white and the hydrochlorothiazide layer being red, marked BOEHRINGER INGELHEIM logo and "H8" on the white layer, contains: telmisartan 80 mg and hydrochlorothiazide 12.5 mg. Nonmedicinal ingredients: iron oxide red, lactose monohydrate, magnesium stearate, maize starch, meglumine, microcrystalline cellulose, povidone, sodium hydroxide, sodium starch glycolate and sorbitol. Individually blister-sealed cartons of 28 (4 cards of 7 tablets each).

80/25 mg: Each bilayered, oblong-shaped, uncoated tablet, the telmisartan layer being white and the hydrochlorothiazide layer being yellow, marked BOEHRINGER INGELHEIM logo and "H9" on the white layer, contains: telmisartan 80 mg and hydrochlorothiazide 25 mg. Nonmedicinal ingredients: iron oxide yellow, lactose monohydrate, magnesium stearate, maize starch, meglumine, microcrystalline cellulose, povidone, sodium hydroxide, sodium starch glycolate and sorbitol. Individually blister-sealed cartons of 28 (4 cards of 7 tablets each).

(Shown in Product Identification Section)

Micatin®
miconazole nitrate
Topical Antifungal

WellSpring

Date of Preparation: September 25, 2008

PHARMACOLOGY: Miconazole exhibits broad spectrum in vitro fungistatic activity; e.g., against species of the genus Candida. Studies with *C. albicans* indicate that at low concentrations, miconazole acts primarily on the yeast cell membrane resulting in selective inhibition of the uptake of precursors of RNA and DNA (purines) and mucopolysaccharide (glutamine).

In addition, in vitro antibacterial activity has been reported with Gram-positive bacilli and cocci.

INDICATIONS: MICATIN is indicated for the topical treatment of dermatophytes and Candida infections and also lesions caused by mixed infections involving susceptible fungi. It has been clinically effective in treating tinea pedis (athlete's foot), tinea cruris, tinea corporis and tinea versicolor caused by dermatophytes.

MICATIN is also effective in cutaneous candidiasis, excluding moderate to severe candidal paronychia. Among the organisms against which MICATIN has been found to be effective are *T. rubrum, T. mentagrophytes, T. interdigitale, E. floccosum, M. canis, M. gypseum*, species of Candida (including *C. albicans*) and *M. furfur*.

CONTRAINDICATIONS: None known.

PRECAUTIONS: If irritation occurs, or there is no improvement following the full treatment period (see Dosage), discontinue use and see a doctor. Avoid contact with the eyes; if this happens, rinse thoroughly with water. For external use only. Do not use in children under 2 years of age unless directed by a doctor. Do not use for infections of the nails.

ADVERSE EFFECTS: On rare occasions it has been reported that patients treated with MICATIN experience mild pruritus, irritation and burning at the site of application.

OVERDOSE:
None known.

> For management of a suspected drug overdose, CPhA recommends that you contact your regional Poison Control Centre. See the *CPS* Directory section for a list of Poison Control Centres.

DOSAGE: Cleanse skin with soap and water and dry thoroughly. Apply (or spray) a thin layer over the affected area morning and night for the full treatment period. If there is no improvement within 2 weeks a physician should be consulted. Otherwise, continue treatment for 1-2 weeks after symptoms have disappeared up to a maximum of 4 weeks. Jock itch and ringworm usually require 2 weeks to resolve, while athlete's foot may require 4 weeks.

When treating athlete's foot pay special attention to the spaces between toes; wear well fitting, ventilated shoes and cotton socks.

MICATIN Cream should be applied sparingly and smoothed in well to avoid maceration effects. The treated area should be massaged gently until the MICATIN Cream disappears.

Early clinical improvement (1-2 weeks) has been seen in the treatment of infections caused by common dermatophytes and Candida species, but resistant lesions may take longer to clear. Candida infections should be treated for 2 weeks.

If a patient shows no clinical improvement after the full treatment period, the diagnosis should be reconsidered.

SUPPLIED: Cream: Each tube of cream contains: miconazole nitrate 2% in a water miscible, white to off-white cream base. Nonmedicinal ingredients: benzoic acid, butylated hydroxyanisole, mineral oil, peglicol 5 oleate, pegoxol 7 stearate and purified water. Tubes of 30 g. Store at controlled room temperature (15-30°C).
Spray: Each can contains: miconazole nitrate 2% (as a percent of nonvolatile ingredients). Nonmedicinal ingredients: alcohol, hydrocarbon propellant, stearalkonium hectorite, sorbitan sesquioleate and talc. Cans of 85 g. Store at controlled room temperature (15-30°C).

Micozole
miconazole nitrate
Antifungal

Taro

SUPPLIED: Each g of vaginal cream contains: miconazole nitrate 2%. Nonmedicinal ingredients: apricot kernel oil/PEG-6, benzoic acid, butylated hydroxytoluene, mineral oil, PEG-6-32 stearate/glycol stearate and purified water. Tubes of 45 g sufficient for a 7-day course of therapy. Packages include a consumer information leaflet and 7 disposable applicators. Each tube of vaginal cream has sufficient cream for the treatment period and sufficient cream for extravaginal use, if necessary. Each full applicator supplies miconazole nitrate 100 mg in 5 g cream. Store at 15 to 30°C. Protect from freezing.

Micro-K Extencaps®
potassium chloride
Potassium Supplement

Paladin

Date of Revision: August 21, 2008

PHARMACOLOGY: Potassium ions participate in a number of physiological processes including the maintenance of intracellular tonicity; the transmission of nerve impulses; the contraction of cardiac, skeletal and smooth muscle; and the maintenance of normal renal function. Depletion may occur whenever the rate of potassium loss through renal excretion and/or loss from the gastrointestinal tract exceeds the rate of potassium intake.

Micro-K Extencaps are hard gelatin capsules containing small, microencapsulated, crystalline, dispersible particles of potassium chloride. Micro-K Extencaps contain 600 mg (8 mEq K^+) of potassium chloride. Each particle is microencapsulated with a polymeric coating which allows for controlled release of potassium and chloride ions. The dispersibility of the microcapsules and the controlled release of ions are intended to minimize the likelihood of high localized concentrations of potassium chloride and resultant mucosal ulceration within the gastrointestinal tract.

The polymeric coating forming the microcapsules functions as a water-permeable membrane. Fluids pass through the membrane and gradually dissolve the potassium chloride. In this manner, slow and sustained release of potassium chloride from the coated particles into the gastrointestinal tract occurs over a period of 4 to 8 hours.

INDICATIONS: Micro-K is indicated for the prevention of potassium depletion when the dietary intake of potassium is inadequate for this purpose. Micro-K is also indicated for the treatment of potassium depletion in patients with hypokalemia and metabolic alkalosis, and in the treatment of chronic digitalis intoxication.

The prophylactic administration of potassium may be indicated in patients receiving digitalis and diuretics for the treatment of congestive heart failure and hepatic cirrhosis with ascites. Micro-K may be indicated in selected patients with hypertension on long-term diuretic therapy, hyperaldosteronism states with normal renal function, the nephrotic syndrome and certain diarrheal states.

CONTRAINDICATIONS: Potassium supplements are contraindicated in patients with hyperkalemia since a further increase in serum potassium concentration in such patients can produce cardiac arrest. hyperkalemia may complicate any of the following conditions: acute and chronic renal failure, systemic acidosis such as diabetic acidosis, acute dehydration, extensive tissue breakdown as in severe burns, adrenal insufficiency, or the administration of a potassium-sparing diuretic (e.g. spironolactone, triamterene), or other drugs causing hyperkalemia such as captopril and enalapril.

Patients with renal impairment with oliguria or azotemia.

Patients who may have an increased sensitivity to potassium administration, e.g., in congenital paramyotonia, or adynamia episodica hereditaria.

All solid dosage forms of potassium supplements are contraindicated in any patient in whom there is cause for arrest or delay in tablet passage through the gastrointestinal tract. In these instances, potassium supplementation should be with a liquid preparation. Long-acting potassium chloride preparations have produced esophageal ulceration in certain cardiac patients with esophageal compression due to an enlarged left atrium. Micro-K Extencaps are therefore contraindicated in such patients as well as in patients with dysphagia.

WARNINGS: In patients with impaired mechanisms for excreting potassium, the administration of potassium salts can produce hyperkalemia and cardiac arrest. This occurs most commonly in patients given potassium by the intravenous route but may also occur in patients given potassium orally. Potentially fatal hyperkalemia can develop rapidly and be asymptomatic. The use of potassium salts in patients with chronic renal disease, or any other condition which impairs potassium excretion, requires particularly careful monitoring of the serum potassium concentration and appropriate dosage adjustment. Hypokalaemia has the potential to promote quinidine toxicity (see Contraindications).

Hypokalemia should not be treated by the concomitant administration of potassium salts and a potassium-sparing diuretic (e.g. spironolactone, triamterene) or other drugs causing hyperkalemia such as captopril or enalapril, since the simultaneous administration of these agents can produce severe hyperkalemia. Hypokalemia in patients with metabolic acidosis should be treated with an alkalinizing potassium salt such as potassium acetate, potassium bicarbonate or potassium citrate (see Contraindications).

Potassium chloride tablets have produced stenotic and/or ulcerative lesions of the small bowel, and deaths. These lesions are caused by a high localized concentration of potassium ion in the region of a rapidly dissolving tablet, which injures the bowel wall and thereby produces obstruction, hemorrhage or perforation. Micro-K is formulated from microencapsulated crystalline particles of potassium chloride. The sustained release of potassium chloride from the microcaps is intended to minimize the possibility of a high local concentration of potassium ion near the bowel wall. Micro-K should be discontinued immediately and the possibility of bowel obstruction or perforation considered if severe vomiting, abdominal pain, distention or gastrointestinal bleeding occurs (see Contraindications).

All oral potassium preparations should be prescribed with particular caution in patients with a history of peptic ulcer.

PRECAUTIONS: The treatment of potassium depletion, particularly in the presence of cardiac disease, renal disease or acidosis, requires careful attention to acid-base balance and appropriate monitoring of serum electrolytes, the electrocardiogram and the clinical status of the patient.

Potassium supplements should be used with caution in diseases associated with heart block since increased serum potassium may increase the degree of block.

Since anticholinergic agents have the potential to slow gastrointestinal motility, caution should be exercised when prescribing solid oral potassium preparations to patients concurrently receiving anticholinergic agents (see Contraindications and Warnings).
Pregnancy: Because of gastrointestinal hypomotility associated with pregnancy, solid oral potassium supplements should be given to pregnant women only if clearly needed.
Children: Safety and effectiveness in children have not been established. Keep out of reach of children.

ADVERSE EFFECTS: The most common adverse reactions are nausea, vomiting, diarrhea and abdominal discomfort. These symptoms are due to irritation of the GI tract and can be reduced by increasing fluid intake when possible, by taking the dose with meals or by reducing the dose. One of the most severe adverse effects of potassium supplementation is hyperkalemia. Skin rash has been reported rarely. Intestinal bleeding, ulceration, perforation and stenosis have been reported in patients treated with solid dosage forms of potassium salts, but there appears to be less likelihood of this occurring with Micro-K.

OVERDOSE:
Overdosage from therapeutic doses of solid oral potassium salts in persons with normal excretory mechanism rarely occurs; however, if excretory mechanisms are impaired, potentially fatal hyperkalemia may occur. Acute (accidental or intentional) overdosages of solid oral potassium salts have resulted in severe and/or fatal hyperkalemia.

Symptoms: Overdosage with potassium is characterized chiefly by cardiovascular, neuromuscular and gastrointestinal disturbances.
Cardiovascular: ECG changes, hypotension and shock, bundle-branch block, ventricular arrhythmias, ventricular fibrillation leading possibly to cardiac arrest.
Neuromuscular: paresthesia, areflexia, convulsions, flaccid paralysis of striated muscle leading possibly to respiratory paralysis.
Gastrointestinal: nausea, vomiting, diarrhea and abdominal cramp.

It is important to recognize that hyperkalemia is usually asymptomatic and may be manifested only by an increased serum potassium concentration and characteristic electrocardiographic changes, which include increased amplitude and peaking of the T wave, and flattening or absence of P wave. As hyperkalemia worsens, prolongation of the P-R interval, widening of the QRS complex with S-T segment depression and arrhythmias may develop.

Widening of the QRS complex is one of the most ominous signs and indicates the need for aggressive treatment.

Treatment: The plasma concentration and electrocardiogram must be monitored in every case of potassium overdosage, as well as serum electrolytes, BUN, glucose and arterial blood gases.

Electrocardiographic signs of hyperkalemia (tall peaked T waves, P-R prolongation, disappearance of P waves, QRS widening, heart block) are indications for immediate treatment.

In severe hyperkalemia (plasma potassium exceeds 8 mEq/L or ECG abnormalities include absence of P wave, presence of widened QRS complex or ventricular arrhythmia): Administer intravenously 300 to 500 mL/h of 10% dextrose solution containing 10-20 units of insulin per 1000 mL.

Correct acidosis, if present, with intravenous sodium bicarbonate (44 to 132 mEq/L of glucose solution).

Administer 10 to 30 mL of 10% calcium gluconate i.v. over 1 to 5 minutes under continuous ECG monitoring.

Administer cation exchange resin by high retention enema.

100 mL of warm aqueous solution of sorbitol containing 30 to 50 g of sodium polystyrene sulfonate should be kept in the sigmoid colon for several hours, if possible. The colon is then irrigated with a non-sodium containing solution to remove the resin. Repeated enemas can be administered, or the resin given repeatedly by mouth, to maintain a physiologic potassium concentration.

Hemodialysis or peritoneal dialysis may be of use, particularly in patients with renal failure.

In moderately severe hyperkalemia (plasma potassium between 6.5 and 8 mEq/L or ECG peaking of T wave): Administer intravenously 300 to 500 mL/h of 10% dextrose solution containing 10-20 units insulin per 1000 mL.

Correct acidosis, if present, with intravenous sodium bicarbonate (44 to 132 mEq/L of glucose solution).

Correct hyponatremia and hypovolemia, if present.

Once the patient's cardiac state has been stabilized, in the case of a recent **acute** ingestion of Micro-K, consideration should be given to the evacuation of the stomach. When overdosage is the result of **chronic** therapeutic ingestion, Micro-K should be discontinued immediately as well as potassium containing foods and medications and also potassium-sparing diuretics.

> For management of a suspected drug overdose, CPhA recommends that you contact your **regional Poison Control Centre**. See the *CPS* Directory section for a list of Poison Control Centres.

DOSAGE: The usual dietary intake of potassium by the average adult is 40 to 80 mEq per day. Potassium depletion sufficient to cause hypokalemia usually requires the loss of 200 or more mEq of potassium from the total body store.

Dosage must be adjusted to the individual needs of each patient but typically is approximately 20 mEq per day for the prevention of hypokalemia and 40 to 100 mEq per day for the treatment of potassium depletion (see Table 1).

Table 1: Micro-K Extencaps Dosage

	For Prevention	For Treatment
Micro-K Extencaps (8 mEq K^+)	2 or 3 Extencaps/day (16–24 mEq K^+)	5 to 12 Extencaps/day (40–96 mEq K^+)

If more than 2 Extencaps are prescribed per day, the total daily dosage should be divided into two or more separate doses. These capsules should not be crushed or chewed, but administered whole and taken with water. Those patients having difficulty swallowing the capsules may be advised to sprinkle the contents onto a spoonful of soft food to facilitate ingestion.

SUPPLIED: Each hard gelatin capsule, opaque pale orange body and cap, monogrammed with a Paladin shield and "Micro-K" in black ink, contains: microencapsulated potassium chloride 600 mg (8 mEq K^+). Bottles of 100 and 500. Nonmedicinal ingredients: magnesium stearate and sodium lauryl sulfate. Sodium: <1 mmol (0.048 mg). Alcohol-, gluten-, lactose-, parabens-, sugars-, sulfites- and tartrazine-free.

(Shown in Product Identification Section)

Microlax®

glycerin—sodium citrate—sodium lauryl sulfoacetate—sorbic acid—sorbitol

Micro-enema

McNeil Consumer Healthcare

Date of Revision: May 5, 2008

INDICATIONS: Rectal constipation; or, as directed by a physician, to facilitate rectoscopic or sigmoidoscopic examination.

CONTRAINDICATIONS: No data supplied by the manufacturer.

WARNINGS: No data supplied by the manufacturer.

PRECAUTIONS: No data supplied by the manufacturer.

ADVERSE EFFECTS: No severe reactions have been reported. Very occasionally slight cramps or tenesmus may occur.

OVERDOSE:

No data supplied by the manufacturer.

> For management of a suspected drug overdose, CPhA recommends that you contact your **regional Poison Control Centre**. See the *CPS* Directory section for a list of Poison Control Centres.

DOSAGE: Adults and children: the contents of 1 tube (5 mL) administered rectally is usually sufficient but a second tube may be needed in severe cases. 1. Remove the nozzle cap by twisting the seal of the nozzle. 2. Squeeze the tube slightly so that a drop of Microlax smears the tip and thus makes insertion easier. 3. Insert the nozzle fully into the rectum. Note: In children under 3 years of age, insert only half the length of the nozzle (see indication on the nozzle). 4. Squeeze out the contents fully by squeezing the shoulder of the tube. 5. Withdraw the nozzle still squeezing tightly. Defecation can normally be expected within 5 to 20 minutes.

SUPPLIED: Each mL contains: sodium citrate, sodium lauryl sulfoacetate, glycerin, sorbitol, sorbic acid, and purified water q.s. in a disposable plastic tube fitted with a flexible enema tip about 5 cm long. Tubes of 5 mL. Boxes of 12 and 50.

Micronor® Pr

norethindrone

Oral Contraceptive

Janssen-Ortho

Date of Preparation: April 1972
Date of Revision: June 18, 2010

PHARMACOLOGY: The mechanism of contraception action of MICRONOR tablets is multicausal, primarily at the local pelvic level and secondarily at the systemic level. The hormonal effect is mainly progestational.

Pelvic effects include changes in the cervical mucus and endometrium. Systemic effects involve mainly the inhibition of secretion of pituitary gonadotrophins which in turn prevents follicular maturation and ovulation.

Studies by Moghissi, Beck, Fortier and Lefebvre, and others suggest the following priority of causes:

1. Inhibitory cervical mucus changes including increased viscosity and cell content, with inhibition of sperm transport or migration. Changes in cervical mucus reach their peak 3 to 4 hours after MICRONOR pill intake and the possibility of sperm penetration remains low for 16 to 19 hours.
2. Suppression of FSH levels and the LH surge.
3. Abnormal ovulation and deficient corpus luteum function. (Serum progesterone levels may be suppressed in the second half of the menstrual cycle when they are usually low, i.e., dysphasic.) Serum estrogens may be increased above normal early in the cycle.
4. Endometrial changes (progestational), unfavourable to implantation.

INDICATIONS: Conception control.

MICRONOR tablets contain a low dosage of norethindrone without the addition of an estrogen agent. Progestin-only pills are often called "Progestin-only pills" or the "Mini-pill".

CONTRAINDICATIONS: Progestin-only pills should not be used by women who currently have the following conditions:

1. when pregnancy is suspected or diagnosed;
2. active liver disease or history of/or actual benign or malignant liver tumours;
3. known or suspected carcinoma of the breast;
4. undiagnosed abnormal vaginal bleeding;
5. hypersensitivity to any component of this product.

WARNINGS: Progestin-only pills have less progestin than the combined birth control pill (or "the Pill") which contains both an estrogen and a progestin. Therefore, this product monograph does not discuss the serious health risks that have been associated with the estrogen component of combined oral contraceptives.

> Cigarette smoking increases the risk of serious adverse effects on the heart and blood vessels. This risk increases with age and becomes significant in oral contraceptive users over 35 years of age. Women should be counselled not to smoke.

Ectopic Pregnancy: The incidence of ectopic pregnancies for progestin-only oral contraceptive users is 5 per 1000 woman-years. Up to 10% of pregnancies reported in clinical studies of progestin-only oral contraceptive users are extrauterine. Although symptoms of ectopic pregnancy should be watched for, a history of ectopic pregnancy need not be considered a contraindication to use of this contraceptive method. Health providers should be alert to the possibility of an ectopic pregnancy in women who become pregnant or complain of lower abdominal pain while on progestin-only oral contraceptives.

Delayed Follicular Atresia/Ovarian Cysts: If follicular development occurs, atresia of the follicle is sometimes delayed and the follicle may continue to grow beyond the size it would attain in a normal cycle. Generally these enlarged follicles disappear spontaneously. Often they are asymptomatic; in some cases they are associated with mild abdominal pain. Rarely they may twist or rupture, requiring surgical intervention.

Carcinoma of the Breast and Reproductive Organs: Some epidemiological studies of oral contraceptive users have reported an increased relative risk of developing breast cancer, particularly at a younger age and apparently related to duration of use. These studies have predominantly involved combined oral contraceptives and there is insufficient data to determine whether the use of progestin-only pills similarly increases the risk. Women with breast cancer should not use oral contraceptives because the role of female hormones in breast cancer has not been fully determined.

Some studies suggest that oral contraceptive use has been associated with an increase in the risk of cervical intraepithelial neoplasia in some populations of women. However, there continues to be controversy about the extent to which such findings may be due to differences in sexual behaviour and other factors. There is insufficient data to determine whether the use of progestin-only pills increases the risk of developing cervical intraepithelial neoplasia.

Headache: Discontinue medication at the earliest manifestation of severe headache of unknown etiology or worsening of pre-existing migraine headache.

Vaginal Bleeding: Irregular menstrual patterns are common among women using progestin-only oral contraceptives. If genital bleeding is suggestive of infection, malignancy or other abnormal conditions, such nonpharmacologic causes should be ruled out. If prolonged amenorrhea occurs, the possibility of pregnancy should be evaluated.

PRECAUTIONS:

> **Sexually Transmitted Infections:** Birth control pills **do not protect** against sexually transmitted infections (STIs), including HIV/AIDS. For protection against STIs, it is advisable to use latex or polyurethane condoms **in combination with** birth control pills.

Physical Examination and Follow-up: Before oral contraceptives are used, a thorough history and physical examination should be performed, including a blood pressure determination. Breasts, liver, extremities, and pelvic organs should be examined. A Papanicolaou smear should be taken if the patient has been sexually active.

The first follow-up visit should be done 3 months after oral contraceptives are prescribed. Thereafter, examinations should be performed at least once a year, or more frequently if indicated. At each annual visit, examination should include those procedures that were done at the initial visit as outlined above or per recommendations of the Canadian Workshop on Screening for Cancer of the Cervix. Their suggestion was that, for women who had 2 consecutive negative Pap smears, screening could be continued every 3 years up to the age of 69.

Pregnancy: Oral contraceptives should not be taken by pregnant women. However, if conception accidentally occurs while taking the pill, there is no conclusive evidence that the progestin contained in the oral contraceptive will damage the developing child.

Lactation: In most women, progestin-only contraceptives, such as MICRONOR, do not affect the quantity and quality of breast milk or length of lactation. However, isolated post-marketing cases of decreased milk production have been reported. Studies with various orally administered progestin-only contraceptives have shown that small amounts of progestins pass into the breast milk of nursing mothers resulting in detectable steroid levels in infant plasma.

No adverse effects have been found on the health, growth or development of the infant.

Hepatic Neoplasia: The incidence of both benign and malignant liver tumours (hepatic adenomas and hepatocellular carcinomas) is rare. Case-control studies have indicated that the risk of these tumours may increase in association with the use and duration of use of oral contraceptives. Rupture of benign, hepatic adenomas may cause death through intra-abdominal hemorrhage. There is insufficient data to determine whether progestin-only pills increase the risk of developing hepatic neoplasia.

Migraine and Headache: The onset or exacerbation of migraine or the development of headache of a new pattern which is recurrent, persistent or severe, requires discontinuation of oral contraceptives and evaluation of the cause.

Carbohydrate and Lipid Metabolism: Some users may experience slight deterioration in glucose tolerance, with increases in plasma insulin, but women with diabetes mellitus who use progestin-only oral contraceptives do not generally experience changes in their insulin requirements. Nonetheless, prediabetic and diabetic women in particular should be carefully monitored while taking progestin-only pills.

Lipid metabolism is occasionally affected in that HDL, HDL_2, and apolipoprotein A-I and A-II may be decreased; hepatic lipase may be increased. There is usually no effect on total cholesterol, HDL_3, LDL, or VLDL.

Emotional Disorders: Patients with a history of emotional disturbances, especially the depressive type, may be more prone to have a recurrence of depression while taking oral contraceptives. In cases of a serious recurrence, a trial of an alternative method of contraception should be made which may help to clarify the possible relationship. Women with premenstrual syndrome (PMS) may have a varied response to oral contraceptives, ranging from symptomatic improvement to worsening of the condition.

Laboratory Tests: The following endocrine tests may be affected by progestin-only oral contraceptive use:

- sex hormone-binding globulin (SHBG) concentrations may be decreased;
- thyroxine concentrations may be decreased, due to a decrease in thyroid-binding globulin (TBG).

Results of laboratory tests should be interpreted in light of the fact that the patient is on oral contraceptives. LH and FSH levels are suppressed by the use of oral contraceptives. Wait 2 weeks after discontinuing the use of oral contraceptives before measurements are made.

Tissue Specimens: Pathologists should be advised of oral contraceptive therapy when specimens obtained from surgical procedures and Pap smears are submitted for examination.

Return to Fertility: The limited available data indicate a rapid return of normal ovulation and no delay to fertility following discontinuation of progestin-only oral contraceptives.

Amenorrhea: Women having a history of oligomenorrhea, secondary amenorrhea, or irregular cycles may remain anovulatory or become amenorrheic following discontinuation of progestin therapy. Amenorrhea, especially if associated with breast secretion, that continues for 6 months or more after withdrawal, warrants a careful assessment of hypothalamic-pituitary function.

Drug Interactions: It is important to ascertain all drugs that a patient is taking, both prescription and non-prescription, including herbal preparations/remedies, before oral contraceptives are prescribed.

If a woman on norethindrone takes a drug or herbal product that induces an enzyme(s) that metabolizes norethindrone, particularly CYP3A4, she should be counselled to use additional contraception or a different method of contraception. Drugs that induce such enzymes may decrease the plasma concentrations of norethindrone, and may decrease the effectiveness of norethindrone or increase breakthrough bleeding. See Table 1 for a list of drugs that may decrease the efficacy of MICRONOR.

Some anti-epileptic drugs are known to induce or inhibit a number of hepatic enzymes in the cytochrome P450 system. In drug interaction studies with combined oral contraceptives containing norethindrone, the administration of topiramate (50 mg/day to 800 mg/day) did not significantly affect the exposure to norethindrone.

Significant changes (increase or decrease) in the plasma levels of norethindrone have been noted in some cases of co-administration of HIV protease inhibitors and non-nucleoside reverse transcriptase inhibitors.

In vitro studies suggest that activated charcoal binds to norethindrone; however, the therapeutic effect of norethindrone is not affected when activated charcoal is administered 3 hours after the previous dose or 12 hours before the next dose.

No significant interaction has been found with broad-spectrum antibiotics.

Refer to Oral Contraceptives 1994 (Chapter 8), Health Canada, for other possible drug interactions with OCs which is adapted from Dickey RP, ed.: Managing Contraceptive Pill Patients, 5th edition, EMIS Inc. Medical Publishers 1987.

Table 1: MICRONOR

Drugs That May Decrease the Efficacy of Oral Contraceptives

Class of Compound	Drug	Proposed Mechanism	Suggested Management
Anticonvulsants	Carbamazepine ethosuximide phenobarbital phenytoin primidone	Induction of hepatic microsomal enzymes: Increased binding of progestin to SHBG.	Use higher dose OCs (50 µg ethinyl estradiol), another drug or another method.
Antituberculosis	Rifampin	Increased metabolism of progestins.	Use another method.
Antifungals	Griseofulvin	Stimulation of hepatic metabolism of contraceptive steroids may occur.	Use another method.
Sedatives and Hypnotics	benzodiazepines barbiturates chloral hydrate glutethimide meprobamate	Induction of hepatic microsomal enzymes.	For short course, use additional method or another drug. For long course, use another method or higher dose OCs.
Other Drugs	Bosentan	Induction of hepatic microsomal enzymes.	Consider switching to a non-hormonal contraceptive method or adding a barrier method to oral contraceptive therapy.

Drug-Herb Interactions: Herbal products containing St. John's wort (hypericum perforatum) may induce hepatic enzymes (cytochrome P450) and p-glycoprotein transporter and may reduce the effectiveness of contraceptive steroids. This may also result in breakthrough bleeding.

ADVERSE EFFECTS: Adverse reactions reported with the use of progestin-only pills include:

- Menstrual irregularity is the most frequently reported side effect.
- Frequent and irregular bleeding are common, while long duration of bleeding episodes and amenorrhea are less likely.

- Headache, breast tenderness, nausea, and dizziness are increased among progestin-only oral contraceptive users in some studies.
- Androgenic side effects such as acne, hirsutism, and weight gain occur rarely.
- Decreased lactation has been reported very rarely.

OVERDOSE:

Treatment: In case of overdose or accidental ingestion by children, the physician should observe the patient closely although generally no treatment is required. Gastric lavage may be utilized if considered necessary. There have been no reports of serious ill effects from overdosage. Overdosage may cause nausea and vomiting and withdrawal bleeding may occur in females. There are no antidotes and treatment should be symptomatic.

> For management of a suspected drug overdose, contact your regional Poison Control Centre. See the *CPS* Directory section for a list of Poison Control Centres.

DOSAGE: MICRONOR 28-Tablet Regimen: The dosage of MICRONOR tablets is one tablet daily without interruption for 28 days.

Starting Progestin-Only Pills

1. For the initial cycle of therapy, patients should start treatment on the first day of their menstrual period (Day 1).* Then they should continue taking one tablet every day until their package is empty. Without missing a day, they should start taking MICRONOR from a new package.
2. If the patient has had a miscarriage or an abortion, she can start progestin-only pills the next day.
3. Patients should take one pill at the same time every day for 28 days. After finishing a pack, they should begin a new pack the next day, **not missing any days on the pills**. Their period should occur during the last seven days of using the pill pack. MICRONOR tablets are taken every day, even when patients are having some menstrual bleeding.

Breast-feeding:

1. **For women who are fully breast-feeding** (not giving their babies any food or formula), they may start taking MICRONOR tablets 6 weeks after delivery.
2. **For women who are partially breast-feeding** (giving their babies some food or formula), they should start taking MICRONOR tablets 3 weeks after delivery.

Switching pills:

1. To switch from 21-Day combined oral contraceptive pills to progestin-only pills, patients should start taking their first MICRONOR tablet (progestin-only pill) the day after they finish the last **active** combined pill.

   To switch from a 28-Day combined oral contraceptive regimen, patients should not take any of the 7 **inactive** pills from the combined pill pack.

   Many women have irregular periods after switching to progestin-only pills, but this is normal and to be expected.
2. For women who switch from progestin-only pills to combined pills, the first **active** combined pill is taken on the first day of their period, even if their progestin-only pill pack is not finished.
3. If the patient is breast-feeding, she can switch to another method of birth control at any time, except she should not switch to the combined pills until she has stopped breast-feeding or at least until 6 months after delivery.

Administration: It is recommended that MICRONOR tablets be taken at the same time every day until the pack is empty. Progestin-only pills must be taken at the same time every day since their action is time dependent.

When the pack is finished after 28 days, the next pack is started **on the next day**. Women are not to wait any days between packs.

Vomiting and/or diarrhea may reduce absorption of oral contraceptives resulting in decreased serum concentrations and therefore may reduce contraceptive efficacy. Physicians should advise patients of the need for a back-up contraceptive method in the case of such gastrointestinal symptoms.

For women who take other drugs or herbal products concurrently, the pill may not work as well. See Drug Interactions, for a list of drugs that may decrease the effectiveness of MICRONOR or increase breakthrough bleeding. They should be advised to use a back-up method, until they can check for possible drug interactions with their doctor or clinic.

Missed Dose: If a patient is more than 3 hours late taking her progestin-only pill, she should take the missed pill as soon as she remembers then go back to taking progestin-only pills at her regular time.

Inform patients to use a back-up method, every time they have sex, for 48 hours after missing a pill.

If patients forget more than one pill two months in a row, talk to them about ways to make pill-taking easier or about using another method of birth control.

Counselling Issues: The following points should be discussed with prospective users before prescribing progestin-only oral contraceptives:

- the necessity of taking pills at the same time every day, including throughout all bleeding episodes;
- the need to use a back-up method such as condoms and spermicides for the next 48 hours whenever a progestin-only oral contraceptive is taken 3 or more hours late;
- the potential side effects of progestin-only oral contraceptives, particularly menstrual irregularities;
- the need to inform the clinician of prolonged episodes of bleeding, amenorrhea or severe abdominal pain;
- the importance of using an effective barrier method in addition to progestin-only oral contraceptives if a woman is at risk of contracting or transmitting STIs/HIV.

INFORMATION FOR THE PATIENT: Published in e-CPS, available by subscription at www.e-cps.ca.

SUPPLIED: Each green, unscored tablet, with ORTHO 0.35 engraved on each side, contains: norethindrone 0.35 mg. Nonmedicinal ingredients: D&C Green No. 5, D&C Yellow No. 10, lactose, magnesium stearate, polyvinylpyrrolidone and starch. A 28-day DISCREET Package contains a 4-week supply of tablets. Store between 15 and 30°C. Leave contents in protective packaging until time of use.

(Shown in Product Identification Section)

Midazolam

CPhA Monograph

see *Benzodiazepines*

Midazolam Injection (Sandoz Standard)

midazolam

Premedicant—Sedative—Anesthetic

Sandoz

SUPPLIED: 1 mg/mL: Each mL of sterile aqueous solution contains: midazolam 1 mg (hydrochloric acid added for solubilization). Nonmedicinal ingredients: benzyl alcohol as a preservative, disodium edetate, sodium chloride for tonicity, sodium hydroxide and/or hydrochloric acid to adjust pH and water for injection. Multidose vials of 2, 5 and 10 mL, boxes of 10. Discard unused portion 28 days after initial puncture. Store between 15 and 30°C. Protect from light.

5 mg/mL: Each mL of sterile aqueous solution contains: midazolam 5 mg (hydrochloric acid added for solubilization). Nonmedicinal ingredients: benzyl alcohol as a preservative, disodium edetate, sodium chloride for tonicity, sodium hydroxide and/or hydrochloric acid to adjust pH and water for injection. Multidose vials of 1, 2 and 10 mL, boxes of 10. Discard unused portion 28 days after initial puncture. Pharmacy bulk vials of 50 mL, boxes of 1, intended for single puncture, multiple dispensing. Discard unused portion. Store between 15 and 30°C. Protect from light.

* If the first progestin-only pill is taken on another day, it is recommended that an additional method of birth control (such as latex or polyurethane condoms and spermicidal foam or gel) be used every time the patient has sex during the next 48 hours.

Midol® PMS Complete

acetaminophen—pamabrom—pyrilamine maleate

Premenstrual Syndrome Therapy

Bayer Consumer Care

Midol® Menstrual Complete

acetaminophen—caffeine—pyrilamine maleate

Analgesic

Bayer Consumer Care

Midol® Teen Complete

acetaminophen—caffeine—pyrilamine maleate

Analgesic

Bayer Consumer Care

Midol® Night-Time

acetaminophen—methocarbamol

Analgesic—Muscle Relaxant

Bayer Consumer Care

SUPPLIED: PMS Complete: Each white caplet, with MIDOL in orange on one side, contains: acetaminophen 500 mg, pamabrom 25 mg and pyrilamine maleate 15 mg. Nonmedicinal ingredients: carnauba wax, croscarmellose sodium, D&C Red #30, D&C Yellow #10, hypromellose, magnesium stearate, microcrystalline cellulose, pregelatinized starch, propylene glycol, shellac, titanium dioxide and triacetin. Lactose-, paraben- and sucrose-free. Blister packages of 16. Bottles of 32.

Menstrual Complete: Each film-coated, white caplet printed in blue ink on one face with MIDOL with a score on each end, contains: acetaminophen 500 mg, caffeine 60 mg and pyrilamine maleate 15 mg. Nonmedicinal ingredients: butyl alcohol, carnauba wax, croscarmellose sodium, dehydrated alcohol, FD&C Blue #2, hypromellose, isopropyl alcohol, magnesium stearate, microcrystalline cellulose, pregelatinized starch, propylene glycol, shellac, sodium hydroxide, titanium dioxide and triacetin. Lactose- and tartrazine-free. Blister packages of 16. Bottles of 32.

Teen Complete: Each white caplet, engraved MIDOL on one side of the caplet, contains: acetaminophen 325 mg, caffeine 60 mg and pyrilamine maleate 15 mg. Nonmedicinal ingredients: croscarmellose sodium, hypromellose, magnesium stearate, microcrystalline cellulose, pregelatinized starch and triacetin. Blister packages of 16.

Night-Time: Each blue caplet with "MIDOL" engraved on one side contains: acetaminophen 500 mg and methocarbamol 400 mg. Nonmedicinal ingredients: cornstarch, D&C Red #27, FD&C Blue #2, magnesium stearate, microcrystalline cellulose, polyethylene glycol, polyvinyl alcohol, povidone, silicon dioxide, sodium starch glycolate, stearic acid, talc and titanium dioxide. Bottles of 20.

Migranal®

dihydroergotamine mesylate

Migraine Therapy

SteriMax

SUPPLIED: Each mL of clear, colourless to faintly yellow solution contains: dihydroergotamine mesylate USP 4 mg. Nonmedicinal ingredients: caffeine, dextrose and water. Cartons of 3 units, each consisting of 1 bottle and 1 sprayer. Store at room temperature (15 to 25°C).

Milk of Magnesia USP

magnesium hydroxide

Antacid—Laxative

Rougier Pharma

SUPPLIED: Regular: Each mL of white, more or less viscous suspension contains: magnesium hydroxide 77.5 mg. Nonmedicinal ingredients: potassium sorbate and purified water. Partial settling on standing. Bottles of 500 mL. Keep out of reach of children. Store between 15-30°C.

Mint Flavoured: Each mL of white, more or less viscous suspension contains: magnesium hydroxide 80 mg. Nonmedicinal ingredients: glycerine, menthol, peppermint oil, potassium sorbate, propylene glycol, purified water and sorbitol. Partial settling on standing. Bottles of 500 mL. Keep out of reach of children. Store between 15-30°C.

Milrinone Lactate Injection

milrinone lactate

Inotrope—Vasodilator

Sandoz

SUPPLIED: Each mL of sterile solution contains: milrinone (as lactate) 1 mg. Nonmedicinal ingredients: anhydrous dextrose, lactic acid and/or sodium hydroxide for pH adjustment and water for injection. Clear single use vials of 10 and 20 mL, boxes of 10. Discard unused portion. Store between 15 and 30 °C. Protect from light. Protect from freezing.

Minirin® Ⓟ
desmopressin acetate
Antidiuretic

Ferring

Date of Preparation: July 13, 2001
Date of Revision: February 24, 2006

SUMMARY PRODUCT INFORMATION:

Route of Administration	Dosage Form/Strength	Clinically Relevant Nonmedicinal Ingredients
Oral	Tablet, 0.1 mg	Lactose, potato starch, povidone, magnesium stearate For a complete listing see Dosage Forms, Composition and Packaging.

INDICATIONS AND CLINICAL USE: Minirin Tablets are indicated for:
- Treatment of nocturia in adults.

CONTRAINDICATIONS:
- Hypersensitivity to desmopressin acetate or to any ingredient in the formulation or component of the container. For complete listing, see Dosage Forms, Composition and Packaging.
- Known hyponatraemia, severe liver disease, nephrosis or any other condition associated with impaired water excretion, cardiac insufficiency, chronic renal insufficiency, congestive heart failure, habitual or psychogenic polydypsia.
- Existing medical conditions, which lead to sodium losing states such as nausea, bulimia, anorexia nervosa, chronic vomiting, diarrhoea and adrenocortical insufficiency as well as salt losing nephropathies, are contraindicated for use of desmopressin acetate.
- Because of the risk of platelet aggregation and thrombocytopenia, the drug should not be used in patients with type IIB or platelet-type (pseudo) von Willebrand's disease.

WARNINGS AND PRECAUTIONS: General: Desmopressin acetate is not effective in controlling polyuria caused by renal disease, nephrogenic diabetes insipidus, diabetes mellitus, psychogenic polydypsia, hypokalaemia or hypercalcaemia.

Desmopressin should not be administered to dehydrated patients until water balance has been adequately restored.

Fluid intake should be adjusted to reduce the possibility of water intoxication and hyponatraemia.

The initiation of treatment in patients 65 years and older is not recommended [see Special Populations, Geriatrics (≥65 years of age)].

Patients treated with diuretics for fluid retention should not be treated with antidiuretics.

Desmopressin should be used with caution in patients with cystic fibrosis because these patients are prone to hyponatremia.

Treatment with desmopressin should be interrupted during acute inter-current illnesses characterized by fluid and/or electrolyte imbalance (such as systemic infections, fever, gastroenteritis).

Precautions to avoid hyponatraemia must be taken in:
- conditions characterised by fluid and/or electrolyte imbalance (such as systemic infections, fever, and SIADH (Syndrome of Inappropriate ADH secretion) and in patients with high intra-cranial pressure
- cases of concomitant treatment with drugs which are known to induce SIADH, e.g. tricyclic antidepressants (amitriptyline, nortriptyline), selective serotonin reuptake inhibitor antidepressants (fluoxetine, paroxetine, sertraline, fluvoxamine, citalopram), chlorpromazine and carbamazepine
- cases of concomitant treatment with NSAIDs, including COX-2 inhibitors

In general, both hyponatraemia and SIADH respond to fluid intake limitation and restriction in the range of 1000 to 1200 mL per day. Physicians should not use hypertonic saline infusion for rapid correction of severe hyponatraemia as this may lead to severe sequelae.

Cardiovascular: Intranasal formulation of desmopressin acetate at high dosage (40 µg or more) has occasionally produced a slight elevation of blood pressure, which disappeared with a reduction in dosage. The drug should be used with caution in patients with coronary artery insufficiency and/or hypertensive cardiovascular disease because of possible tachycardia and changes in blood pressure.

Genitourinary: Severe bladder dysfunction and outlet obstruction should be considered before starting treatment.

Sensitivity/Resistance: There are reports of changes in response over time, usually when the drug has been administered for periods longer than 6 months. Some patients may show decreased responsiveness, others a shortened duration of effect. There is no evidence that this effect is due to the development of binding antibodies, but may be due to local inactivation of the peptide.

Special Populations: Pregnant Women: Reproductive studies performed in rats and rabbits have revealed no evidence of harm to the fetus by desmopressin. The use of desmopressin acetate in pregnant women with no harm to the fetus has been reported.

No controlled studies in pregnant women have been carried out. However, as with all medications used during pregnancy, the physician should weigh possible therapeutic advantages against potential risks in each case.

Nursing Women: There have been no controlled studies in nursing mothers. A single study on a post-partum woman demonstrated a marked change in maternal plasma desmopressin acetate level following an intranasal dose of 10 µg, but little desmopressin was detectable in breast milk.

Geriatrics (≥65 years of age): The initiation of treatment in patients 65 years and older is not recommended due to the increased risk of hyponatremia in this population.

Should physicians decide to initiate desmopressin treatment in these patients then serum sodium should be measured before beginning treatment, 3 days after the start of therapy and 3 days following a change of dose. If the serum sodium level is below normal limits, or has significantly decreased from baseline, a repeat serum sodium should be obtained within 3 to 4 days. If Minirin Tablets (desmopressin acetate) are being used long-term, a further sodium test at one month should be taken. If Minirin Tablets are being used long term and the patient shows a tendency to hyponatraemia, the sodium should be measured every month. If there is no tendency to hyponatraemia, then measuring the sodium every 2 to 3 months is appropriate. In the event serum sodium levels are not within normal limits, or have not stabilized, the patient should be discontinued from further treatment.

Geriatric patients should be closely observed for possible water retention due to over-ingestion of fluids. When fluid intake is not excessive, there is little danger of water intoxication and hyponatraemia. Fluid intake should be carefully adjusted to prevent over-hydration.

Monitoring and Laboratory Tests: In nocturia patients, a frequency/volume chart should be used to diagnose nocturnal polyuria for at least two days before starting treatment. A night-time urine production exceeding the functional bladder capacity or exceeding 20% in the young, 27% in the middle age and 33 % in the elderly of the 24 hour urine production is regarded as nocturnal polyuria.

Serum sodium should be measured before beginning the treatment, 3 days after initiation of therapy or increase in dosage and at other times during treatment as deemed necessary by the treating physician.

ADVERSE REACTIONS: Clinical Trial Adverse Drug Reactions: Because clinical trials are conducted under very specific conditions the adverse reaction rates observed in the clinical trials may not reflect the rates observed in practice and should not be compared to the rates in the clinical trials of another drug. Adverse drug reaction information from clinical trials is useful for identifying drug-related adverse events and for approximating rates.

Two clinical studies in patients with nocturia were conducted. The two clinical trials (male and female studies) were identical in design. They were randomized, double blind, placebo-controlled, parallel group, multicentre investigations in adult males or females aged ≥18 years. The patients had an average of ≥2 nocturnal voids. Exclusion criteria were adopted to ensure that the presence of Nocturia was not due to other well-defined causes of increased urinary frequency as multiple sclerosis, urge incontinence, diabetes insipidus or polydipsia. Patients with cardiac insufficiency, those requiring diuretic therapy and those with any other medical condition characterized by a fluid or electrolyte imbalance, were also excluded. Patients receiving diuretics, tricyclic antidepressants, indomethacin, carbamazepine, or chlorpromamide were excluded. Antihypertensives were permitted providing that no dose adjustments occurred in the previous 3 months and patients were receiving long-term treatment.

The studies commenced with a 1-week screening period to establish baseline. In week 1, patients received daily one 0.1 mg Minirin Tablet at bedtime for seven days. If necessary, medication was increased in week 2 to one 0.2 mg tablet daily for seven days and again in week 3 to two 0.2 mg tablets (i.e., 0.4 mg) daily for an additional seven days. If patient obtained zero nocturnal voids during the dose-titration week, this dose was chosen as the optimal dose for the double-blind treatment period and the patient would not proceed to the next dose level. In patients not achieving zero nocturnal voids with any of the doses, the tolerated dose giving the lowest nocturnal diuresis was selected. The double-blind period commenced after the seven-day wash-out period. Patients were randomly assigned to their optimal dose of Minirin tablets or placebo. The treatment period was five weeks, giving a total of 6-8 weeks depending on the length of the titration period.

Table 1 summarizes the incidence of related adverse events with an occurrence rate of at least 1% in both the male and female study. The majority of adverse events were seen in the dose titration phase (see Table 2).

Apart from hyponatraemia, there were no differences between Minirin tablets and placebo with respect to number of abnormal laboratory values, or changes in vital sign measurements from baseline to study end. The most commonly used concomitant medication was anti-thrombotic agents.

Clinical Trial Adverse Drug Reactions (Frequency ≥1%): See Table 1.

Table 1: Minirin

Incidence of Related Adverse Events with Occurrence Rate of at Least 1% in the Male and Female Studies

	Male Study[a]			Female Study[a]		
	Titration	Double-Blind		Titration	Double-Blind	
	Desmopressin (N=224) %	Desmopressin (N=86) %	Placebo (N=65) %	Desmopressin (N=224) %	Desmopressin (N=72) %	Placebo (N=72) %
Body as a Whole						
Headache	12	2	2	22	10	7
Abdominal Pain	3			4		
Fatigue	2	1		3		
Back Pain						1
Nervous System						
Dizziness	4			3		
Insomnia	<1			2		
Somnolence	1					
Gastrointestinal						
Nausea	4			8		1
Dry Mouth	3	1		4		
Diarrhea	4			1		
Dyspepsia	1		2	<1		
Flatulence				2		
Vomiting	<1	1		1		
Constipation		1		1		
Cardiovascular						
Hypertension	1			2		
Arrhythmia		1				
Urogenital						
Micturation Frequency	1			4		
Urinary Incontinence					1	
Metabolic						
Oedema Peripheral	1	1	3	3		
Musculoskeletal						
Cramp Legs				2		
Blood Disorders						
Thrombocytopenia			2			
Laboratory Changes						
Hyponatraemia	4			6		
ALT Incr.			2	<1		
Creatine Phosphokinase Incr.	<1	1		1		

[a] In both the male and female studies there was an open dose titration arm, where the optimal dose was determined. The double blind period commenced after a 7 day wash out period. Patients were assigned to their optimal dose, as determined in the titration phase of desmopressin or to a placebo in a randomized fashion. Most AEs were reported during the dose titration phase.

Male Study: A total of 237 adverse events in 107 (48%) patients occurred during the dose titration and wash out periods. Treatment related events were reported in 60 (27%) patients during the dose-titration period. In the double-blind period: 12 patients experienced at least one related event; six (7%) patients on desmopressin and six (9%) patients on the placebo.

Female Study: Three hundred ninety eight (398) adverse events were reported in 158 (71%) patients in the dose titration and wash out periods. Two hundred thirty one (231) related adverse events occurred in 109 (49%) patients during the dose-titration period. In the double-blind period, fifteen patients experienced at least one related adverse event; 9 (13%) patients on desmopressin and 6 (8%) on placebo.

A summary of the most frequently reported (>3%) related adverse events during the dose titration phase is listed in Table 2.

Table 2: Minirin

Summary of Treatment Related Adverse Events >3% During the Dose Titration Phase

	Male Study		Female Study	
	N (%)	E	N (%)	E
Patient Exposed	224 (100)		224 (100)	
Total Adverse Events	107 (48)	237	158 (71)	398
Adverse Events Related to Study Medication	60 (27)	139	109 (49)	231
Body as a Whole				
Headache	26 (12)	32	50 (22)	63
Abdominal Pain			9 (4)	10
Fatigue			7(3)	8
Nervous System				
Dizziness	9 (4)	10	7 (3)	7
Gastrointestinal				
Diarrhea	9 (4)	10		
Nausea	10 (4)	11	17 (8)	18
Dry Mouth			9 (4)	9
Urogenital				
Micturation Frequency			8 (4)	9
Metabolic				
Peripheral Edema			7 (3)	9
Laboratory Changes				
Hyponatraemia	8 (4)	8	14 (6)	15

Legend: N=number of patients with event; %=proportion of patients with event; E=number of events.

Frequency of Adverse Events: Male Study: The most frequently reported adverse events during the dose titration period were headache (12%), followed by diarrhea, nausea, dizziness, and hyponatraemia (all 4%). The adverse event with the highest frequency during the double blind period was headache: 4% (2% of desmopressin treated group and 2% of placebo treated group).

Female Study: The most frequently reported adverse events during the dose titration were headache (22%), followed by nausea (8%), hyponatraemia (6%), abdominal pain, dry mouth, and micturation frequency (all 4%), and fatigue, dizziness and peripheral edema (all 3%). In the double blind period, the most frequent adverse event related to desmopressin was headache which was reported in 10% of desmopressin treated patients and 7% of placebo treated patients.

DRUG INTERACTIONS: Overview: Clofibrate, chlorpropamide and carbamazepine may potentiate the antidiuretic activity of desmopressin while demeclocycline, lithium and norepinephrine may decrease its activity.

Substances which are known to induce Syndrome of Inappropriate Antidiuretic Hormone secretion (SIADH), e.g. tricyclic antidepressants (amitriptyline, nortriptyline), selective serotonin reuptake inhibitor antidepressants (fluoxetine, paroxetine, sertraline, fluvoxamine, citalopram), chlorpromazine and carbamazepine may cause an additive antidiuretic effect leading to an increased risk of water retention/hyponatraemia.

Concomitant use of non-steroidal anti-inflammatory drugs (NSAIDs) such as etodolac, ibuprofen and naproxen, and including COX-2 Inhibitors such as celecoxib may induce water retention/hyponatraemia.

Patients treated with diuretics for fluid retention should not be treated with antidiuretics.

Concomitant treatment with opiates such as loperamide may result in a 3-fold increase of plasma desmopressin concentrations which may lead to water retention and hyponatremia. Although not investigated, other drugs slowing gastrointestinal motility, or disease characterized by impaired gastrointestinal motility (e.g. diabetic gastroparesis), may increase exposure to desmopressin.

Clinically significant inhibition of desmopressin metabolism by other drugs is unlikely. Desmopressin is a peptide analogue of vasopressin and its in vivo inactivation occurs via disulfide reductases, aminopeptidases, and serine proteases, similar to the inactivation of vasopressin. However, the structural modifications to the molecule render desmopressin less susceptible to inactivation by these enzymes compared with vasopressin. Furthermore, in vitro human liver microsome metabolism of desmopressin has shown that no significant amount is metabolized in the liver, and thus human liver metabolism in vivo is not likely to occur. The relative resistance to usual peptide inactivation pathways and the lack of oxidative metabolism are supported by the observation that desmopressin is excreted largely unchanged in the urine. No in vitro inhibition of human Cytochrome P450 enzymes could be demonstrated. Desmopressin did not show any effect on any of the nine Cytochrome P450 subtypes. In vivo drug-drug interactions based on activation or inhibition of Cytochrome P450 are therefore very unlikely.

The precise relationship between increased exposure to desmopressin, prolongation of effect, and the development of hyponatraemia, has not been determined. However, clinical data suggest the approach to treating Nocturia with desmopressin is to initiate therapy at a low dose and titrate upward according to tolerability and response.

Although the pressor activity of desmopressin acetate is very low compared with the anti-diuretic activity, use of large doses of desmopressin with other pressor agents should be done only with careful monitoring.

Drug-Food Interactions: Intake of a standardized meal with oral desmopressin resulted in a significant decrease in bioavailability compared to the fasting condition. This is hypothesized to be due to reduced absorption from the gastrointestinal tract. However no effect on dynamics was observed.

The clinical impact of decreased exposure to desmopressin when administered with a meal, or following a meal, is likely to be inconsequential because pharmacodynamic response to desmopressin is similar in either feeding regimen. Furthermore, the intended bedtime administration of desmopressin is not typically the time of a meal.

Drug-Herb Interactions: There are no known drug-herb interactions. It is unlikely that herbal medicines which may act on the cytochrome P450 system interact with desmopressin, since desmopressin seems not to undergo a significant hepatic metabolism.

Drug-Laboratory Test Interactions: There are no known drug-laboratory interactions.

DOSAGE AND ADMINISTRATION:

Dosing Considerations: The dosage of Minirin tablets (desmopressin acetate) must be determined for each individual patient and adjusted according to response. Response should be measured by reduction of nocturnal voids and an increase mean duration of first undisturbed sleep by two hours.

The initiation of treatment to patients 65 years and older is not recommended due to increased risk of hyponatraemia in this population. [see Warnings and Precautions, Geriatrics (≥65 years of age)].

In the event of signs and symptoms of water retention and hyponatraemia (headache, nausea/vomiting, weight gain, and, in severe cases, convulsions) treatment should be discontinued.

Recommended Dose and Dosage Adjustment: The treatment with Minirin Tablets begins with a 3 week period of titration to establish the optimal dose. In this period, Minirin Tablets are taken orally once daily at bedtime.

The recommended initial dose is 0.1 mg at bedtime. The dose may be titrated up to 0.4 mg to achieve the desired response using the following dosage plan:

In the first week, the patient takes one 0.1 mg tablet daily for seven nights and if necessary increasing in week 2 to one 0.2 mg tablet (0.2) daily for seven nights, and again in week 3 to two 0.2 mg tablets (0.4) daily for seven nights. If the patient obtains zero nocturnal voids during a dose-titration week, this dose is chosen as the optimal dose. If a patient is not achieving zero nocturnal voids on any of the doses, the tolerated dose giving the lowest nocturnal diuresis is selected. After the 3 week period of titration, the patient continues treatment with the established dosage.

The maximum recommended dose is 0.4 mg per day.

Missed Dose: If the patient misses a dose, the patient should be advised not to take the missed dose.

Administration: Restricted fluid intake is recommended a few hours before administration, especially one hour before, and until the next morning (at least 8 hours) after administration. As well, during the evening, the amount of alcohol and caffeine intake should be limited.

OVERDOSAGE:

Overdosage of desmopressin acetate may lead to an increased duration of action. This will increase the risk of fluid retention and symptoms which include headaches, abdominal cramps, nausea, and facial flushing. There is no known antidote. Dosage and frequency of administration should be reduced, or the drug withdrawn, according to severity of the condition.

If hyponatraemia occurs following medication or excessive fluid intake, treatment should be discontinued and fluid intake restricted until serum sodium is normalized. In most cases this is sufficient. In cases with severe symptoms, [e.g., those associated with the central nervous system (CNS) such as unconsciousness], a slow normalization of serum sodium is required to avoid additional complications. Intensive fluid intake regulation may be required in these cases.

Water retention can be controlled by decreasing the dosage of desmopressin; severe water retention caused by overdosage maybe treated with a diuretic such as furosemide.

For management of a suspected drug overdose, CPhA recommends that you contact your **regional Poison Control Centre**. See the *CPS* Directory section for a list of Poison Control Centres.

ACTION AND CLINICAL PHARMACOLOGY: Mechanism of Action: Desmopressin acetate is a synthetic structural analogue of the antidiuretic hormone, arginine vasopressin, which alters the permeability of the renal tubule to increase resorption of water. The increase in the permeability of both the distal tubules and collecting ducts appears to be mediated by a stimulation of the adenylcyclase activity in the renal tubules.

The bioavailability of orally ingested desmopressin has been found to be approximately 0.08%, sufficient to induce antidiuresis (urine osmolality greater than 400 mOsm/kg) lasting 7 to 9 hours in healthy subjects and in patients with diabetes insipidus. Recent clinical studies of the pharmacokinetics and pharmacodynamics of desmopressin showed that desmopressin has longer antidiuretic action than previously reported. Plasma desmopressin concentrations from healthy volunteers were analysed using a new and sensitive bioassay with a low limit of quantification (LLOQ) of 0.8 ng/L. Desmopressin in-vivo potency was found to be 1.64 ng/L based on urine osmolality of 200 mOsm/kg. Given the high variability in absorption, the pharmacological antidiuretic effects of desmopressin can be expected to last from 6 hours up to 14 hours.

Onset of action, as determined by decreased urine volume and increased urine osmolality, is within one hour. Mean maximum plasma concentrations in the range 6.57-16.6 pg/mL (0.2 mg dose) to 31.4-51.6 pg/mL (0.4 mg dose) are reached within 2 hours (t_{max} 0.75-1.9 hours). The oral mean terminal half-life varies between 2.0 and 3.2 hours. Intra- and inter-individual variability of about 30% in absorption of desmopressin is apparent. However, the plasma levels obtained are well above the amount required for a maximal antidiuretic effect, even for a prolonged period.

In both adults and children, there is a log linear relationship between desmopressin acetate doses and maximal urine osmolality and duration of antidiuresis within the dose range 12.5 to 400 µg. Measurements of plasma desmopressin concentrations after peroral desmopressin acetate administration show a linear relationship between amounts of desmopressin acetate absorbed and dose, but with great inter-individual differences.

Pharmacodynamics: Clinical studies have demonstrated that peroral administration of desmopressin acetate is active in eliciting an antidiuretic effect in humans, be they normal subjects, or adults and children suffering from central diabetes insipidus (CDI) of various etiologies, or from nocturnal enuresis. The synthetic analogue exhibits a greater antidiuretic potency, as well as a longer half-life and duration of action, as compared to endogenous antidiuretic hormone.

When administered as a solution (20-200 µg per 50 mL water), desmopressin acetate produced a dose dependent effect both on the magnitude and the duration of the antidiuretic response as determined by measurements of urine osmolality, urine volume and free water clearance. Administration of desmopressin acetate through a duodenal tube caused similar antidiuretic effects, indicating that the intact peptide can be absorbed from the gastrointestinal mucosa. Onset of action was approximately one hour.

Desmopressin acetate does not directly affect urinary sodium or potassium excretion, or serum sodium, potassium, or creatinine concentrations. It does not stimulate uterine contractions, adrenocorticotropic hormone release or increase plasma cortisol concentrations.

Currently available information indicates that although absorption of desmopressin is low after oral administration, sufficient quantities are available to be clinically effective. The only recognized pharmacodynamic actions detected after orally administered desmopressin are reduction in urine flow and increase in urine osmolality. A number of studies have examined dose-, and concentration-effect relationships of desmopressin with respect to its antidiuretic effects. Some studies show clear dose- and concentration-effect relationships, while others do not.

To explore the pharmacology of desmopressin, two Phase II dose ranging studies have been conducted with oral desmopressin tablets. The target populations were women with nocturia and elderly subjects with nocturnal polyuria. The efficacy criteria for both studies included change in nocturnal micturition episodes.

In one of the phase II studies a dose-titration phase was used before randomization to either desmopressin or placebo. The population was considered to likely benefit from desmopressin treatment, i.e. elderly subjects with nocturia with a polyuric component (defined as urine production ≥0.9 mL/min) and without daytime urinary symptoms. The study showed that desmopressin decreased nocturnal diuresis as well as the frequency of nocturnal voidings in patients included in the study, in a statistically significant manner compared with placebo treatment (see Table 3 and Table 4). A decrease in diuresis compared with baseline could be seen at the 0.1 mg dose. Most patients (10 of 17) experienced the best effect on diuresis at 0.2 mg, while 0.4 mg provided the best reduction in only three patients. There was no significant difference between treatments in 24 h diuresis (see Table 5).

Table 3: Minirin

Nocturnal Diuresis Measured After 2 Weeks of Treatment

	Mean		Mean Difference[a]	p-values from ANOVA		
Population	**Desmopressin**	**Placebo**	**(95% CI)**	**Treatment**	**Sequence**	**Period**
APT	1 mL/min	1.6 mL/min	−0.59 (−0.85 to −0.33)	0.0002[b]	0.5463	0.5862
PP	0.9 mL/min	1.4 mL/min	−0.48 (−0.76 to −0.19)	0.0033[b]	0.6314	0.6719

[a] Least square means from ANOVA.
[b] Statistically significant effect (p<0.05).
Legend: PP=per protocol; APT=all patients treated.

Table 4: Minirin

Number of Nocturnal Voids During Second Week of Treatment

Population	Mean Desmopressin	Mean Placebo	Mean Difference[a] (95% CI)	p-values from ANOVA Treatment	Sequence	Period
APT	1.1	1.7	−0.59 (−0.85 to −0.32)	0.0003[b]	0.8219	0.921
PP	0.9	1.5	−0.54 (−0.84 to −0.24)	0.0022[b]	0.4612	0.8974

[a] Least square means from the ANOVA.
[b] Statistically significant effect (p<0.05).
Legend: PP=per protocol; APT=all patients treated.

Secondary to the decrease in nocturnal micturition episodes, the maximum duration of sleep between nocturnal voidings was significantly longer for desmopressin compared with placebo (5.4 h versus 4.0 h; mean difference 1.31 (95% CI 0.7-1.9) (see Table 5).

Table 5: Minirin

24 h Diuresis Measured After 2 Weeks of Treatment

Population	Mean Desmopressin	Mean Placebo	Mean Difference[a] (95% CI)	p-values from ANOVA Treatment	Sequence	Period
APT	1.3 mL/min	1.4 mL/min	−0.12 (−0.33 to 0.09)	0.2220	0.4144	0.3869
PP	1.2 mL/min	1.2 mL/min	−0.11 (−0.34 to 0.13)	0.7977	0.8431	0.5839

[a] Least square means from the ANOVA.
Legend: PP=per protocol; APT=all patients treated.

A third Phase II study was an exploratory epidemiological survey of nocturia in three parts, during which subjects with Nocturia aged 65 years and over were treated with 0.2 mg oral desmopressin.

The aim was to mimic clinical practice, namely, treatment of elderly subjects with nocturia on an unselected basis.

Part A: A questionnaire was sent to all inhabitants aged 65 years in a defined area (Tierp) in Sweden. A response was obtained from 2866 subjects.

Part B: A frequency B volume chart was sent to all consenting nocturics and non-nocturics from part A; a response was obtained from 159 nocturics and 131 non-nocturics.

Part C: A short therapeutic trial where all patients received 0.2 mg desmopressin for three consecutive nights; 72 subjects were included.

One hundred percent of the nocturic subjects (nocturia defined as ≥2 voids/night) had a nocturia index >1, i.e. a urine production exceeding bladder capacity. The need to void at night could be explained, at least partly, by a polyuric component to their condition. When treated with desmopressin, 78% of subjects showed a response in terms of decreased nocturnal urine production (≥20% decrease from baseline). The mean number of nocturnal voids was 1.6 during treatment compared to 2.6 at baseline and the mean change in nocturnal urine output was 286 mL (95% CI 336 to 237 mL). The mean time from bedtime to the first void increased from 2.8 hours at baseline to 4.6 hours during treatment.

Pharmacokinetics: Human pharmacokinetic studies have been conducted on desmopressin using the oral and intravenous formulations. Three studies enrolled healthy volunteers. Two additional studies were conducted in elderly male subjects, considered to represent an element of the population for Nocturia. The studies are summarized below (see Table 6). The pharmacokinetic profile of oral desmopressin is summarized in Table 7.

Absorption: Orally administered desmopressin is poorly absorbed (see Table 7). The oral mean terminal half-life varies between 2.0 and 3.2 hours. Intra- and inter-individual variability of about 30% in absorption of desmopressin is apparent, probably due to the low absorption after oral administration. However, the plasma levels obtained are well above the amount required for a maximal antidiuretic effect even for a prolonged period.

Table 7: Minirin

Pharmacokinetic Profile of Oral Desmopressin

Parameter	0.2 mg dose	0.4 mg dose
Average absolute bioavailability (%)	0.08	0.16
C_{max} range (pg/mL)	6.57–16.6	31.4–51.6
T_{max} range (h)	0.75–1.9	

Food Effects

Parameter	Desmopressin acetate 400 µg po Estimate	CV%	Desmopressin acetate and concomitant meal Estimate	CV%
AUC_{inf} (pg·h/mL)	80.0 (68.6–93.1)	49	45.2 (38.8–52.6)	22
AUC_{last} (pg·h/mL)	63.1 (53.5–74.6)	51	33.1 (28.0–39.1)	26
C_{max} (pg/mL)	24.8 (19.9–31.0)	67	11.8 (9.5–11.8)	28
$T_{½}$ (h)	2.3 (2.1–2.5)	21	2.4 (2.2–2.7)	21
T_{max} (h)	1.0 (0.05–3.0)	52	1.5 (0.8–2.5)	38

Intake of a standardized meal with oral desmopressin resulted in a significant decrease in bioavailability compared to the fasting condition (see Table 7). The pharmacodynamic action of desmopressin appears to be unaffected by food as assessed by urine volume and urine osmolality for at least 4 hours post-dose. The degree of antidiuresis was similar in the absence of food and when the drug was taken with or 1.5 hours after food.

After daytime administration of desmopressin, the mean urine volume gradually decreased from about 130 mL/h to a level of approximately 70 mL/h during the first collection period (see Figure 1). A minimum level of approximately 50 mL/h was achieved during the second collection period. During the subsequent collection periods the urine production returned to pre-dose levels. When desmopressin was given perorally in the evening, the mean urine production decreased from about 115 mL/h to approximately 50 mL/h during the night (see Figure 2). There was a slight increase in the morning values to a level of about 60 mL/h.

Urine osmolality increased after daytime administration from a mean value of about 610 mOsm/L to a maximum level of 780 mOsm/L, which was achieved during the second collection period. During the subsequent collection periods the urine osmolality decreased to below pre-dose levels. During the night, urine osmolality increased from a mean per-dose value of 540 mOsm/L to about 700 mOsm/L during the night. This osmolality level was also seen in the urine produced the subsequent morning.

In a recently conducted study, healthy subjects were water loaded to suppress endogenous vasopressin levels. The aim of the study was to investigate the antidiuretic effectiveness of five low doses of desmopressin and placebo. Due to wide inter- and intra-individual variations seen with the oral route, an intravenous infusion study was designed to minimize the variations. The study provided information about the pharmacokinetic and pharmacodynamic (PK/PD) relationship of low doses of desmopressin levels and their duration of antidiuretic action. Combining this new insight into the correlation between plasma desmopressin levels and antidiuretic effects of desmopressin with plasma concentration-time profiles after oral administration of desmopressin, showed that desmopressin is a potent compound with EC_{50} value of 1.6 pg/mL.

Thus desmopressin can be expected to have a continued effect even at a very low plasma level of 1 pg/mL. After oral administration, an effect lasting from 6 to 14 hours can be expected.

Table 6: Minirin

Summary of Pharmacokinetic Data

Duration	Dose/Dosage form	Exposure	T_{max} (h)	C_{max} (pg/mL)	AUC (pg·h/mL)	t ½ (h)	t ½ λ2 (h)	Vss (L)	Cl (L/h)
Desmopressin was administered both orally and intravenously, both during the day and in the night, yielding 4 different sessions:	0.2 mg tablet per oral desmopressin	night p.o. day p.o.	1.9 1.4	6.21 6.57	22.9 21.3				
Day p.o. Day i.v. Night p.o. Night i.v. During each session, volunteers were hospitalized for 12 hours. Between each session, there was a washout period of at least 2 days. All four sessions were performed within one month.	2 g i.v. desmopressin	night i.v. day i.v.	— —	18.1 20.4	2.84 2.69	0.25 0.22	3.09 2.77	25.7 24.2	6.6 7.2
3 single doses with at least 7 days washout between doses.	2×0.2 mg tablet	Period 1 2 3	 1.0 — 1.0	 27.6 29.8 34.4	 79.6 90.3 99.5	 0.34 0.34 0.35	 B	 —	 —
Erythromycin—4 times daily (7, 13 and 18 and at bed time) with the first dose in the morning 3 days before the study day and the last one 1 hour before intake of desmopressin. Loperamide at 24, 12 and 1 hour before intake of desmopressin	2×0.2 mg tablet	A B C	1.3 2.0 0.9	25.4 58.4 19.2	90.4[a] 280.0[a] 70.4[a] 75.6[b] 239.0[b] 58.7[b]	2.4 2.5 2.4	0.3 H 0.2 H 0.2 H	 —	
A single oral dose of 0.4 mg (2 tablets of 0.2 mg) will be used at PK day 2. Oral dose of 0.4 mg (2 tablets at 0.2 mg each) at bedtime during the placebo controlled effect evaluation period of 2×3 days.	0.4 mg (2×0.2 mg) tablet	N/A	—	15.91	76.62[c] 61.24[d]	—	3.11	 —	—
Single Dose	0.4 mg (2×0.2 mg) tablet	with food 1.5 h after food without food	1.5 1.5 1.0	11.8 13.4 24.8	45.2 47.5 80.0	2.4 2.1 2.3	0.5 I 0.5 I 0.25	— —	— —

[a] AUC (pg·h/mL).
[b] AUCt (pg·h/mL).
[c] AUC_{inf}.
[d] AUC_{o-t}.
Legend: A=desmopressin alone; B=loperamide/desmopressin; C=erythromycin/desmopressin; H=these T values refer to T lag; I= t_{lag} (h); $t_{½}λ_2$; (h)=terminal half-life.

Figure 1: Minirin

Mean (±SD) Day-time Diuresis in Each Collection Period (Time) Before and After Day Administration (Desmopressin Given at 11.00 h)

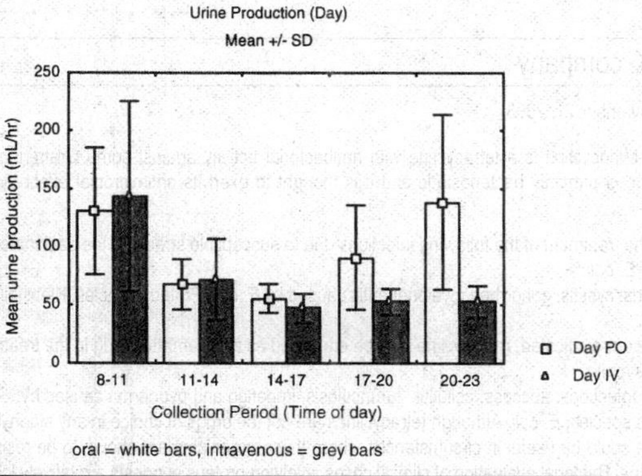

Figure 2: Minirin

Mean (±SD) Night-time Diuresis in Each Collection Period (Time) Before and After Day Administration (Desmopressin Given at 22.00 h)

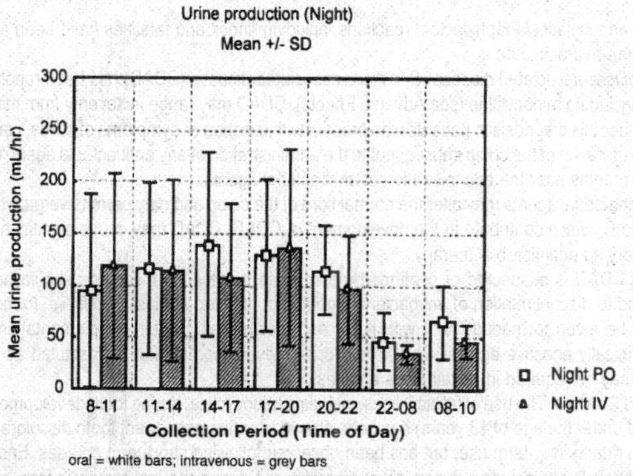

Seventy two over-hydrated non smoking male subjects participated in a phase I study investigating the antidiuretic effect and pharmacokinetics of 30, 60, 125, 250 and 500 ng desmopressin and placebo infused intravenously at a constant rate for two hours. A clear positive dose-response slope was seen between duration of antidiuretic action (primary endpoint) and dose of desmopressin (placebo included as zero), independent of the cut-off level (either 200 mOsm/kg or 400 mOsm/kg. No placebo response was seen, and very limited response was seen with 30 ng desmopressin. An increase in duration of antidiuretic action (DOA) with increasing dose of desmopressin was statistically significant for most pair-wise comparisons. In the 250 ng and 500 ng desmopressin groups the median DOA was 5.36 hours (range: 0.75-10.64 hours) and 8.00 hours (range: 4.45-11.66 hours), respectively, when using 200 mOsm/kg as cut-off, while it was 3.94 hours (range: 0-7.56 hours) and 6.27 hours (range: 4.35-8.28 hours), respectively, when using 400 mOsm/kg as cut-off. The dose-response curve for the DOA did not flatten out within the dose range of 0-500 ng desmopressin for either cut-off (200 or 400 mOsm/kg), i.e. the plateau of the curve was not observed. This indicates that further increase in dosage (>500 ng) may increase duration of antidiuretic action. Linear relationship between DOA and log (dose) among the dose range of 30-500 ng desmopressin was observed with the statistically significant slope, independent of cut-off level (either 200mOsm/kg or 400mOsm/kg). No serious adverse events were seen with any of the desmopressin doses administered.

The analysis of other pharmacodynamic endpoints (maximum osmolality, AUC 0-6 hour for osmolality, AUC 0-6 hour for absolute change from dosing in osmolality) showed a clear positive dose-response relationship. The median maximum osmolality in the placebo group was 80 mOsm/kg (range: 55-183 mOsm/kg), while desmopressin was 830 mOsm/kg (range: 762-1052 mOsm/kg) in the 500 ng desmopressin group.

Twenty-eight non-smoking healthy (n=14 male and n=14 female) subjects took part in a single-centre, open-labelled, randomised, study investigating the antidiuretic effect and pharmacokinetics of two doses of the currently marketed desmopressin tablet (2×200 μg). Blood samples for plasma concentrations of desmopressin were collected according to the following schedule: pre-dose (i.e. 0-30 minutes pre-dosing), 15, 30 min 1, 1.5, 2, 3, 4, 6, 8, 9, 10, 11, 12, 13 and 14 hours after dosing. The concentration of desmopressin in plasma was determined by a validated RIA method. The lower limit of quantification (LLOQ) of the assay was 0.8 pg/mL. After administration of DDAVP tablets, the geometric mean t_{max} was observed at 1.0 hour after dosing, the geometric mean value for C_{max} was 20.8 (CV =60%) pg/mL, the geometric mean value for AUC_t was 71.8 (CV=57%) (hr·pg/mL), and the geometric value for AUC was 77.2 (CV=55%) (hr·pg/mL).

Sixty four percent (64%) of the subjects had plasma desmopressin concentration above 1 pg/mL at 12 hours post dose. No safety concerns were observed.

Distribution: The distribution of desmopressin has not been fully characterized. It is not known if desmopressin crosses the placenta. The drug may be distributed into milk. The metabolic fate of desmopressin is unknown. Unlike vasopressin, desmopressin apparently is not degraded by aminopeptidases or other peptidases that cleave oxytocin and endogenous vasopressin in the plasma during pregnancy.

Metabolism: In vitro human liver microsome metabolism of desmopressin has shown that no significant amount is metabolised in the liver, and thus human liver metabolism in vivo is not likely to occur. Furthermore, no in vitro inhibition of human Cytochrome P450 enzymes could be demonstrated. Desmopressin did not show any effect on any of the nine Cytochrome P450 subtypes. In vivo drug-drug interactions based on activation or inhibition of Cytochrome P450 are therefore very unlikely.

Excretion: Urinary clearance in 6 hydrated volunteers was calculated to be 0.514 mL/min/kg body weight and the amount of peptide excreted in the urine during the 6-hour observation period constituted 16.4% of the amount absorbed from the intestine over the same period of time. Urinary clearance for desmopressin is thus smaller than reported for vasopressin.

Special Populations and Conditions: The pharmacokinetics of desmopressin acetate in the nocturia population do not differ from those in healthy subjects. A pooled data analysis demonstrated no significant correlation between age and pharmacokinetics, and no gender-related difference in AUC_{inf} could be found. In very elderly patients, a decrease in the renal elimination of desmopressin could be expected. The results of a small pharmacokinetics study (n=8) indicated that in patients on chronic haemodialysis because of end stage renal failure, total clearance of desmopressin administered intravenously was lower and the half-life was longer compared with values previously observed in normal subjects.

STORAGE AND STABILITY: Store between 15 and 25°C in a dry place. Keep the container tightly closed. Keep in a safe place out of reach of children and pets.

SPECIAL HANDLING INSTRUCTIONS: No special requirement.

INFORMATION FOR THE PATIENT: Published in e-CPS, available by subscription at www.e-cps.ca.

DOSAGE FORMS, COMPOSITION AND PACKAGING: Each white, oval, uncoated tablet, marked with "0.1" on one side contains: desmopressin acetate 0.1 mg. Nonmedicinal ingredients: lactose monohydrate, magnesium stearate, potato starch and povidone. Bottles of 100.

Minitran™

nitroglycerin

Antianginal

Graceway

PHARMACOLOGY: The principal pharmacological action of nitroglycerin is relaxation of vascular smooth muscle and consequent dilation of both peripheral arteries and veins, with more prominent effects on the latter. Dilation of the postcapillary vessels, including large veins, promotes peripheral pooling of blood and decreases venous return to the heart, thereby reducing left ventricular end-diastolic pressure (preload). Arteriolar relaxation reduces systemic vascular resistance and arterial pressure (afterload). Dilation of the coronary arteries also occurs. The relative importance of preload reduction, afterload reduction, and coronary dilation remains undefined.

When Minitran is applied to the skin, nitroglycerin is absorbed continuously through the skin into the systemic circulation. Thus, the active drug reaches target sites before inactivation by the liver. Nitroglycerin is rapidly metabolized, principally by a liver reductase, to form glycerol nitrate metabolites and inorganic nitrate. Two active major metabolites, 1,2- and 1,3-dinitroglycerols, the products of hydrolysis, appear to be less potent than nitroglycerin as vasodilators but have longer plasma half-lives. The dinitrates are further metabolized to mononitrates (biologically inactive with respect to cardiovascular effects) and ultimately to glycerol and carbon dioxide. There is extensive first-pass deactivation by the liver following gastrointestinal absorption.

In healthy volunteers, steady-state plasma concentrations of nitroglycerin were reached within 2 hours after application of the patch and were maintained at the same level for the duration of the study (24 hours). Upon removal of the patch, plasma concentrations decline rapidly.

Dosing regimens for most chronically used drugs are designed to provide plasma concentrations that are continuously greater than a minimally effective concentration. This strategy is probably inappropriate for organic nitrates. Some controlled clinical trials using exercise tolerance testing have shown maintenance of effectiveness when patches are worn continuously. The large majority of such controlled trials, however, has shown the development of tolerance (i.e., complete loss of effect as measured by exercise testing) within the first day. Tolerance has occurred even when doses greater than 4 mg/h were delivered continuously. This dose is far in excess of the effective dose of 0.2 to 0.8 mg/h delivered intermittently.

Efficacy of organic nitrates is restored after a period of absence of nitrates from the body. Drug-free intervals of 10 to 12 hours are known to be sufficient to restore response. Several studies have demonstrated that when nitroglycerin is administered according to an intermittent regimen, doses of nitroglycerin 0.4 to 0.8 mg/h (20 to 40 cm²) have increased exercise capacity for up to 8 hours, with a trend of increased exercise capacity to 12 hours.

The results of one controlled clinical trial suggests that the intermittent use of nitrates may be associated with decreased exercise tolerance during the last part of the nitrate-free interval, in comparison to placebo. The clinical relevance of this observation is unknown.

In another clinical trial, there was an increase in nocturnal angina attacks during the drug-free period in some patients treated with nitroglycerin as compared to placebo; therefore, the possibility of increased frequency of severity of angina during the nitrate-free interval should be considered. However, in one controlled clinical study involving 291 patients with angina, involving exercise tolerance testing at 4 hours duration post-dosing, Minitran did not demonstrate any significant evidence of vascular tolerance or rebound angina attacks during long-term intermittent treatment.

INDICATIONS: Used intermittently (see Pharmacology) for the prevention of anginal attacks in patients with stable angina pectoris associated with coronary artery disease. It can be used in conjunction with other antianginal agents such as beta-blockers and/or calcium antagonists.

Minitran is not intended for the immediate relief of acute attacks of angina pectoris. Sublingual nitroglycerin preparations should be used for this purpose.

CONTRAINDICATIONS: Known hypersensitivity to nitroglycerin or other nitrates or nitrites. Known or suspected hypersensitivity to components of the patch. Acute circulatory failure associated with marked hypotension (shock and states of collapse). Concomitant use of Minitran, either regularly and/or intermittently, with sildenafil citrate is absolutely contraindicated. Postural hypotension; Myocardial insufficiency due to obstruction (e.g., in the presence of aortic or mitral stenosis or constrictive pericarditis); Increased intracranial pressure; Increased intraocular pressure; Severe anemia.

WARNINGS: The benefits and safety of transdermal nitroglycerin in patients with acute myocardial infarction or congestive heart failure have not been established. If one elects to use Minitran in these conditions, careful clinical or hemodynamic monitoring must be used to avoid the hazards of hypotension and tachycardia.

Minitran must be removed before cardioversion or DC defibrillation is attempted, as well as before applying diathermy treatment, since it may be associated with damage to the paddles and burns to the patient.

PRECAUTIONS: Headaches or symptoms of hypotension, such as weakness or dizziness, particularly when arising suddenly from a recumbent position, may occur. A reduction in dose or discontinuation of treatment may be necessary.

Caution should be exercised when using nitroglycerin in patients prone to, or who might be affected by hypotension. The drug therefore should be used with caution in patients who may have volume depletion from diuretic therapy or in patients who have low systolic blood pressure (e.g., below 90 mm Hg). Paradoxical bradycardia and increased angina pectoris may accompany nitroglycerin-induced hypotension.

Nitrate therapy may aggravate the angina caused by hypertrophic cardiomyopathy.

In industrial workers who have had long-term exposure to unknown (presumably high) doses of nitroglycerin, tolerance clearly occurs. There is moreover, physical dependence since chest pain, acute myocardial infarction, and even sudden death have occurred during temporary withdrawal of nitroglycerin from these workers. In clinical trials of angina patients, there are reports of anginal attacks being more easily provoked and of rebound in the hemodynamic effects soon after nitrate withdrawal. The importance of these observations to the routine clinical use of nitroglycerin has not been fully elucidated, but patients should be monitored closely for increased anginal symptoms during drug-free periods.

Caution should be exercised in patients with arterial hypoxemia due to anemia (see Contraindications), because in such patients the biotransformation of nitroglycerin is reduced. Similarly, caution is called for in patients with hypoxemia and a ventilation/perfusion imbalance due to lung disease or ischemic heart failure. Patients with angina pectoris, myocardial infarction, or cerebral ischemia frequently suffer from abnormalities of the small airways (especially alveolar hypoxia). Under these circumstances vasoconstriction occurs within the lung to shift perfusion from areas of alveolar hypoxia to better ventilated regions of the lung. As a potent vasodilator, nitroglycerin could reverse this protective vasoconstriction and thus result in increased perfusion to poorly ventilated areas, worsening of the ventilation/perfusion imbalance, and a further decrease in the arterial partial pressure of oxygen.

Tolerance to nitroglycerin with cross tolerance to other nitrates of nitrites may occur (see Pharmacology). Coadministration of other long-acting nitrates could jeopardize the integrity of the nitrate-free interval and therefore must be avoided. As tolerance to nitroglycerin patches develops, the effect of sublingual nitroglycerin on exercise tolerance, although still observable, is somewhat blunted.

Occupational Hazards: As patients may experience faintness and/or dizziness, reaction time when driving or operating machinery may be impaired, especially at the start of treatment.

Pregnancy: It is not known whether nitroglycerin can cause fetal harm when administered to pregnant women or if it can affect reproductive capacity. Therefore, use only if the potential benefit justifies the risk to the fetus.

Lactation: It is not known whether nitroglycerin is excreted in human milk. Benefits to the mother must be weighed against the risk to the infant.

Children: Safety and effectiveness of use in children have not been established.

Drug Interactions: Concomitant treatment with other vasodilators, calcium channel blockers, ACE inhibitors, beta-blockers, diuretics, antihypertensives, tricyclic antidepressants and major tranquilizers may potentiate the blood pressure lowering effect of Minitran. Dose adjustment may be necessary.

Concomitant use of Minitran and sildenafil citrate can potentiate the hypotensive effect of Minitran. This could result in life-threatening hypotension with syncope or myocardial infarction and death. Therefore, sildenafil citrate should not be given to patients receiving Minitran therapy.

Alcohol may enhance sensitivity to the hypotensive effects of nitrates.

Marked symptomatic orthostatic hypotension has been reported when calcium channel blockers and organic nitrates were used in combination. Dosage adjustments of either class of agents may be necessary.

Concurrent administration of Minitran with dihydroergotamine may increase the bioavailability of dihydroergotamine. Special attention should be paid to this point in patients with coronary artery disease, because dihydroergotamine antagonizes the effect of nitroglycerin and may lead to coronary vasoconstriction.

The possibility that the ingestion of ASA and NSAIDs might diminish the therapeutic response to nitrates and nitroglycerin cannot be excluded.

Information to Be Provided to the Patient: Daily headaches sometimes accompany treatment with nitroglycerin. In patients who get these headaches, the headaches may be a marker of the activity of the drug. Patients should resist the temptation to avoid headaches by altering the schedule of their treatment with nitroglycerin, since loss of headache may be associated with simultaneous loss of antianginal efficacy.

Treatment with nitroglycerin may be associated with lightheadedness on standing, especially just after rising from a recumbent or seated position. This effect may be more frequent in patients who have also consumed alcohol.

After normal use, there is enough residual nitroglycerin in discarded patches that they are a potential hazard to children and pets.

A patient leaflet is supplied with the patches (see Information for the Patient).

ADVERSE EFFECTS: Headache, which may be severe, is the most commonly reported side effect. Headache may be recurrent with each daily dose, especially at high doses of nitroglycerin. Headaches may be treated with concomitant administration of mild analgesics. If such headaches are unresponsive to treatment, the nitroglycerin dosage should be reduced or the product discontinued. Transient episodes of lightheadedness, occasionally related to blood pressure changes, may also occur. Hypotension occurs infrequently, but in some patients it may be severe enough to warrant discontinuation of therapy.

Reddening of the skin, with or without a mild local itching or burning sensation, as well as allergic contact dermatitis may occasionally occur. Upon removal of the patch, any slight reddening of the skin will usually disappear within a few hours. The application site should be changed regularly to prevent local irritation.

Less frequently reported adverse reactions include dizziness, faintness, facial flushing and postural hypotension which may be associated with reflex tachycardia. Syncope, crescendo angina and rebound hypertension have been reported but are uncommon. Nausea and vomiting have been reported rarely.

OVERDOSE:

Symptoms: Nitroglycerin overdose may result in severe hypotension, persistent throbbing headache, vertigo, palpitations, visual disturbances, flushing, and perspiring skin (later becoming cold and cyanotic), nausea and vomiting (possibly with colic and even bloody diarrhea), syncope (especially in the upright posture), methemoglobinemia with cyanosis, initial hyperpnea, dyspnea, and slow breathing, slow pulse (dicrotic and intermittent), heart block, and bradycardia, increased intracranial pressure with cerebral symptoms of fever, confusion and coma possibly followed by paralysis, clonic convulsions and death due to circulatory collapse.

Treatment: Keep the patient recumbent in a shock position and comfortably warm. Remove all nitroglycerin patches. Passive movement of the extremities may aid venous return. Administer oxygen and artificially ventilate if necessary. Epinephrine is ineffective in reversing the severe hypotensive events associated with overdose; it and related compounds are contraindicated in this situation.

I.V. infusion of normal saline or similar fluid may also be required to produce sufficient central volume expansion. However, in patients with renal disease or congestive heart failure, therapy resulting in central volume expansion is not without hazard. Treatment of nitroglycerin overdose in these patients may be subtle and difficult, and invasive monitoring may be required.

Methemoglobinemia:

Case reports of clinically significant methemoglobinemia are rare at conventional doses of nitroglycerin. The formation of methemoglobin is dose-related, and in the case of genetic abnormalities of hemoglobin that favor methemoglobin formation, even conventional doses of organic nitrates can produce harmful concentrations of methemoglobin. Methemoglobin levels are available from most clinical laboratories. The diagnosis should be suspected in patients who exhibit signs of impaired oxygen delivery despite adequate cardiac output and adequate arterial pO_2.

Classically, methemoglobinemic blood is described as chocolate brown, without color change on exposure to air. If methemoglobinemia is present, i.v. administration of 1 to 2 mg/kg methylene blue 1% solution for injection may be required.

For management of a suspected drug overdose, CPhA recommends that you contact your **regional Poison Control Centre**. See the *CPS* Directory section for a list of Poison Control Centres.

DOSAGE: Daily Dosage Schedule: The daily dosage schedule is based on intermittent therapy to prevent the development of tolerance to nitroglycerin. The optimal dose should be selected based upon the clinical response, side effects and the effects of therapy on blood pressure.

The suggested starting dose is between 0.2 and 0.4 mg/h. Doses between 0.2 and 0.8 mg/h have shown continued effectiveness for 12 hours daily for at least 1 month (the longest period of studies) of intermittent administration. Although the minimum nitrate-free interval has not been defined, data show that a nitrate-free interval of 10 to 12 hours is sufficient (see Pharmacology). Thus, an appropriate dosing schedule for nitroglycerin patches would include a daily patch-on period of 12 to 14 hours during waking hours and a patch-off period of 10 to 12 hours, usually overnight.

Prevention of Tolerance: Although some controlled clinical trials using exercise tolerance testing have shown maintenance of effectiveness when patches are worn continuously, the large majority of such controlled trials have shown the development of tolerance (i.e., complete loss of effect) within the first 24 hours after therapy was initiated. Dose adjustments, even to levels much higher than generally used, did not prevent the development of tolerance.

Tolerance can be prevented or attenuated by use of an intermittent dosage schedule. Although the minimum nitrate-free interval has not been defined, clinical trials have demonstrated that an appropriate dosing schedule for nitroglycerin patches would provide for a daily patch-on period of 12 to 14 hours and a daily patch-off period of 10 to 12 hours. The patch-free time should coincide with the period in which angina pectoris is least likely to occur (usually at night). Patients should be watched carefully for an increase of angina pectoris during the patch-free period. Adjustment of background medication may be required.

The dose of Minitran should be periodically reviewed in relation to continuing antianginal control.

Site of Application: Minitran should be applied to the chest, shoulders, upper arm or back and should not be applied to the distal extremities. The skin area should be free of hair in order to provide direct contact of the patch to the skin. If hair is likely to interfere with adhesion of the patch, the area may be lightly shaved. The skin area should be clean, dry and free of irritation or cuts. A different skin site should be used each time a new Minitran patch is applied. It may be necessary to apply more than 1 patch in order to achieve the optimal dose level. Following use, the patch should be discarded in a manner that prevents accidental application or ingestion by curious children or others.

INFORMATION FOR THE PATIENT: Published in e-CPS, available by subscription at www.e-cps.ca.

SUPPLIED: The Minitran transdermal delivery system is a unit designed to provide continuous controlled release of nitroglycerin through intact skin. The rate of release of nitroglycerin is linearly dependent upon the area of the applied system; each cm^2 of applied system delivers approximately 0.03 mg of nitroglycerin per hour. Thus, the 6.7, 13.3, and 20 cm^2 systems deliver approximately 0.2, 0.4, and 0.6 mg of nitroglycerin per hour, respectively (see Table 1).

The remainder of the nitroglycerin in each system serves as a reservoir and is not delivered in normal use. After 12 hours, for example, each system has delivered about 14% of its original content of nitroglycerin.

The Minitran transdermal delivery system contains nitroglycerin in a hypoallergenic, medical grade, acrylate-based polymer adhesive. Each patch is packaged in foil/polymer film laminate. Cartons of 30 and 100.

Store at controlled room temperature 15 to 30°C. Extremes of temperature and/or humidity should be avoided.

Table 1: Minitran

Minitran Systems

Related Release in vivo (mg/h)	System Size (cm^2)	Nitroglycerin in System (mg)
0.2	6.7	18
0.4	13.3	36
0.6	20.0	54

Can't find information on a particular drug? Consult the CPhA Monograph Index in the front pages of the *CPS*. The CPhA monographs are compiled by the editorial staff of the Canadian Pharmacists Association and reviewed by expert Canadian physicians and pharmacists.

Minocin® Ⓟ

minocycline HCl

Antibiotic

Stiefel, a GSK company

Date of Revision: November 21, 2008

PHARMACOLOGY: Minocycline is a tetracycline with antibacterial activity against some Gram-negative and Gram-positive organisms. The action is primarily bacteriostatic and it is thought to exert its antimicrobial effect by the inhibition of protein synthesis.

INDICATIONS: For the treatment of the following infections due to susceptible strains of the designated organisms: gallbladder infections caused by *E. coli*.

Urinary Tract Infections: cystitis, gonorrhea, pyelonephritis caused by *E. coli*, Proteus species, Klebsiella species, *E. aerogenes*, *N. gonorrhea*.

When penicillin is contraindicated, minocycline may be employed as an alternative drug in the treatment of anal and pharyngeal gonorrhea and syphilis.

Skin and Soft Tissue Infections: abscess, cellulitis, furunculosis, impetigo and pyoderma caused by: *S. epidermidis*, *S. aureus*, *S. pyogenes*, Proteus species, *E. coli*. Although tetracyclines are not the drugs of choice in any staphylococcal or streptococcal infection, minocycline could be useful in circumstances where these organisms are shown to be resistant to other agents but sensitive to minocycline. Bacterial evaluation of clinical cases involving proteus suggests a relatively lower success rate may be expected where these organisms are concerned.

Respiratory Tract Infections: Bronchitis, pharyngitis, pneumonia, bronchopneumonia, sinusitis and tonsillitis caused by: *H. influenzae*, Klebsiella species, Enterobacter species. Tetracyclines should not be prescribed for acute throat infections.

CONTRAINDICATIONS: History of hypersensitivity to minocycline or any other tetracycline.

WARNINGS: Rarely, anaphylactic/anaphylactoid reactions including shock and fatalities have been associated with the administration of minocycline hydrochloride.

Gastrointestinal: *C. difficile*-associated disease: *C. difficile*-associated disease (CDAD) has been reported with the use of many antibacterial agents, including minocycline (see Adverse Effects). CDAD may range in severity from mild diarrhea to fatal colitis. It is important to consider this diagnosis in patients who present with diarrhea or symptoms of colitis, pseudomembranous colitis, toxic megacolon, or perforation of the colon subsequent to the administration of any antibacterial agent. CDAD has been reported to occur more than 2 months after the administration of antibacterial agents.

Treatment with antibacterial agents may alter the normal flora of the colon and may permit overgrowth of *C. difficile*. *C. difficile* produces toxins A and B, which contribute to the development of CDAD. CDAD may cause significant morbidity and mortality. CDAD can be refractory, to antimicrobial therapy.

If the diagnosis of CDAD is suspected or confirmed, appropriate therapeutic measures should be initiated. Mild cases of CDAD usually respond to discontinuation of antibacterial agents not directed against *C. difficile*. In moderate to severe cases, consideration should be given to management with fluids and electrolytes, protein supplementation, and treatment with an antibacterial agent clinically effective against *C. difficile*. Surgical evaluation should be instituted as clinically indicated since surgical intervention may be required in certain severe cases.

Newborns, Infants and Children: The use of tetracyclines, including minocycline, during tooth development (last half of pregnancy, infancy and childhood under the age of 13 years) has been shown to cause permanent tooth discoloration (yellow-grey-brown). This is more common during long-term use, but has been observed following short-term courses. Enamel hypoplasia has also been reported. All tetracyclines, including minocycline, administered during the last trimester form a stable calcium complex throughout the human fetal skeleton. A decrease in the fibula growth rate has been observed in premature human infants given oral tetracycline in doses of 25 mg/kg every 6 hours. This appeared to be reversible when the drug was discontinued. Minocycline should not be used in such patients unless other drugs are ineffective or are contraindicated.

Congenital anomalies including limb reductions have been reported in post-marketing experience.

Pregnancy: Tetracyclines, including minocycline, are not recommended during pregnancy and lactation because of possible adverse effects on developing bones and teeth of the fetus and neonate. Results of animal studies indicate that tetracyclines cross the placenta, are found in fetal tissues and can have toxic effects on the developing fetus (often related to retardation of skeletal development). If minocycline hydrochloride is used during pregnancy or if the patient becomes pregnant while taking this drug, the patient should be apprised of the potential hazard to the fetus.

Evidence of embryotoxicity has also been noted in animals treated early in pregnancy. The safety of minocycline for use during pregnancy has not been established.

Tetracyclines, including minocycline, are excreted in the milk of lactating women; therefore, a decision should be made whether to discontinue breast-feeding or to discontinue minocycline.

Lactation: See Pregnancy.

It is advisable to avoid giving minocycline in conjunction with penicillin since some bacteriostatic drugs may interfere with the bactericidal action of penicillin.

Minocycline should not be used for the treatment of streptococcal diseases unless the organism is demonstrated to be sensitive, since most streptococci have been found to be resistant to tetracycline drugs. If it is deemed necessary that infection due to Group A beta-hemolytic streptococci be treated with minocycline, then such treatment should be continued for at least 10 days.

In the presence of significant renal impairment, usual oral doses may lead to excessive systemic accumulations of minocycline and possible liver toxicity. Under such conditions, lower than usual doses may be indicated. After initial therapy, and if therapy is prolonged, serum level determinations of the drug are advisable.

The anti-anabolic action of tetracyclines can also produce dose-related increases in BUN; consequently, in patients with significant renal impairment, elevated serum minocycline levels can lead to azotemia, hypophosphatemia and acidosis.

Renal failure, including interstitial nephritis has been reported rarely.

Minocycline is capable of aggravating the symptoms associated with lupus erythematosus. Therefore, caution should be taken when administering the drug to patients with this disease.

Minocycline has been shown to depress plasma prothrombin activity. Therefore, patients who are on anticoagulant therapy should be monitored regularly and may require downward adjustment of their anticoagulant dosage. Interference with vitamin K synthesis by microorganisms in the gut has been reported.

Cross-sensitization among the various tetracyclines is extremely common.

Pigmentation of skin, thyroid, bone and teeth have been reported occasionally in persons receiving minocycline usually for extended periods of time. The pigmentation may be irreversible.

Reduced efficacy and increased incidence of breakthrough bleeding has been suggested with concomitant use of tetracycline and oral contraceptive preparations.

PRECAUTIONS: The administration of minocycline to children under 13 years of age is not recommended.

Very rare, serious events have occurred with minocycline hydrochloride including Stevens-Johnson Syndrome and toxic epidermal necrolysis. Minocycline hydrochloride should be discontinued if either of these serious skin reactions is suspected.

Bulging fontanelles have been reported in young infants following full therapeutic dosage of tetracyclines including minocycline. Pseudotumor cerebri (benign intracranial hypertension) has very rarely been reported in adults (see Adverse Effects). The usual clinical manifestations are headache and blurred vision. While both of these conditions and related symptoms usually resolve after discontinuation of the tetracycline, the possibility of permanent sequelae exists.

Patients should be warned to avoid exposure to direct sunlight and/or ultraviolet light while under treatment with minocycline or other tetracycline drugs, and treatment should be discontinued at the first evidence of skin erythema or discomfort. Photosensitivity manifested by an exaggerated sunburn reaction has been observed in some individuals taking tetracyclines. Studies to date indicate that photosensitivity is rarely reported with minocycline.

Occupational Hazards: Patients treated with minocycline may suffer from headaches, light-headedness, dizziness or vertigo. Decreased hearing has been rarely reported in patients on minocycline. Administration in excess of the recommended dosage can increase the frequency and severity of these CNS symptoms. Patients should be cautioned about driving vehicles or using hazardous machinery while on minocycline therapy. These symptoms may disappear during therapy and usually disappear rapidly when the drug is discontinued.

As with other antibiotics, therapy may result in overgrowth of non-susceptible organisms (including fungi). If superinfection occurs, minocycline should be discontinued and appropriate therapy instituted.

The development of cross-resistance to many antibiotics can develop rapidly in several species of microorganisms. The clinician should bear this in mind if minocycline is not achieving expected results.

The frequency of resistance to minocycline in hemolytic streptococci is highest in strains from infections of the ear, wounds and skin. Culture and sensitivity studies should be performed whenever feasible and routinely in suspected streptococcal infections. Since sensitivity reactions are more likely to occur in persons with a history of allergy, asthma, hay fever, or urticaria, minocycline should be used with caution in such individuals.

Before treating patients with gonorrhea, a darkfield examination should be made from any lesion suggestive of concurrent syphilis. Serological tests for syphilis should be repeated monthly for at least 4 months.

Hepatotoxicity has been reported with minocycline hydrochloride; therefore, minocycline hydrochloride should be used with caution in patients with hepatic dysfunction and in conjunction with alcohol or other hepatotoxic drugs.

Periodic laboratory evaluation of organ systems, including hematopoietic, renal and hepatic studies, should be performed.

Minocycline has been shown to depress plasma prothrombin activity. Therefore, patients who are on anticoagulant therapy should be monitored regularly and may require downward adjustment of their anticoagulant dosage. Interference with vitamin K synthesis by microorganisms in the gut has been reported.

Antacids containing aluminum, calcium or magnesium and oral iron preparations impair absorption and should not be given to patients taking oral minocycline.

Food and/or milk reduce the absorption of tetracycline. Minocycline is not affected to the same extent.

In a study by Leyden, the absorption of a single 100 mg dose of minocycline was inhibited by the ingestion of solid food by 13% (as measured by a reduction in mean serum concentration), and the absorption of a single 250 mg dose of tetracycline was inhibited by 46% when that antibiotic was administered with solid food. When administered with milk, the mean serum concentration of minocycline was reduced by 27% and that of tetracycline, by 65%. The clinical significance of such declines in serum levels is not known.

The concurrent use of tetracyclines with oral contraceptives may render oral contraceptives less effective.

Administration of isotretinoin or other systemic retinoids or retinol should be avoided shortly before, during, and shortly after minocycline therapy. Each of these agents used alone has been associated with pseudotumor cerebri.

Increased risk of ergotism when ergot alkaloids or their derivatives are given with tetracyclines.

The following syndromes have been reported. In some cases involving these syndromes, death has been reported. As with other serious adverse reactions, if any of these syndromes are recognized, the drug should be discontinued immediately:

- Hypersensitivity syndrome consisting of cutaneous reaction (such as rash or exfoliative dermatitis), eosinophilia, and one or more of the following: hepatitis, pneumonitis, nephritis, myocarditis, pericarditis. Fever and lymphadenopathy may be present.
- Lupus-like syndrome consisting of positive antinuclear antibody; arthralgia, arthritis, joint stiffness, or joint swelling; and one or more of the following: fever, myalgia, hepatitis, rash, vasculitis.
- Serum sickness-like syndrome consisting of fever; urticaria or rash; and arthralgia, arthritis, joint stiffness, or joint swelling. Eosinophilia may be present.

ADVERSE EFFECTS: The following adverse reactions have been reported with the tetracycline analogues including minocycline:

Central Nervous System: increased intracranial pressure, light-headedness, dizziness or vertigo and, rarely, fainting spells have been reported with a variable but overall incidence of approximately 7% in patients treated. These symptoms usually disappear rapidly when the drug is discontinued. Impaired hearing, tinnitus, headache, convulsions, sedation, hypesthesia or paresthesia have also been reported.

Gastrointestinal: anorexia, nausea, vomiting, diarrhea, stomatitis, glossitis, enterocolitis, pancreatitis, pruritus ani, constipation, dyspepsia, dysphagia, inflammatory lesions (with monilial overgrowth) in the anogenital region, increases in liver enzymes, and rarely hepatitis and acute liver failure have been reported. Rare instances of esophagitis and esophageal ulcerations have been reported in patients taking the tetracycline-class antibiotics in capsule and tablet form. Most of these patients took the medication immediately before going to bed. Very rare incidence of pseudomembranous colitis has been reported.

Teeth and Bone: Dental staining (yellow-gray-brown) has been reported in children of mothers given tetracyclines, including minocycline, during the latter half of pregnancy, and in children given the drug during the neonatal period, infancy and childhood to age of 13 years. Enamel hypoplasia has also been reported. Discoloration of bones and teeth has been documented to occur rarely in adolescents and adults upon extended treatment. The effects may be irreversible. At present the mechanism of staining, although not completely elucidated, appears to be mediated by the formation of a stable iron complex. Very rarely arthritis, joint stiffness and joint swelling have been reported.

Renal: Rise in BUN has been reported and is apparently dose-related. Increased excretion of nitrogen and sodium has also been reported. Acute renal failure, including interstitial nephritis has been reported rarely.

Skin: maculopapular and erythematous rashes. Rarely reported: alopecia, fixed drug eruption, photosensitivity, pruritus, rash, urticaria, onycholysis, discolouration of the nails, tongue, gum and lip, pigmentation of the skin and mucous membrane, erythema multiforme, erythema nodosum. Lesions occurring on the glans penis have caused balanitis.

Very rare, serious events have occurred with minocycline hydrochloride including angioedema, exfoliative dermatitis, hyperpigmentation of nails, Stevens-Johnson Syndrome, vasculitis and toxic epidermal necrolysis. Minocycline hydrochloride should be discontinued if either of these serious skin reactions is suspected.

Hypersensitivity Reactions: urticaria, angioneurotic edema, polyarthralgia, anaphylaxis/anaphylactoid reactions (including shocks and fatalities), hypersensitivity, anaphylactoid purpura, pericarditis and exacerbation of systemic lupus erythematosus. Myalgia and myocarditis have also been rarely reported.

Pseudotumor cerebri (benign intracranial hypertension) in adults has been associated with the use of tetracyclines. The usual clinical manifestations are headache and blurred vision. Bulging fontanels have been associated with the use of tetracyclines in infants. While both of these conditions and related symptoms usually resolve soon after discontinuation of the tetracycline, the possibility for permanent sequelae exists.

Respiratory: Rarely: cough and dyspnea; very rarely: bronchospasm, exacerbation of asthma and pulmonary eosinophilia and undetermined frequency of pneumonitis have been reported.

Other: fever, elevated liver enzymes including AST or ALT values, hepatic cholestasis, hepatic failure (including fatalities) hyperbilirubinemia, jaundice, autoimmune hepatitis, hemolytic anemia, leukopenia, neutropenia, thrombocytopenia, eosinophilia and pancytopenia and agranulocytosis. When given over prolonged periods, minocycline, like other tetracyclines, has been reported to produce brown-black microscopic discolouration of the thyroid gland. Abnormalities of thyroid function have not been shown to date. If adverse reactions or idiosyncrasy occur, the administration of minocycline should be discontinued and appropriate alternate therapy instituted. Very rare incidence of oral and anogenital candidiasis and vulvovaginitis have also been reported.

Very rarely: Discoloration of secretions have been reported.

OVERDOSE:

Symptoms: Dizziness, nausea, vomiting, abdominal pain, intestinal hemorrhage, hypotension, lethargy, coma, acidosis, azotemia without a concomitant rise in creatinine.

Treatment: Specific antidote: none. General antidotes: antacids (e.g., calcium carbonate or lactate, milk of magnesia, aluminum hydroxide) which form relatively insoluble complexes with minocycline. (Calcium Solution 5%: 50 g calcium carbonate or lactate dissolved in 1000 mL water, yields a 5% solution). Gastric lavage, if necessary.

For management of a suspected drug overdose, contact your regional Poison Control Centre. See the *CPS* Directory section for a list of Poison Control Centres.

DOSAGE: Children (13 years of age or older): The usual dosage is 4 mg/kg initially followed by 2 mg/kg every 12 hours. Tetracyclines are not recommended in children under 13 years of age (see Warnings).

Adults: The usual oral dosage is 100 or 200 mg initially, followed by 100 mg every 12 hours. Alternatively, if more frequent doses are preferred, 2 or 4 doses of 50 mg may be given initially, followed by one 50 mg dose every 6 hours. Therapy should be continued for 1 or 2 days beyond the time when characteristic symptoms or fever have subsided.

For treatment of syphilis, therapy should be administered over a period of 10 or 15 days. Close follow-up, including laboratory tests, is recommended.

Concomitant Therapy: Antacids containing aluminum, calcium or magnesium and/or iron preparations impair absorption and should not be given to patients taking minocycline.

Dose selection for an elderly patient should be cautious, usually starting at the low end of the dosing range, reflecting the greater frequency of decreased hepatic, renal, or cardiac function, and of concomitant disease or other drug therapy.

SUPPLIED: 50 mg: Each orange, hard shell, pellet-filled capsule, printed "Stiefel" and "MINOCIN 50 mg", contains: minocycline HCl equivalent to minocycline 50 mg. Nonmedicinal ingredients: microcrystalline cellulose; empty capsule: FD&C Blue No. 1, FD&C Yellow No. 6, gelatin, silicon dioxide, sodium lauryl sulfate and titanium dioxide. Tartrazine-free. Bottles of 100 and 500.

100 mg: Each orange-purple, hard shell, pellet-filled capsule, printed "Stiefel" and "MINOCIN 100 mg", contains: minocycline HCl equivalent to minocycline 100 mg. Nonmedicinal ingredients: microcrystalline cellulose; empty capsule: FD&C Blue No. 1, FD&C Red No. 3, FD&C Yellow No. 6, gelatin, silicon dioxide, sodium lauryl sulfate and titanium dioxide. Tartrazine-free. Bottles of 100 and 500.

Minocycline Ⓟ

CPhA Monograph

see *Tetracyclines*

Min-Ovral® 21 Ⓟ

levonorgestrel—ethinyl estradiol

Oral Contraceptive

Pfizer

Min-Ovral® 28 Ⓟ

levonorgestrel—ethinyl estradiol

Oral Contraceptive

Pfizer

SUPPLIED: Min-Ovral 21: Each white tablet, engraved W on one face and "M-O" on the other, contains: levonorgestrel 150 µg and ethinyl estradiol 30 µg. Nonmedicinal ingredients: lactose, magnesium stearate, microcrystalline cellulose and polacrilin potassium. Energy: 1.67 kJ (0.40 kcal). Gluten- and tartrazine-free. Blister packages of 21 tablets. Store at 15-30°C. Should be protected from light once opened using the protective covering provided. Keep out of reach of children.

Min-Ovral 28: Each white tablet, engraved W on one face and "M-O" on the other, contains: levonorgestrel 150 µg and ethinyl estradiol 30 µg. Nonmedicinal ingredients: lactose, magnesium stearate, microcrystalline cellulose and polacrilin potassium. In addition, inert tablets contain FD&C Red No. 3 Lake. Energy: 1.67 kJ (0.40 kcal). Gluten- and tartrazine-free. Blister packages of 28 tablets (21 white Min-Ovral tablets and 7 pink inert tablets). Store at 15-30°C. Should be protected from light once opened using the protective covering provided. Keep out of reach of children.

(Shown in Product Identification Section)

Miochol-E® Ⓟ

acetylcholine chloride—electrolytes

Miotic

Novartis Pharmaceuticals

PHARMACOLOGY: Acetylcholine is a naturally occurring neurohormone which mediates nerve impulse transmission at all cholinergic sites involving somatic and autonomic nerves. After release from the nerve ending, acetylcholine is rapidly inactivated by the enzyme acetylcholinesterase by hydrolysis to acetic acid and choline.

Direct application of acetylcholine to the iris will cause rapid miosis of short duration. Topical ocular instillation of acetylcholine to the intact eye causes no discernible response as cholinesterase destroys the molecule more rapidly than it can penetrate the cornea.

INDICATIONS: To obtain miosis of the iris in seconds after delivery of the lens in cataract surgery, in penetrating keratoplasty, iridectomy and other anterior segment surgery where rapid miosis may be required.

CONTRAINDICATIONS: None known.

WARNINGS: Do not gas sterilize. If blister or peelable backing is damaged or broken, sterility of the enclosed bottle cannot be assured. Open under aseptic conditions only.

PRECAUTIONS: General: In the reconstitution of the solution, as described under Directions for Using Univial, if the centre rubber plug seal in the univial does not go down or is down, do not use the vial.

If miosis is to be obtained quickly with Miochol-E, anatomical hindrances to miosis, such as anterior or posterior synechiae, must be released prior to administration. During cataract surgery, use Miochol-E only after delivery of the lens.

Aqueous solutions of acetylcholine are unstable. Prepare solution immediately before use. Do not use solution which is not clear and colorless. Discard any solution that has not been used.

Drug Interactions: Although clinical studies with acetylcholine and animal studies with acetylcholine or carbachol revealed no interference, and there is no known pharmacological basis for an interaction, there have been reports that acetylcholine and carbachol have been ineffective when used in patients treated with topical nonsteroidal anti-inflammatory agents.

Children: Safety and effectiveness in children have not been established.

ADVERSE EFFECTS: Infrequent cases of corneal edema, corneal clouding and corneal decompensation have been reported with the use of intraocular acetylcholine.

Adverse reactions have been reported rarely which are indicative of systemic absorption. These include bradycardia, hypotension, flushing, breathing difficulties and sweating.

OVERDOSE:

Treatment: Atropine sulfate (0.5 to 1 mg) should be given i.m. or i.v. and should be readily available to counteract possible overdosage. Epinephrine (0.1 to 1 mg s.c.) is also of value in overcoming severe cardiovascular or bronchoconstrictor responses.

For management of a suspected drug overdose, CPhA recommends that you contact your **regional Poison Control Centre**. See the *CPS* Directory section for a list of Poison Control Centres.

DOSAGE: With a new needle of sturdy gauge, 18 to 20, draw all the solution into a dry, sterile syringe. Replace needle with a suitable atraumatic cannulae for intraocular irrigation.

The Miochol-E solution is instilled into the anterior chamber before or after securing one or more sutures. Instillation should be gentle and parallel to the iris face and tangential to pupil border.

If there are no mechanical hindrances, the pupil starts to constrict in seconds and the peripheral iris is drawn away from the angle of the anterior chamber. Any anatomical hindrance to miosis must be released to permit the desired effect of the drug. In most cases, 0.5 to 2 mL produces satisfactory miosis.

In cataract surgery, use Miochol-E only after delivery of the lens.

Aqueous solutions of acetylcholine are unstable. Prepare solution immediately before use. Do not use solution which is not clear and colorless. Discard any solution that has not been used.

Directions for using the univial: **Sterile unless package open or broken.**

1. Inspect univial while inside unopened blister. Diluent must be in upper chamber.
2. Peel open blister.
3. Aseptically transfer univial to sterile field. Maintain sterility of outer container during preparation of solution.
4. Immediately before use, give plunger-stopper a quarter turn and press to force diluent and centre plug into lower chamber.
5. Shake gently to dissolve drug.
6. Discard univial and any unused solution.

SUPPLIED: Each univial (two chamber vial) contains: acetylcholine chloride 20 mg and mannitol 56 mg (lower chamber) and electrolyte diluent 2 mL (upper chamber). The reconstituted solution provides acetylcholine chloride 10 mg/mL. Nonmedicinal ingredients: calcium chloride dihydrate, magnesium chloride hexahydrate, mannitol, potassium chloride, sodium acetate trihydrate and sterile water for injection. Store at 4 to 25°C. **Keep from freezing.**

Miostat® ℞

carbachol

Miotic

Alcon

SUPPLIED: Each glass vial contains: a sterile buffered solution of carbachol 0.01%. Nonmedicinal ingredients: calcium chloride, hydrochloric acid, magnesium chloride, potassium chloride, purified water, sodium acetate, sodium chloride, sodium citrate and sodium hydroxide. Preservative-free. Glass vials of 1.5 mL, cartons of 12.

Mirapex® ℞

pramipexole dihydrochloride

Antiparkinsonian Agent—Dopamine Agonist

Boehringer Ingelheim

Date of Revision: February 17, 2009

SUMMARY PRODUCT INFORMATION:

Route of Administration	Dosage Form/ Strength	All Nonmedicinal Ingredients
Oral	Tablets 0.125 mg, 0.25 mg, 0.5 mg, 1 mg and 1.5 mg	Colloidal silicon dioxide, corn starch, magnesium stearate, mannitol, povidone.

INDICATIONS AND CLINICAL USE: Adults: MIRAPEX (pramipexole dihydrochloride monohydrate) is indicated for:

- treatment of the signs and symptoms of idiopathic Parkinson's disease. MIRAPEX may be used both as early therapy, without concomitant levodopa, and as an adjunct to levodopa.
- symptomatic treatment of moderate to severe idiopathic Restless Legs Syndrome. The effectiveness of MIRAPEX used for longer than 12 weeks has not been systematically evaluated in controlled trials for Restless Legs Syndrome. The physician who elects to prescribe MIRAPEX for an extended time should periodically re-evaluate the long-term usefulness for the individual patient.

Geriatrics (>65 years of age): The majority of pramipexole (88%) is cleared via renal secretion. Due to age-related reduction in renal function, the elderly have a slower clearance of pramipexole (approximately 25-30% lower). The efficacy and safety appear to be unaffected, except the relative risk of hallucination is higher. (See Warnings and Precautions, Special Populations, Geriatrics (>65 years of age).)

Pediatrics: The safety and efficacy of MIRAPEX have not been established in children less than 18 years of age, therefore MIRAPEX is not recommended in this patient population.

CONTRAINDICATIONS:

- MIRAPEX (pramipexole dihydrochloride monohydrate) is contraindicated in patients who have demonstrated hypersensitivity to pramipexole or the excipients of the drug product (see Dosage Forms, Composition and Packaging).

WARNINGS AND PRECAUTIONS:

Serious Warnings and Precautions

Sudden Onset of Sleep: Patients receiving treatment with MIRAPEX (pramipexole dihydrochloride monohydrate) and other dopaminergic agents have reported suddenly falling asleep while engaged in activities of daily living, including operating a motor vehicle, which sometimes resulted in accidents. Although some of the patients reported somnolence while on MIRAPEX, others perceived that they had no warning signs, such as excessive drowsiness, and believed that they were alert immediately prior to the event.

Physicians should alert patients of the reported cases of sudden onset of sleep, bearing in mind that these events are **not** limited to initiation of therapy. Patients should also be advised that sudden onset of sleep has occurred without warning signs. If drowsiness or sudden onset of sleep should occur, patients should immediately contact their physician.

Until further information is available on the management of this unpredictable and serious adverse event, patients should be warned not to drive or engage in other activities where impaired alertness could put themselves and others at risk of serious injury or death (e.g., operating machines). Substituting other dopamine agonists may not alleviate these symptoms, as episodes of falling asleep while engaged in activities of daily living have also been reported in patients taking these products.

While dose reduction clearly reduces the degree of somnolence, there is insufficient information to establish that dose reduction will eliminate episodes of falling asleep while engaged in activities of daily living.

Presently, the precise cause of this event is unknown. It is known that many Parkinson's disease patients experience alterations in sleep architecture, which results in excessive daytime sleepiness or spontaneous dozing, and that dopaminergic agents can also induce sleepiness.

The following Warnings and Precautions are listed in alphabetical order.

Carcinogenesis and Mutagenesis: Two-year carcinogenicity studies have been conducted with pramipexole in mice and rats. In rats, pramipexole was administered in the diet, at doses of 0.3, 2 and 8 mg/kg/day. The highest dose corresponded to 12.5 times the highest recommended clinical dose (1.5 mg t.i.d.) based on comparative AUC values. No significant increases in tumours occurred.

Testicular Leydig cell adenomas were found in male rats as follows: 13 of 50 control group A males, 9 of 60 control group B males, 17 of 50 males given 0.3 mg/kg/day, 22 of 50 males given 2 mg/kg/day, and 22 of 50 males given 8 mg/kg/day. Leydig cell hyperplasia and increased numbers of adenomas are attributed to pramipexole-induced decreases in serum prolactin levels, causing a down-regulation of Leydig cell luteinizing hormone (LH) receptors and a compensatory elevation of LH secretion by the pituitary gland. The endocrine mechanisms believed to be involved in rats are not relevant to humans.

In mice, pramipexole was administered in the diet, at doses of 0.3, 2 and 10 mg/kg/day. The highest dose corresponded to 11 times the highest recommended clinical dose on a mg/m^2 basis. No significant increases in tumours occurred.

Pramipexole was not mutagenic in a battery of in vitro and in vivo assays including the Ames assay and the in vivo mouse micronucleus assay.

Cardiovascular: Hypotension: In case of severe cardiovascular disease, care should be taken. Dopamine agonists appear to impair the systemic regulation of blood pressure with resulting postural (orthostatic) hypotension, especially during dose escalation. Postural (orthostatic) hypotension has been observed in patients treated with MIRAPEX (pramipexole dihydrochloride monohydrate). Therefore, patients should be carefully monitored for signs and symptoms of orthostatic hypotension especially during dose escalation (see Dosage and Administration) and should be informed of this risk (see Information for the Patient).

In clinical trials of MIRAPEX, however, and despite clear orthostatic effects in normal volunteers, the reported incidence of clinically significant orthostatic hypotension was not greater among those assigned to MIRAPEX than among those assigned to placebo. This result is clearly unexpected in light of the previous experience with the risks of dopamine agonist therapy.

While this finding could reflect a unique property of MIRAPEX, it might also be explained by the conditions of the study and the nature of the population enrolled in the clinical trials. Patients were very carefully titrated, and patients with active cardiovascular disease or significant orthostatic hypotension at baseline were excluded.

Connective Tissue: Fibrotic Complications: Although not reported with pramipexole in the clinical development program, cases of retroperitoneal fibrosis, pulmonary infiltrates, pleural effusion, pleural thickening, pericarditis, and cardiac valvulopathy have been reported in some patients treated with ergot-derived dopaminergic agents. While these complications may resolve when the drug is discontinued, complete resolution does not always occur.

Although these adverse events are believed to be related to the ergoline structure of these compounds, whether other, non-ergot derived dopamine agonists can cause them is unknown.

A small number of reports have been received of possible fibrotic complications, including peritoneal fibrosis, pleural fibrosis, and pulmonary fibrosis, in the postmarketing experience for MIRAPEX. While the evidence is not sufficient to establish a causal relationship between MIRAPEX and these fibrotic complications, a contribution of MIRAPEX cannot be completely ruled out in rare cases.

Dependence/Tolerance: MIRAPEX has not been systematically studied in animals or humans for its potential for abuse, tolerance, or physical dependence. However, in a rat model on cocaine self-administration, MIRAPEX had little or no effect.

Neurologic: Augmentation and Rebound in Restless Legs Syndrome: Reports in the literature indicate treatment of RLS with dopaminergic medications can result in a worsening of symptoms in the early morning hours, referred to as rebound. Reports in the literature also indicate treatment of RLS with dopaminergic medications can result in augmentation. Augmentation refers to the earlier onset of symptoms in the evening (or even the afternoon), increase in symptoms, and spread of symptoms to involve other extremities. Spontaneous reports of augmentation were uncommon in the RLS development programme. The frequency of augmentation and/or rebound after longer use of MIRAPEX and the appropriate management of these events have not been evaluated in controlled clinical trials.

Drug Withdrawal Effects in Restless Legs Syndrome: In RLS clinical trials, some patients have reported worsening of the RLS symptoms following abrupt discontinuation of MIRAPEX treatment. The worsening of symptoms was independent of the MIRAPEX dosage and generally resolved within one week. Tapering is recommended whenever possible if discontinuation is necessary.

Dyskinesia: MIRAPEX may potentiate the dopaminergic side effects of levodopa and may cause or exacerbate pre-existing dyskinesia. Decreasing the dose of levodopa may ameliorate this side effect.

Neuroleptic Malignant Syndrome: A symptom complex resembling the neuroleptic malignant syndrome (characterized by elevated temperature, muscular rigidity, altered consciousness, and autonomic instability), with no other obvious etiology, has been reported in association with rapid dose reduction, withdrawal of, or changes in anti-Parkinsonian therapy, including MIRAPEX. (See Dosage and Administration for dose tapering.)

Ophthalmologic: Retinal Pathology in Albino Rats: Pathologic changes (degeneration and loss of photoreceptor cells) were observed in the retina of albino rats in the 2-year carcinogenicity study with pramipexole. These findings were first observed during week 76 and were dose-dependant in animals receiving 2 mg/kg/day (25/50 male rats, 10/50 female rats) and 8 mg/kg/day (44/50 male rats, 37/50 female rats). Plasma AUCs at these doses were 2.5 and 12.5 times the AUC seen in humans at the maximal recommended dose of 4.5 mg per day. Similar findings were not present in either control rats, or in rats receiving 0.3 mg/kg/day of pramipexole (0.3 times the AUC seen in humans at the 4.5 mg per day dose).

Studies demonstrated that pramipexole at very high dose (25 mg/kg/day) reduced the rate of disk shedding from the photoreceptor rod cells of the retina in albino rats; this reduction was associated with enhanced sensitivity to the damaging effects of light. In a comparative study, degeneration and loss of photoreceptor cells occurred in albino rats after 13 weeks of treatment with 25 mg/kg/day of pramipexole (54 times the highest clinical dose on an mg/m basis) and constant light (100 lux) but not in Brown-Norway rats exposed to the same dose and higher light intensities (500 lux).

The albino rats seem to be more susceptible than pigmented rats to the damaging effect of pramipexole and light. While the potential significance of this effect on humans has not been established, it cannot be excluded that human albinos (or people who suffer from albinismus oculi) might have an increased susceptibility to pramipexole compared to normally pigmented people. Therefore, such patients should take MIRAPEX only under ophthalmological monitoring.

Psychiatric: Behavioural Changes: Patients and caregivers should be aware of the fact that abnormal behaviour (reflecting symptoms of impulse control disorders and compulsive behaviours) such as pathological gambling, increased libido, hypersexuality, binge eating or compulsive shopping have been reported in patients treated with dopaminergic drugs. Dose reduction/tapered discontinuation should be considered.

Hallucinations: Hallucinations and confusion are known side effects of treatment with dopamine agonist and levodopa. Hallucinations were more frequent when MIRAPEX was given in combination with levodopa in patients with advanced disease than in monotherapy in patients with early disease. Patients should be aware of the fact that hallucinations (mostly visual) can occur.

In the double-blind, placebo-controlled trials in early Parkinson's disease, hallucinations were observed in 9% (35 of 388) of patients receiving MIRAPEX, compared with 2.6% (6 of 235) of patients receiving placebo. In the double-blind, placebo-controlled trials in advanced Parkinson's disease, where patients received MIRAPEX and concomitant levodopa, hallucinations were observed in 16.5% (43 of 260) of patients receiving MIRAPEX compared with 3.8% (10 of 264) of patients receiving placebo. Hallucinations were of sufficient severity to cause discontinuation of treatment in 3.1% of the early Parkinson's disease patients and 2.7% of the advanced Parkinson's disease patients compared with about 0.4% of placebo patients in both populations.

Age appears to increase the risk of hallucinations. In patients with early Parkinson's disease, the risk of hallucinations was 1.9 times and 6.8 times greater in MIRAPEX patients than placebo patients <65 years old, and >65 years old, respectively. In patients with advanced Parkinson's disease, the risk of hallucinations was 3.5 times and 5.2 times greater in MIRAPEX patients than placebo patients <65 years old, and >65 years old, respectively.

In the RLS clinical program, one pramipexole-treated patient (of 889) reported hallucinations; this patient discontinued treatment and the symptoms resolved.

Renal: Since MIRAPEX (pramipexole dihydrochloride monohydrate) is eliminated through the kidneys, caution should be exercised when prescribing MIRAPEX to patients with renal insufficiency (see Action and Clinical Pharmacology, Pharmacokinetics and Dosage and Administration).

Skeletal Muscular: Rhabdomyolysis: A single case of rhabdomyolysis occurred in a 49-year old male with advanced Parkinson's disease treated with MIRAPEX. The patient was hospitalized with an elevated CPK (10.631 IU/L). The symptoms resolved with discontinuation of the medication.

Skin: Melanoma: Epidemiological studies have shown that patients with Parkinson's disease have a higher risk (2- to approximately 6-fold higher) of developing melanoma that the general population. Whether the increased risk observed was due to Parkinson's disease or other factors, such as drugs used to treat Parkinson's disease, is unclear.

For the reasons stated above, patients and health-care providers are advised to monitor for melanomas frequently and on a regular basis when using MIRAPEX for any indication. Ideally, periodic skin examination should be performed by appropriately qualified individuals (e.g. dermatologists).

Sexual Function/Reproduction: In rat fertility studies, pramipexole at a dose of 2.5 mg/kg/day, prolonged the estrus cycle and inhibited implantation. These effects were associated with a reduction in serum levels of prolactin, a hormone necessary for implantation and maintenance of early pregnancy in rats.

Pramipexole, at a dose of 2.5 mg/kg/day inhibited implantation. Pramipexole, at a dose of 1.5 mg/kg/day (4.3 times the AUC observed in humans at the maximal recommended clinical dose of 1.5 mg t.i.d.) resulted in a high incidence of total resorption of embryos. This finding is thought to be due to the prolactin lowering effect of pramipexole. Prolactin is necessary for implantation and maintenance of early pregnancy in rats, but not in rabbits and humans. Because of pregnancy disruption and early embryonic loss, the teratogenic potential of pramipexole could not be assessed adequately. In pregnant rabbits which received doses up to 10 mg/kg/day during organogenesis (plasma AUC 71 times that seen in humans at the 1.5 mg t.i.d. dose), there was no evidence of adverse effects on embryo-fetal development. Postnatal growth was inhibited in the offspring of rats treated with a 0.5 mg/kg/day dose of pramipexole during the latter part of pregnancy and throughout lactation.

Special Populations: Pregnant Women: There are no studies of MIRAPEX in pregnant women. Because animal reproduction studies are not always predictive of human response, MIRAPEX should be used during pregnancy only if the potential benefit outweighs the potential risk to the fetus.

Nursing Women: The excretion of pramipexole into breast milk has not been studied in women. Since MIRAPEX suppresses lactation, it should not be administered to mothers who wish to breast-feed infants.

A single-dose, radio-labelled study showed that drug-related materials were excreted into the breast milk of lactating rats. Concentrations of radioactivity in milk were three to six times higher than concentrations in plasma at equivalent time points.

Geriatrics (>65 years of age): MIRAPEX total oral clearance was approximately 25 to 30% lower in the elderly (aged 65 years and older) as a result of a decline in pramipexole renal clearance due to an age-related reduction in renal function. This resulted in an increase in elimination half-life from approximately 8.5 hours to 12 hours (see Action and Clinical Pharmacology, Pharmacokinetics).

In clinical studies, 40.8% (699 of 1715) of patients were between the ages of 65 and 75 years, and 6.5% (112 of 1715) of patients were >75 years old. There were no apparent differences in efficacy or safety between older and younger patients, except that the relative risk of hallucination associated with the use of MIRAPEX was increased in the elderly.

Pediatrics: The safety and efficacy of MIRAPEX in children under 18 years of age have not been established.

Monitoring and Laboratory Tests: There are no specific laboratory tests recommended for the management of patients receiving MIRAPEX.

ADVERSE REACTIONS: Parkinson's Disease: Adverse Drug Reaction Overview: During the premarketing development of MIRAPEX (pramipexole dihydrochloride monohydrate), patients enrolled in clinical trials had either early or advanced Parkinson's disease. Apart from the severity and duration of their disease, the two populations differed in their use of concomitant levodopa therapy. Namely, patients with early disease did not receive concomitant levodopa therapy during treatment with MIRAPEX, while those with advanced Parkinson's disease did.

Because these two populations may have differential risk for various adverse events, adverse event data will be presented for both populations.

All controlled clinical trials performed during premarketing development (except one fixed dose study) used a titration design. Consequently, it was impossible to adequately evaluate the effects of a given dose on the incidence of adverse events.

Clinical Trial Adverse Drug Reactions: Because clinical trials are conducted under very specific conditions the adverse reaction rates observed in the clinical trials may not reflect the rates observed in practice and should not be compared to the rates in the clinical trials of another drug. Adverse drug reaction information from clinical trials is useful for identifying drug-related adverse events and for approximating rates.

Adverse Reactions Leading to Discontinuation of Treatment: Early Parkinson's Disease: Approximately 12% of 388 patients treated with MIRAPEX and 11% of 235 patients treated with placebo discontinued treatment due to adverse events. The events most commonly causing discontinuation of treatment were related to the nervous system, namely hallucinations (3.1% on MIRAPEX vs 0.4% on placebo), dizziness (2.1% on MIRAPEX vs 1.0% on placebo), somnolence (1.6% on MIRAPEX vs 0% on placebo), headache and confusion (1.3% and 1.0%, respectively, on MIRAPEX vs 0% on placebo), and to the gastrointestinal system (nausea 12.1% on MIRAPEX vs 0.4% on placebo).

Advanced Parkinson's Disease: Approximately 12% of 260 patients treated with MIRAPEX and 16% of 264 patients treated with placebo discontinued treatment due to adverse events. The events most commonly causing discontinuation of treatment were related to the nervous system, namely hallucinations (2.7% on MIRAPEX vs 0.4% on placebo), dyskinesia (1.9% on MIRAPEX vs 0.8% on placebo), dizziness (1.2% on MIRAPEX vs 1.5% on placebo), confusion (1.2% on MIRAPEX vs 2.3% on placebo, and to the cardiovascular system (postural [orthostatic] hypotension (2.3% on MIRAPEX vs 1.1% on placebo).

Most Frequent Adverse Events: Adverse events occurring with an incidence of greater than, or equal to, 10% and listed in decreasing order of frequency, were as follows:

Early Parkinson's disease: nausea, dizziness, somnolence, insomnia, asthenia and constipation.

Advanced Parkinson's disease: postural [orthostatic] hypotension, dyskinesia, insomnia, dizziness, hallucinations, accidental injury, dream abnormalities, constipation and confusion.

Incidence of Adverse Events in Placebo Controlled Trials: Table 1 lists treatment-emergent adverse events that were reported in the double-blind, placebo-controlled studies by ≥1% of patients treated with MIRAPEX and were numerically more frequent than in the placebo group. Adverse events were usually mild or moderate in intensity.

Table 1: MIRAPEX

Adverse Events from Placebo-Controlled Early and Adjunct Therapy Studies (incidence of events ≥1% in patients[a] treated with MIRAPEX and numerically more frequent than in patients treated with placebo)

	Early Therapy		Advanced Therapy	
Body System/Adverse Event	**MIRAPEX N=388 % occurrence**	**Placebo N=235 % occurrence**	**MIRAPEX[b] N=260 % occurrence**	**Placebo[b] N=264 % occurrence**
Body as a Whole				
Asthenia	14	12	10	8
General Edema	5	3	4	3
Malaise	2	1	3	2
Reaction Unevaluable	2	1	—	—
Fever	1	0	—	—
Chest Pain	—	—	3	2
Accidental Injury	—	—	17	15
Cardiovascular System				
Postural Hypotension	—	—	53	48
Digestive System				
Nausea	28	18	—	—
Constipation	14	6	10	9
Anorexia	4	2	—	—
Dysphagia	2	0	—	—
Dry Mouth	—	—	7	3
Metabolic and Nutritional System				
Peripheral Edema	5	4	2	1
Decreased Weight	2	0	—	—
Increased Creatine PK	—	—	1	0
Musculoskeletal System				
Arthritis	—	—	3	1
Twitching	—	—	2	0
Bursitis	—	—	2	0
Myasthenia	—	—	1	0
Nervous System				
Dizziness	25	24	26	25
Somnolence	22	9	9	6
Insomnia	17	12	27	22
Hallucinations	9	3	17	4
Confusion	4	1	10	7
Amnesia	4	2	6	4
Hyperesthesia	3	1	—	—
Dystonia	2	1	8	7
Thinking Abnormalities	2	0	3	2
Decreased Libido	1	0	—	—
Myoclonus	1	0	—	—
Hypertonia	—	—	7	6
Paranoid Reaction	—	—	2	0
Delusions	—	—	1	0
Sleep Disorders	—	—	1	0
Dyskinesia	—	—	47	31
Gait Abnormalities	—	—	7	5
Dream Abnormalities	—	—	11	10
Respiratory System				
Dyspnea	—	—	4	3
Rhinitis	—	—	3	1
Pneumonia	—	—	2	0
Skin and Appendages				
Skin Disorders	—	—	2	1
Special Senses				
Vision Abnormalities	3	0	3	1
Accommodation Abnormalities	—	—	4	2
Diplopia	—	—	1	0
Urogenital System				
Impotence	2	1	—	—
Urinary Frequency	—	—	6	3
Urinary Tract Infection	—	—	4	3
Urinary Incontinence	—	—	2	1

[a] Patients may have reported multiple adverse experiences during the study or at discontinuation, thus, patients may be included in more than one category.

[b] Patients received concomitant levodopa.

Other Clinical Trial Adverse Drug Reactions (≥1%): Other events reported by 1% or more of patients treated with MIRAPEX but reported equally or more frequently in the placebo group were as follows:

Early Parkinson's Disease: Infection, accidental injury, headache, pain, tremor, back pain, syncope, postural hypotension, hypertonia, diarrhoea, rash, ataxia, dry mouth, leg cramps, twitching, pharyngitis, sinusitis, sweating, rhinitis, urinary tract infection, vasodilation, flu syndrome, increased saliva, tooth disease, dyspnoea, increased cough, gait abnormalities, urinary frequency, vomiting, allergic reaction, hypertension, pruritis, hypokinesia, increased creatine PK, nervousness, dream abnormalities, chest pain, neck pain, paresthesia, tachycardia, vertigo, voice alteration, conjunctivitis, paralysis, accommodation abnormalities, tinnitus, diplopia, and taste perversions.

Advanced Parkinson's Disease: Nausea, pain, infection, headache, depression, tremor, hypokinesia, anorexia, back pain, dyspepsia, flatulence, ataxia, flu syndrome, sinusitis, diarrhoea, myalgia, abdominal pain, anxiety, rash, paresthesia, hypertension, increased saliva, tooth disorder, apathy, hypotension, sweating, vasodilation, vomiting, increased cough, nervousness, pruritus, hyperesthesia, neck pain, syncope, arthralgia, dysphagia, palpitations, pharyngitis, vertigo, leg cramps, conjunctivitis, and lacrimation.

Adverse Events: Relationship to Age, Gender and Race: Among the treatment-emergent adverse events in patients treated with MIRAPEX, hallucinations appeared to exhibit a positive relationship to age. No gender-related differences were observed. Only a small percentage (4%) of patients enrolled were non-Caucasian, therefore, an evaluation of adverse events related to race is not possible.

Other Adverse Events Observed During all Phase 2 and 3 Clinical Trials: MIRAPEX has been administered to 1,715 subjects during the premarketing development program, 782 of who participated in double-blind, controlled studies. During these trials, all adverse events were recorded by the clinical investigators using terminology of their own choosing. To provide a meaningful estimate of the proportion of individuals having adverse events, similar types of events were grouped into a smaller number of standardized categories using modified COSTART dictionary terminology. These categories are used in the listing below.

The events listed below occurred in less than 1% of the 1,715 subjects exposed to MIRAPEX. All reported events, except those already listed above, are included, without regard to determination of a causal relationship to MIRAPEX.

Events are listed within body-system categories in order of decreasing frequency.

Body as a Whole: fever, enlarged abdomen, rigid neck, no drug effect.

Cardiovascular System: palpitations, angina pectoris, atrial arrhythmia, peripheral vascular disease.

Digestive System: tongue discoloration, GI hemorrhage, fecal incontinence.

Endocrine System: diabetes mellitus.

Hemic and Lymphatic System: ecchymosis.
Metabolic and Nutritional System: gout.
Musculoskeletal System: bursitis, myasthenia.
Nervous System: apathy, libido decrease, paranoid reaction, akinesia, coordination abnormalities, speech disorder, hyperkinesia, neuralgia.
Respiratory System: voice alteration, asthma, hemoptysis.
Skin and Appendages: skin disorder, herpes simplex.
Special Senses: tinnitus, taste perversion, otitis media, dry eye, ear disorder, hemianopia.
Urogenital System: urinary incontinence, dysuria, prostate disorder, kidney calculus.

In individual patients, hypotension may occur at the beginning of treatment, especially if MIRAPEX is titrated too rapidly.

Restless Legs Syndrome: MIRAPEX (pramipexole dihydrochloride monohydrate) Tablets for treatment of RLS has been evaluated for safety in 889 patients, including 427 treated for over six months and 75 for over one year. The overall safety assessment focuses on the results of three double-blind, placebo-controlled trials, in which 575 patients with RLS were treated with MIRAPEX for 3-12 weeks. The most commonly observed adverse events with MIRAPEX in the treatment of RLS (observed in >5% of pramipexole treated patients and at a rate at least twice that observed in placebo-treated patients) were nausea and somnolence. Occurrences of nausea and somnolence in clinical trials were generally mild and transient.

Approximately 7% of 575 patients treated with MIRAPEX during the double-blind periods of three placebo-controlled trials discontinued treatment due to adverse events compared to 5% of 223 patients who received placebo. The adverse event most commonly causing discontinuation of treatment was nausea (1%).

Clinical Trial Adverse Drug Reactions: Because clinical trials are conducted under very specific conditions the adverse reaction rates observed in the clinical trials may not reflect the rates observed in practice and should not be compared to the rates in the clinical trials of another drug. Adverse drug reaction information from clinical trials is useful for identifying drug-related adverse events and for approximating rates. See Table 2.

Table 2: MIRAPEX

Treatment-Emergent Adverse-Event[a] Incidence in Double-Blind, Placebo-Controlled Trials in Restless Legs Syndrome (events ≥2% of patients treated with MIRAPEX and numerically more frequent than in the placebo group)

Body System/Adverse Event	MIRAPEX 0.125–0.75 mg/day (N=575) %	Placebo (N=223) %
Gastrointestinal Disorders		
Nausea	16	5
Constipation	4	1
Diarrhoea	3	1
Dry Mouth	3	1
General Disorders and Administration Site Conditions		
Fatigue	9	7
Infections and Infestations		
Influenza	3	1
Nervous System Disorders		
Headache	16	15
Somnolence	6	3

[a] Patients may have reported multiple adverse experiences during the study or at discontinuation; thus, patients may be included in more than one category.

In general, the frequency of nausea and fatigue was reduced with continued MIRAPEX therapy. Other events reported by 2% or more of RLS patients treated with MIRAPEX but equally or more frequently in the placebo group, were: vomiting, nasopharyngitis, back pain, pain in extremity, dizziness, and insomnia.

Table 3 summarizes data for adverse events that appeared to be dose related in the 12-week fixed dose study.

Table 3: MIRAPEX

Dose Related Adverse Events in a 12-Week Double-Blind, Placebo-Controlled Fixed Dose Study in Restless Legs Syndrome (occurring in ≥5% of all patients in the treatment phase)

Body System/ Adverse Event	MIRAPEX 0.25 mg (N=88) %	MIRAPEX 0.5 mg (N=80) %	MIRAPEX 0.75 mg (N=90) %	Placebo (n=86) %
Gastrointestinal Disorders				
Nausea	11.4	18.8	26.7	4.7
Diarrhoea	3.4	1.3	6.7	0
Dyspepsia	3.4	1.3	4.4	7
Infections and Infestations				
Influenza	1.1	3.8	6.7	1.2
General Disorders and Administration Site Conditions				
Fatigue	3.4	5.0	6.7	4.7
Psychiatric Disorders				
Insomnia	9.1	8.8	13.3	9.3
Abnormal Dreams	2.3	1.3	7.8	2.3
Respiratory, Thoracic and Mediastinal Disorders				
Nasal Congestion	0.0	2.5	5.6	1.2
Musculoskeletal and Connective Tissue Disorders				
Pain in Extremity	3.4	2.5	6.7	1.2

(cont'd)

Table 3: MIRAPEX *(cont'd)*

Adverse Events: Relationship to Age, Gender and Race: Although no gender-related differences were observed in Parkinson's disease patients, nausea and fatigue, both generally transient, were more frequently reported by female than male RLS patients. Less than 4% of patients enrolled were non-Caucasian, therefore, an evaluation of adverse events related to race in not possible.

Other Adverse Events Observed During Phase 2 and 3 Clinical Trials: MIRAPEX Tablets have been administered to 889 individuals in RLS clinical trials. During these trials, all adverse events were recorded by the clinical investigators using terminology of their own choosing; similar types of events were grouped into a smaller number of standardized categories using MedDRA dictionary terminology. These categories are used in the listing below. The events listed below occurred on at least two occasions (on one occasion if the event was serious) within the 889 individuals exposed to MIRAPEX. All reported events, except those already listed above, are included, without regard to determination of a causal relationship to MIRAPEX.

Blood and Lymphatic System Disorders: anaemia.
Cardiac Disorders: arrhythmia, coronary artery disease, myocardial infarction, myocardial ischemia, palpitations, tachycardia.
Congenital, Familial, and Genetic Disorders: congenital atrial septal defect.
Ear and Labyrinth Disorders: tinnitus, vertigo.
Endocrine Disorders: goiter, hypothyroidism.
Eye Disorders: conjunctivitis, dry eye, eye irritation, eyelid edema, vision blurred, visual acuity reduced, visual disturbance.
Gastrointestinal Disorders: abdominal discomfort, abdominal distension, abdominal pain, dyspepsia, enteritis, flatulence, gastroesophageal reflux disease, gastritis, haemorrhoids, inguinal hernia, irritable bowel syndrome, loose stools, toothache, umbilical hernia.
General Disorders and Administration Site Conditions: alcohol interaction, asthenia, chest pain, peripheral edema, feeling cold, feeling hot, inflammation localized, influenza-like illness, malaise, pain, pitting edema, pyrexia, thirst.
Hepatobiliary Disorders: biliary colic, cholecystitis, cholelithiasis.
Immune System Disorders: hypersensitivity, seasonal allergy.
Infections and Infestations: Borrelia infection, bronchitis, cystitis, ear infection, fungal infection, gastroenteritis, herpes simplex, herpes zoster, hordeolum, laryngitis, localized infection, onychomycosis, otitis (externa and media), paronychia, pharyngitis, pneumonia, rhinitis, sinusitis, tonsillitis, tooth infection, urinary tract infection, vaginitis, viral infection.
Injury, Poisoning and Procedural Complication: contusion, epicondylitis, failure of implant, fall, foot fracture, fractured sacrum, hip fracture, joint injury, joint sprain, limb injury, muscle strain, open fracture, radius fracture, sunburn, tendon rupture, thermal burn, wound, wrist fracture.
Investigations: alanine aminotransferase increased, aspartate aminotransferase increased, blood glucose increased, blood pressure increased, blood triglycerides increased, gammaglutamyltransferase increased, heart rate increased, heart rate irregular, weight decreased, weight increased.
Metabolism and Nutrition Disorders: anorexia, decreased appetite, hypercholesterolemia, hyperlipidemia, hypocalcaemia, increased appetite.
Musculoskeletal and Connective Tissue Disorders: arthralgia, bursitis, cervical spinal stenosis, intervertebral disc protrusion, intervertebral discitis, joint stiffness, localized osteoarthritis, lumbar spinal stenosis, muscle cramps, musculoskeletal stiffness, neck pain, myalgia, osteoporosis, sensation of heaviness, spinal osteoarthritis, tendonitis, toe deformity.
Neoplasms Benign, Malignant and Unspecified: lung cancer metastatic, metastases to lung, ovarian cancer, prostatic adenoma, renal neoplasm, squamous cell carcinoma.
Nervous System Disorders: balance disorder, carpal tunnel syndrome, cerebral ischemia, cervicobrachial syndrome, disturbance in attention, dizziness postural, dysgeusia, hypoesthesia, memory impairment, migraine, nerve compression, paraesthesia, Restless Legs Syndrome, sciatica, sedation, sinus headache, sudden onset of sleep, syncope, tension headache, transient ischemic attack, tremor.
Psychiatric Disorders: abnormal dreams, agitation, anxiety, confusional state, depression, irritability, libido decreased, mood altered, nervousness, nightmare, restlessness, sleep disorder, stress symptoms.
Renal and Urinary Disorders: nocturia, pollakiuria, polyuria, renal colic.
Reproductive System and Breast Disorders: dysmenorrhoea, menopausal symptoms, sexual dysfunction.
Respiratory, Thoracic and Mediastinal Disorders: asthma, chronic obstructive airways disease (including exacerbation), cough, dyspnoea, exertional dyspnoea, epistaxis, nasal congestion, nasal septum deviation, pharyngolaryngeal pain, respiratory tract infection, sinus congestion, snoring.
Skin and Subcutaneous Tissue Disorders: acne, eczema, erythema, hyperhidrosis, night sweats, photosensitivity allergic reaction, pruritus, rash, rosacea, seborrheic dermatitis.
Surgical and Medical Procedures: hysterectomy.
Vascular Disorders: flushing, haematoma, hypertension, hypotension, orthostatic hypotension.

Post-Market Adverse Drug Reactions: In addition to the adverse events reported during clinical trials, the following adverse reactions have been identified (essentially in Parkinson's disease patients) during post-approval use of MIRAPEX. Because these reactions are reported voluntarily from a population of uncertain size, it is not always possible to reliably estimate their frequency or establish a causal relationship to drug exposure.

Sudden Onset on Sleep: Patients treated with MIRAPEX have rarely reported suddenly falling asleep while engaged in activities of daily living; including operation of motor vehicles which has sometimes resulted in accidents (see Warnings and Precautions).

Abnormal Behaviour: Post marketing experience suggests MIRAPEX may be associated with increase or decrease of libido and hypersexuality.

Pathological (compulsive) gambling has been described in the literature for some dopamine agonists used in the treatment of Parkinson's disease. Cases of pathological (compulsive) gambling have been reported in patients treated with MIRAPEX, especially at high doses. Pathological gambling, increased libido and hypersexuality were generally reversible upon dose reduction or treatment discontinuation.

Abnormal behaviour (reflecting symptoms of impulse control disorders and compulsions), abnormal dreams, amnesia, delusion, hyperkinesias, paranoia, increased eating (binge eating, hyperphagia), compulsive shopping, restlessness, visual disturbance including vision blurred and visual acuity reduced, vomiting, weight decrease, and weight increase have been observed.

Insomnia and peripheral edema have been reported.

DRUG INTERACTIONS: Drug-Drug Interactions: The drugs listed in Table 4 are based on information collected in clinical studies, interaction case reports, or pharmacological properties of the drug that may be used. See Action and Clinical Pharmacology, Drug-Drug Interactions for more information.

MIRAPEX is bound to plasma proteins to a very low extent (<20%) and little biotransformation is seen in humans. Therefore, interactions with other medication affecting plasma protein binding or elimination by biotransformation are unlikely. Medication that inhibit the active renal tubular secretion of basic (cationic) drugs or are themselves eliminated by active renal tubular secretion may interact with MIRAPEX resulting in reduced clearance of either or both medications.

Drug-Food Interactions: Interactions with food have not been established.
Drug-Herb Interactions: Interactions with herbal products have not been established.
Drug-Laboratory Interactions: There are no known interactions between MIRAPEX and laboratory tests.

Table 4: MIRAPEX

Established or Potential Pharmacokinetic Interactions

MIRAPEX	Effect	Clinical Comment
Antiparkinsonian Drugs		
Levodopa/Carbidopa	Pramipexole increases levodopa C_{max} by about 40% and reduces T_{max} from 2.5 to 0.5 hours. No change in total exposure (AUC) was observed. Levodopa/carbidopa has no effect on the pharmacokinetics of pramipexole in healthy volunteers.	The combined use of pramipexole and levodopa increases the frequency of hallucination. Dosage adjustment, even discontinuation, may be necessary. While increasing the dose of MIRAPEX in Parkinson's disease patients it is recommended that the dosage of levodopa is reduced and the dosage of other anti-parkinsonian medication is kept constant.
Selegiline	Selegiline has no effect on the pharmacokinetics of pramipexole in volunteers.	
Amantadine	Amantadine inhibits the renal cationic transport system. Amantadine might alter the clearance of pramipexole.	Dosage adjustment may be necessary. See below.
Anticholinergics		
Anticholinergics	As anticholinergics are mainly eliminated by hepatic metabolism, pharmacokinetic drug-drug interactions with pramipexole are rather unlikely.	
Other Drugs Eliminated via Renal Secretion		
Drugs eliminate via the renal cationic transport system Amantadine Cimetidine Ranitidine Diltiazem Triamterene Verapamil Quinidine Quinine	These drugs inhibit the renal tubular secretion of organic bases via the cationic transport system. They reduce the renal clearance of pramipexole to various degrees.	Dosage adjustment should be considered if concomitant treatment is necessary. Dosage reduction is necessary if adverse reactions, such as dyskinesia, agitation, or hallucination, are observed.
Drugs eliminate via the renal anionic transport system Probenecid Cephalosporins Penicillins Indomethacin Hydrochlorothiazide Chloropramide	These drugs inhibit the renal tubular secretion of organic bases via the anionic transport system. They are unlikely to reduce the renal clearance of pramipexole.	Dosage adjustment is not necessary.
Interactions Mediated by CYP Isoenzymes		
Drugs metabolized by CYP isoenzymes	Inhibitors of CYP isoenzymes are not expected to affect the elimination of pramipexole. Pramipexole has no inhibitory action on CYP1A2, CYP2C9, CYP2C19, CYP2E1, and CYP3A4. Inhibition of CYP2D6 is observed with an apparent Ki of 30 µM, suggesting that MIRAPEX will not inhibit CYP enzymes at plasma concentrations following the highest recommended clinical dose (1.5 mg tid).	
Dopamine Antagonists		
Neuroleptics, e.g. phenothiazines, butyrophenones, thioxathines Metoclopramide	Pramipexole is a dopamine agonist. Dopamine antagonists reduce its therapeutic effects.	Concurrent use is not recommended. Pramipexole can exacerbate psychotic symptoms.
Miscellaneous		
Sedating medication or alcohol	Possible additive effects.	Because of possible additive effects, caution should be advised when patients are taking other sedating medication or alcohol in combination with MIRAPEX.

DOSAGE AND ADMINISTRATION: Parkinson's Disease: MIRAPEX (pramipexole dihydrochloride monohydrate) should be taken orally, three times daily. The tablets can be taken with or without food.

Missed Dose: Patients should be advised that if a dose is missed, they should not take a double dose, but continue with the regular treatment schedule.

Dosing Considerations: Adults: In all clinical studies, dosage was initiated at a subtherapeutic level to avoid orthostatic hypotension and severe adverse effects. MIRAPEX should be titrated gradually in all patients. The dosage should be increased to achieve maximal therapeutic effect, balanced against the principal adverse reactions of dyskinesia, nausea, dizziness and hallucinations.

Initial Treatment: Dosages should be increased gradually from a starting dose of 0.375 mg/day given in three divided doses and should not be increased more frequently than every 5 to 7 days. A suggested ascending dosage schedule that was used in clinical studies is shown in Table 5.

Maintenance Treatment: MIRAPEX was effective and well-tolerated over a dosage range of 1.5 to 4.5 mg/day, administered in equally divided doses three times per day, as monotherapy or in combination with levodopa (approximately 800 mg/day). In a fixed-dose study in patients with early Parkinson's disease, MIRAPEX at doses of 3, 4.5 and 6 mg/day was not shown to provide any significant benefit beyond that achieved at a daily dose of 1.5 mg/day. For individual patients who have not achieved efficacy at 1.5 mg/day, higher doses can result in additional therapeutic benefit.

When MIRAPEX is used in combination with levodopa, a reduction of the levodopa dosage should be considered. In the controlled study in advanced Parkinson's disease, the dosage of levodopa was reduced by an average of 27% from baseline.

Table 5: MIRAPEX

Ascending-Dose Schedule of MIRAPEX

Week	Dosage (mg)	Total Daily Dose (mg)
1	0.125 t.i.d.	0.375
2	0.25 t.i.d.	0.75
3	0.50 t.i.d.	1.5
4	0.75 t.i.d.	2.25
5	1.00 t.i.d.	3.0
6	1.25 t.i.d.	3.75
7	1.50 t.i.d.	4.5

Discontinuation of Treatment: It is recommended that MIRAPEX be discontinued over a period of one week.

Recommended Dose and Dosage Adjustment: The maximal recommended dose of MIRAPEX is 4.5 mg per day. MIRAPEX is not recommended at the 6 mg per day dose since the incidence of some adverse reactions is higher.

Dosing in Patients with Concomitant Levodopa Therapy: In patients with concomitant levodopa therapy it is recommended that the dosage of levodopa is reduced during both dose escalation and maintenance treatment with MIRAPEX. This may be necessary in order to avoid excessive dopaminergic stimulation.

Patients with Renal Impairment: Since the clearance of MIRAPEX is reduced in patients with renal impairment (see Action and Clinical Pharmacology, Pharmacokinetics), the following dosage recommendation should be considered (see Table 6).

Table 6: MIRAPEX

MIRAPEX Dosage in Renal Impairment

Renal Status	Starting Dose (mg)	Maximum Dose (mg)
Mild Impairment (Creatinine Cl >60 mL/min)	0.125 t.i.d.	1.5 t.i.d.
Moderate Impairment (Creatinine Cl=35 to 59 mL/min)	0.125 b.i.d.	1.5 b.i.d.
Severe Impairment (Creatinine Cl=15 to 34 mL/min)	0.125 qd	1.5 qd
Very Severe Impairment (Creatinine Cl <15 mL/min and hemodialysis patients)	MIRAPEX has not been adequately studied in this group and its administration to patients with end stage renal disease is not recommended.	

Patients with a creatinine clearance above 50 mL/min require no reduction in daily dose.

If renal function declines during maintenance therapy reduce MIRAPEX daily dose by same percentage as decline in creatinine clearance, i.e. if creatinine clearance declines by 30%, then reduce MIRAPEX daily dose by 30%. The daily dose can be administered in two divided doses if creatinine clearance is between 20 and 50 mL/min and as a single daily dose if creatinine clearance is less than 20 mL/min.

Patients with Hepatic Impairment: Dose reduction not considered necessary.

Restless Legs Syndrome: Adults: The tablets should be taken orally, swallowed with water, and can be taken either with or without food.

The recommended starting dose of MIRAPEX is 0.125 mg taken once daily 2-3 hours before bedtime. For patients requiring additional symptomatic relief, the dose may be increased every 4-7 days to 0.50 mg per day (as shown in Table 7):

Table 7: MIRAPEX

Ascending-Dose Schedule of MIRAPEX

Titration Step	Once Daily Evening Dose (mg)
1	0.125
2[a]	0.25
3[a]	0.50

[a] If needed.

Some patients may find optimal relief at 0.75 mg per day, albeit with a higher rate of adverse reactions. Intermediate doses (such as 0.375 mg or 0.625 mg per day) may be used. Patients should be re-assessed periodically, and the dose adjusted accordingly.

Treatment Discontinuation: Due to the chronic and fluctuating nature of RLS, continuous treatment may not be necessary. If discontinuation is desirable, tapering in 4-7 day intervals is recommended whenever possible.

Dosing in Patients with Renal Impairment: The duration between up titration steps should be increased to 14 days in RLS patients with severe and moderately severe renal impairment (creatinine clearance 20-60 mL/min). (See Action and Clinical Pharmacology, Renal Insufficiency).

Dosing in Patients with Hepatic Impairment: Dose reduction is not considered necessary in patients with hepatic impairment, as approx. 90% of absorbed drug is excreted through the kidneys.

Dosing in Children and Adolescents: Safety and efficacy of MIRAPEX have not been established in children and adolescents up to 18 years of age.

OVERDOSAGE:

Signs and Symptoms: There is no clinical experience with massive overdosage. The expected adverse events are those related to the pharmacodynamic profile of a dopamine agonist including nausea, vomiting, hyperkinesia, hallucinations, agitation and hypotension.

One patient with a 10-year history of schizophrenia (who participated in a schizophrenia study) took 11 mg/day of MIRAPEX (pramipexole dihydrochloride monohydrate) for two days; this was two to three times the daily dose recommended in the protocol. No adverse events were reported related to the increased dose. The blood pressure remained stable although pulse rates increased to between 100 and 120 beats/minute. The patient withdrew from the study at the end of week 2 due to lack of efficacy.

Recommended Management: There is no known antidote for overdosage of a dopamine agonist. If signs of central nervous system stimulation are present, a phenothiazine or other butyrophenone neuroleptic agent may be indicated; the efficacy of such drugs in reversing the effects of overdosage has not been assessed. Management of the overdose may require general supportive measures along with gastric lavage, intravenous fluids, and electrocardiogram monitoring. Haemodialysis has not been shown to be helpful.

> For management of a suspected drug overdose, CPhA recommends that you contact your **regional Poison Control Centre**. See the *CPS* Directory section for a list of Poison Control Centres.

ACTION AND CLINICAL PHARMACOLOGY: Mechanism of Action: MIRAPEX (pramipexole dihydrochloride monohydrate) is a non ergot dopamine agonist with high in vitro specificity at the D_2 subfamily of dopamine receptors. Pramipexole is a full agonist and exhibits higher affinity to the D_3 receptor subtypes (which are in prominent distribution within the mesolimbic area) than to D_2 or D_4 receptor subtypes. While MIRAPEX exhibits high affinity for the dopamine D_2 receptor subfamily, it has low affinity for α_2 adrenergic receptors and negligible or undetectable affinity for other dopaminergic, adrenergic, histaminergic, adenosine and benzodiazepine receptors.

The ability of pramipexole to alleviate the signs and symptoms of Parkinson's disease is believed to be related to its ability to stimulate dopamine receptors in the striatum. This assumption is supported by a dose-dependent antagonism of Parkinsonian symptoms in rhesus monkeys pre-treated with the neurotoxin N-methyl-4-phenyl-1,2,3,6-tetrahydropyridine (MPTP) which destroys dopamine cell bodies in the substantia nigra.

The precise mechanism of action of MIRAPEX as a treatment for Restless Legs Syndrome is not known. Although the pathophysiology of Restless Legs Syndrome is largely unknown, neuropharmacological evidence suggests primary dopaminergic system involvement. Positron emission tomographic (PET) studies suggest that a mild striatal presynaptic dopaminergic dysfunction may be involved in the pathogenesis of Restless Legs Syndrome.

In human volunteers a dose-dependent decrease in prolactin was observed.

Pharmacokinetics: Absorption: Following oral administration, pramipexole is rapidly absorbed reaching peak concentrations between 1 and 3 hours. The absolute bioavailability of pramipexole is greater than 90%. Pramipexole can be administered with or without food. A high-fat meal did not affect the extent of pramipexole absorption (AUC and C_{max}) in healthy volunteers, although the time to maximal plasma concentration (T_{max}) was increased by about 1 hour.

Pramipexole displays linear pharmacokinetics over the range of doses that are recommended for patients with Parkinson's disease.

Distribution: Pramipexole is extensively distributed, having a volume of distribution of about 500 L. Protein binding is less than 20% in plasma; with albumin accounting for most of the protein binding in human serum. Pramipexole distributes into red blood cells as indicated by an erythrocyte to plasma ratio of approximately 2.0 and a blood to plasma ratio of approximately 1.5. Consistent with the large volume of distribution in humans, whole body autoradiography and brain tissue levels in rats indicated that pramipexole was widely distributed throughout the body, including the brain.

Metabolism and Excretion: Urinary excretion is the major route of pramipexole elimination. Approximately 88% of a 14C-labelled dose was recovered in the urine and less than 2% in the faeces following single intravenous and oral doses in healthy volunteers. The terminal elimination half-life was about 8.5 hours in young volunteers (mean age 30 years) and about 12 hours in elderly volunteers (mean age 70 years). Approximately 90% of the recovered 14C-labelled dose was unchanged drug; with no specific metabolites having been identified in the remaining 10% of the recovered radio-labelled dose. Pramipexole is the levorotational (−) enantiomer, and no measurable chiral inversion or racemization occurs in vivo.

The renal clearance of pramipexole is approximately 400 mL/min, approximately three times higher than the glomerular filtration rate. Thus, pramipexole is secreted by the renal tubules, probably by the organic cation transport system.

Special Populations and Conditions: Because therapy with pramipexole is initiated at a subtherapeutic dose and gradually titrated according to clinical tolerability to obtain optimal therapeutic effect, adjustment of the initial dose based on gender, weight, or age is not necessary. However, renal insufficiency, which can cause a large decrease in the ability to eliminate pramipexole, may necessitate dosage adjustment.

Early vs Advanced Parkinson's Disease Patients: The pharmacokinetics of pramipexole was comparable between early and advanced Parkinson's disease patients.

Restless Legs Syndrome Patients: A cross-study comparison of data suggests that the pharmacokinetic profile of pramipexole administered once daily in RLS patients is generally consistent with the pharmacokinetic profile of pramipexole in healthy volunteers.

Pediatrics: The pharmacokinetics of pramipexole in the pediatric population has not been evaluated.

Geriatrics: Renal function declines with age. Since pramipexole clearance is correlated with renal function, the drug's total oral clearance was approximately 25% to 30% lower in elderly (aged 65 years or older) compared with young healthy volunteers (aged less than 40 years). The decline in clearance resulted in an increase in elimination half-life from approximately 8.5 hours in young volunteers (mean age 30 years) to 12 hours in elderly volunteers (mean age 70 years).

Gender: Pramipexole renal clearance is about 30% lower in women than in men, most of this difference can be accounted for by differences in body weight. The reduced clearance resulted in a 16 to 42% increase in AUC and a 2 to 10% increase in C_{max}. The differences remained constant over the age range of 20 to 80 years. The difference in pramipexole half-life between males and females was less than 10%.

Race: The potential influence of race on pramipexole pharmacokinetics has not been evaluated.

Hepatic Insufficiency: The potential influence of hepatic insufficiency on pramipexole pharmacokinetics has not been evaluated; however, it is considered to be small. Since approximately 90% of the recovered 14C-labelled dose was excreted in the urine as unchanged drug, hepatic impairment would not be expected to have a significant effect on pramipexole elimination.

Renal Insufficiency: The clearance of pramipexole was about 75% lower in patients with severe renal impairment (creatinine clearance approximately 20 mL/min) and about 60% lower in patients with moderate impairment (creatinine clearance approximately 40 mL/min) compared with healthy volunteers. A lower starting and maintenance dose is recommended in patients with renal impairment (see Dosage and Administration). In patients with varying degrees of renal impairment, pramipexole clearance correlates well with creatinine clearance. Therefore, creatinine clearance can be used as a predictor of the extent of decrease in pramipexole clearance. As pramipexole clearance is reduced even more in dialysis patients (N=7), than in patients with severe renal impairment, the administration of pramipexole to patients with end stage renal disease is not recommended.

Drug-Drug Interactions: Anticholinergics: As anticholinergics are mainly eliminated by hepatic metabolism, pharmacokinetic drug-drug interactions with pramipexole are rather unlikely.

Antiparkinsonian Drugs: In volunteers (N=11), selegiline did not influence the pharmacokinetics of pramipexole. Population pharmacokinetic analysis suggests that amantadine may alter the oral clearance of pramipexole (N=54). Levodopa/carbidopa did not influence the pharmacokinetics of pramipexole in volunteers (N=10). Pramipexole did not alter the extent of absorption (AUC) or elimination of levodopa/carbidopa, although it increased levodopa C_{max} by about 40%, and decreased T_{max} from 2.5 to 0.5 hours. While increasing the dose of MIRAPEX in Parkinson's disease patients it is recommended that the dosage of levodopa is reduced and the dosage of other antiparkinsonian medication is kept constant.

Cimetidine: Cimetidine, a known inhibitor of renal tubular secretion of organic bases via the cationic transport system, increased MIRAPEX AUC by 50% and increased its half-life by 40% in volunteers (N=12).

Probenecid: Probenecid, a known inhibitor of renal tubular secretion of organic acids via the anionic transport system, did not influence the pharmacokinetics of MIRAPEX in volunteers (N=12).

Other Drugs Eliminated via Renal Secretion: Concomitant therapy with drugs secreted by the renal cationic transport system (e.g., amantadine, cimetidine, ranitidine, diltiazem, triamterene, verapamil, quinidine, and quinine), may decrease the oral clearance of MIRAPEX and thus, may necessitate an adjustment in the dosage of MIRAPEX. In case of concomitant treatment with these kinds of drugs (incl. amantadine) attention should be paid to signs of dopamine overstimulation, such as dyskinesias, agitation or hallucinations. In such cases a dose reduction is necessary. Concomitant therapy with drugs secreted by the renal anionic transport system (e.g., cephalosporins, penicillins, indomethacin, hydrochlorothiazide and chlorpropamide) are not likely to have any effect on the oral clearance of MIRAPEX.

CYP Interactions: Inhibitors of cytochrome P450 enzymes would not be expected to affect MIRAPEX elimination because MIRAPEX is not appreciably metabolized by these enzymes in vivo or in vitro. MIRAPEX does not inhibit CYP1A2, CYP2C9, CYP2C19, CYP2E1, and CYP3A4. Inhibition of CYP2D6 was observed with an apparent Ki of 30 µM, suggesting that MIRAPEX will not inhibit CYP enzymes at plasma concentrations observed following the highest recommended clinical dose (1.5 mg tid).

Dopamine Antagonists: Since MIRAPEX is a dopamine agonist, dopamine antagonists such as the neuroleptics (phenothiazines, butyrophenones, thioxanthines) or metoclopramide may diminish the effectiveness of MIRAPEX and should ordinarily not be administered concurrently.

Miscellaneous: Because of possible additive effects, caution should be advised when patients are taking other sedating medication or alcohol in combination with MIRAPEX and when taking concomitant medication that increase plasma levels of pramipexole (e.g. cimetidine).

STORAGE AND STABILITY: Store at controlled room temperature of 15 to 30°C.

SPECIAL HANDLING INSTRUCTIONS: The product should be dispensed in the original container. The product should be protected from light.

INFORMATION FOR THE PATIENT: Published in e-CPS, available by subscription at www.e-cps.ca.

DOSAGE FORMS, COMPOSITION AND PACKAGING: 0.125 mg: Each white, round tablet, both faces flat with bevelled edges, one side imprinted with the symbol P6, the other side imprinted with the Boehringer Ingelheim company symbol, contains: pramipexole dihydrochloride monohydrate 0.125 mg. Nonmedicinal ingredients: colloidal silicon dioxide, cornstarch, magnesium stearate, mannitol and povidone. Blister packs of 30.

0.25 mg: Each white, oval tablet, both faces flat with beveled edges, one side has a deep break score and is imprinted with the symbol P7 on either side of the score, the other side is also scored and imprinted with the Boehringer Ingelheim company symbol on either side of the score, contains: pramipexole dihydrochloride monohydrate 0.25 mg. Nonmedicinal ingredients: colloidal silicon dioxide, cornstarch, magnesium stearate, mannitol and povidone. Bottles of 90.

0.5 mg: Each white, oval tablet, both faces flat with beveled edges, one side has a deep break score and is imprinted with the symbol P8 on either side of the score, the other side is also scored and imprinted with the Boehringer Ingelheim company symbol on either side of the score, contains: pramipexole dihydrochloride monohydrate 0.5 mg. Nonmedicinal ingredients: colloidal silicon dioxide, cornstarch, magnesium stearate, mannitol and povidone. Bottles of 90.

1 mg: Each white, round tablet, both faces flat with beveled edges, one side has a deep break score and is imprinted with the symbol P9 on either side of the score, the other side is also scored and imprinted with the Boehringer Ingelheim company symbol on either side of the score, contains: pramipexole dihydrochloride monohydrate 1 mg. Nonmedicinal ingredients: colloidal silicon dioxide, cornstarch, magnesium stearate, mannitol and povidone. Bottles of 90.

1.5 mg: Each white, round tablet, both faces flat with beveled edges, one side has a deep break score and is imprinted with the symbol P11 on either side of the score, the other side is also scored and imprinted with the Boehringer Ingelheim company symbol on either side of the score, contains: pramipexole dihydrochloride monohydrate 1.5 mg. Nonmedicinal ingredients: colloidal silicon dioxide, cornstarch, magnesium stearate, mannitol and povidone. Bottles of 90.

(Shown in Product Identification Section)

Mirena® Ⓟ
levonorgestrel
Progestogen

Bayer

Date of Revision: May 11, 2010

SUMMARY PRODUCT INFORMATION:

Route of Administration	Dosage Form/ Strength	Clinically Relevant Nonmedicinal Ingredients
Intrauterine	Intrauterine system/ 52 mg levonorgestrel	Barium sulphate, iron oxide, polydimethylsiloxane, polyethylene, silica For a complete listing see Dosage Forms, Composition and Packaging.

INDICATIONS AND CLINICAL USE: MIRENA (levonorgestrel-releasing intrauterine system) is indicated for:

- conception control for maximum up to 5 years
- treatment of idiopathic menorrhagia following appropriate diagnostic investigation in women accepting the contraceptive effect of MIRENA

CONTRAINDICATIONS: MIRENA (levonorgestrel-releasing intrauterine system) is contraindicated in patients with the following conditions:

- known or suspected pregnancy
- current or recurrent pelvic inflammatory disease
- lower genital tract infection
- postpartum endometritis
- undiagnosed abnormal uterine bleeding
- uterine anomalies including fibroids if they distort the uterine cavity
- uterine or cervical malignancy
- known or suspected progestin-dependent neoplasia, including breast cancer
- cervicitis
- cervical dysplasia
- active liver disease or dysfunction
- actual benign or malignant liver tumors
- septic abortion within the previous three months
- hypersensitivity to levonorgestrel or any of the other ingredients in the formulation or component of the container components of MIRENA. For a complete listing, see Dosage Forms, Composition and Packaging.
- bacterial endocarditis
- established immunodeficiency
- acute malignancies affecting blood or leukemias
- recent trophoblastic disease while hCG levels are elevated

WARNINGS AND PRECAUTIONS:

> **Serious Warnings and Precautions**
> Hormonal contraceptives **do not protect** against Sexually Transmitted Infections (STIs) including HIV/AIDS. For protection against STIs, it is advisable to use latex or polyurethane condoms **in combination with MIRENA.**
> Cigarette smoking increases the risk of serious adverse effects on the heart and blood vessels. Women should be counseled not to smoke (see Cardiovascular).
> **Uterine Perforation may occur with the use of intrauterine contraceptives including MIRENA (see Uterine Perforation).**

General: MIRENA should be used with caution in women who have migraine, focal migraine with asymmetrical visual loss or other symptoms indicating transient cerebral ischemia, severe headache, marked increase in blood pressure or confirmed or suspected hormone dependent neoplasia including breast cancer, or active or previous severe arterial disease such as stroke or myocardial infarction (see Warnings and Precautions, Cardiovascular; Hematologic; Neurologic). Removal of MIRENA should be considered if any of the above conditions occur during use.

Cases of breast cancer have been reported in users of MIRENA (see Warnings and Precautions, Carcinogensis and Mutagenesis).

MIRENA is not the contraceptive method of first choice for young, nulligravid women. Controlled clinical trials were done in previously parous women aged mainly over 18 years.

MIRENA is intended for use only in women of child-bearing age.

MIRENA is not suitable for use as a post-coital contraceptive.

Insertion Removal and Replacement Precautions: See Dosage and Administration, Insertion, Removal and Replacement and Insertion Instructions.

Carcinogensis and Mutagenesis: Breast Cancer: Cases of breast cancer have been reported in users of MIRENA (see Adverse Reactions).

The incidence rate of breast cancer in association with MIRENA use has been analyzed in a large Finnish epidemiological study using hospital registry data and cancer diagnoses derived from the Finnish Cancer Registry. In this study, the incidence rate of breast cancer in 17 360 MIRENA users (a total of >58 000 women years with MIRENA, and >150 000 women years of follow-up) was not statistically significantly different compared to the occurrence of breast cancer in 4863 control women. In addition, the incidence rate of breast cancer among these MIRENA users has been compared to the average breast cancer incidence rates in Finland. There was no indication of a statistically significant difference between the MIRENA users and average

Finnish female population in any of the age group of women studied (30-54 years). Although these studies do not support a causal relationship between MIRENA and the development of breast cancer, an elevated breast cancer risk cannot be totally excluded, since these studies did not control for confounding factors such as use of oral hormonal contraception by control subjects, genetics and lifestyle and environmental factors such as smoking and alcohol.

Increasing age, inherited mutations, and a strong family history are the most significant risk factors for the development of breast cancer. Other established risk factors include nulliparity, first full-term pregnancy after the age of 30, menarche before the age of 12, never breast-fed a child, and daily alcohol consumption. In some women, the use of hormonal contraceptives may accelerate the growth of an existing but undiagnosed breast cancer. More thorough studies are needed to determine the definitive link between hormonal contraceptive use and the potential risk of breast cancer. There is currently no conclusive evidence of an association between MIRENA use and development of breast cancer or progression of subclinical breast cancer. There is no reason to change prescribing habits at present.

Breast self-examination should be discussed with women receiving hormonal contraceptives. Women should be instructed to notify their physicians whenever any masses are detected.

Cardiovascular: An individual benefit-risk assessment in relation to continued use of MIRENA should be carried out in the event of arterial thrombosis. In particular, removal of MIRENA should be considered if severe arterial disease such as stroke or myocardial infarction occurs. In addition, MIRENA should be used with caution in patients with a previous history of severe arterial disease such as stroke or myocardial infarction. Women with a history of thromboembolic disorders should be made aware of the possibility of a recurrence (see Warnings and Precautions, Hematologic and Adverse Reactions, Post-Market Adverse Drug Reactions). There have been postmarket reports of cardiovascular events, including myocardial infarction and stroke in women using MIRENA, although a causal relationship with MIRENA could not be clearly established in these cases.

Predisposing Factors for Coronary Artery Disease: Cigarette smoking increases the risk of serious cardiovascular side effects and mortality. Hormonal contraceptives increase this risk, especially with increasing age.

Other women who are independently at high risk for cardiovascular disease include those with diabetes, hypertension, abnormal lipid profile, or a family history of these risk factors.

Hypertension: If a significant elevation of blood pressure in previously normotensive or hypertensive subjects occurs at any time during MIRENA use, MIRENA removal should be considered.

Congenital or Valvular Heart Disease: MIRENA should be used with caution in women with congenital or valvular heart disease who are at risk of infective endocarditis. Antibiotic prophylaxis should be administered to such patients when inserting or removing MIRENA.

Endocrine and Metabolism: Glucose Tolerance: Combination and progestogen-only oral contraceptives, including those containing levonorgestrel, may affect glucose tolerance in some users. Diabetic patients, and those with a family history of diabetes, should be observed closely to detect any alterations in carbohydrate metabolism. Young diabetic patients whose disease is of recent origin, well-controlled and not associated with hypertension or other signs of vascular disease such as ocular fundal changes, should be closely observed. One published clinical study indicated no change in mean daily insulin requirements in women with Type 1 diabetes using MIRENA over a 12-month period.

Genitourinary: Bleeding Irregularities: Because irregular menstrual bleeding or spotting is common during the first few months of use, endometrial pathology should be excluded prior to insertion of MIRENA. Irregular bleeding patterns in users of MIRENA could mask the signs and symptoms of cervical or endometrial cancer. If bleeding irregularities develop after prolonged use, appropriate diagnostic measures should be undertaken.

Prolonged menstrual bleeding may occur during the first few months, however with continued use, bleeding patterns vary from regular scanty menstruation in some women to oligomenorrhea or amenorrhea in others. Oligomenorrhea or amenorrhea develop gradually in about 20% of users. Reduced bleeding increases the level of blood hemoglobin.

The possibility of pregnancy should be considered if menstruation does not occur after six weeks or more of amenorrhea, following a pattern of regular menses. A pregnancy test is not necessary in amenorrheic women unless indicated by other symptoms.

Hematologic: An individual benefit-risk assessment in relation to continued use of MIRENA should be carried out in the event of thrombosis. In particular, removal of MIRENA should be considered if venous thromboembolic disease such as deep vein thrombosis or pulmonary embolism occurs. Women with a history of thromboembolic disorders should be made aware of the possibility of a recurrence (see Warnings and Precautions, Cardiovascular and Adverse Reactions, Post-Market Adverse Drug Reactions). There have been postmarketing reports of arterial and venous thromboembolism (ATE, VTE) in women using MIRENA, although a causal relationship with MIRENA could not be clearly established in such cases. Epidemiological studies have indicated that women using progestogen-only oral contraceptives may have a slightly increased risk of venous thromboembolism; however, the results are not statistically significant.

Appropriate diagnostic and therapeutic measures should be undertaken immediately if there are symptoms or signs of thrombosis in users of MIRENA. Symptoms of thromboembolism include: unilateral leg pain and/or swelling, sudden severe pain in the chest whether or not it radiates to the left arm, sudden breathlessness, sudden onset of coughing, any unusual severe prolonged headache, sudden partial or complete loss of vision, diplopia, slurred speech or aphasia, vertigo, collapse with or without focal seizure, weakness or very marked numbness suddenly affecting one side or part of the body, motor disturbances and acute abdomen. Symptoms or signs of retinal thrombosis are: unexplained partial or complete loss of vision, onset of proptosis or diplopia, papilledema, or retinal vascular lesions.

Other Risk Factors for Venous Thromboembolism: Other generalized risk factors for venous thromboembolism include but are not limited to a personal history, a family history (the occurrence of VTE in a direct relative at a relatively early age may indicate genetic predisposition), severe obesity (body mass index ≥30 kg/m²) and systemic lupus erythematosus. The risk of VTE also increases with age and smoking. The risk of VTE may be temporarily increased with prolonged immobilization, major surgery, or trauma. Also patients with varicose veins and leg cast should be closely monitored.

Hepatic/Biliary/Pancreatic: Steroid hormones may be poorly metabolized in patients with impaired liver function. Acute or chronic disturbances of liver function may necessitate the discontinuation of hormonal contraceptive use until markers of liver function return to normal (see Contraindications).

To date, no studies have examined whether the avoidance of the first-pass effect through the liver, as with non-oral hormonal contraceptives, lessens concerns in women with liver conditions.

Jaundice: Patients who have had jaundice should be given hormonal contraceptives only with great care and under close observation. If jaundice develops in a patient using MIRENA, consideration should be given to removing the system. Hormonal contraceptive-related cholestasis has been described in women with a history of pregnancy-related cholestasis. This condition may recur with subsequent hormonal contraceptive use (see Contraindications).

Neurologic: Headache: MIRENA should be used with caution in women with a history of migraine headache, including migraine with focal neurological symptoms. The onset or exacerbation of migraine or the development of headaches with a new pattern that is recurrent, persistent or severe requires evaluation of the cause and consideration to remove MIRENA (see Warnings and Precautions, General; Cardiovascular).

Ophthalmologic: Contact Lenses: Visual changes or changes in contact lens tolerance may occur in users of MIRENA. If this occurs, an ophthalmologist should be consulted. Temporary or permanent cessation of wear may be advised.

Peri-Operative Considerations: Thromboembolic Complications—Post-surgery: Women using MIRENA who require surgery associated with prolonged immobilization should be followed closely for signs and symptoms of thromboembolism.

Psychiatric: Patients with a history of emotional disturbances, especially the depressive type, may be more prone to have a recurrence of depression while using MIRENA. In cases of a serious recurrence, consideration should be given to removing MIRENA, since the depression may be drug-related.

Sexual Function/Reproduction: Ovarian Cysts (Delayed Follicular Atresia): Since the contraceptive action of MIRENA is due mainly to its local effect on the uterus, ovulatory cycles with follicular rupture usually occur in women of fertile age. Sometimes atresia of the follicle is delayed and folliculogenesis may continue. These enlarged follicles cannot be distinguished clinically from ovarian cysts.

Enlarged follicles were diagnosed in about 12% of women using MIRENA in one study involving 50 women. In a larger clinical trial (n=2246), the rate of functional ovarian cysts was 1.2 per 100 woman-years. Cysts are usually small and disappear spontaneously within a few months.

Most of these follicles are asymptomatic, although some may be accompanied by pelvic pain or dyspareunia. In most cases, the enlarged follicles disappear spontaneously over a two to three month period. Should this not occur, continued ultrasound monitoring and other diagnostic or therapeutic measures are recommended. Rarely, surgical intervention may be required.

Ectopic Pregnancy: Women with a previous history of ectopic pregnancy, tubal surgery or pelvic infection carry a higher risk of ectopic pregnancy. Carefully consider the possibility of an ectopic pregnancy in women who become pregnant while having MIRENA in place. Pregnancies with MIRENA use are rare, however, when a woman becomes pregnant with MIRENA in situ, the relative likelihood of ectopic pregnancy is increased. Up to half of the pregnancies that occur with MIRENA in place are ectopic. The possibility of ectopic pregnancy should be considered in the case of lower abdominal pain, especially in association with missed periods, or if an amenorrheic woman starts bleeding.

Women who choose MIRENA should be told about the risk of ectopic pregnancy, including the possibility of impaired fertility or loss of fertility. Educate women to recognize and report to their physician any signs and symptoms of ectopic pregnancy.

Combined data from prospective clinical trials with MIRENA reveal an overall rate of ectopic pregnancy of 0.06 per 100 woman-years. A similar ectopic pregnancy rate has been reported in a postmarketing surveillance study with data from over 17 000 women using MIRENA.

Pelvic Infection: The inserter provided with MIRENA helps protect the system from contamination with micro-organisms during insertion, thereby minimizing the risk of pelvic infection. The exposed product should be handled with aseptic precautions (see Dosage and Administration, Insertion Instructions). Known risk factors for pelvic inflammatory disease include multiple sexual partners, frequent intercourse and young age. Less common causes of pelvic inflammatory disease include pelvic actinomycosis and pelvic tuberculosis, both of which are extremely rare. There is an increased risk of PID during 20 days following the insertion of IUDs related to the insertion procedure. Thereafter, the risk of PID during the use of IUDs or MIRENA is small. Patients should be advised to report to their physicians promptly if they experience symptoms suggestive of PID.

If recurrent endometritis or pelvic infections are experienced, or if an acute infection does not respond to treatment within a few days, MIRENA must be removed.

Sepsis: There have been very rare postmarket reports of Group A streptococcal sepsis temporally associated with MIRENA insertion.

Uterine Perforation: Partial perforation (uterine embedment) or complete perforation of the uterus wall or cervix (occurring at a rate of between 1/1000 and 1/10 000) may occur during insertion, although the perforation may not be detected until later. Pregnancy may result from partial or complete perforation. If partial or complete perforation occurs, MIRENA must be located and removed; surgery may be required. Partial perforation (uterine embedment) can result in difficult removal. Delayed detection of perforation may result in complications (eg, adhesions, peritonitis, intestinal perforation and obstruction, abscesses and erosion of adjacent viscera). The number of uterine perforations is linked to the experience of the person inserting the system. Removal of a perforated IUS was associated (in a few cases) with sliding/separating of the hormone cylinder.

The risk of perforation may be increased in lactating women, women with abnormal uterine anatomy or with fixed retroverted uteri and postpartum insertions. To reduce the possibility of perforation postpartum, MIRENA insertion should be delayed a minimum of 6 weeks after delivery or until uterine involution is complete. If involution is delayed, consider waiting until 12 weeks postpartum. Inserting MIRENA immediately after first trimester abortion is not known to increase the risk of perforation, but insertion after second trimester abortion should be delayed until uterine involution is complete.

To reduce the possibility of perforation, it is important to follow the recommended insertion technique. (See Dosage and Administration, Insertion Instructions.)

Inform patients before the procedure about the risk of uterine perforation and educate them on possible signs of this complication, including, but not limited to, severe low abdominal pain, which may be associated with bleeding after the procedure, loss of threads, or change in thread length.

Uterine Embedment: Embedment of MIRENA in the myometrium may occur. Embedment may decrease contraceptive effectiveness and result in pregnancy. An embedded MIRENA must be removed. Embedment can result in difficult removal, and may require surgery.

MIRENA Expulsion: See Dosage and Administration, Expulsion.

Special Populations: Pregnant Women/Intrauterine Pregnancy: MIRENA is not to be used during an existing or suspected pregnancy. If pregnancy occurs with MIRENA in place, MIRENA should be removed since any intrauterine system left in place may increase the risk of abortion and preterm labour. Removal of MIRENA or probing of the uterus may result in spontaneous abortion. In the event of an intrauterine pregnancy with MIRENA in place, consider the following:

a) Risk of septic abortion.

b) Continuation of pregnancy: If MIRENA cannot be removed or the woman chooses not to have it removed, she should be warned that failure to remove MIRENA increases the risk of miscarriage, sepsis, premature labor, and premature delivery. Ectopic pregnancy should be excluded. The woman should be followed closely and advised to report any abnormal symptoms, such as fever, chill, cramping, abdominal pain, bleeding, vaginal discharge, or leakage of fluid.

c) Long-term effects and congenital anomalies: When pregnancy continues with MIRENA in place, long-term effects on the offspring are unknown. Congenital anomalies in live births have occurred infrequently. No clear trend towards specific anomalies has been observed. Because of the intrauterine administration of levonorgestrel and local exposure of the fetus to the hormone, the possibility of teratogenicity following exposure to MIRENA cannot be completely excluded. Some observational data support a small increased risk of masculinization of the external genitalia of the female fetus following exposure to progestins at doses greater than those currently used for oral contraception. Whether these data apply to MIRENA is unknown.

Nursing Women: Hormonal contraceptives are not recommended as the contraceptive method of first choice in breast-feeding women. A published study indicated that during lactation, 0.1% of the daily maternal dose of levonorgestrel could be transferred to the newborn via milk. Although levonorgestrel has been found in the breast milk of women using MIRENA, there does not appear to be a detrimental effect on growth or development of breast-fed infants whose mothers started using the product after six weeks postpartum. Progestogen-only contraceptive methods do not appear to affect the quantity and quality of breast milk.

Pediatrics (<18 years of age): MIRENA is not the contraceptive method of first choice for young, nulligravid women. Controlled clinical trials were done in previously parous women aged mainly over 18 years. Use of this product before menarche is not indicated.

Geriatrics: MIRENA is not indicated for use in postmenopausal women.

Monitoring and Laboratory Tests: Physical Examination and Follow-up: Before insertion, the woman must be informed of the efficacy, risks, and side effects of MIRENA. As well, before MIRENA is inserted, a thorough history and physical examination should be performed, including a blood pressure determination. Breasts, liver, extremities, and pelvic organs should be examined. A Papanicolaou smear should be taken if the patient has been sexually active. Pregnancy and sexually transmitted diseases should be excluded, and genital infections have to be successfully treated.

Women should be re-examined 4 to 12 weeks after insertion and at least once a year thereafter, or more frequently if clinically indicated. At each annual visit, examination should include those procedures that were done at the initial visit as outlined above or per recommendations of the Canadian Task Force on the Periodic Health Examination.

See also Dosage and Administration, Medical Examination/Consultation.

ADVERSE REACTIONS: Adverse Drug Reaction Overview: The most commonly occurring adverse events (ie, in greater than 10% of users) that are observed post-marketing with MIRENA (levonorgestrel-releasing intrauterine system) are uterine/vaginal bleeding (including frequent, prolonged or heavy bleeding, spotting, oligomenorrhea, amenorrhea) and benign ovarian cysts.

Clinical Trial Adverse Drug Reactions: Because clinical trials are conducted under very specific conditions the adverse drug reaction rates observed in the clinical trials may not reflect the rates observed in practice and should not be compared to the rates in the clinical trials of another drug. Adverse drug reaction information from clinical trials is useful for identifying drug-related adverse events and for approximating rates.

Adverse drug reactions (ADRs) were collected from a total of 3754 subjects using MIRENA during 9 clinical trials in contraception (n=3422) and 10 clinical trials in menorrhagia (n=332), worldwide. The length of treatment varied between studies: from 3 months to 5 years in the MIRENA menorrhagia studies and from 1.5 months to 5 years in the MIRENA contraception studies.

ADRs were more common during the first months after insertion of MIRENA, and then gradually decreased over time. The ADR safety profile was consistent across the two indications. See Table 1.

Post-Market Adverse Drug Reactions: Based on approximately 12.7 million insertions, the reporting rate for suspected uterine perforation with MIRENA is 0.21 per 1000 insertions.

Undesirable effects are more common during the first months after insertion and subside during prolonged use. In addition to the adverse events observed in clinical trials, the following undesirable effects have been reported in users of MIRENA, although a causal relationship with MIRENA could not always be confirmed. See Table 2.

Device breakage has been reported with the use of MIRENA. This can occur with MIRENA in place or during its removal. The broken pieces should be located and removed; surgery may be required. Check device integrity when removing MIRENA.

DRUG INTERACTIONS: Drug-Drug Interactions: The effect of hormonal contraceptives may be impaired by drugs which induce liver enzymes, including primidone, barbiturates, phenytoin, carbamazepine, rifampicin and griseofulvin. The influence of these drugs on the efficacy of MIRENA (levonorgestrel-releasing intrauterine system) has not been studied, but it is not believed to be of major importance due to the local action of MIRENA.

Drug-Food Interactions: Interactions with food have not been established.

Drug-Herb Interactions: Interactions with herbal products have not been established.

Drug-Laboratory Test Interactions: Interactions with laboratory tests have not been established.

Tissue Specimens: Pathologists should be advised of MIRENA therapy when specimens obtained from surgical procedures and Pap smears are submitted for examination.

Drug-Lifestyle Interactions: The effect of MIRENA on the ability to drive or to use machines has not been studied. Patients should be advised not to drive or use machines until they know how they react to MIRENA.

Table 1: MIRENA

Number and Percentage of Subjects (≥1.0%) with Treatment-related AEs (ADRs) by Preferred Team[a]—FAS for all Contraception and Menorrhagia Studies with MIRENA

System Organ Class	N=3754 Very Common (≥10%)	N=3754 Common (≥1% to <10%)
Gastrointestinal Disorders		Abdominal pain Nausea Pelvic pain
General Disorders		Pain
Infections and Infestations		Vaginal infection
Injury, Poisoning, and Procedural Complications		Procedural pain
Investigations		Weight increased
Musculoskeletal and Connective Tissue Disorders		Back pain
Nervous System Disorders		Headache
Psychiatric Disorders		Depression Libido decreased Nervousness
Reproductive System and Breast Disorders	Amenorrhea Hypomenorrhea Menstrual disorder Metrorrhagia	Breast pain Breast tenderness Dysmenorrhea Genital hemorrhage IUD complication Menometrorrhagia Menorrhagia Menstruation irregular Oligomenorrhea Ovarian cyst Polymenorrhea Vaginal/genital discharge
Skin and Subcutaneous Tissue Disorders		Skin disorder

[a] MedDRA Version 11.0 coding.
Legend: N=total number of subjects.
Note: In original study reports causalities of related AEs are defined as 'Yes', 'Possible', 'Probable', or 'Certain'.

Table 2: MIRENA

Adverse Reactions Identified in Postmarketing Surveillance

Gastrointestinal Disorders	Abdominal bloating
General Disorders and Administration Site Conditions	Expulsion, device breakage
Reproductive System and Breast Disorders	Breast cancer, breast tension, mastalgia, pelvic pain, uterine perforation
Skin and Subcutaneous Disorders	Chloasma, hirsutism, rash, urticaria

DOSAGE AND ADMINISTRATION: Recommended Dose: Following insertion into the uterine cavity, MIRENA (levonorgestrel-releasing intrauterine system) is effective for up to five years. The in vivo dissolution rate is approximately 20 μg levonorgestrel per day initially, and diminishes over time to approximately 10 μg per day after five years. The mean dissolution rate is approximately 14 μg per day over five years.

If after 5 years, continued use of MIRENA is desired a new MIRENA system should be inserted immediately after the old one is removed.

Administration: Medical Examination/Consultation: Before insertion, the patient must be informed of the efficacy, risks and side effects of MIRENA. A physical examination including pelvic examination, examination of the breasts and cervical smear should be performed. Pregnancy and sexually transmitted diseases should be excluded and any genital infections must be successfully treated. The position of the uterus and the size of the uterine cavity should be determined. Fundal positioning of MIRENA is particularly important in order to ensure uniform exposure of the endometrium to the progestogen, prevent expulsion and maximize efficacy. The instructions for insertion should be followed carefully. The patient should be re-examined 4 to 12 weeks after insertion and once-a-year thereafter, or more frequently if clinically indicated.

Insertion, Removal and Replacement: In women of fertile age, MIRENA should be inserted within seven days of the onset of menstruation. MIRENA may be replaced by a new system at any time during the cycle. The system can also be inserted immediately after first trimester abortion. Postpartum insertions should be postponed until the uterus is fully involuted, and not earlier than six weeks after delivery. If involution is substantially delayed, consider waiting until 12 weeks postpartum. In case of a difficult insertion and/or exceptional pain or bleeding during or after insertion, physical examination and ultrasound should be performed immediately to exclude perforation.

MIRENA is not suitable for use as a post-coital contraceptive.

Because irregular bleeding is common during the first months of therapy, it is recommended to exclude endometrial pathology before insertion of MIRENA. If bleeding irregularities develop during prolonged treatment, appropriate diagnostic measures should be undertaken.

MIRENA can be removed by gently pulling on the removal threads with forceps. If the threads are not visible and the system is in the uterine cavity, it may be removed using a narrow tenaculum. This may require dilatation of the cervical canal.

After removal of MIRENA, verify that the system is intact. During difficult removals (ie, removal through a tight cervical canal or surgical removal after perforation), the hormone cylinder may slide over and cover the horizontal arms. This situation generally does not require further intervention once the system is verified to be intact. The reporting rate for hormone cylinder dislocation/shifting with MIRENA is approximately 7 per 1 million insertions.

The system should be removed after five years of use. If the patient wishes to continue using MIRENA, a new system can be inserted at the time of removal of the old one. If pregnancy is not desired, removal should be carried out during menstruation in women of fertile age provided that there appears to be a menstrual cycle. If the system is removed mid-cycle and the patient has had intercourse within a week, she is at risk of pregnancy unless a new system is inserted immediately following removal.

Insertion and removal may be associated with some pain and bleeding. The procedure may cause a fainting spell or precipitate a seizure in an epileptic patient. It is recommended to wait 24 to 48 hours before having sexual intercourse in the event of general discomfort after insertion of MIRENA.

Expulsion: Symptoms of the partial or complete expulsion of MIRENA may include bleeding or pain, however, a system may be expelled from the uterine cavity without the patient noticing it. Partial expulsion may decrease the effectiveness of MIRENA. Since MIRENA decreases menstrual flow, an increase in menstrual flow may indicate an expulsion. A displaced system should be removed. A new system can be inserted at that time and the patient should be advised on how to check for the presence of the system by feeling for the removal threads.

In a five-year clinical trial, the net cumulative expulsion rate ranged from 3.4 per 100 women in year one to 4.9 in year five. Expulsion rates for MIRENA are comparable to those observed for copper IUDs.

In the same clinical trial, the net cumulative removal rate due to pain ranged from 1.6 per 100 women in the first year to 4.2 in the fifth year.

Lost Removal Threads: If the threads are not visible upon follow-up examination, they may have retracted into the uterus or broken, or MIRENA may have broken, perforated the uterus, or been expelled. If the length of the threads has changed from the length at the time of insertion, the system may have become displaced (see Expulsion). Pregnancy must be excluded and the location of MIRENA must be verified by sonography, X-ray (MIRENA is radiopaque), or by gentle exploration of the uterine cavity with a probe. If MIRENA is displaced, remove it. A new MIRENA may be inserted at that time or during the next menses if it is certain that conception has not occurred.

Missed Dose: MIRENA should be removed after 5 years. If the user wishes to continue using MIRENA, a new system can be inserted replacing the old system. If the system has been used for a longer period of time than 5 years, pregnancy should be ruled out before insertion of a new system.

Insertion Instructions:

Because the insertion technique is different from other intrauterine devices, it is important that physicians receive training on the correct insertion technique.

Physicians should become thoroughly familiar with the insertion instructions in their entirety before insertion of MIRENA.

MIRENA is supplied in a sterile pouch which should not be opened until required for insertion. It is sterilized with ethylene oxide. Do not resterilize. For single use only. Do not use if the seal of the sterile pouch is broken, or if the pouch is damaged or opened. The exposed product should be handled with aseptic precautions. Insert before the date indicated on the label.

MIRENA is inserted into the uterine cavity using the enclosed inserter within seven days of the onset of menstruation by carefully following these insertion instructions. It can be replaced by a new system at any time during the menstrual cycle.

Conduct a gynecological examination of the patient to establish the size and position of the uterus and to exclude pregnancy or other genital tract contraindications for the use of MIRENA.

Preparation for Insertion:

1. Visualize the cervix with the aid of a speculum and thoroughly cleanse the cervix and vagina with a suitable antiseptic solution.
2. Grasp the upper lip of the cervix with a suitable holding forceps. Gentle traction on the holding forceps has been shown to align the cervical canal with the uterine cavity. The forceps should remain in position throughout the insertion procedure to maintain gentle traction on the cervix to facilitate insertion.
3. Gently move a uterine sound into the uterine cavity to the fundus to determine the direction of the cervical canal and the depth of the uterine cavity (sound measure), and to exclude a uterine septum, synechiae or submucosal fibroids. It is important not to force the insertion. Should the cervical canal be too narrow, consider the need for dilatation and the use of analgesics or paracervical block.

Insertion: Step 1—Opening of the sterile package:

- Open the sterile package completely.
- Place sterile gloves on your hands.
- Pick up the handle of the inserter containing MIRENA and carefully release the threads so that they hang freely.

Place your thumb or forefinger on the slider. Make sure that the slider is in the furthest position away from you, for example, at the top of the handle towards the insertion tube.

Note: Keep your thumb or forefinger on the slider until insertion is complete.

- With the centimeter scale of the insertion tube facing up, check that the arms of MIRENA are in a horizontal position. If they are not, align them on a flat, sterile surface, for example, the sterile package.

Step 2—Load MIRENA into the insertion tube:

- Holding the slider in the furthest position, pull on both threads to load MIRENA into the insertion tube.
- Note that the knobs at the ends of the arms now meet to close the open end of the insertion tube.

If the knobs do not meet properly: If the knobs do not meet properly, release the arms by pulling the slider back to the mark (raised horizontal line on the handle). Re-load MIRENA by aligning the open arms on a sterile surface. Return the slider to its furthermost position and pull on both threads. Check for proper loading.

Step 3—Secure the threads: Secure the threads in the cleft at the bottom end of the handle to keep MIRENA in the loaded position.

Step 4—Setting the flange: Set the upper edge of the flange to the depth measured during the uterine sounding.

Step 5—MIRENA is now ready to be inserted:

- Continue to hold the slider with the thumb or forefinger firmly in the furthermost position. Grasp the tenaculum forceps with your other hand and apply gentle traction to align the cervical canal with the uterine cavity.
- While maintaining traction on the cervix, gently advance the insertion tube through the cervical canal and into the uterine cavity **until the flange is 1.5 to 2 cm from the external cervical os.**
- **Caution: do not advance flange to the cervix at this step.** Maintaining the flange 1.5 to 2 cm from the cervical os allows sufficient space for the arms to open (when released) within the uterine cavity.

Note: Do not force the inserter. If necessary, dilate the cervical canal.

Step 6—Release the arms:

- While holding the inserter steady, release the arms of MIRENA by pulling the slider back until the top of the slider reaches the mark (raised horizontal line on the handle).
- Wait approximately 10 seconds to allow the horizontal arms of MIRENA to open and regain its T-shape.

Step 7—Advance to fundal position: Gently advance the inserter into the uterine cavity until the flange meets the cervix and you feel fundal resistance. MIRENA should now be in the desired fundal position.

Step 8—Release MIRENA and withdraw the inserter:

- While holding the inserter steady, pull the slider all the way down to release MIRENA from the insertion tube. The threads will release automatically from the cleft.
- Check that the threads are hanging freely and gently withdraw the inserter from the uterus. Be careful not to pull on the threads as this will displace MIRENA.

Step 9—Cut the threads:

- Cut the threads perpendicular to the thread length, for example, with sterile curved scissors, leaving about 3 cm visible outside the cervix.

Note: Cutting threads at an angle may leave sharp ends.

MIRENA insertion is now complete.

In case difficulties arise during insertion, the patient complains of pain, or if there is any doubt that the system is not in the correct position, verify with ultrasound or X-ray. Remove the system if it is not positioned properly in the intrauterine cavity, and insert a new one. A removed system must never be reinserted.

Patients should be re-examined 4 to 12 weeks after insertion and once a year thereafter, or more frequently if clinically indicated.

Use of Sanitary Pads: The use of sanitary pads is recommended. If tampons are used, they should be changed carefully to avoid inadvertently pulling the MIRENA removal threads.

Removal of MIRENA: MIRENA can be removed by pulling the threads with forceps.

A MIRENA system should not remain in the uterus longer than 5 years.

OVERDOSAGE:

Not applicable. MIRENA is an intrauterine system.

For management of a suspected drug overdose, CPhA recommends that you contact your **regional Poison Control Centre**. See the *CPS Directory* section for a list of Poison Control Centres.

ACTION AND CLINICAL PHARMACOLOGY: Mechanism of Action: MIRENA (levonorgestrel-releasing intrauterine system) consists of a small polyethylene T-shaped frame with a cylindrical reservoir containing levonorgestrel around the vertical arm of the T frame. After insertion into the uterus, MIRENA releases levonorgestrel continuously for up to five years. Intrauterine administration allows a very low daily dosage, as the hormone is released directly to the target organ. MIRENA contains a total of 52 mg levonorgestrel and has an initial intrauterine release rate of 20 µg per day that diminishes over time to approximately 10 µg per day after 5 years.

Pharmacodynamics: The contraceptive action of MIRENA is due mainly to the local progestogenic effect of levonorgestrel on the uterine cavity. It produces a strong antiproliferative effect on the endometrium and causes a thickening of the cervical mucus which prevents passage of sperm through the cervical canal. Ovulation is inhibited in some women. Clinical trials with MIRENA were performed in parous women mainly over the age of 18 years; results from these studies involving more than 7600 woman-years of use indicate an overall Pearl index of 0.11. The 5-year cumulative gross pregnancy rates in these trials ranged from 0 to 1.2 per 100 women.

Normal menstruation returns quickly after removal of MIRENA. After five years of use in clinical trials, the return of normal cyclical endometrial morphology was observed to occur from one to three months after removal of MIRENA. The use of MIRENA does not alter the course of future fertility; nearly 90% of women wishing to become pregnant conceive within 24 months after removal of the system.

The duration and volume of menstrual bleeding and menstrual blood loss gradually decreases during the first few months of use. With continued use, bleeding patterns vary from regular scanty menstruation in some women to oligomenorrhea or amenorrhea in others.

The menstrual bleeding patterns of 1495 women enrolled in a clinical trial were examined for the first 12 months after MIRENA insertion. The number of combined days of vaginal bleeding or spotting decreased from a mean of 16.1 days during the first month, to a mean of 3.8 days during the 12th month (see Table 3).

Table 3: MIRENA

Number of Combined Vaginal Bleeding/Spotting Days During the First 12 Months After MIRENA Insertion

	Interval (in 30-Day segments) Days											
	1–30	31–60	61–90	91–120	121–150	151–180	181–210	211–240	241–270	271–300	301–330	331–360
N	1495	1472	1422	1297	1237	1199	1168	1142	1113	1079	1055	988
Mean	16.1	11.2	8.5	7.1	6.4	5.8	5.2	4.8	4.5	4.3	4.1	3.8

The altered menstrual bleeding pattern that occurs with MIRENA use is a result of the direct action of levonorgestrel on the endometrium and is not due to the suppression of the ovulatory cycle. There is no clear difference in follicle development, ovulation, or estradiol and progesterone production in women with different bleeding patterns. Ovarian function is normal and estradiol levels are maintained even when users of MIRENA are amenorrheic.

The effect of MIRENA on ovarian function depends on plasma levonorgestrel levels achieved. While marked interindividual variation is observed, plasma concentrations are relatively constant within each individual. Patterns of ovarian function in women using MIRENA include normal ovulatory cycles, anovulatory cycles with some inhibition of estradiol production, anovulation with high follicular activity and ovulation with an inadequate luteal phase. In general, anovulatory cycles correlate with higher plasma levels of levonorgestrel, and are more frequent in the first year of MIRENA use. Functional ovarian cysts may occur in relation to pre-ovulatory arrest of follicular development in any woman, and are associated with progestogen-only methods of contraception.

Endometrial histology has been investigated in clinical studies examining the intrauterine release of levonorgestrel at rates ranging from 10 to 40 µg/day. Subjects with anywhere from 3 to 84 months of exposure to continuous levonorgestrel release showed endometrial glandular atrophy and decidualized stroma throughout the period. Local inflammation and focal necrosis compatible with the intrauterine mode of administration were observed.

In one study, cervical histology was evaluated by examining cervical smears from 1355 women using MIRENA over a period of five years. A total of twelve smears indicated moderate to severe cervical dysplasia. Large multi-centre studies have not detected differences in cervical cytology between women using MIRENA and those using copper IUDs.

Pharmacokinetics: Absorption: The intrauterine release of levonorgestrel results in the absorption of the drug into the systemic circulation.

Distribution: The drug can be detected in plasma within 15 minutes of insertion and maximum concentrations are seen within a few hours. Following intrauterine insertion of MIRENA, the initial release rate of levonorgestrel is 20 µg per day. This provides stable plasma levonorgestrel concentrations which, after the first few weeks, stabilize at between 150 to 200 pg/mL in women of fertile age. After 12, 24, and 60 months of use in young women, plasma levonorgestrel concentrations of 180±66 pg/mL, 192±140 pg/mL, and 159±60 pg/mL were observed, respectively. Because of the low drug levels in plasma, the systemic effects of the progestogen are minimized.

Orally administered levonorgestrel is rapidly and completely absorbed and the absolute bioavailability is about 90%. Levonorgestrel is bound to serum albumin and to sex hormone-binding globulin (SHBG). The relative distribution (free, albumin-bound, SHBG-bound) depends on the SHBG concentration in the serum. Only about 2.5% of the total serum drug levels are present as free steroid, but 47.5% and 50% are bound to SHBG and albumin, respectively. For levonorgestrel, a mean volume of distribution of approximately 137 L and a metabolic clearance rate from serum of about 5.7 L/hr were reported.

Metabolism and Excretion: The terminal half-life in serum is in the range of 14 to 20 hours after single-dose administration.

Levonorgestrel is excreted as metabolites at about equal proportion in urine and feces. The metabolites have little or no pharmacological activity. The principal metabolite in urine is tetrahydronorgestrel which accounts for approximately 25% of the radioactivity recovered from the urine after administration of radiolabeled levonorgestrel. A published study indicated that during lactation, 0.1% of the daily maternal dose of levonorgestrel could be transferred to the newborn via milk.

STORAGE AND STABILITY: Store at room temperature (between 15 and 30°C). Protect from moisture and direct sunlight. Keep out of reach of children and pets.

SPECIAL HANDLING INSTRUCTIONS: MIRENA (levonorgestrel-releasing intrauterine system) should be handled with aseptic precautions. Used MIRENA systems should be considered biohazardous waste and disposed of accordingly. Care should be taken to ensure the remaining hormonal ingredients are not introduced into water/sewer systems.

INFORMATION FOR THE PATIENT: Published in e-CPS, available by subscription at www.e-cps.ca.

DOSAGE FORMS, COMPOSITION AND PACKAGING: Each sterile intrauterine system contains: levonorgestrel USP 52 mg in a cylindrical-shaped reservoir composed of a matrix of levonorgestrel and polydimethylsiloxane. The reservoir is mounted on the vertical arm of a T-shaped frame made of polyethylene and covered with a rate-controlling membrane of polydimethylsiloxane and silica. The T-frame is pigmented with barium sulphate. The polyethylene removal threads attached to the T-frame are pigmented with black iron oxide. Pouches containing the sterile intrauterine system within an inserter, cartons of 1.

(Shown in Product Identification Section)

Misoprostol

Mucosal Protective Agent

CPhA Monograph

Date of Preparation: November 2004
Date of Revision: October 2008

This monograph has been compiled by CPhA and reviewed by experts. It may contain information different from that found in Health Canada-approved Product Monographs. The reader is referred to the *CPS* Editorial Policy for more information.

SUMMARY PRODUCT INFORMATION:

Route of Administration	Dosage Form	Product Strength
Oral	Tablet	100 µg, 200 µg

INDICATIONS AND CLINICAL USE: Misoprostol is indicated for:

- the treatment and prevention of NSAID-induced gastroduodenal ulcers; the risk of developing an NSAID-induced ulcer is greater in persons over the age of 65, and with use of more than one NSAID, higher doses of NSAIDs, concomitant use of steroids or anticoagulants, a past history of ulcer disease and coexisting ischemic heart disease.
- the treatment of duodenal ulcers caused by peptic ulcer disease.

Uses Not Approved in Canada: The Society of Obstetricians and Gynecologists of Canada (SOGC) Guidelines for Induced Abortion 2006, recommend misoprostol as an option in the following situations: medical abortion alone or in combination with methotrexate; cervical ripening prior to surgical abortion; evacuation of the uterus in the case of miscarriage or fetal demise. An international joint policy statement, "Management of the Third Stage of Labour to Prevent Postpartum Hemorrhage" endorsed by the SOGC in 2003 includes misoprostol as an option for prevention of postpartum hemorrhage. Misoprostol has been studied for induction of labour at term. It has also been used to facilitate transcervical procedures including dilatation and curettage, hysteroscopy and intrauterine device insertion. Misoprostol is not recommended as a method of induction or cervical ripening in women who have had a previous caesarian delivery, due to an increased risk of uterine rupture.

Pediatrics: Safety and efficacy of misoprostol in children below the age of 18 have not been established.

CONTRAINDICATIONS: Patients who are hypersensitive to misoprostol or prostaglandins or to any ingredient in the various formulations.

Because of its abortifacient properties, misoprostol should not be used to reduce the risk of NSAID-induced ulcers in pregnant women. Furthermore, it may cause congenital anomalies in the fetus. Malformations are thought to be due to a disturbed blood supply to the developing embryo during misoprostol induced uterine contractions [*Int J Gynaecol Obstet* 2007;99(Suppl 2):S160-7].

Misoprostol should not be used to reduce the risk of NSAID-induced ulcers in women of childbearing potential unless the benefits outweigh the risk as determined by the patient and physician. In such situations, misoprostol should not be initiated until the possibility of pregnancy has been excluded and an effective method of contraception started. A reliable blood pregnancy test should be performed within 2 weeks prior to the start of misoprostol therapy. The medication should not be provided to the patient until the pregnancy test is reported as negative. In addition, written and oral information about the medication should be given to the patient. Initiation of therapy should begin on the 2nd or 3rd day of the next normal menstrual period.

WARNINGS AND PRECAUTIONS: Gastrointestinal: Reports of profound diarrhea such as voluminous, watery diarrhea resulting in severe dehydration have been documented. Such diarrhea has resulted in severe metabolic acidosis and can be life-threatening. Patients with inflammatory bowel disease may be at increased risk of developing diarrhea. Misoprostol can also exacerbate intestinal inflammation in these patients; careful monitoring is essential in this patient population.

Special Populations: Pregnant Women: Misoprostol is a potent uterine stimulant that induces abortion in early pregnancy, and labour in advanced pregnancy. Premature labor or birth defects can also result when misoprostol is administered to pregnant women. See Contraindications.

Nursing Women: To date, there have been no studies evaluating the passage of misoprostol or its active metabolite, misoprostol acid, into breast milk. Because of the potential for severe, drug-induced diarrhea in the nursing infant, a decision should be made whether to discontinue nursing, or the drug, taking into account the importance of the drug to the mother.

ADVERSE REACTIONS: More Common Adverse Drug Reactions: General: The most common adverse drug reactions encountered with misoprostol are gastrointestinal. Mild dose-related diarrhea occurs in 14-40% of patients. Onset is about two weeks after starting misoprostol and it usually resolves within a week. Diarrhea can be minimized by administering divided doses after meals and at bedtime, or starting with a low dose and titrating up. Abdominal pain has been reported in 7-20% of patients. Headache occurs in approximately 2% of patients.

Obstetric/Gynecologic Use: When used for uterine evacuation in medical termination of pregnancy or pregnancy failure, vaginal bleeding and uterine cramping (possibly heavy and severe) are expected side effects. Soaking of 2 pads per hour for 2 hours in a row should be a trigger for the patient to call the health care provider [*Obstet Gynecol* 2005;106(4):871-82]. Chills are a common side effect but are transient. Fever can also occur and is more common with higher doses and shorter intervals and with oral or sublingual administration. If fever or chills persist beyond 24 hours after misoprostol, the possibility of infection should be investigated. Analgesics including NSAIDs may be given for cramping, fever and chills without affecting misoprostol's efficacy. Nausea and vomiting may occur but will resolve within 2-6 hours after misoprostol. Diarrhea may also occur following misoprostol administration, but should resolve within one day.

Less Common Adverse Drug Reactions: General: Reported rarely and not necessarily causally linked to misoprostol are: anaphylaxis, anxiety, appetite changes, arrhythmia, arterial thrombosis, bronchospasm, confusion, cramps, depression, drowsiness, edema, fever, GI bleeding, GI inflammation, gingivitis, gout, hypertension, hypotension, impotence, loss of libido, menstrual irregularities, MI, neuropathy, neurosis, pulmonary embolism, purpura, rash, reflux, rigors, thrombocytopenia, weakness, and weight change.

Obstetric/Gynecologic Use: When tablets are used sublingually or buccally unpleasant taste has been reported. Sense of numbness over the mouth and throat has been reported with sublingual use. Skin rash occurs occasionally and usually resolves within several hours. Uterine rupture is a rare complication reported mostly when misoprostol is used for medical termination of pregnancy between 13 and 26 weeks gestation, and may even occur in women who do not have a uterine scar.

DRUG INTERACTIONS: Overview: Misoprostol is rapidly de-esterified in the liver to its active metabolite, misoprostol acid. It is not metabolized by the hepatic CYP450 enzyme system and neither induces or inhibits it. See Table 1.

Drug-Drug Interactions: See Table 1.

Table 1: Misoprostol

Drug-Drug Interactions

Interacting Drug	Effect	Clinical Comment
Antacids	Possibly decreases the rate of absorption resulting in delayed and decreased peak plasma concentrations of misoprostol acid. Magnesium-containing antacids may increase the incidence of misoprostol-induced diarrhea.	Decreased oral bioavailability of misoprostol. May not be clinically important since misoprostol's activity in protecting the GI mucosa appears to be local rather than systemic. If concomitant administration of an antacid is necessary, avoid magnesium-containing or other laxative-containing antacids. Use a constipating (e.g., aluminum-containing) antacid instead.
Oxytocin	Enhanced therapeutic effect of oxytocin.	The oxytocic activity of oxytocin may be augmented by agents used to promote cervical ripening and uterine contractions (including misoprostol). Caution is advised.

Drug-Food Interactions: Food slows the absorption of misoprostol, reducing the peak concentration (C_{max}) and increasing the time to reach C_{max} after a 400 µg dose. This interaction is clinically insignificant since misoprostol's ability to protect the GI mucosa appears to be local rather than systemic.

DOSAGE AND ADMINISTRATION: Dosing Considerations: Administer with food to minimize the incidence of diarrhea.

In older adults, start slow and titrate up to avoid the potential for diarrhea. The following recommendation can be made: start at 100 µg/day orally and increase by 100 µg/day at 3-day intervals until the desired dose is achieved.

No dosage adjustment is necessary in renal impairment. If the dose is not tolerated, the dose may be reduced. Alternatively, start slow (100 µg four times daily) and titrate up.

For obstetric/gynecologic use, choice of route of administration may depend on clinical situation. (See Action and Clinical Pharmacology, Pharmacokinetics.)

Recommended Dosing (see also Indications and Clinical Use): Treatment and Prevention of NSAID-induced Gastroduodenal Ulcers and Treatment of Duodenal Ulcers Caused by Peptic Ulcer Disease: 200 µg orally 4 times daily with food. The last dose of the day should be taken at bedtime. If not tolerated, may decrease dose to 100 µg 4 times daily or 200 µg twice daily. Alternatively, start slow and titrate up to a tolerable therapeutic dose. Administer for the duration of NSAID therapy.

Medical Termination of Pregnancy: In combination with methotrexate up to 56 days gestation: 800 µg vaginal misoprostol 5-7 days after methotrexate 50 mg/m² orally or intramuscularly, may repeat misoprostol dose in 24 h if needed. Misoprostol alone up to 56 days gestation: 800 µg vaginally Q24-48H max 3 doses. Second trimester termination by induction of labour: 200 µg vaginally Q12H for up to 48 h [*SOGC Induced Abortion Guidelines* 2006].

Cervical Ripening Prior to Surgical Abortion: ≤13 weeks gestation: 400 µg oral or vaginal misoprostol 4-12 h prior to procedure; for gestations 14-16 weeks 600 µg buccally 2-4 h prior to procedure (if misoprostol is administered vaginally more than 4 h prior to procedure there is potential for unexpected and therefore unsupervised delivery) [*SOGC Induced Abortion Guidelines* 2006].

Evacuation of the Uterus Due to Miscarriage or Fetal Demise: 200 µg vaginally Q12H up to 48 h [*SOGC Induced Abortion Guidelines* 2006].

Prevention of Postpartum Hemorrhage: 600 µg orally or sublingually to be given immediately after delivery of the baby only in situations in which use of injectable oxytocin or ergot alkaloids is not possible. In the event of continued hemorrhage, a minimum of 2 hours should elapse before a second dose is given. This interval should be increased to 6 hours if the initial dose was associated with pyrexia or marked shivering. [*Int J Gynaecol Obstet* 2007;99(Suppl 2):S198-201].

Induction of Labour at Term: The Federation of International Gynecologists and Obstetricians (FIGO) suggests the following dosage options: 25 µg misoprostol vaginally Q4H (max 6 doses), 50 µg misoprostol orally Q4H (max 6 doses), 20 µg misoprostol solution (made by dissolving tablet in water) orally Q2H (max 12 doses). Contraindicated in women with previous caesarean sections due to reports of uterine rupture [*Int J Gynaecol Obstet* 2007;99(Suppl 2):S194-7].

Facilitation of Transcervical Procedures: For cervical priming prior to instrumentation (e.g., dilatation and curettage, hysteroscopy, intrauterine device insertion) FIGO suggests 400 µg misoprostol vaginally or sublingually 3 hours before the procedure [*Int J Gynaecol Obstet* 2007;99(Suppl 2):S168-71].

Administration (see also Indications and Clinical Use): Oral: Tablets should be swallowed whole. Misoprostol may be administered with meals.

Vaginal: Oral tablets placed high in the vagina. Studies have shown that moistening the tablets prior to insertion does not improve efficacy.

Sublingual: Oral tablets are kept under the tongue until dissolved or for at least 20 minutes and then swallowed. Some patients have reported unpleasant taste and sense of numbness across mouth and throat with this route.

Buccal: Oral tablets are placed between the teeth and cheek and allowed to dissolve (usually 10-20 minutes).

Rectal: Oral tablets are placed in the rectum and allowed to dissolve.

OVERDOSAGE:

For management of a suspected drug overdose, CPhA recommends that you contact your **regional Poison Control Centre**. See the *CPS* Directory section for a list of Poison Control Centres.

ACTION AND CLINICAL PHARMACOLOGY: Misoprostol, a synthetic analogue of prostaglandin E_1, is rapidly de-esterified to misoprostol acid in the stomach upon oral administration. The active metabolite then binds to specific prostaglandin receptors on the gastric parietal cells thus inhibiting acid production. Though the mechanism of gastrointestinal mucosal protective effect is not well understood, it is thought that misoprostol may increase mucus production, increase bicarbonate secretion in the duodenum, increase mucosal blood flow, decrease vascular permeability, increase cellular proliferation and migration and restore gastric potential difference. It also replaces prostaglandins that have been depleted due to various insults in the area.

Misoprostol has been shown to be an effective myometrial stimulant of the pregnant uterus, selectively binding to EP-2/EP-3 prostanoid receptors. Studies show that the initial effect of increased uterine tonus is replaced by regular uterine contractions after 1-2 hours when a very low, but sustained serum level of misoprostol is maintained. (See Pharmacokinetics.) This is complicated by the fact that the sensitivity of the uterus to prostaglandins increases with gestation. Misoprostol has also exhibited a significant cervical priming effect in the pregnant state. There is evidence suggesting that misoprostol's effects on the uterus and cervix may also be seen in the non-pregnant state.

Pharmacokinetics: General: Absorption: Misoprostol, an ester, undergoes rapid de-esterification to its pharmacologically active metabolite, misoprostol acid, in the stomach after oral administration. Absorption of misoprostol acid is rapid, with peak plasma concentrations occurring within 15 to 30 minutes and rapidly declining within 120 minutes. The plasma half-life of the acid is 13 to 40 minutes. Plasma steady state is achieved within 2 days. Misoprostol acid does not accumulate when misoprostol is taken chronically.

Distribution: Only 7% of the dose is systemically bioavailable as the acid following oral administration. Approximately 85% of the misoprostol acid is bound to serum albumin.

Metabolism: Misoprostol acid is metabolized by the liver but it does not inhibit or induce the hepatic CYP450 system.

Excretion: Inactive metabolites are secreted in the urine.

Obstetrics and Gynecology: The pharmacokinetic profile of the various routes of administration is important when using misoprostol for obstetric/gynecologic applications. Sublingual administration has the shortest T_{max} (30 min) and is perhaps useful in situations where a fast onset of action is required such as postpartum hemorrhage or cervical priming. Vaginal misoprostol exhibits longer T_{max} (75 min), but high bioavailability and sustained serum levels (≥6 hours) making it useful for situations that require long duration of effect such as medical abortion.

Mitoxantrone Injection USP Ⓟ

mitoxantrone HCl

Antineoplastic

Hospira

SUPPLIED: Each mL of clear, dark blue sterile aqueous solution contains: 2 mg mitoxantrone HCl equivalent to mitoxantrone (free base). Nonmedicinal ingredients: acetic acid 0.46 mg, sodium acetate 0.05 mg and sodium chloride 8.0 mg. Sodium metabisulfite is used during production but does not appear in the final product. Must be diluted before use. Single use vials of 10 mL. Store between 15 and 25°C. Protect from light and freezing. Keep out of reach of children. Discard unused portion.

M-M-R® II

measles, mumps and rubella virus vaccine, live, attenuated, Merck Frosst Std.

Active Immunizing Agent

Merck Frosst

Date of Revision: February 26, 2009

SUMMARY PRODUCT INFORMATION:

Route of Administration	Dosage Form/ Strength	Clinically Relevant Nonmedicinal Ingredients
Subcutaneous	Lyophilized powder for injection 0.5 mL dose after reconstitution Measles: ≥1000 $CCID_{50}$ Mumps: ≥5000 $CCID_{50}$ Rubella: ≥1000 $CCID_{50}$	Gelatin, neomycin, recombinant human albumin For a complete listing see Dosage Forms, Composition and Packaging.

DESCRIPTION: M-M-R II (measles, mumps and rubella virus vaccine, live, attenuated, Merck Frosst Std.) is a sterile lyophilized preparation of (1) ATTENUVAX (measles virus vaccine, live, attenuated, Merck Frosst Std.), a more attenuated line of measles virus, derived from Enders' attenuated Edmonston strain and propagated in chick embryo cell culture; (2) MUMPSVAX (mumps virus vaccine, live, attenuated, Merck Frosst Std.), the Jeryl Lynn (B level) strain of mumps virus propagated in chick embryo cell cultures; and (3) MERUVAX II (rubella virus vaccine, live, attenuated, Merck Frosst Std.), the Wistar RA 27/3 strain of live attenuated rubella virus propagated in human diploid lung fibroblasts (see Warnings and Precautions, Immune and Hypersensitivity).

The growth medium for measles and mumps is Medium 199 (a buffered salt solution containing vitamins and amino acids and supplemented with fetal bovine serum) containing SPGA (sucrose, phosphate, glutamate, and recombinant human albumin) as stabilizer and neomycin.

The growth medium for rubella is Minimum Essential Medium (MEM) (a buffered salt solution containing vitamins and amino acids and supplemented with fetal bovine serum) containing recombinant human albumin and neomycin. Sorbitol and hydrolyzed gelatin stabilizer are added to the individual virus harvests.

The cells, virus pools and fetal bovine serum are all screened for the absence of adventitious agents.

INDICATIONS AND CLINICAL USE: M-M-R II is indicated for simultaneous vaccination against measles, mumps, and rubella in persons 12 months of age or older. A second dose of M-M-R II is recommended (see Dosage and Administration, Revaccination).

Infants who are less than 12 months of age may fail to respond to the measles component of the vaccine due to presence in the circulation of residual measles antibody of maternal origin; the younger the infant, the lower the likelihood of seroconversion. In geographically isolated or other relatively inaccessible populations for whom immunization programs are logistically difficult, and in population groups in which wild-type measles infection may occur in a significant proportion of infants before one year of age, it may be desirable to give the vaccine to infants during their first year of life. Infants vaccinated under these conditions at less than 12 months of age should be revaccinated (two additional doses) after reaching 12 months of age. There is some evidence to suggest that infants who are born to mothers who had wild-type measles and who are vaccinated at less than one year of age may not develop sustained antibody levels when later revaccinated. The advantage of early protection must be weighed against the chance for failure to respond adequately on reimmunization.

Previously unvaccinated children older than 12 months who are in contact with susceptible pregnant women should receive live attenuated rubella vaccine (such as that contained in monovalent vaccine or in M-M-R II) to reduce the risk of exposure of the pregnant woman.

Individuals planning travel abroad, if not immune, can acquire measles, mumps, or rubella and import these diseases to their country. Therefore, prior to international travel, individuals known to be susceptible to one or more of these diseases can receive either a monovalent vaccine (measles, mumps or rubella), or a combination vaccine as appropriate. However, M-M-R II is preferred for persons likely to be susceptible to mumps and rubella; and if monovalent measles vaccine is not readily available, travelers should receive M-M-R II regardless of their immune status to mumps or rubella.

Vaccination has been recommended for susceptible individuals in high-risk groups such as students at post-secondary institutions, health care workers and military personnel.

Passively acquired antibody can interfere with the response to live, attenuated-virus vaccines. Therefore, administration of M-M-R II should be deferred until approximately three months after passive immunization.

CONTRAINDICATIONS: Hypersensitivity to any component of the vaccine including gelatin. For a complete listing, see Dosage Forms, Composition and Packaging.

Do not give M-M-R II to pregnant females; the possible effects of the vaccine on fetal development are unknown at this time. If vaccination of post-pubertal females is undertaken, pregnancy must be avoided by medically acceptable methods for three months following vaccination (see Warnings and Precautions, Pregnant Women).

Histologic changes, similar to those seen in gestational rubella, have been observed and rubella virus has been recovered from decidua following vaccination of pregnant women with live attenuated rubella vaccine. These vaccines may thus constitute a risk to the fetus.

Anaphylactic or anaphylactoid reactions to neomycin. Each dose of reconstituted vaccine contains approximately 25 µg neomycin.

Any febrile respiratory illness or other active febrile infection.

Active untreated tuberculosis.

Patients receiving immunosuppressive therapy with ACTH, corticosteroids, irradiation, alkylating agents or antimetabolites. This contraindication does not apply to patients who are receiving corticosteroids as replacement therapy, e.g., for Addison's disease.

Individuals with blood dyscrasias, leukemia, lymphomas of any type, or other malignant neoplasms affecting the bone marrow or lymphatic systems.

Primary and acquired immunodeficiency states, including patients who are immunosuppressed in association with AIDS or other clinical manifestation of infection with human immunodeficiency viruses; cellular immune deficiencies, hypogammaglobulinemic and dysgammaglobulinemic states. Measles inclusion body encephalitis (MIBE), pneumonitis and death as a direct consequence of disseminated measles vaccine virus infection has been reported in severely immunocompromised individuals inadvertently vaccinated with measles-containing vaccine. M-M-R II is recommended for asymptomatic HIV-infected individuals. M-M-R II is not normally recommended for symptomatic HIV-infected individuals because safety and immunogenicity data are not yet available. If there is a known exposure to measles, measles-immune globulin (IG) should be given within 6 days whether or not the individual has been vaccinated, although the efficacy of IG for passive immunoprophylaxis of measles in HIV-infected individuals is uncertain.

Individuals with a family history of congenital or hereditary immunodeficiency, until the immune competence of the potential vaccine recipient is demonstrated.

WARNINGS AND PRECAUTIONS: Severe allergic reactions including anaphylaxis can occur after administration of M-M-R II (see Post-Market Adverse Drug Reactions).

General: Administer M-M-R II subcutaneously; **do not give intravascularly**.

Adequate treatment provisions including epinephrine injection (1:1000) should be available for immediate use in case an anaphylactic or anaphylactoid reaction occurs.

Due caution should be employed in administration of M-M-R II to persons with individual or family histories of convulsions, a history of cerebral injury or any other condition in which stress due to fever should be avoided. The physician should be alert to the temperature elevation which may occur 5 to 12 days following vaccination (see Adverse Reactions).

Children and young adults who are known to be infected with human immunodeficiency viruses and are not immunosuppressed may be vaccinated. However, the vaccinees who are infected with HIV should be monitored closely for vaccine-preventable diseases because immunization may be less effective than for uninfected persons (see Contraindications).

Excretion of small amounts of the live attenuated rubella virus from the nose or throat has occurred in the majority of susceptible individuals 7 to 28 days after vaccination. There is no confirmed evidence to indicate that such virus is transmitted to susceptible persons who are in contact with the vaccinated individuals. Consequently, transmission, while accepted as a theoretical possibility, is not regarded as a significant risk. However, transmission of the rubella vaccine virus to infants via breast milk has been documented (see Nursing Women).

There are no reports of transmission of live attenuated measles or mumps viruses from vaccinees to susceptible contacts.

This product contains a trace amount ($<1\times10^{-6}$ mg/dose) of albumin, a derivative of human blood. Although there is a theoretical risk for transmission of Creutzfeldt-Jakob disease (CJD) or its variant (vCJD), no cases of transmission of CJD, vCJD, or viral diseases have ever been identified that were associated with the use of albumin.

As for any vaccine, vaccination with M-M-R II may not result in protection in 100% of vaccinees.

Hematologic: Thrombocytopenia: Individuals with current thrombocytopenia may develop more severe thrombocytopenia following vaccination. In addition, individuals who experienced thrombocytopenia with the first dose of M-M-R II (or its component vaccines) may develop thrombocytopenia with repeat doses. Serologic status may be evaluated to determine whether or not additional doses of vaccine are needed. The potential risk to benefit ratio should be carefully evaluated before considering vaccination in such cases (see Adverse Reactions).

Immune and Hypersensitivity: Live measles vaccine and live mumps vaccine are produced in chick embryo cell culture. Persons with a history of anaphylactic, anaphylactoid or other immediate reactions (e.g., hives, swelling of the mouth and throat, difficulty breathing, hypotension, or shock) subsequent to egg ingestion may be at an enhanced risk of immediate-type hypersensitivity reactions after receiving vaccines containing traces of chick embryo antigen. The potential risk to benefit ratio should be carefully evaluated before considering vaccination in such cases. Such individuals may be vaccinated with extreme caution, having adequate treatment on hand should a reaction occur.

According to the National Advisory Committee on Immunization (NACI), "anaphylaxis after measles vaccination is rare. It has been reported both in people with anaphylactic hypersensitivity to eggs and in those with no history of egg allergy. In some of these instances it is hypersensitivity to gelatin that is responsible for the anaphylactic reaction. As well, allergy to other components of the vaccine, such as neomycin, has been hypothesized but not proven. The minute quantity of egg proteins contained in measles-mumps-rubella vaccines (MMR) seems to be insufficient to cause an allergic reaction in egg-allergic people."

"Several studies have reported uneventful routine MMR immunization in egg-allergic people and in those with positive MMR skin tests, whereas others have reported occasional adverse reactions despite the use of MMR skin testing and graded challenge vaccination. Therefore the use of skin testing with MMR vaccines in egg-allergic individuals is no longer recommended."

"In view of the cumulative data indicating the safety of MMR immunization in people with a history of anaphylactic hypersensitivity to hens' eggs and the lack of evidence of the predictive value of MMR skin testing, NACI does not recommend routine MMR skin testing or any special precaution in these individuals. As for all vaccines, NACI recommends immunization by personnel with the capability and facilities to manage adverse events following immunization such as anaphylaxis."

Special Populations: Pregnant Women: Animal reproduction studies have not been conducted with M-M-R II. It is also not known whether M-M-R II can cause fetal harm when administered to a pregnant woman or can affect reproduction capacity. Therefore, the vaccine should not be administered to pregnant females; furthermore, pregnancy should be avoided for three months following vaccination (see Contraindications).

In counseling women who are inadvertently vaccinated when pregnant or who become pregnant within 3 months of vaccination, the physician should be aware of the following: (1) In a 10-year survey involving over 700 pregnant women who received rubella vaccine within 3 months before or after conception (of whom 189 received the Wistar RA 27/3 strain), none of the newborns had abnormalities compatible with congenital rubella syndrome; (2) Mumps infection during the first trimester of pregnancy may increase the rate of spontaneous abortion. Although mumps vaccine virus has been shown to infect the placenta and fetus, there is no good evidence that it causes congenital malformations in humans; and (3) Reports have indicated that contracting of wild-type measles during pregnancy enhances fetal risk. Increased rates of spontaneous abortion, stillbirth, congenital defects and prematurity have been observed subsequent to infection with wild-type measles during pregnancy. There are no adequate studies of the attenuated (vaccine) strain of measles virus in pregnancy. However, it would be prudent to assume that the vaccine strain of virus is also capable of inducing adverse fetal effects.

Nursing Women: It is not known whether measles or mumps vaccine virus is secreted in human milk. Recent studies have shown that lactating postpartum women immunized with live attenuated rubella vaccine may secrete the virus in breast milk and transmit it to breast-fed infants. In the infants with serological evidence of rubella infection, none exhibited severe disease; however, one exhibited mild clinical illness typical of acquired rubella. Caution should be exercised when M-M-R II is administered to a nursing woman.

Pediatrics (<12 months): Safety and effectiveness of measles vaccine in infants below the age of 6 months have not been established. Safety and effectiveness of mumps and rubella vaccine in infants less than 12 months of age have not been established.

Monitoring and Laboratory Tests: It has been reported that live attenuated measles, mumps and rubella virus vaccines given individually may result in a temporary depression of tuberculin skin sensitivity. Therefore, if a tuberculin test is to be done, it should be administered either before or simultaneously with M-M-R II.

Children under treatment for tuberculosis have not experienced exacerbation of the disease when immunized with live measles virus vaccine; no studies have been reported to date of the effect of measles virus vaccines on untreated tuberculous children.

ADVERSE REACTIONS: A clinical trial comparing the safety and immunogenicity of M-M-R II manufactured with recombinant human albumin (rHA) and M-M-R II manufactured with human serum albumin (HSA) was conducted in 1279 children. Clinical follow-up was obtained for 634/641 (98.9%) subjects who received M-M-R II with rHA and 632/638 (99.1%) subjects who received M-M-R II with HSA.

The number and percentage of subjects who reported specific systemic adverse experiences with an incidence of ≥1% in either treatment group during Days 1 to 42 postvaccination are presented by body system and treatment group in Table 1.

Table 1: M-M-R II

Number (%) of Subjects with Specific Systemic Clinical Adverse Experiences (Incidence ≥1% in One or More Treatment Groups) by Body System (Days 1 to 42 Following Vaccination)

	M-M-R II with rHA (N=641)				M-M-R II with HSA (N=638)			
	All Adverse Experiences		VR		All Adverse Experi-ences		VR	
	n	(%)	n	(%)	n	(%)	n	(%)
Number of subjects	641				638			
Number of subjects without follow-up	7				6			
Number of subjects with follow-up	634				632			
Number (%) of subjects with one or more systemic adverse experiences	469	(74.0)			465	(73.6)		
Number (%) of subjects with no systemic adverse experience	165	(26.0)			167	(26.4)		
Ear and Labyrinth Disorders	**11**	**(1.7)**			**7**	**(1.1)**		
Ear pain	7	(1.1)			2	(0.3)		
Eye Disorders	**27**	**(4.3)**			**14**	**(2.2)**	**4**	**(0.6)**
Conjunctivitis	22	(3.5)			10	(1.6)	2	(0.3)
Gastrointestinal Disorders	**99**	**(15.6)**	**8**	**(1.3)**	**110**	**(17.4)**	**14**	(2.2)
Constipation	5	(0.8)			7	(1.1)		
Diarrhea NOS	45	(7.1)	4	(0.6)	41	(6.5)	6	(0.9)
Loose stools	8	(1.3)	1	(0.2)	9	(1.4)	2	(0.3)
Teething	11	(1.7)			9	(1.4)		
Vomiting NOS	35	(5.5)	3	(0.5)	41	(6.5)	5	(0.8)
General Disorders and Administration Site Conditions	**158**	**(24.9)**	**61**	**(9.6)**	**149**	**(23.6)**	**69**	**(10.9)**
Pain NOS	10	(1.6)	4	(0.6)	4	(0.6)	2	(0.3)
Pyrexia	144	(22.7)	56	(8.8)	138	(21.8)	63	(10)
Immune System Disorders	**6**	**(0.9)**			**8**	**(1.3)**	**1**	**(0.2)**
Hypersensitivity NOS	2	(0.3)			8	(1.3)	1	(0.2)
Infections and Infestations	**279**	**(44)**	**15**	**(2.4)**	**256**	**(40.5)**	**17**	**(2.7)**

(cont'd)

Table 1: M-M-R II *(cont'd)*

Number (%) of Subjects with Specific Systemic Clinical Adverse Experiences (Incidence ≥1% in One or More Treatment Groups) by Body System (Days 1 to 42 Following Vaccination)

	M-M-R II with rHA (N=641)				M-M-R II with HSA (N=638)			
	All Adverse Experiences		VR		All Adverse Experi-ences		VR	
	n	(%)	n	(%)	n	(%)	n	(%)
Croup infectious	8	(1.3)			5	(0.8)		
Ear infection NOS	23	(3.6)	1	(0.2)	18	(2.8)	1	(0.2)
Gastroenteritis NOS	11	(1.7)	1	(0.2)	12	(1.9)		
Nasopharyngitis	80	(12.6)	4	(0.6)	84	(13.3)	5	(0.8)
Otitis media NOS	79	(12.5)	1	(0.2)	65	(10.3)	3	(0.5)
Sinusitis NOS	5	(0.8)			13	(2.1)		
Upper respiratory tract infection NOS	98	(15.5)	3	(0.5)	87	(13.8)	5	(0.8)
Upper respiratory tract infection viral NOS	8	(1.3)			3	(0.5)		
Viral infection NOS	25	(3.9)	2	(0.3)	17	(2.7)		
Viral rash NOS	14	(2.2)	3	(0.5)	14	(2.2)	5	(0.8)
Injury, Poisoning and Procedural Complications	**33**	**(5.2)**			**25**	**(4.0)**	**1**	**(0.2)**
Arthropod bite	15	(2.4)			8	(1.3)	1	(0.2)
Metabolism and Nutrition Disorders	**7**	**(1.1)**			**5**	**(0.8)**		
Nervous System Disorders	**7**	**(1.1)**	**1**	**(0.2)**	**6**	**(0.9)**	**3**	**(0.5)**
Psychiatric Disorders	**53**	**(8.4)**	**27**	**(4.3)**	**48**	**(7.6)**	**26**	**(4.1)**
Insomnia	7	(1.1)	1	(0.2)	0	(0)		
Irritability	49	(7.7)	27	(4.3)	47	(7.4)	25	(4.0)
Respiratory, Thoracic and Mediastinal Disorders	**109**	**(17.2)**	**4**	**(0.6)**	**121**	**(19.1)**	**11**	**(1.7)**
Cough	41	(6.5)	1	(0.2)	43	(6.8)	1	(0.2)
Nasal congestion	22	(3.5)			30	(4.7)	3	(0.5)
Rhinitis NOS	6	(0.9)			12	(1.9)	1	(0.2)
Rhinorrhoea	41	(6.5)	3	(0.5)	41	(6.5)	4	(0.6)
Wheezing	15	(2.4)	1	(0.2)	12	(1.9)	1	(0.2)
Skin and Subcutaneous Tissue Disorders	**162**	**(25.6)**	**50**	**(7.9)**	**142**	**(22.5)**	**41**	**(6.5)**
Dermatitis diaper	31	(4.9)	1	(0.2)	32	(5.1)	1	(0.2)
Eczema	10	(1.6)			15	(2.4)		
Heat rash	25	(3.9)	4	(0.6)	8	(1.3)	1	(0.2)
Rash morbilliform	20	(3.2)	20	(3.2)	11	(1.7)	10	(1.6)
Rash NOS	53	(8.4)	20	(3.2)	47	(7.4)	19	(3.0)
Urticaria NOS	8	(1.3)	3	(0.5)	8	(1.3)	3	(0.5)

Percentages are calculated based on the number of subjects with follow-up.
Although a subject may have had 2 or more systemic adverse experiences, the subject is counted only once in the overall total.
Adverse experience terms are from MedDRA Version 6.0.
Legend : N=Number of subjects vaccinated in each treatment group; VR=Vaccine-related. Entries in this column refer to the number (%) of subjects with systemic adverse experiences that were determined by the investigator to be possibly, probably, or definitely related to the vaccine; rHA=Recombinant human albumin; HSA=Human serum albumin.

Potential Undesirable Effects: Additional clinical and post marketing data from previous formulations of monovalent and of the combined measles, mumps, and rubella vaccines manufactured by Merck & Co., Inc. without regard to causality or frequency are available and are summarized below. These data were reported based on more than 400 million doses distributed worldwide. Potential undesirable effects already provided in the previous section (related to the clinical experience with M-M-R II with rHA) are excluded from the data provided below.

Common: burning and/or stinging of short duration at the injection site.

Occasional: Body as a Whole: fever (38.3°C or higher).

Skin: rash, or measles-like rash, usually minimal but may be generalized. Generally, fever, rash, or both appear between the 5th and the 12th day.

Rare: Body as a Whole: mild local reactions such as erythema, induration and tenderness; sore throat, malaise, atypical measles, syncope, irritability.

Cardiovascular: vasculitis.

Digestive: parotitis, nausea, vomiting, diarrhea.

Hematologic/Lymphatic: regional lymphadenopathy, thrombocytopenia, purpura.

Hypersensitivity: allergic reactions such as wheal and flare at injection site, anaphylaxis and anaphylactoid reactions, as well as related phenomena such as angioneurotic edema (including peripheral or facial edema) and bronchial spasm, urticaria in individuals with or without an allergic history.

Musculoskeletal: arthralgia and/or arthritis (usually transient and rarely chronic [see Other]), myalgia.

Nervous/Psychiatric: febrile convulsions in children, afebrile convulsions or seizures, headache, dizziness, paresthesia, polyneuritis, polyneuropathy, Guillain-Barré syndrome, ataxia, aseptic meningitis (see below), measles inclusion body encephalitis (MIBE) (see Contraindications). Encephalitis/encephalopathy have been reported approximately once for every three million doses. In no case has it been shown that reactions were actually caused by vaccine. The risk of such serious neurological disorders following live measles virus vaccine administration remains far less than that for encephalitis and encephalopathy with wild-type measles (one per two thousand reported cases).

Respiratory System: pneumonia, pneumonitis (see Contraindications), cough, rhinitis.

Skin: erythema multiforme, Stevens-Johnson syndrome, vesiculation at injection site, swelling, pruritis.

Special Senses: forms of optic neuritis, including retrobulbar neuritis, papillitis, and retinitis; ocular palsies, otitis media, nerve deafness, conjunctivitis.

Urogenital: epididymitis, orchitis.

Other: Death from various, and in some cases unknown, causes has been reported rarely following vaccination with measles, mumps, and rubella vaccines; however, a causal relationship has not been established in healthy individuals (see Contraindications). No deaths or permanent sequelae were reported in a published post-marketing surveillance study in Finland involving 1.5 million children and adults who were vaccinated with M-M-R II during 1982 to 1993.

Arthralgia and/or arthritis (usually transient and rarely chronic), and polyneuritis are features of infection with wild-type rubella and vary in frequency and severity with age and sex, being greatest in adult females and least in prepubertal children.

Chronic arthritis has been associated with wild-type rubella infection and has been related to persistent virus and/or viral antigen isolated from body tissues. Only rarely have vaccine recipients developed chronic joint symptoms.

Following vaccination in children, reactions in joints are uncommon and generally of brief duration. In women, incidence rates for arthritis and arthralgia are generally higher than those seen in children (children: 0-3%; women: 12-20%), and the reactions tend to be more marked and of longer duration. Symptoms may persist for a matter of months or on rare occasions for years. In adolescent girls, the reactions appear to be intermediate in incidence between those seen in children and in adult women. Even in older women (35 to 45 years), these reactions are generally well tolerated and rarely interfere with normal activities.

Post-Market Adverse Drug Reactions: Post-marketing surveillance of the more than 200 million doses of M-M-R II that have been distributed worldwide over 25 years (1971 to 1996) indicates that serious adverse events such as encephalitis and encephalopathy continue to be rarely reported.

There have been reports of subacute sclerosing panencephalitis (SSPE) in children who did not have a history of infection with wild-type measles but did receive measles vaccine. Some of these cases may have resulted from unrecognized measles in the first year of life or possibly from the measles vaccination. Based on estimated nationwide measles vaccine distribution, the association of SSPE cases to measles vaccination is about one case per million vaccine doses distributed. This is far less than the association with infection with wild-type measles, 6-22 cases of SSPE per million cases of measles. The results of a retrospective case-controlled study conducted by the Centers for Disease Control and Prevention suggest that the overall effect of measles vaccine has been to protect against SSPE by preventing measles with its inherent higher risk of SSPE.

Cases of aseptic meningitis have been reported following measles, mumps, and rubella vaccination. A causal relationship between the Urabe strain of mumps vaccine and aseptic meningitis has been shown. Although a temporal association has been observed between the administration of M-M-R II and rare cases of aseptic meningitis, there is no laboratory-confirmed evidence to link Jeryl Lynn mumps vaccine to aseptic meningitis.

Panniculitis has been reported rarely following administration of measles vaccine.

Cases of severe allergic reaction including anaphylaxis have been reported shortly after the administration of M-M-R II.

DRUG INTERACTIONS: Administration of immune globulins concurrently with M-M-R II may interfere with the expected immune response. Vaccination should be deferred for 3 months or longer following administration of immune globulin (human) and blood or plasma transfusions.

DOSAGE AND ADMINISTRATION:

Recommended Dose and Dosage Adjustment: The dosage of M-M-R II is the same for all persons.

After suitably cleansing the immunization site, inject the total volume of the single-dose vial (about 0.5 mL) of reconstituted vaccine subcutaneously, preferably into the outer aspect of the upper arm.

Revaccination: Children vaccinated when younger than 12 months of age should be revaccinated (two additional doses) after reaching 12 months of age (see Indications and Clinical Use).

A number of national, governmental vaccine authorities, the American Academy of Pediatrics (AAP), the Advisory Committee on Immunization Practices (ACIP) and the National Advisory Committee on Immunization (NACI) have recommended guidelines for routine revaccination and to help control measles and mumps outbreaks.*

A second dose of measles-containing vaccine should be deferred for HIV-infected persons with moderate or advanced immunodeficiency. Measles revaccination may still be appropriate for HIV-infected persons with moderate immunodeficiency if, there is a high risk of wild strain measles in the local community, or travel to an area where measles is endemic.

If the prevention of sporadic measles outbreaks is the sole objective, revaccination with a measles-containing vaccine should be considered (see appropriate Product Monograph). If concern also exists about immune status regarding mumps or rubella, revaccination with appropriate mumps- or rubella-containing vaccine should be considered after consulting the appropriate Product Monographs. Unnecessary doses of a vaccine are best avoided by ensuring that written documentation of vaccination is preserved and a copy given to each vaccinee's parent or guardian.

Non-Pregnant Adolescent and Adult Females: Immunization of susceptible non-pregnant adolescent and adult females of childbearing age with live attenuated rubella virus vaccine is indicated if certain precautions are observed (see Warnings and Precautions, Pregnant Women). In view of the importance of protecting this age group against rubella, reasonable precautions in a rubella immunization program include asking females if they are pregnant, excluding those who say they are, and explaining the theoretical risks to the others. Vaccinating susceptible postpubertal females confers individual protection against subsequently acquiring rubella infection during pregnancy, which in turn prevents infection of the fetus and consequent congenital rubella injury.

Women of childbearing age should be advised not to become pregnant for three months after vaccination and should be informed on the reasons for this precaution.

It is recommended, when feasible, that rubella susceptibility be determined by serologic testing prior to immunization. Since serologic testing is expensive and not always accurate, rubella vaccination of a woman who is not known to be pregnant and has no history of vaccination is justifiable without serologic testing. If immune, as evidenced by a specific rubella antibody titer of 1:8 or greater (hemagglutination-inhibition test), vaccination is unnecessary. Congenital malformations do occur in up to seven percent of all live births. Their chance appearance after vaccination could lead to misinterpretation of the cause, particularly if the prior rubella-immune status of vaccinees is unknown.

Postpubertal females should be informed of the frequent occurrence of generally self-limited arthralgia and/or possible arthritis beginning 2 to 4 weeks after vaccination (see Adverse Reactions).

Postpartum Women: It has been found convenient in many instances to vaccinate rubella-susceptible women in the immediate postpartum period (see Warnings and Precautions, Nursing Women).

Use with Other Vaccines: M-M-R II should be given concomitantly, or one month before or after administration of other live attenuated viral vaccines.

In combined clinical studies involving 1107 children 12 to 36 months of age, 680 received varicella vaccine (Oka/Merck) and M-M-R II concomitantly at separate sites and 427 received the vaccines six weeks apart. Seroconversion rates and antibody levels were comparable between the two groups at approximately six weeks postvaccination to each of the virus vaccine components. No differences were noted in adverse reactions reported in those who received varicella vaccine (Oka/Merck) concomitantly with M-M-R II at separate sites and those who received varicella vaccine (Oka/Merck) and M-M-R II at different times.

In a clinical study involving 609 children 12 months to 23 months of age, 305 received varicella vaccine (Oka/Merck), M-M-R II, and Tetramune (*H. influenzae* type b, diphtheria, tetanus, and pertussis vaccines) concomitantly at separate sites and 304 received M-M-R II and Tetramune given concomitantly at separate sites followed by varicella vaccine (Oka/Merck) 6 weeks later. At six weeks postvaccination, seroconversion rates for measles, mumps, rubella, and varicella were similar between the two groups. Compared to prevaccination GMTs, the six week postvaccination boost in GMTs for *H. influenzae* type b, diphtheria, tetanus and pertussis was similar between the two groups. GMTs for all antigens were similar except for varicella which was lower when varicella vaccine (Oka/Merck) was administered concomitantly with M-M-R II and Tetramune but within the range of GMTs seen in previous clinical experience when varicella vaccine (Oka/Merck) was administered alone. At 1 year postvaccination, GMTs for measles, mumps, rubella, varicella and *H. influenzae* type b were similar between the two groups. All three vaccines were well tolerated regardless of whether they were administered concomitantly at separate sites or 6 weeks apart. There were no clinically important differences in reaction rates when the three vaccines were administered concomitantly versus 6 weeks apart.

* Note: A primary difference among these recommendations is the timing of revaccination: The NACI recommends routine revaccination at least one month after the first dose, or at 18 months, or with entry into daycare or school. The AAP and ACIP recommend routine revaccination at 4 to 6 years of age. In addition, some public health jurisdictions mandate the age for revaccination. The complete text of applicable guidelines should be consulted.

† 50% cell culture infectious dose.

M-M-R II has been administered concurrently with other vaccines (i.e., live attenuated varicella, DTaP [or DTwP], IPV [or OPV], Hib with or without Hepatitis B vaccine) using separate injection sites and syringes. No impairment of immune response to individual tested vaccine antigens was demonstrated. The type, frequency, and severity of adverse experiences observed with M-M-R II were similar to those seen when each vaccine was given alone.

Administration: Do not inject M-M-R II intravascularly. **Do not give immune globulin (IG) concurrently with M-M-R II** (see Drug Interactions).

Caution: A sterile syringe free of preservatives, antiseptics, and detergents should be used for each injection and/or reconstitution of the vaccine because these substances may inactivate the live virus vaccine. A 25 gauge, 15 mm needle is recommended.

Prior to Administration: Inspect the reconstituted solution for particulate matter and discoloration. The reconstituted solution should be **clear yellow**. Should complete dissolution not occur within two minutes, do not use and return for reimbursement.

It is important to use a separate sterile syringe and needle for each individual patient to prevent transmission of hepatitis B and other infectious agents from one person to another.

Reconstitution: Prior to Reconstitution: Check the appearance of the content of each vial of vaccine. The content should be a light yellow solid mass ("plug") of powder which fills the bottom of each vial.

To reconstitute, use only the diluent supplied, since it is free of preservatives or other antiviral substances which might inactivate the vaccine.

First withdraw the entire volume of diluent (0.7 mL) into the syringe to be used for reconstitution. Inject all the diluent in the syringe into the vial of lyophilized vaccine, and agitate to mix thoroughly. Withdraw the entire contents into a syringe and inject the total volume of restored vaccine subcutaneously.

Vial Size	Volume of Diluent to be Added to Vial	Number of Doses Available
Single-dose	0.7 mL	1 (0.5 mL/dose)

OVERDOSAGE:

Overdosage has been reported rarely and was not associated with any serious adverse events.

For management of a suspected drug overdose, CPhA recommends that you contact your **regional Poison Control Centre**. See the *CPS* Directory section for a list of Poison Control Centres.

ACTION AND CLINICAL PHARMACOLOGY: M-M-R II is a live, attenuated vaccine for immunization against measles (rubeola), mumps, and rubella (German measles).

Measles, mumps, and rubella are three common childhood diseases, caused by measles virus, mumps virus (paramyxoviruses), and rubella virus (togavirus), respectively, that may be associated with serious complications and/or death. For example, pneumonia and encephalitis are caused by measles. Mumps is associated with aseptic meningitis, deafness and orchitis; and rubella during pregnancy may cause congenital rubella syndrome in the infants of infected mothers.

Clinical studies of 284 triple seronegative children, 11 months to 7 years of age, demonstrated that M-M-R II is highly immunogenic and generally well tolerated. In these studies, a single injection of the vaccine induced measles hemagglutination-inhibition (HI) antibodies in 95%, mumps neutralizing antibodies in 96%, and rubella HI antibodies in 99% of susceptible persons. However, a small percentage (1-5%) of vaccinees may fail to seroconvert after the primary dose.

The RA 27/3 rubella strain in M-M-R II elicits higher immediate post-vaccination HI, complement-fixing and neutralizing antibody levels than other strains of rubella vaccine 27-33 and has been shown to induce a broader profile of circulating antibodies including anti-theta and anti-iota precipitating antibodies. The RA 27/3 rubella strain immunologically simulates natural infection more closely than other rubella vaccine viruses. The increased levels and broader profile of antibodies produced by RA 27/3 strain rubella virus vaccine appear to correlate with greater resistance to subclinical reinfection with the wild virus, and provide greater confidence for lasting immunity.

Following vaccination, antibodies associated with protection can be measured by neutralization assays, HI, or ELISA (enzyme linked immunosorbent assay) tests. Neutralizing and ELISA antibodies to measles, mumps, and rubella viruses are still detectable in most individuals 11 to 13 years after primary vaccination.

STORAGE AND STABILITY: During shipment, to ensure that there is no loss of potency, the vaccine must be maintained at a temperature of 10°C or colder. Freezing during shipment will not affect potency of the vaccine. Protect the vaccine from light at all times, since such exposure may inactivate the viruses.

Before reconstitution, store the vial of lyophilized vaccine at 2 to 8°C or colder. The diluent may be stored in the refrigerator with the lyophilized vaccine or separately at room temperature. **Do not freeze the diluent.**

Reconstituted Solutions: To maintain the potency, it is imperative that only the sterile diluent for Merck & Co., Inc. live, attenuated virus vaccines (Sterile Water) be used for reconstitution and injection.

Use **as soon as possible** after reconstitution. Store reconstituted vaccine in the vaccine vial in a dark place at 2 to 8°C. Discard if not used **within 8 hours**.

INFORMATION FOR THE PATIENT: Published in e-CPS, available by subscription at www.e-cps.ca.

DOSAGE FORMS, COMPOSITION AND PACKAGING: M-M-R II (measles, mumps and rubella virus vaccine, live, attenuated, Merck Frosst Std.) is supplied as a sterile, lyophilized, light yellow compact crystalline plug in a single-dose vial. The diluent (Sterile Diluent for Merck & Co., Inc., live, attenuated virus vaccines) is a sterile, clear, colourless fluid supplied separately in a single-dose vial. After reconstitution, M-M-R II is a clear yellow liquid.

When reconstituted as directed, each single dose (0.5 mL) contains: measles virus, Enders' Edmonston strain (live, attenuated) not less than 1000 $CCID_{50}$†, mumps virus, Jeryl Lynn (B level) strain (live, attenuated) not less than 5000 $CCID_{50}$, rubella virus, Wistar RA 27/3 strain (live, attenuated) not less than 1000 $CCID_{50}$. Nonmedicinal ingredients: hydrolyzed gelatin, medium 199 with Hank's salts, minimum essential medium Eagle, monosodium L-glutamate monohydrate, neomycin, phenol red, potassium phosphate dibasic (anhydrous), potassium phosphate monobasic, sodium bicarbonate, sodium phosphate dibasic (anhydrous), sodium phosphate monobasic, sorbitol, sucrose and water for injection. Manufacturing process residuals: recombinant human albumin, fetal bovine serum. Preservative-free. The diluent is sterile water for injection. Single-dose Type I glass vials of 3 mL. Each vial contains one dose of lyophilized vaccine (approximately 0.5 mL when reconstituted as directed). The diluent (0.7 mL) is supplied separately in 3 mL single-dose Type I glass vials. The container closure systems of M-M-R II and the diluent are free of latex. M-M-R II is available in packages of 10 single-dose vials. The diluent is also available in packages of 10 single-dose vials.

Mobicox® Ⓟ

meloxicam

Anti-inflammatory—Analgesic

Boehringer Ingelheim

Date of Revision: May 28, 2008

SUMMARY PRODUCT INFORMATION:

Route of Administration	Dosage Form/ Strength	Clinically Relevant Nonmedicinal Ingredients
Oral	Tablet, 7.5 mg and 15 mg	Anhydrous colloidal silica, crospolyvidone, lactose, magnesium stearate, microcrystalline cellulose, polyvidone, sodium citrate

INDICATIONS AND CLINICAL USE: MOBICOX (meloxicam) is indicated for the symptomatic treatment of:

- Rheumatoid arthritis in adults and
- Painful osteoarthritis (arthrosis, degenerative joint disease) in adults.

Throughout this document, the term NSAIDs refers to both non-selective NSAIDs and selective COX-2 inhibitor NSAIDs, unless otherwise indicated.

For patients with an increased risk of developing CV and/or GI adverse events, other management strategies that do not include the use of NSAIDs should be considered first. (See Contraindications and Warnings and Precautions.)

Use of MOBICOX should be limited to the lowest effective dose for the shortest possible duration of treatment in order to minimize the potential risk for cardiovascular or gastrointestinal adverse events. (See Contraindications and Warnings and Precautions.)

MOBICOX, as a NSAID, does **not** treat clinical disease or prevent its progression.

MOBICOX, as a NSAID, only relieves symptoms and decreases inflammation for as long as the patient continues to take it.

Geriatrics (>65 years of age): Evidence from clinical studies and postmarket experience suggests that use in the geriatric population is associated with differences in safety. (See Warnings and Precautions, Special Populations, Geriatrics (>65 years of age) and Dosage and Administration, Recommended Dose and Dosage Adjustment, Geriatrics (>65 years of age)).

Pediatrics (<18 years of age): Safety and efficacy have not been established in the pediatric population. (See Contraindications.)

CONTRAINDICATIONS: MOBICOX is contraindicated in:

- the peri-operative setting of coronary artery bypass graft surgery (CABG). Although MOBICOX has **not** been studied in this patient population, a selective COX-2 inhibitor NSAID studied in such a setting has led to an increased incidence of cardiovascular/thromboembolic events, deep surgical infections and sternal wound complications;
- pregnancy. The risks during the third trimester are premature closure of the ductus arteriosus and prolonged parturition (see Warnings and Precautions, Special Populations, Pregnant Women);
- women who are breastfeeding because of the potential for serious adverse reactions in nursing infants. NSAIDs are known to pass into mother's milk;
- severe uncontrolled heart failure;
- known or suspected hypersensitivity to meloxicam or to any of the components/excipients;
- history of acute asthmatic attacks or symptoms of asthma, urticaria, nasal polyps, anaphylaxis, rhinitis, angioedema or other allergic manifestations that are precipitated by ASA or other NSAIDs, since cross-sensitivity may exist. Fatal anaphylactoid reactions may occur in such individuals. Individuals with the above medical problem are at risk of a severe reaction even if they have taken NSAIDs in the past without any adverse reaction (see Warnings and Precautions, Hypersensitivity Reactions, Anaphylactoid Reactions, ASA-Intolerance);
- active or recent gastro-intestinal/gastric/duodenal/peptic ulceration/perforation, active GI bleeding;
- cerebrovascular bleeding or other bleeding disorders;
- inflammatory bowel disease (Crohn's Disease or Ulcerative Colitis);
- severe liver impairment or active liver disease;
- severe renal impairment (creatinine clearance <30 mL/min or 0.5 mL/sec) or deteriorating renal disease (individuals with lesser degrees of renal impairment are at risk of deterioration of their renal function when prescribed NSAIDs and must be monitored) (see Warnings and Precautions, Renal);
- known hyperkalemia (see Warnings and Precautions, Renal, Fluid and Electrolyte Balance);
- children and adolescents aged less than 18 years.

In case of rare hereditary conditions that may be incompatible with an excipient of the product (see Warnings and Precautions) the use of the product is contraindicated.

WARNINGS AND PRECAUTIONS:

Risk of Cardiovascular (CV) Adverse Events: Ischemic Heart Disease, Cerebrovascular Disease, Congestive Heart Failure (NYHA II-IV) (see Warnings and Precautions, Cardiovascular): MOBICOX is a non-steroidal anti-inflammatory drug (NSAID). Use of some NSAIDs is associated with an increased incidence of cardiovascular adverse events (such as myocardial infarction, stroke or thrombotic events) which can be fatal. The risk may increase with duration of use. Patients with cardiovascular disease or risk factors for cardiovascular disease may be at greater risk.

Caution should be exercised in prescribing MOBICOX to any patient with ischemic heart disease (including but not limited to acute myocardial infarction, history of myocardial infarction and/or angina), cerebrovascular disease (including but not limited to stroke, cerebrovascular accident, transient ischemic attacks and/or amaurosis fugax) and/or congestive heart failure (NYHA II-IV).

Use of NSAIDs, such as MOBICOX, can promote sodium retention in a dose-dependent manner, through a renal mechanism, which can result in increased blood pressure and/or exacerbation of congestive heart failure. (See Warnings and Precautions, Renal, Fluid and Electrolyte Balance.)

Randomized clinical trials with MOBICOX have not been designed to detect differences in cardiovascular events in a chronic setting. Therefore, caution should be exercised when prescribing MOBICOX.

Risk of Gastrointestinal (GI) Adverse Events (see Warnings and Precautions, Gastrointestinal (GI)): Use of NSAIDs, such as MOBICOX, is associated with an increased incidence of gastrointestinal adverse events (such as peptic/duodenal ulceration, perforation, obstruction and gastrointestinal bleeding).

General: For relevant drug interactions that require particular attention, see Drug Interactions.

Frail or debilitated patients may tolerate side effects less well and therefore special care should be taken in treating this population. **To minimize the potential risk for an adverse event, the lowest effective dose should be used for the shortest possible duration.** As with other NSAIDs, caution should be used in the treatment of elderly patients who are more likely to be suffering from impaired renal, hepatic or cardiac function. For high risk patients, alternate therapies that do not involve NSAIDs should be considered.

MOBICOX is **not** recommended for use with other NSAIDs, with the exception of low-dose ASA for cardiovascular prophylaxis, because of the absence of any evidence demonstrating synergistic benefits and the potential for additive adverse reactions. (See Drug Interactions, Drug/Drug Interactions, Acetylsalicylic Acid (ASA) or Other NSAIDs.)

MOBICOX tablets 7.5 mg contains 47 mg lactose per maximum recommended daily dose. Patients with rare hereditary problems of galactose intolerance, the Lapp-lactase deficiency or glucose-galactose malabsorption should not take this medicine.

MOBICOX tablets 15 mg contains 20 mg lactose per maximum recommended daily dose. Patients with rare hereditary problems of galactose intolerance, the Lapp-lactase deficiency or glucose-galactose malabsorption should not take this medicine.

Cardiovascular: MOBICOX is a non-steroidal anti-inflammatory drug (NSAID). Use of some NSAIDs is associated with an increased incidence of cardiovascular adverse events (such as myocardial infarction, stroke or thrombotic events) which can be fatal. The risk may increase with duration of use. Patients with cardiovascular disease or risk factors for cardiovascular disease may be at greater risk.

Caution should be exercised in prescribing MOBICOX to patients with risk factors for cardiovascular disease, cerebrovascular disease or renal disease, such as any of the following (not an exhaustive list): hypertension; dyslipidemia/hyperlipidemia; diabetes mellitus; congestive heart failure (NYHA I); coronary artery disease (atherosclerosis); peripheral arterial disease; smoking; creatinine clearance (<60 mL/min or 1 mL/sec).

Use of NSAIDs, such as MOBICOX, can lead to new hypertension or can worsen pre-existing hypertension, either of which may increase the risk of cardiovascular events as described above. Thus blood pressure should be monitored regularly. Consideration should be given to discontinuing MOBICOX should hypertension either develop or worsen with its use.

Use of NSAIDs, such as MOBICOX, can induce fluid retention and edema, and may exacerbate congestive heart failure, through a renally-mediated mechanism. (See Warnings and Precautions, Renal, Fluid and Electrolyte Balance.)

For patients with a high risk of developing an adverse CV event, other management strategies that do **not** include the use of NSAIDs should be considered first. **To minimize the potential risk for an adverse CV event, the lowest effective dose should be used for the shortest possible duration.**

Endocrine and Metabolism: Corticosteroids: MOBICOX (meloxicam) is **not** a substitute for corticosteroids. It does **not** treat corticosteroid insufficiency. Abrupt discontinuation of corticosteroids may lead to exacerbation of corticosteroid responsive illness. Patients on prolonged corticosteroid therapy should have their therapy tapered slowly if a decision is made to discontinue corticosteroids. (See Drug Interactions, Drug-Drug Interactions, Glucocorticoids.)

Gastrointestinal (GI): Serious GI toxicity (sometimes fatal), such as peptic/duodenal ulceration, inflammation, perforation, obstruction and gastrointestinal bleeding, can occur at any time, with or without warning symptoms in patients treated with NSAIDs, such as MOBICOX. Minor upper GI problems, such as dyspepsia, commonly occur at any time. Health care providers should remain alert for ulceration and bleeding in patients treated with MOBICOX, even in the absence of previous GI tract symptoms. Most spontaneous reports of fatal GI events are in elderly or debilitated patients and therefore special care should be taken in treating this population. **To minimize the potential risk for an adverse GI event, the lowest effective dose should be used for the shortest possible duration.** For high risk patients, alternate therapies that do not involve NSAIDs should be considered. (See Warnings and Precautions, Special Populations, Geriatrics (>65 years of age).)

Patients should be informed about the signs and/or symptoms of serious GI toxicity and instructed to discontinue using MOBICOX and seek emergency medical attention if they experience any such symptoms. The utility of periodic laboratory monitoring has **not** been demonstrated, nor has it been adequately assessed. Most patients who develop a serious upper GI adverse event on NSAID therapy have no symptoms. Upper GI ulcers, gross bleeding or perforation, caused by NSAIDs, appear to occur in approximately 1% of patients treated for 3-6 months, and in about 2-4% of patients treated for one year. These trends continue, thus increasing the likelihood of developing a serious GI event at some time during the course of therapy. Even short-term therapy has its risks.

Caution should be taken if prescribing MOBICOX to patients with a prior history of peptic/duodenal ulcer disease or gastrointestinal bleeding as these individuals have a greater than 10-fold higher risk for developing a GI bleed when taking a NSAID than patients with neither of these risk factors. Other risk factors for GI ulceration and bleeding include the following: *H. pylori* infection, increased age, prolonged use of NSAID therapy, excess alcohol intake, smoking, poor general health status or concomitant therapy with any of the following: anti-coagulants (e.g. warfarin); antiplatelet agent (e.g. ASA, clopidogrel); oral corticosteroids (e.g. prednisone); Selective Serotonin Reuptake Inhibitors (SSRIs) (e.g. citalopram, fluoxetine, paroxetine, sertraline).

Prospective, long-term studies required to compare the incidence of serious clinically significant upper gastrointestinal adverse events among patients taking meloxicam versus other NSAID products have not been performed.

There is no definitive evidence that the concomitant administration of histamine H_2 receptor antagonists and/or antacids will either prevent the occurrence of gastrointestinal adverse events or allow continuation of therapy when and if these adverse reactions appear.

Genitourinary: Some NSAIDs are associated with persistent urinary symptoms (bladder pain, dysuria, urinary frequency), hematuria or cystitis. The onset of these symptoms may occur at any time after the initiation of therapy with a NSAID.

Should urinary symptoms occur, in the absence of an alternate explanation, treatment with MOBICOX should be stopped to ascertain if symptoms disappear. This should be done before any urological investigations or treatments are carried out.

Hematologic: NSAIDs inhibiting prostaglandin biosynthesis interfere with platelet function to varying degrees; patients who may be adversely affected by such an action, such as those on anti-coagulants or suffering from hemophilia or platelet disorders should be carefully observed when MOBICOX is administered.

Anti-coagulants: Numerous studies have shown that the concomitant use of NSAIDs and anti-coagulants increases the risk of bleeding. Concurrent therapy of MOBICOX with warfarin requires close monitoring of the international normalized ratio (INR).

Even with therapeutic INR monitoring, increased bleeding may occur. (See Drug Interactions, Drug-Drug Interactions, Anti-coagulants.)

Anti-platelet Effects: NSAIDs inhibit platelet aggregation and have been shown to prolong bleeding time in some patients. Unlike acetylsalicylic acid (ASA) their effect on platelet function is quantitatively less, or of shorter duration, and reversible.

MOBICOX and other NSAIDs have no proven efficacy as anti-platelet agents and should **not** be used as a substitute for ASA or other anti-platelet agents for prophylaxis of cardiovascular thromboembolic diseases. Anti-platelet therapies (e.g. ASA) should **not** be discontinued. There is some evidence that use of NSAIDs with ASA can markedly attenuate the cardioprotective effects of ASA. (See Drug Interactions, Drug-Drug Interactions, Acetylsalicylic Acid (ASA) or Other NSAIDs.)

Concomitant administration of MOBICOX with low dose ASA increases the risk of GI ulceration and associated complications.

For information on interaction between low dose ASA and MOBICOX and any other interaction, see Drug Interactions, Acetylsalicylic Acid (ASA) or Other NSAIDs.

Blood Dyscrasias: Blood dyscrasias (such as neutropenia, leukopenia, thrombocytopenia, aplastic anemia, and agranulocytosis) associated with the use of NSAIDs are rare, but can occur with severe consequences.

Anemia is sometimes seen in patients receiving NSAIDs, including MOBICOX. This may be due to fluid retention, GI blood loss, or an incompletely described effect upon erythropoiesis. Patients on long-term treatment with NSAIDs, including MOBICOX, should have their hemoglobin or hematocrit checked if they exhibit any signs or symptoms of anemia or blood loss.

The incidence of treatment-related anemia is more frequent than 1%. The incidence of disturbances of blood count, including differential white cell count, leukopenia and thrombocytopenia, is between 0.1 and 1%.

Concomitant administration of a potentially myelotoxic drug, in particular methotrexate, appears to be a predisposing factor to the onset of a cytopenia.

Hepatic/Biliary/Pancreatic: As with other NSAIDs, borderline elevations of one or more liver enzyme tests (AST, ALT, alkaline phosphatase) may occur in up to 15% of patients. These abnormalities may progress, may remain essentially unchanged, or may be transient with continued therapy. Notable elevations of ALT or AST (approximately three or more times the upper limit of normal) have been reported in approximately 1% of patients in clinical trials with NSAIDs.

A patient with signs and/or symptoms suggesting liver dysfunction, or in whom an abnormal liver function test has occurred, should be evaluated for evidence of the development of a more severe hepatic reaction while on therapy with MOBICOX. Severe hepatic reactions including jaundice and cases of fatal hepatitis, liver necrosis and hepatic failure, some of them with fatal outcomes, have been reported with NSAIDs.

Although such reactions are rare, if abnormal liver tests persist or worsen, if clinical signs and symptoms consistent with liver disease develop (e.g. jaundice), or if systemic manifestations occur (e.g., eosinophilia, associated with rash, etc.), MOBICOX should be discontinued.

If there is a need to prescribe MOBICOX in the presence of impaired liver function, it must be done under strict observation.

Hypersensitivity Reactions: Anaphylactoid Reactions: As with NSAIDs in general, anaphylactoid reactions have occurred in patients without known prior exposure to MOBICOX. In post-marketing experience, rare cases of anaphylactic/anaphylactoid reactions and angioedema have been reported in patients receiving MOBICOX. MOBICOX should **not** be given to patients with the ASA-triad. This symptom complex typically occurs in asthmatic patients who experience rhinitis with or without nasal polyps, or who exhibit severe, potentially fatal bronchospasm after taking ASA or other NSAIDs (see Contraindications). Emergency help should be sought in cases where anaphylactoid reaction occurs.

ASA-Intolerance: MOBICOX should **not** be given to patients with complete or partial syndrome of ASA-intolerance (rhinosinusitis, urticaria/angioedema, nasal polyps, asthma) in whom asthma, anaphylaxis, urticaria/angioedema, rhinitis or other allergic manifestations are precipitated by ASA or other NSAIDs. Fatal anaphylactoid reactions have occurred in such individuals. As well, individuals with the above medical problems are at risk of a severe fatal reaction even if they have taken NSAIDs in the past without any adverse reaction. (See Contraindications.)

Cross-sensitivity: Patients sensitive to any one of the NSAIDs may be sensitive to any of the other NSAIDs as well.

Serious Skin Reactions: See Warnings and Precautions, Skin.

Immune: See Warnings and Precautions, Infection, Aseptic Meningitis.

Infection: MOBICOX, in common with other NSAIDs, may mask signs and symptoms of an underlying infectious disease.

Aseptic Meningitis: Rarely, with some NSAIDs, the symptoms of aseptic meningitis (stiff neck, severe headaches, nausea and vomiting, fever or clouding of consciousness) have been observed. Patients with autoimmune disorders (systemic lupus erythematosus, mixed connective tissues diseases, etc.) seem to be pre-disposed. Therefore, in such patients, the health care provider must be vigilant to the development of this complication.

Neurologic: Some patients may experience drowsiness, dizziness, blurred vision, vertigo, tinnitus, hearing loss, insomnia or depression with the use of NSAIDs, such as MOBICOX. If patients experience these side effects, they should exercise caution in carrying out activities that require alertness.

Ophthalmologic: Blurred and/or diminished vision has been reported with the use of NSAIDs. If such symptoms develop MOBICOX should be discontinued and an ophthalmologic examination performed. Ophthalmologic examination should be carried out at periodic intervals in any patient receiving MOBICOX for an extended period of time.

Peri-Operative Considerations: See Contraindications, Coronary Artery Bypass Graft Surgery.

Psychiatric: See Warnings and Precautions, Neurologic.

Renal: Long-term administration of NSAIDs to animals has resulted in renal papillary necrosis and other abnormal renal pathology. In humans, there have been reports of acute interstitial nephritis, hematuria, low grade proteinuria, glomerulonephritis, renal medullary necrosis and occasionally nephrotic syndrome.

Renal insufficiency due to NSAID use is seen in patients with pre-renal conditions leading to reduction in renal blood flow or blood volume. Under these circumstances, renal prostaglandins help maintain renal perfusion and glomerular filtration rate (GFR). In these patients, administration of a NSAID may cause a reduction in prostaglandin synthesis leading to impaired renal function. Patients at greatest risk of this reaction are those with pre-existing renal insufficiency (GFR <60 mL/min or 1 mL/s), dehydrated patients, patients on salt restricted diets, those with congestive heart failure, cirrhosis, liver dysfunction, taking angiotensin-converting enzyme inhibitors, angiotensin-II receptor blockers, cyclosporine, diuretics and those who are elderly. Serious or life-threatening renal failure has been reported in patients with normal or impaired renal function after short-term therapy with NSAIDs. Even patients at risk who demonstrate the ability to tolerate a NSAID under stable conditions may decompensate during periods of added stress (e.g. dehydration due to gastroenteritis). Discontinuation of NSAIDs is usually followed by recovery to the pre-treatment state.

The extent to which metabolites may accumulate in patients with renal failure has not been studied with MOBICOX. As with other NSAIDs, metabolites of which are excreted by the kidney, patients with significantly impaired renal function should be more closely monitored.

Caution should be used when initiating treatment with NSAIDs, such as MOBICOX, in patients with considerable dehydration. Such patients should be rehydrated prior to initiation of therapy. Caution is also recommended in patients with pre-existing kidney disease. No dose reduction is required in patients with mild or moderate renal impairment (i.e. in patients with a creatinine clearance of greater than 15 mL/min or 0.25 mL/s).

Advanced Renal Disease: See Contraindications.

Fluid and Electrolyte Balance: Use of NSAIDs, such as MOBICOX, can promote sodium retention in a dose-dependent manner, which can lead to fluid retention and edema, and consequences of increased blood pressure and exacerbation of congestive heart failure. Thus, caution should be exercised in prescribing MOBICOX in patients with a history of congestive heart failure, compromised cardiac function, hypertension, increased age or other conditions predisposing to fluid retention. For patients at risk, clinical monitoring is recommended. (See Warnings and Precautions, Cardiovascular.)

Use of NSAIDs, such as MOBICOX, can increase the risk of hyperkalemia, especially in patients with diabetes mellitus, renal failure, increased age, or those receiving concomitant therapy with adrenergic blockers, angiotensin-converting enzyme inhibitors, angiotensin-II receptor antagonists, cyclosporine, or some diuretics.

Electrolytes should be monitored periodically. (See Contraindications.)

Respiratory: ASA-induced asthma is an uncommon but very important indication of ASA and NSAID sensitivity. It occurs more frequently in patients with asthma who have nasal polyps.

Sexual Function/Reproduction: The use of MOBICOX, as with any drug known to inhibit cyclooxygenase/prostaglandin synthesis, may impair fertility and is not recommended in women attempting to conceive. Therefore, in women who have difficulties conceiving, or who are undergoing investigation of infertility, withdrawal of meloxicam should be considered.

Skin: In rare cases, serious skin reactions such as Stevens-Johnson syndrome, toxic epidermal necrolysis, exfoliative dermatitis and erythema multiforme have been associated with the use of some NSAIDs. Because the rate of these reactions is low, they have usually been noted during post-marketing surveillance in patients taking other medications also associated with the potential development of these serious skin reactions. Thus, causality is **not** clear. These reactions are potentially life threatening but may be reversible if the causative agent is discontinued and appropriate treatment instituted. Patients appear to be at highest risk of these reactions early in the course of therapy, the onset of the reaction occurring in the majority of cases within the first month of treatment. MOBICOX should be discontinued at the first appearance of skin rash, mucosal lesions, or any other sign of hypersensitivity. Patients should be advised that if they experience a skin rash they should discontinue their NSAID and contact their physician for assessment and advice, including which additional therapies to discontinue.

Special Populations: Pregnant Women: MOBICOX is contraindicated in for use during pregnancy. The risks during the third trimester are premature closure of the ductus arteriosus and prolonged parturition.

Inhibition of prostaglandin-synthesis may adversely affect pregnancy and/or the embryo-foetal development. Data from epidemiological studies suggest an increased risk of miscarriage and of cardiac malformation and gastroschisis after use of a prostaglandin synthesis inhibitor in early pregnancy. The absolute risk for cardiovascular malformation was increased from less than 1%, up to approximately 1.5 %. The risk is believed to increase with dose and duration of therapy.

In animals, administration of a prostaglandin synthesis inhibitor has been shown to result in increased pre- and post-implantation loss and embryo-foetal lethality. In addition, increased incidences of various malformations, including cardiovascular, have been reported in animals given a prostaglandin synthesis inhibitor during the organogenetic period.

During the third trimester of pregnancy all prostaglandin-synthesis inhibitors may expose the foetus to: cardiopulmonary toxicity (with premature closure of the ductus arteriosus and pulmonary hypertension); renal dysfunction, which may progress to renal failure with oligo-hydroamniosis; the mother and the neonate, at the end of pregnancy, to: possible prolongation of bleeding time, an anti-aggregating effect which may occur even at very low doses; inhibition of uterine contractions resulting in delayed or prolonged labour.

See Contraindications.

Nursing Women: MOBICOX is **contraindicated** in nursing women.

MOBICOX is contraindicated for use in women who are breastfeeding because of the potential for serious adverse reactions in nursing infants. NSAIDs are known to pass into mother's milk.

Pediatrics (<18 years of age): See Contraindications.

Safety and effectiveness of MOBICOX in pediatric patients below the age of 18 years have not been evaluated.

Geriatrics (>65 years of age): Patients older than 65 years (hereafter referred to as older or elderly) and frail or debilitated patients are more susceptible to a variety of adverse reactions from NSAIDs. The incidence of these adverse reactions increases with dose and duration of treatment. In addition, these patients are less tolerant to ulceration and bleeding. Most reports of fatal GI events are in this population. Older patients are also at risk of a lower esophageal injury including ulceration and bleeding. For such patients, consideration should be given to a starting dose lower than the one usually recommended, with individual adjustment when necessary and under close supervision.

Monitoring and Laboratory Tests: The following monitoring criteria and laboratory tests are recommended for patients taking MOBICOX. This is not an exhaustive list.

Laboratory Testing:

- Potassium (Renal function, Hyperkalemia)
- INR/effects of anti-coagulants (co-prescription of oral anti-coagulants)
- Serum transaminases and other liver function tests (liver function)
- Renal function parameters such as serum creatinine and serum urea (in case of Methotrexate, Diuretics, Cyclosporine, ACE-Inhibitor or ARB co-prescription, and in susceptible patients re: the renal effects of meloxicam, e.g. impaired renal function or dehydration)
- Lithium plasma concentrations (in case of Lithium co-prescription)
- Blood cell count, including differential white cell count (in case of Methotrexate co-prescription)

Monitoring Activities:

- Patients with GI symptoms
- Patients with oral anticoagulation (see above)
- Blood pressure (in case of Anti-hypertensives co-prescription, and in susceptible patients with fluid retention)
- Periodic ophthalmologic evaluation (in patients on extended treatment).

For more information, please refer to the Warnings and Precautions and Drug Interactions.

ADVERSE REACTIONS: Adverse Drug Reaction Overview: The information to compile the following data is based on clinical trials involving 14 325 patients who have been treated with daily oral doses of 7.5 and 15 mg MOBICOX tablets or capsules. In these clinical trials, the following indications were studied: osteoarthritis and rheumatoid arthritis (approved indications); ankylosing spondylitis, sciatica and low back pain (unapproved indications).

In the overall clinical trial database of 14 325 patients, treatment exposure up to 6 weeks was obtained in 14 313* patients, while exposure up to 3 months was in 2185 patients. Exposure up to 6 months was in 1642 patients, exposure up to one year was obtained in 1031 patients and 471 patients were exposed for more than one year to meloxicam.

Frequent Adverse Events: The following adverse events, which may be causally related to the administration of MOBICOX, have a frequency of ≥1%.

Gastrointestinal: dyspepsia, nausea, abdominal pain, diarrhoea.

Skin and Appendages: skin rash.

Central Nervous System: light-headedness, headache.

Serious Adverse Drug Reactions: The following serious adverse drug reactions have been reported in association with MOBICOX use:

- Gastrointestinal ulceration, perforation or bleeding (see Warnings and Precautions, Gastrointestinal (GI) and Drug Interactions, Drug-Drug Interactions, Selective Serotonin Reuptake Inhibitors (SSRIs);
- Asthma, bronchospasm (see Warnings and Precautions, Hypersensitivity Reactions, Anaphylactoid Reactions and Warnings and Precautions, Respiratory);
- Hypersensitivity reactions including angioedema, skin rash, pruritus (see Warnings and Precautions, Hypersensitivity Reactions, Anaphylactoid Reactions and Skin);
- Renal failure, hematuria (see Warnings and Precautions, Genitourinary and Renal, Drug Interactions, Drug-Drug Interactions, Anti-Hypertensives, Cyclosporine or Tacrolimus, Diuretics and Methotrexate);
- Visual disturbances including blurred vision (see Warnings and Precautions, Neurologic and Ophthalmologic);
- Vomiting or persistent dyspepsia, nausea, abdominal pain or diarrhea (see Warnings and Precautions, Gastrointestinal (GI) and Infection, Aseptic Meningitis);
- Micturition disorders;
- Oedema (see Warnings and Precautions, Cardiovascular and Renal, Fluid and Electrolyte Balance);
- Jaundice (see Warnings and Precautions, Hepatic/Biliary/Pancreatic);
- Malaise, fatigue;
- Aseptic meningitis (see Warnings and Precautions, Infection, Aseptic Meningitis);
- Confusion, depression, lightheadedness (see Warnings and Precautions, Neurologic);
- Tinnitus (see Warnings and Precautions, Neurologic).

Clinical Trial Adverse Drug Reactions: Because clinical trials are conducted under very specific conditions the adverse reaction rates observed in the clinical trials may not reflect the rates observed in practice and should not be compared to the rates in the clinical trials of another drug. Adverse drug reaction information from clinical trials is useful for identifying drug-related adverse events and for approximating rates.

Adverse drug reactions (ADRs) occurring with a frequency of ≥1% in a 12 week, double-blind, randomized, placebo- and active-controlled clinical trial in osteoarthritis (Study 107.181) are presented in Table 1. Diclofenac was used as a comparator in a dose of 100 mg/day.

Adverse drug reactions (ADRs) occurring with a frequency of ≥1% in a 12-week, double-blind, randomized, placebo- and active-controlled trial in rheumatoid arthritis (Study 107.183) are presented in Table 2. Diclofenac was used as a comparator in a dose of 150 mg/day (n=182).

* For 12 patients treated with meloxicam, information is missing to categorize the duration of exposure.

Table 1: MOBICOX

Adverse Drug Reactions in a Placebo- and Active-controlled Trial in Osteoarthritis (107.181) with Incidence ≥1% in Any Treatment Displayed on Preferred Term Level

	Treatment at Onset											
	Placebo		Meloxicam 3.75 mg		Meloxicam 7.5 mg		Meloxicam 15 mg		Diclofenac 100 mg		Total	
MedDRA system organ class **MedDRA preferred term**	**N**	**%**	**N**	**%**	**N**	**%**	**N**	**%**	**N**	**%**	**N**	**%**
Summary Data												
Total Treated	157	100	154	100	154	100	156	100	153	100	774	100
Total with any Adverse Event	28	17.8	34	22.1	31	20.1	26	16.7	34	22.2	153	19.8
Ear and Labyrinth Disorders	1	0.6	1	0.6	1	0.6	1	0.6	2	1.3	6	0.8
Tinnitus	1	0.6	1	0.6	0	0.0	0	0.0	2	1.3	4	0.5
Gastrointestinal Disorders	15	9.6	19	12.3	21	13.6	14	9	22	14.4	91	11.8
Abdominal pain	3	1.9	2	1.3	2	1.3	3	1.9	2	1.3	12	1.6
Constipation	3	1.9	1	0.6	2	1.3	0	0	4	2.6	10	1.3
Diarrhea	4	2.5	1	0.6	8	5.2	2	1.3	4	2.6	19	2.5
Dry mouth	0	0.0	1	0.6	0	0.0	0	0.0	2	1.3	3	0.4
Dyspepsia	5	3.2	6	3.9	5	3.2	6	3.8	6	3.9	28	3.6
Flatulence	5	3.2	5	3.2	4	2.6	3	1.9	4	2.6	21	2.7
Gastroesophageal reflux disease	0	0.0	0	0.0	1	0.6	3	1.9	2	1.3	6	0.8
Nausea	0	0.0	7	4.5	4	2.6	1	0.6	5	3.3	17	2.2
General Disorders and Administration Site Conditions	4	2.5	3	1.9	4	2.6	5	3.2	4	2.6	20	2.6
Gravitational oedema	1	0.6	1	0.6	0	0	2	1.3	1	0.7	5	0.6
Oedema peripheral	0	0.0	0	0.0	1	0.6	2	1.3	0	0.0	3	0.4

(cont'd)

Table 1: MOBICOX *(cont'd)*

Adverse Drug Reactions in a Placebo- and Active-controlled Trial in Osteoarthritis (107.181) with Incidence ≥1% in Any Treatment Displayed on Preferred Term Level

MedDRA system organ class MedDRA preferred term	Treatment at Onset											
	Placebo		Meloxicam 3.75 mg		Meloxicam 7.5 mg		Meloxicam 15 mg		Diclofenac 100 mg		Total	
	N	%	N	%	N	%	N	%	N	%	N	%
Metabolism and Nutrition Disorders	2	1.3	1	0.6	2	1.3	2	1.3	1	0.7	8	1
Increased appetite	1	0.6	1	0.6	0	0.0	2	1.3	0	0.0	4	0.5
Musculoskeletal and Connective Tissue Disorders	2	1.3	4	2.6	1	0.6	2	1.3	1	0.7	10	1.3
Arthralgia	0	0.0	2	1.3	0	0.0	1	0.6	1	0.7	4	0.5
Nervous System Disorders	9	5.7	9	5.8	5	3.2	5	3.2	5	3.3	33	4.3
Dizziness	3	1.9	3	1.9	1	0.6	2	1.3	1	0.7	10	1.3
Headache	6	3.8	4	2.6	1	0.6	1	0.6	3	2	15	1.9
Skin and Subcutaneous Tissue Disorders	2	1.3	3	1.9	4	2.6	5	3.2	2	1.3	16	2.1
Hyperhidrosis	0	0.0	1	0.6	0	0	2	1.3	0	0.0	3	0.4
Rash	1	0.6	1	0.6	2	1.3	0	0	0	0.0	4	0.5
Vascular Disorders	2	1.3	1	0.6	0	0	2	1.3	1	0.7	6	0.8
Hypertension	2	1.3	1	0.6	0	0	1	0.6	0	0.0	4	0.5

Table 2: MOBICOX

Adverse Drug Reactions in a Placebo- and Active-controlled Trial in Rheumatoid Arthritis (107.183) with Incidence ≥1% in Any Treatment Displayed on Preferred Term Level

MedDRA system organ class MedDRA preferred term	Treatment at Onset											
	Placebo		Meloxicam 7.5 mg		Meloxicam 15 mg		Meloxicam 22.5 mg		Diclofenac 150 mg		Total	
	N	%	N	%	N	%	N	%	N	%	N	%
Summary Data												
Total Treated	178	100.0	176	100.0	185	100.0	177	100.0	182	100.0	898	100.0
Total with any Adverse Event	34	19.1	38	21.6	38	20.5	31	17.5	40	22.0	181	20.2
Blood and Lymphatic System Disorders	1	0.6	0	0.0	2	1.1	0	0.0	0	0.0	3	0.3
Red blood cell abnormality	1	0.6	0	0.0	2	1.1	0	0.0	0	0.0	3	0.3
Ear and Labyrinth Disorders	0	0.0	0	0.0	2	1.1	1	0.6	0	0.0	3	0.3
Tinnitus	0	0.0	0	0.0	2	1.1	1	0.6	0	0.0	3	0.3
Eye Disorders	2	1.1	0	0.0	1	0.5	1	0.6	1	0.5	5	0.6
Visual disturbance	2	1.1	0	0.0	0	0.0	1	0.6	0	0.0	3	0.3
Gastrointestinal Disorders	21	11.8	27	15.3	25	13.5	22	12.4	29	15.9	124	13.8
Abdominal pain	2	1.1	8	4.5	5	2.7	2	1.1	6	3.3	23	2.6
Constipation	1	0.6	2	1.1	3	1.6	2	1.1	4	2.2	12	1.3
Diarrhea	8	4.5	6	3.4	9	4.9	2	1.1	6	3.3	31	3.5
Dyspepsia	6	3.4	9	5.1	5	2.7	5	2.8	6	3.3	31	3.5
Flatulence	2	1.1	3	1.7	6	3.2	7	4	6	3.3	24	2.7
Gastritis	0	0.0	0	0.0	0	0.0	1	0.6	3	1.6	4	0.4
Gastrointestinal hemorrhage	0	0.0	2	1.1	1	0.5	0	0.0	1	0.5	4	0.4
Melena	0	0.0	2	1.1	1	0.5	0	0.0	0	0.0	3	0.3
Mouth ulceration	0	0.0	0	0.0	0	0.0	4	2.3	0	0.0	4	0.4
Nausea	4	2.2	7	4	7	3.8	1	0.6	3	1.6	22	2.4
Vomiting	2	1.1	0	0.0	1	0.5	0	0.0	0	0.0	3	0.3
General Disorders and Administration Site Conditions	3	1.7	4	2.3	3	1.6	4	2.3	7	3.8	21	2.3
Fatigue	0	0.0	1	0.6	0	0.0	0	0.0	4	2.2	5	0.6
Gravitational edema	0	0.0	1	0.6	0	0.0	2	1.1	1	0.5	4	0.4
Hepatobiliary Disorders	0	0.0	0	0.0	0	0.0	1	0.6	2	1.1	3	0.3
Hepatic function abnormal	0	0.0	0	0.0	0	0.0	1	0.6	2	1.1	3	0.3
Investigations	1	0.6	0	0.0	2	1.1	3	1.7	2	1.1	8	0.9

(cont'd)

Table 2: MOBICOX *(cont'd)*

Adverse Drug Reactions in a Placebo- and Active-controlled Trial in Rheumatoid Arthritis (107.183) with Incidence ≥1% in Any Treatment Displayed on Preferred Term Level

MedDRA system organ class MedDRA preferred term	Treatment at Onset											
	Placebo		Meloxicam 7.5 mg		Meloxicam 15 mg		Meloxicam 22.5 mg		Diclofenac 150 mg		Total	
	N	%	N	%	N	%	N	%	N	%	N	%
Blood urea increased	0	0.0	0	0.0	1	0.5	1	0.6	2	1.1	4	0.4
Creatinine renal clearance decreased	0	0.0	0	0.0	1	0.5	2	1.1	0	0.0	3	0.3
Nervous System Disorders	8	4.5	8	4.5	4	2.2	2	1.1	7	3.8	29	3.2
Dizziness	4	2.2	4	2.3	1	0.5	0	0.0	1	0.5	10	1.1
Headache	6	3.4	2	1.1	3	1.6	0	0.0	4	2.2	15	1.7
Somnolence	0	0.0	0	0.0	0	0.0	1	0.6	2	1.1	3	0.3
Psychiatric Disorders	0	0.0	2	1.1	1	0.5	0	0.0	0	0.0	3	0.3
Insomnia	0	0.0	2	1.1	1	0.5	0	0.0	0	0.0	3	0.3
Skin and Subcutaneous Tissue Disorders	2	1.1	8	4.5	5	2.7	2	1.1	3	1.6	20	2.2
Hyperhidrosis	0	0.0	2	1.1	0	0.0	0	0.0	0	0.0	2	0.2
Rash	1	0.6	2	1.1	5	2.7	0	0.0	1	0.5	9	1
Rash erythematous	0	0.0	2	1.1	0	0.0	1	0.6	0	0.0	3	0.3
Vascular Disorders	1	0.6	0	0.0	1	0.5	1	0.6	2	1.1	5	0.6
Hypertension	1	0.6	0	0.0	1	0.5	1	0.6	2	1.1	5	0.6

Less Common Clinical Trial Adverse Drug Reactions (<1%): The following is a list of adverse drug reactions regardless of causality occurring in <1% of patients receiving 7.5 or 15 mg MOBICOX in clinical trials involving approximately 14 325 patients. In these clinical trials, the following indications were studied: osteoarthritis and rheumatoid arthritis (approved indications); ankylosing spondylitis, sciatica and low back pain (unapproved indications).

Body as a Whole: allergic reaction, face edema, fatigue, fever, hot flushes, malaise, syncope, weight decrease, weight increase.

Cardiovascular: angina pectoris, cardiac failure, hypertension (increase of blood pressure), hypotension, myocardial infarction, vasculitis, edema, flushes.

Heart Rate and Rhythm: arrhythmia, palpitation, tachycardia.

Central and Peripheral Nervous System: convulsions, dizziness, paresthesia, tremor, vertigo, tinnitus, drowsiness.

Psychiatric Disorders: abnormal dreaming, anxiety, appetite increased, confusion, depression, nervousness, somnolence.

Gastrointestinal: colitis, dry mouth, duodenal ulcer, eructation, esophagitis, gastric ulcer, gastritis, gastroesophageal reflux, gastrointestinal hemorrhage (occult or macroscopic gastro-intestinal bleeding), hematemesis, hemorrhagic duodenal ulcer, hemorrhagic gastric ulcer, gastro-intestinal perforation, melena, pancreatitis, perforated duodenal ulcer, perforated gastric ulcer, stomatitis ulcerative, vomiting, constipation, flatulence, gastroduodenal ulcer.

Gastrointestinal bleeding, ulceration or perforation may potentially be fatal (see Warnings and Precautions, Gastrointestinal (GI)).

Hematologic: disturbances of blood count, including differential white cell count, leukopenia, purpura, thrombocytopenia and anemia.

Liver and Biliary System: hepatitis, liver function test abnormal (e.g. raised transaminases or bilirubin).

Metabolic and Nutritional: dehydration.

Respiratory: asthma, bronchospasm, dyspnea.

Skin and Appendages: alopecia, angioedema, bullous eruption, dermatitis bullous, photosensitivity reaction (photosensitisation), pruritus, sweating increased, stomatitis, urticaria.

Special Senses: abnormal vision (including blurred vision), conjunctivitis, taste perversion, tinnitus.

Urinary System: albuminuria, abnormal renal function parameters (increased serum creatinine and/or serum urea), hematuria, acute renal failure.

Abnormal Hematologic and Clinical Chemistry Findings: Few patients in clinical trials in osteoarthritis (study 107.181) and rheumatoid arthritis (study 107.183) experienced abnormal hematologic or clinical chemistry findings with potential clinical significance. There were a few instances of decreased red blood cells in both meloxicam-treated (1.1%) and placebo-treated patients (0.7%). Increased red blood cells were experienced in placebo-treated patients (0.7%). Increased serum potassium was experienced in both meloxicam-treated patients (7.5 mg-0.7%, 15 mg-1.7%) and placebo-treated patients (1.3%). Increased blood urea nitrogen and increased serum creatinine was experienced in meloxicam-treated patients (1.3% and 2.0% respectively).

Post-Market Adverse Drug Reactions: Additional reports of serious adverse events temporally associated with MOBICOX during worldwide post-marketing experience are included below. Because these events are reported voluntarily from a population of uncertain size, it is not always possible to reliably estimate their frequency or clearly establish a causal relationship to MOBICOX exposure.

Gastrointestinal: hepatitis, gastritis.

Hematologic: agranulocytosis.

Liver and Biliary System: jaundice, liver failure.

Dermatological: bullous reactions, erythema multiforme, Stevens-Johnson syndrome, toxic epidermal necrolysis.

Respiratory: asthma, in individuals allergic to aspirin or other NSAIDs.

Central Nervous System: confusion and disorientation, alteration of mood.

Genitourinary: acute renal failure, interstitial nephritis, micturition disorders, acute urinary retention.

Vision Disorders: conjunctivitis, visual disturbances including blurred vision.

Hypersensitivity Reactions: angio-oedema and immediate hypersensitivity reactions, including anaphylactoid/anaphylactic reactions including shock.

DRUG INTERACTIONS: Overview: Cytochrome P450 Interactions: Meloxicam is eliminated almost entirely by hepatic metabolism, of which approximately two thirds are mediated by cytochrome (CYP) P450 enzymes (CYP 2C9 major pathway and CYP 3A4 minor pathway) and one-third by other pathways, such as peroxidase oxidation. The potential for a pharmacokinetic interaction should be taken into account when meloxicam and drugs known to inhibit, or to be metabolised by, CYP 2C9 and/or CYP 3A4 are administered concurrently.

Drug-Drug Interactions: Acetylsalicylic Acid (ASA) or Other NSAIDs: Concomitant administration of aspirin (1000 mg TID) to healthy volunteers tended to increase the AUC (10%) and C_{max} (24%) of meloxicam. The clinical significance of this interaction is not known.

The use of MOBICOX in addition to any other NSAID, including over-the-counter ones (such as ASA and ibuprofen) for analgesic and/or anti-inflammatory effect is **not** recommended because of the absence of any evidence demonstrating synergistic benefits and the potential for additive adverse reactions (e.g. increased risk of gastro-intestinal ulcers and bleeding).

The exception is the use of low dose ASA for cardiovascular protection, when another NSAID is being used for its analgesic/anti-inflammatory effect, keeping in mind that combination NSAID therapy is associated with additive adverse reactions. Concomitant administration of low-dose aspirin with MOBICOX may result in an increased rate of GI ulceration or other complications, compared to use of MOBICOX alone. MOBICOX is not a substitute for aspirin for cardiovascular prophylaxis.

Some NSAIDs (e.g. ibuprofen) may interfere with the antiplatelet effects of low dose ASA, possibly by competing with ASA for access to the active site of cyclooxygenase-1.

Antacids: No pharmacokinetic interaction was detected with concomitant administration of antacids. MOBICOX tablets can be administered without regard to timing of antacids. (See Action and Clinical Pharmacology, Pharmacokinetics.)

Anti-coagulants: Anticoagulant activity should be monitored, particularly in the first few days after initiating or changing MOBICOX therapy in patients receiving warfarin or similar agents, since these patients are at an increased risk of bleeding. The effect of meloxicam on the anticoagulant effect of warfarin was studied in a group of healthy subjects receiving daily doses of warfarin that produced an INR (International Normalized Ratio) between 1.2 and 1.8. In these subjects, meloxicam did not alter warfarin pharmacokinetics and the average anticoagulant effect of warfarin as determined by prothrombin time. However, one subject showed an increase in INR from 1.5 to 2.1. Caution should be used when administering MOBICOX with warfarin since patients on warfarin may experience changes in INR and an increased risk of bleeding complications when a new medication is introduced. (See Warnings and Precautions, Hematologic, Anti-coagulants.)

Anti-Hypertensives: NSAIDs may diminish the anti-hypertensive effect of Angiotensin Converting Enzyme (ACE) inhibitors.

Combinations of ACE inhibitors, angiotensin-II antagonists, diuretics and NSAIDs might have an increased risk for acute renal failure and hyperkalemia. Blood pressure and renal function (including electrolytes) should be monitored more closely in this situation, as occasionally there can be a substantial increase in blood pressure.

NSAIDs and ACE Inhibitors or angiotensin-II receptor antagonists exert a synergistic effect on the decrease of glomerular filtration. In patients with pre-existing renal impairment this may lead to acute renal failure.

Anti-Platelet Agents (including ASA): There is an increased risk of bleeding, via inhibition of platelet function, when anti-platelet agents, oral anti-coagulants, systemically administered heparin and thrombolytics are combined with NSAIDs, such as MOBICOX. If such co-prescribing cannot be avoided, close monitoring of the effects of anti-coagulants is required. (See Warnings and Precautions, Hematologic.)

Cholestyramine: Pretreatment for four days with cholestyramine significantly increased the clearance of meloxicam by 50%. This resulted in a decrease in $t_{1/2}$, from 19.2 hours to 12.5 hours, and a 35% reduction in AUC. This suggests the existence of a recirculation pathway for meloxicam in the gastrointestinal tract. The clinical relevance of this interaction has not been established.

Cimetidine: Concomitant administration of 200 mg cimetidine QID did not alter the single-dose pharmacokinetics of 30 mg meloxicam.

Cyclosporine or Tacrolimus: Nephrotoxicity of cyclosporine or tacrolimus may be enhanced by NSAIDs via renal prostaglandin mediated effects. During combined treatment with either of these drugs, renal function should be monitored.

Digoxin: Meloxicam 15 mg once daily for 7 days did not alter the plasma concentration profile of digoxin after b-acetyldigoxin administration for 7 days at clinical doses. In vitro testing found no protein binding drug interaction between digoxin and meloxicam.

Diuretics: Clinical studies, as well as post-marketing observations, have shown that NSAIDs can reduce the natriuretic effect of furosemide and thiazide diuretics in some patients. This effect has been attributed to inhibition of renal prostaglandin synthesis. Studies with furosemide agents and meloxicam have not demonstrated a reduction in natriuretic effect. Furosemide single and multiple dose pharmacodynamics and pharmacokinetics are not affected by multiple doses of meloxicam. Nevertheless, during concomitant therapy with furosemide and MOBICOX, patients should be observed closely for signs of declining renal function (see Warnings and Precautions, Renal), as well as to assure diuretic efficacy.

Glucocorticoids: Some studies have shown that the concomitant use of NSAIDs and oral glucocorticoids increases the risk of GI adverse events such as ulceration and bleeding via a synergistic effect. This is especially the case in older (>65 years of age) individuals.

Lithium: Monitoring of plasma lithium concentrations is advised when stopping or starting a NSAID, as increased lithium concentrations can occur.

In clinical trials, NSAIDs have produced a reduction in renal lithium clearance and an elevation of plasma lithium levels, which may reach toxic values. The concomitant use of lithium and NSAIDs is not recommended. In a study conducted in healthy subjects, mean pre-dose lithium concentration and AUC were increased by 21% in subjects receiving lithium doses ranging from 804 to 1072 mg BID with meloxicam 15 mg QD as compared to subjects receiving lithium alone. These effects have been attributed to inhibition of renal prostaglandin synthesis by MOBICOX. If this combination appears necessary, lithium plasma concentrations should be monitored carefully during the initiation, adjustment and withdrawal of meloxicam treatment.

Methotrexate: A study in 13 rheumatoid arthritis (RA) patients evaluated the effects of multiple doses of meloxicam on the pharmacokinetics of methotrexate taken once weekly. Meloxicam did not have a significant effect on the pharmacokinetics of single doses of methotrexate. In vitro, methotrexate did not displace meloxicam from its human serum binding sites.

In case combination treatment with methotrexate and NSAIDs is necessary, blood cell count and the renal function should be monitored. Caution should be taken in case both NSAID and methotrexate are given within 3 days, in which case the plasma level of methotrexate may increase and cause increased toxicity. Although the pharmacokinetics of methotrexate (15 mg/week) were not relevantly affected by concomitant meloxicam treatment, it should be considered that the hematological toxicity of methotrexate can be amplified by treatment with NSAID drugs.

Concomitant administration of NSAIDs with a potentially myelotoxic drug, such as methotrexate, appears to be a predisposing factor to the onset of a cytopenia.

NSAIDs can reduce the tubular secretion of methotrexate thereby increasing the plasma concentrations of methotrexate. For this reason, for patients on high dosages of methotrexate (more than 15 mg/week) the concomitant use of NSAIDs is not recommended. The risk of an interaction between NSAID preparations and methotrexate, should be considered also in patients on low dosage of methotrexate, especially in patients with impaired renal function.

Oral Contraceptives: No drug interaction information is available for MOBICOX coadministered with oral contraceptives. A decrease of the efficacy of intrauterine devices by NSAIDs has been previously reported but needs further confirmation.

Oral Hypoglycemics: An interaction with oral hypoglycemic agents has been noted with some NSAIDs, however no interaction data is available for the co-administration of these agents with MOBICOX.

Selective Serotonin Reuptake Inhibitors (SSRIs): Concomitant administration of NSAIDs and SSRIs may increase the risk of gastrointestinal ulceration and bleeding. (See Warnings and Precautions, Gastrointestinal (GI).)

Other Drug Interactions: A population kinetics study with MOBICOX indicated a lack of relevant interaction of sulfasalazine, gold compounds and glucocorticoids on the pharmacokinetics of MOBICOX. No drug interaction data is available for MOBICOX and the coadministration of the following products: phenytoin, acetaminophen, alcohol, aminoglycosides, butemide, colchicine, cyclosporin, indapamide, insulin, nephrotoxic agents, NSAIDs (other than ASA), oral contraceptives, potassium supplements, probenicid, valproic acid, zidovudine.

Drug-Food Interactions: Interactions with food have not been established.

Drug-Herb Interactions: Interactions with herbal products have not been established.

Drug-Laboratory Test Interactions: Interactions with laboratory tests have not been established.

Drug-Lifestyle Interactions: There are no specific studies about effects on the ability to drive vehicles and to use machinery. Patients who experience visual disturbances, drowsiness or other central nervous system disturbances should refrain from these activities.

DOSAGE AND ADMINISTRATION:

Dosing Considerations: In patients with increased risks of adverse reactions, treatment should be started at the dose of 7.5 mg once daily.

The maximum recommended daily dose of MOBICOX (meloxicam) tablets is 15 mg.

Recommended Dose and Dosage Adjustment: Use of MOBICOX is restricted to adults 18 years of age and older and should be limited to the lowest effective dose for the shortest possible duration of treatment. (See Contraindications and Warnings and Precautions.)

Osteoarthritis: 7.5 mg once daily. If necessary, the dose may be increased to 15 mg once daily.

Rheumatoid Arthritis: 15 mg once daily. According to the therapeutic response, the dose may be reduced to 7.5 mg once daily.

MOBICOX may be taken without regard to timing of meals.

Hepatic Impairment: No dose adjustment is necessary in patients with mild to moderate hepatic insufficiency.

No dose reduction is required in patients with clinically stable liver cirrhosis.

MOBICOX is contraindicated in patients with severe liver impairment or active liver disease.

See Contraindications; Warnings and Precautions, Hepatic/Biliary/Pancreatic and Action and Clinical Pharmacology, Special Populations and Conditions, Hepatic Insufficiency.

Renal Impairment: No dose reduction is required in patients with mild or moderate renal impairment (i.e., in patients with creatinine clearance of greater than 15 mL/min or 0.25 mL/s).

In dialysis patients with severe renal failure, the dose should not exceed 7.5 mg/day.

MOBICOX is contraindicated in patients with severe renal impairment (creatinine clearance <30 mL/min or 0.5 mL/sec) or deteriorating renal disease.

See Contraindications; Warnings and Precautions, Renal and Action And Clinical Pharmacology, Special Populations and Conditions, Renal Insufficiency.

Geriatrics (>65 years of age): For elderly, frail or debilitated patients, consideration should be given to a starting dose lower than the one usually recommended, with individual adjustment when necessary and under close supervision.

See Contraindications; Warnings and Precautions, General and Special Populations, Geriatrics (>65 years of age) and Action and Clinical Pharmacology, Special Populations and Conditions, Geriatrics.

Missed Dose: If a dose is missed, the usual schedule must be resumed the following day. An extra dose must not be taken.

OVERDOSAGE:

There is limited experience with meloxicam overdose. Four cases have taken 6 to 11 times the highest recommended dose; all recovered. Cholestyramine is known to accelerate the clearance of meloxicam.

Symptoms following acute NSAID overdose are usually limited to lethargy, drowsiness, nausea, vomiting, and epigastric pain, which are generally reversible with supportive care. Gastrointestinal bleeding can occur. Severe poisoning may result in hypertension, acute renal failure, hepatic dysfunction, respiratory depression, coma, convulsions, cardiovascular collapse, and cardiac arrest. Anaphylactoid reactions have been reported with therapeutic ingestion of NSAIDs, and may occur following an overdose.

Patients should be managed with symptomatic and supportive care following an NSAID overdose. In cases of acute overdose, gastric lavage followed by activated charcoal is recommended. Gastric lavage performed more than one hour after overdose has little benefit in the treatment of overdose. Administration of activated charcoal is recommended for patients who present 1-2 hours after overdose. For substantial overdose or severely symptomatic patients, activated charcoal may be administered repeatedly. Accelerated removal of meloxicam by 4 g oral doses of cholestyramine given three times a day was demonstrated in a clinical trial. Administration of cholestyramine may be useful following an overdose. Forced diuresis, alkalinization of urine, hemodialysis, or hemoperfusion may not be useful due to high protein binding.

> For management of a suspected drug overdose, CPhA recommends that you contact your **regional Poison Control Centre**. See the *CPS* Directory section for a list of Poison Control Centres.

ACTION AND CLINICAL PHARMACOLOGY:

Mechanism of Action: Meloxicam is a nonsteroidal anti-inflammatory drug (NSAID) that exhibits anti-inflammatory, analgesic, and antipyretic properties in animals. Meloxicam showed potent anti-inflammatory activity in all standard models of inflammation. NSAIDs are believed to exert their pharmacologic effects primarily through inhibition of the enzyme cyclooxygenase (COX). In turn, inhibition of this enzyme leads to an inhibition of biosynthesis of prostaglandins and other autacoids, substances which are potent biological mediators involved in diverse physiologic functions as well as pathologic conditions.

To date, two isozymes of COX have been identified and characterized, namely, COX-1 and COX-2 which have different intrinsic properties, expression controls and localization. COX-1, the constitutive form, has been described as a constitutive enzyme occurring in many tissues including the gastrointestinal tract, kidney, lungs, brain and platelets. COX-1 is found in blood vessels, platelets, stomach and kidney. In contrast, COX-2, the inducible form, is mostly an inducible enzyme, limited in distribution and expressed in high levels in inflamed tissues. COX-2 is thought to be involved in inflammatory responses. Recent studies have shown that differential inhibition of these two isozymes is associated with a different biological profile. Meloxicam has shown a selective inhibition of COX-2 in several in vitro test systems, as demonstrated by a greater dose dependent inhibition of COX-2 over COX-1 at levels similar to those seen in plasma at therapeutic steady state concentrations. The prostaglandins produced by the cyclooxygenases are not the only factors involved in the protection of the gastric mucosa.

A human pharmacology study compared the effects of meloxicam 7.5 mg once daily and indomethacin 25 mg three times daily on platelet aggregation and platelet thromboxane formation, which are exclusively COX-1 dependent, and renal prostaglandin (PGE_2) excretion. Platelet aggregation and thromboxane formation were almost completely inhibited by indomethacin but remained unaffected by meloxicam. Meloxicam showed no significant effects on urinary PGE_2 excretion whereas indomethacin reduced urinary PGE_2 excretion by 43%.

In another study, meloxicam (7.5 and 15 mg) demonstrated a greater inhibition of COX-2 ex vivo, as demonstrated by a greater inhibition of lipopolysaccharide-stimulated PGE_2 production (COX-2) as compared with serum thromboxane production (COX-1).

Meloxicam has been shown to inhibit COX-2 in several in vitro and ex vivo test systems. The inhibition of thromboxane in platelets, and consequently platelet aggregation, occurs via inhibition of COX-1. Meloxicam inhibition of thromboxane in platelets (via COX-1) is dose dependent and incomplete at anti-inflammatory doses. No significant inhibition of platelet aggregation has been observed with meloxicam at the recommended therapeutic doses of 7.5 and 15 mg once daily.

Inhibition of COX-2 also inhibits the production of systemic prostacyclin. Inhibition of prostacyclin may have a pro-thrombotic effect.

Prospective, controlled, long-term (>3 months) studies required to establish the clinical significance of these results have not been performed.

Pharmacodynamics: See Action and Clinical Pharmacology, Mechanism of Action.

Pharmacokinetics: Absorption: The absolute bioavailability of meloxicam capsules was 89% following a single oral dose of 30 mg compared with 30 mg IV bolus injection. Meloxicam capsules have been shown to be bioequivalent to MOBICOX tablets. Following single intravenous doses, dose-proportional pharmacokinetics were shown in the range of 5 mg to 60 mg. After multiple oral doses the pharmacokinetics of meloxicam capsules were dose-proportional over the range of 7.5 mg to 15 mg. Mean C_{max} was achieved within four to five hours after a 7.5 mg meloxicam tablet was taken under fasted conditions, indicating a prolonged drug absorption. The rate or extent of absorption was not affected by multiple dose administration, suggesting linear pharmacokinetics. With multiple dosing, steady state conditions were reached by day 5. A second meloxicam concentration peak occurs around 12 to 14 hours post-dose suggesting gastrointestinal recirculation.

Once daily dosing leads to drug plasma concentrations with a relatively small peak-trough fluctuation in the range of 0.4-1.0 μg/mL for 7.5 mg doses and 0.8-2.0 μg/mL for 15 mg doses, respectively (C_{min} and C_{max} at steady state, respectively).

Continuous treatment for longer periods (e.g. six months) did not point to any changes in pharmacokinetics compared to steady state pharmacokinetics after two weeks of oral treatment with 15 mg meloxicam/day. Any differences after treatment longer than six months are thus rather unlikely.

Table 3: MOBICOX

Single Dose and Steady-state Pharmacokinetic Parameters for Oral 15 mg Meloxicam (Mean and % CV)[a]

Pharmacokinetic Parameters (% CV)		Steady State						Single Dose			
		Healthy Male Adults (Fed)[b]		Elderly Males (Fed)[b]		Elderly Females (Fed)[b]		Renal Failure (Fasted)		Hepatic Insufficiency (Fasted)	
		15 mg[c]		15 mg		15 mg		15 mg		15 mg	
N		24		5		8		12		12	
C_{max}	(μg/mL)	1.9	−25	2.3	−59	3.2	−24	0.59	−36	0.84	−29
t_{max}	(h)	6.5	−37	5	−12	6	−27	4	−65	10	−87
$t_{½}$	(h)	15	−45	21	−34	24	−34	18	−46	16	−29
CL/f	(mL/min)	8.3	−32	9.9	−76	5.1	−22	19	−43	11	−44
Vz/f[d]	(L)	10	−36	15	−42	10	−30	26	−44	14	−29

a The parameter values in the table are from various studies.
b Not under high fat conditions.
c MOBICOX tablets.
d Vz/f=Dose/(AUC·Kel).

Food and Antacid Effects: Drug intake after a high fat breakfast (75 g of fat) did not affect extent of absorption of meloxicam capsules, but led to 22% higher C_{max} values. Mean C_{max} values were achieved between five and six hours. No pharmacokinetic interaction was detected with concomitant administration of antacids. MOBICOX tablets can be administered without regard to timing of meals and antacids.

Distribution: The mean volume of distribution (Vss) of meloxicam is approximately 10 L. Meloxicam is ~99.4% bound to human plasma proteins (primarily albumin) within the therapeutic dose range. The fraction of protein binding is independent of drug concentration, over the clinically relevant concentration range, but decreases to ~99% in patients with renal disease. Meloxicam penetration into human red blood cells, after oral dosing, is less than 10%. Following a radiolabeled dose, over 90% of the radioactivity detected in the plasma was present as unchanged meloxicam.

Meloxicam concentrations in synovial fluid, after a single oral dose, range from 40% to 50% of those in plasma. The free fraction in synovial fluid is 2.5 times higher than in plasma, due to the lower albumin content in synovial fluid as compared to plasma. The significance of this penetration is unknown.

Metabolism: Meloxicam is almost completely metabolized to four pharmacologically inactive metabolites. The major metabolite, 5′-carboxy meloxicam (60% of dose), from P450 mediated metabolism was formed by oxidation of an intermediate metabolite 5′-hydroxymethyl meloxicam which is also excreted to a lesser extent (9% of dose). In vitro studies indicate that cytochrome P450 2C9 plays an important role in this metabolic pathway with a minor contribution of the CYP 3A4 isozyme. Patients' peroxidase activity is probably responsible for the other two metabolites which account for 16% and 4% of the administered dose, respectively.

Excretion: Meloxicam excretion is predominantly in the form of metabolites, and occurs to equal extents in the urine and feces. Only traces of the unchanged parent compound are excreted in the urine (0.2%) and feces (1.6%). The extent of the urinary excretion was confirmed for unlabeled multiple 7.5 mg doses: 0.5%, 6% and 13% of the dose were found in urine in the form of meloxicam, and the 5′-hydroxymethyl and 5′-carboxy metabolites, respectively. There is significant biliary and/or enteral secretion of the drug. This was demonstrated when oral administration of cholestyramine following a single IV dose of meloxicam decreased the AUC of meloxicam by 50%.

The mean elimination half-life ($t_{1/2}$) ranges from 15 hours to 20 hours. The elimination half-life is constant across dose levels indicating linear metabolism within the therapeutic dose range. Plasma clearance ranges from 7 to 9 mL/min.

Special Populations and Conditions: Pediatrics: In a study of 36 children, kinetic measurements were made in 18 children at doses of 0.25 mg/kg BW. Maximum plasma concentration C_{max} (−34%) as well as $AUC0_{0-\infty}$ (−28%) tended to be lower in the younger age group (aged 2 to 6 years, n=7) as compared to the older age group (7 to 14 years, n=11) while weight normalized clearance appeared to be higher in the younger age group. A historical comparison with adults revealed that plasma concentrations were at least similar for older children and adults. Plasma elimination half-lives (13 h) were similar for both groups and tended to be shorter than in adults (15-20 h).

Geriatrics: Elderly males (≥65 years of age) exhibited meloxicam plasma concentrations and steady state pharmacokinetics similar to young males. Elderly females (≥65 years of age) had a 47% higher AUC_{ss} and 32% higher $C_{max\ ss}$ as compared to younger females (<55 years of age) after body weight normalization. Despite the increased total concentrations in the elderly females, the adverse event profile was comparable for both elderly patient populations. A smaller free fraction was found in elderly female patients in comparison to elderly male patients.

Mean plasma clearance at steady state in elderly subjects was slightly lower than that reported for younger subjects.

Gender: Young females exhibited slightly lower plasma concentrations relative to young males. After single doses of 7.5 mg MOBICOX, the mean elimination half-life was 19.5 hours for the female group as compared to 23.4 hours for the male group. At steady state, the data were similar (17.9 hours vs 21.4 hours). This pharmacokinetic difference due to gender is likely to be of little clinical importance. There was linearity of pharmacokinetics and no appreciable difference in the C_{max} or T_{max} across genders.

Race: Pharmacokinetic data in Japanese subjects suggest a lower clearance of meloxicam in comparison to Caucasian subjects, but is not considered to require dose-adjustment due to the high intra-individual variability observed.

Hepatic Insufficiency: Following a single 15 mg dose of meloxicam there was no marked difference in plasma concentrations in subjects with mild (Child-Pugh Class I) and moderate (Child-Pugh Class II) hepatic impairment compared to healthy volunteers. Protein binding of meloxicam was not affected by hepatic insufficiency. No dose adjustment is necessary in mild to moderate hepatic insufficiency. Patients with severe hepatic impairment (Child-Pugh Class III) have not been adequately studied.

Renal Insufficiency: Meloxicam pharmacokinetics have been investigated in subjects with different degrees of renal insufficiency. Total drug plasma concentrations decreased with the degree of renal impairment while free AUC values were similar. Total clearance of meloxicam increased in these patients probably due to the increase in free fraction leading to an increased metabolic clearance. There is no need for dose adjustment in patients with mild to moderate renal failure (CrCL >15 mL/min or >0.25 mL/s). Patients with severe renal insufficiency have not been adequately studied. The use of MOBICOX in subjects with severe renal impairment is not recommended (see Warnings and Precautions, Advanced Renal Disease).

In terminal renal failure, the increase in the volume of distribution may result in higher free meloxicam concentrations, and a daily dose of 7.5 mg must not be exceeded.

Hemodialysis: Following a single dose of meloxicam, the free C_{max} plasma concentrations were higher in patients with renal failure on chronic hemodialysis (1% free fraction) in comparison to healthy volunteers (0.3% free fraction). Hemodialysis did not lower the total drug concentration in plasma; therefore, additional doses are not necessary after hemodialysis. Meloxicam is not dialyzable.

STORAGE AND STABILITY: Store at controlled room temperature (15-30°C), safely out of the reach of children. Store in a dry place.

INFORMATION FOR THE PATIENT: Published in e-CPS, available by subscription at www.e-cps.ca.

DOSAGE FORMS, COMPOSITION AND PACKAGING: 7.5 mg: Each round, biconvex, pastel yellow tablet, identified with "M" on one side and the company logo on the other side, contains: meloxicam 7.5 mg. Nonmedicinal ingredients: anhydrous colloidal silica, crospolyvidone, lactose, magnesium stearate, microcrystalline cellulose, polyvidone and sodium citrate. Bottles of 100 and 500.

15 mg: Each round, pastel yellow, snap-tab tablet , impressed with the code "77C" on both sides of a broad score line on its concave side and the Boehringer company log on its convex side, contains: meloxicam 15 mg. Nonmedicinal ingredients: anhydrous colloidal silica, crospolyvidone, lactose, magnesium stearate, microcrystalline cellulose, polyvidone and sodium citrate. Bottles of 100 and 500.

(Shown in Product Identification Section)

Moclobemide

Antidepressant—Reversible Inhibitor of Monoamine Oxidase-A

CPhA Monograph

Date of Preparation: October 2005

This monograph has been compiled by CPhA and reviewed by experts. It may contain information different from that found in Health Canada-approved Product Monographs. The reader is referred to the *CPS* Editorial Policy for more information.

SUMMARY PRODUCT INFORMATION:

Route of Administration	Dosage Form	Strength
Oral	Immediate-release tablet	100 mg, 150 mg, 300 mg

INDICATIONS AND CLINICAL USE: Moclobemide is indicated for:

- Management of depressive illness

Moclobemide has been used as a second-line agent in the management of social anxiety disorder and in the management of bipolar disorder.

CONTRAINDICATIONS:

- Patients who are hypersensitive to moclobemide or to any ingredient in the formulation or component of the container.
- Patients taking tricyclic antidepressants, SSRIs, other MAO inhibitors, meperidine or thioridazine.

WARNINGS AND PRECAUTIONS: Endocrine and Metabolism: Caution is advised in prescribing moclobemide to patients with thyrotoxicosis or pheochromocytoma, as conventional (irreversible, nonselective) MAO inhibitors may precipitate a hypertensive crisis in these patients.

Perioperative Considerations: Moclobemide should be discontinued at least 2 days prior to administration of anesthetic agents, particularly local or spinal anesthesia that includes epinephrine.

Psychiatric: The possibility of suicide in depressed patients should always be taken into consideration. Therapy with moclobemide should be appropriately monitored and potentially suicidal patients should be prescribed limited quantities of moclobemide at a time.

Special Populations: Pregnant Women: There is very little published information on the use of moclobemide during pregnancy. One case report described no harmful effects on the fetus following moclobemide 300 mg/day taken throughout pregnancy. As with any antidepressant, the possible risk of using moclobemide during pregnancy must be weighed against the potential effects of untreated depression on both mother and fetus.

Nursing Women: Moclobemide is excreted in small amounts in breast milk. Levels in milk are highest 3 hours following a dose and undetectable after 12 hours. Clinical effects on the nursing infant are not known. If breast-feeding is continued during moclobemide therapy, it should be timed to minimize exposure of the infant to the drug.

Occupational Hazards: Patients should be advised not to drive or perform other hazardous tasks while taking moclobemide until they are certain of how the drug affects them.

ADVERSE REACTIONS: More Common Adverse Drug Reactions (≥1%): See Table 1.

Table 1: Moclobemide

More Common Adverse Drug Reactions (≥1%)

Body System	Effect	Clinical Comment
Cardiovascular	Tachycardia/palpitations (3.8%), hypotension (3%)	May be dose-related
Central Nervous System	Headache (8%), insomnia (7.3%), dizziness (5.1%), tremor (5%), agitation (4.5%), restlessness (4.1%), sedation (3.7%)	May be dose-related; in clinical trials, the incidences of headache, dizziness and sedation were higher in the placebo group
Dermatologic	Sweating (2.4%)	
Gastrointestinal	Dry mouth (9.2%), nausea (5.2%), constipation (3.9%), epigastric pain (2.3%), diarrhea (1.8%), vomiting (1.6%)	May be dose-related; in clinical trials the incidences of dry mouth and epigastric pain were higher in the placebo group
Ophthalmologic	Blurred vision (1.8%)	May be dose-related

DRUG INTERACTIONS: Drug-Drug Interactions: See Table 2.

Table 2: Moclobemide

Drug-Drug Interactions

Interacting Drug	Effect	Clinical Comment
Alpha/beta agonists (e.g., pseudoephedrine, ephedrine), $alpha_1$ agonists (e.g., midodrine, phenylephrine), amphetamines (e.g., dextroamphetamine, phentermine), buspirone, methylphenidate, reserpine	Possible increased hypertensive effect of interacting drug	Avoid combination
Antipsychotic Agents	Increase in psychotic symptoms in depressed patients with schizophrenia or schizoaffective disorder	Monitor psychiatric symptoms during concomitant therapy
CNS Depressants (e.g., alcohol, benzodiazepines, opioids)	Additive CNS depressant effects	Avoid excessive alcohol consumption; monitor for additive effects; caution patients about potential effect on ability to perform hazardous tasks such as driving
Serotonergic drugs such as dextromethorphan, ergotamine, L-tryptophan, mirtazapine, pethidine (meperidine), sibutramine, SSRIs, SNRIs (duloxetine, venlafaxine), TCAs, triptans (except eletriptan, naratriptan)	Increased serotonergic effect of interacting drug (possible serotonin syndrome)	Avoid combination; allow 2 week wash out period between drugs, 5 weeks after discontinuing fluoxetine
Atomoxetine, bupropion	Potential increased neurotoxicity of interacting drug	Avoid combination; mechanism may involve increased dopaminergic activity
Inhibitors of CYP2D6 (e.g., cimetidine, fluoxetine, itraconazole, ketoconazole, paroxetine, ritonavir) or CYP2C19 (e.g., fluvoxamine)	Decreased clearance of moclobemide	Consider alternative therapy to avoid moclobemide toxicity, or monitor closely for increased effects of moclobemide and reduce dose if indicated; if taken concurrently with cimetidine, use half the usual moclobemide dose
Inducers of CYP2D6 or CYP2C19 (e.g., carbamazepine, phenytoin, rifampin)	Increased clearance of moclobemide	Consider alternative therapy to avoid therapeutic failure of moclobemide or monitor for inadequate moclobemide response
Levodopa	Increased adverse effects of levodopa (e.g., headache, insomnia, nausea)	Monitor for adverse effects of levodopa, including hypertension

Legend:
SSRIs=selective serotonin reuptake inhibitors.
SNRIs=serotonin/norepinephrine reuptake inhibitors.
TCAs=tricyclic antidepressants.

Drug-Food Interactions: Treatment with moclobemide does not necessitate the special dietary restrictions associated with irreversible MAO inhibitor use. Moclobemide should be given immediately after meals to minimize tyramine potentiation.

Drug-Herb Interactions: St. John's Wort: Concurrent administration of moclobemide and St. John's wort may result in excessive serotonergic effects or serotonin syndrome. Combination therapy should be avoided.

DOSAGE AND ADMINISTRATION: Recommended Dose and Dosage Adjustment: Adults: See Table 3.

Table 3: Moclobemide

Dose in Adult Patients

Indication	Route	Initial Dose	Dose Titration	Usual Dose	Maximum Dose	Duration of Therapy	Clinical Comment
Depression	Oral	150 mg BID	Starting at least 1 week after therapy initiated, increase dose gradually as needed	450 mg/day	600 mg/day	Several weeks to months or years, depending on response and whether depressive episode is initial or recurrent	For older individuals, use adult dosing regimen

Hepatic Impairement: Patients with severe hepatic dysfunction should receive one-third to one-half the usual dose.

Renal Impairement: Caution is advised. Dosage adjustment is not routinely recommended.

Mixed Dose: Missed doses should be taken as soon as possible unless it is close to the time for the next scheduled dose.

Administration: Moclobemide should be taken immediately after a meal.

OVERDOSAGE:

Signs and Symptoms: Clinical effects of excessive MAO inhibition result from accumulation of amines such as serotonin and norepinephrine. Initial symptoms include hypertension, drowsiness, dizziness, confusion, tremors and headache, which may progress to agitation, muscle rigidity and seizures. Dysrhythmias, sweating, chills and hyperthermia can also occur. Late phase symptoms include hypotension, bradycardia, cardiovascular collapse, respiratory depression, pulmonary edema and coma. Potential complications are rhabdomyolysis, hemolysis, disseminated intravascular coagulation, acute renal failure (secondary to hypotension or rhabdomyolysis) and hypertensive crisis.

The risk of hypertensive crisis is increased in the presence of drugs such as amphetamines, cocaine, decongestants (e.g., pseudoephedrine, phenylephrine) or foods containing tyramine (e.g., aged cheese, smoked meats, red wine and beer). Other overdose symptoms may be exacerbated by co-ingestion of serotonergic drugs such as dextromethorphan, ergotamine, L-tryptophan, mirtazapine, pethidine (meperidine), sibutramine, SSRIs, SNRIs (duloxetine, venlafaxine), TCAs, triptans (except eletriptan, naratriptan).

Although reversible MAO inhibitors such as moclobemide are considered to be less toxic in overdose than their irreversible counterparts, at least one fatality attributed to a single ingestion of moclobemide has been reported.

Recommended Management: Initial management should focus first on establishing the airway and stabilizing the heart rate and blood pressure, and subsequently on management of rhabdomyolysis, hyperthermia, seizures and muscle rigidity. Gut decontamination can take place after the patient is stabilized.

Because severe hypertension is often short-lived, it is important to use agents with a shorter duration of action such as nitroprusside, nitroglycerin or phentolamine. These drugs should be titrated to response. Beta-blockers should not be used.

Hyperthermia should be aggressively managed using ice baths, cold water and fans. Benzodiazepines are useful for muscle rigidity, seizures and agitation. Dysrhythmias should be treated with lidocaine or procainamide. Once the patient is stable, a dose of activated charcoal 1 g/kg should be given. If the time of stabilization is within one hour post-ingestion, gastric lavage should be considered.

Consideration should be given to the possibility of mixed overdose and its potential medical implications.

For management of a suspected drug overdose, CPhA recommends that you contact your **regional Poison Control Centre**. See the *CPS* Directory section for a list of Poison Control Centres.

ACTION AND CLINICAL PHARMACOLOGY: Mechanism of Action: Moclobemide binds to monoamine oxidase-A (MAO-A) in a competitive (reversible) manner, allowing for repletion of deactivated MAO within hours, as opposed to days for irreversible MAO inhibitors. Inhibition of MAO-A results in decreased metabolism of norepinephrine, serotonin and dopamine in neuronal cells and synapses.

Pharmacokinetics: Adults: Absorption: Moclobemide is well absorbed (> 95%) from the gastrointestinal tract. First-pass hepatic metabolism reduces the bioavailability of single doses to 45 to 70%, but with ongoing administration, first-pass metabolism becomes saturated and bioavailability stabilizes at around 80%.

Distribution: Maximal plasma concentration is achieved within 1 to 2 hours after oral administration. Moclobemide is approximately 50% protein bound and is distributed extensively to tissues.

Metabolism: Moclobemide is extensively metabolized in the liver primarily by acetylation. Some metabolites may possess pharmacologic activity. The elimination half-life of moclobemide is approximately 1 to 2 hours.

Excretion: Metabolites are excreted in the urine.

STORAGE AND STABILITY: Moclobemide tablets should be stored at 15 to 30°C.

Modecate® Concentrate ℞
fluphenazine decanoate
Antipsychotic

Bristol-Myers Squibb

Date of Preparation: July 22, 1980
Date of Revision: July 23, 2009

PHARMACOLOGY: The effects of fluphenazine decanoate are the same as those of fluphenazine HCl; however, the slow release of the decanoate derivative of fluphenazine from the site of injection results in a prolonged duration of action. Once released in the blood, fluphenazine decanoate is rapidly hydrolyzed by blood esterases with no attenuation of its antipsychotic action. The onset of action generally appears between 24 to 72 hours after injection, and the effects of the drug on psychotic symptoms become significant within 48 to 96 hours. Amelioration of symptoms then continues for 1 to 8 weeks with an average duration of 3 to 4 weeks. There is considerable variation in the individual response of patients to this depot fluphenazine and its use for maintenance therapy requires careful supervision.

Like other phenothiazines fluphenazine exerts activity at various levels of the CNS as well as on peripheral organ systems which accounts for its antipsychotic action and side effects common to this class of drugs. Indirect evidence indicates that the antipsychotic effects of phenothiazines are linked to their effect in blocking dopamine and other catecholamine receptor sites.

Fluphenazine differs from some phenothiazine derivatives in several respects: it has less potentiating effect on CNS depressants and anesthetics than do some of the phenothiazines and appears to be less sedating. While hypotension may occur less frequently than with other phenothiazines, appropriate precautions should be observed when using fluphenazine decanoate (see Precautions). Fluphenazine however, is among the group of phenothiazines which exhibit a greater propensity for producing extrapyramidal reactions.

Pharmacokinetics: As with all antipsychotic drugs, fluphenazine is characterized by inter-individual variability in pharmacokinetics.

Fluphenazine is extensively metabolized, undergoing "first pass" metabolism by the liver, and is excreted in both the urine and the feces. Fluphenazine is highly protein-bound (greater than 90 %) in plasma.

Esterification of fluphenazine with a long-chain fatty acid and dissolving it in a sesame seed oil vehicle delays diffusion and availability of free drug released from the oily deposit site. Peak plasma concentration occurs within the first 24-hours after intramuscular injection of fluphenazine decanoate. The onset of action is generally between 24 and 72 hours after injection of fluphenazine decanoate, and the effects of drug on psychotic symptoms become significant within 48 to 96 hours. The serum half-life is approximately 7-10 days.

Phenothiazines cross the blood-brain barrier, cross the placenta easily, and cannot be removed by dialysis. It is not known whether fluphenazine is present in breast milk. However, other phenothiazines have been shown to be excreted in human breast milk.

INDICATIONS: Adults: MODECATE CONCENTRATE (fluphenazine decanoate) is a long-acting parenteral preparation, indicated in the management of manifestations of schizophrenia (see Dosage).

Fluphenazine decanoate is not indicated for the management of severely agitated psychotic patients or psychoneurotic patients.

Geriatrics (≥65 years of age): Fluphenazine decanoate is not indicated for the management of geriatric patients with confusion or agitation.

Pediatrics (<18 years of age): Fluphenazine decanoate is not intended for use in children under 18 years of age.

CONTRAINDICATIONS: MODECATE (fluphenazine decanoate) is contraindicated in:
- Patients with a history of hypersensitivity to the active or inactive ingredients.
- Patients, who have shown hypersensitivity to other phenothiazines, including fluphenazine, should not be given fluphenazine decanoate as cross-sensitivity reactions may occur.
- Patients with marked cerebral atherosclerosis, suspected or established subcortical brain damage, with or without hypothalamic damage, since a hyperthermic reaction with temperatures above 40°C may occur, sometimes not until 14-16 hours after drug administration.
- Patients with renal insufficiency, pheochromocytoma, or in patients with severe cardiovascular disorders.
- Patients who are comatose.
- Patients with severe CNS depression.
- Patients receiving large doses of CNS depressant medications (e.g., alcohol, barbiturates, narcotics, hypnotics, etc).
- Patients with blood dyscrasias.
- Patients with liver damage.

WARNINGS: Severe adverse reactions requiring immediate medical attention may occur and are difficult to predict. Therefore, the evaluation of tolerance and response, and establishment of adequate maintenance therapy, require careful stabilization of each patient under continuous, close medical observation and supervision.

Occupational Hazards: The use of this drug may impair the mental and physical abilities required for driving a car or operating heavy machinery particularly during the first days of therapy. Potentiation of the effects of alcohol may also occur.

Prolongation of the QT Interval: As with other neuroleptics, very rare cases of QT interval prolongation have been reported with MODECATE. Neuroleptic phenothiazines may potentiate QT interval prolongation, which increases the risk of onset of serious ventricular arrhythmias of the torsades de pointes type, which is potentially fatal (sudden death). QT prolongation is exacerbated, in particular, in the presence of bradycardia, hypokalemia, and congenital or acquired (i.e., drug induced) QT prolongation (see also Adverse Events, Prolongation of the QT Interval). As well, concomitant treatment with other drugs known to cause QT prolongation should be avoided (for more information, see Drug Interactions, Medicines that Prolong the QT Interval).

Pregnancy: The safety of use in pregnant women has not been established. Therefore, MODECATE CONCENTRATE (fluphenazine decanoate) should not be administered to women of childbearing potential, particularly during the first trimester of pregnancy, unless, in the opinion of the physician, the expected benefit to the patient outweighs the potential risk to the fetus.

Children: The safety and efficacy of fluphenazine decanoate in children have not been established. Therefore, fluphenazine decanoate is not indicated for use in the pediatric age group (see Indications).

Tardive Dyskinesia: Tardive dyskinesia (TD) is a syndrome of involuntary hyperkinetic abnormal movements that occur in predisposed individuals during or following the cessation of long-term neuroleptic drug therapy including fluphenazine. TD is characterized by involuntary, repetitive, purposeless hyperkinetic movements that involve the tongue, face, mouth, lips or jaw, trunk and extremities. The prevalence of TD greatly varies; when the mildest symptoms are included, prevalence can be 70%, whereas severe symptom rates are around 2.5%. The frequency and severity of TD increases with age, particularly in females.

The mechanism of TD is not known; though dopamine dysfunction is believed to underlie TD, it may be necessary but not sufficient to explain this complex disorder. Both the risk of developing the syndrome and the likelihood that it will become irreversible are believed to increase as the duration of treatment and the total cumulative dose of neuroleptic drugs administered to the patient increase. However, the syndrome can develop, although much less commonly, after relatively brief treatment periods at low doses.

There is no known treatment for established cases of TD, although the syndrome may remit, partially or completely, if neuroleptic treatment is withdrawn. However, neuroleptic treatment itself suppresses the signs and symptoms of the syndrome thereby masking the underlying disease process.

Given these considerations, neuroleptic drugs should be prescribed in a manner that is most likely to minimize the occurrence of TD. Reducing the dose to the lowest effective level or discontinuing the drug for as long as possible continues to be the most rational approach. In patients who require chronic treatment, the smallest dose and the shortest duration of treatment producing a satisfactory clinical response should be sought. The need for continued treatment should be reassessed periodically.

If signs and symptoms of tardive dyskinesia appear in a patient on neuroleptics, drug discontinuation should be considered. However, some patients may require treatment despite the presence of the syndrome.

Neuroleptic Malignant Syndrome (Hyperthermia with Extrapyramidal and Autonomic Disturbances; Neuroleptic-Induced Hyperpyrexia): Neuroleptic malignant syndrome is a potentially fatal symptom complex that has been reported in association with antipsychotic drugs.

Clinical manifestations of NMS are hyperpyrexia, muscle rigidity, altered mental status, and evidence of autonomic instability (irregular pulse or blood pressure, tachycardia, diaphoresis, and cardiac dysrhythmia). Additional signs may include elevated creatine phosphokinase, myoglobinuria (rhabdomyolysis), and acute renal failure.

In arriving at a diagnosis, it is important to identify cases where the clinical presentation includes both serious medical illness (e.g., pneumonia, systemic infection, etc.), and untreated or inadequately treated extrapyramidal signs and symptoms (EPS). Other important considerations in the differential diagnosis include central anticholinergic toxicity, heat stroke, drug fever, and primary central nervous system pathology.

The management of NMS should include 1) immediate discontinuation of all antipsychotic drugs including MODECATE CONCENTRATE and other drugs not essential to therapy; 2), intensive symptomatic treatment and medical monitoring; and 3) treatment of any concomitant serious medical problems for which specific treatments are available. There is no general agreement about specific pharmacological treatment for uncomplicated NMS.

If a patient requires antipsychotic drug treatment after recovery from NMS, the potential re-introduction of therapy should be very carefully considered. The patient should be carefully monitored, since recurrence of NMS has been reported.

Cerebrovascular Events, Including Stroke, in Elderly Patients with Dementia: Elderly patients with dementia treated with certain atypical antipsychotic drugs are at an increased risk of Cerebrovascular Adverse Events (CVAEs) such as stroke and transient ischemic attacks, as well as death, compared to placebo. The mechanism of this increased risk is not known. As an increase in the risk with other antipsychotic drugs cannot be excluded, fluphenazine should be used with caution in the elderly with dementia.

Other Warnings: The use of this drug may impair the mental and physical abilities required for driving or operating heavy machinery, particularly during the first days of therapy. Potentiation of the effects of alcohol may occur with the use of this drug (see Precautions, Information to Be Provided to the Patient).

PRECAUTIONS: Autonomic Nervous System Effects, including Blood Pressure Changes and Paralytic Ileus: (See also Adverse Events, Autonomic Nervous System.)

Since hypotension and electrocardiographic changes suggestive of myocardial ischemia have been associated with the administration of phenothiazines, fluphenazine decanoate should be used with caution in patients with compensated cardiovascular or cerebrovascular disorders.

Hypotensive phenomena may develop in phenothiazine-treated patients who are undergoing surgery. Careful observation is necessary and anesthetic or central nervous system depressant dosages may have to be reduced.

The effects of anticholinergics may be potentiated in patients receiving fluphenazine because of added anticholinergic effects. Paralytic ileus, even resulting in death, may occur especially in the elderly. Fluphenazine decanoate should be used cautiously in patients exposed to extreme heat or phosphorus insecticides.

Fluphenazine should be used cautiously in patients exposed to extreme heat or phosphorous insecticides; in patients with a history of convulsive disorders (since grand mal convulsions have been known to occur in patients on therapy with fluphenazine); and in patients with special medical disorders, such as mitral insufficiency or other cardiovascular diseases, or pheochromocytoma.

Blood Dyscrasias, Liver Damage: (See also Adverse Effects, Hematologic and Hepatic.)

Particularly during the first few months of therapy routine blood counts and hepatic function tests are advised as blood dyscrasias and liver damage, manifested by cholestatic jaundice, may occur. In patients on long-term therapy, renal function should be monitored; if BUN (blood urea nitrogen) becomes abnormal, treatment should be discontinued.

The possibility of liver damage, lenticular and corneal deposits, pigmentary retinopathy, and the development of irreversible dyskinesia should be borne in mind when patients are on prolonged therapy.

Alterations in Cephalin flocculation, alkaline phosphatase, sometimes accompanied by abnormalities in other liver function tests, have been reported in patients receiving esterified fluphenazine who have had no clinical evidence of liver damage. This, however, is not uncommon with phenothiazine therapy.

Convulsions: Phenothiazines, particularly those with a long duration of action, should be used with caution in patients with a history of convulsive disorders since grand mal convulsions have been known to occur.

Allergic Cross-Sensitivity: Because of the possibility of cross-sensitivity, MODECATE CONCENTRATE (fluphenazine decanoate) should be used with caution in patients who have developed cholestatic jaundice, and dermatoses or other allergic reactions to phenothiazine derivatives.

Silent Pneumonia: As with other antipsychotic agents, the physician should be alert to the possible development of silent pneumonias in patients under treatment with phenothiazines.

Elevated Prolactin Levels: Neuroleptic drugs elevate prolactin levels; the elevation persists during chronic administration. An increase in mammary neoplasms has been found in rodents after chronic administration of neuroleptic drugs. Neither clinical studies nor epidemiologic studies conducted to date, however, have shown an association between chronic administration of these drugs and mammary tumorigenesis.

Drug Interactions: Medicines that Prolong the QT Interval: Medicines that can prolong the QT interval should be avoided, as should any medicine that can cause electrolyte imbalance or an increase in the concentration of fluphenazine in the blood (see Warnings and Adverse Effects). Medications that prolong the QT interval include dofetilide, sotalol, quinidine, other Class Ia and III anti-arrhythmias, some other antipsychotics (e.g. mesoridazine, thioridazine, chlorpromazine, droperidol, pimozide), sparfloxacin, gatifloxacin, moxifloxacin, halofantrine, mefloquine, pentamidine, arsenic trioxide, levomethadyl acetate, dolasetron mesylate, probucol or tacrolimus. MODECATE should not be given with drugs that have demonstrated QT prolongation as one of their pharmacodynamic effects and have this effect described in their respective Product Monograph as a contraindication or a warning.

CNS Depressants/Alcohol/Analgesics: The patient's response to alcohol and other CNS depressants such as hypnotics, sedatives or strong analgesics, may be exaggerated while taking MODECATE CONCENTRATE. Combined use with narcotic analgesics may cause hypotension as well as CNS or respiratory depression (see Contraindications).

Tricyclic Antidepressants: Phenothiazines impair the metabolism of tricyclic antidepressants. Serum concentrations of both the tricyclic and phenothiazine are increased. Sedative and antimuscarinic effects may be potentiated or prolonged. Tricyclics may increase potential for arrhythmia.

Lithium: Neurotoxicity has been reported rarely when used concomitantly with fluphenazine.

ACE inhibitors/Thiazide Diuretics: Hypotension may result via additive or synergistic pharmacological activity.

Antihypertensives: The antihypertensive action of guanethidine, clonidine and possibly other adrenegic-blocking antihypertensive agents may be blocked. Clonidine may decrease the antipsychotic activity of phenothiazine.

Beta Blockers: Plasma levels of both drugs may be increased. Dosage reduction of both drugs is recommended.

Metrizamide: Phenothiazines may predispose patients to metrizamide-induced seizures. Discontinue for 48 hours prior to and for at least 24 hours after myelography.

Epinephrine and Other Sympathomimetics: Phenothiazines may antagonize the action of adrenaline and other sympathomimetics and may cause severe hypotension.

Antiparkinsonian Medications: Phenothiazines may impair the anti-Parkinson effect of dopaminergic antiparkinsonian medications such as dopamine agonists and L-Dopa.

Anticholinergics/Antimuscarinics: Cholinergic blockade may be exaggerated when MODECATE CONCENTRATE is administered with anticholinergic agents, especially in older patients. Antimuscarinic effects may be potentiated or prolonged. Close supervision and careful dosage adjustment are required when MODECATE CONCENTRATE is used with other anticholinergic or antimuscarinic drugs.

Anticonvulsants: Anticonvulsant action may be impaired by MODECATE CONCENTRATE.

Anticoagulants: Phenothiazines may alter the effects of anticoagulants.

Antidiabetics: Phenothiazines have been associated rarely with loss of blood glucose control in patients with diabetes.

Cimetidine: Cimetidine may reduce plasma concentrations of phenothiazines.

Antacids/Antidiarrheal Agents: Concurrent administration may interfere with absorption. Administration of antacids should be spaced at least 1 hour before or 2-3 hours after fluphenazine dose.

Amphetamine/Anorectic Agents: Concurrent administration may produce antagonistic pharmacologic effects.

Abrupt Withdrawal: In general, phenothiazines do not produce psychic dependence; however, gastritis, nausea and vomiting, dizziness, and tremulousness have been reported following abrupt cessation of high-dose therapy. Reports suggest that these symptoms can be reduced if concomitant antiparkinson agents are continued for several weeks after the phenothiazine is withdrawn.

Geriatrics: Antipsychotic drugs should be used with care in elderly patients (>60 years old), as these patients have a greater potential for adverse effects.

Doses in the lower range (¼ to ⅓ of those in younger adults) should be sufficient for most elderly patients. Response should be monitored and dose adjusted. If an increase is necessary, doses should be gradually increased (see Dosage).

Information to Be Provided to the Patient: Given the likelihood that some patients exposed chronically to neuroleptics will develop tardive dyskinesia, it is advised that all patients in whom chronic use is contemplated be given, if possible, full information about this risk. The decision to inform patients and/or their guardians must obviously take into account the clinical circumstances and the competency of the patient to understand the information provided.

Patients should also be warned that fluphenazine may 1) impair their ability to perform activities requiring mental alertness or physical coordination, 2) enhance their response to alcohol, barbiturates or other CNS depressants, and 3) increase their vulnerability when exposed to temperature extremes, possibly resulting in hyperthermia or hypothermia.

ADVERSE EFFECTS: Central Nervous System: Extrapyramidal Symptoms: The adverse effects most frequently reported with phenothiazine compounds are extrapyramidal symptoms including pseudoparkinsonism (tremor, rigidity, etc.), dystonia, dyskinesia, akathisia, oculogyric crises, opisthotonos, and hyperreflexia. Most often these extrapyramidal symptoms are reversible; however, they may be persistent. With any given phenothiazine derivative, the incidence and severity of such events depend more on individual patient sensitivity than on other factors, but dosage level and patient age are also determinants.

MODECATE CONCENTRATE (fluphenazine decanoate) produces a higher incidence of extrapyramidal reactions than the less potent piperazine derivatives or the straight-chain phenothiazines such as chlorpromazine. Extrapyramidal reactions tend to occur in the first few days after an injection of fluphenazine decanoate. Caution should be exercised in those who have marked extrapyramidal reactions to oral phenothiazines or similar drugs, particularly elderly females. Extrapyramidal reactions may be alarming, and the patient should be forewarned and reassured. These symptoms can usually be controlled by administration of anticholinergic or antiparkinson drugs (such as benztropine mesylate) and by subsequent reduction in dosage.

The use of prophylactic antiparkinson medication may be considered, although its therapeutic value has not yet been established.

Tardive Dyskinesia: (see Warnings, Tardive Dyskinesia). The syndrome is characterized by rhythmical involuntary movements of the tongue, face, mouth, or jaw (e.g., protrusion of tongue, puffing of cheeks, puckering of mouth, chewing movements). These may be accompanied by involuntary movements of the trunk and the extremities. The severity of the syndrome and the degree of impairment produced vary widely.

As with all antipsychotic agents, tardive dyskinesia may appear in some patients on long-term therapy or may occur upon dosage reduction or after drug therapy has been discontinued. The risk seems to be greater in elderly patients on high dose therapy, especially females. The symptoms are persistent and in some patients appear to be irreversible.

There is no known effective treatment for tardive dyskinesia; antiparkinsonian agents usually do not alleviate the symptoms of this syndrome.

Neuroleptic drugs should be prescribed in a manner that is most likely to minimize the occurrence of tardive dyskinesia. Reducing the dose to the lowest effective level or discontinuing the drug for as long as possible continues to be the most rational approach. In patients who require chronic treatment, the smallest dose and the shortest duration of treatment producing a satisfactory clinical response should be sought. The need for continued treatment should be reassessed periodically.

Other CNS Effects: Drowsiness or lethargy, if they occur, may necessitate a reduction in dosage; the induction of a catatonic-like state has been known to occur with high dosages of fluphenazine. As with other phenothiazine compounds, reactivation or aggravation of psychotic processes may be encountered. In some patients, phenothiazine derivatives have been known to cause restlessness, excitement, or bizarre dreams.

Rare occurrences of **neuroleptic malignant syndrome (NMS)** have been reported in patients on neuroleptic therapy. The syndrome is characterized by hyperthermia, muscular rigidity, autonomic instability (labile blood pressure, tachycardia, diaphoresis), akinesia, and altered consciousness, sometimes progressing to stupor or coma. Leukocytosis, fever, elevated CPK, liver function abnormalities, and acute renal failure may also occur with NMS. Neuroleptic therapy should be discontinued immediately and vigorous symptomatic treatment implemented since the syndrome is potentially fatal (see Warnings, Neuroleptic Malignant Syndrome (Hyperthermia with Extrapyramidal and Autonomic Disturbances; Neuroleptic-Induced Hyperpyrexia).

Prolongation of the QT Interval: QT prolongation, ventricular arrhythmias, ventricular fibrillation, ventricular tachycardia, cardiac arrest, torsades de pointes and sudden unexplained death are class effects of phenothiazines. (See Warnings, Prolongation of the QT Interval, and Precautions, Drug Interactions.)

Cerebrovascular Stroke-like Events: An approximately 3-fold increased risk, compared to placebo, of cerebrovascular adverse events, such as stroke and transient ischemic attacks as well as death, has been seen in randomized, placebo-controlled clinical trials, in the dementia population with some atypical antipsychotics. Fluphenazine should be used with caution in the elderly with dementia. (See Warnings, Cerebrovascular Events, Including Stroke, in Elderly Patients with Dementia.)

Autonomic Nervous System: (See also Warnings.) Hypotension, hypertension and fluctuations in blood pressure have been reported with fluphenazine.

Patients with pheochromocytoma, cerebral vascular or renal insufficiency, or a severe cardiac reserve deficiency such as mitral insufficiency, appear to be particularly prone to hypotensive reactions with phenothiazine compounds and should therefore be observed closely when the drug is administered.

Autonomic reactions including nausea and loss of appetite, salivation, polyuria, perspiration, dry mouth, headache, and constipation may occur. Autonomic effects can usually be controlled by reducing or temporarily discontinuing dosage.

In some patients, phenothiazine derivatives have caused blurred vision, glaucoma, bladder paralysis, fecal impaction, paralytic ileus, tachycardia, or nasal congestion.

Metabolic and Endocrine: Weight change, peripheral edema, hyponatremia, syndrome of inappropriate antidiuretic hormone secretion, abnormal lactation, gynecomastia, menstrual irregularities, false pregnancy test results, impotency in men and libido changes in women have all been known to occur in some patients on phenothiazine therapy.

Allergic Reactions: Skin disorders such as itching, erythema, urticaria, seborrhea, photosensitivity, eczema and exfoliative dermatitis have been reported with phenothiazine derivatives. The possibility of anaphylactoid reactions should be borne in mind.

Hematologic: Leukopenia, agranulocytosis, thrombocytopenic or nonthrombocytopenic purpura, eosinophilia, and pancytopenia have been observed with phenothiazine derivatives. If any soreness of the mouth, gums or throat or any symptoms of upper respiratory infection occur and confirmatory leukocyte count indicates cellular depression, therapy should be discontinued and other appropriate measures instituted immediately.

Hepatic: Liver damage as manifested by cholestatic jaundice may be encountered, particularly during the first months of therapy; treatment should be discontinued if this occurs. An increase in cephalin flocculation, sometimes accompanied by alterations in other liver function tests and hepatitis, has been reported in patients receiving the enanthate ester of fluphenazine (a closely related compound).

Others: Sudden, unexpected and unexplained deaths have been reported in hospitalized psychotic patients receiving phenothiazines. Previous brain damage or seizures may be predisposing factors; high doses should be avoided in known seizure patients. Several patients have shown flare-ups of psychotic behaviour patterns shortly before death. Autopsy findings have usually revealed acute fulminating pneumonia or pneumonitis, aspiration of gastric contents or intramyocardial lesions.

Potentiation of central nervous system depressants (opiates, analgesics, antihistamines, barbiturates, alcohol) may occur (see Contraindications).

The following adverse reactions have also occurred with phenothiazine derivatives: fever, vomiting, systemic lupus erythematosus like syndrome, hypotension severe enough to cause fatal cardiac arrest, altered ECG and EEG tracings, altered CSF proteins, cerebral edema, asthma, disturbances of body temperature (hypo- or hyperthermia), laryngeal edema, and angioneurotic edema. Skin pigmentation, and lenticular and corneal opacities have been seen with long-term use.

Injections of fluphenazine decanoate are well tolerated, local tissue reactions occur only rarely.

OVERDOSE:

Symptoms : Symptoms of overdose will likely be manifested as severe extrapyramidal reactions, hypotension or sedation. CNS depression may progress to coma with areflexia. Restlessness, confusion and excitement may occur with early or mild intoxication.

Treatment: The drug should be withdrawn and the symptoms of overdose treated supportively. Initial hospitalization may be required in cases of large overdose and close medical supervision should be maintained throughout the duration of drug action. Up to several hours after an oral overdose, gastric lavage should be attempted, followed by activated charcoal and then cathartics.

An airway should be maintained. If severe hypotension should occur, supportive measures including the use of intravenous vasopressor drugs should be instituted immediately. Levarterenol bitartrate Injection, U.S.P. is the most suitable drug for this purpose; **epinephrine should not be used** since phenothiazine derivatives have been found to reverse its action, resulting in a further lowering of blood pressure.

Extrapyramidal symptoms may be treated with antiparkinsonian agents, and should be continued for several weeks. Antiparkinson medication should be withdrawn gradually to avoid the emergence of rebound extrapyramidal symptoms.

Limited experience indicates that phenothiazines are not dialyzable. Hemodialysis, peritoneal dialysis, exchange transfusions, and forced diuresis are ineffective in phenothiazine poisoning.

> For management of a suspected drug overdose, contact your regional Poison Control Centre. See the *CPS* Directory section for a list of Poison Control Centres.

DOSAGE: MODECATE CONCENTRATE (fluphenazine decanoate) is usually given as an intramuscular injection preferably in the gluteus maximus, although it may also be administered subcutaneously. MODECATE CONCENTRATE is not for intravenous use.

A dry syringe with a needle of at least 21 gauge should be used to inject MODECATE CONCENTRATE. Use of a wet needle or syringe may cause the solution to become cloudy.

As a long-acting depot fluphenazine, fluphenazine decanoate has been found useful in the maintenance treatment of non-agitated, chronic schizophrenic patients who have been stabilized with short-acting neuroleptics and might benefit from transfer to longer-acting injectable medication. The changeover of medication should aim at maintaining a clinical outcome similar to, or better than, that obtained with the previous therapy. To achieve and maintain the optimum dose, the changeover from other neuroleptic medication should proceed gradually and constant supervision is required during the period of dosage adjustment in order to minimize the risk of overdosage or insufficient suppression of psychotic symptoms before the next injection.

Adults: The initial recommended dose is 2.5 mg to 12.5 mg. An initial dose of 12.5 mg is usually well tolerated.

The onset of action generally appears between 24 to 72 hours after injection, and the effects of the drug on psychotic symptoms become significant within 48 to 96 hours.

Discontinuation of oral neuroleptic medication has been recommended for up to 1 week prior to initiation of depot fluphenazine therapy.

Subsequent doses and frequency of administration must be determined for each patient. There is no reliable dosage comparability between a short-acting neuroleptic and depot fluphenazine and, therefore, the dosage of the long-acting drug must be individualized. Except in particularly sensitive patients, a second dose of 12.5 mg or 25 mg can be given 4 to 10 days after the initial injection. Subsequent dosage adjustments are made in accordance with the clinical circumstances and the response of the patient. Patients can usually be controlled with 25 mg or less, every 2 to 3 weeks. Although doses greater than 50 mg are usually not deemed necessary, doses up to 100 mg have been used in some patients. If doses greater than 50 mg are necessary, the next dose and succeeding doses should be increased in increments of 12.5 mg. While the response to a single injection lasts usually 2 to 3 weeks, it may last for 4 weeks or more.

After an appropriate dosage adjustment is achieved, regular and continuous supervision and reassessment is considered essential in order to permit any further dosage adjustments that might be required to ensure use of the lowest effective individual dose and avoid troublesome side effects.

Since higher doses increase the incidence of extrapyramidal reactions and other adverse effects, the amount of drug used should not be increased in order to prolong the intervals between injections. With higher doses, there is also more variability in the action of depot fluphenazine.

MODECATE CONCENTRATE (100 mg/mL) may be administered in patients who complain of discomfort with a large injection volume or when a smaller injection volume is desirable.

Geriatrics: The suggested initial test dose is 2.5 mg, gradually adjusted according to the response of the patient. Maintenance doses in the lower range (¼ to ⅓ of those in younger adults) may be sufficient for most elderly patients.

"Poor Risk" Patients: MODECATE is contraindicated in patients with known hypersensitivity to phenothiazines (see Contraindications). For patients with disorders that predispose to undue reactions (see Warnings and Precautions), therapy may be initiated cautiously with oral or parenteral fluphenazine hydrochloride. When the pharmacologic effects and an appropriate dosage are apparent, an equivalent dose of MODECATE may be administered. Subsequent dosage adjustments are made in accordance with the response of the patient.

INFORMATION FOR THE PATIENT: Published in e-CPS, available by subscription at www.e-cps.ca.

SUPPLIED: Each mL of injectable solution contains: fluphenazine decanoate 100 mg. Nonmedicinal ingredients: benzyl alcohol 1.5% w/v (preservative) and sesame oil. Ampuls of 1 mL. Store at room temperature and protect from light. Avoid freezing and extreme heat.

Modulon®

trimebutine maleate

Lower Gastrointestinal Tract Motility Regulator

Axcan Pharma

PHARMACOLOGY: MODULON (trimebutine maleate) is a noncompetitive spasmolytic agent. It possesses moderate opiate receptor affinity and has marked antiserotonin activity especially on "M" receptors. It induces regulation of spontaneous activity and increases synchronization between electrophysiological spikes and contractions in isolated guinea pig strips of colon and ileum. However, it does not alter normal motility, but regulates abnormal intestinal activity.

INDICATIONS: For the treatment and relief of symptoms associated with the irritable bowel syndrome (spastic colon). In post-operative paralytic ileus in order to accelerate the resumption of the intestinal transit following abdominal surgery.

CONTRAINDICATIONS: MODULON (trimebutine maleate) is contraindicated in patients with known hypersensitivity to trimebutine or any of the excipients.

No other contraindications have been identified at this time.

WARNINGS: *Pregnancy:* Although teratological studies have not shown any drug related adverse effects on the course and outcome of pregnancy in laboratory animals by both oral and parenteral routes, the use of MODULON (trimebutine maleate) in pregnant women is not recommended.

Children: Not recommended for use in children under 12 years of age.

PRECAUTIONS: *Drug Interactions:* Animal studies have shown that trimebutine maleate increases the duration of d-tubocurarine-induced curarization. No other drug interactions have been observed during clinical trials or otherwise reported.

ADVERSE EFFECTS: In clinical studies, adverse effects of mild to moderate nature occurred in 7% of the patients treated with MODULON (trimebutine maleate). No single side effect occurred in more than 1.8% of the patients and some of these might have been related to the patient's condition rather than the medication. The commonly reported adverse effects are as follows:

Gastrointestinal: Dry mouth, foul taste, diarrhea, dyspepsia, epigastric pain, nausea and constipation were reported in a total of 3.1% of the patient population.

Central Nervous System: Drowsiness, fatigue, dizziness, hot/cold sensations and headaches were reported in 3.3%.

Allergic: rash in 0.4% of the patients.

Miscellaneous: Menstrual problems, painful enlargement of breasts, anxiety, urine retention and slight deafness were also infrequently reported.

OVERDOSE:

Treatment: No evidence of overdosage have been reported to date. However, if overdosage should occur following oral administration of MODULON (trimebutine maleate), gastric lavage is recommended. Treatment should be made according to the symptoms observed.

> For management of a suspected drug overdose, CPhA recommends that you contact your **regional Poison Control Centre**. See the *CPS* Directory section for a list of Poison Control Centres.

DOSAGE: The adult recommended dose is up to 600 mg daily in divided doses. It is administered as one 200 mg tablet three times daily before meals.

SUPPLIED: Each white, round, biconvex tablet, bisected on one side, contains: trimebutine maleate 200 mg. Nonmedicinal ingredients: lactose, magnesium stearate, microcrystalline cellulose, povidone, silicon dioxide and sodium starch glycolate. Bottles of 100. Store at room temperature (15 to 30°C).

(Shown in Product Identification Section)

Mogadon®

nitrazepam

Hypnotic—Anticonvulsant

Valeant

Date of Revision: June 29, 2009

PHARMACOLOGY: Nitrazepam is a benzodiazepine with hypnotic and anticonvulsant properties.

In sleep laboratory studies, nitrazepam decreased sleep latency, increased total sleep time and decreased awake time. There is delay in the onset, and decrease in the duration of REM sleep. Nitrazepam is reported to significantly decrease stage 1, 3 and 4 sleep and to increase stage 2. Following discontinuation of the drug, REM sleep rebound has been reported in some studies. Nitrazepam has been shown to raise the seizure threshold.

General Benzodiazepine: The duration of hypnotic effect and the profile of unwanted effects may be influenced by the alpha (distribution) and beta (elimination) half-lives of the administered drug and any active metabolites formed. When half-lives are long, the drug or metabolite may accumulate during periods of nightly administration and be associated with impairments of cognitive and motor performance during waking hours. If half-lives are short, the drug and metabolites will be cleared before the next dose is ingested, and carry-over effects related to sedation or CNS depression should be minimal or absent. However, during nightly use and for an extended period, pharmacodynamic tolerance or adaptation to some effects of benzodiazepine hypnotics may develop. If the drug has a very short elimination half-life, it is possible that a relative deficiency (i.e., in relation to the receptor site) may occur at some point in the interval between each night's use. This sequence of events may account for 2 clinical findings reported to occur after several weeks of nightly use of rapidly eliminated benzodiazepine hypnotics: 1) increased wakefulness during the last third of the night; and 2) the appearance of increased daytime anxiety (see Warnings).

Nitrazepam has an intermediate half-life.

Pharmacokinetics: Nitrazepam is rapidly absorbed from the gastrointestinal tract. Bioavailability after an oral dose averages about 80%. Peak blood concentrations after oral administration are observed in approximately 3 hours.

Following the administration of single oral doses of 5 or 10 mg nitrazepam to healthy volunteers, mean peak plasma concentrations ranged between 23 to 66 ng/mL and 55 to 107 ng/mL, respectively. In elderly patients suffering from various debilitating diseases, a mean peak plasma concentration of 22 ng/mL was observed after a single dose of 5 mg nitrazepam. Steady-state plasma concentrations following administration of 5 mg nitrazepam once daily were reached after approximately 4 days. Steady-state plasma concentrations of nitrazepam were approximately 40 ng/mL.

Nitrazepam is a lipophilic drug and crosses the membrane barriers of the body readily. The concentrations in cerebrospinal fluid, about 10% of the total plasma level, are similar to the protein free fraction of plasma. Following oral administration, mean volumes of distribution were greater in elderly patients than in young volunteers (4.8±1.7 vs 2.4±0.8 L/kg, respectively). Total clearance was not significantly different in the two groups (78±25 and 68±33 mL/min, respectively).

Nitrazepam has no clinically active metabolites. The drug is excreted in human urine mainly as conjugated and nonconjugated aminonitrazepam and aceta-midonitrazepam. When given orally, 65 to 71% of the dose eventually appears in the urine and 14 to 20% in the feces. Only about 1% of the administered dose is excreted in the urine as unchanged nitrazepam. The major pathway involves hepatic nitroreduction.

The half-life of nitrazepam in healthy young volunteers is approximately 30 hours (range 18 to 57 hours). Elderly, ill patients showed a prolonged half-life of approximately 40 hours. Due to its slow elimination, nitrazepam accumulates when taken every night.

Approximately 87% of unchanged nitrazepam is bound to plasma proteins. In patients with liver cirrhosis, protein binding was significantly less than in healthy subjects (19 vs 14% unbound). In patients with mild to moderate renal insufficiency, protein binding was somewhat less than in healthy volunteers (16.8 vs 15.0% unbound).

Nitrazepam crosses the placental barrier and is excreted in maternal milk. Milk nitrazepam concentrations increased significantly from the first (30 nmol/L) to the fifth morning (48 nmol/L) in nursing mothers receiving 5 mg nitrazepam at night. The milk to plasma ratio of nitrazepam was 0.27 after 7 hours and did not vary from day 1 to day 5.

INDICATIONS: Sleep disturbance may be the presenting manifestation of a physical and/or psychiatric disorder. Consequently, a decision to initiate symptomatic treatment of insomnia should only be made after the patient has been carefully evaluated.

Nitrazepam is indicated for the short-term treatment and symptomatic relief of insomnia characterized by difficulty in falling asleep, frequent nocturnal awakenings, and/or early morning awakenings.

Treatment with nitrazepam should usually not exceed 7 to 10 consecutive days. Use for more than 2 to 3 consecutive weeks requires complete re-evaluation of the patient. Prescriptions for nitrazepam should be written for short-term use (7 to 10 days) and it should not be prescribed in quantities exceeding a 1-month supply.

The use of hypnotics should be restricted for insomnia where disturbed sleep results in impaired daytime functioning.

Nitrazepam is also useful for the management of myoclonic seizures.

CONTRAINDICATIONS: In patients with known hypersensitivity to benzodiazepines, any component to its formulation, and in those with severe impairment of respiratory function, e.g., significant sleep apnea syndrome.

Nitrazepam is contraindicated in patients who have myasthenia gravis or severe hepatic insufficiency. Nitrazepam is contraindicated in children when used as a hypnotic.

WARNINGS: General: Benzodiazepines should be used with extreme caution in patients with a history of substance or alcohol abuse.

Geriatrics: The smallest possible effective dose should be prescribed for elderly patients. Inappropriate, heavy sedation in the elderly, may result in accidental events/falls.

The failure of insomnia to remit after 7 to 10 days of treatment may indicate the presence of a primary psychiatric and/or medical illness or the presence of sleep state misperception.

Worsening of insomnia or the emergence of new abnormalities of thinking or behaviour may be the consequence of an unrecognized psychiatric or physical disorder. These have also been reported to occur in association with the use of drugs that act at the benzodiazepine receptors. Nitrazepam should be used with caution in patients who in the past manifested paradoxical reactions to alcohol and/or sedative medications.

Pregnancy: The use of nitrazepam during pregnancy is not recommended. Benzodiazepines may cause fetal damage when administered during pregnancy. During the first trimester of pregnancy, several studies have suggested an increased risk of congenital malformations associated with the use of benzodiazepines. During the last weeks of pregnancy, ingestion of therapeutic doses of a benzodiazepine hypnotic has resulted in neonatal CNS depression due to transplacental distribution. If nitrazepam is prescribed to women of childbearing potential, the patient should be warned of the potential risk to a fetus and advised to consult her physician regarding the discontinuation of the drug if she intends to become pregnant or suspects that she might be pregnant.

Memory Disturbance: Anterograde amnesia of varying severity has been reported following therapeutic doses of benzodiazepines. The event is rare with nitrazepam. Anterograde amnesia is a dose-related phenomenon and elderly subjects may be at particular risk.

Cases of transient global amnesia and "traveller's amnesia" have also been reported in association with benzodiazepines, the latter in individuals who have taken benzodiazepines, often in the middle of the night, to induce sleep while travelling. Transient global amnesia and traveller's amnesia are unpredictable and not necessarily dose-related phenomena. Patients should be warned not to take nitrazepam under circumstances in which a full night's sleep and clearance of the drug from the body are not possible before they need again to resume full activity.

Abnormal thinking and psychotic behavioural changes have been reported to occur in association with the use of benzodiazepines, including nitrazepam, although rarely. Some of the changes may be characterized by decreased inhibition, e.g., aggressiveness or extroversion that seem excessive, similar to that seen with alcohol and other CNS depressants (e.g., sedative/hypnotics). Particular caution is warranted in patients with a history of violent behaviour and a history of unusual reactions to sedatives including alcohol and the benzodiazepines. Psychotic behavioural changes that have been reported with benzodiazepines include bizarre behaviour, hallucinations, and depersonalization. Abnormal behaviours associated with the use of benzodiazepines have been reported more with chronic use and/or high doses but they may occur during the acute, maintenance or withdrawal phases of treatment.

It can rarely be determined with certainty whether a particular instance of abnormal behaviours listed above is drug induced, spontaneous in origin, or a result of an underlying psychiatric disorder. Nevertheless, the emergence of any new behavioural sign or symptom of concern requires careful and immediate evaluation.

Confusion: The benzodiazepines affect mental efficiency, e.g., concentration, attention and vigilance. The risk of confusion is greater in the elderly and in patients with cerebral impairment.

Anxiety, Restlessness: An increase in daytime anxiety and/or restlessness have been observed during treatment with short half-life benzodiazepines although the syndrome can apply on occasion to drugs with longer elimination half-lives as well. Nitrazepam has an intermediate half-life.

Depression: Caution should be exercised if nitrazepam is prescribed to patients with signs or symptoms of depression that could be intensified by hypnotic drugs. The potential for self-harm (e.g., intentional overdose) is high in patients with depression and thus, the least amount of drug that is feasible should be available to them at any one time.

Complex Sleep-related Behaviours: Complex sleep-related behaviours such as "sleep-driving" (i.e., driving while not fully awake after ingestion of a sedative-hypnotic, with amnesia for the event) have been reported in patients who have taken nitrazepam. Other potentially dangerous behaviours have been reported in patients who got out of bed after taking a sedative-hypnotic and were not fully awake, including preparing and eating food, making phone calls, leaving the house, etc. As with "sleep-driving", patients usually do not remember these events. The use of alcohol and other CNS-depressants with nitrazepam appears to increase the risk of such behaviours, as does the use of nitrazepam at doses exceeding the maximum recommended dose. Nitrazepam is not to be taken with alcohol. Caution is needed with concomitant use of other CNS depressant drugs. Due to the risk to the patient and the community, discontinuation of nitrazepam should be strongly considered for patients who report any such sleep-related behaviours.

Severe Anaphylactic and Anaphylactoid Reactions: Rare cases of angioedema involving the tongue, glottis or larynx have been reported in patients after taking the first or subsequent doses of sedative-hypnotics, including nitrazepam. Some patients have had additional symptoms such as dyspnea, throat closing or nausea and vomiting that suggest anaphylaxis. Some patients have required medical therapy in the emergency department. If angioedema involves the throat, glottis or larynx, airway obstruction may occur and be fatal. Patients who develop angioedema after treatment with nitrazepam should not be rechallenged with the drug.

PRECAUTIONS: *Drug Interactions:* Nitrazepam may produce additive CNS depressant effects when coadministered with alcohol, sedative antihistamines, narcotic analgesics, anticonvulsants, antipsychotics (neuroleptics), anesthetics, or antidepressant agents or psychotropic medications which themselves can produce CNS depression. In the case of narcotic analgesics, enhancement of the euphoria may also occur leading to an increase in psychological dependence.

Compounds which inhibit certain hepatic enzymes (particularly cytochrome P450) may enhance the activity of benzodiazepines and benzodiazepine-like agents. Examples include cimetidine or erythromycin.

Tolerance: Some tolerance to the hypnotic effects of benzodiazepines may develop after repeated use.

Drug Abuse, Dependence and Withdrawal: Withdrawal symptoms, similar in character to those noted with barbiturates and alcohol (convulsions, tremor, abdominal and muscle cramps, vomiting, sweating, dysphoria, perceptual disturbances and insomnia, headache, extreme anxiety, tension, restlessness, confusion and irritability) have occurred following abrupt discontinuation of benzodiazepines, and may follow the discontinuation of nitrazepam. In severe cases, the following symptoms may occur: derealization, depersonalization, hyperacusis, numbness and tingling of the extremities, hypersensitivity to light, noise and physical contact, hallucinations and epileptic seizures. The more severe symptoms are usually associated with higher dosages and longer usage, although patients given therapeutic dosages for as few as 1 to 2 weeks can also have withdrawal symptoms including daytime anxiety between nightly doses. Consequently, abrupt discontinuation should be avoided and a gradual dosage tapering schedule is recommended in any patient taking more than the lowest dose for more than a few weeks. The recommendation for tapering is particularly important in patients with a history of seizures.

The risk of dependence is increased in patients with a history of alcoholism, drug abuse, or in patients with marked personality disorders. Caution must be exercised if it is at all necessary to administer nitrazepam to these individuals.

As with all hypnotics, repeat prescriptions should be limited to those who are under medical supervision.

It may be useful to inform the patient when treatment is started that it will be of limited duration and to explain precisely how the dosage will be progressively decreased. Moreover, it is important that the patient should be aware of the possibility of rebound phenomena, thereby minimizing anxiety over such symptoms should they occur while the medicinal product is being discontinued.

Rebound Insomnia: A transient syndrome whereby the symptoms that led to treatment with a benzodiazepine or benzodiazepine-like agent recur in an enhanced form, may occur on withdrawal of hypnotic treatment. It may be accompanied by other reactions including mood changes, anxiety and restlessness.

Patients with Specific Conditions: Nitrazepam should be given with caution to patients with impaired hepatic or renal function, and is contraindicated in patients with severe impairment of hepatic or respiratory function. Respiratory depression has been reported in patients with compromised respiratory function. A lower dose is also recommended for patients with chronic respiratory insufficiency due to the risk of respiratory depression. Benzodiazepines are not recommended for the primary treatment of psychotic illnesses.

Occupational Hazards: Because of nitrazepam's CNS depressant effect, patients receiving the drug should be cautioned against engaging in hazardous occupations requiring complete mental alertness such as operating machinery or driving a motor vehicle. For the same reason, patients should be warned against the concomitant ingestion of nitrazepam and alcohol or CNS depressant drugs.

Bronchial Hypersecretion, Excessive Salivation: In infants and young children, as well as elderly, bedridden patients, bronchial hypersecretion and excessive salivation leading to aspiration/pneumonia may occur on rare occasions.

Pregnancy: Nitrazepam is not recommended for use during pregnancy. For teratogenic effects see Warnings. Nonteratogenic effects: a child born to a mother who is on benzodiazepines may be at risk for withdrawal symptoms from the drug during the postnatal period. Also, neonatal flaccidity has been reported in an infant born to a mother who had been receiving benzodiazepines.

Lactation: Since nitrazepam is excreted in maternal milk, nursing should not be undertaken while the patient is taking nitrazepam.

Children: The safety and effectiveness of nitrazepam as a hypnotic in children below the age of 18 have not been established (see Contraindications).

Geriatrics: Elderly patients are especially susceptible to dose-related adverse effects, such as drowsiness, dizziness, or impaired coordination. Inappropriate, heavy sedation may result in accidental events/falls. Therefore, the lowest possible dose should be used in these subjects.

ADVERSE EFFECTS: The most common adverse reactions are fatigue, dizziness, lightheadedness, drowsiness, lethargy, mental confusion, staggering, ataxia and falling. These phenomena occur predominantly at the start of therapy and usually disappear with repeated administration.

Depressed dreaming and nightmares have also been reported.

Sedative effects can often be decreased by a reduction in dosage.

Children, the elderly and/or debilitated patients are more susceptible to sedative effects and paradoxical reactions. Therefore, these patients should be carefully screened before they are given hypnotics and the lowest effective dose should be used. Paradoxical reactions such as agitation, hyperactivity, excitement, hallucinations, increased muscle spasticity, aggressiveness, irritability, rages, psychoses and violent behaviour have been reported in rare instances when using drugs that act at the benzodiazepine receptors. Should these occur, the drug should be discontinued.

Hangover, disorientation, severe sedation, hypotension, signs and symptoms of withdrawal including delirium tremens, and cutaneous reactions have been reported. Headache, heartburn, upset stomach, diarrhea, constipation, nausea, vomiting, weakness, faintness, palpitations, blurred vision, dyspnea, nervousness, apprehension, depression, numbed emotions, changes in libido, inappropriate behaviour, altered hepatic function tests and, in rare instances, leukopenia and granulocytopenia have been reported with this drug or other drugs of this class.

OVERDOSE:

Symptoms: The cardinal manifestations are drowsiness, confusion, reduced reflexes, increasing sedation, and coma. Effects on respiration, pulse and blood pressure are noticed with large overdoses. Patients exhibit some jitteriness and overstimulation usually when the effects of the drug begin to wear off.

Treatment: In the management of overdose with any medicinal product, it should be borne in mind that multiple agents may have been taken. Following overdose with nitrazepam vomiting should be induced (within 1 hour) if the patient is conscious or gastric lavage undertaken with the airway protected if the patient is unconscious. If there is no advantage in emptying the stomach, activated charcoal should be given to reduce absorption. If respiratory depression and/or coma are observed, the presence of other CNS depressants should be suspected. Respiration, pulse and blood pressure should be monitored. General supportive measures aimed at maintaining cardiopulmonary function should be instituted and administration of i.v. fluids started. Hypotension and CNS depression are managed by the usual means. Dialysis is usually of little value.

Reversal Agent: The benzodiazepine antagonist, flumazenil is a specific antidote in known or suspected benzodiazepine overdose. (For conditions of use see Anexate Product Monograph.)

The use of flumazenil is not recommended in epileptic patients who have been treated with nitrazepam (or any other benzodiazepine). The reversal of the benzodiazepine effect could induce convulsions in such patients.

For management of a suspected drug overdose, CPhA recommends that you contact your **regional Poison Control Centre**. See the *CPS* Directory section for a list of Poison Control Centres.

DOSAGE: The lowest effective dose should be used. Treatment should be as short as possible, and should usually not exceed 7 to 10 consecutive days. Use for more than 2 to 3 consecutive weeks requires complete re-evaluation of the patient. Nitrazepam should be withdrawn for a treatment-free period at regular intervals to ascertain whether the therapy needs to be continued.

Dosage should be individualized for maximal beneficial effect.

Nitrazepam tablets may be swallowed whole, chewed or dissolved in liquid.

Insomnia: Adults: The usual adult dose is 5 or 10 mg before retiring.

Elderly and/or Debilitated Patients: It is recommended that in these patients therapy be initiated with 2.5 mg until individual responses are determined. Doses higher than 5 mg are not usually recommended in the elderly.

Myoclonic Seizures: Children (up to 30 kg of body weight): between 0.3 and 1.0 mg/kg/day given in 3 divided doses. Treatment should be initiated with a lower dose than the usual recommended dosage range in order to determine tolerance and response. If a dose within the recommended dosage range does not control the condition, a higher dosage may be gradually attempted. Higher doses may cause excessive drowsiness, and may cause bronchial hypersecretion in infants with epilepsy. The use of nitrazepam in infants with epilepsy must be examined before treatment is started in order to determine whether the upper airways are clear. Whenever possible the daily dosage should be divided into 3 equal doses. If doses are not equally divided, the larger dose should be given before retiring. In some patients tolerance develops to the effects of nitrazepam.

The use of multiple anticonvulsants may result in an increase of CNS depressant adverse effects. This should be borne in mind whenever nitrazepam is added to an already existing anticonvulsant regimen.

INFORMATION FOR THE PATIENT: Published in e-CPS, available by subscription at www.e-cps.ca.

SUPPLIED: 5 mg: Each white cylindrical, bi-plane scored tablet, contains: nitrazepam 5 mg. Energy: 1.68 kJ (0.4 kcal). Nonmedicinal ingredients: croscarmellose sodium, lactose, magnesium stearate and microcrystalline cellulose. Bottles of 100. Gluten-, paraben-, sodium-, sulfite- and tartrazine-free. Store at 15 to 30°C. Protect from light. The medicine should not be used after the expiry date (EXP) shown on the pack.

10 mg: Each white, cylindrical, bi-plane, scored tablet, contains: nitrazepam 10 mg. Energy: 3.2 kJ (0.8 kcal). Nonmedicinal ingredients: croscarmellose sodium, lactose, magnesium stearate and microcrystalline cellulose. Bottles of 100. Gluten-, paraben-, sodium-, sulfite- and tartrazine-free. Store at 15 to 30°C. Protect from light. The medicine should not be used after the expiry date (EXP) shown on the pack.

Mometasone Ⓟ

CPhA Monograph

see *Corticosteroids: Eye Ear Nose*

see *Corticosteroids: Topical*

Monistat® 7 Vaginal Cream
miconazole nitrate
Antifungal

Johnson & Johnson

Monistat® 7 Dual-Pak® Package (Combination Packs)
miconazole nitrate
Antifungal

Johnson & Johnson

Monistat® Derm Cream
miconazole nitrate
Antifungal

Johnson & Johnson

Monistat® 3 Vaginal Cream
miconazole nitrate
Antifungal

Johnson & Johnson

Monistat® 3 Dual-Pak® Package (Combination Packs)
miconazole nitrate
Antifungal

Johnson & Johnson

Monistat® 3 Vaginal Ovules
miconazole nitrate
Antifungal

Johnson & Johnson

Monistat® 1 Vaginal Ovule
miconazole nitrate
Antifungal

Johnson & Johnson

Monistat® 1 Combination Pack
miconazole nitrate
Antifungal

Johnson & Johnson

Date of Revision: June 2, 2008

PHARMACOLOGY: Depending upon concentration, miconazole exhibits broad spectrum in vitro fungistatic or fungicidal activity against species of the genus Candida. Miconazole also inhibits several other genera of fungi, including dermatophytes and yeasts, as well as Gram-positive bacteria.

Miconazole inhibits the biosynthesis of ergosterol or other sterols, damaging the fungal cell wall membrane and altering its permeability. In fungi, it also inhibits biosynthesis of triglycerides and phospholipids as well as oxidative and peroxidative enzymes. The latter action results in intracellular buildup of toxic concentrations of hydrogen peroxide, which may contribute to deterioration of subcellular organelles and cellular necrosis.

C. albicans cells have been observed to exhibit progressive cytoplasmic deterioration and prominent shape changes resulting in complete cell necrosis depending on the dose and duration of exposure to miconazole. The sequence of morphologic alterations induced by miconazole at fungistatic doses (10^{-6} M) are lysis of cytoplasmic organelles, focal to complete loss of cell plasmalemma and irregular thickening of the cell wall containing multiple inclusions. Administration of fungicidal doses (10^{-4} M) induces a completely necrotic cell interior with an unaltered cell wall.

In *C. albicans*, miconazole inhibits the transformation of blastospores into invasive mycelial form. Not all species or strains of a particular organism may be susceptible to miconazole.

To date, no wild strains or fungal mutants with substantial acquired resistance to miconazole have been reported; however, miconazole resistant *C. albicans* has been isolated from an infant following bladder irrigation with miconazole for the treatment of urinary candidiasis.

INDICATIONS: Monistat 7 Vaginal Cream, Monistat 3 Vaginal Cream, Monistat 3 Vaginal Ovules and Monistat 1 Vaginal Ovule: For the local treatment of vulvovaginal candidiasis (moniliasis).

Monistat 7 Dual-Pak, Monistat 3 Dual-Pak and Monistat 1 Combination Pack: For the local treatment of vulvovaginal candidiasis (moniliasis) and for the relief of particularly severe external itching and irritation associated with vulvovaginal candidiasis.

Monistat 1 Vaginal Ovule and Monistat 1 Combination Pack is indicated for use during the day or at bedtime. No statistically significant differences in therapeutic, mycological or clinical cure rates were noted between patients treating during the daytime and those treating before bedtime. Additionally, no statistically significant difference in therapeutic cure rate was seen between patients treating prior to bedtime and daytime patients who participated in physical activity (mild, moderate or vigorous) up to four hours post-ovule administration.

Although vulvovaginal candidiasis may be more difficult to cure during pregnancy, pregnant patients can be treated with the same regimen as nonpregnant patients. The 3-day regimen is preferred, with the 1- or 7-day regimen providing an effective alternative.

No significant difference in therapeutic cure rate (therapeutic cure includes both symptomatic and microbiological cure) was reported between the pregnant and nonpregnant patient groups who participated in clinical evaluations of the 3-day (ovules) or 7-day (suppositories + cream) treatment regimens.

Similarly, users and non-users of oral contraceptives who participated in these clinical evaluations experienced therapeutic cure rates which did not differ significantly.

In addition, no statistically significant differences in therapeutic cure rates were noted between patients undergoing dosage regimens of varying duration (1, 3, 7, 10 and 14 day).

Monistat Derm Cream: Used clinically in conjunction with vaginal ovules or suppositories in Monistat 1 Combination Pack, Monistat 3 and Monistat 7 Dual-Paks, when symptoms of vulvovaginal candidiasis are particularly extensive.

CONTRAINDICATIONS: Hypersensitivity to this drug or any of its ingredients.

WARNINGS: No data supplied by the manufacturer.

PRECAUTIONS: Patients should not use vaginal preparations for self-medication if vaginal pruritus or discomfort is occurring for the first time. In this instance, a physician must be consulted to establish the diagnosis of vulvovaginal candidiasis.

Patients should not use vaginal preparations for self-medication if fever, nausea, unexplained pain in the lower back, lower abdomen, or either shoulder or a foul-smelling vaginal discharge are present, as a condition more serious than vulvovaginal candidiasis may exist.

Patients should discontinue medication if sensitization or other signs of irritation (skin rash, hives, burning, blistering, redness) not present before therapy occur from intravaginal or topical use.

Intractable candidiasis may be the presenting symptom of unrecognized diabetes; thus appropriate urine/blood studies may be indicated in patients not responding to treatment. In any case if a patient is unresponsive to therapy, repeat appropriate microbiological studies to confirm the diagnosis of vulvovaginal candidiasis and to rule out other pathogens.

Pregnancy: Advise pregnant patients either to exercise caution in the insertion of the applicator during vaginal therapy or to insert the suppository or ovule digitally.

Follow-up reports on infants born to 26 pregnant patients who participated in European and North American clinical evaluations of miconazole nitrate 100 mg suppositories and on infants born to 167 of 263 pregnant patients (some follow-up reports are not yet available) who participated in North American clinical evaluations of miconazole nitrate 2% cream administered in a 14-day regimen, described no complications or adverse effects attributed to this therapeutic agent. Nevertheless, since miconazole nitrate is absorbed in small amounts from the human vagina, Monistat vaginal preparations should not be used by pregnant or nursing women unless the physician considers it essential to the welfare of the patient.

Lactation: See Pregnancy.

During therapy it may be advisable to instruct patients to refrain from intercourse.

Miconazole nitrate preparations reduce the effectiveness of latex condoms and diaphragms. Therefore concurrent use of the suppository, ovule or cream prefilled applicator with natural rubber products, such as vaginal diaphragms or condoms, is not recommended.

Drug Interactions: Miconazole administered systemically is known to inhibit CYP3A4/2C9. Due to the limited systemic availability after vaginal application, clinically relevant interactions occur very rarely. Patients taking prescription blood thinners, such as warfarin, should talk to their physician or pharmacist before using Monistat due to the risk of bleeding and bruising. Caution should be exercised and the anticoagulant effect should be monitored.

ADVERSE EFFECTS: The standard for defining frequency terms will be based on the Council for International Organizations of Medical Science (CIOMS) convention. Specifically: Very common: ≥1/10 (≥10%). Common: ≥1/100 and <1/10 (≥1% and <10%). Uncommon: ≥1/1000 and <1/100 (≥0.1% and <1%). Rare: ≥1/10 000 and <1/1000 (≥0.01% and <0.1%). Very rare: <1/10 000, including isolated reports (<0.01%).

In general, the complaints reported with miconazole therapy involved vulvovaginal burning, itching, irritation, pelvic cramping, edema as well as hives, rash and headache.

A total of 1089 patients participated in clinical evaluations of miconazole nitrate 2% vaginal cream administered in dosage regimens of varying duration. Of these, 59 patients reported reactions which were possibly drug related but not severe enough to cause discontinuation of therapy, 4 patients discontinued therapy due to vulvovaginal burning and itching, and 1 patient discontinued therapy due to hives.

A total of 1724 patients participated in clinical evaluations of miconazole nitrate 100 mg vaginal suppositories administered in dosage regimens of varying duration. Of these, 3 patients reported reactions which were interpreted as minor treatment emergent signs and symptoms (burning, itching, edema) and considered by the investigators to be nontherapy related. No patients were reported to have discontinued therapy due to drug related reasons.

The 3-day treatment with miconazole nitrate 400 mg vaginal ovules was exceptionally well tolerated by a total of 410 patients in 3 clinical studies, without any related side effects. However, the generally reported complaints referred to above could be expected with this dosage form and regimen as well.

A randomized clinical study involving 278 patients comparing one-day treatment with Monistat 1 to the 7-day cream treatment indicated that generally both products were equally well tolerated.

A randomized clinical study involving 570 patients comparing one-day treatment administered during the day to one day treatment administered at bedtime indicated that treatment emergent adverse events observed between the two groups were similar and were consistent with the known safety profile of miconazole nitrate.

Adverse events, regardless of causality, reported in 2 Phase 3 clinical trials are shown in Table 1. A total of 537 women with microbiologically confirmed candidiasis and symptoms (e.g. vulvovaginal itching, burning/irritation), or signs of vulvar erythema, edema, excoriation, or vaginal erythema or edema were treated with miconazole intravaginally: randomly assigned to either a single 1200 mg capsule, or a 7-day application of 2% vaginal cream. There was no placebo reference. Safety was self-assessed daily on a diary card. Included in the table are adverse events reported by >5% of subjects in either treatment group.

Table 1: Monistat

Adverse Events, Regardless of Causality, Reported in 2 Phase 3 Clinical Trials

System Organ Class Adverse Event	% of Patients on Miconazole (2% Cream, 7-day) Reporting AEs During Trial (n=265)	% of Patients on Miconazole (1200 mg Capsule) Reporting AEs During Trial (n=272)
Overall Adverse Events	64	70
Nervous System Disorders		
Headache	18.9	17.6
Renal and Urinary Disorders		
Urinary tract infection NOS	—	5.1

(cont'd)

Table 1: Monistat *(cont'd)*

Adverse Events, Regardless of Causality, Reported in 2 Phase 3 Clinical Trials

System Organ Class Adverse Event	% of Patients on Miconazole (2% Cream, 7-day) Reporting AEs During Trial (n=265)	% of Patients on Miconazole (1200 mg Capsule) Reporting AEs During Trial (n=272)
Reproductive System and Breast Disorders		
Genital pruritus female	26.8	19.1
Genital burning sensation	23.8	26.1
Vaginal irritation	15.5	20.2
Vaginal discharge	4.5	10.3

Two randomized clinical studies involving over 500 patients, comparing 3-day treatment with Monistat 3 Vaginal Cream (4%) to the 7-day cream treatment with Monistat 7 Vaginal Cream (2%), indicated that, generally, both products were equally well tolerated. Both studies were double-blind, randomized, controlled, parallel group, comparative, multi-centre, Phase III studies of patients with documented vulvovaginal candidiasis. The most frequent adverse experiences reported in both treatment groups from either study were external genital pruritus, genital burning, headache, genital irritation, genital discharge, respiratory congestion, dysmenorrhea, abdominal pain, nausea and upper respiratory infection. For each study, body systems with the highest incidence of adverse experience reporting (greater than 10% in either treatment group) were determined. Results from each study were combined and are displayed in Table 2.

Table 2: Monistat

Results From Two Randomized Clinical Studies Comparing 3-day Treatment with Monistat 3 Vaginal Cream (4%) to the 7-day Cream Treatment with Monistat 7 Vaginal Cream (2%)

System Organ Class Adverse Event	% Patients on Miconazole (2% Cream, 7 Day) Reporting AEs During 2 Trials (n=274)	% of Patients on Miconazole (4% Cream, 3 Day) Reporting AEs During 2 Trials (n=272)
Overall Adverse Events	—	—
Nervous System Disorders	22.1	19.0
Reproductive System and Breast Disorders	46.0	46.7
Gastrointestinal System Disorders	14.7	11.3
Respiratory System Disorders	11.4	10.9

Postmarketing Data: Adverse events which may be causally related to the administration of Monistat that have come to light as a result of reports received in relation to administration of the marketed product are provided in this section. Because these reactions are reported voluntarily from a population of uncertain size, it is not always possible to reliably estimate their frequency or establish a causal relationship to drug exposure.

Immune System Disorders: allergic conditions, including anaphylactic and anaphylactoid reactions, angioneurotic edema.

Skin and Subcutaneous Tissue Disorders: urticaria, pruritus, rash.

Reproductive System and Breast Disorders: pelvic pain (cramping), genital burning sensation, genital pruritus female, vaginal irritation, vaginal discharge.

General Disorders and Administration Site Conditions: Application site reactions: The combination pack products combine a small amount (9 g) of miconazole nitrate 2% cream to be applied externally during a course of therapy with miconazole nitrate vaginal suppositories or ovules so a similar safety and efficacy profile, as with each individually, could be expected.

OVERDOSE:

Monistat products are intended for local application and not for oral use.

Symptoms: Each Monistat 3 and Monistat 1 Dual-Pak contains 1380 mg of miconazole nitrate, which represents the greatest possible quantity in any one package. Approximately 50% of an oral dose is absorbed from the gastrointestinal tract. Hence, the maximum possible systemic exposure, if the entire contents of the Monistat 3 or Monistat 1 Dual-Pak were to be accidentally or deliberately ingested would be equivalent to 690 mg. This represents the lowest dose administered i.v. to adults (600 to 1800 mg) and compares favorably to the i.v. dose that would be administered to a 1-year-old child (400 mg). Consequently, the possibility of acute overdosage is remote. However, although unlikely to occur, in the case of a substantial overdose and if taken concomitantly with other drugs (e.g., coumarin derivatives, oral hypoglycemics or phenytoin), the effects and side effects of the other drugs can be increased.

For management of a suspected drug overdose, CPhA recommends that you contact your **regional Poison Control Centre**. See the *CPS* Directory section for a list of Poison Control Centres.

DOSAGE: **Monistat 7 Vaginal Cream:** Administer one 5 g applicatorful intravaginally once daily at bedtime for 7 consecutive days. The course of therapy may be repeated if the patient remains symptomatic and it has been determined by appropriate smears and cultures that the infecting organism is still miconazole-susceptible Candida.

Monistat 3 Vaginal Cream: Administer one 5 g applicator intravaginally once daily at bedtime for 3 consecutive days. The course of therapy may be repeated if the patient remains symptomatic and it has been determined by appropriate smears and cultures that the infecting organism is still miconazole-susceptible Candida.

Monistat 3 Vaginal Ovules: Administer 1 ovule intravaginally once daily at bedtime for 3 consecutive days. The course of therapy may be repeated if the patient remains symptomatic and it has been determined by appropriate smears and cultures that the infecting organism is still miconazole-susceptible Candida.

Monistat 1 Vaginal Ovule: Administer 1 ovule intravaginally once during the day or at bedtime for 1 day. The course of therapy may be repeated if the patient remains symptomatic and it has been determined by appropriate smears and cultures that the infecting organism is still miconazole-susceptible Candida.

Monistat 1 Combination Pack (to be used when symptoms are particularly extensive): One 1200 mg ovule administered intravaginally once during the day or at bedtime for 1 day. Apply a thin layer of cream to external areas twice daily, in the morning and evening. Massage gently until cream disappears. Apply cream as required for external itching for up to 7 days.

The course of therapy may be repeated if the patient remains symptomatic and it has been determined by appropriate smears and cultures that the infecting organism is still miconazole-susceptible Candida.

Monistat 7, Monistat 3 Dual-Paks (to be used when symptoms are particularly extensive): One 100 mg suppository or one 400 mg ovule administered intravaginally once daily at bedtime for 7 (Monistat 7) or 3 (Monistat 3) consecutive days, respectively. Apply a thin layer of cream to external areas twice daily, in the morning and evening. Massage gently until cream disappears. Apply cream as required for external itching for up to 7 days.

The course of therapy may be repeated if the patient remains symptomatic and it has been determined by appropriate smears and cultures that the infecting organism is still miconazole-susceptible Candida.

Monistat Derm Cream: Apply a thin layer of cream topically to cover the affected area once or twice per day, if needed. Massage gently until cream disappears.

SUPPLIED: **Monistat 7 Vaginal Cream:** Each package contains: 7 prefilled disposable applicators of white, water miscible cream containing miconazole nitrate 2%, sufficient for one 7-day course of therapy, and a consumer information leaflet. Nonmedicinal ingredients: benzoic acid, cetyl alcohol, isopropyl myristate, polysorbate 60, potassium hydroxide, propylene glycol, purified water and stearyl alcohol.

Monistat 7 Dual-Pak Package: Each package contains: 7 white, egg shaped vaginal suppositories each containing 100 mg miconazole nitrate sufficient for one 7-day course of therapy, a vaginal applicator and a 9 g tube of Monistat Derm Cream, along with a consumer information leaflet. Also known as Combination Packs. Nonmedicinal ingredients: hydrogenated vegetable oil base.

Monistat Derm Cream: Each tube contains: miconazole nitrate 2%. Tubes of 15 and 30 g. Nonmedicinal ingredients: benzoic acid, cetyl alcohol, isopropyl myristate, polysorbate 60, potassium hydroxide, propylene glycol, purified water and stearyl alcohol.

Monistat 3 Dual-Pak Package: Each package contains: 3 Monistat 3 vaginal ovules sufficient for one 3-day course of therapy, 3 vaginal applicators and a 9 g tube of Monistat Derm Cream, along with a consumer information leaflet. Also known as Combination Packs.

Monistat 3 Vaginal Cream: Each package contains: 3 prefilled disposable applicators of white, water-miscible cream containing miconazole nitrate 4%, sufficient for one 3-day course of therapy, and a consumer information leaflet. Nonmedicinal ingredients: benzoic acid, cetyl alcohol, isopropyl myristate, polysorbate 60, potassium hydroxide, propylene glycol, purified water and stearyl alcohol.

Monistat 3 Vaginal Ovules: Each package contains: 3 soft, gelatin ovules filled with a suspension of miconazole nitrate 400 mg, sufficient for one 3-day course of therapy, 3 vaginal applicators and a consumer information leaflet. Nonmedicinal ingredients: gelatin, glycerin, mineral oil, sodium ethylparaben, sodium propylparaben, titanium dioxide and white petrolatum.

Monistat 1 Vaginal Ovule: Each package contains: 1 soft, gelatin ovule filled with a suspension of miconazole nitrate 1200 mg, sufficient for one 1-day course of therapy, a vaginal applicator and a consumer information leaflet. Nonmedicinal ingredients: gelatin, glycerin, lecithin, mineral oil, sodium ethylparaben, sodium propylparaben, titanium dioxide and white petrolatum.

Monistat 1 Combination Pack: Each package contains: 1 Monistat 1 vaginal ovule, sufficient for one 1-day course of therapy, a vaginal applicator and a 9 g tube of Monistat Derm Cream, along with a consumer information leaflet.

The reader is invited to consult CPhA's monograph **ACE Inhibitors**.

Monopril™ Ⓟ

fosinopril sodium

Angiotensin Converting Enzyme Inhibitor

Bristol-Myers Squibb

Date of Preparation: April 6, 1992
Date of Revision: November 8, 2006

PHARMACOLOGY: Fosinopril is an angiotensin converting enzyme (ACE) inhibitor which is used in the treatment of mild to moderate essential hypertension and in the management of symptomatic congestive heart failure.

Following oral administration, fosinopril, an ester prodrug, is rapidly hydrolyzed to fosinoprilat, its principal active metabolite.

ACE is a peptidyl dipeptidase that catalyzes the conversion of angiotensin I to the vasoconstrictor substance, angiotensin II. Angiotensin II also stimulates aldosterone secretion by the adrenal cortex. Inhibition of ACE activity leads to decreased levels of angiotensin II thereby resulting in decreased vasoconstriction and decreased aldosterone secretion. The latter decrease may result in a small increase in serum potassium. Decreased levels of angiotensin II and the accompanying lack of negative feedback on renal renin secretion results in increases in plasma renin activity.

ACE is identical to kininase II. Thus, fosinopril may interfere with the degradation of bradykinin, a potent peptide vasodilator. However, it is not known whether this contributes to the therapeutic effects of fosinopril.

While the mechanism through which fosinopril lowers blood pressure appears to result primarily from suppression of the renin-angiotensin-aldosterone system, fosinopril has an antihypertensive effect even in patients with low-renin hypertension.

The antihypertensive effect of angiotensin converting enzyme inhibitors is generally lower in black patients than in non-blacks.

Pharmacokinetics: Following oral administration, fosinopril (the prodrug) is absorbed slowly. The absolute absorption of fosinopril averaged 36% of an oral dose. The primary site of absorption is the proximal small intestine (duodenum/jejunum). While the rate of absorption may be slowed by the presence of food in the gastrointestinal tract, the extent of absorption of fosinopril is essentially unaffected. The bioavailability of fosinoprilat is reduced by about 20%.

Hydrolysis of fosinopril to the active fosinoprilat is rapid and complete. This biotransformation probably occurs in the gastrointestinal mucosa and liver.

After an oral dose of radiolabeled fosinopril to healthy subjects, 75% of radioactivity in plasma was present as active fosinoprilat, 20 to 30% as a glucuronide conjugate of fosinoprilat, and 1 to 5% as a p-hydroxy metabolite of fosinoprilat. In urine, 75% of the drug excreted was fosinoprilat, the remainder consisted primarily of the glucuronide conjugate of fosinoprilat. In rats, the para-hydroxy metabolite of fosinoprilat is as potent an inhibitor of ACE as fosinoprilat; the glucuronide conjugate of fosinoprilat is devoid of ACE inhibitor activity.

After single and repeated doses, areas under serum concentration-time curves (AUCs) and peak concentrations (C_{max}) were directly proportional to the dose of fosinopril. The time to reach peak concentrations (T_{max}) was independent of dose and achieved in approximately 3 hours.

In hypertensive patients with normal renal and hepatic function, who received repeated doses of fosinopril, the effective half-life for accumulation of fosinoprilat averaged 11.5 hours, while in patients with heart failure, the effective half-life was 14 hours. Fosinoprilat is highly protein-bound (≥95%), has a relatively small volume of distribution, and negligible binding to cellular components in blood.

After i.v. administration, elimination of fosinoprilat was shared equally by the liver and kidney. After an oral dose of radiolabeled fosinopril, approximately half of the absorbed dose was excreted in urine and the remainder was excreted in the feces. In normal subjects, the mean body clearance of i.v. fosinoprilat was between 26 and 39 mL/min.

In patients with renal insufficiency, pharmacokinetic parameters (including absorption, bioavailability, protein binding, and biotransformation/metabolism) were not appreciably altered by reduced renal function. The total body clearance of fosinoprilat in patients with impaired renal function (creatinine clearance <80 mL/min/1.73 m²) was approximately 50% slower than in patients with normal renal function. Since hepatobiliary elimination partially compensates for diminished renal elimination, the body clearance of fosinoprilat does not appreciably differ with any degree of renal insufficiency including end-stage renal failure (creatinine clearance values <10 mL/min/1.73 m²). A modest increase in plasma AUC levels (<2 times that in normals) was observed in patients with various degrees of renal insufficiency, including end stage renal failure (see Dosage).

Clearance of fosinoprilat by hemodialysis and peritoneal dialysis averages 2% and 7%, respectively, of urea clearances.

In patients with hepatic insufficiency (alcoholic or biliary cirrhosis), the extent of absorption was not affected. In single and multiple dose pharmacokinetic studies, the mean AUC for fosinoprilat was markedly increased (50 to 100%) as compared to that of patients with normal liver functions. The extent of hydrolysis of fosinopril was not appreciably reduced although the rate may be slowed. Patients with hepatic insufficiency could develop elevated plasma levels of unchanged fosinopril.

In elderly (male) subjects (65 to 74 years old) with clinically normal renal and hepatic function, there were no significant differences in the pharmacokinetic parameters of fosinoprilat as compared to those in younger subjects (20 to 35 years old).

Fosinoprilat was found to cross the placenta of pregnant animals.

Studies in animals indicate that fosinopril and fosinoprilat do not cross the blood-brain barrier.

Pharmacodynamics: Administration of fosinopril to patients with mild to moderate essential hypertension has reduced both supine and standing blood pressures with minimal effect on heart rate. Following administration of a single dose, the onset of an antihypertensive effect is seen within 1 hour with peak blood pressure reduction usually achieved by 3 to 6 hours after dosing. Achievement of maximum blood pressure lowering effect may require several weeks of therapy in some patients. At the recommended doses, antihypertensive effects are maintained throughout the 24-hour dosing interval in most patients. The effectiveness of fosinopril appears to be similar in the elderly (over 65 years of age) and younger adult patients given the same daily dosages.

The antihypertensive effect of fosinopril and thiazide diuretics used concurrently is greater than that seen with either agent alone.

Abrupt withdrawal of fosinopril has not resulted in rapid increase in blood pressure.

In hemodynamic study involving patients with mild to moderate hypertension, after 3 months of therapy, responses (changes in blood pressure, heart rate, cardiac index and peripheral vascular resistance) to various stimuli (e.g., isometric exercise, 45 degree head-up tilt and mental challenge) were unchanged compared to baseline, suggesting that fosinopril does not affect the activity of the sympathetic nervous system. Reduction in systemic blood pressure appears to have been mediated by a decrease in peripheral vascular resistance without reflex cardiac effects. Similarly, renal, splanchnic, cerebral and skeletal muscle blood flow were unchanged compared to baseline, as was glomerular filtration rate.

Administration of fosinopril to patients with congestive heart failure reduces afterload and preload of the heart, resulting in an increase in cardiac output, without reflex tachycardia. At the recommended doses, the hemodynamic effects are maintained throughout the 24-hour dosing interval in most patients.

Administration of fosinopril to hypertensive patients with proteinuria and microalbuminuria has resulted in significant reductions of urinary albumin excretion.

INDICATIONS: In the treatment of mild to moderate essential hypertension. It may be used alone or in association with thiazide diuretics.

In using fosinopril consideration should be given to the risk of angioedema (see Warnings).

Fosinopril should normally be used in those patients in whom treatment with a diuretic or a beta-blocker was found ineffective or has been associated with unacceptable adverse effects.

Fosinopril can also be tried as an initial agent in those patients in whom use of diuretics and/or beta-blockers is contraindicated or in patients with medical conditions in which these drugs frequently cause serious adverse effects.

The safety and efficacy of fosinopril in renovascular hypertension have not been established and therefore, its use in this condition is not recommended.

The safety and efficacy of concurrent use of fosinopril with antihypertensive agents other than thiazide diuretics have not been established.

In the management of symptomatic congestive heart failure as adjunctive treatment with diuretics, and where appropriate, digoxin. Treatment with fosinopril should be initiated under medical supervision.

CONTRAINDICATIONS: Patients who are hypersensitive to this product and in patients with a history of angioedema related to previous treatment with an angiotensin converting enzyme inhibitor.

WARNINGS:

Serious Warning
When used in pregnancy, angiotensin converting enzyme (ACE) inhibitors can cause injury or even death of the developing fetus. When pregnancy is detected, MONOPRIL should be discontinued as soon as possible.

Angioedema: Angioedema has been reported in patients treated with ACE inhibitors, including fosinopril. Angioedema associated with laryngeal involvement may be fatal. If laryngeal stridor or angioedema of the face, tongue, or glottis occurs, fosinopril should be discontinued immediately, the patient treated appropriately in accordance with accepted medical care, and carefully observed until the swelling disappears. In instances where swelling is confined to the face and lips, the condition generally resolves without treatment, although antihistamines may be useful in relieving symptoms. Where there is involvement of the tongue, glottis or larynx, likely to cause airway obstruction, appropriate therapy (including but not limited to 0.3 to 0.5 mL of s.c. epinephrine solution 1:1000) should be administered promptly (see Adverse Effects).

The incidence of angioedema during ACE inhibitor therapy has been reported to be higher in black than in non-black patients.

Patients with a history of angioedema unrelated to ACE inhibitor therapy may be at increased risk of angioedema while receiving an ACE inhibitor (see Contraindications).

Hypotension: Symptomatic hypotension has occurred after administration of fosinopril, usually after the first or second dose or when the dose was increased. It is more likely to occur in patients who are volume depleted by diuretic therapy, dietary salt restriction, dialysis, diarrhea or vomiting. Volume and/or salt depletion should be corrected before initiating therapy with fosinopril.

In patients with severe congestive heart failure, with or without associated renal insufficiency, ACE inhibitor therapy may cause excessive hypotension and has been associated with oliguria and/or progressive azotemia, and rarely, with acute renal failure and/or death. In patients with ischemic heart or cerebrovascular disease, an excessive fall in blood pressure could result in a myocardial infarction or cerebrovascular accident (see Adverse Effects). Because of the potential fall in blood pressure in these patients, therapy with fosinopril should be started under close medical supervision. Such patients should be followed closely for the first weeks of treatment and whenever the dose of fosinopril or diuretic is increased. Consideration should be given to reducing the diuretic dose in patients with normal or low blood pressure who have been treated vigorously with diuretics or who are hyponatremic.

If hypotension occurs, the patient should be placed in a supine position, and, if necessary, receive an i.v. infusion of 0.9% sodium chloride. A transient hypotensive response is not a contraindication to further doses which usually can be given without difficulty once the blood pressure has increased after volume expansion. However, lower doses of fosinopril and/or reduced concomitant diuretic therapy should be considered.

Neutropenia/Agranulocytosis: Agranulocytosis and bone marrow depression have been caused by ACE inhibitors. Current experience with fosinopril shows the incidence to be rare and a causal relationship to the administration of fosinopril has not been established. Periodic monitoring of white blood cell counts should be considered, especially in patients with collagen vascular disease and/or renal disease.

Pregnancy: ACE inhibitors can cause fetal and neonatal morbidity and mortality when administered to pregnant women. When pregnancy is detected, fosinopril should be discontinued as soon as possible.

The use of ACE inhibitors during the second and third trimesters of pregnancy has been associated with fetal and neonatal injury including hypotension, neonatal skull hypoplasia, anuria, reversible or irreversible renal failure, and death. Oligohydramnios has also been reported, presumably resulting from decreased fetal renal function, associated with fetal limb contractures, craniofacial deformation, and hypoplastic lung development.

Prematurity, patent ductus arteriosus, and other structural cardiac malformations, as well as neurologic malformations, have also been reported following exposure in the first trimester of pregnancy.

Infants with a history of in utero exposure to ACE inhibitors should be closely observed for hypotension, oliguria, and hyperkalemia. If oliguria occurs, attention should be directed toward support of blood pressure and renal perfusion. Exchange transfusion or dialysis may be required as a means of reversing hypotension and/or substituting for impaired renal function, however, limited experience with those procedures has not been associated with significant clinical benefit.

Clearance of fosinoprilat by hemodialysis and peritoneal dialysis averages 2% and 7%, respectively of urea clearance.

Animal Data: In pregnant rabbits, maternal toxicity was evident at doses ranging from 2.5 to 40 mg/kg/day (approximately 3 to 50 times the maximum human dose). Fosinopril was embryocidal in rabbits at 10 and 40 mg/kg/day (approximately 12 and 50 times the maximum human dose). These effects were probably due to marked decreases in blood pressure caused by ACE inhibition in this species. There were no teratogenic effects in rabbits at any dose level tested.

In pregnant rats, there was evidence of maternal toxicity at all dose levels tested, i.e. 25 to 400 mg/kg/day (about 30 to 500 times the maximum human dose). Slight reductions in placental weights and degree of skeletal ossification were observed at all dose levels, and fetal body weights were reduced in the high-dose group. Three similar orofacial malformations and one fetus with situs inversus occurred in fosinopril-treated animals. The association of these anomalies with treatment is uncertain.

Lactation: The presence of concentrations of ACE inhibitor have been reported in human milk. Use of ACE inhibitors is not recommended during breat-feeding.

PRECAUTIONS: Renal Impairment: As a consequence of inhibiting the renin-angiotensin-aldosterone system, changes in renal function have been seen in susceptible individuals. In patients whose renal function may depend on the activity of the renin-angiotensin-aldosterone system, such as patients with bilateral renal artery stenosis, unilateral renal artery stenosis to a solitary kidney, or severe congestive heart failure, treatment with agents that inhibit this system has been associated with oliguria, progressive azotemia, and rarely, acute renal failure and/or death. In susceptible patients, concomitant diuretic use may further increase risk.

Use of fosinopril should include appropriate assessment of renal function.

Surgery/Anesthesia: ACE inhibitors may augment the hypotensive effects of anesthetics and analgesics. In patients undergoing surgery or during anesthesia with agents that produce hypotension, fosinopril will block the angiotensin II formation that could otherwise occur secondary to compensatory renin release. Hypotension that occurs as a result of this mechanism can be corrected by volume expansion.

Hyperkalemia and Potassium-Sparing Diuretics: In clinical trials, elevated serum potassium (greater than 5.5 mEq/L) was observed in approximately 2.6% of hypertensive patients receiving fosinopril. In most cases these were isolated values which resolved despite continued therapy. Hyperkalemia was a cause of discontinuation of therapy in less than 0.1% of hypertensive patients. Risk factors for the development of hyperkalemia may include renal insufficiency, diabetes mellitus, and the concomitant use of agents to treat hypokalemia or other drugs associated with increases in serum potassium (e.g., heparin) (see Precautions, Drug Interactions and Adverse Effects).

Anaphylactoid Reactions During Membrane Exposure: Anaphylactoid reactions have been reported in patients dialysed with high-flux membranes (e.g., polyacrylonitrile (PAN) and treated concomitantly with an ACE inhibitor. Dialysis should be stopped immediately if symptoms such as nausea, abdominal cramps, burning, angioedema, shortness of breath and severe hypotension occur. Symptoms are not relieved by antihistamines. In these patients consideration should be given to using a different type of dialysis membrane or a different class of antihypertensive agents.

Anaphylactoid Reactions During Desensitization: There have been isolated reports of patients experiencing sustained life threatening anaphylactoid reactions while receiving ACE inhibitors during desensitizing treatment with hymenoptera (bees, wasps) venom. In the same patients, these reactions have been avoided when ACE inhibitors were temporarily withheld for at least 24 hours, but they have reappeared upon inadvertent rechallenge.

Valvular Stenosis: There is concern on theoretical grounds that patients with aortic stenosis might be at particular risk of decreased coronary perfusion when treated with vasodilators because they do not develop as much afterload reduction.

Patients with Impaired Liver Function: Hepatitis (hepatocellular and/or cholestatic), elevations of liver enzymes and/or serum bilirubin have occurred during therapy with ACE inhibitors including fosinopril, in patients with or without pre-existing liver abnormalities (see Adverse Effects). Fosinopril therapy was discontinued because of serum transaminase elevations in 0.7% of patients. In most cases the changes were reversed on discontinuation of the drug.

Should the patients receiving fosinopril experience any unexplained symptoms particularly during the first weeks or months of treatment, it is recommended that a full set of liver function tests and any other necessary investigation be carried out. Discontinuation of fosinopril should be considered when appropriate.

Fosinopril should be used with particular caution in patients with pre-existing liver abnormalities. In such patients baseline liver function tests should be obtained before administration of the drug and close monitoring of response and metabolic effects should apply.

Cough: Cough has been reported with the use of fosinopril. Characteristically, ACE-inhibitor induced cough is non productive, persistent and resolves after discontinuation of therapy or lowering of the dose. Fosinopril induced cough should be considered as part of the differential diagnosis of the cough.

Children: The safety and effectiveness of fosinopril in children have not been established, therefore, its use in this age group is not recommended.

Geriatrics: Although clinical experience has not identified differences in response between the elderly and younger patients, greater sensitivity of some older individuals cannot be ruled out.

Drug Interactions: Concomitant Diuretic Therapy: Patients concomitantly taking ACE inhibitors and diuretics, and especially those in whom diuretic therapy was recently instituted, may occasionally experience an excessive reduction of blood pressure after initiation of therapy. The possibility of hypotensive effects after the first dose of fosinopril can be minimized by either discontinuing the diuretic or increasing the salt intake prior to initiation of treatment with fosinopril. If it is not possible to discontinue the diuretic, the starting dose can be reduced, and the patient should be closely observed for several hours following an initial dose and until blood pressure has stabilized (see Warnings and Dosage).

Decreases in serum sodium and increases in serum creatinine occurred more frequently in patients on concomitant diuretics than in those treated with fosinopril alone (see Adverse Effects, Laboratory Test Abnormalities).

Agents Increasing Serum Potassium: Since fosinopril decreases aldosterone production, elevation of serum potassium may occur. Potassium sparing diuretics such as spironolactone, triamterene or amiloride, or potassium supplements should be given only for documented hypokalemia and with caution and frequent monitoring of serum potassium, since they may lead to a significant increase in serum potassium. Salt substitutes which contain potassium should also be used with caution.

Agents Causing Renin Release: The antihypertensive effect of fosinopril is augmented by antihypertensive agents that cause renin release (e.g., diuretics).

With Lithium: Increased serum lithium levels and symptoms of lithium toxicity have been reported in patients receiving concomitant lithium and ACE inhibitor therapy. These drugs should be coadministered with caution and frequent monitoring of serum lithium levels is recommended. If a diuretic is also used, it may increase the risk of lithium toxicity.

With Antacids: In a clinical pharmacology study, coadministration of an antacid (aluminum hydroxide, magnesium hydroxide and simethicone) with fosinopril reduced serum levels and urinary excretion of fosinoprilat as compared with fosinopril administered alone, suggesting that antacids may impair absorption of fosinopril. Therefore, if concomitant administration of these agents is indicated, dosing should be separated by 2 hours.

With ASA: In a study with concomitant administration of ASA and fosinopril the bioavailability of unbound fosinoprilat was not altered. Since it is believed that it is free fosinoprilat that inhibits ACE, the reduced bioavailability (30 to 40%) of bound fosinoprilat would not be expected to have a significant effect on the antihypertensive effects of fosinopril.

With Digoxin: In a study with concomitant administration of digoxin and fosinopril, the bioavailability of fosinoprilat was not altered. The bioavailability of digoxin (i.e. AUC and C_{max}) appeared to be reduced slightly in the presence of fosinopril. This reduction, of less than 20%, is considered to have little or no clinical relevance.

With Furosemide: In a steady-state pharmacokinetic study, coadministration of furosemide with fosinopril increased the AUC of fosinoprilat by 26% and C_{max} by 25%. Furosemide levels were decreased.

With Warfarin: In a pharmacokinetic interaction study with warfarin, bioavailability parameters, the degree of protein binding and the anticoagulant effect (measured by prothrombin time) of warfarin were not significantly changed. The bioavailability of fosinoprilat was not altered by coadministration of fosinopril with warfarin.

Other: In separate single or multiple dose pharmacokinetic interaction studies with chlorthalidone, nifedipine, propranolol, hydrochlorothiazide, cimetidine, metoclopramide and propantheline, the bioavailability of fosinoprilat was not altered by coadministration of fosinopril with any one of these drugs.

Drug/Laboratory Test Interactions: Fosinopril may cause a false low measurement of serum digoxin levels with the Digi-Tab RIA kit for digoxin. Other kits such as the Coat-A-Count RIA kit may be used.

Information to Be Provided to the Patient: **Pregnancy: Patients should be told that taking fosinopril during pregnancy can cause injury and even death to the developing fetus. Patients should be advised to stop taking the medication and to contact their physician as soon as possible if they become pregnant while taking fosinopril.**

Breast-feeding: Patients should be advised that fosinopril may pass into breast milk and that they should not breast-feed while taking fosinopril.

Angioedema: Angioedema, including laryngeal edema, may occur especially following the first dose of fosinopril. Patients should be so advised and told to report immediately any signs or symptoms suggesting angioedema (swelling of face, eyes, lips, tongue, difficulty in swallowing or breathing); they should immediately stop taking fosinopril and consult with their physician (see Warnings).

Hypotension: Patients should be cautioned to report light-headedness, especially during the first few days of fosinopril therapy. If actual syncope occurs, the patients should be told to discontinue the drug and consult with their physician.

All patients should be cautioned that excessive perspiration and dehydration may lead to an excessive fall in blood pressure because of reduction in fluid volume. Other causes of volume depletion such as vomiting or diarrhea may also lead to a fall in blood pressure; patients should be advised to consult with their physician.

Neutropenia: Patients should be advised to report promptly any signs or symptoms of infection (e.g., pharyngitis, fever) since these may be an early indicator of neutropenia (see Warnings and Adverse Effects).

Impaired Liver Function: Patients should be advised to return to the physician if he/she experiences any symptoms possibly related to liver dysfunction. This would include "viral-like symptoms" in the first weeks to months of therapy (such as fever, malaise, muscle pain, rash or adenopathy which are possible indicators of hypersensitivity reactions), or if abdominal pain, nausea or vomiting, loss of appetite, jaundice, itching or any other unexplained symptoms occur during therapy.

Hyperkalemia: Patients should be advised not to use potassium supplements or salt substitutes containing potassium without consulting their physician (see Precautions and Adverse Effects).

ADVERSE EFFECTS: Fosinopril has been evaluated for safety in 1548 hypertensive patients. Of these, 1479 patients participated in controlled clinical trials, including 1048 who were treated with fosinopril monotherapy. In heart failure trials, 516 patients were treated with fosinopril including 316 who participated in placebo-controlled trials. Fosinopril has been evaluated for long-term safety in approximately 519 patients treated for 1 year or more.

Severe adverse reactions occurring in hypertensive patients treated with fosinopril were: angioedema (1 case) and orthostatic hypotension (2.7%). Myocardial infarction (2 cases) and cerebrovascular accident (4 cases) occurred, possibly secondary to excessive hypotension in high risk patients (see Warnings). In 516 heart failure patients, the severe adverse reaction occurring with the highest frequency was angina pectoris (1.6%).

In placebo-controlled hypertensive trials, the most frequent adverse experiences were: nausea/vomiting, diarrhea, fatigue, musculoskeletal pain, headache, dizziness and cough. Discontinuation of therapy due to adverse events was required in 4.1% of the 688 patients. Cough was the cause for discontinuation of therapy in 0.4% of these patients.

In placebo-controlled heart failure trials, the most frequent adverse reactions were: dizziness, cough, headache and fatigue. Significant hypotension after the first dose of fosinopril occurred in 2.4% of patients, while 0.8% discontinued due to first dose hypotension (see Warnings, Hypotension). Discontinuation of therapy due to adverse events was required in 7.8% of the 361 patients. Cough was the cause for discontinuation of therapy in 0.8% of these patients.

Adverse reactions occurring in 1% or more of the 1048 hypertensive and 361 congestive heart failure patients in controlled clinical trials who were treated with fosinopril monotherapy are listed in Table 1.

Table 1: Monopril
Adverse Reactions

Body System/Reaction	Hypertension[a] N=1048 %	Heart Failure[b] N=361 %
Cardiovascular		
Hypotension	—	4.4
Orthostatic hypotension	1.4	1.9
Palpitation	—	1.4
Angina pectoris	—	1.1
Edema	—	1.1
Dermatologic		
Rash	1.0	1.4
Endocrine/Metabolic		
Sexual dysfunction	1.7	—
Gastrointestinal		
Nausea/Vomiting	1.4	2.2
Diarrhea	1.4	2.2
Pyrosis	1.0	—
Dry mouth	1.0	—
Abdominal pain	—	1.4
General		
Fatigue	2.8	4.7
Chest pain (noncardiac)	—	2.2
Weakness	—	1.4
Musculoskeletal/Connective Tissue		
Musculoskeletal pain	—	3.3
Muscle cramp	—	1.4
Nervous System		
Headache	4.6	3.6
Dizziness	3.8	11.9
Insomnia	—	1.1
Respiratory		
Cough	4.0	9.7
Dyspnea	—	4.4
Upper respiratory infection	—	2.2

[a] Placebo and active controlled trials.
[b] Placebo controlled trials.

Clinical adverse reactions occurring in less than 1% of the 1479 hypertensive patients and 516 heart failure patients treated with fosinopril in controlled clinical trials are listed below by body system:
Cardiovascular: angina/myocardial infarction, cerebrovascular accidents, palpitations, syncope, edema, tachycardia, flushing, cardiac chest pain, hypertension, rhythm disturbances, heart failure, peripheral vascular disease of arteries, cardiac tamponade, coronary artery disease, hypertensive crisis, sudden death, cardiorespiratory arrest, shock, atrial rhythm disturbance, nonanginal chest pain, edema lower extremity, conduction disorder and bradycardia.
Dermatologic: pruritus, dermatitis, skin induration, skin dryness, urticaria, skin eschar, photosensitivity, pruritic rash and nail abnormality. Pemphigus and Stevens-Johnson syndrome have been reported with other ACE inhibitors and may occur rarely with fosinopril as well.
Endocrine/Metabolic: gout, libido change, breast disorder and menstrual disorder.
Gastrointestinal: upper abdominal pain, abdominal distention, appetite change, constipation, flatulence, dysphagia, pancreatitis, hepatitis, tongue lesion and hepatomegaly.
General: pain, excess sweating, change in weight, volume depletion, influenza, fever, hyperhidrosis and sensation of cold.
Hematologic: lymphadenopathy, leukopenia, neutropenia (see Warnings), eosinophilia and hemolytic anemia.
Immunology/Sensitivity Disorders: angioedema.
Musculoskeletal/Connective Tissues: arthralgia, muscle ache, swelling extremity, and weakness extremity.
Nervous System: sleep disturbance, stress, paresthesia, mood change, equilibrium disturbance, drowsiness, tremor, cerebrovascular accident, mental activity disorder, memory disturbance, cranial nerve disorder, confusion, vertigo, cerebral infarction, transient ischemic attack, depression, numbness and behavior change.
Renal/Genitourinary: renal insufficiency, change in urinary frequency, abnormal urination and kidney pain.
Respiratory: sinus abnormality, pharyngitis, rhinitis, epistaxis, hoarseness, laryngitis, breathing abnormality, asthma, bronchospasm, sinusitis, abnormal vocalization, tracheobronchitis and pleuritic chest pain. A symptom-complex of cough, bronchospasm and eosinophilia has been observed in 2 hypertensive patients treated with fosinopril.
Special Senses: eye irritation, vision disturbance, tinnitus, taste disturbance, ear pain, abnormal visual field and abnormal intraocular pressure.

As with other ACE inhibitors, a syndrome has been reported which includes: fever, myalgia, arthralgia, rash or other dermatologic manifestations, eosinophilia and an elevated ESR. Findings have usually resolved with discontinuation of treatment.

Laboratory Test Findings: Serum Electrolytes: hyperkalemia (see Precautions), Hyponatremia (see Precautions, Drug Interactions, Diuretics).
BUN/Serum Creatinine: Elevations, usually transient and minor, of BUN or serum creatinine have been observed. In placebo-controlled clinical trials, there were no significant differences in the number of patients experiencing increases in serum creatinine (outside the normal range or 1.33 times the pretreatment value) between the fosinopril and placebo treatment groups.
Urinary Albumin: In placebo-controlled trials, a urinary albumin (2 consecutive dip-stick values greater than 3+ or ≥2 times the pretreatment value) unassociated with a rise in serum creatinine was seen in 0.4% of fosinopril-treatment patients without pre-existing renal disease. Increases in urinary albumin usually developed in patients with pre-existing proteinuria or diabetes mellitus. In the majority of these patients, values returned to baseline despite continuation of therapy.
Hematology: In controlled trials, a mean hemoglobin decrease of 0.1 g/dL was observed in fosinopril-treated patients. In individual patients decreases in hemoglobin or hematocrit were usually transient, small, and not associated with symptoms. No patient was discontinued from therapy due to the development of anemia.
Liver Function Tests: Elevations of transaminases, LDH, alkaline phosphatase and serum bilirubin have been reported.

OVERDOSE:

Symptoms: No data are available regarding overdosage of fosinopril in humans. The most likely clinical manifestation would be symptoms attributable to severe hypotension, which should be normally treated by i.v. volume expansion with 0.9% sodium chloride. Hemodialysis and peritoneal dialysis have little effect on the elimination of fosinoprilat.

Treatment: See Symptoms.

> For management of a suspected drug overdose, CPhA recommends that you contact your **regional Poison Control Centre**. See the *CPS* Directory section for a list of Poison Control Centres.

DOSAGE: Dosage must be individualized.
Hypertension: Initiation of therapy requires consideration of recent antihypertensive drug treatment, the extent of blood pressure elevation and salt restriction. The dosage of other antihypertensive agents being used with fosinopril may need to be adjusted.
Monotherapy: The recommended initial dose is 10 mg once daily. Dosage should be adjusted according to blood pressure response, generally, at intervals of at least 2 weeks. The usual maintenance dose is 20 mg daily administered in a single daily dose. No additional blood pressure lowering effects were achieved with doses greater than 40 mg daily. A dose of 40 mg daily should not be exceeded.

In most patients, the antihypertensive effect of fosinopril is maintained with a once daily dosage regimen. In some patients treated once daily, the antihypertensive effect may diminish towards the end of the dosing interval. This can be evaluated by measuring blood pressure just prior to dosing to determine whether satisfactory control is being maintained for 24 hours. If it is not, either twice daily administration with the same total daily dose, or an increase in dose should be considered. If blood pressure is not controlled with fosinopril alone, a diuretic may be added. After the addition of a diuretic, it may be possible to reduce the dose of fosinopril.
Concomitant Diuretic Therapy: Symptomatic hypotension occasionally may occur following the initial dose of fosinopril and is more likely in patients who are currently being treated with a diuretic. The diuretic should, if possible, be discontinued for 2 to 3 days before beginning therapy with fosinopril to reduce the likelihood of hypotension (see Warnings). If the diuretic cannot be discontinued, an initial dose of 10 mg fosinopril should be used with careful medical supervision for several hours and until blood pressure has stabilized. The dosage of fosinopril should subsequently be titrated to the optimal response.
Heart Failure: Fosinopril is generally used in conjunction with a diuretic, with or without digoxin. Blood pressure and renal function should be monitored, both before and during treatment with fosinopril, because severe hypotension, and more rarely renal failure, have been reported (see Warnings, Hypotension and Precautions, Renal Impairment).

Initiation of therapy requires consideration of recent diuretic therapy, and the possibility of severe salt/volume depletion. If possible, the dose of diuretic should be reduced before beginning treatment to reduce the likelihood of hypotension (see Precautions, Drug Interactions).

In patients with heart failure, the recommended initial dose is 10 mg once daily, initiated under close medical supervision. If the initial dose is well tolerated, the dose should be titrated over 1 to 3 weeks to 20 to 40 mg once daily. The occurrence of hypotension after the initial dose may not preclude careful dose titration with fosinopril following effective management of hypotension.

In patients with severe congestive heart failure with or without renal insufficiency, therapy with fosinopril should be initiated with caution (see Warnings, Hypotension). A lower starting dose should be considered.
Renal Impairment: In hypertensive patients with renal impairment and normal liver function no dosage adjustment is necessary. The recommended initial dose of fosinopril is 10 mg once daily. Depending on the response, the dose should then be titrated, to achieve the optimal response (see Pharmacology, Pharmacokinetics and Precautions). In such patients with heart failure, therapy should be initiated with caution.
Hepatic Impairment: In hypertensive patients with hepatic impairment and normal renal function no dosage adjustment is necessary. The recommended initial dose of fosinopril is 10 mg once daily. Depending on the response, the dose should then be titrated to achieve the optimal response (see Pharmacology, Pharmacokinetics). In such patients with heart failure, therapy should be initiated with caution.

SUPPLIED: 10 mg: Each white to off-white, flat end diamond-shaped, compressed tablet, with a partial bisect bar engraved with BMS on one side and MONOPRIL 10 on the other, contains: fosinopril sodium 10 mg. Nonmedicinal ingredients: crospovidone, lactose, microcrystalline cellulose, povidone and sodium stearyl fumarate. Bottles of 100. Blister strips of 30.
20 mg: Each white to off-white, oval-shaped, compressed tablet, engraved with BMS on one side and MONOPRIL 20 on the other, contains: fosinopril sodium 20 mg. Nonmedicinal ingredients: crospovidone, lactose, microcrystalline cellulose, povidone and sodium stearyl fumarate. Bottles of 100. Blister strips of 30.

Store at room temperature (15 to 30°C). Keep container tightly closed. Protect from high humidity.

(Shown in Product Identification Section)

Monovisc™
sodium hyaluronate
Synovial Fluid Replacement/Replenishment

Helix Biopharma

DESCRIPTION: MONOVISC is a sterile, non-pyrogenic, translucent sodium hyaluronate solution, lightly cross-linked with a proprietary chemical cross-linker. MONOVISC contains nominal 20 mg/mL of lightly cross-linked sodium hyaluronate (NaHA) dissolved in phosphate buffered saline at physiological pH and osmolality. MONOVISC is manufactured from ultra pure, high molecular weight sodium hyaluronate produced by bacterial fermentation. Hyaluronic acid is a natural complex polysaccharide of the glycosaminoglycan family.
Characteristics: Sodium Hyaluronate is a high molecular weight polysaccharide composed of sodium glucuronate and N-acetyl-glucosamine. The sodium hyaluronate in MONOVISC is derived from bacterial fermentation. Hyaluronic acid is ubiquitously distributed throughout the tissue of the body and is present in high concentrations in such tissues as vitreous humor, synovial fluid, umbilical cord and dermis. Sodium hyaluronate functions as a tissue lubricant and is thought to play an important role in modulating the interactions between adjacent tissues. It can also act as a viscoelastic support maintaining a separation between tissues. Different sodium hyaluronate preparations may have different molecular weights, but have the same chemical structure. The MONOVISC cross-linked sodium hyaluronate injection is biocompatible, non-inflammatory and non-pyrogenic. Sodium hyaluronate preparations have been shown to be well tolerated in osteoarthritic synovial joints.
Application: MONOVISC Cross-Linked Sodium Hyaluronate Injection is a single, intra-articular injection of cross-linked sodium hyaluronate designed to treat the symptoms of osteoarthritis.

INDICATIONS: MONOVISC is indicated in the treatment of pain in osteoarthritis (OA) of the knee in patients who have failed to respond to adequately to conservative non-pharmacologic therapy and to simple analgesics, e.g., acetaminophen.

CONTRAINDICATIONS: MONOVISC is composed of cross-linked sodium hyaluronate and may contain trace amounts of gram positive bacterial proteins. The following pre-existing conditions may constitute relative or absolute contraindications to the use of MONOVISC:

- Known sensitivity to hyaluronic acid based products
- Pre-existing infections of the skin region of the intended injection site

- Known infection of the index joint
- Known systemic bleeding disorders
- Known sensitivity to any of the materials contained in MONOVISC

PRECAUTIONS:
- Those precautions normally considered during injection of substances into joints are recommended.
- Only medical professionals trained in accepted injection techniques for delivering agents to joint spaces should inject sodium hyaluronate for this application.
- The amount of MONOVISC necessary to be injected depends on specific site and patient anatomy and needs to be defined by the medical professional performing the procedure. An excess quantity of sodium hyaluronate should not be used and the patient should be monitored closely.
- The synovial space should not be overfilled.
- If pain increased during the injection procedure, the injection should be stopped and the needle withdrawn.
- The safety and effectiveness of MONOVISC concomitantly with other intra-articular injectables have not been tested.
- MONOVISC has not been tested in pregnant or lactating women or in children.
- The effect of repeated injections of MONOVISC has not been tested.

ADVERSE EFFECTS: Hyaluronic acid is a natural component of the tissues of the body. MONOVISC is thoroughly tested to determine that each batch conforms to the product quality attributes. MONOVISC is proven to be non-inflammatory by biocompatibility testing.

Mild to moderate episodes of transient swelling and discomfort have occasionally been observed following intra-articular injection of sodium hyaluronate preparations. General risks associated with the procedure of injecting substances into joints may include infections and bleeding.

OVERDOSE:

For management of a suspected drug overdose, CPhA recommends that you contact your **regional Poison Control Centre**. See the *CPS* Directory section for a list of Poison Control Centres.

DOSAGE: MONOVISC is a single dose preparation. The recommended dose is 4 mL (one syringe) per knee joint.
Directions for Use: The required amount of MONOVISC is injected through a sterile, disposable, hypodermic needle of suitable gauge into the selected joint space. The sterile needle should be attached to the MONOVISC syringe by a health care professional using a health care facility-approved aseptic technique. Common needle gauges for injections into the knee are 18-21 gauge. The final needle selection for any procedure is determined by the physician. The health care provider should ensure proper penetration into joint synovial space prior to injecting MONOVISC. The syringe is intended for single injection only; any unused product should be discarded per health care facility approved procedures.

SUPPLIED: Each mL of sterile viscoelastic preparation contains: 20 mg of lightly cross-linked sodium hyaluronate (NaHA) dissolved in phosphate buffered saline. Disposable glass syringes delivering 4 mL. **For intra-articular use. Store at 2 to 25°C. Protect from freezing. Caution:** This device is restricted to sale and use by or under the supervision of a physician.

Morphine Ⓝ

CPhA Monograph

see *Opioids*

Morphine HP® Injection Ⓝ

morphine sulfate

Opioid Analgesic

Sandoz

PHARMACOLOGY: Morphine exerts its main actions by acting as an opioid agonist at specific opioid receptor sites in the CNS and other tissues.

Morphine produces many effects including analgesia, decreased gastrointestinal motility, respiratory depression, nausea, vomiting, drowsiness, changes in mood and alterations of the endocrine and autonomic nervous system.

Maximum analgesia occurs within 50 to 90 minutes after SC administration, 30 to 60 minutes after IM administration and 20 minutes after IV administration. Analgesia persists for 2.5 to 7 hours.

Morphine is rapidly metabolized by the liver and excreted in the urine primarily as the active metabolite, morphine-6-glucuronide. The half-life of morphine in young adults is about 2 hours; the half-life of morphine-6-glucuronide is somewhat longer. In older patients, the volume of distribution is considerably smaller and initial concentrations of morphine are correspondingly higher.

INDICATIONS: Morphine HP 25 and Morphine HP 50 (Morphine Sulfate Injection USP), used **without dilution**, are indicated exclusively for the symptomatic relief of moderate to severe pain in patients who require opioids in doses higher than those usually needed.

Furthermore, since Morphine Sulfate Injection USP contains either 25 mg or 50 mg of morphine sulfate pentahydrate per mL, it provides a smaller injection volume, thus reducing the discomfort associated with large volume subcutaneous or intramuscular injection. Morphine Sulfate Injection USP may also be diluted for intravenous infusion.

CONTRAINDICATIONS: Hypersensitivity to morphine; respiratory insufficiency or depression; severe CNS depression; attack of bronchial asthma; heart failure secondary to chronic lung disease; cardiac arrhythmias; increased intracranial or cerebrospinal pressure; head injuries, brain tumor; acute alcoholism; delirium tremens; convulsive disorders; after biliary tract surgery; suspected surgical abdomen; surgical anastomosis; concomitantly with MAO inhibitors or within 14 days of such treatment.

WARNINGS: Morphine Sulfate Injection USP used without dilution should be used specifically for patients who are already receiving large doses of opioids. This strength of morphine undiluted is indicated for relief of severe pain in opioid-tolerant patients. The inadvertent administration of this strength of morphine to patients requiring standard dosage strengths may lead to overdose or death.
Drug Dependence: As with other opioids, tolerance and physical dependence tend to develop upon repeated administration of morphine and there is potential for abuse of the drug and for development of strong psychological dependence. Morphine should therefore be prescribed and handled with the high degree of caution appropriate to the use of a drug with strong abuse potential. Drug abuse is not, however, a problem in patients with severe pain in which morphine is appropriately indicated.

On the other hand, in the absence of a clear indication for a strong opioid analgesic, drug-seeking behaviour must be suspected and resisted, particularly in individuals with a history of, or propensity for drug abuse. Withdrawal symptoms may occur following abrupt discontinuation of morphine therapy or upon administration of an opioid antagonist. Therefore, a patient on prolonged therapy should be withdrawn gradually from the drug if it is no longer required for pain control.

Morphine should be used with caution and in reduced dosage in patients who are concurrently receiving other opioid analgesics, general anesthetics, phenothiazines and other tranquillizers, sedative-hypnotics, tricyclic antidepressants and other CNS depressants (including alcohol). Respiratory depression, hypotension and profound sedation or coma may result.

The respiratory depressant effects of morphine and its capacity to elevate cerebrospinal fluid pressure may be greatly increased in the presence of an already elevated intracranial pressure produced by trauma. Also, morphine may produce confusion, miosis, vomiting and other side effects which obscure the clinical course of patients with head injury. In such patients, morphine must be used with extreme caution and only if its use is judged essential.

Morphine should also be used with extreme caution in patients having an acute asthmatic attack, patients with chronic obstructive pulmonary disease or cor pulmonale, patients having a substantially decreased respiratory reserve and patients with preexisting respiratory depression, hypoxia or hypercapnia. In such patients, even usual therapeutic doses of opioids may decrease respiratory drive while simultaneously increasing airway resistance to the point of apnea.

PRECAUTIONS: Acute Abdominal Condition: The administration of morphine or other opioids may obscure the diagnosis or clinical course in patients with acute abdominal conditions.

Special Risk Groups: Morphine should be administered with caution, and in reduced dosages, to elderly or debilitated patients, and to patients with severe impairment of hepatic or renal function, hypothyroidism, Addison's disease, prostatic hypertrophy or urethral stricture.

Morphine should be used with extreme caution in patients with disorders characterized by hypoxia, since even usual therapeutic doses of opioids may decrease respiratory drive to the point of apnea while simultaneously increasing airway resistance.
Hypotensive Effect: Morphine, like other opioids, may produce orthostatic hypotension in ambulatory patients. The administration of morphine may result in severe hypotension in the postoperative patient, or any individual whose ability to maintain blood pressure has been compromised by a depleted blood volume or the administration of drugs such as the phenothiazines or certain anesthetics.
Supraventricular Tachycardias: Because of possible vagolytic action that may produce a significant increase in the ventricular response rate, morphine should be used with caution in patients with atrial flutter and other supraventricular tachycardias.
Convulsions: Morphine may exacerbate preexisting convulsions in patients with convulsive disorders. If dosage is escalated substantially above recommended levels because of tolerance development, convulsions may occur in individuals without a history of convulsive disorders.
Kidney or Liver Dysfunction: Morphine may have a prolonged duration and cumulative effect in patients with kidney or liver dysfunction. In these patients, analgesia may last for 6, 8 or even up to 24 hours following a standard dose. Continuous infusions should be avoided.
Patients in Shock: Impaired blood perfusion may prevent complete absorption following SC or IM injection of morphine. Repeated administration may result in overdosage due to an excessive amount of morphine suddenly being absorbed when circulation is restored.
Drug Interactions: Generally, the effects of morphine may be antagonized by acidifying agents and potentiated by alkalizing agents.

The analgesic effect of morphine is potentiated by amphetamines, chlorpromazine and methocarbamol. CNS depressants, such as other opioids, anesthetics, sedatives, hypnotics, barbiturates, phenothiazines, chloral hydrate and glutethimide may enhance the depressant effects of morphine. MAO inhibitors (including procarbazine), pyrazolidone antihistamines, beta-blockers and alcohol may also enhance the depressant effect of morphine.

Morphine may increase the anticoagulant activity of coumarin and other anticoagulants.
Carcinogenesis, Mutagenesis, Impairment of Fertility: Morphine has no known carcinogenic or mutagenic potential. However, no long-term animal study is available to support this observation.
Pregnancy: Animal reproduction studies have not been conducted with morphine. It is not known whether morphine can cause fetal harm when administered to a pregnant woman or can affect reproduction capacity. On the basis of the historical use of morphine during all stages of pregnancy, there is no known risk of fetal abnormality. Morphine should not be given to pregnant women unless it is clearly necessary and when the anticipated benefits outweigh the potential risks to the fetus.
Labor and Delivery: Morphine should not be used in pregnant women prior to labor unless the potential benefits outweigh the possible hazards. The use of morphine in obstetrics may prolong labor. Morphine crosses the placental barrier and may produce respiratory depression in the newborn. For resuscitation and in severe depression, the administration of an opioid antagonist such as naloxone may be required.
Lactation: Morphine sulfate appears in the milk of nursing mothers. Breast feeding should be discontinued if morphine is required.
Children: Safety and efficacy of morphine in neonates and children has not been established.
Information to Be Provided to the Patient: Occupational Hazards: Morphine may impair the mental and/or physical abilities required for the performance of potentially hazardous tasks, such as driving a motor vehicle or operating machinery. Morphine, in combination with other opioid analgesics, general anesthetics, phenothiazines, tranquillizers, sedative-hypnotics or other CNS depressants (including alcohol) has additive depressant effects. The patient should be cautioned accordingly.

ADVERSE EFFECTS: The major hazards of morphine, as with other opioid analgesics, are respiratory depression and, to a lesser degree, circulatory depression; respiratory arrest, shock and cardiac arrest have occurred. The most frequently observed adverse reactions include: light-headedness, dizziness, sedation, nausea, vomiting, constipation and sweating. These effects seem to be more prominent in ambulatory patients and in those who are not experiencing severe pain. In such individuals, lower doses are advisable. Some adverse reactions in ambulatory patients may be alleviated if the patient lies down.

Rapid IV injection of the drug may result in an increased frequency of opioid-induced adverse effects: severe respiratory depression, apnea, hypotension, peripheral circulatory collapse, chest wall rigidity, cardiac arrest and possible anaphylactoid reactions.
Most Common Adverse Effects Requiring Medical Attention: The most frequently observed side effects of opioid analgesics, such as morphine, are sedation, nausea and vomiting, constipation and sweating.
Sedation: Most patients experience initial drowsiness partly for pharmacokinetic reasons and partly because patients with chronic pain often recuperate from prolonged fatigue after the relief of persistent pain. Drowsiness usually clears in 3 to 5 days and is usually not a reason for concern providing that it is not excessive, or associated with unsteadiness or confusional symptoms.
Nausea and Vomiting: Nausea and vomiting occur frequently after single doses of opioids or as an early unwanted effect of regular opioid therapy. When instituting prolonged therapy for chronic pain the routine prescription of an antiemetic should be considered. Patients taking a single dose of 20 mg or more of morphine usually require an antiemetic during early therapy. Small doses of prochlorperazine or haloperidol are the most frequently prescribed antiemetics. Nausea and vomiting tend to lessen in a week or so but may persist due to opioid-induced gastric stasis. In such patients, metoclopramide is often useful.
Constipation: Practically all patients become constipated while taking opioids on a persistent basis. In some instances, particularly the elderly or bedridden, patients may become impacted. It is essential to caution the patients in this regard and to institute an appropriate regimen of bowel management at the start of prolonged opioid therapy. In addition to ample intake of fluid, stool softeners, laxatives and other appropriate measures should be used as required.
Other Adverse Reactions:
Central Nervous System: euphoria, dysphoria, weakness, headache, insomnia, agitation, tremor, uncoordinated muscle movements, transient hallucinations, disorientation and visual disturbances.
Gastrointestinal: dry mouth, anorexia, constipation, cramps, taste alterations and biliary tract spasm.
Cardiovascular: flushing of the face, tachycardia, bradycardia, palpitation, faintness and syncope.
Genitourinary: urinary retention or hesitance, antidiuretic effect and reduced libido or potency.
Allergic: pruritus, urticaria, other skin rashes, edema and rarely hemorrhagic urticaria, wheal and flare over the vein with IV injection.
Endocrine: A syndrome of inappropriate antidiuretic hormone secretion characterized by hyponatremia secondary to decreased free-water excretion may be prominent (monitoring of electrolytes may be necessary).
Withdrawal (Abstinence) Syndrome: Physical dependence with or without psychological dependence tends to occur on chronic administration. An abstinence syndrome may be precipitated when opioid administration is discontinued or opioid antagonists administered. The following withdrawal symptoms may be observed after opioids are discontinued: body aches, diarrhea, gooseflesh, loss of appetite, nervousness or restlessness, runny nose, sneezing, tremors or shivering, stomach cramps, nausea, trouble with sleeping, unusual increase in sweating and yawning, weakness, tachycardia and unexplained fever. With appropriate medical use of opioids and gradual withdrawal from the drug, these symptoms are usually mild.
Other: pain at injection site; local tissue irritation and induration following SC injection, particularly when repeated.

OVERDOSE:

Symptoms: Serious morphine overdosage is characterized by respiratory depression (reduced respiratory rate and/or tidal volume, Cheyne-Stokes respiration, cyanosis), extreme somnolence progressing to stupor or coma, skeletal muscle flaccidity, cold or clammy skin, and sometimes bradycardia and hypotension. Severe overdosage may result in apnea, circulatory collapse, cardiac arrest and death.

Treatment: Primary attention should be given to the establishment of adequate respiratory exchange through the provision of a patent airway and controlled or assisted ventilation. The opioid antagonist, naloxone, is a specific antidote against respiratory depression due to overdosage or resulting from an unusual sensitivity to morphine. Therefore, an appropriate dose of this antagonist should be administered, preferably by the IV route. The usual initial IV adult dose of naloxone is 0.4 mg or higher. Concomitant efforts at respiratory resuscitation should be carried out.

Since the duration of action of morphine may exceed that of the antagonist, the patient should be under continued surveillance and doses of the antagonist should be repeated as needed to maintain adequate respiration.

An antagonist should not be administered in the absence of clinically significant respiratory or cardiovascular depression. Oxygen, IV fluids, vasopressors and other supportive measures should be employed as indicated.

In an individual physically dependent on opioids, the administration of the usual dose of opioid antagonist will precipitate an acute withdrawal syndrome. The severity of this syndrome will depend on the degree of physical dependence and the dose of antagonist administered. The use of an opioid antagonist in such individuals should be avoided if possible. If an opioid antagonist must be used to treat serious respiratory depression in the physically dependent patient, the antagonist should be administered with extreme care by using dosage titration, commencing with 10 to 20% of the usual recommended initial dose.

For management of a suspected drug overdose, CPhA recommends that you contact your **regional Poison Control Centre**. See the *CPS* Directory section for a list of Poison Control Centres.

DOSAGE: Morphine Sulfate Injection USP (25 mg/mL or 50 mg/mL) used without dilution is not to be given to patients who are not already receiving large doses of opioids. These strengths of morphine are indicated exclusively for pain relief in opioid tolerant patients.

Administration and dosing of morphine should be individualized bearing in mind the properties of the drug. In addition, the nature and severity of the pain or pains experienced, and the total condition of the patient must be taken into account. Of special importance is other medication given previously or concurrently.

As with other strong opioid analgesics, use of morphine for the management of persistent pain should be preceded by a thorough assessment of the patient and diagnosis of the specific pain or pains and their causes. Use of opioids for the relief of chronic pain, including cancer pain, all important as it may be, should be only one part of a comprehensive approach to pain control including other treatment modalities of drug therapy, nondrug measures and psychosocial support.

Individual dosing requirements vary considerably based on each patient's age, weight, severity of pain, and medical and analgesic history.

Orally administered morphine should be used in preference to parenteral morphine whenever adequate pain control can be achieved by this route. However oral morphine is often inadequate or impractical in the terminally ill patient.

Patients being converted from oral morphine to concentrated morphine sulfate injection require dosage reduction (about half), since about 66% of oral morphine is metabolized in first pass metabolism. If the patient has been treated previously with a lower strength of parenteral morphine, similar doses would be given initially, and then titrated according to the patient's clinical response.

Morphine Sulfate Injection USP should be given regularly around the clock, in most instances every 4 hours. The basis of pain control with morphine sulfate injection should be regular scheduling rather than on an "as required" or PRN opioid order. Patients requiring high doses of morphine usually need to be awakened for medication during the night to prevent morning pain.

Patients over the age of 50 tend to require much lower doses of morphine than in the younger age group. In elderly and debilitated patients and those with impaired respiratory function or significantly decreased renal function, the initial dose should be one half the usual recommended dose.

For patients who are receiving an alternate opioid, the "oral morphine sulfate equivalent" of the analgesic presently being used should be determined. Having determined the total daily dosage of the present analgesic, Table 1 can be used to calculate the approximate daily morphine sulfate dosage that should provide equivalent analgesia.

Table 1: Morphine HP Injection

Opioid Analgesics: Approximate Analgesic Equivalences[a]

Drug	Equivalent Dose (mg)[b] (compared to morphine 10 mg IM) — Parenteral	Oral	Duration of Action (hours)
Strong Opioid Agonists:			
Morphine (single dose)	10	60	3–4
Morphine (chronic dose)	10	20–30[c]	3–4
Hydromorphone	1.5–2	6–7.5	2–4
Anileridine	25	75	2–3
Levorphanol	2	4	4–8
Meperidine[d]	75	300	1–3
Oxymorphone	1.5	5 (rectal)	3–4
Methadone[e]			
Heroin	5–8	10–15	3–4
Weak Opioid Agonists:			
Codeine	120	200	3–4
Oxycodone	5–10	10–15	2–4
Propoxyphene	50	100	2–4
Mixed Agonist-Antagonists:[f]			
Pentazocine[d]	60	180	3–4
Nalbuphine	10		3–6
Butorphanol	2		3–4

[a] References:
Cancer Pain: A Monograph on the Management of Cancer Pain, Health and Welfare Canada, 1984.
Foley, K.M., New Engl. J. Med. 313: 84-95, 1985.
Aronoff, G.M. and Evans,W.O., In: Evaluation and Treatment of Chronic Pain, 2nd Ed., G.M. Aronoff (Ed.), Williams and Wilkins, Baltimore, pp. 359-368, 1992.
Cherny, N.I. and Portenoy, R.K., In: Textbook of Pain, 3rd Ed., P.D.Wall and R. Melzack (Eds.), Churchill Livingstone, London, pp. 1437-1467, 1994.

[b] Most of these data were derived from single-dose, acute pain studies and should be considered an approximation for selection of doses when treating chronic pain.

[c] For acute pain, the oral dose of morphine is six times the injectable dose. However, for chronic dosing, this ratio becomes 2 or 3:1, possibly due to the accumulation of active metabolites.

[d] These drugs are not recommended for the management of chronic pain.

[e] Extremely variable equianalgesic dose. Patients should undergo personalized titration starting at an equivalent to 1/10 of the morphine dose.

[f] Mixed agonist-antagonists can precipitate withdrawal in patients on pure opioid agonists.

Dose Titration: In patients with chronic pain, dose titration is the key to success with morphine therapy. Proper optimization of doses scaled to the relief of the individual's pain should aim at the **regular** administration of the lowest dose of morphine which will maintain the patient free of pain at all times. Dose adjustments should be based on the patient's clinical response. Higher doses may be justified in some patients to cover periods of physical activity.

Morphine Dosage Reduction: During the first two to three days of effective pain relief, the patient may sleep for many hours. This can be misinterpreted as the effect of excessive analgesic dosing rather than the first sign of relief in a pain exhausted patient. The dose, therefore, should be maintained for about 3 days before reduction, if respiratory activity and other vital signs are adequate.

Following successful relief of severe pain, periodic attempts to reduce the opioid dose should be made. Lower doses or complete discontinuation of the opioid analgesic may become feasible due to a physiological change or the improved mental state of the patient.

Morphine Dosage Increase: Dosage increases should not be made more frequently than every 24 hours, since it will take approximately 4 to 5 morphine half-lives to attain a new steady-state concentration in a patient with normal liver and kidney function.

Following all dosage increases, the patient must be monitored closely for side effects, the most common being sedation, nausea, vomiting, constipation and hypotension.

Opioid agents do not relieve effectively dysesthetic pain, post-herpetic neuralgia, stabbing pains, activity-related pain, and some forms of headache. This is not to say that patients with advanced cancer suffering from some of these forms of pain should not be given an adequate trial of opioid analgesics, but it may be necessary to refer such patients at an early time for other forms of pain therapy. Pain without nociception is usually not opioid-responsive.

SC or IM Injection: The SC route of injection is preferred over the IM route in terminal cancer patients. **In any case, IV or SC infusion is preferred over injection because of the risks of accidental overdose with direct injection.**

IV Infusion with Dilution: Morphine Sulfate Injection USP may be diluted in a parenteral solution (5% Dextrose Injection in water or 0.9% Sodium Chloride Injection) to the desired concentration (usually 0.1 to 0.5 mg/mL) and administered by IV infusion as required. **It is recommended that an opioid antagonist and equipment for artificial ventilation be available.**

SC Infusion: If a patient has low muscle mass, is cachectic or has no accessible peripheral veins, Morphine Sulfate Injection USP may be given by SC infusion using a portable pump. When switching from IV to SC infusion, use the same dose and monitor the same parameters. The maximum dose that can be safely given has not been defined but doses as high as 480 mg/24 hours have been administered. The infusion rate tolerated by patients is variable. Most patients can tolerate 10 mL/hour subcutaneously, and some may tolerate higher infusion rates. When an infusion rate is excessive there may be leakage at the infusion site. This is most likely to occur at lower infusion rates in severely cachectic patients who have minimal SC tissue. In such cases, higher strength solutions or potent opioids will permit lower infusion rates and minimize the chance of leakage.

Erythema, bruising, induration or tenderness around the injection site may occur. The injection site must be inspected daily for these effects, and for infection or leakage of medication. The needle site should be changed periodically (every 7 to 10 days, although some clinicians prefer every 48 hours).

Morphine Sulfate Injection USP and dilutions of Morphine Sulfate Injection USP in 5% Dextrose Injection or 0.9% Sodium Chloride Injection can be stored in portable infusion pump cassettes, syringes, and PVC minibags. Protected from light, they will stay stable for 31 days at room temperature (15 to 30°C). Appropriate aseptic techniques must be used in order to minimize contamination of the solution.

Warnings: As with all parenteral drug products, IV admixtures should be inspected visually for clarity, particulate matter, precipitation and leakage prior to administration, whenever solution and container permit. Solutions showing haziness, particulate matter, precipitate or leakage should not be used. Development of a yellow colour in morphine solutions does not indicate toxicity nor loss of potency or efficacy.

SUPPLIED: 25 mg/mL: Each mL of clear, colourless or yellow isotonic, sterile, and preservative free solution contains: morphine sulfate pentahydrate 25 mg. Nonmedicinal ingredients: sodium chloride for tonicity, sulfuric acid and/or sodium hydroxide to adjust pH and water for injection. Single use amber vials of 1 mL, boxes of 10. Single use amber vials of 4 mL, boxes of 5. Latex-free stopper: Stoppers contain no dry natural rubber. Store between 15 and 30°C. Protect from light. Discard unused portion. Do not autoclave. **No loss of analgesic potency and no increase in toxicity have ever been demonstrated for discoloured solutions.**

50 mg/mL: Each mL of clear, colourless or yellow isotonic, sterile, and preservative free solution contains: morphine sulfate pentahydrate 50 mg. Nonmedicinal ingredients: sodium chloride for tonicity, sulfuric acid and/or sodium hydroxide to adjust pH and water for injection. Single use amber vials of 1 mL, boxes of 10. Single use amber vials of 5 mL, boxes of 5. Single use amber vials of 10 mL, boxes of 5. Single use amber vials of 50 mL, boxes of 1. Latex-free stopper: Stoppers contain no dry natural rubber. Store between 15 and 30°C. Protect from light. Discard unused portion. Do not autoclave. **No loss of analgesic potency and no increase in toxicity have ever been demonstrated for discoloured solutions.**

Morphine LP® Epidural Ⓝ

morphine sulfate

Opioid Analgesic

Sandoz

SUPPLIED: 0.5 mg/mL: Each mL of sterile, isotonic solution free of antioxidants or preservatives contains: morphine sulfate 0.5 mg. Nonmedicinal ingredients: sodium chloride 9 mg for isotonicity, sulfuric acid and/or sodium hydroxide to adjust pH and water for injection. Single use vials of 10 mL, boxes of 5. Do not autoclave. Store between 15 and 30°C. Protect from light. Discard unused portion. Latex-free stoppers: Stoppers contain no dry natural rubber.

1 mg/mL: Each mL of sterile, isotonic solution free of antioxidants or preservatives contains: morphine sulfate 1 mg. Nonmedicinal ingredients: sodium chloride 9 mg for isotonicity, sulfuric acid and/or sodium hydroxide to adjust pH, and water for injection. Single use vials of 5 mL, boxes of 5. Do not autoclave. Store between 15 and 30°C. Protect from light. Discard unused portion. Latex-free stoppers: Stoppers contain no dry natural rubber.

Morphine Sulfate Ⓝ

morphine sulfate

Opioid Analgesic

Hospira

SUPPLIED: Each mL contains: morphine sulfate 1 or 5 mg. Also contains citric acid, sodium chloride, sodium citrate, sodium metabisulfite and water for injection. Cartridges (single dose vials) of 30 mL for Patient-Controlled-Analgesia infusor (PCA), cases of 10.

Morphine Sulfate Injection USP Ⓝ

morphine sulfate

Opioid Analgesic

Sandoz

SUPPLIED: 1 mg/mL: Each mL of clear, colourless or pale yellow, isotonic, sterile solution contains: morphine sulfate·$5H_2O$ 1 mg. Nonmedicinal ingredients: sodium chloride for isotonicity, sodium metabisulfite, sulfuric acid and/or sodium hydroxide to adjust pH and water for injection. Single use vials of 10 mL, boxes of 5. Discard unused portion. Do not use if the solution is darker than pale yellow, is discoloured in any other way or contains a precipitate. Store between 15 and 30°C. Protect from light.

2 mg/mL (ampoules): Each mL of clear, colourless or pale yellow, isotonic, sterile solution contains: morphine sulfate·$5H_2O$ 2 mg. Nonmedicinal ingredients: sodium chloride for isotonicity, sodium metabisulfite, sulfuric acid and/or sodium hydroxide to adjust pH and water for injection. Ampoules of 1 mL, boxes of 10. Discard unused portion. Do not use if the solution is darker than pale yellow, is discoloured in any other way or contains a precipitate. Store between 15 and 30°C. Protect from light.

2 mg/mL (50 mL vial): Each mL of clear, colourless or pale yellow, isotonic, sterile solution contains: morphine sulfate·$5H_2O$ 2 mg. Nonmedicinal ingredients: anhydrous citric acid, sodium chloride for isotonicity, sodium citrate ·$2H_2O$, sodium metabisulfite and water for injection. Single use vials of 50 mL, boxes of 10. Discard unused portion. Do not use if the solution is darker than pale yellow, is discoloured in any other way or contains a precipitate. Store between 15 and 30°C. Protect from light.

5 mg/mL: Each mL of clear, colourless or pale yellow, isotonic, sterile solution contains: morphine sulfate·$5H_2O$ 5 mg. Nonmedicinal ingredients: anhydrous citric acid, sodium chloride for isotonicity, sodium citrate ·$2H_2O$, sodium metabisulfite and water for injection. Single use vials of 30 mL, boxes of 10. Discard unused portion. Do not use if the solution is darker than pale yellow, is discoloured in any other way or contains a precipitate. Store between 15 and 30°C. Protect from light.

10 mg/mL: Each mL of clear, colourless or pale yellow, sterile solution contains: morphine sulfate·$5H_2O$ 10 mg. Nonmedicinal ingredients: sodium metabisulfite, sulfuric acid and/or sodium hydroxide to adjust pH and water for injection. Ampoules of 1 mL, boxes of 10. Do not use if the solution is darker than pale yellow, is discoloured in any other way or contains a precipitate. Store between 15 and 30°C. Protect from light.

15 mg/mL: Each mL of clear, colourless or pale yellow, sterile solution contains: morphine sulfate·$5H_2O$ 15 mg. Nonmedicinal ingredients: sodium metabisulfite, sulfuric acid and/or sodium hydroxide to adjust pH and water for injection. Multidose vials (30 mL) of Morphine Sulfate Injection USP 15 mg/mL also contain benzyl alcohol 1% as preservative. Ampoules of 1 mL, boxes of 10. Multidose vials of 30 mL, boxes of 1. Do not use if the solution is darker than pale yellow, is discoloured in any other way or contains a precipitate. Store between 15 and 30°C. Protect from light.

M.O.S.® Ⓝ
morphine HCl
Opioid Analgesic

Valeant

M.O.S.-SR® Ⓝ
morphine HCl
Opioid Analgesic

Valeant

SUPPLIED: M.O.S.: Concentrate: M.O.S.–20: Each mL of clear, yellow-colored, unflavored, syrupy liquid contains: morphine HCl BP 20 mg. Nonmedicinal ingredients: citric acid, FD&C Yellow No. 6, fructose, propylene glycol, sodium benzoate, sodium cyclamate, sodium metabisulfite and sorbitol. Alcohol-free. Graduated, opaque brown glass bottles of 50 mL with graduated syringe.
M.O.S.–50: Each mL of clear, yellow-colored, unflavored, syrupy liquid contains: morphine HCl BP 50 mg. Nonmedicinal ingredients: citric acid, FD&C Yellow No. 6, propylene glycol, sodium benzoate, sodium metabisulfite and sorbitol. Alcohol-free. Graduated, opaque brown glass bottles of 50 mL with graduated syringe.
Syrup: M.O.S.–1: Each mL of clear, yellow-colored, orange-flavored (alcohol 5%) syrupy liquid contains: morphine HCl BP 1 mg. Nonmedicinal ingredients: citric acid, ethyl alcohol, FD&C Yellow No. 6, fructose, propylene glycol, sodium benzoate, sodium cyclamate, sodium metabisulfite and sorbitol. Graduated, opaque brown plastic bottles of 250 and 500 mL.
M.O.S.–5: Each mL of clear, yellow-colored, orange-flavored (alcohol 5%) syrupy liquid contains: morphine HCl BP 5 mg. Nonmedicinal ingredients: citric acid, ethyl alcohol, D&C Yellow No. 10, FD&C Yellow No. 6, fructose, propylene glycol, sodium benzoate, sodium cyclamate, sodium metabisulfite and sorbitol. Graduated, opaque brown plastic bottles of 250 and 500 mL.
M.O.S.–10: Each mL of clear, yellow-colored, orange-flavored, syrupy liquid (alcohol 5%) contains: morphine HCl BP 10 mg. Nonmedicinal ingredients: citric acid, ethyl alcohol, FD&C Yellow No. 6, fructose, propylene glycol, sodium benzoate, sodium cyclamate, sodium metabisulfite and sorbitol. Graduated, opaque brown plastic bottles of 250 mL.
Tablets: M.O.S.–10: Each round, beige, film-coated tablet, contains: morphine HCl BP 10 mg. Nonmedicinal ingredients: croscarmellose sodium, isopropyl alcohol, lactose, microcrystalline cellulose, magnesium stearate, povidone, starch and talc. Bottles of 100.
M.O.S.–20: Each round, salmon-pink, film-coated tablet, contains: morphine HCl BP 20 mg. Nonmedicinal ingredients: croscarmellose sodium, isopropyl alcohol, lactose, microcrystalline cellulose, magnesium stearate, povidone, starch and talc. Bottles of 100.
M.O.S.–40: Each round, blue, film-coated tablet, contains: morphine HCl BP 40 mg. Nonmedicinal ingredients: croscarmellose sodium, isopropyl alcohol, lactose, microcrystalline cellulose, magnesium stearate, povidone, starch and talc. Bottles of 100.
M.O.S.–60: Each round, yellow, film-coated tablet, contains: morphine HCl BP 60 mg. Nonmedicinal ingredients: croscarmellose sodium, isopropyl alcohol, lactose, microcrystalline cellulose, magnesium stearate, povidone, starch and talc. Bottles of 100.
M.O.S.-SR: M.O.S.-SR-30: Each blue, round, biconvex, film-coated, slow release tablet printed 30 on one side, contains: morphine HCl 30 mg. Nonmedicinal ingredients: microcrystalline cellulose, magnesium stearate, simetry and talc. Bottles of 50. Store below 30°C. Protect from light.
M.O.S.-SR-60: Each red, round, biconvex film-coated, slow release tablet printed 60 on one side, contains: morphine HCl 60 mg. Nonmedicinal ingredients: microcrystalline cellulose, magnesium stearate, simetry and talc. Bottles of 50. Store below 30°C. Protect from light.

M.O.S.®-Sulfate Ⓝ
morphine sulfate
Opioid Analgesic

Valeant

SUPPLIED: M.O.S.-Sulfate 5: Each round, green tablet contains: morphine sulfate, USP (pentahydrate) 5 mg. Nonmedicinal ingredients: cornstarch, croscarmellose sodium, D&C Yellow #10, FD&C Blue #1, isopropyl alcohol, lactose, magnesium stearate, microcrystalline cellulose, povidone and talc. Bottles of 100.
M.O.S.-Sulfate 10: Each round, blue tablet contains: morphine sulfate, USP (pentahydrate) 10 mg. Nonmedicinal ingredients: as in 5 mg tablets, but FD&C Blue #1 only. Bottles of 100.
M.O.S.-Sulfate 25: Each round, pink tablet contains: morphine sulfate, USP (pentahydrate) 25 mg. Nonmedicinal ingredients: as in 5 and 10 mg tablets, but FD&C Red #40 only. Bottles of 100.
M.O.S.-Sulfate 50: Each round, orange tablet contains: morphine sulfate, USP (pentahydrate) 50 mg. Nonmedicinal ingredients: as in 5, 10 and 25 mg tablets, but FD&C Yellow #6 only. Bottles of 100.
Store below 30°C. Keep containers well closed. Protect from light. Keep out of reach of children.

Motrin® (Children's)
ibuprofen
Analgesic—Antipyretic

McNeil Consumer Healthcare

Date of Revision: August 28, 2008

SUMMARY PRODUCT INFORMATION:

Route of Administration	Dosage Form/ Strength	Clinically Relevant Nonmedicinal Ingredients
Oral	100 mg/5 mL ibuprofen oral suspension	None For a complete listing see Dosage Forms, Composition and Packaging.
	40 mg/mL ibuprofen oral suspension	None For a complete listing see Dosage Forms, Composition and Packaging.
	50 mg and 100 mg ibuprofen tablets	None For a complete listing see Dosage Forms, Composition and Packaging.

INDICATIONS AND CLINICAL USE: Children's MOTRIN (ibuprofen) is indicated for:
- Temporary relief of minor aches and pains in muscles, bones and joints, headache, fever, the aches and fever due to the common cold or flu, immunizations, toothache (dental pain), sore throat, earache. (Arthritis Advisory Committee; 1983, Proceeding of Joint Meeting of Arthritis Drug Advisory Committee & Nonprescription Drug Advisory Committee; 1995)

CONTRAINDICATIONS: Children's MOTRIN (ibuprofen) should not be used in patients:
- who have previously exhibited hypersensitivity to it or in individuals who are known to have a sensitivity (manifested as asthma, bronchospasm, hypotension, angioedema, laryngeal edema, swelling, shock or urticaria) to acetylsalicylic acid or other nonsteroidal anti-inflammatory drugs (Arthritis Advisory Committee; 1983).
- with acute peptic ulcer or gastrointestinal bleeding.
- during pregnancy or in nursing mothers because its safety under these conditions has not been established.
- with Systemic Lupus Erythematosus as an anaphylaxis like reaction with fever may occur, particularly when ibuprofen has been administered previously. Aseptic meningitis has also been reported.
- who are children and are suffering from dehydration as a result of acute diarrhea, vomiting or lack of fluid intake

WARNINGS AND PRECAUTIONS: General: Several medical conditions which can predispose patients to the adverse effects of nonsteroidal anti-inflammatory drugs in general may be applicable to ibuprofen.

Patients taking Children's MOTRIN should be cautioned to report to their physician unusual signs or symptoms which might be a manifestation of GI ulceration or bleeding, blurred vision or other ocular symptoms, skin rash, tinnitus, dizziness, weight gain, edema or respiratory difficulties.

Children's MOTRIN should be used with caution in patients with a history of cardiac failure or kidney disease because of the possibility of aggravating pre-existing states of fluid-retention or edema (Arthritis Advisory Committee; 1983). Mild impairment of renal function (decreased renal blood flow and glomerular filtration rate) can occur at maximal doses of ibuprofen. Renal papillary necrosis has been reported.

Also, patients with underlying medical or pharmacologically-induced hemostatic defects could also experience further prolongation of bleeding time through the inhibition of platelet aggregation induced to varying degrees by this class of drugs (Arthritis Advisory Committee; 1983).

Long-term ingestion of combinations of analgesics has been associated with the condition analgesic nephropathy. It is therefore appropriate that patients be discouraged from long-term unsupervised consumption of analgesics, particularly in combination. Patients should be directed to consult a physician if their underlying condition requires administration of Children's MOTRIN for more than 3 days for fever or 5 days for pain, nor should Children's MOTRIN usually be administered with acetaminophen or acetylsalicylic acid (Arthritis Advisory Committee; 1983).

A general precaution seems appropriate for patients with any serious medical condition to consult a physician before using Children's MOTRIN as an analgesic or antipyretic (Arthritis Advisory Committee; 1983).

Cardiovascular: Conditions such as congestive heart failure and hypertension may be aggravated by sodium retention and edema caused by ibuprofen in such patients.

Endocrine and Metabolism: If Children's MOTRIN is taken in conjection with prolonged corticosteroid therapy and it is decided to discontinue this therapy, the corticosteroid should be tapered slowly to avoid exacerbation of disease or adrenal insufficiency.

Gastrointestinal: Gastrointestinal side effects to ibuprofen have been reported including dyspepsia, heartburn, nausea, vomiting, anorexia, diarrhea, constipation, stomatitis, flatulence, bloating, epigastric pain, abdominal pain, and peptic ulcer with GI bleeding or perforation which could have a fatal outcome (Arthritis Advisory Committee; 1983). Children's MOTRIN ibuprofen should therefore be given only under close supervision to patients with a history of upper gastrointestinal tract disease.

Occasionally serious gastrointestinal side effects have been associated with the anti-inflammatory uses of ibuprofen. Minor gastrointestinal complaints have also been reported during the clinical use of ibuprofen at analgesic doses. Therefore, if occasional and mild heartburn, upset stomach or stomach pain were to occur with its use, the administration of Children's MOTRIN with food or milk is recommended. Patients should be advised to seek the consultation of a physician if gastrointestinal side effects occur, persist or appear to worsen (Arthritis Advisory Committee; 1983).

Hematologic: Children's MOTRIN ibuprofen, like other nonsteroidal anti-inflammatory agents, can inhibit platelet aggregation but the effect is quantitatively less than that seen with acetylsalicylic acid. Ibuprofen has been shown to prolong bleeding time (but within the normal range) in normal subjects. Because this prolonged bleeding effect may be exaggerated in patients with underlying haemostatis defects, Children's MOTRIN ibuprofen should be avoided by persons with intrinsic coagulation defects and by those on anticoagulant therapy.

Immune: Anaphylactoid reactions have occurred after administration of ibuprofen to patients with known acetylsalicylic acid or other NSAID sensitivity manifested as asthma, swelling, shock or hives (Arthritis Advisory Committee; 1983).

Ophthalmologic: Tinnitus, blurred and/or diminished vision, scotoma, and/or changes in colour vision have been reported. If a patient develops such complaints while taking Children's MOTRIN, the drug should be discontinued. Patients with any visual disturbances or eye complaints during therapy should have an ophthalmologic examination.

Renal: Like other nonsteroidal anti-inflammatory agents, ibuprofen inhibits renal prostaglandin synthesis which may decrease renal function and cause sodium retention.

Advanced age, hypertension, use of diuretics, diabetes, atherosclerotic cardiovascular disease, chronic renal failure, cirrhosis and conditions which may be associated with dehydration appear to increase the risk of renal toxicity. Children's MOTRIN should therefore be used with caution when these risk factors are present.

Respiratory: Ibuprofen may elicit an asthma attack in individuals with a history of asthma, but who have no history of allergy or asthma induced by aspirin and other NSAIDs (Antonicelli & Tagliabracci; 1995, Ayres et al.; 1987, Friedlander et al.; 1994).

Special Populations: Pregnant Women: No evidence specifically identifies exposure to analgesic doses of ibuprofen as a cause of harm to either mother or fetus during pregnancy (Arthritis Advisory Committee, 1983; Barry et. al., 1984). Nonsteroidal anti-inflammatory drugs in general, however, are known to affect the action of prostaglandin synthetase which could alter a variety of the physiological functions of prostaglandins or platelets during delivery such as facilitating uterine contraction in the mother, closure of the ductus arteriosus in the fetus, and platelet-related haemostasis. Patients should therefore be advised not to use Children's MOTRIN during pregnancy without the advice of a physician, particularly during the last trimester (Arthritis Advisory Committee; 1983). Clinical information is limited on the effects of ibuprofen in pregnancy.

Nursing Women: Pharmacokinetic studies indicated that following oral administration of ibuprofen 400 mg the level of drug which appeared in breast milk was below detection levels of 1 µg/mL. The amount of ibuprofen to which an infant would be exposed through this source was considered negligible (Albert & Gernaat; 1984). However, since the absolute safety of ibuprofen ingested under these circumstances has not been determined, nursing mothers should be advised to consult a physician before using Children's MOTRIN (Arthritis Advisory Committee; 1983).

Geriatrics: Although Children's MOTRIN is labelled specifically for children, particular caution should be observed should it be administered to elderly patients, as they are more likely to be taking other medications or have pre-existing disease states which can increase the likelihood of the complications that have been associated with ibuprofen. Elderly patients appear to be more susceptible to the central nervous system disease reactions; cognitive dysfunction (forgetfulness, inability to concentrate, a feeling of separation from the surroundings) in such patients has been reported.

ADVERSE REACTIONS: Adverse Drug Reaction Overview: Experience reported with prescription use of ibuprofen has included the following adverse reactions. Note: Reactions listed below under Causal Relationship Unknown are those where a causal relationship could not be established; however, in these rarely reported events, the possibility of a relationship to ibuprofen also cannot be excluded. The adverse reactions most frequently seen with ibuprofen therapy involve the gastrointestinal system.

Clinical Trial Adverse Drug Reactions: Because clinical trials are conducted under very specific conditions the adverse reaction rates observed in the clinical trials may not reflect the rates observed in practice and should not be compared to the rates in the clinical trials of another drug. Adverse drug reaction information from clinical trials is useful for identifying drug-related adverse events and for approximating rates.

Table 1: Motrin (Children's)

Incidence of Adverse Events Attributed to Ibuprofen

Adverse Effect	Incidence 3–9%	Incidence 1–3%
Gastrointestinal	nausea epigastric pain heartburn	diarrhea abdominal distress nausea and vomiting indigestion constipation abdominal cramps and pain gastrointestinal tract fullness (bloating or flatulence)

(cont'd)

Table 1: Motrin (Children's) *(cont'd)*

Incidence of Adverse Events Attributed to Ibuprofen

Adverse Effect	Incidence 3–9%	Incidence 1–3%
CNS	dizziness	headache nervousness
Dermatologic	rash (including maculopapular type)	pruritus
Special Senses		tinnitus
Metabolic		decreased appetite edema fluid retention (generally responds promptly to drug discontinuation)

Less Common Clinical Trial Adverse Drug Reactions (<1%): Gastrointestinal: gastric or duodenal ulcer with bleeding and/or perforation, gastrointestinal hemorrhage, melena, hepatitis, jaundice, abnormal liver function (AST, serum bilirubin and alkaline phosphatase).

Central Nervous System: depression, insomnia.

Dermatologic: vesiculobullous eruptions, urticaria, erythema multiforme.

Special Senses: amblyopia (blurred and/or diminished vision, scotomata and/or changes in colour vision).

Cardiovascular: congestive heart failure in patients with marginal cardiac function, elevated blood pressure.

Allergic: anaphylaxis.

Hematologic: leukopenia and decreases in haemoglobin and hematocrit.

Reports with an Unknown Causal Relationship: Central Nervous System: paresthesias; hallucinations; dream abnormalities; aseptic meningitis has been reported in patients with systemic lupus erythematosus or other connective tissue disease; aseptic meningitis and meningoencephalitis, in one case accompanied by eosinophilia in the cerebrospinal fluids, has been reported in patients who took ibuprofen intermittently and did not have any connective tissue disease; cognitive dysfunction has been observed in elderly patients who took ibuprofen.

Dermatologic: alopecia, Stevens-Johnson syndrome have been reported.

Special Senses: conjunctivitis, diplopia; optic neuritis.

Hematologic: hemolytic anemia; thrombocytopenia; granulocytopenia; bleeding episodes (e.g. purpura, epistaxis, hematuria, menorrhagia); auto-immune hematological anemia occurred in one patient taking 400 mg of ibuprofen three times a day for ten days; fatal aplastic anemia was reported in one patient who took 600 mg per day for 8 months.

Cardiovascular: arrhythmias (sinus tachycardia, sinus bradycardia, palpitations).

Allergic: fever, serum sickness, lupus erythematosus syndrome.

Endocrine: gynecomastia; hypoglycemic reaction; menstrual delays of up to two weeks and dysfunctional uterine bleeding; occurred in nine patients taking ibuprofen 400 mg three times a day for three days before menses.

Renal: decreased creatinine clearance, polyuria, azotemia.

Abnormal Hematologic and Clinical Chemistry Findings: Gastrointestinal: The generally modest elevations of serum transaminase activity that has been observed are usually without clinical sequelae but severe, potentially fatal toxic hepatitis can occur.

Renal: Renal blood flow glomerular filtration rate decreased in patients with mild impairment of renal functions who took 1200 mg/day of ibuprofen for one week. Renal papillary necrosis has been reported. A number of factors appear to increase the risk of renal toxicity.

DRUG INTERACTIONS: Overview: Although ibuprofen binds to a significant extent to plasma proteins, interactions with other protein-bound drugs occur uncommonly. Nevertheless, caution should be observed when other drugs also having a high affinity for protein binding sites are used concurrently. Some observations have suggested a potential for ibuprofen to interact with digoxin, methotrexate, phenytoin and lithium salts. However, the mechanisms and clinical significance of these observations are presently not known.

A general precaution is appropriate for patients to assure the compatibility of Children's MOTRIN with their other prescribed medications through consultation with a physician (Arthritis Advisory Committee; 1983).

Drug-Drug Interactions: Coumarin Type Anticoagulants: Several short-term controlled studies failed to show that ibuprofen significantly affected prothrombin time or a variety of other clotting factors when administered to individuals on Coumarin-type anticoagulants. However, bleeding has been reported when ibuprofen and other NSAID agents have been administered to patients on Coumarin-type anticoagulants. The use of Children's MOTRIN in patients who are taking anticoagulants should therefore be avoided because of the possibility of enhanced GI bleeding or an additive effect due to ibuprofen's reversible anti-platelet action.

Acetylsalicylic Acid: Animal studies show that ASA given with NSAIDs, including ibuprofen, yields a net decrease in anti-inflammatory activity with lowered blood levels of the non-ASA drug. Single dose bioavailability studies in normal volunteers have failed to show an effect of ASA on ibuprofen blood levels. Correlative clinical studies have not been done.

Since there have been no controlled trials to demonstrate whether there is any beneficial or harmful interaction with use of ibuprofen in conjunction with ASA, the combination can not be recommended.

The platelet inhibiting effects of ibuprofen, although less potent and of shorter duration than those induced by acetylsalicylic acid, warrant cautionary supervision by a physician before co-administration of Children's MOTRIN and anti-coagulants.

Other Anti-Inflammatory Agents (NSAIDs): The addition of Children's MOTRIN to a pre-existent prescribed NSAID regimen in patients with a condition such as rheumatoid arthritis may result in increased risk of adverse effects.

Diuretics: Ibuprofen, because of its fluid retention properties, can decrease the diuretic and anti-hypertensive effects of diuretics, and increased diuretic dosage may be needed. Patients with impaired renal function taking potassium-sparing diuretics who develop ibuprofen-induced renal insufficiency might be in serious danger of fatal hyperkalemia.

Acetaminophen: Although interactions have not been reported, concurrent use with Children's MOTRIN is not advisable.

DOSAGE AND ADMINISTRATION: Recommended Dose and Dosage Adjustment: Prescribed Dosage and Administration: Fever Reduction: For reduction of fever in children up to 12 years of age, the dosage should be adjusted on the basis of the initial temperature level. The recommended dose is 5 mg/kg if the baseline temperature is less than 39.1°C or 10 mg/kg if the baseline temperature is 39.1°C or greater. The duration of fever reduction is generally 6 to 8 hours. The recommended maximum daily dose is 40 mg/kg.

Analgesia: For relief of mild to moderate pain in children up to 12 years of age, the recommended dosage is 10 mg/kg, every 6 to 8 hours. The recommended maximum daily dose is 40 mg/kg. Doses should be given so as not to disturb the child's sleep pattern.

Individualization of Dosage: The dose of Children's MOTRIN should be tailored to each patient, and may be lowered or raised from the suggested doses depending on the severity of symptoms either at the time of initiating drug therapy or as the patient responds or fails to responds.

Limited data suggests that, after the initial dose of Children's MOTRIN, subsequent doses may be lowered and still provide adequate fever control (McEnvoy; 1997). In a situation when lower fever would require the Children's MOTRIN 5 mg/kg dose in a child with pain, the dose that will effectively treat the predominant symptom should be chosen.

OTC Dosage and Administration: Mild to Moderate pain or fever: The OTC Dosing recommendation is based on a single dose of ibuprofen of approximately 7.5 mg/kg for either pain or fever.

Adults: MOTRIN brand of ibuprofen is available for adults in table/caplet/gelcap form. The equivalent adult dosage of Children's MOTRIN Suspension (100 mg/5 mL) is 200-400 mg (2 to 4 teaspoons or 10-20 mL) as required every 4 to 6 hours, not to exceed 1200 mg (12 teaspoons or 60 mL) in 24 hours unless directed by a physician.

Children: See Table 2.

Do not take for fever for more than 3 days or pain for more than 5 days unless directed by a physician. If the painful area is red or swollen, if condition deteriorates or new symptoms occur, consult a physician.

Administration: Take with food or milk if mild upset stomach occurs with use.

Table 2: Motrin (Children's)

Children's MOTRIN Ibuprofen

	Weight		Single Dose[a]			
Age	**lbs**	**kg**	**Suspension: 100 mg/5 mL**	**Infant's Suspension Drops: 40 mg/mL**	**Tablets: 50 mg**	**Tablets: 100 mg**
0 to 3 mos[c]	6 to 11	2.5 to 5.4		Calculate based on weight and target dose 7.5 mg/kg 0.625 mL=25 mg 1.25 mL=50 mg		
4 to 11 mos[b]	12 to 17	5.5 to 7.9	½ tsp= 2.5 mL=50 mg	1.25 mL=50 mg		
12 to 23 mos[b]	18 to 23	8 to 10.9	¾ tsp= 3.75 mL=75 mg	1.875 mL=75 mg		
2 to 3 yrs	24 to 35	11 to 15.9	1 tsp= 5 mL=100 mg		2 tablets= 100 mg	1 tablet= 100 mg
4 to 5 yrs	36 to 47	16 to 21.9	1 ½ tsp= 7.5 mL=150 mg		3 tablets= 150 mg	1 ½ tablets= 150 mg
6 to 8 yrs	48 to 59	22 to 26.9	2 tsp= 10 mL=200 mg		4 tablets= 200 mg	2 tablets= 200 mg
9 to 10 yrs	60 to 71	27 to 31.9	2 ½ tsp= 12.5 mL=250 mg		5 tablets= 250 mg	2 ½ tablets= 250 mg
11 yrs	72 to 95	32 to 43.9	3 tsp= 15 mL=300 mg		6 tablets= 300 mg	3 tablets= 300 mg

[a] Single dose may be given every 6 to 8 hours as needed but do not exceed 4 doses per day unless advised by your doctor.
[b] Only Infant's MOTRIN Suspension Drops are labelled for children under 2 years of age. Consumer labelling for Children's MOTRIN Suspension 100 mg/5 mL does not offer dosing for children under 2 years of age; therefore these doses are provided as a guide for professional recommendations to consumers.
[c] Infant's MOTRIN Suspension Drops 40 mg/mL are labelled "as directed by a doctor" for children under 4 months of age.

OVERDOSAGE:

Clinical Features: A clear pattern of clinical features associated with accidental or intentional overdose of ibuprofen has not been established. Reported cases of overdose have often been complicated by co-ingestions or additional suicidal gestures. The range of symptoms observed has included nausea, vomiting, abdominal pain, drowsiness, nystagmus, diplopia, headache, tinnitus, impaired renal function, coma and hypotension. A review of 4 fatalities associated with ibuprofen overdose indicates other contributing factors co-existed so it would be difficult to identify the toxicity of ibuprofen as a specific cause of death. (Barry et al.; 1984, Court et al.; 1984).

Post-ingestion blood levels may be useful to confirm a diagnosis and to quantify the degree of exposure but otherwise have not been helpful in predicting clinical outcome. Generally, full recovery can be expected with appropriate symptomatic management.

The following cases of overdose have been reported: A 19 month old child, 1-1/2 hours after the ingestion of 7 to 10×400 mg tablets of ibuprofen presented apnea, cyanosis and responded only to painful stimuli. After treatment with O_2, $NaHCO_3$, infusion of dextrose and normal saline, the child was responsive and 12 hours after ingestion appeared completely recovered. Blood levels of ibuprofen reached 102.9 µg/mL, 8-1/2 hours after the accident. Two other children weighing approximately 10 kg, had taken an estimated 120 mg/kg. There were no signs of acute intoxication or late sequelae. In 1 child the ibuprofen blood level at 90 minutes after ingestion was approximately 700 µg/mL. A 19 year old male who ingested 8000 mg of ibuprofen reported dizziness and nystagmus was noted. He recovered with no reported sequelae after parenteral hydration and 3 days of bed rest.

Management of Overdose: General measures to reduce absorption such as gastric lavage, administration of activated charcoal or ipecac-induced emesis are appropriate particularly within 1 to 4 hours of ingestion. Routine symptomatic and supportive treatment is then recommended as follow-up (Court et al.; 1984).

For management of a suspected drug overdose, CPhA recommends that you contact your **regional Poison Control Centre**. See the *CPS* Directory section for a list of Poison Control Centres.

ACTION AND CLINICAL PHARMACOLOGY: Mechanism of Action: The basic mechanism of the pharmacological actions of ibuprofen, like other NSAID's, has not been precisely determined. It is generally thought to be related to the inhibition of prostaglandin synthesis (Flower et al.; 1985).

Pharmacodynamics: Ibuprofen: Ibuprofen is a member of the class of agents commonly known as nonsteroidal anti-inflammatory drugs (NSAID). Consistent with this classification, ibuprofen exhibits anti-inflammatory activity at higher dosage ranges (Brooks et al.; 1973). At lower adult single doses (200-400 mg) relevant to the non-prescription analgesic/antipyretic indications and dosage strength, ibuprofen relieves pain of mild to moderate intensity (Cooper et al.; 1977, Gollardo & Rossi; 1980, Jain et al.; 1984, Vecchio et al.; 1983, Ihles; 1980) and reduces fever (Gaitonde et al.; 1973, Sheth et al.; 1973, Sheth et al.; 1980, Simila et al.; 1976). Clinical studies have also confirmed the analgesic (Bertin et al.; 1991, Schachtel & Thoden; 1993) and antipyretic (Walson et al.; 1989, Wilson et al.; 1991) effects of ibuprofen in children. Analogous to acetylsalicylic acid, the prototype of this class, this analgesic/antipyretic activity of ibuprofen occurs at lower doses than necessary for anti-inflammatory effects which are thought to require sustained administration of higher individual doses (Flower et al.; 1985).

Pharmacokinetics: Absorption: Ibuprofen is rapidly absorbed after oral administration with peak plasma levels usually occurring within 1 to 2 hours. Oral absorption is estimated to be 80% of the dose. Both the rate of ibuprofen absorption and peak plasma concentrations are reduced when the drug is taken with food, but, bioavailability as measured by total area under the concentration-time curve is minimally altered.

A single 200 mg oral dose study in 6 fasting healthy men produced a peak plasma concentration of 15.0 µg/mL at 0.75 hr (Adams et al.; 1967). Another study using a single oral 400 mg dose in humans produced a peak serum level of 31.9±8.8 µg/mL 0.5 hours after ingestion, and at 16 hours serum concentrations had dropped to 1 µg/mL (Kaiser & Martin; 1978). Comparable serum levels and time to peak within 1-2 hours were confirmed by other investigations with 200 mg and 400 mg solid doses (Kaiser & Vangiessen; 1974, Glass & Swannell; 1978). A multiple dose study of administration of a 200 mg ibuprofen tablet three times a day for 2 weeks showed no evidence of accumulation of ibuprofen (Mills et al.; 1973). As is true with most tablet and suspension formulations, Children's MOTRIN Suspension is absorbed somewhat faster than a tablet with a time to peak generally within one hour.

Distribution: Clinical studies indicate a duration of clinical effect for up to 8 hours. Ibuprofen like most drugs of its class, is highly protein bound (>99% bound at 20 µg/mL) (Mills et al.; 1973, Kober & Sjoholm; 1980). Based on oral dosing data there is an age- or fever-related change in volume of distribution for ibuprofen. Febrile children <11 years old have a volume of approximately 0.2 L/kg while adults have a volume of approximately 0.12 L/kg. The clinical significance of these findings is unknown (McEnvoy; 1997). Tissue distribution of ibuprofen is also extensive in humans. Studies comparing synovial fluid levels with serum concentrations indicated that equilibration time post-ingestion occurred within approximately 3 to 5 hours (Glass & Swannell; 1978).

Metabolism: Ibuprofen is rapidly metabolized through oxidation and glucuronic acid conjugation with urinary excretion of the inactive metabolites usually complete with 24 hours. In humans, ibuprofen is extensively metabolized with approximately 84% recoverable in the urine, primarily as conjugated hydroxyl- and carboxy- metabolites, with only approximately 1% excreted unchanged

(Albert & Gernaat; 1984). Less than 10% is excreted unchanged in the urine (Albert & Gernaat; 1984). The 2 major metabolites of ibuprofen in humans have been found to have no activity in the ultraviolet erythema test in guinea pigs and in the acetylcholine-induced mouse writhing test at doses of 10 mg/kg and 15 mg/kg respectively (Adams, Cliffe et al.; 1969).

Excretion: Ibuprofen is rapidly metabolized and eliminated in the urine. The excretion of ibuprofen is virtually complete 24 hours after the last dose. It has a biphasic plasma elimination time curve with a half-life of approximately 2.0 hours. There is no difference in the observed terminal elimination rate or half-life between children and adults, however, there is an age- or fever-related change in total clearance (McEnvoy; 1997). This suggests that the observed difference in clearance is due to differences in the volume of distribution of ibuprofen, as described above. The clinical relevance of these differences in clearance is unknown, although extensive clinical experience with ibuprofen in children at the pertinent dosage range (5-10 mg/kg) indicates a wide margin of safety.

Special Populations and Conditions: Pediatrics: The pharmacokinetics of ibuprofen has also been studied in humans. Although there is little evidence of clinically significant age depenent kinetics in febrile children ages 3 months to 12 years (Kauffman et al.; 1989), some differences in the pharmacokinetic parameters of volume of distribution and clearance have been observed between adults and children (McEnvoy; 1997). Controlled clinical trials comparing doses between 5 and 10 mg/kg of ibuprofen and 10-15 mg/kg of acetaminophen have been conducted in children 6 months to 12 years of age with fever primarily due to viral illnesses. In these studies, there were few differences between treatments in fever reduction in the first hour and maximum fever reduction occurred between 2 and 4 hours. There was some evidence that the higher dosage range of ibuprofen (10 mg/kg) resulted in a prolonged duration of effect (from 6 to 8 hours) and that it was more effective for children with higher baseline temperatures (above 39.1°C but the numbers of patients were not adequate to draw definitive conclusions. In children with baseline temperatures at or below 39.1°C both ibuprofen doses and acetaminophen were equally effective in their maximum effect.

Geriatrics: Studies demonstrate no significant alterations in ibuprofen pharmacokinetics in the elderly or in children (Albert et al.; 1984, Kauffman et al.; 1989).

Hepatic Insufficiency: Ibuprofen pharmacokinetics has also been studied in patients with alcoholic liver disease who have been assessed to have fair to poor hepatic function. Results suggest despite the liver being the primary organ of metabolism of ibuprofen, its kinetic parameters are not substantially altered by this condition (Juhl et al.; 1983).

STORAGE AND STABILITY: Suspension/Suspension Drops: Store in tightly closed container at room temperature; 15 to 30°C. Avoid high humidity and excessive heat (40°C).

Tablets/Caplets: Store at room temperature; 15 to 30°C.

SPECIAL HANDLING INSTRUCTIONS: None.

INFORMATION FOR THE PATIENT: Published in e-CPS, available by subscription at www.e-cps.ca.

DOSAGE FORMS, COMPOSITION AND PACKAGING: Children's Chewable Tablets (Grape): Each round, purple tablet having a grape odor, debossed with "MO" and "50" on one side and scored on the other side, contains: ibuprofen 50 mg. Nonmedicinal ingredients: acesulfame potassium, aspartame, citric acid, D&C Red No. 7 calcium lake, D&C Red No. 30 aluminum lake, FD&C Blue No.1 aluminum lake, flavor, fumaric acid, hydroxyethyl cellulose, hypromellose, magnesium stearate, mannitol, microcrystalline cellulose, povidone, sodium lauryl sulfate and sodium starch glycolate. Energy: 3.9 kJ (0.93 kcal). Sodium: 0 mmol (0 mg). Gluten-, lactose-, sulfite-, sucrose- and tartrazine-free. Bottles of 24*.

Children's Chewable Tablets (Orange): Each round, light orange tablet having an orange odor, debossed with "MO" and "50" on one side and scored on the other side, contains: ibuprofen 50 mg. Nonmedicinal ingredients: acesulfame potassium, aspartame, citric acid, FD&C yellow no. 6 aluminum lake, flavor, fumaric acid, hydroxyethyl cellulose, hypromellose, magnesium stearate, mannitol, microcrystalline cellulose, povidone, sodium lauryl sulfate and sodium starch glycolate. Energy: 4.4 kJ (1.0 kcal). Sodium: <1 mmol (0.09 mg). Gluten-, lactose-, sulfite-, sucrose- and tartrazine-free. Bottles of 24*.

Children's Suspension Liquid (Berry): Each 5 mL of orange liquid suspension with a distinct berry odor contains: ibuprofen 100 mg. Nonmedicinal ingredients: acesulfame potassium, citric acid, D&C Yellow No. 10, FD&C Red No. 40, flavor, glycerin, hydroxypropyl distarch phosphate, polysorbate 80, purified water, sodium benzoate, sucrose and xanthan gum. Energy: 34.7 kJ (8.3 kcal). Sodium: <1 mmol (1.6 mg). Gluten-, lactose-, sulfite- and tartrazine-free. Bottles of 120* mL.

Children's Suspension Liquid (Bubblegum): Each 5 mL of pink liquid suspension with a distinct bubblegum odor contains: ibuprofen 100 mg. Nonmedicinal ingredients: acesulfame potassium, citric acid, FD&C Red No. 40, flavor, glycerin, hydroxypropyl distarch phosphate, polysorbate 80, purified water, sodium benzoate, sucrose and xanthan gum. Energy: 34.7 kJ (8.3 kcal). Sodium: <1 mmol (1.6 mg). Gluten-, lactose-, sulfite- and tartrazine-free. Bottles of 120* mL.

Children's Suspension Liquid (Dye-Free): Each 5 mL of white liquid suspension with a distinct berry odor contains: ibuprofen 100 mg. Nonmedicinal ingredients: acesulfame potassium, citric acid, flavor, glycerin, hydroxypropyl distarch phosphate, polysorbate 80, purified water, sodium benzoate, sucrose and xanthan gum. Energy: 34.7 kJ (8.3 kcal). Sodium: <1 mmol (1.6 mg). Gluten-, lactose-, sulfite- and tartrazine-free. Bottles of 120* mL.

Children's Suspension Liquid (Grape): Each 5 mL of purple liquid suspension with a distinct grape odor contains: ibuprofen 100 mg. Nonmedicinal ingredients: acesulfame potassium, citric acid, D&C Red No. 33, FD&C Blue No. 1, FD&C Red No. 40, flavor, glycerin, hydroxypropyl distarch phosphate, polysorbate 80, purified water, sodium benzoate, sucrose and xanthan gum. Energy: 34.7 kJ (8.3 kcal). Sodium: <1 mmol (1.6 mg). Gluten-, lactose-, sulfite- and tartrazine-free. Bottles of 120* mL.

Children's Suspension Liquid (Tropical Punch): Each 5 mL of red liquid suspension with a distinct tropical punch odor contains: ibuprofen 100 mg. Nonmedicinal ingredients: acesulfame potassium, citric acid, FD&C Red No. 40, flavor, glycerin, hydroxypropyl distarch phosphate, polysorbate 80, potassium sorbate, purified water, sodium benzoate, sucralose, sucrose and xanthan gum. Energy: 34.7 kJ (8.3 kcal). Sodium: <1 mmol (1.6 mg). Gluten-, lactose-, sulfite- and tartrazine-free. Bottles of 120* mL.

Infants Suspension Drops (Berry): Each mL of pink-colored, berry-flavored liquid suspension contains: ibuprofen 40 mg. Nonmedicinal ingredients: citric acid, cornstarch, FD&C Red No. 40, flavor, glycerin, polysorbate 80, purified water, sodium benzoate, sorbitol, sucrose and xanthan gum. Energy: 7.1 kJ (1.7 kcal). Sodium: <1 mmol (0.32 mg). Gluten-, lactose-, sulfite- and tartrazine-free. Bottles of 15* and 30* mL.

Infants Suspension Drops (Berry Dye-Free): Each mL of white-colored, berry-flavored liquid suspension contains: ibuprofen 40 mg. Nonmedicinal ingredients: citric acid, cornstarch, flavor, glycerin, polysorbate 80, purified water, sodium benzoate, sorbitol, sucrose and xanthan gum. Energy: 7.1 kJ (1.7 kcal). Sodium: <1 mmol (0.32 mg). Gluten-, lactose-, sulfite- and tartrazine-free. Bottles of 7.5*, 15* and 30* mL.

Junior Strength Chewable Tablets (Grape): Each round, purple tablet having a grape odor, debossed with "MO" and "100" on one side and scored on the other side, contains: ibuprofen 100 mg. Nonmedicinal ingredients: acesulfame potassium, aspartame, citric acid, D&C Red No. 7 calcium lake, D&C Red. No. 30 aluminum lake, FD&C Blue No. 1 aluminum lake, flavor, fumaric acid, hydroxyethyl cellulose, hypromellose, magnesium stearate, mannitol, microcrystalline cellulose, povidone, sodium lauryl sulfate and sodium starch glycolate. Energy: 7.8 kJ (1.87 kcal). Sodium: 0 mmol (0 mg). Gluten-, lactose-, sulfite-, sucrose- and tartrazine-free. Bottles of 24* and in pouches of 2.

Junior Strength Chewable Tablets (Orange): Each round, light orange tablet having an orange odor, debossed with "MO" and "100" on one side and scored on the other side, contains: ibuprofen 100 mg. Nonmedicinal ingredients: acesulfame potassium, aspartame, citric acid, FD&C Yellow No. 6 aluminum lake, flavor, fumaric acid, hydroxyethyl cellulose, hypromellose, magnesium stearate, mannitol, microcrystalline cellulose, povidone, sodium lauryl sulfate and sodium starch glycolate. Energy: 7.8 kJ (1.87 kcal). Sodium: 0 mmol (0 mg). Gluten-, lactose-, sulfite-, sucrose- and tartrazine-free. Bottles of 24*.

* Containers provided with a child-resistant closure. All packages are safety sealed.

Motrin® IB
ibuprofen
Analgesic—Antipyretic

McNeil Consumer Healthcare

Motrin® IB Extra Strength
ibuprofen
Analgesic—Antipyretic

McNeil Consumer Healthcare

Motrin® IB Super Strength
ibuprofen
Analgesic—Antipyretic

McNeil Consumer Healthcare

Date of Revision: June 14, 2005

SUMMARY PRODUCT INFORMATION:

Route of Administration	Dosage Form/ Strength	Clinically Relevant Nonmedicinal Ingredients
Oral	Tablet 200 mg	None For a complete listing see Dosage Forms, Composition and Packaging.
	Tablet 300 mg	None For a complete listing see Dosage Forms, Composition and Packaging.
	Tablet 400 mg	None For a complete listing see Dosage Forms, Composition and Packaging.

INDICATIONS AND CLINICAL USE: MOTRIN IB ibuprofen is indicated for fast and effective relief of:

- headache pain (including mild to moderate migraine and tension headache)
- menstrual pain
- toothache (dental pain)
- pain from inflammation associated with conditions including:
  - arthritis
  - physical or athletic overexertion, (e.g. sprains or strains)
- minor aches and pains in muscles, bones and joints
- backache
- the aches and pain due to the common cold and flu
- reduction of fever

Geriatrics (>65 years of age): Evidence from clinical studies and experience suggest that use in the geriatric population is associated with differences in safety or effectiveness and a brief discussion can be found in the appropriate sections (e.g., Warnings and Precautions).

Pediatrics (<12 years of age): Children's MOTRIN formulations are available to treat children under 12 years of age (see Children's MOTRIN Product Monograph).

CONTRAINDICATIONS: The following are contraindications to the use of MOTRIN IB:

- Patients who are hypersensitive to ibuprofen, other nonsteroidal anti-inflammatory drugs (NSAIDs), or to any ingredient in the formulation. For a complete listing of ingredients, see Dosage Forms, Composition and Packaging. The potential for cross-reactivity between different NSAIDs must be kept in mind.
- Ibuprofen should not be used in patients with the complete or partial syndrome of acetylsalicylic acid (ASA) intolerance (rhinosinusitis, urticaria/angioedema, nasal polyps, asthma) in whom asthma, anaphylaxis, urticaria/angioedema, rhinitis or other allergic manifestations are precipitated by ASA or other nonsteroidal anti-inflammatory agents. Fatal anaphylactoid reactions have occurred in such individuals. As well, individuals with the above medical problems are at risk of a severe reaction even if they have taken NSAIDs in the past without any adverse effects.
- Active gastric or duodenal ulcer, a history of recurrent ulceration, gastrointestinal bleeding, or active inflammatory disease of the gastrointestinal system.
- Significant hepatic impairment or active liver disease.
- Severely impaired or deteriorating renal function (creatinine clearance <30 mL/min).
- Ibuprofen should not be used in the presence of known hyperkalemia (also see Warnings and Precautions, Renal).
- Children with kidney disease and/or who have suffered significant fluid loss.
- Ibuprofen is contraindicated in patients with systemic lupus erythematosus as an anaphylaxis-like reaction with fever may occur, particularly when ibuprofen has been administered previously.
- Ibuprofen should not be used during pregnancy.

WARNINGS AND PRECAUTIONS:

- Patients with heart disease and high blood pressure should not take this drug unless directed by a physician.
- Caution in patients with heart failure, hypertension or other conditions predisposing to fluid retention.
- Caution in patients prone to gastrointestinal tract irritation, particularly those with a history of peptic ulcer, diverticulosis or other inflammatory disease of the gastrointestinal tract such as ulcerative colitis and Crohn's disease.
- The elderly and patients with impaired renal function, heart failure, liver dysfunction, and those taking diuretics are at increased risk of renal toxicity.
- If persistent urinary symptoms (bladder pain, dysuria, urinary frequency), hematuria and cystitis occur, the drug should be stopped immediately.
- Ibuprofen use during nursing should be avoided.

General: Several medical conditions that can predispose patients to the adverse effects of nonsteroidal anti-inflammatory drugs in general may be applicable to ibuprofen.

Patients with any serious medical condition should consult a physician before using ibuprofen as an analgesic or antipyretic. In common with other anti-inflammatory drugs, ibuprofen may suppress fever.

Cardiovascular: Some patients with pre-existing hypertension may develop worsening of blood pressure control when placed on an NSAID and regular monitoring of blood pressure should be performed under such circumstances. NSAIDs may exacerbate congestive heart failure.

Patients who are taking low-dose ASA as cardio protective therapy should consult with a health professional prior to taking ibuprofen (see also Drug Interactions, Acetylsalicylic Acid (ASA) or Other NSAIDs).

Gastrointestinal: Serious GI toxicity, such as ulceration, perforation, obstruction and gastrointestinal bleeding, sometimes severe and occasionally fatal, can occur at any time, with or without symptoms in patients treated with nonsteroidal anti-inflammatory drugs (NSAIDs) including ibuprofen.

GI symptoms, such as dyspepsia, are common, usually developing early in therapy. Health providers should remain alert for ulceration and bleeding in patients treated with nonsteroidal anti-inflammatory drugs, even in the absence of previous GI tract symptoms.

In patients observed in clinical trials of such agents, symptomatic upper GI ulcers, gross bleeding, or perforation occur in approximately 1% of patients treated for 3-6 months and in about 2-4% of patients treated for one year. The risk continues beyond one year. The incidence of these complications is related to dose, past history of known ulcer disease, and advanced age (see Special Populations). Studies have shown that the use of oral corticosteroids increases the risk of upper gastrointestinal complications associated with NSAIDs.

Ibuprofen should be given under close medical supervision to patients with a history of ulcer of the upper gastrointestinal tract or inflammatory disease of the gastrointestinal tract such as ulcerative colitis and Crohn's disease. In these cases the health provider must weigh the benefits of treatment against the possible hazards.

Health providers should inform patients about the signs and symptoms of serious GI toxicity and instruct them to contact a health provider immediately if they experience persistent dyspepsia or other symptoms or signs suggestive of gastrointestinal ulceration or bleeding.

Because serious GI tract ulceration and bleeding can occur without warning symptoms, health providers should follow chronically treated patients and watch for the signs and symptoms of ulceration and bleeding and should inform the patients of the importance of this follow-up.

If ulceration is suspected or confirmed, or if GI bleeding occurs ibuprofen should be discontinued immediately, appropriate treatment instituted and the patient monitored closely.

No studies, to date, have identified any group of patients **not** at risk of developing ulceration and bleeding. The major risk factors are a prior history of serious GI events and increasing age. Possible risk factors include *H. pylori* infection, excess alcohol intake, smoking, and concomitant oral steroids, anti-coagulants, anti-platelet agents (including ASA), or selective serotonin reuptake inhibitors (SSRIs).

The administration of ibuprofen with food or milk is recommended since occasional and mild heartburn, upset stomach or stomach pain may occur with its use. Patients should be advised to seek the consultation of a physician if gastrointestinal side effects occur consistently, persist, or appear to worsen.

Genitourinary: Some NSAIDs are associated with persistent urinary symptoms (bladder pain, dysuria, urinary frequency), hematuria or cystitis. The onset of these symptoms may occur at any time after the initiation of therapy with an NSAID. Should urinary symptoms occur, in the absence of an alternate explanation, treatment with ibuprofen should be stopped to ascertain if symptoms disappear. This should be done before urological investigations or treatments are considered.

Hematologic: Ibuprofen, like other nonsteroidal anti-inflammatory agents, can inhibit platelet aggregation but the effect is quantitatively less than that seen with acetylsalicylic acid. Ibuprofen has been shown to prolong bleeding time (but within the normal range) in normal subjects. Because this prolonged bleeding effect may be exaggerated in patients with underlying haemostatic defects, ibuprofen should be avoided by persons with intrinsic coagulation defects and by those on anticoagulant therapy. Concurrent therapy of ibuprofen with warfarin requires close monitoring of INR (see Drug Interactions).

Also, patients with underlying medical or pharmacologically-induced haemostatic defects could experience further prolongation of bleeding time through the inhibition of platelet aggregation induced to varying degrees by this class of drugs.

Blood dyscrasias (such as neutropenia, leukopenia, thrombocytopenia, aplastic anemia and agranulocytosis) associated with the use of nonsteroidal anti-inflammatory drugs are rare, but could occur with severe consequences.

Hepatic: As with other nonsteroidal anti-inflammatory drugs, borderline elevations of one or more liver enzyme tests (AST, ALT, ALP) may occur in up to 15% of patients. These abnormalities may progress, may remain essentially unchanged, or may be transient with continued therapy.

A patient with symptoms and/or signs suggesting liver dysfunction, or in whom an abnormal liver test has occurred, should be evaluated for evidence of the development of a more severe hepatic reaction while on therapy with this drug. Severe hepatic reactions including jaundice and cases of fatal hepatitis have been reported with nonsteroidal anti-inflammatory drugs.

Although such reactions are rare, if abnormal liver tests persist or worsen, if clinical signs and symptoms consistent with liver disease develop (e.g. jaundice), or if systemic manifestations occur (e.g. eosinophilia, associated with rash, etc.), this drug should be discontinued.

If there is a need to prescribe this drug in the presence of impaired liver function, it must be done under strict observation.

Immune: Patients sensitive to any one of the nonsteroidal anti-inflammatory drugs may be sensitive to any of the other NSAIDs also.

As with NSAIDs in general, some patients may experience urticaria and angioedema upon exposure to ibuprofen. Ibuprofen should not be given to patients with the complete or partial syndrome of ASA-intolerance (see Contraindications).

Neurologic: Some patients may experience drowsiness, dizziness, vertigo, tinnitus or hearing loss with the use of ibuprofen. If patients experience these side effects, they should exercise caution in carrying out activities that require alertness.

In occasional rare cases, with some NSAIDs, the symptoms of aseptic meningitis (stiff neck, severe headaches, nausea and vomiting, fever or clouding of consciousness) have been observed. Patients with autoimmune disorders (systemic lupus erythematosus, mixed connective tissues diseases, etc.) seem to be pre-disposed. Therefore, in such patients, the health provider must be vigilant to the development of this complication.

Ophthalmologic: Blurred and/or diminished vision, scotoma, and/or changes in colour vision have been reported. If a patient develops such complaints while taking ibuprofen, the drug should be discontinued. Patients with any visual disturbances should have an ophthalmologic examination.

Peri-Operative Considerations: In general, NSAIDs should be discontinued prior to surgeries to decrease the risk of postoperative bleeding.

Renal: Long-term administration of nonsteroidal anti-inflammatory drugs to animals has resulted in renal papillary necrosis and other abnormal renal pathology. In humans, there have been reports of acute interstitial nephritis with hematuria, proteinuria, and occasionally nephrotic syndrome.

A second form of renal toxicity has been seen in patients with pre-renal conditions leading to reduction in renal blood flow or blood volume, where the renal prostaglandins have a supportive role in the maintenance of renal perfusion. In these patients, administration of a nonsteroidal anti-inflammatory drug may cause a dose dependent reduction in prostaglandin formation and may precipitate overt renal decompensation. Patients at greatest risk of this reaction are those with impaired renal function (Glomerular Filtration Rate (GFR) <60 mL/min or 1 mL/sec), patients on salt restricted diets, those with congestive heart failure, cirrhosis, liver dysfunction, those taking diuretics, angiotensin-converting enzyme inhibitors, angiotensin-II receptor blockers, cyclosporin, ASA and the elderly. Serious or life-threatening renal failure has been reported in patients with normal or impaired renal function after short-term therapy with NSAIDs. Even patients at risk who demonstrate the ability to tolerate an NSAID under stable conditions may decompensate during periods of added stress, for example during states of fluid restriction as can occur during gastroenteritis. Discontinuation of nonsteroidal anti-inflammatory therapy is usually followed by recovery to the pretreatment state.

NSAIDs can increase the risk of hyperkalemia. In patients on dialysis, NSAIDs should be used with caution.

Fluid retention and edema have been observed in patients treated with ibuprofen. Therefore, as with many other NSAIDs, the possibility of precipitating congestive heart failure in elderly patients or those with compromised cardiac function should be borne in mind. Ibuprofen should be used with caution in patients with heart failure, hypertension or other conditions predisposing to fluid retention. Ask patients who are on chronic therapy and at risk for fluid retention to weigh themselves at regular intervals to assist in monitoring for fluid accumulation.

With nonsteroidal anti-inflammatory treatment there is a potential risk of hyperkalemia, particularly in patients with conditions such as diabetes mellitus or renal failure; elderly patients; or in patients receiving concomitant therapy with angiotensin-II receptor antagonists, adrenergic blockers, angiotensin-converting enzyme inhibitors or some diuretics. Patients at risk should be monitored periodically during long-term therapy.

Respiratory: ASA-induced asthma is an uncommon but very important indication of ASA and NSAID sensitivity. It occurs more frequently in patients with asthma who have nasal polyps.

Skin: In rare cases, serious skin reactions such as Stevens-Johnson syndrome, toxic epidermal necrolysis, exfoliative dermatitis and erythema multiforme have been associated with the use of some NSAIDs. Because the rate of these reactions is low, they have usually been noted during post-marketing surveillance in patients taking other medications also associated with the potential development of these serious skin reactions. Thus, causality is not clear. These reactions are potentially life threatening but may be reversible if the causative agent is discontinued and appropriate treatment instituted. Patients should be advised that if they experience a skin rash they should discontinue their NSAID and contact their physician for assessment and advice, including which additional therapies to discontinue.

Special Populations: Pregnant Women: No evidence specifically identifies exposure to analgesic doses of ibuprofen as a cause of harm to either mother or fetus during pregnancy. Nonsteroidal anti-inflammatory drugs in general, however, are known to affect the action of prostaglandin synthetase which could alter a variety of the physiological functions of prostaglandins or platelets during delivery such as facilitating uterine contraction in the mother, closure of the ductus arteriosus in the fetus, and platelet-related haemostasis. Patients should therefore be advised not to use ibuprofen during pregnancy without the advice of a physician, particularly during the last trimester. Clinical information is limited on the effects of ibuprofen in pregnancy.

Nursing Women: Pharmacokinetic studies indicated that following oral administration of ibuprofen 400 mg the level of drug that appeared in breast milk was below detection levels of 1 µg/mL. The amount of ibuprofen to which an infant would be exposed through this source was considered negligible. However, since the absolute safety of ibuprofen ingested under these circumstances has not been determined, nursing mothers should be advised to consult a physician before using ibuprofen.

Geriatrics (>65 years of age): Patients older than 65 years and frail or debilitated patients are most susceptible to a variety of adverse reactions from nonsteroidal anti-inflammatory drugs (NSAIDs); the incidence of these adverse reactions increases with dose and duration of treatment. In addition, these patients are less tolerant to ulceration and bleeding. Most reports of fatal GI events are in this population, especially those with cardiovascular disease. Older patients are also at risk of lower esophageal ulceration and bleeding. Elderly patients appear to be more susceptible to the central nervous system reactions; cognitive dysfunction (forgetfulness, inability to concentrate, a feeling of separation from the surroundings) in such patients has been reported.

For such patients, consideration should be given to a starting dose lower than the one usually recommended, with individual adjustment when necessary and under close supervision.

ADVERSE REACTIONS: Post-Market Adverse Drug Reactions: The most common adverse reactions encountered with nonsteroidal anti-inflammatory drugs are gastrointestinal, of which gastric or duodenal ulcer, with or without bleeding, is the most severe. Fatalities have occurred, particularly in the elderly.

Experience reported with prescription use of ibuprofen has included the following adverse reactions (see Table 1). **Note:** Reactions listed below under Causal Relationship Unknown are those where a causal relationship could not be established; however, in these rarely reported events, the possibility of a relationship to ibuprofen also cannot be excluded.

Table 1: MOTRIN IB

Adverse Effects

Adverse Effect	Common (>1% but <10%)		
	Incidence 3–9%	**Incidence 1–3%**	**Less Common (<1%)**
Allergic			• anaphylaxis (See Contraindications)
	Also reported but with unknown causal relationship, rarely: • fever • serum sickness • lupus erythematosus syndrome		
Cardiovascular			• congestive heart failure in patients with marginal cardiac function • elevated blood pressure Conditions such as congestive heart failure and hypertension may be aggravated by sodium retention and edema caused by ibuprofen in such patients.
	Also reported but with unknown causal relationship, rare cases of: • arrhythmias (sinus tachycardia, sinus bradycardia, palpitations)		
Central Nervous System	• dizziness	• headache • nervousness	• depression • insomnia
	Also reported but with unknown causal relationship: • paresthesias • hallucinations • dream abnormalities • aseptic meningitis has been reported in patients with systemic lupus erythematosus or other connective tissue disease • aseptic meningitis and meningioencephalitis, in one case accompanied by eosinophilia in the cerebrospinal fluids, has been reported in patients who took ibuprofen intermittently and did not have any connective tissue disease • cognitive dysfunction has been observed in elderly patients who took ibuprofen		
Dermatologic	• rash (including maculopapular type)	• pruritus	• vesiculobullous eruptions • urticaria • erythema multiforme
	Also reported but with unknown causal relationship: • alopecia • Stevens-Johnson Syndrome		
Endocrine	Also reported but with unknown causal relationship, rare cases of: • gynecomastia • hypoglycemic reaction • menstrual delays of up to two weeks and dysfunctional uterine bleeding occurred in nine patients taking ibuprofen 400 mg three times a day for three days before menses		
Gastrointestinal	• nausea • epigastric pain • heartburn	• diarrhea • abdominal distress • nausea and vomiting • indigestion • constipation • abdominal cramps and pain • gastrointestinal tract fullness (bloating or flatulence)	• gastric or duodenal ulcer with bleeding and/or perforation • gastrointestinal hemorrhage • melena • hepatitis • jaundice • abnormal liver function (AST, serum bilirubin and alkaline phosphatase)
	The generally modest elevations of serum transaminase activity that has been observed are usually without clinical sequelae but severe, potentially fatal toxic hepatitis can occur.		
Hematologic			• leukopenia and decreases in hemoglobin and hematocrit
	Also reported but with unknown causal relationship, rare cases of: • hemolytic anemia • thrombocytopenia • granulocytopenia • bleeding episodes (e.g. prupura, epistaxis, hematuria, menorrhagia) • auto-immune hematological anemia occurred in one patient taking 400 mg of ibuprofen three times a day for ten days • fatal aplastic anemia was reported in one patient who took 600 mg per day for eight months		

(cont'd)

Table 1: **MOTRIN IB** *(cont'd)*

Adverse Effects

Adverse Effect	Common (>1% but <10%) Incidence 3–9%	Incidence 1–3%	Less Common (<1%)
Metabolic		• decreased appetite • edema • fluid retention	
	Fluid retention generally responds promptly to drug discontinuation.		
Renal	Also reported but with unknown causal relationship: • decreased creatinine clearance • polyuria • azotemia Like other nonsteroidal anti-inflammatory agents, ibuprofen inhibits renal prostaglandin synthesis that may decrease renal function and cause sodium retention. Renal blood flow glomerular filtration rate decreased in patients with mild impairment of renal functions who took 1200 mg/day of ibuprofen for one week. • Renal papillary necrosis has been reported. A number of factors appear to increase the risk of renal toxicity (see Warnings and Precautions)		
Special Senses		• tinnitus	• amblyopia (blurred and/or diminished vision, scotomata and/or changes in color vision) Any patient with eye complaints during ibuprofen therapy should have an ophthalmological examination.
	Also reported but with unknown causal relationship: • conjunctivitis • diplopia • optic neuritis		

DRUG INTERACTIONS: Serious Drug Interactions:
- Use with acetylsalicylic acid (ASA) or other NSAIDs, including ibuprofen, may result in possible additive adverse side effects.
- Use with acetaminophen, may increase the risk of adverse renal effect.
- Use with anticoagulants may increase the risk of GI adverse events (e.g., bleeding).
- Use with hypoglycemic agents (oral agents and insulin) may increase the risk of hypoglycaemia.
- Use with antihypertensives may interfere with circulatory control.
- Use with diuretics may reduce the diuretic effect.
- Use with methotrexate may increase the risk of methotrexate toxicity.
- Use with lithium may increase the risk of lithium toxicity.

Acetylsalicylic Acid (ASA) or Other NSAIDs: The use of ibuprofen in addition to any other NSAID is not recommended because of the absence of any evidence demonstrating synergistic benefits and the potential for additive side effects.

Animal studies show that ASA given with NSAID agents, including ibuprofen, yield a net decrease in anti-inflammatory activity with lowered blood levels of the non-ASA drug. Single dose bioavailability studies in normal volunteers have failed to show an effect of ASA on ibuprofen blood levels. Correlative clinical studies have not been done.

Also, some NSAIDs may interfere with the anti-platelet effects of low dose ASA, possibly by competing with ASA for access to the active site of cyclooxygenase-I.

The concomitant administration of ibuprofen but not acetaminophen has been shown to antagonize the irreversible platelet inhibition induced by ASA. Regular use of ibuprofen in patients with increased cardiovascular risk may limit the cardio protective effects of ASA.

Anti-Platelet Agents (including ASA): See Warnings and Precautions, Hematologic.

Anticoagulants: See Warnings and Precautions, Hematologic.

Coumarin Type Anticoagulants: Several short-term controlled studies failed to show that ibuprofen significantly affected prothrombin time or a variety of other clotting factors when administered to individuals on coumarin-type anticoagulants. However, bleeding has been reported when ibuprofen and other NSAID agents have been administered to patients on coumarin-type anticoagulants. The use of ibuprofen in patients who are taking anticoagulants should therefore be avoided because of the possibility of enhanced GI bleeding or an additive effect due to ibuprofen's reversible anti-platelet actions.

Oral Hypoglycemics: Ibuprofen may increase the hypoglycemic effects of oral sulfonylurea hypoglycemic agents.

Anti-Hypertensives: NSAIDs may diminish the antihypertensive effect of Angiotensin Converting Enzyme (ACE) inhibitors.

Combinations of ACE inhibitors, diuretics and NSAIDs might have an increased risk for acute renal failure and hyperkalemia. In longer term therapy blood pressure and kidney function should be monitored more closely, as occasionally there can be a substantial increase in blood pressure.

Diuretics: Ibuprofen, because of its fluid retention properties, can decrease the diuretic and anti-hypertensive effects of diuretics, and increased diuretic dosage may be needed. Patients with impaired renal function taking potassium-sparing diuretics who develop ibuprofen-induced renal insufficiency might be in serious danger of fatal hyperkalemia.

Glucocorticoids: Some studies have shown that the concomitant use of NSAIDs and oral glucocorticoids increases the risk of GI side effects such as ulceration and bleeding. This is especially the case in older (>65 years of age) individuals.

Lithium: Monitoring of plasma lithium concentrations is advised when stopping or starting an NSAID, as increased lithium concentrations can occur.

Other Drug Interactions: Although ibuprofen binds to a significant extent to plasma proteins, interactions with other protein-bound drugs occur uncommonly. Nevertheless, caution should be observed when other drugs also having a high affinity for protein binding sites are used concurrently. Some observations have suggested a potential for ibuprofen to interact with digoxin, methotrexate, and phenytoin. However, the mechanisms and clinical significance of these observations are presently not known.

Patients taking other prescribed medications should consult a physician before using ibuprofen to assure its compatibility with the other medications.

DOSAGE AND ADMINISTRATION: Dosing Considerations: Do not take for pain for more than 5 consecutive days or fever for more than 3 days unless directed by a physician.

If your condition deteriorates or new symptoms occur (such as the painful area becomes unusually red, swollen or tender), consult a physician.

Individuals older than 65 years who are frail or debilitated should be given a starting dose lower than the one usually recommended, with individual adjustments when necessary.

Missed Dose: If you miss a dose, take the missed dose as soon as you remember. If it is almost time for your next dose, wait until then to take your medicine and skip the missed dose. Do not take two doses at the same time.

Recommended Dose: Mild to moderate pain or fever.

Adults: Single oral dose may be taken every 4-6 hours, as required, not to exceed the maximum daily dose (1200 mg) in 24 hours unless directed by a physician.

Product	Strength (Ibuprofen mg/tablet)	Single Oral Dose	Maximum Daily Dose (1200 mg)
MOTRIN IB	200 mg	1 or 2 tablets	6 tablets
Extra Strength MOTRIN IB	300 mg	1 tablet	4 tablets
Super Strength MOTRIN IB	400 mg	1 tablet	3 tablets

Children: Children's MOTRIN formulations are available to treat children under 12 years of age. Children's MOTRIN Suspensions may be also used for adults requiring liquid dosage forms (see Children's MOTRIN Product Monograph).

OVERDOSAGE:

Clinical Features: A clear pattern of clinical features associated with accidental or intentional overdose of ibuprofen has not been established. Reported cases of overdose have often been complicated by co-ingestions or additional suicidal gestures. The range of symptoms observed has included nausea, vomiting, abdominal pain, drowsiness, nystagmus, diplopia, headache, tinnitus, impaired renal function, coma and hypotension. A review of four fatalities associated with ibuprofen overdose indicates other contributing factors co-existed so it would be difficult to identify the toxicity of ibuprofen as a specific cause of death.

Post-ingestion blood levels may be useful to confirm a diagnosis and to quantify the degree of exposure but otherwise have not been helpful in predicting clinical outcome. Generally, full recovery can be expected with appropriate symptomatic management.

The following cases of overdose have been reported. A 19-month-old child, 1½ hours after the ingestion of seven to ten 400 mg tablets of ibuprofen presented apnea, cyanosis and responded only to painful stimuli. After treatment with O_2, $NaHCO_3$, infusion of dextrose and normal saline, the child was responsive and 12 hours after ingestion appeared completely recovered. Blood levels of ibuprofen reached 102.9 µg/mL, 8½ hours after the accident. Two other children weighing approximately 10 kg had taken an estimated 120 mg/kg. There were no signs of acute intoxication or late sequelae. In one child the ibuprofen blood level at 90 minutes after ingestion was approximately 700 µg/mL. A nineteen-year-old male who ingested 8000 mg of ibuprofen reported dizziness and nystagmus was noted. He recovered with no reported sequelae after parenteral hydration and 3 days of bed rest.

For perspective, a single 200 mg oral dose study in 6 fasting healthy men produced a peak plasma concentration of 15.0 µg/mL at 0.75 hr. Another study using a single oral 400 mg dose in humans produced a peak serum level of 31.9±8.8 µg/mL 0.5 hour after ingestion, and at 16 hours serum concentrations had dropped to 1 µg/mL.

Management of Overdose: Appropriate interventions to decontaminate the gastrointestinal tract may be beneficial within the first four hours after ingestion. Routine symptomatic and supportive treatment is then recommended. Physicians should contact the Regional Poison Control Centre for additional guidance about ibuprofen overdose management.

> For management of a suspected drug overdose, CPhA recommends that you contact your **regional Poison Control Centre**. See the *CPS* Directory section for a list of Poison Control Centres.

ACTION AND CLINICAL PHARMACOLOGY: Mechanism of Action: Ibuprofen is a member of the class of agents commonly known as nonsteroidal anti-inflammatory drugs (NSAID). Like all NSAIDs, ibuprofen is an analgesic, antipyretic, and anti-inflammatory medication.

It is generally accepted that the basic mechanism of pharmacological action of ibuprofen, and other NSAIDs, is the inhibition of prostaglandin synthesis.

Nonselective NSAIDs (such as ibuprofen) and ASA act by inhibiting systemic (peripheral and central) prostaglandin G/H synthase isoenzymes, also known as cyclooxygenase-1 (COX-1) and cyclooxygenase-2 (COX-2). These isoenzymes are responsible for the conversion of arachidonic acid to various tissue specific prostaglandins and thromboxanes. COX-1 is constitutively expressed in all tissues and is responsible for generating prostaglandins that maintain organ function, protect the integrity of the gastric mucosa and generate platelet-derived thromboxane responsible for platelet aggregation and vasoconstriction. During the inflammatory process COX-2 is induced, generating prostaglandins that mediate pain and inflammation. COX-2 is also present constitutively in the kidneys and vascular endothelium. Reported adverse experiences with ASA and other NSAIDs can be understood on the basis of this mechanism of action.

Pharmacodynamics: Consistent with the NSAID classification, ibuprofen exhibits anti-inflammatory activity at higher dosage ranges. At lower adult single doses relevant to a nonprescription dosage (200 mg to 400 mg) ibuprofen relieves pain of mild to moderate intensity and reduces fever. Analogous to acetylsalicylic acid, the prototype of this class, this analgesic/antipyretic activity of ibuprofen occurs at lower doses than necessary for anti-inflammatory effects, which are thought to require sustained administration of higher individual doses.

Clinical studies indicate a duration of clinical effect for up to 8 hours for fever and up to 6 hours for pain.

Pharmacokinetics: Absorption: Ibuprofen is rapidly absorbed after oral administration, with peak serum or plasma levels generally appearing within 1 to 2 hours. Oral absorption is estimated to be 80% of the dose. Both the rate of absorption and peak plasma concentrations are reduced when the drug is taken with food, but bioavailability as measured by total area under the concentration-time curve is minimally altered.

Distribution: Ibuprofen, like most drugs of its class, is highly protein bound (>99% bound at 20 µg/mL). Tissue distribution of ibuprofen is also extensive in humans. Studies comparing synovial fluid levels with serum concentrations indicated that equilibration time post ingestion occurred within approximately 3 to 5 hours.

Metabolism: It is rapidly metabolized through oxidation and glucuronic acid conjugation with urinary excretion of the inactive metabolites usually complete within 24 hours. Less than 10% is excreted unchanged in the urine.

Excretion: Ibuprofen has an elimination half-life of approximately two hours.

Special Populations and Conditions: Geriatrics: Studies demonstrate no apparent clinically significant alterations in ibuprofen pharmacokinetics in the elderly.

Hepatic Insufficiency: Ibuprofen pharmacokinetics have also been studied in patients with alcoholic liver disease who have been assessed to have fair to poor hepatic function. Results suggest that, despite the liver being the primary organ of metabolism of ibuprofen, its kinetic parameters are not substantially altered by this condition.

STORAGE AND STABILITY: Store away from heat and direct light.

INFORMATION FOR THE PATIENT: Published in e-CPS, available by subscription at www.e-cps.ca.

DOSAGE FORMS, COMPOSITION AND PACKAGING: MOTRIN IB: Each white, sweet-coated biconvex tablet, with "Motrin IB" printed in black ink, contains: ibuprofen 200 mg. Nonmedicinal ingredients: colloidal silicon dioxide, cornstarch, hypromellose, iron oxide black, polyethylene glycol, pregelatinized starch, propylene glycol, sodium cyclamate, sodium starch glycolate, stearic acid and titanium dioxide. Gluten-, lactose-, paraben-, sulfite- and tartrazine-free. Bottles of 10*, 24*, 50*, 100 and 150†.

Extra Strength MOTRIN IB: Each solid, light orange colored, round, biconvex, sweet-coated tablet, with "MOTRIN 300 mg" printed in black ink, contains: ibuprofen 300 mg. Nonmedicinal ingredients: carnauba wax, colloidal silicon dioxide, cornstarch, FD&C Yellow no. 6, hypromellose, iron oxide black, polydextrose, polyethylene glycol, propylene glycol, sodium cyclamate, sodium starch glycolate, stearic acid and titanium dioxide. Gluten- and lactose-free. Bottles of 20* and 65*.

Super Strength MOTRIN IB: Each solid, orange colored, round, biconvex, sweet-coated tablet, with "MOTRIN 400 mg" printed in black ink, contains: ibuprofen 400 mg. Nonmedicinal ingredients: carnauba wax, colloidal silicon dioxide, cornstarch, FD&C Yellow No. 6, hypromellose, iron oxide black, polydextrose, polyethylene glycol, propylene glycol, sodium cyclamate, sodium starch glycolate, stearic acid and titanium dioxide. Gluten- and lactose-free. Pouches of 1. Bottles of 16* and 50*.

For all preparations, keep out of the reach of children.

All packages are safety sealed.

Motrin® IB Liquid Gels

ibuprofen

Analgesic—Antipyretic

McNeil Consumer Healthcare

Date of Preparation: July 20, 2006
Date of Revision: June 12, 2007

SUMMARY PRODUCT INFORMATION:

Route of Administration	Dosage Form/ Strength	Clinically Relevant Nonmedicinal Ingredients
Oral	Capsule/200 mg	None For a complete listing see Dosage Forms, Composition and Packaging.

* Containers provided with a child-resistant closure.
† Easy-to-open container.

INDICATIONS AND CLINICAL USE: Adults Over 12 Years: MOTRIN IB LIQUID GELS (Ibuprofen) is indicated for treatment of pain associated with migraine.

MOTRIN IB LIQUID GELS is also indicated for headaches and the temporary relief of menstrual pain (dysmenorrhea), toothache (dental pain), minor aches and pains in muscles, bones and joints and for reduction of fever and for temporary relief of mild to moderate pain.

There is considerable evidence in the world literature documenting the efficacy of 200 to 400 mg doses of ibuprofen in the treatment of mild to moderate pain in a broad range of pain models.

Geriatrics: Patients older than 65 years and frail or debilitated patients are most susceptible to a variety of adverse reactions from nonsteroidal anti-inflammatory drugs (NSAIDs): the incidence of these adverse reactions increases with dose and duration of treatment. In addition, these patients are less tolerant to ulceration and bleeding. Most reports of fatal GI events are in this population. Older patients are also at risk of lower oesophageal ulceration and bleeding.

For such patients, consideration should be given to a starting dose lower than the one usually recommended, with individual adjustment when necessary and under close supervision. See Warnings and Precautions, Gastrointestinal for further advice.

Pediatrics: Studies conducted to date have **not** demonstrated pediatric-specific problems that would limit the usefulness of ibuprofen in children 6 months and older.

Ibuprofen is not recommended for use in patients under 2 months of age since safety and effectiveness have not been established.

Sore Throat Pain: A double-blind, randomized study showed that ibuprofen 400 mg relieved sore throat pain significantly better than placebo and acetaminophen.

Headache: A double-blind, randomized study showed that ibuprofen 400 mg relieved headache pain significantly better than acetaminophen 1000 mg and placebo. Another double-blind, placebo-controlled, randomized study showed that ibuprofen 400 mg began to exert a significant analgesic effect on headache within 30 minutes after dosing.

Dental Pain: A double-blind, randomized study showed that ibuprofen 400 mg relieved dental pain following removal of impacted third molars significantly better than acetaminophen and placebo. Several other comparative dental studies have described similar results.

Muscle Aches: A double-blind, randomized study showed that ibuprofen 400 mg every four hours for a total of three doses relieved muscle soreness following exercise significantly better than acetaminophen 1000 mg and placebo every four hours.

Dysmenorrhea: Several studies demonstrate the significant effect of ibuprofen compared to placebo or other active analgesics on uterine pain and cramping.

Fever: The antipyretic efficacy of ibuprofen has been demonstrated in adult.

CONTRAINDICATIONS: The following are contraindications to the use of MOTRIN IB LIQUID GELS (Ibuprofen):

1. Active peptic ulcer, a history of recurrent ulceration or active inflammatory disease of the gastrointestinal system.
2. Known or suspected hypersensitivity to the drug or other nonsteroidal anti-inflammatory drugs. The potential for cross-reactivity between different NSAIDs must be kept in mind.

   MOTRIN IB LIQUID GELS should not be used in patients with the complete or partial syndrome of nasal polyps, or in whom asthma, anaphylaxis, urticaria, rhinitis or other allergic manifestations are precipitated by ASA or other nonsteroidal anti-inflammatory agents. Fatal anaphylactoid reactions have occurred in such individuals. As well, individuals with the above medical problems are at risk of a severe reaction even if they have taken NSAIDs in the past without any adverse effects.
3. Significant hepatic impairment or active liver disease.
4. Severely impaired or deteriorating renal function (creatinine clearance <30 mL/min). Individuals with lesser degrees of renal impairment are at risk of deterioration of their renal function when prescribed NSAIDs and must be monitored.
5. Ibuprofen is not recommended for use with other NSAIDs because of the absence of any evidence demonstrating synergistic benefits and the potential for additive side effects.
6. Children with kidney disease and children who have suffered significant fluid loss should not be given ibuprofen.
7. Patients who are hypersensitive to the drug or to any ingredients in the formulation or component of the container. For a complete listing, see Dosage Forms, Composition and Packaging.

WARNINGS AND PRECAUTIONS:

> **Serious Warnings and Precautions**
> **History of peptic ulcers, gastrointestinal bleeding or other diseases of the gastrointestinal tract.**

General: In common with other anti-inflammatory drugs, ibuprofen may mask the usual signs of infection.

Cardiovascular: Congestive heart failure in patients with marginal cardiac function, elevated blood pressure and palpitations.

Endocrine and Metabolism: Fluid retention and oedema have been observed in patients treated with ibuprofen. Therefore, as with many other nonsteroidal anti-inflammatory drugs, the possibility of precipitating congestive heart failure in elderly patients or those with compromised cardiac function should be borne in mind. MOTRIN IB LIQUID GELS (Ibuprofen) should be used with caution in patients with heart failure, hypertension or other conditions predisposing to fluid retention.

With nonsteroidal anti-inflammatory treatment there is a potential risk of hyperkalemia, particularly in patients with conditions such as diabetes mellitus or renal failure; elderly patients; or in patients receiving concomitant therapy with B-adrenergic blockers, angiotensin converting enzyme inhibitors or some diuretics. Serum electrolytes should be monitored periodically during long-term therapy, especially in those patients who are at risk.

Gastrointestinal: Serious GI toxicity, such as peptic ulceration, perforation and gastrointestinal bleeding, **sometimes severe and occasionally fatal**, can occur at any time, with or without symptoms in patients treated with NSAIDs including ibuprofen.

Minor upper GI problems, such as dyspepsia, are common, usually developing early in therapy. Physicians should remain alert for ulceration and bleeding in patients treated with nonsteroidal anti-inflammatory drugs, even in the absence of previous GI tract symptoms.

In patients observed in clinical trials of such agents, symptomatic upper GI ulcers, gross bleeding, or perforation appear to occur in approximately 1% of patients treated for 3-6 months and in about 2-4% of patients treated for one year. The risk continues beyond one year and possibly increases. The incidence of these complications increases with increasing dose.

MOTRIN IB LIQUID GELS should be given under close medical supervision to patients prone to gastrointestinal tract irritation, particularly those with a history of peptic ulcer, diverticulosis or other inflammatory disease of the gastrointestinal tract such as ulcerative colitis and Crohn's disease. In these cases the physician must weigh the benefits of treatment against the possible hazards.

Physicians should inform patients about the signs and/or symptoms of serious GI toxicity and instruct them to contact a physician immediately if they experience persistent dyspepsia or other symptoms or signs suggestive of gastrointestinal ulceration or bleeding. Because serious GI tract ulceration and bleeding can occur without warning symptoms, physicians should follow chronically treated patients by checking their haemoglobin periodically and by being vigilant for the signs and symptoms of ulceration and bleeding and should inform the patients of the importance of this follow-up.

If ulceration is suspected or confirmed, or if GI bleeding occurs, MOTRIN IB LIQUID GELS should be discontinued immediately, appropriate treatment instituted and the patient monitored closely.

No studies, to date, have identified any group of patients not at risk of developing ulceration and bleeding. A prior history of serious GI events and other factors such as excess alcohol intake, smoking, age, female gender and concomitant oral steroid and anticoagulant use have been associated with increased risk. Studies to date show that all NSAIDs can cause GI tract adverse events. Although existing data does not clearly identify differences in risk between various NSAIDs, this may be shown in the future.

There is no definitive evidence that the concomitant administration of histamine H2-receptor antagonists and/or antacids will either prevent the occurrence of gastrointestinal side effects or allow the continuation of MOTRIN IB LIQUID GELS therapy when and if these adverse reactions appear.

Genitourinary: Some NSAIDs are known to cause persistent urinary symptoms (bladder pain, dysuria, urinary frequency), hematuria or cystitis. The onset of these symptoms may occur at any time after the initiation of therapy with an NSAID. Some cases have become severe on continued treatment. Should urinary symptoms occur, treatment with MOTRIN IB LIQUID GELS **must be stopped immediately** to obtain recovery. This should be done before any urological investigations or treatments are carried out.

Hematologic: Drugs inhibiting prostaglandin biosynthesis do interfere with platelet function to varying degrees; therefore, patients who may be adversely affected by such an action should be carefully observed when ibuprofen is administered.

Blood dyscrasias (such as neutropenia, leukopenia, thrombocytopenia, aplastic anaemia and agranulocytosis) associated with the use of nonsteroidal anti-inflammatory drugs are rare, but could occur with severe consequences.

Hepatic/Biliary/Pancreatic: As with other nonsteroidal anti-inflammatory drugs, borderline elevations of one or more liver function tests may occur in up to 15% of patients. These abnormalities may progress, may remain essentially unchanged, or may be transient with continued therapy. A patient with symptoms and/or signs suggesting liver dysfunction, or in whom an abnormal liver test has occurred, should be evaluated for evidence of the development of more severe hepatic reaction while on therapy with this drug. Severe hepatic reactions including jaundice and cases of fatal hepatitis have been reported with nonsteroidal anti-inflammatory drugs.

Although such reactions are rare, if abnormal liver tests persist or worsen, if clinical signs and symptoms consistent with liver disease develop, or if systemic manifestations occur (e.g. eosinophilia, rash, etc.), this drug should be discontinued.

During long-term therapy, liver function tests should be monitored periodically. If there is a need to prescribe this drug in the presence of impaired liver function, it must be done under strict observation.

The frequency of acute liver injury among 625 307 people who received NSAIDs in England and Wales between 1987 and 1991, was examined. There were 311 716 patients who were prescribed ibuprofen. The incidence of acute liver injury among ibuprofen users was 1.6/100 000; this was the lowest incidence among the 8 NSAIDs studied and was significantly lower than the incidence among users of ketoprofen, piroxicam, fenbrufen, or sulindac. For NSAID users as a group, the only factors that had an independent effect on the occurrence of acute liver injury were the simultaneous use of hepatotoxic medication or the presence of rheumatoid arthritis. Based on these data, the short-term use of ibuprofen as an analgesic/antipyretic should not be of concern regarding the development of liver disease.

Immune: In occasional cases, with some NSAIDs, the symptoms of aseptic meningitis (stiff neck, severe headaches, nausea and vomiting, fever or clouding of consciousness) have been observed. Patients with autoimmune disorders (systemic lupus erythematosus, mixed connective tissue diseases, etc.) seem to be pre-disposed. Therefore, in such patients, the physician must be vigilant to the development of this complication.

Skin: Some people may become more sensitive to sunlight than they are normally. Brief exposure to sunlight or sunlamps may cause sunburn, blisters on the skin, skin rash, redness, itching or discoloration or vision changes.

Neurologic: Some patients may experience drowsiness, dizziness, vertigo, insomnia or depression with the use of ibuprofen. If patients experience these side effects, they should exercise caution in carrying out activities that require alertness.

Ophthalmologic: Blurred and/or diminished vision has been reported with the use of ibuprofen and other nonsteroidal anti-inflammatory drugs. If such symptoms develop this drug should be discontinued and an ophthalmologic examination performed; ophthalmic examination should be carried out at periodic intervals in any patient receiving this drug for an extended period of time.

Renal: Long term administration of nonsteroidal anti-inflammatory drugs to animals has resulted in renal papillary necrosis and other abnormal renal pathology. In humans, there have been reports of acute interstitial nephritis with hematuria, proteinuria, and occasionally nephrotic syndrome.

A second form of renal toxicity has been seen in patients with prerenal conditions leading to the reduction in renal blood flow or blood volume, where the renal prostaglandins have a supportive role in the maintenance of renal perfusion. In these patients, administration of a nonsteroidal anti-inflammatory drug may cause a dose dependent reduction in prostaglandin formation and may precipitate overt renal decompensation. Patients at greatest risk of this reaction are those with impaired renal function, heart failure, liver dysfunction, those taking diuretics, and the elderly. Discontinuation of nonsteroidal anti-inflammatory therapy is usually followed by recovery to the pre-treatment state.

Ibuprofen and its metabolites are eliminated primarily by the kidneys; therefore the drug should be used with great caution in patients with impaired renal function. In these cases, utilisation of lower doses of MOTRIN IB LIQUID GELS should be considered and patients carefully monitored.

During long-term therapy kidney function should be monitored periodically.

Sensitivity/Resistance: Patients sensitive to any one of the nonsteroidal anti-inflammatory drugs may be sensitive to any of the other NSAIDs also.

Special Populations: Pregnant Women: Reproductive studies conducted in rats and rabbits have not demonstrated evidence of developmental abnormalities. However, animal reproduction studies are not always predictive of human response. Because of the known effects of NSAIDs on the fetal cardiovascular system, use of ibuprofen during late pregnancy should be avoided. As with other drugs known to inhibit prostaglandin synthesis, an increased incidence of dystocia and delayed parturition occurred in rats. Administration of ibuprofen is not recommended during pregnancy.

Nursing Women: The high protein binding and lower pH of breast milk versus plasma tend to inhibit the excretion of ibuprofen into breast milk. One study showed an ibuprofen concentration of 13 ng/mL 30 minutes after ingesting 400 mg. The milk: plasma ratio was 1:126. This translates to an infant exposure of 0.0008% of the maternal dose. It is not known to what extent, if any, ibuprofen crosses the human placenta.

ADVERSE REACTIONS: Prescription Experience: The following adverse reactions have been noted in patients treated with prescription doses (≥1200 mg/day).

Note: Reactions listed below under Causal Relationship Unknown are those which occurred under circumstances where a causal relationship could not be established. However, in these rarely reported events, the possibility of a relationship to ibuprofen cannot be excluded.

Gastrointestinal: The adverse reactions most frequently seen with prescribed ibuprofen therapy involve the gastrointestinal system.

Incidence 3 to 9%: nausea, epigastric pain, heartburn.

Incidence 1 to 3%: diarrhoea, abdominal distress, nausea and vomiting, indigestion, constipation, abdominal cramps or pain, fullness of the gastrointestinal tract (bloating or flatulence).

Incidence less than 1%: gastric or duodenal ulcer with bleeding and/or perforation, gastrointestinal haemorrhage, melena, hepatitis, jaundice, abnormal liver function (AST, serum bilirubin and alkaline phosphatase).

Allergic: Incidence less than 1%: anaphylaxis (see Contraindications).

Causal relationship unknown: fever, serum sickness, lupus erythematosus.

Central Nervous System: Incidence 3 to 9%: dizziness.

Incidence 1 to 3%: headache, nervousness.

Incidence less than 1%: depression, insomnia.

Causal relationship unknown: paresthesias, hallucinations, dream abnormalities.

Aseptic meningitis and meningoencephalitis, in one case accompanied by eosinophilia in the cerebrospinal fluid, have been reported in patients who took ibuprofen intermittently and did not have any connective tissue disease.

Dermatologic: Incidence 3 to 9%: rash (including maculopapular type).

Incidence 1 to 3%: pruritus.

Incidence less than 1%: vesiculobullous eruptions, urticaria, erythema multiforme.

Causal relationship unknown: alopecia, Stevens-Johnson syndrome.

Cardiovascular: Incidence less than 1%: congestive heart failure in patients with marginal cardiac function, elevated blood pressure.

Causal relationship unknown: arrhythmias (sinus tachycardia, sinus bradycardia, palpitations).

Special Senses: Incidence 1 to 3%: tinnitus.

Incidence less than 1%: amblyopia (blurred and/or diminished vision, scotomata and/or changes in colour vision). Any patient with eye complaints during ibuprofen therapy should have an ophthalmological examination.

Causal relationship unknown: conjunctivitis, diplopia, optic neuritis.

Hematologic: Incidence less than 1%: leukopenia, and decreases in haemoglobin and hematocrit.

Causal relationship unknown: haemolytic anaemia, thrombocytopenia, granulocytopenia, bleeding episodes (e.g., purpura, epistaxis, hematuria, menorrhagia).

Renal: Causal relationship unknown: decreased creatinine clearance, polyuria, azotemia.

Like other nonsteroidal anti-inflammatory drugs, ibuprofen inhibits renal prostaglandin synthesis, which may decrease renal function and cause sodium retention. Renal blood flow and glomerular filtration rate decreased in patients with mild impairment of renal function who took 1200 mg/day of ibuprofen for one week. Renal papillary necrosis has been reported. A number of factors appear to increase the risk of renal toxicity.

Hepatic: Incidence less than 1%: hepatitis, jaundice, abnormal liver function (AST, serum bilirubin, and alkaline phosphatase).

Endocrine: Causal relationship unknown: gynecomastia, hypoglycaemic reaction.

Menstrual delays of up to two weeks and dysfunctional uterine bleeding occurred in nine patients taking ibuprofen, 400 mg t.i.d., for three days before menses.

Metabolic: Incidence 1 to 3%: decreased appetite, oedema, fluid retention.

Fluid retention generally responds promptly to drug discontinuation (see Warnings and Precautions).

Non-Prescription Experience: Literature (at dosages ≤1200 mg/day): One researcher conducted an extensive analysis of published data concerning the relative safety of non-prescription doses of ibuprofen and acetaminophen. Of a total of 96 randomized and blinded trials, there were 10 trials of seven days' duration or less where the safety of both drugs was directly compared. In three of these trials, the incidence of adverse events was higher with acetaminophen; there were no reported adverse events in six trials; and one trial reported a higher incidence with ibuprofen. In this subset of 10 studies, it was reported that gastrointestinal adverse events were found to be the most common type of event reported and were predominantly dyspepsia, nausea, or vomiting. None of the GI events appeared to warrant follow-up from which the author inferred there were no serious gastrointestinal events.

It was concluded: "Although we recognise that the above mentioned data are very selective and are based on information derived from a variety of trial designs and populations, it is nonetheless instructive for indicating a relatively low incidence of severe adverse reactions with both drugs when taken at their respective non-prescription dosages."

A double-blind, placebo-controlled study (N=1246) was conducted to prospectively evaluate the gastrointestinal tolerability, as compared to placebo, of the maximum non-prescription dose and duration (1200 mg/day for 10 consecutive days) of ibuprofen use in healthy subjects representative of a non-prescription analgesic user population. Gastrointestinal adverse experiences were similar in the placebo and ibuprofen groups (67 out of 413, 16% with placebo vs. 161 out of 833, 19% with ibuprofen). There was no difference between the two groups in the proportion of discontinuing due to a gastrointestinal event. Gastrointestinal adverse experiences reported by ≥1% of subjects were: dyspepsia, abdominal pain, nausea, diarrhoea, flatulence, and constipation. Seventeen (1.4%) subjects had positive occult blood tests: their frequency was comparable between treatments. When used as directed to treat episodic pain, nonprescription ibuprofen at the maximum dose of 1200 mg/day for 10 days, is well-tolerated.

In two multitrial analyses, a meta analysis, and a literature review, single doses of ibuprofen had a low incidence of gastrointestinal drug reactions, comparable to that of acetaminophen and placebo. Reports from spontaneous reporting systems in the United Kingdom, France and the United States, where a prescription is not needed for ibuprofen at a daily dose up to 1200 mg, confirm the medication's gastrointestinal safety and acceptability. A recently-completed large-scale randomised trial comparing nonprescription doses of acetylsalicylic acid, acetaminophen, and ibuprofen in 8677 adults found that the rates of significant adverse reactions were: aspirin 18.7%, ibuprofen 13.7%, and acetaminophen 14.5%. Ibuprofen was not statistically different from acetaminophen. Total gastrointestinal events (including dyspepsia) and abdominal pain were less frequent with ibuprofen (4% and 2.8%, respectively) than with acetaminophen (5.3% and 3.9%) or aspirin (7.1% and 6.8%) [all p<0.035]. It was concluded that "The overall tolerability of ibuprofen in this large-scale study was equivalent to that of paracetamol and better than that of [ASA]."

DRUG INTERACTIONS: Drug-Drug Interactions: Acetylsalicylic acid (ASA) or other NSAIDs: The use of MOTRIN IB LIQUID GELS (Ibuprofen) in addition to any other NSAID, including ASA, is not recommended due to the possibility of additive side effects. Animal studies show that aspirin given with NSAIDs, including ibuprofen, yields a net decrease in anti-inflammatory activity with lowered blood levels of the non-aspirin drug. Single-dose bioavailability studies in normal volunteers have failed to show an effect of aspirin on ibuprofen blood levels. Correlative clinical studies have not been conducted.

Acetaminophen: Although interactions have not been reported, concurrent use with MOTRIN IB LIQUID GELS is not advisable: it may increase the risk of adverse renal effect.

Digoxin: Ibuprofen has been shown to increase serum digoxin concentration. Increased monitoring and dosage adjustments of digitalis glycoside may be necessary during and following concurrent ibuprofen therapy.

Coumarin-type: Numerous studies have shown that the concomitant use of NSAIDs and anticoagulants increases the risk of GI adverse events such as ulceration and bleeding. Because prostaglandins play an important role in hemostasis, and NSAIDs affect platelet function, concurrent therapy of ibuprofen with warfarin requires close monitoring to be certain that no change in anticoagulant dosage is necessary. Several short-term controlled studies failed to show that ibuprofen significantly affected prothrombin time or a variety of other clotting factors when administered to individuals on coumarin-type anticoagulants. Nevertheless, the physician, should be cautious when administering MOTRIN IB LIQUID GELS to patients on anticoagulants.

Hypoglycaemic Agents: Ibuprofen may increase hypoglycaemic effects of oral antidiabetic agents and insulin.

Antihypertensives: Prostaglandins are an important factor in cardiovascular homeostasis and inhibition of their synthesis by NSAIDs may interfere with circulatory control. NSAIDs may elevate blood pressure in patients receiving antihypertensive medication. Two meta analyses have observed this relationship for NSAIDs as a class and for certain NSAIDs in particular, but ibuprofen did not significantly affect blood pressure in either meta analysis. Consistent with this lack of effect, a study by Davies et al showed that ibuprofen 1600 mg/day for 14 days did not attenuate the antihypertensive effect of two β-adrenergic blockers. Houston et al. showed no effect of three weeks' therapy with ibuprofen on the antihypertensive efficacy of verapamil, but it is not known whether this lack of interaction extends to other classes of calcium channel blockers.

When renal perfusion pressure is reduced both prostaglandins and angiotensin II are important mediators of renal autoregulation. As a class, the combination of an NSAID and angiotensin converting enzyme inhibitor theoretically may have the potential to decrease renal function. One study found a clinically significant decrease in renal function in 4 of 17 patients treated with hydrochlorothiazide and fosinopril who received ibuprofen 2400 mg/day for one month. In contrast, Minuz found no effect on the antihypertensive effect of enalapril or on plasma renin or aldosterone following two days' treatment with ibuprofen 1200 mg/day.

The relationship of ibuprofen and antihypertensives is clearly not well defined. The benefits of concomitant medication should be analysed and compared to the potential risks before being prescribed. If ibuprofen is being recommended for **long-term** use, then periodic monitoring of blood pressure may be useful. Blood pressure monitoring is not necessary if ibuprofen is being recommended for **short-term** use as an analgesic.

Diuretics: Clinical studies, as well as random observations, have shown that ibuprofen can reduce the natriuretic effect of furosemide and thiazides in some patients. This response has been attributed to inhibition of renal prostaglandin synthesis. During concomitant therapy with ibuprofen, the patient should be observed closely for signs of renal failure as well as to assure diuretic efficacy.

Antacids: A bioavailability study has shown that there was no interference with the absorption of ibuprofen when given in conjunction with an antacid containing aluminium hydroxide and magnesium hydroxide.

H-2 antagonists: In studies with human volunteers, coadministration of cimetidine or ranitidine with ibuprofen had no substantive effect on ibuprofen serum concentrations.

Methotrexate: Ibuprofen as well as other NSAIDs has been reported to competitively inhibit methotrexate accumulation in rabbit kidney slices. This may indicate that ibuprofen could enhance the toxicity of methotrexate. Caution should be used when ibuprofen is administered concomitantly with methotrexate.

Lithium: Ibuprofen produced an elevation of plasma lithium levels and a reduction in renal lithium clearance in a study of eleven normal volunteers. The mean minimum lithium concentration increased 15% and the renal clearance of lithium was decreased by 19% during this period of concomitant drug administration. This effect has been attributed to inhibition of renal prostaglandin synthesis by ibuprofen. Thus, when ibuprofen and lithium are administered concurrently, subjects should be observed carefully for signs of lithium toxicity.

Other Drugs: Although ibuprofen binds extensively to plasma proteins, interactions with other protein-bound drugs occur rarely. Nevertheless, caution should be observed when other drugs, also having a high affinity for protein binding sites, are used concurrently. No interactions have been reported when ibuprofen has been used in conjunction with probenecid, thyroxine, steroids, antibiotics or benzodiazepines.

Drug-Food Interactions: Interactions with food have not been established.

Drug-Herb Interactions: Interactions with herbal products have not been established.

Drug-Laboratory Test Interactions: Interactions with laboratory tests have not been established.

DOSAGE AND ADMINISTRATION: Adults and Children Over 12: Take 1 or 2 capsules every four hours as needed. Do not exceed six capsules in 24 hours, unless directed by a physician.

OVERDOSAGE:
Symptoms of Overdose : The toxicity of ibuprofen overdose is dependent upon the amount of drug ingested and the time elapsed since ingestion; individual responses may vary, thus making it necessary to evaluate each case separately. Although uncommon, serious toxicity and death have been reported with ibuprofen overdosage. The most frequently reported symptoms of ibuprofen overdose include abdominal pain, nausea, vomiting, lethargy and drowsiness. Other CNS symptoms include headache, tinnitus, CNS depression and seizures. Metabolic acidosis, coma, acute renal failure and apnoea (primarily in very young pediatric patients) may rarely occur. Cardiovascular toxicity, including hypotension, bradycardia, tachycardia and atrial fibrillation, also have been reported.

Treatment of Overdose: In cases of acute overdose, the stomach should be emptied through induction of emesis (in alert patients only) or gastric lavage. Emesis is most effective if initiated within 30 minutes of ingestion. Orally administered activated charcoal may help in reducing the absorption of ibuprofen when given less than 2 hours following ingestion. There is some evidence that repeated administration of activated charcoal may bind the medication that has diffused from the circulation. Inducing diuresis may be helpful. The treatment of acute overdose is primarily supportive. Management of hypotension, acidosis and gastrointestinal bleeding may be necessary.

In pediatric patients, the estimated amount of ibuprofen ingested per body weight may be helpful to predict the potential for development of toxicity although each case must be evaluated. Ingestion of less than 100 mg/kg is unlikely to produce toxicity. Pediatric patients ingesting 100 to 200 mg/kg may be managed with induced emesis and a minimal observation time of at least four hours. Pediatric patients ingesting 200 to 400 mg/kg of ibuprofen should have immediate gastric emptying and at least four hours observation. Pediatric patients ingesting greater than 400 mg/kg require immediate medical referral, careful observation and appropriate supportive therapy. Induced emesis is not recommended in overdoses greater than 400 mg/kg because of the risk for convulsions and the potential for aspiration of gastric contents.

In adult patients, the dose reportedly ingested does not appear to be predictive of toxicity. The need for referral and follow-up must be judged by the circumstances at the time of the overdose ingestion. Symptomatic adults should be carefully evaluated, observed and supported.

Examples of Ibuprofen Overdose: A 41-year-old man with multiple medical problems, including long-term renal insufficiency, developed near-fatal acute renal failure after ingestion of a massive dose (36 g) of ibuprofen. He required dialysis for several months, at which point his renal function improved.

In children, ibuprofen overdoses less than 100 mg/kg are unlikely to produce toxicity. In adults, the dose of ibuprofen reportedly ingested does not appear to be predictive of toxicity.

With electrolyte replacement and other intensive measures, a 21-month-old child recovered within 5 days after accidental ingestion of 8 g of ibuprofen. A 2-year-old child who ingested approximately 8 g of ibuprofen was treated with activated charcoal, developed metabolic acidosis and acute renal insufficiency, and recovered within 72 hours. A 6-year-old child became comatose after ingesting 6 g of ibuprofen. He was treated with gastric lavage, charcoal, and various supportive measures and recovered within 24 hours.

> For management of a suspected drug overdose, CPhA recommends that you contact your **regional Poison Control Centre**. See the *CPS* Directory section for a list of Poison Control Centres.

ACTION AND CLINICAL PHARMACOLOGY: Mechanism of Action: Ibuprofen, like all nonsteroidal anti-inflammatory drugs (NSAIDs), is an analgesic, antipyretic, and anti-inflammatory medication. There is strong evidence to support the view that the main mechanism of action of ibuprofen (like other NSAIDs) is related to decreasing prostaglandin biosynthesis.

Prostaglandins are naturally-occurring fatty acid derivatives that are widely distributed in the tissues. They are believed to be a common factor in the production of pain, fever, and inflammation. Prostaglandins are believed to sensitise tissues to pain- and inflammation-producing mediators such as histamine, 5-hydroxytryptamine, and kinins. The enzyme catalysing the committed step in prostaglandin biosynthesis is prostaglandin endoperoxide synthase, also know as cyclooxygenase.

There is significant evidence that the main mechanism of analgesic/antipyretic action of NSAIDs is prostaglandin biosynthesis inhibition. Other pharmacologic effects such as lysosome and plasma membrane stabilisation have been observed, but the potential relevance of these effects to ibuprofen-induced analgesia and antipyresis is unclear.

A recent study confirmed that ibuprofen 400 mg provided a significantly faster onset of relief as measured by first perceptible relief, meaningful relief, per cent attaining complete relief, and superior overall analgesic efficacy compared to acetaminophen 1000 mg for relief of episodic tension-type headache.

Pharmacokinetics: Absorption: Ibuprofen is rapidly and almost completely absorbed. Peak serum concentration occurs within 1-2 hours in adults. Ibuprofen capsules contain solubilized ibuprofen which has peak serum concentrations within 36-42 minutes. In febrile children ages 3 months to <12 years, the time of peak serum concentration was 1.60 and 1.54 hours for ibuprofen 5 mg/kg and 10 mg/kg, respectively. Nahata found a time to peak concentration of 1.1 and 1.2 hours for these respective doses. A similar study in febrile children by Walson which used an ibuprofen suspension showed a time of peak serum concentration of 1.3 and 1.7 hours for ibuprofen 5 mg/kg and 10 mg/kg, respectively. Walson also found that mean ibuprofen plasma concentration at one hour was 21.7±6.7 and 28.4±15.2 μg/mL for 5 mg/kg and 10 mg/kg, respectively. Food decreases the rate but not the extent of absorption.

Distribution: The volume of distribution in adults after oral administration is 0.1-0.2 L/kg. In febrile children the volume of distribution is 0.18 and 0.22 L/kg for ibuprofen 5 mg/kg and 10 mg/kg, respectively.

At therapeutic concentrations ibuprofen is highly bound to whole human plasma and to site II of purified albumin. There is no appreciable plasma accumulation of ibuprofen or its metabolites with repeated doses.

Metabolism: Ibuprofen is a racemic mixture of R-(-) ibuprofen and S-(+) ibuprofen. R-(-) ibuprofen undergoes extensive enantiomeric conversion to S-(+) ibuprofen in humans, averaging between 53% and 65%. S-(+) ibuprofen is believed to be the pharmacologically more active enantiomer. Two major metabolites, 2-[4-(2-carboxypropyl)phenyl] propionic acid and 2-[4-(2-hydroxy-2-methylpropyl]propionic acid, have been identified in plasma and urine. The metabolites 1-hydroxyibuprofen and 3-hydroxyibuprofen have also been found in urine in very small concentrations. Cytochrome P450 (CYP) 2C9 has been identified as the most important catalyst for formation of all oxidative metabolites of R-(-) and S-(+) ibuprofen. Approximately 80% of a dose is recovered in urine, primarily as carboxymetabolites and conjugated hydroxymetabolites. Ibuprofen does not appear to induce the formation of drug metabolising enzymes in the rat.

Excretion: Ibuprofen's plasma half-life in adults is 1.5-2.0 hours. In febrile children the plasma half-life is 1.65 and 1.48 hours for ibuprofen 5 mg/kg and 10 mg/kg, respectively. Parent drug and metabolites are primarily excreted in the urine; bile and faeces are relatively minor elimination routes. Total recovery in urine is between 70% and 90% of the administered dose within 24 hours.

There is no evidence of a differential metabolism or elimination of ibuprofen in the elderly. A pharmacokinetic evaluation of ibuprofen in geriatric subjects (65 to 78 years) compared with young adult subjects (22 to 35 years) found that there was no clinically significant difference in the kinetic profiles of ibuprofen for these age groups. Furthermore, there was no statistically significant difference between the two populations in the urinary excretion pattern of the drug and its major metabolites.

The pharmacokinetics of ibuprofen have also been evaluated in children, in whom the metabolism has been shown to be similar to that reported for adults. Walson reported that for ibuprofen 10 mg/kg given to children under 12 years of age, peak plasma concentration occurred at 1.5 hours and then declined with a plasma half-life of 1.8 hours. Thus, ibuprofen appears to exhibit a similar pharmacokinetic profile in all age groups examined.

Special Populations and Conditions: Breast Milk and Placental Transport: Ibuprofen excretion in breast milk following ingestion of one 400 mg ibuprofen tablet every 6 hours for five doses was below the level (i.e., 1 μg/mL) of detection. However, a later study using a more sensitive assay showed ibuprofen to be rapidly excreted in breast milk 30 minutes following oral ingestion of 400 mg of ibuprofen at a concentration of 13 ng/mL. A milk: plasma ratio of 1:126 was determined and the exposure of a suckling infant was calculated to be approximately 0.0008% of the maternal dose. It is not known whether ibuprofen crosses the placenta.

STORAGE AND STABILITY: MOTRIN IB LIQUID GELS should be stored at room temperature (15-30°C). Protect from heat and humidity.

INFORMATION FOR THE PATIENT: Published in e-CPS, available by subscription at www.e-cps.ca.

DOSAGE FORMS, COMPOSITION AND PACKAGING: Each capsule of a clear, colourless to pale yellow solution in a clear oblong gelatin shell, printed with the "M200" logo in black ink contains: ibuprofen 200 mg. Nonmedicinal ingredients: castor oil, gelatin, PEG-40 hydrogenated castor oil, povidone, purified water, sorbitan, sorbitol and titanium dioxide. Bottles of 16 and 72.

Moxifloxacin Ⓟ

CPhA Monograph

see *Fluoroquinolones*

MS Contin® Ⓝ

morphine sulfate

Opioid Analgesic

Purdue Pharma

Date of Revision: August 25, 2009

PHARMACOLOGY: Morphine is an opioid analgesic which exerts an agonist effect at specific, saturable opioid receptors in the CNS and other tissues. In man, morphine produces a variety of effects including analgesia, constipation from decreased gastrointestinal motility, suppression of the cough reflex, respiratory depression from reduced responsiveness of the respiratory center to CO_2, nausea and vomiting via stimulation of the CTZ, changes in mood including euphoria and dysphoria, sedation, mental clouding, and alterations of the endocrine and autonomic nervous systems.

Morphine is readily absorbed when given orally, rectally or by s.c. or i.m. injection. Due to "first-pass" metabolism in the liver, the effect of an oral dose is less than after parenteral administration. With repeated regular dosing, oral morphine is about 1/3 as potent as when given by intramuscular injection. Morphine is primarily excreted in the urine as morphine-3-glucuronide. About 7 to 10% of a dose of morphine is excreted in the feces via the bile.

When administered every 12 hours, the sustained-release tablets provide equivalent analgesia to morphine oral solution given 4 hourly. In most cases, administration on a twelve hourly schedule produces equivalent pain control to eight hourly administration.

Absorption of the sustained-release tablets is equivalent to that of immediate-release tablet or liquid formulations and is not significantly affected by administration with food. At steady-state, the sustained-release tablets produce peak morphine levels approximately 4 to 5 hours post-dose and therapeutic levels persist for a 12 hour period.

The relationship between mean plasma concentration and dose has been shown to be linear over a dosage range of 60-600 mg/day in the case of the MS Contin tablets.

INDICATIONS: MS Contin (morphine sulfate sustained release) is indicated for the relief of severe pain requiring the prolonged use of an opioid analgesic preparation.

CONTRAINDICATIONS: MS Contin (morphine sulfate sustained release) should not be given to patients with: hypersensitivity to opioid analgesics, morphine or any other component of the product; acute asthma or other obstructive airway disease and acute respiratory depression; cor pulmonale; cardiac arrhythmias; acute alcoholism; delirium tremens; severe CNS depression; convulsive disorders; increased cerebrospinal or intracranial pressure; head injury; brain tumor; suspected surgical abdomen (e.g., paralytic ileus); concomitant MAO inhibitors (or within 14 days of such therapy).

WARNINGS: MS Contin (morphine sulfate sustained release tablets) 15, 30, 60 and 100 mg tablets must be swallowed whole, and must not be chewed, dissolved or crushed. Taking broken, chewed, dissolved or crushed tablets could lead to the rapid release and absorption of a potentially fatal dose of morphine. Only the 200 mg tablet is scored and may be broken in half. The half tablet should also be swallowed intact.

MS Contin 100 mg and 200 mg tablets are for use in opioid tolerant patients only (see also Dosage). These tablet strengths may cause fatal respiratory depression if administered to patients not previously exposed to daily morphine equivalent dosages of 200 mg or more. Care should be taken in the prescribing of these tablet strengths.

Patients should be instructed not to give MS Contin to anyone other than for whom it was prescribed, as such, inappropriate use may have severe medical consequences, including death.

Patients should be cautioned not to consume alcohol while taking MS Contin, as it may increase the chance of experiencing dangerous side effects (see Precautions, Drug Interactions).

MS Contin is not recommended for preoperative use or postoperatively within the first 24 hours.

Abuse of Opioid Formulations: MS Contin consists of a polymer matrix intended for oral use only. Abuse can lead to overdose and death. This risk is increased when the tablets are crushed, broken, dissolved or chewed, and with concurrent consumption of alcohol or other CNS depressants. With parenteral abuse, the tablet excipients, especially talc, can be expected to result in local tissue necrosis, infection, pulmonary granulomas, and increased risk of endocarditis and valvular heart injury.

Drug Dependence: As with other opioids, tolerance and physical dependence tend to develop upon repeated administration of morphine and there is potential for abuse of the drug and for development of strong psychological dependence. MS Contin should therefore be prescribed and handled with the high degree of caution appropriate to the use of a drug with strong abuse potential. Drug abuse is not usually a problem in patients with severe pain in which morphine is appropriately indicated. However, in the absence of a clear indication for a strong opioid analgesic, drug-seeking behaviour must be suspected and resisted, particularly in individuals with a history of, or propensity for drug abuse. Withdrawal symptoms may occur following abrupt discontinuation of morphine therapy or upon administration of an opioid antagonist. Therefore, patients on prolonged therapy should be withdrawn gradually from the drug if it is no longer required for pain control.

Use in Drug and Alcohol Addiction: MS Contin is an opioid with no approved use in the management of addictive disorders. Its proper usage in individuals with drug or alcohol dependence, either active or in remission is for the management of pain requiring opioid analgesia.

CNS Depression: Morphine should be used only with caution and in reduced dosage during concomitant administration of other opioid analgesics, general anaesthetics, phenothiazines and other tranquilizers, sedative-hypnotics, tricyclic antidepressants and other CNS depressants (including alcohol). Respiratory depression, hypotension and profound sedation or coma may result.

Severe pain antagonizes the subjective and respiratory depressant actions of morphine. Should pain suddenly subside, these effects may rapidly become manifest. Patients who are scheduled for cordotomy or other interruption of pain transmission pathways should not receive MS Contin within 24 hours of the procedure.

Pregnancy: Animal studies with morphine and other opioids have indicated the possibility of teratogenic effect. In humans, it is not known whether morphine can cause fetal harm when administered during pregnancy or can affect reproductive capacity. MS Contin should be given to pregnant patients only if clearly needed and when the anticipated benefits outweigh the potential risks to the fetus.

PRECAUTIONS: Respiratory Depression: Morphine should be used with extreme caution in patients with substantially decreased respiratory reserve, pre-existing respiratory depression, hypoxia or hypercapnia. Such patients are often less sensitive to the stimulatory effects of carbon dioxide on the respiratory center and the respiratory depressant effects of morphine may reduce respiratory drive to the point of apnea.

Head Injury: The respiratory depressant effects of morphine, and the capacity to elevate cerebrospinal fluid pressure, may be greatly increased in the presence of an already elevated intracranial pressure produced by trauma. Also, morphine may produce confusion, miosis, vomiting and other side effects which obscure the clinical course of patients with head injury. In such patients, morphine must be used with extreme caution and only if it is judged essential.

Hypotension: Morphine administration may result in severe hypotension in patients whose ability to maintain adequate blood pressure is compromised by reduced blood volume, or concurrent administration of such drugs as phenothiazines or certain anaesthetics.

Acute Abdominal Conditions: Morphine (and other morphine-like opioids) has been shown to decrease bowel motility. Morphine may obscure the diagnosis or clinical course of patients with acute abdominal conditions.

Special Risk Groups: Morphine should be administered with caution, and in reduced dosages, to elderly or debilitated patients, to patients with severely reduced hepatic or renal function, and to patients with adrenocortical insufficiency (e.g., Addison's disease), biliary tract disorders, hypothyroidism, pancreatitis, prostatic hypertrophy or urethral stricture.

Morphine should not be used where there is the possibility of paralytic ileus occurring.

Morphine may lower the seizure threshold in patients with a history of epilepsy.

Labor/Delivery: Morphine crosses the placental barrier and its administration during labour can produce respiratory depression in the neonate.

Lactation: Morphine has been detected in human breast milk. Caution should be exercised if morphine is administered to a nursing mother.

Occupational Hazards: Driving and Operating Dangerous Machinery: Morphine may impair the mental and/or physical abilities needed for certain potentially hazardous activities such as driving a car or operating machinery. Patients should be cautioned accordingly.

Patients should also be cautioned about the combined effects of morphine with other CNS depressants, including other opioids, phenothiazines, sedative/hypnotics and alcohol.

Drug Interactions: Generally, the effects of morphine may be antagonized by acidifying agents and potentiated by alkalizing agents.

The analgesic effect of morphine is potentiated by amphetamines, chlorpromazine and methocarbamol. CNS depressants, such as other opioids, anaesthetics, sedatives, hypnotics, barbiturates, phenothiazines, other tranquilizers, chloral hydrate, glutethimide or gabapentin, may enhance the depressant effect of morphine and may result with respiratory depression, hypotension, profound sedation or coma. Monoamine oxidase inhibitors (including procarbazine hydrochloride) should not be taken within two weeks of use. Pyrazolidone antihistamines, beta-blockers and alcohol may also enhance the depressant effect of morphine. When combined therapy is contemplated, the dose of one or both agents should be reduced.

"In Vitro" Dissolution Studies of Interaction with Alcohol: Increasing concentrations of alcohol in the dissolution medium resulted in a decrease in the rate of release of morphine from MS Contin tablets. The clinical significance of these findings is unknown.

Mixed agonist/antagonist opioid analgesics (i.e., pentazocine, nalbuphine, butorphanol, and buprenorphine) should be administered with caution to a patient who has received or is receiving a course of therapy with a pure opioid agonist analgesic such as morphine. In this situation, mixed agonist/antagonist analgesics may reduce the analgesic effect of morphine and/or may precipitate withdrawal symptoms in these patients.

Morphine may increase the anticoagulant activity of coumarin and other anticoagulants.

ADVERSE EFFECTS: The major hazards associated with morphine, as with other opioid analgesics, are respiratory depression and, to a lesser degree, circulatory depression. Respiratory arrest, shock and cardiac arrest have occurred following oral or parenteral use of morphine.

Most Common Adverse Effects Requiring Medical Attention: The most frequently observed side effects of opioid analgesics such as morphine are sedation, nausea, vomiting, constipation, lightheadedness, dizziness and hyperhidrosis.

Sedation: Some degree of sedation is experienced by most patients upon initiation of therapy. This may be at least partly because patients often recuperate from prolonged fatigue after the relief of persistent pain. Drowsiness usually clears in three to five days and is usually not a reason for concern providing that it is not excessive, or associated with unsteadiness or confusion. If excessive sedation persists, the reason for it must be sought. Some of these are: concomitant sedative medications, hepatic or renal failure, exacerbated respiratory failure, higher doses than tolerated in an older patient, or the patient is actually more severely ill than realized. If it is necessary to reduce the dose, it can be carefully increased again after three or four days if it is obvious that the pain is not being well controlled. Dizziness and unsteadiness may be caused by postural hypotension particularly in elderly or debilitated patients. It can be alleviated if the patient lies down. Because of the slower clearance in patients over 50 years of age, an appropriate dose in this age group may be as low as half or less the usual dose in the younger age group.

Nausea and Vomiting: Nausea and vomiting occur frequently after single doses of opioids or as an early unwanted effect of regular opioid therapy. When instituting prolonged therapy for chronic pain, the routine prescription of an antiemetic should be considered. Patients taking the equivalent of 20 mg or more of oral morphine every four hours (60 mg q12h of MS Contin [morphine sulfate sustained release]) usually require an antiemetic during early therapy. Small doses of prochlorperazine or haloperidol are the most frequently prescribed antiemetics. Nausea and vomiting tend to lessen in a week or so but may persist due to opioid-induced gastric stasis. In such patients, metoclopramide is often useful.

Constipation: Practically all patients become constipated while taking opioids on a persistent basis. In some patients, particularly the elderly or bedridden, fecal impaction may result. It is essential to caution the patients in this regard and to institute an appropriate regimen of bowel management at the start of prolonged opioid therapy. Stool softeners, stimulant laxatives and other appropriate measures should be used as required.

Other Adverse Reactions Include: Cardiovascular: faintness, hypotension, palpitations, syncope and supraventricular tachycardia .

CNS: agitation, confusion, convulsions, dizziness, dysphoria, euphoria, hallucinations, headache, insomnia, involuntary muscle contractions, malaise, mood altered, paresthesia, somnolence, thinking disturbances, vertigo, visual disturbances and weakness.

Dermatologic: edema, other skin rashes, pruritus, and urticaria.

Endocrine: a syndrome of inappropriate antidiuretic hormone secretion characterized by hyponatremia secondary to decreased free-water excretion may be prominent (monitoring of electrolytes may be necessary).

Gastrointestinal: abdominal pain, anorexia, biliary tract spasm, constipation, cramps, dry mouth, dyspepsia, gastrointestinal disorders, ileus, increased hepatic enzymes, nausea, taste perversion and vomiting.

General: allergic reaction, anaphylactic reaction, anaphylactoid reaction, asthenia, drug dependence, drug tolerance, drug withdrawal syndrome, facial flushing, hyperhidrosis, hypertonia and miosis.

Genitourinary: amenorrhea, decreased libido or potency, erectile dysfunction, urinary retention or hesitance.

Metabolic and Nutritional: peripheral edema.

Respiratory: bronchospasm, cough decreased, pulmonary edema and respiratory depression.

Withdrawal (Abstinence) Syndrome: Physical dependence with or without psychological dependence tends to occur with chronic administration. An abstinence syndrome may be precipitated when opioid administration is discontinued or opioid antagonists administered. The following withdrawal symptoms may be observed after opioids are discontinued: body aches, diarrhea, gooseflesh, loss of appetite, nausea, nervousness or restlessness, runny nose, sneezing, stomach cramps, tachycardia, tremors or shivering, trouble with sleeping, unexplained fever, hyperhidrosis, weakness and yawning. With appropriate medical use of opioids and gradual withdrawal from the drug, these symptoms are usually mild.

OVERDOSE:

Symptoms: Serious morphine overdosage is characterized by respiratory depression (reduced respiratory rate and/or tidal volume; Cheyne-Stokes respiration; cyanosis), extreme somnolence progressing to stupor or coma, rhabdomyolysis progressing to renal failure, flaccidity of skeletal muscle, cold or clammy skin, and sometimes hypotension and bradycardia. Pinpoint pupils are a sign of narcotic overdose, but are not pathognomonic (e.g., pontine lesions of hemorrhagic or ischemic origin may produce similar findings). Marked mydriasis rather than miosis may be seen with hypoxia in the setting of morphine overdose. Severe overdosage may result in apnea, circulatory collapse, cardiac arrest and death.

Treatment: Primary attention should be given to the establishment of adequate respiratory exchange through the provision of a patent airway and controlled or assisted ventilation. The opioid antagonist naloxone hydrochloride is a specific antidote against respiratory depression due to overdosage or as a result of unusual sensitivity to morphine. An appropriate dose of one of the antagonists should therefore be administered, preferably by the intravenous route. The usual initial i.v. adult dose of naloxone is 0.4 mg or higher. Concomitant efforts at respiratory resuscitation should be carried out. Since the duration of action of morphine, particularly sustained release formulations, may exceed that of the antagonist, the patient should be under continued surveillance and doses of the antagonist should be repeated as needed to maintain adequate respiration.

An antagonist should not be administered in the absence of clinically significant respiratory or cardiovascular depression. Oxygen, intravenous fluids, vasopressors and other supportive measures should be used as indicated.

In an individual physically dependent on opioids, the administration of the usual dose of opioid antagonist will precipitate an acute withdrawal syndrome. The severity of this syndrome will depend on the degree of physical dependence and the dose of antagonist administered. The use of opioid antagonists in such individuals should be avoided if possible. If an opioid antagonist must be used to treat serious respiratory depression in the physically dependent patient, the antagonist should be administered with extreme care by using dosage titration, commencing with 10 to 20% of the usual recommended initial dose.

Evacuation of gastric contents may be useful in removing unabsorbed drug, particularly when a sustained release oral formulation has been taken.

> For management of a suspected drug overdose, contact your **regional Poison Control Centre**. See the *CPS* Directory section for a list of Poison Control Centres.

DOSAGE: MS Contin 15, 30, 60 and 100 mg tablets must be swallowed intact, not chewed, dissolved or crushed. Taking broken, chewed, dissolved or crushed tablets could lead to the rapid release and absorption of a potentially fatal dose of morphine. Only the 200 mg tablet is scored and may be broken in half. The half tablet should also be swallowed intact.

Administration and dosing of morphine should be individualized bearing in mind the properties of the drug. In addition, the nature and severity of the pain or pains experienced, and the total condition of the patient must be taken into account. Of special importance is other medication given previously or concurrently.

As with other strong opioid analgesics, use of morphine for the management of persistent pain should be preceded by a thorough assessment of the patient and diagnosis of the specific pain or pains and their causes. Use of opioids for the relief of chronic pain, including cancer pain, all important as it may be, should be only one part of a comprehensive approach to pain control including other treatment modalities or drug therapy, non-drug measures and psychosocial support.

For essential information on the important details of the management of cancer pain, the reader may wish to consult the following resources: Cancer pain: a monograph on the management of cancer pain. Ministry of Supplies and Services Canada, 1987. Cat. No. H42-2/5-1984E. Twycross RG, Lack SA. Symptom control in far advanced cancer: pain relief. London: Pitman, 1983.

Adult Dose: Individual dosing requirements vary considerably based on each patient's age, weight, severity of pain, and medical and analgesic history.

The most frequent initial dose is 30 mg orally every 12 hours.

Patients over the age of 50 tend to require much lower doses of morphine than in the younger age group. In elderly and debilitated patients and those with impaired respiratory function or significantly decreased renal function, the initial dose should be one half of the usual recommended dose.

Patients Currently Receiving Opioids: Patients currently receiving other oral morphine formulations may be transferred to MS Contin at the same total daily morphine dosage, equally divided into two 12 hourly MS Contin doses.

For patients who are receiving an alternate opioid, the "oral morphine sulfate equivalent" of the analgesic presently being used should be determined. Having determined the total daily dosage of the present analgesic, the following equivalence table (see Table 1) can be used to calculate the approximate daily oral morphine sulfate dosage that should provide equivalent analgesia. This total daily oral morphine dosage should then be equally divided into two 12 hourly MS Contin doses. Some patients may require a lower dose on initial conversion, followed by further titration during chronic dosing, to maintain optimal analgesia.

Dose Titration: Dose titration is the key to success with morphine therapy. **Proper optimization of doses scaled to the relief of the individual's pain should aim at regular administration of the lowest dose of sustained release morphine (MS Contin) which will achieve the overall treatment goal of satisfactory pain relief with acceptable side effects.**

Dose adjustments should be based on the patient's clinical response. Higher doses, at certain times, may be justified in some patients to cover periods of physical activity.

Because of the sustained release properties of MS Contin, dosage adjustments should generally be separated by 48 hours. If dose increments turn out to be required, they should be proportionately greater at the lower dose level (in terms of percentage of previous dose), than when adjusting a higher dose. The usual recommended dose (q12h) increments for MS Contin tablets are 15, 30, 45, 60, 90, 120, 150, 180 and 200 mg. Above the 200 mg/dose (400 mg/day) increments should be by 30-60 mg/dose.

MS Contin is designed to allow 12 hourly dosing. If "breakthrough" pain repeatedly occurs at the end of a dose interval, it is generally an indication for a dosage increase, **not** more frequent administration of sustained release morphine (MS Contin). However, where judged necessary for optimization of drug effects, MS Contin tablets may be administered q8h. More frequent (than q8h) administration is not recommended.

Adjustment or Reduction of Dosage: Following successful relief of severe pain, periodic attempts to reduce the opioid dose should be made. Smaller doses or complete discontinuation may become feasible due to a change in the patient's condition or improved mental state. If treatment discontinuation is required, the dose of opioid may be decreased as follows: one-half of the previous daily dose given q12h for the first two days, followed thereafter by a 25% reduction every two days.

Opioid analgesics may only be partially effective in relieving dysesthetic pain, postherpetic neuralgia, stabbing pains, activity-related pain and some forms of headache. That is not to say that patients with advanced cancer suffering from some of these forms of pain should not be given an adequate trial of opioid analgesics, but it may be necessary to refer such patients at an early time to other forms of pain therapy.

Table 1: MS Contin

Opioid Analgesics: Approximate Analgesic Equivalences[a]

Drug	Equivalent Dose (mg)[b] (compared to morphine 10 mg IM)		Duration of Action (hours)
	Parenteral	Oral	
Strong Opioid Agonists			
Morphine	10[c]	60[c]	3–4
Hydromorphone	1.5	7.5	2–4
Anileridine	25	75	2–3
Levorphanol	2	4	4–8
Meperidine[d]	75	300	1–3
Oxymorphone	1.5	5 (rectal)	3–4
Methadone[e]	—	—	—
Heroin	5–8	10–15	3–4
Weak Opioid Agonists			
Codeine	120	200	3–4
Oxycodone	—	10–15[f]	2–4
Propoxyphene	50	100	2–4
Mixed Agonist-Antagonists[g]			
Pentazocine[d]	60	180	3–4
Nalbuphine	10	—	3–6
Butorphanol	2	—	3–4

[a] References:
Expert Advisory Committee on the Management of Severe Chronic Pain in Cancer Patients, Health and Welfare Canada. Cancer pain: A monograph on the management of cancer pain. Ministry of Supplies and Services Canada, 1987. Cat. No. H42-2/5-1984E.
Foley KM. The treatment of cancer pain. N Engl J Med 1985;313(2):84-95.
Aronoff GM, Evans WO. Pharmacological management of chronic pain: A review. In: Aronoff GM, editor. Evaluation and treatment of chronic pain. 2nd ed. Baltimore (MD): Williams and Wilkins; 1992. p. 359-68.
Cherny NI, Portenoy RK. Practical issues in the management of cancer pain. In: Wall PD, Melzack R, editors. Textbook of pain. 3rd ed. New York: Churchill Livingstone; 1994. p. 1437-67.

[b] **Most of this data was derived from single-dose, acute pain studies and should be considered an approximation for selection of doses when treating chronic pain.**

[c] **For acute pain, the oral or rectal dose of morphine is six times the injectable dose. However, for chronic dosing, clinical experience indicates that this ratio is 2-3: 1 (i.e., 20-30 mg of oral or rectal morphine is equivalent to 10 mg of parenteral morphine).**

[d] These drugs are not recommended for the management of chronic pain.

[e] Extremely variable equianalgesic dose. Patients should undergo individualized titration starting at an equivalent to 1/10 of the morphine dose.

[f] In combination with acetaminophen or ASA. For acute pain, single entity oral oxycodone is twice as potent as oral morphine.

[g] Mixed agonist-antagonists can precipitate withdrawal in patients on pure opioid agonists.

INFORMATION FOR THE PATIENT: Published in e-CPS, available by subscription at www.e-cps.ca.

SUPPLIED: 15 mg: Each green, round, sustained-release, film-coated, biconvex tablet, imprinted with PF on one side and 15 mg on the other, contains: morphine sulfate 15 mg. Nonmedicinal ingredients: cetostearyl alcohol, hydroxyethyl cellulose, lactose, magnesium stearate and talc; film coating: Opadry OY-8855 Green: D&C Yellow No. 10 Aluminum Lake, FD&C Blue No. 1 Aluminum Lake, FD&C Blue No. 2 Aluminum Lake, hydroxypropyl methylcellulose, polyethylene glycol 400 and titanium dioxide. Alcohol-, gluten-, sulfite- and tartrazine-free. Plastic, opaque bottles of 50. Store at 15 to 30 °C.

30 mg: Each violet, round, sustained-release, film-coated, biconvex tablet, imprinted with PF on one side and 30 mg on the other, contains: morphine sulfate 30 mg. Nonmedicinal ingredients: cetostearyl alcohol, hydroxyethyl cellulose, lactose, magnesium stearate and talc; film coating: Opadry YS-1-4729 Purple: D&C Red No. 7 Calcium Lake, FD&C Blue No. 2 Aluminum Lake, FD&C Yellow No. 6 Aluminum Lake, hydroxypropyl methylcellulose, polyethylene glycol 400, polysorbate 80 and titanium dioxide. Alcohol-, gluten-, sulfite- and tartrazine-free. Plastic, opaque bottles of 50. Store at 15 to 30 °C.

60 mg: Each orange, round, sustained-release, film-coated, biconvex tablet, imprinted with PF on one side and 60 mg on the other, contains: morphine sulfate 60 mg. Nonmedicinal ingredients: cetostearyl alcohol, hydroxyethyl cellulose, lactose, magnesium stearate and talc; film coating: Opadry OY-3508 Orange: D&C Yellow No. 10 Aluminum Lake, FD&C Red No. 3 Aluminum Lake, FD&C Yellow No. 6 Aluminum Lake, hydroxypropyl methylcellulose, polyethylene glycol 400 and titanium dioxide. Alcohol-, gluten-, sulfite- and tartrazine-free. Plastic, opaque bottles of 50. Store at 15 to 30 °C.

100 mg: Each grey, round, sustained-release, film-coated, biconvex tablet, imprinted with PF on one side and 100 mg on the other, contains: morphine sulfate 100 mg. Nonmedicinal ingredients: cetostearyl alcohol, hydroxyethyl cellulose, magnesium stearate and talc; film coating: Opadry OY-8215 Grey: FD&C Blue No. 2 Aluminum Lake, hydroxypropyl methylcellulose, iron oxide, yellow, iron oxide, black, polyethylene glycol 400 and titanium dioxide. Alcohol-, gluten-, lactose-, sulfite- and tartrazine-free. Plastic, opaque bottles of 50. Store at 15 to 30 °C.

200 mg: Each red, scored, caplet-shaped, sustained-release, film-coated, biconvex tablet, imprinted with PF on one side and 200 mg on the other, contains: morphine sulfate 200 mg. Nonmedicinal ingredients: cetostearyl alcohol, hydroxyethyl cellulose, magnesium stearate and talc; film coating: Opadry OY-5970: FD&C Blue No. 2, FD&C Red No. 3, FD&C Yellow No. 6 Aluminum Lake, hydroxypropyl methylcellulose, polyethylene glycol 400 and titanium dioxide. May be broken in half. Alcohol-, gluten-, lactose-, sulfite- and tartrazine-free. Plastic, opaque bottles of 50. Store at 15 to 30 °C.

(Shown in Product Identification Section)

MS•IR® Ⓝ

morphine sulfate

Opioid Analgesic

Purdue Pharma

Date of Revision: August 25, 2009

PHARMACOLOGY: Morphine is an opioid analgesic which exerts an agonist effect at specific, saturable opioid receptors in the CNS and other tissues. In man, morphine produces a variety of effects including analgesia, constipation from decreased gastrointestinal motility, suppression of the cough reflex, respiratory depression from reduced responsiveness of the respiratory centre to CO_2, nausea and vomiting via stimulation of the CTZ, changes in mood including euphoria and dysphoria, sedation, mental clouding, and alterations of the endocrine and autonomic nervous systems.

Morphine is readily absorbed when given orally, rectally or by s.c. or i.m. injection. Due to first-pass metabolism in the liver, the effect of an oral dose is less than after parenteral administration. With repeated regular dosing, oral morphine is about 1/3 as potent as when given by i.m. injection. Morphine is primarily excreted in the urine as morphine-3-glucuronide. About 7 to 10% of a dose of morphine is excreted in the feces via the bile.

INDICATIONS: For the symptomatic relief of severe pain.

CONTRAINDICATIONS: MS•IR (morphine sulfate tablets) should not be given to patients with: hypersensitivity to opioid analgesics morphine or any other component of the product; in acute asthma or other obstructive airway disease and acute respiratory depression; cor pulmonale; cardiac arrhythmias; acute alcoholism; delirium tremens; severe CNS depression; convulsive disorders; increased cerebrospinal or intracranial pressure; head injury; brain tumor; suspected surgical abdomen (e.g., paralytic ileus); concomitant MAO inhibitors (or within 14 days of such therapy).

WARNINGS: Abuse of Opioid Formulations: MS•IR (morphine sulfate tablets) is intended for oral use only. Abuse can lead to overdose and death. This risk is increased if MS•IR is taken with alcohol or other CNS depressants. With parenteral abuse, the tablet excipients, can be expected to result in local tissue necrosis, infection, pulmonary granulomas, and increased risk of endocarditis and valvular heart injury.

Patients should be instructed not to give MS•IR to anyone other than for whom it was prescribed, as such, inappropriate use may have severe medical consequences, including death.

Patients should be cautioned not to consume alcohol while taking MS•IR, as it may increase the chance of experiencing dangerous side effects.

MS•IR should be used with caution preoperatively and within the first 24 hours postoperatively.

Drug Dependence: As with other opioids, tolerance and physical dependence tend to develop upon repeated administration of morphine and there is potential for abuse of the drug and for development of strong psychological dependence. MS•IR should therefore be prescribed and handled with the high degree of caution appropriate to the use of a drug with strong abuse potential. Drug abuse is not usually a problem in patients with severe pain in which morphine is appropriately indicated. However, in the absence of a clear indication for a strong opioid analgesic, drug-seeking behaviour must be suspected and resisted, particularly in individuals with a history of, or propensity for drug abuse. Withdrawal symptoms may occur following abrupt discontinuation of morphine therapy or upon administration of a opioid antagonist. Therefore, patients on prolonged therapy should be withdrawn gradually from the drug if it is no longer required for pain control.

CNS Depression: Morphine should be used only with caution and in reduced dosage during concomitant administration of other opioid analgesics, general anaesthetics, phenothiazines and other tranquilizers, sedative-hypnotics, tricyclic antidepressants and other CNS depressants (including alcohol). Respiratory depression, hypotension and profound sedation or coma may result.

Severe pain antagonizes the subjective and respiratory depressant actions of morphine. Should pain suddenly subside, these effects may rapidly become manifest. Patients who are scheduled for cordotomy or other interruption of pain transmission pathways should not receive MS•IR within 24 hours of the procedure.

Pregnancy: Animal studies with morphine and other opioids have indicated the possibility of teratogenic effect. In humans, it is not known whether morphine can cause fetal harm when administered during pregnancy or can affect reproductive capacity. MS•IR should be given to pregnant patients only if clearly needed and when the anticipated benefits outweigh the risks to the fetus.

PRECAUTIONS: Respiratory Depression: Morphine should be used with extreme caution in patients with substantially decreased respiratory reserve, pre-existing respiratory depression, hypoxia or hypercapnia. Such patients are often less sensitive to the stimulatory effects of carbon dioxide on the respiratory center and the respiratory depressant effects of morphine may reduce respiratory drive to the point of apnea.

Head Injury: The respiratory depressant effects of morphine, and the capacity to elevate cerebrospinal fluid pressure, may be greatly increased in the presence of an already elevated intracranial pressure produced by trauma. Also, morphine may produce confusion, miosis, vomiting and other side effects which obscure the clinical course of patients with head injury. In such patients, morphine must be used with extreme caution and only if it is judged essential.

Hypotension: Morphine administration may result in severe hypotension in patients whose ability to maintain adequate blood pressure is compromised by reduced blood volume, or concurrent administration of such drugs as phenothiazines or certain anaesthetics.

Acute Abdominal Conditions: Morphine has been shown to decrease bowel motility. Morphine may obscure the diagnosis or clinical course of patients with acute abdominal conditions.

Special Risk Groups: Morphine should be administered with caution, and in reduced dosages, to elderly or debilitated patients, to patients with severely reduced hepatic or renal function, and to patients with adrenocortical insufficiency (e.g., Addison's disease), biliary tract disorders, hypothyroidism, pancreatitis, prostatic hypertrophy or urethral stricture.

Morphine should not be used where there is the possibility of paralytic ileus occurring.

Morphine may lower the seizure threshold in patients with a history of epilepsy.

Labor/Delivery: Morphine crosses the placental barrier and its administration during labor can produce respiratory depression in the neonate.

Lactation: Morphine has been detected in human breast milk. Caution should be exercised if morphine is administered to a nursing mother.

Occupational Hazards: Driving and Operating Dangerous Machinery: Morphine may impair the mental and/or physical abilities needed for certain potentially hazardous activities such as driving a car or operating machinery. Patients should be cautioned accordingly.

Patients should also be cautioned about the combined effects of morphine with other CNS depressants, including other opioids, phenothiazines, sedative/hypnotics and alcohol.

Drug Interactions: Generally, the effects of morphine may be antagonized by acidifying agents and potentiated by alkalizing agents. The analgesic effect of morphine is potentiated by amphetamines, chlorpromazine and methocarbamol. CNS depressants, such as other opioids, anaesthetics, sedatives, hypnotics, barbiturates, phenothiazines and other tranquilizers, gabapentin, chloral hydrate and glutethimide may enhance the depressant effect of morphine and may result with respiratory depression, hypotension, profound sedation or coma. Monoamine oxidase inhibitors (including procarbazine hydrochloride) should not be taken within two weeks of use. Pyrazolidone antihistamines, beta-blockers and alcohol may also enhance the depressant effect of morphine. When combined therapy is contemplated, the dose of one or both agents should be reduced.

Mixed agonist/antagonist opioid analgesics (i.e., pentazocine, nalbuphine, butorphanol, and buprenorphine) should be administered with caution to a patient who has received or is receiving a course of therapy with a pure opioid agonist analgesic such as morphine. In this situation, mixed agonist/antagonist analgesics may reduce the analgesic effect of morphine and/or may precipitate withdrawal symptoms in these patients.

Morphine may increase the anticoagulant activity of coumarin and other anticoagulants.

ADVERSE EFFECTS: The major hazards associated with morphine, as with other opioid analgesics, are respiratory depression and, to a lesser degree, circulatory depression. Respiratory arrest, shock and cardiac arrest have occurred following oral or parenteral use of morphine.

The most frequently observed side effects of opioid analgesics such as morphine are sedation, nausea, vomiting, constipation, lightheadedness, dizziness, and hyperhidrosis.
Sedation: Some degree of sedation is experienced by most patients upon initiation of therapy. This may be a least partly because patients often recuperate from prolonged fatigue after the relief of persistent pain. Drowsiness usually clears in three to five days and is usually not a reason for concern providing that it is not excessive, or associated with unsteadiness or confusion. If excessive sedation persists, the reason for it must be sought. Some of these are: concomitant sedative medications, hepatic or renal failure, exacerbated respiratory failure, higher doses than tolerated in an older patients, or the patient is actually more severely ill than realized. If it is necessary to reduce the dose, it can be carefully increased again after three or four days if it is obvious that the pain is not being well controlled. Dizziness and unsteadiness may be caused by postural hypotension particularly in elderly or debilitated patients. It can be alleviated if the patient lies down. Because of the slower clearance in patients over 50 years of age, an appropriate dose in this age group may be as low as half or less the usual dose in the younger age group.
Nausea and Vomiting: Nausea and vomiting occur frequently after single doses of opioids or as an early unwanted effect of regular opioid therapy. When instituting prolonged therapy for chronic pain, the routine prescription of an antiemetic should be considered. Patients taking a single dose of 20 mg or more of oral morphine every four hours usually require an antiemetic during early therapy. Small doses of prochlorperazine or haloperidol are the most frequently prescribed antiemetics. Nausea and vomiting tend to lessen in a week or so but may persist due to opioid-induced gastric stasis. In such patients, metoclopramide is often useful.
Constipation: Practically all patients become constipated while taking opioids on a persistent basis. In some instances, particularly the elderly or bedridden, fecal impaction may result. It is essential to caution the patients in this regard and to institute an appropriate regimen of bowel management at the start of prolonged opioid therapy. Stool softeners, stimulant laxatives and other appropriate measures should be used as required.
Other Adverse Reactions Include: Cardiovascular: faintness, hypotension, palpitations, supraventricular tachycardia and syncope.
Central Nervous System: agitation, confusion, convulsions, dizziness, dysphoria, euphoria, hallucinations, headache, insomnia, involuntary muscle contractions, malaise, mood altered, paresthesia, somnolence, thinking disturbances, vertigo, visual disturbance and weakness.
Dermatologic: edema, pruritus, other skin rashes and urticaria.
Endocrine: a syndrome of inappropriate antidiuretic hormone secretion characterized by hyponatremia secondary to decreased free-water excretion may be prominent (monitoring of electrolytes may be necessary).
Gastrointestinal: abdominal pain, anorexia, biliary tract spasms, constipation, cramps, dry mouth, dyspepsia, gastrointestinal disorders, ileus, increased hepatic enzymes, nausea, taste perversion and vomiting.
General: allergic reaction, anaphylactic reaction, anaphylactoid reaction, asthenia, drug dependence, drug tolerance, drug withdrawal syndrome, facial flushing, hyperhidrosis, hypertonia and miosis.
Genitourinary: amenorrhea, decreased libido or potency, erectile dysfunction, urinary retention or hesitance.
Metabolic and Nutritional: peripheral edema.
Respiratory: bronchospasm, cough decreased, pulmonary edema, and respiratory depression.
Withdrawal (Abstinence) Syndrome: Physical dependence with or without psychological dependence tends to occur with chronic administration. An abstinence syndrome may be precipitated when opioid administration is discontinued or opioid antagonists administered. The following withdrawal symptoms may be observed after opioids are discontinued: body aches, diarrhea, gooseflesh, loss of appetite, nervousness or restlessness, runny nose, sneezing, tremors or shivering, stomach cramps, nausea, trouble with sleeping, hyperhidrosis and yawning, weakness, tachycardia and unexplained fever. With appropriate medical use of opioids and gradual withdrawal from the drug, these symptoms are usually mild.

OVERDOSE:

Symptoms: Serious morphine overdosage is characterized by respiratory depression (reduced respiratory rate and/or tidal volume; Cheyne-Stokes respiration; cyanosis), extreme somnolence progressing to stupor or coma, rhabdomyolysis progressing to renal failure, flaccidity of skeletal muscle, cold or clammy skin, and sometimes hypotension and bradycardia. Pinpoint pupils are a sign of narcotic overdose, but are not pathognomonic (e.g., pontine lesions of hemorrhagic or ischemic origin may produce similar findings). Marked mydriasis rather than miosis may be seen with hypoxia in the setting of morphine overdose. Severe overdosage may result in apnea, circulatory collapse, cardiac arrest and death.

Treatment: Primary attention should be given to the establishment of adequate respiratory exchange through the provision of a patent airway and controlled or assisted ventilation. The opioid antagonist naloxone hydrochloride is a specific antidote against respiratory depression due to overdosage or as a result of unusual sensitivity to morphine. An appropriate dose should therefore be administered, preferably by the intravenous route. The usual initial i.v. adult dose of naloxone is 0.4 mg or higher. Concomitant efforts at respiratory resuscitation should be carried out. Since the duration of action of morphine may exceed that of the antagonist, the patient should be under continued surveillance and doses of the antagonist should be repeated as needed to maintain adequate respiration.

An antagonist should not be administered in the absence of clinically significant respiratory or cardiovascular depression. Oxygen, intravenous fluids, vasopressors and other supportive measures should be used as indicated.

In an individual physically dependent on opioids, the administration of the usual dose of opioid antagonist will precipitate an acute withdrawal syndrome. The severity of this syndrome will depend on the degree of physical dependence and the dose of antagonist administered. The use of opioid antagonists in such individuals should be avoided if possible. If an opioid antagonist must be used to treat serious respiratory depression in the physically dependent patient, the antagonist should be administered with extreme care by using dosage titration, commencing with 10 to 20% of the usual recommended initial dose.

Evacuation of gastric contents may be useful in removing unabsorbed drug.

For management of a suspected drug overdose, contact your **regional Poison Control Centre**. See the *CPS* Directory section for a list of Poison Control Centres.

DOSAGE: Administration and dosing of morphine should be individualized bearing in mind the properties of the drug. In addition, the nature and severity of the pain or pains experienced, and the total condition of the patient must be taken into account. Of special importance is other medication given previously or concurrently.

As with other strong opioid analgesics, use of morphine for the management of persistent pain should be preceded by a thorough assessment of the patient and diagnosis of the specific pain or pains and their causes. Use of opioids for the relief of chronic pain, including cancer pain, all important as it may be, should be only one part of a comprehensive approach to pain control including other treatment modalities or drug therapy, non-drug measures and psychosocial support.
Adult Dose: Individual dosing requirements vary considerably based on each patient's age, weight, severity of pain, and medical and analgesic history.

The most frequent initial dose is 10 mg every 4 hours as needed for acute pain and every 4 hours around the clock for chronic pain, or as directed by a physician. The suppository may be used in situations where the patient cannot tolerate oral dosing, at the same dosage and frequency.

Patients over the age of 50 tend to require much lower doses of morphine than in the younger age group. In elderly and debilitated patients and those with impaired respiratory function or significantly decreased renal function, the initial dose should be one half the usual recommended dose.
Patients Currently Receiving Opioids: For patients who are receiving an alternate opioid, the "oral morphine sulfate equivalent" of the analgesic presently being used should be determined. Having determined the total daily dosage of the present analgesic, Table 1 can be used to calculate the approximate daily oral morphine sulfate dosage that should provide equivalent analgesia.
Dose Titration: Dose titration is the key to success with morphine therapy. **Proper optimization of doses scaled to the relief of the individual's pain should aim at regular administration of the lowest dose of immediate release morphine (MS•IR) which will achieve the overall treatment goal of satisfactory pain relief with acceptable side effects.**

Dose adjustments should be based on the patient's clinical response. Higher doses may be justified in some patients to cover periods of physical activity.
Adjustment or Reduction of Dosage: Following successful relief of severe pain, periodic attempts to reduce the opioid dose should be made. Smaller doses or complete discontinuation may become feasible due to a change in the patient's condition or improved mental state. If treatment discontinuation is required, the dose of opioid may be decreased as follows: one-half of the previous daily dose given q4h for the first two days, followed thereafter by a 25% reduction every two days.

Opioid analgesics may only be partially effective in relieving dysesthetic pain, post-herpetic neuralgia, stabbing pains, activity-related pain, and some forms of headache. This is not to say that patients with advanced cancer suffering from some of these forms of pain should not be given an adequate trial of opiate analgesics, but it may be necessary to refer such patients at an early time for other forms of pain therapy.

Table 1: MS•IR
Opioid Analgesics: Approximate Analgesic Equivalences[a]

Drug	Equivalent Dose (mg)[b] (compared to morphine 10 mg IM)		Duration of Action (hours)
	Parenteral	Oral	
Strong Opioid Agonists			
Morphine	10	60[c]	3–4
Oxycodone	15	30[d]	2–4
Hydromorphone	1.5	7.5	2–4
Anileridine	25	75	2–3
Levorphanol	2	4	4–8
Meperidine[f]	75	300	1–3
Oxymorphone	1.5	5 (rectal)	3–4
Methadone[e]	—	—	—
Heroin	5–8	10–15	3–4
Weak Opioid Agonists			
Codeine	120	200	3–4
Propoxyphene	50	100	2–4
Mixed Agonist-Antagonists[g]			
Pentazocine[f]	60	180	3–4
Nalbuphine	10	—	3–6
Butorphanol	2	—	3–4

[a] References:
Expert Advisory Committee on the Management of Severe Chronic Pain in Cancer Patients, Health and Welfare Canada. Cancer pain: A monograph on the management of cancer pain. Ministry of Supplies and Services Canada, 1987. Cat. No. H42-2/5-1984E.
Foley KM. The treatment of cancer pain. N Engl J Med 1985;313(2):84-95.
Aronoff GM, Evans WO. Pharmacological management of chronic pain: A review. In: Aronoff GM, editor. Evaluation and treatment of chronic pain. 2nd ed. Baltimore (MD): Williams and Wilkins; 1992. p. 359-68.
Cherny NI, Portenoy RK. Practical issues in the management of cancer pain. In: Wall PD, Melzack R, editors. Textbook of pain. 3rd ed. New York: Churchill Livingstone; 1994. p. 1437-67.
[b] **Most of the data were derived from single-dose, acute pain studies and should be considered an approximation for selection of doses when treating chronic pain.**
[c] **For acute pain, the oral or rectal dose of morphine is six times the injectable dose. However, for chronic dosing, clinical experience indicates that this ratio is 2-3: 1 (i.e., 20-30 mg of oral or rectal morphine is equivalent to 10 mg of parenteral morphine).**
[d] Based on single entity oral oxycodone in acute pain.
[e] Extremely variable equianalgesic dose. Patients should undergo individualized titration starting at an equivalent to 1/10 of the morphine dose.
[f] Not recommended for the management of chronic pain.
[g] Mixed agonist-antagonists can precipitate withdrawal in patients on pure opioid agonists.

INFORMATION FOR THE PATIENT: Published in e-CPS, available by subscription at www.e-cps.ca.

SUPPLIED: 5 mg: Each round, white, film-coated, immediate-release tablet, scored with "5" engraved on one side and "PF" on the other, contains: morphine sulfate pentahydrate 5 mg. Nonmedicinal ingredients: croscarmellose sodium, hydroxypropyl methylcellulose, lactose, magnesium stearate, microcrystalline cellulose and polyethylene glycol 400. Opaque plastic bottles of 50. Store at room temperature (15-30° C).
10 mg: Each round, white, film-coated, immediate-release tablet, scored with "10" engraved on one side and "PF" on the other, contains: morphine sulfate pentahydrate 10 mg. Nonmedicinal ingredients: croscarmellose sodium, hydroxypropyl methylcellulose, lactose, magnesium stearate, microcrystalline cellulose and polyethylene glycol 400. Opaque plastic bottles of 50. Store at room temperature (15-30° C).
20 mg: Each caplet-shaped, white, film-coated, immediate-release tablet, scored with "20" engraved on one side and "PF" on the other, contains: morphine sulfate pentahydrate 20 mg. Nonmedicinal ingredients: croscarmellose sodium, hydroxypropyl methylcellulose, lactose, magnesium stearate, microcrystalline cellulose and polyethylene glycol 400. Opaque plastic bottles of 50. Store at room temperature (15-30° C).
30 mg: Each caplet-shaped, white, film-coated, immediate-release tablet, scored with "30" engraved on one side and "PF" on the other, contains: morphine sulfate pentahydrate 30 mg. Nonmedicinal ingredients: croscarmellose sodium, hydroxypropyl methylcellulose, lactose, magnesium stearate, microcrystalline cellulose and polyethylene glycol 400. Opaque plastic bottles of 50. Store at room temperature (15-30° C).

(Shown in Product Identification Section)

Mucomyst®
acetylcysteine
Mucolytic—Antidote for Acetaminophen Poisoning

WellSpring

PHARMACOLOGY: The viscosity of pulmonary mucous secretions depends on the concentrations of mucoprotein and to a lesser extent deoxyribonucleic acid (DNA). The latter increases with increasing purulence owing to cellular debris. The mucolytic action of acetylcysteine is related to the sulfhydryl group in the molecule. This group probably "opens" disulfide linkages in mucus thereby lowering the viscosity. The mucolytic activity of acetylcysteine is unaltered by the presence of DNA, and increases with increasing pH. Significant mucolysis occurs between pH 7 and 9.

Acetaminophen is rapidly absorbed from the upper gastrointestinal tract with peak plasma levels occurring between 30 and 60 minutes after therapeutic doses and usually within 4 hours following an overdose. The parent compound, which is non-toxic, is extensively metabolized in the liver to form principally the sulfate and glucuronide conjugates which are also nontoxic and are rapidly excreted in the urine.

A small fraction of the ingested dose is metabolized in the liver by the cytochrome P-450 mixed function oxidase enzyme system to form a reactive, potentially toxic, intermediate metabolite which preferentially conjugates with hepatic glutathione to form the nontoxic cysteine and mercapturic acid derivatives which are then excreted by the kidney.

Therapeutic doses of acetaminophen do not saturate the glucuronide and sulfate conjugation pathways and do not result in formation of sufficient reactive metabolite to deplete glutathione stores.

However, following ingestion of a large overdose (150 mg/kg or greater) the glucuronide and sulfate conjugation pathways are saturated resulting in a larger fraction of the drug being metabolized via the P-450 pathway. The increased formation of reactive metabolite may deplete the hepatic stores of glutathione with subsequent binding of the metabolite to protein molecules within the hepatocyte resulting in cellular necrosis. Acetylcysteine probably protects the liver by maintaining or restoring the glutathione levels, or by acting as an alternate substrate for conjugation with and thus detoxification of the reactive metabolite.

INDICATIONS: As adjuvant therapy for patients with abnormal, viscid, or inspissated mucous secretions in such conditions as: chronic bronchopulmonary disease (chronic emphysema, emphysema with bronchitis, chronic asthmatic bronchitis, tuberculosis, bronchiectasis and primary amyloidosis of the lung); acute bronchopulmonary disease (pneumonia, bronchitis, tracheobronchitis); pulmonary complications of cystic fibrosis; post-tracheostomy care; pulmonary complications associated with surgery; use during anesthesia; post-traumatic chest conditions; atelectasis due to mucous obstruction; diagnostic bronchial studies (bronchograms, bronchospirometry and bronchial wedge catheterization).

Administered orally or i.v., as an antidote to prevent or lessen hepatic injury which may occur following the ingestion of a potentially hepatotoxic quantity of acetaminophen.

CONTRAINDICATIONS: In those patients who are sensitive or who have developed a sensitivity to it.

There are no contraindications to oral or i.v. administration of acetylcysteine in the treatment of acetaminophen overdose.

WARNINGS: After proper administration of acetylcysteine, an increased volume of liquefied bronchial secretions may occur. When cough is inadequate, the open airway must be maintained by mechanical suction if necessary. When there is a large mechanical block due to foreign body or local accumulation, the airway should be cleared by endotracheal aspiration, with or without bronchoscopy.

Asthmatics under treatment with acetylcysteine should be watched carefully. If bronchospasm progresses, this medication should be immediately discontinued.

Generalized urticaria has been observed rarely in patients receiving oral acetylcysteine for acetaminophen overdose. If this occurs and other allergic symptoms appear, treatment with acetylcysteine should be discontinued unless it is deemed essential and the allergic symptoms cannot be otherwise controlled.

If encephalopathy due to hepatic failure is evident, acetylcysteine treatment should be discontinued to avoid further administration of nitrogenous substances. There are no data indicating acetylcysteine adversely influences hepatic failure; however, this remains a theoretical possibility.

Based on a single reported case, it is recommended that physicians pay particular attention to neurological functions when high-dose N-acetylcysteine is utilized as an antidote in the treatment of acetaminophen poisoning.

PRECAUTIONS: With the administration of acetylcysteine as a mucolytic agent, the patient may initially notice a slight disagreeable odor which soon is not noticeable. With a face mask, there may be a stickiness on the face after nebulization which is easily removed by washing with water.

Acetylcysteine is not compatible with rubber and metals, particularly iron, copper and nickel. Silicone and lacquered rubber and plastic are satisfactory for use with acetylcysteine.

Under certain conditions, a color change may take place in the solution of acetylcysteine in the open vial. The light purple color is the result of a chemical reaction which does not significantly impair the safety or mucolytic efficacy of acetylcysteine.

Continued nebulization of an acetylcysteine solution with a dry gas will result in an increased concentration of the drug in the nebulizer because of evaporation of the solvent. Extreme concentration may impede nebulization and efficient delivery of the drug. Dilution of the nebulizing solution with Sterile Water for Injection USP, as concentration occurs, will obviate this problem.

Occasionally severe and persistent vomiting occurs as a symptom of acute acetaminophen overdose. Treatment with oral acetylcysteine may aggravate the vomiting. Patients at risk of gastric hemorrhage (e.g., esophageal varices, peptic ulcers, etc.) should be evaluated concerning the risk of upper gastrointestinal hemorrhage versus the risk of developing hepatic toxicity, and treatment with acetylcysteine given accordingly. Dilution of the acetylcysteine with cola drinks minimizes the propensity of oral acetylcysteine to aggravate vomiting.

Drug/Laboratory Interaction: Acetylcysteine may cause a false-positive reaction with reagent dipstick tests for urinary ketones.

ADVERSE EFFECTS: Adverse reactions have been included in order of frequency: stomatitis, nausea and rhinorrhea. Sensitivity and sensitization to acetylcysteine have been reported very rarely. A few susceptible patients, particularly asthmatics (see Warnings), may experience varying degrees of bronchospasm associated with the administration of nebulized acetylcysteine. Most patients with such bronchospasm are quickly relieved by the use of a bronchodilator given by nebulization.

Oral or i.v. administration of acetylcysteine, especially in the large doses needed to treat acetaminophen overdose, in order of frequency may result in nausea, vomiting and other gastrointestinal symptoms. Hypersensitivity reactions following the i.v. administration of acetylcysteine have been reported. Symptoms include rashes, facial edema, urticaria, hypotension and bronchospasm.

Compatibility: The physical and chemical compatibility of acetylcysteine solutions with other drugs commonly administered by nebulization, direct instillation, or topical application, has been studied.

Acetylcysteine should not be mixed with all antibiotics. For example, the antibiotics tetracycline HCl, oxytetracycline HCl and erythromycin lactobionate were found to be incompatible when mixed in the same solution. These agents may be administered from separate solutions if administration of these agents is desirable.

OVERDOSE:

No data supplied by the manufacturer.

For management of a suspected drug overdose, CPhA recommends that you contact your **regional Poison Control Centre**. See the *CPS* Directory section for a list of Poison Control Centres.

DOSAGE: As a Mucolytic Agent: The 20% solution may be diluted to a lesser concentration with either sterile normal saline or Sterile Water for Injection, USP. Any unused portion of a vial should be refrigerated and used within 96 hours.

Nebulization-face mask, mouth piece, tracheostomy: When nebulized into a face mask, mouth piece or tracheostomy, 1 to 10 mL of the 20% solution may be given every 2 to 6 hours; the recommended dose for most patients is 3 to 5 mL of the 20% solution 3 to 4 times daily.

Nebulization-tent, croupette: In special circumstances it may be necessary to nebulize into a tent or croupette, and this method of use must be individualized to take into account the available equipment and the patient's particular needs. This form of administration requires very large volumes of the solution, occasionally as much as 300 mL during a single treatment period. If a tent or croupette must be used, the recommended dose is the volume of solution that will maintain a very heavy mist in the tent or croupette for the desired period. Administration for intermittent or continuous prolonged periods, including overnight, may be desirable.

Direct instillation: When used by direct instillation, 1 to 2 mL of a 10 to 20% solution may be given as often as every hour.

When used for the routine nursing care of patients with tracheostomy, 1 to 2 mL of a 10 to 20% solution may be given every 1 to 4 hours by instillation into the tracheostomy.

Acetylcysteine may be introduced directly into a particular segment of the bronchopulmonary tree by inserting (under local anesthesia and direct vision) a small plastic catheter into the trachea. Two to 5 mL of the 20% solution may then be instilled by means of a syringe connected to the catheter.

Acetylcysteine may also be given through a percutaneous intratracheal catheter. One to 2 mL of the 20% solution may be given every 1 to 4 hours by a syringe attached to the catheter.

Diagnostic Bronchograms: For diagnostic bronchial studies, 2 or 3 administrations of 1 to 2 mL of the 20% solution should be given by nebulization or by instillation intratracheally, prior to the procedure.

Administration of Aerosol: Materials: Acetylcysteine may be administered using conventional nebulizers made of plastic or glass. Certain materials used in nebulization equipment react with acetylcysteine. The most reactive of these are certain metals (notably iron and copper), and rubber. Where materials may come into contact with acetylcysteine solution, parts made of the following acceptable materials should be used: glass, plastic, aluminum, anodized aluminum, chromed metal, tantalum, sterling silver or stainless steel. Silver may become tarnished after exposure, but this is not harmful to the drug action or the patient.

Nebulizing Gases: Compressed tank gas (air) or an air compressor should be used to provide pressure for nebulizing the solution. Oxygen may also be used but should be used with usual caution in patients with severe respiratory disease and CO_2 retention.

As an Antidote for Acetaminophen Poisoning: In the case of an overdosage of acetaminophen, acetylcysteine should be administered immediately if 24 hours or less have elapsed from the reported time of ingestion. To be effective in protecting against severe liver damage, therapy with acetylcysteine must be started within 10 hours of acetaminophen ingestion. There is some evidence of progressively diminished efficacy thereafter, possibly lasting up to 24 hours.

It should be borne in mind that after a fatal dose of acetaminophen, the patient may appear relatively well initially and may even continue normal activities for a day or two before the onset of hepatic failure.

The following procedure is recommended:

1. The stomach should be emptied promptly by lavage or by inducing emesis with syrup of ipecac. Syrup of ipecac should be given in a dose of 15 to 30 mL for children and 30 to 45 mL for adults accompanied by drinking copious quantities of water. The dose should be repeated if emesis does not occur in 20 minutes.
2. In the case of a mixed drug overdose activated charcoal may be indicated. However, if activated charcoal has been administered, perform gastric lavage before administering oral acetylcysteine treatment. Activated charcoal will absorb acetylcysteine and reduce its effectiveness.
3. Draw blood for acetaminophen plasma assay and for baseline AST, ALT, bilirubin, prothrombin time, creatinine, BUN, blood sugar and electrolytes. The acetaminophen assay provides a reliable prognostic indication of potential hepatotoxicity and serves as a basis for determining the need for continuing with the maintenance doses of acetylcysteine treatment. The laboratory measurements are used to monitor hepatic and renal function and electrolyte fluid balance.
4. Administer the loading dose of acetylcysteine as outlined in Table 1 or Table 2 according to route of administration employed.
5. For information regarding oral and i.v. maintenance doses, see Table 1 and Table 2.
6. If the patient vomits the oral loading dose or any oral maintenance dose within 1 hour of administration, repeat that dose.
7. If the patient is unable to retain the orally administered acetylcysteine, the antidote may be administered by duodenal intubation or by the i.v. route.
8. Repeat AST, ALT, bilirubin, prothrombin time, creatinine, BUN, blood sugar and electrolytes daily if acetaminophen plasma level is in the potentially toxic range.

Preparation of Solution for Oral Administration: Oral administration requires dilution of the 20% solution with cola drinks, or other soft drinks, to a final concentration of 5% (see Table 1). If administered via gastric tube or Miller-Abbott tube, water may be used as the diluent. The dilutions should be freshly prepared and utilized within 1 hour. Remaining undiluted solutions in opened vials can be stored in the refrigerator up to 96 hours.

Preparation of Solution for I.V. Administration: Acetylcysteine may be used for i.v. administration following acetaminophen overdose according to Dosage Guidelines in Table 2. Dilutions recommended should be prepared with 5% Dextrose and Water, as appropriate. Acetylcysteine for i.v. use should be considered as a single-dose container. Solutions recommended under each column in Table 2 should be freshly prepared and used only over times stated.

Table 1: Mucomyst

Dosage Guide and Preparation for Oral Administration

	Dose of acetylcysteine			
Body Weight (kg)	**Grams Acetylcysteine**	**mLs of 20% Acetylcysteine**	**mLs of diluent**	**Total mLs of 5% solution**
		Loading Dose[a]		
100–110	15	75	225	300
90–100	14	70	210	280
80–90	13	65	195	260
70–80	11	55	165	220
60–70	10	50	150	200
50–60	8	40	120	160
40–50	7	35	105	140
30–40	6	30	90	120
20–30	4	20	60	80
		Maintenance Dose[a]		
100–110	7.5	37	113	150
90–100	7.0	35	105	140
80–90	6.5	33	97	130
70–80	5.5	28	82	110
60–70	5.0	25	75	100
50–60	4.0	20	60	80
40–50	3.5	18	52	70
30–40	3.0	15	45	60
20–30	2.0	10	30	40
4 hours after the loading dose, administer the first maintenance dose (70 mg of acetylcysteine/kg). The maintenance dose is then repeated at 4 hour intervals for a total of 17 doses unless the acetaminophen assay reveals a non-toxic level as discussed above.				

[a] If patient weighs less than 20 kg, usually patients younger than 6 years, calculate the dose of acetylcysteine. Each mL of 20% solution contains 200 mg of acetylcysteine. The loading dose is 140 mg/kg of body weight. The maintenance dose is 70 mg/kg. Three mL of diluent are added to each mL of 20% solution. Do not decrease the proportion of diluent. Increased gastrointestinal irritation is associated with increased concentrations of acetylcysteine.

Table 2: Mucomyst

Dosage Guide and Preparation for I.V. Administration

	Initial Infusion (in 5% dextrose over 15 minutes)		**2nd Infusion (in 500 mL 5% dextrose over 4 hours)**	**3rd Infusion (in 1 L 5% dextrose over 16 hours)**
Body Weight (kg)	**Acetylcysteine (mL)**	**5% Dextrose (mL)**	**Acetylcysteine (mL)**	**Acetylcysteine (mL)**
10–15	11.25	40	3.75	7.50
15–20	15.00	50	5.00	10.00
20–25	18.75	75	6.25	12.50

(cont'd)

Table 2: Mucomyst *(cont'd)*

Dosage Guide and Preparation for I.V. Administration

Initial Infusion (in 5% dextrose over 15 minutes)			2nd Infusion (in 500 mL 5% dextrose over 4 hours)	3rd Infusion (in 1 L 5% dextrose over 16 hours)
Body Weight (kg)	**Acetylcysteine (mL)**	**5% Dextrose (mL)**	**Acetylcysteine (mL)**	**Acetylcysteine (mL)**
25–30	22.50	75	7.50	15.00
30–40	30.00	100	10.00	20.00
40–50	37.50	200	12.50	25.00
50–60	45.00	200	15.00	30.00
60–70	52.50	200	17.50	35.00
70–80	60.00	200	20.00	40.00
80–90	67.50	200	22.50	45.00
90–100	75.00	200	25.00	50.00
100–110	82.50	200	27.50	55.00
The volumes and rates of infusion for children suggested above must be adjusted according to the medical circumstances and restrictions in the volumes of parenteral fluids administered as they apply to each individual patient.				

Supportive Treatment of Acetaminophen Overdose: Maintain fluid and electrolyte balance based on clinical evaluation of state of hydration and serum electrolytes. Treat as necessary for hypoglycemia. Administer vitamin K_1 if prothrombin time ratio exceeds 1.5 or fresh frozen plasma if the prothrombin time ratio exceeds 3.0. Diuretics and forced diuresis should be avoided.

Hemodialysis or peritoneal dialysis have not been found helpful.

SUPPLIED: Each rubber-stoppered, glass vial contains: a sterile 20% solution of acetylcysteine. Vials of 10 and 30 mL.

Multaq™ Ⓟ

dronedarone HCl

Antiarrhythmic Agent

sanofi-aventis

Date of Preparation: July 31, 2009

SUMMARY PRODUCT INFORMATION:

Route of Administration	Dosage Form/ Strength	Clinically Relevant Nonmedicinal Ingredients
Oral	Tablet 400 mg	Lactose monohydrate For a complete listing see Dosage Forms, Composition and Packaging.

INDICATIONS AND CLINICAL USE: MULTAQ is indicated for the treatment of patients with a history of, or current atrial fibrillation to reduce the risk of cardiovascular hospitalization due to atrial fibrillation.

Pediatrics (<18 years of age): No data are available.

CONTRAINDICATIONS: MULTAQ is contraindicated in patients with:

- Severe congestive heart failure (Stage NYHA IV) and other unstable hemodynamic conditions
- Second- or third- degree AV block or sick sinus syndrome (except when used in conjunction with a functioning pacemaker)
- Bradycardia <50 bpm
- Co-administration with strong CYP3A4 inhibitors, such as ketoconazole, itraconazole, voriconazole, cyclosporin, telithromycin, clarithromycin, nefazodone and ritonavir (see Drug Interactions)
- Co-administration with drugs inducing torsades de pointes such as phenothiazines, tricyclic antidepressants, and certain oral macrolides, class I and III antiarrhythmics
- QTc Bazett interval ≥500 msec
- Severe hepatic impairment
- Pregnancy (see Warnings and Precautions, Special Populations) and
- Lactation (see Warnings and Precautions, Special Populations)
- History of hypersensitivity reactions to dronedarone or any of its excipients or component of the container. For a complete listing, see Dosage Forms, Composition and Packaging.

WARNINGS AND PRECAUTIONS: Cardiovascular: QT Prolongation: The pharmacological action of dronedarone may induce a moderate (about 10 msec) QTc Bazett prolongation, related to prolonged repolarization. These changes are linked to the therapeutic effect of dronedarone and do not reflect toxicity. Follow up, including ECG, is recommended during treatment. If QTc Bazett interval is ≥500 msec, dronedarone should be stopped (see Contraindications).

Based on clinical experience, dronedarone has a low pro-arrhythmic effect. However, proarrhythmic effects may occur in particular situations such as concomitant use with drugs favoring arrhythmia and/or electrolytic disorders (see Warnings and Precautions and Drug Interactions).

Congestive Heart Failure (CHF): Dronedarone is contraindicated for use in patients with severe CHF (Stage NYHA IV) (see Contraindications). It should be used with caution in patients with moderate CHF (Stage NYHA III) and only if the benefits are deemed to outweigh the risks involved.

Endocrine and Metabolism: Electrolyte imbalance: Since antiarrhythmic drugs may be ineffective or may be arrhythmogenic in patients with hypokalemia, any potassium or magnesium deficiency should be corrected before initiation and during dronedarone therapy.

Renal: Plasma Creatinine Increase: An increase in plasma creatinine has been observed with dronedarone 400 mg twice daily in healthy subjects and in patients. This increase occurs early after treatment initiation and reaches a plateau after 7 days. Mean increase in Atrial Fibrillation (AF) patients is about 10 µmol/L. Values return to baseline within one week after treatment discontinuation. In a specific study in healthy subjects, this increase was shown to be related to inhibition of creatinine secretion at the tubular level, with no effect on glomerular filtration or on renal blood flow. The same mechanism has also been described with other drugs such as cimetidine, trimethoprime or amiodarone. Increased plasma creatinine could be misinterpreted and lead to inappropriate discontinuation of ACE inhibitors or AIIRAs in patients requiring this treatment (see Warnings and Precautions, Monitoring and Laboratory Tests, Management of Plasma Creatinine Increase).

Special Populations: Pregnant Women (see Contraindications): MULTAQ has been shown to be teratogenic in the rat and is contraindicated in women who are or may become pregnant. Women of childbearing potential should use effective methods of contraception during treatment with MULTAQ. If this drug is used during pregnancy or if the patient becomes pregnant while taking this drug, the patient should be apprised of the potential hazard to the fetus.

MULTAQ can cause fetal harm when administered to pregnant women. In rats, dronedarone caused marked effects on embryo-fetal development at 100 mg/kg/day such as increased post-implantation losses, reduced fetal and placental weights and various external, visceral and skeletal malformations in most fetuses. At lower dosages, up to 50 mg/kg/day (corresponding to 4.5 times the recommended human therapeutic dose), dronedarone had no effects on the litters (with the exception of a transient minor effect on the bodyweight gain of the pups from D1 to D4 post-partum). Dronedarone had no adverse effects on the mothers and their litters up to 30 mg/kg/day. In rabbits, the high dose level (200 mg/kg/day) did not induce any effects to fetuses.

Labor and Delivery: It is not known whether the use of dronedarone during labor or delivery has any immediate or delayed adverse effects. In pre- and post-natal development studies in the rat, at doses up to 50 mg/kg/day, dronedarone induced no effect on the duration of gestation or on parturition.

Nursing Women: Dronedarone and its metabolites are excreted in rat milk. Nursing in lactating rats administered dronedarone was associated with minor reduced body-weight gain in the offspring.

It is not known whether this drug is excreted in human milk. Therefore, when dronedarone therapy is indicated, the mother should be advised to discontinue nursing (see Contraindications).

Pediatrics (<18 years of age): Safety and efficacy in children below the age of 18 years has not been established. Therefore use in these patients is not recommended.

Geriatrics (>65 years of age): A large number of elderly patients with AF or AFL have been included in the MULTAQ clinical program (more than 4500 patients aged 65 years or above, of which more than 2000 patients were 75 years or above). Efficacy and safety was comparable in both elderly and younger patients.

Renal Impairment: Patients with renal impairment were included in clinical studies. Consistent with the minimal renal excretion of dronedarone, no pharmacokinetic modification was observed in patients with renal impairment in particular in patients with severe renal impairment (see Action and Clinical Pharmacology, Pharmacokinetics) and no particular precaution is needed.

Monitoring and Laboratory Tests: Management of Plasma Creatinine Increase: It is recommended that baseline values of plasma creatinine be established 7 days after initiation of treatment with dronedarone.

If the result obtained for the plasma creatinine is above the upper limit of normal as provided by the laboratory, this value should be used as the new reference baseline taking into account that this may be expected with dronedarone, since the drug can affect baseline values. An increase in creatinemia should not necessarily lead to the discontinuation of treatment with dronedarone or discontinuation of treatment with ACE-inhibitors or angiotensin receptor blockers (ARBs) (see Warnings and Precautions, Renal).

Further laboratory testing is at the discretion of the attending physician.

ADVERSE REACTIONS: Adverse Drug Reaction Overview: The safety profile of dronedarone 400 mg twice daily in patients with AF or AFL is based on 5 placebo controlled studies, ATHENA, EURIDIS, ADONIS, ERATO and DAFNE. In these studies, a total of 6285 patients were randomized and treated. Of these, 3282 patients were treated with dronedarone 400 mg twice daily, and 2875 received placebo.

The mean exposure across studies was 12 months. In ATHENA, the maximum follow-up was 30 months.

Assessment of intrinsic factors such as race, gender or age on the incidence of any treatment emergent adverse events did not suggest any excess of adverse events in a particular sub-group.

In pooled clinical trials, premature discontinuation due to adverse reactions occurred in 11.8% of the dronedarone-treated patients and in 7.7% in the placebo-treated group. The most common reasons for discontinuation of therapy with MULTAQ were gastrointestinal disorders (3.2 % of patients versus 1.8% in the placebo group).

The most frequent adverse reactions observed with dronedarone 400 mg twice daily in the 5 studies were diarrhea, nausea and vomiting, fatigue and asthenia.

Clinical Trial Adverse Drug Reactions: Because clinical trials are conducted under very specific conditions the adverse reaction rates observed in the clinical trials may not reflect the rates observed in practice and should not be compared to the rates in the clinical trials of another drug. Adverse drug reaction information from clinical trials is useful for identifying drug-related adverse events and for approximating rates.

Table 1 displays adverse reactions ≥1% associated with dronedarone 400 mg twice daily in AF or AFL patients, presented by system organ class and by decreasing order of frequency. Adverse reactions included in the system organ class "Investigation" are presented separately in Table 2.

Table 1: MULTAQ

Adverse Reactions Occurring ≥ Than 1% of Patients Taking Dronedarone in Placebo-controlled Clinical Trials

	Placebo (N=2875)	Dronedarone 400 mg Twice Daily (N=3282)
Gastrointestinal Disorders		
Diarrhoea	5.8%	9.0%
Nausea	3.1%	4.9%
Abdominal pains	2.8%	3.5%
Vomiting	1.1%	2.0%
Dyspepsia	1.0%	1.5%
General Disorders and Administration Site Conditions		
Fatigue	3.6%	4.3%
Asthenia	1.7%	2.3%
Cardiac Disorders		
Bradycardia	1.3%	3.3%
Skin and Subcutaneous Tissue Disorders		
Rashes (including generalised, macular, maculo-papular)	1.6%	2.7%
Pruritus	0.9%	1.3%

Less Common Clinical Trial Adverse Drug Reactions (<1%): Nervous System Disorders: ageusia and dysgeusia.

Skin and Subcutaneous Tissue Disorders: dermatitis, dermatitis allergic, eczema, erythemas (including erythema and rash erythematous) and photosensitivity reaction.

In addition, the following laboratory data/ECG parameters were reported with dronedarone 400 mg twice daily.

Table 2: MULTAQ

Laboratory Data/ECG Parameters

	Placebo (N=2875)	Dronedarone 400 mg Twice Daily (N=3282)
Blood creatinine increased ≥10% five days after treatment initiation	20.6%	50.9%
QTc Bazett prolonged (>450 msec in male; >470 msec in female)	18.7%	27.6%

DRUG INTERACTIONS: Overview: Dronedarone is primarily metabolized by CYP 3A4 (see Action and Clinical Pharmacology, Pharmacokinetics) and is a moderate inhibitor of CYP 3A4 and a mild inhibitor of CYP 2D6. Therefore, inhibitors and inducers of CYP 3A4 have the potential to interact with dronedarone, and dronedarone has the potential to interact with medicinal products that are substrates of CYP 3A4 and CYP 2D6. It also has the potential to inhibit P-glycoprotein (P-gP) transport. Dronedarone has no significant potential to inhibit CYP1A2, CYP2C9, CYP2C19, CYP2C8 and CYP 2B6.

A potential pharmacodynamic interaction can also be expected with beta-blockers, calcium antagonists and digitalis.

Co-administration of drugs prolonging the QT interval (such as phenothiazines, bepridil, tricyclic antidepressants, certain oral macrolides, Class I and III antiarrhythmics, which may induce torsades de pointes) is contraindicated because of the potential risk of proarrhythmia. (See Contraindications).

In clinical trials, patients treated with dronedarone received a variety of concomitant medications including beta-blockers, digitalis, calcium antagonists (including those with heart rate-lowering effects), statins and oral anticoagulants.

Drug-Drug Interactions: See Table 3.

Table 3: MULTAQ

Established or Potential Drug-Drug Interactions

Agent	Ref	Effect	Clinical Comment
Antidepressants	T	No effect	Dronedarone is a weak inhibitor of CYP2D6 in humans, so it is predicted to have limited interaction on antidepressants that are metabolized by CYP2D6.
		Proarrhythmic effect	Co-administration of dronedarone with tricyclic antidepressants and other medicinal products inducing torsades de pointes is contraindicated (see Contraindications).
Beta-blockers (e.g. metoprolol and propranolol	CT	↑ metoprolol and propranolol exposure	Beta-blockers that are metabolized by CYP 2D6 can have their exposure increased by dronedarone. Moreover, beta-blockers have the potential to interact with dronedarone from a pharmacodynamic point of view. Dronedarone 800 mg daily increased metoprolol exposure by 1.6-fold and propranolol exposure by 1.3-fold (i.e. much below the 6-fold differences observed between poor and extensive CYP 2D6 metabolizers).
	CT	Bradycardia	In clinical trials, bradycardia was more frequently observed when dronedarone was given in combination with beta-blockers. Due to the pharmacokinetic interaction and possible pharmacodynamic interaction, beta-blockers should be used with caution if taken concomitantly with dronedarone.
Calcium antagonists (e.g. verapamil, diltiazem, nifedipine)	CT	↑ dronedarone exposure	Calcium antagonists are substrates and/or moderate inhibitors of CYP3A4. Moreover, calcium antagonists with heart-rate lowering properties have the potential to interact with dronedarone from a pharmacodynamic point of view. Repeated doses of diltiazem (240 mg twice daily), verapamil (240 mg once daily) and nifedipine (20 mg twice daily) resulted in an increase in dronedarone exposure of 1.7-, 1.4-, and 1.2-fold, respectively.
		↑ verapamil and nisoldipine exposure	Calcium antagonists also have their exposure increased by dronedarone (400 mg twice daily) (verapamil by 1.4-fold, and nisoldipine by 1.5-fold). In clinical trials, there was no evidence of safety concerns when dronedarone was co-administered with calcium antagonists with heart rate-lowering effects. Overall, due to the pharmacokinetic interaction and possible pharmacodynamic interaction, calcium antagonists with depressant effects on sinus and atrio-ventricular node such as verapamil and diltiazem should be used with caution when associated with dronedarone.
Digoxin	CT	↑ digoxin exposure	Dronedarone (400 mg twice daily) increased digoxin exposure by 2.5-fold by inhibiting P-gP transporter. Moreover, digitalis has the potential to interact with dronedarone from a pharmacodynamic point of view. In clinical trials, increased levels of digitalis and/or gastrointestinal disorders were observed when dronedarone was co-administered with digitalis. Due to the pharmacokinetic interaction and possible pharmacodynamic interaction, digoxin should be used with caution concomitantly with dronedarone and patients should be closely monitored for serum digoxin levels, especially during the first week of co-administration. Clinical and ECG monitoring are also recommended and the digoxin dose should be adjusted as appropriate.
Drugs prolonging the QT interval (e.g. phenothiazines, bepridil, tricyclic antidepressants, certain oral macrolides, Class I and III antiarrhythmics)	T	Proarrhythmic effect	Co-administration of drugs prolonging the QT interval (inducing torsades de pointes) is contraindicated because of the potential risk of proarrhythmia (see Contraindications).
Losartan (CYP 2C9 substrate)	CT	No effect	Although not considered to be a clinically significant interaction, co-administration of losartan 100 mg once daily for 14 days with dronedarone 400 mg bid decreased the C_{max} of losartan by 18% and the C_{max} and AUC_{0-24} of the active metabolite by 25% and 21% respectively.
Oral contraceptives (e.g. ethinylestradiol and levonorgestrel	CT	No effect	No decreases in ethinylestradiol and levonorgestrel were observed in healthy subjects receiving dronedarone (800 mg twice daily) concomitantly with oral contraceptives. However, an increase of 28% in ethinylestradiol exposure and a 19% increase in levonorgestrel exposure were observed.
Pantoprazole	CT	No effect	Pantoprazole (40 mg once daily), a drug increasing gastric pH without any effect on cytochrome P450, had no significant pharmacokinetic interaction with dronedarone.
P-glycoprotein substrates (e.g. doxorubicin, fexofenadine and talinolol)	T	↑ P-gp plasma concentration	Dronedarone inhibits P-gP, and interactions may therefore occur with doxorubicin, fexofenadine and talinolol.
Potent CYP 3A4 inducers (e.g. rifampicin, phenobarbital, carbamazepine, phenytoin)	CT	↓ dronedarone exposure	Rifampicin (600 mg once daily) decreased dronedarone exposure by 5-fold with no major change in its active metabolite exposure. Co-administration of rifampicin or other potent CYP3A4 inducers are not recommended with dronedarone as they decrease its exposure.
Potent CYP 3A4 inhibitors (e.g. ketoconazole, itraconazole, voriconazole, ritonavir, cyclosporin, telithromycin, clarithromycin)	CT	↑ dronedarone exposure	Repeated doses of ketoconazole (200 mg daily), a strong CYP 3A4 inhibitor, resulted in a 17-fold increase in dronedarone exposure. Concomitant use of ketoconazole as well as other potent CYP 3A4 inhibitors is contraindicated (see Contraindications).
Sirolimus and Tacrolimus (CYP 3A4 substrates)	T	↑ sirolimus and tacrolimus exposure	Dronedarone can increase plasma concentrations of tacrolimus and sirolimus (CYP3A4 substrates) when given orally. Monitoring of their plasma concentrations and appropriate dosage adjustment is recommended when these drugs are co-administered with dronedarone
Statins (Substrates of CYP3A4 and/or P-gP substrates e.g. simvastatin, lovastatin, atorvastatin and pravastatin)	CT	↑ Simvastatin and simvastatin acid exposure	Dronedarone can increase exposure of statins that are substrates of CYP3A4 and/or P-gP substrates. Dronedarone (400 mg twice daily) increased simvastatin and simvastatin acid exposure by 4-fold and 2-fold respectively.
	T	↑ lovastatin, atorvastatin and pravastatin	It is predicted that dronedarone could also increase the exposures of lovastatin, atorvastatin and pravastatin within the same range as simvastatin acid. In clinical trials, there was no evidence of safety concerns when dronedarone was co-administered with statins metabolized by CYP3A4. As high doses of statins increase the risk of myopathy, concomitant use of statins which are CYP3A4 substrates and/or P-gP substrates should be undertaken with caution and patients monitored for clinical signs of muscular toxicity. A significant interaction of dronedarone on statins which are not CYP3A4/P-gP substrates such as fluvastatin and rosuvastatin is unlikely.
Theophylline (CYP 1A2 substrate)	CT	↓ theophylline exposure	Concomitant administration of dronedarone 400 mg bid with theophylline 400 mg bid resulted in decreased theophylline exposure (18% decrease in AUC_{0-12} and a 17% decrease in C_{max} of theophylline).
Warfarin (CYP 2C9 substrate)	CT	↑ S-warfarin exposure	Dronedarone (600 mg twice daily) increased S-warfarin by 1.2-fold with no change in R-warfarin and increased INR by only 1.07-fold. In clinical trials, there was no evidence of safety concerns when dronedarone was co-administered with oral anticoagulants.

Legend: C=case study; CT=clinical trial; T=theoretical.

Drug-Food Interactions: Grapefruit Juice: Repeated doses of 300 mL of grapefruit juice (inhibitor of the CYP3A4) three times daily resulted in a 3-fold increase in dronedarone exposure. Therefore, patients should be warned to avoid grapefruit juice beverages while taking dronedarone.

Drug-Herb Interactions: Co-administration of St John's Wort, a potent CYP3A4 inducer, is not recommended with dronedarone as this herb decreases its exposure.

DOSAGE AND ADMINISTRATION: Recommended Dose and Dosage Adjustment: The recommended dosage is 400 mg twice daily in adults. MULTAQ should be taken as one tablet with the morning meal and one tablet with the evening meal.

Treatment with class I or III antiarrhythmics (such as flecainide, propafenone, quinidine, disopyramide, dofetilide, sotalol, amiodarone) must be stopped before starting MULTAQ.

Treatment with MULTAQ can be initiated in an outpatient setting.

Renal Impairment: No dose adjustment is required in patients with renal impairment (see Warnings and Precautions, Special Populations and Action and Clinical Pharmacology, Pharmacokinetics).

Severe Hepatic Impairment: Multaq is contraindicated in patients with severe hepatic impairment (see Contraindications).

Missed Dose: If a dose of this medication has been missed, the missed dose should be skipped and the patient should go back to the regular dosing schedule. The dose should not be doubled.

OVERDOSAGE:
In the event of overdosage, the patient's cardiac rhythm and blood pressure should be monitored in addition to general supportive measures. Treatment should be supportive and based on symptoms.

It is not known whether dronedarone and/or its metabolites can be removed by dialysis (hemodialysis, peritoneal dialysis or hemofiltration). There is no specific antidote available.

For management of a suspected drug overdose, CPhA recommends that you contact your **regional Poison Control Centre**. See the *CPS* Directory section for a list of Poison Control Centres.

ACTION AND CLINICAL PHARMACOLOGY: Mechanism of Action: In animals, dronedarone prevents atrial fibrillation or restores normal sinus rhythm depending on the model used. It also prevents ventricular tachycardia and ventricular fibrillation in several animal models. These effects most likely result from its electrophysiological properties belonging to all four Vaughan-Williams classes. Dronedarone is a multichannel blocker inhibiting the potassium currents (including $I_{K(Ach)}$, I_{Kur}, I_{Kr}, I_{Ks}) and thus prolonging cardiac action potential and refractory periods (Class III). It also inhibits the sodium currents (Class Ib) and the calcium currents (Class IV). It non-competitively antagonizes adrenergic activities (Class II).
Pharmacodynamics: In animal models, dronedarone reduces heart rate. It prolongs Wenckebach cycle length and AH-, PQ-, QT- intervals; with no marked effect on QTc-, HV- and QRS- intervals. It increases effective refractory periods of the atrium, atrio-ventricular node and ventricle with minimal degree of reverse-use dependency.

Dronedarone decreases arterial blood pressure and myocardial contractility (dP/dt_{max}) with no change in left ventricular ejection fraction and reduces myocardial oxygen consumption.

Dronedarone has vasodilatory properties, more pronounced in coronary arteries (related to the activation of the nitric oxide pathway) than in peripheral arteries.

Dronedarone displays indirect antiadrenergic effects; it reduces alpha-adrenergic blood pressure response to epinephrine and beta1 and beta2 responses to isoproterenol.
Pharmacokinetics: See Table 4.

Table 4: MULTAQ

Summary of MULTAQ's Pharmacokinetic Parameters in Healthy Young Male Subjects

Single Dose Mean	C_{max}	$t_{½}$ (h)	$AUC_{0-\infty}$	Clearance	Volume of Distribution
400 mg	67.2 (36)	17.6 (56)	474 (33)	937 (35)	21 000 (31)

Absorption: Dronedarone should be taken with food. Following oral administration in fed conditions, dronedarone is well absorbed (at least 70 %) from intestines to blood. However due to presystemic first pass metabolism, the absolute bioavailability of dronedarone (given with food) is 15 %. Concomitant intake of food increases dronedarone bioavailability by on average 2- to 4-fold. After oral administration in fed conditions, peak plasma concentrations of dronedarone and the main circulating active metabolite (N-debutyl metabolite) are reached within 3 to 6 hours. After repeated administration of 400 mg twice daily, steady state is reached within 4 to 8 days of treatment and the mean accumulation ratio for dronedarone ranges from 2.6 to 4.5. The steady state mean dronedarone C_{max} is 84-147 ng/mL and the exposure of the main N-debutyl metabolite is similar to that of the parent compound.

The pharmacokinetics of dronedarone and its N-debutyl metabolite both deviate moderately from dose proportionality: a 2-fold increase in dose results in an approximate 2.5- to 3.0-fold increase with respect to C_{max} and AUC.
Distribution: The in vitro plasma protein binding of dronedarone and its N-debutyl metabolite is >98 % and not saturable. Both compounds bind mainly to albumin. After intravenous (IV) administration the volume of distribution at steady state (Vss) ranges from 1200 to 1400 L.
Metabolism: Dronedarone is extensively metabolized, mainly by CYP3A4. The major metabolic pathway includes N-debutylation to form the main circulating active metabolite followed by oxidation, oxidative deamination to form the inactive propanoic acid metabolite, followed by oxidation, and direct oxidation. The N-debutyl metabolite exhibits pharmacodynamic activity but is 3 to 10-times less potent than dronedarone.
Excretion: After oral administration, approximately 6 % of the labeled dose is excreted in urine mainly as metabolites (no unchanged compound excreted in urine) and 84 % are excreted in feces mainly as metabolites. After IV administration the plasma clearance of dronedarone ranges from 130 to 150 L/h. The terminal elimination half-life of dronedarone is around 25-30 hours and that of its N-debutyl metabolite around 20-25 hours. In patients, dronedarone and its metabolite are completely eliminated from the plasma within 2 weeks after the end of a 400 mg twice daily-treatment.
Special Populations and Conditions: The pharmacokinetics of dronedarone in patients with atrial fibrillation is consistent with that in healthy subjects. The main sources of variability in dronedarone exposure (age, gender, bodyweight, concomitant treatment with weak to moderate CYP3A4 inhibitors) remain modest in their magnitude (less than 2-fold).

Assessment of intrinsic factors such as race, gender or age on the incidence of any treatment emergent adverse events did not suggest any excess of adverse events in a particular sub-group.
Gender: In female patients, dronedarone exposures are on average 30% higher as compared to male patients (see Adverse Reactions, Adverse Drug Reaction Overview).
Race: Pharmacokinetic differences due to race were not assessed.
Elderly: Of the total number of subjects in clinical studies of dronedarone, 73% were 65 years of age and over and 34% were 75 and over. In patients aged 65 years old and above, dronedarone exposures are 23% higher in comparison with patients aged below 65 years (see Warnings and Precautions, Special Populations).
Pediatric Population: The pharmacokinetics of dronedarone were not assessed in pediatric patients.
Hepatic Insufficiency: In subjects with moderate hepatic impairment, dronedarone total and unbound exposures are increased by 1.3-fold and by 2-fold respectively. Those of the active metabolite are decreased by 1.6-fold to 1.9-fold. The effect of severe hepatic impairment on the pharmacokinetics of dronedarone was not assessed (see Contraindications).
Renal Insufficiency: Consistent with the very weak renal excretion of dronedarone, no pharmacokinetic modification was observed in patients with renal impairment in particular in patients with severe renal impairment (see Warnings and Precautions, Special Populations).

STORAGE AND STABILITY: Store at 25°C, with excursion permitted between 15 and 30°C.
Store in the original package.

INFORMATION FOR THE PATIENT: Published in e-CPS, available by subscription at www.e-cps.ca.

DOSAGE FORMS, COMPOSITION AND PACKAGING: Each white film-coated tablet for oral administration, oblong-shaped, engraved with a double wave marking on one side and "4142" code on the other side contains: dronedarone hydrochloride equivalent to dronedarone 400 mg. Nonmedicinal ingredients: core: colloidal anhydrous silica, crospovidone, hypromellose, lactose monohydrate, magnesium stearate, maize starch and poloxamer 407; coating/polishing: carnauba wax, hypromellose, macrogol 6000 and titanium dioxide. Bottles of 180. Boxes of 4 blisters (15 tablets per blister).

(Shown in Product Identification Section)

MUSE® Pr

alprostadil
Prostaglandin

Paladin

Date of Preparation: June 5, 2009

PHARMACOLOGY: Actions: Alprostadil is a synthetic prostaglandin with various pharmacological actions that include vasodilation, inhibition of platelet aggregation, inhibition of gastric secretion, stimulation of intestinal smooth muscle and stimulation of uterine smooth muscle.

Prostaglandin E_1 is a naturally occurring acidic lipid that is synthesized from fatty acid precursors by most mammalian tissues and has a variety of pharmacologic effects. Human seminal fluid is a rich source of prostaglandins, including PGE_1 and PGE_2, and the total concentration of prostaglandins in ejaculate has been estimated to be approximately 100-200 µg/mL.

The vasodilatory effects of alprostadil on the cavernosal arteries and the trabecular smooth muscle of the corpora cavernosa result in rapid arterial inflow and expansion of the lacunar spaces within the corpora. As the expanded corporal sinusoids are compressed against the tunica albuginea, venous outflow through subtunical vessels is impeded and penile rigidity develops. This process is referred to as the corporal veno-occlusive mechanism.
Pharmacokinetics: About 80% of alprostadil administered by the MUSE system is absorbed within 10 minutes and is rapidly cleared from the systemic circulation by the lungs, leaving barely detectable systemic blood levels.
Absorption: MUSE alprostadil is designed to deliver alprostadil directly to the urethral lining for transfer via the corpus spongiosum to the corpora cavernosa. Intraurethral administration of MUSE alprostadil is preceded by urination, and the residual urine disperses the medicated pellet, permitting alprostadil to be absorbed by the urethral mucosa. The transurethral absorption of alprostadil after administration is biphasic. Initial absorption is rapid, with approximately 80% of an administered dose absorbed within 10 minutes. The mean time to the maximum plasma PGE_1 concentration after a 1000 µg intraurethral dose of MUSE alprostadil is approximately 16 minutes.
Distribution: Following administration, MUSE alprostadil is absorbed from the urethral mucosa into the corpus spongiosum. A portion of the administered dose is transported to the corpora cavernosa through collateral vessels, while the remainder passes into the pelvic venous circulation through veins draining the corpus spongiosum. The half-life of alprostadil in humans is short, varying between 30 seconds and 10 minutes, depending on the body compartment in which it is measured and the physiological status of the subject. Nearly all of the alprostadil entering the central venous circulation is removed in a single pass through the lungs; thus peripheral venous plasma levels of PGE_1 are low or undetectable (<2 picograms/mL) after MUSE administration. The mean maximum plasma PGE_1 concentration following intraurethral administration of the highest dose of MUSE alprostadil (1000 µg) was barely detectable (11.4 picograms/mL). In a study of 14 subjects, the plasma PGE_1 level was shown to be undetectable within 60 minutes of MUSE alprostadil administration in most subjects.
Metabolism: Alprostadil is rapidly metabolized locally by enzymatic oxidation of the 15-hydroxyl group to 15-keto-PGE_1. The enzyme catalyzing this process has been isolated from many tissues in the lower genitourinary tract including the urethra, prostate, and corpus cavernosum. 15-keto-PGE_1 retains little (1-2%) of the biological activity of PGE_1. 15-keto-PGE_1 is rapidly reduced at the C_{13}-C_{14} position to form the most abundant metabolite in plasma, 13,14-dihydro, 15-keto-PGE_1 (DHK-PGE_1), which is biologically inactive. The majority of DHK-PGE_1 is further metabolized to smaller prostaglandin remnants that are cleared primarily by the kidney and liver. Between 60% and 90% of PGE_1 has been shown to be metabolized after one pass through the pulmonary capillary beds. However, pulmonary clearance of PGE_1 can be affected by disease states such as acute respiratory distress syndrome (ARDS), with a resultant reduction in the pulmonary extraction ratio.
Excretion: After intravenous administration of tritium-labelled alprostadil in man, labelled drug disappears rapidly from the blood in the first 10 minutes, and by 1 hour radioactivity in the blood reaches a low level.

The metabolites of alprostadil are excreted primarily by the kidney, with approximately 90% of an administered intravenous dose excreted in the urine within 24 hours of dosing. The remainder is excreted in the feces. There is no evidence of tissue retention of alprostadil or its metabolites following intravenous administration.
Pharmacokinetics in Special Populations: Pulmonary Disease: The near-complete pulmonary first-pass metabolism of PGE_1 is the primary factor influencing the systemic pharmacokinetics of MUSE alprostadil and is a reason that peripheral venous plasma levels of PGE_1 are low or undetectable (<2 picograms/mL) following administration. Patients with pulmonary disease, therefore, may have a reduced capacity to clear the drug. In patients with the adult respiratory distress syndrome (ARDS), pulmonary extraction of intravescularly administered alprostadil was reduced by approximately 15% compared to a control group of patients with normal respiratory function (66±3.2% vs. 78±2.4%).
Geriatrics: The effects of age on the pharmacokinetics of alprostadil have not been evaluated.
Clinical Experience: The MUSE system was evaluated in 7 placebo-controlled trials of various design in over 2500 patients with a history of erectile dysfunction of various etiologies. These trials assessed erectile function in the clinic and sexual intercourse in outpatient settings.

Studies that established benefit demonstrated improvements in success rates for sexual intercourse compared with similarly administered placebo.

In 2 identical multicentre, double-blind, placebo-controlled, parallel-group studies, 1511 monogamous and heterosexual patients were enrolled and began dose titration in the clinic with doses between 125 µg and 1000 µg. Sixty-six percent of patients (996) completed dose titration and achieved an erection sufficient for intercourse. Couples on active therapy were more likely to have at least one successful sexual intercourse (65% vs. 19%) than were couples on placebo.

Among patients who reported successful intercourse at least once with active treatment, approximately 7 of 10 MUSE systems resulted in successful sexual intercourse.

Results were similar in patients with erectile dysfunction stemming from surgery or trauma, diabetes, vascular disease, or other etiologies. In administrations resulting in sexual intercourse, average erections sufficient for penetration was 16 minutes on active drug. Successful therapy with MUSE alprostadil was associated with improvement in the quality of life measures of "emotional well-being" for patients and "relationship with partner" for both patients and their female partners.

INDICATIONS: MUSE alprostadil is indicated for the treatment of erectile dysfunction. MUSE alprostadil may also be useful as an adjunct to diagnostic tests in the diagnosis of erectile dysfunction.

CONTRAINDICATIONS: MUSE alprostadil is contraindicated in men with any of the following:
1. Known hypersensitivity to alprostadil.
2. Abnormal penile anatomy: MUSE alprostadil is contraindicated in patients with urethral stricture, balanitis (inflammation/infection of the glans of the penis), severe hypospadias and curvatures, and in patients with acute or chronic urethritis.
3. Sickle cell anemia or trait, thrombocythemia, polycythemia, multiple myeloma: MUSE alprostadil is contraindicated in patients who are prone to venous thrombosis or who have a hyperviscosity syndrome and are therefore at increased risk of priapism (rigid erection lasting 6 or more hours).
4. MUSE alprostadil should not be used in men for whom sexual activity is inadvisable (see Precautions, General).
5. MUSE alprostadil should not be used for sexual intercourse with a pregnant woman unless the couple uses a condom barrier.

WARNINGS: Because of the potential for symptomatic hypotension and syncope, which occurred in 3% and 0.4%, respectively, of patients during in-clinic dosing, MUSE titration should be carried out under medical supervision.

There exists a possibility of syncope or fainting occurring within one hour of post-administration of MUSE alprostadil. Patients should be cautioned to avoid activities, such as driving or hazardous tasks, where injury could result if hypotension or syncope were to occur after the administration of MUSE alprostadil.

PRECAUTIONS: General: A complete medical history and physical examination should be undertaken to exclude reversible causes of erectile dysfunction prior to the initiation of MUSE alprostadil therapy. In addition, underlying disorders that might preclude the use of the MUSE system (see Contraindications) should be sought.
Cardiovascular Effects: During in-clinic dosing, patients should be monitored for symptoms of hypotension, and the lowest effective dose of MUSE alprostadil should be prescribed.
Hematologic Effects: Patients administering MUSE alprostadil improperly may be at risk of urethral abrasion resulting in minor bleeding or spotting. Patients on anticoagulant therapy or with bleeding disorders may be at higher risk of bleeding. Patients on anticoagulant therapy have been safely treated with MUSE alprostadil; however, the risk/benefit ratio in these patients should be considered prior to prescribing MUSE alprostadil.
Resumption of Sexual Activity: Sexual intercourse is considered a vigorous physical activity, and it increases heart rate as well as cardiac work. Physicians may want to examine the cardiac fitness of patients prior to treating erectile dysfunction.
Priapism and Prolonged Erection: In clinical trials of MUSE alprostadil, priapism (rigid erection lasting ≥6 hours) and prolonged erection (rigid erection lasting 4 hours and <6 hours) were reported infrequently (<0.1% and 0.3% of patients, respectively). Nevertheless, these events are a potential risk of pharmacologic therapy and can cause penile injury. Physicians should lower the dose or consider discontinuing treatment with MUSE alprostadil in any patient who develops priapism or prolonged erection.
Drug Interactions: Drug-Drug Interactions: Because there are low or undetectable (<2 picograms/mL) amounts of alprostadil found in the peripheral venous circulation following administration, systemic drug-drug interactions with MUSE alprostadil are unlikely. The presence of medications in the circulation that attenuate erectile function, however, may influence the response to MUSE alprostadil.

Although formal studies have not been conducted, the concomitant use of MUSE alprostadil and anti-hypertension medications may increase the risk of hypotension. It is therefore advised that caution be used in the administration of MUSE alprostadil to individuals on anti-hypertensive medications. In addition, the presence of medication in the circulation that attenuate erectile function may influence the response to MUSE alprostadil.
Drug-Device Interactions: Use of the MUSE system in patients with penile implants has not been studied.
Sexual Preference: There is no experience in homosexual men and no experience with other than vaginal intercourse.
Lactation: MUSE alprostadil is not indicated for use in women or children.
Children: See Lactation.

ADVERSE EFFECTS: In-Clinic Titration: In the 2 largest double-blind, parallel, placebo-controlled trials, 1511 patients received MUSE alprostadil at least 1 time in the clinic setting. The most frequently reported drug-related side effects during in-clinic titration included pain in the penis (36%), urethra (13%), or testes (5%). These discomforts were most commonly reported as mild and transient, but about 7% of patients withdrew at this stage because of adverse events. Urethral bleeding/spotting and other minor abrasions to the urethra were reported in approximately 3% of patients.

Symptomatic lowering of blood pressure (hypotension) occurred in 3% of patients. Dizziness was reported in 4% of patients. Syncope (fainting) was reported by 0.4% of patients.

Home Treatment: 996 patients (66% of those who began titration) were studied during the home treatment portion of 2 Phase III placebo-controlled studies. Fewer than 2% of patients discontinued from these studies primarily because of adverse events. Table 1 summarizes the frequency of adverse events reported by patients using MUSE alprostadil or placebo.

Table 1: MUSE

Adverse Events Reported by ≥2% of Patients Treated with MUSE alprostadil and More Common Than on Placebo at Home in Phase III Placebo-Controlled Clinical Studies for up to 3 Months

Event	MUSE n=486	Placebo n=511
Urogenital System		
Penile Pain	32%	3%
Urethral Burning	12%	4%
Minor Urethral Bleeding/Spotting	5%	1%
Testicular Pain	5%	1%
Nervous System		
Dizziness	2%	<1%
Body as a Whole		
Flu symptoms	4%	2%
Headache	3%	2%
Pain	3%	1%
Accidental Injury	3%	2%
Back Pain	2%	1%
Pelvic Pain	2%	<1%
Respiratory		
Rhinitis	2%	<1%
Infection	3%	2%

Other drug-related side effects observed during in-clinic titration and home treatment include swelling of leg veins, leg pain, perineal pain, and rapid pulse, each occurring in <2% of patients.

Female Partner Adverse Events: The most common drug-related adverse event reported by female partners during placebo-controlled clinical studies was vaginal burning/itching, reported by 5.8% of partners of patients on active vs. 0.8% of partners of patients on placebo. It is unknown whether this adverse event experienced by female partners was a result of the medication or a result of resuming sexual intercourse, which occurred much more frequently in partners of patients on active medication.

OVERDOSE:

Symptoms: Overdosage has not been reported with MUSE alprostadil. Overdosage with MUSE alprostadil may result in hypotension, persistent penile pain, and possibly priapism (rigid erection lasting ≥6 h). Priapism can result in permanent worsening of erectile function. Patients suspected of overdosage who develop these symptoms should be kept under medical supervision until systemic or local symptoms have resolved and/or until penile detumescence has occurred. Symptomatic treatment of any systemic symptoms would be appropriate.

Treatment: Patients should be instructed to report any erections persisting for more than 4 hours to a physician. The treatment of priapism/prolonged erection should be according to established medical practice. Physicians may refer to two suggested protocols for detumescence presented below.

Detumescence Protocols:

1. Aspirate 40 to 60 mL from either right or left corpora using vacutainer and holder as for drawing blood. Patient will often detumesce while aspirating. Apply ice for 20 minutes post aspiration if erection remains.
   If 1) unsuccessful then,
2. Have patient in supine position. Dilute 10 mg phenylephrine into 20 mL water for injection (0.05%). With an insulin syringe, inject 0.1 to 0.2 mL (50-100 µg) into the corpora every 2 to 5 minutes, until detumescence occurs. The occasional patient may experience very transient bradycardia and hypertension when given phenylephrine injections, therefore monitor patient's blood pressure and pulse every 10 minutes. Patients at risk include those with cardiac arrhythmias and diabetics. Refer to the prescribing information for phenylephrine before use. **Do not** give to patients on MAO inhibitors. When phenylephrine is used within the first 12 hours of erection, the majority of patients will respond.
3. If the above measures fail to detumesce the patient, a urologist should be consulted as soon as possible, especially if the erection has been present for many hours. If priapism is not treated immediately, penile tissue damage and/or permanent loss of potency may result.

For management of a suspected drug overdose, CPhA recommends that you contact your **regional Poison Control Centre**. See the *CPS* Directory section for a list of Poison Control Centres.

DOSAGE: MUSE alprostadil is a transurethral delivery system available in 3 dosage strengths: 250 µg, 500 µg and 1000 µg. MUSE alprostadil should be administered as needed to achieve an erection. The onset of effect is within 5-10 minutes after administration. The duration of effect is approximately 30-60 minutes. However, the actual duration will vary from patient to patient. Each patient should be instructed by a medical professional on proper technique for administering MUSE alprostadil prior to self-administration. The maximum frequency of use is no more than 2 systems per 24-hour period.

Initiation of Therapy: Dose titration should be undertaken under the supervision of a physician to test a patient's responsiveness to MUSE alprostadil, to demonstrate proper administration technique (see detailed instructions for the administration of MUSE alprostadil in the patient package insert), and to monitor for evidence of hypotension. Patients should be individually titrated to the lowest dose that is sufficient for sexual intercourse. The lower dose of MUSE alprostadil (250 µg) is recommended for initial dosing. If necessary, the dose should be increased on separate occasions in a stepwise manner until the patient achieves an erection that is sufficient for sexual intercourse.

Home Treatment Regimen: MUSE alprostadil should be used as needed to achieve an erection. The maximum frequency of use is 2 administrations per 24-hour period. Each MUSE system is for single-use only and should be properly discarded after use.

INFORMATION FOR THE PATIENT: Published in e-CPS, available by subscription at www.e-cps.ca.

SUPPLIED: Transurethral delivery system contains: alprostadil 250, 500 or 1000 µg. Nonmedicinal ingredients: polyethylene glycol 1450 USP. Store unopened foil pouches in a refrigerator at 2 to 8°C. Do not expose to temperatures above 30°C. May be kept by the patient at room temperature (below 30°C) for up to 14 days prior to use.

Mycamine® Ⓟ

micafungin sodium

Antifungal

Astellas

Date of Revision: September 2, 2008

SUMMARY PRODUCT INFORMATION:

Route of Administration	Dosage Form/ Strength	Clinically Relevant Nonmedicinal Ingredients
Intravenous infusion	Lyophilized Powder for Injection/50 mg vial	Lactose, citric acid and/or sodium hydroxide This is a complete listing of all nonmedicinal ingredients.

INDICATIONS AND CLINICAL USE: Mycamine is indicated for:

- Treatment of patients with Candidemia, Acute Disseminated Candidiasis, Candida Peritonitis and Abscesses infections. Mycamine has not been adequately studied in patients with endocarditis, osteomyelitis and meningitis due to Candida infections.
- Treatment of patients with esophageal candidiasis
- Prophylaxis of Candida infections in patients undergoing hematopoietic stem cell transplantation

Geriatrics (≥65 years of age): No overall differences in safety or effectiveness have been observed between geriatrics subjects (≥65 years) and younger subjects in clinical studies.

Pediatrics (<16 years): The safety and efficacy of Mycamine has not been established in pediatric patients below the age of 16 years.

Note: The efficacy of Mycamine against infections caused by fungi other than Candida has not been established.

CONTRAINDICATIONS: Mycamine is contraindicated in patients with hypersensitivity to micafungin, echinocandins or any component of this drug product. (For a complete listing, see Dosage Forms, Composition and Packaging).

WARNINGS AND PRECAUTIONS: General: Isolated cases of serious hypersensitivity (anaphylaxis and anaphylactoid) reactions (including shock) have been reported in patients receiving Mycamine. If these reactions occur, Mycamine infusion should be discontinued and appropriate treatment administered.

Carcinogenesis, Mutagenesis, Impairment of Fertility: Hepatic carcinomas and adenomas were observed in a 6-month intravenous toxicology study with an 18-month recovery period of micafungin sodium in rats designed to assess the reversibility of hepatocellular lesions.

Rats administered micafungin sodium for 3 months at 32 mg/kg/day (corresponding to 8 times the highest recommended human dose [150 mg/day], based on AUC comparisons), exhibited colored patches/zones, multinucleated hepatocytes and altered hepatocellular foci after 1 or 3 month recovery periods, and adenomas were observed after 20-month recovery period. Rats administered micafungin sodium at the same dose for 6 months exhibited adenomas after a 12-month recovery period; after an 18-month recovery period, an increased incidence of adenomas was observed, and additionally, carcinomas were detected. A lower dose of micafungin sodium (equivalent to 5 times the human AUC) in the 6-month rat study resulted in a lower incidence of adenomas and carcinomas following 18 months recovery. The duration of micafungin dosing in these rat studies (3 or 6 months) exceeds the usual duration of Mycamine dosing in patients, which is typically less than 1 month for treatment of esophageal candidiasis, but dosing may exceed 1 month for Candida prophylaxis.

Although the increase in carcinomas in the 6-month rat study did not reach statistical significance, the persistence of altered hepatocellular foci subsequent to micafungin dosing, and the presence of adenomas and carcinomas in the recovery periods suggest a causal relationship between micafungin sodium, altered hepatocellular foci, and hepatic neoplasms. Whole-life carcinogenicity studies of Mycamine in animals have not been conducted, and it is not known whether the hepatic neoplasms observed in treated rats also occur in other species, or if there is a dose threshold for this effect.

Hepatic Insufficiency: Laboratory abnormalities in liver function tests have been seen in healthy volunteers and patients treated with Mycamine. In some patients with serious underlying conditions who were receiving Mycamine along with multiple concomitant medications, clinical hepatic abnormalities have occurred, and isolated cases of significant hepatic dysfunction, hepatitis, or worsening hepatic failure have been reported. Patients who develop abnormal liver function tests during Mycamine therapy should be monitored for evidence of worsening hepatic function and evaluated for the risk/benefit of continuing Mycamine therapy.

Renal Insufficiency: Elevations in BUN and creatinine, and isolated cases of significant renal dysfunction or acute renal failure have been reported in patients who received Mycamine. In fluconazole-controlled trials, the incidence of drug-related renal adverse events was 0.4% for Mycamine treated patients and 0.5% for fluconazole treated patients. Patients who develop abnormal renal function tests during Mycamine therapy should be monitored for evidence of worsening renal function.

Hematological Effects: Acute intravascular hemolysis and hemoglobinuria were seen in a healthy volunteer during infusion of Mycamine (200 mg) and oral prednisolone (20 mg). This event was transient, and the subject did not develop significant anemia. Isolated cases of significant hemolysis and hemolytic anemia have also been reported in patients treated with Mycamine. Patients who develop clinical or laboratory evidence of hemolysis or hemolytic anemia during Mycamine therapy should be monitored closely for evidence of worsening of these conditions and evaluated for the risk/benefit of continuing Mycamine therapy.

Sexual Function/Reproduction: Male rats treated intravenously with micafungin sodium for 9 weeks showed vacuolation of the epididymal ductal epithelial cells at or above 10 mg/kg (about 0.6 times the recommended clinical dose for esophageal candidiasis, based on body surface area comparisons). Higher doses (about twice the recommended clinical dose, based on body surface area comparisons) resulted in higher epididymis weights and reduced numbers of sperm cells. In a 39-week intravenous study in dogs, seminiferous tubular atrophy and decreased sperm in the epididymis were observed at 10 and 32 mg/kg, doses equal to about 2 and 7 times the recommended clinical dose, based on body surface area comparisons. There was no impairment of fertility in animal studies with micafungin sodium.

Special Populations: Pregnant Women: No adequate, well-controlled studies have been conducted in pregnant women. Mycamine should be used during pregnancy only if the benefits outweigh the potential risks.

Micafungin sodium administration to pregnant rabbits (intravenous dosing on days 6 to 18 of gestation) resulted in visceral abnormalities and abortion at 32 mg/kg, a dose equivalent to about four times the recommended dose based on body surface area comparisons. Visceral abnormalities included abnormal lobation of the lung, levocardia, retrocaval ureter, anomalous right subclavian artery, and dilatation of the ureter. However, animal studies are not always predictive of human response.

Nursing Women: It is not known whether micafungin is excreted in human milk. Micafungin was found in the milk of lactating, drug-treated rats. Caution should be exercised when Mycamine is administered to a nursing woman.

Pediatrics (<16 years): The safety and efficacy of Mycamine has not been established in pediatric patients below the age of 16 years.

Geriatrics (≥65 years of age): A total of 418 subjects in clinical studies of Mycamine were 65 years of age and older, and 124 subjects were 75 years of age and older. No overall differences in safety or effectiveness were observed between these subjects and younger subjects. Other reported clinical experience has not identified differences in responses between the elderly and younger patients, but greater sensitivity of some older individuals cannot be ruled out.

ADVERSE REACTIONS: Adverse Drug Reaction Overview: Possible histamine-mediated symptoms have been reported with Mycamine, including rash, pruritus, facial swelling, and vasodilatation. Serious hypersensitivity (anaphylaxis and anaphylactoid) reactions (including shock) have been reported during administration of Mycamine (micafungin sodium).

Injection site reactions, including phlebitis and thrombophlebitis have been reported, at Mycamine doses of 50-150 mg/day. These events tended to occur more often in patients receiving Mycamine via peripheral intravenous administration.

Clinical Trial Adverse Drug Reactions: Because clinical trials are conducted under very specific conditions, the adverse reaction rates observed in the clinical trials may not reflect the rates observed in practice and should not be compared to the rates in the clinical trials of another drug. Adverse drug reaction information from clinical trials is useful for identifying drug-related adverse events and for approximating rates.

Candidemia and Other Candida Infections: In a phase III, randomized, double-blind study for treatment of candidemia and other Candida infections, treatment emergent adverse events occurred in 183/200 (91.5%), 187/202 (92.6%) and 171/193 (88.6%) patients in the Mycamine 100 mg/day, Mycamine 150 mg/day, and caspofungin (70/50 mg/day) treatment groups, respectively. Treatment emergent adverse events occurring in ≥5% of the patients in any treatment study groups are shown in Table 1.

Table 1: Mycamine

[a]Treatment Emergent Adverse Events in Patients with Candidemia and Other Candida Infections

MedDRA v 5.0 System Organ Class Preferred Term[b]	Micafungin 100 mg (n=200)	Micafungin 150 mg (n=202)	Caspofungin[c] (n=193)
All Systems, Any Adverse Event	183 (91.5)	187 (92.6)	171 (88.6)
Gastrointestinal Disorders	**81 (40.5)**	**89 (44.1)**	**76 (39.4)**
Diarrhea NOS	15 (7.5)	26 (12.9)	14 (7.3)
Nausea	19 (9.5)	15 (7.4)	20 (10.4)
Vomiting NOS	18 (9)	15 (7.4)	16 (8.3)
Abdominal Pain NOS	5 (2.5)	4 (2)	10 (5.2)
Metabolism and Nutrition Disorders	**77 (38.5)**	**83 (41.1)**	**73 (37.8)**
Hypokalemia	28 (14)	34 (16.8)	28 (14.5)
Hypomagnesaemia	11 (5.5)	17 (8.4)	14 (7.3)
Hypoglycemia NOS	12 (6)	14 (6.9)	9 (4.7)
Hypernatremia	8 (4)	13 (6.4)	8 (4.1)
Hyperkalemia	10 (5)	8 (4)	5 (2.6)
Infections and Infestations	**67 (33.5)**	**81 (40.1)**	**59 (30.6)**
Bacteremia	10 (5)	18 (8.9)	11 (5.7)
Septic Shock	15 (7.5)	9 (4.5)	9 (4.7)
Sepsis NOS	11 (5.5)	10 (5)	11 (5.7)
Pneumonia NOS	3 (1.5)	11 (5.4)	4 (2.1)
General Disorders/Administration Site Conditions	**59 (29.5)**	**56 (27.7)**	**51 (26.4)**
Pyrexia	14 (7)	22 (10.9)	15 (7.8)
Edema Peripheral	11 (5.5)	12 (5.9)	14 (7.3)
Vascular Disorders	**43 (21.5)**	**47 (23.3)**	**36 (18.7)**
Hypotension NOS	20 (10)	12 (5.9)	15 (7.8)
Hypertension NOS	6 (3)	10 (5)	12 (6.2)
Investigations	**36 (18)**	**49 (24.3)**	**37 (19.2)**
Blood Alkaline Phosphatase NOS Increased	11 (5.5)	16 (7.9)	8 (4.1)
Blood/Lymphatic System Disorders	**38 (19)**	**45 (22.3)**	**37 (19.2)**
Thrombocytopenia	8 (4)	8 (4)	11 (5.7)
Anemia NOS	5 (2.5)	6 (3)	13 (6.7)
Anemia NOS Aggravated	4 (2)	10 (5)	5 (2.6)
Cardiac Disorders	**35 (17.5)**	**48 (23.8)**	**36 (18.7%)**
Tachycardia NOS	6 (3)	7 (3.5)	13 (6.7%)
Bradycardia NOS	5 (2.5)	10 (5)	8 (4.1%)
Atrial Fibrillation	5 (2.5)	10 (5)	0
Nervous System Disorders	**21 (10.5)**	**42 (20.8)**	**32 (16.6)**
Headache NOS	4 (2)	10 (5)	11 (5.7)
Skin/Subcutaneous Tissue Disorders	**26 (13)**	**34 (16.8)**	**33 (17.1)**
Decubitus Ulcer	9 (4.5)	12 (5.9)	9 (4.7)
Psychiatric Disorders	**31 (15.5)**	**27 (13.4)**	**33 (17.1)**
Insomnia	11 (5.5)	8 (4)	16 (8.3)

[a] During IV treatment+3 days.
[b] Within a system organ class patients may experience more than 1 adverse event.
[c] 70 mg loading dose on day 1 followed by 50 mg/day thereafter (caspofungin).
Patient base: All randomized patients who received at least 1 dose of trial drug.
Common: ≥5% in any treatment arm.

In a second phase III, randomized, double-blind study for treatment of candidemia and other Candida infections, treatment emergent adverse events occurred in 245/264 (92.8%) and 250/265 (94.3%) patients in the Mycamine (100 mg/day) and AmBisome (3 mg/kg/day) treatment groups, respectively. The most common treatment emergent adverse events occurring in ≥5% of the Mycamine-treated patients at least 16 years of age were: pyrexia (15.2% vs. 17%); hypokalemia (16.7% vs. 20.8%); nausea (9.5% vs. 8.3%); diarrhea (10.6% vs. 11.3%) and vomiting (12.9% vs. 9.4%), in the Mycamine and AmBisome treatment groups, respectively. Other important treatment emergent adverse events that occurred at <5% frequency were abnormal liver function tests (4.2% vs. 3%); increased aspartate aminotransferase (2.7% vs. 1.9%), and increased blood alkaline phosphatase (3% vs. 2.3%), in the Mycamine and AmBisome treatment groups, respectively.

Esophageal Candidiasis: In a phase III, randomized, double-blind study for treatment of esophageal candidiasis, a total of 202/260 (77.7%) patients who received Mycamine 150 mg/day and 186/258 (72.1%) patients who received intravenous fluconazole 200 mg/day experienced an adverse event. Treatment emergent adverse events resulting in discontinuation were reported in 17 (6.5%) Mycamine treated patients; and in 12 (4.7%) fluconazole treated patients. Treatment emergent adverse events occurring in ≥5% of the patients in either treatment group are shown in Table 2.

Table 2: Mycamine

[a]Treatment Emergent Adverse Events in Patients with Esophageal Candidiasis

Adverse Events[b] (MedDRA System Organ Class and Preferred Term)	Mycamine 150 mg/day n (%)	Fluconazole 200 mg/day n (%)
Number of Patients	**260**	**258**
All Systems, Any Adverse Event	**202 (77.7)**	**186 (72.1)**
Gastrointestinal Disorders	**84 (32.3)**	**93 (36)**
Diarrhea NOS	27 (10.4)	29 (11.2)
Nausea	20 (7.7)	23 (8.9)
Vomiting NOS	17 (6.5)	17 (6.6)
Abdominal Pain NOS	10 (3.8)	15 (5.8)
General Disorders/Administration Site Conditions	**52 (20)**	**45 (17.4)**
Pyrexia	34 (13.1)	21 (8.1)
Nervous System Disorders	**42 (16.2)**	**40 (15.5)**
Headache NOS	22 (8.5)	20 (7.8)
Blood/Lymphatic System Disorders	**38 (14.6)**	**43 (16.7)**
Anemia NOS	8 (3.1)	16 (6.2)
Vascular Disorders	**54 (20.8)**	**21 (8.1)**
Phlebitis NOS	49 (18.8)	13 (5)
Skin and Subcutaneous Tissue Disorders	**36 (13.8)**	**26 (10.1)**
Rash NOS	14 (5.4)	6 (2.3)
Psychiatric Disorders	**20 (7.7)**	**21 (8.1)**
Insomnia	9 (3.5)	13 (5)

[a] During treatment+3 days.
[b] Within a system organ class patients may experience more than 1 adverse event.
Patient base: All randomized patients who received at least 1 dose of trial drug.
Common: ≥5% in either treatment arm.

Prophylaxis of Candida Infections in Hematopoietic Stem Cell Transplant Recipients: A double-blind, phase III study was conducted in a total of 882 patients scheduled to undergo an autologous or allogeneic hematopoietic stem cell transplant. The median duration of treatment was 18 days (range 1 to 51 days) in both treatment arms.

All patients who received Mycamine (425) and all patients who received fluconazole (457) experienced at least one adverse event during the study. Treatment emergent adverse events resulting in Mycamine discontinuation were reported in 18 (4.2%) patients; while those resulting in fluconazole discontinuation were reported in 33 (7.2%). Treatment emergent adverse events occurring in ≥15% of the patients in either treatment group are shown in Table 3.

Table 3: Mycamine

[a]Treatment Emergent Adverse Events During Prophylaxis of Candida Infection in Hematopoietic Stem Cell Transplant Recipients

Adverse Events[b] (MedDRA System Organ Class and Preferred Term)	Mycamine 50 mg/day n (%)	Fluconazole 400 mg/day n (%)
Number of Patients	**425**	**457**
All Systems, Any Adverse Events	**425 (100)**	**457 (100)**
Gastrointestinal Disorders	**421 (99.1)**	**449 (98.2)**
Diarrhea NOS	302 (71.1)	348 (76.1)
Nausea	296 (69.6)	309 (67.6)
Vomiting NOS	281 (66.1)	307 (67.2)
Constipation	129 (30.4)	143 (31.3)
Dyspepsia	104 (24.5)	122 (26.7)
Abdominal Pain NOS	115 (27.1)	107 (23.4)
General Disorders/Administration Site Conditions	**410 (96.5)**	**440 (96.3)**
Mucosal Inflammation NOS	322 (75.8)	360 (78.8)
Pyrexia	191 (44.9)	218 (47.7)
Fatigue	126 (29.6)	145 (31.7)

(cont'd)

Table 3: Mycamine *(cont'd)*

[a]Treatment Emergent Adverse Events During Prophylaxis of Candida Infection in Hematopoietic Stem Cell Transplant Recipients

Adverse Events[b] (MedDRA System Organ Class and Preferred Term)	Mycamine 50 mg/day n (%)	Fluconazole 400 mg/day n (%)
Rigors	112 (26.4)	118 (25.8)
Edema Peripheral	88 (20.7)	100 (21.9)
Blood and Lymphatic System Disorders	**408 (96)**	**429 (93.9)**
Neutropenia	320 (75.3)	327 (71.6)
Thrombocytopenia	307 (72.2)	304 (66.5)
Anemia NOS	151 (35.5)	173 (37.9)
Febrile Neutropenia	155 (36.5)	166 (36.3)
Metabolism and Nutrition Disorders	**385 (90.6)**	**428 (93.7)**
Hypomagnesaemia	214 (50.4)	256 (56)
Hypokalemia	209 (49.2)	232 (50.8)
Anorexia	116 (27.3)	121 (26.5)
Appetite Decreased NOS	87 (20.5)	93 (20.4)
Fluid Overload	74 (17.4)	96 (21)
Hyperglycemia NOS	68 (16)	92 (20.1)
Hypocalcemia	72 (16.9)	82 (17.9)
Fluid Retention	69 (16.2)	66 (14.4)
Respiratory, Thoracic and Mediastinal Disorders	**291 (68.5)**	**336 (73.5)**
Cough	98 (23.1)	112 (24.5)
Epistaxis	49 (11.5)	84 (18.4)
Dyspnea NOS	54 (12.7)	64 (14)
Skin and Subcutaneous Tissue Disorders	**290 (68.2)**	**316 (69.1)**
Rash NOS	110 (25.9)	102 (22.3)
Pruritus NOS	75 (17.6)	87 (19.)
Erythema	48 (11.3)	71 (15.5)
Nervous System Disorders	**261 (61.4)**	**268 (58.6)**
Headache NOS	179 (42.1)	165 (36.1)
Dizziness	55 (12.9)	83 (18.2)
Psychiatric Disorders	**257 (60.5)**	**249 (54.5)**
Insomnia	152 (35.8)	146 (31.9)
Anxiety	95 (22.4)	92 (20.1)
Vascular Disorders	**224 (52.7)**	**267 (58.4)**
Hypertension NOS	91 (21.4)	113 (24.7)
Hypotension NOS	79 (18.6)	89 (19.5)
Flushing	47 (11.1)	70 (15.3)
Infections and Infestations	**178 (41.9)**	**208 (45.5)**
Bacteremia	66 (15.5)	86 (18.8)
Cardiac Disorders	**147 (34.6)**	**162 (35.4)**
Tachycardia NOS	105 (24.7)	102 (22.3)

[a] During treatment + 3 days.
[b] Within a system organ class patients may experience more than 1 adverse event.
Patient base: All randomized patients who received at least 1 dose of trial drug.
Common: ≥15% in either treatment arm.

Overall Mycamine Safety Experience: The overall safety of Mycamine was assessed in 3083 patients and 501 volunteers in 41 clinical studies, including the invasive candidiasis, esophageal candidiasis and prophylaxis studies, who received single or multiple doses of Mycamine, ranging from 12.5 mg to ≥150 mg/day. Treatment emergent adverse events which occurred in ≥5% of all patients who received Mycamine in these trials are shown in Table 4.

Overall, 2810 of 3083 (91.1%) patients who received Mycamine experienced an adverse event.

Clinically significant adverse events regardless of causality or incidence which occurred in these trials are listed below:

Blood and Lymphatic System Disorders: coagulopathy, febrile neutropenia, hemolysis, hemolytic anemia, pancytopenia, thrombotic thrombocytopenic purpura.

Cardiac Disorders: arrhythmia, atrial fibrillation, cardiac arrest, cyanosis, hypotension, myocardial infarction, tachycardia.

Gastrointestinal Disorders: abdominal pain upper, dyspepsia.

General Disorders and Administration Site Conditions: injection site thrombosis.

Hepatobiliary Disorders: hepatocellular damage, hepatomegaly, jaundice, hepatic failure.

Infections and Infestations: infection, pneumonia, sepsis.

Metabolism and Nutrition Disorders: acidosis, anorexia, hyponatremia.

Musculoskeletal, Connective Tissue and Bone Disorders: arthralgia.

Nervous System Disorders: convulsions, encephalopathy, intracranial hemorrhage.

Psychiatric Disorders: delirium.

Renal and Urinary Disorders: anuria, hemoglobinuria, oliguria, renal failure acute, renal tubular necrosis.

Respiratory, Thoracic and Mediastinal Disorders: apnea, dyspnea, hypoxia, pulmonary embolism.

Skin And Subcutaneous Tissue Disorders: erythema multiforme, skin necrosis, urticaria.

Vascular Disorders: deep venous thrombosis, hypertension.

Table 4: Mycamine

[a]Treatment Emergent Adverse Events in Patients Who Received Mycamine in Clinical Trials

Adverse Events[b] (MedDRA System Organ Class and Preferred Term)	Mycamine n (%)
Number of Patients	**3083**
All Systems, Any Adverse Event	**2810 (91.1)**
Gastrointestinal Disorders	**1764 (57.2)**
Diarrhea NOS	718 (23.3)
Nausea	679 (22)
Vomiting NOS	669 (21.7)
Constipation	341 (11.1)
Abdominal Pain	300 (9.7)
Dyspepsia	176 (5.7)
General Disorders/Administration Site Conditions	**1407 (45.6)**
Pyrexia	618 (20)
Mucosal Inflammation NOS	438 (14.2)
Rigors	281 (9.1)
Edema Peripheral	209 (6.8)
Fatigue	198 (6.4)
Metabolism and Nutrition Disorders	**1316 (42.7)**
Hypokalemia	556 (18)
Hypomagnesemia	409 (13.3)
Hypocalcemia	201 (6.5)
Anorexia	190 (6.2)
Hyperglycemia NOS	173 (5.6)
Fluid Overload	155 (5)
Infections and Infestations	**1227 (39.8)**
Bacteremia	185 (6)
Sepsis NOS	156 (5.1)
Respiratory, Thoracic and Mediastinal Disorders	**1108 (35.9)**
Cough	251 (8.1)
Dyspnea NOS	182 (5.9)
Epistaxis	172 (5.6)
Blood and Lymphatic System Disorders	**1047 (34)**
Thrombocytopenia	474 (15.4)
Neutropenia	436 (14.1)
Anemia NOS	302 (9.8)
Febrile Neutropenia	187 (6.1)
Investigations	**989 (32.1)**
Aspartate Aminotransferase Increased	172 (5.6)
Blood Alkaline Phosphatase NOS Increased	168 (5.4)
Alanine Aminotransferase Increased	165 (5.4%)
Skin and Subcutaneous Tissue Disorders	**940 (30.5)**
Rash NOS	269 (8.7)
Pruritus NOS	187 (6.1)
Nervous System Disorders	**889 (28.8)**
Headache NOS	489 (15.9)

(cont'd)

Table 4: Mycamine *(cont'd)*

[a]Treatment Emergent Adverse Events in Patients Who Received Mycamine in Clinical Trials

Adverse Events[b] (MedDRA System Organ Class and Preferred Term)	Mycamine n (%)
Psychiatric Disorders	**727 (23.6)**
Insomnia	303 (9.8)
Anxiety	198 (6.4)
Vascular Disorders	**867 (28.1)**
Hypotension NOS	279 (9.1)
Hypertension NOS	214 (6.9)
Phlebitis NOS	172 (5.6)
Musculoskeletal and Connective Tissue Disorders	**579 (18.8)**
Back Pain	166 (5.4)
Cardiac Disorders	**563 (18.3)**
Tachycardia NOS	231 (7.5)

[a] During treatment+3 days.
[b] Within a system organ class, patients may experience more than 1 adverse event.
Patient base: All randomized patients who received at least 1 dose of trial drug.
Common: Incidence of adverse event ≥5%.

Post-Market Adverse Drug Reactions: The following adverse events have been identified during the post-approval use of Mycamine for injection. Because these reactions are reported voluntarily from a population of uncertain size, it is not always possible to reliably estimate their frequency. A causal relationship to Mycamine could not be excluded for these adverse events, which included:
Hepatobiliary Disorders: hyperbilirubinemia, hepatic function abnormal, hepatic disorder, hepatocellular damage.
Renal and Urinary Disorders: acute renal failure and renal impairment.
Blood and Lymphatic System Disorders: white blood cell count decreased, hemolytic anemia.
Vascular Disorders: shock.

DRUG INTERACTIONS: Drug-Drug Interactions: A total of 14 clinical drug-drug interaction studies were conducted in healthy volunteers to evaluate the potential for interaction between Mycamine and amphotericin B, mycophenolate mofetil, cyclosporine, tacrolimus, prednisolone, sirolimus, nifedipine, fluconazole, itraconazole, voriconazole, ritonavir, or rifampin. In these studies, no interaction that altered the pharmacokinetics of micafungin was observed.

Co-administration of Mycamine and amphotericin B deoxycholate was associated with a 30% increase in amphotericin B deoxycholate exposure. The clinical significance of this increase is unclear however this co-administration should only be used when the benefits clearly outweigh the risks, with close monitoring of amphotericin B deoxycholate toxicities.

Co-administration of voriconazole with Mycamine was associated with approximately 20% reduction of voriconazole exposure on average. In the same study co-administration of placebo and voriconazole was associated with a similar reduction of voriconazole exposure. When the effect of Mycamine was corrected for the effect of placebo, there was no significant effect of Mycamine on the pharmacokinetics of voriconazole.

There was no effect of a single dose or multiple doses of Mycamine on mycophenolate mofetil, cyclosporine, tacrolimus, prednisolone, voriconazole and fluconazole pharmacokinetics.

Sirolimus AUC was increased by 21% with no effect on C_{max} in the presence of steady-state Mycamine compared with sirolimus alone. Nifedipine AUC and C_{max} were increased by 18% and 42%, respectively, in the presence of steady-state Mycamine compared with nifedipine alone. Itraconazole AUC and C_{max} were increased by 22% and 11%, respectively, in the presence of steady-state Mycamine compared with itraconazole alone. Patients receiving sirolimus, itraconazole or nifedipine in combination with Mycamine should be monitored for sirolimus, itraconazole or nifedipine toxicity. The sirolimus, itraconazole or nifedipine dosage should be reduced if necessary.

Micafungin is not an inhibitor of P-glycoprotein and, therefore, would not be expected to alter P-glycoprotein-mediated drug transport activity.
Drug-Food Interactions: Interactions with food have not been established.
Drug-Herb Interactions: Interactions with herbs have not been established.
Drug-Laboratory Test Interactions: Interactions with laboratory tests have not been established.

DOSAGE AND ADMINISTRATION: Dosing Considerations: Do not mix or co-infuse Mycamine with other medications. Mycamine has been shown to precipitate when mixed directly with a number of other commonly used medications.

Mycamine should be administered by a slow intravenous infusion over the period of 1 hour. More rapid infusions may result in more frequent histamine mediated reactions.
Note: An existing intravenous line should be flushed with 0.9% Sodium Chloride Injection, USP, prior to infusion of Mycamine.
Recommended Dose and Dosage Adjustment: Mycamine Dosage:

Indication	Recommended Dose Adults (mg/day)
Treatment of Candidemia and other Candida infections[a]	100
Prophylaxis of Candida Infections in HSCT Recipients[b]	50
Treatment of Esophageal Candidiasis[c]	150

[a] In patients treated successfully for candidemia and other Candida infections, the mean duration of treatment was 15 days (range 10-47 days).
[b] In hematopoietic stem cell transplant (HSCT) recipients who experienced success of prophylactic therapy, the mean duration of prophylaxis was 19 days (range 6-51 days).
[c] In patients treated successfully for esophageal candidiasis, the mean duration of treatment was 15 days (range 10-30 days).

A loading dose is not required; typically, 85% of the steady-state concentration is achieved after three daily Mycamine doses.

No dosing adjustments are required based on age, race, gender, or in patients with severe renal dysfunction or mild-to-moderate hepatic insufficiency. The effect of severe hepatic impairment on micafungin pharmacokinetics has not been studied. (See Action and Clinical Pharmacology, Special Populations and Conditions.)

No dose adjustment for Mycamine is required with concomitant use of mycophenolate mofetil, cyclosporine, tacrolimus, prednisolone, sirolimus, nifedipine, fluconazole, voriconazole, itraconazole, amphotericin B, ritonavir, or rifampin. (See Drug Interactions.)

Reconstitution: Please read this entire section carefully before beginning reconstitution.

The diluent to be used for reconstitution and dilution is 0.9% Sodium Chloride Injection, USP (without a bacteriostatic agent). Alternatively, 5% Dextrose Injection, USP, may be used for reconstitution and dilution of Mycamine. Solutions for infusion are prepared as follows:
Mycamine 50 mg Vial: Aseptically add 5 mL of 0.9% Sodium Chloride Injection, USP (without a bacteriostatic agent) to each **50 mg vial** to yield a preparation containing approximately **10 mg micafungin/mL**.
Dilution: The diluted solution should be protected from light. It is not necessary to cover the infusion drip chamber or the tubing.

For treatment of Candidemia and other Candida infections: add 100 mg of reconstituted Mycamine (see Reconstitution) into 100 mL of 0.9% Sodium Chloride Injection, USP or 100 mL of 5% Dextrose Injection, USP.
For prophylaxis of Candida infections: add 50 mg of reconstituted Mycamine (see Reconstitution) into 100 mL of 0.9% Sodium Chloride Injection, USP or 100 mL of 5% Dextrose Injection, USP.
For treatment of esophageal candidiasis: add 150 mg of reconstituted Mycamine (see Reconstitution) into 100 mL of 0.9% Sodium Chloride Injection, USP or 100 mL of 5% Dextrose Injection, USP.

Mycamine is preservative-free. Discard partially used vials.

OVERDOSAGE:
Mycamine is highly protein bound and, therefore, is not dialyzable. No cases of Mycamine overdosage have been reported. Repeated daily doses up to 8 mg/kg (maximum total dose of 896 mg) in adult patients have been administered in clinical trials with no reported dose-limiting toxicity. The minimum lethal dose of Mycamine is 125 mg/kg in rats, equivalent to 8.1 times the recommended human clinical dose for esophageal candidiasis based on body surface area comparisons.

For management of a suspected drug overdose, contact your **regional Poison Control Centre**. See the *CPS* Directory section for a list of Poison Control Centres.

ACTION AND CLINICAL PHARMACOLOGY: Mechanism of Action: Micafungin is a semisynthetic lipopeptide (echinocandin) compound synthesized by a chemical modification of a fermentation product of Coleophoma empetri F-11899.

Micafungin is a member of a class of antifungal drugs known as echinocandins. It inhibits the synthesis of 1,3-β-D glucan, an essential component of fungal cell walls, which is not present in mammalian cells.
Pharmacokinetics: The pharmacokinetics of micafungin were determined in healthy subjects, hematopoietic stem cell transplant recipients, and patients with esophageal candidiasis or invasive candidiasis up to a maximum daily dose of 8 mg/kg body weight.

The relationship of area under the concentration-time curve (AUC) to micafungin dose was linear over the daily dose range of 50 mg to 150 mg and 3 mg/kg to 8 mg/kg body weight.

Steady-state pharmacokinetic parameters in relevant patient populations after repeated daily administration are presented in Table 5.

Table 5: Mycamine

Pharmacokinetic Parameters of Micafungin in Adult Patients

Population	N	Dose (mg)	Pharmacokinetic Parameters (Mean±Standard Deviation) C_{max} (μg/mL)	AUC_{0-24}[a] (μg·h/mL)	$T_{1/2}$ (h)	Cl (mL/min/kg)
Patients with IC						
[Day 1]	20	100	5.7±2.2	83±51	14.5±7.0	0.359 ±0.179
[Steady State]	20	100	10.1±4.4	97±29	13.4±2.0	0.298 ±0.115
HIV Positive Patients with EC						
[Day 1]	20	50	4.1±1.4	36±9	14.9±4.3	0.321±0.098
	20	100	8.0±2.4	108±31	13.8±3.0	0.327±0.093
	14	150	11.6±3.1	151±45	14.1±2.6	0.340±0.092
[Day 14 or 21]	20	50	5.1±1.0	54±13	15.6±2.8	0.300±0.063
	20	100	10.1±2.6	115±25	16.9±4.4	0.301±0.086
	14	150	16.4±6.5	167±40	15.2±2.2	0.297±0.081
HSCT Recipients		per kg				
[Day 7]	8	3	21.1±2.84	234±34	14.0±1.4	0.214±0.031
	10	4	29.2±6.2	339±72	14.2±3.2	0.204±0.036
	8	6	38.4±6.9	479±157	14.9±2.6	0.224±0.064
	8	8	60.8±26.9	663±212	17.2±2.3	0.223±0.081

[a] $AUC_{0-infinity}$ is presented for day 1 and AUC_{0-24} is presented for steady state.
Legend: HIV=human immunodeficiency virus; EC=esophageal candidiasis; HSCT=hematopoietic stem cell transplant; IC=Candidemia and other Candida infections; a=n for C_{max} and $T_{½}$; b=n for AUC_{0-24} and Cl.

Distribution: The mean ± standard deviation volume of distribution of micafungin at terminal phase was 0.39±0.11 L/kg body weight when determined in adult patients with esophageal candidiasis at the dose range of 50 mg to 150 mg. Micafungin is highly (>99%) protein bound in vitro, independent of plasma concentrations over the range of 10 to 100 μg/mL. The primary binding protein is albumin; however, micafungin, at therapeutically relevant concentrations, does not competitively displace bilirubin binding to albumin. Micafungin also binds to a lesser extent to α_1-acid-glycoprotein.
Metabolism: Micafungin is metabolized to M-1 (catechol form) by arylsulfatase, with further metabolism to M-2 (methoxy form) by catechol-O-methyltransferase. M-5 is formed by hydroxylation at the side chain (ω-1 position) of micafungin catalyzed by cytochrome P450 (CYP) isozymes. Even though micafungin is a substrate for and a weak inhibitor of CYP3A in vitro, hydroxylation by CYP3A is not a major pathway for micafungin metabolism in vivo. Micafungin is neither a P-glycoprotein substrate nor inhibitor in vitro.

In four healthy volunteer studies, the ratio of metabolite to parent exposure (AUC) at a dose of 150 mg/day was 6% for M-1, 1% for M-2, and 6% for M-5. In patients with esophageal candidiasis, the ratio of metabolite to parent exposure (AUC) at a dose of 150 mg/day was 11% for M-1, 2% for M-2, and 12% for M-5.
Excretion: The excretion of radioactivity following a single intravenous dose of ^{14}C-micafungin sodium for injection (25 mg) was evaluated in healthy volunteers. At 28 days after administration, mean urinary and fecal recovery of total radioactivity accounted for 82.5% (76.4 to 87.9%) of the administered dose. Fecal excretion is the major route of elimination (total radioactivity at 28 days was 71.0% of the administered dose).
Special Populations and Conditions: Mycamine disposition has been studied in a variety of populations as described below.
Geriatrics: The exposure and disposition of a 50 mg Mycamine dose administered as a single 1-hour infusion to 10 healthy subjects aged 66-78 years were not significantly different from those in 10 healthy subjects aged 20-24 years. No dose adjustment is necessary for the elderly.
Race and Gender: No dose adjustment of Mycamine is required based on gender or race. After 14 daily doses of 150 mg to healthy subjects, micafungin AUC in women was greater by approximately 23% compared with men, due to smaller body weight. No notable differences among white, black, and Hispanic subjects were seen. The micafungin AUC was greater by 26% in Japanese subjects compared to blacks, due to smaller body weight.
Renal Insufficiency: Mycamine does not require dose adjustment in patients with renal impairment. A single 1-hour infusion of 100 mg Mycamine was administered to 9 subjects with severe renal dysfunction (creatinine clearance <30 mL/min) and to 9 age-, gender-, and weight-matched subjects with normal renal function (creatinine clearance >80 mL/min). The maximum concentration (C_{max}) and AUC were not significantly altered by severe renal impairment.

Since micafungin is highly protein bound, it is not dialyzable. Supplementary dosing should not be required following hemodialysis.

Hepatic Insufficiency: A single 1-hour infusion of 100 mg Mycamine was administered to 8 subjects with moderate hepatic dysfunction (Child-Pugh score 7-9) and 8 age-, gender-, and weight-matched subjects with normal hepatic function. The C_{max} and AUC values of micafungin were lower by approximately 22% in subjects with moderate hepatic insufficiency. This difference in micafungin exposure does not require dose adjustment of Mycamine in patients with moderate hepatic impairment. The pharmacokinetics of Mycamine have not been studied in patients with severe hepatic insufficiency.

STORAGE AND STABILITY: Stability and Storage Recommendations: Unopened vials of lyophilized material should be stored, protected from light, at controlled room temperature, 15-30°C.

Storage of Reconstituted Product Concentrate: The reconstituted product may be stored in the original vial for up to 24 hours at room temperature, 25°C.

Storage of Diluted Product: The diluted infusion should be protected from light and may be stored for up to 24 hours at room temperature, 25°C.

Note: Mycamine is preservative-free. Discard partially used vials.

SPECIAL HANDLING INSTRUCTIONS: Not applicable.

INFORMATION FOR THE PATIENT: Published in e-CPS, available by subscription at www.e-cps.ca.

DOSAGE FORMS, COMPOSITION AND PACKAGING: Each vial of a sterile, nonpyrogenic, lyophilized powder for intravenous infusion contains: micafungin sodium 50 mg. Nonmedicinal ingredients: citric acid and/or sodium hydroxide (used for pH adjustment) and lactose. Following reconstitution with 0.9% Sodium Chloride for Injection, USP, the resulting pH of the solution is between 5.0-7.0. USP Type 1 glass vials of 10 mL, individual cartons of 10. The glass vials are covered with a light protective film.

Mycobutin® Ⓟ

rifabutin

Antibacterial

Pfizer

Date of Preparation: September 24, 2003
Date of Revision: August 6, 2008

PHARMACOLOGY: Rifabutin is a derivative of rifamycin S, belonging to the class of ansamycins. The rifamycins owe their antimycobacterial efficacy to their ability to penetrate the cell wall and to their ability to complex with and to inhibit DNA-dependent RNA polymerase. Rifabutin has been found to interact with and to penetrate the outer layers of the mycobacterial envelope.

Rifabutin inhibits DNA-dependent RNA polymerase in susceptible strains of *E. coli* and *B. subtilis* but not in mammalian cells. In resistant strains of *E. coli*, rifabutin, like rifampin, did not inhibit this enzyme. It is not known whether rifabutin inhibits DNA-dependent RNA polymerase in *M. avium* or in *M. intracellulare* which constitutes *M. avium* complex (MAC). Rifabutin inhibited incorporation of thymidine into DNA of rifampin-resistant *M. tuberculosis* suggesting that rifabutin may also inhibit DNA synthesis which may explain its activity against rifampin-resistant organisms.

Pharmacokinetics: Following oral administration, at least 53% of rifabutin dose is rapidly absorbed with rifabutin peak plasma concentrations attained in 2 to 4 hours. High-fat meals slow the rate without influencing the extent of absorption of rifabutin from the capsule dosage form.

The mean (±SD) absolute bioavailability assessed in HIV positive patients in a multiple dose study was 20% (±16%, n=5) on day 1 and 12% (±5%, n=7) on day 28.

In healthy adult volunteers administered a single oral dose of 300 mg of rifabutin, the mean (±SD) peak plasma concentration (C_{max}) was 375 (±267) ng/mL (range: 141 to 1033 ng/mL). Mean rifabutin steady-state trough levels (C_p, min^{ss}, 24-hour post dose) ranged from 50 to 65 ng/mL in HIV positive patients and in healthy normal volunteers. Pharmacokinetic dose-proportionality over the 300 to 900 mg single dose range has been demonstrated in early symptomatic HIV positive patients and in healthy normal volunteers over the 300 to 600 mg single dose range.

Rifabutin appears to be widely distributed throughout the body and has been detected in all tissues and body fluids examined. Several times higher concentrations than those achieved in plasma have been observed in lung parenchyma, gall bladder and the small intestinal wall. The apparent volume of distribution at steady-state (V_{ss}) estimated in early symptomatic HIV positive male patients following i.v. dosing was large (8 to 9 L/kg), suggesting extensive distribution of rifabutin into the tissues. About 85% of the drug is bound to plasma proteins over a concentration range of 50 to 1000 ng/mL. Binding is predominantly to human serum albumin, is concentration independent and does not appear to be influenced by renal or hepatic dysfunction.

Rifabutin undergoes extensive oxidative metabolism. Of the 5 metabolites that have been identified, 25-O-deacetyl and 31-hydroxy are the most predominant and show a plasma metabolite:parent area under the curve ratio of 0.10 for 25-O-deacetyl and 0.07 for 31-hydroxy metabolite. The 25-O-deacetyl metabolite has antimycobacterial activity equal to the parent drug and contributes up to 10% to the total antimicrobial activity. The 31-hydroxy metabolite has some antimicrobial activity (1/16 that of parent drug), but, considering its concentration in plasma, it is probably not contributing significantly to the therapeutic activity of rifabutin. Rifabutin can induce its own metabolism on multiple dosing. The area under the plasma concentration-time curve (AUC) following multiple dosing decreased by 38%, but its terminal half-life remained unchanged.

The plasma elimination profile of rifabutin is biphasic with an initial half-life of approximately 4 hours followed by a mean terminal half-life 45 (±17) hours (range: 16 to 69 hours). Mean systemic clearance in healthy adult volunteers following a single oral dose was 0.69 (±0.32) L/hour/kg (range: 0.46 to 1.34 L/hour/kg). Rifabutin is mainly excreted in the urine, primarily as metabolites and to a lesser extent in the feces. Fifty-three percent (53%) of the oral dose of ^{14}C-labelled drug was recovered in the urine by 5 days post-dose and 30% was recovered in the feces over the same period. Renal and biliary excretion of unchanged drug each contribute approximately 5% to the systemic clearance.

The pharmacokinetic profile of rifabutin is not significantly modified by age or by hepatic dysfunction, although the inter-individual variability in elderly subjects (71 to 80 years) was slightly higher. Rifabutin steady-state pharmacokinetics in early symptomatic HIV positive patients are similar to those in healthy normal volunteers but the variability between individuals is higher in the HIV positive patients. Renal insufficiency was correlated to a decrease in rifabutin urinary excretion. Other pharmacokinetic parameters did not appear to differ in a clinically relevant way between patients with various degrees of renal insufficiency and patients with normal renal function. Care is recommended when treating patients with severe renal insufficiency. No rifabutin disposition information is currently available in children or adolescents under 18 years of age.

INDICATIONS: For the prevention of disseminated *M. avium* complex (MAC) disease in patients with advanced HIV infection (CD4+ cell count ≤200/mm³ with an AIDS defining diagnosis, or CD4+ cell count ≤100/mm³ without an AIDS defining diagnosis).

CONTRAINDICATIONS: In patients who have had clinically significant hypersensitivity to this drug, or to any other rifamycins.

WARNINGS: Rifabutin prophylaxis must not be administered to patients with **active** tuberculosis. Among HIV positive patients, tuberculosis is common and may present with atypical or extrapulmonary findings. Patients are likely to have a nonreactive purified protein derivative (PPD) test despite active disease. In addition to chest x-ray and sputum culture, the following studies may be useful in the diagnosis of tuberculosis in the HIV positive patient: blood culture, urine culture, or biopsy of a suspicious lymph node.

Patients who develop signs and symptoms consistent with active tuberculosis while on rifabutin prophylaxis should be evaluated immediately, so that those with active disease may be given an effective combination regimen of antituberculosis medications. Administration of rifabutin, as a single-agent, to patients with active tuberculosis is likely to lead to the development of tuberculosis which is resistant both to rifabutin and to rifampin.

There is no evidence that rifabutin provides effective prophylaxis against *M. tuberculosis* infections. Patients requiring prophylaxis against both *M. tuberculosis* and *M. avium* complex may be given isoniazid and rifabutin concurrently.

C. difficile-associated disease (CDAD) has been reported with use of many antibacterial agents, including rifabutin. CDAD may range in severity from mild diarrhea to fatal colitis. It is important to consider this diagnosis in patients who present with diarrhea, or symptoms of colitis, pseudomembranous colitis, toxic megacolon, or perforation of colon subsequent to the administration of any antibacterial agent. CDAD has been reported to occur over 2 months after the administration of antibacterial agents.

Treatment with antibacterial agents may alter the normal flora of the colon and may permit overgrowth of *C. difficile*. *C. difficile* produces toxins A and B, which contribute to the development of CDAD. CDAD may cause significant morbidity and mortality. CDAD can be refractory to antimicrobial therapy.

If the diagnosis of CDAD is suspected or confirmed, appropriate therapeutic measures should be initiated. Mild cases of CDAD usually respond to discontinuation of antibacterial agents not directed against *C. difficile*. In moderate to severe cases, consideration should be given to management with fluids and electrolytes, protein supplementation, and treatment with an antibacterial agent clinically effective against *C. difficile*. Surgical evaluation should be instituted as clinically indicated, as surgical intervention may be required in certain severe cases.

PRECAUTIONS: General: Because rifabutin may be associated with neutropenia, and more rarely thrombocytopenia, physicians should consider obtaining hematologic studies periodically in patients receiving rifabutin prophylaxis.

Geriatrics: Rifabutin administered as a single dose has been evaluated in 24 healthy, elderly (71 to 80 years) volunteers. The pharmacokinetic profile of rifabutin is not significantly modified by age, although the inter-individual variability in this age group was slightly higher when compared to younger (25 to 37 years) volunteers.

Children: The safety and effectiveness of rifabutin for prophylaxis of MAC disease in children and adolescents under 18 years of age have not been established. However, limited safety data are available from 22 HIV positive children who received rifabutin as treatment for disseminated MAC disease, in combination with at least 2 other antimycobacterials for periods ranging from 1 to 183 weeks.

The mean daily doses (mg/kg) for these children were: infants 1 year of age, 18.5 (range 15.0 to 25.0); children 2 to 10 years, 8.6 (range 4.4 to 18.8); adolescents 14 to 16 years, 4.0 (range 2.8 to 5.4). Rifabutin was generally safe in this treatment group. Adverse experiences were similar to those observed in the adult population, and included leukopenia, neutropenia and skin rash. Doses of rifabutin may be administered mixed with foods such as applesauce.

Pregnancy: There are no adequate and well-controlled studies of rifabutin use in pregnant women. No teratogenic effects were observed in reproduction studies carried out in rats and rabbits. Because animal reproduction studies are not always predictive of human response, rifabutin should be used in pregnant women only if the potential benefit justifies the potential risk to the fetus.

Lactation: It is not known whether rifabutin is excreted in human milk. Because many drugs are excreted in human milk and given the potential for serious adverse reactions in nursing infants, a decision should be made whether to discontinue nursing or discontinue the drug, taking into account the importance of the drug to the nursing mother.

Renal Impairment: In a study of 18 patients with increasing degrees of renal insufficiency, rifabutin was administered as a single 300 mg dose. Renal insufficiency was correlated to a decrease in rifabutin urinary excretion. Other pharmacokinetic parameters did not appear to differ in a clinically relevant way between patients with various degrees of renal insufficiency and patients with normal renal function. Care is recommended when treating patients with severe renal insufficiency.

Hepatic Impairment: The pharmacokinetics of single-dose rifabutin have been studied in 12 patients with alcoholic liver disease. Hepatic impairment did not significantly modify the overall pharmacokinetic profile of rifabutin.

Drug Interactions: In 10 healthy adult volunteers and 8 HIV positive patients, steady-state plasma levels of zidovudine (ZDV), an antiretroviral agent which is metabolized mainly through glucuronidation, were decreased after repeated rifabutin dosing. The mean zidovudine decrease in C_{max} was 48% and in the AUC, 32%. In vitro studies have demonstrated that rifabutin does not affect the inhibition of HIV by ZDV.

Steady-state kinetics in 12 HIV positive patients show that both the rate and extent of systemic availability of didanosine (ddI), was not altered after repeated dosing of rifabutin.

Possible drug-drug interaction between rifabutin and fluconazole was also evaluated in HIV positive patients. Preliminary results from the Phase I study did not show any alterations in the steady-state fluconazole plasma kinetics following multiple rifabutin dosing.

Rifabutin has liver enzyme-inducing properties. The related drug rifampin is known to reduce the activity of a number of drugs, including dapsone, narcotics (including methadone), anticoagulants, corticosteroids, cyclosporine, cardiac glycoside preparations, quinidine, oral contraceptives, oral hypoglycemic agents (sulfonylureas), and analgesics. Rifampin has also been reported to decrease the effects of concurrently administered ketoconazole, barbiturates, diazepam, verapamil, beta-adrenergic blockers, clofibrate, progestins, disopyramide, mexiletine, theophylline, chloramphenicol and anticonvulsants. Because of the structural similarity of rifabutin and rifampin, rifabutin may be expected to have some effect on these drugs as well. However, unlike rifampin, rifabutin appears not to affect the acetylation of isoniazid. When the effects of rifabutin on hepatic microsomal enzyme activity were compared to those of rifampin in a study with 8 healthy normal volunteers, rifabutin appeared to be a less potent enzyme inducer than rifampin. The significance of this finding for clinical drug interactions is not known. **Dosage adjustment of drugs listed above may be necessary if they are given concurrently with rifabutin.**

Patients using oral contraceptives should consider changing to nonhormonal methods of birth control.

Information to Be Provided to the Patient: Mycobutin is used for the prevention of serious disease caused by *M. avium* complex (MAC) organisms in patients with advanced HIV infection. Mycobutin should not be given to patients with active tuberculosis. Patients should ask their physicians to advise them of the signs and symptoms of both MAC disease and tuberculosis. Patients should consult their physician if they develop new complaints suggestive of either MAC disease or tuberculosis.

Mycobutin should be taken as a single dose (two 150 mg capsules) once daily with or without food. For those patients who experience nausea, vomiting or other stomach upsets, it may be useful to split the Mycobutin dose in half (one 150 mg capsule) twice a day with food.

The most common side effect of Mycobutin is that urine may be colored brown-orange. Similar discoloration may affect stools, saliva, sputum, perspiration, tears or the skin. Contact lenses may be permanently stained.

Other side effects associated with Mycobutin include: a reduction in the number of white blood cells which fight infections, skin rashes, and gastrointestinal complaints such as indigestion, belching, flatulence, nausea, vomiting and abdominal pain. Very rarely, Mycobutin may cause muscle aches, inflammation of the inside of the eye (uveitis), and generalized joint pains.

ADVERSE EFFECTS: Rifabutin was generally well tolerated in the controlled clinical trials involving 566 patients treated with rifabutin and 580 patients treated with placebo. The most serious adverse reaction to rifabutin was neutropenia.

The most common adverse events, reported more frequently in the rifabutin treated patients than in the placebo group were: urine discoloration, neutropenia, skin rash, nausea and/or vomiting, and abdominal pain (see Table 1 and Table 2). The incidence of urine discoloration and neutropenia in patients treated with rifabutin were significantly greater than in patients treated with placebo (Fisher's Test, p<0.01 and p=0.03 respectively).

Sixteen percent (16%) of rifabutin treated patients discontinued therapy due to an adverse event as compared to 8% of placebo-treated patients. The primary reasons for discontinuation of rifabutin were: skin rash (4%), gastrointestinal intolerance (3%) and neutropenia (2%).

Table 1 enumerates adverse experiences that occurred at a frequency of 1% or greater among the patients treated with rifabutin and those treated with placebo in the Phase III clinical trials.

Table 1: Mycobutin

Clinical Adverse Experiences Reported in ≥1% of Patients Treated with Mycobutin

Adverse Event	Mycobutin (n=566) %	Placebo (n=580) %
Body as a Whole		
Abdominal Pain	4	3
Headache	3	5
Fever	2	1
Asthenia	1	1
Chest Pain	1	1
Pain	1	2
Digestive System		
Nausea	6	5
Nausea and Vomiting	3	2

(cont'd)

Table 1: Mycobutin *(cont'd)*

Clinical Adverse Experiences Reported in ≥1% of Patients Treated with Mycobutin

Adverse Event	Mycobutin (n=566) %	Placebo (n=580) %
Vomiting	1	1
Diarrhea	3	3
Dyspepsia	3	1
Eructation	3	1
Anorexia	2	2
Flatulence	2	1
Musculoskeletal System		
Myalgia	2	1
Nervous System		
Insomnia	1	1
Skin and Appendages		
Rash	11	8
Pruritus	1	1
Special Senses		
Taste Perversion	3	1
Urogenital System		
Discolored Urine	30	6

Considering data from the Phase III clinical trials, and from other clinical studies, rifabutin appears to be a likely cause of the following adverse events which occurred in less than 1% of the treated patients: arthralgia, chest pressure or pain with dyspnea, hemolysis, hepatitis, myositis, and skin discoloration.

The following adverse events have occurred in more than 1 patient receiving rifabutin, but an etiologic role for rifabutin has not been established: aphasia, confusion, non-specific T wave changes on the ECG, and seizures. The following adverse event has occurred in one patient receiving rifabutin, but an etiologic role for rifabutin has not been established: pseudomembranous colitis.

When rifabutin was administered at doses from 1050 mg/day to 2400 mg/day, generalized arthralgia and uveitis were reported. These adverse experiences abated when rifabutin was discontinued.

Laboratory Test Abnormalities: Table 2 enumerates the changes in laboratory values that were considered as laboratory test abnormalities in the Phase III clinical trials.

Table 2: Mycobutin

Percentage of Patients with Laboratory Abnormalities

Laboratory Test Abnormalities	Mycobutin (n=566) %	Placebo (n=580) %
Chemistry:		
Increased ALT (>150 U/L)	9	11
Increased AST (>150 U/L)	7	12
Increased Alkaline Phosphatase (>450 U/L)	<1	3
Hematology:		
Neutropenia (ANC <750/mm³)	25	20
Leukopenia (WBC <1500/mm³)	17	16
Anemia (Hemoglobin <8.0 g/dL)	6	7
Thrombocytopenia (Platelet count <50 000/mm³)	5	4
Eosinophilia	1	1

Although thrombocytopenia was not significantly more common among rifabutin treated patients in the Phase III trials, rifabutin has been clearly linked to thrombocytopenia in rare cases. One patient in the Phase III trials developed thrombotic thrombocytopenic purpura which was attributed to rifabutin.

OVERDOSE:

Symptoms: No information is available on accidental overdosage in humans.

Treatment: While there is no experience in the treatment of overdose with rifabutin, clinical experience with rifamycins suggest that gastric lavage to evacuate gastric contents (within a few hours of overdose), followed by instillation of an activated charcoal slurry into the stomach, may help absorb any remaining drug from the gastrointestinal tract.

Rifabutin is 85% protein bound, and distributed extensively into tissues (V_{ss}:8 to 9 L/kg). As unchanged drug, rifabutin is not primarily excreted via the urinary route (less than 10%), therefore, neither hemodialysis nor forced diuresis is expected to enhance the systemic elimination of unchanged rifabutin from the body in a patient with rifabutin overdose.

For management of a suspected drug overdose, contact your **regional Poison Control Centre**. See the *CPS* Directory section for a list of Poison Control Centres.

DOSAGE: It is recommended that 300 mg of rifabutin be administered once daily with or without food. For those patients who experience nausea, vomiting or other gastrointestinal upsets, it may be useful to split the rifabutin dose in half (one 150 mg capsule) twice a day with food.

SUPPLIED: Each hard gelatin capsule having an opaque red-brown cap and body, imprinted with PHARMACIA & UPJOHN/MYCOBUTIN, in white ink, contains: rifabutin 150 mg. Nonmedicinal ingredients: microcrystalline cellulose, magnesium stearate, red iron oxide, silica gel, sodium lauryl sulfate, titanium dioxide and edible white ink. Bottles of 100. Store at controlled room temperature, 15 to 30°C. Keep container tightly closed.

(Shown in Product Identification Section)

Mydfrin®
phenylephrine HCl
Vasoconstrictor—Mydriatic

Alcon

SUPPLIED: A sterile, buffered, isotonic 2.5% solution of phenylephrine HCl USP. Preservative: benzalkonium chloride. Nonmedicinal ingredients: boric acid, edetate disodium, hydrochloric acid, purified water, sodium bisulfite and sodium hydroxide. Protect from light and excessive heat. Plastic Drop-Tainer dispensers of 5 mL.

Mydriacyl® Ⓟ
tropicamide
Mydriatic—Cycloplegic—Anticholinergic

Alcon

SUPPLIED: A sterile, buffered, isotonic solution of tropicamide 0.5% or 1%. Preservatives: benzalkonium chloride. Nonmedicinal ingredients: edetate disodium, hydrochloric acid, purified water, sodium chloride and sodium hydroxide. Drop-Tainer dispensers of 15 mL.

Myfortic® Ⓟ
mycophenolate sodium
Immunosuppressant

Novartis Pharmaceuticals

Date of Preparation: February 14, 2005
Date of Revision: June 1, 2010

SUMMARY PRODUCT INFORMATION: MYFORTIC (mycophenolate sodium) Enteric-Coated Tablets, deliver the active moiety mycophenolic acid (MPA), an immunosuppressive agent.

Route of Administration	Dosage Form/ Strength	Clinically Relevant Nonmedicinal Ingredients
Oral	Enteric-Coated Tablets equivalent to mycophenolic acid 180 mg and 360 mg	Colloidal silicon dioxide, crospovidone, lactose anhydrous, magnesium stearate, povidone (K-30) and starch. For a complete listing see Dosage Forms, Composition and Packaging.

INDICATIONS AND CLINICAL USE: MYFORTIC (mycophenolate sodium) Enteric-Coated Tablets are indicated for the prophylaxis of organ rejection in patients receiving allogeneic renal transplants, administered in combination with cyclosporine, and corticosteroids.

CONTRAINDICATIONS: MYFORTIC (mycophenolate sodium) Enteric-Coated Tablets are contraindicated in patients with a hypersensitivity to mycophenolate sodium, mycophenolic acid, mycophenolate mofetil, or to any of its excipients (see Dosage Forms, Composition and Packaging).

WARNINGS AND PRECAUTIONS:

Serious Warnings and Precautions
Increased susceptibility to infection and the possible development of lymphoma and other neoplasms may result from immunosuppression. Only physicians experienced in immunosuppressive therapy and management of solid organ transplant patients should use MYFORTIC (mycophenolate sodium) Enteric-Coated Tablets. Patients receiving the drug should be managed in facilities equipped and staffed with adequate laboratory and supportive medical resources. The physician responsible for maintenance therapy should have complete information requisite for the follow up of the patient.

General: Oversuppression of the immune system can also increase susceptibility to infection, including opportunistic infections, fatal infections, and sepsis.

Patients receiving MYFORTIC should be instructed to immediately report any evidence of infection, unexpected bruising, bleeding, or any other manifestation of bone marrow suppression.

During treatment with MYFORTIC, the use of live attenuated vaccines should be avoided and patients should be advised that vaccinations may be less effective.

Cases of progressive multifocal leukoencephalopathy (PML), sometimes fatal, have been reported in patients treated with mycophenolate sodium (MYFORTIC) and mycophenolate mofetil (MMF) which both metabolize to the same active form of mycophenolic acid (MPA) in the body. Hemiparesis, apathy, confusion, cognitive deficiencies and ataxia were the most frequent clinical features observed. The reported cases generally had risk factors for PML, including treatment with immunosuppressants and impairment of immune functions. In immunosuppressed patients, physicians should consider PML in the differential diagnosis in patients reporting neurological symptoms and consultation with a neurologist should be considered as clinically indicated. Polyomavirus associated nephropathy (PVAN), especially due to BK virus infection (BK virus associated nephropathy [BKVAN]), should be included in the differential diagnosis in immunosuppressed patients with deteriorating renal function (see Adverse Reactions). Consideration should be given to reducing the amount of immunosuppression in patients who develop PML or PVAN. In transplant patients, physicians should also consider the risk that reduced immunosuppression represents to the graft.

PVAN and BKVAN are associated with serious outcomes, sometimes leading to renal graft loss (see Adverse Reactions, Post-Market Adverse Drug Reactions). Patient monitoring may help detect patients at risk for polyomavirus or BK virus-associated nephropathy.

Carcinogenesis and Mutagenesis: Patients receiving immunosuppressive regimens involving combinations of drugs, including MYFORTIC, as part of an immunosuppressive regimen are at an increased risk of developing lymphomas and other malignancies, particularly of the skin. The risk appears to be related to the intensity and duration of immunosuppression rather than to the use of any specific agent. As general advice to minimize the risk for skin cancer, exposure to sunlight and UV light should be limited by wearing protective clothing and using a sunscreen with a high protection factor.

Gastrointestinal: Because mycophenolic acid derivatives have been associated with an increased incidence of digestive system adverse events, including infrequent cases of gastrointestinal tract ulceration, hemorrhage, and perforation, MYFORTIC should be administered with caution in patients with active serious digestive system disease. Gastrointestinal adverse events are common in patients receiving MPA treatment. Gastrointestinal bleeding (requiring hospitalization), gastrointestinal tract ulceration, and perforation have rarely been reported in de novo renal transplant patients or maintenance patients treated with MYFORTIC Enteric-Coated Tablets during clinical trials. Most patients receiving MYFORTIC were also receiving other drugs known to be associated with these complications. Patients with active peptic ulcer disease were excluded from enrollment in studies with MYFORTIC.

Drug Interactions: In view of the significant reduction in the AUC of MPA by cholestyramine, caution should be used in the concomitant administration of MYFORTIC with drugs that interfere with enterohepatic recirculation because of the potential to reduce the efficacy of MYFORTIC.

Hematologic: Patients receiving MYFORTIC should be monitored for blood dyscrasias (e.g. neutropenia or anemia) (see Warnings and Precautions, Monitoring and Laboratory Tests). The development of neutropenia may be related to MYFORTIC itself, concomitant medications, viral infections, or some combination of these events. If blood dyscrasias occur (e.g. neutropenia with absolute neutrophil count [ANC $<1.5\times10^3/\mu L$] or anemia), dosing with MYFORTIC should be interrupted or the dose reduced, appropriate diagnostic tests performed, and the patient managed appropriately (see Dosage and Administration).

Cases of pure red cell aplasia (PRCA) have been reported in patients treated with MYFORTIC or mycophenolate mofetil (MMF) in combination with other immunosuppressive agents (see Adverse Reactions). The mechanism for MYFORTIC or MMF-induced PRCA is unknown; the relative contribution of other immunosuppressants and their combinations in an immunosuppressive regimen is also unknown. In some cases PRCA was found to be reversible with dose reduction or cessation of therapy with MYFORTIC. In transplant patients, however, reduced immunosuppression may place the graft at risk. Changes to MYFORTIC therapy should only be undertaken under appropriate supervision in transplant recipients in order to minimize the risk of graft rejection.

Inborn Disorders of Metabolism: On theoretical grounds, because MYFORTIC is an IMPDH Inhibitor, it should be avoided in patients with rare hereditary deficiency of hypoxanthine-guanine phosphoribosyl-transferase (HGPRT) such as Lesch-Nyhan and Kelley-Seegmiller syndrome.

Renal: Subjects with severe chronic renal impairment (GFR <25 mL/min/1.73 m^2) may present higher plasma MPAG AUCs relative to subjects with lesser degrees of renal impairment or normal healthy volunteers. No data are available on the safety of long-term exposure to these levels of MPAG.

In the de novo study, 18.3% of MYFORTIC patients versus 16.7% in the MMF group experienced delayed graft function (DGF). Patients with DGF experienced a higher incidence of certain adverse events such as anemia, leukopenia, and hyperkalemia than patients without DGF, but these events in DGF patients were not more frequent in patients receiving MYFORTIC than MMF. No dose adjustment is recommended for these patients; however, such patients should be carefully observed (see Dosage and Administration).

Sexual Function/Reproduction: Mycophenolate sodium had no effect on fertility of male rats at oral doses up to 40 mg/kg/day. The systemic exposure at this dose represents approximately 9 times the clinical exposure at the tested clinical dose of 1.44 g/day MYFORTIC. No effects on female fertility were seen up to a dose of 20 mg/kg, a dose at which maternal toxicity and embryotoxicity were already observed and yielding an exposure similar to that observed at the maximum recommended clinical dose.

Special Populations: Pregnant Women: In a teratology study performed with mycophenolate sodium in rats, at a dose as low as 1 mg/kg, malformations in the offspring were observed, including anophthalmia, exencephaly and umbilical hernia. The systemic exposure at this dose represents 0.05 times the clinical exposure at the dose of 1.44 g/day MYFORTIC. In teratology studies in rabbits fetal resorptions and malformations occurred from 80 mg/kg/day, in the absence of maternal toxicity (dose levels are equivalent to about 0.8 times the recommended clinical dose, corrected for BSA). There are no relevant qualitative or quantitative differences in the teratogenic potential of mycophenolate sodium and mycophenolate mofetil.

There are no adequate and well-controlled studies in pregnant women conducted with either MYFORTIC or mycophenolate mofetil. Based on data from the National Transplant Pregnancy Registry (NTPR), congenital disorders (congenital malformations of heart, ear, face, hand, eye, vertebrae, oesophagus, and multiple congenital abnormalities) have been reported in infants of patients exposed to mycophenolate mofetil in combination with other immunosupressants during pregnancy. The postmarketing data of pregnant women exposed to mycophenolate mofetil suggest that use of MPA during pregnancy may be associated with an increased risk of first trimester pregnancy loss. Since MMF is converted to mycophenolic acid following oral or IV administration, the above risks must be taken into account for MYFORTIC as well. Since MPA may cause fetal harm when administered to a pregnant woman, MYFORTIC should not be used in pregnant women unless the potential benefit justifies the potential risk to the fetus.

Women of childbearing potential should have a negative serum or urine pregnancy test with a sensitivity of at least 50 mIU/mL within 1 week prior to beginning therapy. It is recommended that MYFORTIC therapy should not be initiated by the physician until a report of a negative pregnancy test has been obtained.

Effective contraception must be used before beginning MYFORTIC therapy, during therapy, and for 6 weeks following discontinuation of therapy, even where there has been a history of infertility, unless due to hysterectomy. Two reliable forms of contraception must be used simultaneously unless abstinence is the chosen method. If pregnancy does occur during treatment, the patient should inform the physician immediately, and should discuss the potential risk to the fetus with him/her (see Information for the Patient).

Nursing Women: It is not known whether MPA is excreted in human milk. Because of the potential for serious adverse reactions in nursing infants from mycophenolate sodium, a decision should be made whether to discontinue the drug or to discontinue nursing while on treatment or within 6 weeks after stopping therapy, taking into account the importance of the drug to the mother.

Pediatrics: Safety and efficacy in pediatric patients have not been established. Limited pharmacokinetic data are available for pediatric renal transplant patients (see Action and Clinical Pharmacology).

Geriatrics: Patients ≥65 years may generally be at increased risk of adverse drug reactions due to an immunosuppression. Based on the controlled MYFORTIC clinical trials, patients ≥65 receiving MYFORTIC as part of a combination immunosuppressive regimen, did not show an increased risk of adverse reactions, compared to younger patients.

No dose adjustment is required in this patient population.

Monitoring and Laboratory Tests: Complete blood count should be performed weekly during the first month, twice monthly for the second and the third month of treatment, then monthly through the first year. If neutropenia develops (ANC $<1.3\times10^3/\mu L$) dosing with MYFORTIC should be interrupted or the dose reduced, appropriate texts performed, and the patient managed accordingly (see Warnings and Precautions).

ADVERSE REACTIONS: Clinical Trial Adverse Drug Reactions: Because clinical trials are conducted under very specific conditions the adverse reaction rates observed in the clinical trials may not reflect the rates observed in practice and should not be compared to the rates in the clinical trials of another drug. Adverse drug reaction information from clinical trials is useful for identifying drug-related adverse events and for approximating rates.

The most common (≥25%) adverse events from clinical trial data from de novo kidney transplant patients treated with MYFORTIC include constipation, nausea, and urinary tract infection. Clinical trial data from maintenance patients treated with MYFORTIC show that nausea, diarrhea and nasopharyngitis were the most frequently observed adverse reactions (≥15%). Fatal infections were rarely observed in patients receiving MYFORTIC (0.5%) in controlled clinical trials.

The incidence of adverse events for MYFORTIC Enteric-Coated Tablets was determined in randomized, comparative, active-controlled, double-blind, double-dummy trials in prevention of acute rejection in de novo and maintenance kidney transplant patients.

Adverse events reported in ≥10% of patients receiving MYFORTIC or MMF in the 12-months de novo renal study and maintenance renal study, when used in combination with cyclosporine and corticosteroids are listed in Table 1. Adverse event rates were similar between MYFORTIC and MMF in both de novo and maintenance patients.

Table 1: MYFORTIC

Adverse Events (%) in Controlled de novo and Maintenance Renal Studies Reported in ≥10% of Patients

	de novo Renal Study		Maintenance Renal Study	
	MYFORTIC 1.44 g/day (n=213)	MMF 2 g/day (n=210)	MYFORTIC 1.44 g/day (n=159)	MMF 2 g/day (n=163)
Blood and Lymphatic System Disorders				
Anemia	21.6	21.9	—	—
Leukopenia	19.2	20.5	—	—
Gastrointestinal System Disorders				
Constipation	38	39.5	—	—
Nausea	29.1	27.1	24.5	19
Diarrhea	23.5	24.8	21.4	24.5
Vomiting	23	20	15.1	12.9
Dyspepsia	22.5	19	13.8	14.7
Upper abdominal pain	14.1	14.3	—	—
General and Administrative Site Disorders				
Edema	16.9	17.6	—	—
Edema lower limb	15.5	17.1	—	—
Edema peripheral			10.7	12.3
Pyrexia	12.7	18.6	—	—
Pain	13.6	8.6	—	—
Infections and Infestations				
Urinary tract infection	29.1	33.3	10.1	11.7
CMV infection	20.2	18.1	—	—
Nasopharyngitis	—	—	16.4	19.6
Upper respiratory tract infection	—	—	12.6	9.8
Investigations				
Increased blood creatinine	14.6	10	—	—
Metabolism and Nutrition Disorders				
Hypocalcemia	11.3	15.2	—	—
Hyperuricemia	12.7	13.3	—	—
Hyperlipidemia	12.2	9.5	—	—
Hypokalemia	12.7	9	—	—
Hypophosphatemia	10.8	8.6	—	—
Musculoskeletal, Connective Tissue and Bone Disorders				
Back pain	11.7	6.2	—	—
Arthralgia	—	—	13.8	9.8
Nervous System Disorders				
Insomnia	23.5	23.8	—	—
Tremor	11.7	14.3	—	—
Headache	13.1	11	17.6	16.6
Respiratory, Thoracic and Mediastinal Disorders				
Cough	—	—	11.3	8
Surgical and Medical Procedure				
Post-operative pain	23.9	18.6	—	—
Vascular Disorder				
Hypertension	18.3	18.1	—	—

(cont'd)

Table 1: MYFORTIC (cont'd)

Table 2 summarizes the incidence of opportunistic infections in de novo and maintenance transplant patients, which were similar in both treatment groups.

Long-term administration of MYFORTIC (up to 30 months of exposure) did not show any unexpected changes in the pattern of adverse events including infections and malignancies.

The following adverse events were reported between 3% to <10% incidence in de novo and maintenance patients treated with MYFORTIC in combination with cyclosporine and corticosteroids are listed in Table 3.

The following opportunistic infections occurred rarely in the above controlled trials: aspergillus and cryptococcus.

The incidence of malignancies and lymphoma is consistent with that reported in the literature for this patient population. Lymphoma developed in 2 de novo patients (0.9%), (one diagnosed 9 days after treatment initiation) and in 2 maintenance patients (1.3%) (one was AIDS-related), receiving MYFORTIC with other immunosuppressive agents in the 12-month controlled clinical trials. Non-melanoma skin carcinoma occurred in 0.9% de novo and 1.8% maintenance patients. Other types of malignancy occurred in 0.5% de novo and 0.6% maintenance patients.

Table 2: MYFORTIC

Viral and Fungal Infections (%) Reported Over 0–12 Months

	de novo Renal Study		Maintenance Renal Study	
	MYFORTIC 1.44 g/day (n=213) (%)	**MMF 2 g/day (n=210) (%)**	**MYFORTIC 1.44 g/day (n=159) (%)**	**MMF 2 g/day (n=163) (%)**
Any cytomegalovirus	21.6	20.5	1.9	1.8
–Cytomegalovirus disease	4.7	4.3	0	0.6
Herpes simplex	8	6.2	1.3	2.5
Herpes zoster	4.7	3.8	1.9	3.1
Any fungal infection	10.8	11.9	2.5	1.8
–Candida NOS	5.6	6.2	0	1.8
–*C. albicans*	2.3	3.8	0.6	0

Table 3: MYFORTIC

Adverse Events Reported in 3% to <10% of Patients Treated with MYFORTIC in Combination with Cyclosporine and Corticosteroids

	de novo Renal Study	**Maintenance Renal Study**
Blood and Lymphatic Disorders	Lymphocele, thrombocytopenia	Leukopenia, anemia
Cardiac Disorder	Tachycardia	—
Eye Disorder	Vision blurred	—
Endocrine Disorders	Cushingoid, hirsutism	—
Gastrointestinal Disorders	Flatulence, abdominal distension, sore throat, abdominal pain lower, abdominal pain, gingival hyperplasia, loose stool	Abdominal pain, constipation, gastroesophageal reflux disease, loose stool, flatulence, abdominal pain upper
General Disorders and Administration Site Conditions	Fatigue, edema peripheral, chest pain	Fatigue, pyrexia, edema, chest pain
Infections and Infestations	Nasopharyngitis, herpes simplex, upper respiratory tract infection, oral candidiasis, herpes zoster, sinusitis, wound infection, implant infection, pneumonia	Influenza, sinusitis
Injury, Poisoning, and Procedural Complications	Drug toxicity	Post procedural pain
Investigations	Hemoglobin decrease, blood pressure increased, liver function tests abnormal	Blood creatinine increase, weight increase
Metabolism and Nutrition Disorders	Hypercholesterolemia, hyperkalemia, hypomagnesemia, diabetes mellitus, hyperphosphatemia, dehydration, fluid overload, hyperglycemia, hypercalcemia	Dehydration, hypokalemia, hypercholesterolemia
Musculoskeletal and Connective Tissue Disorders	Arthralgia, pain in limb, muscle cramps, myalgia	Pain in limb, back pain, muscle cramps, peripheral swelling, myalgia
Nervous System Disorders	Dizziness (excluding vertigo)	Dizziness
Psychiatric Disorders	Anxiety	Insomnia, depression
Renal and Urinary Disorders	Renal tubular necrosis, renal impairment, dysuria, hematuria, hydronephrosis, bladder spasm, urinary retention	—
Respiratory, Thoracic and Mediastinal Disorders	Cough, dyspnea, dyspnea exertional	Dyspnea, pharyngolaryngeal pain, sinus congestion
Skin and Subcutaneous Tissue Disorders	Acne, pruritus	Rash, contusion
Surgical and Medical Procedures	Complications of transplant surgery, post operative complications, post operative wound complication	—
Vascular Disorders	Hypertension aggravated, hypotension	Hypertension

Adverse Events Associated with MPA: The following additional adverse reactions have been associated with MPA (including MMF):

Gastrointestinal: colitis (sometimes caused by CMV), pancreatitis, esophagitis, intestinal perforation, gastrointestinal hemorrhage, gastric ulcers, duodenal ulcers, and ileus.

Respiratory: Although not reported with MYFORTIC, interstitial lung disorders, including fatal pulmonary fibrosis, have been reported rarely with MPA administered as MMF and should be considered in the differential diagnosis of pulmonary symptoms ranging from dyspnea to respiratory failure in post transplant patients receiving MPA derivatives.

Post-Market Adverse Drug Reactions: Based on data from the National Transplant Pregnancy Registry (NTPR), congenital disorders (congenital malformations of heart, ear, face, hand, eye, vertebrae, oesophagus, and multiple congenital abnormalities) have been reported in infants of patients exposed to mycophenolate mofetil in combination with other immunosupressants during pregnancy. The postmarketing data of pregnant women exposed to mycophenolate mofetil suggest that use of MPA during pregnancy may be associated with an increased risk of first trimester pregnancy loss (see Warnings and Precautions, Special Populations).

Cases of progressive multifocal leukoencephalopathy (PML), sometimes fatal, have been reported in patients treated with mycophenolate sodium (MYFORTIC) and mycophenolate mofetil (MMF) (see Warnings and Precautions, General).

Polyomavirus associated nephropathy (PVAN), especially due to BK virus infection is attributed to mycophenolic acid compounds (including MYFORTIC) as a class effect (see Warnings and Precautions, General).

Cases of pure red cell aplasia (PRCA) have been reported in patients treated with mycophenolic acid compounds (including MYFORTIC*) in combination with other immunosuppressive agents (see Warnings and Precautions, Hematologic).

Rash has been identified as an adverse drug reaction from post-approval clinical trials, postmarketing surveillance and spontaneous reports.

DRUG INTERACTIONS: Overview: MYFORTIC has been administered in combination with the following agents in clinical trials: antilymphocyte/thymocyte immunoglobulin, Simulect (basiliximab), daclizumab, muromonab, cyclosporine, Prograf (tacrolimus) and corticosteroids. The efficacy and safety of the use of MYFORTIC with other immunosuppressive agents have not been studied.

Drug-Drug Interactions: See Table 4.

Table 4: MYFORTIC

Established or Predicted Drug-Drug Interactions

Drug	Reference	Effect	Clinical Comment
Antacids/ Antacids with magnesium and aluminium hydroxides	Single-dose of MYFORTIC administered to 12 stable renal transplant patients alone and in combination with Maalox (30 mL).	Absorption of a single dose of MYFORTIC was decreased when administered in combination with Maalox (30 mL). The C_{max} and $AUC_{(0\text{-}t)}$ for MPA were 25% and 37% lower, respectively, than when MYFORTIC was given alone.	Magnesium-aluminum containing antacids may be used intermittently (several doses/week) for the treatment of occasional dyspepsia. However, the chronic daily use of magnesium-aluminum containing antacids with MYFORTIC is not recommended due to the potential for decreased MPA exposure.
Cyclosporine	Stable renal transplant patients.	Cyclosporine pharmacokinetics were unaffected by steady-state dosing of MYFORTIC.	—
Acyclovir	CellCept Prescribing Information.	Higher plasma concentrations of both MPAG (mycophenolic acid glucuronide) and Acyclovir may occur in the presence of renal impairment.	The potential exists for these two drugs to compete for tubular secretion, resulting in a further increase in the concentration of both MPAG and Acyclovir. In this situation patients should be carefully followed up.
Gancyclovir	CellCept Prescribing Information.	MPA and MPAG pharmacokinetics are unaffected by the addition of Gancyclovir. The clearance of Gancyclovir is unchanged in the setting of therapeutic MPA exposure.	In patients with renal impairment in which MYFORTIC and Gancyclovir are coadministered the dose recommendations for Gancyclovir should be observed and patients monitored carefully.
Tacrolimus/ Neoral	Calcineurin cross-over study in stable renal transplant patients.	Mean MPA AUC was 19% higher and C_{max} approximately 20% lower. Mean MPAG AUC and C_{max} were approximately 30% lower on tacrolimus treatment compared to Neoral treatment.	
Azathioprine/ mycophenolate mofetil	CellCept Prescribing Information.	Inhibition of purine metabolism.	Given that azathioprine and mycophenolate mofetil inhibit purine metabolism, it is recommended that MYFORTIC not be administered concomitantly with azathioprine or mycophenolate mofetil.
Cholestyramine and drugs that bind bile acids	CellCept Prescribing Information.	Concomitant administration of cholestyramine leads to a reduction in the AUC of MPA.	Caution should be used when coadministering drugs or therapies that may bind bile acids, for example bile acid sequestrates or oral activated charcoal, because of the potential to reduce the efficacy of MYFORTIC.
Oral contraceptives	CellCept Prescribing Information.	None	Although not measured in a clinical trial, given the different metabolism of MYFORTIC and oral contraceptives, no drug interaction between these two classes of drug is expected.
Proton Pump inhibitors	Clinical Expert report	In healthy volunteers, no changes in the pharmacokinetics of MPA were observed following concomitant administration of MYFORTIC and pantoprazole.	

Drug-Food Interactions: Compared to the fasting state, administration of MYFORTIC 720 mg with a high fat meal (55 g fat, 1000 calories) had no effect on the systemic exposure (AUC) of MPA. However, there was a 33% decrease in the maximal concentration (C_{max}) of MPA, significant delays in absorption of MPA (T_{max} delayed up to 20 hours) were observed. To avoid variations in MPA absorption between doses, MYFORTIC should be taken on an empty stomach (see Dosage and Administration).

DOSAGE AND ADMINISTRATION: Recommended Dose and Dosage Adjustment: The recommended dose in adult is 720 mg administered twice daily (1.440 g total daily dose).

MYFORTIC (mycophenolic acid as mycophenolate sodium) Enteric-Coated Tablets should be used in combination with cyclosporine and corticosteroid therapy.

MYFORTIC should be taken on an empty stomach, one hour before or two hours after food intake (see Drug Interactions, Drug-Food Interactions).

Patients are to be instructed that MYFORTIC tablets should not be crushed, chewed, or cut prior to ingesting but to be swallowed whole in order to maintain the integrity of the enteric coating.

Dosage Adjustment: Geriatric Use: No dose adjustments are required. The recommended dose is 720 mg administered twice daily.

Pediatric Use: Safety and efficacy in pediatric patients have not been established. Limited pharmacokinetic data are available for pediatric renal transplant patients (see Action and Clinical Pharmacology).

Treatment During Rejection Episodes: Renal transplant rejection does not lead to changes in MPA pharmacokinetics; dosage reduction or interruption of MYFORTIC is not required.

Patients with Renal Impairment: No dose adjustments are needed in patients experiencing delayed renal graft function post-operatively. Patients with severe chronic renal impairment (GFR <25 mL/min/1.73 m^2) should be carefully followed.

Patients with Hepatic Impairment: No dose adjustments are needed for renal transplant patients with hepatic parenchymal disease.

Patients Developing Neutropenia: If neutropenia develops (ANC <1.3×10^3/μL), dosing with MYFORTIC should be interrupted or the dose reduced, appropriate diagnostic tests performed, and the patient managed appropriately (see Warnings and Precautions).

OVERDOSAGE:
There has been no reported experience of acute overdose of MYFORTIC (mycophenolate sodium) Enteric-Coated Tablets in humans.

Possible signs and symptoms of acute overdose could include the following: hematological abnormalities such as leukopenia and neutropenia, and gastrointestinal symptoms such as abdominal pain, diarrhea, nausea and vomiting, and dyspepsia.

General supportive measures and symptomatic treatment should be followed in all cases of overdosage. Although dialysis may be used to remove the inactive metabolite MPAG, it would not be expected to remove clinically significant amounts of the active moiety MPA due to the 98% plasma protein binding of MPA. By interfering with enterohepatic circulation of MPA, activated charcoal or bile acid sequestrants, such as cholestyramine, may reduce the systemic MPA exposure.

> For management of a suspected drug overdose, contact your regional Poison Control Centre. See the *CPS* Directory section for a list of Poison Control Centres.

ACTION AND CLINICAL PHARMACOLOGY: MYFORTIC (mycophenolate sodium) Enteric-Coated Tablets, deliver the active moiety, mycophenolic acid (MPA). MPA is a potent, selective, uncompetitive, and reversible inhibitor of inosine monophosphate dehydrogenase (IMPDH), and therefore inhibits the de novo pathway of guanosine nucleotide synthesis without incorporation to DNA. Because T- and B-lymphocytes are critically dependent for their proliferation on de novo synthesis of purines, whereas other cell types can utilize salvage pathways, MPA has a potent cytostatic effect on lymphocytes. Thus the mode of action is complementary to calcineurin inhibitors which interfere with cytokine transcription and resting T-lymphocytes.

Mycophenolate sodium has been shown to prevent the occurrence of acute rejection in models of kidney allotransplantation, of heart allotransplantation and of heart xenotransplantation associated or not with other immunosuppressive treatment. Mycophenolate sodium also inhibited proliferative arteriopathy in experimental models of aortic allografts in rats as well as antibody production in mice.

Pharmacokinetics:

Table 5: MYFORTIC

Mean (±SD) Pharmacokinetic Parameters for MPA Following Oral Administration of MYFORTIC to Renal Transplant Patients on Cyclosporine Based Immunosuppression

Study Patient	MYFORTIC Dosing	N	Dose (mg)	T_{max}[a] (hr)	C_{max} (ug/mL)	AUC $_{0\text{-}12\ hr}$ (ug·hr/mL)
Adult	Single	24	720	2 (0.8–8)	26.1±12.0	66.5±22.6[b]
Pediatric[c]	Single	10	450/m^2	2.5 (1.5–24)	36.3±20.9	74.3±22.5[b]
Adult	Multiple × 6 days, BID	10	720	2 (1.5–3.0)	37.0±13.3	67.9±20.3
Adult	Multiple × 28 days, BID	36	720	2.5 (1.5–8)	31.2±18.1	71.2±26.3
Adult	Chronic, Multiple dose, BID					
	2 weeks post-transplant	12	720	1.8 (1.0–5.3)	15.0±10.7	28.6±11.5
	3 months post-transplant	12	720	2 (0.5–2.5)	26.2±12.7	52.3±17.4
	6 months post-transplant	12	720	2 (0–3)	24.1±9.6	57.2±15.3
Adult	Chronic, Multiple dose, BID	18	720	1.5 (0–6)	18.9±7.9	57.4±15.0

[a] Median (range).
[b] $AUC_{0-\infty}$.
[c] Age range of 5-16 years.

The mean pharmacokinetic parameters for MPA following the administration of MYFORTIC in renal transplant patients on cyclosporine based immunosuppression are shown in Table 5. Single dose MYFORTIC pharmacokinetics predict multiple dose pharmacokinetics. However, in the early post transplant period, mean MPA AUC and C_{max} were approximately one-half of those measured six months post transplant.

After near equimolar dosing of MYFORTIC (720 mg BID) and MMF (1000 mg BID) in both the single and multiple dose cross-over trials, mean systemic MPA exposure was similar.

Absorption: In vitro studies demonstrated that the MYFORTIC Enteric-Coated Tablet does not release MPA under acidic conditions (pH <5) as in the stomach but is highly soluble in neutral pH conditions as in the intestine. Following MYFORTIC oral administration without food, consistent with its enteric-coated formulation, the median time to maximum concentration (T_{max}) of MPA was 1.5-2.5 hours (range: 1.5 to 8 hours) compared to 1 hour (range: 0.5 to 3 hours) for mycophenolate mofetil (MMF). In stable renal transplant patients on cyclosporine based immunosuppression, gastrointestinal absorption of MPA was 93% and absolute bioavailability 71%. MYFORTIC pharmacokinetics is dose proportional over the dose range of 180 to 2160 mg.

Food Effect: Compared to the fasting state, administration of MYFORTIC 720 mg with a high fat meal (55 g fat, 1000 calories) had no effect on the systemic exposure (AUC) of MPA. However, there was a 33% decrease in the maximal concentration (C_{max}) of MPA, significant delays in absorption of MPA (T_{max} delayed up to 20 hours) were observed. To avoid variations in MPA absorption between doses, MYFORTIC should be taken on an empty stomach (see Dosage and Administration).

Distribution: The volume of distribution at steady-state for MPA is 54.3 (±25.2) L. MPA is highly protein bound to albumin, >98%. The protein binding of mycophenolic acid glucuronide (MPAG) is 82%. The free MPA concentration may increase under conditions of decreased protein binding (uremia, hepatic failure, and hypoalbuminemia). This may put patients at an increased risk of MPA-related adverse events.

Metabolism: The half-life of MPA is 11.7 (±3.2) hours and the clearance is 8.4 (±1.8) L/hr. MPA is metabolized principally by glucuronyl transferase to the phenolic glucuronide of MPA, mycophenolic acid glucuronide (MPAG). MPAG is the predominant metabolite of MPA and does not manifest pharmacological activity. In stable renal transplant patients on cyclosporine based immunosuppression, approximately 28% of the oral MYFORTIC dose is converted to MPAG by pre-systemic metabolism. The half-life of MPAG is longer than MPA, approximately 15.7 (±3.9) hours and its clearance is 0.45 (±0.15) L/hr.

Elimination: The majority of MPA (>60% of the dose) is eliminated in the urine primarily as MPAG and <3% as MPA. MPAG secreted in the bile is available for deconjugation by gut flora. The MPA resulting from this deconjugation may then be reabsorbed. Approximately 6-8 hours after MYFORTIC dosing, a second peak of MPA concentration can be measured which is consistent with reabsorption of the deconjugated MPA.

Special Populations and Conditions: Pediatrics: Limited data are available on the use of MYFORTIC at a dose of 450 mg/m^2 body surface area in children. The mean MPA pharmacokinetic parameters for stable pediatric renal transplant patients, 5-16 years, on cyclosporine are shown in Table 5. At the same dose administered based on body surface area, the respective mean C_{max} and AUC of MPA determined in children were higher by 33% and 18% than those determined for adults. The clinical impact of the increase in MPA exposure is not known.

Geriatrics: Pharmacokinetics in the elderly have not been formally studied.

Gender: There are no significant gender differences in MYFORTIC pharmacokinetics.

Hepatic Insufficiency: In a single dose (1 g MMF) study of 18 volunteers with alcoholic cirrhosis and 6 healthy volunteers, hepatic MPA glucuronidation processes appeared to be relatively unaffected by hepatic parenchymal disease when the pharmacokinetic parameters of healthy volunteers and alcoholic cirrhosis patients within this study were compared. However, it should be noted that for unexplained reasons, the healthy volunteers in this study had about a 50% lower AUC compared to healthy volunteers in other studies, thus making comparison between volunteers with alcoholic cirrhosis and health volunteers difficult. Effects of hepatic disease on this process probably depend on the particular disease. Hepatic disease with other etiologies may show a different effect.

Renal Insufficiency: No specific pharmacokinetic studies in individuals with renal impairment were conducted with MYFORTIC. MPA pharmacokinetic was unchanged over the range of normal to severely impaired renal function based on studies with mycophenolate mofetil. In contrast, MPAG exposure increased with decreased renal function; MPAG exposure being approximately 8 fold higher in the setting of anuria. Although dialysis may be used to remove the inactive metabolite MPAG, it would not be expected to remove clinically significant amounts of the active moiety MPA. This is in large part due to the high plasma protein binding of MPA.

STORAGE AND STABILITY: Store at 15-30°C. Protect from moisture. Dispense in a tight container.

SPECIAL HANDLING INSTRUCTIONS: Tablets should not be crushed or cut.

INFORMATION FOR THE PATIENT: Published in e-CPS, available by subscription at www.e-cps.ca.

DOSAGE FORMS, COMPOSITION AND PACKAGING: 180 mg: Each lime green, film-coated, round tablet with bevelled edges and the imprint (debossing) "C" on one side, contains: mycophenolic acid 180 mg as mycophenolate sodium. Nonmedicinal ingredients: colloidal silicon dioxide, crospovidone, lactose anhydrous, magnesium stearate, povidone (K-30), and starch; enteric coating: hypromellose phthalate, indigotine, iron oxide yellow and titanium dioxide. Unit dose of 10 tablets/blister pack, 12 packs/carton.

360 mg: Each pale orange, red film-coated, ovaloid tablet with imprint (debossing) "CT" on one side, contains: mycophenolic acid 360 mg as mycophenolate sodium. Nonmedicinal ingredients: colloidal silicon dioxide, crospovidone, lactose anhydrous, magnesium stearate, povidone (K-30), and starch; enteric coating: hypromellose phthalate, iron oxide red, iron oxide yellow and titanium dioxide. Unit dose of 10 tablets/blister pack, 12 packs/carton.

(Shown in Product Identification Section)

The reader is invited to consult CPhA's monograph **Corticosteroids: Eye, Ear, Nose.**

Mylan-Beclo AQ. Pr

beclomethasone dipropionate

Corticosteroid

Mylan

PHARMACOLOGY: Beclomethasone is a potent anti-inflammatory steroid with a strong topical and weak systemic activity. When inhaled intranasally in therapeutic doses, it has a direct anti-inflammatory action within the nasal mucosa, the mechanism of which is not yet completely defined. The minute amount absorbed in therapeutic doses has not been shown to exert any apparent clinical systemic effects.

INDICATIONS: The treatment of perennial and seasonal allergic rhinitis unresponsive to conventional treatment.

CONTRAINDICATIONS: In patients with active or quiescent tuberculosis or untreated fungal, bacterial and viral infections.

Mylan-Beclo AQ. is also contraindicated in patients with a history of hypersensitivity to any of its ingredients.

WARNINGS: In patients previously on high doses of systemic steroids, transfer to beclomethasone aqueous suspension may cause withdrawal symptoms such as tiredness, aches and pains and depression. In severe cases, adrenal insufficiency may occur, necessitating the temporary resumption of systemic steroids. Careful attention must be given to patients with asthma and other clinical conditions in whom a rapid decrease in systemic steroid may cause a severe exacerbation of their symptoms.

The safety of beclomethasone in pregnancy has not been established. If used, the expected benefits should be weighed against the potential hazard to the fetus, particularly during the first trimester of pregnancy. Like other glucocorticosteroids, beclomethasone is teratogenic to rodent species. The relevance of these findings to humans has not yet been established. Infants born of mothers who have received substantial doses of glucocorticosteroids during pregnancy should be carefully observed for hypoadrenalism.

PRECAUTIONS: The replacement of a systemic steroid with beclomethasone aqueous suspension has to be gradual and carefully supervised by the physician. The guidelines under Dosage should be followed in all such cases.

Corticosteroids may mask some signs of infection and new infections may appear. A decreased resistance to localized infection has been observed during corticosteroid therapy. During long-term therapy, pituitary-adrenal function and hematological status should be periodically assessed.

Patients should be advised to inform subsequent physicians of the prior use of corticosteroids.

During beclomethasone aqueous suspension therapy, the possibility of atrophic rhinitis, and/or pharyngeal candidiasis should be kept in mind.

With the use of usual doses of nasal beclomethasone, significant suppression of growth has not been strongly documented. If significant systemic absorption of nasal adrenocorticoids occurs, adrenal suppression and growth suppression may result in pediatric patients.

Pregnancy: Adrenocorticoids cross the placenta. Unnecessary administration of drugs during pregnancy is undesirable.

Patients with Special Diseases and Conditions: There is an enhanced effect of corticosteroids on patients with hypothyroidism and in those with cirrhosis.

Drug Interactions: ASA should be used cautiously in conjunction with corticosteroids in hypoprothrombinemia.

Patients should be informed that the full effect of beclomethasone aqueous suspension therapy is not achieved until 2 to 3 days of treatment have been completed. Treatment of seasonal rhinitis should, if possible, start before the exposure to allergens.

Treatment with beclomethasone aqueous suspension should not be stopped abruptly but tapered off gradually.

Because of the inhibitory effect of corticosteroids on wound healing, in patients who have had recent nasal surgery or trauma, a nasal corticosteroid should be used with caution until healing has occurred.

Children: Beclomethasone aqueous suspension is not presently recommended for children younger than 6 years of age.

Lactation: Glucocorticosteroids are secreted in human milk. It is not known whether beclomethasone would be secreted in human milk, but it is suspected to be likely. The use of beclomethasone aqueous suspension in nursing mothers requires that the possible benefits of the drug be weighed against the potential hazards to the infant.

ADVERSE EFFECTS: No major side effects attributable to beclomethasone aqueous suspension have been reported. In controlled clinical trials involving 269 patients the following adverse events and incidences thereof were observed: sneezing 26%, stinging 24%, sore throat 10%, cough 8%, epistaxis 7%, headache 7%, dizziness 6%, nausea 6%, nasal drying/crusting 5%, lethargy 3%, stomach pains 3%.

Rare instances of nasal mucosal ulceration and nasal septum perforation have been reported following intranasal application of aerosol and aqueous corticosteroids. Localized infections of the nose and pharynx with *C. albicans* have occurred rarely (see Precautions). Rare cases of raised intraocular pressure or glaucoma in association with intranasal formulations of beclomethasone have been reported. Immediate and delayed hypersensitivity reactions, including urticaria, angioedema, rash and bronchospasm, have been reported rarely after the use of beclomethasone oral or intranasal inhalers.

When patients are transferred to beclomethasone aqueous suspension from a systemic steroid, allergic conditions such as asthma or eczema may be unmasked.

OVERDOSE:

Symptoms: Like any other nasally administered corticosteroid, acute overdosing is unlikely in view of the amount of active ingredient present. However, when used chronically in excessive doses (above 600 µg or 12 sprays/day of beclomethasone aqueous suspension) or in conjunction with other corticosteroid formulations, systemic corticosteroid effects such as hypercorticism and adrenal suppression may appear. If such changes occur, the dosage of beclomethasone aqueous suspension should be discontinued slowly consistent with accepted procedures for discontinuation of chronic steroid therapy (see Dosage).

The restoration of hypothalamic-pituitary-axis may be slow; during periods of pronounced physical stress (i.e., severe infections, trauma, surgery) a supplement with systemic steroids may be advisable.

Treatment: See Symptoms.

For management of a suspected drug overdose, CPhA recommends that you contact your **regional Poison Control Centre**. See the *CPS* Directory section for a list of Poison Control Centres.

DOSAGE: The usual dose for patients of all ages who received no previous systemic steroid is 2 applications (100 µg of beclomethasone) into each nostril twice daily. Maximum daily dose should not exceed 12 applications (600 µg of beclomethasone) in adults and 8 applications (400 µg of beclomethasone) in children.

When beclomethasone dipropionate aqueous suspension is used concurrently with other beclomethasone dipropionate inhalers, the combined total daily dose should not exceed the maximum daily recommended dose of beclomethasone dipropionate.

The safety and efficacy of beclomethasone aqueous suspension in children under 6 years of age have not been established.

Since the effect of beclomethasone aqueous suspension depends on its regular use, patients must be instructed to take the nasal inhalations at regular intervals and not as with other nasal sprays, as they feel necessary. They should also be instructed in the correct method, which is to blow the nose, then insert the nozzle firmly into the nostril, compress the opposite nostril and actuate the spray while inspiring through the nose, with the mouth closed.

In the presence of excessive nasal mucus secretion or edema of the nasal mucosa, the drug may fail to reach the site of action. In such cases it is advisable to use a nasal vasoconstrictor for 2 to 3 days prior to beclomethasone aqueous suspension.

Careful attention must be given to patients previously treated for prolonged periods with systemic corticosteroids when transferred to beclomethasone aqueous suspension. Initially, beclomethasone aqueous suspension and the systemic corticosteroid must be given concomitantly, while the dose of the latter is gradually decreased. The usual rate of withdrawal of the systemic steroid is the equivalent of 2.5 mg of prednisone every 4 days if the patient is under close supervision. If continuous supervision is not feasible, the withdrawal of the systemic steroid should be slower, approximately 2.5 mg of prednisone (or equivalent) every 10 days. If withdrawal symptoms appear, the previous dose of the systemic steroid should be resumed for a week before further decrease is attempted.

An improvement of symptoms usually becomes apparent within a few days after the start of therapy. However, symptomatic relief may not occur in some patients for as long as 2 weeks. Beclomethasone aqueous suspension should not be continued beyond 3 weeks in the absence of significant symptomatic improvement.

INFORMATION FOR THE PATIENT: Published in e-CPS, available by subscription at www.e-cps.ca.

SUPPLIED: Each spray of suspension delivered by the nasal applicator contains: beclomethasone dipropionate 50 µg. Amber glass bottles of 200 doses fitted with a metering pump and a nasal applicator. Nonmedicinal ingredients: benzalkonium chloride, dextrose, microcrystalline cellulose, phenyl ethanol, polysorbate, purified water and sodium carboxymethyl cellulose. Store between 15 and 30°C. Protect from light. Do not refrigerate.

Mylan-Budesonide AQ. 🅿

budesonide

Glucocorticosteroid

Mylan

SUPPLIED: 64 µg: Each metered dose of a white to off-white, thixotropic aqueous suspension contains: budesonide 64 µg. Nonmedicinal ingredients: Avicel RC-591, dextrose anhydrous, disodium edetate, HCl acid, polysorbate 80, potassium sorbate, purified water. Amber glass bottles of 10 mL (120 doses, provided with a pump spray mechanism, nasal adapter and patient instruction leaflet. Store at room temperature (15 to 30°C).

100 µg: Each metered dose of a white to off-white, thixotropic aqueous suspension contains: budesonide 100 µg. Nonmedicinal ingredients: Avicel RC-591, dextrose, disodium edetate, hydrochloric acid, potassium sorbate, Tween 80 (polysorbate) and water. Amber glass bottles of 10 mL (equivalent to 165 doses minimum), provided with a pump spray mechanism, nasal adapter and patient instruction leaflet. Store between 15 and 30°C.

Mylan-Nifedipine Extended Release 🅿

nifedipine

Antianginal—Antihypertensive

Mylan

SUPPLIED: 30 mg: Each round, biconvex, pink coated extended-release tablet, imprinted in black with a "KU 260" contains: nifedipine 30 mg. Nonmedicinal ingredients: cellulose acetate, colloidal silicon dioxide, glycerol triacetate, hydroxypropylmethylcellulose, iron oxide black, iron oxide red, lactose monohydrate, magnesium stearate, microcrystalline cellulose, polyethylene glycol, polyethylene oxide, polysorbate, povidone, propylene glycol, sodium chloride and titanium dioxide. Bottles of 100. Cartons with blisters of 30 tablets (2×15). Store between 15 and 30°C. Protect from light, humidity and moisture.

60 mg: Each round, biconvex, pink coated extended-release tablet, imprinted in black with a "KU 261" contains: nifedipine 60 mg. Nonmedicinal ingredients: cellulose acetate, colloidal silicon dioxide, glycerol triacetate, hydroxypropylmethylcellulose, iron oxide black, iron oxide red, lactose monohydrate, magnesium stearate, microcrystalline cellulose, polyethylene glycol, polyethylene oxide, polysorbate, povidone, propylene glycol, sodium chloride and titanium dioxide. Bottles of 100. Cartons with blisters of 30 tablets (2×15). Store between 15 and 30°C. Protect from light, humidity and moisture.

Mylan-Nitro

nitroglycerin

Antianginal

Mylan

SUPPLIED: Each metered dose contains: nitroglycerin 0.4 mg. Nonmedicinal ingredients: ethanol, peppermint oil and propellant HFA 134a (1,1,1, 2-tetrafluoroethane). Aerosol canisters delivering 200 metered doses. Store at room temperature (15 to 30°C).

Myleran® 🅿

busulfan

Antileukemic

GlaxoSmithKline

Date of Preparation: September 12, 2001
Date of Revision: July 26, 2004

Caution: Busulfan is a potent cytotoxic drug and should be used only by physicians experienced in the administration of cancer chemotherapeutic drugs. Blood counts should be taken at frequent intervals but minimally once weekly. Therapy should be discontinued or the dosage reduced at the first signs of abnormal depression of bone marrow.

PHARMACOLOGY: Busulfan is a bifunctional alkylating agent. Binding to DNA is believed to play a role in its mode of action, and di-guanyl derivatives have been isolated, but interstrand crosslinking has not been conclusively demonstrated.

The basis for the uniquely selective effect of busulfan on granulocytopoiesis is not fully understood.

Pharmacokinetics: Early pharmacokinetic studies were carried out with radioactively labelled busulfan. More recently, gas liquid chromatography with selected ion monitoring has been used to quantitate busulfan in biological fluids. Absorption of busulfan shows intra-individual variation. Both zero and first-order absorption, one compartment open models have been fitted to pharmacokinetic data. The mean half-life for drug elimination was 2.57 hours.

More recently, automated solid phase extraction with liquid chromatography mass spectrometry analysis has been used to quantitate busulfan in plasma. In a study of 12 patients administered single oral dose of busulfan 4 to 8 mg, the mean (dose adjusted to 4 mg) maximum plasma concentration (68±24 ng/ml) occurred between 0.5 and 2 hours after administration. The mean terminal plasma elimination half-life was 2.7±0.5 hours.

The bioavailability of oral busulfan shows large intra-individual variation ranging from 22% to 120% in adults and children.

The pharmacokinetics of busulfan have also been studied in patients following high-dose administration (1 mg/kg administered orally every 6 hours for 4 days). The mean elimination half-life was 2.3 hours after the final busulfan dose, but 3.4 hours after the first dose. The mean steady-state plasma concentration was 1.1 µg/mL after 2 to 3 doses 6 hours apart. Due to the variable absorption kinetics observed, it was not possible to evaluate the order of kinetics.

The primary mode of elimination of busulfan is through extensive metabolism and very little (1-2%) of the drug is excreted unchanged in the urine. In humans, busulfan is at least partly metabolized via the glutathione route. The urinary metabolites of busulfan have been identified as 3-hydroxysulpholane, tetrahydrothiophene 1-oxide and sulpholane, in patients treated with high-dose busulfan. The clinical activity of these compounds, however, remains unclear.

Busulfan given in high doses has recently been shown to enter the cerebrospinal fluid (CSF) in concentrations comparable to those found in plasma, with a mean CSF:plasma ratio of 1.3:1. The saliva:plasma distribution of busulfan was 1.1:1.

The level of busulfan bound reversibly to plasma proteins has been variably reported to range from insignificant to approximately 55%. Irreversible binding of drug to blood cells and plasma proteins has been reported to be 47% and 32%, respectively.

INDICATIONS: Chronic granulocytic (myelocytic, myeloid) leukemia for the production of remissions. May be used with extreme caution in patients with prior radiation or P_{32} therapy and in those untreated by any other means.

CONTRAINDICATIONS: Busulfan should not be given if neutrophil or platelet counts are depressed.

Busulfan should not be used in patients whose disease has demonstrated resistance to busulfan. Busulfan should not be given to patients with previous hypersensitivity reaction to the drug or any of its components.

WARNINGS: Caution: Busulfan is a potent cytotoxic drug. Blood counts should be taken at frequent intervals and not less than weekly. Therapy should be discontinued or the dosage reduced at the first signs of abnormal depression of bone marrow.

The most frequent, serious side effect of treatment with busulfan is the induction of bone marrow failure (which may or may not be anatomically hypoplastic) resulting in severe pancytopenia. The pancytopenia caused by busulfan may be more prolonged than that induced with other alkylating agents. It is generally felt that the usual cause of busulfan-induced pancytopenia is the failure to stop administration of the drug soon enough; individual idiosyncrasy to the drug does not seem to be an important factor. **Busulfan should be used with extreme caution and exceptional vigilance in patients whose bone marrow reserve may have been compromised by prior irradiation or chemotherapy, or whose marrow function is recovering from previous cytotoxic therapy.** Although recovery from busulfan-induced pancytopenia may take from 1 month to 2 years, this complication is potentially reversible and the patient should be vigorously supported through any period of severe pancytopenia.

A rare, important complication of busulfan therapy is the development of bronchopulmonary dysplasia with pulmonary fibrosis. Symptoms have been reported to occur within 8 months to 10 years after initiation of therapy—the average duration of therapy being 4 years. The histologic findings associated with busulfan lung mimic those seen following pulmonary irradiation. Clinically, patients have reported the insidious onset of cough, dyspnea, and low-grade fever. Pulmonary function studies have revealed diminished diffusion capacity and decreased pulmonary compliance. It is important to exclude more common conditions (such as opportunistic infections or leukemic infiltration of the lungs) with appropriate diagnostic techniques. If measures such as sputum cultures, virologic studies and exfoliative cytology fail to establish an etiology for the pulmonary infiltrates, lung biopsy may be necessary to establish the diagnosis. Treatment of established busulfan-induced pulmonary fibrosis is unsatisfactory; in most cases the patients have died within 6 months after the diagnosis was established. There is no specific therapy for this complication other than the immediate discontinuation of busulfan. The administration of corticosteroids has been suggested, but the results have not been impressive or uniformly successful.

If anesthesia is required in patients with possible pulmonary toxicity, the concentration of inspired oxygen should be kept as low as safely possible and careful attention given to postoperative respiratory care.

Busulfan may cause cellular dysplasia in many organs in addition to the lung. Cytologic abnormalities characterized by giant, hyperchromatic nuclei have been reported in lymph nodes, pancreas, thyroid, adrenal glands, liver, and bone marrow. This cytologic dysplasia may be severe enough to cause difficulty in interpretation of exfoliative cytologic examinations from the lung, bladder, breast and the uterine cervix.

In addition to the widespread epithelial dysplasia that has been observed during busulfan therapy, chromosome aberrations have been reported in cells from patients receiving busulfan.

Busulfan is mutagenic in mice and, possibly in man.

A number of malignant tumors have been reported in patients on busulfan therapy and this drug may be a human carcinogen. Four cases of acute leukemia occurred among 243 patients treated with busulfan as adjuvant chemotherapy following surgical resection of bronchogenic carcinoma. All 4 cases were from a subgroup of 19 of these 243 patients who developed pancytopenia while taking busulfan 5 to 8 years before leukemia became clinically apparent. These findings suggest that busulfan is leukemogenic, although its mode of action is uncertain.

Hepatic veno-occlusive disease, which may be life-threatening, has been reported following the investigational use of very high doses of busulfan in combination with cyclophosphamide or other chemotherapeutic agents prior to bone marrow transplantation. Possible risk factors for the development of hepatic veno-occlusive disease include: total busulfan dose exceeding 16 mg/kg based on the ideal body weight, and concurrent use of multiple alkylating agents.

A clear cause and effect relationship with busulfan has not been demonstrated. Periodic measurement of serum transaminases, alkaline phosphatase, and bilirubin is indicated for early detection of hepatotoxicity. A reduced incidence of hepatic veno-occlusive disease and other regimen-related toxicities have been observed in patients treated with high-dose busulfan and cyclophosphamide when the first dose of cyclophosphamide has been delayed for >24 hours after the last dose of busulfan.

Cardiac tamponade has been reported in a small number of patients with thalassemia (2% in one series) who received high doses of busulfan and cyclophosphamide as the preparatory regimen for bone marrow transplantation. In this series, the cardiac tamponade was often fatal. Abdominal pain and vomiting preceded the tamponade in most patients.

If high-dose busulfan is prescribed, patients should be given prophylactic anticonvulsant therapy, preferably with a benzodiazepine rather than enzyme-inducing anticonvulsants (e.g. phenytoin) (see Precautions, Drug Interactions).

Patients coprescribed systemic itraconazole with busulfan should be monitored for signs of busulfan toxicity (see Precautions, Drug Interactions).

Pregnancy: As with all cytotoxic chemotherapy, adequate contraceptive precautions should be used when either partner is receiving busulfan.

Busulfan may cause fetal harm when administered to a pregnant woman. Although there have been a number of cases reported where apparently normal children have been born after busulfan treatment during pregnancy, one case has been cited where a malformed baby was delivered by a mother treated with busulfan. During the pregnancy that resulted in the malformed infant, the mother received x-ray therapy early in the first trimester, mercaptopurine until the third month, then busulfan until delivery.

When cytotoxic drugs are used in pregnancy, the possible teratogenic effect on the fetus should be kept in mind. Delay treatment as long as possible and certainly until after the first 3 months of pregnancy. Women of childbearing potential should be advised to avoid becoming pregnant. In every individual case the expected benefit of treatment to the mother must be weighed against the possible risks to the fetus.

There is evidence from animal studies that busulfan produces foetal abnormalities and adverse effects on off-spring, including defects of the musculoskeletal system, reduced body weight and size, and impairment of gonadal development and effects on fertility.

In pregnant rats, busulfan produces sterility in both male and female offspring, due to the absence of germinal cells in testes and ovaries. Germinal cell aplasia or sterility in offspring of mothers receiving busulfan during pregnancy has not been reported in humans.

Effects on Fertility: Ovarian suppression and amenorrhea with menopausal symptoms commonly occur during busulfan therapy in premenopausal patients. In very rare cases, recovery of ovarian failure has been reported with continuing treatment. Treatment with high-dose busulfan has been associated with severe and persistent ovarian failure, including failure to achieve puberty after administration to young girls and pre-adolescents. Busulfan interferes with spermatogenesis in experimental animals and there have been clinical reports of sterility, azoospermia and testicular atrophy in male patients.

PRECAUTIONS: General: Use of busulfan should be restricted to patients for whom complete blood counts are available at intervals of at least 1 week. The most careful hematological control is essential since large doses may produce irreversible depression of the bone marrow which may not be obvious for 4 to 6 months.

The most consistent, dose-related toxicity is bone marrow suppression. This may be manifested by anemia, leukopenia, thrombocytopenia or any combination of these. It is imperative that patients be instructed to report promptly the development of fever, sore throat, signs of local infection, bleeding from any site or symptoms suggestive of anemia. Any one of these findings may indicate busulfan toxicity; however, they may also indicate transformation of the disease to an acute blastic form. Since busulfan may have a delayed effect on the bone marrow, it is important to withdraw the medication temporarily at the first sign of an abnormally large or exceptionally rapid fall in any of the formed elements of the blood.

Seizures have been reported in patients receiving very high, investigational doses of busulfan. As with any potentially epileptogenic drug, caution should be exercised when administering very high doses of busulfan to patients with a history of seizure disorder, head trauma, or receiving other potentially epileptogenic drugs. Some investigators have used prophylactic anticonvulsivant therapy in this setting.

Pregnancy: Teratogenic Effects: see Warnings.

Nonteratogenic Effects: There have been reports in the literature of small infants being born after the mothers received busulfan during pregnancy, in particular, during the third trimester. One case was reported where an infant had mild anemia and neutropenia at birth after busulfan was administered to the mother from the eighth week of pregnancy to term.

Lactation: It is not known whether busulfan or its metabolites are excreted in human milk. Mothers receiving busulfan should not breast feed their infants. Because of the potential for tumorigenicity shown in animal and human studies, a decision should be made whether to discontinue nursing or to discontinue the drug, taking into account the importance of the drug to the mother.

Drug Interactions: Busulfan may cause additive pulmonary toxicity when administered with other cytotoxic drugs.

Busulfan may cause additive myelosuppression when used with other myelosuppressive drugs.

The administration of phenytoin to patients receiving high-dose busulfan may result in a decrease in the myeloblative effect, due to increased busulfan clearance.

In one study, 12 of approximately 330 patients receiving continuous busulfan and thioguanine therapy for treatment of chronic myelogenous leukemia were found to have esophageal varices associated with abnormal liver function tests. Subsequent liver biopsies were performed in 4 of these patients, all of which showed evidence of nodular regenerative hyperplasia. Duration of combination therapy prior to the appearance of esophageal varices ranged from 6 to 45 months. However, subsequent large clinical trials have demonstrated increasing evidence that thioguanine alone results in severe liver toxicity, negating the influence of busulfan.

The concomitant systemic administration of itraconazole to patients receiving high-dose busulfan may result in reduced busulfan clearance.

A reduced incidence of hepatic veno-occlusive disease and other regimen-related toxicities have been observed in patients treated with high-dose busulfan and cyclophosphamide when the first dose of cyclophosphamide has been delayed for >24 hours after the last dose of busulfan.

Laboratory Tests: It is recommended that evaluation of the hemoglobin or hematocrit, total white blood cell count and differential count, and quantitative platelet count be obtained weekly while the patient is on busulfan therapy. In cases where the cause of fluctuation in the formed elements of the peripheral blood is obscure, bone marrow examination may be useful for evaluation of marrow status. A decision to increase, decrease, continue, or discontinue a given dose of busulfan should be based not only on the absolute hematologic values, but also on the rapidity with which changes are occurring. The dosage of busulfan may need to be reduced if combined with other drugs whose primary toxicity is myelosuppression. Occasionally, patients may be unusually sensitive to busulfan administered at standard dosages and suffer neutropenia or thrombocytopenia after a relatively short exposure to the drug. Busulfan should not be used where facilities for complete blood counts, including quantitative platelet counts, are not available at weekly (or more frequent) intervals.

Information to Be Provided to the Patient: Patients beginning therapy with busulfan should be informed of the importance of having periodic blood counts and to immediately report any unusual fever or bleeding. Aside from the major toxicity of myelosuppression, patients should be instructed to report any difficulty in breathing, persistent cough or congestion. They should be told that diffuse pulmonary fibrosis is an infrequent but serious and potentially life-threatening complication of long-term busulfan therapy. Patients should be alerted to report any signs of abrupt weakness, unusual fatigue, anorexia, weight loss, nausea and vomiting, and melanoderma that could be associated with a syndrome resembling adrenal insufficiency. Patients should never be allowed to take the drug without medical supervision and they should be informed that other encountered toxicities to busulfan include infertility, amenorrhea, skin hyperpigmentation, drug hypersensitivity, dryness of the mucous membranes and rarely cataract formation. Patients of childbearing potential should be advised to avoid becoming pregnant. Mothers receiving Myleran should not breast feed their infants. The increased risk of a secondary malignancy should be explained to the patient.

ADVERSE REACTIONS: Hematologic: The chief toxic effect is a dosage-related myelosuppression which may cause leukopenia and thrombocytopenia (hemorrhage) and eventually lead to pancytopenia.

Aplastic anemia (sometimes irreversible) has been reported rarely, often following long-term conventional doses and also high doses of busulfan.

Pulmonary: Interstitial pulmonary fibrosis has been reported rarely, but it is a clinically significant adverse effect when observed and calls for immediate discontinuation of further administration of the drug. The role of corticosteroids in arresting or reversing the fibrosis has been reported to be beneficial in some cases and without effect in others.

The lung pathology may be complicated by superimposed infections.

Pulmonary ossification and dystrophic calcification have also been reported.

Metabolic: Hyperuricemia and/or hyperuricosuria are not uncommon in patients with chronic myelogenous leukemia. Additional rapid destruction of granulocytes may accompany the initiation of chemotherapy and increase the urate pool. The risk of uric acid nephropathy can be minimized by increased hydration, urine alkalinization, and the prophylactic administration of a xanthine oxidase inhibitor such as allopurinol.

In a few cases, a clinical syndrome closely resembling adrenal insufficiency and characterized by weakness, severe fatigue, anorexia, weight loss, nausea and vomiting, and melanoderma has developed after prolonged busulfan therapy. The symptoms have sometimes been reversible when busulfan was withdrawn. Adrenal responsiveness to exogenously administered ACTH has usually been normal. However, pituitary function testing with metyrapone revealed a blunted urinary 17-hydroxycorticosteroid excretion in two patients. Following the discontinuation of busulfan (which was associated with clinical improvement), rechallenge with metyrapone revealed normal pituitary-adrenal function.

Cardiac: Cardiac tamponade has been reported in a small number of patients with thalassemia who received high doses of busulfan and cyclophosphamide as the preparatory regimen for bone marrow transplantation (see Warnings).

One case of endocardial fibrosis has been reported in a 79 year-old woman who received a total dose of 7200 mg over a period of 9 years for the management of chronic myelogenous leukemia. At autopsy, she was found to have endocardial fibrosis of the left ventricle in addition to interstitial pulmonary fibrosis.

Ocular: Busulfan is capable of inducing cataracts in rats and there have been several reports indicating that this is a rare complication in humans. In the few cases reported in humans, cataracts have occurred only after prolonged administration of busulfan.

Corneal thinning has been reported with the investigational use of high-dose busulfan prior to bone marrow transplantation.

Dermatologic: Esophageal varices have been reported in patients receiving continuous busulfan and thioguanine therapy for treatment of chronic myelogenous leukemia (see Precautions, Drug Interactions).

Hyperpigmentation is the most common adverse skin reaction and occurs in 5 to 10% of patients, particularly those with a dark complexion. It is often most marked on the neck, upper trunk, nipples, abdomen and palmar creases.

Gastrointestinal and Hepatic: Hyperbilirubinemia, jaundice and hepatic veno-occlusive disease and centrilobular sinusoidal fibrosis with hepatocellular atrophy and necrosis have been observed in patients receiving high dose busulfan (see Warnings).

Miscellaneous: Other complications of therapy include instances of nausea, vomiting, diarrhea, dryness of the oral mucous membranes and cheilosis, glossitis, urticaria, erythema multiforme, erythema nodosum, porphyria cutanea tarda, myasthenia gravis, cholestatic jaundice, impotence, sterility, amenorrhea, gynecomastia, excessive dryness and fragility of the skin with anhidrosis, alopecia and, hemorrhagic cystitis. Seizures have been observed in patients receiving higher than recommended doses of busulfan (see Precautions, General).

OVERDOSE:

There is no known antidote to busulfan. The acute dose-limiting toxicity of busulfan in man is myelosuppression. The main effect of chronic overdosage is bone marrow depression and pancytopenia. Survival after a single dose of 140 mg has been reported in an 18 kg 4 year old child, but hematological toxicity is likely to be more profound with chronic overdosage. If high dose busulfan is used in association with bone marrow transplantation, gastrointestinal toxicity becomes dose limiting with mucositis, nausea, vomiting, diarrhea and anorexia.

Symptoms: Purpuric hemorrhages.

Treatment: The hematologic status should be closely monitored and vigorous supportive measures instituted if necessary. Induction of vomiting or gastric lavage followed by administration of charcoal would be indicated if ingestion were recent.

Dialysis should be considered in the management of overdose as there is one report of successful dialysis of busulfan.

If high-dose busulfan is used in association with bone marrow transplantation, gastrointestinal toxicity becomes dose limiting with mucositis, nausea, vomiting, diarrhea and anorexia.

For management of a suspected drug overdose, CPhA recommends that you contact your **regional Poison Control Centre**. See the *CPS* Directory section for a list of Poison Control Centres.

DOSAGE: Busulfan is administered orally at a dosage of 0.06 mg/kg (1.8 mg/m² body surface area) to a total maximum dose of 4 mg daily, until maximum hematological and clinical improvement is obtained or symptoms of toxicity supervene. During remission, the patient is examined at monthly intervals and the treatment is resumed when the white cell count reaches 50 000/mm³. When remission is shorter than 3 months, maintenance therapy of 1 to 3 mg daily may be advisable in order to keep the hematological status under control and prevent rapid relapse. Discontinue drug or reduce dosage at the first sign of abnormal depression of platelets, hemoglobin, or low white blood cell count.

Special Instructions: All materials which have come in contact with cytotoxic drugs should be segregated and incinerated at 1000°C or more.

Tablets should be returned to the manufacturer for destruction. Proper precautions should be taken in packaging these materials for transport.

Personnel regularly involved in the preparation and handling of cytotoxic agents should have biannual blood examinations.

Care should be taken when handling or halving the tablets so as not to contaminate hands or to inhale the drug.

SUPPLIED: Each white, film-coated, round, biconvex tablet, engraved "GX EF3" on one side and "M" on the other, contains: busulfan 2 mg. Nonmedicinal ingredients: anhydrous lactose, magnesium stearate and pregelatinized starch; film coat: hypromellose (hydroxypropyl methylcellulose), titanium and triacetin. Bottles of 25. Store between 15 and 30°C in a dry place.

(Shown in Product Identification Section)

Myochrysine® ℞

sodium aurothiomalate

Antirheumatic Agent

sanofi-aventis

Date of Revision: November 29, 2007

PHARMACOLOGY: Sodium aurothiomalate exhibits anti-inflammatory, antiarthritic and immunomodulating effects. The predominant clinical effect of sodium aurothiomalate appears to be suppression of the synovitis in the active stage of the rheumatoid disease. The precise mechanism of action is unknown but it has been suggested that the drug may act by inhibiting cell-mediated and humoral immune mechanisms. Additional modes of action include alteration or inhibition of various enzyme systems, suppression of phagocytic activity of macrophage and polymorphonuclear leukocytes, and alteration of collagen biosynthesis.

The metabolic fate of sodium aurothiomalate in humans is unknown but it is believed not to be broken down to elemental gold. It is very highly bound to plasma proteins. Sixty to 90% is excreted very slowly by the renal route while 10 to 40% is eliminated in the feces mostly via biliary secretion. The biologic half-life of gold following a single 50 mg dose of parenteral gold has been reported to range from 6 to 25 days. It increases following successive weekly doses.

The appearance of clinical effect is slow. It may take at least 8 weeks to become significant and the maximum benefits may not be achieved for at least 6 months.

INDICATIONS: In the treatment of both adult and juvenile rheumatoid arthritis.

It may also be of benefit in the treatment of patients with psoriatic arthritis or Felty's syndrome.

It is usually used for treating patients who show evidence of continued or additional disease activity despite conservative drug therapy, e.g., with salicylates or other anti-inflammatory agents. Sodium aurothiomalate may induce partial or complete remission of rheumatoid arthritis. In chronic advanced rheumatoid arthritis, it may prevent further damage to affected joints; however, it does not reverse existing damage.

CONTRAINDICATIONS: In patients with known hypersensitivity to gold.

It is also contraindicated in patients who have experienced the following serious adverse effects with previous gold therapy; bone marrow aplasia or other hematological disorders, exfoliative dermatitis, necrotizing enterocolitis or pulmonary fibrosis.

Pregnancy: While reassuring, the information concerning the administration of gold during pregnancy is sparse and largely anecdotal; there have been no controlled prospective studies of the effect of sodium aurothiomalate on human fetal development.

In rats, gold compounds have been shown to cause hydrocephalus and microphthalmia when administered at a dose of 25 mg/kg per day from day 6 through day 15 of gestation; in rabbits, they caused gastroschisis, umbilical hernia, anomalies of the brain, heart, lung and skeleton, microphthalmia and limb defects when given at 20 to 45 mg/kg per day from day 6 through day 18 of gestation.

Gold is known to cross the placenta and it can reach significant concentrations in the fetus.

Gold therapy is seldom needed during pregnancy. If its use is nevertheless contemplated, the risk/benefit ratio should be considered keeping in mind the potential of sodium aurothiomalate for teratogenicity.

Lactation: Parenterally administered gold is excreted in human breast milk and has been detected in the blood of a nursing infant. Although problems in humans have not been documented, the use of sodium aurothiomalate in nursing mothers is not usually recommended because of the potential for serious adverse effects in the infant.

WARNINGS: The following conditions may aggravate or precipitate adverse reactions to sodium aurothiomalate, or their symptoms may mask the forewarning signs of gold toxicity: blood dyscrasias or a history of agranulocytosis, hemorrhagic diathesis or drug induced granulocytopenia or anemia; renal disease; hepatic dysfunction; systemic lupus erythematosus; significant dermatitis including urticaria or eczema.

Any of the above conditions should be considered as a relative contraindication to the use of sodium aurothiomalate. In such cases, treatment should be initiated with extreme caution and only after careful assessment of expected benefits versus the potential risks.

Rarely, anaphylactic shock, syncope, bradycardia, thickening of the tongue, difficulty in swallowing and breathing, and angioedema may occur in the minutes that follow the injection of Myochrysine. If an anaphylactic reaction occurs, treatment should be discontinued.

A vasomotor (nitritoid) reaction may occur within several minutes of a sodium aurothiomalate injection. The nitritoid reaction is characterized by flushing, tachycardia and faintness. When it occurs, caution should be exercised before resuming therapy in patients with compromised cardiovascular status.

Carcinogenicity/Tumorigenicity: Renal adenoma and adenocarcinoma have been reported in rats after prolonged administration of frequent, high doses of parenteral gold compounds (2 mg/kg/week for 45 weeks followed by 6 mg/kg/day for 47 weeks in one study; 3 mg/kg or 6 mg/kg/day for up to 2 years in a second study). The adenomas were similar to those produced in rats by chronic administration of other heavy metals such as lead or nickel. The relevance of these findings to man is unknown. Renal adenomas have not been reported in humans receiving therapeutic doses of sodium aurothiomalate.

PRECAUTIONS: Sodium aurothiomalate should be administered only to selected patients who are under the supervision of a physician experienced with chrysotherapy and thoroughly familiar with the toxicity and benefits of the drug.

Patient Monitoring: Toxic reactions to sodium aurothiomalate are relatively frequent and, in certain cases, may be quite severe. Thus emphasis should be placed on careful clinical and laboratory monitoring and early detection of adverse reactions.

Baseline evaluation should include a biochemical profile to identify any preexisting conditions. Before receiving gold, patients should also have a complete blood cell count with differential, platelet count, hemoglobin determination and urinalysis for protein, white cells, red cells and casts; these tests should be repeated before each injection and patients should have an examination of the skin and buccal mucosa for skin rash, bruising or mouth ulcers. They should be questioned for the presence of pruritus, rash, stomatitis or metallic taste.

Dermatitis and lesions of the mucous membranes are common and may be serious; pruritus may precede the early development of a skin reaction. Renal toxicity ranges from mild proteinuria to the nephrotic syndrome; prognosis is usually good. Hematologic reactions have been observed rarely but fatalities have ensued. Other severe toxic manifestations include cholestatic jaundice, enterocolitis and interstitial lung disease.

If toxicity develops, sodium aurothiomalate should be discontinued immediately and symptomatic treatment be given as required.

If the reaction to gold therapy is not of a serious type, injections may be cautiously resumed 2 or 3 weeks after the toxic reaction has subsided. In these circumstances, from 5 to 10 mg of gold is administered; if the challenge dose is tolerated, sodium aurothiomalate may be administered cautiously in larger doses on subsequent injections.

Severe reactions are a contraindication to further gold therapy.

Drug Interactions: The concurrent use of D-penicillamine or other drugs with potential bone marrow toxicity may increase the potential for serious hematologic and/or renal adverse reactions.

ADVERSE EFFECTS: The most frequent adverse reactions with sodium aurothiomalate involve the skin (ranging from simple rash to severe exfoliative dermatitis) and mucous membranes (ulcers) and may affect 30% of patients. Renal effects are next in frequency with proteinuria being observed in 10 to 15% of patients.

The severe adverse reactions are those affecting the bone marrow (agranulocytosis, thrombocytopenia and aplastic anemia), exfoliative dermatitis, enterocolitis, liver failure, anaphylactoid reactions and nephropathy; these are rare but may be fatal. It has been proposed that serious reactions may be the result of failure to discontinue therapy when earlier less serious symptoms occur. Close patient monitoring will not eliminate untoward effects but may help reduce their severity (see Precautions).

The following adverse reactions have been reported:

Skin and Mucous Membranes: pruritus and rash (30%) ranging from simple erythema to exfoliative dermatitis, and mucous membrane lesions (20%) including stomatitis.

Hematological: leukopenia (2%), thrombocytopenia (1 to 3%), eosinophilia, agranulocytosis and aplastic anemia.

Renal: proteinuria (10 to 15%), nephrotic syndrome, acute renal failure.

Allergic: anaphylactoid and vasomotor (nitritoid) reactions.

Digestive: metallic taste, diarrhea, enterocolitis, cholestatic jaundice.

Miscellaneous: Other very rare reactions include encephalitis, peripheral neuropathy and pulmonary infiltrates.

Chrysiasis (affecting the skin and mucus membranes) and corneal gold deposits have been noted in some patients.

A transient flare of articular inflammation appearing within 24 hours of injection and lasting 2 or 3 days has also been reported.

OVERDOSE:

Symptoms: Symptoms are those of heavy metal toxicity; they include: pruritus, dermatitis, stomatitis, vague gastrointestinal discomfort, albuminuria with or without a nephrotic syndrome, hematuria, agranulocytosis, thrombocytopenic purpura, and aplastic anemia.

Treatment: Gold therapy should be discontinued promptly and supportive treatments should be given as required for specific complications.

Patients with severe dermatitis may benefit from oral antihistamines, topical corticosteroids or emollients.

For the management of severe renal, hematologic, pulmonary enterocolic or generalized pruritic reactions, moderate to high dose corticosteroid therapy (e.g., prednisone 20 to 100 mg daily in divided doses) reportedly is beneficial.

When high-dose corticosteroid therapy is ineffective or substantial adverse reactions to steroids occur, a chelating agent (e.g., dimercaprol) or a drug such as N-acetylcysteine may be used to enhance the elimination of gold.

For management of a suspected drug overdose, CPhA recommends that you contact your **regional Poison Control Centre**. See the *CPS* Directory section for a list of Poison Control Centres.

DOSAGE: Should be administered by the **i.m. route only**, preferably in the gluteal muscle.

Warning: It is advisable to inject sodium aurothiomalate immediately after transfer into syringe because exposure to daylight will produce a rapid discoloration of the solution.

Do not administer the solution if darker than pale yellow.

Because of the possibility of anaphylactic reaction, it is recommended that patients be kept under medical observation for a period of 30 minutes after the administration of the drug.

Adults: Initial: 10 mg i.m. the first week, 25 mg the second week, then 25 to 50 mg weekly for the next 20 weeks or until toxicity occurs.

At this stage the response to therapy should dictate the future course of treatment. Patients with good to excellent response can go to maintenance therapy. In those with modest improvement a prolonged period of weekly injections may be maintained.

Maintenance: 50 mg i.m. tapered progressively to every 2 to 4 weeks according to clinical response and tolerance, and maintained indefinitely.

Children: 10 mg i.m. the first week followed by 1 mg/kg of body weight/week; do not exceed 50 mg/dose. See adult dosage for intervals between injections.

Note: To reinstitute therapy following mild adverse reactions, see Precautions, Patient Monitoring.

SUPPLIED: Each mL of aqueous solution contains: 10, 25 or 50 mg of sodium aurothiomalate. Nonmedicinal ingredients: chlorocresol and water for injection. Ampoules of 10, 25 and 50 mg/mL, boxes of 5. Store between 15 and 30°C. **Protect from light. Do not use a darkened solution (more than pale yellow).**

Myoflex®

triethanolamine salicylate

Topical Analgesic

Bayer Consumer Care

SUPPLIED: Regular: Each g contains: triethanolamine salicylate 10% w/w in a greaseless, nonstaining, odorless, vanishing cream base. Nonmedicinal ingredients: cetyl alcohol, edetate disodium, lavender oil, propylene glycol, sodium lauryl sulfate, stearyl alcohol and white wax. Tubes of 100 g.

Extra Strength: Each g contains: triethanolamine salicylate 15% w/w in a greaseless, nonstaining, odorless, vanishing cream base. Nonmedicinal ingredients: cetyl alcohol, edetate disodium, lavender oil, propylene glycol, sodium lauryl sulfate, stearyl alcohol and white wax. Tubes of 50 and 100 g.

Maximum Strength: Each g contains: triethanolamine salicylate 20% w/w in a greaseless, nonstaining, odorless, vanishing cream base. Nonmedicinal ingredients: cetyl alcohol, edetate disodium, lavender oil, propylene glycol, sodium lauryl sulfate, stearyl alcohol and white wax. Tubes of 50 and 100 g.

Deep Therapy: Each patch contains: triethanolamine salicylate 12.5% w/w in a greaseless, nonstaining, odorless patch. Nonmedicinal ingredients: glycerin, kaolin, methylparaben, methyl acrylate 2-ethylhexyl acrylate copolymer, polyacrylic acid, polysorbate 80, propylparaben, silicon dioxide, sodium carboxymethylcellulose, sodium polyacrylate, sodium polyacrylate starch, sorbitol, tartaric acid and titanium dioxide. Boxes of 4 patches (10×14 cm).

Myozyme® Ⓟ

alglucosidase alfa

Enzyme Replacement Therapy

Genzyme

Date of Preparation: August 14, 2006
Date of Revision: June 26, 2009

SUMMARY PRODUCT INFORMATION:

Route of Administration	Dosage Form/Strength	Clinically Relevant Nonmedicinal Ingredients
Intravenous infusion	Sterile solution/50 mg	There are no clinically relevant nonmedicinal ingredients. For a complete listing of nonmedicinal ingredients, see Dosage Forms, Composition and Packaging.

DESCRIPTION: MYOZYME (alglucosidase alfa) is a common form of the human enzyme acid α-glucosidase (GAA) that is produced by recombinant DNA technology in a Chinese hamster ovary cell line. Alglucosidase alfa degrades glycogen by catalyzing the hydrolysis of α-1,4- and α-1,6- glycosidic linkages of lysosomal glycogen.

INDICATIONS AND CLINICAL USE: MYOZYME (alglucosidase alfa) is indicated for use in patients with Pompe's Disease (GAA deficiency). MYOZYME has been shown to improve ventilator-free survival in patients with infantile-onset Pompe's Disease as compared to untreated historical controls. MYOZYME has also been shown to stabilize % predicted forced vital capacity in patients with late-onset Pompe's Disease. Ventilation free survival was not evaluated in patients with late-onset Pompe's Disease.

CONTRAINDICATIONS:

- Patients who are hypersensitive to this drug or to any ingredient in the formulation or component of the container. For a complete listing, see Dosage Forms, Composition and Packaging.

WARNINGS AND PRECAUTIONS:

Serious Warnings and Precautions

Risk of Anaphylaxis: Risk of life-threatening anaphylactic reactions, including anaphylactic shock, have been observed in patients during MYOZYME infusion.

Because of the potential for severe infusion reactions, appropriate medical support measures should be readily available when MYOZYME is administered.

Risk of Cardiorespiratory Failure: Infantile-onset patients with compromised cardiac or respiratory function may be at risk of serious acute exacerbation of their cardiac or respiratory compromise due to infusion reactions, and require additional monitoring.

General: Based on experience in clinical studies, patients with an acute underlying illness (for example: acute febrile illness as pneumonia or sepsis, wheezing/bronchospasm, decompensated cardiac failure, etc.) at the time of MYOZYME (alglucosidase alfa) infusion appear to be at greater risk for infusion-associated reactions. Careful consideration should be given to the patient's clinical status prior to administration of MYOZYME.

Carcinogenesis and Mutagenesis: There are no animal or human studies to assess the carcinogenic or mutagenic potential of MYOZYME.

A single study to address the impact of MYOZYME on fertility in mice was not conclusive since decreased fertility was noted in all groups, including vehicle controls.

Cardiac Adverse Events During General Anaesthesia for Central Venous Catheter Placement: Precaution must be observed when administering general anaesthesia to patients with infantile-onset Pompe's Disease. Reports of intraoperative cardiac arrest following anaesthesia induction for invasive procedures have been reported, some of which were fatal. The presence of severe hypertrophic cardiomyopathy in infantile-onset Pompe's Disease may increase the risk of general anaesthesia complications (Ing, 2004, Paediatr Anaesth).

Hypersensitivity Reactions: Significant Hypersensitivity Reactions: In clinical trials and in the post-marketing safety experience with MYOZYME, approximately 1% of patients developed anaphylactic shock and/or cardiac arrest during MYOZYME infusion that required life-support measures. Some of these reactions were IgE-mediated. Additionally, in a randomized, double-blind, placebo controlled study in patients with late-onset Pompe's Disease, 5% of patients (3/60) treated with MYOZYME experienced anaphylactic reactions. Two of which were IgE-mediated.

Eight (8) of approximately 280 patients (3%) treated in clinical trials and expanded access programs with MYOZYME experienced significant hypersensitivity reactions as of April 12, 2006. One of 59 pediatric patients (approximately 2%) experienced a life-threatening hypersensitivity reaction consisting of bronchospasm, oxygen saturation decreased, tachycardia, urticaria, and periorbital edema. Five of the 8 patients had infantile-onset Pompe's Disease and 3 had late-onset disease. Significant hypersensitivity reactions generally consisted of a constellation of signs and symptoms. Symptoms occurring in more than 1 patient included bronchospasm, oxygen saturation decreased, hypotension, and urticaria. Remaining symptoms were single occurrences of periorbital edema, swollen tongue, angioedema, chest discomfort, throat tightness, tachycardia, and rash. Reactions generally occurred within the first 3 months of initiation of treatment; all 8 patients experienced their first reaction between the first and approximately eighth infusion. Time from onset of infusion to onset of the reaction ranged between a few minutes after initiation of the infusion up to and including 20 minutes after completion of the infusion. The majority of the reactions were moderate or severe in intensity. Reactions were primarily managed with infusion rate reduction and/or interruption of the infusion and administration of antihistamines, corticosteroids, bronchodilators (including epinephrine in 2 patients) and/or oxygen. All 8 patients recovered without sequelae from the reactions. In 2 of the 8 patients, infusions were permanently discontinued as a result of the reaction. In the remaining 6 patients, MYOZYME treatment was continued with pre-treatment medication (e.g. antihistamines, corticosteroids and/or acetaminophen) administered for infusion management in 5 patients. Two of the 8 patients experienced anaphylactic reactions of angioedema, throat tightness and chest discomfort in the double-blind, placebo-controlled study of late-onset patients. An additional third patient in the late-onset study experienced an anaphylactic reaction of chest pain and chest discomfort.

Based on experience in clinical studies, patients with acute underlying illness (for example: acute febrile illness as pneumonia or sepsis, wheezing/bronchospasm, decompensated cardiac failure, etc.) at the time of MYOZYME infusion appear to be at greater risk for infusion-associated reactions. Careful consideration should be given to the patient's clinical status prior to administration of MYOZYME (see Warnings and Precautions, General). Patients with advanced Pompe's Disease may have compromised cardiac and respiratory function, which may also predispose them to a higher risk of severe complications from infusion reactions.

Patients should be closely monitored during the MYOZYME infusion. If significant hypersensitivity reactions occur during the MYOZYME infusion, immediate discontinuation of the MYOZYME infusion should be considered and appropriate medical treatment should be initiated. Because of the potential for significant hypersensitivity reactions, appropriate medical support measures, including cardiopulmonary resuscitation equipment, especially for patients with cardiac hypertrophy and patients with significantly compromised respiratory function, should be readily available when MYOZYME is administered. Patients who have experienced hypersensitivity reactions should be closely monitored when MYOZYME is re-administered.

Infusion Reactions: In 3 clinical studies of 59 pediatric patients receiving treatment with MYOZYME (AGLU01602, AGLU01702, AGLU02203), 30 patients (51%) experienced infusion-associated reactions (IARs). Seventeen of the 30 patients (57%) experienced their first infusion-associated reaction within the first 3 months of initiation of treatment. In the remaining patients (43%), the first reaction occurred as late as 95 weeks after initiation of treatment. Twenty-one of the 30 patients (70%) experienced reactions with multiple infusions; the remaining 9 patients experienced reactions with a single infusion. Infusion-associated reactions that occurred in ≥5% of patients included urticaria, rash, rash maculopapular, pyrexia, rigors, oxygen saturation decreased, blood pressure decreased, blood pressure increased, heart rate increased, flushing, hypertension, cough, tachypnea, tachycardia, agitation, irritability, and vomiting (see Adverse Reactions). The majority of infusion-associated reactions were assessed as non-serious and mild or moderate in intensity. Two reactions (heart rate increased and pyrexia) were assessed as severe. Four patients (4/59=7%) experienced serious infusion-associated reactions. Serious infusion-associated reactions included rales, bronchospasm, oxygen saturation decreased, tachypnea, tachycardia, periorbital edema, urticaria, hypertension, heart rate increased and fever. Most infusion-associated reactions requiring intervention were ameliorated with slowing the infusion rate, temporarily stopping the infusion and/or administration of antipyretics, antihistamines or steroids. All patients recovered without sequelae from the reactions.

In clinical trials and expanded access programs with MYOZYME, approximately 92 of 280 (33%) patients treated with MYOZYME have developed infusion reactions as of April 12, 2006.

Approximately 28% of the patients treated with MYOZYME in a double-blind, placebo-controlled study in late-onset patients developed IARs, compared to 23% of placebo-treated patients. The majority of these reactions were mild to moderate and resolved spontaneously. Infusion reactions which were reported in ≥5% of MYOZYME-treated patients included headache, nausea, urticaria, dizziness, chest discomfort, hyperhidrosis, flushing, blood pressure increased, and vomiting.

Based on experience in clinical studies, patients with acute underlying illness (for example: acute febrile illness as pneumonia or sepsis, wheezing/bronchospasm, decompensated cardiac failure, etc.) at the time of MYOZYME infusion appear to be at greater risk for infusion-associated reactions. Careful consideration should be given to the patient's clinical status prior to administration of MYOZYME (see Warnings and Precautions, General). Infusion reactions are also more likely to occur with higher infusion rates. Infantile-onset patients treated with the higher dose (40 mg/kg) generally developed a more robust antibody response and experienced more IARs. Patients with advanced Pompe's Disease may have compromised cardiac and respiratory function, which may also predispose them to a higher risk of severe complications from infusion reactions.

In clinical trials, some patients were pre-treated with antihistamines, antipyretics and/or corticosteroids. Infusion reactions occurred in some patients after receiving antipyretics, antihistamines and/or steroids.

Patients should be closely monitored during the MYOZYME infusion. Infusion reactions may occur at any time during, or shortly after completion of MYOZYME infusion. If the patient experiences an infusion reaction during the MYOZYME infusion, the patient should be managed according to general standards of care consistent with treatment of the presenting symptom(s). Regardless of pre-treatment, reduction of the infusion rate, temporarily interrupting the infusion, and/or administration of antihistamines, antipyretics and/or corticosteroids may ameliorate the symptoms. If severe infusion reactions occur, immediate discontinuation of the MYOZYME infusion should be considered, and appropriate medical support measures should be initiated. Because of the potential for significant hypersensitivity reactions, appropriate medical support measures, including cardiopulmonary resuscitation equipment, should be readily available when MYOZYME is administered. Severe infusion reactions are generally managed with administration of antihistamines, corticosteroids, intravenous fluids, and/or oxygen, when clinically indicated. In some cases of anaphylactic reactions epinephrine was administered. Patients who have experienced infusion reactions should be treated with caution when they are readministered MYOZYME.

Risk of Acute Cardiorespiratory Failure: Acute cardiorespiratory failure requiring intubation and inotropic support has been observed after infusion with MYOZYME in 1 infantile-onset Pompe's Disease patient with underlying cardiac hypertrophy, possibly associated with fluid overload with intravenous administration of MYOZYME. (See Dosage and Administration, Administration, Instructions for Use.) Because of the potential for fluid overload, appropriate medical support measures should be readily available when MYOZYME is administered.

Special Populations: Patients should be informed that a registry for patients with Pompe's Disease has been established in order to better understand the variability and progression of Pompe's Disease and to continue to monitor and evaluate treatments. Patients should be encouraged to participate and advised that their participation may involve long-term follow-up. Information regarding the registry program may be found at www.pomperegistry.com or by calling 1-800-745-4447.

Pregnant Women: Reproduction studies have been performed in mice at doses of MYOZYME up to 40 mg/kg administered daily for 10 days with no evidence of embryo-fetal abnormality.

There are no adequate and well-controlled studies of MYOZYME in pregnant women. Because animal reproduction studies are not always predictive of human response, MYOZYME should be used during pregnancy only if clearly needed.

Women of childbearing potential should be encouraged to enroll in the Pompe patient registry (see Warnings and Precautions, Special Populations).

Nursing Women: It is not known whether MYOZYME is secreted in human milk. Because many drugs are secreted in human milk, caution should be exercised when MYOZYME is administered to a nursing woman. (See Warnings and Precautions, Special Populations regarding a registry program. Nursing women are encouraged to participate in the registry program.)

Pediatrics (<18 years of age): Pediatric patients from 1 month up to 18 years of age at time of first infusion have been treated with MYOZYME in clinical trials.

Geriatrics (>65 years of age): Clinical studies did not include any patients aged 65 years and older.

Monitoring and Laboratory Tests: There are no marketed tests for antibodies against MYOZYME. It is recommended that patients be monitored for IgG antibody formation every 3 months. Patients who experience reactions suggestive of anaphylactic or allergic reactions may also be tested for IgE antibodies to alglucosidase alfa and other mediators of anaphylaxis. If testing is warranted, contact your local Genzyme representative or Genzyme Corporation at 1-800-745-4447.

ADVERSE REACTIONS: Adverse Drug Reaction Overview: The most serious adverse reactions reported in infantile and late-onset patients treated with MYOZYME (alglucosidase alfa) were hypersensitivity reactions (including anaphylactic reactions), acute cardiorespiratory failure, and cardiac arrest. Acute cardiorespiratory failure, possibly associated with fluid overload, has been reported in infantile-onset Pompe disease patients with pre-existing hypertrophic cardiomyopathy (see Warnings and Precautions, Risk of Acute Cardiorespiratory Failure and Warnings and Precautions, Boxed Warning, Risk of Anaphylaxis).

Clinical Trial Adverse Drug Reactions: Because clinical trials are conducted under very specific conditions, the adverse reaction rates observed in the clinical trials may not reflect the rates observed in practice and should not be compared to the rates in the clinical trials of another drug. Adverse drug reaction information from clinical trials is useful for identifying drug-related adverse events and for approximating rates.

Infantile-Onset Pompe's Disease: The data described below reflect exposure of 59 pediatric patients to 20 or 40 mg/kg of MYOZYME administered every other week in three separate clinical trials (AGLU01602, AGLU01702, AGLU02203) for a period of up to 76 weeks. These three studies included a population of patients which ranged in age from 1 month to 16 years at initiation of treatment.

Infusion Reactions: In 3 clinical studies of 59 pediatric patients receiving treatment with MYOZYME, 30 patients (51%) experienced infusion-associated reactions. Infusion-associated reactions that occurred in ≥5% of patients included urticaria, rash, rash maculopapular, pyrexia, rigors, oxygen saturation decreased, blood pressure decreased, blood pressure increased, heart rate increased, flushing, hypertension, cough, tachypnea, tachycardia, agitation, irritability, and vomiting (see Warnings and Precautions, Infusion Reactions).

Table 1 enumerates infusion reactions that occurred in at least 5% of the pediatric patients treated with MYOZYME in clinical trials described above. Reported frequencies of infusion reactions have been classified by MedDRA terms.

Table 1: MYOZYME

Summary of Infusion Reactions by System Organ Class and Preferred Term During Treatment Occurring in at Least 5% of Pediatric Patients Treated with MYOZYME in Clinical Trials

System Organ Class Preferred Term	Number of Patients N=59 n (%)	Number of Reactions N=271
Any Adverse Events	**30 (50.8)**	**271**
Skin and Subcutaneous Tissue Disorders	**17 (28.8)**	**71**
Urticaria	8 (13.6)	28
Rash	6 (10.2)	12
Rash maculopapular	3 (5.1)	5
General Disorders and Administration Site Conditions	**15 (25.4)**	**43**
Pyrexia	13 (22.0)	33
Rigors	3 (5.1)	4
Investigations	**14 (23.7)**	**47**
Oxygen saturation decreased	8 (13.6)	22
Blood pressure decreased	4 (6.8)	5
Blood pressure increased	3 (5.1)	4
Heart rate increased	3 (5.1)	7

(cont'd)

Table 1: MYOZYME *(cont'd)*

Summary of Infusion Reactions by System Organ Class and Preferred Term During Treatment Occurring in at Least 5% of Pediatric Patients Treated with MYOZYME in Clinical Trials

System Organ Class Preferred Term	Number of Patients N=59 n (%)	Number of Reactions N=271
Vascular Disorders	**11 (18.6)**	**29**
Flushing	7 (11.9)	19
Hypertension	4 (6.8)	5
Respiratory, Thoracic and Mediastinal Disorders	**9 (15.3)**	**28**
Cough	5 (8.5)	17
Tachypnoea	5 (8.5)	8
Cardiac Disorders	**6 (10.2)**	**18**
Tachycardia	6 (10.2)	15
Psychiatric Disorders	**6 (10.2)**	**10**
Agitation	3 (5.1)	5
Irritability	3 (5.1)	3
Gastrointestinal Disorders	**4 (6.8)**	**17**
Vomiting	4 (6.8)	9

Infusion associated reactions that occurred with frequency less than 5% of patients (reported in more than 1 patient) based on the MedDRA SOCs of:

Skin and Subcutaneous Tissue Disorders: include hyperhydrosis, livedo reticularis, pruritus and rash macular.
Investigations: include body temperature increased.
Vascular Disorders: include pallor.
Cardiac Disorders: include cyanosis.
Psychiatric Disorders: include restlessness.
Gastrointestinal Disorders: include retching.
Nervous System Disorders: include tremor.

Treatment Emergent Adverse Events: The most common treatment emergent adverse events (occurring in at least 18 of the 59 patients) (regardless of relationship) included upper respiratory tract infection, otitis media, pneumonia cough, respiratory failure, pyrexia, rash, diarrhoea, vomiting, and oxygen saturation decreased.

Table 2 enumerates treatment emergent adverse events (regardless of relationship) that occurred in at least 5% of pediatric patients treated with MYOZYME in clinical trials. Reported frequencies of adverse events have been classified by MedDRA terms.

Table 2: MYOZYME

Summary of Adverse Events by System Organ Class and Preferred Term During Treatment Occurring in at Least 5% of Pediatric Patients Treated with MYOZYME in Clinical Trials

System Organ Class Preferred Term	Number of Patients (N=59) n (%)	Number of Adverse Events N=2725
Any Adverse Events	**58 (98.3)**	**2725**
Infections and Infestations	**54 (91.5)**	**553**
Upper respiratory tract infection	25 (42.4)	58
Otitis media	24 (40.7)	45
Pneumonia	20 (33.9)	49
Viral infection	16 (27.1)	24
Catheter related infection	14 (23.7)	22
Ear infection	14 (23.7)	26
Gastroenteritis	12 (20.3)	12
Nasopharyngitis	12 (20.3)	32
Oral candidiasis	11 (18.6)	13
Pharyngitis	11 (18.6)	19
Bronchiolitis	10 (16.9)	13
Respiratory syncytial virus infection	9 (15.3)	12
Tracheitis	9 (15.3)	31
Gastroenteritis viral	8 (13.6)	8
Influenza	8 (13.6)	17
Bacteraemia	7 (11.9)	11
Candidiasis	7 (11.9)	10
Urinary tract infection	7 (11.9)	8
Otitis media acute	6 (10.2)	11

(cont'd)

Table 2: MYOZYME *(cont'd)*

Summary of Adverse Events by System Organ Class and Preferred Term During Treatment Occurring in at Least 5% of Pediatric Patients Treated with MYOZYME in Clinical Trials

System Organ Class Preferred Term	Number of Patients (N=59) n (%)	Number of Adverse Events N=2725
Bronchopneumonia	5 (8.5)	7
Respiratory tract infection	5 (8.5)	5
Sinusitis	5 (8.5)	6
Bronchitis	4 (6.8)	13
Dental Caries	4 (6.8)	6
Acute tonsillitis	3 (5.1)	5
Bronchitis acute	3 (5.1)	9
Cellulitis	3 (5.1)	4
Fungal skin infection	3 (5.1)	3
Localised infection	3 (5.1)	7
Pharyngitis streptococcal	3 (5.1)	6
Sepsis	3 (5.1)	4
Tonsillitis	3 (5.1)	3
Respiratory, Thoracic and Mediastinal Disorders	**51 (86.4)**	**423**
Cough	20 (33.9)	76
Respiratory failure	18 (30.5)	43
Respiratory distress	16 (27.1)	24
Rhinorrhoea	12 (20.3)	19
Increased bronchial secretion	11 (18.6)	24
Tachypnoea	11 (18.6)	17
Atelectasis	10 (16.9)	23
Upper respiratory tract congestion	9 (15.3)	15
Nasal congestion	8 (13.6)	9
Pharyngolaryngeal pain	8 (13.6)	11
Pneumonia aspiration	8 (13.6)	23
Bronchospasm	6 (10.2)	12
Rhinitis	6 (10.2)	8
Wheezing	6 (10.2)	8
Asthma	5 (8.5)	10
Choking	5 (8.5)	10
Dyspnoea	5 (8.5)	7
Respiratory tract congestion	4 (6.8)	4
Tracheal disorder	4 (6.8)	5
Lung infiltration	3 (5.1)	3
Rhonchi	3 (5.1)	3
General Disorders and Administration Site Conditions	**49 (83.1)**	**369**
Pyrexia	46 (78.0)	252
Catheter related complication	10 (16.9)	22
Granuloma	7 (11.9)	11
Oedema peripheral	7 (11.9)	9
Pain	4 (6.8)	7
Asthenia	3 (5.1)	11
Hyperthermia	3 (5.1)	3
Inflammation localised	3 (5.1)	6
Lethargy	3 (5.1)	6
Oedema	3 (5.1)	3
Rigors	3 (5.1)	4
Skin and Subcutaneous Tissue Disorders	**46 (78.0)**	**232**
Rash	18 (30.5)	46
Dermatitis diaper	17 (28.8)	40
Urticaria	12 (20.3)	32
Erythema	7 (11.9)	11
Hyperhidrosis	6 (10.2)	7
Rash macular	6 (10.2)	18
Dry skin	5 (8.5)	5
Eczema	5 (8.5)	9
Pruritus	5 (8.5)	6
Rash maculopapular	4 (6.8)	8
Rash papular	4 (6.8)	6
Skin irritation	4 (6.8)	4
Skin ulcer	4 (6.8)	4
Face oedema	3 (5.1)	4
Periorbital oedema	3 (5.1)	3
Rash erythematous	3 (5.1)	5
Gastrointestinal Disorders	**44 (74.6)**	**275**
Diarrhoea	28 (47.5)	75
Vomiting	24 (40.7)	74
Constipation	14 (23.7)	21
Gastrooesophageal reflux disease	12 (20.3)	15
Dysphagia	7 (11.9)	9
Teething	6 (10.2)	8
Loose stools	5 (8.5)	8
Abdominal distension	3 (5.1)	3
Abdominal pain	3 (5.1)	3
Nausea	3 (5.1)	4
Toothache	3 (5.1)	3
Investigations	**42 (71.2)**	**251**
Oxygen saturation decreased	21 (35.6)	57
Sputum culture positive	9 (15.3)	56
Heart rate increased	7 (11.9)	15
Blood potassium decreased	6 (10.2)	7
Blood pressure decreased	6 (10.2)	7
Blood creatine phosphokinase MB increased	5 (8.5)	5
Blood creatine phosphokinase increased	5 (8.5)	6
Blood pressure increased	5 (8.5)	6
Blood bicarbonate decreased	4 (6.8)	5
Ejection fraction decreased	4 (6.8)	4
Blood chloride decreased	3 (5.1)	3
Blood phosphorus increased	3 (5.1)	4
Blood pressure systolic increased	3 (5.1)	4
Body temperature increased	3 (5.1)	7
Haemoglobin decreased	3 (5.1)	3

(cont'd)

Table 2: MYOZYME *(cont'd)*

Summary of Adverse Events by System Organ Class and Preferred Term During Treatment Occurring in at Least 5% of Pediatric Patients Treated with MYOZYME in Clinical Trials

System Organ Class Preferred Term	Number of Patients (N=59) n (%)	Number of Adverse Events N=2725
Urine output decreased	3 (5.1)	3
Weight decreased	3 (5.1)	3
White blood cell count increased	3 (5.1)	3
Cardiac Disorders	**34 (57.6)**	**130**
Tachycardia	12 (20.3)	42
Bradycardia	9 (15.3)	20
Cardiac failure	6 (10.2)	6
Cardio-respiratory arrest	5 (8.5)	7
Cyanosis	5 (8.5)	7
Ventricular hypertrophy	4 (6.8)	6
Arrhythmia	3 (5.1)	3
Cardiomegaly	3 (5.1)	3
Cardiomyopathy	3 (5.1)	3
Musculoskeletal and Connective Tissue Disorders	**32 (54.2)**	**54**
Joint contracture	11 (18.6)	15
Osteopenia	10 (16.9)	10
Arthralgia	5 (8.5)	8
Pain in extremity	4 (6.8)	4
Myopathy	3 (5.1)	6
Osteoporosis	3 (5.1)	3
Injury, Poisoning and Procedural Complications	**30 (50.8)**	**94**
Post procedural pain	11 (18.6)	22
Medical device complication	9 (15.3)	28
Excoriation	6 (10.2)	6
Blister	4 (6.8)	4
Fall	4 (6.8)	4
Femur fracture	4 (6.8)	5
Contusion	3 (5.1)	3
Ear and Labyrinth Disorders	**23 (39.0)**	**37**
Hypoacusis	7 (11.9)	11
Middle ear effusion	7 (11.9)	7
Conductive deafness	3 (5.1)	4
Ear pain	3 (5.1)	3
Otorrhoea	3 (5.1)	4
Metabolism and Nutrition Disorders	**22 (37.3)**	**66**
Dehydration	7 (11.9)	7
Feeding disorder	5 (8.5)	6
Hypokalaemia	5 (8.5)	6
Hypoglycaemia	3 (5.1)	3
Blood and Lymphatic System Disorders	**21 (35.6)**	**49**
Anaemia	16 (27.1)	27
Lymphadenopathy	4 (6.8)	8
Vascular Disorders	**19 (32.2)**	**48**
Flushing	8 (13.6)	20
Hypertension	8 (13.6)	10
Hypotension	5 (8.5)	11

(cont'd)

Table 2: MYOZYME *(cont'd)*

Summary of Adverse Events by System Organ Class and Preferred Term During Treatment Occurring in at Least 5% of Pediatric Patients Treated with MYOZYME in Clinical Trials

System Organ Class Preferred Term	Number of Patients (N=59) n (%)	Number of Adverse Events N=2725
Eye Disorders	**16 (27.1)**	**20**
Conjunctivitis	7 (11.9)	8
Eye discharge	3 (5.1)	3
Psychiatric Disorders	**16 (27.1)**	**31**
Insomnia	6 (10.2)	6
Agitation	5 (8.5)	8
Irritability	5 (8.5)	7
Anxiety	3 (5.1)	6
Restlessness	3 (5.1)	3
Renal and Urinary Disorders	**16 (27.1)**	**34**
Haematuria	4 (6.8)	7
Hypercalciuria	4 (6.8)	6
Proteinuria	3 (5.1)	3
Renal insufficiency	3 (5.1)	3
Nervous System Disorders	**13 (22.0)**	**22**
Hypotonia	3 (5.1)	4
Immune System Disorders	**9 (15.3)**	**13**
Drug hypersensitivity	5 (8.5)	8
Congenital, Familial and Genetic Disorders	**7 (11.9)**	**8**
Macroglossia	3 (5.1)	3
Reproductive System and Breast Disorders	**6 (10.2)**	**6**
Endocrine Disorders	**4 (6.8)**	**5**

The adverse events that occurred with frequency less than 5% of patients (reported in more than 1 patient) based on the MedDRA SOCs of:

Infections and Infestations: include bacteriuria, clostridium colitis, eye infection, gastroenteritis rotavirus, infection, lower respiratory tract infection, respiratory tract infection viral, skin infection, viral rash and viral upper respiratory tract infection.
Respiratory, Thoracic and Mediastinal Disorders: include aspiration, epistaxis, hypercapnia, hypoventilation, hypoxia, lung crepitation, lung disorder, pleural effusion, pulmonary congestion, respiratory acidosis, respiratory arrest, respiratory tract irritation, throat secretion increased, and tracheal pain.
General Disorder and Administration Site Conditions: include application site reaction, catheter site related reaction, fatigue, feeling hot, infusion site reaction, and localised oedema.
Skin and Subcutaneous Tissue Disorders: include decubitus ulcer, dermatitis contact, hair growth abnormal, livedo reticularis, skin disorder, and skin lesion.
Gastrointestinal Disorders: include mouth ulceration, regurgitation of food, retching, and upper gastrointestinal haemorrhage.
Investigations: include acoustic stimulation tests abnormal, alanine aminotransferase increased, aspartate aminotransferase increased, blood calcium increased, blood culture positive, blood urea increased, bone density decreased, culture throat positive, eosinophil count increased, gallop rhythm present and heart rate decreased.
Cardiac Disorders: include cardiac arrest, hypertrophic obstructive cardiomyopathy and supraventricular tachycardia.
Injury, Poisoning and Procedural Complications: include arthropod bite.
Musculoskeletal and Connective Tissue Disorders: include scoliosis.
Metabolism and Nutrition Disorders: include electrolyte imbalance, fluid imbalance, hypercalcaemia, hyperuricaemia, hypocalcaemia, hypochloraemia, hypomagnesaemia and metabolic acidosis.
Blood and Lymphatic System Disorders: include eosinophilia and lymphadenitis.
Vascular Disorders: include pallor.
Ear and Labyrinth Disorders: 25 of 39 patients in the infantile-onset pooled population have been tested for hearing disorders. Of these, 15 (60%) patients had hearing loss at Baseline while 10 had normal hearing test results. Among the 10 patients with normal hearing at baseline, 5 (50%) had abnormal hearing test results at Week 26. In many patients, interpretation of hearing test results was complicated by the presence of middle ear dysfunction at Baseline and/or at subsequent time points. These findings suggest that the hearing loss in patients with Pompe's Disease is related to the disease itself and is not a complication of therapy).
Eye Disorders: include blepharitis and keratoconjunctivitis sicca.
Renal and Urinary Disorders: include dysuria, oliguria, and pyuria.
Nervous System Disorders: include areflexia, headache, hypokinesia and tremor.
Immune System Disorders: include hypersensitivity.
Congenital, Familial and Genetic Disorders: include talipes.
Reproductive System and Breast Disorders: include phimosis.
Endocrine Disorders: include hypoparathyroidism.

Immunogenicity: In the 3 pediatric clinical trials (AGLU01602, AGLU01702, AGLU02203), 49 of the 54 evaluable patients (91%) tested positive for IgG antibodies to alglucosidase alfa. The data reflect the percentage of patients whose test results were considered positive using an enzyme-linked immunosorbent assay (ELISA) and radioimmunoprecipitation (RIP) assay for alglucosidase alfa-specific IgG antibodies. The majority of patients (45 of 49 or 92%) developed IgG antibodies within the first 3 months of initiation of treatment. One of the IgG positive patients tested positive for inhibitory effects on in vitro testing. Infusion reactions were reported in 30 of the 59 patients (51%) treated with MYOZYME and appear to be more common in antibody-positive patients; 16 of 20 patients (80%) with high antibody titers (≥12 800) experienced infusion reactions whereas only 1 of the 5 antibody-negative patients (20%) experienced infusion reactions. Patients treated with a higher dose (40 mg/kg) generally developed a more robust antibody response and experienced more infusion reactions.

The effect of antibody development on the long term efficacy of MYOZYME is not fully understood. There is an observation that some patients, including those who possess two null mutations, are developing high and sustained anti-alglucosidase alfa antibody titers. The cause of a poorer clinical response in some of these patients is thought to be multi-factorial.

Patients who experience IARs suggestive of anaphylactic or allergic reactions may also be tested for IgE antibodies to alglucosidase alfa (see Warnings and Precautions, Monitoring and Laboratory Tests).

In clinical trials and expanded access programs of MYOZYME, approximately forty patients with moderate or severe or recurrent infusion reactions have been tested for MYOZYME specific IgE antibodies. A small number of patients tested positive for IgE antibodies, some of whom experienced anaphylactic reactions. Testing was typically performed for IARs, especially moderate to severe or recurrent reactions (see Warnings and Precautions, Hypersensitivity Reactions, Significant Hypersensitivity Reactions). Some patients have been successfully rechallenged using a slower infusion rate at lower initial doses and have and continued to receive treatment with MYOZYME under close clinical supervision.

Late-Onset Pompe's Disease: Five additional pediatric Pompe's Disease patients were evaluated in a single-center, open-label, non-randomized, uncontrolled clinical trial. Patients were ages 5 to 15 years, ambulatory (able to walk at least 10 meters in 6 minutes), and not receiving invasive ventilatory support at study entry. All 5 patients received treatment with 20 mg/kg MYOZYME for 26 weeks. The most common treatment-emergent adverse events (regardless of causality) observed with MYOZYME treatment in this study were headache, pharyngitis, upper abdominal pain, malaise and rhinitis.

The data described below reflect exposure of 90 patients (45 male, 45 female) with late-onset Pompe's Disease, ages 10 to 70 years, to 20 mg/kg of MYOZYME or placebo in a randomized, double-blind, placebo-controlled study. All patients were naïve to enzyme replacement therapy. Patients were randomized in a 2:1 ratio and received MYOZYME or placebo every other week for 78 weeks (18 months). The study population included 34 males and 26 females (N=60) in the MYOZYME group and 11 males and 19 females (N=30) in the placebo group. In the MYOZYME treatment group, 32 patients (53%) experienced adverse reactions and 17 patients (57%) in the Placebo group. The majority of the adverse reactions were characterized as infusion reactions which included 17 patients (28%) in the MYOZYME group and 7 patients (23%) experienced infusion reactions in the Placebo group. Thirteen (22%) patients experienced serious adverse reactions in the MYOZYME group and 6 (20%) patients in the Placebo group.

The most serious adverse reactions reported with MYOZYME in the randomized, double-blind, placebo-controlled study were anaphylactic reactions. Reactions included chest discomfort/pain, throat tightness and angioedema [see Warnings and Precautions, Boxed Warning, Risk of Anaphylaxis and Hypersensitivity Reactions]. Other reported serious adverse reactions included one event of supraventricular tachycardia in a single patient.

The most common adverse reactions observed were infusion reactions. In the randomized, double-blind, placebo-controlled study, infusion reactions occurred in approximately 28% of patients treated with MYOZYME, compared to 23% of placebo-treated patients. The majority of these reactions were mild to moderate and resolved spontaneously. Infusion reactions which were reported in ≥5% of MYOZYME-treated patients included headache, nausea, urticaria, dizziness, chest discomfort, hyperhidrosis, flushing, blood pressure increased, and vomiting. See Table 3.

Table 3: MYOZYME

Summary of IARs Occurring in at Least 5% of Late-Onset Patients in Either Treatment Group

System Organ Class Preferred Term	MYOZYME Patients Number of Patients[a] (N=60) n (%)	Placebo Patients Number of Patients[a] (N=30) n (%)
Any IARs	**17 (28.3)**	**7 (23.3)**
Nervous System Disorders	**9 (15.0)**	**6 (20.0)**
Headache	5 (8.3)	5 (16.7)
Dizziness	4 (6.7)	2 (6.7)
General Disorders and Administration Site Conditions	**10 (16.7)**	**2 (6.7)**
Chest discomfort	4 (6.7)	0
Gastrointestinal Disorders	**8 (13.3)**	**3 (10.0)**
Nausea	5 (8.3)	3 (10.0)
Vomiting	3 (5.0)	0
Skin and Subcutaneous Tissue Disorders	**10 (16.7)**	**0**
Urticaria	5 (8.3)	0
Hyperhidrosis	3 (5.0)	0
Vascular Disorders	**3 (5.0)**	**1 (3.3)**
Flushing	3 (5.0)	0
Investigations	**3 (5.0)**	**0**
Blood pressure increased	3 (5.0)	0

[a] Percentages are based on the total number of patients treated in the study group. A patient experiencing more than 1 IAR within an SOC or preferred term is counted once within that SOC or preferred term. Events occurring in at least 5% of patients in either treatment group are presented; corresponding percentage of patients in alternate treatment group is presented which may represent less than 5% of patients.

Infusion associated reactions that occurred with frequency less than 5% in patients treated with MYOZYME (reported in at least 1 patient) based on the MedDRA SOCs of:

Nervous System Disorders: include paraesthesia, somnolence.

General Disorders and Administration Site Conditions: include pyrexia, local swelling, feeling hot, chills, non-cardiac chest pain, oedema peripheral.

Gastrointestinal Disorders: include lip swelling, oral pruritus, dyspepsia, epigastric discomfort, retching, stomach discomfort, swollen tongue.

Skin and Subcutaneous Tissue Disorders: include pruritus, rash popular, skin nodule, rash macular, cold sweat, rash maculopapular, erythema, rash, rash pruritic, angioneurotic oedema, subcutaneous nodule.

Investigations: include oxygen saturation decreased.

Eye Disorders: include asthenopia, eye pruritus.

Immune System Disorders: include hypersensitivity.

Musculoskeletal and Connective Tissue Disorders: include sensation of heaviness, muscle twitching.

Respiratory, Thoracic and Mediastinal Disorders: include throat tightness, wheezing.

Cardiac Disorders: include sinus tachycardia.

Ear and Labyrinth Disorders: include ear discomfort, auricular swelling.

Table 4 enumerates treatment-emergent adverse reactions that occurred in at least 5% of patients during the randomized, double-blind, placebo-controlled study. Reported adverse reactions have been classified by Medical Dictionary for Regulatory Activities (MedDRA) terminology System Organ Class and Preferred Term.

Adverse reactions that occurred with frequency less than 5% in patients treated with MYOZYME (reported in at least 1 patient) based on the MedDRA SOCs of:

General Disorders And Administration Site Conditions: include local swelling, pyrexia, feeling hot, oedema peripheral, catheter site pain, chills, infusion site bruising, infusion site paraesthesia, malaise, non-cardiac chest pain.

Table 4: MYOZYME

Summary of Adverse Reactions Occurring in ≥5% of Late-Onset Patients by Treatment Group

System Organ Class Preferred Term	MYOZYME N=60 n (%)	Placebo N=30 n (%)
Any Adverse Events	**32 (53.3)**	**17 (56.7)**
General Disorders and Administration Site Conditions	**15 (25.0)**	**7 (23.3)**
Fatigue	3 (5.0)	4 (13.3)
Chest discomfort	4 (6.7)	1 (3.3)
Asthenia	0	2 (6.7)
Nervous System Disorders	**10 (16.7)**	**8 (26.7)**
Headache	5 (8.3)	6 (20.0)
Dizziness	4 (6.7)	2 (6.7)
Skin and Subcutaneous Tissue Disorders	**13 (21.7)**	**4 (13.3)**
Urticaria	5 (8.3)	0
Hyperhidrosis	5 (8.3)	0
Gastrointestinal Disorders	**9 (15.0)**	**4 (13.3)**
Nausea	5 (8.3)	3 (10.0)
Vomiting	3 (5.0)	0
Musculoskeletal and Connective Tissue Disorders	**8 (13.3)**	**2 (6.7)**
Muscle twitching	4 (6.7)	1 (3.3)
Myalgia	3 (5.0)	1 (3.3)
Eye Disorders	**6 (10.0)**	**2 (6.7)**
Cataract	4 (6.7)	1 (3.3)
Ear and Labyrinth Disorders	**4 (6.7)**	**2 (6.7)**
Hypoacusis	2 (3.3)	2 (6.7)
Vascular Disorders	**4 (6.7)**	**2 (6.7)**
Flushing	3 (5.0)	0
Investigations	**4 (6.7)**	**0**
Blood pressure increased	3 (5.0)	0

Nervous System Disorders: include paraesthesia, lethargy, somnolence.

Skin and Subcutaneous Tissue Disorders: include pruritus, rash pruritic, rash, rash papular, skin nodule, rash macular, cold sweat, rash maculopapular, erythema, angioedema, skin odour abnormal, subcutaneous nodule.

Gastrointestinal Disorders: include diarrhea, lip swelling, oral pruritus, abdominal distension, dyspepsia, epigastric discomfort, retching, stomach discomfort, swollen tongue.

Musculoskeletal and Connective Tissue Disorders: include muscle spasms, pain in extremity, sensation of heaviness.

Eye Disorders: include asthenopia, eye pruritus, photophobia.

Ear and Labyrinth Disorders: include hypoacusis, ear discomfort, auricular swelling, tinnitus.

Vascular Disorders: include hot flush.

Cardiac Disorders: include bundle branch block left, buncle branch block right, sinus tachycardia, supraventricular tachycardia.

Investigations: include electrocardiogram QT corrected interval prolonged, oxygen saturation decreased.

Respiratory, Thoracic and Mediastinal Disorders: include throat tightness, wheezing.

Renal and Urinary Disorders: include haematuria, urine odour abnormal.

Immune System Disorders: include hypersensitivity.

Immunogenicity: In the randomized, double-blind, placebo-controlled study, all patients with available samples treated with MYOZYME (N=59, 100%) developed IgG antibodies to alglucosidase alfa. Patients were considered positive for antibodies to alglucosidase alfa using an enzyme-linked immunosorbent assay (ELISA) and confirmed by a radioimmunoprecipitation (RIP) assay for alglucosidase alfa-specific IgG antibodies. All patients who developed IgG antibodies did so within the first 3 months of exposure (median time to seroconversion was 4 weeks).

Patients who developed IgG antibodies to alglucosidase alfa were also evaluated for inhibition of enzyme activity or cellular uptake of enzyme in in vitro assays. None of the 59 evaluable patients tested positive for inhibition of enzyme activity. Ten of 59 patients had antibody titers for uptake inhibition ≥40 at two consecutive time points. An additional 8 patients tested positive for uptake inhibition at least once, but did not have antibody titers for uptake inhibition ≥40 at any two consecutive time points. All other patients tested negative for inhibition of cellular uptake. Patients who were positive for uptake inhibition tended to have higher mean peak IgG titers than patients who tested negative for uptake inhibition. Among the 32 patients with evaluable pharmacokinetic (PK) samples, 5 patients tested positive for uptake inhibition at times corresponding to PK sampling times, and had higher mean clearance, lower mean AUC, and lower mean C_{max} [see Action and Clinical Pharmacology, Pharmacokinetics] as compared to other patients.

Ten patients in the randomized, double-blind, placebo-controlled study underwent testing for alglucosidase alfa-specific IgE antibodies. Testing was performed in patients who experienced moderate to severe or recurrent infusion reactions, for which mast-cell activation was suspected. Two of 10 patients evaluated tested positive for alglucosidase alfa-specific IgE-binding antibodies, both of whom experienced anaphylactic reactions [see Warnings and Precautions, Boxed Warning, Risk of Anaphylaxis and Hypersensitivity Reactions]. One patient who developed IgE antibodies discontinued the study following an anaphylactic reaction. Both IgE positive patients were successfully rechallenged with MYOZYME during or after discontinuation from the study using a slower infusion rate at lower initial doses and have continued to receive treatment under close clinical supervision. Patients who develop IgE antibodies to MYOZYME appear to be at a higher risk for the occurrence of infusion reactions [see Warnings and Precautions, Hypersensitivity Reactions]. Therefore, these patients should be monitored more closely during administration of MYOZYME.

Post-Market Adverse Drug Reactions: Additional IARs reported from worldwide post-marketing sources after marketing approval (including ongoing clinical programs) included: cardiac arrest, bradycardia, angioedema, pharyngeal edema, edema peripheral, chest pain, chest discomfort, dyspnea, muscle spasm, fatigue, and conjunctivitis. Those IARs assessed as severe included cardiac arrest, bradycardia, chest pain, and dyspnea.

Significant hypersensitivity reactions have been reported in both infantile- and late-onset patients treated with MYOZYME. Some patients experienced life-threatening anaphylactic reactions, including anaphylactic shock, some of which were IgE-mediated. Reactions generally occurred shortly after initiation of the infusion. Patients presented with a constellation of signs and symptoms, primarily respiratory, cardiovascular, edematous and/or cutaneous in nature. Reactions included bronchospasm, wheezing, respiratory distress, dyspnea, oxygen saturation decreased, brief episodes of cardiac arrest, hypotension, bradycardia, tachycardia, cyanosis, vasoconstriction, flushing, chest pain, chest discomfort, throat tightness, angioedema **[change in terminology]**, face edema, peripheral edema, urticaria, and rash.

Reactions were generally managed with temporary interruption and/or discontinuation of infusion and administration of antihistamines, corticosteroids, intravenous fluids, and/or oxygen, when clinically indicated. In some cases of anaphylactic reaction and cardiac arrest, epinephrine and/or cardiopulmonary resuscitation were also administered. All patients recovered from the reactions. The majority of patients continued to receive treatment with MYOZYME, some under close clinical supervision.

Early detection of signs and symptoms of hypersensitivity or anaphylactic reactions may assist in effective management of patients and prevent possible significant or irreversible outcomes.

DRUG INTERACTIONS: Drug-Drug Interactions: Interactions with other drugs have not been established.
Drug-Food Interactions: Interactions with food have not been established.
Drug-Herb Interactions: Interactions with herbal products have not been established.
Drug-Laboratory Test Interactions: Interactions with laboratory tests have not been established.

DOSAGE AND ADMINISTRATION: Dosing Considerations:

- MYOZYME (alglucosidase alfa) is intended for long-term, chronic use under the guidance and supervision of a physician.

Recommended Dose and Dosage Adjustment: The recommended dosage regimen of MYOZYME is 20 mg/kg body weight administered every 2 weeks as an intravenous infusion. There was no additional clinical benefit with doses of MYOZYME higher than 20 mg/kg of body weight in clinical trials.

The total volume of infusion is determined by the patient's body weight and should be administered over approximately 4 hours. In the clinical trials, pre-treatment medications were used but not routinely administered to patients.

Infusions should be administered in a step-wise manner using an infusion pump. The initial infusion rate should be no more than 1 mg/kg/h. The infusion rate may be increased by 2 mg/kg/h every 30 minutes, after patient tolerance to the infusion rate is established, until a maximum rate of 7 mg/kg/h is reached. The infusion rate may be slowed and/or temporarily stopped in the event of infusion reactions. See Table 5.

Table 5: MYOZYME

Recommended Administration of MYOZYME

1 mg/kg/h×30 minutes	Obtain vital signs, if stable increase rate to...
3 mg/kg/h×30 minutes	Obtain vital signs, if stable increase rate to...
5 mg/kg/h×30 minutes	Obtain vital signs, if stable increase rate to...
7 mg/kg/h	Administer for the remainder of the infusion

Administration: Instructions for Use: Vials of MYOZYME are stored under refrigerated conditions (at 2-8°C). As MYOZYME does not contain a preservative, strict aseptic techniques are to be used in the preparation of a patient's dose. Once reconstituted, vials of MYOZYME are to be used immediately for dilution into an infusion bag. Diluted MYOZYME into an infusion bag is also to be used immediately (within 3 hours). The reconstituted and diluted infusion solution should be protected from light. Any unused product should be discarded.

MYOZYME should be reconstituted, diluted and administered by a health care professional.

Use aseptic technique during preparation. Do not use filter needles during preparation.

1. Determine the number of vials to be reconstituted based on the individual patient's weight and the recommended dose of 20 mg/kg. Round up to the nearest whole vial. Remove the required number of vials from the refrigerator and allow them to reach room temperature prior to reconstitution (approximately 30 minutes).
   Patient weight (kg)×Dose (mg/kg)=Patient Dose (in mg).
   Patient dose (in mg)÷50 mg/vial = number of vials to reconstitute. If the number of vials includes a fraction, round up to the next whole number.
   Example: Patient Weight (16 kg)×20 mg/kg = Patient Dose (320 mg).
   320 mg÷50 mg/vial = 6.4 vials; therefore, 7 vials should be reconstituted.
2. Reconstitute each MYOZYME vial by **slowly** injecting 10.3 mL of Sterile Water for Injection, USP to the inside wall of each vial. Avoid forceful impact of the water for injection on the powder and avoid foaming. This is done by slow drop-wise addition of the water for injection down the inside of the vial and not directly onto the lyophilized cake. Tilt and roll each vial gently. Do not invert, swirl or shake. Each vial will yield 5 mg/mL. The total extractable dose per vial is 50 mg, 10 mL. The reconstituted MYOZYME should be protected from light.
3. Visually inspect the reconstituted vials. The vials should contain a clear, colorless to pale yellow solution. The reconstituted solution may also contain a few particles in the form of thin white strands or translucent fibers. These particles have been shown to be composed of alglucosidase alfa which can be easily filtered during the infusion. Do not use vials that contain foreign matter or if discolored.
4. Slowly withdraw the reconstituted solution from each vial and further dilute with 0.9 % Sodium Chloride Injection, USP. Avoid foaming in the syringe. The final infusion solution should be prepared to a concentration of 0.5 to 4 mg/mL. Remove airspace from the infusion bag to minimize particle formation due to the sensitivity of MYOZYME to air-liquid interface. Inject the reconstituted MYOZYME solution directly into the sodium chloride solution rather than into the air within the infusion bag. Avoid foaming in the infusion bag. Discard any vial with unused reconstituted solution. The diluted MYOZYME should be protected from light.
   Patient dose (in mg)÷5 mg/mL = number of mL of reconstituted MYOZYME required for patient dose.
   Example: Patient dose = 320 mg.
   320 mg÷5 mg/mL = 64 mL of MYOZYME.
   See Table 6.

Table 6: MYOZYME

Recommended Total Volume

Dose (mg/kg)	Patient Weight Range (kg)	Infusion Volume (mL)
20	1–10	50
20	10.1–20	100
20	20.1–30	150
20	30.1–35	200
20	35.1–50	250
20	50.1–60	300
20	60.1–100	500
20	100.1–120	600
20	120.1–140	700
20	140.1–160	800
20	160.1–180	900
20	180.1–200	1000

5. Gently invert the infusion solution bag to mix. Avoid any vigorous shaking and agitation.
6. MYOZYME should not be infused in the same intravenous line with other products.
7. The diluted solution should be filtered through an in-line, low protein-binding 0.2 ·m filter during administration to remove any visible particles.

OVERDOSAGE:
There have been no reports of overdose with MYOZYME (alglucosidase alfa). In clinical trials, patients received doses up to 40 mg/kg of body weight.

For management of a suspected drug overdose, CPhA recommends that you contact your **regional Poison Control Centre**. See the *CPS* Directory section for a list of Poison Control Centres.

ACTION AND CLINICAL PHARMACOLOGY: Mechanism of Action: Pompe's Disease is an inherited, progressive muscle disease resulting from a deficiency of the lysosomal enzyme GAA. Deficiency of GAA results in the accumulation of organelle-bound (lysosomal) and extra lysosomal glycogen. Alglucosidase alfa degrades glycogen by catalyzing the hydrolysis of α-1,4- and α-1,6- glycosidic linkages of lysosomal glycogen. Glycogen accumulation in Pompe's Disease occurs in various tissues, particularly cardiac, respiratory and skeletal muscle, leading to the development of cardiomyopathy and progressive muscle weakness, including impairment of respiratory function. MYOZYME (alglucosidase alfa) is intended to provide an exogenous source of GAA for patients with Pompe's Disease.

Pharmacodynamics: Pharmacodynamic parameters were evaluated in two studies both of which included patients with infantile-onset Pompe's Disease. Patients in the first study were older (median age of 15.0 months at first infusion) and had signs of more advanced disease than patients in the second study (median age of 5.3 months at first infusion). Pharmacodynamics were evaluated by measuring tissue GAA activity and glycogen content in quadriceps muscle biopsies.

GAA activity in skeletal muscle was measured at baseline and week 12 in both studies and at week 52 in the first study. In both studies, muscle GAA activity increased during treatment with MYOZYME.

Glycogen content was measured both biochemically and histomorphometrically in muscle biopsy specimens obtained from patients at baseline, week 12 (both studies), and week 52 (first study). See Table 7 and Table 8.

Table 7: MYOZYME

GAA Activity and Glycogen Content in Skeletal Muscle Biopsies in Study AGLU01602

				Glycogen Content		Change in Glycogen Content from Baseline to Week 12	
Patient ID	Dose Group (mg/kg)	Visit	GAA Activity (nmol/h/g wet tissue)	Biochem (mg/g tissue)[a]	Histomorph % Tissue Area Mean (SD)	Biochem	Histmorph
1602–301	40	Baseline	BQL	46.5	31.2 (6.19)		
		Week 12	279.5	108.2	58.5 (6.64)	Increase	Increase
1602–302	20	Baseline	8.8	11.9	8.3 (5.05)		
		Week 12	62.3	36.3	20.2 (10.26)	Increase	Stable
1602–303	40	Baseline	BQL	56.4	22.1 (6.39)		
		Week 12	225.1	43.2	25.1 (8.11)	Decrease	Stable
1602–305	20	Baseline	BQL	98.1	38.9 (8.03)		
		Week 12	22.3	99.1	59.9 (5.83)	Stable	Increase
1602–306	20	Baseline	8.5	35.2	45.5 (9.34)		
		Week 12	33.4	74.2	39.4 (6.22)	Increase	Stable

(cont'd)

Table 7: MYOZYME *(cont'd)*

GAA Activity and Glycogen Content in Skeletal Muscle Biopsies in Study AGLU01602

Patient ID	Dose Group (mg/kg)	Visit	GAA Activity (nmol/h/g wet tissue)	Glycogen Content		Change in Glycogen Content from Baseline to Week 12	
				Biochem (mg/g tissue)[a]	Histomorph % Tissue Area Mean (SD)	Biochem	Histmorph
1602–307	40	Baseline	BQL	53.1	20.6 (8.04)		
		Week 12	407.9	24.0	6.6 (4.11)	Decrease	Decrease
1602–308	40	Baseline	BQL	69.7	39.1 (4.91)		
		Week 12	213.4	37.5	31.0 (7.67)	Decrease	Stable
1602–309	20	Baseline	4.6	39.4	16.7 (5.91)		
		Week 12	95.8	18.0	9.9 (3.03)	Decrease	Stable
1602-310	20	Baseline	BQL	37.1	15.7 (9.34)		
		Week 12	82.7	40.3	47.8 (6.62)	Stable	Increase
1602–311	40	Baseline	BQL	85.5	30.2 (11.78)		
		Week 12	228.8	72.3	31.3 (9.75)	Stable	Stable
1602–312	20	Baseline	BQL	96.1	32.2 (9.76)		
		Week 12	39.6	77.1	21.5 (9.21)	Stable	Stable
1602–313	40	Baseline	BQL	21.8	21.0 (4.55)		
		Week 12	638.3	10.0	5.6 (4.31)	Decrease	Decrease
1602–314	20	Baseline	BQL	48.9	17.0 (7.46)		
		Week 12	65.2	24.8	5.9 (2.36)	Decrease	Decrease
1602–315	40	Baseline	BQL	40.0	13.4 (7.38)		
		Week 12	88.6	3.4	0.01 (0.02)	Decrease	Decrease
1602–316	20	Baseline	BQL	34.2	28.1 (6.45)		
		Week 12	79.6	20.5	16.8 (7.23)	Decrease	Stable
1602–317	40	Baseline	BQL	112.9	55.4 (12.57)		
		Week 12	197.1	68.2	51.6 (7.55)	Decrease	Stable
1602–318	40	Baseline	BQL	74.7	42.1 (8.28)		
		Week 12	799.9	47.3	27.6 (12.13)	Decrease	Stable
1602–319	20	Baseline	BQL	57.6	27.6 (5.85)		
		Week 12	428.9	45.9	29.7 (6.65)	Decrease	Stable

[a] To calculate the percentage of wet weight, glycogen content (mg glycogen/g tissue) is divided by 10.
Legend: BQL=below quantifiable levels; Histomorph=histomorphometric.

Table 8: MYOZYME

GAA Activity and Glycogen Content in Skeletal Muscle Biopsies in Study AGLU01702

Patient ID	Visit	GAA Activity (nmol/h/g wet tissue)	Glycogen Content		Change in Glycogen Content from Baseline to Week 52[b]	
			Biochem (mg/g tissue)[a]	Histomorph % Tissue Area Mean (SD)	Biochem	Histomorph
1702–402	Baseline	12.1	46.9	17.41 (2.83)		
	Week 52	101.1	31.6	23.09 (10.87)	Decrease	Stable
1702–403	Baseline	NAV	NAV	53.25 (7.14)		
	Week 52	ND	ND	ND	ND	ND
1702–404	Baseline	8.9	71.4	37.71 (11.26)		
	Week 52	132.6	76.6	71.67 (4.63)	Stable	Increase
1702–405	Baseline	BQL	90.2	64.87 (5.42)		
	Week 52	D	D	D	NA	NA
1702–406	Baseline	9.3	66.9	67.25 (7.17)		
	Week 52[c]	59.6	56.6	61.63 (9.34)	Stable	Stable
1702–407	Baseline	BQL	75.8	42.08 (5.44)		
	Week 52	D	D	D	NA	NA
1702–408	Baseline	23.2	72	62.87 (10.24)		
	Week 52	105.4	43.4	57.56 (9.66)	Decrease	Stable

(cont'd)

Table 8: MYOZYME *(cont'd)*

GAA Activity and Glycogen Content in Skeletal Muscle Biopsies in Study AGLU01702

Patient ID	Visit	GAA Activity (nmol/h/g wet tissue)	Glycogen Content		Change in Glycogen Content from Baseline to Week 52[b]	
			Biochem (mg/g tissue)[a]	Histomorph % Tissue Area Mean (SD)	Biochem	Histomorph
1702–409	Baseline	BQL	79.1	56.06 (14.98)	NA	NA
	Week 52	D	D	D		
1702–410	Baseline	19.8	98.6	58.05 (13.16)	Decrease	Stable
	Week 52	44.6	64.7	45.20 (8.02)		
1702–411	Baseline	4.8	87.9	40.60 (11.93)	Stable	Increase
	Week 52	63.3	76.1	67.02		
1702–412	Baseline	BQL	75.9	53.43 (6.85)	NA	NA
	Week 52	D	D	D		
1702–413	Baseline	BQL	46.3	24.56 (8.31)	Increase	Increase
	Week 52	153.9	89.0	48.17 (8.36)		
1702–414	Baseline	28.0	40.1	36.98 (13.25)	Decrease	Decrease
	Week 52	86.5	BQL	2.59 (2.14)		
1702–415	Baseline	16.8	63.4	30.68 (8.06)	Decrease	Stable
	Week 52	72.9	39.7	47.43 (20.71)		
1702–416	Baseline	7.2	70.9	63.62 (4.68)	ND	Stable
	Week 52	NAV	NAV	58.00 (12.54)		

[a] Divide value by 10 to express glycogen content as percent of wet tissue.
[b] Results are presented only for patients who had data both at Baseline and Week 52 and for both biochemical and histomorphometric methods.
[c] Labeled as a Screening visit in the appendix.
Note: BQL=Below Quantifiable Level; D=deceased; NA = Not Applicable; NAV=Not Available; ND=Not Done.

Pharmacokinetics: The pharmacokinetics of MYOZYME were evaluated in 13 patients with Pompe's Disease (age 1 month to 7 months) who received 20 mg/kg (as an approximate 4-hour infusion) or 40 mg/kg (as an approximate 6.5-hour infusion) of MYOZYME every 2 weeks. The measurement of MYOZYME plasma concentration was based on an activity assay using an artificial substrate. Systemic exposure was approximately dose proportional between the 20 and 40 mg/kg doses (see Table 9).

Table 9: MYOZYME

Pharmacokinetic Parameters (Mean±SD) After Single Intravenous Infusion of MYOZYME (AGLU01602)

Pharmacokinetic Parameter	20 mg/kg (n=5)	40 mg/kg (n=8)
C_{max} (µg/mL)	162±31	276±64
AUC_∞ (µg-h/mL)	811±141	1781±520
CL (mL/h/kg)	25±4	24±7
Vss (mL/kg)	96±16	119±28
$t_{1/2}$ (h)	2.3±0.4	2.9±0.5

Note: With the exception of Cmax, the pharmacokinetic parameters in this table have been estimated by fitting a two-compartment model, with elimination from the central compartment, to the observed data.

The pharmacokinetics of MYOZYME were also evaluated in a separate trial (AGLU01702) in 14 infantile-onset patients with Pompe's Disease (age from 6 months to 3.5 years) who received 20 mg/kg of MYOZYME as an approximate 4-hour infusion every 2 weeks. The pharmacokinetic parameters were similar to those observed for the 20 mg/kg dose group in the trial of patients of age ranging from 1 month to 7 months.

Nineteen of 21 patients who received treatment with MYOZYME in trial AGLU01602 and AGLU01702 and had pharmacokinetics and antibody titer data available at Week 12 developed antibodies to MYOZYME. Five patients with antibody titers ≥12 800 at Week 12 had an average increase in clearance of 50% (range 5% to 90%) from Week 1 to Week 12. The other 14 patients with antibody titers <12 800 at Week 12 had similar average clearance values at Week 1 and Week 12.

The pharmacokinetics of alglucosidase alfa were studied in a population analysis of 32 late-onset Pompe patients from the randomized, double-blind, placebo-controlled study (AGLU02704) ranging in age from 21 to 70 years old who received MYOZYME 20 mg/kg every other week. The measurement of alglucosidase alfa plasma concentration was based on an activity assay using an artificial substrate. AUC and C_{max} were similar at Week 0, 12 and 52 visits indicating alglucosidase alfa pharmacokinetics were not time-dependent (see Table 10).

Table 10: MYOZYME

Alglucosidase Alfa Pharmacokinetics After Single Dose and After 12 and 52 Weeks of Therapy (AGLU02704)

Parameter	Week 0	Week 12	Week 52
C_{max} (µg/mL)	385±106	349±79	370±88
$AUC_{(0-\infty)}$ (µg*h/mL)	2672±1140	2387±555	2700±1000
CL (mL/h)	633±175	700±244	645±198
Vss (L)	69±92	70±91	70±92
Effective Half-life (h)	2.4±0.4	2.4±0.3	2.5±0.4

There was no evidence that IgG antibodies to alglucosidase alfa affected pharmacokinetics. Higher mean clearance, lower mean AUC, and lower mean C_{max} were observed in 5 patients that tested positive for inhibition of cellular uptake of enzyme in the randomized, double-blind, placebo-controlled study (AGLU02704) (see Adverse Reactions, Clinical Trial Adverse Drug Reactions, Late-Onset Pompe's Disease, Immunogenicity).

Effects of Antibodies: Most patients who received infusions of MYOZYME developed antibodies to alglucosidase alfa by week 12.

STORAGE AND STABILITY: Store MYOZYME (alglucosidase alfa) under refrigeration between 2-8°C. **Do not freeze or shake. Do not use MYOZYME** after the expiration date on the vial.

MYOZYME contains no preservatives. Strict aseptic conditions are to be used for the reconstitution of vials and their dilution into the infusion bag. Reconstituted vials should be used immediately for dilution. Administration of the diluted MYOZYME infusion bags should be initiated without delay (within 3 hours). If immediate use is not possible, MYOZYME has been shown to be physically and chemically stable for up to 24 hours at 2-8°C provided that aseptic technique is used throughout the procedure.

Protect reconstituted and diluted MYOZYME from light.

INFORMATION FOR THE PATIENT: Published in e-CPS, available by subscription at www.e-cps.ca.

DOSAGE FORMS, COMPOSITION AND PACKAGING: Myozyme (alglucosidase alfa) is intended for intravenous infusion. It is supplied as a sterile, nonpyrogenic, white to off-white, lyophilized cake or powder for reconstitution with 10.3 mL Sterile Water for Injection, USP. Each 50 mg vial contains: 52.5 mg alglucosidase alfa, 210 mg mannitol, 0.5 mg polysorbate 80, 9.9 mg sodium phosphate dibasic heptahydrate, 31.2 mg sodium phosphate monobasic monohydrate. Following reconstitution as directed, each vial contains 10.5 mL reconstituted solution and a total extractable volume of 10 mL at 5 mg/mL alglucosidase alfa. Preservative-free. Single-use, clear Type I glass 20 mL vials. The closure consists of a siliconized butyl stopper and an aluminum seal with a plastic flip-off cap.

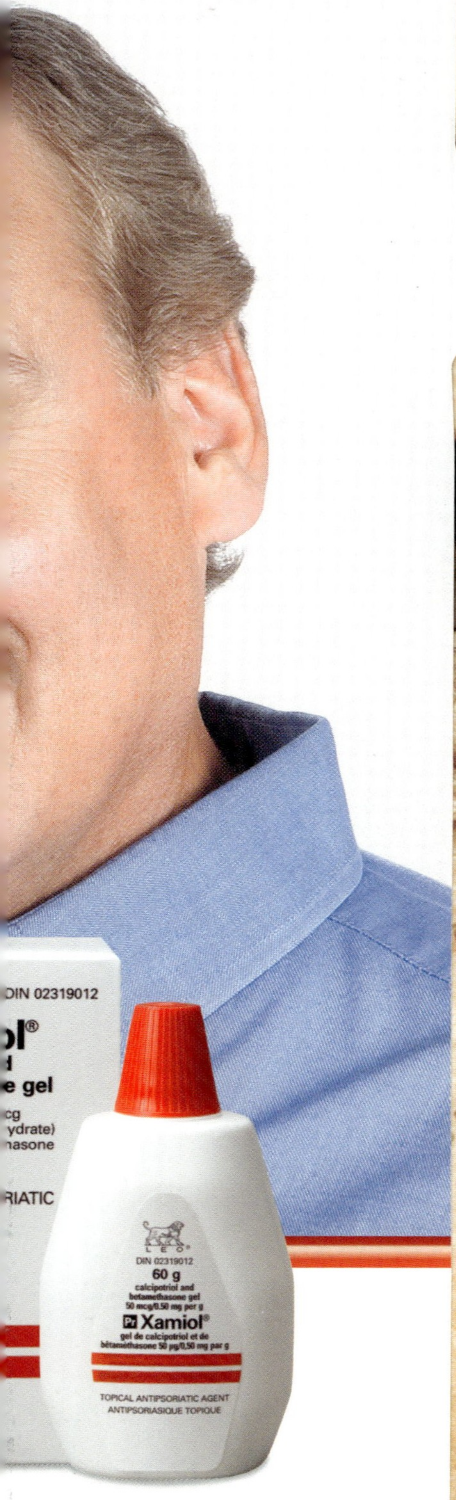

ed areas of the scalp once daily for
ximum daily dose, including other
rrect application and hand washing.
tients at risk, serum calcium levels
this increases systemic absorption
use is not recommended. Not for
to tuberculosis or syphilis, perioral
severe renal insufficiency, hepatic
stular psoriasis. **Adverse reactions:**
, photosensitivity, hypersensitivity.
perioral dermatitis, allergic contact
VR. This potential risk is known from
pply Xamiol® to exposed skin (e.g. a
LEO Pharma Inc., at 1-800-263-4218.

PAAB Member R&D

N

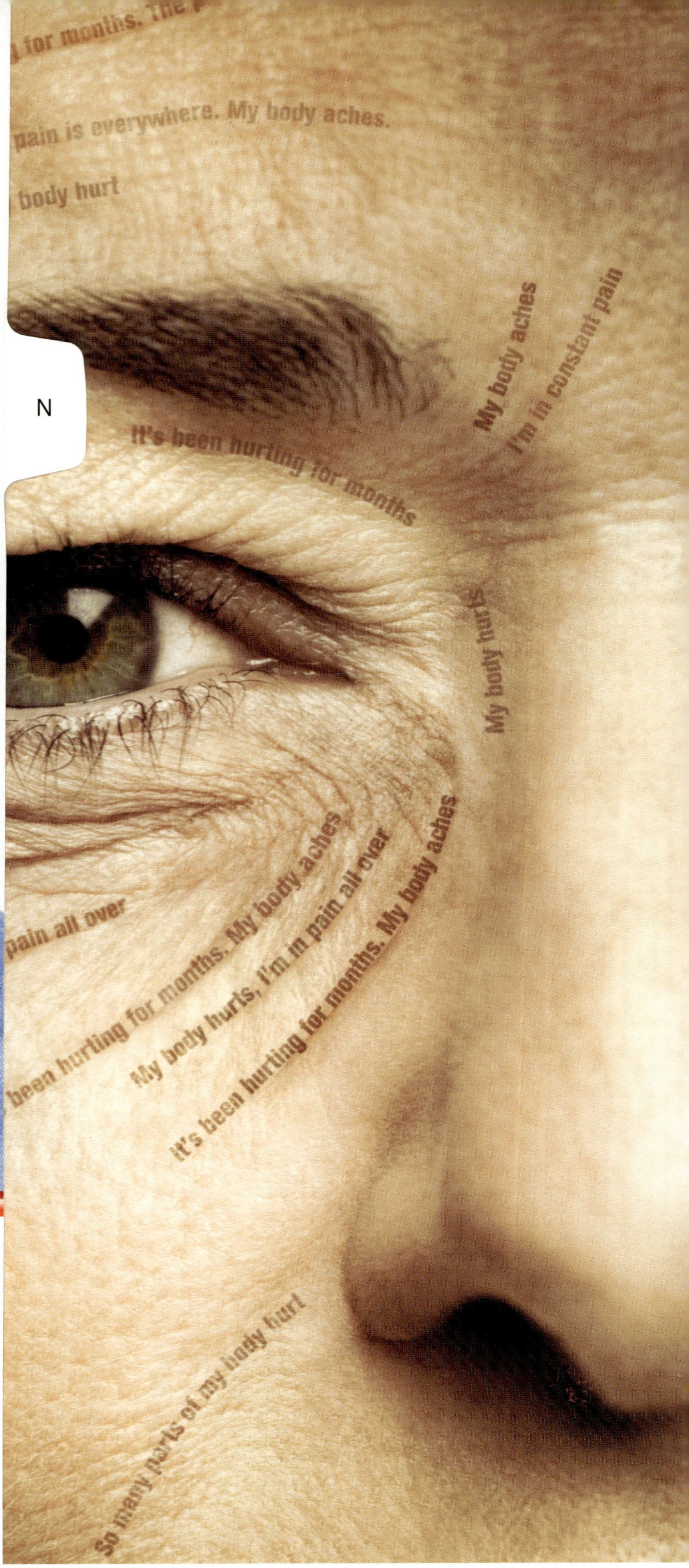

ITH PAIN*

VITH FIBROMYALGIA

Nexium® is indicated in adults for the treatment of conditions where a reduction of gastric acid secretion is required such as: reflux esophagitis, maintenance treatment of patients with reflux esophagitis, nonerosive reflux disease (NERD) (i.e., heartburn and regurgitation), healing* and reduction of risk of gastric ulcers associated with non-steroidal anti-inflammatory drug (NSAID) therapy, treatment of pathological hypersecretory conditions, including Zollinger-Ellison syndrome, and *Helicobacter pylori* eradication.

Nexium® is indicated in children (1-17 years of age) for the treatment of conditions where a reduction of gastric acid secretion is required such as: reflux esophagitis and nonerosive reflux disease (NERD) (i.e., heartburn and regurgitation).

Among reactions which occurred in adults with a frequency of >1% in clinical studies, only headache, diarrhea, flatulence, abdominal pain, nausea, vomiting, dizziness and dry mouth are thought to be associated with the use of Nexium®.

Among reactions which occurred in children (1-11 years of age) with a frequency of >1% in clinical studies, only headache, diarrhea and somnolence are associated with the use of Nexium®. In children (12-17 years of age) the treatment related adverse event profile was found to be consistent with that seen in adults.

*Note: Superiority of Nexium® over ranitidine 150 mg BID with the use of non-selective NSAIDs was demonstrated. Superiority was not established with the use of COX-2 selective NSAIDs alone due to the small number of patients analysed in this subgroup.[1]

Reference: 1. Nexium® Product Monograph. AstraZeneca Canada Inc. Revised December 3, 2008.

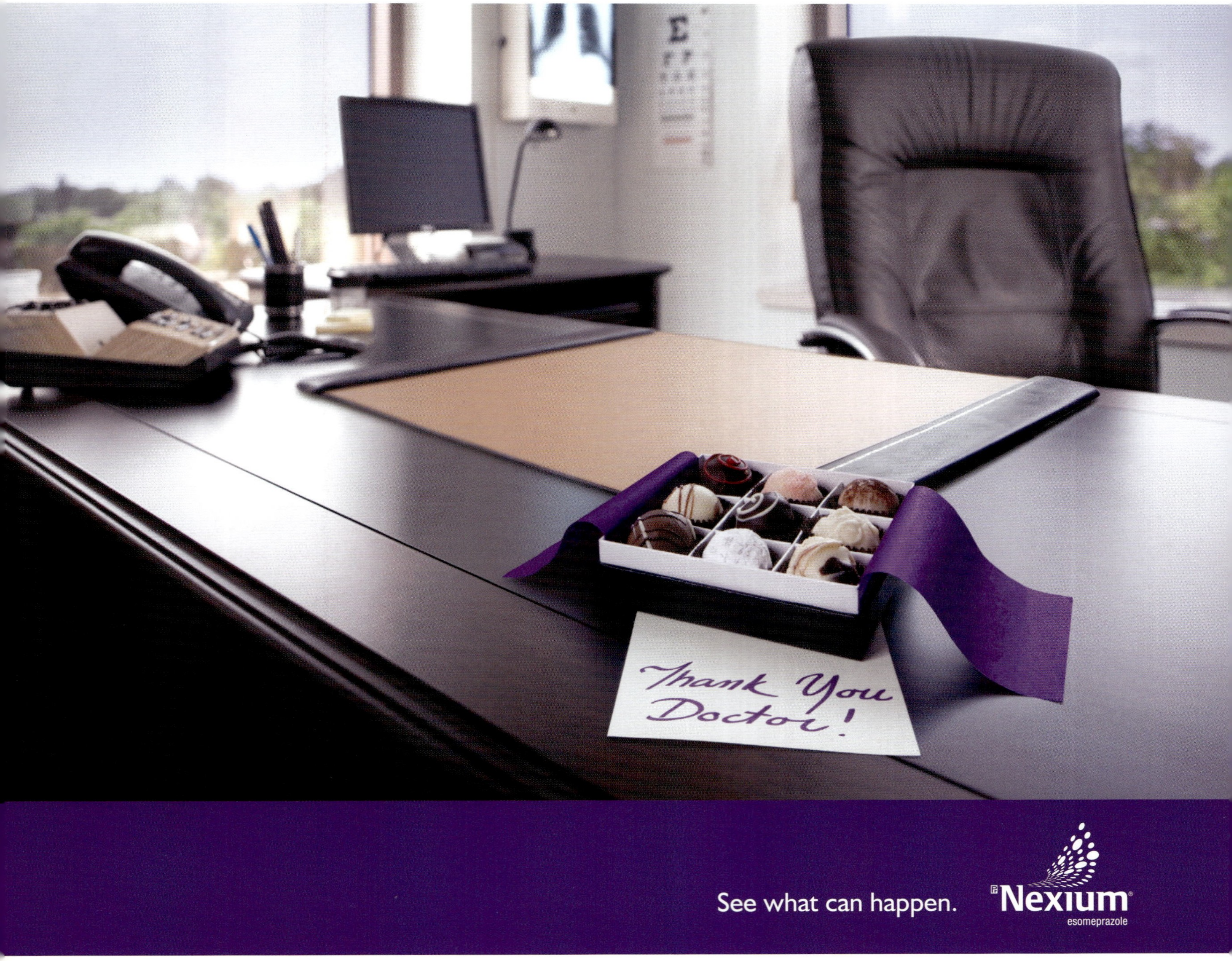

N

Nadolol ℗
Beta-adrenergic Blocking Agent, Nonselective

CPhA Monograph

Date of Preparation: May 2009

This monograph has been compiled by CPhA and reviewed by experts. It may contain information different from that found in Health Canada-approved Product Monographs. The reader is referred to the *CPS* Editorial Policy for more information.

SUMMARY PRODUCT INFORMATION:

Route of Administration	Dosage Form	Strength
Oral	Tablet	40 mg, 80 mg, 160 mg

INDICATIONS AND CLINICAL USE: Nadolol is indicated for:
- treatment of hypertension, either alone or in combination with other antihypertensive agents
- prophylaxis of chronic stable angina pectoris

Other Uses: Nadolol can be used to control heart rate in supraventricular tachycardias. It has been used for the prophylaxis of migraine headaches, as an adjunct in the management of hyperthyroidism and for prevention of variceal bleeding caused by portal hypertension.
Geriatrics: Lower doses should be used in the elderly.
Pediatrics: Experience is limited, but nadolol has been used in children.

CONTRAINDICATIONS:
- Patients who are hypersensitive to nadolol or to any ingredient in the formulation
- Patients with sinus bradycardia or heart block
- Patients with cardiogenic shock or decompensated heart failure
- Some patients with a history of bronchospasm as part of asthma or obstructive airway disease

WARNINGS AND PRECAUTIONS:

Serious Warnings and Precautions
Abrupt discontinuation of nadolol therapy in patients with angina pectoris can lead to exacerbation of angina and in some cases, myocardial infarction. If nadolol is to be discontinued, gradually reduce the dose over a period of 2 weeks and observe the patient closely.

General: Nadolol is well tolerated overall, though significant problems can develop as a result of its beta-adrenergic blocking actions.
Cardiovascular: Nadolol administration can result in bradycardia and hypotension in a dose-related manner. Patients may experience postural hypotension and syncope as a consequence. Heart failure and heart block may occur in predisposed individuals. Reduced peripheral blood flow may result in cold extremities.
Endocrine and Metabolism: Beta-adrenergic blocking drugs can interfere with carbohydrate and insulin regulation with reports of both hypo- and hyperglycemia. This group of drugs can mask some of the symptoms of hypoglycemia such as tachycardia and blood pressure changes, but not dizziness and sweating. Nadolol may mask the signs of hyperthyroidism, including thyroid storm.
Immune: It has been reported that patients with a history of anaphylactic reactions have a more severe response to the allergen if they are receiving beta-adrenergic blocking drugs. The response to epinephrine used to treat the allergic reaction may be attenuated.
Neurologic: Nadolol has a low lipid solubility so may be less likely than some other beta-adrenergic blocking drugs to enter the CNS and produce neurologic effects. However, dizziness, fatigue and other effects have been reported.
Peri-Operative Considerations: The need to discontinue nadolol prior to major surgery is controversial. There have been cases of protracted severe hypotension and difficulty in restarting and maintaining the heartbeat in patients receiving beta-adrenergic blocking agents. If necessary, the effects of nadolol can be reversed with beta-agonists such as dobutamine or isoproterenol.
Renal: Nadolol is partially eliminated from the body through the kidney. The dose should be adjusted in the presence of renal function.
Respiratory: Beta-adrenergic blocking drugs may inhibit bronchodilation and increase airway resistance and bronchospasm. Patients with bronchospastic disease should in general not use nadolol. Use with caution in patients with nonallergic bronchospasm (e.g., chronic bronchitis, emphysema).
Special Populations: Pregnant Women: Use of nadolol during pregnancy is not recommended. If a beta-adrenergic blocking drug is required during pregnancy other members of the class may be safer.
Nursing Women: Nadolol is excreted into breast milk in small amounts. Nursing infants of mothers consuming nadolol should be monitored for effects of beta-adrenergic blockade.
Geriatrics: Lower starting doses of nadolol should be used in the elderly since they may be more sensitive to the adverse effects of the drug.

ADVERSE REACTIONS: Overview: The common adverse effects of nadolol are a consequence of its mechanism of action. These include bradycardia, cold sensations, dizziness, fatigue, heart failure and hypotension. Other important effects include changes in airway reactivity and blood glucose control. Severe adverse reactions may be avoided by careful patient selection.
More Common Adverse Drug Reactions (≥1%): Table 1 lists the more common adverse effects of nadolol.

Table 1: Nadolol

More Common Adverse Drug Reactions (≥1%)

Body System	Effect (% incidence)	Clinical Comment
Cardiovascular	Bradycardia (3%), cold sensations (1%), heart failure (1%), hypotension (1%)	May be mitigated by reducing the dose. Cold sensations may improve if a more cardioselective agent is used.
Central Nervous System	Dizziness (3%), fatigue (2%)	May be mitigated by reducing the dose.

Less Common Adverse Drug Reactions (<1%): Cardiovascular: chest pain, edema, orthostatic hypotension; peripheral vascular insufficiency including intermittent claudication and cold extremities, pulmonary edema; rhythm or conduction disturbances including AV block, bigeminy and Adams-Stokes syndrome, syncope.
Central Nervous System: anxiety, depression, hallucinations, headache, irritability, lethargy, nervousness, paresthesia; short-term memory loss, sleep disturbances including insomnia and nightmares, slurred speech, tinnitus, visual disturbances.
Dermatologic: dry skin, facial swelling, pruritus, rash, reversible alopecia, sweating.
Ear/Nose/Throat: dry mouth, nasal stuffiness.
Endocrine and Metabolism: enlarged thyroid, hypoglycemia, type 2 diabetes mellitus, weight gain.
Gastrointestinal: abdominal pain or pressure, anorexia, constipation, diarrhea, flatulence, gastritis, nausea, vomiting.
Hematologic: agranulocytosis, thrombocytopenic or nonthrombocytopenic purpura.
Immune: fever with aching and sore throat.
Ophthalmologic: blurred vision, conjunctivitis, dry eyes.
Respiratory: bronchospasm, cough.
Sexual Function/Reproduction: impotence or decreased libido.
DRUG INTERACTIONS: Drug-Drug Interactions: Drug-drug interactions involving nadolol are listed in Table 2.

Table 2: Nadolol

Drug-Drug Interactions

Interacting Drug	Effect	Clinical Comment
Amiodarone	Increased bradycardic effect of nadolol	Monitor for bradycardia.
Cholinesterase Inhibitors	Increased bradycardic effect of nadolol	Monitor for bradycardia.
Clonidine	Increased blood pressure due to unopposed alpha activity	Closely monitor blood pressure after initiation or discontinuation of either drug. Discontinue nadolol several days before stopping clonidine.
Digoxin	Bradycardia, heart failure	Monitor for bradycardia.
Diltiazem	Bradycardia, heart failure	Monitor for bradycardia.
Epinephrine	Hypertension and bradycardia	Caution when larger doses used as a local anesthetic.
Ergotamine	Increased vasoconstrictive action of ergotamine	Monitor for signs of peripheral ischemia.
Insulin	Nadolol prolongs and masks the signs of hypoglycemia	Avoid combination or use with caution. Monitor for signs of hypoglycemia not masked by beta-blockers (e.g., sweating).
Lidocaine	Increased effects of lidocaine	Monitor lidocaine levels and adjust if necessary.
Methacholine	Increased effects of methacholine	Avoid combination or use with caution.
NSAIDs	Decreased antihypertensive effect of nadolol	Monitor blood pressure and adjust nadolol dose as necessary when either starting or stopping an NSAID.
Prazosin	Increased hypotension with first prazosin dose	Minimize first prazosin dose.
Verapamil	Increased effects of both drugs	Monitor cardiac function and decrease dose if necessary.

Drug-Food Interactions: Nadolol absorption is not altered by the presence of food.
Drug-Laboratory Interactions: Nadolol may produce hypoglycemia and interfere with glucose tolerance testing. Conflicting reports suggest beta-blockers may alter serum lipids; increasing total cholesterol, LDL and VLDL, decreasing HDL.

DOSAGE AND ADMINISTRATION: Recommended Dose and Dosage Adjustment: Adults: See Table 3.

Table 3: Nadolol

Dose in Adult Patients

Indication	Route	Initial Dose	Dose Titration	Usual Dose	Maximum Dose	Clinical Comment
Angina Pectoris	Oral	40–80 mg/day	40–80 mg every 3–7 days	240 mg/day	640 mg/day	Titrate to tolerated heart rate (between 50 and 60 beats per min).
Arrhythmias	Oral			40–160 mg/day		
Hypertension	Oral	40–80 mg/day	40–80 mg every 3–7 days	320 mg/day	640 mg/day	Titrate to target blood pressure.
Migraine Prophylaxis	Oral			40–160 mg/day	240 mg/day	
Prevention of Bleeding Esophageal Varices	Oral	40 mg/day		80 mg/day		Adjust to maximally tolerated dose.
Thyrotoxicosis	Oral			80–160 mg/day		

Geriatrics: See Table 4.
Pediatrics: See Table 5.
Renal Impairment: See Table 6.
Dosage in Dialysis: Moderately dialyzable (20-50%) via hemodialysis. Administer postdialysis or give a 40 mg supplemental dose. Supplemental doses are not necessary following peritoneal dialysis.
Hepatic Impairment: Reduced dose may be necessary.

Missed Dose: Advise patients to take a missed dose as soon as they remember that a dose has been missed, but not to take a double dose if they do not remember until the next dose is due.

Table 4: Nadolol

Dose in Geriatric Patients

Indication	Route	Initial Dose	Dose Titration	Maximum Dose	Clinical Comment
Angina	Oral	20 mg/day	20 mg every 3–7 days	240 mg/day	Titrate to tolerated heart rate (between 50 and 60 beats per minute).
Hypertension	Oral	20 mg/day	20 mg every 3–7 days	240 mg/day	Titrate to target blood pressure.

Table 5: Nadolol

Dose in Pediatric Patients

Indication	Route	Initial Dose	Dose Titration	Maximum Dose
Hypertension	Oral	1 mg/kg/day	1 mg/kg/day every 3–4 days	4 mg/kg/day or 320 mg whichever is less
Supraventricular Tachycardia	Oral	0.5–1 mg/kg/day		2.5 mg/kg/day

Table 6: Nadolol

Dose in Adult Patients with Renal Impairment

Route	Creatinine Clearance	Dosage Adjustment
Oral	>50 mL/min	Dose given every 24 h
	10–50 mL/min	Dose given every 24–48 h
	<10 mL/min	Dose given every 40–60 h

OVERDOSAGE:

For management of a suspected drug overdose, CPhA recommends that you contact your **regional Poison Control Centre**. See the *CPS* Directory section for a list of Poison Control Centres.

ACTION AND CLINICAL PHARMACOLOGY: Mechanism of Action: Nadolol is a nonselective beta-adrenergic blocking agent. It does not possess membrane stabilizing or intrinsic sympathomimetic (partial agonist) activities.

Nadolol competitively blocks the response to adrenergic stimuli of beta receptors in the myocardium, pancreas, and in bronchial and vascular smooth muscle. In the heart this will reduce heart rate, myocardial contractility, and the rate of conduction of impulses through the conducting system. Effects outside the heart include suppression of adrenergic-induced renin release and lipolysis, increased bronchial resistance and inhibition of catecholamine-induced glucose metabolism.

Pharmacokinetics: Adults: Absorption: Peak plasma concentrations usually occur 2 to 4 hours following oral administration. Oral bioavailability varies between 30 and 40%.

Distribution: Nadolol distributes widely in body tissues. In plasma approximately 30% is protein bound. Nadolol crosses the placenta and is found in breast milk.

Metabolism: Nadolol is not metabolized.

Excretion: Approximately 30% of a dose is excreted by the kidney, the remainder through the bowel. The plasma half-life of nadolol is 10 to 24 h, but is prolonged in the presence of renal impairment. Nadolol is removed by hemodialysis.

Nadroparin ℞

CPhA Monograph

see *Heparins: Low Molecular Weight*

Nalbuphine Ⓒ

CPhA Monograph

see *Opioids*

Nalcrom® ℞

sodium cromoglycate

Antiallergic

sanofi-aventis

Date of Revision: April 26, 2006

PHARMACOLOGY: Sodium cromoglycate is considered to exert a stabilizing effect upon mast cells capable of releasing mediators. In gastrointestinal disease, the release of mediators causes a local inflammation which can either result in gastrointestinal symptoms or may allow absorption of antigenic material leading to systemic allergic reactions.

Sodium cromoglycate has no antihistaminic or anti-inflammatory activity.

In humans, oral administration of sodium cromoglycate was followed by a low rate of urinary excretion. The mean urinary excretion of the administered dose over 24 hours was only 0.5%. This indicates that little of the compound is absorbed from the gastrointestinal tract.

INDICATIONS: Gastrointestinal allergy.

CONTRAINDICATIONS: Hypersensitivity to sodium cromoglycate. Possible immunologic changes resulting in reactions such as, polymyositis, pneumonitis and heart failure, urticaria and anaphylaxis have been reported in conjunction with inhalation of sodium cromoglycate and are being actively investigated.

WARNINGS: *Pregnancy:* Safety in pregnancy, and for the treatment of children under 2 years, has not yet been established.
Children: See Pregnancy.
Withdrawal of Sodium Cromoglycate Therapy: Patients should be warned against suddenly discontinuing therapy when symptoms have been partially or completely controlled.

The optimum dose required to maintain remission will need to be determined for each patient, but it is probably not less than 2 capsules 4 times daily.

Particular care should be taken where steroid and/or sulfasalazine dosage has been reduced during sodium cromoglycate treatment.

PRECAUTIONS: *Pregnancy:* The safety of capsules of granulated sodium cromoglycate (100 mg) in pregnancy, and for the treatment of children under 2 years, has not yet been established. The drug should not be used in such patients unless, in the opinion of the prescribing physician, the potential benefits outweigh the possible hazards.
Children: See Pregnancy.

Experience in patients is limited and patients should be carefully observed while undergoing treatment.

The effect of sodium cromoglycate has been studied with those antibody systems concerned with immunity. To date, no effect was observed.

ADVERSE EFFECTS: Nausea, headache, insomnia, skin rashes and joint pains have been reported in a few cases of Nalcrom treatment.

The most frequently reported adverse reactions attributed to sodium cromoglycate on inhalation (on the basis of recurrence following readministration) involve the respiratory tract and include bronchospasm, cough, laryngeal edema (rare), nasal congestion, pharyngeal irritation and wheezing.

Cases of erythema, urticaria or maculopapular rash have been reported and these have cleared within a few days on withdrawal of the drug. Occasional headache, sneezing, cough and unpleasant taste in the mouth have been reported.

OVERDOSE:

Symptoms: There have been no reported cases in humans of overdosage of the drug.

Treatment: As sodium cromoglycate is absorbed only to a very limited extent, no action other than medical observation should be necessary alone or with symptomatic treatment, if any symptoms appear.

For management of a suspected drug overdose, CPhA recommends that you contact your **regional Poison Control Centre**. See the *CPS* Directory section for a list of Poison Control Centres.

DOSAGE: Chronic Inflammatory Bowel Disease: Initial dose: Adults: 2 capsules 4 times daily before meals.
Initial dose: Children from 2 to 14 years: 1 capsule 4 times daily before meals.
Maintenance Dose: To prevent relapses dosage should be maintained indefinitely at 2 capsules 4 times daily in adults and 1 capsule 4 times daily in children.
Food allergy: Initial dose: Adults: 2 capsules 4 times daily before meals.
Initial dose: Children from 2 to 14 years: 1 capsule 4 times daily before meals.

If satisfactory control of symptoms is not achieved within 2 to 3 weeks the dosage may be doubled but should not exceed 40 mg/kg/day.

Maintenance dose: Once a therapeutic response has been achieved the dose may be reduced to the minimum required to maintain the patient free of symptoms. Patients unable to avoid allergenic foods under certain circumstances may be able to protect themselves against the effect of these foods by taking a single dose 15 minutes before the meal. The optimum dosage will need to be determined for each patient. A suitable starting dose would be 200 mg in adults and 100 mg in children.
Information to Be Provided to the Patient: Swallow the capsules whole or dissolve the contents in a small quantity of very hot water, dilute with cold water to drink. Administration as a solution is probably the method of choice in food allergy.
Concomitant Therapy: May be used in conjunction with steroid therapy and sulphasalazine in the management of ulcerative colitis, proctitis and proctocolitis.

SUPPLIED: Each clear, hard gelatin capsule for oral use, imprinted Sodium Cromoglycate 100 mg in black, contains: sodium cromoglycate 100 mg as a white powder. Nonmedicinal ingredients: gelatin and iron oxide. Sodium: <1 mmol (9.0 mg). Tartrazine-free. Bottles of 100.

(Shown in Product Identification Section)

Naloxone Hydrochloride Injection USP ℞

naloxone HCl

Opioid Antagonist

Sandoz

SUPPLIED: 0.4 mg/mL: Each mL of aqueous injectable solution contains: naloxone HCl 0.4 mg. Nonmedicinal ingredients: hydrochloric acid to adjust pH, methylparaben and propylparaben (as preservatives), sodium chloride and water for injection. Ampoules of 1 mL, boxes of 10 (discard unused portion). Multidose vials of 10 mL, boxes of 1 (discard 28 days after initial use). Store between 15 and 30°C. Protect from light.
1 mg/mL: Each mL of aqueous injectable solution contains: naloxone HCl 1 mg. Nonmedicinal ingredients: hydrochloric acid to adjust pH, methylparaben and propylparaben (as preservatives), sodium chloride and water for injection. Multidose vials of 2 mL, boxes of 10. Discard 28 days after initial use. Store between 15 and 30°C. Protect from light.

Naphcon Forte®

naphazoline HCl

Ophthalmic Vasoconstrictor

Alcon

SUPPLIED: A sterile, buffered solution of naphazoline HCl 0.1% preserved with benzalkonium chloride. Nonmedicinal ingredients: boric acid, edetate disodium, hydrochloric acid, potassium chloride, purified water, sodium carbonate and sodium chloride. Drop-Tainer dispensers of 15 mL.

Naprelan® ℞

naproxen sodium

Nonsteroidal Anti-inflammatory Drug (NSAID)

Sepracor

Date of Preparation: June 16, 2000
Date of Revision: August 21, 2009

SUMMARY PRODUCT INFORMATION:

Route of Administration	Dosage Form/ Strength	Clinically Relevant Nonmedicinal Ingredients
Oral	Controlled release tablet/375 mg, 500 mg	Not applicable For a complete listing see Dosage Forms, Composition and Packaging.

INDICATIONS AND CLINICAL USE: NAPRELAN (naproxen sodium) is indicated for the following:

- management of the signs and symptoms of rheumatoid arthritis and osteoarthritis.

Throughout this document, the term NSAIDs refers to both non-selective NSAIDs and selective COX-2 inhibitor NSAIDs, unless otherwise indicated.

For patients with an increased risk of developing CV and/or GI adverse events, other management strategies that do not include the use of NSAIDs should be considered first. (See Contraindications and Warnings and Precautions.)

Use of NAPRELAN should be limited to the lowest effective dose for the shortest possible duration of treatment in order to minimize the potential risk for cardiovascular or gastrointestinal adverse events. (See Contraindications and Warnings and Precautions.)

NAPRELAN, as a NSAID, does **not** treat clinical disease or prevent its progression.

NAPRELAN, as a NSAID, only relieves symptoms and decreases inflammation for as long as the patient continues to take it.

Geriatrics (>65 years of age): Evidence from clinical studies and postmarket experience suggests that use in the geriatric population is associated with differences in safety (see Warnings and Precautions).

Pediatrics (<18 years of age): NAPRELAN is not recommended for use in patients under 18 years of age since safety and effectiveness have not been established.

CONTRAINDICATIONS: NAPRELAN is contraindicated in:

- the peri-operative setting of coronary artery bypass graft surgery (CABG). Although NAPRELAN has **not** been studied in this patient population, a selective COX-2 inhibitor NSAID studied in such a setting has led to an increased incidence of cardiovascular/thromboembolic events, deep surgical infections and sternal wound complications.
- the third trimester of pregnancy, because of risk of premature closure of the ductus arteriosus and prolonged parturition
- women who are breastfeeding, because of the potential for serious adverse reactions in nursing infants
- severe uncontrolled heart failure
- known hypersensitivity to naproxen or to any of the components/excipients
- history of asthma, urticaria, or allergic-type reactions after taking ASA or other NSAIDs (i.e. complete or partial syndrome of ASA-intolerance—rhinosinusitis, urticaria/angioedema, nasal polyps, asthma). Fatal anaphylactoid reactions have occurred in such individuals. Individuals with the above medical problems are at risk of a severe reaction even if they have taken NSAIDs in the past without any adverse reaction. The potential for cross-reactivity between different NSAIDs must be kept in mind (see Warnings and Precautions, Hypersensitivity Reactions, Anaphylactoid Reactions).
- active gastric/duodenal/peptic ulcer, active GI bleeding.
- cerebrovascular bleeding or other bleeding disorders
- inflammatory bowel disease
- severe liver impairment or active liver disease
- severe renal impairment (creatinine clearance <30 mL/min or 0.5 mL/sec) or deteriorating renal disease (individuals with lesser degrees of renal impairment are at risk of deterioration of their renal function when prescribed NSAIDs and must be monitored) (see Warnings and Precautions, Renal)
- known hyperkalemia (see Warnings and Precautions, Renal, Fluid and Electrolyte Balance)
- children and adolescents less than 18 years of age

WARNINGS AND PRECAUTIONS:

Risk of Cardiovascular (CV) Adverse Events: Ischemic Heart Disease, Cerebrovascular Disease, Congestive Heart Failure (NYHA II-IV) (see Warnings and Precautions, Cardiovascular): NAPRELAN is a nonsteroidal anti-inflammatory drug (NSAID). Use of some NSAIDs is associated with an increased incidence of cardiovascular adverse events (such as myocardial infarction, stroke or thrombotic events) which can be fatal. The risk may increase with duration of use. Patients with cardiovascular disease or risk factors for cardiovascular disease may be at greater risk.

Caution should be exercised in prescribing NAPRELAN to any patient with ischemic heart disease (including but not limited to acute myocardial infarction, history of myocardial infarction and/or angina), cerebrovascular disease (including but not limited to stroke, cerebrovascular accident, transient ischemic attacks and/or amaurosis fugax) and/or congestive heart failure (NYHA II-IV).

Use of NSAIDs, such as NAPRELAN, can promote sodium retention in a dose-dependent manner, through a renal mechanism, which can result in increased blood pressure and/or exacerbation of congestive heart failure (see also Warnings and Precautions, Renal, Fluid and Electrolyte Balance).

Randomized clinical trials with NAPRELAN have not been designed to detect differences in cardiovascular events in a chronic setting. Therefore, caution should be exercised when prescribing NAPRELAN.

Risk of Gastrointestinal (GI) Adverse Events (see Warnings and Precautions, Gastrointestinal (GI)): Use of NSAIDs, such as NAPRELAN, is associated with an increased incidence of gastrointestinal adverse events (such as peptic/duodenal ulceration, perforation, obstruction and gastrointestinal bleeding).

General: Frail or debilitated patients may tolerate side effects less well and therefore special care should be taken in treating this population. **To minimize the potential risk for an adverse event, the lowest effective dose should be used for the shortest possible duration.** As with other NSAIDs, caution should be used in the treatment of elderly patients who are more likely to be suffering from impaired renal, hepatic or cardiac function. For high risk patients, alternate therapies that do not involve NSAIDs should be considered.

NAPRELAN is **not** recommended for use with other NSAIDs, with the exception of low-dose ASA for cardiovascular prophylaxis, because of the absence of any evidence demonstrating synergistic benefits and the potential for additive adverse reactions. (See Drug Interactions, Drug-Drug Interactions, Acetylsalicylic Acid (ASA) or Other NSAIDs.)

NAPRELAN should not be used concomitantly with other naproxen products since they all circulate in the plasma as the naproxen anion.

Cardiovascular: NAPRELAN is a nonsteroidal anti-inflammatory drug (NSAID). Use of some NSAIDs is associated with an increased incidence of cardiovascular adverse events (such as myocardial infarction, stroke or thrombotic events) which can be fatal. The risk may increase with duration of use. Patients with cardiovascular disease or risk factors for cardiovascular disease may be at greater risk.

Caution should be exercised in prescribing NAPRELAN to patients with risk factors for cardiovascular disease, cerebrovascular disease or renal disease, such as any of the following (not an exhaustive list): hypertension; dyslipidemia/hyperlipidemia; diabetes mellitus; congestive heart failure (NYHA I); coronary artery disease (atherosclerosis); peripheral arterial disease; smoking; creatinine clearance <60 ml/min or 1 ml/sec.

Use of NSAIDs, such as NAPRELAN, can lead to new hypertension or can worsen pre-existing hypertension, either of which may increase the risk of cardiovascular events as described above. Thus blood pressure should be monitored regularly. Consideration should be given to discontinuing NAPRELAN should hypertension either develop or worsen with its use.

Use of NSAIDs, such as NAPRELAN, can induce fluid retention and edema, and may exacerbate congestive heart failure, through a renally-mediated mechanism. (See Warnings and Precautions, Renal, Fluid and Electrolyte Balance.)

For patients with a high risk of developing an adverse CV event, other management strategies that do **not** include the use of NSAIDs should be considered first. **To minimize the potential risk for an adverse CV event, the lowest effective dose should be used for the shortest possible duration.**

Endocrine and Metabolism: Corticosteroids: NAPRELAN (naproxen sodium) is **not** a substitute for corticosteroids. It does NOT treat corticosteroid insufficiency. Abrupt discontinuation of corticosteroids may lead to exacerbation of corticosteroid-responsive illness. Patients on prolonged corticosteroid therapy should have their therapy tapered slowly if a decision is made to discontinue corticosteroids. (See Drug Interactions, Drug-Drug Interactions, Glucocorticoids.)

Gastrointestinal (GI): Serious GI toxicity (sometimes fatal), such as peptic/duodenal ulceration, inflammation, perforation, obstruction and gastrointestinal bleeding, can occur at any time, with or without warning symptoms, in patients treated with NSAIDs, such as NAPRELAN. Minor upper GI problems, such as dyspepsia, commonly occur at any time. Health care providers should remain alert for ulceration and bleeding in patients treated with NAPRELAN, even in the absence of previous GI tract symptoms. Most spontaneous reports of fatal GI events are in elderly or debilitated patients and therefore special care should be taken in treating this population. **To minimize the potential risk for an adverse GI event, the lowest effective dose should be used for the shortest possible duration.** For high risk patients, alternate therapies that do not involve NSAIDs should be considered. (See Warnings and Precautions, Special Populations, Geriatrics (>65 years of age).)

Patients should be informed about the signs and/or symptoms of serious GI toxicity and instructed to discontinue using NAPRELAN and seek emergency medical attention if they experience any such symptoms. The utility of periodic laboratory monitoring has **not** been demonstrated, nor has it been adequately assessed. Most patients who develop a serious upper GI adverse event on NSAID therapy have no symptoms. Upper GI ulcers, gross bleeding or perforation, caused by NSAIDs, appear to occur in approximately 1% of patients treated for 3-6 months, and in about 2-4% of patients treated for one year. These trends continue, thus increasing the likelihood of developing a serious GI event at some time during the course of therapy. Even short-term therapy has its risks.

GI adverse reactions reported with NAPRELAN were based on the results from two double-blind clinical trials of three months duration with an additional nine-month open-label extension. During these clinical trials upper GI ulcers and gross bleeding occurred with an incidence of less than 1% with naproxen (see Adverse Reactions). The risk continues beyond one year and possibly increases. The incidence of these complications increases with increasing dose.

Caution should be taken if prescribing NAPRELAN to patients with a prior history of peptic/duodenal ulcer disease or gastrointestinal bleeding as these individuals have a greater than 10-fold higher risk for developing a GI bleed when taking a NSAID than patients with neither of these risk factors. Other risk factors for GI ulceration and bleeding include the following: *H. pylori* infection, increased age, prolonged use of NSAID therapy, excess alcohol intake, smoking, poor general health status or concomitant therapy with any of the following: anti-coagulants (e.g. warfarin); anti-platelet agents (e.g. ASA, clopidogrel); oral corticosteroids (e.g. prednisone); Selective Serotonin Reuptake Inhibitors (SSRIs) (e.g. citalopram, fluoxetine, paroxetine, sertraline).

Genitourinary: Some NSAIDs are associated with persistent urinary symptoms (bladder pain, dysuria, urinary frequency), hematuria or cystitis. The onset of these symptoms may occur at any time after the initiation of therapy with an NSAID. Should urinary symptoms occur, in the absence of an alternate explanation, treatment with NAPRELAN should be stopped to ascertain if symptoms disappear. This should be done before urological investigations or treatments are carried out.

Hematologic: NSAIDs inhibiting prostaglandin biosynthesis interfere with platelet function to varying degrees; patients who may be adversely affected by such an action, such as those on anti-coagulants or suffering from haemophilia or platelet disorders should be carefully observed when NAPRELAN is administered.

Anti-Coagulants: Numerous studies have shown that the concomitant use of NSAIDs and anti-coagulants increases the risk of bleeding. Concurrent therapy of NAPRELAN with warfarin requires close monitoring of the international normalized ratio (INR).

Even with therapeutic INR monitoring, increased bleeding may occur.

Anti-Platelet Effects: NSAIDs inhibit platelet aggregation and have been shown to prolong bleeding time in some patients. Unlike acetylsalicylic acid (ASA), their effect on platelet function is quantitatively less, or of shorter duration, and is reversible.

NAPRELAN and other NSAIDs have no proven efficacy as anti-platelet agents and should **not** be used as a substitute for ASA or other anti-platelet agents for prophylaxis of cardiovascular thromboembolic diseases. Anti-platelet therapies (e.g. ASA) should **not** be discontinued. There is some evidence that use of NSAIDs with ASA can markedly attenuate the cardioprotective effects of ASA. (See Drug Interactions, Drug-Drug Interactions, Acetylsalicylic Acid (ASA) or Other NSAIDs.)

Concomitant administration of NAPRELAN with low dose ASA increases the risk of GI ulceration and associated complications.

Blood Dyscrasias: Blood dyscrasias (such as neutropenia, leukopenia, thrombocytopenia, aplastic anemia and agranulocytosis) associated with the use of NSAIDs are rare, but could occur with severe consequences.

Anemia is sometimes seen in patients receiving NSAIDs, including NAPRELAN. This may be due to fluid retention, GI blood loss, or an incompletely described effect upon erythropoiesis. Patients on long-term treatment with NSAIDs, including NAPRELAN, should have their hemoglobin or hematocrit checked if they exhibit any signs or symptoms of anemia or blood loss.

Hepatic/Biliary/Pancreatic: As with other NSAIDs, borderline elevations of one or more liver enzyme tests (AST, ALT, alkaline phosphatase) may occur in up to 15% of patients (less than 1% with naproxen, see Adverse Reactions). These abnormalities may progress, may remain essentially unchanged, or may be transient with continued therapy.

A patient with symptoms and/or signs suggesting liver dysfunction, or in whom an abnormal liver function test has occurred, should be evaluated for evidence of the development of a more severe hepatic reaction while on therapy with this drug. Severe hepatic reactions including jaundice and cases of fatal hepatitis, liver necrosis and hepatic failure, some of them with fatal outcomes, have been reported with NSAIDs.

Although such reactions are rare, if abnormal liver tests persist or worsen, if clinical signs and symptoms consistent with liver disease develop (e.g. jaundice), or if systemic manifestations occur (e.g. eosinophilia, associated with rash, etc.), this drug should be discontinued.

During long-term therapy, liver function tests should be monitored periodically. If there is a need to prescribe this drug in the presence of impaired liver function, it must be done under strict observation.

Hepatic diseases with decreased or abnormal plasma proteins (albumin) reduce the total plasma concentration of naproxen, but the plasma concentration of unbound naproxen is increased. Caution is advised when high doses are required and some adjustment of dosage may be required in these patients. It is prudent to use the lowest effective dose.

Hypersensitivity Reactions: Anaphylactoid Reactions: As with NSAIDs in general, anaphylactoid reactions have occurred in patients without known prior exposure to NAPRELAN. In post-marketing experience, rare cases of anaphylactic/anaphylactoid reactions and angioedema have been reported in patients receiving naproxen. NAPRELAN should **not** be given to patients with the ASA-triad. This symptom complex typically occurs in asthmatic patients who experience rhinitis with or without nasal polyps, or who exhibit severe, potentially fatal bronchospasm after taking ASA or other NSAIDs (see Contraindications).

ASA-Intolerance: NAPRELAN should **not** be given to patients with complete or partial syndrome of ASA-intolerance (rhinosinusitis, urticaria/angioedema, nasal polyps, asthma) in whom asthma, anaphylaxis, urticaria/angioedema, rhinitis or other allergic manifestations are precipitated by ASA or other NSAIDs. Fatal anaphylactoid reactions have occurred in such individuals. As well, individuals with the above medical problems are at risk of a severe reaction even if they have taken NSAIDs in the past without any adverse reaction (see Contraindications).

Cross-Sensitivity: Patients sensitive to one NSAID may be sensitive to any of the other NSAIDs as well.

Serious Skin Reactions: (See Warnings and Precautions, Skin.)

Immune: (See Warnings and Precautions, Infection, Aseptic Meningitis.)

Infection: NAPRELAN, in common with other NSAIDs, may mask signs and symptoms of an underlying infectious disease.

Aseptic Meningitis: Rarely, with some NSAIDs, the symptoms of aseptic meningitis (stiff neck, severe headaches, nausea and vomiting, fever or clouding of consciousness) have been observed. Patients with autoimmune disorders (systemic lupus erythematosus, mixed connective tissue diseases, etc.) seem to be pre-disposed. Therefore, in such patients, the health care provider must be vigilant to the development of this complication.

Neurologic: Some patients may experience drowsiness, dizziness, blurred vision, vertigo, tinnitus, hearing loss, insomnia or depression with the use of NSAIDs, such as NAPRELAN. If patients experience such adverse reaction(s), they should exercise caution in carrying out activities that require alertness.

Ophthalmologic: Blurred and/or diminished vision has been reported with the use of NSAIDs. In rare cases, adverse ocular disorders including papillitis, retrobulbar optic neuritis and papilledema have been reported in users of NSAIDs including naproxen, although a cause and effect relationship cannot be established. If such symptoms develop NAPRELAN should be discontinued and an ophthalmologic examination performed. Ophthalmologic examination should be carried out at periodic intervals in any patient receiving NAPRELAN for an extended period of time.

The use of NAPRELAN may cause photosensitivity. Exposure to sunlight or sunlamps may cause vision changes. Patients should be advised to contact their physician if they experience ophthalmologic reactions from exposure to the sun.

Peri-Operative Considerations: (See Contraindications, Coronary Artery Bypass Graft Surgery.)

Psychiatric: (See Warnings and Precautions, Neurologic.)

Renal: Long term administration of NSAIDs to animals has resulted in renal papillary necrosis and other abnormal renal pathology. In humans, there have been reports of acute interstitial nephritis, hematuria, low grade proteinuria and occasionally nephrotic syndrome.

Renal insufficiency due to NSAID use is seen in patients with pre-renal conditions leading to reduction in renal blood flow or blood volume. Under these circumstances, renal prostaglandins help maintain renal perfusion and glomerular filtration rate (GFR). In these patients, administration of a NSAID may cause a reduction in prostaglandin synthesis leading to impaired renal function. Patients at greatest risk of this reaction are those with pre-existing renal insufficiency (GFR <60 mL/min or 1 mL/s), dehydrated patients, patients on salt restricted diets, those with congestive heart failure, cirrhosis, liver dysfunction, taking angiotensin-converting enzyme inhibitors, angiotensin-II receptor blockers, cyclosporin, diuretics, and those that are elderly. Serious or life-threatening renal failure has been reported in patients with normal or impaired renal function after short term therapy with NSAIDs. Even patients at risk who demonstrate the ability to tolerate an NSAID under stable conditions may decompensate during periods of added stress (e.g. dehydration due to gastroenteritis). Assessment of renal function in these patients before and during therapy with naproxen is recommended. Discontinuation of NSAIDs is usually followed by recovery to the pre-treatment state.

Caution should be used when initiating treatment with NSAIDs, such as NAPRELAN, in patients with considerable dehydration. Such patients should be rehydrated prior to initiation of therapy. Caution is also recommended in patients with pre-existing kidney disease.

NAPRELAN and its metabolites are eliminated primarily by the kidneys, therefore, the drug should be used with great caution in patients with impaired renal function. In these cases, utilization of lower doses of NAPRELAN should be considered and patients carefully monitored.

During long-term therapy, kidney function should be monitored periodically.

Advanced Renal Disease: (See Contraindications.)

Fluid and Electrolyte Balance: Use of NSAIDs, such as NAPRELAN, can promote sodium retention in a dose-dependent manner, which can lead to fluid retention and edema, and consequences of increased blood pressure and exacerbation of congestive heart failure. Thus, caution should be exercised in prescribing NAPRELAN in patients with a history of congestive heart failure, compromised cardiac function, hypertension, increased age or other conditions predisposing to fluid retention (see Warnings and Precautions, Cardiovascular).

Use of NSAIDs, such as NAPRELAN, can increase the risk of hyperkalemia, especially in patients with diabetes mellitus, renal failure, increased age, or those receiving concomitant therapy with adrenergic blockers, angiotensin-converting enzyme inhibitors, angiotensin-II receptor antagonists, cyclosporin, or some diuretics. Electrolytes should be monitored periodically (see Contraindications).

NAPRELAN tablets contain 37.5 mg or 50 mg of sodium (1.5 mEq or 2.0 mEq respectively). This should be considered in patients whose overall intake of sodium must be severely restricted.

Respiratory: ASA-induced asthma is an uncommon but very important indication of ASA and NSAID sensitivity. It occurs more frequently in patients with asthma who have nasal polyps.

Sexual Function/Reproduction: The use of NAPRELAN, as with any drug known to inhibit cyclooxygenase/prostaglandin synthesis, may impair fertility and is not recommended in women attempting to conceive. Therefore, in women who have difficulties conceiving, or who are undergoing investigation of infertility, withdrawal of NAPRELAN should be considered.

Skin: In rare cases, serious skin reactions such as Stevens-Johnson syndrome, toxic epidermal necrolysis, exfoliative dermatitis and erythema multiforme have been associated with the use of some NSAIDs. Because the rate of these reactions is low, they have usually been noted during post-marketing surveillance in patients taking other medications also associated with the potential development of these serious skin reactions. Thus, causality is **not** clear. These reactions are potentially life threatening but may be reversible if the causative agent is discontinued and appropriate treatment instituted. Patients should be advised that if they experience a skin rash they should discontinue their NSAID and contact their physician for assessment and advice, including which additional therapies to discontinue.

The use of NAPRELAN may cause photosensitivity. Exposure to sunlight or sunlamps may cause sunburn, skin blisters, skin rash, redness, itching, or discoloration. Patients should be advised to contact their physician if they experience a reaction from exposure to sun.

Special Populations: Pregnant Women: NAPRELAN is contraindicated for use during the third trimester of pregnancy because of risk of premature closure of the ductus arteriosus and the potential to prolong parturition.

Caution should be exercised in prescribing NAPRELAN during the first and second trimesters of pregnancy.

Inhibition of prostaglandin synthesis may adversely affect pregnancy and/or the embryo-foetal development. Data from epidemiological studies suggest an increased risk of miscarriage and of cardiac malformation after use of a prostaglandin synthesis inhibitor in early pregnancy.

In animals, administration of a prostaglandin synthesis inhibitor has been shown to result in increased pre- and post-implantation loss and embryo-foetal lethality. In addition, increased incidences of various malformations, including cardiovascular, have been reported in animals given a prostaglandin synthesis inhibitor during the organogenetic period.

Nursing Women: The naproxen anion has been found in the milk of lactating women at a concentration of approximately 1% of that found in the plasma. Because of the possible adverse effects of prostaglandin-inhibiting drugs on neonates, use in nursing mothers should be avoided (see Contraindications).

Pediatrics: No pediatric studies have been performed with NAPRELAN, thus safety of NAPRELAN in pediatric populations has not been established (see Contraindications).

Geriatrics (>65 years of age): Patients older than 65 years (referred to in this document as older or elderly) and frail or debilitated patients are more susceptible to a variety of adverse reactions from NSAIDs. The incidence of these adverse reactions increases with dose and duration of treatment. In addition, these patients are less tolerant to ulceration and bleeding. Most reports of fatal GI events are in this population. Older patients are also at risk of lower esophageal injury including ulceration and bleeding. For such patients, consideration should be given to a starting dose lower than the one usually recommended, with individual adjustment when necessary and under close supervision.

Monitoring and Laboratory Tests: Patients on long-term treatment with NAPRELAN should have their blood pressure monitored regularly and an ophthalmologic examination should be carried out at periodic intervals (see Warnings and Precautions, Cardiovascular and Ophthalmologic).

Hemoglobin, hematocrit, red blood cells (RBCs), white blood cells (WBCs), and platelets should be checked in patients on long-term treatment with NAPRELAN. Additionally, concurrent therapy of NAPRELAN with warfarin requires close monitoring of the international normalized ratio (INR) (see Warnings and Precautions, Hematologic).

Serum transaminases and bilirubin should be monitored regularly during NAPRELAN therapy (see Warnings and Precautions, Hepatic/Biliary/Pancreatic).

Serum creatinine, creatine clearance and serum urea should be checked in patients during therapy with NAPRELAN. Electrolytes, including serum potassium should be monitored periodically (see Warnings and Precautions, Renal).

When stopping or starting NAPRELAN therapy; monitoring of plasma lithium concentrations is advised.

ADVERSE REACTIONS: Adverse Drug Reaction Overview: The most common adverse reactions encountered with nonsteroidal anti-inflammatory drugs are gastrointestinal, of which peptic ulcer, with or without bleeding, is the most severe. Fatalities have occurred particularly in the elderly.

As with all drugs in this class, the frequency and severity of adverse events depends on several factors: the dose of the drug and duration of treatment; the age, the sex, physical condition of the patient; any concurrent medical diagnoses or individual risk factors.

Clinical Trial Adverse Drug Reactions: Because clinical trials are conducted under very specific conditions the adverse reaction rates observed in the clinical trials may not reflect the rates observed in practice and should not be compared to the rates in the clinical trials of another drug. Adverse drug reaction information from clinical trials is useful for identifying drug-related adverse events and for approximating rates.

The adverse reactions reported were based on the results from two double blind controlled clinical trials of three months duration with an additional nine month open label extension. Of these 542 patients, 232 received NAPRELAN tablets, 167 were initially treated with Naprosyn and 143 were initially treated with placebo.

The most frequent adverse events form the double blind and open label clinical trials were headache (15%), followed by dyspepsia (14%) and flu syndrome (10%).

Adverse Events (AEs) reported in combined rheumatoid arthritis (RA) and osteoarthritis (OA) clinical studies*: See Table 1, Table 2 and Table 3.

Adverse Events (AEs) (Incidence between 1% and 9%) that have been reported in clinical trials with naproxen, but were not observed in those patients who received NAPRELAN during the controlled clinical trials described above. In view of the similarity of the two products, these events could potentially occur during the administration of NAPRELAN.

Table 1: NAPRELAN

Adverse Events (AEs): Incidence Between 3% and 9% in RA and OA Clinical Studies

Body System	NAPRELAN	Naprosyn	Placebo
Body as a Whole			
Infection	3–9%	1–3%	1–3%
Pain (back)	3–9%	3–9%	3–9%
Pain	3–9%	3–9%	3–9%
Cardiovascular			
Edema	3–9%	1–3%	1–3%
Dermatologic			
Skin Rash	3–9%	3–9%	3–9%
Gastrointestinal			
Abdominal Pain	3–9%	3–9%	3–9%
Constipation	3–9%	1–3%	3–9%
Diarrhea	3–9%	3–9%	3–9%
Nausea	3–9%	3–9%	1–3%
Renal			
Urinary Tract Infection	3–9%	1–3%	3–9%
Respiratory			
Pharyngitis	3–9%	3–9%	3–9%
Rhinitis	3–9%	3–9%	3–9%
Sinusitis	3–9%	3–9%	3–9%

* **Combined AEs regardless of causality and including AEs reported on active control and/or placebo.**

Table 2: NAPRELAN

Adverse Events (AEs): Incidence Between 1% and <3% in RA and OA Clinical Studies*

Body System	NAPRELAN	Naprosyn	Placebo
Body as a Whole			
Asthenia	<1%	1–3%	0.0%
Fever	1–3%	<1%	1–3%
Injury (accident)	1–3%	1–3%	1–3%
Pain Chest	1–3%	1–3%	1–3%
Cardiovascular			
Hypertension	1–3%	1–3%	
Central Nervous System			
Dizziness	1–3%	1–3%	<1%
Insomnia	1–3%	1–3%	1–3%
Paresthesia	1–3%	1–3%	<1%
Gastrointestinal			
Dysphagia	<1%	1–3%	<1%
Flatulence	1–3%	1–3%	1–3%
Gastritis	<1%	1–3%	1–3%
Vomiting	1–3%	1–3%	<1%
Hematologic			
Anemia	1–3%	1–3%	0.0%
Ecchymosis	<1%	1–3%	1–3%
Metabolic and Nutritional			
Hyperglycemia	<1%	<1%	1–3%
Peripheral Edema	1–3%	1–3%	1–3%
Musculoskeletal			
Arthralgia	1–3%	1–3%	<1%
Cramps (leg)	1–3%	1–3%	1–3%
Joint Disorder	<1%	1–3%	1–3%
Myalgia	1–3%	1–3%	<1%
Tendon Disorder	1–3%	1–3%	0.0%
Renal			
Cystitis	<1%	1–3%	<1%
Respiratory			
Bronchitis	1–3%	1–3%	1–3%
Cough Increased	1–3%	1–3%	1–3%

(cont'd)

Table 3: NAPRELAN

Adverse Events (AEs); Incidence Less Than 1% RA and OA Clinical Studies*

Body as a Whole	Abdomen enlarged, abscess, allergic reaction, carcinoma, cellulitis, edema general, LE syndrome, malaise, monilia, mucous membrane disorder, neck rigid, pain neck, pain pelvic
Cardiovascular	Abnormal electrocardiogram (ECG), angina pectoris, aortic stenosis, arrhythmia, bundle branch block, coronary artery disease, deep thrombophlebitis, heart failure right, hemorrhage, migraine, myocardial infarction, syncope, tachycardia, vascular anomaly, vasculitis, vasodilation
Central Nervous System	Amnesia, anxiety, confusion, co-ordination abnormal, depression, emotional lability, hematoma subdural, hypertonia, nervousness, neuralgia, neuritis, paralysis, vertigo
Dermatologic	Acne, alopecia, dermatitis contact, dry skin, eczema, herpes simplex, herpes zoster, nail disorder, neoplasm skin, pruritus, subcutaneous nodule, ulcer skin, urticaria
Gastrointestinal	Anorexia, cholecystitis, cholelithiasis, colitis, eructation, esophagitis, gastroenteritis, GI disorder, GI hemorrhage, hepatosplenomegaly, liver function abnormality, melena, periodontal abscess, rectal disorder, rectal hemorrhage, stomatitis aphthous, stomatitis ulcer, tooth disorder, ulcer esophagus, ulcer mouth, ulcer stomach, ulcerative stomatitis
Hematologic	Abnormal red blood cell (RBC), abnormal white blood cell (WBC), bleeding time increased, eosinophilia, leukopenia, thrombocytopenia
Metabolic and Nutritional	Albuminuria, alkalosis, blood urea nitrogen (BUN) increased, creatine increase, dehydration, edema, glucose tolerance decrease, glucosuria, hypercholesteremia, hyperuricemia, hypokalemia, serum glutamic oxaloacetic transaminase (AST) increase, serum glutamic pyruvic transaminase (ALT) increase, weight decrease
Musculoskeletal	Bone disorder, bone pain, bursitis, fibrotendinitis, myasthenia, ptosis, spasm general, spontaneous bone fracture
Renal	Carcinoma breast, dysmenorrhea, dysuria, hematuria, kidney calculus, kidney failure, kidney function abnormality, menorrhagia, metrorrhagia, neoplasm breast, nephrosclerosis, nocturia, pain kidney, prostate disorder, pyelonephritis, pyuria, urinary frequency, urinary incontinence, urinary retention, urine abnormal, uterine spasm, vaginitis
Respiratory	Asthma, dyspnea, epistaxis, laryngitis, lung disorder, lung edema, pneumonia, respiratory disorder, respiratory distress
Special Senses	Amblyopia, conjunctivitis, deaf, ear disorder, keratoconjunctivitis, lacrimation disorder, otitis media, pain eye, scleritis, cataract
General	Angioneurotic edema, hypoglycemia

Cardiovascular System: congestive heart failure.
Central Nervous System: aseptic meningitis, cognitive dysfunction, diplopia, dream abnormalities, inability to concentrate, muscle weakness.
Dermatologic: angiodermatitis, epidermal necrolysis, epidermolysis bullosa, erythema multiforme, photosensitive dermatitis, photosensitivity reactions resembling porphyria cutanea tarda, skin necrosis, Stevens-Johnson syndrome, sweating.
Gastrointestinal: cardiospasm, hematemesis, jaundice, necrosis, non-peptic GI ulceration, pancreatitis.
Hematologic: agranulocytosis, aplastic anemia, granulocytopenia, hemolytic anemia.
Renal: glomerular nephritis, hyperkalemia, interstitial nephritis, nephrotic syndrome, renal disease, renal failure, renal papillary necrosis.
Respiratory: eosinophilic pneumonitis.
General: anaphylactoid reactions, menstrual disorders, pyrexia (chills and fevers).

Serious Adverse Events (SAEs) (Incidence <1%) that have been reported in clinical trials with naproxen, but were not observed in patients who received NAPRELAN during the controlled clinical trials described above. In view of the similarity of the two products, these events could potentially occur during the administration of NAPRELAN.
Cardiovascular: palpitations, dyspnea.
Central Nervous System: lightheadedness, drowsiness.
Dermatologic: ecchymoses, purpura, skin eruptions.
Gastrointestinal: heartburn, stomatitis.
Special Senses: hearing disturbances, tinnitus, visual disturbances.
General: thirst.

DRUG INTERACTIONS: Drug-Drug Interactions: Acetaminophen: Prolonged concurrent use of acetaminophen with an NSAID may increase the risk of adverse renal effects. Therefore it is recommended that patients be under close medical supervision while receiving such combined therapy.
Acetylsalicylic Acid (ASA) or Other NSAIDs: The use of NAPRELAN in addition to any other NSAID, including over the counter ones (such as ASA and ibuprofen) for analgesic and/or anti-inflammatory effect is **not** recommended because of the absence of any evidence demonstrating synergistic benefits and the potential for additive adverse reactions.

The exception is the use of low dose ASA for cardiovascular protection, when another NSAID is being used for its analgesic/anti-inflammatory effect, keeping in mind that combination NSAID therapy is associated with additive adverse reactions.

Some NSAIDs (e.g. ibuprofen) may interfere with the anti-platelet effects of low dose ASA, possibly by competing with ASA for access to the active site of cyclooxygenase-1.
Albumin-Bound Drugs: In vitro studies have shown that the naproxen anion, because of its affinity for protein, may displace from their binding sites other drugs which are also albumin-bound (see Action and Clinical Pharmacology, Pharmacokinetics).

Theoretically, the naproxen anion itself could likewise be displaced. Short-term controlled studies failed to show that taking the drug significantly affects prothrombin times when administered to individuals on coumarin-type anticoagulants. Caution is advised nonetheless, since interactions have been seen with other nonsteroidal agents of this class. Similarly, patients receiving the drug and a hydantoin, sulfonamide or sulfonylurea should be observed for signs of toxicity to these drugs.

Concomitant administration of naproxen and ASA is not recommended because naproxen is displaced from its binding sites during the concomitant administration of ASA, resulting in lower plasma concentrations and peak plasma levels.
Antacids: The rate of absorption of naproxen can be altered (increased or decreased) by concomitant administration of antacids but is not adversely influenced by the presence of food.
Anti-Coagulants: (See Warnings and Precautions, Hematologic, Anti-Coagulants.)
Anti-Hypertensives: Naproxen and other NSAIDs may diminish the anti-hypertensive effect of propranolol, other beta blockers and Angiotensin Converting Enzyme (ACE) inhibitors as well as other antihypertensive agents.

Combinations of ACE inhibitors, angiotensin-II antagonists, or diuretics with NSAIDs might have an increased risk for acute renal failure and hyperkalemia. Blood pressure and renal function (including electrolytes) should be monitored more closely in this situation, as occasionally there can be a substantial increase in blood pressure.
Anti-Platelet Agents (including ASA): There is an increased risk of bleeding, via inhibition of platelet function, when anti-platelet agents are combined with NSAIDs, such as NAPRELAN (see Warnings and Precautions, Hematologic, Anti-Platelet Effects).
Cholestyramine: Concomitant administration of cholestyramine can delay the absorption of naproxen, but does not affect its extent.
Cyclosporin: Inhibition of renal prostaglandin activity by NSAIDs may increase the plasma concentration of cyclosporin and/or the risk of cyclosporin-induced nephrotoxicity. Patients should be carefully monitored during concurrent use.
Digoxin: Concomitant administration of an NSAID with digoxin can result in an increase in digoxin concentrations which may result in digitalis toxicity. Increased monitoring and dosage adjustments of digitalis glycosides may be necessary during and following concurrent NSAID therapy.
Diuretics: Clinical studies as well as post-marketing observations have shown that NSAIDs can reduce the effect of diuretics.
Glucocorticoids: Some studies have shown that the concomitant use of NSAIDs and oral glucocorticoids increase the risk of GI adverse events such as ulceration and bleeding. This is especially the case in older (>65 years of age) individuals.
Lithium: Concurrent administration of NSAIDs with lithium may increase plasma lithium concentrations. Monitoring of plasma lithium concentrations is therefore advised when starting or stopping a NSAID.
Methotrexate: Caution is advised in the concomitant administration of naproxen and methotrexate since naproxen and other nonsteroidal anti-inflammatory agents have been reported to reduce the tubular secretion of methotrexate in an animal model, thereby possibly enhancing its toxicity.
Oral Contraceptives: Salicylate effectiveness may be impaired in women taking oral contraceptives. Women taking oral contraceptives may require higher or more frequent aspirin doses for desired clinical effects. Where maintenance of a specific plasma concentration is crucial, salicylate levels should be monitored when oral contraceptives are begun or discontinued.
Oral Hypoglycemics: Caution is advised in concomitant administration of salicylates and sulfonylureas. Some studies show salicylates reduce basal plasma glucose levels, increase glucose tolerances and augment acute insulin response.
Potassium Supplements: Concurrent use of potassium supplements with an NSAID may increase the risk of gastrointestinal side effects including ulceration and hemorrhage.
Probenecid: Probenecid given concurrently increases naproxen anion plasma levels and extends its plasma half-life significantly.
Selective Serotonin Reuptake Inhibitors (SSRIs): Concomitant administration of NSAIDs and SSRIs may increase the risk of gastrointestinal ulceration and bleeding (see Warnings and Precautions, Gastrointestinal (GI)).
Tacrolimus: Although this interaction has not been studied with NAPRELAN, co-administration of tacrolimus and any NSAID may increase the nephrotoxic effect of tacrolimus. Renal function should be monitored when NAPRELAN and tacrolimus are used in combination.
Drug-Food Interactions: Interactions with food have not been established.
Drug-Herb Interactions: Interactions with herbal products have not been established.
Drug-Laboratory Test Interactions: Naproxen may decrease platelet aggregation and prolong bleeding time. This effect should be kept in mind when bleeding times are determined. Other laboratory tests in patients on naproxen therapy have shown sporadic abnormalities but no definite trend was seen that would indicate potential toxicity.

The administration of naproxen may result in increased urinary values for 17-ketogenic steroids because of an interaction between the drug and/or its metabolites with m-di-nitrobenzene used in this assay. Although 17-hydroxy-corticosteroid measurements (Porter-Silber test) do not appear to be artifactually altered, it is suggested that therapy with naproxen be temporarily discontinued 72 hours before adrenal function tests are performed if the Porter-Silber test is to be used. Naproxen may interfere with some urinary assays of 5-hydroxy indoleacetic acid (5HIAA).
Drug-Lifestyle Interactions: Alcohol: Concurrent use of alcohol with an NSAID may increase the risk of gastrointestinal side effects including ulceration and hemorrhage.

DOSAGE AND ADMINISTRATION: Dosing Considerations:
- A lower dose should be considered in patients with renal or hepatic impairment or in elderly patients (see Warnings and Precautions).

Studies indicate that although total plasma concentration of naproxen is unchanged, the unbound plasma fraction of naproxen is increased in the elderly. Caution is advised when high doses are required and some adjustment of dosage may be required in elderly patients. As with other drugs used in the elderly, it is prudent to use the lowest effective dose.
Recommended Dose and Dosage Adjustment: The lowest effective dose of NAPRELAN should be used in every patient. NAPRELAN like other NSAIDs show considerable variation in response. The recommended starting dose of NAPRELAN in adults is two NAPRELAN 375 mg tablets (750 mg) once daily, or two NAPRELAN 500 mg tablets (1000 mg) once daily. Patients already taking naproxen 250 mg, 375 mg or 500 mg twice daily (morning and evening) may have their total daily dose replaced with NAPRELAN as a single daily dose.

During long-term administration, the dose of NAPRELAN may be adjusted depending on the clinical response of the patient.

In patients who tolerate lower doses of NAPRELAN well, the dose may be increased to three NAPRELAN 500 mg tablets (1500 mg) once daily for limited periods when a higher level of anti-inflammatory activity is required. When treating patients, especially at the higher dose levels, the physician should observe sufficient increased clinical benefit to offset the potential increased risk. Symptomatic improvement in arthritis usually begins within one week; however, treatment for two weeks may be required to achieve a therapeutic benefit.

Regardless of indication, the dosage should be individualized to achieve effective dose and minimize adverse events, however the maximum daily dose is three NAPRELAN 500 mg (1500 mg) once daily.

To lessen stomach upset, take this medicine after a meal or with food or milk.
Missed Dose: If a dose of this medication is missed, it is not necessary to make up the missed dose. Skip the missed dose and continue with the next scheduled dose. Do not double doses.

To lessen stomach upset, take this medicine immediately after a meal or with food or milk.

OVERDOSAGE:
Significant naproxen overdosage may be characterized by drowsiness, dizziness, disorientation, heartburn, indigestion, epigastric pain, abdominal discomfort, nausea, vomiting, transient alterations in liver function, hypoprothrombinemia, renal dysfunction, metabolic acidosis and apnea. Because naproxen sodium may be rapidly absorbed, high and early blood levels should be anticipated. A few patients have experienced seizures, but it is not clear whether or not these were drug-related. No evidence of toxicity or late sequelae have been reported five to 15 months after ingestion for three to seven days of doses up to 3000 mg of naproxen. One patient ingested a single dose of 25 g of naproxen and experienced mild nausea and indigestion. It is not known what dose of the drug would be life threatening.

Should a patient ingest a large number of tablets, accidentally or purposefully, the stomach may be emptied and usual supportive care following a NSAID overdose should be employed. Emesis and/or activated charcoal may be indicated following overdose. Hemodialysis does not decrease the plasma concentration of naproxen because of the high degree of its protein binding. However, hemodialysis may still be appropriate in the management of renal failure.

For management of a suspected drug overdose, CPhA recommends that you contact your **regional Poison Control Centre**. See the *CPS* Directory section for a list of Poison Control Centres.

ACTION AND CLINICAL PHARMACOLOGY: Mechanism of Action: NAPRELAN contains naproxen sodium, a member of the arylacetic acid group of NSAIDs.

Naproxen has demonstrated anti-inflammatory, analgesic and antipyretic properties. As with other NSAIDs, its mode of action is not fully understood; however, its ability to inhibit prostaglandin synthesis may be involved in the anti-inflammatory effect.
Pharmacokinetics: NAPRELAN uses the proprietary IPDAS (Intestinal Protective Drug Absorption System) technology. It is a rapidly disintegrating tablet system combining an immediate release component and a sustained release component of microparticles that are widely dispersed allowing absorption of the active ingredient throughout the GI tract, maintaining blood levels over 24 hours.

Although naproxen itself is well absorbed, the sodium salt form is more rapidly absorbed resulting in higher peak plasma levels for a given dose. Approximately 30% of the total naproxen sodium dose in NAPRELAN is present in the dosage form as an immediate release component. The remaining naproxen sodium is coated as microparticles to provide sustained release properties. After oral administration, plasma levels of naproxen are detected within 30 minutes of dosing, with peak plasma levels occurring approximately 5 hours after dosing. The observed terminal elimination half-life of naproxen from both immediate release naproxen sodium and NAPRELAN is approximately 15 hours. Steady state levels of naproxen are achieved in 3 days and the degree of naproxen accumulation in the blood is consistent with this. See Table 4.
Absorption: Naproxen itself is rapidly and completely absorbed from the GI tract with an in vivo bioavailability of 95%. Based on the pharmacokinetic profile, the absorption phase of NAPRELAN occurs in the first 4-6 hours after administration. This coincides with disintegration of the tablet in the stomach, the transit of the sustained release microparticles through the small intestine and into the proximal large intestine. An in vivo imaging study has been performed in healthy volunteers which confirms rapid disintegration of the tablet matrix and dispersion of the microparticles.

The absorption rate from the sustained release particulate component of NAPRELAN is slower than that of conventional naproxen sodium tablets. It is this prolongation of drug absorption processes which maintains plasma levels and allows for once daily dosing.

Food Effects: No significant food effects were observed when twenty-four subjects were given a single dose of NAPRELAN 500 mg either after an overnight fast or 30 minutes after a meal. In common with conventional naproxen and naproxen sodium formulations, food causes a slight decrease in the rate of naproxen absorption following NAPRELAN administration.

Table 4: NAPRELAN

Pharmacokinetic Parameters at Steady State Day 5 (Mean of 24 Subjects)

Parameter (units)	Naproxen 500 mg Tablets Q12h (1000 mg)/5 days			NAPRELAN 2×500 mg Tablets (1000 mg) Q24h/5 days		
	Mean	SD	Range	Mean	SD	Range
AUC_{0-24} (μg×h/mL)	1446	168	1167–1858	1448	145	1173–1174
C_{max} (μg/mL)	95	13	71–117	94	13	74–127
C_{avg} (μg/mL)	60	7	49–77	60	6	49–74
C_{min} (μg/mL)	36	9	13–51	33	7	23–48
T_{max} (h)	3	1	1–4	5	2	2–10

Distribution: Naproxen has a volume of distribution of 0.16 L/kg. At therapeutic levels naproxen is greater than 99% albumin-bound. At doses of naproxen greater than 500 mg/day there is a less than proportional increase in plasma levels due to an increase in clearance caused by saturation of plasma protein binding at higher doses. However the concentration of unbound naproxen continues to increase proportionally to dose. NAPRELAN exhibits similar dose proportional characteristics.

Metabolism: Naproxen is extensively metabolized to 6-O-desmethyl naproxen and neither the parent nor the metabolites induce metabolizing enzymes.

Excretion: The elimination half-life of NAPRELAN and conventional naproxen is approximately 15 hours. Steady state conditions are attained after 2-3 doses of NAPRELAN. Most of the drug is excreted in the urine, primarily as unchanged naproxen (less than 1%), 6-O-desmethyl naproxen (less than 1%) and their glucuronide or other conjugates (66-92%). A small amount (<5%) of the drug is excreted in the feces. The rate of excretion has been found to coincide closely with the rate of clearance from the plasma.

Special Populations and Conditions: Renal Insufficiency: In patients with renal failure metabolites may accumulate.

STORAGE AND STABILITY: Store at room temperature 15-30°C, in well-closed containers. Dispense in a well-closed container with a child-resistant closure.

Keep in a safe place out of the reach of children.

INFORMATION FOR THE PATIENT: Published in e-CPS, available by subscription at www.e-cps.ca.

DOSAGE FORMS, COMPOSITION AND PACKAGING: NAPRELAN 375: Each white, capsule-shaped, film-coated, controlled-release tablet, debossed with N on one side, and "375" on the other, contains: naproxen sodium 412.5 mg equivalent to naproxen 375 mg and sodium 37.5 mg. Nonmedicinal ingredients: ammonio methacrylate copolymer Type A, ammonio methacrylate copolymer Type B, citric acid, crospovidone, magnesium stearate, methacrylic acid copolymer Type A, microcrystalline cellulose, povidone and talc; coating: hydroxypropyl methylcellulose, polyethylene glycol and titanium dioxide. Light-resistant bottles of 75.

NAPRELAN 500: Each white, capsule-shaped, film-coated, controlled-release tablet, debossed with N on one side and "500" on the other, contains: naproxen sodium 550 mg equivalent to naproxen 500 mg and sodium 50 mg. Nonmedicinal ingredients: ammonio methacrylate copolymer Type A, ammonio methacrylate copolymer Type B, citric acid, crospovidone, magnesium stearate, methacrylic acid copolymer Type A, microcrystalline cellulose, povidone and talc; coating: hydroxypropyl methylcellulose, polyethylene glycol and titanium dioxide. Light-resistant bottles of 60.

Naprosyn® Pr

naproxen

Nonsteroidal Anti-inflammatory Drug (NSAID)

Roche

Date of Revision: March 11, 2008

SUMMARY PRODUCT INFORMATION:

Route of Administration	Dosage Form/ Strength	Clinically Relevant Nonmedicinal Ingredients
Oral	250, 375, and 500 mg Enteric-Coated Tablet 750 mg Sustained-Release Tablet 25 mg/mL Suspension	None For a complete listing see Dosage Forms, Composition and Packaging.

INDICATIONS AND CLINICAL USE: NAPROSYN (naproxen) is indicated for:

- The treatment of the signs and symptoms of osteoarthritis, rheumatoid arthritis, ankylosing spondylitis, and juvenile rheumatoid arthritis.
- The relief of minor aches and pains in muscles, bones and joints, mild to moderate pain accompanied by inflammation in musculoskeletal injuries (sprains and strains) and primary dysmenorrhea.

Modified release formulations of naproxen (i.e., enteric coated and sustained release) are not recommended for initial treatment of acute pain because the absorption of naproxen is delayed.

For patients with an increased risk of developing cardiovascular and/or gastrointestinal adverse events, other management strategies that do NOT include the use of NSAIDs should be considered first. (See Contraindications and Warnings and Precautions.)

Use of NAPROSYN should be limited to the lowest effective dose for the shortest possible duration of treatment in order to minimize the potential risk for cardiovascular or gastrointestinal adverse events. (See Contraindications and Warnings and Precautions.)

NAPROSYN, as a NSAID, does **not** treat clinical disease or prevent its progression.

NAPROSYN, as a NSAID, only relieves symptoms and decreases inflammation for as long as the patient continues to take it.

Geriatrics (>65 years of age): Evidence from clinical studies and postmarket experience suggests that use in the geriatric population is associated with differences in safety (see Warnings and Precautions).

Pediatrics (<2 years of age): NAPROSYN should not be used in children under 2 years of age. The safety and efficacy in infants younger than 2 years of age has not been established.

NAPROSYN E and NAPROSYN SR have not been studied in subjects under the age of 18.

CONTRAINDICATIONS: NAPROSYN is contraindicated in:

- the peri-operative setting of coronary artery bypass graft surgery (CABG). Although NAPROSYN has NOT been studied in this patient population, a selective COX-2 inhibitor NSAID studied in such a setting has led to an increased incidence of cardiovascular/thromboembolic events, deep surgical infections and sternal wound complications.
- the third trimester of pregnancy, because of risk of premature closure of the ductus arteriosus and prolonged parturition
- women who are breastfeeding, because of the potential for serious adverse reactions in nursing infants
- severe uncontrolled heart failure
- known hypersensitivity to naproxen or to any of the components/excipients
- history of asthma, urticaria, or allergic-type reactions after taking ASA or other NSAIDs (i.e. complete or partial syndrome of ASA-intolerance - rhinosinusitis, urticaria/angioedema, nasal polyps, asthma). Fatal anaphylactoid reactions have occurred in such individuals. Individuals with the above medical problems are at risk of a severe reaction even if they have taken NSAIDs in the past without any adverse reaction. The potential for cross-reactivity between different NSAIDs must be kept in mind (see Warnings and Precautions, Hypersensitivity Reactions, Anaphylactoid Reactions).
- active gastric/duodenal/peptic ulcer, active GI bleeding.
- cerebrovascular bleeding or other bleeding disorders
- inflammatory bowel disease
- severe liver impairment or active liver disease
- severe renal impairment (creatinine clearance <30 mL/min or 0.5 mL/sec) or deteriorating renal disease (individuals with lesser degrees of renal impairment are at risk of deterioration of their renal function when prescribed NSAIDs and must be monitored) (see Warnings and Precautions, Renal)
- known hyperkalemia (see Warnings and Precautions, Renal, Fluid and Electrolyte Balance)
- children less than 2 years of age

WARNINGS AND PRECAUTIONS:

Serious Warnings and Precautions

Risk of Cardiovascular (CV) Adverse Events: Ischemic Heart Disease, Cerebrovascular Disease, Congestive Heart Failure (NYHA II-IV) (see Warnings and Precautions, Cardiovascular and Cerebrovascular).

NAPROSYN is a nonsteroidal anti-inflammatory drug (NSAID). Use of some NSAIDs is associated with an increased incidence of cardiovascular adverse events (such as myocardial infarction, stroke or thrombotic events) which can be fatal. The risk may increase with duration of use. Patients with cardiovascular disease or risk factors for cardiovascular disease may be at greater risk.

Caution should be exercised in prescribing NAPROSYN to any patient with ischemic heart disease (including but NOT limited to acute myocardial infarction, history of myocardial infarction and/or angina), cerebrovascular disease (including but NOT limited to stroke, cerebrovascular accident, transient ischemic attacks and/or amaurosis fugax) and/or congestive heart failure (NYHA II-IV).

Use of NSAIDs, such as NAPROSYN, can promote sodium retention in a dose-dependent manner, through a renal mechanism, which can result in increased blood pressure and/or exacerbation of congestive heart failure. (See also Warnings and Precautions, Renal, Fluid and Electrolyte Balance.)

Randomized clinical trials with NAPROSYN have not been designed to detect differences in cardiovascular events in a chronic setting. Therefore, caution should be exercised when prescribing NAPROSYN.

Risk of Gastrointestinal (GI) Adverse Events (see Warnings and Precautions, Gastrointestinal).

Use of NSAIDs, such as NAPROSYN, is associated with an increased incidence of gastrointestinal adverse events (such as peptic/duodenal ulceration, perforation, obstruction and gastrointestinal bleeding).

General: Frail or debilitated patients may tolerate side effects less well and therefore special care should be taken in treating this population. **To minimize the potential risk for an adverse event, the lowest effective dose should be used for the shortest possible duration.** As with other NSAIDs, caution should be used in the treatment of elderly patients who are more likely to be suffering from impaired renal, hepatic or cardiac function. For high risk patients, alternate therapies that do not involve NSAIDs should be considered.

NAPROSYN is **not** recommended for use with other NSAIDs, with the exception of low-dose ASA for cardiovascular prophylaxis, because of the absence of any evidence demonstrating synergistic benefits and the potential for additive adverse reactions. (See Drug Interactions, Drug-Drug Interactions, Acetylsalicylic acid (ASA) or other NSAIDs.)

NAPROSYN (naproxen) should not be used concomitantly with the related drug Anaprox (naproxen sodium) since they both circulate in plasma as the naproxen anion.

Carcinogenesis and Mutagenesis: There is no evidence from animal data that NAPROSYN is carcinogenic or mutagenic.

Cardiovascular and Cerebrovascular: NAPROSYN is a nonsteroidal anti-inflammatory drug (NSAID). Use of some NSAIDs is associated with an increased incidence of cardiovascular adverse events (such as myocardial infarction, stroke or thrombotic events) which can be fatal. The risk may increase with duration of use. Patients with cardiovascular disease or risk factors for cardiovascular disease may be at greater risk.

Caution should be exercised in prescribing NAPROSYN to patients with risk factors for cardiovascular disease, cerebrovascular disease or renal disease, such as any of the following (NOT an exhaustive list) :

- **Hypertension**
- **Dyslipidemia / Hyperlipidemia**
- **Diabetes Mellitus**
- **Congestive Heart Failure (NYHA I)**
- **Coronary Artery Disease (Atherosclerosis)**
- **Peripheral Arterial Disease**
- **Smoking**
- **Creatinine Clearance <60 mL/min or 1 mL/sec**

Use of NSAIDs, such as NAPROSYN, can lead to new hypertension or can worsen pre-existing hypertension, either of which may increase the risk of cardiovascular events as described above. Thus blood pressure should be monitored regularly. Consideration should be given to discontinuing NAPROSYN should hypertension either develop or worsen with its use.

Use of NSAIDs, such as NAPROSYN, can induce fluid retention and edema, and may exacerbate congestive heart failure, through a renally-mediated mechanism. (See Warnings and Precautions, Renal, Fluid and Electrolyte Balance.)

For patients with a high risk of developing an adverse CV event, other management strategies that do **not** include the use of NSAIDs should be considered first. **To minimize the potential risk for an adverse CV event, the lowest effective dose should be used for the shortest possible duration.**

Endocrine and Metabolism: Corticosteroids: NAPROSYN (naproxen) is **not** a substitute for corticosteroids. It does **not** treat corticosteroid insufficiency. Abrupt discontinuation of corticosteroids may lead to exacerbation of corticosteroid-responsive illness. Patients on prolonged corticosteroid therapy should have their therapy tapered slowly if a decision is made to discontinue corticosteroids. (See Drug Interactions, Drug-Drug Interactions, Glucocorticoids.)

Gastrointestinal: Serious GI toxicity (sometimes fatal), such as peptic/duodenal ulceration, inflammation, perforation, obstruction and gastrointestinal bleeding, can occur at any time, with or without warning symptoms, in patients treated with NSAIDs, such as NAPROSYN. Minor upper GI problems, such as dyspepsia, commonly occur at any time. Health care providers should remain alert for ulceration and bleeding in patients treated with NAPROSYN, even in the absence of previous GI tract symptoms. Most spontaneous reports of fatal GI events are in elderly or debilitated patients and therefore special care should be taken in treating this population. **To minimize the potential risk for an adverse GI event, the lowest effective dose should be used for the shortest possible duration.** For high risk patients, alternate therapies that do not involve NSAIDs should be considered. (See Warnings and Precautions, Special Populations, Geriatrics.)

Patients should be informed about the signs and/or symptoms of serious GI toxicity and instructed to discontinue using NAPROSYN and seek emergency medical attention if they experience any such symptoms. The utility of periodic laboratory monitoring has **not** been demonstrated, nor has it been adequately assessed. Most patients who develop a serious upper GI adverse event on NSAID therapy have no symptoms. Upper GI ulcers, gross bleeding or perforation, caused by NSAIDs, appear to occur in approximately 1% of patients treated for 3-6 months, and in about 2-4% of patients treated for one year. These trends continue, thus increasing the likelihood of developing a serious GI event at some time during the course of therapy. Even short-term therapy has its risks.

Caution should be taken if prescribing NAPROSYN to patients with a prior history of peptic/duodenal ulcer disease or gastrointestinal bleeding as these individuals have a greater than 10-fold higher risk for developing a GI bleed when taking a NSAID than patients with neither of these risk factors. Other risk factors for GI ulceration and bleeding include the following: *H. pylori* infection, increased age, prolonged use of NSAID therapy, excess alcohol intake, smoking, poor general health status or concomitant therapy with any of the following:

- Anti-coagulants (e.g. warfarin)
- Anti-platelet agents (e.g. ASA, clopidogrel)
- Oral corticosteroids (e.g. prednisone)
- Selective Serotonin Reuptake Inhibitors (SSRIs) (e.g. citalopram, fluoxetine, paroxetine, sertraline)

Genitourinary: Some NSAIDs are associated with persistent urinary symptoms (bladder pain, dysuria, urinary frequency), hematuria or cystitis. The onset of these symptoms may occur at any time after the initiation of therapy with a NSAID. Should urinary symptoms occur, in the absence of an alternate explanation, treatment with NAPROSYN should be stopped to ascertain if symptoms disappear. This should be done before urological investigations or treatments are carried out.

Hematologic: NSAIDs inhibiting prostaglandin biosynthesis interfere with platelet function to varying degrees; patients who may be adversely affected by such an action, such as those on anti-coagulants or suffering from haemophilia or platelet disorders should be carefully observed when NAPROSYN is administered.

Anti-coagulants: Numerous studies have shown that the concomitant use of NSAIDs and anticoagulants increases the risk of bleeding. Concurrent therapy of NAPROSYN with warfarin requires close monitoring of the international normalized ratio (INR).

Even with therapeutic INR monitoring, increased bleeding may occur.

Anti-platelet Effects: NSAIDs inhibit platelet aggregation and have been shown to prolong bleeding time in some patients. Unlike acetylsalicylic acid (ASA), their effect on platelet function is quantitatively less, or of shorter duration, and is reversible.

NAPROSYN and other NSAIDs have no proven efficacy as anti-platelet agents and should **not** be used as a substitute for ASA or other anti-platelet agents for prophylaxis of cardiovascular thromboembolic diseases. Anti-platelet therapies (e.g. ASA) should NOT be discontinued. There is some evidence that use of NSAIDs with ASA can markedly attenuate the cardioprotective effects of ASA. (See Drug Interactions, Drug-Drug Interactions, Acetylsalicylic acid (ASA) or other NSAIDs.)

Concomitant administration of NAPROSYN with low dose ASA increases the risk of GI ulceration and associated complications.

Blood Dyscrasias: Blood dyscrasias (such as neutropenia, leukopenia, thrombocytopenia, aplastic anemia and agranulocytosis) associated with the use of NSAIDs are rare, but could occur with severe consequences.

Anemia is sometimes seen in patients receiving NSAIDs, including NAPROSYN. This may be due to fluid retention, GI blood loss, or an incompletely described effect upon erythropoiesis. Patients on long-term treatment with NSAIDs, including NAPROSYN, should have their hemoglobin or hematocrit checked if they exhibit any signs or symptoms of anemia or blood loss.

Hepatic/Biliary/Pancreatic: As with other NSAIDs, borderline elevations of one or more liver enzyme tests (AST, ALT, alkaline phosphatase) may occur in up to 15% of patients. These abnormalities may progress, may remain essentially unchanged, or may be transient with continued therapy.

Chronic alcoholic liver disease and probably also other forms of cirrhosis reduce the total plasma concentration of naproxen, but the plasma concentration of unbound naproxen is increased. The implication of this finding for naproxen dosing is unknown, but caution is advised when high doses are required. It is prudent to use the lowest effective dose.

A patient with symptoms and/or signs suggesting liver dysfunction, or in whom an abnormal liver function test has occurred, should be evaluated for evidence of the development of a more severe hepatic reaction while on therapy with this drug. Severe hepatic reactions including jaundice and cases of fatal hepatitis, liver necrosis and hepatic failure, some of them with fatal outcomes, have been reported with NSAIDs.

Although such reactions are rare, if abnormal liver tests persist or worsen, if clinical signs and symptoms consistent with liver disease develop (e.g. jaundice), or if systemic manifestations occur (e.g. eosinophilia, associated with rash, etc.), this drug should be discontinued.

If there is a need to prescribe this drug in the presence of impaired liver function, it must be done under strict observation.

Hypersensitivity Reactions: Anaphylactoid Reactions: As with NSAIDs in general, anaphylactoid reactions have occurred in patients without known prior exposure to NAPROSYN. In post-marketing experience, rare cases of anaphylactic/ anaphylactoid reactions and angioedema have been reported in patients receiving NAPROSYN. NAPROSYN should **not** be given to patients with the ASA-triad. This symptom complex typically occurs in asthmatic patients who experience rhinitis with or without nasal polyps, or who exhibit severe, potentially fatal bronchospasm after taking ASA or other NSAIDs (see Contraindications).

ASA-Intolerance: NAPROSYN should **not** be given to patients with complete or partial syndrome of ASA-intolerance (rhinosinusitis, urticaria/angioedema, nasal polyps, asthma) in whom asthma, anaphylaxis, urticaria/angioedema, rhinitis or other allergic manifestations are precipitated by ASA or other NSAIDs. Fatal anaphylactoid reactions have occurred in such individuals. As well, individuals with the above medical problems are at risk of a severe reaction even if they have taken NSAIDs in the past without any adverse reaction (see Contraindications).

Cross-sensitivity: Patients sensitive to one NSAID may be sensitive to any of the other NSAIDs as well.

Serious Skin Reactions: See Warnings and Precautions, Skin.

Immune: See Warnings and Precautions, Infection, Aseptic Meningitis.

Infection: NAPROSYN, in common with other NSAIDs, may mask signs and symptoms of an underlying infectious disease.

Aseptic Meningitis: Rarely, with some NSAIDs, the symptoms of aseptic meningitis (stiff neck, severe headaches, nausea and vomiting, fever or clouding of consciousness) have been observed. Patients with autoimmune disorders (systemic lupus erythematosus, mixed connective tissue diseases, etc.) seem to be pre-disposed. Therefore, in such patients, the health care provider must be vigilant to the development of this complication.

Neurologic: Some patients may experience drowsiness, dizziness, blurred vision, vertigo, tinnitus, hearing loss, insomnia or depression with the use of NSAIDs, such as NAPROSYN. If patients experience such adverse reaction(s), they should exercise caution in carrying out activities that require alertness.

Ophthalmologic: Blurred and/or diminished vision has been reported with the use of NSAIDs. If such symptoms develop NAPROSYN should be discontinued and an ophthalmologic examination performed. Ophthalmologic examination should be carried out at periodic intervals in any patient receiving NAPROSYN for an extended period of time.

Peri-Operative Considerations: See Contraindications, Coronary Artery Bypass Graft Surgery.

Psychiatric: See Warnings and Precautions, Neurologic.

Renal: Long-term administration of NSAIDs to animals has resulted in renal papillary necrosis and other abnormal renal pathology. In humans, there have been reports of acute interstitial nephritis, hematuria, low grade proteinuria and occasionally nephrotic syndrome.

Renal insufficiency due to NSAID use is seen in patients with pre-renal conditions leading to reduction in renal blood flow or blood volume. Under these circumstances, renal prostaglandins help maintain renal perfusion and glomerular filtration rate (GFR). In these patients, administration of a NSAID may cause a reduction in prostaglandin synthesis leading to impaired renal function. Patients at greatest risk of this reaction are those with pre-existing renal insufficiency (GFR <60 mL/min or 1 mL/s), dehydrated patients, patients on salt restricted diets, those with congestive heart failure, cirrhosis, liver dysfunction, taking angiotensin-converting enzyme inhibitors, angiotensin-II receptor blockers, cyclosporin, diuretics, and those who are elderly. Serious or life-threatening renal failure has been reported in patients with normal or impaired renal function after short term therapy with NSAIDs. Even patients at risk who demonstrate the ability to tolerate a NSAID under stable conditions may decompensate during periods of added stress (e.g. dehydration due to gastroenteritis). Discontinuation of NSAIDs is usually followed by recovery to the pre-treatment state.

Caution should be used when initiating treatment with NSAIDs, such as NAPROSYN, in patients with considerable dehydration. Such patients should be rehydrated prior to initiation of therapy. Caution is also recommended in patients with pre-existing kidney disease.

Advanced Renal Disease: See Contraindications.

Fluid and Electrolyte Balance: Use of NSAIDs, such as NAPROSYN, can promote sodium retention in a dose-dependent manner, which can lead to fluid retention and edema, and consequences of increased blood pressure and exacerbation of congestive heart failure. Thus, caution should be exercised in prescribing NAPROSYN in patients with a history of congestive heart failure, compromised cardiac function, hypertension, increased age or other conditions predisposing to fluid retention (see Warnings and Precautions, Cardiovascular and Cerebrovascular).

Use of NSAIDs, such as NAPROSYN, can increase the risk of hyperkalemia, especially in patients with diabetes mellitus, renal failure, increased age, or those receiving concomitant therapy with adrenergic blockers, angiotensin-converting enzyme inhibitors, angiotensin-II receptor antagonists, cyclosporin, or some diuretics.

Electrolytes should be monitored periodically (see Contraindications).

Naproxen formulated as a suspension (25 mg/mL) contains sodium chloride (20 mg/mL). This should be considered in patients whose overall intake of sodium must be restricted.

Respiratory: ASA-induced asthma is an uncommon but very important indication of ASA and NSAID sensitivity. It occurs more frequently in patients with asthma who have nasal polyps.

Sexual Function/Reproduction: The use of NAPROSYN, as with any drug known to inhibit cyclooxygenase/prostaglandin synthesis, may impair fertility and is not recommended in women attempting to conceive. Therefore, in women who have difficulties conceiving, or who are undergoing investigation of infertility, withdrawal of NAPROSYN should be considered.

Skin: In rare cases, serious skin reactions such as Stevens-Johnson syndrome, toxic epidermal necrolysis, exfoliative dermatitis and erythema multiforme have been associated with the use of some NSAIDs. Because the rate of these reactions is low, they have usually been noted during post-marketing surveillance in patients taking other medications also associated with the potential development of these serious skin reactions. Thus, causality is **not** clear. These reactions are potentially life threatening but may be reversible if the causative agent is discontinued and appropriate treatment instituted. Patients should be advised that if they experience a skin rash they should discontinue their NSAID and contact their physician for assessment and advice, including which additional therapies to discontinue.

Special Populations: Pregnant Women: NAPROSYN is CONTRAINDICATED for use during the third trimester of pregnancy because of risk of premature closure of the ductus arteriosus and the potential to prolong parturition.

Caution should be exercised in prescribing NAPROSYN during the first and second trimesters of pregnancy.

Inhibition of prostaglandin synthesis may adversely affect pregnancy and/or the embryo-foetal development. Data from epidemiological studies suggest an increased risk of miscarriage and of cardiac malformation after use of a prostaglandin synthesis inhibitor in early pregnancy.

In animals, administration of a prostaglandin synthesis inhibitor has been shown to result in increased pre- and post-implantation loss and embryo-foetal lethality. In addition, increased incidences of various malformations, including cardiovascular, have been reported in animals given a prostaglandin synthesis inhibitor during the organogenetic period.

NAPROSYN is not recommended in labour and delivery because, through their prostaglandin synthesis inhibitory effect, they may adversely affect fetal circulation and inhibit uterine contractions, thus increasing the risk of uterine hemorrhage.

Nursing Women: See Contraindications.

Pediatrics: See Contraindications.

Geriatrics: Patients older than 65 years (referred to in this document as older or elderly) and frail or debilitated patients are more susceptible to a variety of adverse reactions from NSAIDs. The incidence of these adverse reactions increases with dose and duration of treatment. In addition, these patients are less tolerant to ulceration and bleeding. Most reports of fatal GI events are in this population. Older patients are also at risk of lower esophageal injury including ulceration and bleeding. For such patients, consideration should be given to a starting dose lower than the one usually recommended, with individual adjustment when necessary and under close supervision.

Monitoring and Laboratory Tests: Patients on long-term treatment with NAPROSYN should have their blood pressure monitored regularly and an ophthalmic examination should be carried out at periodic intervals (see Warnings and Precautions, Cardiovascular and Cerebrovascular and Ophthalmologic).

Hemoglobin, hematocrit, red blood cells (RBCs), white blood cells (WBCs), and platelets should be checked in patients on long-term treatment with NAPROSYN. Additionally, concurrent therapy with warfarin requires close monitoring of the international normalized ratio (INR). (See Warnings and Precautions, Hematologic.)

Serum transaminase and bilirubin should be monitored regularly during NAPROSYN therapy (see Warnings and Precautions,Hepatic/Biliary/Pancreatic).

Serum creatinine, creatine clearance and serum urea should be checked in patient during NAPROSYN therapy. Electrolytes including serum potassium should be monitored periodically (see Warnings and Precautions, Renal).

Monitoring of plasma lithium concentration is recommended when stopping or starting NAPROSYN therapy.

ADVERSE REACTIONS: Adverse Drug Reaction Overview: The most common adverse reactions encountered with nonsteroidal anti-inflammatory drugs are gastrointestinal, of which peptic ulcer, with or without bleeding, is the most severe. Fatalities have occurred particularly in the elderly.

As with all drugs in this class, the frequency and severity of adverse events depends on several factors: the dose of the drug and duration of treatment; the age, the sex, physical condition of the patient; any concurrent medical diagnoses or individual risk factors.

Clinical Trial Adverse Drug Reactions: Because clinical trials are conducted under very specific conditions the adverse reaction rates observed in the clinical trials may not reflect the rates observed in practice and should not be compared to the rates in the clinical trials of another drug. Adverse drug reaction information from clinical trials is useful for identifying drug-related adverse events and for approximating rates.

A clinical study found gastrointestinal reactions to be more frequent and more severe in rheumatoid arthritis patients taking daily doses of 1500 mg naproxen compared to those taking 750 mg naproxen.

The adverse reactions in controlled clinical trials in 960 patients with rheumatoid arthritis or osteoarthritis treated with the NAPROSYN (naproxen) standard tablets are listed below.

Table 1: NAPROSYN

Most Common Clinical Trial Adverse Drug Reactions (3-9% and 1-3%)

Body System	Incidence	Adverse Reaction
Gastrointestinal	3-9%	Heartburn, constipation, abdominal pain, nausea
	1-3%	Diarrhea, dyspepsia, stomatitis, diverticulitis, gastrointestinal bleeding
Central Nervous System	3-9%	Headache, dizziness, drowsiness
	1-3%	Lightheadedness, vertigo, depression, fatigue. Occasionally patients had to discontinue treatment because of the severity of some of these complaints (headache and dizziness).
Dermatologic	3-9%	Pruritus, ecchymoses, skin eruptions
	1-3%	Sweating, purpura
Cardiovascular	3-9%	Dyspnea, peripheral edema
	1-3%	Palpitations
Special Senses	3-9%	Tinnitus
	1-3%	Hearing disturbances
General	1-3%	Thirst

Less Common Clinical Trial Adverse Drug Reactions (<1%):

Gastrointestinal	Gastrointestinal bleeding, hematemesis, melena, peptic ulceration with or without bleeding and/or perforation, vomiting, ulcerative stomatitis
Central Nervous System	Inability to concentrate, malaise, myalgia, insomnia and cognitive dysfunction (i.e. decreased attention span, loss of short term memory, difficulty with calculations)
Dermatologic	Alopecia, urticaria, skin rash, erythema multiforme, Stevens-Johnson syndrome, epidermal necrolysis, photosensitive dermatitis, exfoliative dermatitis, erythema nodosum
Hepatic	Abnormal liver function tests, jaundice, cholestasis and hepatitis
Cardiovascular	Congestive heart failure and vasculitis
Renal	Glomerular nephritis, hematuria, interstitial nephritis, nephrotic syndrome, nephropathy and tubular necrosis
Hematologic	Eosinophilia, granulocytopenia, leukopenia, thrombocytopenia, agranulocytosis, aplastic anemia and hemolytic anemia
Special Senses	Hearing impairment and visual disturbances
Reproductive, female	Infertility
General	Muscle weakness, anaphylactoid reactions, menstrual disorders, pyrexia (chills and fever), angioneurotic edema, hyperglycemia, hypoglycemia and eosinophilic pneumonitis

Post-Market Adverse Drug Reactions: The following additional adverse events have been reported with NSAIDs including naproxen and naproxen sodium:

Gastrointestinal	Peptic ulcers, perforation, or GI bleeding, sometimes fatal, particularly in the elderly. Heartburn, nausea, oesophagitis, vomiting, diarrhoea, flatulence, constipation, dyspepsia, abdominal pain, nonpeptic gastrointestinal ulceration, melaena, haematemesis, stomatitis, ulcerative stomatitis, exacerbation of ulcerative colitis and Crohn's disease, pancreatitis, gastritis.

Infections	Aseptic meningitis
Blood and Lymphatic System Disorders	Agranulocytosis, aplastic anaemia, eosinophilia, haemolytic anaemia , leucopoenia, thrombocytopenia
Immune System Disorders	Anaphylactoid reactions
Metabolic and Nutrition Disorders	Hyperkalemia
Psychiatric Disorders	Depression, dream abnormalities, insomnia
Nervous System Disorders	Dizziness, drowsiness, headache, lightheadedness, retrobulbar optic neuritis convulsions, cognitive dysfunction, inability to concentrate
Eye Disorders	Visual disturbances, corneal opacity, papillitis, papilloedema
Ear and LabyrinthDisorders	Hearing impairment, hearing disturbances, tinnitus, vertigo
Cardiac Disorders	Palpitations, cardiac failure has been reported in association with NSAID treatment, congestive heart failure
Vascular Disorders	Hypertension, vasculitis. Clinical trial and epidemiological data suggest that use of coxibs and some NSAIDs (particularly at high doses and in long-term treatment) may be associated with a small increased risk of arterial thrombotic events (for example myocardial infarction or stroke).
Respiratory, Thoracic and Mediastinal Disorders	Dyspnoea, pulmonary oedema, asthma, eosinophilic pneumonitis
Hepatobiliary Disorders	Hepatitis (some cases of hepatitis have been fatal), jaundice
Skin and Subcutaneous Tissue Disorders	Ecchymoses, itching (pruritus), purpura, skin eruptions, sweating, alopecia, epidermal necrolysis, very rarely toxic epidermal necrolysis, erythema multiforme, bullous reactions, including Stevens-Johnson syndrome, erythema nodosum, fixed drug eruption, lichen planus, pustular reaction, skin rashes, SLE, urticaria, photosensitivity reactions, including rare cases resembling porphyria cutanea tarda ("pseudoporphyria") or epidermolysis bullosa and angioneurotic oedema. If skin fragility, blistering or other symptoms suggestive of pseudoporphyria occur, treatment should be discontinued and the patient monitored.
Musculoskeletal and Connective Tissue Disorders	Myalgia, muscle weakness
Renal and Urinary Disorders	Haematuria, interstitial nephritis, nephrotic syndrome, renal disease, renal failure, renal papillary necrosis
Reproductive System and Breast Disorders	Female infertility
General Disorders and Administration Site Conditions	Oedema, thirst, pyrexia (chills and fever), malaise
Investigations	Abnormal liver function tests, raised serum creatinine

DRUG INTERACTIONS: Drug-Drug Interactions: Acetylsalicylic acid (ASA) or other NSAIDs: The use of NAPROSYN in addition to any other NSAID, including over-the-counter ones (such as ASA and ibuprofen) for analgesic and/or anti-inflammatory effects is **not** recommended because of the absence of any evidence demonstrating synergistic benefits and the potential for additive adverse reactions.

The exception is the use of low dose ASA for cardiovascular protection, when another NSAID is being used for its analgesic/anti-inflammatory effect, keeping in mind that combination NSAID therapy is associated with additive adverse reactions.

Some NSAIDs (e.g. ibuprofen) may interfere with the anti-platelet effects of low dose ASA, possibly by competing with ASA for access to the active site of cyclooxygenase-1.

Albumin Bound Drugs: The naproxen anion may displace from their binding sites other drugs which are also albumin-bound and may lead to drug interactions. For example, in patients receiving bishydroxycoumarin or warfarin, the addition of NAPROSYN could prolong the prothrombin time. These patients should, therefore, be under careful observation. Similarly, patients receiving NAPROSYN and a hydantoin, sulfonamide or sulfonylurea should be observed for adjustment of dose if required.

Antacids: The rate of absorption of naproxen is altered by concomitant administration of antacids but is not adversely influenced by the presence of food.

Anti-coagulants: See Warnings and Precautions, Hematologic, Anti-coagulants.

Anti-hypertensives: NSAIDs may diminish the anti-hypertensive effect of Angiotensin Converting Enzyme (ACE) inhibitors.

Combinations of ACE inhibitors, angiotensin-II antagonists, or diuretics with NSAIDs might have an increased risk for acute renal failure and hyperkalemia. Blood pressure and renal function (including electrolytes) should be monitored more closely in this situation, as occasionally there can be a substantial increase in blood pressure.

Naproxen and other non steroidal anti inflammatory drugs can reduce the antihypertensive effect of propranolol and other beta blockers as well as other antihypertensive agents.

Anti-platelet Agents (including ASA: There is an increased risk of bleeding, via inhibition of platelet function, when anti-platelet agents are combined with NSAIDs, such as NAPROSYN. (See Warnings and Precautions, Hematologic, Anti-platelet Effects.)

Cyclosporin: Inhibition of renal prostaglandin activity by NSAIDs may increase the plasma concentration of cyclosporin and/or the risk of cyclosporin induced nephrotoxicity. Patients should be carefully monitored during concurrent use.

Cholestyramine: Concomitant administration of cholestyramine can delay the absorption of naproxen, but does not affect its extent.

Digoxin: Concomitant administration of an NSAID with digoxin can result in an increase in digoxin concentrations which may result in digitalis toxicity. Increased monitoring and dosage adjustments of digitalis glycosides may be necessary during and following concurrent NSAID therapy.

Diuretics: Clinical studies as well as post-marketing observations have shown that NSAIDs can reduce the effect of diuretics.

Glucocorticoids: Some studies have shown that the concomitant use of NSAIDs and oral glucocorticoids increases the risk of GI adverse events such as ulceration and bleeding. This is especially the case in older (>65 years of age) individuals.

Lithium: Monitoring of plasma lithium concentrations is advised when stopping or starting a NSAID, as increased lithium concentrations can occur.

Methotrexate: Caution is advised in the concomitant administration of naproxen and methotrexate since naproxen and other non steroidal anti inflammatory agents have been reported to reduce the tubular secretion of methotrexate in an animal model, thereby possibly enhancing its toxicity.

Probenecid: Probenecid given concurrently increases naproxen anion plasma levels and extends its plasma half-life significantly. Caution is advised when probenecid is administered concurrently.

Selective Serotonin Reuptake Inhibitors (SSRIs): Concomitant administration of NSAIDs and SSRIs may increase the risk of gastrointestinal ulceration and bleeding (see Warnings and Precautions, Gastrointestinal).

Drug-Food Interactions: Concomitant administration of food can delay the absorption of naproxen, but does not affect its extent.

Drug-Herb Interactions: Interactions with herbal products have not been established.

Drug-Laboratory Test Interactions: Interactions with laboratory tests have not been established.

Drug-Lifestyle Interactions: There are no specific studies about effects on the ability to drive vehicles and to use machinery. Patients who experience visual disturbances or other central nervous system disturbances should refrain from these activities.

Concurrent use of alcohol with an NSAID may increase the risk of gastrointestinal side effects, including ulceration and hemorrhage.

DOSAGE AND ADMINISTRATION: Recommended Dose and Dosage Adjustment: Adult: Osteoarthritis/Rheumatoid Arthritis/Ankylosing Spondylitis: Oral: The usual total daily dosage for osteoarthritis, rheumatoid arthritis and ankylosing spondylitis is 500 mg a day in divided doses. It may be increased gradually to 750 or 1000 mg or decreased depending on the patient's response.

Recommended Daily Dosing		
NAPROSYN Enteric Coated Tablets	250 mg or 375 mg or 500 mg	twice daily twice daily twice daily
NAPROSYN Suspension	250 mg (10 mL/2 tsp) or 375 mg (15 mL/3 tsp) or 500 mg (20 mL/4 tsp)	twice daily twice daily twice daily
NAPROSYN Sustained Release Tablet	750 mg	once daily

Studies have not shown any clinically significant benefit in using doses higher than 1000 mg/day. In patients who tolerate lower doses of naproxen well and who exhibit only a partial response to 1000 mg/day, the dose may be increased to 1500 mg/day for **limited periods**. Experience with 1500 mg/day naproxen is limited to using the standard tablets. NAPROSYN tablets should be swallowed with food or milk.

When treating such patients with naproxen 1500 mg/day, the physician should observe sufficient increased clinical benefit to offset the potential increased risk (see Adverse Reactions).

In addition, patients on 1500 mg/day need to be followed closely for the development of any adverse events.

During long-term administration the dose of NAPROSYN may be adjusted up or down depending on the clinical response of the patient. A lower dose may suffice for long-term administration.

Patients with rheumatoid arthritis or osteoarthritis maintained on a dose of 750 or 1000 mg/day in divided doses can be switched to a once daily dose of NAPROSYN SR (naproxen sustained release) 750 mg respectively. The single daily dose of NAPROSYN SR should not be exceeded and can be administered in the morning or evening. NAPROSYN SR tablet should be swallowed whole.

NAPROSYN E and NAPROSYN SR have not been studied in subjects under the age of 18.

Analgesia/Musculoskeletal Injuries: Oral: The recommended dose is 750 mg/day divided into either two or three doses/day. This may be increased to 1000 mg/day if needed. The lowest effective dose should be used.

Modified release formulations of naproxen (i.e., enteric coated and sustained release) are not recommended for initial treatment of acute pain because the absorption of naproxen is delayed.

Dysmenorrhea: Oral: The recommended starting dose is two 250 mg tablets, followed by one 250 mg tablet every 6-8 hours, as required. The total daily dose should not exceed 5 tablets (1250 mg). Alternatively, one 500 mg tablet given twice daily may be used.

Modified release formulations of naproxen (i.e., enteric coated and sustained release) are not recommended for initial treatment of acute pain because the absorption of naproxen is delayed.

Juvenile Rheumatoid Arthritis (2-16 years): The use of NAPROSYN suspension is recommended for juvenile arthritis in children 2 years or older because it allows for more flexible dose titration based on the child's weight. The recommended total daily dose is approximately 10 mg/kg in two divided doses at 12 hour intervals. The following table may be used as a guide:

Child's Weight	Dose
13 kg	2.5 mL (½ tsp) b.i.d.
25 kg	5 mL (1 tsp) b.i.d.
38 kg	7.5 mL (1½ tsp) b.i.d.

Administration of NAPROSYN more frequently than twice daily is not necessary. Clinical experience has shown that steroids can often be decreased and sometimes eliminated when NAPROSYN is administered.

Bottles of NAPROSYN suspension should be shaken gently before use.

Missed Dose: The missed dose should be taken as soon as remembered, and then the regular dosing schedule should be continued. Two doses of NAPROSYN should not be taken at the same time.

OVERDOSAGE:

Symptoms and Signs: Significant overdosage may be characterized by drowsiness, dizziness, disorientation, heartburn, indigestion, epigastric pain, abdominal discomfort, nausea, vomiting, transient alterations in liver function, hypoprothrombinemia, renal dysfunction , metabolic acidosis and apnea. A few patients have experienced convulsions, but it is not clear whether or not these were naproxen related.

Gastrointestinal bleeding may occur. Hypertension, acute renal failure, respiratory depression and coma may occur after the ingestion of NSAIDs but are rare.

Anaphylactoid reactions have been repeated with therapeutic ingestion of NSAIDs, and may occur following an overdose.

Treatment: Patients should be managed by symptomatic and supportive care following NSAIDs overdose. There are no specific antidotes. Prevention of further absorption (e.g. activated charcoal) may be indicated in patients seen within 4 hours of ingestion with symptoms or following a large overdose. Forced diuresis, alkalinization of urine, haemodialysis, or haemoperfusion may not be useful due to high protein binding.

For management of a suspected drug overdose, contact your regional Poison Control Centre. See the *CPS* Directory section for a list of Poison Control Centres.

ACTION AND CLINICAL PHARMACOLOGY: Mechanism of Action: NAPROSYN contains naproxen, a member of the arylacetic acid group of NSAIDs.

Naproxen is a nonsteroidal anti-inflammatory drug (NSAID) with analgesic properties. The mechanism of action of naproxen, like that of other NSAIDs, is not completely understood but may be related to prostaglandin synthetase inhibition.

Pharmacokinetics: Naproxen is rapidly and completely absorbed from the gastro-intestinal tract. After oral administration of naproxen, peak plasma levels of naproxen anion are attained in 2 to 4 hours, with steady state conditions normally achieved after 4-5 doses. Plasma naproxen levels and areas under plasma concentration vs. time curves increased linearly with dose increments up to 500 mg twice a day, but larger doses resulted in a plateau effect. The mean biological half-life of the anion in humans is approximately 13 hours, and at therapeutic levels it is greater than 99% albumin bound. Approximately 95% of the dose is excreted in the urine, primarily as naproxen, 6-0-desmethyl naproxen or their conjugates. The rate of excretion has been found to coincide closely with the rate of drug disappearance from the plasma. The drug does not induce metabolizing enzymes.

In children with rheumatic diseases aged between 5 to 16 years, naproxen reached peak plasma levels 2 to 4 hours following oral dosing and the mean plasma half-life was 11.5 to 14.1 hours. NAPROSYN Suspension was found to have similar bioavailability to the naproxen tablets in two single dose studies done in 24 healthy male volunteers. No clinically significant differences in tolerance were reported between the two dosage forms.

When naproxen is administered in the sustained release form (NAPROSYN SR), the peak plasma levels are delayed and the maximum plasma concentrations are reduced compared to those seen with standard release formulations of naproxen. The minimum plasma concentrations, at steady state, are equivalent between NAPROSYN SR given once a day and the corresponding standard dosage given twice a day. The peak to trough plasma concentration ratio of 2.2 and 2.6 observed with the standard tablet formulation (375 mg b.i.d. and 500 mg b.i.d. respectively) is reduced to 1.6 and 1.8 with the 750 and 1000 mg NAPROSYN SR tablets respectively, resulting in smaller fluctuations in plasma concentrations of naproxen with the NAPROSYN SR tablets.

The average T_{max} of naproxen in subjects receiving the 1000 mg SR tablet immediately after a high fat meal did not differ significantly when compared to the fasting state (7.7 hours post prandial; 9.7 hours fasting). The average C_{max} increased significantly from 63.1 µg/mL (fasting) to 86.1 µg/mL (post-prandial). This increase in C_{max} was still lower than that observed with the 1000 mg dose of standard NAPROSYN tablets. Based upon the 95% confidence interval, the AUC's were equivalent when the SR tablet was administered under fasting and non fasting conditions.

A 28 day study of chromium–51-labeled red blood cell loss in feces was conducted with the 750 mg sustained release naproxen tablets in 20 patients. There was no statistically significant difference in red blood cell loss between patients 60 years of age or younger and those over 60.

Enteric-coated naproxen (NAPROSYN E) is designed to be dispersed and dissolved in the small bowel rather than the stomach, so the absorption is delayed until the stomach is emptied. Naproxen enteric-coated tablets were bioequivalent to the standard 375 mg and 500 mg tablets, except for a substantially increased time to peak plasma concentration (T_{max}). The average maximum plasma concentration (C_{max}) following the 375 mg, 2x250 mg and 500 mg enteric-coated tablets were 47.9, 58.2 and 60.7 µg/mL, while the C_{max} following the 375 mg and 500 mg standard immediate release tablets were 46.6 and 63.1 µg/mL, respectively. The T_{max}'s were 4.5, 4.2 and 4.2 hr for the respective enteric-coated formulations as compared to 2.3 and 2.6 hr after standard naproxen tablets. At steady state (multiple dosing) naproxen enteric coated and naproxen STD were equivalent to each other with respect to C_{max}, C_{ave}, C_{max}/C_{ave}, 0-12 hr AUC and half-life. In addition, fluctuation in plasma levels about C_{ave} were considerably less with naproxen EC as compared to naproxen STD (49.3% vs 85.3%). Administration of 500 mg enteric-coated naproxen tablets with food and antacid did not alter the extent of absorption of naproxen as compared to the fasting condition. However, antacid treatment resulted in a higher C_{max} (70.7 vs 58.5 µg/mL) and earlier T_{max} (5.2 hr vs. 8.7 hr) in comparison to the fasting condition. Relative to the fasting state, the average T_{max} was delayed following a high fat meal (5.6-8.7 hr fasting, 9.2-10.8 hr post prandial) while the average C_{max} and AUC were bioequivalent.

STORAGE AND STABILITY: NAPROSYN SR tablets and NAPROSYN E tablets: Store at room temperature (15 to 30°C). NAPROSYN Suspension: Store at room temperature not exceeding 25°C, with protection from light. Store upright.

Keep out of reach of children.

INFORMATION FOR THE PATIENT: Published in e-CPS, available by subscription at www.e-cps.ca.

DOSAGE FORMS, COMPOSITION AND PACKAGING: NAPROSYN Suspension: Each 5 mL contains: naproxen 125 mg. Nonmedicinal ingredients: FD&C Yellow #6, fumaric acid, imitation orange flavor, imitation pineapple flavor, magnesium aluminum silicate, methylparaben, sodium chloride, sorbitol solution and sucrose. Bottles of 474 mL.

NAPROSYN E Tablets: 250 mg: Each white, round, biconvex, enteric-coated tablet, with one side printed in black NPR EC 250, contains: naproxen 250 mg. Nonmedicinal ingredients: croscarmellose sodium, magnesium stearate and povidone; coating suspension: methacrylic acid copolymer, sodium hydroxide, talc and triethyl citrate; black ink: ferric iron. Bottles of 100.

375 mg: Each white, oval-shaped, enteric-coated tablet, with one side printed in black NPR EC 375, contains: naproxen 375 mg. Nonmedicinal ingredients: croscarmellose sodium, magnesium stearate and povidone; coating suspension: methacrylic acid copolymer, sodium hydroxide, talc and triethyl citrate; black ink: ferric iron. Bottles of 100 and 500.

500 mg: Each white, oblong-shaped, enteric-coated tablet, with one side printed in black NPR EC 500, contains: naproxen 500 mg. Nonmedicinal ingredients: croscarmellose sodium, magnesium stearate and povidone; coating suspension: methacrylic acid copolymer, sodium hydroxide, talc and triethyl citrate; black ink: ferric iron. Bottles of 100.

NAPROSYN SR Tablets: Each peach, ellipsoid shaped, sustained-release tablet, NPR SR 750 engraved on one side, contains: naproxen 750 mg. Nonmedicinal ingredients: FD&C Yellow #6, hydroxypropyl methylcellulose and magnesium stearate. Bottles of 100.

Narcotic Analgesics Ⓝ

CPhA Monograph

see *Opioids*

Naropin®

ropivacaine HCl

Local Anesthetic

AstraZeneca

Date of Preparation: February 10, 2000
Date of Revision: March 7, 2008

SUMMARY PRODUCT INFORMATION:

Route of Administration	Dosage Form/ Strength	Clinically Relevant Nonmedicinal Ingredients
Parenteral	Sterile Solution 2, 5 and 10 mg/mL ropivacaine hydrochloride	For a complete listing see Dosage Forms, Composition and Packaging.

INDICATIONS AND CLINICAL USE: Adults (>18 years of age): NAROPIN (ropivacaine hydrochloride) is indicated for:

Analgesia: Acute pain management in connection with:

- Continuous epidural infusion or intermittent bolus administration e.g. postoperative or labour pain;
- Field block e.g. infiltration.

Anaesthesia: Surgical anaesthesia in connection with:

- Epidural block for surgery, including Caesarean section;
- Major nerve block e.g. brachial plexus block;
- Field block e.g. infiltration.

Geriatrics (>65 years of age): Elderly patients should be given reduced doses of ropivacaine, commensurate with their age and physical condition (see Warnings and Precautions, Geriatrics (>65 years of age) and Dosage and Administration, Special Populations).

Pediatrics (<18 years of age): The safety and efficacy of NAROPIN have not been investigated in children under 18 years of age. NAROPIN is not indicated for use in patients below the age of 18 years (see Warnings and Precautions, Special Populations).

CONTRAINDICATIONS: NAROPIN (ropivacaine hydrochloride) is contraindicated:

- in patients with a hypersensitivity to ropivacaine or any other local anaesthetic agent of the amide type.
- for intravenous regional anaesthesia (Bier block).
- in obstetric paracervical block anaesthesia. Use of other local anaesthetics in this technique has resulted in foetal bradycardia and death.

WARNINGS AND PRECAUTIONS: General: In performing NAROPIN blocks, unintended intravascular or subarachnoid injection is possible and may result in cardiac arrhythmia or cardiac arrest. The potential for successful resuscitation has not been studied in humans.

Local anaesthetics should only be employed by clinicians who are well versed in the diagnosis and management of dose-related toxicity and other acute emergencies which might arise from the block to be employed. For management of toxic reactions and related emergencies, cardiopulmonary resuscitative equipment, oxygen, resuscitative drugs, and personnel resources should be immediately available when any local anaesthetic is used. Delay in proper management of dose-related toxicity, underventilation from any cause and/or altered sensitivity may lead to the development of acidosis, cardiac arrest and, possibly, death (see Adverse Reactions and Overdosage).

Prior to receiving major blocks the general condition of the patient should be optimized and the patient should have an i.v. line inserted. All necessary precautions should be taken to avoid intravascular injection.

NAROPIN should be administered in incremental doses. It is not recommended for emergency situations, where a fast onset of surgical anaesthesia is necessary.

It is essential that aspiration for blood and cerebrospinal fluid be done prior to injecting any local anaesthetic, both for the original dose and all subsequent doses, to avoid intravascular or subarachnoid injection. However, a negative aspiration does not ensure against an intravascular or subarachnoid injection.

Solutions of NAROPIN (ropivacaine hydrochloride) should not be used for the production of retrobulbar block or spinal anaesthesia (subarachnoid block) due to insufficient data to support such use.

For Caesarean section, the 5 mg/mL NAROPIN solution in doses up to 150 mg is recommended. The 10 mg/mL solution should not be used for this indication. Historically, pregnant patients were reported to have a high risk for cardiac arrhythmias, cardiac/circulatory arrest and death when 0.75% bupivacaine (another member of the amino amide class of local anaesthetics) was inadvertently rapidly injected intravenously.

Major peripheral nerve blocks may imply the administration of a large volume of local anaesthetic in highly vascularized areas, often close to large vessels where there is increased risk of intravascular injection and/or rapid systemic absorption, which can lead to high plasma concentrations and serious adverse reactions (see Adverse Reactions).

Local anaesthetic procedures should be performed with care in inflamed regions. Injections should not be performed through inflamed tissue nor when there is sepsis at or near the injection site.

NAROPIN should be used with caution in patients receiving other local anaesthetics or agents structurally related to amide-type local anaesthetics, since the toxic effects are additive (see Drug Interactions).

Patients treated with class III antiarrhythmic drugs (e.g., amiodarone) should be under close surveillance and ECG monitoring, since cardiac effects may be additive (see Drug Interactions).

High Risk Populations: Local anaesthetics should be used with caution in patients in poor general condition due to advanced age, debilitation, or other compromising factors such as partial or complete heart conduction block, advanced liver disease, or severe renal dysfunction (see Dosage and Administration). Patients treated with class III anti-arrhythmic drugs (e.g. amiodarone) should be under close surveillance and ECG monitoring.

There have been rare reports of cardiac arrest during the use of NAROPIN for epidural anaesthesia or peripheral nerve blockade, especially after unintentional accidental intravascular administration in elderly patients or in patients with concomitant heart disease. In some instances, resuscitation has been difficult. Should cardiac arrest occur, prolonged resuscitative efforts may be required to improve the likelihood of a successful outcome.

NAROPIN is possibly porphyrinogenic and should only be prescribed to patients with acute porphyria when no safer alternative is available. Appropriate precautions should be taken in the case of vulnerable patients.

Cardiovascular: There have been rare reports of cardiac arrest during the use of NAROPIN for epidural anaesthesia or peripheral nerve blockade, especially after unintentional accidental intravascular administration in patients with concomitant heart disease (see Warnings and Precautions, High Risk Populations).

Local anaesthetics should be used with caution in patients with impaired cardiovascular function who may be less able to compensate for functional changes associated with prolongation of AV conduction produced by these drugs. Hypotension, hypovolemia, or partial or complete heart block represent risk factors.

Peri-Operative Considerations: The safe and effective use of local anaesthetics depends on proper dosage, correct technique, adequate precautions and readiness for emergencies. Resuscitative equipment, oxygen and resuscitative drugs should be available for immediate use (see Adverse Reactions and Overdosage). During major regional nerve blocks, the patients should be in an optimal condition and have i.v. fluids running via an indwelling catheter to assure a functioning intravenous pathway. The clinician responsible should take the necessary precautions to avoid intravascular injection (see Dosage and Administration) and be trained, and familiar with, the diagnosis and treatment of side effects, systemic toxicity, and other complications. The lowest dosage of local anaesthetics that results in effective anaesthesia should be used. Injections should be made slowly and incrementally. When a continuous catheter technique is used, syringe aspirations should be performed before and during each supplemental injection.

If blood is aspirated, relocate the needle. Inadvertent intravascular injection may cause serious consequences. Absorption is more rapid when injections are made into highly vascular tissues. Administration of higher than recommended doses of NAROPIN to achieve greater motor blockade or increased duration of sensory blockade may pose a particular risk in the event that an inadvertent intravascular injection occurs. In epidural administration, the procedure should be discontinued and re-initiated if the subarachnoid space has been entered, as shown by aspiration of spinal fluid.

Careful and constant monitoring of cardiovascular and respiratory vital signs (adequacy of ventilation) and the patient's state of consciousness should be performed during the anaesthetic procedure. It should be kept in mind at such times that restlessness, anxiety, incoherent speech, lightheadedness, numbness and tingling of the mouth and lips, metallic taste, tinnitus, dizziness, blurred vision, tremors, twitching, depression, or drowsiness may be early warning signs of central nervous system toxicity.

Ropivacaine plasma concentrations may approach the threshold for central nervous system toxicity after the administration of 300 mg of ropivacaine for brachial plexus block. Caution should be exercised when using the 300 mg dose.

Epidural Anaesthesia and Analgesia: A well known risk of epidural anaesthesia is unintentional subarachnoid injection of the local anaesthetic. Two clinical studies have been performed to verify the safety of NAROPIN injected into the subarachnoid space at a volume of 3 mL, selected to be representative of an incremental epidural volume that could be unintentionally injected. The 15 and 22.5 mg doses injected resulted in sensory block levels as high as T5 and T4, respectively. Sensory block started in the sacral dermatomes in 2-3 minutes, extended to the T10 level in 10-13 minutes and lasted for approximately 2 hours. The results of these two clinical studies showed that a 3 mL dose did not produce any serious adverse events when spinal anaesthesia was achieved.

Epidural anaesthesia or analgesia may lead to hypotension and bradycardia. This risk can be reduced either by preloading the circulation or by injecting a vasopressor such as ephedrine 20-40 mg i.m. Hypotension should be treated promptly with e.g. ephedrine 5-10 mg intravenously and repeated as necessary.

During epidural administration, it is recommended that a test dose of a local anaesthetic with a fast onset of action be administered initially. The patient should be monitored for central nervous system and cardiovascular toxicity, as well as for signs of unintended intrathecal administration, before proceeding. When clinical conditions permit, test doses of local anaesthetic solutions which contain epinephrine should be considered because circulatory changes compatible with epinephrine may also serve as a warning sign of unintended intravascular injection. If injected into a blood vessel, this amount of epinephrine is likely to produce a transient "epinephrine response" within 45 seconds, consisting of an increase in heart rate and systolic blood pressure, circumoral pallor, palpitations and nervousness in the unsedated patient. The sedated patient may exhibit only a pulse rate increase of 20 or more beats per minute for 15 or more seconds. Therefore, following the test dose, the heart rate should be continuously monitored. Patients on beta-blockers may not manifest changes in heart rate, but blood pressure monitoring can detect a rise in systolic blood pressure. A test dose of a short-acting amide anaesthetic such as lidocaine (30-40 mg) is recommended to detect an unintentional intrathecal administration. This will be manifested within a few minutes by signs of spinal block (e.g., decreased sensation of the buttocks, paresis of the legs, or, in the sedated patient, absent knee jerk). An intravascular or subarachnoid injection is still possible even if results of the test dose are negative. The test dose itself may produce a systemic toxic reaction, high spinal or epinephrine-induced cardiovascular effects.

During epidural administration, ropivacaine should be administered in incremental doses of 3 to 5 mL with sufficient time between doses to detect toxic manifestations of unintentional intravascular or subarachnoid injection. Frequent aspirations for blood or cerebrospinal fluid (where applicable, i.e. when using a "continuous" intermittent catheter technique) should be performed before and during each supplemental injection because plastic tubing in the epidural space can migrate into a blood vessel or through the dura. A negative aspiration, however, does not ensure against an intravascular or intrathecal injection.

Head and Neck Area: Small doses of local anaesthetics injected into the head and neck area, including dental and stellate ganglion blocks, may produce adverse reactions as a result of inadvertent intra-arterial injection and subsequent retrograde flow to the cerebral circulation. These adverse reactions may be similar to systemic toxicity seen with unintentional intravascular injections of larger doses. Confusion, convulsions, respiratory depression, and/or respiratory arrest, and cardiovascular stimulation or depression have been reported. Patients receiving these blocks should have their circulation and respiration monitored and be constantly observed. Resuscitative equipment and personnel for treating adverse reactions should be immediately available. Dosage recommendations should not be exceeded.

Hepatic/Biliary/Pancreatic: Because amide-type local anaesthetics such as ropivacaine are metabolized by the liver, these drugs, especially repeat doses, should be used cautiously in patients with hepatic disease. Patients with severe hepatic disease, because of their inability to metabolize local anaesthetics normally, are at an increased risk of developing toxic plasma concentrations (see Warnings and Precautions, High Risk Populations, and Dosage and Administration, Special Populations).

Neurologic: Psychomotor Effects: Local anaesthetics may have a dose-dependent effect on mental function and coordination, causing temporary impairment of locomotion and alertness, even in the absence of overt CNS toxicity.

Ophthalmologic: Solutions of NAROPIN should not be used for the production of retrobulbar block due to insufficient data to support such use.

Until appropriate experience is gained, the use of NAROPIN for such surgery is not recommended.

Renal: Local anaesthetics should be used with caution in patients in poor general condition due to severe renal dysfunction (see Dosage and Administration).

Normally there is no need to modify the dose of NAROPIN when used for single dose or short term treatment in patients with impaired renal function. Acidosis and reduced plasma protein concentration, frequently seen in patients with chronic renal failure, may increase the risk of systemic toxicity.

Special Populations: Pregnant Women: Reproduction studies have been performed in rats and rabbits.

No effects on fertility and general reproductive performance were seen in rats over two generations. At the highest dose level, increased pup loss was seen during the first three days post partum, which was considered to be secondary to impaired maternal care of the newborn, due to maternal toxicity.

Teratogenicity studies in rats and rabbits did not show evidence of any adverse effects of ropivacaine on organogenesis or early foetal development. There were no treatment-related effects on late foetal development, parturition, lactation, neonatal viability or growth of the offspring in a perinatal and postnatal study in rats using the maximum tolerated dose.

An additional perinatal and postnatal study in rats, in which ropivacaine was compared with bupivacaine, showed that maternal toxicity was observed at much lower dose levels and at lower unbound plasma concentrations of bupivacaine than of ropivacaine.

There are no clinical studies in preterm pregnant women on the effects of ropivacaine on the developing foetus. Ropivacaine should be used during pregnancy only if the potential benefit justifies the potential risk to the foetus. The use of ropivacaine at term for obstetric anaesthesia or analgesia is well documented.

Labour and Delivery: Local anaesthetics, including NAROPIN, rapidly cross the placenta, and when used for an epidural block, can cause varying degrees of maternal, foetal and neonatal toxicity. The incidence and degree of toxicity depend upon the procedure performed, the type and amount of drug used, and the technique of drug administration. Adverse reactions in the parturient, foetus and neonate involve alterations of the central nervous system, peripheral vascular tone and cardiac function.

Maternal hypotension has resulted from epidural analgesia with NAROPIN for obstetrical pain relief. Elevating the patient's legs and positioning her on her left side will help prevent decreases in blood pressure. The foetal heart rate also should be monitored continuously, and electronic foetal monitoring is highly advisable.

It is extremely important to avoid aorto-caval compression by the gravid uterus during administration of regional block to parturients. The patient should be maintained in the left lateral decubitus position if possible, or manual displacement of the uterus off the great vessels be accomplished.

Nursing Women: The excretion of ropivacaine or its metabolites in human milk has not been studied. Based on the milk/plasma concentration ratio in rats, the estimated daily dose to a pup will be about 4% of the dose given to the mother. Caution should be exercised when NAROPIN is administered to a nursing woman. Assuming that the milk/plasma concentration ratio in humans is of the same order, the total ropivacaine dose to which the baby is exposed by breast-feeding is far lower than by exposure in utero in pregnant women at term.

Pediatrics (<18 years of age): The safety and efficacy of NAROPIN have not been investigated in children under 18 years of age. In children early signs of local anaesthetic toxicity may be difficult to detect in cases where the block is given during general anaesthesia (Overdosage). NAROPIN is not indicated for use in patients below the age of 18 years.

Geriatrics (>65 years of age): Elderly patients should be given reduced doses of ropivacaine, commensurate with their age and physical condition (Dosage and Administration, Special Populations). The risk of hypotension and bradycardia in patients receiving epidural anaesthesia with NAROPIN increases in an age-dependent manner (see Table 5 in Adverse Reactions).

ADVERSE REACTIONS: Reactions to NAROPIN (ropivacaine hydrochloride) are characteristic of those associated with other long-acting local anaesthetics of the amide type.

Clinical Trial Adverse Drug Reactions: In clinical trials, the great majority of adverse events reported with ropivacaine were related to the expected effects of the block and to the clinical situation, rather than reactions to the drug. When all clinical studies were pooled (total n=3056), hypotension and nausea were registered in 41.2% (n=1259) and 28.4% (n=867) of the patients, respectively. Similar incidences were reported for bupivacaine in the double-blind comparisons.

Adverse reactions to local anaesthetics are very rare in the absence of overdose or inadvertent intravascular injection. The effects of systemic overdose and unintentional intravascular injections can be serious, but should be distinguished from the physiological effects of the nerve block itself e.g. a decrease in blood pressure, bradycardia, urinary retention after epidural and intrathecal block, and events caused directly by needle puncture (e.g. spinal haematoma, postdural puncture, headache), or indirectly by introduction of micro-organisms (e.g. meningitis and epidural abscess).

Acute systemic toxicity from local anaesthetics is generally dose-related and due to high plasma levels which may result from overdosage (see Overdosage), rapid absorption from the injection site, diminished tolerance, or from inadvertent intravascular injection. Most commonly, the acute adverse experiences originate from the central nervous and cardiovascular systems.

See Table 1, Table 2, Table 3, Table 4, Table 5, Table 6, Table 7 and Table 8.

Table 1: NAROPIN

Adverse Events Reported in ≥1% of Adult Patients Receiving Regional or Local Anaesthesia (Surgery, Labour, Caesarean Section, Peripheral Nerve Block, Local Infiltration and Post-Operative Pain Management)

	Total Number of Patients=2867							
	2 mg/mL Total n=1360		5 mg/mL Total n=740		7.5 mg/mL Total n=540		10 mg/mL Total n=222	
Adverse Reaction	n	%	n	%	n	%	n	%
Hypotension	641	47.1	224	30.1	174	32.2	116	52.3
Nausea	550	40.4	84	11.3	98	18.1	41	18.5
Fever	281	20.7	11	1.5	6	1.1	6	2.7
Vomiting	272	20.0	41	5.5	43	8.0	16	7.2
Postoperative Complications	204	15.0	21	2.8	3	0.6	3	1.4
Anemia	188	13.8	4	0.5	1	0.2	1	0.5
Bradycardia	140	10.3	48	6.4	82	15.2	35	15.8
Pain	140	10.3	42	5.6	15	2.8	2	0.9
Oliguria	139	10.2						
Dizziness	136	10.0	20	2.7	11	2.0	4	1.8
Pruritus	123	9.0	10	1.3	16	3.0	2	0.9
Hypertension	113	8.3	4	0.5	3	0.6		
Unexpected Therapeutic Effect	108	7.9						
Paresthesia	107	7.9	51	6.8	14	2.6	3	1.4
Hypoxia	86	6.3			2	0.4		
Rigors (chills)	84	6.2	11	1.5	10	1.9	12	5.4
Hypokalemia	79	5.8	2	0.3				
Headache	74	5.4	21	2.8	30	5.6	18	8.1

(cont'd)

Table 1: NAROPIN (cont'd)

Adverse Events Reported in ≥1% of Adult Patients Receiving Regional or Local Anaesthesia (Surgery, Labour, Caesarean Section, Peripheral Nerve Block, Local Infiltration and Post-Operative Pain Management)

	Total Number of Patients=2867							
	2 mg/mL Total n=1360		5 mg/mL Total n=740		7.5 mg/mL Total n=540		10 mg/mL Total n=222	
Adverse Reaction	n	%	n	%	n	%	n	%
Back Pain	74	5.4	31	4.2	33	6.1	24	10.8
Hypoproteinemia	74	5.4						
Diarrhea	66	4.9	1	0.1	1	0.2	1	0.5
Bradycardia Fetal	66	4.9	2	0.3				
Hematuria	63	4.6					2	0.9
Urinary Retention	62	4.6	7	0.9	8	1.5	5	2.3
Hypothermia	62	4.6	1	0.1				
Tachycardia	60	4.4	7	0.9			1	0.5
Constipation	59	4.3	1	0.1	1	0.2		
Abdominal Pain	59	4.3	8	1.1				
Urinary Tract Infection	48	3.5	1	0.1				
Creatine Phosphokinase Increased	46	3.4						
Hypoesthesia	45	3.3	7	0.9	6	1.1	5	2.3
Leukocytosis	44	3.2						
Dyspepsia	42	3.1	1	0.1				
Hypocalcemia	41	3.0						
Urine Abnormal	40	2.9						
Chest Pain	39	2.9	4	0.5	3	0.6	1	0.5
Anxiety	36	2.6	7	0.9	1	0.2	1	0.5
Dyspnea	35	2.6	3	0.4	1	0.2	2	0.9
Hypotension Postural	34	2.5						
Abdomen Enlarged	34	2.5	1	0.1				
Edema Peripheral	33	2.4			3	0.6		
Phosphatase Alkaline Increased	29	2.1						
Injection Site Reaction	28	2.1			1	0.2		
Insomnia	27	2.0						
Thrombocytopenia	27	2.0						
Infection	27	2.0			6	1.1	1	0.5
Pleural Effusion	26	1.9						
Thrombocythemia	26	1.9						
Rash	25	1.8	4	0.5	3	0.6		
AST Increased	25	1.8						
Pyuria	25	1.8						
Confusion	24	1.8	2	0.3	1	0.2		
Fecal Incontinence	24	1.8						
Hyperglycemia	23	1.7						
Arthralgia	22	1.6	4	0.5			1	0.5
Atelectasis	22	1.6						
Bronchospasm	21	1.5	1	0.1				
Rales	21	1.5						
Albuminuria	20	1.5						
Progression of Labour Poor/Failed	20	1.5						
BUN Decreased	19	1.4						

(cont'd)

Table 1: NAROPIN *(cont'd)*

Adverse Events Reported in ≥1% of Adult Patients Receiving Regional or Local Anaesthesia (Surgery, Labour, Caesarean Section, Peripheral Nerve Block, Local Infiltration and Post-Operative Pain Management)

	Total Number of Patients=2867							
	2 mg/mL Total n=1360		5 mg/mL Total n=740		7.5 mg/mL Total n=540		10 mg/mL Total n=222	
Adverse Reaction	n	%	n	%	n	%	n	%
Sweating Increased	18	1.3			2	0.4	1	0.5
Urinary Incontinence	18	1.3	4	0.5	4	0.7	1	0.5
Agitation	18	1.3			1	0.2		
Somnolence	18	1.3			3	0.6		
ALT Increased	18	1.3			1	0.2		
Coughing	18	1.3						
Respiratory Disorder	18	1.3						
Respiratory Insufficiency	18	1.3						
Paresis	17	1.3	1	0.1				
Injection Site Inflammation	16	1.2						
Prothrombin Decreased	16	1.2						
Tremor	15	1.1	5	0.7	1	0.2	2	0.9
Purpura	15	1.1	3	0.4			1	0.5
Application Site Reaction	14	1.0						
Myalgia	14	1.0	1	0.1				
Hepatic Function Abnormal	14	1.0						
Arrhythmia	14	1.0			1	0.2	1	0.5
Micturition Disorder	14	1.0			1	0.2	1	0.5
Dysuria	8	0.6	2	0.3	2	0.4	3	1.4
Jaundice Neonatal	3	0.2	9	1.2				

Table 2: NAROPIN

Adverse Events Reported in ≥1% of Women who Received NAROPIN 5 mg/mL During Cesarean Section

	Total Number of Patients=173[a]	
Adverse Reaction	n	(%)
Hypotension	101	58.4
Paresthesia	44	25.4
Pain	29	16.8
Nausea	27	15.6
Vomiting	10	5.8
Dizziness	7	4.0
Anxiety	7	4.0
Abdominal Pain	7	4.0
Pruritus	5	2.9
Bradycardia	5	2.9
Back Pain	5	2.9
Dyskinesia	4	2.3
Headache	4	2.3
Tachycardia	4	2.3
Hypoesthesia	3	1.7
Tremor	2	1.2
Anemia	2	1.2
Rigors (chills)	2	1.2
Postoperative Complications	2	1.2
Postpartum Hemorrhage	2	1.2

[a] Some patients experienced more than 1 adverse event.

Table 3: NAROPIN

Adverse Events Reported in ≥1% of Fetuses or Neonates of Mothers who Received NAROPIN 5 mg/mL During Cesarean Section

	Total Number of Patients=173[a]	
Adverse Reaction	n	(%)
Jaundice Neonatal	9	5.2
Tachypnoea Neonatal	6	3.5
Respiratory Disorder Neonatal	3	1.7
Bradycardia Fetal	2	1.2

[a] Some patients experienced more than 1 adverse event.

Table 4: NAROPIN

Adverse Events Reported in ≥1% of Women who Received NAROPIN 2 mg/mL During Labour

	Total Number of Patients=231[a]	
Adverse Reaction	n	%
Hypotension	35	15.2
Progression of Labour poor/failed	20	8.7
Paraesthesia	15	6.5
Fever	15	6.5
Back Pain	13	5.6
Nausea	9	3.9
Pain	7	3.0
Vomiting	6	2.6
Rigors (chills)	6	2.6
Bradycardia	5	2.2
Urinary Tract Infection	4	1.7
Dystocia	4	1.7
Urinary Retention	3	1.3
Tachycardia	3	1.3
Jaundice	3	1.3

[a] Some patients experienced more than 1 adverse event.

Table 5: NAROPIN

Adverse Events Reported in ≥1% of Fetuses or Neonates of Mothers who Received NAROPIN 2 mg/mL During Labour

	Total Number of Patients=231[a]	
Adverse Reaction	n	%
Bradycardia Fetal	66	28.6
Fetal Distress	10	4.3
Tachycardia Fetal	7	3.0
Fever Neonatal	6	2.6
Vomiting Neonatal	4	1.7
Apgar Score Low	4	1.7
Jaundice Neonatal	3	1.3
Hypoglycemia Neonatal	3	1.3
Neonatal Complication (Not Other Specified)	3	1.3
Tachypnea Neonatal	3	1.3
Respiratory Disorder Neonatal	3	1.3

[a] Some patients experienced more than 1 adverse event.

Central Nervous System: These are characterized by excitation and/or depression. Restlessness, anxiety, dizziness, tinnitus, blurred vision or tremors may occur, possibly proceeding to convulsions. However, excitement may be transient or absent, with depression being the first manifestation of an adverse reaction. This may quickly be followed by drowsiness merging into unconsciousness and respiratory arrest. Other central nervous system effects may be nausea, vomiting, chills, and constriction of the pupils.

The incidence of convulsions associated with the use of local anaesthetics varies with the procedure used and the total dose administered.

For a detailed description of Central Nervous System toxicity, please refer to Overdosage.

Table 6: NAROPIN

Common Events (Epidural Administration)

	5 mg/mL Total n=256		7.5 mg/mL Total n=297		10 mg/mL Total n=207	
Adverse Reaction	**n**	**(%)**	**n**	**(%)**	**n**	**(%)**
Hypotension	99	(38.7)	146	(49.2)	113	(54.6)
Nausea	34	(13.3)	68	(22.9)	—	—
Bradycardia	29	(11.3)	58	(19.5)	40	(19.3)
Back Pain	18	(7.0)	23	(7.7)	34	(16.4)
Vomiting	18	(7.0)	33	(11.1)	23	(11.1)
Headache	12	(4.7)	20	(6.7)	16	(7.7)
Fever	8	(3.1)	5	(1.7)	18	(8.7)

Table 7: NAROPIN

Most Common Adverse Events by Gender (Epidural Administration) Total n: females=405, males=355

	Female		Male	
Adverse Reaction	**n**	**(%)**	**n**	**(%)**
Hypotension	220	(54.3)	138	(38.9)
Nausea	119	(29.4)	23	(6.5)
Bradycardia	65	(16.0)	56	(15.8)
Vomiting	59	(14.6)	8	(2.3)
Back Pain	41	(10.1)	23	(6.5)
Headache	33	(8.1)	17	(4.8)
Chills	18	(4.4)	5	(1.4)
Fever	16	(4.0)	3	(0.8)
Pruritus	16	(4.0)	1	(0.3)

Table 8: NAROPIN

Incidence of Hypotension in Relation to Age (Epidural Administration) Total n: NAROPIN=760

	NAROPIN					
	5 mg/mL		7.5 mg/mL		10 mg/mL	
Age	**n**	**(%)**	**n**	**(%)**	**n**	**(%)**
<65	68	(32.2)	99	(43.2)	87	(51.5)
≥65	31	(68.9)	47	(69.1)	26	(68.4)

Cardiovascular System: High doses or unintentional intravascular injection may lead to high plasma levels and related depression of the myocardium, decreased cardiac output, heart block, hypotension, bradycardia, ventricular arrhythmias, including ventricular tachycardia and ventricular fibrillation, and cardiac arrest. Reactions due to systemic absorption may be either slow or rapid in onset. Cardiovascular collapse and cardiac arrest can occur rapidly (see Warnings and Precautions, General and Overdosage).

Allergic: Allergic type reactions are rare and may occur as a result of sensitivity to local anaesthetics of the amide-type. These reactions are characterized by signs such as urticaria, pruritus, erythema, angioneurotic oedema (including laryngeal oedema), tachycardia, sneezing, nausea, vomiting, dizziness, syncope, excessive sweating, elevated temperature, and in the most severe instances, anaphylactic shock.

Neurologic: The incidence of adverse neurologic reactions may be related to the total dose of local anaesthetic administered but is also dependent upon the particular drug used, the route of administration and the physical status of the patient. Neuropathy and spinal cord dysfunction (e.g. anterior spinal artery syndrome, arachnoiditis, cauda equina syndrome), have been associated with regional anaesthesia. Neurological effects may be related to local anaesthetic techniques, with or without a contribution from the drug.

During epidural block, occasional unintentional penetration of the subarachnoid space by the catheter or needle may occur. Neurologic effects following unintentional subarachnoid administration during epidural anaesthesia may include spinal block of varying magnitude (including total or high spinal block) and hypotension secondary to spinal block. A high spinal block is characterized by limb paralysis, loss of consciousness, respiratory paralysis and bradycardia.

Other neurological effects following unintentional subarachnoid administration during epidural anaesthesia may include persistent anaesthesia, paraesthesia, weakness, paralysis of the extremities and loss of sphincter control, all of which may have slow, incomplete or no recovery. Urinary retention, loss of bladder and bowel control (faecal and urinary incontinence), and loss of perineal sensation and sexual functions are extremely rare but possible neurotoxic complications. Headache, septic meningitis, meningismus, slowing of labour, increased incidence of forceps delivery, or cranial nerve palsies due to traction on nerves from loss of cerebrospinal fluid have been reported.

Elevation of Body Temperature: Epidural infusion of NAROPIN has, in some cases, been associated with transient elevations in body temperature to >38.5°C. This has occurred more frequently at doses greater than 16 mg/hour. The pyrexia seen in connection with postoperative epidural infusion of ropivacaine is similar to that seen with bupivacaine. Body temperature is not affected by systemic concentrations of ropivacaine.

DRUG INTERACTIONS: Drug-Drug Interactions: Local Anaesthetics and Agents Structurally Related to Amide-type Local Anaesthetics: NAROPIN (ropivacaine hydrochloride) should be used with caution in patients receiving other amide-type local anaesthetics such as lidocaine, bupivacaine, mepivacaine and prilocaine since toxic effects are additive.

Antiarrhythmic Drugs: NAROPIN should also be used with caution with structurally related agents such as the antiarrhythmics procainamide, disopyramide, tocainide, mexiletine and flecainide.

Class III Antiarrhythmic Drugs: Specific interactions studies with ropivacaine and class III anti-arrhythmic drugs (e.g. amiodarone) have not been performed. Caution is advised when using Class III antiarrhythmic drugs concomitantly with ropivacaine due to potential pharmacodynamic or pharmacokinetic interactions, or both (see Warnings and Precautions, High Risk Populations). Patients treated with class III antiarrhythmic drugs should be under close surveillance and ECG monitoring, since cardiac effects may be additive.

Sedatives: If sedatives are employed to reduce patient apprehension, they should be used in reduced doses, since local anaesthetic agents, like sedatives, are central nervous system depressants which in combination may have an additive effect.

Strong Inhibitors of P4501A2: In vitro studies indicate that the cytochrome P4501A2 is involved in the formation of 3-hydroxy-ropivacaine, the major metabolite.

Fluvoxamine and Enoxacin: In healthy volunteers, the plasma clearance of ropivacaine was reduced by up to 77% during co-administration of fluvoxamine, a selective and potent P4501A2 inhibitor. Thus strong inhibitors of cytochrome P4501A2, such as fluvoxamine, and enoxacin, given concomitantly during repeated administration of NAROPIN, can interact with NAROPIN. Prolonged administration should be avoided in patients treated with such strong inhibitors of P4501A2.

Theophylline and Imipramine: Possible interactions with drugs known to be metabolized by P4501A2 via competitive inhibition, such as theophylline and imipramine will occur, but should be of less importance.

Drug-Food Interactions: Interactions of ropivacaine with food have not been established.

Drug-Herb Interactions: Interactions of ropivacaine with herbal products have not been established.

Drug-Laboratory Test Interactions: Interactions of ropivacaine with laboratory tests have not been established.

Drug-Lifestyle Interactions: Interactions of ropivacaine with lifestyle have not been established.

DOSAGE AND ADMINISTRATION: Dosing Considerations: General: NAROPIN (ropivacaine hydrochloride) should only be used by or under the supervision of clinicians experienced in regional anaesthesia.

It is recommended that hospitals using local anaesthetic infusions have a treatment protocol in place for nursing to follow in order to safely monitor the level of the block and for the proper management of complications and/or toxic reactions. If toxic reactions occur, the infusion should be stopped immediately.

NAROPIN should be administered at the smallest dose and the lowest concentration which are consistent with the necessary degree of anaesthesia or analgesia. The rapid injection of a large volume of local anaesthetic solution should be avoided and fractional doses should always be used. In general, surgical anaesthesia, e.g. epidural administration, requires the use of higher concentrations and doses. For analgesia, e.g. epidural administration for acute pain management, lower concentrations and doses are recommended.

The dose of any local anaesthetic administered varies with the anaesthetic procedure, the area to be anaesthetized, the vascularity of the tissues, the number of neuronal segments to be blocked, the depth of anaesthesia and degree of muscle relaxation required, the duration of anaesthesia desired, individual tolerance, and the physical condition of the patient. Patients in poor general condition due to advanced age or other compromising factors such as partial or complete heart conduction block, advanced liver disease or severe renal dysfunction require special attention although regional anaesthesia is frequently indicated in these patients. To reduce the risk of potentially serious adverse reactions, attempts should be made to optimize the patient's condition before major blocks are performed, and the dosage should be adjusted accordingly.

Parenteral drug products should be inspected visually for particulate matter and discolouration prior to administration, whenever solution and container permit. Solutions which are discoloured or which contain particulate matter should not be administered. For specific techniques and procedures, refer to standard contemporary textbooks.

Special Populations: Local anaesthetics should be used with caution in patients in poor general condition due to advanced age, debilitation, or other compromising factors such as partial or complete heart conduction block, advanced liver disease, or severe renal dysfunction.

Elderly and acutely ill patients should be given reduced doses of ropivacaine, commensurate with their age and physical condition.

Recommended Dose and Dosage Adjustment: Adults: The dosages in Table 9 are recommended as a guide for use in the average adult for the more commonly used blocks. The clinician's experience and knowledge of the patient's physical status are of importance in calculating the required dose.

Table 9: NAROPIN

Adult Dosage Recommendations for NAROPIN

Type of Block	Conc. (mg/mL)	Volume (mL)	Dose (mg)
Acute Pain Management			
Lumbar Epidural			
Bolus (initial dose)	2	10–20	20–40
Intermittent injections (top-up) e.g., labour pain management	2	10–15 (minimum interval 30 minutes)	20–30
Continuous infusion e.g., labour pain and postoperative pain management	2	6–14 mL/h	12–28 mg/h
Thoracic Epidural			
Continuous infusion e.g., postoperative pain management	2	6–14 mL/h	12–28 mg/h
Field Block			
e.g., infiltration	2 5	1–100 1–40	2–200 5–200
Surgical Anaesthesia			
Lumbar Epidural			
Surgery	5 10	15–30 15–20	75–150 150–200
Cesarean Section	5	20–30	100–150
Thoracic Epidural			
To establish block for postoperative pain management	5	5–15	25–75
Major Nerve Block			
e.g., brachial plexus block	5	35–50	175–250[a]
Field Block			

(cont'd)

Table 9: NAROPIN *(cont'd)*

Adult Dosage Recommendations for NAROPIN

Type of Block	Conc. (mg/mL)	Volume (mL)	Dose (mg)
e.g., infiltration	5	1–40	5–200

[a] The dose for a major nerve block must be adjusted according to site of administration and patient status. Interscalene and supraclavicular brachial plexus blocks may be associated with a higher frequency of serious adverse reactions, regardless of anaesthetic used.

The doses in the table are those considered to be necessary to produce a successful block and should be regarded as guidelines for use in adults. The figures reflect the expected average dose range needed. For other local anaesthetic techniques standard textbooks should be consulted.

Careful aspiration before and during injection is recommended to prevent intravascular injection. When employing an epidural block, a test dose of 3-5 mL lidocaine (Xylocaine 1-2%) with epinephrine is recommended. An inadvertent intravascular injection may be recognized by a temporary increase in heart rate and an accidental subarachnoid injection by signs of a spinal block. Aspiration should be repeated prior to and during administration of the main dose, which should be injected slowly or in incremental doses, at a rate of 25-50 mg/min, while closely observing the patient's vital functions and maintaining verbal contact. If toxic symptoms occur, the injection should be stopped immediately. The test dose should be repeated if the patient is moved in such a fashion as to have displaced the epidural catheter.

In epidural block for surgery (excluding Caesarean section), single doses of up to 250 mg ropivacaine have been used and are well tolerated.

In epidural block for Caesarean section, an initial epidural dose of up to 150 mg (25 mL NAROPIN 5 mg/mL) injected over 5 minutes is well tolerated (see Warnings and Precautions, Peri-Operative Considerations).

For treatment of postoperative pain, the following technique is recommended: Unless preoperatively instituted, an initial epidural block with NAROPIN 5 mg/mL is induced via an epidural catheter. Analgesia is maintained with NAROPIN 2 mg/mL infusion. Clinical studies have demonstrated that infusion rates of 6-14 mL (12-28 mg) per hour provide adequate analgesia with only slight and non-progressive motor block in most cases of moderate to severe postoperative pain. With this technique, a significant reduction in the need for narcotics has been observed. Clinical experience supports the use of NAROPIN epidural infusions at rates up to 28 mg/h for 72 hours.

When prolonged blocks are used, either through continuous infusion or through repeated bolus administration, the risks of reaching a toxic plasma concentration or inducing local neural injury must be considered. Clinical experience to date indicates that a cumulative dose of up to 770 mg ropivacaine administered over 24 hours and continuous epidural infusion at rates up to 28 mg/h for 72 hours have been well tolerated in adults when used for postoperative pain management (i.e., ≥2000 mg).

The duration and intensity of ropivacaine block are not improved by the addition of epinephrine.

Children: The safety and efficacy of NAROPIN have not been investigated in children under 18 years of age. NAROPIN is not indicated for use in patients below the age of 18 years.

OVERDOSAGE:

Systemic toxic reactions primarily involve the central nervous system and cardiovascular system. Such reactions are caused by high plasma levels encountered during therapeutic use, overdose, or to unintended intravascular or subarachnoid injection (see Adverse Reactions and Warnings and Precautions). CNS reactions are similar for all amide local anaesthetics, while cardiac reactions are more dependent on the drug, both quantitatively and qualitatively.

Symptoms: Accidental intravascular injections may cause immediate (within seconds to a few minutes) toxic effects. In the event of overdose, peak plasma concentrations may not be reached for 1 to 2 hours, depending on the site of injection, with signs of toxicity thus being delayed.

Central nervous system toxicity is a graded response with symptoms and signs of escalating severity. First symptoms are usually light-headedness, circumoral paraesthesia, numbness of the tongue, hyperacusis, tinnitus and visual disturbances. Dysarthria, muscular rigidity and muscular twitching are more serious and may precede the onset of generalized convulsions. These signs must not be mistaken for a neurotic behaviour. Unconsciousness and grand mal convulsions may follow which may last from a few seconds to several minutes. Hypoxia and hypercarbia occur rapidly following convulsions due to the increased muscular activity, together with the interference with normal respiration and loss of the airway. In severe cases apnoea may occur. Acidosis, hyperkalaemia, hypocalcaemia and hypoxia increase and extend the toxic effects of local anaesthetics.

Recovery is due to redistribution and metabolism of the local anaesthetic drug. Recovery may be rapid unless large amounts of the drug have been administered.

Cardiovascular system toxicity indicates a more severe situation and is generally preceded by signs of toxicity in the central nervous system, unless the patient is receiving a general anaesthetic or is heavily sedated with drugs such as a benzodiazepine or barbiturate. Hypotension, bradycardia, arrhythmia and cardiac arrest may occur as a result of high systemic concentrations of local anaesthetic. In volunteers, the intravenous infusion of ropivacaine resulted in signs of depression of conductivity and contractility.

In children early signs of local anaesthetic toxicity may be difficult to detect in cases where the block is given during general anaesthesia. It should be noted that NAROPIN (ropivacaine hydrochloride) is not approved for use in paediatric patients.

Treatment: The first consideration is prevention, best accomplished by incremental injection of NAROPIN, careful and constant monitoring of cardiovascular and respiratory vital signs and the patient's state of consciousness after each local anaesthetic injection and during continuous infusion. At the first sign of change, oxygen should be administered. If signs of acute systemic toxicity appear, injection of the local anaesthetic should be immediately stopped.

The first step in the management of systemic toxic reactions, as well as underventilation or apnoea due to unintentional subarachnoid injection of drug solution, consists of immediate attention to the establishment and maintenance of a patent airway and assisted or controlled ventilation with oxygen and a delivery system capable of permitting immediate positive airway pressure by mask and bag or tracheal intubation. This may prevent convulsions if they have not already occurred.

If necessary, use drugs to control the convulsions. An anticonvulsant should be given i.v. if the convulsions do not stop spontaneously in 15-20 seconds. Thiopental 1-3 mg/kg i.v. will abort the convulsions rapidly. Alternatively diazepam 0.1 mg/kg i.v. may be used, although its action will be slow. Both these drugs, however, depress the central nervous system, respiratory and cardiac function, add to postictal depression, and may result in apnoea. Prolonged convulsions may jeopardize the patient's ventilation and oxygenation. If so, injection of a muscle relaxant such as succinylcholine (1 mg/kg) will stop the muscle convulsions rapidly, so that ventilation and oxygenation can be controlled. Endo-tracheal intubation must be considered in such situations.

If cardiovascular depression is evident (hypotension, bradycardia) administration of intravenous fluids or a vasopressor such as ephedrine or epinephrine may be required.

Should circulatory arrest occur, immediate cardiopulmonary resuscitation should be instituted. Optimal oxygenation and ventilation and circulatory support as well as treatment of acidosis are of vital importance.

Should cardiac arrest occur, prolonged resuscitative efforts may be required to improve the likelihood of a successful outcome.

Clinical data from patients experiencing local anaesthetic-induced convulsions demonstrated rapid development of hypoxia, hypercarbia, and acidosis within a minute of the onset of convulsions. These observations suggest that oxygen consumption and carbon dioxide production are greatly increased during local anaesthetic convulsions and emphasize the importance of immediate and effective ventilation with oxygen which may avoid cardiac arrest.

The supine position is dangerous in pregnant women at term because of aorto-caval compression by the gravid uterus. Therefore, during treatment of systemic toxicity, maternal hypotension or foetal bradycardia following regional block, the parturient should be maintained in the left lateral decubitus position if possible, or manual displacement of the uterus off the great vessels should be accomplished. Resuscitation of obstetrical patients may take longer than resuscitation of non-pregnant patients and closed-chest cardiac compression may be ineffective. Rapid delivery of the foetus may improve the response to resuscitative efforts.

In human volunteers given intravenous NAROPIN, the mean maximum tolerated total and free arterial plasma concentrations were 4.3 and 0.6 μg/mL respectively, at which time moderate CNS symptoms (muscle twitching) were noted.

For management of a suspected drug overdose, CPhA recommends that you contact your **regional Poison Control Centre**. See the *CPS* Directory section for a list of Poison Control Centres.

ACTION AND CLINICAL PHARMACOLOGY: NAROPIN (ropivacaine hydrochloride), a local anaesthetic of the amino amide class, is supplied as the pure S-(-)-enantiomer.

NAROPIN has both local anaesthetic and analgesic effects. At high doses, surgical anaesthesia is achieved. At lower doses, NAROPIN produces sensory block (analgesia) with limited and non-progressive motor block.

Mechanism of Action: NAROPIN, like other local anaesthetics, causes reversible blockade of impulse propagation along nerve fibres by preventing the inward movement of sodium ions through the cell membrane of the nerve fibres.

Onset and Duration of Action: The duration of action of local anaesthetics depends on the injection site, the route of administration, and the concentration and volume of the drug. The duration and intensity of ropivacaine block are not improved by the addition of epinephrine.

After epidural infusion of ropivacaine, the spread of sensory block and the degree of motor block, as well as their subsequent regression, are dose-dependent.

Pharmacodynamics: Ropivacaine, like other local anaesthetics, can also have effects on the central nervous and cardiovascular systems. If excessive amounts of drug reach the systemic circulation, symptoms and signs of central nervous system toxicity and cardiotoxicity may appear.

Signs and symptoms of central nervous system toxicity (see Overdosage) generally occur at lower plasma concentrations than do those of cardiotoxicity. Following systemic absorption, local anaesthetics can produce central nervous system stimulation, depression or both. Apparent central stimulation is usually manifested as restlessness, tremors, and shivering, progressing to convulsions, followed by depression and coma, leading ultimately to respiratory arrest. However, the local anaesthetics have a primary depressant effect on the medulla and on higher centres. The depressed stage may occur without a prior excited stage. High blood concentrations of local anaesthetics resulting from systemic absorption or intravascular injection can depress cardiac conduction and excitability. At toxic levels, atrioventricular block, ventricular arrhythmias, cardiac arrest, and death are possibilities.

Indirect cardiovascular effects (hypotension, bradycardia) may occur after epidural administration, depending on the extent of the concomitant sympathetic block.

In two clinical pharmacology studies (total N=24) ropivacaine and bupivacaine were infused (10 mg/min) in human volunteers until the appearance of CNS symptoms, e.g., visual or hearing disturbances, perioral numbness, tingling and others. Similar symptoms were seen with both drugs. In one study, the mean±SD maximum tolerated intravenous dose of ropivacaine infused (124±38 mg) was significantly higher than that of bupivacaine (99±30 mg), while in the other study the doses were not different (115±29 mg of ropivacaine and 103±30 mg of bupivacaine). In the latter study, the number of subjects reporting each symptom was similar for both drugs with the exception of muscle twitching, which was reported by more subjects with bupivacaine than ropivacaine at comparable intravenous doses. At the end of the infusion, ropivacaine in both studies caused significantly less depression of cardiac conductivity (less QRS widening) than bupivacaine. Ropivacaine and bupivacaine caused evidence of depression of cardiac contractility, but there were no changes in cardiac output.

Pharmacokinetics: Absorption: The systemic concentration of local anaesthetics is dependent upon the total dose and the concentration administered, the route of administration, the patient's hemodynamic/ circulatory condition, and the vascularity of the injection site. Ropivacaine follows linear pharmacokinetics and the maximum plasma concentration is proportional to the dose.

Ropivacaine shows complete and biphasic absorption from the epidural space. The mean half-lives of the two phases are in the order of 14 min and 4 h. The slow absorption is the rate-limiting factor in the elimination of ropivacaine, which explains why the apparent elimination half-life is longer after epidural than after intravenous administration. Ropivacaine shows dose proportionality at epidural doses up to 250 mg and intravenous doses up to 80 mg.

Distribution: Following intravenous administration, the volume of distribution of NAROPIN is approximately 40 L. NAROPIN is extensively bound to alpha$_1$-acid glycoprotein in plasma with an unbound, i.e. pharmacologically active, fraction of about 6%. An increase in total plasma concentration during continuous epidural infusion has been observed in postoperative patients and is related to the postoperative increase of alpha$_1$-acid glycoprotein. Variations in unbound concentration have been much less than in total plasma concentration.

Ropivacaine readily crosses the placenta and equilibrium, in regard to unbound concentration, is rapidly reached. The degree of plasma protein binding in the foetus is less than in the mother, which results in lower total plasma concentrations in the foetus than in the mother. The ratios of umbilical vein to maternal vein total and free concentrations are 0.31 and 0.74, respectively.

Metabolism: Ropivacaine is extensively metabolized in the liver predominantly to 3-hydroxy-ropivacaine by an aromatic hydroxylation process mediated by cytochrome P4501A2 and N-dealkylation to PPX mediated by CYP3A4. Conjugated and unconjugated 3-hydroxy-ropivacaine represent the major urinary metabolites. Urinary excretion of 4-hydroxy-ropivacaine, N-dealkylated pipecoloxylidide (S-PPX) and both the 3-hydroxy and 4-hydroxy N-dealkylated metabolites account for less than 3% of the dose. An additional metabolite, 2-hydroxy-methyl-ropivacaine has been identified, but not quantified in urine. S-PPX and 3-hydroxy-ropivacaine are the major metabolites excreted in the urine during epidural infusion. A total S-PPX concentration in the plasma was about half that of total ropivacaine however, mean unbound concentrations of S-PPX were about 7-9 times higher than that of unbound ropivacaine following continuous epidural infusion up to 72 hours. The threshold for CNS toxicity in rats due to unbound plasma concentrations of PPX is approximately 12 times higher than that of unbound ropivacaine. S-PPX, 3-hydroxy-ropivacaine, and 4-hydroxy-ropivacaine have a pharmacological activity in animal models less than that of ropivacaine.

There is no evidence of in vivo racemization of ropivacaine.

Excretion: After intravascular administration, 86% of the total dose of ropivacaine is excreted in the urine of which approximately 1% is the parent compound and 36% is 3-hydroxy-ropivacaine. Ropivacaine has a mean total plasma clearance in the order of 440 mL/min, an unbound plasma clearance of 8 L/min, a renal clearance of 1 mL/min, and a volume of distribution at steady state of 47 L. Ropivacaine has an intermediate hepatic extraction ratio of about 0.4. The terminal elimination half-life is 1.6 to 1.8 hours after intravenous administration, 4.1-6.5 hours after epidural administration, and 5.7-8.0 hours after brachial plexus block. The total and unbound clearance of epidural ropivacaine at term in pregnancy (223-256 mL/min and 2.8-3.3 L/min, respectively), are lower than that observed in non-pregnant patients.

STORAGE AND STABILITY: Store solutions at 15-30°C.

SPECIAL HANDLING INSTRUCTIONS: Do not freeze. Due to the nature of the Polyamp and the Polybag systems, the containers must not be re-autoclaved.

NAROPIN (ropivacaine hydrochloride) solutions are sterile, without preservative and are for single use only. Discard unused portion.

Drug Compatibilities: NAROPIN for infusion in polypropylene infusion bags (Polybag) is chemically and physically compatible with the following drugs: see Table 10.

Table 10: NAROPIN

Drug Compatibilities

Concentration of NAROPIN: 1–2 mg/mL	
Additive	**Concentration**
Fentanyl citrate	1.0–10.0 μg/mL
Sufentanil citrate	0.4–4.0 μg/mL
Morphine sulphate	20.0–100.0 μg/mL
Clonidine hydrochloride	5.0–50.0 μg/mL

The mixtures should be used immediately. As with all parenteral products, intravenous admixtures should be visually inspected for clarity, particulate matter, precipitate, discoloration and leakage prior to administration, whenever solution and container permit. Solutions showing haziness, particulate matter, precipitate, discoloration or leakage should not be used. Discard unused portions.

Incompatibility: Alkalinization may lead to precipitation since ropivacaine is poorly soluble above pH 6.0

INFORMATION FOR THE PATIENT: Published in e-CPS, available by subscription at www.e-cps.ca.

DOSAGE FORMS, COMPOSITION AND PACKAGING: 2 mg/mL: Each mL of sterile isotonic solution contains: ropivacaine HCl 2 mg. Nonmedicinal ingredients: sodium chloride, sodium hydroxide and/or hydrochloric acid to adjust pH to 4.0 to 6.0 and water for injection. Polybag (polypropylene infusion bags) of 100 and 200 mL packed in a sterile blister pack.

5 mg/mL: Each mL of sterile isotonic solution contains: ropivacaine HCl 5 mg. Nonmedicinal ingredients: sodium chloride, sodium hydroxide and/or hydrochloric acid to adjust pH to 4.0 to 6.0 and water for injection. Polyamp Duofit (polypropylene ampuls suitable for Luer-lock and Luer fit syringes) of 20 mL packed in sterile blister packs.

10 mg/mL: Each mL of sterile isotonic solution contains: ropivacaine HCl 10 mg. Nonmedicinal ingredients: sodium chloride, sodium hydroxide and/or hydrochloric acid to adjust pH to 4.0 to 6.0 and water for injection. Polyamp Duofit (polypropylene ampuls suitable for Luer-lock and Luer fit syringes) of 10 and 20 mL packed in sterile blister packs.

Nasacort® AQ ℞

triamcinolone acetonide

Corticosteroid for Nasal Use

sanofi-aventis

Date of Revision: July 7, 2010

SUMMARY PRODUCT INFORMATION:

Route of Administration	Dosage Form/Strength	Clinically Relevant Nonmedicinal Ingredients
Nasal	Aqueous Nasal Spray 55 µg/Metered Spray	Benzalkonium chloride For a complete listing see Dosage Forms, Composition and Packaging.

INDICATIONS AND CLINICAL USE: NASACORT AQ (triamcinolone acetonide aqueous nasal spray) is indicated in adults, adolescents and children between the ages of 4 and 12 years for the topical treatment of the symptoms of perennial and seasonal allergic rhinitis unresponsive to conventional treatment.

Regular usage is essential since maximum relief may not be obtained until after 2 to 3 days of treatment.

CONTRAINDICATIONS: Hypersensitivity to any of the ingredients of NASACORT AQ (triamcinolone acetonide aqueous nasal spray), and in patients with active or quiescent tuberculosis, or untreated fungal, bacterial and viral infection.

WARNINGS AND PRECAUTIONS: General: The replacement of a systemic steroid with NASACORT AQ (triamcinolone acetonide aqueous nasal spray) has to be gradual and carefully supervised by the physician. The guidelines under "Dosage and Administration" should be followed in all such cases.

Patients should be informed that the full effect of NASACORT AQ therapy is not achieved until 2 to 3 days of treatment have been completed. Treatment of seasonal rhinitis should, if possible, start before the exposure to allergens.

Patients should be advised to inform subsequent physicians of prior use of corticosteroids.

To ensure the proper dosage and administration of the drug, the patient should be instructed by a physician or other health professional in the use of NASACORT AQ (see Information for the Patient).

Dependence/Tolerance: Treatment with NASACORT AQ should not be stopped abruptly but tapered off gradually. In patients previously on prolonged periods or high doses of systemic steroids, the replacement with a topical corticosteroid can be accompanied by symptoms of withdrawal, e.g. joint and/or muscular pain, lassitude, and depression; in severe cases, adrenal insufficiency may occur, necessitating the temporary resumption of systemic steroid therapy. These patients should be carefully monitored for acute adrenal insufficiency in response to stress. Careful attention must be given to patients with asthma or other clinical conditions in whom a rapid decrease in systemic steroids may cause a severe exacerbation of their symptoms.

Ear/Nose/Throat: Because of the inhibitory effect of corticosteroids on wound healing, in patients who have had recent nasal surgery or trauma, a nasal corticosteroid should be used with caution until healing has occurred. As with other nasally inhaled corticosteroids, nasal septal perforations have been reported in rare instances.

The possibility of atrophic rhinitis and/or pharyngeal candidiasis should be kept in mind.

In clinical studies with NASACORT AQ Aqueous nasal spray, the development of localized infections of the nose and pharynx with *C. albicans* has rarely occurred. When such an infection develops it may require treatment with appropriate local or systemic therapy and temporary discontinuation of treatment with NASACORT AQ Aqueous nasal spray. Therefore, patients using NASACORT AQ Nasal Spray over several months or longer should be examined periodically for evidence of Candida infection or other signs of adverse effects on the nasal mucosa.

Endocrine and Metabolism: Osteoporosis is a possible adverse effect associated with a long-term use of large doses of corticosteroids.

Immune: Corticosteroids may mask some signs of infection and new infections may appear. A decreased resistance to localized infections has been observed during corticosteroid therapy; this may require treatment with appropriate therapy or stopping the administration of NASACORT AQ.

Patients who are on immunosuppressant drugs are more susceptible to infections than healthy individuals. Chickenpox and measles, for example, can have a more serious or even fatal course in children or adults on immunosuppressant doses of corticosteroids. In such children, or in adults who have not had these diseases, particular care should be taken to avoid exposure. If exposed, therapy with varicella zoster immune globulin (VZIG) or pooled intravenous immunoglobulin (IVIG), as appropriate, may be indicated. If chickenpox develops, treatment with antiviral agents may be considered.

Effects on Growth : Growth retardation has been reported in children receiving nasal corticosteroids at licensed doses. It is recommended that the height of children receiving prolonged treatment with nasal corticosteroids is regularly monitored. If growth is slowed, therapy should be reviewed with the aim of reducing the dose of nasal corticosteroid if possible, to the lowest dose at which effective control of symptoms is maintained. In addition, consideration should be given to referring the patient to a paediatric specialist. The long-term effects of reduction in growth velocity associated with nasal corticosteroids, including the impact on final adult height are unknown.

Ophthalmologic: Glaucoma and/or cataracts have been reported in patients receiving nasal corticosteroids. Therefore, close monitoring is warranted in patients with a change in vision or with a history of increased intraocular pressure, glaucoma, and/or cataracts.

Sensitivity/Resistance: There is an enhanced effect of corticosteroids on patients with hypothyroidism and in those with cirrhosis. Acetylsalicylic acid should be used cautiously in conjunction with corticosteroids in hypothrombinemia.

The use of NASACORT AQ (triamcinolone acetonide aqueous nasal spray) with alternate day systemic prednisone could increase the likelihood of hypothalamic-pituitary-adrenal (HPA) suppression compared to a therapeutic dose of either one alone. Therefore, NASACORT AQ should be used with caution in patients already receiving alternate-day prednisone treatment for any disease.

Special Populations: Pregnant Women: The safety of NASACORT AQ in pregnancy has not been established. If used, the expected benefits should be weighed against the potential hazard to the fetus, particularly during the first trimester of pregnancy.

Like other glucocorticosteroids, triamcinolone acetonide is teratogenic to rodents and non-human primates. The relevance of these findings to humans has not yet been established. Infants born of mothers who have received substantial doses of glucocorticosteroids during pregnancy should be carefully observed for hypoadrenalism.

Nursing Women: Glucocorticosteroids are excreted in human milk. It is not known whether triamcinolone acetonide would be secreted in human milk, but it is suspected to be likely. The use of NASACORT AQ in nursing mothers, requires that the possible benefits of the drug be weighed against the potential hazards to the infant.

Pediatrics: NASACORT AQ is not presently recommended for children younger than 4 years of age due to limited clinical data in this age group. Oral corticosteroids have been shown to cause growth suppression in children and teenagers, particularly with higher doses over extended periods. If a child or teenager on any corticosteroids appears to have growth suppression, the possibility that they are particularly sensitive to this effect of steroids should be considered.

Monitoring and Laboratory Tests: During long-term therapy pituitary-adrenal function and hematological status should be assessed.

ADVERSE REACTIONS: Adverse Drug Reaction Overview : Systemic and local corticosteroid use may result in the following:

- Epistaxis, ulcerations, *C. albicans* infection, nasal septal perforation, impaired wound healing (see Warnings and Precautions)
- Glaucoma and Cataracts (see Warnings and Precautions)
- Immunosuppression (see Warnings and Precautions)
- Hypothalamic-pituitary-adrenal (HPA) axis effects, including growth reduction (see Warnings and Precautions)

Clinical Trial Adverse Drug Reactions: Because clinical trials are conducted under very specific conditions, the adverse reaction rates observed in the clinical trials may not reflect the rates observed in practice and should not be compared to the rates in the clinical trials of another drug. Adverse drug reaction information from clinical trials is useful for identifying drug-related adverse events and for approximating rates.

In placebo-controlled, double-blind and open-label clinical studies, 1483 adults and children 12 years and older received treatment with NASACORT AQ Nasal Spray. These patients were treated for an average duration of 50.7 days. In the controlled, seasonal trials (2-5 weeks duration) from which the following adverse reaction data is derived, 1394 patients were treated with NASACORT AQ Nasal Spray for an average of 18.7 days. In the long-term, open-label study, the 172 patients enrolled received treatment for an average of 286 days duration.

The most commonly reported adverse reactions included those involving mucous membranes of the nose and throat. The three most prevalent adverse reactions considered to be at least possibly drug-related in adults and children 12 years and older were rhinitis (1.5%), headache (0.7%), and pharyngitis (0.3%), and in children 4 to 12 years were epistaxis (3.1%), rhinitis (1.4%) and headache (1.2%).

Children 4 to 12 years of age (n=622) were studied in 3 controlled clinical trials. Of these, 179 received 110 µg/day and 215 received 220 µg/day of NASACORT AQ Nasal Spray in two, six, or twelve week trials. The longest average duration of treatment for patients receiving 110 µg/day was 76.3 days and 79.6 days for those receiving 220 µg/day.

The incidence of specific nasopharyngeal-related adverse reactions considered drug related is summarized in Table 1.

Table 1: NASACORT AQ
Nasopharyngeal Adverse Reactions

	Placebo (n=176)	NASACORT AQ 110 µg (n=179)	NASACORT AQ 220 µg (n=187)	Placebo (n=626)	NASACORT AQ 27.5–440 µg (n=1068)
Nasal AEs (overall)	15 (8.5%)	8 (4.5%)	12 (6.4%)	20 (3.2%)	31 (2.9%)
Dry Mucous Membranes	0	0	0	2 (0.3%)	3 (0.3%)
Epistaxis	9 (5.1%)	6 (3.4%)	6 (3.2%)	3 (0.5%)	17 (1.6%)
Nasal Irritation	5 (2.8%)	0	2 (1.1%)	3 (0.5%)	9 (0.8%)
Naso-sinus Congestion	0	1 (0.6%)	1 (0.5%)	1 (0.2%)	2 (0.2%)
Sneezing	1 (0.6%)	0	2 (1.1%)	6 (1.0%)	2 (0.2%)
Throat Discomfort	1 (0.6%)	1 (0.6%)	1 (0.5%)	6 (1.0%)	3 (0.3%)

These adverse reactions, with the exception of epistaxis (in adults), and the exception of nasal congestion and sneezing (in children) were reported at approximately the same or lower incidence as placebo treated patients. Only 1% of the patients in the controlled trials discontinued treatment (e.g. pharyngitis, headache). In children, no patient receiving 110 µg/day discontinued due to a serious adverse event and one patient receiving 220 µg/day discontinued due to a serious event that was considered not drug related. Overall, these studies found the adverse experience profile for NASACORT AQ to be similar to placebo.

Table 2 and Table 3 summarize the adverse events (% of patients) present in at least 5% of patients in the double-blind and open label phase studies in adults and in controlled studies in children 4 to 12 years of age.

Table 2: NASACORT AQ
Adverse Events in Adults

	Studies in Adults		
	Double-Blind		Open-Label
Variables	Placebo n=90	NASACORT AQ 220 µg n=88	NASACORT AQ 220/110 µg n=172
Flu Syndrome	5 (5.6%)	5 (5.7%)	17 (9.9%)
Headache	12 (13.3%)	6 (6.8%)	38 (22.1%)
Epistaxis	1 (1.1%)	6 (6.8%)	31 (18.0%)
Pharyngitis	5 (5.6%)	13 (14.8%)	55 (32.0%)
Rhinitis	5 (5.6%)	6 (6.8%)	49 (28.5%)
Injury Accident	—	—	20 (11.6%)
Back Pain	—	—	13 (7.6%)
Cough Increased	—	—	14 (8.1%)
Sinusitis	—	—	27 (15.7%)
Pain	—	—	10 (5.8%)
Diarrhea	—	—	10 (5.8%)

Table 3: NASACORT AQ
Adverse Events in Children

	Studies in Children 4–12 Years of Age			
Variables	Placebo n=202	NASACORT AQ 110 µg n=179	NASACORT AQ 220 µg n=215	NASACORT AQ 440 µg n=26
Fever	11 (5.4%)	8 (4.5%)	12 (5.6%)	2 (7.7%)
Flu Syndrome	15 (7.4%)	16 (8.9%)	4 (1.9%)	0
Headache	22 (10.9%)	18 (10.1%)	16 (7.4%)	4 (15.4%)
Infection	15 (7.4%)	13 (7.3%)	16 (7.4%)	0
Injury Accidental	3 (1.5%)	3 (1.7%)	4 (1.9%)	2 (7.7%)
Cough Increased	13 (6.4%)	15 (8.4%)	15 (7.0%)	0

(cont'd)

Table 3: NASACORT AQ *(cont'd)*

Adverse Events in Children

	Studies in Children 4–12 Years of Age			
Epistaxis	14 (6.9%)	8 (4.5%)	10 (4.7%)	1 (3.8%)
Pharyngitis	13 (6.4%)	14 (7.8%)	16 (7.4%)	2 (7.7%)
Rhinitis	18 (8.9%)	18 (10.1%)	18 (8.4%)	0
Sinusitis	16 (6.4%)	7 (3.9%)	7 (3.3%)	0

In addition, the most frequent (frequencies ≥2%) adverse reactions in adults and children greater than 6 years are: Headache, cough, bronchitis, dyspepsia, rhinitis, pharyngitis, flu syndrome, and tooth disorder.

In patients aged 2 to 5 years, the following adverse reactions have been observed (frequency ≥2%): headache pharyngolaryngeal pain, nasopharyngitis, excoriation, diarrhea, and upper abdominal pain.

In the event of accidental overdose, an increased potential for these adverse experiences may be expected, but systemic adverse experiences are unlikely (see Overdosage).

Hypersensitivity reactions including skin rash and edema of the face or tongue have been reported with other intranasal corticosteroids.

When patients are transferred to NASACORT AQ from a systemic steroid, allergic conditions such as asthma or eczema may be unmasked (see Warnings and Precautions).

Post-Market Adverse Drug Reactions: The following additional adverse reactions have been reported during post-marketing experience; they are derived from spontaneous reports and therefore, the frequency of these adverse reactions is not known: nasal irritation, dry mucous membrane, nasal congestion, sneezing alterations of taste and smell, nausea, insomnia, dizziness, fatigue, dyspnea, decreased blood cortisol, cataract, glaucoma, increased ocular pressure, pruritus, rash, and hypersensitivity.

As with other nasally inhaled corticosteroids, nasal septum perforations have been reported in rare instances.

DOSAGE AND ADMINISTRATION:

Dosing Considerations: See Warnings and Precautions.

NASACORT AQ (triamcinolone acetonide aqueous nasal spray) is not recommended for children under 4 years of age.

Careful attention must be given to patients previously treated for prolonged periods with systemic corticosteroids when transferred to NASACORT AQ. Initially, NASACORT AQ and the systemic corticosteroid must be given concomitantly, while the dose of the latter is gradually decreased. The usual rate of withdrawal of the systemic steroid is the equivalent of 2.5 mg of prednisone every four days if the patient is under close supervision. If continuous supervision is not feasible, the withdrawal of the systemic steroid should be slower, approximately 2.5 mg of prednisone (or equivalent) every ten days. If withdrawal symptoms appear, the previous dose of the systemic steroid should be resumed for a week before further decrease is attempted.

Recommended Dose and Dosage Adjustment: Adults and children 12 years of age and older: The recommended starting dose of NASACORT AQ (triamcinolone acetonide aqueous nasal spray) is 220 µg as two sprays in each nostril once daily.

It is always desirable to titrate an individual patient to the minimum effective dose to reduce the possibility of side effects. Therefore, when the maximum benefit has been achieved and symptoms have been controlled, reducing the dose to 110 µg (one spray in each nostril once per day) has been shown to be effective in maintaining control of the allergic rhinitis symptoms in patients who were initially controlled at 220 µg/day (see Warnings and Precautions; Information for the Patient and Adverse Reactions).

Children 4 to 12 years of age: The recommended starting dose is 110 µg per day given as one spray in each nostril once a day. Patients who do not achieve maximum symptom control may benefit from a dose of 220 µg given as 2 sprays in each nostril once a day. Once symptoms are controlled, patients can be maintained on 110 µg (1 spray in each nostril) once daily.

Administration: The therapeutic effects of corticosteroids, unlike those of decongestants, are not immediate. Since the effect of NASACORT AQ depends on its regular use, patients must be instructed to take the nasal inhalations at regular intervals and not as with other nasal sprays, as they feel necessary.

In the presence of excessive nasal mucus secretion or edema of the nasal mucosa, the drug may fail to reach the site of action. In such cases it is advisable to use a nasal vasoconstrictor for two to three days prior to NASACORT AQ therapy. Patients should be instructed on the correct method of use, which is to blow the nose, then insert the nozzle firmly into the nostril, compress the opposite nostril and actuate the spray while inspiring through the nose, with the mouth closed.

An improvement of symptoms usually becomes apparent within a few days after the start of therapy. However symptomatic relief may not occur in some patients for as long as two weeks. NASACORT AQ should not be continued beyond three weeks in the absence of significant symptomatic improvement.

OVERDOSAGE:

Like any other nasally administered corticosteroid, acute overdosing is unlikely in view of the total amount of active ingredient present. In the event that the entire contents of the bottle were administered all at once, via either oral or nasal application, clinically significant systemic adverse events would most likely not result. The patient may experience some gastrointestinal upset.

However when used chronically in excessive doses or in conjunction with other corticosteroid formulations, systemic corticosteroid effects such as hypercorticism and adrenal suppression may appear. If such changes occur, the dosage of NASACORT AQ (triamcinolone acetonide aqueous nasal spray) should be discontinued slowly consistent with accepted procedures for discontinuation of chronic steroid therapy. (See Dosage and Administration.)

The restoration of hypothalamic-pituitary axis may be slow; during periods of pronounced physical stress (i.e. severe infections, trauma, surgery) a supplement with systemic steroids may be advisable.

> For management of a suspected drug overdose, contact your regional Poison Control Centre. See the *CPS* Directory section for a list of Poison Control Centres.

ACTION AND CLINICAL PHARMACOLOGY: Mechanism of Action: Triamcinolone acetonide is a potent anti-inflammatory steroid with strong topical and weak systemic activity. Triamcinolone acetonide is a more potent derivative of triamcinolone. Although triamcinolone itself is approximately one to two times as potent as prednisone in animal models of inflammation, triamcinolone acetonide is approximately 8 times more potent than prednisone.

When administered intranasally in therapeutic doses, it has a direct anti-inflammatory action on the nasal mucosa, the mechanism of which is not yet completely defined. The minute amount absorbed in therapeutic doses has not been shown to exert any apparent clinical systemic effects.

Corticosteroids are very effective. However, when allergic symptoms are very severe, local treatment with recommended doses (µg) of any available topical corticosteroid are not as effective as treatment with larger doses (mg) of oral or parenteral formulations. Corticosteroids do not have an immediate effect on allergic signs and symptoms. An improvement of symptoms may be seen as early as the first day after initiation of treatment and full benefit may be expected in 3 to 4 days. However, symptomatic relief may not occur in some patients for as long as two weeks. NASACORT AQ should not be continued beyond three weeks in the absence of significant symptomatic improvement.

Pharmacokinetics: Based upon intravenous dosing of triamcinolone acetonide phosphate ester, the half-life of triamcinolone acetonide was reported to be 88 minutes. The volume of distribution (Vd) reported was 99.5 L (SD±27.5) and clearance was 45.2 L/hour (SD±9.1) for triamcinolone acetonide. The plasma half-life of corticosteroids does not correlate well with the biologic half-life.

Pharmacokinetic characterization of the NASACORT AQ Nasal Spray formulation was determined in both normal adult subjects and patients with allergic rhinitis. Single dose intranasal administration of 220 µg of NASACORT AQ in normal adult subjects and patients demonstrated minimal absorption of triamcinolone acetonide. The mean peak plasma concentration was approximately 0.5 ng/mL (range: 0.1 to 1.0 ng/mL) and occurred at 1.5 hours post dose. The mean plasma drug concentration was less than 0.06 ng/mL at 12 hours, and below the assay detection limit at 24 hours. The average terminal half-life was 3.1 hours. Dose proportionality was demonstrated in normal subjects and in patients following a single intranasal dose of 110 µg or 220 µg NASACORT AQ.

Triamcinolone acetonide aqueous administered intranasally has been shown to be minimally absorbed into the systemic circulation in humans. Patients with active rhinitis showed absorption similar to that found in normal volunteers.

In order to determine if systemic absorption plays a role in NASACORT AQ treatment of allergic rhinitis symptoms, a two week double-blind placebo-controlled clinical study was conducted comparing NASACORT AQ, orally ingested triamcinolone acetonide, and placebo in 297 patients with seasonal allergic rhinitis. The study demonstrated that the therapeutic efficacy of NASACORT AQ can be attributed to the topical effects of triamcinolone acetonide.

In order to evaluate the effects of systemic absorption on the Hypothalmic-Pituitary-Adrenal (HPA) axis, a clinical study was performed comparing 220 µg or 440 µg NASACORT AQ, or 10 mg prednisone to placebo for 42 days. Adrenal response to a 6 hour cosyntropin stimulation test clearly indicated that NASACORT AQ administered at doses of 220 µg and 440 µg had no effect on HPA activity versus placebo. Conversely, oral prednisone at 10 mg/day significantly reduced the response to ACTH.

Special Populations: Pediatrics: Following multiple doses in pediatric patients ages 6 to 12 years old receiving 440 µg/day, plasma drug concentration, AUC, C_{max} and T_{max} were similar to those values observed in adult patients.

A six week study was conducted in 80 pediatric patients to evaluate the effect of 220 µg or 440 µg of NASACORT AQ versus placebo on HPA function. No evidence of adrenal axis suppression was observed in the pediatric patients exposed to systemic levels of triamcinolone acetonide higher than the systemic levels observed following administration of the maximum recommended dose of NASACORT AQ Nasal Spray.

STORAGE AND STABILITY: Store at 15-25°C.

INFORMATION FOR THE PATIENT: Published in e-CPS, available by subscription at www.e-cps.ca.

DOSAGE FORMS, COMPOSITION AND PACKAGING: Each actuation releases approximately 55 µg triamcinolone acetonide from the nasal actuator to the patient (estimated from in vitro testing) in an unscented, thixotrophic, water-based spray formulation. Nonmedicinal ingredients: benzalkonium chloride, carboxymethylcellulose sodium, dextrose, edetate disodium, microcrystalline cellulose, polysorbate 80 and purified water. Hydrochloric acid or sodium hydroxide may be added to adjust the pH to between 4.5 and 6.0. Non-chlorofluorocarbon (CFC) containing-metered dose pump spray which will provide 120 actuations. After 120 actuations, the amount delivered per actuation may not be consistent and the unit should be discarded. It is supplied with a nasal adapter and patient instructions. Each bottle contains 9.075 mg triamcinolone acetonide.

Nasonex® Ⓟ

mometasone furoate monohydrate

Corticosteroid

Schering-Plough

Date of Preparation: July 14, 1998
Date of Revision: December 17, 2008

PHARMACOLOGY: Mometasone furoate is a topical glucocorticosteroid with local anti-inflammatory properties at doses that are minimally systemically active. Mometasone furoate, administered as a nasal spray, has negligible (≤0.1%) systemic bioavailability and is generally undetectable in plasma, despite the use of a sensitive assay with a lower quantitation limit of 50 pg/mL; thus, there are no relevant pharmacokinetic data for this dosage form. Mometasone furoate suspension is very poorly absorbed from the gastrointestinal tract, and the small amount that may be swallowed and absorbed undergoes extensive first-pass metabolism prior to excretion in urine and bile.

In two clinical studies utilizing nasal antigen challenge, NASONEX (mometasone furoate monohydrate aqueous nasal spray) has shown anti-inflammatory activity in both the early- and late-phase allergic responses. This has been demonstrated by decreases (vs. placebo) in histamine and eosinophil activity and reductions (vs. baseline) in eosinophils, neutrophils, and epithelial cell adhesion proteins. The clinical significance of these finding is not known.

Two Phase I studies conducted to assess the systemic exposure and tolerability of NASONEX in children aged 3 to 12 years showed no clinically relevant systemic exposure to NASONEX and indicated that NASONEX was well tolerated. A third Phase I study in children aged 6 to12 years showed normal short-term lower leg growth velocity.

The results of Phase II and Phase III studies indicated no evidence of HPA- (hypothalamic-pituitary-adrenal) axis suppression following treatment with NASONEX and demonstrated that NASONEX can alleviate the allergic symptoms in pediatric patients aged 3 to 12 years with seasonal and perennial allergic rhinitis.

In clinical trials with nasal polyposis, NASONEX showed significant improvement when compared to placebo in the clinically relevant endpoints of congestion, and nasal polyp size (see Table 1).

Table 1: NASONEX

Effect of NASONEX in Two Randomized, Placebo-Controlled Trials in Patients with Nasal Polyps

	NASONEX 200 µg od	NASONEX 200 µg bid	Placebo	P Value for NASONEX 200 µg od vs. Placebo	P Value for NASONEX 200 µg bid vs. Placebo
Study P01925	n=115	n=122	n=117		
Baseline bilateral polyp grade[a]	4.21	4.27	4.25		
Mean change from baseline in bilateral polyp grade[c]	−1.15	−0.96	−0.50	<0.001	0.01
Baseline nasal congestion[b]	2.29	2.35	2.28		
Mean change from baseline in nasal congestion[d]	−0.47	−0.61	−0.24	0.001	<0.001
Study P01926	n=102	n=102	n=106		
Baseline bilateral polyp grade[a]	4.00	4.10	4.17		
Mean change from baseline in bilateral polyp grade[c]	−0.78	−0.96	−0.62	0.33	0.04
Baseline nasal congestion[b]	2.23	2.20	2.18		
Mean change from baseline in nasal congestion[d]	−0.42	−0.66	−0.23	0.01	<0.001

[a] Polyps in each nasal fossa were graded by the investigator based on endoscopic visualization, using a scale of 0-3 where 0=no polyps; 1=polyps in the middle meatus, not reaching below the inferior border of the middle turbinate; 2=polyps reaching below the inferior border of the middle turbinate but not the inferior border of the inferior turbinate; 3=polyps reaching to or below the border of the inferior turbinate, or polyps medial to the middle turbinate (score reflects sum of left and right nasal fossa grades).

[b] Nasal congestion/obstruction was scored daily by the patient using a 0-3 categorical scale where 0=no symptoms; 1=mild symptoms; 2=moderate symptoms and 3=severe symptoms.

[c] To the last assessment during the entire four months of the treatment period.

[d] Averaged over the first month of treatment.

In two clinical trials with 1954 patients 12 years of age and older with mild to moderate uncomplicated acute rhinosinusitis, NASONEX 200 µg twice daily was effective in significantly improving symptoms of acute rhinosinusitis compared to placebo as evaluated by the Major Symptom Score (MSS) composite of symptoms (facial pain/pressure/tenderness, sinus headache, rhinorrhea, post nasal drip, and nasal congestion/stuffiness) during the 15 day treatment period (P02683 $p<0.001$; P02692 $p=0.038$). A 500 mg three times a day amoxicillin arm was not significantly different from placebo in reducing symptoms of mild to moderate uncomplicated acute rhinosinusitis as evaluated by the MSS (see Table 2). Fewer subjects treated with NASONEX 200 µg twice daily were considered by the treating physician to be treatment failures than those treated with placebo.

Table 2: NASONEX

Summary Results for the Major-Symptom Score

	MFNS 200 µg OD (A)		**MFNS 200 µg BID (B)**		**Amoxicillin 500 mg TID (C)**		**Placebo (D)**	
	N	**LS Mean[a]**	**N**	**LS Mean[a]**	**N**	**LS Mean[a]**	**N**	**LS Mean[a]**
P02683								
Baseline[b]	243	8.17	234	8.28	251	8.53	252	8.36
Actual Score Days 2–15 (primary assessment)	240	4.16[d]	234	3.80[d,e]	249	4.40	247	4.61
% Change from Baseline Days 2 to 15	240	−4.01 (−49.8%)	233	−4.51[d,f] (−55.6%)	249	−4.13 (−49.3%)	247	−3.75 (−45.6%)
P02692								
Baseline[b]	229	7.69	236	7.70	233	7.55	242	7.72
Actual Score Days 1–15[c]	229	3.99	236	3.95[d]	233	4.17	242	4.36
% Change from Baseline Days 1 to 15[c] (primary assessment)	229	−3.70 (−46.7%)	236	−3.76[d,e] (−48.4%)	233	−3.38 (−42.5%)	242	−3.36 (−41.5%)
Pairwise Comparisons MSS changes from baseline and 95% Confidence Interval								
			A-B	**A-C**	**A-D**	**B-C**	**B-D**	**C-D**
P02683								
Change from Baseline Days 2 to 15			0.5 (0.10, 0.90)	−0.12 (−0.28, 0.51)	−0.26 (−0.66, 0.13)	−0.38 (−0.78, 0.01)	−0.76 (−1.16, −0.36)	−0.38 (−0.76, 0.01)
P02692								
Change from Baseline Days 1 to 15[c] (primary Assessment)			0.06 (−0.32, 0.44)	−0.32 (−0.70, 0.064)	−0.34 (−0.72, 0.04)	−0.38 (−0.76, −0.00)	−0.40 (−0.78, −0.02)	−0.02 (−0.40, 0.36)

[a] LS Means were obtained from the ANOVA model with effects for treatment, site, and duration of symptoms (7 to 14 days or 15 to 28 days).
[b] In Study P02683, Baseline was an in-office evaluation performed jointly by the subject and physician. In Study P02692, Baseline was the mean of three diary evaluations performed by the subject only.
[c] Day 1 includes the PM assessment for subjects in P02692 only.
[d] $P<0.05$ vs. placebo.
[e] $P\leq0.05$ vs. amoxicillin.
[f] $P<0.05$ vs. MFNS 200 µg OD.

In addition, a 14-day post-treatment follow-up period was conducted among the four treatment groups. Study results indicated that the recurrence rate of rhinosinusitis was comparable between treatment groups.

INDICATIONS: NASONEX (mometasone furoate aqueous nasal spray) is indicated for: use in adults, adolescents, and children between the ages of 3 and 11 years to treat the symptoms of seasonal or perennial allergic rhinitis; use in adults and children 12 years of age and older as adjunctive treatment to antibiotics in acute episodes of rhinosinusitis, where signs or symptoms of bacterial infection are present; use in adults and children 12 years of age and older in the treatment of symptoms associated with mild to moderate uncomplicated acute rhinosinusitis where signs or symptoms of bacterial infection are not present; the treatment of nasal polyps in adult patients 18 years of age or older.

CONTRAINDICATIONS: Hypersensitivity to any ingredients of NASONEX.

NASONEX should be used with caution, if at all, in patients with active or quiescent tuberculous infections of the respiratory tract, or in untreated fungal, bacterial, systemic viral infections or ocular herpes simplex.

PRECAUTIONS: General: NASONEX should not be used in the presence of untreated localized infection involving the nasal mucosa.

Because of the inhibitory effect of corticosteroids on wound healing, patients who have experienced recent nasal surgery or trauma should not use a nasal corticosteroid until healing has occurred.

Following 12 months of treatment with NASONEX, there was no evidence of atrophy of the nasal mucosa; also, mometasone furoate tended to reverse the nasal mucosa closer to a normal histologic phenotype. As with any long-term treatment, patients using NASONEX over several months or longer should be examined periodically for possible changes in the nasal mucosa. If localized fungal infection of the nose or pharynx develops, discontinuance of NASONEX therapy or appropriate treatment may be required. Persistence of nasopharyngeal irritation may be an indication for discontinuing NASONEX.

There is no evidence of hypothalamic-pituitary-adrenal (HPA) axis suppression following prolonged (12 months) treatment with NASONEX. However, patients who are transferred from long-term administration of systemically active corticosteroids to NASONEX require careful attention. Systemic corticosteroid withdrawal in such patients may result in adrenal insufficiency for a number of months until recovery of HPA axis function. If these patients exhibit signs and symptoms of adrenal insufficiency, systemic corticosteroid administration should be resumed and other modes of therapy and appropriate measures instituted.

NASONEX permitted normal growth in a placebo-controlled clinical trial in which pediatric patients were administered NASONEX 100 µg daily for one year.

During transfer from systemic corticosteroid to NASONEX, some patients may experience symptoms of withdrawal from systemically active corticosteroids (e.g., joint and/or muscular pain, lassitude, and depression initially) despite relief from nasal symptoms and will require encouragement to continue NASONEX therapy. Such transfer may also unmask pre-existing allergic conditions such as allergic conjunctivitis and eczema, previously suppressed by systemic corticosteroid therapy.

Patients receiving corticosteroids who are potentially immunosuppressed should be warned of the risk of exposure to certain infections (e.g., chickenpox, measles) and of the importance of obtaining medical advice if such exposure occurs.

Following the use of intranasal aerosolized corticosteroids, instances of nasal septum perforation or increased intraocular pressure have been reported very rarely.

Acute Rhinosinusitis: Patients should not use NASONEX without an antibiotic if bacterial infection of the sinuses is present or suspected.

NASONEX is not indicated to treat the symptoms of the common cold. To distinguish mild to moderate acute rhinosinusitis from the common cold, patients should have symptoms of acute rhinosinusitis persisting or increasing for at least seven days before starting NASONEX treatment.

If signs or symptoms of severe bacterial infection are observed during treatment (such as fever, persistent severe unilateral facial/tooth pain, orbital or peri-orbital facial swelling, or worsening of symptoms after an initial improvement), the patient should be advised to consult their physician immediately at which time the physician may advise the patient to stop using NASONEX.

Safety and efficacy of NASONEX as adjunctive treatment to antibiotics in acute episodes of rhinosinusitis in children less than 12 years of age have not been studied.

Safety and efficacy of NASONEX for the treatment of symptoms associated with mild to moderate uncomplicated acute rhinosinusitis in children less than 12 years of age have not been studied.

Safety and efficacy of NASONEX in the treatment of symptoms associated with mild to moderate uncomplicated acute rhinosinusitis beyond 15 days has not been evaluated.

Nasal Polyps: Safety and efficacy of NASONEX for the treatment of nasal polyps in children and adolescents less than 18 years of age have not been studied.

Pregnancy: There are no adequate or well-controlled studies in pregnant or nursing women. Following intranasal administration of the maximal recommended clinical dose to patients, mometasone furoate plasma concentrations are not measurable; thus fetal or breast milk exposure is expected to be negligible and the potential for reproductive or nursing toxicity, very low.

As with other nasal corticosteroid preparations, NASONEX should be used in pregnant women, nursing mothers or women of childbearing age only if the potential benefit justifies the potential risk to the mother, fetus, or infant. Infants born of mothers who received corticosteroids during pregnancy should be observed carefully for hypoadrenalism.

Lactation: See Pregnancy.

Drug Interactions: NASONEX has been administered concomitantly with loratadine with no apparent effect on plasma concentrations of loratadine or its major metabolite. Mometasone furoate plasma concentrations were not detectable. The combination therapy was well tolerated.

ADVERSE EFFECTS: Allergic Rhinitis: Treatment-related local adverse events reported in clinical studies include headache (8%), epistaxis (e.g., frank bleeding, blood-tinged mucus, and blood flecks) (8%), pharyngitis (4%), nasal burning (2%), nasal irritation (2%), and nasal ulceration (1%), which are typically observed with use of a corticosteroid nasal spray.

Epistaxis was generally self-limiting and mild in severity, and occurred at a higher incidence compared to placebo (5%), but at a comparable or lower incidence compared to the active control nasal corticosteroids studied (up to 15%). The incidence of all other effects was comparable with that of placebo.

In the pediatric population, the incidence of adverse effects, e.g. headache (3%), epistaxis (6%), nasal irritation (2%), and sneezing (2%) was comparable to placebo.

Rarely, immediate hypersensitivity reactions (e.g., bronchospasm, dyspnea) may occur after intranasal administration of mometasone furoate monohydrate. Very rarely, anaphylaxis and angioedema have been reported.

Disturbances of taste and smell have been reported very rarely.

Acute Rhinosinusitis as Adjunctive Treatment to Antibiotics: In adults and adolescent patients receiving NASONEX as adjunctive treatment for acute episodes of rhinosinusitis, treatment-related adverse events, which occurred at an incidence comparable to placebo, included headache (2%), pharyngitis (1%), nasal burning (1%), and nasal irritation (1%). Epistaxis was mild in severity and also occurred at an incidence comparable to placebo (5% vs. 4%, respectively).

Mild to Moderate Uncomplicated Acute Rhinosinusitis: In patients treated for mild to moderate acute rhinosinusitis, the overall incidence of adverse events was comparable to placebo and similar to that observed for patients with allergic rhinitis.

Nasal Polyps: In patients treated for nasal polyps, the overall incidence of adverse events was comparable to placebo and similar to that observed for patients with allergic rhinitis.

OVERDOSE:

Treatment: Because of the negligible (≤0.1%) systemic bioavailability of NASONEX, overdose is unlikely to require any therapy other than observation, followed by initiation of the appropriate prescribed dosage.

For management of a suspected drug overdose, CPhA recommends that you contact your **regional Poison Control Centre.** See the *CPS* Directory section for a list of Poison Control Centres.

DOSAGE: The therapeutic effects of corticosteroids, unlike those of decongestants, are not immediate. Since the effect of NASONEX depends on its regular use, patients should be instructed to take the nasal inhalation at regular intervals and not, as with other nasal sprays, as they feel necessary.

After initial priming of the NASONEX nasal pump (usually 10 actuations, until a uniform spray is observed), each actuation delivers approximately 100 mg of mometasone furoate suspension, containing mometasone furoate monohydrate equivalent up to 50 µg mometasone furoate. If the spray pump has not been used for 14 days or longer, it should be reprimed with 2 actuations, until a uniform spray is observed, before next use.

In the presence of excessive nasal mucous secretion or edema of the nasal mucosa, the drug may fail to reach the site of action. In such cases, it is advisable to use a nasal vasoconstrictor for 2 to 3 days prior to starting treatment with NASONEX. Patients should be instructed on the correct method of use, which is to blow the nose, then insert the nozzle carefully into the nostril, compress the opposite nostril and actuate the spray while inspiring through the nose, with the mouth closed.

Shake container well before each use.

Treatment of Seasonal Or Perennial Allergic Rhinitis: Adults (including geriatric patients) and children 12 years of age and older: The usual recommended dose is two sprays (50 µg/spray) in each nostril once daily (total daily dose of 200 µg). Once symptoms are controlled, dose reduction to one spray in each nostril (total daily dose 100 µg) may be effective for maintenance.

If symptoms are inadequately controlled, the dose may be increased to four sprays in each nostril (total daily dose of 400 µg). Dose reduction is recommended following control of symptoms.

Clinically significant onset of action occurs as early as 12 hours after the first dose.

Children between the ages of 3 and 11 years: The usual recommended dose is one spray (50 µg/spray) in each nostril once daily (total daily dose of 100 µg).

Administration to young children should be aided by an adult.

Adjunctive Treatment to Antibiotics in Acute Episodes of Rhinosinusitis: NASONEX should not be used in the presence of untreated localized infection involving the nasal mucosa.

Adults (including geriatric patients) and children 12 years of age and older: The usual recommended dose is two sprays (50 µg/spray) in each nostril twice daily (total daily dose of 400 µg).

If symptoms are inadequately controlled, the dose may be increased to four sprays (50 µg/spray) in each nostril twice daily (total daily dose of 800 µg).

Treatment of Mild to Moderate Uncomplicated Acute Rhinosinusitis: Patients should not use NASONEX without an antibiotic if bacterial infection of the sinuses is present or suspected.

Adults (including geriatric patients) and children 12 years of age and older: The usual recommended dose is two sprays (50 µg/spray) in each nostril twice daily (total daily dose of 400 µg).

If signs or symptoms of severe bacterial infection are observed during treatment (such as fever, persistent severe unilateral facial/tooth pain, orbital or peri-orbital facial swelling, or worsening of symptoms after an initial improvement), the patient should be advised to consult their physician immediately, at which time the physician may advise the patient to stop using NASONEX.

Safety and efficacy of NASONEX in the treatment of symptoms associated with mild to moderate uncomplicated acute rhinosinusitis beyond 15 days have not been evaluated.

Treatment of Nasal Polyps: Adults (including geriatric patients) and adolescents 18 years of age and older: The usual recommended dose is two sprays (50 µg/spray) in each nostril twice daily (total daily dose of 400 µg).

Once the symptoms are controlled, dose reduction to two sprays (50 µg/spray) in each nostril once daily (total daily dose 200 µg) may be effective for continued treatment.

Efficacy and safety studies of NASONEX for the treatment of nasal polyps were four months in duration.

INFORMATION FOR THE PATIENT: Published in e-CPS, available by subscription at www.e-cps.ca.

SUPPLIED: NASONEX is formulated as an aqueous nasal suspension for nasal administration via a metered-dose manual pump spray delivering 140 doses. Each actuation delivers approximately 100 mg of mometasone furoate suspension, containing mometasone furoate monohydrate equivalent to 50 µg mometasone furoate. Nonmedicinal ingredients: benzalkonium chloride, citric acid, dispersible cellulose BP 65 cps (carboxymethylcellulose sodium, microcrystalline cellulose), glycerol, polysorbate 80, purified water and sodium citrate dihydrate. Single packs (1 bottle) or dual packs (2 bottles). A sample size (40 doses) is also available. Store between 2 and 25°C and protect from light. Do not freeze.

Natrecor™ Ⓟ
nesiritide
Recombinant Human B-type Natriuretic Peptide (rhBNP)

Janssen-Ortho

Date of Preparation: November 8, 2007
Date of Revision: June 30, 2009

Conditional market authorization has been issued for NATRECOR for the treatment of hospitalized symptomatic Acute Decompensated Heart Failure (ADHF) patients, presenting with moderate to severe dyspnea. These are patients who present with signs and symptoms of persistent heart failure despite 2 hours of treatment with intravenous loop diuretics. This authorization is conditional upon further confirmation of clinical benefit. Patients should be advised of the conditional nature of the authorization.

SUMMARY PRODUCT INFORMATION:

Route of Administration	Dosage Form/ Strength	Clinically Relevant Nonmedicinal Ingredients
Intravenous infusion only	Lyophilized powder for injection 1.5 mg in a 5 mL vial	None For a complete listing see Dosage Forms, Composition and Packaging.

DESCRIPTION: NATRECOR (nesiritide) is a sterile, purified preparation of a new drug class, human B-type natriuretic peptide (hBNP), and is manufactured from *E. coli* using recombinant DNA technology. Nesiritide has a molecular weight of 3464 g/mol and an empirical formula of $C_{143}H_{244}N_{50}O_{42}S_4$. Nesiritide has the same 32 amino acid sequence as the endogenous peptide, which is produced by the ventricular myocardium.

NATRECOR is formulated as the citrate salt of recombinant hBNP and is provided in a sterile, single-use vial. Each 1.5 mg vial contains a white to off-white lyophilized powder for intravenous (IV) administration after reconstitution.

INDICATIONS AND CLINICAL USE: NATRECOR is indicated for the treatment of hospitalized symptomatic Acute Decompensated Heart Failure (ADHF) patients, presenting with moderate to severe dyspnea. These are patients who present with signs and symptoms of persistent heart failure despite 2 hours of treatment with intravenous loop diuretics.

Additional clinical efficacy parameters are being further assessed in a confirmatory phase III multinational study.

Geriatrics (>65 years of age): No dose adjustment is required in the elderly. Evidence from clinical studies suggests that when using NATRECOR in the geriatric population, no overall differences in effectiveness were observed between these subjects and younger subjects (see Warnings and Precautions, Special Populations, Geriatrics (>65 years of age)).

Pediatrics (<18 years of age): The safety and effectiveness of NATRECOR in pediatric patients have not been established.

CONTRAINDICATIONS: NATRECOR should not be used as primary therapy for patients with cardiogenic shock or in patients with a systolic blood pressure <90 mm Hg.

NATRECOR should not be used in patients who are hypersensitive to this drug or to any ingredient in the formulation or component of the container. For a complete listing, see Dosage Forms, Composition and Packaging.

WARNINGS AND PRECAUTIONS: Administration of NATRECOR should be avoided in patients suspected of having, or known to have, low cardiac filling pressures.

General: Parenteral administration of protein pharmaceuticals or *E. coli*-derived products should be attended by appropriate precautions in case of an allergic or untoward reaction. No serious allergic or anaphylactic reactions have been reported with NATRECOR.

NATRECOR is not recommended for patients for whom vasodilating agents are not appropriate, such as patients with significant valvular stenosis, restrictive or obstructive cardiomyopathy, constrictive pericarditis, pericardial tamponade, or other conditions in which cardiac output is dependent upon venous return, or for patients suspected of having low cardiac filling pressures.

Cardiovascular: As expected with an agent having potent vasodilator properties, NATRECOR may cause hypotension which is dose-dependent. In the VMAC (Vasodilation in the Management of Acute Congestive Heart Failure) trial, in patients given the recommended dose (2 µg/kg bolus followed by a 0.01 µg/kg/min infusion) or the adjustable dose, the incidence of symptomatic hypotension in the first 24 hours was similar for NATRECOR (4%) and IV nitroglycerin (5%). When hypotension occurred, the duration of symptomatic hypotension was longer with NATRECOR (mean duration was 2.2 hours) than with nitroglycerin (mean duration was 0.7 hours). In earlier trials, when NATRECOR was initiated at doses higher than the recommended 2 µg/kg bolus followed by a 0.01 µg/kg/min infusion (i.e. 0.015 and 0.03 µg/kg/min preceded by a small bolus), there were more hypotensive episodes and these were of greater intensity and duration. They were also more often symptomatic and/or more likely to require medical intervention (see Warnings and Precautions, Monitoring and Laboratory Tests and Adverse Reactions). The rate of symptomatic hypotension may be increased in patients with a blood pressure <100 mm Hg at baseline, and NATRECOR should be used cautiously in those patients.

The potential for hypotension may be increased by combining NATRECOR with other drugs that cause hypotension (see Drug Interactions).

Renal: Although NATRECOR is eliminated, in part, through renal clearance, clinical data suggest that dose adjustment is not required in patients with renal insufficiency. The effects of NATRECOR on pulmonary capillary wedge pressure (PCWP), cardiac index (CI), and systolic blood pressure (SBP) were not significantly different in patients with chronic renal insufficiency and patients with normal renal function (see Action and Clinical Pharmacology, Special Populations and Conditions, Renal Insufficiency).

NATRECOR may affect renal function in susceptible individuals. In patients with severe heart failure whose renal function may depend on the activity of the renin-angiotensin-aldosterone system, treatment with NATRECOR may be associated with azotemia.

In the 30-day follow-up period in the VMAC trial, 5 patients in the nitroglycerin group (2%) and 9 patients in the NATRECOR group using the recommended dose (3%) required first-time dialysis.

When NATRECOR was initiated at doses higher than the recommended dose of 0.01 µg/kg/min (0.015 and 0.03 µg/kg/min), there was an increased rate of elevated serum creatinine over baseline compared with standard therapies, although the rate of acute renal failure and need for dialysis was not increased.

Special Populations: Pregnant Women: It is not known whether NATRECOR can cause fetal harm when administered to pregnant women or can affect reproductive capacity. NATRECOR should be used during pregnancy only if the potential benefit to the mother outweighs the theoretical risk to the fetus.

Nursing Women: It is not known whether NATRECOR is excreted in human milk. Therefore, caution should be exercised when NATRECOR is administered to a nursing woman.

Pediatrics (<18 years of age): The safety and effectiveness of NATRECOR in pediatric patients have not been established.

Geriatrics (>65 years of age): NATRECOR has been shown to be well tolerated in patients with a safety profile broadly similar across a wide age range, including those 75 years or older. Of the total number of subjects in clinical trials treated with NATRECOR (n=941), 38% were 65 years or older and 16% were 75 years or older. No overall differences in effectiveness were observed between these subjects and younger subjects and clinical experience has not identified differences in responses between the elderly and younger patients. Some older individuals may experience a higher frequency of hypotension.

Monitoring and Laboratory Tests: NATRECOR should be administered only in settings where blood pressure can be monitored closely, and the dose of NATRECOR should be reduced or the drug discontinued in patients who develop hypotension (see Dosage and Administration). Monitoring of renal function is recommended (see Warnings and Precautions, Renal).

ADVERSE REACTIONS: Adverse Drug Reaction Overview: The overall safety database consists of 941 HF patients that enrolled in IV bolus, short infusion and long infusion studies. The nature and incidence of adverse events (AEs) that occurred during the NATRECOR clinical trial program have been well characterized and are consistent with the expected AE profile for the acutely decompensated HF population.

Patients in these studies had typical comorbidity such as diabetes, hypertension, renal insufficiency, arrhythmia and coronary artery disease. Therefore, NATRECOR has been evaluated in patients who are highly susceptible to adverse events and in whom a high reporting rate would be expected.

For the purposes of assessing the safety profile of NATRECOR, data have been reported at 24 hours and 14 days post-initiation of study medication. Data from the first 24-hour period is considered important since this is the period when treatment is aimed at producing rapid improvements in hemodynamic status and symptoms. Also, this is the time during which NATRECOR is actually being infused. Therefore, AEs during this period provide the clearest profile of drug treatment effect.

Clinical Trial Adverse Drug Reactions: Because clinical trials are conducted under very specific conditions the adverse reaction rates observed in the clinical trials may not reflect the rates observed in practice and should not be compared to the rates in the clinical trials of another drug. Adverse drug reaction information from clinical trials is useful for identifying drug-related adverse events and for approximating rates.

Adverse drug reactions that occurred with at least a 1% frequency during the first 24 hours of NATRECOR infusion are shown in Table 1.

Table 1: NATRECOR
Adverse Drug Reactions That Occurred with ≥1% Frequency During the First 24 Hours of NATRECOR Infusion

	VMAC Trial		Other Long Infusion Trials[b]		
				NATRECOR µg/kg/min	
Undesirable Effect	IV Nitroglycerin (n=216) %	NATRECOR Recommended Dose 0.010 µg/kg/min (n=273) %	Control[a] (n=256) %	0.015 (n=253) %	0.03 (n=246) %
Cardiovascular					
Hypotension	12	11	8	22	35
Symptomatic Hypotension	5	4	3	11	17
Asymptomatic Hypotension	8	8	5	12	20
Bradycardia	<1	1	<1	3	5
Body as a Whole					
Headache	20	8	9	9	7
Nervous					
Dizziness	2	3	3	6	5
Digestive					
Nausea	6	4	5	9	13
Vomiting	2	1	1	2	4
Urogenital					
Creatinine Increased	0	0	<1	2	2
Skin and Appendages					
Sweating	0	<1	<1	2	3
Pruritus	<1	0	<1	2	1
Rash	<1	1	1	0	<1

[a] Includes dobutamine, milrinone, nitroglycerin, placebo, dopamine, nitroprusside, or amrinone.
[b] Trials in which NATRECOR was administered as a continuous infusion for ≥24 hours.

In placebo and active-controlled clinical trials, NATRECOR has not been associated with an increase in atrial or ventricular tachyarrhythmias (VT). In placebo-controlled trials, the incidence of VT in both NATRECOR and placebo patients was 2%. In the PRECEDENT (Prospective Randomized Evaluation of Cardiac Ectopy with Dobutamine or NATRECOR Therapy) trial, the effects of NATRECOR (n=163) and dobutamine (n=83) on the provocation or aggravation of existing ventricular arrhythmias in patients with decompensated CHF was compared using Holter monitoring. Treatment with NATRECOR (0.015 and 0.03 µg/kg/min without an initial bolus) for 24 hours did not aggravate pre-existing VT or the frequency of premature ventricular beats, compared to a baseline 24-hour Holter tape.

Effect on Mortality: NATRECOR has not been studied in a trial designed or powered to assess mortality as a primary or key secondary endpoint.

A large double-blind controlled trial (VMAC) included 273 patients receiving NATRECOR and 216 patients receiving IV nitroglycerin. The mortality rates at thirty days from any cause were 8.1% in the NATRECOR arm and 5.1% in the nitroglycerin arm (hazard ratio of 1.56 [95% CI: 0.75-3.24]). The mortality rates at six months in patients receiving NATRECOR or nitroglycerin were 25.1% and 20.8% respectively (hazard ratio of 1.22 [95% CI: 0.83-1.79]).

In a pooled analysis of adequate and well-controlled clinical trials (Studies 311, 325, 326, 329 [PRECEDENT], 339 [VMAC], 341 [PROACTION], and 348 [FUSION I]), mortality with NATRECOR was compared with control treatment (30 day hazard ratio of 1.34 [95% CI: 0.85-2.11]). Of the 1059 patients treated with NATRECOR in these 7 trials, 58 died at 30 days of any cause (Kaplan-Meier estimate, 5.5%), whereas 28 of the 658 control patients died (Kaplan-Meier estimate, 4.3%).

All-cause mortality from 5 trials (Studies 325, 326, 329 [PRECEDENT], 339 [VMAC] and 341 [PROACTION] where 180-day mortality data were collected showed a 180-day hazard ratio of 1.08 [95% CI: 0.85-1.37]. In this analysis, 178/844 patients treated with NATRECOR (Kaplan-Meier estimate, 21.5%) and 114/560 control patients (Kaplan-Meier estimate, 20.7%) died of any cause.

There were few deaths in these studies, so the confidence limits around the hazard ratios were wide. The studies were small and some potentially important baseline imbalances existed among the treatment groups, the effects of which could not be ascertained.

Abnormal Hematologic and Clinical Chemistry Findings: In the VMAC trial, through day 30, the incidence of elevations in creatinine to >0.5 mg/dL above baseline was 28% and 21% in the NATRECOR (2 µg/kg bolus followed by 0.01 µg/kg/min) and nitroglycerin groups, respectively.

In the PRECEDENT trial, the incidence of elevations in serum creatinine to >0.5 mg/dL above baseline through day 14 was higher in the NATRECOR 0.015 µg/kg/min group (17%) and the NATRECOR 0.03 µg/kg/min group (19%) than with standard therapy (11%).

Post-Market Adverse Drug Reactions: In addition to the previously mentioned clinical trials safety data, spontaneous adverse drug reactions (ADRs) from the worldwide post-marketing experience with NATRECOR are listed below.

The frequency provided is a reflection of reporting rates for spontaneous adverse drug reactions and does not represent true incidence or frequency as seen with clinical trials or epidemiologic studies.

ADRs reported in the post-marketing period by System Organ Class include:
Immune System Disorders: Very rare—hypersensitivity reactions.

DRUG INTERACTIONS: Overview: No trials specifically examining potential drug interactions with NATRECOR were conducted, although many concomitant drugs were used in clinical trials.
Drug-Drug Interactions: During clinical studies, NATRECOR was administered concomitantly with other medications, including: diuretics, digoxin, oral ACE inhibitors, anticoagulants, oral nitrates, 3-hydroxy-3-methylglutaryl coenzyme A (HMG-CoA) reductase inhibitors, class III antiarrhythmics, beta-blockers, dobutamine, calcium channel blockers, angiotensin II receptor antagonists, and dopamine. Although pharmacokinetic (PK) interactions were not specifically assessed, there did not appear to be evidence suggesting any clinically significant PK interaction, except for an increase in symptomatic hypotension in patients receiving oral ACE inhibitors (see Warnings and Precautions, Cardiovascular). The co-administration of NATRECOR with enalapril did not have significant effects on the PK of NATRECOR. The PK effect of co-administration of NATRECOR with other IV vasodilators such as nitroglycerin, nitroprusside, milrinone, or IV ACE inhibitors has not been evaluated.
Drug-Food Interactions: Interactions with food have not been established.
Drug-Herb Interactions: Interactions with herbal products have not been established.
Drug-Laboratory Test Interactions: Interactions with laboratory tests have not been established.
Chemical/Physical Interactions: NATRECOR is physically and/or chemically incompatible with injectable formulations of heparin, insulin, ethacrynate sodium, bumetanide, enalaprilat, hydralazine, and furosemide. These drugs should not be co-administered as infusions with NATRECOR through the same IV catheter. The preservative sodium metabisulfite is incompatible with NATRECOR. Injectable drugs that contain sodium metabisulfite should not be administered in the same infusion line as NATRECOR (see Dosage and Administration, Dosing Instructions, Chemical/Physical Interactions).

DOSAGE AND ADMINISTRATION:

NATRECOR (nesiritide) is for intravenous use only.
Dosing Considerations: The dose-limiting side effect of NATRECOR is hypotension.

NATRECOR should **not** be titrated at frequent intervals as is done with other IV agents that have a shorter half-life.
Recommended Dose and Dosage Adjustment: The NATRECOR bolus must be drawn from the prepared infusion bag.

The recommended dose of NATRECOR is an IV bolus of 2 μg/kg followed by a continuous infusion of 0.01 μg/kg/min. NATRECOR should not be initiated at a dose that is above the recommended dose (see Dosage and Administration, Administration).

The use of NATRECOR at doses higher than recommended is not encouraged. However, in the few cases where, following physician assessment further optimization of clinical status may be required, the NATRECOR infusion dose may be increased or decreased according to hemodynamic and clinical response. If an increase in dose is required, the infusion dose may be increased by 0.005 μg/kg/min (preceded by a bolus of 1 μg/kg) no more frequently than every 3 hours up to a maximum dose of 0.03 μg/kg/min.

Blood pressure should be monitored closely during NATRECOR administration. There is limited experience with administering NATRECOR for longer than 48 hours. If hypotension occurs during the administration of NATRECOR, the dose should be reduced or discontinued and other measures to support blood pressure should be started (IV fluids, changes in body position).

In the VMAC trial, when symptomatic hypotension occurred, NATRECOR was discontinued and subsequently could be restarted at a dose that was reduced by 30% (with no bolus administration) once the patient was stabilized. Because hypotension caused by NATRECOR may be prolonged (up to hours), a period of observation may be necessary before restarting the drug.
Administration: Preparation, Reconstitution and Special Handling Instructions: The NATRECOR bolus must be drawn from the prepared infusion bag.

1. Reconstitute one 1.5 mg vial of NATRECOR by adding 5 mL of diluent removed from a pre-filled 250 mL plastic IV bag containing the diluent of choice. After reconstitution of the vial, each mL contains 0.32 mg of nesiritide. The following preservative-free diluents are recommended for reconstitution: 5% Dextrose Injection (D5W), USP; 0.9% Sodium Chloride Injection, USP; 5% Dextrose and 0.45% Sodium Chloride Injection, USP, or 5% Dextrose and 0.2% Sodium Chloride Injection, USP. Aseptic technique must be used in the reconstitution procedure.
2. Do not shake the vial. Rock the vial gently so that all surfaces, including the stopper, are in contact with the diluent to ensure complete reconstitution. Use only a clear, essentially colourless solution.

   Reconstituted single use vials of NATRECOR should be added to the 250 mL plastic IV bag and used immediately (within 3 hours). If the reconstituted vial is not used right away, store under refrigeration (2-8°C). Do not freeze. Protect from light. As NATRECOR contains no antimicrobial preservative, the storage of the reconstituted vial is not recommended. However, when prepared under aseptic conditions, the chemical and physical stability of the reconstituted vial has been demonstrated for 24 hours at 25°C.
3. **Withdraw the entire contents of the reconstituted NATRECOR vial** and add to the 250 mL plastic IV bag. This will yield a solution with a concentration of NATRECOR of approximately 6 μg/mL. The IV bag should be inverted several times to ensure complete mixing of the solution.
4. Use the reconstituted and diluted solution, to start dosing, immediately (within 3 hours). As NATRECOR contains no antimicrobial preservative, storage of the reconstituted solution is not recommended. However, when prepared under aseptic conditions, the chemical and physical stability of the reconstituted and diluted solution has been demonstrated for 24 hours at 25°C. Parenteral drug products should be inspected visually for particulate matter and discoloration prior to administration, whenever solution and container permit.

Table 2: NATRECOR

Reconstitution and Dilution of NATRECOR

Vial Size	Volume of Diluent to Be Added to Vial	Approximate Available Volume	Nominal Concentration per mL	Concentration per 250 mL Bag
5 mL	5 mL	5 mL	0.32 mg of nesiritide	6 μg/mL

Dosing Instructions: Prime the IV tubing with an infusion of 5 mL prior to connecting to the patient's vascular access port and prior to administering the bolus or starting the infusion.

The administration of the recommended dose of NATRECOR is a two-step process:
Step 1. Administration of the IV Bolus: After preparation of the infusion bag, as described previously, withdraw the bolus volume (see Table 3) from the NATRECOR infusion bag, and administer it over approximately 60 seconds through an IV port in the tubing.

Table 3: NATRECOR

Weight-Adjusted Bolus Volume

Bolus Volume (mL)=Patient Weight (kg)/3
NATRECOR Weight-Adjusted Bolus Volume Administered Over 60 Seconds
(Final Concentration=6 μg/mL)

Patient Weight (kg)	Volume of Bolus (mL=kg/3)
60	20
70	23.3
80	26.7
90	30
100	33.3
110	36.7

Step 2. Administration of the Continuous Infusion: Immediately following the administration of the bolus, infuse NATRECOR at a flow rate of 0.1 mL/kg/hr. This will deliver a NATRECOR infusion dose of 0.01 μg/kg/min. To calculate the infusion flow rate to deliver a 0.01 μg/kg/min dose, use the following formula (see Table 4).

Table 4: NATRECOR

Weight-Adjusted Infusion Flow Rate for Dosing

Infusion Flow Rate (mL/hr)=Patient Weight (kg)×0.1
NATRECOR Weight-Adjusted Infusion Flow Rate for a 0.01 μg/kg/min Dose following Bolus
(Final Concentration=6 μg/mL)

Patient Weight (kg)	Infusion Flow Rate (mL/hr)
60	6
70	7
80	8
90	9
100	10
110	11

Chemical/Physical Interactions: NATRECOR is physically and/or chemically incompatible with injectable formulations of heparin, insulin, ethacrynate sodium, bumetanide, enalaprilat, hydralazine, and furosemide. These drugs should not be co-administered as infusions with NATRECOR through the same IV catheter. The preservative sodium metabisulfite is incompatible with NATRECOR. Injectable drugs that contain sodium metabisulfite should not be administered in the same infusion line as NATRECOR. The catheter must be flushed between administration of NATRECOR and incompatible drugs.

NATRECOR binds to heparin and therefore could bind to the heparin lining of a heparin-coated catheter, decreasing the amount of NATRECOR delivered to the patient for some period of time. Therefore, NATRECOR must **not** be administered through a central heparin-coated catheter. Concomitant administration of a heparin infusion through a separate catheter is acceptable.

OVERDOSAGE:
Overdose with NATRECOR therapy has been reported and is primarily the result of either a miscalculated dose or a mechanical error such as an infusion pump malfunction or an infusion pump programming error. The most frequently reported adverse event with NATRECOR overdose is hypotension, which may be asymptomatic and most often resolves with drug stoppage, although, in some cases, hypotension may persist for several hours after discontinuation (see Warnings and Precautions). Treatment of NATRECOR overdose should include drug discontinuation and the administration of supportive measures.

For management of a suspected drug overdose, CPhA recommends that you contact your **regional Poison Control Centre**. See the *CPS* Directory section for a list of Poison Control Centres.

ACTION AND CLINICAL PHARMACOLOGY: Mechanism of Action: Human BNP (hBNP) acts on the cardio-renal axis by exerting effects on the vasculature, the heart and the kidneys. Human BNP binds to the particulate guanylate cyclase receptor of vascular smooth muscle and endothelial cells, leading to increased intracellular concentrations of guanosine 3'5'-cyclic monophosphate (cGMP) and smooth muscle cell relaxation. Cyclic GMP serves as a second messenger to dilate veins and arteries. Nesiritide has been shown to relax isolated human arterial and venous tissue preparations that were precontracted with either endothelin-1 or the alpha-adrenergic agonist, phenylephrine. hBNP also suppresses the renin-angiotensin-aldosterone system (RAAS) and has natriuretic and diuretic effects.

In human studies, nesiritide produced dose-dependent reductions in pulmonary capillary wedge pressure (PCWP) and systemic arterial pressure in patients with heart failure.

In animals, nesiritide had no effects on cardiac contractility or on measures of cardiac electrophysiology such as atrial and ventricular effective refractory times or atrioventricular node conduction.
Pharmacodynamics: The recommended dosing regimen of NATRECOR is a 2 μg/kg IV bolus followed by an intravenous infusion dose of 0.01 μg/kg/min. With this dosing regimen, 60% of the 3-hour effect on PCWP reduction is achieved within 15 minutes after the bolus, reaching 95% of the 3-hour effect within 1 hour. Approximately 70% of the 3-hour effect on SBP reduction is reached within 15 minutes. The pharmacodynamic half-life of the onset and offset of the hemodynamic effect of NATRECOR is longer than the pharmacokinetic half-life of 18 minutes. In patients who developed symptomatic hypotension in the VMAC trial, half of the recovery of SBP toward the baseline value after discontinuation or reduction of the dose of NATRECOR was observed in about 60 minutes. When higher doses of NATRECOR were infused, the duration of hypotension was sometimes several hours.
Pharmacokinetics: In patients with congestive heart failure (CHF), NATRECOR administered intravenously by infusion or bolus exhibits biphasic disposition from the plasma.

At steady state, plasma BNP levels increase from baseline endogenous levels by approximately 3-fold to 6-fold with NATRECOR infusion doses ranging from 0.01 to 0.03 μg/kg/min. The mean terminal elimination half-life ($t_{1/2}$) of nesiritide is approximately 18 minutes. The mean initial elimination phase was estimated to be approximately 2 minutes. Steady-state volume of distribution, plasma clearance, and terminal elimination half-life were not dose dependent.
Distribution: The mean volume of distribution of the central compartment (V_c) of nesiritide was estimated to be 0.073 (range 0.034 to 0.59) L/kg and the mean steady-state volume of distribution (V_{ss}) was 0.19 (range 0.005 to 0.177) L/kg.
Excretion: Human BNP is cleared from the circulation via the following three independent mechanisms, in order of decreasing importance: 1) binding to cell surface clearance receptors with subsequent cellular internalization and lysosomal proteolysis; 2) proteolytic cleavage of the peptide by endopeptidases, such as neutral endopeptidase, which are present on the vascular lumenal surface; 3) renal filtration.

Nesiritide has a mean terminal elimination half-life of 18 minutes and a mean clearance of 9.2 (range 2.4 to 44.6) mL/min/kg.
Special Populations and Conditions: Pediatrics: There are no pharmacokinetic data in pediatric patients.
Geriatrics: Clearance of nesiritide is not influenced significantly by age. The safety profile in the elderly is consistent with that in the general population, further supporting no requirement for dosage adjustment in the elderly.
Gender and Race: The effects of gender and race on the pharmacokinetics of nesiritide have not been evaluated.
Hepatic Insufficiency: While hepatically impaired patients were not excluded from the clinical program, the effects of hepatic impairment on pharmacokinetic parameters of nesiritide have not been specifically assessed.
Renal Insufficiency: Although nesiritide is eliminated, in part, through renal clearance, clinical data suggest that dose adjustment is not required in patients with renal insufficiency. The effects of nesiritide on PCWP, cardiac index (CI), and systolic blood pressure (SBP) were not significantly different in patients with chronic renal insufficiency (baseline serum creatinine ranging from 2 mg/dL to 4.3 mg/dL), and patients with normal renal function. The population pharmacokinetic (PK) analyses carried out to determine the effects of demographics and clinical variables on PK parameters showed that clearance of nesiritide is proportional to body weight, supporting the administration of weight-adjusted dosing of nesiritide (i.e., administration on a μg/kg/min basis). Clearance was not influenced significantly by age, gender, race/ethnicity, baseline endogenous hBNP concentration, severity of CHF (as indicated by baseline PCWP, baseline CI, or New York Heart Association [NYHA] classification), or concomitant administration of an ACE inhibitor.
STORAGE AND STABILITY: Store NATRECOR at 2-25°C. Do not freeze. Keep in carton until time of use, to protect from light.

For storage of reconstituted vial and reconstituted and diluted solution, see Preparation, Reconstitution and Special Handling Instructions in Dosage and Administration.
INFORMATION FOR THE PATIENT: Published in e-CPS, available by subscription at www.e-cps.ca.
DOSAGE FORMS, COMPOSITION AND PACKAGING: Each vial of sterile, white to off-white, lyophilized powder contains: nesiritide 1.5 mg. Nonmedicinal ingredients: citric acid monohydrate, mannitol and sodium citrate dihydrate. Boxes of 1 single-use 5 mL vial.

(Shown in Product Identification Section)

Navelbine® ℞
vinorelbine tartrate
Antineoplastic

Pierre Fabre Pharma

Caution: Vinorelbine is a cytotoxic drug and should be used only by physicians experienced with cancer chemotherapeutic drugs. Blood counts should be taken prior to each dose. The dosage should be reduced or the drug discontinued upon evidence of abnormal depression of the bone marrow.

This preparation is for intravenous administration only. Intrathecal administration of other vinca alkaloids has resulted in death. Syringes containing this product should be labelled "Warning - for intravenous use only. Fatal if given intrathecally".

PHARMACOLOGY: Vinorelbine is a novel vinca alkaloid which interferes with microtubule assembly. Vinca alkaloids are structurally similar compounds comprising 2 multiringed units, vindoline and catharanthine. Vinorelbine is a vinca alkaloid in which the catharanthine unit is the site of structural modification. This structural change imparts unique pharmacologic properties which may translate into clinical benefits for patients with various malignancies. The antitumor activity of vinorelbine is thought to be due primarily to inhibition of mitosis at metaphase through its interaction with tubulin. Vinorelbine may also interfere with amino acid, cyclic AMP, and glutathione metabolism; calmodulin-dependent Ca^{++}-transport ATPase activity; cellular respiration; and nucleic acid and lipid biosynthesis.

Pharmacokinetics: Following i.v. administration, vinorelbine concentration in plasma decays in a triphasic manner. The initial rapid decline represents distribution of drug to peripheral compartments and metabolism of the drug. The prolonged terminal phase is due to relatively slow efflux of vinorelbine from peripheral compartments. The terminal phase half-life averaged 27.7 to 43.6 hours; the mean plasma clearances ranged from 0.97 to 1.26 L/hr/kg; and steady state volume of distribution (V_{ss}) values ranged from 25.4 to 40.1 L/kg.

The disposition of radiolabeled vinorelbine has been studied in a limited number of patients. Approximately 18% of the administered dose was recovered in the urine and 46% in the feces. Incomplete recovery in humans is consistent with results in animals. A separate study of the urinary excretion of vinorelbine showed that 10.9%±0.7% of a 30 mg/m² i.v. dose was excreted unchanged in the urine.

One metabolite of vinorelbine, deacetylvinorelbine, has been shown to possess antitumor activity. This metabolite has been detected but not quantified in human plasma. The effects of renal or hepatic dysfunction on the disposition of vinorelbine have not been assessed.

The pharmacokinetics of vinorelbine are not influenced by the concurrent administration of cisplatin with vinorelbine (see Precautions, Drug Interactions).

INDICATIONS: In the treatment of advanced non-small cell lung cancer (NSCLC), as a single agent or in combination.

Also indicated for the treatment of patients with metastatic breast cancer who have failed standard first-line chemotherapy for metastatic disease. In addition, vinorelbine is indicated for the treatment of patients with metastatic breast cancer who have relapsed within 6 months of anthracycline-based adjuvant therapy.

CONTRAINDICATIONS: In patients with known hypersensitivity to vinorelbine.

As with other vinca alkaloids, vinorelbine is contraindicated in patients who have drug-induced severe granulocytopenia or severe thrombocytopenia.

WARNINGS: Vinorelbine is a cytotoxic drug and should be used only by physicians experienced with cancer chemotherapeutic drugs. Blood counts should be taken prior to each dose. Discontinue or reduce the dosage upon evidence of abnormal depression of the bone marrow.

Vinorelbine is for i.v. use only. Vinorelbine is a moderate vesicant and can produce phlebitis or extravasation injury. Inadequate flushing of the vein after peripheral administration may increase the risk of phlebitis.

It is extremely important that the needle be properly positioned in the vein before this product is injected. If leakage into surrounding tissue should occur during i.v. administration of vinorelbine, it may cause severe irritation. The injection should be discontinued immediately, and any remaining portion of the dose should then be introduced into another vein.

A low incidence of death (1%) due to neutropenic sepsis has been reported (see Adverse Effects). Bone marrow toxicity, specifically granulocytopenia, is dose-limiting. Complete blood counts with differentials should be performed and results reviewed prior to each dose of vinorelbine. Vinorelbine should not be administered to patients with granulocyte counts <1000 cells/mm³. Patients developing severe granulocytopenia should be monitored carefully for evidence of infection and/or fever (see Dosage).

Pregnancy: There are no studies in pregnant women. Vinorelbine has been shown to be embryotoxic and/or fetotoxic in animals. Vinorelbine should not be used in pregnancy.

Lactation: It is not known whether the drug is excreted in human milk. Because many drugs are excreted in human milk and because of its potential for serious adverse reactions in nursing infants, it is recommended that nursing be discontinued in women who are receiving therapy with vinorelbine.

Children: Safety and effectiveness in children have not been established.

PRECAUTIONS: General: In all instances where the use of vinorelbine is considered for chemotherapy, the physician must evaluate the need and usefulness of the drug against the risk of adverse events. Most drug-related adverse reactions are reversible. If severe adverse events occur, the drug should be reduced in dosage or discontinued and appropriate corrective measures should be taken based on the clinical judgment of the physician. Reinstitution of therapy with vinorelbine should be carried out with caution and alertness as to possible recurrence of toxicity.

Vinorelbine should be used with extreme caution in patients whose bone marrow reserve may have been compromised by prior irradiation or chemotherapy, or whose marrow function is recovering from previous chemotherapy.

Administration of vinorelbine to patients with prior radiation therapy may result in radiation recall reactions (see Adverse Effects and Drug Interactions).

Patients with a prior history of pre-existing neuropathy, regardless of etiology, should be monitored for new or worsening signs and symptoms of neuropathy while receiving vinorelbine.

Acute shortness of breath and severe bronchospasm have been reported infrequently following the administration of vinorelbine and of other vinca alkaloids. These events have been encountered most commonly when the vinca alkaloid was used in combination with mitomycin and may require aggressive treatment, particularly when there is pre-existing pulmonary dysfunction. Bronchodilators, steroids and/or oxygen have produced symptomatic relief.

Care must be exercised to avoid contamination of the eye with vinorelbine. Accidental exposure should be treated immediately with a large volume of irrigation solution (water or sodium chloride).

Geriatrics: Of the total number of patients in North American clinical studies of i.v. vinorelbine, approximately one-third were 65 years of age or greater. No overall differences in effectiveness or safety were observed between these patients and younger patients. Other reported clinical experience has not identified differences in responses between the elderly and younger patients, but greater sensitivity of some older individuals cannot be ruled out.

Pregnancy: See Warnings.

Hematologic: Since dose-limiting clinical toxicity is the result of depression of the white blood cell count, it is imperative that complete blood counts with differentials be obtained prior to each dose of vinorelbine (see Adverse Effects, Hematologic).

Hepatic: There is no evidence that the toxicity of vinorelbine is enhanced in patients with elevated liver enzymes; no data are available for patients with severe baseline cholestasis. However, pharmacologic evidence suggests that the liver plays an important role in the metabolism of vinorelbine. Although there are no data available from patients with severe liver disease, caution should be exercised when administering vinorelbine to patients with severe hepatic injury or impairment.

Drug Interactions: Acute pulmonary reactions have been reported with vinorelbine and other vinca alkaloids used in conjunction with mitomycin (see General). Vinorelbine should be administered with caution in combination with mitomycin. Although the pharmacokinetics of vinorelbine are not influenced by the concurrent administration of cisplatin, the incidence of toxicities, specifically granulocytopenia, high-frequency hearing loss and tinnitus, with the combination of vinorelbine and cisplatin is higher than with single-agent vinorelbine.

Patients who receive vinorelbine and paclitaxel, either concomitantly or sequentially, should be monitored for signs and symptoms of neuropathy. Administration of vinorelbine to patients with prior or concomitant radiation therapy may result in radiosensitizing effects.

Information to Be Provided to the Patient: Patients should be informed that vinorelbine is a vesicant and can produce phlebitis or extravasation injury, and that the major acute toxicities of vinorelbine are related to bone marrow toxicity, specifically granulocytopenia with increased susceptibility to infection, and neuropathy. They should also be advised to report fever or chills immediately. Vinorelbine should not be used in pregnancy unless the physician feels the potential benefit justifies the risk of potential harm to the fetus.

ADVERSE EFFECTS: Data in Table 1 and Table 2 are based on the experience of 365 patients (143 patients with NSCLC; 222 patients with advanced breast cancer) for whom a complete safety database was available and who were treated with vinorelbine as a single agent in 3 North American trials (1 NSCLC trial and 2 advanced breast cancer trials). Patients treated for breast cancer were allowed to have received adjuvant chemotherapy in both trials, and in one, up to 2 prior regimens for advanced disease. The dosing schedule was 30 mg/m² i.v. vinorelbine on a weekly basis.

Table 1: Navelbine

Hematologic Adverse Events and Clinical Chemistry Elevations in 365 Patients Receiving Single-agent Navelbine that are Possibly Attributable to the Study Medication[a,b]

Hematology		ABC (%)	NSCLC (%)
Granulocytopenia	<2000 cells/mm³ <500 cells/mm³	96 41	80 28
Leukopenia	<4000 cells/mm³ <1000 cells/mm³	99 16	81 12
Thrombocytopenia	<100 000 cells/mm³ <50 000 cells/mm³	6 <1	4 1
Anemia	<11 g/dL Hgb <8 g/dL Hgb	87 14	77 1
Hospitalizations due to granulocytopenic complications		9	8

Clinical Chemistry Elevations		% Incidence All Grades		% Incidence Grade 3		% Incidence Grade 4	
		ABC	NSCLC	ABC	NSCLC	ABC	NSCLC
Total Bilirubin							
NSCLC: ABC:	n=137 n=214	14	9	4	3	3	2
AST							
NSCLC: ABC:	n=133 n=213	74	54	7	2	<1	1

[a] Grade based on modified criteria of the National Cancer Institute.
[b] Patients with NSCLC had not received prior chemotherapy. The majority of patients with advanced breast cancer had received prior chemotherapy.

Legend:
ABC=Advanced Breast Cancer.
NSCLC=Non-Small Cell Lung Cancer.

Table 2: Navelbine

Summary of Adverse Events Occurring in ≥5% of 365 Patients Receiving Single-agent Navelbine that are Possibly Attributable to the Study Medication[a,b]

Adverse Event	% Incidence All Grades		% Incidence Grade 3		% Incidence Grade 4	
	ABC n=222	NSCLC n=143	ABC n=222	NSCLC n=143	ABC n=222	NSCLC n=143
General						
Injection Site Reaction	21	38	1	5	0	0
Asthenia	41	25	8	5	0	0
Pain	16	15	3	2	0	0
Pain Injection Site	18	13	3	1	0	0
Fever	19	10	1	0	0	1
Pain Abdomen	12	6	1	1	0	0
Pain Chest	8	5	1	2	0	0
Phlebitis	5	10	0	1	0	0
Digestive						
Nausea	50	33	3	1	0	0
Constipation	38	28	3	2	0	0
Anorexia	19	16	<1	2	0	0
Stomatitis	16	15	0	0	0	0
Vomiting	23	14	2	1	0	0
Diarrhea	20	13	<1	1	0	0
Musculoskeletal						
Myasthenia	9	5	2	1	<1	0

(cont'd)

Table 2: Navelbine *(cont'd)*

Summary of Adverse Events Occurring in ≥5% of 365 Patients Receiving Single-agent Navelbine that are Possibly Attributable to the Study Medication[a,b]

Adverse Event	% Incidence All Grades ABC n=222	% Incidence All Grades NSCLC n=143	% Incidence Grade 3 ABC n=222	% Incidence Grade 3 NSCLC n=143	% Incidence Grade 4 ABC n=222	% Incidence Grade 4 NSCLC n=143
Nervous System						
Paresthesia	20	11	0	1	0	0
Hypesthesia	11	10	<1	0	<1	0
Respiratory						
Dyspnea	9	3	1	2	1	0
Skin and Appendages						
Alopecia	12	12	0	1	0	0
Rash	5	5	0	0	0	0

[a] Grade based on modified criteria of the National Cancer Institute.
[b] Patients with NSCLC had not received prior chemotherapy. The majority of patients with advanced breast cancer had received prior chemotherapy.
Legend:
ABC=Advanced Breast Cancer.
NSCLC=Non-Small Cell Lung Cancer.

Hematologic: Granulocytopenia was the major dose-limiting toxicity with vinorelbine; it was generally reversible and not cumulative over time. Granulocyte nadirs occurred 7 to 10 days after the dose and usually recovered within the following 7 to 14 days. Granulocytopenia resulted in hospitalizations for fever and/or sepsis in 8% of NSCLC and 9% of breast cancer patients. Septic deaths occurred in approximately 1% of patients.

Grade 3 or 4 anemia occurred in 1% of lung cancer and 14% of breast cancer patients. Blood products were administered to 18% of patients who received vinorelbine. The incidence of Grade 3 and 4 thrombocytopenia was less than 1%.

Neurologic: Mild to moderate peripheral neuropathy manifested by paresthesia and hypesthesia were the most frequently reported neurologic toxicities (10 to 20%, see Table 2). Loss of deep tendon reflexes occurred in less than 5% of patients. The development of severe peripheral neuropathy was unusual.

Dermatologic: Alopecia was reported in only 12% of patients and was usually mild.

Vinorelbine is a moderate vesicant. Injection site reactions, including erythema, pain at injection site, and vein discoloration occurred in approximately one-third of all patients; 2% were severe. Chemical phlebitis along the vein proximal to the site of injection was reported.

Gastrointestinal: Mild or moderate nausea occurred in 32% of NSCLC and 47% of breast cancer patients treated with vinorelbine. Severe nausea was infrequent (1% and 3% in NSCLC and breast cancer patients, respectively). Prophylactic administration of antiemetics was not routine in patients treated with single-agent vinorelbine. Constipation occurred in approximately 28% of NSCLC and 38% of breast cancer patients, with paralytic ileus occurring in less than 2% of patients. Vomiting, diarrhea, anorexia and stomatitis were usually mild or moderate and occurred in less than 20% of patients.

Hepatic: Transient elevations of liver enzymes were reported without clinical symptoms.

Cardiovascular: Chest pain was reported in 5% of NSCLC and 8% of breast cancer patients. Most reports of chest pain were in patients who had either a history of cardiovascular disease or tumor within the chest. There have been rare reports of myocardial infarction; however, these have not been shown definitely attributable to vinorelbine.

Pulmonary: Shortness of breath was reported in 3% of NSCLC and 9% of breast cancer patients and was severe in 2% of each patient population. Interstitial pulmonary changes have been documented in a few patients.

Other: Asthenia occurred in approximately 25% of patients with NSCLC and 41% of patients with breast cancer. It was usually mild or moderate but tended to increase with cumulative dosing.

Other toxicities that have been reported in ≤ 5% of patients include jaw pain, myalgia, arthralgia, headache, dysphagia and rash. Hemorrhagic cystitis and the syndrome of inappropriate ADH secretion were reported in <1% of patients. The treatment of these entities are mainly symptomatic. The treatment of hemorrhagic cystitis is i.v. fluids for forced diuresis and/or irrigation of the bladder. For the treatment of SIADH, please refer to the major textbooks of medicine.

Observed During Clinical Practice: In a randomized study in NSCLC patients, 206 patients received treatment with vinorelbine plus cisplatin and 206 patients received single-agent vinorelbine. The incidence of severe nausea and vomiting was 30% for vinorelbine/cisplatin compared to <2% for single-agent vinorelbine. Cisplatin did not appear to increase the incidence of neurotoxicity observed with single-agent vinorelbine. However, myelosuppression, specifically Grade 3 and 4 granulocytopenia, was greater with the combination of vinorelbine/cisplatin (79%) than with single-agent vinorelbine (53%). The incidence of fever and infection may be increased with the combination.

In addition to adverse events reported from clinical trials, the following events have been identified during postmarketing use of vinorelbine. Because they are reported voluntarily from a population of unknown size, estimates of frequency cannot be made. These events have been chosen for inclusion due to combination of their seriousness, frequency of reporting, or potential causal connection to vinorelbine or a combination of these factors.

Body as a Whole: Systemic allergic reactions reported as anaphylaxis, pruritus, urticaria and angioedema, flushing and radiation recall events such as dermatitis and esophagitis (see Precautions) have been reported.

Hematologic: Thromboembolic events including pulmonary embolus and deep venous thrombosis have been reported, primarily in seriously ill and debilitated patients with known predisposing risk factors for these events.

Neurologic: Peripheral neurotoxicities such as, but not limited to, muscle weakness and disturbance of gait have been observed in patients with and without prior symptoms. Vestibular and auditory deficits have been observed with vinorelbine, usually when used in combination with cisplatin. There may be increased potential for neurotoxicity in patients with pre-existing neuropathy, regardless of etiology, who receive vinorelbine. Patients who receive vinorelbine and paclitaxel, either concomitantly or sequentially, should be monitored for signs and symptoms of neuropathy (see Precautions).

Skin: Injection site reactions, including localized rash and urticaria, blister formation and skin sloughing have been observed in clinical practice. Some of these reactions may be delayed in appearance.

Gastrointestinal: Dysphagia and mucositis have been reported.

Cardiovascular: Hypertension, hypotension, vasodilation, tachycardia and pulmonary edema have been reported.

Pulmonary: Pneumonia has been reported.

Vinorelbine can produce acute and subacute pulmonary reactions. The acute reaction usually resembles an allergic event and may respond to bronchodilators. Subacute pulmonary reactions may occur shortly after drug administration and may be characterized by cough, dyspnea, hypoxemia, and interstitial infiltration. Subacute pulmonary reactions may respond to corticosteroid therapy.

Musculoskeletal: Headache has been reported with and without other musculoskeletal aches and pains.

Other: Pain in tumor-containing tissue, back pain and abdominal pain have been reported. Electrolyte abnormalities, including hyponatremia consistent with the syndrome of inappropriate ADH secretion, have been reported in seriously ill and debilitated patients.

Combination Use: Patients with prior exposure to paclitaxel and who have demonstrated neuropathy should be monitored closely for new or worsening neuropathy. Patients who have experienced neuropathy with previous drug regimens should be monitored for symptoms of neuropathy while receiving vinorelbine. Vinorelbine may result in radiosensitizing effects with prior or concomitant radiation therapy (see Precautions).

OVERDOSE:

Symptoms: The primary anticipated complications of overdosage would consist of bone marrow suppression and peripheral neurotoxicity.

Treatment: There is no known antidote for vinorelbine overdosage. Overdoses involving quantities up to 10 times the recommended dose (30 mg/m²) have been reported. The toxicities described were consistent with those listed in the Adverse Effects section including paralytic ileus, stomatitis, and esophagitis. Bone marrow aplasia, sepsis, and paresis have also been reported. Fatalities have occurred following overdose of vinorelbine. If overdosage occurs, general supportive measures together with appropriate blood transfusions, growth factors and antibiotics should be instituted as deemed necessary by the physician.

> For management of a suspected drug overdose, CPhA recommends that you contact your **regional Poison Control Centre**. See the *CPS* Directory section for a list of Poison Control Centres.

DOSAGE: This preparation is for i.v. administration only. It should be administered by individuals experienced in the administration of cancer chemotherapeutic drugs.

The usual initial dose is 30 mg/m² administered weekly. The recommended method of administration is an i.v. injection over 6 to 10 minutes. In controlled trials, single-agent vinorelbine was given weekly until progression or dose-limiting toxicity.

No dose adjustments are required for renal insufficiency. If moderate or severe neurotoxicity develops, vinorelbine should be discontinued. The dosage should be adjusted according to hematologic toxicity or hepatic insufficiency.

Dose Modifications for Hematologic Toxicity: Granulocyte counts should be ≥1000 cells/mm³ prior to the administration of vinorelbine. In the referenced North American trial, in which hematologic adverse events were observed, the dose adjustment scheme in Table 3 was employed and should be followed in patients receiving vinorelbine.

Table 3: Navelbine

Dose Adjustments Based on Granulocyte Counts

Granulocytes (cells/mm³) on days of Treatment	Dose of Navelbine (mg/m²)
≥1500	30
1000 to 1499	15
<1000	Do not administer. Repeat granulocyte count in 1 week. If granulocyte count is <1000 cells/mm³ for >3 weeks, discontinue Navelbine.

Note: For patients who, during treatment with vinorelbine, have experienced fever and/or sepsis while granulocytopenic or required a delay in dosing of up to 3 weeks due to granulocytopenia, the dose of vinorelbine should be: 22.5 mg/m² for granulocytes ≥1500 cells/m³ and 11.25 mg/m² for granulocytes 1000 to 1499 cells/m³.

Vinorelbine should be administered with caution to patients with hepatic insufficiency. In patients who develop hyperbilirubinemia during treatment with vinorelbine, the dose should be adjusted for total bilirubin.

Administration Precautions: Vinorelbine must be administered i.v. It is extremely important that the i.v. needle or catheter be properly positioned before any vinorelbine is injected. Leakage into surrounding tissue during i.v. administration of vinorelbine may cause considerable irritation, local tissue necrosis and/or thrombophlebitis. If extravasation occurs, the injection should be discontinued immediately, and any remaining portion of the dose should then be introduced into another vein. The application of moderate heat to the area of leakage in the form of warm compress applied for 15 to 20 minutes at least 4 times per day for the first 24 to 48 hours in addition to rest and elevation of the affected site for 48-72 hours has been reported to help disperse drug and minimize discomfort associated with the extravasation of other vinca alkaloids.

As with other toxic compounds, caution should be exercised in handling and preparing the solution of vinorelbine. Skin reactions may occur with accidental exposure. The use of gloves is recommended. If the solution of vinorelbine contacts the skin or mucosa, immediately wash the skin or mucosa thoroughly with soap and water. Severe irritation of the eye has been reported with accidental contamination of the eye with another vinca alkaloid. If this happens with vinorelbine, the eye should be washed with water immediately and thoroughly.

Preparation for Administration: Vinorelbine injection must be diluted in either a syringe or i.v. bag using one of the recommended solutions. The diluted vinorelbine should be administered over 6 to 10 minutes into the side port of a free-flowing i.v. followed by flushing with at least 75 to 125 mL of one of the solutions. For diluents that may be used, see Dosage, Reconstituted Solutions.

Syringe: The calculated dose of vinorelbine should be diluted to a concentration between 1.5 and 3 mg/mL.

I.V. Bag: The calculated dose of vinorelbine should be diluted to a concentration between 0.5 and 2 mg/mL.

Reconstituted Solutions: Syringe: Vinorelbine diluted to a concentration between 1.5 and 3 mg/mL may be used for up to 24 hours when stored in polypropylene syringes at 5 to 30°C. The following solutions may be used for dilution: 5% Dextrose Injection, USP; 0.9% Sodium Chloride Injection, USP.

I.V. Bag: Vinorelbine diluted to a concentration between 0.5 and 2 mg/mL may be used for up to 24 hours when stored in polyvinylchloride bags at 5 to 30°C. The following solutions may be used for dilution: 5% Dextrose Injection, USP; 0.9% Sodium Chloride Injection, USP; 0.45% Sodium Chloride Injection, USP; 5% Dextrose and 0.45% Sodium Chloride Injection, USP; Ringer's Injection, USP; Lactated Ringer's Injection, USP.

Potassium chloride injection solutions are found to be compatible with vinorelbine.

As with all the parenteral drug products, i.v. admixtures should be inspected visually for clarity, particulate matter, discoloration and leakage prior to administration, whenever solution and container permit. Any unused portion should be discarded.

Special Instructions: Since vinorelbine is a cytostatic agent, established procedures specific to the handling and use of such agents must be followed.

Vinorelbine injection is initially clear and colorless to pale yellow, but may develop a slightly darker yellow to light amber color in time. This does not indicate a change which should preclude its use. Parenteral drug products should be visually inspected for particulate matter and discoloration prior to administration whenever solution and container permit. If particulate matter is seen, vinorelbine should not be administered.

SUPPLIED: Each mL of clear, colorless to pale yellow aqueous solution contains: vinorelbine tartrate equivalent to vinorelbine base 10 mg. Additive- and preservative-free. Single-dose clear flint glass vials of 1 and 5 mL. Store vials under refrigeration (2 to 8°C) in the original package to protect from light. This product should not be frozen.

NeisVac-C®

meningococcal group C-TT conjugate vaccine, adsorbed

Active Immunizing Agent

GlaxoSmithKline

Date of Revision: June 21, 2010

SUMMARY PRODUCT INFORMATION:

Route of Administration	Dosage Form/ Strength	Clinically Relevant Nonmedicinal Ingredients
Intramuscular	Suspension for injection/10 µg *N. meningitidis* group C polysaccharide[a]	Aluminum hydroxide. For a complete listing see Dosage Forms, Composition and Packaging.

[a] Conjugated to tetanus toxoid carrier protein.

DESCRIPTION: NeisVac-C vaccine (meningococcal group C-TT conjugate vaccine, adsorbed) is a semi-opaque white to off-white suspension presented as a 0.5 mL latex-free pre-filled syringe. NeisVac-C vaccine is composed of a meningococcal group C polysaccharide conjugated to a tetanus toxoid protein, a chemically detoxified form of tetanus toxin, adsorbed onto aluminum hydroxide.

INDICATIONS AND CLINICAL USE: NeisVac-C vaccine (meningococcal group C-TT conjugate vaccine, adsorbed) is indicated for:

- Active immunization of children from 2 months of age, adolescents and adults, for the prevention of meningitis and/or septicemia caused by *N. meningitidis* serogroup C.

Geriatrics: Although the vaccine has been studied in adults, studies have not been conducted in adults 65 years or older.

CONTRAINDICATIONS:

- Known or suspected hypersensitivity to NeisVac-C vaccine (meningococcal group C-TT conjugate vaccine, adsorbed), or to any of its components including tetanus toxoid (see Dosage Forms, Composition and Packaging).

WARNINGS AND PRECAUTIONS:

> **Serious Warnings and Precautions**
> - **NeisVac-C vaccine should under no circumstances be injected intravenously.**

General: NeisVac-C vaccine (meningococcal group C-TT conjugate vaccine, adsorbed) will only confer protection against group C of *N. meningitidis* and may not completely prevent meningococcal group C disease. It will not protect against other groups of *N. meningitidis* or other organisms that cause meningitis or septicaemia.

Adequate medical treatment and provisions should be available for immediate use in the rare event of an anaphylactic reaction. For this reason the subject should remain under supervision for the appropriate length of time after vaccination.

As with any vaccine, administration of NeisVac-C vaccine should be postponed for subjects suffering from acute severe febrile illness.

Immunization with this vaccine does not substitute for routine tetanus immunization.

No data on the applicability of the vaccine in outbreak control are yet available.

There is no evidence that the vaccine causes meningococcal C meningitis. Clinical alertness to the possibility of coincidental meningitis should therefore be maintained.

In the event of petechiae and/or purpura following vaccination, the aetiology should be thoroughly investigated. Both infective and non-infective causes should be considered.

Hematologic: To avoid the possibility of excessive bleeding, the vaccine should be given with caution to individuals with thrombocytopenia or any coagulation disorder. No data are available on subcutaneous administration of NeisVac-C vaccine, therefore the possibility of any toxicity or reduced efficacy is unknown.

Immune: In subjects deficient in producing antibody (e.g., due to genetic defect, HIV infection or immunosuppressive therapy) this vaccine may not induce protective antibody levels following vaccination. Hence, vaccination may not result in an appropriate protective antibody response in all individuals.

It would be anticipated that functionally or anatomically asplenic individuals would mount an immune response to meningococcal C conjugate vaccines; however, there are no specific data available regarding immune responses in these patient groups.

Non-conjugated meningococcal polysaccharide vaccines should not be used for booster vaccination as they may negatively influence the immunologic memory.

Respiratory: The potential risk of apnea and the need for respiratory monitoring for 48-72 hours should be considered when administering the primary immunization series to very premature infants (born ≤28 weeks of gestation) and particularly for those with a previous history of respiratory immaturity.

As the benefit of vaccination is high in this group of infants, vaccination should not be withheld or delayed.

Special Populations: Pregnant Women and Nursing Women: The safety of the vaccine during pregnancy has not been established. The vaccine should not be used during pregnancy unless there is a defined risk of meningococcal C disease, in which case the risk/benefit relationship should be evaluated.

Lactation: The safety of the vaccine during lactation has not been established. The risk/benefit relationship should also be examined before making the decision as to whether to immunize during lactation.

Geriatrics: Although the vaccine has been studied in adults, studies have not been conducted in adults 65 years or older.

ADVERSE REACTIONS: Adverse Drug Reaction Overview: Although very rare, anaphylaxis and serious hypersensitivity reactions have occurred with all injectable vaccines, including NeisVac-C vaccine (meningococcal group C-TT conjugate vaccine, adsorbed). When signs or symptoms of anaphylaxis or hypersensitivity occur (bronchospasm, facial edema, angioedema, rash, hypotension or faints), they usually develop very quickly after the injection is given and while the person affected is still in the clinic or doctor's office.

The most common adverse reactions that have been reported are injection site reactions (redness, tenderness/pain, swelling), headache and fever, drowsiness and somnolence, or impaired sleeping, myalgia in the arms or legs (in all age groups); anorexia, vomiting, nausea or diarrhea, crying and irritability (in infants and/or toddlers); anorexia, vomiting, nausea or diarrhea (in older children).

In rare cases, in patients with pre-existing nephrotic syndrome, reoccurrence has been reported to present within a few months following vaccination with meningococcal group C polysaccharide conjugated vaccines. Signs of reoccurrence include angioedema, proteinurea and/or abnormal weight gain.

In addition, although very rare, other adverse reactions have been reported following product availability (see Post-Market Adverse Drug Reactions (for all age groups)).

Clinical Trial Adverse Drug Reactions: Because clinical trials are conducted under very specific conditions the adverse reaction rates observed in the clinical trials may not reflect the rates observed in practice and should not be compared to the rates in the clinical trials of another drug. Adverse drug reaction information from clinical trials is useful for identifying drug-related adverse events and for approximating rates.

In controlled clinical studies performed in all age groups, signs and symptoms were actively monitored and recorded on diary cards following administration of the vaccine. Of the local solicited symptoms, the most frequently reported were injection-site pain, erythema and swelling. Fevers may also occur following vaccination, but these are rarely severe.

The general symptoms that have been solicited and reported included irritability, somnolence, change in appetite, diarrhea, and fever in infants and younger children. These solicited general symptoms were also reported in the control groups and have been reported when NeisVac-C vaccine was administered concomitantly with other vaccines.

In infants and toddlers, symptoms including crying, irritability, drowsiness, impaired sleeping, anorexia, diarrhea and vomiting were common after vaccination but there was no evidence that these were related to NeisVac-C vaccine rather than concomitant vaccines, particularly DTP.

Commonly reported adverse events include headache (ranging from 1 in 7 secondary school children to 1 in 20 primary school children) and myalgia in adults (1 in 100) and irritability (ranging from 1 in 2 babies to 1 in 25 pre-school children) and somnolence in younger children.

The most common adverse reactions reported in clinical studies are presented in Table 1.

Post-Market Adverse Drug Reactions (for all age groups): The following additional indesirable effects were reported under the spontaneous reporting system:

Blood and Lymphatic System Disorders: lymphadenopathy, idiopathic thrombocytopenic purpura.

Table 1: NeisVac-C

Adverse Reactions

Frequency of Adverse Reactions (AR)	Adverse Reaction (Percent of Subjects with AR[a])
Very Common (more than 10%)	Injection site reactions: redness (5–50%) tenderness/pain (14–71%) swelling (8–31%) Pain in limb (32%) Headache (7–26%) Crying and irritability in infants and toddlers (22–53%) Drowsiness/somnolence/impaired sleeping in infants and toddlers (12–53%) Vomiting/nausea/diarrhea in infants (12%) Loss of appetite in infants (27%)
Common (between 1% and 10%)	Fever (1–7%) Loss of appetite in children (1–7%) Vomiting/nausea/diarrhea in children (3–5%) Muscle pain in older children and adults (6–7%) Pain in limb in children (2%) Drowsiness/somnolence/impaired sleeping (3–8%)

a The range of AR frequency percentages in clinical studies is provided for each AR. Percentages are based on all age groups unless otherwise stated.

Immune System Disorders: anaphylaxis, hypersensitivity reactions including bronchospasm, facial oedema and angioedema.

Nervous System Disorders: dizziness, convulsions including febrile convulsions, faints, hypoaesthesia, and paraesthesia, hypotonia in infants.

There have been very rare reports of seizures following meningococcal group C conjugate vaccine administration. Individuals have usually rapidly recovered. Some of the reported seizures may have been faints. The reporting rate of seizures was below the background rate of epilepsy in children. In infants, seizures were usually associated with fever and were likely to be febrile convulsions.

Respiratory, Thoracic and Mediastinal Disorders: apnea in very premature infants (≤28 weeks of gestation).

Gastrointestinal Disorders: vomiting and nausea.

Skin and Subcutaneous Tissue Disorders: rash, urticaria and pruritus.

Stevens-Johnson syndrome and erythema multiforme have been reported in post-marketing surveillance for other Meningococcal Group C Conjugate Vaccines.

Very rarely petechiae and/or purpura have been reported following vaccination. However, new cases should be investigated for aetiology as recommended under Warnings and Precautions.

Musculoskeletal, Connective Tissue and Bone Disorders: arthralgia.

Renal Disorders: Relapse of nephrotic syndrome has been reported in association with meningococcal group C conjugate vaccines.

All adverse drug reaction reports received under spontaneous reporting conditions (post-marketing surveillance) were at a frequency of very rare (<0.01%) except for the adverse drug reaction of rash which has been a rarely (between ≥0.01% and <0.1%) reported event.

DRUG INTERACTIONS: Drug-Drug Interactions: NeisVac-C vaccine (meningococcal group C-TT conjugate vaccine, adsorbed) must not be mixed with other vaccines in the same syringe. Separate injection sites should be used if more than one vaccine is being administered.

The vaccine can be administered safely at the same time as diphtheria, tetanus and whole cell or acellular pertussis-containing vaccines, e.g., DTP, Td, DT, *H. influenzae* type b conjugate vaccines (Hib), measles, mumps and rubella vaccine (MMR), inactivated polio vaccine (IPV) or pneumococcal conjugate vaccine (7- and 10-valent).

NeisVac-C vaccine administration did not affect antibody responses to diphtheria and tetanus toxoid, Hib conjugate vaccines or MMR.

Administration of meningitis group C-conjugate vaccine at the same time as, but at a separate injection site from, IPV, DTP, Hib, DTaP, DT, Td and MMR vaccines does not reduce the immunologic response to any of these other antigens.

Concomitant administration of NeisVac-C vaccine (2 dose infant schedule) and Infanrix hexa (DTaP-IPV-HBV-Hib) in a 3-dose primary series in infants did not indicate any clinically relevant interference with responses to any of the antigens in the hexavalent vaccine.

Concomitant administration of NeisVac-C with Prevnar, a 7-valent pneumococcal conjugate vaccine, given in infants did not indicate any clinically relevant immunologic interference. Also, concomitant administration with Synflorix, a 10-valent pneumococcal conjugate vaccine did not reveal any evidence of immunologic interference between the two conjugate vaccines after the primary series or after the booster dose.

DOSAGE AND ADMINISTRATION: Recommended Dose and Dosage Adjustment: There are no data on the use of different meningococcal group C conjugate vaccines within the primary series or for boosting. Whenever possible, the same vaccine should be used throughout.

Primary Immunization: Infants From 2 Months of Age up to 12 Months: Two doses, each of 0.5 mL, should be given with an interval of at least two months. Based on findings from effectiveness studies with meningococcal C conjugate vaccines, following their introduction in the United Kingdom, at least one of the doses from the two-dose schedule should be administered when the infant is older than five months of age.

Children 12 Months of Age and Older, Adolescents and Adults: A single 0.5 mL dose.

Booster Doses: Based on findings from effectiveness studies with meningococcal C conjugate vaccines, it is recommended that a booster dose of NeisVac-C vaccine be given to infants who have completed their primary series before the age of 5 months. There are no data available on the most appropriate time point for booster vaccination with NeisVac-C vaccine. It is, however, suggested that when needed, the booster dose should be given within the second year of life, approximately one year after the last dose of the primary vaccination series.

In subjects primed with a single dose (i.e., aged 12 months or more when first immunized), the necessity of a booster dose has not been established.

Administration: The vaccine must not be administered subcutaneously or intravenously.

NeisVac-C vaccine must not be mixed with other vaccines in the same syringe. Separate injection sites should be used if more than one vaccine is being administered on the same day.

NeisVac-C vaccine is for intramuscular injection, preferably in the anterolateral thigh region in infants and the deltoid region in older children, adolescents and adults.

In children 12 to 24 months of age, the vaccine may be administered in the deltoid or the anterolateral thigh.

Upon storage, a white deposit and clear supernatant can be observed. The vaccine should be well shaken in order to obtain a homogenous suspension and visually inspected for any foreign particulate matter and/or any variation of physical aspect prior to administration. In the event of either being observed, discard the vaccine.

OVERDOSAGE:

There is no experience with overdose of NeisVac-C vaccine (meningococcal group C-TT conjugate vaccine, adsorbed). Overdosing with the vaccine is highly unlikely, since it is administered from a single dose syringe by a health care provider.

> For management of a suspected drug overdose, contact your regional Poison Control Centre. See the *CPS* Directory section for a list of Poison Control Centres.

ACTION AND CLINICAL PHARMACOLOGY: Mechanism of Action: NeisVac-C vaccine (meningococcal group C-TT conjugate vaccine, adsorbed) is intended for the prevention of meningitis and/or septicemia caused by *N. meningitidis* group C in infants and older age groups. NeisVac-C vaccine is composed of a meningococcal group C polysaccharide conjugated to a tetanus toxoid protein, a chemically detoxified form of tetanus toxin, adsorbed onto aluminum hydroxide.

In clinical trials, NeisVac-C vaccine was shown to be highly immunogenic in infants, children, adolescents and adults against serogroup C *N. meningitidis*. Immunologic memory was also demonstrated in all age groups.

Pharmacodynamics/Pharmacokinetics: No pharmacodynamics studies and no pharmacokinetics studies have been conducted with NeisVac-C vaccine in accordance with its status as a vaccine.

STORAGE AND STABILITY: Store at 2 to 8°C. Do not freeze. Do not use vaccine after expiration date.

Within the indicated shelf life the product may be stored at room temperature (up to +25°C) for a single period not exceeding 9 months. Record the period of storage at room temperature on the product package. At the end of this period, the product should be used or discarded.

SPECIAL HANDLING INSTRUCTIONS: The vaccine should be well shaken prior to use (see Dosage and Administration).

INFORMATION FOR THE PATIENT: Published in e-CPS, available by subscription at www.e-cps.ca.

DOSAGE FORMS, COMPOSITION AND PACKAGING: Each 0.5 mL dose of semi-opaque white to off-white suspension contains: *N. meningitidis* group C polysaccharide 10 µg, tetanus toxoid 10 to 20 µg, aluminum hydroxide 0.5 mg AL^{3+} and sodium chloride 4.1 mg. Prefilled syringes with a rubber cap and a rubber plunger stopper, packs of 1, 10 and 20.

Neo-Laryngobis
bismuth dipropylacetate
Sore Throat—Loss of Voice Treatment

Rougier Pharma

PHARMACOLOGY: Bismuth dipropylacetate has both antibacterial and anti-inflammatory activity. Once absorbed, it distributes into the lymph ducts and is eliminated from the tonsils into the saliva. Once in the saliva, it acts to disinfect the pharyngeal area. Generally, sore throat symptoms (fever and swallowing pain) will decrease within 24 to 48 hours, and disappear completely within 48 to 72 hours.

INDICATIONS: The treatment of throat infections, more particularly for nondiphtheritic anginas, pharyngitis, tonsillitis, laryngitis and gingivostomatitis.

Also recommended as an adjuvant to the treatment of tonsil phlegmons, Vincent's angina, otitis and sinusitis.

CONTRAINDICATIONS: In the presence of chronic nephritis, albumin deficiency, congestive heart failure, rectal lesions and intolerance towards bismuth.

WARNINGS: No data supplied by the manufacturer.

PRECAUTIONS: No data supplied by the manufacturer.

ADVERSE EFFECTS: No data supplied by the manufacturer.

OVERDOSE:
No data supplied by the manufacturer.

> For management of a suspected drug overdose, CPhA recommends that you contact your **regional Poison Control Centre**. See the *CPS* Directory section for a list of Poison Control Centres.

DOSAGE: Adults: 1 rectal suppository daily. **Not recommended for children under 15 years of age.**

SUPPLIED: Each white to creamy white opaque rectal suppository contains: bismuth dipropylacetate 135 mg (bismuth octanoate). Nonmedicinal ingredients: semisynthetic glycerides. Boxes of 2. Store in a cool place under 30°C. Protect from freezing.

Neo-Medrol® Acne Lotion ℞
methylprednisolone acetate—neomycin sulfate—aluminum chlorhydroxide—sulfur
Acne Therapy

Pfizer

INDICATIONS: For control of acne vulgaris in the adolescent and young adult. Also in some cases of acne rosacea and seborrheic dermatitis.

CONTRAINDICATIONS: In tuberculosis of the skin, herpes simplex, vaccinia, varicella and in other cutaneous infections which do not respond to neomycin. Known hypersensitivity to any of the components.

WARNINGS: No data supplied by the manufacturer.

PRECAUTIONS: Avoid contact with eyes. If signs of irritation or sensitivity develop, application should be discontinued. As with any antibiotic containing product, overgrowth by resistant organisms may occur, particularly monilia. If this occurs, discontinue treatment and institute appropriate measures. Articles in current medical literature indicate an increase in the incidence of patients allergic to neomycin. The possibility of such a reaction should be borne in mind.

If extensive areas are treated or if the occlusion technique is used, the possibility exists of increased absorption of the corticosteroid and suitable precautions should be taken. The prolonged use of antibiotic-containing preparations may result in overgrowth of nonsusceptible organisms, particularly fungi. If new infections appear during treatment, appropriate therapy should be instituted.

Convulsions have been reported with concurrent use of methylprednisolone and cyclosporine. Since concurrent administration of these agents results in a mutual inhibition of metabolism, it is possible that convulsions and other adverse events associated with the individual use of either drug may be more apt to occur.

Ototoxicity and nephrotoxicity have been reported following absorption of topically applied neomycin.

Pregnancy: Although topical steroids have not been reported to have an adverse effect on pregnancy, the safety of their use has not absolutely been established. Therefore, use with care during pregnancy.

Children: When topical corticosteroids are applied for a prolonged period of time, sufficient systemic absorption can suppress the hypothalamic-pituitary-adrenal axis. Growth suppression may also occur.

ADVERSE EFFECTS: The following local adverse reactions have been reported with topical corticosteroids, either with or without occlusive dressings: burning sensation, itching, irritation, dryness, folliculitis, secondary infection, skin atrophy, striae, hypertrichosis, acneiform eruptions, allergic contact dermatitis, laceration of the skin and hypopigmentation.

OVERDOSE:
No data supplied by the manufacturer.

> For management of a suspected drug overdose, CPhA recommends that you contact your **regional Poison Control Centre**. See the *CPS* Directory section for a list of Poison Control Centres.

DOSAGE: After careful cleansing of the affected skin to minimize the possibility of introducing infection, Neo-Medrol Acne Lotion should be applied sparingly to the affected areas once or twice a day initially. Care should be taken to avoid contact with the eyes. The frequency of application will vary from patient to patient, depending on their susceptibility to the drying effect of the lotion, and may have to be reduced to every other day in some patients.

SUPPLIED: Each mL contains: methylprednisolone acetate 2.5 mg, neomycin sulfate 2.5 mg, aluminum chlorhydroxide complex 100 mg and colloidal sulfur 50 mg. Nonmedicinal ingredients: butylparaben, cetyl palmitate, lexemul ar, methylcellulose, methylparaben, perfume oil, polyethylene glycol, polysorbate 80, polysorbate 85 and propylene glycol. Plastic squeeze bottles of 25 and 75 mL.

Neoral® ℞
cyclosporine
Immunosuppressant

Novartis Pharmaceuticals

Sandimmune® I.V. ℞
cyclosporine
Immunosuppressant

Novartis Pharmaceuticals

Date of Preparation: March 23, 1984
Date of Revision: April 26, 2010

SUMMARY PRODUCT INFORMATION:

Route of Administration	Dosage Form/ Strength	Clinically Relevant Nonmedicinal Ingredients
Oral	Soft Gelatin Capsules 10 mg, 25 mg, 50 mg and 100 mg	Ethanol, hydrogenated castor oil, maize oil For a complete listing see Dosage Forms, Composition and Packaging.
Oral	Oral Solution 100 mg/mL	Ethanol, hydrogenated castor oil, maize oil For a complete listing see Dosage Forms, Composition and Packaging.
Intravenous	50 mg/mL concentrate for infusion	Ethanol, polyoxyethylated castor oil For a complete listing see Dosage Forms, Composition and Packaging.

Only physicians experienced in immunosuppressive therapy and management of organ transplant patients should prescribe NEORAL and SANDIMMUNE I.V. (cyclosporine). Patients receiving the drug should be managed in centres staffed with professionals experienced in transplantation and the use of immunosuppressants and equipped with adequate laboratory facilities to monitor cyclosporine levels. The ability to measure cyclosporine blood levels facilitates the management of the patient. The radioimmunoassay (RIA) method has been used most often in clinical trials.

For long-term follow-up, the attending physician should receive complete information from the transplant centre on the patient, to include: recommended NEORAL dosage, target trough levels of cyclosporine and, frequency of determination of these levels. The attending physician should consult with the transplant centre when making dose adjustments to ensure that toxicity is minimized while maintaining adequate immunosuppression. Increased susceptibility to infection and the possible development of lymphoma may result from immunosuppression.

Psoriasis/Rheumatoid Arthritis/Nephrotic Syndrome: Careful monitoring of NEORAL treated patients is mandatory. NEORAL should only be prescribed for psoriasis, rheumatoid arthritis or nephrotic syndrome by physicians experienced with its use. NEORAL is indicated: in patients with severe psoriasis in whom conventional therapy is ineffective or inappropriate and when the psoriasis is of such severity that the risks inherent in treatment with cyclosporine are justified for that patient; for the treatment of severe, active rheumatoid arthritis in patients for whom classical slow-acting antirheumatic agents are inappropriate or ineffective; in patients with steroid dependent and steroid resistant nephrotic syndrome.

INDICATIONS AND CLINICAL USE: Solid Organ Transplantation: NEORAL capsules and oral solution and SANDIMMUNE I.V. (cyclosporine) are indicated in the prevention of graft rejection following solid organ transplantation and in the treatment of transplant rejection in patients previously receiving other immunosuppressive agents.

Bone Marrow Transplantation: NEORAL capsules and oral solution and SANDIMMUNE I.V. (cyclosporine) are indicated in the prevention of graft rejection following bone marrow transplantation and the prevention or treatment of graft-versus-host disease (GVHD).

Psoriasis: NEORAL capsules and oral solution (cyclosporine) are indicated for the treatment of severe psoriasis in patients for whom conventional therapy is ineffective or inappropriate.

Rheumatoid Arthritis: NEORAL capsules and oral solution (cyclosporine) are also indicated for the treatment of severe active rheumatoid arthritis in patients for whom classical slow-acting antirheumatic agents are inappropriate or ineffective.

Nephrotic Syndrome: NEORAL capsules and oral solution (cyclosporine) are indicated in adults and children for steroid dependent and steroid resistant nephrotic syndrome due to glomerular diseases such as minimal change nephropathy; focal and segmental glomerulosclerosis, or membranous glomerulonephritis. NEORAL can be used to induce remissions and to maintain them. It can also be used for maintenance of steroid induced remissions, allowing withdrawal of, or reduction in the dosage of steroids.

CONTRAINDICATIONS:

- Patients who are hypersensitive to cyclosporine or any of its excipients. For a complete listing, see the Dosage Forms, Composition and Packaging.
- NEORAL is also contraindicated in the treatment of psoriasis and rheumatoid arthritis patients under the following circumstances: abnormal renal function; uncontrolled hypertension; malignancy (except non-melanoma skin cancer); uncontrolled infection; primary or secondary immunodeficiency excluding autoimmune disease.

WARNINGS AND PRECAUTIONS: General: Transplantation: NEORAL capsules and oral solution and SANDIMMUNE I.V. (cyclosporine) should be prescribed only by physicians who are experienced in immunosuppressive therapy and management of transplant patients and can provide adequate follow-up, including regular full physical examination, measurement of blood pressure and control of laboratory safety parameters. Patients receiving the drug should be managed in facilities with adequate laboratory and supportive medical resources.

The concentrate for solution for infusion contains polyoxyethylated castor oil which has been reported to cause anaphylactoid reactions. Patients receiving SANDIMMUNE I.V. should be observed continuously for at least 30 minutes following the start of the infusion and at frequent intervals thereafter. (See also Monitoring and Laboratory Tests, Transplant Patient Management.)

Non transplant indications: Patients with impaired renal function (except in nephrotic syndrome patients with a permissible degree of renal impairment), abnormal liver function, uncontrolled hypertension, uncontrolled infections or any kind of malignancy should not receive NEORAL.

Psoriasis: NEORAL should only be prescribed for psoriatic patients by physicians experienced with its use. All patients to be treated with NEORAL for psoriasis must have a pre-treatment physical examination to include blood pressure, renal function and careful examination for tumours, particularly of the skin, to establish accurate baseline values and clinical status.

Skin lesions not typical of psoriasis should be biopsied to exclude skin cancers, mycosis fungoides or other pre-malignant conditions.

Rheumatoid Arthritis: Discontinuation of the drug is recommended if hypertension developing during NEORAL therapy cannot be controlled with appropriate antihypertensive therapy. As with other long-term immunosuppressive treatments, an increased risk of lymphoproliferative disorders must be borne in mind.

Nephrotic Syndrome: NEORAL should only be prescribed by physicians experienced with its use. All patients to be treated with NEORAL for nephrotic syndrome must have a pre-treatment physical examination to include blood pressure, renal function (see Dosage and Administration) and screening for malignancies.

For All Patients: Appropriate patient and laboratory monitoring is essential to prevent, reverse or minimize the following adverse events: nephrotoxicity; hypertension; the development of malignancies and lymphoproliferative disorders; increased risk of infections; hepatotoxicity; lipoprotein abnormalities; neurotoxicity.

Cyclosporine absorption has significant inter-and intra-patient variability. Cyclosporine whole blood concentrations as well as the effectiveness and the adverse events related to cyclosporine should be appropriately monitored in all patients, particularly in de novo patients undergoing any change in their treatment regimen, to ensure maximum safety and optimal clinical outcome.

Carcinogenesis and Mutagenesis: Malignancy and lymphoproliferative disorders have developed, but their incidence and distribution are similar to those in patients on conventional immuno-suppressive therapy. In psoriatic patients on cyclosporine therapy, development of malignancies (in particular of the skin) has been reported. Skin lesions, not typical of psoriasis, but suspected to be malignant or premalignant should be biopsied before starting cyclosporine treatment. Patients with malignant or premalignant alterations of the skin should be treated with cyclosporine only after appropriate treatment of such lesions and if no other option for successful therapy exists. Cyclosporine should be discontinued if malignancy occurs.

In view of the potential risk of skin malignancy, patients on NEORAL or SANDIMMUNE I.V., should be warned to avoid excess ultraviolet light exposure.

Cardiovascular: Hypertension: Patients receiving cyclosporine may develop hypertension, and regular monitoring of blood pressure is required. Caution is advised in choosing an agent to treat this hypertension. Diuretics are not recommended (see Drug Interactions).

In addition, in psoriasis patients; beta-blockers are not generally recommended due to their propensity to exacerbate psoriasis. Only calcium channel blockers which do not interfere with cyclosporine pharmacokinetics are recommended (see Drug Interactions).

Endocrine and Metabolism: Lipoprotein Abnormalities: Many transplant patients have hyperlipidemia and cyclosporine may contribute to the genesis of this problem. It is advisable to perform lipid determination before treatment and after the first month of therapy. If lipids are increased, restriction of dietary fat should be considered. (If the risk benefit ratio warrants, a reduction of NEORAL capsules and oral solution (cyclosporine) dose may also be considered.) Caution is advised in the co-administration of NEORAL or SANDIMMUNE I.V. and the HMG-CoA reductase inhibitor, lovastatin due to the risk of myocyte necrosis. The potential for interaction with other drugs in this class should be considered (see Drug Interactions and Adverse Reactions).

Hyperkalemia/Hyperuricemia/Hypomagnesemia: Cyclosporine enhances the risk of hyperkalemia, especially in patients with renal dysfunction. Caution is also required when cyclosporine is co-administered with potassium sparing diuretics, angiotensin converting enzyme inhibitors, angiotensin II receptor antagonists and potassium containing drugs as well as in patients on a potassium rich diet (see Drug Interactions). Control of potassium levels in these situations is advisable.

Caution is required in treating patients with hyperuricemia (see Drug Interactions).

Cyclosporine enhances the clearance of magnesium. This can lead to symptomatic hypomagnesemia, especially in the peri-transplant period. Control of serum magnesium levels is therefore recommended in the peri-transplant period, particularly in the presence of neurological symptoms/signs. If considered necessary, magnesium supplementation should be given.

Hepatic/Biliary/Pancreatic: Hepatotoxicity: Cyclosporine may also cause dose-dependent, reversible increases in serum bilirubin and, occasionally, in liver enzymes.

Close monitoring of parameters that assess hepatic function is required. Abnormal values may necessitate dose reduction.

Immune: Infection/Immunization: Like other immunosuppressants, cyclosporine, predisposes patients to the development of a variety of bacterial, fungal, parasitic and viral infections, often with opportunistic pathogens. Activation of latent polyomavirus infections that may lead to Polyomavirus associated nephropathy (PVAN), especially to BK virus nephropathy (BKVN), or to JC virus associated progressive multifocal leukoencephalopathy (PML) has been observed in patients receiving cyclosporine. These conditions are often related to a high total immunosuppressive burden and should be considered in the differential diagnosis in immunosuppressed patients with deteriorating renal function or neurological symptoms. Serious and/or fatal outcomes have been reported. Effective pre-emptive and therapeutic strategies should be employed particularly in patients on multiple long-term immunosuppressive therapy.

Vaccination may be less effective and the use of live attenuated vaccines should be avoided.

Neurologic: Cyclosporine has the potential to induce tremor, convulsions and paresthesia in post-transplant recipients. Rarely, more complex neurological abnormalities including motor spinal cord and cerebellar syndromes have been reported in post-transplant patients.

Renal: Cyclosporine may cause increases in serum creatinine and urea levels, even at recommended doses as a result of reduced glomerular filtration rate (GFR). The mechanism leading to these increases is not fully understood. These functional changes are dose dependent and reversible, and usually respond to dose reduction. Although less frequent, some patients may develop structural changes in the kidney (e.g. interstitial fibrosis) during long term treatment. Although these renal changes are less common, they may be irreversible. In renal transplant patients, structural changes in the kidney must be differentiated from organ rejection.

Close monitoring of parameters that assess renal function is required. Abnormal values may necessitate dose reduction.

In elderly patients (>65 years of age), renal function should be monitored more closely. Kidney changes occur both structurally and functionally with aging leading to a natural decrease of renal function. Cyclosporine whole blood concentrations should be closely monitored in this patient group to ensure maximum safety and optimal clinical outcome.

In patients who are treated with cyclosporine for non-transplant indications, the risk of renal structural changes is greater if the serum creatinine level increases more than 30% from the patient's own baseline value. Thus regular measurements of serum creatinine levels must be made (see also Monitoring and Laboratory Tests, Psoriasis/Rheumatoid Arthritis/Nephrotic Syndrome Patient Management).

Special Populations: Pregnant Women: Cyclosporine is not teratogenic in animals, but was shown to be both embryo- and feto-toxic in rats and rabbits at 2 to 5 times the human dose.

To date, information has been received on 514 pregnancies with exposure to SANDIMMUNE. In most patients, the indication for cyclosporine therapy was organ transplantation.

Pregnant women receiving immunosuppressive therapies after transplantation, including cyclosporine and cyclosporine-containing regimens, are at risk of premature delivery (<37 weeks).

Most patients who became pregnant continued cyclosporine therapy throughout pregnancy, usually in combination with other immunosuppressive drugs and further medication.

Fetal loss occurred in 9.1% of the patients, which is within the range found in a normal population. In 4.9% of the patients, the pregnancy was interrupted, either for medical considerations or at the wish of the patient.

The course of pregnancy was often complicated by disorders specific to pregnancy, in particular in renal transplant patients, or by disorders relating to the underlying disease. A large proportion of the pregnancies ended in preterm delivery. Accordingly, the main problems seen in the neonates relate to prematurity, best exemplified by the short median gestation duration of 35.7 weeks in the 439 pregnancies completed, and the low median birth weight, 2291 g, of the 446 babies delivered, including 10 twins.

It appears that premature delivery and the delivery of infants small for their age occur more often in patients who have undergone a renal transplantation.

Out of 102 babies born to mothers treated with SANDIMMUNE, five were born with malformations. It is not clear what role cyclosporine has played in the complications of pregnancy.

Males treated with cyclosporine have fathered normal children.

In pregnant transplant recipients who are being treated with immunosuppressants the risks of premature births is increased.

A limited number of observations in children exposed to cyclosporine in utero is available, up to an age of approximately 7 years. Renal function and blood pressure in these children were normal.

However there are no adequate and well-controlled studies in pregnant women and, therefore, NEORAL or SANDIMMUNE I.V. should **not** be used during pregnancy unless the potential benefit to the mother justifies the potential risk to the foetus.

Nursing Women: As cyclosporine is transferred into breast milk of lactating females, mothers receiving treatment with NEORAL or SANDIMMUNE I.V. should not breast-feed.

Animal studies have shown reproductive toxicity in rats and rabbits.

Pediatrics: Experience with NEORAL in children is still limited. Experience in children is almost entirely based on SANDIMMUNE. In several studies pediatric patients required and tolerated higher doses of SANDIMMUNE per kg body weight than those used in adults.

Geriatrics (>65 years of age): Experience with cyclosporine in the elderly is limited, but no particular problems have been reported following the use of the drug at the recommended dose. However, factors sometimes associated with aging, in particular impaired renal function, necessitate careful supervision and may necessitate dosage adjustment.

In rheumatoid arthritis clinical trials with cyclosporine, 17.5% of patients were age 65 or older. These patients were more likely to develop systolic hypertension on therapy, and more likely to show serum creatinine rises ≥50% above the baseline after 3-4 months of therapy.

Clinical studies of Neoral in transplant and psoriasis patients did not include a sufficient number of subjects aged 65 and over to determine whether they respond differently from younger subjects. Other reported clinical experiences have not identified differences in response between the elderly and younger patients. In general, dose selection for an elderly patient should be cautious, usually starting at the low end of the dosing range, reflecting the greater frequency of decreased hepatic, renal, or cardiac function, and of concomitant disease or other drug therapy.

Monitoring and Laboratory Tests: Transplant Patient Management: Clinical: The concentrate for solution for infusion contains polyoxyethylated castor oil which has been reported to cause anaphylactoid reactions. These reactions can consist of flushing of the face and upper thorax, and non-cardiogenic pulmonary edema with acute respiratory distress, dyspnea, wheezing, and blood pressure changes and tachycardia.

Special caution is therefore necessary in patients who have previously received, by I.V. injection or infusion, preparations containing polyoxyethylated castor oil, or in patients with an allergic predisposition. Thus, patients receiving SANDIMMUNE I.V. should be observed continuously for at least the first 30 minutes following the start of the infusion and at frequent intervals thereafter. If anaphylaxis occurs, the infusion should be discontinued. An aqueous solution of adrenaline 1:1000 and a source of oxygen should be available at the bedside. Prophylactic administration of an antihistamine (H_1+H_2 blocker) prior to SANDIMMUNE I.V. has also been successfully employed to reduce the severity and prevent the occurrence of anaphylactoid reactions. The oral forms of NEORAL (cyclosporine) do not contain polyoxyethylated castor oil.

Laboratory: Accurate and regular monitoring of cyclosporine blood levels in conjunction with other laboratory and clinical parameters is regarded as an essential aid to maintain the trough concentrations within the relatively narrow therapeutic window between efficacy and toxicity.

During the immediate post-operative period, levels should be monitored every 2-3 days.

Monitoring schedules should continue until the patient's clinical condition and NEORAL or SANDIMMUNE I.V. dosage are stable. Following discharge from hospital, cyclosporine levels are determined at each clinic visit, which is usually twice weekly for the first two months, weekly until four months and monthly thereafter for the first year.

The reported therapeutic range for 12 hour trough levels from whole blood which appear to minimize side effects and rejection episodes are between 100-400 ng/mL as measured by the RIA method using specific monoclonal antibody (see Dosage and Administration).

Two methods are available for the specific assay of cyclosporine parent compound: radioimmunoassay (RIA) and high-performance liquid chromatography (HPLC). Comparative findings for the analysis of blood samples by both the RIA method (based on specific monoclonal antibody) and the HPLC method has established that the specific antibody gives a selective measure of the cyclosporine parent compound without significant interference from drug metabolites. Therefore, 12 hour trough levels of the cyclosporine parent compound should routinely be measured using the radioimmunoassay (RIA) kit for cyclosporine based on the specific monoclonal antibody.

Because there is a temperature and time-dependent uptake of cyclosporine by erythrocytes, the concentration of cyclosporine in plasma separated at room temperature and 37°C will differ substantially, the latter being higher. For this reason, it is not recommended to use plasma or serum as the matrix of choice. However, if plasma or serum are used a standard separation protocol (time and temperature) should be followed.

Whole blood is the matrix of choice. Specimens should be collected into tubes containing ethylene diamine tetraacetic acid (EDTA) anticoagulant. Heparin anticoagulation is not recommended because of the tendency to form clots on storage. Samples which are not to be analyzed immediately should be stored in a refrigerator (4°C) and assayed within 7 days; if the samples are to be kept longer they should be deep frozen (−20°C) for up to 6 months.

Psoriasis/Rheumatoid Arthritis/Nephrotic Syndrome Patient Management: Prior to Initiation of NEORAL Therapy: Clinical: Before treatment, the patient should undergo a history and physical examination with investigations as warranted. An initial blood pressure reading should be made on at least two occasions within 2 weeks to establish a baseline. As NEORAL is immunosuppressive, a search should be made for tumours of all kinds, particularly of the skin. Any persistent previously undiagnosed skin lesion should be biopsied for a confirmed diagnosis prior to starting therapy. Female patients should have an examination of the cervix within the first 6 months of therapy, and periodically thereafter, to exclude malignancy.

Laboratory: Prior to therapy, a 12-hour fasting serum creatinine should be measured on at least three occasions within 2 weeks to give an accurate baseline value. A baseline creatinine clearance is also suggested, if possible.

It is recommended that initial investigations should include urinalysis, complete blood count, liver function tests, serum uric acid and serum potassium.

Follow-up during NEORAL Therapy: Clinical: Regular clinical examinations are necessary during treatment with NEORAL. Follow-up assessment of blood pressure should be performed every 2 weeks during the initial 3 months and every month thereafter.

Should hypertension occur, in the majority of patients, elevated blood pressure can be adequately controlled by dose reduction. Should antihypertensive therapy be necessary, diuretics are not recommended. In addition, in psoriasis patients, beta-blockers are not generally recommended due to their propensity to exacerbate psoriasis. Only calcium channel blockers which do not interfere with NEORAL pharmacokinetics are recommended (see Drug Interactions). If hypertension is uncontrolled with antihypertensive treatment, NEORAL should be discontinued. When NEORAL is discontinued, blood pressure returns to normal within 3 months. Development of malignancies has been reported in patients when treated with cyclosporine. In patients with nephrotic syndrome treated with immunosuppressants (including cyclosporine) the occurrence of malignancies (including Hodgkins lymphoma) has occasionally been reported. Careful physical examination should thus be made for malignancies, notably of skin, oral mucosa, major lymph nodes. Psoriatic patients should avoid direct sun exposure as this will increase the risk of skin cancer.

Laboratory:

a. Psoriasis and rheumatoid arthritis: A complete blood count including, differential WBC, platelet counts, liver function tests, urinalysis, serum potassium, uric acid should be measured periodically during treatment with NEORAL. Serum creatinine should be measured every 2 weeks for the initial 3 months (see Dosage and Administration). Thereafter, if creatinine levels remain stable, measurements should be made every 2 months in patients who are receiving up to 2.5 mg/kg/day and every 4 weeks in patients who are receiving higher doses.

   More frequent checks are necessary when the NEORAL dose is increased or concomitant treatment with a non-steroidal anti-inflammatory drug is initiated or the dosage is increased. The same precaution applies to the introduction of any drug known to increase cyclosporine blood levels.

   Routine measurements of cyclosporine blood levels are not necessary because of their poor predictive value, but may be useful in special cases where drug interactions or altered bioavailability are suspected.

b. Nephrotic syndrome: Since cyclosporine can impair renal function, it is necessary to assess renal function frequently and, if the serum creatinine remains increased by more than 30% above baseline at more than one measurement the dosage of NEORAL must be reduced by 25 to 50%.

   In some patients it may be difficult to detect cyclosporine-induced renal dysfunction because of changes in renal function related to the nephrotic syndrome itself. This may explain why, in rare cases, cyclosporine-associated structural kidney alterations have been observed without changes in serum creatinine. Renal biopsy should be considered for patients with steroid-dependent minimal change nephropathy in whom cyclosporine therapy has been maintained for more than one year.

   Periodic monitoring of cyclosporine trough levels is recommended.

Drug Interactions: Caution should be exercised in patients receiving drug treatment with:

- Nephrotoxic Drugs
- Cytotoxic Drugs
- Immunosuppressants or radiation (including PUVA or UVB)
- Drugs affecting metabolism/absorption of cyclosporine.
- Lercanidipine
- Methotrexate

ADVERSE REACTIONS: Adverse Drug Reaction Overview: Despite the increase in C_{max} and AUC seen in patients who are treated with NEORAL capsules and oral solution (cyclosporine), a similar safety profile to the conventional formulation of cyclosporine (SANDIMMUNE capsules and oral solution) has been observed. Studies have reported no significant difference between the two formulations in terms of renal safety, risk of adverse events, or laboratory parameters (eg blood pressure, creatinine clearance, serum levels of urea, creatinine, potassium, cholesterol, triglycerides). Furthermore, there is no indication of a correlation between peak cyclosporine concentration (C_{max}) and changes in renal function.

The following adverse reactions observed with SANDIMMUNE are also likely to occur with NEORAL.

Many side effects associated with cyclosporine therapy are dose-dependent and responsive to dose reduction. In the various indications, the overall spectrum of side effects is essentially the same. There are, however, differences in incidence and severity. As a consequence of the higher initial doses and longer maintenance therapy required after transplantation, side effects are more frequent and usually more severe in transplant patients than in patients treated for other indications.

Anaphylactoid reactions have been observed following i.v. administration (see Warnings and Precautions).

Infections and Infestations: Patients receiving immunosuppressive therapies, including cyclosporine and cyclosporine- containing regimens, are at increased risk of infections (viral, bacterial, fungal, parasitic) (see Warnings and Precautions). Both generalised and localised infections can occur. Pre-existing infections may also be aggravated and reactivation of polyomavirus infections may lead to Polyomavirus associated nephropathy (PVAN) or to JC virus associated progressive multifocal leukoencephalopathy (PML). Serious and/or fatal outcomes have been reported.

Neoplasms Benign, Malignant and Unspecified (including cysts and polyps): Patients receiving immunosuppressive therapies, including cyclosporine and cyclosporine- containing regimens, are at increased risk of developing lymphomas or lymphoproliferative disorders and other malignancies, particularly of the skin. The frequency of malignancies increases with the intensity and duration of therapy (see Warnings and Precautions).

Frequency estimate: very common (≥1/10); common (≥1/100, <1/10); uncommon (≥1/1000, <1/100); rare (≥1/10 000, <1/1000) very rare (<1/10 000), including isolated reports.

Renal and Urinary Disorders: Very common: renal dysfunction (see Warnings and Precautions).

Cardiovascular Disorders: Very common: hypertension (particularly in heart transplant patients).

Nervous System Disorders: Very common: tremor, headache. Common: paresthesia. Uncommon: signs of encephalopathy such as convulsions, confusion, disorientation, decreased responsiveness, agitation, insomnia, visual disturbances, cortical blindness, coma, paresis, cerebellar ataxia. Rare: motor polyneuropathy. Very rare: optic disc edema including papilloedema, with possible visual impairment secondary to benign intracranial hypertension.

Gastrointestinal Tract Disorders: Common: Common: nausea, vomiting, abdominal pain, diarrhea, gingival hyperplasia. Rare: pancreatitis.
Hepatobiliary Disorders: Common: hepatic dysfunction.
Metabolism and Nutrition Disorders: Very common: hyperlipidemia. Common: anorexia, hyperuricemia, hyperkalemia, hypomagnesemia. Rare: hyperglycemia.
Reproductive System and Breast Disorders: Rare: menstrual disturbances, gynecomastia.
Musculoskeletal and Connective Tissue Disorders: Common: muscle cramps, myalgia. Rare: muscle weakness, myopathy.
Blood and Lymphatic System Disorders: Uncommon: anemia, thrombocytopenia. Rare: micro-angiopathic hemolytic anemia, hemolytic uremic syndrome.
Skin and Subcutaneous Tissue Disorders: Common: hypertrichosis. Uncommon: allergic rashes.
General Disorders and Administration Site Conditions: Common: fatigue. Uncommon: edema, weight increase.

Especially in liver transplant patients, signs of encephalopathy, vision and movement disturbances, and impaired consciousness are described. Whether these alterations are caused by cyclosporine, the underlying disease or other conditions remains to be established.

In rare instances, thrombocytopenia, in some patients associated with micro-angiopathic hemolytic anemia and renal failure (hemolytic uremic syndrome), has been observed.

Malignancies and lymphoproliferative disorders have developed, but their incidence and distribution are similar to those in patients on conventional immunosuppressive therapy.

Clinical Trial Adverse Drug Reactions: Because clinical trials are conducted under very specific conditions the adverse reaction rates observed in the clinical trials may not reflect the rates observed in practice and should not be compared to the rates in the clinical trials of another drug. Adverse drug reaction information from clinical trials is useful for identifying drug-related adverse events and for approximating rates.

Transplantation: The following events occurred in patients involved in two clinical trials with NEORAL. The first column reports on a study in which stable renal transplant patients were switched to NEORAL; in the second, de novo renal transplant patients were treated with NEORAL. See Table 1.

Table 1: NEORAL

Adverse Events with NEORAL

Adverse Event	Stable Renal Transplant Patients (N=372)	New Renal Transplant Patients (N=45)
Gingival Hyperplasia	29 (7.8%)	3 (6.7%)
Hypertrichosis	24 (6.5%)	17 (37.8%)
Edema	32 (8.6%)	14 (31.1%)
Tremor	31 (8.3%)	19 (42.2%)
Loss of Muscle Strength	3 (0.8%)	8 (17.8%)
Change in Vegetative Functions	24 (6.5%)	8 (17.8%)
Nausea, Vomiting, Epigastrical Pain	30 (8.1%)	7 (15.6%)
Headache	37 (10.0%)	10 (22.2%)
Paresthesia	16 (4.3%)	5 (11.1%)
Heat Sensations	28 (7.5%)	5 (11.1%)
Others	62 (16.7%)	11 (27.5%)

Psoriasis: In clinical trials, the most frequent side effects associated with the use of cyclosporine in psoriasis were renal dysfunction, hypertension, gastrointestinal disorders, hypertrichosis, paresthesia, headache, influenza-like symptoms, upper-respiratory tract infections, gum hyperplasia, fatigue, hyperuricemia, hypomagnesemia and increase in plasma liquids.

The following events (excluding renal dysfunction, hypertension and malignancies) occurred in 3% or greater of 631 psoriatic patients involved in clinical trials: See Table 2.

Table 2: NEORAL

Adverse Events (Excluding Renal Dysfunction, Hypertension and Malignancies) Occurring in Psoriatic Patients Involved in Clinical Trials

Body System Adverse Event	%
Skin and Appendages	
Hypertrichosis	14.6
Central and Peripheral Nervous System	
Paresthesia	11.4
Headache	9.4
Gastrointestinal Tract	
Nausea	4.8
Gingival Overgrowth	4.6
Gastrointestinal Disorder	3.3
General Disorders	
Fatigue	4.0
E.N.T. and Respiratory Tract	
Influenza-like Symptoms	5.5
Upper Respiratory Tract Infection	4.6

In psoriasis in 1439 patients treated with SANDIMMUNE the following were reported: 21 cases of skin cancer, 17 cases of solid malignant tumours and 6 cases of lymphoproliferative disorders (2 lymphomas).

There is an increased risk of malignancies, particularly skin cancer in psoriasis patients especially when the psoriasis has been previously treated with carcinogens, such as PUVA treatment.

Rheumatoid Arthritis: In clinical trials, the most frequent side effects associated with the use of cyclosporine in rheumatoid arthritis were hypertrichosis; hypertension; nausea; abdominal pain; paresthesia; headache and gum disorders. See Table 3.

Table 3: NEORAL

Adverse Events Associated with the Use of Cyclosporine in Rheumatoid Arthritis in Clinical Trials

Body System Adverse Event	Sandimmune Patients Initial Dose <6 mg/kg/d (n=378) (%)	Placebo-treated Patients (n=176) (%)
Skin Appendages		
Alopecia	3.4	2.3
Hypertrichosis	33.9	5.1
Rash	3.4	6.3
Central and Peripheral		
Cramps	4.0	0.6
Dizziness	4.5	4.5
Headache	15.6	9.7
Paresthesia	15.9	6.3
Tremor	13.5	3.4
Autonomic Nervous		
Flushing	5.0	1.7
Gastrointestinal		
Abdominal Pain	18.8	10.2
Diarrhea	6.1	6.3
Dyspepsia	9.5	5.7
Gum Disorders	11.6	0.6
Nausea	27.2	13.6
Vomiting	8.2	2.3
Body as a Whole		
Fatigue	4.2	4.0
Fever	3.2	2.3
Edema	4.8	2.8
Resistance Change		
Pharyngitis	3.2	2.3

Nephrotic Syndrome: In clinical trials, the most frequent side effects associated with the use of cyclosporine in nephrotic syndrome were: renal dysfunction, hypertrichosis, gingival hyperplasia, hypertension, tremor and paresthesia, and gastrointestinal symptoms.

The following events occurred in 3% or greater of nephrotic syndrome patients involved in clinical trials. See Table 4.

Table 4: NEORAL

Adverse Events Occurring in ≥3% of Nephrotic Syndrome Patients Involved in Clinical Trials

Body System Adverse Event	Sandimmune Patients (n=270) (%)
Skin/Appendages	
Hypertrichosis	31.5%
Hypotrichosis	3.0%
Musculoskeletal	
Muscle Contraction	4.1%
Central and Peripheral Nervous System	
Paresthesia	12.2%
Headache	5.6%
Tremor	5.6%
Psychiatric Disorders	
Weakness	4.8%
Gastrointestinal	
Gingival Hyperplasia	27.0%
Nausea	4.4%

(cont'd)

Table 4: NEORAL *(cont'd)*

Adverse Events Occurring in ≥3% of Nephrotic Syndrome Patients Involved in Clinical Trials

Body System Adverse Event	Sandimmune Patients (n=270) (%)
Gastric Pain	3.7%
Diarrhea	3.3%
Abdominal Pain	3.1%
Liver and Biliary System	
Liver Enzyme Increase	3.3%
Metabolic and Nutritional	
Hypomagnesemia	5.2%
Cardiovascular	
Hypertension	13.7%
Urinary System	
Renal Dysfunction	7.0%

In nephrotic syndrome of 660 patients treated with Sandimmune, malignancies occurred in 5 patients (3 carcinomas, 2 Hodgkins lymphomas).

Post-Market Adverse Drug Reactions: Literature and postmarketing cases of myotoxicity, including muscle pain and weakness, myositis, and rhabdomyolysis, have been reported with concomitant administration of cyclosporine with lovastatin, simvastatin, atorvastatin, pravastatin, and, rarely, fluvastatin.

DRUG INTERACTIONS: Overview: Of the many drugs reported to interact with cyclosporine, those for which the interactions are adequately substantiated and considered to have clinical implications are listed below.

Various agents are known to either increase or decrease plasma or whole blood cyclosporine levels usually by inhibition or induction of enzymes involved in the metabolism of cyclosporine, in particular CYP3A4. Cyclosporine is also an inhibitor of CYP3A4 and of the multidrug efflux transporter P-glycoprotein and may increase plasma levels of comedications that are substrates of this enzyme and/or transporter.

Nonsteroidal Anti-inflammatory Drugs: Nonsteroidal anti-inflammatory drug therapy should be discontinued where possible. As nonsteroidal anti-inflammatory drugs alone can have an adverse effect on renal function, addition of these drugs to NEORAL or SANDIMMUNE I.V. therapy or an increase in their dosage should be accompanied by particular close monitoring of renal function.

Infection/Immunization: During treatment with cyclosporine, vaccination may be less effective; the use of live-attenuated vaccines should be avoided.

HMG-CoA Reductase Inhibitors: In transplant patients who received the HMG-CoA reductase inhibitor lovastatin in combination with cyclosporine and other immunosuppressive drugs, there have been reports of severe rhabdomyolysis that precipitated acute renal failure. The potential for NEORAL or SANDIMMUNE I.V. to interact with drugs in this class should be considered.

Cyclosporine may reduce the clearance of digoxin*, colchicine*, prednisolone*, HMG-CoA reductase inhibitors (statins) and etoposide.

Severe digitalis toxicity has been seen within days of starting cyclosporine in several patients taking digoxin. There are also reports on the potential of cyclosporine to enhance the toxic effects of colchicine such as myopathy and neuropathy, especially in patients with renal dysfunction. If digoxin or colchicine are used concurrently with cyclosporine, close clinical observation is required in order to enable early detection of toxic manifestations of digoxin or colchicine, followed by reduction of dosage or its withdrawal.

Literature and postmarketing cases of myotoxicity, including muscle pain and weakness, myositis, and rhabdomyolysis, have been reported with concomitant administration of cyclosporine with lovastatin, simvastatin, atorvastatin, pravastatin, and, rarely, fluvastatin. When concurrently administered with cyclosporine, the dosage of these statins should be reduced according to label recommendations. Statin therapy needs to be temporarily withheld or discontinued in patients with signs and symptoms of myopathy or those with risk factors predisposing to severe renal injury, including renal failure, secondary to rhabdomyolysis.

Elevations in serum creatinine were observed in the studies using sirolimus in combination with full-dose cyclosporine for microemulsion. This effect is often reversible with cyclosporine dose reduction. Sirolimus had only a minor influence on cyclosporine pharmacokinetics. Co-administration of cyclosporin significantly increases blood levels of sirolimus.

The concomitant use of these drugs with NEORAL capsules and oral solution or SANDIMMUNE I.V. (cyclosporine) should be carefully considered.

In graft recipients there have been isolated reports of considerable but reversible impairment of kidney function (with corresponding increase in serum creatinine) following concomitant administration of fibric acid derivatives (e.g. bezafibrate, fenofibrate). Kidney function must therefore be closely monitored in these patients. In the event of significant impairment of kidney function the comedication should be withdrawn.

Prednisolone and Methylprednisolone: It has been noted that cyclosporine reduces the clearance of prednisolone and conversely, high dose therapy with methylprednisolone can increase the blood concentration of cyclosporine.

Potassium Sparing Drugs and Potassium Containing Drugs: Caution is required for concomitant use of potassium sparing drugs (e.g. potassium sparing diuretics, angiotensin converting enzyme inhibitors, angiotensin II receptor antagonists) or potassium containing drugs since they may lead to significant increases in serum potassium (see Warnings and Precautions).

Cyclosporine may increase the plasma concentrations of repaglinide and thereby increase the risk of hypoglycaemia.

Lercanidipine: Following concomitant administration of cyclosporine and lercanidipine, the AUC of lercanidipine was increased threefold and the AUC of cyclosporine was increased 21%.

Drug-Drug Interactions: The drugs listed in this Table 5 are based on either drug interaction case reports or studies, or potential interactions due to the expected magnitude and seriousness of the interaction.

Concomitant use with tacrolimus should be avoided due to increased potential for nephrotoxicity.

If combined administration is unavoidable, careful monitoring of blood cyclosporine concentration and appropriate modification of NEORAL or SANDIMMUNE I.V. dosage are essential. See Table 6.

Caspofungin: In two clinical studies, cyclosporine (one 4 mg/kg dose or two 3 mg/kg doses) increased the AUC of caspofungin by approximately 35%. Caspofungin did not increase the blood levels of cyclosporine. There were transient increases in liver ALT and AST when caspofungin and cyclosporine were co-administered. Cyclosporine and caspofungin should only be used concomitantly in those patients for whom the potential benefit outweighs the potential risk. Patients who develop abnormal liver function tests during concomitant therapy should be monitored and the risk/benefit of continuing therapy should be evaluated.

Drug-Food Interactions: Grapefruit juice should be avoided owing to its interference with the P450 enzyme system which has been reported to increase the bioavailability of NEORAL.

DOSAGE AND ADMINISTRATION

Dosing Considerations: The dose ranges of NEORAL capsules and oral solution and SANDIMMUNE I.V. given below are intended to serve as guideline only. Routine monitoring of cyclosporine blood levels is required; this can be carried out by means of an RIA method based on monoclonal antibodies. Routine monitoring of cyclosporine blood levels is also required when switching a patient from one oral cyclosporine formulation to another. The results obtained will serve as a guide for determining the actual dosage required to achieve the desired target concentration in individual patients.

* If digoxin, colchicine, or HMG-CoA reductase inhibitors (statins), are used concurrently with cyclosporine, close clinical observation is required in order to enable early detection of toxic manifestations of the drug, followed by reduction of its dosage or its withdrawal.

Recommended Dose and Dosage Adjustment: Solid Organ Transplantation: Treatment with NEORAL may be initiated within 12 hours prior to surgery at a dose of 10 to 15 mg/kg given in two divided doses. This dose should be maintained as the daily dose for one to two weeks post-operatively before being gradually reduced in accordance with blood levels until a maintenance dose of about 2 to 6 mg/kg given in two divided doses is reached. The following Table 7 outlines the recommended steady state therapeutic ranges of cyclosporine 12 hour trough levels (the level immediately before the next dose).

Table 5: NEORAL/SANDIMMUNE I.V.

Summary of Drug Interactions

	Drugs Increasing the Serum Concentration of Cyclosporine	Drugs Decreasing the Serum Concentration of Cyclosporine	Drugs Causing Additive Nephrotoxicity
Substantiated Interactions	Allopurinol Amiodarone Calcium-channel blockers -Diltiazem -Verapamil -Nicardipine Colchicine Cholic acid and derivatives Corticosteroids Fluconazole Imatinib Imipenem Itraconazole Ketoconazole Macrolide antibiotics (erythromycin, azithromycin and clarithromycin) Lercanidipine Metoclopramide Methylprednisolone Norethisterone or danazol Oral contraceptives Protease inhibitors Voriconazole Nefazodone	Barbiturates Bosentan Carbamazepine Hypericum perforatum (St. John's wort) Metamizole Nafcillin Octreotide Orlistat Oxcarbazepine Phenytoin or phenobarbitone Probucol Rifampicin i.v. Sulfadimine i.v. and trimethoprim i.v. Sulfinpyrazone Terbinafine Ticlopidine	Aminoglycosides (incl. gentamycin, tobramycin) Amphotericin B Ciprofloxacin Colchicine Cotrimoxazole or Trimethoprim (+ sulfamethoxazole) Melphalan Methotrexate Vancomycin
Suspected or potential interactions	Acyclovir Androgenic steroids Cephalosporins Furosemide H_2-antagonists Thiazide diuretics Warfarin	Anticonvulsants	Histamine H_2 receptor antagonist (e.g. cimetidine, ranitidine) Nonsteroidal anti-inflammatory drugs (e.g. diclofenac, naproxen, sulindac) Tacrolimus

Table 6: NEORAL/SANDIMMUNE I.V.

Miscellaneous Interactions

Alteration of Immunosuppressive Effect	Interactions with Alcohol Content	Others
Etoposide Propranolol Verapamil	Chlorpropamide Disulfiram Metronidazole	Captopril Caspofungin Colchicine Digoxin HMG-CoA reductase inhibitors Nifedipine[a] Prednisolone Toxoids or vaccines Potassium sparing drugs

[a] Concurrent administration of nifedipine with cyclosporine may result in an increased rate of gingival hyperplasia compared with that observed when cyclosporine is given alone. The concomitant use of nifedipine should be avoided in patients in whom gingival hyperplasia develops as a side-effect of cyclosporine.

Table 7: NEORAL/SANDIMMUNE I.V.

Target Trough Levels

RIA Method	Blood ng/mL	Plasma/ Serum ng/mL
Monoclonal specific[a]	100–400	50–200
Polyclonal non-specific[b]	150–1500	50–300

[a] Values are based on HPLC data and the results of a multi-centre comparison of the monoclonal specific RIA with the polyclonal RIA kit. Plasma serum values are based on separation at 37°C. These values will be lower if plasma/serum is separated at room temperature.

[b] Whole blood values are based on a multiplication factor of 3-5x concentration obtained using plasma/serum values. Plasma/serum values are based on separation at 22°C.

When NEORAL is given with other immunosuppressants (e.g. with corticosteroids or as part of a triple or quadruple drug therapy), lower doses (e.g. 3 to 6 mg/kg given in two divided doses for the initial treatment) may be used.

Recommended Dosage of Concentrate for Solution for Infusion: Patients unable to take NEORAL soft gelatin capsules or oral solution pre- or postoperatively, may be treated with the SANDIMMUNE I.V. at one-third the oral dose.

The initial dose of SANDIMMUNE I.V. is 3 to 5 mg/kg/day. This daily dose is continued post-operatively for up to 2 weeks until the patient can tolerate the NEORAL soft gelatin capsules or oral solution. Patients should be switched to NEORAL as soon as possible after surgery. In pediatric usage, the adult dose and dosing regimen have been used initially and adjusted to target blood levels (see Warnings and Precautions).

Bone Marrow Transplantation: The initial dose should be given on the day before transplantation. In most cases i.v. infusion of SANDIMMUNE is preferred for this purpose (please refer to previous Section). Maintenance treatment with NEORAL is at a daily dose of about 12.5 mg/kg given in two divided doses, and should be continued for at least 3 months (and preferably for 6 months) before the dose is gradually decreased to zero by one year after transplantation. If NEORAL is used to initiate therapy, the recommended daily dose is 12.5 to 15 mg/kg given in two divided doses, starting on the day before transplantation.

Higher doses of NEORAL, or the use of i.v. therapy, may be necessary in the presence of gastrointestinal disturbances which might decrease drug absorption. In some patients, GVHD occurs after discontinuation of cyclosporine treatment, but usually responds favourably to re-introduction of therapy.

Low doses of NEORAL should be used to treat mild, chronic GVHD.

Psoriasis: Dose Titration for Induction of Remission, the recommended initial dose is 2 mg/kg/day given in two divided oral doses.

If there is no improvement after one month, the daily dose may be gradually increased. Dose adjustments should be made in increments of 0.5 to 1 mg/kg/day body weight per month and total daily dose, depending on monitoring of drug tolerance, should not exceed 5 mg/kg/day.

Treatment Discontinuation: Treatment should be discontinued in patients in whom psoriatic lesions do not respond sufficiently within 6 weeks on 5 mg/kg/day, **or in whom the effective dose is not compatible with the safety guidelines given below under Monitoring for Psoriasis Patients**. As skin lesions improve the dose should be reduced in increments of 0.5-1 mg/kg/day per month.

Long-term Goals of Therapy: Psoriasis generally recurs when NEORAL treatment is stopped. The goal of maintenance therapy is to optimize therapy and achieve sustained improvement. That is, to keep the patient's disease controlled with the minimal dose of NEORAL in order to avoid adverse effects. Total clearing of the skin should not always be the ultimate goal.

Maintenance Dose: After reaching a relatively disease-free state, the patient should be given the minimum effective maintenance dose. For maintenance treatment, **doses should be titrated individually to the lowest effective level**, and, depending on monitoring of drug tolerance, should not exceed 5 mg/kg/day.

If a patient experienced a worsening of the condition during maintenance, therapy can be changed to a dose that is sufficient to control psoriasis **while remaining compatible with the safety guidelines**, i.e. maximum 5 mg/kg/day. An attempt should then be made to reduce the dose to the lowest effective level.

Dosage adjustments should follow the guidelines for inducing remission. If no relapse occurs within 6 months, an attempt should be made to wean the patient off NEORAL.

Monitoring for Psoriasis Patients: Since NEORAL can impair renal function, serum creatinine should be measured every 2 weeks for the first 3 months of therapy. Thereafter, if creatinine remains stable, measurements should be done every 2 months in patients who are on up to 2.5 mg/kg/day, and at monthly intervals in patients who require higher doses. The dose must be reduced by 25-50% when serum creatinine increases by more than 30% above the patient's own baseline, even if the values are still within the normal range. If dose reduction is not successful within 1 month, NEORAL treatment should be discontinued.

Discontinuation of NEORAL therapy is also recommended if hypertension developing during NEORAL therapy cannot be controlled with appropriate therapy.

As cyclosporine is an immunosuppressive agent, search should be made for tumours of all kinds, in particular the skin, oral mucosa and major lymph nodes. This physical examination should be made initially at least every 3 months and any skin lesion not typical for psoriasis should be biopsied. NEORAL treatment should be discontinued if a malignancy occurs, and appropriate treatment of the malignancy instituted.

Rheumatoid Arthritis: For the first 6 weeks of treatment, the recommended initial dose is 2 mg/kg/day orally given in two divided doses. If necessary, the daily dose may then be increased gradually as **tolerability** permits (see Warnings and Precautions) but, depending on monitoring of drug tolerance, should not exceed 5 mg/kg/day. Up to 12 weeks of NEORAL therapy may be required before full effectiveness is achieved.

For maintenance therapy, the dose must be titrated individually according to tolerability.

NEORAL may be given in combination with low-dose corticosteroids and/or non-steroidal anti-inflammatory drugs (see Warnings and Precautions).

Monitoring for Rheumatoid Arthritis Patients: Since cyclosporine can impair renal function, a reliable baseline level of serum creatinine should be established by at least two measurements prior to treatment, and serum creatinine should be monitored every 2 weeks during the first 3 months of therapy. Thereafter, if creatinine remains stable, measurements can be made every 4 weeks. More frequent checks are necessary when the dose of NEORAL is increased or concomitant treatment with a non-steroidal anti-inflammatory drug is initiated or its dosage increased. The same precaution applies to the introduction of any drug known to increase cyclosporine blood levels.

Dose adjustment based on creatinine values: If serum creatinine remains increased by more than 30% above baseline at more than one measurement, the dosage of NEORAL should be reduced. If serum creatinine increases by more than 50%, a dosage reduction by 50% is mandatory. These recommendations apply even if the patient's values still lie within the laboratory normal range. If dose reduction is not successful in reducing levels within one month, NEORAL treatment should be discontinued.

Nephrotic Syndrome: Dose Titration for Induction of Remission : For inducing remission, the recommended initial daily dose, given in two divided oral doses, is 3.5 mg/kg for adults and 4.2 mg/kg for children if, except for proteinuria, renal function is normal. In patients with impaired renal function, the initial dose should not exceed 2.5 mg/kg/day.

The combination of NEORAL with low doses of oral corticosteroids is recommended if the effect of NEORAL is not satisfactory, especially in steroid-resistant patients.

Treatment Discontinuation: Treatment should be discontinued if no improvement has been observed after three months' of NEORAL therapy.

Maintenance Dose: The dose must be adjusted individually according to efficacy (proteinuria) and safety (primarily serum creatinine), but, depending on monitoring of drug tolerance, should not exceed 5 mg/kg a day in adults and 6 mg/kg a day in children.

Monitoring for Nephrotic Syndrome Patients: For maintenance treatment, the dose should be slowly reduced to the lowest effective level. Monitoring for Nephrotic Syndrome Patients.

Since NEORAL can impair renal function, it is necessary to assess renal function frequently and if serum creatine remains increased by more than 30% above baseline at more than one measurement, the dosage of NEORAL must be reduced by 25% to 50%.

In some patients it may be difficult to detect cyclosporine-induced renal dysfunction because of changes in renal function related to the nephrotic syndrome itself. Renal biopsy should be considered for patients with steroid-dependent minimal change nephropathy in whom NEORAL therapy has been maintained for more than one year.

Periodic monitoring of cyclosporine trough levels is recommended.

Administration: NEORAL should always be given in two divided doses.

NEORAL soft gelatin capsules: When the blister package is opened, a characteristic smell is noticeable. This is normal and does not mean that there is anything wrong with the capsule.

Capsules should be swallowed whole.

NEORAL solution should be diluted with preferably orange juice or apple juice. Grapefruit juice should be avoided for dilution owing to its possible interference with the P450 enzyme system. Immediately before taking the solution, it should be stirred well. Other drinks such as soft drinks can be used according to individual taste.

The syringe should not come into contact with the diluent. If the syringe is to be cleaned, do not rinse it but wipe the outside with a dry tissue.

SANDIMMUNE I.V. (50 mg/mL Concentrate for Solution for Infusion) is diluted to l:20 to l:l00, immediately prior to use, with 5% glucose or normal saline and administered by slow intravenous infusion over a period of two to six hours (see Warnings and Precautions).

If available, glass containers should be used. Plastic bottles should only be used if they conform to the requirements for "sterile plastic containers for human blood and blood components" respectively to "empty sterile containers of plasticized poly(vinyl chloride) for human blood and blood components" of the current european pharmacopoeia, since polyoxyethylated castor oil contained in the concentrate can cause phathalate stripping from PVC. Containers and stoppers should be free of silicone oil and fatty substances.

OVERDOSAGE:

Experience with acute overdosage of cyclosporine is limited. Oral doses of cyclosporine of up to 10 g (about 150 mg/kg) have been tolerated with relatively minor clinical consequences, such as vomiting, drowsiness, headache, tachycardia, hyperesthesia in the hands and feet, flushing of face, gum soreness and bleeding, and sensation of increased abdominal girth. Although high levels may cause transient hepato- and nephrotoxicity, no permanent residual or long-term sequelae have been reported. However, serious symptoms of intoxication have been reported following accidental parenteral overdosage with cyclosporine in premature neonates.

If overdosage occurs, the patient must be monitored for evidence of toxicity, and standard supportive treatment applied as necessary. Cyclosporine is not dialysable to any great extent nor is it cleared well by charcoal hemoperfusion.

> For management of a suspected drug overdose, contact your regional Poison Control Centre. See the *CPS* Directory section for a list of Poison Control Centres.

ACTION AND CLINICAL PHARMACOLOGY: Mechanism of Action: Cyclosporine is a potent immunosuppressive agent with a narrow therapeutic range which has been shown in man to prolong the survival of allogenic transplants.

NEORAL capsules and oral solution include a microemulsion formulation of cyclosporine. NEORAL provides a more complete and consistent absorption profile and is less influenced by concomitant food intake or by diurnal rhythm than the previously marketed conventional formulation of cyclosporine (SANDIMMUNE capsules and oral solution). These properties combined yield a lower intra-patient variability, as well as in some cases, a lower inter-patient variability in pharmacokinetics of cyclosporine and a stronger correlation between trough concentration and total exposure (AUC_B) for a more accurate targeting of the level of immunosuppression.

As a consequence of these properties, the time schedule of NEORAL administration does not require that meals be considered. In addition, NEORAL produces a more even exposure to cyclosporine throughout the day and from day to day on a maintenance regimen, thereby helping to avoid periods of either under-immunosuppression or over-exposure to the drug.

Cyclosporine is distributed largely outside the blood volume. In the blood, 33 to 47 % is present in plasma, 4 to 9 % in lymphocytes, and 41 to 58 % in erythrocytes. In plasma, approximately 90% is bound to proteins, mostly lipoproteins.

Cyclosporine is extensively biotransformed to approximately 15 metabolites. There is no single major metabolic pathway. Elimination is primarily biliary, with only 6% of the oral dose excreted in the urine; only 0.1 % is excreted in the urine as unchanged drug. The distribution of cyclosporine appears to conform to a multicompartmental model in which continued administration leads to eventual saturation of the peripheral compartment.

The half-life of cyclosporine is approximately 18 hours (range 7.7 to 26.9). However there is a high variability in the data reported on the terminal half-life of cyclosporine depending on the assay applied and on the target population. For example, the terminal half-life ranged from 6.3 hours in healthy volunteers to 20.4 hours in patients with severe liver disease.

The recommended therapeutic range for 12-hour trough (C_0) levels from whole blood which appear to minimize side effects and rejection episodes is between 100-400 ng/mL as measured by the RIA method based on the specific monoclonal antibody (see Dosage and Administration).

It has however been reported that monitoring with the area under the time concentration curve for the first 4 hours ($AUC_{0\text{-}4}$) may provide for a more accurate prediction of optimal Neoral immunosuppression than trough (C_0) monitoring, thereby minimizing the risk of rejection, nephrotoxicity, neurotoxicity, hepatoxicity, and lowering serum creatinine levels.

Reports in the literature further indicate that using a single sampling point at 2 hours post-dose (C_2) best correlates with $AUC_{0\text{-}4}$ and provides for accurate assessment of Neoral absorption and immunosuppression in organ transplant recipients. When compared to C_0 monitoring, Neoral C_2 monitoring provided lower rates of rejection and toxicity in liver and renal transplant patients who attained C_2 target levels.

Pharmacodynamics: NEORAL and SANDIMMUNE I.V. (cyclosporine) strongly suppress cell mediated immunity and are therefore highly effective in preventing allograft rejection. However, interference with the primary activation of T-helper/inducer lymphocytes through the suppression of IL-2 production may be only one of several mechanisms contributing to an immunosuppressed state.

Pharmacokinetics: Bioequivalency of Soft Gelatin Capsules and Oral Solution: In a study of 24 healthy male volunteers it was demonstrated that NEORAL soft gelatin capsules and NEORAL solution are bioequivalent.

Absorption: When NEORAL is given, it provides improved dose linearity in cyclosporine exposure (AUC_B), a more consistent absorption profile and less influence from concomitant food intake and from diurnal rhythm than does SANDIMMUNE. These properties combined yield a lower within-patient variability in pharmacokinetics of cyclosporine and a stronger correlation between trough concentration and total exposure (AUC). As a consequence of these additional advantages, the time schedule of NEORAL administration does not require that meals be considered. In addition, NEORAL produces a more uniform exposure to cyclosporine throughout the day and from day to day on a maintenance regimen.

Compared to other oral forms of SANDIMMUNE, NEORAL capsules and solution is more quickly absorbed (resulting in a 1 hour earlier mean T_{max} and a 59% higher mean C_{max}) and exhibits, on average, a 29 % higher bioavailability.

Distribution: Following intravenous (I.V.) administration, SANDIMMUNE exhibits multi-compartment behaviour. The initial rapid distribution half-life is 0.10 hours, followed by a second slower distribution half-life of 1.1 hours. Continuous administration of the drug leads to eventual saturation of the peripheral compartment. This is reflected clinically by a decreased dosage requirement with long-term administration to maintain constant cyclosporine levels.

In blood, cyclosporine is highly bound to erythrocytes and plasma lipoprotein. However, all cyclosporine metabolites are less bound to plasma lipoprotein than cyclosporine itself. The relative distribution of cyclosporine in blood is a function of drug concentration, hematocrit, temperature and lipoprotein concentration. At a blood concentration of 500 mg/mL, 58 % of the drug is associated with erythrocytes, 4% with granulocytes, 5% with lymphocytes and the remaining 33% is distributed within the plasma. The plasma concentration of cyclosporine increased linearly with whole blood concentrations up to 1000 ng/mL. Above this concentration, the distribution of cyclosporine between blood and plasma is non-linear. Blood cells appear saturated by cyclosporine at concentrations above 500 ng/mL. Above this concentration there is a sharp decrease in the fraction of cyclosporine absorbed by erythrocytes, with a corresponding increase in the fraction of drug in the plasma.

In transplant recipients, low hematocrit (due to chronic disease or intraoperative blood loss) alters cyclosporine distribution between blood and plasma, resulting in higher levels of the drug in the plasma. This effect is temperature-dependent.

In plasma, more than 80% of cyclosporine is bound to lipoproteins. The major lipoprotein fractions involved are high-(HDL) and low-(LDL) density lipoprotein, which bind more than 80% of cyclosporine in plasma. The binding of cyclosporine to plasma protein is independent of concentration between 20 and $20{\times}10^3$ ng/mL. However, binding is markedly influenced by temperature; about 70% of the drug is bound at 4°C, 93% at 20°C and 98% at 37°C.

With a temperature decrease from 37° to 21°C, approximately 50% of cyclosporine diffuses from the plasma to the red blood cells, where it binds to hemoglobin; this process is reversible upon re-equilibration at 37°C for 2 hours.

Consistent with the lipophilic nature of cyclosporine, body fat contains the highest concentration of the drug. Accumulation also occurs in liver, pancreas, lungs, kidneys, adrenal glands, spleen and lymph nodes. Very low levels are found in brain tissues and cerebrospinal fluid suggesting that cyclosporine does not readily cross the blood brain barrier. The large tissue distribution of cyclosporine is consistent with the large apparent volume of distribution of 3.5-9 litres/kg and results from the high lipid solubility of cyclosporine and its ability to diffuse easily through biological membranes.

Metabolism: Cyclosporine is primarily metabolized by the hepatic mono-oxygenase multiple forms of cytochrome P-450. Metabolites and unchanged drug are excreted into bile. Of the 17 suspected metabolites of cyclosporine, 9 have been isolated and identified. All the identified metabolites have the intact cyclic oligopeptide structure of the parent drug. Structural modifications during metabolism include mono- and dihydroxylation as well as N-demethylation, mainly at the N-methyl leucines. Both cyclosporine clearance and half-life are highly variable among patients and seem to be influenced by the type of transplant, age, disease state and concurrent drug therapy.

Since cyclosporine is primarily eliminated by hepatic metabolism, its clearance is impaired in patients with liver disease and in liver transplant recipients in the early post-operative phase. On a bodyweight basis, pediatric patients appear to clear the drug more rapidly as compared to adults. Therefore, children may require more frequent and larger doses of cyclosporine to achieve therapeutic blood levels. The metabolism of cyclosporine is also significantly influenced by changes in the activity of the hepatic drug metabolising system; for example, the induction of the cytochrome P-450 enzyme system by barbiturates, phenytoin and rifampicin markedly accelerated the elimination of cyclosporine, potentially causing inadequate immunosuppression and acute rejection. In contrast, ketoconazole increases cyclosporine levels by inhibiting its metabolism and/or active transport into the bile. A similar interaction is observed with erythromycin.

The administration of high dose methylprednisolone (for acute rejection) and long term steroid therapy may also affect the pharmacokinetics of cyclosporine.

Excretion: The major route of elimination of cyclosporine is through the bile. Less than 1 % of an administered dose of cyclosporine is excreted in the bile as parent drug. More than 44% of a cyclosporine dose appears in the bile as metabolites when measured by RIA.

Enterohepatic recirculation of parent drug is thus very low. Hepatic functional impairment can reduce total clearance of parent drug and/or metabolite. Renal excretion is a minor pathway with only 6 % of an oral dose excreted in urine; only 0. 1 % is excreted as unchanged drug.

STORAGE AND STABILITY: NEORAL Soft Gelatin Capsules: NEORAL capsules should be stored at temperatures between 15 and 25°C and should not be removed from the blister packs until required for use. Occasional increases in temperature up to 30°C do not affect the quality of the product.

NEORAL Solution: Once opened, the contents must be used within 2 months.

NEORAL solution should be stored and dispensed in the original container. Store between 15 and 30°C, preferably not below 20°C for prolonged periods, as it contains oily components of natural origin which tend to solidify at low temperatures. Do not store in the refrigerator and protect from freezing.

A jelly-like formation may occur below 20°C, which is however reversible at temperatures up to 30°C. Minor flakes or a slight sediment may still be observed. These phenomena do not affect the efficacy and safety of the product, and the dosing by means of the syringe remains accurate.

SANDIMMUNE I.V. (concentrate for solution for infusion): Dilution: The concentrate for solution for infusion should be diluted to between 1:20 and 1:100 in 5% glucose or normal saline only, immediately prior to use (see Administration).

Storage: Store the intravenous product, protected from light, between 15 and 30°C. Do not store in the refrigerator and protect from freezing.

INFORMATION FOR THE PATIENT: Published in e-CPS, available by subscription at www.e-cps.ca.

DOSAGE FORMS, COMPOSITION AND PACKAGING: Neoral: Capsules: 10 mg: Each soft gelatin capsule with the imprint NVR 10 mg contains: cyclosporine for microemulsion 10 mg. Nonmedicinal ingredients: dl-α-tocopherol, ethanol, hydrogenated castor oil, maize oil and propylene glycol; shell: gelatin, glycerol and propylene glycol; coloring agents: aluminum chloride, hydroxypropyl methylcellulose, sodium hydroxide and titanium dioxide. Packs of 60 (6 full aluminum blister strips of 10 capsules each).
25 mg: Each soft gelatin capsule with the imprint NVR 25 mg contains: cyclosporine for microemulsion 25 mg. Nonmedicinal ingredients: dl-α-tocopherol, ethanol, hydrogenated castor oil, maize oil and propylene glycol; shell: gelatin, glycerol and propylene glycol; coloring agents: aluminum chloride, carminic acid, hydroxypropyl methylcellulose, iron oxide black, sodium hydroxide and titanium dioxide. Packs of 30 (6 full aluminum blister strips of 5 capsules each).
50 mg: Each soft gelatin capsule with the imprint NVR 50 mg contains: cyclosporine for microemulsion 50 mg. Nonmedicinal ingredients: dl-α-tocopherol, ethanol, hydrogenated castor oil, maize oil and propylene glycol; shell: gelatin, glycerol and propylene glycol; coloring agents: aluminum chloride, hydroxypropyl methylcellulose, sodium hydroxide and titanium dioxide. Packs of 30 (6 full aluminum blister strips of 5 capsules each).
100 mg: Each soft gelatin capsule with the imprint NVR 100 mg contains: cyclosporine for microemulsion 100 mg. Nonmedicinal ingredients: dl-α-tocopherol, ethanol, hydrogenated castor oil, maize oil and propylene glycol; shell: gelatin, glycerol and propylene glycol; coloring agents: aluminum chloride, carminic acid, hydroxypropyl methylcellulose, iron oxide black, sodium hydroxide and titanium dioxide. Packs of 30 (6 full aluminum blister strips of 5 capsules each).
Solution: Each mL contains: cyclosporine for microemulsion 100 mg dissolved. Nonmedicinal ingredients: dl-α-tocopherol, ethanol, hydrogenated castor oil, maize oil and propylene glycol. Bottles of 50 mL. A graduated syringe for dispensing is provided.
Sandimmune I.V. (concentrate for solution for infusion): Each mL contains: cyclosporine 50 mg in a polyoxyethylated castor oil/ethanol vehicle. Ampoules of 1 and 5 mL.

(Shown in Product Identification Section)

Neosporin® Cream

polymyxin B sulfate—neomycin sulfate—gramicidin

Antibacterial

GlaxoSmithKline

Neosporin® Eye and Ear Solution

polymyxin B sulfate—neomycin sulfate—gramicidin

Antibacterial

GlaxoSmithKline

Neosporin® Irrigating Solution

polymyxin B sulfate—neomycin sulfate

Antibacterial

GlaxoSmithKline

Neosporin® Ointment

polymyxin B sulfate—neomycin sulfate—bacitracin zinc

Antibacterial

GlaxoSmithKline

PHARMACOLOGY: The anti-infective components in the combination are included to provide action against specific organisms susceptible to them. Polymyxin B sulfate and neomycin sulfate together are considered active against the following microorganisms: *S. aureus*, *E. coli*, *H. influenzae*, Klebsiella-Enterobacter species, Neisseria species and *P. aeruginosa*. Bacitracin is active against most gram-positive bacteria, pathogenic Neisseria spp and *H. influenzae*. Gramicidin is active against most species of aerobic and anaerobic gram-positive bacteria.

INDICATIONS: Cream: The treatment of infection in dermatologic disorders, particularly where the lesions are moist or weeping; the prophylaxis of bacterial contamination in burns, skin grafts, incisions and other clean lesions; abrasions, minor cuts and wounds, where the cream may prevent infection and permit normal healing.
Ointment: For all lesions which are infected or likely to become infected by bacteria.
Eye and Ear Solution Sterile: For the prophylaxis and treatment of eye and ear infections.
Irrigating Solution: Neosporin irrigating solution is to be diluted and used as a continuous irrigant or rinse for short-term use in the urinary bladder of abacteriuric patients to help prevent bacteriuria and gram-negative rod bacteremia associated with the use of indwelling catheters.

CONTRAINDICATIONS: General: The use of Neosporin is contraindicated in patients who have demonstrated allergic hypersensitivity to any of the components of the preparation or to cross-sensitizing substances such as aminoglycosides and other related antibiotics.

Due to the known ototoxic and nephrotoxic potential of neomycin sulfate, the use of Neosporin in large quantities or on large areas for prolonged periods of time is not recommended in circumstances where significant systemic absorption may occur.

A possibility of increased absorption exists in very young children, thus Neosporin is not recommended for use in neonates and infants (<2 years). In neonates and infants, absorption by immature skin may be enhanced and renal function may be immature.
Cream: Neosporin cream should not be used in the eyes or in the external ear canal if the eardrum is perforated.
Ointment: Neosporin ointment should not be used in the eyes. It should not be used to treat otitis externa in the presence of a perforated tympanic membrane because of the risk of ototoxicity.

The presence of pre-existing nerve deafness is a contraindication to the use of Neosporin ointment or any topical aminoglycoside in circumstances where significant systemic absorption could occur.
Eye and Ear Solution Sterile: For ophthalmic use, Neosporin Eye and Ear Solution Sterile should not be used during surgical procedures or before surgery in circumstances where the product could gain access to intraocular fluids. Due to the risk of absorption of the preservative (benzalkonium chloride), contact lenses should not be worn when using Neosporin (Neomycin and Polymyxin B Sulfates, and Gramicidin) Eye and Ear Solution Sterile, in the eye.

For otic use, Neosporin eye and ear solution sterile is contraindicated in patients in whom perforation of the tympanic membrane is known or suspected and in long-standing cases of chronic otitis media, because of the possibility of ototoxicity caused by neomycin. In otic use, ototoxicity has been reported (see Adverse Effects).

WARNINGS: General: Neomycin sulfate may cause cutaneous sensitization. A precise incidence of hypersensitivity reactions (primarily skin rash) due to topical neomycin is not known.

When using neomycin-containing products to control secondary infection in the chronic dermatoses, such as chronic otitis externa or stasis dermatitis, it should be borne in mind that the skin in these conditions is more liable than is normal skin to become sensitized to many substances including neomycin.

The manifestation of sensitization to neomycin is usually a low-grade reddening with swelling, dry scaling and itching; it may be manifested simply as a failure to heal. Periodic examination for such signs is advisable, and the patient should be told to discontinue the product if they are observed. These symptoms regress quickly on withdrawing the medication. Neomycin-containing applications should be avoided for the patient thereafter.

Following significant systemic absorption: aminoglycosides such as neomycin can cause irreversible ototoxicity; neomycin sulfate, polymyxin B sulfate, and bacitracin zinc have nephrotoxic potential; polymyxin B sulfate has neurotoxic potential.

The concurrent use of other aminoglycoside antibiotics is not recommended in circumstances where significant systemic absorption of neomycin sulfate following topical application could occur.
Irrigating Solution: Prophylactic bladder care with Neosporin irrigating solution should not be given where there is a possibility of systemic absorption.

Neosporin irrigating solution is intended for continuous prophylactic irrigation of the lumen of the intact urinary bladder of patients with indwelling catheters. Patients should be under constant supervision by a physician. Irrigation should be avoided in patients with defects in the bladder mucosa or bladder wall, such as vesical rupture, or in association with operative procedures on the bladder wall, because of the risk of toxicity due to systemic absorption following diffusion into absorptive tissues and spaces.

Neosporin irrigating solution should not be used for irrigation other than for the urinary bladder. Systemic absorption after topical administration of neomycin to open wounds, burns and granulating surfaces is significant and serum concentrations comparable to and often higher than those attained following oral and parenteral therapy have been reported.

Absorption of neomycin from the denuded bladder surface has been reported. However, the likelihood of toxicity following topical irrigation of the intact urinary bladder with Neosporin irrigating solution is low since no appreciable amounts of these antibiotics enter the systemic circulation by this route if irrigation does not exceed 10 days (see Precautions).

When absorbed, neomycin and polymyxin B are nephrotoxic antibiotics, and the nephrotoxic potentials are additive. In addition, both antibiotics, when absorbed, are neurotoxins: neomycin can destroy fibers of the acoustic nerve causing permanent bilateral deafness; neomycin and polymyxin B are additive in their neuromuscular blocking effects, not only in terms of potency and duration but also in terms of characteristics of the blocks produced.

PRECAUTIONS: General: The use of Neosporin should not be continued for more than 7 days without medical supervision. If the infection is not improved after 1 week, cultures and susceptibility tests should be repeated to verify the identity of the organism and to determine whether therapy should be changed (see Warnings).

Articles in current medical literature indicate an increase in the incidence of allergies to neomycin in patients with stasis ulcers or eczema. The possibility of an allergic reaction to neomycin should be borne in mind.

As with other antibiotic preparations, prolonged use may result in overgrowth of nonsusceptible organisms, including fungi. Appropriate measures should be taken if this occurs.

Because of the potential hazard of nephrotoxicity and ototoxicity due to neomycin, care should be exercised when treating extensive burns, trophic ulceration and other extensive conditions where absorption of neomycin is possible.

After a maximal course, treatment should **not** be repeated for at least 3 months.
Eye and Ear Solution: Neosporin eye and ear solution sterile should not be given subconjunctivally or intraocularly, nor should it be used for the irrigation of fistulous tracts in or about the eye or its socket. Treatment should be continued until at least 48 hours after the eye has apparently recovered.
Irrigating Solution: Care should be taken to prevent reflux of Neosporin irrigating solution up to the ureters, since the concentration of neomycin may cause renal toxicity. Ototoxicity, nephrotoxicity, and neuromuscular blockade may occur if the components of the preparation are systemically absorbed (see Warnings). Absorption of neomycin from the denuded bladder surface has been reported. Patients with impaired renal function, dehydrated patients, elderly patients, and patients receiving high doses of prolonged treatment are especially at risk for the development of toxicity.

The safety and effectiveness of the preparation for use in the care of patients with recent lower urinary tract surgery have not been established.

Urine specimens should be collected during prophylactic bladder care for urinalysis, culture, and susceptibility testing. Positive cultures suggest the presence of organisms which are resistant to the bladder rinse antibiotics.
Geriatrics: Neosporin is suitable for use in elderly patients. Caution should be exercised in cases where a decrease in renal function exists and significant systemic absorption of neomycin sulfate may occur (see Dosage).
Children: Neosporin is suitable for use in children (2 years and over) at the same dose as adults. A possibility of increased absorption exists in very young children, thus Neosporin is not recommended for use in neonates and infants (<2 years) (see Contraindications and Dosage).
Pregnancy: There is little information to demonstrate the possible effect of topically applied neomycin in pregnancy. However, neomycin present in maternal blood can cross the placenta and may give rise to a theoretical risk of fetal toxicity, thus use of Neosporin is not recommended in pregnancy.
Lactation: There is little information to demonstrate the possible effect of topically applied neomycin in lactation. Thus, use of Neosporin is not recommended in nursing mothers.
Patients with Special Diseases and Conditions: In renal impairment the plasma clearance of neomycin is reduced (see Dosage).
Drug Interactions: Following significant systemic absorption, both neomycin sulfate and polymyxin B sulfate can intensify and prolong the respiratory depressant effects of neuromuscular blocking agents. However, the neuromuscular blocking activity of neomycin sulfate and polymyxin B sulfate is unlikely to present a hazard during use of Neosporin.

ADVERSE EFFECTS: Adverse reactions have occurred with topical use of antibiotic combination containing neomycin and polymyxin B. Exact incidence figures are not available since no denominator of treated patients is available. The reaction occurring most often is allergic sensitization. In 1 clinical study, using a 20% neomycin patch, neomycin-induced allergic skin reactions occurred in 2 of 2175 (0.09%) individuals in the general population. In another study the incidence was found to be approximately 1%.

Ototoxicity and nephrotoxicity have been reported (see Warnings).

Stinging and burning have been reported rarely when this product has gained access to the middle ear.

The incidence of allergic hypersensitivity reactions to neomycin sulfate in the general population are low. There is, however, an increased incidence of hypersensitivity to neomycin sulfate in certain selected groups of patients in dermatological practice, particularly those with venous stasis eczema and ulceration, and chronic otitis externa.

Allergic hypersensitivity to neomycin following topical use may manifest itself as an eczematous exacerbation with reddening, scaling, swelling and itching of the affected skin, or as a failure of the lesion to heal.

Allergic hypersensitivity reactions following the topical administration of bacitracin zinc and polymyxin B sulfate are rare events.

Anaphylactic reactions following the topical application of bacitracin zinc have been reported, but are rare events.

Reactions occurring most often from the presence of the anti-infective ingredient in ophthalmic use are localized hypersensitivity, including itching, swelling and conjunctival erythema. Local irritation on instillation has also been reported.

Irritation of the urinary bladder mucosa has been reported with use of Neosporin irrigating solution.

OVERDOSE:

Symptoms: No specific symptoms or signs have been associated with excessive use of Neosporin. However, consideration should be given to significant systemic absorption (see Contraindications, Warnings and Precautions).

Following accidental ingestion, minimal absorption is expected.

Treatment: Use of the product should be stopped and the patient's general status, hearing acuity, renal and neuromuscular functions should be monitored.

Blood levels of neomycin sulfate, polymyxin B, and bacitracin zinc should be determined. Hemodialysis may reduce the serum level of neomycin sulfate.

For management of a suspected drug overdose, CPhA recommends that you contact your **regional Poison Control Centre**. See the *CPS* Directory section for a list of Poison Control Centres.

DOSAGE: Treatment should not be continued for more than 7 days without medical supervision.
Adults: Cream: Following any necessary removal of debris, such as pus, crusts, etc., from the affected area, apply a small quantity 2 to 5 times daily, as required. Rub in gently if condition permits.
Ointment: Following any necessary removal of debris, such as pus, crusts, etc., from the affected area, apply a thin film 2 to 5 times daily over the affected area. Cover with dressing or leave exposed. **Do not use in the eyes.**

Eye and Ear Solution: 1 or 2 drops in the affected eye or ear, 2 to 4 times a day, or more frequently as required.
Irrigating Solution: For use with 3-way catheters or with other catheter systems permitting continuous bladder irrigation. Under sterile conditions, add 1 mL of solution to a 1000 mL bottle of isotonic saline solution. Connect this solution to the inflow lumen of the 3-way catheter, which has been inserted with aseptic precautions. The outflow lumen is connected via a sterile disposable plastic hose to a sterile disposable collection bag. The in-flow rate, for most patients, should be adjusted to a slow drip to deliver about 1000 mL every 24 hours. If the patient's urine output exceeds 2 L/day, it is recommended that the in-flow rate should be adjusted to deliver 2000 mL of the solution in a 24-hour period.
Children: Neosporin is suitable for use in children (2 years and over) at the same dose as adults. A possibility of increased absorption exists in very young children, thus Neosporin is not recommended for use in neonates and infants (<2 years) (see Contraindications and Precautions).
Geriatrics: Neosporin is suitable for use in elderly patients. Caution should be exercised in cases where a decrease in renal function exists and significant systemic absorption of neomycin sulfate may occur (see Warnings and Precautions).
Renal Impairment: Dosage should be reduced in patients with reduced renal function (see Precautions).

INFORMATION FOR THE PATIENT: Published in e-CPS, available by subscription at www.e-cps.ca.

SUPPLIED: Neosporin formulations are antibacterial preparations for topical use.

Only Neosporin eye and ear solution is a sterile preparation appropriate for use in the eye.

Cream: Each g contains: polymyxin B sulfate 10 000 units, neomycin sulfate (equiv. to 3.5 mg neomycin base) 5 mg, gramicidin 250 µg in a white vanishing cream base, pH approximately 5.0. Nonmedicinal ingredients: emulsifying wax, methylparaben, mineral oil, poloxamer, propylene glycol and white petrolatum. Tubes of 15 g. Store at 15 to 25°C.

Irrigating Solution: Each mL of sterile, aqueous solution contains: neomycin (as sulfate, 57 mg) 40 mg, polymyxin B (as sulfate) 200 000 units. Nonmedicinal ingredients: methylparaben, sulfuric acid and/or sodium hydroxide, as pH adjusters. Not for injection. Ampuls of 1 mL. Vials of 20 mL. Store at 2 to 8°C.

Ointment: Each g contains: polymyxin B sulfate 5000 units, bacitracin zinc 400 units and neomycin sulfate 5 mg, in a low melting point petrolatum base. Tubes of 15 and 30 g. Store at 15 to 25°C.

Sterile Eye and Ear Solution: Each mL contains: polymyxin B sulfate 10 000 units, neomycin sulfate 2.5 mg, gramicidin 25 µg. Nonmedicinal ingredients: alcohol, benzalkonium chloride, poloxamer and propylene glycol. Plastic dropper bottles of 10 mL. Store at 15 to 25°C. Protect from light.

Except for Neosporin irrigating solution—for which dilution is required for administration—dilution of Neosporin is not recommended; reduction of the antibiotic concentrations may reduce their therapeutic efficacy.

Neostigmine Methylsulfate Injection USP Pr

neostigmine methylsulfate

Parasympathomimetic

Sandoz

SUPPLIED: 0.5 mg/mL: Each mL of solution contains: neostigmine methylsulfate 0.5 mg. Nonmedicinal ingredients: phenol as a preservative, sodium acetate and acetic acid as a buffer to adjust pH and water for injection. Multidose vials of 10 mL, boxes of 10. Store between 15 and 30°C. Protect from light.

1 mg/mL: Each mL of solution contains: neostigmine methylsulfate 1 mg. Nonmedicinal ingredients: phenol as a preservative, sodium acetate and acetic acid as a buffer to adjust pH and water for injection. Multidose vials of 10 mL, boxes of 10. Store between 15 and 30°C. Protect from light.

2.5 mg/mL: Each mL of solution contains: neostigmine methylsulfate 2.5 mg. Nonmedicinal ingredients: phenol as a preservative, sodium acetate and acetic acid as a buffer to adjust pH and water for injection. Multidose vials of 5 mL, boxes of 10. Store between 15 and 30°C. Protect from light.

Neo-Synephrine® Hydrochloride USP

phenylephrine HCl

Vasopressor

Hospira

SUPPLIED: Each mL of 1% solution contains: phenylephrine HCl 10 mg in water for injection. Nonmedicinal ingredients: citric acid monohydrate, sodium chloride, sodium citrate dihydrate and sodium metabisulfite. Ampoules of 1 mL, boxes of 10.

NeoVisc®

sodium hyaluronate

Synovial Fluid Replacement/Replenishment

Stellar

DESCRIPTION: Sodium hyaluronate is a naturally occurring linear polysaccharide composed of repeating disaccharide unit of D-glucuronic acid and N-acetyl-D-glucosamine linked by β1-3 and β1-4 glycosidic bond. Hyaluronate maintains the structure of proteoglycan molecules. Proteoglycans bind hyaluronate chains to form large aggregates in the range of 10^8 Daltons. The linking proteins of aggregates stabilize the macromolecular structures which are deposited within the collagen network of cartilage. Hydration of aggrecan molecules provides resilience and elastic strength to cartilage. Viscoelasticity of synovial fluid is due mainly to rheological properties of hyaluronate solution.

In osteoarthritis, the concentration of hyaluronate is decreased, resulting in a loss of viscoelastic properties of synovial fluid. NeoVisc is a specific high molecular weight hyaluronate, free of avian proteins, in a phosphate-buffered saline for synovial fluid replacement/replenishment.

INDICATIONS: As a replacement/replenishment for synovial fluid, following arthrocentesis.

CONTRAINDICATIONS: No contraindications to hyaluronate solutions have been reported with intra-articular injections.

WARNINGS: Do not inject intra-vascularly. **Do not freeze.**

All medical procedures carry some risk. After intra articular injections of NeoVisc, the injected joint may experience: transient pain, and/or swelling, and/or effusion. In cases of large effusions; it is important to remove and analyze the fluid to rule out infection or crystalline arthropathies. Expect these reactions to abate within a few days, often overnight. After such reactions there may still be clinical benefit from the treatment.

PRECAUTIONS: Do not administer to patients with known hypersensitivity reactions to this solution. Arthrocentesis is strongly recommended as an indicator that the injection location is correct and to reduce pressure caused by added volume in the synovial space.

ADVERSE EFFECTS: Sodium Hyaluronate is naturally occurring in the body. Since it is naturally occurring they are not inflammatory. Transient short duration pain and/or swelling may occur following intra-articular injection.

OVERDOSE:

For management of a suspected drug overdose, CPhA recommends that you contact your **regional Poison Control Centre**. See the *CPS* Directory section for a list of Poison Control Centres.

DOSAGE: 3 × 2 mL: Using aseptic technique, administer 2 mL (20 mg) intra-articularly to the affected joints. Continue with one injection per week for a total of 3 to 5 injections. Repeat every 6 to 8 months, depending on clinical response.

Single Dose 1 × 6 mL: Using aseptic technique, administer 6 mL (60 mg) intra-articularly to the affected joints. Repeat depending on clinical response.

SUPPLIED: 3 × 2 mL: Each mL contains: sodium hyaluronate 10 mg (20 mg/2 mL). Single dose disposable syringes of 2 mL, boxes of 3. Only the contents of the syringe are sterile. Store between 2 to 25°C. **Do not freeze.** Bring contents to room temperature before use.

Single Dose 1 × 6 mL: Each mL contains: sodium hyaluronate 10 mg (60 mg/6 mL). Single dose disposable syringes of 6 mL, boxes of 1. Only the contents of the syringe are sterile. Store between 2 to 25°C. **Do not freeze.** Bring contents to room temperature before use.

Blister Pack Directions: To be opened by a Physician only.

3 × 2 mL: To access syringe, grip tab at top while supporting neighbouring strip and peel off one strip as needed. To separate individual blister packs, fold on perforation and bend back and forth several times prior to tearing.

Single Dose 1 × 6 mL: To access syringe, grip tab at top and peel off the strip.

Nerisalic® Pr

diflucortolone valerate—salicylic acid

Topical Corticosteroid—Keratolytic

Stiefel, a GSK company

PHARMACOLOGY: Nerisalic combines the anti-inflammatory, antipruritic and vasoconstrictive activity of diflucortolone valerate and the keratolytic effects of salicylic acid.

Both diflucortolone valerate and its split ester are topically active.

INDICATIONS: The topical treatment of chronic eczema, psoriasis vulgaris, neuro-dermatitis and scaly crusty dermatoses which respond to corticosteroid therapy.

Nerisalic is not suitable for the treatment of perioral dermatitis and rosacea.

CONTRAINDICATIONS: In patients who have shown hypersensitivity, allergy or intolerance to diflucortolone valerate or other corticosteroids or salicylic acid or to any excipients in the preparation. Nerisalic should not be applied to skin areas with fissures, erosions, scratches or excoriations.

Topical steroids are contraindicated in untreated bacterial and/or fungal skin infections. Topical steroids should not be applied in cases of tuberculosis of the skin, or syphilitic skin infections, chickenpox, eruptions following vaccinations and viral diseases of the skin in general.

WARNINGS: Nerisalic is not for ophthalmic use and, consequently, should not be used in or near the eyes.

Nerisalic should not be applied in rhagades and ulcerations (e.g. lower leg ulcers). Inclusion of salicylic acid in this preparation increases steroid penetration into the viable epidermis thereby increasing the potential for skin atrophy.

Pregnancy: The safety of Nerisalic during pregnancy has not been established. Teratogenic and embryotoxic effects of diflucortolone valerate have been reported following dermal application in animal studies. Nerisalic should be used during pregnancy only if the potential benefits justify the potential risks to the fetus.

Lactation: Systemically administered corticosteroids can appear in human milk and can suppress growth, interfere with endogenous corticosteroid production or cause adverse effects. Caution should be exercised when Nerisalic is administered to a nursing woman since it is not known whether the ingredients of Nerisalic are excreted in human milk.

PRECAUTIONS: Systemic absorption of topical corticosteroids has produced reversible hypothalamic-pituitary-adrenal (HPA) axis suppression, manifestations of Cushing's syndrome, hyperglycemia and glucosuria in some patients.

Significant systemic absorption may occur when steroids are applied over large areas of the body or if used under an occlusive dressing. To minimize this possibility when long-term therapy is anticipated, interrupt treatment periodically or treat one area of the body at a time. It is recommended that patients receiving a large dose of a potent topical steroid applied over a large surface area be evaluated periodically for evidence of HPA axis suppression by using the urinary free cortisol and ACTH stimulation tests. If HPA axis inhibition is observed, an attempt should be made to withdraw the drug, to reduce the frequency of application or substitute a less potent steroid. Recovery of HPA axis function is generally prompt and complete upon discontinuation of the drug. Infrequently, signs and symptoms of steroid withdrawal may occur, requiring supplemental systemic corticosteroids.

If irritation or hypersensitivity reactions develop, Nerisalic should be discontinued and appropriate therapy initiated.

Prolonged use of topical corticosteroid products may produce atrophy of the skin and of s.c. tissues, particularly on flexor surfaces and on the face, telangiectasias, hirsutism and steroid induced acne. If this is noted, discontinue use of the product. Long-term therapy with Nerisalic should be avoided.

In cases of bacterial or fungal skin infections, appropriate antibacterial agents should be used as primary therapy. If it is considered necessary, Nerisalic may be used as an adjunct to control inflammation, erythema and itching.

Nerisalic should be used with caution in patients with stasis dermatitis and other skin diseases associated with impaired circulation, on extremities of diabetics with impaired circulation or on patients with inherent compromised cardiovascular circulatory problems.

Patients should be advised to inform subsequent physicians of the prior use of corticosteroids.

Systemic absorption of the corticosteroid and salicylic acid may be increased with elevated body temperature or occlusive dressings. Patients with elevated temperatures should be monitored for HPA axis effects and occlusive dressings should not be used.

Occlusive dressings should not be applied if there is an elevation of body temperature.

Because of the risk of salicylate intoxication, long term or large area and occlusive use of Nerisalic should be avoided in patients with impaired renal function.

Since salicylic acid is absorbed almost completely, the simultaneous topical or internal use of other preparations containing salicylic acid or salicylate is inadvisable. The concentration of salicylic acid contained in the preparation is not high enough for the treatment of secondary skin diseases caused by bacteria or fungi. Additional antibacterial or antimycotic therapy is recommended in these cases.

Children: Due to their larger skin surface area to body weight ratio, children may demonstrate a greater susceptibility to the topical corticosteroid-induced HPA axis suppression and Cushing's syndrome than mature patients.

Suppression of the HPA axis, Cushing's syndrome and intracranial hypertension have been reported in children receiving topical corticosteroids. Manifestations of adrenal suppression in children include linear growth retardation, delayed weight gain, low plasma cortisol levels and absence of response to ACTH stimulation. Manifestations of intracranial hypertension include bulging fontanelles, headaches and bilateral papilledema.

Administration of topical corticosteroid to children should be limited to the least amount compatible with an effective therapeutic regimen. Chronic corticosteroid therapy may interfere with the growth and development of the children.

The following tests may be helpful in evaluating HPA axis suppression due to corticosteroid component: urinary free cortisol test and ACTH stimulation test.

Because of the risk, of salicylate intoxication, long term or large area and occlusive use of Nerisalic should be avoided in babies, infants and in children.

ADVERSE EFFECTS: The following local adverse reactions are reported when topical corticosteroids are used as recommended. These reactions are listed in an approximate decreasing order of occurrence: burning, itching, irritation, dryness folliculitis, hypertrichosis, acneiform eruptions, hypopigmentation, perioral dermatitis, allergic contact dermatitis, maceration of the skin, secondary infection, skin atrophy, telangiectasia, striae and miliaria. Hypothalamic-pituitary-adrenal axis suppression have also been reported following topical corticosteroid therapy.

Posterior sub-capsular cataracts have been reported following systemic use of corticosteroids.

In addition, the salicylic acid contained in the preparation may produce some desquamation, local reddening of the skin, pruritus, burning, pain and stinging. Hypersensitivity to salicylic acid may occur. If this occurs, discontinue use.

OVERDOSE:

Symptoms: Percutaneous absorption of corticosteroids can occur when large amounts of corticosteroids are applied. Toxic effects may include ecchymosis of skin, peptic ulceration, hypertension, aggravation of infection, hirsutism, acne, edema and muscle weakness due to protein depletion.

High levels of salicylates may cause temporary hearing or visual disturbance, drowsiness and nausea.

Treatment: No specific antidote is available. Treatment should be symptomatic.

Appropriate symptomatic treatment of corticosteroid and/or salicylic acid overdosage is indicated. Acute hypercorticoid symptoms are usually reversible. Treat electrolyte imbalance, if necessary. In cases of chronic toxicity, slow withdrawal of corticosteroid is advised.

For management of a suspected drug overdose, CPhA recommends that you contact your **regional Poison Control Centre**. See the *CPS* Directory section for a list of Poison Control Centres.

DOSAGE: Nerisalic should be applied as a thin film to diseased areas 2 to 3 times daily in the first week of treatment. During subsequent weeks, 1 or 2 applications/day are sufficient. The duration of the treatment should not exceed a total of 4 weeks.

The total dose applied weekly should not exceed 100 g.

If improvement is not noted within a few days to a week, the local application of Nerisalic should be discontinued and the patient re-evaluated.

SUPPLIED: Each g of oily cream contains: diflucortolone-21-valerate 0.1% and salicylic acid 3% in a water-in-oil emulsion. Nonmedicinal ingredients: hydrocarbons (white petrolatum, paraffin), white wax and dehymuls E. There is no preservative. Tubes of 30 g. Store at 15 to 30°C.

The reader is invited to consult CPhA's monograph **Corticosteroids: Topical**.

Nerisone®

diflucortolone valerate

Topical Corticosteroid

Stiefel, a GSK company

SUPPLIED: Cream: Each g of oil-in-water emulsion contains: diflucortolone valerate 1 mg (0.1%). Nonmedicinal ingredients: carbomer 934, edetate disodium, methyl paraben, mineral oil, polyoxyl 40 stearate, propyl paraben, purified water, sodium hydroxide, stearyl alcohol and white petrolatum. Tubes of 30 g. Store between 15 and 30°C.

Oily Cream: Each g of water-in-oil emulsion contains: diflucortolone valerate 1 mg (0.1%). Nonmedicinal ingredients: Dehymuls E, mineral oil, purified water, white petrolatum and white wax. There is no preservative. Tubes of 30 and 60 g. Store between 15 and 30°C.

Ointment: Each g of single-phase fatty ointment contains: diflucortolone valerate 1 mg (0.1%). Nonmedicinal ingredients: hydrogenated castor oil, microcrystalline wax, mineral oil and white petrolatum. There is no preservative. Tubes of 30 g. Store between 15 and 30°C.

Nesacaine®-CE

chloroprocaine HCl

Local Anesthetic

AstraZeneca

Date of Preparation: April 12, 2000
Date of Revision: June 29, 2006

PHARMACOLOGY: Mechanism of Action: Chloroprocaine stabilizes the neuronal membrane and prevents the initiation and transmission of nerve impulses, thereby effecting local anesthetic action.

Onset of Action: The onset of action is rapid (usually within 6 to 12 minutes). The duration of anesthesia depends on the procedure and the amount used, but could last up to 60 minutes.

Pharmacokinetics: Chloroprocaine is rapidly hydrolyzed in plasma by pseudocholinesterase. This hydrolysis results in the formation of β-diethylaminoethanol and 2-chloro-4 aminobenzoic acid which inhibits the action of sulfonamides (see Precautions).

Solutions of chloroprocaine do not injure nervous tissue and are not irritating to other tissues in the recommended concentrations.

INDICATIONS: For the production of local anesthesia by infiltration and regional nerve block, including caudal and epidural blocks. Any unused portion should be discarded. Chloroprocaine should not be used for spinal anesthesia.

CONTRAINDICATIONS: Hypersensitive (allergic) to drugs of the PABA ester group.

Although CNS disease is generally considered a contraindication to caudal or epidural nerve block, it is not a contraindication to peripheral nerve block. Pathologic changes of the vertebral column may make epidural puncture impossible or inadvisable.

WARNINGS: Local anesthetics should only be employed by clinicians who are well versed in diagnosis and management of dose related toxicity and other acute emergencies which might arise from the block to be employed, and then only after ensuring the immediate availability of oxygen, other resuscitative drugs, cardiopulmonary resuscitative equipment, and the personnel resources needed for proper management of toxic reactions and related emergencies (see also Adverse Effects and Precautions). Delay in proper management of dose related toxicity, underventilation from any cause and/or altered sensitivity may lead to the development of acidosis, cardiac arrest and possibly, death.

Vasopressors should not be used in the presence of ergot-type oxytocic drugs, since a severe persistent hypertension may occur. To avoid **intravascular injection**, aspiration should be performed before the anesthetic solution is injected. The needle must be repositioned until no blood return can be elicited. However, the absence of blood in the syringe does not guarantee that intravascular injection has been avoided.

There are no data concerning use of chloroprocaine for **obstetrical paracervical block** when **toxemia of pregnancy** is present or when **fetal distress or prematurity** is anticipated in advance of the block; such use is, therefore, not recommended. The following information should be considered by clinicians who select chloroprocaine for obstetrical paracervical block anesthesia:

Fetal bradycardia (generally a heart rate of less than 120 per minute for more than 2 minutes) has been noted by electronic monitoring in about 5% to 10% of the cases (various studies) where initial total doses of 120 mg to 400 mg of chloroprocaine were employed. The incidence of bradycardia, within this dose range, might not be dose related.

Fetal acidosis has not been demonstrated by blood gas monitoring around the time of bradycardia or afterwards. These data are limited and are generally restricted to non-toxemic cases where fetal distress or prematurity was not anticipated in advance of the block.

No intact chloroprocaine and only trace quantities of a hydrolysis product, 2-chloro-4 aminobenzoic acid have been demonstrated in umbilical cord arterial or venous plasma following properly administered paracervical block with chloroprocaine.

The role of drug factors and non-drug factors associated with fetal bradycardia following paracervical block are unexplained at this time.

PRECAUTIONS: The safety and effectiveness of chloroprocaine injections depend upon proper dosage, correct technique, adequate precautions and readiness for emergencies.

The lowest dosage that results in effective anesthesia should be used to avoid high plasma levels and serious undesirable systemic side effects. Tolerance varies with the status of the patient. Debilitated patients, elderly patients, acutely ill patients and children should be given reduced doses commensurate with their age and physical status.

Solutions containing vasoconstrictors should be used cautiously in the presence of disease which may adversely affect the patient's cardiovascular system.

Since ester-type local anesthetics are hydrolyzed by plasma cholinesterase produced by the liver, chloroprocaine should be used cautiously in patients with hepatic disease.

Injections should always be made slowly and with frequent aspirations to avoid inadvertent rapid intravascular administration which can produce systemic toxicity.

Chloroprocaine should be employed cautiously in persons with known drug allergies or sensitivities.

Injection of solutions containing epinephrine (see Dosage) in areas where the blood supply is limited (i.e., ears, nose, digits, etc.) or when peripheral vascular disease is present should be used cautiously.

Drug Interactions: Serious cardiac arrhythmias may occur if preparations containing a vasopressor are employed in patients during or following the administration of chloroform, halothane, cyclopropane, trichloroethylene, or other related agents. The para-aminobenzoic acid metabolite of chloroprocaine inhibits the action of sulfonamides. Therefore, chloroprocaine should not be used in any condition in which a sulfonamide drug is being employed.

In obstetrics, if vasoconstrictor drugs are used either to correct hypotension or are added to the local anesthetic solution, the obstetrician should be warned that some oxytocic drugs may cause severe persistent hypertension and even rupture of a cerebral blood vessel may occur during the postpartum period.

Solutions containing vasoconstrictors, particularly epinephrine and norepinephrine, should be used with extreme caution in patients receiving certain antidepressants, such as MAO inhibitors and tricyclic compounds, since severe prolonged hypertension may occur.

Carcinogenesis, Mutagenesis and Impairment of Fertility: Long-term studies in animals to evaluate carcinogenic potential and reproduction studies to evaluate mutagenesis or impairment of fertility have not been conducted with chloroprocaine.

Pregnancy: Safe use of chloroprocaine has not been established with respect to adverse effects upon fetal development. This fact should be carefully considered before administering this drug to women of childbearing potential, particularly during early pregnancy. This does not preclude the use of the drug at term for obstetrical analgesia. Adverse effects on the fetus, course of labor, or delivery have rarely been observed when proper dosage and proper technique have been employed.

Labor and Delivery: Local anesthetics rapidly cross the placenta, and when used for epidural, paracervical, pudendal or caudal block anesthesia, can cause varying degrees of maternal, fetal and neonatal toxicity.

The incidence and degree of toxicity depend upon the procedure performed, the type and amount of drug used, and the technique of drug administration. Adverse reactions in the parturient, fetus and neonate involve alterations of the CNS, peripheral vascular tone and cardiac function.

Maternal hypotension has resulted from regional anesthesia. Local anesthetics produce vasodilation by blocking sympathetic nerves. Elevating the patient's legs and positioning her on her left side will help prevent decreases in blood pressure. The fetal heart rate should also be monitored continuously, and electronic fetal monitoring is highly advisable.

Lactation: It is not known whether this drug is excreted in human milk. Because many drugs are excreted in human milk, caution should be exercised when chloroprocaine is administered to a nursing mother.

ADVERSE EFFECTS: Systemic: Systemic adverse reactions result from high plasma levels due to rapid absorption, inadvertent intravascular injection or excessive dosage. Hypersensitivity, idiosyncrasy, or diminished tolerance (as in patients with plasma cholinesterase deficiency) are other causes of reactions. Reactions due to overdosage (high plasma levels) are systemic and involve the CNS and the cardiovascular system.

Central Nervous System: These are characterized by excitation and/or depression. Restlessness, anxiety, dizziness, tinnitus, blurred vision or tremors may occur, possibly proceeding to convulsions. However, excitement may be transient or absent, with depression the first manifestation of an adverse reaction. This may quickly be followed by drowsiness merging into unconsciousness and respiratory arrest.

Cardiovascular: High doses or unintended intravascular injection may cause depression of the myocardium manifested by an initial episode of hypotension and bradycardia and even cardiac arrest.

Allergic: Allergic reactions are rare and may occur as a result of sensitivity to chloroprocaine and are characterized by cutaneous lesions, urticaria, edema and anaphylactoid type symptomatology. These allergic reactions should be managed by conventional means. The detection of potential sensitivity by skin testing has not been fully established.

Neurologic: In the practice of epidural block, occasional inadvertent penetration of the subarachnoid space by the catheter may occur. The subsequent reactions depend on the amount of drug administered subdurally and may include, among others, spinal block of varying magnitude, loss of bowel and bladder control, loss of perineal sensation and sexual function. Persistent neurological deficit of some lower spinal segments with slow recovery (several months) has been reported in rare instances (see Dosage, Caudal and Epidural Block). Backache and headache have also been noted following lumbar epidural or caudal block.

OVERDOSE:

Symptoms: Acute emergencies from local anesthetics are generally related to high plasma levels encountered during therapeutic use of local anesthetics or to unintended subarachnoid injection of local anesthetic solution (see Adverse Effects, Warnings, and Precautions).

Treatment of a patient with toxic manifestations consists of assuring and maintaining a patent airway and supporting ventilation with oxygen and assisted or controlled ventilation (respiration) as required. This usually will be sufficient in the management of most reactions. Should a convulsion persist despite ventilatory therapy, small increments of anticonvulsive agents may be given i.v. such as a benzodiazepine (e.g. diazepam), or an ultra-short acting barbiturate (e.g. thiopental or thiamylal) or a short-acting barbiturate (e.g. pentobarbital or secobarbital). Cardiovascular depression may require circulatory assistance with i.v. fluids and/or vasopressors (e.g. ephedrine) as dictated by the clinical situation.

If not treated immediately, both convulsions and cardiovascular depression can result in hypoxia, acidosis, bradycardia, arrhythmias and cardiac arrest. If cardiac arrest should occur, standard cardiopulmonary resuscitative measures should be instituted. Recovery has been reported after prolonged resuscitative efforts.

Treatment: See Symptoms.

For management of a suspected drug overdose, CPhA recommends that you contact your **regional Poison Control Centre**. See the *CPS* Directory section for a list of Poison Control Centres.

DOSAGE: The lowest dose needed to provide effective anesthesia should be administered. As with all local anesthetics, the dosage varies and depends upon the area to be anesthetized, vascularity of the tissues, number of neuronal segments to be blocked, individual tolerance and the technique employed.

Dosages should be reduced for children, elderly or debilitated patients, and in patients with cardiac and/or liver disease. For specific techniques and procedures, refer to standard textbooks.

Preparation of Epinephrine Solution: To prepare a 1:200 000 epinephrine-chloroprocaine HCl solution add 0.1 mL of a 1:1000 epinephrine injection USP to 20 mL of Nesacaine-CE. Please consult package insert text for epinephrine for Contraindications, Warnings and Precautions.

As a guide for some routine procedures, suggested doses are given below:

1. Infiltration and Nerve Block: Local Infiltration: Quantity depends on the concentration of chloroprocaine, the site to be infiltrated and the discretion of the operator (see Table 1).

Table 1: Nesacaine-CE

Nerve Blocks

Type of Block	Volume (mL)	Concentration	Total Dose (mg)
Mandibular	2 to 3	2%	40–60
Infraorbital	0.5 to 1	2%	10–20
Brachial Plexus	30 to 40	2%	600–800
Pudendal Block for obstetrics	10 mL each side	2%	400

2. Caudal and Epidural Block: Caudal Anesthesia: The initial dose is 15 to 25 mL of chloroprocaine 2%. This volume should not be exceeded. Repeated doses may be given at 40 to 60 minute intervals.

Epidural Anesthesia: The recommended total volume of chloroprocaine for the main dose in epidural anesthesia is 15 to 25 mL, and this volume should not be exceeded. Furthermore, a local anesthetic agent other than chloroprocaine, such as Xylocaine Parenteral Solution for infiltration and nerve block, should be used for skin and needle tract infiltration. Repeated doses 2 to 6 mL less than the original dose may be given at 40 to 50 minute intervals.

In order to guard against possible adverse reactions resulting from inadvertent penetration of the subarachnoid space, the following procedures are recommended:

1. Use of an adequate (in the case of Nesacaine-CE, approximately 5 mL of 2%) test dose prior to induction of complete block. This test dose should be repeated if the patient is moved in such a fashion as to have displaced the epidural catheter. At least 5 minutes should elapse after each test dose prior to proceeding further.
2. Injection of a large, single therapeutic dose through a catheter should be avoided; instead, repeated fractional doses are advocated.
3. In the event of the known injection of a large volume of Nesacaine-CE into the subarachnoid space, an appropriate amount of cerebrospinal fluid (such as 10 mL) should be withdrawn through the catheter or by separate lumbar puncture.

Maximum Dosage: Adults: The maximum single recommended doses of chloroprocaine in adults are: without epinephrine, 11 mg/kg body weight, not to exceed 800 mg; and with epinephrine (1:200 000), 14 mg/kg body weight, not to exceed 1000 mg. For caudal and lumbar epidural anesthesia, a total of 25 mL of solution should not be exceeded.

Sterilization, Storage and Technical Procedures: As with other anesthetics having a free aromatic amino group, Nesacaine-CE solutions are slightly photosensitive and may become discolored after prolonged exposure to light. It is recommended that these vials be stored in the original outer containers, protected from direct sunlight. Discolored solution should not be administered. If exposed to low temperatures, Nesacaine-CE may deposit crystals of chloroprocaine HCl, which will redissolve with shaking when returned to room temperature. The product should not be used if it contains undissolved material.

Nesacaine solutions should not be resterilized by autoclaving. Sterilization of vials with ethylene oxide is not recommended, since absorption through the closure may occur.

Chloroprocaine is incompatible with caustic alkalis and their carbonates, soaps, silver salts, iodine and iodides.

SUPPLIED: Each mL contains: chloroprocaine HCl 20 mg (2%). Also contains sodium chloride, water for injection, hydrochloric acid and/or sodium hydroxide to adjust pH to 2.7 to 4.0. Single use vials of 20 mL, packages of 10. Keep from freezing. Protect from light. Store at controlled room temperature 15 to 30°C.

Neulasta® Ⓟ

pegfilgrastim

Hematopoietic Agent—Granulocyte Colony-stimulating Factor

Amgen

Date of Revision: January 25, 2010

SUMMARY PRODUCT INFORMATION:

Route of Administration	Dosage Form/ Strength	Clinically Relevant Nonmedicinal Ingredients
Subcutaneous	Sterile Solution for Injection/ 6 mg (10 mg/mL)	Not applicable For a complete listing see Dosage Forms, Composition and Packaging.

DESCRIPTION: Neulasta (pegfilgrastim) is a long-acting form of recombinant human granulocyte colony-stimulating factor (r-metHuG-CSF) or filgrastim. Neulasta is composed of filgrastim with a 20 000 dalton polyethylene glycol (PEG) molecule covalently bound to the N-terminal methionine residue. Filgrastim is a 175 amino acid protein with a molecular weight of 18 800 daltons; Neulasta has a total molecular weight of 39 000 daltons.

INDICATIONS AND CLINICAL USE: Neulasta (pegfilgrastim) is indicated to decrease the incidence of infection, as manifested by febrile neutropenia, in patients with non-myeloid malignancies receiving myelosuppressive anti-neoplastic drugs.

Pediatrics (<18 years of age): The safety and effectiveness of Neulasta in pediatric patients have not been established.

CONTRAINDICATIONS: Neulasta (pegfilgrastim) is contraindicated in patients with known hypersensitivity to *E. coli*-derived proteins, pegfilgrastim, filgrastim, or any other component of the product. For a complete listing of the components, see Dosage Forms, Composition and Packaging.

WARNINGS AND PRECAUTIONS:

Serious Warnings and Precautions

- Splenic rupture, including fatal cases, has been reported following the administration of Neulasta (pegfilgrastim) and its parent compound, filgrastim (see Warnings and Precautions, General).
- Severe sickle cell crises have been associated with the use of Neulasta in patients with sickle cell disorders. Severe sickle cell crises, in some cases resulting in death, have also been associated with filgrastim, the parent compound of pegfilgrastim (see Warnings and Precautions, Hematologic (Sickle Cell Disorders)).

General: Neulasta (pegfilgrastim) has not been evaluated for PBPC (peripheral blood progenitor cell) mobilization. Therefore, it should not be used in that setting.

Splenic Rupture: Splenic rupture, including fatal cases, has been reported following the administration of Neulasta (pegfilgrastim) and its parent compound, filgrastim. Patients receiving Neulasta who report left upper abdominal and/or shoulder tip pain should be evaluated for an enlarged spleen or splenic rupture.

Simultaneous Use with Chemotherapy and Radiation Therapy: The safety and efficacy of Neulasta administered concurrently with cytotoxic chemotherapy have not been established. Because of the potential for an increase in sensitivity of rapidly dividing myeloid cells to cytotoxic chemotherapy, Neulasta should not be administered in the period between 14 days before and 24 hours after administration of cytotoxic chemotherapy (see Dosage and Administration).

The safety and efficacy of Neulasta have not been evaluated in patients receiving chemotherapy associated with delayed myelosuppression (e.g., nitrosoureas), mitomycin C, or myelosuppressive doses of anti-metabolites such as 5-fluorouracil (5-FU). Concomitant use of Neulasta with 5-FU or other anti-metabolites has not been evaluated in humans, although it has been studied and shown to potentiate myelosuppression in animal models.

The safety and efficacy of Neulasta have not been evaluated in patients receiving radiation therapy.

Carcinogenesis and Mutagenesis: No carcinogenesis or mutagenesis studies were conducted with Neulasta.

Potential Effect on Malignant Cells: Neulasta (pegfilgrastim) and filgrastim are growth factors that primarily stimulate production of neutrophils and neutrophil precursors by binding to the G-CSF receptor. Overall, the possibility that Neulasta can act as a growth factor for any tumour type cannot be excluded. Randomized studies have demonstrated that treatment with filgrastim following chemotherapy for AML does not adversely influence the outcome of treatment. The use of Neulasta in AML, chronic myeloid leukemia (CML) and myelodysplasia (MDS) has not been studied.

Hematologic (Sickle Cell Disorders): Severe sickle cell crises have been associated with the use of Neulasta in patients with sickle cell disorders. Severe sickle cell crises, in some cases resulting in death, have also been associated with filgrastim, the parent compound of pegfilgrastim. Only physicians qualified by specialized training or experience in the treatment of patients with sickle cell disorders should prescribe Neulasta for such patients, and only after careful consideration of the potential risks and benefits.

Hypersensitivity/Allergic Reactions: Allergic-type reactions, including anaphylaxis, skin rash, urticaria and erythema/flushing occurring on initial or subsequent treatment have been reported both with Neulasta and filgrastim. In some cases, symptoms have recurred with rechallenge, suggesting a causal relationship. In rare cases, allergic reactions including anaphylaxis, recurred within days after initial anti-allergic treatment was discontinued. If a serious allergic reaction or an anaphylactic reaction occurs, appropriate therapy should be administered and further use of Neulasta should be discontinued. Antibodies to filgrastim or pegfilgrastim have been reported, although no neutralizing antibodies have been reported (see Adverse Reactions, Immunogenicity).

Leukocytosis: In clinical studies with Neulasta, white blood cell counts of 100×10^9/L or greater have been reported in less than 1% of patients with cancer receiving myelosuppressive chemotherapy (n=930), and were not associated with any reported adverse clinical effects.

In studies of Neulasta administration after chemotherapy, most reported side effects were consistent with those usually seen as a result of cytotoxic chemotherapy (see Adverse Reactions). Because of the potential for patients to receive full doses of chemotherapy on the prescribed schedule, patients may be at greater risk of thrombocytopenia, anemia, and non-hematologic consequences of increased chemotherapy doses (please refer to the prescribing information for specific chemotherapy agents). Regular monitoring of hematocrit value and platelet count is recommended. Furthermore, care should be exercised in the administration of Neulasta in conjunction with drugs known to lower platelet count.

Respiratory: Acute respiratory distress syndrome (ARDS) has been reported following administration of Neulasta and is postulated to be secondary to an influx of neutrophils to sites of inflammation in the lungs. Neutropenic patients receiving Neulasta who develop fever, lung infiltrates, or respiratory distress should be evaluated for the possibility of ARDS. In the event that ARDS occurs, Neulasta should be discontinued and/or withheld until resolution of ARDS and patients should receive appropriate medical management for this condition.

Sexual Function/Reproduction: No studies evaluating sexual function or reproduction in humans were conducted with Neulasta.

Special Populations: Pregnant Women: There were no pregnant women exposed to Neulasta in clinical trials. Neulasta should be used during pregnancy only if the potential benefit outweighs the risk to the fetus.

Nursing Women: It is not known whether Neulasta is excreted in human milk. Because many drugs are excreted in human milk, Neulasta is not recommended for women who are breast feeding. Neulasta should only be administered to a nursing woman if the potential benefit outweighs the risk.

Pediatrics (<18 years of age): The safety and effectiveness of Neulasta in pediatric patients have not been established.

Geriatrics (>65 years of age): Of the total number of subjects with cancer who received Neulasta in clinical studies (n=930), 139 subjects (15%) were 65 years or older and 18 subjects (2%) were 75 years or older. No overall differences in safety or effectiveness were observed between these patients and younger patients, and other reported clinical experience has not identified differences in responses between the elderly and younger patients; however, due to the small number of elderly subjects, small but clinically relevant differences cannot be excluded.

Monitoring and Laboratory Tests: To assess a patient's hematologic status and ability to tolerate myelosuppressive chemotherapy, a complete blood count (CBC) and platelet count should be obtained before chemotherapy is administered. Neulasta produced ANC (absolute neutrophil count) profiles similar to daily filgrastim, including earlier ANC nadir, shorter duration of severe neutropenia, and accelerated ANC recovery, compared with ANC profiles observed without growth factor support. Regular monitoring of hematocrit value, white blood cell count and platelet count, as clinically indicated, is recommended.

ADVERSE REACTIONS: Adverse Drug Reaction Overview: See Warnings and Precautions regarding Splenic Rupture, ARDS, Allergic Reactions and Sickle Cell Disease.

Clinical Trial Adverse Drug Reactions: Because clinical trials are conducted under very specific conditions the adverse reaction rates observed in the clinical trials may not reflect the rates observed in practice and should not be compared to the rates in the clinical trials of another drug. Adverse drug reaction information from clinical trials is useful for identifying drug-related adverse events and for approximating rates.

Safety data are based on 7 randomized clinical trials involving 932 patients with lymphoma and solid tumours (breast and thoracic) who received Neulasta (pegfilgrastim) after non-myeloablative cytotoxic chemotherapy. Common adverse events occurred at similar rates between the treatment arms in both the filgrastim-controlled trials (Neulasta, n=465; filgrastim, n=331) and the placebo-controlled trial (Neulasta, n=467; placebo, n=461). Most adverse experiences were attributed by the investigator as the sequelae of the underlying malignancy or cytotoxic chemotherapy. In the filgrastim-controlled trials, these adverse experiences occurred at rates between 15% and 72% and included: nausea, fatigue, alopecia, diarrhea, vomiting, constipation, fever, anorexia, skeletal pain, headache, taste perversion, dyspepsia, myalgia, insomnia, abdominal pain, arthralgia, generalized weakness, peripheral edema, dizziness, granulocytopenia, stomatitis, mucositis and neutropenic fever. A summary of the most frequently reported adverse reactions in these randomized clinical trials can be found in Table 1 and Table 2.

In clinical trials comparing Neulasta to filgrastim, medullary bone pain was reported in 26% of Neulasta-treated patients, which was comparable to the incidence in filgrastim-treated patients. In the study comparing Neulasta to placebo, the incidence of bone pain was 23% vs. 16%, respectively. This bone pain was generally reported to be of mild-to-moderate severity. Approximately 17% (for all bone pain type AEs; 10% for specifically "bone pain") of all subjects utilized non narcotic analgesics and less than 6% utilized narcotic analgesics in association with bone pain. No patient withdrew from study due to bone pain.

Across all studies, no life-threatening or fatal adverse events were attributed to Neulasta. There was only one serious adverse event (dyspnea) reported as possibly related to Neulasta in a single patient. No events of pleuritis, pericarditis, or other major systemic reactions to Neulasta were reported.

No clinically significant changes in vital signs were observed. No evidence of interaction of Neulasta with other drugs was observed in the course of clinical trials (see Warnings and Precautions).

Table 1: Neulasta

Most Frequently[a] Reported Adverse Reactions in Randomized Clinical Trials with Filgrastim as Comparator

Body System and Preferred Term	Neulasta (pegfilgrastim) (n=465)	Filgrastim (n=331)
Application Site		
Injection Site Pain	16 (3%)	9 (3%)
Body as a Whole		
Pain	8 (2%)	4 (1%)
Chest Pain (non-cardiac)	4 (1%)	3 (1%)
Edema Periorbital	3 (1%)	0 (0%)
Fever	3 (1%)	4 (1%)
CNS/PNS		
Headache	20 (4%)	12 (4%)
Musculoskeletal		
Skeletal Pain	96 (21%)	89 (27%)
Myalgia	32 (7%)	25 (8%)
Arthralgia	27 (6%)	19 (6%)
Back Pain	19 (4%)	26 (8%)
Limb Pain	12 (3%)	7 (2%)
Musculoskeletal Pain	5 (1%)	4 (1%)
Neck Pain	4 (1%)	3 (1%)

[a] Most frequently reported events were considered to be those events reported in ≥1% of the patients in the Neulasta group.

Table 2: Neulasta

Most Frequently[a] Reported Adverse Reactions in Randomized Clinical Trials with Placebo Control

Body System and Preferred Term	Neulasta (pegfilgrastim) (n=467)	Placebo (n=461)
Blood and Lymphatic System Disorders		
Leukocytosis	5 (1%)	1 (0%)
Gastrointestinal Disorders		
Diarrhea	9 (2%)	10 (2%)
General Disorders and Administration Site Conditions		
Pyrexia	8 (2%)	9 (2%)
Fatigue	3 (1%)	5 (1%)
Infections and Infestations		
Influenza	6 (1%)	5 (1%)
Musculoskeletal and Connective Tissue Disorders		
Bone Pain	62 (13%)	41 (9%)
Myalgia	26 (6%)	23 (5%)
Arthralgia	32 (7%)	19 (4%)

(cont'd)

Table 2: Neulasta *(cont'd)*

Most Frequently[a] Reported Adverse Reactions in Randomized Clinical Trials with Placebo Control

Body System and Preferred Term	Neulasta (pegfilgrastim) (n=467)	Placebo (n=461)
Polymyalgia	8 (2%)	7 (2%)
Musculoskeletal Pain	14 (3%)	5 (1%)
Pain in Limb	11 (2%)	5 (1%)
Back Pain	8 (2%)	4 (1%)
Polyarthralgia	5 (1%)	0 (0%)
Nervous System Disorders		
Headache	6 (1%)	2 (0%)
Skin and Subcutaneous Tissue Disorders		
Alopecia	8 (2%)	9 (2%)

a Most frequently reported events were considered to be those events reported in ≥1% of the patients in the Neulasta group.

Less Common Clinical Trial Adverse Drug Reactions (<1%): The following adverse drug reactions were reported at an incidence of <1% in controlled clinical studies (occurring in more than 1 patient, with higher frequency than filgrastim):
General Disorders and Administration Site Conditions: injection site bruising.
Infections and Infestations: rhinitis.
Nervous System Disorders: hypertonia.
Skin and Subcutaneous Tissue Disorders: periorbital edema.

The following adverse drug reactions were reported at an incidence of <1% in controlled clinical studies (occurring in more than 1 patient, with higher frequency than placebo):
General Disorders and Administration Site Conditions: chest pain, pain.
Abnormal Hematologic and Clinical Chemistry Findings: Spontaneously reversible elevations in LDH, alkaline phosphatase, and uric acid of mild-to-moderate severity were observed. Most changes have been attributed to post-cytokine bone marrow expansion as well as to chemotherapy and metastatic disease. The incidences of these changes, presented for Neulasta versus filgrastim and placebo, were: LDH (18% versus 29% and 18%), alkaline phosphatase (11% versus 16% and 12%), and uric acid (10% versus 9% and 13% [1% of uric acid reported cases for filgrastim and Neulasta treatment groups were classified as severe]).

In clinical studies with Neulasta, white blood cell counts of 100×10^9/L or greater have been reported in less than 1% of patients with cancer receiving myelosuppressive chemotherapy (n=930), and were not associated with any reported adverse clinical effects.
Immunogenicity: As with all therapeutic proteins, there is a potential for immunogenicity. The incidence of antibody development in patients receiving Neulasta has not been adequately determined. While available data suggest that a small proportion of patients developed binding antibodies to filgrastim or Neulasta, the nature and specificity of these antibodies has not been adequately studied. No neutralizing antibodies have been detected using a cell based bioassay in 46 (9%, n=534) patients who apparently developed binding antibodies. The detection of antibody formation is highly dependent on the sensitivity and specificity of the assay, and the observed incidence of antibody positivity in an assay may be influenced by several factors including sample handling, concomitant medications, and underlying disease. Therefore, comparison of the incidence of antibodies to Neulasta with the incidence of antibodies to other products may be misleading.

Cytopenias resulting from an antibody response to exogenous growth factors have been reported on rare occasions in patients treated with other recombinant growth factors. There is a theoretical possibility that an antibody directed against Neulasta may cross react with endogenous G-CSF, resulting in immune mediated neutropenia, but this has not been observed in clinical studies.
Post-Market Adverse Drug Reactions: In addition to the events listed above, reports of adverse reactions have been identified post-market in patients receiving Neulasta, including:

- Splenic rupture (see Warnings and Precautions, Splenic Rupture)
- Acute respiratory distress syndrome (ARDS) (see Warnings and Precautions, Respiratory)
- Allergic reactions (see Warnings and Precautions, Hypersensitivity/Allergic Reactions)
- Sickle cell crisis (see Warnings and Precautions, Hematologic (Sickle Cell Disorders))
- Injection site reactions (pain, induration, and local erythema)
- Generalized erythema and flushing
- Sweet's syndrome (acute febrile neutrophilic dermatosis)

DRUG INTERACTIONS: Overview: Drug interactions between Neulasta (pegfilgrastim) and other drugs have not been studied. Drugs such as lithium that may potentiate the release of neutrophils should be used with caution; such patients should have more frequent monitoring of their neutrophil counts.
Drug-Drug Interactions: Interactions with other drugs have not been established.
Drug-Food Interactions: Interactions with food have not been established.
Drug-Herb Interactions: Interactions with herbal products have not been established.
Drug-Laboratory Test Interactions: Increased hematopoietic activity of the bone marrow in response to growth factor therapy has been associated with transient positive bone-imaging changes. This should be considered when interpreting bone-imaging results.

DOSAGE AND ADMINISTRATION: Dosing Considerations: Neulasta (pegfilgrastim) should be administered no sooner than 24 hours after the administration of cytotoxic chemotherapy (see Warnings and Precautions).

Renal impairment, including end-stage renal disease, appears to have no effect on the pharmacokinetics of Neulasta and no dosage adjustment is required.
Recommended Dose and Dosage Adjustment: The recommended dosage of Neulasta is a single subcutaneous injection of 6 mg, administered once per cycle of chemotherapy. Neulasta should be administered no sooner than 24 hours after the administration of cytotoxic chemotherapy (see Warnings and Precautions).
Missed Dose: If a scheduled dose is missed, Neulasta should not be administered less than 14 days before subsequent administration of cytotoxic chemotherapy.
Administration: Neulasta is intended for subcutaneous injection only and should not be given by any other route of administration. Neulasta should not be mixed with any diluents.

Neulasta should not be vigorously shaken.

Following administration of Neulasta from the single-use prefilled syringe, the patient should activate the UltraSafe Needle Guard by placing their hands behind the needle, grasping the guard with one hand, and sliding the guard forward until the needle is completely covered and the guard clicks into place. **Note:** If an audible click is not heard, the needle guard may not be completely activated.

OVERDOSAGE:
The maximum tolerated dose of Neulasta (pegfilgrastim) has not been determined in humans. Neulasta administered at a dose of 300 µg/kg (n=12), approximately three times the recommended dose, exhibited an adverse event profile similar to that observed at the recommended dose.

For management of a suspected drug overdose, CPhA recommends that you contact your **regional Poison Control Centre**. See the *CPS* Directory section for a list of Poison Control Centres.

ACTION AND CLINICAL PHARMACOLOGY: Mechanism of Action: Both Neulasta (pegfilgrastim) and filgrastim are colony-stimulating factors that act on hematopoietic cells by binding to specific cell surface receptors thereby stimulating proliferation, differentiation, commitment, and end cell functional activation. Studies on cellular proliferation, receptor binding, and neutrophil function demonstrate that filgrastim and pegfilgrastim have the same mechanism of action. Pegfilgrastim has reduced renal clearance and prolonged persistence in vivo as compared to filgrastim.
Pharmacodynamics: See Pharmacokinetics.
Pharmacokinetics: The pharmacokinetics and pharmacodynamics of Neulasta (pegfilgrastim) were studied in patients with cancer. The pharmacokinetics of pegfilgrastim were nonlinear in cancer patients and clearance decreased with increases in dose. Neutrophil-mediated clearance is an important component of the clearance of pegfilgrastim, and serum clearance is related to the number of neutrophils. For example, the concentration of pegfilgrastim declined rapidly at the onset of neutrophil recovery that followed myelosuppressive chemotherapy. In addition to numbers of neutrophils, body weight appeared to be a factor. Patients with higher body weights experienced higher systemic exposure to pegfilgrastim after receiving a dose normalized for body weight. A large variability in the pharmacokinetics of pegfilgrastim was observed in cancer patients. The half-life of pegfilgrastim ranged from 25 to 49 hours after SC injection.

Table 3: Neulasta

Summary of Pharmacokinetic Parameters of pegfilgrastim in Cancer Patients After SC Administration

	C_{max}	$t_{½}$	$AUC_{0-\infty}$	Clearance
Single dose[a] Median	78.3–175 ng/mL	25–49 h	5640–15 000 ng·h/mL	6.68–17.7 mL/h/kg

a Doses de 100 µg/kg et 6 mg.

Special Populations and Conditions: No gender-related differences were observed in the pharmacokinetics of Neulasta (pegfilgrastim), and no differences were observed in the pharmacokinetics of geriatric patients with cancer (≥65 years of age) compared to younger patients (<65 years of age) (see Warnings and Precautions, Special Populations, Geriatrics (>65 years of age)). Renal impairment, including end-stage renal disease, appears to have no effects on the pharmacokinetics of pegfilgrastim. The pharmacokinetic profile in pediatric populations or in patients with hepatic insufficiency has not been assessed. The effect of race on pharmacokinetics has not been adequately assessed.
STORAGE AND STABILITY: Neulasta (pegfilgrastim) should be stored refrigerated at 2 to 8°C and protected from light. Before injection, Neulasta may be allowed to reach room temperature for a maximum of 72 hours. Neulasta left at room temperature for more than 72 hours should be discarded. Freezing should be avoided; however, if accidentally frozen Neulasta should be allowed to thaw in the refrigerator before administration. If frozen a second time, Neulasta should be discarded.

Neulasta should be visually inspected for discolouration and particulate matter before administration. Neulasta should not be administered if discolouration or particulates are observed.
SPECIAL HANDLING INSTRUCTIONS: Neulasta (pegfilgrastim) should not be vigorously shaken.
INFORMATION FOR THE PATIENT: Published in e-CPS, available by subscription at www.e-cps.ca.
DOSAGE FORMS, COMPOSITION AND PACKAGING: Each single-use syringe of sterile, clear, colourless, preservative-free liquid for SC administration, contains: pegfilgrastim 6 mg (based on protein mass only). Nonmedicinal ingredients: polysorbate 20, sodium acetate, sorbitol and water for injection USP. pH: 4.0. Single-dose syringes of 0.6 mL with a 27 gauge, 1/2 inch needle, with an UltraSafe Needle Guard. Dispensing packs containing one syringe.

The needle cover on the single-use prefilled syringe contains dry natural rubber (a derivative of latex), which may cause allergic reactions and should not be handled by individuals who are sensitive to latex.

To reduce the risk of accidental needle sticks to users, each single-use prefilled syringe is equipped with an UltraSafe Needle Guard that is manually activated to cover the needle during disposal.

Neupogen® Pr

filgrastim

Hematopoietic Agent—Granulocyte Colony Stimulating Factor

Amgen

Date of Revision: March 3, 2010

SUMMARY PRODUCT INFORMATION:

Route of Administration	Dosage Form/ Strength	Clinically Relevant Nonmedicinal Ingredients
Subcutaneous (SC) or Intravenous (IV)	Sterile Solution for Injection/300 µg/mL	Not Applicable For a complete listing see Dosage Forms, Composition and Packaging.

DESCRIPTION: NEUPOGEN (filgrastim) is a recombinant methionyl human granulocyte colony stimulating factor (r-metHuG-CSF) produced by recombinant DNA technology. Filgrastim is a 175 amino acid protein produced by Escherichia coli (*E. coli*) bacteria into which has been inserted the human granulocyte colony stimulating factor gene. Filgrastim has a molecular weight of 18 800 Daltons. The protein has an amino acid sequence that is identical to the natural sequence predicted from human DNA sequence analysis, except for the addition of an N-terminal methionine necessary for expression in *E. coli*.
INDICATIONS AND CLINICAL USE: NEUPOGEN (filgrastim) is indicated for the following:

1. **Cancer Patients Receiving Myelosuppressive Chemotherapy**
NEUPOGEN (filgrastim) is indicated to decrease the incidence of infection, as manifested by febrile neutropenia, in patients with non-myeloid malignancies (see Patients with Acute Myeloid Leukemia) receiving myelosuppressive anti-neoplastic drugs.
NEUPOGEN is indicated in adult and pediatric patients with cancer receiving myelosuppressive chemotherapy.
A complete blood count (CBC) and platelet count should be obtained prior to chemotherapy, and twice per week (see Warnings and Precautions, Monitoring and Laboratory Tests) during NEUPOGEN therapy to avoid leukocytosis and to monitor the neutrophil count. In phase 3 clinical studies, NEUPOGEN therapy was discontinued when the ANC was $>10 \times 10^9$/L after expected chemotherapy-induced nadir.
2. **Patients with Acute Myeloid Leukemia**
NEUPOGEN is indicated for the reduction in the duration of neutropenia, fever, antibiotic use and hospitalization, following induction and consolidation treatment for acute myeloid leukemia.
3. **Cancer Patients Receiving Myeloablative Chemotherapy Followed by Bone Marrow Transplantation**
NEUPOGEN is indicated to reduce the duration of neutropenia and neutropenia-related clinical sequelae, e.g., febrile neutropenia, in patients undergoing myeloablative therapy followed by bone marrow transplantation.
A CBC and platelet count should be obtained at a minimum of 3 times per week following marrow infusion to monitor marrow reconstitution (see Warnings and Precautions, Monitoring and Laboratory Tests).
4. **Cancer Patients Undergoing Peripheral Blood Progenitor Cell (PBPC) Collection and Therapy**
NEUPOGEN is indicated for the mobilization of autologous peripheral blood progenitor cells in order to accelerate haematopoietic recovery by infusion of such cells, supported by NEUPOGEN, after myelosuppressive or myeloablative chemotherapy.
5. **Patients with Severe Chronic Neutropenia**
NEUPOGEN is indicated for chronic administration to increase neutrophil counts and to reduce the incidence and duration of infection in patients with a diagnosis of congenital, cyclic or idiopathic neutropenia.
6. **Patients with HIV Infection**
NEUPOGEN is indicated in patients with HIV infection for the prevention and treatment of neutropenia, to maintain a normal ANC (e.g., between 2×10^9 and 10×10^9/L). NEUPOGEN therapy reduces the clinical sequelae associated with neutropenia (e.g., bacterial infections) and increases the ability to deliver myelosuppressive medications used for the treatment of HIV and its associated complications. It is recommended that complete blood counts and platelet counts be monitored at regular intervals (e.g., initially twice weekly for 2 weeks, once weekly for an additional 2 weeks, then once monthly thereafter, or as clinically indicated) during NEUPOGEN therapy (see Warnings and Precautions, Monitoring and Laboratory Tests).

CONTRAINDICATIONS: NEUPOGEN (filgrastim) is contraindicated in patients with known hypersensitivity to *E. coli*-derived products or to any component of the product. For a complete listing of the components, see Dosage Forms, Composition and Packaging.

WARNINGS AND PRECAUTIONS:

> **Serious Warnings and Precautions**
> - Splenic rupture, including fatal cases, has been reported following the administration of NEUPOGEN (see Warnings and Precautions, General).
> - Severe sickle cell crises, in some cases resulting in death, have been associated with the use of NEUPOGEN in patients with sickle cell disorders (see Warnings and Precautions, Hematologic).

General: Splenic Rupture: Splenic rupture, including fatal cases, has been reported following the administration of NEUPOGEN. Patients receiving NEUPOGEN who report left upper abdominal and/or shoulder tip pain should be evaluated for an enlarged spleen or splenic rupture.

Simultaneous Use with Chemotherapy: The safety and efficacy of NEUPOGEN (filgrastim) given simultaneously with cytotoxic chemotherapy have not been established. Studies in adult patients showed that an interaction between concurrent NEUPOGEN and 5-fluorouracil (5-FU) is possible and can result in a paradoxical fall in ANC. Because of the potential sensitivity of rapidly dividing myeloid cells to cytotoxic chemotherapy, do not use NEUPOGEN in the period 24 hours before through 24 hours after the administration of cytotoxic chemotherapy (see Dosage and Administration).

The efficacy of NEUPOGEN has not been evaluated in patients receiving chemotherapy associated with delayed myelosuppression (e.g., nitrosoureas) or with mitomycin C or with myelosuppressive doses of anti-metabolites such as 5-FU or cytosine arabinoside.

The safety and efficacy of NEUPOGEN have not been evaluated in patients receiving concurrent radiation therapy. Simultaneous use of NEUPOGEN with chemotherapy and radiation therapy should be avoided.

Carcinogenesis and Mutagenesis: The carcinogenic potential of NEUPOGEN has not been studied. NEUPOGEN failed to induce bacterial gene mutations in either the presence or absence of a drug metabolizing enzyme system. NEUPOGEN had no observed effect on the fertility of male or female rats, or on gestation at doses up to 500 µg/kg.

Growth Factor Potential: NEUPOGEN is a growth factor that primarily stimulates production of neutrophils. However, the possibility that NEUPOGEN can act as a growth factor for certain tumor types cannot be excluded. Randomized studies have demonstrated that treatment with NEUPOGEN following chemotherapy for acute myeloid leukemia does not adversely influence the outcome of treatment. The use of NEUPOGEN in chronic myeloid leukemia (CML) and myelodysplasia (MDS) has not been fully investigated, and caution should be exercised in using this drug in patients with CML or MDS.

Tumor cells may be collected in the leukapheresis product, following PBPC mobilization by NEUPOGEN. The clinical significance and the effect of reinfusion of tumor cells with the leukapheresis product are still unknown and the possible contribution of clonogenic tumor cells to an eventual relapse has not been determined.

Acute myeloid leukaemia (AML) has been reported to occur in the natural history of severe chronic neutropenia without cytokine therapy. It is not known what, if any, additional risk may be imposed by NEUPOGEN therapy.

Cardiovascular: Cardiac events (myocardial infarctions, arrhythmias) have been reported in 11 of 375 cancer patients receiving NEUPOGEN in clinical studies; the relationship to NEUPOGEN therapy is unknown. However, patients with pre-existing cardiac conditions receiving NEUPOGEN should be monitored closely.

Hematologic: Severe sickle cell crises, in some cases resulting in death, have been associated with the use of NEUPOGEN in patients with sickle cell disorders. Only physicians qualified by specialized training or experience in the treatment of patients with sickle cell disorders should prescribe NEUPOGEN for such patients, and only after careful consideration of the potential risks and benefits.

The response to NEUPOGEN may be diminished in patients with reduced neutrophil precursors such as those previously treated with extensive dose chemotherapy or radiotherapy.

In studies of NEUPOGEN administration following chemotherapy, most reported side effects were consistent with those usually seen as a result of cytotoxic chemotherapy (see Adverse Reactions). As a result of the potential of receiving higher doses of chemotherapy (i.e., full doses on the prescribed schedule), the patient may be at greater risk of thrombocytopenia, anemia, and non-haematological consequences of increased chemotherapy doses (please refer to the prescribing information of the specific chemotherapy agents used). Regular monitoring of the hematocrit and platelet count is recommended.

Leukocytosis: Cancer Patients Receiving Myelosuppressive Chemotherapy: In all studies, including phase 1/2 dose ranging studies, WBC counts of 100×10^9/L or greater were observed in approximately 2% of patients receiving NEUPOGEN at doses above 5 and up to 115 µg/kg/day. There were no reports of adverse events associated with this degree of leukocytosis. In order to avoid the potential complications of excessive leukocytosis, a complete blood count (CBC) is recommended twice per week during NEUPOGEN therapy (see Warnings and Precautions, Monitoring and Laboratory Tests).

Hypersensitivity/Allergic Reactions: Allergic-type reactions occurring on initial or subsequent treatment have been reported in <1 in 4000 patients treated with NEUPOGEN. These have generally been characterized by systemic symptoms involving at least 2 body systems, most often skin (rash, urticaria, facial edema), respiratory (wheezing, dyspnea), and cardiovascular (hypotension, tachycardia). Some reactions occurred on initial exposure. Reactions tended to occur within the first 30 minutes after administration and appeared to occur more frequently in patients receiving NEUPOGEN intravenously. Rapid resolution of symptoms occurred in most cases after administration of antihistamines, steroids, bronchodilators, and/or epinephrine. Symptoms recurred in more than half the patients who were rechallenged.

Cutaneous Vasculitis: Cutaneous vasculitis has been reported in patients treated with NEUPOGEN. In most cases, the severity of cutaneous vasculitis was moderate or severe. Most of the reports involved patients with SCN receiving long-term NEUPOGEN therapy. Symptoms of vasculitis generally developed simultaneously with an increase in the ANC and abated when the ANC decreased. Many patients were able to continue NEUPOGEN at a reduced dose.

Immune: As with all therapeutic proteins, there is a potential for immunogenicity. The incidence of antibody development in patients receiving NEUPOGEN has not been adequately determined. While available data suggest that a small proportion of patients developed binding antibodies to filgrastim, the nature and specificity of these antibodies has not been adequately studied. In clinical studies comparing NEUPOGEN and Neulasta, the incidence of antibodies binding to NEUPOGEN was 3% (11/333). In these 11 patients, no evidence of a neutralizing response was observed using a cell-based bioassay. The detection of antibody formation is highly dependent on the sensitivity and specificity of the assay, and the observed incidence of antibody positivity in an assay may be influenced by several factors including timing of sampling, sample handling, concomitant medications, and underlying disease. Therefore, comparison of the incidence of antibodies to NEUPOGEN with the incidence of antibodies to other products may be misleading.

Cytopenias resulting from an antibody response to exogenous growth factors have been reported on rare occasions in patients treated with other recombinant growth factors. There is a theoretical possibility that an antibody directed against filgrastim may crossreact with endogenous G-CSF, resulting in immune-mediated neutropenia; however, this has not been reported in clinical studies or in post-marketing experience. Patients who develop hypersensitivity to filgrastim (NEUPOGEN) may have allergic or hypersensitivity reactions to other *E.coli*-derived proteins.

Respiratory: Acute respiratory distress syndrome (ARDS) has been reported in patients receiving NEUPOGEN, and is postulated to be secondary to an influx of neutrophils to sites of inflammation in the lungs. Patients receiving NEUPOGEN who develop fever, lung infiltrates, or respiratory distress should be evaluated for the possibility of ARDS. In the event that ARDS occurs, NEUPOGEN should be withheld until resolution of ARDS or discontinued. Patients should receive appropriate medical management for this condition.

Alveolar hemorrhage manifesting as pulmonary infiltrates and hemoptysis requiring hospitalization has been reported in healthy donors undergoing peripheral blood progenitor cell (PBPC) mobilization. Hemoptysis resolved with discontinuation of NEUPOGEN. The use of NEUPOGEN for PBPC mobilization in healthy donors is not an approved indication.

Other: Cancer Patients Receiving Myelosuppressive Chemotherapy: Premature Discontinuation of NEUPOGEN Therapy: A transient increase in neutrophil counts is typically seen 1 to 2 days after initiation of NEUPOGEN therapy. However, for a sustained therapeutic response, NEUPOGEN therapy should be continued following chemotherapy until the post nadir ANC reaches 10×10^9/L. Therefore, the premature discontinuation of NEUPOGEN therapy, prior to the time of recovery from the expected neutrophil nadir, is generally not recommended (see Dosage and Administration).

Risks Associated with Increased Doses of Chemotherapy: Intensified doses of chemotherapeutic agents may lead to increased toxicities associated with these agents, including cardiac, pulmonary, neurologic and dermatologic effects (please refer to the product monograph of the specific chemotherapy agents used). Increased exposure to alkylating agents, particularly if combined with radiotherapy, is known to be associated with the genesis of secondary malignancies. When considering chemotherapy dose intensification with NEUPOGEN support, clinicians should weigh the risk of secondary malignancy against the potential benefits of improved primary disease outcome.

Patients with Severe Chronic Neutropenia: Diagnosis of Congenital, Cyclic or Idiopathic Neutropenia: Care should be taken to confirm the diagnosis of congenital, cyclic or idiopathic neutropenia, which may be difficult to distinguish from myelodysplasia, before initiating NEUPOGEN therapy. The safety and efficacy of NEUPOGEN in the treatment of neutropenia or pancytopenia due to other haematopoietic disorders (e.g., myelodysplastic syndrome) has not been established.

It is, therefore, essential that serial complete blood counts with differential and platelet counts, and an evaluation of bone marrow morphology and karyotype, be performed prior to initiation of NEUPOGEN therapy.

Myelodysplasia (MDS), and acute myeloid leukemia (AML) have been reported to occur in the natural history of congenital neutropenia without cytokine therapy. Cytogenetic abnormalities, transformation to MDS, and AML have been observed in patients treated with NEUPOGEN for severe chronic neutropenia (SCN). Based on available data, the risk of developing MDS, and AML has been confined to the subset of patients with congenital neutropenia. Abnormal cytogenetics has been associated with the eventual development of myeloid leukaemia. The effect of continued NEUPOGEN administration in patients with abnormal cytogenetics is unknown. If a patient with SCN develops abnormal cytogenetics, the risks and benefits of continuing NEUPOGEN should be carefully considered (see Adverse Reactions).

Chronic Administration: The safety and efficacy of chronic daily administration of NEUPOGEN in patients with SCN have been established in phase 1/2 clinical trials of 74 patients treated for up to 4.5 years, and in a phase 3 trial of 123 patients treated for up to 3.5 years.

Although the relationship to NEUPOGEN is unclear, osteoporosis has been reported in approximately 7% of patients receiving NEUPOGEN therapy for up to 4.5 years in clinical trials in patients with SCN. Patients with SCN, particularly those with congenital neutropenia and those with underlying osteoporotic bone disease, should be monitored for the possible occurrence of bone density changes while on long-term NEUPOGEN therapy. Other infrequently observed adverse events included exacerbation of some pre-existing skin disorders (e.g., psoriasis), cutaneous vasculitis (leukocytoclastic), alopecia, haematuria/proteinuria, thrombocytopenia (platelets $<50\times10^9$/L).

Patients with HIV Infection: Risks Associated with Increased Doses of Myelosuppressive Medications: Treatment with NEUPOGEN alone does not preclude thrombocytopenia and anemia due to myelosuppressive medications. As a result of the potential to receive higher doses or a greater number of these medications with NEUPOGEN therapy, the patient may be at higher risk of developing thrombocytopenia (see Adverse Reactions) and anemia. Regular monitoring of blood counts is recommended.

Infections Causing Myelosuppression: Neutropenia may be due to bone marrow infiltrating opportunistic infections such as *M. avium* complex or malignancies such as lymphoma. In patients with known bone marrow infiltrating infection or malignancy, consideration should be given to appropriate therapy for treatment of the underlying condition, in addition to administration of NEUPOGEN for treatment of neutropenia.

Special Populations: Pregnant Women: NEUPOGEN has been shown to cause adverse effects in pregnant rabbits when given in doses 2 to 10 times the human dose.

In rabbits, increased abortion and embryolethality were observed in animals treated with NEUPOGEN at 80 µg/kg/day. NEUPOGEN administered to pregnant rabbits at doses of 80 µg/kg/day during the period of organogenesis was associated with increased fetal resorption, genitourinary bleeding, developmental abnormalities, and decreased body weight, live births, and food consumption. External abnormalities were not observed in the fetuses of dams treated at 80 µg/kg/day. Reproductive studies in pregnant rats have shown that NEUPOGEN was not associated with lethal, teratogenic, or behavioral effects on fetuses when administered by daily intravenous injection during the period of organogenesis at dose levels up to 575 µg/kg/day.

In Segment III studies in rats, offspring of dams treated at greater than 20 µg/kg/day exhibited a delay in external differentiation (detachment of auricles and descent of testes) and slight growth retardation, possibly due to lower body weight of females during rearing and nursing. Offspring of dams treated at 100 µg/kg/day exhibited decreased body weights at birth, and a slightly reduced 4 day survival rate.

There are cases in the literature where the transplacental passage of NEUPOGEN has been demonstrated. NEUPOGEN should be used during pregnancy only if the potential benefit justifies any potential theoretical risk to the fetus.

Nursing Women: It is not known whether NEUPOGEN is excreted in human milk, therefore, NEUPOGEN is not recommended for use in nursing women.

Neonates: The safety and efficacy of NEUPOGEN in neonates have not been established.

Pediatrics (<18 years of age): Cancer Patients Receiving Myelosuppressive Chemotherapy: Data from clinical studies in pediatric patients indicate that the safety of NEUPOGEN is similar in both adults and children receiving cytotoxic chemotherapy.

Twelve pediatric patients with neuroblastoma have received up to 6 cycles of cyclophosphamide, cisplatin, doxorubicin, and etoposide chemotherapy concurrently with NEUPOGEN. In this population, NEUPOGEN was well tolerated. There was one report of palpable splenomegaly associated with NEUPOGEN therapy, however, the only consistently reported adverse event was musculoskeletal pain, which is no different from the experience in the adult population.

Patients with Acute Myeloid Leukemia: Published experience with the administration of NEUPOGEN post-chemotherapy in pediatric patients with AML has included 136 patients. This interim analysis included children receiving intensive induction chemotherapy with NEUPOGEN, and demonstrated that it had no detrimental impact on disease outcome in comparison to a similarly-treated historical control group.

Patients with Severe Chronic Neutropenia: NEUPOGEN is indicated for chronic administration to adults and pediatric patients with SCN to reduce the incidence and duration of the sequelae of neutropenia. In a phase 3 study, 120 patients with a median age of 12 years (range 1 to 76 years) were treated; 12 of these were infants (1 month to 2 years of age), 47 were children (2 to 12 years of age), and 9 were adolescents (12 to 16 years of age) (see Indications and Clinical Use; Warnings and Precautions, Monitoring and Laboratory Tests; Dosage and Administration).

The most commonly reported adverse event in clinical trials was bone pain; splenomegaly has also been reported with chronic administration (see Adverse Reactions). Pediatric patients with congenital types of neutropenia have been reported to develop MDS/AML or cytogenetic abnormalities while receiving chronic NEUPOGEN treatment. The relationship of these events to NEUPOGEN administration is unknown (see Warnings and Precautions, Adverse Reactions).

Other serious long-term risks associated with daily administration of NEUPOGEN have not been identified in pediatric patients (ages 1 month to 17 years) with SCN. Regarding growth and development, long term follow-up data from the post-marketing surveillance study suggest that height and weight are not adversely affected in patients who received up to 5 years of NEUPOGEN treatment. Limited data from patients who were followed in the phase 3 study for 1.5 years did not suggest alterations in sexual maturation, or endocrine function.

The safety and efficacy in neonates and patients with autoimmune neutropenia of infancy have not been established.

Monitoring and Laboratory Tests: Cancer Patients Receiving Myelosuppressive Chemotherapy: A complete blood count (CBC) and platelet count should be obtained prior to chemotherapy, and at regular intervals (twice per week) during NEUPOGEN therapy. Following cytotoxic chemotherapy, the neutrophil nadir occurred earlier during cycles when NEUPOGEN was administered, and white blood cell (WBC) differentials demonstrated a left shift, including the appearance of promyelocytes and myeloblasts. In addition, the duration of severe neutropenia was reduced, and was followed by an accelerated recovery in the neutrophil counts. Therefore, regular monitoring of WBC counts, particularly at the time of the recovery from the post chemotherapy nadir, is recommended in order to avoid excessive leukocytosis.

Cancer Patients Receiving Myeloablative Chemotherapy Followed by Bone Marrow Transplantation: A CBC and platelet count should be obtained at regular intervals (3 times per week during NEUPOGEN therapy) following marrow infusion.

Cancer Patients Undergoing Peripheral Blood Progenitor Cell (PBPC) Collection and Therapy: After 4 days of NEUPOGEN treatment for PBPC mobilization, neutrophil counts should be monitored. Monitoring of platelet and red blood cell counts is recommended during the leukapheresis period. Frequent CBCs and platelet counts are recommended (at least 3 times per week) following PBPC reinfusion.

Patients with Severe Chronic Neutropenia: During the initial 4 weeks of NEUPOGEN therapy, and for 2 weeks following any dose adjustment, a CBC with differential and platelet determination should be performed twice weekly. Once a patient is clinically stable, a CBC with differential and platelet determination should be performed monthly during the first year of treatment. Thereafter, if clinically stable, routine monitoring with regular CBCs (i.e., as clinically indicated but at least quarterly) is recommended. Additionally, for those patients with congenital neutropenia, annual bone marrow and cytogenetic evaluations should be performed throughout the duration of treatment.

In clinical trials, the following laboratory results were observed:

- Cyclic fluctuations in the neutrophil counts were frequently observed in patients with congenital or idiopathic neutropenia after initiation of NEUPOGEN therapy,
- Platelet counts were generally at the upper limits of normal prior to NEUPOGEN therapy. With NEUPOGEN therapy, platelet counts decreased but generally remained within normal limits (see Adverse Reactions),
- Early myeloid forms were noted in the peripheral blood in most patients, including the appearance of metamyelocytes and myelocytes. Promyelocytes and myeloblasts were noted in some patients,
- Relative increases were occasionally noted in the number of circulating eosinophils and basophils. No consistent increases were observed with NEUPOGEN therapy,
- As in other trials, increases were observed in serum uric acid, lactic dehydrogenase, and serum alkaline phosphatase.

Patients with HIV Infection: A CBC and platelet count should be obtained prior to starting NEUPOGEN therapy and at regular intervals (e.g., initially twice weekly for 2 weeks, once weekly for an additional 2 weeks, then once monthly thereafter, or as clinically indicated) during NEUPOGEN therapy. Some patients may respond very rapidly and with a considerable increase in neutrophil count to the initial doses of NEUPOGEN. It is recommended that blood samples be drawn for ANC measurement prior to any scheduled dosing with NEUPOGEN.

ADVERSE REACTIONS: Adverse Drug Reaction Overview: See Warnings and Precautions regarding Splenic Rupture, ARDS, Allergic Reactions and Sickle Cell Disease.

Clinical Trial Adverse Drug Reactions: Because clinical trials are conducted under very specific conditions the adverse reaction rates observed in the clinical trials may not reflect the rates observed in practice and should not be compared to the rates in the clinical trials of another drug. Adverse drug reaction information from clinical trials is useful for identifying drug-related adverse events and for approximating rates.

Cancer Patients Receiving Myelosuppressive Chemotherapy: In clinical trials involving over 350 patients receiving NEUPOGEN (filgrastim) following cytotoxic chemotherapy, most adverse experiences were the sequelae of the underlying malignancy or cytotoxic chemotherapy. In all phase 2 and 3 trials, medullary bone pain, reported in 24% of patients, was the only consistently observed adverse reaction attributed to NEUPOGEN therapy. This bone pain was generally reported to be of mild-to-moderate severity, and could be controlled in most patients with non-narcotic analgesics. Infrequently, bone pain was severe enough to require narcotic analgesics. Bone pain was reported more frequently in patients treated with higher doses (20 to 100 µg/kg/day) administered intravenously, and less frequently in patients treated with lower subcutaneous doses of NEUPOGEN (3 to 10 µg/kg/day).

In the randomized, double-blind, placebo-controlled trial of NEUPOGEN therapy following combination chemotherapy in patients (n=207) with small cell lung cancer, the following adverse events were reported during blinded cycles of study medication (placebo or NEUPOGEN at 4 to 8 µg/kg/day). Events are reported as exposure adjusted since patients remained on double-blind NEUPOGEN a median of 3 cycles versus 1 cycle for placebo. See Table 1.

Table 1: NEUPOGEN

Adverse Effects

Event	% of Blinded Cycles with Events	
	NEUPOGEN Patient Cycles N=384	Placebo Patient Cycles N=257
Nausea/Vomiting	57	64
Skeletal Pain	22	11
Alopecia	18	27
Diarrhea	14	23
Neutropenic Fever	13	35
Mucositis	12	20
Fever	12	11
Fatigue	11	16
Anorexia	9	11
Dyspnea	9	11
Headache	7	9
Cough	6	8
Skin Rash	6	9
Chest Pain	5	6
Generalized Weakness	4	7
Sore Throat	4	9
Stomatitis	5	10
Constipation	5	10
Pain (Unspecified)	2	7

In this study, there were no serious, life-threatening, or fatal adverse reactions attributed to NEUPOGEN therapy. Specifically, there were no reports of flu-like symptoms, pleuritis, pericarditis, or other major systemic reactions to NEUPOGEN.

Spontaneously reversible elevations in uric acid, lactate dehydrogenase, and alkaline phosphatase occurred in 27% to 58% of 98 patients receiving blinded NEUPOGEN therapy following cytotoxic chemotherapy. Increases were generally mild-to-moderate. Transient decreases in blood pressure (<90/60 mmHg) which did not require clinical treatment, were reported in 7 of 176 patients in phase 3 clinical studies following administration of NEUPOGEN. No evidence of interaction of NEUPOGEN with other drugs was observed in the course of clinical trials (see Warnings and Precautions, General, Simultaneous Use with Chemotherapy).

The safety profile of NEUPOGEN in the pediatric population is comparable to that seen in adult cancer patients receiving cytotoxic chemotherapy. Adverse events considered related to NEUPOGEN administration by the investigators of 3 non-blinded studies included application site disorders, haematologic disorders (including thrombocytopenia), musculoskeletal disorders, and a single case of vasculitis. Of these, musculoskeletal disorders are the most consistent adverse events seen in other NEUPOGEN studies.

Patients with Acute Myeloid Leukemia: In a randomized phase 3 clinical trial involving 521 patients with de novo AML, 259 patients received NEUPOGEN post-chemotherapy and 262 patients received placebo. NEUPOGEN was generally well tolerated, and most adverse experiences were considered to be the sequelae of the underlying malignancy or cytotoxic chemotherapy. The most frequently reported events were diarrhea, rash, and petechiae, and there were no significant differences between the treatment groups.

Cancer Patients Receiving Myeloablative Chemotherapy Followed by Bone Marrow Transplantation: In clinical trials, the reported adverse effects were those typically seen in patients receiving intensive chemotherapy followed by bone marrow transplantation. The most common events reported in both control and treatment groups included stomatitis, nausea and vomiting, generally of mild-to-moderate severity and were considered unrelated to NEUPOGEN. In the randomized studies of BMT involving 167 patients who received study drug, the following events occurred more frequently in patients treated with NEUPOGEN than in controls: nausea (10% vs. 4%), vomiting (7% vs. 3%), hypertension (4% vs. 0%), rash (12% vs. 10%), and peritonitis (2% vs. 0%). None of these events were reported by the investigator to be related to NEUPOGEN. One event of erythema nodosum was reported moderate in severity and possibly related to NEUPOGEN.

Cancer Patients Undergoing Peripheral Blood Progenitor Cell (PBPC) Collection and Therapy: NEUPOGEN Mobilized PBPC Collection: In clinical trials, 126 patients have received NEUPOGEN for mobilization of PBPC. During the mobilization period, adverse events related to NEUPOGEN consisted primarily of mild-to-moderate musculoskeletal symptoms, reported in 44% of patients. These symptoms were predominantly events of medullary bone pain (38%). Headache was reported related to NEUPOGEN in 7% of patients. Mild-to-moderate transient increases in alkaline phosphatase levels were reported related to NEUPOGEN in 21% of the patients who had serum chemistries evaluated during the mobilization phase.

All patients had increases in neutrophil counts consistent with the biological effects of NEUPOGEN. Two patients had a WBC count greater than 100×10^9/L with WBC count increases during the mobilization period ranging from 16.7×10^9/L to 138×10^9/L above baseline. Eighty-eight percent of patients had an increase in WBC count between 10×10^9/L and 70×10^9/L above baseline. No clinical sequelae were associated with any grade of leukocytosis.

Sixty-five percent of patients had mild-to-moderate anemia and 97% of patients had decreases in platelet counts possibly related to the leukapheresis procedure. Only 5 patients had platelet counts $<50\times10^9$/L.

PBPC Transplantation Followed by NEUPOGEN: During the period of NEUPOGEN administration post PBPC transplant, NEUPOGEN was administered to 110 patients as supportive therapy and adverse events were consistent with those expected after high dose chemotherapy. Mild-to-moderate musculoskeletal pain was the most frequently reported adverse event related to NEUPOGEN reported in 15% of patients.

Patients with Severe Chronic Neutropenia: Mild-to-moderate bone pain was reported in approximately 33% of patients in clinical trials. This symptom was usually readily controlled with mild analgesics. General musculoskeletal pain was also noted in higher frequency in patients treated with NEUPOGEN. Palpable splenomegaly was observed in approximately 30% of patients. Abdominal or flank pain was seen infrequently and thrombocytopenia ($<50\times10^9$/L) was noted in 12% of patients with palpable spleens. Less than 3% of all patients underwent splenectomy, and most of these had a pre-study history of splenomegaly. Approximately 7% of patients had thrombocytopenia ($<50\times10^9$/L) during NEUPOGEN therapy, most of whom had a pre-study history. In most cases, thrombocytopenia was managed by NEUPOGEN dose reduction or interruption. There were no associated, serious haemorrhagic sequelae in these patients. Epistaxis was noted in 15% of patients treated with NEUPOGEN, but was associated with thrombocytopenia in only 2% of patients. Anemia was reported in approximately 10% of patients, but in most cases appeared to be related to frequent diagnostic phlebotomy, chronic illness or concomitant medications.

Cytogenetic abnormalities, transformation to MDS, and AML have been observed in patients treated with NEUPOGEN for SCN (see Warnings and Precautions, Patients with Severe Chronic Neutropenia). As of December 31, 1997, data were available from a post-marketing surveillance study of 531 SCN patients with an average follow-up of 4.0 years. Of these 531 patients, 32 were infants (1 month to 2 years of age), 200 were children (2 to 12 years of age), and 68 were adolescents (12 to 16 years of age). Based on analysis of these data, the risk of developing MDS, and AML was confined to the subset of patients with congenital neutropenia (Kostmann's syndrome, congenital agranulocytosis, and Shwachman-Diamond syndrome). A life table analysis of these data revealed that the cumulative risk of developing leukemia or MDS by the end of the eighth year of NEUPOGEN treatment in a patient with congenital neutropenia was 16.5% (95% C.I.=9.8% to 23.3%); this represents an annual rate of approximately 2%. Leukemic transformation has also been documented in congenital neutropenia patients who have never received NEUPOGEN; it is unknown if the rate of conversion in untreated patients is different from that of treated patients. Cytogenetic abnormalities, including monosomy 7, have been reported in patients treated with NEUPOGEN who had previously documented normal cytogenetic evaluations. It is unknown whether the development of cytogenetic abnormalities, MDS, or AML is related to chronic daily NEUPOGEN administration or to the natural history of SCN. Routine monitoring through regular CBCs is recommended for all patients with SCN.

Additionally, annual bone marrow and cytogenetic evaluations are recommended in all patients with congenital neutropenia (see Warnings and Precautions, Monitoring and Laboratory Tests).

Other adverse events infrequently observed and possibly related to NEUPOGEN therapy were: injection site reaction, headache, hepatomegaly, arthralgia, osteoporosis, rash, alopecia, and haematuria/proteinuria.

Patients with HIV Infection: In the multicenter, randomized, controlled trial, 172 of 258 patients were treated with NEUPOGEN. NEUPOGEN was generally well tolerated. The most frequently reported treatment-related adverse events in the 24-week treatment period were skeletal pain (14.5%), headache (6.4%), back pain and myalgia (5.8% each), and increased alkaline phosphatase (5.2%).

There were no new or unexpected treatment-related events seen in NEUPOGEN-treated patients. Adverse events observed in clinical trials were consistent with progression of HIV disease or events observed in other clinical settings.

There was no apparent increase or decrease in HIV replication and viral load as measured by quantitative reverse transcriptase polymerase chain reaction (RT-PCR). Although prior in vitro and in vivo studies have not shown any increase in viral load following use of NEUPOGEN in HIV-infected patients. The randomized study was not powered to address this issue and the possibility of an effect due to NEUPOGEN on HIV replication cannot be entirely excluded.

As of 31 January 1996, an estimated 1.2 million patients worldwide have received NEUPOGEN therapy across all indications. Of an estimated 150 000 HIV-infected patients receiving NEUPOGEN to date, there have been 106 spontaneous adverse event reports received worldwide. No new adverse event patterns were identified in adults or children receiving NEUPOGEN for neutropenia associated with HIV infection. Five deaths were reported in 106 post-marketing reports in patients receiving NEUPOGEN for HIV infection. Three of 5 deaths were attributed to various manifestations of HIV disease progression. In the fourth case, the cause of death was not reported. In the fifth case, the physician reported that death in the context of ARDS occurred in the absence of fever and microbiological cause and was typical of bleomycin pulmonary toxicity. However, the physician reported that this may have been enhanced by NEUPOGEN. It is notable, however, that randomized trials, and non-randomized trials demonstrated no increase in the known pulmonary toxicity of bleomycin when NEUPOGEN was added to treatment.

In the randomized controlled study, the overall incidence of thrombocytopenia was 9.9% in the NEUPOGEN-treated groups compared with 8.1% in the control group. Severe thrombocytopenia occurred in 7% of the NEUPOGEN-treated patients and 3.5% of control patients in the controlled, randomized study. During this study, mean platelet count decreased at week 2 in the NEUPOGEN-treated patients, but returned to baseline by week 3 and remained stable thereafter. In the post-marketing experience of HIV-infected patients which includes an estimated 150 000 patients worldwide, 10 of 106 spontaneous reports of adverse reactions were for thrombocytopenia. Of these, 3 cases were reported as serious.

Because adverse events of thrombocytopenia in HIV-infected individuals are multifactorial and may be attributed to the natural progression of HIV disease and associated infections, and because of the inconsistent occurrence of thrombocytopenia in a small number of patients in the aforementioned clinical trials, no definitive relationship between NEUPOGEN therapy in HIV-infected patients and thrombocytopenia can be established.

In one study, 16 of 24 patients (66.7%) were reported to have splenomegaly during an observation period of 49-701 days. However, no baseline measurements of spleen size were made for comparison to on-study values. In 3 other uncontrolled clinical trials, only 1 of 297 patients (0.3%) had a report of splenomegaly. Since splenomegaly is a common clinical finding in 72% of patients with AIDS sometime during the course of their disease, it is likely that the observed splenomegaly was associated with HIV disease and not related to NEUPOGEN.

Post-Market Adverse Drug Reactions: In addition to the events listed above, reports of serious adverse reactions have been identified post-market in patients receiving NEUPOGEN, including:

- Splenic rupture (see Warnings and Precautions, Splenic Rupture)
- Acute respiratory distress syndrome (ARDS) (see Warnings and Precautions, Respiratory)
- Alveolar hemorrhage and hemoptysis (see Warnings and Precautions, Respiratory)
- Allergic reactions (see Warnings and Precautions, Hypersensitivity/Allergic Reactions)
- Sickle cell crisis (see Warnings and Precautions, Hematologic)
- Cutaneous vasculitis (see Warnings and Precautions, Cutaneous Vasculitis)
- Sweet's syndrome (acute febrile neutrophilic dermatosis)
- Pseudogout (in patients treated with cancer)

DRUG INTERACTIONS: Overview: Interactions of NEUPOGEN with other cytokines, including haematopoietic growth factors, have been observed in animal studies. The safety, efficacy, and possible interactions of NEUPOGEN used in combination with other cytokines have not been characterized in clinical trials. Drugs which may potentiate the release of neutrophils, such as lithium, should be used with caution.

Drug-Drug Interactions: Interactions with other drugs have not been established.

Drug-Food Interactions: Interactions with food have not been established.

Drug-Herb Interactions: Interactions with herbal products have not been established.

Drug-Laboratory Test Interactions: Increased hematopoietic activity of the bone marrow in response to growth factor therapy has been associated with transient positive bone-imaging changes. This should be considered when interpreting bone-imaging results.

DOSAGE AND ADMINISTRATION: Dosing Considerations: Cancer Patients Receiving Myelosuppressive Chemotherapy: NEUPOGEN should be administered no earlier than 24 hours after the administration of cytotoxic chemotherapy. NEUPOGEN should not be administered in the period 24 hours before the administration of chemotherapy (see Warnings and Precautions).

Cancer Patients Receiving Myeloablative Chemotherapy Followed by Bone Marrow Transplantation: NEUPOGEN should be administered no earlier than 24 hours after the administration of cytotoxic chemotherapy and at least 24 hours after bone marrow infusion.

Cancer Patients Undergoing Peripheral Blood Progenitor Cell (PBPC) Collection and Therapy: The first dose should be administered at least 24 hours after cytotoxic chemotherapy and at least 24 hours after PBPC infusion.

Recommended Dose and Dosage Adjustment: Cancer Patients Receiving Myelosuppressive Chemotherapy: The recommended starting dose of NEUPOGEN (filgrastim) in adult patients is 5 µg/kg/day, administered as a single daily injection by subcutaneous bolus injection, by short intravenous infusion (15 to 30 minutes), or by continuous subcutaneous or continuous intravenous infusion.

The recommended dose in pediatric oncology patients is 5 µg/kg/day administered subcutaneously.

A CBC and platelet count should be obtained before instituting NEUPOGEN therapy, and monitored twice weekly during therapy. Doses may be increased in increments of 5 µg/kg for each chemotherapy cycle, according to the duration and severity of the ANC nadir. Therapy should be discontinued if the ANC surpasses 10×10^9/L after the ANC nadir has occurred.

NEUPOGEN should be administered daily for up to 2 weeks, until the ANC has reached 10×10^9/L following the expected chemotherapy-induced neutrophil nadir. The duration of NEUPOGEN therapy needed to attenuate chemotherapy-induced neutropenia may be dependent on the myelosuppressive potential of the chemotherapy regimen employed. NEUPOGEN therapy should be discontinued if the ANC surpasses 10×10^9/L after the expected chemotherapy-induced neutrophil nadir (see Warnings and Precautions). In phase 3 trials, efficacy was observed at doses of 4 to 8 µg/kg/day.

Cancer Patients Receiving Myeloablative Chemotherapy Followed by Bone Marrow Transplantation: The recommended dose of NEUPOGEN following bone marrow transplant is 10 µg/kg/day given as an intravenous infusion of 4 or 24 hours, or as a continuous 24-hour subcutaneous infusion. During the period of neutrophil recovery, the daily dose of NEUPOGEN should be titrated against the neutrophil response as follows: see Table 2.

Table 2: NEUPOGEN

Dose Adjustment

Absolute Neutrophil Count	NEUPOGEN Dose Adjustment
When ANC $>1.0\times10^9$/L for 3 consecutive days	Reduce to 5 µg/kg/day[a]
then:	
If ANC remains $>1.0\times10^9$/L for 3 more consecutive days	Discontinue NEUPOGEN
If ANC decreases to $<1.0\times10^9$/L	Resume at 5 µg/kg/day

[a] If ANC decreases to $<1.0\times10^9$/L at any time during the 5 µg/kg/day administration, NEUPOGEN should be increased to 10 µg/kg/day, and the above steps should then be followed.

Cancer Patients Undergoing Peripheral Blood Progenitor Cell (PBPC) Collection and Therapy: The recommended dose of NEUPOGEN for PBPC mobilization is 10 µg/kg/day given as a single daily subcutaneous injection or a continuous 24-hour infusion. NEUPOGEN therapy should be given for at least 4 days before the first leukapheresis procedure, and should be continued through to the day of the last leukapheresis procedure. Collections should be commenced on day 5 and continued on consecutive days until the desired yield of haematopoietic progenitor cells is obtained. For peripheral blood progenitor cells mobilized with NEUPOGEN, a schedule of leukapheresis collections on days 5, 6, and 7 of a 7-day treatment regimen has been found to be effective.

The target number of progenitor cells to be collected and reinfused is to be determined by the treating physician. The following should be considered:

- A minimum or optimal number of progenitor cells in the leukapheresis product, needed for adequate haematopoietic reconstitution, have not been determined. However, studies indicate that the infusion of higher numbers of progenitor cells appears to be associated with a shorter time to neutrophil and platelet recovery,
- Tests for quantifying the number of progenitor cells, measured as $CD34^+$ or GM-CFU, are not standardized and variations may exist between laboratories, and
- Factors other than NEUPOGEN dosage, such as prior cytotoxic chemo- or radiotherapy, may affect the number and quality of progenitor cells mobilized and collected by leukapheresis.

The recommended dose of NEUPOGEN following PBPC transplant is 5 µg/kg/day given either subcutaneously or as an intravenous infusion. The daily dose of NEUPOGEN should be titrated according to the schedule provided above (Cancer Patients Receiving Myeloablative Chemotherapy Followed by Bone Marrow Transplantation).

Patients with HIV Infection: The recommended starting dose of NEUPOGEN is 1 µg/kg/day or 300 µg 3 times per week by subcutaneous injection until a normal neutrophil count is reached and can be maintained (ANC $\geq2\times10^9$/L). Dose adjustments may be necessary as determined by the patient's ANC to maintain the ANC between 2×10^9 and 10×10^9/L.

When reversal of neutropenia has been achieved, the minimal effective dose to maintain a normal neutrophil count should be established. An initial dose of 300 µg 3 times per week by subcutaneous injection is recommended. A further dose adjustment may be necessary to maintain the ANC between 2×10^9 and 10×10^9/L.

In clinical trials, the maximum NEUPOGEN dose did not exceed 10 µg/kg/day.

Patients with Severe Chronic Neutropenia: Starting Dose: Congenital Neutropenia: The recommended daily starting dose is 12 µg/kg subcutaneously (single or divided dose).

Idiopathic or Cyclic Neutropenia: The recommended daily starting dose is 5 µg/kg subcutaneously (single or divided dose).

Dose Adjustments: NEUPOGEN may be administered subcutaneously as a single daily injection to increase and sustain the ANC above 1.5×10^9/L. Chronic daily administration is required to maintain an adequate neutrophil count. After 1 to 2 weeks of therapy, the initial dose may be doubled or halved. Subsequently, the dose may be individually adjusted not more than every 1 to 2 weeks to maintain the ANC between 1.5×10^9/L and 10×10^9/L. WBC/ANC monitoring should be done more frequently (e.g., every other day) if the ANC reaches values above 25×10^9/L, and the dose reduced if the ANC remains greater than 25×10^9/L for 1 week. In the SCN post-marketing surveillance study, the median daily doses of NEUPOGEN reported (median duration 4.4 years) were: Congenital Neutropenia 6.9 µg/kg; Cyclic Neutropenia 2.1 µg/kg; Idiopathic Neutropenia 1.2 µg/kg.

In clinical trials in patients with SCN, 91% of patients who responded to NEUPOGEN therapy responded at doses of ≤12 µg/kg/day. Ninety seven percent of patients responded at doses of ≤24 µg/kg/day. Therefore, patients with SCN who do not respond to the recommended starting dose should be treated with up to 24 µg/kg/day in order to determine if they will respond. In some cases, where higher doses were tried, an improvement in the ANC and the clinical condition was seen with a few patients only.

Administration: NEUPOGEN is intended for subcutaneous injection or intravenous use and should not be given by any other route of administration.

NEUPOGEN should not be vigorously shaken.

In those situations in which the physician determines that the patient can safely and effectively self-administer NEUPOGEN, the patient should be instructed as to the proper dosage and administration. If home use is prescribed, patients should be thoroughly instructed in the importance of proper disposal and cautioned against the reuse of needles, syringes, or drug product. A puncture-resistant container for the disposal of used syringes and needles should be available to the patient. The full container should be disposed of according to the directions provided by the physician.

Dilution: If required, NEUPOGEN may be diluted in 5% dextrose. NEUPOGEN diluted to a concentration between 5 and 15 µg/mL should be protected from adsorption to plastic materials by the addition of Albumin (Human) at a concentration of 2.0 mg/mL. When diluted in 5% dextrose or 5% dextrose plus Albumin (Human), NEUPOGEN is compatible with glass bottles, PVC and polyolefin intravenous bags and polypropylene syringes.

Dilution of NEUPOGEN to a final concentration of <5 µg/mL even in the presence of Albumin (Human) is not recommended at any time. **Do not dilute with saline at any time: product may precipitate.**

OVERDOSAGE:

The maximum tolerated dose of NEUPOGEN (filgrastim) has not been determined. In dose ranging studies, 5 of 16 patients given ≥69 µg/kg/day were withdrawn due to adverse experiences. In these and other clinical trials, only 2 of 253 patients on lower doses were withdrawn due to adverse events.

In NEUPOGEN clinical trials of cancer patients receiving myelosuppressive chemotherapy, WBC counts $>100\times10^9$/L have been reported in less than 2% of patients and were not associated with any reported adverse clinical effects.

It is recommended, to avoid the potential risks of excessive leukocytosis, that NEUPOGEN therapy should be discontinued if the ANC surpasses 10×10^9/L after the chemotherapy-induced ANC nadir has occurred.

In cancer patients receiving myelosuppressive chemotherapy, discontinuation of NEUPOGEN therapy usually results in a 50% decrease in circulating neutrophils within 1 to 2 days, with a return to pretreatment levels in 1 to 7 days.

> For management of a suspected drug overdose, CPhA recommends that you contact your **regional Poison Control Centre**. See the *CPS* Directory section for a list of Poison Control Centres.

ACTION AND CLINICAL PHARMACOLOGY: Mechanism of Action: Filgrastim is a human granulocyte colony stimulating factor (G-CSF) produced by recombinant DNA technology. G-CSF regulates the production of neutrophils within the bone marrow; endogenous G-CSF is a glycoprotein produced by monocytes, fibroblasts, and endothelial cells. G-CSF is a colony stimulating factor which has been shown to have minimal direct in vivo or in vitro effects on the production of other haematopoietic cell types. NEUPOGEN (filgrastim) is the name for recombinant methionyl human granulocyte colony stimulating factor (r-metHuG-CSF).

Pharmacodynamics: In phase 1 studies involving 96 patients with various non-myeloid malignancies, NEUPOGEN administration resulted in a dose-dependent increase in neutrophil counts over the dose range of 1 to 70 µg/kg/day. This increase in neutrophil counts was observed whether NEUPOGEN was administered intravenously (1 to 70 µg/kg twice daily), subcutaneously (1 to 3 µg/kg once daily), or by continuous subcutaneous infusion (3 to 11 µg/kg/day). With discontinuation of NEUPOGEN therapy, neutrophil counts returned to baseline, in most cases within 4 days. Isolated neutrophils displayed normal phagocytic (measured by zymosan-stimulated chemoluminescence) and chemotactic [measured by migration under agarose using N-formyl-methionyl-leucyl-phenylalanine (fMLP) as the chemotaxin] activity in vitro.

The absolute monocyte count was reported to increase in a dose-dependent manner in most patients receiving NEUPOGEN, however, the percentage of monocytes in the differential count remained within the normal range. In all studies to date, absolute counts of both eosinophils and basophils did not change and were within the normal range following administration of NEUPOGEN. Increases in lymphocyte counts following NEUPOGEN administration have been reported in some normal subjects and cancer patients.

White blood cell (WBC) differentials obtained during clinical trials have demonstrated a shift towards granulocyte progenitor cells (left shift), including the appearance of promyelocytes and myeloblasts, usually during neutrophil recovery following the chemotherapy-induced nadir. In addition, Dohle bodies, increased granulocyte granulation, as well as hypersegmented neutrophils have been observed. Such changes were transient, and were not associated with clinical sequelae nor were they necessarily associated with infection.

Pharmacokinetics: Absorption and clearance of NEUPOGEN follows first-order pharmacokinetic modeling without apparent concentration dependence. A positive linear correlation occurred between the parenteral dose and both the serum concentration and area under the concentration-time curves. Continuous intravenous infusion of 20 µg/kg of NEUPOGEN over 24 hours resulted in mean and median serum concentrations of approximately 48 and 56 ng/mL, respectively.

Subcutaneous administration of 3.45 µg/kg and 11.5 µg/kg resulted in maximum serum concentrations of 4 and 49 ng/mL, respectively, within 2 to 8 hours. The volume of distribution averaged 150 mL/kg in normal subjects and cancer patients. The elimination half-life, in both normal subjects and cancer patients, was approximately 3.5 hours. Clearance rates of NEUPOGEN were approximately 0.5 to 0.7 mL/min/kg. Single parenteral doses or daily intravenous doses, over a 14 day period, resulted in comparable half-lives. The half-lives were similar for intravenous administration (231 minutes, following NEUPOGEN doses of 34.5 µg/kg) and for subcutaneous administration (210 minutes, following NEUPOGEN doses of 3.45 µg/kg). Continuous 24-hour intravenous infusions of 20 µg/kg over an 11 to 20 day period produced steady state serum concentrations of NEUPOGEN with no evidence of drug accumulation over the time period investigated.

Special Populations and Conditions: Pediatrics: In a study of 15 children with neuroblastoma, 5 children were treated at each of the 3 dose levels; 5, 10, and 15 µg/kg/day NEUPOGEN subcutaneously for 10 days. Peak concentrations of NEUPOGEN of 3 to 117 ng/mL were reached after 4 to 12 hours with measurable NEUPOGEN concentrations for the entire 24-hour dosing interval. Mean elimination half-life of 5.8 hours and 4.5 hours were found on day 1 and on day 10, respectively.

Geriatrics: Pharmacokinetic data in geriatric patients (>65 years) are not available.

STORAGE AND STABILITY: NEUPOGEN should be stored in the refrigerator at 2 to 8°C. Avoid vigorous shaking.

Accidental exposure to room temperature (up to 30°C) or exposure to freezing temperatures does not adversely affect the stability of the product.

Prior to injection, NEUPOGEN may be allowed to reach room temperature for a maximum of 24 hours. Any vial left at room temperature for greater than 24 hours should be discarded.

Parenteral drug products should be inspected visually for particulate matter and discoloration prior to administration, whenever solution and container permit.

SPECIAL HANDLING INSTRUCTIONS: NEUPOGEN should not be vigorously shaken.

INFORMATION FOR THE PATIENT: Published in e-CPS, available by subscription at www.e-cps.ca.

DOSAGE FORMS, COMPOSITION AND PACKAGING: Each mL of sterile, clear, colourless, preservative-free liquid for parenteral administration contains: filgrastim 300 µg (3×10^7 units/mL) formulated in a 10 mM sodium acetate buffer at pH 4.0, containing 5% sorbitol and 0.004% Tween 80. Single use, preservative-free vials of 1 mL (filgrastim 300 µg) and 1.6 mL (filgrastim 480 µg). Boxes of 10.

Use only 1 dose per vial; do not re-enter the vial. Discard unused portions. Do not save unused drug for later administration.

Neurontin® Pr

gabapentin

Antiepileptic

Pfizer

Date of Revision: November 9, 2009

SUMMARY PRODUCT INFORMATION:

Route of Administration	Dosage Form/ Strength	Nonmedicinal Ingredients
Oral	Capsules 100 mg, 300 mg and 400 mg	Corn starch, lactose and talc. Capsule shells may contain: FD&C Blue No. 2, gelatin, red iron oxide, silicon dioxide, sodium lauryl sulfate, titanium dioxide and yellow iron oxide
Oral	Tablets 600 mg and 800 mg	Candelilla wax, copolyvidone, corn starch, hydroxypropylcellulose, poloxamer 407 NF, magnesium stearate and talc. Ink: 600 mg tablets—ammonium hydroxide and black iron oxide; 800 mg tablets—hypromellose, red and yellow iron oxides

INDICATIONS AND CLINICAL USE: Adults: Neurontin (gabapentin) is indicated as adjunctive therapy for the management of patients with epilepsy who are not satisfactorily controlled by conventional therapy.

Geriatrics (>65 years of age): Systematic studies in geriatric patients have not been conducted. (See Warnings and Precautions, Special Populations.)

Pediatrics (<18 years of age): The safety and efficacy in patients under the age of 18 have not been established. (See Warnings and Precautions, Special Populations.)

CONTRAINDICATIONS: Hypersensitivity: Neurontin (gabapentin) is contraindicated in patients who have demonstrated hypersensitivity to the drug or to any of the components of the formulation.

WARNINGS AND PRECAUTIONS: General: Neurontin (gabapentin) is not considered effective in the treatment of absence seizures and should therefore be used with caution in patients who have mixed seizure disorders that include absence seizures.

Discontinuation of Treatment with Neurontin: As with other anticonvulsant agents, abrupt withdrawal is not recommended because of the possibility of increased seizure frequency. There have been post-marketing reports of adverse events such as anxiety, insomnia, nausea, pain and sweating following abrupt discontinuation of treatment. (See Adverse Reactions, Post-market Adverse Drug Reactions.) When in the judgement of the clinician there is a need for dose reduction, discontinuation or substitution with an alternative medication, this should be done gradually over a minimum of 1 week (a longer period may be needed at the discretion of the prescriber).

Concomitant Use with Morphine: Patients who require concomitant treatment with morphine may experience increases in gabapentin concentrations. Patients should be carefully observed for signs and symptoms of CNS depression, such as somnolence, and the dose of gabapentin or morphine should be reduced appropriately. (See Drug Interactions.)

Psychomotor Impairment: Patients with uncontrolled epilepsy should not drive or handle potentially dangerous machinery. During clinical trials, the most common adverse reactions observed were somnolence, ataxia, fatigue, and nystagmus. Patients should be advised to refrain from activities requiring mental alertness or physical coordination until they are sure that Neurontin does not affect them adversely.

Carcinogenesis and Mutagenesis: Gabapentin produced an increased incidence of acinar cell adenomas and carcinomas in the pancreas of male rats, but not female rats or in mice, in oncogenic studies with doses of 2000 mg/kg which resulted in plasma concentrations 14 times higher than those occurring in humans at a dose of 2400 mg/day. The relevance of these pancreatic acinar cell tumours in male rats to humans is unknown, particularly since tumours of ductal rather than acinar cell origin are the predominant form of human pancreatic cancer.

Dependence/Tolerance: The abuse and dependence potential of gabapentin has not been evaluated in human studies. As with any CNS active drug, however, physicians should carefully evaluate patients for history of drug abuse and follow such patients closely, observing them for signs of abuse or misuse of Neurontin.

Special Populations: Pregnant Women: No evidence of impaired fertility or harm to the fetus due to gabapentin administration was revealed in reproduction studies in mice at doses up to 62 times, and in rats and rabbits at doses up to 31 times the human dose of 2400 mg/day.

There are no adequate and well-controlled studies to establish the safety of gabapentin in pregnant women. Gabapentin should only be used during pregnancy if the potential benefit to the mother outweighs the potential risk to the fetus.

Nursing Women: Gabapentin is excreted in human milk. Because the effect on the nursing infant is unknown, caution should be exercised when gabapentin is administered to a nursing mother. Gabapentin should be used in nursing mothers only if the potential benefit to the mother outweighs the potential risks to the fetus.

Pediatrics: The safety and efficacy in patients under the age of 18 have not been established. Data in 39 patients between the ages of 12 and 18 years included in the double-blind, placebo-controlled trials showed that, at doses of 900 to 1200 mg/day, gabapentin was superior to placebo in reducing seizure frequency. Doses above 1200 mg/day have not been investigated. Safety data showed that the incidence of adverse events in this group of patients was similar to that observed in older individuals.

In controlled clinical trials involving patients, 3 to 12 years of age (N=323), psychiatric adverse events such as emotional lability, hostility, hyperkinesia and thought disorder were reported at a higher frequency in patients treated with gabapentin compared to placebo.

Geriatrics: Systematic studies in geriatric patients have not been conducted. Adverse clinical events reported among 59 patients over the age of 65 years treated with Neurontin did not differ from those reported for younger individuals. The small number of individuals evaluated and the limited duration of exposure limits the strength of any conclusions reached about the influence of age, if any, on the kind and incidence of adverse events associated with the use of Neurontin.

As Neurontin is eliminated primarily by renal excretion, dosage adjustment may be required in elderly patients because of declining renal function. (See Dosage and Administration, Dosing Considerations; Action and Clinical Pharmacology, Special Populations and Conditions.)

Monitoring and Laboratory Tests: Clinical trials data do not indicate that routine monitoring of clinical laboratory parameters is necessary for the safe use of Neurontin. Neurontin may be used in combination with other commonly used antiepileptic drugs without concern for alteration of the blood concentrations of gabapentin or other antiepileptic drugs.

ADVERSE REACTIONS: Adverse Drug Reaction Overview: Commonly Observed Adverse Events: The most commonly observed adverse events associated with the use of Neurontin (gabapentin) in combination with other antiepileptic drugs, not seen at an equivalent frequency in placebo-treated patients, were somnolence, dizziness, ataxia, fatigue, nystagmus and tremor (see Table 1).

Adverse Events Leading to Discontinuation of Treatment: Approximately 6.4% of the 543 patients who received Neurontin in the placebo-controlled studies withdrew due to adverse events. In comparison, approximately 4.5% of the 378 placebo-controlled participants withdrew due to adverse events during these studies. The adverse events most commonly associated with withdrawal were somnolence (1.2%), ataxia (0.8%), fatigue, nausea and/or vomiting and dizziness (all at 0.6%).

Clinical Trial Adverse Drug Reactions: Because clinical trials are conducted under very specific conditions the adverse reaction rates observed in the clinical trials may not reflect the rates observed in practice and should not be compared to the rates in the clinical trials of another drug. Adverse drug reaction information from clinical trials is useful for identifying drug-related adverse events and for approximating rates.

Incidence in Controlled Clinical Trials: Adults: Multiple doses of Neurontin were administered to 543 subjects with partial seizures in placebo controlled clinical trials of 12 weeks duration. In these studies, either Neurontin (at doses of 600, 900, 1200 or 1800 mg/day) or placebo was added to the patient's current antiepileptic drug therapy. Treatment-emergent signs and symptoms that occurred in at least 1% of patients participating in these studies are listed in Table 1.

Table 1: Neurontin

Treatment-emergent Adverse Event Incidence in Placebo-controlled Add-on Trials (Events in at Least 1% of Neurontin Patients and Numerically More Frequent Than in the Placebo Group)

	Neurontin[a] n=543 %	Placebo[a] n=378 %
Body as a Whole		
Fatigue	11.0	5.0
Weight Increase	2.9	1.6
Back Pain	1.8	0.5
Peripheral Edema	1.7	0.5
Cardiovascular		
Vasodilatation	1.1	0.3
Digestive System		
Dyspepsia	2.2	0.5
Mouth or Throat Dry	1.7	0.5
Constipation	1.5	0.8
Dental Abnormalities	1.5	0.3
Increased Appetite	1.1	0.8
Hematologic and Lymphatic Systems		
Leukopenia	1.1	0.5

(cont'd)

Table 1: Neurontin *(cont'd)*

Treatment-emergent Adverse Event Incidence in Placebo-controlled Add-on Trials (Events in at Least 1% of Neurontin Patients and Numerically More Frequent Than in the Placebo Group)

	Neurontin[a] n=543 %	Placebo[a] n=378 %
Musculoskeletal		
Myalgia	2.0	1.9
Fracture	1.1	0.8
Nervous System		
Somnolence	19.3	8.7
Dizziness	17.1	6.9
Ataxia	12.5	5.6
Nystagmus	8.3	4.0
Tremor	6.8	3.2
Nervousness	2.4	1.9
Dysarthria	2.4	0.5
Amnesia	2.2	0.0
Depression	1.8	1.1
Thinking Abnormal	1.7	1.3
Twitching	1.3	0.5
Coordination Abnormal	1.1	0.3
Respiratory System		
Rhinitis	4.1	3.7
Pharyngitis	2.8	1.6
Coughing	1.8	1.3
Skin and Appendages		
Abrasion	1.3	0.0
Pruritus	1.3	0.5
Urogenital System		
Impotence	1.5	1.1
Special Senses		
Diplopia	5.9	1.9
Amblyopia	4.2	1.1
Laboratory Deviations		
WBC Decreased	1.1	0.5

[a] Plus background antiepileptic drug therapy.

Since Neurontin was administered most often in combination with other antiepileptic agents, it was not possible to determine which agent(s) was associated with adverse events.

Dose-related Treatment-emergent Adverse Events: Among the treatment-emergent adverse events occurring in Neurontin-treated patients, somnolence and ataxia appeared to exhibit a positive dose-response relationship. Patients treated with 1800 mg/day (n=54, from one controlled study) experienced approximately a two-fold increase, as compared to patients on lower doses of 600 to 1200 mg/day (n=489, from several controlled studies), in the incidence of nystagmus (20.4%), tremor (14.8%), rhinitis (13%), peripheral edema (7.4%), coordination abnormal, depression and myalgia (all at 5.6%). Adverse events were usually mild to moderate in intensity, with a median time to resolution of 2 weeks.

Data from long-term, open, uncontrolled studies shows that Neurontin treatment does not result in any new or unusual adverse events.

Other Adverse Events Observed in All Clinical Trials: Adverse events that occurred in at least 1% of the 2074 individuals who participated in all clinical trials, only some of which were placebo-controlled, are described below. During these trials, all adverse events were recorded by the clinical investigators using terminology of their own choosing. To provide a meaningful estimate of the proportion of individuals having adverse events, similar types of events were grouped into a smaller number of standardized categories using modified COSTART dictionary terminology. These categories are used in the listing below. The frequencies presented represent the proportion of the 2074 patients exposed to Neurontin who experienced an event of the type cited on at least one occasion while receiving Neurontin. All reported events are included except those already listed in Table 1, those too general to be informative, and those not reasonably associated with the use of the drug.

Events are further classified within body system categories and enumerated in order of decreasing frequency using the following definitions: frequent adverse events are defined as those occurring in at least 1/100 patients; infrequent adverse events are those occurring in 1/100 to 1/1000 patients; rare events are those occurring in fewer than 1/1000 patients.

Body as a Whole: Frequent: asthenia, malaise, face edema; Infrequent: allergy, generalized edema, weight decrease, chill; Rare: strange feelings, lassitude, alcohol intolerance, hangover effect.

Cardiovascular System: Frequent: hypertension; Infrequent: hypotension, angina pectoris, peripheral vascular disorder, palpitation, tachycardia, migraine, murmur; Rare: atrial fibrillation, heart failure, thrombophlebitis, deep thrombophlebitis, myocardial infarction, cerebrovascular accident, pulmonary thrombosis, ventricular extrasystoles, bradycardia, premature atrial contraction, pericardial rub, heart block, pulmonary embolus, hyperlipidemia, hypercholesterolemia, pericardial effusion, pericarditis.

Digestive System: Frequent: anorexia, flatulence, gingivitis; Infrequent: glossitis, gum hemorrhage, thirst, stomatitis, increased salivation, gastroenteritis, hemorrhoids, bloody stools, fecal incontinence, hepatomegaly; Rare: dysphagia, eructation, pancreatitis, peptic ulcer, colitis, blisters in mouth, tooth discolor, perlèche, salivary gland enlarged, lip hemorrhage, esophagitis, hiatal hernia, hematemesis, proctitis, irritable bowel syndrome, rectal hemorrhage, esophageal spasm.

Endocrine System: Rare: hyperthyroid, hypothyroid, goiter, hypoestrogen, ovarian failure, epididymitis, swollen testicle, cushingoid appearance.
Hematologic and Lymphatic Systems: Frequent: purpura most often described as bruises resulting from physical trauma; Infrequent: anemia, thrombocytopenia, lymphadenopathy; Rare: WBC count increased, lymphocytosis, non-Hodgkin's lymphoma, bleeding time increased.
Musculoskeletal System: Frequent: arthralgia; Infrequent: tendinitis, arthritis, joint stiffness, joint swelling, positive Romberg test; Rare: costochondritis, osteoporosis, bursitis, contracture.
Nervous System: Frequent: vertigo, hyperkinesia, paresthesia, decreased or absent reflexes, increased reflexes, anxiety, hostility; Infrequent: CNS tumors, syncope, dreaming abnormal, aphasia, hypesthesia, intracranial hemorrhage, hypotonia, dysesthesia, paresis, dystonia, hemiplegia, facial paralysis, stupor, cerebellar dysfunction, positive Babinski sign, decreased position sense, subdural hematoma, apathy, hallucination, decrease or loss of libido, agitation, paranoia, depersonalization, euphoria, feeling high, doped-up sensation, suicide attempt, psychosis; Rare: choreoathetosis, orofacial dyskinesia, encephalopathy, nerve palsy, personality disorder, increased libido, subdued temperament, apraxia, fine motor control disorder, meningismus, local myoclonus, hyperesthesia, hypokinesia, mania, neurosis, hysteria, antisocial reaction, suicide.
Respiratory System: Frequent: pneumonia; Infrequent: epistaxis, dyspnea, apnea; Rare: mucositis, aspiration pneumonia, hyperventilation, hiccup, laryngitis, nasal obstruction, snoring, bronchospasm, hypoventilation, lung edema.
Dermatological: Infrequent: alopecia, eczema, dry skin, increased sweating, urticaria, hirsutism, seborrhea, cyst, herpes simplex; Rare: herpes zoster, skin discolor, skin papules, photosensitive reaction, leg ulcer, scalp seborrhea, psoriasis, desquamation, maceration, skin nodules, subcutaneous nodule, melanosis, skin necrosis, local swelling.
Urogenital System: Infrequent: hematuria, dysuria, urination frequency, cystitis, urinary retention, urinary incontinence, vaginal hemorrhage, amenorrhea, dysmenorrhea, menorrhagia, breast cancer, unable to climax, ejaculation abnormal; Rare: kidney pain, leukorrhea, pruritus genital, renal stone, acute renal failure, anuria, glycosuria, nephrosis, nocturia, pyuria, urination urgency, vaginal pain, breast pain, testicle pain.
Special Senses: Frequent: abnormal vision; Infrequent: cataract, conjunctivitis, eyes dry, eye pain, visual field defect, photophobia, bilateral or unilateral ptosis, eye hemorrhage, hordeolum, hearing loss, earache, tinnitus, inner ear infection, otitis, taste loss, unusual taste, eye twitching, ear fullness; Rare: eye itching, abnormal accommodation, perforated ear drum, sensitivity to noise, eye focusing problem, watery eyes, retinopathy, glaucoma, iritis, corneal disorders, lacrimal dysfunction, degenerative eye changes, blindness, retinal degeneration, miosis, chorioretinitis, strabismus, eustachian tube dysfunction, labyrinthitis, otitis externa, odd smell.
Post-market Adverse Drug Reactions: Sudden, unexplained deaths in patients with epilepsy have been reported where a causal relationship to treatment with gabapentin has not been established.

Post-marketing adverse events that have been reported, that may have no causal relationship to gabapentin, include:
Blood and Lymphatic System Disorders: thrombocytopenia.
Cardiac Disorders: palpitation.
Ear and Labyrinth Disorders: tinnitus.
Gastrointestinal Disorders: abdominal pain, diarrhea, nausea and/or vomiting, pancreatitis.
General Disorders: chest pain, fever, peripheral edema.
Hepatobiliary Disorders: rare or very rare cases of hepatic events including hepatitis sometimes associated with elevated liver function tests (LFTs) and jaundice. Isolated reports have been received for hepatic function abnormal, hepatitis cholestatic, liver failure, and hepatitis fulminant. In most of these reports, patients taking multiple medications, including those known to be potentially hepatotoxic, while being treated with Neurontin.
Immune System Disorders: allergic reaction including anaphylactic reaction and urticaria, hypersensitivity including systemic reactions.
Infections and Infestations: viral infection.
Investigations: blood glucose fluctuations in patients with diabetes.
Metabolism and Nutrition Disorders: hyponatremia.
Nervous System Disorders: headache, movement disorders such as choreoathetosis, dyskinesia, dystonia.
Psychiatric Disorders: confusion, emotional lability, hallucinations, insomnia.
Renal and Urinary Disorders: acute kidney failure, urinary incontinence.
Reproductive: breast hypertrophy, gynecomastia.
Respiratory, Thoracic and Mediastinal Disorders: pulmonary edema.
Skin and Subcutaneous Tissue Disorders: acne, alopecia, angioedema, erythema muiltiforme, rash, Stevens-Johnson syndrome.

Adverse events following the abrupt discontinuation of gabapentin have also been reported during postmarketing experience. The most frequently reported events were anxiety, insomnia, nausea, pain and sweating.

DRUG INTERACTIONS: Overview: In vitro studies were performed to investigate the potential of gabapentin to inhibit the major cytochrome P450 enzymes (CYP1A2, CYP2A6, CYP2C9, CYP2C19, CYP2D6, CYP2E1, and CYP3A4) that mediate drug and xenobiotic metabolism, using isoform selective marker substrates and human liver microsomal preparations. Only at the highest concentration tested (171 µg/mL; 1 mM) was a slight degree of inhibition (14% to 30%) observed with isoform CYP2A6. No inhibition was observed with any of the other isoforms tested at gabapentin concentrations up to 171 µg/mL (approximately 15 times the C_{max} at 3600 mg/day). Gabapentin is not an inducer of cytochrome P450 enzymes.

At plasma concentrations associated with doses up to 3600 mg/day (C_{max} 11.6 µg/mL), the highest recommended daily dose, a metabolically-based interaction between gabapentin and a drug whose clearance is dependent upon the major cytochrome P450 enzymes is unlikely.

Gabapentin is not metabolized to a significant extent in humans and does not interfere with the metabolism of commonly administered antiepileptic drugs. (See Drug Interactions, Drug-Drug Interactions, Antiepileptic Agents). Gabapentin also shows a low level of binding to plasma proteins (approximately 3%) and is eliminated solely by renal excretion as unchanged drug. (See Action and Clinical Pharmacology.) Consequently, there have been few drug interactions described in which the pharmacokinetics of gabapentin or other coadministered drugs were affected to an appreciable extent.

Drug-Drug Interactions: The drug interaction data described in this subsection were obtained from studies involving healthy adults and adult patients with epilepsy:
Antiepileptic Agents: There is no interaction between Neurontin (gabapentin) and phenytoin, valproic acid, carbamazepine, or phenobarbital. Consequently, Neurontin may be used in combination with other commonly used antiepileptic drugs without concern for alteration of the plasma concentrations of gabapentin or the other antiepileptic drugs.
Hydrocodone: Coadministration of single doses of gabapentin (125 mg to 500 mg; N=48) and hydrocodone (10 mg; N=50) decreased the C_{max} and AUC values of hydrocodone in a dose-dependent manner relative to administration of hydrocodone alone. The C_{max} and AUC values for hydrocodone were 2% and 4% lower, respectively, after administration of 125 mg gabapentin and 16% and 22% lower, respectively, after administration of 500 mg gabapentin. The mechanism for this interaction is unknown. Hydrocodone increased gabapentin AUC values by 14%. The magnitude of interaction with higher doses of gabapentin is not known.
Morphine: A literature article reported that when a 60 mg controlled release morphine capsule was administered 2 hours prior to a 600 mg gabapentin capsule in healthy volunteers (N=12), mean gabapentin AUC increased by 44% compared to gabapentin administered without morphine. Morphine pharmacokinetic parameter values were not affected by administration of gabapentin 2 hours after morphine in this study. Because this was a single dose study, the magnitude of the interaction at steady state and at higher doses of gabapentin are not known.
Naproxen: In healthy adult volunteers (N=18), the coadministration of single doses of naproxen sodium capsules (250 mg) and gabapentin (125 mg) increased the amount of gabapentin absorbed by 12% to 15%. Gabapentin did not affect naproxen pharmacokinetic parameters in this study. These doses are lower than the therapeutic doses for both drugs. Therefore, the magnitude of interaction at steady state and within the recommended dose ranges of either drug is not known.
Oral Contraceptives: Coadministration of gabapentin with the oral contraceptive Norlestrin does not influence the steady-state pharmacokinetics of norethindrone or ethinyl estradiol.
Antacids: Coadministration of gabapentin with an aluminum and magnesium-based antacid reduces gabapentin bioavailability by up to 20%. Although the clinical significance of this decrease is not known, coadministration of similar antacids and gabapentin is not recommended.
Cimetidine: A slight decrease in renal excretion of gabapentin observed when it is coadministered with cimetidine is not expected to be of clinical importance. The effect of gabapentin on cimetidine has not been evaluated.
Probenecid: Renal excretion of gabapentin is unaltered by probenecid.
Drug-Food Interactions: Neurontin is given orally with or without food.
Drug-Herb Interactions: Interactions with herbal products have not been established.
Drug-Laboratory Interactions: For urinary protein determination the sulfosalicylic acid precipitation procedure is recommended, as false positive readings were reported with the Ames N-Multistix SG dipstick test, when gabapentin or placebo was added to other anticonvulsant drugs.

DOSAGE AND ADMINISTRATION: Dosing Considerations: Because Neurontin is eliminated solely by renal excretion, dosage adjustments are recommended for patients with renal impairment (including elderly patients with declining renal function) and patients undergoing hemodialysis. (See Dosage and Administration, Special Patient Populations, Table 2.)
Adults: Neurontin (gabapentin) is given orally with or without food.
Initial Dose: The starting dose is 300 mg three times a day.
Dose Range: The dose may be increased, depending on the response and tolerance of the patient, using 300 or 400 mg capsules, or 600 or 800 mg tablets 3 times a day up to 1800 mg/day. In clinical trials, the effective dosage range was 900 to 1800 mg/day, given 3 times a day using 300 mg or 400 mg capsules, or 600 mg or 800 mg tablets. Dosages up to 2400 mg/day have been well tolerated in long-term open-label clinical studies. Doses of 3600 mg/day have also been administered to a small number of patients for a relatively short duration and have been well tolerated.

Although data from clinical trials suggest that doses higher than 1200 mg/day may have increased efficacy in some patients, higher doses may also increase the incidence of adverse events. (See Adverse Reactions.)
Maintenance: Daily maintenance doses should be given in three equally divided doses, and the maximum time between doses in a three times daily schedule should not exceed 12 hours to prevent breakthrough convulsions. It is not necessary to monitor gabapentin plasma concentrations in order to optimize Neurontin therapy. Further, as there are no drug interactions with commonly used antiepileptic drugs, Neurontin may be used in combination with these drugs without concern for alteration of plasma concentrations of either gabapentin or other antiepileptic drugs.
Discontinuation of Treatment, Dose Reduction or Initiation of Adjunctive Antiepileptic Therapy: If Neurontin dose is reduced, discontinued or substituted with an alternate anticonvulsant or an alternate anticonvulsant is added to Neurontin therapy, this should be done gradually over a minimum of 1 week (a longer period may be needed at the discretion of the prescriber. (See Warnings and Precautions.)
Special Patient Populations: Geriatrics and Renal Impairment: Due to the primarily renal excretion of Neurontin, the following dosage adjustments are recommended for elderly patients with declining renal function, patients with renal impairment and patients undergoing hemodialysis (see Dosage and Administration, Dosing Considerations; Action and Clinical Pharmacology, Special Populations and Conditions).

Table 2: Neurontin

Dosage of Neurontin in Adults Based on Renal Function

Renal Function Creatinine Clearance (mL/min)	Total Daily Dose Range[a] (mg/day)	Dose Regimen[b]
≥60	900–3600	Total daily dose (mg/day) should be divided by 3 and administered three times daily (TID)
>30–59	400–1400	Total daily dose (mg/day) should be divided by 2 and administered twice daily (BID)
>15–29	200–700	Total daily dose (mg/day) should be administered once daily (QD)
15	100–300	Total daily dose (mg/day) should be administered once daily (QD) For patients with creatinine clearance <15 mL/min, reduce daily dose in proportion to creatinine clearance (e.g., patients with a creatinine clearance of 7.5 mL/min should receive one-half the daily dose that patients with a creatinine clearance of 15 mL/min receive).
Post-hemodialysis Supplemental Dose (mg)		
Hemodialysis	125–350	Patients on hemodialysis should receive maintenance doses as indicated and an additional post hemodialysis dose administered after each 4 hours of hemodialysis.

[a] The table lists the recommended dose to be administered. When the recommended dose is unobtainable with the available dosage strengths, in these cases, dose selection should be based on available dosage strengths, clinical judgement and tolerability.
[b] Physician should administer the dose regimen according to the response and tolerance of the patient.

Pediatrics: Neurontin is not indicated for use in children under 18 years of age. (See Indications and Clinical Use; Warnings and Precautions, Special Populations.)
Hepatic Impairment: Because gabapentin is not metabolized to a significant extent in humans, no studies have been performed in patients with hepatic impairment.
Missed Dose: Physicians should instruct their patients that if a dose is missed, the next one should be taken as soon as possible. However, if it is within 4 hours of the next dose, the missed dose is not to be taken and the patient should return to the regular dosing schedule. To avoid breakthrough convulsions the maximum time between doses should not exceed 12 hours.

OVERDOSAGE:
Symptoms of Overdosage: Acute, life-threatening toxicity has not been observed with Neurontin (gabapentin) overdoses of up to 49 g ingested at one time. In these cases, dizziness, double vision, slurred speech, drowsiness, lethargy and mild diarrhea were observed. All patients recovered with supportive care.

An oral lethal dose of gabapentin was not identified in mice and rats given doses as high as 8000 mg/kg. Signs of acute toxicity in animals included ataxia, laboured breathing, ptosis, hypoactivity, or excitation.
Treatment of Overdosage: Gabapentin can be removed by hemodialysis. Although hemodialysis has not been performed in the few overdose cases reported, it may be indicated by the patient's clinical state or in patients with significant renal impairment.

Reduced absorption of gabapentin at higher doses may limit drug absorption at the time of overdosing and, hence, reduce toxicity from overdoses.

In managing overdosage, consider the possibility of multiple drug involvement. The physician should consider contacting a poison control center for additional information on the treatment of overdosage.

> For management of a suspected drug overdose, CPhA recommends that you contact your **regional Poison Control Centre**. See the *CPS* Directory section for a list of Poison Control Centres.

ACTION AND CLINICAL PHARMACOLOGY: Mechanism of Action: Neurontin (gabapentin) exhibits antiseizure activity in mice and rats both in the maximal electroshock and in the pentylenetetrazol seizure models.

Gabapentin is structurally related to the neurotransmitter GABA (gamma-aminobutyric acid) but does not interact with GABA receptors, it is not metabolized to GABA or to GABA agonists, and it is not an inhibitor of GABA uptake or degradation. Gabapentin at concentrations up to 100 µM did not demonstrate affinity for other receptor sites such as benzodiazepine, glutamate, glycine or N-methyl-D-aspartate receptors nor does it interact with neuronal sodium channels or L-type calcium channels.

The mechanism of action of gabapentin has not yet been established, however, it is unlike that of the commonly used anticonvulsant drugs.

In vitro studies with radiolabelled gabapentin have revealed a gabapentin binding site in rat brain tissues including neocortex and hippocampus. The identity and function of this binding site remain to be elucidated.
Pharmacokinetics: All pharmacological actions following gabapentin administration are due to the activity of the parent compound; gabapentin is not metabolized to a significant extent in humans.

Plasma gabapentin concentrations are dose-proportional at doses of 300 to 400 mg q8h, ranging between 1 µg/mL and 10 µg/mL, but are less than dose-proportional above the clinical range (>600 mg q8h). There is no correlation between plasma levels and efficacy.

Gabapentin pharmacokinetics are not affected by repeated administration, and steady state plasma concentrations are predictable from single dose data. Gabapentin steady-state pharmacokinetics are similar for healthy subjects and patients with epilepsy receiving antiepileptic agents.

Absorption: Following oral administration of Neurontin (gabapentin), peak plasma concentrations are observed within 2 to 3 hours. Absolute bioavailability of a 300 mg dose of Neurontin capsules is approximately 59%. At doses of 300 and 400 mg, gabapentin bioavailability is unchanged following multiple dose administration.

Food has no effect on the rate or extent of absorption of gabapentin.

Distribution: Less than 3% of gabapentin is bound to plasma proteins. The apparent volume of distribution of gabapentin after 150 mg intravenous administration is 58±6 L (Mean±SD). In patients with epilepsy, gabapentin concentrations in cerebrospinal fluid are approximately 20% of corresponding steady-state trough plasma concentrations.

Metabolism: Gabapentin is not appreciably metabolized to a significant extent in humans. Gabapentin does not induce or inhibit hepatic mixed function oxidase enzymes responsible for drug metabolism and does not interfere with the metabolism of commonly coadministered antiepileptic drugs.

Excretion: Gabapentin is eliminated solely by renal excretion as unchanged drug, and can be removed from plasma by hemodialysis. Gabapentin elimination rate constant, plasma clearance and renal clearance are directly proportional to creatinine clearance. The elimination half-life of gabapentin is independent of dose and averages 5 to 7 hours in subjects with normal renal function.

Table 3 summarizes the mean steady-state pharmacokinetic parameters of Neurontin capsules.

Table 3: Neurontin

Summary of Neurontin (gabapentin) Mean Steady-state Pharmacokinetic Parameters in Adults Following q8h Administration

Pharmacokinetic Parameter	300 mg (N=7)	400 mg (N=11)
C_{max} (μg/mL)	4.02	5.50
t_{max} (h)	2.7	2.1
t½ (h)	5.2	6.1
AUC $(_{0-\infty})$ (μg·h/mL)	24.8	33.3
AE%[a]	NA	63.6

[a] Amount excreted in urine (% of dose).
Legend: NA=not available.

Bioequivalence of Dosage Forms: Neurontin 600 mg and 800 mg tablets are bioequivalent to two 300 mg capsules and two 400 mg capsules, respectively. The results of a single-dose, two-way crossover, comparative bioavailability study in the fasted state comparing Neurontin 600 mg tablets and 2×300 mg Neurontin capsules are summarized in Table 4.

Table 4: Neurontin

Summary Table of the Comparative Bioavailability Data Neurontin 600 mg Tablets and Neurontin 2×300 mg Capsules

	Neurontin				
	600 mg Tablets		2×300 mg Capsules		
	Arithmetic (CV%)	Geometric	Arithmetic (CV%)	Geometric	% Ratio of Geometric Means
Parameter	Mean Values From Measured Data				
AUC_T (μg·h/mL)	51.3 (31.8)	48.9	46.8 (28.4)	45.2	108
AUC_I (μg·h/mL)	52.5 (30.2)	50.4	47.7 (27.1)	46.1	109
C_{max} (μg/mL)	4.94 (30.9)	4.71	4.48 (25.9)	4.35	108
T_{max} (h)	3.2 (27.3)	—	3.5 (34.1)	—	—
$T_{1/2}$ (h)	15.6 (88.2)	—	15.4 (90.5)	—	—

Special Populations and Conditions: Pediatrics: There are no pharmacokinetic data available in children under 18 years of age.

Geriatrics: Apparent oral clearance (CL/F) of gabapentin decreased as age increased, from about 225 mL/min in subjects under 30 years of age to about 125 mL/min in subjects over 70 years of age. Renal clearance (CLr) of gabapentin also declined with age; however, this decrease can largely be explained by the decline in renal function. Reduction of gabapentin dose may be required in patients who have age-related compromised renal function. (See Dosage and Administration, Dosing Considerations.)

Hepatic Insufficiency: Because gabapentin is not metabolized to a significant extent in humans, no study was performed in patients with hepatic impairment.

Renal Insufficiency: In patients with impaired renal function, gabapentin clearance is markedly reduced and dosage adjustment is necessary. (See Dosage and Administration, Dosing Considerations and Special Patient Populations, Table 2.)

Hemodialysis: In a study in anuric subjects (N=11), the apparent elimination half-life of gabapentin on non-dialysis days was about 132 hours; during dialysis the apparent half-life of gabapentin was reduced to 3.8 hours. Hemodialysis thus has a significant effect on gabapentin elimination in anuric subjects.

Dosage adjustment in patients undergoing hemodialysis is necessary. (See Dosage and Administration, Dosing Considerations and Special Patient Populations, Table 2.)

STORAGE AND STABILITY: Capsules: Store at controlled room temperature, 15-30°C.
Tablets: Store at controlled room temperature, 20-25°C.

INFORMATION FOR THE PATIENT: Published in e-CPS, available by subscription at www.e-cps.ca.

DOSAGE FORMS, COMPOSITION AND PACKAGING: Capsules: 100 mg: Each hard gelatin CONI-SNAP capsule, with white opaque body and cap printed with "PD" on one side and "Neurontin/100 mg" on the other, contains: gabapentin 100 mg. Nonmedicinal ingredients: cornstarch, lactose and talc; capsule shell may contain: FD&C Blue No. 2, gelatin, red iron oxide, silicon dioxide, sodium lauryl sulfate, titanium dioxide and yellow iron oxide. Bottles of 100.

300 mg: Each hard gelatin CONI-SNAP capsule, with yellow opaque body and cap printed with "PD" on one side and "Neurontin/300 mg" on the other, contains: gabapentin 300 mg. Nonmedicinal ingredients: cornstarch, lactose and talc; capsule shell may contain: FD&C Blue No. 2, gelatin, red iron oxide, silicon dioxide, sodium lauryl sulfate, titanium dioxide and yellow iron oxide. Bottles of 100.

400 mg: Each hard gelatin CONI-SNAP capsule, with orange opaque body and cap printed with "PD" on one side and "Neurontin/400 mg" on the other, contains: gabapentin 400 mg. Nonmedicinal ingredients: cornstarch, lactose and talc; capsule shell may contain: FD&C Blue No. 2, gelatin, red iron oxide, silicon dioxide, sodium lauryl sulfate, titanium dioxide and yellow iron oxide. Bottles of 100.

Tablets: 600 mg: Each white, elliptical, film-coated tablet, with "Neurontin 600" printed on one side contains: gabapentin 600 mg. Nonmedicinal ingredients: ammonium hydroxide, black iron oxide, candelilla wax, copolyvidone, cornstarch, hydroxypropylcellulose, magnesium stearate, poloxamer 407 NF and talc. Bottles of 100.

800 mg: Each white, elliptical, film-coated tablet, with "Neurontin 800" printed on one side contains: gabapentin 800 mg. Nonmedicinal ingredients: candelilla wax, copolyvidone, cornstarch, hydroxypropylcellulose, hypromellose, magnesium stearate, poloxamer 407 NF, red iron oxide, yellow iron oxide and talc. Bottles of 100.

(Shown in Product Identification Section)

Nevanac® 🅿

nepafenac

Nonsteroidal Anti-inflammatory Agent

Alcon

Date of Preparation: April 16, 2008
Date of Revision: July 8, 2008

SUMMARY PRODUCT INFORMATION:

Route of Administration	Dosage Form/ Strength	Clinically Relevant Nonmedicinal Ingredients
Ophthalmic (topical)	Suspension 0.1%	For a complete listing see Dosage Forms, Composition and Packaging.

INDICATIONS AND CLINICAL USE: NEVANAC (nepafenac) Ophthalmic Suspension is indicated for management of pain and inflammation associated with cataract surgery.

Geriatrics (>65 years of age): No overall differences in safety and effectiveness have been observed between elderly and younger patients.

Pediatrics (<18 years of age): The safety and effectiveness of NEVANAC Suspension in pediatric patients have not been established. Its use is not recommended in these patients until further data become available.

CONTRAINDICATIONS: NEVANAC (nepafenac) Ophthalmic Suspension is contraindicated in patients who are hypersensitive to nepafenac, to any ingredient in the formulation or component of the container (for a complete listing see the Dosage Forms, Composition and Packaging), or to other nonsteroidal anti-inflammatory drugs (NSAIDs).

WARNINGS AND PRECAUTIONS: General: There is a potential for cross-sensitivity of nepafenac to acetylsalicylic acid, phenylacetic acid derivatives, and other NSAIDs. Therefore, caution should be used when treating individuals who have previously exhibited sensitivities to these drugs.

Topical NSAIDs may slow or delay healing. Topical corticosteroids are also known to slow or delay healing. Concomitant use of topical NSAIDs and topical steroids may increase the potential for healing problems.

Hematologic: With some NSAIDs, including NEVANAC Suspension, the potential exists for increased bleeding time due to interference with thrombocyte aggregation. There have been reports that ophthalmic NSAIDs may cause increased bleeding of ocular tissues (including hyphemas) in conjunction with ocular surgery.

It is recommended that NEVANAC Suspension be used with caution in patients with known bleeding tendencies or who are receiving medications which may prolong bleeding time.

Ophthalmologic: Use of topical NSAIDs may result in keratitis. In some susceptible patients, continued use of topical NSAIDs may result in epithelial breakdown, corneal thinning, corneal erosion, corneal ulceration or corneal perforation. These events may be sight-threatening. Patients with evidence of corneal epithelial breakdown should immediately discontinue use of NEVANAC Suspension and should be closely monitored for corneal health.

Postmarketing experience with topical NSAIDs suggests that patients with complicated ocular surgeries, corneal denervation, corneal epithelial defects, diabetes mellitus, ocular surface diseases (e.g., dry eye syndrome), rheumatoid arthritis, or repeat ocular surgeries within a short period of time may be at increased risk for corneal adverse events which may become sight-threatening. Topical NSAIDs should be used with caution in these patients. Postmarketing experience also suggests that prolonged use of topical NSAIDs may increase patient risk for occurrence and severity of corneal adverse reactions.

Contact lens wear is not recommended during the postoperative period following cataract surgery; therefore, contact lenses should not be worn during treatment with NEVANAC Suspension.

Sexual Function/Reproduction: Nepafenac did not impair fertility when administered orally to male and female rats at 3 mg/kg (approximately 90 and 380 times the plasma exposure to the parent drug, nepafenac, and the active metabolite, amfenac, respectively, at the recommended human topical ophthalmic dose).

Special Populations: Pregnant Women: No adequate and well-controlled studies have been conducted in pregnant women. Because animal reproduction studies are not always predictive of human response, NEVANAC Suspension should be used during pregnancy only if the potential benefit justifies the potential risk to the fetus.

Because of the known effects of prostaglandin biosynthesis inhibiting drugs on the fetal cardiovascular system (closure of the ductus arteriosus), the use of NEVANAC Suspension during late pregnancy should be avoided.

Reproduction studies performed with nepafenac in rabbits and rats at oral doses up to 10 mg/kg/day have revealed no evidence of teratogenicity due to nepafenac, despite the induction of maternal toxicity. At this dose, the animal plasma exposure to nepafenac and amfenac was approximately 260 and 2400 times human plasma exposure at the recommended human topical ophthalmic dose for rats and 80 and 680 times human plasma exposure for rabbits, respectively. In rats, maternally toxic doses ≥10 mg/kg were associated with dystocia, increased postimplantation loss, reduced fetal weights and growth, and reduced fetal survival. Nepafenac has been shown to cross the placental barrier in rats.

Nursing Women: It is unknown whether nepafenac is excreted in human milk. Animal studies have shown excretion of nepafenac in the milk of pregnant rats. Caution should be exercised when NEVANAC Suspension is administered to a nursing woman.

Pediatrics: The safety and effectiveness of NEVANAC Suspension in pediatric patients have not been established. Its use is not recommended in these patients until further data become available.

Geriatrics: No overall differences in safety and effectiveness have been observed between elderly and younger patients.

ADVERSE REACTIONS: Adverse Drug Reaction Overview: In clinical studies with over 800 patients receiving NEVANAC (nepafenac) Ophthalmic Suspension, approximately 5% of patients experienced adverse reactions. These events led to discontinuation in 0.5% of patients, which was less than placebo-treated patients (1.3%) in these same studies. No serious adverse events related to NEVANAC Suspension were reported in these studies.

Clinical Trial Adverse Drug Reactions: Because clinical trials are conducted under very specific conditions the adverse reaction rates observed in the clinical trials may not reflect the rates observed in practice and should not be compared to the rates in the clinical trials of another drug. Adverse drug reaction information from clinical trials is useful for identifying drug-related adverse events and for approximating rates.

In 11 clinical studies, NEVANAC Suspension was administered to 811 patients at a dose of one drop one, two, three or four times daily. The most frequent adverse drug reactions (>0.1%) in patients with exposure to NEVANAC Suspension are presented in Table 1. No treatment-related adverse drug reactions were reported at a frequency of ≥1% in patients with exposure to NEVANAC Suspension.

Table 1: NEVANAC

Treatment-Related Adverse Drug Reactions >0.1%

MedDRA Preferred Term (Version 9.0)	NEVANAC 0.1% n=811 (%)	Placebo n=529 (%)	Ketorolac 0.5% n=73 (%)	Ketorolac 0.4% n=163 (%)	Diclofenac 0.1% n=44 (%)
Eye Disorders					
Eyelid margin crusting	0.6		1.4		
Eye pain	0.5	0.9		2.5	
Punctate keratitis	0.5	0.6	1.4		
Vision blurred	0.5	0.2			
Foreign body sensation	0.4	1.5			

(cont'd)

Table 1: NEVANAC (cont'd)

Treatment-Related Adverse Drug Reactions >0.1%

MedDRA Preferred Term (Version 9.0)	NEVANAC 0.1% n=811 (%)	Placebo n=529 (%)	Ketorolac 0.5% n=73 (%)	Ketorolac 0.4% n=163 (%)	Diclofenac 0.1% n=44 (%)
Dry eye	0.4	0.2			
Eye pruritus	0.4				
Lacrimation increased	0.2	0.2			
Nervous System Disorders					
Headache	0.4				

Less Common Clinical Trial Adverse Drug Reactions (≤0.1%): Eye Disorders: allergic conjunctivitis, choroidal effusion, conjunctival hyperaemia, corneal deposits, eye discharge, eye irritation, eyelid disorder, iritis, keratitis, ocular discomfort, photophobia.

Gastrointestinal Disorders: dry mouth, nausea.

Immune System Disorders: hypersensitivity.

Abnormal Hematologic and Clinical Chemistry Findings: NEVANAC Suspension had no clinically relevant effect on laboratory parameters.

Post-Market Adverse Drug Reactions: Adverse reactions identified from postmarketing experience that have not been reported previously in clinical trials with NEVANAC Suspension include the following: ulcerative keratitis, corneal epithelium defect/disorder, corneal abrasion, anterior chamber inflammation, impaired healing (cornea), reduced visual acuity, corneal scar, corneal opacity.

DRUG INTERACTIONS: Overview: Neither nepafenac nor amfenac inhibits any of the major human cytochrome P450 (CYP1A2, CYP2C9, CYP2C19, CYP2D6, CYP2E1, and CYP3A4) metabolic activities in vitro at concentrations up to 300 ng/mL. Therefore, drug-drug interactions involving CYP-mediated metabolism of concomitantly administered drugs are unlikely. Drug-drug interactions mediated by protein binding are also unlikely.

Drug-Drug Interactions: NEVANAC (nepafenac) Ophthalmic Suspension may be administered in conjunction with other topical ophthalmic medications such as beta-blockers, carbonic anhydrase inhibitors, alpha-agonists, cycloplegics, and mydriatics.

The administration of NEVANAC Suspension in conjunction with prostaglandin analogues was not evaluated in clinical trials. Interactions between NEVANAC Suspension and prostaglandin analogues are not anticipated following topical ocular administration.

There is a potential cross-sensitivity to acetylsalicylic acid, phenylacetic acid derivatives, and other nonsteroidal anti-inflammatory agents.

Drug-Food Interactions: Interactions with food are not anticipated following topical ocular administration.

Drug-Herb Interactions: Interactions with herbal products are not anticipated following topical ocular administration.

Drug-Laboratory Test Interactions: Interactions with laboratory tests are not anticipated following topical ocular administration.

DOSAGE AND ADMINISTRATION: Dosing Considerations: NEVANAC (nepafenac) Ophthalmic Suspension has not been studied in patients with hepatic disease or renal impairment. Nepafenac is eliminated primarily through biotransformation and the systemic exposure is very low following topical ocular administration. No dose adjustment is warranted in these patients.

Recommended Dose and Dosage Adjustment: Shake well before use. One drop of NEVANAC Suspension should be applied to the affected eye(s) three-times-daily beginning 1 day prior to cataract surgery, and continued on the day of surgery and through the first 2 weeks of the postoperative period.

Missed Dose: If a dose is missed, a single drop should be applied as soon as possible before reverting to regular routine. Do not use a double dose to make up for the one missed.

Administration: NEVANAC Suspension has been safely administered in conjunction with other ophthalmic medications such as antibiotics, anesthetics, beta-blockers, carbonic anhydrase inhibitors, alpha-agonists, cycloplegics, and mydriatics. Because the administration of NEVANAC Suspension in conjunction with prostaglandin analogues has not been studied, use only if the benefit outweighs any potential risk.

If more than one topical ophthalmic medication is being used, the medicines must be administered at least 5 minutes apart.

Contact lens wear is not recommended during the postoperative period following cataract surgery; therefore, contact lenses should not be worn during treatment with NEVANAC Suspension.

To prevent contamination of the dropper tip and solution, care must be taken not to touch the eyelids, surrounding areas or other surfaces with the dropper tip of the bottle. Keep bottle tightly closed when not in use.

OVERDOSAGE:

A topical overdosage may be flushed from the eye(s) with warm tap water.

There is minimal risk of adverse effects due to accidental ingestion of a 5 mL bottle of NEVANAC (nepafenac) Ophthalmic Suspension (total dose of 5 mg) by a child. The recommended adult dose of amfenac sodium (FENAZOX), marketed in Japan since 1986, is one to four 50 mg tablets daily. This translates to 1 to 4 mg/kg per day for a 50 kg person. If a 20 kg child ingested the entire contents of a 5 mL bottle of NEVANAC Suspension, it would translate to a dose of 0.25 mg/kg or only 6% to 25% of the recommended adult dose.

For management of a suspected drug overdose, CPhA recommends that you contact your **regional Poison Control Centre**. See the *CPS* Directory section for a list of Poison Control Centres.

ACTION AND CLINICAL PHARMACOLOGY: Mechanism of Action: Nepafenac is a nonsteroidal anti-inflammatory and analgesic prodrug. After topical ocular dosing, nepafenac penetrates the cornea and is converted by ocular tissue hydrolases to amfenac, a nonsteroidal anti-inflammatory drug. Amfenac inhibits the action of prostaglandin H synthase (cyclooxygenase), an enzyme required for prostaglandin production.

Pharmacodynamics: In rabbits, nepafenac has been shown to inhibit blood-retinal-barrier breakdown, concomitant with suppression of PGE_2 synthesis. Ex vivo, a single topical ocular dose of nepafenac was shown to inhibit prostaglandin synthesis in the iris/ciliary body (85%-95%) and the retina/choroid (55%) for up to 6 hours and 4 hours, respectively. Topical nepafenac inhibits choroidal neovascularisation and ischemia induced retinal neovascularisation. A decreased production of vascular endothelial growth factor was noted in these studies.

The majority of hydrolytic conversion is in the retina/choroid followed by the iris/ciliary body and cornea consistent with the degree of vascularised tissue. The enhanced permeability of nepafenac, combined with rapid bioactivation, make it a target-specific NSAID for inhibiting prostaglandin formation in the anterior and posterior segments of the eye.

Results from clinical studies indicate the NEVANAC (nepafenac) Ophthalmic Suspension has no significant effect on intraocular pressure.

Pharmacokinetics:

	C_{max} (ng/mL)	T_{max} (h)	AUC_{0-8} (ng·h/mL)	$t_{½}$ (h)
Nepafenac	0.310±0.104	0.25±0.10	0.368±0.106	0.9±0.2
Amfenac	0.422±0.121	0.55±0.14	0.976±0.284	1.6±0.3

Absorption: Following bilateral topical ocular three-times-daily dosing of NEVANAC Suspension, low but quantifiable plasma drug concentrations were observed in the majority of subjects at 2 hours (nepafenac) and 5 hours (amfenac) post-dose. The mean steady-state plasma C_{max} for nepafenac and for amfenac were 0.310±0.104 ng/mL and 0.422±0.121 ng/mL, respectively, following ocular administration.

Distribution: Amfenac has high affinity toward serum albumin proteins. In vitro, the percent bound to human albumin and human serum was 95.4% and 99.1%, respectively.

Studies in rats have shown that radioactive drug-related materials distribute widely in the body following single and multiple oral doses of ^{14}C-nepafenac.

Metabolism: Nepafenac undergoes relatively rapid bioactivation to amfenac via intraocular hydrolases. Subsequently, amfenac undergoes extensive metabolism to more polar metabolites involving hydroxylation of the aromatic ring leading to glucuronide conjugate formation. Radiochromatographic analyses before and after β-glucuronidase hydrolysis indicated that all metabolites were in the form of glucuronide conjugates, with the exception of amfenac. Amfenac was the major metabolite in plasma, representing approximately 13% of total plasma radioactivity. The second most abundant plasma metabolite was identified as 5-hydroxy nepafenac, representing approximately 9% of total radioactivity at C_{max}.

Excretion: After oral administration of ^{14}C-nepafenac to healthy volunteers, urinary excretion was found to be the major route of radioactivity elimination, accounting for approximately 85% of the dose while fecal excretion represented approximately 6% of the dose. Nepafenac and amfenac were not quantifiable in the urine.

Special Populations and Conditions: Pediatrics: NEVANAC Suspension has not been evaluated in the pediatric population.

Geriatrics: No overall differences in safety and effectiveness have been observed between elderly and younger patients.

Gender: Gender differences in the plasma pharmacokinetics of nepafenac and amfenac were small and not clinically relevant.

Race: A comparison of the single- and steady-state pharmacokinetic data for nepafenac and amfenac in healthy Japanese and non-Japanese subjects indicate that there are no clinically meaningful ethnic differences in the systemic exposure of either nepafenac or amfenac following topical ocular administration of NEVANAC Suspension.

Hepatic or Renal Insufficiency: NEVANAC Suspension has not been studied in patients with hepatic disease or renal impairment. The systemic exposure is very low following topical ocular administration and no dose adjustment is warranted in these patients.

STORAGE AND STABILITY: Store at 2-30°C. Discard 28 days after opening.

SPECIAL HANDLING INSTRUCTIONS: None.

INFORMATION FOR THE PATIENT: Published in e-CPS, available by subscription at www.e-cps.ca.

DOSAGE FORMS, COMPOSITION AND PACKAGING: Each mL of ophthalmic suspension contains: nepafenac 1 mg (0.1%). Nonmedicinal ingredients: benzalkonium chloride as a preservative 0.005%, carbomer 974P, edetate disodium, mannitol, purified water, sodium chloride, sodium hydroxide and/or hydrochloric acid (to adjust pH) and tyloxapol. Round low density polyethylene bottles of 8 mL with a natural low density polyethylene dispensing plug and white polypropylene cap. Tamper evidence is provided by a closure with an extended skirt that locks to the bottle finish on application and breaks away from the closure on opening. Net contents are 5 mL supplied in an 8 mL bottle.

Nexavar® Pr

sorafenib

Multikinase Inhibitor—Antineoplastic

Bayer

Date of Revision: October 15, 2009

SUMMARY PRODUCT INFORMATION:

Route of Administration	Dosage Form/ Strength	Clinically Relevant Nonmedicinal Ingredients
Oral	Film-coated tablets, 200 mg sorafenib (as 274 mg sorafenib tosylate)	None For a complete list of ingredients see Dosage Forms, Composition and Packaging.

INDICATIONS AND CLINICAL USE: NEXAVAR (sorafenib tablets) is indicated for:

- treatment of patients with unresectable hepatocellular carcinoma (HCC)
  There are limited safety data available for Child-Pugh Class B patients.
- treatment of locally advanced/metastatic Renal Cell (clear cell) Carcinoma (RCC) in patients who failed or are intolerant to prior systemic therapy.

Approval of NEXAVAR for locally advanced/metastatic Renal Cell (clear cell) Carcinoma (RCC) is based on progression-free survival [PFS] in low and intermediate risk [MSKCC prognostic criteria] patients without brain metastasis. Prolongation of overall survival has not been established for NEXAVAR in RCC. The quality of life was not significantly different in the pivotal clinical trial comparing NEXAVAR to placebo.

NEXAVAR should be prescribed by a qualified healthcare professional who is experienced in the use of antineoplastic therapy.

Geriatrics (≥65 years of age): Analyses of data by age demographics suggest that no dose adjustment is required on the basis of patient age (65 years or older). No differences in safety or efficacy were observed between older and younger patients.

Pediatrics (<18 years of age): The safety and effectiveness of sorafenib in pediatric patients has not been established.

CONTRAINDICATIONS: NEXAVAR (sorafenib tablets) is contraindicated in patients who are hypersensitive to this drug or to any ingredient in the formulation or component of the container. For a complete listing of ingredients, see Dosage Forms, Composition and Packaging.

WARNINGS AND PRECAUTIONS:

Serious Warnings and Precautions

NEXAVAR (sorafenib tablets) should be prescribed by a qualified healthcare professional who is experienced in the use of antineoplastic therapy.

NEXAVAR has not been studied in patients with severe hepatic impairment.

The following are clinically significant adverse events:

- Hypertension (see Warnings and Precautions, Cardiovascular)
- Hemorrhage (including gastrointestinal and respiratory tracts) (see Warnings and Precautions, Hematologic)
- Cardiac ischemia/infarction (see Warnings and Precautions, Cardiovascular)
- Gastrointestinal perforation (see Warnings and Precautions, Gastrointestinal)

General: Drug-Drug Interactions: Caution is recommended when administering sorafenib together with compounds that are metabolized/eliminated predominantly by the UGT1A1 and UGT1A9 pathways (e.g., irinotecan) (see Drug Interactions).

Caution is recommended if sorafenib has to be coadministered with docetaxel as it may result in an increase in docetaxel AUC (see Drug Interactions).

Coadministration of neomycin may cause a decrease in sorafenib bioavailability (see Drug Interactions).

Warfarin: Infrequent bleeding events or elevations in the International Normalized Ratio (INR) have been reported in some patients taking warfarin while on sorafenib therapy (see Monitoring and Laboratory Tests and Adverse Reactions).

Wound Healing Complications: No formal studies of the effect of sorafenib on wound healing have been conducted. In patients undergoing major surgical procedures, temporary interruption of sorafenib therapy is recommended for precautionary reasons. There is limited clinical experience regarding the timing of reinitiation of therapy following major surgical intervention. Therefore, the decision to resume sorafenib therapy following a major surgical intervention should be based on clinical judgment of adequate wound healing.

Carcinogenesis and Mutagenesis: Carcinogenicity studies have not been performed with NEXAVAR.

Positive genotoxic effects were obtained for sorafenib in an in vitro mammalian cell assay (Chinese hamster ovary) for clastogenicity (chromosome aberrations) in the presence of metabolic activation. One intermediate in the manufacturing process, which is also present in the final drug substance (<0.15%), was positive for mutagenesis in an in vitro bacterial cell assay (Ames test). Sorafenib was not genotoxic in the Ames test (the material contained the intermediate at 0.34%) and in an in vivo mouse micronucleus assay.

Cardiovascular: QT Interval Prolongation: The effect of sorafenib on QT interval is unknown at this time. Sorafenib should be administered with caution in patients who have or may develop prolongation of the QT interval. These include patients with hypokalemia or hypomagnesemia, patients with congenital long QT syndrome and patients taking anti-arrhythmic medicines or other medicinal products that lead to QT interval prolongation.

Cardiac Ischemia and/or Infarction: Cardiac ischemia and/or infarction were reported as common adverse events in subjects treated with NEXAVAR. The incidence rates were higher in NEXAVAR-treated patients than those treated with the placebo in both RCC and HCC pivotal trials (see Adverse Reactions). Patients with unstable coronary artery disease or recent myocardial infarction (within 6 months) were excluded from these studies. Temporary or permanent discontinuation of NEXAVAR should be considered in patients who develop cardiac ischemia and/or infarction.

Hypertension: An increased incidence of hypertension was observed in sorafenib-treated patients. In the phase III NEXAVAR RCC clinical trial, treatment-emergent hypertension was reported in 17% of sorafenib treated patients and in 2% of patients in the placebo group prior to the crossover event in the trial. Patients randomized to sorafenib were permitted to continue sorafenib after the crossover. In these patients the overall rate of treatment-emergent hypertension was reported as 22% (see Adverse Reactions). Hypertension was usually mild to moderate, occurred early in the course of treatment, and was amenable to management with standard antihypertensive therapy. In cases of severe or persistent hypertension, or hypertensive crisis despite adequate antihypertensive therapy, permanent discontinuation of sorafenib should be considered. At the beginning of therapy, blood pressure should be monitored on a weekly basis and thereafter should be monitored regularly and treated, if required, in accordance with standard medical practice (see Monitoring and Laboratory Tests and Adverse Reactions).

Gastrointestinal: Gastrointestinal Perforation: Gastrointestinal perforation is an uncommon event and has been reported in less than 1% of patients taking NEXAVAR. In some cases, this was not associated with apparent intra-abdominal tumour. NEXAVAR therapy should be discontinued in the event of gastrointestinal perforation.

Hematologic: Hemorrhage: An increase in the risk of bleeding may occur following sorafenib administration. In the phase III NEXAVAR RCC clinical trial, bleeding, regardless of the cause, was found in 15% of sorafenib- treated patients and in 8% of patients in the placebo group. Pulmonary hemorrhages were observed in 4.7% of the placebo group and in 4.4% of the sorafenib group. Gastrointestinal hemorrhages were reported in 0.9% of the placebo group (and in 3.8% of the sorafenib-treated patients).

In the phase III NEXAVAR HCC clinical trial, the incidence of hemorrhagic events was reported in 18.2% of sorafenib-treated patients and in 19.9% of patients in the placebo group. Pulmonary hemorrhages were observed in 4.0% of the placebo group and in 5.2 % of the sorafenib group. Gastrointestinal hemorrhages were reported in 14.6% of the placebo group and in 11.6% of the sorafenib-treated patients. The reported incidence of hemorrhagic events assessed as drug related by the reporting investigator was 7.1% in sorafenib-treated patients and 3.6% in the placebo arm.

The incidence of severe bleeding events is uncommon. Cerebral hemorrhages have been reported in patients with RCC and HCC receiving sorafenib and placebo at similar rates. These events are uncommon.

If any bleeding event necessitates medical intervention, it is recommended that permanent discontinuation of sorafenib should be considered (see Adverse Reactions).

Hepatic/Biliary/Pancreatic: Hepatic Impairment: In vitro and in vivo data indicate that sorafenib is primarily metabolized by the liver. Based on the results from one phase II study, $AUC_{0\text{-}8}$ and C_{max} in patients with Child-Pugh B hepatic impairment were greater than the corresponding parameters in patients with Child-Pugh A hepatic impairment. NEXAVAR has not been studied in patients with Child-Pugh C hepatic impairment (see Action and Clinical Pharmacology, Special Populations and Conditions). There are limited safety data available for Child-Pugh Class B patients.

Pancreatitis: In both HCC and RCC NEXAVAR clinical trials elevated serum lipase was common in sorafenib-treated and placebo-treated groups (see Adverse Reactions). The diagnosis of pancreatitis should not be made on the basis of laboratory abnormalities alone. In the RCC NEXAVAR clinical trial, clinical evidence of pancreatitis was reported in 4 (0.9%) patients in the sorafenib group (2 grade 4; 2 grade 1 or 2) and in 1 patient (grade 2) in the placebo group prior to the crossover event in the trial. Patients randomized to sorafenib were permitted to continue sorafenib after the crossover. In these patients the overall rate of treatment-emergent pancreatitis was reported as 1.1% (5 patients—2 grade 4 and 3 grade 1 or 2). In the HCC NEXAVAR clinical trial, clinical pancreatitis was reported in 1 sorafenib-treated patient (see Adverse Reactions).

Infections: Infection-related events (all grade), were reported more frequently in sorafenib-treated patients than in placebo-treated patients. Similarly, grade 3 to 5 infection-related events were reported more frequently in sorafenib-treated patients than in placebo-treated patients (see Adverse Reactions).

Neurologic: In the RCC NEXAVAR clinical trial, sensory neuropathy was reported in 67 (14.8%) of patients with sorafenib and 32 (7.1%) of patients receiving placebo. This event was usually considered to be mild or moderate (grade 1 or 2) and tended to occur in the first few cycles of therapy.

Renal: No dose adjustment is required in patients with mild, moderate, or severe renal impairment not requiring dialysis. Sorafenib has not been studied in patients undergoing dialysis (see Dosage and Administration).

Monitoring of fluid balance and electrolytes in patients at risk of renal dysfunction is advised.

Sexual Function/Reproduction: Results from animal studies indicate that sorafenib can impair male and female fertility.

Skin: Hand-foot skin reaction (palmar-plantar erythrodysesthesia) and rash represent the most common adverse drug reactions with sorafenib. Rash and hand-foot skin reaction are usually CTC (National Cancer Institute Common Terminology Criteria) grade 1 and 2 and generally appear during the first two cycles (12 weeks) of treatment with sorafenib. Dermatologic toxicities are generally easily managed and may include topical therapies for symptomatic relief, temporary treatment interruption and/or dose modification of sorafenib, or in severe or persistent cases, permanent discontinuation of sorafenib (see Adverse Reactions).

Special Populations: Pregnant Women: There are no adequate and well-controlled studies in pregnant women using sorafenib. In animals, sorafenib has been shown to be teratogenic and embryotoxic.

Adequate contraception should be used during therapy and for at least 2 weeks after completion of therapy. Women of child-bearing potential must be apprised of the potential hazard to the fetus, which includes severe malformation (teratogenicity), failure to thrive and fetal death (embryotoxicity).

Sorafenib should not be used during pregnancy. Prescribers may only consider the use of sorafenib in pregnant women if the potential benefits justify the potential risks to the fetus.

Nursing Women: It is not known whether sorafenib is excreted in human milk. In animals, sorafenib and/or its metabolites were excreted in milk. Because many drugs are excreted in human milk and because the effects of sorafenib on infants have not been studied, woman should discontinue breast-feeding during sorafenib treatment.

Pediatrics (<18 years of age): The safety and effectiveness of sorafenib in pediatric patients has not been established.

Geriatrics (≥65 years of age): Analyses of data by demographics suggest that no dose adjustment is required on the basis of patient age (≥65 years of age). No differences in safety or efficacy were observed between older and younger patients.

Monitoring and Laboratory Tests: Patients taking warfarin concurrently with sorafenib should be monitored regularly for changes in prothrombin time, INR, and for clinical bleeding episodes.

Complete blood counts [CBC] should be performed and phosphate, lipase and amylase levels should be measured at the beginning of treatment and at regular intervals thereafter.

At the beginning of therapy, blood pressure should be monitored on a weekly basis and thereafter should be monitored regularly and treated, if required, in accordance with standard medical practice.

ADVERSE REACTIONS: Adverse Drug Reaction Overview: The data described in this section reflects exposure to NEXAVAR in 748 patients who participated in placebo-controlled studies in hepatocellular carcinoma (n=297) or locally advanced/metastatic renal cell carcinoma (n=451).

The most common adverse events (≥20%) which were considered to be related to NEXAVAR in patients with HCC or RCC are fatigue, weight loss, rash/desquamation, hand-foot skin reaction, alopecia, diarrhea, anorexia, nausea, and abdominal pain.

In addition, the following medically significant adverse events were reported infrequently during clinical trials of NEXAVAR: cerebral hemorrhage, transient ischemic attack, cardiac failure, arrhythmia, and thromboembolism. For these events, the causal relationship to NEXAVAR has not been established.

An increased incidence of hypertension was observed in sorafenib-treated patients. Hypertension was usually mild to moderate, occurred early in the course of treatment, and was amenable to management with standard antihypertensive therapy (see Warnings and Precautions).

Hand-foot skin reaction (palmar-plantar erythrodysesthesia) and rash represent the most common adverse drug reactions with sorafenib. Rash and hand-foot skin reaction are usually CTC (National Cancer Institute Common Terminology Criteria) grade 1 and 2 and generally appear during the first 12 weeks of treatment with sorafenib (see Warnings and Precautions and Dosage and Administration).

Clinical Trial Adverse Drug Reactions in Hepatocellular Carcinoma (HCC): Table 1 shows the percentage of HCC patients experiencing adverse events that were reported in at least 10% of patients and at a higher rate in the NEXAVAR arm than the placebo arm in Study 100554. The reported adverse events are listed according to CTCAE Version 3.0.

CTCAE grade 3 adverse events were reported in 39% of patients receiving NEXAVAR compared to 24% of patients receiving placebo. CTCAE grade 4 adverse events were reported in 6% of patients receiving NEXAVAR compared to 8% of patients receiving placebo.

Hypertension was reported in 9% of patients treated with NEXAVAR and 4% of those treated with placebo. CTCAE grade 3 hypertension was reported in 4% of NEXAVAR treated patients and 1% of placebo-treated patients. No patients were reported with CTCAE grade 4 events in either treatment group.

Hemorrhage/bleeding was reported in 18% of NEXAVAR treated patients and 20% of placebo treated patients. The rates of CTCAE grade 3 and 4 bleeding were also higher in the placebo group (CTCAE grade 3 in 3% NEXAVAR and 5% placebo and CTCAE grade 4 in 2% NEXAVAR and 4% placebo). Bleeding from esophageal varices was reported in 2% of NEXAVAR-treated patients and 4% of placebo-treated patients.

Table 1: NEXAVAR

Incidence of Adverse Events Reported in at Least 10% of Patients and at a Higher Rate in the NEXAVAR Arm Than the Placebo Arm—Study 100554 (HCC)

Adverse Event[a] NCI- CTCAE v3 Category/Term	NEXAVAR N=297			Placebo N=302		
	All Grades %	Grade 3 %	Grade 4 %	All Grades %	Grade 3 %	Grade 4 %
Any Event	98	39	6	96	24	8
Cardiac, General						
Any event	17	2	<1	8	5	1
Constitutional Symptoms						
Any event	62	13	1	57	15	3
Fatigue	46	9	1	45	12	2
Weight loss	30	2	0	10	1	0
Dermatology/Skin						
Any event	52	10	0	32	1	0
Rash/desquamation	19	1	0	14	0	0
Pruritus	14	<1	0	11	<1	0
Hand-foot skin reaction	21	8	0	3	<1	0
Dry skin	10	0	0	6	0	0
Alopecia	14	0	0	2	0	0
Gastrointestinal						
Any event	82	23	<1	62	18	1
Diarrhea	55	10	<1	25	2	0
Anorexia[b]	29	3	0	18	3	<1
Nausea	24	1	0	20	3	0
Vomiting	15	2	0	11	2	0
Constipation	14	0	0	10	0	0
Mucositis/stomatitis	11	<1	0	5	<1	0
Hepatobiliary/Pancreas						
Any event	18	5	3	17	5	2
Liver dysfunction[c]	11	2	1	8	2	1
Infection						
Any event	24	4	0	19	3	1
Musculoskeletal/Soft Tissue						
Any event	15	3	<1	9	2	1
Pain						
Any event	60	16	<1	54	12	2
Pain, abdomen	31	9	0	26	5	1
Pulmonary Upper Respiratory						
Any event	27	4	0	18	3	<1

a In Study 100554 (HCC), the rate of ascites was similar in both NEXAVAR and placebo groups.
b Grade 5 events were reported in 0.7% of NEXAVAR-treated patients and 0% of placebo-treated patients.
c Grade 5 events were reported in 3.7% of NEXAVAR-treated patients and 2.3% of placebo-treated patients.

Cardiac ischemia/infarction was reported as an adverse event in 8 (2.7%) subjects in the sorafenib group and 4 (1.3%) subjects in the placebo group.

Renal failure was reported in 0.3% of those patients receiving NEXAVAR and 2.6% of placebo patients.

Neurology (adverse events reported regardless of causality): Mood alteration depression was reported in 4% of those patients receiving NEXAVAR and 2% of placebo patients. The rates of CTCAE grade 3 were <1% and 0% in NEXAVAR and placebo, respectively. No CTCAE grade 4 was reported in either group. In the NEXAVAR treatment group, one subject had a CTCAE grade 5 event (suicide). Four (1%) subjects experienced CTCAE grade 3 syncope in the NEXAVAR treatment group. Incidence of similar events in the placebo arm was 0%.

Pulmonary/upper respiratory (adverse events reported regardless of causality): Dyspnea was reported in 9% (grade 3: 3%) and 8% (grade 3:2%) of patients in the NEXAVAR and placebo treatment arms respectively.

Cough was reported in 8% (grade 3: <1%) and 5% (grade 3: 0%) of patients in the NEXAVAR and placebo treatment arms respectively.

Pleural effusion was reported in 4% (grade 3: 1%) and 2% (grade 3: <1%) of patients in the NEXAVAR and placebo treatment arms respectively.

Voice changes were reported in 9% (grade 3: <1%) and 1% (grade 3: 0%) of patients in the NEXAVAR and placebo treatment arms respectively.

No patients were reported with CTCAE grade 4 events in any of the above categories in either treatment group.

Abnormal Hematologic and Clinical Chemistry Findings—HCC: Incidence of abnormal hematologic and clinical chemistry findings reported in at least 10% of patients and at a higher rate in the NEXAVAR arm is summarised in Table 2.

Table 2: NEXAVAR

Treatment-Emergent Laboratory Abnormalities in ≥10% of Patients—Study 100554 (HCC)

	NEXAVAR n=297		Placebo n=302	
	All Grades %	Grade 3/4 %	All Grades %	Grade 3/4 %
Lipase	40	9	37	9
Amylase	34	2	29	3
Hypophosphatemia	35	11	11	3
ALT	69	3	68	8
AST	94	16	91	17
Bilirubin	47	10	45	11
Hypoalbuminemia	59	0	47	0
Alkaline Phosphatase	82	6	83	8
INR	42	4	34	2
Lymphopenia	47	6	42	6
Neutropenia	11	1	14	<1
Hemoglobin	59	3	64	3
Platelets	46	4	41	<1

Legend: ALT: alanine aminotransferase; AST: aspartate aminotransferase; INR: international normalized ratio.

Elevated lipase was observed in 40% of patients treated with NEXAVAR compared to 37% of patients in the placebo group. CTCAE grade 3 or 4 lipase elevations occurred in 9% of patients in each group. Elevated amylase was observed in 34% of patients treated with NEXAVAR compared to 29% of patients in the placebo group. CTCAE grade 3 or 4 amylase elevations were reported in 2% of NEXAVAR-treated patients and 3% of placebo-treated patients. Many of the lipase and amylase elevations were transient, and in the majority of cases NEXAVAR treatment was not interrupted. Clinical pancreatitis was reported in 1 of 297 NEXAVAR-treated patients (CTCAE grade 2).

Hypophosphatemia was a common laboratory finding, observed in 35% of NEXAVAR-treated patients compared to 11% of placebo patients; CTCAE grade 3 hypophosphatemia (1-2 mg/dL) occurred in 11% of NEXAVAR-treated patients and 3% of patients in the placebo group; there was 1 case of CTCAE grade 4 hypophosphatemia (<1 mg/dL) reported in the placebo group. The etiology of hypophosphatemia associated with NEXAVAR is not known.

Elevations in liver function tests were comparable between the 2 arms of the study. Elevated AST was observed in 94% of NEXAVAR-treated patients and 91% of placebo-treated patients; CTCAE grade 3 or 4 AST elevations were reported in 16% of NEXAVAR-treated patients and 17% of patients in the placebo group. ALT elevations were observed in 69% of NEXAVAR-treated patients and 68% of placebo patients; CTCAE grade 3 or 4 ALT elevations were reported in 3% of NEXAVAR-treated patients and 8% of placebo-treated patients. Elevated bilirubin was observed in 47% of NEXAVAR-treated patients and 45% of placebo patients; CTCAE grade 3 or 4 bilirubin elevations were reported in 10% of NEXAVAR-treated patients and 11% of placebo-treated patients. Hypoalbuminemia was observed in 59% of NEXAVAR-treated patients and 47% of placebo patients; no CTCAE grade 3 or 4 hypoalbuminemia was observed in either group.

Alkaline phosphatase elevations were observed in 82% of NEXAVAR-treated patients and 83% of placebo patients; CTCAE grade 3 alkaline phosphatase elevations were reported in 6% of NEXAVAR-treated patients and 8% of placebo-treated patients; no CTCAE grade 4 alkaline phosphatase elevation was observed in either group.

INR elevations were observed in 42% of NEXAVAR-treated patients and 34% of placebo-treated patients; CTCAE grade 3 INR elevations were reported in 4% of NEXAVAR-treated patients and 2% of placebo patients; there was no CTCAE grade 4 INR elevation in either group.

Lymphopenia was observed in 47% of NEXAVAR-treated patients and 42% of placebo patients; CTCAE grade 3 or 4 lymphopenia was reported in 6% of patients in each group. Neutropenia was observed in 11% of NEXAVAR-treated patients and 14% of placebo patients; CTCAE grade 3 or 4 neutropenia was reported in 1% of patients in each group.

Anemia was observed in 59% of NEXAVAR-treated patients and 64% of placebo patients; CTCAE grade 3 or 4 anemia was reported in 3% of patients in each group.

Thrombocytopenia was observed in 46% of NEXAVAR-treated patients and 41% of placebo patients; CTCAE grade 3 or 4 thrombocytopenia was reported in 4% of NEXAVAR-treated patients and less than 1% of placebo patients.

Of the hematological laboratory abnormalities outlined in Table 2, some were also reported as adverse events. The overall treatment-emergent hematologic event rate reported was 13% and 12% in the sorafenib and placebo treatment groups respectively. Of these adverse events, 3% (sorafenib-treated patients) and 2% (placebo-treated patients) were reported as serious treatment-emergent events.

Treatment-emergent decreased hemoglobin adverse events were reported in 9% and 8% of sorafenib and placebo treatment groups, respectively. Of these adverse events, the reporting investigator reported 4% (sorafenib-treated patients) and 2% (placebo-treated patients) as being drug related.

Clinical Trial Adverse Drug Reactions in Renal Cell Carcinoma (RCC): In the pivotal study, 11213, based on the results of the planned PFS analysis, a decision was made to allow crossover of patients from the placebo arm to the sorafenib arm of the trial. The safety data from that analysis allow comparison between the placebo and sorafenib arms of the trial.

Table 3 includes all treatment-emergent adverse events that were reported in at least 10% of patients in the phase III NEXAVAR clinical trial at the time of crossover.

Table 3: NEXAVAR

Treatment-Emergent Adverse Events Reported in at Least 10% of NEXAVAR-Treated Patients—Study 11213

Adverse Event NCI- CTCAE v3 Category/Term	NEXAVAR N=451			Placebo N=451		
	All Grades %	Grade 3 %	Grade 4 %	All Grades %	Grade 3 %	Grade 4 %
Any Event	95	31	7	86	22	6
Cardiovascular, General						
Hypertension	17	3	<1	2	<1	0
Constitutional Symptoms						
Fatigue	37	5	<1	28	3	<1
Weight loss	10	<1	0	6	0	0
Dermatology/Skin						
Rash/desquamation	40	<1	0	16	<1	0
Hand-foot skin reaction	30	6	0	7	0	0
Alopecia	27	<1	0	3	0	0
Pruritus	19	<1	0	6	0	0
Dry skin	11	0	0	4	0	0
Gastrointestinal Symptoms						
Diarrhea	43	2	0	13	<1	0
Nausea	23	<1	0	19	<1	0
Anorexia	16	<1	0	13	1	0
Vomiting	16	<1	0	12	1	0
Constipation	15	<1	0	11	<1	0
Hemorrhage/Bleeding						
Hemorrhage—all sites	15	2	0	8	1	<1
Infection						
Any event	23	4	<1	15	2	0
Neurology						
Neuropathy-sensory	13	<1	0	6	<1	0
Pain						
Pain, abdomen	11	2	0	9	2	0
Pain, joint	10	2	0	6	<1	0
Pain, headache	10	<1	0	6	<1	0
Pulmonary						
Dyspnea	14	3	<1	12	2	<1
Cough	13	<1	0	14	<1	0

The incidence of treatment-emergent cardiac ischemia/infarction events was higher in the NEXAVAR group (2.9%) compared with the placebo group (0.4%).

The rate of adverse events (including events associated with progressive disease) resulting in permanent discontinuation was similar in both the NEXAVAR and placebo groups (10% of NEXAVAR patients and 8% of placebo patients).

Based on the results from the interim PFS analysis, patients randomised to placebo were permitted to crossover to NEXAVAR treatment. Patients demonstrating clinical benefit from sorafenib treatment were permitted to continue treatment after progression of disease. Follow up of these patients continued to the planned duration of the trial for final assessment of all other study endpoints, including overall survival. In the final analysis dataset of the clinical study in locally advanced/metastatic RCC, 216 subjects originally randomized to placebo had crossed over to sorafenib treatment after the PFS analysis.

Table 4 summarizes data from the final dataset for treatment-emergent adverse events reported in at least 10% of patients who were randomized to sorafenib treatment (N=451) prior to crossover.

At the time of the postcrossover final dataset, treatment-emergent adverse events were reported in 442 (97.8%) of patients randomized to sorafenib and 212 (98.1%) of the 216 patients that crossed over from placebo to sorafenib. The incidence of grade 3 and 4 treatment-emergent adverse events was also similar in both of these 2 groups of patients. Adverse events attributed by the investigator as related to study drug were reported in 392 subjects randomized to sorafenib (86.7%) and 173 crossover subjects (80.1%). Both groups of patients, sorafenib and placebo patients that crossed over, had a median treatment duration of 40.1 weeks. The median duration of treatment of placebo subjects prior to crossover was 12 weeks. As expected, due to increased time on sorafenib therapy, more toxicities reached the 10% threshold compared to the safety profile at the time of the PFS analysis (see Table 3).

Table 4: NEXAVAR

Treatment-Emergent Adverse Events from Postcrossover Final Analysis Dataset Reported in at Least 10% of NEXAVAR-Treated Patients—Study 11213

Adverse Event NCI-CTCAE v3 Category/Term	NEXAVAR N=451		
	All Grades %	Grade 3 %	Grade 4 %
Any Event	98	36	11
Blood/Bone Marrow	18	4	2
Hemoglobin	14	3	2

(cont'd)

Table 4: NEXAVAR *(cont'd)*

Treatment-Emergent Adverse Events from Postcrossover Final Analysis Dataset Reported in at Least 10% of NEXAVAR-Treated Patients—Study 11213

Adverse Event NCI-CTCAE v3 Category/Term	NEXAVAR N=451		
	All Grades %	Grade 3 %	Grade 4 %
Cardiovascular, General	31	5	3
Hypertension	22	4	1
Constitutional Symptoms	68	11	1
Fatigue	49	8	1
Weight loss	21	2	0
Fever	12	0	0
Dermatology/Skin	75	9	0
Rash/desquamation	43	1	0
Hand-foot-skin reaction	34	6	0
Alopecia	32	0	0
Pruritus	20	0	0
Dry skin	14	0	0
Gastrointestinal Symptoms	76	11	1
Diarrhea	54	4	0
Nausea	27	1	0
Anorexia	24	1	0
Vomiting	20	1	0
Constipation	18	1	0
Hemorrhage/Bleeding	22	3	0
Hemorrhage—all sites	22	3	0
Infection	29	6	0
Any event	29	6	0
Neurology	37	7	2
Neuropathy-sensory	15	0	0
Pain	68	17	0
Pain, abdomen	15	2	0
Pain, joint	13	2	0
Pain, headache	12	0	0
Pain, bone	13	4	0
Pain, back	12	2	0
Pain, muscle	11	1	0
Pulmonary	44	8	2
Dyspnea	23	5	1
Cough	20	1	0

Abnormal Hematologic and Clinical Chemistry Findings—RCC: Elevated lipase and amylase levels were very commonly reported. In the pivotal study in advanced RCC prior to crossover, CTCAE grade 3 or 4 lipase elevations occurred in 12% of patients in the sorafenib group compared to 7% of patients in the placebo group. CTCAE grade 3 or 4 amylase elevations were reported in 1% of patients in the sorafenib group compared to 3% of patients in the placebo group prior to crossover. Postcrossover, grade 3 or 4 lipase and amylase elevations in patients treated with sorafenib were 13% and 3%, respectively (see Warnings and Precautions, Hepatic/Biliary/Pancreatic, Pancreatitis).

Hypophosphataemia was observed prior to crossover in 45% of sorafenib-treated patients compared to 11% of placebo patients. Postcrossover, hypophosphatemia was observed in 50% of sorafenib-treated patients in which grade 3 hypophosphatemia (0.3 to 0.6 mmol/L) occurred in 19% of sorafenib-treated patients. There were no cases of grade 4 hypophosphatemia (<0.3 mmol/L) reported.

Grade 3 or 4 events were reported for lymphopenia in 13% of sorafenib-treated patients and 7% of placebo patients, for neutropenia in 5% of sorafenib-treated patients and 2% of placebo patients, for anaemia in 2% of sorafenib-treated patients and 4% of placebo patients and for thrombocytopenia in 1% of sorafenib-treated patients and 0% of placebo patients.

Table 5: NEXAVAR

Treatment-Emergent Laboratory Abnormalities Reported in at least 10% of Patients—Study 11213

Time of Analysis:	Prior to Crossover				Postcrossover	
	Sorafenib n=451		Placebo n=451		Sorafenib n=451	
	All Grades (%)	Grade 3 and 4 (%)	All Grades (%)	Grade 3 and 4 (%)	All Grades (%)	Grade 3 and 4 (%)
Hypophosphatemia	45	13[a]	11	3[a]	50	19[a]
Hyponatremia	35	6	38	5[a]	41	7
Hypocalcemia	12	2	8	<1	18	3
Hyperkalemia	15	5	11	3	19	7
Lymphopenia	23	13	13	7	27	14
Leukocytes	25	3[a]	14	<1	28	3[a]
Neutropenia	18	5	10	2	19	5
Hemoglobin	44	2	49	3	51	5
Platelets	11	1	5	0	13	1
INR	23	5[a]	22	7	22	1[a]
Hypoalbuminemia	27	<1[a]	24	<1[a]	35	1[a]
Alkaline Phosphatase	30	<1[a]	22	1[a]	38	1[a]
ALT	30	<1[a]	22	<1[a]	35	<1[a]
AST	26	<1[a]	15	<1[a]	32	<1[a]
Bilirubin	8	<1	7	<1	10	1
Amylase	30	1[a]	23	3	33	3
Lipase	41	12	30	7	43	13
Creatinine	17	0	18	<1	19	<1[a]
Hyperglycemia[b]	72	3	70	5	76	4

[a] No grade 4 events were reported.
[b] Plasma collection was random for glucose test.

Drug-Related Adverse Events from Multiple Clinical Trials: The following drug-related adverse events and laboratory abnormalities were reported from clinical trials of NEXAVAR (very common 10% or greater, common 1 to less than 10%, uncommon 0.1% to less than 1%) (see Table 6).

Table 6: NEXAVAR

Drug-Related Clinical Trial Adverse Events and Laboratory Abnormalities

Blood and Lymphatic System Disorders	Very common: lymphopenia, leucopenia. Common: neutropenia, anemia, thrombocytopenia
Cardiac Disorders	Common: myocardial ischemia and/or infarction[a], congestive heart failure[a]
Ear and Labyrinth Disorders	Uncommon: tinnitus
Endocrine Disorders	Uncommon: hypothyroidism
Gastrointestinal Disorders	Very common: diarrhea, nausea, vomiting. Common: constipation, stomatitis (including dry mouth and glossodynia), dyspepsia, dysphagia, mucositis oral. Uncommon: gastro-esophageal reflux disease, pancreatitis, gastritis, gastrointestinal perforations[a]
General Disorders and Administration Site Conditions	Very common: asthenia, fatigue, pain (including mouth, abdominal, bone, tumour pain and headache). Common: fever, influenza-like illness
Hepatobiliary Disorders	Common: cholecystitis, cholangitis. Uncommon: increase in bilirubin, jaundice
Immune System Disorders	Uncommon: hypersensitivity reactions (including skin reactions and urticaria)
Infections and Infestations	Uncommon: folliculitis, infection
Investigations	Very common: increased amylase, increased lipase. Common: weight decreased, transient increase in transaminases. Uncommon: transient increase in blood alkaline phosphatase, INR abnormal, prothrombin level abnormal (Note that elevations in lipase are very common (41%); a diagnosis of pancreatitis should not be made solely on the basis of abnormal laboratory values.)
Metabolism and Nutrition Disorders	Very common: hypophosphatemia. Common: anorexia. Uncommon: hyponatremia, dehydration
Musculoskeletal and Connective Tissue Disorders	Common: arthralgia, myalgia
Nervous System Disorders	Common: peripheral sensory neuropathy. Uncommon: reversible posterior leukoencephalopathy[a]
Psychiatric Disorders	Common: depression

(cont'd)

Table 6: NEXAVAR *(cont'd)*

Drug-Related Clinical Trial Adverse Events and Laboratory Abnormalities

Renal and Urinary Disorders	Common: renal failure[b]
Reproductive System and Breast Disorders	Common: erectile dysfunction. Uncommon: gynaecomastia
Respiratory, Thoracic and Mediastinal Disorders	Common: hoarseness. Uncommon: rhinorrhea
Skin and Subcutaneous Tissue Disorders	Very common: rash, alopecia, hand-foot syndrome, pruritus, erythema. Common: dry skin, dermatitis exfoliative, acne, skin desquamation. Uncommon: eczema, erythema multiforme, keratoacanthomas/squamous cell cancer of the skin
Vascular Disorders	Very common: bleeding events (hemorrhage including hematoma, epistaxis, mouth, pulmonary[a] and respiratory tract[a], GI tract[a], and uncommon cases of cerebral hemorrhage[a]), hypertension. Common: flushing. Uncommon: hypertensive crisis[a]

[a] Events may have a life-threatening or fatal outcome. Such events are uncommon.
[b] Including prerenal, renal and postrenal causes, and including cases of proteinuria, nephrotic syndrome and acute interstitial nephritis.

Further Information on Selected Adverse Drug Reactions: Congestive Heart Failure—in company-sponsored clinical trials congestive heart failure was reported as an adverse event in 1.9% of patients treated with sorafenib (N=2276). In study 11213 (RCC), adverse events consistent with congestive heart failure were reported in 1.7% of those treated with sorafenib and in 0.7% receiving placebo. In study 100554 (HCC), 0.99% of those treated with sorafenib and 1.1 % receiving placebo were reported with these events.

In a randomized controlled trial comparing a chemotherapy regimen (carboplatin and paclitaxel) plus or minus sorafenib in chemonaive patients with Stage IIIB-IV Non-Small-Cell Lung Cancer (NSCLC), higher mortality was observed in the subset of patients with squamous cell carcinoma treated with sorafenib plus carboplatin and paclitaxel versus those treated with carboplatin and paclitaxel alone (HR 1.81, 95% CI 1.19-2.74). This trial was stopped early because it was unlikely to demonstrate an improvement in overall survival.

Post-Market Adverse Drug Reactions: The following events have been observed in postmarketing experience: Cardiac failure, cardiac ischemia and infarction, Stevens-Johnson syndrome, hyperthyroidism, allergic reaction, angioedema and interstitial lung disease-like events (includes reports of pneumonitis, radiation pneumonitis, acute respiratory distress, interstitial pneumonia, pulmonitis and lung inflammation).

DRUG INTERACTIONS: Overview: Sorafenib is metabolized primarily in the liver undergoing oxidative metabolism mediated by CYP3A4 as well as glucuronidation mediated by UGT1A9.

Drug-Drug Interactions: CYP3A4 Inducers: Chronic concomitant administration of rifampin with a single dose of sorafenib resulted in a 24% decrease in the combined AUC of sorafenib and its active primary metabolite when rifampin was coadministered with sorafenib. The clinical significance of this overall decrease in drug exposure is unknown. Other inducers of CYP3A4 activity (eg, hypericum perforatum [also known as St. John's wort], phenytoin, carbamazepine, phenobarbital, and dexamethasone) may also increase the metabolism of sorafenib and decrease its exposure.

CYP3A4 Inhibitors: Ketoconazole, a potent inhibitor of CYP3A4 administered once daily for 7 days to healthy male volunteers did not alter the mean AUC of a single subclinical dose (50 mg) of sorafenib.

CYP2C9 Substrates: The possible effect of sorafenib on warfarin, a CYP2C9 substrate, was assessed in sorafenib-treated patients compared to placebo-treated patients. The concomitant treatment with sorafenib and warfarin did not result in changes in mean PT-INR compared to placebo. However, patients taking warfarin should have their INR checked regularly (see Warnings and Precautions).

CYP Isoform-Selective Substrates: Concomitant administration of sorafenib and midazolam, dextromethorphan or omeprazole, which are substrates of cytochromes CYP3A4, CYP2D6 and CYP2C19, respectively, following 4 weeks of sorafenib administration did not alter the exposure of these agents. This indicates that sorafenib is neither an inhibitor nor an inducer of these cytochrome P450 isoenzymes. Therefore, clinical pharmacokinetic interactions of sorafenib with substrates of these enzymes are unlikely.

UGT1A9 Inhibitors: An in vitro study has revealed a number of drugs affected UGT1A9-mediated sorafenib glucuronidation with an IC50 value below 100 μM. They were atorvastatin (IC50=67 μM), ketoconazole (87 μM), mefenamic acid (28 μM), erlotinib (69 μM), and niflumic acid (1.2 μM). The clinical relevance of these drug interactions has not been tested.

Combination with Other Antineoplastic Agents: NEXAVAR is only approved as monotherapy in the treatment of RCC and HCC (see Indications and Clinical Use).

In clinical studies, sorafenib has been administered together with a variety of other antineoplastic agents at their commonly-used dosing regimens, including gemcitabine, oxaliplatin, doxorubicin, and irinotecan. Sorafenib had no effect on the pharmacokinetics of gemcitabine or oxaliplatin. Concomitant treatment with sorafenib resulted in a 21% increase in the AUC of doxorubicin. When administered with irinotecan, whose active metabolite SN-38 is further metabolized by the UGT1A1 pathway, there was a 67%-120% increase in the AUC of SN-38 and a 26%-42% increase in the AUC of irinotecan. The clinical significance of these findings is unknown (see Warnings and Precautions).

A clinical study has revealed that administration of sorafenib with a 3-day break in dosing around administration of docetaxel resulted in a 36%-80% increase in docetaxel AUC and a 16%-32% increase in docetaxel C_{max} (see Warnings and Precautions).

Neomycin: Coadministration of neomycin, a nonsystemic antimicrobial agent used to eradicate GI flora, interferes with the enterohepatic recycling of sorafenib (see Action And Clinical Pharmacology, Metabolism and Excretion), resulting in decreased sorafenib exposure. In healthy volunteers treated with a 5-day regimen of neomycin, the average bioavailability of sorafenib decreased by 54%. The clinical significance of these findings is unknown. Effects of other antibiotics have not been studied, but will likely depend on their ability to decrease glucuronidase activity (see Warnings and Precautions).

In Vitro Studies on Enzyme Inhibition: Sorafenib inhibits glucuronidation by the UGT1A1 and UGT1A9 pathways. Systemic exposure to substrates of UGT1A1 and UGT1A9 may be increased when coadministered with sorafenib. Sorafenib inhibits CYP2B6 and CYP2C8 in vitro with Ki values of 6 and 1-2 μM, respectively. Systemic exposure to substrates of CYP2B6 and CYP2C8 may increase when coadministered with sorafenib.

In Vitro Studies of CYP Enzyme Induction: CYP1A2 and CYP3A4 activities were not altered after treatment of cultured human hepatocytes with sorafenib, indicating that sorafenib is unlikely to be an inducer of CYP1A2 and CYP3A4.

Drug-Food Interactions: It is recommended that sorafenib be administered without food or together with a low-fat or moderate-fat meal. Following oral administration, sorafenib reaches peak plasma levels in approximately 3 hours. When given with a moderate-fat meal, bioavailability is similar to that in the fasted state. With a high-fat meal, sorafenib bioavailability is reduced by 29% compared to administration in the fasted state (see Dosage and Administration).

Drug-Herb Interactions: Interactions with herbal products have not been established. St. John's wort (an inducer of CYP3A4 activity) may increase metabolism of sorafenib and thus decrease sorafenib concentrations.

Drug-Laboratory Test Interactions: Interactions with results of laboratory tests have not been established.

Drug-Lifestyle Interactions: No studies on the effects of sorafenib on the ability to drive or use machines have been performed. There is no evidence that sorafenib affects the ability to drive or operate machinery.

DOSAGE AND ADMINISTRATION: Dosing Considerations:

- No dose adjustment is required on the basis of patient age (65 years or above), gender, or body weight.
- The safety and effectiveness of sorafenib in pediatric patients has not been established.
- Based on the results from one phase II study, subjects with Child-Pugh B hepatic impairment had greater systemic exposure than those with Child-Pugh A hepatic impairment (see Action and Clinical Pharmacology, Special Populations and Conditions). Sorafenib has not been studied in patients with Child-Pugh C hepatic impairment.
- No dose adjustment is required in patients with mild, moderate, or severe renal impairment not requiring dialysis. Sorafenib has not been studied in patients undergoing dialysis.

Recommended Dose and Dosage Adjustment: The recommended daily dose of NEXAVAR (sorafenib tablets) is 400 mg (2×200 mg tablets) taken twice a day (equivalent to total daily dose of 800 mg) without food or with a low-fat or moderate-fat meal. Treatment should be continued until the patient is no longer clinically benefiting from therapy or until unacceptable toxicity occurs.

Management of suspected adverse drug reactions may require temporary interruption and/or dose reduction of sorafenib therapy. When dose reduction is necessary, the sorafenib dose should be reduced to 400 mg daily (see Table 7 and Warnings and Precautions).

Table 7: NEXAVAR

Suggested Dose Modification for Skin Toxicity

Grade	Occurrence	NEXAVAR Dose Modification
1	Any	Institute supportive measures immediately and continue NEXAVAR treatment.
2	First	Institute supportive measures immediately and consider a decrease in NEXAVAR dose to 400 mg daily for 28 days. If toxicity returns to grade 0-1 after dose reduction, increase NEXAVAR to full dose after 28 days. If toxicity does not return to grade 0-1 despite dose reduction, interrupt NEXAVAR treatment for a minimum of 7 days until toxicity has resolved to grade 0-1. When resuming treatment after dose interruption, resume NEXAVAR at a reduced dose of 400 mg daily for 28 days. If toxicity is maintained at grade 0-1 at reduced dose, increase NEXAVAR to full dose after 28 days.
	Second or third	As for first occurrence, but upon resuming NEXAVAR treatment, decrease dose to 400 mg daily indefinitely.
	Fourth	Decision whether to discontinue NEXAVAR treatment should be made based on clinical judgment and patient preference.
3	First	Institute supportive measures immediately and interrupt NEXAVAR treatment for a minimum of 7 days and until toxicity has resolved to grade 0-1. When resuming treatment after dose interruption, resume NEXAVAR at reduced dose of 400 mg daily for 28 days. If toxicity is maintained at grade 0-1 at reduced dose, increase NEXAVAR to full dose after 28 days.
	Second	As for first occurrence, but upon resuming NEXAVAR treatment, decrease dose to 400 mg daily indefinitely.
	Third	Decision whether to discontinue NEXAVAR treatment should be made based on clinical judgement and patient preference.

Missed Dose: The missed dose should be taken as soon as the patient remembers. However, if it is almost time for the next dose, the missed dose should be skipped and the patient should take his/her next dose as scheduled. A double dose should not be administered to make up for forgotten individual doses.

Administration: For oral use. To be swallowed with a glass of water.

OVERDOSAGE:

The highest dose of sorafenib studied clinically is 800 mg twice daily. The adverse reactions observed at this dose were primarily diarrhea, grade 3 hypertension, dyspnea, and dermatologic events (rash/desquamation).

There is no specific treatment for sorafenib overdose.

In the event of suspected overdose, sorafenib should be withheld and supportive care instituted. Vital signs, complete blood count (CBC) with differential and platelet count should be monitored periodically. Fluid and electrolyte status should be monitored in patients with vomiting and diarrhea. Serum lipase should be monitored in patients with abdominal pain. Administration of activated charcoal may be appropriate in some cases.

> For management of a suspected drug overdose, contact your **regional Poison Control Centre**. See the *CPS* Directory section for a list of Poison Control Centres.

ACTION AND CLINICAL PHARMACOLOGY: Mechanism of Action: Sorafenib was shown to inhibit multiple intracellular (c-CRAF, BRAF and mutant BRAF) and cell surface kinases (KIT, FLT-3, RET, VEGFR-1, VEGFR-2, VEGFR-3, and PDGFR-β). Several of these kinases are thought to be involved in tumour cell signaling, angiogenesis, and apoptosis. Sorafenib inhibited cell proliferation of the human hepatocellular carcinoma PLC/PRF/5 and HepG2 cell lines, and renal cell carcinoma (786-O cell line), and tumour growth of several human tumour xenografts (PLC/PRF/5 cell line) in immunocompromised mice. A reduction in tumour angiogenesis and increases in tumour apoptosis was seen in the xenograft models of human hepatocellular and renal cell carcinoma cell lines. Additionally, a reduction in Raf/MEK/ERK signaling was seen in human hepatocellular carcinoma PLC/PRF/5 and HepG2 cell lines.

Pharmacokinetics: Absorption and Distribution: After administration of sorafenib tablets, the mean relative bioavailability is 38-49% when compared to an oral solution.

Following oral administration, sorafenib reaches peak plasma levels in approximately 3 hours. When given with a moderate-fat meal (30% fat; 700 calories), bioavailability is similar to that in the fasted state. With a high-fat meal (50% fat; 900 calories), sorafenib bioavailability is reduced by 29% compared to administration in the fasted state.

Mean C_{max} and AUC increase less than proportionally beyond doses of 400 mg administered orally twice daily.

Multiple dosing of sorafenib for 7 days results in a 2.5-fold to 7-fold accumulation compared to single-dose administration. Steady-state plasma sorafenib concentrations are achieved within 7 days, with a peak-to-trough ratio of mean concentrations of less than 2. In vitro binding of sorafenib to human plasma proteins is 99.5%.

Metabolism and Excretion: Sorafenib is metabolized primarily in the liver undergoing oxidative metabolism mediated by CYP3A4 as well as glucuronidation mediated by UGT1A9.

Sorafenib accounts for approximately 70%-85% of the circulating analytes in plasma at steady state. Eight metabolites of sorafenib have been identified, of which 5 have been detected in plasma. The main circulating metabolite of sorafenib in plasma, the pyridine N-oxide, shows in vitro potency similar to that of sorafenib and comprises approximately 9%-16% of circulating analytes at steady state.

Following oral administration of a 100 mg dose of a solution formulation of sorafenib, 96% of the dose was recovered within 14 days, with 77% of the dose excreted in feces, and 19% of the dose excreted in urine as glucuronidated metabolites. Unchanged sorafenib, accounting for 51% of the dose, was found in feces but not in urine.

The elimination half-life of sorafenib is approximately 25-48 hours.

Special Populations and Conditions: Gender: Analyses of pharmacokinetic and safety data in male and female subgroups suggest that no dose adjustments are necessary based on patient gender.

Geriatrics (≥65 years of age): Analyses of data suggest that no dose adjustments are necessary based on patient age.

Pediatrics (<18 years of age): There are no pharmacokinetic data in pediatric patients.

Hepatic Insufficiency: Sorafenib is cleared primarily by the liver. The results of one phase II study revealed 36% and 54% higher $AUC_{0\text{-}8}$ and C_{max} in patients with Child-Pugh B hepatic impairment (n=6) compared to patients with Child-Pugh A hepatic impairment (n=14) in subjects administered 400 mg bid NEXAVAR (see Table 8). The pharmacokinetics of sorafenib has not been studied in patients with severe (Child-Pugh C) hepatic impairment (see Warnings and Precautions).

Renal Insufficiency: In a clinical pharmacology study, the pharmacokinetics of sorafenib were evaluated following administration of a single 400 mg dose to subjects with normal renal function and in subjects with mild (Cl_{cr} 50-80 mL/min), moderate (Cl_{cr} 30 to <50 mL/min), or severe (Cl_{cr} <30 mL/min) renal impairment, not requiring dialysis. There was no relationship observed between sorafenib exposure and renal function. No dosage adjustment is necessary based on mild, moderate or severe renal impairment not requiring dialysis (see Warnings and Precautions).

Table 8: NEXAVAR

Pharmacokinetic Parameters in Child Pugh A and B Patients—Phase II Study 10874

	Child Pugh A [n=14]		Child Pugh B [n=6]		Ratio [A/B]
$AUC_{(0-8)}$, mg*h/L (CV%)	23.3	(36.7)	31.6	(71.2)	1.36
C_{max}, mg/L (CV%)	4.4	(32.6)	6.8	(67.8)	1.54

STORAGE AND STABILITY: Store at controlled room temperature (15-30°C) in a dry place. Do not use after the expiry date stated on bottle.

Medicines should not be disposed of via wastewater or household waste. Ask your pharmacist how to dispose of medicines no longer required. These measures will help to protect the environment.

Keep out of the reach and sight of children and pets.

INFORMATION FOR THE PATIENT: Published in e-CPS, available by subscription at www.e-cps.ca.

DOSAGE FORMS, COMPOSITION AND PACKAGING: Each round, biconvex, red, film-coated tablet, debossed with the "Bayer cross" on one side and "200" on the other side, contains: sorafenib 200 mg (as sorafenib tosylate 274 mg). Nonmedicinal ingredients: tablet core: croscarmellose sodium, hydroxypropylmethyl cellulose, magnesium stearate, microcrystalline cellulose and sodium lauryl sulfate; film-coat: hydroxypropylmethyl cellulose, ferric oxide red, macrogol and titanium dioxide. Bottles of 120.

(Shown in Product Identification Section)

Nexium® Ⓟ

esomeprazole magnesium trihydrate

H+, K+-ATPase Inhibitor

AstraZeneca

Date of Revision: December 3, 2008

SUMMARY PRODUCT INFORMATION:

Route of Administration	Dosage Form/ Strength	Clinically Relevant Nonmedicinal Ingredients
Oral	Tablet/20 mg and 40 mg esomeprazole	None For a complete listing see Dosage Forms, Composition and Packaging.
Oral	Granules for oral suspension/ 10 mg esomeprazole per sachet	None For a complete listing see Dosage Forms, Composition and Packaging.

INDICATIONS AND CLINICAL USE: Adults: NEXIUM (esomeprazole) is indicated for treatment of conditions where a reduction in gastric acid secretion is required such as:
- reflux esophagitis
- maintenance treatment of patients with reflux esophagitis
- nonerosive reflux disease (NERD) (i.e. heartburn and regurgitation)
- healing of NSAID*-associated gastric ulcers
- reduction of risk of NSAID-associated gastric ulcers
- treatment of pathological hypersecretory conditions, including Zollinger-Ellison syndrome
- *H. pylori* eradication

NEXIUM, in combination with clarithromycin and amoxicillin, is indicated for the treatment of patients with duodenal ulcer disease associated with *H. pylori* infection to eradicate the *H. pylori* and heal ulcers. Eradication of *H. pylori* has been shown to reduce the risk of duodenal ulcer recurrence.

Pediatrics (1-17 Years of Age): NEXIUM (esomeprazole) is indicated for treatment of conditions where a reduction in gastric acid secretion is required such as:
- reflux esophagitis.
- nonerosive reflux disease (NERD) (i.e. heartburn and regurgitation).

CONTRAINDICATIONS:
- Hypersensitivity to esomeprazole, substituted benzimidazoles or any of the components of this medication (see Dosage Forms, Composition and Packaging).
- When used for eradication of *H. pylori*, the contraindications for amoxicillin and clarithromycin as found in the corresponding Product Monographs should be taken into consideration.

WARNINGS AND PRECAUTIONS: General: In the presence of any alarm symptom (e.g., significant unintentional weight loss, recurrent vomiting, dysphagia, hematemesis or melena), and/or when gastric ulcer is suspected or present, malignancy should be excluded, as treatment may alleviate symptoms and delay diagnosis.

Pseudomembranous colitis has been reported with nearly all antibacterial agents, including clarithromycin and amoxicillin, and may range in severity from mild to life threatening. Therefore, it is important to consider this diagnosis in patients who present with diarrhea subsequent to the administration of antibacterial agents.

Treatment with antibacterial agents alters the normal flora of the colon and may permit overgrowth of Clostridia. Studies indicate that a toxin produced by *C. difficile* is a primary cause of "antibiotic-associated colitis".

After the diagnosis of pseudomembranous colitis has been established, therapeutic measures should be initiated. Mild cases of pseudomembranous colitis usually respond to discontinuation of the drug alone. In moderate to severe cases, consideration should be given to management with fluids and electrolytes, protein supplementation, and treatment with an antibacterial drug clinically effective against *C. difficile* colitis.

Concomitant administration with atazanavir or nelfinavir is not recommended (see Drug Interactions).

Carcinogenesis and Mutagenesis: Long-term toxicity studies of omeprazole, revealed the gastric mucosa as the target organ. The carcinogenic potential of esomeprazole was assessed using omeprazole studies. In the rat carcinogenicity study (24 months), ECL-cell carcinoids were found in some animals treated with 14-140 mg/kg/day for their normal life span. ECL-cell carcinoids were seen in a background of ECL-cell hyperplasia. No ECL-cell carcinoids were identified in the carcinogenicity study in mice or in long-term (up to 7 years) general toxicity studies in dogs.

A vast number of studies have revealed that pronounced and sustained hypergastrinemia is the mechanism behind the development of the gastric ECL-cell carcinoids in the rat. Such ECL carcinoids have been seen in rats after life-long treatment with other inhibitors of acid secretion such as H2-receptor blockers and other proton pump inhibitors. Partial fundectomy in rats results in hypergastrinemia and gastric ECL-cell carcinoids in the remaining part of the fundic mucosa, towards the end of the rats' life span.

Treatment with NEXIUM (esomeprazole) for up to 1 year in more than 800 patients has not resulted in any significant pathological changes in the gastric oxyntic endocrine cells. Short-term treatment and long-term treatment with the racemate, omeprazole, capsules in a limited number of patients for up to 11 years have not resulted in any significant pathological changes in gastric oxyntic endocrine cells.

* Note: Superiority of NEXIUM over ranitidine 150 mg BID with the use of non-selective NSAIDs was demonstrated. Superiority was not established with the use of COX-2 selective NSAIDs alone due to the small number of patients analysed in this subgroup.

During treatment with all antisecretory drugs serum gastrin increases in response to the decreased acid secretion. The effect of NEXIUM on serum gastrin concentrations was evaluated in approximately 2700 patients in clinical trials up to 8 weeks and in over 1300 patients for up to 6-12 months (daily doses of either 20 or 40 mg). The mean fasting gastrin level increased in a dose-related manner. This increase reached a plateau (approximately 100 pg/mL) within two to three months of therapy and returned to baseline levels (approximately 30-40 pg/mL) within four weeks after discontinuation of therapy.

Special Populations: Pregnant Women: The safety of NEXIUM in pregnancy has not been established. NEXIUM should not be administered to pregnant women unless the expected benefits outweigh the potential risks.

Nursing Women: It has not been investigated whether or not esomeprazole is excreted in human breast milk. No studies in lactating women have been performed. Therefore, NEXIUM should not be given to nursing mothers unless its use is considered essential.

Pediatrics (1-17 years of age): The use of NEXIUM in pediatric patients (1 to 17 years of age) for the short term treatment (up to 8 weeks) of GERD is supported by extrapolation of results already included in the currently approved labelling from a) adequate and well-controlled studies in adults that supported the approval of NEXIUM for adults, and additionally from b) safety and a pharmacokinetic study performed in pediatric patients (see Adverse Reactions, Clinical Trial Adverse Drug Reactions, Pediatrics (1-17 Years of Age) and Action and Clinical Pharmacology, Pharmacokinetics, Special Populations and Conditions, Pediatrics (1-17 Years of Age)).

No data is currently available in children (1-11 years of age) with hepatic insufficiency (see Dosage and Administration).

The safety and effectiveness of NEXIUM have not yet been established in pediatric patients <1 years of age.

Geriatrics (>71 years of age): The metabolism of NEXIUM is not significantly changed in elderly subjects. Following repeated oral dosing with 40 mg NEXIUM in healthy elderly subjects (6 males, 8 females; 71 to 80 years of age), AUC and C_{max} values measured were similar to those previously measured in young GERD patients (ratio of AUC values in elderly vs GERD subjects: 1.25; ratio of C_{max} values: 1.18). Therefore, dose adjustment is not required in the elderly.

Gender: The AUC and C_{max} values were slightly higher (13%) in females than in males at steady state. Dosage adjustment based on gender is not necessary.

Hepatic Insufficiency: The metabolism of esomeprazole magnesium in patients with mild to moderate liver dysfunction (Child Pugh Class A or B), is similar to that in patients with symptoms of GERD with normal liver function. Metabolism of esomeprazole is decreased in patients with severe liver dysfunction (Child Pugh Class C) resulting in a doubling of the area under the plasma concentration-time curve of esomeprazole. The plasma elimination half-life in patients with severe liver dysfunction is still very short (3 hours) relative to the dosing interval (24 hours). Esomeprazole and its major metabolites do not show any tendency to accumulate with once-daily dosing. Dose adjustment is not required in patients with mild to moderate liver impairment. A daily dose of 20 mg in patients with severe liver disease should not, as a rule, be exceeded (see Dosage and Administration).

Renal Insufficiency: Since the kidney is responsible for the excretion of metabolites of esomeprazole but not for the elimination of the parent compound, the metabolism of esomeprazole is not expected to be changed in patients with impaired renal function. Esomeprazole is extensively protein-bound and is, therefore, not expected to be readily dialyzable. Dose adjustment is not required in patients with impaired renal function (see Dosage and Administration).

Poor Metabolizers: The CYP 2C19 and CYP 3A4 isozymes are responsible for metabolism of esomeprazole. CYP 2C19, which is involved in the metabolism of all available proton pump inhibitors, exhibits polymorphism. Approximately 3% of Caucasians and 15-20% of Asians lack CYP 2C19 and are termed "poor metabolizers". At steady state, the ratio of AUC in poor metabolizers to AUC in the rest of the population is approximately 2. Dosage adjustment of NEXIUM based on CYP 2C19 status is not necessary.

Monitoring and Laboratory Tests: The clinical documentation for NEXIUM does not support the need for routine laboratory monitoring of response to therapy. (See Warnings and Precautions, Carcinogenesis and Mutagenesis for effects of NEXIUM on serum gastrin levels and Adverse Reactions, Post-Market Adverse Drug Reactions for effects on liver functioning.)

ADVERSE REACTIONS: Adverse Drug Reaction Overview: NEXIUM (esomeprazole) is well-tolerated. Most adverse reactions have been mild and transient, showing no consistent relationship with treatment.

Adverse reactions have been recorded during controlled clinical investigations in >8500 adult patients exposed to NEXIUM. Additionally >1200 adult subjects/patients were exposed to NEXIUM in Phase I studies. Among reactions which occurred with a frequency of >1% in clinical studies, only headache, diarrhea, flatulence, abdominal pain, nausea, vomiting, dizziness and dry mouth are thought to be associated with the use of NEXIUM.

Adverse reactions have been recorded during a clinical investigation in 109 pediatric patients (1-11 years of age) exposed to NEXIUM. Among reactions which occurred with a frequency of >1% in clinical studies, only diarrhea, headache and somnolence are associated with the use of NEXIUM. No new safety concerns were identified. Adverse reactions have also been recorded during a clinical investigation in 149 pediatric patients (12-17 years of age) exposed to NEXIUM. The treatment related adverse event profile was found to be consistent with that seen in adults.

Clinical Trial Adverse Drug Reactions: Because clinical trials are conducted under very specific conditions the adverse reaction rates observed in the clinical trials may not reflect the rates observed in practice and should not be compared to the rates in the clinical trials of another drug. Adverse drug reaction information from clinical trials is useful for identifying drug-related adverse events and for approximating rates.

Adults: The following adverse reactions, irrespective of causal relationship, were reported (at a rate of more than 1%) in controlled short-term (up to 8 weeks) clinical trials involving 5668 patients (see Table 1):

Table 1: NEXIUM

Percentage of Patients Reporting Adverse Reactions, Irrespective of Causal Relationship, (at a Rate of More than 1%) in Short Term Clinical Trials (up to 8 Weeks) Treated with NEXIUM

	All Studies	Placebo Controlled Studies	
Adverse Reaction	NEXIUM (20 & 40 mg) n=5668 (%)	NEXIUM (20 & 40 mg) n=470 (%)	Placebo n=240 (%)
Body as a Whole			
Headache	8.4	6.6	7.5
Gastrointestinal			
Diarrhea	5.7	5.7	4.2
Abdominal Pain	3.6	5.7	2.5
Nausea	3.5	5.1	5.4
Flatulence	3.3	3.2	—
Gastritis	2.1	—	—
Constipation	1.6	1.7	1.3
Vomiting	1.4	1.1	1.7
Mouth Dry	1.3	1.3	—
Respiratory			
Respiratory Infection	3.8	1.9	3.8
Sinusitis	1.7	2.8	2.5
Pharyngitis	1.3	0.4	1.3

(cont'd)

Table 1: NEXIUM *(cont'd)*

Percentage of Patients Reporting Adverse Reactions, Irrespective of Causal Relationship, (at a Rate of More than 1%) in Short Term Clinical Trials (up to 8 Weeks) Treated with NEXIUM

Adverse Reaction	All Studies NEXIUM (20 & 40 mg) n=5668 (%)	Placebo Controlled Studies NEXIUM (20 & 40 mg) n=470 (%)	Placebo n=240 (%)
Nervous System			
Dizziness	1.2	0.9	1.7
Resistance Mechanism			
Viral Infection	1.1	—	0.4

In clinical trials up to 6 months' duration, the following adverse events were reported (see Table 2).

Table 2: NEXIUM

Percentage of Patients Reporting Adverse Reactions, Irrespective of Causal Relationship, (at a Rate of More than 3%) in Clinical Trials up to 6 Months' Duration Treated with NEXIUM

Adverse Reaction	NEXIUM (10, 20 and 40 mg) n=519 (%)	Placebo n=169 (%)
Body as a Whole		
Headache	6.6	4.1
Gastrointestinal		
Gastritis/Gastritis Aggravated[a]	6.2	5.3
Flatulence	5.0	1.8
Diarrhea	6.7	3.0
Abdominal Pain	3.7	2.4
Nausea/Nausea Aggravated	4.8	2.4
Vomiting/Vomiting Aggravated	3.3	1.2
Respiratory		
Respiratory Infection	8.5	3.0
Sinusitis	4.2	1.8
Resistance Mechanism		
Viral Infection	3.7	1.8
Miscellaneous		
Accident and/or Injury	3.7	1.8

[a] Endoscopic assessment.

Additionally, the following adverse reactions (irrespective of causality) were each reported at a rate of >1% with NEXIUM in these same long-term studies (n=519): rash, fracture, hernia, dizziness, duodenitis, dyspepsia, epigastric pain, serum gastrin increased, gastroenteritis, GI mucosal discoloration, esophageal disorder, tooth disorder, ALT (alanine transferase) increased, hypertension, coughing, rhinitis, anemia, benign GI neoplasm, back pain, chest pain, and fatigue.

Clinical experience for up to one year in over 800 patients with doses of NEXIUM of 40 mg have shown a similar adverse reaction pattern to that seen in short-term trials. In addition to the adverse reactions listed above, the following adverse reactions were reported (at a rate of more than 1%), irrespective of causal relationship (mean duration of treatment=294 days): accident/injury (7.6%), pain (4.3%), urinary tract infection (3.7%), bronchitis (3.6%), arthralgia (2.9%), hypertension (2.6%), allergy (2.1%), insomnia (2.1%), hypercholesterolemia (2.0%), anxiety (1.7%), gastroesophageal reflux (1.6%), fever (1.5%), ear infection (1.5%), flu-like disorder (1.4%), myalgia (1.2%), arthropathy (1.1%), dyspnea (1.1%), overdose (1.1%).

***H. pylori* Eradication Combination Therapy:** In clinical studies, a total of 446 patients received NEXIUM in combination with amoxicillin and clarithromycin for 7 days. The following adverse reactions were reported (at a rate of more than 1%), irrespective of causal relationship: diarrhea (21.5%), taste perversion (12.6%), headache (3.6%), dry mouth (3.4%), ALT increased (1.8%), flatulence (1.6%), nausea (1.3%), stomatitis (1.3%), vomiting (1.1%) and pharyngitis (1.1%). However, it should be noted that taste perversion is commonly associated with clarithromycin treatment and diarrhea is commonly associated with antibiotic treatment.

When NEXIUM is used in combination with amoxicillin and clarithromycin, the Product Monographs for those agents must be consulted and followed.

Healing of Gastric Ulcers Associated with NSAID Therapy: The data presented in this section is derived from two short-term gastric ulcer healing studies comprising 836 patients.

Table 3: NEXIUM

Percentage of Patients Reporting Adverse Reactions that were Assessed by the Investigator to Have a Reasonable Causal Relationship with Treatment (at a Rate of >1%) in Short Term Clinical Trials (up to 8 Weeks), for the Healing of Gastric Ulcers Associated with NSAID Therapy

Adverse Reaction	NEXIUM (20 & 40 mg qd) n=556 (%)	Ranitidine (150 mg bid) n=280 (%)
Gastrointestinal		
Flatulence	2.5	3.6
Gastritis	1.8	0.7
Diarrhea	1.6	0.7
Dyspepsia/Dyspepsia Aggravated	1.6	2.5

The following adverse reactions occurred (<1% for NEXIUM) in clinical trials for the healing of gastric ulcers associated with NSAID therapy, and were considered causally related by the investigator:

Gastrointestinal: abdominal pain, epigastric pain, gastric retention, gastric ulcer, gastroesophageal reflux, nausea, peptic ulcer aggravated.
Liver and Biliary: abnormal hepatic function, increased AST, increased ALT.
Metabolic & Nutritional: increased phosphatase alkaline.
Nervous System: headache.
Psychiatric: insomnia.
Special Senses: taste perversion.

The following adverse events (considered unrelated to esomeprazole by the investigator) were each reported at a frequency of >1% in clinical trials for the healing of gastric ulcers; gastric ulcer aggravated, mucosal discoloration GI, gastrointestinal symptoms NOS, esophageal stricture, esophagitis, vomiting, constipation, duodenitis, rash, anxiety, pharyngitis, respiratory infection, sinusitis, urinary tract infection, accident and/or injury, and back pain.

In addition, the following adverse events of a potentially severe nature (considered unrelated to esomeprazole by the investigator) were reported in these same studies; cardiac failure aggravated, hypertension/hypertension aggravated, syncope, arrhythmia, bradycardia, atrial fibrillation, palpitation/palpitation aggravated.

Risk-reduction of Gastric Ulcers Associated with NSAID Therapy: The data presented in this section is derived from two long-term ulcer risk-reduction studies comprising 1390 patients.

Table 4: NEXIUM

Percentage of Patients Reporting Adverse Reactions that were Assessed by the Investigator to have a Reasonable Causal Relationship with Treatment (at a Rate of >1%) in Long Term Clinical Trials (up to 6 Months), for the Risk-reduction of Gastric Ulcers Associated with NSAID Therapy

Adverse Reaction	NEXIUM (20 & 40 mg qd) n=936 (%)	Placebo n=454 (%)
Gastrointestinal		
Flatulence	4.0	3.7
Gastritis/Gastritis Aggravated	2.2	2.9
Gastrointestinal Symptoms	2.0	2.6
Gastroesophageal Reflux	1.9	3.5
Dyspepsia/Dyspepsia Aggravated	1.9	3.7
Nausea/Nausea Aggravated	1.7	2.0
Abdominal Pain	1.4	0.9
Diarrhea	1.1	0.9

The following adverse reactions occurred (<1% for NEXIUM) in clinical trials for the risk-reduction of gastric ulcers associated with NSAID therapy, and were considered causally related by the investigator:

Body as a Whole: asthenia, back pain.
Blood System: anemia, leukopenia, thrombocytopenia.
Gastrointestinal: constipation, defecation urge, duodenitis, epigastric pain, eructation, gastric retention, gastric ulcer, dry mouth, mucosal discolouration GI, frequent stools, vomiting.
Liver and Biliary: hepatic enzymes increased NOS, increased AST, increased ALT.
Metabolic & Nutritional: dehydration, weight decrease, weight increase.
Neoplasms: GI neoplasm.
Nervous System: dizziness, headache, hyperesthesia, vertigo.
Psychiatric: anorexia, increased appetite, insomnia, sleep disorder.
Resistance Mechanism: herpes simplex.
Skin: rash.
Special Senses: taste perversion.

The following adverse events (considered unrelated to esomeprazole by the investigator) were each reported at a frequency of >1% in clinical trials for the risk-reduction of gastric ulcers; arthralgia, arthrosis, aggravated rheumatoid arthritis, cramps, myalgia, rash, urticaria, dizziness, headache, neuropathy, insomnia, constipation, duodenitis, epigastric pain, gastric mucosal lesion NOS, mucosal discoloration GI, esophageal disorder, esophagitis, vomiting, dry mouth, increased AST, increased ALT, bronchitis, coughing, dyspnoea, pharyngitis, respiratory infection, sinusitis, anemia, thrombocythemia, micturation frequency, urinary tract infection, benign GI neoplasm, accident/or injury, back pain, chest pain, fatigue, peripheral edema, pain, and postoperative complications.

In addition, the following adverse events of a potentially severe nature (considered unrelated to esomeprazole by the investigator) were reported in these same studies; cardiac failure, hypertension/hypertension aggravated, tachycardia, palpitation, atrial fibrillation, extrasystoles, bradycardia, arrhythmia, myocardial fibrosis, coronary artery disorder, syncope, thrombocytopenia, leucopenia, and cholelithiasis.

Zollinger-Ellison Syndrome: In an open label, 12 month clinical study conducted in 21 patients with either Zollinger-Ellison syndrome or idiopathic hypersecretion, single cases of the following adverse events, not previously listed under other indications, were reported with NEXIUM use, irrespective of causality: abdominal rigidity, asthma, Barrett's esophagus, carcinoid tumour of the stomach, carpal tunnel syndrome, depression, erosive gastritis, gingival abscess, hematuria, hyperparathyroidism, hypoesthesia, hypokalemia, hypomagnesemia, hypothyroidism, mean cell volume decreased, melena, muscle spasms, neoplasm progression, osteoporosis, parathesia, pharyngolaryngeal pain, postoperative pain, proteinuria, pruritus, rhinorrhea.

Less Common Clinical Trial Adverse Drug Reactions (<1%): Skin: dermatitis, pruritus and urticaria.
Nervous System: paresthesia.
Rare Clinical Trial Adverse Drug Reactions (<0.1%): Body as a Whole: malaise.
Metabolic and Nutritional: hyponatremia.
Very Rare Clinical Trial Adverse Drug Reactions (<0.01%): Body as a Whole: muscular weakness.
Hepatic and Biliary: hepatic encephalopathy.
Abnormal Hematologic and Clinical Chemistry Findings: See Adverse Reactions, Post-Market Adverse Drug Reactions, and Warnings and Precautions, Carcinogenesis and Mutagenesis.

Pediatrics (1-17 Years of Age): In Children (1-11 Years) with Gastroesophageal Reflux Disease (GERD): Adverse reactions have been recorded during a clinical investigation in 109 pediatric patients (1-11 years of age) exposed to NEXIUM. There was an increase number of adverse events reported (irrespective of causality) in the >20 kg treatment groups (mean age of 8.4 years old) versus the <20 kg treatment group (mean age 2.3 years old), however there was no difference in the character of the adverse events reported by age group or dosing group. The most common reactions (irrespective of causality) which occurred with a frequency of >1% in clinical studies included vomiting, pyrexia, diarrhea and cough. The most frequently reported (at least 1%) treatment-related adverse events were diarrhea (2.8%), headache (1.9%) and somnolence (1.9%). No new safety concerns were identified.

In this study there were some inconsistent and minor changes (i.e. <5 mmHg) in blood pressure (BP) which were not considered to be a drug effect. For most dosing groups there was a slight increase in mean systolic and diastolic BP values (<5 mmHg) while for the 20 mg dosing group there was a slight decrease in mean systolic BP (<1 mmHg). Overall, the mean BP values remained within normal limits. The interpretation of these inconsistent and minor changes is uncertain due to the lack of a placebo arm in this study.

No clinically important changes or trends were noted over time in clinical chemistry that were different from those already listed from adult studies (see Adults, Abnormal Hematologic and Clinical Chemistry Findings).

In Children (12-17 Years) with Gastroesophageal Reflux Disease (GERD): In a multicentre, randomized, double-blind, parallel-group safety and tolerability study in 149 pediatric patients (12-17 years of age; 89 female, 124 Caucasian, 15 Black, 10 Other) with clinically diagnosed GERD), adverse events were recorded after exposure to NEXIUM 20 mg and 40 mg once daily for up to 8 weeks. Patients were not endoscopically characterized as to the presence or absence of erosive esophagitis.

The observed adverse event profile was found to be consistent with that seen in adults, with treatment related events of headache (8.1%), abdominal pain (2.7%), diarrhea (2.0%), and nausea (2.0%) commonly reported. No new safety concerns were identified for this population.

Post-Market Adverse Drug Reactions: From post-marketing experience there have been uncommon reports (<1%) of peripheral edema, insomnia, paresthesia, somnolence, vertigo, increased liver enzymes.

There have been rare reports (<0.1%) of blurred vision, hypersensitivity reactions (e.g. angioedema, anaphylactic reaction/shock), myalgia, leukopenia, thrombocytopenia, depression, alopecia, hepatitis with or without jaundice, hyponatremia, agitation, confusion, taste disturbance, bronchospasm, stomatitis, GI candidiasis, rash, dermatitis photosensitivity, arthralgia, malaise, and hyperhidrosis.

Very rarely (<0.01%) agranulocytosis, erythema multiforme, Stevens-Johnson syndrome, toxic epidermal necrolysis, pancytopenia, aggression, hallucination, hepatic failure, hepatic encephalopathy, intestinal nephritis, muscular weakness and gynecomastia have been reported.

As of 25 July 2007, AstraZeneca's post-marketing safety database has received 28 medically confirmed case reports with 59 adverse events in children between 1 and 11 years of age. All cases constituted off-label use. An overall assessment of the adverse events reported in children ages 1-11 years raised no safety concerns with esomeprazole treatment in this age group.

As of 25 June 2007, AstraZeneca's post-marketing safety database has received 48 medically confirmed case reports with 84 adverse events in children between 12 and 17 years of age. Five of the 48 cases were reported within approved label use, while 43 cases constituted off-label use. An overall assessment of the adverse events reported after within-label and off-label use in children ages 12-17 years raised no safety concerns with esomeprazole treatment in this age group.

DRUG INTERACTIONS: Overview: Esomeprazole magnesium is metabolized by the cytochrome P-450 system (CYP), mainly in the liver, through CYP 2C19 and CYP 3A4. There are no clinically significant interactions between esomeprazole and diazepam, phenytoin, warfarin, quinidine or cisapride†.

With on-demand therapy, the implications for interactions with other pharmaceuticals, due to fluctuating plasma concentrations of esomeprazole, should be considered when NEXIUM is prescribed in this manner (see Dosage and Administration).

Drug-Drug Interactions: Diazepam: Concomitant administration of NEXIUM (30 mg once daily for 5 days) resulted in a 45% decrease in the clearance of diazepam in healthy male volunteers. Studies in females have not been conducted. Increased levels of diazepam were seen some 12 hours after dosing and later when the plasma levels of diazepam were below its therapeutic range. Therefore, this interaction is unlikely to be of clinical significance.

Warfarin: Concomitant administration of 40 mg NEXIUM (once daily for 3 weeks) to male and female patients on stable anticoagulation therapy with warfarin, resulted in a 13% increase in trough plasma levels of R-warfarin (the less potent enantiomer) while that of S-warfarin was unchanged. Coagulation times were stable throughout the entire study period. No clinically significant interaction was observed. However, from post marketed use, cases of elevated international normalized ratio (INR) of clinical significance have been reported during concomitant treatment with warfarin. Close monitoring is recommended when initiating and ending treatment with warfarin or other coumarin derivatives (please refer to approved Product Monograph for warfarin or relevant coumarin derivative).

Phenytoin: Concomitant administration of 40 mg NEXIUM (once daily for 2 weeks) to male and female epileptic patients stabilized on phenytoin, resulted in a 13% increase in trough plasma levels of phenytoin. This minor interaction is unlikely to be of clinical relevance as dose reduction was not required in any patient nor was the profile and frequency of adverse events affected.

Results from a range of interaction studies with NEXIUM versus other drugs indicate that daily doses of 40 mg NEXIUM, given for 5 to 21 days in male and/or female subjects, has no clinically relevant interactions with CYP 1A2 (caffeine), CYP 2C9 (S-warfarin), and CYP 3A (quinidine, estradiol and cisapride†).

Antiretroviral Drugs: Omeprazole, like other acid-reducing agents, has been reported to interact with some antiretroviral drugs. The clinical importance and the mechanisms behind these interactions are not always known. A change in gastric pH may change the absorption of the antiretroviral drug. Other possible interaction mechanisms are via CYP 2C19.

Reports indicate that omeprazole has a significant impact on atazanavir exposure, decreasing AUC, C_{max} and C_{min}. This interaction is only partially overcome by the addition of ritonavir to the atazanavir treatment regimen. Similarly, decreased serum levels of nelfinavir have also been reported when given together with omeprazole. Concomitant administration of omeprazole with atazanavir and nelfinavir is therefore not recommended. For other antiretroviral drugs, such as saquinavir, increased serum levels have been reported. There are also some antiretroviral drugs where unchanged serum levels have been reported when given with omeprazole. Due to the similar pharmacodynamic effects and pharmacokinetic properties of omeprazole and esomeprazole, concomitant administration with esomeprazole and antiretroviral drugs such as atazanavir and nelfinavir is not recommended (see Warnings and Precautions).

Voriconazole: Concomitant administration of esomeprazole with a combined inhibitor of CYP 2C19 and CYP 3A4 may result in more than double the levels of esomeprazole exposure.

As with all drugs that reduce gastric acidity, changes in plasma levels of other drugs whose absorption is pH dependent (e.g. ketoconazole or itraconazole) must be taken into account when they are co-administered with esomeprazole.

Drug-Food Interactions: Food intake delays and decreases the absorption of esomeprazole although this has no significant influence on the effect of esomeprazole on intragastric acidity.

Other Interactions: As demonstrated with other PPIs, prolonged use may impair the absorption of protein-bound Vitamin B_{12} and may contribute to the development of Vitamin B_{12} deficiency.

DOSAGE AND ADMINISTRATION: **Dosing Considerations: Tablets:**

- The tablets should be swallowed whole with sufficient water.
- The tablets may also be dispersed in half a glass of non-carbonated water. No other liquids should be used as the enteric coating may be dissolved. Stir until the tablets disintegrate and drink the liquid with the pellets immediately or within 30 minutes. Rinse the glass with half a glass of water and drink. The pellets must not be chewed or crushed.
- Dispersed tablets can also be administered via naso-gastric feeding tubes (8-20 French) using a 25 to 60 mL disposable syringe. The type of syringe used should ensure a secure fit with the feeding tube. Each NEXIUM tablet should be dispersed in 50 mL of water and passed through the tube into the stomach. After administering the suspension, the naso-gastric tube may be flushed with an additional 25-50 mL of water to clear the syringe and tube. In larger naso-gastric feeding tubes (i.e. 14 French or larger), the dispersion volume may be reduced to 25 mL.

Granules for Oral Suspension (Sachet):

- The contents of each sachet should be emptied into a container containing 1 tablespoon (15 mL) of water. Stir the contents and leave for a few minutes to thicken. Stir again and drink within 30 minutes. If any material remains after drinking, add more water stir and drink immediately.
- For patients who have a naso-gastric or gastric tube in place, the contents of the sachet can be added to a syringe containing 15 mL of water. Immediately shake the syringe and leave for a few minutes to thicken. Shake the syringe and inject through the nasogastric or gastric tube within 30 minutes. Refill the syringe with an equal amount of water and shake and flush any remaining contents from the nasogastric tube into the stomach.

† No longer marketed in Canada.

Recommended Dose and Dosage Adjustment: Adults: Treatment of Conditions Where a Reduction of Gastric Acid Secretion is Required: Reflux Esophagitis: The recommended dose in patients with reflux esophagitis is 40 mg NEXIUM once daily for 4 to 8 weeks in order to optimize the healing rate and symptom resolution. Healing occurs in the majority of patients within 4 weeks. Sustained freedom from symptoms is achieved rapidly for most patients. An additional 4 weeks of treatment is recommended for patients in whom esophagitis has not healed or who have persistent symptoms.

Maintenance of Healing of Erosive Esophagitis: For the long-term treatment of patients whose reflux esophagitis has been healed with acid suppression therapy, the recommended dose is 20 mg NEXIUM once daily. Controlled studies do not extend beyond 6 months.

Nonerosive Reflux Disease: In patients with heartburn and/or acid regurgitation, without esophagitis, the recommended dose is 20 mg NEXIUM once daily for 2 to 4 weeks. If symptom control is not achieved after 4 weeks of treatment, further investigation is recommended.

Maintenance Treatment of NERD (On-demand): For the maintenance of symptom relief in patients whose symptoms were initially controlled after daily doses for 2 to 4 weeks, the recommended dose is 20 mg NEXIUM once daily taken as needed. Despite treatment, the possibility for development of esophagitis in patients cannot be excluded.

Healing of Gastric Ulcers Associated with NSAID Therapy: In patients requiring NSAID therapy, the recommended dose is 20 mg NEXIUM once daily for 4 to 8 weeks. No additional clinical benefit was observed for the 40 mg dose over the 20 mg dose.

Risk-reduction of Gastric Ulcers Associated with NSAID Therapy: In patients requiring NSAID therapy who are at risk of gastric ulcers, the recommended dose is 20 mg NEXIUM once daily. No additional clinical benefit was observed for the 40 mg dose over the 20 mg dose. Controlled studies did not extend beyond 6 months.

Zollinger-Ellison Syndrome: The dosage in patients with pathological hypersecretory conditions varies with each individual. The recommended initial dosage is 40 mg NEXIUM twice a day. Dosages should then be adjusted to individual patient's needs and treatment should continue as long as clinically indicated. A small number of patients have been treated with doses up to 80 mg t.i.d. In a clinical study, 90% of patients (19 out of 21) with a hypersecretory condition such as Zollinger-Ellison syndrome had gastric acid outputs appropriately controlled at various doses and were maintained through 12 months. Safety information is limited in doses above 80 mg a day.

H. pylori **Eradication: In Patients with *H. pylori*-associated Active Duodenal Ulcer:** The recommended dose is NEXIUM 20 mg, amoxicillin 1000 mg and clarithromycin 500 mg, all twice daily for seven days. No further treatment with NEXIUM is required to ensure healing and/or symptom control. This dosing regimen can also be known as NEXIUM 1-2-3 A.

In Patients with a History of Duodenal Ulcer: The recommended dose is NEXIUM 20 mg, amoxicillin 1000 mg and clarithromycin 500 mg, all twice daily for seven days. This dosing regimen can also be known as NEXIUM 1-2-3 A. Eradication of *H. pylori* has been shown to reduce the risk of duodenal ulcer recurrence.

Pediatrics (1-17 Years of Age): Treatment of Conditions Where a Reduction of Gastric Acid Secretion is Required: Children (1-11 Years of Age): Reflux Esophagitis: The recommended dose in patients with reflux esophagitis is:

Weight <20 kg:	10 mg NEXIUM once daily for 8 weeks
Weight ≥20 kg:	10 mg or 20 mg NEXIUM once daily for 8 weeks

Safety studies do not extend beyond 8 weeks.

Nonerosive Reflux Disease (NERD): In children with heartburn and/or acid regurgitation, without esophagitis, the recommended dose is 10 mg NEXIUM once daily for up to 8 weeks. Safety studies do not extend beyond 8 weeks.

Doses over 1 mg/kg/day have not been studied. There are currently no data on appropriate doses for children with hepatic impairment (see also Warnings and Precautions).

Children (12-17 Years of Age): No dose adjustment is required (see Warnings and Precautions and Action and Clinical Pharmacology, Pharmacokinetics, Special Populations and Conditions, Pediatrics (1-17 Years of Age)).

Reflux Esophagitis: The recommended dose in patients with reflux esophagitis is 20 mg or 40 mg NEXIUM once daily for 4 to 8 weeks. Safety studies do not extend beyond 8 weeks.

Nonerosive Reflux Disease (NERD): In patients with heartburn and/or acid regurgitation, without esophagitis, the recommended dose is 20 mg NEXIUM once daily for 2 to 4 weeks. If symptom control is not achieved after 4 weeks of treatment, further investigation is recommended. Safety studies do not extend beyond 8 weeks.

Missed Dose: A missed dose should be taken as soon as possible within 12 hours. If more than 12 hours have passed, then the next scheduled dose should be taken at the appropriate time.

Administration: Special Populations: When used in combination with amoxicillin and clarithromycin, please refer to the Product Monographs of these drugs for prescribing information regarding Contraindications, Warnings and Dosing (in elderly and patients with renal and hepatic insufficiency).

Patients with Renal Insufficiency: No dose adjustment is required (see Warnings and Precautions).

Patients with Hepatic Insufficiency: No dose adjustment is required for patients with mild to moderate hepatic impairment. The daily doses of 20 mg in patients with severe hepatic impairment should not, as a rule, be exceeded (see Warnings and Precautions).

Elderly Patients: No dose adjustment is required (see Warnings and Precautions).

OVERDOSAGE:

Limited information is available on the effects of higher doses in man, and specific recommendations for treatment cannot be given. Experience from a patient who deliberately ingested an overdose of esomeprazole (280 mg), demonstrated symptoms that were transient, and included weakness, loose stools and nausea. Single doses of 80 mg NEXIUM (esomeprazole) have been shown to be uneventful. No specific antidote is known. Esomeprazole is extensively protein-bound and is therefore not readily dialyzable. Treatment should be symptomatic and general supportive measures should be utilized.

The maximum non-lethal oral dose in male and female rats ranged from 240 to 480 mg/kg.

When used in combination with antibiotics, the Prescribing Information/Product Monograph for those antibiotics should be consulted.

> For management of a suspected drug overdose, contact your **regional Poison Control Centre**. See the *CPS* Directory section for a list of Poison Control Centres.

ACTION AND CLINICAL PHARMACOLOGY: Mechanism of Action: NEXIUM (esomeprazole) delayed release tablets and granules for oral suspension contain esomeprazole (the S-isomer of omeprazole). Esomeprazole is acid labile and therefore is administered orally as enteric-coated granules compressed into a tablet or as enteric-coated granules in an oral suspension.

Esomeprazole magnesium (a substituted benzimidazole), reduces gastric acid secretion through a highly targeted mechanism of action. It is a specific inhibitor of the gastric enzyme H^+,K^+-ATPase (the proton pump) which is responsible for acid secretion by the parietal cells of the stomach.

Pharmacodynamics: Esomeprazole accumulates in the acidic environment of the parietal cells after absorption, where it is converted into the active form. This active sulphenamide specifically binds the H^+, K^+-ATPase (proton pump), to block the final step in acid production, thus reducing gastric acidity. Esomeprazole is effective in the inhibition of both basal acid secretion and stimulated acid secretion.

In healthy male subjects (n=12), repeated administration with 20 mg NEXIUM once daily for 5 days, decreased mean peak acid output after pentagastrin stimulation by 90% when measured 6 to 7 hours after dosing.

The effect of antisecretory therapy can be predicted from the duration of suppression of intragastric acidity to above pH 4.0 achieved by each drug regimen, and the length of treatment.

The antisecretory activity of esomeprazole magnesium was studied in patients with nonerosive reflux disease. NEXIUM 20 and 40 mg tablets were administered over 5 days and the proportion of time when intragastric pH was >4 over a 24 hour period was assessed on Day 5, as shown in Table 5.

Table 5: NEXIUM

Effect on Intragastric pH on Day 5 (n=36)

Parameter	NEXIUM 40 mg	NEXIUM 20 mg
% Time gastric pH >4[a] (h)	70%[b] (16.8 h)	53% (12.7 h)
Coefficient of variation	26%	37%

(cont'd)

Table 5: NEXIUM *(cont'd)*

Effect on Intragastric pH on Day 5 (n=36)

Parameter	NEXIUM 40 mg	NEXIUM 20 mg
Median 24-hour pH	4.9[b]	4.1
Coefficient of variation	16%	27%

[a] Gastric pH was measured over a 24-hour period.
[b] p<0.01 NEXIUM 40 mg vs NEXIUM 20 mg.

Eradication of *H. pylori*: Infection with *H. pylori* is associated with peptic ulcer disease and is a major factor in the development of gastritis. Approximately 90 to 100% of patients with duodenal ulcers, and 80% of patients with gastric ulcer, are infected with *H. pylori*. Treatment with NEXIUM alone has been shown to suppress, but not eradicate *H. pylori*.

Eradication of *H. pylori* with triple therapy consisting of NEXIUM and clarithromycin/amoxicillin for seven days is associated with healing and improvement of symptoms of duodenal ulcers.

Pharmacokinetics: Absorption of esomeprazole in healthy subjects results in peak plasma levels occurring 1 to 2 hours after dosing. The systemic bioavailability is 64% after a single 40 mg dose and 89% after repeated once daily oral administration (40 mg for 5 days). The apparent volume of distribution at steady state in healthy subjects is approximately 0.22 L/kg body weight. Esomeprazole is 97% protein bound and optically stable in vivo, with negligible inversion to the other isomer.

A pharmacokinetic profile of esomeprazole was studied in 36 patients with NERD after repeated once daily administration of 20 mg and 40 mg. See Table 6.

Table 6: NEXIUM

Pharmacokinetic Parameters of Esomeprazole After Oral Administration for 5 Days. Mean (% CV)

Parameter	NEXIUM 40 mg	NEXIUM 20 mg
$AUC_{(tot)}$ (μmol·h/L)	12.6 (42%)	4.2 (59%)
C_{max} (μmol/L)	4.7 (37%)	2.1 (45%)
T_{max} (h)	1.6 (50%)	1.6 (86%)
$t_{1/2}$ (h)	1.5 (32%)	1.2 (37%)

Values represent geometric mean except the T_{max}, which is the arithmetic mean.

Food intake delays and decreases the absorption of esomeprazole although this has no significant influence on the effect of esomeprazole on intragastric acidity.

Pharmacokinetics in Combination with Antibiotics: Interactions between esomeprazole (20 mg b.i.d.), amoxicillin (1 g b.i.d.) and clarithromycin (500 mg b.i.d.), were evaluated in a 4-way cross-over study (each study period was 7 days). When given as the triple combination, the bioavailability (AUC and C_{max}) of amoxicillin and clarithromycin were not significantly changed in healthy volunteers, compared with either drug given alone. The AUC and C_{max} of the 14-hydroxyclarithromycin metabolite were both increased by 53% during dosing with the triple combination, compared to values following dosing with clarithromycin alone. There were also significant increases in the AUC (two-fold increase) and C_{max} (39%) values for esomeprazole during concomitant administration with the antibiotic drugs, compared with esomeprazole alone.

Metabolism: Esomeprazole is completely metabolized by the cytochrome P-450 system, mainly in the liver (via CYP 2C19 and CYP 3A4). The major metabolites of esomeprazole (hydroxy and desmethyl metabolites) have no effect on gastric acid secretion. The CYP 2C19 isozyme, which is involved in the metabolism of all available proton pump inhibitors, exhibits polymorphism. Some 3% of Caucasians and 15-20% of Asians lack CYP 2C19 and are termed "poor metabolizers". At steady state (40 mg for 5 days), the ratio of AUC in poor metabolizers to AUC in the rest of the population is approximately 2. Dosage adjustment of NEXIUM based on CYP 2C19 status is not necessary.

Almost 80% of an oral dose of esomeprazole is excreted as metabolites in urine with the remainder recovered in feces. Less than 1% of the parent drug is found in urine. Total recovery from urine and feces is 92 to 96% within 48 hours of a single oral dose.

Special Populations and Conditions: Pediatrics (1-17 Years of Age): Children (1-11 Years of Age): The pharmacokinetics of esomeprazole were studied in 31 pediatric patients with GERD 1 to 11 years of age inclusive, in a single centre study. Patients were divided into 2 subgroups by age. For ages 1 to 5, patients received esomeprazole 5 mg or 10 mg once daily for 5 days. For ages 6 to 11 years, patients received esomeprazole 10 mg or 20 mg once daily for 5 days.

Following repeated dose administration of esomeprazole 10 mg and 20 mg, the total exposure (AUC) and the time to reach maximum plasma drug concentration (t_{max}) for the 10 mg dose was similar across the 1-11 year-olds and similar to the total exposure seen with the 20 mg dose in adults. The 20 mg dose resulted in higher exposure in 6-11 year-olds compared to adults.

Repeated dose administration of 5 mg esomeprazole resulted in insufficient exposure in 1-5 year-olds. See Table 7.

Table 7: NEXIUM

Summary of Pharmacokinetic Parameters in 1-11 Year-olds with GERD Following of 5-Days of Once-daily Oral Esomeprazole Treatment

	1 to 5 Year-olds		6 to 11 Year-olds	
	5 mg (n=6)	10 mg (n=8)	10 mg (n=7)	20 mg (n=6)
$AUC_{(tot)}$ (μmol·h/L)	0.74	4.83	3.7	6.28
C_{max} (μmol/L)	0.62	2.98	1.77	3.73
T_{max} (h)	1.33	1.44	1.79	1.75
$t_{1/2}$ (h)	0.42	0.74	0.88	0.73
Cl/F (L/h)	19.44	5.99	7.84	9.22

Values represent geometric mean except the T_{max}, which is the arithmetic mean.

(See Dosage and Administration and Warnings and Precautions.)

Children (12-17 Years of Age): The pharmacokinetics of esomeprazole were studied in 28 pediatric patients with GERD aged 12 to 17 years, in a single centre randomized study. Patients received esomeprazole 20 mg or 40 mg once daily for 8 days. Mean C_{max} and AUC values of esomeprazole were not affected by body weight or age. More than dose-proportional increases in mean C_{max} and AUC values were observed between the two groups in the study. Overall, esomeprazole pharmacokinetics in pediatric patients aged 12 to 17 years were similar to those observed in adult patients with NERD. See Table 8.

Geriatrics: The metabolism of NEXIUM is not significantly changed in elderly subjects. Following repeated oral dosing with 40 mg NEXIUM in healthy elderly subjects (6 males, 8 females; 71 to 80 years of age), AUC and C_{max} values measured were similar to those previously measured in young GERD patients (ratio of AUC values in elderly vs GERD subjects: 1.25; ratio of C_{max} values: 1.18).

Gender: The AUC and C_{max} values were slightly higher (13%) in females than in males at steady state. Dosage adjustment based on gender is not necessary.

Hepatic Insufficiency: (See Dosage and Administration and Warnings and Precautions.)

Renal Insufficiency: (See Dosage and Administration and Warnings and Precautions.)

Poor Metabolizers: (See Dosage and Administration and Warnings and Precautions.)

Table 8: NEXIUM

Comparison of Pharmacokinetic Parameters in 12-17 Year-olds with GERD and Adults with NERD Following Esomeprazole Daily Repeated Oral Dosing[a]

	Pediatrics (aged 12-17 years) (n=28)		Adults (≥18 years) (n=36)	
Pharmacokinetic Parameter	20 mg	40 mg	20 mg	40 mg
AUC (μmol·h/L)	3.65	13.86	4.2	12.6
C_{max}(μmol/L)	1.45	5.13	2.1	4.7
t_{max}(h)	2	1.75	1.6	1.6
$t_{1/2\ \lambda z}$ (h)	0.82	1.22	1.2	1.5

[a] Data presented are geometric means for AUC, C_{max} and $t_{1/2\ \lambda z}$ and median value for t_{max}. Duration of treatment for 12-17 year olds and adults were 8 days and 5 days, respectively. Data were obtained from two independent studies.

STORAGE AND STABILITY: Temperature: Store in a dry place at controlled room temperature (15-30°C).

Moisture: NEXIUM (esomeprazole) delayed release tablets and delayed release granules for oral suspension are moisture-sensitive and are therefore provided in blister compliance packages and aluminum sachets, suitable for direct distribution to the patient.

Others: Keep in a safe place out of reach of children.

INFORMATION FOR THE PATIENT: Published in e-CPS, available by subscription at www.e-cps.ca.

DOSAGE FORMS, COMPOSITION AND PACKAGING: Granules: Each unit-dose sachet of fine, pale yellow, delayed release granules for oral suspension contains: esomeprazole 10 mg. Brownish granules may also be visible. Nonmedicinal ingredients: citric acid, crospovidone, dextrose, glycerol monostearate, hydroxypropyl cellulose, hypromellose, iron oxide, magnesium stearate, methacrylic acid copolymer type C, polysorbate, sugar spheres, talc, triethyl citrate and xanthan gum. Cartons of 30.

Tablets: 20 mg: Each light pink, oblong and biconvex, delayed-release tablet, engraved with "20 mg" on one side and "$\hat{\text{EH}}$" on the other side, contains: esomeprazole 20 mg equivalent to esomeprazole magnesium trihydrate 22.3 mg. Nonmedicinal ingredients: cellulose microcrystalline, crospovidone, glyceryl monostearate, hydroxypropyl cellulose, hypromellose, iron oxide, magnesium stearate, methacrylic acid ethylacrylate copolymer, polyethylene glycol, polysorbate, sodium stearyl fumarate, sugar spheres, synthetic paraffin, talc, titanium dioxide and triethyl citrate. Press-through blister compliance strips, cartons of 30.

40 mg: Each pink, oblong and biconvex, delayed-release tablet, engraved with "40 mg" on one side and "$\hat{\text{EI}}$" on the other side, contains: esomeprazole 40 mg equivalent to esomeprazole magnesium trihydrate 44.5 mg. Nonmedicinal ingredients: cellulose microcrystalline, crospovidone, glyceryl monostearate, hydroxypropylcellulose, hypromellose, iron oxide, magnesium stearate, methacrylic acid ethylacrylate copolymer, polyethylene glycol, polysorbate, sodium stearyl fumarate, sugar spheres, synthetic paraffin, talc, titanium dioxide and triethyl citrate. Press-through blister compliance strips, cartons of 30 and 60. HDPE bottles of 100.

(Shown in Product Identification Section)

Nexium 1-2-3 A®

esomeprazole magnesium trihydrate—amoxicillin—clarithromycin

H. pylori Associated Peptic Ulcer Disease

AstraZeneca

Note: Regimen consists of esomeprazole magnesium trihydrate 20 mg, amoxicillin 1000 mg and clarithromycin 500 mg. All twice daily for 7 days. For further details on this triple therapy for treatment of *H. pylori* eradication, consult the Nexium product monograph. For additional safety information on amoxicillin and clarithromycin, consult the product monographs.

Niacin

Vitamin

CPhA Monograph

Niacinamide

Vitamin

CPhA Monograph

Date of Revision: August 2009

This monograph has been compiled by CPhA and reviewed by experts. It may contain information different from that found in Health Canada-approved Product Monographs. The reader is referred to the *CPS* Editorial Policy for more information.

SUMMARY PRODUCT INFORMATION:

Drugs[a]	Route of Administration	Dosage Form	Strength
Niacin	Oral	Immediate release tablet or capsule[b]	100 mg, 500 mg
		Extended release tablet	500 mg, 750 mg, 1000 mg
Niacinamide	Oral	Tablet	100 mg
		Capsule	500 mg

[a] Table includes single entity niacin or niacinamide products only. For specific product information consult Health Canada's Drug Product Database [www.hc-sc.gc.ca/dhp-mps/prodpharma/databasdon/index_e.html].
[b] Some products may contain niacin in the form of inositol nicotinate.

PHARMACOLOGY: Niacin (nicotinic acid or vitamin B_3) and niacinamide (or nicotinamide) are water-soluble B complex vitamins. Inositol nicotinate is metabolised in the body to release inositol and niacin. In vivo, niacin is converted to niacinamide, a constituent of nicotinamide adenine dinucleotide (NAD) and nicotinamide adenine dinucleotide phosphate (NADP), which are coenzymes involved in glycogenolysis, tissue respiration and lipid metabolism. Deficiency of niacin or tryptophan, its precursor, results in pellagra, a chronic wasting disease characterized by dermatitis, dementia and diarrhea. As niacin equivalents, 1 mg of niacin is equivalent to approximately 60 mg of tryptophan. Some causes of niacin deficiency include nutritional deficiencies, chronic alcoholism, malabsorption syndromes, carcinoid tumors, isoniazid therapy or Hartnup disease (impaired tryptophan transport).

When larger pharmacologic doses are used, niacin has the following properties that are distinct from niacinamide: Niacin produces peripheral vasodilation, a process believed to be mediated by prostacyclin, which affects the cutaneous vessels of the upper body. Tolerance to this effect usually develops after about 2 weeks of treatment.

Niacin decreases the rate of hepatic synthesis of very low-density lipoprotein (VLDL) and low-density lipoprotein (LDL) while raising high-density lipoprotein (HDL) in serum, both in normal individuals and patients with type II, III, IV or V dyslipidemia. The exact mechanism for the beneficial effects on serum lipids remains unknown, but the main antilipemic effect seems to result from decreased VLDL-cholesterol production. Partial inhibition of free fatty acid release from adipose tissue, decreased delivery of free fatty acids to the liver and a decrease in triglyceride synthesis and VLDL-triglyceride transport may explain this decreased production. Clearance of VLDL-cholesterol and chylomicron triglycerides may also be increased, possibly due to enhanced lipoprotein lipase activity. This has led to a lowering of LDL-C by 5 to 25% and triglycerides by 20 to 50%. Niacin raises HDL-C by 15 to 35% with most of the rise occurring at daily doses of 1 to 1.5 g. It also lowers the lipoprotein Lp(a) by nearly 30%, though the clinical significance of lowering Lp(a) is not yet known.

Pharmacokinetics: Niacin and niacinamide are readily absorbed from the gastrointestinal tract.

When taken in physiologic doses niacin is metabolized in the liver to niacinamide. When therapeutic doses are taken, only a portion is converted to niacinamide. The remainder is eventually excreted unchanged in the urine. Niacinamide is widely distributed in the body and is further metabolized in the liver before being excreted in the urine.

INDICATIONS:

- Niacin and niacinamide are used in the prevention and treatment of pellagra.
- Niacin is used as an adjunct to therapeutic lifestyle changes (e.g., diet, weight control, physical activity) for the reduction of elevated total cholesterol, LDL-C and TG levels and to increase HDL-C levels in patients with primary hypercholesterolemia, mixed dyslipidemia (Fredickson Type IIa and IIb) and hypertriglyceridemia (Fredickson Type IV and V). It may be used alone or in combination with other agents for additive effects. Canadian guidelines for the diagnosis and treatment of dyslipidemia have been published [*Can J Cardiol* 2006;22(11):913-27].
- **Niacinamide is not effective in the management of dyslipidemia and should not be used as a substitute.**

CONTRAINDICATIONS:

- Patients with a known hypersensitivity to niacin or niacinamide or to any ingredient in the formulation or component of the container.
- Patients with active liver disease, peptic ulcer disease, hyperuricemia with a history of gouty arthritis or uncontrolled hyperglycemia.
- Niacin specifically is contraindicated in patients with severe hypotension.

WARNINGS AND PRECAUTIONS: Endocrine and Metabolism: Mean changes in fasting blood glucose levels in well-controlled clinical trials were generally transient and modest. In patients with diabetes, an adjustment or change in diet and/or hypoglycemic treatment may be necessary for blood glucose control. Patients with impaired fasting glucose may require initiation of hypoglycemic treatment if they develop diabetes. Periodic monitoring of blood glucose concentration during niacin or niacinamide therapy is advised especially in the early phase of treatment.

Hyperuricemia may occur during niacin treatment and in general, once it occurs, it may remain during the duration of the treatment. Periodic monitoring of uric acid is advised. Niacin must be used with caution in patients predisposed to gout (see Contraindications).

Hepatic/Biliary/Pancreatic: Patients with gallbladder disease, history of jaundice or liver disease should be monitored closely while on niacin or niacinamide. Liver function tests (LFTs) should be conducted at baseline, and every 6 to 12 weeks during the first year, then periodically thereafter. If there are persistent unexplained elevations in serum transaminases more than 3 times the upper limit of normal or if the LFTs are associated with fever, nausea and/or malaise, therapy should be discontinued.

Musculoskeletal: A small number of cases of myopathy with niacin monotherapy have been reported. Myopathy and rhabdomyolysis have also been reported with concurrent statin therapy. The true incidence of muscle side effects is unknown.

Special Populations: *Pregnant Women:* Niacin and probably niacinamide are compatible with pregnancy when the recommended daily allowance is used; however, safety of niacin, used at higher doses in lowering elevated serum cholesterol in pregnancy, has not been established. Fetal abnormalities have not been reported. Animal reproduction or teratology studies have not been conducted and thus it is unknown if fetal harm can occur using niacin at doses used for lipid disorders.

Nursing Women: Niacin and niacinamide distribute into breast milk. Problems have not been reported with intake of normal daily requirements, but there is no information pertaining to higher doses used in the treatment of dyslipidemia.

Drug Interactions: Due to potential of hypotensive effect, postural hypotension may occur when niacin is administered with vasoactive drugs or ganglionic blocking agents.

Although sometimes used in combination, there have been isolated reports of rhabdomyolysis in patients taking niacin and lovastatin. A causal relationship with niacin has not been established. It is not known if there is an interaction with other HMG-CoA reductase inhibitors. Patients should be advised to report unexplained muscle pain, tenderness or weakness to their physician.

Because niacin can cause hyperglycemia, dosage adjustment of insulin or oral antihyperglycemic therapy may be required in diabetic patients.

Niacinamide has been reported to increase the blood levels of primidone and carbamazepine when taken concurrently.

Drug-Laboratory Interactions: Niacin may cause false elevation in fluorometric determinations of urinary catecholamines and false-positive results may be obtained for urinary glucose when Benedict's reagent is used. Niacin has also been reported to cause false-positive results for blood bilirubin tests.

ADVERSE REACTIONS: More Common Adverse Drug Reactions Associated with Niacin: See Table 1.

Table 1: Niacin

Adverse Drug Reactions with Incidence ≥1%

Body System	Effect (estimated % incidence)	Clinical Comment
Cardiovascular	Flushing (90)	Flushing starts in the face and is accompanied by an intense feeling of warmth and itching. It may spread to the arms and chest and occasionally down to the legs and feet. Flushing may be accompanied by burning, stinging or tingling sensations, increase in skin temperature, gastrointestinal symptoms, pruritus and hypotension. Following oral administration, niacin-induced vasodilation occurs within 20 min and may persist for 20 to 60 min. The frequency and severity of flushing usually subsides with continued therapy. Administration of reduced doses or on a full stomach may decrease flushing. If not contraindicated, pretreatment with a nonsteroidal prostaglandin inhibitor (e.g., ASA) may reduce flushing. Less flushing episodes are associated with Niaspan, an extended-release formulation. Avoid concomitant alcohol, spicy foods, hot beverages or hot showers.
Central Nervous System	Headache (7)	
Dermatologic	Pruritus and rash (12)	
Gastrointestinal	Diarrhea (10), nausea (5), vomiting (5)	
Hepatic	Increased serum aminotransferase concentrations (1–50)	Hepatotoxicity has been reported more frequently with sustained-release formulations. It is usually dose related and reversible (see Warnings and Precautions).

Adverse Drug Reactions Associated with Niacin (incidence unknown): **Cardiovascular**: arrhythmias, edema, hypotension, orthostasis, vasovagal attacks.

Gastrointestinal: abdominal pain, anorexia, constipation, flatulence, heartburn, activation of peptic ulcers and or peptic ulceration.

Dermatologic: acanthosis nigricans, dry skin, hyperpigmentation, urticaria, sweating.

Endocrine and Metabolism: decreased glucose tolerance, hyperuricemia, gout.

Central Nervous System: asthenia, dizziness, fatigue, insomnia, migraine.

Musculoskeletal: myopathy, myositis, rhabdomyolysis (see Warnings and Precautions).

Neurologic: paresthesia.

Ophthalmic: blurred vision, proptosis.

Adverse Drug Reactions Associated with Niacinamide: Niacinamide lacks vasodilating effects but is not effective in the management of dyslipidemia. Parenteral solutions of B complex vitamins containing niacinamide may cause flushing, itching or burning of the skin in patients susceptible to the effects of niacinamide. Niacinamide has also caused hyperhidrosis, nausea and abdominal cramps. Abnormal liver function test results have been reported.

OVERDOSE:

For management of a suspected drug overdose, CPhA recommends that you contact your **regional Poison Control Centre**. See the *CPS* Directory section for a list of Poison Control Centres.

DOSAGE AND ADMINISTRATION: To prevent deficiency, adequate dietary intake is preferred over supplementation whenever possible. Food sources include meat, poultry, fish (e.g., cod, halibut, salmon), dairy products (e.g., milk), eggs, whole grains, enriched flour and cereals.

Dosage of niacin and niacinamide must be carefully adjusted according to the patient's response and tolerance (see Table 2).

Table 2: Niacin/Niacinamide

Dose in Adult Patients

Indication	Drug	Dose	Clinical Comment
Pellagra	Niacin/ Niacinamide	300–500 mg po daily in divided doses; maximum daily dose is 500 mg. Children: 100–300 mg daily in divided doses.	In the treatment and prevention of pellagra, either niacin or niacinamide can be administered.
Dyslipidemia	Niacin, immediate release	Initial dose: 50 mg po TID. May double the dose q5days to 1.5–2.0 g/day. If tolerated, maximum daily dose is 4 g.	Starting at a low dose and titrating up slowly may reduce potential adverse reactions and achieve treatment goals by improving adherence to the regimen. Cholesterol and triglyceride concentrations should be determined prior to initiation of therapy and regularly during treatment. Monitor blood glucose, uric acid and liver transaminases at baseline and every 6 to 8 weeks during dose titration, then periodically thereafter. Administration of doses on a full stomach may reduce gastrointestinal distress. Flushing abates with time (see Adverse Reactions) as tachyphylaxis occurs.
	Niacin, extended release	Initial dose: 500 mg po HS after a low fat snack for 4 weeks. May ↑ by 500 mg q4weeks to a maximum daily dose of 2000 mg po HS, if required.	Bedtime dosing minimizes flushing during the day.

Dosage in Renal Impairment: Dose adjustment is recommended for niacin (see Table 3), but is not required for niacinamide.

Table 3: Niacin

Dose in Adult Patients with Renal Impairment

Creatinine Clearance	Dose Adjustment
>50 mL/min	usual dose
10–50 mL/min	50% of total daily dose, administered in divided doses.
<10 mL/min	25% of total daily dose, administered in divided doses.

The reader is invited to consult CPhA's monograph **Niacin/Niacinamide.**

Niaspan® Pr

niacin

Lipid Metabolism Regulator

Sepracor

Date of Revision: April 13, 2010

SUMMARY PRODUCT INFORMATION:

Route of Administration	Dosage Form/Strength	Clinically Relevant Nonmedicinal Ingredients
Oral	500 mg, 750 mg, 1000 mg extended-release tablets	Methylcellulose, povidone, stearic acid

INDICATIONS AND CLINICAL USE: NIASPAN (extended-release niacin) is indicated as an adjunct to diet for reduction of elevated total cholesterol (TC), low-density lipoprotein cholesterol (LDL-C), apolipoprotein B (Apo B) and triglyceride (TG) levels, and to increase high-density lipoprotein cholesterol (HDL-C) in patients with primary hypercholesterolaemia (heterozygous familial and nonfamilial) and mixed dyslipidaemia (Frederickson Types IIa and IIb), when the response to an appropriate diet and other non-pharmacological measures have been inadequate.

Therapy with NIASPAN should be only one component of multiple risk factor intervention in individuals at significantly increased risk for atherosclerotic vascular disease due to hypercholesterolemia. Prior to initiating therapy with NIASPAN, secondary causes for hypercholesterolemia (e.g., poorly controlled diabetes mellitus, hypothyroidism, nephrotic syndrome, dysproteinemias, obstructive liver disease, other drug therapy, alcoholism) should be excluded, and a lipid profile obtained to measure TC, HDL-C, and TG.

Pediatrics: No studies in patients under 21 years of age have been conducted with NIASPAN.

CONTRAINDICATIONS:

- NIASPAN (extended-release niacin) is contraindicated in patients with a known hypersensitivity to niacin or any component of this medication (see Dosage Forms, Composition and Packaging).
- Active liver disease or unexplained persistent elevations of serum transaminases, active peptic ulcer, or active bleeding.

WARNINGS AND PRECAUTIONS:

> **Serious Warnings and Precautions**
> - NIASPAN (extended-release niacin) preparations should not be substituted for equivalent doses of immediate-release (crystalline) niacin or nicotinic acid. For patients switching from immediate-release niacin or nicotinic acid to NIASPAN, therapy with NIASPAN should be initiated with low doses (i.e., 500 mg qhs) and the NIASPAN dose should then be titrated to the desired therapeutic response.
> - Cases of severe hepatic toxicity, including fulminant hepatic necrosis, have occurred in patients who have substituted sustained-release (modified-release, timed-release) niacin products for immediate-release (crystalline) niacin at equivalent doses.

Clinically significant warnings and precautions are listed below in alphabetical order.

General: Before instituting therapy with NIASPAN, an attempt should be made to control hyperlipidaemia with appropriate diet, exercise, and weight reduction in obese patients, and to treat other underlying medical problems (see Indications and Clinical Use).

While pretreatment with acetylsalicylic acid (ASA) or other non-steroidal anti-inflammatory drugs (NSAIDs) may reduce flushing of the skin, some patients should not take these medications (e.g., patients who have peptic ulcer or active inflammatory disease of the gastrointestinal system or ASA hypersensitivity; refer to the Product Monograph for the NSAID product).

Cardiovascular: Data on the safety and efficacy of NIASPAN in patients with unstable angina or in the acute phase of myocardial infarction are not available. Therefore, caution should be used when NIASPAN is used, particularly when such patients are also receiving vasodilator agents.

Endocrine and Metabolism: Elevated uric acid levels have occurred with niacin therapy, therefore use with caution in patients predisposed to gout.

In placebo-controlled trials, NIASPAN has been associated with small but statistically significant, dose-related reductions in phosphorus levels (mean of −13% with 2000 mg). Although these reductions were transient, phosphorus levels should be monitored periodically in patients at risk for hypophosphatemia.

Periodic serum creatine phosphokinase (CPK) and potassium determinations should be carried out.

Gastrointestinal: Patients with a past history of jaundice or peptic ulcer should be observed closely during NIASPAN therapy.

Hematologic: NIASPAN has been associated with small, but statistically significant dose-related reductions in platelet count (mean of −11% with 2000 mg). In addition, NIASPAN has been associated with small but statistically significant increases in prothrombin time (mean of approximately +4% with 2000 mg); accordingly, patients undergoing surgery should be carefully evaluated. Caution should be observed when NIASPAN is administered concomitantly with anticoagulants; prothrombin time and platelet counts should be monitored closely in such patients.

Hepatic/Biliary/Pancreatic: No clinical studies have been carried out in patients with impaired liver function.

Patients with a past history of jaundice, hepatobiliary disease, or peptic ulcer should be observed closely during NIASPAN therapy. Frequent monitoring of liver function tests and blood glucose should be performed.

NIASPAN should be used with caution in patients who consume substantial quantities of alcohol and/or have a past history of liver disease.

Niacin preparations have been associated with abnormal liver tests. In three placebo-controlled clinical trials involving titration to final daily NIASPAN doses ranging from 500 to 3000 mg, 245 patients received NIASPAN for a mean duration of 17 weeks and no patient with normal serum transaminase levels (AST, ALT) at baseline experienced elevations to more than 3 times the upper limit of normal (ULN). In these studies, fewer than 1% (2/245) of NIASPAN patients discontinued due to transaminase elevations greater than 2 times the ULN.

In three safety and efficacy studies with a combination tablet of NIASPAN and lovastatin involving titration to final daily doses (expressed as mg of extended-release niacin/mg of lovastatin) 500 mg/10 mg to 2500 mg/40 mg, ten of 1028 patients (1.0%) experienced reversible elevations in AST/ALT to more than 3 times the upper limit of normal (ULN). Three of ten elevations occurred at doses outside the recommended dosing limit of 2000 mg/40 mg; no patient receiving 1000 mg/20 mg had 3-fold elevations in AST/ALT.

In the placebo-controlled clinical trials and the long-term extension study, elevations in transaminases did not appear to be related to treatment duration. However, elevations in AST levels did appear to be dose related. Transaminase elevations were reversible upon discontinuation of NIASPAN.

Diabetic patients may experience a dose-related rise in glucose tolerance. Diabetic or potentially diabetic patients with hypercholesterolaemia should be observed closely. Adjustment of diet and/or hypoglycemic therapy may be necessary.

Renal: No clinical studies have been carried out in patients with impaired renal function. Niacin and its metabolites are excreted through the kidneys. NIASPAN should be used with caution in patients with renal dysfunction.

Skeletal Muscle: Rare cases of rhabdomyolysis have been associated with concomitant administration of lipid-altering doses (≥1 g/day) of niacin and HMG-CoA reductase inhibitors. In clinical studies with a combination tablet of NIASPAN and lovastatin, no cases of rhabdomyolysis and one suspected case of myopathy have been reported in 1079 patients who were treated with doses up to 2000 mg of NIASPAN and 40 mg of lovastatin daily for periods up to 2 years. Physicians contemplating combined therapy with HMG-CoA reductase inhibitors and NIASPAN should carefully weigh the potential benefits and risks and should carefully monitor patients for any signs and symptoms of muscle pain, tenderness, or weakness, particularly during the initial months of therapy and during any periods of upward dosage titration of either drug. Periodic serum creatine phosphokinase (CPK) and potassium determinations should be considered in such situations, but there is no assurance that such monitoring will prevent the occurrence of severe myopathy.

Special Populations: Pregnant Women: No information is available on the safety of NIASPAN in pregnant women. Animal reproduction studies have not been conducted with niacin or with NIASPAN. It is not known whether niacin at doses used for lipid disorders can cause fetal harm when administered to pregnant women or whether it can affect reproductive capacity. If a woman receiving treatment with NIASPAN becomes pregnant, the drug should be discontinued.

Nursing Women: No information is available on the safety of NIASPAN in nursing women. Niacin has been reported to be excreted in human milk. Because of the potential for serious adverse reactions in nursing infants, a decision should be made whether to discontinue nursing or to discontinue the drug.

Pediatrics: Safety and effectiveness of niacin therapy in pediatric patients have not been established. No studies in patients under 21 years of age have been conducted with NIASPAN.

Geriatrics: No formal studies have been carried out in elderly patients. Patients up to 75 years of age participated in controlled clinical trials of NIASPAN.

Monitoring and Laboratory Tests: Liver tests should be performed on all patients during therapy with NIASPAN. Serum transaminase levels, including AST and ALT, should be monitored before treatment begins, every 6 to 12 weeks for the first year, and periodically thereafter (e.g., at 6 month intervals. Special attention should be paid to patients who develop elevated serum transaminase levels. In these patients, measurements should be repeated promptly and then performed more frequently. If the transaminase levels show evidence of progression, particularly if they rise to 3 times ULN and are persistent, or if they are associated with symptoms of nausea, fever, and/or malaise, the drug should be discontinued.

ADVERSE REACTIONS: Adverse Drug Reaction Overview: The most frequently-reported events with NIASPAN (extended-release niacin) are flushing episodes, which generally become less common as treatment progresses and which may be reduced by concomitant acetylsalicylic acid (ASA) therapy and by following the recommended dose titration schedule (see Warnings and Precautions, General).

In the placebo-controlled clinical trials, flushing episodes (i.e., warmth, redness, itching and/or tingling) were the most common treatment-emergent adverse events for NIASPAN, reported in up to 88% of patients. Spontaneous reports suggest that flushing may also be accompanied by symptoms of dizziness, tachycardia, palpitations, shortness of breath, sweating, chills, and/or edema, which in rare cases may lead to syncope. In pivotal studies, fewer than 6% (14/245) of NIASPAN patients discontinued due to flushing. Following 4 weeks of maintenance therapy with NIASPAN at daily doses of 1500 mg, the incidence of flushing over the 4-week period averaged 8.56 events per patient for IR niacin versus 1.88 events per NIASPAN patient.

Other commonly-reported non-serious events include gastrointestinal symptoms and rash. The majority of adverse events reported were mild and transient.

In general, the incidence of adverse events was higher in women compared to men.

Niacin therapy has been associated with abnormalities of liver function. In patients receiving NIASPAN, liver function should be periodically monitored.

Clinical Trial Adverse Drug Reactions: Because clinical trials are conducted under very specific conditions the adverse reaction rates observed in the clinical trials may not reflect the rates observed in practice and should not be compared to the rates in the clinical trials of another drug. Adverse drug reaction information from clinical trials is useful for identifying drug-related adverse events and for approximating rates.

Based on the experience in a total of 723 patients, of whom 477 were treated with NIASPAN for one year (48 weeks) and 379 for 2 years (96 weeks), the majority of adverse events were mild and transient.

Adverse events occurring at an incidence of ≥2% in patients treated with NIASPAN during premarketing controlled studies are shown in Table 1 by body system.

Less Common Adverse Drug Reactions (<2%): The following adverse events have been reported with NIASPAN or other niacin products, either during clinical trials or in routine patient management, irrespective of causality.

Table 1: NIASPAN

Treatment-emergent Adverse Events by Dose Level in ≥2% of Patients and at an Incidence Greater than Placebo, Regardless of Causality

	Placebo-controlled Studies	
	Placebo	**NIASPAN (All Doses)**
Total # of Patients	157	245
Body as a Whole		
Asthenia	3%	4%
Chills	1%	3%
Fever	3%	7%
Flu Syndrome	5%	7%
Pain, Abdominal	6%	8%
Pain, Back	7%	9%
Pain, Chest	2%	6%
Surgical Procedure	1%	2%
Cardiovascular System		
Migraine	1%	2%
Palpitation	1%	3%
Tachycardia	0%	2%
Digestive System		
Diarrhea	13%	20%
Dyspepsia	12%	13%
Eructation	1%	2%
Nausea	7%	13%
Vomiting	4%	7%
Metabolism & Nutritional Disorders		
Edema	1%	2%
Edema, Peripheral	0%	2%
Musculoskeletal System		
Arthralgia	0%	3%
Arthritis	2%	3%
Nervous System		
Dry Mouth	0%	2%
Somnolence	1%	2%
Respiratory System		
Cough, Increase	6%	7%
Rhinitis	31%	34%
Skin & Appendages		
Pruritus	2%	6%
Rash	1%	7%
Skin Discoloration	1%	3%
Sweating	1%	2%
Urticaria	1%	2%
Special Senses		

(cont'd)

Table 1: NIASPAN *(cont'd)*

Treatment-emergent Adverse Events by Dose Level in ≥2% of Patients and at an Incidence Greater than Placebo, Regardless of Causality

	Placebo-controlled Studies	
	Placebo	**NIASPAN (All Doses)**
Tinnitus	1%	2%

Body as a Whole: enlarged abdomen, cyst, hernia, mucous membrane disorder, face edema.
Cardiovascular: angina pectoris, cardiovascular disorder, hemorrhage, atrial fibrillation and other cardiac arrhythmias, hypotension, orthostasis, syncope.
Digestive: cholelith, dysphagia, esophagitis, GI hemorrhage, fecal incontinence, stomatitis, tongue disorder, flatulence, activation of peptic ulcers and peptic ulceration, jaundice.
Hemic and Lymphatic: leucopenia.
Hypersensitivity Reactions: An apparent hypersensitivity reaction has been reported rarely that has included one or more of the following features: anaphylaxis, angioedema, urticaria, flushing, dyspnea, tongue edema, larynx edema, face edema, peripheral edema, laryngismus, and vesiculobullous rash, hypotension and circulatory collapse.
Metabolism and Nutritional Disorders: bilirubinemia, xanthoma, decreased glucose tolerance, anorexia, gout.
Musculoskeletal: bone disorder, bursitis, myasthenia, rhabdomyolysis, myalgia, myopathy.
Nervous: hypertonia, hypesthesia, hypokinesia, increased libido, twitch, vertigo, leg cramps, nervousness, paresthesia, dizziness, headache, insomnia.
Respiratory: bronchitis, hemoptysis, hyperventilation, laryngitis, lung disorder, dyspnea.
Skin and Appendages: acne, alopecia, application site reaction, contact dermatitis, fungal dermatitis, eczema, herpes zoster, skin neoplasm, vesiculobullous rash, dry skin, skin ulcer, general exanthema, hyperpigmentation, acanthosis nigricans, maculopapular rash.
Special Senses: eye disorder, glaucoma, vision abnormal, toxic amblyopia, cystoid macular edema.
Urogenital: impotence, breast pain, polyuria, prostatic disorder, UG disorder, urinary retention, vaginitis.
Abnormal Hematologic and Clinical Chemistry Findings: Chemistry: Elevations in serum transaminases (see Warnings and Precautions, Hepatic/Biliary/Pancreatic), LDH, fasting glucose, uric acid, total bilirubin, and amylase; reductions in phosphorus. Hematology: Slight reductions in platelet counts and prolongation in prothrombin time (see Warnings and Precautions, Hematologic).
Post-market Adverse Drug Reactions: In post-market safety surveillance, flushing, headache, tachycardia, asthenia, insomnia, and maculopapular rash were the most frequently reported non-serious adverse events.

DRUG INTERACTIONS: Overview: HMG-CoA Reductase Inhibitors: Rhabdomyolysis has been rarely reported in patients receiving niacin concomitantly with an HMG-CoA reductase inhibitor (statin) (see Warnings and Precautions).

Alcohol or **hot drinks** taken at the time of NIASPAN (extended-release niacin) administration may worsen the flushing response and pruritus.

Antihypertensive Therapy: Niacin may potentiate the effects of ganglionic blocking agents and vasoactive drugs resulting in postural hypotension.

Acetylsalicylic acid (ASA): Concomitant administration of ASA may decrease the metabolic clearance of niacin (see Warnings and Precautions, General).

Bile-Acid Sequestrants: An interval of 4 to 6 hours, or as great an interval as possible, should elapse between the ingestion of bile acid-binding resins and the administration of NIASPAN. An in vitro study showed that about 98% of available niacin was bound to colestipol, and 10 to 30% was bound to cholestyramine.

Other: Vitamins or other nutritional supplements containing large doses of niacin or related compounds such as nicotinamide may potentiate the adverse effects of NIASPAN.

Drug-Food Interactions: Concomitant alcohol or hot drinks may increase the side effects of flushing and pruritus and should be avoided around the time of NIASPAN ingestion.

Drug-Herb Interactions: Interactions with herbal products have not been studied.

Drug-Laboratory Test Interactions: Niacin may produce false elevations in some fluorometric determinations of plasma or urinary catecholamines. Niacin may also give false-positive reactions with cupric sulfate solution (Benedict's reagent) in urine glucose tests.

DOSAGE AND ADMINISTRATION: Patients should be placed on a standard cholesterol-lowering diet at least equivalent to the NCEP Adult Treatment Panel III TLC diet before receiving NIASPAN (extended-release niacin) and should continue on this diet during treatment with NIASPAN. If appropriate, a program of weight control and physical exercise should be implemented.

Dosing Considerations:
- Equivalent doses of NIASPAN should not be substituted for immediate-release (crystalline) niacin.
- NIASPAN tablet strengths are not interchangeable.
- If lipid response to NIASPAN alone is insufficient, or if higher doses of NIASPAN are not well tolerated, some patients may benefit from combination therapy with a bile acid binding resin or an HMG-CoA reductase inhibitor.
- Patients already receiving a stable dose of a statin who require further TG lowering or HDL raising, may receive concomitant NIASPAN administered according to the initial titration schedule.
- Women may respond at lower NIASPAN doses than men.
- Flushing of the skin may be reduced in frequency or severity by pretreatment with acetylsalicylic acid and avoiding administration on an empty stomach (see Warnings and Precautions, General).
- NIASPAN is contraindicated in patients with significant or unexplained hepatic dysfunction.
- No information is available on the safety of NIASPAN in patients with renal insufficiency.

Recommended Dose and Dosage Adjustment: NIASPAN should be taken at bedtime, after a low-fat snack, and doses should be individualized according to patient response. Therapy with NIASPAN must be initiated at 500 mg at bedtime, in order to reduce the incidence and severity of side effects which may occur during early therapy. The recommended dose escalation is shown in Table 2.

Table 2: NIASPAN

Recommended Dosing

	Week(s)	Daily Dose
Initial Titration Schedule	1 to 4	500 mg
	5 to 8	1000 mg
Further Titration Schedule[a]	After Week 8	1500 mg
		2000 mg

[a] After Week 8, titrate to patient response and tolerance. If response to 1000 mg daily is inadequate, increase dose to 1500 mg daily; may subsequently increase dose to 2000 mg daily. Daily dose should not be increased more than 500 mg in a 4-week period, and doses above 2000 mg daily are not recommended.

Maintenance Dose: The daily dosage of NIASPAN should not be increased by more than 500 mg in any 4-week period. The initial recommended maintenance dose is 1000 mg once daily at bedtime with further titration to 2000 mg depending on patient response. Doses greater than 2000 mg daily are not recommended.

The tablet strengths of NIASPAN are not interchangeable. Do not alternate between different strengths to provide the same daily dosage. The physician should specify the tablet strengths that the patient should use during titration and continue to use for maintenance therapy.

Women may respond at lower NIASPAN doses than men (see Action and Clinical Pharmacology, Special Populations and Conditions, Sex).

If lipid response to NIASPAN alone is insufficient or if higher doses of NIASPAN are not well tolerated, some patients may benefit from combination therapy with a bile acid binding resin or an HMG CoA reductase inhibitor (see Drug Interactions).

Flushing of the skin (see Adverse Reactions) may be reduced in frequency or severity by pretreatment with ASA (taken 30 minutes prior to NIASPAN dose) or non-steroidal anti-inflammatory drugs. Tolerance to this flushing develops rapidly over the course of several weeks. Flushing, pruritus, and gastrointestinal distress are also greatly reduced by slowly increasing the dose of NIASPAN and avoiding administration on an empty stomach (see Warning and Precautions, General).

Equivalent doses of NIASPAN should not be substituted for sustained-release (modified-release, timed-release) niacin preparations or immediate-release (crystalline) niacin and visa versa (see Warnings and Precautions). This should be explained to patients. Patients previously receiving other niacin products should be started with the recommended NIASPAN titration schedule (see Table 2).

If NIASPAN therapy is discontinued for an extended period, reinstitution of therapy should include a titration phase (see Table 2).

Dosage in Patients with Renal Insufficiency: Use of NIASPAN in patients with renal insufficiency has not been studied. No information is available regarding the safety of NIASPAN use in patients with renal insufficiency.

Dosage in Patients with Hepatic Insufficiency: Use of NIASPAN in patients with hepatic insufficiency has not been studied. NIASPAN is contraindicated in patients with significant or unexplained hepatic dysfunction (see Contraindications).

Missed Dose: If a dose of this medication is missed, it is not necessary to make up the missed dose. Skip the missed dose and continue with the next scheduled dose. Do not double doses.

Administration: NIASPAN tablets should be taken whole and should not be broken, crushed or chewed before swallowing.

OVERDOSAGE:
Supportive measures should be undertaken in the event of an overdose.

For management of a suspected drug overdose, CPhA recommends that you contact your **regional Poison Control Centre**. See the *CPS* Directory section for a list of Poison Control Centres.

ACTION AND CLINICAL PHARMACOLOGY: Mechanism of Action: The mechanism by which niacin alters lipid profiles has not been well defined. It may involve several actions including partial inhibition of release of free fatty acids from adipose tissue, and increased lipoprotein lipase activity, which may increase the rate of chylomicron triglyceride removal from plasma. Niacin decreases the rate of hepatic synthesis of VLDL and LDL, and does not appear to affect fecal excretion of fats, sterols, or bile acids.

Pharmacodynamics: Niacin functions in the body after conversion to nicotinamide adenine dinucleotide (NAD) in the NAD coenzyme system. Niacin (but **not** nicotinamide) in gram doses reduces TC, LDL-C and TG, and increases HDL-C. The magnitude of individual lipid and lipoprotein responses may be influenced by the severity and type of underlying lipid abnormality. The increase in HDL-C is associated with an increase in apolipoprotein A-I (Apo A-I) and a shift in the distribution of HDL subfractions. These shifts include an increase in the HDL_2:HDL_3 ratio, and an elevation in lipoprotein A-I (Lp A-I, an HDL particle containing only Apo A-I). Niacin treatment also decreases serum levels of Apo B, the major protein component of the VLDL and LDL fractions, and of lipoprotein a (Lp(a)), a variant form of LDL independently associated with coronary risk. In addition, niacin has been shown to cause favourable transformations in LDL particle size subclass distribution, converting the pattern B phenotype (characterised by a predominance of triglyceride-rich, small dense LDL) to pattern A (characterised by a predominance of large buoyant LDL) or the intermediate AB phenotype. Pattern B LDL phenotype is one manifestation of what has been termed the Atherogenic Lipoprotein Profile (ALP), a Mendelian dominant inherited condition which also includes low levels of HDL-C, raised triglyceride, and insulin resistance.

Epidemiologic, clinical and experimental studies have established that high LDL cholesterol (LDL-C), low High Density Lipoprotein cholesterol (HDL-C) and high plasma triglycerides (TG) promote human atherosclerosis and are risk factors for developing cardiovascular disease. Some studies have also shown that the total cholesterol (TC):HDL-C ratio (TC:HDL-C) is the best predictor of coronary artery disease. In addition, increased levels of HDL-C are associated with decreased cardiovascular risk. Drug therapies that reduce levels of LDL-C or decrease TG while simultaneously increasing HDL-C have demonstrated reductions in rates of cardiovascular mortality and morbidity.

Pharmacokinetics: Absorption: Niacin is rapidly and extensively absorbed (at least 60 to 76% of dose) when administered orally. To maximize bioavailability, administration of NIASPAN (extended-release niacin) with a low-fat meal or snack is recommended.

Single-dose bioavailability studies have demonstrated that NIASPAN tablet strengths are not interchangeable.

Distribution: Studies using radiolabeled niacin in mice showed that niacin and its metabolites concentrate in the liver, kidney and adipose tissue.

Metabolism: The pharmacokinetic profile of niacin is complicated due to rapid and extensive first-pass metabolism, which is species and dose-rate specific. In humans, one pathway is through a simple conjugation step with glycine to form nicotinuric acid which is then excreted in the urine, although there may be a small amount of reversible metabolism back to niacin. The other pathway results in the formation of nicotine adenine dinucleotide (NAD). It is unclear whether nicotinamide is formed as a precursor to, or following the synthesis of NAD. Nicotinamide is further metabolized to at least N-methylnicotinamide (MNA) and nicotinamide-N-oxide. MNA is further metabolized to two other compounds, N-methyl-2-pyridone-5-carboxamide (2PY) and N-methyl-4-pyridone-5-carboxamide (4PY). The formation of 2PY appears to predominate over 4PY in humans. At the doses used to treat hyperlipidaemia, these metabolic pathways are saturable, which explains the nonlinear relationship between niacin dose and plasma concentrations following multiple-dose NIASPAN administration (Table 3).

Table 3: NIASPAN

Mean Steady-state Pharmacokinetic Parameters for Plasma Niacin

NIASPAN		Niacin		
Dose/Day	**Given as**	**Peak Concentration (µg/mL)**	**Time to Peak (h)**	**AUC (µg·h/mL)**
1000 mg	2×500 mg	0.6	5	0.6
1500 mg	2×750 mg	4.9	4	9.1
2000 mg	2×1000 mg	15.5	5	46.2

Nicotinamide does not have hypolipidaemic activity; the activity of the other metabolites is unknown.

Excretion: Niacin and its metabolites are rapidly eliminated in the urine. Following single and multiple doses, approximately 60 to 75% of the niacin dose administered as NIASPAN was recovered in urine as niacin and metabolites; up to 12% was recovered as unchanged niacin after multiple dosing. The ratio of metabolites recovered in the urine was dependent on the dose administered.

Special Populations and Conditions: Pediatrics: No studies in patients under 21 years of age have been conducted with NIASPAN.

Geriatrics: No data is available.

Sex: Steady-state plasma concentrations of niacin and metabolites after administration of NIASPAN are generally higher in women than in men. Recovery of niacin and metabolites in urine, however, is generally similar for men and women, indicating that absorption is similar for both sexes. Data from the clinical trials suggest that women have a greater hypolipidaemic response than men at equivalent doses of NIASPAN.

Hepatic Insufficiency: No studies have been performed. NIASPAN should be used with caution in patients with a past history of liver disease, who consume substantial quantities of alcohol. NIASPAN is contraindicated in patients with active liver disease or unexplained transaminase elevations (see Contraindications, and Warnings and Precautions, Hepatic/Biliary/Pancreatic).

Renal Insufficiency: There are no data available on the use of NIASPAN in patients with impaired renal function (see Warnings and Precautions).

STORAGE AND STABILITY: Temperature: Store at room temperature, (15 to 30°C).

Others: Keep in a safe place out of the reach of children.

INFORMATION FOR THE PATIENT: Published in e-CPS, available by subscription at www.e-cps.ca.

DOSAGE FORMS, COMPOSITION AND PACKAGING: 500 mg: Each unscored, off-white, capsule-shaped, extended-release tablet, debossed with 500 on one side, contains niacin 500 mg. Nonmedicinal ingredients: methylcellulose, povidone and stearic acid. Bottles of 100.
750 mg: Each unscored, off-white, capsule-shaped, extended-release tablet, debossed with 750 on one side, contains niacin 750 mg. Nonmedicinal ingredients: methylcellulose, povidone and stearic acid. Bottles of 100.
1000 mg: Each unscored, off-white, capsule-shaped, extended-release tablet, debossed with 1000 on one side, contains niacin 1000 mg. Nonmedicinal ingredients: methylcellulose, povidone and stearic acid. Bottles of 100.

The reader is invited to consult CPhA's monograph **Niacin/Niacinamide**.

Niaspan FCT® ℞

niacin

Lipid Metabolism Regulator

Sepracor

Date of Preparation: August 18, 2009

SUMMARY PRODUCT INFORMATION:

Route of Administration	Dosage Form/ Strength	Clinically Relevant Nonmedicinal Ingredients
Oral	500 mg, 750 mg, 1000 mg extended-release film coated tablets	Methylcellulose, povidone, stearic acid

INDICATIONS AND CLINICAL USE: NIASPAN FCT (extended-release niacin) is indicated as an adjunct to diet for reduction of elevated total cholesterol (TC), low-density lipoprotein cholesterol (LDL-C), apolipoprotein B (Apo B) and triglyceride (TG) levels, and to increase high-density lipoprotein cholesterol (HDL-C) in patients with primary hypercholesterolaemia (heterozygous familial and nonfamilial) and mixed dyslipidaemia (Fredrickson Types IIa and IIb), when the response to an appropriate diet and other non-pharmacological measures have been inadequate.

Therapy with NIASPAN FCT should be only one component of multiple risk factor intervention in individuals at significantly increased risk for atherosclerotic vascular disease due to hypercholesterolemia. Prior to initiating therapy with NIASPAN FCT, secondary causes for hypercholesterolemia (e.g., poorly controlled diabetes mellitus, hypothyroidism, nephrotic syndrome, dysproteinemias, obstructive liver disease, other drug therapy, alcoholism) should be excluded, and a lipid profile obtained to measure TC, HDL-C, and TG.

Pediatrics: No studies in patients under 21 years of age have been conducted with NIASPAN FCT.

CONTRAINDICATIONS:

- NIASPAN FCT (extended-release niacin) is contraindicated in patients with a known hypersensitivity to niacin or any component of this medication (see Dosage Forms, Composition and Packaging).
- Active liver disease or unexplained persistent elevations of serum transaminases, active peptic ulcer, or active bleeding.

WARNINGS AND PRECAUTIONS:

Serious Warnings and Precautions

- NIASPAN FCT (extended-release niacin) preparations should not be substituted for equivalent doses of immediate-release (crystalline) niacin or nicotinic acid. For patients switching from immediate-release niacin or nicotinic acid to NIASPAN FCT, therapy with NIASPAN FCT should be initiated with low doses (i.e., 500 mg qhs) and the NIASPAN FCT dose should then be titrated to the desired therapeutic response.
- Cases of severe hepatic toxicity, including fulminant hepatic necrosis, have occurred in patients who have substituted sustained-release (modified-release, timed-release) niacin products for immediate-release (crystalline) niacin at equivalent doses.

Clinically significant warnings and precautions are listed below in alphabetical order.

General: Before instituting therapy with NIASPAN FCT, an attempt should be made to control hyperlipidaemia with appropriate diet, exercise, and weight reduction in obese patients, and to treat other underlying medical problems (see Indications and Clinical Use).

While pretreatment with acetylsalicylic acid (ASA) or other non-steroidal anti-inflammatory drugs (NSAIDs) may reduce flushing of the skin, some patients should not take these medications (e.g., patients who have peptic ulcer or active inflammatory disease of the gastrointestinal system or ASA hypersensitivity; refer to the Product Monograph for the NSAID product).

Cardiovascular: Data on the safety and efficacy of NIASPAN FCT in patients with unstable angina or in the acute phase of myocardial infarction are not available. Therefore, caution should be used when NIASPAN FCT is used, particularly when such patients are also receiving vasodilator agents.

Endocrine and Metabolism: Elevated uric acid levels have occurred with niacin therapy, therefore use with caution in patients predisposed to gout.

In placebo-controlled trials, extended-release niacin has been associated with small but statistically significant, dose-related reductions in phosphorus levels (mean of −13% with 2000 mg). Although these reductions were transient, phosphorus levels should be monitored periodically in patients at risk for hypophosphatemia.

Periodic serum creatine phosphokinase (CPK) and potassium determinations should be carried out.

Gastrointestinal: Patients with a past history of jaundice or peptic ulcer should be observed closely during NIASPAN FCT therapy.

Hematologic: Extended-release niacin has been associated with small, but statistically significant dose-related reductions in platelet count (mean of −11% with 2000 mg). In addition, extended-release niacin has been associated with small but statistically significant increases in prothrombin time (mean of approximately +4% with 2000 mg); accordingly, patients undergoing surgery should be carefully evaluated. Caution should be observed when NIASPAN FCT is administered concomitantly with anticoagulants; prothrombin time and platelet counts should be monitored closely in such patients.

Hepatic/Biliary/Pancreatic: No clinical studies have been carried out in patients with impaired liver function.

Patients with a past history of jaundice, hepatobiliary disease, or peptic ulcer should be observed closely during NIASPAN FCT therapy. Frequent monitoring of liver function tests and blood glucose should be performed.

NIASPAN FCT should be used with caution in patients who consume substantial quantities of alcohol and/or have a past history of liver disease.

Niacin preparations have been associated with abnormal liver tests. In three placebo-controlled clinical trials involving titration to final daily extended-release niacin doses ranging from 500 to 3000 mg, 245 patients received extended-release niacin for a mean duration of 17 weeks and no patient with normal serum transaminase levels (AST, ALT) at baseline experienced elevations to more than 3 times the upper limit of normal (ULN). In these studies, fewer than 1% (2/245) of extended-release niacin patients discontinued due to transaminase elevations greater than 2 times the ULN.

In three safety and efficacy studies with a combination tablet of extended-release niacin and lovastatin involving titration to final daily doses (expressed as mg of extended-release niacin/mg of lovastatin) 500 mg/10 mg to 2500 mg/40 mg, ten of 1028 patients (1.0%) experienced reversible elevations in AST/ALT to more than 3 times the upper limit of normal (ULN). Three of ten elevations occurred at doses outside the recommended dosing limit of 2000 mg/40 mg; no patient receiving 1000 mg/20 mg had 3-fold elevations in AST/ALT.

In the placebo-controlled clinical trials and the long-term extension study, elevations in transaminases did not appear to be related to treatment duration. However, elevations in AST levels did appear to be dose related. Transaminase elevations were reversible upon discontinuation of extended-release niacin.

Diabetic patients may experience a dose-related rise in glucose tolerance. Diabetic or potentially diabetic patients with hypercholesterolaemia should be observed closely. Adjustment of diet and/or hypoglycemic therapy may be necessary.

Renal: No clinical studies have been carried out in patients with impaired renal function. Niacin and its metabolites are excreted through the kidneys. NIASPAN FCT should be used with caution in patients with renal dysfunction.

Skeletal Muscle: Rare cases of rhabdomyolysis have been associated with concomitant administration of lipid-altering doses (≥1 g/day) of niacin and HMG-CoA reductase inhibitors. In clinical studies with a combination tablet of extended-release niacin and lovastatin, no cases of rhabdomyolysis and one suspected case of myopathy have been reported in 1079 patients who were treated with doses up to 2000 mg of extended-release niacin and 40 mg of lovastatin daily for periods up to 2 years. Physicians contemplating combined therapy with HMG-CoA reductase inhibitors and NIASPAN FCT should carefully weigh the potential benefits and risks and should carefully monitor patients for any signs and symptoms of muscle pain, tenderness, or weakness, particularly during the initial months of therapy and during any periods of upward dosage titration of either drug. Periodic serum creatine phosphokinase (CPK) and potassium determinations should be considered in such situations, but there is no assurance that such monitoring will prevent the occurrence of severe myopathy.

Special Populations: Pregnant Women: No information is available on the safety of NIASPAN FCT in pregnant women. Animal reproduction studies have not been conducted with niacin or with NIASPAN FCT. It is not known whether niacin at doses used for lipid disorders can cause fetal harm when administered to pregnant women or whether it can affect reproductive capacity. If a woman receiving treatment with NIASPAN FCT becomes pregnant, the drug should be discontinued.

Nursing Women: No information is available on the safety of NIASPAN FCT in nursing women. Niacin has been reported to be excreted in human milk. Because of the potential for serious adverse reactions in nursing infants, a decision should be made whether to discontinue nursing or to discontinue the drug.

Pediatrics: Safety and effectiveness of niacin therapy in pediatric patients have not been established. No studies in patients under 21 years of age have been conducted with NIASPAN FCT.

Geriatrics: No formal studies have been carried out in elderly patients. Patients up to 75 years of age participated in controlled clinical trials of NIASPAN FCT.

Monitoring and Laboratory Tests: Liver tests should be performed on all patients during therapy with NIASPAN FCT. Serum transaminase levels, including AST and ALT, should be monitored before treatment begins, every 6 to 12 weeks for the first year, and periodically thereafter (e.g., at 6 month intervals). Special attention should be paid to patients who develop elevated serum transaminase levels. In these patients, measurements should be repeated promptly and then performed more frequently. If the transaminase levels show evidence of progression, particularly if they rise to 3 times ULN and are persistent, or if they are associated with symptoms of nausea, fever, and/or malaise, the drug should be discontinued.

ADVERSE REACTIONS: Adverse Drug Reaction Overview: The most frequently-reported events with NIASPAN FCT (extended-release niacin) are flushing episodes, which generally become less common as treatment progresses and which may be reduced by concomitant acetylsalicylic acid (ASA) therapy and by following the recommended dose titration schedule (see Warnings and Precautions, General).

In the placebo-controlled clinical trials, flushing episodes (i.e., warmth, redness, itching and/or tingling) were the most common treatment-emergent adverse events for extended-release niacin, reported in up to 88% of patients. Spontaneous reports suggest that flushing may also be accompanied by symptoms of dizziness, tachycardia, palpitations, shortness of breath, sweating, chills, and/or edema, which in rare cases may lead to syncope. In pivotal studies, fewer than 6% (14/245) of extended-release niacin patients discontinued due to flushing. Following 4 weeks of maintenance therapy with extended-release niacin at daily doses of 1500 mg, the incidence of flushing over the 4-week period averaged 8.56 events per patient for IR niacin versus 1.88 events per extended-release niacin patient.

Other commonly reported non-serious events include gastrointestinal symptoms and rash. The majority of adverse events reported were mild and transient.

In general, the incidence of adverse events was higher in women compared to men.

Niacin therapy has been associated with abnormalities of liver function. In patients receiving NIASPAN FCT, liver function should be periodically monitored.

Clinical Trial Adverse Drug Reactions: Because clinical trials are conducted under very specific conditions the adverse reaction rates observed in the clinical trials may not reflect the rates observed in practice and should not be compared to the rates in the clinical trials of another drug. Adverse drug reaction information from clinical trials is useful for identifying drug-related adverse events and for approximating rates.

Based on the experience in a total of 723 patients, of whom 477 were treated with extended-release niacin for one year (48 weeks) and 379 for 2 years (96 weeks), the majority of adverse events were mild and transient.

Adverse events occurring at an incidence of ≥2% in patients treated with extended-release niacin during premarketing controlled studies are shown in Table 1 by body system.

Table 1: NIASPAN FCT

Treatment-Emergent Adverse Events by Dose Level in ≥2% of Patients and at an Incidence Greater than Placebo, Regardless of Causality

Placebo-Controlled Studies		
	Placebo	Extended-release Niacin (All Doses)
Total # of Patients	157	245
Body As a Whole		
Asthenia	3%	4%
Chills	1%	3%
Fever	3%	7%
Flu Syndrome	5%	7%
Pain, Abdominal	6%	8%
Pain, Back	7%	9%
Pain, Chest	2%	6%
Surgical Procedure	1%	2%
Cardiovascular System		
Migraine	1%	2%
Palpitation	1%	3%
Tachycardia	0	2%
Digestive System		
Diarrhea	13%	20%
Dyspepsia	12%	13%
Eructation	1%	2%
Nausea	7%	13%
Vomiting	4%	7%

(cont'd)

Table 1: NIASPAN FCT *(cont'd)*

Treatment-Emergent Adverse Events by Dose Level in ≥2% of Patients and at an Incidence Greater than Placebo, Regardless of Causality

	Placebo-Controlled Studies	
	Placebo	**Extended-release Niacin (All Doses)**
Metabolism & Nutritional Disorders		
Edema	1%	2%
Edema, Peripheral	0	2%
Musculoskeletal System		
Arthralgia	0	3%
Arthritis	2%	3%
Nervous System		
Dry Mouth	0	2%
Somnolence	1%	2%
Respiratory System		
Cough, Increase	6%	7%
Rhinitis	31%	34%
Skin & Appendages		
Pruritus	2%	6%
Rash	1%	7%
Skin Discoloration	1%	3%
Sweating	1%	2%
Urticaria	1%	2%
Special Senses		
Tinnitus	1%	2%

Less Common Clinical Trial Adverse Drug Reactions (<2%): The following adverse events have been reported with extended-release niacin or other niacin products, either during clinical trials or in routine patient management, irrespective of causality.
Body as a Whole: enlarged abdomen, cyst, hernia, mucous membrane disorder, face edema.
Cardiovascular: angina pectoris, cardiovascular disorder, hemorrhage, atrial fibrillation and other cardiac arrhythmias, hypotension, orthostasis, syncope.
Digestive: cholelith, dysphagia, esophagitis, GI hemorrhage, fecal incontinence, stomatitis, tongue disorder, flatulence, activation of peptic ulcers and peptic ulceration, jaundice.
Hemic and Lymphatic: leucopenia.
Hypersensitivity Reactions: An apparent hypersensitivity reaction has been reported rarely that has included one or more of the following features: anaphylaxis, angioedema, urticaria, flushing, dyspnea, tongue edema, larynx edema, face edema, peripheral edema, laryngismus, and vesiculobullous rash, hypotension and circulatory collapse.
Metabolism and Nutritional Disorders: bilirubinemia, xanthoma, decreased glucose tolerance, anorexia, gout.
Musculoskeletal: bone disorder, bursitis, myasthenia, rhabdomyolysis, myalgia, myopathy.
Nervous: hypertonia, hypesthesia, hypokinesia, increased libido, twitch, vertigo, leg cramps; nervousness; paresthesia, dizziness, headache, insomnia.
Respiratory: bronchitis, hemoptysis, hyperventilation, laryngitis, lung disorder, dyspnea.
Skin and Appendages: acne, alopecia, application site reaction, contact dermatitis, fungal dermatitis, eczema, herpes zoster, skin neoplasm, vesiculobullous rash, dry skin, skin ulcer, general exanthema, hyperpigmentation, acanthosis nigricans, maculopapular rash.
Special Senses: eye disorder, glaucoma, vision abnormal, toxic amblyopia, cystoid macular edema.
Urogenital: impotence, breast pain, polyuria, prostatic disorder, UG disorder, urinary retention, vaginitis.
Abnormal Hematologic and Clinical Chemistry Findings: Chemistry: elevations in serum transaminases (see Warnings and Precautions, Hepatic/Biliary/Pancreatic), LDH, fasting glucose, uric acid, total bilirubin, and amylase; reductions in phosphorus.
Hematology: slight reductions in platelet counts and prolongation in prothrombin time (see Warnings and Precautions, Hematologic).
Post-Market Adverse Drug Reactions: In post-market safety surveillance, flushing, headache, tachycardia, asthenia, insomnia, and maculopapular rash were the most frequently reported non-serious adverse events.
DRUG INTERACTIONS: Overview: HMG-CoA Reductase Inhibitors: Rhabdomyolysis has been rarely reported in patients receiving niacin concomitantly with an HMG-CoA reductase inhibitor (statin) (see Warnings and Precautions).
Alcohol or **hot drinks** taken at the time of NIASPAN FCT (extended-release niacin) administration may worsen the flushing response and pruritus.
Antihypertensive Therapy: Niacin may potentiate the effects of ganglionic blocking agents and vasoactive drugs resulting in postural hypotension.
Acetylsalicylic acid (ASA): Concomitant administration of ASA may decrease the metabolic clearance of niacin (see Warnings and Precautions, General).
Bile-Acid Sequestrants: An interval of 4 to 6 hours, or as great an interval as possible, should elapse between the ingestion of bile acid-binding resins and the administration of NIASPAN FCT. An in vitro study showed that about 98% of available niacin was bound to colestipol, and 10 to 30% was bound to cholestyramine.
Other: Vitamins or other nutritional supplements containing large doses of niacin or related compounds such as nicotinamide may potentiate the adverse effects of NIASPAN FCT.
Drug-Food Interactions: Concomitant alcohol or hot drinks may increase the side effects of flushing and pruritus and should be avoided around the time of NIASPAN FCT ingestion.
Drug-Herb Interactions: Interactions with herbal products have not been studied.
Drug-Laboratory Test Interactions: Niacin may produce false elevations in some fluorometric determinations of plasma or urinary catecholamines. Niacin may also give false-positive reactions with cupric sulfate solution (Benedict's reagent) in urine glucose tests.

DOSAGE AND ADMINISTRATION:

Patients should be placed on a standard cholesterol-lowering diet at least equivalent to the NCEP Adult Treatment Panel III TLC diet before receiving NIASPAN FCT (extended-release niacin) and should continue on this diet during treatment with NIASPAN FCT. If appropriate, a program of weight control and physical exercise should be implemented.

Dosing Considerations:
- Equivalent doses of NIASPAN FCT should not be substituted for immediate-release (crystalline) niacin.
- If lipid response to NIASPAN FCT alone is insufficient, or if higher doses of NIASPAN FCT are not well tolerated, some patients may benefit from combination therapy with a bile acid binding resin or an HMG-CoA reductase inhibitor.
- Patients already receiving a stable dose of a statin who require further TG lowering or HDL raising, may receive concomitant NIASPAN FCT administered according to the initial titration schedule.
- Women may respond at lower NIASPAN FCT doses than men.
- Flushing of the skin may be reduced in frequency or severity by pretreatment with acetylsalicylic acid and avoiding administration on an empty stomach (see Warnings and Precautions, General).
- NIASPAN FCT is contraindicated in patients with significant or unexplained hepatic dysfunction.
- No information is available on the safety of NIASPAN FCT in patients with renal insufficiency.

Recommended Dose and Dosage Adjustment: NIASPAN FCT should be taken only once per day in the evening or before bedtime, after a low-fat snack, and doses should be individualized according to patient response. Therapy with NIASPAN FCT must be initiated at 500 mg, in order to reduce the incidence and severity of side effects which may occur during early therapy. The recommended dose escalation is shown in Table 2.

Table 2: NIASPAN FCT

Recommended Dosing

	Week(s)	Daily Dose
Titration Schedule	1 to 4 5 to 8	500 mg 1000 mg
Further Titration Schedule[a]	After Week 8	1500 mg 2000 mg

[a] After Week 8, titrate to patient response and tolerance. If response to 1000 mg daily is inadequate, increase dose to 1500 mg daily; may subsequently increase dose to 2000 mg daily. Daily dose should not be increased more than 500 mg in a 4-week period, and doses above 2000 mg daily are not recommended.

Maintenance Dose: The daily dosage of NIASPAN FCT should not be increased by more than 500 mg in any 4-week period. The recommended maintenance dose is 1000 mg once daily in the evening or at bedtime with further titration to 2000 mg depending on patient response. Doses greater than 2000 mg daily are not recommended.

Single-dose bioavailability studies have demonstrated that two of the 500 mg and one of the 1000 mg tablet strengths are interchangeable but three of the 500 mg and two of the 750 mg tablet strengths are not interchangeable. The physician should specify the tablet strengths that the patient should use during titration and continue to use for maintenance therapy, accordingly.

Women may respond at lower NIASPAN FCT doses than men (see Action And Clinical Pharmacology, Special Populations and Conditions, Gender).

If lipid response to NIASPAN FCT alone is insufficient or if higher doses of NIASPAN FCT are not well tolerated, some patients may benefit from combination therapy with a bile acid binding resin or an HMG CoA reductase inhibitor (see Drug Interactions).

Flushing of the skin (see Adverse Reactions) may be reduced in frequency or severity by pretreatment with ASA (taken 30 minutes prior to NIASPAN FCT dose) or non-steroidal anti-inflammatory drugs. Tolerance to this flushing develops rapidly over the course of several weeks. Flushing, pruritus, and gastrointestinal distress are also greatly reduced by slowly increasing the dose of NIASPAN FCT and avoiding administration on an empty stomach (see Warning and Precautions, General).

Equivalent doses of NIASPAN FCT should not be substituted for sustained-release (modified-release, timed-release) niacin preparations or immediate-release (crystalline) niacin and visa versa (see Warnings and Precautions). This should be explained to patients. Patients previously receiving other niacin products should be started with the recommended NIASPAN FCT titration schedule (see Table 2).

If NIASPAN FCT therapy is discontinued for an extended period, reinstitution of therapy should include a titration phase (see Table 2).

Dosage in Patients with Renal Insufficiency: Use of NIASPAN FCT in patients with renal insufficiency has not been studied. No information is available regarding the safety of NIASPAN FCT use in patients with renal insufficiency.
Dosage in Patients with Hepatic Insufficiency: Use of NIASPAN FCT in patients with hepatic insufficiency has not been studied. NIASPAN FCT is contraindicated in patients with significant or unexplained hepatic dysfunction (see Contraindications).
Missed Dose: If a dose of this medication is missed, it is not necessary to make up the missed dose. Skip the missed dose and continue with the next scheduled dose. Do not double doses.
Administration: NIASPAN FCT tablets should be taken whole and should not be broken, crushed or chewed before swallowing.

OVERDOSAGE:
Supportive measures should be undertaken in the event of an overdose.

For management of a suspected drug overdose, CPhA recommends that you contact your **regional Poison Control Centre**. See the *CPS* Directory section for a list of Poison Control Centres.

ACTION AND CLINICAL PHARMACOLOGY: Mechanism of Action: The mechanism by which niacin alters lipid profiles has not been well defined. It may involve several actions including partial inhibition of release of free fatty acids from adipose tissue, and increased lipoprotein lipase activity, which may increase the rate of chylomicron triglyceride removal from plasma. Niacin decreases the rate of hepatic synthesis of VLDL and LDL, and does not appear to affect fecal excretion of fats, sterols, or bile acids.
Pharmacodynamics: Niacin functions in the body after conversion to nicotinamide adenine dinucleotide (NAD) in the NAD coenzyme system. Niacin (but **not** nicotinamide) in gram doses reduces TC, LDL-C and TG, and increases HDL-C. The magnitude of individual lipid and lipoprotein responses may be influenced by the severity and type of underlying lipid abnormality. The increase in HDL-C is associated with an increase in apolipoprotein A-I (Apo A-I) and a shift in the distribution of HDL subfractions. These shifts include an increase in the HDL_2:HDL_3 ratio, and an elevation in lipoprotein A-I (Lp A-I, an HDL particle containing only Apo A-I). Niacin treatment also decreases serum levels of Apo B, the major protein component of the VLDL and LDL fractions, and of lipoprotein a (Lp(a)), a variant form of LDL independently associated with coronary risk. In addition, niacin has been shown to cause favourable transformations in LDL particle size subclass distribution, converting the pattern B phenotype (characterised by a predominance of triglyceride-rich, small dense LDL) to pattern A (characterised by a predominance of large buoyant LDL) or the intermediate AB phenotype. Pattern B LDL phenotype is one manifestation of what has been termed the Atherogenic Lipoprotein Profile (ALP), a Mendelian dominant inherited condition which also includes low levels of HDL-C, raised triglyceride, and insulin resistance.

Epidemiologic, clinical and experimental studies have established that high LDL cholesterol (LDL-C), low High Density Lipoprotein cholesterol (HDL-C) and high plasma trigylcerides (TG) promote human atherosclerosis and are risk factors for developing cardiovascular disease. Some studies have also shown that the total cholesterol (TC):HDL-C ratio (TC:HDL-C) is the best predictor of coronary artery disease. In addition, increased levels of HDL-C are associated with decreased cardiovascular risk. Drug therapies that reduce levels of LDL-C or decrease TG while simultaneously increasing HDL-C have demonstrated reductions in rates of cardiovascular mortality and morbidity.
Pharmacokinetics: Absorption: Niacin is rapidly and extensively absorbed (at least 60 to 76% of dose) when administered orally. To maximize bioavailability, administration of NIASPAN FCT (extended-release niacin) with a low-fat meal or snack is recommended.
Distribution: Studies using radiolabeled niacin in mice showed that niacin and its metabolites concentrate in the liver, kidney and adipose tissue.
Metabolism: The pharmacokinetic profile of niacin is complicated due to rapid and extensive first-pass metabolism, which is species and dose-rate specific. In humans, one pathway is through a simple conjugation step with glycine to form nicotinuric acid which is then excreted in the urine, although there may be a small amount of reversible metabolism back to niacin. The other pathway results in the formation of nicotine adenine dinucleotide (NAD). It is unclear whether nicotinamide is formed as a precursor to, or following the synthesis of NAD. Nicotinamide is further metabolized to at least N-methylnicotinamide (MNA) and nicotinamide-N-oxide. MNA is further metabolized to two other compounds, N-methyl-2-pyridone-5-carboxamide (2PY) and

N-methyl-4-pyridone-5-carboxamide (4PY). The formation of 2PY appears to predominate over 4PY in humans. At the doses used to treat hyperlipidaemia, these metabolic pathways are saturable, which explains the nonlinear relationship between niacin dose and plasma concentrations following multiple-dose extended-release niacin administration (Table 3).

Table 3: NIASPAN FCT

Mean Steady-State Pharmacokinetic Parameters for Plasma Niacin

Extended-release Niacin		Niacin		
Dose/day	**given as**	**Peak Concentration (μg/mL)**	**Time to Peak (hr)**	**AUC (μg·hr/mL)**
1000 mg	2×500 mg	0.6	5	0.6
1500 mg	2×750 mg	4.9	4	9.1
2000 mg	2×1000 mg	15.5	5	46.2

Nicotinamide does not have hypolipidaemic activity; the activity of the other metabolites is unknown.

Excretion: Niacin and its metabolites are rapidly eliminated in the urine. Following single and multiple doses, approximately 60 to 75% of the niacin dose administered as extended-release niacin was recovered in urine as niacin and metabolites; up to 12% was recovered as unchanged niacin after multiple dosing. The ratio of metabolites recovered in the urine was dependent on the dose administered.

Special Populations and Conditions: Pediatrics: No studies in patients under 21 years of age have been conducted with NIASPAN FCT.

Geriatrics: No data is available.

Gender: Steady-state plasma concentrations of niacin and metabolites after administration of extended-release niacin are generally higher in women than in men. Recovery of niacin and metabolites in urine, however, is generally similar for men and women, indicating that absorption is similar for both sexes. Data from the clinical trials suggest that women have a greater hypolipidaemic response than men at equivalent doses of extended-release niacin.

Hepatic Insufficiency: No studies have been performed. NIASPAN FCT should be used with caution in patients with a past history of liver disease, who consume substantial quantities of alcohol. NIASPAN FCT is contraindicated in patients with active liver disease or unexplained transaminase elevations (see Contraindications, and Warnings and Precautions, Hepatic/Biliary/Pancreatic).

Renal Insufficiency: There are no data available on the use of NIASPAN FCT in patients with impaired renal function (see Warnings and Precautions).

STORAGE AND STABILITY: Temperature: Store at room temperature, (15 to 30°C).

Others: Keep in a safe place out of the reach of children.

INFORMATION FOR THE PATIENT: Published in e-CPS, available by subscription at www.e-cps.ca.

DOSAGE FORMS, COMPOSITION AND PACKAGING: 500 mg: Each unscored, medium-orange, extended-release, film coated tablet for oral administration, debossed with 500 on one side, contains: extended-release niacin 500 mg. Nonmedicinal ingredients: methylcellulose, polyethylene glycol, povidone, stearic acid, titanium dioxide and the following coloring agents: FD&C yellow #6/sunset yellow FCF Aluminum Lake, synthetic red and yellow iron oxides. Bottles of 90.

750 mg: Each unscored, medium-orange, extended-release, film coated tablet for oral administration, debossed with 750 on one side, contains: extended-release niacin 750 mg. Nonmedicinal ingredients: methylcellulose, polyethylene glycol, povidone, stearic acid, titanium dioxide and the following coloring agents: FD&C yellow #6/sunset yellow FCF Aluminum Lake, synthetic red and yellow iron oxides. Bottles of 90.

1000 mg: Each unscored, medium-orange, extended-release, film coated tablet for oral administration, debossed with 1000 on one side, contains: extended-release niacin 1000 mg. Nonmedicinal ingredients: methylcellulose, polyethylene glycol, povidone, stearic acid, titanium dioxide and the following coloring agents: FD&C yellow #6/sunset yellow FCF Aluminum Lake, synthetic red and yellow iron oxides. Bottles of 90.

NiaStase RT®

eptacog alfa (activated)

Coagulation Factor

Novo Nordisk

Date of Preparation: March 18, 2010

SUMMARY PRODUCT INFORMATION:

Route of Administration	Dosage Form/ Strength	Clinically Relevant Nonmedicinal Ingredients
Intravenous bolus injection	Lyophilized powder to be reconstituted for injection/ 1.0 mg (50 KIU) 2.0 mg (100 KIU) 5.0 mg (250 KIU)	Calcium chloride dihydrate, glycylglycine, mannitol, methionine, polysorbate 80, sodium chloride, sucrose The solvent for reconstitution of NiaStase RT contains histidine in water for injections. For a complete listing of nonmedicinal ingredients see Dosage Forms, Composition and Packaging.

DESCRIPTION: NiaStase RT (eptacog alfa, activated) contains activated recombinant human blood coagulation Factor VII (rFVIIa) (eptacog alfa, activated). Recombinant Factor VII is a vitamin K-dependent glycoprotein consisting of 406 amino acids (MW approximately 50 K Dalton), which is structurally similar to human plasma-derived Factor VIIa.

INDICATIONS AND CLINICAL USE: NiaStase RT (eptacog alfa, activated) is indicated:

- in hemophilia A/B patients with inhibitors to FVIII or FIX, respectively, for the treatment of bleeding episodes (including treatment and prevention of those occurring during and after surgery).

Based on the data obtained so far with rFVIIa in the treatment of hemophilia patients with inhibitors, the apparent lack of anamnestic response during and after exposure to rFVIIa makes it suitable for use in all inhibitor patients.

CONTRAINDICATIONS: Known hypersensitivity to the active substance, the excipients, or to mouse, hamster or bovine protein may be a contraindication to the use of NiaStase RT (eptacog alfa, activated).

WARNINGS AND PRECAUTIONS:

Serious Warnings and Precautions

- Both arterial and venous thromboembolic adverse events have been reported after treatment with rFVIIa, mostly in patients with predisposing concurrent risk factors. (See General under Warnings and Precautions; Pharmacodynamics, under Action and Clinical Pharmacology; Adverse Reactions.)
- Patients with inherent Factor VII deficiency may have pre-existing or may develop anti-Factor VII antibodies during therapy with NiaStase RT. The clinical significance of these antibodies is unknown. See Adverse Reactions.

General: The extent of the risk of thrombotic adverse events after treatment with rFVIIa in patients with hemophilia and inhibitors is not known, but is considered to be low.

Patients with disseminated intravascular coagulation (DIC), advanced atherosclerotic disease, crush injury, septicemia, or concomitant treatment with aPCCs/PCCs (activated or non-activated prothrombin complex concentrates) may have an increased risk of developing thrombotic events due to their underlying condition or concomitant treatment. Because the risk of thromboembolic complications, caution should be exercised when administering NiaStase RT (eptacog alfa, activated) to patients with a history of coronary heart disease, to patients with liver disease, to patients immobilized post-operatively, to neonates, or to patients at risk of thrombolembolic phenomena or disseminated intravascular coagulation. In each of these situations, the potential benefit of treatment with NiaStase RT should be weighed against the risk of these complications.

Clinical studies in non hemophilia patients indicated an increased risk of arterial thromboembolic adverse events with the use of rFVIIa including myocardial infarction, myocardial ischemia, cerebral infarction and cerebral ischemia.

Patients who receive NiaStase RT should be kept under close observation for signs and symptoms of unfavourable activation of the coagulation system or thrombosis. When there is laboratory confirmation of intravascular coagulation or presence of clinical thrombosis, the NiaStase RT dosage should be reduced or treatment stopped, depending on the patient's symptoms.

Patients self-administering NiaStase RT at home should be instructed not to exceed three doses. The duration of the ambulatory treatment should not exceed 24 hours. Patients should seek medical attention if bleeding is not controlled or if any unusual symptoms are experienced.

Patients receiving NiaStase RT should be directed in its appropriate use and informed of the benefits and risks associated with treatment. If home use is prescribed, a puncture-resistant container for the disposal of used syringes and needles should be supplied to the patient, and patients should be thoroughly instructed in the importance of proper disposal and cautioned against reuse of syringes and needles.

Hypersensitivity and anaphylaxis reactions have rarely been reported with the use of rFVIIa. Initial treatment with NiaStase RT would always be under medical supervision, where emergency treatment for anaphylaxis can be rapidly applied. Patients should be monitored and warned about the early signs of hypersensitivity reactions and anaphylaxis, and asked to contact a physician if needed.

As recombinant coagulation factor VIIa, NiaStase RT, may contain trace amounts of mouse IgG, bovine IgG and other residual culture proteins (hamster and bovine serum proteins), the remote possibility exists that patients treated with the product may develop hypersensitivity to these proteins. In such cases, treatment with i.v. antihistamines should be considered.

If allergic or anaphylactic-type reactions occur, the administration should be discontinued immediately. In case of shock, standard medical treatment for shock should be implemented. Patients should be informed of the early signs of hypersensitivity reactions. If such symptoms occur, the patient should be advised to discontinue use of the product immediately and contact their physician.

Carcinogenesis and Mutagenesis: No chronic carcinogenicity studies have been performed with NiaStase RT. Two mutagenicity studies have given no indication of carcinogenic potential for rFVIIa.

Special Populations: Pregnant Women: As a precautionary measure it is preferable to avoid the use of NiaStase RT during pregnancy. Data on a limited number of exposed pregnancies indicate no adverse effects of rFVIIa on pregnancy or on the health of the fetus/new-born child. To date, no other relevant epidemiological data are available. Animal studies do not indicate direct or indirect harmful effects with respect to pregnancy, embryonal/fetal development, parturition or postnatal development.

In patients receiving rFVIIa during delivery or post partum, thrombotic events such as myocardial infarction, pulmonary embolism, deep venous thrombosis, retinal artery occlusion, or cerebral ischemia were observed. In this period, patients are at increased risk for thrombotic complications. It is not known to which extent rFVIIa contributes to the occurrence of these events. No specific preventive actions can be recommended.

Nursing Women: It is unknown whether rFVIIa is excreted in human breast milk. The excretion of rFVIIa in milk has not been studied in animals. A decision on whether to continue/discontinue breast-feeding or to continue/discontinue therapy with NiaStase RT should be made taking into account the benefit of breast-feeding to the child and the benefit of NiaStase RT therapy to the woman.

Pediatrics (birth to 16 years of age): Evidence for the safety and effectiveness of rFVIIa has been obtained in the age groups up to adolescence (up to 16 years of age). When dosed on a body weight basis, the efficacy and safety of rFVIIa appear to be comparable in adult and pediatric patients. Available clinical trials and post marketing data show a faster clearance of FVII in children. However, the data are insufficient to support the recommendation of higher doses in children (see Action and Clinical Pharmacology, Pharmacokinetics).

Geriatrics (≥65 years of age): Clinical studies in hemophilia did not enrol geriatric patients.

Monitoring and Laboratory Tests: It should be noted that the therapeutic range of rFVIIa for hemostasis has not been identified in tests for prothrombin time (PT), aPTT, and plasma FVII clotting activity (FVII:C). For these reasons, coagulation parameters should be used only as an adjunct to the evaluation of clinical hemostasis to monitor the effectiveness and treatment schedule of NiaStase RT in patients.

Monitoring the effectiveness of therapy, the need for additional doses of NiaStase RT or a change to alternative therapy should be based on the changes in the clinical parameters of pain, swelling and joint mobility compared to baseline or, if following improvement in any of the above parameters; symptoms of a rebleed are present. See Table 1.

Table 1: NiaStase RT

Criteria for Administration of Additional Treatment

Subjects with persistent moderate or severe pain following rFVIIa treatment	Subjects with persistent mild pain following rFVIIa treatment
One or more of the clinical assessments (1 to 4) is fulfilled	Two or more of the clinical assessments (1 to 4) are fulfilled
1. Pain judged same/worse. 2. Swelling (evident before treatment as compared to baseline) judged same/worse. 3. Joint mobility (evident before treatment as compared to baseline) judged same/worse. 4. Following improvement in either pain, swelling or joint mobility; signs or symptoms of a rebleed are present.	

There is no requirement for monitoring of NiaStase RT therapy. Severity of bleeding condition and clinical response to NiaStase RT administration must guide dosing requirements.

After administration of rFVIIa, prothrombin time (PT) and activated partial thromboplastin time (aPTT) have been shown to shorten, however, no correlation has been demonstrated between PT and aPTT and clinical efficacy of rFVIIa.

ADVERSE REACTIONS: Adverse Drug Reaction Overview: The most serious adverse drug reactions observed in patients receiving rFVIIa are thrombotic events, however the extent of the risk of thrombotic adverse events after treatment with rFVIIa in individuals with hemophilia and inhibitors is considered to be low.

The most common adverse drug reactions observed for the labelled indication of rFVIIa are pyrexia, injection site reaction, headache, hypertension, hypotension, nausea, vomiting, pain, oedema and rash. See Warnings and Precautions.

Patients who receive NiaStase RT (eptacog alfa, activated) should be kept under close observation for signs and symptoms of unfavourable activation of the coagulation system or thrombosis.

Clinical Trial Adverse Drug Reactions in the Hemophiliac Population: Because clinical trials are conducted under very specific conditions the adverse reaction rates observed in the clinical trials may not reflect the rates observed in practice and should not be compared to the rates in the clinical trials of another drug. Adverse drug reaction information from clinical trials is useful for identifying drug-related adverse events and for approximating rates.

During clinical studies in 298 hemophilia A/B patients with inhibitors involving 1,939 bleeding episodes, there were 182 adverse reactions that were possibly related or of unknown relationship to rFVIIa. Of these, there were 21 serious adverse reactions that were possibly related or of unknown relation to treatment reported in 14 patients, and included 6 deaths. During the clinical program, 4 episodes of clinical or laboratory evidence of DIC were documented in hemophilia patients with inhibitors.

In the clinical studies, thrombogenicity has been associated rarely with the use of rFVIIa (11 events out of 1939 treatment episodes for an incidence of <1%). Thrombosis was reported in two of the 298 patients with hemophilia.

In 175 surgical procedures with rFVIIa, three thrombotic events occurred—one thrombosis, one episode of phlebitis and one patient with a large abscess and sepsis died of DIC. In the clinical testing program, isolated cases of antibody development have been reported in FVII deficient patients after treatment with rFVIIa.

No severe allergic reactions have occurred in hemophilia patients receiving rFVIIa. Additionally, the potential for development of antibodies towards rFVIIa has been followed in hemophilia A/B patients and in none of these cases have antibodies towards rFVIIa or other potentially antigenic components of the drug product (BHK-cell protein, murine IgG, or bovine serum) been detected.

In a clinical study comparing the safety and efficacy of rFVIIa when administered through bolus injection versus continuous infusion to hemophiliacs with inhibitors during and after surgery, seven of 24 patients had serious adverse events (4 for bolus injection, 3 for continuous infusion). There were 4 serious adverse events which were considered probably or possibly related to rFVIIa treatment (2 events of decreased therapeutic response in each treatment arm). No deaths occurred during the study period. See Table 2.

Table 2: NiaStase RT

Adverse Events That Were Reported in ≥1% of rFVIIa Treatment Episodes and Were Considered to be Possibly Related to rFVIIa Administration

Body System	Number of Adverse Events Reported n=1939 Treatments (%)
Body as a Whole	(2)
Fever	16 (1)
Platelets, Bleeding, and Clotting	(3)
Hemorrhage NOS	15 (1)
Fibrinogen plasma decreased	10 (1)
Skin and Musculoskeletal	(2)
Hemarthrosis	14 (1)
Nervous System	15 (1)
Cardiovascular	18 (1)

Less Common Clinical Trial Adverse Drug Reactions (<1%): Gastrointestinal: <1%.
Liver and Biliary: <1%.
Metabolic and Endocrine: <1%.
Respiratory: <1%.
Urinary: <1%.
Application Site: <1%.
Resistance Mechanism: <1%.
Other: <1%.
Abnormal Hematologic and Clinical Chemistry Findings: See Table 3 and Table 4.

Table 3: NiaStase RT

Coagulation Parameter Shifts in Hemophilia A/B Patients with Inhibitors

Parameter	Shift[a]	No. of Treatment Episodes Experiencing Shift (%)	Total No. of Treatment Episodes Evaluated
D-Dimer	Normal to High	17 (15)	112
Fibrinogen	Normal to Low High to Low	27 (9)	288
Platelets	Normal to Low High to Low	28 (8)	365

[a] Refers to potential clinically significant shift during the study. A shift to D-dimer values higher than the normal range may be clinically significant, while a shift to fibrinogen and platelet values lower than normal range may be clinically significant.

Table 4: NiaStase RT

Clinical Chemistry Parameter Shifts in Hemophilia A/B Patients with Inhibitors

Parameter	Shift[a]	No. of Treatment Episodes Experiencing Shift (%)	Total No. of Treatment Episodes Evaluated
Alkaline Phosphatase	Normal to High	14 (12)	112
ALT	Normal to High	12 (12)	102
AST	Normal to High	11 (10)	108
LDH	Normal to High	8 (9)	85
Creatinine	Normal to High	4 (3)	137

[a] Refers to potential clinically significant shift during the study. Increases to values above the normal range in alkaline phosphatase, ALT, AST and LDH may indicate changes in liver function, while increase in creatinine may indicate renal function changes.

Adverse Drug Reaction Overview in Clinical Trials using NiaStase RT: The safety profile of NiaStase RT administered to achieve or maintain hemostasis has not been assessed in clinical trials. However, the short term safety profile and the tolerability of a single dose of NiaStase RT were investigated in the NN1007-1744 and NN1007-1862 trials, which included non-bleeding healthy subjects and patients with hemophilia, respectively. A total of 25 subjects were exposed to a single dose of NiaStase RT (24 subjects) and/or NiaStase (24 subjects) in the NN1007-1744 trial. A total of 24 patients with hemophilia were exposed to a single dose of NiaStase RT in the NN1007-1862 trial.

Overall, the results of the clinical trials do not suggest any alteration to the established rFVIIa safety profile, or any additional risk of thromboembolic complications or antibody formation. There were no clinically relevant findings in other safety parameters including local tolerability, physical examination, vital signs and laboratory parameters. In addition, the documented equivalence of the pharmacokinetic profiles substantiates equivalent or similar safety of NiaStase RT and NiaStase.

Post-Market Adverse Drug Reactions: The following post-marketing adverse drug reactions are reported voluntarily from a population of uncertain size; hence, it is not possible to estimate their frequency or establish a causal relationship to exposure.

Based on post-marketing experience adverse drug reactions are rare (<1 per 1000 standard doses). When analyzed by system organ classes, the reporting rates of adverse drug reactions during the post-marketing period, including both serious and non-serious reactions, are as indicated in Table 5.

Adverse Drug Reaction Reporting and Re-Issuance of the Product Monograph: Healthcare providers are encouraged to report Adverse Drug Reactions associated with normal use of these and all drug products to Health Canada's Health Product Safety Information Division at 1-866-234-2345. The Product Monograph will be re-issued in the event of serious safety concerns previously unidentified or at such time as the sponsor provides the additional data in support of the product's clinical benefit.

DRUG INTERACTIONS:

Serious Drug Interactions
- NiaStase RT (eptacog alfa, activated) should not be mixed with infusion solutions or be given in a drip.
- Simultaneous use of prothrombin complex concentrates, activated or not, should be avoided.

Overview: The risk of a potential interaction between NiaStase RT and coagulation factor concentrates is unknown.

Anti-fibrinolytics have been reported to reduce blood loss in association with surgery in hemophilia patients, especially in orthopaedic surgery and surgery in regions rich in fibrinolytic activity, such as the oral cavity. Experience with concomitant administration of anti-fibrinolytics and rFVIIa treatment is, however, limited.

Drug-Drug Interactions: Interactions with other drugs have not been established.
Drug-Food Interactions: Interactions with food have not been established.
Drug-Herb Interactions: Interactions with herbal products have not been established.
Drug-Laboratory Test Interactions: Changes in D-Dimer, Fibrinogen, Platelets, Alkaline Phosphatase, ALT, AST, LDH and Creatinine were seen in clinical trials. See Adverse Reactions, Abnormal Hematologic and Clinical Chemistry Findings.

Table 5: NiaStase RT

Reporting Rates of Post-Marketing Adverse Drug Reactions

	Post-Market Adverse Drug Reactions
Blood and Lymphatic Disorders	
Very rare (<1/10 000)	- Disseminated intravascular coagulation - Coagulopathy
Gastrointestinal Disorders	
Very rare (<1/10 000)	- Nausea - Vomiting
General Disorders and Administration Site Conditions	
Rare (>1/10 000, <1/1000)	- Therapeutic response decreased* - Pyrexia - Injection site reaction including bruising and swelling * Lack of efficacy (therapeutic response decreased) has been reported. It is important that the dosage regimen of NiaStase RT is compliant with the recommended dosage as stated. See Dosage and Administration.
Immune System Disorders	
Very rare (<1/10 000)	- Immune mediated reactions including anaphylactic reaction, and hypersensitivity
Investigations	
Very rare (<1/10 000)	- Fibrin D-dimer increased - Thrombin-antithrombin III complex increased Increased troponin I and troponin T - Anti FVII antibodies have only been seen in patients with FVII deficiency. There have been no confirmed reports of antibodies against factor VII in hemophilia A or hemophilia B patients.
Nervous System Disorders	
Very rare (<1/10 000)	- Headache - Paresthesia
Skin and Subcutaneous Tissue Disorders	
Very rare (<1/10 000)	- Skin rashes including rash, maculopapular rash, urticaria and pruritus
Vascular Disorders	
Very rare (<1/10 000)	- Venous thrombotic events including portal vein thrombosis, pulmonary embolism, deep vein thrombosis, sub clavian vein thrombosis, jugular vein thrombosis, superior vena caval occlusion, renal vein thrombosis, thrombophlebitis and venous thrombosis limb - Arterial thromboembolic events including myocardial infarction and ischemia, cerebral infarction, cerebral ischemia, cerebrovascular disorders, ischemic stroke, thrombotic stroke, transient ischemic attack, renal artery thrombosis and intestinal ischemia - Mixed thromboembolic events including intracardiac thrombosis and thrombosis - Flushing Incidents of hemorrhage have been reported. NiaStase RT is not expected to precipitate hemorrhage, but pre-existing hemorrhage may continue in case of insufficient efficacy or sub-optimal dosage regimen.

DOSAGE AND ADMINISTRATION: Dosing Considerations:
- Treatment should be initiated under the supervision of a physician experienced in the treatment of hemophilia and/or bleeding disorders.
- Hemostasis evaluation should be used to determine the effectiveness of NiaStase RT (eptacog alfa, activated) and to provide a basis for modification of the NiaStase RT treatment schedule.
- NiaStase RT should be given as early as possible after the start of a bleeding episode. Following the initial dose of NiaStase RT further injections may be repeated. The duration of treatment and the interval between injections will vary with the severity of the hemorrhage, the invasive procedures or surgery being performed.
- In hereditary severe FVII-deficient patients, replacement therapy with NiaStase RT in doses of 15 to 30 µg/kg at 4 to 6 hour intervals has been shown to significantly shorten or normalize prothrombin time. However, no correlation has been demonstrated between PT and aPTT and clinical efficacy of NiaStase RT.

Recommended Dose and Dosage Adjustment: NiaStase RT is intended for intravenous bolus administration only. The recommended dose range, dose, frequency, and duration of NiaStase RT administration as a single agent are outlined below. Coagulation parameters should not be used to evaluate NiaStase RT effectiveness. See Table 6.

Reconstitution: Calculate the NiaStase RT dosage you will need and select the appropriate NiaStase RT vial package. The selected package contains 1 vial of NiaStase RT powder and 1 vial of histidine solvent, which is required to prepare and reconstitute the NiaStase RT powder. Reconstitute only with the histidine solvent provided with NiaStase RT. **Do not reconstitute with sterile water or other solvents.**

The specified volume of histidine solvent corresponding to the amount of NiaStase RT is as follows: see Table 7.

For detailed instructions on how to reconstitute NiaStase RT refer to Information for the Patient.

Administration: Administration should take place immediately. If not used immediately after reconstitution, the vial may be stored at room temperature (below 30°C) or refrigerated for up to 3 hours. Any unused solution should be discarded. Do not freeze reconstituted NiaStase RT or store in syringes.

NiaStase RT is intended for intravenous bolus injection only and should not be mixed with infusion solutions or be given in a drip. Parenteral drug products should be inspected visually for particulate matter and discolouration prior to administration, whenever the solution and container permit. Do not use if particulate matter or discolouration is observed.

For detailed instructions on how to administer NiaStase RT refer to Information for the Patient.

Table 6: NiaStase RT

NiaStase RT Dosage

Indication	Recommended Dose	Frequency and Duration
Bleeding Episodes	90 µg/kg[a]	• An initial dose of 90 µg/kg is recommended. • Dose may vary depending on bleed severity (see dose range). • Administer every 2 hours until clinical improvement is observed. • If continued therapy is required, the dosage interval may be increased from 2 to 6 hours depending on the period of time the treatment is judged to be indicated.
Surgery	90 µg/kg	• An initial dose of 90 µg/kg is recommended. • Dose may vary depending on surgery type (see dose range). • Administer prior to surgery and at least every 2 hours during the procedure. • Dosing should be repeated every 2 hours for the first 24-48 hours after surgery, depending on the surgery performed and the clinical status of the patient. • Dosing may be repeated once during the 2-hour interval after surgery depending on the clinical status of the patient. • If continued therapy is required, the dosage interval may be increased from 2 to 6 hours depending on the period of time the treatment is judged to be indicated.

[a] Doses between 35 and 120 µg/kg have been used successfully in clinical trials for hemophilia A or B patients with inhibitors, and both the dose and administration interval may be adjusted based on the severity of the bleeding and degree of hemostasis achieved.

Table 7: NiaStase RT

Parenteral Products

NiaStase RT Vial Size (mg)	Volume of Histidine Solvent to be Added to Vial (mL)	Approximate Concentration of rFVIIa After Reconstitution (mg per mL)
1.0	1.1	1.0
2.0	2.1	1.0
5.0	5.2	1.0

OVERDOSAGE:

Dose limiting toxicities of rFVIIa have not been investigated in clinical trials.

The following are examples of accidental overdose. One hemophilia B patient (16 years of age, 68 kg) received a single dose of 352 µg/kg, and one hemophilia A patient (2 years of age, 14.6 kg) received doses ranging from 246 µg/kg to 986 µg/kg on five consecutive days. There were no reported complications in either case. One newborn female congenital FVII-deficient patient (7 weeks of age, 3 kg) received one dose of 800 µg/kg and 8 doses of 400 µg/kg and subsequently developed antibodies to FVII. No thrombotic complications as a result of the overdosages were reported.

A Factor VII deficient male (83 years of age, 111.1 kg) received two doses of 324 µg/kg (10-20 times the recommended dose) and experienced a thrombotic event (occipital stroke). In addition, the development of antibodies against rFVIIa and FVII, has been associated with overdose in patients with factor VII deficiency.

In addition, 16 normal volunteers in a dose escalation study received doses up to 320 µg/kg without serious adverse reactions.

The recommended dose schedule should not be intentionally increased, even in the case of lack of effect, due to the absence of information on the additional risk that may be incurred.

For management of a suspected drug overdose, CPhA recommends that you contact your **regional Poison Control Centre**. See the *CPS* Directory section for a list of Poison Control Centres.

ACTION AND CLINICAL PHARMACOLOGY: Pharmacodynamics: NiaStase RT (eptacog alfa, activated), when complexed with tissue factor at the site of injury, activates coagulation Factor X (to Factor Xa), as well as coagulation Factor IX (to Factor IXa). Factor Xa then converts prothrombin to thrombin. Thrombin leads to the activation of platelets and factors V and VIII at the site of injury and to the formation of the hemostatic plug by converting fibrinogen into fibrin. Pharmacological doses of NiaStase RT activate factor X directly on the surface of activated platelets, localized to the site of injury, independently of tissue factor. This results in the conversion of prothrombin into large amounts of thrombin independently of tissue factor. Accordingly, the pharmacodynamic effect of factor VIIa gives rise to an increased local formation of factor Xa, thrombin and fibrin. Because NiaStase RT can activate Factor X independent of Factor VIII and IX activity, it can be used for the management of bleeding episodes and surgery in patients with inhibitors to coagulation Factors VIII or IX.

A theoretical risk for the development of systemic activation of the coagulation system in patients suffering from underlying diseases predisposing them to DIC cannot be totally excluded.

Pharmacokinetics: Healthy Subjects: Using the FVII clotting assay, the pharmacokinetics of rFVIIa were investigated in 35 healthy Caucasian and Japanese subjects in a dose-escalation study. Subjects were stratified according to gender and ethnic group and dosed with 40, 80 and 160 µg rFVIIa per kg body weight and/or placebo (3 doses each). The pharmacokinetic profiles indicated dose proportionality. The pharmacokinetics were similar across gender and ethnic groups. The mean steady state volume of distribution ranged from 130 to 165 mL/kg, the mean values of clearance ranged from 33.3 to 37.2 mL/kg.h, and the mean terminal half-life ranged from 3.9 to 6.0 hours.

Hemophilia A and B with Inhibitors: Using the FVIIa assay, the pharmacokinetic properties of rFVIIa were studied in 12 pediatric and 5 adult patients. Dose proportionality was established for the investigated doses of 90 and 180 µg per kg body weight, which is in accordance with previous findings at lower doses (17.5-70 µg per kg body weight). Mean clearance was approximately 50% higher in pediatric patients relative to adults (78 versus 53 mL kg^{-1} h^{-1}), whereas the mean terminal half life was determined to 2.3 hours in both groups. Mean volume of distribution at steady state was 196 mL kg^{-1} in pediatric patients versus 159 mL kg^{-1} in adults.

STORAGE AND STABILITY: Prior to reconstitution, keep NiaStase RT powder and the histidine solvent refrigerated or store between 2 to 30°C. Do not freeze. Protect powder and solvent from light. Do not use past the expiration date.

After reconstitution, NiaStase RT may be stored either at room temperature (below 30°C) or refrigerated for up to 3 hours. Do not freeze reconstituted NiaStase RT or store it in syringes.

INFORMATION FOR THE PATIENT: Published in e-CPS, available by subscription at www.e-cps.ca.

DOSAGE FORMS, COMPOSITION AND PACKAGING: Each vial of sterile, white lyophilized powder for reconstitution, contains: 1.0 mg (50 KIU), 2.0 mg (100 KIU) or 5.0 mg (250 KIU) of eptacog alfa activated. Nonmedicinal ingredients: calcium chloride dihydrate, glycylglycine, mannitol, methionine, polysorbate 80, sodium chloride and sucrose. After reconstitution 1 mL of solution contains 10 mg of sucrose. Single-use vials, packages of 1. The vials are made of Type 1 glass, closed with a latex-free, chlorobutyl rubber stopper, and covered with an aluminum cap. The vials are equipped with a tamper-evident snap-off polypropylene cap.

Histidine Solvent: The solvent for reconstitution of NiaStase RT is a 10 mmol solution of histidine in water for injection and is supplied as a clear colourless solution. The vials are made of Type 1 glass, closed with a latex-free, chlorobutyl rubber stopper, and covered with an aluminum cap. The vials are equipped with a tamper-evident snap-off polypropylene cap.

Nicoderm®

nicotine transdermal system

Smoking Cessation Aid

McNeil Consumer Healthcare

PHARMACOLOGY: Nicoderm (nicotine transdermal system) is a multilayered rectangular film containing nicotine as the active ingredient. It provides 24 hour rate-controlled delivery of nicotine following its application to intact skin. Nicoderm reduces the withdrawal symptoms associated with smoking cessation and thus increases the success rate of smoking cessation programs.

INDICATIONS: As an aid to smoking cessation for partial relief of nicotine withdrawal symptoms. This treatment should be used as part of a comprehensive behavioral smoking-cessation program.

CONTRAINDICATIONS: In patients with hypersensitivity or allergy to nicotine or the components of the transdermal system. Patients with acute hypersensitivity reactions should discontinue use of Nicoderm and should be advised of the possibility of acute hypersensitivity reactions to other forms of nicotine, including cigarettes.

In non-smokers or occasional smokers.

In children under 18 years of age (see Precautions).

In patients during the immediate post-myocardial infarction period, in patients with life-threatening arrhythmias, in patients with severe or worsening angina pectoris and in patients who have had a recent cerebral vascular accident (see Warnings).

In pregnant women (see Precautions), in nursing mothers, and in patients with generalized skin disorders.

WARNINGS: Nicotine from any source can be toxic and addictive. The amounts of nicotine that are tolerated by adult smokers can produce symptoms of poisoning and could prove fatal if the Nicoderm system is applied or ingested by children or pets. Used Nicoderm systems contain approximately 70% of their initial drug content. Therefore, patients should be cautioned to keep both the used and unused Nicoderm systems out of the reach of children and pets.

Cardiovascular or Peripheral Vascular Disease: The risks of nicotine replacement in patients with certain cardiovascular and peripheral vascular diseases should be weighed against the benefits of including nicotine replacement in a smoking-cessation program for them. Specifically, patients with coronary heart disease (history of myocardial infarction and/or angina pectoris), serious cardiac arrhythmias, or vasospastic diseases (Buerger's disease, Prinzmetal's variant angina) should be carefully screened and evaluated before nicotine replacement is prescribed.

Tachycardia occurring in association with the use of Nicoderm therapy has been reported occasionally. If serious cardiovascular symptoms occur with the use of Nicoderm therapy, it should be discontinued.

PRECAUTIONS: General: The patient should be urged to stop smoking completely when initiating Nicoderm therapy (see Dosage). Patients should be informed that if they continue to smoke while using Nicoderm systems, they may experience adverse effects due to peak nicotine levels higher than those experienced from smoking alone. If there is a clinically significant increase in cardiovascular or other effects attributable to nicotine, the Nicoderm dose should be reduced or Nicoderm treatment discontinued (see Warnings). The use of Nicoderm systems beyond 3 months by patients who stop smoking should be discouraged. If the patient continues to smoke, treatment should be discontinued after 4 weeks.

Pregnancy: Women of childbearing age should be advised to take adequate precautions to avoid becoming pregnant while using Nicoderm. Nicoderm therapy should be discontinued if pregnancy is suspected (see Contraindications).

Drug Interactions: Physicians should anticipate that the pharmacokinetics of certain concomitant medications may be altered by smoking cessation with or without nicotine replacement. Therefore the dosage of certain concomitant medications may require adjustment (see Table 1).

Table 1: Nicoderm

Dose Adjustment of Concomitant Medications

May require a decrease in dose at cessation of smoking	Possible Mechanism
Acetaminophen, caffeine, imipramine, oxazepam, pentazocine, propranolol, theophylline	Deinduction of hepatic enzymes on smoking cessation
Insulin	Increase in s.c. insulin absorption with smoking cessation
Adrenergic antagonists (e.g. prazosin, labetalol)	Decrease in circulating catecholamines with smoking cessation
May require an increase in dose at cessation of smoking	**Possible Mechanism**
Adrenergic agonists (e.g. isoproterenol, phenylephrine)	Decrease in circulating catecholamines with smoking cessation

Allergic Reactions: Patients should be instructed to promptly discontinue the use of Nicoderm systems and contact their physicians if they experience severe or persistent local skin reactions (e.g., severe erythema, pruritus, or edema) at the site of application or a generalized skin reaction (e.g., urticaria, hives, or generalized rash). Patients using Nicoderm therapy concurrently with other transdermal systems may exhibit local reactions at both application sites. In such patients use of one or both systems may have to be discontinued.

Skin Disease: Nicoderm systems are usually well tolerated by patients with normal skin, but may be irritating for patients with some skin disorders (atopic or eczematous dermatitis).

Renal or Hepatic Insufficiency: The pharmacokinetics of nicotine have not been studied in the elderly or in patients with renal or hepatic impairment; however, given that nicotine is extensively metabolized and that its total system clearance is dependent on liver blood flow, some influence of hepatic impairment on drug kinetics (reduced clearance) should be anticipated. Only severe renal impairment would be expected to affect the clearance of nicotine or its metabolites from the circulation.

Endocrine Diseases: Nicoderm therapy should be used with caution in patients with hyperthyroidism, pheochromocytoma, or insulin-dependent diabetes since nicotine causes the release of catecholamines by the adrenal medulla.

Peptic Ulcer Disease: Nicotine delays healing in peptic ulcer disease; therefore, Nicoderm therapy should be used with caution in patients with active peptic ulcers and only when the benefits of including nicotine replacement in a smoking-cessation program outweigh the risks.

Accelerated Hypertension: Nicotine therapy constitutes a risk factor for development of malignant hypertension in patients with accelerated hypertension; therefore, Nicoderm therapy should be used with caution in these patients and only when the benefits of including nicotine replacement in a smoking-cessation program outweigh the risks.

Children and Geriatrics: Nicoderm therapy is not recommended for use in children under 18 years of age, because its safety and effectiveness in children and adolescents who smoke has not been evaluated. In clinical trials Nicoderm therapy appeared to be as effective in the over 60 age group as in younger adult smokers. However, asthenia, various body aches and dizziness occurred slightly more often in patients over 60 years of age.

Drug Dependency: Nicoderm therapy is likely to have a low abuse potential based on differences between it and cigarettes in 4 characteristics commonly considered important in contributing to abuse: much slower absorption, much smaller fluctuations in blood levels, lower blood levels of nicotine, and less frequent use (i.e., once daily).

Dependence on nicotine polacrilex chewing gum replacement therapy has been reported. Such dependence might also occur from transference to Nicoderm systems of tobacco-based nicotine dependence. The use of the system beyond 3 months has not been evaluated and should be discouraged. To minimize the risk of dependence, patients should be encouraged to withdraw gradually from Nicoderm treatment after 4 to 8 weeks of use. Recommended dose reduction is to progressively decrease the dose every 2 to 4 weeks (see Dosage).

Strenuous Exercise: Preliminary evidence suggests that wearing a nicotine transdermal patch during periods of strenuous exercise may lead to nicotine toxicity as a result of increased absorption of nicotine from the depot of nicotine in the skin under the patch, due to increased skin temperature and increased cutaneous vasodilation and perfusion from exercising. Three cases illustrating this phenomenon were described in Health Canada Adverse Reaction Newsletter, Volume 6, Number 1, January, 1996. Advice to remove the nicotine patch before engaging in strenuous exercise was recommended by W. Dafoe and P. Huston. Until definitive studies have been undertaken to clarify this hazard, it is advisable to remove the nicotine patch prior to engaging in prolonged strenuous activity.

ADVERSE EFFECTS: Assessment of adverse events in patients who participated in controlled clinical trials is complicated by the occurrence of GI and CNS effects of nicotine withdrawal as well as nicotine excess. The actual incidence of both is confounded by concurrent smoking by many of the patients. When reporting adverse events in the clinical trials, the clinical investigators did not attempt to identify the cause of the symptom.

The most common adverse event associated with Nicoderm is a short-lived erythema, pruritus and/or burning at the application site, which was seen at least once in 47% of patients on the Nicoderm system in the clinical trials. Local erythema after system removal was noted at least once in 14% of patients and local edema in 3%. Erythema generally resolved within 24 hours. Cutaneous hypersensitivity (contact sensitization) occurred in 2% of patients on Nicoderm systems (see Precautions).

Table 2 presents the number of patients reporting adverse events at a frequency greater than 1% in placebo-controlled clinical trials.

Table 2: Nicoderm

Number (%) of Patients Reporting Adverse Events (Patients-Treatment N=1080[a]) (Patients N=1061)

Adverse Event[a]	Nicoderm (n=744)	Placebo (n=336)
Body as a Whole		
Headache	118 (15.9%)	52 (15.5%)
Asthenia	38 (5.1%)	15 (4.5%)
Flu Syndrome	26 (3.5%)	10 (3.0%)
Pain	21 (2.8%)	6 (1.8%)
Abdominal Pain	13 (1.7%)	4 (1.2%)
Cardiovascular		
Palpitations	11 (1.5%)	3 (0.9%)
Tachycardia	9 (1.2%)	1 (0.3%)
Digestive		
Dyspepsia	43 (5.8%)	10 (3.0%)
Nausea	40 (5.4%)	18 (5.4%)
Diarrhea	17 (2.3%)	9 (2.7%)
Constipation	16 (2.2%)	5 (1.5%)
Dry Mouth	13 (1.7%)	2 (0.6%)
Nausea and Vomiting	10 (1.3%)	3 (0.9%)
Flatulence	10 (1.3%)	4 (1.2%)
Stomatitis	8 (1.1%)	5 (1.5%)
Musculoskeletal		
Myalgia	26 (3.5%)	3 (0.9%)
Nervous System		
Insomnia	117 (15.7%)	38 (11.3%)
Dizziness	53 (7.1%)	25 (7.4%)
Abnormal Dreams	47 (6.3%)	4 (1.2%)
Nervousness	23 (3.1%)	8 (2.4%)
Depression	23 (3.1%)	15 (4.5%)
Hypertonia	11 (1.5%)	3 (0.9%)
Somnolence	11 (1.5%)	13 (3.9%)
Paresthesia	10 (1.3%)	4 (1.2%)
Respiratory		
Cough Increased	21 (2.8%)	4 (1.2%)
Pharyngitis	19 (2.6%)	4 (1.2%)
Rhinitis	10 (1.3%)	3 (0.9%)
Dyspnea	8 (1.1%)	7 (2.1%)
Skin and Appendages		
Rash	15 (2.0%)	5 (1.5%)
Sweating	12 (1.6%)	3 (0.9%)
Special Senses		
Taste Perversion	23 (3.1%)	10 (3.0%)

[a] 19 patients were in more than one Nicoderm treatment group.

OVERDOSE:

Symptoms: Treatment of overdosage generally involves symptomatic and supportive care; there is no specific antidote for nicotine intoxication. Signs and symptoms of an overdose from a Nicoderm system are generally the same as those of acute nicotine poisoning, including pallor, cold sweat, nausea, salivation, vomiting, abdominal pain, diarrhea, headache, dizziness, disturbed hearing and vision, tremor, mental confusion and weakness. Prostration, hypotension and respiratory failure may ensue with large overdoses. Lethal doses of nicotine produce convulsions quickly and death follows as a result of peripheral or central respiratory paralysis or, less frequently, cardiac failure. The oral minimum single acute lethal dose for nicotine in human adults is reported to be 40 to 60 mg (<1 mg/kg). Much lower doses have been reported to be toxic in children.

Treatment: The Nicoderm system should be removed immediately if the patient shows signs of overdosage, and the patient should seek immediate medical care, by contacting a physician or local Poison Control Centre. The skin surface should be flushed with water and dried. Soap must not be used since it may increase nicotine absorption. Nicotine will continue to be delivered into the bloodstream for several hours after removal of the system because of a depot of nicotine in the skin.

Persons ingesting Nicoderm systems should be referred to a health care facility for management. Due to the possibility of nicotine-induced seizures, activated charcoal should be administered. In unconscious patients with a secure airway, instill activated charcoal via a nasogastric tube. Repeated doses of activated charcoal should be administered as long as the system remains in the gastrointestinal tract since it will continue to release nicotine for many hours. A saline cathartic or sorbitol added to the first dose of activated charcoal may speed gastrointestinal passage of the system.

Other supportive measures include diazepam or barbiturates for seizures, atropine for excessive bronchial secretions or diarrhea, respiratory support for respiratory failure, and vigorous fluid support for hypotension and cardiovascular collapse.

> For management of a suspected drug overdose, CPhA recommends that you contact your **regional Poison Control Centre**. See the *CPS* Directory section for a list of Poison Control Centres.

DOSAGE: Patients must desire to stop smoking and should be instructed to stop smoking immediately as they begin using Nicoderm therapy. The patient should read the patient instruction booklet (User's Guide) on Nicoderm therapy and be encouraged to ask questions.

Therapy should begin with the Nicoderm 21 mg/day system and continue for 6 weeks. The patient should stop smoking cigarettes completely during this period. If the patient is unable to stop smoking within 4 weeks, Nicoderm therapy should be stopped, since few additional patients in clinical trials were able to quit after this time. Patients who have successfully abstained from smoking should have their dose of Nicoderm reduced after 6 weeks of treatment. Treatment with Nicoderm 14 mg/day should then be initiated for 2 weeks followed by 2 weeks on Nicoderm 7 mg/day. For patients who have cardiovascular disease, who weigh less than 45 kg or who smoke less than ½ pack of cigarettes a day, treatment should be started with Nicoderm 14 mg/day for 6 weeks. The dose should then be decreased to Nicoderm 7 mg/day for the final 2 to 4 weeks of treatment.

In all patients the need for dosage adjustment should be assessed during the first 2 weeks of therapy. The entire course of nicotine replacement and gradual withdrawal should take 8 to 12 weeks, depending on the size of the initial dose.

As the use of Nicoderm beyond 3 months has not been studied, this duration of treatment should not be exceeded.

The Nicoderm system should be applied promptly upon its removal from the protective pouch to prevent evaporative loss of nicotine from the system. Nicoderm systems should be used only when the pouch is intact to assure that the product has not been tampered with.

Nicoderm systems should be applied only once a day to a non-hairy, clean, dry skin site on the upper body or outer upper arm. After 24 hours, the used Nicoderm system should be removed and a new system applied to an alternate skin site. Skin sites should not be reused for at least a week. Patients should be cautioned not to continue to use the same system for more than 24 hours.

Safety and Handling: The Nicoderm system can be a dermal irritant and can cause contact sensitization. Patients should be instructed in the proper use of Nicoderm systems by using demonstration systems. Although exposure of health care workers to nicotine from Nicoderm systems should be minimal, care should be taken to avoid unnecessary contact with active systems. When handling active systems, wash with water alone, since soap may increase nicotine absorption. Do not touch the eyes.

Disposal: When the used system is removed from the skin, it should be folded over and placed in the protective pouch that contained the new system. The used system should be immediately disposed of in such a way as to prevent its access by children or pets. See Information for the Patient for further directions on handling and disposal.

INFORMATION FOR THE PATIENT: Published in e-CPS, available by subscription at www.e-cps.ca

SUPPLIED: Each Nicoderm (nicotine transdermal system) contains nicotine base in an ethylene-vinyl acetate copolymer matrix. Proceeding from the visible surface toward the surface attached to the skin are (1) an occlusive backing (Original: polyethylene/aluminum/polyester/ethylene-vinyl acetate copolymer; Clear: polyester/ethylene-vinyl acetate copolymer); (2) a drug reservoir containing nicotine (in an ethylene-vinyl acetate copolymer matrix); (3) a rate-controlling membrane (polyethylene); (4) a polyisobutylene adhesive; and (5) a protective liner that covers the adhesive layer and which must be removed before application to the skin.

21 mg/day: Each rectangular 22 cm^2 system contains: nicotine 114 mg and provides 24-hour rate-controlled delivery of 21 mg/day to the patient. Nonmedicinal ingredients: ethylene vinyl acetate copolymer, polyisobutylene and high density polyethylene between polyester backings. Boxes of 7 and 14 with user's guide. Available in Original and Clear patches.

14 mg/day: Each rectangular 15 cm^2 system contains: nicotine 78 mg and provides 24-hour rate-controlled delivery of 14 mg/day to the patient. Nonmedicinal ingredients: ethylene vinyl acetate copolymer, polyisobutylene and high density polyethylene between polyester backings. Boxes of 7 with user's guide. Available in Original and Clear patches.

7 mg/day: Each rectangular 7 cm^2 system contains: nicotine 36 mg and provides 24-hour rate-controlled delivery of 7 mg/day to the patient. Nonmedicinal ingredients: ethylene vinyl acetate copolymer, polyisobutylene and high density polyethylene between polyester backings. Boxes of 7 with user's guide. Available in Original and Clear patches.

Store at room temperature, between 15 and 30°C. Apply immediately upon removal from pouch, and do not store after the pouch has been opened.

Nicorette® Gum

nicotine

Stop Smoking Aid

McNeil Consumer Healthcare

Date of Revision: March 7, 2007

SUMMARY PRODUCT INFORMATION:

Route of Administration	Dosage Form/ Strength	Clinically Relevant Nonmedicinal Ingredients
Buccal	Gum 2 mg, 4 mg	For a complete listing see Dosage Forms, Composition and Packaging.

INDICATIONS AND CLINICAL USE: Nicorette Gum (nicotine polacrilex) is a stop smoking aid designed to provide partial substitution for the nicotine in cigarette smoke and is intended as a temporary aid in cushioning the patient against the psychopharmacological effects of nicotine withdrawal symptoms.

Nicorette Gum is indicated in:

1. Smoking Cessation: Nicorette Gum can be used as an adjunct to a smoking cessation program. It can be used in the following ways:
   A. Quitting Abruptly (Stop-to-Quit): Smokers set a quit date and use Nicorette Gum to control their nicotine cravings and withdrawal symptoms.
   B. Quitting Gradually (Reduce-to-Quit): For smokers unable or not ready to quit abruptly, Nicorette Gum can be used to gradually reduce the number of cigarettes smoked per day prior to making a quit attempt.
2. Temporary Abstinence from Smoking: Although smoking cessation is preferable, Nicorette Gum can also be used in cases in which a smoker temporarily refrains from smoking. Nicorette Gum can be used during smoke free periods, for example in smoke free areas or in other situations when the patient wishes to avoid smoking.

Before initiating treatment with Nicorette Gum, the physician or pharmacist should determine the patient's level of nicotine dependence using the Fagerström Nicotine Tolerance Scale shown in Table 1.

Instructions for Use of the Fagerström Scale: Assign the appropriate score indicated in each column according to the patient's answer to the questions (note that not all questions have an answer in Column C). The highest possible score is 11.

If the score is 6 or less, Nicorette Gum (2 mg) is recommended for use. If the score is 7 or greater, Nicorette Gum (4 mg) should be used.

Table 1: Nicorette Gum

The Fagerström Nicotine Tolerance Scale

	A=0 points	B=1 point	C=2 points	Score
How soon after you wake do you smoke your first cigarette?	After 30 minutes	Within 30 minutes		
How many cigarettes a day do you smoke?	1–15	16–25	more than 26	
Does the brand you smoke have a low, medium or high nicotine content?	Low, less than 0.4 mg	Medium, between 0.5–0.8 mg	High, greater than 0.9 mg	
Which of all the cigarettes you smoke a day is the most satisfying one?	Any other than the first one in the morning	The first one in the morning		
Do you smoke more during the morning than during the rest of the day?	No	Yes		
Do you smoke when you are so ill that you are in bed most of the day?	No	Yes		
Do you find it difficult to refrain from smoking in places where it is forbidden, such as the library, theatre, doctor's office?	No	Yes		
How often do you inhale smoke from your cigarette?	Never	Sometimes	Always	
			Score	

CONTRAINDICATIONS:

- Patients who are hypersensitive to this drug or to any ingredient in the formulation or component of the container. For a complete listing, see Dosage Forms, Composition and Packaging.
- Patients in the immediate post-myocardial infarction period, patients with life-threatening arrhythmias, and patients with severe or worsening angina pectoris.
- Patients with active temporomandibular joint disease.
- Pregnant women (see Warnings and Precautions).
- Breast feeding mothers, as nicotine is excreted in breast milk (see Warnings and Precautions).
- Non-smokers and children under 18 years of age (see Warnings and Precautions).

WARNINGS AND PRECAUTIONS: General: The amounts of nicotine that are tolerated by adult smokers can produce symptoms of poisoning and could prove fatal if ingested by children or pets. Patients should be warned to keep Nicorette Gum out of the reach of children and pets.

Simultaneous smoking and chewing of Nicorette Gum should be avoided.

Nicorette Gum should be used with caution in patients with oral or pharyngeal inflammation and in patients with a history of esophagitis or peptic ulcer.

The Nicorette Gum dosage form dictates that it be used with caution in patients whose dental problems might be exacerbated by chewing gum. In such patients, prior dental evaluation may be advisable.

Nicorette Gum is sucrose-free (sweetened with xylitol and acesulfame potassium) and has been formulated to minimize stickiness. As with other gums, however, the degree to which Nicorette Gum may stick to dentures, dental caps or partial dentures may depend on the materials from which they are made and other factors such as amount of saliva produced, possible interaction with denture adhesives, denture cleaning compounds, dryness of mouth due to other causes and salivary constituents. Should an excessive degree of adherence to dental work occur, there is the possibility that as with other gums Nicorette Gum may damage dental work. If this should occur, the patient should discontinue its use and consult a physician or dentist.

Carcinogenesis and Mutagenesis: Nicotine was not mutagenic in the Ames Salmonella test. Literature reports indicate that nicotine is neither an initiator nor a tumour-promoter in mice, and there is inconclusive evidence to suggest that cotinine, an oxidized metabolite of nicotine, may be carcinogenic in rats. Cotinine was not mutagenic in the Ames Salmonella test.

Studies have shown a decrease of litter size in rats treated with nicotine during the time of fertilization.

Cardiovascular: In patients with certain cardiovascular and endocrine diseases, the risks of using nicotine should be carefully weighed against the benefits of including Nicorette Gum in a smoking cessation program.

Patients with coronary heart disease (history of myocardial infarction and/or angina pectoris), serious cardiac arrhythmias, or vasospastic diseases (Buerger's disease, Prinzmetal variant angina) should be carefully screened and evaluated before Nicorette Gum is used. Occasional reports of tachyarrhythmias occurring in association with the use of Nicorette Gum have been reported; therefore, if an increase in cardiovascular symptoms occurs with the use of Nicorette Gum it should be discontinued.

Cigarette smoking is felt to play a perpetuating role in hypertension. Therefore, Nicorette Gum should be used in patients with systemic hypertension only when the benefits of including Nicorette Gum in a smoking cessation program outweigh the risks.

Dependence/Tolerance: The sustained use of Nicorette Gum by former smokers is not to be encouraged because the chronic consumption of nicotine is toxic and addicting. The relative risks of a possible return to smoking should however be weighed against the continued long-term use of Nicorette Gum.

Endocrine and Metabolism: As the action of nicotine on the adrenal medulla (release of catecholamines) does not appear to be affected by tolerance, Nicorette Gum should be used with caution in patients with hyperthyroidism, pheochromocytoma or insulin-dependent diabetes.

Gastrointestinal: Cigarette smoking is felt to play a perpetuating role in peptic ulcer disease. Therefore, Nicorette Gum should be used in patients with peptic ulcer (active or inactive) only when the benefits of including Nicorette Gum in a smoking cessation program outweigh the risks.

Renal: Nicorette Gum should be used with caution in patients with severe renal insufficiency.

Special Populations: Pregnant Women: Use of cigarettes or Nicorette Gum during the last trimester has been associated with a decrease in fetal breathing movements. These effects may be the result of decreased placental perfusion caused by nicotine. Rare reports of miscarriages have been received, and a relationship to drug therapy as a contributing factor cannot be excluded. Studies in pregnant rhesus monkeys have shown that maternal nicotine administration produced acidosis, hypoxia and hypercarbia in the fetus.

Nicorette Gum, therefore, should generally not be used in women who are or may become pregnant, and female patients should be advised to take adequate precautions to avoid becoming pregnant. If this drug is used during pregnancy, or if the patient becomes pregnant while taking this drug, the patient should be apprised of the potential hazard to the fetus.

Nursing Women: Nicotine passes freely into the breast milk. Because of the potential for serious adverse reactions from nicotine in nursing infants, a decision should be made whether to discontinue nursing or to discontinue the drug, taking into account the importance of the drug to the mother. (See Contraindications.)

Pediatrics: Safety and effectiveness in children and adolescents who smoke have not been evaluated. The use of Nicorette Gum is not recommended in smokers under 18 years of age. (See Contraindications.)

ADVERSE REACTIONS: Adverse Drug Reaction Overview: Adverse reactions reported in association with the use of Nicorette Gum include both local effects and systemic effects representing the pharmacological action of nicotine.

Clinical Trial Adverse Drug Reactions: Because clinical trials are conducted under very specific conditions the adverse reaction rates observed in the clinical trials may not reflect the rates observed in practice and should not be compared to the rates in the clinical trials of another drug. Adverse drug reaction information from clinical trials is useful for identifying drug-related adverse events and for approximating rates.

Cessation Studies: Local Side Effects—Nicorette Gum (2 mg) and Nicorette Gum (4 mg): Mechanical effects of gum chewing include traumatic injury to oral mucosa or teeth, adhesion to dentures/teeth, jaw ache, and eructation secondary to air swallowing. These side effects may be minimized by modifying chewing technique. Oral mucosa changes such as stomatitis and throat irritation, glossitis, gingivitis, pharyngitis, and aphthous ulcers, in addition to changes in taste perception, can occur during smoking cessation efforts with or without the use of Nicorette Gum.

Oral adverse events occurring with a frequency of 1% or greater in 1801 patients using Nicorette Gum (4 mg) in two clinical trials were throat irritation 5%, stomatitis (excluding aphthous and ulcerative stomatitis) 4%, taste perversion 3%, tooth disorder (e.g., occlusal stress as a result of chewing, loosening of fillings, gum sticking to dentures, etc.) 2%, aphthous stomatitis 2%, gingivitis 1% and glossitis 1%.

Other oral events reported were gingival bleeding, taste loss, tongue discoloration and tongue ulceration.

Systemic Side Effects—Nicorette Gum (2 mg): Although the types of systemic adverse drug effects seen in clinical trials are similar from one trial to the other, the incidence of individual effects varies considerably from trial to trial. In two well-controlled clinical trials (one performed in the United States and one in England) designed to evaluate the safety and efficacy of Nicorette Gum (2 mg) this variation was evident (see Table 2).

Table 2: Nicorette Gum

Adverse Event Incidence in Clinical Trials Performed in the U.S. and England

Body System Event/ Number of Subjects	Number of Subjects U.S. Trial (N=94) %	British Trial (N=58) %
Autonomic		
Excessive Salivation	2.1	—
CNS		
Insomnia	1.1	—
Dizziness/Lightheadedness	2.1	19.0
Irritable/Fussy	1.1	—
Headache	1.1	24.1
Gastrointestinal		
Nonspecific GI Distress	9.6	—
Eructation	6.4	—
Indigestion	—	41.4
Nausea/Vomiting	18.1	31.0
Reactions Referable to Mouth, Jaw or Teeth		
Mouth or Throat Soreness	37.2	56.9
Jaw Muscle Ache	18.1	44.8
Others		
Anorexia	1.1	—
Hiccups	14.9	22.4

Due to its inherent variability, the list of adverse event incidences can be used only as an indication of the relative frequency of adverse events reported in representative clinical trials. It cannot predict expected incidences of these effects during the course of usual medical practice.

Systemic Side Effects—Nicorette Gum (2 mg): Adverse events that occurred in 1801 patients who participated in two clinical trials of Nicorette Gum (4 mg) are listed by body system. Incidences of 1% or greater are shown in brackets.

Cardiovascular: chest pain (1%).

CNS: headache (11%), dizziness (4%), insomnia (2%), fatigue (1%), abnormal dreaming, agitation, anxiety, apathy, depersonalization, drug dependence, emotional lability, hypoesthesia, impaired concentration, irritability, light-headedness, migraine, nervousness, nightmare, sleep disorder, tremor.

Dermatologic: acne, pruritus.

Gastrointestinal: dyspepsia (9%), nausea (9%), abdominal pain (1%), diarrhea (1%), eructation (1%), flatulence (1%), vomiting (1%), abdominal distension, colitis, diverticulitis, gastritis, gastroesophageal reflux, increased salivation, non-specific gastrointestinal distress, peptic ulcer, ulcer.

Respiratory: cough (1%), bronchitis, bronchospasm, congestion, epistaxis, laryngitis, nasal irritation, rhinitis, rhinorrhea, sinusitis.

Other: hiccups (10%), pain (2%), dry mouth (1%), malaise (1%), abnormal lacrimation, abnormal serum folate test, allergic reaction, anorexia, arthralgia, back pain, dehydration, dysmenorrhea, dysphagia, dysphonia, earache, ear disorder, fever, halitosis, hot flushes, hypothyroidism, leg cramps, lymphadenopathy, mucus membrane disorder, myalgia, nail disorder, oliguria, sweating, thirst, vision abnormality.

Post-Market Adverse Drug Reactions: In addition to the reported effects in clinical trials, the following events have been reported:

Cardiovascular: edema, flushing, hypertension, palpitations, tachyarrhythmias, tachycardia.

CNS: confusion, convulsions, depression, euphoria, numbness, paraesthesia, syncope, tinnitus, weakness.

Dermatologic: erythema, itching, rash, urticaria.

Gastrointestinal: alteration of liver function tests, constipation, diarrhea.

Respiratory: breathing difficulty, hoarseness, sneezing, wheezing.

Other: dry mouth, systemic nicotine intoxication.

Reports of myocardial infarction, congestive heart failure, cerebrovascular accident and cardiac arrest, including death have been received. A cause and effect relationship between these reports and the use of Nicorette Gum has not been established.

Rare reports of miscarriage have been received and a relationship to drug therapy as a contributing factor cannot be excluded.

In addition, rare reports of an apparent severe allergic reaction have been received.

Reduction Studies: The placebo-controlled studies of Nicorette Gum performed to reduce smoking indicate that smoking concomitantly with use of nicotine gum is well tolerated for up to 12 or 18 months.

In these studies, a total of 1001 subjects were allocated to active treatment and 995 to placebo. The subjects in the active groups reported a total of 1846 adverse events of which 38% were assessed as mild, 35% as moderate and 27% as severe. The 995 subjects in the placebo groups reported a total of 1465 adverse events of which 35% were assessed as mild, 39% as moderate and 26% as severe.

Common Adverse Events: Adverse events in the studies of Nicorette Gum to reduce smoking did not substantially differ from those seen in smoking cessation studies. The most commonly reported events were headache, influenza-like symptoms, dyspepsia and nausea/vomiting.

Nausea and/or vomiting, hiccups and dyspepsia are mainly related to nicotine gum use. Nausea and/or vomiting were seen in 56/995 (5.6%) and 132/1020 (13%) subjects in the placebo and active treatment groups respectively. Dyspepsia was reported by 49/995 (4.9%) subjects in the placebo group and 87/1020 (8.5%) subjects in the active treatment group. Hiccups were reported by 5/995 (0.5%) subjects in the placebo group compared to 88/1020 (8.6%) in the active treatment group. Throat irritation was reported more frequently in the active group; 49/1020 (4.8%) compared to 7/995 (0.7%) in the placebo group.

Palpitation, a possible sign of systemic nicotine overdose, was reported by less than 1% of subjects who used active treatment, supporting smoking reduction with gum as a safe intervention.

DRUG INTERACTIONS: Overview: The pharmacokinetics of certain concomitant medications may be altered by smoking cessation with or without nicotine replacement. Therefore, the dosage of certain concomitant medications may require adjustment in ex-smokers.

Drug-Drug Interactions: See Table 3.

Table 3: Nicorette Gum

Established or Potential Drug-Drug Interactions

Proper name	Ref	Effect	Clinical comment
Acetaminophen, caffeine, imipramine (and other tricyclic antidepressants), oxazepam (and other benzodiazepines), pentazocine, propranolol, theophylline	T	Possible mechanism: de-induction of hepatic enzymes on smoking cessation	May require a decrease in dose at cessation of smoking
insulin	T	Possible mechanism: increase in subcutaneous insulin absorption with smoking cessation	May require a decrease in dose at cessation of smoking
adrenergic antagonists (e.g. prazosin, labetolol)	T	Possible mechanism: decrease in circulating catecholamines with smoking cessation	May require a decrease in dose at cessation of smoking
propoxyphene	T	Possible mechanism: "first pass" metabolism decreased	May require a decrease in dose at cessation of smoking
adrenergic agonists (e.g. isoproterenol, phenylephrine)	T	Possible mechanism: decrease in circulating catecholamines with smoking cessation	May require an increase in dose at cessation of smoking

Legend:
C=Case Study;
CT=Clinical Trial;
T=Theoretical.

Both smoking and other forms of nicotine can increase circulating cortisol and catecholamines. Therefore, drugs affected by cortisol or catecholamines, such as insulin, may need to be adjusted according to changes in nicotine therapy or smoking status.

Other reported effects of smoking, which do not involve enzyme induction, include reduced diuretic effects of furosemide and decreased cardiac output, and reduced effect on blood pressure with propranolol, which may also relate to the hormonal effects of nicotine. Smoking cessation may reverse these actions.

Drug-Food Interactions: Patients should be advised not to consume liquids while chewing Nicorette Gum as the pH of the oral cavity may be reduced and interfere with absorption of nicotine.

Drug-Lifestyle Interactions: Weight Gain: Weight gain is commonly associated with abstention from smoking. The mechanism for this is believed to be a combination of the abstention from the oral habit of cigarette smoking and its replacement by increased intake of food and reduced GI motility due to the absence of the stimulant nicotine. Patients who quit smoking should always be monitored for weight gain.

DOSAGE AND ADMINISTRATION: Dosing Considerations: Nicorette Gum is an adjunct to smoking cessation (quitting abruptly and quitting gradually) and dosage should be individualized. Although smoking cessation is preferable, Nicorette Gum can also be used in cases in which a smoker temporarily refrains from smoking; Nicorette Gum can be used during smoke-free periods, for example in smoke-free areas or in other situations when the patient wishes to avoid smoking.

Each piece should be chewed slowly and intermittently for about 30 minutes. The aim of this chewing is to promote even, slow, buccal absorption of the nicotine released from the buffered gum. Chewing quickly can release the nicotine too rapidly, leading to effects similar to over-smoking, e.g. nausea, hiccups or irritation of the throat.

As the nature of adverse effects experienced by an individual patient will be primarily related to the balance between the degree of nicotine tolerance and the rate and degree of absorption of nicotine from the gum, it is important for the patient to learn to chew the gum slowly and to self-titrate the nicotine dose, in order to minimize side effects.

Recommended Dose and Dosage Adjustment: Quitting Abruptly (Stop-to-Quit): A patient who is a candidate for this program must desire to quit smoking and should be instructed to stop smoking immediately.

For optimum results, the initial treatment should be based on the patient's level of nicotine dependence, which can be determined by using the Fagerström Nicotine Tolerance Scale (See Indications and Clinical Use).

If the score is 6 or less, Nicorette Gum (2 mg) is recommended for use. If the score is 7 or greater or for patients who have cravings with the use of Nicorette Gum (2 mg), Nicorette Gum (4 mg) should be used.

Patients should chew one piece of gum whenever they have a craving to smoke.

Most patients require approximately 10 to 12 pieces of gum per day during the first month of treatment. For the first month, about one piece per hour is common for a pack a day smoker.

Patients should be instructed not to exceed 20 pieces of Nicorette Gum per day.

With Nicorette Gum, as with cigarette smoking, the abrupt cessation of nicotine may result in withdrawal symptoms that may lead to a return to smoking. Therefore, Nicorette Gum dosing should be gradually reduced. The suggested procedures for a gradual reduction of Nicorette Gum include, but are not limited to, the following: decrease the total number of pieces of Nicorette Gum used per day by one or more pieces every 4 to 7 days, substitute one or more pieces of sugarless gum for an equal number of pieces of Nicorette Gum. The number of pieces of sugarless gum substituted for Nicorette Gum should be increased every 4 to 7 days.

As guidance, Nicorette Gum may be chewed every 2 to 4 hours during the second month. During the third month, Nicorette Gum may be chewed every 4 to 8 hours.

Combination or modification of the above procedures may be adjusted to the individual patient. Nicorette Gum consumption should be terminated once the patient has successfully broken the smoking habit. This can take up to 6 months in some smokers. It is strongly recommended that Nicorette Gum pieces be carried by the patient for up to three months following cigarette abstention in case a sudden overpowering urge to smoke occurs.

Successful abstainers at three months should stop using gum or gradually withdraw from gum usage. Gradual withdrawal from Nicorette Gum should be initiated after 3 months' usage and completed by 6 months. Patients who chew gum beyond a 3-month period should be considered as possibly using Nicorette Gum as a substitute source of nicotine for their nicotine dependence. The use of Nicorette Gum beyond 6 months in the Quitting Abruptly program is not recommended.

Nicorette Gum dosing may be stopped when usage has been reduced to one or two pieces per day.

Most patients in Nicorette Gum assisted programs who resumed smoking have done so within 6 months of treatment. If necessary, a separate course of Nicorette Gum may be prescribed at a later time for patients who continue or resume smoking.

Quitting Gradually (i.e. Reduce-to-Quit): For patients who are not ready or unable to quit abruptly, Nicorette Gum can be used to facilitate smoking reduction prior to making a quit attempt.

Patients should use Nicorette Gum whenever they have a craving to smoke in order to prolong smoke-free intervals for as long as possible, with the goal of achieving 50% reduction in daily cigarette consumption between 6 weeks and 4 months of treatment. If such a reduction has not been achieved by 4 months, the patient should be further counselled and/or re-evaluated.

The initial dosage of Nicorette Gum is individualized. Patients may self-titrate to the level of nicotine they require to reduce the withdrawal symptoms. Patients should be instructed to use a sufficient number of gum pieces each day but not to exceed 20 pieces of Nicorette Gum.

A reduction of cigarette consumption should be continued until complete cessation can be attempted.

A quit attempt should be made as soon as the patient feels ready but not later than 6 months after the start of treatment. When a patient is ready to make a quit attempt, the instructions outlined under the "Quitting Abruptly" program should be followed.

Regular use of the gum beyond 12 months in the Quitting Gradually program is generally not recommended.

OVERDOSAGE:

Overdosage could occur if many pieces were chewed simultaneously or in rapid succession. The risk of poisoning by swallowing the gum is small because absorption in the absence of chewing is slow and incomplete. The consequences of overdosage will most likely be minimized by the early nausea and vomiting known to occur with excessive nicotine intake. Should an overdosage occur the symptoms would be those of acute nicotine poisoning.

Symptoms: Symptoms and signs include nausea, salivation, abdominal pain, vomiting, diarrhea, cold sweat, headache, dizziness, disturbed hearing and vision, mental confusion and marked weakness. Faintness and prostration will likely ensue and hypotension may occur, breathing is difficult; the pulse may be rapid, weak and irregular, circulatory collapse may be followed by terminal convulsions. Death may result within a few minutes from respiratory failure caused by paralysis of the respiratory muscles.

The oral minimum acute lethal dose for nicotine in human adults is 40 to 60 mg. In human volunteer studies, ten 4 mg nicotine polacrilex pieces were deliberately swallowed and blood nicotine levels followed over a 24-hour period. At no time did the blood nicotine level exceed 5 ng/mL in that period, a level that is considerably less than that produced by smoking a mild cigarette. An analysis of the nicotine polacrilex pieces recovered from the feces of the volunteers showed that only 32% of the original nicotine content had been released.

Treatment: In view of the lack of actual experience in the treatment of Nicorette Gum overdose, the procedures recommended are those that have been suggested for the treatment of acute nicotine poisoning.

In a conscious, alert patient, prompt evacuation of the stomach should be performed. When evacuation is complete, activated charcoal may be administered by mouth, if necessary. A saline cathartic will speed gastrointestinal passage of the gum.

In comatose patients, a clear airway must be established immediately and ventilator support may be required. Mechanical ventilation for respiratory paralysis may be necessary in severe nicotine poisoning. Other therapeutic measures are purely symptomatic and should be conducted according to the attending physician's assessment of the patient.

When the patient's clinical status stabilizes, consideration may be given to gastric lavage and administration of activated charcoal. Hypotension and/or cardiovascular collapse may occur and should be treated vigorously.

For management of a suspected drug overdose, CPhA recommends that you contact your **regional Poison Control Centre**. See the *CPS* Directory section for a list of Poison Control Centres.

ACTION AND CLINICAL PHARMACOLOGY: Mechanism of Action: The active component of Nicorette Gum is nicotine in the form of a natural extract from the tobacco plant.

Pharmacodynamics: In small doses, nicotine stimulates autonomic ganglia. Larger doses of the drug result in a blockage of the ganglia. The effects on autonomic ganglia vary according to the degree of tolerance to nicotine. The major cardiovascular effects of nicotine are vasoconstriction, tachycardia and elevated blood pressure resulting from stimulation of sympathetic ganglia and the adrenal medulla as well as from the activation of chemoreceptors of aortic and carotid bodies.

Pharmacokinetics: Absorption: The pharmacokinetics of nicotine favour buccal (rather than gastrointestinal) absorption. Absorption from the mouth is more rapid than from the stomach and the absorbed nicotine avoids immediate and rapid inactivation by the liver (first pass effect).

Nicorette Gum is formulated to provide blood nicotine levels via buccal absorption that will approximate those produced by the inhalation of tobacco smoke. The nicotine in Nicorette Gum is bound to an ion exchange resin and is released only during chewing. The rate of release of nicotine and, as a consequence, nicotine blood levels, are related to the rate and vigour with which Nicorette Gum is chewed. The chewing of a Nicorette Gum 2 mg piece over a 30 minute period on a one-time-only basis produces peak blood nicotine levels of 5 ng/mL. The chewing of a Nicorette Gum 4 mg piece over a 30 minute period on a one-time-only basis produces peak blood nicotine levels of 10 ng/mL. This peak is reached by about the 25th minute and compares with a peak of 16 to 35 ng/mL reached within 5 minutes from smoking a cigarette of mild to moderate nicotine content. Blood nicotine levels increase and stabilize at 25 ng/mL following repeated administration of Nicorette Gum 2 mg at half-hourly intervals. Blood nicotine levels increase and stabilize at 50 ng/mL following repeated administration of Nicorette Gum 4 mg at half-hourly intervals. Thus, with Nicorette Gum, it is possible to produce nicotine blood levels of the same order as those produced by smoking cigarettes.

Metabolism: Nicotine is metabolized mainly by the liver, but may also be metabolized to a lesser extent by the kidney and the lung. The principal metabolites are cotinine and nicotine-1'-N-oxide. The elimination half-life of nicotine in plasma is 120 minutes.

Excretion: Both nicotine and its metabolites are excreted through the kidneys with about 10 to 20% of absorbed nicotine excreted unchanged in the urine. Excretion of nicotine is increased in acid urine and by high urine output. Serum nicotine concentrations have been reported to be significantly higher in patients with severe renal failure compared to healthy subjects.

STORAGE AND STABILITY: Store Nicorette Gum at room temperature, between 15 and 30°C. Protect Nicorette Gum from light.

INFORMATION FOR THE PATIENT: Published in e-CPS, available by subscription at www.e-cps.ca.

DOSAGE FORMS, COMPOSITION AND PACKAGING: Available in fresh mint, ice mint and fruit flavours.

2 mg: Each off-white square contains: nicotine 2 mg. Nonmedicinal ingredients (fresh mint flavoured): gum base, magnesium oxide, menthol, peppermint oil, sodium bicarbonate and sodium carbonate. Sweetened with xylitol and acesulfame potassium. Contains sodium. Nonmedicinal ingredients (ice mint flavoured): acacia, gum base, magnesium oxide, menthol, peppermint oil, sodium bicarbonate, sodium carbonate, titanium dioxide and wax. Sweetened with xylitol and acesulfame potassium. Contains sodium. Nonmedicinal ingredients (fresh fruit flavoured): acacia, flavour, gum base, hypromellose, magnesium oxide, menthol, peppermint oil, polysorbate, sodium bicarbonate, sodium carbonate, sucralose, titanium dioxide and wax. Sweetened with xylitol and acesulfame potassium. Contains sodium. Blister packs of 30 and 105 pieces.

4 mg: Each yellow square contains: nicotine 4 mg. Nonmedicinal ingredients (fresh mint flavoured): D&C Yellow No. 10, gum base, magnesium oxide, menthol, peppermint oil and sodium carbonate. Sweetened with xylitol and acesulfame potassium. Contains sodium. Nonmedicinal ingredients (ice mint flavoured): acacia, D&C Yellow No. 10, gum base, magnesium oxide, menthol, peppermint oil, sodium carbonate, titanium dioxide and wax. Sweetened with xylitol and acesulfame potassium. Contains sodium. Nonmedicinal ingredients (fresh fruit flavoured): acacia, D&C Yellow No. 10, flavour, gum base, magnesium oxide, menthol, peppermint oil, polysorbate, sodium carbonate, sucralose, titanium dioxide and wax. Sweetened with xylitol and acesulfame potassium. Contains sodium. Blister packs of 30 and 105 pieces.

Nicorette® Inhaler

nicotine inhalation system

Stop Smoking Aid

McNeil Consumer Healthcare

Date of Preparation: October 10, 2003

PHARMACOLOGY: Nicotine is the active ingredient in Nicorette Inhaler (nicotine inhalation system). Nicorette Inhaler releases 4 mg of nicotine in the form of vapor when air is inhaled through the inhaler. Clinical studies have shown that nicotine replacement from nicotine containing products can help people give up smoking by relief of abstinence symptoms associated with smoking cessation.

The cardiovascular effects of nicotine include peripheral vasoconstriction, tachycardia, and elevated blood pressure. Acute and chronic tolerance to nicotine develops from smoking tobacco or ingesting nicotine preparations. Acute tolerance (a reduction in response for a given dose) develops rapidly (less than 1 hour), but not at the same rate for different physiologic effects (skin temperature, heart rate, subjective effects). Withdrawal symptoms such as cigarette craving can be reduced in most individuals by plasma nicotine levels lower than those achieved from smoking.

Withdrawal from nicotine in addicted individuals can be characterized by craving, nervousness, restlessness, irritability, mood lability, anxiety, drowsiness, sleep disturbances, impaired concentration, increased appetite, minor somatic complaints (headache, myalgia, constipation, fatigue), and weight gain. Nicotine toxicity is characterized by nausea, salivation, abdominal pain, vomiting, diarrhea, diaphoresis, flushing, dizziness, disturbed hearing and vision, confusion, weakness, palpitations, prostration, altered respiration and hypotension.

The major fraction of the nicotine in Nicorette Inhaler is deposited in the oral cavity. Continuous, rapid inhalation over 20 minutes releases up to 40% (4 mg) of the nicotine from each cartridge and about 50% of the released nicotine is systemically available, i.e. about 2 mg. Absorption of nicotine through the buccal mucosa is slow and does not produce the high and rapid nicotine plasma concentrations seen with cigarette smoking. Self-administration (ad lib. at clinical use) typically produces nicotine plasma levels of 6-8 ng/mL, which are only about 1/3 of those achieved with cigarette smoking. The plasma levels following clinical use correspond to once hourly chewing of Nicorette chewing gum 2 mg. One puff of 50 mL contains approximately 15 µg of nicotine. Maximal plasma concentrations are reached within 15 minutes after forced inhalation for 20 minutes.

Steady state plasma levels of approximately 20-25 ng/mL are achieved with continuous, rapid inhalations during 20 minutes per hour for 12 hours at ambient room temperature in a laboratory setting. The release of nicotine from the Nicorette Inhaler is temperature dependent. Average peak plasma nicotine concentrations achieved after forced inhalation were 22.5 ng/mL at 20°C, 29.7 ng/mL at 30°C and 34.0 ng/mL at 40°C.

The therapeutic blood concentrations of nicotine, i.e. the blood levels which relieve craving, are individual, based on the patient's nicotine dependence.

The volume of distribution following i.v. administration of nicotine is approximately 2 to 3 L/kg and the half-life ranges from 1 to 2 hours. The major eliminating organ is the liver, and average plasma clearance is about 1.2 L/min; the kidney and lung also metabolize nicotine. More than 20 metabolites of nicotine have been identified, all of which are believed to be less active than nicotine. The primary metabolite of nicotine is cotinine, which has a half-life of 15 to 20 hours and reaches concentrations that exceed those of nicotine by 10-fold. The plasma protein binding of nicotine is less than 5%. Other diseases or concomitant use of other drugs would not be expected to have a significant effect on nicotine kinetics. The primary urinary metabolites are cotinine (15% of the dose) and trans-3-hydroxycotinine (45% of the dose). About 10% of the nicotine is excreted unchanged in the urine. As much as 30% may be excreted in the urine with high urine flow rates and acidification below pH 5.

There are no differences in nicotine kinetics between men and women.

Pharmacokinetic differences due to age have not been identified.

Severe renal impairment would be expected to affect the clearance of nicotine and its metabolites. In smoking patients undergoing hemodialysis, elevated nicotine levels have been seen.

INDICATIONS: Nicorette Inhaler (nicotine inhalation system) is indicated as an aid to smoking cessation for the relief of nicotine withdrawal symptoms. Nicorette Inhaler provides the smoker with adequate amounts of nicotine to reduce the urge to smoke, and may provide some degree of comfort by providing a hand-to-mouth ritual similar to smoking, although the importance of such an effect in smoking cessation is, as yet, unknown. Nicorette Inhaler treatment should be used as part of a comprehensive behavioral smoking-cessation program.

CONTRAINDICATIONS: The use of Nicorette Inhaler (nicotine inhalation system) is contraindicated in the following:

1. Patients with hypersensitivity or allergy to nicotine or to menthol. Patients with acute hypersensitivity reactions should discontinue use of Nicorette Inhaler and should be advised of the possibility of acute hypersensitivity reactions to other forms of nicotine, including cigarettes;
2. Non-smokers or occasional smokers;
3. Persons under 18 years of age (see Warnings);
4. Pregnant women or nursing mothers (see Warnings); and
5. Patients during the immediate post-myocardial infarction period, patients with life-threatening arrhythmias, patients with severe or worsening angina pectoris and patients who have had a recent cerebral vascular accident (see Warnings).

WARNINGS: General: Nicotine from any source can be toxic and addictive. For any smoker, with or without concomitant disease, the risk of nicotine replacement in a smoking cessation program should be weighed against the hazard of continued smoking, and the likelihood of achieving cessation of smoking without nicotine replacement.

Safety Note Concerning Children and Pets: **The amounts of nicotine that are tolerated by adult smokers can cause severe poisoning if a child or pet swallows, chews or sucks on the nicotine cartridge. The risk of poisoning also exists if a child sucks on an inhaler containing the nicotine cartridge. Therefore, patients should be cautioned to keep both the used and unused Nicorette Inhaler (nicotine inhalation system) out of the reach of children and pets.**

All components of the Nicorette Inhaler system should also be kept out of the reach of children and pets to avoid accidental swallowing and choking.

Pediatric: Nicorette Inhaler is not to be used by persons under 18 years of age. The use of Nicorette Inhaler in children and adolescents who smoke has not been evaluated (see Contraindications). However, no specific medical risk is known or expected in nicotine dependent adolescents. Nicorette Inhaler should be used for the treatment of tobacco dependence in the older adolescent only if the potential benefit justifies the potential risk.

Pregnancy: Tobacco smoke, which has been shown to be harmful to the fetus, contains nicotine, hydrogen cyanide, and carbon monoxide. The Nicorette Inhaler does not deliver hydrogen cyanide and carbon monoxide. However, nicotine has been shown in animal studies to cause fetal harm. It is therefore presumed that Nicorette Inhaler can cause fetal harm when administered to a pregnant woman. The effect of nicotine delivery by Nicorette Inhaler has not been examined in pregnancy (see Contraindications). **Therefore, pregnant smokers should be encouraged to attempt cessation using educational and behavioral interventions before using pharmacological approaches.**

Women of child-bearing potential should be advised to take adequate precautions to avoid becoming pregnant while using the Nicorette Inhaler.

Lactation: The safety of Nicorette Inhaler therapy in nursing infants has not been examined. Nicotine passes freely into breast milk; the milk to plasma ratio averages 2.9. Nicotine is absorbed orally (see Contraindications). Nicotine concentrations in milk can be expected to be lower with Nicorette Inhaler when used as recommended than with cigarette smoking, as plasma nicotine concentrations are generally reduced with nicotine replacement. The risk of exposure of the infant to nicotine from Nicorette Inhaler therapy should be weighed against the risk associated with the infant's exposure to nicotine from continued smoking by the mother (passive smoke exposure and contamination of breast milk with other components of tobacco smoke).

Cardiovascular or Peripheral Vascular Disease: The risks of nicotine replacement in patients with certain cardiovascular and peripheral vascular diseases should be weighed against the benefits of including nicotine replacement in a smoking cessation program for them. Specifically, patients with coronary heart disease (history of myocardial infarction and/or angina pectoris), serious cardiac arrhythmias, or vasospastic diseases (Buerger's disease, Prinzmetal's variant angina) should be carefully screened and evaluated before nicotine replacement is recommended.

Palpitations have been reported occasionally with the use of Nicorette Inhaler as well as with other nicotine replacement therapies. No serious cardiovascular events were reported in clinical studies with Nicorette Inhaler, but if such symptoms occur, its use should be discontinued.

Accelerated Hypertension: Nicorette Inhaler therapy should be used with caution in these patients and only when the benefits of including nicotine replacement in a smoking-cessation program outweigh the risks.

Peptic Ulcer Disease: Nicotine delays healing in peptic ulcer disease; therefore, Nicorette Inhaler therapy should be used with caution in patients with active peptic ulcers and only when the benefits of including nicotine replacement in a smoking-cessation program are considered to outweigh the risks.

PRECAUTIONS: General: The patient should stop smoking completely when initiating Nicorette Inhaler therapy (nicotine inhalation system) (see Dosage). Patients should be informed that they should not continue to smoke while using Nicorette Inhaler, because they may experience adverse effects due to peak nicotine levels higher than those experienced from smoking alone. If there is a clinically significant increase in cardiovascular or other effects attributable to nicotine, the Nicorette Inhaler dose should be reduced or treatment discontinued (see Warnings). The use of Nicorette Inhaler beyond 6 months by patients who stop smoking has not been studied and is not recommended.

Bronchospastic Disease: Nicorette Inhaler has not been specifically studied in asthma or chronic obstructive pulmonary disease. Nicotine is an airway irritant and might cause bronchospasm. Nicorette Inhaler should be used with caution in patients with bronchospastic disease. Other forms of nicotine replacement might be preferable in patients with severe bronchospastic airway disease.

Geriatrics: One hundred and thirty-two patients over the age of 60 participated in clinical trials of Nicorette Inhaler therapy. Nicorette Inhaler appeared to be as effective in this age group as in younger smokers. The initial dose in elderly patients may have to be adjusted because their concomitant diseases may increase risk.

Endocrine Diseases: Nicorette Inhaler therapy should be used with caution in patients with hyperthyroidism pheochromocytoma, or insulin-dependent diabetes since nicotine causes the release of catecholamines by the adrenal medulla.

Renal or Hepatic Insufficiency: The pharmacokinetics of nicotine have not been studied in the elderly or in patients with renal or hepatic impairment; however, given that nicotine is extensively metabolized and that its total systemic clearance is dependent on liver blood flow, some influence of hepatic impairment on drug kinetics (reduced clearance) should be anticipated. Only severe renal impairment would be expected to affect the clearance of nicotine or its metabolites from the circulation.

Drug Interactions: Physicians should anticipate that the pharmacokinetics of certain concomitant medications may be altered by smoking cessation with or without nicotine replacement. Smoking is associated with increased CYP1A2 activity. Upon smoking cessation, reduced clearance of substrates for this enzyme may occur. This may lead to an increase in plasma levels for some medicinal products. Of potential clinical importance are products with a narrow therapeutic window, such as theophylline, tacrine and clozapine.

Upon smoking cessation, the plasma concentration of other medications, such as imipramine, olanzapine, clomipramine and fluvoxamine, which are partially metabolized by CYP1A2, may also be increased. However, data that supports this occurrence is not available, and its possible clinical significance is unknown.

Drug Dependency: Nicorette Inhaler therapy is likely to have a low abuse potential based on differences between it and cigarettes in three characteristics commonly considered important in contributing to abuse: much slower absorption causing a slower rise in blood nicotine levels, lower blood levels of nicotine and over time the amount of use/day declines. Nicorette Inhaler does not produce arterial concentrations similar to cigarettes.

The use of the inhaler beyond 6 months has not been evaluated in clinical trials and is not recommended. To minimize the risk of dependence, patients should be encouraged to withdraw gradually from Nicorette Inhaler therapy after 3 months of usage (see Dosage). If necessary, dose reduction can be achieved by gradual reduction of the dose over a 6 to 12 week period.

Information to Be Provided to the Patient: A separate User Guide is included in the package of Nicorette Inhaler (see Information for the Patient). It contains important information on how to use and dispose of Nicorette Inhaler. Patients should be encouraged to ask questions to ensure they understand the instructions. **Patients must be advised to keep both used and unused cartridges as well as the plastic Nicorette Inhaler out of the reach of children and pets.**

ADVERSE EFFECTS: Assessment of adverse events in the 1439 patients (730 on active drug) who participated in controlled clinical trials is complicated by the occurrence of signs and symptoms of nicotine withdrawal in some patients and nicotine excess in others. The incidence of adverse events is confounded by: (1) the many minor complaints that smokers commonly have, (2) continued smoking by many patients and (3) the local irritation from both the active drug and the placebo.

Local Irritation: Nicorette Inhaler (nicotine inhalation system) and the placebo were both associated with local irritant side effects occurring most often in the early stages of treatment. The most frequent complaints from local side effects were cough, irritation in throat, pharyngitis, stomatitis and rhinitis. Overall, these complaints were rated as mild. Coughing was reported by 27% in the active group and by 8% in the placebo group, irritation in the throat was reported by 24% active versus 7% placebo, pharyngitis by 15% active versus 8% placebo, stomatitis by 15% active and 8% placebo, and rhinitis by 18% active and 13% placebo (see Table 1). The frequency of cough, and mouth and throat irritation declined with continued use of Nicorette Inhaler.

Systemic Effects: The most frequent complaints were headache, dyspepsia and nausea. Headache was reported by 26% in the active group and by 20% in the placebo group, dyspepsia was reported by 14% and 8%, respectively, and nausea was reported by 10% and 7%, respectively (see Table 1).

Table 1: Nicorette Inhaler

Adverse Reactions in Placebo-controlled Clinical Trials

	Inhaler Treatment Groups	
Adverse Event	**Nicorette Inhaler (%) n=730**	**Placebo (%) n=709**
Systemic Effects		
Headache	190 (26)	143 (20)
Dyspepsia	100 (14)	54 (8)
Nausea	72 (10)	47 (7)
Chest Pain	35 (5)	20 (3)
Diarrhea	31 (4)	19 (3)
Flatulence	31 (4)	17 (2)
Vomiting	16 (2)	5 (1)
Dyspnea	14 (2)	10 (1)
Hiccup	14 (2)	1 (0.1)
Thirst	12 (2)	6 (1)
Local Effects		
Coughing	199 (27)	62 (8)
Throat Irritation	178 (24)	51 (7)
Pharyngitis	111 (15)	59 (8)
Stomatitis	110 (15)	56 (8)
Rhinitis	135 (18)	90 (13)
Sinusitis	57 (8)	50 (7)
Mouth Dry	53 (7)	45 (6)
Local Paresthesia	33 (4)	6 (1)
Gingival Irritation	13 (2)	7 (1)

Withdrawal: Symptoms of withdrawal were common in both active and placebo groups. Common withdrawal symptoms seen in over 3% of patients on active drug included dizziness, anxiety, sleep disorder and depression.

A complete overview of spontaneous adverse drug event reports from the market since the introduction of the Nicorette Inhaler in many countries worldwide has not revealed any change in the adverse drug event profile nor the incidence of adverse drug events.

OVERDOSE:

Symptoms: Signs and symptoms of an overdose from a Nicorette Inhaler (nicotine inhalation system) are expected to be the same as those of acute nicotine poisoning, including: pallor, cold sweat, nausea, salivation, vomiting, abdominal pain, diarrhea, flushing, palpitations, headache, dizziness, disturbed hearing and vision, tremor, mental confusion and weakness. Prostration, hypotension, and respiratory failure may ensue with large overdoses. Lethal doses of nicotine produce convulsions quickly and death follows as a result of peripheral or central respiratory paralysis or, less frequently, cardiac failure. The acute, minimal, oral lethal dose of nicotine in human adults is believed to be 40 to 60 mg (<1 mg/kg). Much lower doses have been reported to be toxic in children. The effects of using several cartridges in rapid succession are unknown. One cartridge of Nicorette Inhaler contains 10 mg nicotine, of which, approximately 4 mg is delivered nicotine. It is unlikely that an excessive nicotine overdose will occur via inhalation, but should such an overdose occur, the signs would be that of acute nicotine poisoning.

Treatment: Nicorette Inhaler should be stopped immediately if the patient shows signs of overdosage and the patient should seek immediate medical care by contacting a physician or local poison-control centre. Persons ingesting nicotine cartridges should be referred to a health care facility for management. Due to the possibility of nicotine-induced seizures, activated charcoal should be administered. In unconscious patients with a secure airway, instill activated charcoal via a nasogastric tube. Repeated doses of activated charcoal should be administered as long as the cartridge remains in the gastrointestinal tract since it will continue to release nicotine for many hours. The Nicorette Inhaler cartridges can be identified with a radiogram. A saline cathartic or sorbitol added to the first dose of activated charcoal may speed gastrointestinal passage of the cartridge.

Other supportive measures include diazepam or barbiturates for seizures, atropine for excessive bronchial secretions or diarrhea, respiratory support for respiratory failure, and vigorous fluid support for hypotension and cardiovascular collapse.

For management of a suspected drug overdose, CPhA recommends that you contact your **regional Poison Control Centre**. See the *CPS* Directory section for a list of Poison Control Centres.

DOSAGE: Patients must desire to stop smoking and should be instructed to **stop smoking completely** as they begin using the Nicorette Inhaler therapy (nicotine inhalation system). If a patient is unable to stop smoking by the fourth week of therapy, treatment should probably be discontinued.

The initial dosage of Nicorette Inhaler is individualized. Patients may self-titrate to the level of nicotine they require to reduce the abstinence symptoms. Most successful patients in the clinical trials used between 6 and 12 cartridges a day. The best effect was achieved by frequent continuous puffing (20 minutes). Nicotine is released in the form of a vapor when air is inhaled through the inhaler.

The recommended duration of treatment is 3 months, after which patients may be weaned from the Nicorette Inhaler by gradual reduction of the daily dose over the following 6 to 12 weeks. When daily use is reduced to 1-2 cartridges, the use of Inhaler should be stopped. The safety and efficacy of the continued use of Nicorette Inhaler for periods longer than 6 months have not been studied and such use in not recommended.

Dosing recommendations are summarized in Table 2.

Table 2: Nicorette Inhaler

Recommended Dosing

	Duration	Recommended cartridges/day
Initial treatment	Up to 12 weeks	6–12
Gradual reduction (if needed)	6–12 weeks	No tapering strategy has been shown to be superior to any other in clinical studies.

In order to ensure optimal efficacy and safety of the Nicorette Inhaler, patients should be advised to use the Nicorette Inhaler only at room temperature (15-30°C).

Initial Treatment (Up to 12 Weeks): For best results, patients should be encouraged to use at least 6 cartridges per day at least for the first 3 to 6 weeks of treatment. In clinical trials, the average daily dose was >6 cartridges for patients who successfully quit smoking. Additional doses may be needed to control the urge to smoke with a maximum of 12 cartridges daily for up to 12 weeks. Regular use of Nicorette Inhaler during the first week of treatment may help patients adapt to the irritant effects of the product.

Dosage can be adjusted in those patients with signs or symptoms of nicotine withdrawal or excess. The symptoms of nicotine withdrawal overlap those of nicotine excess. Since patients using the Nicorette Inhaler may also smoke intermittently, it is sometimes difficult to determine if they are experiencing nicotine withdrawal or nicotine excess. Controlled clinical trials of nicotine products suggest that palpitations, nausea and sweating are more often symptoms of nicotine excess, whereas anxiety, nervousness and irritability are more often symptoms of nicotine withdrawal.

Gradual Reduction of Dose (Up to 12 Weeks): Most patients will need to gradually discontinue the use of Nicorette Inhaler after the initial treatment period. Gradual reduction of the dose may begin after 12 weeks of initial treatment and may last for up to 12 weeks. Recommended strategies for discontinuing use include suggesting to patients that they use the product less frequently, keeping a tally of daily usage, trying to meet a steadily reducing target or setting a planned quit date for stopping use of the product. Some patients may not require gradual reduction of dosage and may abruptly stop treatment successfully. The safe use of this product for longer than 6 months has not been established.

Smoking cessation should be accompanied by a behavioral support program.

Special Instructions: After using the Nicorette Inhaler, carefully separate the mouthpiece and remove the used cartridge. The used cartridge should be disposed of immediately in such a way as to prevent its access by children or pets (see Information for the Patient leaflet for further directions on handling and disposal). The mouthpiece is reusable and should be cleaned regularly with soap and water.

INFORMATION FOR THE PATIENT: Published in e-CPS, available by subscription at www.e-cps.ca.

SUPPLIED: Nicorette Inhaler (nicotine inhalation system) consists of a mouthpiece and a plastic cartridge delivering 4 mg of nicotine from a porous polyethylene plug containing 10 mg nicotine. Nicotine is the active ingredient. Inactive components of the product are menthol, ethanol, and a porous plug which are pharmacologically inactive. Store at room temperature (15-30°C). Protect cartridges from light and humidity.

Package Size	Description
6 cartridges (Professional Sample only)	Each unit consists of 1 mouthpiece, 1 Plastic Storage Case and 1 storage tray containing 6 cartridges.
30 cartridges starter pack	Each unit consists of 1 mouthpiece, 1 Plastic Storage Case and 5 storage trays each containing 6 cartridges.
42 cartridges refill pack	Each unit consists of 1 mouthpiece and 7 storage trays each containing 6 cartridges.

Nicorette® Lozenge

nicotine polacrilex

Smoking Cessation Aid

McNeil Consumer Healthcare

Date of Revision: October 4, 2007

SUMMARY PRODUCT INFORMATION:

Route of Administration	Dosage Form/ Strength	Clinically Relevant Nonmedicinal Ingredients
Buccal	2 mg, 4 mg nicotine (as nicotine polacrilex)	For a complete listing see Dosage Forms, Composition and Packaging.

INDICATIONS AND CLINICAL USE: Nicorette Lozenge (nicotine polacrilex) is indicated for the reduction of nicotine withdrawal symptoms including cravings associated with smoking cessation. If possible, when stopping smoking, Nicorette Lozenge should be used in conjunction with a behavioural support program.

CONTRAINDICATIONS:

- Patients who are hypersensitive to this drug or to any ingredient in the formulation or component of the container. For a complete listing, see Dosage Forms, Composition and Packaging.
- In patients during the immediate post-myocardial infarction period, patients with life-threatening arrhythmias and in patients with severe or worsening angina pectoris.
- In pregnant women
- In breast-feeding mothers, as nicotine is excreted in breast milk (see Warnings and Precautions)
- In non-smokers and children under 18 years of age (see Warnings and Precautions)

WARNINGS AND PRECAUTIONS: General: The amounts of nicotine that are tolerated by adult smokers can cause poisoning and even prove fatal if ingested by children or pets. Patients should therefore be warned to keep Nicorette Lozenge (nicotine polacrilex) out of the reach of children or pets.

Patients should not smoke, use nicotine patches or any other form of nicotine while using Nicorette Lozenge.

Nicorette Lozenge, mint flavour, is sucrose free, but contains aspartame, which metabolizes to phenylalanine, of relevance for those with phenylketonuria.

Keep safely away from children.

Cardiovascular: In patients with certain cardiovascular diseases, the risks of using nicotine should be carefully weighted against the benefits of including Nicorette Lozenge in a smoking cessation program.

Patients with coronary heart disease (history of myocardial infarction and/or angina pectoris), heart failure, cerebrovascular disease, serious cardiac arrhythmia, vasospastic diseases (Buerger's disease, Prinzmetal variant angina) or severe peripheral vascular disease should be carefully screened and evaluated before Nicorette Lozenge is used.

Cigarette smoking is felt to play a perpetuating role in hypertension. Therefore, Nicorette Lozenge should be used in patients with systemic hypertension only when the benefits of including Nicorette Lozenge in a smoking cessation program outweigh the risks.

Dependence/Tolerance: Nicorette Lozenge therapy has a low abuse potential when compared to d-amphetamine and similar low abuse potential when compared to nicotine gum. To minimize the risk of dependence, therapy should not exceed 24 weeks (6 months).

Endocrine and Metabolism: In patients with certain endocrine diseases, the risks of using nicotine should be carefully weighted against the benefits of including Nicorette Lozenge in a smoking cessation program.

Nicotine causes the release of catecholamines by the adrenal medulla. Therefore, Nicorette Lozenge should be used with caution in patients with hyperthyroidism, pheochromocytoma or insulin-dependent diabetes.

Gastrointestinal: Cigarette smoking is felt to play a perpetuating role in peptic ulcer disease. Therefore, Nicorette Lozenge should be used in patients with peptic ulcer (active or inactive) only when the benefits of including Nicorette Lozenge in a smoking cessation program outweigh the risks.

Hepatic/Biliary/Pancreatic: The pharmacokinetics of nicotine have not been studied in patients with renal or hepatic impairment; however, given that nicotine is extensively metabolized and that its total system clearance is dependent on liver blood flow, some influence of hepatic impairment on drug kinetics (reduced clearance) should be anticipated.

Renal: Only severe renal impairment would be expected to affect the clearance of nicotine or its metabolites from the circulation.

Special Populations: Pregnant Women: Nicotine and its major metabolite, cotinine, are transferred to the human fetus, placenta and amniotic fluid of smoking mothers. Nicotine concentrations in the placenta (3.3-28 ng/g), amniotic fluid (1.5-23 ng/mL) and in fetal serum (0.5-25 ng/mL) are all higher than the corresponding maternal serum values, presumably because alkaline nicotine ions are trapped in these compartments.

Because of the possible effects of nicotine on the fetus, Nicorette Lozenge therefore should generally not be used in women who are or may become pregnant, and female patients should be advised to take adequate precautions to avoid becoming pregnant. If this drug is used during pregnancy, or if the patient becomes pregnant while taking this drug, the patient should be apprised of the potential hazard to the fetus.

Nursing Women: Nicotine crosses the placenta and is distributed into breast milk with average milk to placenta ratio of 2.9. For this reason, the advice regarding use of Nicorette Lozenge during lactation should be subject to a risk/benefit assessment of the physician.

Pediatrics: Nicorette Lozenge is not to be used by persons under 18 years of age. The use of Nicorette Lozenge in children and adolescents who smoke has not been evaluated. However, no specific medical risk is known or expected in nicotine dependent adolescents. Nicorette Lozenge should be used for the treatment of tobacco dependence in the older adolescent only if the potential benefit justifies the potential risk.

Geriatrics: Nicorette Lozenge has been used in individuals in clinical trials up to 79 years of age. Of the 1818 randomized subjects in the pivotal safety and efficacy clinical trial, 302 (16.6%) were ≥55 years of age. The overall adverse event profile was comparable to that of the younger patients.

ADVERSE REACTIONS: Adverse Drug Reaction Overview: Nicorette Lozenge (nicotine polacrilex) can cause adverse reactions similar to those associated with nicotine administered in other ways. Common adverse events reported in clinical trials include nausea, heartburn or reflux symptoms, oral- or throat-related irritations, headache, flatulence, hiccup and diarrhea.

Clinical Trial Adverse Drug Reactions: Because clinical trials are conducted under very specific conditions the adverse reaction rates observed in the clinical trials may not reflect the rates observed in practice and should not be compared to the rates in the clinical trials of another drug. Adverse drug reaction information from clinical trials is useful for identifying drug-related adverse events and for approximating rates.

Adverse Events Leading to Subject Withdrawal: Adverse events associated with therapy were generally not serious. Only 7% of subjects in the placebo controlled safety and efficacy trial (n=1818) discontinued because of treatment-emergent adverse events, demonstrating that the events were tolerated by most subjects. Sixty-four (64) subjects who received placebo lozenges (16 and 48 from the 2 and 4 mg groups, respectively) and 64 subjects who received nicotine lozenges (31 and 33 from the 2 and 4 mg groups, respectively) discontinued treatment because of an adverse event. Nausea, mouth soreness, diarrhea/flatus, and heartburn were the most frequent reasons for discontinuation.

Most Commonly Observed Adverse Events: The adverse events most commonly observed in clinical studies included primarily gastrointestinal system events such as nausea (9.2% vs 5.1% with placebo), heartburn (5.4% vs 1.5%), hiccup (4.5% vs 0%) and flatulence (5% vs 6.2%). Headache (6.5% vs 4.6%) and respiratory events such as coughing (4.8% vs 2.8%) also commonly occurred. All of these adverse events are similar to those seen with other oral nicotine replacement therapies.

Adverse Events Observed at an Incidence of >1% in the Controlled Clinical Trial: Table 1 and Table 2 list the treatment-emergent adverse events by body system that were observed among the intent-to-treat population who received nicotine polacrilex lozenges in the placebo-controlled pivotal clinical trial.

Table 1: Nicorette Lozenge

Proportion of Subjects Reporting Treatment-Emergent Adverse Events by Body System: ITT Population

	Number (%) of Subjects[a]			
	2 mg		4 mg	
Body System	Nicotine n=459	Placebo n=458	Nicotine n=450	Placebo n=451
Application Site Disorders	2 (0.4%)	2 (0.4%)	1 (0.2%)	0

(cont'd)

Table 1: Nicorette Lozenge *(cont'd)*

Proportion of Subjects Reporting Treatment-Emergent Adverse Events by Body System: ITT Population

Body System	Number (%) of Subjects[a]			
	2 mg		4 mg	
	Nicotine n=459	Placebo n=458	Nicotine n=450	Placebo n=451
Body as a Whole-General Disorders	**41 (8.9%)**	**28 (6.1%)**	**47 (10.4%)**	**28 (6.2%)**
Cardiovascular Disorders, General	8 (1.7%)	3 (0.7%)	9 (2.0%)	6 (1.3%)
Central and Peripheral Nervous Systems Disorders	**50 (10.9%)**	**53 (11.6%)**	**67 (14.9%)**	**49 (10.9%)**
Endocrine Disorders	1 (0.2%)	1 (0.2%)	2 (0.4%)	0
Fetal Disorders	2 (0.4%)	0	1 (0.2%)	0
Gastrointestinal System Disorders	**195 (42.5%)**	**130 (28.4%)**	**215 (47.8%)**	**128 (28.4%)**
Hearing and Vestibular Disorders	1 (0.2%)	3 (0.7%)	1 (0.2%)	0
Heart Rate and Rhythm Disorders	6 (1.3%)	2 (0.4%)	3 (0.7%)	4 (0.9%)
Liver and Biliary System Disorders	0	2 (0.4%)	0	0
Metabolic and Nutritional Disorders	8 (1.7%)	3 (0.7%)	11 (2.4%)	10 (2.2%)
Musculoskeletal System Disorders	16 (3.5%)	17 (3.7%)	14 (3.1%)	15 (3.3%)
Myo Endo Pericardial & Valve Disorders	1 (0.2%)	0	3 (0.7%)	1 (0.2%)
Neoplasm	6 (1.3%)	1 (0.2%)	2 (0.4%)	1 (0.2%)
Platelet, Bleeding & Clotting Disorders	5 (1.1%)	5 (1.1%)	11 (2.4%)	6 (1.3%)
Poison Specific Terms	0	1 (0.2%)	0	0
Psychiatric Disorders	**77 (16.8%)**	**67 (14.6%)**	**66 (14.7%)**	**42 (9.3%)**
Female Reproductive Disorders	5 (1.1%)	4 (0.9%)	10 (2.2%)	1 (0.2%)
Male Reproductive Disorders	1 (0.2%)	0	0	0
Resistance Mechanism Disorders	**35 (7.6%)**	**20 (4.4%)**	**30 (6.7%)**	**15 (3.3%)**
Respiratory System Disorders	**112 (24.4%)**	**90 (19.7%)**	**116 (25.8%)**	**65 (14.4%)**
Secondary Terms	17 (3.7%)	11 (2.4%)	17 (3.8%)	11 (2.4%)
Skin and Appendages Disorders	15 (3.3%)	16 (3.5%)	22 (4.9%)	20 (4.4%)
Special Senses: Others Disorders	5 (1.1%)	4 (0.9%)	4 (0.9%)	2 (0.4%)
Urinary System Disorders	6 (1.3%)	2 (0.4%)	6 (1.3%)	2 (0.4%)
Vascular (extra cardiac) Disorders	4 (0.9%)	0	3 (0.7%)	0
Vision Disorders	4 (0.9%)	0	2 (0.4%)	4 (0.9%)
White Cell and Reticuloendothelial System Disorders	1 (0.2%)	0	2 (0.4%)	1 (0.2%)

[a] Displayed in bold characters when the proportion of subjects reporting the adverse event was ≥5% in any treatment group.

Table 2: Nicorette Lozenge

Treatment-emergent Adverse Events Occurring in ≥1% of Subjects in Any Treatment Group: ITT Population

Body System	Number (%) of Subjects[a]			
	2 mg		4 mg	
	Nicotine n=459	Placebo n=458	Nicotine n=450	Placebo n=451
Body as a Whole—General Disorders				
Back pain	4 (0.9%)	3 (0.7%)	**7 (1.6%)**	1 (0.2%)
Chest pain	**5 (1.1%)**	1 (0.2%)	3 (0.7%)	2 (0.4%)
Influenza-like symptoms	**7 (1.5%)**	3 (0.7%)	**6 (1.3%)**	3 (0.7%)
Pain	**10 (2.2%)**	**6 (1.3%)**	**9 (2.0%)**	**7 (1.6%)**
Tiredness	3 (0.7%)	1 (0.2%)	**6 (1.3%)**	**6 (1.3%)**
Cardiovascular Disorders—General				
Hypertension	**5 (1.1%)**	2 (0.4%)	3 (0.7%)	1 (0.2%)
Central and Peripheral Nervous Systems Disorders				
Dizziness	**6 (1.3%)**	7 (1.5%)	10 (2.2%)	8 (1.8%)

(cont'd)

Table 2: Nicorette Lozenge *(cont'd)*

Treatment-emergent Adverse Events Occurring in ≥1% of Subjects in Any Treatment Group: ITT Population

Body System	Number (%) of Subjects[a]			
	2 mg		4 mg	
	Nicotine n=459	Placebo n=458	Nicotine n=450	Placebo n=451
Headache	**23 (5.0%)**	**27 (5.9%)**	**36 (8.0%)**[a]	**15 (3.3%)**
Light-headed feeling	**6 (1.3%)**	2 (0.4%)	3 (0.7%)	6 (1.3%)
Paresthesia circumoral	**5 (1.1%)**	**5 (1.1 %)**	**7 (1.6%)**	**12 (2.7%)**
Gastrointestinal System Disorders				
Abdominal pain	**5 (1.1%)**	**6 (1.3%)**	4 (0.9%)	3 (0.7%)
Belching	**7 (1.5%)**	2 (0.4%)	**6 (1.3%)**	1 (0.2%)
Bloating	3 (0.7%)	4 (0.9%)	**9 (2.0%)**	3 (0.7%)
Constipation	**10 (2.2%)**	**10 (2.2%)**	**11 (2.4%)**	**9 (2.0%)**
Diarrhoea	**16 (3.5%)**	**10 (2.2%)**	**24 (5.3%)**	**17 (3.8%)**
Dyspepsia	**8 (1.7%)**	1 (0.2%)	**5 (1.1%)**	2 (0.4%)
Dysphagia	1 (0.2%)	0	**6 (1.3%)**	0
Flatulence	**42 (9.2%)**	**33 (7.2%)**	**35 (7.8%)**	**23 (5.1%)**
Flatus	**3 (0.7%)**	**7 (1.5%)**	**13 (2.9%)**	**13 (2.9%)**
Heartburn	**23 (5.0%)**[a]	**10 (2.2%)**	**26 (5.8%)**[a]	**5 (1.1%)**
Hiccough	1 (0.2%)	0	**13 (2.9%)**	0
Hiccup	**15 (3.3%)**	0	**26 (5.8%)**[a]	0
Indigestion	**10 (2.2%)**	4 (0.9%)	**15 (3.3%)**	2 (0.4%)
Mouth dry	**7 (1.5%)**	**14 (3.1%)**	**11 (2.4%)**	**6 (1.3%)**
Mouth irritation	**18 (3.9%)**	**13 (2.8%)**	**15 (3.3%)**	**12 (2.7%)**
Mouth ulceration	**16 (3.5%)**	**10 (2.2%)**	**22 (4.9%)**	**13 (2.9%)**
Nausea	**56 (12.2%)**[a]	**22 (4.8%)**	**69 (15.3%)**[a]	**24 (5.3%)**
Singultus	3 (0.7%)	1 (0.2%)	**8 (1.8%)**	0
Stomach upset	**5 (1.1%)**	**10 (2.2%)**	**5 (1.1%)**	**8 (1.8%)**
Stools loose	1 (0.2%)	4 (0.9%)	4 (0.9%)	**5 (1.1%)**
Tongue ulceration	**6 (1.3%)**	1 (0.2%)	**6 (1.3%)**	4 (0.9%)
Tooth ache	3 (0.7%)	**6 (1.3%)**	4 (0.9%)	**5 (1.1%)**
Vomiting	**15 (3.3%)**	**6 (1.3%)**	**12 (2.7%)**	**12 (2.7%)**
Musculoskeletal Disorders				
Bone fracture spontaneous	2 (0.4%)	**5 (1.1%)**	2 (0.4%)	1 (0.2%)
Platelet, Bleeding & Clotting Disorders				
Gingival bleeding	2 (0.4%)	1 (0.2%)	**5 (1.1%)**	1 (0.2%)
Psychiatric Disorders				
Anxiety	**9 (2.0%)**	7 (1.5%)	6 (1.3%)	2 (0.4%)
Appetite increased	**15 (3.3%)**	**15 (3.3%)**	4 (0.9%)	4 (0.9%)
Depression	**10 (2.2%)**	5 (1.1%)	**15 (3.3%)**	3 (0.7%)
Insomnia	**12 (2.6%)**	5 (1.1%)	**15 (3.3%)**	**6 (1.3%)**
Irritability	**13 (2.8%)**	**13 (2.8%)**	6 (1.3%)	4 (0.9%)
Sleep disturbed	**17 (3.7%)**	**15 (3.3%)**	4 (0.9%)	**8 (1.8%)**
Resistance Mechanism Disorders				
Abscess	4 (0.9%)	1 (0.2%)	3 (0.7%)	**6 (1.3%)**
Infection viral	**19 (4.1%)**	**13 (2.8%)**	**17 (3.8%)**	**6 (1.3%)**
Otitis media	**5 (1.1%)**	2 (0.4%)	2 (0.4%)	0
Respiratory System Disorders				
Breath shortness	0	0	**6 (1.3%)**	1 (0.2%)
Bronchitis	**7 (1.5%)**	3 (0.7%)	4 (0.9%)	3 (0.7%)

(cont'd)

Table 2: Nicorette Lozenge *(cont'd)*

Treatment-emergent Adverse Events Occurring in ≥1% of Subjects in Any Treatment Group: ITT Population

	Number (%) of Subjects[a]			
	2 mg		4 mg	
Body System	**Nicotine n=459**	**Placebo n=458**	**Nicotine n=450**	**Placebo n=451**
Coughing	**19 (4.1%)**	13 (2.8%)	**26 (5.8%)**[a]	12 (2.7%)
Pharyngitis	**11 (2.4%)**	0	**6 (1.3%)**	0
Respiratory disorder	2 (0.4%)	2 (0.4%)	**10 (2.2%)**	3 (0.7%)
Sinus congestion	2 (0.4%)	2 (0.4%)	**9 (2.0%)**	1 (0.2%)
Sinusitis	**13 (2.8%)**	**12 (2.6%)**	**10 (2.2%)**	1 (0.2%)
Sore throat	**13 (2.8%)**	**12 (2.6%)**	**24 (5.3%)**	**18 (4.0%)**
Upper respiratory tract infection	**58 (12.6%)**	**47 (10.3%)**	**45 (10.0%)**	**29 (6.4%)**
Secondary Terms				
Surgical intervention	**12 (2.6%)**	**5 (1.1%)**	**10 (2.2%)**	**7 (1.6%)**

[a] Statistically significantly different from placebo ($p<0.05$).

Certain symptoms which have been reported, such as depression, insomnia, increased appetite, irritability, anxiety, difficulty concentrating and restlessness may be related to withdrawal symptoms associated with smoking cessation. Subjects quitting smoking by any means could expect to suffer from headache, dizziness, increased coughing or a cold.

DRUG INTERACTIONS: Overview: Although no drug-drug interaction studies have been conducted with the Nicorette Lozenge, concomitant medication may need dose adjustment due to reduced nicotine levels; caffeine, theophylline, imipramine, pentazocine, phenylbutazone, insulin, clomipramine, propoxyphene, adrenergic blockers may need dose decrease; adrenergic agonists may need dose increase.

DOSAGE AND ADMINISTRATION: Dosing Considerations:

- Nicorette Lozenge nicotine 2 mg (as nicotine polacrilex) is to be used in patients who smoke their first cigarette more than 30 minutes after waking up.
- Nicorette Lozenge nicotine 4 mg (as nicotine polacrilex) is to be used in patients who smoke their first cigarette within 30 minutes of waking up.

Recommended Dose and Dosage Adjustment: The recommended dosage is 1 lozenge to be dissolved slowly in the mouth as needed to reduce smoking withdrawal symptoms, with a recommendation to repeat use at intervals ranging from every 1.5 to 8 hours depending on the phase of use (see below), and not to exceed a maximum dosage of 15 lozenges per day.

One lozenge should be placed in the mouth and allowed to dissolve. Periodically, the lozenge should be moved from one side of the mouth to the other, and repeated, until the lozenge is completely dissolved (approximately 20-30 minutes). The lozenge should not be chewed or swallowed whole. Users should not eat or drink while a lozenge is in the mouth. Users should follow the schedule of treatment below:

Step 1 Weeks 1 to 6	**Step 2 Weeks 7 to 9**	**Step 3 Weeks 10 to 12**	
Initial treatment period	Step down treatment period	Step down treatment period	To help stay smoke free over the next 12 weeks: use 1-2 lozenges per day only on occasions when strongly tempted to smoke
1 lozenge every 1 to 2 hours	1 lozenge every 2 to 4 hours	1 lozenge every 4 to 8 hours	

During weeks 1 to 6, it is recommended that users take a minimum of 8 lozenges per day.

The recommended schedule of treatment is 12 weeks. Lozenges should not be used for more than 24 weeks (6 months). If users still feel the need for treatment, a physician should be consulted.

Children and Adolescents: Safety and effectiveness in children and adolescents who smoke have not been evaluated. Nicorette Lozenge is not recommended for use in children. Nicorette Lozenge should only be used in adolescents (12-17 years) with advice from a doctor.

OVERDOSAGE:

Even small quantities of nicotine may be dangerous in children. If poisoning is suspected in a child, a doctor must be consulted immediately.

Overdose with Nicorette Lozenge (nicotine polacrilex) may occur if too many lozenges are ingested.

Signs and symptoms of an overdose would be expected to be the same as those of acute nicotine poisoning, including pallor, cold sweat, nausea, salivation, vomiting, abdominal pain, diarrhea, headache, dizziness, disturbed hearing and vision, tremor, mental confusion and weakness.

There has been no experience of overdosage with the Nicorette Lozenge. Nicotine overdose can cause severe clinical problems in children and nicotine-naive individuals. However, experience with other nicotine replacement therapies have demonstrated that an accidental overdose usually results in only mild to moderate symptoms that resolve in a few hours.

Prostration, hypotension and respiratory failure may ensue with large overdoses. Lethal doses in animals produce convulsions quickly and death follows as a result of peripheral and central respiratory paralysis, or less frequently, cardiac failure.

Treatment of Overdose: In the event of overdosage in a conscious, alert patient, vomiting should be induced with syrup of ipecac or gastric lavage carried out with a wide bore tube. A suspension of activated charcoal should then be passed through the tube and left in the stomach. Artificial respiration with oxygen should be instituted if needed and continued for as long as necessary. Other therapy, including treatment of shock, is purely symptomatic.

In comatose patients, a clear airway must be established immediately and ventilatory support may be required. Mechanical ventilation for respiratory paralysis may be necessary in severe nicotine poisoning. Other therapeutic measures are purely symptomatic and should be conducted according to the attending physician's assessment of the patient. When the patient's clinical status stabilizes, consideration may be given to gastric lavage and administration of activated charcoal. Hypotension and/or cardiovascular collapse may occur and should be treated vigorously.

For management of a suspected drug overdose, CPhA recommends that you contact your **regional Poison Control Centre**. See the *CPS* Directory section for a list of Poison Control Centres.

ACTION AND CLINICAL PHARMACOLOGY: Mechanism of Action: Nicotine, the chief alkaloid in tobacco products and a naturally occurring autonomic drug, is an agonist at nicotine receptors in the peripheral and central nervous systems and has pronounced CNS and cardiovascular effects.

Pharmacodynamics: The pharmacological effects of nicotine are generally dose related. Low doses of nicotine cause ganglionic stimulation and high doses cause ganglionic blockade following brief stimulation. At low doses, such as those associated with smoking cigarettes, the cardiovascular effects of nicotine appear to be mediated by the central nervous system through activation of chemoreceptors, afferent pathways or by direct effect on the brain stem. The result is sympathetic neural discharge of adrenaline resulting in an increase in blood pressure, heart rate, stroke volume and myocardial contractility. These effects result in increased myocardial oxygen demand. At high doses, nicotine is thought to act directly on the peripheral nervous system, producing ganglionic stimulation and the release of adrenal catecholamines with resultant hypotension and bradycardia. When consumed in tobacco products, nicotine has been shown to be addictive; abstinence is linked to craving and withdrawal symptoms, which include: urge to smoke, depressed mood, insomnia, irritability, frustration or anger, anxiety, difficulty in concentrating, restlessness and increased appetite or weight gain. The lozenges replace some of the nicotine provided by tobacco and help reduce the severity of these nicotine craving and withdrawal symptoms.

Pharmacokinetics: Absorption: Nicorette Lozenge (nicotine polacrilex) completely dissolves in the mouth, and the entire amount of nicotine contained in the lozenge becomes available for buccal absorption or ingestion (swallowing). The complete dissolution of Nicorette Lozenge is typically achieved in 20-30 minutes. The peak plasma concentrations of nicotine achieved after single doses of 2 mg or 4 mg are approximately 4.4 and 10.8 ng/mL, respectively. When dosed every 1.5 hours, the steady state peak and trough concentrations for the 2 mg lozenge are 12.7 and 9.4 ng/mL, respectively and for the 4 mg lozenge are 26.0 and 19.7 ng/mL, respectively. Ingestion of Nicorette Lozenge without following the dosing instructions (chewed, retained in the mouth, and swallowed; chewed and immediately swallowed) does not result in faster or higher absorption, but a substantial amount of nicotine (80-93%) is still absorbed.

Distribution: As the plasma protein binding of nicotine is low (4.9-20%), the volume of distribution of nicotine is large (2.51 L/kg). The distribution of nicotine to tissue is pH-dependent, with the highest concentrations of nicotine found in the brain, stomach, kidney and liver.

Metabolism: Nicotine is extensively metabolized to a number of metabolites, all of which are less active than the parent compound. The metabolism of nicotine primarily occurs in the liver, but also in the lung and kidney. Nicotine is metabolized primarily to cotinine but also to nicotine N'-oxide. Cotinine has a half-life of 15-20 hours and its blood levels are ten times higher than those of nicotine. Cotinine is further oxidized to trans-3'-hydroxycotinine, which is the most abundant metabolite of nicotine in the urine. Both nicotine and cotinine undergo glucuronidation.

Excretion: The elimination half-life of nicotine is approximately 2 hours (range 1-4 hours). Total clearance for nicotine ranges from approximately 62 to 89 L/hr. Non-renal clearance for nicotine is estimated to be about 75% of total clearance. Nicotine and its metabolites are excreted almost exclusively in the urine. The renal excretion of unchanged nicotine is highly dependent on urinary pH, with greater excretion occurring at acidic pH.

STORAGE AND STABILITY: Store Nicorette Lozenge (nicotine polacrilex) between 15 and 30°C. Protect from light. Keep container tightly closed.

INFORMATION FOR THE PATIENT: Published in e-CPS, available by subscription at www.e-cps.ca.

DOSAGE FORMS, COMPOSITION AND PACKAGING: 2 mg: Mint: Each white, round lozenge with convex surfaces, embossed with "NL2S" on one side, contains: nicotine polacrilex equivalent to nicotine 2 mg. Nonmedicinal ingredients: acacia, aspartame (contains phenylalanine), calcium polycarbophil, corn syrup solids, flavours, lactose, magnesium stearate, maltodextrin, mannitol, potassium bicarbonate, sodium alginate, sodium carbonate, soy protein, triethyl citrate and xanthan gum. Twenty-four-count cylindrical, flip-top polypropylene vials, packages of 24, 48 and 72.

Cherry: Each white, round lozenge with convex surfaces, embossed with "NL2C" on one side, contains: nicotine polacrilex equivalent to nicotine 2 mg. Nonmedicinal ingredients: acesulfame potassium, calcium polycarbophil, benzyl alcohol, butylhydroxy toluene, coconut and/or palm kernel oil, eugenol, flavours, magnesium stearate, maltodextrin, mannitol, modified corn starch, potassium bicarbonate, sodium alginate, sodium carbonate and xanthan gum. Twenty-four-count cylindrical, flip-top polypropylene vials, packages of 24, 48 and 72.

4 mg: Mint: Each white, round lozenge with convex surfaces, embossed with "NL4S" on one side, contains: nicotine polacrilex equivalent to nicotine 4 mg. Nonmedicinal ingredients: acacia, aspartame (contains phenylalanine), calcium polycarbophil, corn syrup solids, flavours, lactose, magnesium stearate, maltodextrin, mannitol, potassium bicarbonate, sodium alginate, sodium carbonate, soy protein, triethyl citrate and xanthan gum. 24-count cylindrical, flip-top polypropylene vials, packages of 24, 48 and 72.

Cherry: Each white, round lozenge with convex surfaces, embossed with "NL4C" on one side, contains: nicotine polacrilex equivalent to nicotine 4 mg. Nonmedicinal ingredients: acesulfame potassium, calcium polycarbophil, benzyl alcohol, butylhydroxy toluene, coconut and/or palm kernel oil, eugenol, flavours, magnesium stearate, maltodextrin, mannitol, modified corn starch, potassium bicarbonate, sodium alginate, sodium carbonate and xanthan gum. 24-count cylindrical, flip-top polypropylene vials, packages of 24, 48 and 72.

Nicorette® Patch

nicotine transdermal system

Stop Smoking Aid

McNeil Consumer Healthcare

Date of Preparation: May 20, 2008
Date of Revision: July 8, 2009

SUMMARY PRODUCT INFORMATION:

Route of Administration	**Dosage Form/ Strength**	**Clinically Relevant Nonmedicinal Ingredients**
Transdermal	Patch, 15 mg, 10 mg, 5 mg	For a complete listing see Dosage Forms, Composition and Packaging.

INDICATIONS AND CLINICAL USE: The NICORETTE Patch (Nicotine Transdermal System), is applied while patients are awake, is indicated as a temporary aid to facilitate smoking cessation in smokers with a strong desire to quit and to provide partial substitution for the nicotine in cigarettes in order to lessen withdrawal symptoms of smoking cessation. NICORETTE Patch treatment should be used as part of a comprehensive behavioral smoking-cessation program.

The NICORETTE Patch, when used up to 15 mg per patch, may be used alone or in combination with NICORETTE Gum 2 mg. Combination treatment may be needed by some patients who have relapsed with the patch in the past or in cases of breakthrough cravings. Combination treatment may also be used when there is difficulty controlling cravings for cigarettes while on the patch alone.

Geriatrics (>60 years of age): Based on limited evidence from clinical trials NICORETTE Patch therapy appeared to be as effective in this age group as in younger smokers. The initial dose in elderly patients may have to be adjusted because their concomitant diseases may increase risk (see Warnings and Precautions and Action and Clinical Pharmacology).

Pediatrics (<18 years of age): NICORETTE PATCH is contraindicated in persons under 18 years of age (see Warnings and Precautions).

CONTRAINDICATIONS:

- Patients who are hypersensitive to nicotine or to any ingredient in the formulation or component of the transdermal system. (For a complete listing, see Dosage Forms, Composition and Packaging.) Patients with acute hypersensitivity reactions should discontinue use of NICORETTE Patch and should be advised of the possibility of acute hypersensitivity reactions to other forms of nicotine, including cigarettes;
- Patients with generalized skin disorders;
- Non-smokers or occasional smokers;
- Persons under 18 years of age (see Warnings and Precautions);
- Pregnant women or nursing mothers (see Warnings and Precautions); and
- Patients during the immediate post-myocardial infarction period, patients with life-threatening arrhythmias, patients with severe or worsening angina pectoris and patients who have had a recent cerebral vascular accident (see Warnings and Precautions).

WARNINGS AND PRECAUTIONS: General: Nicotine from any source can be toxic and addictive. For any smoker, with or without concomitant disease, the risk of nicotine replacement in a smoking cessation program should be weighed against the hazard of continued smoking.

The patient should stop smoking completely when initiating NICORETTE Patch therapy (Nicotine Transdermal System) (see Dosage and Administration). Patients should be informed that they should not continue to smoke while using NICORETTE Patch systems, because they may experience adverse effects due to peak nicotine levels higher than those experienced from smoking alone. If there is a clinically significant increase in cardiovascular or other effects attributable to nicotine, the NICORETTE Patch

dose should be reduced or NICORETTE Patch treatment discontinued. The use of NICORETTE Patch systems beyond 10 weeks by patients who stop smoking should be discouraged because the chronic consumption of nicotine by any route can be harmful and addicting. If the patient continues to smoke, treatment should be discontinued.

Strenuous Exercise: Preliminary evidence suggests that wearing a nicotine transdermal patch during periods of strenuous exercise may lead to nicotine toxicity as a result of increased absorption of nicotine from the depot of nicotine in the skin under the patch, due to increased skin temperature and increased cutaneous vasodilation and perfusion from exercising. Three cases illustrating this phenomenon were described in Health Canada Adverse Reaction Newsletter, Volume 6, Number 1, January, 1996. Advice to remove the nicotine patch before engaging in strenuous exercise was recommended by; W. Dafoe and P. Huston, Current Trends in Cardiac Rehabilitation, Canadian Medical Association Journal, February 15, 1997;156(4):527-532. Until definitive studies have been undertaken to clarify this hazard, it is advisable to remove the nicotine patch prior to engaging in strenuous activity.

Cardiovascular: The risks of nicotine replacement in patients with certain cardiovascular and peripheral vascular diseases should be weighed against the benefits of including nicotine replacement in a smoking-cessation program for them. Specifically, patients with coronary heart disease (history of myocardial infarction and/or angina pectoris), serious cardiac arrhythmias, or vasospastic diseases (Buerger's disease, Prinzmetal's variant angina) should be carefully screened and evaluated before nicotine replacement is recommended.

Palpitations occurring in association with the use of NICORETTE Patch therapy have been reported occasionally. If serious cardiovascular symptoms occur with the use of NICORETTE Patch it should be discontinued. NICORETTE Patch therapy should be used with caution in patients with accelerated hypertension only when the benefits of including nicotine replacement in a smoking-cessation program outweigh the risks.

Dependence/Tolerance: NICORETTE Patch therapy is likely to have a low abuse potential based on differences between it and cigarettes in four characteristics commonly considered important in contributing to abuse: much slower absorption, much smaller fluctuations in blood levels, lower blood levels of nicotine, and less frequent use (i.e., once daily). Dependency on NICORETTE Patch has not been reported.

To minimize the risk of dependence, therapy should not exceed 10 weeks (see Dosage and Administration).

Endocrine and Metabolism: NICORETTE Patch therapy should be used with caution in patients with hyperthyroidism pheochromocytoma, or insulin-dependent diabetes since nicotine causes the release of catecholamines by the adrenal medulla.

Gastrointestinal: Nicotine delays healing in peptic ulcer disease; therefore, NICORETTE Patch therapy should be used with caution in patients with active peptic ulcers and only when the benefits of including nicotine replacement in a smoking-cessation program are considered to outweigh the risks.

Hepatic/Biliary/Pancreatic: The pharmacokinetics of nicotine have not been studied in the elderly or in patients with hepatic impairment); however, given that nicotine is extensively metabolized and that its total system clearance is dependent on liver blood flow, some influence of hepatic impairment on drug kinetics (reduced clearance) should be anticipated.

Renal: The pharmacokinetics of nicotine have not been studied in the elderly or in patients with renal impairment; however, given that nicotine is extensively metabolized and that its total system clearance is dependent on liver blood flow, some influence of hepatic impairment on drug kinetics (reduced clearance) should be anticipated. Only severe renal impairment would be expected to affect the clearance of nicotine or its metabolites from the circulation.

Sensitivity/Resistance: Patients with acute hypersensitivity reactions should discontinue use of NICORETTE Patch and should be advised of the possibility of acute hypersensitivity reactions to other forms of nicotine, including cigarettes.

Skin: NICORETTE Patch systems are usually well tolerated by patients with normal skin, but may be irritating for patients with some skin disorders (atopic or eczematous dermatitis). Patients should be instructed to discontinue promptly the use of NICORETTE Patch systems and contact their physician if they experience severe or persistent local skin reactions (e.g. urticaria, hives, or generalized rash). Patients using NICORETTE Patch therapy concurrently with other transdermal systems may exhibit local reactions at both application sites. In such patients use of one or both systems may have to be discontinued. Serious allergic reactions may occur rarely. About 1% of patients dropped out of clinical trials due to skin reactions; none had classical contact sensitization.

Special Populations: Pregnant Women: Pregnant smokers should be encouraged to attempt cessation using educational and behavioral interventions before using pharmacological approaches.

Tobacco smoke (containing nicotine, hydrogen cyanide and carbon monoxide) has been shown to be harmful to the fetus. Nicotine has been shown in animal studies to cause fetal harm. There is a possibility that nicotine from NICORETTE Patch systems can cause fetal harm when administered to a pregnant woman. Women of child-bearing potential should be advised to take adequate precautions to avoid becoming pregnant while using NICORETTE Patch (see Contraindications).

Nursing Women: The safety of NICORETTE Patch therapy in nursing infants has not been examined. Nicotine passes freely into breast milk; the milk to plasma ratio averages 2.9. Nicotine is absorbed orally (see Contraindications).

Pediatrics (<18 years of age): NICORETTE Patch is not to be used by persons under 18 years of age. The use of NICORETTE Patch in children and adolescents who smoke has not been evaluated (see Contraindications).

Geriatrics (>60 years of age): The initial dose in elderly patients may have to be adjusted because their concomitant diseases may increase risk (see Action and Clinical Pharmacology, Special Populations and Conditions).

Safety Note Concerning Children and Pets: The amounts of nicotine that are tolerated by adult smokers can cause severe poisoning and even prove fatal if the NICORETTE Patch system (Nicotine Transdermal System) is applied or ingested by children or pets. Used NICORETTE Patch systems contain approximately 40% of their initial nicotine content. Therefore, patients should be cautioned to keep both the used and unused NICORETTE Patch systems out of the reach of children and pets.

Monitoring and Laboratory Tests: No specific monitoring or laboratory tests are required while using NICORETTE Patch.

ADVERSE REACTIONS: Adverse Drug Reaction Overview: Assessment of adverse events in patients who participated in controlled clinical trials is complicated by the occurrence of GI and CNS effects of nicotine withdrawal as well as nicotine excess. The actual incidences of both effects are confounded by concurrent smoking by many of the patients. When reporting adverse events in the clinical trials, the clinical investigators did not attempt to identify the cause of the symptom.

The most common adverse event associated with NICORETTE Patch (Nicotine Transdermal System) is a mild, short-lived erythema and/or pruritus at the application site. Erythema and/or pruritus were seen at least once in 47% of patients on the NICORETTE Patch system (versus 45% of patients on placebo) in the clinical efficacy trials. These signs were not considered clinically relevant and usually disappeared within one hour. After removal of the system, local erythema was noted at least once in 7% of patients and local edema in 3% of patients.

Erythema generally resolved within 24 hours. About 1% of patients dropped out of the clinical trials due to skin reactions. None of these were classified as contact sensitization reactions.

In the prescription to OTC switch trials approximately 32% of reported events were skin reactions.

Clinical Trial Adverse Drug Reactions: Because clinical trials are conducted under very specific conditions the adverse reaction rates observed in the clinical trials may not reflect the rates observed in practice and should not be compared to the rates in the clinical trials of another drug. Adverse drug reaction information from clinical trials is useful for identifying drug-related adverse events and for approximating rates.

Patch-Only Trials: Table 1 summarizes the adverse events with an incidence of greater than 1% in 2 placebo-controlled clinical trials and two prescription to OTC switch trials.

Table 1: NICORETTE Patch

Adverse Reactions Reported (%) with an Incidence of >1% in Placebo-Controlled Clinical Trials and Prescription to OTC Switch Trials

Body System/ Adverse Event	Prescription Treatment Groups: NICORETTE (n=258)	Prescription Treatment Groups: Placebo (n=251)	Prescription to OTC Switch: NICORETTE (n=3885)
CNS			
Headache	5.4	4.0	3.3
Vertigo	3.1	0.8	—
Digestive			
Nausea	3.5	4.0	2.4
Flatulence	2.7	2.4	—
Diarrhea	1.9	1.6	—
Taste Perversion	1.9	1.6	—
Mouth Ulceration	1.6	0.4	—
Heartburn/Indigestion	1.2	2.4	—
Tongue Disorder	1.2	0.4	—
Musculoskeletal			
Myalgia	3.1	3.1	—
Skin (Not Application Site)			
Rash/Pruritus/Tingling/Edema	1.9	1.2	—
Acne	1.2	0.0	—
Body as a Whole			
Pain	—	—	2.1

Patch + Gum Combination Treatment Trials: Table 2 summarizes the adverse events with an incidence of greater than 1% in 2 patch + gum combination treatment trials.

Table 2: NICORETTE Patch

Adverse Event Incidence for Combination Treatment with NICORETTE 15 mg/16 h Patch Plus NICORETTE Gum 2 mg in Clinical Trials Performed in the Belgium and Finland

	Belgium Trial (Kornitzer) n/N (%)	Finland Trial (Puska) n/N (%)
CNS		
Insomnia	2/149 (1.34)	10/150 (6.66)
Dizziness/Light-headedness	8/149 (5.36)	—
Vertigo	5/149 (3.36)	2/150 (1.33)
Irritable/Fussy	—	—
Headache	9/149 (6.0)	5/150 (3.33)
Gastrointestinal		
Non-Specific GI Distress	—	—
Indigestion=Dyspepsia/Constipation	23/149 (15.4)	3/150 (2)
Flatulence	—	2/150 (1.33)
Nausea/Vomiting	4/149 (2.68)	2/150 (1.33)
Diarrhea	5/149 (3.35)	—
Gastritis	2/149 (1.34)	—
Local		
Pruritus/Itching	16/147 (10.9) (first week)	46/150 (30.7)
Erythema/Rash	15/147 (10.2) (first week)	10/150 (6.7)
Stomatitis	10/149 (6.7)	4/150 (0.66)
Throat Irritation	10/149 (6.7)	—
Hiccups	11/149 (7.38)	—

In the Kornitzer study, in Table 2 (combination nicotine replacement therapy patch + gum) versus patch alone versus placebo), the incidence of local reactions was higher in both the groups that used NICORETTE Patch than in the placebo group. However, there was no significant difference between the patch + gum and patch alone groups. The incidence of local oral effects was: stomatitis 6.7% (Combination), 10% (patch alone) and 2.7% (placebo); throat irritation 6.7%, 5.3% and 2.7%, respectively and hiccup 7.4%, 0.7% and 0%, respectively. The incidence of local skin reactions after one week of treatment was: erythema 10.1%, 10.1% and 8%, respectively, and itching 10.7%, 10.7% and 1.3%, respectively. The frequency of AEs was highest in the first week, reflecting the higher compliance to treatment at the beginning of the study. The incidence of moderate (which were in a majority) or severe systemic AEs was 20.1%, 20% and 18.7% in the combination group, patch alone group and placebo, respectively during the course of the study. However, there were few withdrawals due to AEs.

In the Puska study, in Table 2 (combination patch + gum versus gum alone) a total of 138/150 (92%) of subjects in the patch + gum group and 136/150 (90.61%) in the gum alone group reported one or more AE. These were mild in the majority of cases (60% in the patch + gum group and 53.3% in gum alone group). The only difference between patch + gum and single gum alone was the incidence of itching (30.7% versus 11.3%, respectively). Erythema was reported by 6.7 and 7.3% of subjects in both groups respectively. The frequency of local oral AEs did not differ significantly between the combination patch + gum group than single gum alone group: sore throat 1.3% and 4%, respectively, sore mouth 3.3% and 4.7%, respectively and throat irritation 0% and 2%, respectively and stomatitis 2.7 and 2.7 respectively. The majority of AEs were mild in intensity.

In the pharmacokinetic study (980 CHC 9134-001) there were no serious AEs or withdrawals due to AEs. There were no unexpected findings. In the clinical pharmacology study [Fagerström et al 1993]), there were no withdrawals due to AEs. No other safety data are presented in the publication.

The data from these studies suggest that safety risk is similar in the group that receive combination patch + gum therapy to that noted in the group receiving single therapy with either patch alone or gum alone. Although ex-smokers using the combination of the patch and the gum may develop both groups of AEs that are formulation specific i.e. application site reactions for the patch and gastrointestinal events for the gum, the data from these studies do not suggest that this is a problem in clinical usage. The majority of AEs are mild and few patients discontinue usage due to AEs.

Post-Market Adverse Drug Reactions: In addition to the reported effects in clinical trials, the following events have been reported:

Cardiovascular: chest pain, edema, flushing, palpitations, arrhythmias, tachycardia.
Dermatologic: erythema, itching, rash, urticaria, pruritus, hypersensitivity; application site swelling and irritation.
Gastrointestinal: nausea.
CNS: numbness, paresthesia, syncope, dizziness, vertigo.
Respiratory: throat tightness.

Reports of myocardial infarction, cardiac arrest and cerebral hemorrhage including death have been received and a relationship to drug therapy as a contributing factor cannot be excluded.

Rare reports of miscarriage and fetal abnormalities have been received and a relationship to drug therapy as a contributing factor cannot be excluded.

DRUG INTERACTIONS: Overview: Physicians should anticipate that the pharmacokinetics of certain concomitant medications may be altered by smoking cessation with or without nicotine replacement. Therefore the dosage of certain concomitant medications may require adjustment. Refer to Table 3.

Drug-Drug Interactions:

Table 3: NICORETTE Patch

Established or Potential Drug-Drug Interactions

Proper Name of Drug	Ref	Effect	Clinical Comment
Acetaminophen, caffeine, imipramine, oxazepam, pentazocine, propranolol, theophylline	T	Deinduction of hepatic enzymes on smoking cessation	May require a **decrease** in dose at cessation of smoking
Insulin	T	Increase in subcutaneous insulin absorption with smoking cessation	May require a **decrease** in dose at cessation of smoking
Adrenergic antagonists (e.g. prazosin, labetalol)	T	Decrease in circulating catecholamines with smoking cessation	May require a **decrease** in dose at cessation of smoking
Adrenergic agonists (e.g. isoproterenol, phenylephrine)	T	Decrease in circulating catecholamines with smoking cessation	May require an **increase** in dose at cessation of smoking

Legend: C=Case Study; CT=Clinical Trial; T=Theoretical.

Drug-Food Interactions: Interactions with food have not been established.
Drug-Herb Interactions: Interactions with herbal products have not been established.
Drug-Laboratory Test Interactions: Interactions with laboratory tests have not been established.

DOSAGE AND ADMINISTRATION: Dosing Considerations:

- Patients must desire to stop smoking and should be instructed to stop smoking immediately as they begin using NICORETTE Patch (Nicotine Transdermal System) therapy.
- If the patient is unable to avoid cigarette smoking within 2 weeks of starting treatment, NICORETTE Patch therapy should be stopped, since few additional patients in clinical trials were able to quit after this time. The duration of treatment should not exceed 10 weeks.
- The patient should be told to read the consumer information leaflet (see Information for the Patient) on NICORETTE Patch therapy and should be encouraged to ask questions.
- Smoking cessation should be accompanied by a behavioral support program.

Recommended Dose and Dosage Adjustment: Patch Treatment:

- Use one 15 mg patch daily for up to 6 weeks.
- NICORETTE Patch should be applied promptly upon its removal from the protective pouch to prevent loss of nicotine from the system. NICORETTE Patch should be applied only once a day to a non-hairy, clean, and dry skin site on the upper arm or the hip. A different site of application should be chosen each day. Each day a new NICORETTE Patch system should be applied upon waking and removed at bedtime. It should not be worn for more than 16 hours/day.

For patients who wish to wean themselves rather than abruptly stop, follow the regimen outlined in Table 4.

Table 4: NICORETTE Patch

Recommended Dosage of NICORETTE Patches

Dose	Duration
NICORETTE 15 mg/16 hours	First 6 weeks
NICORETTE 10 mg/16 hours	Next 2 weeks
NICORETTE 5 mg/16 hours	Last 2 weeks

Patch Treatment Used in Combination with NICORETTE Gum 2 mg: The NICORETTE Patch (up to 15 mg **only**) can be used in combination with NICORETTE Gum 2 mg if breakthrough cravings are experienced or there is difficulty in controlling cravings for cigarettes. When used in combination with NICORETTE Patch, NICORETTE Gum 2 mg should be taken as required, when cravings occur. It is recommended that a minimum of 5-6 pieces of gum are used daily. The maximum number of gums used in conjunction with the patch is 15 pieces per day.

Combination treatment should be used for 6-10 weeks, including a weaning period.

When NICORETTE Patch and 2 mg Gum are used in combination, weaning can be done by either (see Table 5):

1. Using the NICORETTE Patch 10 mg/16 hour for 2 weeks and then the NICORETTE Patch 5 mg/16 hour for 2 weeks while maintaining the number of pieces of 2 mg Gum that have been routinely used. Then when a patch is no longer used, the number of pieces of gum can be gradually reduced.

or

2. Stopping use of the NICORETTE Patch 15 mg/16 hour and then gradually reducing the number of pieces of NICORETTE Gum 2 mg that are being used.

Missed Dose: If a dose is missed, the patch should be applied immediately and removed at bedtime. A new patch should be applied the next morning.

OVERDOSAGE:

There have been two reported cases of applying several nicotine patches simultaneously. Both people were attempting suicide and combined several nicotine patches, 21 mg, with other drugs. No serious effects resulted from either attempt.

Signs and symptoms of an overdose from NICORETTE Patch (Nicotine Transdermal System) are expected to be the same as those of acute nicotine poisoning, including: pallor, cold sweat, nausea, salivation, vomiting, abdominal pain, diarrhea, headache, dizziness, disturbed hearing and vision, tremor, mental confusion and weakness. Prostration, hypotension, and respiratory failure may ensue with large overdoses. Lethal doses of nicotine produce convulsions quickly and death follows as a result of peripheral or central respiratory paralysis or, less frequently, cardiac failure. The acute, minimal, oral lethal dose of nicotine in human adults is believed to be 40 to 60 mg (<1 mg/kg). Much lower doses have been reported to be toxic in children.

Table 5: NICORETTE Patch

Recommended Dosage for Combination Treatment

	Patch	Gum
Initial Treatment Period		
First 6 weeks	1 patch 15 mg/16 hours per day	Ad libitum Recommended 5–6 gums per day Maximum 15 gums per day
Weaning Period—Alternative 1		
Next 4 weeks	1 patch 10 mg/16 hours per day for 2 weeks Followed by 1 patch 5 mg/16 hours per day for 2 weeks	Ad libitum Recommended 5–6 gums per day Maximum 15 gums per day
From then up to 6 months	Do not use the patch.	Ad libitum Recommended 5–6 gums per day Maximum 15 gums per day
Up to 12 months	Do not use the patch.	Gradually wean from gum use
Weaning Period—Alternative 2		
During the next 12 months	Do not use the patch.	Gradually wean from gum use

Treatment: The NICORETTE Patch system should be removed immediately if the patient shows signs of overdosage and the patient should seek immediate medical care by contacting a physician or local poison-control centre. The skin surface should be flushed with water and dried. **Soap must NOT be used since it may increase nicotine absorption.** Nicotine will continue to be delivered into the bloodstream for several hours after removal of the system because of a depot of nicotine in the skin.

Persons ingesting NICORETTE Patch systems should be referred to a health care facility for management. Due to the possibility of nicotine-induced seizures, activated charcoal should be administered. In unconscious patients with a secure airway, instill activated charcoal via a nasogastric tube. Repeated doses of activated charcoal should be administered as long as the system remains in the gastrointestinal tract since it will continue to release nicotine for many hours. A saline cathartic or sorbitol added to the first dose of activated charcoal may speed gastrointestinal passage of the system.

Other supportive measures include diazepam or barbiturates for seizures, atropine for excessive bronchial secretions or diarrhea, respiratory support for respiratory failure, and vigorous fluid support for hypotension and cardiovascular collapse.

Combination Treatment: The signs and symptoms associated with over dosage with the combined used of NICORETTE Patch and 2 mg Gum product are likely to be no different to those associated with the patch itself.

For management of a suspected drug overdose, contact your **regional Poison Control Centre**. See the *CPS* Directory section for a list of Poison Control Centres.

ACTION AND CLINICAL PHARMACOLOGY: Mechanism of Action: NICORETTE Patch (Nicotine Transdermal System) is a multilayered, laminated, flexible thin film patch containing nicotine as the active ingredient. NICORETTE Patch has been specifically designed to provide a 16-hour rate-controlled delivery of nicotine following its application to intact skin. It is intended to be applied during the day and removed at night prior to sleeping, thus minimizing the potential for any sleep disturbances. NICORETTE Patch provides nicotine without the other ingredients in tobacco smoke (e.g. tar, carbon monoxide, hydrogen cyanide) thereby attenuating abstinence symptoms associated with nicotine withdrawal during the cessation of smoking. NICORETTE Patch increases the success rate of cessation in smokers who are motivated to quit.

Pharmacodynamics: Nicotine, the chief alkaloid in tobacco products, stereo-selectively binds to acetylcholine receptors at the autonomic ganglia, in the adrenal medulla, at neuromuscular junctions, and in the brain. Two types of central nervous system effects are believed to be responsible for nicotine's positively reinforcing properties. A stimulating effect, exerted mainly in the cortex via the locus ceruleus, produces increased alertness and cognitive performance. A "reward" effect via the "pleasure system" in the brain is exerted in the limbic system. At low doses the stimulant effects predominate while at high doses the reward effects predominate. Intermittent intravenous administration of nicotine activates neurohormonal pathways, releasing acetylcholine, norepinephrine, dopamine, serotonin, vasopressin, beta-endorphin, growth hormone and ACTH.

The cardiovascular effects of nicotine include peripheral vasoconstriction, tachycardia, and elevated blood pressure. Acute and chronic tolerance to nicotine develops from smoking tobacco or ingesting nicotine preparations. Acute tolerance (a reduction in response for a given dose) develops rapidly (less than one hour), but at distinct rates for different physiologic effects (skin temperature, heart rate, subjective effects). Withdrawal symptoms, such as cigarette craving, can be reduced in most individuals by plasma nicotine levels lower than those for smoking.

Withdrawal from nicotine in addicted individuals is characterized by craving, nervousness, restlessness, irritability, mood lability, anxiety, drowsiness, sleep disturbances, impaired concentration, increased appetite, minor somatic complaints (headache, myalgia, constipation, fatigue), and weight gain. Nicotine toxicity is dose-related and characterized by nausea, abdominal pain, vomiting, diarrhea, diaphoresis, flushing, dizziness, disturbed hearing and vision, confusion, weakness, palpitations, altered respiration, and hypotension.

Both smoking and nicotine can increase circulating cortisol and catecholamines, and tolerance does not develop to the catecholamine-releasing effects of nicotine.

Pharmacokinetics: The average amount of nicotine delivered to the patient from each NICORETTE Patch system (31 μg/cm²/hr) is approximately proportional to the surface area and results in systemic absorption of 5, 10 and 15 mg/day, respectively from each of the 3 patches over a 16-hour period as shown in Table 6.

The dose of nicotine absorbed from the NICORETTE Patch systems represents approximately 95% of the amount released in 16 hours. The remainder is lost via evaporation from the edge. About 40% of the total amount of nicotine remains in the system 16 hours after application.

Table 6: NICORETTE Patch

Composition of NICORETTE Patch Systems

NICORETTE Dose	Dose Absorbed (mg/16 hours)	System Surface Area (cm²)	Total Nicotine Content (mg)
Treatment Dose	15	30	24.9
First Weaning Dose	10	20	16.6
Second Weaning Dose	5	10	8.3

Following the first application of a NICORETTE Patch system, plasma nicotine concentrations gradually increase to reach peak levels within 5-10 hours and then slowly decline until the system is removed, after which the terminal elimination half-life of nicotine is about 4 hours. The mean peak plasma level of nicotine achieved with the 15 mg/day system is 9-15 ng/mL.

After repeated application of NICORETTE Patch systems, plasma nicotine concentrations were not significantly higher than those after a single application, indicating no accumulation (see Table 7).

Table 7: NICORETTE Patch

Pharmacokinetics After Repeated Administration

Day (15 mg/16 hour system)	AUC (ng·h/mL)	AUC_{Inf} (ng·h/mL)	C_{MAX} (ng/mL)	$t_{½}$ (h)	T_{MAX} (h)
1	12.2	13	13	3.7	8
6	12.2	12.9	14.2	3.4	6

Plasma nicotine concentrations show a slight deviation from dose proportionality for the three NICORETTE Patch doses: with increasing system size the increase in concentration is somewhat less than expected. Nicotine kinetics are similar following application of the patch on the arm and hip.

Combination Patch + Gum Treatment: The plasma levels achieved when administering the maximum daily dosage of NICORETTE Patch (15 mg/16 hour) in combination with NICORETTE Gum 2 mg (24 pieces in 15 hours) were similar to those seen after administration of a maximum daily dose of NICORETTE 4 mg gum (19 pieces in 15 hours). The C_{trough} max value for the combination treatment (Patch + 2 mg Gum) was 39.4 ng/mL as compared to 38.1 ng/mL for the reference group (4 mg gum). Also, the maximum and minimum concentrations during the intense sampling time interval were similar for the combination treatment (38.3 and 35.4 ng/mL, respectively for Patch + Gum) and the reference treatment (40.0 and 33·4 ng/mL, respectively).

The total amount of nicotine released from the combined administration of maximum daily dosages of the patch (15 mg/16 hour) and 2 mg gum (24 pieces in 15 hours) was somewhat lower than from the administration of 19 NICORETTE 4 mg gum over 15 hours (49.1 and 55.1 ng·mL respectively).

Absorption: Following removal of the NICORETTE Patch system after 16 hours of wear, plasma nicotine concentrations decline in an apparently exponential fashion. The half-life after removal was about twice that observed after intravenous infusion, suggesting continued absorption from the skin depot. Patients had non-detectable nicotine concentrations within 10 to 12 hours after removing the system.

The average plasma nicotine level is about 20 to 36 ng/mL in moderate to heavy smokers. In comparison, the average plasma nicotine concentration in subjects delivered from NICORETTE Patch 15 mg/16 hour system is about 9 ng/mL.

Table 8: NICORETTE Patch

Steady State Nicotine Pharmacokinetic Parameters for NICORETTE Patch Applied for 16 Hours (N=12)

	Mean ± SD (Range of Delivery Rate) (mg/day)		
	15[a]	10	5
C_{max} (ng/mL)	13.0±3.1 (7.8–17.9)	6.9±2.0 (4.8–10.0)	3.5±0.7 (2.7–4.7)
C_{avg} 16 (ng/mL)	9.4±2.4 (5.3–13.3)	4.9±1.2 (3.0–6.8)	2.7±0.5 (2.0–3.6)
C_{avg} 24 (ng/mL)	8.7±2.1 (5.2–11.8)	4.8±1.0 (3.3–6.3)	2.7±0.4 (2.1–3.3)
C_{min} (ng/mL)	2.5±0.8 (1.2–4.1)	1.4±0.5 (0.5–2.4)	0.8±0.3 (0.3–1.2)
T_{max} (hrs)	8±3 (4–16)	9±4 (6–16)	9±4 (3–16)

[a] Data for 15 mg system are derived from a different study than the 5 and 10 mg systems.

Legend: C_{max}=maximum observed plasma concentration; C_{avg} 16=estimated average plasma concentration during the 0 to 16 hour period, calculated as AUC (0-16)/16; C_{avg} 24=average plasma concentration calculated over 24 hrs; C_{min}=minimum observed plasma concentration; T_{max}=time of maximum plasma concentration.

There are no differences in nicotine kinetics between men and women using NICORETTE Patch systems. Linear regression of both AUC and C_{max} versus total body weight shows the expected inverse relationship. Men and women having low body weight are expected to have higher AUC and C_{max} values.

Distribution: The volume of distribution following i.v. administration of nicotine is approximately 2 to 3 L/kg and the half-life ranges from 1 to 2 hours. Plasma protein binding of nicotine is <5%. Therefore, changes in nicotine binding from use of concomitant drugs or alterations of plasma proteins by disease states would not be expected to have significant effects on nicotine kinetics.

Metabolism: The major elimination organ is the liver, and average plasma clearance is about 1.2 L/min; the kidney and lung also metabolize nicotine. There is no significant skin metabolism of nicotine. More than 20 metabolites of nicotine have been identified, all of which are believed to be less active than the parent compound. The primary metabolite of nicotine in plasma, cotinine, has a half-life of 15 to 20 hours and concentrations that exceed nicotine by 10-fold.

Excretion: The primary urinary metabolites are cotinine (15% of the dose) and trans-3-hydroxycotinine (45% of the dose). Usually about 10% of nicotine is excreted unchanged in the urine. As much as 30% may be excreted unchanged in the urine with high urine flow rates and acidification below pH 5.

Special Populations and Conditions: Pediatrics: NICORETTE Patches are contraindicated in persons under 18 years of age.

Geriatrics: The initial dose in elderly patients may have to be adjusted because concomitant diseases may increase risk. The pharmacokinetics of nicotine have not been studied in the elderly; however, given that nicotine is extensively metabolized and that its total system clearance is dependent on liver blood flow, some influence of hepatic impairment on drug kinetics (reduced clearance) should be anticipated. Only severe renal impairment would be expected to affect the clearance of nicotine or its metabolites from the circulation.

Gender: There are no differences in nicotine kinetics between men and women using NICORETTE Patch. Linear regression of both AUC and C_{max} versus total body weight shows the expected inverse relationship. Men and women having low body weight are expected to have higher AUC and C_{max}.

STORAGE AND STABILITY: Do not store above 25° C. Protect from light.

Once removed from the protective pouch, NICORETTE Patch (Nicotine Transdermal System) should be applied promptly since nicotine is volatile and the system may lose strength.

SPECIAL HANDLING INSTRUCTIONS: The amounts of nicotine that are tolerated by adult smokers can cause severe poisoning and even prove fatal if the NICORETTE Patch system is applied or ingested by children or pets. Used NICORETTE Patch systems contain approximately 40% of their initial nicotine content. Therefore, patients should be cautioned to keep both the used and unused NICORETTE Patch systems out of the reach of children and pets.

NICORETTE Patch systems can be a dermal irritant and can cause contact sensitization. Care should be taken to avoid unnecessary contact with active systems. If you do handle active systems, wash with water alone since soap may increase nicotine absorption. Do not touch your eyes.

Disposal of Used Patches: When the used system is removed from the skin, it should be folded over and placed in its pouch. The used system should be disposed of immediately in such a way as to prevent its access by children or pets (see Information for the Patient for further directions on handling and disposal).

INFORMATION FOR THE PATIENT: Published in e-CPS, available by subscription at www.e-cps.ca.

DOSAGE FORMS, COMPOSITION AND PACKAGING: NICORETTE Patch (Nicotine Transdermal System) is a multilayered, rectangular-shaped, laminated thin film containing nicotine as the active ingredient. Proceeding from the visible surface toward the surface attached to the skin, there are 3 distinct layers. These include (1) an outer backing layer composed of a laminated polyester film, (2) a middle layer which contains an adhesive, a structural non-woven material and nicotine; the adhesive controls the rate of delivery of nicotine to the skin, and (3) a third layer comprised of a disposable liner that protects the systems; the liner is removed prior to use.

NICORETTE Patches are available in three strengths/sizes. The average amount of nicotine delivered to the patient from each NICORETTE Patch system is approximately proportional to the surface area of each system and results in systemic absorption of 5 mg (10 cm²), 10 mg (20 cm²) and 15 mg (30 cm²), respectively, from each of the patches over a 16 hour period as shown in Table 9. Each patch contains nicotine at a concentration of 0.83 mg/cm². Other ingredients are polyester (non woven), polybutene and polyisobutylene.

A single patch comes in a foil pouch. NICORETTE Patch (Nicotine Transdermal System) are labeled with the average amount of nicotine absorbed by the patient over 16 hours and are available in packages of 7 and 14 patches.

Table 9: NICORETTE Patch

Composition of NICORETTE Patch Systems

NICORETTE Dose	Dose Absorbed (mg/16 hours)	System Surface Area (cm²)	Total Nicotine Content (mg)
Treatment Dose	15	30	24.9
First Weaning Dose	10	20	16.6
Second Weaning Dose	5	10	8.3

Table 10: NICORETTE Patch

Availability of NICORETTE

Strength	Size	Total Amount of Nicotine	Patch Imprint
15 mg/16 hours system	30 cm²	24.9 mg	NICORETTE 15 mg
10 mg/16 hours system	20 cm²	16.6 mg	NICORETTE 10 mg
5 mg/16 hours system	10 cm²	8.3 mg	NICORETTE 5 mg

Nicotinamide

CPhA Monograph

see *Niacin/Niacinamide*

Nicotinic Acid

CPhA Monograph

see *Niacin/Niacinamide*

Nicoumalone ℞

acenocoumarol

Oral Anticoagulant

CPhA Monograph

Date of Preparation: November 2008

This monograph has been compiled by CPhA and reviewed by experts. It may contain information different from that found in Health Canada-approved Product Monographs. The reader is referred to the *CPS* Editorial Policy for more information.

SUMMARY PRODUCT INFORMATION:

Route of Administration	Dosage Form	Strength
Oral	Tablet	1 mg, 4 mg

INDICATIONS AND CLINICAL USE: Nicoumalone (also known as acenocoumarol) is indicated for:

- primary and secondary prevention of venous thromboembolism
- prevention of systemic embolism in patients with prosthetic heart valves or atrial fibrillation
- prevention of acute myocardial infarction in patients with peripheral arterial disease
- prevention of stroke, recurrent infarction or death in patients after acute myocardial infarction.

When a rapid anticoagulant effect is required, for example in the setting of acute venous thromboembolism, both heparin and an oral anticoagulant should be administered initially and heparin discontinued after the international normalized ratio (INR) is in the therapeutic range for at least 2 days, after which time the oral anticoagulant is continued alone.

Achievement and maintenance of the target INR is an important determinant of the efficacy and safety of oral anticoagulation therapy. The INR may be influenced by drugs or illnesses that alter the metabolism of anticoagulants, and dietary and gastrointestinal factors that affect the synthesis or metabolism of vitamin K-dependent coagulation factors. See Adverse Reactions, Abnormal Hematologic and Clinical Chemistry Findings. There are also well described genetic polymorphisms that influence the pharmacokinetics of oral anticoagulants. See Dosage and Administration, Recommended Dose and Dosage Adjustment, Genetic Polymorphism.

Geriatrics: In general the dose of an oral anticoagulant required to maintain a therapeutic INR decreases with age.

Pediatrics: Nicoumalone is not approved for the treatment of children; however, the drug has been studied in children aged 2 months to 18 years for the purpose of determining age-appropriate dosing recommendations. The dose required to achieve a therapeutic INR declined with age and was significantly higher in neonates and infants aged 2 months to 1 year than in older children. Similarly the dose required to achieve a therapeutic INR was significantly higher in children aged >1 to 5 years when compared with adolescents and young adults aged 11 to 18 years [*J Thromb Haemost* 2003;1(8):1740-3]. See Dosage and Administration, Recommended Dose and Dosage Adjustment.

CONTRAINDICATIONS:

- Patients who are hypersensitive to nicoumalone
- Patients in whom the risk of hemorrhage exceeds the possible therapeutic benefit, for example patients with a hemorrhagic diathesis or low platelet counts; recent surgery of the CNS or eye, or extensive surgery for trauma; active bleeding of the gastrointestinal, genitourinary or respiratory tracts; cerebrovascular hemorrhage or aneurysm; aortic dissection, pericardial effusion or pericarditis; subacute bacterial endocarditis
- Pregnancy
- Severe uncontrolled hypertension
- Severe liver dysfunction

WARNINGS AND PRECAUTIONS:

Serious Warnings and Precautions

- Patients receiving oral anticoagulants are at increased risk of hemorrhage, which can be severe and life threatening. Therefore, nicoumalone should not be administered to patients with active bleeding.
- The dose of nicoumalone must be individualized according to the INR.
- Many drugs alter the pharmacokinetics of nicoumalone. If undetected, such drug interactions can negate the potential benefit of nicoumalone treatment or, alternatively, increase the risk of hemorrhage. Vigilance on the part of the patient and the physician, more frequent monitoring of the INR, and possible dose adjustments are required when initiating or discontinuing another drug in a patient stabilized on nicoumalone.
- Abrupt changes in vitamin K intake can alter the pharmacokinetics of nicoumalone.
- Elderly patients are at greater risk of hemorrhagic adverse events.
- Patients with liver dysfunction are at increased risk of adverse events during treatment with oral anticoagulants, because clotting factors are produced in the liver and these drugs are eliminated by hepatic metabolism.
- Avoid intramuscular injections because of the risk of hematoma.

Dermatologic: Skin necrosis is an uncommon but potentially serious complication of oral anticoagulant therapy that is more common in women than in men and tends to occur early during the course of therapy (days 1 to 10) at sites where fat is deposited (abdomen, breast, buttocks, thighs). Skin necrosis may be accompanied by infection and may require surgical debridement. Patients with protein C or protein S deficiencies may be at increased risk of skin necrosis, although deficiencies in these factors are not prerequisites for this adverse event.

Oral anticoagulants can precipitate a rare condition known as "purple toes syndrome", which usually manifests later in the course of therapy than skin necrosis (i.e., 3 to 10 weeks or later) and may be due to cholesterol microembolization. Affected areas tend to have a mottled purplish appearance and may be painful or tender.

Hemorrhagic Complications: The severity of hemorrhage ranges from minor to severe and life threatening. Hemorrhage may occur when the INR is in the therapeutic range and may be occult. Risk factors for hemorrhage during treatment with an oral anticoagulant include prolonged treatment, a high (>4) or variable INR, age >65 years, hypertension, cerebrovascular disease, serious heart disease, history of gastrointestinal bleeding, anemia, trauma, malignancy, renal dysfunction, and/or treatment with drugs that increase the INR (see Drug Interactions).

Perioperative/Periprocedural Considerations: Patients receiving nicoumalone are at increased risk of bleeding should they undergo invasive diagnostic or therapeutic interventions (e.g., angiography, lumbar puncture, minor surgical procedures). If a procedure involves a high risk of bleeding the anticoagulant should be discontinued 3 to 5 days before the procedure. Treatment with the oral anticoagulant can be resumed on the day of the procedure because it will take several days to re-establish the therapeutic INR [Thrombosis Interest Group of Canada. Available from: www.tigc.org/eguidelines/warfarin05.htm].

Renal: Patients with severe renal dysfunction may be at increased risk of hemorrhage due to impaired platelet function.

Special Populations: Pregnant Women: Use of nicoumalone is contraindicated during pregnancy. Heparin is the anticoagulant of choice in this setting.

Nursing Women: Oral anticoagulants including nicoumalone are highly bound to plasma proteins and only a small amount partitions into breast milk. Exposure to oral anticoagulants is low in nursing infants; thus, use of these drugs is considered to be compatible with breast-feeding. Moreover, administration of low doses of vitamin K to nursing infants will negate the effects of any oral anticoagulant that is absorbed from breast milk.

Monitoring and Laboratory Tests: The efficacy of oral anticoagulants is measured by determining the prothrombin time (PT), which reflects the activity of factors II, VII and X. Since the responsiveness of thromboplastin (a reagent used in the PT test) varies, the sensitivity of the reagent must be taken into consideration. For this reason the results of the assay are reported as the INR. The intensity of anticoagulation is determined by regular monitoring of the INR. Monitoring of the hemoglobin level and hematocrit may be useful for the detection of occult bleeding.

Liver function tests should be done before initiating therapy and periodically during treatment with an oral anticoagulant.

ADVERSE REACTIONS: Adverse Drug Reactions Overview: The most prominent complication of nicoumalone therapy is bleeding, the probability of which is directly related to the intensity of anticoagulation as indicated by the INR.

More Common Adverse Drug Reactions: See Table 1.

Table 1: Nicoumalone

More Common Adverse Drug Reactions (≥1%)

Body System	Effect	Clinical Comment
Hematological	Hemorrhage	Bleeding may occur in sites such as the gastrointestinal tract (as evidenced by melena), brain (hemorrhagic stroke), urogenital tract (macroscopic and microscopic hematuria), the uterus (metrorrhagia and menorrhagia) and the eye
Gastrointestinal	Loss of appetite, nausea, diarrhea, vomiting	Some GI symptoms may be mitigated by adjusting administration time (e.g., evening dose instead of daytime)

Less Common Adverse Drug Reactions (<1%): Dermatologic: allergic reactions (urticaria, dermatitis and fever), alopecia.

Abnormal Hematologic and Clinical Chemistry Findings: See Table 2. The PT, and hence the INR, is influenced by a wide range of endogenous and exogenous factors. These factors must be kept in mind when assessing the dose requirements and/or therapeutic response of any patient receiving nicoumalone.

Endogenous factors that can prolong the PT (increase the INR) and predispose patients to bleeding include: cancer, collagen disease, congestive heart failure, diarrhea, fever, hepatic dysfunction, hyperthyroidism, malnutrition, steatorrhea, and/or vitamin K deficiency.

Endogenous factors that can shorten the PT (decrease the INR) and may predispose patients to thromboembolic events include: edema, genetic (hereditary) factors, and hypothyroidism.

Exogenous factors that can prolong the prothrombin time (increase the INR) and predispose patients to bleeding include Drug Interactions which are discussed below.

Exogenous factors that can shorten the prothrombin time (decrease the INR) and may predispose patients to thromboembolic events include: high dietary intake of vitamin K (in green leafy vegetables or in food supplements containing vitamin K) and Drug Interactions which are discussed below.

Table 2: Nicoumalone

Abnormal Hematologic and Clinical Chemistry Findings

Test	Effect	Clinical Comment
INR	Increase	Monitor frequently upon initiation of therapy and at regular intervals in patients on stable doses (at least once a month) Monitor before and after adding or discontinuing a medication, especially those known to alter the effect of nicoumalone

DRUG INTERACTIONS:

Serious Drug Interactions

- Oral anticoagulants including nicoumalone are subject to a large number of potential drug interactions involving drugs that inhibit or induce their metabolism. Depending on the circumstances many of these potential interactions can result in serious harm.
- Other drugs that affect hemostasis (i.e., antiplatelet agents, anticoagulants, fibrinolytic agents) can increase the hemorrhagic potential of oral anticoagulants including nicoumalone.

Overview: Nicoumalone is metabolized via hepatic cytochrome P450 2C9 (CYP2C9). Any drug that inhibits or induces this isoenzyme has the potential to alter the metabolism of nicoumalone and hence the dose required to maintain the INR within the recommended range. The Thrombosis Interest Group of Canada advises that almost any drug can be used safely with an oral anticoagulant provided that the INR is monitored at the beginning of therapy (i.e., 4 to 6 days after the addition of any drug to an ongoing anticoagulant regimen). Exceptions to this rule include amiodarone, which has a very long half-life, and drugs such as NSAIDs which may increase the risk of bleeding without altering the INR. For amiodarone, the INR should be monitored more frequently for several months after initiating therapy in patients taking nicoumalone [Thrombosis Interest Group of Canada. Available from: www.tigc.org/eguidelines/warfarin05.htm].

Many drugs have been reported to interact with oral anticoagulants although the quality of the reports varies widely. For the drugs listed in Table 3 and Table 4, an interaction with warfarin (an oral anticoagulant that is chemically similar to nicoumalone) was considered probable or highly probable in a systematic review [*Arch Intern Med* 2005;165(10):1095-106].

Alcohol can alter the elimination of oral anticoagulants leading to fluctuations in the INR. Alcohol consumption is best avoided, or limited to one or two alcoholic drinks per day.

Drug-Drug Interactions: See Table 3 and Table 4.

Table 3: Nicoumalone

Drugs that Potentiate the Anticoagulant Effects and/or Increase the INR[a]

Class	Drugs
Anti-inflammatories/Analgesics	
Analgesics	Acetaminophen (at doses >2 g/day), dextropropoxyphene, tramadol
Anti-inflammatories	ASA, celecoxib, phenylbutazone, piroxicam, sulfinpyrazone
Antimicrobials	
Azole Antifungals	Fluconazole, itraconazole, miconazole (including vaginal preparations), voriconazole
Fluoroquinolones	Ciprofloxacin, levofloxacin
Macrolides	Azithromycin, clarithromycin, erythromycin
Other	Amoxicillin/clavulanate, sulfamethoxazole/trimethoprim, isoniazid, metronidazole, ritonavir, tetracycline
Cardiovascular Drugs	
Fibrates	Fenofibrate
Statins	Fluvastatin, simvastatin
Other	Amiodarone, diltiazem, propafenone, propranolol, quinidine
CNS Drugs	
Antiparkinsonian Drugs	Entacapone, ropinirole
Antidepressants	Citalopram, fluvoxamine, sertraline
Other	Alcohol (large amounts; patients with liver disease), chloral hydrate, disulfiram, phenytoin
Various Agents	
Antineoplastic Agents	Fluorouracil, gemcitabine, paclitaxel, tamoxifen,
Gastrointestinal Drugs	Cimetidine, omeprazole
Immunologics	Interferon
Other	Anabolic steroids, tolterodine

[a] Clinical significance rated as highly probable or probable according to a systematic review of drug interactions involving warfarin (a chemically similar anticoagulant) [*Arch Intern Med* 2005;165(10):1095-106].

Table 4: Nicoumalone

Drugs that Diminish the Anticoagulant Effect and Decrease the INR[a]

Class	Drugs
Antimicrobials	Griseofulvin, ribavirin, rifampin, ritonavir
Cardiovascular Drugs	Bosentan, cholestyramine
CNS Drugs	Barbiturates, carbamazepine, chlordiazepoxide
Gastrointestinal Drugs	Azathioprine, 5-ASA, sucralfate
Other	Chelation therapy, influenza vaccine, mercaptopurine, raloxifene

[a] Clinical significance rated as highly probable or probable according to a systematic review of drug interactions involving warfarin (a chemically similar anticoagulant) [*Arch Intern Med* 2005;165(10):1095-106].

Drug-Food Interactions: Foods, enteral feeds or multivitamins that contain vitamin K have the potential to reduce the therapeutic effects of nicoumalone and increase the dosage required to maintain a therapeutic INR. Other foods such as fish oil, avocado, grapefruit juice and mango fruit may also alter the response to anticoagulants through diverse mechanisms [*Arch Intern Med* 2005;165(10):1095-106].

Drug-Herb Interactions: Ginseng has been reported to reduce the therapeutic effects of warfarin. Herbal products reported to potentiate the effects of warfarin include Boldo-fenugreek, a herbal combination of boldo, (*Peumus boldus*) and fenugreek, (*Trigonella foenum-graecum*); Danshen, a Chinese medicine derived from *Salvia miltiorrhiza*; Dong quai, a Chinese medicine derived from Chinese Angelica (*Angelica sinensis*); *Lycium barbarum*; PC-SPES; and Guilinggao, a Chinese medicine that contains several herbs (the composition varies between manufacturers). Use of these substances should be avoided in patients receiving nicoumalone, because of the close chemical similarity between nicoumalone and warfarin.

DOSAGE AND ADMINISTRATION:

Dosing Considerations: Before starting nicoumalone, the INR, a platelet count, and liver function tests should be performed. If the baseline INR is greater than 1.4, the patient should be screened for coagulopathies.

The dose of nicoumalone must be individualized for each patient on the basis of the INR. The optimal intensity of anticoagulation varies with the indication. Before starting therapy patients must be assessed to determine whether they have the capacity to comply with the practical demands of oral anticoagulation therapy. This includes confirming that the patient understands the benefits and risks of therapy, is likely to comply with the regimen, and is willing to return for laboratory monitoring.

The antithrombotic effect of vitamin K antagonists depends most on depletion of factor II (prothrombin), which typically has a biological half-life of 60 to 72 hours. On this basis it is recommended that when treating patients with acute thrombosis, administration of nicoumalone overlap with heparin for at least 4 or 5 days and until the INR is in the therapeutic range for 2 successive days.

For most indications a moderate intensity of anticoagulation indicated by a target INR of 2.5 (range 2 to 3) is sufficient to balance efficacy with the risk of hemorrhage. The exception is patients with mechanical prosthetic heart valves in whom the recommended target INR ranges vary by the type of valve and the presence of risk factors. The recommended INR is 2 to 3 in patients receiving aortic valves if no risk factors are present, these being atrial fibrillation, prior thromboembolic event, left ventricular dysfunction and a hypercoagulable state. In patients with risk factors and in those receiving mechanical mitral valves the recommended INR range is 2.5 to 3.5 [*Chest* 2004;126(3 Suppl):457S-482S; *J Am Coll Cardiol* 2006;48(3):e1-148].

Fixed dose therapy with nicoumalone is not recommended.

Lower initial doses are recommended in the elderly, in patients who are malnourished and in those with liver disease or heart failure.

It is unnecessary to determine the INR on a daily basis especially in outpatients. When initiating therapy the INR should be determined initially on the day of the third or fourth dose and twice per week during the first one or two weeks of treatment. If the desired INR is maintained then the duration between tests can be extended to a maximum of 4 to 5 weeks [Thrombosis Interest Group of Canada. Available from: www.tigc.org/eguidelines/warfarin05.htm].

Recommended Dose and Dosage Adjustment: Nicoumalone is approximately twice as potent as warfarin; thus, if switching a patient from warfarin to nicoumalone, the initial dose should be 50% of the warfarin dose. After initiating nicoumalone the INR should be monitored and the dose adjusted to maintain the target INR [Thrombosis Interest Group of Canada. Available from: www.tigc.org/eguidelines/warfarin05.htm].

In patients in whom oral anticoagulation is being initiated for a non-acute indication, for example atrial fibrillation, nicoumalone may be initiated at a low dose (e.g., 1 mg daily) to avoid the possibility of over-anticoagulation.

When a rapid anticoagulant effect is required, for example in the setting of acute venous thromboembolism, heparin is preferred over oral anticoagulants as initial therapy because of its rapid onset of action. If long-term anticoagulation will be required then it is recommended that treatment with an oral anticoagulant be initiated concurrent with heparin and that heparin be discontinued after the INR has been in the therapeutic range for at least 2 days. The recommended initial dose of nicoumalone is 8 to 12 mg on the first day and 4 to 8 mg on the second day. Subsequent doses are determined by the INR.

Pediatrics: Pediatric doses are outlined in Table 5 [*J Thromb Haemost* 2003;1(8):1740-3].

Table 5: Nicoumalone

Dose in Pediatric Patients

Route	Age	Initial Dose	Clinical Comment
Oral	<1 year	0.20 mg/kg	Monitor the INR and adjust the dose to achieve the target INR
	1 to 5 years	0.09 mg/kg	
	6 to 10 years	0.07 mg/kg	
	11 to 18 years	0.06 mg/kg	

Hepatic Impairment: Patients with hepatic impairment require lower doses of oral anticoagulants to achieve a therapeutic INR.

Genetic Polymorphism: A genetic polymorphism in the CYP2C9-mediated metabolism of nicoumalone is responsible for 14% of the interindividual variability in the pharmacodynamic response to nicoumalone. Patients who are homozygous for the CYP2C9*3 allele are at increased risk of being over-anticoagulated at the start of treatment and of bleeding complications during maintenance treatment.

Missed Dose: Advise patients to take a missed dose as soon as they remember that a dose has been missed, but not to take a double dose if they do not remember until the next dose is due.

Administration: Nicoumalone may be taken with or without meals. The drug should be taken in a consistent manner with respect to meals and time of day.

OVERDOSAGE:

For management of a suspected drug overdose, CPhA recommends that you contact your **regional Poison Control Centre**. See the *CPS* Directory section for a list of Poison Control Centres.

ACTION AND CLINICAL PHARMACOLOGY: Mechanism of Action: Like all vitamin K antagonists nicoumalone interferes with the interconversion of vitamin K and its 2,3-epoxide metabolite by inhibiting vitamin K epoxide reductase. This prevents carboxylation of glutamate residues on the N-terminus of vitamin K-dependent coagulation factors (II, VII, IX and X). Carboxylation is a prerequisite for the calcium-dependent conformational change that allows these proteins to bind to cofactors on phospholipid surfaces. Vitamin K antagonists also inhibit carboxylation of protein C and protein S which are natural anticoagulants. The net effect is an altered balance between anticoagulation mediated by inhibition of factors II, VII, IX and X, and procoagulation mediated by inhibition of proteins C and S. Under most situations the anticoagulant effect dominates.

The antithrombotic effect of vitamin K antagonists depends to the greatest extent on depletion of factor II (prothrombin), which typically has a biological half-life of 60 to 72 hours.

The R(+) and S(−) enantiomers of nicoumalone produce comparable anticoagulant effects.

Pharmacokinetics: Adults: Absorption: Peak plasma concentrations of nicoumalone are achieved within 1 to 3 hours after oral administration. The oral bioavailability of nicoumalone is at least 60%. Peak plasma concentrations and the area under the plasma-concentration versus time curve (AUC) are dose-proportional over the range of 8 to 16 mg.

Distribution: Nicoumalone is highly bound (98.7%) to plasma proteins. Hence the drug has a high apparent volume of distribution: (0.16 L/kg for the R(+) enantiomer and 0.22 to 0.34 L/kg for the S(−) enantiomer). The drug crosses the placenta and is distributed into breast milk.

Metabolism: Nicoumalone is extensively metabolized by cytochrome P450 (CYP)-mediated hepatic metabolism. The parent drug is converted to two different hydroxy metabolites by oxidative metabolism. Two further metabolites are formed by reduction of the keto function to an alcohol group. Another metabolic pathway involves reduction of the nitro group to form an amino metabolite which is then converted to an acetamido metabolite.

CYP2C9 is primarily responsible for metabolism of the S(−) enantiomer; CYP1A2, CYP2C19 and CYP3A4 are involved in the metabolism of the R(+) enantiomer.

Excretion: The elimination half-life of nicoumalone is 8 to 11 hours. The bulk of an administered dose is excreted as metabolites in the urine and feces. Only 0.1% to 0.3% of an orally administered dose is excreted unchanged in urine.

NidaGel™ Ⓟ

metronidazole

Antibacterial

Graceway

PHARMACOLOGY: Metronidazole demonstrates antibacterial activity against bacteria classified as obligate anaerobes including Bacteroides and to a lesser extent against anaerobic gram-positive rods. The nitro group of the drug is thought to be reduced in the target cell leading to the production of cytotoxic metabolites.

Bioavailability studies on the administration of a single 5 g dose of NidaGel into the vaginas of 12 normal subjects showed a mean maximum serum concentration of 237 ng/mL. This is approximately 2% of the mean maximum serum concentration afforded by a single 500 mg tablet of metronidazole taken orally (mean C_{max} = 12 785 ng/mL). Therefore, under normal usage levels, the formulation affords minimal serum concentrations of metronidazole.

INDICATIONS: For the treatment of bacterial vaginosis (formerly called nonspecific vaginitis, *G. vaginalis* or Haemophilus vaginitis).

A clinical diagnosis of bacterial vaginosis is usually defined by the presence of a homogenous vaginal discharge that: has a pH of greater than 4.5; emits a fishy amine odor when mixed with a 10% KOH solution; contains clue cells on microscopic examination.

Other pathogens commonly associated with vulvovaginitis, e.g., *T. vaginalis*, *C. trachomatis*, *N. gonorrhoeae*, *C. albicans* and herpes simplex virus should be ruled out.

Use of metronidazole during menses is not recommended.

CONTRAINDICATIONS: Patients with a prior history of hypersensitivity to metronidazole, parabens, other ingredients of the formulation or other nitroimidazole derivatives.

Pregnancy: Metronidazole is contraindicated during the first trimester of pregnancy (see Precautions).

WARNINGS: Convulsive seizures and peripheral neuropathy, the latter characterized mainly by numbness or paresthesia of an extremity, have been reported in patients treated with oral metronidazole. The appearance of abnormal neurologic signs demands the prompt discontinuation of metronidazole therapy. It should be administered with caution to patients with CNS diseases. Psychotic reactions to oral metronidazole have been reported in alcoholic patients who are using metronidazole and disulfiram concurrently.

PRECAUTIONS: NidaGel affords minimal serum levels of metronidazole compared to oral metronidazole therapy. Although these lower serum levels are less likely to produce the common reactions seen with oral metronidazole, the possibility of these and other reactions cannot be excluded.

General: Patients with severe hepatic disease metabolize metronidazole slowly, with resultant accumulation of metronidazole and its metabolites in the plasma. Accordingly, for such patients, metronidazole should be administered cautiously.

Known or previously unrecognized candidiasis may present more prominent symptoms during therapy with metronidazole and requires treatment with a candicidal agent.

No reports of alcohol interaction were received during clinical studies with metronidazole. Despite the relatively low serum levels of metronidazole afforded by NidaGel, the possibility of a disulfiram-like reaction to alcohol while on metronidazole therapy cannot be excluded. Patients should be advised to abstain from alcohol during therapy and for 1 day following therapy.

Hematologic Effects: Metronidazole is a nitroimidazole and should be used with care in patients with evidence of or history of blood dyscrasia. A mild transient leukopenia has been observed during oral metronidazole administration.

In clinical studies with 0.75% metronidazole vaginal gel a mild, clinically insignificant leukopenia was observed in some patients. Relationship to therapy could not be determined.

Drug Interactions: Oral metronidazole has been reported to potentiate the anticoagulant effect of warfarin and other coumarin anticoagulants, resulting in a prolongation of prothrombin time. This possible drug interaction should be considered when metronidazole is prescribed for patients on this type of anticoagulant therapy.

Laboratory Test Interactions: Metronidazole may interfere with certain types of determinations of serum chemistry values, such as aspartate aminotransferase (AST), alanine aminotransferase (ALT), lactate dehydrogenase (LDH), triglycerides and hexokinase glucose. These determinations are based on the decrease in ultraviolet absorbance which occurs when NADH is oxidized to NAD. Metronidazole causes an increase in absorbance at the peak of NADH (340 nm) resulting in falsely decreased values.

Carcinogenicity: Metronidazole has shown evidence of carcinogenic activity following chronic oral administration in mice and rats. Pulmonary tumorigenesis has been reported in mice, and significant increases in the incidence of mammary and hepatic tumors have been found in female rats. Lifetime tumorigenicity studies in hamsters have given negative results.

These studies were conducted with orally administered metronidazole which results in significantly higher systemic blood levels than those obtained after use of 0.75% metronidazole vaginal gel.

Pregnancy: There has been no experience to date with the use of NidaGel in pregnant patients. Metronidazole crosses the placental barrier and enters the fetal circulation rapidly. It should not be used during the first trimester of pregnancy. Use of metronidazole for bacterial vaginosis in the second and third trimesters should be restricted to those patients in whom local palliative treatment has been inadequate to control symptoms. No fetotoxicity was observed after oral metronidazole in pregnant rats or mice. Because animal reproduction studies are not always predictive of human response, this drug should be used during pregnancy only if clearly needed (see Contraindications).

Lactation: NidaGel blood levels are significantly lower than those achieved with oral metronidazole. After oral administration metronidazole has been shown to be secreted in breast milk in concentrations similar to those found in plasma. If the use of metronidazole is considered to be necessary in nursing mothers, the potential benefits must be weighed against the possible risks to the infant.

Children: Safety and effectiveness in children have not been established.

ADVERSE EFFECTS: Based on a multicenter clinical trial involving 505 patients, comparing NidaGel twice-daily dosing to once-daily dosing, adverse event experiences are listed below, in descending order of frequency: vaginal discharge, descriptions of which varied in both color and consistency (12%), yeast infection (9%), vulva/vaginal irritative symptoms (9%), gastrointestinal discomfort which included patient descriptions of abdominal or stomach cramping, pain and discomfort (7%), headache (5%), nausea and vomiting (4%), pelvic discomfort (3%). The following reactions were seen at a frequency of 2%: unusual taste, dizziness, cramping, undocumented or self-diagnosed yeast infections. The following reactions were seen at a frequency of 1%: decreased appetite, diarrhea/loose stools, fatigue, medication leakage, urinary tract infection symptoms. The following reactions were seen at a frequency of <1%: abdominal bloating/gas, constipation, thirst/dry mouth, depression, irritability, menstrual discomfort, menstrual irregularities, vaginal numbness, vaginal spotting/bleeding, itching, darkened urine.

Other reactions noted with oral metronidazole therapy include anorexia, epigastric distress, nausea, vomiting, furry tongue, dry mouth, metallic taste, transient eosinophilia or neutropenia, convulsive seizures, peripheral neuropathy, vertigo, incoordination, ataxia, confusion, insomnia, flushing, headache, dryness of the vagina, dysuria, darkened urine, modification of taste of alcoholic beverages, rash, pruritus, palpitation and chest pain.

OVERDOSE:

Symptoms: There is no human experience with overdosage of metronidazole. Massive ingestion may produce vomiting and slight disorientation.

Treatment: Early gastric lavage may remove a large amount of the drug; otherwise, treatment should be symptomatic.

For management of a suspected drug overdose, CPhA recommends that you contact your **regional Poison Control Centre**. See the *CPS* Directory section for a list of Poison Control Centres.

DOSAGE: One applicator full (approximately 5 g) of vaginal gel should be inserted into the vagina once daily at bedtime for 5 days, or twice daily at morning and bedtime for 5 days. Controlled studies with alternate dosage schedules have not been conducted. If patients do not respond to initial therapy, it is recommended that appropriate laboratory measures be used to rule out other conditions before retreating with metronidazole.

Pregnancy: Pregnant patients should not be treated during the first trimester of pregnancy (see Contraindications and Precautions).

Use during menses is not recommended.

INFORMATION FOR THE PATIENT: Published in e-CPS, available by subscription at www.e-cps.ca.

SUPPLIED: Each g of colorless to straw-colored, slightly hazy gel contains: metronidazole 7.5 mg. Nonmedicinal ingredients: carbomer 934P, edetate disodium, methylparaben, propylene glycol, propylparaben, purified water and sodium hydroxide to adjust the pH to 4. Aluminum tubes of 70 g, packaged with five, 5 g vaginal applicators. Store between 15 and 25°C.

Nifedipine Ⓟ

CPhA Monograph

see *Calcium Channel Blockers*

Nimbex®

cisatracurium besylate

Nondepolarizing Skeletal Neuromuscular Blocking Agent

Abbott

Date of Preparation: May 6, 1999
Date of Revision: November 12, 2008

This drug should be administered only by adequately trained professionals familiar with its actions, characteristics, and hazards.

SUMMARY PRODUCT INFORMATION:

Route of Administration	Dosage Form/ Strength	Clinically Relevant Nonmedicinal Ingredients
Intravenous	Solution for injection/2 mg/mL	Benzyl alcohol, benzenesulfonic acid, water for injection. For a complete listing see Dosage Forms, Composition and Packaging.

INDICATIONS AND CLINICAL USE: NIMBEX (cisatracurium besylate injection) is a non-depolarizing neuromuscular blocking agent with an intermediate onset and duration of action indicated as an adjunct to general anesthesia, to facilitate non-emergency endotracheal intubation, and to provide skeletal muscle relaxation during surgery or mechanical ventilation.

Geriatrics (>65 years of age): The time to maximum block is about 1 minute slower in the elderly. For details, see Dosage and Administration, Recommended Dose and Dosage Adjustment, Elderly and Renal Failure Patients.

Pediatrics (≤12 years of age): For children 2 to 12 years of age, dosage adjustment is required, see Dosage and Administration, Recommended Dose and Dosage Adjustment, Children, Initial Doses. NIMBEX has not been studied in children less than 2 years old.

CONTRAINDICATIONS: NIMBEX (cisatracurium besylate injection) is contraindicated in:

- Patients who are hypersensitive to NIMBEX (cisatracurium besylate injection) or to any ingredient in the formulation or component of the container. For a complete listing, see Dosage Forms, Composition and Packaging.
- Patients who are hypersensitive to TRACRIUM or other bis-benzylisoquinolinium agents.
- Patients with a known hypersensitivity to benzyl alcohol, which is used as a preservative.

The NIMBEX formulation from the multiple-dose vials contains benzyl alcohol. It should not be used in neonates (infants less than 1 month of age) who are susceptible to the adverse effects of benzyl alcohol (see Warnings and Precautions, Special Populations, Pediatrics (≤12 years of age)).

WARNINGS AND PRECAUTIONS:

> **Serious Warnings and Precautions**
> NIMBEX (cisatracurium besylate injection) should be administered in carefully adjusted dosage by or under the supervision of experienced clinicians who are familiar with the drug's actions and the possible complications of its use. The drug should not be administered unless personnel and facilities for resuscitation and life support (tracheal intubation, artificial ventilation, oxygen therapy), and an antagonist of cisatracurium besylate are immediately available. It is recommended that a peripheral nerve stimulator be used to measure neuromuscular function during the administration of cisatracurium besylate in order to monitor drug effect, determine the need for additional doses, and confirm recovery from neuromuscular block.
> NIMBEX has no known effect on consciousness, pain threshold, thinking, or memory. To avoid distress to the patient, neuromuscular block should not be induced before unconsciousness.

General: Because of its intermediate onset of action, NIMBEX (cisatracurium besylate injection) is not recommended for rapid sequence endotracheal intubation.

Patients subjected to hypothermia may necessitate a reduction in the rate of infusion of NIMBEX (see Dosage and Administration).

Acid-base and/or serum electrolyte abnormalities may potentiate or antagonize the action of neuromuscular blocking agents. The action of neuromuscular blocking agents may be enhanced by magnesium salts administered for the management of pre-eclampsia or eclampsia.

As NIMBEX has not been studied in patients with asthma or a history of severe anaphylactic reactions, it should be administered with caution to these patient groups.

No data are available to support the use of NIMBEX by intramuscular injection.

NIMBEX is acidic (pH 3.25 to 3.65) and should not be mixed with alkaline solutions having a pH greater than 8.5 (e.g., barbiturate solutions). NIMBEX is also hypotonic and must not be administered into the infusion line of a blood transfusion.

Burns: Patients with burns have been shown to develop resistance to non-depolarizing neuromuscular blocking agents, including atracurium. The extent of altered response depends upon the size of the burn and the time elapsed since the burn injury. NIMBEX has not been studied in patients with burns; however, based on its structural similarity to atracurium, the possibility of increased dosing requirements and shortened duration of action must be considered if NIMBEX is administered to burn patients.

Malignant Hyperthermia (MH): In a study of MH-susceptible pigs, cisatracurium besylate did not trigger MH. NIMBEX has not been studied in MH-susceptible patients. Because MH can develop in the absence of established triggering agents, the clinician should be prepared to recognize and treat MH in any patient undergoing general anesthesia.

Carcinogenesis and Mutagenesis: Long-term studies in animals have not been performed to evaluate the carcinogenic potential of cisatracurium besylate.

Cisatracurium besylate was evaluated in a battery of four short-term mutagenicity tests. It was non-mutagenic in the Ames Salmonella assay, a rat bone marrow cytogenic assay, and in in vitro human lymphocyte cytogenetics assay. As was the case with atracurium, the mouse lymphoma assay was positive both in the presence and absence of exogenous metabolic activation (rat live S-9). In the absence of S-9, cisatracurium besylate was positive at in vitro cisatracurium concentrations of 40 µg/mL and higher. In the presence of S-9, cisatracurium besylate was positive at a cisatracurium concentration of 300 µg/mL but not at lower or higher concentrations.

Cardiovascular: Recommended doses of NIMBEX have no clinically significant effects on heart rate; therefore, NIMBEX will not counteract the bradycardia produced by many anesthetic agents or by vagal stimulation.

Neurologic: Patients with hemiparesis or paraparesis also may demonstrate resistance to non-depolarizing neuromuscular blocking agents in affected limbs. To avoid inaccurate dosing, neuromuscular monitoring should be performed on the non-paretic limb.

In patients with neuromuscular disease such as myasthenia gravis or myasthenic (Eaton-Lambert) syndrome, small doses of non-depolarizing neuromuscular blocking agents may have profound effects. In these patients, and patients with conditions in which prolonged neuromuscular blockade is a possibility (e.g. neuromuscular disease, carcinomatosis, severe cachexia or debilitation), the use of a peripheral nerve stimulator and a first dose of not more than 0.02 mg/kg NIMBEX is recommended to assess the level of neuromuscular block and to monitor dosage requirements.

Renal and Hepatic: Cisatracurium undergoes degradation in the body at physiological pH and temperature by organ-independent Hofmann elimination to form laudanosine and the monoquaternary acrylate metabolite. No clinically significant alterations in the recovery profile were observed in patients with renal impairment or hepatic impairment following a 0.1 mg/kg (2×ED_{95}; twice the dose required to produce 95% suppression of the adductor polices muscle twitch response to ulnar nerve stimulation) dose of cisatracurium. The onset time was approximately 1 minute faster in patients with end-stage liver disease and approximately 1 minute slower in patients with renal dysfunction than in healthy adult control patients.

Intensive Care Unit (ICU): Whenever the use of NIMBEX, or any neuromuscular blocking agent, is contemplated in the ICU, it is recommended that a peripheral nerve stimulator be used to continuously monitor neuromuscular transmission during administration and recovery. Additional doses of NIMBEX or any other neuromuscular blocking agent should not be given before there is evidence of the return of the first twitch response to peripheral nerve stimulation. If no response is elicited, the infusion should be discontinued until a response returns.

Long-Term Use in the ICU: To reduce the possibility of prolonged neuromuscular blockade and other complications that might occur following long-term use in the ICU, NIMBEX, or any other neuromuscular relaxant, should be administered in carefully adjusted doses by or under the supervision of experienced clinicians who are familiar with its actions and with appropriate peripheral nerve stimulator muscle monitoring techniques.

Continuous infusion or intermittent bolus dosing to support long-term mechanical ventilation has not been studied sufficiently to support dosage recommendations. There is limited information regarding the safety and efficacy of long-term infusion of cisatracurium besylate during mechanical ventilation in the ICU (up to 2 days n=37, 2 to 4 days n=19, 4 to 6 days n=12) and no information on its use beyond 6 days. Thus dosage recommendations cannot be made at this time. In rare cases, long-term use of neuromuscular blocking drugs to facilitate mechanical ventilation in ICU settings has been associated with prolonged paralysis and/or skeletal muscle weakness that is first noted during attempts to wean patients from the ventilator. In these patients, the actions of the neuromuscular blocking agent may be enhanced by other drugs (e.g., broad spectrum antibiotics, narcotics and/or steroids) or by conditions such as acid-base or electrolyte imbalance, hypoxic episodes of varying duration, or extreme debilitation. Additionally patients immobilized for extended periods frequently develop symptoms consistent with disuse muscle atrophy Recovery may vary from regaining movement and strength in all muscles to initial recovery of movement of the facial muscles and small muscles of the extremities then to the remaining muscles. In rare cases, recovery may involve an extended period of time or even require rehabilitation. Therefore, when there is a need for long-term mechanical ventilation, the benefits to risk ratio of neuromuscular blockade must be considered. The syndrome of critical illness polyneuropathy associated with sepsis and multiorgan failure may be associated with prolonged muscle paralysis, but can also occur without the use of muscle relaxants. Thus, the role of muscle relaxants in the etiology of prolonged paralysis in the ICU is not known with certainty.

Special Populations: Pregnant Women: Teratology testing in rats revealed no maternal or fetal toxicity or teratogenic effects. There are no adequate and well-controlled studies of NIMBEX in pregnant women. Because animal studies are not always predictive of human response, NIMBEX should be used during pregnancy only if clearly needed.

Labor and Delivery: The use of NIMBEX during labor, vaginal delivery, or cesarean section has not been studied in humans and it is not known whether cisatracurium besylate administered to the mother has effects on the fetus. Doses of 0.2 or 0.4 mg/kg (4× or 8× human ED_{95}) cisatracurium besylate given to female beagles undergoing cesarean section resulted in negligible levels of cisatracurium besylate in umbilical vessel blood of neonates and no deleterious effects on the pups.

Nursing Women: It is not known whether cisatracurium besylate is excreted in human milk. Because many drugs are excreted in human milk, caution should be exercised following administration of NIMBEX to a nursing woman.

Pediatrics (≤12 years of age): For children 2-12 years of age, a lower dose should be used. NIMBEX has not been studied in children under 2 years of age (see Action and Clinical Pharmacology for clinical experience and Dosage and Administration for recommendations for use in children 2 to 12 years of age).

NIMBEX contains benzyl alcohol as a preservative. In neonates (infants less than 1 month of age), benzyl alcohol has been associated with an increased incidence of neurological and other complications which are sometimes fatal. NIMBEX should not be used in neonates (see Contraindications).

Geriatrics (≥65 years of age): NIMBEX was safely administered during clinical trials to 130 elderly (≥65 years) patients, including a subset of patients with significant cardiovascular disease (see Warnings and Precautions, General).

Minor differences in the pharmacokinetics of cisatracurium between elderly and young adult patients are not associated with clinically significant differences in the recovery profile of cisatracurium following a single 0.1 mg/kg (2×ED_{95}) dose; however, the time to maximum block is approximately one minute slower in elderly patients (see Action and Clinical Pharmacology, Pharmacokinetics).

The effects of hemofiltration, hemodialysis, and hemoperfusion on plasma levels of cisatracurium besylate and its metabolites are unknown.

ADVERSE REACTIONS: Clinical Trial Adverse Drug Reactions: Because clinical trials are conducted under very specific conditions the adverse reaction rates observed in the clinical trials may not reflect the rates observed in practice and should not be compared to the rates in the clinical trials of another drug. Adverse drug reaction information from clinical trials is useful for identifying drug-related adverse events and for approximating rates.

Adverse experiences were uncommon among the 908 surgical patients who received NIMBEX (cisatracurium besylate injection) in conjunction with other drugs in U.S. and European clinical studies in the course of a wide variety of procedures in patients receiving opioid, propofol, or inhalation anesthesia.

Less Common Clinical Trial Adverse Drug Reactions (<1%): The following adverse experiences were judged by investigators during the clinical trials to have a possible causal relationship to NIMBEX (cisatracurium besylate injection) (incidence less than 1%):

Cardiovascular System: flushing (0.2%), hypotension (0.2%), bradycardia (0.4%).

Respiratory System: bronchospasm (0.2%).

Skin and Appendages: rash (0.1%).

Post-Market Adverse Drug Reactions: In addition to events reported from clinical trials, the following events have been identified during post-approval use of NIMBEX in conjunction with one or more anesthetic agents in clinical practice. Because they are reported voluntarily from a population of unknown size, estimates of frequency cannot be made. These events are reported due to their seriousness, frequency of reporting, or potential causal relationship to NIMBEX.

General: hypersensitivity reactions including anaphylactic or anaphylactoid responses which, in some cases were severe.

Musculoskeletal System: prolonged neuromuscular block, inadequate neuromuscular block.

DRUG INTERACTIONS: Drug-Drug Interactions: Succinylcholine: The use of NIMBEX (cisatracurium besylate injection) prior to succinylcholine, for the purpose of attenuating succinylcholine-induced side effects, has not been studied. The use of NIMBEX following varying degrees of recovery from succinylcholine-induced neuromuscular block has been assessed in a limited number of patients. Administration of 0.1 mg/kg (2×ED_{95}) cisatracurium at 10% (n=15) or 95% recovery (n=15) following an intubating dose of succinylcholine (1 mg/kg) produced ≥95% neuromuscular block. The time of onset of maximum block following NIMBEX is approximately 2 minutes faster with prior administration of succinylcholine. Prior administration of succinylcholine had no effect on the duration of neuromuscular block following initial or maintenance bolus doses of NIMBEX. Cisatracurium besylate infusion requirements were comparable or slightly greater in patients who received succinylcholine prior to the cisatracurium besylate infusions, in contrast to patients who did not receive succinylcholine.

Other non-depolarizing Muscle Relaxants: Although not studied systematically in clinical trials, no drug interactions were observed when vecuronium, pancuronium, or atracurium were administered following varying degrees of recovery from single doses or infusions of NIMBEX.

Inhalation Anesthetics: Inhalational anesthetics may prolong the clinically effective duration of action of initial and maintenance doses of NIMBEX, and decrease the average infusion rate of NIMBEX. The magnitude of these effects may depend on the duration of administration of the volatile agents (see Dosage and Administration, Maintenance Doses and Action and Clinical Pharmacology).

Intravenous Anesthetics: In clinical studies, propofol had no effect on the duration of action or dosing requirements for NIMBEX.

Anticonvulsants: Resistance to the neuromuscular blocking action of non-depolarizing neuromuscular blocking agents has been demonstrated in patients chronically administered phenytoin or carbamazepine. While the effects of chronic phenytoin or carbamazepine therapy on the action of cisatracurium besylate are unknown, slightly shorter durations of neuromuscular block may be anticipated and infusion rate requirements may be higher.

Other Drugs: The neuromuscular blocking action of non-depolarizing agents such as cisatracurium besylate may be enhanced by certain antibiotics (e.g., aminoglycosides, tetracyclines, bacitracin, polymyxins, lincomycin, clindamycin, colistin, and sodium colistemethate), magnesium salts, lithium, local anesthetics, procainamide, and quinidine.

Drug-Laboratory Test Interactions: There are no known drug-laboratory interactions.

DOSAGE AND ADMINISTRATION: Dosing Considerations: NIMBEX (cisatracurium besylate injection) should be administered only by intravenous route. This drug should be administered by or under the supervision of experienced clinicians familiar with the use of neuromuscular blocking agents. Dosage must be individualized in each case.

To avoid patient distress, NIMBEX should **not** be administered prior to the induction of unconsciousness. It should **not** be mixed in the same syringe or administered simultaneously through the same needle with alkaline solutions (e.g. barbiturate solutions).

Recommended Dose and Dosage Adjustment: The dosage information provided below is intended as a guide only. Doses of NIMBEX should be individualized and a peripheral nerve stimulator should be used to measure neuromuscular function during administration of NIMBEX in order to monitor drug effect, to determine the need for additional doses, and to confirm recovery from neuromuscular block. The use of a peripheral nerve stimulator will permit the most advantageous use of NIMBEX, minimize the possibility of overdosage or underdosage, and assist in the evaluation of recovery.

Adults: Initial Doses: One of two intubating doses of cisatracurium may be chosen, based on the desired time to intubation and the anticipated length of surgery. Doses of 0.15 mg/kg (3×ED_{95}) and 0.20 mg/kg (4×ED_{95}) cisatracurium, as components of a propofol/nitrous oxide/oxygen induction-intubation technique, each may produce generally good or excellent conditions for intratracheal intubation in 1.5 to 2.0 minutes. The clinically effective durations of action for 0.15 and 0.20 mg/kg cisatracurium during propofol anesthesia are 55 minutes (range: 44 to 74 min) and 61 minutes (range: 41 to 81 min), respectively. Lower doses may result in a longer time for the development of satisfactory intubation conditions. In addition to the dose of the neuromuscular blocking agent, the presence of co-induction agents (e.g., fentanyl and midazolam) and the depth of anesthesia are factors that can influence intubation conditions. Doses of cisatracurium up to 8 times the ED_{95} (0.40 mg/kg) have been administered to a limited number of healthy adult patients (n=15) and patients with serious cardiovascular disease (n=31). These larger doses are associated with a longer clinically effective duration of action (see Action and Clinical Pharmacology).

Cardiovascular Disease: NIMBEX doses of up to 0.30 mg/kg (6×ED_{95}) cisatracurium were found to have no significant hemodynamic effects in patients with cardiovascular disease (New York Heart Association Class I-III). There are limited data for doses above 0.30 mg/kg in this patient population. At a dose of 0.10 mg/kg an extension of the interval between administration of NIMBEX and the intubation attempt may be required to achieve satisfactory intubation conditions.

Elderly and Renal Failure Patients: Because a slower time to onset of complete neuromuscular block was observed in elderly patients and in patients with renal failure, extending the interval between administration of NIMBEX and the intubation attempt for these patients may be required to achieve adequate intubation conditions.

Maintenance Doses: A dose of 0.03 mg/kg cisatracurium is recommended for maintenance of neuromuscular block during prolonged surgical procedures. Maintenance doses of 0.03 mg/kg each sustain neuromuscular block for approximately 20 minutes. Although maintenance dosing is generally required 40 to 50 minutes following an initial dose of 0.15 mg/kg (3×ED_{95}) cisatracurium besylate injection and 50 to 60 minutes following an initial dose of 0.20 mg/kg (4×ED_{95}) cisatracurium besylate injection, the need for maintenance doses should be determined by clinical criteria. For a shorter or longer duration of action, smaller or larger maintenance doses may be administered.

Isoflurane or enflurane administered with nitrous oxide/oxygen to achieve 1.25 MAC (Minimum Alveolar Concentration) may prolong the clinically effective duration of action of initial and maintenance doses. The magnitude of these effects may depend on the duration of administration of the volatile agents. Fifteen to 30 minutes of exposure to 1.25 MAC isoflurane or enflurane had minimal effects on the duration of action of initial doses of NIMBEX; therefore, no adjustment to the initial dose should be necessary when NIMBEX is administered shortly after initiation of volatile agents. In long surgical procedures during enflurane or isoflurane anesthesia, less frequent maintenance dosing or lower maintenance doses of NIMBEX may be necessary.

No adjustments to the initial dose of NIMBEX are required when used in patients receiving propofol anesthesia.

Children: Initial Doses: The recommended dose of NIMBEX for children 2 to 12 years of age is 0.10 mg/kg of cisatracurium administered over 5 to 10 seconds during either halothane or opioid anesthesia. When administered during stable opioid/nitrous oxide/oxygen anesthesia, 0.10 mg/kg cisatracurium produces maximum neuromuscular block in an average of 2.8 minutes (range: 1.8 to 6.7 min) and clinically effective block for an average of 28 minutes (range: 21 to 38 min). NIMBEX has not been studied in children under 2 years of age.

Special Conditions: Based on the known action of cisatracurium besylate and other neuromuscular blocking agents, the following factors should be considered when administering NIMBEX:

Renal and Hepatic Disease: Doses for patients with renal or hepatic impairment are as recommended for healthy adult patients. However, the onset time may be slightly faster in patients with liver impairment and slightly slower in patients with renal impairment (see Warnings and Precautions, Renal and Hepatic).

Drugs or Conditions Causing Potentiation of, or Resistance to, Neuromuscular Block: Patients with hemiparesis or paraparesis may be more resistant to cisatracurium, whereas those with myasthenia, myasthenic syndrome, or some other neuromuscular diseases may be more susceptible to the effect of cisatracurium (see Warnings and Precautions, Neurologic).

Patients with burns have been shown to develop resistance to non-depolarizing neuromuscular blocking agents, and may require adjustment to dosing (see Warnings and Precautions, Burns).

Concomitant use of cisatracurium with anticonvulsants, certain antibiotics, magnesium salts, lithium, local anesthetics, procainamide, and quinidine may affect the action of duration of cisatracurium (see Drug Interactions, Drug-Drug Interactions).

Hypothermia: The rate of infusion of atracurium required to maintain adequate surgical relaxation in patients undergoing coronary artery bypass surgery with induced hypothermia (25 to 28°C) is approximately half the rate required during normothermia. Based on the structural similarity between cisatracurium besylate and atracurium, a similar effect on the infusion rate of NIMBEX may be expected.

Use by Continuous Infusion: Infusion in the Operating Room (OR): After administration of an initial bolus dose of NIMBEX, a diluted solution of NIMBEX can be administered by continuous infusion to adults and children (≥2 years of age) for maintenance of neuromuscular block during extended surgical procedures. Infusion of cisatracurium besylate should be individualized for each patient. The rate of administration should be adjusted according to the patient's response as determined by peripheral nerve stimulation. Accurate dosing is best achieved using a precision infusion device.

Infusion of cisatracurium besylate should be initiated only after early evidence of spontaneous recovery from the initial bolus dose. An initial infusion rate of 3 µg/kg/min cisatracurium may be required to rapidly counteract the spontaneous recovery of neuromuscular function. Thereafter, a rate of 1 to 2 µg/kg/min should be adequate to maintain continuous neuromuscular block in the range of 89% to 99% in most pediatric and adult patients under opioid/nitrous oxide/oxygen anesthesia.

Reduction of the infusion rate by up to 30% to 40% should be considered when cisatracurium besylate is administered during stable isoflurane or enflurane anesthesia (administered with nitrous oxide/oxygen to achieve 1.25 MAC). Greater reductions in the infusion rate of cisatracurium besylate may be required with longer durations of administration of isoflurane or enflurane.

Spontaneous recovery from neuromuscular block following discontinuation of cisatracurium besylate infusion may be expected to proceed at a rate comparable to that following administration of a single bolus dose.

Infusion Rate Tables: The amount of infusion solution required per minute will depend upon the concentration of cisatracurium besylate in the infusion solution, the desired dose of cisatracurium besylate, and the patient's weight. The contribution of the infusion solution to the fluid requirements of the patient also must be considered. Table 1 and Table 2 provide guidelines for delivery in mL/hr (equivalent to microdrops/min when 60 microdrops=1 mL) of cisatracurium besylate solutions in concentrations of 0.1 mg/mL (10 mg/100 mL) or 0.4 mg/mL (40 mg/100 mL) of cisatracurium.

Table 1: NIMBEX

NIMBEX Infusion Rates for Maintenance of Neuromuscular Block During Opioid/Nitrous Oxide/Oxygen Anesthesia Using Cisatracurium at a Concentration of 0.1 mg/mL

Patient Weight (kg)	Cisatracurium Delivery Rate (µg/kg/min)				
	1	1.5	2	3	5
	Infusion Delivery Rate (mL/h)				
10	6	9	12	18	30
45	27	41	54	81	135
70	42	63	84	126	210
100	60	90	120	180	300

Special Considerations for Administration: Y-site Administration: NIMBEX (cisatracurium besylate injection) is acidic (pH=3.25 to 3.65) and may not be compatible with alkaline solution having a pH greater than 8.5 (e.g., barbiturate solutions).

Studies have shown that NIMBEX is compatible with:

- 5% Dextrose Injection USP
- 0.9% Sodium Chloride Injection USP
- 5% Dextrose and 0.9% Sodium Chloride Injection USP
- Sufentanil Citrate Injection (such as SUFENTA), diluted as directed
- alfentanil hydrochloride injection (such as ALFENTA), diluted as directed
- fentanyl citrate injection, diluted as directed
- Midazolam hydrochloride injection, diluted as directed
- Droperidol Injection USP, diluted as directed

NIMBEX is not compatible with propofol injection (such as DIPRIVAN) or ketorolac tromethamine injection (such as TORADOL) for Y-site administration. Studies of other parenteral products have not been conducted.

Antagonism of Neuromuscular Block: Antagonists (such as neostigmine and edrophonium) should not be administered when complete neuromuscular block is evident or suspected. The use of a peripheral nerve stimulator to evaluate recovery and antagonism of neuromuscular block is recommended. The time required for anticholinesterase mediated recovery is longer for reversals attempted at deeper levels of blockade.

Table 2: NIMBEX

NIMBEX Infusion Rates for Maintenance of Neuromuscular Block During Opioid/Nitrous Oxide/Oxygen Anesthesia Using Cisatracurium at a Concentration of 0.4 mg/mL

Patient Weight (kg)	Cisatracurium Delivery Rate (µg/kg/min)				
	1	1.5	2	3	5
	Infusion Delivery Rate (mL/h)				
10	1.5	2.3	3	4.5	7.5
45	6.8	10.1	13.5	20.3	33.8
70	10.5	15.8	21	31.5	52.5
100	15	22.5	30	45	75

Administration of 0.04 to 0.07 mg/kg neostigmine at approximately 10% recovery from neuromuscular block (range: 0% to 15%) produced 95% recovery of the muscle twitch response and a T_4:T_1 ratio ≥70% in an average of 9 to 10 minutes. The time from 25% recovery of the muscle twitch response to a T_4:T_1 ratio ≥70% following these doses of neostigmine averaged 7 minutes. The mean 25 to 75% recovery index following reversal was 3 to 4 minutes.

Administration of 1.0 mg/kg edrophonium at approximately 25% recovery from neuromuscular block (range: 16% to 30%) produced 95% recovery and a T_4:T_1 ratio ≥70% in an average of 3 to 5 minutes.

Patients administered antagonists should be evaluated for evidence of adequate clinical recovery (e.g., 5-second head lift and grip strength). Ventilation must be supported until no longer required.

The onset of antagonism may be delayed in the presence of debilitation, cachexia, carcinomatosis, and the concomitant use of certain broad spectrum antibiotics, or anesthetic agents and other drugs which enhance neuromuscular block or separately cause respiratory depression (see Drug Interactions). Under such circumstances the management is the same as that of prolonged neuromuscular block (see Overdosage).

OVERDOSAGE:

Overdosage with neuromuscular blocking agents may result in neuromuscular block beyond the time needed for surgery and anesthesia. The primary treatment is maintenance of a patent airway and controlled ventilation until recovery of normal neuromuscular function is assured. Once recovery from neuromuscular block begins, further recovery may be facilitated by administration of an anticholinesterase agent (e.g., neostigmine, edrophonium) in conjunction with an appropriate anticholinergic agent (see Dosage and Administration, Antagonism of Neuromuscular Block). A peripheral nerve stimulator should be used to monitor recovery.

For management of a suspected drug overdose, CPhA recommends that you contact your **regional Poison Control Centre**. See the *CPS* Directory section for a list of Poison Control Centres.

ACTION AND CLINICAL PHARMACOLOGY: Mechanism of Action: NIMBEX (cisatracurium besylate injection) is an intermediate-acting, non-depolarizing neuromuscular blocking agent for intravenous administration. Cisatracurium besylate, one of 10 isomers of atracurium besylate (TRACRIUM), constitutes approximately 15% of atracurium bysylate. Cisatracurium besylate binds competitively to cholinergic receptors on the motor end-plate to antagonize the action of acetylcholine, resulting in block of neuromuscular transmission. This action is antagonized by acetylcholinesterase inhibitors such as neostigmine and edrophonium.

Pharmacodynamics: The average ED_{95} (dose required to produce 95% suppression of the adductor pollices muscle twitch response to ulnar nerve stimulation) of cisatracurium is 0.05 mg/kg (range: 0.048 to 0.053 mg/kg) in adults receiving opioid/nitrous oxide/oxygen anesthesia. For comparison, the average ED_{95} for atracurium when also expressed as the parent biscation is 0.17 mg/kg under similar anesthetic conditions. When the dose of cisatracurium is doubled, the clinically effective duration of block increased by approximately 25 to 35 minutes. Once recovery begins, the rate of recovery is independent of dose.

The pharmacodynamics of 2 to 8 times the ED_{95} (0.1 to 0.4 mg/kg) of cisatracurium administered over 5 to 10 seconds during opioid/nitrous oxide/oxygen anesthesia are summarized in Table 3.

The neuromuscular blocking potency of cisatracurium besylate is approximately three-fold that of atracurium besylate. At equipotent doses, the time to maximum block of cisatracurium besylate is up to 2 minutes longer than that of atracurium besylate. The clinically effective duration of action and rate of spontaneous recovery from equipotent doses of cisatracurium besylate and atracurium besylate are similar.

The neuromuscular blocking effect of cisatracurium besylate administered by infusion is potentiated by potent inhalation anesthetics. Isoflurane or enflurane administered with nitrous oxide/oxygen to achieve 1.25 MAC may prolong the clinically effective duration of action of initial and maintenance doses, and decrease the average infusion rate requirement of cisatracurium besylate. The magnitude of these effects may depend on the duration of administration of the volatile agents. Fifteen to 30 minutes of exposure to 1.25 MAC isoflurane or enflurane had minimal effects on the duration of action of initial doses of cisatracurium besylate and therefore, no adjustment to the initial dose should be necessary when cisatracurium besylate is administered shortly after initiation of volatile agents. In long surgical procedures during enflurane or isoflurane anesthesia, less frequent maintenance dosing, lower maintenance doses, or reduced infusion rates of cisatracurium besylate may be necessary. As for atracurium, the average infusion rate requirement for cisatracurium besylate may be decreased under these circumstances by as much as 30% to 40%.

The onset, duration of action, and recovery profiles of cisatracurium besylate during propofol/oxygen or propofol/nitrous oxide/oxygen anesthesia are similar to those during opioid/nitrous oxide/oxygen anesthesia.

Table 3: NIMBEX

Pharmacodynamic Dose Response[a] of NIMBEX Administered Over 5 to 10 Seconds During Opioid/Nitrous Oxide/Oxygen Anesthesia

Initial Dose of Cisatracurium (mg/kg)	Time to 90% Block (min)	Time to Maximum Block (min)	Time to Spontaneous Recovery[g]				25–75% Recovery Index (min)
			5% Recovery (min)	25% Recovery[b] (min)	95% Recovery (min)	T_4:T_1 Ratio[c] ≥70% (min)	
Adults							
0.1 (2×ED_{95}) n[d]=98	3.3 (1.0–8.7)	5.0 (1.2–17.2)	33 (15–51)	42 (22–63)	64 (25–93)	64 (32–91)	13 (5–30)
0.15[e] (3×ED_{95}) n=39	2.6 (1.0–4.4)	3.5 (1.6–6.8)	46 (28–65)	55 (44–74)	76 (60–103)	75 (63–98)	13 (11–16)
0.2 (4×ED_{95}) n=30	2.4 (1.5–4.5)	2.9 (1.9–5.2)	59 (31–103)	65 (43–103)	81 (53–114)	85 (55–114)	12 (2–30)

(cont'd)

Table 3: NIMBEX *(cont'd)*

Pharmacodynamic Dose Response[a] of NIMBEX Administered Over 5 to 10 Seconds During Opioid/Nitrous Oxide/Oxygen Anesthesia

			Time to Spontaneous Recovery[g]				
Initial Dose of Cisatracurium (mg/kg)	**Time to 90% Block (min)**	**Time to Maximum Block (min)**	**5% Recovery (min)**	**25% Recovery[b] (min)**	**95% Recovery (min)**	**T_4:T_1 Ratio[c] ≥70% (min)**	**25–75% Recovery Index (min)**
0.25 (5×ED_{95}) n=15	1.6 (0.8–3.3)	2.0 (1.2–3.7)	70 (58–85)	78 (66–86)	91 (76–109)	97 (82–113)	8 (5–12)
0.4 (8×ED_{95}) n=15	1.5 (1.3–1.8)	1.9 (1.4–2.3)	83 (37–103)	91 (59–107)	121 (110–134)	126 (115–137)	14 (10–18)
Children (2–12 years)							
0.08[f] (2×ED_{95}) n=60	2.2 (1.2–6.8)	3.3 (1.7–9.7)	22 (11–38)	29 (20–46)	52 (37–64)	50 (37–62)	11 (7–15)
0.1 n=16	1.7 (1.3–2.7)	2.8 (1.8–6.7)	21 (13–31)	28 (21–38)	46 (37–58)	44 (36–58)	10 (7–12)

[a] Values shown are medians of means from individual studies. Values in parentheses are ranges of individual patient values.
[b] Clinically effective duration of block.
[c] Train-of-four ratio.
[d] n=the number of patients with Time to Maximum Block data.
[e] Propofol anesthesia.
[f] Halothane anesthesia.
[g] Not all patients (~50%) were evaluated for spontaneous recovery parameters.

Intubation Conditions: When administered during the induction of adequate anesthesia using propofol, nitrous oxide/oxygen, and co-induction agents (e.g., fentanyl, midazolam), good or excellent conditions for tracheal intubation occurred in 67/71 (94%) patients in 1.5 to 2.0 minutes following 0.15 mg/kg (3×ED_{95}) cisatracurium and in 69/80 (87%) patients in 1.5 minutes following 0.2 mg/kg (4×ED_{95}) cisatracurium. Favourable intubation conditions, within 2.0 minutes, were achieved less frequently with a cisatracurium dose of 0.1 mg/kg (2×ED_{95}).

Maintenance Doses: Repeated administration of maintenance doses or a continuous infusion of cisatracurium besylate for up to 3 hours is not associated with development of tachyphylaxis or cumulative neuromuscular blocking effects. The time needed to recover from successive maintenance doses does not change with the number of doses administered as long as partial recovery is allowed to occur between doses. Maintenance doses can therefore be administered at relatively regular intervals with predictable results. The rate of spontaneous recovery of neuromuscular function after infusion is independent of the duration of infusion and comparable to the rate of recovery following initial doses (see Table 3).

Anticholinesterase Antagonism: The neuromuscular block produced by cisatracurium besylate is readily antagonized by anticholinesterase agents once recovery has started. As with other non-depolarizing neuromuscular blocking agents, the more profound the neuromuscular block at the time of reversal, the longer the time required for recovery of neuromuscular function.

Pediatrics: In children (2 to 12 years of age) cisatracurium has a lower ED_{95} than in adults (0.04 mg/kg, halothane/nitrous oxide/oxygen anesthesia). At 0.1 mg/kg during opioid anesthesia, cisatracurium had a faster onset and shorter duration of action in children than in adults (see Table 3). Recovery following reversal is faster in children than in adults.

Hemodynamics Profile: No dose-related effects were observed on mean arterial blood pressure (MAP) or heart rate following doses of cisatracurium ranging from 2 to 8×ED_{95} (0.1 mg/kg to 0.4 mg/kg), administered over 5 to 10 seconds, in healthy adult patients, or in patients with serious cardiovascular disease.

A total of 141 patients undergoing coronary artery bypass grafting (CABG) have been administered cisatracurium in three active controlled clinical trials and have received doses ranging from 2 to 8×ED_{95} (0.10 mg/kg to 0.40 mg/kg). While the hemodynamic profile was comparable in cisatracurium besylate and active control groups, data for doses above 0.3 mg/kg in this population are limited.

Cisatracurium, at therapeutic doses of 2 to 8 times the ED_{95} (0.10 to 0.40 mg/kg), administered over 5 to 10 seconds, does not cause dose-related elevations in mean plasma histamine concentration.

No clinically significant changes in Mean Arterial Pressure (MAP) or Heart Rate (HR) were observed following administration of doses up to 0.10 mg/kg cisatracurium over 5 to 10 seconds in children (2 to 12 years of age) receiving either halothane/nitrous oxide/oxygen or opioid/nitrous oxide/oxygen anesthesia.

Pharmacokinetics: Following i.v. administration of cisatracurium besylate, plasma concentrations of cisatracurium are best described by a two-compartment open model. Cisatracurium undergoes degradation in the body at physiological pH and temperature by organ-independent Hofmann elimination to form laudanosine and the monoquaternary acrylate metabolite. Laudanosine is further metabolized to many components which are eliminated in the urine. The monoquaternary acrylate metabolite undergoes hydrolysis by non-specific plasma esterases to form the monoquaternary alcohol metabolite. Cisatracurium does not appear to undergo direct hydrolysis by non-specific plasma esterases. Organ-independent Hofmann elimination appears to be the predominant pathway for the elimination of cisatracurium.

Plasma cisatracurium concentrations and neuromuscular block data from 261 patients in six studies were combined to develop population estimates of the pharmacokinetic/pharmacodynamic parameters for cisatracurium in healthy adult patients. The plasma clearance was 4.6 mL/min/kg and the volume of distribution at steady state was 145 mL/kg in healthy adult patients receiving opioid/nitrous oxide/oxygen anesthesia. Results from population pharmacokinetic/pharmacodynamic analyses and from conventional pharmacokinetic analyses of cisatracurium in healthy adult patients and in patient subpopulations (e.g., geriatric, pediatric, obese) are described in Special Populations and Conditions.

Dose Proportionality: Conventional pharmacokinetic analysis from a study of 10 healthy adult patients receiving 0.10 mg/kg (2×ED_{95}) cisatracurium besylate and 10 healthy adult patients receiving 0.20 mg/kg (4×ED_{95}) cisatracurium besylate showed no statistically significant differences in the pharmacokinetic parameters between the two groups (see Table 4). In addition, population pharmacokinetic/pharmacodynamic analyses revealed no statistically significant effect of dose on plasma clearance between 0.10 mg/kg and 0.40 mg/kg (2× to 8×ED_{95}) doses of cisatracurium. The pharmacokinetics are linear between these doses of cisatracurium (i.e., plasma concentrations are approximately proportional to dose).

Table 4: NIMBEX

Pharmacokinetic Parameters[a] of Cisatracurium in Healthy Adult Patients (Opioid/Nitrous Oxide/Oxygen Anesthesia)

	Initial Dose of NIMBEX (mg/kg)	
Parameter	**0.1 (2×ED_{95}) n=10**	**0.2 (4×ED_{95}) n=10**
Elimination $t_{1/2\beta}$ (min)	22.4±2.7	25.5±4.1
Volume of Distribution at Steady-state (mL/kg)	144±34	121±22
Plasma Clearance (mL/min/kg)	5.3±1.2	4.7±0.7

[a] Values presented are mean±Standard Deviation (SD).

Absorption: Not applicable.

Distribution: The volume of distribution at steady state was 145 mL/kg in healthy adult patients receiving opioid/nitrous oxide/oxygen anesthesia.

Metabolism: Tests in which the monoquaternary alcohol metabolite or the monoquaternary acrylate was administered to cats suggest that metabolites are unlikely to produce clinically significant neuromuscular, autonomic, or cardiovascular effects following administration of cisatracurium besylate. Laudanosine, a biologically active metabolite of cisatracurium besylate without neuromuscular blocking activity, produces transient hypotension and, in higher concentrations, cerebral excitatory effects when administered in several species of animals. The relationship between CNS excitation and laudanosine concentrations in humans has not been established. Because cisatracurium is three times more potent than atracurium and lower doses are required, maximum concentrations of laudanosine following infusions of cisatracurium besylate to surgical patients were lower (5- to 8-fold) than following atracurium besylate. After adjusting for differences in doses, the area under the curve for laudanosine was significantly lower following cisatracurium besylate administration than following atracurium besylate administration (i.e., less laudanosine may be formed following cisatracurium besylate than following atracurium besylate). The clinical relevance of this finding is unknown.

Excretion: The liver and the kidney play a minor role in the elimination of cisatracurium but are primary routes for elimination of the metabolites.

Special Populations and Conditions: Pediatrics: Population pharmacokinetic analysis of cisatracurium revealed a plasma clearance of 5.9 mL/kg/min and a volume of distribution at steady-state of 125 mL/kg in 20 healthy pediatric patients during halothane anesthesia. These minor differences were associated with a faster time to onset and a shorter duration of cisatracurium induced neuromuscular block in pediatric patients.

Geriatrics: The results of conventional pharmacokinetic analysis from a study of 12 healthy elderly patients (≥65 years) and 12 healthy young adult patients (18 to 50 years of age) receiving a single i.v. of 0.10 mg/kg (2×ED_{95}) cisatracurium besylate are summarized in Table 5. Plasma clearance of cisatracurium was not affected by age; however, the volume of distribution was slightly larger in elderly patients than in young patients, resulting in a slightly longer $t_{½}$ for cisatracurium. The time to maximum block was approximately one minute slower in elderly patients than in young patients. These minor differences in pharmacokinetics of cisatracurium besylate between elderly and young adult patients were not associated with clinically significant differences in the recovery profile of cisatracurium.

Table 5: NIMBEX

Pharmacokinetic Parameters[a] of Cisatracurium in Healthy Elderly and Young Adult Patients Following 0.1 mg/kg (2×ED_{95}) NIMBEX (Isoflurane/Nitrous Oxide/Oxygen Anesthesia)

Parameter	Elderly Patients n=12	Young Adult Patients n=12
Elimination $t_{1/2\beta}$ (min)	25.8±3.6[b]	22.1±2.5
Volume of Distribution at Steady State (mL/kg)	156±17[b]	133±15
Plasma Clearance (mL/min/kg)	5.7±1.0	5.3±0.9

[a] Values presented are mean±S.D.
[b] $p<0.05$ for comparisons between the two groups.

Gender and Obesity: Population pharmacokinetic/pharmacodynamic analysis revealed that gender and obesity were associated with statistically significant effects on the pharmacokinetics and/or pharmacodynamics of cisatracurium; these factors were not associated with clinically significant alterations in the predicted onset or recovery profile of cisatracurium.

Hepatic Insufficiency: Organ-independent Hofmann elimination is the predominant pathway for the elimination of cisatracurium. Table 6 summarizes the conventional pharmacokinetic analysis from a study of 13 patients with end-stage liver disease undergoing liver transplantation and 11 healthy adult patients undergoing elective surgery. The slightly larger volume of distribution in liver transplant patients was associated with slightly higher plasma clearance of cisatracurium. The parallel changes in these parameters resulted in no difference in t½. The time to maximum block was approximately one minute faster in liver transplant patients than in healthy adult patients. These minor differences in pharmacokinetics were not associated with clinically significant changes in the recovery profile of cisatracurium.

The $t_{1/2\beta}$ values of metabolites are longer in patients with hepatic disease and concentrations may be higher after long-term administration.

Table 6: NIMBEX

Pharmacokinetic Parameters[a] of Cisatracurium in Healthy Adult Patients and in Patients Undergoing Liver Transplantation Following 0.1 mg/kg (2×ED_{95}) NIMBEX (Isoflurane/Nitrous Oxide/Oxygen Anesthesia)

Parameter	Healthy Adult Patients	Liver Transplant Patients
Elimination $t_{1/2\beta}$ (min)	23.5±3.5	24.4±2.9
Volume of Distribution at Steady State (mL/kg)	161±23	195±38[b]
Plasma Clearance (mL/min/kg)	5.7±0.8	6.6±1.1[b]

[a] Values presented are mean±S.D.
[b] $p<0.05$ for comparisons between liver transplant patients and healthy adult patients.

Renal Insufficiency: Results from a conventional pharmacokinetic study of 13 healthy adult patients and 15 patients with end-stage renal disease (ESRD) undergoing elective surgery are summarized in Table 7. The pharmacokinetics of cisatracurium were similar in healthy adult patients and ESRD patients.

Table 7: NIMBEX

Pharmacokinetic Parameters[a] for Cisatracurium in Healthy Adult Patients and in Patients with End-stage Renal Disease (ESRD) Receiving 0.1 mg/kg (2×ED_{95}) NIMBEX (Opioid/Nitrous Oxide/Oxygen Anesthesia)

Parameter	Healthy Adult Patients	ESRD Patients
Elimination $t_{1/2\beta}$ (min)	29.4±4.1	32.3±6.3
Volume of distribution at steady state (mL/kg)	149±35	160±32
Plasma Clearance (mL/min/kg)	4.66±0.86	4.26±0.62

[a] Values presented are mean±S.D.

The time to 90% block was approximately one minute slower in ESRD patients following 0.10 mg/kg cisatracurium. There was no difference in the duration or rate of recovery between ESRD and healthy adult patients.

The $t_{1/2\beta}$ values of metabolites are longer in patients with renal failure and concentrations may be higher after long-term administration.

Population pharmacokinetic analysis revealed that patients with creatinine clearances ≤70 mL/min had a slower rate of equilibration between plasma concentrations and neuromuscular block than patients with normal renal function; therefore, the predicted time to 90% T_1 suppression may be slightly slower in patients with renal dysfunction. There was no clinically significant alteration in the recovery profile of cisatracurium in patients with renal dysfunction.

Other Patient Factors: The use of inhalation anesthesia (i.e., enflurane or isoflurane) was associated with statistically significant effects on the pharmacokinetics and pharmacodynamics of cisatracurium. These changes were associated with a slightly faster predicted time to 90% suppression for patients under inhalation anesthesia, but there were no clinically significant alterations in the predicted recovery profile of cisatracurium.

STORAGE AND STABILITY: NIMBEX (cisatracurium besylate injection) slowly loses potency with time at a rate of approximately 5% per year under refrigeration (5°C). NIMBEX **should be stored under refrigeration (2 to 8°C)** and protected from light to preserve potency. **Protect from freezing.**

The rate of loss in potency increases to approximately 5% per month at 25°C. If removed from refrigeration to room temperature storage (25°C), NIMBEX must be used within 21 days, even if re-refrigerated.

Dilution Stability: NIMBEX diluted to 0.1 mg/mL in 5% Dextrose Injection USP, 0.9% Sodium Chloride Injection USP, or 5% Dextrose and 0.9% Sodium Chloride Injection USP, may be stored either under refrigeration or at room temperature for 24 hours without significant loss of potency. Dilutions to 0.1 mg/mL in 5% Dextrose and Lactated Ringer's Injection may be stored under refrigeration for 24 hours.

NIMBEX should not be diluted in Lactated Ringer's Injection USP due to chemical instability.

SPECIAL HANDLING INSTRUCTIONS: Parenteral drug products should be inspected visually for particulate matter and discoloration prior to administration whenever solution and container permit. Solutions which are not clear, or contain visible particulates, should not be used.

INFORMATION FOR THE PATIENT: Published in e-CPS, available by subscription at www.e-cps.ca.

DOSAGE FORMS, COMPOSITION AND PACKAGING: Each mL of a sterile, non-pyrogenic, aqueous, colorless to slightly yellow or greenish-yellow solution contains: cisatracurium 2 mg (as 2.81 mg cisatracurium besylate). Nonmedicinal ingredients: benzenesulfonic acid, benzyl alcohol and water for injection. Since NIMBEX contains benzyl alcohol, it should not be used in neonates (see Contraindications). The pH is adjusted to 3.25 to 3.65 with benzenesulfonic acid. Multidose vials of 10 mL.

Nimodipine ℞

CPhA Monograph

see *Calcium Channel Blockers*

The reader is invited to consult CPhA's monograph **Calcium Channel Blockers**.

Nimotop® Tablets ℞

nimodipine

Adjunct in the Management of Subarachnoid Hemorrhage —Calcium Channel Blocking Agent

Bayer

Date of Preparation: April 28, 2009

SUMMARY PRODUCT INFORMATION:

Route of Administration	Dosage Form/ Strength	All Nonmedicinal Ingredients
Oral	Tablets, 30 mg	Crospovidone, ferric oxide yellow, hypromellose, macrogol, magnesium stearate, maize starch, microcrystalline cellulose, povidone, and titanium dioxide

INDICATIONS AND CLINICAL USE: Adults: NIMOTOP Tablets (nimodipine tablets) may be useful as an adjunct to improve the neurologic outcome following subarachnoid hemorrhage (SAH) from ruptured intracranial aneurysm.

Geriatrics (>65 years of age): Clinical studies of nimodipine did not include sufficient numbers of subjects aged 65 and over to determine whether they respond differently from younger subjects. Other reported clinical experience has not identified differences in responses between elderly and younger patients. In general, dosing for elderly patients should be cautious, reflecting the greater frequency of decreased hepatic, renal, or cardiac function, and of concomitant disease or other drug therapy.

Pediatrics (<18 years of age): The safety and effectiveness of nimodipine in children have not been established.

CONTRAINDICATIONS:

- Hypersensitivity to nimodipine or to any ingredient of the drug product.
- The concomitant use of oral nimodipine and the antiepileptic drugs phenobarbital, phenytoin, or carbamazepine is contraindicated, as the efficacy of nimodipine tablets could be significantly reduced.
- The use of nimodipine in combination with rifampin is contraindicated, as the efficacy of nimodipine tablets could be significantly reduced when concomitantly administered with rifampin.

WARNINGS AND PRECAUTIONS: General: NIMOTOP Tablets (nimodipine tablets) should only be used with great caution when cerebral edema or severely raised intracranial pressure is present. Although treatment with nimodipine has not been shown to be associated with increases in intracranial pressure, close monitoring is recommended in these cases or when the water content of the brain tissue is elevated (generalized cerebral edema).

NIMOTOP should not be used in patients with traumatic subarachnoid hemorrhage as a positive benefit to risk ratio has not been established and the specific patient groups that might benefit cannot be identified for this indication.

Caution is required in patients with hypotension (systolic blood pressure lower than 100 mm Hg) (see Warnings and Precautions, Cardiovascular).

NIMOTOP is metabolized via the cytochrome P450 3A4 system. Drugs that are known to either inhibit or induce this enzymatic system may therefore alter the first pass or the clearance of nimodipine. Drugs known to inhibit the cytochrome P450 3A4 system and therefore may lead to increased plasma concentrations of nimodipine are:

- antidepressants (eg, nefazodone and fluoxetine)
- azole antimycotics (eg, ketoconazole)
- cimetidine
- HIV protease inhibitors (eg, ritonavir)
- macrolide antibiotics (eg, erythromycin)
- valproic acid

Upon coadministration with these drugs, blood pressure should be monitored and, if necessary, a reduction of the nimodipine dose should be considered (see Drug Interactions).

Intestinal pseudo-obstruction (paralytic ileus) has been reported rarely. A causal relationship to NIMOTOP Tablets (nimodipine tablets) cannot be ruled out. In three cases, the condition responded to conservative management, but a fourth patient required surgical decompression of the extremely distended colon.

Cardiovascular: NIMOTOP Tablets (nimodipine tablets) have the hemodynamic effects of a calcium channel blocker. In the course of clinical studies in patients with SAH, hypotension was reported in 6.6% of patients with Hunt and Hess grades III to V given 90 mg doses (n=91), and in 7.5% of patients with grades I and II using 30 to 60 mg doses (n=255). A fall in blood pressure requiring discontinuation of the drug was reported in 2.2% of the patients in the former group. Hypertensive patients may be more susceptible to a lowering of the blood pressure. Blood pressure should, nevertheless, always be carefully monitored during treatment with nimodipine. The use of nimodipine is, however, not generally recommended in patients taking antihypertensive drugs, including other calcium channel blockers, since it may potentiate the effects of these medications (see Drug Interactions, Drug-Drug Interactions, Blood Pressure Lowering Drugs).

Since there has not been a study of NIMOTOP in acute myocardial infarction reported, similar effects of NIMOTOP to that of immediate-release nifedipine cannot be excluded in acute myocardial infarction. Immediate-release nifedipine is contraindicated in acute myocardial infarction.

Some clinical trials have shown that treatment with the immediate-release formulation of the dihydropyridine, nifedipine, in patients with unstable angina, increases the risk of myocardial infarction and recurrent ischemia.

Effect on Ability to Drive and Operate Machinery: Reactions to nimodipine, which vary in intensity from individual to individual, can impair the ability to drive or to operate machinery. This is most prevalent at the start of the treatment, upon changing the medication, or in combination with alcohol.

Hepatic/Biliary/Pancreatic: The metabolism of nimodipine is decreased in patients with impaired hepatic function. Such patients should be given lower doses of the drug and their blood pressure and pulse should be closely monitored.

In Vitro Fertilization: In single cases of in vitro fertilization, calcium antagonists have been associated with reversible biochemical changes in the spermatozoa's head section that may result in impaired sperm function.

Renal: There are insufficient data on patients with impaired renal function.

Special Populations: Pregnant Women: The safety of nimodipine with respect to adverse effects on human fetal development has not been established.

Nimodipine has been shown to have a teratogenic effect in rabbits and to be embryotoxic, causing resorption, stunted growth, and higher incidence of skeletal variations in rats.

Nimodipine should, therefore, not be used during pregnancy unless the potential benefits are considered to justify the potential risk to the fetus.

Pediatrics (<18 years of age): The safety and effectiveness of nimodipine in children less than 18 years of age has not been established. Therefore, NIMOTOP is not recommended for use in this patient population.

Geriatrics (>65 years of age): Clinical studies of nimodipine did not include sufficient numbers of subjects aged 65 and over to determine whether they respond differently from younger subjects. Other reported clinical experience has not identified differences in responses between elderly and younger patients. In general, dosing for elderly patients should be cautious, reflecting the greater frequency of decreased hepatic, renal, or cardiac function, and of concomitant disease or other drug therapy.

ADVERSE REACTIONS: Adverse Drug Reaction Overview: Adverse drug reactions (ADRs) based on placebo-controlled clinical trials with nimodipine have been evaluated in 1395 patients with subarachnoid hemorrhage. In these studies, 703 patients received oral doses of nimodipine and 692 patients received placebo.

Clinical Trial Adverse Drug Reactions: Because clinical trials are conducted under very specific conditions the adverse reaction rates observed in the clinical trials may not reflect the rates observed in practice and should not be compared to the rates in the clinical trials of another drug. Adverse drug reaction information from clinical trials is useful for identifying drug-related adverse events and for approximating rates.

The following are common and less common adverse drug reactions reported by patients in the double-blind, placebo-controlled clinical trial (British Aneurysm and Nimodipine Trial [BRANT Study]): See Table 1.

Table 1: NIMOTOP Tablets

Adverse Drug Reactions

Sign/Symptom	Nimodipine (2×30 mg q4h) 60 mg (N=278) n (%)	Placebo (N=276) n (%)
Blood and Bone Marrow		
Anemia	1 (0.4%)	0
Colonic Bleed	1 (0.4%)	0
Hematoma	1 (0.4%)	0
Thrombocytopenia	1 (0.4%)	0
Cardiovascular		
Headache	3 (1.1%)	1 (0.4%)
Hypertension	1 (0.4%)	0
Hypotension	1 (0.4%)	2 (0.7%)
Vasodilation (Flushing)	1 (0.4%)	0
Gastrointestinal Tract		
Nausea	1 (0.4%)	0
Liver and Biliary System		
Jaundice	2 (0.7%)	1 (0.4%)
Liver Function Test Abnormal	2 (0.7%)	4 (1.4%)
Respiratory System		
Bronchospasm	0	1 (0.4%)
Skin		
Rash	2 (0.7%)	1 (0.4%)

Legend: N=number of patients; n=number of patients with specific event.

Other uncommon or rare adverse drug reactions reported by patients in other SAH clinical trials include allergic reaction, bradycardia, ileus and tachycardia.

In severely ill patients, there was an overall increased mortality rate in the nimodipine group using the 90 mg q4h dose as compared to placebo.

Adverse events known to be associated with calcium channel blockers should be appropriately monitored.

Post-Market Adverse Drug Reactions: Gastrointestinal Disorders: nausea, vomiting.

Nervous System Disorders: headache.

Vascular Disorders: hypotension.

Abnormal Hematologic and Clinical Chemistry Findings: Isolated cases of nonfasting elevated serum glucose levels (0.8%), elevated LDH levels (0.4%), decreased platelet counts (0.3%), elevated alkaline phosphatase levels (0.2%), and elevated ALT levels (0.2%) have been reported rarely.

DRUG INTERACTIONS:

Serious Drug Interactions

- **The concomitant use of oral nimodipine and the antiepileptic drugs phenobarbital, phenytoin, or carbamazepine is contraindicated, as the efficacy of nimodipine tablets could be significantly reduced.**
- **The use of nimodipine in combination with rifampin is contraindicated, as the efficacy of nimodipine tablets could be significantly reduced when concomitantly administered with rifampin.**

Overview: As with all drugs, care should be exercised when treating patients with multiple medications. Dihydropyridine calcium channel blockers undergo biotransformation by the cytochrome P450 system, mainly via the CYP3A4 isoenzyme. Coadministration of nimodipine with other drugs which follow the same route of biotransformation may result in altered bioavailability. Dosages of similarly metabolized drugs, particularly those of low therapeutic ratio, and especially in patients with renal and/or hepatic impairment, may require adjustment when starting or stopping concomitantly administered nimodipine to maintain optimum therapeutic blood levels.

Drugs which are known inhibitors of the cytochrome P450 system and therefore may lead to increased plasma concentrations of nimodipine include: azole antifungals, HIV protease inhibitors, fluoxetine, nefazodone, cimetidine, macrolide antibiotics (eg, erythromycin), quinidine and valproic acid. Upon coadministration of nimodipine with these drugs, blood pressure should be monitored and, if necessary, a reduction of the nimodipine dosage should be considered. Consumption of grapefruit juice, a CYP3A4 inhibitor, prior to or during treatment with nimodipine should be avoided.

The extent as well as the duration of interactions should be taken into account when administering nimodipine together with drugs known to be inducers of the cytochrome P450 system. Concomitant use of nimodipine and phenobarbital, phenytoin, carbamazepine, or rifampin is contraindicated (see Contraindications). Other CYP3A4 inducers include dexamethasone, rifabutin, and St. John's Wort.

Drug-Drug Interactions: See Table 2.

Table 2: NIMOTOP Tablets

Established or Potential Drug-Drug Interactions

Proper Name	Ref	Effect	Clinical Comment
Alcohol	T	↑ NIMOTOP	Concomitant use of alcohol may potentiate the effect of nimodipine by lowering blood pressure and causing dizziness.
Anticoagulant: warfarin	CT	No effect on NIMOTOP	An interaction study with nimodipine and warfarin has shown no clinically significant interactions between these drugs.
Anticonvulsant: valproic acid	CT	↑ NIMOTOP	In a pharmacokinetic study in epileptic patients receiving long-term treatment concomitant administration of sodium valproate and oral nimodipine resulted in a 50% increase in the bioavailability of nimodipine. Therefore, the simultaneous administration of the anticonvulsant valproic acid can lead to an increase in the plasma nimodipine concentration.
Antidepressant (SSRI): fluoxetine	CT	↑ NIMOTOP	In 39 elderly patients (57-75 years of age) treated with 30 mg nimodipine tid, for at least 3 months, concomitant administration of fluoxetine (20 mg/day for 14 days) resulted in a 50% increase in nimodipine steady-state plasma concentrations. In these patients, fluoxetine plasma concentrations were decreased by approximately 20%, while those of its active metabolite, norfluxetine, were not significantly affected. In patients receiving fluoxetine, a reduction in nimodipine dosage may be required.
Antidepressant (Tricyclic Antidepressant): nortriptyline	CT	No effect on NIMOTOP	In 12 elderly patients treated with nimodipine (30 mg tid), for at least 3 months, coadministration of nortriptyline (10 mg tid) for 7 days resulted in nonsignificant decreases in nimodipine with $AUC_{(0-24h)}$ of 10% and C_{max} of 17% at steady state. The pharmacokinetics of nortriptyline were not affected by nimodipine.
Antiepileptic: phenobarbital, phenytoin and/or carbamazepine	CT	↓ NIMOTOP/ ↑ NIMOTOP	A pharmacokinetic study in epileptic patients receiving long-term treatment has shown that concurrent administration of oral nimodipine and CYP450 enzyme-inducer antiepileptic drugs (phenobarbital, phenytoin and/or carbamazepine) reduces the bioavailability of nimodipine by about 80%. Concomitant use of nimodipine and phenobarbital, phenytoin, or carbamazepine is contraindicated (see Contraindications).
Antipsychotic: haloperidol	CT	No effect on NIMOTOP	In 12 elderly patients (60-80 years of age) receiving haloperidol with an individual but constant dosing (0.7-23.0 mg/day depending on individual need) for at least one month, treatment with 30 mg tid nimodipine for 7 days did not affect the pharmacokinetics of haloperidol.
Anxiolytic, sedative: diazepam	CT	No effect on NIMOTOP	An interaction study with nimodipine and diazepam has shown no clinically significant interactions between these drugs.
Azole Antifungals: ketoconazole	T	↑ NIMOTOP	A formal interaction study investigating the potential drug interaction between nimodipine and ketoconazole has not been performed. Azole antifungals are known to inhibit the CYP3A4 system, and various interactions have been reported for other dihydropyridine calcium antagonists. Therefore, when administered together with oral nimodipine, a substantial increase in systemic bioavailibility of nimodipine due to a decreased first-pass metabolism cannot be excluded.
H_2-receptor antagonist: cimetidine	CT	↑ NIMOTOP	A pharmacokinetic study has shown that concurrent administration of cimetidine and oral nimodipine results in an almost doubling of the area under the nimodipine plasma concentration curve and about a 50% increase in the peak nimodipine plasma concentration. Patients receiving the two drugs concomitantly should be watched carefully for the possible exaggeration of the effects of nimodipine. It may be necessary to adjust the dosage of nimodipine.
HIV Protease Inhibitors: ritonavir	T	↑ NIMOTOP	No formal studies have been performed to investigate the potential interaction between nimodipine and HIV protease inhibitors. Drugs of this class have been reported to be potent inhibitors of the cytochrome P450 3A4 system. Therefore, the potential for a marked and clinically relevant increase in nimodipine plasma concentrations upon coadministration with these protease inhibitors cannot be excluded.
Macrolide Antibiotics: erythromycin	T	↑ NIMOTOP	No interaction studies have been carried out between nimodipine and macrolide antibiotics. Certain macrolide antibiotics are known to inhibit the cytochrome P450 3A4 system and the potential for drug interaction cannot be ruled out. Therefore, macrolide antibiotics should not be used in combination with nimodipine.

Legend: CT=clinical trial; T=theoretical.

Blood Pressure Lowering Drugs: Nimodipine may increase the blood-pressure-lowering effect of concomitantly administered antihypertensives, such as A1-antagonists, ACE inhibitors, alpha-adrenergic blocking agents, methyldopa, beta-blockers, diuretics, PDE5 inhibitors, and other calcium antagonists. If coadministration with these drugs is unavoidable, careful monitoring of the patient is necessary (see Warnings and Precautions, Cardiovascular).

In addition to the effect on blood pressure, verapamil and diltiazem are also CYP3A4 inhibitors and may decrease clearance of nimodipine.

Simultaneous intravenous administration of beta blockers can lead to mutual potentiation of negative inotropic effects and even to decompensated heart failure.

Drug-Food Interactions: The effects of a standard breakfast on the bioavailability of nimodipine tablets were investigated in two separate studies. From the results it was concluded that, although the rate of absorption is delayed as evidenced by the decrease in C_{max} (approximately 40%) and the increase in T_{max} (approximately 100%) the presence of food does not alter the extent of absorption of nimodipne tablets.

Patients should be advised to be consistent in the timing of nimodipine tablet administration, either with or without food.

Published data indicate that through inhibition of cytochrome P450, grapefruit juice can increase plasma levels and augment pharmacodynamic effects of some dihydropyridine calcium channel blockers. As a consequence, the blood-pressure-lowering effect may be increased. This effect may last for at least 4 days after the last ingestion of grapefruit juice. Therefore, consumption of grapefruit juice prior to or during treatment with nimodipine should be avoided.

Drug-Herb Interactions: Herbal products containing St. John's Wort (hypericum perforatum) may lead to a decreased nimodipine plasma concentration. Strong CYP3A4 inducers should be administered with caution in combination with NIMOTOP Tablets.

DOSAGE AND ADMINISTRATION:

Dosing Considerations: NIMOTOP Tablets (nimodipine tablets) contain 30 mg of the active ingredient nimodipine which is consistent with NIMOTOP 30 mg capsules. The 30 mg nimodipine tablet has been shown to provide the same AUC exposure as the 30 mg nimodipine capsule (see Action and Clinical Pharmacology, Pharmacokinetics, Absorption).

NIMOTOP Tablets should not be dissolved in any type of liquid solution (eg, water, saline) for administration by way of intravenous injection or other parenteral routes.

Recommended Dose and Dosage Adjustment: For the management of neurological deficits following subarachnoid hemorrhage (SAH), NIMOTOP Tablets (nimodipine tablets) therapy should commence as soon as possible or within 4 days of the diagnosis of SAH.

The recommended dosage of NIMOTOP Tablets (nimodipine tablets) is 60 mg (two tablets of 30 mg) administered **orally** every 4 hours for 21 consecutive days after diagnosis of SAH. Doses of up to 90 mg every 4 hours have been used in some patients, although the safety of higher doses in severely ill patients has not been well established (see Adverse Reactions).

Due to the possibility of hydrolysis in high alkaline pH, alkaline mixtures should not be given for 2 hours before or after administering NIMOTOP tablets.

NIMOTOP may be used during anesthesia or surgical procedures. In the event of surgical intervention, administration of NIMOTOP should be continued, with dosages as above, to complete the 21-day period.

Drug effects should be carefully monitored in all patients, particularly if higher doses are used.

Special Populations: Hepatic Impairment: Patients with hepatic insufficiency may have substantially reduced clearance and approximately doubled maximum plasma concentration; accordingly, the dosage should be reduced to one 30 mg NIMOTOP tablet every 4 hours in these patients.

Renal Impairment: There are insufficient data on patients with impaired renal function.

Geriatrics (>65 years of age): Clinical studies of nimodipine did not include sufficient numbers of subjects aged 65 and over to determine whether they respond differently from younger subjects.

In a single parallel-group study involving 24 elderly subjects (aged 59-79) and 24 younger subjects (aged 22-40), the observed AUC and C_{max} of nimodipine was approximately 2-fold higher in the elderly population compared to the younger study subjects following oral administration (given as a single dose of 30 mg and dosed to steady state with 30 mg tid for 6 days). The clinical response to these age-related pharmacokinetic differences, however, was not considered significant.

In general, dosing for elderly patients should be cautious, reflecting the greater frequency of decreased hepatic, renal or cardiac function, and of concomitant disease or other drug therapy.

Pediatrics (<18 years of age): The safety and effectiveness of nimodipine in children less than 18 years of age has not been established. Therefore, NIMOTOP is not recommended for use in this patient population.

Missed Dose: If the patient has forgotten to take a dose, they should be instructed to take it as soon as they remember. The patient should carry on with the remaining days' tablets at the normal four-hour intervals.

A double dose should not be taken to make up for a forgotten tablet.

Administration: The tablets should be swallowed whole with plenty of fluid (preferably a glass of water), independent of meal times. NIMOTOP Tablets should not be crushed as this may result in reduced bioavailability and clinical effectiveness. Tablets should not be taken while lying down. Grapefruit juice is to be avoided. The interval between successive doses should not be less than 4 hours.

OVERDOSAGE:

Symptoms of Intoxication: Symptoms of acute overdosage would be related to cardiovascular effects and the patient may experience marked systemic hypotension, tachycardia or bradycardia, flushing, headache, and gastrointestinal complaints and nausea.

Treatment of Intoxication: Clinically significant hypotension due to NIMOTOP overdosage may require active cardiovascular support and should include close monitoring of cardiac and respiratory function. In the event of acute overdose, treatment with NIMOTOP must be discontinued immediately. Symptoms of acute overdose are marked lowering of blood pressure, tachycardia or bradycardia, and gastrointestinal complaints and nausea.

Emergency measures should be governed by the symptoms. Gastric lavage with addition of charcoal should be considered as an emergency therapeutic measure. If there is a marked fall in blood pressure, dopamine or noradrenaline can be administered intravenously. Since no specific antidote is known, subsequent treatment for other side effects should be aimed at the most prominent symptoms. Since nimodipine is 99% bound to serum protein, dialysis is not likely to be of benefit.

> For management of a suspected drug overdose, contact your **regional Poison Control Centre**. See the *CPS* Directory section for a list of Poison Control Centres.

ACTION AND CLINICAL PHARMACOLOGY: Mechanism of Action: Delayed neurological deterioration secondary to cerebral ischemic deficits is believed to be a major determinant of outcome in patients who survive their initial subarachnoid hemorrhage (SAH). NIMOTOP (nimodipine) is a calcium channel blocker of the dihydropyridine group. It appears to have a more marked effect on the cerebral circulation than on the peripheral circulation. Since it acts on the vascular smooth muscle tone by modifying the contractile process which is dependent upon the movement of extracellular calcium into the cells during depolarization, it was tested in patients with SAH in an effort to improve the neurologic outcome in these patients. Clinical studies with nimodipine support its usefulness as an adjunct in the management of some patients with SAH from ruptured aneurysm by improving their neurologic outcome, particularly in Hunt and Hess grades 1 to 3 patients.

The actual mechanism of the possible beneficial effect of nimodipine is, however, unknown. The original rationale for using nimodipine after SAH was to reduce cerebral arterial spasm, but available evidence indicates that nimodipine does not reduce the incidence or severity of cerebral spasm as seen on angiography.

Pharmacokinetics: Absorption: The orally administered active substance nimodipine is almost completely absorbed. The unchanged active substance and its early "first pass" metabolites are detected in plasma as little as 10 to 15 minutes after the ingestion of the tablet. Following multiple-dose oral administration (3×30 mg/day), the mean peak plasma concentrations (C_{max}) are 7.3 to 43.2 ng/mL in elderly individuals, these being reached after 0.6 to 1.6 h (T_{max}). Single dosing of 30 mg and 60 mg in young subjects results in mean peak plasma concentrations of 16±8 ng/mL and 31±12 ng/mL, respectively. The peak plasma concentration and the area under the curve increase proportionally to the dose, up to the highest dose under test (90 mg).

A study was conducted to investigate the bioequivalency of NIMOTOP Tablets (nimodipine tablets) and NIMOTOP (Nimodipine Capsules). From the results, it was concluded that the AUCs for the tablet versus the capsules were comparable, 91.1 nanogram hours per millilitre (ng.h/mL) and 103.5 ng.h/mL, respectively, resulting in a ratio of mean AUCs of tablet to capsule of 0.88 (90% two-sided confidence interval (CI): 80% to 97%). The C_{max} for the tablet was lower than that of the capsule (45.6 ng/mL and 69.1 ng/mL, respectively), with a mean ratio of 0.66 (90% two-sided CI: 55% to 79%). The T_{max} for the tablet (0.77 h) was longer than that of the capsule (0.59 h). The ratio of the mean T_{max} for the tablet compared to the capsule was 1.31 with a 90% two-sided CI of 111% to 154%.

The effects of a standard breakfast on the bioavailability of nimodipine tablets were investigated in two separate studies. From the results, it was concluded that although the rate of absorption is delayed as evidenced by the decrease in C_{max} (approximately 40%) and the increase of T_{max} (approximately 100%), the presence of food does not alter the extent of absorption of nimodipine tablets.

Distribution: Studies in animals indicate that nimodipine is widely distributed into body tissues after oral administration. Nimodipine is 97%-99 % bound to plasma proteins.

Nimodipine appears to distribute to a limited extent into cerebrospinal fluid (CSF). After oral administration of nimodipine 0.35 mg/kg every 4 hours for 3 weeks, mean CSF and plasma nimodipine concentrations were 0.77 and 6.9 ng/mL, respectively. However, concentrations as high as 12.5 ng/mL reportedly have been detected in the CSF of nimodipine-treated SAH patients.

Nimodipine and/or its metabolites have been shown to appear in rat milk at concentration much higher than in maternal plasma. Nimodipine itself has been shown to appear in human breast milk: the concentrations were lower than in maternal plasma.

Metabolism: Nimodipine undergoes extensive first pass metabolism in the liver via the cytochrome P450 3A4 system. The mean bioavailability of nimodipine tablets ranges from ±3% to 12% in healthy individuals to 16% (range 3-30%) in patients with SAH.

Bioavailability is significantly increased in patients with hepatic disease (eg, cirrhosis) with C_{max} approximately double that in normal patients, which necessitates lowering the dose in this patient population (see Dosage and Administration, Special Populations, Hepatic Impairment).

Excretion: Nimodipine and its metabolites have a dual route of elimination. Approximately 50% of the metabolites undergo renal excretion while 30% are excreted in the feces due to biliary excretion. The metabolites of nimodipine are believed to be either inactive or considerably less active than the parent compound. The elimination kinetics are linear. The half-life for nimodipine is between 1.1 and 1.7 hours and the terminal half-life is approximately 5 to 10 hours and dose-independent.

Nimodipine is eliminated almost exclusively in the form of metabolites and less than 1% is recovered in the urine as unchanged drug. There were no signs of accumulation in patients receiving 40 mg nimodipine three times daily for seven days.

Special Populations and Conditions: Pediatrics (<18 years of age): The safety and effectiveness of nimodipine in children have not been established.

Geriatrics (>65 years of age): In a single, parallel-group study involving 24 elderly subjects (aged 59-79) and 24 younger subjects (aged 22-40), the observed AUC and C_{max} of nimodipine were approximately 2-fold higher in the elderly population compared to the younger study subjects following oral administration (given as a single dose of 30 mg and dosed to steady state with 30 mg tid for 6 days). The clinical response to these age-related pharmacokinetic differences, however, was not considered significant.

Clinical studies of nimodipine did not include sufficient numbers of subjects aged 65 and over to determine whether they respond differently from younger subjects. In general, dosing for elderly patients should be cautious, reflecting the greater frequency of decreased hepatic, renal, or cardiac function, and of concomitant disease or other drug therapy.

Hepatic Insufficiency: Patients with hepatic insufficiency may have substantially reduced clearance and approximately doubled maximum plasma concentration: accordingly, the dosage should be reduced to one 30 mg NIMOTOP tablet every 4 hours in these patients.

Renal Insufficiency: There are insufficient data on patients with impaired renal function.

STORAGE AND STABILITY: NIMOTOP tablets should be stored in original packaging between 15 and 30°C. Protect from humidity.

Keep out of reach of children.

INFORMATION FOR THE PATIENT: Published in e-CPS, available by subscription at www.e-cps.ca.

DOSAGE FORMS, COMPOSITION AND PACKAGING: Each yellow, film-coated, round tablet, embossed with "BAYER" cross on one side and "SK" on the other side, contains: nimodipine 30 mg. Nonmedicinal ingredients: crospovidone, ferric oxide yellow, hypromellose, macrogol, magnesium stearate, maize starch, microcrystalline cellulose, povidone and titanium dioxide. Blister packs of 100.

(Shown in Product Identification Section)

The reader is invited to consult CPhA's monograph **Niacin/Niacinamide**.

Ni-odan™ Extended Release Formula

niacin

Vitamin

Odan

SUPPLIED: Each white, caplet-shaped, unscored, time-release (extended-release) tablet, engraved N-500 on one side, contains: niacin (nicotinic acid) 500 mg. Nonmedicinal ingredients: methylcellulose, povidone and stearic acid (plant source). Formulated to release the niacin gradually over a period of eight hours. This product is free from artificial colours, flavours and preservatives, corn, starch, gluten, lactose, sugar, yeast, soy and animal by-products. Bottles of 100. Store at room temperature (15 to 30°C) in a dark dry place. Keep out of reach of children.

Nipride® Ⓟ

sodium nitroprusside

Antihypertensive

Hospira

SUPPLIED: Each vial of sterile powder contains: the equivalent of sodium nitroprusside 50 mg. Nonmedicinal ingredients: none. Single use amber vials of 50 mg, packs of 5. Store the powder at 15 to 30°C. Protect the reconstituted powder and i.v. infusion fluid from light. Discard unused portion.

Nitoman® Ⓟ

tetrabenazine

Monoamine Depleting Agent

Biovail Pharmaceuticals

Date of Revision: July 16, 2009

PHARMACOLOGY: The central effects of Nitoman (tetrabenazine) closely resemble those of reserpine, but it differs from the latter in having less peripheral activity and in being much shorter acting. In laboratory animals, tetrabenazine interferes with vesicular storage of biogenic amines, including dopamine as well as serotonin and norepinephrine; this effect is mainly limited to the brain. Hydroxytetrabenazine is believed to be the principle active moiety, and it is thought that its clinical activity in movement disorders results from its action on monoamine storage in the brain. The duration of action of tetrabenazine ranges from 16 to 24 hours.

Tetrabenazine also has dopamine antagonistic effects, such as displacing ^{3}H-spiperone from striatal binding sites in vitro, and blocking dopaminergic inhibition of prolactin release in vitro and in vivo.

Pharmacokinetics: Tetrabenazine has a low and erratic bioavailability. It is extensively metabolised by first-pass metabolism. Little to no unchanged tetrabenazine can be detected in the urine. The major metabolite, hydroxytetrabenazine, is formed by reduction. Following i.v. administration of radiolabelled tetrabenazine to humans, the radioactivity decreased to minimal levels within 10 hours and could not be detected 3 days later. Forty percent (40%) of total activity was found in the urine within 24 hours and 2.5% in the feces. Fifty four percent (54%) of the total activity was excreted after 48 hours.

INDICATIONS: Nitoman (tetrabenazine) has been found useful in the treatment of hyperkinetic movement disorders such as Huntington's chorea, Hemiballismus, Senile Chorea, Tic and Gille's de la Tourette Syndrome and Tardive Dyskinesia.

Tetrabenazine is not indicated for the treatment of levodopa-induced dyskinetic/choreiform movements (see Warnings).

Tetrabenazine should only be used by (or in consultation with) physicians who are experienced in the treatment of hyperkinetic movement disorders.

CONTRAINDICATIONS: Nitoman (tetrabenazine) is contraindicated in patients with a known hypersensitivity to the drug or to any of the components of the formulation.

Nitoman is contraindicated in patients with a current episode or a history of clinical depression (see Warnings).

Nitoman should not be administered together with a monoamine oxidase inhibitor (MAOI). At least 14 days should elapse between the discontinuation of an MAOI and initiation of treatment with Nitoman, as well as between the discontinuation of Nitoman and the initiation of treatment with an MAOI (see Precautions, Drug Interactions).

WARNINGS: Depression: Nitoman may cause depression. Recognition of depression may be difficult because this condition may often be disguised by somatic complaints. The drug should be stopped immediately at the first signs or symptoms of depression. The depression can be profound, and the possibility of suicide should be kept in mind until the depression clears. There is no information on the safety or efficacy of antidepressant drug treatment in Nitoman-induced depression.

Parkinsonism: Nitoman can induce symptoms of Parkinsonism, which are seen more frequently in the elderly and at relatively low doses. Nitoman dosage should be adjusted as tolerated and needed. Levodopa-induced dyskinetic/choreiform movements should be treated by reducing the dose of levodopa, and not by giving Nitoman, since the latter exacerbates Parkinsonian symptoms.

PRECAUTIONS: General: Occupational Hazards: Tetrabenazine may cause drowsiness and orthostatic hypotension. Therefore caution is recommended when driving, operating machinery, or performing other skilled tasks until the effect of Nitoman is known.

Pregnancy: Animal reproductive studies have not been performed with Nitoman. There is no information on the safety of the drug in human pregnancy. However, tetrabenazine has been used for many years and no cases of malformation have been reported.

Lactation: Limited information indicates that Nitoman is excreted in milk, therefore it should be avoided in breast-feeding mothers.

Drug Interactions: CYP2D6 Inhibitors: In vitro and in vivo studies indicate that the tetrabenazine metabolites α-DTBZ and β-DTBZ are substrates for CYP2D6. Caution should be used when adding a CYP2D6 inhibitor (such as fluoxetine, paroxetine, quinidine, duloxetine, terbinafine, amiodarone, or sertraline) to a patient already receiving a stable dose of tetrabenazine and a reduction in the dose of tetrabenazine should be considered.

Levodopa: Tetrabenazine exacerbates Parkinsonian symptoms, and thereby attenuates the effect of levodopa (see Warnings).

Antidepressants and Monoamine Oxidase Inhibitors (MAOIs): Central excitation and possibly hypertension have occurred when tetrabenazine was added to existing therapy with desipramine or MAOIs.

There is no information on the safety and efficacy of antidepressant drugs, including MAOIs, in the treatment of tetrabenazine-induced depression (see Contraindications).

Neuroleptic Agents: There is a potential for severe manifestations of dopamine deficiency, when administering Nitoman concomitantly with neuroleptic agents (e.g., haloperidol, chlorpromazine, metoclopramide, etc.). Neuroleptic malignant syndrome has been observed in isolated cases.

ADVERSE EFFECTS: The most commonly observed adverse reactions with Nitoman (tetrabenazine) include, in decreasing order of frequency and observed during clinical use of the drug: signs and symptoms of Parkinsonism; drowsiness, fatigue, weakness; depression; anxiety, nervousness; insomnia; restlessness, akathisia; drooling; irritability, agitation; nausea, vomiting, epigastric pain; confusion, disorientation; hypotension; dizziness.

Although Nitoman has been in clinical use for a number of years, controlled clinical trials with the drug are limited.

OVERDOSE:

Symptoms: Signs and symptoms of overdosage may include drowsiness, sweating, hypotension and hypothermia.

Treatment: Treatment is symptomatic.

For management of a suspected drug overdose, CPhA recommends that you contact your **regional Poison Control Centre**. See the *CPS* Directory section for a list of Poison Control Centres.

DOSAGE: General: The initial dose should be low, and dosage should be titrated slowly according to the tolerance and responsiveness of the individual patient.

Adults: An initial starting dose of 12.5 mg 2 to 3 times a day is recommended. This can be increased by 12.5 mg a day every 3 to 5 days until the maximal tolerated and effective dose is reached for the individual, and may have to be up/down titrated depending on individual tolerance. In most cases the maximal tolerated dose will be 25 mg t.i.d. In very rare cases, a 200 mg dose has been reached (the maximum recommended dose in some publications).

If there is no improvement at the maximal tolerated dose in 7 days, it is unlikely that Nitoman will be of benefit to the patient, either by increasing the dose or by extending the duration of treatment.

Geriatrics and Debilitated Patients: No adequately controlled clinical studies have been performed in the elderly and/or debilitated patients. Clinical experience suggests that a reduced initial and maintenance dose should be used. Parkinsonian-like adverse reactions are relatively common in these patients and may be dose-limiting.

Children: No adequately controlled clinical studies have been performed in children. Limited clinical experience suggests that treatment should be started at approximately half the adult dose, and titrated slowly and carefully according to tolerance and individual response.

SUPPLIED: Each round, yellowish-buff tablet, with CL25 imprinted across one face and a single break bar on the other, contains: tetrabenazine 25 mg. Nonmedicinal ingredients: iron oxide, lactose, magnesium stearate, starch maize white and talc. Bottles of 112. Store in well-closed containers. Store at 15 to 30°C.

(Shown in Product Identification Section)

Nitrates

isosorbide dinitrate

isosorbide-5-mononitrate

nitroglycerin

Antianginal—Antihypertensive

CPhA Monograph

Date of Revision: February 2010

This monograph has been compiled by CPhA and reviewed by experts. It may contain information different from that found in Health Canada-approved Product Monographs. The reader is referred to the *CPS* Editorial Policy for more information.

SUMMARY PRODUCT INFORMATION:

Drug	Route of Administration	Dosage Form	Strength
Isosorbide dinitrate	Oral or Sublingual[a]	Tablet	5 mg, 10 mg, 30 mg
Isosorbide-5-mononitrate	Oral	Extended release tablet	60 mg
Nitroglycerin	Transdermal	Patch	0.2 mg/h, 0.4 mg/h, 0.6 mg/h, 0.8 mg/h
		Ointment	2% ointment
	Oral, sublingual	Pumpspray	0.4 mg/metered dose
		Sublingual tablet	0.3 mg, 0.6 mg
	Intravenous	Ampoules, vials	1 mg/mL, 5 mg/mL
		Solution	100 µg/mL, 200 µg/mL, 400 µg/mL

[a] Some brands formulated for sublingual use

PHARMACOLOGY: The organic nitrates are esters of nitrous or nitric acid that are rendered nonexplosive by the addition of inert excipients such as lactose. The organic nitrates are prodrugs and must be denitrated to exert their therapeutic effects. Denitration liberates nitric oxide which is also known as endothelium-derived relaxing factor. Nitric oxide stimulates guanylyl cyclase leading to the conversion of guanosine triphosphate to cyclic guanosine monophosphate, which causes vasodilation.

In addition to the relaxation of vascular smooth muscle, these drugs relax bronchial, biliary, gastrointestinal, ureteral and uterine smooth muscle as well.

The hemodynamic and antianginal actions of the organic nitrates result from vasodilation of capacitance veins and conductive arteries. Dilation of capacitance veins reduces ventricular volume and preload. To a lesser extent, afterload is reduced through a combination of the reduction in left ventricular volume and dilation of systemic conductive arteries. Nitrates also dilate epicardial coronary arteries and collateral vessels, improving blood flow to ischemic areas. The net result of these actions is a favourable effect on the imbalance between myocardial oxygen supply and demand in patients with coronary artery disease.

Tolerance to the antianginal and hemodynamic effects of nitrates develops during therapy and is more likely to occur at higher doses and with formulations that have longer half-lives. It is common in patients being treated with topical, transdermal or continuous iv infusions and is not as likely to develop with the use of short-acting preparations.

Efficacy of organic nitrates is restored after a drug-free interval of 10 to 12 hours. The intermittent use of nitrates may be associated with decreased exercise tolerance during the last part of the nitrate-free interval; the clinical relevance of this observation is unknown. There may also be an increased frequency of angina during the drug-free period in some patients. Therefore, the possibility of increased frequency or severity of angina during the nitrate-free interval should be considered.

Pharmacokinetics: The organic nitrates are well absorbed from the gastrointestinal tract. Nitroglycerin is well absorbed through intact skin as well.

Nitrates undergo first pass denitration in the liver. Nitroglycerin is metabolized to 1,3- and 1,2-glyceryl dinitrate which are active metabolites with lower potency than nitroglycerin itself. Inactive metabolites are also produced. Further metabolism of these compounds yields glycerol and carbon dioxide. Isosorbide dinitrate is metabolized to isosorbide 2- and 5-mononitrate, the latter being available commercially as isosorbide mononitrate. Both are further metabolized and excreted in the urine.

Table 1 provides information on the pharmacokinetics of various dosage forms of nitrates.

Table 1: Nitrates

Pharmacokinetics

Dosage Form	Onset of Action	Duration of Action
Isosorbide Dinitrate		
Sublingual tablets	2 to 5 min	1 to 3 h
Oral tablets	20 to 40 min	4 to 6 h
Isosorbide Mononitrate		
Oral sustained-release tablets	up to 4 h	10 to 12 h
Nitroglycerin		
IV infusion	1 to 2 min	3 to 5 min[a]
Sublingual tablets	1 to 3 min	10 to 30 min
Translingual spray	2 to 4 min	10 to 30 min
Transdermal patch	2 h[b]	24 h[b]
Topical ointment	30 to 60 min	4 to 8 h

[a] After infusion discontinued.

[b] Steady-state serum concentrations are reached in approximately 2 hours and are maintained through constant drug delivery for as long as the patch is worn, up to 24 hours or slightly longer. Once the patch is removed, the serum concentration decreases to undetectable levels within 2 hours.

INDICATIONS: Health Canada-approved indications include:

- acute symptomatic relief of angina pectoris and prophylactic management in situations likely to provoke angina attacks
- long-term prophylactic management of stable angina
- perioperative hypertension

Uses Without Health Canada Approval: Nitrates are used to treat chest pain during acute coronary syndromes [*Circulation* 2004;110:e82-e293; *Circulation* 2000;102:1193-1209] and in the management of acute and chronic heart failure [*Can J Cardiol* 2006;22(1):23-45]. Nitroglycerin has been used as an intravenous antihypertensive in infants and children.

CONTRAINDICATIONS: Nitrates should not be administered to individuals with: a known hypersensitivity or idiosyncratic reaction to organic nitrates; severe anemia (because of potential methemoglobin formation and resulting impaired oxygen delivery); hypotension or uncorrected hypovolemia, as the use of nitrates in such states could produce severe hypotension or shock; head trauma or cerebral hemorrhage (to avoid increased intracranial pressure); constrictive pericarditis and pericardial tamponade. Long-acting dosage forms should be avoided in the treatment of acute coronary syndromes.

WARNINGS AND PRECAUTIONS: The use of nitroglycerin in acute MI or heart failure requires careful clinical and/or hemodynamic monitoring and appropriate patient selection, to avoid excessive hypotension.

Nitrate dependence may occur in patients with chronic use. In industry workers continuously exposed to nitrates, chest pain, acute MI and even sudden death have occurred during temporary withdrawal of nitrate exposure. To avoid possible withdrawal effects, nitrates should be tapered gradually.

Nitroglycerin ointment, transdermal patches or oral nitrate tablets are not intended for immediate relief of acute attacks of angina pectoris. Sublingual tablets or translingual spray should be used for this purpose.

Caution should be exercised in using nitrates in patients who are volume depleted or have low blood pressure. Severe hypotension, especially postural, may occur.

Nitrates should be used with caution in patients with severe liver or renal disease. Avoid extended-release oral preparations in patients with gastrointestinal hypermotility or malabsorption syndrome.

Headaches or symptoms of hypotension, such as weakness or dizziness, particularly when arising suddenly from a recumbent position, may be due to overdosage. If this occurs the dose should be reduced or the frequency of topical application should be reduced.

Cardioversion: Transdermal nitroglycerin patches should be removed prior to cardioversion to avoid formation of electrical arc.

Hypotension: Nitrates can cause sudden severe hypotension. Excessive hypotension, especially for prolonged periods of time, must be avoided because of possible deleterious effects on the brain, heart, liver and kidneys from poor perfusion and attendant risk of ischemia, thrombosis and altered function of these organs. Paradoxical bradycardia and increased angina pectoris may accompany nitroglycerin-induced hypotension. Patients with normal or low pulmonary capillary wedge pressure are especially sensitive to the hypotensive effects of nitroglycerin. A fall in pulmonary capillary wedge pressure precedes the onset of arterial hypotension and is thus a useful guide to safe titration of the drug.

Tolerance: The smallest dose required for effective relief of the acute anginal attack should be prescribed. Excessive use may lead to the development of tolerance. Tolerance to nitrates (especially with transdermal, sustained-release and iv preparations) and cross tolerance among nitrates may occur. A minimum interval of 10 to 12 hours per day without the transdermal patch in place is required for continued effectiveness when using this dosage form. With the chronic use of nitrates, there have been reports of anginal attacks being more easily provoked, as well as reports of rebound in hemodynamic effects, occurring soon after nitrate withdrawal.

Drug Interactions: Alcohol: Alcohol and nitrates may have additive vasodilatory effects possibly resulting in hypotension. Use caution with this combination.

Ergot Alkaloids: The effect of nitrates is antagonized by ergot alkaloids, which may precipitate angina.

Heparin: Heparin resistance has been encountered with concurrent use of iv nitroglycerin. APTT should be monitored when nitroglycerin is added or discontinued in patients receiving heparin. The dose of heparin may need to be adjusted.

Hypotensive Agents: Patients receiving antihypertensive agents and nitrates should be monitored for possible additive hypotensive effects.

Phosphodiesterase 5 Inhibitors: Systolic and diastolic blood pressure may be significantly reduced following coadministration of nitrates and sildenafil, tadalafil or vardenafil. Avoid this combination. Separate doses by at least 24 hours.

Pregnancy: Limited experience with the use of nitroglycerin as a tocolytic agent in preterm labor or version has not shown any risk to the fetus. Further study is required to establish the safety and efficacy of nitroglycerin during pregnancy, especially in the 1st trimester. There is little or no data regarding isosorbide mono- or dinitrate use during pregnancy.

Lactation: It is likely that the nitrates distribute into human breast milk, though no data are available. They are probably compatible with breast feeding.

Pediatrics: The safety and efficacy of nitroglycerin has not been studied as extensively in children as in adults. The recommended doses are estimates from medical literature and have been reasonably studied.

Geriatrics: The elderly may be more sensitive to the hypotensive effects of nitrates so lower initial doses should be used.

ADVERSE EFFECTS: The most frequent adverse reaction to nitrates is headache, which occurs in up to 50% of patients at the beginning of therapy as a result of dilation of cerebral vessels. Headache usually disappears within several days with continued treatment. Acetaminophen may be used to treat nitrate headaches.

Other adverse reactions occurring in less than 1% of patients are:

Allergic: itching, wheezing, tracheobronchitis; contact dermatitis with topical dosage forms.

Cardiovascular: hypotension, reflex tachycardia, paradoxical increase of anginal pain, palpitations and bradycardia. Syncope due to nitrate vasodilation, although rare, has been reported.

Central Nervous System: headache, weakness, dizziness, apprehension and restlessness.

Dermatologic: exfoliative dermatitis, cutaneous vasodilation, crusty skin lesions, pruritus, rash.

Gastrointestinal: nausea, vomiting, diarrhea and abdominal pain.

Genitourinary: dysuria, urinary frequency, impotence.

Metabolic: methemoglobinemia, especially in the presence of methemoglobin reductase deficiencies or in congenital hemoglobin variants.

Musculoskeletal: arthralgia, muscle twitching.

Ophthalmologic: blurred vision.

OVERDOSE:

For management of a suspected drug overdose, CPhA recommends that you contact your **regional Poison Control Centre**. See the *CPS* Directory section for a list of Poison Control Centres.

DOSAGE: Prevention of Tolerance: Tolerance can be prevented or attenuated by the use of an intermittent dosage schedule. An appropriate dosing schedule for nitrates should provide for a nitrate-free period of 10 to 12 hours daily. The drug-free time should coincide with the period in which angina pectoris is least likely to occur (usually at night). Monitor patients carefully for an increase of angina pectoris during the nitrate-free period. Adjustment of other cardiovascular medication may be required.

Nitroglycerin: Ointment: May be applied every 6 to 8 hours if necessary, and wiped off at bedtime to provide a nitrate-free interval. Some patients may require as much as 10 to 12.5 cm and/or application every 4 hours.

Any nonhairy skin area may be used; some patients psychologically prefer the chest. The dose is measured onto the skin using a specially designed paper applicator/ruler which is then used to spread out the dose over an area of at least 5×7.5 cm. The applicator can then be taped in place covering the ointment, to protect clothing. The ratio of dose to area of application should be kept constant.

The dose and frequency of application should be adjusted to meet the individual patient's needs.

Transdermal: Patient instructions provided with the product should be consulted for each individual product. Generally a patch is applied to a hairless, clean area of skin that is not subject to excessive movement (e.g., trunk). Patches should not be applied to areas with cuts, burns or abrasions or used on distal parts of extremities (e.g., forearms). For successive applications, a different site should be used.

Spray: For an acute attack of angina pectoris or for prophylaxis 5 to 10 minutes before planned exercise: 1 or 2 metered doses (0.4 or 0.8 mg nitroglycerin) administered onto or under the tongue, **without inhaling**. The mouth must be closed immediately after each dose. If there is no relief of chest pain after one dose, instruct the patient to call 911 or contact a physician. The patient can take another dose every 5 minutes if needed (up to three doses total) until the ambulance arrives.

Sublingual Tablets: One tablet should be dissolved under the tongue or in the buccal pouch immediately upon indication of an acute anginal attack. If there is no relief of chest pain after one dose, instruct the patient to call 911 or contact a physician. For prophylactic use, 1 sublingual tablet can be taken 5 to 10 minutes before engaging in activities that might precipitate an anginal event.

Storage: Store at room temperature, below 30°C. To prevent loss of potency, the tablets should be dispensed and kept in tight amber glass containers. The container should be closed tightly immediately after each use. No more than 100 tablets should be packaged in a container.

Repeated opening of the container may shorten the period of potency of sublingual tablets. Replacement of tablet stock is recommended 6 months after opening the bottle. Specific manufacturers may have different recommendations. The stabilized sublingual tablets are designed to maintain potency for longer periods (until the printed expiry dates), but must be properly stored. Whether the tablet stings or tingles when placed under the tongue is not an indication of potency and should not be used to assess whether the tablets will work or not.

IV: Not for direct iv injection. Nitroglycerin must be diluted in dextrose 5% injection USP or sodium chloride 0.9% injection USP, prior to infusion. Nitroglycerin should not be mixed with other drugs.

Caution: Several preparations of nitroglycerin for injection are available which differ in concentration and/or vial volume. When switching from one product to another, attention must be paid to the dilution, dosage and administration instructions.

Table 2: Nitrates

Dose in Adult Patients

Indication	Drug	Route	Initial Dose	Usual Dose	Clinical Comment
Acute angina	Isosorbide dinitrate	Sublingual	5 or 10 mg	3 doses at 5- to 10-minute intervals	If relief is not obtained within 5 min of 1 dose, a physician should be contacted
	Nitroglycerin	Sublingual tablet	0.3 or 0.6 mg		
		Sublingual spray	0.4 or 0.8 mg		
Stable angina	Isosorbide dinitrate	Oral	10 mg 3 times daily	10 to 30 mg 3 times daily	Last dose at 7 pm to provide nitrate free interval
	Isosorbide mononitrate		30 mg once daily	60 to 240 mg once daily	Give dose in the morning
	Nitroglycerin	Transdermal	0.2 mg/h patch once daily	0.2 to 0.8 mg/h patch once daily	Apply the patch once daily (usually in the morning), leave on for 12 to 14 hours, then remove.
			1.25 cm ointment	2.5 to 5 cm 2 or 3 times daily	Titrate to side-effects (usually headache)

(cont'd)

Table 2: Nitrates *(cont'd)*

Dose in Adult Patients

Indication	Drug	Route	Initial Dose	Usual Dose	Clinical Comment
Heart failure (Not an approved use in Canada)	Isosorbide dinitrate	Oral	10 mg 3 times daily	20 to 40 mg 3 times daily	Maintenance therapy in combination with hydralazine if first-line agents not tolerated
	Nitroglycerin	Intravenous	5 to 10 µg/min	5 to 200 µg/min	For symptom control in acute heart failure
Acute coronary syndromes (Not an approved use in Canada)	Isosorbide dinitrate	Oral	10 mg 3 times daily	10 to 30 mg 3 times daily	May be needed if chest pain returns once intravenous nitroglycerin stopped
	Isosorbide mononitrate	Oral		30 to 60 mg once daily	
	Nitroglycerin	Intravenous	5 to 10 µg/min	5 to 200 µg/min	Used in select patients for the first 24 to 48 h following an acute coronary event
		Transdermal	0.2 mg/h patch once daily	0.2 to 0.8 mg/h patch per day	Alternative to oral route
Perioperative hypertension	Nitroglycerin	Intravenous	5 to 10 µg/min	5 to 200 µg/min	See Dosage section for parameters

Table 3: Nitrates

Dose in Pediatric Patients

Indication	Drug	Route	Age/Weight	Usual Dose
Hypertension (Not an approved use in Canada)	Nitroglycerin	Intravenous	1 month to 16 yrs	0.5 to 10 µg/kg/min

Because of alterations to the amount of nitroglycerin delivered to the patient caused by variations in administration sets and pumps, and the great variations in responsiveness of individual patients to nitroglycerin, there is no fixed optimum dose of nitroglycerin. Each patient must be titrated to the desired level of hemodynamic function.

Initial dosage should be 5 to 10 µg/min delivered through an infusion pump capable of exact and constant delivery of the drug. Subsequent titration must be adjusted to the clinical situation, with dose increments becoming more cautious as partial hemodynamic response is seen. Initial titration should be in 5 µg/min increments with increases every 3 to 5 minutes until some response is noted. If no response is seen at 20 µg/min, increments of 10 to 20 µg/min can be used. Once a partial blood pressure response is observed, the dose increase should be reduced and the interval between increments should be lengthened. Some patients with normal or low left ventricular filling pressure or pulmonary capillary wedge pressure (e.g., angina patients without other complications) may respond fully to doses as small as 5 µg/min. These patients require especially careful titration and monitoring.

Nitrazadon®

nitrazepam

Hypnotic—Anticonvulsant

Valeant

SUPPLIED: 5 mg: Each white, round, scored tablet, imprinted "N21", contains: nitrazepam BP 5 mg. Nonmedicinal ingredients: croscarmellose sodium, lactose, magnesium stearate and microcrystalline cellulose. Bottles of 100 and 500.

10 mg: Each white, round, scored tablet, imprinted "N22", contains: nitrazepam BP 10 mg. Nonmedicinal ingredients: croscarmellose sodium, lactose, magnesium stearate and microcrystalline cellulose. Bottles of 100 and 500.

Nitrazepam

CPhA Monograph

see *Benzodiazepines*

Nitro-Dur®

nitroglycerin

Antianginal

Schering-Plough

PHARMACOLOGY: The principal pharmacological action of nitroglycerin is relaxation of vascular smooth muscle and consequent dilation of both peripheral arteries and veins, with more prominent effects on the latter. Dilation of the post-capillary vessels, including large veins, promotes peripheral pooling of blood and decreases venous return to the heart, thereby reducing left ventricular end-diastolic pressure (preload). Arteriolar relaxation reduces systemic vascular resistance and arterial pressure (afterload). Dilation of the coronary arteries also occurs. The relative importance of preload reduction, afterload reduction, and coronary dilation remains undefined.

When NITRO-DUR is applied to the skin, nitroglycerin is absorbed continuously through the skin into the systemic circulation. Thus, the active drug reaches target sites before inactivation by the liver. Nitroglycerin is rapidly metabolized, principally by a liver reductase, to form glycerol nitrate metabolites and inorganic nitrate. Two active major metabolites, the 1,2- and 1,3-dinitroglycerols, the products of hydrolysis, appear to be less potent than nitroglycerin as vasodilators but have longer plasma half-lives. The dinitrates are further metabolized to mononitrates (biologically inactive with respect to cardiovascular effects) and ultimately to glycerol and carbon dioxide. There is extensive first-pass deactivation by the liver following gastrointestinal absorption.

In healthy volunteers, steady-state plasma concentrations of nitroglycerin were reached within one-half hour after application of the patch and were maintained at the same level for the duration of the study (24 hours). Between 2 and 24 hours, the mean steady-state concentration was 0.224 ng/mL (20 cm^2 patch); the total amount of nitroglycerin delivered in 24 hours was 5.11±1.69 mg, 10.67±4.78 mg and 17.85±7.40 mg from 10 cm^2, 20 cm^2, and 40 cm^2 patches, respectively, indicating that the dose delivered is proportional to the surface area of the patch. Within 1 hour of removal of the patch, the plasma concentration declines to about 50% of steady-state concentration and to undetectable concentrations by 2 hours.

Dosing regimens for most chronically used drugs are designed to provide plasma concentrations that are continuously greater than a minimally effective concentration. This strategy is probably inappropriate for organic nitrates. Some well-controlled clinical trials using exercise tolerance testing have shown maintenance of effectiveness when patches are worn continuously. The large majority of such controlled trials, however, have shown the development of tolerance (i.e. complete loss of effect as measured by exercise testing) within the first day. Tolerance has occurred even when doses greater than 4 mg/hour were delivered continuously. This dose is far in excess of the effective dose of 0.2 to 0.8 mg/hour delivered intermittently.

Efficacy of organic nitrates is restored after a period of absence of nitrates from the body. Drug-free intervals of 10 to 12 hours are known to be sufficient to restore response. Several studies have demonstrated that when nitroglycerin is administered according to an intermittent regimen, doses of nitroglycerin 0.4 to 0.8 mg/hour (20 to 40 cm^2) have increased exercise capacity for up to 8 hours, with a trend of increased exercise capacity for up to 12 hours. One controlled clinical trial suggested that the intermittent use of nitrates may be associated with a decreased, in comparison to placebo, exercise tolerance during the last part of the nitrate-free interval; the clinical relevance of this observation is unknown. In another clinical trial there was an increase in nocturnal angina attacks during the drug-free period in some patients treated with nitroglycerin as compared to placebo. Therefore the possibility of increased frequency or severity of angina during the nitrate-free interval should be considered.

INDICATIONS: NITRO-DUR (nitroglycerin) used intermittently (see Pharmacology), is indicated for the prevention of anginal attacks in patients with stable angina pectoris associated with coronary artery disease. It can be used in conjunction with other antianginal agents such as beta-blockers and/or calcium antagonists.

NITRO-DUR is not intended for the immediate relief of acute attacks of angina pectoris. Sublingual nitroglycerin preparations should be used for this purpose.

CONTRAINDICATIONS: Known hypersensitivity or idiosyncrasy to nitroglycerin or other nitrates or nitrites. Allergy to the adhesive used in nitroglycerin patches has been reported and constitutes a contraindication to the use of this product. Acute circulatory failure associated with marked hypotension (shock and states of collapse). Postural hypotension. Myocardial insufficiency due to obstruction (e.g. in the presence of aortic or mitral stenosis or of constrictive pericarditis). Increased intracranial pressure. Increased intraocular pressure. Severe anemia.

Concomitant use of NITRO-DUR (nitroglycerin) either regularly and/or intermittently, with a phosphodiesterase inhibitor (e.g. sildenafil citrate, tadalafil) is absolutely contraindicated.

WARNINGS: The benefits and safety of transdermal nitroglycerin in patients with acute myocardial infarction or congestive heart failure have not been established. If one elects to use NITRO-DUR in these conditions, careful clinical or hemodynamic monitoring must be used to avoid the hazards of hypotension and tachycardia.

NITRO-DUR must be removed before cardioversion or DC defibrillation is attempted, as well as before applying diathermy treatment, since it may be associated with damage to the paddles and burns to the patient.

PRECAUTIONS: Headaches or symptoms of hypotension, such as weakness or dizziness, particularly when arising suddenly from a recumbent position, may occur. A reduction in dose or discontinuation of treatment may be necessary.

Caution should be exercised when using nitroglycerin in patients prone to, or who might be affected by hypotension. The drug therefore should be used with caution in patients who may have volume depletion from diuretic therapy or in patients who have low systolic blood pressure (e.g. below 90 mmHg). Paradoxical bradycardia and increased angina pectoris may accompany nitroglycerin-induced hypotension.

Nitrate therapy may aggravate the angina caused by hyperthrophic cardiomyopathy.

In industrial workers who have had long-term exposure to unknown (presumably high) doses of nitroglycerin, tolerance clearly occurs. There is moreover, physical dependence since chest pain, acute myocardial infarction, and even sudden death have occurred during temporary withdrawal of nitroglycerin from these workers. In clinical trials of angina patients, there are reports of anginal attacks being more easily provoked and of rebound in the hemodynamic effects soon after nitrate withdrawal.

The importance of these observations to the routine clinical use of nitroglycerin has not been fully elucidated, but patients should be monitored closely for increased anginal symptoms during drug-free periods.

Caution should be exercised in patients with arterial hypoxemia due to anemia (see Contraindications), because in such patients the biotransformation of nitroglycerin is reduced. Similarly, caution is called for in patients with hypoxemia and a ventilation/perfusion imbalance due to lung disease or ischemic heart failure. Patients with angina pectoris, myocardial infarction, or cerebral ischemia frequently suffer from abnormalities of the small airways (especially alveolar hypoxia). Under these circumstances vasoconstriction occurs within the lung to shift perfusion from areas of alveolar hypoxia to better ventilated regions of the lung. As a potent vasodilator, nitroglycerin could reverse this protective vasoconstriction and thus result in increased perfusion to poorly ventilated areas, worsening of the ventilation/perfusion imbalance, and a further decrease in the arterial partial pressure of oxygen.

Tolerance to nitroglycerin with cross tolerance to other nitrates or nitrites may occur (see Pharmacology). As tolerance to nitroglycerin patches develops, the effect of sublingual nitroglycerin on exercise tolerance, although still observable, is somewhat blunted.

Occupational Hazards: As patients may experience faintness and/or dizziness, reaction time when driving or operating machinery may be impaired, especially at the start of treatment.

Pregnancy: It is not known whether NITRO-DUR can cause fetal harm when administered to pregnant women or can affect reproductive capacity. Therefore, use NITRO-DUR only if the potential benefit justifies the risk to the fetus.

Lactation: It is not known whether nitroglycerin is excreted in human milk. Benefits to the mother must be weighed against the risk to the infant.

Children: Safety and effectiveness in children have not been established.

Drug Interactions: Concomitant treatment with other vasodilators, calcium antagonists, ACE inhibitors, beta-blockers, diuretics, antihypertensives, tricyclic antidepressants and major tranquilizers may potentiate the blood pressure lowering effect of nitroglycerin. Dose adjustment may be necessary.

Nitroglycerin acts directly on vascular muscles. Therefore, any other agent that directly or indirectly acts on vascular smooth muscle may have decreased or increased effect depending upon the agent.

Alcohol may enhance sensitivity to the hypotensive effects of nitrates.

Concomitant use of NITRO-DUR (nitroglycerin) with a phosphodiester inhibitor (e.g. sildenafil citrate, tadalafil) can potentiate the hypotensive effect of NITRO-DUR. This could result in life-threatening hypotension with syncope or myocardial infarction and death. Therefore, phosphodiesterase inhibitor drugs should not be given to patients receiving NITRO-DUR therapy.

Concurrent administration of NITRO-DUR with dihydroergotamine may increase the bioavailability of dihydroergotamine. Special attention should be paid to this point in patients with coronary artery disease, because dihydroergotamine antagonizes the effect of nitroglycerin and may lead to coronary vasconstriction.

The possibility that the ingestion of ASA and nonsteroidal anti-inflammatory drugs might diminish the therapeutic response to nitrates and nitroglycerin cannot be excluded.

ADVERSE EFFECTS: Headache, which may be severe, is the most commonly reported side effect. Headache may be recurrent with each daily dose, especially at higher doses of nitroglycerin. Headaches may be treated with concomitant administration of mild analgesics. If such headaches are unresponsive to treatment, the nitroglycerin dosage should be reduced or the product discontinued. Transient episodes of lightheadedness, occasionally related to blood pressure changes, may also occur. Hypotension occurs infrequently, but in some patients it may be severe enough to warrant discontinuation of therapy.

Reddening of the skin, with or without a mild local itching or burning sensation, as well as allergic contact dermatitis may occasionally occur. Upon removal of the patch, any slight reddening of the skin will usually disappear within a few hours. The application site should be changed regularly to prevent local irritation.

Less frequently reported adverse reactions include dizziness, faintness, facial flushing, postural hypotension which may be associated with reflex tachycardia. Syncope, crescendo angina and rebound hypertension have been reported but are uncommon. Nausea and vomiting have been reported rarely.

OVERDOSE:

Symptoms: Nitroglycerin overdose may result in severe hypotension, persistent throbbing headache, vertigo, palpitations, visual disturbances, flushing and perspiring skin (later becoming cold and cyanotic), nausea and vomiting (possibly with colic and even bloody diarrhea), syncope (especially in the upright posture), methemoglobinemia with cyanosis, initial hyperpnea, dyspnea, and slow breathing, slow pulse (dicrotic and intermittent), heart block, increased intracranial pressure with cerebral symptoms of confusion and moderate fever, paralysis, coma, clonic convulsions and death due to circulatory collapse.

The patch should be removed immediately and the underlying skin scrubbed thoroughly. No specific antagonist to the vasodilator effects of nitroglycerin is known, and no intervention has been subject to controlled study as a therapy of nitroglycerin overdose. Because the hypotension associated with nitroglycerin overdose is the result of venodilation and arterial hypovolemia, prudent therapy in this situation should be directed toward increase in central fluid volume. Specific elements of such therapy might include any or all of the following: elevation of the patient's legs, passive motion of the patient's extremities, and i.v. infusion of normal saline or similar fluid. In patients with renal disease or congestive heart failure, central volume expansion is not without hazard. Treatment of nitroglycerin overdose in these patients may be subtle and difficult, and invasive monitoring may be required.

Treatment: Keep the patient recumbent in a shock position and comfortably warm. Remove the NITRO-DUR patch. Passive movement of the extremities may aid venous return. Administer oxygen and artificial ventilation if necessary. Epinephrine is ineffective in reversing the severe hypotensive events associated with overdose; it and related compounds are contraindicated in this situation.

Methemoglobinemia: Case reports of clinically significant methemoglobinemia are rare at conventional doses of nitroglycerin. The formation of methemoglobin is dose-related, and in the case of genetic abnormalities of hemoglobin that favor methemoglobin formation, even conventional doses of organic nitrates can produce harmful concentrations of methemoglobin.

Methemoglobinemia should be treated with methylene blue if the patient develops cardiac or CNS effects of hypoxia. The initial dose is 1-2 mg/kg infused intravenously over 5 minutes. Repeat methemoglobin levels should be obtained 30 minutes later and a repeat dose of 0.5-1.0 mg/kg may be used if the level remains elevated and the patient is still symptomatic. Relative contraindications for methylene blue include known NADH methemoglobin reductase or G-6-PD deficiency. Infants under the age of 4 months may not respond to methylene blue due to immature NADH methemoglobin reductase. Exchange transfusion has been used successfully in critically ill patients when methemoglobinemia is refractory to treatment.

> For management of a suspected drug overdose, CPhA recommends that you contact your **regional Poison Control Centre**. See the *CPS* Directory section for a list of Poison Control Centres.

DOSAGE: Daily Dosage Schedule: The daily dosage schedule is based on intermittent therapy to prevent the development of tolerance to nitroglycerin. The optimal dose should be selected based upon the clinical response, side effects, and the effects of therapy on blood pressure.

Starting dose is 1 NITRO-DUR 0.2 patch (10 cm^2), usually applied in the morning. If 0.2 mg/hour (10 cm^2) is well tolerated, the dose can be increased to 0.4 mg/hour (20 cm^2) if required. A maximum of 0.8 mg/hour (40 cm^2) may be used.

Prevention of Tolerance: Although some controlled clinical trials using exercise tolerance testing have shown maintenance of effectiveness when patches are worn continuously, the large majority of such controlled trials have shown the development of tolerance (i.e. complete loss of effect) within the first 24 hours after therapy was initiated. Dose adjustments even to levels much higher than generally used did not prevent the development of tolerance.

Tolerance can be prevented or attenuated by use of an intermittent dosage schedule. Although the minimum nitrate-free interval has not been defined, clinical trials have demonstrated that an appropriate dosing schedule for nitroglycerin patches would provide for a daily patch-on period of 12 to 14 hours and a daily patch-off period of 10 to 12 hours. The patch-free time should coincide with the period in which angina pectoris is least likely to occur (usually at night). Patients should be watched carefully for an increase of angina pectoris during the patch-free period. Adjustment of background medication may be required.

The dose of NITRO-DUR should be periodically reviewed in relation to continuing antianginal control.

Site of Application: The NITRO-DUR nitroglycerin transdermal system may be applied to any convenient skin area; a recommended site of application is the arm or chest. Application sites should be rotated. A suitable area may be shaved if necessary. Do not apply NITRO-DUR to the distal part of the extremities. Hands should be washed thoroughly after application. Following use, the patch should be discarded in a manner that prevents accidental application or ingestion by curious children or others.

INFORMATION FOR THE PATIENT: Published in e-CPS, available by subscription at www.e-cps.ca.

SUPPLIED: The NITRO-DUR Nitroglycerin Transdermal System is a flat unit designed to provide continuous controlled release of nitroglycerin through intact skin. The rate of release of nitroglycerin is linearly dependent upon the area of the applied system; each cm^2 of applied system delivers approximately 0.02 mg of nitroglycerin per hour. Thus, the 10-, 20-, 30- and 40-cm^2 systems deliver approximately 0.2, 0.4, 0.6 and 0.8 mg of nitroglycerin per hour, respectively. The remainder of the nitroglycerin in each system serves as a reservoir and is not delivered in normal use.

The NITRO-DUR transdermal system contains nitroglycerin in acrylic-based polymer adhesives with a resinous cross-linking agent to provide a continuous source of active ingredient.

NITRO-DUR 0.2 (0.2 mg/hour): Each 10 cm^2 patch contains: nitroglycerin 40 mg.
NITRO-DUR 0.4 (0.4 mg/hour): Each 20 cm^2 patch contains: nitroglycerin 80 mg.
NITRO-DUR 0.6 (0.6 mg/hour): Each 30 cm^2 patch contains: nitroglycerin 120 mg.
NITRO-DUR 0.8 (0.8 mg/hour): Each 40 cm^2 patch contains: nitroglycerin 160 mg.

Each unit is sealed in a paper polyethylene-foil pouch. Retail unit dose boxes of 30. Hospital unit dose boxes of 100. Store between 15 to 30°C. Do not refrigerate.

(Shown in Product Identification Section)

Nitroglycerin

CPhA Monograph

see *Nitrates*

Nitroglycerin in 5% Dextrose Injection

nitroglycerin—dextrose

Vasodilator

Baxter

SUPPLIED: Each mL of clear, practically colorless, sterile, nonpyrogenic solution contains: nitroglycerin in 5% dextrose. Nonmedicinal ingredients: alcohol USP, citric acid hydrous USP, hydrochloric acid, propylene glycol, sodium hydroxide and water for injection USP. pH 4.0 (3.0 to 5.0). Osmolarity: 428, 440 and 465 mOsmol/L (calc), respectively. Glass, single dose bottles in the following sizes and concentrations: see Table 1.

Table 1: Nitroglycerin in 5% Dextrose Injection

Supplied

Total Volume (mL)	Total Nitroglycerin Content (mg)	Nitroglycerin Concentration (mg/mL)
250	25	0.1
250	50	0.2
250	100	0.4

Store between 15 and 25°C. Protect from light and freezing. Do not use unless vacuum is present and solution is clear.

Nitrol®

nitroglycerin

Antianginal—Vasodilator

Paladin

SUPPLIED: Each tube of ointment contains: 2% nitroglycerin. Nonmedicinal ingredients: lactose, lanolin, petrolatum and purified water (all USP standard). Tubes of 30 and 60 g. Keep tube tightly closed and store at room temperature (15 to 30°C).

Nitrolingual® Pumpspray

nitroglycerin

Antianginal

sanofi-aventis

Date of Revision: May 9, 2007

SUMMARY PRODUCT INFORMATION:

Route of Administration	Dosage Form/ Strength	Clinically Relevant Nonmedicinal Ingredients
Oral (Sublingual)	spray, 0.4 mg per metered dose	For a complete listing see Dosage Forms, Composition and Packaging.

INDICATIONS AND CLINICAL USE: NITROLINGUAL PUMPSPRAY (nitroglycerin) is indicated for:
- the management and treatment of acute attacks of angina pectoris.

CONTRAINDICATIONS: NITROLINGUAL PUMPSPRAY (nitroglycerin) is contraindicated in:
- Patients with known hypersensitivity to nitroglycerin or any of the excipients, or with previous idiosyncratic reaction to organic nitrates. For a complete listing, see Dosage Forms, Composition and Packaging.
- Patients with severe anemia;
- Patients with closed angle glaucoma;
- Patients with increased intracranial pressure;
- Patients with myocardial infarction;
- Patients with acute circulatory failure (cardiogenic shock, severe hypovolemia or severe hypotension)
- Patients with heart failure (aortic or mitral stenosis, constrictive pericarditis or hypertrophic obstructive cardiomyopathy).

Concomitant use of NITROLINGUAL PUMPSPRAY (nitroglycerin) either regularly and/or intermittently, with phosphodiesterase type 5 (PDE5) inhibitors such as VIAGRA (sildenafil), CIALIS (tadalafil) and LEVITRA (vardenafil) is absolutely contraindicated, because PDE5 inhibitors amplify the vasodilatory effects of NITROLINGUAL PUMPSPRAY (nitroglycerin) which can lead to severe hypotension.

WARNINGS AND PRECAUTIONS: Headaches or symptoms of hypotension, such as weakness or dizziness, particularly when arising suddenly from a recumbent position, may be due to overdosage. When they occur, the dose or frequency of application of NITROLINGUAL PUMPSPRAY (nitroglycerin) should be reduced.

In cases where cyanosis should develop during high-dose treatment, work-up must include search for methemoglobinemia.

Cardiovascular: Nitroglycerin is a potent vasodilator and causes a slight decrease in mean blood pressure (approximately 10-15 mmHg) in some patients when used in therapeutic dosages. Caution should be exercised in using the drug in patients who are prone to, or who might be affected by hypotension.

Dependence/Tolerance: Tolerance to this drug and cross-tolerance to other nitrates or nitrites may occur. Physical dependence has also been described. With the chronic use of nitrates, there have been reports of anginal attacks being more easily provoked as well as reports of rebound in hemodynamic effects, occurring soon after nitrate withdrawal.

Driving a Vehicle or Performing on Hazardous Tasks: Especially during treatment start, nitroglycerin may induce symptoms related to orthostatic hypotension such as dizziness, which can possibly impact the ability to drive or use machines (See Adverse Reactions).

Special Populations: Pregnant Women: Animal reproduction studies have not been conducted with nitroglycerin. It is not known whether nitroglycerin can cause fetal harm when administered to a pregnant woman. Therefore use NITROLINGUAL PUMPSPRAY only if the potential benefit justifies the risk to the fetus.

Nursing Women: It is not known whether nitroglycerin is excreted into breast milk. Benefits to the mother must be weighed against the risks to the child.

Pediatrics: The safety and effectiveness of nitroglycerin in children have not been established.

Geriatrics: The safety and effectiveness of nitroglycerin in the elderly population have not been established.

Monitoring and Laboratory Tests: The use of nitroglycerin in patients with congestive heart failure requires careful clinical and/or hemodynamic monitoring.

ADVERSE REACTIONS: Adverse Drug Reaction Overview: Adverse reactions to NITROLINGUAL PUMPSPRAY (nitroglycerin) are generally dose-related. In a clinical trial studying patients with chronic stable angina, the following adverse events were reported during the use of NITROLINGUAL PUMPSPRAY: headache, dizziness, paresthesia and dyspnea. All adverse events were mild to moderate.

Clinical Trial Adverse Drug Reactions: Because clinical trials are conducted under very specific conditions the adverse reactions rates observed in the clinical trials may not reflect the rates observed in practice and should not be compared to the rates in the clinical trials of another drug. Adverse drug reaction information from clinical trials is useful for identifying drug-related adverse events and for approximating rates.

The safety of NITROLINGUAL PUMPSPRAY was assessed in a double-blind, randomized, single-dose, 5-period crossover study involving patients with chronic, stable angina pectoris, who were known to be acutely responsive to sublingual nitroglycerin. The effects of varying doses (0.2 mg, 0.4 mg 0.8 mg and 1.6 mg) were assessed. The following adverse effects have been observed: headache, which may be severe and persistent, is the most commonly reported side effect of nitroglycerin. Occasionally, an individual may exhibit marked sensitivity to the hypotensive effects of nitrates and severe responses (nausea, vomiting, weakness, restlessness, pallor, retrosternal discomfort, perspiration and collapse) may occur even with therapeutic doses (see Less Common Clinical Trial Adverse Drug Reactions).

Common adverse events considered related to the drug are shown in Table 1.

Table 1: NITROLINGUAL PUMPSPRAY

Common Adverse Drug Reactions to NITROLINGUAL PUMPSPRAY in Patients with Angina

System Organ Class Adverse Event	Frequency	
	Nitrolingual Pumpspray 0.4–1.6 mg n=51 %	Placebo n=49 %
Gastrointestinal disorders		
Abdominal Pain	2	0
Stomatitis	0	2
General disorders and Administration Site Conditions		
Asthenia	2	0
Peripheral Edema	2	0
Infections and Infestations		
Pharyngitis	4	0

(cont'd)

Table 1: NITROLINGUAL PUMPSPRAY *(cont'd)*

Common Adverse Drug Reactions to NITROLINGUAL PUMPSPRAY in Patients with Angina

System Organ Class Adverse Event	Frequency Nitrolingual Pumpspray 0.4–1.6 mg n=51 %	Placebo n=49 %
Rhinitis	2	2
Nervous System disorders		
Headache	16	0
Dizziness	6	2
Paresthesia	4	0
Respiratory, Thoracic and Mediastinal disorders		
Dyspnea	4	0
Vascular disorders		
Vasodilatation	2	0

Less Common Clinical Trial Adverse Drug Reactions: Blood and Lymphatic System Disorders: Clinically significant methemoglobinemia is rare at conventional doses, but may occur, especially in patients with genetic hemoglobin abnormalities.
Cardiac Disorders: tachycardia.
Gastrointestinal Disorders: nausea, vomiting.
General Disorders and Administration Site Conditions: retrosternal discomfort, weakness.
Psychiatric Disorders: restlessness.
Skin and Subcutaneous Tissue Disorders: exfoliative dermatitis, perspiration, rash.
Vascular Disorders: collapse, flushing, pallor, postural hypotension.

DRUG INTERACTIONS:

> **Serious Drug Interactions**
> **PDE5 Inhibitors:** Concomitant use of NITROLINGUAL PUMPSPRAY and sildenafil, tadalafil, vardenafil or any other cGMP-specific phosphodiesterase Type 5 (PDE5) inhibitor could result in life-threatening hypotension with syncope or myocardial infarction and death.

Overview: Alcohol may enhance sensitivity to the hypotensive effects of nitrates.
Drug-Drug Interactions: The drugs listed in Table 2 are based on either drug interaction case reports or studies, or potential interactions due to the unexpected magnitude and seriousness of the interaction (i.e., those identified as contraindicated).

Table 2: NITROLINGUAL PUMPSPRAY

Established or Potential Drug-Drug Interactions

Proper Name	Ref	Effect	Clinical comment
CGMP-specific Phosphodiesterase Type 5 (PDE5) Inhibitors			
Sildenafil citrate	CT		The hypotensive effects of nitrates or nitric oxide donors are potentiated by PDE5 inhibitors. Concomitant use with NITROLINGUAL PUMPSPRAY could result in life-threatening hypotension with syncope or myocardial infarction and death. Concomitant administration of NITROLINGUAL PUMPSPRAY with PDE5 inhibitors is absolutely contraindicated (see Contraindications). If a patient treated with any PDE5 inhibitor needs a rapidly effective nitrate (e.g. in case of an acute angina pectoris attack) he/she the patient must be hospitalized immediately.
Tadalafil	T		Please see comments for sildenafil citrate.
Vardenafil	T		Please see comments for sildenafil citrate.

Interactions with other drugs have not been established.
Drug-Food Interactions: Interactions with food have not been established.
Drug-Herb Interactions: Interactions with herbal products have not been established.
Drug-Laboratory Test Interactions: Interactions with laboratory tests have not been established.
Drug-Lifestyle Interactions: Interactions with lifestyle have not been established.

DOSAGE AND ADMINISTRATION: Dosing Considerations:

- The spray should not be inhaled.
- The spray should be kept away from eyes.
- This spray formulation is intended to be applied and absorbed on or under the tongue.

Recommended Dose and Dosage Adjustment: Upon initiating therapy with NITROLINGUAL PUMPSPRAY (nitroglycerin), especially when changing from another form of nitroglycerin administration, patients should be followed closely by their physicians in order to determine the minimal effective dose for each patient.

Each metered dose contains 0.4 mg nitroglycerin. With the onset of an acute attack of angina pectoris, 1 or 2 metered doses (0.4 or 0.8 mg of nitroglycerin), as determined by experience, may be administered onto or under the tongue,**without inhaling.** The optimal dose may be repeated twice at 5 10 minute intervals. Dosage must be individualized and should be sufficient to provide relief without producing untoward reactions.

Administration: During administration the patient should be at rest, ideally in the sitting position, and the container kept vertical with the nozzle head up. The opening in the nozzle head should be kept as close to the mouth as possible. Patients should familiarize themselves with the position of the spray orifice, identified by the finger rest on top of the valve, in order to facilitate administration at night.

OVERDOSAGE:

Symptoms: Symptoms of overdosage are primarily related to vasodilation, that could lead to severe hypotension and possible reflex tachycardia. These include cutaneous flushing, headache, nausea, dizziness, and hypotension. Methemoglobinemia has been reported in association with high dose of glyceryl nitrate therapy. This may possibly be clinically significant, especially in the context of hemoglobin reductase deficiencies or in congenital methemoglobin variants.
Treatment: No specific antidote is available. Treatment should be symptomatic and supportive.

> For management of a suspected drug overdose, CPhA recommends that you contact your **regional Poison Control Centre**. See the *CPS* Directory section for a list of Poison Control Centres.

ACTION AND CLINICAL PHARMACOLOGY: Mechanism of Action: The principal action of NITROLINGUAL PUMPSPRAY (nitroglycerin) is that of all nitrates, namely, relaxation of vascular smooth muscle. Nitrates act primarily by reducing myocardial oxygen demand rather than increasing its oxygen supply. This effect is thought to be brought about predominantly by peripheral action. Although venous effects predominate, nitroglycerin produces, in a dose-related manner, dilation of both arterial and venous beds. Dilation of the post capillary vessels, including large veins, promotes peripheral pooling of blood and decreases venous return to the heart, reducing left ventricular end-diastolic pressure (pre-load). Arteriolar relaxation reduces systemic vascular resistance and arterial pressure (after-load). Left ventricular end-diastolic pressure and volume are decreased, resulting in reduction of ventricular size and wall tension. The reduction in ventricular wall tension results in a net decrease in myocardial oxygen consumption and a favorable net balance between myocardial oxygen supply and demand.
Pharmacodynamics: No data available.
Pharmacokinetics: Absorption: In a pharmacokinetic study when a single 0.8 mg dose of NITROLINGUAL PUMPSPRAY (nitroglycerin) was administered to 24 healthy volunteers, the mean C_{max} and t_{max} were 1.04 ng/mL and 7.5 min, respectively. Additionally, in these subjects the mean AUC was 12.8 ng.min/mL.
Distribution: Nitroglycerin and its major metabolites are approximately 60% protein bound.
Metabolism: Nitroglycerin is rapidly metabolized in the liver by hepatic enzymes. The two active major metabolites are the hydrolysis products, 1,3- and 1,2-dinitro-glycerols. There are also two inactive minor metabolites, the 1- and 2-mononitroglycerols, which are considered biologically inactive.
Excretion: Nitroglycerin is excreted by the renal route primarily as the two dinitro-metabolites, which have an excretion half-life of approximately 3-4 hours.

STORAGE AND STABILITY: NITROLINGUAL PUMPSPRAY (nitroglycerin) should be stored at room temperature: 15 to 30°C.
SPECIAL HANDLING INSTRUCTIONS: Do not place NITROLINGUAL PUMPSPRAY in hot water or near radiators, stoves or other sources of heat. Do not open forcefully or incinerate container or expose to temperature over 40°C.
INFORMATION FOR THE PATIENT: Published in e-CPS, available by subscription at www.e-cps.ca.
DOSAGE FORMS, COMPOSITION AND PACKAGING: Each metered dose contains: nitroglycerin 0.4 mg in an aromatized oily solution. Nonmedicinal ingredients: ethanol anhydrous, medium chained partial glycerides, medium chained triglycerides and peppermint oil. Spray bottles delivering 75 (hospital trade pack) or 200 metered doses.

Nitrostat™
nitroglycerin
Vasodilator

Pfizer

Date of Preparation: January 19, 2001
Date of Revision: February 21, 2005

PHARMACOLOGY: The principal pharmacological action of nitroglycerin is relaxation of vascular smooth muscle. Although venous effects predominate, nitroglycerin produces, in a dose-related manner, dilation of both arterial and venous beds. Dilation of postcapillary vessels, including large veins, promotes peripheral pooling of blood, decreases venous return to the heart, and reduces left ventricular end-diastolic pressure (preload). Nitroglycerin also produces arteriolar relaxation, thereby reducing peripheral vascular resistance and arterial pressure (afterload), and dilates large epicardial coronary arteries; however, the extent to which this latter effect contributes to the relief of exertional angina is unclear.

Therapeutic doses of nitroglycerin may reduce systolic, diastolic, and mean arterial blood pressure. Effective coronary perfusion pressure is usually maintained, but can be compromised if blood pressure falls excessively or increased heart rate decreases diastolic filling time.

Elevated central venous and pulmonary capillary wedge pressures, and pulmonary and systemic vascular resistance are also reduced by nitroglycerin therapy. Heart rate is usually slightly increased, presumably due to a compensatory response to the fall in blood pressure. Cardiac index may be increased, decreased, or unchanged. Myocardial oxygen consumption or demand (as measured by the pressure-rate product, tension-time index, and stroke-work index) is decreased and a more favorable supply-demand ratio can be achieved. Patients with elevated left ventricular filling pressures and increased systemic vascular resistance in association with a depressed cardiac index are likely to experience an improvement in cardiac index. In contrast, when filling pressures and cardiac index are normal, cardiac index may be slightly reduced following nitroglycerin administration.
Mechanism of Action: Nitroglycerin forms free radical nitric oxide (NO) which activates guanylate cyclase, resulting in an increase of guanosine 3'5' monophosphate (cyclic GMP) in smooth muscle and other tissues. These events lead to dephosphorylation of myosin light chains, which regulate the contractile state in smooth muscle, and result in vasodilatation.
Pharmacodynamics: Consistent with the symptomatic relief of angina, digital plethysmography indicates that onset of the vasodilatory effect occurs approximately 1 to 3 minutes after sublingual nitroglycerin administration and reaches a maximum by 5 minutes postdose. Effects persist for at least 25 minutes following NITROSTAT administration.
Pharmacokinetics: Absorption: Nitroglycerin is rapidly absorbed following sublingual administration of NITROSTAT (nitroglycerin tablets). Mean peak nitroglycerin plasma concentrations occur at a mean time of approximately 6 to 7 minutes postdose (Table 1). Maximum plasma nitroglycerin concentrations (C_{max}) and area under the plasma concentration-time curves (AUC) increase dose-proportionally following 0.3 to 0.6 mg NITROSTAT. The absolute bioavailability of nitroglycerin from NITROSTAT tablets is approximately 40% but tends to be variable due to factors influencing drug absorption such as sublingual hydration and mucosal metabolism.

Table 1: NITROSTAT

Pharmacokinetics

Parameters	Mean Nitroglycerin (SD) Values 2×0.3 mg NITROSTAT Tablets	1×0.6 mg NITROSTAT Tablets
C_{max}, ng/mL	2.3 (1.7)	2.1 (1.5)
t_{max}, min	6.4 (2.5)	7.2 (3.2)
$AUC_{(0-\infty)}$, ng/mL·min	14.9 (8.2)	14.9 (11.4)
$t_{1/2}$, min	2.8 (1.1)	2.6 (0.6)

Distribution: The volume of distribution (V_{Area}) of nitroglycerin following intravenous administration is 3.3 L/kg. At plasma concentrations between 50 and 500 ng/mL, the binding of nitroglycerin to plasma proteins is approximately 60%, while that of 1,2- and 1,3-dinitroglycerin is 60% and 30%, respectively.
Metabolism: A liver reductase enzyme is of primary importance in the metabolism of nitroglycerin to glycerol di- and mononitrate metabolites and ultimately to glycerol and organic nitrate. Known sites of extrahepatic metabolism include red blood cells and vascular walls. In addition to nitroglycerin, 2 major metabolites 1,2- and 1,3-dinitroglycerin, are found in plasma. Mean peak 1,2- and 1,3-dinitroglycerin plasma concentrations occur at approximately 15 minutes postdose. The elimination half-life of 1,2- and 1,3-dinitroglycerin is 36 and 32 minutes, respectively. The 1,2- and 1,3 dinitroglycerin metabolites have been reported to possess approximately 2% and 10% of the pharmacological activity of nitroglycerin. Higher plasma concentrations of the dinitro metabolites, along with their nearly 10-fold longer elimination half-lives, may contribute significantly to the duration of pharmacologic effect. Glycerol mononitrate metabolites of nitroglycerin are biologically inactive.
Elimination: Nitroglycerin plasma concentrations decrease rapidly with a mean elimination half-life of 2 to 3 minutes. Half-life values range from 1.5 to 7.5 minutes. Clearance (13.6 L/min) greatly exceeds hepatic blood flow. Metabolism is the primary route of drug elimination.

INDICATIONS: NITROSTAT (nitroglycerin tablets) are indicated for the acute relief of an attack or acute prophylaxis of angina pectoris due to coronary artery disease.

CONTRAINDICATIONS: Sublingual nitroglycerin therapy is contraindicated in patients with early myocardial infarction, severe anemia, increased intracranial pressure, and those with a known sensitivity or hypersensitivity to nitroglycerin or its ingredients, or other nitrates or nitrites.

Concomitant use of NITROSTAT (nitroglycerin tablets) either regularly and/or intermittently, with phosphodiesterase type 5 (PDE5) inhibitors such as sildenafil citrate (VIAGRA) is absolutely contraindicated since sildenafil citrate has been shown to potentiate the hypotensive effects of nitrates.

WARNINGS: The benefits of sublingual nitroglycerin in patients with acute myocardial infarction or congestive heart failure have not been established. If one elects to use nitroglycerin in these conditions, careful clinical or hemodynamic monitoring must be used because of the possibility of hypotension and tachycardia.

PRECAUTIONS: General: Only the smallest dose required for effective relief of the acute anginal attack should be used. Excessive use may lead to the development of tolerance. NITROSTAT (nitroglycerin tablets) are intended for sublingual or buccal administration and should not be swallowed.

Severe hypotension, particularly with upright posture, may occur with small doses of nitroglycerin. This drug should therefore be used with caution in patients who may be volume-depleted or who, for whatever reason, are already hypotensive. Hypotension induced by nitroglycerin may be accompanied by paradoxical bradycardia and increased angina pectoris.

Nitrate therapy may aggravate the angina caused by hypertrophic cardiomyopathy.

As tolerance to other forms of nitroglycerin develops, the effects of sublingual nitroglycerin on exercise tolerance, although still observable, is blunted.

In industrial workers who have had long-term exposure to unknown (presumably high) doses of organic nitrates, tolerance rarely occurs. Chest pain, acute myocardial infraction, and even sudden death have occurred during temporary withdrawal of nitrates from these workers, demonstrating the existence of true physical dependence.

Several clinical trials of nitroglycerin patches or infusions in patients with angina pectoris have evaluated regimens which incorporated a 10 to 12 hour nitrate free interval. In some of these trials, an increase in the frequency of anginal attacks during the nitrate free interval was observed in a small number of patients. In one trial, patients had decreased exercise tolerance at the end of the nitrate interval. Hemodynamic rebound has been observed only rarely; on the other hand, few studies were so designed that rebound, if it had occurred, would have been detected.

Nitrate tolerance as a result of sublingual nitroglycerin administration is probably possible, but only in patients who maintain high continuous nitrate levels for more than 10 or 12 hours daily. Such use of sublingual nitroglycerin would entail administration of scores of tablets daily and is not recommended.

The drug should be discontinued if blurring of vision or drying of the mouth occurs. Excessive dosage of nitroglycerin may produce severe headaches.

Pregnancy: There are no adequate and well-controlled studies in pregnant women. Nitroglycerin should be given to a pregnant woman only if clearly needed.

Lactation: It is not known whether nitroglycerin is excreted in human milk. Because many drugs are excreted in human milk, caution should be exercised when nitroglycerin is administered to a nursing woman.

Children: Safety and effectiveness of nitroglycerin in children have not been established.

Geriatrics: Clinical studies of NITROSTAT did not include sufficient numbers of subjects aged 65 and over to determine whether they respond differently from younger subjects. Other reported clinical experience has not identified differences in responses between the elderly and younger patients. In general, dose selection for an elderly patient should be cautious, usually starting at the low end of the dosing range, reflecting the greater frequency of decreased hepatic, renal, or cardiac function, and of concomitant disease or other drug therapy.

Drug Interactions: Hypotensive Agents: Patients receiving antihypertensive drugs, beta-adrenergic blockers, or phenothiazines and nitrates should be observed for possible additive hypotensive effects. Marked orthostatic hypotension has been reported when calcium channel blockers and organic nitrates were used concomitantly.

Alcohol: Concomitant use of nitrates and alcohol may cause hypotension.

ASA: The vasodilatory and hemodynamic effects of nitroglycerin may be enhanced by concomitant administration of ASA.

Alteplase: Intravenous administration of nitroglycerin decreases the thrombolytic effect of alteplase. Therefore, caution should be observed in patients receiving sublingual nitroglycerin during alteplase therapy.

Heparin: Intravenous nitroglycerin reduces the anticoagulant effect of heparin and activated partial thromboplastin times (APTT) should be monitored in patients receiving heparin and intravenous nitroglycerin. It is not known if this effect occurs following single sublingual nitroglycerin doses.

Anticholinergic Agents: Tricyclic antidepressants (amitriptyline, desipramine, doxepin, others) and anticholinergic drugs may cause dry mouth and diminished salivary secretions. This may make dissolution of sublingual nitroglycerin difficult. Increasing salivation with chewing gum or artificial saliva products may prove useful in aiding dissolution of sublingual nitroglycerin.

Ergot Alkaloids: Oral administration of nitroglycerin markedly decreases the first-pass metabolism of dihydroergotamine and subsequently increases its oral bioavailability. Ergotamine is known to precipitate angina pectoris. Therefore, patients receiving sublingual nitroglycerin should avoid ergotamine and related drugs or be monitored for symptoms of ergotism if this is not possible.

Nitrates: A decrease in therapeutic effect of sublingual nitroglycerin may result from use of long-acting nitrates.

Phosphodiesterase Type 5 (PDE5) Inhibitors: Concomitant use of NITROSTAT (nitroglycerin) and phophodiesterase type 5 (PDE5) inhibitors such as sildenafil citrate (VIAGRA) has been shown to potentiate the hypotensive effect of NITROSTAT (nitroglycerin). This could result in life-threatening hypotension with syncope or myocardial infarction and death. Therefore, VIAGRA (sildenafil citrate) should not be given to patients receiving NITROSTAT (nitroglycerin).

Drug/Laboratory Test Interactions: Nitrates may interfere with the Zlatkis-Zak color reaction causing a false report of decreased serum cholesterol.

Information to Be Provided to the Patient: The healthcare professional should communicate the following information to the patient.

This product is not intended for oral ingestion. It is intended for buccal or sublingual use only. If possible, patients should sit down when taking NITROSTAT (nitroglycerin tablets). This eliminates the possibility of falling due to lightheadedness or dizziness. There is a possibility of a headache (possibly severe) shortly after taking this medication (see Precautions).

Nitroglycerin may cause dizziness, vertigo and syncope. Patients with marked sensitivity to the vasodilatory effects of nitroglycerin should avoid potentially hazardous task such as driving or operating machinery unless it is known that this medication does not affect their ability to engage in these activities.

Patients using NITROSTAT (nitroglycerin) must not take phosphodiesterase type 5 (PDE5) inhibitors such as sildenafil citrate (VIAGRA). Such a combination can produce severe lowering of blood pressure, loss of consciousness, heart attack or death.

Nitroglycerin may produce a burning or tingling sensation when administered sublingually; however the ability to produce a burning or tingling sensation should not be considered a reliable method for determining the potency of the tablets.

Nitroglycerin should be kept in the original glass container, tightly capped, at controlled room temperature between 15-30°C. The cotton should be discarded once the bottle is opened.

ADVERSE EFFECTS: Headache, which may be severe and persistent may occur immediately after use. Vertigo, dizziness, weakness, palpitation, and other manifestations of postural hypotension may develop occasionally, particularly in erect, immobile patients. Marked sensitivity to the hypotensive effects of nitrates (manifested by nausea, vomiting, weakness, diaphoresis, pallor and collapse) may occur at therapeutic doses. Syncope due to nitrate vasodilation has been reported. Flushing, drug rash, exfoliative dermatitis, and urticaria have been reported in patients receiving nitrate therapy. Paradoxical bradycardia and increased angina pectoris may accompany nitroglycerin induced hypotension (see Precautions).

OVERDOSE:

Symptoms: Hemodynamic Effects: The effects of nitroglycerin overdose are generally the results of nitroglycerin's capacity to induce vasodilatation, venous pooling, reduced cardiac output, and hypotension. These hemodynamic changes may have protean manifestations, including increased intracranial pressure, with any or all of persistent throbbing headache, confusion, and moderate fever; vertigo; palpitations; tachycardia; visual disturbances; nausea and vomiting (possibly with colic and even bloody diarrhea); syncope (especially in the upright posture); dyspnea, later followed by reduced ventilatory effort, diaphoresis, with the skin either flushed or cold and clammy; heart block and bradycardia; paralysis; coma; seizures; and death.

No specific antagonist to the vasodilator effects of nitroglycerin is known, and no intervention has been subject to controlled study as a therapy of nitroglycerin overdose. Because the hypotension associated with nitroglycerin overdose is the result of venodilatation and arterial hypovolemia, prudent therapy in this situation should be directed toward increase in central fluid volume. Passive elevation of the patient's legs may be sufficient, but intravenous infusion of normal saline or similar fluid may also be necessary.

The use of epinephrine or other arterial vasoconstrictors in this setting is likely to do more harm than good.

In patients with renal disease or congestive heart failure, therapy resulting in central volume expansion is not without hazard. Treatment of nitroglycerin overdose in these patients may be subtle and difficult, and invasive monitoring may be required.

Methemoglobinemia: Methemoglobinemia has been rarely reported in association with organic nitrates. The diagnosis should be suspected in patients who exhibit signs of impaired oxygen delivery despite adequate cardiac output and adequate arterial PO_2. Classically, methemoglobinemic blood is described as chocolate brown, without color change on exposure to air.

If methemoglobinemia is present, intravenous administration of methylene blue, 1 to 2 mg/kg of body weight, may be required.

Treatment: See Symptoms.

> For management of a suspected drug overdose, CPhA recommends that you contact your **regional Poison Control Centre**. See the *CPS* Directory section for a list of Poison Control Centres.

DOSAGE: Usual adult dosage ranges from 0.3 to 0.6 mg.

One tablet should be dissolved under the tongue or in the buccal pouch at the first sign of an acute anginal attack. The dose may be repeated approximately every five minutes, until relief is obtained. If the pain persists after a total of 3 tablets in a 15-minute period, prompt medical attention is recommended. NITROSTAT (nitroglycerin tablets) may be used prophylactically five to ten minutes prior to engaging in activities which might precipitate an acute attack.

During administration for an acute angina attack, the patient should rest, preferably in the sitting position.

No dosage adjustment is required in patients with renal failure.

SUPPLIED: 0.3 mg: Each small, round, white sublingual tablet, marked with "N" on one side and the number "3" on the other side, contains: nitroglycerin 0.3 mg. Nonmedicinal ingredients: calcium stearate, glyceryl monostearate, lactose monohydrate, pregelatinized starch and silicon dioxide. Gluten-, paraben-, sodium-, sulfite- and tartrazine-free. Amber glass bottles of 100.

0.6 mg: Each small, round, white sublingual tablet, marked with "N" on one side and the number "6" on the other side, contains: nitroglycerin 0.6 mg. Nonmedicinal ingredients: calcium stearate, glyceryl monostearate, lactose monohydrate, pregelatinized starch and silicon dioxide. Gluten-, paraben-, sodium-, sulfite- and tartrazine-free. Amber glass bottles of 100.

Store at controlled room temperature, 15 to 30°C.

(Shown in Product Identification Section)

Nix® Creme Rinse

permethrin

Topical Pediculicide—Ovicide

Insight Pharma

PHARMACOLOGY: Permethrin is a synthetic pyrethroid, active against a broad range of pests including lice, ticks, fleas, mites, and other arthropods. It acts on the nerve cell membrane to disrupt the sodium channel current by which the polarization of the membrane is regulated. Delayed repolarization and paralysis of the pests are the consequences of this disturbance.

In vitro data indicate that permethrin has excellent pediculicidal and ovicidal activity against Pediculus humanus var. capitis. The high cure rate of permethrin in patients with head lice following a single application is attributable to a combination of its pediculicidal and ovicidal activities and its residual persistence on the hair which may also prevent reinfestation.

Permethrin is rapidly metabolized by ester hydrolysis to inactive metabolites which are excreted primarily in the urine. Although the amount of permethrin absorbed after a single application of the 1% cream rinse has not been determined precisely, preliminary data suggest it is less than 2% of the amount applied. Residual persistence of permethrin is detectable on the hair for at least 10 days following a single application.

INDICATIONS: For the single-application treatment of infestation with Pediculus humanus var. capitis (the head louse) and its nits (eggs). Retreatment for recurrences is required in less than 1% of patients since the ovicidal activity may be supplemented by residual persistence of permethrin in the hair. If live lice are observed after at least 7 days following the initial application, a second application can be given.

CONTRAINDICATIONS: In patients with known hypersensitivity to any of its components, to any synthetic pyrethroid or pyrethrin, or to chrysanthemums.

WARNINGS: If hypersensitivity to permethrin occurs, discontinue use.

PRECAUTIONS: Head lice infestation is often accompanied by pruritus, erythema and edema. Treatment with permethrin may temporarily exacerbate these conditions.

Pregnancy: Reproduction studies have been performed in mice, rats and rabbits and have revealed no evidence of impaired fertility or harm to the fetus due to permethrin. There are, however, no adequate and well-controlled studies in pregnant women. Because animal reproduction studies are not always predictive of human response, this drug should be used during pregnancy only if clearly needed.

Lactation: It is not known whether this drug is excreted in human milk. Because many drugs are excreted in human milk, and because of the evidence for tumorigenic potential of permethrin in animal studies, consideration should be given to discontinuing nursing temporarily or withholding the drug while the mother is nursing.

Children: Permethrin is safe and effective in children 2 years of age and older. Safety and effectiveness in children less than 2 years of age have not been established.

ADVERSE EFFECTS: The most frequent adverse reaction to permethrin is pruritus. This is usually a consequence of head lice infestation itself, but may be temporarily aggravated following treatment with permethrin. Mild temporary itching was experienced by 5.9% of patients enrolled in clinical studies; 3.4% experienced mild transient burning/stinging, tingling, numbness or scalp discomfort; and 2.1% experienced mild transient erythema, edema or rash of the scalp.

OVERDOSE:

No instance of accidental ingestion has been reported.

Treatment: If ingested, gastric lavage and general supportive measures should be employed.

> For management of a suspected drug overdose, CPhA recommends that you contact your **regional Poison Control Centre**. See the *CPS* Directory section for a list of Poison Control Centres.

DOSAGE: Adults and Children: For use after the hair has been washed with conditioner-free shampoo, rinsed with water and towel dried. Apply a sufficient volume of permethrin to saturate the hair and scalp. It should remain on the hair for 10 minutes before being rinsed off with water. A single treatment is sufficient to eliminate head lice infestation. Remove nits using a fine toothed (nit) comb.

Shake well before using.

INFORMATION FOR THE PATIENT: Published in e-CPS, available by subscription at www.e-cps.ca.

SUPPLIED: Each g of creme rinse contains: permethrin 1% w/w. Nonmedicinal ingredients: balsam Canada, cetyl alcohol, citric acid, FD&C Yellow No. 6, hydrolyzed animal protein, hydroxyethylcellulose, isopropyl alcohol, methylparaben , perfume, polyoxyethylene 10 cetyl ether, propylene glycol, propylparaben, stearalkonium chloride and water. Plastic squeeze bottles of 56 g (59 mL) including nit removal combs. Store at 15 to 25°C.

Nix® Dermal Cream

permethrin

Topical Scabicide

GlaxoSmithKline Consumer Healthcare

PHARMACOLOGY: Permethrin is a synthetic pyrethroid which is active against a broad range of pests including lice, ticks, fleas, mites, and other arthropods. It acts on the nerve cell membrane to disrupt the sodium channel current by which the polarization of the membrane is regulated. Delayed repolarization and paralysis of the pests are the consequences of this disturbance.

A very small amount (<2%) of topically administered permethrin is absorbed through the skin. This contrasts to the 32% absorption seen after ingestion. The maximum absorption occurs during the first 48 hours following application. Permethrin is metabolized by ester hydrolysis to dichlorovinyl acid derivatives (DCVAs). Blood levels of metabolites were still quantifiable after 28 days in one-third of test samples. The main route of excretion is via the kidneys.

Lag time for penetration of permethrin through the skin ranged from 1.3 to 4 hours for cis-permethrin and 2.6 to 4.8 hours for trans-permethrin. Male patients excreted more DCVA than female patients. Excretion of trans-DCVA in the urine was 4 to 5 times faster than cis-DCVA, reflecting its greater concentration and more rapid rate of metabolism. Presence of esterase in skin could account for observed differences in the amount of DCVA excreted in urine of male and female patients.

There was no evidence of contact sensitization to permethrin during induction or challenge phases of maximization testing. No reactions were observed during phototoxicity testing.

INDICATIONS: For the treatment of infestation with *S. scabiei* (scabies). If live mites or new lesions appear, a second treatment may be necessary 7 to 10 days after the first treatment.

CONTRAINDICATIONS: Patients with known hypersensitivity to any of its components, to any synthetic pyrethroid or pyrethrins, or to chrysanthemums.

WARNINGS: If hypersensitivity to the dermal cream occurs, discontinue use.

PRECAUTIONS: General: Scabies infestation is often accompanied by pruritus, edema and erythema. Treatment with permethrin may temporarily exacerbate these conditions. Pruritus caused by an acquired sensitivity to mites and their products frequently persists for one to several weeks following treatment; this reaction does not indicate treatment failure.

Information to Be Provided to the Patient: Patients with scabies should be advised that itching, mild burning and/or stinging may occur after application of permethrin. In clinical trials, approximately 75% of patients treated with permethrin who continued to manifest pruritus at 2 weeks had cessation by 4 weeks. If irritation persists, they should consult their physician. Permethrin cream may cause marked irritation to the eyes. Patients should be advised to avoid contact with eyes during application and to flush with plenty of water or, if readily available, normal saline immediately if the cream gets in the eyes.

Pregnancy: Teratogenic Effects: Reproduction studies have been performed in mice, rats, and rabbits (200 to 400 mg/kg/day orally) and have revealed no evidence of impaired fertility or harm to the fetus due to permethrin. Negative in vivo genotoxicity tests and the very low mammalian toxicity would suggest that any risk to the fetus following treatment with permethrin dermal cream is minimal. There are, however, no adequate and well-controlled studies in pregnant women. Because animal reproduction studies are not always predictive of human response, this drug should be used during pregnancy only if clearly needed.

Lactation: It is not known whether this drug is excreted in human milk. Because many drugs are excreted in human milk and because of the evidence for tumorigenic potential of permethrin in some animal species, consideration should be given to discontinuing nursing temporarily or withholding the drug while the mother is nursing.

Children: Permethrin is safe and effective in children 2 years of age and older. Safety and effectiveness in children between 2 and 23 months of age are limited. This product should therefore only be used in this age group on the advice and supervision of a physician.

Drug Interactions: The treatment of eczematous-like reactions with corticosteroids should be withheld prior to treatment with permethrin, as there is a risk of exacerbating the scabies infestation by reducing the immune response to the mite. The likelihood of interactions between the two treatments leading to potential adverse reactions or reduced efficacy is, however, small.

ADVERSE EFFECTS: Ten percent of patients in clinical trials experienced generally mild and transient burning and stinging following application of the dermal cream. This was associated with the severity of infestation. Pruritus was reported in 7% of patients at various times post-application. Erythema, numbness, tingling and rash were reported in up to 2% of patients. Eczema and edema were also reported.

OVERDOSE:

Symptoms: There are no reports of overdosage with permethrin.

It is possible that excessive application of permethrin might result in localized adverse reactions or more severe skin reactions.

Treatment: Symptomatic treatment is indicated should hypersensitivity-type reactions occur.

In the event of accidental ingestion, gastric lavage should be considered if consultation is within 2 hours of ingestion.

For management of a suspected drug overdose, CPhA recommends that you contact your **regional Poison Control Centre**. See the *CPS* Directory section for a list of Poison Control Centres.

DOSAGE: Adults and Children over 12 Years: Approximately one 30 g tube/½ of a 60 g tube. 5 to 12 years: Approximately ½ of a 30 g tube/¼ of a 60 g tube. 2 to 4 years: Approximately ¼ of a 30 g tube/⅛ of a 60 g tube.

In view of the great individual variability in body area and skin types precise recommendations are not possible.

Usually 30 g is sufficient for an average adult. A few adults may need to use an additional 30 g.

It is recommended that family members and close contacts, including sexual partners, be treated with permethrin to reduce the risk of transmission or eliminate reinfestation.

Administration: In cases where the head, neck, scalp and outer ears are treated the dosage may be increased to ensure total body coverage.

Adults and Children (≥2 years): Thoroughly massage the dermal cream into the skin from the head to the soles of the feet paying particular attention to the areas between the fingers and toes, wrists, axillae (arm pits), external genitalia (external sexual organs), buttocks and under the finger area and toe nails. Reapply to the hands if washed off with soap and water within 8 hours of application. It is **not necessary** to apply a thick visible layer of cream into the skin as it disappears on application. Scabies rarely infests the scalp of adults, although the hairline, neck, temple and forehead may be infested in geriatric patients. Children should be supervised by an adult.

The dermal cream should be removed by washing (shower or bath) after 12 to 14 hours.

In the majority of individuals, the scabies infestation is cleared with a single application of the cream. If necessary, a second application may be given 7 to 10 days after the first, but only if live mites can be demonstrated or new lesions appear.

To prevent reinfestations all clothing and bed linens used within 2 days prior to treatment should be machine-washed in hot water and dried in the dryer for at least 20 minutes, or dry cleaned.

Persistent pruritus after treatment is not an indication for retreatment (see Precautions).

Children Aged 2 to 23 Months: Children aged between 2 and 23 months should be treated only under medical supervision. The dose required is usually between ⅛ and ¼ of a 30 g tube. The cream should be massaged thoroughly into the skin from the head to the soles of the feet, as directed for adults and older children, but should include the face, neck. Infants should also be treated on the scalp, outer ears, temples and forehead. Care must be taken to avoid the vicinity of the mouth where it could be licked off, and areas close to eyes.

INFORMATION FOR THE PATIENT: Published in e-CPS, available by subscription at www.e-cps.ca.

SUPPLIED: Each g of off-white, vanishing dermal cream contains: permethrin 50 mg (5%). Nonmedicinal ingredients: butylated hydroxytoluene, carbomer 934P, coconut oil, glycerin, glyceryl monostearate, isopropyl myristate, lanolin alcohols, mineral oil, polyoxyethylene cetyl ethers, purified water and sodium hydroxide. Formaldehyde 1 mg (0.1%) added as preservative. Tubes of 30 and 60 g. Store between 15 and 25°C.

Nizatidine Ⓟ

Histamine H2-Receptor Antagonist

CPhA Monograph

Date of Preparation: October 2006

This monograph has been compiled by CPhA and reviewed by experts. It may contain information different from that found in Health Canada-approved Product Monographs. The reader is referred to the *CPS* Editorial Policy for more information.

SUMMARY PRODUCT INFORMATION:

Route of Administration	Dosage Form	Strength
Oral	Capsule	150 mg, 300 mg

INDICATIONS AND CLINICAL USE: Nizatidine is indicated for:

- treatment of acute duodenal ulcer, acute benign gastric ulcer, and esophagitis associated with gastroesophageal reflux.
- prevention of recurrent duodenal ulcers and reflux esophagitis.

Pediatrics: Nizatidine has been used in infants aged ≥5 days and children aged <18 years for the treatment of gastroesophageal reflux.

CONTRAINDICATIONS:

- Patients who are hypersensitive to nizatidine, other H_2 receptor antagonists, or to any ingredient in the formulation. Cross-sensitivity between nizatidine and ranitidine has been reported.

WARNINGS AND PRECAUTIONS: Gastrointestinal: Nizatidine may mask the symptoms of gastric malignancy.

Respiratory: Acid-suppressive therapy may increase the risk of community-acquired pneumonia.

Special Populations: Pregnant Women: There is limited human data regarding the safety of nizatidine during pregnancy. Reproductive studies in rats and rabbits at doses of up to 1500 mg/kg/day and 275 mg/kg/day, respectively, have revealed no evidence of teratogenecity. A placental perfusion model revealed that about 40% of freely diffusible nizatidine crosses the placenta. In a prospective study of 178 women exposed to histamine H_2 antagonists, including nizatidine, during the first trimester of pregnancy there was no increase in major fetal malformations compared with matched controls.

Nursing Women: Less than 0.1% of a 150 mg dose of nizatidine was excreted into the breast milk of 5 lactating women during a 12 hour period.

ADVERSE REACTIONS: More Common Adverse Drug Reactions: Placebo-controlled clinical trials in North America, which included over 2600 patients given nizatidine and over 1700 patients given placebo, reported the following common adverse events: see Table 1.

Table 1: Nizatidine

More Common Adverse Drug Reactions in Clinical Trials (≥1%)[a]

Body System	Effect	Clinical Comment
Body as a whole	Headache, pain, asthenia, chest pain, infection, accident	The incidence of adverse events in recipients of nizatidine and placebo was generally similar.
CNS	Dizziness, somnolence anxiety, nervousness	
Gastrointestinal	Diarrhea, dry mouth	
Respiratory	Rhinitis, pharyngitis, sinusitis	
Skin	Pruritus	

[a] Based on an analysis of treatment-emergent adverse events reported in 2694 nizatidine recipients and 1729 placebo recipients enrolled in controlled clinical trials conducted in Canada and the US. Events included are those for which the incidence in nizatidine recipients exceeded that in placebo recipients.

Less Common Adverse Drug Reactions (<1%): Cardiovascular: asymptomatic ventricular tachycardia.

Central Nervous System: reversible mental confusion.

Dermatologic: urticaria (significantly more common in nizatidine than placebo recipients), exfoliative dermatitis.

Endocrine and Metabolism: impotence and decreased libido (similar incidence to placebo), gynecomastia.

Gastrointestinal: nausea, vomiting, abdominal discomfort, constipation, flatulence, dyspepsia, dry mouth, anorexia (similar incidence to placebo).

Hematologic: anemia (significantly more common in nizatidine than placebo recipients), thrombocytopenic purpura.

Hepatic: reversible increase in serum AST, ALT and/or alkaline phosphatase, hepatitis, jaundice; reversible cholestatic or mixed cholestatic hepatocellular injury with jaundice.

DRUG INTERACTIONS: Overview: Nizatidine does not inhibit cytochrome P450 isozymes. As a result, drug interactions linked to inhibition of hepatic metabolism are not expected. Nizatidine significantly raises gastric pH; thus, it has the potential to modify the pharmacokinetic profile of drugs that are dependent on gastric acidity for dissolution and/or absorption from the gastrointestinal tract.

Drug-Drug Interactions: See Table 2.

Table 2: Nizatidine

Drug-Drug Interactions

Interacting Drug	Effect	Clinical Comment
ASA	↑ serum salicylate concentration	With high doses of ASA (3.9 g); possibly due to inhibition of renal salicylate excretion
Atazanavir	↓ Atazanavir plasma concentrations	Separate administration of the two drugs by ≥12 hours.
Cefuroxime axetil	↓ bioavailability of cefuroxime	Separate administration by ≥2 hours.
Cyclosporine	May ↑ serum cyclosporine concentrations.	Monitor serum cyclosporine concentration.
Gefitinib	↓ absorption of gefitinib	Clinical implications are unclear.
Imidazole antifungal agents	↓ bioavailability of ketoconazole and itraconazole	Consider using a non-interacting antifungal agent (e.g., fluconazole).

Drug-Food Interactions: Nizatidine prepared as an extemporaneous solution in apple juice has a much lower bioavailability than the capsule dosage form.

Drug-Laboratory Interactions: Multistix test for urobilinogen may produce false positive results.

DOSAGE AND ADMINISTRATION: Recommended Dose and Dosage Adjustment: Adults: See Table 3.

Table 3: Nizatidine

Dose in Adult Patients

Indication	Usual Dose	Duration of Therapy	Clinical Comment
Treatment of duodenal ulcers	300 mg qhs or 150 mg BID	4–8 weeks	In most patients, healing occurs within 4 weeks.
Maintenance therapy for prevention of duodenal ulcer recurrence	150 mg qhs	6–12 months	
Treatment of gastric ulcers	300 mg qhs or 150 mg BID	8 weeks	

(cont'd)

Table 3: Nizatidine *(cont'd)*

Dose in Adult Patients

Indication	Usual Dose	Duration of Therapy	Clinical Comment
Gastroesophageal reflux	150 mg BID	12 weeks	

Pediatrics: See Table 4.

Table 4: Nizatidine

Dose in Pediatric Patients

Indication	Age/ Weight	Usual Dose	Maximum Dose	Duration of Therapy
Gastroesophageal reflux	≥12 years	150 mg BID	300 mg/day	8 weeks
	<12 years	5–10 mg/kg/day divided BID	Do not exceed 300 mg daily	8 weeks

Renal Impairement: See Table 5.

Table 5: Nizatidine

Dose in Adult Patients with Renal Impairment

Renal Function	Creatinine Clearance	Dosage Adjustment: Acute	Dosage Adjustment: Maintenance
Normal	>50 mL/min	300 mg/day	150 mg/day
Moderate Impairment	20–50 mL/min	150 mg/day	150 mg every other day
Severe Impairment	<20 mL/min	150 mg every other day	150 mg q3days

Hepatic Impairment: No dosage adjustment is required in patients with hepatic impairment.
Administration: Nizatidine may be administered concomitantly with antacids. The effect of food on the pharmacokinetics of nizatidine is not clinically significant.

OVERDOSAGE:

For management of a suspected drug overdose, CPhA recommends that you contact your **regional Poison Control Centre**. See the *CPS* Directory section for a list of Poison Control Centres.

ACTION AND CLINICAL PHARMACOLOGY: Mechanism of Action: Nizatidine competitively inhibits histamine at the H_2 receptor on parietal cells resulting in decreased basal acid secretion and, to a smaller degree, decreased stimulated acid production. The extent and duration of gastric acid suppression is directly correlated with the dose of nizatidine. A 300 mg dose of nizatidine inhibited 90% of nocturnal gastric acid secretion for up to 10 hours and 97% of meal-stimulated secretion for up to 4 hours.

Nizatidine has no anticholinergic properties and has no effect on gastric motility or lower esophageal sphincter pressure.
Pharmacokinetics: Adults: See Table 6.

Table 6: Nizatidine

Summary of Pharmacokinetic Parameters

C_{max}	Duration of Action	Elimination $t_{½}$	Clearance	Volume of Distribution
0.5–3 h	8–12 h	1–2 h	40–60 L/h	0.8–1.5 L/kg

Absorption: Nizatidine is rapidly absorbed from the gastrointestinal tract with absolute bioavailability of about 70%. Food increases the bioavailability of nizatidine to a small degree. Single oral doses of 150 and 300 mg achieved peak plasma concentrations of 700-1800 and 1400-3600 ng/mL, respectively.
Distribution: Nizatidine is widely distributed into body fluids. Approximately 35% of the drug in the circulation is bound to plasma proteins, primarily $α_1$-acid glycoprotein.
Metabolism: About 10 to 35% of the drug is metabolized by the liver to N-desmethylnizatidine, nizatidine N-oxide, and nizatidine sulfoxide. Only N-desmethylnizatidine has H_2 receptor blocking activity, which corresponds to about 60% of the parent drug. First pass metabolism is not significant. The remainder of a dose is excreted unchanged in the urine.
Excretion: Nizatidine is excreted by the kidneys via glomerular filtration and tubular secretion. Dosage adjustments are required in patients with renal impairment. In patients with creatinine clearance <10 mL/min, the elimination half-life ranged from 3.5 to 11 hours and the plasma clearance was estimated to be 7 to 14 L/h.
Special Populations: Pediatrics: In children with a mean age of 8 years given a single oral dose of nizatidine 5 mg/kg, the apparent terminal elimination rate was virtually identical to that reported in adults. Estimates of nizatidine pharmacokinetic parameters (e.g., C_{max}, CL/F, Vss/F) in children were also similar to those in adults administered similar oral doses of the drug.

Nizoral® Shampoo

ketoconazole

Topical Antifungal

Johnson & Johnson

Date of Revision: October 19, 2010

PHARMACOLOGY: In vitro studies suggest that the antifungal properties of NIZORAL (ketoconazole) may be related to its ability to impair the synthesis of ergosterol, a component of fungal and yeast cell membranes. Without the availability of this essential sterol, there are morphological alterations of the fungal and yeast cell membranes manifested as abnormal membranous inclusions between the cell wall and the plasma membrane. The inhibition of ergosterol synthesis has been attributed to interference with the reactions involved in the removal of the 14-α-methyl group of the precursor of ergosterol, lanosterol.

Except for its specific pharmacologic effect, i.e., a sporicidal or fungicidal activity, ketoconazole when formulated in a 2% shampoo is not expected to exert any other pharmacodynamic effect when applied topically on the skin or hair.
INDICATIONS: NIZORAL (ketoconazole) 2% shampoo is indicated for the topical treatment and prophylaxis of conditions in which the yeast Pityrosporum is involved, such as pityriasis capitis (dandruff). NIZORAL shampoo is also indicated for seborrheic dermatitis.
CONTRAINDICATIONS: NIZORAL (ketoconazole) 2% shampoo is contraindicated in persons who have shown hypersensitivity to the active or excipient ingredients of this formulation.

WARNINGS: Irritation may occur when NIZORAL (ketoconazole) 2% shampoo is used immediately after prolonged treatment with topical corticosteroids. To prevent a rebound effect after stopping a prolonged treatment with topical corticosteroids, it is recommended to continue applying a mild topical corticosteroid at the onset of treatment with NIZORAL shampoo, and to subsequently and gradually withdraw the steroid therapy over a period of 2-3 weeks.

PRECAUTIONS: If a reaction suggesting sensitivity or chemical irritation should occur, use of NIZORAL (ketoconazole) 2% shampoo should be discontinued.
Pregnancy: There are no adequate and well-controlled studies in pregnant or lactating women. NIZORAL shampoo does not produce detectable blood levels after topical application to the scalp. Plasma levels were detected after topical administration of NIZORAL shampoo on the whole body. There are no known risks associated with the use of NIZORAL shampoo 2% in pregnancy or lactation. There were reports of spontaneous abortion and anencephaly after exposure to NIZORAL shampoo during pregnancy, although there is insufficient information to confirm any association between NIZORAL shampoo and these abnormal pregnancy outcomes. However, due to the teratogenic nature of the active ingredient, ketoconazole, the use of NIZORAL shampoo is not recommended in pregnant or nursing women except under the advice of a physician.
Lactation: See Pregnancy.
Pediatrics: Clinical data on the use of NIZORAL shampoo in children under 12 are not available; therefore, such use is not recommended except under the advice of a physician.

ADVERSE EFFECTS: Clinical Trial Data: The safety of NIZORAL Shampoo 2% was evaluated in 2890 subjects in 22 clinical trials where NIZORAL Shampoo 2% was administered topically to the scalp and/or skin. No adverse drug reactions (ADRs) were reported in ≥1% of NIZORAL Shampoo 2%-treated subjects. Adverse drug reactions that occurred in <1% of NIZORAL Shampoo 2%-treated subjects in the clinical datasets are listed in Table 1.

Table 1: NIZORAL Shampoo

Adverse Drug Reactions Reported in <1% of 2890 NIZORAL Shampoo 2%-treated Subjects in 22 Clinical Trials

System Organ Class	Preferred Term
Eye Disorders	Eye irritation Increased lacrimation
General Disorders and Administration Site Conditions	Application site erythema Application site irritation Application site hypersensitivity Application site pruritus Application site pustules Application site reaction
Immune System Disorders	Hypersensitivity
Infections and Infestations	Folliculitis
Nervous System Disorders	Dysgeusia
Skin and Subcutaneous Tissue Disorders	Acne Alopecia Dermatitis contact Dry skin Hair texture abnormal Rash Skin burning sensation Skin disorder Skin exfoliation

Post-marketing Experience: Adverse drug reactions first identified during post-marketing experience with NIZORAL Shampoo 2% are included in Table 2. In this table, the frequencies are provided according to the following convention: Very common ≥1/10; Common ≥1/100 and <1/10; Uncommon ≥1/1000 and <1/100; Rare ≥1/10 000 and <1/1000; Very rare <1/10 000, including isolated reports.

In Table 2, ADRs are presented by frequency category based on spontaneous reporting rates.

Table 2: NIZORAL Shampoo

Adverse Drug Reactions Identified During Post-Marketing Experience with NIZORAL Shampoo 2% by Frequency Category Estimated from Spontaneous Reporting Rates

	Post-Market Adverse Reaction
Skin and Subcutaneous Tissue Disorders	Very rare: Angioedema, urticaria, hair colour changes

OVERDOSE:
Symptoms: Oral ingestion is usually followed by nausea and vomiting due to the detergent. In the event of accidental ingestion, supportive and symptomatic measures should be carried out. In order to avoid aspiration, neither emesis nor gastric lavage should be performed. It has been reported that ketoconazole cannot be removed by hemodialysis.

For management of a suspected drug overdose, CPhA recommends that you contact your **regional Poison Control Centre**. See the *CPS* Directory section for a list of Poison Control Centres.

DOSAGE: Adults and children over 12 years of age: NIZORAL (ketoconazole) 2% shampoo (5 to 10 mL) should be applied to the wet scalp, worked into a lather and left on for 3-5 minutes before rinsing with water. As with other shampoos, care should be taken to keep the shampoo out of the eyes and off the eyelids.
Treatment: Twice weekly for 2 to 4 weeks.
Prophylaxis: Once every one or two weeks.

SUPPLIED: Each mL of pink-orange, viscous shampoo with an herbal bouquet contains: ketoconazole 2% (20 mg/g). Nonmedicinal ingredients: coconut fatty acid diethanolamide, disodium laureth sulfosuccinate, erythrosin, hydrochloric acid, imidurea, laurdimonium hydrolyzed animal collagen, macrogol 120 methyl glucose dioleate, perfume bouquet, sodium chloride, sodium hydroxide, sodium laureth sulfate and water. HDPE bottles of 60 and 120 mL. Store at or below 25°C.

Nolvadex®-D

tamoxifen citrate

Antineoplastic

AstraZeneca

Date of Revision: September 2, 2010

Tamoxifen therapy was associated with serious and life-threatening events including uterine malignancies, stroke, pulmonary embolism, and deep vein thrombosis in the NSABP P-1 trial for the prevention of breast cancer. The use of Nolvadex for breast cancer prevention in not an approved indication in Canada. In the NSABP P-1 trial, the relative risk of tamoxifen compared to placebo was 3.1 for endometrial cancer, 4.0 for uterine sarcomas, 1.6 for stroke, 3.0 for pulmonary embolism, and 1.6 for deep vein thrombosis. These events were fatal in some patients. Health care providers should be aware of the possible risks associated with tamoxifen therapy and should discuss them with their patients.

The benefits of tamoxifen therapy outweigh the risks in the majority of women being treated according to the approved Canadian indication for the treatment of breast cancer.

PHARMACOLOGY: Tamoxifen, the active ingredient, is a non-steroidal agent which has demonstrated potent antiestrogenic properties in animal test systems. The antiestrogenic effects are related to its ability to compete with estrogen for binding sites in target tissues such as breast and uterus. Tamoxifen inhibits the induction of rat mammary carcinoma induced by dimethylbenzanthracene (DMBA), and causes the regression of already established DMBA-induced tumours. In this rat model, tamoxifen appears to exert its antitumour effects by binding to estrogen receptors.

In cytosols derived from human endometrium and human breast and uterine adenocarcinomas, tamoxifen competes with estradiol for estrogen receptor protein.

In women with estrogen receptor-positive/unknown breast tumours, adjuvant tamoxifen has been shown to significantly reduce recurrence of the disease and improve 10-year survival, achieving a significantly greater effect with five years treatment than with 1 or 2 years treatment. These benefits appear to be largely irrespective of age, menopausal status, tamoxifen dose and additional chemotherapy.

Ranges as large as 0 to 300 fmol/mg protein have been reported in histologically comparable portions of the same tumour. In addition, the collection, transport and storage of tumour specimens can affect the validity of current estrogen receptor assays.

The apparent discrepancy in correlation between estrogen receptor status and clinical response may also be explained by recent in vitro evidence indicating that not all of the growth inhibiting effects of tamoxifen are mediated through the estrogen receptor. Tamoxifen has been shown to have a low affinity for the androgen receptor and on a binding site distinct from the estrogen receptor. The possibility also exists that tamoxifen interferes with the action of hormonal steroids on cell growth, that it could modulate the action of peptide hormones at their receptors by effects on cell membranes, and that it inhibits prostaglandin synthetase thereby having the potential to limit tumour growth. It is recognized that tamoxifen also displays estrogenic-like effects on several body systems including the endometrium, bone and blood lipids.

INDICATIONS: Tamoxifen is indicated for the adjuvant treatment of early breast cancer in women with estrogen receptor positive tumors.

Tamoxifen is indicated for the treatment of women with hormone responsive locally advanced/metastatic breast cancer.

CONTRAINDICATIONS: Tamoxifen is contraindicated in patients with hypersensitivity to the product or any of its components.

Pregnancy: Tamoxifen must not be given during pregnancy. There have been a small number of reports of spontaneous abortions, birth defects and fetal deaths after women have taken tamoxifen, although no causal relationship has been established.

Reproductive toxicology studies in rats, rabbits and monkeys have shown no teratogenic potential.

In rodent models of fetal reproductive tract development, tamoxifen was associated with changes similar to those caused by estradiol, ethynylestradiol, clomiphene and diethylstilboestrol (DES). Although the clinical relevance of these changes is unknown, some of them, especially vaginal adenosis, are similar to those seen in young women who were exposed to DES in utero and who have a 1 in 1000 risk of developing clear-cell carcinoma of the vagina or cervix. Only a small number of pregnant women have been exposed to tamoxifen. Such exposure has not been reported to cause subsequent vaginal adenosis or clear-cell carcinoma of the vagina or cervix in young women exposed in utero to tamoxifen.

Women should be advised not to become pregnant while taking tamoxifen and should use barrier or other nonhormonal contraceptive methods if sexually active. Premenopausal patients must be carefully examined before treatment to exclude the possibility of pregnancy. Women should be informed of the potential risks to the fetus, should they become pregnant while taking tamoxifen or within 2 months of cessation of therapy.

When used in the prevention setting (an indication not approved in Canada), tamoxifen is contraindicated in patients with a history of stroke, deep venous thrombosis or pulmonary embolism, and in patients who are at an increased risk of developing endometrial cancer.

WARNINGS: Tamoxifen should be used only for the conditions listed under the Indications.

An increased incidence of uterine malignancies has been reported in association with tamoxifen treatment. The underlying mechanism is unknown, but may be related to the estrogen-like effect of tamoxifen. Most uterine malignancies seen in association with tamoxifen are classified as adenocarcinoma of the endometrium. However, rare uterine sarcomas, including malignant mixed Mullerian tumors, have also been reported. Uterine sarcoma is generally associated with a higher FIGO stage (III/IV) at diagnosis, poorer prognosis, and shorter survival. Uterine sarcoma has been reported to occur more frequently among long-term users (≥2 years) of tamoxifen than non-users.

There is evidence of an increased incidence of thromboembolic events, including deep vein thrombosis and pulmonary embolism, during tamoxifen therapy. When tamoxifen is co-administered with chemotherapy, there may be a further increase in the incidence of thromboembolic effects. For treatment of breast cancer, the risks and benefits of tamoxifen should be carefully considered in women with a history of thromboembolic events.

An increased risk of stroke has been found to be associated with tamoxifen therapy in high-risk patients being treated for the prevention of breast cancer. The use of tamoxifen for the prevention of breast cancer is not an approved indication in Canada.

Incidence rates for the above events were estimated from a long-term clinical study called the National Surgical Adjuvant Breast and Bowel Project Breast Cancer Prevention (NSABP P-1) Trial. In this trial, high-risk patients were randomized to either tamoxifen therapy or placebo, for the prevention of breast cancer. Uterine malignancies were separated into cases of endometrial adenocarcinomas and uterine sarcomas. The relative risk of tamoxifen compared to placebo was 3.1 for endometrial cancer, 4.0 for uterine sarcomas, 1.6 for stroke, 3.0 for pulmonary embolism, and 1.6 for deep vein thrombosis.

Disturbances of menstrual function, including oligomenorrhea and amenorrhea, have been reported in a proportion of premenopausal women receiving tamoxifen for the treatment of breast cancer. Available information indicates that in those women receiving tamoxifen for up to 2 years for the treatment of early breast cancer who develop disturbances of menstrual function on treatment, a proportion return to normal cyclical bleeding on cessation of therapy.

Hepatocellular carcinomas have been reported in the 2-year oncogenicity study in rats receiving tamoxifen. In addition, gonadal tumors have been reported in mice receiving tamoxifen in long-term studies. The clinical relevance of these findings has not been established.

Cataracts were also reported in the 2 year oncogenicity study in rats, and since then it has been established that treatment with tamoxifen has been associated with an increased incidence of cataracts.

A number of second primary tumours, occurring at sites other than the endometrium and the opposite breast, have been reported in clinical trials, following the treatment of breast cancer patients with tamoxifen. No causal link has been established and the clinical significance of these observations remains unclear.

Nolvadex is a pro-drug requiring metabolic activation by CYP2D6. Low CYP2D6 activity that occurs in patients harbouring certain CYP2D6 alleles (i.e. *4) or from the chronic use of CYP2D6 inhibitors can lead to persistent reductions in plasma concentrations of an active metabolite of Nolvadex (endoxifen). Reduced efficacy on tamoxifen has been reported with concomitant usage of some selective serotonin reuptake inhibitor (SSRI) antidepressants (e.g. paroxetine, a known CYP2D6 inhibitor). Concurrent chronic use of CYP2D6 inhibitors that may affect tamoxifen efficacy should be avoided if possible (see also Precautions, Drug Interactions).

PRECAUTIONS: Tamoxifen should be used cautiously in patients with existing thrombocytopenia or leukopenia. Decreases in platelet counts, usually to 50 000 to 100 000/mm³, infrequently lower, have been observed occasionally during treatment with tamoxifen. However, no hemorrhagic tendency has been reported, and the platelet counts returned to normal levels even though treatment with tamoxifen was continued.

Transient decreases in leukocytes also have been observed occasionally during treatment. Although it was uncertain if these occasional incidences of leukopenia and thrombocytopenia were due to tamoxifen therapy, complete blood counts, including platelet counts, should be obtained periodically.

As with other additive hormonal therapy (estrogens and androgens), hypercalcemia has been reported in some breast cancer patients with bone metastases within a few weeks of starting treatment with tamoxifen. Any symptoms suggestive of hypercalcemia should be evaluated promptly. Patients who have metastatic bone disease should have periodic serum calcium determinations during the first few weeks of tamoxifen therapy. If hypercalcemia is present, appropriate measures should be taken and, if severe, tamoxifen should be discontinued.

The first patient follow-up should be done within 1 month following initiation of treatment. Thereafter, examinations may be performed at 1- to 2-month intervals.

Bone pain, if it should occur, may require the use of analgesics.

An increased incidence of endometrial cancer and uterine sarcoma (mostly malignant mixed Mullerian tumors) has been reported in association with tamoxifen treatment. The incidence and pattern of this increase suggest that the underlying mechanism may be related to estrogenic properties of tamoxifen. Any patients receiving tamoxifen or having previously received tamoxifen who report abnormal gynecological symptoms, especially vaginal bleeding, should be promptly investigated.

In clinical studies, the median duration of treatment before the onset of a definite objective response has been 2 months. However, approximately 25% of patients who eventually responded were treated for 4 or more months before a definite objective response was recorded.

The duration of treatment with tamoxifen will depend on the patient's response. The drug should be continued as long as there is a favourable response (see Dosage).

With obvious disease progression, the drug should be discontinued. However, because an occasional patient will have a local disease flare (see Adverse Effects) or an increase in bone pain shortly after starting tamoxifen, it is sometimes difficult during the first few weeks of treatment to determine whether the patient's disease is progressing or whether it will stabilize or respond to continued treatment. There are data to suggest that, if possible, treatment should not be discontinued before a minimum of 3 to 4 weeks.

Drug Interactions: When tamoxifen is used in combination with coumarin-type anticoagulants, a significant increase in anticoagulant effect may occur. Where such coadministration exists, careful monitoring of the patient's prothrombin time is recommended.

When tamoxifen is used in combination with cytotoxic agents, there is increased risk of thromboembolic events occurring.

The use of tamoxifen in combination with an aromatase inhibitor as adjuvant therapy has not shown improved efficacy compared with tamoxifen alone.

The known principal pathway for tamoxifen metabolism in humans is demethylation, catalyzed by CYP3A4 enzymes. A pharmacokinetic interaction with the CYP3A4 inducing agent rifampicin, involving a reduction in tamoxifen plasma levels, has been reported in the literature. The relevance of this to clinical practice is not known.

Pharmacokinetic interaction with CYP2D6 inhibitors, showing a reduction in plasma level of an active tamoxifen metabolite, 4-hydroxy-N-desmethyltamoxifen (endoxifen), has been reported in the literature. Chronic use of CYP2D6 inhibitors can lead to reduced plasma concentrations of an active metabolite. Reduced efficacy on tamoxifen has been reported with concomitant usage of some SSRI antidepressants (e.g. paroxetine) (see Warnings).

Pediatric: The use of tamoxifen is not recommended in children, as safety and efficacy have not been established.

Lactation: It is not known if tamoxifen is excreted in human milk and, therefore, the drug is not recommended during lactation. The decision either to discontinue nursing or discontinue tamoxifen should take into account the importance of the drug to the mother.

Occupational Hazards: Effect on Ability to Drive and Use Machinery: There is no evidence that tamoxifen results in impairment of these activities.

ADVERSE EFFECTS: Side effects can be classified as either due to the pharmacological action of the drug, e.g., hot flushes, vaginal discharge, pruritus vulvae, or those requiring further investigations, such as vaginal bleeding (to exclude the possibility of endometrial malignancy) and tumor flare (to exclude the possibility of progressive disease). Side effects can also be classified as more general in nature such as gastrointestinal intolerance (including such events as nausea, vomiting, constipation and diarrhea), headache, light-headedness and occasionally fluid retention and alopecia. When such side effects are severe, it may be possible to control them by a simple reduction of dosage (within the recommended dose range) without loss of control of the disease (see Table 1).

Skin rashes (including isolated reports of erythema multiforme, Stevens-Johnson syndrome, cutaneous vasculitis, and bullous pemphigoid) and rare hypersensitivity reactions, including angioedema have been reported.

Increased bone and tumour pain and also local disease flare have occurred. These are sometimes associated with a good tumour response. Patients with soft tissue disease may have sudden increases in the size of pre-existing lesions, sometimes associated with marked erythema within and surrounding the lesions, and/or the development of new lesions. When they occur, the bone pain or disease flare are seen shortly after starting tamoxifen and generally subside rapidly. A small number of patients with bony metastases have developed hypercalcaemia on initiation of therapy.

A number of cases of visual disturbances, including retinal crystals, macular oedema, keratopathy, infrequent reports of corneal changes and retinopathy have been described in patients receiving Nolvadex therapy. An increased incidence of cataracts has been reported in association with the administration of Nolvadex. Cases of optic neuropathy and optic neuritis have been reported in patients receiving tamoxifen and, in a small number of cases, blindness has occurred.

Uterine fibroids, endometriosis and other endometrial changes including hyperplasia and polyps have been reported.

Falls in platelet count, usually only to 80 000 to 90 000 per cu mm but occasionally lower, have been reported in patients taking tamoxifen.

Leukopenia has been observed following the administration of tamoxifen, sometimes in association with anemia and/or thrombocytopenia. Neutropenia has been reported on rare occasions; this can sometimes be severe, and cases of agranulocytosis have been reported.

There is evidence of an increased incidence of ischemic cerebrovascular events, thromboembolic events, including deep vein thrombosis and pulmonary embolism, during tamoxifen therapy (see Warnings). In the prevention setting, treatment with tamoxifen has been associated with an increased risk of stroke (see Warnings). When tamoxifen is used in combination with cytotoxic agents, there is an increased risk of thromboembolic events occurring.

Leg cramps have been reported commonly in patients receiving tamoxifen.

Very rarely, cases of interstitial pneumonitis have been reported.

Elevation of alanine aminotransferase (ALT), aspartate aminotransferase (AST) and gamma-glutamyl transpeptidase (GGT) levels has been reported infrequently during tamoxifen citrate therapy, and on rare occasions with a spectrum of more severe liver abnormalities, including fatty liver, cholestasis and hepatitis. Very rarely, cases of hepatic cyst and peliosis hepatitis have also been reported.

Rarely, elevation of serum triglyceride levels, in some cases with pancreatitis, may be associated with the use of tamoxifen.

Cystic ovarian swellings have occasionally been observed in premenopausal women receiving tamoxifen.

An increased incidence of endometrial cancer and uterine sarcoma (mostly malignant mixed Mullerian tumors) has been reported in association with tamoxifen treatment.

Other adverse reactions which are seen infrequently are depression and distaste for food.

OVERDOSE:

Symptoms: Acute overdosage in humans has not been reported. Possible overdosage effects might include hot flashes, nausea, vomiting and vaginal bleeding.

There have been reports in the literature that tamoxifen given at several times the standard dose may be associated with prolongation of the QT interval of the ECG.

Treatment: No specific treatment for overdosage is known and treatment must be symptomatic.

In the case of accidental ingestion by a child, gastric emptying is suggested.

For management of a suspected drug overdose, contact your regional Poison Control Centre. See the *CPS* Directory section for a list of Poison Control Centres.

DOSAGE: The recommended daily dose is 20 to 40 mg in a single or two divided doses. The lowest effective dose should be used. In early disease, the recommended duration of therapy is 5 years. The optimal duration of therapy remains to be determined.

Pediatric: The use of tamoxifen is not recommended in children, as safety and efficacy have not been established.

Table 1: Nolvadex-D
Adverse Drug Reactions (ADR) Seen with Nolvadex-D

Frequency	System	ADR
Very common	Vascular	Hot flushes
Common	Vascular	Ischemic cerebrovascular events Thromboembolic events, including deep vein thrombosis and pulmonary embolism
	Reproductive and Breast	Vaginal bleeding Vaginal discharge Pruritus vulvae Endometrial changes (including hyperplasia and polyps)
	Gastrointestinal	Gastrointestinal intolerance
	Dermatologic	Alopecia Skin rash
	Nervous	Headache Light-headedness
	General	Tumor flare Fluid retention
	Musculoskeletal	Leg cramps
Uncommon	Ophthalmologic	Cataracts Retinopathy
	Reproductive and Breast	Uterine fibroids Endometrial cancer
	General	Hypersensitivity, including angioedema
	Investigations	Thrombocytopenia Leukopenia Neutropenia Anaemia Changes in liver enzymes Elevated triglycerides
Rare	Dermatologic	Cutaneous vasculitis[a]
	Ophthalmologic	Corneal changes Optic neuropathy Optic neuritis
	Reproductive and Breast	Uterine sarcoma (mostly malignant mixed Mullerian tumors) Endometriosis Ovarian cysts
	Gastrointestinal	Pancreatitis
	Hepatic and Biliary	Fatty liver Cholestasis Hepatitis
	Investigations	Hypercalcaemia (not including tumor flare) Agranulocytosis[a]
Very rare	Pulmonary	Interstitial pneumonitis
	Dermatologic	Erythema multiforme Stevens-Johnson syndrome Bullous pemphigoid

[a] Exact frequency not known but known to occur at ≤0.1% from the ATAC study (A Randomized, Double Blind Trial Comparing Arimidex to Nolvadex).

The frequency definitions are: Very common (>10%); Common (>1–≤10%); Uncommon (>0.1%–≤1%), Rare (>0.01–≤0.1%); Very rare (≤0.01%).

INFORMATION FOR THE PATIENT: Published in e-CPS, available by subscription at www.e-cps.ca.

SUPPLIED: Each off-white to white, octagonal, film-coated, biconvex tablet, intagliated with NOLVADEX-D on one face and plain on the reverse, contains: tamoxifen citrate 30.4 mg equivalent to 20 mg of tamoxifen. Nonmedicinal ingredients: cornstarch, croscarmellose sodium, gelatin, lactose, macrogol 300, magnesium stearate, methylhydroxypropylcellulose and titanium dioxide. Blister packs of 30. Store at room temperature (15 to 30°C) protected from light.

Norepinephrine Bitartrate Injection USP

norepinephrine bitartrate

Sympathomimetic

Sandoz

SUPPLIED: Each mL of solution contains: norepinephrine base 1 mg (norepinephrine bitartrate 1.88 mg). Nonmedicinal ingredients: hydrochloric acid and/or sodium hydroxide to adjust pH, sodium chloride for isotonicity, sodium metabisulfite and water for injection. Single use vials of 4 mL, boxes of 10. Store between 15 and 30°C.

Norflex™

orphenadrine citrate

Skeletal Muscle Relaxant

Graceway

PHARMACOLOGY: The mode of therapeutic action has not been clearly identified but may be related to its analgesic properties. Orphenadrine citrate also possesses anticholinergic actions. Norflex is an extended release formulation that gives a peak level of 60 ng/mL at 8 hours following a 100 mg dose, as opposed to an immediate release product that gives a peak of 100 ng/mL at 3 hours following the same dose. The apparent half-life of Norflex is 18 hours.

INDICATIONS: Acute skeletal muscle spasm.

CONTRAINDICATIONS: Stenosing peptic ulcers, prostatic hypertrophy, glaucoma, pyloric or duodenal obstruction, bladder neck obstruction, cardiospasm and myasthenia gravis. Hypersensitivity to orphenadrine.

WARNINGS: No data supplied by the manufacturer.

PRECAUTIONS: Use with caution in patients with cardiac decompensation, coronary insufficiency, cardiac arrhythmias and tachycardia. The concurrent use of orphenadrine and propoxyphene need not be avoided when indicated. If toxic CNS effects occur, they are probably due to either drug alone and require a reduction in the dose or discontinuation of one or both agents.

Safety of continuous long-term therapy with orphenadrine has not been established. Therefore, if orphenadrine is prescribed for prolonged use, periodic monitoring of blood, urine and liver values is recommended.

Occupational Hazards: Some patients may experience transient episodes of light-headedness, dizziness or syncope. Orphenadrine may impair the ability of the patient to engage in potentially hazardous activities such as operating machinery or driving a motor vehicle; ambulatory patients should therefore be cautioned accordingly.

Pregnancy: Safe use of orphenadrine has not been established with respect to adverse effects upon fetal development. Therefore, orphenadrine should be used in women of childbearing potential and particularly during early pregnancy only when the potential benefits outweigh the possible hazards.

Children: Safety and effectiveness in children have not been established; therefore, this drug is not recommended for use in the pediatric age group.

ADVERSE EFFECTS: Mainly due to the mild anticholinergic action of orphenadrine, and are usually associated with higher dosage. Dryness of the mouth is the first untoward effect to appear. When the daily dose is increased, possible adverse effects include: tachycardia, palpitation, urinary hesitancy or retention, blurred vision, dilatation of the pupil, increased ocular tension, weakness, nausea, vomiting, headache, dizziness, constipation and drowsiness and rarely, urticaria and other dermatoses. Infrequently, an elderly patient may experience some degree of mental confusion. These adverse effects can usually be eliminated by reduction in the dosage. Two cases of aplastic anemia associated with the use of orphenadrine citrate tablets have been reported. No causal relationship has been established.

OVERDOSE:
No data supplied by the manufacturer.

> For management of a suspected drug overdose, CPhA recommends that you contact your **regional Poison Control Centre**. See the *CPS* Directory section for a list of Poison Control Centres.

DOSAGE: Average adult dose, 60 mg i.v. or i.m. Orally, 100 mg twice daily.

SUPPLIED: Ampuls: Each 2 mL ampul contains: orphenadrine citrate 60 mg. Nonmedicinal ingredients: sodium bisulfite, sodium chloride, sodium hydroxide and water for injection, USP. Ampuls of 2 mL, boxes of 6.

Tablets: Each white, unscored tablet, imprinted with "3M" on one side and "221" imprinted on the other side, contains: orphenadrine citrate 100 mg in an extended release formulation. Nonmedicinal ingredients: calcium stearate, ethylcellulose and lactose. Tartrazine-free. Bottles of 100 and 500.

Store at controlled room temperature (15 to 30°C).

Norfloxacin Ⓟ

CPhA Monograph

see *Fluoroquinolones*

Noritate® Ⓟ

metronidazole

Antirosacea Agent

sanofi-aventis

Date of Revision: September 29, 2008

PHARMACOLOGY: Metronidazole topical cream is particularly effective against the inflammatory papulopustular component of rosacea. The mechanisms by which metronidazole acts in reducing inflammatory lesions of rosacea are unknown, but may include an antibacterial and/or an anti-inflammatory effect.

INDICATIONS: For topical application in the treatment of inflammatory papules, pustules and erythema of rosacea.

CONTRAINDICATIONS: In individuals with a history of hypersensitivity to metronidazole, parabens or other ingredients of the formulation.

WARNINGS: Avoid contact with eyes.

Studies in rats and mice have provided some evidence that metronidazole may cause tumors in these species when administered orally for a long period at high doses. The relevance of these findings in humans undergoing topical treatment with metronidazole is not known.

The mutagenic potential of metronidazole was tested in two ways: the dominant lethal test in mammalian germ cells, which yielded negative results, and a test using a bacterial indicator strain, which yielded positive results. The inherent antimicrobial property of metronidazole complicates the interpretation of this result with respect to any possible risk to humans.

Children: Safety and effectiveness in children have not been established.

Pregnancy: There has been no experience to date with the use of Noritate in pregnant patients. Systemically administered metronidazole crosses the placental barrier and enters the fetal circulation rapidly. No fetotoxicity was observed after oral administration of metronidazole in rats or mice. However, because animal reproduction studies are not always predictive of the human response, this drug should be used during pregnancy only after careful assessment of the risk/benefit ratio.

Lactation: Even though metronidazole blood levels are significantly lower after topical than after oral administration, a decision should be made whether to discontinue nursing or to discontinue the drug, taking into account the importance of the drug to the mother. After oral administration, metronidazole is secreted in breast milk in concentrations similar to those found in plasma.

PRECAUTIONS: Because of the minimal absorption of metronidazole and consequently its insignificant plasma concentration after topical administration, the adverse experiences reported with the oral form of the drug have not been reported with Noritate.

General: Metronidazole has been reported to cause tearing of the eyes. Therefore, contact with the eyes should be avoided. If a reaction suggesting local irritation occurs, patients should be directed to use the medication less frequently, discontinue use temporarily or discontinue use until further instructions. Metronidazole is a nitroimidazole and should be used with care in patients with evidence of, or a history of, blood dyscrasia. Although rosacea is a chronic disease, data on the long-term use of metronidazole in rosacea are not available. In controlled clinical trials, patients were treated for a maximum 2 months (see Dosage).

Drug Interactions: Drug interactions are less likely with topical administration, but should be kept in mind when metronidazole is prescribed for patients who are receiving anticoagulant treatment. Oral metronidazole has been reported to potentiate the anticoagulant effect of coumarin and warfarin resulting in a prolongation of prothrombin time. Oral metronidazole also interacts with alcohol, producing a disulfiram-like reaction. Although this response has never been reported with topically applied metronidazole, an interaction with alcohol may be a possibility.

Dermatological Sensitivity: During clinical trials, there were 3 reports of possible contact dermatitis during treatment with metronidazole. Sensitivity to metronidazole was confirmed in only 1 of these patients by re-challenging with the product. In the other patients, a clear causal relationship could not be established. Nevertheless, physicians should be aware of the possibility of skin sensitivity reactions to metronidazole and/or of cross-sensitization with other imidazole preparations, such as clotrimazole and tioconazole.

ADVERSE EFFECTS: Adverse conditions reported included transient skin irritation, dryness and stinging, as well as three cases of possible contact dermatitis. The incidence of these dermatological effects was about 3 to 4% during clinical trials.

Watering or tearing eyes may also occur if metronidazole is applied too closely to this area.

Gastrointestinal side effects (nausea, constipation, gastrointestinal upset) were reported in 7 patients (less than 2% of the total clinical experience with Noritate).

Table 1 provides specific information about the adverse effects observed during the two controlled clinical trials in which a total of 99 patients received metronidazole.

Table 1: Noritate

Adverse Effects Observed During Controlled Clinical Trials

Body System/Adverse Effect	Severity	Incidence (No. of Patients)	Course of Action Taken
Skin			
Burning Sensation	Mild Moderate	1 1	None required None required
Pruritus	Mild	2	None required
Pruritus/Erythema/Burning	Mild/Moderate	1	None required
Erythema	Mild	1	None required
Oily Skin	Mild	1	None required
Photosensitivity	Moderate	1	None required
Papular Rash	Mild	1	Drug discontinued
Contact Dermatitis	Moderate Severe	1 2	Drug discontinued Drug discontinued
Gastrointestinal			
Nausea	Mild Moderate	1 1	None required None required
Burping	Mild	1	None required
Gastrointestinal Upset	Mild Severe	1 2	None required Drug discontinued[a]
Gastrointestinal Cramps/Anorexia	Moderate/Severe	1	Drug discontinued[b]

[a] One of these patients likely received an oral antibiotic.
[b] Patient predisposed to stomach ailments.

OVERDOSE:
There is no human experience with overdosage of topically applied metronidazole cream.

Symptoms: Massive ingestion may produce vomiting and slight disorientation.

Treatment: There is no specific antidote. Ipecac syrup or gastric lavage; then activated charcoal followed by a saline cathartic is suggested. Treatment should include symptomatic and supportive therapy.

For management of a suspected drug overdose, CPhA recommends that you contact your **regional Poison Control Centre**. See the *CPS* Directory section for a list of Poison Control Centres.

DOSAGE: Cleanse all affected areas of the skin. Then, squeeze out approximately ½ cm of metronidazole cream and apply to the entire affected areas twice daily, morning and evening. Rub in lightly.

Significant therapeutic results should be evident within the first month of treatment and controlled clinical studies have demonstrated continuing improvement through 8 weeks of therapy. The dosage required for long-term administration is uncertain (see Precautions).

Patients may use cosmetics after application of metronidazole.

SUPPLIED: Each g of white to slightly off-white soft cream, contains: metronidazole 10 mg (1% w/w). Nonmedicinal ingredients: glycerin, glyceryl monostearate, methylparaben, propylparaben, purified water, stearic acid and triethanolamine. Aluminum tubes of 45 g. Store at room temperature (15 to 30°C).

NorLevo®

levonorgestrel

Emergency Contraception

HRA Pharma

Date of Revision: November 23, 2009

SUMMARY PRODUCT INFORMATION:

Route of Administration	Dosage Form/ Strength	Clinically Relevant Nonmedicinal Ingredients
Oral	Tablets 0.75 mg	Lactose monohydrate, maize starch, povidone For a complete listing see Dosage Forms, Composition and Packaging.

INDICATIONS AND CLINICAL USE: NorLevo (levonorgestrel 0.75 mg tablets) is an emergency contraceptive intended to be used within 72 hours following known or suspected contraceptive failure or unprotected intercourse such as:

- ruptured or forgotten condom;
- missed oral contraceptive pill;
- expelled intrauterine device;
- early removal or dislodgment of a vaginal diaphragm or of a contraceptive cap;
- failure of the coitus interruptus method;
- sexual intercourse during the supposedly fertile period when relying on periodic abstinence (temperature method);
- rape.

Treatment should not be delayed as efficacy declines with an increased interval between intercourse and the start of the treatment. When initiated within 24 hours of unprotected intercourse NorLevo prevents 95% of expected pregnancies. When initiated within 24-48 h or 48-72 hours, it prevents 85 % and 58% of expected pregnancies, respectively. Efficacy after 72 hours is unknown.

The pregnancy rate of levonorgestrel 0.75 mg tablets is calculated for a single use. If NorLevo is used on more than one occasion, the cumulative pregnancy rate may be higher. NorLevo is not recommended for routine use as a contraceptive.

NorLevo will not prevent pregnancy from future acts of unprotected intercourse. Following use of this product, the woman should either abstain or use an alternative contraceptive method until her next menstrual cycle.

Note to Pharmacist: If you judge that a woman is a repeat user of Emergency Contraception (defined as use more than once a month on a regular basis) or that NorLevo has been used within the past cycle, you should consider discussing other, more effective contraceptive methods with the woman, as well as encouraging her to see her physician or other health care provider for contraceptive counselling services and advise on other methods of contraception and prevention of sexually transmitted infections. NorLevo should be dispensed if indicated.

Geriatrics: NorLevo has not been studied in this population.

Pediatrics: NorLevo has not been studied in this population.

CONTRAINDICATIONS:

- NorLevo is contraindicated in women with hypersensitivity to the active substance levonorgestrel or any of the excipients. For a complete listing, see Dosage Forms, Composition and Packaging.
- NorLevo (levonorgestrel tablets) 0.75 mg is contraindicated in women with known or suspected pregnancy. If there is a doubt regarding pregnancy following a previous act of intercourse, especially if there is recent abnormal bleeding, a pregnancy test should be performed before taking NorLevo.

Progestin-only oral contraceptives are used as a routine method of birth control over longer periods of time, and are contraindicated in some conditions (acute liver disease or history of or actual benign or malignant liver tumors, known or suspected carcinoma of the breast and undiagnosed abnormal vaginal bleeding). It is not known whether these same conditions apply to the NorLevo regimen consisting of the emergency use of two progestin pills, but these risks should be considered if NorLevo needs to be administered several times.

WARNINGS AND PRECAUTIONS: General: NorLevo is not effective in terminating an existing pregnancy.

Emergency contraception is an **occasional** method. It should in no instance replace a regular contraceptive method. Repeated administration within a menstrual cycle is not advisable, because of an undesirable high load of hormones for the patient and the possibility of severe disturbances of the cycle. Emergency contraception does not prevent a pregnancy from occurring in every instance, especially if uncertain about the timing of the unprotected intercourse.

The use of NorLevo does not protect against HIV infections (AIDS) and other sexually transmitted diseases.

The use of cyclic combination oral contraceptives containing estrogen and progestin is associated with increased risks of several serious conditions including hepatic neoplasia and gallbladder disease. NorLevo does not contain estrogen. While these conditions have not been associated with the routine use of progestin-only oral contraceptives, it is unknown if the use of short-term high-dose progestin-only contraceptives (a single 1.5 mg dose of levonorgestrel) would accentuate the risk.

Cardiovascular: The use of cyclic combination oral contraceptives containing estrogen and progestin is also associated with increased risks of thromboembolic and cardiovascular disorders (e.g. thrombophlebitis, pulmonary embolism, cerebrovascular disorders, myocardial ischemia, mesenteric thrombosis, and retinal thrombosis).

NorLevo does not contain estrogen. These conditions have not been associated with the routine use of progestin-only oral contraceptives, but whether short-term use of high-dose progestin-only contraceptives (2 doses of 0.75 mg levonorgestrel, taken at once) would accentuate the risk is unknown. Controlled clinical trials using levonorgestrel for postcoital and emergency contraception have not identified any serious cardiovascular adverse reactions. There have been reports of thrombotic events during the postmarketing period, however a causal relationship with NorLevo treatment has not been determined.

Sexual Function/Reproduction: Effects on Menses: Some women may experience spotting a few days after taking levonorgestrel as an emergency contraceptive. At the time of expected menses, approximately 75% of women using levonorgestrel had vaginal bleeding similar to their normal menses, 12-13% bled more than usual, and 12% bled less than usual. Approximately 75 % of women had their next menstrual period earlier than expected, on time, or just slightly later than expected. However, in 19.9 % of women, menses was delayed by more than 7 days. **If there is a delay in the onset of menses beyond 5-7 days, a pregnancy test is recommended.**

Ectopic Pregnancy: Ectopic pregnancies account for approximately 2% of reported pregnancies. It is not known to what extent NorLevo prevents implantation of an ectopic pregnancy and one cannot exclude that an ectopic pregnancy continues to develop despite the occurrence of uterine bleeding. Therefore, NorLevo is not recommended for patients who are at risk of ectopic pregnancy (previous history of salpingitis or of ectopic pregnancy). Physicians should be alert to the possibility of an ectopic pregnancy in women who become pregnant or complain of lower abdominal pain after taking NorLevo.

Suspected Pregnancy: A pregnancy test and/or a physical examination are warranted if pregnancy is suspected (see Effects on Menses). Women should be counselled to abstain from sexual intercourse or use an alternative contraceptive method until the onset of their next normal menstrual period after NorLevo intake. If a normal menstrual period is delayed by more than 5-7 days of its expected date, after NorLevo has been used, a pregnancy test should be performed. Counseling on routine contraception for future use should be provided as appropriate.

Special Populations: Pregnant Women: This medicinal product is not indicated in case of pre-existing pregnancy and cannot interrupt it. Several epidemiological studies have shown no increase in congenital malformation risk after failure of regular contraceptive pills, some of which contained levonorgestrel. In case of failure of this treatment with persisting pregnancy, only few pregnancies brought to term and documented were available and no increased risk of congenital abnormalities was observed.

Nursing Women: Levonorgestrel is secreted into breast milk. Therefore, it is suggested to breastfeed immediately before taking the NorLevo tablets and to skip the nursing following NorLevo administration for at least 8 hours. Discard the extracted milk during this period.

Pediatrics: NorLevo has not been studied in this population.

Geriatrics: NorLevo has not been studied in this population.

Monitoring and Laboratory Tests: Pathologists should be advised about recent oral contraceptive therapy when specimens obtained from Pap smears are submitted for examination.

ADVERSE REACTIONS: Adverse Drug Reaction Overview: The most frequent undesirable effects are nausea, low abdominal pain, headache, fatigue and dizziness. Vomiting is reported in less than 8 percent of women. These effects usually disappear within 48 hours after levonorgestrel intake. Breast tenderness is reported in 5 to 21 percent of patients, bleeding (including spotting) is reported in 28 to 31 percent of patients; both can last until the next menstrual period. Delayed menses (greater than 7 days) is reported in up to 24 % of patients.

Cutaneous hypersensitivity revealed by common rash (urticaria, erythema, scaling irritation), pruritus or rare severe allergic reactions (acute angioedema, extensive urticaria, mouth oedema) have been reported after the intake of NorLevo.

Clinical Trial Adverse Drug Reactions: Because clinical trials are conducted under very specific conditions the adverse reaction rates observed in the clinical trials may not reflect the rates observed in practice and should not be compared to the rates in the clinical trials of another drug. Adverse drug reaction information from clinical trials is useful for identifying drug-related adverse events and for approximating rates.

Table 1 gives the frequency of undesirable effects reported in two clinical trials and two post-marketing observational (Actual Use) studies.

Table 1: NorLevo

Percent of Women with Undesirable Effects After the Intake of 1.5 mg of Levonorgestrel in a Single Administration

	Clinical Trials		Post-marketing Observational Studies	
Effect	**Trial 1 n=544[a]**	**Trial 2 n=1359[b]**	**Observational Study 1 n=242[c]**	**Observational Study 2 n=299[d]**
Nausea	24.3%	14%	19%	13%
Low abdominal pain	15.6%	14%	29%	17%
Fatigue	NR	14%	28%	20%
Headache	21.3%	10%	22%	25%

(cont'd)

Table 1: NorLevo *(cont'd)*

Percent of Women with Undesirable Effects After the Intake of 1.5 mg of Levonorgestrel in a Single Administration

Effect	Clinical Trials		Post-marketing Observational Studies	
	Trial 1 n=544[a]	Trial 2 n=1359[b]	Observational Study 1 n=242[c]	Observational Study 2 n=299[d]
Dizziness	12.6%	10%	NR	NR
Breast tenderness	12.9%	8%	21%	5%
Vomiting	7.8%	1%	NR	2%
Heavy menses	15.5%	NR	NR	NR
Diarrhea	NR	4%	NR	7%
Bleeding	NR	31%	28%	28%
Delay of menses	19.9%[e]	5%	18%	24%
Sun sensitivity	NR	NR	3%	NR
Paresthesia of the lower limbs	NR	NR	4%	5%

[a] 1062 women have been evaluated for the adverse events, of these 1062 women, only 544 received a single dose of 1.5 mg of levonorgestrel.
[b] 4071 women participated in this study, of these 4071 women, only 1359 women received a single dose of 1.5 mg of levonorgestrel.
[c] 528 women were interviewed (data from pharmacies), of these 528 women, only 242 women received a single dose of 1.5 mg of levonorgestrel.
[d] 409 women were interviewed (data from family planning organisations), of these 409 women, only 299 women received a single dose of 1.5 mg of levonorgestrel.
[e] Delay defined as more than 7 days.
Legend: NR: No record.

The safety data analysis of reported side effects from the efficacy studies indicates that levonorgestrel is safe with an acceptable number of mild to moderate undesirable experiences. The most frequent adverse experiences were nausea, vomiting, dizziness, fatigue and headache. The incidence of adverse events was lower in the levonorgestrel groups than in the Yuzpe regimen groups. However, some adverse events such as breast tenderness and inter-menstrual bleeding or spotting were found with similar incidence in both groups. In the Grimes 1998 WHO study, one case of fatal meningitis was reported without any relationship to levonorgestrel.

In the WHO study comparing the two regimens of levonorgestrel (second intake 12 hours and 24 hours after the first intake), the occurrence of diarrhoea and breast tenderness was more frequent in the 12-hour group ($p<0.05$). The incidence of the other side effects was otherwise similar between the two groups.

An open labelled study was performed in Edinburg (UK). The primary end-point was the tolerance to NorLevo when used in regular clinical settings. Women were eligible as long as they requested an Emergency Contraception, and were not pregnant. After treatment with NorLevo (one 0.75 mg tablet to be repeated 12 hours later) women were asked to fill a diary card during the 7 days post treatment. They were asked to attend a control visit after the expected date of the next menstrual periods.

Of the 400 enrolled, 286 women accepted to fill the diary card. The frequency range of the reported symptoms during the first 4 days were: nausea (4.2-21%), fatigue (6.6-17.5%), headache (4.9-11.5%), tender breast (4.9-7.3%), dizziness (0.7-5.9%) and spotting (2.4-4.2%). The incidence of vomiting was very low. The mean length of the cycle was 28 days. In only 15 percent of the women, the onset of menstrual periods was delayed by more than 5 days. No other specific side effect was reported during this study.

In a double-blind study, the two-dose regimen levonorgestrel 0.75 mg taken 12 h apart (group A) and levonorgestrel 1.5 mg taken in a single dose administration (group B) were studied in 1118 volunteers for emergency contraception. From the 1118 women analyzed, only 1062 subjects (518 in group A and 544 in group B) provided enough information to be assessed for side effects and timing of next menses. The side effects observed after treatment were nausea, vomiting, headache, breast tenderness, lower abdominal pain, and menorrhagia. Women in group A had more frequent vomiting, dizziness and lower abdominal pain and less nausea, headache, breast tenderness, and increased menstrual flow than those in group B.

In a double-blind WHO study compared the efficacy and safety of a single 10 mg dose of mifepristone (group A), two 0.75 mg doses of levonorgestrel 12 hours apart (group B) and a single dose of 1.5 mg levonorgestrel (group C) in 4136 healthy women. There are no significant difference between the side-effects observed in group B and C.

From all of these studies, no embryo or fetal disorders were reported in the women who continued their pregnancy and for whom follow-up information was available.

Post-Market Adverse Drug Reactions: The safety profile of NorLevo, based on the post-marketing spontaneous reports, does not differ from the one observed in the clinical trials. In the last periodic safety update report (April 17, 2005–April 16, 2008), the most commonly spontaneously reported adverse drug reactions were: unintended pregnancy, metrorrhagia, nausea, fatigue, menstruation delayed, dizziness, abdominal pain and headache.

There have been reports of thrombotic events (e.g. venous thromboembolism, pulmonary embolism) during the postmarketing period, however a causal relationship with NorLevo treatment has not been determined.

DRUG INTERACTIONS: Overview: The metabolism of levonorgestrel is enhanced by the concomitant use of liver enzyme inducers: anticonvulsant (phenobarbital, phenytoin, primidone, carbamazepine); rifabutin; rifampicin; griseofulvin; ritonavir; Hypericum perforatum (St. John's wort). As the efficacy of NorLevo may be decreased in case of concomitant intake of these drugs, it is recommended that patients perform a pregnancy test 2 to 3 weeks after NorLevo intake.

Drug-Drug Interactions: As mentioned in the overview above, the metabolism of levonorgestrel is enhanced by the concomitant use of certain drugs such as anticonvulsant (phenobarbital, phenytoin, primidone, carbamazepine), rifabutin, rifampicin, griseofulvin and ritonavir. Acetaminophen was tested for potential interactions but none were observed with levonorgestrel.

As the efficacy of NorLevo may be decreased in case of concomitant intake of these drugs, it is recommended that patients perform a pregnancy test 2 to 3 weeks after NorLevo intake.

Drug-Food Interactions: No formal pharmacokinetic studies of the effects of food have been performed. Efficacy is presumed to be independent of the timing of meals.

Drug-Herb Interactions: The concomitant use of Hypericum perforatum (St. John's wort) can decrease the efficacy of NorLevo.

As the efficacy of NorLevo may be decreased in case of concomitant intake of these drugs, it is recommended that patients perform a pregnancy test if there is a delay in the onset of menses beyond 5-7 days.

Drug-Laboratory Test Interactions: Interactions between laboratory tests and levonorgestrel have not been established.

Use of oral contraceptives can modify the results of laboratory tests. Laboratory test should therefore be done prior to dosing or more than 3 days after dosing to avoid misinterpretation of the results. Pathologists should be advised about oral contraceptive therapy when specimens obtained from Pap smears are submitted for examination.

DOSAGE AND ADMINISTRATION: Dosing Considerations: NorLevo can be taken at any moment during the menstrual cycle.

Recommended Dose and Dosage Adjustment: Two tablets of NorLevo (0.75 mg levonorgestrel) should be taken simultaneously for a total dose of 1.5 mg levonorgestrel. The efficacy of the treatment is higher the sooner after the unprotected intercourse it is initiated. Therefore, the tablets must be taken **as soon as possible, preferably within 12 hours, after the unprotected intercourse** and no longer than 72 hours (3 days) after the intercourse.

In case of vomiting taking place within three hours after intake of NorLevo, the patient should make sure that the two tablets are found in the content of the vomit. If this is the case, and only then, it is recommended that an additional dose (2 tablets) be taken immediately.

After using an emergency contraception, it is recommended to use a barrier contraceptive method (condom, spermicide, cervical cap) until the next menstrual period resumes (see Warnings and Precautions). The use of NorLevo does not contraindicate the continuation of regular hormonal contraception.

OVERDOSAGE:
Serious effects have not been reported following acute ingestion of large doses of oral contraceptives. Overdose may cause nausea and withdrawal bleeding may occur. There are no specific antidotes and treatment should be symptomatic.

> For management of a suspected drug overdose, CPhA recommends that you contact your **regional Poison Control Centre**. See the *CPS* Directory section for a list of Poison Control Centres.

ACTION AND CLINICAL PHARMACOLOGY: Mechanism of Action: The precise mode of action of levonorgestrel is not fully understood. Published studies suggest that at the regimen of two 0.75 mg tablets, taken in a single administration, levonorgestrel acts mainly by suppressing or delaying ovulation thus preventing fertilization if the intercourse has taken place in the preovulatory phase when the likelihood of fertilization is the highest. It is not effective once the process of implantation has begun. Other mechanisms may also be involved.

Pharmacokinetics: The absolute bioavailability of levonorgestrel in humans has not been specifically investigated. However, levonorgestrel is reported in the literature to be rapidly and completely absorbed following oral administration and does not undergo first pass metabolism. In the plasma, it is strongly bound to SHBG. Levonorgestrel is hydroxylated in the liver, and its metabolites are excreted as glucuronide and sulphate conjugates eliminated mostly in urine and, to a lesser extent, in feces.

A pharmacokinetic study with levonorgestrel was performed to compare its plasma profile relative to different dosing regimen. This open observer-blind randomized study was performed on 24 healthy Caucasian female volunteers. The latter were randomized into three groups of eight women taking either a single 0.75 mg levonorgestrel tablet (Group B) or two 0.75 mg levonorgestrel tablets 12 hours (Group A) or 24 hours apart (Group C). Plasma levels of levonorgestrel were measured from the time of intake up to 36 hours after this initial intake. Plasma sampling began at the time of intake.

The results showed T_{max} and C_{max} values of 2.50 hr, 2.30 hr, 2.06 hr and 33.1 nmol/L, 30.7 nmol/L, 27.2 nmol/L, for groups A, B and C, respectively. The results of this study also indicated that the absorption, distribution and elimination profiles of levonorgestrel between the different treatments were similar. The maximal concentration of all groups combined was reached within 2.27 hours (±1.17 hr). The plasma half-life was estimated to be approximately 22 hours. The mean plasma concentration of levonorgestrel 24 hours after the first tablet intake was 6.2 nmol/L±5.46 (in both groups B and C combined). Also it indicates that 12 or 24 hours after administration, levonorgestrel plasma levels remain significant.

In another similar pharmacokinetic study, five healthy women received NorLevo tablets in a cross-over fashion according to different schemes. Each woman participated in the three arms of the study with a washout period between treatments of 27-28 days. The treatments were: A: two doses of 0.75 mg levonorgestrel given 12 hours apart; B: two doses of 0.75 mg levonorgestrel given 24 hours apart; C: a single dose of 1.5 mg levonorgestrel (two 0.75 mg tablets).

Maximum concentration levels of approximately 27 nmol/L (for group A and B) and 40 nmol/L (for group C) of levonorgestrel were reached between 1.54 and 1.8 hours (for group A and B) and 2.6 hours (for group C). The peak plasma concentration observed following the second dose, 12 or 24 hours later, was slightly higher than that following first dose (32.8 vs 29.5 nmol/L and 30.0 vs 27.2 nmol/L respectively). By 48 hours, all treatment arms had very similar levonorgestrel levels (6.2-7.4 nmol/L). The total area under the curve (AUC_{total}) was similar for treatment A and B (443.6 vs 432.5 nmol/h) and significantly higher for treatment C (925.0 nmol/h) ($p=0.0003$).

Lactation: A pharmacokinetic study was performed in healthy lactating women volunteers to assay levonorgestrel (LNG) concentrations in plasma and milk following the intake of NorLevo (single tablet containing 1.5 mg levonorgestrel).

Twelve healthy lactating women volunteers on average 25 years old and 11 weeks post-partum participated in the study. Following a screening visit, they pumped breast milk (450 mL per kilogram infant bodyweight) and conserved it frozen to use to feed their babies during the first 72 hours after dosing. Women reported to the clinic with their infants at 08.00-10.00 am the day of the scheduled treatment phase. After collection of pre-dose blood and milk samples, women received one tablet of Norlevo (1.5 mg LNG) with 240 ml water. Milk and plasma LNG levels were measured at 1 (plasma only), 2, 4, 6, 8, 24, 48, 72, 96 and 120 hours after dosing. Plasma sex hormone binding globulin (SHBG) was performed prior to dosing and at 1, 24, 48, 72, 96 and 120 hours post-dosing.

LNG milk concentrations paralleled those of plasma but were lower than plasma concentrations, with an overall mean milk-to-plasma ratio of 0.23±0.09. LNG concentrations increased after dosing to reach a peak between 1 and 4 h in plasma and between 2 and 4 h in milk. The mean LNG concentrations were 15.4 and 6.9 ng/mL in plasma and milk, respectively. The mean terminal half-life of LNG was 29 h in plasma and 26 h in milk. At 120 h after dosing, plasma concentrations (mean±SD) of LNG were still above the lower limit of quantification for all subjects (0.23±0.07 ng/mL), while milk concentrations were very low (0.06±0.4 ng/mL) and reached undetectable levels for two subjects out of twelve.

The amount of LNG excreted in milk over the first 24 h was 0.09% of the dose administered. This amount decreased rapidly with time, with only 0.01% of the given dose recovered in milk over the 49-72 h interval. The concentration of LNG (mean±SD) measured in pooled milk samples was 1.56±0.41 ng/mL on the first day, decreasing to 0.34±0.20 ng/mL on the second day and to 0.20±0.13 ng/mL on the third day. Based on AUC per 24-hour interval, the estimated mean amount of progestin potentially absorbed by an infant suckling about 800 mL of milk per day was 1.6 µg in the 0-24 h interval after dosing (1.0 µg in the first eight hours and 0.6 µg in the interval 8 to 24 hours after dosing), 0.3 µg in the 24-48 h interval and 0.2 µg in the 48-72 h interval. The mean total amount of LNG excreted in milk was 1830±522 ng over the three days following the administration of 1.5 mg LNG.

On average, plasma SHBG concentrations remained essentially unchanged 1 h after LNG dosing (56.3±21.5 nmol/L to 57.5±23.0 nmol/L) and then decreased consistently for all subjects over the 120 h sampling time period to a mean of 35.9±12.8 nmol/L at the 120 h time-point, which corresponds to a mean of 64% of pre-dose values.

These suggest that to limit infant exposure to the period of maximum levonorgestrel excretion in milk, mothers should discontinue nursing for at least 8 h, but not more than 24 h, after emergency contraception.

Special Populations and Conditions: Pediatrics: Due to the nature of the product, no studies have been performed on pediatrics population.

Geriatrics: Due to the nature of the product, no studies have been performed on geriatrics population.

Gender: Studies have been performed with women only.

Race: No differences in safety or efficacy relative to ethnicity have been observed.

Hepatic and Renal Insufficiency: No formal studies have been conducted in patients with hepatic or renal insufficiency. Due to the sporadic administration of NorLevo there are no concerns about the potential accumulation that may occur in patients with hepatic or renal insufficiency.

STORAGE AND STABILITY: NorLevo is stable at room temperature (15-30°C) for the period indicated on the label. Protect from light.

INFORMATION FOR THE PATIENT: Published in e-CPS, available by subscription at www.e-cps.ca.

DOSAGE FORMS, COMPOSITION AND PACKAGING: Each white, round, biconvex tablet with no marking contains: levonorgestrel 0.75 mg. Nonmedicinal ingredients: anhydrous colloidal silica, lactose monohydrate, magnesium stearate, maize starch and povidone. PVC/PE/PVDC/Aluminum blisters of 2 tablets. Pack sizes of 10, 20, 50 or 100 tablets presented in blisters of 2 tablets are available for hospital use.

Normacol®

sterculia

Bulk Laxative

Helix Biopharma

SUPPLIED: Each 7 g sachet of granules contains: sterculia gum equivalent to sterculia BP 62% w/w. Nonmedicinal ingredients: paraffin, sodium bicarbonate, sucrose, talc, titanium dioxide and vanillin. Sucrose: 1.72 g per sachet. Boxes of 30. Store in a cool dry place below 25°C.

Norprolac® ℞
quinagolide HCl
Prolactin Inhibitor

Ferring

Date of Preparation: June 13, 2005
Date of Revision: January 12, 2006

SUMMARY PRODUCT INFORMATION:

Route of Administration	Dosage Form/Strength	Clinically Relevant Nonmedicinal Ingredients
Oral	Tablet 0.025 mg, 0.050 mg, 0.075 mg and 0.150 mg	Silica (colloidal anhydrous), magnesium stearate, methylhydroxy propylcellulose, maize starch, cellulose (microcrystalline), lactose

INDICATIONS AND CLINICAL USE: NORPROLAC is indicated for the treatment of hyperprolactinemia (idiopathic or originating from a prolactin-secreting pituitary microadenoma or macroadenoma).

CONTRAINDICATIONS: Hypersensitivity to the drug and impaired hepatic or renal function. For procedure during pregnancy, see Warnings and Precautions, Pregnant Women.

WARNINGS AND PRECAUTIONS: Warnings: Fertility may be restored in patients receiving treatment with NORPROLAC (quinagolide hydrochloride). Women of child-bearing age who do not wish to conceive should therefore be advised to practice a reliable method of contraception.

Treatment with NORPROLAC may effectively lower prolactin levels in patients with pituitary tumours but does not obviate the necessity for radiotherapy or surgical intervention where appropriate.

Caution should be exercised when administering NORPROLAC to patients with a history of psychotic disorders due to its stimulant effect on D_2 receptors. In a few isolated cases, treatment with NORPROLAC has been associated with the occurrence of acute psychosis, reversible upon discontinuation.

NORPROLAC has been associated with somnolence, and episodes of sudden sleep onset, particularly in patients with Parkinson's disease. Patients must be informed of this and advised not to drive or operate machines if they experience any episodes of sudden sleep onset. Furthermore, if sudden onset of sleep does develop, a reduction of dosage or termination or therapy may be necessary.

Effects on Ability to Drive and Use Machines: Patients being treated with NORPROLAC and presenting with somnolence and/or sudden sleep episodes, must be advised not to drive or engage in activities where impaired alertness may put themselves or others at risk of serious injury or death (e.g. operating machines) until such recurrent episodes and somnolence have resolved.

Precautions: General: Hypotensive reactions may occur during the first few days of treatment with NORPROLAC (quinagolide hydrochloride) and patients should be cautious when driving a vehicle or operating machinery. Since, on rare occasions, orthostatic hypotension may result in syncope, it is recommended to check blood pressure during the first few days of therapy.

Carcinogenesis and Mutagenesis: A 2-year carcinogenicity study was conducted in rats using dietary levels of quinagolide hydrochloride equivalent to oral doses of 0.01, 0.06 and 0.2 mg/kg/day. A 90-week study in mice was conducted using dietary levels equivalent to oral doses of 0.02, 0.1 and 0.4 mg/kg/day. The highest doses tested in rats and mice were approximately 10 and 20 times the maximum human oral dose administered in controlled clinical trials (0.9 mg/day equivalent to 0.02 mg/kg/day).

A low incidence of Leydig-cell adenomas in male rats and mesenchymal uterine tumours in mice was observed. The occurrence of these neoplasms is probably attributable to the high luteinizing hormone secretion and estrogen/progesterone ratio that would occur in rodents as a result of the prolactin-inhibiting action of quinagolide. In addition, quinagolide showed no mutagenic or genotoxic potential in various assay systems investigated. The findings in rats and mice were not shown to be relevant for humans due to the fundamental difference in the regulation of the endocrine system between rodents and humans. However, even though there is no known correlation between testicular tumours and uterine malignancies occurring in quinagolide-treated rodents and human risk, there are no human data to substantiate this conclusion.

Quinagolide was not embryotoxic or teratogenic in rats and rabbits. Hypoprolactinemia was associated with reduced pregnancy rate and inhibition of lactation of rat dams and slightly retarded but otherwise normal development of rat pups.

Special Populations: Pregnant Women: Animal data provide no evidence that NORPROLAC has any embryotoxic or teratogenic potential, but experience in pregnant women is still limited. In patients wishing to conceive, NORPROLAC should be discontinued when pregnancy is confirmed, unless there is a medical reason for continuing therapy. So far, no increased incidence of abortion has been observed following withdrawal of the drug during pregnancy.

If pregnancy occurs in the presence of a pituitary adenoma and NORPROLAC treatment has been stopped, close supervision throughout pregnancy is essential. In patients who show symptoms of tumour enlargement, e.g. visual field deterioration or headache, NORPROLAC treatment may be re-instituted or surgery may be appropriate.

Nursing Women: Owing to its inhibitory effect on prolactin secretion, NORPROLAC suppresses lactation. Therefore, mothers receiving the drug cannot breast-feed.

Pediatrics: Safety and effectiveness in children has not been established.

Monitoring and Laboratory Tests: No specific laboratory tests are deemed essential for the management of patients on NORPROLAC (quinagolide hydrochloride). Periodic routine evaluation of all patients, however, is appropriate.

ADVERSE REACTIONS: The adverse reactions reported with the use of NORPROLAC (quinagolide hydrochloride) are characteristic for dopamine receptor agonist therapy. The most commonly observed adverse events (>10%) reported during clinical trials with NORPROLAC were: nausea, vomiting, headache, dizziness and fatigue. Most of these adverse events occur predominantly during the first few days of the initial treatment or, as a mostly transient event, following dosage increase and are usually not sufficiently serious to require discontinuation of treatment and tend to disappear with continued treatment.

Nausea and Vomiting: Nausea and vomiting may be prevented by the intake of a peripheral dopaminergic antagonist, such as domperidone, for a few days, at least 1 hour before the ingestion of NORPROLAC.

Less frequent side effects (1 to 10%) include anorexia, abdominal pain, constipation or diarrhoea, insomnia, oedema, flushing, nasal congestion and hypotension. Orthostatic hypotension may result in faintness or syncope (see Warnings and Precautions).

In rare cases NORPROLAC has been associated with somnolence.

Relative to the occurrence of the above-mentioned reactions the following adverse reactions have been less frequently observed in clinical trials involving 549 patients during the first month of treatment. Incidence between 0.5 and 3.5%:

Musculoskeletal: painful extremities (0.6%).

Respiratory: nasal congestion (2.4%).

Cardiovascular: hypotension (1.3%), syncope (0.9%), palpitation (0.7%), flushing (0.6%).

Gastrointestinal: constipation (3.4%), abdominal pain (3.3%), dyspepsia (1.5%), abdominal discomfort (3.3%), diarrhoea (0.9%).

Central Nervous System: asthenia (2.9%), anorexia (2.4%), insomnia (2.0%), eye disorders (1.5%), malaise (1.1%), reduced concentration (0.6%).

Miscellaneous: oedema (1.5%), breast pain (0.9%), mood lability (0.9%), sedation (3.3%), weight gain (0.6%).

Abnormal Hematologic and Clinical Chemistry Findings: Laboratory parameters may be affected during treatment with NORPROLAC, but the changes are usually not considered serious. Among the laboratory changes that were reported during clinical trials were increases in bilirubin, serum transaminases, CPK (creatine phosphokinase), potassium, triglycerides and decreases in hematocrit and hemoglobin. These changes were usually transient and rarely of clinical significance.

Only five patients (0.5 %) had to be discontinued from therapy because of laboratory adverse experiences, including one case of neutropenia.

Other: In a few isolated cases, treatment with NORPROLAC has been associated with acute psychosis, reversible upon discontinuation.

Approximately 200 patients have been treated with NORPROLAC for longer than four years. There is no evidence that any type of adverse event occurs more frequently with prolonged treatment.

DRUG INTERACTIONS: No interactions between NORPROLAC and other drugs have so far been reported. On theoretical grounds, a reduction of the prolactin-lowering effect could be expected when drugs (e.g. neuroleptic agents) with strong dopamine antagonist properties are used concomitantly.

NORPROLAC administered concomitantly with antihypertensive agents may have an additive effect on lowering blood pressure. In patients with angina or arrhythmias using antihypertensives, this additional hypotensive effect should be taken into consideration. The tolerability of NORPROLAC may be reduced by alcohol.

DOSAGE AND ADMINISTRATION: NORPROLAC (quinagolide hydrochloride) tablets should be taken once a day at bedtime with a snack. The optimal dose must be titrated individually on the basis of the prolactin-lowering effect and patient tolerability.

Dosing Considerations: Most adverse events occur predominantly during the first few days of treatment, are usually not sufficiently serious to require discontinuation of treatment and tend to disappear with continued treatment.

There is no evidence of reduced tolerance or altered dosage requirements in elderly patients.

Recommended Dose and Dosage Adjustment: With the "starter pack", treatment begins with 0.025 mg/day for the first 3 days, followed by 0.050 mg/day for a further 3 days. From day 7 onwards, the recommended dose is 0.075 mg/day. If necessary, the daily dose may then be increased stepwise at intervals not shorter than 1 week until the optimal individual response is attained. The usual maintenance dosage is 0.075 to 0.150 mg/day. Daily doses of 0.300 mg or higher doses are required in less than one-third of patients. In such cases, the daily dosage may be increased by increments of 0.075 to 0.150 mg at intervals not shorter than 4 weeks. The maximum dose evaluated in efficacy studies was 0.900 mg.

OVERDOSAGE:
No data are available in regard to overdosage in humans with NORPROLAC (quinagolide hydrochloride). However, based on the pharmacological properties of quinagolide, gastrointestinal (nausea, vomiting), CNS (headache, dizziness, drowsiness, hallucinations) and cardiovascular effects (hypotension) might possibly occur. In the event of overdosage, treatment should be symptomatic and supportive.

For management of a suspected drug overdose, CPhA recommends that you contact your **regional Poison Control Centre**. See the *CPS* Directory section for a list of Poison Control Centres.

ACTION AND CLINICAL PHARMACOLOGY: NORPROLAC (quinagolide hydrochloride) is a selective dopamine D2 receptor agonist not belonging to the chemical classes of ergot or ergoline compounds.

NORPROLAC exerts a strong and specific inhibitory effect on prolactin release by acting directly on the prolactin-secreting cells of the anterior pituitary without reducing the levels of other pituitary hormones. In some patients the reduction of prolactin secretion may be accompanied by short-lasting, small increases in plasma growth hormone levels, the clinical significance of which is unknown.

As a specific inhibitor of prolactin secretion with a prolonged duration of action (greater than 24 hours), NORPROLAC has been shown to be effective for once-a-day oral treatment of patients presenting with hyperprolactinemia and its clinical manifestations. This includes patients in whom treatment with other dopamine agonists was found ineffective or has been associated with unacceptable adverse effects.

Long-term treatment with NORPROLAC was found to reduce the size or limit the growth of prolactin-secreting pituitary macroadenomas.

Quinagolide is rapidly absorbed following oral administration of radiolabelled drug. Quinagolide has an apparent volume of distribution of 100 L. The terminal half-life for parent drug was 11.5 hours following single dose and 17 hours at steady state.

Quinagolide undergoes extensive first pass metabolism. Studies performed with ^{3}H-labelled quinagolide revealed that more than 95% of the drug is excreted as metabolites. Almost equal amounts of total radioactivity were found in faeces (40%) and urine (50%).

In blood, quinagolide and its N-desethyl analogue are the biologically active but minor components. Their sulfate or glucuronide conjugates represent the major circulating metabolites. In urine, the main metabolites are the glucuronide and sulfate conjugates of quinagolide and the N-desethyl, N, N,-didesethyl analogues. In faeces the unconjugated forms of the three compounds were found. The major metabolites in the blood are the N-desethyl and N, N-bidesethyl analogues.

Quinagolide is approximately 90% bound to plasma proteins.

Pharmacodynamic studies using plasma prolactin levels as a reliable marker of drug activity showed that the prolactin-lowering effect of quinagolide at recommended therapeutic doses occurs within 2 hours after ingestion reaches a maximum within 4 to 6 hours and is maintained for at least 24 hours.

In healthy volunteers, the duration of the prolactin-lowering effect is proportional to the dose of quinagolide.

Pharmacokinetics: Quinagolide is rapidly and almost completely absorbed in animals. Almost dose-proportional blood or plasma levels of parent compound and metabolites were observed after single and multiple oral dosing, indicating linear pharmacokinetics. The pharmacokinetics are species-dependent with a terminal half-life varying between 8 hours (rabbit) and 59 hours (dog).

In rats and mice, quinagolide and/or its metabolites were extensively distributed in the extravascular compartment. Target organs were liver, kidneys, salivary glands and pituitary. In pregnant animals the fetal exposure was low due to a limited placental transfer. Elimination of radioactivity from the tissues was rapid and no retention of drug derived material was observed. Quinagolide-derived material was rapidly excreted in all species after single and multiple oral doses. Recovery of drug-derived material is almost complete within 4 days post single dose.

In healthy volunteers, single oral doses of radiolabelled quinagolide (0.025 and 0.05 mg) were rapidly ($t_{1/2}$ absorption=0.1 h) and almost completely absorbed (>95 % of dose). The absolute bioavailability was low (4 %) due to presystemic metabolism. Peak levels of radioactivity and parent drug were achieved at 0.5-1 hour post-dose. The elimination was biphasic with a terminal half-life of 12 h for parent drug and 24 h for radioactivity. Elimination occurred almost equally via the urine (50 %) and bile (40%). The pharmacokinetics of quinagolide were not altered after repeated administration of 0.075 mg/day for 5 days and an accumulation factor of less than 2 was calculated for parent drug and radioactivity.

STORAGE AND STABILITY: Store between 15 to 30°C. Protect from light and humidity.

INFORMATION FOR THE PATIENT: Published in e-CPS, available by subscription at www.e-cps.ca.

DOSAGE FORMS, COMPOSITION AND PACKAGING: 0.025 mg: Each light pink with pigment spots, circular, flat, bevelled edge tablet, engraved "25" on one side and "NORPROLAC" on the other, contains: quinagolide 0.025 mg (as the hydrochloride salt). Nonmedicinal ingredients: cellulose (microcrystalline), iron oxide red, lactose, magnesium stearate, maize starch, methylhydroxy propylcellulose and silica (colloidal anhydrous). Blister packs of a total of 30 tablets: 3×0.025 mg tablets, 3×0.050 mg tablets and 24×0.075 mg tablets (Starter Packs).

0.050 mg: Each pale blue with pigment spots, circular, flat bevelled edge tablet, engraved "50" on one side and "NORPROLAC" on the other, contains: quinagolide 0.050 mg (as the hydrochloride salt). Nonmedicinal ingredients: cellulose (microcrystalline), indigotin lake, lactose, magnesium stearate, maize starch, methylhydroxy propylcellulose and silica (colloidal anhydrous). Blister packs of a total of 30 tablets: 3×0.025 mg tablets, 3×0.050 mg tablets and 24×0.075 mg tablets (Starter Packs).

0.075 mg: Each whitish, circular, flat bevelled edge tablet, engraved "75" on one side and "NORPROLAC" on the other, contains: quinagolide 0.075 mg (as the hydrochloride salt). Nonmedicinal ingredients: cellulose (microcrystalline), lactose, magnesium stearate, maize starch, methylhydroxy propylcellulose and silica (colloidal anhydrous). Blister packs of 30 (packages intended for maintenance therapy).

0.150 mg: Each whitish, circular, flat bevelled edge tablet, engraved "150" on one side and "NORPROLAC" on the other, contains 0.150 mg quinagolide (as the hydrochloride salt). Nonmedicinal ingredients: cellulose (microcrystalline), lactose, magnesium stearate, maize starch, methylhydroxy propylcellulose and silica (colloidal anhydrous). Blister packs of 30 (packages intended for maintenance therapy).

Nortriptyline ℞
Antidepressant

CPhA Monograph

Date of Preparation: November 2003
Date of Revision: November 2009

This monograph has been compiled by CPhA and reviewed by experts. It may contain information different from that found in Health Canada-approved Product Monographs. The reader is referred to the *CPS* Editorial Policy for more information.

PHARMACOLOGY: Nortriptyline is a dibenzocycloheptene-derivative tricyclic antidepressant (TCA), and is the active metabolite of amitriptyline. The mechanism of action of TCAs believed to be related to their inhibition of the presynaptic reuptake of neurotransmitters, including serotonin and norepinephrine, which potentiates the effects of the neurotransmitters. As with other antidepressants, several weeks of therapy may be required in order to realize the full antidepressant effect of nortriptyline.

Pharmacokinetics: Nortriptyline is well absorbed from the gastrointestinal tract with peak plasma concentrations occurring between 2 and 8 hours after administration. Bioavailability is about 30 to 70%, with extensive first-pass hepatic metabolism. Nortriptyline is approximately 90% protein bound, and is a substrate of CYP1A2 and CYP2D6. Its inactive metabolites are excreted in the urine.

The average elimination half-life of nortriptyline in adults is 30 hours with a range of 18 to 56 hours. The mean half-life in children is 18 hours. The therapeutic serum concentration is considered to be in the range of 190 to 570 nmol/L. Routine serum drug concentration monitoring is not warranted but may be useful in assessing adherence, suspected toxicity or lack of effect. Recommended therapeutic trough levels range from 170 to 495 nmol/L. Ideally, the trough level should be taken 12 hours following administration of the last dose.

INDICATIONS: Nortriptyline is used in the pharmacologic management of depressive illness. It has also been used in the management of neuropathic pain, chronic pain and smoking cessation.

CONTRAINDICATIONS: Nortriptyline is contraindicated in patients who have known hypersensitivity to the drug. Cross-sensitivity between nortriptyline and related TCAs is possible.

Hypertension, tachycardia, confusion, hyperpyretic crisis, severe seizures and death have occurred in patients receiving TCAs and MAO inhibiting drugs simultaneously. Normally, when nortriptyline must be substituted for an MAO inhibitor or vice versa, a minimum of 14 days should elapse after the initial drug is discontinued before the new drug is cautiously started; however, patients with refractory depression have received combination therapy without significant adverse effects, under certain strict conditions and under the supervision of prescribers experienced with such therapy.

Nortriptyline is not recommended during the acute recovery phase following myocardial infarction or in the presence of congestive heart failure (see Warnings).

WARNINGS: Cardiovascular: Orthostatic hypotension, arrhythmias and conduction abnormalities have occurred during therapy with TCAs. An increased incidence of sudden death has been reported in cardiac patients receiving therapeutic doses of tricyclic antidepressants. Caution is advised if TCAs are used in patients with pre-existing cardiovascular disease.

Sedation: Patients should be warned about the possible sedation and mental or motor impairment associated with nortriptyline therapy and advised of the potential danger of operating machinery or driving a motor vehicle if this occurs.

Suicide: The potential for attempted suicide must always be considered in depressed patients. It is considered prudent to provide a limited supply of nortriptyline to patients considered to be at high risk for attempted suicide.

PRECAUTIONS: Bipolar Disorder: The use of antidepressants during the depressed phase of bipolar disorder may precipitate a hypomanic or manic state.

Cardiovascular: TCAs can have significant effects on the cardiovascular system (see Adverse Effects). Patients with a history of cardiovascular disease who require treatment with nortriptyline should be started on a low dose which may be cautiously increased over time. These patients also require close monitoring, including periodic ECG tracings. In addition, all patients receiving higher than usual dosage should have periodic ECG tracings, whether or not cardiac abnormalities were present prior to treatment. Lying and standing blood pressure should be checked.

Central Nervous System: Sedation is the most common CNS effect of TCAs. Other reactions have occurred such as agitation, confusion (i.e., delirium, hallucinations), nightmares, restlessness, hostility, exacerbation of psychosis and extrapyramidal symptoms. Elderly patients may be more susceptible to these effects.

TCAs can lower the seizure threshold and should be used with caution in patients with a history of seizures or those who may be predisposed to seizures.

Elective Surgery: Temporary discontinuation of nortriptyline may be considered prior to elective surgery. Patients receiving nortriptyline in the perioperative period may be predisposed to intraoperative arrhythmias. Risks of temporary discontinuation must be weighed against those of continued therapy throughout the perioperative period. If therapy is to be interrupted, nortriptyline should be stopped approximately 10 days prior to surgery. If the patient is at risk of experiencing withdrawal symptoms, consideration should be given to tapering the dose (see Adverse Effects).

Hematologic: Rarely, blood dyscrasias have occurred in patients taking TCAs. A leukocyte and differential count should be performed in patients who develop symptoms such as sore throat and fever while taking these drugs.

Hypersensitivity: Allergic reactions have included rash, edema, drug fever and photosensitivity. The possibility of cross-sensitivity among the tricyclic agents must be considered.

Endocrine: TCAs should be used with caution in patients who are hyperthyroid or receiving thyroid medication, because of the possibility of cardiac arrhythmias.

Withdrawal: Nortriptyline therapy should be gradually rather than abruptly discontinued, especially after prolonged use of higher doses, to avoid withdrawal symptoms such as sleep disturbances, gastrointestinal discomfort, flu-like symptoms, anxiety, depression, hypomania, mania, panic and depersonalization, delirium, dizziness, tremor, muscle twitching and, rarely, dyskinesia. These usually occur within 1 to 3 days of discontinuation, are mild and self-limiting and resolve within 2 weeks. Very rarely, cardiac disturbances may also occur.

Drug Interactions: Anticholinergics: Concurrent use of TCAs and other drugs with anticholinergic activity may necessitate dosage adjustments to minimize the additive effects. Hyperpyrexia has been reported when TCAs are administered with other anticholinergic agents, particularly during hot weather. Elderly patients may be particularly susceptible to anticholinergic effects, especially delirium, constipation and urinary retention.

Antihypertensives: TCAs may antagonize the antihypertensive effects of clonidine or guanethidine.

Hepatic Enzyme Inducers: Plasma concentrations of nortriptyline may be decreased when it is used concurrently with inducers of CYP1A2 and/or CYP2D6 such as barbiturates, carbamazepine, phenytoin or rifampin.

Hepatic Enzyme Inhibitors: Plasma concentrations of nortriptyline may be increased when it is used concurrently with inhibitors of CYP1A2 or CYP2D6 such as amiodarone, celecoxib, chloroquine, cimetidine, ciprofloxacin, clarithromycin, erythromycin, ethinyl estradiol, isoniazid, ketoconazole, methadone, mexiletine, propranolol and quinidine. See also SSRIs.

CNS Depressants: The concomitant use of TCAs and other CNS depressants may result in additive depressant effects.

Lithium: There is some evidence that concurrent use of lithium and TCAs may increase the risk of neurotoxicity, particularly in the elderly. It has been suggested that reducing the dose of lithium in elderly patients may reduce the risk of neurotoxicity without compromising its clinical effect. Elderly patients should be monitored carefully for signs of neurotoxicity (e.g., tremor, ataxia, seizures) when on combined therapy.

MAO Inhibitors: Because of the additive serotonergic effects, combination therapy with TCAs and MAO inhibitors is not recommended, except under certain conditions (see Contraindications).

Sympathomimetics: TCAs can significantly enhance the pressor response to norepinephrine and may potentiate the cardiovascular effects (e.g., arrhythmia) of sympathomimetics in general.

Selective Serotonin Reuptake Inhibitors (SSRIs): Nortriptyline toxicity may occur if used concurrently with fluoxetine, because of inhibition of CYP2D6. Reduction of nortriptyline dose by as much as 75% may be necessary. The potential for this interaction occurring with other SSRIs must be considered. Because of the extremely long elimination half-life of fluoxetine, the potential for interacting with other drugs remains for several weeks after its discontinuation.

Serotonin syndrome has also been reported rarely following combination of TCAs and SSRIs. The reader is referred to the SSRI general monograph for more information on the serotonin syndrome.

Thyroid Hormones: Concomitant use of nortriptyline and levothyroxine may potentiate the cardiovascular effects (e.g., arrhythmias) of both drugs.

Drug-Herb Interactions: It has been recommended that, although the clinical significance of any interaction is not known, concurrent administration of the following herbs with nortriptyline be avoided: essiac, kava, marshmallow, St. John's wort, Indian snake root, rhubarb root and valerian.

Pregnancy: Nortriptyline has not been associated with an increased risk of fetal malformations or other long-term effects on exposed fetuses. Antidepressant therapy is often continued during pregnancy because of the known risks of untreated depression. The decision to use nortriptyline during pregnancy must be based on an assessment of the potential risks/benefits for each patient.

Lactation: Nortriptyline is excreted into breast milk in small quantities. It should be used with caution in breast-feeding mothers.

Geriatrics: Elderly patients may be more susceptible to the anticholinergic, cardiovascular and CNS effects of TCAs. Nortriptyline has a lower propensity to cause anticholinergic side effects (e.g., dry mouth, decreased perspiration, visual disturbances, urinary retention), orthostatic hypotension and sedation than many other TCAs. When nortriptyline is prescribed to an older patient, lower initial dosages with more gradual increases are recommended.

ADVERSE EFFECTS: Note: Included in this listing are some adverse reactions reported with TCAs but not necessarily with nortriptyline specifically. Pharmacologic similarities among the TCAs require that each reaction be considered when nortriptyline is administered.

Cardiovascular: Frequently: hypotension, particularly orthostatic hypotension (although nortriptyline causes less orthostasis than many other TCAs) with associated dizziness/lightheadedness, tachycardia, ECG changes including flattening or inversion of T waves. Occasionally: arrhythmia, disturbances in cardiac conduction, palpitation, syncope. In isolated cases: hypertension, congestive heart failure, myocardial infarction, heart block, asystole, stroke, peripheral vasospastic reactions.

Central Nervous System: Frequently: drowsiness, fatigue, tremors (although nortriptyline causes less sedation than many other TCAs). Occasionally: insomnia, dizziness, headache, paresthesia (numbness, tingling sensation, symptoms suggestive of peripheral neuropathy). Rarely: seizures. In isolated cases: tinnitus, incoordination, ataxia, alterations in EEG patterns, extrapyramidal symptoms, myoclonus, speech disorders.

Endocrine: Frequently: weight gain. Occasionally: increased or decreased libido, impotence. In isolated cases: gynecomastia in the male, breast enlargement and galactorrhea in the female, testicular swelling, elevation or depression of blood sugar levels, weight loss, syndrome of inappropriate antidiuretic hormone secretion (SIADH).

Hypersensitivity: Occasionally: skin rash, urticaria. In isolated cases: petechiae, itching, photosensitization (avoid excessive exposure to sunlight), edema (general or of face and tongue), drug fever, obstructive jaundice, nasal congestion, alopecia, allergic alveolitis (pneumonia) with or without eosinophilia.

Hematologic: In isolated cases: agranulocytosis, eosinophilia, leukopenia, purpura and thrombocytopenia may occur as an idiosyncratic response.

Gastrointestinal: Occasionally: nausea, vomiting, anorexia. Rarely: elevated transaminases. In isolated cases: diarrhea, bitter taste, stomatitis, epigastric distress, abdominal cramps, black tongue, dysphagia, increased salivation, hepatitis with or without jaundice.

Genitourinary: Urinary retention.

OVERDOSE:

Symptoms: Nortriptyline and other TCAs are extremely toxic in overdose. Consultation with a Poison Control Centre is recommended. See the *CPS* Directory section for contact numbers.

Cardiac arrhythmias and CNS involvement pose the greatest threat and may occur suddenly even when initial symptoms appear to be mild. The toxic dose is variable but, in general, acute ingestion of 10 to 20 mg/kg may result in serious toxicity and may be lethal. TCA overdose has one of the highest mortality rates of any type of ingestion. Toxicity most commonly begins within two hours of ingestion. The onset of symptoms is frequently precipitous, with patients progressing from a wakeful, interactive state to having severe CNS and cardiac involvement within a matter of minutes.

Peripheral anticholinergic symptoms may include urinary retention, dry mucous membranes, mydriasis, constipation, and occasionally adynamic ileus. Patients may also be hyperpyrexic. CNS signs and symptoms can be highly variable and may range from somnolence to agitation, irritability, confusion, delirium, and hallucinations. In severe cases, patients may display extreme drowsiness, areflexia, respiratory depression, and coma. Patients may occasionally become hypothermic. Seizures are common and may precipitate cardiac toxicity.

Cardiac irregularities are frequent. Sinus tachycardia is common. Its presence is not a reliable predictor of serious toxicity, and its absence does not ensure a benign clinical course. An effect on cardiac conduction similar to that of quinidine may be seen with slowing of conduction, widening of the QRS complex, rightward shift in the axis of the terminal 40 milliseconds of the QRS complex, prolongation of the PR and QT intervals, right bundle branch and AV block, ventricular tachyarrhythmias (including torsades de pointes and fibrillation), and death. Prolongation of the QRS duration to more than 0.1 seconds is generally associated with more severe toxicity. Bradycardia may be seen in severely poisoned patients. Hypotension is common and may be severe, resulting from vasodilation, central and peripheral alpha-adrenergic blockade, and myocardial depression. Metabolic and/or respiratory acidosis may occur secondary to seizures, poor tissue perfusion, respiratory depression or poor gas exchange. In an otherwise healthy young person, prolonged resuscitation may be required.

Treatment: All cases of accidental pediatric exposure or adult overdose should be monitored at a health care facility. Asymptomatic cases without ECG abnormalities should be monitored for a minimum of 6 hours. Plasma concentrations of nortriptyline are of little use and should not guide management of the patient. In managing overdose, consider the possibility of multiple drug overdose, interactions among drugs and altered pharmacokinetics, including delayed absorption. Protect the patient's airway and support ventilation and perfusion. Closely monitor and maintain the patient's vital signs, ECG, blood gases, serum electrolytes, and acid-base balance. Minimize external stimulation to reduce the risk of seizures.

Consultation with a regional poison centre is advisable in all patients with TCA overdose. Activated charcoal (1 gram per kilogram) may reduce absorption of drug from the gastrointestinal tract, and should be considered in patients who present within 2 hours of ingestion. This can be given through a nasogastric tube if necessary. Although it should not be routinely performed, gastric lavage may be considered in the unusual case where a patient presents within 30 to 60 minutes of a massive TCA overdose, but only on the advice of a Poison Control Centre. If performed, gastric lavage should be followed by administration of activated charcoal. If the patient has a decreased level of consciousness, consideration should be given to placement of an endotracheal tube with cuff inflated before beginning the lavage procedure, to lessen the likelihood of aspiration of gastric contents.

Hypotension should be promptly corrected. If hypotension does not respond to a rapid isotonic fluid bolus and the patient has a widened QRS interval (> 0.1 seconds), sodium bicarbonate boluses should be administered at a dose of 1 to 2 mmol/kg (an average adult would typically receive 1 to 3 ampoules of 50 mmol/50 mL). If hypotension still hasn't responded, vasopressors should be employed, with a direct-acting agonist such as norepinephrine being the drug of choice.

Widened QRS intervals (> 0.14 seconds) and ventricular arrhythmias should be treated with iv sodium bicarbonate. An iv bolus of 1 to 2 mmol/kg (typically 1 to 3 ampoules of 50 mmol/50 mL) should be administered and repeated if necessary to achieve a serum pH of 7.45 to 7.55. Maintain the pH between 7.45 and 7.55. Do not exceed pH 7.6. Monitor for hypokalemia and fluid overload. Hyperventilation may also be used to maintain alkalemia.

Ventricular arrhythmias refractory to sodium bicarbonate may respond to lidocaine. Quinidine, procainamide and other type IA or IC antiarrhythmics should not be used because they may exacerbate arrhythmias and conduction slowing due to the overdosage. Overdrive pacing should be considered in patients whose arrhythmias are not responsive to drug therapy.

In patients with severe/refractory toxicity, consideration should be given to the use of intravenous lipid emulsion. Consult a toxicologist.

Seizures should be aggressively treated with iv benzodiazepines such as lorazepam or diazepam. If this is unsuccessful, barbiturates and other measures should be employed as for status epilepticus. However, phenytoin is no longer recommended for the treatment of TCA-induced seizures.

Diuresis, hemoperfusion and dialysis are not helpful in TCA overdose.

Flumazenil is contraindicated in any patient with an altered level of consciousness who has or may have taken a TCA or any drug that can cause seizures or arrhythmias, as it may precipitate seizures or even cardiac arrest. This is true even in cases of mixed overdose where the patient is known to have coingested benzodiazepines.

> For management of a suspected drug overdose, CPhA recommends that you contact your **regional Poison Control Centre**. See the *CPS* Directory section for a list of Poison Control Centres.

DOSAGE: Depression: Dosage should be initiated at a low level and increased gradually, noting carefully the clinical response and any evidence of adverse effects. In the treatment of depression, it may take several weeks to obtain full therapeutic effect. It is generally recommended that therapy for depression be continued for a year for first episodes and for at least two years for subsequent episodes. Some experts recommend lifelong therapy for patients who have had more than two episodes.

Adults: Initial dose: 25 to 50 mg/day. The dose may be gradually increased, if necessary, to the dose providing maximal clinical benefit with minimal adverse effects (usual maximum 200 mg daily).

Geriatrics: Recommended initial dose is 10 to 25 mg at bedtime. May be increased by 10 to 25 mg daily, at weekly intervals; usual maintenance dose is 50 to 75 mg daily.

Children 6 to 12 years: 10 to 20 mg/day in divided doses.

Adolescents: 30 to 50 mg/day in divided doses; usual maximum: 150 mg/day.

Neuropathic Pain: Adults: Initial dose is 10 to 25 mg at bedtime; increase by 10 to 25 mg daily, at weekly intervals, until relief of pain or side effects occur (not to exceed 200 mg).

SUPPLIED: Nortriptyline is available as a 10 or 25 mg oral capsule.

The reader is invited to consult CPhA's monograph **Calcium Channel Blockers**.

Norvasc™ 🅿

amlodipine besylate

Antihypertensive—Antianginal

Pfizer

Date of Preparation: June 23, 1992
Date of Revision: June 8, 2005

PHARMACOLOGY: NORVASC (amlodipine besylate) is a calcium ion influx inhibitor (calcium entry blocker or calcium ion antagonist). Amlodipine is a member of the dihydropyridine class of calcium antagonists.

Mechanism of Action: The therapeutic effect of this group of drugs is believed to be related to their specific cellular action of selectively inhibiting transmembrane influx of calcium ions into vascular smooth muscle and cardiac muscle. The contractile processes of these tissues are dependent upon the movement of extracellular calcium ions into these cells through specific ion channels. Amlodipine inhibits calcium ion influx across cell membranes selectively, with a greater effect on vascular smooth muscle cells than on cardiac muscle cells. Serum calcium concentration is not affected by amlodipine. Within the physiologic pH range, amlodipine is an ionized compound and its kinetic interaction with the calcium channel receptor is characterized by the gradual association and dissociation with the receptor binding site. Experimental data suggest that amlodipine binds to both dihydropyridine and nondihydropyridine binding sites.

Hypertension: The mechanism by which amlodipine reduces arterial blood pressure involves direct peripheral arterial vasodilation and reduction in peripheral vascular resistance.

Angina: The precise mechanism by which amlodipine relieves angina has not been fully delineated. Amlodipine is a dilator of peripheral arteries and arterioles which reduces the total peripheral resistance and, therefore, reduces the workload of the heart (afterload). The unloading of the heart is thought to decrease ischemia and relieve effort angina by reducing myocardial energy oxygen consumption and oxygen requirements.

Pharmacokinetics: After oral administration of therapeutic doses of amlodipine, absorption occurs gradually with peak plasma concentration reached between 6 and 12 hours. Absolute bioavailability has been estimated to be between 64 and 90%. The bioavailability of amlodipine is not altered by the presence of food.

Amlodipine is metabolized through the cytochrome P450 system, mainly via CYP 3A4 isoenzyme. Amlodipine is extensively (about 90%) converted to inactive metabolites (via hepatic metabolism) with 10% of the parent compound and 60% of the metabolites excreted in the urine. Ex vivo studies have shown that approximately 93% of the circulating drug is bound to plasma proteins in hypertensive patients. Elimination from the plasma is biphasic with a terminal elimination half-life of about 35-50 hours. Steady state plasma levels of amlodipine are reached after 7 to 8 days of consecutive daily dosing.

The pharmacokinetics of amlodipine are not significantly influenced by renal impairment. Plasma concentrations in the patients with moderate to severe renal failure were higher than in the normal subjects. Accumulation and mean elimination half-life in all patients were within the range of those observed in other pharmacokinetic studies with amlodipine in normal subjects.

In elderly hypertensive patients (mean age 69 years) there was a decrease in clearance of amlodipine from plasma as compared to young volunteers (mean age 36 years) with a resulting increase in the area under the curve (AUC) of about 60%.

Following single oral administration of 5 mg of amlodipine, patients with chronic mild-moderate hepatic insufficiency showed about 40% increase in AUC of amlodipine as compared to normal volunteers. This was presumably due to a reduction in clearance of amlodipine as the terminal elimination half-life was prolonged from 34 hrs in young normal subjects to 56 hrs in the elderly patients with hepatic insufficiency.

Following oral administration of 10 mg amlodipine to 20 male volunteers, pharmacokinetics of amlodipine were similar when amlodipine was administered with and without grapefruit juice. Geometric mean Cmax of amlodipine was 6.2 ng/mL when the drug was administered with grapefruit juice and 5.8 ng/mL when administered with water. Mean Tmax of amlodipine was 7.6 hours with grapefruit juice and 7.9 hours with water. Geometric mean $AUC_{0-\infty}$ was 315 ng/h/mL with grapefruit juice and 293 ng/h/mL with water. Geometric mean bioavailability of amlodipine was 85% when administered with grapefruit juice and 81% when administered with water.

Pediatric Patients: Two studies were conducted to evaluate the use of NORVASC in a pediatric population. In one study (pharmacokinetic), sixty-two hypertensive patients aged greater than 6 years received doses of NORVASC between 1.25 mg and 20 mg. Weight-adjusted clearance and volume of distribution were similar to values in adults (see Dosage). The mean absorption rate constant (K_a) in children (0.85 h^{-1}) is approximately 50% higher than that in healthy adults (0.55 h^{-1}, range of 0.28-1.09 h^{-1}).

Gender effect: In a second trial (clinical), a pattern of greater reductions in both systolic and diastolic blood pressure in females than in males was observed. Mean change in systolic blood pressure from baseline to end of study: amlodipine 2.5 mg: males, −6.9 mmHg (n=51); females, −8.9 mmHg (n=32); amlodipine 5.0 mg: males, −6.6 mmHg (n=63); females, −14.0 mmHg (n=23); placebo males, −2.5 mmHg (n=54), females, −3.8 mmHg (n=33).

Pharmacodynamics: Hemodynamics: Following administration of recommended doses to patients with hypertension, amlodipine produces vasodilation resulting in a reduction of supine and standing blood pressures. These decreases in blood pressure are not accompanied by any significant change in heart rate or plasma catecholamine levels with chronic dosing. With chronic once daily oral administration (5 and 10 mg once daily), antihypertensive effectiveness is maintained throughout the 24 hours dose interval with minimal peak to trough differences in blood pressure reduction. Since the vasodilation induced by amlodipine is gradual in onset, acute hypotension has rarely been reported after oral administration of amlodipine. In normotensive patients with angina amlodipine has not been associated with any clinically significant reductions in blood pressure or changes in heart rate.

Negative inotropic effects have not been observed when amlodipine was administered at the recommended doses to man, but has been demonstrated in animal models. Hemodynamic measurements of cardiac function at rest and during exercise (or pacing) in angina patients with normal ventricular function have generally demonstrated a small increase in cardiac index without significant influence on dP/dt or on left ventricular end diastolic pressure or volume.

In hypertensive patients with normal renal function, therapeutic doses of amlodipine resulted in a decrease in renal vascular resistance and an increase in glomerular filtration rate and effective renal plasma flow without change in filtration fraction.

Electrophysiologic Effects: Amlodipine does not change sinoatrial nodal function or atrioventricular conduction in intact animals, or man. In patients with chronic stable angina, intravenous administration of 10 mg of amlodipine and a further 10 mg of amlodipine after a 30 min. interval produced peripheral vasodilation and afterload reduction, but did not significantly alter A-H and H-V conduction and sinus node recovery time after pacing. Similar results were obtained in patients receiving amlodipine and concomitant beta-blockers. In clinical studies in which amlodipine was administered in combination with beta-blockers to patients with either hypertension or angina, no adverse effects on electrocardiographic parameters were observed. In clinical trials with angina patients, amlodipine as monotherapy did not alter electrocardiographic intervals.

Effects in Hypertension: Pediatric Patients: Two hundred sixty-eight hypertensive patients aged 6 to 17 years were randomized first to NORVASC 2.5 or 5 mg once daily for 4 weeks and then randomized again to the same dose or to placebo for another 4 weeks. Patients receiving 5 mg at the end of 8 weeks had lower blood pressure than those secondarily randomized to placebo. The magnitude of the treatment effect is difficult to interpret, but it is probably less than 5 mmHg systolic on the 5 mg dose. Adverse events were similar to those seen in adults.

Pediatric safety and efficacy studies beyond 8 weeks of duration have not been conducted. In addition, the long-term effect of amlodipine on growth and development, myocardial growth and vascular smooth muscles has not been studied.

INDICATIONS: Hypertension: NORVASC (amlodipine besylate) is indicated in the treatment of mild to moderate essential hypertension.

Combination of NORVASC with a diuretic, a beta-blocking agent, or an angiotensin converting enzyme inhibitor has been found to be compatible and showed additive antihypertensive effect.

Chronic Stable Angina: NORVASC is indicated for the management of chronic stable angina (effort-associated angina) in patients who remain symptomatic despite adequate doses of beta-blockers and/or organic nitrates or who cannot tolerate those agents.

NORVASC may be tried in combination with beta-blockers in chronic stable angina in patients with normal ventricular function. When such concomitant therapy is introduced, care must be taken to monitor blood pressure closely since hypotension can occur from the combined effects of the drugs.

CONTRAINDICATIONS: NORVASC (amlodipine besylate) is contraindicated in patients with hypersensitivity to the drug or other dihydropyridines and in patients with severe hypotension (less than 90 mmHg systolic).

WARNINGS: Increased Angina and/or Myocardial Infarction: Rarely, patients, particularly those with severe obstructive coronary artery disease, have developed documented increased frequency, duration and/or severity of angina or acute myocardial infarction on starting calcium channel blocker therapy or at the time of dosage increase. The mechanism of this effect has not been elucidated.

Outflow Obstruction (Aortic Stenosis): NORVASC (amlodipine besylate) should be used with caution in a presence of fixed left ventricular outflow obstruction (aortic stenosis).

Use in Patients with Impaired Hepatic Function: There are no adequate studies in patients with liver dysfunction and dosage recommendations have not been established. In a small number of patients with mild to moderate hepatic impairment given single dose of 5 mg, amlodipine half-life has been prolonged (see Pharmacology, Pharmacokinetics). NORVASC should, therefore, be administered with caution in these patients and careful monitoring should be performed. A lower starting dose may be required (see Dosage).

Beta-blocker Withdrawal: NORVASC gives no protection against the dangers of abrupt beta-blocker withdrawal and such withdrawal should be done by the gradual reduction of the dose of beta-blocker.

PRECAUTIONS: Use in Patients with Congestive Heart Failure: Although generally calcium channel blockers should only be used with caution in patients with heart failure, it has been observed that NORVASC (amlodipine besylate) had no overall deleterious effect on survival and cardiovascular morbidity in both short-term and long-term clinical trials in these patients. While a significant proportion of the patients in these studies had a history of ischemic heart disease, angina or hypertension, the studies were not designed to evaluate the treatment of angina or hypertension in patients with concomitant heart failure.

Hypotension: NORVASC may occasionally precipitate symptomatic hypotension. Careful monitoring of blood pressure is recommended, especially in patients with a history of cerebrovascular insufficiency, and those taking medications known to lower blood pressure.

Peripheral Edema: Mild to moderate peripheral edema was the most common adverse event in the clinical trials (see Adverse Effects). The incidence of peripheral edema was dose-dependent and ranged in frequency from 3.0 to 10.8% in 5 to 10 mg dose range. Care should be taken to differentiate this peripheral edema from the effects of increasing left ventricular dysfunction.

Pregnancy: Although amlodipine was not teratogenic in the rat and rabbit some dihydropyridine compounds have been found to be teratogenic in animals. In rats, amlodipine has been shown to prolong both the gestation period and the duration of labor. There is no clinical experience with NORVASC in pregnant women. NORVASC should be used during pregnancy only if the potential benefit outweighs the potential risk to the mother and fetus.

Lactation: It is not known whether amlodipine is excreted in human milk. Since amlodipine safety in newborns has not been established, NORVASC should not be given to nursing mothers.

Children: The use of NORVASC is not recommended in patients less than 6 years of age since safety and efficacy have not been established in that population. Pediatric safety and efficacy studies beyond 8 weeks of duration have not been conducted.

The effect of NORVASC on blood pressure in patients less than 6 years of age is not known. The pediatric administration should be based on a careful risk/benefit assessment of the limited available information. The risk/benefit assessment should be conducted by a qualified physician.

Geriatrics: In elderly patients (>65 years) clearance of amlodipine is decreased with a resulting increase in AUC (see Pharmacology, Pharmacokinetics). In clinical trials the incidence of adverse reactions in elderly patients was approximately 6% higher than that of younger population (<65 years). Adverse reactions include edema, muscle cramps and dizziness. NORVASC should be used cautiously in elderly patients. Dosage adjustment is advisable (see Dosage).

Interaction with Grapefruit Juice: Published data indicate that through inhibition of the cytochrome P450 system, grapefruit juice can increase plasma levels and augment pharmacodynamic effects of some dihydropyridine calcium channel blockers. Following oral administration of 10 mg amlodipine to 20 male volunteers, pharmacokinetics of amlodipine were similar when amlodipine was administered with and without grapefruit juice (see Pharmacology, Pharmacokinetics).

Drug Interactions: As with all drugs, care should be exercised when treating patients with multiple medications. Dihydropyridine calcium channel blockers undergo biotransformation by the cytochrome P450 system, mainly via CYP 3A4 isoenzyme. Coadministration of amlodipine with other drugs which follow the same route of biotransformation may result in altered bioavailability of amlodipine or these drugs. Dosages of similarly metabolized drugs, particularly those of low therapeutic ratio, and especially in patients with renal and/or hepatic impairment, may require adjustment when starting or stopping concomitantly administered amlodipine to maintain optimum therapeutic blood levels.

Drugs known to be inhibitors of the cytochrome P450 system include: azole antifungals, cimetidine, cyclosporine, erythromycin, quinidine, terfenadine, warfarin.

Drugs known to be inducers of the cytochrome P450 system include: phenobarbital, phenytoin, rifampin.

Drugs known to be biotransformed via P450 include: benzodiazepines, flecainide, imipramine, propafenone, theophylline.

Amlodipine has a low (rate of first-pass) hepatic clearance and consequent high bioavailability, and thus, may be expected to have a low potential for clinically relevant effects associated with elevation of amlodipine plasma levels when used concomitantly with drugs that compete for or inhibit the cytochrome P450 system.

Cimetidine, Warfarin, Cyclosporin, Digoxin: Pharmacokinetic interaction studies with amlodipine in healthy volunteers have indicated:

- **cimetidine** did not alter the pharmacokinetics of amlodipine.
- amlodipine did not change **warfarin**-induced prothrombin response time.
- amlodipine does not significantly alter the pharmacokinetics of **cyclosporin**.
- amlodipine did not change serum **digoxin** levels or **digoxin** renal clearance.

Antacids: Concomitant administration of Maalox had no effect on the disposition of a single 5 mg dose of amlodipine in 24 subjects.

Beta-blockers: When beta-adrenergic receptor blocking drugs are administered concomitantly with NORVASC, patients should be carefully monitored since blood pressure lowering effect of beta-blockers may be augmented by amlodipine's reduction in peripheral vascular resistance.

Sildenafil: A single 100 mg dose of sildenafil (VIAGRA) in subjects with essential hypertension had no effect on AUC_t or C_{max} of amlodipine. When sildenafil (100 mg) was co-administered with amlodipine, 5 or 10 mg in hypertensive patients, the mean additional reduction of supine blood pressure was 8 mm Hg systolic and 7 mm Hg diastolic.

Special Studies: Effect of NORVASC on other agents.

Atorvastatin: In healthy volunteers, co-administration of multiple 10 mg doses of NORVASC with 80 mg of atorvastatin resulted in no significant change in the AUC_t or C_{max} or T_{max} of atorvastatin.

ADVERSE EFFECTS: NORVASC (amlodipine besylate) has been administered to 1714 patients (805 hypertensive and 909 angina patients) in controlled clinical trials (vs placebo alone and with active comparative agents). Most adverse reactions reported during therapy were of mild to moderate severity.

Hypertension: In the 805 hypertensive patients treated with NORVASC in controlled clinical trials, adverse effects were reported in 29.9% of patients and required discontinuation of therapy due to side effects in 1.9% of patients. The most common adverse reactions in controlled clinical trials were: edema (8.9%), and headache (8.3%).

The following adverse reactions were reported with an incidence of >0.5% in the controlled clinical trials program (n=805):
Cardiovascular: edema (8.9%), palpitations (2.0%), tachycardia (0.7%), postural dizziness (0.5%).
Skin and Appendages: pruritus (0.7%).
Musculoskeletal: muscle cramps (0.5%).
Central and Peripheral Nervous Systems: headache (8.3%), dizziness (3.0%), paresthesia (0.5%).
Autonomic Nervous System: flushing (3.1%), increased sweating (0.9%), dry mouth (0.7%).
Psychiatric: somnolence (1.4%).
Gastrointestinal: nausea (2.4%), abdominal pain (1.1%), dyspepsia (0.6%), constipation (0.5%).
General: fatigue (4.1%), pain (0.5%).

Angina: In the controlled clinical trials in 909 angina patients treated with NORVASC, adverse effects were reported in 30.5% of patients and required discontinuation of therapy due to side effects in 0.6% of patients. The most common adverse reactions reported in controlled clinical trials were: edema (9.9%) and headache (7.8%).

The following adverse reactions occurred at an incidence of >0.5% in the controlled clinical trials program (n=909):
Cardiovascular: edema (9.9%), palpitations (2.0%), postural dizziness (0.6%).
Skin and Appendages: rash (1.0%), pruritus (0.8%).
Musculoskeletal: muscle cramps (1.0%).
Central and Peripheral Nervous Systems: headache (7.8%), dizziness (4.5%), paresthesia (1.0%), hypoesthesia (0.9%).
Autonomic Nervous System: flushing (1.9%).
Psychiatric: somnolence (1.2%), insomnia (0.9%), nervousness (0.7%).
Gastrointestinal: nausea (4.2%), abdominal pain (2.2%), dyspepsia (1.4%), diarrhea (1.1%), flatulence (1.0%), constipation (0.9%).
Respiratory: dyspnea (1.1%).
Special Senses: vision abnormal (1.3%), tinnitus (0.6%).

General: fatigue (4.8%), pain (1.0%), asthenia (1.0%).

NORVASC has been evaluated for safety in about 11,000 patients with hypertension and angina. The following events occurred in <1% but >0.1% of patients in comparative clinical trials (double-blind comparative vs placebo or active agents; n=2615) or under conditions of open trials or marketing experience where a causal relationship is uncertain.

Cardiovascular: arrhythmia (including ventricular tachycardia and atrial fibrillation), bradycardia, hypotension, peripheral ischemia, syncope, tachycardia, postural dizziness, postural hypotension, vasculitis.

Central and Peripheral Nervous Systems: hypoesthesia, peripheral neuropathy, tremor, vertigo.

Gastrointestinal: anorexia, constipation, dysphagia, vomiting, gingival hyperplasia.

General: allergic reaction, asthenia*, back pain, hot flushes, malaise, rigors, weight gain.

Musculoskeletal: arthralgia, arthrosis, myalgia.

Psychiatric: sexual dysfunction (male* and female), insomnia, nervousness, depression, abnormal dreams, anxiety, depersonalization.

Respiratory: epistaxis.

Skin and Appendages: pruritus*, rash erythematous, rash maculopapular, erythema multiforme.

Special Senses: conjunctivitis, diplopia, eye pain, tinnitus.

Urinary: micturition frequency, micturition disorder, nocturia.

Autonomic Nervous System: dry mouth, sweating increased.

Metabolic and Nutritional: hyperglycemia, thirst.

Hemopoietic: leukopenia, purpura, thrombocytopenia.

The following events occurred in <0.1% of patients: cardiac failure, skin discoloration, urticaria, skin dryness, Stevens-Johnson syndrome, alopecia, twitching, ataxia, hypertonia, migraine, apathy, amnesia, gastritis, pancreatitis, increased appetite, coughing, rhinitis, parosmia, taste perversion, and xerophthalmia.

Isolated cases of angioedema have been reported. Angioedema may be accompanied by breathing difficulty.

In postmarketing experience, jaundice and hepatic enzyme elevations (mostly consistent with cholestasis or hepatitis) in some cases severe enough to require hospitalization have been reported in association with use of amlodipine.

OVERDOSE:

Symptoms: Overdosage can cause excessive peripheral vasodilation with marked and probably prolonged hypotension and possibly a reflex tachycardia. In humans, experience with overdosage of NORVASC (amlodipine besylate) is limited. When amlodipine was ingested at doses of 105-250 mg some patients remained normotensive with or without gastric lavage while another patient experienced hypotension (90/50 mmHg) which normalized following plasma expansion. A patient who took 70 mg of amlodipine with benzodiazepine developed shock which was refractory to treatment and died. In a 19 month old child who ingested 30 mg of amlodipine (about 2 mg/kg) there was no evidence of hypotension but tachycardia (180 bpm) was observed. Ipecac was administered 3.5 hours after ingestion and on subsequent observation (overnight) no sequelae were noted.

Treatment: Clinically significant hypotension due to overdosage requires active cardiovascular support including frequent monitoring of cardiac and respiratory function, elevation of extremities, and attention to circulating fluid volume and urine output. A vasoconstrictor (such as norepinephrine) may be helpful in restoring vascular tone and blood pressure, provided that there is no contraindication to its use. As NORVASC is highly protein bound, hemodialysis is not likely to be of benefit. Intravenous calcium gluconate may be beneficial in reversing the effects of calcium channel blockade. Clearance of amlodipine is prolonged in elderly patients and in patients with impaired liver function. Since amlodipine absorption is slow, gastric lavage may be worthwhile in some cases.

> For management of a suspected drug overdose, CPhA recommends that you contact your **regional Poison Control Centre**. See the *CPS* Directory section for a list of Poison Control Centres.

DOSAGE: Dosage should be individualized depending on patient's tolerance and responsiveness.

For both hypertension and angina, the recommended initial dose of NORVASC (amlodipine besylate) is 5 mg once daily. If necessary, dose can be increased after 1-2 weeks to a maximum dose of 10 mg once daily.

Geriatrics or Patients with Impaired Renal Function: The recommended initial dose in patients over 65 years of age or patients with impaired renal function is 5 mg once daily. If required, increasing in the dose should be done gradually and with caution (see Precautions).

Patients with Impaired Hepatic Function: Dosage requirements have not been established in patients with impaired hepatic function. When NORVASC is used in these patients, the dosage should be carefully and gradually adjusted depending on patients tolerance and response. A lower starting dose of 2.5 mg once daily should be considered (see Warnings).

Children: The effective antihypertensive oral dose in pediatric patients ages 6-17 years is 2.5 mg to 5 mg once daily. Doses in excess of 5 mg daily have not been studied; dose should be determined based upon the medical need of the patients. See Pharmacology.

SUPPLIED: 5 mg: Each white, octagonal tablet, scored, debossed on one face as "NRV 5" with "Pfizer" on the opposite face, contains: amlodipine besylate equivalent to amlodipine 5 mg. Nonmedicinal ingredients: dibasic calcium phosphate anhydrous, magnesium stearate, microcrystalline cellulose and sodium starch glycolate. White plastic (high density polyethylene) bottles of 100 and 250. Store at 15 to 30°C. Protect from light.

10 mg: Each white, octagonal tablet, debossed on one face as "NRV 10" with "Pfizer" on the opposite face, contains: amlodipine besylate equivalent to amlodipine 10 mg. Nonmedicinal ingredients: dibasic calcium phosphate anhydrous, magnesium stearate, microcrystalline cellulose and sodium starch glycolate. White plastic (high density polyethylene) bottles of 100 and 250. Store at 15 to 30°C. Protect from light.

(Shown in Product Identification Section)

Norvir® Pr
ritonavir
Human Immunodeficiency Virus (HIV) Protease Inhibitor

Abbott

Norvir® SEC Pr
ritonavir
Human Immunodeficiency Virus (HIV) Protease Inhibitor

Abbott

Date of Preparation: August 9, 1996
Date of Revision: August 19, 2009

SUMMARY PRODUCT INFORMATION:

Route of Administration	Dosage Form/ Strength	Clinically Relevant Nonmedicinal Ingredients
Oral	Oral Solution: 80 mg/mL	Ethanol, polyoxyl 35 castor oil, propylene glycol
	Soft Elastic Capsules: 100 mg	Ethanol, polyoxyl 35 castor oil For a complete listing, see Dosage Forms, Composition and Packaging.

INDICATIONS AND CLINICAL USE: NORVIR (ritonavir oral solution) and NORVIR SEC (ritonavir soft elastic capsules) are indicated in combination with other antiretroviral agents for:

* These events occurred in less than 1% in placebo controlled trials, but the incidence of these side effects was between 1% and 2% in all multiple dose studies.

- the treatment of HIV infection when therapy is warranted.

For patients with advanced HIV disease, this indication is based on the results from a study that showed a reduction in both mortality and AIDS-defining clinical events for patients who received ritonavir. Median duration of follow-up in this study was 6 months. The clinical benefit from ritonavir therapy for longer periods of treatment is unknown.

For patients with less advanced disease, this indication is based on changes in surrogate markers in studies evaluating patients who received ritonavir alone or in combination with other antiretroviral agents.

Geriatrics (>65 years of age): Clinical studies of ritonavir did not include sufficient numbers of subjects aged 65 and over to determine whether they respond differently from younger subjects. In general, appropriate caution should be exercised in the administration and monitoring of ritonavir in elderly patients reflecting the greater frequency of decreased hepatic, renal, or cardiac function, and of concomitant disease or other drug therapy.

Pediatrics (2 to 16 years of age): The safety and effectiveness of ritonavir in pediatric patients below the age of 2 years have not been established. Although the database in HIV-infected patients age 2 to 16 years is much smaller, the adverse event profile seen during a clinical trial and post-marketing experience was similar to that observed for adult patients.

CONTRAINDICATIONS:

- NORVIR (ritonavir oral solution) and NORVIR SEC (ritonavir soft elastic capsules) are contraindicated in patients with known hypersensitivity to ritonavir or any of its ingredients. For a complete listing, see Dosage Forms, Composition and Packaging.
- Co-administration of ritonavir is contraindicated with the drugs listed in Table 1 (see also Drug Interactions, Serious Drug Interactions Box) because competition for primarily CYP3A by ritonavir could result in inhibition of the metabolism of these drugs and create the potential for serious and/or life-threatening reactions such as cardiac arrhythmias, prolonged or increased sedation, and respiratory depression.

Table 1: NORVIR/NORVIR SEC

Drugs That Are Contraindicated with Ritonavir

Drug Class	Drugs Within Class That Are Contraindicated with Ritonavir	Clinical Comment
$Alpha_1$-Adrenoreceptor Antagonist	alfuzosin	**Contraindicated** due to potential for serious reactions such as hypotension (see Drug Interactions, Drug-Drug Interactions, Effect of Ritonavir on Co-Administered Drugs).
Antiarrhythmics	amiodarone, bepridil, flecainide, propafenone, quinidine	**Contraindicated** due to potential for serious and/or life-threatening reactions such as cardiac arrhythmias.
Antifungal	voriconazole	**Contraindicated** due to a significant reduction in voriconazole plasma concentrations and possible loss of effect (see Drug Interactions, Drug-Drug Interactions, Effect of Ritonavir on Co-Administered Drugs).
Antihistamines	astemizole[a], terfenadine[a]	**Contraindicated** due to potential for serious and/or life-threatening reactions such as cardiac arrhythmias.
Ergot Derivatives	dihydroergotamine, ergonovine, ergotamine, methylergonovine	**Contraindicated** due to potential for serious and/or life-threatening reactions such as acute ergot toxicity characterized by vasospasm and tissue ischemia.
GI Motility Agent	cisapride[a]	**Contraindicated** due to potential for serious and/or life-threatening reactions such as cardiac arrhythmias.
Herbal Products	St. John's wort (Hypericum perforatum)	**Contraindicated:** May lead to loss of virologic response and possible resistance to ritonavir or to the class of protease inhibitors.
HMG-CoA Reductase Inhibitors	lovastatin, simvastatin	**Contraindicated:** Potential for serious reactions such as risk of myopathy including rhabdomyolysis.
Long Acting Beta-Adrenoceptor	salmeterol	**Contraindicated:** May result in potential increased risk of cardiovascular adverse events associated with salmeterol.
Neuroleptic	pimozide	**Contraindicated** due to potential for serious and/or life-threatening reactions such as cardiac arrhythmias.
PDE5 Inhibitors	vardenafil, sildenafil[b], only when used for the treatment of pulmonary arterial hypertension (PAH)	**Contraindicated** due to potential increase in PDE5 inhibitor associated adverse reactions including hypotension, syncope, visual changes and prolonged erection.
Sedative/Hypnotics	midazolam, triazolam	**Contraindicated** due to potential for serious and/or life-threatening reactions such as prolonged or increased sedation or respiratory depression.

[a] Product no longer marketed in Canada.
[b] See Warnings and Precautions and Drug Interactions for co-administration of sildenafil in patients with erectile dysfunction.

WARNINGS AND PRECAUTIONS:

> **Serious Warnings and Precautions**
> Pancreatitis should be considered if clinical symptoms (nausea, vomiting, abdominal pain) or abnormalities in laboratory values (such as increased serum lipase or amylase values) suggestive of pancreatitis should occur. Patients who exhibit these signs or symptoms should be evaluated and ritonavir therapy should be discontinued if a diagnosis of pancreatitis is made (see Warnings and Precautions, Hepatic/Biliary/Pancreatic).

General: Co-administration of NORVIR (ritonavir oral solution) or NORVIR SEC (ritonavir soft elastic capsules) with certain nonsedating antihistamines, sedative hypnotics, or antiarrhythmics may result in potentially serious and/or life-threatening adverse events due to possible effects of ritonavir on the hepatic metabolism of certain drugs. See Contraindications and Drug Interactions.

Ritonavir is an inhibitor of cytochrome P450 3A (CYP3A) both in vitro and in vivo. Ritonavir also inhibits CYP2D6 in vitro, but to a lesser extent than CYP3A. Co-administration of ritonavir and drugs primarily metabolized by CYP3A or CYP2D6 may result in increased plasma concentrations of other drugs that could increase or prolong its therapeutic and adverse effects (see Contraindications, Table 1 and Drug Interactions, Table 4, Table 5 and Table 6).

The magnitude of the interactions and therapeutic consequences between ritonavir and the drugs listed in Drug Interactions, Table 7 (Predicted Drug Interactions: Use with Caution) cannot be predicted with any certainty. When co-administering ritonavir with any agent listed in Table 7, special attention is warranted.

Cardiac and neurologic events have been reported with ritonavir when co-administered with disopyramide, mexiletine, nefazodone, fluoxetine and beta blockers. The possibility of drug interactions cannot be excluded.

There have been post-marketing reports of drug interactions, including increased itraconazole levels, when ritonavir and itraconazole were co-administered.

Antimycobacterial: Saquinavir/ritonavir should not be given together with rifampin, due to the risk of severe hepatotoxicity (presenting as increased hepatic transaminases) if the three drugs are given together.

Corticosteroids: A drug interaction study in healthy subjects has shown that ritonavir significantly increases plasma fluticasone propionate exposures, resulting in significantly decreased serum cortisol concentrations. Systemic corticosteroid effects, including Cushing's syndrome and adrenal suppression have been reported during postmarketing use in patients receiving ritonavir and inhaled or intranasally administered fluticasone propionate. Therefore, co-administration of fluticasone propionate and ritonavir is not recommended unless the potential benefit to the patient outweighs the risk of systemic corticosteroid side effects (see Drug Interactions).

Erectile Dysfunction Agents: Particular caution should be used when prescribing sildenafil or tadalafil for the treatment of erectile dysfunction in patients receiving ritonavir. Co-administration of ritonavir with these drugs is expected to substantially increase their concentrations and may result in increased associated adverse events, such as hypotension, syncope, visual changes, and prolonged erection. Concomitant use of sildenafil with ritonavir is contraindicated in pulmonary arterial hypertension patients. Concomitant use of vardenafil with ritonavir is contraindicated. (See Contraindications and Drug Interactions, Table 6.)

HMG-CoA Reductase Inhibitors: Concomitant use of ritonavir with lovastatin and simvastatin is contraindicated (see Contraindications). Caution should be exercised if HIV protease inhibitors, including ritonavir, are used concurrently with other HMG-CoA reductase inhibitors that are also metabolized by the CYP3A4 pathway (e.g., atorvastatin). While rosuvastatin elimination is not dependent on CYP3A, an elevation of rosuvastatin exposure has been reported with ritonavir co-administration. The risk of myopathy including rhabdomyolysis may be increased when HIV protease inhibitors, including ritonavir, are used in combination with these drugs.

Allergic Reactions: Allergic reactions including urticaria, mild skin eruptions, bronchospasm, and angioedema have been reported. Rare cases of anaphylaxis and Stevens-Johnson syndrome have also been reported.

Organ Targets for Toxicity: Toxicological studies in laboratory animals identified various organs as targets for toxicity at drug exposures below or approaching those achieved in patients participating in clinical trials with ritonavir. Because no safety margin or a small safety margin has been demonstrated in long-term studies, these organs should be assessed periodically or if clinical signs and symptoms occur during therapy.

Co-Administration with Tipranavir: Co-administration of tipranavir with 200 mg ritonavir has been associated with reports of clinical hepatitis and hepatic decompensation including some fatalities (see Drug Interactions). Refer to the APTIVUS (tipranavir) Product Monograph for more information.

Extra vigilance is warranted in patients with chronic hepatitis B or hepatitis C co-infection, as these patients have an increased risk of hepatotoxicity.

Diabetes Mellitus/Hyperglycemia: New onset diabetes mellitus, exacerbation of pre-existing diabetes mellitus and hyperglycemia have been reported during post-marketing surveillance in HIV-infected patients receiving protease inhibitor therapy. Some patients required either initiation or dose adjustments of insulin or oral hypoglycemic agents for treatment of these events. In some cases diabetic ketoacidosis has occurred. In those patients who discontinue protease inhibitor therapy, hyperglycemia persisted in some cases. Because these events have been reported voluntarily during clinical practice, estimates of frequency cannot be made and a causal relationship between protease inhibitor therapy and these events has not been established.

Fat Redistribution/Accumulation: Redistribution/accumulation of body fat including central obesity, dorsocervical fat enlargement (buffalo hump), peripheral wasting, facial wasting, breast enlargement, and "cushingoid appearance" have been observed in patients receiving antiretroviral therapy. The mechanism and long-term consequences of these events are currently unknown. A causal relationship has not been established.

Hematologic: There have been reports of increased bleeding, including spontaneous skin hematomas and hemarthrosis, in patients with Hemophilia Type A and Type B treated with protease inhibitors. In some patients, additional Factor VIII was given. In more than half of the reported cases, treatment with protease inhibitors was continued or re-introduced. There is no proven relationship between protease inhibitors and such bleeding, however, the frequency of bleeding episodes should be closely monitored in patients on ritonavir.

Hepatic/Biliary/Pancreatic: Impaired Hepatic Function: Ritonavir is principally metabolized by the liver. Pre-clinical studies have identified the liver as a toxicity target. Therefore, appropriate tests should be performed at treatment initiation and at periodic intervals to assess hepatic function.

Caution should be exercised when administering ritonavir to patients with impaired hepatic function.

Hepatic Reactions: Hepatic transaminase elevations exceeding 5 times the upper limit of normal, clinical hepatitis, and jaundice have occurred in patients receiving ritonavir alone or in combination with other antiretroviral drugs (see Adverse Reactions, Table 3). There may be an increased risk for transaminase elevations in patients with underlying hepatitis B or C. Therefore, caution should be exercised when administering ritonavir to patients with pre-existing liver disease, liver enzyme abnormalities, or hepatitis.

There have been post-marketing reports of hepatic dysfunction, including some fatalities. These have generally occurred in patients taking multiple concomitant medications and/or with advanced AIDS.

Pancreatitis: Pancreatitis has been observed in patients receiving ritonavir therapy, including those who developed hypertriglyceridemia. In some cases fatalities have been observed. Patients with advanced HIV disease may be at increased risk of elevated triglycerides and pancreatitis.

Pancreatitis should be considered if clinical symptoms (nausea, vomiting, abdominal pain) or abnormalities in laboratory values (such as increased serum lipase or amylase values) suggestive of pancreatitis should occur. Patients who exhibit these signs or symptoms should be evaluated and ritonavir therapy should be discontinued if a diagnosis of pancreatitis is made.

Immune Reconstitution Syndrome: Immune reconstitution syndrome has been reported in HIV-infected patients treated with combination antiretroviral therapy, including ritonavir. During the initial phase of treatment, patients responding to antiretroviral therapy may develop an inflammatory response to indolent or residual opportunistic infections (such as *M. avium* infection, cytomegalovirus, *P. jiroveci* pneumonia, or tuberculosis), which may necessitate further evaluation and treatment.

Cardiovascular: PR Interval Prolongation: Ritonavir has been shown to cause asymptomatic prolongation of the PR interval in some patients. Reports of second or third degree atrioventricular block in patients with underlying structural heart disease and preexisting conduction system abnormalities or in patients receiving drugs known to prolong the PR interval (such as verapamil or atazanavir) have been reported in patients receiving ritonavir. Ritonavir should be used with caution in such patients. (See Action and Clinical Pharmacology, Pharmacodynamics, Effects on the Electrocardiogram.)

Lipid Disorders: Treatment with ritonavir therapy alone or in combination with saquinavir has resulted in substantial increases in the concentration of total triglycerides and cholesterol (see Adverse Reactions, Abnormal Hematologic and Clinical Chemistry Findings). Triglycerides and cholesterol testing should be performed prior to initiating ritonavir therapy and at periodic intervals during therapy. Lipid disorders should be managed as clinically appropriate.

Neurologic: CNS penetration of ritonavir has not been established.

Sensitivity/Resistance: Resistance: HIV-1 isolates with reduced susceptibility to ritonavir have been selected in vitro. Genotypic analysis of these isolates showed mutations in the HIV protease gene at amino acid positions 84 (Ile to Val), 82 (Val to Phe), 71 (Ala to Val), and 46 (Met to Ile). Phenotypic (n=18) and genotypic (n=44) changes in HIV isolates from selected patients treated with ritonavir were monitored in Phase I/II trials over a period of 3 to 32 weeks. Mutations associated with the HIV viral protease in isolates obtained from 41 patients appeared to occur in a stepwise and ordered fashion; in sequence, these mutations were position 82 (Val to Ala/Phe), 54 (Ile to Val), 71 (Ala to Val/Thr), and 36 (Ile to Leu), followed by combinations of mutations at an additional 5 specific amino acid positions.

Of 18 patients for which both phenotypic and genotypic analysis were performed on free virus isolated from plasma, 12 showed reduced susceptibility to ritonavir in vitro. All 18 patients possessed one or more mutations in the viral protease gene. The 82 mutation appeared to be necessary but not sufficient to confer phenotypic resistance. Phenotypic resistance was defined as a ≥5-fold decrease in viral sensitivity in vitro from baseline. The clinical relevance of phenotypic and genotypic changes associated with ritonavir therapy has not been established.

Cross-Resistance: Among protease inhibitors variable cross-resistance has been recognized. Serial HIV isolates obtained from six patients during ritonavir therapy showed a decrease in ritonavir susceptibility in vitro but did not demonstrate a concordant decrease in susceptibility to saquinavir in vitro when compared to matched baseline isolates. However, isolates from two of these patients demonstrated decreased susceptibility to indinavir in vitro (8-fold). Isolates from 5 patients were also tested for cross-resistance to amprenavir and nelfinavir; isolates from 2 patients had a decrease in susceptibility to nelfinavir (12- to 14-fold), and none to amprenavir. Cross-resistance between ritonavir and reverse transcriptase inhibitors is unlikely because of the different enzyme targets involved. One ZDV-resistant HIV isolate tested in vitro retained full susceptibility to ritonavir.

Special Populations: Pregnant Women: There are no adequate and well-controlled studies in pregnant women. Because animal reproduction studies are not always predictive of human response, this drug should be used during pregnancy only if clearly needed.

In rat fertility studies, hepatic toxicity precluded drug exposures equal to those achieved with the proposed human therapeutic dose. No effects on fertility in rats were produced at drug exposures approximately 40% (male) and 60% (female) of that achieved with the proposed human therapeutic dose.

No treatment-related malformations were observed when ritonavir was administered to pregnant rats or rabbits. Developmental toxicity observed in rats (early resorptions, decreased fetal body weight and ossification delays and developmental variations) occurred at a maternally toxic dosage at an exposure equivalent to approximately 30% of that achieved with the proposed therapeutic dose. A slight increase in the incidence of cryptorchidism was also noted in rats at an exposure approximately 22% of that achieved with the proposed therapeutic dose.

Developmental toxicity observed in rabbits (resorptions, decreased litter size and decreased fetal weights) also occurred at a maternally toxic dosage equivalent to 1.8 times the proposed therapeutic dose based on a body surface area conversion factor.

Antiretroviral Pregnancy Registry: To monitor maternal-fetal outcomes of pregnant women exposed to ritonavir, an Antiretroviral Pregnancy Registry has been established. Physicians are encouraged to register patients by calling 1-800-258-4263.

Nursing Women: The Centers for Disease Control and Prevention recommend that HIV-infected mothers not breast-feed their infants to avoid risking postnatal transmission of HIV. It is not known whether ritonavir is secreted in human milk. Because of both the potential for HIV transmission and the potential for serious adverse reactions in nursing infants, mothers should be instructed **not to breast-feed if they are receiving NORVIR or NORVIR SEC.**

Pediatrics (2 to 16 years of age): The safety and effectiveness of ritonavir in pediatric patients below the age of 2 years have not been established. Although the database in HIV-infected patients age 2 to 16 years is much smaller, the adverse event profile seen during a clinical trial and post-marketing experience was similar to that observed for adult patients.

Geriatrics (> 65 years of age): Clinical studies of ritonavir did not include sufficient numbers of subjects aged 65 and over to determine whether they respond differently from younger subjects. In general, appropriate caution should be exercised in the administration and monitoring of ritonavir in elderly patients reflecting the greater frequency of decreased hepatic, renal, or cardiac function, and of concomitant disease or other drug therapy.

Monitoring and Laboratory Tests: Ritonavir has been associated with elevations in cholesterol, triglycerides, AST, ALT, GGT, CK, and uric acid. Appropriate laboratory testing should be performed prior to initiating ritonavir therapy and at periodic intervals or if any clinical signs or symptoms occur during therapy. For comprehensive information concerning laboratory test alterations associated with other antiretroviral agents, physicians should refer to the complete product information for each of these drugs.

ADVERSE REACTIONS: Clinical Trial Adverse Drug Reactions: Because clinical trials are conducted under very specific conditions the adverse reaction rates observed in the clinical trials may not reflect the rates observed in practice and should not be compared to the rates in the clinical trials of another drug. Adverse drug reaction information from clinical trials is useful for identifying drug-related adverse events and for approximating rates.

The safety of NORVIR (ritonavir) alone and in combination with nucleoside reverse transcriptase inhibitors was studied in 1270 adult patients. Table 2 lists treatment-emergent adverse events (at least possibly related and of at least moderate intensity) that occurred in 2% or greater of adult patients receiving ritonavir alone or in combination with nucleoside reverse transcriptase inhibitors in Study 245 or Study 247 and in combination with saquinavir in Study 462. In that study, 141 protease inhibitor-naïve, HIV-infected patients with mean baseline CD_4 of 300 cells/μL were randomized to one of four regimens of ritonavir + saquinavir, including ritonavir 400 mg twice-daily + saquinavir 400 mg twice-daily. Overall, the most frequently reported clinical adverse events, other than asthenia, among patients receiving ritonavir were gastrointestinal and neurological disturbances including nausea, diarrhea, vomiting, anorexia, abdominal pain, taste perversion, and circumoral and peripheral paresthesias. Similar adverse event profiles were reported in adult patients receiving ritonavir in other trials.

Table 2: NORVIR/NORVIR SEC

Percentage of Patients with Treatment-Emergent Adverse Events[a] of Moderate or Severe Intensity Occurring in ≥2% of Adult Patients Receiving NORVIR (ritonavir)

	Study 245 Naïve Patients[b]			Study 247 Advanced Patients[c]		Study 462 PI-Naïve Patients[d]
Adverse Events	**NORVIR+ ZDV n=116**	**NORVIR n=117**	**ZDV n=119**	**NORVIR n=541**	**Placebo n=545**	**NORVIR+ Saquinavir n=141**
Body as a Whole						
Abdominal Pain	5.2	6.0	5.9	8.3	5.1	2.1
Asthenia	28.4	10.3	11.8	15.3	6.4	16.3
Fever	1.7	0.9	1.7	5.0	2.4	0.7
Headache	7.8	6.0	6.7	6.5	5.7	4.3
Malaise	5.2	1.7	3.4	0.7	0.2	2.8
Pain (unspecified)	0.9	1.7	0.8	2.2	1.8	4.3
Cardiovascular						
Syncope	0.9	1.7	0.8	0.6	0.0	2.1
Vasodilation	3.4	1.7	0.8	1.7	0.0	3.5
Digestive						
Anorexia	8.6	1.7	4.2	7.8	4.2	4.3
Constipation	3.4	0.0	0.8	0.2	0.4	1.4
Diarrhea	25.0	15.4	2.5	23.3	7.9	22.7
Dyspepsia	2.6	0.0	1.7	5.9	1.5	0.7
Fecal Incontinence	0.0	0.0	0.0	0.0	0.0	2.8
Flatulence	2.6	0.9	1.7	1.7	0.7	3.5
Liver Function Tests Abnormal	2.6	1.7	1.7	3.3	0.9	5.0
Local Throat Irritation	0.9	1.7	0.8	2.8	0.4	1.4
Nausea	46.6	25.6	26.1	29.8	8.4	18.4
Vomiting	23.3	13.7	12.6	17.4	4.4	7.1
Metabolic and Nutritional						
Creatinine Phosphokinase (CK) Increase	4.3	3.4	3.4	0.9	0.2	N/A
Hyperlipidemia	2.6	1.7	0.0	5.7	0.2	3.5

(cont'd)

Table 2: NORVIR/NORVIR SEC *(cont'd)*

Percentage of Patients with Treatment-Emergent Adverse Events[a] of Moderate or Severe Intensity Occurring in ≥2% of Adult Patients Receiving NORVIR (ritonavir)

Adverse Events	Study 245 Naïve Patients[b]			Study 247 Advanced Patients[c]		Study 462 PI-Naïve Patients[d]
	NORVIR+ ZDV n=116	NORVIR n=117	ZDV n=119	NORVIR n=541	Placebo n=545	NORVIR+ Saquinavir n=141
Weight Loss	0.0	0.0	0.0	2.4	1.7	0.0
Musculoskeletal						
Arthralgia	0.0	0.0	0.0	1.7	0.7	2.1
Myalgia	1.7	1.7	0.8	2.4	1.1	2.1
Nervous						
Anxiety	0.9	0.0	0.8	1.7	0.9	2.1
Circumoral Paresthesia	5.2	3.4	0.0	6.7	0.4	6.4
Confusion	0.0	0.9	0.0	0.6	0.6	2.1
Depression	1.7	1.7	2.5	1.7	0.7	7.1
Dizziness	5.2	2.6	3.4	3.9	1.1	8.5
Insomnia	3.4	2.6	0.8	2.0	1.8	2.8
Paresthesia	5.2	2.6	0.0	3.0	0.4	2.1
Peripheral Paresthesia	0.0	6.0	0.8	5.0	1.1	5.7
Somnolence	2.6	2.6	0.0	2.4	0.2	0.0
Thinking Abnormal	2.6	0.0	0.8	0.9	0.4	0.7
Respiratory						
Pharyngitis	0.9	2.6	0.0	0.4	0.4	1.4
Skin and Appendages						
Rash	0.9	0.0	0.8	3.5	1.5	0.7
Sweating	3.4	2.6	1.7	1.7	1.1	2.8
Special Senses						
Taste Perversion	17.2	11.1	8.4	7.0	2.2	5.0
Urogenital						
Nocturia	0.0	0.0	0.0	0.2	0.0	2.8

[a] Includes those adverse events at least possibly related to study drug or of unknown relationship and excludes concurrent HIV conditions.
[b] The median duration of treatment for patients randomized to regimens containing ritonavir in Study 245 was 9.1 months.
[c] The median duration of treatment for patients randomized to regimens containing ritonavir in Study 247 was 9.4 months.
[d] The median duration of treatment for patients in Study 462 was 48 weeks.
Legend: N/A=not available.

Less Common Clinical Trial Adverse Drug Reactions (<2%): Adverse events occurring in less than 2% of adult patients receiving ritonavir in all Phase II/Phase III studies and considered at least possibly related or of unknown relationship to treatment and of at least moderate intensity are listed below by body system.

Body as a Whole: abdomen enlarged, accidental injury, allergic reaction, back pain, cachexia, chest pain, chills, facial edema, facial pain, flu syndrome, hormone level altered, hypothermia, kidney pain, neck pain, neck rigidity, pelvic pain, photosensitivity reaction, and substernal chest pain.

Cardiovascular System: cardiovascular disorder, cerebral ischemia, cerebral venous thrombosis, hemorrhage, hypertension, hypotension, migraine, myocardial infarct, palpitation, peripheral vascular disorder, phlebitis, postural hypotension, tachycardia, and vasospasm.

Digestive System: abnormal stools, bloody diarrhea, cheilitis, cholangitis, cholestatic jaundice, colitis, dry mouth, dysphagia, eructation, esophageal ulcer, esophagitis, gastritis, gastroenteritis, gastrointestinal disorder, gastrointestinal hemorrhage, gingivitis, hepatic coma, hepatitis, hepatomegaly, hepatosplenomegaly, ileitis, ileus, liver damage, melena, mouth ulcer, oral moniliasis, pancreatitis, periodontal abscess, pseudomembranous colitis, rectal disorder, rectal hemorrhage, sialadenitis, stomatitis, tenesmus, thirst, tongue edema, and ulcerative colitis.

Endocrine System: adrenal cortex insufficiency and diabetes mellitus.

Hemic and Lymphatic System: acute myeloblastic leukemia, anemia, ecchymosis, leukopenia, lymphadenopathy, lymphocytosis, myeloproliferative disorder, and thrombocytopenia.

Metabolic and Nutritional Disorders: albuminuria, alcohol intolerance, avitaminosis, BUN increased, dehydration, edema, enzymatic abnormality, glycosuria, gout, hypercholesteremia, peripheral edema, and xanthomatosis.

Musculoskeletal System: arthritis, arthrosis, bone disorder, bone pain, extraocular palsy, joint disorder, leg cramps, muscle cramps, muscle weakness, myositis, and twitching.

Nervous System: abnormal dreams, abnormal gait, agitation, amnesia, aphasia, ataxia, coma, convulsion, dementia, depersonalization, diplopia, emotional lability, euphoria, grand mal convulsion, hallucinations, hyperesthesia, hyperkinesia, hypesthesia, incoordination, libido decreased, manic reaction, nervousness, neuralgia, neuropathy, paralysis, peripheral neuropathic pain, peripheral neuropathy, peripheral sensory neuropathy, personality disorder, sleep disorder, speech disorder, stupor, subdural hematoma, tremor, urinary retention, vertigo, and vestibular disorder.

Respiratory System: asthma, bronchitis, dyspnea, epistaxis, hiccup, hypoventilation, increased cough, interstitial pneumonia, larynx edema, lung disorder, rhinitis, and sinusitis.

Skin and Appendages: acne, contact dermatitis, dry skin, eczema, erythema multiforme, exfoliative dermatitis, folliculitis, fungal dermatitis, furunculosis, maculopapular rash, molluscum contagiosum, onychomycosis, pruritus, psoriasis, pustular rash, seborrhea, skin discoloration, skin disorder, skin hypertrophy, skin melanoma, urticaria, and vesiculobullous rash.

Special Senses: abnormal electro-oculogram, abnormal electroretinogram, abnormal vision, amblyopia/blurred vision, blepharitis, conjunctivitis, ear pain, eye disorder, eye pain, hearing impairment, increased cerumen, iritis, parosmia, photophobia, taste loss, tinnitus, uveitis, visual field defect, and vitreous disorder.

Urogenital System: acute kidney failure, breast pain, cystitis, dysuria, hematuria, impotence, kidney calculus, kidney failure, kidney function abnormal, kidney pain, menorrhagia, penis disorder, polyuria, pyelonephritis, urethritis, urinary frequency, urinary tract infection, and vaginitis.

Abnormal Hematologic and Clinical Chemistry Findings: Table 3 shows the percentage of adult patients who developed marked laboratory abnormalities.

Table 3: NORVIR/NORVIR SEC

Percentage of Adult Patients, by Study and Treatment Group, with Chemistry and Hematology Abnormalities Occurring in ≥2% of Patients Receiving NORVIR

Variable	Limit	Study 245 Naïve Patients			Study 247 Advanced Patients		Study 462 PI-Naïve Patients
		NORVIR+ ZDV	NORVIR	ZDV	NORVIR	Placebo	NORVIR+ Saquinavir
Chemistry	**High**						
Alkaline Phosphatase	>550 IU/L	—	0.9	—	2.3	2.2	—
Cholesterol	>6.22 mmol/L	30.7	44.8	9.3	36.5	8.0	65.2
CK	>1000 IU/L	9.6	12.1	11.0	9.1	6.3	9.9
GGT	>300 IU/L	1.8	5.2	1.7	19.6	11.3	9.2
Glucose	>13.88 mmol/L	2.6	0.9	0.8	0.9	1.3	0.7
AST	>180 IU/L	5.3	9.5	2.5	6.4	7.0	7.8
ALT	>215 IU/L	5.3	7.8	3.4	8.5	4.4	9.2
Total Bilirubin	>61.56 µmol/L	—	0.9	0.8	1.3	0.2	2.1
Triglycerides	>9.04 mmol/L	9.6	17.2	3.4	33.6	9.4	23.4
Triglycerides	>16.95 mmol/L	1.8	2.6	—	12.6	0.4	11.3
Triglycerides Fasting	>16.95 mmol/L	1.5	1.3	—	9.9	0.3	—
Uric Acid	>713.76 µmol/L	—	—	—	3.8	0.2	1.4
Chemistry	**Low**						
Potassium	<3.0 mEq/L	—	1.7	—	3.0	2.0	2.1
Hematology	**High**						
Eosinophils	>1.0×10^{9}/L	—	2.6	1.7	2.6	3.3	0.7
Neutrophils	>20×10^{9}/L	—	—	—	2.3	1.3	—
Hematology	**Low**						
Hematocrit	<30%	2.6	—	0.8	17.3	22.0	0.7
Hemoglobin	<80 g/L	0.9	—	—	3.8	3.9	—
Neutrophils	≤0.5×10^{9}/L	—	—	—	6.0	8.3	—
RBC	<3.0×10^{12}/L	1.8	—	5.9	18.6	24.4	—
WBC	<2.5×10^{9}/L	—	0.9	6.8	36.9	59.4	3.5

Legend: — Indicates no events reported.

Post-Market Adverse Drug Reactions: The following adverse events have been reported during post-marketing use of ritonavir. Because these reactions are reported voluntarily from a population of unknown size, it is not possible to reliably estimate their frequency or establish a causal relationship to ritonavir exposure.

Cardiovascular System: Myocardial infarction has been reported. Cardiac and neurologic events have been reported when ritonavir has been co-administered with disopyramide, mexiletine, nefazodone, fluoxetine, and beta blockers. The possibility of drug interaction cannot be excluded.

Endocrine System: Hyperglycemia has been reported in individuals with and without a known history of diabetes.

Cushing's syndrome and adrenal suppression have been reported when ritonavir has been co-administered with fluticasone propionate.

Hemic and Lymphatic System: There have been reports of increased bleeding in patients with hemophilia A or B (see Warnings and Precautions, Hematologic).

Metabolism and Nutrition Disorders: Redistribution/accumulation of body fat has been reported (see Warnings and Precautions). Dehydration, usually associated with gastrointestinal symptoms, and sometimes resulting in hypotension, syncope, or renal insufficiency has been reported. Syncope, orthostatic hypotension and renal insufficiency have also been reported without known dehydration.

Co-administration of ritonavir with ergotamine or dihydroergotamine has been associated with acute ergot toxicity characterized by vasospasm and ischemia of the extremities and other tissues including the central nervous system.

Nervous System Disorders: There have been post-marketing reports of seizure. Cause and effect relationship has not been established.

Reproductive System and Breast Disorders: Menorrhagia has been reported.

DRUG INTERACTIONS:

Serious Drug Interactions

- See Contraindications.
- **Co-administration** (saquinavir/rifampin/ritonavir): Saquinavir and ritonavir should not be given together with rifampin due to risk of severe hepatotoxicity (presenting as increased transaminases) if the three drugs are given together.
- **Co-administration** (tipranavir/ritonavir): Tipranavir co-administered with 200 mg of ritonavir has been associated with reports of clinical hepatitis and hepatic decompensation including some fatalities. Extra vigilance is warranted in patients with chronic hepatitis B or hepatitis C co-infection, as these patients have an increased risk of hepatotoxicity.

Overview: Agents which increase CYP3A activity (e.g., phenobarbital, carbamazepine, dexamethasone, phenytoin, rifampin, and rifabutin) would be expected to increase the clearance of ritonavir resulting in decreased ritonavir plasma concentrations. Tobacco use is associated with an 18% decrease in the AUC of ritonavir.

Ritonavir can produce large increases in plasma concentrations of certain highly metabolized drugs. Ritonavir has a high affinity for several cytochrome P450 (CYP) isoforms with the following rank order: CYP3A >CYP2D6 >CYP2C9, CYP2C19 >>CYP2A6, CYP1A2, CYP2E1. There is some evidence that ritonavir may increase the activity of glucuronosyltransferases; thus, loss of therapeutic effects from directly glucuronidated agents during ritonavir therapy may signify the need for dosage alteration of these agents.

A systematic review of over 200 medications prescribed to HIV-infected patients was performed to identify potential drug interactions with ritonavir. There are a number of agents in which CYP3A or CYP2D6 partially contribute to the metabolism of the agent. In these cases, the magnitude of the interaction and therapeutic consequences cannot be predicted with any certainty.

When co-administering ritonavir with calcium channel blockers, immunosuppressants, some HMG-CoA reductase inhibitors (see Warnings and Precautions and Contraindications), some steroids, or other substrates of CYP3A, or most antidepressants, certain antiarrhythmics, and some narcotic analgesics which are partially mediated by CYP2D6 metabolism, it is possible that substantial increases in concentrations of these other agents may occur, possibly requiring a dosage reduction (>50%); Examples are listed in Drug Interactions, Table 7 (Predicted Drug Interactions: Use with Caution, Dose **Decrease** May Be Needed).

When co-administering ritonavir with any agent having a narrow therapeutic margin, such as anticoagulants, anticonvulsants, and antiarrhythmics, special attention is warranted. With some agents, the metabolism may be induced, resulting in decreased concentrations (see Drug Interactions, Table 7 [Predicted Drug Interactions: Use with Caution, Dose **Increase** May Be Needed]).

Drug-Drug Interactions: Table 4 and Table 5 summarize the effects on AUC and C_{max} with 95% confidence intervals (95% CI) around the mean differences, of the co-administration of ritonavir with a variety of drugs. For information about clinical recommendations, see Drug Interactions, Table 6 and Table 7.

Effect of Co-Administered Drugs on Ritonavir:

Table 4: NORVIR/NORVIR SEC

Drug Interactions: Pharmacokinetic Parameters (AUC and C_{max}) for Ritonavir in the Presence of the Co-Administered Drug (see Drug Interactions, Table 6 and Table 7 for Recommended Alterations in Dose or Regimen)

Co-Administered Drug	Dose of Co-Administered Drug	Ritonavir Dosage	n	AUC % (95% CI)	C_{max} % (95% CI)	C_{min} % (95% CI)
Clarithromycin	500 mg q12h 4 days	200 mg q8h 4 days	22	↑ 12% (2, 23%)	↑ 15% (2, 28%)	↑ 14% (−3, 36%)
Didanosine	200 mg q12h 4 days, about 2.5 hrs before ritonavir	600 mg q12h 4 days	12	↔	↔	↔
Fluconazole	400 mg Day 1, 200 mg daily 4 days	200 mg q6h 4 days	8	↑ 12% (5, 20%)	↑ 15% (7, 22%)	↑ 14% (0, 26%)
Fluoxetine	30 mg q12h 8 days	600 mg single dose	16	↑ 19% (7, 34%)	↔	ND
Ketoconazole	200 mg daily 7 days	500 mg q12h 10 days	12	↑ 18% (−3, 52%)	↑ 10% (−11, 36%)	ND
Rifampin	600 mg or 300 mg daily 10 days	500 mg q12h 20 days	7,9[a]	↓ 35% (7, 55%)	↓ 25% (−5, 46%)	↓ 49% (−14, 91%)
Voriconazole	400 mg q12h, 1 day; then 200 mg q12h 8 days	400 mg q12h 9 days	17	↔	↔	ND
Zidovudine	200 mg q8h 4 days	300 mg q6h 4 days	10	↔	↔	ND

[a] Parallel group design; entries are subjects receiving combination and control regimens, respectively.
Legend: ↑ Indicates increase; ↓ indicates decrease; ↔ indicates no change.

Effect of Ritonavir on Co-Administered Drugs:

Table 5: NORVIR/NORVIR SEC

Drug Interactions: Pharmacokinetic Parameters (AUC and C_{max}) for Co-Administered Drug in the Presence of Ritonavir (see Drug Interactions, Table 6 and Table 7 for Recommended Alterations in Dose or Regimen)

Co-Administered Drug	Dose of Co-Administered Drug	Ritonavir Dosage	n	AUC % (95% CI)	C_{max} % (95% CI)	C_{min} % (95% CI)
HIV-Antiviral Agents						
Atazanavir	300 mg q24h days 1 to 20	100 mg q24h days 11 to 20	28	↑ 3.4-fold	↑ 1.9-fold	↑ 11.9-fold
Darunavir	800 mg single dose	Titrated: 300 to 600 mg q12h over 6 days	8	↑ 9.2-fold	↑ 2-fold	not reported
Indinavir[a]	400 mg q12h 15 days	400 mg q12h 15 days	10			
Day 14				↑ 6% (−14, 29%)	↓ 51% (40, 61%)	↑ 4-fold (2.8, 6.8X)
Day 15				↓ 7% (−22, 28%)	↓ 62% (52, 70%)	↑ 4-fold (2.5, 6.5X)
Saquinavir[b]	400 mg q12h steady-state	400 mg q12h steady-state	7	↑ 17-fold (9, 31X)	↑ 14-fold (7, 28X)	ND
Maraviroc	100 mg q12h	100 mg q12h	8	↑ 28%	↑ 161%	not reported
Other Agents						
Alprazolam	1 mg single dose	500 mg q12h 10 days	12	↓ 12% (−5, 30%)	↓ 16% (5, 27%)	ND
Clarithromycin	500 mg q12h 4 days	200 mg q8h 4 days	22	↑ 77% (56, 103%)	↑ 31% (15, 51%)	↑ 2.8-fold (2.4, 3.3X)

(cont'd)

Table 5: NORVIR/NORVIR SEC *(cont'd)*

Drug Interactions: Pharmacokinetic Parameters (AUC and C_{max}) for Co-Administered Drug in the Presence of Ritonavir (see Drug Interactions, Table 6 and Table 7 for Recommended Alterations in Dose or Regimen)

Co-Administered Drug	Dose of Co-Administered Drug	Ritonavir Dosage	n	AUC % (95% CI)	C_{max} % (95% CI)	C_{min} % (95% CI)
14-OH clarithromycin metabolite				↓100%	↓ 99%	↓ 100%
Desipramine	100 mg single dose	500 mg q12h 12 days	14	↑ 145% (103, 211%)	↑ 22% (12, 35%)	ND
2-OH desipramine metabolite				↓ 15% (3, 26%)	↓ 67% (62, 72%)	ND
Didanosine	200 mg q12h 4 days, about 2.5 hrs before ritonavir	600 mg q12h 4 days	12	↓ 13% (0, 23%)	↓ 16% (5, 26%)	↔
Ethinyl estradiol	50 µg single dose	500 mg q12h 16 days	23	↓ 40% (31, 49%)	↓ 32% (24, 39%)	ND
Fluticasone propionate aqueous nasal spray	200 µg daily 7 days	100 mg q12h 7 days	18	↑ approx. 350-fold[f]	↑ approx. 25-fold[f]	
Ketoconazole	200 mg daily 7 days	500 mg q12h 10 days	12	↑ 3.4-fold (2.8, 4.3X)	↑ 55% (40, 72%)	ND
Meperidine	50 mg oral single dose	500 mg q12h 10 days	8	↓ 62% (59, 65%)	↓ 59% (42, 72%)	ND
Normeperidine metabolite			6	↑ 47% (−24, 345%)	↑ 87% (42, 147%)	ND
Methadone[c]	5 mg single dose	500 mg q12h 15 days	11	↓ 36% (16, 52%)	↓ 38% (28, 46%)	ND
Rifabutin	150 mg daily 16 days	500 mg q12h 10 days	5,11[g]	↑ 4-fold (2.8, 6.1X)	↑ 2.5-fold (1.9, 3.4X)	↑ 6-fold (3.5, 18.3X)
25-O-desacetyl rifabutin metabolite				↑ 38-fold (28, 56X)	↑ 16-fold (13, 20X)	↑ 181-fold (ND)
Sildenafil	100 mg single dose	500 mg b.i.d.[h] 8 days	28	↑ 11-fold	↑ 4-fold	ND
Sulfamethoxazole[d]	800 mg single dose	500 mg q12h 12 days	15	↓ 20% (16, 23%)	↔	ND
Tadalafil	20 mg single dose	200 mg q12h		↑ 124%	↔	ND
Theophylline	3 mg/kg q8h 15 days	500 mg q12h 10 days	13, 11[g]	↓ 43% (42, 45%)	↓ 32% (29, 34%)	↓ 57% (55, 59%)
Trazodone	50 mg single dose	200 mg q12h 10 days	10	↑ 2.4-fold	↑ 34%	
Trimethoprim[d]	160 mg single dose	500 mg q12h 12 days	15	↑ 20% (3, 43%)	↔	ND
Vardenafil	5 mg	600 mg q12h		↑ 49-fold	↑ 13-fold	ND
Voriconazole	400 mg q12h, 1 day; then 200 mg q12h 8 days	400 mg q12h 9 days	17	↓ 82%	↓ 66%	
Warfarin	5 mg single dose	400 mg q12h 12 days	12			
S-Warfarin				↑ 9% (−17, 44%)[e]	↓ 9% (−16, −2%)[e]	ND
R-Warfarin				↓ 33% (−38, −27%)[e]	↔	ND
Zidovudine	200 mg q8h 4 days	300 mg q6h 4 days	9	↓ 25% (15, 34%)	↓ 27% (4, 45%)	ND

[a] Ritonavir and indinavir were co-administered for 15 days; Day 14 doses were administered after a 15%-fat breakfast (757 Kcal) and 9%-fat evening snack (236 Kcal), and Day 15 doses were administered after a 15%-fat breakfast (757 Kcal) and 32%-fat dinner (815 Kcal). Indinavir C_{min} was also increased 4-fold. Effects were assessed relative to an indinavir 800 mg q8h regimen under fasting conditions.
[b] Comparison to a standard saquinavir 600 mg q8h regimen (n=114).
[c] Effects were assessed on a dose normalized comparison to a methadone 20 mg single dose.
[d] Sulfamethoxazole and trimethoprim taken as single combination tablet.
[e] 90% CI presented for R- and S-warfarin AUC and C_{max} ratios.
[f] This significant increase in plasma fluticasone propionate exposure resulted in a significant decrease (86%) in plasma cortisol AUC.
[g] Parallel group design; entries are subjects receiving combination and control regimens, respectively.
[h] b.i.d.=twice daily.
Legend: ↑ Indicates increase; ↓ indicates decrease; ↔ indicates no change.

Alfuzosin: Based on results of a drug interaction study with ketoconazole, another potent inhibitor of CYP3A4, and alfuzosin, a significant increase in alfuzosin exposure is expected in the presence of ritonavir (600 mg twice daily). Therefore, alfuzosin should not be co-administered with ritonavir.

Amprenavir: Literature reports have shown that concentrations of the HIV-protease inhibitor, amprenavir, are increased when co-administered with ritonavir.

Digoxin: A literature report has shown that co-administration of ritonavir (300 mg every 12 hours) and digoxin resulted in significantly increased digoxin levels. Caution should be exercised when co-administrating ritonavir and digoxin, with appropriate monitoring of serum levels.

Efavirenz: In healthy volunteers receiving 500 mg ritonavir twice daily with efavirenz 600 mg once daily, the steady-state AUC was increased by 21%. An associated increase in the AUC of ritonavir of 17% was observed.

Tenofovir: Lopinavir/ritonavir has been shown to increase tenofovir concentrations. Higher tenofovir concentrations could potentiate tenofovir-associated adverse events, including renal disorders. Patients receiving ritonavir and tenofovir disoproxil fumarate should be monitored for tenofovir-associated adverse events. Refer to the VIREAD (tenofovir) Product Monograph for more information.

Possible Dose Adjustments Based on Drug-Drug Interactions:

Table 6: NORVIR/NORVIR SEC

Established Drug Interactions: Alteration in Dose or Regimen Recommended Based on Drug Interaction Studies or Predicted Interaction (see Drug Interactions, Table 4 and Table 5 for Magnitude of Interaction)

Concomitant Drug Class: Drug Name	Effect on Concentration of Ritonavir or Concomitant Drug	Clinical Comment
HIV-Antiviral Agents		
HIV Protease Inhibitor: atazanavir	When co-administered with reduced doses of atazanavir and ritonavir ↑ atazanavir (↑ AUC, ↑ C_{max}, ↑ C_{min})	Atazanavir plasma concentrations achieved with atazanavir 300 mg once daily and ritonavir 100 mg once daily are higher than those achieved with atazanavir 400 mg once daily. Refer to the atazanavir Product Monograph for details on co-administration of atazanavir 300 mg once daily, with ritonavir 100 mg once daily.
HIV Protease Inhibitor: darunavir	When co-administered with reduced doses of ritonavir ↑ darunavir (↑ AUC, ↑ C_{max}, ↑ C_{min})	Refer to the darunavir Product Monograph for details on co-administration darunavir 600 mg twice daily with ritonavir 100 mg twice daily.
HIV Protease Inhibitor: fosamprenavir	When co-administered with ritonavir ↑ amprenavir (↑ AUC, ↑ C_{max})	Refer to the fosamprenavir Product Monograph for details on co-administration fosamprenavir 700 mg twice daily with ritonavir 100 mg twice daily or fosamprenavir 1400 mg once daily with ritonavir 200 mg once daily.
HIV Protease Inhibitor: indinavir	When co-administered with reduced doses of indinavir and ritonavir ↑ indinavir (↔ AUC, ↓ C_{max}, ↑ C_{min})	Alterations in concentrations are noted when reduced doses of indinavir are co-administered with ritonavir. The safety and efficacy of this combination have not yet been established. The risk of nephroliathiasis may be increased when doses of indinavir equal to or greater than 800 mg b.i.d.[a] are given with ritonavir. Adequate hydration and monitoring of the patients is warranted.
HIV Protease Inhibitor: saquinavir	When co-administered with reduced doses of saquinavir and ritonavir ↑ saquinavir (↑ AUC, ↑ C_{max}, ↑ C_{min})	The recommended dosage regimen is saquinavir 1000 mg with ritonavir 100 mg twice daily taken within 2 hours after a meal. Dose adjustment may be needed if other HIV-protease inhibitors are used in combination with saquinavir and ritonavir. Saquinavir and ritonavir should not be given together with rifampin due to risk of severe hepatotoxicity (presenting as increased hepatic transaminases) if the three drugs are given together. In some cases, co-administration of saquinavir and ritonavir has led to severe adverse events, mainly diabetic ketoacidosis and liver disorders, especially in patients with pre-existing liver disease. Refer to the INVIRASE Product Monograph for prescribing information.
HIV Protease Inhibitor: nelfinavir	↑ M8 (major active metabolite of nelfinavir; ↑ AUC)	Interactions between ritonavir and nelfinavir are likely to involve cytochrome P450 inhibition and induction.
HIV Protease Inhibitor: tipranavir	When co-administered with ritonavir ↑ tipranavir (↑ AUC, ↑ C_{max}, ↑ C_{min})	Refer to the tipranavir Product Monograph for details on co-administration of tipranavir 500 mg twice daily with ritonavir 200 mg twice daily.
Nucleoside Reverse Transcriptase Inhibitor: didanosine		Dosing of didanosine and ritonavir should be separated by 2.5 hours to avoid formulation incompatibility.
Non-Nucleoside Reverse Transcriptase Inhibitor: delavirdine	↑ ritonavir (↑ AUC, ↑ C_{max}, ↑ C_{min})	When used in combination with delavirdine, a dose reduction of ritonavir should be considered. Based on comparison to historical data, the pharmacokinetics of delavirdine did not appear to be affected by ritonavir. The safety and efficacy of this combination (delavirdine/ritonavir) have not been established.
CCR5 Antagonist: maraviroc	When co-administered with reduced dose of ritonavir ↑ maraviroc (↑ AUC, ↑ C_{max})	Refer to the maraviroc Product Monograph for details on co-administration of maraviroc 150 mg twice daily with ritonavir.
Other Agents		
Anesthetic: meperidine	↓ meperidine ↑ normeperidine (metabolite)	Dosage increase and long-term use of meperidine with ritonavir are not recommended due to the increased concentrations of the metabolite normeperidine which has both analgesic activity and CNS stimulant activity (e.g., seizures).
Antialcoholics: disulfiram/metronidazole		Ritonavir formulations contain alcohol, which can produce disulfiram-like reactions when co-administered with disulfiram or other drugs that produce this reaction (e.g., metronidazole).

(cont'd)

Table 6: NORVIR/NORVIR SEC *(cont'd)*

Established Drug Interactions: Alteration in Dose or Regimen Recommended Based on Drug Interaction Studies or Predicted Interaction (see Drug Interactions, Table 4 and Table 5 for Magnitude of Interaction)

Concomitant Drug Class: Drug Name	Effect on Concentration of Ritonavir or Concomitant Drug	Clinical Comment
Antibacterial: fusidic acid	↑ fusidic acid ↑ ritonavir	
Anticancer agents: vincristine, vinblastine	↑ Anticancer agents	Serum concentrations may be increased when co-administered with ritonavir resulting in the potential for increased incidence of adverse events.
Anticoagulant: warfarin	↓ R-warfarin ↓ ↑ S-warfarin	Initial frequent monitoring of the INR during ritonavir and warfarin co-administration is indicated.
Antidepressant: desipramine	↑ desipramine	Dosage reduction and concentration monitoring of desipramine is recommended.
Antidepressant: bupropion	↓ bupropion	Bupropion is primarily metabolized by CYP2B6. Concurrent administration of bupropion with repeated doses of ritonavir is expected to decrease bupropion levels.
Antidepressant: trazodone	↑ trazodone	Concomitant use of ritonavir and trazodone increases concentrations of trazodone. Adverse events of nausea, dizziness, hypertension and syncope have been observed. If trazodone is used with a CYP3A4 inhibitor such as ritonavir, the combination should be used with caution and a lower dose of trazodone should be considered.
Antifungal: ketoconazole, itraconazole	↑ ketoconazole ↑ itraconazole	High doses of ketoconazole or itraconazole (>200 mg/day) are not recommended.
Anti-infective: clarithromycin	↑ clarithromycin	For patients with renal impairment, the following dosage adjustments should be considered: For patients with CL_{CR} 30 to 60 mL/min, the dose of clarithromycin should be reduced by 50%. For patients with CL_{CR} <30 mL/min, the dose of clarithromycin should be reduced by 75%. No dose adjustment for patients with normal renal function is necessary.
Antimycobacterial: rifabutin	↑ rifabutin and rifabutin metabolite	Dosage reduction of rifabutin by at least three-quarters of the usual dose of 300 mg/day is recommended (e.g., 150 mg every other day or three times a week). Further dosage reduction may be necessary.
Antimycobacterial: rifampin	↓ ritonavir	May lead to loss of virologic response. Alternate antimycobacterial agents such as rifabutin should be considered (see Antimycobacterial: rifabutin, for dose reduction recommendations).
Bronchodilator: theophylline	↓ theophylline	Increased dosage of theophylline may be required; therapeutic monitoring should be considered.
Erectile Dysfunction (PDE5 Inhibitors): sildenafil	↑ sildenafil	Sildenafil should be used with caution and should not exceed a maximum single dose of 25 mg in a 48-hour period (see Warnings and Precautions). Concomitant use of sildenafil with ritonavir is contraindicated in patients with pulmonary arterial hypertension (see Contraindications and Warnings and Precautions).
Tadalafil	↑ tadalafil	Tadalafil may be used with caution at reduced doses of no more than 10 mg every 72 hours with increased monitoring for adverse events.
Vardenafil	↑ vardenafil	Concomitant use of vardenafil with ritonavir is contraindicated.
Hypolipidemics, HMG-CoA Reductase Inhibitors: atorvastatin, rosuvastatin	↑ atorvastatin ↑ rosuvastatin	Co-administration with lovastatin and simvastatin is not recommended (see Contraindications and Warnings and Precautions, General, HMG-CoA Reductase Inhibitors). Use the lowest possible dose of atorvastatin or rosuvastatin with careful monitoring or consider other HMG-CoA reductase inhibitors such as pravastatin or fluvastatin in combination with ritonavir.
Immunosuppressants: cyclosporine, everolimus, tacrolimus, rapamycin	↑ immunosuppressants	Therapeutic concentration monitoring is recommended for immunosuppressant agents when co-administered with ritonavir.
Inhaled Steroid: fluticasone propionate	↑ fluticasone	Concomitant use of fluticasone propionate and ritonavir may significantly increase fluticasone propionate plasma concentrations and reduce serum cortisol concentrations. Co-administration of fluticasone propionate and ritonavir is not recommended unless the potential benefit to the patient outweighs the risk of systemic corticosteroid side effects. Consider alternatives to fluticasone propionate, particularly for long-term use (see Warnings and Precautions, General, Corticosteroids).

(cont'd)

Table 6: NORVIR/NORVIR SEC *(cont'd)*

Established Drug Interactions: Alteration in Dose or Regimen Recommended Based on Drug Interaction Studies or Predicted Interaction (see Drug Interactions, Table 4 and Table 5 for Magnitude of Interaction)

Concomitant Drug Class: Drug Name	Effect on Concentration of Ritonavir or Concomitant Drug	Clinical Comment
Narcotic Analgesic: methadone	↓ methadone	Dosage increase of methadone may be considered.
Oral Contraceptive or Patch Contraceptive: ethinyl estradiol	↓ ethinyl estradiol	Dosage increase or alternate contraceptive measures should be considered.

[a] b.i.d.=twice daily.

Possible Dose Adjustments Based on Predicted Drug-Drug Interactions:

Table 7: NORVIR/NORVIR SEC

Predicted Drug Interactions: Use with Caution, Dose Adjustment of Co-Administered Drug May Be Needed (see Warnings and Precautions)

Drug Class	Examples of Drugs
Examples of Drugs in Which Plasma Concentrations May Be Increased by Co-Administration with Ritonavir Dose Decrease of Co-Administered Drug May Be Needed	
Analgesics, narcotics	tramadol, propoxyphene
Antiarrhythmics	disopyramide, lidocaine, mexiletine
Anticonvulsants	carbamazepine, clonazepam, ethosuximide
Antidepressants, tricyclic	amitriptyline, clomipramine, imipramine, maprotiline, nortriptyline, trimipramine
Antidepressants, SSRIs and non-tricyclics	nefazodone, sertraline, fluoxetine, paroxetine, venlafaxine
Antiemetics	dronabinol
Antiparasitics	quinine
Beta-blockers	metoprolol, timolol
Calcium channel blockers	diltiazem, nifedipine, verapamil
Neuroleptics	perphenazine, risperidone, thioridazine
Sedative/hypnotics	buspirone, clorazepate, diazepam, estazolam, flurazepam, zolpidem
Steroids	dexamethasone, prednisone
Stimulants	methamphetamine
HIV Antivirals	atazanavir, darunavir, (fos)amprenavir, tipranavir, maraviroc
Examples of Drugs in Which Plasma Concentrations may be Decreased by Co-Administration with Ritonavir Dose Increase of Co-Administered Drug May Be Needed	
Anticonvulsants	divalproex, lamotrigine, phenytoin
Antiparasitics	atovaquone

Drug-Food Interactions: It is recommended that ritonavir be taken with meals, if possible. Refer to Action and Clinical Pharmacology, Absorption for information on the effect of food of ritonavir pharmacokinetics.
Drug-Herb Interactions: St-John's Wort: Concomitant use of ritonavir and St. John's wort (Hypericum perforatum) or products containing St. John's wort is not recommended. Co-administration of protease inhibitors, including ritonavir, with St. John's wort is expected to substantially decrease protease inhibitor concentrations and may result in sub-optimal levels of ritonavir and lead to loss of virologic response and possible resistance to ritonavir or to the class of protease inhibitors (see Contraindications).
Drug-Laboratory Test Interactions: Interactions with laboratory tests have not been established.

DOSAGE AND ADMINISTRATION:

Dosing Considerations: Patients should be aware that frequently observed adverse events, such as mild to moderate gastrointestinal disturbances and paraesthesias, may diminish as therapy is continued. In addition, patients initiating combination regimens with ritonavir and other antiretroviral agents may improve gastrointestinal tolerance by initiating ritonavir alone and subsequently adding the other antiretroviral agents before completing two weeks of ritonavir monotherapy. The long-term effects of dose escalation on efficacy have not been established.
Recommended Dose and Dosage Adjustment: Adult Patients: The recommended dosage of ritonavir is 600 mg (6 capsules or 7.5 mL) twice daily orally. Some patients experience nausea upon initiation of 600 mg twice daily dosing. Use of a dose titration schedule may help to reduce treatment-emergent adverse events while maintaining appropriate ritonavir plasma levels. Ritonavir should be started at no less than 300 mg twice daily and increased by 100 mg twice daily increments up to 600 mg twice daily. The titration period should not exceed 14 days.
Pediatric Patients: Ritonavir should be used in combination with other antiretroviral agents. The recommended dosage of ritonavir is 400 mg/m² of body surface area twice daily by mouth and should not exceed 600 mg twice daily (see Table 8). Ritonavir should be started at 250 mg/m² twice daily and increased at 2- to 3-day intervals by 50 mg/m² twice daily, as tolerated. If patients do not tolerate 400 mg/m² twice daily due to adverse events, the highest tolerated dose should be used for maintenance therapy in combination with other antiretroviral agents. When possible, doses should be administered using a calibrated dosing syringe.

Table 8: NORVIR/NORVIR SEC

Pediatric Dosage Guidelines

Body Surface Area[a] (m²)	Twice Daily Dose 250 mg/m²	Twice Daily Dose 300 mg/m²	Twice Daily Dose 350 mg/m²	Twice Daily Dose 400 mg/m²
0.25	0.8 mL (62.5 mg)	0.9 mL (75 mg)	1.1 mL (87.5 mg)	1.25 mL (100 mg)
0.50	1.6 mL (125 mg)	1.9 mL (150 mg)	2.2 mL (175 mg)	2.5 mL (200 mg)
0.75	2.3 mL (187.5 mg)	2.8 mL (225 mg)	3.3 mL (262.5 mg)	3.75 mL (300 mg)
1.00	3.1 mL (250 mg)	3.75 mL (300 mg)	4.4 mL (350 mg)	5 mL (400 mg)
1.25	3.9 mL (312.5 mg)	4.7 mL (375 mg)	5.5 mL (437.5 mg)	6.25 mL (500 mg)
1.50	4.7 mL (375 mg)	5.6 mL (450 mg)	6.6 mL (525 mg)	7.5 mL (600 mg)

[a] Body surface area can be calculated with the following equation:

$$BSA\ (m^2) = \sqrt{\frac{\text{Height (cm)} \times \text{Weight (kg)}}{3600}}$$

Missed Dose: If a dose of ritonavir is missed, patients should take the dose as soon as possible and then return to their normal schedule. However, if a dose is skipped, the patient should not double the next dose.
Administration: NORVIR (ritonavir oral solution) and NORVIR SEC (ritonavir soft elastic capsules) are administered orally. It is recommended that ritonavir be taken with meals if possible. Patients may improve the taste of ritonavir oral solution by mixing with chocolate milk or ENSURE within one hour of dosing. The effects of antacids on the absorption of ritonavir have not been studied.

The ritonavir solution dosage cup should be cleaned immediately with hot water and dish soap after use. When cleaned immediately, drug residue is removed. The dosage cup **must** be dry prior to use.

OVERDOSAGE:
Acute Overdosage: Human Overdose Experience: Human experience of acute overdose with NORVIR (ritonavir oral solution) and NORVIR SEC (ritonavir soft elastic capsules) is limited. One patient in clinical trials took ritonavir 1500 mg/day for two days. The patient reported paresthesias which resolved after the dose was decreased.

A post-marketing case of renal failure with eosinophilia has been reported with ritonavir overdose.
Management of Overdosage: Administration of activated charcoal may be used to aid in removal of unabsorbed drug. Treatment of overdose with ritonavir consists of general supportive measures including monitoring of vital signs and observation of the clinical status of the patient. There is no specific antidote for overdose with ritonavir. Since ritonavir is extensively metabolized by the liver and is highly protein-bound, dialysis is unlikely to be beneficial in significant removal of the drug. A Certified Poison Control Centre should be consulted for up-to-date information on the management of overdose with ritonavir.

NORVIR Oral Solution contains 43% alcohol by volume. Accidental ingestion of the product by a young child could result in significant alcohol-related toxicity and could approach the potential lethal dose of alcohol.

> For management of a suspected drug overdose, contact your regional Poison Control Centre. See the *CPS* Directory section for a list of Poison Control Centres.

ACTION AND CLINICAL PHARMACOLOGY: Mechanism of Action: Ritonavir is an inhibitor of HIV protease with activity against the Human Immunodeficiency Virus (HIV).

Ritonavir is an orally active peptidomimetic inhibitor of both the HIV-1 and HIV-2 proteases. Inhibition of HIV protease renders the enzyme incapable of processing the gag-pol polyprotein precursor which leads to the production of HIV particles with immature morphology that are unable to initiate new rounds of infection. Ritonavir has selective affinity for the HIV protease and has little inhibitory activity against human aspartyl proteases.
Antiviral Activity in vitro: The activity of ritonavir was assessed in vitro in acutely infected lymphoblastoid cell lines and in peripheral blood lymphocytes. The concentration of drug that inhibits 50% (EC_{50}) of viral replication ranged from 3.8 to 153 nM depending upon the HIV-1 isolate and the cells employed. The average EC_{50} for low passage clinical isolates was 22 nM (n=13). In MT_4 cells, ritonavir demonstrated additive effects against HIV-1 in combination with either zidovudine (ZDV) or didanosine (ddI). Studies which measured cytotoxicity of ritonavir on several cell lines showed that >20 μM was required to inhibit cellular growth by 50% resulting in an in vitro therapeutic index of at least 1000.
Resistance: HIV-1 isolates with reduced susceptibility to ritonavir have been selected in vitro. The clinical relevance of phenotypic and genotypic changes associated with ritonavir therapy has not been established (see Warnings and Precautions).
Cross-Resistance to Other Antiretrovirals: Among protease inhibitors variable cross-resistance has been recognized (see Warnings and Precautions).

Cross-resistance between ritonavir and reverse transcriptase inhibitors is unlikely because of the different enzyme targets involved. One ZDV-resistant HIV isolate tested in vitro retained full susceptibility to ritonavir.
Pharmacodynamics: In vitro data indicate that ritonavir is active against all strains of HIV tested in a variety of transformed and primary human cell lines. The concentration of drug that inhibits 50% and 90% (EC_{50}, EC_{90}) of viral replication is approximately 0.02 and 0.11 μM, respectively. Studies which measured direct cell toxicity of ritonavir on several cell lines showed no direct toxicity at concentrations up to 25 μM, with a resulting in vitro therapeutic index of at least 1000.
Pharmacokinetics: The pharmacokinetics of ritonavir have been studied in healthy volunteers and HIV-infected patients (CD_4 ≥50 cells/μL). See Table 9 for ritonavir pharmacokinetic characteristics.

Table 9: NORVIR/NORVIR SEC

Ritonavir Pharmacokinetic Characteristics

Parameter	n	Values (Mean±SD)
C_{max} SS[a]	10	11.2±3.6 μg/mL
C_{trough} SS[a]	10	3.7±2.6 μg/mL
$V_β$/F[b]	91	0.41±0.25 L/kg
$t_{1/2}$		3 to 5 h
CL/F SS[a]	10	8.8±3.2 L/h
CL/F[b]	91	4.6±1.6 L/h
CL_R	62	<0.1 L/h
RBC/Plasma Ratio		0.14
Percent Bound[c]		98 to 99%

[a] SS=steady-state; patients taking ritonavir 600 mg q12h.
[b] Single ritonavir 600 mg dose.
[c] Primarily bound to human serum albumin and alpha-1 acid glycoprotein over the ritonavir concentration range of 0.01 to 30 μg/mL.

Absorption: The absolute bioavailability of ritonavir has not been determined. After a 600 mg dose of oral solution, peak concentrations of ritonavir were achieved approximately 2 hours and 4 hours after dosing under fasting and non-fasting (514 KCal; 9% fat, 12% protein, and 79% carbohydrate) conditions, respectively.
Effect of Food on Oral Absorption: When the oral solution was given under non-fasting conditions, peak ritonavir concentrations decreased 23% and the extent of absorption decreased 7% relative to fasting conditions. Dilution of oral solution, within one hour of administration, with 240 mL of chocolate milk, ADVERA or ENSURE did not significantly affect the extent and rate of ritonavir absorption. After a single 600 mg dose under non-fasting conditions, in two separate studies, the capsule (n=21) and

oral solution (n=18) formulations yielded mean±SD areas under the plasma concentration-time curve (AUCs) of 129.5±47.1 and 129.0±39.3 μg·h/mL, respectively. Relative to fasting conditions, the extent of absorption of ritonavir from the capsule formulation was 15% higher when administered with a meal (771 KCal; 46% fat, 18% protein, and 37% carbohydrate).

Distribution: The protein binding of ritonavir in human plasma was noted to be approximately 98 to 99%. Ritonavir binds to both human α-1-acid glycoprotein (AAG) and human serum albumin (HSA) with comparable affinities. Total plasma protein binding is constant over the concentration range of 1-100 μg/mL.

Tissue distribution studies with ^{14}C-labeled ritonavir in rats showed the liver, adrenals, pancreas, kidneys and thyroid to have the highest concentrations of drug. Tissue to plasma ratios of approximately one, measured in rat lymph nodes, suggests that ritonavir distributes into lymphatic tissue. Ritonavir penetrates minimally into the brain.

Metabolism: Nearly all of the plasma radioactivity after a single oral 600 mg dose of ^{14}C-ritonavir oral solution (n=5) was attributed to unchanged ritonavir. Five ritonavir metabolites have been identified in human urine and feces. The isopropyl thiazole oxidation metabolite (M-2) is the major metabolite and has antiviral activity similar to that of parent drug; however, the concentrations of this metabolite in plasma are low. Studies utilizing human liver microsomes have demonstrated that cytochrome P450 3A (CYP3A) is the major isoform involved in ritonavir metabolism, although CYP2D6 also contributes to the formation of M-2.

Excretion: In a study of five subjects receiving a 600 mg dose of ^{14}C-ritonavir oral solution, 11.3±2.8% of the dose was excreted into the urine, with 3.5±1.8% of the dose excreted as unchanged parent drug. In that study, 86.4±2.9% of the dose was excreted in the feces with 33.8±10.8% of the dose excreted as unchanged parent drug. Upon multiple dosing, ritonavir accumulation is less than predicted from a single dose possibly due to a time and dose-related increase in clearance.

Effects on the Electrocardiogram: QTcF interval was evaluated in a randomized, placebo and active (moxifloxacin 400 mg once-daily) controlled cross-over study in 45 healthy adults, with 10 measurements over 12 hours on Day 3. The maximum mean (95% upper confidence bound) difference in QTcF from placebo was 5.5 (7.6) msec for 400 mg twice-daily ritonavir. The Day 3 ritonavir exposure was approximately 1.5 fold higher than that observed with the 600 mg twice-daily dose at steady-state. No subject experienced an increase in QTcF of ≥60 msec from baseline or a QTcF interval exceeding the potentially clinically relevant threshold of 500 msec.

Mean change from baseline in PR interval of 11.0-24.0 msec was also noted in subjects receiving ritonavir in the same study on Day 3. Maximum PR interval was 252 msec and no second or third degree heart block was observed. (See Warnings and Precautions.)

Special Populations and Conditions: Pediatrics: The pharmacokinetic profile of ritonavir in pediatric patients below the age of 2 years has not been established. Steady-state pharmacokinetics were evaluated in 37 HIV-infected patients ages 2 to 14 years receiving doses ranging from 250 mg/m² twice daily to 400 mg/m² twice daily. Across dose groups, ritonavir steady-state oral clearance (CL/F/m²) was approximately 1.5 times faster in pediatric patients than in adult subjects. Ritonavir concentrations obtained after 350 to 400 mg/m² twice daily in pediatric patients were comparable to those obtained in adults receiving 600 mg (approximately 330 mg/m²) twice daily.

Geriatrics: No age-related pharmacokinetic differences have been observed in adult patients (18 to 63 years). Ritonavir pharmacokinetics have not been studied in older patients.

Gender: A study of ritonavir pharmacokinetics in healthy males and females showed no statistically significant differences in the pharmacokinetics of ritonavir.

Race: Pharmacokinetic differences due to race have not been identified.

Weight: Ritonavir pharmacokinetic parameters were not statistically significantly associated with body weight or lean body mass.

Hepatic Insufficiency: In six HIV-infected adult subjects with mild hepatic insufficiency dosed with ritonavir 400 mg twice daily, ritonavir exposures were similar to control subjects dosed with 500 mg twice daily. Results indicate that dose adjustment is not required in patients with mild hepatic impairment. Adequate pharmacokinetic data are not available for patients with moderate hepatic impairment. Protein binding of ritonavir was not statistically significantly affected by mild or moderately impaired hepatic function.

Renal Insufficiency: Ritonavir pharmacokinetics have not been studied in patients with renal insufficiency; however, since renal clearance is negligible, a decrease in total body clearance is not expected in patients with renal insufficiency.

Because ritonavir is highly protein bound it is unlikely that ritonavir will be significantly removed by dialysis (see Overdosage).

STORAGE AND STABILITY: Soft Elastic Capsules: Store NORVIR SEC (soft elastic capsules) in the refrigerator between 2 and 8°C until dispensed. Refrigeration of NORVIR SEC by the patient is recommended, but not required if used within 30 days and stored below 25°C. Protect from light. Avoid exposure to excessive heat. Product must be stored and dispensed in the original container.

Oral Solution: Store NORVIR (ritonavir oral solution) at room temperature, between 20 and 25°C. **Do not refrigerate. Shake well before each use.** Product must be stored and dispensed in the original container. Avoid exposure to excessive heat. Keep cap tightly closed. Use by product expiration date.

The ritonavir oral solution dosage cup should be cleaned immediately with hot water and dish soap after use. When cleaned immediately, drug residue is removed. The dosage cup **must** be dry prior to use.

INFORMATION FOR THE PATIENT: Published in e-CPS, available by subscription at www.e-cps.ca.

DOSAGE FORMS, COMPOSITION AND PACKAGING: NORVIR: Each mL of orange-colored oral solution, in a peppermint and caramel-flavored vehicle, contains: ritonavir 80 mg. Nonmedicinal ingredients: anhydrous citric acid (to adjust pH), creamy caramel flavoring, ethanol, FD&C Yellow No. 6, peppermint oil, polyoxyl 35 castor oil, propylene glycol, saccharin sodium and water. Amber-colored, multidose bottles of 240 mL with marked dosage cup of 7.5 mL (600 mg/7.5 mL).

NORVIR SEC: Each white, oblong, soft elastic capsule, imprinted with the Abbott logo, 100, and the Abbo-Code DS, contains: ritonavir 100 mg. Nonmedicinal ingredients: black opacode ink (iron oxide), butylated hydroxytoluene, ethanol, gelatin, glycerin, oleic acid, polyoxyl 35 castor oil, purified water, sorbitol and titanium dioxide. HDPE bottles of 120.

Novahistex® DH Ⓝ
hydrocodone bitartrate—phenylephrine HCl
Antitussive—Decongestant

sanofi-aventis

SUPPLIED: Each 5 mL of red, raspberry flavored liquid contains: hydrocodone bitartrate 5 mg and phenylephrine HCl 20 mg. Nonmedicinal ingredients: amaranth color, artificial raspberry flavor, artificial taste modified, citric acid, glucose (liquid), glycerin, menthol, propylene glycol, purified water, sodium benzoate, sodium chloride, sodium citrate, sodium cyclamate and xylitol. Alcohol- and sucrose-free. Bottles of 100 and 500 mL.

Novahistine® DH Ⓝ
hydrocodone bitartrate—phenylephrine HCl
Antitussive—Decongestant

sanofi-aventis

SUPPLIED: Each 5 mL of purple, grape-flavored liquid contains: hydrocodone bitartrate 1.7 mg and phenylephrine HCl 10 mg. Nonmedicinal ingredients: artificial and natural grape flavor, citric acid, D&C Green #5, D&C Red #33, glucose, sodium benzoate, sodium chloride, sodium citrate, sodium cyclamate and xylitol. Alcohol- and sucrose-free. Bottles of 100 and 500 mL.

NovoFine® 32G Tip
disposable needles
Insulin Delivery Device

Novo Nordisk

NovoFine® 30G
disposable needles
Insulin Delivery Device

Novo Nordisk

SUPPLIED: NovoFine 32G Tip (0.23/0.25×6 mm), NovoFine 30G (0.3×8 mm) and NovoFine 30G (0.3×6 mm) needles are intended for single use. Sterile, nontoxic, nonpyrogenic, sterilized with ethylene oxide. NovoFine needles should not be used after the expiry date printed on the protective tab. Sterility is guaranteed until expiry date if needle seal is unbroken.

Use once and destroy. Do not use needles where the protective tab is missing or damaged.

NovoFine needles are specifically designed for use with all Novo Nordisk Insulin Delivery Devices (see Novolin-Pen 4 and Innovo). NovoFine needles offer the added safety of Function Check capability when used with Novo Nordisk Insulin Delivery Devices and Penfill cartridges as part of The All-In-One System.

The NovoFine needles should be removed from the Novo Nordisk Insulin Delivery Device after each injection. If the needle is not removed, changes in ambient temperature can result in some liquid being expelled from the cartridge. In the case of insulin suspensions, removal of supernatant liquid can cause an increase in insulin concentration (i.e., strength) remaining in the cartridge.

Consult Insulin Delivery System Instruction Manual for information on assembly; injection and Function Check capability.

Novolin®ge (30/70, 40/60, 50/50)
insulin regular (human biosynthetic)—insulin NPH (human biosynthetic)
Antidiabetic

Novo Nordisk

Novolin®ge NPH
insulin NPH (human biosynthetic)
Antidiabetic

Novo Nordisk

Novolin®ge Toronto
insulin regular (human biosynthetic)
Antidiabetic

Novo Nordisk

Date of Revision: March 14, 2008

SUMMARY PRODUCT INFORMATION:

Route of Administration	Dosage Form/ Strength	Clinically Relevant Nonmedicinal Ingredients
Novolin ge Toronto subcutaneous, intramuscular, or intravenous injection	Injectable solution 3.5 mg (100 IU)	Zinc chloride, glycerol, metacresol, sodium hydroxide and/or hydrochloric acid, water for injections For a complete listing see Dosage Forms, Composition and Packaging.
Novolin ge NPH Subcutaneous injection	Injectable suspension 3.5 mg (100 IU)	Zinc chloride, glycerol, metacresol, phenol, disodium phosphate dihydrate, sodium hydroxide and/or hydrochloric acid, protamine sulphate, water for injections For a complete listing see Dosage Forms, Composition and Packaging.
Novolin ge 30/70 **Novolin ge 40/60** **Novolin ge 50/50** Subcutaneous injection	Injectable suspension 3.5 mg (100 IU)	Zinc chloride, glycerol, metacresol, phenol, disodium phosphate dihydrate, sodium hydroxide and/or hydrochloric acid, protamine sulphate, water for injections For a complete listing see Dosage Forms, Composition and Packaging.

DESCRIPTION: The active substance in Novolin **ge**, Insulin, Human Biosynthetic, is a polypeptide that is structurally identical to natural human insulin. Insulin human is produced by recombinant DNA technology in *S. cerevisiae*.

INDICATIONS AND CLINICAL USE: Novolin **ge** (Insulin, Human Biosynthetic) is indicated for:
- treatment of patients with diabetes mellitus who require insulin for the control of hyperglycemia

When administered in appropriate regular doses to patients with diabetes mellitus and who follow a controlled diet and exercise program, Novolin **ge** (Insulin, Human Biosynthetic) temporarily restores their ability to metabolize carbohydrates, protein and fats.

The Novolin **ge** formulations differ with respect to onset, peak and duration of action. These times reflect averages and can vary depending upon the individual patient. The standard time action characteristics are as follows:

Novolin **ge** Toronto (Insulin Injection, Human Biosynthetic) is a clear, colourless neutral solution of human insulin with a short duration of action. The effect of Novolin **ge** Toronto after subcutaneous administration begins after approximately ½ hour, is maximal between 2½ and 5 hours and terminates after approximately 8 hours.

Novolin **ge** NPH (Insulin Isophane, Human Biosynthetic) is a cloudy neutral suspension of human isophane insulin with an intermediate duration of action. The effect of Novolin **ge** NPH begins after approximately 1½ hours, is maximal between 4 and 12 hours and terminates after approximately 24 hours.

Novolin **ge** Premixed Insulin Preparations: Novolin **ge** 30/70, Novolin **ge** 40/60, Novolin **ge** 50/50 are a series of Insulin, Human Biosynthetic mixtures containing Novolin **ge** Toronto and Novolin **ge** NPH, respectively, in the proportions indicated by the ratio in the product name. The Novolin **ge** Premixed Insulin Preparations are dual-acting insulins. They have a biphasic formulation containing fast-acting and intermediate-acting insulin. The mixtures are cloudy, neutral suspensions with an intermediate duration of action. The strength of the initial effect is dependent on the amount of Novolin **ge** Toronto in the mixture. The effect of Novolin **ge** mixtures begins after approximately ½ hour, is maximal between 2 and about 12 hours and terminates after approximately 24 hours. Premixed insulin preparations are usually given once or twice daily when a rapid initial effect together with a more prolonged effect is desired.

Novolin **ge** NPH insulin in vials may be mixed with Novolin **ge** Toronto in order to meet the requirements of individual diabetics as determined by the physician.

Only Novolin **ge** Toronto, using intravenous administration, should be used for the treatment of emergencies, such as diabetic coma and pre-coma, and in diabetics undergoing surgery. (See also Contraindications.)

Geriatrics: No data is available.

Pediatrics: No data is available.

CONTRAINDICATIONS:
- Patients who are hypersensitive to human insulin or to any ingredient in the formulation or component of the container. For a complete listing, see Dosage Forms, Composition and Packaging.
- During episodes of hypoglycemia
- Novolin **ge** NPH (Insulin Isophane, Human Biosynthetic) and Novolin **ge** (Insulin, Human Biosynthetic) Premixed Insulin Preparations are never to be administered intravenously, or intramuscularly

- Novolin **ge** NPH (Insulin Isophane, Human Biosynthetic) and Novolin **ge** (Insulin, Human Biosynthetic) Premixed Insulin Preparations are not suitable for the treatment of diabetic coma

WARNINGS AND PRECAUTIONS:

Serious Warnings and Precautions
- Novolin **ge** Toronto should not be used if it is not water-clear and colourless. Due to the risk of precipitation in some pump catheters, Novolin **ge** Toronto is not recommended for use in insulin pumps.
- Insulin suspensions are never to be administered intravenously.
- Insulin suspensions are not to be used in insulin infusion pumps.

General: As with all insulins, the duration of Novolin **ge** NPH, Novolin **ge** Toronto and Novolin **ge** Premixed Insulin preparations may vary in different individuals or in the same individual according to dose, injection site, blood flow, temperature and level of physical activity. Novolin **ge** NPH and Novolin **ge** Premixed Insulin suspensions should not be used if the precipitate has become lumpy or granular in appearance or has formed a deposit of solid particles on the wall of the vial or cartridge. These insulin suspensions should also not be used if the contents remain clear after the vial or cartridge has been shaken carefully.

To avoid possible transmission of disease, Penfill cartridge must not be used by more than one person.

Insulin should not be used after the expiration date printed on the package.

Stress or illness may increase insulin requirements. In these instances, patients should contact their physicians and carefully control their blood glucose.

An insulin reaction (hypoglycemia) may occur if the patient takes too much insulin, misses a meal or exercises more than usual (see Overdosage).

Diabetic patients should be instructed to carry a few lumps of sugar, candies or biscuits to prevent the progression of a hypoglycemic reaction, should one occur. The diabetic should make relatives and close work-mates aware that he/she is diabetic and instruct them regarding assistance in the event of a hypoglycemic reaction. An unconscious person should not be given anything to eat or drink as choking is possible.

Inadequate dosage or discontinuation of treatment, especially in type 1 diabetes, may lead to hyperglycaemia. Inadequate dosage could occur due to increased insulin demand during illness or infection, neglect of diet, omission or mal-administration of prescribed insulin doses. A developing ketoacidosis will be revealed by urine tests which show large amounts of sugar and acetone. The symptoms of thirst, large urine volumes, loss of appetite, fatigue, dry skin and deep and rapid breathing come on gradually, usually over a period of some hours or days. If hyperglycemia is not treated, it can cause diabetic coma or death.

Hypokalemia is among the potential clinical adverse effects associated with the use of all insulins. This potential clinical adverse effect may be relevant in patients who are on potassium lowering drugs.

Patients whose blood glucose control is greatly improved e.g. by intensified insulin therapy, may experience a change in their usual warning symptoms of hypoglycaemia and should be advised accordingly.

Before travelling between different time zones, the patient should seek the doctor's advice, since this may mean that the patient has to take insulin and meals at different times.

Omission of a meal or unplanned, strenuous physical exercise may lead to hypoglycaemia.

Patients should be advised to take precautions to avoid hypoglycemia while driving. This is particularly important in those who have reduced or absent awareness of the warning signs of hypoglycemia or have frequent episodes of hypoglycemia. The advisability of driving should be considered in these circumstances.

Any change of insulin dose should be made cautiously and under medical supervision. Changes in insulin strength, manufacturer, type (e.g. regular, NPH, analog), species (animal, human), or method of manufacture (rDNA versus animal-source insulin) may result in the need for a change in dosage.

Concomitant illness, especially infections, usually increase the patient's insulin requirements.

Endocrine and Metabolism: Hypoglycaemia: In certain cases (long duration of diabetes, diabetic nerve disease, intensified diabetes control, or use of medications such as beta blocking agents), the nature and intensity of early warning symptoms of hypoglycaemia may change or be less pronounced.

Hypoglycaemia is the most frequently occurring undesirable effect of insulin therapy. Such reactions following treatment with Novolin **ge** NPH, Novolin **ge** Toronto or Novolin **ge** Premixed Insulin preparations are mostly mild and easily managed.

Severe hypoglycaemia can result in temporary or permanent impairment of brain function and death.

Changes in insulin therapy or changes in life style (i.e. diet, exercise/physical activity) may require a change in dosage. Inadequate dosing or discontinuation of insulin treatment may lead to hyperglycaemias and diabetic ketoacidosis. Severe sustained hyperglycaemia may result in diabetic coma and death.

Glucose monitoring is recommended for all patients with diabetes. The patient's ability to concentrate and react may be impaired as a result of hypoglycemia. This may constitute a risk in situations where these abilities are of special importance (e.g. driving a car or operating machinery).

Hepatic/Biliary/Pancreatic: Hepatic impairment may reduce insulin requirements.

Immune: Human insulin is known to be antigenic, with low titres of antibodies developing in most patients (up to 80%). The effect of insulin antibodies on insulin pharmacokinetics, with the presence of binding IgG in serum, may delay time to peak levels of free insulin. Antibodies may be cross-reactive to both insulin aspart and human insulin.

Renal: Renal impairment may reduce insulin requirements.

Sexual Function/Reproduction: There in no information available on teratogenicity of human insulin products.

Skin: Local Allergic Reaction: As with other insulins, patients may experience redness, swelling or itching at the site of injection. These minor reactions usually resolve in a few days to a few weeks. They may occur if the injection is not properly made, or if the patient is allergic to the insulin or any excipients.

Lipodystrophy may occur at the injection site as a consequence of failure to rotate injection sites within an area.

Systemic Allergic Reaction: Systemic allergic reactions have rarely occurred with human insulin products. These reactions may be characterized by generalized skin rash, itching, seating, gastrointestinal upset, angioneurotic oedema, difficulties in breathing, palpitation, reduction in blood pressure and loss of consciousness. Severe cases of generalized allergy include anaphylactic reaction may be life threatening.

Special Populations: Pregnant Women: During pregnancy and lactation, diabetes may become more difficult to manage. However, optimal metabolic control not only during pregnancy, but also prior to conception has proven to be beneficial in reducing the risk of miscarriage and malformation of the fetus. Diabetics who have become pregnant or desiring to become pregnant should consult their doctor for advice. Insulin ingested with the mother's milk has not been associated with any risk for the baby.

Nursing Women: There are no restrictions on the treatment of diabetes with Novolin **ge** Toronto, Novolin **ge** NPH, or Novolin **ge** Premixed Insulin Preparations during lactation. Insulin treatment of the nursing mother presents no risk to the baby. However, the dosage of Novolin **ge** Toronto, Novolin **ge** NPH, or Novolin **ge** Premixed Insulin Preparations and/or diet may need to be adjusted.

Pediatrics: No data is available.

Geriatrics: No data is available.

Monitoring and Laboratory Tests: In patients with diabetes mellitus optimised metabolic control delays the onset and slows the progression of late diabetic complications. Optimised metabolic control, including glucose monitoring, is therefore recommended.

ADVERSE REACTIONS: Adverse Drug Reaction Overview: At institution of insulin therapy, edema and refraction anomalies may occur. These conditions are usually of a transitory nature.

Occasionally, transitory redness, swelling, and itching at the injection site can either be caused by the insulin as such or the preservative used in the preparation. These reactions will often be of a non-specific and transitory nature. In very rare cases, lipoatrophy or lipohypotrophy can develop at the injection site. Patients should rotate the injection site to avoid this side effect.

If, in exceptional cases, redness at the injection site quickly spreads as rash and blisters over the whole body, immediate medical attention is required. This is extremely rare with the use of Novolin **ge** (Insulin, Human Biosynthetic).

Hypoglycemia is the most frequent undesirable effect. It may occur if the insulin dose is too high in relation to the insulin requirement. In clinical trials and during marketed use, the frequency varies with patient population and dose regimes. Therefore, no specific frequency can be presented. Severe hypoglycaemia may lead to unconsciousness and/or convulsions and may result in temporary or permanent impairment of brain function or even death.

Clinical Trial Adverse Drug Reactions: Because clinical trials are conducted under very specific conditions the adverse reaction rates observed in the clinical trials may not reflect the rates observed in practice and should not be compared to the rates in the clinical trials of another drug. Adverse drug reaction information from clinical trials is useful for identifying drug-related adverse events and for approximating rates.

Adverse events were reported in three comparative studies. In one study, one patient in the Novolin **ge** treatment group experienced pain at the injection site. In one study, two patients in the Novolin **ge** treatment group had suspected insulin allergy. However, skin tests showed no evidence of a response to either Novolin **ge** or Novolin, Insulin Human Semi-synthetic (ss). One patient receiving Novolin **ge** was hospitalized with mild ketoacidosis but fully recovered after hospital treatment. In one study seven patients receiving Novolin **ge** and two Novolin (ss) reported headaches. There was no clear etiology for these. In addition, eight patients receiving Novolin **ge** and one receiving Novolin (ss) experienced pain and burning after injection. These latter findings are difficult to interpret as they are currently seen in clinical practice. They were not related to insulin allergy except in one patient who tested positive to protamine.

Less Common Clinical Trial Adverse Drug Reactions (<1%): No clinical trials, where human insulin has been used as the primary investigational medicinal products (IMP), have been conducted recently. However, human insulin has been used as comparator or concomitant medication in clinical trials where other products have been the IMP.

The overall profile of adverse events—frequency, severity or type of adverse events—reported on human insulin during these clinical trials, has not caused any safety concern. No specific clustering of less common adverse drug reactions have been seen and no changes to the core safety information have been necessary for safety reasons.

Post-Market Adverse Drug Reactions: The following are adverse drug reactions based on post-marketing experience.

Metabolism and Nutrition Disorders: Rare (<1/1000): Change in blood glucose: Hypoglycemia/hyperglycemia.

Hypoglycemia: Symptoms of hypoglycemia usually occur suddenly. They may include cold sweats; cool pale skin; fatigue; nervousness or tremor; anxiousness; unusual tiredness or weakness; confusion; difficulty in concentration; drowsiness; excessive hunger; vision changes; headache; nausea and palpitation. Severe hypoglycemia may lead to unconsciousness and/or convulsions and may result in temporary or permanent impairment of brain function or even death.

Hyperglycemia: Usually the first symptoms of hyperglycaemia set in gradually, over a period of hours or days. They include thirst; increased frequency of urination; nausea; vomiting; drowsiness; flushed dry skin; dry mouth; loss of appetite as well as acetone odour of breath.

In type 1 diabetes, untreated hyperglycaemic events eventually lead to diabetic ketoacidosis which is potentially lethal.

Immune System Disorders: Uncommon (>1/1000, <1/100): urticaria, rash. Very rare (<1/10 000): anaphylactic reactions. Symptoms of generalized hypersensitivity may include generalized skin rash; itching; sweating; gastrointestinal upset; angioneurotic oedema; difficulties in breathing; palpitation; reduction in blood pressure and fainting/loss of consciousness. Generalized hypersensitivity reactions are potentially life threatening.

Nervous System Disorders: Uncommon (>1/1000, <1/100): peripheral neuropathy for Novolin **ge** Toronto and Novolin **ge** Premix Insulin. Very rare (<1/10 000): peripheral neuropathy for Novolin **ge** NPH. Fast improvement in blood glucose control may be associated with a condition termed "acute painful neuropathy", which is usually reversible.

Eye Disorders: Uncommon (>1/1000, <1/100): diabetic retinopathy for Novolin **ge** NPH and Novolin **ge** Premix Insulin. Very rare (<1/10 000): diabetic retinopathy for Novolin **ge** Toronto. Long-term improved glycemic control decreases the risk of progression of diabetic retinopathy. However, intensification of insulin therapy with abrupt improvement in glycaemic control may be associated with temporary worsening of diabetic retinopathy.

Very rare (<1/10 000): refraction disorders for Novolin **ge** NPH and Novolin **ge** Premix Insulin. Uncommon (>1/1000, <1/100): refraction disorders for Novolin **ge** Toronto. Refraction anomalies may occur upon initiation of insulin therapy. These symptoms are usually transitory in nature.

Skin and Subcutaneous Tissue Disorders: Uncommon (>1/1000, <1/100): lipodystrophy. Lipodystrophy may occur at the injection site as a consequence of failure to rotate injection sites within an area.

General Disorders and Administration Site Conditions: Uncommon (>1/1000, <1/100): injection site reactions. Injection site reactions (redness, swelling, itching, pain and haematoma at the injection site) may occur during treatment with insulin. Most reactions are usually transitory and disappear during continued treatment.

Uncommon (>1/1000, <1/100): oedema. Oedema may occur upon initiation of insulin therapy. These symptoms are usually of transitory in nature.

DRUG INTERACTIONS: Overview: A number of medicinal products are known to interact with the glucose metabolism. The physician must therefore take possible interactions into account and should always ask their patients about any medicinal products they take.

Insulin suspensions should not be added to infusion fluids. Medicinal products added to the insulin solution may cause degradation of the insulin, e.g. if the medicinal products contain thiols or sulphites.

However, when mixing Novolin **ge** Toronto and Novolin **ge** NPH the blunting effect is not observed and the rapid onset of Novolin **ge** Toronto is preserved.

Drug-Drug Interactions: The drugs listed in Table 1 are based on either drug interaction case reports or studies, or potential interactions due to the expected magnitude and seriousness of the interaction (i.e., those identified as contraindicated).

Table 1: Novolin ge

Established or Potential Drug-Drug Interactions

Drug Class	Ref	Effect	Clinical Comment
Oral hypoglycemic agents (OHA), monoamine oxidase inhibitors (MAOI), non-selective beta-blocking agents, angiotensin converting enzyme (ACE) inhibitors, salicylates, alcohol, anabolic steroids and sulphonamides	C	May reduce insulin requirement	Therapeutic concentration monitoring is recommended
Oral contraceptives, thiazides, glucocorticoids, thyroid hormones and beta-sympathomimetics, growth hormone and danazol	C	May increased insulin requirement	Therapeutic concentration monitoring is recommended
Beta-blocking agents	C	May mask the symptoms of hypoglycemia and delay recovery from hypoglycemia	Therapeutic concentration monitoring is recommended
Octreotide/lanreotide	C	May both decrease and increase insulin requirement	Therapeutic concentration monitoring is recommended

Legend: C=case study; CT=clinical trial; T=theoretical.

Drug-Food Interactions: Please refer to Dosage and Administration for more information. Alcohol may intensify and prolong the hypoglycaemic effect of insulin.

Drug-Herb Interactions: Interactions with herbal products have not been established.

Drug-Laboratory Test Interactions: Interactions with laboratory tests have not been established.

Drug-Lifestyle Interactions: Changes in insulin therapy or changes in lifestyle (i.e. diet, exercise/physical activity) may require a change in dosage.

DOSAGE AND ADMINISTRATION: Dosing Considerations:

- Concomitant stress or illness, especially infections and feverish conditions, usually increases the patient's insulin requirement. In these instances, patients should contact their physicians and carefully control their blood glucose.

Recommended Dose and Dosage Adjustment: Novolin **ge** (Insulin, Human Biosynthetic) is made in one strength in Canada, 100 units per mL. The dosage is determined by the physician in accordance with the needs of the patient.

The individual insulin requirement is usually between 0.3 and 1 IU/kg/day. The daily insulin requirement may be higher in patients with insulin resistance (e.g. during puberty in the young or due to obesity) and lower in patients with residual, endogenous insulin production.

Novolin ge Toronto: Novolin **ge** Toronto when used alone is usually given three or more times daily. Novolin **ge** Toronto may also be used in combination with longer-acting insulins of equal purity to suit the needs of the individual patients. It may be given subcutaneously, intramuscularly or intravenously. The injection of Novolin **ge** Toronto should be followed by a meal no later than 30 minutes after injection.

Novolin ge NPH: Novolin **ge** NPH is usually given once or twice daily. It is administered by subcutaneous injection.

Novolin **ge** NPH may be used alone or mixed with fast-acting soluble insulin. In intensive insulin therapy the suspensions may be used as basal insulin (evening and/or morning injection) with fast-acting or rapid-acting insulin given at meals.

Novolin ge Premixed Insulin Preparations: Novolin **ge** 30/70, Novolin **ge** 40/60, Novolin **ge** 50/50 are usually given once or twice daily, especially when a strong initial effect is desired. They are administered by subcutaneous injection. The injection of Novolin **ge** Premixed Insulins Preparations should be followed by a meal no later than 30 minutes after injection.

Dosage Adjustments:
- Renal or hepatic impairment may reduce insulin requirement.
- Adjustment of dosage may also be necessary if patients undertake increased physical activity or change their usual diet.
- In insulin resistance, e.g. during puberty or due to obesity, the daily insulin requirement may be substantially higher.

The following are general prescribing guidelines:

New Patients: Although each patient must be assessed individually, initial stabilization on multiple injections of Novolin **ge** Toronto is recommended. Following this, most patients will respond well to a regimen of Novolin **ge** NPH once or twice daily. Usually small amounts of Novolin **ge** Toronto are added to cover the morning and evening meals.

Alternatively, Novolin **ge** Premixed Insulin Preparations may be given once or twice daily.

Transfer of Patients: When patients are transferred from other insulins to Novolin **ge**, the change should be made as directed by the physician according to the following general guidelines:
- Transferring a patient to another type or brand name of insulin should be done under strict medical supervision. Changes in strength, brand (manufacturer), type (fast-, dual-, intermediate- and long-acting insulin etc.), origin (animal, human, human insulin human insulin analogue) and/or method of manufacture (recombinant DNA versus animal source insulin) may result in a need for a change in dosage.

If an adjustment is needed when switching the patients to Novolin **ge** Toronto, Novolin **ge** NPH, or Novolin **ge** Premixed Insulin Preparations, it may occur with the first dose or during the first several weeks or months.

Patients currently on self-prepared mixtures should be transferred to the closest available Novolin **ge** fixed mixture preparation.

Any patient on a total daily dose of greater than 100 units of insulin may need to be closely monitored by the physician when transferring to a different insulin preparation, preferably in hospital.

Administration: Before each injection, check that the right preparation is being used.

Novolin ge in Vials: A U-100 syringe should always be used. Failure to use the correct syringe can lead to dosage errors. Insulin should only be mixed as directed by the physician. Novolin **ge** Toronto should be mixed in the syringe with insulin of equal purity (e.g., Novolin **ge** NPH). The order of mixing and brand or model of syringe should be specified by the physician. In general, when longer-acting insulin are mixed with short-acting soluble insulins, the short-acting insulin should be drawn into the syringe first.

Novolin ge Toronto: Insulin solution should not be used if it does not appear water-clear and colourless.

Novolin ge NPH and Novolin ge Premixed Insulin Preparations: An insulin suspension should not be used if it does not appear uniformly white and cloudy after re-suspension.

Routine Injection Procedure: Syringes: If sterile disposable syringes and needles are not used, sterile glass syringes and appropriate sterile needles may be used.

1. The surface of the vial-stopper and the site of injection should be wiped with a suitable antiseptic, such as alcohol, and allowed to dry.
2. If only one insulin type is used, a volume of air equal to the dose of insulin to be injected is drawn into the syringe, then introduced into the vial. The vial and syringe is turned upside down and the correct insulin dose is drawn into the syringe. Then the needle is removed from the vial, any air is expelled from the syringe and the dose is checked.
3. Insulins of different types should be mixed only on the recommendation of the physician. The order of mixing of insulins and brand or model of syringe should not be changed, otherwise dosage errors may result. This is because insulin hypodermic syringes may vary in the amount of space between the bottom line and the needle (dead space).
4. The skin is pinched between the thumb and forefinger and the needle pushed into the fold at an angle of approximately 45 degrees. The insulin is injected under the skin (subcutaneously). Care should be taken not to inject into a muscle or vein. The needle is removed and the injection spot pressed gently for a few seconds to prevent any insulin seeping out.
5. Successive injections at any one site should be avoided. The site of injection should be altered routinely as advised by the physician.

Insulin suspensions should be carefully shaken to ensure that the contents are uniformly mixed before injecting each dose.

Novo Nordisk Insulin Delivery Devices: Penfill cartridges are only for use in Novolin-Pen Novo Nordisk insulin delivery devices described in Dosage Forms, Composition and Packaging. If treatment involves two insulins in Penfill cartridges, a separate Novolin-Pen Novo Nordisk Insulin Delivery Device should be used for each type of insulin.

Novolin **ge** Penfill must not be refilled.

1. Before use check that the Penfill cartridge is intact (e.g., no cracks). Do not use Penfill if any damage is seen, or if more of the rubber stopper (piston) is visible than equal to the width of the white bar code band.
2. Check that sufficient insulin remains in the cartridge, prefilled syringe or delivery system to complete the injection and that the insulin is the correct preparation.
3. Wipe the rubber membrane of the Penfill cartridge and the site of injection with a suitable antiseptic, such as alcohol, and allow to dry.
4. Remove the protective disc from a NovoFine needle and screw it firmly onto the Novo Nordisk Insulin Delivery Device. Pull off the outer and inner needle caps.
5. For insulin suspensions, before insertion into Novo Nordisk Insulin Delivery Device, the Penfill cartridge should be carefully shaken up and down at least 10 times (except for Novolin **ge** Toronto Penfill which is a clear solution), until the liquid appears uniformly white and cloudy. The glass ball inside the cartridge should move from one end to the other during mixing.

   Before each injection, Novo Nordisk Insulin Delivery Device with the inserted cartridge should be carefully shaken up and down at least 10 times (except for Novolin **ge** Toronto which is a clear solution), until the liquid appears uniformly white and cloudy. The glass ball inside the cartridge should move from one end of the cartridge to the other during mixing.
6. When making an injection using a Novo Nordisk insulin delivery device, allow the needle to remain under the skin for at least 6 seconds. Keep the push button fully depressed until after the needle has been withdrawn from the skin. This will ensure correct delivery and limit possible flow of blood or other body fluids into the needle or insulin reservoir.
7. NovoFine needles should be removed after each injection. If the needle is not removed, changes in ambient temperature can result in some liquid being expelled from the cartridge. In the case of insulin suspensions, removal of supernatant liquid can cause an increase in insulin concentration (i.e., strength) within the cartridge, which can cause inaccurate dosing.

Use only Novolin **ge** Penfill cartridges and NovoFine needles with Novolin-Pen systems.

Use only NovoFine needles with Novo Nordisk Insulin Delivery Devices.

Novolin **ge** Toronto is usually administered subcutaneously in the abdominal wall. The thigh, the buttocks or the deltoid region may also be used. Subcutaneous injection into the abdominal wall ensures a faster absorption than from other injection sites.

Novolin **ge** NPH are usually administered subcutaneously in the thigh. If convenient, the abdominal wall, the buttocks or the deltoid region may also be used. Subcutaneous injection into the thigh results in a slower and less variable absorption compared to the other injection sites.

Novolin **ge** Premixed Insulin Preparations are usually administered subcutaneously in the thigh or abdominal wall. If convenient, the buttocks or the deltoid region may also be used. Subcutaneous injection into the abdominal wall ensures a faster absorption than from other injection sites.

OVERDOSAGE:

Hypoglycemia may occur if the diabetic administers too much insulin, misses a meal or exercises more than usual. The first symptoms can come on suddenly and may include cold sweat, rapid heart beat, nervousness or shakiness. If untreated, the situation may progress to unconsciousness. In rare cases, the nature and intensity of hypoglycemia warning symptoms may change. This has been observed in patients with long duration of diabetes (with diabetic neuropathy), after changes of regimen and in patients on strict metabolic control. However, if severe hypoglycemia is not treated it can cause temporary or permanent brain damage or death.

In the event of an overdose, glucose should be given orally if the patient is conscious. Where the patient is unconscious, an intramuscular, subcutaneous or intravenous injection of glucagon should be given and oral carbohydrate administered when the patient responds. Alternatively, intravenous glucose may be administered; it **must** be given if there is no response to glucagon within 10 to 15 minutes.

For management of a suspected drug overdose, CPhA recommends that you contact your **regional Poison Control Centre**. See the *CPS* Directory section for a list of Poison Control Centres.

ACTION AND CLINICAL PHARMACOLOGY: Mechanism of Action: The primary activity of Novolin **ge** Toronto, Novolin **ge** NPH, Novolin **ge** 30/70, Novolin **ge** 40/60 and Novolin **ge** 50/50 is the regulation of glucose metabolism. The blood glucose lowering effect of insulins, including Novolin **ge** Toronto, Novolin **ge** NPH, Novolin **ge** 30/70, Novolin **ge** 40/60 and Novolin **ge** 50/50 is due to the facilitated uptake of glucose following binding of insulin to receptors on muscle and fat cells and to the simultaneous inhibition of glucose output from the liver.

Pharmacodynamics: Novolin **ge** Toronto: fast-acting insulin. Onset of action is within ½ hour, reaches maximum effect within 1.5-3.5 hours and entire time of duration is approximately 7-8 hours.

Novolin **ge** NPH: intermediate-acting insulin. Onset of action is within 1½ hour, reaches maximum effect within 4-12 hours and the entire time of duration is approximately 24 hours.

Novolin **ge** Premixes: dual-acting insulin. Onset of action is within ½ hour, reaches a maximum effect within 2-8 hours and the entire time of duration is up to 24 hours.

This profile is similar in children and adolescents.

Pharmacokinetics: Insulin in the blood stream has a half-life of a few minutes. Consequently, the time-action profile of an insulin preparation is determined solely by its absorption characteristics.

This process is influenced by several factors (e.g. insulin dosage, injection route and site, thickness of subcutaneous fat, type of diabetes). The pharmacokinetics of insulin is are therefore affected by significant intra- and inter-individual variation.

In general, the absorption after subcutaneous administration of Novolin **ge** products is different, dependant on the injection site. The absorption is fastest from the abdomen and slowest from the thigh. An approximate action profile following subcutaneous administration indicates:

	Novolin ge Toronto	Novolin ge NPH	Novolin ge Premixed
Onset	0.5 hour	1.5 hours	0.5 hour
Maximum	1.5–3.5 hours	4–12 hours	2–8 hours
Duration	approx. 7–8 hrs	approx. 24 hours	up to 24 hours

Absorption: Novolin ge Toronto: The maximum plasma concentration is reached within 1.5-2. 5 hours after subcutaneous administration.

Novolin ge NPH: The maximum plasma concentration of the insulin is reached within 2-18 hours after subcutaneous administration.

Novolin ge Premixed Insulin Preparations: The absorption profile is due to the product being a mixture of insulins with fast and protracted absorption respectively. The maximum plasma concentration of the fast-acting insulin is reached within 1.5-2.5 hours after subcutaneous administration.

Distribution: Novolin **ge** Toronto, Novolin **ge** NPH, Novolin **ge** Premixed Insulin Preparations: No profound binding to plasma proteins, except circulating insulin antibodies (if present) has been observed.

Metabolism: Novolin **ge** Toronto, Novolin **ge** NPH, Novolin **ge** Premixed Insulin Preparations: Human insulin is reported to be degraded by insulin protease or insulin-degrading enzymes and possibly protein disulfide isomerase. A number of cleavage (hydrolysis) sites on the human insulin molecule have been proposed; none of the metabolites formed following the cleavage are active.

Excretion: The terminal half-life is determined by the rate of absorption from the subcutaneous tissue. The terminal half-life ($t_{1/2}$) is therefore a measure of the terminal absorption rather than of the elimination per se of insulin from plasma (insulin in the blood stream has a $t_{1/2}$ of a few minutes).

Novolin ge Toronto: Trials have indicated a $t_{1/2}$ of about 2-5 hours.

Novolin ge NPH and Premixed Insulin Preparations: Trials have indicated a $t_{1/2}$ of about 5-10 hours.

Special Populations and Conditions: No specific pharmacokinetic data on Novolin **ge** products in special patient populations are available. The approved indication covers "Treatment of insulin requiring diabetics" (see Indications and Clinical Use) without any restrictions regarding age, gender or ethnicity of the diabetes patients.

Dosage is individual and is determined by the physician in accordance with the needs of the patients. However, renal or hepatic impairment may reduce insulin requirements.

STORAGE AND STABILITY: Temperature: Novolin **ge** that is not being used should be stored in a refrigerator between 2-10°C not in or too near the freezer section or cooling element. Do not freeze. Insulin preparations which have been frozen must not be used.

After removing the vial of Novolin **ge** NPH and Novolin **ge** 30/70 from the refrigerator it is recommended to allow it to reach room temperature before resuspending the insulin as instructed for first time use.

After removing the Novolin **ge** NPH Penfill cartridge and Novolin **ge** Penfill cartridge Premixed insulin preparation, (Novolin **ge** 30/70, Novolin **ge** 40/60, Novolin **ge** 50/50) from the refrigerator it is recommended to allow it to reach room temperature before resusspending the insulin as instructed for first time use.

During use: Do not refrigerate. Do not store Novolin **ge** above 25°C (vial) or 30°C (Penfill).

Novolin **ge** Penfill when used in Novolin-Pen can be in-use or carried as a spare for up to one month at room temperature (not above 30°C). When in use, Novo Nordisk insulin delivery devices are to be maintained at room temperature.

Light: Keep the vial or cartridge in the outer carton in order to protect the insulin from light. Keep the pen cap on Penfill in order to protect the insulin from light. Protect from excessive heat and sunlight.

Others: Insulin should not be used after the expiry date printed on the package.

INFORMATION FOR THE PATIENT: Published in e-CPS, available by subscription at www.e-cps.ca.

DOSAGE FORMS, COMPOSITION AND PACKAGING: Vials of 10 mL and Penfill cartridges of 3 mL. All in a strength of 100 units/mL. Novolin **ge** preparations are available in the following presentations (see Table 2).

Table 2: Novolin ge Preparations

Availability of Novolin ge Preparations

10 mL vials	3 mL Penfill cartridges
Novolin **ge** Toronto	Novolin **ge** Toronto
Novolin **ge** NPH	Novolin **ge** NPH
Novolin **ge** 30/70	Novolin **ge** 30/70
	Novolin **ge** 40/60
	Novolin **ge** 50/50

Novolin-Pen systems are insulin delivery devices designed for use with Novolin **ge** Penfill insulin cartridges and NovoFine needles.

The following nonmedicinal ingredients are found in Novolin **ge** Toronto: glycerol, hydrochloric acid and/or sodium hydroxide (for pH adjustment), metacresol, water for injection, zinc chloride.

The following nonmedicinal ingredients are found in Novolin **ge** NPH and Novolin **ge** Premixed Insulin Preparations: disodium phosphate dihydrate, glycerol, hydrochloric acid and/or sodium hydroxide, metacresol, phenol, protamine sulphate, water for injection, zinc chloride.

Novolin-Pen® 4

insulin delivery device

Insulin Delivery Device

Novo Nordisk

SUPPLIED: In appearance Novolin-Pen 4 resembles a cartridge pen. The device is loaded with a Penfill cartridge containing 3 mL of U100 human insulin (Novolin**ge** Toronto, NPH, 10/90, 20/80, 30/70, 40/60, or 50/50), NovoRapid (insulin aspart) or Levemir (insulin detemir). Novolin-Pen 4 is a dial-a-dose injection device capable of delivering 1 to 60 units of insulin, delivered in increments of 1 unit, with a single depression of the push button.

The product is designed for use with Novolin**ge** Penfill insulin preparations, NovoRapid or Levemir and NovoFine needles. See Novolin**ge** and NovoRapid.

The NovoFine needle should be removed after each injection. If the needle is not removed, changes in ambient temperature can result in some liquid being expelled from the cartridge. In the case of insulin suspensions, removal of supernatant liquid can cause an increase in insulin concentration (i.e., strength) remaining in the cartridge.

Novo Nordisk cannot be held responsible for malfunctions as a consequence of using Novolin-Pen 4 in combination with products that do not meet the same specifications or quality standards as Novolin**ge** Penfill 3 mL insulin preparations, NovoRapid Penfill 3 mL or Levemir Penfill 3 mL and NovoFine needles.

Consult the manufacturer for instructions for use.

NovoMix® 30

insulin aspart—insulin aspart protamine crystals

Antidiabetic Agent

Novo Nordisk

Date of Preparation: February 25, 2005

PHARMACOLOGY: NovoMix 30 (30% soluble insulin aspart and 70% insulin aspart protamine crystals) is a dual-release human insulin analogue suspension containing 30% soluble insulin aspart and 70% insulin aspart protamine crystals. The rapid absorption characteristics of NovoRapid are maintained by NovoMix 30. The insulin aspart in the soluble component of NovoMix 30 is absorbed more rapidly from the subcutaneous layer than regular human insulin. The remaining 70% is in crystalline form as insulin aspart protamine which has a prolonged absorption profile after subcutaneous injection.

The primary activity of NovoMix 30 is the regulation of glucose metabolism. Insulins, including NovoMix 30, bind to the insulin receptors on muscle and fat cells and lower blood glucose by facilitating the cellular uptake of glucose—and simultaneously inhibit the output of glucose from the liver.

The effect of NovoMix 30 is more rapid in onset compared to biphasic human insulin 30/70 (i.e. Novolin ge 30/70, insulin, human biosynthetic) due to the faster absorption of the soluble component after subcutaneous injection.

Pharmacokinetics: Bioavailability and Absorption of NovoMix 30: The rapid absorption characteristics of NovoRapid are maintained by NovoMix 30. The insulin aspart in the soluble component of NovoMix 30 is absorbed more rapidly from the subcutaneous layer than regular soluble human insulin. The remaining 70% is in crystalline form as insulin aspart protamine that has a prolonged absorption profile after subcutaneous injection.

The relative bioavailability of NovoMix 30 compared to premixed human insulin 30/70 indicates that they are absorbed to similar degrees.

The maximum serum insulin concentration (C_{max}) for NovoMix 30 is, on average, 50% higher than with biphasic human insulin 30/70 (p=0.000). The time to maximum concentration (T_{max}) is, on average, half that for biphasic human insulin 30/70 (p=0.000). In healthy volunteers, a mean maximum serum concentration of 23.4±5.3 mU/L was reached about 60 minutes after a subcutaneous dose of 0.2 U/kg body weight versus 15.5±3.7 mU/L at about 130 minutes for biphasic human insulin 30/70. The mean half life ($t_{½}$) of NovoMix 30, reflecting the absorption rate of the protamine bound fraction, was about 8-9 hours. Serum insulin levels returned to baseline about 15-18 hours after a subcutaneous dose. In type 2 diabetic patients, the maximum concentration was reached about 95 minutes after dosing.

Pharmacokinetic Profiles of NovoMix 30 and Biphasic Human Insulin 30/70: See Figure 1.

Figure 1: NovoMix 30

Mean Serum Insulin Concentration Following a Single Subcutaneous Dose (0.2 U/kg body weight) of NovoMix 30 (solid line) and Biphasic Human Insulin 30/70 (hatched line) in Healthy Subjects

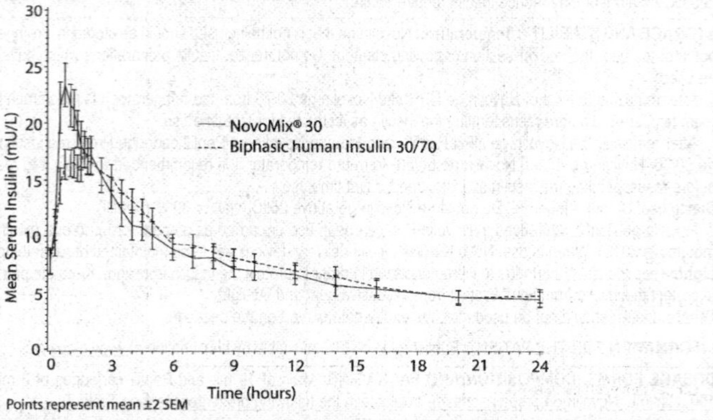

Distribution and Elimination: Insulin aspart has a low binding to plasma proteins, 0-9%. After subcutaneous administration, insulin aspart was more rapidly eliminated than regular human insulin with an average apparent half life of 81 minutes compared to 141 minutes for regular human insulin.

Pharmacodynamics: NovoMix 30: NovoMix 30 (30% soluble insulin aspart and 70% insulin aspart protamine crystals) is a dual-release human insulin analogue suspension containing 30% soluble insulin aspart. This has a rapid onset of action, thus allowing it to be given closer to a meal when compared to soluble human insulin. The crystalline phase (70%) consists of insulin aspart protamine, which has an activity profile similar to that of human NPH insulin.

The pharmacodynamic response to a single dose of 0.3 U/kg NovoMix 30 and premixed human insulin 30/70 was investigated in 24 healthy subjects using the hyperinsulinaemic euglycemic clamp method. NovoMix 30 shows a significantly greater metabolic effect in the first 4 hours after subcutaneous injection than the premixed human insulin 30/70 (see Figure 2). When NovoMix 30 is injected subcutaneously, the onset of action will occur within 10 to 20 minutes of injection. The maximum effect is exerted between 1 and 4 hours after injection. The duration of action is up to 24 hours.

Figure 2: NovoMix 30

Pharmacodynamic Activity Profile of NovoMix 30 and Biphasic Human Insulin 30/70 in Healthy Subjects

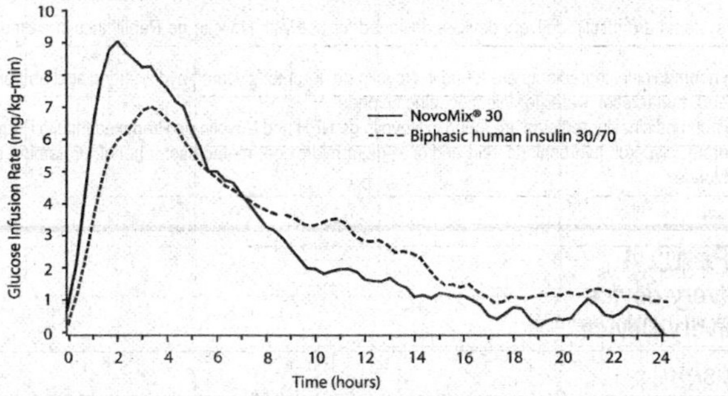

In a randomized, double-blind, two-way cross-over trial comparing NovoMix 30 and biphasic human insulin 30/70 in patients with type 2 diabetes, the therapeutic response was evaluated following two 2-week treatment periods where insulin was administered in a twice daily dose regimen; immediately before breakfast and dinner. The shape of the 24-hour total serum glucose concentration-time profiles were statistically significantly different between treatments over time (see Figure 3). Although there was no difference detected between treatments with respect to average serum glucose levels over 24 hours, the estimated mean time-action curves shown below indicate that postprandial glucose control was superior with NovoMix 30 compared to biphasic human insulin 30/70, following dinner and breakfast but higher after lunch.

Estimated Mean 24-hour Serum Glucose Profiles: See Figure 3.

Figure 3: NovoMix 30

Estimated Serum Glucose Levels Following Twice Daily Injection (immediately before breakfast and dinner) of NovoMix 30 (BIAsp 30) or Biphasic Human Insulin (BHI 30) in 13 Patients with Type 2 Diabetes.

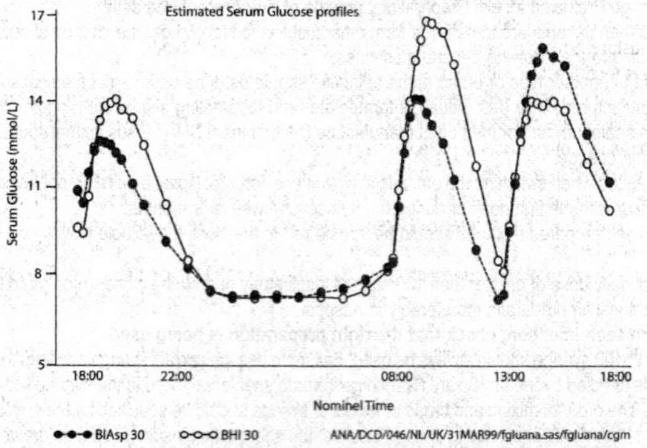

In a 3 month, multicentre, open-labelled, randomized, parallel group study, NovoMix 30 was as effective as biphasic human insulin 30/70 (Novolin ge 30/70) in long-term glycemic control, based on HbA_{1C} levels. Mealtime blood glucose increment averaged over the three main meals was statistically significantly different (29% lower) in the NovoMix 30 group (p<0.02) and statistically significant differences (approximately 1 mmol/L lower) were observed in mean blood glucose levels after breakfast, before lunch, after dinner and at bedtime (p<0.02-0.05). Improvements in postprandial glycemic control did not increase the risk of hypoglycemia. Patients wishing to continue in an extension of this study were followed for an additional 21 month period on either NovoMix 30 or Novolin ge 30/70. At the end of the 24 month period of treatment, glycemic control, as measured by HbA_{1c}, was similar in the two groups.

With similar levels of glycemic control (as assessed by HbA_{1c}), the number and rate of hypoglycemic episodes was similar in patients with Type 1 diabetes. However, for patients with type 2 diabetes, those treated with NovoMix 30 had a lower frequency of major hypoglycemia than those receiving Novolin ge 30/70 and during the last six months of the study, no patients treated with NovoMix 30 experienced major hypoglycemia.

In a clinical trial, 61 subjects with type 2 diabetes received a single dose of NovoMix 30, Humalog Mix25 and Novolin ge 30/70 (insulin, human biosynthetic) on three separate occasions in a cross-over trial. Postprandial glycemic control, as assessed by the 5-hour post meal serum glucose excursion was statistically significantly improved (a 10% reduction, p<0.05) with NovoMix 30 over Humalog Mix25 and Novolin ge 30/70 (a 17% reduction, p<0.001). For NovoMix 30 versus Novolin ge 30/70, maximum glucose concentration was reduced and occurred earlier. Compared to Humalog Mix25 there was a shorter time to maximum glucose concentration.

One hundred and fifty-one type 2 patients inadequately treated with oral diabetes medication (metformin with/without insulin secretagogues) were entered into a clinical trial. During the first 4 weeks of the trial, patients were titrated to target with metformin only. Those patients who did not achieve fasting glycemic levels within the target range of 5-7 mmol/L (n=140) were initiated on insulin therapy in a randomized fashion to receive one of three insulin treatment regimens once a day in combination with the metformin therapy: NovoMix 30 (at dinner), Novolin ge 30/70 (at dinner) or Novolin ge NPH (before bed). There were no statistically significant differences between treatment groups for long term glycemic control; mean HbA_{1c} levels were reduced from baseline by 1.1-1.3% with 12 weeks of treatment. There was no significant difference in reporting of hypoglycemic events among the three groups although fewer patients reported nocturnal hypoglycemic events in the NovoMix 30 group than in the other groups. At the end of the study, the final fasting plasma glucose fell within target range (5-7 mmol/L) for 9 subjects in the NovoMix 30 group, 9 subjects in the Novolin ge NPH group and 8 subjects in the Novolin ge 30/70 group. The mean decrease in HbA_{1c} values experienced by these subjects (−2.3%, −1.9% and −1.8% respectively) were greater than observed for the total study population.

Metformin-treated patients with type 2 diabetes (n=341) were randomized to receive NovoMix 30 monotherapy BID, NovoMix 30 BID with existing metformin or sulphonylurea therapy with existing metformin. In the total population, the mean difference in HbA_{1c} levels was statistically significant only for subjects receiving NovoMix 30 plus metformin versus NovoMix 30 monotherapy (p=0.004). Mean decrease in HbA_{1c} during the study was 1.5-1.8% in all groups. In 193 patients with poorly controlled diabetes at the start of the trial (HbA_{1c} ≥9.0%), the mean difference in HbA_{1c} was statistically significant in the NovoMix 30 plus metformin group versus the NovoMix 30 monotherapy group (p=0.037) and the sulphonylurea plus metformin group (p=0.033) after 16 weeks of treatment. Mean HbA_{1c} decrease during the study was 1.9 to 2.4% in all groups.

The efficacy and safety of NovoMix 30 in NovoMix 30 FlexPen was compared with Humalog Mix25 in Humalog Mix25 Pen in 132 insulin-treated patients with type 2 diabetes in a open-label, two-period crossover design trial. Following a 2-week run-in period on NovoMix 30, patients began the first 12-week treatment period on either NovoMix 30 or Humalog Mix25. At the last visit of the first treatment period, the patients completed pen device questionnaires and the WHO Diabetes Treatment Satisfaction Questionnaire (DTSQ) and then changed to the alternate insulin treatment. At the end of the 2nd 12-week treatment period, patients again completed the pen device questionnaires, the DTSQ and a comparative questionnaire asking which device they would prefer to continue to use after the trial. Treatment with NovoMix 30 and Humalog Mix25 were comparable with respect to HbA_{1c}, prandial blood glucose increment, postprandial blood glucose and episodes of hypoglycemia at the end of the trial. Patient treatment satisfaction, as measured by DTSQ was similar for both groups. For the device specific questionnaires, NovoMix 30 FlexPen was evaluated as slightly superior to Humalog Mix25 Pen in 15 of 16 device features assessed (all p<0.001). Approximately 75% of patients preferred to continue with NovoMix 30 FlexPen after the trial was completed.

Special Populations: Age and Gender: Children and adolescents: The safety and efficacy of NovoMix 30 were compared to biphasic human insulin 30/70 (BHI 30) in a double-blind crossover trial in 54 children, aged 6-12 years. The incidence of all hypoglycemic episodes was significantly lower for NovoMix 30 than for BHI 30 by approximately 10%. No safety concerns were raised during the trial. However, after 12 weeks of treatment it could not be demonstrated, that treatment with NovoMix 30 was non-inferior to treatment with BHI 30 with respect to HbA_{1c} and serum fructosamine. The data available are inadequate to establish the effectiveness in children.

Geriatrics: The effect of age on the pharmacokinetics and pharmacodynamics of NovoMix 30 has not been studied.

Gender: The effect of gender on the pharmacokinetics and pharmacodynamics of NovoMix 30 in diabetic patients has not been studied.

Obesity: The effect of obesity on the pharmacokinetics and pharmacodynamics of NovoMix 30 has not been studied.

Ethnic Origin: The effect of ethnic origin on the pharmacokinetics and pharmacodynamics of NovoMix 30 has not been studied.

Smoking: The effect of smoking on the pharmacokinetics and pharmacodynamics of NovoMix 30 has not been studied.

INDICATIONS: NovoMix 30 (30% soluble insulin aspart and 70% insulin aspart protamine crystals) is indicated for the treatment of adult patients with diabetes mellitus who require insulin for the maintenance of normal glucose homeostasis.

CONTRAINDICATIONS: NovoMix 30 (30% soluble insulin aspart and 70% insulin aspart protamine crystals) is contraindicated during episodes of hypoglycemia (see Overdose) and in patients hypersensitive to insulin aspart or any of the excipients they contain.

WARNINGS: Insulin aspart differs from regular human insulin by its rapid onset and shorter duration of action. Because of the fast onset of action, the injection of NovoMix 30 (30% soluble insulin aspart and 70% insulin aspart protamine crystals) should immediately be followed by a meal. To avoid possible transmission of disease, a Penfill cartridge must not be used by more than one person.

PRECAUTIONS: General: As with all insulins, the duration of action of NovoMix 30 (30% soluble insulin aspart and 70% insulin aspart protamine crystals) may vary in different individuals or in the same individual according to dose, injection site, blood flow, temperature and level of physical activity.

Hypokalemia is among the potential clinical adverse effect associated with the use of all insulins. This potential clinical adverse effect may be relevant in patients who are on potassium lowering drugs.

Stress or illness may change insulin requirements. In these instances, patients should contact their physician and carefully control their blood glucose.

Hypoglycemia: In certain cases (long duration of diabetes, diabetic nerve disease, intensified diabetes control, or use of medications such as beta blocking agents), the nature and intensity of early warning symptoms of hypoglycemia may change or be less pronounced.

Hypoglycemia is the most frequently occurring undesirable effect of insulin therapy. Such reactions following treatment with NovoMix 30 are mostly mild and easily managed.

Severe hypoglycemia can result in temporary or permanent impairment of brain function and death.

Changes in insulin therapy or changes in life style (i.e. diet, exercise/physical activity) may require a change in dosage. Inadequate dosing or discontinuation of insulin treatment, especially in type 1 diabetes, may lead to hyperglycemia and diabetic ketoacidosis. Severe sustained hyperglycemia may result in diabetic coma and death.

Glucose monitoring is recommended for all patients with diabetes.

The patient's ability to concentrate and react may be impaired as a result of hypoglycemia. This may constitute a risk in situations where these abilities are of special importance (e.g., driving a car or operating machinery).

Local Allergic Reaction: As with other insulins, patients may experience redness, swelling or itching at the site of injection. These minor reactions usually resolve in a few days to a few weeks. They may occur if the injection is not properly made, or if the patient is allergic to the insulin or any excipients. Few local injection site reactions were observed with NovoMix 30 in the clinical development program and there was no difference in frequency when compared to human insulin.

Systemic Allergic Reaction: Systemic allergic reaction have not been reported during the clinical development of NovoMix 30. Systemic allergic reactions have rarely occurred with NovoMix 30 as with other insulin treatment. These reactions may be characterized by a generalized rash (with pruritus), shortness of breath, wheezing and drop in blood pressure. Severe cases of generalized allergy including anaphylactic reaction may be life threatening.

Antibody Production: Insulin antibodies may develop during treatment with insulin. Insulin antibody production was fmonitored during the clinical development program for NovoMix 30. A transitory 11.2% increase in cross-reactive antibodies observed during the initial 3 months of treatment with BIAsp 30 in the phase III trial was followed by a significant decrease from month 3 to 12. This decrease was maintained between months 12 and 24, where concentrations were constant at about 5 absolute percentage points above baseline for the type 2 diabetic subjects and 7.02% for the total population (type 1 and 2 diabetic subjects). No relationship between cross-reactive antibody level and metabolic control, insulin dose requirements or adverse events has been observed.

Renal Impairment: There is no experience of treatment with insulin aspart in patients with renal impairment. As with other insulins, NovoMix 30 requirement may be reduced in patients with renal impairment.

Hepatic Impairment: There is no experience of treatment with insulin aspart in patients with hepatic impairment. As with other insulins, NovoMix 30 requirement may need to be adjusted in patients with hepatic impairment.

Use in Women: Teratogenicity: There is no information on teratogenicity of insulin aspart in humans. In rabbit trials, insulin aspart did not exert any direct adverse effect on fertility, mating performance, reproductive capacity or embryo-fetal development and did not differ from human insulin.

Pregnancy: Reproduction studies have been performed in rats and rabbits at doses up to 16-32 times the human dose and have revealed no evidence of impaired fertility or harm to the fetus due to insulin aspart . There are, however, no adequate and well-controlled studies in pregnant women. Because animal reproduction studies are not always predictive of human response, this drug should be used during pregnancy only if clearly needed.

Although there are no clinical studies of the use of NovoMix 30 in pregnancy, published studies with human insulin suggest that optimizing overall glycemic control, including postprandial control, before conception and during pregnancy improves fetal outcome. Although the fetal complications of maternal hyperglycemia have been well documented, fetal toxicity also has been reported with maternal hypoglycemia. Insulin requirements usually fall during the first trimester and increase during the second and third trimesters. Careful monitoring of the patient is required throughout pregnancy. During the perinatal period, careful monitoring of infants born to mothers with diabetes is warranted.

Lactation: It is unknown whether NovoMix 30 is excreted in significant amounts in human milk. For this reason, caution should be exercised when NovoMix 30 is administered to a nursing mother. Patients with diabetes who are lactating may require adjustments in insulin dose, meal plan or both.

Children: The data available are inadequate to establish the efficacy of NovoMix 30 in children (see Special Populations, Children and adolescents).

Self-Monitoring of Blood Glucose: As with all insulin therapy the need for regular blood glucose self-monitoring should be considered when using NovoMix 30 to obtain optimal glycemic control.

Drug Interactions: Concomitant use of other drugs may influence insulin requirements. The following substances may reduce the insulin requirements: oral hypoglycemic agents (OHA), octreotide, monoamine oxidase inhibitors (MAOI), non-selective beta adrenergic blocking agents, angiotensin converting enzyme (ACE) inhibitors, salicylates, alcohol, and anabolic steroids.

Other drugs may increase insulin requirements: oral contraceptives, thiazides, glucocorticosteroids, thyroid hormones, sympathomimetics and danazol.Beta blocking agents may mask the symptoms of hypoglycemia. Alcohol may intensify and prolong the hypoglycemic effect of insulin.

Transferring Patients from Other Insulins: When patients are transferred between different types of insulin products, the early warning symptoms of hypoglycaemia may change or become less pronounced than those experienced with their previous insulin. Transferring a patient to a new type or brand of insulin should be done under strict medical supervision. Changes in strength, brand, type, species (animal, human, human insulin analogue), and/or method of manufacture may result in the need for a change in dosage. Patients taking NovoMix 30 may need a change in dosage from that used with their usual insulins. If an adjustment is needed, it may be done with the first dose or during the first few weeks or months.

Information to Be Provided to the Patient: Patients should be informed about potential advantages and disadvantages of NovoMix 30 therapy including the possible side effects. Patients should also be offered continued education and advice on insulin therapies, life-style management, self-monitoring, complications of insulin therapy, timing of dosage, instruction for use of injection devices and storage of insulin.

The need for regular blood glucose self-monitoring should be considered when using any insulin therapy to obtain optimal glycemic control.

Female patients should be advised to discuss with their physician if they intend to or if they become pregnant.

Mixing of Insulins: NovoMix 30 should not be mixed with any other insulin product.

ADVERSE EFFECTS: Clinical trials comparing NovoRapid (insulin aspart) with regular human insulin did not demonstrate any differences in frequency of adverse events between the aspart formulations and their human insulin counterparts.

Adverse events can be categorized into the following areas:

Body as a Whole: (see Precautions).

Skin Reactions: (see Precautions, Local Allergic Reaction).

Other; Hypoglycemia: (see Warnings, Precautions and below).

The serious and important Adverse Drug Reactions associated with insulin treatment are events of hypoglycemia, hypoglycemic coma, poor blood glucose control, and the most frequent event hyperglycemia (see Overdose).

Table 1 provides the distribution of all Adverse Events (greater than 1%) occurring in >1% of subjects in a 24 month study for NovoMix.

Table 1: NovoMix 30

Commonly Report Adverse Events Occurring in >1% of Patients

	BIAsp 30 N=101		BHI 30 N=103	
Respiratory System Disorders				
Upper resp tract infection	46	46%	35	34%
Pharyngitis	16	16%	10	10%
Coughing	12	12%	8	8%
Rhinitis	10	10%	9	9%

(cont'd)

Table 1: NovoMix 30 *(cont'd)*

Commonly Report Adverse Events Occurring in >1% of Patients

	BIAsp 30 N=101		BHI 30 N=103	
Sinusitis	5	5%	3	3%
Bronchitis	4	4%	3	3%
Dyspnoea	2	2%	3	3%
Pneumonia			2	2%
Pulmonary oedema			2	2%
Chronic obstructive airways disease			2	2%
Central & Peripheral Nervous System Disorders				
Headache	29	29%	1712	17%
Sensory disturbance	10	10%	9	12%
Hyporeflexia	9	9%	8	9%
Neuropathy	8	8%	4	8%
Migraine	3	3%	2	4%
Cramps legs	3	3%	3	2%
Dizziness	2	2%	1	3%
Vertigo	2	2%	3	<1%
Neuralgia	1	<1%		3%
Body as a Whole—General Disorders				
Influenza-like symptoms	21	21%	205	19%
Back pain	11	11%	4	5%
Leg pain	5	5%	3	4%
Allergic reaction	4	4%	1	3%
Headache	4	4%	2	<1%
Fatigue	2	2%	1	2%
Allergy	2	2%	1	<1%
Pain	2	2%		<1%
Malaise	2	2%		
Nasal polyp	2	2%	5	
Chest pain	1	<1%	2	5%
Carpal tunnel syndrome				2%
Gastro-Intestinal System Disorders				
Dyspepsia	13	13%	9	9%
Diarrhea	12	12%	13	13%
Abdominal pain	8	8%	5	5%
Tooth ache	6	6%	4	4%
Nausea	5	5%	7	7%
Gastroenteritis	4	4%	1	<1%
Vomiting	3	3%	9	9%
Constipation	3	3%	4	4%
Gingivitis	2	2%	2	2%
Tooth disorder	2	2%	2	2%
Oesophagitis	2	2%		
Gastritis			4	4%
Gastro-intestinal disorder nos			2	2%
Musculo-Skeletal System Disorders				
Arthralgia	9	9%	6	6%
Skeletal pain	8	8%	7	7%
Back pain	7	7%	3	3%

(cont'd)

Table 1: NovoMix 30 *(cont'd)*

Commonly Report Adverse Events Occurring in >1% of Patients

	BIAsp 30 N=101		BHI 30 N=103	
Myalgia	7	7%	1	<1%
Arthropathy	3	3%	3	3%
Arthritis	2	2%	3	3%
Arthrosis	2	2%	2	2%
Bone disorder	2	2%	1	<1%
Ischias			3	3%
Resistance Mechanism Disorders				
Infection	15	15%	17	17%
Infection fungal	4	4%	4	4%
Moniliasis	3	3%	4	4%
Infection viral	2	2%	2	2%
Abscess	2	2%	1	<1%
Herpes simplex	2	2%		
Infection wound	1	<1%	3	3%
Upper resp tract infection	1	<1%	2	2%
Skin and Appendages Disorders				
Skin disorder	5	5%	4	4%
Rash	4	4%	4	4%
Skin ulceration	3	3%	4	4%
Eczema	3	3%	3	3%
Dermatitis fungal	3	3%		
Urticaria	3	3%		
Hyperkeratosis	2	2%	1	<1%
Seborrhoea	2	2%	1	<1%
Skin dry	2	2%	1	<1%
Pruritus	1	<1%	2	2%
Metabolic and Nutritional Disorders				
Hypercholesterolaemia	7	7%	2	2%
Hyperlipaemia	4	4%	5	5%
Lipid metabolism disorder nos	3	3%		
Diabetes mellitus aggravated	2	2%		
Gout	2	2%		
Weight decrease	2	2%		
Hyperglycaemia	1	<1%	3	3%
Hypoglycaemia	1	<1%	2	2%
Oedema leg				2%
Cardiovascular Disorders, General				
Hypertension	16	16%	14	14%
Cardiac failure	3	3%	3	3%
Heart murmur	1	<1%	2	2%
Oedema dependent			2	2%
Secondary Terms				
Injury accidental	12	12%	15	15%
Vision Disorders				
Retinal disorder	5	5%	4	4%
Conjunctivitis	2	2%	1	<1%
Retinal hemorrhage	2	2%	1	<1%

(cont'd)

Table 1: NovoMix 30 *(cont'd)*

Commonly Report Adverse Events Occurring in >1% of Patients

	BIAsp 30 N=101		BHI 30 N=103	
Vision abnormal	2	2%	1	<1%
Eye abnormality			3	3%
Urinary System Disorders				
Urinary tract infection	5	5%	9	9%
Cystitis	2	2%	2	2%
Albuminuria	2	2%	1	<1%
Haematuria			3	3%
Renal function abnormal			2	2%
Liver and Biliary System Disorders				
Hepatic enzymes increased	4	4%		
Cholecystitis			2	2%
Psychiatric Disorders				
Depression	3	3%	3	3%
Anxiety	2	2%	4	4%
Impotence	2	2%		
Vascular (Extracardiac) Disorders				
Peripheral ischaemia	3	3%	1	<1%
Vascular disorder	1	<1%	3	3%
Myo Endo Pericardial & Valve Disorders				
Myocardial ischaemia	4	4%		
Angina pectoris	2	2%	3	3%
Coronary artery disorder	1	<1%	2	2%
Myocardial infarction			2	2%
Neoplasm				
Pulmonary carcinoma	2	2%		
Application Site Disorders				
Fibrous nodule	2	2%		
Reproductive Disorders, Female				
Dysmenorrhoea	2	2%	2	2%
Heart Rate and Rhythm Disorders				
Arrhythmia	2	2%	1	<1%
Red Blood Cell Disorders				
Erythrocytes abnormal	2	2%		
Anaemia secondary terms			3	3%
Injury accidental				
Hearing and Vestibular Disorders				
Earache	2	2%	2	2%

Legend:
N=number of subjects with event.
%=proportion of exposed subjects having the event.

Other: Small elevations in alkaline phosphatase were observed in patients treated with NovoMix 30 in controlled clinical trials. Some patients initially had normal levels of alkaline phosphatase, which subsequently rose above normal range. There have been no clinical consequences of these findings.

OVERDOSE:

Treatment: Hypoglycemia and Treatment of Overdosage: Overdose may cause hypoglycemia. Omission of a meal or unplanned strenuous physical exercise may lead to hypoglycemia. Symptoms of hypoglycemia may occur suddenly. They may include cold sweat, cool pale skin, fatigue, nervousness or tremor, anxious feeling, unusual tiredness or weakness, confusion, difficulty in concentration, drowsiness, excessive hunger, vision changes, headache, nausea and palpitation. Severe hypoglycemia may lead to unconsciousness and/or convulsions and may be fatal.

Mild episodes of hypoglycemia can be treated by oral administration of glucose or sugary products. It is therefore recommended that patients with diabetes always carry some sugar candy.

Severe hypoglycemic episodes, where the patient has become unconscious, can be treated with glucagon (0.5 to 1 mg) given intramuscularly or subcutaneously by a trained person or glucose given intravenously by a medical professional. Glucose must also be given intravenously if the patient does not respond to glucagon within 10 to 15 minutes. Upon regaining consciousness, administration of an oral carbohydrate is recommended for the patient in order to prevent relapse.

For management of a suspected drug overdose, CPhA recommends that you contact your **regional Poison Control Centre**. See the *CPS* Directory section for a list of Poison Control Centres.

DOSAGE: NovoMix 30 (30% soluble insulin aspart and 70% insulin aspart protamine crystals) should generally be given immediately before a meal because of the fast onset of action (start of the meal should be not more than 5-10 minutes after injection). When necessary NovoMix 30 may be given immediately after the meal.

Dosage of any insulin is individual and determined, based on the physician's advice, in accordance with the needs of the patient. The individual insulin requirement is usually between 0.5-1.0 units/kg/day. In a meal-related treatment, 50-70% of this requirement may be provided by NovoRapid and the remainder provided by an intermediate-acting or long-acting insulin. In a premixed insulin regimen, the total daily dose can be provided by NovoMix 30.

The dosing of any insulin should be regularly adjusted according to blood glucose measurements.

New Patients: Patients being initiated on insulin for the first time can be started on NovoMix 30 in the same manner as they would be on animal-source or human insulin.

Transfer Patients: When patients are transferred from other insulin to NovoMix 30, the change should be made as directed by the physician.

In clinical trials of NovoMix 30, patients were transferred on a unit to unit basis from human premixed 30/70 or human NPH to NovoMix 30 with doses subsequently adjusted according to individual patient needs.

Administration: NovoMix 30 (30% soluble insulin aspart and 70% insulin aspart protamine crystals) is administered subcutaneously in the abdominal wall, the thigh, the upper arm or the buttock. Care should be taken to avoid entry into a blood vessel. Injection sites should be rotated within the same region. As with all insulins, the duration of action will vary according to the dose, injection site, blood flow, temperature and level of physical activity.

NovoMix 30: NovoMix 30 is a white suspension. The carton contains a package leaflet with instructions for use and handling. The necessity of properly resuspending NovoMix 30 immediately before use should be stressed to the patient. The resuspended liquid must appear uniformly white and cloudy. NovoMix 30 should not be used after it's expiration date. NovoMix 30 should not be injected intravenously.

In patients with diabetes mellitus, optimized metabolic control effectively delays the onset and slows the progression of late diabetic complications. Optimized metabolic control, including glucose monitoring is therefore recommended.

INFORMATION FOR THE PATIENT: Published in e-CPS, available by subscription at www.e-cps.ca.

SUPPLIED: Each mL of sterile, uniform, white suspension that contains: insulin aspart (B28 asp regular human insulin analogue) 100 units. Nonmedicinal ingredients: disodium hydrogen phosphate dihydrate, mannitol, metacresol, phenol, protamine sulfate, sodium chloride and zinc. pH:7.20-7.44. Penfill cartridges of 3 mL, cartons of 5. NovoMix 30 Penfill cartridges are designed for use Novo Nordisk Insulin Delivery Devices and NovoFine needles. Store between 2 and 10°C. Do not freeze. Cartridges in use or carried as a spare may be kept at room temperature (not above 30°C) for up to 4 weeks, but should not be exposed to excessive heat or sunlight. Do not use after the expiry date printed on the package.

NovoRapid®

insulin aspart

Antidiabetic

Novo Nordisk

Date of Revision: October 24, 2005

PHARMACOLOGY: Insulin aspart is a unique human insulin analogue of rDNA origin that rapidly lowers blood glucose. Insulin aspart is homologous with regular human insulin with the exception of a substitution of the amino acid proline with aspartic acid in position B28. The substitution of the amino acid proline with aspartic acid at position B28 in insulin aspart reduces the tendency to form hexamers as observed with regular human insulin. Insulin aspart is therefore more rapidly absorbed from the s.c. layer compared to regular human insulin.

The primary activity of insulin aspart is the regulation of glucose metabolism. Insulins, including insulin aspart, bind to the insulin receptors on muscle and fat cells and lower blood glucose by facilitating the cellular uptake of glucose and simultaneously inhibit the output of glucose from the liver.

Insulin aspart is equipotent to regular human insulin on a molar basis.

Insulin aspart produces a more rapid and more pronounced blood glucose lowering effect than regular human insulin, due to a faster absorption from the injection site.

When administered immediately before a meal, the effect of insulin aspart more closely mimics normal physiological postprandial insulin release than regular human insulin used as replacement therapy. This effect leads to reduced postprandial variability in blood glucose concentration.

Pharmacokinetics: Bioavailability and Absorption: Insulin aspart has a faster absorption, a faster onset and a shorter duration of action than regular human insulin (see Figure 1 and Figure 2). The relative bioavailability of insulin aspart to regular human insulin indicates that the two insulins are absorbed to a similar extent.

In clinical trials in healthy volunteers and Type 1 diabetic patients, insulin aspart consistently reached maximum serum concentration at least twice as fast as regular human insulin. The average median time to maximum serum concentration was 40 to 50 minutes for insulin aspart versus 80 to 120 minutes for regular human insulin. The intra-individual variability in time to maximum concentration was significantly less for insulin aspart than for regular human insulin.

Figure 1: NovoRapid

Mean serum insulin concentration following a single pre-meal s.c. dose (0.15 U/kg body weight) of NovoRapid injected immediately before a meal (solid line) or regular human insulin administered s.c. 30 minutes before a meal (hatched line) in 22 patients with Type 1 diabetes.

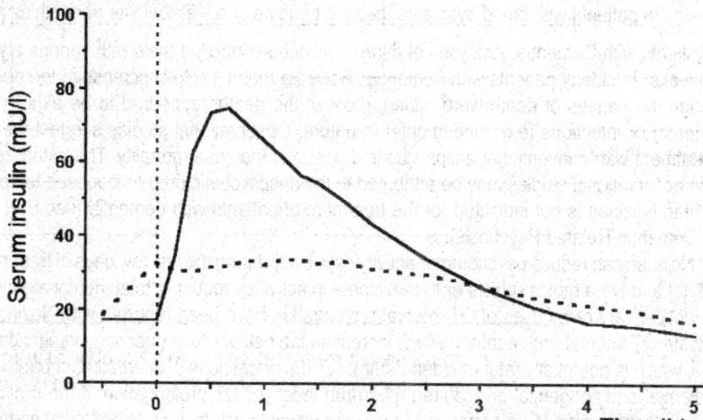

The pharmacokinetics following a single 0.15 U/kg dose of insulin aspart just before a standard meal or of regular human insulin 30 minutes before a standard meal were compared in Type 1 diabetic subjects (see Figure 1). Insulin aspart was rapidly absorbed after s.c. administration. There was a significant difference between C_{max} for insulin aspart and regular human insulin (mean maximum concentrations 82.1 mU/l and 35.9 mU/l respectively).

In healthy subjects, the pharmacokinetic differences between insulin aspart and regular human insulin, were maintained independent of the injection site (abdomen, thigh or deltoid).

Distribution and Elimination: Insulin aspart has a low binding to plasma proteins, 0 to 9%. After s.c. administration, insulin aspart was more rapidly eliminated than regular human insulin with an average apparent half-life of 81 minutes compared to 141 minutes for regular human insulin.

Pharmacodynamics: Insulin aspart produces a more rapid and pronounced blood glucose regulating effect than regular human insulin, due to the fast onset of action.

When compared to regular human insulin on an equimolar basis, insulin aspart produces significantly superior control of blood glucose following a meal as assessed by excursion of blood glucose during the first 4 hours after a meal (see Figure 2). When injected s.c. into the abdomen, the onset of action will occur from 10 minutes after injection. The maximum effect is exerted between 1 to 3 hours after s.c. injection. The duration of action for insulin aspart is 3 to 5 hours compared to 5 to 8 hours for regular human insulin. In this trial, subjects were clamped from the evening before the trial product administration in order to obtain a blood glucose concentration of 5 to 8 mmol/L.

The mean serum glucose profiles in Figure 2 show the superior postprandial glucose control obtained with insulin aspart compared to human insulin during the first 4 hours postdosing. This was confirmed by the significantly lower postprandial glucose excursion (EXC) for insulin aspart than for regular human insulin (p=0.015).

Figure 2: NovoRapid

Mean blood glucose levels following a single pre-meal s.c. dose (0.15 U/kg) of NovoRapid injected immediately before a meal (solid line) or regular human insulin administered 30 minutes before a meal (hatched line) in 22 patients with Type 1 diabetes.

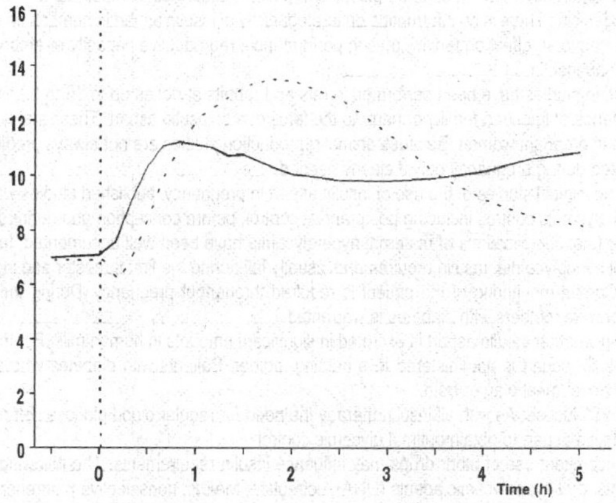

The effect of insulin aspart given in a meal related regimen on 23-hour glucose control was studied in 104 Type 1 diabetic patients. After 4 weeks of treatment, the instances of blood glucose levels outside the normal range (4 to 7 mmol/L or 72 to 126 mg/dL) were significantly lower with insulin aspart than with regular human insulin.

Long-term metabolic control, assessed by HbA_{1C} was studied in 882 Type 1 diabetic patients in one trial and 1065 Type 1 diabetic patients in another trial, on a meal-related insulin regimen. With insulin aspart, significantly improved long-term metabolic control was obtained compared to regular human insulin after 6 months treatment, the values being 7.78±0.03% for insulin aspart and 7.93±0.05% (p<0.01) for regular human insulin in one trial and correspondingly 7.88±0.03% and 8.00±0.04% (p<0.02) in the other trial. Furthermore, this improvement in glycemic control was achieved without increasing the risk of hypoglycemic events.

In 182 Type 2 diabetic patients treated with insulin aspart in a meal-related regimen for 6 months, the pharmacodynamic properties of insulin aspart were shown to be not different than regular human insulin with respect to metabolic control as assessed by insulin dose (meal related and NPH).

To evaluate the use of NovoRapid by continuous subcutaneous insulin infusion (CSII) with an external pump, one open-label, randomized, parallel design study, 16 weeks [n=118) compared NovoRapid versus Humalog (insulin lispro) in patients with Type 1 diabetes. Glycaemic control (as measured by HbA_{1C}) and rates of hypoglycemia were comparable. Patients with Type 2 diabetes were also studied in an open-label, randomized, parallel design trial (24 weeks [n=127]). NovoRapid by CSII was compared to a basal/bolus regimen of pre-prandial NovoRapid and basal Novolinge NPH injections. Reductions in HbA_{1C} and rates of hypoglycemia were comparable. In the study (NovoRapid versus Humalog), the rate of clogging or blockage events was similar between NovoRapid and Humalog.

Special Populations: Age and Gender: Children and adolescents: The pharmacokinetic properties of insulin aspart and regular human insulin were investigated in 18 children (6 to 12 years, n=9) and adolescents (13 to 17 years, n=9) with Type 1 diabetes. The relative difference in pharmacokinetics and pharmacodynamics in Type 1 diabetic children and adolescents between insulin aspart and regular human insulin correlated well with those in healthy adult subjects and Type 1 diabetic adults.

Geriatrics: In the clinical development program, 226 patients aged 50 years and older (including 35 patients above the age of 65) were treated with insulin aspart for up to 6 months. No differences in dose, efficacy or adverse events were observed between these patients and younger population.

Gender: There was no significant difference in pharmacokinetics in a trial in Type 2 diabetic patients. No significant difference in efficacy, as assessed by HbA_{1C}, was found between genders in a trial in Type 1 diabetic patients.

Obesity: The influence of obesity and/or s.c. fat thickness on the pharmacokinetics and glucodynamics of insulin aspart has not been studied. Patients with a body mass index (BMI) up to 40 kg/m^2 were treated with insulin aspart. No difference was observed in efficacy and safety compared to leaner patients.

Ethnic Origin: There was no difference in efficacy in terms of blood glucose control as measured by HbA_{1C} or safety in terms of adverse events between African Americans, Hispanics and Caucasian patients.

Smoking: The effect of smoking on the pharmacokinetics and pharmacodynamics of insulin aspart has not been studied. However, metabolic control was similar in smokers and non-smokers after 6 months treatment with insulin aspart in the clinical development program.

INDICATIONS: For the treatment of patients with diabetes mellitus who require insulin for the maintenance of normal glucose homeostasis. Insulin aspart should normally be used in regimens together with an intermediate or long-acting insulin.

NovoRapid (10 mL vial) may also be used for continuous subcutaneous insulin infusion (CSII) in pump systems which are licensed in Canada for insulin infusion.

CONTRAINDICATIONS: During episodes of hypoglycemia (see Hypoglycemia and Overdose: Treatment) and in patients hypersensitive to insulin aspart or one of its excipients.

WARNINGS: Insulin aspart differs from regular human insulin by its rapid onset and shorter duration of action. Because of the fast onset of action, the injection of insulin aspart should immediately be followed by a meal.

PRECAUTIONS: General: As with all insulins, the duration of action of insulin aspart may vary in different individuals or in the same individual according to dose, injection site, blood flow, temperature and level of physical activity.

Hypokalemia is among the potential clinical adverse effects associated with the use of all insulins. This potential clinical adverse effect may be relevant in patients who are on potassium lowering drugs.

Stress or illness may increase insulin requirements. In these instances, patients should contact their physician and carefully control their blood glucose.

Hypoglycemia: In certain cases (long duration of diabetes, diabetic nerve disease, intensified diabetes control, or use of medications such as β blocking agents), the nature and intensity of early warning symptoms of hypoglycemia may change or be less pronounced.

Hypoglycemia is the most frequently occurring undesirable effect of insulin therapy. Such reactions following treatment with insulin aspart are mostly mild and easily managed. The frequency of hypoglycemia observed in clinical trials is similar to that observed with regular human insulin.

Severe hypoglycemia can result in temporary or permanent impairment of brain function and death.

Changes in insulin therapy or changes in life style (i.e. diet, exercise/physical activity) may require a change in dosage. Inadequate dosing or discontinuation of insulin treatment, especially in Type 1 diabetes, may lead to hyperglycemia and diabetic ketoacidosis. Severe sustained hyperglycemia may result in diabetic coma and death.

Glucose monitoring is recommended for all patients with diabetes.

Local Allergic Reaction: As with other insulins, patients may experience redness, swelling or itching at the site of injection. These minor reactions usually resolve in a few days to a few weeks. They may occur if the injection is not properly made, or if the patient is allergic to the insulin or any excipients. Few local injection site reactions were observed with insulin aspart in the clinical development program and there was no difference in frequency when compared to regular human insulin.

Systemic Allergic Reaction: Systemic allergic reactions have not been reported during the clinical development of insulin aspart. Systemic allergic reactions have rarely occurred with other insulin treatment. These reactions may be characterized by a generalized rash (with pruritus), shortness of breath, wheezing and drop in blood pressure. Severe cases of generalized allergy including anaphylactic reaction may be life threatening.

Antibody Production: Insulin antibodies may develop during treatment with insulin. In the clinical development program, insulin aspart-specific, regular human insulin-specific and cross reactive antibodies were analyzed. Antibody production was monitored in 665 patients for 12 months. After a transient statistically significant increase in cross-reacting antibodies from baseline to 3 months for insulin aspart compared to human insulin, cross-reacting antibody levels returned to baseline levels in the insulin aspart group and were not different from the human insulin group. No adverse effects could be attributed to patients producing cross reactive antibodies as compared to those who did not. There was no correlation between the extent of antibody formation and the insulin dose needed, level of glycemic control attained or adverse event reporting after 12 months of treatment. No systemic allergic reactions were observed.

Renal Impairment: There is no experience of treatment with insulin aspart in patients with renal impairment. As with other insulins, insulin aspart requirement may be reduced in patients with renal impairment.

Hepatic Impairment: There is no experience of treatment with insulin aspart in patients with hepatic impairment. As with other insulins, insulin aspart requirement may need to be adjusted in patients with hepatic impairment.

Use in Women: Teratogenicity: There is no information on teratogenicity of insulin aspart in humans. In rabbit trials, insulin aspart did not exert any direct adverse effect on fertility, mating performance, reproductive capacity or embryo-fetal development and did not differ from human insulin.

Pregnancy: Reproduction studies have been performed in rats and rabbits at doses up to 16 to 32 times the human dose and have revealed no evidence of impaired fertility or harm to the fetus due to insulin aspart. There are, however, no adequate and well-controlled studies in pregnant women. Because animal reproduction studies are not always predictive of human response, this drug should be used during pregnancy only if clearly needed.

Although there are no clinical studies of the use of insulin aspart in pregnancy, published studies with human insulin suggest that optimizing overall glycemic control, including postprandial control, before conception and during pregnancy improves fetal outcome. Although the fetal complications of maternal hyperglycemia have been well documented, fetal toxicity also has been reported with maternal hypoglycemia. Insulin requirements usually fall during the first trimester and increase during the second and third trimesters. Careful monitoring of the patient is required throughout pregnancy. During the perinatal period, careful monitoring of infants born to mothers with diabetes is warranted.

Lactation: It is unknown whether insulin aspart is excreted in significant amounts in human milk. For this reason, caution should be exercised when insulin aspart is administered to a nursing mother. Patients with diabetes who are lactating may require adjustments in insulin dose, meal plan or both.

Self-monitoring of Blood Glucose: As with all insulin therapy the need for regular blood glucose self-monitoring should be considered when using insulin aspart to obtain optimal glycemic control.

Drug Interactions: Concomitant use of other drugs may influence insulin requirements. The following substances may reduce the insulin requirements: oral hypoglycemic agents (OHA), octreotide, MAOIs, nonselective β adrenergic blocking agents, ACE inhibitors, salicylates, alcohol, and anabolic steroids.

Other drugs may increase insulin requirements: oral contraceptives, thiazides, glucocorticosteroids, thyroid hormones, sympathomimetics and danazol.

β blocking agents may mask the symptoms of hypoglycemia.

Alcohol may intensify and prolong the hypoglycemic effect of insulin.

Information to Be Provided to the Patient: Patients should be informed about potential advantages and disadvantages of insulin aspart therapy including the possible side effects. Patients should also be offered continued education and advice on insulin therapies, life-style management, self-monitoring, complications of insulin therapy, timing of dosage, instruction for use of injection devices and storage of insulin.

The need for regular blood glucose self-monitoring should be considered when using insulin aspart to obtain optimal glycemic control.

Female patients should be advised to discuss with their physician if they intend to or if they become pregnant.

Patients administering NovoRapid by CSII must have alternative insulin available in case of pump system failure.

Mixing of Insulins: If insulin aspart is mixed with an intermediate-acting or long-acting insulin, insulin aspart should be drawn into the syringe first. The injection should be made immediately after mixing. Pharmacodynamic trials conducted in pigs showed bioequivalence between separate injections of insulin aspart. These injections included neutral protamine hagedorn (NPH) human insulin and insulin aspart injected separately and a mix of insulin aspart and neutral protamine hagedorn (NPH) human insulin injected 5 minutes after mixing.

The effect of mixing insulin aspart with either animal-source insulins or human insulin preparations produced by other manufacturers have not been studied. This practice is not recommended.

NovoRapid should never be mixed with any other insulin when used in a pump.

ADVERSE EFFECTS: Clinical trials comparing insulin aspart with regular human insulin did not demonstrate any differences in frequency of adverse events. Adverse events can be categorized into the following areas:

Body as a Whole: (see Precautions).

Skin Reactions: (see Precautions, Local Allergic Reactions).

Other: Hypoglycemia (see Warnings).

Clinical Trial Adverse Drug Reactions: Because clinical trials are conducted under very specific conditions, the adverse drug reaction rates observed in the clinical trials may not reflect the rates observed in practice and should not be compared to the rates in the clinical trials of another drug. Adverse drug reaction information from clinical trials is useful for identifying drug-related adverse events and for approximating rates.

Adverse Drug Events Overview for a Post-marketing CSII Trial: A 4 month post-marketing study in 511 subjects with type 1 and insulin-requiring type 2 diabetes mellitus was conducted as a preference trial to assess the treatment satisfaction of NovoRapid and insulin lispro during CSII pump therapy. Adverse drug events were recorded when spontaneously reported by the patients in the study. The only adverse drug event reported at an incidence 1% was upper respiratory tract infection (incidence of 1.3% in the NovoRapid group).

Less Common Adverse Drug Events (<1%) in a Post-marketing CSII Trial: In addition, the following adverse drug events were reported at an incidence of <1% for NovoRapid or insulin lispro in this study (in more than 1 patient in each treatment group), regardless of drug relationship.

Gastrointestinal Disorders: vomiting, nausea.

Infections and Infestations: viral infection, urinary tract infection, sinusitis, onychomycosis, nasopharyngitis, bronchitis.

Metabolism and Nutrition Disorders: hypoglycemia, hyperglycemia, diabetic ketoacidosis.

Musculoskeletal and Connective Tissue Disorders: pain in extremity, back pain, arthralgia.

Nervous System Disorders: neuropathy.

Respiratory, Thoracic and Mediastinal Disorders: nasal congestion.

The following serious adverse events were reported in more than 1 patient but at an incidence of <1% for NovoRapid in Study 2190:

Metabolic and Nutritional Disorders: hypoglycemia (4 episodes) and diabetic ketoacidosis (2 episodes).

Hypoglycemia as an Adverse Drug Reaction in a Post-maketing CSII Trial: The reporting of hypoglycemia was not a specific safety endpoint in this trial. Hypoglycemic episodes were recorded only if spontaneously reported by the subject as adverse drug reactions. Consequently, data on hypoglycemia is limited from this study. There were only seven episodes of hypoglycemia reported during the four-month trial with over 500 patients. As such, the incidence of hypoglycemia was calculated to be <1% of the patient treated with either NovoRapid or insulin lispro and does not reflect real-life occurence of hypoglycemia in diabetes patients.

OVERDOSE:

Treatment: Hypoglycemia and Overdose: Overdose may cause hypoglycemia. Omission of a meal or unplanned strenuous physical exercise may lead to hypoglycemia. Symptoms of hypoglycemia may occur suddenly. They may include cold sweat, cool pale skin, fatigue, nervousness or tremor, anxious feeling, unusual tiredness or weakness, confusion, difficulty in concentration, drowsiness, excessive hunger, vision changes, headache, nausea and palpitation. Severe hypoglycemia may lead to unconsciousness and/or convulsions and may be fatal.

Mild episodes of hypoglycemia can be treated by oral administration of glucose or sugary products. It is therefore recommended that patients with diabetes always carry some sugar candy.

Severe hypoglycemic episodes, where the patient has become unconscious, can be treated with glucagon (0.5 to 1 mg) given i.m. or s.c. by a trained person or glucose given i.v. by a medical professional. Glucose must also be given i.v. if the patient does not respond to glucagon within 10 to 15 minutes. Upon regaining consciousness, administration of an oral carbohydrate is recommended for the patient in order to prevent relapse.

For management of a suspected drug overdose, CPhA recommends that you contact your **regional Poison Control Centre**. See the *CPS* Directory section for a list of Poison Control Centres.

DOSAGE: Insulin aspart should generally be given immediately before a meal. When necessary insulin aspart may be given immediately after the meal.

Dosage of insulin aspart is individual and determined, based on the physician's advice, in accordance with the needs of the patient. The individual insulin requirement is usually between 0.5 and 1 unit/kg/day. In a meal-related treatment, 50 to 70% of this requirement may be provided by insulin aspart and the remainder provided by an intermediate-acting or long-acting insulin.

Because of the fast onset of action of insulin aspart, it should be given close to a meal (start of the meal should be not more than 5 to 10 minutes after injection). The dosing of insulin aspart should be regularly adjusted according to blood glucose measurements.

New Patients: Patients being initiated on insulin for the first time can be started on insulin aspart in the same manner as they would be on animal-source or human insulin.

Transfer Patients: When patients are transferred from other insulin to insulin aspart, the change should be made as directed by the physician.

In clinical trials, patients were transferred on a unit to unit basis from Novolinge Toronto (regular insulin) to insulin aspart and then the doses of meal-related and basal insulin were changed according to the patients' needs and local practice.

Administration: Insulin aspart is administered s.c. in the abdominal wall, the thigh "buttock," or the upper arm. Injection sites should be rotated within the same region. Insulin aspart retains its more rapid onset and shorter duration of action irrespective of the injection site used (abdomen, thigh, upper arm). As with all insulins, the duration of action will vary according to the dose, injection site, blood flow, temperature and level of physical activity.

Parenteral drug products should be inspected visually for particulate matter and discoloration prior to administration, whenever solution and container permit. Never use insulin aspart if it has become viscous (thickened) or cloudy; use it only if it is clear and colorless. Insulin aspart should not be used after its expiration date.

If insulin aspart is mixed with an intermediate-acting or long-acting insulin, insulin aspart should be drawn into the syringe first. The injection should be made immediately after mixing. The effect of mixing insulin aspart with either animal-source insulins or human insulin preparations produced by other manufacturers have not been studied. This practice is not recommended.

In patients with diabetes mellitus, optimized metabolic control effectively delays the onset and slows the progression of late diabetic complications. Optimized metabolic control, including glucose monitoring is therefore recommended.

NovoRapid (10 mL vial) may be used for Continuous Subcutaneous Insulin Infusion (CSII) in pump systems licenced for insulin infusion. Patients using CSII should be comprehensively instructed in the use of the pump system. The infusion and reservoir set should be changed according to the pump manufacturer's instructions. Patients administering NovoRapid by CSII must have an alternate insulin delivery device available in case of pump system failure.

INFORMATION FOR THE PATIENT: Published in e-CPS, available by subscription at www.e-cps.ca.

SUPPLIED: Each mL of sterile, aqueous, clear, colorless solution contains: insulin aspart 100 units. Nonmedicinal ingredients: disodium hydrogen phosphate dihydrate, glycerin, metacresol, phenol, sodium chloride and zinc. pH: 7.2 to 7.6. Penfill cartridges of 3 mL, cartons of 5. Vials of 10 mL, cartons of 1.

NovoRapid Penfill cartridges are designed for use with Novo Nordisk Insulin Delivery Devices and NovoFine needles.

Insulin aspart should be stored between 2 and 10°C. Do not freeze. Cartridges in use or carried as a spare may be kept at ambient temperature for up to 4 weeks, but should not be exposed to excessive heat or sunlight. Insulin aspart should not be used after the expiry date printed on the package.

(Shown in Product Identification Section)

Nozinan® Ⓟ
methotrimeprazine HCl
Neuroleptic

sanofi-aventis

Date of Revision: March 19, 2010

PHARMACOLOGY: Nozinan possesses antipsychotic, tranquilizing, anxiolytic, sedative and analgesic properties and it is also a potent potentiator of anesthetics.

Nozinan possesses strong sedative properties. It potentiates ether and hexobarbital anesthesia as well as morphine analgesia. It also exerts a potent anti-apomorphine effect, a hypothermic action 3 times more potent than that of chlorpromazine and strong antispasmodic and anti-histaminic effects.

Nozinan is capable of reversing epinephrine-induced hypertension but has practically no effect against norepinephrine and acetylcholine. It readily protects rats against traumatic shock and produces deep local anesthesia following parasciatic injections.

INDICATIONS: Psychotic disturbances: acute and chronic schizophrenias, senile psychoses, manic-depressive syndromes.

Conditions associated with anxiety and tension: autonomic disturbances, personality disturbances, emotional troubles secondary to such physical conditions as resistant pruritus, etc.

Nozinan is also employed: As an analgesic: In pain due to cancer, zona, trigeminal neuralgia and neurocostal neuralgia and in phantom limb pains and muscular discomforts.

As a potentiator of anesthetics: In general anesthesia where it can be used as both a pre- and postoperative sedative and analgesic.

As an antiemetic: For the treatment of nausea and vomiting of central origin.

As a sedative: For the management of insomnia.

CONTRAINDICATIONS: In cases of coma or CNS depression due to alcohol, hypnotics, analgesics or narcotics.

It is also contraindicated in patients with blood dyscrasia, hepatic troubles or a sensitivity to phenothiazines.

WARNINGS: Elderly Patients with Dementia: Analyses of thirteen placebo-controlled trials with various atypical antipsychotics (modal duration of 10 weeks) in elderly patients with dementia showed a mean 1.6 fold increase in the death rate in the drug-treated patients. Although the causes of deaths were varied, most of the deaths appeared to be either cardiovascular (e.g., heart failure, sudden death) or infectious (e.g., pneumonia) in nature. Observational studies suggest that, similar to atypical antipsychotic drugs, treatment with conventional antipsychotic drugs may increase mortality. The extent to which the findings of increased mortality in observational studies may be attributed to the antipsychotic drug as opposed to some characteristic(s) of the patients is not clear. Nozinan is not indicated for the treatment of patients with dementia (see Precautions, Mortality in Geriatric Patients with Dementia-Related Psychosis).

Occupational Hazards: Nozinan can reduce psychomotor activity especially during the first few days of treatment. Patients should therefore be cautioned not to drive a motor vehicle or to participate in activities requiring total mental alertness.

As with other neuroleptics, very rare cases of QT interval prolongation have been reported with Nozinan. Neuroleptic phenothiazines may potentiate QT interval prolongation, which increases the risk of onset of serious ventricular arrhythmias of the torsade de pointes type, which is potentially fatal (sudden death). QT prolongation is exacerbated, in particular, in the presence of bradycardia, hypokalemia, and congenital or acquired (i.e., drug induced) QT prolongation. If the clinical situation permits, medical and laboratory evaluations should be performed to rule out possible risk factors before initiating treatment with a neuroleptic agent and as deemed necessary during treatment (see also Adverse Effects and Precautions, Drug Interactions).

Tardive Dyskinesia: As with all antipsychotic agents, tardive dyskinesia may appear in some patients on long-term therapy or after drug discontinuation. The syndrome is mainly characterized by rhythmical involuntary movements of the tongue, face, mouth or jaw. The manifestations may be permanent in some patients. The syndrome may be masked when treatment is reinstituted, when the dosage is increased or when a switch is made to a different antipsychotic drug. Nozinan should be prescribed in a manner that is most likely to minimize the risk of tardive dyskinesia. The lowest effective dose and the shortest duration of treatment should be used, and treatment should be discontinued at the earliest opportunity, or if a satisfactory response cannot be obtained. If the signs and symptoms of tardive dyskinesia appear during treatment, discontinuation of Nozinan should be considered.

Neuroleptic Malignant Syndrome: Neuroleptic malignant syndrome (NMS) may occur in patients receiving antipsychotic drugs. NMS is characterized by hyperthermia, muscle rigidity, altered consciousness, and signs of autonomic instability including irregular blood pressure, tachycardia, cardiac arrhythmias and diaphoresis. Additional signs may include elevated serum creatine kinase, myoglobinuria (rhabdomyolysis), acute renal failure and leukocytosis. Hyperthermia is often an early sign of this syndrome. Antipsychotic treatment should be withdrawn immediately and appropriate supportive therapy and careful monitoring instituted.

Elderly patients with dementia treated with certain atypical antipsychotic drugs are at an increased risk of Cerebrovascular Adverse Events (CVAEs) such as stroke and transient ischemic attacks, as well as death, compared to placebo. The mechanism of this increased risk is not known. As an increase in the risk with other antipsychotic drugs cannot be excluded, Nozinan should be used with caution in the elderly with dementia.

As with other psychotropic drugs, rare cases of priapism have been reported. This reaction did not appear to be dose-dependent and did not correlate with the duration of treatment. The most likely mechanism of action of priapism is a relative decrease in sympathetic tone.

Cases of venous thromboembolism, sometimes fatal, have been reported with antipsychotic drugs. Therefore, Nozinan should be used with caution in patients with risk factors for thromboembolism (see Adverse Effects).

Pregnancy: The drug should be used with caution in pregnant women, particularly during the first trimester, unless the benefit to the patient outweighs any possible risk to the fetus.

PRECAUTIONS: In high parenteral doses, orthostatic hypotension may be encountered at the start of treatment. Patients whose treatment is started by the parenteral route should be kept in bed during the first few days.

Nozinan therapy should be initiated at low doses in patients with arteriosclerosis or cardiovascular problems.

Because of its anticholinergic effects, Nozinan must be administered with caution in patients with glaucoma or prostatic hypertrophy.

During long-term therapy, periodic liver function tests should be performed. In addition, blood counts should be conducted regularly, particularly during the first 2 or 3 months of treatment, and physicians should watch for any signs of blood dyscrasia.

Nozinan does not alter EEG activity. Nevertheless, since phenothiazines can lower the threshold of cortical excitation, it is advisable to administer an appropriate anticonvulsant medication to epileptic patients receiving Nozinan therapy.

Drug Interactions: Nozinan potentiates the action of other phenothiazines and CNS depressants (barbiturates, analgesics, narcotics and antihistaminics). The usual doses of these agents should be reduced by half if they are to be given concomitantly with Nozinan until the dosage of the latter has been established.

Nozinan and its non-hydroxylated metabolites are reported to be inhibitors of cytochrome P450 2D6. Coadministration of Nozinan and drugs primarily metabolized by the cytochrome P450 2D6 enzyme system may result in increased plasma concentrations of these drugs.

Neuroleptic phenothiazines may potentiate QT interval prolongation. QT prolongation is exacerbated, in particular, in the presence of bradycardia, hypokalemia, and congenital or acquired (i.e., drug induced) QT prolongation (see also Warnings and Precautions).

Hyperglycaemia or intolerance to glucose has been reported in patients treated with Nozinan. Patients with an established diagnosis of diabetes mellitus or with risk factors for the development of diabetes who are started on Nozinan, should get appropriate glycaemic monitoring during treatment (see Adverse Effects).

Drug-Laboratory Interactions: False positive or negative pregnancy tests have occurred in patients receiving phenothiazine therapy.

Mortality in Geriatric Patients with Dementia-Related Psychosis: In elderly patients with dementia-related psychosis, the efficacy and safety of Nozinan has not been studied. Observational studies suggest that elderly patients with dementia-related psychosis treated with antipsychotic drugs are at an increased risk of death. Nozinan is not indicated for the treatment of patients with dementia-related psychosis.

Cerebrovascular Adverse Events (CVAEs) Including Stroke in Elderly Patients with Dementia: An increased risk of cerebrovascular adverse events has been seen in the dementia population in clinical trials with some atypical antipsychotics. The mechanism for this increased risk is not known. There is insufficient data to know if there is an increased risk of cerebrovascular events associated with Nozinan. An increased risk however cannot be excluded. Nozinan is not indicated in elderly patients with dementia.

Vascular Disease: Nozinan should be used with caution in patients with risk factors for stroke or with a history of stroke.

ADVERSE EFFECTS: May be classified as follows:

CNS: Drowsiness may appear early in treatment but will gradually disappear during the first weeks or with an adjustment in the dosage.

Extrapyramidal effects are rare and usually appear only after prolonged therapy at high doses. These reactions may be corrected either by reducing the dose of Nozinan or by administering an antiparkinsonian agent.

Autonomic Nervous System: dryness of the mouth and, in older patients occasional urinary retention, constipation and tachycardia.

Cardiovascular: Orthostatic hypotension may be encountered at the start of treatment by the parenteral route. Very rare cases of QT interval prolongation have been reported. There have been isolated reports of sudden death, with possible causes of cardiac origin (see Warnings and Precautions, Drug Interactions), as well as cases of unexplained sudden death, in patients receiving neuroleptic phenothiazines.

Vascular Disorder: Cases of venous thromboembolism, including cases of pulmonary embolism, sometimes fatal, and cases of deep vein thrombosis have been reported with antipsychotic drugs (see Warnings).

Blood: Rare instances of agranulocytosis have been reported.

Endocrine: Weight gain has been occasionally reported in patients during prolonged treatment with high doses.

Gastrointestinal: Rare cases of cholestatic jaundice without liver damage have been observed. Necrotizing enterocolitis, which can be fatal, has been very rarely reported in patients treated with Nozinan.

Skin Reactions: Skin reactions due to photosensitivity or allergies are extremely rare.

Urogenital System: Priapism has been very rarely reported.

Hyperglycaemia or intolerance to glucose has been reported in patients treated with Nozinan (see Precautions).

OVERDOSE:

Symptoms: Symptoms of acute intoxication may include: simple CNS depression, spasms, tremor or tonic and clonic convulsions, coma accompanied by hypotension and respiratory depression.

Treatment: There is no specific antidote. After gastric lavage, treatment is symptomatic. Centrally acting emetics are ineffective because of the antiemetic action of Nozinan.

Hypotension: A 5% glucose solution may be administered. If a hypertensive agent is required, norepinephrine or phenylephrine may be used, but not epinephrine which can aggravate hypotension.

Respiratory Depression: oxygen by inhalation or controlled respiration after tracheal intubation.

Respiratory Infection: wide spectrum antibiotics.

Extrapyramidal Reactions: An antiparkinsonian agent or chloral hydrate, however the latter must be used with caution because of its depressant effect on respiration.

Any CNS stimulant should be used with caution.

For management of a suspected drug overdose, contact your regional Poison Control Centre. See the *CPS* Directory section for a list of Poison Control Centres.

DOSAGE: Dosage must be adjusted according to the indication and individual needs of the patient. If sedation during the day is too pronounced, lower doses may be given during the day and higher doses at night.

Adults: Parenteral: I.M.: To be used primarily for the initial treatment of psychoses for certain severe pain as a premedication or for the treatment of postoperative pain. In psychoses and pain, doses vary from 75 to 100 mg given as 3 or 4 deep i.m. injections in a large muscle. When given as a premedication or post-operative analgesic, the average dose varies from 10 to 25 mg every 8 hours, which is equivalent to 20 to 40 mg given orally. The last dose during premedication, given 1 hour before surgery, can be 25 to 50 mg i.m.

I.V.: To be used primarily as an infusion during surgery or labour. The dose may range from 10 to 25 mg in 500 mL of a 5% glucose solution administered at a rate of 20 to 40 drops/minute. If Nozinan is administered with a barbiturate or narcotic, the doses of the latter must be reduced by at least one-half.

Children: Parenteral: I.M.: A dose of 1/16 to 1/8 mg/kg/day in one or divided among several injections. Oral medication should be substituted as soon as possible.

I.V.: In anesthesia, 1/16 mg/kg in 250 mL of a 5% glucose solution may be administered as a slow infusion (20 to 40 drops per minute) during surgery.

INFORMATION FOR THE PATIENT: Published in e-CPS, available by subscription at www.e-cps.ca.

SUPPLIED: Each mL contains: methotrimeprazine base 25 mg (as the hydrochloride). Nonmedicinal ingredients: ascorbic acid, sodium chloride, sodium sulfite and water for injection. Amber glass ampouls of 1 mL, boxes of 10. Store at 15 to 30°C. Protect from light.

Nplate™ Ⓟ

romiplostim

Thrombopoiesis-Stimulating Protein

Amgen

Date of Preparation: February 19, 2009

SUMMARY PRODUCT INFORMATION:

Route of Administration	Dosage Form/ Strength	Clinically Relevant Nonmedicinal Ingredients
Subcutaneous	Lyophilized powder for solution for injection/ 250 µg/0.5 mL and 500 µg/1 mL	Nplate contains small amounts of sugar (mannitol 4% and sucrose 2%). For a complete listing see Dosage Forms, Composition and Packaging.

DESCRIPTION: Nplate (romiplostim), a member of the TPO mimetic class, is an Fc-peptide fusion protein (peptibody) that activates intracellular transcriptional pathways to increase platelet production via the thrombopoietin (TPO) receptor (also known as cMpl).

The peptibody molecule is comprised of a human immunoglobulin IgG1 Fc domain, with each single-chain subunit covalently linked at the C-terminus to a peptide chain containing two thrombopoietin receptor-binding domains. Nplate has no amino acid sequence homology to endogenous thrombopoietin (eTPO). Nplate is produced by recombinant DNA technology in *Escherichia coli* (*E. coli*).

Nplate is to be administered by subcutaneous injection. Nplate is supplied as a sterile, preservative-free, lyophilized solid white powder for reconstitution. Nplate (500 µg) is reconstituted with 1.2 mL of Sterile Water for Injection, USP and Nplate (250 µg) is reconstituted with 0.72 mL of Sterile Water for Injection, USP. Reconstitution yields a clear, colorless, iso-osmotic solution of Nplate.

INDICATIONS AND CLINICAL USE: Nplate (romiplostim) is indicated to increase the platelet levels in adult patients with chronic immune (idiopathic) thrombocytopenic purpura (ITP):

- who are nonsplenectomized and have had an inadequate response or are intolerant to corticosteroids and/or immunoglobulins;
- who are splenectomized and have had an inadequate response to splenectomy.

Nplate has been used alone or in combination with other ITP therapies such as corticosteroids, azathioprine, or danazol.

CONTRAINDICATIONS: Nplate (romiplostim) is contraindicated in patients who are hypersensitive to this drug or to any ingredient in the formulation or component of the container, or with a known history of sensitivity or allergy to any *E. coli*-derived product. For a complete listing of ingredients, see Dosage Forms, Composition and Packaging.

WARNINGS AND PRECAUTIONS:

Serious Warnings and Precautions

- Nplate should not be used in patients with myelodysplastic syndromes, outside of a clinical research study, because of the possibility of potentiating the development of myeloid leukemia in such patients.
- Despite ongoing treatment with Nplate, serious bleeding could occur and patients should be closely monitored during treatment. Rescue medications including platelet transfusions might be required, especially for patients with unstable platelet counts.
- Recurrence of thrombocytopenia, sometimes markedly below pre-treatment baseline levels, and serious life-threatening or fatal bleeding after discontinuation of Nplate have been reported.

The following warnings and precautions are observed or theoretical class effects of TPO receptor stimulators.

General: Nplate (romiplostim) should be prescribed and monitored only by qualified healthcare providers.

- Nplate should be used only in patients with ITP whose degree of thrombocytopenia and clinical condition increase the risk for bleeding.
- Nplate should not be used in an attempt to normalize platelet counts.

Increased Bone Marrow Reticulin and Risk for Bone Marrow Fibrosis: Nplate administration increases the risk for development or progression of reticulin fiber deposition within the bone marrow. Overall, in clinical studies, 10 of 271 (3.7%) were observed to have reticulin in the bone marrow. Nplate was discontinued in 4 of the 271 (1.5%) patients because of bone marrow reticulin deposition. Six (2.2%) additional patients had reticulin observed upon bone marrow biopsy. All 10 patients with bone marrow reticulin deposition had received Nplate doses ≥5 µg/kg and six had received doses ≥10 µg/kg. Progression to marrow fibrosis with cytopenias was not reported in the controlled clinical studies. In the extension study, one patient with ITP and hemolytic anemia developed marrow fibrosis with collagen during Nplate therapy. Clinical studies have not excluded a risk of bone marrow fibrosis with cytopenias with Nplate.

Following identification of a stable Nplate dose, examine peripheral blood smears and complete blood counts (CBCs) monthly for new or worsening morphological abnormalities (e.g., teardrop and nucleated red blood cells, immature white blood cells) or cytopenia(s). If the patient develops new or worsening morphological abnormalities or cytopenia(s), discontinue treatment with Nplate and consider a bone marrow biopsy, including staining for fibrosis.

The long term risk for progression to myelofibrosis is unknown.

Recurrence of Thrombocytopenia and Bleeding After Cessation of Treatment: Thrombocytopenia is likely to recur upon discontinuation of Nplate. There is an increased risk for bleeding if Nplate is discontinued in the presence of anticoagulants or anti-platelet agents. Patients should be closely monitored for a decrease in platelet count and medically managed to avoid bleeding upon discontinuation of Nplate. It is recommended that, if treatment with Nplate is discontinued, weekly platelet counts should be obtained for at least two weeks and ITP treatment should be restarted according to current treatment guidelines. Additional medical management may include cessation of anticoagulant and/or antiplatelet therapy, reversal of anticoagulation, or platelet support.

In clinical studies of patients with chronic ITP who had Nplate discontinued, four of 57 patients developed thrombocytopenia of greater severity than was present prior to Nplate therapy. This worsened thrombocytopenia resolved within 14 days; rescue treatments were required to resolve it.

Thrombotic/Thromboembolic Complications: Thrombotic/thromboembolic complications may result from excessive increases in platelet counts. Excessive doses of Nplate or medication errors that result in excessive Nplate doses may produce thrombocytosis and thrombotic/thromboembolic complications. In controlled clinical studies, the incidence of thrombotic/thromboembolic complications was 2.4% in both Nplate and placebo. To minimize the risk for thrombocytosis, do not use Nplate in an attempt to "normalize" platelet counts. Follow the dose adjustment guidelines to achieve and maintain a platelet count of $\geq 50\times10^9$/L see Dosage and Administration.

Of the 271 patients who received Nplate in ITP clinical studies, the study duration adjusted thrombotic/thromboembolic rate in subjects with age 65 and over was 22.9 per 100-subject year compared with 4.1 per 100-subject year in the <65 years age group (see Special Populations, Geriatrics).

As a note the venous thrombotic/thromboembolic event ratios between age 65 and over vs younger are in line with general population.

Lack or Loss of Response to Nplate: Hyporesponsiveness or failure to maintain a platelet response with Nplate within the recommended dosing range should prompt a search for causative factors including immunogenicity and increased bone marrow reticulin (see Adverse Reactions, Immunogenicity and Warnings and Precautions, Increased Bone Marrow Reticulin and Risk for Bone Marrow Fibrosis). Discontinue Nplate if the platelet count does not increase to $\geq 50\times10^9$/L or to a level sufficient to avoid clinically important bleeding after four weeks at the highest weekly dose of 10 µg/kg (see Dosage and Administration, Treatment Discontinuation).

Malignancies and Progression of Malignancies: Stimulation of the thrombopoietin (TPO) receptor on the surface of hematopoietic cells may increase the risk for hematologic malignancies. In controlled clinical studies among patients with chronic ITP, the incidence of hematologic malignancy was 1.2 % in Nplate-treated patients versus 2.4 % in patients treated with placebo. In a separate single-arm clinical study of 44 patients with myelodysplastic syndromes (MDS), 11 patients were reported as having possible disease progression, among whom 4 patients had confirmation of acute myelogenous leukemia (AML) during follow-up. Nplate is not indicated for the treatment of thrombocytopenia due to MDS or any cause of thrombocytopenia other than chronic ITP.

Monitoring and Laboratory Tests: Monitor CBCs, including platelet counts, prior to initiation, throughout and following discontinuation of Nplate therapy. Prior to the initiation of Nplate, examine the peripheral blood differential to establish the baseline extent of red and white blood cell abnormalities. Obtain CBCs, including platelet counts, weekly during the dose adjustment phase of Nplate therapy and then monthly following establishment of a stable Nplate dose. Obtain CBCs, including platelet counts weekly for at least two weeks following discontinuation of Nplate.

Special Populations: Pregnant Women: There are no adequate and well-controlled studies of Nplate in pregnant women. Nplate should not be used during pregnancy unless the potential benefit to the mother justifies the potential risk to the fetus or embryo.

Nursing Women: It is not known whether Nplate is excreted in human milk. Caution should be exercised when Nplate is administered to women who are breast-feeding. Because many drugs are excreted into human milk and because of the potential for serious adverse reactions in nursing infants from Nplate, a decision should be made whether to discontinue nursing or to discontinue the drug, taking into account the importance of the drug to the mother and the known benefits of breast-feeding.

Pediatrics: The safety and effectiveness of Nplate in pediatric patients (<18 years) have not been established.

Geriatrics: Of the 271 patients who received Nplate in ITP clinical studies, 55 (20%) were age 65 and over, and 27 (10%) were 75 and over. Due to the limited number of older patients, no definitive conclusions can be made with regards to the impact of age on efficacy or safety. The study duration adjusted thrombotic/thromboembolic rate in subjects with age 65 and over was 22.9 per 100-subject year compared with 4.1 per 100-subject year in the <65 years age group. As a note the venous thrombotic/thromboembolic event ratios between age 65 and over vs younger are in line with general population.

Hepatic Impairment: Experience is limited in patients with severe hepatic impairment. Nplate should be used with caution in this population.

Renal Impairment: Experience is limited in patients with severe renal impairment. Nplate should be used with caution in this population.

ADVERSE REACTIONS: Adverse Drug Reaction Overview: Thrombocytopenia is likely to recur upon discontinuation of Nplate (romiplostim). Patients should be closely monitored for a decrease in platelet count and medically managed to avoid bleeding. Increased bone marrow reticulin has been observed in some ITP patients treated with Nplate. This finding may be suggested by morphological changes in the peripheral blood cells and can be detected by bone marrow biopsy. Platelet counts above the normal range present a theoretical risk for thrombotic/thromboembolic complications; dose adjustment guidelines should be followed. Please see Warnings and Precautions, Thrombotic/Thromboembolic Complications.

In the Phase 3, placebo-controlled trials, the most common adverse drug reactions were headache, arthralgia, dizziness, insomnia, myalgia, pain in extremity, abdominal pain, shoulder pain, dyspepsia, paresthesia.

Clinical Trial Adverse Drug Reactions: Because clinical trials are conducted under very specific conditions, the adverse reaction rates observed in the clinical trials may not reflect the rates observed in practice and should not be compared to the rates in the clinical trials of another drug. Adverse drug reaction information from clinical trials is useful for identifying drug-related adverse events and for approximating rates.

Serious adverse reactions associated with Nplate in clinical studies were bone marrow reticulin deposition and worsening thrombocytopenia after Nplate discontinuation.

The data described below reflect Nplate exposure to 271 patients with chronic ITP, age 18 to 88, of whom 62% were female. Nplate was studied in two randomized, placebo-controlled, double-blind studies that were identical in design, with the exception that Study 1 (Table 1 and Table 3) evaluated nonsplenectomized patients with ITP and Study 2 (Table 2 and Table 4) evaluated splenectomized patients with ITP. Data are also reported from an open label, single arm study in which patients received Nplate over an extended period of time. Overall, Nplate was administered to 114 patients for at least 52 weeks and 53 patients for at least 96 weeks.

In the placebo-controlled studies, headache was the most commonly reported adverse drug reaction. In nonsplenectomized patients, headaches occurred in 26% of patients receiving Nplate and 30% of patients receiving placebo. In splenectomized patients, headaches occurred in 43% of patients receiving Nplate and 33% of patients receiving placebo. Headaches were usually of mild or moderate severity.

Adverse Reactions from Nplate Phase 3 Placebo Controlled ITP Studies: Table 1 and Table 2 present adverse drug reactions from the two Phase 3 placebo-controlled studies (Study 1 and Study 2; n=125) at a frequency ≥1%. The majority of these adverse drug reactions were mild to moderate in severity. Table 3 and Table 4 present adverse events with a ≥2% difference (Nplate verses placebo) in nonsplenectomized (Study 1) and splenectomized (Study 2) patients.

Table 1: Nplate

Adverse Drug Reactions ≥1% Identified in Study 1 (Nonsplenectomized Patients)

Preferred Term	Nplate (N=42) n (%)	Placebo (N=20) n (%)
Headache	11 (26.2)	6 (30.0)
Arthralgia	10 (23.8)	5 (25.0)
Pain in extremity	8 (19.0)	2 (10.0)
Dizziness	7 (16.7)	0 (0)
Insomnia	5 (11.9)	2 (10.0)
Abdominal pain	5 (11.9)	0 (0)
Shoulder pain	5 (11.9)	0 (0)
Myalgia	3 (7.1)	1 (5.0)
Dyspepsia	2 (4.8)	0 (0)
Paresthesia	2 (4.8)	0 (0)

Note: One patient randomized to placebo in Study S1 (212) actually received Nplate and is included in the Nplate group.

Table 2: Nplate

Adverse Drug Reactions ≥1% Identified in Study 2 (Splenectomized Patients)

Preferred Term	Nplate (N=42) n (%)	Placebo (N=21) n (%)
Headache	18 (42.9)	7 (33.3)
Arthralgia	12 (28.6)	3 (14.3)
Myalgia	9 (21.4)	0 (0)
Insomnia	8 (19.0)	1 (4.8)
Dizziness	7 (16.7)	0 (0)
Abdominal pain	4 (9.5)	0 (0)
Dyspepsia	4 (9.5)	0 (0)
Pain in extremity	3 (7.1)	0 (0)
Paresthesia	3 (7.1)	0 (0)
Shoulder pain	2 (4.8)	0 (0)
Bone marrow disorder[a]	1 (2.4)	0 (0)

[a] Actual frequency is unknown since routine bone marrow biopsies were not performed, see Warnings and Precautions, Increased Bone Marrow Reticulin and Risk for Bone Marrow Fibrosis.

Table 3: Nplate

Adverse Events with ≥2% difference (Nplate vs Placebo) in Study 1 (Nonsplenectomized Patients)

Preferred Term	Nplate (N=42) n (%)	Placebo (N=20) n (%)
Epistaxis	11 (26.2)	3 (15.0)
Pain in extremity	8 (19.0)	2 (10.0)
Dizziness	7 (16.7)	0 (0)
Nausea	6 (14.3)	2 (10.0)
Upper respiratory tract infection	6 (14.3)	2 (10.0)
Back pain	6 (14.3)	1 (5.0)
Gingival bleeding	5 (11.9)	1 (5.0)
Injection site bruising	5 (11.9)	1 (5.0)
Abdominal pain	5 (11.9)	0 (0)
Shoulder pain	5 (11.9)	0 (0)
Myalgia	3 (7.1)	1 (5.0)
Anemia	3 (7.1)	0 (0)
Excoriation	3 (7.1)	0 (0)
Pruritus	3 (7.1)	0 (0)
Depression	2 (4.8)	0 (0)
Dysarthria	2 (4.8)	0 (0)
Dyspepsia	2 (4.8)	0 (0)
Flatulence	2 (4.8)	0 (0)
Herpes simplex	2 (4.8)	0 (0)
Hydronephrosis	2 (4.8)	0 (0)
Paresthesia	2 (4.8)	0 (0)
Splenomegaly	2 (4.8)	0 (0)
Allergic sinusitis	1 (2.4)	0 (0)
Anal fissure	1 (2.4)	0 (0)
Arthritis	1 (2.4)	0 (0)
B-cell lymphoma	1 (2.4)	0 (0)
Basal cell carcinoma	1 (2.4)	0 (0)
Bladder pain	1 (2.4)	0 (0)
Blood pressure increased	1 (2.4)	0 (0)
Bone pain	1 (2.4)	0 (0)
Burning sensation	1 (2.4)	0 (0)
Carotid bruit	1 (2.4)	0 (0)
Cerebrovascular accident	1 (2.4)	0 (0)
Chest pain	1 (2.4)	0 (0)
Coccydynia	1 (2.4)	0 (0)
Confusional state	1 (2.4)	0 (0)

(cont'd)

Table 3: Nplate *(cont'd)*

Adverse Events with ≥2% difference (Nplate vs Placebo) in Study 1 (Nonsplenectomized Patients)

Preferred Term	Nplate (N=42) n (%)	Placebo (N=20) n (%)
Conjunctivitis infective	1 (2.4)	0 (0)
Constipation	1 (2.4)	0 (0)
Dental caries	1 (2.4)	0 (0)
Diabetes mellitus	1 (2.4)	0 (0)
Dysphonia	1 (2.4)	0 (0)
Dyspnea exertional	1 (2.4)	0 (0)
Ear congestion	1 (2.4)	0 (0)
Ear infection	1 (2.4)	0 (0)
Erythema	1 (2.4)	0 (0)
Eye pruritus	1 (2.4)	0 (0)
Gastritis	1 (2.4)	0 (0)
Gastroenteritis viral	1 (2.4)	0 (0)
Gastrointestinal hemorrhage	1 (2.4)	0 (0)
Genital infection fungal	1 (2.4)	0 (0)
Hematochezia	1 (2.4)	0 (0)
Hemoptysis	1 (2.4)	0 (0)
Hemorrhage intracranial	1 (2.4)	0 (0)
Head injury	1 (2.4)	0 (0)
Hepatic steatosis	1 (2.4)	0 (0)
Hiatus hernia	1 (2.4)	0 (0)
Hot flush	1 (2.4)	0 (0)
Hypersensitivity	1 (2.4)	0 (0)
Hypertension	1 (2.4)	0 (0)
Hypertensive crisis	1 (2.4)	0 (0)
Hypothyroidism	1 (2.4)	0 (0)
Hypotrichosis	1 (2.4)	0 (0)
Increased appetite	1 (2.4)	0 (0)
Influenza like illness	1 (2.4)	0 (0)
Injection site discomfort	1 (2.4)	0 (0)
Injection site pain	1 (2.4)	0 (0)
Joint stiffness	1 (2.4)	0 (0)
Keratoconjunctivitis sicca	1 (2.4)	0 (0)
Lethargy	1 (2.4)	0 (0)
Lip hemorrhage	1 (2.4)	0 (0)
Muscle strain	1 (2.4)	0 (0)
Muscular weakness	1 (2.4)	0 (0)
Musculoskeletal chest pain	1 (2.4)	0 (0)
Musculoskeletal pain	1 (2.4)	0 (0)
Musculoskeletal stiffness	1 (2.4)	0 (0)
Non-cardiac chest pain	1 (2.4)	0 (0)
Edema peripheral	1 (2.4)	0 (0)
Oral infection	1 (2.4)	0 (0)
Pericardial effusion	1 (2.4)	0 (0)
Pleural effusion	1 (2.4)	0 (0)
Pollakiuria	1 (2.4)	0 (0)
Renal artery stenosis	1 (2.4)	0 (0)
Road traffic accident	1 (2.4)	0 (0)

(cont'd)

Table 3: Nplate *(cont'd)*

Adverse Events with ≥2% difference (Nplate vs Placebo) in Study 1 (Nonsplenectomized Patients)

Preferred Term	Nplate (N=42) n (%)	Placebo (N=20) n (%)
Sciatica	1 (2.4)	0 (0)
Scratch	1 (2.4)	0 (0)
Sinus headache	1 (2.4)	0 (0)
Skin discolouration	1 (2.4)	0 (0)
Skin warm	1 (2.4)	0 (0)
Sternal fracture	1 (2.4)	0 (0)
Suicidal ideation	1 (2.4)	0 (0)
Tendonitis	1 (2.4)	0 (0)
Thermal burn	1 (2.4)	0 (0)
Tremor	1 (2.4)	0 (0)
Umbilical hernia	1 (2.4)	0 (0)
Urinary hesitation	1 (2.4)	0 (0)
Urine abnormality	1 (2.4)	0 (0)
Viral infection	1 (2.4)	0 (0)
Vision blurred	1 (2.4)	0 (0)
Weight increased	1 (2.4)	0 (0)
Wound	1 (2.4)	0 (0)

Table 4: Nplate

Adverse Events with ≥2% difference (Nplate vs Placebo) in Study 2 (Splenectomized Patients)

Preferred Term	Nplate (N=42) n (%)	Placebo (N=21) n (%)
Headache	18 (42.9)	7 (33.3)
Epistaxis	16 (38.1)	7 (33.3)
Fatigue	13 (31.0)	5 (23.8)
Arthralgia	12 (28.6)	3 (14.3)
Diarrhea	9 (21.4)	2 (9.5)
Myalgia	9 (21.4)	0 (0)
Contusion	8 (19.0)	3 (14.3)
Upper respiratory tract infection	8 (19.0)	3 (14.3)
Insomnia	8 (19.0)	1 (4.8)
Cough	7 (16.7)	3 (14.3)
Dizziness	7 (16.7)	0 (0)
Pain	6 (14.3)	2 (9.5)
Pharyngolaryngeal pain	6 (14.3)	0 (0)
Pyrexia	6 (14.3)	0 (0)
Muscle spasms	5 (11.9)	2 (9.5)
Nausea	5 (11.9)	2 (9.5)
Edema peripheral	5 (11.9)	2 (9.5)
Oral mucosal blistering	5 (11.9)	2 (9.5)
Asthenia	5 (11.9)	1 (4.8)
Injection site pain	4 (9.5)	1 (4.8)
Vomiting	4 (9.5)	1 (4.8)
Abdominal pain	4 (9.5)	0 (0)
Dyspepsia	4 (9.5)	0 (0)
Hematoma	4 (9.5)	0 (0)
Alopecia	3 (7.1)	1 (4.8)
Influenza	3 (7.1)	1 (4.8)

(cont'd)

Table 4: Nplate *(cont'd)*

Adverse Events with ≥2% difference (Nplate vs Placebo) in Study 2 (Splenectomized Patients)

Preferred Term	Nplate (N=42) n (%)	Placebo (N=21) n (%)
Injection site bruising	3 (7.1)	1 (4.8)
Chills	3 (7.1)	0 (0)
Musculoskeletal chest pain	3 (7.1)	0 (0)
Pain in extremity	3 (7.1)	0 (0)
Paresthesia	3 (7.1)	0 (0)
Rhinitis allergic	3 (7.1)	0 (0)
Viral upper respiratory tract infection	3 (7.1)	0 (0)
Weight increased	3 (7.1)	0 (0)
Abdominal pain upper	2 (4.8)	0 (0)
Acne	2 (4.8)	0 (0)
Angina pectoris	2 (4.8)	0 (0)
Blood pressure increased	2 (4.8)	0 (0)
Bone pain	2 (4.8)	0 (0)
Bronchitis	2 (4.8)	0 (0)
Candidiasis	2 (4.8)	0 (0)
Flushing	2 (4.8)	0 (0)
Hematochezia	2 (4.8)	0 (0)
Hemoptysis	2 (4.8)	0 (0)
Hot flush	2 (4.8)	0 (0)
Lacrimation increased	2 (4.8)	0 (0)
Menorrhagia	2 (4.8)	0 (0)
Metrorrhagia	2 (4.8)	0 (0)
Migraine	2 (4.8)	0 (0)
Muscular weakness	2 (4.8)	0 (0)
Nasal congestion	2 (4.8)	0 (0)
Edema	2 (4.8)	0 (0)
Shoulder pain	2 (4.8)	0 (0)
Skin hemorrhage	2 (4.8)	0 (0)
Sleep apnea syndrome	2 (4.8)	0 (0)
Thrombocytopenia	2 (4.8)	0 (0)
Acarodermatitis	1 (2.4)	0 (0)
Alanine aminotransferase increased	1 (2.4)	0 (0)
Allergic sinusitis	1 (2.4)	0 (0)
Angioneurotic edema	1 (2.4)	0 (0)
Aphthous stomatitis	1 (2.4)	0 (0)
Appendicitis	1 (2.4)	0 (0)
Aspartate aminotransferase increased	1 (2.4)	0 (0)
Body tinea	1 (2.4)	0 (0)
Bone marrow disorder	1 (2.4)	0 (0)
Breath odour	1 (2.4)	0 (0)
Cardiac failure congestive	1 (2.4)	0 (0)
Cellulitis	1 (2.4)	0 (0)
Cholelithiasis	1 (2.4)	0 (0)
Constipation	1 (2.4)	0 (0)
Dehydration	1 (2.4)	0 (0)
Dermal cyst	1 (2.4)	0 (0)
Disturbance in attention	1 (2.4)	0 (0)

(cont'd)

Table 4: Nplate *(cont'd)*

Adverse Events with ≥2% difference (Nplate vs Placebo) in Study 2 (Splenectomized Patients)

Preferred Term	Nplate (N=42) n (%)	Placebo (N=21) n (%)
Dry skin	1 (2.4)	0 (0)
Dry throat	1 (2.4)	0 (0)
Dysgeusia	1 (2.4)	0 (0)
Dysmenorrhea	1 (2.4)	0 (0)
Dysphonia	1 (2.4)	0 (0)
Ear hemorrhage	1 (2.4)	0 (0)
Excoriation	1 (2.4)	0 (0)
Extrasystoles	1 (2.4)	0 (0)
Face edema	1 (2.4)	0 (0)
Fall	1 (2.4)	0 (0)
Fungal infection	1 (2.4)	0 (0)
Gastroenteritis	1 (2.4)	0 (0)
Gastrointestinal infection	1 (2.4)	0 (0)
Goitre	1 (2.4)	0 (0)
Gynecomastia	1 (2.4)	0 (0)
Hair growth abnormal	1 (2.4)	0 (0)
Heart rate increased	1 (2.4)	0 (0)
Hepatitis C antibody positive	1 (2.4)	0 (0)
Herpes simplex	1 (2.4)	0 (0)
Hypersensitivity	1 (2.4)	0 (0)
Hypoesthesia	1 (2.4)	0 (0)
Hypokalemia	1 (2.4)	0 (0)
Hypovolemia	1 (2.4)	0 (0)
Idiopathic thrombocytopenic purpura	1 (2.4)	0 (0)
Influenza like illness	1 (2.4)	0 (0)
Injection site swelling	1 (2.4)	0 (0)
Intervertebral disc protrusion	1 (2.4)	0 (0)
Lip blister	1 (2.4)	0 (0)
Mouth hemorrhage	1 (2.4)	0 (0)
Musculoskeletal stiffness	1 (2.4)	0 (0)
Nail disorder	1 (2.4)	0 (0)
Nightmare	1 (2.4)	0 (0)
Ocular hyperaemia	1 (2.4)	0 (0)
Oral candidiasis	1 (2.4)	0 (0)
Paranasal sinus hypersecretion	1 (2.4)	0 (0)
Peripheral embolism	1 (2.4)	0 (0)
Peripheral ischemia	1 (2.4)	0 (0)
Petit mal epilepsy	1 (2.4)	0 (0)
Pharyngitis	1 (2.4)	0 (0)
Photosensitivity reaction	1 (2.4)	0 (0)
Pleural effusion	1 (2.4)	0 (0)
Postmenopausal hemorrhage	1 (2.4)	0 (0)
Prurigo	1 (2.4)	0 (0)
Psychomotor hyperactivity	1 (2.4)	0 (0)
Rash papular	1 (2.4)	0 (0)
Rectal hemorrhage	1 (2.4)	0 (0)
Scleral hemorrhage	1 (2.4)	0 (0)

(cont'd)

Table 4: Nplate *(cont'd)*

Adverse Events with ≥2% difference (Nplate vs Placebo) in Study 2 (Splenectomized Patients)

Preferred Term	Nplate (N=42) n (%)	Placebo (N=21) n (%)
Seasonal allergy	1 (2.4)	0 (0)
Skin infection	1 (2.4)	0 (0)
Skin lesion	1 (2.4)	0 (0)
Skin odour abnormal	1 (2.4)	0 (0)
Soft tissue injury	1 (2.4)	0 (0)
Sputum discoloured	1 (2.4)	0 (0)
Stomach discomfort	1 (2.4)	0 (0)
Suicide attempt	1 (2.4)	0 (0)
Syncope	1 (2.4)	0 (0)
Tendonitis	1 (2.4)	0 (0)
Tension headache	1 (2.4)	0 (0)
Tinnitus	1 (2.4)	0 (0)
Tongue injury	1 (2.4)	0 (0)
Tooth discolouration	1 (2.4)	0 (0)
Tooth infection	1 (2.4)	0 (0)
Uterine polyp	1 (2.4)	0 (0)
Vaginal hemorrhage	1 (2.4)	0 (0)
Viral infection	1 (2.4)	0 (0)
Visual disturbance	1 (2.4)	0 (0)
Visual field defect	1 (2.4)	0 (0)
Vitamin B12 deficiency	1 (2.4)	0 (0)
Vulvovaginal mycotic infection	1 (2.4)	0 (0)
Weight decreased	1 (2.4)	0 (0)
Wound	1 (2.4)	0 (0)

Long-Term ITP Extension Study: An interim analysis was done for subjects from 6 ITP studies who completed their parent study and entered the ongoing open label extension study 20030213. A total of 137 subjects were enrolled, and 136 subjects received at least 1 dose of Nplate. At the time of the interim analysis, the mean time on study for the 136 subjects in the safety analysis set was 45 weeks (SD, 34.7 weeks; range, 1 to 122 weeks).

Adverse events with a subject incidence ≥10% were headache (30.9%), contusion (26.5%), fatigue (24.3%), diarrhea (23.5%), epistaxis (22.8%), nasopharyngitis (21.3%), arthralgia (19.9%), upper respiratory tract infection (17.6%), cough (16.2%), nausea (15.4%), back pain (14.7%), petechiae (14.0%), dizziness (12.5%), pain in extremity (12.5%), peripheral edema (11.8%), oral mucosal blistering (11.8%), gingival bleeding (11.0%), hematoma (11.0%), and rash (11.0%).

Adverse events were reported as treatment-related for 47 subjects (34.6%). Serious adverse events were reported for 35 subjects (25.7%). Adverse events leading to study withdrawal were reported for 8 (5.9%) subjects.

Nine serious thrombotic or thromboembolic events were reported in 6 subjects (6/136=4.4%). Reports that mentioned fibrosis or reticulin in the bone marrow were received for 7 subjects. In addition, bone marrow reticulin was noted in reports of adverse events in 2 other subjects. Three subjects died during this study. None of the deaths were considered treatment related.

Table 5, Table 6, Table 7 and Table 8 present Adverse Drug Reactions with a subject incidence ≥1%; Adverse Events with a subject incidence ≥2%; Serious Adverse Events; and Adverse Events leading to study withdrawal, respectively, for the long term ITP extension study.

Table 5: Nplate

Subject Incidence of Adverse Drug Reactions with Subject Incidence ≥1%

Preferred Term	Nplate (N=136) n (%)
Headache	42 (30.9)
Arthralgia	27 (19.9)
Dizziness	17 (12.5)
Pain in extremity	17 (12.5)
Abdominal pain	13 (9.6)
Insomnia	13 (9.6)
Myalgia	9 (6.6)
Paresthesia	9 (6.6)
Dyspepsia	6 (4.4)
Bone marrow disorder	4 (2.9)
Shoulder pain	3 (2.2)

Table 6: Nplate

Subject Incidence of Adverse Events With Subject Incidence ≥2%

Preferred Term	Nplate (N=136) n (%)
Headache	42 (30.9)
Contusion	36 (26.5)
Fatigue	33 (24.3)
Diarrhea	32 (23.5)
Epistaxis	31 (22.8)
Nasopharyngitis	29 (21.3)
Arthralgia	27 (19.9)
Upper respiratory tract infection	24 (17.6)
Cough	22 (16.2)
Nausea	21 (15.4)
Back pain	20 (14.7)
Petechiae	19 (14.0)
Dizziness	17 (12.5)
Pain in extremity	17 (12.5)
Edema peripheral	16 (11.8)
Oral mucosal blistering	16 (11.8)
Gingival bleeding	15 (11.0)
Hematoma	15 (11.0)
Rash	15 (11.0)
Abdominal pain	13 (9.6)
Insomnia	13 (9.6)
Muscle spasms	13 (9.6)
Pain	13 (9.6)
Pharyngolaryngeal pain	13 (9.6)
Sinusitis	13 (9.6)
Rhinorrhea	12 (8.8)
Injection site bruising	11 (8.1)
Pyrexia	11 (8.1)
Vomiting	11 (8.1)
Depression	9 (6.6)
Myalgia	9 (6.6)
Paresthesia	9 (6.6)
Thrombocytopenia	9 (6.6)
Constipation	8 (5.9)
Ecchymosis	8 (5.9)
Sinus headache	8 (5.9)
Urinary tract infection	8 (5.9)
Asthenia	7 (5.1)
Dyspnea	7 (5.1)
Procedural pain	7 (5.1)
Pruritus	7 (5.1)
Abdominal discomfort	6 (4.4)
Dyspepsia	6 (4.4)
Injection site pain	6 (4.4)
Joint swelling	6 (4.4)
Abdominal pain upper	5 (3.7)

(cont'd)

Table 6: Nplate *(cont'd)*

Subject Incidence of Adverse Events With Subject Incidence ≥2%

Preferred Term	Nplate (N=136) n (%)
Anxiety	5 (3.7)
Chills	5 (3.7)
Dysuria	5 (3.7)
Ear infection	5 (3.7)
Eczema	5 (3.7)
Herpes simplex	5 (3.7)
Joint sprain	5 (3.7)
Migraine	5 (3.7)
Mouth hemorrhage	5 (3.7)
Nasal congestion	5 (3.7)
Pharyngitis	5 (3.7)
Purpura	5 (3.7)
Skin lesion	5 (3.7)
Toothache	5 (3.7)
Vaginal hemorrhage	5 (3.7)
Bone marrow disorder	4 (2.9)
Cardiac failure congestive	4 (2.9)
Conjunctival hemorrhage	4 (2.9)
Dehydration	4 (2.9)
Excoriation	4 (2.9)
Fall	4 (2.9)
Gastroenteritis	4 (2.9)
Hemorrhage	4 (2.9)
Hypersensitivity	4 (2.9)
Hypertension	4 (2.9)
Hypoesthesia	4 (2.9)
Influenza	4 (2.9)
Menorrhagia	4 (2.9)
Musculoskeletal chest pain	4 (2.9)
Sciatica	4 (2.9)
Seasonal allergy	4 (2.9)
Stomatitis	4 (2.9)
Swelling face	4 (2.9)
Viral upper respiratory tract infection	4 (2.9)
Anemia	3 (2.2)
Arthropod bite	3 (2.2)
Asthma	3 (2.2)
Chest discomfort	3 (2.2)
Cystitis	3 (2.2)
Dyspnea exertional	3 (2.2)
Ear hemorrhage	3 (2.2)
Ear pain	3 (2.2)
Erythema	3 (2.2)
Eye pain	3 (2.2)
Hemoptysis	3 (2.2)
Influenza like illness	3 (2.2)
Limb injury	3 (2.2)

(cont'd)

Table 6: Nplate *(cont'd)*

Subject Incidence of Adverse Events With Subject Incidence ≥2%

Preferred Term	Nplate (N=136) n (%)
Malaise	3 (2.2)
Metrorrhagia	3 (2.2)
Musculoskeletal stiffness	3 (2.2)
Neck pain	3 (2.2)
Oral mucosal petechiae	3 (2.2)
Osteoarthritis	3 (2.2)
Pneumonia	3 (2.2)
Renal failure	3 (2.2)
Rhinitis	3 (2.2)
Shoulder pain	3 (2.2)
Urticaria	3 (2.2)
Vision blurred	3 (2.2)

Table 7: Nplate

Subject Incidence of Serious Adverse Events

Preferred Term	Nplate (N=136) n (%)
Thrombocytopenia	8 (5.9)
Bone marrow disorder	3 (2.2)
Abdominal pain	2 (1.5)
Cardiac failure congestive	2 (1.5)
Gingival bleeding	2 (1.5)
Platelet count increased	2 (1.5)
Pneumonia	2 (1.5)
Pyrexia	2 (1.5)
Renal failure	2 (1.5)
Thrombosis	2 (1.5)
Acute myocardial infarction	1 (0.7)
Adverse drug reaction	1 (0.7)
Anemia	1 (0.7)
Anal fistula	1 (0.7)
Anxiety	1 (0.7)
Asthma	1 (0.7)
Atrial fibrillation	1 (0.7)
Blindness	1 (0.7)
Cardiac arrest	1 (0.7)
Catheter related infection	1 (0.7)
Cerebral thrombosis	1 (0.7)
Cholecystitis	1 (0.7)
Deep vein thrombosis	1 (0.7)
Dehydration	1 (0.7)
Device related infection	1 (0.7)
Dyspnea	1 (0.7)
Epistaxis	1 (0.7)

(cont'd)

Table 7: Nplate *(cont'd)*

Subject Incidence of Serious Adverse Events

Preferred Term	Nplate (N=136) n (%)
Evan's syndrome	1 (0.7)
Gastric ulcer hemorrhage	1 (0.7)
Gastritis	1 (0.7)
Gastrointestinal hemorrhage	1 (0.7)
Hematoma	1 (0.7)
Hemoptysis	1 (0.7)
Headache	1 (0.7)
Hepatic failure	1 (0.7)
Hepatic neoplasm malignant	1 (0.7)
Hepatitis	1 (0.7)
Hypertension	1 (0.7)
Idiopathic thrombocytopenic purpura	1 (0.7)
Knee arthroplasty	1 (0.7)
Mechanical complication of implant	1 (0.7)
Melaena	1 (0.7)
Metrorrhagia	1 (0.7)
Multiple myeloma	1 (0.7)
Multiple sclerosis relapse	1 (0.7)
Myelofibrosis	1 (0.7)
Oral mucosal petechiae	1 (0.7)
Osteoarthritis	1 (0.7)
Papilloedema	1 (0.7)
Petechiae	1 (0.7)
Plastic surgery	1 (0.7)
Platelet count decreased	1 (0.7)
Pneumonia pneumococcal	1 (0.7)
Portal vein thrombosis	1 (0.7)
Post procedural cellulitis	1 (0.7)
Renal failure acute	1 (0.7)
Salpingo-oophorectomy	1 (0.7)
Surgery	1 (0.7)
Thrombophlebitis septic	1 (0.7)
Transient ischemic attack	1 (0.7)
Upper gastrointestinal hemorrhage	1 (0.7)
Urosepsis	1 (0.7)
Vaginal hemorrhage	1 (0.7)

Table 8: Nplate

Subject Incidence of Adverse Events Leading to Study Withdrawal

Preferred Term	Nplate (N=136) n (%)
Cardiac arrest	1 (0.7)
Headache	1 (0.7)
Hepatic failure	1 (0.7)
Multiple myeloma	1 (0.7)
Musculoskeletal pain	1 (0.7)
Myelofibrosis	1 (0.7)
Pneumonia pneumococcal	1 (0.7)
Renal failure	1 (0.7)
Thrombophlebitis septic	1 (0.7)
Vaginal hemorrhage	1 (0.7)

Bleeding Events: Across the entire ITP clinical programme, an inverse relationship between bleeding events and platelet counts was observed. All clinically significant (≥ grade 3) bleeding events occurred at platelet counts $<30\times10^9$/L. All bleeding events ≥ grade 2 occurred at platelet counts $<50\times10^9$/L.

In the Phase 3 studies, 9 patients reported a bleeding event that was considered serious (5 [6.0%] Nplate, 4 [9.8%] placebo). When adjusted for study duration, serious bleeding events were reported at 16.6 and 26.9 per 100 patient-years for Nplate and placebo, respectively.

Bleeding events that were grade 2 or higher were reported by 15% of patients treated with Nplate and 34% of patients treated with placebo. When adjusted for study duration, bleeding events grade 2 or higher were reported at 118.4 per and 134.4 per 100 patient-years for Nplate and placebo, respectively.

In the Phase 3 ITP long-term safety set, the study duration adjusted event rate of grade 2 or higher bleeding events was 71 per 100 patient-years for patients treated with Nplate and 132 per 100 patient-years for placebo treated patients.

Bleeding Events in Subjects with Variable Platelet Counts (Unstable Platelet Counts): Nine (7%) subjects in the pivotal studies had platelet counts that rose and fell to extreme levels within short periods of time; these subjects' course on study often included multiple rescue medications and numerous Nplate dose adjustments. Among these subjects 6 were treated with Nplate and 3 were treated with placebo. In addition 7 of the 9 subjects had been splenectomized. Nplate treated subjects had wider platelet count ranges with higher upper limits compared to those with placebo, possibly due to the effect of Nplate alone or synergistic effect with rescue medications.

As a result of the many severe declines in platelet count, these subjects experienced numerous bleeding events, including severe and serious bleeding events, and a life threatening hemorrhage. These 9 subjects highlight the individual variability that is found in ITP and the challenges of managing patients whose platelet counts cannot be stabilized, in contrast to subjects who were able to achieve a stable response.

Figure 1 and Figure 2 provide a representation of two individual subjects treated with Nplate who experienced stable and unstable platelet counts, respectively.

Figure 1: Nplate

Individual Platelet Count and Cumulative Dose Over Time: Durable Responder

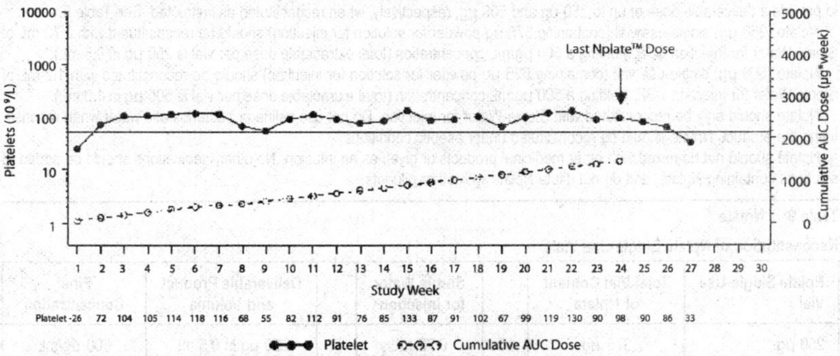

Only rescue medication use in Weeks 1-24 have been included. Severity of bleeding event is represented by the length of the vertical line segment. Rescue medications are indicated by the following: P=Prednisone, I=Immunoglobulins, B=Platelets, Human Blood, and O=Other.

Figure 2: Nplate

Individual Platelet Count and Cumulative Dose Over Time: Non-Durable Responder

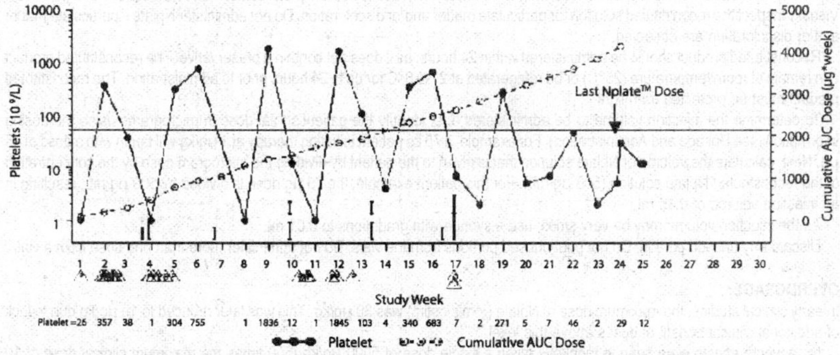

Only rescue medication use in Weeks 1-24 have been included. Severity of bleeding event is represented by the length of the vertical line segment. Rescue medications are indicated by the following: P=Prednisone, I=Immunoglobulins, B=Platelets, Human Blood, and O=Other.

Immunogenicity: As with all therapeutic proteins, patients may develop antibodies to the therapeutic protein. Patients were screened for immunogenicity to romiplostim using a Biacore-based biosensor immunoassay. This assay is capable of detecting both high and low affinity binding antibodies that bind to romiplostim and cross-react with TPO. The samples from patients that tested positive for binding antibodies were further evaluated for neutralizing capacity using a cell-based bioassay.

In clinical studies, the incidence of pre-existing antibodies to romiplostim was 8% (17/225) and the incidence of binding antibody development during Nplate treatment was 10% (23/225). The incidence of pre-existing antibodies to endogenous TPO was 5% (12/225) and the incidence of binding antibody development to endogenous TPO during Nplate treatment was 5% (12/225). Of the patients with positive antibodies to romiplostim or to TPO, 1 (0.4%) patient had neutralizing activity to romiplostim and none had neutralizing activity to TPO. There was no correlation of antibody activity and either clinical effectiveness or safety.

Immunogenicity assay results are highly dependent on the sensitivity and specificity of the assay used in detection and may be influenced by several factors, including sample handling, concomitant medications, and underlying disease. For these reasons, comparison of incidence of antibodies to romiplostim with the incidence of antibodies to other products may be misleading.

If formation of neutralizing antibodies is suspected, Amgen Canada Medical Information (1-866-502-6436) may be contacted for information on antibody testing.

DRUG INTERACTIONS: No formal drug-drug interaction studies of Nplate (romiplostim) have been performed.

ITP medical therapies used in combination with Nplate in clinical studies included corticosteroids, danazol, and/or azathioprine, intravenous immunoglobulins (IVIG), and anti-D immunoglobulin. When combining Nplate with other ITP medical therapies, platelet counts should be monitored in order to manage unexpected changes (see Dosage and Administration).

DOSAGE AND ADMINISTRATION: **Dosing Considerations:** Treatment should be prescribed and monitored only by qualified healthcare providers.

Nplate (romiplostim) is administered subcutaneously.

Use the lowest dose of Nplate necessary to achieve and maintain a platelet count ≥50×10⁹/L. Administer Nplate as a weekly subcutaneous (SC) injection with dose adjustments based upon the platelet count response. Nplate should not be used in an attempt to normalize platelet counts.

The prescribed Nplate dose may consist of a very small volume (for example, 0.15 mL). As the Nplate volume may be very small, a syringe with 0.01 mL graduations may be necessary.

Recommended Dose and Dosage Adjustment: Recommended Initial Dose: The recommended initial dose for Nplate is 1 µg/kg based on actual body weight, administered once weekly as a subcutaneous (SC) injection. All dosing calculations should be based on actual body weight at initiation of treatment.

Dose Adjustments: Use the actual body weight at initiation of therapy, then adjust the weekly dose of Nplate by increments of 1 µg/kg until the patient achieves a platelet count ≥50×10⁹/L. Assess the platelet count weekly until a stable platelet count (≥50×10⁹/L for at least 4 weeks without dose adjustment) has been achieved. Obtain platelet counts monthly thereafter. Do not exceed a maximum weekly dose of 10 µg/kg.

Adjust the dose as follows:

- If the platelet count is <50×10⁹/L, increase the dose by 1 µg/kg every 1-2 weeks.
- If platelet count is >200×10⁹/L for 2 consecutive weeks, reduce the dose by 1 µg/kg every 2 weeks.
- If platelet count is >400×10⁹/L, do not dose. Continue to assess the platelet count weekly. After the platelet count has fallen to <200×10⁹/L, resume Nplate at a dose reduced by 1 µg/kg.

Treatment Discontinuation: The recurrence of thrombocytopenia should be expected upon discontinuation of treatment (see Warnings and Precautions). Patients should be clinically evaluated periodically and continuation of treatment should be decided on an individual basis by the treating physician.

Discontinue Nplate if the platelet count does not increase to a level of 50×10⁹/L or to a level sufficient to avoid clinically important bleeding after four weeks at the highest weekly dose of 10 µg/kg. Dosing requirements should be individualized according to the needs of each ITP patient. During the placebo controlled studies, 3 µg/kg (25th-75th percentile: 1-4 µg/kg) was the median most frequent dose administered to both splenectomized and nonsplenectomized patients to achieve a platelet count ≥50×10⁹/L. In an open label study of refractory patients with ITP who had failed numerous prior ITP therapies, 7 µg/kg (25th-75th percentile: 5-9.5 µg/kg) was the median most frequent dose administered to achieve the same platelet level. Therefore, while doses higher than 7 µg/kg are not required for most patients, a subgroup of the most severely ill patients may require higher maximum doses. Doses higher than 10 µg/kg should not be exceeded.

Use of Nplate with Concomitant Medical ITP Therapies: Medical ITP therapies used in combination with Nplate in clinical studies included corticosteroids, danazol, azathioprine, intravenous immunoglobulin (IVIG), and anti-D immunoglobulin. Corticosteroids, danazol, and azathioprine were reduced or discontinued when given in combination with Nplate. If the patient's platelet count is ≥50×10⁹/L, medical ITP therapies may be reduced or discontinued.

Physician knowledge of platelet response may have had an impact on the differential reduction of concomitant medications and administration of rescue medications observed in clinical studies.

Rescue medications including platelet transfusions might be required during treatment with Nplate.

Administration: Nplate should be administered by subcutaneous injection.

Reconstitution: Nplate is supplied in two vial presentations: 250 µg/vial and 500 µg/vial. Each vial contains sufficient product to provide a deliverable dose of up to 250 µg and 500 µg, respectively, when reconstituted as instructed. See Table 9.

Nplate (250 µg) single-use vial (containing 375 µg powder for solution for injection) should be reconstituted with 0.72 mL of Sterile Water for Injection USP, yielding a 500 µg/mL concentration (total extractable dose per vial is 250 µg in 0.5 mL).

Nplate (500 µg) single-use vial (containing 625 µg powder for solution for injection) should be reconstituted with 1.2 mL of Sterile Water for Injection USP, yielding a 500 µg/mL concentration (total extractable dose per vial is 500 µg in 1.0 mL).

Nplate should only be reconstituted with Sterile Water for Injection. Do not use saline or bacteriostatic water when reconstituting the product. Nplate should be reconstituted under aseptic conditions.

Nplate should not be mixed with other medicinal products or given as an infusion. No other medications should be added to solutions containing Nplate, and do not dilute Nplate with other diluents.

Table 9: Nplate

Reconstitution of Nplate Single-Use Vials

Nplate Single-Use Vial	Total Vial Content of Nplate		Sterile Water for Injection[a]		Deliverable Product and Volume	Final Concentration
250 µg	375 µg	add	0.72 mL	=	250 µg in 0.5 mL	500 µg/mL
500 µg	625 µg	add	1.2 mL	=	500 µg in 1 mL	500 µg/mL

[a] Use Sterile Water for Injection.

During reconstitution, the vial contents may be gently swirled and inverted. Avoid excess or vigorous agitation: **do not shake**. Generally, dissolution of Nplate takes less than 2 minutes. The reconstituted Nplate solution should be clear and colorless. Visually inspect the reconstituted solution for particulate matter and/or discoloration. Do not administer Nplate if particulate matter and/or discoloration are observed.

Reconstituted product should be administered within 24 hours, as it does not contain a preservative. The reconstituted product can remain at room temperature (25°C) or be refrigerated at 2° to 8°C for up to 24 hours prior to administration. The reconstituted product must be protected from light.

To determine the injection volume to be administered, first identify the patient's total dose in micrograms using the dosing information (see Dosage and Administration). For example, a 75 kg patient initiating therapy at 1 µg/kg will begin with a dose of 75 µg. Next, calculate the volume of Nplate solution that is given to the patient by dividing the microgram dose by the concentration of the reconstituted Nplate solution (500 µg/mL). For this patient example, the 75 µg dose is divided by 500 µg/mL, resulting in an injection volume of 0.15 mL.

As the injection volume may be very small, use a syringe with gradations to 0.01 mL.

Discard any unused portion. Do not pool unused portions from the vials. Do not administer more than one dose from a vial.

OVERDOSAGE:

In early clinical studies, the maximum dose of Nplate (romiplostim) was 30 µg/kg. This was later reduced to 10 µg/kg due to lack of additional clinical benefit of doses above this level.

No adverse effects were seen in monkeys given a single dose of 5000 µg/kg (500 times the maximum clinical dose of 10 µg/kg).

In the event of overdose, platelet counts may increase above the normal range. In this case, discontinue Nplate and monitor platelet counts. Reinitiate treatment with Nplate in accordance with dosing and administration recommendations.

> For management of a suspected drug overdose, CPhA recommends that you contact your **regional Poison Control Centre**. See the *CPS* Directory section for a list of Poison Control Centres.

ACTION AND CLINICAL PHARMACOLOGY: Mechanism of Action: Nplate (romiplostim) increases platelet production through binding and activation of the thrombopoietin receptor, a mechanism analogous to endogenous thrombopoietin (eTPO).

Pharmacodynamics: Among all ITP patients treated with Nplate in study S1 (212) and S2 (105), during the 24-week treatment period the mean (SD) number of weeks with platelet response (platelet count ≥50×10⁹/L without rescue therapy within 8 weeks) was 15 (7.5) for non-splenectomized patients and 12 (7.9) for splenectomized patients.

Pharmacokinetics: In the long-term extension study in patients with ITP (n=20) receiving weekly treatment of Nplate subcutaneously, the pharmacokinetics of Nplate over the dose range of 3 to 15 µg/kg (Table 10) indicated that peak serum concentrations were observed about 7 to 50 hours postdose (median, 14 hours) with half-life values ranging from 1 to 34 days (median, 3.5 days). The serum concentrations varied among patients and did not correlate with the dose administered. The elimination of serum Nplate is in part dependent on the TPO receptor on platelets. As a result, for a given dose, high platelet counts in patients are associated with low serum concentrations and vice versa. The relationship between the exposure (AUC or C_{max}) and the predose platelet count was nonlinear, however, it is approximately linear in log-log scale. In another ITP clinical study, no accumulation in serum concentrations was observed after 6 weekly doses of Nplate (3 µg/kg). The potential for accumulation at higher dose of Nplate is unknown.

Table 10: Nplate

PK Parameters of Nplate Following 2 Consecutive Weekly Subcutaneous Doses in Subjects with ITP After Chronic Weekly Treatment in the Long-Term Extension Study

		AUC_{0-7}day (pg*hr/mL)		C_{max} (pg/mL)		t_{max} (hour)		$t_{1/2}$ (hour)		Predose Platelet Count (×10⁹/L)	
Subject	Dose µg/kg	Week 1	Week 2	Week 1	Week 2	Week 1	Week 2	Week 1	Week 2	Week 1	Week 2
1	3	2970	NA	37.8	NA	24	NA	47	NA	304	216
2	4	8880	9400	71.8	90.8	36	24	826	207	195	84
3	4	6240	6830	45.1	56	23	23	172	102	144	99
4	4	—[a]	—	—	—	—	—	—	—	194	131
5	4	14 500	7180	289	124	12	11	24	38	124	151
6	5	18 800	18 900	390	338	12	12	53	131	99	94
7	5	11 700	21 400	192	303	8	24	183	60	131	104
8	5	10 400	4830	162	52.4	12	24	145	29	102	144
9	5	5040	5090	94.3	67.2	11	24	415	51	257	326
10	7	7290	5260	105	37.1	7	24	39	153	100	333
11	8	117 000	94 100	1510	1310	12	11	67	91	74	74
12	8	13 700	8660	197	74.2	12	36	115	127	37	115
13	8	12 400	10 400	149	88.5	24	24	70	125	182	214
14	10	66 300	18 300	1440	159	24	22	78	124	78	152
15	15	305 000	209 000	8580	7550	12	12	68	109	5	5

[a] All samples from this subject were below the limit of quantification.

Data from 5 subjects were not included due to incomplete concentration time profile or dose change; AUC_{0-7day}=the area under the Nplate serum concentration-time curve over 7 days; C_{max}=the maximum serum concentration; t_{max}=the time of C_{max}; $t_{1/2}$=the half-life, probably represents the absorption rate due to flip-flop kinetics; NA=not available.

STORAGE AND STABILITY: Nplate (romiplostim) should be stored refrigerated at 2° to 8°C; the vial should be kept in the carton to protect from light until time of use. Do not freeze.

INFORMATION FOR THE PATIENT: Published in e-CPS, available by subscription at www.e-cps.ca.

DOSAGE FORMS, COMPOSITION AND PACKAGING: 250 µg/0.5 mL: Each vial of sterile lyophilized solid white powder contains: romiplostim 375 µg. Nonmedicinal ingredients: dilute hydrochloric acid (for pH adjustment), L-histidine, mannitol, polysorbate 20 and sucrose (15 mg). Each vial has a rubber stopper, an aluminum seal and a plastic flip-off cap. Dispensing packs of 1 single-dose vial for reconstitution.

500 µg/1 mL: Each vial of sterile lyophilized solid white powder contains: romiplostim 625 µg. Nonmedicinal ingredients: dilute hydrochloric acid (for pH adjustment), L-histidine, mannitol, polysorbate 20 and sucrose (25 mg). Each vial has a rubber stopper, an aluminum seal and a plastic flip-off cap. Dispensing packs of 1 single-dose vial for reconstitution.

Nu-Acebutolol 🄿

acebutolol HCl

Antihypertensive—Antianginal

Nu-Pharm

SUPPLIED: 100 mg: Each white, round, biconvex, film-coated tablet, scored and identified NU over 100 on one side, contains: acebutolol HCl equivalent to acebutolol 100 mg. Nonmedicinal ingredients: carnauba wax, colloidal silicon dioxide, dextrates, hydroxypropyl methylcellulose, magnesium stearate, polyethylene glycol (carbowax) and titanium dioxide. Energy: <1 kJ (0.10 kcal). Gluten-, sodium- and tartrazine-free. Bottles of 100.

200 mg: Each white, oval, biconvex, film-coated tablet, scored and identified NU 200 on one side, contains: acebutolol HCl equivalent to acebutolol 200 mg. Nonmedicinal ingredients: carnauba wax, colloidal silicon dioxide, dextrates, hydroxypropyl methylcellulose, magnesium stearate, polyethylene glycol (carbowax) and titanium dioxide. Energy: <1 kJ (0.21 kcal). Gluten-, sodium- and tartrazine-free. Bottles of 100.

400 mg: Each white, capsule-shaped, biconvex, film-coated tablet, scored and identified NU 400 on one side, contains: acebutolol HCl equivalent to acebutolol 400 mg. Nonmedicinal ingredients: carnauba wax, colloidal silicon dioxide, dextrates, hydroxypropyl methylcellulose, magnesium stearate, polyethylene glycol (carbowax) and titanium dioxide. Energy: <1.73 kJ (0.41 kcal). Gluten-, sodium- and tartrazine-free. Bottles of 100.

Store at room temperature (15 to 30°C). Protect from light.

Nu-Acyclovir 🄿

acyclovir

Antiviral Agent

Nu-Pharm

SUPPLIED: 200 mg: Each blue, round, flat-faced, beveled-edged tablet, identified NU over 200 on one side, contains: acyclovir 200 mg. Nonmedicinal ingredients: colloidal silicon dioxide, croscarmellose sodium, indigotine (FD&C blue #2), lactose, magnesium stearate and microcrystalline cellulose. Gluten- and tartrazine-free. Bottles of 100.

400 mg: Each pink, round, flat-faced, beveled-edged tablet, identified NU over 400 on one side, contains: acyclovir 400 mg. Nonmedicinal ingredients: colloidal silicon dioxide, croscarmellose sodium, magnesium stearate, microcrystalline cellulose and red ferric oxide. Gluten- and tartrazine-free. Bottles of 100.
800 mg: Each blue, oval, biconvex tablet, scored and identified NU 800 on one side, contains: acyclovir 800 mg. Nonmedicinal ingredients: brilliant blue FCF aluminum lake 12% (FD&C blue #1), colloidal silicon dioxide, croscarmellose sodium, indigotine (FD&C blue #2), magnesium stearate and microcrystalline cellulose. Gluten- and tartrazine-free. Bottles of 100.

Store at room temperature (15 to 30°C). Protect from light.

The reader is invited to consult CPhA's monograph **Thiazide Diuretics**.

Nu-Amilzide ℞
amiloride HCl—hydrochlorothiazide
Diuretic—Antihypertensive

Nu-Pharm

SUPPLIED: Each peach-colored, diamond-shaped, biconvex tablet, scored and identified NU above the score, 5/50 below the score contains: hydrochlorothiazide 50 mg and amiloride HCl equivalent to amiloride 5 mg. Nonmedicinal ingredients: colloidal silicon dioxide, croscarmellose sodium, lactose monohydrate, magnesium stearate, microcrystalline cellulose, sodium bicarbonate and sunset yellow aluminum lake 40% (FD&C yellow #6). Energy: 2.9 kJ (0.69 kcal). Sodium: <1 mmol (2.93 mg). Gluten- and tartrazine-free. Bottles of 100 and 1000.

Nu-Amoxi ℞
amoxicillin trihydrate
Antibiotic

Nu-Pharm

SUPPLIED: Capsules: 250 mg: Each scarlet red and gold No. 2 capsule, identified NU 250, contains: amoxicillin trihydrate equivalent to amoxicillin 250 mg. Nonmedicinal ingredients: colloidal silicon dioxide, croscarmellose sodium, D&C red #28, D&C red #40, D&C yellow #10, FD&C Blue #1, FD&C yellow #6, gelatin, silicon dioxide, sodium lauryl sulfate, stearic acid and titanium dioxide. Energy: <1 kJ (0.21 kcal). Gluten- and tartrazine-free. Bottles of 500 and 1 000.
500 mg: Each scarlet red and gold No. 0 capsule, identified NU 500, contains: amoxicillin trihydrate equivalent to amoxicillin 500 mg. Nonmedicinal ingredients: colloidal silicon dioxide, croscarmellose sodium, D&C red #28, D&C red #40, D&C yellow #10, FD&C Blue #1, FD&C yellow #6, gelatin, silicon dioxide, sodium lauryl sulfate, stearic acid and titanium dioxide. Energy: 1.52 kJ (0.36 kcal). Gluten- and tartrazine-free. Bottles of 500.
Suspensions: 125 mg: After reconstitution each 5 mL of strawberry-flavored suspension contains: amoxicillin trihydrate equivalent to amoxicillin 125 mg. Nonmedicinal ingredients: artificial strawberry flavoring, guar gum, sodium benzoate, sodium citrate and sucrose. Energy: 38.21 kJ (9.12 kcal)/5 mL. Sodium: <1 mmol (2.18 mg)/5 mL. Paraben-, sulfite- and tartrazine-free. Bottles of 100 and 150 mL.
250 mg: After reconstitution each 5 mL of banana-flavored suspension contains: amoxicillin trihydrate equivalent to amoxicillin 250 mg. Nonmedicinal ingredients: artificial banana flavoring, D&C yellow #10 aluminum lake 16%, guar gum, sodium benzoate, sodium citrate and sucrose. Energy: 37.3 kJ (8.91 kcal)/5 mL. Sodium: <1 mmol (2.6 mg)/5 mL. Paraben-, sulfite- and tartrazine-free. Bottles of 100 and 150 mL.

The reconstituted suspension is stable for 7 days at room temperature (15 to 30°C) or 14 days when refrigerated (4.5°C). Keep bottles tightly closed and shake thoroughly to obtain a uniform suspension.

Nubain® Ⓒ
nalbuphine HCl
Opioid Analgesic—Component to Balance Anesthesia

Sandoz

PHARMACOLOGY: Nubain (nalbuphine hydrochloride) is a synthetic opioid agonist-antagonist analgesic for parenteral use, related chemically to the opioid oxymorphone, and to the opioid antagonist naloxone. Nalbuphine has an analgesic (agonist action) potency equivalent to that of morphine on a milligram basis. Receptor studies show that nalbuphine binds to mu, kappa, and delta receptors, but not to sigma receptors. Nalbuphine is primarily a kappa agonist/mu antagonist analgesic. Nalbuphine has an antagonist activity (reversal of major effects of opioids drugs) about one-fourth of that of nalorphine and 10 times that of pentazocine. The onset of action of nalbuphine occurs within 2 to 3 minutes after intravenous administration, and in less than 15 minutes following subcutaneous or intramuscular injection. The plasma half-life of nalbuphine is 5 hours and in clinical studies the duration of analgesic activity has been reported to range from 3 to 6 hours.

At the usual adult dose of 10 mg/70 kg, nalbuphine may produce respiratory depression equivalent to that of equianalgesic doses of morphine. However, Nubain exhibits a ceiling effect such that increases in dose greater than 30 mg do not produce further respiratory depression.

Nalbuphine by itself has potent opioid antagonist activity at doses equal to or lower than its analgesic dose. When administered following or concurrent with mu agonist opioid analgesics (e.g. morphine, oxymorphone, fentanyl), nalbuphine may partially reverse or block opioid-induced respiratory depression from the mu agonist analgesic. Nalbuphine may precipitate withdrawal in patients dependent on opioid drugs. Nalbuphine should be used with caution in patients who have been receiving mu opioid analgesics on a regular basis.

INDICATIONS: Nubain (nalbuphine hydrochloride) is indicated for the relief of moderate to severe pain. Clinical studies indicate that it can also be used for preoperative analgesia, as a supplement to surgical anesthesia and for obstetrical analgesia during labour.

CONTRAINDICATIONS: Nubain (nalbuphine hydrochloride) should not be administered to patients who are hypersensitive to nalbuphine hydrochloride or to any of the other ingredients in Nubain (see Supplied).

WARNINGS: In patients physically dependent on opiate drugs, Nubain (nalbuphine hydrochloride) should not be given prior to detoxification since withdrawal symptoms are likely to be produced.

Nubain should be administered as a supplement to surgical anesthesia only by persons specifically trained in the use of intravenous anesthetics and management of the respiratory effects of potent opioids.

Naloxone, resuscitative and intubation equipment and oxygen should be readily available.

Drug Dependence: On the basis of behavioural, substitution and direct addiction studies in humans, Nubain has been shown to have low abuse potential. When compared with drugs that are not mixed agonists-antagonists, it has been reported that nalbuphine's potential for abuse may be less than that of codeine or propoxyphene. Drug abuse has been reported relatively infrequently. Psychological and physical dependence and tolerance may follow the abuse or misuse of Nubain. Therefore, caution should be observed in prescribing it for emotionally unstable patients or for individuals with a history of opioid abuse. Such patients should be closely supervised when long-term therapy is contemplated.

Care should be taken to avoid increases in dosage or frequency of administration which in susceptible individuals might result in physical dependence.

Abrupt discontinuation of Nubain following prolonged use has been followed by symptoms of opioid withdrawal, such as abdominal cramps, nausea and vomiting, rhinorrhea, lacrimation, restlessness, anxiety, elevated temperature and piloerection.

Use in Ambulatory Patients: Nubain may impair the mental or physical abilities required for the performance of potentially dangerous tasks such as driving a car or operating machinery. Therefore, Nubain should be administered with caution to ambulatory patients, who should be warned to avoid such hazards until recovered from the effects of the drug.

Interaction with Other Central Nervous System Depressants: Although Nubain possesses opioid antagonist activity, there is evidence that in non-dependent patients it may not antagonize an opioid analgesic administered just before, concurrently, or just after an injection of Nubain. Therefore, patients receiving opioid analgesics, general anesthetics, phenothiazines or other tranquilizers, sedatives, hypnotics or other CNS depressants (including alcohol) concomitantly with Nubain may exhibit an additive effect. When such combined therapy is contemplated, the dose of one or both agents should be reduced.

Children: Because clinical experience in children under the age of 12 years is limited, the administration of Nubain in this age group is not recommended.

Pregnancy: (Other than labour): Safe use of Nubain in pregnancy (other than labour) has not been established. Although animal reproductive studies have not revealed teratogenic or embryotoxic effects, Nubain should only be administered to pregnant women, when in the judgment of the physician, the potential benefits outweigh the possible hazards.

Use in Labour and Delivery: Since Nubain can produce respiratory depression in the neonate, it should be administered with caution to women delivering premature infants. The placental transfer of nalbuphine is high, relatively rapid and variable with a maternal to fetal ratio ranging from 1:0.37 to 1:6.03. Fetal and neonatal adverse effects that have been reported following the administration of nalbuphine to the mother during labour include fetal bradycardia, respiratory depression at birth, apnea, cyanosis, and hypotonia. Maternal administration of naloxone during labour has normalized these effects in some cases. Severe and prolonged fetal bradycardia has been reported. Permanent neurological damage attributed to fetal bradycardia has occurred. A sinusoidal fetal heart rate pattern associated with the use of nalbuphine has also been reported. Nubain should be used with caution in women during labour and delivery, and newborns should be monitored for respiratory depression, apnea, bradycardia, and arrythmias if Nubain has been administered.

Head Injury and Increased Intracranial Pressure: The possible respiratory depressant effects and the potential of potent analgesics to elevate cerebrospinal fluid pressure (resulting from vasolidation following CO_2 retention) may be markedly exaggerated in the presence of head injury, intracranial lesions, or a preexisting increase in intracranial pressure. Furthermore, potent analgesics can produce effects which may obscure the clinical course of patients with head injuries. Therefore, Nubain should be administered in these circumstances only when essential, and with extreme caution.

Laboratory Tests: Nubain may interfere with enzymatic methods for the detection of opioids depending on the specificity/sensitivity of the tests. Please consult the test manufacturer for specific details.

PRECAUTIONS: Impaired Respiration: At the usual adult dose of 10 mg/70 kg, Nubain (nalbuphine hydrochloride) may produce respiratory depression equivalent to that of equianalgesic doses of morphine. Caution should be observed when administering Nubain to patients with impaired respiration, or who are receiving other medications which produce respiratory depression. In the presence of bronchial asthma, uremia, severe infection, cyanosis, or respiratory obstruction, Nubain should be administered only with great caution and in reduced doses. Respiratory depression induced by Nubain can be reversed by the administration of Naloxone Hydrochloride for Injection USP.

Impaired Renal or Hepatic Function: Because Nubain is metabolized in the liver and excreted by the kidneys, patients with renal or liver dysfunction may show an exaggerated response to customary doses. Therefore, in these individuals Nubain should be used with caution and administered in reduced amounts.

Myocardial Infarction: As with all potent analgesics, Nubain should be used with caution in patients with myocardial infarction who have nausea or vomiting. Hemodynamic studies in patients with severe arteriosclerotic heart changes reveal that Nubain has circulatory effects similar to those of morphine, i.e. a minimal decrease in oxygen consumption, cardiac index, left ventricular end-diastolic pressure and cardiac work.

Biliary Tract Surgery: As with all opioid analgesics, Nubain should be used with caution in patients about to undergo surgery of the biliary tract since it may cause spasm of the sphincter of Oddi.

Cardiovascular System: During evaluation of Nubain in anesthesia, a higher incidence of bradycardia has been reported in patients who did not receive atropine preoperatively.

Carcinogenesis, Mutagenesis, Impairment of Fertility: No evidence of carcinogenicity was found in a 24-month carcinogenicity study in rats and an 18-month carcinogenicity study in mice at oral doses as high as the equivalent of approximately three times the maximum recommended therapeutic dose. No evidence of a mutagenic/genotoxic potential to Nubain was found in the Ames, Chinese Hamster Ovary HGPRT, and Sister Chromatid Exchange, mouse micronucleus, and rat bone marrow cytogenicity assays. Nalbuphine induces an increased frequency of mutation in mouse lymphoma cells.

Pregnancy: Teratogenic Effects: Reproduction studies have been performed in rabbits and in rats at dosages as high as approximately 14 and 31 times respectively the maximum recommended daily dose and revealed no evidence of impaired fertility or harm to the fetus due to Nubain. There are, however, no adequate and well-controlled studies in pregnant women. Because animal reproduction studies are not always predictive of human response, this drug should be used during pregnancy only if, in the judgment of the physician, the potential benefits outweigh the possible risks (see Warnings).

Non-Teratogenic Effects: Neonatal body weight and survival was reduced when Nubain was subcutaneously administered to female rats prior to mating and throughout gestation and lactation or to pregnant rats during the last third of gestation and throughout lactation at doses approximately 8 to 17 times the maximum recommended therapeutic dose. The clinical significance of this effect is unknown (see Warnings).

Lactation: Limited data suggest that Nubain is excreted in maternal milk in small amounts (less than 1% of the administered dose) considered clinically insignificant. Caution should be exercised when Nubain is administered to a nursing mother.

Patients Dependent on Opioids: Patients who have been taking opioids chronically may experience withdrawal symptoms upon the administration of Nubain. Unduly troublesome opioid withdrawal symptoms may be controlled by the slow intravenous administration of small increments of morphine, until relief occurs.

ADVERSE EFFECTS: In clinical trials with Nubain (nalbuphine hydrochloride) the most frequently reported side effects were: sedation (36% of 1066 patients treated), sweaty or clammy (9%), nausea or vomiting (6%), dizziness or vertigo (5%), dry mouth (4%) and headache (3%). Other adverse reactions which occurred (reported incidence of 1% or less) were:

Central Nervous System: nervousness, crying, depression, restlessness, euphoria, hostility, confusion, faintness, floating, unusual dreams, numbness, feeling of heaviness and psychotomimetic effects such as hallucinations, feeling of unreality and dysphoria.

The incidence of psychomimetic effects, such as unreality, depersonalization, delusions, dysphoria and hallucination has been shown to be less than that which occurs with pentazocine.

Cardiovascular: hypertension, hypotension, bradycardia, tachycardia.
Gastrointestinal: cramps, dyspepsia, bitter taste.
Respiratory: depression, dyspnea, asthma.
Dermatological: itching, burning, urticaria.
Miscellaneous: speech difficulty, urinary urgency, blurred vision, flushing and warmth.
Allergic Reactions: Anaphylactic/anaphylactoid and other serious hypersensitivity reactions have been reported following the use of nalbuphine and may require immediate, supportive medical treatment. These reactions may include shock, respiratory distress, respiratory arrest, bradycardia, cardiac arrest, hypotension, or laryngeal edema. Other allergic-type reactions reported with patients using Nubain include stridor, bronchospasm, wheezing, edema, rash, pruritus, nausea, vomiting, diaphoresis, weakness, and shakiness.
Postmarketing: Other reports include pulmonary edema, agitation and injection site reactions such as pain, swelling, redness, burning and hot sensations.

OVERDOSE:

Symptoms: These are expected to be similar to those of other drugs of this class. The administration of single intramuscular doses of 72 mg of Nubain (nalbuphine hydrochloride) to 8 normal subjects has been reported to have resulted primarily in symptoms of sleepiness and mild dysphoria.

Treatment: Naloxone hydrochloride administered intravenously is a specific antidote for Nubain. Since the duration of action of Nubain may exceed that of naloxone hydrochloride, the patient should be kept under continued surveillance and repeated doses of naloxone hydrochloride should be administered as necessary. Oxygen, intravenous fluids, vasopressors and other supportive measures should be employed as indicated.

For management of a suspected drug overdose, CPhA recommends that you contact your **regional Poison Control Centre**. See the *CPS* Directory section for a list of Poison Control Centres.

DOSAGE: The usual recommended dose of Nubain (nalbuphine hydrochloride) is 10 mg for a 70 kg individual, administered subcutaneously, intramuscularly or intravenously. This dose may be repeated every 3 to 6 hours as required. The recommended dosage range is 10 to 20 mg, with a maximum single dose of 20 mg and a maximum total daily dose of 160 mg. Dosage should be adjusted according to the severity of the pain, physical status of the patient, and other medications which the patient may be receiving. (See Interaction with Other Central Nervous System Depressants under Warnings.)

Nubain is physically incompatible with nafcillin and ketorolac. Solutions of these drugs should not be mixed. Patients who have been taking opioids chronically for pain under medical supervision, may experience withdrawal symptoms upon the administration of Nubain. If Nubain is administered to those patients, as an analgesic, it should be introduced gradually (see Patients Dependent on Opioids under Precautions). Nubain should not be used as a substitute for other opioids or for withdrawal purposes in individuals dependent on these drugs. See Table 1.

Table 1: Nubain

Opioids Analgesics—Approximate Analgesic Equivalences

Drug	Equivalent Dose (mg) (compared to morphine 10 mg IM)		Duration of Action (hours)
	Parenteral	Oral	
Strong Opioid Agonists:			
Morphine (single dose)	10	60	3–4
Morphine (chronic dose)	10	20–30	3–4
Hydromorphone	1.5–2	6–7.5	2–4
Anileridine	25	75	2–3
Levorphanol	2	4	4–8
Meperidine	75	300	1–3
Oxymorphone	1.5	5 (rectal)	3–4
Heroin	5–8	10–15	3–4
Weak Opioid Agonists:			
Codeine	120	200	3–4
Oxycodone	5–10	10–15	2–4
Propoxyphene	50	100	2–4
Mixed Agonist-Antagonists:			
Pentazocine	60	180	3–4
Nalbuphine	10		3–6
Butorphanol	2		3–4

SUPPLIED: 10 mg/mL: Each mL contains: nalbuphine hydrochloride 10 mg, sodium chloride 2 mg, sodium citrate dihydrate 9.41 mg, and citric acid 12.62 mg; pH adjusted with hydrochloric acid. Ampoules of 1 mL, boxes of 10. Store at controlled room temperature (15 to 30°C). Protect from excessive light. Store in carton until contents have been used. Parenteral drug products should be inspected visually for particulate matter and discolouration prior to administration whenever solution and container permit.
20 mg/mL: Each mL contains: nalbuphine hydrochloride 20 mg, sodium citrate dihydrate 9.41 mg, and citric acid 12.62 mg; pH adjusted with hydrochloric acid. Ampoules of 1 mL, boxes of 10. Store at controlled room temperature (15 to 30°C). Protect from excessive light. Store in carton until contents have been used. Parenteral drug products should be inspected visually for particulate matter and discolouration prior to administration whenever solution and container permit.

Nu-Cal
calcium carbonate
Calcium Supplement

Odan

Nu-Cal D
calcium carbonate—vitamin D
Calcium Supplement—Vitamin D Supplement

Odan

Nu-Cal D 400
calcium carbonate—vitamin D
Calcium Supplement—Vitamin D Supplement

Odan

SUPPLIED: Nu-Cal: Each light green, capsule-shaped, coated tablet contains: calcium carbonate 1250 mg from oyster shell which provides 500 mg (25 mEq) elemental calcium. Nonmedicinal ingredients: acacia gum, carnauba wax, croscarmellose sodium, FD&C blue No. 1, hypromellose, magnesium stearate, maltodextrin, riboflavin, sodium lauryl sulfate, titanium dioxide and triacetin. Contains no preservatives, artificial flavor, lactose, yeast or gluten. Packages of 100 and 500.
Nu-Cal D: Each shiny grey, capsule-shaped, coated tablet contains: calcium carbonate 1250 mg from oyster shell which provides 500 mg (25 mEq) elemental calcium and vitamin D_3 125 IU (3.13 µg). Nonmedicinal ingredients: acacia gum, alpha tocopherol, calcium silicate, carnauba wax, corn starch, distilled monoglycerides, hypromellose, magnesium stearate, maltodextrin, medium chain triglycerides, microcrystalline cellulose, polyethylene glycol, propylene glycol monoesters, sodium lauryl sulfate, sodium starch glycolate, sodium stearoyl lactylate and sucrose. Contains no preservatives, artificial flavor, lactose, yeast, or gluten. Packages of 100 and 500.
Nu-Cal D 400: Each light blue, capsule-shaped, coated tablet contains: calcium carbonate 1250 mg from oyster shell which provides 500 mg (25 mEq) elemental calcium and vitamin D_3 400 IU (10 µg). Nonmedicinal ingredients: acacia gum, alpha tocopherol, carnauba wax, croscarmellose sodium, FD&C blue No. 2, corn starch, hypromellose, magnesium stearate, maltodextrin, medium chain triglycerides, silicone dioxide, sodium ascorbate, sodium lauryl sulfate, sucrose, titanium dioxide and triacetin. Contains no preservatives, artificial flavor, lactose yeast or gluten. Packages of 100 and 500.

Nu-Cephalex ℞
cephalexin
Antibiotic

Nu-Pharm

SUPPLIED: 250 mg: Each orange, capsule-shaped, biconvex, film-coated tablet, identified NU-250 on one side, contains: cephalexin 250 mg. Nonmedicinal ingredients: carnauba wax, colloidal silicon dioxide, hydroxypropyl methylcellulose, magnesium stearate, microcrystalline cellulose, polyethylene glycol, stearic acid, sunset yellow aluminum lake 40% (FD&C yellow #6), sunset yellow lake 16% and titanium dioxide. Energy: 2.14 kJ (0.51 kcal). Gluten-, sodium- and tartrazine-free. Bottles of 100 and 1000.
500 mg: Each orange, capsule-shaped, biconvex, film-coated tablet, scored and identified NU 500 on one side, contains: cephalexin 500 mg. Nonmedicinal ingredients: carnauba wax, colloidal silicon dioxide, hydroxypropyl methylcellulose, magnesium stearate, microcrystalline cellulose, polyethylene glycol, stearic acid, sunset yellow aluminum lake 40% (FD&C yellow #6), sunset yellow lake 16% and titanium dioxide. Energy: 4.18 kJ (1.02 kcal). Gluten-, sodium- and tartrazine-free. Bottles of 100 and 500.
Store at room temperature (15 to 30°C).

Nu-Cimet ℞
cimetidine
Histamine H2-Receptor Inhibitor

Nu-Pharm

SUPPLIED: 200 mg: Each pale green, round, biconvex, film-coated tablet, identified NU over 200 on one side, contains: cimetidine 200 mg. Nonmedicinal ingredients: carnauba wax, colloidal silicon dioxide, croscarmellose sodium, D&C yellow #10 aluminum lake 16%, ferric ferrous oxide, hydroxypropyl methylcellulose, magnesium stearate, microcrystalline cellulose, polyethylene glycol and titanium dioxide. Energy: 3.11 kJ (0.74 kcal). Sodium: <1 mmol (0.11 mg). Gluten- and tartrazine-free. Bottles of 500.
300 mg: Each pale green, round, biconvex, film-coated tablet, identified NU over 300 on one side, contains: cimetidine 300 mg. Nonmedicinal ingredients: carnauba wax, colloidal silicon dioxide, croscarmellose sodium, D&C yellow #10 aluminum lake 16%, ferric ferrous oxide, hydroxypropyl methylcellulose, magnesium stearate, microcrystalline cellulose, polyethylene glycol and titanium dioxide. Energy: 3.59 kJ (0.86 kcal). Sodium: <1 mmol (0.17 mg). Gluten- and tartrazine-free. Bottles of 1000.
400 mg: Each pale green, oblong-shaped, biconvex, film-coated tablet, identified NU-400 on one side, contains: cimetidine 400 mg. Nonmedicinal ingredients: carnauba wax, colloidal silicon dioxide, croscarmellose sodium, D&C yellow #10 aluminum lake 16%, ferric ferrous oxide, hydroxypropyl methylcellulose, magnesium stearate, microcrystalline cellulose, polyethylene glycol and titanium dioxide. Energy: 4.26 kJ (1.02 kcal). Sodium: <1 mmol (0.23 mg). Gluten- and tartrazine-free. Bottles of 100 and 500.
600 mg: Each pale green, oblong-shaped, biconvex, film-coated tablet, identified NU-600 on one side, contains: cimetidine 600 mg. Nonmedicinal ingredients: carnauba wax, colloidal silicon dioxide, croscarmellose sodium, D&C yellow #10 aluminum lake 16%, ferric ferrous oxide, hydroxypropyl methylcellulose, magnesium stearate, microcrystalline cellulose, polyethylene glycol and titanium dioxide. Energy: 5.85 kJ (1.40 kcal). Sodium: <1 mmol (0.34 mg). Gluten- and tartrazine-free. Bottles of 100 and 500.

Nu-Cotrimox ℞
sulfamethoxazole—trimethoprim
Antibacterial

Nu-Pharm

SUPPLIED: Adult Tablets: Each white, round tablet, one side convex, scored and identified NU over 400-80, other side flat-faced with beveled edges, contains: sulfamethoxazole 400 mg and trimethoprim 80 mg. Nonmedicinal ingredients: colloidal silicon dioxide, croscarmellose sodium, magnesium stearate and methylcellulose. Energy: <1 kJ (0.15 kcal). Sodium: <1 mmol (0.25 mg). Gluten- and tartrazine-free. Bottles of 500.
DS Tablets: Each white, capsule-shaped, biconvex tablet, partially scored and identified NU-DS on one side, contains: sulfamethoxazole 800 mg and trimethoprim 160 mg. Nonmedicinal ingredients: colloidal silicon dioxide, croscarmellose sodium, magnesium stearate and methylcellulose. Energy: 1.27 kJ (0.3 kcal). Sodium: <1 mmol (0.15 mg). Gluten- and tartrazine-free. Bottles of 100 and 500.
Oral Suspension: Each 5 mL of pink, cherry-flavored suspension contains: sulfamethoxazole 200 mg and trimethoprim 40 mg. Nonmedicinal ingredients: artificial cherry flavor, carboxymethylcellulose, carboxymethylcellulose sodium, FD&C red #2, FD&C yellow #6, glycerin, methylparaben, microcrystalline cellulose, polysorbate, sodium cyclamate, sorbitol and water. Energy: 51.67 kJ (12.34 kcal)/5 mL. Sodium: 4 mmol (0.93 mg)/5 mL. Paraben-, sugar-, sulfite- and tartrazine-free. Bottles of 400 mL. Store at room temperature (15 to 30°C).

Nu-Diclo ℞
diclofenac sodium
Anti-inflammatory—Analgesic

Nu-Pharm

SUPPLIED: 25 mg: Each yellow, round, biconvex, enteric-coated tablet, identified 25 on one side, contains: diclofenac sodium 25 mg. Nonmedicinal ingredients: colloidal silicon dioxide, D&C yellow #10 aluminum lake, dextrates, hydroxypropyl methylcellulose, magnesium stearate, methylcellulose, polyethylene glycol, polyvinyl acetate phthalate, stearic acid, sunset yellow aluminum lake 40% (FD&C yellow #6), titanium dioxide, triethyl citrate and yellow ferric oxide. Energy: 1.99 kJ (0.47 kcal). Sodium: <1 mmol (1.81 mg). Gluten- and tartrazine-free. Bottles of 100 and 500.
50 mg: Each light brown, round, biconvex, enteric-coated tablet, identified 50 on one side, contains: diclofenac sodium 50 mg. Nonmedicinal ingredients: colloidal silicon dioxide, D&C yellow #10 aluminum lake, dextrates, hydroxypropyl methylcellulose, magnesium stearate, methylcellulose, polyethylene glycol, polyvinyl acetate phthalate, stearic acid, sunset yellow aluminum lake 40% (FD&C yellow #6), titanium dioxide, triethyl citrate and yellow ferric oxide. Energy: 3.97 kJ (0.95 kcal). Sodium: <1 mmol (3.62 mg). Gluten- and tartrazine-free. Bottles of 100 and 500.
Store at room temperature (15 to 30°C). Protect from humidity.

Nu-Diclo-SR ℞
diclofenac sodium
Anti-inflammatory—Analgesic

Nu-Pharm

SUPPLIED: 75 mg: Each light pink, triangular, biconvex, film-coated, slow-release tablet, identified NU over 75 on one side, contains: diclofenac sodium 75 mg. Nonmedicinal ingredients: carnauba wax, dextrates, hydroxyethyl cellulose, hydroxypropyl methylcellulose, magnesium stearate, microcrystalline cellulose, polyethylene glycol, red ferric oxide and titanium dioxide. Gluten-, lactose- and tartrazine-free. Bottles of 100.

100 mg: Each pink, round, biconvex, film-coated, slow-release tablet, identified NU over 100 on one side, contains: diclofenac sodium 100 mg. Nonmedicinal ingredients: carnauba wax, dextrates, hydroxyethyl cellulose, hydroxypropyl methylcellulose, magnesium stearate, microcrystalline cellulose, polyethylene glycol, red ferric oxide and titanium dioxide. Gluten-, lactose- and tartrazine-free. Bottles of 100.

Store at room temperature (15 to 30°C). Protect from light.

The reader is invited to consult CPhA's monograph **Calcium Channel Blockers**.

Nu-Diltiaz

diltiazem HCl

Antianginal

Nu-Pharm

SUPPLIED: 30 mg: Each light green, round, biconvex, film-coated tablet, identified NU over 30 on one side, contains: diltiazem HCl 30 mg. Nonmedicinal ingredients: brilliant blue FCF aluminum lake 12% (FD&C blue #1), carnauba wax, colloidal silicon dioxide, D&C yellow #10 aluminum lake 16%, hydroxypropyl methylcellulose, lactose, magnesium stearate, polyethylene glycol and titanium dioxide. Energy: 2.91 kJ (0.69 kcal). Gluten-, sodium- and tartrazine-free. Bottles of 100 and 500.
60 mg: Each yellow, round, biconvex, film-coated tablet, scored and identified NU over 60 on one side, contains: diltiazem HCl 60 mg. Nonmedicinal ingredients: carnauba wax, colloidal silicon dioxide, D&C yellow #10 aluminum lake 16%, hydroxypropyl methylcellulose, lactose, magnesium stearate, polyethylene glycol, sunset yellow aluminum lake 40% (FD&C yellow #6) and titanium dioxide. Energy: 5.82 kJ (1.39 kcal). Gluten-, sodium- and tartrazine-free. Bottles of 100 and 500.

The reader is invited to consult CPhA's monograph **Calcium Channel Blockers**.

Nu-Diltiaz-CD

diltiazem HCl

Antihypertensive—Antianginal

Nu-Pharm

SUPPLIED: 120 mg: Each turquoise No. 2, controlled delivery capsule, identified NU 120, contains: diltiazem HCl 120 mg. Nonmedicinal ingredients: eudragit, FD&C blue #1, gelatin, methylcellulose, microcrystalline cellulose, polysorbate, silicon dioxide, sodium lauryl sulfate, talc, titanium dioxide and tributyl citrate. Gluten- and tartrazine-free. Bottles of 100.
180 mg: Each turquoise and dark blue No. 1, controlled delivery capsule, identified NU 180, contains: diltiazem HCl 180 mg. Nonmedicinal ingredients: eudragit, FD&C blue #1, gelatin, methylcellulose, microcrystalline cellulose, polysorbate, silicon dioxide, sodium lauryl sulfate, talc, titanium dioxide and tributyl citrate. Gluten- and tartrazine-free. Bottles of 100.
240 mg: Each blue No. 0, controlled delivery capsule, identified NU 240, contains: diltiazem HCl 240 mg. Nonmedicinal ingredients: eudragit, FD&C blue #1, gelatin, methylcellulose, microcrystalline cellulose, polysorbate, silicon dioxide, sodium lauryl sulfate, talc, titanium dioxide and tributyl citrate. Gluten- and tartrazine-free. Bottles of 100.

Store at room temperature (15 to 30°C).

Nu-Divalproex

divalproex sodium

Anticonvulsant

Nu-Pharm

SUPPLIED: 125 mg: Each red, oblong, enteric-coated tablet, identified 125 on one side, contains: divalproex sodium equivalent to valproic acid 125 mg. Nonmedicinal ingredients: D&C red No. 30 aluminum lake, eudragit FD&C yellow #6, guar gum, hydroxypropylcellulose, hydroxypropyl methylcellulose, microcrystalline cellulose, polyethylene glycol, talc, titanium dioxide and triethyl citrate. Gluten- and tartrazine-free. Bottles of 100.
250 mg: Each peach, oblong, enteric-coated tablet, identified 250 on one side, contains: divalproex sodium equivalent to valproic acid 250 mg. Nonmedicinal ingredients: eudragit FD&C yellow #6, guar gum, hydroxypropylcellulose, hydroxypropyl methylcellulose, microcrystalline cellulose, polyethylene glycol, talc, titanium dioxide and triethyl citrate. Gluten- and tartrazine-free. Bottles of 100 and 500.
500 mg: Each pink, oblong, enteric-coated tablet, identified 500 on one side, contains: divalproex sodium equivalent to valproic acid 500 mg. Nonmedicinal ingredients: D&C red No. 33, eudragit, guar gum, hydroxypropylcellulose, hydroxypropyl methylcellulose, microcrystalline cellulose, polyethylene glycol, red ferric oxide, talc, titanium dioxide and triethyl citrate. Gluten- and tartrazine-free. Bottles of 100 and 500.

Store at room temperature (15 to 30°C). Protect from light.

The reader is invited to consult CPhA's monograph **Tetracyclines**.

Nu-Doxycycline

doxycycline hyclate

Antibiotic

Nu-Pharm

SUPPLIED: Capsules: Each blue, No. 2 capsule, identified NU 100, contains: doxycycline hyclate equivalent to doxycycline base 100 mg. Nonmedicinal ingredients: croscarmellose sodium, FD&C Blue No. 1, gelatin, lactose, magnesium stearate, silicon dioxide, sodium lauryl sulfate, stearic acid, talc and titanium dioxide. Energy: 3.09 kJ (0.74 kcal). Sodium: <1 mmol (0.25 mg). Gluten- and tartrazine-free. Bottles of 100.
Tablets: Each orange, round, biconvex, film-coated tablet, identified NU over 100 on one side, contains: doxycycline hyclate equivalent to doxycycline base 100 mg. Nonmedicinal ingredients: carnauba wax, colloidal silicon dioxide, croscarmellose sodium, magnesium stearate, microcrystalline cellulose, hydroxypropyl methylcellulose, polyethylene glycol, sunset yellow aluminum lake 40% (FD&C yellow #6) and titanium dioxide. Energy: ≤3.62 kJ (≤0.87 kcal). Sodium: <1 mmol (0.19 mg). Gluten- and tartrazine-free. Bottles of 100.

Nu-Famotidine

famotidine

Histamine H2-Receptor Antagonist

Nu-Pharm

SUPPLIED: 20 mg: Each beige, D-shaped, film-coated tablet, identified NU over 20 on one side, contains: famotidine 20 mg. Nonmedicinal ingredients: carnauba wax, colloidal silicon dioxide, croscarmellose sodium, hydroxypropyl methylcellulose, lactose, magnesium stearate, microcrystalline cellulose, polyethylene glycol, red ferric oxide, stearic acid, titanium dioxide and yellow ferric oxide. Energy: 3.23 kJ (0.77 kcal). Sodium: <1 mmol (0.44 mg). Gluten- and tartrazine-free. Bottles of 100 and 500.
40 mg: Each light brown, D-shaped, film-coated tablet, identified NU over 40 on one side, contains: famotidine 40 mg. Nonmedicinal ingredients: carnauba wax, colloidal silicon dioxide, croscarmellose sodium, hydroxypropyl methylcellulose, lactose, magnesium stearate, microcrystalline cellulose, polyethylene glycol, red ferric oxide, stearic acid, titanium dioxide and yellow ferric oxide. Energy: 2.9 kJ (0.69 kcal). Sodium: <1 mmol (0.44 mg). Gluten- and tartrazine-free. Bottles of 100.

Store at room temperature (15 to 30°C). Protect from light and moisture.

The reader is invited to consult CPhA's monograph **Selective Serotonin Reuptake Inhibitors**.

Nu-Fluoxetine

fluoxetine HCl

Antidepressant—Antiobsessional—Antibulimic

Nu-Pharm

SUPPLIED: 10 mg: Each green and grey, No. 4 capsule, identified NU 10, contains: fluoxetine HCl equivalent to fluoxetine 10 mg. Nonmedicinal ingredients: cornstarch, D&C yellow #10, FD&C blue #1, FD&C yellow #6, gelatin, lactose, Sicomet-85 black iron oxide, silicon dioxide, sodium lauryl sulfate, stearic acid, talc and titanium dioxide. Gluten- and tartrazine-free. Bottles of 100.
20 mg: Each green and ivory, No. 3 capsule, identified NU 20, contains: fluoxetine HCl equivalent to fluoxetine 20 mg. Nonmedicinal ingredients: cornstarch, D&C yellow #10, FD&C blue #1, FD&C yellow #6, gelatin, lactose, silicon dioxide, sodium lauryl sulfate, stearic acid, talc and titanium dioxide. Gluten- and tartrazine-free. Bottles of 100 and 500.

Store at room temperature (15 to 30°C) in tightly-closed containers. Protect from light.

The reader is invited to consult CPhA's monograph **Sulfonylureas**.

Nu-Glyburide

glyburide

Oral Hypoglycemic Agent

Nu-Pharm

SUPPLIED: 2.5 mg: Each white, round, flat-faced, beveled-edged tablet, scored and identified NU over 2.5 on one side, contains: glyburide 2.5 mg. Nonmedicinal ingredients: croscarmellose sodium, lactose, magnesium stearate and microcrystalline cellulose. Energy: 1.3 kJ (0.31 kcal). Sodium: <1 mmol (0.13 mg). Gluten- and tartrazine-free. Bottles of 100.
5 mg: Each white, capsule-shaped, flat-faced, beveled-edged tablet, scored on one side and identified NU 5 on the other side, contains: glyburide 5 mg. Nonmedicinal ingredients: croscarmellose sodium, lactose, magnesium stearate and microcrystalline cellulose. Energy: 2.59 kJ (0.62 kcal). Sodium: <1 mmol (0.25 mg). Gluten- and tartrazine-free. Bottles of 500.

Store at room temperature (15 to 30°C).

Nu-Indo

indomethacin

Anti-inflammatory—Analgesic

Nu-Pharm

SUPPLIED: 25 mg: Each blue and white No. 3 capsule, identified NU 25, contains: indomethacin 25 mg. Nonmedicinal ingredients: cornstarch, D&C Red No. 28, FD&C Blue No. 1, FD&C Red No. 40, gelatin, lactose, silicon dioxide, sodium lauryl sulfate, stearic acid, talc and titanium dioxide. Energy: 3.45 kJ (0.82 kcal). Gluten-, sodium- and tartrazine-free. Bottles of 100 and 1000.
50 mg: Each blue and white No. 1 capsule, identified NU 50, contains: indomethacin 50 mg. Nonmedicinal ingredients: cornstarch, D&C Red No. 28, FD&C Blue No. 1, FD&C Red No. 40, gelatin, lactose, silicon dioxide, sodium lauryl sulfate, stearic acid, talc and titanium dioxide. Energy: 7.55 kJ (1.8 kcal). Gluten-, sodium- and tartrazine-free. Bottles of 100 and 500.

The reader is invited to consult CPhA's monograph **HMG-CoA Reductase Inhibitors**.

Nu-Lovastatin

lovastatin

Lipid Metabolism Regulator

Nu-Pharm

SUPPLIED: 20 mg: Each light blue, octagonal, flat-faced, beveled-edged tablet, engraved NU on one side, scored and engraved LOVA over 20 on the other side, contains: lovastatin 20 mg. Nonmedicinal ingredients: croscarmellose sodium, FD&C Blue #1 aluminum lake, FD&C Blue #2 aluminum lake, lactose, magnesium stearate and microcrystalline cellulose. Bottles of 100. Store at room temperature (15 to 30°C). Protect from light.
40 mg: Each light green, octagonal, flat-faced, beveled-edged tablet, engraved NU on one side and LOVA over 40 on the other side, contains: lovastatin 40 mg. Nonmedicinal ingredients: croscarmellose sodium, D&C yellow #10 aluminum lake, FD&C Blue #2 aluminum lake, lactose, magnesium stearate and microcrystalline cellulose. Bottles of 100. Store at room temperature (15 to 30°C). Protect from light.

Nu-Metformin

metformin HCl

Antihyperglycemic

Nu-Pharm

SUPPLIED: 500 mg: Each white, round, flat-faced, beveled-edged tablet, scored and identified NU over M500 on one side, contains: metformin HCl 500 mg. Nonmedicinal ingredients: magnesium stearate and methylcellulose. Gluten-, sodium- and tartrazine-free. Bottles of 100 and 500.
850 mg: Each white, capsule-shaped, biconvex tablet, identified NU on one side and 850 on the other, contains: metformin HCl 850 mg. Nonmedicinal ingredients: magnesium stearate and methylcellulose. Gluten-, sodium- and tartrazine-free. Bottles of 100.

Store at room temperature (15 to 30°C).

Nu-Metoclopramide ℞
metoclopramide HCl
Modifier of Upper Gastrointestinal Motility—Antiemetic

Nu-Pharm

SUPPLIED: 5 mg: Each white, square, biconvex tablet, identified NU over M5 on one side, contains: metoclopramide HCl equivalent to metoclopramide 5 mg. Nonmedicinal ingredients: croscarmellose sodium, lactose, magnesium stearate and microcrystalline cellulose. Energy: 1.58 kJ (0.38 kcal). Sodium: <1 mmol (0.06 mg). Gluten- and tartrazine-free. Bottles of 100.
10 mg: Each white, round, biconvex tablet, scored and identified NU over M10 on one side, contains: metoclopramide HCl equivalent to metoclopramide 10 mg. Nonmedicinal ingredients: croscarmellose sodium, lactose, magnesium stearate and microcrystalline cellulose. Energy: 3.16 kJ (0.76 kcal). Sodium: <1 mmol (0.11 mg). Gluten- and tartrazine-free. Bottles of 100.
Store at room temperature (15 to 30°C).

Nu-Metop ℞
metoprolol tartrate
Antianginal—Antihypertensive

Nu-Pharm

SUPPLIED: 50 mg: Each pink, capsule-shaped, biconvex, film-coated tablet, scored on one side and identified 50 on the other, contains: metoprolol tartrate 50 mg. Nonmedicinal ingredients: carnauba wax, colloidal silicon dioxide, croscarmellose sodium, D&C Red #30 aluminum lake, FD&C Yellow #6 (sunset yellow aluminum lake), hydroxypropyl methylcellulose, lactose, magnesium stearate, microcrystalline cellulose, polyethylene glycol 3350 (carbowax) and titanium dioxide. Energy: 1.74 kJ (0.41 kcal). Sodium: <1 mmol (0.81 mg). Gluten- and tartrazine-free. Bottles of 100 and 1000.
100 mg: Each blue, capsule-shaped, biconvex, film-coated tablet, scored on one side and identified 100 on the other, contains: metoprolol tartrate 100 mg. Nonmedicinal ingredients: carnauba wax, croscarmellose sodium, indigotine aluminum lake (FD&C Blue #2), hydroxypropyl methylcellulose, lactose, magnesium stearate, microcrystalline cellulose, polydextrose, polyethylene glycol 3350 (carbowax) and titanium dioxide. Energy: 3.5 kJ (0.84 kcal). Sodium: <1 mmol (1.72 mg). Gluten- and tartrazine-free. Bottles of 100.

Nu-Moclobemide ℞
moclobemide
Antidepressant

Nu-Pharm

SUPPLIED: 100 mg: Each orange, oval, biconvex, film-coated tablet, scored on one side and identified NU over 100 on the other side, contains: moclobemide 100 mg. Nonmedicinal ingredients: carnauba wax, colloidal silicon dioxide, croscarmellose sodium, dextrates, hydroxypropyl methylcellulose, magnesium stearate, polydextrose, polyethylene glycol, red ferric oxide, titanium dioxide and yellow ferric oxide. Bottles of 100.
150 mg: Each pale yellow, oval, biconvex, film-coated tablet, scored on one side, identified NU over 150 on the other side, contains: moclobemide 150 mg. Nonmedicinal ingredients: carnauba wax, colloidal silicon dioxide, croscarmellose sodium, dextrates, hydroxypropyl methylcellulose, magnesium stearate, polydextrose, polyethylene glycol, titanium dioxide and yellow ferric oxide. Bottles of 100.
Store at room temperature (15 to 30°C).

Nu-Naprox ℞
naproxen
Anti-inflammatory—Analgesic

Nu-Pharm

SUPPLIED: 125 mg: Each light green, oval, biconvex tablet, identified NU-125 on one side, contains: naproxen 125 mg. Nonmedicinal ingredients: colloidal silicon dioxide, croscarmellose sodium, D&C yellow #10 aluminum lake 16%, indigotine aluminum lake 13% (FD&C blue #2), magnesium stearate and methylcellose. Energy: <1 kJ (0.19 kcal). Sodium: <1 mmol (0.17 mg). Gluten- and tartrazine-free. Bottles of 500.
250 mg: Each yellow, oval, biconvex tablet, identified NU-250 on one side, contains: naproxen 250 mg. Nonmedicinal ingredients: colloidal silicon dioxide, croscarmellose sodium, D&C yellow #10 aluminum lake 16%, magnesium stearate, methylcellulose and sunset yellow aluminum lake 40% (FD&C yellow #6). Energy: 1.6 kJ (0.38 kcal). Sodium: <1 mmol (0.34 mg). Gluten- and tartrazine-free. Bottles of 100 and 1000.
375 mg: Each peach-colored, capsule-shaped, biconvex tablet, scored and identified NU 375 on one side, contains: naproxen 375 mg. Nonmedicinal ingredients: colloidal silicon dioxide, croscarmellose sodium, magnesium stearate, methylcellulose and sunset yellow aluminum lake 40% (FD&C yellow #6). Energy: 2.43 kJ (0.58 kcal). Sodium: <1 mmol (0.51 mg). Gluten- and tartrazine-free. Bottles of 100 and 500.
500 mg: Each yellow, capsule-shaped, biconvex tablet, scored and identified NU 500 on one side, contains: naproxen 500 mg. Nonmedicinal ingredients: colloidal silicon dioxide, croscarmellose sodium, D&C yellow #10 aluminum lake 16%, magnesium stearate, methylcellulose and sunset yellow aluminum lake 40% (FD&C yellow #6). Energy: 3.2 kJ (0.76 kcal). Sodium: <1 mmol (0.68 mg). Gluten- and tartrazine-free. Bottles of 100 and 500.

Nu-Oxybutyn ℞
oxybutynin chloride
Anticholinergic—Antispasmodic

Nu-Pharm

SUPPLIED: Each blue, round, biconvex tablet, scored and identified NU over 5 on one side, contains: oxybutynin chloride 5 mg. Nonmedicinal ingredients: brilliant blue FCF aluminum lake 12% (FD&C blue #1), lactose, magnesium stearate and microcrystalline cellulose. Gluten- and tartrazine-free. Bottles of 100 and 500. Store at room temperature (15 to 30°C), in a tight, light resistant container.

Nu-Pindol ℞
pindolol
Antihypertensive—Antianginal

Nu-Pharm

SUPPLIED: 5 mg: Each white, round, flat-faced, beveled-edged tablet, scored and identified NU over 5 on one side, contains: pindolol 5 mg. Nonmedicinal ingredients: croscarmellose sodium, lactose, magnesium stearate and microcrystalline cellulose. Energy: 1.25 kJ (0.3 kcal). Sodium: <1 mmol (0.09 mg). Gluten- and tartrazine-free. Bottles of 100.
10 mg: Each white, round, biconvex tablet, scored and identified NU over 10 on one side, contains: pindolol 10 mg. Nonmedicinal ingredients: croscarmellose sodium, lactose, magnesium stearate and microcrystalline cellulose. Energy: 2.49 kJ (0.6 kcal). Sodium: <1 mmol (0.07 mg). Gluten- and tartrazine-free. Bottles of 100.
15 mg: Each white, round, flat-faced, beveled-edged tablet, scored and identified NU over 15 on one side, contains: pindolol 15 mg. Nonmedicinal ingredients: croscarmellose sodium, lactose, magnesium stearate and microcrystalline cellulose. Energy: 3.74 kJ (0.89 kcal). Sodium: <1 mmol (0.27 mg). Gluten- and tartrazine-free. Bottles of 100.

The reader is invited to consult CPhA's monograph **HMG-CoA Reductase Inhibitors**.

Nu-Pravastatin ℞
pravastatin sodium
Lipid Metabolism Regulator

Nu-Pharm

SUPPLIED: 10 mg: Each pink to peach, rounded, rectangular-shaped, biconvex tablet, identified "PRA" over "10" on one side, contains: pravastatin sodium 10 mg. Nonmedicinal ingredients: croscarmellose sodium, lactose monohydrate, magnesium stearate, microcrystalline cellulose and red ferric oxide. Bottles of 100.
20 mg: Each yellow, rounded, rectangular-shaped, biconvex tablet, identified "PRA" over "20" on one side, contains: pravastatin sodium 20 mg. Nonmedicinal ingredients: croscarmellose sodium, lactose monohydrate, magnesium stearate, microcrystalline cellulose and yellow ferric oxide. Bottles of 100 and 500.
40 mg: Each green, rounded, rectangular-shaped, biconvex tablet, identified "PRA" over "40" on one side, contains: pravastatin sodium 40 mg. Nonmedicinal ingredients: Brilliant Blue FCF aluminium lake 12% (FD&C Blue nº 1), croscarmellose sodium, D&C Yellow Nº 10 aluminum lake 16%, lactose monohydrate, magnesium stearate and microcrystalline cellulose. Bottles of 100.
Store at room temperature (15 to 30°C). Protect from moisture and light.

Nu-Ranit ℞
ranitidine HCl
Histamine H2-Receptor Antagonist

Nu-Pharm

SUPPLIED: 150 mg: Each white, round, biconvex, film-coated tablet, identified NU over 150 on one side, contains: ranitidine 150 mg (as the HCl). Nonmedicinal ingredients: carnauba wax, colloidal silicon dioxide, croscarmellose sodium, hydroxypropyl methylcellulose, magnesium stearate, microcrystalline cellulose, polydextrose, polyethylene glycol, titanium dioxide and vanillin. Energy: 2.54 kJ (0.61 kcal). Sodium: <1 mmol (0.37 mg). Gluten- and tartrazine-free. Bottles of 100 and 500.
300 mg: Each white, capsule-shaped, biconvex, film-coated tablet, identified NU 300 on one side, contains: ranitidine 300 mg (as the HCl). Nonmedicinal ingredients: carnauba wax, colloidal silicon dioxide, croscarmellose sodium, hydroxypropyl methylcellulose, magnesium stearate, microcrystalline cellulose, polydextrose, polyethylene glycol, titanium dioxide and vanillin. Energy: 5.07 kJ (1.21 kcal). Sodium: <1 mmol (0.73 mg). Gluten- and tartrazine-free. Bottles of 100 and 500.

Nu-Sertraline ℞
sertraline HCl
Antidepressant

Nu-Pharm

SUPPLIED: 25 mg: Each yellow, size 4 capsule, imprinted "NU 25" contains: sertraline HCl equivalent to 25 mg of sertraline. Nonmedicinal ingredients: colloidal silicon dioxide, cornstarch, croscarmellose sodium, stearic acid and talc; capsule shell: D&C Yellow #10, FC&C Yellow #6, gelatin and titanium dioxide; edible black ink: ammonium hydroxide, black iron oxide, ethyl alcohol, isopropyl alcohol, n-butyl alcohol, pharmaceutical shellac and propylene glycol, may contain: potassium hydroxide, FD&C Blue #1 aluminum lake, FD&C Blue #2 aluminum lake, D&C Yellow #10 aluminum lake, FD&C Red #40 aluminum lake. Bottles of 100. Store at room temperature (15 to 30°C).
50 mg: Each white and yellow, size 4 capsule, imprinted "NU 50", contains: sertraline HCl equivalent to 50 mg of sertraline. Nonmedicinal ingredients: colloidal silicon dioxide, cornstarch, croscarmellose sodium, stearic acid and talc; capsule shell: D&C Yellow #10, FD&C Yellow #6, gelatin and titanium dioxide; edible black ink: D&C Yellow #10 aluminum lake, FD&C Blue #1 aluminum lake, FD&C Blue #2 aluminum lake, FD&C Red #40 aluminum lake, pharmaceutical glaze and synthetic black iron oxide, may contain: n-butyl alcohol, propylene glycol, SDA-3A alcohol. Bottles of 100. Store at room temperature (15 to 30°C).
100 mg: Each orange, size 2 capsule, imprinted "NU 100", contains: sertraline HCl equivalent to 100 mg of sertraline. Nonmedicinal ingredients: colloidal silicon dioxide, cornstarch, croscarmellose sodium, stearic acid and talc; capsule shell: D&C Yellow #10, FD&C Red #40, gelatin and titanium dioxide; edible black ink: D&C Yellow #10 aluminum lake, FD&C Blue #1 aluminum lake, FD&C Blue #2 aluminum lake, FD&C Red #40 aluminum lake, pharmaceutical glaze and synthetic black iron oxide, may contain: n-butyl alcohol, propylene glycol, SDA-3A alcohol. Bottles of 100. Store at room temperature (15 to 30°C).

Nu-Sucralfate ℞
sucralfate
Gastroduodenal Cytoprotective Agent

Nu-Pharm

SUPPLIED: Each white, capsule-shaped tablet, partially scored on both sides, one side convex, other side flat-faced, scored and identified NU-1g, contains: sucralfate 1 g. Nonmedicinal ingredients: colloidal silicon dioxide, croscarmellose sodium and magnesium stearate. Energy: <1 kJ (0.05 kcal). Sodium: <1 mmol (0.76 mg). Gluten- and tartrazine-free. Bottles of 100 and 500. Store at room temperature (15 to 30°C) and protect from light in tightly closed container.

The reader is invited to consult CPhA's monograph **Tetracyclines**.

Nu-Tetra ℞
tetracycline HCl
Antibiotic

Nu-Pharm

SUPPLIED: Each yellow and orange No. 2 capsule, identified NU 250, contains: tetracycline HCl 250 mg. Nonmedicinal ingredients: black ink (black iron oxide, may contain pharmaceutical glaze, FD&C Blue #2 aluminum lake, FD&C Red #40 aluminum lake, n-butyl alcohol, propylene glycol, SDA-3A alcohol, isopropyl alcohol, ammonium hydroxide, potassium hydroxide) D&C Yellow #10, FD&C Red #40, FD&C Yellow #6, gelatin, silicon dioxide, sodium lauryl sulfate, stearic acid, talc and titanium dioxide. Energy: 1 kJ (0.21 kcal). Gluten- and tartrazine-free. Bottles of 1000.

Nu-Ticlopidine ℞
ticlopidine HCl
Inhibitor of Platelet Function

Nu-Pharm

SUPPLIED: Each white, oval-shaped, biconvex, film-coated tablet, identified NU on one side and 250 on the other, contains: ticlopidine HCl 250 mg. Nonmedicinal ingredients: carnauba wax, croscarmellose sodium, hydroxypropyl methylcellulose, microcrystalline cellulose, polyethylene glycol, stearic acid and titanium dioxide. Gluten- and tartrazine-free. Bottles of 100. Store at room temperature (15 to 30°C).

The reader is invited to consult CPhA's monograph **Thiazide Diuretics**.

Nu-Triazide ℞
triamterene—hydrochlorothiazide
Diuretic—Antihypertensive

Nu-Pharm

SUPPLIED: Each yellow-orange, round, flat-faced, beveled-edged tablet, scored and identified NU over T on one side, contains: triamterene 50 mg and hydrochlorothiazide 25 mg. Nonmedicinal ingredients: colloidal silicon dioxide, croscarmellose sodium, lactose, magnesium stearate and sunset yellow aluminum lake 40% (FD&C yellow #6). Energy: 3.69 kJ (0.88 kcal). Sodium: <1 mmol (1.52 mg). Gluten- and tartrazine-free. Bottles of 1000.

Nutropin® ℞
somatropin
Growth Hormone

Roche

Nutropin AQ® ℞
somatropin
Growth Hormone

Roche

Nutropin AQ Pen® Cartridge ℞
somatropin
Growth Hormone

Roche

Date of Preparation: October 15, 1996
Date of Revision: August 23, 2006

SUMMARY PRODUCT INFORMATION:

Route of Administration	Dosage Form/ Strength	Clinically Relevant Nonmedicinal Ingredients
Intramuscular, subcutaneous	Lyophilized powder for injection; 5 mg/vial and 10 mg/vial	Mannitol Note: The Bacteriostatic Water for Injection, supplied with NUTROPIN (somatropin for injection) contains a preservative, benzyl alcohol. (See Warnings and Precautions, General, Pediatrics.)
Intramuscular, subcutaneous	Solution; 10 mg/2 mL vial	None
Subcutaneous	Solution; 10 mg/2 mL pen cartridge	None

For a complete listing of nonmedicinal ingredients see Dosage Forms, Composition and Packaging.

DESCRIPTION: Somatropin is a single-chain protein of 191 amino acids, including four cysteine residues present as two intrachain disulfides. Somatropin is synthesized in a specific laboratory strain of *E. coli* bacteria (which has been modified by the addition of a plasmid coding for hGH) as a precursor consisting of the rhGH molecule preceded by the secretion signal from an *E. coli* protein. This precursor is then cleaved in the plasma membrane of the cell. The native protein is secreted into the periplasm where it is folded appropriately. The primary and secondary structures of somatropin are identical with pituitary-derived human growth hormone.

INDICATIONS AND CLINICAL USE: Pediatric Patients: NUTROPIN (somatropin) is indicated for:
- the long-term treatment of children who have growth failure due to growth hormone inadequacy.
- the treatment of children who have growth failure associated with chronic renal insufficiency up to the time of renal transplantation. Therapy with NUTROPIN should be used in conjunction with optimal management of chronic renal insufficiency.
- the long-term treatment of short stature associated with Turner syndrome.

Adults Patients: NUTROPIN (somatropin) is indicated for:
- the replacement of endogenous growth hormone (GH) in patients with adult GH deficiency (GHD) who meet both of the following two criteria:
  1. Biochemical diagnosis of adult GH deficiency by means of a subnormal response to a standard growth hormone stimulation test (peak GH ≤5µg/L), and
  2. Adult-onset: Patients who have adult GH deficiency either alone or with multiple hormone deficiencies (hypopituitarism) as a result of pituitary disease, hypothalmic disease, surgery, radiation therapy, or trauma; or
  3. Childhood-onset: Patients who were GH deficient during childhood, confirmed as an adult before replacement therapy with NUTROPIN is started

CONTRAINDICATIONS:
- NUTROPIN (somatropin) is contraindicated in patients who are hypersensitive to somatropin or to any ingredient in the formulation. For a complete listing, see Dosage Forms, Composition and Packaging.
- Growth hormone should not be initiated to treat patients with acute critical illness due to the complications following open heart or abdominal surgery, multiple accidental trauma or to patients having acute respiratory failure. (See Warnings and Precautions.)
- NUTROPIN should not be used in pediatric patients with closed epiphyses.
- NUTROPIN should not be used in patients with active neoplasia. Growth hormone therapy should be discontinued if evidence of neoplasia develops.
- NUTROPIN (somatropin for injection) lyophilized powder, when reconstituted with Bacteriostatic Water for Injection, USP (benzyl alcohol preserved), should not be used in newborns or in patients with a known sensitivity to benzyl alcohol. (See Warnings and Precautions.)
- Growth hormone is contraindicated in patients with Prader-Willi syndrome who are severely obese or have severe respiratory impairment. (See Warnings and Precautions.)
- Unless patients with Prader-Willi syndrome also have a diagnosis of growth hormone deficiency, NUTROPIN is not indicated for the long-term treatment of pediatric patients who have growth failure due to genetically confirmed Prader-Willi syndrome.

WARNINGS AND PRECAUTIONS: General: In two placebo controlled clinical trials in non-growth hormone deficient adult patients (n=522) a significant increase in mortality has been reported among somatropin treated patients with acute critical illnesses in intensive care units due to complications following open heart surgery or abdominal surgery, multiple accidental trauma, or to patients having acute respiratory failure (41.9%) compared to those receiving placebo (19.3%). Doses of 5.3-8 mg/day were given. The safety of continuing growth hormone treatment in patients receiving replacement doses for approved indications who concurrently develop these illnesses has not been established. Therefore, the potential benefit of treatment continuation with growth hormone in patients having an acute critical illness should be weighed against the potential risk.

There have been reports of fatalities after initiating therapy with growth hormone in pediatric patients with Prader-Willi syndrome who had one or more of the following risk factors: severe obesity, history of upper airway obstruction or sleep apnea, or unidentified respiratory infection. Male patients with one or more of these factors may be at greater risk than females. Patients with Prader-Willi syndrome should be evaluated for signs of upper airway obstruction and sleep apnea before initiation of treatment with growth hormone. If during treatment with growth hormone, patients show signs of upper airway obstruction (including onset of or increased snoring) and/or new onset of sleep apnea, treatment should be interrupted. All patients with Prader-Willi syndrome treated with growth hormone should also have effective weight control and be monitored for signs of respiratory infection, which should be diagnosed as early as possible and treated aggressively. (See Contraindications.) Unless patients with Prader-Willi syndrome also have a diagnosis of growth hormone deficiency, NUTROPIN (somatropin) is not indicated for the long-term treatment of pediatric patients who have growth failure due to genetically confirmed Prader-Willi syndrome.

NUTROPIN should be prescribed by physicians experienced in the diagnosis and management of patients with growth failure, Turner syndrome, or chronic renal insufficiency (CRI). No studies have been performed with NUTROPIN in children who have received renal transplants.

Benzyl alcohol as a preservative in Bacteriostatic Water for Injection, USP has been associated with toxicity in newborns. When administering NUTROPIN (somatropin for injection) lyophilized powder in newborns or in patients sensitive to benzyl alcohol, reconstitute with Sterile Water for Injection, USP. When Sterile Water for Injection, USP is used, **use only one dose of NUTROPIN per vial and discard the unused portion**. (See Dosage and Administration, Administration.)

Carcinogenesis and Mutagenesis: Carcinogenicity and mutagenicity studies have not been conducted with NUTROPIN. Patients developing neoplasia should be reported to the Health Products and Food Branch (HPFB) by the treating physician.

Endocrine and Metabolism: Because NUTROPIN may induce a state of **insulin resistance**, patients should be observed for evidence of glucose intolerance.

For patients with diabetes mellitus, the insulin dose may require adjustment when GH therapy is instituted. Because GH may reduce insulin sensitivity, particularly in obese individuals, patients should be observed for evidence of glucose intolerance. Patients with diabetes or glucose intolerance should be monitored closely during GH therapy.

Therapy with NUTROPIN in adults with GHD of adult onset was associated with an increase of median fasting insulin in the NUTROPIN 0.0125 mg/kg/day group from 9.0 µU/mL at baseline to 13.0 µU/mL at Month 12 with a return to the baseline median after a 3-week post-washout period off GH therapy. In the placebo group there was no change from 8.0 µU/mL at baseline to Month 12, and after the post-washout the median was 9.0 µU/mL. The between-treatment-groups difference in change from baseline to Month 12 was significant, p<0.0001. In childhood onset subjects there was a change of median fasting insulin in the NUTROPIN 0.025 mg/kg/day group from 11.0 µU/mL at baseline to 20.0 µU/mL at Month 12, in the NUTROPIN 0.0125 mg/kg/day group from 8.5 µU/mL to 11.0 µU/mL and in the placebo group from 7.0 µU/mL to 8.0 µU/mL. The between-treatment-groups difference for these changes was significant, p=0.0007.

In subjects with adult onset GHD there was no between treatment group difference in changes from baseline to Month 12 in mean HbA1c, p=0.08. In childhood onset mean HbA1c increased in the NUTROPIN 0.025 mg/kg/day group from 5.2% at baseline to 5.5% at Month 12, and did not change in the NUTROPIN 0.0125 mg/kg/day group from 5.1% at baseline or in the placebo group from 5.3% at baseline. The between-treatment-groups difference was significant, p=0.009.

Immune: Local or systemic **allergic reactions** may occur. Parents/Patients should be informed that such reactions are possible and that prompt medical attention should be sought if allergic reactions occur.

Musculoskeletal: Patients with growth failure secondary to chronic renal insufficiency should be examined periodically for evidence of progression of renal **osteodystrophy**. Slipped capital femoral epiphysis or avascular necrosis of the femoral head may be seen in children with advanced renal osteodystrophy, and it is uncertain whether these problems are affected by growth hormone therapy. X-rays of the hips should be obtained prior to initiating therapy for CRI patients. Children with chronic renal insufficiency receiving growth hormone should be serially monitored for avascular necrosis, slipped capital femoral epiphysis and renal osteodystrophy with serial radiographs and appropriate clinical chemistry tests.

Slipped capital femoral epiphysis may also occur more frequently in patients with endocrine disorders or in patients undergoing rapid growth. Therefore, physicians and parents should be alert to the development of a limp or complaints of hip or knee pain in both GHI and CRI patients treated with NUTROPIN.

Patients with Turner syndrome should be evaluated carefully for otitis media and other ear disorders. In a randomized-controlled trial, there was a statistically significant increase, as compared to untreated controls, in otitis media (43% vs. 26%) and ear disorders (18% vs. 5%) in patients receiving GH. In addition, patients with Turner syndrome should be monitored closely for cardiovascular disorders (e.g. stroke, aortic aneurysm, hypertension) as these patients are also at risk for these conditions.

Progression of **scoliosis** can occur in children who experience rapid growth. Because growth hormone increases growth rate, patients with a history of scoliosis who are treated with growth hormone should be monitored for progression of scoliosis. Growth hormone has not been shown to increase the incidence of scoliosis.

Patients with epiphyseal closure who were treated with GH replacement therapy in childhood should be re-evaluated according to the criteria in the Indications and Clinical Use section before continuation of GH therapy at the reduced dose level recommended for GH-deficient adults.

Neurologic: Patients with a history of an **intracranial lesion** should be examined frequently for progression or recurrence of the lesion.

Intracranial hypertension (IH) with papilledema, visual changes, headache, nausea and/or vomiting has been reported in a small number of patients treated with growth hormone products. Symptoms usually occurred within the first eight (8) weeks of the initiation of the growth hormone therapy. In all reported cases, IH-associated signs and symptoms resolved after termination of therapy or a reduction of the growth hormone dose. Funduscopic examination of patients is recommended at the initiation and periodically during the course of growth hormone therapy. Patients with Turner syndrome and CRI may be at increased risk for development of IH.

Special Populations: Pregnant Women: Reproduction studies have not been conducted with NUTROPIN. It is also not known whether NUTROPIN can cause fetal harm when administered to a pregnant woman or can affect reproduction capacity. NUTROPIN should be given to a pregnant woman only if clearly needed.

Nursing Women: It is not known whether somatropin is excreted in human milk. Because many drugs are excreted in human milk, caution should be exercised when NUTROPIN is administered to a nursing mother.

Pediatrics (6 months-3 years of age): Prudence is indicated for children aged 6 months to 3 years, when administering NUTROPIN (somatropin for injection) lyophilized powder reconstituted in Bacteriostatic Water for Injection, USP (benzyl alcohol preserved); although there is no information on the toxicity of benzyl alcohol for this age group, the toxic dose for premature neonates is in the range of 100 to 250 mg/kg per day.

Geriatrics (>65 years of age): Clinical studies of NUTROPIN did not include sufficient numbers of elderly subjects to determine whether they respond differently from younger subjects. Other reported clinical experience has not identified differences in responses between the elderly and younger patients. In general, dose selection for an elderly patient should be cautious, usually starting at the low end of the dosing range, reflecting the greater frequency of decreased hepatic, renal or cardiac function, and of concomitant disease or other drug therapy. Experience with prolonged rhGH treatment in adults is limited.

Monitoring and Laboratory Tests: Serum levels of **inorganic phosphorous, alkaline phosphatase**, and **parathyroid hormone** may increase with therapy with NUTROPIN. Changes in **thyroid hormone** laboratory measurements may develop during growth hormone treatment of children who lack adequate endogenous growth hormone secretion. As untreated hypothyroidism prevents optimal response to NUTROPIN, patients should have periodic thyroid function tests and should be treated with thyroid hormone when indicated. Patients with Turner syndrome have an inherently increased risk of developing autoimmune thyroid disease.

Information to Be Provided to the Patient: Patients being treated with growth hormone and/or their parents should be informed regarding the potential benefits and risks associated with treatment. If home use is determined to be desirable by the physician, instructions on appropriate use should be given, including a review of the contents of the "Information for the Patient/Parent"

Insert (see Information for the Patient, Proper Use of This Medication, Information for the Patient/Parent). This information is intended to aid in the safe and effective administration of the medication. It is not a disclosure of all possible adverse or unintended effects.

If home use is prescribed, a puncture resistant container for the disposal of used syringes and needles should be recommended to the patient. Patients and/or parents should be thoroughly instructed in the importance of proper disposal and cautioned against any reuse of needles and syringes (see Information for the Patient, Proper Use of This Medication, Information for the Patient/Parent).

ADVERSE REACTIONS: Adverse Drug Reaction Overview: The adverse event data reflect the clinical trial and post-marketing experience of using NUTROPIN (somatropin).

Clinical Trial Adverse Drug Reactions: Because clinical trials are conducted under very specific conditions the adverse reaction rates observed in the clinical trials may not reflect the rates observed in practice and should not be compared to the rates in the clinical trials of another drug. Adverse drug reaction information from clinical trials is useful for identifying drug-related adverse events and for approximating rates.

A small percentage of patients may develop antibodies to the growth hormone protein. Growth hormone antibody binding capacities below 2 mg/L have not been associated with growth attenuation. In some cases when binding capacity exceeds 2 mg/L during growth hormone treatment, growth attenuation has been observed.

In clinical studies of patients treated with NUTROPIN (somatropin for injection) lyophilized powder for the first time, 0/107 growth hormone inadequate (GHI) patients and 0/125 chronic renal insufficiency (CRI) patients screened for antibody production developed antibodies with binding capacities ≥2 mg/L at six months.

In a clinical study of naive patients who were treated with NUTROPIN AQ, (somatropin injection) 0/60 GHD patients, who were screened for development of antibodies throughout 15 months of treatment, developed antibodies with binding capacities above 2 mg/L.

Short-term immunologic and renal function studies were carried out in a group of patients with chronic renal insufficiency after approximately one year of growth hormone treatment to detect potential adverse effects of antibodies to growth hormone. Testing included measurements of Clq, C3, C4, rheumatoid factor, creatinine, creatinine clearance and blood urea nitrogen (BUN). No adverse effects of growth hormone antibodies were noted.

In addition to an evaluation of compliance with the treatment program and thyroid status, testing for antibodies to human growth hormone should be carried out in any patient who fails to respond to therapy.

Leukemia has been reported in a small number of growth hormone deficient patients treated with growth hormone. It is uncertain whether this increased risk is related to the pathology of growth hormone deficiency itself, growth hormone therapy or other associated treatments, such as radiation therapy for intracranial tumours. On the basis of current evidence, experts cannot conclude that growth hormone therapy is responsible for these occurrences. The risk to GHI, Turner syndrome, and CRI patients, if any, remains to be established.

In studies of children treated with NUTROPIN, injection site pain was reported infrequently.

Adverse drug reactions which have been reported infrequently (<1%) in growth hormone-treated children include mild and transient peripheral edema. In GHD adults, edema or peripheral edema was reported in 41% of GH-treated patients and 25% of placebo-treated patients. In GHD adults, arthralgias and joint disorders were reported in 27% of GH-treated patients and 15% of placebo-treated patients.

Other rare (< 0.1%) adverse drug reactions reported in growth hormone-treated patients include the following:

Musculoskeletal: arthralgias; carpal tunnel syndrome.

Skin: increased growth of pre-existing nevi (malignant nevi transformation has not been reported).

Endocrine: gynecomastia and pancreatitis.

Post-Market Adverse Drug Reactions: Adverse events that have been observed during the post-marketing period are similar to those seen in clinical trials with NUTROPIN.

DRUG INTERACTIONS: Overview: Concomitant glucocorticoid therapy may inhibit the growth promoting effect of NUTROPIN (somatropin). If glucocorticoid replacement is required, the glucocorticoid dose should be carefully adjusted. The use of NUTROPIN in patients with chronic renal insufficiency (CRI) receiving glucocorticoid therapy has not been evaluated.

There was no evidence in the controlled studies of somatropin's interaction with drugs commonly used in patients. However, formal drug interaction studies have not been conducted.

DOSAGE AND ADMINISTRATION: Dosing Considerations: The dosage and administration schedule of NUTROPIN (somatropin) should be individualized for each patient.

Recommended Dose and Dosage Adjustment: Pediatric Growth Hormone Deficiency: A somatropin dose of up to 0.3 mg/kg/week (approximately 0.90 IU/kg/wk) administered in divided daily doses by subcutaneous or intramuscular injection is recommended.

The total number of mg per daily dose is calculated as follows: Dose (mg) per injection=Patient weight (kg)×up to 0.043 (mg/kg).

In pubertal patients, a weekly dosage of up to 0.7 mg/kg divided daily may be used.

The total number of mg per daily dose is calculated as follows: Dose (mg) per injection=Patient weight (kg)×up to 0.1 (mg/kg).

Therapy should not be continued if final desired height is achieved or epiphyseal fusion occurs. Patients who fail to respond adequately while on therapy with NUTROPIN should be evaluated to determine the cause of unresponsiveness.

Turner Syndrome: A weekly dosage of up to 0.375 mg/kg/week divided into equal doses 3 to 7 times per week by subcutaneous injection is recommended.

The total number of mg per daily dose is calculated as follows: Dose (mg) per injection=Patient weight (kg)×up to 0.054 (mg/kg).

For administration three times a week, the total number of mg per dose is calculated as follows: Dose (mg) per injection Patient weight (kg)×up to 0.125 (mg/kg).

Therapy should not be continued if final desired height is achieved or epiphyseal fusion occurs. Patients who fail to respond adequately while on therapy with NUTROPIN should be evaluated to determine the cause of unresponsiveness.

Chronic Renal Insufficiency: A somatropin dose of up to 0.35 mg/kg/week (approximately 1.05 IU/kg/wk) administered in divided daily doses by subcutaneous or intramuscular injection is recommended.

The total number of mg per daily dose is calculated as follows: Dose (mg) per injection=Patient weight (kg)×up to 0.05 (mg/kg).

Therapy may be continued up to the time of renal transplantation. Therapy should not be continued if final height is achieved or epiphyseal fusion occurs. Patients who fail to respond adequately while on therapy with NUTROPIN should be evaluated to determine the cause of unresponsiveness.

In order to optimize therapy for CRI patients who require dialysis, the following guidelines for selecting the injection schedule are recommended:

1. Hemodialysis patients should receive their injection at night just prior to going to sleep or at least 3-4 hours after their hemodialysis to prevent hematoma formation due to heparin.
2. Chronic Cycling Peritoneal Dialysis patients should receive their injection in the morning after they have completed dialysis.
3. Chronic Ambulatory Peritoneal Dialysis patients should receive their injection in the evening at the time of the overnight exchange.

Adult Growth Hormone Deficiency: The recommended dosage at the start of therapy is not more than 0.042 mg/kg/week given as a daily subcutaneous injection. The dose may be increased according to individual patient requirements to a maximum of 0.175 mg/kg /week in patients under 35 years and to a maximum of 0.0875 mg/kg/week in patients over 35 years.

Starting Dose: The total number of mg per daily dose for adult patients is calculated as follows: Dose (mg) per injection=Patient weight (kg)×0.006 (mg/kg).

Maximum Dose: For patients under 35 years, the total number of mg per daily dose is calculated as follows: Dose (mg) per injection=Patient weight (kg)×up to 0.025 (mg/kg).

For patients over 35 years, the total number of mg per daily dose is calculated as follows: Dose (mg) per injection=Patient weight (kg)×up to 0.0125 (mg/kg).

To minimize the occurrence of adverse events in older or overweight patients, lower doses may be necessary. During therapy, dosage should be decreased if required by the occurrence of side effects or excessive insulin-like growth factor I [IGF-I] levels.

Missed Dose: Patients who miss a dose of NUTROPIN should contact their physician for instructions.

Administration: NUTROPIN (somatropin for injection)—Vials of 5 mg and 10 mg: Reconstitution: NUTROPIN (somatropin for injection) lyophilized powder is dispensed in vials of 5 mg and 10 mg.

- A 5 mg vial of NUTROPIN lyophilized powder should be reconstituted with 1 to 5 mL of Bacteriostatic Water for Injection, USP (benzyl alcohol preserved). (For example, a 5 mg vial of NUTROPIN lyophilized powder reconstituted with 5 mL of Bacteriostatic Water will be reconstituted to a concentration of 1 mg somatropin/mL Bacteriostatic Water.)
- A 10 mg vial of NUTROPIN lyophilized powder should be reconstituted with 1 to 10 mL of Bacteriostatic Water for Injection, USP (benzyl alcohol preserved). (For example, a 10 mg vial of NUTROPIN lyophilized powder reconstituted with 10 mL of Bacteriostatic Water will be reconstituted to a concentration of 1 mg somatropin/mL Bacteriostatic Water.)

When NUTROPIN lyophilized powder is reconstituted to 1 mg somatropin per mL, the recommended daily somatropin dose of 0.05 mg/kg for treatment of chronic renal insufficiency contains 0.45 mg/kg benzyl alcohol while the recommended daily somatropin dose of 0.043 mg/kg for treatment of growth hormone deficiency contains 0.387 mg/kg benzyl alcohol. The recommended daily somatropin dose of 0.1 mg/kg for treatment of growth hormone deficiency for pubertal patients contains 0.09 mg/kg benzyl alcohol. The recommended daily dose of 0.054 mg/kg for Turner's syndrome contains 0.486 mg/kg benzyl alcohol, while the three dose a week regimen contains 1.134 mg/kg benzyl alcohol in each dose.

See Warnings and Precautions, General, Pediatrics for **use in newborns**, persons sensitive to benzyl alcohol and for use in children aged 6 months to 3 years. When Sterile Water for Injection, USP is used **use only one dose of NUTROPIN per vial and discard the unused portion**.

To prepare the NUTROPIN solution, slowly inject the Bacteriostatic Water for Injection, USP into the NUTROPIN vial, aiming the stream of liquid against the glass wall of the vial. Then swirl the NUTROPIN vial with a **gentle** rotary motion until the contents are completely dissolved. **Do not shake.** Because NUTROPIN is a protein, shaking can result in a cloudy solution. After reconstitution, the NUTROPIN solution should be clear, ie. it should not have any solid particles floating on the surface. If you notice lumps or solid particles of powder, continue to gently swirl the solution until all of the powder has dissolved. If the solution does not become clear, **do not** inject it. Note also that occasionally, after refrigeration, small colourless particles of protein may be present in the NUTROPIN solution. This is not unusual for solutions containing proteins. Allow the vial to come to room temperature and gently swirl until the solution is clear. If the solution remains cloudy or hazy, **do not** inject it.

NUTROPIN AQ (somatropin injection)—Vials of 10 mg: The vials contain a solution ready for injection. No reconstitution or preparation is required.

Injection: Before needle insertion, wipe the septum of all vials to be used, both the NUTROPIN and diluent vials, with rubbing alcohol or an antiseptic solution to prevent contamination of the contents by microorganisms that may be introduced by repeated needle insertions. NUTROPIN must be administered using sterile, disposable syringes and needles. The syringes should be of small enough volume that the prescribed dose can be drawn from the vial with reasonable accuracy. If the route of injection selected is intramuscular, the needle should be of sufficient length [usually 2.5 cm (1 inch) or more)] to ensure that the injection reaches the muscular layer. The site of injection should be rotated each time NUTROPIN is administered. Recommended injection sites include upper arm, abdomen, and thigh.

NUTROPIN AQ PEN Cartridge (somatropin injection) of 10 mg: The NUTROPIN AQ PEN Cartridge is intended for use **only** with the NUTROPIN AQ PEN. The pen cartridges contain a solution ready for injection. No reconstitution or preparation is required.

Injection: Before needle insertion, wipe the septum of the cartridge with rubbing alcohol or an antiseptic solution to prevent contamination of the contents by microorganisms that may be introduced by repeated needle insertions. Load the pen cartridge into the NUTROPIN AQ PEN barrel and attach the needle. Push the button on the side of the pen opposite the digital display, which releases a spring-loaded "knob" at the top of the pen. The "knob" is then twisted in a clockwise direction that brings the desired dose into the dose selection window. Once the dose is selected, remove the needle cap, insert the needle into the injection site, and depress the "knob" located at the top of the pen. This advances the plunger to displace the selected dose. After the injection, the needle is removed from the pen and discarded. NUTROPIN AQ must be administered using sterile, disposable needles. The NUTROPIN AQ PEN allows for administration of a minimum dose of 0.1 mg to a maximum dose of 4.0 mg, in 0.1 mg increments. Detailed instructions on how to use the NUTROPIN AQ PEN are provided in the Information for the Parent/Patient Guide (see Information for the Patient, Proper Use of This Medication).

OVERDOSAGE:

Theoretical risks of long-term human growth hormone treatment with doses exceeding the recommended dosage are signs and symptoms of gigantism and/or acromegaly. If any signs of overdosage occur, treatment should be discontinued.

For management of a suspected drug overdose, CPhA recommends that you contact your **regional Poison Control Centre**. See the *CPS* Directory section for a list of Poison Control Centres.

ACTION AND CLINICAL PHARMACOLOGY: Mechanism of Action: General: NUTROPIN (somatropin) is a human growth hormone (hGH) produced by recombinant DNA technology. The amino acid sequence of the somatropin protein is identical to that of pituitary-derived human growth hormone. In vitro and in vivo preclinical testing, and clinical testing have demonstrated that NUTROPIN is therapeutically equivalent to pituitary-derived human growth hormone in pharmacokinetics, in stimulation of linear growth and in other actions.

Treatment of children who lack adequate secretion of endogenous growth hormone with NUTROPIN results in an increase in growth rate and an increase in insulin-like growth factor-I [IGF-I], similar to that seen with pituitary-derived human growth hormone.

Treatment with NUTROPIN in children with Turner's syndrome (a condition without a deficiency of GH) results in an increase in growth rate and an overall increase in cumulative growth, as compared with Historical Controls.

Treatment with NUTROPIN of children with chronic renal insufficiency results in improved growth rate and height standard deviation and an overall increase in cumulative growth, as compared to placebo-treated children with chronic renal insufficiency. Adults with growth hormone deficiency acquired during childhood or adulthood treated with NUTROPIN show an improvement in body fat mass and lean mass. Adults with growth hormone deficiency acquired during childhood treated with NUTROPIN also show an improvement in bone mineral density.

Actions that have been demonstrated for NUTROPIN and/or pituitary-derived human growth hormone include:

Tissue Growth: Skeletal Growth: NUTROPIN stimulates skeletal growth in children with growth failure due to a lack of adequate secretion of endogenous growth hormone and in children with growth failure secondary to chronic renal insufficiency. Skeletal growth is accomplished at the epiphyseal plates at the ends of a growing long bone. Growth and metabolism of epiphyseal plate cells are directly stimulated by growth hormone and one of its mediators, IGF-I. Serum levels of IGF-I are low in children and adolescents who are growth hormone deficient, but increase during treatment with NUTROPIN. New bone is formed at the epiphyses in response to growth hormone. This results in linear growth until these growth plates fuse at the end of puberty.

The clinical effect of the skeletal growth action of somatropin has been observed in well-controlled clinical trials with NUTROPIN in the treatment of growth hormone inadequacy, chronic renal insufficiency patients, and patients with Turner syndrome. Limited data regarding the clinical post-transplant growth effect of treatment with NUTROPIN administered prior to transplant is available.

Cell Growth: Treatment with pituitary-derived human growth hormone results in an increase in both the number and the size of skeletal muscle cells.

Organ Growth: Growth hormone of human pituitary origin influences the size of internal organs, including kidneys, and increases red cell mass. Treatment of hypophysectomized or genetic dwarf rats with somatropin results in organ growth that is proportional to the overall body growth. In normal rats subjected to nephrectomy-induced uremia, somatropin promoted skeletal and body growth.

Protein Metabolism: Linear growth is facilitated in part by growth hormone-stimulated protein synthesis. This is reflected by nitrogen retention as demonstrated by a decline in urinary nitrogen excretion and blood urea nitrogen concentration during growth hormone therapy.

Carbohydrate Metabolism: Growth hormone is a modulator of carbohydrate metabolism. For example, patients with inadequate secretion of growth hormone sometimes experience fasting hypoglycemia which is improved by treatment with growth hormone. Growth hormone therapy may decrease glucose tolerance. Untreated patients with chronic renal insufficiency and Turner syndrome have an increased incidence of glucose intolerance. Administration of NUTROPIN to normal adults, patients who lack adequate secretion of endogenous growth hormone and patients with chronic renal insufficiency resulted in increases in mean serum fasting and postprandial insulin levels. However, mean fasting and postprandial glucose levels and mean hemoglobin A1C levels remained within the normal range. There were no clinically significant persistent abnormalities in any of these measurements of glucose regulation that were related to growth hormone treatment.

Lipid Metabolism: Acute administration of pituitary derived human growth hormone to humans results in lipid mobilization. Nonesterified fatty acids increase in plasma within two hours of pituitary-derived human growth hormone administration. In growth hormone deficient patients, long-term growth hormone administration often decreases body fat. Mean cholesterol levels decreased in patients treated with NUTROPIN.

Mineral Metabolism: The retention of total body potassium in response to growth hormone administration is thought to result from cellular growth. Serum levels of inorganic phosphorus may increase slightly in patients with inadequate secretion of endogenous growth hormone, chronic renal insufficiency, or patients with Turner syndrome, after growth hormone therapy due to the metabolic activity associated with bone growth as well as increased tubular reabsorption of phosphate by the kidney. Serum calcium is not significantly altered in these patients. Sodium retention also occurs. Adults with childhood-onset GH deficiency show low bone mineral density (BMD). GH therapy results in increases in serum alkaline phosphatase. (See Warnings and Precautions, Monitoring and Laboratory Tests.)

Connective Tissue Metabolism: Growth hormone stimulates the synthesis of chondroitin sulfate and collagen as well as the urinary excretion of hydroxyproline.

Pharmacokinetics: See Table 1 and Table 2.

Table 1: NUTROPIN

Summary of Pharmacokinetic Parameters of NUTROPIN in Healthy Adult Males 0.1 mg (approximately 0.3 IU[a])/kg SC

	C_{max} (µg/L)	$t_{½}$ (h)	$AUC_{0-\infty}$ (µg·h/L)	Clearance (mL/[h·kg])	Volume of Distribution (mL/kg)
Single dose mean[b]	56.1	7.5	626[c]	116–174[d]	50

[a] Based on current International Standard of 3 IU=1 mg.
[b] n=36.
[c] Compares with that of somatrem (590 ng·h/mL); the AUC of NUTROPIN somatropin is similar regardless of site of injection.
[d] In healthy adults and children.

Table 2: NUTROPIN AQ

Summary of Pharmacokinetic Parameters of NUTROPIN AQ in Healthy Adult Males 0.1 mg (approximately 0.3 IU[a])/kg SC

	C_{max} (µg/L)	$t_{½}$ (h)	$AUC_{0-\infty}$ (µg·h/L)	Clearance (mL/[h·kg])	Volume of Distribution (mL/kg)
Single dose mean[b]	71.1	3.9	673[c]	116–174[d]	50

[a] Based on current International Standard of 3 IU=1 mg.
[b] n=36.
[c] Comparable with that of NUTROPIN lyophilized powder. NUTROPIN AQ was bioequivalent to NUTROPIN lyophilized powder after subcutaneous administration based on the statistical evaluation of the ratios of the geometric mean of log transformed AUC and C_{max}.
[d] In healthy adults and children.

In both normal and growth hormone deficient adults and children, the intramuscular and subcutaneous pharmacokinetic profiles of somatropin are similar regardless of growth hormone or dosing regimen used. Growth hormone localizes to highly perfused organs, particularly the liver and kidney. Both the liver and kidney have been shown to be important metabolizing organs for pituitary-derived human growth hormone.

Special Populations and Conditions: Pediatrics: Available literature data suggests that rhGH clearances are similar in adults and children.

Gender: No data is available for rhGH. Available data for methionyl human growth hormone and pituitary-derived human growth hormone suggests that there are no consistent gender-based differences in rhGH clearance.

Race: No data is available.

Hepatic Insufficiency: A reduction in rhGH clearance has been noted in patients with severe liver dysfunction. The clinical significance of this decrease is unknown.

Renal Insufficiency: Children and adults with chronic renal failure (CRF) tend to have decreased clearance as compared to normals. However, no rhGH accumulation has been reported in children with CRF or end-stage renal disease dosed with current regimens.

Turner Syndrome: No pharmacokinetic data are available for exogenously administered rhGH. However, reported half-lives, and elimination rates of endogenous GH in this population are similar to the ranges observed for normal subjects and GHD populations.

Growth Hormone Insufficiency (GHI): Reported values for clearance of rhGH in adults and children with GHI range from 138-245 mL/h/kg and are similar to those observed in healthy adults and children. Mean terminal $t_{1/2}$ values following intravenous and subcutaneous administration in GHI patients are also similar to those observed in healthy adult males.

STORAGE AND STABILITY: NUTROPIN (somatropin for injection): Before Reconstitution: NUTROPIN (somatropin for injection) lyophilized powder and Bacteriostatic Water for Injection, USP (benzyl alcohol preserved) must be refrigerated at 2 to 8°C. **Avoid freezing the vials of NUTROPIN and Bacteriostatic Water for Injection, USP (benzyl alcohol preserved).** Expiration dates are stated on the labels.

After Reconstitution: Vial contents are stable for 14 days when reconstituted with Bacteriostatic Water for Injection, USP (benzyl alcohol preserved) and refrigerated at 2 to 8°C. Discard the unused portion after 14 days. **Do not freeze** the reconstituted vial of NUTROPIN.

The remaining Bacteriostatic Water for Injection, USP in the multiple use vial must be refrigerated at 2 to 8°C, and may be used for 14 days after first entry. **Avoid freezing the Bacteriostatic Water for Injection, USP (benzyl alcohol preserved).**

Unusual Handling Conditions: Vials of unreconstituted NUTROPIN lyophilized powder may be held at ambient temperature (not to exceed 37°C) for a total time not to exceed seven days. Vials of reconstituted NUTROPIN lyophilized powder should not be exposed to temperatures greater than 25°C for more than 24 hours in total.

NUTROPIN AQ (somatropin injection): Store under refrigeration at 2 to 8°C. Do not freeze.

NUTROPIN AQ PEN Cartridge: Do not freeze. Protect from light. When not in use, store under refrigeration at 2 to 8°C. NUTROPIN AQ PEN Cartridges should be discarded after 28 days of the first use.

INFORMATION FOR THE PATIENT: Published in e-CPS, available by subscription at www.e-cps.ca.

DOSAGE FORMS, COMPOSITION AND PACKAGING: NUTROPIN: 5 mg: Each vial of sterile, white, lyophilized powder contains: somatropin 5 mg (approximately 15 IU). Nonmedicinal ingredients: glycine, mannitol,sodium phosphate dibasic and sodium phosphate monobasic; diluent contains: Bacteriostatic Water for Injection USP and each mL contains 0.9% benzyl alcohol as an antimicrobial preservative. After reconstitution, the resultant solutionis nearly isotonic at a concentration of 5 mg growth hormone/mL and has a pH of approximately 7.4. Cartons of six 5 mg vials of NUTROPIN and six 10 mL multiple use vials of Bacteriostatic Water for Injection, USP (benzyl alcohol preserved).

10 mg: Each vial of sterile, white, lyophilized powder contains: somatropin 10 mg (approximately 30 IU). Nonmedicinal ingredients: glycine, mannitol, sodium phosphate dibasic and sodium phosphate monobasic; diluent contains: Bacteriostatic Water for Injection USP and each mL contains 0.9% benzyl alcohol as an antimicrobial preservative. After reconstitution, the resultant solution is nearly isotonic at a concentration of 5 mg growth hormone/mL and has a pH of approximately 7.4. Cartons of one 10 mg vial of NUTROPIN and one 10 mL multiple use vial of Bacteriostatic Water for Injection, USP (benzyl alcohol preserved).

NUTROPIN AQ: Each mL of clear, sterile, nearly isotonic solution contains: somatropin 5 mg. Nonmedicinal ingredients: phenol, polysorbate 20, sodium chloride and sodium citrate. The solution has a pH of approximately 6. Vials of 2 mL (10 mg, approximately 30 IU), packs of 6.

NUTROPIN AQ Pen Cartridge: Each mL of clear, sterile, nearly isotonic solution contains: somatropin 5 mg. Nonmedicinal ingredients: phenol, polysorbate 20, sodium chloride and sodium citrate. Pen cartridges of 10 mg (approximately 30 IU) containing 2 mL of somatropin solution, packs of 1.

NuvaRing® Ⓟ

etonogestrel—ethinyl estradiol

Contraceptive Vaginal Ring

Schering-Plough

Date of Revision: February 19, 2009

SUMMARY PRODUCT INFORMATION:

Route of Administration	Dosage Form/ Strength	Clinically Relevant Nonmedicinal Ingredients
Vaginal	Slow release vaginal ring, 11.4 mg etonogestrel/ 2.6 mg ethinyl estradiol (120 µg etonogestrel/ 15 µg ethinyl estradiol per day)	Ethylene vinylacetate copolymers For a complete listing see Dosage Forms, Composition and Packaging.

INDICATIONS AND CLINICAL USE: NuvaRing is indicated for: Conception control.

CONTRAINDICATIONS:

- Hypersensitivity to NuvaRing (etonogestrel/ethinyl estradiol slow release vaginal ring) or to any ingredient in the formulation or component of the container. For a complete listing, see Dosage Forms, Composition and Packaging.
- History of/or actual thrombophlebitis or thromboembolic disorders.
- History of/or actual cerebrovascular disorders.
- History of/or actual myocardial infarction or coronary arterial disease.
- Active liver disease or history of/or actual benign or malignant liver tumours.
- Known or suspected carcinoma of the breast.
- Known or suspected estrogen-dependent neoplasia.
- Undiagnosed abnormal vaginal bleeding.
- Any ocular lesion arising from ophthalmic vascular disease, such as partial or complete loss of vision or defect in visual fields.
- When pregnancy is suspected or diagnosed.

WARNINGS AND PRECAUTIONS:

> **Serious Warnings and Precautions**
> **Women using NuvaRing (etonogestrel/ethinyl estradiol slow release vaginal ring) should be counselled that this product (as with other combined hormonal contraceptives) DOES NOT PROTECT against HIV infection (AIDS) and other sexually transmitted diseases (STDs). For protection against STDs, it is advisable to use latex condoms IN COMBINATION WITH this product.**
> Cigarette smoking increases the risk of serious adverse effects on the heart and blood vessels. This risk increases with age and becomes significant in oral contraceptive-users over 35 years of age. Women who use combination hormonal contraceptives (including NuvaRing [etonogestrel/ethinyl estradiol slow release vaginal ring]) should be counselled not to smoke.

General: NuvaRing (etonogestrel/ethinyl estradiol slow release vaginal ring) and other contraceptives that contain both an estrogen and a progestin are called combination hormonal contraceptives. Most of the warnings below are based on data obtained from the oral route of administration. There is no epidemiologic data available to determine whether the safety with the vaginal route of administration of combined hormonal contraceptives (such as NuvaRing) would be different than the oral route, and, in the absence of these comparable data, associated risks should be assumed to be similar for use through both routes.

Carcinogenesis and Mutagenesis: Breast Cancer: Increasing age and a strong family history are the most significant risk factors for the development of breast cancer. Other established risk factors include obesity, nulliparity and late age at first full-term pregnancy. The identified groups of women that may be at increased risk of developing breast cancer before menopause are long-term users (more than 8 years) of combination hormonal contraceptives (including NuvaRing) and starters at early age. In a few women, the use of combination hormonal contraceptives (including NuvaRing) may accelerate the growth of an existing but undiagnosed breast cancer. Since any potential increased risk related to combination hormonal contraceptives (including NuvaRing) use is small, there is no reason to change prescribing habits at present.

Women receiving combination hormonal contraceptives (including NuvaRing) should be instructed in self-examination of their breasts. Their physicians should be notified whenever any masses are detected. A yearly clinical breast examination is also recommended because, if a breast cancer should develop, estrogen-containing drugs may cause a rapid progression.

Cervical Cancer: Persistent infection with the Human Papilloma Virus (HPV) is believed to be the most important risk factor for cervical cancer. Some epidemiological studies indicated that long-term use of combination oral contraceptives (COCs) may further contribute to this increased risk, but there continues to be controversy about the extent to which this finding may be confounded by other factors, e.g., cervical screening bias and sexual behaviour. It is unknown how this effect relates to NuvaRing.

Cardiovascular: Predisposing Factors for Coronary Artery Disease: Cigarette smoking increases the risk of serious cardiovascular side effects and mortality. Combination hormonal contraceptives (including NuvaRing), increase this risk, especially with increasing age.

Convincing data are available to support an upper age limit of 35 years for combination hormonal contraceptives use in women who smoke.

Other women who are independently at high risk for cardiovascular disease include those with diabetes, hypertension, abnormal lipid profile, or a family history of these. Whether combination hormonal contraceptives, accentuate this risk is unclear.

In low risk, non-smoking women of any age, the benefits of combination hormonal contraceptives use outweigh the possible cardiovascular risks associated with low dose formulations.

Consequently, combination hormonal contraceptives may be prescribed for these women up to the age of menopause.

Hypertension: Patients with essential hypertension whose blood pressure is well-controlled may be prescribed combination hormonal contraceptives (including NuvaRing) but only under close supervision. If a significant elevation of blood pressure in previously normotensive or hypertensive subjects occurs at any time during the administration of the drug, cessation of medication is necessary.

Endocrine and Metabolism: Diabetes: Current low dose combination hormonal contraceptives (including NuvaRing) exert minimal impact on glucose metabolism. Diabetic patients, or those with a family history of diabetes, should be observed closely to detect any worsening of carbohydrate metabolism. Patients predisposed to diabetes who can be kept under close supervision may be given combination hormonal contraceptives. Young diabetic patients whose disease is of recent origin, well-controlled, and not associated with hypertension or other signs of vascular disease such as ocular fundal changes, should be monitored more frequently while using combination hormonal contraceptives.

Bone Mineral Density: A controlled open-label, multicenter trial was conducted to evaluate the effects of NuvaRing on bone mineral density (BMD) in healthy young women (n=105; 76 completers) over a 2 year period (26 cycles). The control group (n=39; 31 completers) consisted of women who did not use a hormonal method of contraception, and an IUD was offered as trial medication. The mean age of subjects was 27 years in the NuvaRing group and 29 years in the control group.

For the NuvaRing group, the BMD for lumbar spine and femoral neck were not statistically different from baseline after two years of follow-up (change in z-score was −0.093 and −0.048, respectively). In the control group, a slight increase of BMD for both the lumbar spine and femoral neck was observed (change in z-score of 0.257 and 0.223, respectively). At the end of 2 years, there was a statistically significant difference in the change of BMD from baseline, between the Nuvaring group and the control group.

Genitourinary: Vaginal Bleeding: Persistent irregular vaginal bleeding requires assessment to exclude underlying pathology.

NuvaRing may not be suitable for women with conditions that make the vagina more susceptible to vaginal irritation or ulceration. In some cases, vaginal (fibrous) tissue may grow over the ring, necessitating removal by a healthcare provider.

Urethra: Very rarely it has been reported that NuvaRing was inadvertently inserted in the urethra and possibly ended up in the bladder. Healthcare providers should assess for incorrect placement of NuvaRing in the urethra or bladder in those users presenting with persistent urinary symptoms and who are unable to locate the ring.

Disconnected Ring: On rare occasions, NuvaRing has been reported to disconnect at the weld joint. Since the core of NuvaRing is solid, its contents will remain intact and release of hormone is unlikely to occur. In the event of a disconnected ring, expulsion (slipping out) is likely to occur (see Drug Interactions, Drug-Lifestyle Interactions, Expulsion). If a woman discovers that her NuvaRing has disconnected, she should discard the ring and replace it with a new ring.

Fibroids: Patients with fibroids (leiomyomata) should be carefully observed. Sudden enlargement, pain, or tenderness require discontinuation of the use of combination hormonal contraceptives (including NuvaRing).

Hematologic: Epidemiological studies have suggested an association between the use of combination oral contraceptives (COCs) and an increased risk of venous thrombotic and thromboembolic diseases.

As NuvaRing is a new contraceptive product with a new (vaginal) route of administration delivering ethinyl estradiol and etonogestrel (the biological active metabolite of desogestrel) the following should be noted:

- Venous thromboembolism (VTE), manifesting as deep vein thrombosis and/or pulmonary embolism, may occur during the use of all combined hormonal contraceptives, including NuvaRing. The approximate incidence of VTE in users of low estrogen dose (<0.05 mg EE) oral contraceptives is up to 4 per 10 000 woman years compared to 0.5-3 per 10 000 woman years in non-oral contraceptive users. The incidence of VTE associated with pregnancy is 6 per 10 000 woman years.
- Several epidemiological studies indicate that third generation oral contraceptives, including those containing desogestrel (etonogestrel, the progestin component released by NuvaRing is the biologically active metabolite of desogestrel) are associated with a higher risk of venous thromboembolism than certain second generation oral contraceptives. These studies indicate an approximately 2-fold difference in risk, which corresponds to 1-2 cases of venous thromboembolism per 10 000 women-years of use. However, data from additional studies have not shown this difference in risk. It should be noted, however, that the incidence of venous thromboembolism in oral contraceptive users is rare.

Hepatic/Biliary/Pancreatic: Jaundice: Patients who have had jaundice including a history of cholestatic jaundice during pregnancy should be given combination hormonal contraceptives (including NuvaRing) with great care and under close observation.

The development of severe generalized pruritus or icterus requires that the medication be withdrawn until the problem is resolved.

If the jaundice should prove to be cholestatic in type, the use of combination hormonal contraceptives should not be resumed. In patients taking combination hormonal contraceptives, changes in the composition of the bile may occur and an increased incidence of gallstones has been reported.

Liver Disorders: Hepatic nodules (adenoma and focal nodular hyperplasia) have been reported, particularly in long-term users of combination hormonal contraceptives. Although these lesions are extremely rare, they have caused fatal intra-abdominal hemorrhage and should be considered in women presenting with an abdominal mass, acute abdominal pain, or evidence of intra-abdominal bleeding.

Neurologic: Migraine and Headache: The onset or exacerbation of migraine or the development of headache of a new pattern which is recurrent, persistent or severe, requires discontinuation of combination hormonal contraceptives (including NuvaRing) and evaluation of the cause.

Ophthalmologic: Ocular Disease: Patients who are pregnant or are using combination hormonal contraceptives (including NuvaRing), may experience corneal edema that may cause visual disturbances and changes in tolerance to contact lenses, especially of the rigid type. Soft contact lenses usually do not cause disturbances. If visual changes or alterations in tolerance to contact lenses occur, temporary or permanent cessation of wear may be advised.

Peri-Operative Considerations: Thromboembolic Complications—Post-surgery: There is an increased risk of post-surgery thromboembolic complications in combination hormonal contraceptive (including NuvaRing) users, after major surgery. If feasible, combination hormonal contraceptives should be discontinued and an alternative method substituted at least one month prior to **major** elective surgery. Combination hormonal contraceptives should not be resumed until the first menstrual period after hospital discharge following surgery.

Psychiatric: Emotional Disorders: Patients with a history of emotional disturbances, especially the depressive type, may be more prone to have a recurrence of depression while using combination hormonal contraceptives (including NuvaRing). In cases of a serious recurrence, a trial of an alternate method of contraception should be made which may help to clarify the possible relationship. Women with premenstrual syndrome (PMS) may have a varied response to combination hormonal contraceptives, ranging from symptomatic improvement to worsening of the condition.

Sexual Function/Reproduction: Return to Fertility: After discontinuing combination hormonal contraceptive (including NuvaRing) therapy, the patient should delay pregnancy until at least one normal spontaneous cycle has occurred in order to date the pregnancy. An alternate contraceptive method should be used during this time.

Amenorrhea: Women having a history of oligomenorrhea, secondary amenorrhea, or irregular cycles may remain anovulatory or become amenorrheic following discontinuation of estrogen-progestin combination therapy.

Amenorrhea, especially if associated with breast secretion, that continues for six months or more after withdrawal, warrants a careful assessment of hypothalamic-pituitary function.

Special Populations: Pregnant Women: Combination hormonal contraceptives (including NuvaRing) should not be used by pregnant women. However, if conception accidentally occurs while using combination hormonal contraceptives, there is no conclusive evidence that the estrogen and progestin contained in combination hormonal contraceptives will damage the developing child.

The extent of exposure in pregnancy during clinical trials: Very Limited: individual cases only.

Nursing Women: The effects of NuvaRing in nursing mothers have not been evaluated and are unknown. In breast-feeding women, the use of combination hormonal contraceptives results in the hormonal components being excreted in breast milk and may reduce its quantity and quality. If the use of combination hormonal contraceptives is initiated after the establishment of lactation, there does not appear to be any effect on the quantity and quality of the milk. There is no evidence that low dose combination hormonal contraceptives are harmful to the nursing infant. However, women who are breast feeding should be advised not to use CHC's (including NuvaRing) but to use other forms of contraception until the child is weaned.

Risk to the Partner: The extent and possible pharmacological role of exposure of male sexual partners to ethinyl estradiol and etonogestrel through absorption through the penis have not been determined.

Monitoring and Laboratory Tests: Physical Examination and Follow-up: Before combination hormonal contraceptives (including NuvaRing) are used, a thorough history and physical examination should be performed, including a blood pressure determination. Breasts, liver, extremities and pelvic organs should be examined. A Papanicolaou smear should be taken if the patient has been sexually active.

The first follow-up visit should be done three months after combination hormonal contraceptives are prescribed. Thereafter, examinations should be performed at least once a year or more frequently if indicated. At each annual visit, examination should include those procedures that were done at the initial visit as outlined above or per recommendations of the Canadian Task Force on the Periodic Health Examination.

Discontinue medication at the earliest manifestation of:

A. **Thromboembolic and Cardiovascular Disorders** such as: thrombophlebitis, pulmonary embolism, cerebrovascular disorders, myocardial ischemia, mesenteric thrombosis, and retinal thrombosis.
B. **Conditions which predispose to venous stasis and to vascular thrombosis**, e.g. immobilization after accidents or confinement to bed during long-term illness. Other non-hormonal methods of contraception should be used until regular activities are resumed. For use of combination hormonal contraceptives when surgery is contemplated, see Peri-Operative Considerations.
C. **Visual Defects, Partial or Complete.**
D. **Papilledema, or Ophthalmic Vascular Lesions.**
E. **Severe Headache of Unknown Etiology or Worsening of Pre-existing Migraine Headache.**

ADVERSE REACTIONS: Adverse Drug Reaction Overview: An increased risk of the following serious adverse reactions has been associated with the use of combination hormonal contraceptives (including NuvaRing [etonogestrel/ethinyl estradiol slow release vaginal ring]): thrombophlebitis; pulmonary embolism; mesenteric thrombosis; neuro-ocular lesions, e.g., retinal thrombosis; myocardial infarction; cerebral thrombosis; cerebral hemorrhage; hypertension; benign hepatic tumours; gallbladder disease; congenital anomalies.

The following adverse reactions also have been reported in patients receiving combination hormonal contraceptives: Nausea and vomiting, usually the most common adverse reaction, occurs in approximately 10% or less of patients during the first cycle. Other reactions, as a general rule, are seen less frequently or only occasionally, as follows: gastrointestinal symptoms (such as abdominal cramps and bloating); breakthrough bleeding; spotting; change in menstrual flow; dysmenorrhea; amenorrhea during and after treatment; temporary infertility after discontinuance of treatment; edema; chloasma or melasma which may persist; breast changes: tenderness, enlargement, and secretion; change in weight (increase [5%] or decrease [0.1%]); endocervical hyperplasias; possible diminution in lactation when given immediately post-partum; cholestatic jaundice; migraine; increase in size of uterine leiomyomata; rash (allergic); mental depression; reduced tolerance to carbohydrates; vaginal candidiasis; premenstrual-like syndrome; intolerance to contact lenses; change in corneal curvature (steepening); cataracts; optic neuritis; retinal thrombosis; changes in libido; chorea; changes in appetite; cystitis-like syndrome; rhinitis; headache; nervousness; dizziness; hirsutism; loss of scalp hair; erythema multiforme; erythema nodosum; hemorrhagic eruption; vaginitis; porphyria; impaired renal function; Raynaud's phenomenon; auditory disturbances; hemolytic uremic syndrome; pancreatitis.

Clinical Trial Adverse Drug Reactions: Because clinical trials are conducted under very specific conditions the adverse reaction rates observed in the clinical trials may not reflect the rates observed in practice and should not be compared to the rates in the clinical trials of another drug. Adverse drug reaction information from clinical trials is useful for identifying drug-related adverse events and for approximating rates.

The most common treatment related AEs seen in all adequate and well controlled pivotal clinical studies were headache, vaginitis, and leukorrhea (Table 1). These adverse events as well as the incidence of acne, breast tenderness, and nausea which are typical of contraceptives were low.

Table 1: NuvaRing

Adverse Events Occurring in ≥1% of Subjects in All Adequate and Well Controlled Pivotal Clinical Studies

System Organ Class	Adverse Event	n[a]	%
Skin and Appendages Disorders	Acne	46	2.0
Central & Peripheral Nervous System Disorders	Headache	135	5.8
	Migraine	24	1.0
Psychiatric Disorders	Emotional Lability	64	2.8
	Libido Decreased	31	1.3
	Depression	33	1.4
Gastrointestinal System Disorders	Nausea	74	3.2
	Abdominal Pain	24	1.0
Metabolic and Nutritional Disorders	Weight Increase	93	4.0
Reproductive Disorders, female	Vaginitis	130	5.6
	Leukorrhea	111	4.8
	Device Related Problems	103	4.4
	Breast Pain (female)	61	2.6
	Dysmenorrhea	60	2.6
	Vaginal Discomfort	56	2.4
	Abdominal Pain (gynecological)	36	1.6

[a] Total n=2322 subjects.

Cervical cytology was assessed in 2039 women during treatment with NuvaRing. For the majority of subjects, the cervical Pap smear result was Pap I at screening and at last assessment. A small number of subjects had a change from normal (Pap smear result of I, IIa, or IIb) at screening to a Pap result of III or IIIa at last assessment (n=33, 1.3%). Clinically relevant shifts of particular note occurred for 7 subjects with a Pap result of I at screening to a Pap result of IIIb/IV (high grade SIL) at last assessment. In summary, changes to abnormal cervical cytology occurred in a low percentage of the subjects.

The incidence of adverse events was similar for the NuvaRing and COC groups (57.9% and 54.0%, respectively). The incidence of drug related AEs was higher in the NuvaRing group than in the COC group (33.9% and 24.6%, respectively), partly due to the AEs device related events and vaginal discomfort, which were only reported in the NuvaRing group. Medical and gynecologic examinations performed before and after the studies showed no clinically relevant changes in either group. Heart rate and blood pressure did not change significantly from baseline in either group. Overall, the tolerability of both contraceptives was good (Table 2).

Table 2: NuvaRing

Adverse Events (at least possibly related) Occurring in ≥2%—Metabolic Studies (NuvaRing n=121; COC n=126)

Adverse Event	NuvaRing n (%)	COC n (%)
Acne	2 (1.7)	3 (2.4)
Breast Tenderness	5 (4.1)	5 (4.0)
Decreased Libido	10 (8.3)	0 (0.0)
Depression	0 (0.0)	6 (4.8)
Device Related Events[a]	3 (2.5)	NA[b]
Headache	4 (3.3)	3 (2.4)
Leukorrhea	3 (2.5)	0 (0.0)
Nausea	6 (5.0)	4 (3.2)
Nervousness	3 (2.5)	2 (1.6)
Weight Increase	4 (3.3)	2 (1.6)
Vaginal Discomfort	3 (2.5)	0 (0.0)
Vaginitis	5 (4.1)	2 (1.6)

[a] Comprising foreign body feeling, coital problems, and expulsion (WHO terms).
[b] NA= Not applicable.

Less Common Clinical Trial Adverse Drug Reactions (<1% at least possibly related): Other rare adverse events which were observed in clinical trials were as follows:

Skin and Appendages: alopecia, dermatitis fungal, eczema, photosensitivity reaction, pigmentation abnormal, pruritus, pruritus genital, rash, rash maculo-papular, seborrhea, skin discolouration, skin disorder, skin dry.

Musculoskeletal System Disorders: arthralgia, muscle weakness.

Central and Peripheral Nervous System Disorder: aphasia, cramps legs, dizziness, dysaesthesia, hypoaesthesia, migraine aggravated, paraesthesia, vertigo.

Vision Disorders: conjunctivitis, vision abnormal.

Psychiatric Disorders: aggressive reaction, agitation, anorexia, anxiety, apathy, appetite increased, concentration impaired, depression aggravated, hallucination, insomnia, libido increased, nervousness.

Gastrointestinal System Disorders: anus disorder, change in bowel habits, colitis ulcerative aggravated, constipation, diarrhoea, dyspepsia, flatulence, haemorrhoids, rectal disorder, tenesmus, vomiting.

Liver and Biliary System Disorders: cholelithiasis, AST increased.

Metabolic and Nutritional Disorders: dehydration, hypercholesterolaemia, hypertriglyceridaemia, oedema generalised, xerophthalmia.

Endocrine Disorders: estrogens increased, glucocorticoids increased, hypothyroidism.

Cardiovascular Disorders, general: hypertension, hypotension, oedema dependent.

Heart Rate and Rhythm Disorders: palpitation.

Vascular (extracardiac) Disorders: thrombophlebitis, thrombophlebitis deep, thrombophlebitis superficial.
Respiratory System Disorders: asthma, dyspnoea, rhinitis.
Red Blood Cell Disorders: anaemia.
Platelet, Bleeding and Clotting Disorders: haematoma, purpura.
Urinary System Disorders: bladder discomfort, cystitis, dysuria, micturition frequency, micturition urgency, strangury, urinary incontinence, urinary tract infection.
Reproductive Disorders, male: device related problems, penis disorders including pain, rash, bruises and abrasions.
Reproductive Disorders, female: amenorrhoea, bleeding irregularity, breast enlargement, cervical dysplasia, cervicitis, cervix lesion, ectopy, endometritis, lactation nonpuerperal, mastitis, ovarian disorder, ovarian mass, ovarian pain, pelvic inflammation, premenstrual tension, uterine disorder nos, vulva discomfort, vulva disorder.
Neoplasm: breast fibroadenosis, breast neoplasm benign female, cervical smear test positive, cervical uterine polyp, haemangioma acquired, ovarian cyst, uterine fibroid, vaginal neoplasm benign.
Body as a Whole: abdomen enlarged, allergic reaction, asthenia, back pain, chest pain, fatigue, hot flushes, influenza-like symptoms, leg pain, malaise, oedema, oedema peripheral, pain, temperature changed sensation.
Application Site Disorders: skin nodule.
Resistance Mechanism Disorders: infection viral.
Secondary Terms: cervical smear test PAP II.
Undefined System-Organ Class: cervical smear PAP II.
Post-Market Adverse Drug Reactions: In general, post-marketing data are in agreement with the expectations and conclusions based on the clinical development program, except for some unanticipated reports related to disconnected rings (<0.005%, see Warning and Precautions, Genitourinary).

DRUG INTERACTIONS: Overview: The concurrent administration of combination hormonal contraceptives (including NuvaRing [etonogestrel/ethinyl estradiol slow release vaginal ring]) with other drugs may result in an altered response to either agent (Table 3 and Table 4). Reduced effectiveness of combination hormonal contraceptives (including NuvaRing), is more likely with the low dose formulations. This could result in unintended pregnancy or breakthrough bleeding. It is important to ascertain all drugs that a patient is taking, both prescription and non-prescription, before combination hormonal contraceptives (including NuvaRing) are prescribed.

Table 3: NuvaRing

Drugs Which May Decrease the Efficacy of Combination Hormonal Contraceptives (CHC)

Class of Compound	Drug	Proposed Mechanism	Suggested Management
Anti-convulsants	Carbamazepine Ethosuximide Phenobarbital Phenytoin Primidone	Induction of hepatic microsomal enzymes: Rapid metabolism of estrogen and increased binding of progestin and ethinyl estradiol to SHBG.	Use higher dose CHC (50 µg ethinyl estradiol) another drug or another method.
Antibiotics	Ampicillin Cotrimoxazole Penicillin	Enterohepatic circulation disturbance, intestinal hurry.	For short course, use additional method or use another drug. For long course, use another method.
	Rifampicin	Increased metabolism of progestins. Suspected acceleration of estrogen metabolism.	Use another method.
	Chloramphenicol Metronidazole Neomycin Nitrofurantoin Sulfonamides Tetracyclines	Induction of hepatic microsomal enzymes. Also disturbance of enterohepatic circulation.	For short course, use additional method or use another drug. For long course, use another method.
	Troleandomycin	May retard metabolism of CHC increasing the risk of cholestatic jaundice.	
Antifungal	Griseofulvin	Stimulation of hepatic metabolism of contraceptive steroids may occur.	Use another method.
Sedatives and Hypnotics	Benzodiazepines Barbiturates Chloral Hydrate Glutethimide Meprobamate	Induction of hepatic microsomal enzymes.	For short course, use additional method or another drug. For long course use another method or higher dose oral contraceptive.
Antacids		Decreased intestinal absorption of progestins.	
Other Drugs	Phenylbutazone Antihistamines Analgesics Antimigraine preparations Vitamin E	Reduced contraceptive efficacy has been reported. Remains to be confirmed.	

Table 4: NuvaRing

Modification of Other Drug Action by Oral Contraceptives

Class of Compound	Drug	Modification of Other Drug Action	Suggested Management
Alcohol		Possible increased levels of ethanol or acetaldehyde.	Use with caution.
Alpha-II Adrenoreceptor Agents	Clonidine	Sedation effect increased.	Use with caution.
Anti-coagulants	All	CHCs increase clotting factors, decrease efficacy. However CHC may potentiate action in some patients.	Use another method.
Anti-convulsants	All	Fluid retention may increase risk of seizures.	Use another method.
Anti-diabetic Drugs	Oral hypoglycemics and insulin	CHCs may impair glucose tolerance and increase blood glucose.	Use low dose estrogen and progestin CHC or another method. Monitor blood glucose.
Anti-hypertensive Agents	Guanethidine and methyldopa	Estrogen component cause sodium retention, progestin has no effect.	Use low estrogen CHC or use another method.
	Beta blockers	Increased drug effect (decreased metabolism).	Adjust dose of drug if necessary. Monitor cardiovascular status.
Antipyretics	Acetaminophen	Increased renal clearance.	Dose of drug may have to be increased.
	Antipyridine	Impaired metabolism.	Decrease dose of drug.
	ASA	Effects of ASA may be decreased by the short term use of CHCs.	Patients on chronic ASA therapy may require an increase in ASA dosage.
Aminocaproic Acid		Theoretically, a hypercoagulable state may occur because CHCs augment clotting factors.	Avoid concomitant use.
Betamimetic Agents	Isoproterenol	Estrogen causes decreased response to these drugs.	Adjust dose of drug as necessary. Discontinuing CHCs can result in excessive drug activity.
Caffeine		The actions of caffeine may be enhanced as CHCs may impair the hepatic metabolism of caffeine.	Use with caution.
Cholesterol Lowering Agents	Clofibrate	CHCs may increase the clearance of clofibrate leading to decreased level of clofibrate.	Use with caution.
Corticosteroids	Prednisone	Markedly increased serum levels.	Possible need for decrease in dose.
Cyclosporine		May lead to an increase in cyclosporine levels and hepatotoxicity.	Monitor hepatic function. The cyclosporine dose may have to be decreased.
Folic Acid		CHCs have been reported to impair folate metabolism.	
Meperidine		Possible increased analgesia and CNS depression due to decreased metabolism of meperidine.	Use combination with caution.
Phenothiazine Tranquilizers	All phenothiazines, reserpine and similar drugs.	Estrogen potentiates the hyperprolactinemia effect of these drugs.	Use other drugs or lower dose CHCs. If galactorrhea or hyperprolactinemia, occurs use other method.
Sedatives and Hypnotics	Chlordiazepoxide Lorazepam Oxazepam Diazepam	Increased effect (increased metabolism).	Use with caution.
Theophylline	All	Decreased oxidation, leading to possible toxicity.	Use with caution. Monitor theophylline levels.
Tricyclic Antidepressants	Clomipramine (possibly others)	Increased side effects; i.e. depression.	Use with caution.
Vitamin B_{12}		CHCs have been reported to reduce serum levels of Vitamin B_{12}.	

Several of the anti-HIV protease inhibitors have been studied with coadministration of oral combination hormonal contraceptives; significant changes (increase and decrease) in the mean AUC of the estrogen and progestin have been noted in some cases. The efficacy and safety of oral contraceptive products may be affected; it is unknown whether this applies to NuvaRing. Healthcare providers should refer to the label of the individual anti-HIV protease inhibitors for further drug-drug interaction information.

Drug-Drug Interactions: Interactions between contraceptive steroids and other drugs have been reported in the literature (see Overview).

The serum concentrations of etonogestrel and ethinyl estradiol were not affected by concomitant administration of oral amoxicillin or doxycycline in standard dosages during 10 days of antibiotic treatment.

The pharmacokinetics of NuvaRing were evaluated in one cycle in 24 healthy female subjects randomized to a single-dose vaginal administration on Day 8 of 100 mg of a nonoxynol-9 spermicide gel or a 1200 mg miconazole nitrate antimycotic capsule.

The single dose of 100 mg vaginally administered, water-based nonoxyl-9 gel did not affect the serum concentrations of etonogestrel or ethinyl estradiol.

The single dose of 1200 mg vaginally-administered, oil-based miconazole nitrate capsule increased the serum concentrations of etonogestrel and ethinyl estradiol by approximately 17% and 16% respectively. The clinical significance of these findings is unknown; however the contraceptive effectiveness of NuvaRing is not expected to change.

In a separate trial, the pharmacokinetics of NuvaRing were evaluated in one cycle in 12 healthy female subjects randomized to 3 doses of an oil-based 200 mg miconazole nitrate antimycotic suppository or a water-based 200 mg miconazole nitrate antimycotic vaginal cream on Days 8, 9, and 10 of the NuvaRing cycle. Following multiple doses, the mean serum concentrations of etonogestrel and ethinyl estradiol remained elevated compared to the concentrations on the first day of interaction treatment, and were elevated by up to 40%. This effect was more pronounced with the oil-based suppository treatment than in the water-based cream treatment.

The effects of chronic administration of these products with NuvaRing are unknown.

Drug-Food Interactions: Interactions with food have not been established.

Drug-Herb Interactions: Herbal products containing St. John's Wort (hypericum perforatum) may induce hepatic enzymes (cytochrome P450) and p-glycoprotein transporter and may reduce the effectiveness of contraceptive steroids. This may also result in breakthrough bleeding. Physicians and other health care providers should be made aware of the non-prescription products concomitantly used by the patient, including herbal and natural products.

Drug-Laboratory Test Interactions: Results of laboratory tests should be interpreted in the light that the patient is on combination hormonal contraceptives (including NuvaRing). The following laboratory tests are modified.

A. Liver function tests: Aspartate serum transaminase (AST)—variously reported elevations. Alkaline phosphatase and gamma glutamine transaminase (GGT)—slightly elevated.

B. Coagulation tests: Minimal elevation of test values reported for such parameters as prothrombin and Factors VII, VIII, IX and X.

C. Thyroid function tests: Protein binding of thyroxine is increased as indicated by increased total serum thyroxine concentrations and decreased T_3 resin uptake.

D. Lipoproteins: Small changes of unproven clinical significance may occur in lipoprotein cholesterol fractions.

E. Gonadotropins: LH and FSH levels are suppressed by the use of oral contraceptives. Wait two weeks after discontinuing the use of oral contraceptives before measurements are made.

Tissue Specimens: Pathologists should be advised of combination hormonal contraceptives (including NuvaRing) therapy when specimens obtained from surgical procedures and Pap smears are submitted for examination.

Drug-Lifestyle Interactions: Vaginal Use: NuvaRing is designed to be a once-a-month contraceptive regimen, therefore NuvaRing should be left in the vagina for a continuous period of 3 weeks. Some women are aware of the ring at random times during the 21 days of use or during intercourse. During intercourse some sexual partners may feel NuvaRing in the vagina. However, clinical studies revealed that 90% of couples did not find this to be a problem. NuvaRing should not be removed during intercourse.

NuvaRing may interfere with the correct placement and position of a diaphragm or cervical cap. A diaphragm or cervical cap is therefore not recommended as a back-up method with NuvaRing use.

Expulsion: NuvaRing can be accidentally expelled, for example, when it has not been inserted properly, or while removing a tampon, during intercourse, or with straining during a bowel movement.

Clinical trial data indicate that expulsion of NuvaRing is most common in the first few cycles of use when women are becoming accustomed to this method of contraception. In a retrospective analysis of four one-year NuvaRing trials it was found that expulsion occurred in 0.5% of cycles (N=33 462) and this percentage decreased to zero with duration of use (1.1% at cycle 1; N=3228 and 0% at cycle 13; N=2071). Overall, 2.3% of subjects (N=3333) experienced expulsion over 13 cycles of use.

If the ring is accidentally expelled and is left outside of the vagina for less than 3 hours, contraceptive efficacy is not reduced. The vaginal ring can be rinsed with cool to lukewarm (not hot) water and re-inserted as soon as possible, but at the latest within 3 hours (see Dosage and Administration, Missed Dose and Information for the Patient, Missed Dose). If NuvaRing is lost, a new vaginal ring should be inserted and the regimen should be continued without alteration.

If the ring has been out of the vagina for more than three hours during the 1st or 2nd week, contraceptive effectiveness may be reduced. The woman should reinsert the ring as soon as she remembers and an additional barrier method of contraception, such as condoms and/or spermicide, **must** be used until the ring has been used **continuously for seven days**. The longer the time NuvaRing has been out of the vagina and the closer this is to the ring free interval, the higher the risk of a pregnancy.

If NuvaRing has been out of the vagina for more than 3 hours during the 3rd week of the three-week use period contraceptive efficacy may be reduced. The woman should discard that ring, and one of the following two options should be chosen:

1. Insert a new ring immediately. Note: Inserting a new ring will start the next three-week use period. The woman may not experience a withdrawal bleed from her previous cycle. However, breakthrough spotting or bleeding may occur.
2. Have a withdrawal bleeding and insert a new ring no later than 7 days (7×24 hours) from the time the previous ring was removed or expelled. Note: This option should only be chosen if the ring was used continuously for the preceding 7 days.

Women with conditions affecting the vagina, such as a prolapsed uterus, may be more likely to have NuvaRing slip out of the vagina.

Tampon Use: The pharmacokinetics of NuvaRing was evaluated in one cycle in 10 healthy female subjects randomized to tampon use (Kotex, regular strength) on Day 8, 9, 10 of the NuvaRing cycle. The use of tampons had no effect on serum concentrations of etonogestrel and ethinyl estradiol during use of NuvaRing. It is unknown how this affects the safety and efficacy of NuvaRing.

Non-contraceptive benefits of combination hormonal contraceptives (including NuvaRing): Several health advantages other than contraception have been reported.

1. Combination hormonal contraceptives (including NuvaRing) reduce the incidence of cancer of the endometrium and ovaries.
2. Combination hormonal contraceptives (including NuvaRing) reduce the likelihood of developing benign breast disease and as a result decrease the incidence of breast biopsies.
3. Combination hormonal contraceptives (including NuvaRing) reduce the likelihood of development of functional ovarian cysts.
4. Combination hormonal contraceptive (including NuvaRing) users have less menstrual blood loss and have more regular cycles, thereby reducing the chance of developing iron-deficiency anemia.
5. The use of combination hormonal contraceptives (including NuvaRing) may decrease the severity of dysmenorrhea and premenstrual syndrome and may improve acne vulgaris, hirsutism and other androgen-mediated disorders.
6. Combination hormonal contraceptives (including NuvaRing) decrease the incidence of acute pelvic inflammatory disease and thereby reduce as well the incidence of ectopic pregnancy.
7. Combination hormonal contraceptives (including NuvaRing) have potential beneficial effects on endometriosis.

DOSAGE AND ADMINISTRATION:

Recommended Dose and Dosage Adjustment: To achieve maximum contraceptive effectiveness, NuvaRing (etonogestrel/ethinyl estradiol slow release vaginal ring) must be used as directed (see When to Start NuvaRing). One NuvaRing is inserted in the vagina by the woman herself. As NuvaRing is designed to be a once-a-month contraceptive regimen the **ring is to remain in place continuously for three weeks**. It is a good habit for the woman to regularly verify the presence of NuvaRing. It is removed for a one-week break, during which a withdrawal bleed usually occurs. A new ring is inserted no more than one week after removal of the last ring.

Missed Dose: Inadvertent removal, expulsion, or prolonged ring-free interval: NuvaRing should be left in the vagina for a continuous period of 3 weeks. If the ring is accidentally expelled and is left outside of the vagina for less than 3 hours contraceptive efficacy is not reduced i.e. the woman should still be protected from pregnancy. NuvaRing should be rinsed with cool to lukewarm (not hot) water and re-inserted as soon as possible, but at the latest within 3 hours. If NuvaRing is lost, a new vaginal ring should be inserted and the regimen should be continued without alteration.

If NuvaRing is out of the vagina for more than 3 continuous hours: During Weeks 1 and 2: If NuvaRing has been out of the vagina for more than 3 continuous hours during the 1st or 2nd week of use, contraceptive efficacy may be reduced. The woman should reinsert the ring as soon as she remembers. A barrier method, such as condoms and/or spermicide, must be used in addition until NuvaRing has been in the vagina continuously for 7 days. The longer the time NuvaRing has been out of the vagina and the closer this is to the ring-free interval, the higher the risk of pregnancy.

During Week 3: If NuvaRing has been out of the vagina for more than 3 continuous hours during the 3rd week of the three-week use period, contraceptive efficacy may be reduced. The woman should discard that ring, and one of the following two options should be chosen:

1. Insert a new ring immediately. Inserting a new ring will start the next three-week use period. The woman may not experience a withdrawal bleed from her previous cycle. However, breakthrough spotting or bleeding may occur.
2. Have a withdrawal bleeding and insert a new ring no later than 7 days (7×24 hours) from the time the previous ring was removed or expelled. This option should only be chosen if the ring was used continuously for the preceding 7 days.

A barrier method such as condoms and/or spermicides must be used until the new ring has been used continuously for seven days.

If the ring-free interval has been extended beyond one week, the possibility of pregnancy should be considered, and an additional method of contraception, such as condoms and/or spermicide, **must** be used until NuvaRing has been used **continuously for seven days**. The longer the ring-free interval, the higher the risk of pregnancy.

Administration: The user can choose the insertion position that is most comfortable to her, for example, standing with one leg up, squatting, or lying down. The ring is to be compressed and inserted into the vagina until it feels comfortable. The exact position of NuvaRing inside the vagina is not critical for the contraceptive effect of the ring. The vaginal ring must be inserted on the appropriate day and left in place for three consecutive weeks. This means that the ring is removed three weeks later on the same day of the week as it was inserted and at about the same time. NuvaRing can be removed by hooking the index finger under the forward rim or by grasping the rim between the index and middle finger and pulling it out. The used ring should be placed in the sachet (foil pouch) and discarded in a waste receptacle out of the reach of children and pets (do not flush in toilet). The withdrawal bleeding usually starts 2-3 days after removal of the ring and may not have finished before the next ring is inserted. In order to maintain contraceptive effectiveness, the new ring must be inserted one week after the previous one was removed even if menstrual bleeding has not finished. For example, if NuvaRing is inserted on Wednesday at 22:00 h the ring should be removed again on the Wednesday 3 weeks later at about 22:00 h. The following Wednesday a new ring should be inserted.

When to Start NuvaRing: Important: The possibility of ovulation and conception prior to the first use of NuvaRing should be considered.

No hormonal contraceptive use in the preceding cycle: The woman may start using NuvaRing within the first five days of her natural cycle. (i.e. Day 1-5 of her menstrual bleeding). During the first seven days of NuvaRing use in the first cycle, an additional barrier method, such as male condoms or spermicide, is recommended.

Switching from another combination hormonal contraceptive : The woman may switch from her previous combined hormonal contraceptive on any day of the cycle, if she has been using this method consistently and correctly, and if it is reasonably certain that she is not pregnant. Otherwise, the woman should insert NuvaRing at the latest on the day following the usual tablet-free, patch-free or placebo tablet interval of her previous combined hormonal contraceptive. The hormone-free interval of the previous method should never be extended beyond its recommended length.

Switching from a progestin-only method: There are several types of progestin-only methods. Women should insert the first NuvaRing as follows:

- Any day of the month when switching from a progestin-only pill; do not skip any days between the last pill and the first day of NuvaRing use.
- On the same day as contraceptive implant removal.
- On the same day as removal of a progestin-containing IUD, or
- On the day when the next contraceptive injection would be due.

In all of these cases, the patient should be advised to use an additional method of contraception, such as condoms and/or spermicide, for the first seven days after insertion of the ring.

Following complete first trimester abortion: The woman may start using NuvaRing within the first five days following a complete first trimester abortion and does not need to use an additional method of contraception. If use of NuvaRing is not started within five days following a first trimester abortion, the patient should follow the instructions for "No hormonal contraceptive use in the preceding cycle." In the meantime she should be advised to use a non-hormonal contraceptive method.

Following delivery or second trimester abortion: The use of NuvaRing for contraception may be initiated four weeks after a second trimester abortion or four weeks postpartum in women who elect not to breastfeed. When NuvaRing is used postpartum or postabortion, the increased risk of thromboembolic disease must be considered (See Contraindications and Warnings and Precautions, Hematologic concerning thromboembolic disease. Also see Warnings and Precautions for Special Populations: Nursing Women regarding breast-feeding.) If a woman begins using NuvaRing postpartum, she should be instructed to use an additional method of contraception, such as male condoms or spermicide for the first seven days. If she has not yet had a period, the possibility of ovulation and conception occurring prior to initiation of NuvaRing should be considered.

Deviations from the Recommended Regimen: To prevent loss of contraceptive efficacy patients should not deviate from the recommended regimen.

Prolonged Use of NuvaRing: If NuvaRing has been left in place for up to one extra week (i.e., up to four weeks total), the woman will remain protected. NuvaRing should be removed and the woman should insert a new ring after a one-week ring-free interval. The mean serum etonogestrel concentration during the fourth week of continuous use of NuvaRing was 1272±311 pg/mL compared to a mean concentration range of 1578±408 to 1374±328 pg/mL during weeks one to three. The mean serum ethinyl estradiol concentration during the fourth week of continuous use of NuvaRing was 16.8±4.6 pg/mL compared to a mean concentration range of 19.1±4.5 to 17.6±4.3 pg/mL during weeks one to three. If NuvaRing has been left in place for longer than four weeks, contraceptive efficacy may be reduced. Pregnancy should be ruled out before inserting a new NuvaRing, and an additional method of contraception, such as condoms and/or spermicide, **must** be used until a new NuvaRing has been used **continuously for seven days**.

In the Event of a Missed Menstrual Period:

1. If the patient has not adhered to the prescribed regimen (NuvaRing has been out of the vagina for more than three hours or the preceding ring-free interval was extended beyond one week) the possibility of pregnancy should be considered at the time of the first missed period and NuvaRing use should be discontinued if pregnancy is confirmed.
2. If the patient has adhered to the prescribed regimen and misses two consecutive periods, pregnancy should be ruled out.
3. If the patient has retained one NuvaRing for longer than four weeks, pregnancy should be ruled out.

How to Change the NuvaRing Start Day to Another Day of the Week: If the woman wishes to change the day on which she starts a new NuvaRing cycle, she should complete the current cycle, removing NuvaRing on the same day of the week as the one on which she started. During the ring-free period, a new start day may be selected by inserting the new NuvaRing on the first occurrence of the desired day. In no case should there be more than 7 consecutive ring-free days. The shorter the ring-free interval, the higher the risk that she does not have a withdrawal bleed and may experience breakthrough bleeding and spotting during the use of the next ring. This practice is for a one-time only change and should not to be used as a standard dosing regimen, as there are no long-term safety data available on the continuous use of NuvaRing.

OVERDOSAGE:

Overdosage of combination hormonal contraceptives may cause nausea, vomiting, vaginal bleeding, or other menstrual irregularities. Given the nature and design of NuvaRing (etonogestrel/ethinyl estradiol slow release vaginal ring) it is unlikely that overdosage will occur. If NuvaRing is broken, it does not release a higher dose of hormones. Serious ill effects have not been reported following acute ingestion of large doses of oral contraceptives by young children. There are no antidotes and further treatment should be symptomatic.

> For management of a suspected drug overdose, CPhA recommends that you contact your **regional Poison Control Centre**. See the *CPS* Directory section for a list of Poison Control Centres.

ACTION AND CLINICAL PHARMACOLOGY: NuvaRing (etonogestrel/ethinyl estradiol slow release vaginal ring) is a non-biodegradable, flexible, transparent, colorless to almost colorless, combination contraceptive vaginal ring containing two active components, a progestin, etonogestrel and an estrogen, ethinyl estradiol. When placed in the vagina, each ring releases on average 120 µg/day of etonogestrel and 15 µg/day of ethinyl estradiol over a three week period of use. NuvaRing is made of ethylene vinylacetate copolymers and magnesium stearate and contains 11.4 mg etonogestrel and 2.6 mg ethinyl estradiol. NuvaRing has an outer diameter of 54 mm and a cross-sectional diameter of 4 mm. It does not contain any latex.

Mechanism of Action: Combination hormonal contraceptives (including NuvaRing) act by suppression of gonadotropins. Although the primary mechanism of this action is inhibition of ovulation, other alterations include changes in the cervical mucus (which increase the difficulty of sperm entry into the uterus) and the endometrium (which reduces the likelihood of implantation).

Pharmacodynamics: Etonogestrel, the progestogen component of NuvaRing, displays low androgenic activity in relation to its progestogenic effects and may increase the HDL_1-, HDL_2-, and HDL_3-cholesterol and apoprotein A-1/B ratio without affecting LDL. Like other hormonal contraceptives, these changes in lipid profile can be associated with an increase in triglycerides.

Pharmacokinetics: The pharmacokinetic parameters of etonogestrel and ethinyl estradiol were determined during one cycle of NuvaRing use in 16 healthy female subjects and are summarized in Table 5.

Table 5: NuvaRing

Summary of NuvaRing's Pharmacokinetic Parameters in 16 Healthy Female Subjects

	C_{max} mean (SD) pg/mL	$t_{½}$ (h)	T_{max} (h)	Clearance (L/h)
Etonogestrel	1716 (445)	29.3 (6.1)	200.3 (69.9)	3.4 (0.8)
Ethinyl Estradiol	34.7 (17.5)	44.7 (28.8)	59.3 (67.5)	34.8 (11.6)

Legend: C_{max}=maximum serum drug concentration; T_{max}=time at which maximum serum drug concentration occurs; $t_{1/2}$=elimination half-life, calculated by $0.693/K_{elim}$; CL=apparent clearance.

Absorption: Etonogestrel: Etonogestrel released by NuvaRing is rapidly absorbed. Bioavailability of etonogestrel after vaginal administration is approximately 100%. The serum etonogestrel and ethinyl estradiol concentrations (pg/mL) observed during three weeks of NuvaRing use are summarized in Table 6.

Ethinyl Estradiol: Ethinyl estradiol released by NuvaRing is rapidly absorbed. Bioavailability of ethinyl estradiol after vaginal administration is approximately 55.6%, which is comparable to that with oral administration of ethinyl estradiol. However, the overall systemic exposure to ethinyl estradiol with NuvaRing was approximately 50% of that for a 30 µg oral contraceptive reflecting the difference in daily doses (15 µg vs 30 µg). The serum ethinyl estradiol concentrations observed during three weeks of NuvaRing use are summarized in Table 6.

Table 6: NuvaRing

Mean (SD) Serum Etonogestrel and Ethinyl Estradiol Concentrations (n=16)

	1 week	2 weeks	3 weeks
Etonogestrel (pg/mL)	1578 (408)	1476 (362)	1374 (328)
Ethinyl Estradiol (pg/mL)	19.1 (4.5)	18.3 (4.3)	17.6 (4.3)

The pharmacokinetic profile of etonogestrel and ethinyl estradiol during use of NuvaRing is shown in Figure 1.

Figure 1: NuvaRing

Mean Serum Concentration-Time Profile of Etonogestrel and Ethinyl Estradiol During Three Weeks of NuvaRing Use

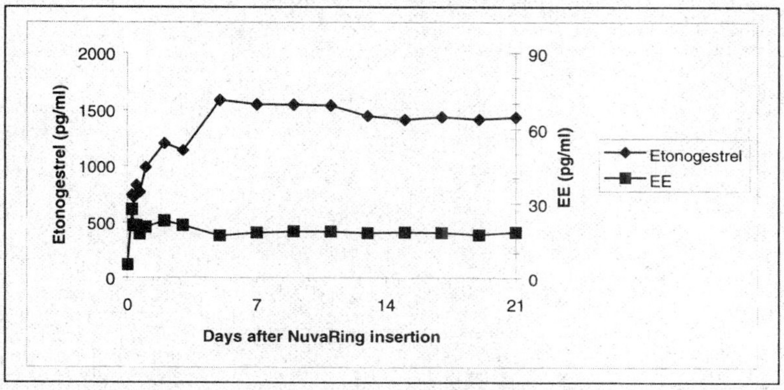

Serum ethinyl estradiol levels were measured in a comparative randomized trial (n=24) with NuvaRing (daily vaginal EE release of 0.015 mg), a transdermal patch (norelgestromin/EE; daily EE release of 0.020 mg) and a COC (levonorgestrel/EE; daily EE release of 0.030 mg) during one cycle in healthy female subjects. The monthly systemic ethinyl estradiol exposure ($AUC_{0-\infty}$) of NuvaRing was 10.9 ng·h/mL.

Distribution: Etonogestrel: Etonogestrel: Etonogestrel was found to be 98% protein bound, primarily to albumin and sex hormone-binding globulin (SHBG). The apparent volume of distribution of etonogestrel is 2.3 L/kg.

Ethinyl Estradiol: Ethinyl estradiol is highly but not specifically bound to serum albumin (approximately 98.5%) and induces an increase in the serum concentrations of SHBG. An apparent volume of distribution of about 15 L/kg has been determined.

Metabolism: In vitro data shows that both etonogestrel and ethinyl estradiol are metabolized in liver microsomes by the cytochrome P450 3A4 isoenzyme. Ethinyl estradiol is primarily metabolized by aromatic hydroxylation, but a wide variety of hydroxylated and methylated metabolites are formed. These are present as free metabolites and as sulfate and glucuronide conjugates. The hydroxylated ethinyl estradiol metabolites have weak estrogenic activity. The biological activity of etonogestrel metabolites is unknown.

Excretion: Etonogestrel and ethinyl estradiol are primarily eliminated in urine, bile and feces.

Special Populations and Conditions: Race: No formal studies were conducted to evaluate the effect of race on the pharmacokinetics of NuvaRing.

Hepatic Insufficiency: No formal studies were conducted to evaluate the effect of hepatic disease on the pharmacokinetics, safety, and efficacy of NuvaRing. However, steroid hormones may be poorly metabolized in patients with impaired liver function (see Warnings and Precautions).

Renal Insufficiency: No formal studies were conducted to evaluate the effect of renal disease on the pharmacokinetics, safety, and efficacy of NuvaRing.

STORAGE AND STABILITY: Prior to dispensing to the user, store refrigerated at 2-8°C. After dispensing to the user, NuvaRing (etonogestrel/ethinyl estradiol slow release vaginal ring) can be stored for up to 4 months at 2-30°C. Avoid storing NuvaRing in direct sunlight or at temperatures above 30°C .

For the Dispenser: When NuvaRing is dispensed to the user, place an expiration date on the label. The date should not exceed either 4 months from the date of dispensing or the expiration date, whichever comes first. Store between 2-30°C.

Keep in a safe place out of the reach of children and pets.

SPECIAL HANDLING INSTRUCTIONS: NuvaRing (etonogestrel/ethinyl estradiol slow release vaginal ring) does not contain any latex.

INFORMATION FOR THE PATIENT: Published in e-CPS, available by subscription at www.e-cps.ca.

DOSAGE FORMS, COMPOSITION AND PACKAGING: Each slow release vaginal ring contains: etonogestrel 11.4 mg and ethinyl estradiol Ph.Eur. 2.6 mg to deliver 120 µg of etonogestrel and 15 µg of ethinyl estradiol per day. NuvaRing also contains ethylene vinylacetate copolymers (28% and 9% vinylacetate) and magnesium stearate. Each NuvaRing is individually packaged in a reclosable aluminum laminate sachet consisting of three layers, from outside to inside: polyethylene terephthalate (PET), aluminum foil, and low-density polyethylene. The ring should be replaced in this reclosable sachet after use for convenient disposal. NuvaRing has an outer diameter of 54 mm and a cross-sectional diameter of 4 mm. Boxes of 3 sachets. Boxes of 1 sachet.

(Shown in Product Identification Section)

The reader is invited to consult CPhA's monograph **Calcium Channel Blockers**.

Nu-Verap

verapamil HCl

Antianginal—Antiarrhythmic—Antihypertensive

Nu-Pharm

SUPPLIED: 80 mg: Each yellow, round, biconvex, film-coated tablet, identified NU over 80 on one side, contains: verapamil HCl 80 mg. Nonmedicinal ingredients: carnauba wax, colloidal silicon dioxide, croscarmellose sodium, D&C yellow #10 aluminum lake 16%, hydroxypropyl methylcellulose, lactose, magnesium stearate, microcrystalline cellulose, polyethylene glycol, sunset yellow aluminum lake 40% (FD&C yellow #6) and titanium dioxide. Energy: 3.07 kJ (0.73 kcal). Sodium: <1 mmol (0.19 mg). Gluten- and tartrazine-free. Bottles of 100 and 500.

120 mg: Each white, round, biconvex, film-coated tablet, identified NU over 120 on one side, contains: verapamil HCl 120 mg. Nonmedicinal ingredients: carnauba wax, colloidal silicon dioxide, croscarmellose sodium, hydroxypropyl methylcellulose, lactose, magnesium stearate, microcrystalline cellulose, polyethylene glycol and titanium dioxide. Energy: 4.59 kJ (1.1 kcal). Sodium: <1 mmol (0.29 mg). Gluten- and tartrazine-free. Bottles of 100.

Nyaderm

nystatin

Antifungal—Antibiotic

Taro

SUPPLIED: Topical Cream: Each g of aqueous, perfumed vanishing cream base contains: nystatin USP 100 000 units. Nonmedicinal ingredients: aluminum hydroxide gel, ceteareth-15, glyceryl monostearate, methylparaben, perfume 9128-Y, polyethylene glycol-400 monostearate, propylene glycol, propylparaben, purified water, simethicone emulsion, sodium hydroxide, sorbitol solution, titanium dioxide and white petrolatum. Tubes of 30 g. Jars of 454 g. Store at room temperature (15-30°C).

Vaginal Cream: Each g contains: nystatin USP 25 000 units. Nonmedicinal ingredients: aluminum hydroxide gel, methylparaben, promulgen-D, propylene glycol, propylparaben, purified water, simethicone emulsion and white petrolatum. Sodium hydroxide and hydrochloric acid to adjust the pH. Tubes of 120 g with applicator designed to deliver a 4 g dose (100 000 units). Store at room temperature (15-30°C).

Nytol® Extra Strength

diphenhydramine HCl

Sleep Aid

GlaxoSmithKline Consumer Healthcare

SUPPLIED: Caplets: Each blue, coated caplet, imprinted with "Nytol" on one side, contains: diphenhydramine HCl 50 mg. Packages of 20.

Capsules: Quick Gels: Each clear, light yellow soft gel capsule, imprinted with a white "N" on one side, contains: diphenhydramine HCl 50 mg. Blister strips of 8, 2 per box (16 capsules).

Tablets: Each blue, uncoated tablet, imprinted with a "N" on one side, contains: diphenhydramine HCl 50 mg. Packages of 20.

NEW PrPRADAX™ 150 mg BID

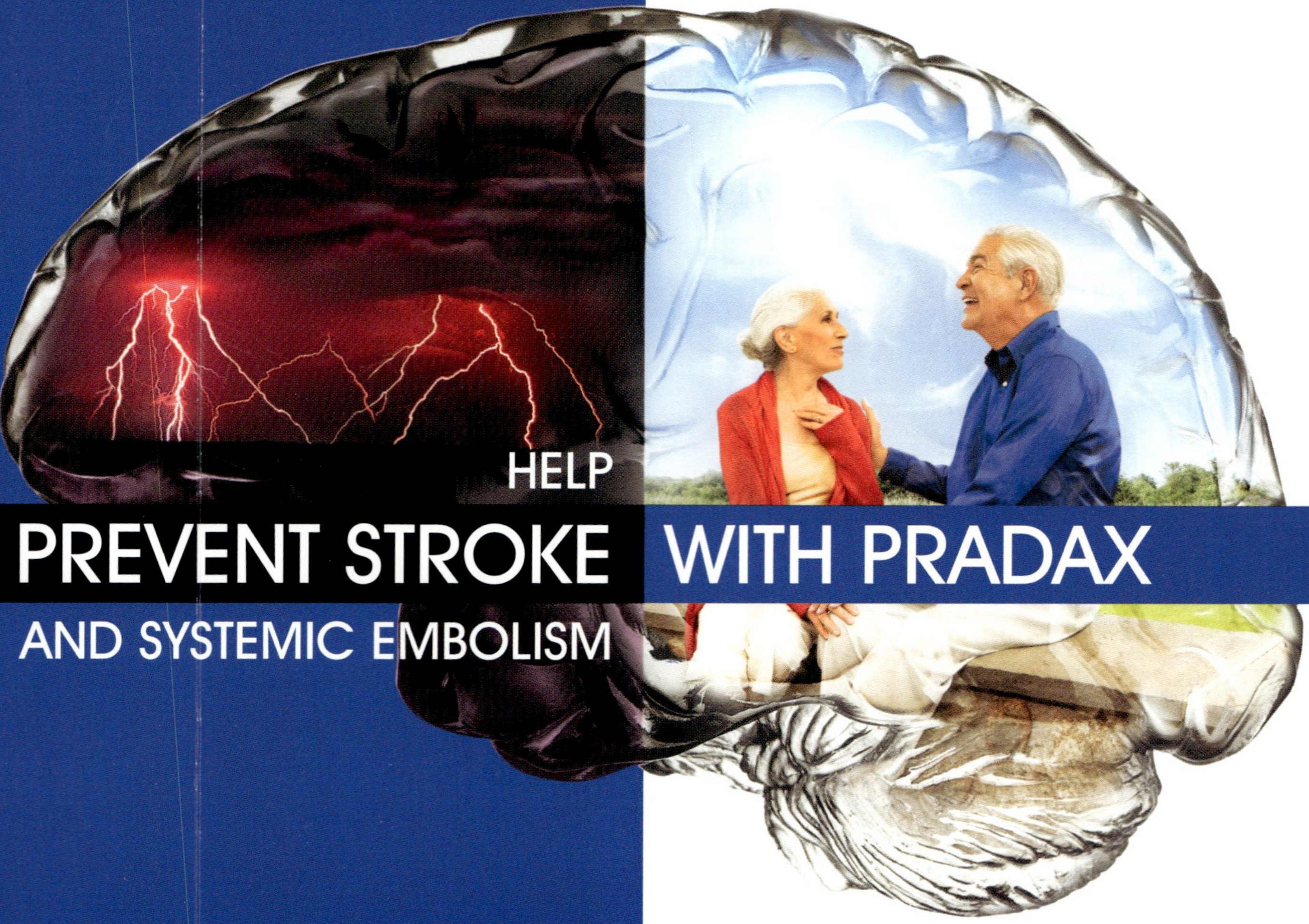

HELP PREVENT STROKE WITH PRADAX AND SYSTEMIC EMBOLISM

PRADAX (dabigatran etexilate) is indicated for the prevention of stroke and systemic embolism in patients with atrial fibrillation, in whom anticoagulation is appropriate.

PRADAX is contraindicated in patients with: severe renal impairment (CrCL <30 mL/min); hemorrhagic manifestations, bleeding diathesis, or patients with spontaneous or pharmacological impairment of hemostasis; lesions at risk of clinically significant bleeding, e.g. extensive cerebral infarction (hemorrhagic or ischemic) within the last 6 months, active peptic ulcer disease with recent bleeding; concomitant treatment with the strong P-glycoprotein (P-gp) inhibitors, i.e. oral ketoconazole, and with known hypersensitivity to dabigatran, dabigatran etexilate or to any ingredient in the formulation or component of the container.

Bleeding is the most relevant side effect of PRADAX; bleeding of any type or severity occurred in long-term treatment in 16.5% of patients with atrial fibrillation treated for the prevention of stroke and systemic embolism. As with all anticoagulants, PRADAX should be used with caution in circumstances associated with an increased risk of bleeding. Bleeding can occur at any site during therapy with PRADAX. An unexplained fall in hemoglobin and/or hematocrit or blood pressure should lead to a search for a bleeding site. Patients at high risk of bleeding should not be prescribed PRADAX. Close clinical surveillance (looking for signs of bleeding or anemia) is recommended throughout the treatment period, especially if risk factors are combined. **Should severe bleeding occur, treatment with PRADAX must be discontinued and the source of bleeding investigated promptly.** Patients who develop acute renal failure must discontinue PRADAX. In patients who are bleeding, an aPTT test may be useful to assist in determining an excess of anticoagulant activity, despite its limited sensitivity. An aPTT >80 sec at trough, i.e. when the next dose is due, is associated with a higher risk of bleeding.

Agents that may enhance the risk of hemorrhage should not be administered concomitantly with PRADAX, or, if necessary, should only be administered with caution. **Treatments that should NOT be administered concomitantly with PRADAX due to increase in bleeding risk include: unfractionated heparin and heparin derivatives, low molecular weight heparins (LMWH), fondaparinux, bivalirudin, thrombolytic agents, GPIIb/IIIa receptor antagonists, ticlopidine, sulfinpyrazone and vitamin K antagonists such as warfarin. The concomitant use of PRADAX with the following treatments has not been studied and may increase the risk of bleeding: rivaroxaban, prasugrel and the strong P-gp inhibitors itraconazole, tacrolimus, cyclosporine, ritonavir, tipranavir, nelfinavir and saquinavir.** Unfractionated heparin may be administered at doses necessary to maintain a patent central venous or arterial catheter. In patients with atrial fibrillation treated for the prevention of stroke and systemic embolism, the co-administration of oral anti-platelet (including ASA and clopidogrel) and NSAID therapies increases the risk of bleeding by about two-fold (see ACTION and CLINICAL PHARMACOLOGY, Special Populations, Pharmacokinetic Interactions). If necessary, co-administration of low-dose ASA, i.e. ≤100 mg daily with PRADAX may be considered for other indications than stroke prevention in atrial fibrillation. The concomitant use of PRADAX with the strong P-gp inducer, rifampicin, reduces

O

octaplex®

human prothrombin complex, freeze dried

Coagulation Factors

Octapharma

Date of Revision: August 6, 2009

SUMMARY PRODUCT INFORMATION:

Route of Administration	Dosage Form/ Strength		Clinically Relevant Nonmedicinal Ingredients
Intravenous injection	Powder and solvent for solution for injection/ Per 20 mL vial:		Heparin (80–310 IU) Sodium Citrate (17.0–27.0 mmol/L) Solvent (Water for Injections 20 mL)
	Human Coagulation Factor II	280–760 IU	For a complete listing see Dosage Forms, Composition and Packaging.
	Human Coagulation Factor VII	180–480 IU	
	Human Coagulation Factor IX	500 IU	
	Human Coagulation Factor X	360–600 IU	
	Protein C	140–620 IU	
	Protein S	140–640 IU	
	Factor IX specific activity is ≥0.6 IU/ mg proteins.		

DESCRIPTION: octaplex is a human prothrombin complex (PCC) containing the coagulation factors II, VII, IX, and X and Proteins C and S in the amounts listed in the table Summary Product Information.

The octaplex manufacturing process has the capability to reduce viruses by way of a solvent/detergent (S/D) viral inactivation process and a virus removal nanofiltration step. The capacity to remove prions has been assessed in a three-step approach for the process: QAE-Sephadex A-50, S/D+DEAE Sepharose FF Chromatography and Nanofiltration. The preparation complies with the monograph on Human Prothrombin Complex (freeze-dried) of the European Pharmacopoeia (2005:0554). Other precautions against viral transmission include: selection of plasma donors, screening of donations and plasma pool, as well as quality control measurements of the final product.

As with any blood product, a potential problem with PCC preparations is the transmission of blood borne pathogens including those of hitherto unknown origin. When medicinal products prepared from human blood or plasma are given to a patient, the transmission of infectious agents cannot be totally excluded. This applies also to hitherto unknown pathogens. This product is prepared from large pools of human plasma, which may contain the causative agents of hepatitis and other viral diseases (see Warnings and Precautions).

INDICATIONS AND CLINICAL USE: octaplex is indicated for:

- Treatment of bleeding and perioperative prophylaxis of bleeding in acquired deficiency of the prothrombin complex coagulation factors, such as deficiency caused by treatment with vitamin K antagonists, or in case of overdose of vitamin K antagonists, when rapid correction of the deficiency is required.

Human prothrombin complex concentrates (PCCs) contain the coagulation factors II, VII, IX and X. In principle, they are indicated for prophylaxis and treatment of acquired deficiencies of one or more of these factors.

In acquired deficiencies, PCCs have been used for the reversal of oral anticoagulation due to overdose or in case of emergency surgical interventions; in bleedings due to vitamin K deficiency; and for the treatment of bleeding disorders after major liver surgery, in severe liver diseases or oesophageal varices.

For the reversal of oral anticoagulant therapy, the administration of PCCs is indicated only when the desired increase in prothrombin complex factor activity cannot efficiently or adequately be achieved through other therapeutic measures. PCC is not indicated in cases where the prothrombin time can be normalised in time by discontinuing oral anticoagulants or by vitamin K administration. Overdose of oral anticoagulants or reversal of such therapy in case of emergency situations, liver cirrhosis and neonatal vitamin K deficiency are frequent causes of acquired prothrombin complex factor deficiencies. There are no data available regarding the use of octaplex in children.

Bleeding episodes are common adverse events of oral anticoagulant therapy that frequently depend on the duration and intensity of treatment. Major bleeding events, particularly intracerebral haemorrhages, are serious complications that require the rapid reversal of anticoagulation. Urgent correction of the coagulation defect is also indicated when emergency surgery is necessary. In addition to vitamin K supplementation, the administration of PCCs is the most effective measure for the rapid reversal of the anticoagulation therapy. Due to the time-consuming administration and increased risk of volume overload, the administration of fresh frozen plasma (FFP) is less advisable in such instances. However, the application of PCCs requires a precautious risk-benefit evaluation, including an estimation of contraindications and repeated laboratory monitoring for dose adjustment.

In patients with acquired deficiency of the vitamin K dependent coagulation factors (e.g. as induced by treatment with vitamin K antagonists), octaplex should only be used when rapid correction of prothrombin complex levels is necessary, such as major bleeding or emergency surgery. In other cases, reduction of the dose of the vitamin K antagonist and/or administration of vitamin K is usually sufficient.

octaplex should be administered under the supervision of a qualified health professional that is experienced in the use of anticoagulation agents and in the management of coagulation disorders. Appropriate management of therapy and complications is only possible when adequate diagnostic and treatment facilities are readily available.

Geriatrics (>65 years of age): Many of the patients in clinical trials with octaplex were over the age of 65. There is no evidence to suggest that use in the geriatric population is associated with differences in safety or effectiveness.

Pediatrics (6-16 years of age): No data are available.

No data are available regarding the use of octaplex in case of perinatal bleeding due to vitamin K deficiency in the newborn or due to deficiency of factors of the prothrombin complex.

CONTRAINDICATIONS:

- octaplex is contraindicated for patients who are hypersensitive to this drug or to any ingredient in the formulation or component of the container. For a complete listing, see Dosage Forms, Composition and Packaging.
- Since octaplex contains up to 310 IU of heparin, it should not be given to patients suffering from heparin-induced thrombocytopenia type II or with known allergies to heparin. Even if the antibody against the heparin-protein complex cannot be demonstrated, the administration of octaplex may cause a booster effect with an immediate generation of the antibody.
- octaplex should not be used in patients with recent myocardial infarction, with a high risk of thrombosis or with angina pectoris with the exception of life-threatening bleeds due to overdose of oral anticoagulants, or when an emergency surgical procedure is indicated in patients on vitamin K antagonists and an INR (International normalised ratio) >3.
- In patients suffering from disseminated intravascular coagulation (DIC), the administration of octaplex is principally not recommended because of the pro-coagulant capacity of the product. However, for life-threatening events when the substitution by FFP is not sufficient enough or if FFP cannot be given because of a threat of hypervolaemia, octaplex might be used after interrupting the cause of DIC. Under these circumstances it is important to administer antithrombin (AT) and heparin before the administration of a PCC.
- In patients treated for coagulation disorders because of chronic liver disease or because of liver transplantation, AT levels should be monitored and an AT concentrate should be given concomitantly if an AT deficiency is present. No clinical data are available for octaplex for the treatment of bleeding disorders because of liver parenchyme disorders or oesophageal varices or because of major liver surgery. For these indications, treatment with FFP is preferable and octaplex cannot be recommended.

WARNINGS AND PRECAUTIONS:

> **Serious Warnings and Precautions**
> This product is prepared from large pools of human plasma, which may contain the causative agents of hepatitis and other viral diseases. The physician should discuss the risks and benefits of this product with the patient before prescribing or administering to the patient (see Warnings and Precautions, General).

General: It is strongly recommended that every time that octaplex is administered to a patient, the name and batch number of the product are recorded in order to maintain a link between the patient and the batch of the product.

Products made from human plasma may contain infectious agents, such as viruses, that can cause disease. The risk that such products will transmit an infectious agent has been reduced by screening plasma donors for prior exposure to certain viruses, by testing for the presence of certain current virus infections, and by inactivating and/or removing certain viruses. The measures taken are considered effective for enveloped viruses such as Human Immunodeficiency Virus (HIV), Hepatitis B Virus (HBV) and Hepatitis C Virus (HCV). The measures taken may be of limited value against non-enveloped viruses such as Hepatitis A Virus (HAV) or parvovirus B19. Parvovirus B19 infection may be serious for pregnant women (foetal infection) and for individuals with immunodeficiency or increased red cell production (e.g. haemolytic anaemia). Despite these measures, such products can still potentially transmit disease. There is also the possibility that unknown infectious agents may be present in such products. Individuals who receive infusions of blood or plasma products may develop signs and/or symptoms of some viral infections. The prion issue is more complicated to address. The prion of major concern is the one causing vCJD, and so far, no prion protein has been found in the plasma from even clinical cases of this disease. The capacity to remove prions has been assessed in a three-step approach for the process with an actual removal log of 5.18 $\log_{10}$:

- Step A: Cryoprecipitation and Capture of the Prothrombin Complex by QAE-Sephadex A-50
- Step B: Step S/D+DEAE Sepharose FF Chromatography
- Step C: Nanofiltration

The studies were performed with PrPSc (hamster-adapted scrapie 263K).

In patients with acquired deficiency of the vitamin K dependent coagulation factors (e.g. as induced by treatment with vitamin K antagonists), octaplex should only be used when rapid correction of prothrombin complex levels is necessary, such as major bleeding or emergency surgery. In other cases, reduction of the dose of the vitamin K antagonist and/or administration of vitamin K is usually sufficient. Patients receiving a vitamin K antagonist may have an underlying hypercoaguable state and infusion of prothrombin complex concentrate may exacerbate this. The long term and repeat use safety of octaplex has not been established in controlled clinical studies.

Appropriate vaccination (hepatitis A and B) is recommended for patients in regular/repeated receipt of human plasma-derived prothrombin complex products.

Hematologic: Treatment with plasma-derived products that contain factors II, VII, IX, and X has been associated with thrombosis and may be associated with an increased risk of DIC, thromboembolic complications including myocardial infarction. There is a risk of thrombosis or disseminated intravascular coagulation when patients, with either acquired or congenital deficiency, are treated with human prothrombin complex, particularly with repeated dosing. The risk may be higher in treatment of isolated factor VII deficiency, since the other vitamin K dependant coagulation factors, with longer half-lives, may accumulate to levels considerably higher than normal.

Patients given human prothrombin complex should be observed closely for signs or symptoms of intravascular coagulation or thrombosis. Because of the risk of thromboembolic complications, close monitoring should be exercised when administering human prothrombin complex to patients with a history of coronary heart disease, myocardial infarction, to patients with liver disease, to peri- or postoperative patients, to neonates, or to patients at risk of thromboembolic events or disseminated intravascular coagulation. In each of these situations, the potential benefit of treatment should be weighed against the risk of these complications. Where adequate, a previous administration of AT concentrate is indicated.

In case of consumptive coagulation and hyperfibrinolysis, octaplex should only be administered after the disruption of the consumption process by appropriate means (e.g. by heparin, AT, antifibrinolytics).

Immune: Replacement therapy may rarely lead to the formation of circulating antibodies inhibiting one or more of the human prothrombin complex factors. If such inhibitors occur, the condition will manifest itself as a poor clinical response. The occurrence of inhibitor formation was evaluated in one clinical trial (LEX 201) but the rate could not be established, due to the very small number of patients in the trial (9 only).

In patients with a known predisposition to allergies, prophylactic anti-allergic medications should be considered. If allergic or anaphylactic reactions occur, the injection must be stopped immediately. Mild reactions may be controlled with glucocorticoids and/or antihistamines. For severe disorders, such as shock, the current standard medical treatment should be implemented.

Special Populations: Pregnant Women: The safety of octaplex for use in human pregnancy and during lactation has not been established in controlled clinical trials.

A study of the embryotoxic and teratogenic properties of TNBP and Octoxynol (Triton X-100) was carried out in rats and rabbits at dose levels of 50 to 900 µg/kg BM/day for TNBP and 250 to 4,500 µg/kg BM/day for Octoxynol (Triton X-100). No test was made of the fertility and breeding efficiency, or the peri- and post-natal development since there was no evidence of any effect on the reproductive organs by the substances. In rats, some malformations occurred, but these were of a type commonly occurring in control animals of this species. No malformations were seen in the rabbits. Pre-natal development was not affected in the rats, although in the high-dose group in the rabbit, the resorption rate was slightly increased and body weight of the foetus was moderately and significantly decreased.

The risk of parvovirus B19 infection on pregnant woman and foetus are well known. Although no harmful effects on mother, embryo, foetus, or child were reported in the three clinical trials, octaplex should be used during pregnancy and lactation only if the benefit outweighs the potential risk.

Nursing Women: See Pregnant Women.

Pediatrics: No data are available.

Geriatrics (>65 years of age): Many of the patients in clinical trials with octaplex were over the age of 65. There is no evidence to suggest that use in the geriatric population is associated with differences in safety or effectiveness.

Monitoring and Laboratory Tests: Prior to the treatment with octaplex, blood coagulation should be monitored if possible using appropriate coagulation assays, at least the Quick test should be determined. When performing clotting tests, which are sensitive to heparin in patients receiving high doses of human prothrombin complex, the heparin as a constituent of the administered product must be taken into account.

In case of major surgical interventions, precise monitoring of the substitution therapy by means of coagulation assays is essential (specific coagulation factor assays and/or global tests for prothrombin complex levels).

ADVERSE REACTIONS: Adverse Drug Reaction Overview: PCCs are known to carry a risk of thromboembolic complications and disseminated intravascular coagulation (DIC). Currently available high-purity FIX concentrates for the treatment of haemophilia B have been reported to have a significantly lower thrombogenic potential than PCCs. It is generally accepted that a suitable PCC preparation should contain all of the 4 coagulation factors in a well-balanced proportion and that it also should contain protein C (PC) and protein S (PS). Additionally, the concentration of activated coagulation factors should be kept at a minimum. Some preparations also contain small amounts of antithrombin (AT) and heparin in order to reduce the thrombotic risk after treatment with PCC.

Other adverse drug reactions of these preparations are related to acute tolerability. Rarely, antibodies (inhibitors) against the proteins administered are seen with PCCs.

Only very few clinical ADRs have been seen with octaplex to date. Nevertheless, all potential side effects seen for other compounds of this class are mentioned in the product monograph.

Immune System Disorders: Replacement therapy may rarely lead to the formation of circulating antibodies inhibiting one or more of the human prothrombin complex factors. If such inhibitors occur, the condition will manifest itself as a poor clinical response (see Warnings and Precautions).

Allergic or anaphylactic-type reactions and an increase in body temperature have not been observed in clinical studies with octaplex but may rarely occur (see Warnings and Precautions).

Nervous System Disorders: Headache may rarely occur.

Vascular Disorders: There is a risk of thromboembolic episodes following the administration of human prothrombin complex (see Warnings and Precautions).

General Disorders and Administration Site Conditions: Increase in body temperature has not been observed but may rarely occur.

Investigations: A transient increase in liver transaminases has been rarely observed.

While the development of antibodies (inhibitors) against coagulation factors is a common feature in haemophilia treatment, it seems to be a very rare event after the administration of the less purified PCCs. A final statement on the development of inhibitors in previously treated patients cannot be made. Data on the occurrence of inhibitors in previously untreated patients are not available.

Clinical Trial Adverse Drug Reactions: Because clinical trials are conducted under very specific conditions, the adverse drug reaction (ADR) rates observed in the clinical trials may not reflect the rates observed in practice and should not be compared to the rates in the clinical trials of another drug. Adverse drug reaction information from clinical trials is useful for identifying drug-related adverse events and for approximating rates.

Three clinical studies with octaplex have been conducted. In total, 90 patients have been enrolled and the patients received a total of about 569 000 IU of octaplex. Eight ADRs in 7 patients, all graded as mild, were assessed as possibly related to octaplex treatment, i.e. headache occurring twice in 1 individual, a transient increase in liver transaminases (alanine aminotransferase (ALAT), aspartate aminotransferase (ASAT)), 3 parvovirus B19 seroconversions, an injection site burning, and an aggravation of arterial hypertension. See Table 1.

Table 1: octaplex

Adverse Drug Reactions

Body System	Adverse Event	Severity/Causality	No. of Episodes
Nervous System Disorders	Headache	Mild/possible	2
Vascular Disorders	Hypertension	Mild/possible	1
General Disorders and Administration Site Conditions	Injection site burning	Mild/possible	1
Investigations	Hepatic Function Abnormal	Mild/possible	1
	Parvovirus B19 serology positive	Mild/possible	3

Study I (LEX-201): This was a prospective, non-randomised, non-controlled, open-labelled, multi-centre study conducted in 2 experienced haemophilia treatment centres in Poland and Hungary. Previously treated patients suffering from severe prothrombin complex factor deficiencies were treated for a period of 6 months. At baseline and after 6 months of regular treatment with octaplex a full pharmacokinetic investigation was performed including assessment of viral markers, inhibitor activity and thrombogenicity markers. After 3 months recovery including inhibitor activity and thrombogenicity markers were assessed.

Ten patients were enrolled in study LEX-201, 6 patients were suffering from haemophilia B and 4 from FVII deficiency. Out of 4 AEs reported in 3 patients, 2 were assessed as possibly related to octaplex administration. Both events occurred in 1 patient, who experienced mild headache 2 and 8 hours after injection. After analgesic treatment, the patient recovered.

Study II (LEX-202): This was a prospective, non-randomised, non-controlled, open-labelled, multi-centre study conducted in 6 centres in Israel and Russia. The primary objective of the study was to assess the efficacy of octaplex in patients suffering from major bleeds or who had to undergo emergency surgical procedures during treatment with anticoagulants of coumarin or indandion type.

Twenty patients were enrolled in Study LEX-202, 10 patients were enrolled because of bleeds and 10 because of surgical interventions. In total, 4 patients experienced 8 AEs; only one, a transient increase in liver transaminases (ALAT, ASAT), was assessed as possibly related to octaplex administration. This patient had transient increases of ALAT and ASAT 12 hours after the last octaplex infusion. Five days after infusion the laboratory tests were back to normal.

Study III (LEX-203): This was a prospective, non-randomised, non-controlled, open-labelled, multi-centre study conducted in 9 centres in Germany and Israel. The primary objective of the study was to investigate the efficacy of octaplex in patients undergoing surgical or invasive procedures being under treatment with anticoagulants.

Sixty patients were enrolled in the study and 56 patients were analysed per protocol. A total of 126 AEs were documented in 40 patients. Most AEs were related to the underlying diseases and the clinical status of the patients, and only 3 events were assessed as possibly related to study treatment: a parovirus B19 seroconversion, an injection site burning, and an aggravation of arterial hypertension.

Relative Frequency of Adverse Drug Reactions: Due to the small number of patient enrolled in clinical trials and the low number of ADRs no meaningful statement on the relative frequency can be made for each potential ADR.

Less Common Clinical Trial Adverse Drug Reactions: Due to the small number of patient enrolled in clinical trials and the low number of ADRs no meaningful statement on the relative frequency can be made for each potential ADR.

Abnormal Hematologic and Clinical Chemistry Findings: During the pharmacokinetic investigation in LEX-201 laboratory markers for coagulation activation and fibrinolysis were monitored (i.e. prothrombin fragment F1+2, thrombin-antithrombin III complex, fibrin monomers, d-dimers plasma levels, Prothrombin time (PT) and Activated partial thromboplastin time (aPTT)). No pattern of elevated markers was seen that could have been induced by the administration of octaplex.

In LEX-202, one patient had transient increases of ALAT and ASAT 12 hours after the last octaplex infusion. Five days after infusion the laboratory tests were back to normal. Otherwise, safety laboratory findings were not altered by octaplex injections.

In LEX-203, a slight decrease over time could be seen for haematological parameters (haematokrit, haemoglobin, blood cell count). Due to the main inclusion criteria for this study being the preparation of a surgical intervention or to control bleedings and the patient population studied (patients under oral anticoagulant therapy), almost all patients showed abnormal haematological values at baseline and during the subsequent sampling period. None of the clinical chemistry parameters seemed to be affected by the study medication.

Post-Market Adverse Drug Reactions: In course of a self-sufficiency programme, octaplex is used in Norway produced from Norwegian plasma for several FVII deficient patients and for a large number of patients in whom a rapid reversal of oral anticoagulant therapy was required. No ADRs have been reported, neither to the Norwegian health authority nor to the company.

Within the framework of post-marketing surveillance, 2 ADRs have been reported so far.

A 80-year-old patient with an INR of 7.8 and an acute bleed received 4000 IU of octaplex. One day later, he developed a peripheral ischemia and a transient ischemic attack.

The second case concerns a patient who received octaplex and red blood concentrate and developed restlessness, nausea and urticaria. Investigations revealed that the patient had HLA antibodies with a wide specificity. The reporter considered the causal relationship to octaplex as unlikely.

There have been no spontaneously reported cases in the post-marketing period that changed the risk/benefit ratio of the product.

DRUG INTERACTIONS: Overview: Human prothrombin complex products neutralise the effect of vitamin K antagonist treatment, but no interactions with other medicinal products are known. Nonetheless, octaplex should not be mixed with other medication during injection.

Interference with Biological Testing: When performing clotting tests, which are sensitive to heparin in patients receiving high doses of human prothrombin complex, the heparin as a constituent of the administered product must be taken into account.

Components used in the packaging of octaplex are latex-free.

Drug-Drug Interactions: Interactions with other drugs have not been established.

Drug-Food Interactions: Interactions with food have not been established.

Drug-Herb Interactions: Interactions with herbal products have not been established.

Drug-Laboratory Test Interactions: Interactions with laboratory tests have not been established.

DOSAGE AND ADMINISTRATION: Dosing Considerations:

- Classical dose-response studies were not performed due to the human origin of the product. Dose recommendations for single factor deficiencies are based on the required level, on the body weight (BW) of the patient and the activity increase per unit of the respective factor administered. For acquired deficiencies, dosing should also be individualised and preferably be accompanied by laboratory analysis of global and single coagulation parameters.
- Because of the risk of thromboembolic complications, close monitoring should be exercised when administering human prothrombin complex to patients with a history of coronary heart disease, myocardial infarction, to patients with liver disease, to peri- or postoperative patients, to neonates, or to patients at risk of thromboembolic events or disseminated intravascular coagulation (see Warnings and Precautions).

Recommended Dose and Dosage Adjustment: Only general dosage guidelines are given below. Treatment should be initiated under the supervision of a physician experienced in the treatment of coagulation disorders. The dosage and duration of the substitution therapy depend on the severity of the disorder, on the location and extent of the bleeding and on the patient's clinical condition.

The amount and the frequency of administration should be calculated on an individual patient basis. Dosage intervals must be adapted to the different circulating half-life of the different coagulation factors in the prothrombin complex.

Individual dosage requirements can only be identified on the basis of regular determinations of the individual plasma levels of the coagulation factors of interest, or on global tests of the prothrombin complex levels (prothrombin time, INR), and continuous monitoring of the clinical condition of the patient.

In case of major surgical interventions precise monitoring of the substitution therapy by means of coagulation assays is essential (specific coagulation factor assays and/or global tests for prothrombin complex levels).

Acquired Deficiencies: Bleeding and Perioperative Prophylaxis of Bleeding During Vitamin K Antagonist Treatment: The dose will depend on the INR before treatment and the targeted INR. In Table 2 approximate doses (mL/kg body weight of the reconstituted product) required for normalisation of INR (≤1.2 within 1 hour) at different initial INR levels are given.

Table 2: octaplex

Approximate Doses of octaplex Required for Normalization of INR

Initial INR	2–2.5	2.5–3	3–3.5	>3.5
Approximate dose[a] (mL octaplex/kg body weight)	0.9–1.3	1.3–1.6	1.6–1.9	>1.9

[a] The single dose should not exceed 3.000 IU (120 mL octaplex).

The correction of the vitamin K antagonist induced impairment of haemostasis persists for approximately 6-8 hours. However, the effects of vitamin K, if administered simultaneously, are usually achieved within 4-6 hours. Thus, repeated treatment with human prothrombin complex is not usually required when vitamin K has been administered.

As these recommendations are empirical and recovery and the duration of effect may vary, monitoring of INR treatment is mandatory.

Missed Dose: Acquired Deficiencies: Not applicable because in acquired deficiencies octaplex is administered in a hospital setting by health care professionals.

Administration: Dissolve the product (see Dosage and Administration, Reconstitution).

octaplex should be administered intravenously. The infusion should start at a speed of 1 mL per minute, followed by 2-3 mL per minute, using an aseptic technique.

As a precautionary measure, the patient's pulse rate should be measured before and during the injection. If a marked increase in the pulse rate occurs, the injection speed must be reduced or the administration must be interrupted.

Reconstitution: Please read all the instructions and follow them carefully.

During the procedure described below, aseptic technique must be maintained.

The product reconstitutes quickly at room temperature.

The solution should be colourless to slightly blue. Do not use solutions that are cloudy or have deposits. Reconstituted products should be inspected visually for particulate matter and discolouration prior to administration. A blue colour is not interpreted as discolouration.

Instructions for Reconstitution:

1. Warm the octaplex powder and water for injection (WFI) in the closed vials up to room temperature (maximum 37°C). This temperature should be maintained during reconstitution.
2. Remove the flip caps from the octaplex vial and the WFI vial and clean the rubber stoppers with an alcohol swab.
3. Peel away the lid of the outer package of the Mix2Vial transfer set. Place the WFI vial on an even surface and hold the vial firmly. Take the Mix2Vial together with its outer package and invert it. Push the blue plastic cannula of the Mix2Vial firmly through the rubber stopper of the WFI vial. While holding onto the WFI vial, carefully remove the outer package from the Mix2Vial, being careful to leave the Mix2Vial attached firmly to the WFI vial.
4. With the octaplex vial held firmly on an even surface, quickly invert the WFI vial (with the Mix2Vial attached) and push the transparent plastic cannula end of the Mix2Vial firmly through the stopper of the octaplex vial. The WFI will be drawn into the octaplex vial by vacuum.
5. With both vials still attached, slowly rotate the octaplex vial to ensure the product is fully dissolved to a clear or slightly opalescent solution. Once the contents of the octaplex vial are dissolved, firmly hold both the transparent and blue parts of the Mix2Vial. Unscrew the Mix2Vial into two separate pieces with the vials still attached) and discard the empty WFI vial and the blue part of the Mix2Vial.
6. Attach a plastic sterile disposable 20 mL syringe to the transparent part of Mix2Vial. Invert the system and draw the reconstituted octaplex into the syringe.
7. Once the octaplex solution has been transferred into the syringe, firmly hold the barrel of the syringe (keeping it facing down) and detach the Mix2Vial from the syringe. Discard the Mix2Vial (transparent plastic part) and the empty octaplex vial.

Incompatibility: octaplex should not be mixed with other medication in the same infusion set.

OVERDOSAGE:

The use of high doses of human prothrombin complex products has been associated with instances of myocardial infarction, disseminated intravascular coagulation (DIC), venous thrombosis and pulmonary embolism. Therefore, in case of overdose, the risk of development of thromboembolic complications or DIC is enhanced.

For management of a suspected drug overdose, CPhA recommends that you contact your **regional Poison Control Centre**. See the *CPS* Directory section for a list of Poison Control Centres.

ACTION AND CLINICAL PHARMACOLOGY: Mechanism of Action: The coagulation factors II, VII, IX and X, which are synthesised in the liver with the help of vitamin K, are commonly called the Prothrombin Complex. FII, FIX and FX are components of the intrinsic coagulation pathway, FVII is a component of the extrinsic pathway. These factors are synthesised in the liver in a vitamin K dependent way. Together they form the prothrombin complex. If one or more of these factors is deficient, the blood coagulation is impaired to such an extent that, depending on coagulation analysis, appropriate substitution therapy may be necessary.

The administration of human prothrombin complex provides an increase in plasma levels of the vitamin K dependent coagulation factors, and can temporarily correct the coagulation defect of patients with deficiency of one or several of these factors. octaplex contains, in addition to FII, FVII, FIX and FX, therapeutically effective concentrations of Protein C and Protein S, inhibitory enzymes of the coagulation pathway. Like the prothrombin complex factors, they are synthesised in the liver.

Acquired deficiency of the vitamin K dependant coagulation factors occurs during treatment with vitamin K antagonists. If the deficiency becomes severe, a severe bleeding tendency results, characterised by retroperitoneal or cerebral bleeds rather than muscle and joint haemorrhage. Severe hepatic insufficiency also results in markedly reduced levels of the vitamin K dependant coagulation factors and a clinical bleeding tendency which, however, is often complex due to a simultaneous ongoing low-grade intravascular coagulation, low platelet levels, deficiency of coagulation inhibitors and disturbed fibrinolysis.

The same mechanism of action applies for bleedings due to vitamin K deficiency, caused by disorders in vitamin K resorption because of biliary tract or pancreas disorders, persisting diarrhoea or massive antibiotic therapy. Therefore, octaplex can also be recommended for this indication.

Factor VII is the zymogen of the active serine protease factor VIIa by which the extrinsic pathway of blood coagulation is initiated. The tissue factor-factor VIIa complex activates coagulation factors X and IX, whereby factor IXa and Xa are formed. With further activation of the coagulation cascade, prothrombin (factor II) is activated and transformed to thrombin. By the action of thrombin, fibrinogen is converted to fibrin, which results in clot formation. The normal generation of thrombin is also of vital importance for platelet function as a part of the primary haemostasis.

Pharmacodynamics: Pharmacotherapeutic group: antihaemorrhagics, blood coagulation factors IX, II, VII, and X in combination. ATC code: B02BD01.

Classical dose-response studies were not performed due to the human origin of the product (see Action and Clinical Pharmacology, Mechanism of Action).

Pharmacokinetics: Absorption, Distribution, Metabolism, and Excretion: octaplex is administered intravenously and therefore immediately available in the organism.

The coagulation factors contained in octaplex are most likely removed by the hepatic reticuloendothelial system followed by degradation to individual amino acids by the normal intracellular processes of proteolytic hydrolysis.

STORAGE AND STABILITY: 2 years shelf-life. After reconstitution the solution must be used immediately.

Store at room temperature (+2 to +25°C). Do not freeze.

Protect from exposure to light.

SPECIAL HANDLING INSTRUCTIONS: Any unused product or waste material should be disposed of in accordance with local requirements.

INFORMATION FOR THE PATIENT: Published in e-CPS, available by subscription at www.e-cps.ca.

DOSAGE FORMS, COMPOSITION AND PACKAGING: Powder and solvent for solution for injection. octaplex nominally contains the components listed in Table 3.

Table 3: octaplex

Composition

Name of Ingredient	octaplex Quantity Per Vial (20 mL)	octaplex Quantity per mL Reconstituted Solution
Total protein	260–820 mg	13–41 mg/mL
Active Substances		
Human coagulation factor II	280–760 IU	14–38 IU/ mL
Human coagulation factor VII	180–480 IU	9–24 IU/ mL
Human coagulation factor IX	500 IU	25 IU/ mL
Human coagulation factor X	360–600 IU	18–30 IU/ mL
Further Active Ingredients		
Protein C	140–620 IU	7–31 IU/ mL
Protein S	140–640 IU	7–32 IU/ mL
Excipients		
Heparin	80–310 IU	4–15.5 IU/ mL
Sodium Citrate	17.0–27.0 mmol/L	

Factor IX specific activity is ≥0.6 IU/ mg proteins.
Further excipient: Solvent (Water for Injections).
Small amounts of the S/D reagents TNBP (≤5 µg/mL) and Polysorbate 80 (≤50 µg/mL) may remain in the finished product. These substances are added during the manufacturing process because of their capacity to inactivate lipid-enveloped viruses.

Nature and Contents of Kit: One package of octaplex contains: powder in a vial (type I glass) with a stopper (halobutyl rubber) and a flip off cap (aluminium); 20 mL of solvent in a vial (type I glass) with a stopper (halobutyl rubber) and a flip off cap (aluminium); Mix2Vial transfer set with integrated filter.

Octostim®

desmopressin acetate

Antihemorrhagic

Ferring

Date of Revision: December 7, 2009

SUMMARY PRODUCT INFORMATION:

Route of Administration	Dosage Form/ Strength	Nonmedicinal Ingredients
Intravenous	15 µg/mL	Hydrochloric acid, purified water, sodium chloride
Intranasal	1.5 mg/mL (each metered dose delivers 150 µg/spray)	Benzalkonium chloride solution, citric acid monohydrate, disodium phosphate dihydrate, purified water, sodium chloride

INDICATIONS AND CLINICAL USE: OCTOSTIM injection and nasal spray are indicated for:

- The prevention of bleeding in patients with mild hemophilia A and mild von Willebrand's disease Type I.

OCTOSTIM injection is indicated for:

- The prevention or treatment of bleeding in patients with uremia.

Hemophilia A: OCTOSTIM is indicated for patients with hemophilia A with Factor VIII levels greater than 5%.

OCTOSTIM will often maintain hemostasis in patients with hemophilia A during surgical procedures and postoperatively, when injected 30 minutes prior to or administered by nasal spray 2 hours prior to the scheduled procedure.

OCTOSTIM will also stop bleeding in hemophilia A patients with episodes of spontaneous or trauma-induced injuries such as hemarthroses, intramuscular hematomas or mucosal bleeding. In certain clinical situations, it may be justified to try OCTOSTIM in patients with Factor VIII levels between 2-5%, however, these patients should be carefully monitored.

Von Willebrand's Disease (Type I): OCTOSTIM injection is indicated for patients with mild to moderate classic von Willebrand's Disease (Type I) with Factor VIII levels greater than 5%. OCTOSTIM will often maintain hemostasis in surgical procedures and postoperatively when administered 30 minutes prior to, or administered by nasal spray 2 hours prior to the scheduled procedure.

OCTOSTIM will usually stop bleeding in mild to moderate von Willebrand's patients with episodes of spontaneous or trauma-induced injuries such as hemarthroses, intramuscular hematomas or mucosal bleeding.

Those von Willebrand's disease patients who are least likely to respond are those with severe homozygous von Willebrand's disease with Factor VIII antigen and von Willebrand's Factor (ristocetin cofactor) activities less than 1%. Other patients may respond in a variable fashion depending on the type of molecular defect they have. Bleeding time and Factor VIII coagulant activity, Factor VIII antigen and von Willebrand's Factor activities should be checked during administration of OCTOSTIM to ensure that adequate levels are being achieved.

OCTOSTIM is not indicated for the treatment of severe classic Type I von Willebrand's disease and Type II B and when there is evidence of an abnormal molecular form of Factor VIII antigen (see Contraindications).

Other Hemostatic Disorders: OCTOSTIM injection is indicated for the treatment of prolonged bleeding time in patients with uremia. It will assist in the maintenance of hemostasis in such patients during surgical procedures and post operatively when administered prior to the procedure.

Therapeutic efficacy (i.e. normalization of bleeding time) should be established in individual patients at the time of diagnosis of the bleeding disorder, or at least 72 hours prior to an elective treatment, by administration of a test dose of OCTOSTIM (see Warnings and Precautions, Monitoring and Laboratory Tests).

CONTRAINDICATIONS: OCTOSTIM is contraindicated in patients with known hypersensitivity to desmopressin acetate, the nasal spray is also contraindicated patients with known hypersensitivity to the preservative.

Because of the risk of platelet aggregation and thrombocytopenia, OCTOSTIM should not be used patients with type II B or platelet-type (pseudo) von Willebrand's disease.

OCTOSTIM should not be used in patients with cardiac insufficiency, or other conditions requiring treatment with diuretic agents.

OCTOSTIM nasal spray should not be used in cases of habitual and psychogenic polydipsia.

WARNINGS AND PRECAUTIONS: OCTOSTIM (desmopressin acetate) treatment without concomitant restriction of water intake may lead to water retention with accompanying signs and symptoms (reduced serum sodium, weight gain, and, in serious cases, convulsions). Other signs include persistent headache and nausea. If these symptoms are present, serum sodium must be checked. Should there be a decrease of serum sodium to below 130 mmol/L or plasma osmolality to below 270 mOsm/kg body weight, the fluid intake must be reduced drastically and the administration of OCTOSTIM interrupted.

Precautions to prevent fluid overload must be taken in:

- the very young and elderly patients
- conditions characterized by fluid and/or electrolyte imbalance
- patients at risk for increased intracranial pressure

Particular attention should be paid to the possibility of the rare occurrence of an extreme decrease in plasma osmolality that may result in seizures, which could lead to coma.

OCTOSTIM must be used with caution in patients prone to vascular headaches, and patients with coronary insufficiency and hypertensive cardiovascular diseases because of possible changes in blood pressure and tachycardia.

Rapid infusion rates may result in severe hypotension; therefore, the speed of intravenous infusion of OCTOSTIM should not be shorter than 20-30 minutes. A maximum dose of 0.3 µg/kg should not be exceeded.

Lack of therapeutic effect has been noted in patients who have been febrile or otherwise "stressed" for several days. Whenever possible, therapeutic efficacy (i.e., Factor VIII response in hemophilia and bleeding time correction in other disorders) should be established in individual patients prior to use and followed throughout the course of treatment. The coincident use of anti-fibrinolytic agents to counteract desmopressin-induced plasminogen activator release has been recommended, however, benefit has not been clearly established.

OCTOSTIM should not be used to treat patients with Type IIB von Willebrand's disease since platelet aggregation may be induced (see Contraindications).

OCTOSTIM should not be used in patients with Hemophilia B because it has no effect on Factor IX levels.

OCTOSTIM has no therapeutic effect in Glazmann's thrombaesthenia.

OCTOSTIM does not reduce prolonged bleeding time in thrombocytopenia.

OCTOSTIM spray should not be used when the intranasal route may be compromised. These situations include changes in the nasal mucosa such as scarring, edema, nasal congestion and blockage, nasal discharge, atrophy of nasal mucosa, and severe atrophic rhinitis. These conditions may lead to unreliable absorption. Intranasal delivery may also be inappropriate where there is an impaired level of consciousness. For such situations, OCTOSTIM injection should be used.

Tachyphylaxis may develop with repeated use.

There have been rare reports of thrombotic events (thrombosis, acute cerebrovascular thrombosis, acute myocardial infarction) following desmopressin acetate injection in patients predisposed to thrombus formation. No causality has been determined; however, the drug should be used with caution in these patients.

Severe allergic reactions have been reported rarely. Fatal anaphylaxis has been reported in one patient who received intravenous OCTOSTIM. It is not known whether antibodies to desmopressin acetate are produced after repeated administration.

OCTOSTIM has an antidiuretic effect. Patients receiving this drug should be cautioned to reduce their ingestion of fluids for at least 6 hours after receiving the drug. Patients receiving intravenous fluids must be placed on fluid input/output monitoring.

Safety and effectiveness of OCTOSTIM Spray in children under 11 months has not been demonstrated.

It is not known whether this drug is excreted in human milk. Because many drugs are excreted in human milk, caution should be exercised when OCTOSTIM spray is administered to a nursing woman.

General: OCTOSTIM (desmopressin acetate) produces changes in blood pressure; either an elevation or a decrease and a compensatory tachycardia. Subcutaneous and intranasal administration usually results in a slight change that is transient. Greater changes may occur with intravenous infusion, especially if administered rapidly (see Warnings and Precautions). It should, therefore, be used with caution in patients with coronary artery insufficiency and/or hypertensive cardiovascular disease.

Before the initial therapeutic administration of OCTOSTIM Spray, the physician should establish that the patient shows an appropriate change in the coagulation profile following a test dose of intranasal administration of OCTOSTIM Spray.

OCTOSTIM should not be administered to dehydrated patients until water balance has been adequately restored.

OCTOSTIM should be used with caution in patients with cystic fibrosis because these patients are prone to hyponatremia. Children and geriatric patients should be closely observed for possible water retention due to over ingestion of fluids.

Special Populations: Pregnant Women: There are no adequate and well-controlled studies in pregnant women. Published reports stress that, as opposed to preparations containing the natural hormone, desmopressin acetate in antidiuretic doses has no uterotonic action, but the physician will have to weigh the possible therapeutic advantage against potential danger in each case.

Reproduction studies performed in rats and rabbits have revealed no evidence of harm to the fetus due desmopressin acetate. Subcutaneous doses up to 4 times the human dose for Factor VIII stimulation on a mg/m² basis (or 12.5 times the human dose on a mg/kg basis) and doses up to 4 times the human dose for diabetes insipidus on a mg/m² basis (or 12.5 times the human dose on a mg/kg basis) were studied. There are several publications of management of diabetes insipidus in pregnant women with no harm to the fetus reported.

Published data on a limited number (n=53) of exposed pregnancies in women with diabetes insipidus indicate no adverse effects of desmopressin on pregnancy or on the health of the foetus/newborn child. To date, no other relevant epidemiological data are available. Animal studies do not indicate direct or indirect harmful effects with respect to pregnancy, embryonal/foetal development, parturition or postnatal development.

Caution should be exercised when prescribing to pregnant women.

Nursing Women: There have been not controlled studies in nursing mothers. A single study on a post-partum woman demonstrated a marked change in plasma desmopressin acetate level following an intranasal dose of 10 µg, but little drug was detectable in breast milk. (See Warnings and Precautions.)

Results from analyses of milk from nursing mothers receiving a high dose of desmopressin (300 µg intranasally), indicate that the amounts of desmopressin that may be transferred to the child are considerably less than the amounts required to influence diuresis.

Pediatrics: No controlled trials have been conducted in children with renal insufficiency.

Use in infants and children will require careful fluid intake restriction to prevent possible hyponatremia and water intoxication. No controlled trials have been conducted in infants under 3 months of age with von Willebrand's disease or Hemophilia A. The physician should weigh possible therapeutic advantages against potential risks in each case. OCTOSTIM Spray should not be used in infants younger than 11 months in the treatment of hemophilia A or von Willebrand's disease.

Monitoring and Laboratory Tests: Hemophilia A: Laboratory tests for assessing patient status include levels of Factor VIII coagulant, Factor VIII antigen and Factor VIII ristocetin cofactor (von Willebrand factor) as well as activated partial thromboplastin time. Factor VIII coagulant activity should be determined before giving OCTOSTIM for hemostasis. If Factor VIII coagulant activity is present at less than 5% of normal, OCTOSTIM should not be relied upon alone.

von Willebrand's Disease: Laboratory tests for assessing patient status include levels of Factor VIII coagulant, Factor VIII antigen and Factor VIII ristocetin cofactor (von Willebrand factor). The skin bleeding time may be helpful in following these patients and should always be assessed pre-operatively.

Uremia: A test dose of OCTOSTIM should be administered at the time of diagnosis of the bleeding disorder, or at least 72 hours prior to an elective treatment. The skin bleeding times should be measured before and 1 hour after OCTOSTIM administration.

ADVERSE REACTIONS: Adverse Drug Reaction Overview: OCTOSTIM has produced transient headache, nausea, facial flushing, tachycardia, hypotention, oliguria, abdominal cramps and vulvar pain. Nasal congestion and rhinitis have also been reported with the nasal spray formulation. The frequency varies with the dosage and the route of administration.

Side effects following intravenous administration to 297 patients included transient facial flushing (approximately 18%), fatigue (3%), headache (2%), and oliguria (1%). Other effects reported at a frequency of less than 1% included nausea, dizziness, syncope and abdominal cramping.

Side effects following subcutaneous administration to 190 subjects included transient facial flushing (7%). Other effects reported at a frequency of less than 1% included hypotension, transient headache, abdominal tension, nausea, tachycardia and discomfort at the injection site.

Side effects following intranasal administration to 78 patients included facial flushing and warmth (24%), dizziness or headache (13%), palpitations (9%), nausea (6%), fatigue (6%), red eyes (4%), decreased diuresis (3%), nasal congestion, rhinitis, tachycardia. Other effects reported at a frequency of less than 1% include abdominal cramps, allergic reactions both to desmopressin and to the preservative, somnolence.

Severe hypotension was observed in some patients who received OCTOSTIM intravenously during cardiac surgical procedures and this may have resulted from rapid infusion rates. A dosage of 0.3 µg/kg should not be exceeded, and the infusion rate of 20 to 30 minutes should not be exceeded.

See Warnings and Precautions for the possibility of water intoxication and hyponatremia. Very occasionally, intravenous injection of OCTOSTIM has produced local erythema, swelling or burning pain along the course of the vein.

DRUG INTERACTIONS: Overview: Although the pressor activity of desmopressin acetate is very low, its use with other pressor agents should be done only with careful patient monitoring.

DDAVP (desmopressin acetate) injection has been used with epsilon aminocaproic acid without adverse events.

Substances which are known to release antidiuretic hormone, e.g., tricyclic antidepressants, chlorpromazine, carbamazepine, chlorpropamide, urea, fludrocortisone, may cause an additive antidiuretic effect and increase the risk of water retention. Desmopressin should be used cautiously in patients who are receiving lithium, large doses of epinephrine, demeclocycline, heparin or alcohol, because the antidiuretic response to desmopressin may be decreased.

Concurrent administration of clofibrate with desmopressin reportedly potentiates and prolongs the antidiuretic effect of desmopressin.

Indomethacin may augment the magnitude but not the duration of the response to desmopressin.

DOSAGE AND ADMINISTRATION: Administration: OCTOSTIM injection is administered by subcutaneous injection or as an intravenous infusion over 20 to 30 minutes to provide a dose of 0.3 µg/kg. The maximum intravenous dose is 20 µg. If OCTOSTIM injection is used pre-operatively, it should be administered 30 minutes prior to the scheduled procedure. The peak effect is obtained one hour after administration. Response is immediate for bleeding time reduction.

Dilution for Infusion: Dilute in sterile physiological saline and infuse slowly over 20 to 30 minutes. In adults and children weighing more than 10 kg, 50 mL of diluent is used; in children weighing 10 kg or less, 10 mL of diluent is used.

OCTOSTIM spray is administered by nasal inhalation, one spray per nostril, to provide a total dose of 300 µg. In patients weighing less than 50 kg, 150 µg is administered as a single spray to provide the expected effect on Factor VIII coagulant activity, Factory VIII ristocetin cofactor activity and skin bleeding time. If OCTOSTIM spray is used pre-operatively, it should be administered 2 hours prior to the scheduled procedure.

The necessity for repeat administration of OCTOSTIM or use of any blood products for hemostasis should be determined by laboratory response, as well as the clinical condition of the patient. The tendency toward tachyphylaxis (lessening of response) with repeated administration, given more frequently than every 48 hours should be considered in treating each patient.

OVERDOSAGE:

OCTOSTIM (desmopressin acetate) at excessive doses may cause headaches, abdominal cramps, nausea and facial flushing. In such cases the dosage should be reduced, frequency of administration decreased, or the drug withdrawn according to the severity of the condition. Rapid intravenous infusion may cause hypotension. A maximum intravenous dose of 0.3 µg/kg should not be exceeded. The infusion rate of 20 to 30 minutes should not be exceeded.

There is no known specific antidote for OCTOSTIM. Water intoxication responds rapidly to diuretic therapy (e.g., furosemide) and appropriate replacement fluid support, without interference with hemostatic effects.

Overdosage increases the risk of fluid retention and hyponatremia. Although the treatment of hyponatremia should be individualized, the following general recommendations can be given. Asymptomatic hyponatremia is treated with discontinuation of desmopressin treatment and fluid restriction. Infusion of isotonic or hypertonic sodium chloride may be added in cases with symptoms. When fluid retention is serious (convulsions and unconsciousness), treatment with furosemide should be added.

For management of a suspected drug overdose, contact your regional Poison Control Centre. See the *CPS* Directory section for a list of Poison Control Centres.

ACTION AND CLINICAL PHARMACOLOGY: Mechanism of Action: OCTOSTIM (desmopressin acetate) is a synthetic structural analogue of the natural human hormone, arginine vasopressin with deamination of 1-cysteine and substitution of 8-L-arginine by 8-D-arginine.

OCTOSTIM administration causes a transient increase in all components of the Factor VIII complex (Factor VIII coagulant activity, Factor VIII related antigen, and ristocetin cofactor) and in plasminogen activator. Either directly or indirectly, OCTOSTIM causes these factors to be released very rapidly from their endothelial cell storage sites. In addition, OCTOSTIM may have a direct effect on the vessel wall, with increased platelet spreading and adhesion at injury sites.

A second dose given before endothelial cell stores are replenished will not have as great an effect as the initial dose. Responses as great as the initial one usually are seen if 48 hours or more have elapsed between doses.

The pharmacokinetic and pharmacodynamic profiles after subcutaneous or intravenous administration to healthy volunteers are equivalent. The plasma half-life following subcutaneous, intravenous and intranasal administration ranges from 3.2 to 3.6 hours.

Pharmacodynamics: Desmopressin causes a dose-dependent increase in plasma Factor VIII (antihemophilic factor), plasminogen activator, and, to a smaller degree, Factor VIII-related antigen and ristocetin cofactor activities. The mechanism by which desmopressin lowers bleeding time remains speculative.

Structural modifications of vasopressin present in desmopressin result in reduced smooth muscle contracting and vasopressor properties compared with vasopressin and lypressin. Initial studies of intranasal desmopressin at a subtherapeutic dose of 20 µg resulted in no effect on blood pressure or pulse rate, but mean arterial pressure increases as much as 15 mm Hg were observed with doses of 40 µg or more. In the therapeutic dose range, cardiovascular changes in normal, healthy volunteers were not considered to be clinically meaningful, but 27 of 32 volunteers had notable changes in systolic and/or diastolic blood pressure, and 8 had notable changes in pulse. Some volunteers experienced increases in diastolic blood pressure of greater than or equal to 20%; one volunteer experienced an increase in systolic blood pressure of 35% (40 mm Hg); and others experienced decreases in diastolic blood pressure, in some cases with compensatory tachycardia.

Desmopressin has been shown to interact with renal (V_2) vasopressin receptors which mediate its antidiuretic effect on renal tubes. The extrarenal effects of desmopressin in normal persons, which include stimulation of the release of Factor VIII coagulant and von Willebrand factory (ristocetin cofactor) and a decrease in blood pressure, may be mediated by interaction with receptors in other tissues which are similar to the renal V_2 receptors.

Desmopressin has not been reported to stimulate uterine contractions.

Injection: Dose-response studies were performed in healthy persons, using doses of 0.1 to 0.4 µg/kg. OCTOSTIM provokes an average increase in Factor VIII coagulant activity two to five times baseline levels.

Plasminogen activator activity increases about threefold, after OCTOSTIM infusion, but is of such short duration of action that there has been no clinically significant fibrinolysis in patients treated with OCTOSTIM. The Factor VIII related antigen and ristocetin cofactor activity were also increased to a smaller degree, but still were dose dependent. The above responses reach a maximum at a point ranging from one to two hours.

The effect of repeated OCTOSTIM administration when doses were given every 12 to 24 hours has generally shown a gradual diminution of the Factor VIII activity increase, noted with a single dose. The initial dose is reproducible in any particular patient if there are 2 or 3 days between administration, when endothelial cell storage sites are replenished.

The percentage increase of Factor VIII levels in patient with mild haemophilia A and von Willebrand's disease was not significantly different from that observed in normal healthy individuals when treated with 0.3 µg/kg of OCTOSTIM infused over 10 minutes.

Desmopressin has also reportedly increased Factor VIII activity and to a lesser extent, Factor VIII related antigen and ristocetin cofactor in patients with uremia; these changes were accompanied by a shortening of bleeding time. In addition, the drug induced release into the plasma of the larger multimers of Factor VIII/von Willebrand factor in these patients.

Nasal Spray: Dose-response studies were performed in healthy persons using doses of 150 to 450 µg administered as one to three sprays. The response is dose-related, with maximal plasma levels of 150 to 250 percent of initial concentration achieved for both Factor VIII and von Willebrand factor. The increase is rapid and evident within 30 minutes, reaching a maximum at about 1.5 hours.

In patients with von Willebrand's disease, levels of Factor VIII coagulant activity and von Willebrand's factor antigen remained greater than 30 U/dL for 8 hours after a 300 µg dose of OCTOSTIM spray.

After 300 µg of OCTOSTIM spray, the percentage increase of Factor VIII and von Willebrand factor levels in patients with mild hemophilia A and von Willebrand's disease was less than observed after 0.3 µg/kg of intravenous OCTOSTIM.

In a trial comparing intranasal and intravenous Desmopressin in patients with mild/moderate hemophilia A or von Willebrand's disease, an intranasal dose of 300 µg desmopressin resulted in a 54% and 75% respective increase in Factor VIII:C and von Willebrand antigen, compared to intravenous desmopressin. The mean maximum percent decrease in bleeding time following intranasal desmopressin was 1.5 times that observed following intravenous desmopressin.

Intranasal desmopressin was tested for prevention and therapy of bleeding complications in mild Factor VIII deficiency when these individuals were undergoing various procedures (surgery, dental extraction etc.), Factor VIII:C levels increased above baseline after intranasal administration of desmopressin. The change in levels was evident after 15 minutes, and peaked at 2 hours after dosing.

Desmopressin 300 µg intranasally generally leads to at least a twofold increase in plasma of factor VIII coagulant activity (VIII:C). Also the content of von Willebrand factor-antigen (vWF:Ag) increases, but to a lesser extent. At the same time there is a release of plasminogen activator (PA).

A prolonged bleeding time is shortened to the same extent after doses of either 300 µg desmopressin intranasally, or intravenous doses of 0.3 µg/kg body weight.

Pharmacokinetics: Injection: Following IV infusion of desmopressin, the increase in plasma Factor VIII activity occurs within 15-30 minutes and peaks between 90 minutes and 3 hours after administration; the increase in Factor VIII activity is dose dependent, with a 300-400% maximum increase reportedly occurring after IV infusion of 0.4 µg/kg dose. Plasma Factor VIII-related antigen activity has also been reported to peak within 3 hours after IV infusion of the drug. The subcutaneous route of OCTOSTIM administered has been compared with the intravenous route in healthy volunteers and found to produce a bioequivalent response in terms of pharmacokinetic profile.

Desmopressin acetate was administered to 10 healthy volunteers in a randomized cross-over study at a dose of 0.4 µg/kg by intravenous infusion and subcutaneous injection. The pharmacokinetic data are summarized in Table 1.

Table 1: OCTOSTIM

Pharmacokinetics of OCTOSTIM after Subcutaneous and Intravenous Administration to 10 Healthy Volunteers. Mean±S.D.

Dose and Route of Administration	AUC (pg/h/mL^{-1})	C_{max} (pg/mL)	T_{max} (min)	Half-life (min^{-1})
0.4 µg/kg i.v.	3109±1056			3.62±0.42
0.4 µg/kg s.c. (4 µg/mL ampoule)	3492±659	568±203	87±66	3.50±0.39
0.4 µg/kg s.c. (40 µg/mL ampoule)	3164±393	544±46	60±7	3.17±0.33

Subcutaneous administration of OCTOSTIM showed the same plasma half-life, from 3.2 to 3.6 hours, as intravenous OCTOSTIM. The plasma profile indicates that the elimination of OCTOSTIM from plasma follow first order kinetics. There is no significant difference in AUC between subcutaneous and intravenous OCTOSTIM. A similar study in 14 hemophiliac patients also showed that the subcutaneous route of administration is bioequivalent to the intravenous route.

Nasal Spray: The bioavailability relative to intravenous administration is about 3-5%. Maximum plasma concentration following a dose of 300 µg is reached after approximately 1 hour and amounts to 400 pg/mL on average. The half-life of OCTOSTIM spray was between 3.3 and 3.5 hours, over the range of intranasal doses, 150 to 450 µg. Plasma concentrations of OCTOSTIM spray were maximal, approximately 40 to 45 minutes after dosing.

STORAGE AND STABILITY: OCTOSTIM injection should be stored at refrigerator temperature 2-8°C. Do not freeze.

OCTOSTIM spray should be stored at 15-25°C. Do not freeze.

SPECIAL HANDLING INSTRUCTIONS: Diluted Solutions: Continuous Intravenous Infusion: For intravenous infusion of OCTOSTIM in adults and children weighing 10 kg or more, a dose of 0.3 µg/kg should be drawn up into a syringe, and added to an IV bag containing 50 mL of sterile physiological saline.

For children weighing less than 10 kg, a dose of 0.3 µg/kg should be added to 10 mL of sterile physiological saline.

It is recommended that the storage of the diluted solutions at room temperature does not exceed 24 hours.

INFORMATION FOR THE PATIENT: Published in e-CPS, available by subscription at www.e-cps.ca.

DOSAGE FORMS, COMPOSITION AND PACKAGING: Injection: Each mL contains: desmopressin acetate 15 µg with sodium chloride and hydrochloric acid to adjust the pH to 3.5, in water for injection. Clear glass ampoules of 1 mL, with a red identification ring and a blue dot indicating the cut area, cartons of 10.

Instructions for Opening Ampoules:

1. Hold ampoule with blue dot pointing upwards. Shake or tap ampoule to empty the tip.
2. With blue dot pointing upwards, snap off tip by forcing it downwards.

Spray: Each mL contains: desmopressin acetate 1.5 mg, benzalkonium chloride (preservative), citric acid monohydrate, disodium phosphate dihydrate, purified water, and sodium chloride. Glass bottles of 2.5 mL furnished with a pre-compression pump with applicator and protective cap. The spray pump is designed to give 100 µL (0.1 mL or 150 µg desmopressin acetate) per activation. The nasal pump can only deliver doses of 150 µg or multiple doses of 150 µg. If doses other than these are required, the injection may be used.

The reader is invited to consult CPhA's monograph **Fluoroquinolones**.

Ocuflox™ Ⓟ

ofloxacin

Antibacterial

Allergan

PHARMACOLOGY: The primary mechanism of action of ofloxacin appears to be the specific inhibition of DNA gyrase (topoisomerase II). This enzyme is responsible for the negative supercoiling of bacterial DNA and consequently for its topological configuration, governing functions such as RNA transcription, protein synthesis, DNA replication and repair functions.

INDICATIONS: For the treatment of conjunctivitis when caused by susceptible strains of the following bacteria: Gram-positive bacteria: *S. aureus*, *S. epidermidis*, *S. pneumoniae*. Gram-negative bacteria: *H. influenzae*.

CONTRAINDICATIONS: In patients with a history of hypersensitivity to ofloxacin or to any of the components of this medication. A history of hypersensitivity to other quinolones also contraindicates use of ofloxacin.

WARNINGS: Ofloxacin ophthalmic solution is not for injection into the eye.

PRECAUTIONS: General: Prolonged use of ofloxacin ophthalmic solution may result in overgrowth of nonsusceptible organisms, including fungi. Whenever clinical judgment dictates, the patient should be examined with the aid of magnification, such as slit lamp biomicroscopy and, where appropriate, fluorescein staining.

In patients receiving systemic quinolone therapy, serious and occasionally fatal hypersensitivity (anaphylactic) reactions, some following the first dose, have been reported. Some reactions were accompanied by cardiovascular collapse, loss of consciousness, tingling, angioedema (including laryngeal, pharyngeal or facial edema), airway obstruction, dyspnea, urticaria, and itching. Only a few patients had a history of hypersensitivity reactions. Serious anaphylactic reactions may require immediate emergency treatment with epinephrine. Oxygen, i.v. steroids and airway management, including intubation, should be administered as clinically indicated.

The systemic administration of quinolones has led to lesions or erosions of the cartilage in weight-bearing joints and other signs of arthropathy in immature animals of various species. Ofloxacin, administered systemically at 10 mg/kg/day in young dogs (equivalent to 150 times the maximum recommended daily adult ophthalmic dose), has been associated with these types of effects.

Pregnancy: There have been no adequate and well-controlled studies performed in pregnant women. Since systemic quinolones have been shown to cause arthropathy in immature animals, ofloxacin should be used during pregnancy only if the potential benefit justifies the potential risk to the fetus.

Lactation: Because ofloxacin taken systemically is excreted in breast milk, and there is potential for harm to nursing infants, a decison should be made whether to temporarily discontinue nursing during therapy or not to administer the drug, taking into account the importance of the drug to the mother.

Children: Safety and effectiveness of ofloxacin in children have not been established.

Geriatrics: No comparative data are available with topical ofloxacin therapy in this age category versus other age groups.

Drug Interactions: Specific drug interaction studies have not been conducted with ofloxacin ophthalmic solution. Interactions between ofloxacin and caffeine have not been detected. Systemic use of ofloxacin with nonsteroidal anti-inflammatory drugs has shown that the risk of CNS stimulation and convulsive seizures may increase. A pharmacokinetic study in 15 healthy males has shown that the steady-state peak theophylline concentration increased by an average of approximately 9% and the AUC increased by an average of approximately 13% when oral ofloxacin and theophylline were administered concurrently.

ADVERSE EFFECTS: Ophthalmic Use of Ofloxacin: The most frequently reported drug-related adverse reaction was transient ocular burning or discomfort. Other reported reactions were ocular redness, stinging, itching, photophobia, tearing and dryness. One report of dizziness, one report of headache and one spontaneous report of toxic epidermal necrolyis have also been received.

Systemic Effects of Ofloxacin: As with all topical ophthalmic drugs, the potential exists for systemic effects. Ofloxacin used systemically has rarely been associated with serious side effects. Serious reactions reported for systemic dosing of ofloxacin include convulsions and increased intracranial pressure. For the oral dosage form of ofloxacin, gastrointestinal symptoms, mainly nausea/vomiting, pain/discomfort, diarrhea and anorexia, were reported most frequently, followed by CNS events (such as dizziness and headaches) and dermatological or hypersensitivity reactions. Photophobia was reported rarely in clinical trials with systemic ofloxacin and phototoxicity has been reported with other drugs in this class.

OVERDOSE:

Symptoms: In the event of accidental ingestion of 10 mL of ofloxacin ophthalmic solution 0.3%, only 30 mg of ofloxacin would be ingested. Although this amount may not be clinically significant in terms of overdosage, there could be an increased potential for systemic reactions.

A topical overdosage of ofloxacin ophthalmic solution is considered a remote possibility. Discontinue medication if heavy or protracted use is suspected. In the event of a topical overdose, flush the eye with a topical ocular irrigant.

Treatment: See Symptoms.

> For management of a suspected drug overdose, CPhA recommends that you contact your **regional Poison Control Centre**. See the *CPS* Directory section for a list of Poison Control Centres.

DOSAGE: 1 to 2 drops every 2 to 4 hours for the first 2 days, and then 4 times daily in the affected eye(s) for 8 days.

If superinfection occurs or if clinical improvement is not noted with 7 days, discontinue use and institute appropriate therapy.

Patients should be advised to avoid contamination of the dropper tip.

Use while wearing contact lenses: The use of ofloxacin ophthalmic solution while wearing contact lenses has not been studied. Therefore, its use is not recommended while the lens is on the eye.

INFORMATION FOR THE PATIENT: Published in e-CPS, available by subscription at www.e-cps.ca.

SUPPLIED: Each bottle contains: ofloxacin 0.3% as a sterile, ophthalmic solution. Nonmedicinal ingredients: benzalkonium chloride 0.005% (as preservative), sodium chloride, hydrochloric acid and/or sodium hydroxide to adjust the pH and purified water. Plastic dropper bottles of 5 mL. Ofloxacin ophthalmic solution is sterile in the unopened package, and is stable for 24 months when stored at 15 to 25°C.

Odan K-20

potassium chloride

Potassium Supplement

Odan

SUPPLIED: Each sustained-release, capsule-shaped, white to off-white tablet imprinted "O-K20" on one side, contains: potassium chloride 1500 mg (20 mEq). Nonmedicinal ingredients: acrylates copolymer, colloidal silicon dioxide, hypromellose, polyethylene glycol, polysorbate 80, polyvinyl alcohol, sodium bicarbonate, sodium lauryl sulfate, stearic acid and talc. Contains no preservatives, artificial flavor, lactose, yeast, sugar, starch, gluten or tartrazine. Plastic bottles of 100 and 500. Keep tightly closed. Store at room temperature (15 to 30°C).

Oesclim® Ⓟ

estradiol hemihydrate

Estrogen

Triton Pharma

SUPPLIED: Oesclim 25: Each rectangular (11 cm²) transdermal system, with rounded corners, consisting of a transparent adhesive layer laminated onto a beige foam backing, contains: estradiol hemidydrate corresponding to 5 mg estradiol for delivery of estradiol 25 µg/24 h. Nonmedicinal ingredients (adhesive formulation containing estradiol): dipropylene glycol, ethylcellulose, ethylene/vinyl acetate copolymer and octyl dodecanol. Patient Packs of 8 systems.

Oesclim 50: Each rectangular (22 cm²) transdermal system, with rounded corners, consisting of a transparent adhesive layer laminated onto a beige foam backing, contains: estradiol hemidydrate corresponding to 10 mg estradiol for delivery of estradiol 50 µg/24 h. Nonmedicinal ingredients (adhesive formulation containing estradiol): dipropylene glycol, ethylcellulose, ethylene/vinyl acetate copolymer and octyl dodecanol. Patient Packs of 8 systems.

Oesclim patches are made up of a self-adhesive polymer matrix, which contains the estradiol, backed onto a rectangular foam mounting with rounded corners. The adhesive surface is covered by a transparent silicone-treated protective film which must be removed before use (peelable release liner). This system provides excellent local tolerability and adhesion.

The active component of the system is estradiol. The drug matrix provides a source for continuous delivery of drug for at least 4 days. The composition of each of the systems per unit area is identical.

Store at room temperature (15 to 25°C). Avoid freezing. Do not store unpouched. Apply immediately upon removal from the protective pouch. Keep out of the reach of children both before and after use. After removal of the patch fold it in half, with the adhesive side inwards, before discarding.

Ofloxacin Ⓟ

CPhA Monograph

see *Fluoroquinolones*

Ogen® Ⓟ

estropipate

Estrogen

Pfizer

Date of Revision: May 25, 2009

SUMMARY PRODUCT INFORMATION:

Route of Administration	Dosage Form/ Strength	Clinically Relevant Nonmedicinal Ingredients
Oral	Tablets/0.75 mg, 1.5 mg, 3 mg	Lactose (see Warnings and Precautions, Endocrine and Metabolism, Other Conditions).

INDICATIONS AND CLINICAL USE: OGEN (estropipate, USP) is indicated for the treatment of menopausal and post-menopausal symptoms. OGEN should be prescribed with an appropriate dosage of a progestin for women with intact uteri in order to prevent endometrial hyperplasia/carcinoma.

Pediatrics (<16 years of age): Safety and effectiveness of OGEN in paediatric patients have not been established (see Warnings and Precautions, Special Populations, Pediatrics).

CONTRAINDICATIONS: Estrogen & Estrogen/Progestin combinations are contraindicated in patients with any of the following disorders:

- Liver dysfunction or disease as long as liver function tests have failed to return to normal.
- Known or suspected estrogen-dependent or progestin-dependent malignant neoplasia (e.g. endometrial cancer).
- Known, suspected, or past history of breast cancer.
- Endometrial hyperplasia.
- Undiagnosed abnormal genital bleeding.
- Known or suspected pregnancy.
- Active or past history of arterial thomboembolic disease (e.g., stroke, myocardial infarction, coronary heart disease).
- Classical migraine.
- Active or past history of confirmed venous thromboembolism (such as deep venous thrombosis or pulmonary embolism) or active thrombophlebitis.
- Partial or complete loss of vision due to ophthalmic vascular disease.
- Hypersensitivity to this drug or to any ingredient in the formulation or component of the container. For a complete listing, see Dosage Forms, Composition and Packaging.

WARNINGS AND PRECAUTIONS:

> **Serious Warnings and Precautions**
>
> The Women's Health Initiative (WHI) trial examined the health benefits and risks of oral combined estrogen plus progestin therapy (n=16 608) and oral estrogen-alone therapy (n=10 739) in postmenopausal women aged 50 to 79 years.
>
> The estrogen plus progestin arm of the WHI trial (mean age 63.3 years) indicated an increased risk of **myocardial infarction (MI), stroke, invasive breast cancer, pulmonary emboli** and **deep vein thrombosis** in postmenopausal women receiving treatment with combined conjugated equine estrogens (CEE, 0.625 mg/day) and medroxyprogesterone acetate (MPA, 2.5 mg/day) for 5.2 years compared to those receiving placebo.
>
> The estrogen-alone arm of the WHI trial (mean age 63.6 years) indicated an increased risk of **stroke** and **deep vein thrombosis** in hysterectomized women treated with CEE-alone (0.625 mg/day) for 6.8 years compared to those receiving placebo.
>
> Therefore, the following should be given serious consideration at the time of prescribing:
>
> - Estrogens with or without progestins **should not** be prescribed for primary or secondary prevention of cardiovascular diseases.
> - Estrogens with or without progestins should be prescribed at the **lowest effective dose** for the approved indication.
> - Estrogens with or without progestins should be prescribed for the **shortest period possible** for the approved indication.

Carcinogenesis and Mutagenesis: Breast Cancer: Available epidemiological data indicate that the use of combined estrogen plus progestin by postmenopausal women is associated with an increased risk of invasive breast cancer. In the estrogen plus progestin arm of the WHI trial, among 10 000 women over a one-year period, there were:

- 8 more cases of invasive breast cancer (38 on combined HRT versus 30 on placebo).

The WHI study reported that the invasive breast cancers diagnosed in the estrogen plus progestin group were similar in histology but were larger (mean [SD], 1.7 cm [1.1] vs 1.5 cm [0.9], respectively; P=0.04) and were at a more advanced stage compared with those diagnosed in the placebo group.

The percentage of women with abnormal mammograms (recommendations for short-interval follow-up, a suspicious abnormality, or highly suggestive of malignancy) was significantly higher in the estrogen plus progestin group versus the placebo group. This difference appeared at year one and persisted in each year thereafter.

In the estrogen-alone arm of the WHI trial, there was no statistically significant difference in the rate of invasive breast cancer in hysterectomized women treated with conjugated equine estrogens versus women treated with placebo.

It is recommended that estrogens not be given to women with existing breast cancer or those with a previous history of the disease (see Contraindications). There is a need for caution in prescribing estrogens for women with known risk factors associated with the development of breast cancer, such as strong family history of breast cancer (first degree relative) or who present a breast condition with an increased risk (abnormal mammograms and/or atypical hyperplasia at breast biopsy). Other known risk factors for the development of breast cancer such as nulliparity, obesity, early menarche, late age at first full term pregnancy and at menopause should also be evaluated.

It is recommended that women undergo mammography prior to the start of HRT treatment and at regular intervals during treatment, as deemed appropriate by the treating physician and according to the perceived risks for each patient.

The overall benefits and possible risks of hormone replacement therapy should be fully considered and discussed with patients. It is important that the modest increased risk of being diagnosed with breast cancer after 4 years of treatment with combined estrogen plus progestin HRT (as reported in the results of WHI-trial) be discussed with the patient and weighed against its known benefits.

Instructions for regular self-examination of the breasts should be included in this counselling.

Endometrial Hyperplasia & Endometrial Carcinoma: Estrogen-only HRT increases the risk of endometrial hyperplasia/carcinoma (if taken by women with intact uteri). OGEN should be prescribed with an appropriate dosage of a progestin for women with intact uteri in order to prevent endometrial hyperplasia/carcinoma.

Ovarian Cancer: Some recent epidemiologic studies have found that the use of hormone replacement therapy (estrogen-alone and estrogen plus progestin therapies), in particular for five or more years, has been associated with an increased risk of ovarian cancer.

Cardiovascular: The results of the Heart and Estrogen/progestin Replacement Studies (HERS and HERS II) and the Women's Health Initiative (WHI) trial indicate that the use of estrogen plus progestin is associated with an increased risk of coronary heart disease (CHD) in postmenopausal women. The results of the WHI trial indicate that the use of estrogen-alone and estrogen plus progestin is associated with an increased risk of stroke in postmenopausal women.

WHI Trial Findings: In the combined estrogen plus progestin arm of the WHI trial, among 10 000 women over a one-year period, there were:

- 8 more cases of stroke (29 on combined HRT versus 21 on placebo)
- 7 more cases of CHD (37 on combined HRT versus 30 on placebo)

In the estrogen-alone arm of the WHI trial of women with prior hysterectomy, among 10 000 women over a one-year period, there were/was:

- 12 more cases of stroke (44 on estrogen-alone therapy versus 32 on placebo)
- no statistically significant difference in the rate of CHD.

HERS and HERS II Findings: In the Heart and Estrogen/progestin Replacement Study (HERS) of postmenopausal women with documented heart disease (n=2763, average age 66.7 years), a randomized placebo-controlled clinical trial of secondary prevention of coronary heart disease (CHD), treatment with 0.625 mg/day oral conjugated equine estrogen (CEE) plus 2.5 mg medroxyprogesterone acetate (MPA) demonstrated no cardiovascular benefit. Specifically, during an average follow-up of 4.1 years, treatment with CEE plus MPA did not reduce the overall rate of CHD events in postmenopausal women with established coronary heart disease. There were more CHD events in the hormone-treated group than in the placebo group in year 1, but not during the subsequent years.

From the original HERS trial, 2321 women consented to participate in an open label extension of HERS known as HERS II. Average follow-up in HERS II was an additional 2.7 years, for a total of 6.8 years overall. After 6.8 years, hormone therapy did not reduce the risk of cardiovascular events in women with CHD.

Blood Pressure: Women using hormonal replacement therapy (HRT) sometimes experience increased blood pressure. Blood pressure should be monitored with HRT use. Elevation of blood pressure in previously normotensive or hypertensive patients should be investigated and HRT therapy may have to be discontinued.

Ear/Nose/Throat: Otosclerosis: Estrogens should be used with caution in patients with otosclerosis.

Endocrine and Metabolism: Glucose and Lipid Metabolism: A worsening of glucose tolerance and lipid metabolism has been observed in a significant percentage of peri- and post-menopausal patients. Therefore, diabetic patients or those with a predisposition to diabetes should be observed closely to detect any alterations in carbohydrate or lipid metabolism, especially in triglyceride blood levels.

Women with familial hypertriglyceridemia need special surveillance. Lipid-lowering measures are recommended additionally, before treatment is started.

Heme Metabolism: Women with porphyria need special surveillance.

Calcium and Phosphorus Metabolism: Because the prolonged use of estrogens influences the metabolism of calcium and phosphorus, estrogens should be used with caution in patients with metabolic and malignant bone diseases associated with hypercalcemia and in patients with renal insufficiency.

Hypothyroidism: Patients who require thyroid hormone replacement therapy and who are also taking estrogen should have their thyroid function monitored regularly to assure that thyroid hormone levels remain in an acceptable range (see Drug Interactions, Drug-Laboratory Test Interactions).

Other Conditions: OGEN contains lactose. In patients with rare hereditary galactose intolerance, lactase deficiency or glucose-galactose malabsorption, the severity of the condition should be taken into careful consideration before prescribing OGEN. The patients should be closely monitored.

Genitourinary: Vaginal Bleeding: Abnormal vaginal bleeding, due to its prolongation, irregularity or heaviness, occurring during therapy should prompt diagnostic measures to rule out the possibility of uterine malignancy and the treatment should be re-evaluated.

Uterine Leiomyomata: Pre-existing uterine leiomyoma may increase in size during estrogen use. Growth, pain or tenderness of uterine leiomyoma requires discontinuation of medication and appropriate investigation.

Endometriosis: Symptoms and physical findings associated with a previous diagnosis of endometriosis may reappear or become aggravated with estrogen use.

Hematologic: Venous Thromboembolism: Available epidemiological data indicate that use of estrogen with or without progestin by postmenauposal women is associated with an increased risk of developing venous thromboembolism (VTE).

In the estrogen plus progestin arm of the WHI trial, among 10 000 women on combined HRT over a one-year period, there were 18 more cases of venous thromboembolism, including 8 more cases of pulmonary embolism.

In the estrogen-alone arm of the WHI trial, among 10 000 women on estrogen therapy over a one-year period, there were 7 more cases of venous thromboembolism, although there was no statistically significant difference in the rate of pulmonary embolism.

Generally recognized risk factors for VTE include a personal history, a family history (the occurrence of VTE in a direct relative at a relatively early age may indicate genetic predisposition) and severe obesity (body mass index >30 kg/m²) and systemic lupus erythematosus. The risk of VTE also increases with age and smoking.

The risk of VTE may be temporarily increased with prolonged immobilization, major surgery or trauma. In women on HRT, attention should be given to prophylactic measures to prevent VTE following surgery. Also, patients with varicose veins should be closely supervised. The physician should be alert to the earliest manifestations of thrombotic disorders (thrombophlebitis, retinal thrombosis, cerebral embolism and pulmonary embolism). If these occur or are suspected, hormone therapy should be discontinued immediately, given the risks of long-term disability or fatality.

If feasible, estrogens with or without progestins should be discontinued at least 4 weeks before major surgery which may be associated with an increased risk of thromboembolism, or during periods of prolonged immobilization.

Hepatic/Biliary/Pancreatic: Gallbladder Diseases: A 2- to 4-fold increase in the risk of gallbladder disease requiring surgery in women receiving postmenopausal estrogens has been reported.

Hepatic Hemangioma: Particular caution is indicated in women with hepatic hemangiomas as estrogens may cause an exacerbation of this condition.

Jaundice: Caution is advised in patients with a history of liver and/or biliary disorders. If cholestatic jaundice develops during treatment, the treatment should be discontinued and appropriate investigations carried out.

Liver Function Tests: Liver function tests should be done periodically in subjects who are suspected of having hepatic disease. For information on endocrine and liver function tests, see Monitoring and Laboratory Tests.

Immune: Angioedema: Estrogens may induce or exacerbate symptoms of angioedema, in particular in women with hereditary angioedema.

Systemic Lupus Erythematosus: Particular caution is indicated in women with systemic lupus erythematosus.

Neurologic: Cerebrovascular Insufficiency: Patients who develop visual disturbances, classical migraine, transient aphasia, paralysis, or loss of consciousness should discontinue medication.

Dementia: Available epidemiological data indicate that the use of combined estrogen plus progestin in women age 65 and over may increase the risk of developing probable dementia.

The Women's Health Initiative Memory Study (WHIMS), a clinical substudy of the WHI, was designed to assess whether postmenopausal hormone replacement therapy (oral estrogen plus progestin or oral estrogen-alone) reduces the risk of dementia in women aged 65 and over (age range 65-79 years) and free of dementia at baseline.

In the estrogen plus progestin arm of the WHIMS (n=4532), women with intact uteri were treated with daily 0.625 mg conjugated equine estrogens (CEE) plus 2.5 mg medroxyprogesterone acetate (MPA) or placebo for an average of 4.05 years. The results, when extrapolated to 10 000 women treated over a one-year period showed:

- 23 more cases of probable dementia (45 on combined HRT versus 22 on placebo).

In the estrogen-alone arm of the WHIMS (n=2947), women with prior hysterectomy were treated with daily 0.625 mg CEE or placebo for an average of 5.21 years. The results, when extrapolated to 10 000 women treated over a one-year period showed:

- 12 more cases of probable dementia (37 on estrogen-alone versus 25 on placebo), although this difference did not reach statistical significance.

When data from the estrogen plus progestin arm of the WHIMS and the estrogen alone arm of the WHIMS were combined, as per the original WHIMS protocol, in 10 000 women over a one-year period, there were:

- 18 more cases of probable dementia (41 on estrogen plus progestin or estrogen-alone versus 23 on placebo)

Epilepsy: Particular caution is indicated in women with epilepsy, as estrogens with or without progestins may cause an exacerbation of this condition. Treatment should be stopped if there is an increase in epileptic seizures.

Renal: Fluid Retention: Estrogens may cause fluid retention. Therefore, particular caution is indicated in cardiac or renal dysfunction or asthma. If, in any of the above-mentioned conditions, a worsening of the underlying disease is diagnosed or suspected during treatment, the benefits and risks of treatment should be reassessed based on the individual case.

Special Populations: Nursing Women: Estrogen administration in lactating women has been shown to decrease the quantity and quality of the milk. Detectable amounts of estrogens have been identified in the milk of women receiving OGEN. The use of OGEN in lactating women is not recommended.

Pediatrics: Safety and effectiveness of OGEN in paediatric patients have not been established.

Monitoring and Laboratory Tests: Before OGEN (estropipate, USP) is administered, the patient should have a complete physical examination including a blood pressure determination. Breasts and pelvic organs should be appropriately examined and a Papanicolaou smear should be performed. Endometrial biopsy should be done only when indicated. Baseline tests should include mammography, measurements of blood glucose, calcium, triglycerides and cholesterol, and liver function tests.

The first follow-up examination should be done within 3-6 months after initiation of treatment to assess response to treatment. Thereafter, examinations should be made at intervals at least once a year. Appropriate investigations should be arranged at regular intervals as determined by the physician.

The importance of regular self-examination of the breasts should be discussed with the patient.

ADVERSE REACTIONS: Adverse Drug Reaction Overview: See Warnings and Precautions regarding potential induction of malignant neoplasms and adverse effects similar to those of oral contraceptives. The following adverse reactions have been reported with estrogen/progestin combination in general:

Blood and Lymphatic System Disorders: Altered coagulation tests (see Warnings and Precautions, Drug Interactions, Drug-Laboratory Test Interactions).

Cardiac Disorders: palpitations; increase in blood pressure (see Warnings and Precautions); coronary thrombosis.

Endocrine Disorders: increased blood sugar levels; decreased glucose tolerance.

Eye Disorders: neuro-ocular lesions (e.g. retinal thrombosis, optic neuritis); visual disturbances; steepening of the corneal curvature; intolerance to contact lenses.

Gastrointestinal Disorders: nausea; vomiting; abdominal discomfort (cramps, pressure, pain, bloating).

General Disorders and Administration Site Conditions: fatigue; changes in appetite; changes in body weight; change in libido.

Hepatobiliary Disorders: gallbladder disorder; asymptomatic impaired liver function; cholestatic jaundice.

Musculoskeletal and Connective Tissue Disorders: Musculoskeletal pain including leg pain not related to thromboembolic disease (usually transient, lasting 3-6 weeks) may occur.

Nervous System Disorders: aggravation of migraine episodes; headaches; dizziness; neuritis.

Psychiatric Disorders: mental depression; nervousness; irritability.

Renal and Urinary Disorders: cystitis; dysuria; sodium retention; edema.

Reproductive System and Breast Disorders: breakthrough bleeding; spotting; change in menstrual flow; dysmenorrhea; vaginal itching/discharge; dyspareunia; endometrial hyperplasia; pre-menstrual-like syndrome; reactivation of endometriosis; changes in cervical erosion and amount of cervical secretion; breast swelling and tenderness.

Skin and Subcutaneous Tissue Disorders: chloasma or melasma, which may persist when drug is discontinued; erythema multiform; erythema nodosum; haemorrhagic eruption; loss of scalp hair; hirsutism and acne.

Vascular Disorders: Isolated cases of: thrombophlebitis; thromboembolic disorders.

Clinical Trial Adverse Drug Reactions: No data are available.

Less Common Clinical Trial Adverse Drug Reactions: No data are available.

Abnormal Hematologic and Clinical Chemistry Findings: No data are available.

Post-Market Adverse Drug Reactions: The following events have been reported in patients who have received OGEN: mouth ulceration, tongue ulceration, gait disturbance, hyperglycaemia, mobility decreased, cognitive disorder, convulsion, eating disorder, incontinence, dyspnoea and pruritus. It should be noted that the uncontrolled nature of post-marketing surveillance makes it difficult to determine definitively if a reported event was actually caused by OGEN, or to reliably assess causation in individual cases.

If adverse symptoms persist, the prescription of HRT should be re-considered.

DRUG INTERACTIONS: Overview: Estrogens may diminish the effectiveness of anticoagulant, antidiabetic and antihypertensive agents.

Preparations inducing liver enzymes (e.g., barbiturates, hydantoins, carbamazepine, meprobamates, phenylbutazone or rifampicin) may interfere with the activity of orally administered estrogens.

Drug-Drug Interactions: The following section contains information on drug interactions with ethinyl estradiol containing products (specifically, oral contraceptives) that have been reported in the published literature. It is unknown whether such interactions occur with drug products containing other forms of estrogens. Drug monitoring is recommended.

1. The metabolism of ethinyl estradiol is increased by rifampin and anticonvulsants such as phenobarbital, phenytoin and carbamazepine. Coadministration of troglitazone and certain ethinyl estradiol containing drug products (e.g., oral contraceptives containing ethinyl estradiol) reduce the plasma concentrations of ethinyl estradiol by 30 percent.

   Ascorbic acid and acetaminophen may increase AUC and/or plasma concentrations of ethinyl estradiol. Coadministration of atorvastatin and certain ethinyl estradiol containing drug products (e.g., oral contraceptives containing ethinyl estradiol) increase AUC values for ethinyl estradiol by 20 percent.

   Clinical pharmacokinetic studies have not demonstrated any consistent effect of antibiotics (other than rifampin) on plasma concentrations of synthetic steroids.
2. Drug products containing ethinyl estradiol may inhibit the metabolism of other compounds. Increased plasma concentrations of cyclosporin, prednisolone, and theophylline have been reported with concomitant administration of certain drugs containing ethinyl estradiol (e.g., oral contraceptives containing ethinyl estradiol). In addition, these drugs containing ethinyl estradiol may induce the conjugation of other compounds.

   Decreased plasma concentrations of acetaminophen and increased clearance of temazepam, salicylic acid, morphine and clofibric acid have been noted when these drugs were administered with certain ethinyl estradiol containing drug products (e.g., oral contraceptives containing ethinyl estradiol).

Drug-Food Interactions: No Drug-Food interaction studies were conducted on OGEN. However, it is known that CYP3A4 inhibitors such as grapefruit juice may increase plasma concentrations of 17β-estradiol and may result in side effects.

Drug-Herb Interactions: It was found that some herbal products (e.g. St. John's wort) which are available as over-the-counter (OTC) products might interfere with steroid metabolism and therefore alter the efficacy and safety of estrogen/progestin products.

Physicians and other health care providers should be aware of other non-prescription products concomitantly used by the patient, including herbal and natural products, obtained from the widely spread Health Stores.

Drug-Laboratory Test Interactions: The results of certain endocrine and liver function tests may be affected by estrogen-containing products:

- increased prothrombin time and partial thromboplastin time; increased levels of fibrinogen and fibrinogen activity; increased coagulation factors VII, VIII, IX, X; increased norepinephrine-induced platelet aggregability; decreased antithrombin III.
- increased thyroxine-binding globulin (TBG), leading to increased circulating total thyroid hormone (T_4) as measured by column or radioimmunoassay; T3 resin uptake is decreased, reflecting the elevated TBG; free T_4 concentration is unaltered;
- other binding proteins may be elevated in serum i.e., corticosteroid binding globulin (CBG), sex-hormone binding globulin (SHBG), leading to increased circulating corticosteroids and sex steroids respectively; free or biologically active hormone concentrations are unchanged.
- impaired glucose tolerance
- increased serum triglycerides and phospholipids concentration

The results of the above laboratory tests should not be considered reliable unless therapy has been discontinued for two to four weeks. The pathologist should be informed that the patient is receiving HRT therapy when relevant specimens are submitted.

Drug-Lifestyle Interactions: Acute alcohol ingestion during HRT may lead to elevations in circulating estradiol levels.

DOSAGE AND ADMINISTRATION:

Dosing Considerations: In general, estrogen should be given cyclically (21 to 25 days followed by a 5 to 7 day rest period) with progestogen in women with intact uteri in order to reduce endometrial hyperplasia/carcinoma. Withdrawal bleeding commonly occurs toward the end of the rest period. The addition of sufficient progestogen to promote conversion of the endometrium is mandatory in those patients who are receiving sufficient unopposed estrogen to cause vaginal bleeding or endometrial hyperplasia. Obviously, abnormal vaginal bleeding in such patients is an indication for prompt diagnostic measures.

Recommended Dose and Dosage Adjustment: As with most drugs, the dosage should be adjusted to the minimum required to control symptoms and the requirement for estrogen therapy should be reassessed periodically.

OGEN (estropipate, USP) is indicated for a variety of estrogen deficiency states. The usual daily dose is 0.75 mg to 3 mg estropipate (OGEN calculated as sodium estrone sulphate). Titrate dosage as necessary according to the individual patient's clinical response.

OGEN should be prescribed with an appropriate dosage of a progestin for women with intact uteri in order to prevent endometrial hyperplasia/carcinoma. Progestin therapy is not required as part of hormone replacement therapy in women who have had a previous hysterectomy

Missed Dose: If a dose of this medication has been missed, it should be taken as soon as possible. However, if it is almost time for the next dose, skip the missed dose and go back to the regular dosing schedule. Do not double doses.

Administration: OGEN (estropipate, USP) is administered orally.

OVERDOSAGE:

Symptoms: Numerous reports of ingestion of large doses of estrogen products and estrogen- containing oral contraceptives by young children have not revealed acute serious ill effects. Over dosage with estrogen may cause nausea, breast discomfort, fluid retention, bloating or vaginal bleeding in women.

Treatment: Give symptomatic treatment.

> For management of a suspected drug overdose, contact your **regional Poison Control Centre**. See the *CPS* Directory section for a list of Poison Control Centres.

ACTION AND CLINICAL PHARMACOLOGY: Mechanism of Action: OGEN (estropipate, USP) owes it therapeutic action to estrone, one of the three principal estrogenic steroid hormones of humans: estradiol, estrone and estriol. Estradiol is rapidly hydrolysed in the body to estrone, which in turn may be hydrated to the less active estriol. These transformations occur readily, mainly in the liver, where there is also free interconversion between estrone and estradiol.

Estrogens act by regulating the transcription of a limited number of genes. Estrogens diffuse through cell membranes, distribute themselves throughout the cell, and bind to and activate the nuclear estrogen receptor, a DNA-binding protein which is found in estrogen-responsive tissues. The activated estrogen receptor binds to specific DNA sequences, or hormone-response elements, which enhance the transcription of adjacent genes and in turn lead to the observed effects. Estrogen receptors have been identified in tissues of the reproductive tract, breast, pituitary, hypothalamus, liver, and bone of women.

Pharmacodynamics: Estrogens are important in the development and maintenance of the female reproductive system and secondary sex characteristics. They promote growth and development of the vagina, uterus, and fallopian tubes, and enlargement of the breasts. Indirectly, they contribute to the shaping of the skeleton, maintenance of tone and elasticity of urogenital structures, changes in the epiphyses of the long bones that allow for the pubertal growth spurt and its termination, growth of axillary and pubic hair, and pigmentation of the nipples and genitals. Along with other hormones such as progesterone, estrogens are intricately involved in the process of menstruation. Estrogens also affect the release of pituitary gonadotropins.

A depletion of endogenous estrogens occurs postmenopausally as a result of a decline in ovarian function, and may cause symptomatic vulvovaginal atrophy.

Pharmacokinetics: Absorption: Gastrointestinal absorption of orally administered estrogens is usually prompt and complete.

In a cross-over, randomized study of eight post-menopausal women aged 51-60, the pharmacokinetics of piperazine estrone sulphate 2.5 mg/day was compared to estradiol valerate 2.0 mg/day. Blood sampling was carried out on days 1 and 21. Levels of estrone (E_1), estradiol (E_2), estrone sulphate (E_1S), estradiol sulphate (E_2S) and estriol sulphate (E_3S) were measured by RIA. On average, the time required to obtain a maximum concentration of estrone (E_1), estradiol (E_2), estrone sulphate (E_1S), estradiol sulphate (E_2S) and estriol sulphate (E_3S) in the circulation is between 4.4 and 9.8 hours. Following a single dose of 2.5 mg piperazine estrone sulphate E_1, E_2 concentrations, measured by RIA, increase for approximately 6.4-9.8 hours to reach peak plasma concentrations of 1.3 to and 0.25 nmol/L respectively.

Distribution: Estrone is 50-80% bound to protein as it circulates in the blood, usually as a conjugate with sulphate.

Metabolism: Inactivation of estrogens in the body occurs mainly in the liver. During cyclic passage through the liver, estrogens are degraded to less active estrogenic compounds and conjugated with sulphuric and glucuronic acids.

Excretion: In the normal menstrual cycle, the mean daily excretion of endogenous estrogens at the midovulatory maximum has been found to be 29 µg of estriol, 21 µg of estrone and 8 µg of estradiol (total, 58 µg). In normal women, after menopause, the average daily excretion of these three estrogens totals only 6 µg.

During the first 24 hours, 50% of estrone or estradiol is excreted via the kidney, 10% is found in the feces and the rest is reabsorbed.

The plasma elimination half-lives of estrone (E_1), estradiol (E_2) and estrone sulphate (E_1S) are 18.5, 34.7, 11.8 hours respectively.

Estrogen Pharmacology: OGEN (estropipate, USP) is a natural estrogenic substance prepared from purified crystalline estrone, solubilized as the sulphate and stabilized with piperazine. It is appreciably soluble in water and has almost no odour or taste. The amount of piperazine in OGEN is not sufficient to exert a pharmacological action. Its addition ensures solubility, stability and uniform potency of the estrone sulphate.

After menopause, when the ovaries have ceased to function, only small amounts of estradiol-17β are still produced, i.e. from the aromatization of androstenedione to estrone and to a lesser extent, testosterone to estradiol-17β. Estrone is transformed to estradiol-17β by the enzyme 17β-hydroxysteroid-dehydrogenase. Both enzymes prevail in fat, liver and muscle tissue. In premenopausal women, the ratio of estradiol-17β (E_2) to estrone (E_1) (i.e. E_2/E_1 ratio) in the plasma is in the range of 0.5 to 2, depending on the phase of the menstrual cycle. The E_2/E_1 ratio for untreated postmenopausal women is below 0.5.

Loss of the ovarian estradiol-17β production after menopause can result in the following: instability of thermoregulation causing hot flushes associated with sleep disturbance and excessive sweating; accelerated loss of bone matrix and mineral, resulting in osteoporosis; alterations in lipid metabolism; urogenital atrophy, causing dyspareunia and urinary incontinence.

The protection against endometrial hyperplasia in women with intact uteri is necessary during long-term therapy. Published data suggest that 12 to 14 days of sequential progestin treatment during estrogen replacement therapy reduces the occurrence of endometrial hyperplasia, and thereby irregular bleeding and endometrial carcinoma, compared to estrogen treatment alone.

STORAGE AND STABILITY: Store at controlled room temperature, 15-30°C.

SPECIAL HANDLING INSTRUCTIONS: Not applicable.

INFORMATION FOR THE PATIENT: Published in e-CPS, available by subscription at www.e-cps.ca.

DOSAGE FORMS, COMPOSITION AND PACKAGING: 0.75 mg: Each yellow-coloured, oval tablet, scored, embossed with "U" and "3772" on left and right halves, contains: estropipate 0.75 mg calculated as sodium estrone sulfate 0.625 mg. Nonmedicinal ingredients: alcohol, colloidal silicon dioxide, FD&C Yellow No. 6, FD&C Yellow No. 10, hydrogenated vegetable oil wax, hydroxypropyl cellulose, lactose monohydrate and/or lactose anhydrous, magnesium stearate, microcrystalline cellulose, potassium phosphate dibasic, purified water, sodium starch glycolate and tromethamine. Bottles of 100.

1.5 mg: Each peach-coloured oval tablet, scored, embossed with "U" and "3773" on left and right halves, contains: estropipate 1.5 mg calculated as sodium estrone sulfate 1.25 mg. Nonmedicinal ingredients: alcohol, colloidal silicon dioxide, FD&C Yellow No. 6, hydrogenated vegetable oil wax, hydroxypropyl cellulose, lactose monohydrate and/or lactose anhydrous, magnesium stearate, microcrystalline cellulose, potassium phosphate dibasic, purified water, sodium starch glycolate and tromethamine. Blisters of 20, cartons of 5 blisters. Bottles of 100.

3 mg: Each blue-coloured, oval tablet, scored, embossed with "U" and "3774" on left and right halves, contains: estropipate 3 mg calculated as sodium estrone sulfate 2.5 mg. Nonmedicinal ingredients: alcohol, colloidal silicon dioxide, FD&C Blue No. 2, hydrogenated vegetable oil wax, hydroxypropyl cellulose, lactose monohydrate and/or lactose anhydrous, magnesium stearate, microcrystalline cellulose, potassium phosphate dibasic, purified water, sodium starch glycolate and tromethamine. Blisters of 20, cartons of 5 blisters. Bottles of 100.

(Shown in Product Identification Section)

Oilatum® Dermatological Shower and Bath Oil

liquid paraffin

Antipruritic—Emollient

Stiefel, a GSK company

SUPPLIED: Each mL of oil contains: light liquid paraffin 63.4%. Nonmedicinal ingredients: fragrance floral-spice, isopropyl palmitate, lanolin alcohol acetylated, PEG 40 sorbitan peroleate and polyethylene glycol 400. Bottles of 250 mL.

Olmetec® Pr

olmesartan medoxomil

Angiotensin II AT1 Receptor Blocker

Schering-Plough

Date of Preparation: October 27, 2008

SUMMARY PRODUCT INFORMATION:

Route of Administration	Dosage Form/ Strength	Clinically Relevant Nonmedicinal Ingredients
Oral	Tablet/20 mg and 40 mg	Lactose (see Dosage Forms, Composition and Packaging).

INDICATIONS AND CLINICAL USE: OLMETEC (olmesartan medoxomil) is indicated for the treatment of mild to moderate essential hypertension.

OLMETEC may be used alone or in combination with thiazide diuretic.

Geriatrics (≥65 years of age): No overall differences in effectiveness or safety were observed between elderly patients and younger patients. Other reported clinical experience has not identified differences in responses between these subjects, however, greater sensitivity of some older individuals cannot be ruled out.

Pediatrics (<18 years of age): The safety and effectiveness in pediatric patients have not been established.

CONTRAINDICATIONS:

- Patients who are hypersensitive to this drug or to any ingredient in the formulation or component of the container. For a complete listing, see Dosage Forms, Composition and Packaging.

WARNINGS AND PRECAUTIONS:

> **Serious Warnings and Precautions**
> When used in pregnancy, angiotensin receptor (AT_1) blockers (ARB) can cause injury or even death of the developing fetus. When pregnancy is detected, OLMETEC (olmesartan medoxomil) should be discontinued as soon as possible (see Warnings and Precautions, Special Populations).

Cardiovascular: Hypotension in Volume- or Salt-Depleted Patients: In patients with an activated renin-angiotensin system, such as volume- and/or salt-depleted patients (e.g., those being treated with high doses of diuretics), symptomatic hypotension may occur after initiation of treatment with OLMETEC. Treatment should start under close medical supervision. Similar considerations apply to patients with ischemic heart or cerebrovascular disease, in whom an excessive fall in blood pressure could result in myocardial infarction or cerebrovascular accident. If hypotension does occur, the patient should be placed in the supine position and, if necessary, given an intravenous infusion of normal saline (see Dosage and Administration). A transient hypotensive response is not a contraindication to further treatment, which usually can be continued without difficulty once the blood pressure has stabilized.

Valvular Stenosis: There is concern on theoretical grounds that patients with aortic stenosis might be at a particular risk of decreased coronary perfusion, because they do not develop as much afterload reduction.

Hepatic/Biliary/Pancreatic: No adjustment of dosage is required for patients with mild hepatic impairment. Data is lacking with respect to the use of 20 mg and 40 mg olmesartan medoxomil; therefore, a lower starting dose is recommended in patients with moderate liver disease, and the maximum dose of 20 mg olmesartan medoxomil daily should not be exceeded. Care should be exercised in patients with liver disease, especially in those patients with biliary obstructive disorders, as the majority of olmesartan is eliminated in the bile. No information is available in patients with severe liver disease; therefore, use of OLMETEC in this group of patients is not recommended (see Action and Clinical Pharmacology, Pharmacokinetics).

Renal: Impaired Renal Function: As a consequence of inhibiting the renin-angiotensin-aldosterone system, changes in renal function may be anticipated in susceptible individuals. In patients whose renal function may depend upon the activity of the renin-angiotensin-aldosterone system (e.g. patients with severe congestive heart failure), treatment with angiotensin converting enzyme inhibitors and angiotensin receptor antagonists has been associated with oliguria, progressive azotemia and (rarely) with acute renal failure and/or death. Similar results may be anticipated in patients treated with olmesartan medoxomil (see Action and Clinical Pharmacology, Special Populations and Conditions).

In studies of ACE inhibitors in patients with unilateral or bilateral renal artery stenosis, increases in serum creatinine or blood urea nitrogen (BUN) have been reported. There has been no long-term use of olmesartan medoxomil in patients with unilateral or bilateral renal artery stenosis, but similar results may be expected.

Use of olmesartan medoxomil should include appropriate assessment of renal function.

Special Populations: Pregnant Women: Drugs that act directly on the renin-angiotensin-aldosterone-system (RAAS) can cause fetal and neonatal morbidity and death when administered to pregnant women. When pregnancy is detected, OLMETEC should be discontinued as soon as possible.

The use of ARB is not recommended during pregnancy. Epidemiological evidence regarding the risk of teratogenicity following exposure to angiotensin converting enzyme inhibitors (another class of therapeutic products interfering with the RAAS) during the first trimester of pregnancy has not been conclusive; however a small increase in risk cannot be excluded. Given the current evidence available on the risk with ARB, similar risks may exist for this class of drugs. Patients planning pregnancy should be changed to alternative antihypertensive treatments which have an established safety profile for use in pregnancy. When pregnancy is diagnosed, treatment with angiotensin II antagonists should be stopped immediately, and, if appropriate, alternative therapy should be started.

The use of ARBs during the second and third trimesters is known to induce human fetotoxicity (decreased renal function, oligohydramnios, skull ossification retardation) and neonatal toxicity (renal failure, hypotension, hyperkalaemia).

Infants with a history of in utero exposure to ARBs should be closely observed for hypotension, oliguria, and hyperkalemia. If oliguria occurs, attention should be directed toward support of blood pressure and renal perfusion. Exchange transfusion or dialysis may be required as a means of reversing hypotension and/or substituting for impaired renal function; however, limited experience with those procedures has not been associated with significant clinical benefit.

It is not known if olmesartan can be removed from the body by hemodialysis.

Animal Data: No teratogenic effects were observed when olmesartan medoxomil was administered to pregnant rats at oral doses up to 1000 mg/kg/day (240 times the maximum recommended human dose [MRHD] of olmesartan medoxomil on a mg/m² basis) pregnant rabbits at oral doses up to 1 mg/kg/day (half the MRHD on a mg/m² basis; higher doses could not be evaluated for effects on fetal development as they were lethal to the does). In rats, significant decreases in pup birth weight and weight gain were observed at doses ≥1.6 mg/kg/day, and delays in developmental milestones and dose-dependent increases in the incidence of dilation of the renal pelvis were observed at doses ≥8 mg/kg/day. The no observed effect dose for developmental toxicity in rats is 0.3 mg/kg/day, about one-tenth the MRHD of 40 mg/day.

Nursing Women: It is not known whether olmesartan is excreted in human milk, but olmesartan is secreted at low concentration in the milk of lactating rats. Because many drugs are excreted in human milk and because of their potential for affecting the nursing infant adversely, a decision should be made whether to discontinue nursing or discontinue the drug, taking into account the importance of the drug to the mother.

Pediatrics (<18 years of age): The safety and effectiveness in pediatric patients have not been established.

Geriatrics (≥65 years of age): No overall differences in effectiveness or safety were observed between elderly patients and younger patients. Other reported clinical experience has not identified differences in responses between these subjects, however, greater sensitivity of some older individuals cannot be ruled out.

ADVERSE REACTIONS: Adverse Drug Reaction Overview: OLMETEC (olmesartan medoxomil) has been evaluated for safety in 3825 patients/subjects treated for essential hypertension, including 900 patients treated for at least 6 months and more than 525 for at least 1 year. Of these, 3275 patients were treated with olmesartan medoxomil monotherapy in controlled clinical trials.

In controlled clinical trials, discontinuation of therapy due to clinical adverse experiences occurred in 2.4% (79/3278) and 2.7% (i.e. 32/1179) of patients treated with OLMETEC and placebo or active control, respectively.

Treatment with OLMETEC was well tolerated, with an incidence of adverse events similar to placebo. Events generally were mild, transient and had no relationship to the dose of olmesartan medoxomil. The following potentially serious adverse reactions have been reported with OLMETEC/OLMETEC PLUS in controlled trials: syncope, hypotension.

Clinical Trial Adverse Drug Reactions: Because clinical trials are conducted under very specific conditions the adverse reaction rates observed in the clinical trials may not reflect the rates observed in practice and should not be compared to the rates in the clinical trials of another drug. Adverse drug reaction information from clinical trials is useful for identifying drug-related adverse events and for approximating rates.

In double-blind placebo-controlled clinical trials, the following adverse events were reported with OLMETEC occurring in >1% of patients, irrespective of relationship to study drug. See Table 1.

Table 1: OLMETEC

Adverse Events Occurring >1% in Placebo-controlled Monotherapy Studies[a]

System Organ Class (SOC) MedDRA Preferred term	Placebo N=555		Total Olmesartan Medoxomil N=2540	
	N	%	N	%
Gastrointestinal Disorders				
Diarrhea	4	(0.7)	27	(1.1)
General Disorders and Administration Site Conditions				
Influenza like illness	16	(2.9)	79	(3.1)

(cont'd)

Table 1: OLMETEC *(cont'd)*

Adverse Events Occurring >1% in Placebo-controlled Monotherapy Studies[a]

System Organ Class (SOC) MedDRA Preferred term	Placebo N=555 N	%	Total Olmesartan Medoxomil N=2540 N	%
Infections and Infestations				
Upper respiratory tract infection	27	(4.9)	83	(3.3)
Bronchitis	10	(1.8)	51	(2.0)
Rhinitis	9	(1.6)	40	(1.6)
Pharyngitis	6	(1.1)	33	(1.3)
Sinusitis	11	(2.0)	29	(1.1)
Injury, Poisoning and Procedural Complications				
Injury	7	(1.3)	34	(1.3)
Metabolism and Nutrition Disorders				
Hyperglycemia	15	(2.7)	32	(1.3)
Hypertriglyceridemia	6	(1.1)	29	(1.1)
Musculoskeletal and Connective Tissue Disorders				
Back pain	8	(1.4)	41	(1.6)
Nervous System Disorders				
Headache	40	(7.2)	141	(5.6)
Dizziness	5	(0.9)	70	(2.8)
Renal and Urinary Disorders				
Hematuria	10	(1.8)	49	(1.9)

[a] Body systems in which patients in either treatment group experienced events and in which at least one event was reported in >1% of patients in either treatment group.

Less Common Clinical Trial Adverse Drug Reactions (<1%): Other (potentially important) adverse events that have been reported in controlled or open-label trials with an incidence of greater than 0.5%, regardless of causality:
Cardiac Disorders: tachycardia.
Ear and Labyrinth Disorders: vertigo.
Gastrointestinal Disorders: abdominal pain, dyspepsia, nausea.
General Disorders and Administration Site Conditions: chest pain, edema peripheral.
Infections and Infestations: gastroenteritis.
Metabolism and Nutrition Disorders: hypercholesterolemia, hyperlipidemia, hyperuricaemia.
Musculoskeletal and Connective Tissue Disorders: arthralgia, arthritis, myalgia.
Renal and Urinary Disorders: albuminuria.
Respiratory, Thoracic and Mediastinal Disorders: cough.
Skin and Subcutaneous Tissue Disorders: rash.

Facial edema was reported in 5 patients receiving olmesartan medoxomil. Angioedema has been reported with other angiotensin II antagonists.

Abnormal Hematologic and Clinical Chemistry Findings: In controlled clinical trials, clinically important changes in standard laboratory parameters were rarely associated with administration of olmesartan medoxomil.

Hemoglobin and Hematocrit: Small decreases in hemoglobin and hematocrit (mean decreases of approximately 0.3 g/dL and 0.3 volume percent, respectively) were observed.

Liver Function Tests: Elevations of liver enzymes and/or serum bilirubin were observed infrequently.

	Placebo (n=555)	Total Olmesartan Medoxomil (n=2450)
γGT increased	13 (2.3%)	57 (2.2%)
CPK increased	6 (1.1%)	40 (1.6%)
ALT increased	9 (1.6%)	33 (1.3%)
AST increased	6 (1.1%)	25 (1.0%)

Post-Market Adverse Drug Reactions: Other adverse events reported rarely in post-marketing use include: asthenia, angioedema, vomiting, hyperkalemia, rhabdomyolysis, renal failure acute, blood creatinine increased, alopecia, pruritus, urticaria, palpitations, syncope, and blood uric acid increased.

DRUG INTERACTIONS: Drug-Drug Interactions: Diuretics: Patients on diuretics, and especially those in whom diuretic therapy was recently instituted, may occasionally experience an excessive reduction in blood pressure after initiation of therapy with OLMETEC. The possibility of symptomatic hypotension with the use of OLMETEC can be minimized by discontinuing the diuretic prior to initiation of treatment (see Warnings and Precautions, Cardiovascular, Hypotension in Volume- or Salt-Depleted Patients). No drug interaction of clinical significance has been identified with thiazide diuretics.

Agents Increasing Serum Potassium: Since OLMETEC decreases the production of aldosterone, potassium-sparing diuretics or potassium supplements should be given only for documented hypokalemia and with frequent monitoring of serum potassium. Potassium-containing salt substitutes should also be used with caution.

Pravastatin: OLMETEC decreased the C_{max} and AUC of pravastatin by approximately 25% and 21%, respectively. Since there is a high degree of variability in the bioavailability of pravastatin, this finding is not considered to be clinically relevant.

Warfarin: There was no effect on either the pharmacokinetics or pharmacodynamics of warfarin when co-administered with OLMETEC (olmesartan medoxomil) in healthy volunteers.

Digoxin: No pharmacokinetics or pharmacodynamics effects were reported when OLMETEC was co-administered with digoxin in healthy volunteers.

Antacids: The bioavailability of olmesartan was not significantly altered when co-administered with antacids [$Al(OH)_3$/$Mg(OH)_2$].

Cytochrome P450 Enzyme System: Unlike some other angiotensin II receptor blockers, olmesartan medoxomil is not metabolized by cytochrome P450 enzymes. Interactions with drugs that inhibit, induce or are metabolized by these enzymes are not expected.

Lithium Salts: As with other drugs which eliminate sodium, lithium clearance may be reduced in the presence of olmesartan. Therefore, serum lithium levels should be monitored carefully if lithium salts are to be administered with olmesartan medoxomil. Lithium generally should not be given with diuretics. Diuretic agents reduce the renal clearance of lithium and add a high risk of lithium toxicity.

Drug-Food Interactions: OLMETEC may be administered with or without food.

Drug-Herb Interactions: Interactions with herbal products have not been established.

Drug-Laboratory Test Interactions: Interactions with laboratory tests have not been established.

DOSAGE AND ADMINISTRATION: Dosing Considerations:

- **Elderly:** No adjustment of dosage is generally required in elderly patients (see below for dose recommendations in patients with renal impairment). If up-titration to the maximum dose of 40 mg daily is required, blood pressure should be closely monitored (see Action and Clinical Pharmacology, Special Populations and Conditions).
- **Hepatic Impairment:** No adjustment of dosage is required for patients with mild hepatic impairment. Data is lacking with respect to the use of 20 mg and 40 mg olmesartan medoxomil; therefore, a lower starting dose is recommended in patients with moderate liver disease, and the maximum dose of 20 mg olmesartan medoxomil daily should not be exceeded. Care should be exercised in patients with liver disease, especially in those patients with biliary obstructive disorders, as the majority of olmesartan is eliminated in the bile. No information is available in patients with severe liver disease; therefore, use of OLMETEC in this group of patients is not recommended (see Action and Clinical Pharmacology, Pharmacokinetics).
- **Renal Impairment:** Owing to limited experience of higher dosages in this patient group, the maximum dose in patients with mild to moderate renal impairment is 20 mg olmesartan medoxomil once daily. The use of olmesartan medoxomil in patients with severe renal impairment is not recommended, since there is only limited experience in this patient group.
- For patients with possible depletion of intravascular volume (e.g., patients treated with diuretics, particularly those with impaired renal function), OLMETEC should be initiated under close medical supervision and consideration should be given to use of a lower starting dose (see Warnings and Precautions, Renal).

Recommended Dose and Dosage Adjustment: Dosage must be individualized.

The usual recommended starting dose of OLMETEC (olmesartan medoxomil) is 20 mg once daily when used as monotherapy in patients who are not volume-contracted. For patients requiring further reduction in blood pressure after 2 weeks of therapy, the dose of OLMETEC may be increased to 40 mg. Doses above 40 mg do not appear to have greater effect. Twice-daily dosing offers no advantage over the same total dose given once daily.

OLMETEC may be administered with or without food.

Concomitant Diuretic Therapy: If blood pressure is not controlled by OLMETEC alone, a thiazide diuretic may be added.

Missed Dose: If patients miss a dose, they should wait until their next scheduled dose. Patients should not double their dose.

OVERDOSAGE:
Limited data are available in regard to overdosage in humans. The most likely manifestations of overdosage would be hypotension and tachycardia; bradycardia could be encountered if parasympathetic (vagal) stimulation occurs. If symptomatic hypotension should occur, supportive treatment should be initiated. The dialyzability of olmesartan is unknown.

For management of a suspected drug overdose, CPhA recommends that you contact your **regional Poison Control Centre**. See the *CPS* Directory section for a list of Poison Control Centres.

ACTION AND CLINICAL PHARMACOLOGY: Mechanism of Action: Olmesartan medoxomil, a prodrug, is hydrolyzed to olmesartan during absorption from the gastrointestinal tract. Olmesartan is a selective AT_1 subtype angiotensin II receptor antagonist.

Angiotensin II is formed from angiotensin I in a reaction catalyzed by angiotensin converting enzyme (ACE, kininase II). Angiotensin II is the principal pressor agent of the renin-angiotensin system, with effects that include vasoconstriction, stimulation of synthesis and release of aldosterone, cardiac stimulation and renal reabsorption of sodium. Olmesartan blocks the vasoconstrictor effects of angiotensin II by selectively blocking the binding of angiotensin II to the AT_1 receptor in vascular smooth muscle. Its action is, therefore, independent of the pathways for angiotensin II synthesis.

An AT_2 receptor is found also in many tissues, but this receptor is not known to be associated with cardiovascular homeostasis. Olmesartan has more than a 12 500-fold greater affinity for the AT_1 receptor than for the AT_2 receptor.

Blockade of the renin-angiotensin system with ACE inhibitors, which inhibit the biosynthesis of angiotensin II from angiotensin I, is a mechanism of many drugs used to treat hypertension. ACE inhibitors also inhibit the degradation of bradykinin, a reaction also catalyzed by ACE. Because olmesartan does not inhibit ACE (kininase II), it does not affect the response to bradykinin. Whether this difference has clinical relevance is not yet known.

Blockade of the angiotensin II receptor inhibits the negative regulatory feedback of angiotensin II on renin secretion, but the resulting increased plasma renin activity and circulating angiotensin II levels do not overcome the effect of olmesartan on blood pressure.

Pharmacodynamics: Olmesartan medoxomil inhibits the pressor effect of an angiotensin II infusion in a dose-dependent manner at doses of 2.5 to 40 mg. The inhibition was 90% at doses of olmesartan medoxomil >40 mg 24 hours post dose.

Plasma concentrations of angiotensin I and angiotensin II and plasma renin activity (PRA) increased after single and repeated administration of olmesartan medoxomil to healthy subjects and hypertensive patients. Repeated administration of up to 80 mg olmesartan medoxomil had minimal influence on aldosterone levels and no effect on serum potassium.

Pharmacokinetics: Absorption: Olmesartan medoxomil is rapidly and completely bioactivated by ester hydrolysis to olmesartan during absorption from the gastrointestinal tract. Olmesartan appears to be eliminated in a biphasic manner with a terminal elimination half-life of approximately 13 hours. Olmesartan shows linear pharmacokinetics following single oral doses of up to 320 mg and multiple oral doses of up to 80 mg. Steady-state levels of olmesartan are achieved within 3 to 5 days and no accumulation in plasma occurs with once-daily dosing.

The absolute bioavailability of olmesartan is approximately 26%. After oral administration, the peak plasma concentration (C_{max}) of olmesartan is reached after 1 to 2 hours. Food does not affect the bioavailability of olmesartan.

Distribution: The volume of distribution of olmesartan is approximately 17 L. Olmesartan is highly bound to plasma proteins (99%) and does not penetrate red blood cells. The protein binding is constant at plasma olmesartan concentrations well above the range achieved with recommended doses.

In rats, olmesartan crossed the blood-brain barrier poorly, if at all. Olmesartan passed across the placental barrier in rats and was distributed to the fetus. Olmesartan was distributed to milk at low levels in rats.

Metabolism and Excretion: Following the rapid and complete conversion of olmesartan medoxomil to olmesartan during absorption, there is virtually no further metabolism of olmesartan. Total plasma clearance of olmesartan is 1.3 L/h with a renal clearance of 0.6 L/h. Approximately 35% to 50% of the absorbed dose is recovered in urine while the remainder is eliminated in feces via the bile.

Special Populations and Conditions: Pediatrics (<18 years of age): The pharmacokinetics of olmesartan have not been investigated in patients <18 years of age.

Geriatrics (≥65 years of age): The pharmacokinetics of olmesartan was studied in the elderly (≥65 years). Overall, maximum plasma concentrations of olmesartan were similar in young adults and the elderly. Modest but statistically significant accumulation of olmesartan was observed in the elderly with repeated dosing; $AUC_{ss,t}$ was 33% higher in elderly patients, corresponding to an approximate 30% reduction in CL_R. However, the clinical relevance is unknown.

Gender: Minor differences were observed in the pharmacokinetics of olmesartan in women compared to men. AUC and C_{max} were 10-15% higher in women than in men.

Race: The antihypertensive effect of olmesartan was smaller in Black patients (usually a low-renin population), as has been seen with other ACE inhibitors, angiotensin receptor blockers and beta-blockers.

Hepatic Insufficiency: Increases in $AUC_{0-\infty}$ and C_{max} were observed in patients with moderate hepatic impairment compared to those in matched controls, with an increase in AUC of about 60%.

Renal Insufficiency: In patients with renal insufficiency, serum concentrations of olmesartan were elevated compared to subjects with normal renal function. After repeated dosing, the AUC was approximately tripled in patients with severe renal impairment (creatinine clearance <20 mL/min). The pharmacokinetics of olmesartan in patients undergoing hemodialysis has not been studied.

STORAGE AND STABILITY: Store at 15-30°C.

INFORMATION FOR THE PATIENT: Published in e-CPS, available by subscription at www.e-cps.ca.

DOSAGE FORMS, COMPOSITION AND PACKAGING: 20 mg: Each white, round-shaped, film-coated tablet, debossed with C14 on one side contains: olmesartan medoxomil 20 mg. Nonmedicinal ingredients: hydroxypropylcellulose, hydroxypropylmethylcellulose, lactose, low-substituted hydroxypropylcellulose, magnesium stearate, microcrystalline cellulose, talc and titanium dioxide. Blister cards of 7 tablets, cartons of 4 cards.

40 mg: Each white, oval-shaped, film-coated tablet, debossed with C15 on one side contains: olmesartan medoxomil 40 mg. Nonmedicinal ingredients: hydroxypropylcellulose, hydroxypropylmethylcellulose, lactose, low-substituted hydroxypropylcellulose, magnesium stearate, microcrystalline cellulose, talc and titanium dioxide. Blister cards of 7 tablets, cartons of 4 cards.

(Shown in Product Identification Section)

Olmetec Plus® Ⓟ

olmesartan medoxomil—hydrochlorothiazide

Angiotensin II AT1 Receptor Blocker—Diuretic

Schering-Plough

Date of Preparation: November 18, 2008

SUMMARY PRODUCT INFORMATION:

Route of Administration	Dosage Form/ Strength	Clinically Relevant Nonmedicinal Ingredients
Oral	Tablet/20 mg/12.5 mg, 40 mg/12.5 mg, and 40 mg/25 mg	Lactose (see Dosage Forms, Composition and Packaging).

INDICATIONS AND CLINICAL USE: OLMETEC PLUS is indicated for the treatment of mild to moderate essential hypertension in patients for whom combination therapy is appropriate.

OLMETEC PLUS is not indicated for initial therapy (see Dosage and Administration).

Geriatrics (≥65 years of age): Reported clinical experience has not identified differences in responses between elderly and younger patients, however, greater sensitivity of some older individuals cannot be ruled out. (See Dosage and Administration.)

Pediatrics (<18 years of age): The safety and effectiveness in pediatric patients have not been established.

CONTRAINDICATIONS:

- Patients who are hypersensitive to this drug or to any ingredient in the formulation or component of the container. For a complete listing, see the Dosage Forms, Composition and Packaging.
- Because of the hydrochlorothiazide component, OLMETEC PLUS (olmesartan medoxomil and hydrochlorothiazide) is contraindicated in patients with anuria, and in patients who are hypersensitive to other sulfonamide-derived drugs.

WARNINGS AND PRECAUTIONS:

> **Serious Warnings and Precautions**
> When used in pregnancy, angiotensin receptor (AT_1) blockers (ARB) can cause injury or even death of the developing fetus. When pregnancy is detected, OLMETEC PLUS (olmesartan medoxomil and hydrochlorothiazide) should be discontinued as soon as possible (see Warnings and Precautions, Special Populations).

Cardiovascular: Hypotension in Volume- or Salt-Depleted Patients: In patients with an activated renin-angiotensin system, such as volume- or salt-depleted patients (e.g., those being treated with high doses of diuretics), symptomatic hypotension may occur after initiation of treatment with OLMETEC PLUS. Treatment should start under close medical supervision. Similar considerations apply to patients with ischemic heart or cerebrovascular disease, in whom an excessive fall in blood pressure could result in myocardial infarction or cerebrovascular accident. If hypotension does occur, the patient should be placed in the supine position and, if necessary, given an intravenous infusion of normal saline (see Dosage and Administration). When electrolyte and fluid imbalances have been corrected, therapy usually can be continued without difficulty. A transient hypotensive response is not a contraindication to further treatment.

Valvular Stenosis: There is concern on theoretical grounds that patients with aortic stenosis might be at a particular risk of decreased coronary perfusion, because they do not develop as much afterload reduction.

Endocrine and Metabolism: Periodic determinations of serum electrolytes to detect possible electrolyte imbalance should be performed at appropriate intervals. All patients receiving thiazide therapy should be observed for clinical signs of fluid or electrolyte imbalance: hyponatremia, hypochloremic alkalosis and hypokalemia. Serum and urine electrolyte determinations are important when the patient is vomiting excessively or receiving parenteral fluids. Warning signs or symptoms of fluid and electrolyte imbalance, irrespective of cause, include dryness of mouth, thirst, weakness, lethargy, drowsiness, restlessness, confusion, seizures, muscle pains or cramps, muscular fatigue, hypotension, oliguria, tachycardia and gastrointestinal disturbances such as nausea and vomiting.

Hypokalemia may develop, especially with brisk diuresis, when severe cirrhosis is present, or after prolonged therapy.

Interference with adequate oral electrolyte intake will also contribute to hypokalemia. Hypokalemia may cause cardiac arrhythmia and may also sensitize or exaggerate the response of the heart to the toxic effects of digitalis (e.g., increased ventricular irritability).

Although any chloride deficit during thiazide therapy is generally mild and usually does not require specific treatment except under extraordinary circumstances (as in liver disease or renal disease), chloride replacement may be required in the treatment of metabolic alkalosis.

Dilutional hyponatremia may occur in edematous patients in hot weather. Appropriate therapy is water restriction rather than administration of salt, except in rare instances, when the hyponatremia is life threatening. In actual salt depletion, appropriate replacement is the therapy of choice.

Thiazides have been shown to increase the urinary excretion of magnesium; this may result in hypomagnesemia.

Hyperuricemia may occur or acute gout may be precipitated in certain patients receiving thiazide therapy.

Increases in cholesterol and triglyceride levels may be associated with thiazide diuretic therapy.

Thiazides may decrease urinary calcium excretion. Thiazides may cause intermittent and slight elevation of serum calcium in the absence of known disorders of calcium metabolism. Marked hypercalcemia may be evidence of hidden hyperparathyroidism. Thiazides should be discontinued before carrying out tests for parathyroid function.

Thiazides may decrease PBI levels without signs of thyroid disturbance.

Hyperglycemia may occur with thiazide diuretics. Insulin or oral hypoglycemic agents requirements in diabetic patients may be altered and latent diabetes mellitus may become manifest during thiazide diuretic therapy.

Hepatic/Biliary/Pancreatic: No adjustment of dosage is required for patients with mild hepatic impairment. Data is lacking with respect to the use of 20 mg and 40 mg olmesartan medoxomil; therefore a lower starting dose is recommended in patients with moderate liver disease, and the maximum dose of 20 mg/12.5 mg olmesartan medoxomil-hydrochlorothiazide daily should not be exceeded. Care should be exercised in patients with liver disease, especially in those patients with biliary obstructive disorders, as the majority of olmesartan is eliminated in the bile. No information is available in patients with severe liver disease; therefore, use of OLMETEC in this group of patients is not recommended (see Action and Clinical Pharmacology, Pharmacokinetics).

Thiazides should be used with caution in patients with impaired hepatic function or progressive liver disease, since minor alterations of fluid and electrolyte balance may precipitate hepatic coma.

Renal: Impaired Renal Function: As a consequence of inhibiting the renin-angiotensin-aldosterone system, changes in renal function may be anticipated in susceptible individuals treated with olmesartan medoxomil. In patients whose renal function may depend upon the activity of the renin-angiotensin-aldosterone system (e.g., patients with severe congestive heart failure), treatment with angiotensin converting enzyme inhibitors and angiotensin receptor antagonists has been associated with oliguria and/or progressive azotemia and rarely, acute renal failure and/or death. Similar results may be anticipated in patients treated with olmesartan medoxomil (see Action and Clinical Pharmacology, Special Populations and Conditions).

In studies of ACE inhibitors in patients with unilateral or bilateral renal artery stenosis, increases in serum creatinine or blood urea nitrogen (BUN) have been reported. There has been no long-term use of olmesartan medoxomil in patients with unilateral or bilateral renal artery stenosis, but similar results may be expected.

Thiazides should be used with caution in severe renal disease. In patients with renal disease, thiazides may precipitate azotemia. Cumulative effects of the drug may develop in patients with impaired renal function.

If progressive renal impairment becomes evident consider withholding or discontinuing diuretic therapy.

Sensitivity/Resistance: Hypersensitivity reactions to hydrochlorothiazide may occur in patients with or without a history of allergy or bronchial asthma, but are more likely in patients with such a history.

Thiazide diuretics have been reported to cause exacerbation or activation of systemic lupus erythematosus.

Special Populations: Pregnant Women: Drugs that act directly on the renin-angiotensin-aldosterone-system (RAAS) can cause fetal and neonatal morbidity and death when administered to pregnant women. When pregnancy is detected, OLMETEC PLUS should be discontinued as soon as possible.

The use of ARBs is not recommended during pregnancy. Epidemiological evidence regarding the risk of teratogenicity following exposure to angiotensin converting enzyme inhibitors (another class of therapeutic products interfering with the RAAS) during the first trimester of pregnancy has not been conclusive; however a small increase in risk cannot be excluded. Given the current evidence available on the risk with ARB, similar risks may exist for this class of drugs. Patients planning pregnancy should be changed to alternative antihypertensive treatments which have an established safety profile for use in pregnancy. When pregnancy is diagnosed, treatment with angiotensin II antagonists should be stopped immediately, and, if appropriate, alternative therapy should be started.

The use of ARBs during the second and third trimesters is known to induce human fetotoxicity (decreased renal function, oligohydramnios, skull ossification retardation) and neonatal toxicity (renal failure, hypotension, hyperkalemia).

Infants with a history of in utero exposure to ARBs should be closely observed for hypotension, oliguria, and hyperkalemia. If oliguria occurs, attention should be directed toward support of blood pressure and renal perfusion. Exchange transfusion or dialysis may be required as a means of reversing hypotension and/or substituting for impaired renal function; however, limited experience with those procedures has not been associated with significant clinical benefit.

It is not known if olmesartan can be removed from the body by hemodialysis.

Thiazides cross the placental barrier and appear in cord blood. The routine use of diuretics in otherwise healthy pregnant women is not recommended and exposes mother and fetus to unnecessary hazard including fetal or neonatal jaundice, thrombocytopenia and possibly other adverse reactions that have occurred in adults.

Animal Data: No teratogenic effects were observed when 1.6:1 combinations of olmesartan medoxomil and hydrochlorothiazide were administered to pregnant mice at oral doses up to 1625 mg/kg/day (122 times the maximum recommended human dose [MRHD] on a mg/m² basis) or pregnant rats at oral doses up to 1625 mg/kg/day (280 times the MRHD on a mg/m² basis). In rats, however, fetal body weights at 1625 mg/kg/day (a toxic, sometimes lethal dose in the dams) were significantly lower than control. The no observed effect dose for developmental toxicity in rats, 162.5 mg/kg/day, is about 28 times, on a mg/m² basis, the MRHD of OLMETEC PLUS (40 mg olmesartan medoxomil/25 mg hydrochlorothiazide/day).

Nursing Women: It is not known whether olmesartan is excreted in human milk, but olmesartan is secreted at low concentration in the milk of lactating rats. Thiazides appear in human milk. A decision should be made whether to discontinue nursing or discontinue the drug, taking into account the importance of the drug to the mother.

Pediatrics (<18 years of age): The safety and effectiveness in pediatric patients have not been established.

Geriatrics (≥65 years of age): Reported clinical experience has not identified differences in responses between elderly and younger patients, however, greater sensitivity of some older individuals cannot be ruled out.

ADVERSE REACTIONS: Adverse Drug Reaction Overview: Olmesartan Medoxomil-Hydrochlorothiazide: Olmesartan medoxomil-hydrochlorothiazide has been evaluated for safety in 1243 patients treated for essential hypertension. Treatment with olmesartan medoxomil-hydrochlorothiazide was well tolerated, with an incidence of adverse events similar to placebo. Events generally were mild, transient and had no relationship to the dose of olmesartan medoxomil-hydrochlorothiazide.

In the clinical trials, the overall frequency of adverse events was not dose-related. Analysis of gender, age and race groups demonstrated no differences between olmesartan medoxomil-hydrochlorothiazide and placebo-treated patients. The rate of discontinuations due to adverse events in all trials of hypertensive patients was 2.0% (25/1243) of patients treated with olmesartan medoxomil-hydrochlorothiazide and 2.0% (7/342) of patients treated with placebo. The following potentially serious adverse reactions have been reported with OLMETEC/OLMETEC PLUS in controlled trials: syncope, hypotension.

Clinical Trial Adverse Drug Reactions: Because clinical trials are conducted under very specific conditions the adverse reaction rates observed in the clinical trials may not reflect the rates observed in practice and should not be compared to the rates in the clinical trials of another drug. Adverse drug reaction information from clinical trials is useful for identifying drug-related adverse events and for approximating rates.

In a placebo-controlled clinical trial, the following adverse events were reported with olmesartan medoxomil-hydrochlorothiazide in >1% of patients (Table 1).

Table 1: OLMETEC PLUS

Adverse Events[a] Occurring >1% in Placebo-controlled Cohort

System Organ Class (SOC) MedDRA Preferred Term	Total Placebo ALONE (N=42) N (%)	Total HCTZ ALONE (N=88) N (%)	Total Olmesartan Medoxomil ALONE (N=125) N (%)	Total Olmesartan Medoxomil+HCTZ (N=247) N (%)
Ear and Labyrinth Disorders				
Ear disorder	0 (0.0%)	0 (0.0%)	0 (0.0%)	5 (2.0%)
Gastrointestinal Disorders				
Nausea	0 (0.0%)	1 (1.1%)	2 (1.6%)	7 (2.8%)
Abdominal pain	1 (2.4%)	1 (1.1%)	4 (3.2%)	5 (2.0%)
Dyspepsia	0 (0.0%)	4 (4.5%)	2 (1.6%)	5 (2.0%)
Diarrhea	1 (2.4%)	2 (2.3%)	4 (3.2%)	4 (1.6%)
Gastroenteritis	1 (2.4%)	0 (0.0%)	0 (0.0%)	3 (1.2%)
General Disorders and Administration Site Conditions				
Fatigue	0 (0.0%)	1 (1.1%)	3 (2.4%)	5 (2.0%)
Influenza like illness	0 (0.0%)	1 (1.1%)	1 (0.8%)	3 (1.2%)
Immune System Disorders				
Hypersensitivity	0 (0.0%)	1 (1.1%)	1 (0.8%)	3 (1.2%)
Infections and Infestations				
Upper respiratory tract infection	0 (0.0%)	6 (6.8%)	8 (6.4%)	16 (6.5%)
Urinary tract infections	1 (2.4%)	1 (1.1%)	1 (0.8%)	8 (3.2%)
Pharyngitis	0 (0.0%)	1 (1.1%)	1 (0.8%)	4 (1.6%)
Rhinitis	2 (4.8%)	0 (0.0%)	3 (2.4%)	4 (1.6%)
Sinusitis	1 (2.4%)	2 (2.3%)	3 (2.4%)	3 (1.2%)

(cont'd)

Table 1: OLMETEC PLUS *(cont'd)*
Adverse Events[a] Occurring >1% in Placebo-controlled Cohort

System Organ Class (SOC) MedDRA Preferred Term	Total Placebo ALONE (N=42) N (%)	Total HCTZ ALONE (N=88) N (%)	Total Olmesartan Medoxomil ALONE (N=125) N (%)	Total Olmesartan Medoxomil+HCTZ (N=247) N (%)
Injury, Poisoning and Procedural Complications				
Injury	0 (0.0%)	3 (3.4%)	1 (0.8%)	6 (2.4%)
Metabolism and Nutrition Disorders				
Hyperuricemia	1 (2.4%)	2 (2.3%)	0 (0.0%)	10 (4.0%)
Hyperglycemia	1 (2.4%)	2 (2.3%)	0 (0.0%)	5 (2.0%)
Hyperlipemia	0 (0.0%)	1 (1.1%)	1 (0.8%)	4 (1.6%)
BUN increased	0 (0.0%)	0 (0.0%)	0 (0.0%)	4 (1.6%)
Musculoskeletal and Connective Tissue Disorders				
Back pain	1 (2.4%)	2 (2.3%)	3 (2.4%)	5 (2.0%)
Myalgia	0 (0.0%)	1 (1.1%)	4 (3.2%)	5 (2.0%)
Nervous System Disorders				
Dizziness	1 (2.4%)	7 (8.0%)	1 (0.8%)	23 (9.3%)
Headache	3 (7.1%)	4 (4.5%)	11 (8.8%)	13 (5.3%)
Renal and Urinary Disorders				
Hematuria	0 (0.0%)	0 (0.0%)	0 (0.0%)	6 (2.4%)
Pyuria	0 (0.0%)	1 (1.1%)	1 (0.8%)	4 (1.6%)
Urine analysis abnormal	0 (0.0%)	0 (0.0%)	0 (0.0%)	4 (1.6%)
Respiratory, Thoracic and Mediastinal Disorders				
Cough	0 (0.0%)	0 (0.0%)	2 (1.6%)	5 (2.0%)
Vascular Disorders				
Hypotension	0 (0.0%)	0 (0.0%)	0 (0.0%)	3 (1.2%)

[a] Adverse events reported in >1% of patients in the Total Olmesartan Medoxomil+HCTZ treatment group.

Other adverse events that have been reported with an incidence of greater than 1.0%, whether or not attributed to treatment, in the more than 1200 hypertensive patients treated with olmesartan medoxomil-hydrochlorothiazide in controlled or open-label trials are listed below.

Gastrointestinal Disorders: abdominal pain, dyspepsia, diarrhea.
General Disorders and Administration Site Conditions: chest pain, edema peripheral.
Infections and Infestations: gastroenteritis.
Investigations: alanine aminotransferase increased, aspartate aminotransferase increased, creatine phosphokinase increased, gamma-glutamyltransferase increased.
Musculoskeletal and Connective Tissue Disorders: arthritis, arthralgia, back pain, myalgia.
Nervous System Disorders: vertigo.
Renal and Urinary Disorders: hematuria.
Respiratory, Thoracic and Mediastinal Disorders: cough.
Skin and Subcutaneous Tissue Disorders: rash.

Less Common Clinical Trial Adverse Drug Reactions (<1%): Facial edema was reported in 2/1243 patients receiving olmesartan medoxomil-hydrochlorothiazide. Angioedema has been reported with angiotensin II receptor antagonists.

Abnormal Hematologic and Clinical Chemistry Findings: In controlled clinical trials, clinically important changes in standard laboratory parameters were rarely associated with administration of olmesartan medoxomil-hydrochlorothiazide.

Liver Functions Tests: Elevations of liver enzymes and/or serum bilirubin were observed infrequently.

	Placebo (n=42)	HCTZ (n=88)	Olmesartan Medoxomil (n=125)	Olmesartan Medoxomil+HCTZ (n=247)
CPK increased	2 (4.8%)	2 (2.3%)	3 (2.4%)	4 (1.6%)
γGT increased	1 (2.4%)	1 (1.1%)	3 (2.4%)	3 (1.2%)
ALT increased	2 (4.8%)	1 (1.1%)	3 (2.4%)	3 (1.2%)
AST increased	1 (2.4%)	1 (1.1%)	3 (2.4%)	3 (1.2%)

Creatinine, Blood Urea Nitrogen: Increases in blood urea nitrogen (BUN) and serum creatinine of >50% were observed in 1.3% of patients. No patients were discontinued from clinical trials of olmesartan medoxomil-hydrochlorothiazide due to increased BUN or creatinine.

Hemoglobin and Hematocrit: A greater than 20% decrease in hemoglobin and hematocrit was observed in 0.0 % and 0.4% (one patient), respectively, of olmesartan medoxomil-hydrochlorothiazide patients, compared with 0.0% and 0.0%, respectively, in placebo-treated patients. No patients were discontinued due to anemia.

Post-Market Adverse Drug Reactions: Other adverse events reported rarely in post-marketing use include: asthenia, angioedema, vomiting, hyperkalemia, rhabdomyolysis, renal failure acute, blood creatinine increased, alopecia, pruritus, urticaria, palpitations, syncope, and blood uric acid increased.

DRUG INTERACTIONS: Drug-Drug Interactions: Olmesartan Medoxomil: Diuretics: Patients on diuretics, and especially those in whom diuretic therapy was recently instituted, may occasionally experience an excessive reduction in blood pressure after initiation of therapy with olmesartan. The possibility of symptomatic hypotension with the use of olmesartan can be minimized by discontinuing the diuretic prior to initiation of treatment (see Warnings and Precautions, Cardiovascular, Hypotension in Volume- or Salt-Depleted Patients). No drug interaction of clinical significance has been identified with thiazide diuretics.

Warfarin: There was no effect on either the pharmacokinetics or pharmacodynamics of warfarin when co-administered with olmesartan medoxomil in healthy volunteers.

Digoxin: No pharmacokinetics or pharmacodynamics effects were reported when olmesartan medoxomil was co-administered with digoxin in healthy volunteers.

Antacids: The bioavailability of olmesartan was not significantly altered when co-administered with antacids [$Al(OH)_3$/$Mg(OH)_2$].

Cytochrome P450 Enzyme System: Unlike some other angiotensin II receptor blockers, olmesartan medoxomil is not metabolized by cytochrome P450 enzymes. Interactions with drugs that inhibit, induce or are metabolized by these enzymes are not expected.

Hydrochlorothiazide: When administered concurrently the following drugs may interact with thiazide diuretics:

Agents Increasing Serum Potassium: Concomitant use of potassium-sparing diuretics (e.g., spironolactone, triamterene, amiloride), potassium supplements, or salt substitutes containing potassium may lead to increase in serum potassium.

Since olmesartan decreases the production of aldosterone, potassium-sparing diuretics or potassium supplements should be given only for documented hypokalemia and with frequent monitoring of serum potassium when olmesartan medoxomil therapy is initiated. Potassium-containing salt substitutes should also be used with caution. Concomitant thiazide diuretic use may attenuate any effect that olmesartan may have on serum potassium.

Alcohol, Barbiturates, or Narcotics: Potentiation of orthostatic hypotension may occur.

Antidiabetic Drugs (oral agents and insulin): Due to the potential for hyperglycemia in patients on thiazides, dosage adjustment of the antidiabetic drug may be required.

Cholestyramine and Colestipol Resins: Absorption of hydrochlorothiazide is impaired in the presence of anionic exchange resins. Single doses of either cholestyramine or colestipol resins bind the hydrochlorothiazide and reduce its absorption from the gastrointestinal tract by up to 85 and 43 percent, respectively.

Corticosteroids, ACTH: Intensified electrolyte depletion, particularly hypokalemia may occur.

Lithium Salts: As with other drugs which eliminate sodium, lithium clearance may be reduced in the presence of olmesartan. Therefore, serum lithium levels should be monitored carefully if lithium salts are to be administered with olmesartan medoxomil. Lithium generally should not be given with diuretics. Diuretic agents reduce the renal clearance of lithium and add a high risk of lithium toxicity.

Non-steroidal Anti-inflammatory Drugs (NSAIDs): The administration of a non-steroidal anti-inflammatory agent can reduce the diuretic, natriuretic and antihypertensive effects of loop, potassium-sparing and thiazide diuretics. Therefore, when OLMETEC PLUS and NSAID agents are used concomitantly, the patients should be observed closely to determine if the desired effect of the diuretic is obtained.

Other Antihypertensive Drugs: Diuretic additive effect or potentiation of anti-hypertensive effect may occur.

Pressor Amines (e.g., Norepinephrine): In the presence of diuretics, possible decreased response to pressor amines may occur but the effect is not sufficient to preclude their use.

Skeletal Muscle Relaxants, Non depolarizing (e.g., Tubocurarine): Thiazide drugs may increase responsiveness to the muscle relaxant.

Drug-Food Interactions: OLMETEC PLUS may be administered with or without food.
Drug-Herb Interactions: Interactions with herbal products have not been established.
Drug-Laboratory Test Interactions: Interactions with laboratory tests have not been established.

DOSAGE AND ADMINISTRATION: Dosing Considerations:

- OLMETEC PLUS (olmesartan medoxomil and hydrochlorothiazide) is not for initial therapy.
- The dosage must be individualized.
- To minimize dose-independent side effects, it is usually appropriate to begin combination therapy only after a patient has failed to achieve the desired effect with monotherapy.
- The dose of OLMETEC PLUS should be determined by the titration of the individual components.

Recommended Dose and Dosage Adjustment: Replacement Therapy: Once the patient has been stabilized on the individual components as described below, OLMETEC PLUS may be substituted if the doses on which the patient was stabilized are the same as those in the fixed combination.

Dose Titration by Clinical Effect: OLMETEC PLUS is available in strengths of 20 mg/12.5 mg, 40 mg/12.5 mg and 40 mg/25 mg. A patient whose blood pressure is inadequately controlled by olmesartan medoxomil or hydrochlorothiazide alone may be switched to once daily OLMETEC PLUS. Dosage should be individualized. Depending on the blood pressure response, the dose may be titrated at intervals of 2-4 weeks.

The antihypertensive effect of OLMETEC PLUS is related to the dose of both components over the range of 10 mg/12.5 mg to 40 mg/25 mg (see Action and Clinical Pharmacology). The dose of OLMETEC PLUS is one tablet once daily. More than one tablet daily is not recommended.

- **Elderly:** No adjustment of dose is generally required in elderly patients (see below for dose recommendation in patients with renal impairment). If up-titration to the maximum dose of 40 mg/25 mg daily is required, blood pressure should be closely monitored (see Action and Clinical Pharmacology, Special Populations and Conditions).
- **Hepatic Impairment:** No adjustment of dosage is required for patients with mild hepatic impairment. Data is lacking with respect to the use of 20 mg and 40 mg olmesartan medoxomil; therefore, a lower starting dose is recommended in patients with moderate liver disease, and the maximum dose of 20 mg/12.5 mg olmesartan medoxomil-hydrochlorothiazide daily should not be exceeded. Care should be exercised in patients with liver disease, especially in those patients with biliary obstructive disorders, as the majority of olmesartan is eliminated in the bile. No information is available in patients with severe liver disease; therefore, use of OLMETEC in this group of patients is not recommended (see Action and Clinical Pharmacology, Pharmacokinetics).
- **Renal Impairment:** Owing to the limited experience of higher dosages in this patient group, the maximum dose in patients with mild to moderate renal impairment is 20 mg/12.5 mg once daily. The use of olmesartan medoxomil in patients with severe renal impairment is not recommended, since there is only limited experience in this patient group. In patients with more severe renal impairment, loop diuretics are preferred to thiazides, so OLMETEC PLUS is not recommended.

For patients with possible depletion of intravascular volume (e.g., patients treated with diuretics, particularly those with impaired renal function), OLMETEC PLUS should be initiated under close medical supervision and consideration should be given to use of a lower starting dose (see Warnings and Precautions, Renal).

The side effects (see Warnings and Precautions) of olmesartan medoxomil are generally rare and independent of dose; those of hydrochlorothiazide are most typically dose-dependent (primarily hypokalemia). Some dose-independent phenomena (e.g., pancreatitis) do occur with hydrochlorothiazide. Therapy with any combination of olmesartan medoxomil and hydrochlorothiazide will be associated with both sets of dose-independent side effects. To minimize dose-independent side effects, it is usually appropriate to begin combination therapy only after a patient has failed to achieve the desired effect with monotherapy.

Olmesartan Medoxomil Monotherapy: The usual recommended starting dose of olmesartan medoxomil monotherapy is 20 mg once daily in patients who are not volume-contracted. For patients requiring further reduction in blood pressure after 2 weeks of therapy, the dose may be increased to 40 mg. Doses above 40 mg do not appear to have greater effect. Twice-daily dosing offers no advantage over the same total dose given once daily.

- **Elderly:** No adjustment of dose is generally required in elderly patients (see below for dose recommendation in patients with renal impairment). If up-titration to the maximum dose of 40 mg daily is required, blood pressure should be closely monitored (see Action and Clinical Pharmacology, Special Populations and Conditions).
- **Hepatic Impairment:** No adjustment of dosage is required for patients with mild hepatic impairment. Data is lacking with respect to the use of 20 mg and 40 mg olmesartan medoxomil; therefore, a lower starting dose is recommended in patients with moderate liver disease, and the maximum dose of 20 mg/12.5 mg olmesartan medoxomil-hydrochlorothiazide daily should not be exceeded. Care should be exercised in patients with liver disease, especially in those patients with biliary obstructive disorders, as the majority of olmesartan is eliminated in the bile. No information is available in patients with severe liver disease; therefore, use of OLMETEC in this group of patients is not recommended (see Action and Clinical Pharmacology, Pharmacokinetics).
- **Renal Impairment:** Owing to the limited experience of higher dosages in this patient group, the maximum dose in patients with mild to moderate renal impairment is 20 mg olmesartan medoxomil once daily. The use of olmesartan medoxomil in patients with severe renal impairment is not recommended, since there is only limited experience in this patient group.

For patients with possible depletion of intravascular volume (e.g., patients treated with diuretics, particularly those with impaired renal function), OLMETEC PLUS should be initiated under close medical supervision and consideration should be given to use of a lower starting dose (see Warnings and Precautions, Renal).

If blood pressure is not controlled by olmesartan medoxomil alone, hydrochlorothiazide may be added starting with a dose of 12.5 mg and later titrated to 25 mg once daily.

Hydrochlorothiazide is effective in doses between 12.5 mg and 50 mg once daily. If a patient is taking hydrochlorothiazide, olmesartan medoxomil may be added starting with a dose of 20 mg once daily and titrated to 40 mg, for inadequate blood pressure control. If large doses of hydrochlorothiazide have been used as monotherapy and volume depletion or hyponatremia is present, caution should be used when adding olmesartan medoxomil or switching to OLMETEC PLUS as marked decreases in blood pressure may occur (see Warnings and Precautions, Renal). Consideration should be given to reducing the dose of hydrochlorothiazide to 12.5 mg before adding olmesartan medoxomil.

Missed Dose: If patients miss a dose, they should wait until their next scheduled dose. Patients should not double their dose.

OVERDOSAGE:

Olmesartan Medoxomil: Limited data are available related to overdosage in humans. The most likely manifestations of overdosage would be hypotension and tachycardia; bradycardia could be encountered if parasympathetic (vagal) stimulation occurs. If symptomatic hypotension should occur, supportive treatment should be initiated. The dialyzability of olmesartan is unknown.

Hydrochlorothiazide: The most common signs and symptoms of overdose observed in humans are those caused by electrolyte depletion (hypokalemia, hypochloremia, hyponatremia) and dehydration resulting from excessive diuresis. If digitalis has also been administered, hypokalemia may accentuate cardiac arrhythmias. The degree to which hydrochlorothiazide is removed by hemodialysis has not been established.

> For management of a suspected drug overdose, CPhA recommends that you contact your **regional Poison Control Centre**. See the *CPS* Directory section for a list of Poison Control Centres.

ACTION AND CLINICAL PHARMACOLOGY: Mechanism of Action: Olmesartan Medoxomil : Olmesartan medoxomil, a prodrug, is hydrolyzed to olmesartan during absorption from the gastrointestinal tract.

Angiotensin II is formed from angiotensin I in a reaction catalyzed by angiotensin converting enzyme (ACE, kininase II). Angiotensin II is the principal pressor agent of the renin-angiotensin system, with effects that include vasoconstriction, stimulation of synthesis and release of aldosterone, cardiac stimulation and renal reabsorption of sodium. Olmesartan blocks the vasoconstrictor effects of angiotensin II by selectively blocking the binding of angiotensin II to the AT_1 receptor in vascular smooth muscle. Its action is, therefore, independent of the pathways for angiotensin II synthesis.

An AT_2 receptor is found also in many tissues, but this receptor is not known to be associated with cardiovascular homeostasis. Olmesartan has more than a 12 500-fold greater affinity for the AT_1 receptor than for the AT_2 receptor.

Blockade of the renin-angiotensin system with ACE inhibitors, which inhibit the biosynthesis of angiotensin II from angiotensin I, is a mechanism of many drugs used to treat hypertension. ACE inhibitors also inhibit the degradation of bradykinin, a reaction also catalyzed by ACE. Because olmesartan does not inhibit ACE (kininase II), it does not affect the response to bradykinin. Whether this difference has clinical relevance is not yet known.

Blockade of the angiotensin II receptor inhibits the negative regulatory feedback of angiotensin II on renin secretion, but the resulting increased plasma renin activity and circulating angiotensin II levels do not overcome the effect of olmesartan on blood pressure.

Hydrochlorothiazide: Hydrochlorothiazide is a thiazide diuretic. Thiazides affect the renal tubular mechanisms of electrolyte reabsorption, directly increasing excretion of sodium and chloride in approximately equivalent amounts. Indirectly, the diuretic action of hydrochlorothiazide reduces plasma volume, with consequent increases in plasma renin activity, increases in aldosterone secretion, increases in urinary potassium loss, and decreases in serum potassium. The renin-aldosterone link is mediated by angiotensin II, so co-administration of an angiotensin II receptor antagonist tends to reverse the potassium loss associated with these diuretics.

The mechanism of the antihypertensive effect of thiazides is not fully understood.

Pharmacodynamics: Olmesartan Medoxomil: Olmesartan medoxomil doses of 2.5 to 40 mg inhibit the pressor effects of angiotensin I infusion. The duration of the inhibitory effect was related to dose, with doses of olmesartan medoxomil >40 mg giving >90% inhibition at 24 hours.

Plasma concentrations of angiotensin I and angiotensin II and plasma renin activity (PRA) increase after single and repeated administration of olmesartan medoxomil to healthy subjects and hypertensive patients. Repeated administration of up to 80 mg olmesartan medoxomil had minimal influence on aldosterone levels and no effect on serum potassium.

Hydrochlorothiazide: After oral administration of hydrochlorothiazide, diuresis begins within 2 hours, peaks in about 4 hours and lasts about 6 to 12 hours.

Pharmacokinetics: Absorption: Olmesartan Medoxomil: Olmesartan medoxomil is rapidly and completely bioactivated by ester hydrolysis to olmesartan during absorption from the gastrointestinal tract. Olmesartan appears to be eliminated in a biphasic manner with a terminal elimination half-life of approximately 13 hours. Olmesartan shows linear pharmacokinetics following single oral doses of up to 320 mg and multiple oral doses of up to 80 mg. Steady-state levels of olmesartan are achieved within 3 to 5 days and no accumulation in plasma occurs with once-daily dosing.

The absolute bioavailability of olmesartan is approximately 26%. After oral administration, the peak plasma concentration (C_{max}) of olmesartan is reached after 1 to 2 hours. Food does not affect the bioavailability of olmesartan.

Hydrochlorothiazide: When plasma levels have been followed for at least 24 hours, the plasma half-life has been observed to vary between 5.6 and 14.8 hours.

Distribution: Olmesartan: The volume of distribution of olmesartan is approximately 17 L. Olmesartan is highly bound to plasma proteins (99%) and does not penetrate red blood cells. The protein binding is constant at plasma olmesartan concentrations well above the range achieved with recommended doses.

In rats, olmesartan crossed the blood-brain barrier poorly, if at all. Olmesartan passed across the placental barrier in rats and was distributed to the fetus. Olmesartan was distributed to milk at low levels in rats.

Hydrochlorothiazide: Hydrochlorothiazide crosses the placental but not the blood-brain barrier and is excreted in breast milk.

Metabolism and Excretion: Olmesartan Medoxomil : Following the rapid and complete conversion of olmesartan medoxomil to olmesartan during absorption, there is virtually no further metabolism of olmesartan. Total plasma clearance of olmesartan is 1.3 L/h, with a renal clearance of 0.6 L/h. Approximately 35% to 50% of the absorbed dose is recovered in urine while the remainder is eliminated in feces via the bile.

Hydrochlorothiazide: Hydrochlorothiazide is not metabolized but is eliminated rapidly by the kidney. At least 61% of the oral dose is eliminated unchanged within 24 hours.

Special Populations and Conditions: Pediatrics (<18 years of age): The pharmacokinetics of olmesartan have not been investigated in patients <18 years of age.

Geriatrics (≥65 years of age): The pharmacokinetics of olmesartan were studied in the elderly (≥65 years). Overall, maximum plasma concentrations of olmesartan were similar in young adults and the elderly. Modest but statistically significant accumulation of olmesartan was observed in the elderly with repeated dosing; $AUC_{ss,t}$ was 33% higher in elderly patients, corresponding to an approximate 30% reduction in CL_R. However, the clinical relevance is unknown.

Gender: Minor differences were observed in the pharmacokinetics of olmesartan in women compared to men. AUC and C_{max} were 10-15% higher in women than in men.

Race: The antihypertensive effect of olmesartan was smaller in Black patients (usually a low-renin population), as has been seen with other ACE inhibitors, angiotensin receptor blockers and beta-blockers.

Hepatic Insufficiency: Increases in $AUC_{0-\infty}$ and C_{max} for olmesartan were observed in patients with moderate hepatic impairment compared to those in matched controls, with an increase in AUC of about 60%.

Renal Insufficiency: In patients with renal insufficiency, serum concentrations of olmesartan were elevated compared to subjects with normal renal function. After repeated dosing, the AUC was approximately tripled in patients with severe renal impairment (creatinine clearance <20 mL/min). The pharmacokinetics of olmesartan in patients undergoing hemodialysis has not been studied.

STORAGE AND STABILITY: Store at 15-30°C.

INFORMATION FOR THE PATIENT: Published in e-CPS, available by subscription at www.e-cps.ca.

DOSAGE FORMS, COMPOSITION AND PACKAGING: 20 mg/12.5 mg: Each reddish-yellow, circular, film-coated tablet, approximately 8.5 mm in diameter, with "C22" debossed on one side, contains: olmesartan medoxomil 20 mg and hydrochlorothiazide 12.5 mg. Nonmedicinal ingredients: hydroxypropylcellulose, hypromellose, lactose, low-substituted hydroxypropylcellulose, magnesium stearate, microcrystalline cellulose, red iron oxide, talc, titanium dioxide and yellow iron oxide. Blister cards of 7 tablets, cartons of 4 cards.

40 mg/12.5 mg: Each reddish-yellow, oval, film-coated tablet, approximately 15×7 mm, with "C23" debossed on one side contains: olmesartan medoxomil 40 mg and hydrochlorothiazide 12.5 mg. Nonmedicinal ingredients: hydroxypropylcellulose, hypromellose, lactose, low-substituted hydroxypropylcellulose, magnesium stearate, microcrystalline cellulose, red iron oxide, talc, titanium dioxide and yellow iron oxide. Blister cards of 7 tablets, cartons of 4 cards.

40 mg/25 mg: Each pink, oval, film-coated tablet, approximately 15×7 mm, with "C25" debossed on one side contains: olmesartan medoxomil 40 mg and hydrochlorothiazide 25 mg. Nonmedicinal ingredients: hydroxypropylcellulose, hypromellose, lactose, low-substituted hydroxypropylcellulose, magnesium stearate, microcrystalline cellulose, red iron oxide, talc, titanium dioxide and yellow iron oxide. Blister cards of 7 tablets, cartons of 4 cards.

(Shown in Product Identification Section)

> The reader is invited to consult CPhA's monograph **Corticosteroids: Eye, Ear, Nose.**

Omnaris™ Ⓟ

ciclesonide

Corticosteroid for Nasal Use

Nycomed

Date of Revision: April 23, 2008

SUMMARY PRODUCT INFORMATION:

Route of Administration	Dosage Form/ Strength	Clinically Relevant Nonmedicinal Ingredients
Nasal	Spray 50 µg/spray	For a complete listing see Dosage Forms, Composition and Packaging.

INDICATIONS AND CLINICAL USE: OMNARIS (ciclesonide nasal spray) is indicated for:

- the treatment of seasonal allergic rhinitis, including hayfever, and perennial allergic rhinitis in adults and adolescents 12 years of age and older.

Geriatrics (>65 years of age): A total of 31 patients 65 years of age and older (age range 65 to 75 years) have been treated with OMNARIS 200 µg/day for up to 1 year. The adverse reactions reported in this population were similar in type and incidence to those reported by younger patients, but greater sensitivity of some older individuals cannot be ruled out. Based on available data for OMNARIS, no adjustment of dosage of OMNARIS in geriatric patients is warranted.

Pediatrics: OMNARIS is not presently approved for use in patients younger than 12 years of age. A total of 91 patients 12-17 years of age were treated with OMNARIS for up to one year. No differences in the rate or incidence of adverse events were observed.

CONTRAINDICATIONS:

- OMNARIS is contraindicated in patients with a hypersensitivity to any of the ingredients. For a complete listing see Dosage Forms, Composition and Packaging.
- OMNARIS should be used with caution, if at all, in patients with active or quiescent tuberculosis infections of the respiratory tract.

WARNINGS AND PRECAUTIONS: Immune: Patients who are on drugs that suppress the immune system are more susceptible to infections than healthy individuals. Chickenpox and measles, for example, can have a more serious or even fatal course in children or adults on corticosteroids. In children or adults who have not had these diseases, particular care should be taken to avoid exposure. How the dose, route, and duration of corticosteroid administration affects the risk of developing a disseminated infection is not known. The contribution of the underlying disease and/or prior corticosteroid treatment to the risk is also not known. If exposed to chickenpox, prophylaxis with varicella zoster immune globulin (VZIG) may be indicated. If exposed to measles, prophylaxis with pooled intramuscular immunoglobulin (IG) may be indicated. If chickenpox develops, treatment with antiviral agents may be considered.

Because of the inhibitory effect of corticosteroids on wound healing, patients who have experienced recent nasal septal ulcers, nasal surgery, or nasal trauma should not use a nasal corticosteroid until healing has occurred.

Infection: In clinical studies with corticosteroids administered intranasally, the development of localized infections of the nose and pharynx with *C. albicans* have been reported only rarely.

When such an infection develops, it may require treatment with appropriate local therapy and discontinuation of treatment with the intranasal steroid. Therefore, patients using intranasal corticosteroids over several months or longer should be examined periodically for evidence of Candida infection or other signs of adverse effects on the nasal mucosa.

OMNARIS should be used with caution, if at all, in patients with untreated local or systemic fungal or bacterial infections; systemic viral or parasitic infections; or ocular herpes simplex.

Systemic Effects: Rarely, immediate hypersensitivity reactions or contact dermatitis may occur after the administration of intranasal corticosteroids. Rare instances of wheezing, nasal septum perforation, cataracts, glaucoma, and increased intraocular pressure have been reported following the intranasal application of corticosteroids. The risk of glaucoma was evaluated by assessments of intraocular pressure in 390 adolescent or adult patients receiving treatment with OMNARIS 200 µg daily for up to 52 weeks. In this trial, no significant differences in intraocular pressure changes were observed between OMNARIS and placebo-treated patients. Additionally, no significant differences between OMNARIS 200 µg and placebo-treated patients were noted during the 52-week study of 577 patients in which thorough ophthalmologic assessments were performed including evaluation of cataract formation using slit lamp examinations.

Although systemic effects have been minimal with recommended doses of OMNARIS, any such effect is likely to be dose dependent. Therefore, larger than recommended doses of OMNARIS should be avoided. When used at excessive doses, systemic corticosteroid effects such as hypercorticism and adrenal suppression may occur. If such changes occur, the dosage of OMNARIS should be discontinued slowly, consistent with accepted procedures for discontinuing oral corticosteroid therapy.

Physicians should closely follow the growth of children and adolescents taking corticosteroids by any route, and weigh the benefits of corticosteroid therapy against the possibility of growth suppression if growth appears slowed. To minimize the systemic effects of intranasal corticosteroids each patient should be titrated to his/her lowest effective dose.

Systemic Steroid Replacement by a Topical Steroid: The replacement of a systemic corticosteroid with a topical corticosteroid can be accompanied by signs of adrenal insufficiency. In addition, some patients may experience symptoms of corticosteroid withdrawal, e.g., joint and/or muscular pain, lassitude, and depression. Patients previously treated for prolonged periods with systemic corticosteroids and transferred to topical corticosteroids should be carefully monitored for acute adrenal insufficiency in response to stress. In those patients who have asthma or other clinical conditions requiring long-term systemic corticosteroid treatment, rapid decreases in systemic corticosteroid dosages may cause a severe exacerbation of their symptoms.

Special Populations: Pregnant Women: There are no adequate and well-controlled studies with OMNARIS in pregnant women. As with other corticosteroids, ciclesonide should only be used during pregnancy when the potential benefit to the mother justifies the potential risk to the mother, fetus or infant. Infants born to mothers who received corticosteroids during pregnancy should be observed carefully for hypoadrenalism.

The extent of exposure in pregnancy during clinical trials: Very Limited: individual cases only.

Nursing Women: It is unknown if ciclesonide is excreted in human milk. As with other corticosteroids, OMNARIS should only be used in nursing women when the potential benefit to the mother justifies the potential risk to the mother and/or infant.

Pediatrics: OMNARIS is not presently approved for use in patients younger than 12 years of age. A total of 91 patients 12-17 years of age were treated with OMNARIS for up to one year. No differences in the rate or incidence of adverse events were observed.

Geriatrics (>65 years of age): A total of 31 patients above 65 years of age (age range 65 to 75 years) have been treated with OMNARIS 200 µg/day for up to 1 year. The adverse reactions reported in this population were similar in type and incidence to those reported by younger patients, but greater sensitivity of some older individuals cannot be ruled out. Based on available data for OMNARIS, no adjustment of dosage of OMNARIS in geriatric patients is warranted.

Monitoring and Laboratory Tests: As with any long-term treatment, patients using OMNARIS over several months or longer should be examined periodically for possible changes in the nasal mucosa.

ADVERSE REACTIONS: Clinical Trial Adverse Drug Reactions: Because clinical trials are conducted under very specific conditions the adverse reaction rates observed in the clinical trials may not reflect the rates observed in practice and should not be compared to the rates in the clinical trials of another drug. Adverse drug reaction information from clinical trials is useful for identifying drug-related adverse events and for approximating rates.

In controlled clinical studies, a total of 2013 patients ages 12 years and older received treatment with OMNARIS. In studies of 2 to 6-weeks duration, 677 patients were treated with OMNARIS 200 µg daily, and in a study of up to one year in duration, 441 patients were treated with OMNARIS 200 µg daily. The overall incidence of adverse events for patients treated with OMNARIS was comparable to that in patients treated with the placebo. Approximately 2% of patients treated with OMNARIS 200 µg in clinical trials discontinued because of adverse events; this rate was similar for patients treated with placebo.

Table 1 displays adverse events, assessed as likely or definitely related to treatment by the investigator, that occurred with an incidence of 1% or greater in clinical trials of 2 to 6-weeks in duration.

Table 1: OMNARIS

Common Adverse Reactions[a] (1-10%) in Controlled Clinical Trials 2 to 6-weeks in Duration in Patients 12 Years of Age and Older with Seasonal or Perennial Allergic Rhinitis

Adverse Reaction	OMNARIS 200 μg n=677 (%)	Placebo n=674 (%)
Epistaxis[b]	2.7	2.1
Nasal Passage Irritation[c]	2.4	2.2
Headache	1.3	0.7

[a] Assessed as likely or definitely related to the treatment by investigator.
[b] Epistaxis (e.g. frank bleeding, blood-tinged mucus and blood flecks).
[c] Nasal passage irritation includes nasal discomfort.

In a 52-week long-term safety trial that included 663 adolescent and adult patients (227 males and 436 females) with perennial allergic rhinitis, the adverse event profile over the treatment period was similar to the adverse event profile in trials of shorter duration. Adverse events considered likely or definitely related to OMNARIS that were reported at an incidence of 1% or greater are presented in Table 2. No patient experienced a nasal septal perforation or nasal ulcer during long-term use of OMNARIS nor was there any evidence of HPA-axis suppression in this study.

Table 2: OMNARIS

Common Adverse Reactions[a] (1-10%) in a 52-week Study in Adult and Adolescent Patients with Perennial Allergic Rhinitis

Adverse Reaction	OMNARIS 200 μg n=441 (%)	Placebo n=222 (%)
Epistaxis[b]	8.4	6.3
Nasal passage irritation[c]	4.3	3.6
Headache	1.6	0.5

[a] Assessed as likely or definitely related to the treatment by investigator.
[b] Epistaxis (e.g. frank bleeding, blood-tinged mucus and blood flecks).
[c] Nasal passage irritation includes nasal discomfort.

The following less common adverse reactions (assessed as possibly related to treatment by the investigator) were reported in controlled clinical trials 2 to 52 weeks in duration in patients 12 years of age and older with Seasonal Allergic or Perennial Allergic Rhinitis treated with OMNARIS 200 μg:

Less Common Clinical Trial Adverse Drug Reactions (≥0.1% to <1%): Gastrointestinal: dry mouth (0.2%), dyspepsia (0.2%).
Infections: candidiasis (0.2%), rhinitis (0.2%).
Investigations: laboratory test abnormal NOS (0.2%), white blood cell count increased (0.3%).
Nervous System: dysgeusia (0.2%).
Respiratory, Thoracic and Mediastinal: nasal dryness (0.4%), pharyngolaryngeal pain (0.4%), rhinorrhoea* (0.3%), nasal septum disorder (0.2%), throat irritation* (0.2%).
Special Populations: The incidence of adverse events did not differ appreciably based on age, gender or race.
Abnormal Hematologic and Clinical Chemistry Findings: Examination of the percentage of patients with normal values at baseline and values above or below the normal range at the end of treatment did not demonstrate any trends with respect to changes in hematology and biochemistry values, see Less Common Clinical Trial Adverse Drug Reactions (≥0.1% to <1%).

DRUG INTERACTIONS: Overview: In vitro data indicate that cytochrome P 450 3A4 is the major enzyme involved in the metabolism of the active metabolite of ciclesonide (M1) in man.

Based on in vitro studies in human liver microsomes, the active metabolite (M1) did not significantly inhibit or induce the metabolism of other drugs. Based on in vitro human hepatocyte studies, ciclesonide and M1 had no significant effect on the induction of major cytochrome P 450 isozymes. In vitro studies also demonstrated that the plasma protein binding of des-ciclesonide was not affected by warfarin or salicylic acid, indicating that protein binding-based drug interactions are unlikely.

The serum levels of ciclesonide and its active metabolite M1, are negligible following administration of ciclesonide nasal spray. Therefore, the potential for clinically relevant drug-drug interactions is very low. However, co-administration with potent inhibitors of the cytochrome P 450 3A4 system (e.g. protease inhibitors for the treatment of HIV infections such as, ritonavir or nelfinavir) should be considered with caution because there might be an increase in systemic drug levels of the active metabolite M1.

Drug-Drug Interactions: A drug interaction study with orally inhaled ciclesonide and oral erythromycin, a substrate and weak inhibitor of cytochrome P 450 3A4, had no relevant effect on the pharmacokinetics of either M1 or erythromycin. In a drug interaction study at steady state with orally inhaled ciclesonide and oral ketoconazole, a potent cytochrome P 450 3A4 inhibitor, the exposure of the active metabolite M1 increased approximately 3.5-fold, while levels of ciclesonide remained unchanged. Due to the low systemic exposure of intranasal ciclesonide relative to orally inhaled ciclesonide, clinically relevant drug interactions with OMNARIS, except with very potent inhibitors of the cytochrome P450 3A4 system, are not expected.
Drug-Food Interactions: Interactions with food have not been established. Drug-food interactions are unlikely for intranasal corticosteroids.
Drug-Herb Interactions: Interactions with herbal products have not been established.
Drug-Laboratory Test Interactions: Interactions with laboratory tests have not been established. Drug-laboratory interactions are unlikely for intranasal corticosteroids.

DOSAGE AND ADMINISTRATION: Dosing Considerations: The therapeutic effects of corticosteroids, unlike those of decongestants, are not immediate. Since the effect of OMNARIS depends on its regular use, patients should be instructed to use the nasal inhalation at regular intervals and not, as with other nasal sprays, as they feel necessary.
Recommended Dose and Dosage Adjustment: Adults and Adolescents (12 Years of Age and Older): The recommended dose of OMNARIS is 200 μg per day administered as 2 sprays (50 μg/spray) in each nostril once daily.

The maximum total daily dosage should not exceed 2 sprays in each nostril (200 μg/day).
Missed Dose: It is very important that OMNARIS is used regularly. If a dose is missed, the next dose should be taken when it is due and patients should not exceed the prescribed daily dosage.
Administration: Prior to initial use, OMNARIS must be shaken gently and then the pump must be primed by actuating 8 times. If not used for 4 or more consecutive days, it should be shaken gently and reprimed with 1 spray or until a fine spray appears. It is recommended that the applicator tip be wiped with a clean tissue following daily use. It is also recommended that the applicator be cleaned weekly using warm water and reprimed with one spray or until a fine mist appears.

OMNARIS delivers 50 μg of ciclesonide per spray. Each bottle of OMNARIS contains 120 metered sprays after initial priming. The bottle should be discarded after 120 sprays following initial priming, since the amount of ciclesonide delivered per spray thereafter may be substantially less than the labeled dose. If more than 6 months have elapsed since the bottle was removed from the foil pouch, it should be discarded.

Do not spray in eyes.

OVERDOSAGE:
Acute overdosage with this dosage form is unlikely since one 120 spray bottle of OMNARIS only contains approximately 9.6 mg of ciclesonide. A single oral dose of up to 10 mg of ciclesonide in healthy volunteers was well tolerated and serum cortisol levels were virtually unchanged in comparison with placebo treatment. Considering the low systemic availability of ciclesonide administered intranasally or orally, systemic effects following an overdose are unlikely.

* Occurred at rates ≤placebo.

For management of a suspected drug overdose, CPhA recommends that you contact your **regional Poison Control Centre**. See the *CPS* Directory section for a list of Poison Control Centres.

ACTION AND CLINICAL PHARMACOLOGY: Mechanism of Action: Ciclesonide is a pro-drug with a low glucocorticoid receptor affinity and is pharmacologically inactive. Following intranasal application, ciclesonide is enzymatically converted by esterases in the nasal mucosa to the pharmacologically active metabolite, 21 des-methylpropionyl-ciclesonide (des-CIC, M1). M1 has potent anti-inflammatory activity with affinity for the glucocorticoid receptor that is 120 times higher than the parent compound and 12 times higher than dexamethasone.

The primary mechanism of corticosteroid action in allergic rhinitis is considered due to anti-inflammation. Corticosteroids have been shown to have a wide range of effects on multiple cell types (e.g., mast cells, eosinophils, neutrophils, macrophages, and lymphocytes) and mediators (e.g., histamine, eicosanoids, leukotrienes, and cytokines) involved in allergic inflammation. The anti-inflammatory properties of ciclesonide and M1 were shown in several in vitro and in vivo investigations, including experiments using a guinea pig model of allergic rhinitis and several investigations in primary human nasal epithelial cells, bronchial epithelial and smooth muscle cells.
Pharmacodynamics: Ciclesonide is a topical glucocorticosteroid delivered in a unique hypotonic suspension that has local anti-inflammatory properties at doses that are minimally systemically active. The effects of ciclesonide nasal spray on the HPA (hypothalamic-pituitary-adrenal) axis were investigated in several Phase III clinical trials up to one-year in duration and no appreciable effects of intranasally administered ciclesonide on serum or urinary cortisol levels were detected. This pharmacodynamic finding is consistent with the negligible systemic bioavailability of ciclesonide following intranasal administration.
Pharmacokinetics: Absorption: Ciclesonide and des-ciclesonide (M1) have negligible oral bioavailability (both less than 1%) due to low gastrointestinal absorption and high first-pass metabolism. The intranasal administration of ciclesonide at recommended doses results in negligible serum concentrations of ciclesonide and its active metabolite (M1) in adult and pediatric subjects using a sensitive bioanalytical assay with a lower limit of quantification of 25 pg/mL and 10 pg/mL for ciclesonide and M1, respectively. Due to the negligible serum concentrations following intranasal administration of ciclesonide, pharmacokinetic calculations could not be performed.
Distribution: The volumes of distribution of ciclesonide and M1 following i.v. administration were approximately 2.9 L/kg and 12.1L/kg, respectively. The percentage of ciclesonide and the active metabolite M1 bound to human plasma proteins averaged ≥99% each. Only the unbound drug in the systemic circulation (approximately 1%) is available for further systemic pharmacodynamic effect. M1 is not significantly bound to human transcortin.
Metabolism: Intranasal ciclesonide is primarily hydrolyzed to its biologically active metabolite, M1, by esterases in the nasal mucosa (primarily by carboxylesterases and cholinesterases). M1 is metabolized in the liver to inactive metabolites mainly by the CYP 3A4 isozyme. Furthermore, inactive fatty acid ester conjugates of M1 in human nasal epithelial cells were detected in vitro for up to 24 hours, providing a reversible depot of M1 due to gradual hydrolysis by lipases.
Excretion: After oral and intravenous administration, ciclesonide is predominantly excreted via the feces (66%), indicating that excretion via the bile is the major route of elimination.
Special Populations and Conditions: The pharmacokinetics of intranasally administered ciclesonide have not been assessed in patient subpopulations because the resulting blood levels are insufficient for pharmacokinetic calculations. However, the pharmacokinetic characteristics of M1 after oral inhalation of ciclesonide were not appreciably influenced by a variety of subject/patient characteristics such as body weight, advanced age, race, gender and liver impairment. Studies in renal impaired patients were not conducted since renal excretion of M1 is a minor route of elimination (≤20%). Because the systemic exposure of intranasally administered ciclesonide is much lower than that of orally inhaled ciclesonide, it is not likely that these special populations will experience clinically relevant changes in the pharmacokinetics of intranasally administered ciclesonide.

STORAGE AND STABILITY: Store at room temperature (15-30°C) with the valve up. Do not freeze. Shake gently.

SPECIAL HANDLING INSTRUCTIONS: The ciclesonide nasal spray device is packaged within a tamper resistant foil pouch to protect the product from oxygen absorption. In addition, a sachet containing beads of iron powder/zeolites is contained within the overwrap to absorb atmospheric oxygen. OMNARIS should be stored in the foil pouch and only removed immediately before first use. OMNARIS should be discarded 6 months after removal from pouch.

INFORMATION FOR THE PATIENT: Published in e-CPS, available by subscription at www.e-cps.ca.

DOSAGE FORMS, COMPOSITION AND PACKAGING: OMNARIS is an unscented, metered-dose, manual-pump spray formulation containing a hypotonic aqueous suspension of ciclesonide. OMNARIS also contains disodium edetate, hydroxypropyl methylcellulose, microcrystalline cellulose and carboxymethylcellulose sodium, potassium sorbate and purified water; hydrochloric acid may be added to adjust the pH to a target 4.5.

OMNARIS is contained within an amber glass bottle within a protective plastic sleeve and shrink wrap label and provides for nasal delivery with a manual metered pump. OMNARIS provides 120-metered sprays after initial priming; net fill weight 12.5 g. The OMNARIS bottle has been filled with an excess to accommodate the priming activity. The bottle should be discarded after 120 sprays following initial priming, since the amount of ciclesonide delivered per spray thereafter may be substantially less than the labeled dose. Each spray delivers 50 μg of ciclesonide to the patient.

(Shown in Product Identification Section)

Omnitrope™ Ⓟ

somatropin

Human Growth Hormone

Sandoz

SUMMARY PRODUCT INFORMATION:

Route of Administration	Dosage Form/ Strength	Clinically Relevant Nonmedicinal Ingredients
Subcutaneous injection	Solution: 5 mg/1.5 mL (3.3 mg/mL) and 10 mg/1.5 mL (6.7 mg/mL)	5 mg/1.5 mL: mannitol, benzyl alcohol (as preservative) 10 mg/1.5 mL: phenol (as preservative) For a complete listing see Dosage Forms, Composition and Packaging.

DESCRIPTION: Omnitrope (somatropin for injection) is a polypeptide hormone of recombinant DNA origin. It has 191 amino acid residues and a molecular weight of 22 125 daltons. The amino acid sequence of the product is identical to that of human growth hormone of pituitary origin (somatropin). Omnitrope is synthesized in a strain of *E. coli* which has been modified by the addition of the human growth hormone gene.

INDICATIONS AND CLINICAL USE: Pediatric Indication: Omnitrope (somatropin for injection) is indicated for:
- **Growth Hormone Deficiency (GHD) in Children:** Long-term treatment of children with growth failure due to an inadequate secretion of endogenous growth hormone. Other causes of short stature should be excluded.

Adult Indication: Omnitrope (somatropin for injection) is indicated for:
- **Adult Growth Hormone Deficiency (GHD):** Long-term replacement therapy in adults with growth hormone deficiency due to underlying hypothalamic or pituitary disease or who were growth deficient during childhood. Growth hormone deficiency should be confirmed by an appropriate growth hormone stimulation test. Patients who were diagnosed as growth hormone deficient during childhood must be retested before treatment starts.

Geriatrics (>65 years of age): The safety and efficacy of Omnitrope in patients aged 65 and over has not been evaluated in clinical studies.
Pediatrics (<3 years of age): The safety and efficacy of Omnitrope in pediatric patients under the age of 3 years has not been evaluated in clinical studies.

CONTRAINDICATIONS: Omnitrope (somatropin for injection) should not be used when there is any evidence of **neoplastic activity**. Intracranial lesions must be inactive and antitumour therapy complete prior to the institution of therapy. Treatment with Omnitrope should be discontinued if there is evidence of tumour growth.

Omnitrope should not be used for growth promotion in pediatric patients with **closed epiphyses**.

Omnitrope should not be used in patients with **acute critical illness** following cardiac surgery, abdominal surgery, multiple trauma, or acute respiratory failure. Clinical studies demonstrated that high doses of another somatropin, were associated with a significantly increased morbidity and mortality in those patients (see Warnings and Precautions).

Growth hormone is contraindicated in patients with **Prader-Willi Syndrome** who are severely obese or have severe respiratory impairment (see Warnings and Precautions).

Omnitrope 5 mg/1.5 mL solution which contains the preservative benzyl alcohol, should not be administered in newborns or in patients with a known sensitivity to benzyl alcohol (see Warnings and Precautions).

Omnitrope is contraindicated in patients who are hypersensitive to somatropin or to any ingredient in the formulation. For a complete listing, see Dosage Forms, Composition and Packaging.

WARNINGS AND PRECAUTIONS:

Serious Warnings and Precautions

- **There have been reports of fatalities associated with the use of growth hormone in pediatric patients with Prader-Willi Syndrome who have one or more of the following risk factors: severe obesity, history of respiratory impairment or sleep apnea or unidentified respiratory infection (see Warnings and Precautions, Congenital Disorders).**
- **Patients with acute critical illness suffering complications following open-heart surgery, abdominal surgery, multiple accidental trauma, acute respiratory failure or similar conditions should not be treated with somatropin (see Warnings and Precautions, Peri-Operative Considerations).**

General: Treatment with Omnitrope (somatropin for injection), as with other growth hormone preparations, should be directed by physicians who are experienced in the diagnosis and management of patients with growth hormone deficiency.

Patients and caregivers who will administer Omnitrope in medically unsupervised situations should receive appropriate training and instruction on the proper use of Omnitrope from the physician or other suitably qualified health professionals.

Carcinogenesis and Mutagenesis: Mutagenicity or carcinogenicity studies have not been conducted with Omnitrope.

Congenital Disorders: Prader-Willi Syndrome (see Contraindications): There have been reports of fatalities after initiating therapy with growth hormone in pediatric patients with Prader-Willi Syndrome who had one or more of the following risk factors: severe obesity, history of upper airway obstruction or sleep apnea, or unidentified infection. Male patients with one or more of these factors may be at greater risk than females.

Endocrine and Metabolism: For patients with **diabetes mellitus**, caution should be used if growth hormone is administered and insulin dosage may need to be adjusted when Omnitrope is instituted. Patients with diabetes or glucose intolerance should be monitored closely during treatment with Omnitrope. Patients with risk factors for glucose intolerance, such as obesity or a family history of Type II diabetes, should be monitored closely as well. Growth hormone may induce a state of insulin resistance, therefore patients should be observed for evidence of glucose intolerance.

In patients with hypopituitarism (multiple hormonal deficiencies) standard hormonal replacement therapy should be monitored closely when treatment with Omnitrope is instituted. Hypothyroidism may develop during treatment with Omnitrope, and inadequate treatment of hypothyroidism may prevent optimal response to Omnitrope. Therefore, patients should have periodic thyroid function tests and be treated with thyroid hormone when indicated.

Hematologic: Serum levels of inorganic phosphorous, alkaline phosphatase and Insulin-like Growth Factor 1 (IGF-1) may increase with growth hormone therapy.

Immune: Local or systemic allergic reactions may occur. Parents and/or patients should be informed that such reactions are possible and that prompt medical attention should be sought if allergic reactions occur.

Musculoskeletal: Pediatric patients with endocrine disorders, including growth hormone deficiency, have a higher incidence of **slipped capital femoral epiphyses**. Any pediatric patient with the onset of a limp or complaints of hip or knee pain during growth hormone therapy should be evaluated.

Progression of **scoliosis** can occur in patients who experience rapid growth. Because growth hormone increases growth rate, patients with a history of scoliosis who are treated with growth hormone should be monitored for progression of scoliosis. However, growth hormone has not been shown to increase the incidence of scoliosis.

Neurologic: Patients with growth hormone deficiency secondary to an **intracranial lesion** should be examined frequently for progression or recurrence of the underlying disease process.

Intracranial hypertension (IH) with papilledema, visual changes, headache, nausea and/or vomiting has been reported in a small number of patients treated with growth hormone products. Symptoms usually occurred within the first eight (8) weeks of the initiation of growth hormone therapy. In all reported cases, IH-associated signs and symptoms resolved after termination of therapy or a reduction of the growth hormone dose. Funduscopic examination of patients is recommended at the initiation, and periodically during the course of growth hormone therapy.

Peri-Operative Considerations: See Contraindications for information on increased mortality in patients with **acute critical illnesses** in intensive care units due to complications following open-heart or abdominal surgery, multiple accidental traumas, or with acute respiratory failure. The safety of continuing growth hormone treatment in patients receiving replacement doses for approved indications who concurrently develop these illnesses has not been established. Therefore, the potential benefit of treatment continuation with growth hormone in patients having acute critical illnesses should be weighed against the potential risk.

Sensitivity/Resistance: Patients with known sensitivities to benzyl alcohol should not use the Omnitrope 5 mg/1.5 mL as the formulation contains benzyl alcohol as a preservative. It must not be used in newborns.

Special Populations: Pregnant Women: Reproduction studies have not been conducted with Omnitrope. It is also not known whether Omnitrope can cause fetal harm when administered to a pregnant woman or affect reproduction capacity. Omnitrope should only be given to a pregnant woman if the benefits outweigh the risks.

Nursing Women: There have been no studies conducted with Omnitrope in nursing mothers. It is not known whether this drug is excreted in human milk. Because many drugs are excreted in human milk, caution should be exercised when Omnitrope is administered to a nursing woman.

Pediatrics (<3 years of age): The safety and efficacy of Omnitrope in pediatric patients under the age of 3 years has not been evaluated in clinical studies. Prudence is indicated for children under age of 3 years, when administering Omnitrope 5 mg/1.5 mL solution (benzyl alcohol preserved); although there is no information on the toxicity of benzyl alcohol for this age group, the toxic dose for premature neonates is in the range of 100 to 250 mg/kg per day.

Adult Patients–Post-Pubertal GHD Patients: Before continuing treatment as an adult, a post-pubertal growth hormone deficient patient who received growth hormone replacement therapy in childhood should be re-evaluated with proper testing as described in Indications and Clinical Use. If continued treatment is appropriate, Omnitrope should be administered at the reduced dose level recommended for adults GHD patients.

Geriatrics (>65 years of age): The safety and effectiveness of Omnitrope in patients aged 65 and over has not been evaluated in clinical studies. Elderly patients may be more sensitive to the action of Omnitrope and may be more prone to develop adverse reactions.

Renal or Hepatic Impairment: No studies have been conducted with Omnitrope in these patient populations.

Monitoring and Laboratory Tests: See Hematologic, Endocrine and Metabolism, and Musculoskeletal.

ADVERSE REACTIONS: Adverse Drug Reaction Overview: Two serious adverse drug reactions (1%) on worsening of a preexisting scoliosis were reported in clinical trials with Omnitrope in the pediatric population.

Most frequent adverse drug reactions (>5%) reported in clinical trials with Omnitrope Powder in the pediatric population were injection site reaction (12%), eosinophilia (9%) and headache (6%). Most frequent adverse drug reactions (>5%) reported in clinical trials with Omnitrope Solution in the pediatric population were glycosylated hemoglobin A1c (HbA1c) increased (9%), eosinophilia (7%) and injection site reaction (7%).

Adverse drug reactions that most commonly result in clinical intervention with Omnitrope Powder in the pediatric population were hypothyroidism (3%) and headache (2%). Adverse drug reactions that most commonly resulted in clinical intervention with Omnitrope Solution in the pediatric population were headache (4%) and upper respiratory tract infections (2%).

The following events were observed in patients using somatropins (see also Warnings and Precautions).

- Short-term local injection site reactions, such as pain, numbness, redness and swelling. The subcutaneous administration of growth hormone at the same injection site over a long period may result in local lipoatrophy.
- Disturbances in fluid balance (swelling), joint pain, muscle pain, stiffness of the hands and feet, numbness. In general, these undesirable effects occur at the beginning of therapy with growth hormones and also depend on the dose. They are common in adult patients, but uncommon in children.
- Carpal tunnel syndrome in adults.
- Benign intracranial hypertension, diabetes mellitus.

Due to the content of benzyl alcohol in Omnitrope, rare general hypersensitivity reactions are possible. No case was observed during the clinical trials.

Leukemia was reported in a small number of pediatric patients who were treated with growth hormone, including growth hormone of pituitary origin and recombinant growth hormone. The relationship, if any, between leukemia and growth hormone therapy is uncertain.

Clinical Trial Adverse Drug Reactions: Because clinical trials are conducted under very specific conditions the adverse reaction rates observed in the clinical trials may not reflect the rates observed in practice and should not be compared to the rates in the clinical trials of another drug. Adverse drug reaction information from clinical trials is useful for identifying drug-related adverse events and for approximating rates.

Adverse Drug Reactions Reported From Omnitrope Clinical Trials: As with all protein drugs, a small number of patients may develop antibodies to the protein. Growth hormone antibody with binding capacity lower than 2 mg/L has not been associated with growth attenuation. In some cases when binding capacity is >2 mg/L, interference with growth response has been observed.

Preparations of Omnitrope contain a small amount of host cell *E. coli* peptides (HCP). Anti-HCP antibodies are found in a small number of patients treated with Omnitrope, but these appear to be of no clinical significance.

The following events were observed during the Omnitrope clinical studies conducted in children with growth hormone deficiency (GHD): Most Common Adverse Drug Reactions (≥1%) for Omnitrope and Genotropin (see Table 1, Table 2, Table 3 and Table 4).

Table 1: Omnitrope

Incidence of Drug-related[a] Adverse Events Occurring in ≥1% Pediatric Patients with GHD (Studies EP2K-99-PhIII/EP2K-00-PhIIIFo)

Preferred Term	Omnitrope Lyophilizate COV[b] N=44 N (%)	Genotropin N=45 N (%)
Abdominal pain	1 (2%)	0 (0%)
Anaemia	1 (2%)	0 (0%)
Anorexia	1 (2%)	1 (2%)
Arthralgia	1 (2%)	0 (0%)
Coma	1 (2%)	0 (0%)
Conjunctivitis	0 (0%)	1 (2%)
Elevated HbA1c	4 (9%)	3 (7%)
Eosinophilia	5 (11%)	3 (7%)
Face oedema	1 (2%)	0 (0%)
Fever	1 (2%)	0 (0%)
Haematoma	4 (9%)	5 (11%)
Headache	3 (7%)	3 (7%)
Heart-murmur	1 (2%)	0 (0%)
Hypercholesterolaemia	1 (2%)	0 (0%)
Hyperglycaemia	1 (2%)	0 (0%)
Hypertriglyceridaemia	2 (5%)	2 (4%)
Hypothyroidism	6 (14%)	2 (4%)
Injection site pain	0 (0%)	1 (2%)
Leg pain	1 (2%)	1 (2%)
Pain	1 (2%)	0 (0%)
Pharyngitis	0 (0%)	1 (2%)
Polyuria	0 (0%)	1 (2%)
Pruritus	1 (2%)	0 (0%)
Purpura	0 (0%)	1 (2%)
Scoliosis	0 (0%)	1 (2%)
AST increased	0 (0%)	1 (2%)
ALT increased	0 (0%)	1 (2%)
T4 decreased	0 (0%)	1 (2%)
TSH decreased	0 (0%)	2 (4%)
Vision abnormal	0 (0%)	1 (2%)

[a] Drug-related=possible, probable or unclassified relationship to study drug.
[b] Not marketed material.
Legend: N=number of patients.

Table 2: Omnitrope

Incidence of Drug-related[a] Adverse Events Occurring in ≥1% Pediatric Patients with GHD (Study EP2K-00-PhIIIAQ Part A)

Preferred Term	Omnitrope Lyophilizate N=44 N (%)	Omnitrope Liquid N=45 N (%)
Arthralgia	0 (0%)	1 (2%)
Bronchitis	0 (0%)	1 (2%)
Elevated HbA1c	0 (0%)	3 (7%)

(cont'd)

Table 2: Omnitrope *(cont'd)*

Incidence of Drug-related[a] Adverse Events Occurring in ≥1% Pediatric Patients with GHD (Study EP2K-00-PhIIIAQ Part A)

Preferred Term	Omnitrope Lyophilizate N=44 N (%)	Omnitrope Liquid N=45 N (%)
Eosinophilia	2 (5%)	3 (7%)
Haematoma	2 (5%)	1 (2%)
Headache	2 (5%)	2 (4%)
Hypercholesterolaemia	1 (2%)	1 (2%)
Hypertriglyceridaemia	1 (2%)	1 (2%)
Hypothyroidism	0 (0%)	1 (2%)
Leg pain	1 (2%)	1 (2%)
Scoliosis	0 (0%)	1 (2%)

[a] Drug-related=possible, probable or unclassified relationship to study drug.
Legend: N=number of patients.

Table 3: Omnitrope

Incidence of Drug-related[a] Adverse Events Occurring in ≥1% Pediatric Patients with GHD (Study EP2K-00-PhIIIAQ Part B)

Preferred Term	Omnitrope Liquid N=89 N (%)
Bilirubinaemia	1 (1%)
Convulsions	1 (1%)
Elevated HbA1c	10 (11%)
Endocrine disorder NOS	1 (1%)
Eosinophilia	8 (9%)
Haematoma	7 (8%)
Headache	3 (3%)
Hyperglycaemia	2 (2%)
Hypertriglyceridaemia	1 (1%)
Hypocholesterolaemia	1 (1%)
Hypothyroidism	1 (1%)
Leg pain	2 (2%)
Leucopaenia	2 (2%)
Leukocytosis	1 (1%)
Pain	1 (1%)
Phosphatase alkaline increased	4 (4%)
Scoliosis	1 (1%)
TSH decreased	2 (2%)

[a] Drug-related=possible, probable or unclassified relationship to study drug.
Legend: N=number of patients.

Table 4: Omnitrope

Incidence of Drug-related[a] Adverse Events Occurring in ≥1% Pediatric Patients with GHD (Studies EP2K-02-PhII-Lyo and EP2K-00-PhIIIb-E)

Preferred Term	EP2K-02-PhII-Lyo[b] N=51 N (%)	EP2K-00-PhIIIb-E[c] N=50 N (%)
Abdominal pain	1 (2 %)	0 (0%)
Antibody test abnormal	0 (0%)	2 (4 %)
Arthralgia	1 (2 %)	0 (0%)
Blood alkaline phosphatase increased	1 (2 %)	0 (0%)
Contusion	1 (2 %)	0 (0%)
Dermatitis	0 (0%)	1 (2 %)
Eosinophilia	6 (12 %)	0 (0%)
Fatigue	1 (2 %)	0 (0%)
Fundoscopy abnormal	1 (2 %)	0 (0%)
Glycosylated haemoglobin increased	1 (2 %)	0 (0%)
Headache	4 (8 %)	1 (2 %)
Hypothyroidism	4 (8 %)	0 (0%)
Injection site erythema	1 (2 %)	0 (0%)
Injection site haemorrhage	5 (10 %)	0 (0%)
Injection site inflammation	1 (2 %)	0 (0%)
Injection site oedema	1 (2 %)	0 (0%)
Injection site pain	0 (0%)	1 (2 %)
Injection site reaction	1 (2 %)	0 (0%)
Lipodystrophy acquired	1 (2 %)	0 (0%)
Migraine	0 (0%)	1 (2 %)
Myopia	1 (2 %)	0 (0%)
Nasopharyngitis	1 (2 %)	0 (0%)
Neck pain	1 (2 %)	0 (0%)
Pain in extremity	1 (2 %)	0 (0%)
Pyrexia	1 (2 %)	0 (0%)
Scoliosis	3 (6 %)	0 (0%)
Tendonitis	0 (0%)	1 (2 %)
Viral pharyngitis	0 (0%)	1 (2 %)
Vomiting	0 (0%)	1 (2 %)

[a] Drug-related=possible, probable or unclassified relationship to study drug.
[b] 24 months.
[c] Up to 30 months.
Legend: N=number of patients.

Less Common Clinical Trial Adverse Drug Reactions (<1%): The following list provides the incidence of drug-related adverse events occurring in pediatric patients with GHD (<1%): hypothyroidism, scoliosis, arthralgia, hypercholesterolemia, hypertriglyceridemia, pharyngitis, pain, bronchitis, convulsions, endocrine disorders, bilirubinaemia, leucocytosis, vomiting, tendonitis, migraine, dermatitis.

Regarding the adverse drug reactions reported from somatropin products in adults, replacement therapy in growth hormone deficient adult patients is often accompanied by signs and symptoms of fluid retention, such as edema, arthralgia and paraesthesia. Musculo-skeletal pain and/or stiffness may also occur. These events usually have an early onset after initiation of treatment with a reduction in incidence and prevalence over time. In most cases the severity is mild or moderate. One patient developed diabetes mellitus during Genotropin therapy, which was probably attributable to treatment. The following events were also reported infrequently: carpal tunnel syndrome, headache, back pain, myalgia, hypoesthesia.

Post-Market Adverse Drug Reactions: The postmarketing data available for Omnitrope did not reveal any unexpected adverse drug reactions.

DRUG INTERACTIONS: Drug-Drug Interactions: No studies on the interaction of Omnitrope with other drugs have been performed.

Concomitant glucocorticoid treatment may inhibit the growth-promoting effect of human growth hormone. Pediatric growth hormone-deficient patients with coexisting Adrenocorticotropic Hormone (ACTH) deficiency should have their glucocorticoid replacement dose carefully adjusted to avoid an inhibitory effect on growth (see also Warnings and Precautions, Endocrine and Metabolism).

Limited published data indicate that growth hormone treatment increases cytochrome P450 (CP450) mediated antipyrine clearance in man. These data suggest that growth hormone administration may alter the clearance of compounds known to be metabolized by CP450 liver enzymes (e.g. corticosteroids, sex steroids, anticonvulsants, cyclosporine). Careful monitoring is advisable when growth hormone is administered in combination with other drugs known to be metabolized by CP450 liver enzymes. See Table 5

Table 5: Omnitrope

Established or Potential Drug-Drug Interactions with Omnitrope

Therapeutic Class	Effect	Clinical Comment
Glucocorticoids	Concomitant glucocorticoid treatment may inhibit the growth promoting effect of human growth hormone.	Patients with coexisting ACTH deficiency should have their glucocorticoid replacement dose carefully adjusted to avoid an inhibitory effect on growth.
Cytochrome P450	Somatropin may be an inducer of CP450 34A when administered in combination with drugs known to be metobolized by CP450 liver enzymes.	Patients should be monitored for clinical effectiveness of such drugs.

Legend: ACTH=Adrenocorticotropic Hormone.

Drug-Food Interactions: Interactions with food have not been established.
Drug-Herb Interactions: Interactions with herbal products have not been established.
Drug-Laboratory Test Interactions: Interactions with laboratory tests have not been established.

DOSAGE AND ADMINISTRATION: Recommended Dose and Dosage Adjustment: The dosage and administration schedule of Omnitrope (somatropin for injection) should be individualized for each patient. The doses should be given by **subcutaneous** injections (administered preferably in the evening). Omnitrope may be given in the thigh, buttocks, or abdomen; the site of subcutaneous injections should be rotated daily to help prevent lipoatrophy.

Growth Disturbance in Children Due to Inadequate Endogenous Growth Hormone Secretion: Generally a dose of 0.025-0.035 mg/kg body weight daily is recommended.

Growth Hormone Deficiency In Adult Patients: The recommended starting dose is 0.15-0.3 mg/day. The final dose should be individually increased as required with respect to age and gender to a maximum daily maintenance dose of 1.33 mg. Women may require higher doses than men. As normal physiological growth hormone production decreases with age, dose requirements may be reduced. Clinical response, side effects and determination of IGF-1 in serum may be used as guidance for dose titration. The level of IGF-1 should not exceed the upper limit of normal IGF-1 levels matched to age and sex.

Missed Dose: For patients who miss a dose of Omnitrope, it is not recommended to double the next dose. Administer the regular dose at the next scheduled dosage time. Patients should contact their physician for instructions.

Administration: Omnitrope (somatropin for injection)—5 mg/1.5 mL; 10 mg/1.5 mL Cartridges: Omnitrope 5 mg/1.5 mL and 10 mg/1.5 mL solutions for injection, are sterile, ready-to-use solutions filled in pen cartridges.

Both presentations are indicated for multiple use. They should only be administered with the Omnitrope Pen 5 and Omnitrope Pen 10 pen injection devices specifically developed for use with Omnitrope 5 mg/1.5 mL and Omnitrope 10 mg/1.5 mL, respectively. The solutions must be administered using sterile, disposable pen needles. The solution must be clear prior to insertion of the cartridge into the Pen. Do not inject if the solution is cloudy. Patients and caregivers have to receive appropriate training and instruction on the proper use of the Omnitrope cartridges and pens from the physician or other suitable qualified healthcare professionals.

After the first injection, the content of the cartridge must be used within 28 days. The cartridge should remain in the pen and be refrigerated between 2 and 8°C. Do not freeze. Protect from light.

The following is a general description of the administration process. The manufacturer's instructions provided with the pens must be followed for loading the cartridge, attaching the injection needle and for the administration.

Wash your hands.

1. Ensure that the solution in the cartridge is clear and colourless prior to inserting the cartridge into the Pen. Do not use if the solution is cloudy or contains particulate matter.
2. Disinfect the rubber membrane of the cartridge with an alcohol swab.
3. Insert the cartridge into the Omnitrope Pen following the instructions for use provided with the pen.
4. Clean the site of injection with an alcohol swab.
5. Administer the appropriate dose by subcutaneous injection using a sterile pen needle. The sites of injection should be rotated each time Omnitrope is administered to avoid lipoatrophy.
6. Remove the pen needle and dispose of it in accordance with local requirements.

OVERDOSAGE:

There is little information on acute or chronic overdosage with Omnitrope. Intravenously administered growth hormone has been shown to result in an acute decrease in plasma glucose and subsequently to hyperglycemia. It is thought that the same effect might occur on rare occasions with high dosages of Omnitrope administered subcutaneously. Long-term overdosage may result in signs and symptoms of acromegaly, consistent with overproduction of human growth hormone.

> For management of a suspected drug overdose, CPhA recommends that you contact your **regional Poison Control Centre**. See the *CPS* Directory section for a list of Poison Control Centres.

ACTION AND CLINICAL PHARMACOLOGY: Mechanism of Action: Omnitrope (somatropin for injection) is a human growth hormone (hGH) produced by recombinant DNA technology. The amino acid sequence of the somatropin protein is identical to that of the human growth hormone of pituitary origin.

In vitro, preclinical, and clinical tests have demonstrated that somatropins are therapeutically equivalent to human growth hormone of pituitary origin and achieve similar pharmacokinetic profiles in normal adults. In pediatric patients who have growth hormone deficiency (GHD), treatment with somatropin stimulates linear growth and normalizes concentrations of Insulin-like Growth Factor -I (IGF-I).

In adults with GHD, treatment with somatropin results in reduced fat mass, increased lean body mass, metabolic alterations that include beneficial changes in lipid metabolism, and normalization of IGF-I concentrations.

In addition, the following actions have been demonstrated for Omnitrope (somatropin for injection) and/or human growth hormone of pituitary origin.

Tissue Growth:

- Skeletal Growth: Somatropin stimulates skeletal growth in children with growth failure due to inadequate secretion of endogenous growth hormone. The measurable increase in body length after administration of somatropin results from an effect on the epiphyseal plates of long bones. Concentrations of IGF-I, which may play a role in skeletal growth, are generally low in the serum of pediatric patients with growth hormone deficiency, but tend to increase during treatment with Omnitrope. Elevations in mean serum alkaline phosphatase concentration are also seen.
- Cell Growth: It has been shown that there are fewer skeletal muscle cells in short-statured children who lack endogenous growth hormone as compared with the normal pediatric population. Treatment with somatropin for injection results in an increase in both the number and size of skeletal muscle cells.

Protein Metabolism: Linear growth is facilitated in part by increased cellular protein synthesis. Nitrogen retention, as demonstrated by decreased urinary nitrogen excretion and serum urea nitrogen, follows the initiation of therapy with somatropin.

Carbohydrate Metabolism: Pediatric patients with hypopituitarism sometimes experience fasting hypoglycemia, which is improved by treatment with somatropin. Large doses of growth hormone may impair glucose tolerance.

Lipid Metabolism: In growth hormone-deficient patients, administration of recombinant somatropin has resulted in lipid mobilization, reduction in body fat stores, and increased plasma fatty acids.

Mineral Metabolism: Retention of sodium, potassium, and phosphorus is induced by pituitary growth hormone in children. Serum concentrations of inorganic phosphate are increased in patients with growth hormone deficiency after therapy with somatropin. Serum calcium is not significantly altered in patients treated with somatropin. Growth hormone could increase calciuria.

Body Composition: Adult growth hormone-deficient patients treated with somatropin at the recommended adult dose (see Dosage and Administration) demonstrate a decrease in fat mass and an increase in lean body mass. When these alterations are coupled with the increase in total body water, the overall effect of somatropin is to modify body composition, an effect that is maintained with continued treatment.

Pharmacodynamics: See Table 6 and Table 7.

Table 6: Omnitrope

Pharmacodynamic Parameters After a Single SC Administration of 5 mg Omnitrope Powder for Solution for Injection (5.8 mg/vial) and of 5 mg Omnitrope 10 mg/1.5 mL Solution for Injection

IGF-1	**5 mg of Omnitrope Powder for Solution for Injection; 5.8 mg/vial (N=32)**	**5 mg of Omnitrope 10 mg/1.5 mL Solution for Injection (N=32)**
$AUEC_{last}$ [h·µg/L]	20 355±5067	19 829±5107
E_{max} [µg/L]	267±64	265±68
$t_{max,E}$ [h]	24[a] (16–48)	24[a] (16–24)
IGFBP-3	**5 mg of Omnitrope Powder for Solution for Injection; 5.8 mg/vial (N=32)**	**5 mg of Omnitrope 10 mg/1.5 mL Solution for Injection (N=32)**
$AUEC_{last}$ [h·mg/L]	471±70	468±67
E_{max} [mg/L]	5.4±0.8	5.4±0.8
$t_{max,E}$ [h]	48[a] (16–96)	48[a] (0–72)

(cont'd)

Table 6: Omnitrope *(cont'd)*

Pharmacodynamic Parameters After a Single SC Administration of 5 mg Omnitrope Powder for Solution for Injection (5.8 mg/vial) and of 5 mg Omnitrope 10 mg/1.5 mL Solution for Injection

NEFA	**5 mg of Omnitrope Powder for Solution for Injection; 5.8 mg/vial (N=32)**	**5 mg of Omnitrope 10 mg/1.5 mL Solution for Injection (N=32)**
$AUEC_{last}$ [h·mmol/L]	13.1±3.8	12.8±3.7
E_{max} [mmol/L]	1.1±0.3	1.1±0.3
$t_{max,E}$ [h]	3[a] (1–16)	3[a] (2–16)

[a] Median value (min-max) for $t_{max,E}$.

Legend: IGF-1=Insulin-like Growth Factor 1; IGFBP=Insulin-like Growth Factor Binding Protein 3; NEFA=Nonesterified Fatty Acids.

Results are presented as mean±SD.

Table 7: Omnitrope

Pharmacodynamic Parameters after a Single SC Administration of 5 mg Omnitrope Powder for Solution for Injection (5.8 mg/vial) and of 5 mg Omnitrope 5 mg/1.5 mL Solution for Injection

IGF-1	**5 mg of Omnitrope Powder for Solution for Injection; 5.8 mg/vial (N=35)**	**5 mg of Omnitrope 5 mg/1.5 mL Solution for Injection (N=35)**
$AUEC_{last}$ [h·µg/L]	16 712±3847	16 295±3664
E_{max} [µg/L]	218±56	213±49
$t_{max,E}$ [h]	24[a] (12–48)	24[a] (12–48)
IGFBP-3	**5 mg of Omnitrope Powder for Solution for Injection; 5.8 mg/vial (N=35)**	**5 mg of Omnitrope 5 mg/1.5 mL Solution for Injection (N=35)**
$AUEC_{last}$ [h·mg/L]	430±61	427±56
E_{max} [mg/L]	4.9±0.7	4.9±0.6
$t_{max,E}$ [h]	48[a] (24–96)	48[a] (12–96)
NEFA	**5 mg of Omnitrope Powder for Solution for Injection; 5.8 mg/vial (N=35)**	**5 mg of Omnitrope 5 mg/1.5 mL Solution for Injection (N=35)**
$AUEC_{last}$ [h·mmol/L]	15.3±4.9	14.8±3.8
E_{max} [mmol/L]	1.3±0.3	1.2±0.3
$t_{max,E}$ [h]	2[a] (0–16)	2[a] (1–24)

[a] Median value (min-max) for $t_{max,E}$.

Results are presented as mean±SD.

Pharmacokinetics: See Table 8 and Table 9.

Table 8: Omnitrope

Pharmacokinetic Parameters After a Single SC Administration of 5 mg of Omnitrope Powder for Solution for Injection (5.8 mg/vial) and 5 mg of Omnitrope 10 mg/1.5 mL Solution for Injection

	5 mg of Omnitrope Powder for Solution for Injection; 5.8 mg/vial (N=32)	**5 mg of Omnitrope 10 mg/1.5 mL Solution for Injection (N=32)**
AUC_T [h·µg/L]	550±96	558±115
AUC_I [h·µg/L]	555±96	561±114
C_{max} [µg/L]	69±16	74±22
t_{max} [h]	4.0[a] (2.0–6.0)	4.0[a] (2.0–6.0)
$t_{1/2}$ [h]	2.9±0.5	2.5±0.7

[a] Median value (min-max).

Results are presented as mean±SD.

Table 9: Omnitrope

Pharmacokinetic Parameters After a Single SC Administration of 5 mg of Omnitrope Powder for Solution for Injection (5.8 mg/vial) and 5 mg of Omnitrope 5 mg/1.5 mL Solution for Injection

	5 mg of Omnitrope Powder for Solution for Injection; 5.8 mg/vial (N=35)	**5 mg of Omnitrope 5 mg/1.5 mL Solution for Injection (N=35)**
AUC_T [h·µg/L]	559±148	542±141
AUC_I [h·µg/L]	566±147	546±140
C_{max} [µg/L]	71±24	72±28
t_{max} [h]	4.0[a] (2.0–6.0)	4.0[a] (2.0–8.0)
$t_{1/2}$ [h]	3.2±0.7	2.8±0.7

[a] Median value (min-max).

Results are presented as mean±SD (n=35).

Absorption: The bioavailability of subcutaneously administered somatropin is approximately 80% in both healthy subjects and growth hormone deficient patients. A subcutaneous dose of 5 mg of Omnitrope (5 mg/1.5 mL Solution for Injection) in healthy adults results in plasma C_{max} and t_{max} values of 72±28 µg/L and 4.0±2.0 hours, respectively. Following SC injection, maximum serum growth hormone concentrations are reached approximately 4 hours (range 2 to 8 hours) and growth hormone serum concentrations return to baseline within 24 hours.

Metabolism: Extensive metabolism studies have not been conducted. The metabolic fate of somatropin involves classical protein catabolism in both the liver and kidneys.

Excretion: The mean terminal half-life of somatropin after intravenous administration in growth hormone deficient adults is about 0.4 hours. However, after subcutaneous administration of Omnitrope in healthy adults, a half-life of approximately 3 hours is estimated. The longer half-life observed after subcutaneous administration is an example of 'flip-flop' pharmacokinetics, such that the estimated elimination rate is actually the absorption rate from the site of administration. The mean metabolic clearance of Omnitrope, subcutaneously administered in healthy adults, is 0.14 (±0.04) L/hr·kg.

Subpopulations: The absolute bioavailability of somatropin seems to be similar in males and females following subcutaneous administration.

Information about the pharmacokinetics of somatropin in geriatric and pediatric populations, in different races and in patients with renal, hepatic or cardiac insufficiency is either lacking or incomplete.

Special Populations and Conditions: Pediatrics: No studies to estimate recombinant human Growth Hormone (rhGH) clearance have been conducted with Omnitrope in these patient populations.

Gender: No gender studies have been performed in pediatric patients; however, following a subcutaneous injection of 5 mg Omnitrope to healthy adult volunteers, gender had no effect on the pharmacokinetic parameters of Omnitrope (C_{max} and t_{max}).

Race: No studies have been conducted with Omnitrope to assess pharmacokinetic differences among races.

Elderly, Renal, Hepatic or Cardiac Insufficiency: No studies have been conducted with Omnitrope in these patient populations.

STORAGE AND STABILITY: Omnitrope (Somatropin For Injection) 5 mg/1.5 mL, 10 mg/1.5 mL: Omnitrope pen cartridges for use with Pen 5 and Pen 10.

- Keep out of reach and sight of children.
- Store in the original package in order to protect from light.
- Store between 2 and 8°C (in a refrigerator). Do not freeze.
- Use a cool box for transporting the package(s) if you are travelling.
- After the first injection, the cartridge should remain in the pen injector and has to be kept in a refrigerator between 2 to 8°C for a maximum of 28 days.
- Do not use after the expiry date stated on the label and carton.
- Do not use Omnitrope if it was frozen or subject to high temperatures.
- Do not use Omnitrope if you notice that the solution is cloudy or contains particles.

DOSAGE FORMS, COMPOSITION AND PACKAGING: 5 mg/1.5 mL: Each 1.5 mL pen cartridge contains: 5 mg of somatropin (15 IU/1.5 mL), 1.3 mg disodium hydrogen phosphate heptahydrate, 1.6 mg sodium dihydrogen phosphate dihydrate, 3 mg poloxamer 188, 13.5 mg benzyl alcohol, 52.5 mg mannitol and water for injection. Phosphoric acid and/or sodium hydroxide may have been used to adjust pH. Cartons of 1 and 5 cartridges.

10 mg/1.5 mL: Each 1.5 mL pen cartridge contains: 10 mg of somatropin (30 IU/1.5 mL), 1.7 mg disodium hydrogen phosphate heptahydrate, 1.35 mg sodium dihydrogen phosphate dihydrate, 3 mg poloxamer 188, 4.5 mg phenol, 27.75 mg gylcine and water for injection. Phosphoric acid and/or sodium hydroxide may have been used to adjust pH. Cartons of 1 and 5 cartridges.

OncoTICE® Ⓟ

Bacillus Calmette-Guérin (BCG), strain TICE

Antineoplastic

Schering-Plough

Date of Revision: April 9, 2010

SUMMARY PRODUCT INFORMATION:

Route of Administration	Dosage Form/ Strength	Clinically Relevant Nonmedicinal Ingredients
Intravesicular	Powder for solution; 50 mg wet weight equivalent to approximately 1 to 8×10⁸ colony forming units (CFU) of TICE BCG/vial	Not applicable For a complete listing see Dosage Forms, Composition and Packaging.

DESCRIPTION: OncoTICE, [Bacillus Calmette-Guérin (BCG), strain TICE], is a freeze-dried preparation containing Bacillus Calmette and Guérin (BCG), strain TICE which is a live, attenuated strain of *M. bovis.* The culture medium from which the freeze-dried cake is prepared has the following relative composition: lactose 150 grams, Sauton medium 250 mL and water 750 mL. The freeze-dried BCG preparation is delivered in vials, each containing 1 to $8{\times}10^8$ colony forming units (CFU) of TICE BCG which is equivalent to approximately 50 mg wet weight. No preservatives have been added.

INDICATIONS AND CLINICAL USE: OncoTICE (Bacillus Calmette-Guérin (BCG), Strain TICE) is indicated for treatment of primary or relapsing flat urothelial cell carcinoma in situ (CIS) of the urinary bladder, and as a adjuvant therapy after TUR of a primary or relapsing superficial papillary urothelial cell carcinoma of the bladder stage T_A (grade 2 or 3) or T_1 (grade 1, 2, or 3). It is only recommended for stage T_A grade 1 papillary tumors, when there is judged to be a high risk of tumor recurrence.

OncoTICE is not indicated for the treatment of invasive bladder cancer. It is not recommended for papillary tumors of stages higher than T_1.

Geriatrics: OncoTICE can be used in geriatric patients (see Dosage and Administration and Warnings and Precautions).

Pediatrics (<18 years of age): No studies with OncoTICE have been performed in pediatric patients.

CONTRAINDICATIONS:

- OncoTICE is not indicated for the treatment of invasive bladder cancer.
- Patients who are hypersensitive to this drug or to any ingredient in the formulation or component of the container. For a complete listing, see Dosage Forms, Composition and Packaging.
- OncoTICE should not be used in patients with impaired immune response irrespective of whether this impairment is congenital or caused by disease, drugs, or other therapy.
- OncoTICE should be avoided in patients with a positive HIV serology.
- OncoTICE is contraindicated during pregnancy and lactation (see Warnings and Precautions).
- Clinical evidence of existing active tuberculosis should be ruled out in individuals who are purified protein derivative (PPD) positive before starting treatment with OncoTICE.
- OncoTICE should not be used concomitantly with antituberculosis drugs like streptomycin, para-amino-salicylic acid (PAS), isoniazid (INH), rifampicin and ethambutol because a potential loss of the antitumor activity of BCG may result.
- In patients with urinary tract infections, therapy with OncoTICE should be postponed or interrupted until the bacterial culture from urine becomes negative and the therapy with antibiotics and/or urinary antiseptics is stopped.
- In case of gross hematuria, OncoTICE therapy should be stopped or postponed until the hematuria has been successfully treated or has resolved.

WARNINGS AND PRECAUTIONS: General: OncoTICE should not be administered intravenously, subcutaneously or intramuscularly.

OncoTICE is not for oral or intradermal use.

OncoTICE is not a vaccine for the prevention of cancer, or for the prevention of tuberculosis. Physicians that use this product should be familiar with the literature on the prevention and treatment of BCG related complications and should be prepared in such emergencies to contact, when appropriate, infectious disease specialists with experience in treating the infectious complications of intravesical BCG. The treatment of infectious complications of BCG requires long term, multiple-drug antibiotic therapy.

OncoTICE contains live, potentially pathogenic bacteria. Reconstitution, preparation of the OncoTICE suspension for instillation and administration should be performed under aseptic conditions. Unused OncoTICE and all equipment, supplies, and receptacles in contact with OncoTICE should be handled and disposed of as biohazardous.

Patients should be monitored for the presence of symptoms of systemic BCG infection and for signs of toxicity after each intravesical treatment as death has been reported as a result of systemic BCG infections and sepsis.

In order to protect the partner, the patient should be recommended to either refrain from intercourse within one week after OncoTICE instillation, or to use a condom.

Transurethral resection (TUR): When used as an adjuvant therapy after TUR of a superficial urothelial cell carcinoma of the bladder (see Indications and Clinical Use), treatment with OncoTICE should be started between 10 and 15 days after performing the TUR. Treatment should not be started until mucosal lesions after TUR have healed.

Genitourinary: Care should be taken not to traumatize the urinary tract. Seven to 14 days should elapse before OncoTICE is administered following TUR, biopsy, or traumatic catheterization.

Traumatic catheterization or other injuries to the urethra or bladder mucosa can promote systemic BCG infection. Delaying OncoTICE administration should be considered in such patients until mucosal damage has healed.

Sensitivity: The use of OncoTICE may sensitize patients to tuberculin resulting in a positive reaction to PPD, therefore determination of tuberculin reactivity by PPD skin testing should be performed before starting the treatment with OncoTICE.

Special Populations: Pregnant Women: Animal reproduction studies have not been conducted with OncoTICE. It is also not known whether OncoTICE can cause fetal harm when administered to a pregnant woman or can affect reproductive capacity. OncoTICE should be given to a pregnant woman only if clearly needed. Women should be advised not to become pregnant while on therapy.

Nursing Women: It is not known whether OncoTICE is excreted in human milk. Because many drugs are excreted in human milk and because of the potential for serious adverse reactions from OncoTICE in nursing infants, a decision should be made whether to discontinue nursing or to discontinue the drug, taking into account the importance of the drug to the mother.

Pediatrics (<18 years of age): Safety and effectiveness of OncoTICE for the treatment of superficial bladder cancer in children have not been established.

Geriatrics: OncoTICE can be used in geriatric patients (see Dosage and Administration and Warnings and Precautions).

Monitoring and Laboratory Tests: In patients with known risk factors for HIV infection, it is recommended to perform adequate HIV assays prior to therapy.

Before the first intravesical instillation of OncoTICE, a Mantoux test (PPD) should be performed. In the event that this test is positive, the intravesical instillation of OncoTICE is contraindicated only if there is supplementary medical evidence for an active tuberculosis infection.

ADVERSE REACTIONS: Adverse Drug Reaction Overview: Adverse reactions are often localized to the bladder but may be accompanied by systemic manifestations.

Toxicity and side-effects appear to be directly related to the cumulative CFU count of BCG administered with the various instillations. Approximately 90% of patients develop local irritative symptoms in the bladder. Pollakiuria and dysuria are reported very frequently. The cystitis and typical inflammatory reactions (granulomas) which occur in the mucosa of the bladder after instillation of BCG, and which cause these symptoms, may be an essential part of the anti-tumor activity of the BCG. In most cases, the symptoms disappear within two days after instillation and the cystitis does not require treatment. During maintenance treatment with BCG, the symptoms of cystitis may be more pronounced and prolonged. Generally there are no long-term urinary complications.

Irritative bladder adverse effects associated with OncoTICE administration have been managed symptomatically with pyridium, propantheline bromide or oxybutinin chloride, and acetaminophen or ibuprofen.

Also commonly observed is malaise, a low to medium grade fever and/or influenza-like symptoms (fever, rigors, malaise and myalgia). These symptoms usually appear within 4 hours after instillation and last for 24 to 48 hours. Fever higher than 39°C typically resolves within 24 to 48 hours when treated with antipyretics (preferably paracetamol) and fluids. However, it is frequently not possible to distinguish these uncomplicated febrile reactions from early systemic BCG infections. Therefore, it is recommended that fever above 39.0°C that does not resolve within 12 hours despite antipyretic therapy must be considered as systemic BCG-infection, necessitating clinical confirmatory diagnosis and treatment (see Warnings and Precautions, General).

Systemic adverse effects such as malaise, fever, and chills may reflect hypersensitivity reactions and can be treated with antihistamines. The "flu-like" syndrome of 1-2 day's duration that frequently accompanies OncoTICE administration should be treated symptomatically. Systemic BCG infections could be due to traumatic catheterization, bladder perforation or premature BCG instillation after extensive TUR of a superficial carcinoma of the bladder (see Warnings and Precautions, Genitourinary). These systemic infections may be manifested initially by pneumonitis, hepatitis and/or cytopenia after a period of fever and malaise during which symptoms progressively increase.

Patients with manifest symptoms of therapy-induced BCG infections should be adequately treated with anti-tuberculous agents following regular treatment schedules used for tuberculosis infections: when systemic infection is present, the triple drug therapy (isoniazid-rifampicin-ethambutol) with or without cycloserine is given first for several weeks and is followed by therapy with isoniazid and rifampicin; rifampicin plus isoniazid are given when there are signs of an active BCG infection without systemic involvement. In these cases, further installations of OncoTICE are contra-indicated.

Deaths have been reported as a result of systemic BCG infections and sepsis. There have been two cases of nephrogenic adenoma, a benign lesion of bladder epithelium, associated with intravesical BCG therapy.

In general, the adverse effects of BCG therapy in bladder carcinoma have been of short duration and moderate morbidity. The side effects of intravesical OncoTICE therapy are generally mild and transient.

Clinical Trial Adverse Drug Reactions: Because clinical trials are conducted under very specific conditions the adverse reaction rates observed in the clinical trials may not reflect the rates observed in practice and should not be compared to the rates in the clinical trials of another drug. Adverse drug reaction information from clinical trials is useful for identifying drug-related adverse events and for approximating rates.

A summary of the incidence and severity of adverse effects observed in a study of 674 patients with superficial bladder cancer, treated intravesically with OncoTICE is presented in Table 1. The adverse events reported in other studies have been similar.

Table 1: OncoTICE
Adverse Effects

Local Adverse Effects	Incidence (%)	Severe (%)
Dysuria	59.5	10.7
Urinary Frequency	40.4	7.4
Hematuria	26.0	7.4
Cystitis	5.9	1.9
Urgency	5.8	1.3
Nocturia	4.5	0.6
Cramps/Pain	4.0	0.9
Urinary Incontinence	2.4	—
Urinary Debris	2.2	0.4
Genital Inflammation/Abscess	1.8	0.4
Urinary Tract Infection	1.5	0.9
Urethritis	1.2	—
Pyuria	0.7	0.1
Epididymitis/Prostatitis	0.3	—
Urinary Obstruction	0.3	—

(cont'd)

Table 1: OncoTICE *(cont'd)*

Adverse Effects		
Contracted Bladder	0.2	
Orchitis	0.2	
Systemic Adverse Effects	**Incidence (%)**	**Severe (%)**
Fever	19.9	7.6
Malaise/Fatigue	7.4	—
Shaking Chills	3.3	1.0
Nausea/Vomiting	3.0	0.3
Arthritis/Myalgia	2.7	0.4
Headache/Dizziness	2.4	—
Anorexia/Weight Loss	2.2	0.1
Allergic	2.1	0.4
Cardiac	1.9	1.3
Respiratory (Unclassified)	1.6	0.2
Abdominal Pain	1.5	0.6
Anemia	1.3	0.4
Diarrhea	1.2	0.1
Pneumonitis	1.2	0.6
Gastrointestinal (Unclassified)	1.0	—
Neurologic	0.9	0.3
Rash	0.6	0.2
BCG Sepsis	0.4	0.4
Coagulopathy	0.3	0.3
Leukopenia	0.3	—
Thrombocytopenia	0.3	—
Hepatic Granuloma	0.2	0.2
Hepatitis	0.2	0.2

Flu-like syndrome (which includes fever, shaking chills, malaise and myalgia) had an incidence of 33.2% of which 9.0% were severe.

Severe was ECOG Grade 3 or 4.

Post-Market Adverse Drug Reactions: The following adverse reactions (Table 2) are reported from the post-market surveillance as serious and unexpected. This information is based on experience and clinical data published.

DRUG INTERACTIONS: Overview: Immunosuppressants and/or bone marrow depressants and/or radiation may interfere with the development of the immune response and thus with the anti-tumour efficacy and should, therefore, not be used in combination with OncoTICE.

Drug-Drug Interactions: OncoTICE is sensitive to most antibiotics and, in particular, to the routinely used anti-tuberculous agents, like streptomycin, para-aminosalicylic acid (PAS), isoniazid (INH), rifampicin and ethambutol except for pyrazinamide. Therefore, the anti-tumour activity of OncoTICE may be decreased by concomitant therapy with antibiotics. If a patient is being treated with antibiotic it is recommended to postpone the intravesical instillation until the end of the antibiotic treatment (see also Contraindications).

Drug-Food Interactions: Interactions with food have not been established.

Drug-Herb Interactions: Interactions with drug-herb have not been established.

Drug-Laboratory Test Interactions: No data has been established.

Drug-Lifestyle Interactions: Based on the pharmacodynamic profile of OncoTICE, it is assumed that the product will not affect the ability to drive and to use machines.

DOSAGE AND ADMINISTRATION: Dosing Considerations: For each instillation, the contents of one vial of OncoTICE, [Bacillus Calmette-Guérin (BCG), strain TICE], reconstituted and diluted as indicated, are instilled into the urinary bladder.

OncoTICE must not be administered intravenously, subcutaneously or intramuscularly.

Induction Treatment: Weekly instillation with OncoTICE for 6 consecutive weeks.

Maintenance Treatment: Additional instillations of OncoTICE at week 8 and 12 and monthly from months 4 to 12.

Missed Dose: No data established.

Administration: Insert a catheter via the urethra into the bladder and drain the bladder completely. Connect the 50 mL syringe containing the prepared OncoTICE suspension to the catheter, and instill the suspension into the bladder.

After instillation, remove the catheter.

The instilled OncoTICE suspension must remain in the bladder for a period of 2 hours. After two hours, have the patient void the instilled suspension in a sitting position.

Note: The patient is not allowed to ingest any fluid during a period of 4 hours prior to instillation, or during the time that the OncoTICE suspension remains in the bladder after instillation (2 hrs).

If a spill or contamination occurs, area should be cleaned by covering the area with paper towels soaked with tuberculocidal disinfectant for at least 10 minutes. Wastes should be treated as biohazardous and disposed of accordingly (see Special Handling Instructions).

Perform the following procedures under aseptic conditions:

Reconstitution-Suspension for Bladder Instillation: Add 1 mL of a sterile, pyrogen-free and preservative-free physiological saline solution by means of a sterile syringe and allow standing for a few minutes. Then gently swirl the vial until a homogeneous suspension is obtained. (Caution: avoid forceful agitation).

Preparation of the Dolution for Instillation: Transfer the suspension from the vial into a sterile 50 mL syringe. Rinse the vial with another 1 mL of sterile, pyrogen-free and preservative-free physiological saline. Add the rinse fluid to the suspension in the 50 mL syringe. Finally dilute the contents of this syringe (1 mL OncoTICE suspension+1 mL rinse fluid) by adding sterile, pyrogen-free and preservative-free physiological saline solution up to a total volume of 50 mL. Mix the suspension carefully.

Note: The suspension must **not** be filtered.

This suspension is now ready for instillation; it contains a total of 1 to 8×10^8 CFU of TICE BCG.

Table 2: OncoTICE
Adverse Reactions

Occurrence	MedDRA System Organ Class	Preferred Terms
Rare (>1/10 000, <1/1000)	Respiratory, Thoracic and Mediastinal Disorders	Cough
	Reproductive System and Breast Disorders	Epididymitis
Very rare (<1/10 000)	Infections and Infestations	Pharyngitis, orchitis, Reiter's syndrome, Lupus vulgaris
	Blood and Lymphatic System Disorders	Lymphadenopathy
	Metabolism and Nutrition Disorders	Anorexia
	Psychiatric Disorders	Confusional state
	Nervous System Disorders	Dizziness, dysaesthesia[a], hyperaesthesia[a], paresthesia, somnolence, headache, hypertonia, neuralgia[a]
	Eye Disorders	Conjunctivitis
	Ear and Labyrinth Disorders	Vertigo[a]
	Vascular Disorders	Hypotension
	Respiratory, Thoracic and Mediastinal Disorders	Bronchitis, dyspnea, rhinitis
	Gastrointestinal Disorders	Dyspepsia[a], flatulence[a]
	Skin and Subcutaneous Tissue Disorders	Alopecia, hyperhidrosis
	Musculoskeletal and Connective Tissue Disorders	Back pain
	Renal and Urinary Disorders	Renal failure acute
	Reproductive System and Breast Disorders	Balanoposthitis, prostatitis, vulvovaginal discomfort[a]
	General Disorders and Administration Site Conditions	Chest pain, edema peripheral, granuloma[b]
	Investigations	Prostatic specific antigen increased, weight decreased

[a] Only isolated cases reported during post-marketing surveillance.
[b] Granuloma NOS has been observed in various organs including the aorta, bladder, epididymis, gastrointestinal tract, kidney, liver, lungs, lymph nodes, peritoneum, prostate.

Incompatibilities: OncoTICE is incompatible with hypotonic and hypertonic solutions. OncoTICE should be mixed with physiological saline as described above under Reconstitution-Suspension for Bladder Instillation. Other incompatibility studies have not been performed.

OVERDOSAGE:
Overdosage occurs if more than one vial of OncoTICE, is administered per instillation. The patient should be closely monitored for signs of systemic BCG infection and treated with anti-tuberculous medication (see Adverse Reactions).

For management of a suspected drug overdose, contact your regional Poison Control Centre. See the *CPS* Directory section for a list of Poison Control Centres.

ACTION AND CLINICAL PHARMACOLOGY: Mechanism of Action: It has anti-tumor activity, but the exact mechanism of action is not known. Study data suggest that an active nonspecific immune response takes place. BCG invokes a local inflammatory response involving a variety of immune cells, such as macrophages, natural killer cells and T cells.

Pharmacodynamics: OncoTICE is an immunostimulating agent (ATC code L 03AX03).

Pharmacokinetics: For the treatment and recurrence prophylaxis of bladder cancer, the attachment of BCG to the bladder wall after voiding has been shown to be important. This allows a targeted pharmacological effect at the site of application. It is known that Tice BCG can bind specifically to fibronectin in the bladder wall. However, most instilled OncoTICE will be excreted with the first urine void two hours after the instillation.

STORAGE AND STABILITY: Intact OncoTICE vials containing freeze-dried BCG, must be stored at 2-8°C and protected from light. The expiry date indicated on the label of the vials only applies if the vials are stored under these conditions.

The reconstituted solution for bladder instillation can be stored for up to **2 hours** when refrigerated at 2-8°C and protected from light. Unused solution should be discarded after **2 hours**.

SPECIAL HANDLING INSTRUCTIONS: OncoTICE contains live attenuated mycobacteria. Reconstitution, preparation of the OncoTICE suspension for instillation and administration should be performed under aseptic conditions.

Spillage of OncoTICE suspension may cause TICE BCG contamination. Any spilled OncoTICE suspension should be cleaned by covering the area with paper towels soaked with tuberculocidal disinfectant for at least 10 minutes. Unused OncoTICE and all equipment, supplies, and receptacles in contact with OncoTICE should be handled and disposed of as bio-hazardous.

Accidental exposure to OncoTICE could occur through self-innoculation, by dermal exposure through an open wound or by ingestion of OncoTICE suspension. OncoTICE exposure should not produce significant adverse health outcomes in healthy individuals. However, in case of suspected, accidental self-innoculation, PPD skin testing is advised at the time of the accident and six weeks later to detect skin test conversion.

INFORMATION FOR THE PATIENT: Published in e-CPS, available by subscription at www.e-cps.ca.

DOSAGE FORMS, COMPOSITION AND PACKAGING: Each vial of freeze-dried preparation contains: 1 to 8×10^8 CFU of TICE BCG which is equivalent to approximately 50 mg wet weight. Vials of 2 mL, boxes of 1.

Ondansetron Injection USP ℞

ondansetron HCl dihydrate

Antiemetic

Sandoz

SUPPLIED: 2 mg/mL (preservative-free): Each mL contains: ondansetron (as HCl dihydrate) 2 mg. Nonmedicinal ingredients: citric acid monohydrate, sodium chloride (for tonicity), sodium citrate and water for injection. Single use vials of 2 mL, boxes of 10 and single use vials of 4 mL, boxes of 5. Store between 2 and 30°C. Protect from light and freezing. Intended for single use only. Do not autoclave. Discard unused portion.

2 mg/mL (with preservative): Each mL contains: ondansetron (as HCl dihydrate) 2 mg. Nonmedicinal ingredients: citric acid monohydrate, methylparaben and propylparaben (as preservatives), sodium chloride (for tonicity), sodium citrate and water for injection. Multidose vials of 20 mL, boxes of 1. Store between 2 and 30°C. Protect from light. Protect from freezing. Do not autoclave. Discard 28 days after initial puncture.

Ondansetron-Odan ℞

ondansetron HCl dihydrate

Antiemetic

Odan

SUPPLIED: 4 mg: Each oval shaped, yellow, film-coated tablet, marked "ON" on one side and "4" on the other, contains: ondansetron 4 mg (as ondansetron hydrochloride dihydrate). Nonmedicinal ingredients: croscarmellose sodium, hydroxypropyl methylcellulose, iron oxide yellow, lactose, magnesium stearate, microcrystalline cellulose, pregelatinized starch, titanium dioxide and triacetin. Plastic bottles of 100. Blisters of 10. Store in a dry place and at room temperature (15 to 30°C).

8 mg: Each oval shaped, yellow, film-coated tablet, marked "ON" on one side and "8" on the other, contains: ondansetron 8 mg (as ondansetron hydrochloride dihydrate). Nonmedicinal ingredients: croscarmellose sodium, hydroxypropyl methylcellulose, iron oxide yellow, lactose, magnesium stearate, microcrystalline cellulose, pregelatinized starch, titanium dioxide and triacetin. Plastic bottles of 100. Blisters of 10. Store in a dry place and at room temperature (15 to 30°C).

One A Day®

multiple vitamins and minerals

Vitamin—Mineral Supplement

Bayer Consumer Care

SUPPLIED: One A Day Women 50 Plus: Each dark red tablet, embossed ONE A DAY on one side contains: vitamin A (as acetate) 750 µg (2500 IU), beta-carotene (a source of vitamin A) 750 µg (2500 IU), thiamine (vitamin B_1) (thiamine mononitrate) 1.5 mg, riboflavin (vitamin B_2) (riboflavin) 1.7 mg, vitamin B_6 (pyridoxine hydrochloride) 2 mg, vitamin B_{12} (cyanocobalamin) 6 µg, biotin (biotin) 30 µg, vitamin C (ascorbic acid) 60 mg, vitamin D (cholecalciferol) 10 µg (400 IU), vitamin E (dl-alpha tocopheryl acetate) 13.5 mg (30 IU), folate (folic acid) 0.4 mg, niacinamide (niacinamide) 20 mg, pantothenic acid (calcium d-pantothenate) 10 mg, calcium (calcium phosphate, dibasic) 130 mg, chlorine (potassium chloride) 34 mg, chromium (chromium yeast) 10 µg, copper (cupric sulfate) 2 mg, iodine (potassium iodide) 0.15 mg, iron (ferrous fumarate) 18 mg, magnesium (magnesium oxide) 100 mg, manganese (manganese sulfate), 2.5 mg, molybdenum (molybdenum yeast) 10 µg, potassium (potassium chloride) 37.5 mg, selenium (selenium yeast) 10 µg and zinc (zinc sulfate) 15 mg. Nonmedicinal ingredients: ascorbic palmitate, brewers yeast, butylated hydroxytoluene, calcium silicate, cellulose, croscarmellose sodium, dextrin, dextrose, dicalcium phosphate, FD&C Blue #2, FD&C Red #40, gelatin, hypromellose, lecithin, magnesium stearate, partially hydrogenated soybean oil, polyethylene glycol, resin, silicon dioxide, sodium ascorbate, sodium carboxymethylcellulose, sodium citrate, sodium starch glycolate, starch, stearic acid, sucrose and titanium dioxide. Bottles of 90.

One A Day Men 50 Plus: Each dark orange tablet, embossed ONE A DAY on one side contains: vitamin A (as acetate) 900 µg (3000 IU), beta-carotene (a source of vitamin A) 1800 µg (3000 IU), thiamine (vitamin B_1) (thiamine mononitrate) 4.5 mg, riboflavin (vitamin B_2) (riboflavin) 3.4 mg, vitamin B_6 (pyridoxine hydrochloride) 6 mg, vitamin B_{12} (cyanocobalamin) 25 µg, biotin (biotin) 30 µg, vitamin C (ascorbic acid) 120 mg, vitamin D (cholecalciferol) 10 µg (400 IU), vitamin E (dl-alpha tocopheryl acetate) 27 mg (60 IU), folate (folic acid) 0.4 mg, niacinamide (niacinamide ascorbate) 20 mg, pantothenic acid (calcium d-pantothenate) 20 mg, calcium (calcium carbonate) 220 mg, chlorine (potassium chloride) 34 mg, chromium (chromium yeast) 10 µg, copper (cupric sulfate) 2 mg, iodine (potassium iodide) 0.15 mg, magnesium (magnesium oxide) 100 mg, manganese (manganese sulfate) 2.5 mg, molybdenum (molybdenum yeast) 10 µg, potassium (potassium chloride) 37.5 mg, selenium (selenium yeast) 10 µg and zinc (zinc sulfate) 15 mg. Nonmedicinal ingredients: acacia, ascorbic palmitate, brewers yeast, butylated hydroxytoluene, calcium silicate, cellulose, croscarmellose sodium, crospovidone, dextrin, dextrose, dicalcium phosphate, FD&C Yellow #6, gelatin, hypromellose, lecithin, magnesium stearate, maltodextrin, mineral oil, partially hydrogenated soybean oil, polyethylene glycol, resin, silicon dioxide, sodium ascorbate, sodium carboxymethylcellulose, sodium citrate, sodium starch glycolate, starch, sucrose and titanium dioxide. Bottles of 90.

One A Day Women: Each cream colored tablet, embossed ONE A DAY on one side contains: vitamin A (as acetate) 600 µg (2000 IU), beta-carotene (a source of vitamin A) 150 µg (500 IU), thiamine (vitamin B_1) (thiamine mononitrate) 1.5 mg, riboflavin (vitamin B_2) (riboflavin) 1.7 mg, vitamin B_6 (pyridoxine hydrochloride) 2 mg, vitamin B_{12} (cyanocobalamin) 10 µg, vitamin C (ascorbic acid) 60 mg, vitamin D (cholecalciferol) 5 µg (200 IU), vitamin E (dl-alpha tocopheryl acetate) 11.25 mg (25 IU), folate (folic acid) 0.4 mg, niacinamide (niacinamide) 14 mg, pantothenic acid (calcium d-pantothenate) 10 mg, calcium (calcium carbonate) 400 mg, iron (ferrous fumarate) 10 mg and magnesium (magnesium oxide) 50 mg. Nonmedicinal ingredients: acacia, ascorbic palmitate, butylated hydroxytoluene, calcium silicate, cellulose, croscarmellose sodium, dextrin, dextrose, FD&C Blue #2, FD&C Yellow #5, FD&C Yellow #6, gelatin, hypromellose, lecithin, magnesium stearate, maltodextrin, partially hydrogenated soybean oil, polyethylene glycol, resin, silicone dioxide, sodium ascorbate, sodium carboxymethylcellulose, sodium citrate dihydrate, sodium lauryl sulfate, starch, stearic acid, sucrose and titanium dioxide. Bottles of 90 and 200.

One A Day Men: Each light orange tablet, embossed ONE A DAY on one side contains: vitamin A (as acetate) 1200 µg (4000 IU), beta-carotene (a source of vitamin A) 300 µg (1000 IU), thiamine (vitamin B_1) (thiamine mononitrate) 2.25 mg, riboflavin (vitamin B_2) (riboflavin) 2.55 mg, vitamin B_6 (pyridoxine hydrochloride) 3 mg, vitamin B_{12} (cyanocobalamin) 9 µg, vitamin C (ascorbic acid) 90 mg, vitamin D (cholecalciferol) 10 µg (400 IU), vitamin E (dl-alpha tocopheryl acetate) 20.25 mg (45 IU), folate (folic acid) 0.4 mg, niacinamide (niacinamide ascorbate) 20 mg, pantothenic acid (calcium d-pantothenate) 10 mg, chlorine (potassium chloride) 34 mg, chromium (chromium chloride) 150 µg, copper (cupric sulfate) 2 mg, iodine (potassium iodide) 0.15 mg, magnesium (magnesium oxide) 100 mg, manganese (manganese sulfate) 3.5 mg, molybdenum (sodium molybdate) 42 µg, potassium (potassium chloride) 37.5 mg, selenium (sodium selenate) 87.5 µg and zinc (zinc sulfate) 15 mg. Nonmedicinal ingredients: ascorbic palmitate, brewers yeast, butylated hydroxytoluene, cellulose, croscarmellose sodium, crospovidone, dextrin, dextrose, dicalcium phosphate, FD&C Blue #2, FD&C Yellow #5, FD&C Yellow #6, gelatin, hypromellose, lecithin, magnesium stearate, partially hydrogenated soybean oil, polyethylene glycol, resin, silicone dioxide, sodium ascorbate, sodium benzoate, sorbic acid, starch, stearic acid, sucrose and titanium dioxide. Bottles of 90 and 200.

One-Alpha® ℞

alfacalcidol

Vitamin D Analogue

LEO Pharma

PHARMACOLOGY: 1α-hydroxyvitamin D_3(1α-OHD_3) stimulates intestinal calcium and phosphorus absorption, the reabsorption of calcium from bone and possibly the renal reabsorption of calcium.

To be effective in disorders resulting from vitamin D deficiency, vitamin D must undergo 2 metabolic conversions, first in the liver to 25-hydroxyvitamin D and then in the kidney to the physiologically active metabolite, 1,25-dihydroxyvitamin D_3 (1,25-$(OH)_2D_3$). In patients with chronic renal failure, progressive nephron destruction blocks the production of 1,25-$(OH)_2D_3$ by the kidneys resulting in diminished serum levels of this metabolite.

When alfacalcidol is administered in this clinical situation, it is rapidly converted to 1,25-$(OH)_2D_3$ in the liver, effectively bypassing the critical renal metabolic conversion. This hepatic conversion of alfacalcidol is accomplished very rapidly, before any stimulation of the intestine or bone occurs.

The biological half-life of alfacalcidol has been shown to be approximately 3 hours in the presence of renal insufficiency. However, serum levels of 1,25-$(OH)_2D_3$ peak approximately 12 hours after a single dose of oral alfacalcidol and approximately 4 hours after a single dose of i.v. alfacalcidol. Levels of 1,25-$(OH)_2D_3$ remain measurable for at least 48 hours. The effect of 1 µg of oral alfacalcidol on intestinal calcium absorption has been observed within 6 hours of ingestion and was maximal at 24 hours. There is evidence that vitamin D, its 1α-hydroxylated metabolites and analogues are extensively bound to a serum binding protein of the α-globulin fraction. 1,25-$(OH)_2D_3$ appears to function in the intestine and bone by a receptor-nuclear activation mechanism.

One of the first abnormalities to be observed in patients with chronic renal failure is the disturbance of calcium metabolism due to increased phosphate retention and impaired production of 1,25-$(OH)_2D_3$. Because calcium metabolism and production of 1,25-$(OH)_2D_3$ is at least partially mediated by the parathyroid glands, hypocalcemia leads to increased parathyroid hormone (PTH) secretion and high plasma PTH levels. Therefore, the patients with renal bone disease most likely to benefit from alfacalcidol therapy are those characterized by abnormally low plasma calcium levels, elevated alkaline phosphatase and PTH levels and histological evidence of osteitic fibrosa and osteomalacia.

In the majority of patients treated with alfacalcidol, clinical symptoms of bone pain and muscle weakness begin to remit promptly, within 2 weeks to 3 months of the start of therapy. Malabsorption of calcium is rapidly corrected. In patients on daily oral therapy, plasma alkaline phosphatase and PTH levels generally begin to fall within 3 months, but plasma calcium levels may not normalize for several months. This delay should not necessarily be construed as a poor response but may indicate that calcium is being utilized for bone mineralization. The decrease in PTH levels may be more rapid in patients on intermittent i.v. therapy, with significant reductions being achieved within 3 months of therapy.

By contrast, hypercalcemia may occur at any stage of treatment, the risk being higher just after treatment is started and later when the plasma alkaline phosphatase level falls towards normal (see Precautions).

Because of a modest action on intestinal phosphorus absorption, alfacalcidol may elevate plasma phosphorus levels even further in patients with renal osteodystrophy and this may require increasing the dose of phosphate binding agents.

Normalization of plasma PTH levels frequently correlates well with healing of osteitis fibrosa, but radiographic improvement can occur without significant changes in plasma PTH concentrations. After 3 to 6 months of treatment, radiological evidence of healing is generally apparent. Histological responses, such as a decrease in the surface of bone undergoing resorption and a decrease in the volume of osteoid, are often much slower.

The beneficial effect of alfacalcidol on the development of renal bone disease in patients with renal failure not yet undergoing dialysis has been demonstrated in a large, randomized, placebo controlled study. Long-term administration of oral alfacalcidol (maximum dose of 1 µg/day for up to 2 years) improved bone histology and halted the progression of changes in serum alkaline phosphatase activity and parathyroid hormone levels compared to placebo. Long-term administration of alfacalcidol proved to be well tolerated and had no adverse effect on renal function in patients for whom the dose was titrated to prevent persistent hypercalcemia. Although elevation of serum calcium was observed, marked hypercalcemia (>3 mmol/L) was uncommon (4.5% of patients) and readily responded to decreases in drug dosage.

INDICATIONS: Management of hypocalcemia, secondary hyperparathyroidism, and osteodystrophy in patients with chronic renal failure.

CONTRAINDICATIONS: Known hypersensitivity to 1α-hydroxyvitamin D_3, vitamin D or any of its analogues and derivatives. Biochemical evidence of hypercalcemia, hyperphosphatemia or of vitamin D overdose.

WARNINGS: Alfacalcidol is a potent cholecalciferol derivative with a profound positive effect on intestinal absorption of dietary calcium. The effect of alfacalcidol on inorganic phosphorus absorption is less marked, although it is important to recognize that the drug may increase plasma phosphorus concentrations, which may increase the requirements for phosphate binding agents.

Alfacalcidol should not be used concomitantly with other vitamin D products or derivatives.

As with all vitamin D preparations and metabolites, hypercalcemia must be anticipated when using alfacalcidol. Regular monitoring of plasma calcium is essential. Indeed, alfacalcidol should only be used when adequate facilities are available for monitoring of blood and urine chemistries on a regular basis.

During treatment with alfacalcidol, progressive hypercalcemia either due to hyperresponsiveness or overdose may become so severe as to require emergency treatment.

Chronic hypercalcemia can lead to generalized vascular calcification, nephrocalcinosis or calcifications of the cornea or other soft tissues. During treatment with alfacalcidol, the **total serum calcium** (mg/dL) **times serum inorganic phosphate** (mg/dL) product (Ca×P) **should be maintained at accepted levels**. A dialysate calcium level of 1.75 mmol/L or above, in addition to excess dietary calcium supplements may lead to frequent episodes of hypercalcemia.

To control serum inorganic phosphate levels and dietary phosphate absorption, appropriate oral phosphate binding agents in association with a low phosphate diet may be necessary to prevent hyperphosphatemia and extra-skeletal calcifications. Serum phosphate levels were maintained below 2 mmol/L in the study that demonstrated the benefits of daily oral alfacalcidol on the development of bone disease in pre-dialysis patients.

Antacids containing magnesium should be avoided as they may contribute towards hypermagnesemia.

In patients on digitalis, hypercalcemia may precipitate cardiac arrhythmias. In such patients alfacalcidol should be used with extreme caution.

Pregnancy: The safety of alfacalcidol in women who are or may become pregnant has not been established; use of the alfacalcidol in these cases may be considered only when the potential benefits have been weighed against possible hazards to mother and fetus.

Lactation: Alfacalcidol may be excreted in human milk, therefore, breast-feeding during treatment should be avoided.

PRECAUTIONS: Patient Selection and Follow-up: The therapeutic margin with alfacalcidol is narrow; the optimal daily dose must be carefully titrated for each individual patient (see Dosage).

The occurrence of hypercalcemia depends on such factors as the degree of bone mineralization, the state of renal function and the dose of alfacalcidol. Excessive doses of the drug induce hypercalcemia and hypercalciuria.

Pre-Dialysis Administration of Alfacalcidol: Serum calcium and phosphate levels should be monitored at monthly intervals or as is considered necessary if hypercalcemia develops.

If hypercalcemia develops at any time during treatment then the dose of alfacalcidol should be reduced by 50% and all calcium supplements stopped until calcium levels return to normal.

Administration of Alfacalcidol to Patients Undergoing Dialysis: Plasma calcium should be measured at weekly intervals depending on the progress of the patient. In early treatment during dosage adjustment, serum calcium should be determined at least twice weekly. In the later stages of treatment when there is evidence of bone healing (e.g., when the plasma alkaline phosphatase level falls toward normal), weekly estimations are recommended.

If hypercalcemia occurs, alfacalcidol should be discontinued immediately. Upon discontinuation of the drug, serum calcium levels generally normalize within a few days to a week. Calcium levels should be rechecked in another week and if still at normal levels, alfacalcidol may be reinstituted at half the previous dose.

Patients with renal bone disease and a relatively high initial plasma calcium and "autonomous" hyperparathyroidism are liable to early hypercalcemia, as are the minority of dialysis patients with low plasma alkaline phosphatase.

Essential Laboratory Tests: Laboratory tests considered essential for adequate patient monitoring include: serum calcium, inorganic phosphorus, magnesium, alkaline phosphatase, creatinine, BUN and protein (for correction of plasma calcium in instances of hypercalcemia). For pre-dialysis patients treated with alfacalcidol, serum calcium and phosphate levels should be monitored at monthly intervals or as is considered necessary if hypercalcemia develops. For patients undergoing dialysis serum calcium should be determined at least twice weekly during dose titration. During maintenance therapy with alfacalcidol, 24-hour urinary calcium and phosphorus should be determined periodically.

Periodic ophthalmological examinations and radiological evaluation of suspected anatomical regions for early detection of ectopic calcifications are advisable.

Drug Interactions: Alfacalcidol should be used with extreme caution in patients on digitalis, as hypercalcemia may trigger cardiac arrhythmias.

Resins such as cholestyramine and mineral oil used as a laxative may interfere with the intestinal absorption of alfacalcidol.

Patients concurrently treated with barbiturates and other anticonvulsant drugs may require higher doses of alfacalcidol, as these drugs may interfere with the action of vitamin D.

Information to Be Provided to the Patient: Patients and their immediate relatives should be informed about the need for compliance with the dosage instructions, strict adherence to prescribed calcium intake (dietary and supplementary) and avoidance of unapproved non-prescription drugs or medications.

Patients should be made aware of symptoms of hypercalcemia and should be instructed to seek medical attention if such symptoms appear (see Adverse Effects).

Children: The safety and efficacy of alfacalcidol in children have not been established.

ADVERSE EFFECTS: In general, the adverse effects of alfacalcidol are similar to those encountered with excessive vitamin D intake.

The early and late signs and symptoms associated with vitamin D intoxication and hypercalcemia may include: a) Early: pruritus, weakness, headache, "red-eyes", somnolence, nausea, cardiac arrhythmia, vomiting, excessive thirst, dry mouth, constipation, muscle pain, bone pain and metallic taste. b) Late: polyuria, polydipsia, anorexia, weight loss, nocturia, conjunctivitis, corneal calcification, photophobia, rhinorrhea, pancreatitis, pruritus, hyperthermia, decreased libido, elevated BUN, albuminuria, hypercholesterolemia, elevated AST and ALT, ectopic calcification, hypertension, cardiac arrhythmias and, rarely, overt psychosis.

Hypercalcemia and possibly an exacerbation of hyperphosphatemia are the most frequent adverse reactions that have been reported with alfacalcidol in patients with renal osteodystrophy. Elevated levels of calcium and phosphorus increase the risk of metastatic calcification and may accelerate the decline in renal function in some patients with chronic renal failure.

OVERDOSE:

Symptoms: Dosages of alfacalcidol in excess of daily requirements can cause hypercalcemia, hypercalciuria and hyperphosphatemia. Conversely, a high intake of calcium and phosphate concomitantly with therapeutic doses of alfacalcidol may cause similar abnormalities.

Treatment: Treatment of Hypercalcemia Due to Overdose: General treatment of serum calcium levels more than 1 mg/dL or 0.25 mmol/L above the upper limit of the normal range (usually 8.0 to 10.4 mg/dL or 2.2 to 2.6 mmol/L) consists of immediate discontinuation of alfacalcidol, institution of a low calcium diet and withdrawal of calcium supplements. Serum calcium levels should be determined daily until the patient achieves normocalcemia. Hypercalcemia frequently resolves in 2 to 7 days. Alfacalcidol therapy can be reinstituted at half the previous dose when serum calcium levels have returned to within normal limits. Serum calcium levels should be carefully monitored (at least twice weekly) during this period of dosage adjustment and subsequent dosage titration. Persistent or markedly elevated serum calcium levels in hemodialysis patients may be corrected by dialysis against a calcium free dialysate.

Treatment of Accidental Overdosage: General supportive measures. If drug ingestion is discovered within a relatively short time, induction of emesis or gastric lavage may be of benefit in preventing further absorption. If the drug has passed through the stomach, the administration of mineral oil may promote its fecal elimination. Serial serum electrolyte determinations (especially calcium ion), rate of urinary calcium excretion and assessment of electrocardiographic abnormalities due to hypercalcemia should be obtained. Such monitoring is critical in patients receiving digitalis. Discontinuation of supplemental calcium and low calcium diet are also indicated in accidental overdosage. Due to the relatively short pharmacological action of alfacalcidol, further measures are probably unnecessary. However, if persistent and markedly elevated serum calcium levels occur, there are a variety of therapeutic alternatives which may be considered depending on the underlying condition of the patient. These include the use of drugs such as phosphates and corticosteroids as well as measures to induce an appropriate forced diuresis. The use of dialysis against a calcium free dialysate has also been reported.

For management of a suspected drug overdose, CPhA recommends that you contact your **regional Poison Control Centre**. See the *CPS* Directory section for a list of Poison Control Centres.

DOSAGE: The daily dose must be carefully individualized and titrated according to such factors as the state of renal function, degree of bone mineralization and initial plasma calcium and alkaline phosphatase concentrations. Other factors which may be taken into account are urinary calcium excretion, plasma PTH and phosphorus.

The success of alfacalcidol is also based on the assumption that the patient is receiving an adequate daily intake of calcium during treatment. The recommended daily allowance of calcium in adults is about 800 to 1000 mg (from all sources such as dialysate, diet and calcium supplements). The physician should ensure that each patient receives an adequate daily intake of calcium by prescribing a calcium supplement or instructing the patients in appropriate dietary measures.

Dose Titration: Pre-Dialysis Patients on Daily Oral Therapy: A dose of alfacalcidol that maintains serum calcium (adjusted for albumin concentration) within the normal range should be selected. An initial dose of 0.25 µg/day is recommended, followed by dose adjustment until an appropriate dose is achieved. Alfacalcidol has been shown to be safe and effective in the prevention of renal bone disease when doses were maintained at or below 1 µg/day. Alfacalcidol is usually administered as a single dose each day taken with food.

The following protocol for dosage adjustment is suggested: An initial dose of 0.25 µg/day should be administered for 2 months, unless hypercalcemia develops. If hypercalcemia occurs then the dose should be reduced to 0.25 µg on alternate days. If serum calcium is below the desired range, the dose may be adjusted in increments of 0.25 µg/day every 2 months. Most patients will be maintained on a dose of 0.5 µg/day. However, doses up to 1 µg/day may be necessary to maintain serum calcium within the desired range. If hypercalcemia develops at any time during treatment then the dose of alfacalcidol should be reduced by 50% and all calcium supplements stopped until calcium levels return to normal.

Serum calcium and phosphate levels should be monitored at monthly intervals or as is considered necessary if hypercalcemia develops. Calcium supplements should not exceed 500 mg of elemental calcium per day.

Dose Titration: Dialysis Patients on Daily Oral Therapy: The recommended initial dose is 1 µg daily. If a satisfactory response in the biochemical parameters and clinical manifestations is not observed within 4 weeks, the daily dose may be increased by 0.5 µg every 2 to 4 weeks. Most patients respond eventually to a dose of between 1 and 2 µg/day. Only, exceptionally, a dose of 3 µg is required. During this titration period, serum calcium levels should be obtained at least twice weekly and, if hypercalcemia is noted, the drug should be discontinued immediately until serum calcium levels normalize.

Maintenance Doses: Dialysis Patients on Daily Oral Therapy: Once serum calcium levels are normalized or only slightly reduced, the dose requirement of alfacalcidol generally decreases. Maintenance doses usually range from 0.25 to 1.0 µg/day. If this small maintenance dose still proves too high, adequate control can usually be achieved by giving the dose on alternate days or even less frequently.

Dose Titration: Dialysis Patients on Intermittent I.V. Therapy: A dose of alfacalcidol that maintains total serum calcium in the upper half of the normal range should be selected. Calcium levels should be measured weekly during the dose titration period. The recommended initial dose of alfacalcidol is 1 µg per dialysis (2 to 3 times a weekly). If a satisfactory response in biochemical parameters is not observed within 1 week, the dose may be increased in weekly increments of 1 µg per dialysis to a maximum of 12 µg/week. The total dose titration period should not exceed 6 weeks. If hypercalcemia is noted, the drug should be discontinued immediately until serum calcium levels normalize. Once calcium levels return to the normal range, alfacalcidol should be reintroduced at lower doses.

Maintenance Doses: Dialysis Patients on Intermittent I.V. Therapy: Doses required to maintain serum calcium levels in the upper half of the normal range are usually around 6 µg/week but can range from 1.5 to 12 µg/week. Serum calcium and phosphate levels should be monitored every other week or as is considered necessary if hypercalcemia is noted. If hypercalcemia develops, adequate control can usually be achieved by temporarily stopping treatment. Once calcium levels normalize, alfacalcidol should be reintroduced at lower doses.

INFORMATION FOR THE PATIENT: Published in e-CPS, available by subscription at www.e-cps.ca.

SUPPLIED: Soft Gel Capsules: 0.25 µg: Each cream-coloured egg-shaped soft gelatin capsule contains: alfacalcidol 0.25 µg. Nonmedicinal ingredients: sesame oil and α-tocopherol; in the shell: gelatin, glycerol (85%), potassium sorbate and titanium dioxide. Tropical blisters of 100. Protect from direct sunlight. Store at 15 to 25°C.

1 µg: Each brown egg-shaped soft gelatin capsule contains: alfacalcidol 1 µg. Nonmedicinal ingredients: sesame oil and α-tocopherol; in the shell: gelatin, glycerol (85%), potassium sorbate, red iron oxide E172 and black iron oxide E172. Tropical blisters of 100. Protect from direct sunlight. Store at 15 to 25°C.

Drops: Each mL of clear or slightly opalescent colorless solution contains: alfacalcidol 2 µg. Nonmedicinal ingredients: citric acid monohydrate, ethanol, methyl parahydroxybenzoate, polyoxyl 40 hydrogenated castor oil, purified water, sodium citrate, sorbitol and α-tocopherol. Amber glass bottles of 10 mL fitted with a polyethylene dropping device. Protect from direct sunlight. Keep refrigerated (2 to 8°C). Drop size: 1 drop equals 0.1 µg alfacalcidol.

Injection: Each mL of i.v. injection contains: alfacalcidol 2 µg. Nonmedicinal ingredients: citric acid monohydrate, ethanol, propylene glycol, sodium citrate and water. Amber glass ampoules containing unit doses of 1 µg/0.5 mL or 2 µg/1 mL, cartons of 10. Single use ampoules—discard unused portion. Shake well before use. Keep ampoules in outer carton to protect from light. Keep refrigerated (2 to 8°C).

Onglyza™ Ⓟ

saxagliptin HCl

Oral Antihyperglycemic Agent—DPP-4 Inhibitor—Incretin Enhancer

Bristol-Myers Squibb/AstraZeneca

Date of Preparation: September 14, 2009

SUMMARY PRODUCT INFORMATION:

Route of Administration	Dosage Form/ Strength	Clinically Relevant Nonmedicinal Ingredients
Oral	Tablet 5 mg	For a complete listing see Dosage Forms, Composition and Packaging.

INDICATIONS AND CLINICAL USE: ONGLYZA (saxagliptin) is indicated in patients with type 2 diabetes mellitus to improve glycemic control in combination with metformin or a sulfonylurea, when metformin or the sulfonylurea used alone, with diet and exercise, does not provide adequate glycemic control.

Geriatrics (≥65 years of age): No dosage adjustment is required based on age, however greater sensitivity of some older individuals cannot be ruled out (see Warnings and Precautions, Dosage and Administration and Action and Clinical Pharmacology).

Pediatrics (<18 years of age): Safety and effectiveness of ONGLYZA in pediatric patients have not been established. Therefore, ONGLYZA should not be used in this patient population.

CONTRAINDICATIONS: Patients who have had a history of any serious hypersensitivity to this drug or to any ingredient in the formulation or to another DPP-4 inhibitor. For a complete listing, see Dosage Forms, Composition and Packaging.

WARNINGS AND PRECAUTIONS: General: ONGLYZA (saxagliptin) should not be used in patients with type 1 diabetes or for the treatment of diabetic ketoacidosis.

Endocrine and Metabolism: A lower dose of sulfonylurea may be required to reduce the risk of hypoglycemia when used in combination with ONGLYZA (see Adverse Reactions, Clinical Trial Adverse Drug Reactions and Dosage and Administration).

Special Populations: Pregnant Women: There are no adequate and well-controlled studies in pregnant women. As animal reproduction studies are not always predictive of human response, ONGLYZA is not recommended for use in pregnancy.

Nursing Women: Saxagliptin is secreted in the milk of lactating rats. It is not known whether saxagliptin is excreted in human milk. Therefore, ONGLYZA should not be used by a woman who is nursing.

Pediatrics (<18 years of age): Safety and effectiveness of ONGLYZA in pediatric patients have not been established. Therefore, ONGLYZA should not be used in this patient population.

Geriatrics (≥65 years of age): Of the total number of subjects (N=4148) studied in controlled clinical safety and efficacy studies of ONGLYZA, 634 (15.3%) patients were 65 years and over, of which 59 (1.4%) patients were 75 years and over. No overall differences in safety or effectiveness were observed between subjects 65 years and over and younger subjects. While this clinical experience has not identified differences in responses between the elderly and younger patients, greater sensitivity of some older individuals cannot be ruled out.

Saxagliptin and its major metabolite are known to be eliminated in part by the kidney. Renal function should be assessed prior to initiating ONGLYZA and periodically thereafter in geriatric patients because they are more likely to have decreased renal function. Care should be taken in prescribing ONGLYZA in this population based on renal function (see Warnings and Precautions, Dosage and Administration and Action and Clinical Pharmacology).

Cardiovascular—Patients with Congestive Heart Failure: A limited number of patients with history of congestive heart failure participated in clinical studies with ONGLYZA. In clinical trials, ONGLYZA patients with NYHA Class III or IV congestive heart failure were excluded. Patients with history of congestive heart failure were included in small number (in total: 2% of patients exposed to ONGLYZA in clinical trials). Use in this population is not recommended.

Hepatic Insufficiency: There are limited clinical data in patients with hepatic impairment taking multiple doses of ONGLYZA. The use of ONGLYZA in patients with moderate to severe hepatic impairment is not recommended (see Action and Clinical Pharmacology).

Renal Impairment: No dosage adjustment is recommended for patients with mild renal impairment.

Clinical experience with ONGLYZA in patients with moderate or severe renal insufficiency including those with end-stage renal disease (ESRD) requiring hemodialysis is limited. Use in these patients is not recommended. Assessment of renal function is recommended prior to initiation of ONGLYZA, and periodically thereafter (see Dosage and Administration and Action and Clinical Pharmacology).

Monitoring and Laboratory Tests: Response should be monitored by periodic measurements of blood glucose and HbA1c levels. Assessment of renal function is recommended prior to initiation of ONGLYZA and periodically thereafter.

ADVERSE REACTIONS: Adverse Drug Reaction Overview: ONGLYZA (saxagliptin) was generally well tolerated in controlled clinical studies as an add-on to metformin and as an add-on to sulfonylurea with the overall incidence of adverse events similar to that reported with placebo.

In a placebo-controlled clinical study of patients receiving ONGLYZA 5 mg or placebo as an add-on to metformin, the incidence of serious adverse events was 9.9% and 5.6% respectively. The most commonly reported adverse events, reported regardless of causality and more common with ONGLYZA than placebo, were nasopharyngitis and bronchitis. Discontinuation of therapy due to adverse events occurred in 7.3% and 4.5% of patients, respectively.

In a placebo-controlled clinical study of patients receiving ONGLYZA 5 mg or placebo as an add-on to sulfonylurea (glyburide), the incidence of serious adverse events was 3.6% and 5.6% respectively. The most commonly reported adverse events, reported regardless of causality and more common with ONGLYZA than placebo, were hypoglycaemia and urinary tract infection. Discontinuation of therapy due to adverse events occurred in 4.7% and 3.4% of patients, respectively.

Clinical Trial Adverse Drug Reactions: Because clinical trials are conducted under very specific conditions the adverse reaction rates observed in the clinical trials may not reflect the rates observed in practice and should not be compared to the rates in the clinical trials of another drug. Adverse drug reaction information from clinical trials is useful for identifying drug-related adverse events and for approximating rates.

The incidence of adverse reactions, reported regardless of causality assessment, in ≥2% of patients treated with either ONGLYZA 5 mg or placebo as an add-on to metformin or add-on to sulfonylurea (glyburide) are shown in Table 1.

Table 1: ONGLYZA

Adverse Reactions (Regardless of Investigator Assessment of Causality) in the Add-on to Metformin[a] Study and in Add-on to Sulfonylurea[b] Study (24-week Short Term Study and the Long Term Extension) Reported in ≥2% of Patients Treated with Either ONGLYZA 5 mg or Placebo in at Least One Study

	Number of Patients (%) Add-on to Metformin		Number of Patients (%) Add-on to Sulfonylurea	
Body System/Organ Class Adverse Event	Saxagliptin 5 mg N=191	Placebo N=179	Saxagliptin 5 mg N=253	Placebo N=267
Blood and Lymphatic System Disorders				
Anemia	11 (5.8)	3 (1.7)	2 (0.8)	3 (1.1)
Eosinophilia	6 (3.1)	0	1 (0.4)	1 (0.4)
Cardiac Disorders				
Coronary artery disease	4 (2.1)	0	1 (0.4)	1 (0.4)
Gastrointestinal Disorders				
Diarrhea	14 (7.3)	23 (12.8)	13 (5.1)	23 (8.6)
Dyspepsia	11 (5.8)	8 (4.5)	9 (3.6)	7 (2.6)
Toothache	8 (4.2)	11 (6.1)	8 (3.2)	8 (3.0)
Abdominal pain	7 (3.7)	2 (1.1)	6 (2.4)	4 (1.5)

(cont'd)

Table 1: ONGLYZA *(cont'd)*

Adverse Reactions (Regardless of Investigator Assessment of Causality) in the Add-on to Metformin[a] Study and in Add-on to Sulfonylurea[b] Study (24-week Short Term Study and the Long Term Extension) Reported in ≥2% of Patients Treated with Either ONGLYZA 5 mg or Placebo in at Least One Study

Body System/Organ Class Adverse Event	Number of Patients (%) Add-on to Metformin		Number of Patients (%) Add-on to Sulfonylurea	
	Saxagliptin 5 mg N=191	Placebo N=179	Saxagliptin 5 mg N=253	Placebo N=267
Abdominal pain upper	7 (3.7)	5 (2.8)	10 (4.0)	8 (3.0)
Nausea	7 (3.7)	8 (4.5)	4 (1.6)	4 (1.5)
Vomiting	7 (3.7)	7 (3.9)	4 (1.6)	4 (1.5)
Constipation	5 (2.6)	3 (1.7)	2 (0.8)	3 (1.1)
Gastroesophageal reflux disease	4 (2.1)	1 (0.6)	2 (0.8)	6 (2.2)
Gastritis	2 (1.0)	2 (1.1)	5 (2.0)	8 (3.0)
General Disorders and Administration Site Conditions				
Edema peripheral	11 (5.8)	9 (5.0)	5 (2.0)	7 (2.6)
Chest pain	5 (2.6)	2 (1.1)	4 (1.6)	3 (1.1)
Fatigue	5 (2.6)	7 (3.9)	8 (3.2)	3 (1.1)
Asthenia	0	2 (1.1)	5 (2.0)	8 (3.0)
Infections and Infestations				
Influenza	22 (11.5)	23 (12.8)	16 (6.3)	26 (9.7)
Nasopharyngitis	21 (11.0)	19 (10.6)	24 (9.5)	27 (10.1)
Bronchitis	18 (9.4)	11 (6.1)	8 (3.2)	7 (2.6)
Upper respiratory tract infection	17 (8.9)	14 (7.8)	22 (8.7)	22 (8.2)
Urinary tract infection	15 (7.9)	12 (6.7)	35 (13.8)	29 (10.9)
Sinusitis	10 (5.2)	9 (5.0)	4 (1.6)	3 (1.1)
Gastroenteritis	5 (2.6)	3 (1.7)	7 (2.8)	7 (2.6)
Tooth infection	5 (2.6)	3 (1.7)	2 (0.8)	2 (0.7)
Gastroenteritis viral	4 (2.1)	2 (1.1)	1 (0.4)	1 (0.4)
Pharyngitis	2 (1.0)	4 (2.2)	19 (7.5)	14 (5.2)
Viral infection	1 (0.5)	4 (2.2)	4 (1.6)	6 (2.2)
Pharyngotonsillitis	1 (0.5)	1 (0.6)	5 (2.0)	10 (3.7)
Injury, Poisoning, and Procedural Complications				
Limb injury	3 (1.6)	1 (0.6)	0	7 (2.6)
Investigations				
Blood creatine phosphokinase increased	4 (2.1)	2 (1.1)	8 (3.2)	4 (1.5)
Alanine aminotransferase increased	1 (0.5)	4 (2.2)	4 (1.6)	3 (1.1)
Metabolism and Nutrition Disorders				
Hypoglycemia	17 (8.9)	18 (10.1)	50 (19.8)	49 (18.4)
Hypertriglyceridemia	6 (3.1)	2 (1.1)	9 (3.6)	5 (1.9)
Dyslipidemia	3 (1.6)	4 (2.2)	11 (4.3)	10 (3.7)
Musculoskeletal and Connective Tissue Disorders				
Arthralgia	16 (8.4)	9 (5.0)	17 (6.7)	20 (7.5)
Back pain	15 (7.9)	16 (8.9)	16 (6.3)	17 (6.4)
Osteoarthritis	8 (4.2)	4 (2.2)	2 (0.8)	7 (2.6)
Myalgia	6 (3.1)	4 (2.2)	6 (2.4)	5 (1.9)
Pain in extremity	6 (3.1)	13 (7.3)	12 (4.7)	18 (6.7)
Exostosis	4 (2.1)	2 (1.1)	1 (0.4)	1 (0.4)
Musculoskeletal pain	4 (2.1)	9 (5.0)	4 (1.6)	9 (3.4)
Muscle spasms	3 (1.6)	4 (2.2)	3 (1.2)	4 (1.5)
Nervous System Disorders				

(cont'd)

Table 1: ONGLYZA *(cont'd)*

Adverse Reactions (Regardless of Investigator Assessment of Causality) in the Add-on to Metformin[a] Study and in Add-on to Sulfonylurea[b] Study (24-week Short Term Study and the Long Term Extension) Reported in ≥2% of Patients Treated with Either ONGLYZA 5 mg or Placebo in at Least One Study

Body System/Organ Class Adverse Event	Number of Patients (%) Add-on to Metformin		Number of Patients (%) Add-on to Sulfonylurea	
	Saxagliptin 5 mg N=191	Placebo N=179	Saxagliptin 5 mg N=253	Placebo N=267
Headache	17 (8.9)	20 (11.2)	25 (9.9)	19 (7.1)
Dizziness	8 (4.2)	9 (5.0)	3 (1.2)	11 (4.1)
Parasthesia	0	2 (1.1)	1 (0.4)	6 (2.2)
Psychiatric Disorders				
Anxiety	8 (4.2)	5 (2.8)	5 (2.0)	4 (1.5)
Depression	6 (3.1)	4 (2.2)	6 (2.4)	2 (0.7)
Renal and Urinary Disorders				
Microalbuminuria	5 (2.6)	4 (2.2)	3 (1.2)	2 (0.7)
Nephrolithiasis	4 (2.1)	3 (1.7)	0	4 (1.5)
Dysuria	0	4 (2.2)	5 (2.0)	7 (2.6)
Respiratory, Thoracic, and Mediastinal Disorders				
Cough	7 (3.7)	9 (5.0)	14 (5.5)	16 (6.0)
Pharyngolaryngeal pain	5 (2.6)	3 (1.7)	3 (1.2)	4 (1.5)
Skin and Subcutaneous Tissue Disorders				
Rash	6 (3.1)	5 (2.8)	1 (0.4)	2 (0.7)
Alopecia	4 (2.1)	0	0	1 (0.4)
Pruritus	3 (1.6)	1 (0.6)	2 (0.8)	6 (2.2)
Vascular Disorders				
Hypertension	9 (4.7)	12 (6.7)	21 (8.3)	13 (4.9)

[a] The mean duration of exposure to double-blind study medication, including exposure after the initiation of rescue medication, was 75 weeks (Standard Deviation=34) for ONGLYZA 5 mg plus metformin and 68 weeks (Standard Deviation=35) for placebo plus metformin groups.

[b] The mean duration of exposure to double-blind study medication, including exposure after the initiation of rescue medication, was 50 weeks (Standard Deviation=17) for ONGLYZA 5 mg plus glyburide and 48 weeks (Standard Deviation=17) for placebo plus uptitrated glyburide groups.

Rash-related adverse events in the add-on to metformin study (24-week short-term and long-term extension) were reported in 4.2% and 2.8% of patients who received ONGLYZA 5 mg and placebo, respectively. In the add-on to sulfonylurea study (24-week short-term and long-term extension) rash-related events were reported in 1.6 % and 1.1% of patients who received ONGLYZA 5 mg and placebo, respectively.

In a pooled analysis of the 24-week placebo-controlled clinical trials, hypersensitivity-related events, such as urticaria and facial edema were reported in 1.5% and 0.4% of patients who received ONGLYZA 5 mg and placebo, respectively. None of these events in patients who received ONGLYZA required hospitalization or were reported as life-threatening by the investigators. One ONGLYZA-treated patient in this pooled analysis discontinued due to generalized urticaria and facial edema.

In the short-term 24-week add-on to sulfonylurea study (glyburide 7.5 mg), the overall incidence of hypoglycemia was higher for ONGLYZA 5 mg versus placebo (14.6% versus 10.1%). The incidence of confirmed hypoglycemic events, defined as symptoms of hypoglycemia accompanied by a fingerstick glucose value of ≤2.8 mmol/L, was similar for ONGLYZA 5 mg treated group (0.8%) and placebo group (0.7%). In the long-term extension of the add-on to sulfonylurea study, the overall incidence of hypoglycemia was similar for ONGLYZA 5 mg (19.8%) versus uptitrated sulfonylurea plus placebo (19.8% versus 18.4%).

The adverse event of hypertension was reported in more patients on ONGLYZA 5 mg plus glyburide (8.3%) versus placebo plus glyburide (4.9%) in the add-on to sulfonylurea trial. Analysis of the mean systolic and diastolic blood pressure values did not reveal clinically meaningful changes.

Serious Adverse Reactions (reported in <2% of patients) and Adverse Reactions of Interest* (reported in <2% of patients and in at least 2 patients), Regardless of Investigator Assessment of Causality and Frequency > Placebo, in the Add-on to Metformin and Add-on to Sulfonylurea Studies (24-week short-term and the long-term extensions).

Blood and Lymphatic System Disorders*: eosinophilia, lymphopenia, iron deficiency anemia, normochromic normocytic anemia.

Cardiac Disorders*: coronary artery disease, left ventricular hypertrophy, atrioventricular block first degree, bundle branch block left, mitral valve incompetence, myocardial ischemia, palpitations, ventricular extrasystoles, acute myocardial infarction, atrioventricular block complete, cardiac failure congestive, cardiogenic shock.

Gastrointestinal Disorders: abdominal pain, diarrhea, salivary gland mass, vomiting.

Hepatobiliary Disorders: cholecystitis acute, cholecystitis.

Immune System Disorders*: hypersensitivity, sarcoidosis.

Infections and Infestations: cellulitis orbital, *C. difficile* colitis, urosepsis, diverticulitis.

Injury, Poisoning and Procedural Complications: road traffic accident, ankle fracture, fall, gastrointestinal injury, incisional hernia, limb injury, skin laceration.

Investigations*: aspartate aminotransferase increased, c-reactive protein increased, electrocardiogram repolarisation abnormality, blood cholesterol increased, blood pressure increased, electrocardiogram abnormal, lymphocyte count decreased.

Metabolism and Nutrition Disorders: dehydration.

Musculoskeletal and Connective Tissue Disorders: arthralgia, osteoarthritis.

Neoplasms Benign, Malignant and Unspecified (incl cysts and polyps): myelodysplastic syndrome.

Nervous System Disorders: altered state of consciousness, dizziness.

Renal and Urinary Disorders: calculus ureteric, calculus urinary.

Respiratory, Thoracic and Mediastinal Disorders: hemoptysis, pulmonary embolism.

Skin and Subcutaneous Tissue Disorders*: rash, alopecia, dermatitis atopic, hyperhidrosis, rash papular, skin lesion, dermatitis contact, dermatitis, dry skin, seborrhoeic dermatitis, urticaria.

Surgical and Medical Procedures: sterilisation.

* System Organ Classes were considered to be of interest based on the adverse event profile of the DPP-4 inhibitor class of drugs, non-clinical data for saxagliptin, as well as the patient population.

Abnormal Hematologic and Clinical Chemistry Findings: Absolute Lymphocyte Counts: A dose-related mean decrease in absolute lymphocyte count was observed with ONGLYZA. From a baseline absolute lymphocyte count of approximately 2200 cells/µL, a mean decrease of approximately 100 cells/µL relative to placebo was observed in a pooled analysis of the placebo-controlled clinical studies. The proportion of patients who were reported to have a lymphocyte count ≤750 cells/µL was 1.5% in the ONGLYZA 5 mg group and 0.4% in the placebo group. The decreases in lymphocyte count were not associated with clinically relevant adverse reactions. When clinically indicated, such as in settings of unusual or prolonged infection, lymphocyte count should be measured. The effect of ONGLYZA on lymphocyte counts in patients with lymphocyte abnormalities (e.g. human immunodeficiency virus) is unknown.

Platelets: ONGLYZA did not demonstrate a clinically meaningful or consistent effect on platelet count in the double-blind, controlled clinical safety and efficacy trials. An event of thrombocytopenia, consistent with a diagnosis of idiopathic thrombocytopenic purpura, was observed in the clinical program. The relationship of this event to ONGLYZA is not known.

DRUG INTERACTIONS: The metabolism of saxagliptin is primarily mediated by P450 3A4/5 (CYP3A4/5).

In in vitro studies, saxagliptin and its major pharmacologically active metabolite neither inhibited nor induced CYP3A4. In addition, in in vitro studies, saxagliptin and its major pharmacologically active metabolite neither inhibited CYP1A2, 2A6, 2B6, 2C9, 2C19, 2D6, 2E1, nor induced CYP1A2, 2B6, 2C9. Therefore, saxagliptin is unlikely to alter the metabolic clearance of coadministered drugs that are metabolized by these enzymes. Saxagliptin is neither a significant inhibitor of P-glycoprotein (P-gp) nor an inducer of P-gp, and is unlikely to cause interactions with drugs that utilize these pathways.

The in vitro protein binding of saxagliptin and its major metabolite in human serum is below measurable levels. Thus, protein binding would not have a meaningful influence on the pharmacokinetics of saxagliptin or other drugs.

Drug-Drug Interactions: Effect of Other Drugs on Saxagliptin: In studies conducted in healthy subjects as described below, the pharmacokinetics of saxagliptin and its major metabolite were not meaningfully altered by metformin, glyburide, pioglitazone, digoxin, simvastatin, diltiazem, ketoconazole, omeprazole, aluminum hydroxide + magnesium hydroxide + simethicone combination, or famotidine. These drugs are considered unlikely to cause a clinically meaningful interaction with ONGLYZA.

Metformin: Coadministration of a single dose of saxagliptin (100 mg) and metformin (1000 mg), an OCT-1 and OCT-2 substrate, decreased the C_{max} of saxagliptin by 21%; however, the AUC was unchanged. Therefore, metformin is considered unlikely to cause a clinically meaningful interaction with ONGLYZA. Meaningful interactions of ONGLYZA with other OCT-1 and OCT-2 substrates would not be expected.

Glyburide: Coadministration of a single dose of saxagliptin (10 mg) and glyburide (5 mg), a CYP2C9 substrate, did not affect the pharmacokinetics of saxagliptin. Therefore, glyburide is considered unlikely to cause a clinically meaningful interaction with ONGLYZA. Meaningful interactions of ONGLYZA with other CYP2C9 substrates would not be expected.

Pioglitazone: Coadministration of multiple once-daily doses of saxagliptin (10 mg) and pioglitazone (45 mg), a CYP2C8 (major) and CYP3A4 (minor) substrate, did not alter the pharmacokinetics of saxagliptin. Therefore, pioglitazone is considered unlikely to cause a clinically meaningful interaction with ONGLYZA. Meaningful interactions of ONGLYZA with other CYP2C8 substrates would not be expected.

Digoxin: Coadministration of multiple once-daily doses of saxagliptin (10 mg) and digoxin (0.25 mg), a P-gp substrate, did not alter the pharmacokinetics of saxagliptin. Therefore, digoxin is considered unlikely to cause a clinically meaningful interaction with ONGLYZA. Meaningful interactions of ONGLYZA with other P-gp substrates would not be expected.

Simvastatin: Coadministration of multiple once-daily doses of saxagliptin (10 mg) and simvastatin (40 mg), a CYP3A4/5 substrate, increased the C_{max} of saxagliptin by 21%; however, the AUC of saxagliptin was unchanged. Therefore, simvastatin is considered unlikely to cause a clinically meaningful interaction with ONGLYZA. Meaningful interactions of ONGLYZA would not be expected with other substrates of CYP3A4/5.

Diltiazem: Coadministration of a single dose of saxagliptin (10 mg) and diltiazem (360 mg long-acting formulation at steady state), a moderate inhibitor of CYP3A4/5, increased the C_{max} and AUC for saxagliptin by 63% and 109%, respectively. This coadministration was also associated with 44% and 34% decreases in C_{max} and AUC(INF) values, respectively of its major metabolite. Therefore, diltiazem is considered unlikely to cause a clinically meaningful interaction with ONGLYZA. Meaningful interactions of ONGLYZA with other moderate CYP3A4/5 inhibitors would not be expected.

Ketoconazole: Coadministration of a single dose of saxagliptin (100 mg) and ketoconazole (200 mg every 12 hours at steady state), a potent inhibitor of CYP3A4/5 and P-gp, increased the C_{max} and AUC for saxagliptin by 62% and 145 % respectively. This coadministration was also associated with 95% and 88% decreases in C_{max} and AUC(INF) values, respectively of its major metabolite.

Following coadministration of a single dose of saxagliptin at 20 times the recommended dose (100 mg) with ketoconazole, transient flu-like symptoms and a transient decrease in absolute lymphocyte count were observed. Additionally, transient decreases in absolute lymphocyte count were observed without any flu-like symptoms following coadministration of a single dose of saxagliptin at 4 times the recommended dose (20 mg) with ketoconazole.

CYP3A4/5 Inducers: The effects of CYP3A4/5 inducers on the pharmacokinetics of saxagliptin have not been studied. However, the coadministration of saxagliptin and CYP3A4/5 inducers such as carbamazepine, dexamethasone, phenobarbital, phenytoin, and rifampin may result in decreased plasma concentrations of saxagliptin and increased concentrations of its major metabolite.

Omeprazole: Coadministration of multiple once-daily doses of saxagliptin (10 mg) and omeprazole (40 mg), a CYP2C19 (major) and CYP3A4 substrate, an inhibitor of CYP2C19, and an inducer of MRP-3, did not alter the pharmacokinetics of saxagliptin. Therefore, omeprazole is considered unlikely to cause a clinically meaningful interaction with ONGLYZA. Meaningful interactions of ONGLYZA with other CYP2C19 inhibitors or MRP-3 inducers would not be expected.

Aluminum Hydroxide + Magnesium Hydroxide + Simethicone: Coadministration of a single dose of saxagliptin (10 mg) and a liquid containing aluminum hydroxide (2400 mg), magnesium hydroxide (2400 mg), and simethicone (240 mg) decreased the C_{max} of saxagliptin by 26%; however, the AUC of saxagliptin was unchanged. Therefore, meaningful interactions of ONGLYZA with antacid and antigas formulations of this type would not be expected.

Famotidine: Administration of a single dose of saxagliptin (10 mg) three hours after a single dose of famotidine (40 mg), an inhibitor of hOCT-1, hOCT-2, and hOCT-3, increased the C_{max} of saxagliptin by 14%; however, the AUC of saxagliptin was unchanged. Therefore, famotidine is considered unlikely to cause a clinically meaningful interaction with ONGLYZA. Meaningful interactions of ONGLYZA would not be expected with other inhibitors of hOCT-1, hOCT-2, and hOCT-3.

Effect of Saxagliptin on Other Drugs: In studies conducted in healthy subjects, as described below, saxagliptin did not meaningfully alter the pharmacokinetics of metformin, glyburide, pioglitazone, digoxin, simvastatin, diltiazem, or ketoconazole. ONGLYZA is considered unlikely to cause a clinically meaningful interaction with these drugs.

Metformin: Coadministration of a single dose of saxagliptin (100 mg) and metformin (1000 mg), an OCT-1 and OCT-2 substrate, did not alter the pharmacokinetics of metformin in healthy subjects. Therefore, ONGLYZA is considered unlikely to cause a clinically meaningful interaction with metformin. ONGLYZA is not an inhibitor of OCT-1 and OCT-2- mediated transport.

Glyburide: Coadministration of a single dose of saxagliptin (10 mg) and glyburide (5 mg), a CYP2C9 substrate, increased the plasma C_{max} of glyburide by 16%; however, the AUC of glyburide was unchanged. Therefore, ONGLYZA is considered unlikely to cause a clinically meaningful interaction with glyburide. ONGLYZA does not meaningfully inhibit CYP2C9-mediated metabolism.

Pioglitazone: Coadministration of multiple once-daily doses of saxagliptin (10 mg) and pioglitazone (45 mg), a CYP2C8 substrate, increased the plasma C_{max} of pioglitazone by 14%; however, the AUC of pioglitazone was unchanged. Therefore, ONGLYZA is considered unlikely to cause a clinically meaningful interaction with pioglitazone. ONGLYZA does not meaningfully inhibit or induce CYP2C8-mediated metabolism.

Digoxin: Coadministration of multiple once-daily doses of saxagliptin (10 mg) and digoxin (0.25 mg), a P-gp substrate, did not alter the pharmacokinetics of digoxin. Therefore, ONGLYZA is considered unlikely to cause a clinically meaningful interaction with digoxin. ONGLYZA is not an inhibitor or inducer of P-gp-mediated transport.

Simvastatin: Coadministration of multiple once-daily doses of saxagliptin (10 mg) and simvastatin (40 mg), a CP3A4/5 substrate, did not alter the pharmacokinetics of simvastatin. Therefore, ONGLYZA is considered unlikely to cause a clinically meaningful interaction with simvastatin. ONGLYZA is not an inhibitor or inducer of CYP3A4/5-mediated metabolism.

Diltiazem: Coadministration of multiple once-daily doses of saxagliptin (10 mg) and diltiazem (360 mg long-acting formulation at steady state), a moderate inhibitor of CYP3A4/5, increased the plasma C_{max} of diltiazem by 16%; however, the AUC of diltiazem was unchanged. Therefore, ONGLYZA is considered unlikely to cause a clinically meaningful interaction with diltiazem.

Ketoconazole: Coadministration of a single dose of saxagliptin (100 mg) and multiple doses of ketoconazole (200 mg every 12 hours at steady state), a potent inhibitor of CYP3A4/5 and P-gp, decreased the geometric means for C_{max} and AUC(INF) of ketoconazole by 16 % and by 13% respectively, relative to those observed following administration of 200 mg ketoconazole q 12 h alone.

Drug-Food Interactions: There are no known interactions with food. Grapefruit juice being a weak inhibitor of CYP3A4 gut wall metabolism may give rise to modest increases in plasma levels of saxagliptin.

Drug-Herb Interactions: Interactions with herbal products have not been established.

Drug-Laboratory Test Interactions: Interactions with laboratory tests have not been established.

Drug-Lifestyle Interactions: No studies of the effects of ONGLYZA on the ability to drive and use machines have been performed. However, ONGLYZA is not expected to affect the ability to drive and use machines.

DOSAGE AND ADMINISTRATION:

Dosing Considerations: ONGLYZA (saxagliptin) may be taken with or without food.

Recommended Dose and Dosage Adjustment: The recommended dose of ONGLYZA is 5 mg once daily.

Renal Impairment: Use of ONGLYZA in patients with moderate to severe renal impairment, including patients with end stage renal disease requiring hemodialysis is not recommended.

Hepatic Impairment: Use of ONGLYZA in patients with moderate to severe hepatic impairment is not recommended due to lack of clinical experience with this patient population.

Pediatrics (<18 years of age): Safety and effectiveness of ONGLYZA in pediatric patients have not been established. Therefore, ONGLYZA should not be used in this patient population.

Geriatrics (≥65 years of age): No dosage adjustment for ONGLYZA is required based solely on age (see Warnings and Precautions and Action and Clinical Pharmacology).

Missed Dose: If a dose of ONGLYZA is missed, it should be taken as soon as the patient remembers. A double dose of ONGLYZA should not be taken on the same day.

OVERDOSAGE:

In the event of an overdose, appropriate supportive treatment should be initiated as dictated by the patient's clinical status. Saxagliptin and its major metabolite are removed by hemodialysis (23% of dose over 4 hours).

For management of a suspected drug overdose, contact your **regional Poison Control Centre**. See the *CPS* Directory section for a list of Poison Control Centres.

ACTION AND CLINICAL PHARMACOLOGY: Mechanism of Action: Saxagliptin is a potent, selective, reversible, competitive, DPP-4 inhibitor. Saxagliptin demonstrates selectivity for DPP-4 versus other DPP enzymes, including DPP-8 and DPP-9. Saxagliptin has extended binding to the DPP-4 active site, prolonging its inhibition of DPP-4. Saxagliptin exerts its actions in patients with type 2 diabetes by slowing the inactivation of incretin hormones, including glucagon-like peptide-1 (GLP-1). The concentration of active (intact) GLP-1 incretin hormone is increased.

Incretin hormones are released by the intestine throughout the day and concentrations are increased in response to a meal. These hormones are rapidly inactivated by the enzyme DPP-4. The incretins are part of an endogenous system involved in the physiologic regulation of glucose homeostasis. When blood glucose concentrations are elevated, GLP-1 and GIP increase insulin synthesis and release from pancreatic beta cells. GLP-1 also lowers glucagon secretion from pancreatic alpha cells, leading to reduced hepatic glucose production.

The concentration of GLP-1 is reduced in patients with type 2 diabetes, but saxagliptin increases active GLP-1 concentration. By increasing active GLP-1 concentration, saxagliptin increases postprandial insulin release and decreases postprandial glucagon concentrations in the circulation in a glucose-dependent manner. In patients with type 2 diabetes with hyperglycemia, these changes in insulin and glucagon levels may lead to lower hemoglobin A1c (HbA1c) and lower fasting and postprandial glucose concentrations.

Pharmacodynamics: In patients with type 2 diabetes, administration of ONGLYZA led to dose-dependent inhibition of DPP-4 enzyme activity for a 24-hour period. After an oral glucose load or a meal, this DPP-4 inhibition resulted in a 2- to 3-fold increase in circulating levels of active GLP-1, decreased postprandial glucagon concentrations, and increased glucose-dependent beta cell responsiveness with higher postprandial insulin and C-peptide concentrations. The rise in insulin and decrease in glucagon were associated with lower fasting glucose concentrations and reduced glucose excursion following an oral glucose load or a meal.

Cardiac Electrophysiology: In a randomized, double-blind, placebo-controlled, 4-way crossover, active comparator study, 40 healthy subjects were administered saxagliptin 40 mg (8 times the RHD), saxagliptin 10 mg (2 times the RHD), or placebo once daily for 4 days, or a single dose of moxifloxacin 400 mg as a positive control. The saxagliptin 10 mg and 40 mg treatments were not associated with any prolongation of the QTc, QRS, or PR intervals. In the saxagliptin 10 mg treatment a significant increase in heart rate was observed at 0.5, 1, 1.5, 4, and 12 h post-dosing, with a maximum placebo- and baseline-corrected mean increase of 3.75 (90% 1.55, 5.95) beats per minute at 0.5 post-dosing when the baseline-corrected change in the placebo treatment at this time was -1.4 (90% CI -3.0, 0.1) beats per minute. Significant increases in heart rate were also observed in the saxagliptin 40 mg treatment at 0.5, 4, and 12 hours post-dosing, with a maximum placebo- and baseline-corrected mean increase of 4.5 (90% CI 2.23, 6.82) beats per minute at 4 hours post-dose dose when the baseline-corrected change in the placebo treatment at this time was -3.3 (90% CI -5.0, -1.6) beats per minute. The effect of the recommended 5 mg dose was not investigated in this study.

Pharmacokinetics: The pharmacokinetics of saxagliptin has been extensively characterized in healthy subjects and patients with type 2 diabetes (Table 2).

Table 2: ONGLYZA

Summary of Saxagliptin's Pharmacokinetic Parameters in Healthy Subjects

	C_{max} (ng/mL)	$t_{1/2}$ (h)	AUC ng·h/mL	Renal Clearance (mL/min)
Single oral dose (5 mg) mean	24	2.5	78	230

Saxagliptin was rapidly absorbed after oral administration, with maximum saxagliptin plasma concentrations (C_{max}) usually attained within two hours after administration in the fasted state. The C_{max} and AUC values increased proportionally to the increment in the saxagliptin dose. Following a 5 mg single oral dose of saxagliptin to healthy subjects, the mean plasma AUC(INF) values for saxagliptin and its major metabolite were 78 ng·h/mL and 214 ng·h/mL, respectively. The corresponding plasma C_{max} values were 24 ng/mL and 47 ng/mL, respectively. The intra-subject coefficients of variation for saxagliptin C_{max} and AUC were less than 12%.

Following a single oral dose of 5 mg saxagliptin to healthy subjects, the mean plasma terminal half-life ($t_{½}$) for saxagliptin was 2.5 hours, and the mean $t_{½}$ value for plasma DPP-4 inhibition was 26.9 hours. The inhibition of plasma DPP-4 activity by saxagliptin occurs for at least 24-hours after oral administration of ONGLYZA. No appreciable accumulation was observed with repeated once-daily dosing at any dose level. No dose- and time-dependence was observed in the clearance of saxagliptin and its major metabolite over 14 days of once-daily dosing with saxagliptin at doses ranging from 2.5 mg to 400 mg. Results from population-based exposure modeling suggest that the pharmacokinetics of saxagliptin and its major metabolite were similar in healthy subjects and in patients with type 2 diabetes.

Absorption: ONGLYZA may be administered with or without food. The amount of saxagliptin absorbed following an oral dose is at least 75%. Food had relatively modest effects on the pharmacokinetics of saxagliptin in healthy subjects. Administration with a high-fat meal resulted in no change in saxagliptin C_{max} and a 27% increase in AUC compared with the fasted state. The time for saxagliptin to reach C_{max} (T_{max}) was increased by approximately 0.5 hours with food compared with the fasted state. These changes were not considered to be clinically meaningful.

Distribution: The in vitro protein binding of saxagliptin and its major metabolite in human serum is below measurable levels. Thus, changes in blood protein levels in various disease states (e.g., renal or hepatic impairment) are not expected to alter the disposition of saxagliptin.

Metabolism: The metabolism of saxagliptin is primarily mediated by cytochrome P450 3A4/5 (CYP3A4/5). The major metabolite of saxagliptin is also a selective, reversible, competitive DPP-4 inhibitor, half as potent as saxagliptin.

Excretion: Saxagliptin is eliminated by both renal and hepatic pathways. Following a single 50 mg dose of ^{14}C-saxagliptin, 24%, 36%, and 75% of the dose was excreted in the urine as saxagliptin, its major metabolite, and total radioactivity, respectively. The average renal clearance of saxagliptin (~230 mL/min) was greater than the average estimated glomerular filtration rate (~120 mL/min), suggesting some active renal excretion. For the major metabolite, renal clearance values were comparable to estimated glomerular filtration rate. A total of 22% of the administered radioactivity was recovered in feces representing the fraction of the saxagliptin dose excreted in bile and/or unabsorbed drug from the gastrointestinal tract.

Pharmacokinetics of the Major Metabolite: The C_{max} and AUC values for the major metabolite of saxagliptin increased proportionally to the increment in the saxagliptin dose. Following single oral doses of 2.5 mg to 400 mg saxagliptin in the fed or fasted states, the mean AUC values for the major metabolite ranged from 2- and 7 times higher than the parent saxagliptin exposures on a molar basis. Following a single oral dose of 10 mg saxagliptin in the fasted state, the mean terminal half-life ($t_{½}$) value for the major metabolite was 3.1 hours and no appreciable accumulation was observed upon repeated once-daily dosing at any dose.

Special Populations and Conditions: Pediatrics (<18 years of age) : Pharmacokinetics in the pediatric population have not been studied. Therefore, ONGLYZA should not be used in this patient population.

Geriatrics (≥65 years of age): No dosage adjustment is necessary based on age alone. Elderly subjects (65-80 years) had 23% and 59% higher geometric mean C_{max} and geometric mean AUC values, respectively, for parent saxagliptin than young subjects (18-40 years). Differences in major metabolite pharmacokinetics between elderly and young subjects generally reflected the differences observed in parent saxagliptin pharmacokinetics. The difference between the pharmacokinetics of saxagliptin and the major metabolite in young and elderly subjects is likely to be due to multiple factors including declining renal function and metabolic capacity with increasing age.
Gender: No dosage adjustment is necessary based on gender. There were no differences observed in saxagliptin pharmacokinetics between males and females. Compared to males, females had approximately 25% higher exposure values for the major metabolite than males, but the clinical relevance of this difference is unknown.
Race: No dosage adjustment is necessary based on race. An exposure modeling analysis compared the pharmacokinetics of saxagliptin and its major metabolite in 309 white subjects with 105 non-white subjects (consisting of 6 race groups). No significant difference in the pharmacokinetics of saxagliptin and its major metabolite were detected between these two populations.
Body Mass Index: No dosage adjustment is recommended based on body mass index (BMI).
Renal Insufficiency: A single-dose, open-label study was conducted to evaluate the pharmacokinetics of saxagliptin (10 mg dose) in subjects (n=8 in each group) with varying degrees of chronic renal impairment compared to subjects with normal renal function. The study included patients with renal impairment classified on the basis of creatinine clearance as mild (>50 to ≤80 mL/min), moderate (30 to ≤50 mL/min), and severe (<30 mL/min), as well as patients with ESRD on hemodialysis. Creatinine clearance was estimated from serum creatinine based on the Cockcroft-Gault formula:

$$CrCl = \frac{[140\text{-age (years)}] \times \text{weight [kg]} \ \{\times 0.85 \text{ for female patients}\}}{[72 \times \text{serum creatinine (mg/dL)}]}$$

In subjects with mild renal impairment, the AUC values of saxagliptin and its major metabolite were 1.2- and 1.7-fold higher, respectively, than AUC values in subjects with normal renal function. Because increases of this magnitude are not clinically relevant, dosage adjustment in patients with mild renal impairment is not recommended.

In subjects with moderate or severe renal impairment or in subjects with ESRD on hemodialysis, the AUC values of saxagliptin and its major metabolite were up to 2.1- and 4.5-fold higher, respectively, than AUC values in subjects with normal renal function. Therefore use in this population is not recommended.
Hepatic Insufficiency: In subjects with hepatic impairment (Child-Pugh classes A, B, and C), mean C_{max} and AUC of saxagliptin were up to 8% and 77% higher, respectively, compared to healthy matched controls following administration of a single 10 mg dose of saxagliptin. The corresponding C_{max} and AUC of the major metabolite were up to 59% and 33% lower, respectively, compared to healthy matched controls. Use in moderate to severe hepatic impairment is not recommended.
STORAGE AND STABILITY: Temperature: Store at room temperature (15-30°C).
Others: Keep in a safe place out of reach of children.
INFORMATION FOR THE PATIENT: Published in e-CPS, available by subscription at www.e-cps.ca.
DOSAGE FORMS, COMPOSITION AND PACKAGING: Each pink, biconvex, round, film-coated tablet with "5" printed on one side and "4215" printed on the reverse side, in blue ink contains: saxagliptin 5 mg (as saxagliptin hydrochloride). Nonmedicinal ingredients: croscarmellose sodium, lactose monohydrate, magnesium stearate and microcrystalline cellulose; film coating: iron oxides, polyethylene glycol, polyvinyl alcohol, talc and titanium dioxide; printing ink: FD&C Blue #2 and shellac glaze. Blisters in cartons of 30 or 100. Information for the patient is provided as a package insert in the ONGLYZA packages.

(Shown in Product Identification Section)

Opioids

alfentanil HCl
buprenorphine HCl
butorphanol tartrate
codeine phosphate
fentanyl
fentanyl citrate
hydrocodone bitartrate
hydromorphone HCl
methadone HCl
morphine HCl
morphine sulfate
nalbuphine HCl
oxycodone HCl
pentazocine HCl
pentazocine lactate
pethidine HCl
propoxyphene HCl
propoxyphene napsylate
sufentanil citrate
tramadol HCl

Analgesic

CPhA Monograph

Date of Revision: May 2010

This monograph has been compiled by CPhA and reviewed by experts. It may contain information different from that found in Health Canada-approved Product Monographs. The reader is referred to the *CPS* Editorial Policy for more information.

SUMMARY PRODUCT INFORMATION:

Drug	Route of Administration	Dosage Form	Strength
AlfentanilⓃ	IV	Injectable solution	500 µg/mL
BuprenorphineⓃ[a]	SL	Tablet	0.4 mg, 2 mg, 8 mg
			2 mg in combination with naloxone 0.5 mg 8 mg in combination with naloxone 2 mg
ButorphanolⓃ	Nasal	Spray	10 mg/mL
CodeineⓃ[b]	Oral	Immediate-release tablet	15 mg, 30 mg
		Controlled-release tablet	50 mg, 100 mg, 150 mg, 200 mg
		Syrup	5 mg/mL
	IM, SC	Injectable solution	30 mg/mL, 60 mg/mL
FentanylⓃ	Transdermal	Patch	Delivers 12 µg, 25 µg, 50 µg, 75 µg or 100 µg per hour
	Epidural, IM, IV	Injectable solution	50 µg/mL
HydrocodoneⓃ[c]	Oral	Immediate-release tablet	5 mg
	Oral	Syrup	1 mg/mL
HydromorphoneⓃ	Oral	Immediate-release tablet	1 mg, 2 mg, 4 mg, 8 mg
		Controlled-release capsule	3 mg, 6 mg, 12 mg, 18 mg, 24 mg, 30 mg
		Syrup	1 mg/mL
	Rectal	Suppository	3 mg
	IM, IV, SC	Injectable solution	2 mg/mL, 10 mg/mL, 20 mg/mL, 50 mg/mL
	IM, IV, SC	Sterile powder for reconstitution	250 mg
MethadoneⓃ[d]	Oral	Tablet	1 mg, 5 mg, 10 mg, 25 mg
		Solution	1 mg/mL, 10 mg/mL
MorphineⓃ	Oral	Immediate-release tablet	10 mg, 20 mg, 25 mg, 30 mg, 40 mg, 50 mg, 60 mg
		Controlled-release capsule	10 mg, 15 mg, 20 mg, 30 mg, 50 mg, 60 mg, 100 mg, 200 mg
		Extended-release tablet	15 mg, 30 mg, 60 mg, 100 mg, 200 mg
		Drops	50 mg/mL
		Syrup	1 mg/mL, 5 mg/mL, 20 mg/mL
	Rectal	Suppository	5 mg, 10 mg, 20 mg, 30 mg
	IV, IM, SC	Injectable solution	1 mg/mL, 2 mg/mL, 5 mg/mL, 10 mg/mL, 15 mg/mL, 25 mg/mL, 50 mg/mL
	Epidural	Injectable solution	0.5 mg/mL, 1 mg/mL
Nalbuphine◈	IV, IM, SC	Injectable solution	10 mg/mL, 20 mg/mL
OxycodoneⓃ	Oral	Immediate-release tablet	5 mg, 10 mg, 20 mg 5 mg in combination with ASA or acetaminophen 325 mg 2.5 mg in combination with acetaminophen 325 mg
		Sustained-release tablet	5 mg, 10 mg, 20 mg, 40 mg, 80 mg
	Rectal	Suppository	10 mg, 20 mg
PentazocineⓃ[d]	Oral	Tablet	50 mg
	IV, IM, SC	Injectable solution	30 mg/mL
PethidineⓃ (meperidine)	Oral	Tablet	50 mg
	IV, IM, SC	Injectable solution	10 mg/mL, 15 mg/mL, 25 mg/mL, 50 mg/mL, 75 mg/mL, 100 mg/mL
PropoxypheneⓃ	Oral	Tablet	65 mg
		Capsule	100 mg
SufentanilⓃ	IV, Epidural	Injectable solution	50 µg/mL
TramadolPr	Oral	Immediate-release tablet	37.5 mg in combination with acetaminophen 325 mg
		Controlled-release tablet	100 mg, 150 mg, 200 mg, 300 mg, 400 mg

[a] Single entity buprenorphine is available only through the Special Access Programme, Health Canada; see also Indications.
[b] Codeine is also available in various combinations with nonopioid analgesics, caffeine, muscle relaxants, cough and cold preparations and/or barbiturates. For more information visit Health Canada's Drug Product Database at www.hc-sc.gc.ca/dhp-mps/prodpharma/databasdon/index-eng.php.
[c] Hydrocodone is also available in various combinations with antihistamines, decongestants, antitussives and/or expectorants. For more information visit Health Canada's Drug Product Database at www.hc-sc.gc.ca/dhp-mps/prodpharma/databasdon/index-eng.php.
[d] Methadone prescribing requires special authorization from Health Canada; see Indications.

PHARMACOLOGY: Opioid analgesics act primarily on the CNS and the intestines. The perception of and emotional response to pain are modified when opioid analgesics bind with stereospecific receptors in the CNS. The most studied subtypes of opioid receptors are mu (μ), delta (δ) and kappa (κ). Pure opioid agonists such as morphine act primarily at the mu receptor. Mixed agonist-antagonists such as butorphanol, nalbuphine and pentazocine are most active at the kappa receptor. Buprenorphine is a partial agonist at the mu receptor and an antagonist at the kappa receptor.

In addition to analgesia, opioid agonist activity in the CNS may cause suppression of the cough reflex, respiratory depression, changes in mood such as euphoria or dysphoria, and EEG changes. Nausea and vomiting, probably caused by stimulation of the chemoreceptor trigger zone, can also occur. Peripheral vasodilation, reduced peripheral resistance and the inhibition of baroreceptors can result in orthostatic hypotension and fainting.

Effects of opioids on the gastrointestinal tract include decreased gastric, biliary and pancreatic secretions, as well as increased rectal smooth muscle tone and inhibition of peristalsis, which can lead to constipation. Opioids can increase smooth muscle tone in the urinary tract, leading to dysuria or urinary retention.

Methadone: Methadone is a synthetic diphenylheptane-derivative opioid agonist with pharmacologic properties qualitatively similar to those of morphine. In equianalgesic doses, methadone may produce a similar or slightly higher degree of respiratory depression and less sedation, euphoria and constipation than morphine. Methadone prevents withdrawal symptoms and reduces opioid cravings in individuals who are opioid-dependent.

Pharmacokinetics: Specific opioid analgesics are absorbed after administration by many different routes including the oral, rectal, intramuscular, intravenous, epidural, intrathecal, subcutaneous, intranasal and transdermal routes. They are metabolized by the liver and eliminated primarily by the kidney. Dosage adjustment in the presence of renal or hepatic disease is usually indicated. A comparison of pharmacokinetic parameters can be found in Table 1.

INDICATIONS: Opioids are used in the symptomatic treatment of acute or chronic pain associated with surgery or medical conditions such as trauma, myocardial infarction or terminal cancer. They have also been used to manage dyspnea associated with respiratory secretions in patients with chronic lung disease or terminal cancer.

Other uses include codeine and hydrocodone as antitussives and alfentanil and sufentanil as adjunctive or primary anesthetic agents.

Buprenorphine: Prescribing of buprenorphine in the management of opioid dependence requires specialized physician education, in accordance with the approved product labelling. Detailed requirements for the prescribing, dispensing, supervision and monitoring of buprenorphine therapy are outlined in the product monograph. For buprenorphine in combination with naloxone, physicians or other health professionals should contact their respective licensing bodies for information on their province's practice requirements concerning buprenorphine. Single entity buprenorphine is available only through Health Canada's Special Access Programme (see Appendix 2).

Table 1: Opioids

Pharmacokinetics

Drug	Route	Onset of Action (minutes)	Duration of Action (hours)	Cytochrome P450 Metabolism (where applicable)
Agonists				
Alfentanil	IV	Immediate	0.5 to 1	CYP3A4
Codeine[a]	PO, SC	15 to 30	4 to 6	CYP2D6, CYP3A4
	IM	10 to 30	4 to 6	
Fentanyl	IM	7 to 15	1 to 2	CYP3A4
	IV	Almost immediate	0.5 to 1	
	Transdermal	Continuously released to maintain consistent serum concentration		
Hydrocodone	PO	10 to 20[b]	4 to 6[c]	CYP2D6
Hydromorphone	PO	30	>5	
	Parenteral	15	>5	
Methadone	PO	30 to 60	24 to 48[d]	CYP1A2, CYP2D6, CYP3A4
Morphine	PO (immediate-release dosage forms)	60	4 to 5	CYP2D6
	SC	50 to 90	4 to 5	
	IM	30 to 60	4 to 5	
	IV	20	4 to 5	
	Epidural	15 to 60	≤24	
Oxycodone	PO	10 to 15	3 to 6	CYP2D6
Pethidine (meperidine)	PO	15	2 to 4	CYP2D6
	IM, SC	10 to 15	2 to 4	
	IV	1	2 to 4	
Propoxyphene	PO	15 to 60	4 to 6	CYP2D6
Sufentanil	IV	1.3 to 4	NA[e]	CYP3A4
	Epidural	10	1 to 2	
Tramadol	PO	1	3 to 6	CYP2D6 (converts tramadol to its only active metabolite)[f]
Agonist-Antagonists				
Buprenorphine	SL	30–60	24[g]	CYP3A4
Butorphanol	Intranasal	30	3 to 4	—
Nalbuphine	SC, IM	15	3 to 6	—
	IV	2 to 3	3 to 6	
Pentazocine	PO	15 to 30	≥3	CYP2D6
	IM, SC	15 to 20	2	
	IV	2 to 3	1	

(cont'd)

Table 1: Opioids *(cont'd)*

[a] Codeine is converted to morphine by CYP2D6. Patients with two or more copies of the variant CYP2D6*2 allele may produce higher amounts of morphine and experience increased opioid effects. See Warnings and Precautions. Conversely, approximately 5-10% of Caucasians do not convert codeine to morphine sufficiently to benefit from the analgesic effect of the drug.
[b] For analgesic effect. No data available for onset of antitussive action.
[c] For antitussive effect.
[d] With repeated dosing.
[e] No data available.
[f] Tramadol and its active metabolite are metabolized in the liver through demethylation and glucuronidation or sulfation.
[g] When used daily for maintenance therapy in opioid dependence.

Methadone: In Canada, methadone is used in the detoxification or maintenance treatment of opioid-dependent individuals and as an analgesic in acute cancer pain, palliative care and chronic pain disorders. Physicians who wish to prescribe or administer methadone must obtain an exemption from the Minister of Health (or designate) at the Office of Controlled Substances, 613-946-5139 or 1-866-358-0453. In British Columbia, Manitoba, Ontario and Québec, the Methadone Program is administered by the respective College of Physicians and Surgeons; after reviewing physicians' requests, the respective College would recommend to the Minister that they be granted an exemption under section 56 of the *Controlled Drugs and Substances Act*, with respect to methadone.

Guidelines have been developed or endorsed by health professional licensing authorities in some provinces, to assist their members in the prescribing or dispensing of methadone. Practitioners should contact their respective licensing authority for more information.

CONTRAINDICATIONS: Hypersensitivity to opioid analgesics. Diarrhea caused by poisoning, until the toxic substance has been eliminated from the gastrointestinal tract. Acute respiratory depression, acute asthma attack, and upper airway obstruction.

Epidural or Intrathecal Use: Infection at or near site of administration, clotting defects due to anticoagulant therapy or hematologic disorders.

See individual product monographs for comprehensive information, with attention to the following: Morphine or pethidine should not be used concurrently or within 2 weeks of MAO inhibitor therapy; fentanyl transdermal patches are contraindicated for opioid-naïve patients and are not recommended for children.

WARNINGS: Opioid analgesics have the potential for abuse. Psychological dependence or physical dependence and tolerance may follow repeated administration. Opioid analgesics should be prescribed and administered with caution, especially in cases of severe hepatic insufficiency, severe CNS depression or coma, in patients with head injuries or conditions in which intracranial pressure is increased, myxedema, Addison's disease, acute alcohol intoxication, delirium tremens, convulsive disorders and in patients taking MAO inhibitors. Opioid analgesics can cause severe hypotension in individuals whose circulation is already compromised by hypovolemia, shock, drugs producing hypotension or other conditions that interfere with ability to maintain normal blood pressure. These drugs may produce orthostatic hypotension in the ambulatory patient.

Rapid iv injection of opioid analgesics increases incidence of adverse reactions such as severe respiratory depression, apnea, hypotension, peripheral circulatory collapse and cardiac arrest. The patient should be lying down during iv administration. These drugs should not be administered iv unless an opioid antagonist and the facilities for assisted or controlled respiration are immediately available.

Opioid analgesics should be used with extreme caution in patients with chronic obstructive pulmonary disease or cor pulmonale, patients having a substantially decreased respiratory reserve and patients with preexisting respiratory depression, hypoxia or hypercapnia. Refer to individual product monographs for specific warnings with attention to the following:

Buprenorphine: IV misuse of buprenorphine has been associated with local reactions (some involving infection) and acute hepatitis. Refer to the product monograph for detailed prescribing information.

Codeine: Some individuals may be ultra-rapid metabolizers of codeine due to a specific CYP2D6 genotype that leads to increased production of morphine for a given dose of codeine. Such individuals may experience toxicity manifested as extreme sedation, confusion and/or shallow breathing. See also Precautions, Lactation.

Fentanyl Transdermal Patches: Fentanyl transdermal patches are generally contraindicated for opioid-naive patients and are not recommended for children; fever or external heat sources can significantly increase absorption; a considerable amount of drug remains in patches after 3 days of use; both used and unused patches should be properly disposed of to prevent diversion or accidental poisoning (i.e., they should *not* be placed in garbage receptacles). The product monograph recommends that used patches be folded (adhesive side in) and flushed in the toilet immediately after removal from the site of application.

Long-acting Oral Formulations: Alcohol (including prescription or nonprescription drug formulations that contain alcohol) may interact with slow-release opioid formulations, potentially resulting in toxicity due to rapid release of the opioid from its slow-release formulation ("dose-dumping").

Methadone: Overdose and death can occur when methadone is ingested by individuals for whom it has not been prescribed, or who are not opioid-dependent.

Nalbuphine: Commercial preparation contains sodium metabisulfite which may cause allergic reactions (e.g., hives, itching, wheezing, anaphylaxis) in susceptible individuals. Prevalence of sensitivity in the general population is probably low; it is seen more frequently in asthmatics or atopic non-asthmatic patients.

Pentazocine: Acute CNS manifestations (e.g., hallucinations, disorientation, confusion) have been reported in patients receiving therapeutic doses.

Tramadol: Seizures have occurred in patients taking therapeutic doses of tramadol. The risk of seizures is greater in patients taking higher than recommended doses or concurrent medications that also lower the seizure threshold (see Drug Interactions).

PRECAUTIONS: General: Opioid analgesics should be used with caution in elderly and debilitated individuals because of the danger of cardiac or respiratory depression, as well as those patients with hemorrhage and those with severe impairment of hepatic, pulmonary or renal function. Careful consideration should be given before using opioid analgesics in the presence of the following conditions: myxedema or hypothyroidism (increased risk of CNS and respiratory depression); adrenocortical insufficiency; toxic psychosis; CNS depression; prostatic hypertrophy or urethral stricture; kyphoscoliosis; acute alcohol intoxication and delirium tremens; severe inflammatory bowel disease; gallbladder disease. Due to their cholinergic effects, opioid analgesics should be used with caution in patients with cardiac arrhythmias.

Opioid analgesics may obscure the diagnosis or clinical course in patients with acute abdominal conditions and may induce or exacerbate seizures.

Hypersensitivity: Opioids cause histamine release from mast cells in blood and tissues to varying degrees. Histamine release seems to be related to the dose and route of administration of the opioid, with the oral, rectal and transdermal routes less likely than parenteral administration to result in a reaction. The propensity for an individual opioid to cause anaphylactoid or anaphylactic reactions appears to be related (inversely) to its analgesic potency, rather than to its chemical structure. Pethidine (meperidine) has a higher propensity to cause histamine release than does fentanyl, for example. Switching to a structurally unrelated opioid is not helpful in preventing subsequent reactions.

It is important to determine the exact nature of the reaction in patients reporting allergy to opioids, as many patients believe they are allergic after experiencing an exaggerated pharmacologic response to opioids such as nausea, drowsiness or constipation.

Methadone: Patients established on methadone maintenance therapy for opioid dependence develop tolerance to the analgesic, sedative and euphoric effects of methadone. The established maintenance dose of methadone in these patients will consistently prevent withdrawal symptoms, but will not, by itself, meet their analgesic requirements in the event of surgery or pain of another cause. If pain is not severe, nonopioid analgesics such as NSAIDs can be used. For severe pain, pure opioid agonists may be used. The use of agonist-antagonists should be avoided because of the possibility of precipitating withdrawal. See Table 1 for a list of opioid agonists and agonist-antagonists.

The use of opioid analgesics in patients on methadone maintenance must be closely supervised, with appropriately frequent reassessment of their pain control needs. Similar precautions are recommended for the use of drugs such as benzodiazepines or CNS stimulants in these patients.

Drug Interactions: Alcohol: Alcohol (including prescription or nonprescription drug formulations that contain alcohol) may interact with slow-release opioid formulations, potentially resulting in toxicity due to rapid release of the opioid from its slow-release formulation ("dose-dumping").

Anticholinergics: Concomitant use of drugs with antimuscarinic activity may increase the risk of severe constipation and/or urinary retention.

CNS Agents: Concomitant administration of other CNS drugs such as sedatives, hypnotics, phenothiazines, anesthetics and alcohol may increase the sedative and depressant effects of opioid analgesics. If the concomitant use of these drugs is considered necessary, their doses should be reduced accordingly. See also Warnings.

Inducers of Cytochrome P450 Enzymes: Enzyme inducers (e.g., barbiturates, carbamazepine, phenytoin, rifampin) may increase the clearance of certain opioids (see Table 1). Monitor for therapeutic failure of the opioid and adjust the dose as appropriate.

Inhibitors of Cytochrome P450 Enzymes: Enzyme inhibitors (e.g., cimetidine, erythromycin, fluconazole, fluvoxamine, isoniazid, itraconazole, ketoconazole, paroxetine, sertraline) may decrease the clearance of certain opioids (see Table 1). Monitor for increased therapeutic and adverse effects of the opioid and adjust the dose as appropriate.

MAO Inhibitors: Serious adverse reactions have been reported in patients who receive MAO inhibitors with pethidine. Other opioid analgesics should be used with extreme caution in patients taking MAO Inhibitors (including selegiline) or within 14 days of such therapy.

Neuromuscular Blocking Agents: Opioid analgesics may enhance the effects of neuromuscular blocking agents resulting in increased respiratory depression.

Opioid Antagonists: Naltrexone and agonist-antagonist opioid analgesics (i.e., pentazocine, nalbuphine, butorphanol) should not be administered to a patient who has received or is receiving a course of therapy with a pure opioid agonist analgesic. In these patients, mixed agonist-antagonists may reduce the analgesic effect or may precipitate withdrawal symptoms.

Other Opioids: The use of more than one opioid agonist at a time is usually inappropriate; additive CNS depressant, respiratory depressant and hypotensive effects may occur if 2 or more agonists are used concurrently. Potentiation of effects may occur with a previously administered long-acting opioid analgesic.

Tramadol: The risk of seizures with tramadol is increased with concurrent use of other medications that lower the seizure threshold, such as tricyclic antidepressants, SSRIs and antipsychotics.

Tricyclic Antidepressants: Tricyclic antidepressants may enhance opioid-induced respiratory depression.

Warfarin: Opioid agonists may potentiate the anticoagulant effects of coumarin anticoagulants.

Drug-Laboratory Test Interactions: Opioid analgesics may interfere with certain diagnostic procedures, by increasing plasma amylase and lipase concentrations and by increasing CSF pressure. Gastric emptying is delayed by these drugs so gastric emptying studies will not be valid.

Pregnancy: Although safety for use in pregnancy has not been established, opioids have not been associated with an increased risk of congenital malformations. Certain opioid analgesics are sometimes used to relieve pain during labor and delivery.

As opioid analgesics cross the placental barrier, potential benefits must be weighed against possible hazards. Babies born to mothers who have been taking opioids regularly prior to delivery will be physically dependent. Withdrawal signs include: irritability and excessive crying, tremors, hyperactive reflexes, increased respiratory rate, increased stools, sneezing, yawning, vomiting and fever.

Methadone: Methadone is sometimes used during pregnancy in opioid-dependent women, even though the fetus will be exposed to the drug and may experience withdrawal after delivery. The use of methadone in pregnancy is often considered to be a safer and more manageable option than the possibility of continued illicit drug use, especially if the mother is likely to engage in high-risk behaviors associated with procuring and using street drugs.

Lactation: The extent to which opioids are excreted in breast milk is controversial. This should be taken into consideration when breast-feeding. Withdrawal symptoms can occur in breast-feeding infants when maternal administration of morphine is stopped.

Codeine: Some individuals are ultra-rapid metabolizers of codeine due to a specific CYP2D6 genotype. This can lead to increased morphine production for a given dose of codeine, compared to individuals without this genotype. Breast-fed babies whose mothers are ultra-rapid metabolizers may be at risk of excessive serum morphine levels due to higher levels of morphine in the mother's milk. Mothers using codeine should be aware of the signs and symptoms of morphine toxicity for themselves (constipation, oversedation) or their babies (drowsiness or sedation, difficulty breast-feeding, breathing difficulties and/or decreased muscular tone). Codeine-containing products should be prescribed at the lowest effective dose for the shortest possible period of time.

Methadone: Methadone is distributed into breast milk in variable amounts but is generally considered to be compatible with breast-feeding.

Children: Opioids are used in children of all ages for the management of pain associated with medical or surgical procedures, as an adjunct to general anesthesia, for postoperative pain and for the treatment of painful medical conditions. Fentanyl transdermal patches are not recommended for the pediatric population (see Warnings). Specialized references should be consulted for specific information on dosage and management of adverse effects.

Neonates: Agents known to compromise respiratory function should be administered only by persons experienced in neonatal airway management and in settings with the capacity for continuous monitoring.

Geriatrics: Elderly patients may be more susceptible to adverse effects, especially respiratory depression and constipation. Caution is advised; the initial dose should be reduced and effects monitored. Elimination and metabolism may be slowed; lower doses or longer dosing intervals may be required.

Pethidine (meperidine) is converted to an active metabolite that can accumulate in the elderly or in patients with renal impairment. Pethidine should be used with caution in older patients.

Occupational Hazards: Patients should be warned against driving or operating machinery if they become drowsy or show impaired mental and/or physical abilities.

Headache: Limited clinical experience appears to suggest patients with migraine headache may be more susceptible to adverse reactions with butorphanol use.

Myocardial Infarction: Opioid analgesics must be used with caution in patients with MI who are experiencing nausea or vomiting.

ADVERSE EFFECTS: Major: respiratory depression and respiratory arrest. To a lesser degree circulatory depression, shock and cardiac arrest (see Warnings and Precautions).

Most Commonly Requiring Medical Attention: sedation, nausea and vomiting, constipation and sweating. These effects seem to be more prominent in ambulatory patients and in those not experiencing severe pain. In such individuals, lower doses are advisable. Some adverse reactions may be alleviated if the patient lies down.

Cardiovascular: supraventricular tachycardia, bradycardia, palpitations, faintness, syncope, postural hypotension, hypertension, and phlebitis following iv injection.

Methadone: Dose-related prolongation of the QTc interval can occur during methadone therapy. Very high dose therapy may be associated with torsades de pointes.

Central Nervous System: drowsiness, sedation, euphoria, dysphoria, weakness, headache, agitation, seizures, myoclonus, uncoordinated muscle movements, alterations of mood, dreams, hallucinations and disorientation, visual disturbances, insomnia, miosis, toxic psychoses.

Constipation: Practically all patients become constipated while taking opioid analgesics on a persistent basis. In some instances, particularly the elderly or bedridden, patients may become impacted. It is essential to caution patients in this regard and to institute an appropriate regimen of bowel management at the start of prolonged therapy.

Gastrointestinal: dry mouth, nausea, vomiting, constipation, biliary tract spasm, anorexia, diarrhea, cramps, dyspepsia, taste alterations.

Genitourinary: urinary retention or hesitance, antidiuretic effect, reduced libido and/or potency.

Hypersensitivity: See Precautions.

Nausea and Vomiting: Occur frequently after single doses of opioids or as an early unwanted effect of regular opioid analgesic therapy.

Withdrawal Syndrome: Physical dependence with or without psychological dependence tends to occur with chronic administration. An abstinence syndrome may be precipitated when an opioid analgesic is abruptly discontinued or opioid antagonists are administered. The following withdrawal symptoms may be observed after abrupt discontinuation of an opioid analgesic: body aches, diarrhea, gooseflesh, loss of appetite, nervousness or restlessness, runny nose, sneezing, tremors or shivering, stomach cramps, nausea, sleep disturbances, unusual increase in sweating and yawning, weakness, tachycardia and unexplained fever. With appropriate medical use and gradual withdrawal from opioid analgesics, these symptoms are usually mild.

Other: abnormal liver function test results (propoxyphene), flushing/warmth, pain at injection site, local tissue irritation and induration following sc injection, particularly when repeated.

OVERDOSE:

Symptoms: Respiratory depression (reduced respiratory rate and/or tidal volume, Cheyne-Stokes respiration, cyanosis), extreme somnolence progressing to stupor or coma, skeletal muscle flaccidity, cold or clammy skin, and sometimes hypotension and bradycardia. Severe overdosage may result in apnea, circulatory collapse, cardiac arrest and death. Miosis can be one characteristic of morphine derivative overdose. Mydriasis can take place in terminal narcosis, severe hypoxia or as a toxic effect of pethidine.

In addition to the effects of opioid analgesic overdose in general, focal and generalized seizures constitute a prominent feature in most cases of severe propoxyphene poisoning. Nephrogenic diabetes insipidus and ECG abnormalities may also occur.

Treatment: In cases of oral ingestion, administer activated charcoal. Do not induce vomiting because of the risk of rapid onset of CNS depression. Establish adequate respiratory exchange through the provision of a patent airway and institution of assisted or controlled ventilation. Naloxone, a pure opioid antagonist, is used as a specific antidote to reverse the effects of opioid agonists and agonist-antagonists. An appropriate dose of naloxone should be administered, preferably by the iv route, simultaneously with efforts at respiratory resuscitation. The usual initial adult dose of naloxone is 0.4 to 2 mg iv; children: 0.01 mg/kg iv (see product monograph). Since the duration of action of the opioid may exceed that of the antagonist, the patient should be under surveillance and doses of the antagonist should be repeated as needed to maintain adequate respiration. A neuromuscular blocking agent may be required if respiratory depression is related to muscular rigidity.

Naloxone only partially reverses the symptoms of tramadol overdose and can increase the risk of tramadol-associated seizures.

Long-acting opioid antagonists such as naltrexone are **not** used in initial opioid reversal because of the risk of precipitating an unrelenting withdrawal syndrome.

In propoxyphene overdose, in addition to the use of an opioid antagonist, the patient may require careful titration with an anticonvulsant such as diazepam, bearing in mind the potential additive respiratory depressant effects.

Naloxone **should not** be administered in the absence of clinically significant respiratory or cardiovascular depression. Oxygen, iv fluids, vasopressors and other supportive measures should be used as indicated. In an individual physically dependent on opioids, the administration of the usual dose of opioid antagonist will precipitate an acute withdrawal syndrome, the severity of which is determined by the degree of physical dependence and the dose of antagonist administered. The use of opioid antagonists in such individuals should be avoided if possible. If an opioid antagonist must be used to treat serious respiratory depression in patients with physical dependence on opioids, the antagonist should be administered with extreme care by using dosage titration, commencing with 10 to 20% of the usual recommended initial dose.

Methadone: The relatively long duration of action of methadone compared to that of naloxone may necessitate repeated doses of naloxone to counteract respiratory depression. A continuous iv infusion of naloxone may be used following the initial bolus, at a rate of two-thirds the bolus dose per hour.

The possibility of precipitating withdrawal must also be considered. Naloxone should not be used in the absence of clinically significant respiratory or cardiovascular depression.

> For management of a suspected drug overdose, CPhA recommends that you contact your **regional Poison Control Centre**. See the *CPS* Directory section for a list of Poison Control Centres.

DOSAGE: Dosing and administration of all opioids should be individualized taking into account the following: the nature and severity of pain and medical status of the patient (e.g., renal and hepatic function), daily dose and potency of other opioids or other medication given previously or concurrently, and the degree of tolerance experienced. The use of potent opioid analgesics for the management of persistent pain should be preceded by a thorough assessment of the patient and diagnosis of the pain and its cause. Basic analgesic dosing information on morphine and methadone is provided in this monograph. Specific product monographs should be consulted for more detailed information. See Table 2 for approximate analgesic equivalences.

Buprenorphine: See Indications. Initial dosing of buprenorphine in opioid-dependent patients, including those already stabilized on methadone, must be individualized. Consult the product monograph and/or other references for detailed dosing recommendations.

Fentanyl Transdermal Patch: Initial dosing must be calculated based on the patient's current opioid dose. Consult the product monograph for specific dosage conversion tables.

Morphine: Adults: (Note: Lower doses may be required for frail older individuals) Oral: 10 to 30 mg every 4 hours; Extended-release: dose should be individualized in the treatment of cancer pain or chronic pain.

Rectal: 10 to 20 mg every 4 hours.

IM or SC: 5 to 20 mg every 4 hours.

IV: 2.5 to 10 mg every 4 hours, injected over 4 to 5 minutes.

Epidural: Usual initial dose for once daily intermittent injection: 5 mg.

Intrathecal: Initially 0.2 to 1 mg daily.

N.B. Morphine may be administered by iv, sc, intrathecal or epidural infusion. Nebulized morphine can be administered via inhalation (see Indications). Additional references should be consulted for specific information on dosage and administration in these situations.

Infants and Children: Oral/rectal: 0.2 to 0.4 mg/kg every 4 hours.

IM/IV/SC: 0.05 to 0.1 mg/kg every 2 to 4 hours; maximum 15 mg/dose.

Continuous iv or sc infusion: 0.01 to 0.04 mg/kg/h.

Neonates: IV: 0.05 to 0.1 mg/kg every 4 to 8 hours. Continuous iv infusion: 0.005 to 0.01 mg/kg/h.

Methadone: Adults: The specific Canadian regulations pertaining to the importation, distribution, prescribing and dispensing of **methadone** are contained within the *Controlled Drugs and Substances Act* and the *Narcotic Control Regulations*. See Indications.

The dosage of methadone in opioid dependence must be individualized, with the aim of controlling abstinence symptoms without causing respiratory depression or excessive sedation. Generally, initial dosage ranges from 15 to 30 mg once daily. Maintenance dosage is usually in the range of 50 to 120 mg daily, but may be higher or lower in some patients.

The usual oral dose of methadone for the relief of severe pain ranges from 5 to 20 mg every 4 to 8 hours. Dosage should be individualized and some patients may require dosages outside that range. When switching from other opioids to methadone in the management of severe pain, careful consideration of the methadone dosage is recommended. Several studies have reported that methadone's relative analgesic potency may be significantly higher than previously believed and that the appropriate dose of methadone, when switching from other opioids, can vary greatly depending on the patient's previous opioid dosage.

Table 2: Opioids

Approximate Analgesic Equivalences[a]

Drug	Approximate Equivalent Dose (mg; compared to morphine 10 mg im)	
Agonists	**Parenteral**	**Oral**
Alfentanil	0.4–0.8	NA[b]
Codeine	120	200
Fentanyl[c]	0.1–0.2	NA[b]
Hydromorphone	2	4–6
Morphine	10	30[d]
Oxycodone	NA[b]	30
Pethidine (Meperidine)	75	300

(cont'd)

Table 2: Opioids *(cont'd)*

Approximate Analgesic Equivalences[a]

Drug	Approximate Equivalent Dose (mg; compared to morphine 10 mg im)	
Propoxyphene	50	100
Sufentanil	0.01–0.04	NA[b]
Tramadol	NA[e]	NA[e]
Agonist-Antagonists	**Parenteral**	**Oral**
Buprenorphine	NA[f]	NA[f]
Butorphanol	2	NA[b]
Nalbuphine	10	NA[b]
Pentazocine	60	180

[a] From single dose studies using immediate-release dosage forms. These approximate analgesic equivalences should be used only as a guide for estimating equivalent doses when switching from one opioid to another. Additional references should be consulted to verify appropriate dosing of individual agents.
[b] Route of administration not applicable.
[c] For initial dosing of fentanyl transdermal patches in patients currently receiving other opioids, consult specific dosing conversion tables in the product monograph.
[d] With repeated dosing.
[e] Tramadol's precise analgesic potency relative to morphine is not established. Consult the product monograph for dosing recommendations.
[f] Buprenorphine is not used as an analgesic in Canada. Consult appropriate references for dosing and other prescribing information. See also Indications.

The reader is referred to individual product monographs for more specific dosing information.

Opticrom®
sodium cromoglycate
Antiallergic

Allergan

PHARMACOLOGY: In the immediate reaction (Type I), the union of antigen with reaginic antibody leads to the formation and release of mediators of the local anaphylactic reaction. The principal effect of sodium cromoglycate is its specific ability to stabilize the membrane of the mast cell and thus prevent the release of mediators of anaphylaxis. The action appears to be specific for reaginic (immediate type) antigen/antibody reactions. No direct effect has been demonstrated on other types of immune reactions (Type II, III, and IV).

Sodium cromoglycate has no vasoconstriction, antihistaminic or anti-inflammatory activity. Within 2 to 3 days of commencing treatment one can expect improvement in the signs and symptoms of seasonal allergic conjunctivitis (itching, tearing, congestion, etc.) in most patients. Continued therapy will usually keep the patient free from ophthalmic allergy symptoms during the challenge period.

INDICATIONS: To help relieve and prevent symptoms associated with allergic conjunctivitis or hay fever conjunctivitis.

CONTRAINDICATIONS: Those patients who have shown hypersensitivity to sodium cromoglycate or to benzalkonium chloride.

WARNINGS: The recommended frequency of administration should not be exceeded.

Sodium cromoglycate should only be used for allergic conditions of the eye. In some instances irritation or redness may be due to serious eye conditions such as infection, foreign body in the eye, or other mechanical or chemical corneal trauma requiring the attention of a doctor. If you experience eye pain, changes in vision, pain on exposure to light, acute redness of the eye, excessive discharge, abnormal pupils, if condition worsens or if relief is not obtained within 72 hours consult your doctor immediately.

Any remaining contents should be discarded 4 weeks after opening. Do not touch dropper tip to any surface since this may contaminate the solution.

PRECAUTIONS: During treatment with sodium cromoglycate solution, soft contact lenses should not be worn.

Children: Safety and effectiveness in children below the age of 5 years has not been established.

Pregnancy: There has been to date, no adequate and well controlled studies in pregnant women.

Lactation: It is not known whether this drug is excreted in human milk. Because many drugs are excreted in human milk, caution should be exercised when sodium cromoglycate is administered to a nursing woman.

Drug Interactions: Sodium cromoglycate has been used in association with other ophthalmic solutions in the rabbit including mydriatics, antibiotics, steroids, vasoconstrictors and astringents. No drug-drug interactions have been observed in the rabbit eyes.

ADVERSE EFFECTS: The most frequently reported adverse reaction attributed to the use of sodium cromoglycate on the basis of reoccurrence following administration is transient ocular stinging or burning upon instillation.

The following adverse reactions have been reported as infrequent events; conjunctival injection, watery eyes, itchy eyes, dryness around the eye, puffy eyes, eye irritation and sties. It is unclear whether they are attributable to the drug.

OVERDOSE:

There have been no reported cases in humans of overdosage of the drug.

Treatment: Symptomatic treatment is suggested should accidental ingestion occur.

For management of a suspected drug overdose, CPhA recommends that you contact your **regional Poison Control Centre**. See the *CPS* Directory section for a list of Poison Control Centres.

DOSAGE: The effect of therapy is dependent upon its administration at regular intervals as directed in the labelling.

Symptomatic response to treatment (decreased itching, tearing, redness and discharge) is usually evident within 2 to 3 days. Once symptomatic improvement has been established, therapy should be continued for as long as needed to sustain improvement.

Adults and Children Over 5 Years: 2 drops in each eye 4 times daily at regular intervals. One drop contains approximately 0.8 mg of sodium cromoglycate.

INFORMATION FOR THE PATIENT: Published in e-CPS, available by subscription at www.e-cps.ca.

SUPPLIED: Each plastic dropper bottle of a clear, colorless to pale yellow sterile solution, contains: sodium cromoglycate 2% w/v. Nonmedicinal ingredients: benzalkonium chloride as a preservative and edetate disodium. Bottles of 5 and 10 mL. Store at 15 to 30°C. Protect from direct sunlight. Discard opened bottle after 4 weeks.

OptiMARK® Pr
gadoversetamide
Paramagnetic, Intravascular Contrast Agent for MRI

tyco Healthcare

Date of Revision: March 31, 2010

SUMMARY PRODUCT INFORMATION:

Route of Administration	Dosage Form/ Strength	Clinically Relevant Nonmedicinal Ingredients
Intravenous injection	Solution containing 330.9 mg/mL of gadoversetamide	Solution containing 25.4 mg/mL of versetamide, 3.7 mg/mL of calcium hydroxide and 0.74 mg/mL of calcium chloride dehydrate. Sodium hydroxide and hydrochloride acid may be added for pH adjustment. For a complete listing see Dosage Forms, Composition and Packaging.

INDICATIONS AND CLINICAL USE: Gadoversetamide is indicated for:

Adults: Gadoversetamide is indicated for use with magnetic resonance imaging (MRI) in adults to provide contrast enhancement in those intracranial lesions with abnormal vascularity or those thought to cause abnormalities in the blood-brain barrier. Gadoversetamide has been shown to facilitate visualization of intracranial lesions including but not limited to tumors.

Gadoversetamide is also indicated for use with MRI in adults to provide contrast enhancement and facilitate visualization of lesions of the spine and associated tissues.

Gadoversetamide is also indicated for use with MRI in adults to provide contrast enhancement and facilitate visualization of lesions in the liver.

Geriatrics (>65 years): There was no effect of age in adult patients on the kinetics or elimination of OptiMARK injection. (See Contraindications, Serious Warnings and Precautions, General, Skin and Renal).

Pediatrics (0-18 years): Gadoversetamide Injection is not recommended for use in children below the age of two years as the safety, efficacy and impact of immature kidney function have not been studied in this age group.

Safety, efficacy and pharmacokinetics in pediatric patients (2-18 years of age) have not been established.

CONTRAINDICATIONS: Gadoversetamide Injection (Optimark) is contraindicated in patients at risk for Nephrogenic Systemic Fibrosis (NSF). This includes patients with acute or chronic severe renal insufficiency (glomerular filtration rate <30 mL/min/1.73m²) and patients with acute renal insufficiency of any severity due to the hepato-renal syndrome or in the perioperative liver transplantation period. In these patients, avoid use of other gadolinium-based contrast agents unless the diagnostic information is essential and not available with non-contrast enhanced MRI. If a contrast-enhanced MRI is essential for a patient at risk for NSF, then a gadolinium-based contrast agent other than Gadoversetamide Injection should be considered.

- Patients who are hypersensitive to this drug or to any ingredient in the formulation or component of the container. For a complete listing, see Dosage Forms, Composition and Packaging.
- Gadoversetamide is contraindicated in patients with known allergic or hypersensitivity reactions to gadolinium, versetamide or any of the inert ingredients.

WARNINGS AND PRECAUTIONS:

Warning: Nephrogenic Systemic Fibrosis

Gadolinium-based contrast agents (GBCAs) increase the risk for Nephrogenic Systemic Fibrosis (NSF) in patients with:

- acute or chronic severe renal insufficiency (glomerular filtration rate <30 mL/min/1.73 m²), or
- acute renal insufficiency of any severity due to the hepato-renal syndrome or in the perioperative liver transplantation period.

Optimark is contraindicated in this patient population and Optimark should not be used with patients at risk of NSF.

In these patients, avoid use of GBCAs unless the diagnostic information is essential and not available with non-contrast enhanced magnetic resonance imaging (MRI). NSF may result in fatal or debilitating systemic fibrosis affecting the skin, muscle and internal organs. Screen all patients for renal dysfunction by obtaining a history and laboratory tests. When administering a GBCA, do not exceed the recommended dose and allow a sufficient period of time for elimination of the agent from the body prior to any re-administration. (See Contraindications, General, Skin, Renal and Post-Market Adverse Drug Reactions.)

Serious Warnings and Precautions

- Patients with history of allergy or drug reaction should be observed for several hours after drug administration.
- The possibility of a reaction, including serious, life threatening, fatal anaphylactoid or cardiovascular reactions or other idiosyncratic reactions should always be considered (see Adverse Reactions) especially in those patients with a known clinical hypersensitivity.
- Repeat procedures: The safety of repeated doses has not been studied. If the physician determines sequential repeat examinations are required, a suitable interval of time between administrations should be observed to allow for normal clearance of the drug from the body. A period of at least 7 days should elapse if a repeat scan is considered.

OptiMARK may be associated with QT/QTc interval prolongation. Many drugs that cause QT/QTc prolongation are suspected to increase the risk of a rare polymorphic ventricular tachyarrhythmia known as torsade de pointes. Torsade de pointes may be asymptomatic or experienced by the patient as dizziness, palpitations, syncope or seizures. If sustained, torsade de points can progress to ventricular fibrillation and sudden cardiac death. The risk of torsade de points during treatment with a QT/QTc prolonging drug is increased in patients who are female or elderly (≥65 years).

Particular care should be exercised when administering OptiMARK in patients who are at an increased risk of experiencing torsade de points. Risk factors for torsade de points include, but are not limited to, the following: female; age (≥65 years); presence of genetic variants affecting cardiac ion channels or regulatory proteins, especially congenital long QT syndrome (eg. Romano-Ward syndrome, Jervell and Lange-Nielsen syndrome, Anderson syndrome); family history of sudden cardiac death at <50 years; cardiac disease (eg. myocardial ischemia or infarction, congestive heart failure, left ventricular hypertrophy, cardiomyopathy); demonstrated history of arrhythmias (especially ventricular arrhythmias, atrial fibrillation, or recent conversion from atrial fibrillation; bradycardia (<50 beats per minute); acute neurological events (e.g. intracranial or subarachnoid hemorrhage, stroke, intracranial trauma); electrolyte disturbances (e.g. hypokalemia, hypomagnesia, hypocalcemia); nutritional deficits (e.g. eating disorders, extreme diets); diabetes mellitus; autonomic neuropathy; hepatic or renal function, if relevant to the elimination of the drug.

(See also Drug Interactions, Drug-Drug Interactions.)

Physicians who prescribe drugs that prolong the QT/QTc interval should counsel their patients concerning the nature and implications of the EKG changes, underlying diseases and disorders that are considered to represent risk factors, demonstrated and predicted drug-drug interactions, symptoms of arrhythmias, risk management strategies, and other information relative to the use of the drug.

General: Diagnostic procedures involving the use of MRI contrast agents should be conducted under supervision of a physician with the prerequisite training and a thorough knowledge of the procedure to be performed. Appropriate facilities should be available for coping with any complications of the procedure, as well as for emergency treatment of severe reactions to the contrast itself.

Patients should remain under observation for at least one hour after OptiMARK administration.

Nephrogenic Systemic Fibrosis (NSF): Gadolinium-based contrast agents (GBCAs) increase the risk for Nephrogenic Systemic Fibrosis (NSF) in patients with acute or chronic severe renal insufficiency (glomerular filtration rate <30 mL/min/1.73 m²), and in patients with acute renal insufficiency of any severity due to the hepato-renal syndrome or in the perioperative liver transplantation period. The risk for the development of NSF in patients with moderate renal impairment is unknown, therefore OptiMARK should only be used after careful risk-benefit evaluation in patients with moderate renal impairment (GFR 30-59 mL/min/1.73m²). OptiMARK is contraindicated and should not be used in patients at risk for NSF (see Contraindications).

In these patients, avoid use of GBCAs unless the diagnostic information is essential and not available with non-contrast enhanced magnetic resonance imaging (MRI). For patients receiving hemodialysis, healthcare professionals may consider prompt hemodialysis following GBCA administration in order to enchance the contrast agent's elimination. However, it is unknown if hemodialysis prevents NSF.

Among the factors that may increase the risk for NSF are repeated or higher than recommended doses of a GBCA and the degree of renal function impairment at the time of exposure.

NSF development is considered a potential class-related effect of all GBCAs.

Post-marketing reports have identified the development of NSF following single and multiple administrations of GBCAs. These reports have not always identified a specific agent. Where a specific agent was identified, the most commonly reported agent was gadodiamide (Omniscan), followed by gadopentetate dimeglumine (Magnevist) and Gadoversetamide (OptiMARK). NSF has also developed following the sequential administration of gadodiamide with gadobenate dimeglumine (MultiHance) or gadoteridol (ProHance). The number of post-marketing reports is subject to change over time and may not reflect the true proportion of cases associated with any specific GBCA.

The extent of risk for NSF following exposure to any specific GBCA is unknown and may vary among the agents. Published reports are limited and predominantly estimate NSF risks with gadodiamide. In one retrospective study of 370 patients with 370 patients with severe renal insufficiency who received gadodiamide, the estimated risk for development of NSF was 4% (J Am Soc Nephrol 2006;17:2359). The risk, if any for the development of NSF among patients with mild to moderate renal insufficiency or normal renal function is unknown, and the cautious utilization of the lowest possible dose of GBCA is preferable.

Screen all patients for renal dysfunction by obtaining a history and laboratory tests. When administering a GBCA, do not exceed the recommended dose and allow a sufficient period of time for elimination of the agent from the body prior to any re-administration. (See Action and Clinical Pharmacology and Dosage and Administration.)

A skin biopsy is necessary in order to exclude the diagnosis of similarly presenting skin disorders (e.g. scleromyxedema). (See Serious Warnings and Precautions, Renal, Skin and Post-Market Adverse Drug Reactions.)

Cardiovascular: See Table 1 and Adverse Reactions.

The most prevalant extreme cardiac event prior to and after the administration of OptiMARK was a prolonged PR interval (>200 msec). After the injection of OptiMARK, the frequency of prolonged PR intervals showed no dose-response relationship to the amount of contrast administered.

Dependence/Tolerance: The safety of repeated doses has not been studied.

Ear/Nose/Throat: See Table 1 and Adverse Reactions.

Endocrine and Metabolism: Genetic polymorphism with this product has not been studied.

Gastrointestinal: See Table 1 and Adverse Reactions.

Genitourinary: See Adverse Reactions.

Hematologic: Deoxygenated sickle erythrocytes have been shown in vitro studies to align perpendicular to a magnetic field which may result in vaso-occlusive complications in vivo. The enhancement of magnetic moment by gadoversetamide may possible potentiate sickle erythrocyte alignment. Gadoversetamide in patient with sickle cell anemia and other hemoglobinopathies has not been studied.

Patients with other hemolytic anemias have not been adequately evaluated following administration of gadoversetamide to exclude the possibility of increased hemolysis. See Table 2 for abnormal hematologic and clinical chemistry findings.

Hepatic/Biliary/Pancreatic: An alternate route of excretion frequently observed in patients with severe renal impairment receiving iodinated contrast media is the hepatobiliary enteric pathway. This has not been demonstrated with gadoversetamide in humans but the existence of this pathway has been demonstrated in animals. Gadoversetamide has been shown to be removed from the body by hemodialysis.

Immune: See Warnings and Precautions.

Neurologic: See Table 1 and Adverse Reactions.

Ophthalmologic: No data available.

Perioperative Considerations: No data available.

Psychiatric: No data available.

Renal: Since gadoversetamide is cleared from the body by glomerular filtration, caution should be exercised in patients with impaired renal function. Dose adjustments in renal impairment have not been studied.

- Exposure to GBCAs increases the risk for NSF and OptiMARK is contraindicated in patients with:
  - acute or chronic severe renal insufficiency (glomerular filtration rate <30 mL/min/1.73m²), or
  - acute renal insufficiency of any severity due to the hepato-renal syndrome or in the perioperative liver transplantation period.
- Screen all patients for renal dysfunction by obtaining a history and laboratory tests.
- The risk, if any for the development of NSF among patients with mild to moderate renal insufficiency or normal renal function is unknown, and the cautious utilization of the lowest possible dose of GBCA is preferable. OptiMARK should only be used after careful risk-benefit evaluation in patients with moderate renal impairment (GFR 30-59 mL/min/1.73m²).

(See Contraindications, Serious Warnings and Precautions, Nephrogenic Systemic Fibrosis (NSF), Skin and Post-Market Adverse Drug Reactions.)

Respiratory: See Table 1 and Adverse Reactions.

Sensitivity/Resistance: No data available.

Skin: See Adverse Reactions.

NSF was first identified in 1997 and has so far, been observed only in patients with renal disease. This is a systemic disorder with the most prominent and visible effects on the skin. Cutaneous lesions associated with this disorder are caused by excessive fibrosis and are usually symmetrically distributed on the limbs and trunk. Involved skin becomes thickened which may inhibit flexion and extension of joints and result in severe contractures. The fibrosis associated with NSF can extend beyond dermis and involve subcutaneous tissues, striated muscles, diaphragm, pleura, pericardium, and myocardium. NSF may be fatal. (See Serious Warnings and Precautions, General, Renal, and Post-Market Adverse Drug Reactions.)

Special Populations: Pregnant Women: Gadoversetamide was shown to cause a slight growth retardation in offspring of rats that received doses of 0.5 mmol/kg/day (1980 mg/m²) (0.8 times the clinical dose of 2442 mg/m², 5 times the recommended human dose of 0.1 mmol/kg) for 5 weeks. Gadoversetamide has been shown to cause a slight increase in visceral abnormalities in the offspring of rabbits at doses of 0.4 and 1.6 mmol/kg/day (2904 and 11616 mg/m²) for 12 days (1.2 and 4.8 times the clinical dose of 2442 mg/m²; 4 and 16 times the recommended human dose of 0.1 mmol/kg). The incidence of these abnormalities was comparable to that of historical control levels.

There are no adequate and well-controlled studies in pregnant women. Gadoversetamide should be used during pregnancy only if the potential benefit justifies the potential risk to the fetus.

Nursing Women: ^{153}Gd-labelled gadoversetamide was administered intravenously to lactating rats at a dose of 0.1 mmol/kg. A low but measurable lacteal transfer occurred in rats in a 24-hour period. The concentrations of radioactivity contained in the milk were low and decreased over time. It is not known whether this drug is excreted in human milk. Because many drugs are excreted in human milk, caution should be exercised when gadoversetamide is administered to a nursing woman and it is recommended to discontinue breast feeding for a period of 24 hours after gadoversetamide administration. (See Serious Warnings and Precautions, General, Skin and Renal.)

Pediatrics (0-18 years): Gadoversetamide Injection is not recommended for use in children below the age of two years as the safety, efficacy and impact of immature kidney function have not been studied in this age group.

Safety, efficacy and pharmacokinetics in pediatric patients (2-18 years of age) have not been established.

Monitoring and Laboratory Tests: Blood pressure, laboratory or other tests are required to monitor response to therapy and possible adverse reactions. Please refer to Warnings and Precautions above.

ADVERSE REACTIONS: Adverse Drug Reaction Overview (from Clinical Trials): Because clinical trials are conducted under very specific conditions, the adverse drug reaction rates observed in the clinical trials may not reflect the rates observed in practice and should not be compared to the rates in the clinical trials of another drug. Adverse drug reaction information from clinical trials is useful for identifying drug-related adverse events and for approximating rates.

In clinical trials, a total of 2038 doses were administered. The Phase 2 studies were designed as pseudo cross over studies in which patients received two separate and different doses of gadoversetamide. All safety data is presented by dose, therefore these patients are counted twice, resulting in 2038 subjects and patients studied; 1663 subjects and patients received gadoversetamide (all doses combined), 329 patients received Magnevist, and 46 subjects received placebo (saline). Of the 1663 subjects and patients who received gadoversetamide, 841 (52%) were men and 822 (48%) were women with a mean age of 49 years (range 12-85 years). In this population, there were 1407 (85%) white, 145 (9%) black, 37 (2%) Asian and 74 (4%) subjects and patients of other racial groups.

In the clinical trials there were 8 serious adverse events and 1 death. All serious adverse events were unrelated to gadoversetamide. The one death occurred in a patient with advanced multisystem disease (end-stage AIDS) and was attributed to the underlying disorders and not gadoversetamide.

For all gadoversetamide subjects/patients, regardless of dose (dose range 0.1 to 0.7 mmol/kg), 510 of 1663 patients (30.7%) reported a total of 997 adverse events; 114 (34.7%) of the 329 patients dosed with Magnevist reported a total of 215 adverse events and 22 (47.8%) of the 46 subjects reported a total of 81 adverse events.

The most commonly noted adverse experiences were headache (8.4%), taste perversion (4.4%), dizziness (3.1%), nausea (3.0%), vasodilation (2.3%) and paresthesia (2.1%). All adverse events reported in 1% or greater of all patients are listed in Table 1.

Of the subjects and patients who experienced adverse events, 95.8% of the adverse events were of mild or moderate intensity after dosing with gadoversetamide (all doses combined). The listings below include all adverse events that occurred following the administration of gadoversetamide, regardless of their attributibility to the drug or to the procedure.

In Phase 3 pivotal clinical studies, the principal investigators considered that 5.6% of all adverse events were considered to be related to the administration of gadoversetamide.

There was no demographic association in the reporting of adverse events.

Table 1: OptiMARK

Summary of Adverse Events Experienced by ≥1% of Patients by Dose and Treatment Group n(%)

Body System or Event Type	OptiMARK 0.1 mmol/kg (n=1663)[a]	OptiMARK All Doses (n=1663)[a]	Magnevist 0.1 mmol/kg (n=329)
Number of patients with one or more adverse events	281 (29.3)	510 (30.7)	114 (34.7)
Total number of adverse events	199 (20.8)	997	215
Patients with any injection associated with discomfort	199 (20.8)	382 (23.0)	75 (22.8)
Body as a Whole	141 (14.7)	217 (13.0)	63 (19.1)
Headache	81 (8.4)	124 (7.5)	31 (9.4)
Pain Abdomen	17 (1.8)	24 (1.4)	4 (1.2)
Asthenia	13 (1.4)	20 (1.2)	8 (2.4)
Injection Site Reaction	16 (1.0)	20 (1.2)	10 (3.0)
Pain Back	9 (0.9)	16 (1.0)	3 (0.9)
Pain	8 (0.8)	13 (0.8)	13 (3.6)
Cardiovascular	38 (4.0)	109 (6.6)	10 (3.0)
Vasodilation	22 (2.3)	90 (5.4)	6 (1.8)
Digestive	58 (6.0)	106 (6.4)	20 (6.1)
Nausea	29 (3.0)	43 (2.6)	8 (2.4)
Diarrhea	12 (1.3)	29 (1.7)	3 (0.9)
Dyspepsia	7 (0.7)	16 (1.0)	2 (0.6)
Hemic and Lymphatic	5 (0.5)	13 (0.8)	5 (1.5)
Ecchymosis	5 (0.5)	11 (0.7)	5 (1.5)
Musculoskeletal	14 (1.5)	19 (1.1)	3 (0.9)
Nervous	66 (6.9)	114 (6.9)	20 (6.1)
Dizziness	30 (3.1)	50 (3.0)	7 (2.1)
Paresthesia	20 (2.1)	30 (1.8)	7 (2.1)
Respiratory	29 (3.0)	47 (2.8)	10 (3.0)
Rhinitis	16 (1.7)	20 (1.2)	4 (1.2)
Skin and Appendages	20 (2.1)	39 (2.3)	13 (4.0)
Rash	6 (0.6)	15 (0.9)	7 (2.1)
Special Senses	53 (5.5)	111 (6.7)	20 (6.1)
Taste Perversion	42 (4.4)	95 (5.7)	16 (4.9)

[a] Gadoversetamide doses of 0.1, 0.2, 0.3, 0.4, 0.5 and 0.7 mmol/kg were evaluated in 18 clinical studies.

Less Common Clinical Trial Adverse Drug Reactions (<1%): Body as a Whole: abdomen enlarge, allergic reaction, edema face, edema injection site, fever, flu syndrome, accidental injury, inflammation injection site, lab test abnormality, malaise, mucous membrane discharge, neck rigidity, chest pain, neck pain, pain pelvic.

Cardiovascular: arrhythmia, hemorrhage, hypertension, hypotension, pallor, palpitation, peripheral vascular disease, syncope, tachycardia, thrombophlebitis, vasospasm.

Digestive: anorexia, increased appetite, constipation, bloody diarrhea, dry mouth, dysphagia, eructation, flatulence, gastrointestinal perforation, hemorrhage—ulcer stomach liver tenderness, increased salivation, melena, tenesmus, rectal disorder, thirst, tongue disorder, vomit.

Hemic and Lymphatic: lymphoadenopathy, thrombocytopenia.

Metabolic and Nutritional: increased creatinine, edema, hypercalcemia, hyperglycemia, hypoglycemia, hyponatremia.

Musculoskeletal: arthralgia, athrosis, leg cramps, myalgia, myasthenia, spasm.

Nervous System: agitation, amnesia, anxiety, confusion, convulsion, depersonalization, diplopia, dystonia, emotional liability, hallucinations, hypertonia, hypesthesia, insomnia, meningitis, nervousness, decreased reflexes, increased reflexes, sleep disorder, somnolence, tremor, vertigo.

Respiratory System: asthma, bronchiectasis, cough, dyspnea, epistaxis, hemoptysis, laryngimus, pharyngitis, pneumonia, sinusitis, voice alteration.

Skin and Appendages: application site reaction, erythema multiforme, hair disorder, herpes simplex, pruritus, rash macular-papular and vesicullous bullous, skin dry, increased sweating, urticaria.

Special Senses: amblyopia, conjunctivitis, hyperacusis, ear pain, eye pain, parosmia, tinnitus.

Urogenital: dysmenorrhea, dysuria, vaginal hemorrhage, urinary tract infection, metrorrhagia, oliguria, breast pain, urine abnormality, urine frequency.

Hypocalcemia: occurred in the clinical trial: the causality has not been established.

Clinical Laboratory Evaluations: Table 2 presents a descriptive summary of the changes from baseline for chemistry and haematology that are statistically significant from baseline.

The urinalysis parameters that were measured in all treated study participants in the Phase III trials are: pH, specific gravity, creatinine clearance, urine iron and urine zinc. No significant changes in the mean values for the urinalysis parameters occurred during the 72 hours of patient evaluation after injection and were comparable in all groups.

Post-Market Adverse Drug Reactions: Post-marketing surveillance reports have identified cases of seizure.

Post-marketing reports have identified the development of NSF following single and multiple administrations of GBCAs. These reports have not always identified a specific agent. Where a specific agent was identified, the most commonly reported agent was gadodiamide (Omniscan), followed by gadopentetate dimeglumine (Magnevist) and Gadoversetamide (OptiMARK). NSF has also developed following the sequential administration of gadodiamide with gadobenate dimeglumine (MultiHance) or gadoteridol (ProHance). The number of post-marketing reports is subject to change over time and may not reflect the true proportion of cases associated with any specific GBCA.

Table 2: OptiMARK

Significant Changes (±SD) from Baseline for Laboratory Parameters for Patients Dosed with 0.1 mmol/kg OptiMARK or Magnevist in Pivotal Phase 3 Studies by Time Period and Treatment

	OptiMARK		Magnevist	
Parameter	N	Mean Change from Baseline (SD)[a]	N	Mean Change from Baseline (SD)[a]
2 Hours Post-dosing				
Alkaline phosphatase	455	−5.52 (18.1)		
Glucose	455	46.66 (112.9)	323	62.66 (106.7)
Iron			319	9.49 (20.5)
Iron saturation	425	−6.92 (19.4)	299	13.17 (25.4)
TIBC	450	13.54 (16.7)		
Monocytes	425	−8.85 (33.4)	303	−9.28 (35.7)
WBC			306	5.34 (21.2)
24 Hours Post-dosing				
AST			321	−8.31 (43.1)
Ferritin			318	5.68 (35.5)
Glucose	453	15.38 (96.3)	322	22.91 (100.0)
LDH	451	−7.08 (44.1)	321	−8.93 (35.6)
72 Hours Post-dosing				
Glucose	439	16.12 (100.2)	313	26.68 (105.3)
LDH	437	−8.22 (44.0)	312	−7.68 (44.6)

[a] Note: Mean change from baseline=(post-contrast standardized value—baseline standardized value); empty cells=change not significant

The extent of risk for NSF following exposure to any specific GBCA is unknown and may vary among the agents. Published reports are limited and predominantly estimate NSF risks with gadodiamide. In one retrospective study of 370 patients with 370 patients with severe renal insufficiency who received gadodiamide, the estimated risk for development of NSF was 4% (J Am Soc Nephrol 2006;17:2359). The risk, if any for the development of NSF among patients with mild to moderate renal insufficiency or normal renal function is unknown, and the cautious utilization of the lowest possible dose of GBCA is preferable. (See Contraindications, Serious Warnings and Precautions, General, Skin and Renal.)

DRUG INTERACTIONS: Drug-Drug Interactions: Drug interactions with other contrast agents, other drugs were not studied. Pharmacokinetic studies were performed with non-fasted volunteers or patients.

Pharmacokinetic studies between OptiMARK and other drugs that prolong the QT interval have not been performed. An interaction between these drugs and OptiMARK can not be excluded. Drugs that have been associated with QT/QTc prolongation and/or torsade de pointes include, but are not limited to, the examples in the following list. Chemical/pharmacological classes are listed if some, though not necessarily all, class members have been implicated in QT/QTc prolongation and/or torsade de pointes:

- Class IA antiarrhythmics (e.g. quinidine, procainamide, disopyramide)
- Class III antiarrhythmics (e.g. amiodarone, sotalol, ibutilide)
- Class IC antiarrhythmics (e.g. flecanide, propafenone)
- antipsychotics (e.g. chlorpromazine, pimozide, haloperidol, droperidol)
- tricyclic/tetracyclic antidepressants (e.g. amitripyline, imipramine, maprotiline)
- fluoxetine
- venlafaxine
- methadone
- macrolide antibiotics and analogues (e.g. erythromycin, clarithromycin, telithromycin)
- fluoroquinolone antibiotics (e.g. moxifloxacin, gatifloxacin)
- pentamide
- antimalarials (e.g. halofantrine, quinine)
- azole antifungals (e.g. ketoconazole, fluconazole, voriconazole)
- domperidone
- 5-HT3 antagonists (e.g. dolasetron, ondansetron)
- tacrolimus

OptiMARK should be used with caution with drugs that can disrupt electrolyte levels, including, but not limited to, the following:

- loop, thiazide, and related diuretics
- amphotericin B
- high dose corticosteroids

The above lists of potentially interacting drugs are not comprehensive. Current scientific literature should be consulted for newly approved drugs that prolong the QT/QTc interval or cause electrolyte disturbances, as well for older drugs for which these effects have recently been established.

Drug-Food Interactions: Not applicable for this product.

Drug-Herb Interactions: Not applicable for this product.

Drug-Laboratory Test Interactions: Transient changes in serum iron, calcium, copper and zinc parameters have been observed. The clinical significance is unknown. OptiMARK injection has been shown to cause colorimetric interference with the determination of calcium that results in an apparent decrease in serum concentrations.

Drug-Lifestyle Interactions: Not applicable for this product.

DOSAGE AND ADMINISTRATION:
(Please see Storage and Stability and Dosage Forms, Composition and Packaging.)

Dosing Considerations: See Table 3.

Table 3: OptiMARK

Dosage Chart for Gadoversetamide

Body Weight (kg)	0.1 mmol/kg (0.2 mL/kg)
40	8 mL
50	10 mL
60	12 mL
70	14 mL
80	16 mL
90	18 mL
100	20 mL
110	22 mL
120	24 mL
130	26 mL
140	28 mL
150	30 mL

Concurrent medications should not be physically mixed with contrast agents because of the potential for chemical incompatibility.

Parenteral products should be inspected visually for particulate matter and discoloration prior to administration. Do not use the solution if it is discolored or particulate matter is present.

Recommended Dose and Dosage Adjustment: Gadoversetamide should be administered as a bolus peripheral intravenous injection at a dose of 0.2 mL (0.1 mmol/kg), and at a rate of 1-2 mL/sec, delivered by manual or by power injector.

Gadoversetamide should be drawn into the syringe and administered using sterile technique. If nondisposable equipment is used, scrupulous care should be taken to prevent residual contamination with traces of cleansing agents. To ensure complete injection of the contrast medium the injection should be followed by a 5 mL normal saline flush. Unused portions of the drug must be discarded.

The imaging procedure should be completed within 1 hour of the injection of gadoversetamide.

The safety of repeat doses has not been studied. (See Pharmacodynamics.)

Missed Dose: Not applicable for this product.

Administration: According to the patient weight, the solution of OptiMARK may be taken from one vial or from one prefill syringe and the solution delivered intravenously by manual or power injector.

Parenteral Products: Direct intravenous injection.

Vial Size	Volume of Diluent	Available Volume	Nominal Concentration 330.9 mg/mL of Gadoversetamide
5 to 20 mL vial or 50 mL	N/A	According to patient weight	Manual injection
10–30 mL prefill syringe	N/A	According to patient weight	Injection with manual or power injector

OVERDOSAGE:

Clinical consequences of overdosage with gadoversetamide have not been reported. Treatment of an overdose is directed toward the support of all vital functions and prompt institution of symptomatic therapy.

Gadoversetamide has been shown to be dialyzable in a clinical study. Gadoversetamide does not undergo protein binding in vitro.

For management of a suspected drug overdose, CPhA recommends that you contact your **regional Poison Control Centre**. See the *CPS* Directory section for a list of Poison Control Centres.

ACTION AND CLINICAL PHARMACOLOGY: Mechanism of Action: OptiMARK Injection contains gadoversetamide, a complex formed between a chelating agent (versetamide) and a paramagnetic ion, gadolinium (III). Gadoversetamide is a paramagnetic agent, which develops a magnetic moment when placed in a magnetic field. The relatively large magnetic moment can enhance the relaxation rates of water protons in its vicinity, leading to an increase in signal intensity (brightness) of tissues.

Gadoversetamide conforms to a two-compartment model as the mean of all distribution and elimination half lives, reported as the mean±SD is 13.3±6.8 and 103±19.5 minutes. Gadoversetamide does not undergo metabolic degradation. It is eliminated by the kidneys by glomerular filtration. The kinetics of gadoversetamide appear to be linear; protein binding appears to be absent. In pregnant rats, only minimal levels of radioactivity were detected in the placenta and the fetus.

Pharmacodynamics: In magnetic resonance imaging (MRI), visualization of normal and pathological brain, spinal and hepatic tissue depends in part on variations in the radiofrequency signal intensity that occurs with: 1) changes in proton density; 2) alterations of the spin-lattice or longitudinal relaxation time (T1); and 3) variation of the spin-spin or transverse relaxation time (T2). When placed in a magnetic field, gadoversetamide decreases T1 and T2 relaxation times in tissues where it accumulates. At usual doses the effect is primarily on T1 relaxation time, and produces an increase in signal intensity (brightness).

Gadoversetamide does not cross the blood brain barrier, and, therefore, does not accumulate in the normal brain or in lesions that do not have abnormal blood-brain barrier or abnormal vascularity (e.g., cysts, mature post-operative scars, etc). However, disruption of the blood-brain barrier or abnormal vascularity allows accumulation of gadoversetamide in the interstitial spaces of lesions such as neoplasms, abscesses, and subacute infarcts. The pharmacokinetic parameters of gadoversetamide in various lesions are not known.

A dose-related increase in T1-signal intensity was seen in both CNS and liver studies.

Pharmacokinetics: Summary of OptiMARK's (Gadoversetamide) Pharmacokinetic Parameters in Study 1177-01 and 433 (see Table 4 and Table 5).

Table 4: OptiMARK

Recalculated Non-compartmental PK Parameters—Study 1177-01 (Japan)

Subject	Dose (mmol/kg)	K_{el} (L/hr)	$T_{1/2}$ (h)	AUC (µg Gd h/mL)	CT_T (mL/h/kg)	V_{DSS} (mL/kg)
A	0.05	0.575	1.2	63.4	123.9	193.6
B	0.05	0.47	1.47	79.8	98.6	182.2
D	0.05	0.5	1.26	68.9	114.1	177.9
E	0.05	0.544	1.27	70.8	111	174.5
Mean	0.05	0.522	1.3	70.7	111.9	182.1

(cont'd)

Table 4: OptiMARK *(cont'd)*

Recalculated Non-compartmental PK Parameters—Study 1177-01 (Japan)

Subject	Dose (mmol/kg)	K_{el} (L/hr)	$T_{1/2}$ (h)	AUC (µg Gd h/mL)	CT_T (mL/h/kg)	V_{DSS} (mL/kg)
SD		0.046	0.12	6.8	10.4	8.3
A	0.1	0.437	1.59	162	97	183.7
C	0.1	0.551	1.26	132	119.1	182.4
D	0.1	0.455	1.52	136.1	115.5	208.2
E	0.1	0.468	1.48	137.4	114.4	210
Mean	0.1	0.478	1.46	141.9	111.5	196.1
SD		0.05	0.14	13.6	9.9	15.1
A	0.3	0.43	1.61	483.2	97.6	195.8
B	0.3	0.521	1.33	443.9	106.3	172.4
C	0.3	0.433	1.6	420.7	112.1	226.4
E	0.3	0.46	1.51	476.7	98.7	177.8
Mean	0.3	0.461	1.51	456	103.7	193.1
SD		0.042	0.13	29.2	6.8	24.3
B	0.5	0.429	1.62	1079	72.9	147.7
C	0.5	0.445	1.56	902.7	87.1	170
D	0.5	0.475	1.46	1051	74.8	139.1
E	0.5	0.451	1.54	1217	63	118.6
Mean	0.5	0.45	1.55	1062	74.5	143.9
SD		0.019	0.07	129	10	21.3

(Parameters estimated in WinNonlin 1.1–Model 201.)

Table 5: OptiMARK

Recalculated Non-compartmental PK Parameters—Study 433 (USA)

Subject	Dose (mmol/kg)	K_{el} (L/h)	$T_{1/2}$ (h)	AUC (µg Gd h/mL)	CT_T (mL/h/kg)	V_{DSS} (mL/kg)
104	0.1	0.43	1.61	166.7	94.2	184.4
106	0.1	0.604	1.15	156.6	100	173.2
107	0.1	0.481	1.44	151	104.1	205.2
108	0.1	0.402	1.72	186.1	84.5	178.1
Mean	0.1	0.479	1.48	165	95.7	185.2
SD		0.089	0.25	15.4	8.5	14.1
122	0.7	0.426	1.63	1177	93.5	213.7
123	0.7	0.519	1.34	1108	99.3	184.5
125	0.7	0.478	1.45	934	117.8	215.2
126	0.7	0.438	1.58	1174	93.7	182.6
Mean	0.7	0.465	1.5	1098	101.1	199
SD		0.042	0.13	114	11	17.9

(Parameters estimated in WinNonlin 1.1–Model 201.)

Absorption: In all groups, gadoversetamide was observed to distribute rapidly into the extracellular fluid volume following an intravenous bolus dose. The pharmacokinetics of intravenously administered gadoversetamide in normal subjects conforms to a two-compartment open-model.

Distribution: Gadoversetamide does not undergo protein binding in vitro. In pregnant rats who received ^{153}Gd-labelled gadoversetamide, minimal levels of radioactivity were detected in the placenta and fetus. The volume of distribution at steady state of gadoversetamide in normal subjects is 162±25 mL/kg, roughly equivalent to that of extracellular water. (See Warnings and Precautions, Pregnant Women.)

Metabolism: There is no detectable biotransformation or decomposition of gadoversetamide.

Excretion: Gadoversetamide injection (0.1 mmol/kg) is eliminated primarily in the urine with 95.5±17.4% (mean±SD) of the administered dose eliminated by 24 hours. The renal and plasma clearance rates of gadoversetamide are essentially identical (69±15.4 and 72±16.3 mL/h/kg, respectively) in normal subjects indicating that the drug is essentially cleared through the kidneys via glomerular filtration. There was no systematic difference in any of the kinetic parameters as a function of dose level (0.1 to 0.7 mmol/kg). Therefore, within this dose range the kinetics of gadoversetamide appear to be linear. The mean terminal elimination half-life in normal subjects was 1.73 hours.

Gadoversetamide is removed from the body by hemodialysis. Approximately 98% of the administered dose (0.1 mmol/kg) was cleared from the circulation over the three dialysis sessions.

The mean dialysis clearance of gadoversetamide was 93.2±17.1 mL/min., or 48% of the creatinine clearance (194±18.6 mL/min.), using a high flux PMMA membrane. (See Table 6.)

Special Populations and Conditions: Pediatrics: Optimark is not recommended for use in children below the age of two years as the safety, efficacy and impact of immature kidney function have not been studied in this age group. Safety, efficacy and pharmacokinetics in pediatric patients (2-18 years of age) have not been established.

Geriatrics: Safety and pharmacokinetics in patients more than 76 years of age have not been established.

Gender: There were no statistically significant differences in the elimination half-lives between men or women who were either healthy or who had renal or hepatic impairment (see Table 6).

Table 6: OptiMARK

Elimination Profiles of Normal, Renally Impaired and Hepatically Impaired Men and Women (mean±SD)

Population	Elimination $T_{1/2}$ (hours)	
	Men	Women
Healthy Volunteers	1.73±0.31	1.73±0.40
Normal Patients	1.90±0.50	1.88±0.47
Renally Impaired	8.74±5.14	6.91±2.46
Hepatically Impaired	2.09±0.03	2.35±1.09

Race: Pharmacokinetic differences due to race after intravenous gadoversetamide were not studied.

Hepatic Insufficiency: A single intravenous dose of 0.1 mmol/kg of gadoversetamide was administered to 5 subjects with impaired hepatic function (3 men and 2 women). Two patients had concurrent renal impairment. There was no difference in the plasma kinetics (see Table 6), when compared to normal subjects for patients with hepatic impairment.

Renal Insufficiency: A single intravenous dose of 0.1 mmol/kg of gadoversetamide was administered to 28 subjects with impaired renal function (17 men and 11 women). Sixteen patients had concurrent CNS or liver pathology. Renal impairment was demonstrated to delay the elimination of gadoversetamide (see Table 6). The mean cumulative urinary excretion of gadoversetamide at 72 hours was approximately 93.5% for renal impaired patients and 95.8% for subjects with normal renal function.

Genetic Polymorphism: Special studies on genetic polymorphism have not been done.

STORAGE AND STABILITY: Gadoversetamide should be stored at controlled room temperature, 20 to 25°C and protected from light and freezing. Its shelf life is 2 years.

SPECIAL HANDLING INSTRUCTIONS: Shipped product must be kept in controlled temperature between 20 to 25°C and protected from freezing.

INFORMATION FOR THE PATIENT: Published in e-CPS, available by subscription at www.e-cps.ca.

DOSAGE FORMS, COMPOSITION AND PACKAGING: Vials: 10 mL: Each mL of sterile, nonpyrogenic, clear, colorless to pale yellow aqueous solution, contains: gadoversetamide 330.9 mg. Nonmedicinal ingredients: calcium chloride dihydrate, calcium hydroxide, sodium hydroxide and hydrochloric acid may be added for pH adjustment, versetamide and water for injection. Preservative-free. Single dose rubber stoppered vials of 5 and 10 mL with an aluminum seal.

20 mL: Each mL of sterile, nonpyrogenic, clear, colorless to pale yellow aqueous solution, contains: gadoversetamide 330.9 mg. Nonmedicinal ingredients: calcium chloride dihydrate, calcium hydroxide, sodium hydroxide and hydrochloric acid may be added for pH adjustment, versetamide and water for injection. Preservative-free. Single dose rubber stoppered vials of 15 and 20 mL with an aluminum seal.

Pharmacy Bulk Package: 50 mL vial for multiple dispensing. **This pharmacy bulk package is not for direct infusion.** This Pharmacy Bulk Package is intended for multiple dispensing for i.v. use only, it must be spiked only once.

Directions for Use: Use proper aseptic techniques when handling injection device for maintenance of sterility during multiple dispensing contrast agent at room temperature.

The availability of the Pharmacy Bulk Package is restricted to hospitals with a recognized intravenous admixture program for multiple dispensing.

Once the bottle has been penetrated, withdrawal of contents should be completed without delay. Discard the container no later than 4 hours after initial entry.

Optimyxin® Ophthalmic Ointment

polymyxin B sulfate—bacitracin zinc

Antibiotic

Sandoz

Optimyxin® Eye/Ear Solution

polymyxin B sulfate—gramicidin

Antibiotic

Sandoz

Optimyxin Plus® Eye/Ear Solution Ⓟ

polymyxin B sulfate—gramicidin—neomycin sulfate

Antibiotic

Sandoz

SUPPLIED: Optimyxin: Ophthalmic Ointment: Each g of ophthalmic ointment contains: polymyxin B (as sulfate) 10 000 units and bacitracin (as zinc) 500 units. Tubes of 3.5 g. Store between 15 and 30°C. Discard within 30 days from opening.

Eye/Ear Solution: Each mL of eye/ear solution contains: polymyxin B (as sulfate) 10 000 units and gramicidin 0.025 mg. Also contains ethyl alcohol and benzalkonium chloride 0.005% (as preservative). Thimerosal-free. Plastic dropper bottles of 10 mL. Store between 15 and 30°C.

Optimyxin Plus: Each mL of eye/ear solution contains: polymyxin B (as sulfate) 10 000 units, gramicidin 0.025 mg and neomycin (as sulfate) 1.75 mg. Also contains ethyl alcohol and benzalkonium chloride 0.005% (as preservative). Plastic dropper bottles of 10 mL. Store between 15 and 30°C.

Optiray®

ioversol

Radiopaque Medium

tyco Healthcare

Date of Revision: March 10, 2004

PHARMACOLOGY: General: The pharmacokinetics of ioversol in normal subjects conform to an open 2 compartment model with first order elimination (a rapid alpha phase 6.8 minutes, for drug distribution and a slower beta phase 92 minutes, for drug elimination). Based on the blood clearance curves for 12 healthy volunteers (6 receiving 50 mL and 6 receiving 150 mL of Optiray 320), the biological half-life was 1.5 hours for both dose levels and there was no evidence of any dose related difference in the rate of elimination. The mean half-life for urinary excretion following a 50 mL dose was 118 minutes (105 to 156) and following a 150 mL dose was 105 minutes.

Ioversol is excreted mainly through the kidneys following intravascular administration. Fecal elimination is 3 to 9%. Approximately 50% of the injected dose is excreted at 1.5 hours and 86% at 48 hours; about 1.5% is retained, mostly by the thyroid and liver. In patients with impaired renal function and in infants with immature kidneys, the elimination half-life is prolonged. In patients with severe renal disease, excretion does not occur.

Ioversol does not notably bind to serum or plasma proteins to any marked extent and no significant metabolism, deionization or biotransformation occurs.

Ioversol, like all other contrast media, may induce changes in thyroid function in some patients, and elevation of thyroxine and/or TSH may be observed.

Ioversol, like other nonionic contrast media, has an insignificant effect on blood coagulation (as shown by slightly increased prothrombin time and partial thromboplastin time, and delayed platelet aggregation) and does not possess the anticoagulant properties of ionic contrast media.

Ioversol causes concentration-dependent hemolysis, aggregation and crenation of red blood cells.

Elevations of several laboratory parameters (AST, ALT, LDH, bilirubin, creatinine, BUN) following intravascular administration have been reported in several patients which were not considered clinically significant.

Intravascular: Intravascular injection of ioversol opacifies those vessels in the path of flow of the contract bolus, permitting their radiographic visualization.

Following i.v. contrast medium administration, the increase in density in non-neural tissue is dependent on the presence of iodine in the vascular and extravascular (extra cellular) compartments. This is related to the rate and amount of contrast material administered, blood flow, vascularity, capillary permeability, extravascular effusion and renal filtration.

Peak iodine blood levels occur immediately following rapid i.v. administration, then fall rapidly as the contrast medium is diluted in the plasma volume and diffuses from the vascular into the extravascular spaces. Equilibration between plasma and extravascular iodine concentration occurs within a few minutes.

Contrast enhancement (increase in the **difference** in density between adjacent tissues) is the result of differential vascular and extravascular iodine concentration between normal and abnormal tissues, which may accentuate inherent differences in pre-existent tissue density. With contrast enhancement a pathological lesion may demonstrate increased or decreased density compared to the surrounding normal tissue. Some lesions, however, will remain or become isodense and thus undetectable by attempted contrast enhancement. Contrast enhancement in most cases is greatest immediately after bolus injection.

Ioversol may be visualized in the renal parenchyma within 30 to 60 seconds following rapid i.v. injection. Opacification of the calyces and pelves in patients with normal renal function becomes apparent within 1 to 3 minutes, with optimum contrast occurring within 5 to 15 minutes.

In nephropathic conditions, particularly when excretory capacity has been altered, the rate of excretion varies unpredictably, and opacification may be delayed for up to several hours after injection. Severe renal impairment may result in a lack of diagnostic opacification of the urinary tract, and depending on the degree of renal impairment, prolonged plasma ioversol levels may be anticipated in these patients as well as in infants with immature kidneys.

Ioversol (33%) was compared in intra-carotid studies in 45 anesthetized rats to iopamidol (32%) and iohexol (30%). There was no detectable damage to the blood-brain barrier with any of these substances.

Generally, less warmth and pain are associated with the injection of ioversol than with conventional ionic media. Comparative studies using diatrizoate and iothalamate showed significantly less heat sensation and pain with ioversol. Other non-ionic agents, iohexol and iopamidol, gave results similar to ioversol.

Ioversol had significantly less effect on cardiovascular and ECG parameters than did diatrizoate. For example, it produced significantly less bradycardia, tachycardia, T-wave changes, ST depression, ST elevation and hypotension than were seen with diatrizoate.

Subarachnoid: Following its injection into the subarachnoid space, ioversol mixes readily with the cerebrospinal fluid (CSF) and diffuses into root sleeves and upward in the spinal and intracranial subarachnoid spaces. The time it takes ioversol to reach the cervical and intracranial subarachnoid spaces will depend to a large degree on the patient's position and movements. As it diffuses upward, its concentration decreases.

Following lumbar subarachnoid injection, conventional radiography will continue to provide good diagnostic degree of contrast for at least 30 minutes. At about 1 hour, a diagnostic degree of contrast will usually not be available due to diffusion through the CSF and transfer to the general circulation.

Computerized Tomography: CT Scanning of the Head: In brain scanning, the contrast medium does not accumulate in normal brain tissue due to the presence of the blood-brain barrier. The increase in x-ray absorption in the normal brain is due to the presence of the contrast agent within the blood pool. A break in the blood-brain barrier, such as occurs in malignant tumors of the brain, allows accumulation of the contrast medium within the interstitial tumor tissue; adjacent normal brain tissue does not retain the contrast medium.

Rapid infusion of the dose yields peak blood iodine concentrations immediately following infusion (within 15 to 120 seconds), which fall rapidly over the next 5 to 10 minutes.

Diagnostic contrast enhancement images of the brain have been obtained up to 1 hour after i.v. bolus administration.

CT Scanning of the Body: During CT of the body, ioversol diffuses rapidly from the vascular to the extravascular space. Increase in x-ray absorption is related to blood flow, concentration of the contrast medium and extraction of the contrast medium by interstitial tissue. Contrast enhancement is thus due to the relative differences in extravascular diffusion between normal and abnormal tissue—a situation quite different from that in the brain.

Contrast enhancement appears to be greatest immediately after bolus infusion (15 to 120 seconds).

Utilization of a continuous scanning technique (dynamic CT scanning) may improve enhancement of tumor and other lesions, such as an abscess.

INDICATIONS: Intravascular: Optiray 160: Adults: For use in **adults** for intra-arterial digital subtraction angiography.

Optiray 240: Adults: For use in **adults** for cerebral angiography, venography, excretory urography and for contrast enhanced computed tomographic imaging of the head and body.

Optiray 300: Adults: For use in **adults** for cerebral angiography, aortography, peripheral and visceral arteriography, i.v. contrast enhancement of computed tomography of the brain and body, excretory urography, i.v. digital subtraction angiography and venography.

Children: In **children** 1 year of age or over for i.v. excretory urography and intra-arterial digital subtraction angiography.

Optiray 320: For angiography throughout the cardiovascular system in **adults**. The uses include cerebral, coronary, peripheral, visceral and renal arteriography, aortography and left ventriculography. Optiray 320 is also recommended for contrast enhanced computed tomographic imaging of the head and body and in excretory urography.

Children: In children one year of age or over for angiocardiography, contrast enhanced computed tomography of the head and body and for excretory urography.

Optiray 350: Adults: In **adults** for coronary arteriography and ventriculography, peripheral and visceral arteriography, i.v. contrast enhancement in computed tomography of the head and body, excretory urography, i.v. digital subtraction angiography and venography.

Children: For angiocardiography.

Subarachnoid: Optiray 240: Adults: For subarachnoid administration in adults for lumbar, thoracic and cervical myelography.

CONTRAINDICATIONS: Should not be administered to patients with known or suspected hypersensitivity to ioversol or in cases of clinically significant impairment of both hepatic and renal function.

WARNINGS: Use the recommended ioversol concentration for the particular procedure to be undertaken.

General: Serious or fatal reactions have been associated with the administration of all iodine-containing radiopaque media, including ioversol. It is of utmost importance that a course of action be carefully planned in advance for immediate treatment of serious reactions, and that adequate facilities and appropriate personnel be readily available in case a severe reaction should occur.

A previous reaction to a contrast medium of different chemical structure or a history of iodine sensitivity is not an absolute contraindication to the use of ioversol. However, extreme caution should be exercised in injecting these patients and prophylactic therapy (as with corticosteroids, for example) should be considered (see Precautions, General).

There must be a clear indication for performing procedures involving the administration of contrast agents in all patients.

Patients with a history of allergy, bronchial asthma or other allergic manifestations, combined renal and hepatic disease, the elderly, debilitated or severely ill patients, those with homo cystinuria, endotoxemia, elevated body temperature, severe hypertension or congestive heart failure, other cardiovascular disease, hyperthyroidism and recent renal transplant recipients, as well as patients sensitive to iodine, present an additional risk and call for careful evaluation of the risks involved against the benefits expected.

Patients with a serum creatinine level above 3 mg/dL should not undergo excretory urography or other radiological procedures unless the benefits clearly outweigh the risks incurred.

In patients with advanced renal disease, iodinated contrast media should be used with caution and only when the examination is essential since excretion of the medium is impaired. Use of ioversol is not recommended in patients with anuria or severe oliguria.

Administration of radiopaque materials to patients known or suspected to have pheochromocytoma should be performed with extreme caution if, in the opinion of the physician, the possible benefits of such procedures outweigh the considered risks. The amount of radiopaque medium injected should be kept to an absolute minimum. The blood pressure should be assessed throughout the procedure, and measures for treatment of a hypertensive crisis should be available.

General anesthesia may be indicated in some procedures; however, one should be aware of possible increased incidence of adverse reactions in such circumstances.

Vascular Use: Intravascularly administered iodine-containing contrast media are potentially hazardous.

Non-ionic iodinated contrast media, including ioversol, inhibit blood coagulation less than ionic contrast media. Clotting has been reported when blood remains in contact with syringes, catheters or tubes containing non-ionic contrast media. Serious, rarely fatal, thromboembolic events causing myocardial infarction and stroke have been reported during angiographic procedures with non-ionic and also with ionic contrast media. Therefore, meticulous intravascular administration technique is necessary, particularly during angiographic procedures, to minimize thromboembolic events. Numerous factors, including length of procedure, number of injections, catheter and syringe material, underlying disease state and concomitant medications may contribute to the development of thromboembolic events. For these reasons, meticulous angiographic techniques are recommended including close attention to keeping guidewires, catheters and all angiographic equipment free of blood, use of manifold systems and/or three way stopcocks, frequent catheter flushing with heparinized saline solutions and minimizing the length of the procedure. Non-ionic iodinated contrast media are not recommended as flush solutions. The use of plastic syringes in place of glass syringes has been reported to decrease but not eliminate the likelihood of clotting.

In patients who are known to have multiple myeloma and other paraproteinemias, because of the risk of inducing transient to fatal renal failure, extreme caution should be used. In these instances, anuria has developed resulting in progressive uremia, renal failure and eventually death. A minimal diagnostic dose should be employed and renal function, as well as extent of urinary precipitation of the myelomatous protein, should be monitored for a few days subsequent to the procedure. The patients should be normally hydrated for the examination since dehydration may predispose to precipitation of myeloma protein in the renal tubules. No form of therapy, including dialysis, has been successful in reversing the effect.

Intravascular administration of contrast media may promote sickling in individuals who are homozygous for sickle cell disease. Fluid restriction is not advised in these patients.

As with any contrast medium, including ioversol, serious neurologic sequelae, including permanent paralysis, can occur following cerebral arteriography and injection into vessels supplying the spinal cord. The injection of a contrast medium should never be made following the administration of vasopressors since they strongly potentiate neurologic effects.

Subarachnoid Use: Myelography should not be performed when lumbar puncture is contraindicated as in the presence of local or systemic infection where bacteremia is likely.

Myelography should be performed only in hospitalized patients under close medical supervision, which is to be continued for 24 hours following the procedure.

Patients receiving anticonvulsants should be maintained on this therapy. Should a seizure occur, i.v. diazepam or phenobarbital is recommended. In patients with a history of seizure activity who are not on anticonvulsant therapy, premedication with barbiturates should be considered. Ioversol should be used in epileptics only if a water soluble contrast medium is considered essential.

Prophylactic anticonvulsant treatment with barbiturates should be considered in patients with evidence of inadvertent intracranial entry of a large bolus of contrast medium, since there may be increased risk of seizure in such cases.

Gravitational displacement of a concentrated bolus of ioversol above the level of C_1 and especially into the intracranial subarachnoid spaces is to be avoided.

PRECAUTIONS: General: All procedures utilizing contrast media carry a definite risk of producing severe, life-threatening and fatal reactions. Therefore, the need for the examination should always be carefully assessed and the risk-benefit factor should always be carefully evaluated before such a procedure is undertaken.

At all times a fully equipped emergency cart, or equivalent supplies and equipment, and personnel competent in recognizing and treating adverse reactions of all severity, or situations which may arise as a result of the procedure, should be immediately available. If a serious reaction should occur, immediately discontinue administration and institute appropriate treatment. Since severe delayed reactions have been known to occur, emergency facilities and competent personnel should be available for at least 30 to 60 minutes after administration.

The reported incidences of adverse reactions to contrast media are twice as high in patients with a history of allergy than in the general population. Patients with a history of previous reactions to a contrast medium or iodine are 3 times more susceptible than other patients. Most adverse reactions to intravascularly injected contrast agents appear within 1 to 30 minutes after the start of injection, but delayed reactions may occur.

Before a contrast medium is injected, the patient should be questioned for a history of bronchial asthma or allergy.

Although a history of allergy may imply a greater than usual risk, it does not arbitrarily contraindicate the use of the medium. Premedication with corticosteroids to avoid or minimize possible allergic reactions may be considered.

The possibility of an idiosyncratic reaction in patients who have previously received a contrast medium without ill effect should always be considered. A positive history of bronchial asthma or allergy, a family history of allergy, or a previous reaction of hypersensitivity to another contrast agent warrant special attention. Such a history, by suggesting proneness to reactions, may be more accurate than pre-testing in predicting the potential for reaction, although not necessarily the severity or type of reaction in the individual case. A positive history of this type does not arbitrarily contraindicate the use of a contrast agent, when a diagnostic procedure is thought essential, but calls for caution.

The sensitivity test most often performed is the slow injection of 0.5 to 1 mL of the radiopaque medium, administered i.v., prior to injection of the full dose. It should be noted that the absence of a reaction to the test dose does not preclude the possibility of a reaction to the full dose. Severe reactions and fatalities have occurred with the full dose after a non-reactive test dose, and with or without a history of allergy.

Prophylactic therapy with corticosteroids should be considered for patients who present with a strong allergic history, a previous reaction to a contrast medium, or a positive pretest (since in these patients the incidence of reaction is 2 to 3 times that of the general population). Adequate doses of corticosteroids should be started early enough prior to contrast medium injection to be effective and should continue through the time of injection and for 24 hours after injection. Corticosteroids should not be mixed in the same syringe with the contrast medium because of chemical incompatibility.

Renal failure has been reported in patients with liver dysfunction who were given an oral cholecystographic agent followed by an intravascular iodinated radiopaque agent and also in patients with occult renal disease, notably diabetics and hypertensives. Administration of ioversol should be postponed in patients with hepatic or biliary disorder who have recently taken a cholecystographic agent. An interval of at least 48 hours should be allowed between examinations, especially in patients with reduced renal reserve. Especially in these classes of patients there should be no fluid restriction and every attempt made to maintain normal hydration, prior to contrast medium administration, since dehydration is the single most important factor influencing further renal impairment.

Acute renal failure has been reported in patients with diabetic nephropathy and in susceptible nondiabetic patients (often elderly with pre-existing renal disease) following administration of iodinated contrast agents. Careful consideration of the potential risks should be given before performing radiographic procedures with ioversol in these patients.

Intravascular: Diagnostic procedures which involve the use of iodinated intravascular contrast agents should be carried out under the direction of a physician skilled and experienced in the particular procedure to be performed.

Reports of thyroid storm occurring following intravascular use of iodinated radiopaque agents in patients with hyperthyroidism or with an autonomously functioning thyroid nodule suggest that this additional risk be carefully evaluated in such patients before use of ioversol.

Special precaution is advised in patients with increased intracranial pressure, cerebral thrombosis or embolism, primary or metastatic cerebral lesions, subarachnoid hemorrhage, arterial spasm, transient ischemic attacks, and in any condition when the blood-brain barrier is breached or the transit time of the contrast agent material through the cerebral vasculature is prolonged, since clinical deterioration, convulsions and serious temporary or permanent neurological complications (including stroke, aphasia, cortical blindness, etc.) may occur following i.v. or intra-arterial injection of relatively large doses of contrast media. Such patients, and patients in clinically unstable or critical condition, should undergo examinations with intravascular contrast media only if in the opinion of the physician the expected benefits outweigh the potential risks, and the dose should be kept to the absolute minimum.

When considering the use of high doses of contrast media, caution should be exercised in patients with congestive heart failure because of the transitory increase in circulatory osmotic load, and such patients should be kept under surveillance for several hours in order to detect delayed hemodynamic disturbances.

There have been reports in the literature indicating that patients on adrenergic beta-blockers may be more prone to severe adverse reactions to contrast media. At the same time, treatment of allergic-anaphylactoid reactions in these patients is more difficult. Epinephrine should be administered with caution since it may not exert its usual effects. On the one hand larger doses of epinephrine may be needed to overcome the bronchospasm, while on the other, these doses can be associated with excessive alpha adrenergic stimulation with consequent hypertension, reflex bradycardia and heart block and possible potentiation of bronchospasm. Alternatives to the use of large doses of epinephrine include vigorous supportive care such as fluids and the use of beta agonists including parenteral salbutamol or isoproterenol to overcome bronchospasm and norepinephrine to overcome hypotension.

In angiography procedures, the presence of a vigorous pulsatile flow should be established before using a catheter or pressure injection technique. A small pilot dose of about 1 to 2 mL should be administered to locate the exact site of needle or catheter tip to help prevent injection of the main dose into a branch of the aorta or intramurally. Great care should be taken to avoid the entry of a large concentrated bolus into an aortic branch.

Mesenteric necrosis, acute pancreatitis, renal shutdown, and serious neurologic complications including spinal cord damage and hemiplegia or quadriplegia have been reported following inadvertent injection of a large part of the aortic dose of contrast media into an aortic branch or arterial trunks providing spinal or cerebral artery branches.

Pulsation must be present in the artery to be injected. Extreme caution is advised in considering peripheral angiography in patients suspected of having thromboangiitis obliterans (Buerger's disease) since any procedure (even insertion of needle or catheter) may induce a severe arterial or venous spasm. Caution is also advisable in patients with severe ischemia associated with ascending infection. Special care is required in patients with suspected thrombosis, ischemic disease, local infection or a significantly obstructed vascular system. Occasional serious neurologic complications, including paraplegia, have been reported in patients with aorto-iliac or femoral artery bed obstruction, abdominal compression, hypotension, and hypertension and following injection of vasopressors.

When large individual doses are administered, an appropriate time interval should be permitted to elapse between injections to allow for subsidence of hemodynamic disturbances. Angiography should be avoided whenever possible in patients with homocystinuria because of the risk of inducing thrombosis and embolism.

Following catheter procedures, gentle pressure hemostasis is advised followed by immobilization of the limb for several hours to prevent hemorrhage from the site of arterial puncture.

I.V. Contrast Enhancement in Computed Tomography: Following injection of relatively large doses of contrast media used in the procedure, transient or permanent neurological changes have been reported.

Pregnancy: No teratogenic effects attributable to ioversol have been observed to date in studies performed in animals. There are no studies on the use of ioversol in pregnant women. Many injectable contrast media cross the placental barrier in humans and appear to enter fetal tissue passively. Ioversol probably crosses the placental barrier in humans by simple diffusion to reach fetal tissue. Ioversol should be used during pregnancy only if the benefit to the mother clearly outweighs the risk to the fetus. It should be borne in mind that x-ray procedures involve a certain risk related to exposure of the fetus.

Lactation: Because contrast media are secreted in human milk, if the administration of ioversol is considered to be essential, breast-feeding should be discontinued for at least 48 hours following the procedure.

Children: Some pediatric patients have a higher risk of adverse reactions to contrast media. Such patients may include those with sensitivity to allergens, including other drugs, those with asthma, congestive heart failure, a serum creatinine >1.5 mg/dL, or ages under 12 months.

Geriatrics: The tolerance of elderly patients to drugs in general is diminished. These patients may have reduced renal reserve and impaired general health and may be taking medication (e.g., adrenergic β-blockers) which make them more susceptible to the potentially harmful effects of procedures involving the use of contrast media. The need for and the expected benefits of the procedure have to be carefully evaluated and dosage should be very conservative.

Drug Interactions: **Drugs which lower seizure threshold**, especially phenothiazine derivatives, including those used for their antihistaminic or antinauseant properties, should not be used with ioversol.

Renal toxicity has been reported in a few patients with liver dysfunction who were given oral cholecystographic agents followed by intravascular contrast agents. Therefore administration of a contrast agent should be postponed by at least 48 hours following use of an oral cholecystographic agent.

Subarachnoid: Elderly patients may present a greater risk following myelography. The need for the procedure in these patients should be evaluated carefully. Special attention must be given not to exceed the recommended dose of the contrast medium, to see that the patient is sufficiently hydrated and to ensure proper and sterile radiographic technique.

If grossly bloody CFS is encountered, the possible benefits of a myelographic procedure should be considered in terms of the risk to the patient.

Any intrathecally administered medication including non-ionic contrast media such as ioversol can enter the brain substance which may increase the risk of adverse effects associated with the procedure. Such adverse reactions may be delayed and, in extremely rare cases, may be life-threatening. Careful patient and dose selection and proper patient management before, during and after the procedure are therefore imperative. Care is required in patient management to prevent inadvertent intracranial entry of a large bolus of contrast medium. Also, effort should be directed to avoid rapid dispersion of the medium (i.e., by active patient movement).

Experience with the use of water-soluble contrast media in myelography indicates that in most cases of major motor seizure one or more of the following factors were present, and should therefore, be avoided: deviations from recommended procedure on myelographic management; use in patients with a history of epilepsy; inadvertent overdosage; intracranial entry of a bolus or premature diffusion of a high concentration of the medium; medication with neuroleptic drugs or phenothiazine antinauseants; failure to maintain elevation of the head during and after the procedure; active patient movement or straining.

Repeat Procedures: If in the clinical judgment of the physician a repeat examination is required, an interval of 5 days between procedures is recommended.

Special Precautions to be observed with performing specific diagnostic procedures are listed in the Dosage section, under individual paragraphs pertaining to said specific procedures.

ADVERSE EFFECTS: Since ioversol is an iodinated contrast agent with an adverse reaction profile similar to other non-ionic contrast media, all known adverse effects associated with the use of any contrast agent can occur with ioversol.

Most adverse reactions following the use of ioversol are of mild or moderate intensity, however, serious, life-threatening and fatal adverse reactions, mostly of cardiovascular origin, have been reported.

It should be kept in mind that, although most adverse reactions occur soon after the administration of the contrast medium, some adverse reactions can be delayed and can be of long-lasting nature.

The reported incidence of adverse reactions to contrast media in patients with a history of allergy is twice that of the general population. Patients with a history of previous reactions to a contrast medium are 3 times more susceptible than other patients.

The incidence of serious adverse reactions is higher with coronary arteriography than with other procedures. In those patients only who had coronary arteriography with ioversol, the incidence of angina was 1.2%. Cardiac decompensation, serious arrhythmias, myocardial ischemia or myocardial infarction may occur during coronary arteriography and left ventriculography.

In a controlled clinical trial involving 30 pediatric patients undergoing angiocardiography, no adverse reactions were reported.

Table 1 is based upon clinical trials with Optiray formulations in 1 506 patients, regardless of their direct attributability to the drug or the procedure.

Adverse reactions to specific procedures are also dealt with under Dosage.

Table 1: Optiray

Adverse Reactions seen with Optiray

	Adverse Reactions	
System	**>1%**	**≤1%**
Cardiovascular	none	angina pectoris, hypotension, blood pressure fluctuation, arterial spasm, bradycardia, conduction defect, false aneurysm, hypertension, transient arrhythmia, vascular trauma
Digestive	none	nausea, vomiting
Nervous	none	cerebral infarct, headache, blurred vision, vertigo, lightheadedness, vasovagal reaction, disorientation, paresthesia, dysphasia, muscle spasm, syncope, visual hallucination
Respiratory	none	laryngeal edema, pulmonary edema, sneezing, nasal congestion, coughing, shortness of breath, hypoxia
Skin	none	periorbital edema, urticaria, facial edema, flush, pruritus
Miscellaneous	none	extravasation, hematoma, shaking chills, bad taste, general pain

In addition to the reported reactions in Table 1, the following may occur with any contrast agent including ioversol: Cardiovascular: hypoxia, heart block, bundle branch block, coronary thrombosis, cyanosis, hypertensive crisis, peripheral vasodilation, acute vascular insufficiency, circulatory collapse, hypotensive shock and cardiogenic shock.

Central Nervous System: photomas, persistent blindness, taste perversion, anxiety, tinnitus, motor dysfunction, convulsion, somnolence, confusion, psychotic reaction, stiff neck, hemiparesis, hemiplegia, nystagmus, restlessness, tremors, aphasia, paralysis, coma and death.

Allergic Type Reaction: purpura, conjunctivitis, lacrimation, erythematous, bullous or pleomorphic rashes, laryngospasm, bronchospasm, apnea, cyanosis, edema of glottis, laryngeal edema, angioneurotic edema, peripheral edema, anaphylactic shock. These allergic type reactions can progress into anaphylaxis, coma and death.

Renal: transient proteinuria, hematuria and rarely oliguria, anuria and renal failure.

Other Reactions: diarrhea, dry mouth, pallor, venous and arterial thrombosis and rarely thrombophlebitis, rare cases of disseminated intravascular coagulation, neutropenia.

Children: In controlled clinical trials involving 128 patients for pediatric angiocardiography, contrast enhanced computed tomography of the head and body and i.v. excretory urography, adverse reactions following the use of Optiray 320 were generally less than with adults. Adverse reactions reported were as follows: fever 1.6%, nausea 0.8%, muscle spasm 0.8%, LV pressure change 0.8%.

Related to Procedure: extravasation, perforation, rupture, dissection of blood vessels, hemorrhage, hematoma, false aneurysm, muscle spasm, arterial spasm, vascular trauma, ecchymosis and tissue necrosis, dislodgment of atheromatous plaques, thrombophlebitis, thrombosis embolization, injury to nerves and neighboring organs, brachial plexus palsy following axillary artery injections.

Treatment of Adverse Effects: Contrast media should be administered only by physicians thoroughly familiar with the emergency treatment of all adverse reactions to contrast media. The assistance of other trained personnel such as cardiologists, internists and anesthetists is required in the management of severe reactions.

A guideline for the treatment of adverse reactions is presented below. This outline is not intended to be a complete manual on the treatment of adverse reactions to contrast media or on cardiopulmonary resuscitation. The physician should refer to the appropriate texts on the subject.

It is also realized that institutions or individual practitioners will already have appropriate systems in effect and that circumstances may dictate the use of additional or different measures.

Minor Allergic Reactions: (if considered necessary). The i.v or i.m. administration of an antihistamine such as diphenhydramine HCl 25 to 50 mg is generally sufficient (contraindicated in epileptics). The resulting drowsiness makes it imperative to ensure that outpatients do not drive or go home unaccompanied.

Major or Life-threatening Reactions: A major reaction may be manifested by signs and symptoms of cardiovascular collapse, severe respiratory difficulty and nervous system dysfunction. Convulsions, coma and cardiorespiratory arrest may ensue.

The following measures should be considered:

1. Start emergency therapy immediately, carefully monitoring vital signs. 2. Have emergency resuscitation team summoned—do not leave patient unattended. 3. Ensure patent airway: guard against aspiration. 4. Commence artificial respiration if patient is not breathing. 5. Administer oxygen, if necessary. 6. Start external cardiac massage in the event of cardiac arrest. 7. Establish route for i.v. medication by starting infusion of appropriate solution (5% dextrose in water). 8. Judiciously administer specific drug therapy as indicated by the type and severity of the reaction. Careful monitoring is mandatory to detect adverse reactions of all drugs administered. (a) Soluble hydrocortisone 500 to 1 000 mg i.v. for all acute allergic-anaphylactic reactions. (b) Epinephrine 1:1 000 solution (in the presence of anoxia it may cause ventricular fibrillation; **caution** in patients on adrenergic beta blockers. See Precautions). i) 0.2 to 0.4 mL s.c. for severe allergic reactions; ii) in extreme emergency 0.1 mL/minute, appropriately diluted, may be given i.v. until desired effect is obtained. Do not exceed 0.4 mL; iii) in case of cardiac arrest 0.1 to 0.2 mL, appropriately diluted, may be given intracardially. (c) In hypotension (carefully monitoring blood pressure): i) phenylephrine HCl 0.1 to 0.5 mg appropriately diluted slowly i.v. or by slow infusion **or** ii) norepinephrine 4 mL of 0.2% solution in 1 000 mL of 5% dextrose by slow drip infusion. (d) Sodium bicarbonate 5%, 50 mL i.v. every 10 minutes as needed to combat post-arrest acidosis. (e) Atropine 0.4 to 0.6 mg i.v. to increase heart rate in sinus bradycardia. May reverse 2nd or 3rd degree block. (f) To control convulsions: i) pentobarbital sodium 50 mg in fractional doses slowly i.v. (contraindicated if cyanosis is present) **or** ii) diazepam 5 to 10 mg slowly i.v. titrating the dose to the response of the patient. 9. Defibrillation, administration of antiarrhythmics and additional emergency measures and drugs may be required. 10. The patient should be transferred to the intensive care unit when feasible for further monitoring and treatment.

OVERDOSE:

Symptoms: The adverse effects of overdosage are life-threatening and affect mainly the pulmonary, cardiovascular and central nervous systems.

Treatment: Treatment of an overdosage is directed toward the support of all vital functions, and prompt institution of specific therapy.

Ioversol does not bind to plasma or serum proteins and is therefore dialyzable.

> For management of a suspected drug overdose, CPhA recommends that you contact your **regional Poison Control Centre**. See the *CPS* Directory section for a list of Poison Control Centres.

DOSAGE: General: Only the lowest dose necessary to obtain adequate visualization should be used.

Use only the recommended concentration for the particular procedure to be undertaken.

Patients should be well hydrated prior to and following administration of ioversol.

Do **not** dehydrate patients for any procedure.

Ioversol should be inspected visually for particulate matter and discoloration prior to administration. If either is present the vial should be discarded.

Ioversol should not be transferred into other delivery systems except immediately before use and should be used immediately once the seal has been punctured.

It is advisable that ioversol be at or close to body temperature when injected.

Under no circumstances should other drugs be administered concomitantly in the same syringe or i.v. administration set as ioversol because of a potential for chemical incompatibility.

Patency of the vessel and the position of the catheter tip or needle should be checked with a small pilot dose of ioversol before injecting the full dose. The catheter tip should be kept free of aspirated blood. Prolonged contact of the contrast medium with blood must be avoided because of potential thromboembolic complications.

The volume of each individual injection is a more important consideration than the total dose used. When large individual volumes are administered, sufficient time should be permitted to elapse between each injection to allow for subsidence of hemodynamic disturbances.

Any unused portion of one container should be discarded.

Intravascular Dosage and Administration: Cerebral Angiography: Optiray 320, 300 or 240 may be used to visualize the cerebral vasculature.

Patient Preparation: Suitable premedication may be given. Introduction of the catheter or needle is normally performed with local anesthesia. General anesthesia is rarely required (see Precautions, General).

Precautions: In addition to the general precautions previously described, cerebral angiography with ioversol should be performed with special caution in elderly patients, patients in poor clinical condition, patients with advanced arteriosclerosis, severe hypertension, cardiac decompensation, senility, recent cerebral thrombosis, embolism or subarachnoid hemorrhage, following a recent attack of migraine, and in any condition compromising the integrity of the blood brain barrier, and only if the examination is considered to be necessary for the welfare of the patient. The patient should be watched carefully for possible adverse reactions.

Adverse Reactions: The major sources of cerebral arteriographic adverse reactions to ioversol appear to be related to repeated injections of the contrast material, administration of doses higher than those recommended, the presence of occlusive atherosclerotic vascular disease and the method and technique of injection.

Since nonionic contrast media have no significant anticoagulant properties, meticulous technique is necessary to avoid thromboembolic complications (see Warnings).

A feeling of warmth in the face and neck is frequently experienced. Infrequently, a more severe burning discomfort is observed. Transient visual hallucinations have been reported.

Serious neurological reactions that have been associated with cerebral angiography include stroke, seizures, amnesia, hemiparesis, visual field loss, cortical blindness, aphasia, confusion, disorientation, hallucination, convulsions, coma and death.

Cardiovascular reactions that may occur with some frequency, but not necessarily with ioversol, are bradycardia, arrhythmia, either an increase or decrease in systemic blood pressure, and ECG changes.

Note: The EEG changes associated with the use of contrast media, including ioversol, for cerebral arteriography are not infrequent: ioversol can be expected to have the same effect on the electrophysiology of the brain, but this has not been systematically assessed.

Usual Adult Dosage: Either Optiray 240, Optiray 300 or Optiray 320 may be used for cerebral angiography. The usual adult dosage of ioversol employed varies with the site and method of injection and the age and condition of the patient. The usual adult dose range for common carotid arteriography is 5 to 10 mL; for vertebral arteriography 4 to 8 mL. For aortic arch injection (4 vessel studies) the usual dose for Optiray 320 is 15 to 25 mL, and for Optiray 240 is 15 to 40 mL. Injections should be made at rates approximately equal to the flow rate of the vessel being injected.

These doses may be repeated if indicated. The total dose per procedure should be limited to the smallest volume necessary to achieve a diagnostic examination and should not exceed 200 mL.

Intra-arterial Digital Subtraction Arteriography: Optiray 160 and Optiray 300 are suitable agents for intra-arterial digital subtraction angiography (IA-DSA). With this technique lower iodine concentrations can yield diagnostic images. Other advantages of the procedure are the use of less contrast medium and a decreased need for selective arterial catheterization. However, with aortic injection, visualization of small vessels may be insufficient.

Patient Preparation: No special patient preparation is required for IA-DSA. However, patients should be normally hydrated prior to examination.

Precautions: In addition to the general precautions already described, the risks and adverse reactions associated with IA-DSA are those usually associated with the conventional procedure performed in the area of the specific vessel.

In IA-DSA of the distal aorta great care is necessary to avoid entry of a large aortic bolus into an aortic branch since this could cause deleterious effects on the organs supplied by the branch. Patient motion, including respiration and swallowing, can result in misregistration leading to image degradation and nondiagnostic studies.

Adverse Reactions: Adverse reactions seen with IA-DSA are similar to those observed during peripheral arteriography. They may sometimes occur due to trauma during the procedure.

Adverse reactions reported with the use of iodinated contrast media include hypotension, soreness in extremities, transient arterial spasm, gangrene, perforation of vessels, extravasation, hemorrhage, hematoma formation with tamponade, injury to nerves and other structures in close proximity to the artery, thrombosis, dissecting aneurysm, arteriovenous fistula, dislodgment of atheromatous plaques, subintimal injection and transient leg pain from contraction of calf muscles in femoral arteriography.

Usual Adult Dosage Using Optiray 160: As a general rule, the volume and concentration used for IA-DSA are about 50%, or less, of that used for conventional procedures. The actual dosage and flow rate will vary depending on the selectivity of the injection site and the area being examined. The following suggested volumes per injection are intended as a guide (see Table 2). Injections may be repeated if necessary. It is advisable to inject at rates approximately equal to the flow rate of the vessel being injected.

Table 2: Optiray 160

Usual Adult Dosage

Carotid Arteries	5–10 mL
Vertebral Arteries	4–8 mL
Aortic Arch	25–50 mL
Distal Aorta	25–50 mL
Iliac Arteries	6–15 mL

Dosage should not usually exceed 250 mL.

Usual Dose in Children 1 Year of Age and Over Using Optiray 300: The usual dose is 1 to 3 mL/kg, depending on the area to be examined.

Peripheral Arteriography: Optiray 300, Optiray 320 or Optiray 350 may be used for arteriograms of the lower extremities.

Patient Preparation: The procedure is normally performed with local anesthesia. General anesthesia usually is not required (see Precautions, General).

Precautions: In addition to the general precautions previously described, moderate decreases in blood pressure occur frequently with intra-arterial injections. This change is usually transient; however, the blood pressure should be monitored for approximately 10 minutes following injection.

Injection of ioversol in patients with severe arterial disease (e.g., thromboangiitis obliterans, severe atherosclerosis, ischemia, thrombosis, significant obstruction) should be undertaken with extreme caution and only when absolutely necessary.

When injections are being made in the distal aorta for aorto-iliac run-off studies, the possibility of inadvertent injection of a large dose into a branch of the aorta or intramural dissection should be considered.

To prevent extravasation or subintimal injection, the position of the catheter tip or needle should be carefully evaluated. Fluoroscopy is recommended. **Pulsation must be present in the artery to be injected.** A small dose of 1 to 2 mL should be administered to locate the exact site of the needle or catheter tip. Great care is necessary to avoid entry of a large bolus into an aortic branch.

Severe pain, paresthesia or peripheral muscle spasm during injection may require discontinuance of the procedure and a re-evaluation of the catheter tip or needle placement.

Following catheter procedures, gentle pressure hemostasis is advised, followed by observation and immobilization of the limb for several hours to prevent hemorrhage from the site of arterial puncture.

Adverse Reactions: Adverse reactions observed during peripheral arteriography may be due to trauma during the procedure or to the injection of the contrast material. Adverse reactions reported with the use of iodinated contrast media include hypotension, soreness in extremities, transient arterial spasm, contrast medium induced thrombosis, embolism, gangrene, perforation of vessels, extravasation, hemorrhage, hematoma formation with tamponade, injury to spinal cord and nerves and other structures in close proximity to the artery; transverse myelitis, thrombosis, dissecting aneurysm, arteriovenous fistula, dislodgment of atheromatous plaques, subintimal injection, leg pain, renal damage including infarction and tubular necrosis due to accidental filling of the renal arteries.

Usual Adult Dosage: The usual single adult dose for aorto-iliac run-off studies is 20 to 50 mL; for iliac and femoral arteries 10 to 30 mL. These doses may be repeated as indicated. The total procedural dose should be limited to the smallest volume required to obtain a diagnostic examination and should not usually exceed 250 mL.

Selective Coronary Arteriography with or without Left Ventriculography: Either Optiray 320 or Optiray 350 is recommended for this procedure.

Precautions: Since the risk in coronary arteriography is increased if the procedure is performed shortly after acute myocardial infarction, some physicians recommend that this procedure should not be performed for approximately 4 weeks following the diagnosis of myocardial infarction. Mandatory prerequisites to the procedure are experienced personnel, ECG monitoring apparatus and adequate facilities for immediate resuscitation and cardioversion.

Patients should be monitored continuously by ECG and vital signs throughout the procedure. The injection of relatively large volumes of hypertonic solutions (e.g., contrast media) into the heart chambers can cause significant hemodynamic disturbances. Caution is advised especially in patients with incipient heart failure because of the possibility of aggravating the pre-existing condition. Hypotension should be corrected promptly since it may induce serious arrhythmias.

Adverse Reactions: Most patients will have transient ECG changes during the procedure. The following adverse effects have occurred in conjunction with the administration of iodinated intravascular contrast agents for this purpose: hypotension, shock, anginal pain, coronary thrombosis, myocardial infarction, cardiac arrhythmias (bradycardia, ventricular tachycardia, heart block, ventricular fibrillation), cardiac arrest and death.

Severe adverse reactions, especially arrhythmias, are likely to occur with greater frequency following right coronary artery injection. Fatalities have been reported. Complications to the procedures include dissection of coronary arteries, dislodgment of atheromatous plaques, embolization from the catheter, perforation of heart chambers or coronary arteries with cardiac tamponade, hemorrhage and thrombosis.

Usual Adult Dosage: The usual adult dose range with Optiray 320 or Optiray 350 for left coronary arteriography is 2 to 10 mL and for right coronary arteriography is 2 to 6 mL. For left ventriculography, the usual single adult dose is 30 to 40 mL. These doses may be repeated if indicated; however, several minutes should be allowed to elapse between injections to allow for subsidence of hemodynamic disturbance, and the total procedural dose should be limited to the smallest volume necessary to obtain a diagnostic examination. The total procedural dose should not exceed 250 mL.

Children: Optiray 320 and Optiray 350 are recommended for this procedure in children 1 year of age and over. The usual single injection dose of Optiray 320 and Optiray 350 is 1.25 mL/kg of body weight with a range of 1 mL/kg to 1.5 mL/kg. When multiple injections are given, the total administered dose should not exceed 5 mL/kg up to a total volume of 250 mL.

Aortography and Visceral Arteriography: Optiray 300, 320 or 350 is recommended for this procedure. Great care is necessary to avoid all entry of a large bolus into an aortic branch. Mesenteric necrosis, acute pancreatitis, renal infarction, acute tubular necrosis, renal shutdown and serious neurologic complications, including paraplegia and quadriplegia, have been reported and may be attributable to an excessive dose being injected into an aortic branch or arterial trunks supplying the spinal arteries or to prolonged contact time of the concentrated contrast medium on the CNS tissue. Conditions which can contribute to prolonged contact time include decreased circulation, aortic stenosis or partial occlusions distal to the site of injection, abdominal compression, hypotension, general anesthesia or the administration of vasopressors. When these conditions exist or occur, the necessity of performing or continuing the procedure should be carefully evaluated and the dose and number of repeat injections should be maintained at a minimum with appropriate intervals between injections.

Adverse Reactions: With aortic injection, depending on the technique employed, the risks of this procedure also include the following: injury to the aorta and neighboring organs, pleural puncture, renal damage including infarction and acute tubular necrosis with oliguria and anuria due to accidental filling of the renal arteries, retroperitoneal hemorrhage from the translumbar approach and spinal cord injury and pathology associated with the syndrome of transverse myelitis. Occasional serious neurological complications including paraplegia have been reported in patients with aorto-iliac or femoral artery obstruction, abdominal compression, hypotension, hypertension, spinal anesthesia and injection of vasopressor drugs to enhance contrast. In such patients, the concentration, volume and number of injections should be kept to a minimum.

Adult Dosage: Optiray 300, Optiray 320 or Optiray 350 is recommended for this procedure. The usual individual injection volumes are as follows: abdominal aorta 20 to 50 mL, superior mesenteric artery 20 to 40 mL and renal artery 4 to 10 mL.

Total procedural dose should not exceed 250 mL.

I.V. Contrast Enhancement in Computed Tomography (CT): Because unenhanced scanning may provide adequate information in the individual patient and the injection of contrast media may obscure certain lesions visible on the plain scan, contrast enhancement is usually performed only if the unenhanced scan has not provided sufficient information. The decision to employ contrast enhancement, which is associated with additional risk and increased radiation exposure, should be based upon a careful evaluation of the patient's clinical condition, renal and cardiac reserve, the status of the blood-brain barrier and other radiological and unenhanced CT findings.

Warnings: Patients with diabetes mellitus, impaired renal function and congestive heart failure are considered to be at greater risk of developing acute renal failure following injection of large doses of contrast media required for contrast enhancement in CT scanning.

Convulsions and other serious neurologic complications including stroke have occurred in patients with primary or metastatic cerebral lesions or breached blood-brain barrier or slowed cerebral circulation following the administration of iodine-containing radiopaque media for enhancement of CT brain images.

Patient Preparation: No special patient preparation is required for contrast enhancement in computerized tomography. **However, it has to be insured that patients are well hydrated prior to examination.** In patients undergoing abdominal or pelvic examination, opacification of the bowel by dilute oral contrast medium may be valuable in scan interpretation.

Precautions: Patient motion, including respiration, can markedly affect image quality, therefore patient cooperation is essential.

The use of an intravascular contrast medium can obscure some tumors in patients undergoing CT evaluation, resulting in a false negative diagnosis.

Computed Tomography of the Head: Neoplastic Conditions: Optiray 240, Optiray 300, Optiray 320 or Optiray 350 may be used to enhance the demonstration of the presence and extent of certain primary or metastatic malignancies.

The usefulness of contrast enhancement for the investigation of the retrobulbar space and in cases of low grade or infiltrative glioma has not been demonstrated.

In cases where lesions have calcified, there is less likelihood of enhancement. Following therapy, tumors may show decreased or no enhancement. Maximum contrast enhancement of certain tumors may be delayed necessitating delayed scans.

Non-neoplastic Conditions: The use of Optiray 240, Optiray 300, Optiray 320 or Optiray 350 may be beneficial in the image enhancement of non-neoplastic lesions, such as cerebral infarctions of recent onset; however, some infarctions are obscured if contrast media are used.

Arteriovenous malformations and aneurysms will show contrast enhancement. In the case of these vascular lesions, the enhancement is probably dependent on the iodine content of the circulating blood pool.

Hematomas and intraparenchymal bleeders seldom demonstrate any contrast enhancement. However, in cases of intraparenchymal clot, for which there is no obvious clinical explanation, contrast medium administration may be helpful in ruling out the possibility of associated arteriovenous malformation (see Precautions).

The opacification of the inferior vermis following contrast medium administration has resulted in false positive diagnoses in a number of normal studies.

Usual Adult Dosage: For adults the usual dosage of Optiray 300, 320 or 350 is 50 to 100 mL; of Optiray 240, 100 to 250 mL. A maximum dose of 150 mL of Optiray 320 or 350 should not be exceeded. For Optiray 240 the maximum dose is 250 mL. Scanning is usually performed immediately after injection.

Children: The dose recommended for use in children 1 year of age and over is 1 to 3 mL/kg of Optiray 320.

Body Computed Tomography: Optiray 240, 300, 320 or 350 may be administered for contrast enhancement of the organs, tissues and larger blood vessels of the chest, abdomen and pelvis.

Continuous or multiple scans separated by intervals of 1 to 3 seconds during the first 30 to 90 seconds postinjection of the contrast medium (dynamic CT scanning) are required to demonstrate enhanceable lesions not seen with CT alone. Subsets of patients in whom delayed body CT scans might be helpful have not been identified.

Inconsistent results have been reported and abnormal and normal tissues are usually isodense during the time frame used for delayed CT scanning. At present, consistent results have been documented using dynamic CT techniques only.

Usual Adult Dosage: Optiray 240, 300, 320 or 350 may be administered by bolus injection, rapid infusion or by a combination of both. Depending on the area to be examined, the usual dose range is 30 to 100 mL. When prolonged enhancement is required, 25 to 50 mL may be given as a rapid bolus and the remainder as an infusion. The total dose should not exceed 150 mL of Optiray 300, 320 or 350 or 200 mL of Optiray 240. Scanning is usually performed immediately after injection.

Children: The dose recommended for use in children 1 year of age and over is 1 to 3 mL/kg body weight of Optiray 320 with a usual dose of 2 mL/kg.

Venography: Optiray 240, 300 or 350 may be used to visualize the peripheral venous circulation. Venograms are obtained by injection or infusion into an appropriate vein in the lower extremity.

Precautions: In addition to the general precautions previously described, specific caution is advised when venography is required in patients with suspected thrombosis, phlebitis, severe ischemic disease, local infection or a significantly obstructed venous system.

Extreme caution is necessary to avoid extravasation and fluoroscopy is recommended. This is especially important in patients with severe venous disease.

Adverse Reactions: Complications of the procedure include bleeding, thrombosis, embolism, contrast medium-induced thrombophlebitis, gangrene and major systemic adverse reactions.

Usual Adult Dosage: The usual adult dose of Optiray 240, 300 or 350 will range from 20 to 100 mL for the lower extremity.

Following the procedure, the venous system should be flushed with normal or heparinized saline solution. Massage and elevation of the leg are also helpful for clearing the contrast medium from the extremity to prevent post-procedural thrombophlebitis. The maximum dose should not usually exceed 250 mL.

Excretory Urography: Optiray 240, 300, 320 or 350 may be used for excretory urography. Following i.v. injection in patients with normal renal function, Optiray is excreted mostly by the kidneys. Maximum radiographic density in the calyces and pelves occurs in most instances within 5 to 15 minutes after injection.

In patients with severe renal impairment, contrast visualization may be substantially delayed, or may not occur at all.

Patient Preparation: A low residue diet the day preceding the examination, and a laxative the evening before the examination, may be given unless contraindicated. **Partial dehydration is dangerous and may contribute to acute renal failure.** Maintenance of normal hydration is desirable.

Precautions: Adequate renal function must be present. Dehydration will not improve contrast quality in patients with impaired renal function and will increase the risk of contrast induced renal damage. The examination should not be repeated for at least 72 hours because of the potential of additive renal damage (see Warnings and Precautions).

Adverse Reactions: All adverse reactions known to occur with the i.v. use of ioversol can also occur with excretory urography (see Adverse Effects).

Usual Adult Dosage: The usual adult dose of Optiray 300, Optiray 320 or Optiray 350 is 50 mL in the average normal adult. With Optiray 240 the equivalent dose is 65 mL in the average normal adult. In these patients, high dose urography may be preferred using Optiray 320 at a dose of 1.5-2 mL/kg. The dose is injected intravenously, usually within 1-3 minutes. Maximum doses of 200 mL of Optiray 240, 150 mL of Optiray 300 or 320 and 140 mL of Optiray 350 should not be exceeded.

Children: Optiray 300 and 320 at doses of 0.5 mL/kg to 3 mL/kg of body weight has produced diagnostic opacification of the urinary tract. The usual dose for children is 1 mL/kg. Dosage for children over 1 year of age should be administered in proportion to age and body weight. The total administered dose should not exceed 3 mL/kg.

Table 3: Optiray
Adult Intravascular Dosage Table

Procedure	Conc. of Solution (mgI/mL)	Usual Recommended Single Dose (mL)
Cerebral Angiography	320	
	300	
	240	
Common Carotid		5–10
Vertebral		4–8
Aortic Arch		15–25 (Optiray 320)
		15–40 (Optiray 240)
Intra-arterial Digital Subtraction Angiography	160	
Common Carotid		5–10
Vertebral Arteries		4–8
Aortic Arch		20–35
Distal Aorta		20–45
Iliac Arteries		6–15
Peripheral Arteriography	350	
	320	
	300	
Aorto-iliac Run-off		20–50
Iliac and Femoral Arteries		10–30
Selective Coronary Arteriography	320	
	350	
Left Coronary		2–10
Right Coronary		2–6
Left Ventriculography		30–40
Aortography and Visceral Arteriography	300	
	320	
	350	
Abdominal Aorta		20–50
Superior Mesenteric Artery		20–40
Renal Artery		4–10
Intravenous Contrast Enhanced CT	240	
	300	
	320	
	350	
Heat CT		50–100
Body CT		30–100 (infusion)
		25–50 (bolus)
Venography	240	
	300	20–100
	350	
Excretory Urography	240	65
	300	50
	320	50
	350	50

Table 4: Optiray
Pediatric Intravascular Dosage Table

Procedure	Conc. of Solution (mgI/mL)	Usual Recommended Single Dose (mL/kg body weight)
Excretory Urography	300	>1 year old: 2 mL/kg
	320	>1 year old: 1–1.5 mL/kg
Intra-Arterial Digital Subtraction Angiography	300	1–3 mL/kg
Pediatric Angiocardiography	320	1–1.5 mL/kg
	350	
Computed Tomography of the Head	320	1–3 mL/kg
Computed Tomography of the Body	320	1–3 mL/kg

Subarachnoid: Precautions: Optiray 240 is recommended for the examination of lumbar, thoracic and cervical regions in adults by lumbar injection. Myelography should not be performed in the presence of significant local or systemic infec tion where bacteremia is likely or when lumbar or cervical puncture is contraindicated.

The volume and concentration of Optiray 240 to be administered will depend on the degree and extent of contrast required within the recommended dose range in the area under examination, and on the equipment and technique employed. Optiray 240 is slightly hypertonic to CSF.

A total dose of 3600 mg (15 mL) iodine should not be exceeded in adults. As in all diagnostic procedures, the minimum volume and dose to produce adequate visualization should be used. Most procedures do not require the total maximum dose.

Anesthesia is not necessary. Patients should be well hydrated. Seizure-prone patients should be maintained on anticonvulsant medication.

Adverse Reactions: Any adverse reactions known to occur with the i.v. use of ioversol can also occur during myelography, especially those which originate in the CNS. The most commonly observed adverse reaction was headache, which had an incidence of 8.6%.

Rate of injection: To avoid excessive mixing with CSF and consequent dilution of contrast, injection should be made slowly, over 1 to 2 minutes.

Depending on the estimated volume of ioversol which may be required for the procedure, a small amount of CSF may be removed to minimize distension of the subarachnoid spaces, unless contraindicated.

The spinal puncture needle may be removed immediately following injection because it is not usually necessary to remove ioversol after injection into the subarachnoid space.

If, in the clinical judgment of the physician, a repeat examination is required, an interval of 5 days between procedures is recommended.

Adults: Usual Dose: The usual recommended total dose of Optiray 240 for use in lumbar myelography is 10 mL and for thoracic and cervical myelography 15 mL. Table 5 indicates these dosages.

Table 5: Optiray 240
Dosages

Procedure	Optiray Concentration	Concentration (mgI/mL)	Volume (mL)
Lumbar Myelography	Optiray 240	240	10
Thoracic Myelography	Optiray 240	240	15
Cervical Myelography	Optiray 240	240	15

If computerized tomography is to follow, it should be deferred for 2 to 6 hours to allow the amount of contrast to decrease. Computerized tomography shows CSF contrast enhancement in the thoracic region in about 1 hour.

Patient Management—Subarachnoid Administration: Good patient management should be exercised at all times to minimize the potential for complications.

Pre-procedure: Discontinue neuroleptic drugs (including phenothiazines, e.g., chlorpromazine, prochlorperazine and promethazine) at least 48 hours beforehand. Maintain normal diet up to 2 hours before procedure. Premedication is not usually considered necessary. Should myelography be necessary in patients with a history of seizures, such patients should be maintained on their anticonvulsant medication.

During Procedure: Use minimum dose required for satisfactory contrast (see Dosage). In all positioning techniques keep the patient's head elevated above highest level of spine. Do not lower head of table more than 15° during examination. In patients with excessive lordosis consider lateral position for injection. Inject slowly (over 1 to 2 minutes) to avoid excessive mixing. Move medium within the spinal subarachnoid space under fluoroscopic monitoring. Avoid intracranial entry of a bolus. Avoid early and high cephalad dispersion of the medium. Avoid abrupt or active patient movement to minimize excessive mixing with CSF. Instruct patient to remain passive. Move patient slowly and only as necessary.

Post-procedure: Following myelography move contrast medium to low lumbosacral area by upright positioning of the patient, for a few minutes. Raise head of stretcher to at least 30° before moving patient onto it. Movement onto and off the stretcher should be done slowly with patient completely passive, maintaining **head-up** position.

Before moving patient onto bed, raise head of bed 30 to 45°. Some clinicians advise patients to remain still in bed, in head-up position or in the semi-sitting position, especially in the first few hours. Others have encouraged their patients to be fully ambulatory and have noted a reduction in the incidence of headache, nausea and vomiting. Maintain close observation and head-up position for at least 24 hours after myelogram. Obtain visitors' cooperation in keeping the patient quiet and in **head-up** position, especially in first few hours. Encourage oral fluids. Diet as tolerated. **If nausea or vomiting** occur do not use phenothiazine antinauseants. Persistent nausea and vomiting will result in dehydration. Therefore prompt consideration of replacement by i.v. fluids is recommended.

It is advisable that sterile Optiray products in vials, bottles or in Ultraject syringes be at or close to body temperature when infused.

SUPPLIED: Optiray 160: Each mL of clear, colorless to pale yellow, sterile, nonpyrogenic aqueous solution (ioversol injection 34%) contains: ioversol 339 mg with tromethamine 3.6 mg as a buffer and edetate calcium disodium 0.2 mg as a stabilizer. Optiray 160 provides 16% (160 mg/mL) of organically bound iodine. Osmolality (mOsm/kg water): 355. Viscosity (cps): 2.7 (25°C) and 1.9 (37°C). Vials of 50 mL, boxes of 10 and 25. Bottles of 100 mL fill/100 mL, boxes of 12. Ultraject prefilled syringes 50/125 mL power injector and 125 mL power injector, boxes of 20.

Optiray 240: Each mL of clear, colorless to pale yellow, sterile, nonpyrogenic aqueous solution (ioversol injection 51%) contains: ioversol 509 mg with tromethamine 3.6 mg as a buffer and edetate calcium disodium 0.2 mg as a stabilizer. Optiray 240 provides 24% (240 mg/mL) organically bound iodine. Osmolality (mOsm/kg water): 502. Viscosity (cps): 4.0 (25°C) and 3.0 (37°C). Vials of 15 mL fill/20 mL, boxes of 10, vials of 50 mL, boxes of 10 and 25. Bottles of 100 mL fill/55 mL, boxes of 12. Bottles of 100 mL fill/65 mL, boxes of 12. Bottles of 100 mL fill/100 mL, boxes of 12. Bottles of 200 mL fill/250 mL, boxes of 6 and 12. Ultraject prefilled syringes 50 mL hand-held, 75 mL fill/125 mL power injector; 100 mL fill/125 mL power injector and 125 mL power injector, boxes of 20.

Optiray 300: Each mL of clear, colorless to pale yellow, sterile nonpyrogenic aqueous solution (ioversol injection 64%) contains: ioversol 636 mg with tromethamine 3.6 mg as a buffer and edetate calcium disodium 0.2 mg as a stabilizer. Optiray 300 provides 30% (300 mg/mL) organically bound iodine. Osmolality (mOsm/kg water): 651. Viscosity (cps): 8.2 (25°C) and 5.5 (37°C). Vials of 30 mL, boxes of 25. Vials of 50 mL, boxes of 25. Bottles of 100 mL fill/55 mL, boxes of 12. Bottles of 100 mL fill/65 mL, boxes of 12. Bottles of 100 mL fill/100 mL, boxes of 12. Ultraject prefilled syringes 30 and 50 mL, hand-held 50 mL fill/125 mL power injector, 100 mL fill/125 mL power injector; 125 mL power injector, boxes of 20.

Optiray 320: Each mL of clear, colorless to pale yellow, sterile, nonpyrogenic aqueous solution (ioversol injection 68%) contains: ioversol 678 mg with tromethamine 3.6 mg as a buffer and edetate calcium disodium 0.2 mg as a stabilizer. Optiray 320 provides 32% (320 mg/mL) organically bound iodine. Osmolality (mOsm/kg water): 702. Viscosity (cps): 9.9 (25°C) and 5.8 (37°C). Vials of 20 mL, boxes of 10 and 25. Vials of 30 mL, boxes of 10 and 25. Vials of 50 mL, boxes of 10 and 25. Bottles of 100 mL fill/55 mL, boxes of 12. Bottles of 100 mL fill/65 mL, boxes of 12. Bottles of 100 mL fill/100 mL, boxes of 12. Bottles of 150 mL, boxes of 6 and 12. Bottles of 200 mL fill/250 mL, boxes of 6 and 12. Ultraject prefilled syringes 30 mL and 50 mL hand-held, 50 mL fill/125 mL power injector, 75 mL fill/125 mL power injector; 100/125 mL power injector; 125 mL power injector, boxes of 20. Pharmacy Bulk Vial: Multi-dispensing bottles of 500 mL, boxes of 12.

Optiray 350: Each mL of clear, colorless to pale yellow, sterile nonpyrogenic aqueous solution (ioversol injection 74%) contains: ioversol 741 mg with tromethamine 3.6 mg as a buffer and edetate calcium disodium 0.2 mg as a stabilizer. Optiray 350 provides 35% (350 mg/mL) organically bound iodine. Osmolality (mOsm/kg water): 792. Viscosity (cps): 14.3 (25°C) and 9.0 (37°C). Vials of 30 mL, boxes of 25. Vials of 50 mL, boxes of 25. Bottles of 75 mL fill/150 mL, boxes of 12. Bottles of 100 mL fill/55 mL, boxes of 12. Bottles of 100 mL fill/65 mL, boxes of 12. Bottles of 100 mL fill/100 mL, boxes of 12. Bottles of 150 mL, boxes of 12. Bottles of 200 mL fill 250/mL, boxes of 12. Ultraject prefilled syringes 30 and 50 mL hand-held; 50 mL fill/125 mL power injector, 75 mL fill/125 mL power injector; 100 mL fill/125 mL power injector; 125 mL power injector, boxes of 20. Pharmacy Bulk Vial: Multi-dispensing bottles of 500 mL, boxes of 12.

Pharmacy Bulk Vial for Optiray 320 and Optiray 350 (500 mL bottle): For Multiple Dispensing: This Bulk Pharmacy Vial is intended for multiple dispensing for intravenous use only, it must be spiked only once.

Directions for Use: Use proper aseptic techniques when handling injection device for maintenance of sterility during multiple dispensing contrast agent at room temperature. **The availability of the Bulk Pharmacy Vial is restricted to hospitals with a recognized intravenous admixture program for multiple dispensing or for use of diluted solution.** Once punctured, use the contents of the Pharmacy Bulk Vial within 4 hours and diluted solutions within 24 hours if kept at room temperature, and 72 hours if refrigerated from the time of initial puncture.

The pH of the formulations is adjusted between 6.0 and 7.4 with hydrochloric acid or sodium hydroxide. The product does not contain a preservative and is intended for single dose use only. Store between 15 and 30°C. Discard unused portion. Submersion of syringes in water is not recommended. Do not re-autoclave plastic container because of possible damage to syringe. Protect from light. Protect from freezing.

Optomega

Cucurbita pepo—Curcuma longa—Helianthus annus—Linum usitatissimum—Olea europaea—Rosmarinus officinalis

Herbal Product

USANA Health Sciences

SUPPLIED: Each dosage unit contains: Cucurbita pepo 185 mg, Curcuma longa 9.3 µg, Helianthus annus 1.01 g, Linum usitatissimum 7.95 g, Olea europaea 93 mg, Rosmarinus officinalis 0.56 mg. Nonmedicinal ingredients: tocopherols excipient NF.

(Shown in Product Identification Section)

Oracort Ⓟ

triamcinolone acetonide

Dental Corticosteroid

Taro

SUPPLIED: Each g of dental paste contains: triamcinolone acetonide 1 mg (0.1%) in a protective emollient vehicle containing gelatin powder, pectin and sodium carboxymethylcellulose in a polyethylene and mineral oil gel base. Tubes of 7.5 g. Store at room temperature (15-30°C). Keep tightly closed.

Orencia™ Ⓟ

abatacept

Selective Co-stimulation Modulator

Bristol-Myers Squibb

Date of Preparation: June 29, 2006
Date of Revision: February 17, 2010

SUMMARY PRODUCT INFORMATION:

Route of Administration	Dosage Form/ Strength	Clinically Relevant Nonmedicinal Ingredients
Intravenous	Vials 250 mg/15 mL	See Dosage Forms, Composition and Packaging

DESCRIPTION: ORENCIA (abatacept), a selective co-stimulation modulator, selectively modulates a key co-stimulatory signal required for full activation of T lymphocytes expressing CD28 (see Action and Clinical Pharmacology). It is a soluble fusion protein that consists of the extracellular domain of human cytotoxic T-lymphocyte-associated antigen 4 (CTLA-4) linked to the modified Fc (hinge, CH2, and CH3 domains) portion of human immunoglobulin G1. ORENCIA is produced by recombinant DNA technology in a mammalian cell expression system.

INDICATIONS AND CLINICAL USE: Adult Rheumatoid Arthritis (RA): ORENCIA (abatacept) is indicated for reducing signs and symptoms, inducing clinical responses, inhibiting the progression of structural damage, and improving physical function in adult patients with moderately to severely active rheumatoid arthritis who have had an inadequate response to one or more DMARDs or to TNF antagonists or to both.

ORENCIA may be used as monotherapy or in combination with DMARD therapy.

When used as first-line treatment in recently diagnosed patients who have not been previously treated with methotrexate (MTX), ORENCIA should be given in combination with MTX.

Juvenile Idiopathic Arthritis (JIA)/Juvenile Rheumatoid Arthritis (JRA): ORENCIA is indicated for reducing signs and symptoms of moderately to severely active polyarticular juvenile idiopathic arthritis/juvenile rheumatoid arthritis in pediatric patients 6 years of age and older who have had an inadequate response to one or more DMARDs, such as MTX. ORENCIA has not been studied in children less than 6 years of age.

CONTRAINDICATIONS: ORENCIA (abatacept) should not be administered to:

- Patients with known hypersensitivity to ORENCIA or any of its components.
- Patients with, or at risk of, sepsis syndrome, such as immunocompromised and HIV+ patients (see Warnings and Precautions, Infections).

WARNINGS AND PRECAUTIONS:

> **Serious Warnings and Precautions**
> Infections:
> - Treatment with ORENCIA should not be initiated in patients with active infections including chronic or localized infections.
> - Treatment with ORENCIA also should not be initiated in patients with chronic or latent infections.
> - Administration of ORENCIA should be discontinued if a patient develops a serious infection.
> - Physicians should exercise caution when considering the use of ORENCIA in patients with a history of recurrent infection or underlying conditions which may predispose them to infections, such as immunodeficiency disorders, or who have resided in regions where tuberculosis and histoplasmosis are endemic.
> - If active tuberculosis is diagnosed, ORENCIA therapy should not be initiated. If inactive ('latent') tuberculosis is diagnosed, treatment for latent tuberculosis should be started with anti-tuberculosis therapy before the initiation of ORENCIA.
> - Physicians should monitor patients receiving ORENCIA for signs and symptoms of active tuberculosis, including patients who tested negative for latent tuberculosis infection.

Combination with Biologic Rheumatoid Arthritis Therapy: Concurrent therapy with ORENCIA (abatacept) and a biologic RA agent is not recommended. While transitioning from biologic RA therapy to ORENCIA therapy, patients should be monitored for signs of infection. There is limited experience with the use of ORENCIA in combination with biologic RA agents (i.e., adalimumab, anakinra, etanercept, infliximab). In controlled clinical trials, compared to patients treated with biologic RA agents and placebo, patients with adult RA receiving combination biologic RA therapy with ORENCIA experienced an increase in overall infections (63.7% vs 43.3%) and serious infections (4.4% vs 1.5%). These studies did not provide sufficient data to complete a benefit and risk assessment of combination of ORENCIA with biologic rheumatoid arthritis agents. There is insufficient experience to assess the safety and efficacy of ORENCIA administered concurrently with anakinra, and therefore such use is not recommended.

Hypersensitivity: As with any other biologic RA therapy, patients should be monitored for allergic reactions. Such reactions have been observed with ORENCIA. In clinical trials with ORENCIA, patients were not pretreated to prevent hypersensitivity reactions. In patients treated with ORENCIA in controlled and open-label clinical trials, the events of hypersensitivity, anaphylaxis, and drug hypersensitivity were rarely reported. Other events potentially associated with drug hypersensitivity, such as hypotension, urticaria, and dyspnea, that occurred within 24 hours of ORENCIA infusion, were uncommon. Medications for the treatment of hypersensitivity reactions (e.g., acetaminophen, antihistamines, corticosteroids, and/or epinephrine) should be available for immediate use in the event of a reaction (see Adverse Reactions, Infusion-related Reactions).

Infections: Serious infections, including sepsis and pneumonia, have been reported in patients receiving ORENCIA. Some of these infections have been fatal. Many of the serious infections have occurred in patients on concomitant immunosuppressive therapy which in addition to their underlying disease, could further predispose them to infections.

Treatment with ORENCIA should not be initiated in patients with active systemic or localized infections. Treatment with ORENCIA also should not be initiated in patients with chronic or latent infections. Patients who develop a new infection while undergoing treatment with ORENCIA should be monitored closely. Administration of ORENCIA should be discontinued if a patient develops a serious infection. Physicians should exercise caution when considering the use of ORENCIA in patients with a history of recurrent infection or underlying conditions which may predispose them to infections, such as immunodeficiency disorders, or who have resided in regions where tuberculosis and histoplasmosis are endemic (see Adverse Reactions, Infections).

Prior to treating patients with therapies that modulate the immune system, including ORENCIA, it is appropriate to screen patients for tuberculosis. Should a patient test positive for tuberculosis screening, the patient should be treated in accordance with standard medical practice prior to therapy with ORENCIA.

Anti-rheumatic therapies have been associated with hepatitis B reactivation. Therefore, screening for viral hepatitis should be performed in accordance with published guidelines before starting therapy with ORENCIA. In clinical studies with ORENCIA, patients who screened positive for hepatitis were excluded from study.

In clinical trials in adult RA patients, the incidence of infections did not appear to increase in the open-label period compared to the double-blind period (see Adverse Reactions, Infections).

During the pediatric clinical trial, there were two cases of varicella and three cases of herpes simplex. All cases resolved appropriately without sequelae.

Blood Glucose Testing: The glucose dehydrogenase pyrroloquinolinequinone (GDH-PQQ) based glucose monitoring systems may react with the maltose present in ORENCIA, resulting in falsely elevated blood glucose readings on the day of infusion. Patients that require blood glucose monitoring should be advised to consider methods that do not react with maltose (see Drug Interactions, Drug-Laboratory Test Interactions).

Immunizations: Live vaccines should not be given concurrently with ORENCIA or within 3 months of discontinuation. No data are available on the effects of vaccinations in patients receiving ORENCIA. It is possible that ORENCIA may blunt the effectiveness of some immunizations. No data are available on the secondary transmission of infections by live vaccines to patients receiving ORENCIA.

It is recommended that JIA/JRA patients be brought up to date with all immunizations in agreement with current immunization guidelines prior to initiating ORENCIA therapy.

Use in Patients with Chronic Obstructive Pulmonary Disease (COPD): Adult COPD patients treated with ORENCIA developed adverse events more frequently than those treated with placebo, including COPD exacerbations, cough, rhonchi, and dyspnea. Use of ORENCIA in patients with rheumatoid arthritis and COPD should be undertaken with caution and such patients should be monitored for worsening of their respiratory status (see Adverse Reactions, Adverse Reactions in Adult Patients with COPD).

Information to Be Provided to the Patient: Patients should be provided with the Information for the Patient of this Product Monograph. Caution should be exercised in administering ORENCIA to patients with clinically important active infections and patients should be assessed accordingly prior to infusion.

Special Populations: Pregnant Women: There are no adequate and well-controlled studies in pregnant women. ORENCIA should not be administered to pregnant women unless the benefits outweigh the potential risks. Reproductive studies have been conducted with abatacept in mice, rats, and rabbits. Abatacept was shown to cross the placenta.

Pregnancy Registry: To monitor maternal-fetal outcomes of pregnant women exposed to ORENCIA, a pregnancy registry has been established. Healthcare professionals are encouraged to register patients by calling 1-877-311-8972.

Nursing Women: It is not known whether abatacept is excreted in human milk or absorbed systemically after ingestion. Because many drugs are excreted in human milk, and because of the potential for serious adverse reactions in nursing infants from ORENCIA, a decision has to be made on whether to discontinue nursing or to discontinue the medication, taking into account the importance of the medication to the mother.

Pediatrics: ORENCIA is indicated for reducing signs and symptoms of moderately to severely active polyarticular juvenile idiopathic arthritis/juvenile rheumatoid arthritis in pediatric patients 6 years of age and older who have had an inadequate response to one or more DMARDs, such as MTX. ORENCIA has not been studied in children <6 years of age.

The long-term effects of ORENCIA therapy on skeletal, behavioral, cognitive, sexual and immune maturation and development in children are unknown.

Geriatrics: A total of 323 patients 65 years of age or older, including 53 patients 75 years and older received ORENCIA in clinical trials. Similar efficacy was observed in these patients and younger patients. The frequency of serious infection and malignancy among ORENCIA-treated patients over age 65 was higher than for those under age 65. As there is a higher incidence of infections and malignancies in the elderly population in general, caution should be used when treating the elderly.

Malignancies: The potential role of ORENCIA in the development of malignancies and lymphomas in humans is unknown. The frequencies of malignancies in the placebo-controlled clinical trials in patients with adult RA were similar for ORENCIA and placebo treated patients (1.3% and 1.1% respectively). There were no studies conducted to date to evaluate the benefit and risk profile of ORENCIA in patients with existing malignancies or a history of lymphoma.

In clinical trials in adult RA patients, the incidence of malignant neoplasms did not appear to increase in the open-label period compared to the double-blind period (see Adverse Reactions, Malignancies).

ADVERSE REACTIONS: Adverse Drug Reaction Overview: In patients with adult RA, the most serious adverse reactions were serious infections and malignancies (see Adverse Reactions, Infections and Adverse Reactions, Malignancies).

The most commonly reported adverse events (occurring in ≥10% of adult RA patients treated with ORENCIA (abatacept)) were headache, upper respiratory tract infection, nasopharyngitis, and nausea.

In patients with adult RA, the adverse events most frequently resulting in clinical intervention (interruption or discontinuation of ORENCIA) were due to infection. The most frequently reported infections resulting in dose interruption were upper respiratory tract infection (1.0%), bronchitis (0.7%), and herpes zoster (0.7%). The most frequent infections resulting in discontinuation were pneumonia (0.2%), localized infection (0.2%), and bronchitis (0.1%).

Clinical Trial Adverse Drug Reactions in Adult RA: Because clinical trials are conducted under very specific conditions, the adverse reaction rates observed in the clinical trials may not reflect the rates observed in practice and should not be compared to the rates in the clinical trials of another drug. Adverse drug reaction information from clinical trials is useful for identifying drug-related adverse events and for approximating rates.

The data described herein reflect exposure to ORENCIA in patients with active RA in placebo-controlled studies (1955 patients with ORENCIA, 989 with placebo). The studies had either a double-blind, placebo-controlled period of 6 months (258 patients with ORENCIA, 133 with placebo) or 1 year (1697 patients with ORENCIA, 856 with placebo). A subset of these patients received concomitant biologic RA therapy, such as a TNF blocking agent (204 patients with ORENCIA, 134 with placebo).

Table 1 lists the adverse drug reactions (ADRs—adverse events at least possibly causally-related to treatment) occurring in ≥1% of patients treated with ORENCIA during placebo-controlled double-blind rheumatoid arthritis studies.

Table 1: ORENCIA

Adverse Drug Reactions (ADRs) Occurring in ≥1% of Patients Treated with ORENCIA During Placebo-Controlled Double-Blind Rheumatoid Arthritis Studies

Related Adverse Event (Preferred Term)	ORENCIA[c] n=1955[a] %	Placebo[c] n=989[b] %
Gastrointestinal Disorders		
Nausea	6.0	5.1
Diarrhea	3.5	3.0
Dyspepsia	1.3	0.9
Abdominal Pain	1.2	0.9
Vomiting	1.2	1.4
General Disorders and Administration Site Conditions		
Fatigue	3.5	3.2
Asthenia	1.5	1.3
Pyrexia	1.4	1.5
Infections and Infestations		
Upper Respiratory Tract Infection	4.8	3.9
Nasopharyngitis	3.2	1.9
Sinusitis	2.8	2.7
Bronchitis	2.2	1.6
Urinary Tract Infection	2.1	1.3
Influenza	1.6	1.7
Pharyngitis	1.3	1.1
Herpes simplex	1.2	0.5
Herpes zoster	1.0	1.1
Rhinitis	1.0	0.4
Investigations		
Blood Pressure Increased	1.5	0.5
Musculoskeletal, Connective Tissues and Bone Disorders		
Myalgia	1.0	1.0
Nervous System Disorders		
Headache	10.0	6.3
Dizziness	4.6	3.5
Somnolence	1.9	2.0
Respiratory, Thoracic and Mediastinal Disorders		
Cough	2.4	1.0
Pharyngolaryngeal Pain	1.0	1.1
Skin and Subcutaneous Tissue Disorders		
Rash	2.1	1.6
Vascular Disorders		
Flushing	1.0	0.5
Hypertension	2.1	1.1

[a] Includes 204 patients on concomitant biologic RA agents (adalimumab, anakinra, etanercept, or infliximab).
[b] Includes 134 patients on concomitant biologic RA agents (adalimumab, anakinra, etanercept, or infliximab).
[c] All patients were on concomitant DMARDs.

Less Common Clinical Trial Adverse Drug Reactions (<1.0%): ADRs reported in less than 1% of patients receiving ORENCIA in the double-blind clinical trials (n=1955) and not listed in Table 1 are listed below by body system.

Blood and Lymphatic System Disorders: leukopenia, anaemia, neutropenia, thrombocytopenia, lymphadenopathy, eosinophilia, lymphopenia, thrombocythaemia, bone marrow depression, iron deficiency anaemia, lymph node pain, lymphocytosis, monocytopenia.

Cardiac Disorders: palpitations, tachycardia, bradycardia, sinus bradycardia, arrhythmia, atrioventricular block first degree, cyanosis, pericarditis, sinus tachycardia, supraventricular extrasystoles, ventricular extrasystoles.

Ear and Labyrinth Disorders: vertigo, tinnitus, vertigo positional, hypoacusis, motion sickness, deafness bilateral, ear congestion, eustachian tube obstruction, sensation of pressure in ear.

Endocrine Disorders: goitre.

Eye Disorders: conjunctivitis, dry eye, visual acuity reduced, lacrimation increased, blepharitis, eye irritation, conjunctivitis allergic, vision blurred, visual disturbance, eye pruritus, blindness unilateral, conjunctival haemorrhage, conjunctival hyperaemia, corneal ulcer, eye haemorrhage, eye inflammation, eye pain, eye redness, eye swelling, keratitis, madarosis, photophobia, retinal vein occlusion, retinopathy hypertensive, scotoma.

Gastrointestinal Disorders: mouth ulceration, abdominal pain upper, aphthous stomatitis, constipation, stomatitis, gastritis, tongue ulceration, loose stools, dry mouth, haemorrhoids, abdominal tenderness, gingivitis, gastroesophageal reflux disease, toothache, aptyalism, abdominal distension, abnormal faeces, diverticulum, epigastric discomfort, oral discomfort, tongue blistering, dysphagia, stomach discomfort, colitis, glossitis, irritable bowel syndrome, oral pain, duodenitis, enteritis, faeces discoloured, frequent bowel movements, gastrointestinal disorder, gastroesophagitis, gingival bleeding, gingival ulceration, glossodynia, infrequent bowel movements, intestinal haemorrhage, lip pain, odynophagia, oral mucosal blistering, pancreatic mass, pancreatitis, parotid gland enlargement, proctalgia, pruritus ani, salivary gland enlargement, salivary hypersecretion, steatorrhoea, upper gastrointestinal haemorrhage.

General Disorders and Administration Site Conditions: chills, oedema peripheral, malaise, influenza like illness, chest pain, chest discomfort, pain, injection site reaction, feeling cold, infusion site pain, injection site pain, nodule, injection site erythema, mucosal inflammation, non-cardiac chest pain, feeling hot, infusion site burning, infusion site swelling, injection site pruritus, inflammation, infusion site rash, infusion site reaction, local swelling, inflammation localised, infusion related reaction, injection site haemorrhage, sensation of foreign body, application site pain, facial pain, generalised oedema, impaired healing, infusion site inflammation, injection site hypersensitivity, injection site phlebitis, injection site thrombosis, mucosal ulceration, oedema, pitting oedema, sluggishness, ulcer.

Hepatobiliary Disorders: hepatitis.

Immune System Disorders: rheumatoid nodule, hypersensitivity, drug hypersensitivity, hypogammaglobulinaemia, rheumatoid vasculitis.

Infections and Infestations: pneumonia, fungal skin infection, bronchitis acute, ear infection, respiratory tract infection, cellulitis, laryngitis, localised infection, lower respiratory tract infection, gastroenteritis, fungal infection, cystitis, vaginal mycosis, tooth infection, folliculitis, herpes virus infection, viral upper respiratory tract infection, infected skin ulcer, onychomycosis, tracheitis, tooth abscess, skin infection, tinea versicolour, furuncle, diverticulitis, gingival infection, body tinea, oral fungal infection, paronychia, tonsillitis, hordeolum, pharyngitis bacterial, postoperative infection, soft tissue infection, bronchopneumonia, dental caries, eye infection, genital infection fungal, nail infection, pneumonia bacterial, pulpitis dental, pyelonephritis, pyelonephritis acute, tracheobronchitis, urinary tract infection bacterial, viral infection, vaginal candidiasis, oral candidiasis, candidiasis, erysipelas, pharyngotonsillitis, vaginitis, bacterial infection, conjunctivitis viral, gastroenteritis viral, oropharyngeal candidiasis, otitis media, subcutaneous abscess, tuberculosis, wound infection, abscess, abscess intestinal, abscess oral, acute sinusitis, arthritis bacterial, bacteraemia, blister infected, borrelia infection, bronchopulmonary aspergillosis, bursitis infective, cellulitis staphylococcal, cervicitis, conjunctivitis bacterial, ear lobe infection, empyema, enterobiasis, escherichia urinary tract infection, eyelid infection, gastrointestinal infection, gingival abscess, groin abscess, hepatitis E, infected bunion, infection, labyrinthitis, laryngopharyngitis, laryngotracheo bronchitis, lobar pneumonia, mycetoma mycotic, oral pustule, papilloma viral infection, peridiverticular abscess, pharyngitis streptococcal, pneumonia haemophilus, pneumonia influenzal, rash pustular, respiratory tract infection bacterial, sepsis, skin bacterial infection, streptococcal sepsis, superinfection, urosepsis, vaginal infection, vaginitis bacterial, varicella, wound infection staphylococcal.

Injury, Poisoning and Procedural Complications: contusion, fall, excoriation, joint dislocation, compression fracture, injury asphyxiation, joint injury, limb traumatic amputation, neck injury.

Investigations: alanine aminotransferase increased, blood pressure decreased, weight increased, aspartate aminotransferase increased, hepatic enzyme increased; gamma-glutamyltransferase increased, white blood cell count decreased, blood pressure diastolic increased, antinuclear antibody positive, blood pressure diastolic decreased, blood pressure systolic decreased, weight decreased, liver function test abnormal, haemoglobin decreased, white blood cell count increased, blood pressure systolic increased, body temperature increased, heart rate increased, mean cell volume increased, transaminases increased, DNA antibody positive, blood creatinine increased, electrocardiogram T wave abnormal, bacterial culture positive, blood glucose increased, blood immunoglobulin G decreased, blood immunoglobulin M decreased, blood iron decreased, blood phosphorus increased, blood potassium increased, blood sodium decreased, electrocardiogram repolarisation abnormality, haematocrit decreased, heart rate irregular, platelet count decreased, platelet count increased, red blood cell count decreased, respiratory rate increased, white blood cells urine positive.

Metabolism and Nutrition Disorders: fluid retention, increased appetite, anorexia, decreased appetite, dehydration, glucose tolerance impaired, hyperlipidaemia, hyperuricaemia, hypoalbuminaemia, hypocalcaemia.

Musculoskeletal and Connective Tissue Disorders: pain in extremity, arthralgia, back pain, rheumatoid arthritis, muscle cramp, musculoskeletal pain, bone pain, musculoskeletal stiffness, neck pain, flank pain, muscle spasms, muscular weakness, nodule on extremity, bursitis, musculoskeletal chest pain, myofascial pain syndrome, night cramps, chest wall pain, fibromyalgia, joint swelling, lupus-like syndrome, muscle contracture, muscle fatigue, myositis, neck mass, pain in jaw, sensation of heaviness, systemic lupus erythematosus, tendonitis.

Neoplasms Benign, Malignant and Unspecified (incl cysts and polyps): skin papilloma, basal cell carcinoma, fibroadenoma of breast, intraductal papilloma of breast, lung neoplasm malignant, lymphoma, renal cell carcinoma stage unspecified, seborrhoeic keratosis, squamous cell carcinoma of skin.

Nervous System Disorders: paraesthesia, dysgeusia, migraine, tremor, hypoaesthesia, lethargy, hypersomnia, dyskinesia, paraesthesia oral, restless legs syndrome, syncope vasovagal, amnesia, anosmia, facial palsy, reflex sympathetic dystrophy, complex partial seizures, disturbance in attention, formication, hyperaesthesia, loss of consciousness, migraine with aura, neuralgia, neuromyopathy, neuropathy peripheral, sedation, sensory disturbance, syncope, tension headache.

Psychiatric Disorders: insomnia, depression, anxiety, irritability, nervousness, euphoric mood, agitation, depressed mood, elevated mood, listless, nightmare, restlessness, screaming, sleep disorder.

Renal and Urinary Disorders: dysuria, polyuria, pollakiuria, renal colic, haematuria, proteinuria, pyuria, renal failure, urinary incontinence.

Reproductive System and Breast Disorders: amenorrhoea, menorrhagia, metrorrhagia, breast pain, genital discharge, breast cyst, breast mass, genital pruritus female, menstruation irregular, vaginal discharge, breast hyperplasia, erectile dysfunction, menopausal symptoms, oligomenorrhoea, pelvic pain.

Respiratory, Thoracic and Mediastinal Disorders: dyspnoea, nasal congestion, sinus congestion, throat irritation, epistaxis, productive cough, rhinorrhoea, rhinitis allergic, wheezing, chronic obstructive airways disease exacerbated, crackles lung, pleural effusion, asthma, bronchospasm, hoarseness, lung crepitation, respiratory tract congestion, throat tightness, rales, allergic bronchitis, nasal discomfort, paranasal sinus hypersecretion, pleurisy, rhonchi, sneezing, bronchial polyp, chronic obstructive airways disease, dry throat, dyspnoea exacerbated, haemoptysis, nasal ulcer, pulmonary embolism, respiratory failure, rhinitis seasonal, sinus pain, upper respiratory tract congestion.

Skin and Subcutaneous Tissue Disorders: pruritus, alopecia, hyperhidrosis, erythema, urticaria, dermatitis, dry skin, ecchymosis, dermatitis allergic, eczema, rash macular, skin lesion, increased tendency to bruise, rash erythematous, acne, dermal cyst, psoriasis, rash maculo-papular, dermatosis, photosensitivity reaction, rash vesicular, swelling face, actinic keratosis, erythema multiforme, rash papular, skin burning sensation, pruritus generalised, skin ulcer, face oedema, night sweats, cold sweat, hair texture abnormal, hyperkeratosis, leukocytoclastic vasculitis, purpura, rash scaly, dermatitis acneiform, dermatitis atopic, dermatitis bullous, dermatitis psoriasiform, dyshidrosis, ephelides, exanthem, localised exfoliation, nail disorder, onychorrhexis, panniculitis, pigmentation disorder, pityriasis, pyoderma, rash pruritic, scar, seborrhoea, skin desquamation, skin discolouration, skin induration, skin nodule, vasculitic rash.

Surgical and Medical Procedures: hormone replacement therapy.

Vascular Disorders: hypotension, hot flush, blood pressure inadequately controlled, systolic hypertension, vasculitis, vein pain, capillary fragility, deep vein thrombosis, infarction, peripheral coldness, peripheral ischaemia, petechiae, phlebitis, vascular rupture, vasculitis necrotising.

Infections: In placebo-controlled trials, infections were reported in 53.8% of ORENCIA treated patients and 48.3% of placebo patients. Serious infections were reported in 3.0% of patients treated with ORENCIA and 1.9% of patients treated with placebo.

Serious infections reported (≥0.2%) with ORENCIA versus placebo were pneumonia (0.5% vs 0.5%), cellulitis (0.3% vs 0.2%), urinary tract infection (0.2% vs 0.1%), bronchitis (0.2% vs 0%), diverticulitis (0.2% vs 0%), and acute pyelonephritis (0.2% vs 0%) (see Warnings and Precautions, Infections).

Other infections reported with a higher frequency (>0.5%) with ORENCIA compared to placebo, were rhinitis (2.7% vs 1.7%), herpes simplex (1.9% vs 1.0%) and pneumonia (1.7% vs 0.8%).

In controlled clinical studies of 1955 ORENCIA patients and 989 placebo patients there were two reported cases of tuberculosis, one each in the ORENCIA and placebo groups. These cases were not confirmed by smear, stain or culture.

During continued extensions of open-label clinical trials in adult RA patients (combined double-blind and open-label mean exposure 22.7-38.8 months), the incidence of infections did not appear to increase compared to the double-blind period (see Warnings and Precautions, Infections).

Malignancies: In placebo-controlled clinical trials (1688 patient-years), the frequency of malignancies was similar in ORENCIA and placebo treated patients (1.3% and 1.1%, respectively). However, more cases of lung cancer were observed in ORENCIA-treated patients (4, 0.2%) than placebo-treated patients (0). Other malignancies included skin, breast, bladder, lymphoma, ovarian, prostate, and thyroid cancers.

In double-blind and open-label clinical trials in 4149 patients treated with ORENCIA during 10,365 patient-years, the incidence rate of malignancy was 1.41 per 100 patient-years. The incidence rates per 100 patient-years were 0.74 for non-melanomatous skin cancer, 0.59 for solid malignancies and 0.12 for hematologic malignancies. The most frequently reported solid organ cancer was lung cancer (0.16 per 100 patient-years), and the most common hematologic malignancy was lymphoma (0.07 per 100 patient-years). The incidence rate did not increase for malignancies overall, by major type (non-melanomatous skin cancer, solid tumors, and hematologic malignancies), or for individual tumor types in the double-blind and open label period compared to the double-blind experience. The number incidence rate of observed malignancies was consistent with that expected in an age- and gender-matched rheumatoid arthritis population.

Compared with the general population based on the U.S. Surveillance, Epidemiology, and End Results Database, patients with rheumatoid arthritis are at a higher risk for the development of lymphoma. The impact of ORENCIA on malignancies in humans is unknown.

During continued extensions of open-label clinical trials in adult RA patients (combined double-blind and open-label mean exposure 22.7-38.8 months), the incidence of malignant neoplasms did not appear to increase compared to the double-blind period (see Warnings and Precautions, Malignancies).

Infusion-related Reactions: In the clinical studies with ORENCIA, pre-medication to prevent hypersensitivity was not required. Acute infusion-related events (reported within 1 hour of the start of the infusion) in the phase III studies (Studies AIM, ATTAIN, ASSURE) were more common in the ORENCIA-treated patients than the placebo patients (8.9% vs 5.5%, respectively). The most frequently reported events (>1.0%) with ORENCIA vs placebo were dizziness (2.1% vs 1.3%), headache (1.8% vs 1.2%), and hypertension (1.2% vs 0.4%). In the AGREE trial, acute infusion-related events were also more common in the ORENCIA-treated patients than the placebo patients (6.3% in ABA+MTX vs. 2% placebo+MTX).

Acute infusion-related events that were reported in >0.1% and ≤1% of patients treated with ORENCIA included cardiopulmonary symptoms such as hypotension, blood pressure decrease, blood pressure increase, and dyspnea; other symptoms included nausea, flushing, urticaria, cough, hypersensitivity, pruritus, rash, and wheezing. Most of these reactions were mild to moderate.

In patients treated with ORENCIA in controlled and open-label clinical trials, the events of hypersensitivity, anaphylaxis, and drug hypersensitivity were rarely reported. Other events potentially associated with drug hypersensitivity, such as hypotension, urticaria, and dyspnea, that occurred within 24 hours of ORENCIA infusion, were uncommon. (See Warnings and Precautions, Hypersensitivity.)

A small proportion of patients in both the ORENCIA and placebo groups discontinued due to an acute infusion-related event (0.4% for ORENCIA, 0.2% for placebo).

Autoantibodies: In controlled trials, 9.7% of ORENCIA treated patients and 10.8% of placebo patients that had negative antinuclear antibody titers at baseline developed positive titers at 12 months. Newly detected anti-dsDNA antibodies were observed in 2.7% of ORENCIA treated patients and 4.7% of placebo patients.

Immunogenicity: Patients with rheumatoid arthritis were tested for antibodies to ORENCIA at multiple time points. Antibodies to the entire abatacept molecule or to the CTLA-4 portion of abatacept were measured. Binding antibodies were detected in 2.8 % of 2237 patients tested over a period of up to 3 years. No apparent correlation of antibody development to clinical response or adverse events was observed, but due to the small number of patients across studies who developed an immune response, conclusions concerning the impact of immunogenicity on safety and efficacy cannot be made.

Adverse Reactions in Adult Patients with COPD: In the ASSURE study, there were 37 patients with chronic obstructive pulmonary disease (COPD) who were treated with ORENCIA and 17 COPD patients who were treated with placebo. The COPD patients treated with ORENCIA developed adverse events more frequently than those treated with placebo (97% vs 88%, respectively). Respiratory disorders occurred more frequently in ORENCIA-treated patients compared to placebo-treated patients (43% vs 24%, respectively) including COPD exacerbation, cough, rhonchi, and dyspnea. A greater percentage of ORENCIA-treated patients developed a serious adverse event compared to placebo-treated patients (27% vs 6%), including COPD exacerbation (3 of 37 patients [8%]) and pneumonia (1 of 37 patients [3%]).

Clinical Trial Adverse Drug Reactions in MTX-Naive Patients: The AGREE (IM101023) study was an active-controlled clinical trial in MTX-naive patients. Subjects were randomized to receive abatacept or placebo for the first 12 months of treatment. In addition both groups received MTX. The adverse reaction profile observed in patients receiving ORENCIA plus MTX was generally comparable to that in patients receiving MTX alone except for the acute infusion-related events (see Infusion-related Reactions). Among MTX-naïve patients treated in AGREE, deaths occurred in 2 (0.8%) subjects in the ORENCIA plus MTX group and 4 (1.6%) subjects in the Placebo plus MTX group.

Table 2 lists the adverse drug reactions (ADRs - adverse events at least possibly causally-related to treatment) occurring in ≥1% of patients treated with ORENCIA+MTX in AGREE (IM101023).

Table 2: ORENCIA

Adverse Drug Reactions (ADRs) Occurring in ≥1% of Patients in the ORENCIA+MTX in AGREE (IM101023)

Related Adverse Event (Preferred Term)	ORENCIA+MTX n = 256 %	Placebo+MTX n = 253 %
Infections and Infestations		
Bronchitis	3.9	1.2
Nasopharyngitis	3.1	2.0
Urinary Tract Infection	2.3	2.8
Upper Respiratory Tract Infection	2.3	2.4
Oral Herpes	2.0	1.2
Pharyngitis	2.0	0.4
Influenza	1.6	2.8
Herpes zoster	1.2	1.2
Gastrointestinal Disorders		
Nausea	4.3	4.3
Mouth Ulceration	1.6	0.4
Diarrhoea	1.2	2.4
Nervous System Disorders		
Headache	3.5	3.6
Dizziness	3.5	2.4
Investigations		
Alanine Aminotransferase Increased	3.1	2.4
Aspartate aminotransferase Increased	2.0	1.6
Weight Increased	1.2	0
Respiratory, Thoracic and Mediastinal Disorders		
Cough	2.7	1.6
General Disorders and Administration Site Conditions		
Fatigue	1.2	1.2
Vascular Disorders		
Hypertension	1.2	1.6

(cont'd)

Table 2: ORENCIA *(cont'd)*

Less common Clinical Trial Adverse Drug Reactions (<1.0%): ADRs reported in less than 1% of patients receiving ORENCIA+MTX in the AGREE Trial and not listed in Table 2 are listed below by body system.

Blood and Lymphatic System Disorders: anaemia.

Ear and Labyrinth Disorders: vertigo.

Eye Disorders: eye irritation, presbyopia.

Gastrointestinal Disorders: vomiting, abdominal pain upper, dry mouth, dyspepsia, abdominal pain, gastritis, gastrointestinal haemorrhage, gastrointestinal pain, gingival ulceration, lip dry.

General Disorders and Administration Site Conditions: malaise, chest pain, asthenia, chest discomfort, axillary pain, chills, feeling hot, infusion related reaction, infusion site erythema, infusion site pain, sudden death.

Hepatobiliary Disorders: hepatic function abnormal.

Immune System Disorders: hypersensitivity.

Infections and Infestations: gastroenteritis, tooth abscess, pneumonia, respiratory tract infection, sinusitis, tonsillitis, viral upper respiratory tract infection, acariasis, furuncle, genital herpes, tinea pedis, acarodermatitis, bacterial infection, bronchopneumonia, cystitis, ear infection, fungal rash, laryngitis, lung infection pseudomonal, rhinitis, sepsis, soft tissue infection, tinea versicolour, vaginal infection.

Injury, Poisoning and Procedural Complications: contusion.

Investigations: transaminases increased, gamma-glutamyltransferase increased, blood alkaline phosphatase increased, blood pressure increased.

Metabolism and Nutrition Disorders: diabetes mellitus.

Musculoskeletal and Connective Tissue Disorders: back pain, joint swelling, ligament disorder, musculoskeletal stiffness, pain in extremity, systemic lupus erythematosus.

Neoplasms Benign, Malignant and Unspecified (incl cysts and polyps): lung neoplasm, skin papilloma.

Nervous System Disorders: dysgeusia, paraesthesia.

Psychiatric Disorders: depression, insomnia, nervousness.

Reproductive System and Breast Disorders: breast mass, breast pain.

Respiratory, Thoracic and Mediastinal Disorders: nasal congestion, pharyngolaryngeal pain, rhinorrhoea, sinus congestion, dyspnoea exertional, nasal discomfort, nasal dryness.

Skin and Subcutaneous Tissue Disorders: rash, alopecia, urticaria, acne, eczema, nail dystrophy, pruritus, psoriasis, skin lesion.

Vascular Disorders: flushing, hyperaemia, hypotension.

Clinical Trial Adverse Drug Reactions in JIA/JRA: In general, the adverse events in pediatric and adolescent patients were similar in frequency and type to those seen in adult patients, and the majority of the adverse events were mild or moderate in intensity (see Warnings and Precautions and Adverse Reactions, Clinical Trial Adverse Drug Reactions in Adult RA).

Overall frequency of adverse events in the 4-month, lead-in, open-label period was 70.0%; infections occurred at a frequency of 35.8%. The most common infections were upper respiratory tract infection and nasopharyngitis. The types of infections reported in JIA/JRA patients were generally mild or moderate, resolved without sequelae, and were consistent with those commonly seen in outpatient pediatric and adolescent populations. Other events that occurred at a prevalence of at least 5% were headache, nausea, diarrhea, cough, pyrexia, and abdominal pain.

A total of 6 serious adverse events (acute lymphocytic leukemia, ovarian cyst, varicella infection, disease flare [2], and joint wear) were reported in 190 JIA/JRA patients aged 6 to 17 years treated during the 4-month, lead-in, open-label period.

For the 122 patients who responded in the lead-in period and entered the placebo-controlled, 6-month, withdrawal phase, there were no serious adverse events in 60 ORENCIA-treated patients and 3 serious adverse events in 2 of the 62 placebo-treated patients (hematoma in one patient, varicella and encephalitis in the other).

Upon continued treatment in the open-label extension period, the types of adverse events were consistent with those observed in the double-blind phase, and were similar in frequency and type to those seen in adult patients except for a single patient diagnosed with multiple sclerosis while on open-label treatment. The majority of the adverse events were mild or moderate in intensity.

Table 3 lists the adverse drug reactions (ADRs—adverse events at least possibly causally-related to treatment) occurring in ≥1% of pediatric patients receiving ORENCIA in period A (open label, abatacept lead-in portion) of the three part study conducted in children with polyarticular JIA.

Table 3: ORENCIA

Adverse Drug Reactions (ADRs) Occurring in ≥1% of Patients Treated with ORENCIA During Period A (Open label, abatacept lead-in portion) of the Juvenile Idiopathic Arthritis Study

Related Adverse Event (Preferred Term)	ORENCIA n=190 %
Blood and Lymphatic System Disorders	
Leukopenia	1.6
Gastrointestinal Disorders	
Nausea	2.1
Abdominal Pain	1.1
Aphthous Stomatitis	1.1

(cont'd)

Table 3: ORENCIA *(cont'd)*

Adverse Drug Reactions (ADRs) Occurring in ≥1% of Patients Treated with ORENCIA During Period A (Open label, abatacept lead-in portion) of the Juvenile Idiopathic Arthritis Study

Related Adverse Event (Preferred Term)	ORENCIA n=190 %
Diarrhea	1.1
Mouth Ulceration	1.1
Vomiting	1.1
General Disorders and Administration Site Conditions	
Asthenia	1.1
Fatigue	1.1
Pyrexia	1.1
Infections and Infestations	
Sinusitis	2.1
Upper respiratory tract infection	1.6
Nasopharyngitis	1.1
Acute otitis media	1.1
Rhinitis	1.1
Nervous System Disorders	
Headache	5.3
Dizziness	2.6
Renal and Urinary Disorders	
Hematuria	1.1
Skin and Subcutaneous Tissue Disorders	
Pruritus	1.1
Rash	1.1
Vascular Disorders	
Flushing	1.1

Table 4 lists the adverse drug reactions (ADRs—adverse events at least possibly causally-related to treatment) occurring in ≥1% of pediatric patients receiving ORENCIA in period B (double-blind phase) of the three part study conducted in children with polyarticular JIA.

Table 4: ORENCIA

Adverse Drug Reactions (ADRs) Occurring in ≥1% of Patients Treated with ORENCIA During Period B (Double-blind, placebo-controlled portion) of the Juvenile Idiopathic Arthritis Study

Related Adverse Event (Preferred Term)	ORENCIA n=60 %	Placebo n=62 %
Blood and Lymphatic System Disorders		
Leukopenia	0	3.2
Eosinophillia	0	1.6
Neutropenia	0	1.6
Gastrointestinal Disorders		
Abdominal Pain	1.7	1.6
Nausea	1.7	1.6
Aphthous Stomatitis	1.7	0
Gingival Hyperplasia	0	1.6
General Disorders and Administration Site Conditions		
Pyrexia	0	1.6
Infections and Infestations		
Sinusitis	1.7	3.2
Influenza	1.7	1.6
Rhinitis	1.7	1.6
Tinea versicolor	1.7	1.6
Upper respiratory tract infection	1.7	1.6
Bacteriuria	1.7	0
Otitis externa	1.7	0
Acute otitis media	0	1.6
Skin candida	0	1.6
Varicella	0	1.6
Neoplasms Benign, Malignant and Unspecified (Including Cysts and Polyps)		
Skin papilloma	0	1.6
Reproductive System and Breast Disorders		
Vaginal discharge	0	1.6
Nervous System Disorders		
Headache	1.7	1.6
Encephalitis	0	1.6
Renal and Urinary Disorders		
Leukocyturia	1.7	0
Skin and Subcutaneous Tissue Disorders		
Pityriasis	1.7	0
Skin lesion	1.7	0
Atopic dermatitis	0	1.6
Eczema	0	1.6
Vascular Disorders		
Hypotension	1.7	0

Table 5 lists the adverse drug reactions (ADRs—adverse events at least possibly causally-related to treatment) occurring in ≥1% of pediatric patients receiving ORENCIA in period C (open label extension phase) of the three part study conducted in children with polyarticular JIA.

Table 5: ORENCIA

Adverse Drug Reactions (ADRs) Occurring in ≥1% of Patients Treated with ORENCIA During Open Label Period (Period) C of the Juvenile Idiopathic Arthritis Study

Related Adverse Event (Preferred Term)	ORENCIA n=153 %
Blood and Lymphatic System Disorders	
Eosinophilia	3.9
Leukopenia	2.6
Eye Disorders	
Conjunctivitis	1.3
Gastrointestinal Disorders	
Abdominal Pain	2.0
Nausea	2.0
Vomiting	1.3
General Disorders and Administration Site Conditions	
Infusion related reaction	1.3
Infections and Infestations	
Upper respiratory tract infection	5.9
Sinusitis	3.3
Rhinitis	2.0
Bacteriuria	1.3
Herpes simplex	1.3
Otitis media	1.3
Tonsillitis	1.3

(cont'd)

Table 5: ORENCIA *(cont'd)*

Adverse Drug Reactions (ADRs) Occurring in ≥1% of Patients Treated with ORENCIA During Open Label Period (Period) C of the Juvenile Idiopathic Arthritis Study

Related Adverse Event (Preferred Term)	ORENCIA n=153 %
Vulvovaginitis	1.3
Nervous System Disorders	
Dizziness	1.3
Renal and Urinary Disorders	
Hematuria	1.3
Respiratory, Thoracic and Mediastinal Disorders	
Cough	2.6
Pharyngolaryngeal Pain	1.3
Skin and Subcutaneous Tissue Disorders	
Skin lesion	1.3
Urticaria	1.3

Less Common Clinical Trial Adverse Reactions (<1%): In Periods A and C of the pediatric trial, the list of less common Adverse Drug Reactions (<1 %) are represented by no more than a single case (by Phase). In the double-blind Period B, where a single ADR case yields an incidence of 1.7%, no ADR with a frequency of less than 1% was reported.

ADRs reported in less than 1% of patients receiving ORENCIA in open-label Phases A and C of the pediatric clinical trial and not listed in Table 3 and Table 5 are listed below by body system.

Blood and Lymphatic System Disorders: anaemia, lymphopenia, monocytosis.

Gastrointestinal Disorders: abdominal discomfort, abdominal pain upper, gastritis, intestinal villi atrophy, stomach discomfort.

General Disorders and Administration Site Conditions: chest pain, chills, influenza like illness, infusion site pain, injection site duration, injection site pain, malaise, pain.

Infections and Infestations: body tinea, bronchitis, bronchitis acute, fungal skin infection, furuncle, gastroenteritis, gastroenteritis viral, giardiasis, helicobacter infection, influenza, nail infection, otitis externa, parasitic infection intestinal, paronychia, pharyngitis, pharyngotonsillitis, staphylococcal infection, tinea cruris, tooth abscess, tracheobronchitis, urinary tract infection, varicella, viral infection.

Immune System Disorders: hypersensitivity.

Injury, Poisoning and Procedural Complications: seroma.

Investigations: alanine aminotransferase increased, antinuclear antibody positive, DNA antibody positive, white blood cell count decreased.

Musculoskeletal and Connective Tissue Disorders: arthralgia, joint swelling, nodule on extremity.

Neoplasms Benign, Malignant and Unspecified (Including Cysts and Polyps): skin papilloma.

Nervous System Disorders: tremor.

Renal and Urinary Disorders: leukocyturia, proteinuria.

Reproductive System and Breast Disorders: breast swelling, breast tenderness, genital discharge, vaginal discharge.

Skin and Subcutaneous Tissue Disorders: ecchymosis, eczema, erythema elevatum diutinum, ingrowing nail, rash macular, rash papular, skin hypopigmentation, vitiligo, yellow skin.

Vascular Disorders: orthostatic hypotension, pallor.

Infections: Adverse events of infections were reported in 36% of patients in the 4-month, lead-in, open-label period. The most common infections were upper respiratory tract infections [14 (7.4%)] and nasopharyngitis [11 (5.8%)]. Other than upper respiratory tract infections and nasopharyngitis, few infectious adverse events were reported. No pneumonias or opportunistic infections were observed.

During the double-blind phase, adverse events of infections were reported in the abatacept and placebo groups [45% and 44%]; influenza 5 [8.3%] vs 4 [6.5%], bacteriuria 4 [6.7%] vs 0 [0%], nasopharyngitis 4 [6.7%] vs 3 [4.8%], and upper respiratory tract infections 4 [6.7%] vs 5 [8.1%], were the most frequently reported events.

Infusion-related Reactions: In the open-label lead-in phase of the study, eight (4.2%) patients experienced acute infusional adverse events; all but one was mild in intensity and none was serious. Most infusional adverse events were reported as single events in one patient each with no recurrences; headache and dizziness occurred in four and two patients, respectively. During the double-blind phase, acute infusional adverse events were reported in 1.7% and 3.2% of the abatacept and placebo groups, respectively; all were either mild or moderate in intensity and none were serious.

Autoantibodies: In Period A of the pediatric clinical trial, 10.6% of ORENCIA treated patients that had negative antinuclear antibody titers at baseline had positive titers at Day 113. In Period B, 5.9% of ORENCIA treated patients and 4.0% of placebo patients that had negative antinuclear antibody titers at baseline had positive titers at Day 169.

In Period A, newly detected anti-dsDNA antibodies were observed in 6.2% of ORENCIA treated patients at Day 113. In Period B, newly detected anti-dsDNA antibodies were observed in 2.3% of ORENCIA treated patients and 0% of placebo patients at Day 169.

Immunogenicity : Antibodies directed against the entire abatacept molecule or to the CTLA-4 portion of abatacept were assessed by ELISA assays in JIA/JRA patients following repeated treatment with ORENCIA throughout the open-label period. For patients who were withdrawn from therapy for up to 6 months during the double-blind period, the rate of antibody formation to the CTLA-4 portion of the molecule was 40.7% (22/54), while for those who remained on therapy the rate was 13.0% (7/54).

The long-term immunogenicity of ORENCIA is unknown.

Malignancies: A single case of acute lymphocytic leukemia was reported in the pediatric trial. No other malignancies were reported.

DRUG INTERACTIONS: Formal drug interaction studies have not been conducted with ORENCIA (abatacept). However, population pharmacokinetic analyses revealed that MTX, non steroidal anti-inflammatory drugs (NSAIDs), corticosteroids, and TNF blocking agents did not influence abatacept clearance. The majority of patients received one or more of the following concomitant medications with ORENCIA: MTX, NSAIDs, corticosteroids, TNF blocking agents, azathioprine, chloroquine, gold, hydroxychloroquine, leflunomide, sulfasalazine, and anakinra.

Drug-Laboratory Test Interactions: Blood Glucose Testing: Parenteral drug products containing maltose can interfere with the readings of blood glucose monitors that use test strips with glucose dehydrogenase pyrroloquinolinequinone (GDH-PQQ). The GDH-PQQ based glucose monitoring systems may react with the maltose present in ORENCIA, resulting in falsely elevated blood glucose readings on the day of infusion. When receiving ORENCIA, patients that require blood glucose monitoring should be advised to consider methods that do not react with maltose, such as those based on glucose dehydrogenase nicotine adenine dinucleotide (GDH-NAD), glucose oxidase, or glucose hexokinase test methods (see Warnings and Precautions, Blood Glucose Testing).

DOSAGE AND ADMINISTRATION: Adult Rheumatoid Arthritis: For adult patients with RA, ORENCIA (abatacept) should be administered as a 30-minute intravenous infusion utilizing the weight range-based dosing specified in Table 6. ORENCIA should be given at 2 and 4 weeks after the first infusion, and every 4 weeks thereafter. ORENCIA may be used as monotherapy or concomitantly with DMARDs.

Table 6: ORENCIA

Dose of ORENCIA in Adult RA

Body Weight of Patient	Dose	Number of Vials[a]
<60 kg	500 mg	2
60 to 100 kg	750 mg	3
>100 kg	1 g	4

[a] Each vial provides 250 mg of abatacept for administration.

Juvenile Idiopathic Arthritis/Juvenile Rheumatoid Arthritis: For pediatric and adolescent patients with juvenile idiopathic arthritis (JIA)/juvenile rheumatoid arthritis (JRA), a dose specifically calculated based on each patient's body weight is used.

The recommended dose of ORENCIA for patients 6 to 17 years of age with juvenile idiopathic arthritis who weigh less than 75 kg is 10 mg/kg calculated based on the patient's body weight at each administration. Pediatric patients weighing 75 kg or more should be administered ORENCIA following the adult dosing regimen, not to exceed a maximum dose of 1000 mg. ORENCIA should be administered as a 30-minute intravenous infusion. Following the initial administration, ORENCIA should be given at 2 and 4 weeks after the first infusion and every 4 weeks thereafter.

Any unused portions in the vials must be immediately discarded.

Preparation and Administration Instructions: Use aseptic technique.

ORENCIA is provided as a lyophilized powder in preservative-free, single-use vials. Each vial of ORENCIA must be reconstituted with 10 mL of Sterile Water for Injection, USP. After reconstitution, the concentration of abatacept in the vial will be 25 mg/mL. Immediately after reconstitution, the product must be further diluted to 100 mL with 0.9% Sodium Chloride Injection, USP. The infusion of the fully diluted ORENCIA solution must be completed within 24 hours of preparation. The fully diluted ORENCIA solution may be stored at room temperature or refrigerated at 2-8°C before use.

1. Each ORENCIA vial provides 250 mg of abatacept for administration.
2. Reconstitute the ORENCIA powder in each vial with 10 mL of Sterile Water for Injection, USP, using a **silicone-free disposable syringe provided with each vial** and a 18-21-gauge needle. Remove the flip-top from the vial and wipe the top with an alcohol swab. Insert the syringe needle into the vial through the center of the rubber stopper and direct the stream of Sterile Water for Injection, USP, to the glass wall of the vial. Do not use the vial if the vacuum is not present. To minimize foam formation in solutions of ORENCIA, the vial should be rotated with gentle swirling until the contents are completely dissolved. **As with any protein, prolonged or vigorous agitation should be avoided. Do not shake.** Upon complete dissolution of the lyophilized powder, the vial should be vented with a needle to dissipate any foam that may be present.
   The solution should be clear, colorless to pale yellow. Do not use if opaque particles, discoloration, or other foreign particles are present.
3. The reconstituted ORENCIA solution must be further diluted to 100 mL as follows. From a 100 mL infusion bag or bottle, withdraw a volume of 0.9% Sodium Chloride Injection, USP equal to the volume of the reconstituted ORENCIA solution required for the patient's dose. Slowly add the reconstituted ORENCIA solution to the infusion bag or bottle using a **silicone-free disposable syringe provided with each vial**. Gently mix. **Do not shake the bag or bottle.** The final concentration of abatacept in the bag or bottle will depend upon the amount of drug added, but will be no more than 10 mg/mL.
4. Prior to administration, parenteral drug products should be inspected visually for particulate matter and discoloration whenever solution and container permit. The solution should be clear, colorless to pale yellow. Do not use if opaque particles, discoloration, or other foreign particles are present.
5. The entire, fully diluted ORENCIA solution should be administered over a period of 30 minutes and must be administered with an infusion set and a sterile, non-pyrogenic, **low-protein-binding filter** (pore size of 1.2 µm or less).
6. ORENCIA should not be infused concomitantly in the same intravenous line with other agents. No physical biochemical compatibility studies have been conducted to evaluate the coadministration of ORENCIA with other agents.

OVERDOSAGE:

ORENCIA (abatacept) is administered as an intravenous infusion. Doses up to 50 mg/kg have been administered without apparent toxic effect. In case of overdosage, it is recommended that the patient be monitored for any signs or symptoms of adverse reactions and appropriate symptomatic treatment instituted.

For management of a suspected drug overdose, CPhA recommends that you contact your **regional Poison Control Centre**. See the *CPS* Directory section for a list of Poison Control Centres.

ACTION AND CLINICAL PHARMACOLOGY: General: Abatacept, a selective co-stimulation modulator, selectively modulates a key co-stimulatory signal required for full activation of T lymphocytes expressing CD28. Activated T lymphocytes are found in the synovium of patients with rheumatoid arthritis (RA). They contribute to the pathogenesis of rheumatoid arthritis and other autoimmune diseases. Full activation of T lymphocytes requires two signals provided by antigen presenting cells: recognition of a specific antigen by a T cell receptor (signal 1) and a second, co-stimulatory signal. A major co-stimulatory pathway involves the binding of CD80 and CD86 molecules on the surface of antigen presenting cells to the CD28 receptor on T lymphocytes (signal 2). Abatacept binds specifically to CD80 and CD86 selectively inhibiting this co-stimulatory pathway. Studies indicate that naive T lymphocyte responses are more affected by abatacept than memory T lymphocyte responses.

Studies in vitro and in animal models demonstrate that abatacept attenuates T lymphocyte dependent antibody responses and inflammation. In vitro, abatacept attenuates T lymphocyte activation as measured by decreased proliferation and cytokine production in human lymphocytes. Abatacept decreases antigen specific tumour necrosis factor alpha (TNFα), interferon-γ and interleukin-2 production by T lymphocytes. In a rat collagen induced arthritis model, abatacept suppresses inflammation, decreases anti-collagen antibody production and reduces antigen specific production of interferon-γ.

Pharmacodynamics: Dose finding studies were conducted with abatacept monotherapy (placebo, 0.5 mg/kg, 2 mg/kg, and 10 mg/kg) and in combination with methotrexate (MTX) (placebo, 2 mg/kg, and 10 mg/kg). In both studies, the ACR response rates increased with increasing doses at 2 mg/kg and 10 mg/kg. In clinical trials with ORENCIA (abatacept) using doses approximating 10 mg/kg, inhibition of T lymphocyte activation, decreases in products of macrophages, fibroblast-like synoviocytes, and B cells, and reductions in acute phase reactants of inflammation were observed.

Decreases were seen in: serum levels of soluble interleukin-2 receptor, a marker of T lymphocyte activation; serum interleukin-6, a product of activated macrophages and fibroblast-like synoviocytes; rheumatoid factor, an autoantibody produced by plasma cells; and C-reactive protein (CRP), an acute phase reactant of inflammation. In addition, serum levels of matrix metalloproteinase-3, which produces cartilage destruction and tissue remodeling, were decreased. Reductions in serum TNFα were also observed. These changes are consistent with the mechanism of action of ORENCIA which modulates upstream events in the inflammatory cascade, preventing downstream production of cytokines or other inflammatory mediators.

Pharmacokinetics: Healthy Adult Subjects: Following a single intravenous dose of 10 mg/kg of abatacept in healthy adult subjects, the mean terminal half-life was 16.7 days, ranging from 12 to 23 days. The systemic clearance of abatacept was approximately 0.23 mL/hr/kg. The distribution volume (Vss) ranged from 0.06 to 0.13 L/kg. The maximum serum concentration (C_{max}) of abatacept following this dose was approximately 290 µg/mL.

Adult Rheumatoid Arthritis Patients: The pharmacokinetics of abatacept in rheumatoid arthritis patients and healthy subjects appeared to be comparable. After multiple intravenous infusions (days 1, 15, 30, and monthly thereafter), the pharmacokinetics of abatacept in rheumatoid arthritis patients showed proportional increases of C_{max} and AUC over the dose range of 2 mg/kg to 10 mg/kg. At 10 mg/kg, the following pharmacokinetic parameters were observed: See Table 7.

Table 7: ORENCIA

Pharmacokinetic Parameters

Parameter	Value	Range
Mean terminal half-life (t½)	13.1 days	8–25 days
Mean distribution volume (Vss)	0.07 L/kg	0.02–0.13 L/kg

(cont'd)

Table 7: ORENCIA *(cont'd)*

Pharmacokinetic Parameters

Parameter	Value	Range
Systemic clearance	~0.22 mL/h/kg	0.13–0.47 mL/h/kg
Mean steady-state trough concentrations	~25 µg/mL	22–29 µg/mL
Mean C_{max} concentrations	~290 µg/mL	171–398 µg/mL

No systemic accumulation of abatacept occurred upon continued repeated treatment with 10 mg/kg at monthly intervals in rheumatoid arthritis patients.

Population pharmacokinetic analyses in RA patients revealed that there was a trend toward higher clearance of abatacept with increasing body weight. Age and gender (when corrected for body weight), did not affect clearance. Concomitant methotrexate (MTX), nonsteroidal anti-inflammatory drugs (NSAIDs), corticosteroids, and TNF blocking agents did not influence abatacept clearance.

No studies have been conducted to examine the effects of either renal or hepatic impairment on the pharmacokinetics of abatacept.

JIA/JRA: Serum concentrations of abatacept in children and adolescents (aged 6 to 17 years; n=186) with JIA/JRA were measured following intravenous administration of 10 mg/kg abatacept on Days 1, 15, and 29, and every 28 days thereafter for up to 40 weeks. The mean (range) trough serum concentration of abatacept at steady-state was 11.9 (0.15 to 44.6) µg/mL. Population pharmacokinetic analyses of the serum concentration data showed that clearance of abatacept increased with baseline body weight. The estimated mean (range) clearance of abatacept in the JIA/JRA patients was 0.40 (0.20 to 1.12) mL/h/kg. After accounting for the effect of body weight, the clearance of abatacept was not related to age and gender. Concomitant methotrexate, corticosteroids, and NSAIDs were also shown not to influence abatacept clearance.

STORAGE AND STABILITY: ORENCIA (abatacept) lyophilized powder must be refrigerated at 2 to 8°C. Do not use beyond the expiration date. Protect the vials from light by storing in the original package until time of use (see Dosage and Administration).

SPECIAL HANDLING INSTRUCTIONS: Not applicable.

INFORMATION FOR THE PATIENT: Published in e-CPS, available by subscription at www.e-cps.ca.

DOSAGE FORMS, COMPOSITION AND PACKAGING: Each vial of sterile, white, preservative-free, lyophilized powder for intravenous administration contains: abatacept 250 mg. Nonmedicinal ingredients: maltose 500 mg, sodium chloride 14.6 mg and sodium phosphate monobasic 17.2 mg. Following reconstitution with 10 mL of Sterile Water for Injection, USP, the solution is clear, colorless to pale yellow, with a pH range of 7.0 to 8.0. Individually packaged single-use vials of 15 mL with a silicone-free disposable syringe.

Orfenace

orphenadrine citrate

Skeletal Muscle Relaxant

SteriMax

SUPPLIED: Each white, round, biconvex tablet contains: orphenadrine citrate 100 mg. Nonmedicinal ingredients: calcium stearate, colloidal silicon dioxide, lactose and microcrystalline cellulose. Bottles of 100. Store at room temperature, protect from moisture.

Orgalutran® Ⓟ

ganirelix acetate

Gonadotropin-releasing Hormone (GnRH) Antagonist

Schering-Plough

Date of Preparation: January 5, 2010

PHARMACOLOGY: The pulsatile release of GnRH stimulates the synthesis and secretion of luteinizing hormone (LH) and follicle-stimulating hormone (FSH). The frequency of LH pulses in the mid and late follicular phase is approximately 1 pulse/hour. These pulses can be detected as transient rises in serum LH. At midcycle, a large increase in GnRH release results in an LH surge. The midcycle LH surge initiates several physiologic actions including: ovulation, resumption of meiosis in the oocyte, and luteinization. Luteinization results in a rise in serum progesterone with an accompanying decrease in estradiol levels.

Ganirelix acts by competitively blocking the GnRH receptors on the pituitary gonadotroph and subsequent transduction pathway. It induces a rapid, reversible suppression of gonadotropin secretion. The suppression of pituitary LH secretion by ganirelix is more pronounced than that of FSH. An initial release of endogenous gonadotropins has not been detected with ganirelix, which is consistent with an antagonistic effect.

Ganirelix may be displaced during competition for the GnRH receptor by GnRH agonists. This may result in the stimulation of significant LH release and, thus, trigger an LH surge. Upon discontinuation of ganirelix, pituitary LH and FSH levels are fully recovered within 48 hours.

Pharmacokinetics: The pharmacokinetic parameters of single and multiple injections of ganirelix in healthy adult females are summarized in Table 1. Steady-state serum concentrations were reached after 2 to 3 days of treatment. The pharmacokinetics are dose proportional in the dose range of 125 to 500 µg.

Table 1: Orgalutran

Mean (SD) Pharmacokinetic Parameters of 250 µg of Orgalutran Following a Single S.C. Injection (N=15) and Daily S.C. Injections (N=15) for 7 Days

	t_{max} h	$t_{1/2}$ h	C_{max} ng/mL	AUC ng·h/mL	Cl L/h	Vd L
Orgalutran Single Dose	1.1 (0.3)	12.8 (4.3)	14.8 (3.2)	96 (12)	2.4 (0.2)[a]	43.7 (11.4)[a]
Orgalutran Multiple Dose	1.1 (0.2)	16.2 (1.6)	11.2 (2.4)	77.1 (9.8)	3.3 (0.4)[b]	76.5 (10.3)

[a] Based on i.v. administration.

[b] Apparent clearance.

Legend: t_{max}=time to maximum concentration; $t_{1/2}$=elimination half-life; C_{max}=maximum serum concentration; AUC=area under the curve; single dose: $AUC_{0-\infty}$; multiple dose: AUC_{0-24}; Cl=clearance=dose/$AUC_{0-\infty}$; Vd=volume of distribution.

Absorption: The geometric mean absolute bioavailability of ganirelix injection following a single 250 µg s.c. injection to healthy female volunteers is 91.1%. Maximum serum concentrations [C_{max} (SD)] following 250 µg of ganirelix acetate were 14.8 (3.2) and 11.2 (2.4) ng/mL for single and multiple doses, respectively. T_{max} is approximately 1 hour after s.c. injection.

Distribution: The mean (SD) volume of distribution of ganirelix in healthy females following i.v. administration of a single 250 µg dose is 43.7 (11.4) L. The apparent volume of distribution (SD) following a s.c. injection of 250 µg daily for 7 days is 76.5 (10.3) L. In vitro protein binding to human plasma was 81.9%.

Metabolism: Following i.v. administration of radiolabeled ganirelix to healthy female volunteers, ganirelix injection was the major compound present in the plasma (50 to 70% of administered dose) and urine (17.0 to 18.4% of administered dose) up to 4 hours after a single dose. There was no ganirelix found in the feces. The 1 to 4 peptide metabolite of ganirelix was the primary compound observed in the feces.

Elimination: The elimination half-life [$t_{1/2}$ (SD)] following a single 250 µg s.c. dose of ganirelix to healthy female subjects was 12.8 (4.3) hours. The $t_{1/2}$ (SD) following daily 250 µg s.c. doses of ganirelix for 7 days was 16.2 (1.6) hours. The apparent clearance (SD) following daily 250 µg s.c. doses of ganirelix for 7 days was 3.3 (0.4) L/h. Approximately 90% of radiolabeled ganirelix was excreted in the urine and feces within 192 hours following a single i.v. dose. On average, 97.2% of the total ganirelix dose administered was recovered in the feces and urine (75.1% and 22.1%, respectively).

INDICATIONS: For the prevention of premature LH surges in women undergoing controlled ovarian hyperstimulation (COH).

CONTRAINDICATIONS: Known hypersensitivity to ganirelix, any of its components, or to any similar peptide (such as GnRH or other GnRH analog); known or suspected pregnancy, moderate or severe impairment of hepatic or renal function.

WARNINGS: Ganirelix injection should be prescribed by physicians who are experienced in infertility treatment. Before starting treatment with ganirelix injection, pregnancy must be excluded. Safe use of ganirelix injection during pregnancy has not been established (see Contraindications).

Ganirelix injection may cause fetal harm when administered to a pregnant woman. No teratogenic effects were observed in rats or rabbits, although, at higher concentrations (≥10 µg/kg/day in rats and ≥30 µg/kg/day in rabbits), an increase in the extent of litter resorption was observed. No treatment-related changes in fertility, physical, or behavioral characteristics were observed in the offspring of female rats treated with ganirelix during pregnancy and lactation. Use of ganirelix injection in human pregnancy has not been studied. Because animal reproduction studies are not always predictive of human response, this drug should not be used during pregnancy. If this drug is used during pregnancy, the patient should be apprised of the potential hazard to the fetus.

PRECAUTIONS: General: Caution is advised in patients with hypersensitivity to GnRH or other GnRH analogs. These patients should be carefully monitored after the first injection. Neither anaphylactic reactions nor anti-ganirelix antibody formation have been reported with the use of ganirelix injection. However, hypersensitivity, antibody formation, and acute anaphylactic reactions have been reported with other GnRH analogs.

Use of ganirelix injection in patients with current allergic symptoms has not been evaluated, therefore, special care should be taken for these patients. The packaging of this product contains natural rubber latex which may cause allergic reactions.

Efficacy and safety of ganirelix injection have not been established in women weighing >90 kg or <50 kg.

Efficacy and safety of ganirelix injection have not been studied in women for more than 3 consecutive cycles.

Laboratory Tests: The only relevant abnormal laboratory value was a neutrophil count ≥8.3 (*10^9/L) in 11.9% of the subjects. In addition, downward shifts within the ganirelix injection group were observed for hematocrit and total bilirubin. The clinical significance of these findings was not determined.

Drug Interactions: Formal in vivo or in vitro drug-drug interaction studies have not been conducted. Since ganirelix injection can suppress the secretion of pituitary gonadotropins, dose adjustments of exogenous gonadotropins may be necessary when used during COH.

Lactation: Ganirelix injection should not be used by lactating women. It is not known whether this drug is excreted in human milk.

Children: Safety and efficacy in pediatric patients have not been established.

Geriatrics: Clinical studies of ganirelix injection did not include a sufficient number of subjects aged 65 and over.

ADVERSE EFFECTS: The safety of ganirelix injection was evaluated in 2 randomized, parallel-group, multicentre controlled clinical studies. Treatment duration for ganirelix injection ranged from 1 to 14 days. Table 2 represents maternal adverse events (AEs) from first day of ganirelix injection administration until confirmation of pregnancy by ultrasound at an incidence of ≥1% in ganirelix injection treated subjects without regard to causality.

Table 2: Orgalutran

Incidence of common AEs (Incidence ≥1% in Orgalutran-treated subjects) (All-subjects-treated group)

	Group	
	Orgalutran (N=872)	**Buserelin (N=236)**
WHO System-Organ Class Preferred Term	**All n (%)**	**All n (%)**
Reproductive Disorders, Female		
Abdominal Pain-Gynecological	38 (4.4)	8 (3.4)
Ovarian Hyperstimulation Syndrome	19 (2.2)	14 (5.9)
Vaginal Bleeding	14 (1.6)	8 (3.4)
Dysmenorrhea	0	8 (3.4)
Central and Peripheral Nervous System Disorders		
Headache	71 (8.1)	23 (9.7)
Dizziness	19 (2.2)	3 (1.3)
Fetal Disorders		
Death Fetal	29 (3.3)	13 (5.5)
Abortion Missed	7 (0.8)	3 (1.3)
GI System Disorders		
Nausea	22 (2.5)	4 (1.7)
Abdominal Pain	16 (1.8)	4 (1.7)
Body as a Whole—General Disorders		
Fever	4 (0.5)	3 (1.3)
Fatigue	23 (2.6)	2 (0.8)
Pain	10 (1.1)	1 (0.4)
Hot Flushes	15 (1.7)	3 (1.3)
Respiratory System Disorders		
Upper Respiratory Tract Infection	6 (0.7)	4 (1.7)
Rhinitis	9 (1.0)	1 (0.4)
Application Site Disorders		
Injection Site Reaction	37 (4.2)	5 (2.1)

(cont'd)

Table 2: Orgalutran *(cont'd)*

Incidence of common AEs (Incidence ≥1% in Orgalutran-treated subjects) (All-subjects-treated group)

	Group	
	Orgalutran (N=872)	**Buserelin (N=236)**
WHO System-Organ Class Preferred Term	**All n (%)**	**All n (%)**
Red Blood Cell Disorder		
Anemia	1 (0.1)	3 (1.3)

Legend: n=number of subjects with AEs or drug-related AEs; N=total number of subjects in the group.

Drug Abuse and Dependence: There have been no reports of abuse or dependence of ganirelix injection.

OVERDOSE:

There have been no reports of overdosage with ganirelix injection in humans.

For management of a suspected drug overdose, CPhA recommends that you contact your **regional Poison Control Centre**. See the *CPS* Directory section for a list of Poison Control Centres.

DOSAGE: Prior to therapy with ganirelix injection, patients should be informed of the length of treatment and monitoring procedures that will be required. The risk of possible reactions to the drug should be discussed (see Adverse Effects).

After initiating FSH therapy on Day 2 or 3 of the cycle, ganirelix injection 250 µg should be administered s.c. once daily during the early to mid follicular phase to take advantage of endogenous pituitary FSH secretion and therefore to potentially reduce the requirement for exogenously administered FSH. Treatment with ganirelix injection should be continued daily until the day of hCG administration. In normal practice, this period is usually around 5 days, although ganirelix injection treatment has ranged from 1 to 19 days in clinical trials. When an appropriate number of follicles of adequate size (≥17 mm in diameter) are present, as assessed by ultrasound, final maturation of follicles could be induced by administering hCG.

The time between two ganirelix injections as well as between the last ganirelix injection and the hCG injection should not exceed 30 hours, otherwise a premature ovulation may occur. Therefore, if the patient normally injects ganirelix injection in the morning, the last of the ganirelix injections in the series should be given on the same day as the hCG is given. If the patient normally injects ganirelix injection in the afternoon, the last ganirelix injection should be given in the afternoon prior to the day the hCG is given.

The administration of hCG should be withheld in cases where the ovaries are abnormally enlarged on the last day of FSH therapy. This will reduce the chance of developing OHSS.

INFORMATION FOR THE PATIENT: Published in e-CPS, available by subscription at www.e-cps.ca.

SUPPLIED: Each prefilled syringe of colorless, sterile, ready-to-use, aqueous solution intended for **s.c.** administration only contains: ganirelix acetate equivalent to ganirelix 250 µg/0.5 mL. Nonmedicinal ingredients: acetic acid and/or sodium hydroxide to adjust pH to 5.0, glacial acetic acid, mannitol and water for injection. Disposable prefilled 1 mL glass syringes affixed with a 27 gauge × ½ inch needle. Blister packed. **Single use only.** The packaging of this product contains natural rubber latex which may cause allergic reactions. Store between 15-30°C. Protect from light.

Orgaran®-DVT

danaparoid sodium

Anticoagulant—Antithrombotic (Heparinoid)-Deep Vein Thrombosis (DVT)

Schering-Plough

PHARMACOLOGY: ORGARAN (danaparoid sodium) is a mixture of non-heparin low molecular weight sulfated glycosaminoglycuronans derived from porcine intestinal mucosa. Its average molecular weight is 4000 to 8000 D and the molecular weights of the fractions range from <2000 to >10 000 D. ORGARAN consists of heparan sulfate with low affinity for antithrombin (AT) (about 80%), heparan sulfate with high affinity for AT (about 4%), dermatan sulfate (8 to 16%) and chondroitin sulfate (<8.5%). ORGARAN is devoid of heparin or heparin fragments. It has been shown both in animal models and in human studies to possess antithrombotic action.

Compared to heparin, ORGARAN has a much higher anti-factor Xa/anti-IIa ratio (more than 20:1). Its anti-Xa activity is 11 to 17 U/mg and its anti-IIa activity ≤0.5 U/mg. ORGARAN exerts a stronger catalytic effect on the inactivation of factor Xa than on the inactivation of thrombin. The anti-Xa activity is mediated by AT and is not inactivated by endogenous heparin neutralizing factors. The anti-thrombin activity is mediated by both AT and heparin cofactor II.

LMW heparins and heparinoids are not measured directly in the bloodstream; instead the effect on clotting mechanisms is measured. ORGARAN inhibits thrombus formation with approximately the same potency as heparin in animal models but shows greater efficacy at inhibiting extension of preformed thrombi. The APTT may not be significantly prolonged relative to unfractionated heparin. In clinical trials, ORGARAN showed improved antithrombotic activity when compared to heparin. Both of the heparan sulfate fractions, the high- and low-affinity for AT, contribute to the antithrombotic activity. ORGARAN has minimal or no effect on platelet function. It produces less bleeding-enhancing activity than heparin in experimental models at equipotent antithrombotic doses. ORGARAN does not inhibit platelet deposition at therapeutic doses and has only minimal effects on platelet degranulation during hemostatic plug formation. In experimental models, the antithrombotic activity of ORGARAN is more persistent and the hemorrhagic effects less persistent than those of heparin.

Pharmacokinetics: The absolute bioavailability of danaparoid after subcutaneous administration approaches 100% and the time to reach peak plasma anti-Xa activity levels is approximately 4 to 5 hours.

The half-lives of elimination of anti-Xa and thrombin generation inhibiting activities are approximately 25 hours and 7 hours respectively, after both subcutaneous and intravenous administration. Steady-state levels of plasma anti-Xa activity are usually reached within 4 to 5 days of dosing. Measured by thrombin generation inhibiting activity steady-state levels are reached earlier, i.e. within 1 to 2 days.

ORGARAN is mainly eliminated by renal excretion and animal experiments indicate that the liver is not involved in its metabolism. In patients with severely impaired renal function the half-life of elimination of plasma anti-factor Xa activity may be prolonged.

INDICATIONS: ORGARAN (danaparoid sodium) is indicated in the prevention of deep vein thrombosis (DVT) following orthopedic, major abdominal and thoracic surgery. Patients with a positive diagnosis of non-haemorrhagic stroke may also be treated with ORGARAN. ORGARAN is also indicated for the treatment of patients with an acute episode of Heparin-Induced Thrombocytopenia (HIT), and for prophylaxis in patients with a history of HIT (see Product Monograph for Orgaran-HIT).

CONTRAINDICATIONS: Danaparoid must not be administered by the intramuscular route or in patients with:

- acute or subacute bacterial endocarditis
- major blood clotting disorders
- history of thrombocytopenia with ORGARAN or in patients in whom an in vitro, platelet aggregation test in the presence of ORGARAN is positive
- active gastric or duodenal ulcer
- haemorrhagic cerebrovascular accident (except if there are systemic emboli)
- severe untreated hypertension
- diabetic or hemorrhagic retinopathy
- surgery involving brain, spinal cord, eyes or ears
- severe haemorrhagic diathesis
- haemorrhagic stroke in the acute phase
- uncontrollable active bleeding state
- hypersensitivity to ORGARAN or any of its components including sulphite
- other conditions or diseases involving an increased risk of haemorrhage

WARNINGS: ORGARAN (danaparoid sodium) should be used with care in patients with hepatic insufficiency, renal insufficiency, or a history of gastrointestinal ulceration.

Determination of anti-factor Xa levels in plasma is the only method available for monitoring danaparoid sodium activity. Anticoagulant activity is characterized by a very flat dose response curve in clotting assays such as prothrombin time, activated partial thromboplastin time, kaolin cephalin clotting time and thrombin clotting time, therefore, these routine clotting assays are unsuitable for monitoring its anticoagulant activity.

Anti-Xa units of ORGARAN have a different relationship to clinical efficacy than those of heparin and low molecular weight heparins. The plasma anti-Xa activity induced by ORGARAN is not neutralised by circulating proteins such as PF4 and histidine rich glycoprotein. Also, ORGARAN has been shown to induce three major biochemical responses in the circulation: anti-Xa activity, antithrombin activity and thrombin generation inhibitory activity, all of which have different half-lives following i.v. injection (25 hours, 4 hours, and 7 hours, respectively). Therefore, at different times after the injection of ORGARAN, different ratios of the various activities will be found and these will have a bearing on the clinical efficacy and safety of ORGARAN. Thus, there is no clear relationship between anti-Xa units and efficacy.

There is a better relationship to clinical efficacy with the actual dose of ORGARAN than with the plasma anti-Xa activity since a single dose can result in a range of plasma anti-Xa activity levels. This variation is caused by factors such as time of blood sampling, body weight, body mass index, renal function and other (unknown) factors.

Protamine is not a neutralizing agent for the activity of ORGARAN. However, in emergency, plasmapheresis has been shown to effectively reduce the plasma anti-Xa levels.

There have been cases of intra-spinal hematomas with the concurrent use of low molecular weight heparins and spinal/epidural anesthesia resulting in transient or permanent paralysis. The risk of these events may be higher with the prolonged use of post-operative indwelling epidural catheters or by the concomitant use of drugs affecting haemostasis; nonsteroidal anti-inflammatory drugs (NSAIDs), platelet inhibitors, or other drugs affecting coagulation. The risk is also increased by traumatic or repeated epidural or spinal procedure. Although these effects have until now not been documented with the concomitant use of ORGARAN and spinal/epidural anesthesia, the potential risk cannot be ruled out. Therefore, ORGARAN should only be used concurrently with spinal/epidural anesthesia when the therapeutic benefits to the patients outweigh the possible risks. When used concurrently, no spinal invasion should be performed for 12 hours following the last dose of ORGARAN, and the next dose should be held until at least 2 hours after the anesthesia procedure. The same rules apply to the withdrawal or manipulation of the catheter. Careful vigilance for neurological signs is recommended with rapid diagnosis and treatment, if signs occur. See also Adverse Effects.

ORGARAN should be carefully monitored in patients with severely impaired renal function because the main route of elimination is via the kidney. The half-life for anti-Xa activity in patients with impaired renal function is longer than for people with normal renal function (29 to 35 hours in patients with renal impairment vs 25 hours in normal patients). In studies with renal failure patients, it was observed that the individual pharmacokinetics of plasma anti-Xa effect is not readily predictable and may show widely different patterns of interpatient variability. The plasma anti-Xa activity may show accumulation between dialysis periods unless the predialysis bolus is suitably adjusted. The dose of ORGARAN for DVT prophylaxis needs to be individualized and possibly decreased for patients on the drug for long-term dialysis.

Except under special circumstances ORGARAN should not be used when abortion is imminent or threatened. It may be used in such cases only when, in the opinion of the physician, the increased risk of bleeding is outweighed by the risk of thrombosis and thromboembolism.

ORGARAN contains sodium sulphite, which may cause allergic reactions including anaphylactic symptoms and life-threatening or less severe asthmatic episodes in certain susceptible people. The overall prevalence of sulphite sensitivity in the general population is unknown. Sulphite sensitivity is seen more frequently in asthmatics than in nonasthmatics.

Use in Patients with Prosthetic Heart Valves: ORGARAN should not be used to prevent thromboembolism in patients with prosthetic heart valves because there is inadequate data to assess the safety and effectiveness in these patients. Adequate studies have not been completed to establish the conditions of use (e.g., the dosage). There have been cases of thrombosis in aortic and mitral prosthetic valves, some of which have resulted in death (see also Pregnancy).

Pregnancy: Pregnancy and Children: The safety of ORGARAN in pregnant women and children has not been established. Animal studies have not demonstrated any teratogenic effects or placental transfer of ORGARAN. The use of ORGARAN in pregnancy has only been studied incidentally. Observations in pregnant women in the last trimesters have so far given no indication that the use of ORGARAN during pregnancy leads to fetal abnormalities or to exacerbation of bleeding in mother or infant during delivery. ORGARAN should not be used in pregnant women and children unless the therapeutic benefits to the patients outweigh the possible risks.

ORGARAN should not be used to prevent thromboembolism in pregnant women with prosthetic heart valves, **unless the patient has HIT**. There has been very limited use of ORGARAN in this patient population for the management of HIT Type II. In patients treated with LMW heparins, clots have developed that resulted in blockage of the valve and death. There is inadequate data to ascertain the safety, effectiveness or dosage in pregnant women with prosthetic heart valves.

Lactation: There has been no experience with ORGARAN during human lactation. Mothers receiving ORGARAN should avoid breast-feeding.

Knee Surgery: The risk of bleeding in knee surgery patients receiving LMW heparins or heparinoids such as ORGARAN may be greater than in other orthopedic surgical procedures. It should be noted that hemarthrosis is a serious complication of knee surgery. The physician should weigh the potential risks with the potential benefits to the patient in determining whether to administer a low molecular weight heparin or heparinoid in this patient population.

PRECAUTIONS: ORGARAN (danaparoid sodium) cannot be used interchangeably (unit for unit) with unfractionated heparin or low molecular weight heparins (LMWHs) as they differ in their manufacturing process, molecular weight distribution, anti-Xa and anti-IIa activities, units dosages and mode of action. Special attention and compliance with instructions for use of each specific product is required during any change in treatment.

In stroke patients, intracranial/intracerebral haemorrhage (haemorrhagic stroke) should be excluded by CT scan prior to the administration of ORGARAN.

Biochemical Monitoring: ORGARAN has only a moderate prolonging effect on clotting time assays such as APTT or thrombin time. For lab monitoring of effect, plasma anti-Xa activity using amidolytic methods are recommended. For all assay methods, ORGARAN should be used as the calibrator for the reference standard. Dose increases aimed at prolonging APTT to the same extent as with unfractionated heparin could cause overdose and bleeding.

ORGARAN is administered subcutaneously, and therefore, the individual patient's antifactor Xa activity level will not remain within the range that would be expected with unfractionated heparin by continuous i.v. infusion throughout the entire dosing interval. The peak plasma antifactor Xa level occurs 4 hours after subcutaneous administration. Administration of single doses of up to 3200 U ORGARAN produce levels of less than 0.5 U/mL anti-Xa activity. ORGARAN administered as a bolus dose of 4000 to 4800 U produces mean anti-Xa levels of greater than 0.5 U/mL. Steady state plasma anti-Xa levels are reached at day 4 to 5. ORGARAN should be administered as directed in Dosage.

Patient Monitoring: As with all antithrombotic agents, there is a risk of systemic bleeding with ORGARAN administration.

After treatment is initiated, patients should be carefully monitored for bleeding complications. This may be done by regular physical examination of patients, close observation of the surgical drain and periodic measurements of haemoglobin, and anti-factor Xa determinations. Bleeding complications may be considered major if haemoglobin is decreased by 2 g/dL or if a transfusion of 2 or more units has been required. With normal prophylactic doses, ORGARAN does not modify global clotting tests of activated partial thromboplastin time (APTT), prothrombin time (PT) and thrombin clotting time (TT). Therefore, treatment can not be monitored with these tests.

Measurement of the Quick, INR, PT may not be reliable within the first 5 hours of a ORGARAN injection. Since the INR depends on PT and/or TT, this cannot be measured accurately within the first 5 hours of the overlap of OAC's and danaparoid.

ORGARAN is administered subcutaneously, and therefore, the individual patient's antifactor Xa activity level will not remain within the range that would be expected with unfractionated heparin by continuous i.v. infusion throughout the entire dosing interval. Mean plasma anti-Xa levels, measured 10 minutes after a single i.v. injection of 1500 to 1600 U, 3000 to 3200 U or 6400 U were as follows: 0.4, 0.9 and 1.6 anti-Xa U/mL, respectively. When ORGARAN was administered at steady state in doses of 800, 1600, 2400 and 3200 U, anti-Xa levels 5 minutes after injection were found to be 0.3, 0.58, 1.07 and 1.14 U/mL, respectively. Pharmacokinetic analysis shows linearity of the kinetics of anti-Xa effect after multiple i.v. bolus injections. (See also Biochemical Monitoring.) ORGARAN should be administered as directed in the Dosage section.

Platelets: Platelet counts should be determined prior to commencement of therapy with ORGARAN and, subsequently, every other day during the first week, twice a week during the 2 weeks thereafter, and after 3 weeks once a week.

Caution is recommended when administering ORGARAN to patients with congenital or drug induced thrombocytopenia, or platelet defects.

Treatment of Patients with a History of (suspected) HIT: Patients with a history of HIT should be tested for cross-reactivity with ORGARAN before routine DVT prophylaxis. If positive then ORGARAN should only be used if no other reasonable alternative is available. If under these circumstances ORGARAN is used, then the following clinical signs should be looked for as possible indications of clinical cross-reactivity: platelet count reduction (more than expected after surgery) and/or a thrombotic event. If either is noted then ORGARAN must be immediately discontinued and a laboratory test must be performed to look for evidence of a ORGARAN activated antiplatelet antibody (i.e. a positive cross-reactivity test). Only if the test is negative may ORGARAN prophylaxis be resumed if still necessary. Please refer to Product Monograph for Orgaran-HIT.

In exceptional circumstances, e.g. very high risk or heavy patients, it may be necessary to initiate ORGARAN prophylaxis with an i.v. bolus dose followed by subcutaneous dosing.

Selection of General Surgery Patients: Risk factors associated with postoperative venous thromboembolism following general surgery include history of venous thromboembolism, varicose veins, obesity, heart failure, malignancy, previous long bone fracture of a lower limb, bed rest for more than 5 days prior to surgery, predicted duration of surgery of more than 30 minutes, age 60 years or above.

Geriatrics: Age is highly correlated to risk of thrombosis. No increased bleeding tendency has been observed in the clinical studies with ORGARAN in elderly patients with normal kidney and liver function. No dose reduction should be necessary unless kidney or liver function is impaired.

Drug Interactions: In clinical studies no clinically significant interactions with other medications have been found. In general, combination with antithrombotics that act by other mechanisms such as oral anticoagulants or ASA would be additive. ORGARAN may be used together with oral anticoagulants or drugs which interfere with platelet function, such as aspirin and non-steroidal anti-inflammatory drugs, but caution remains necessary. Monitoring of anticoagulant activity of oral anticoagulants by prothrombin time and Thrombotest is unreliable within 5 hours after ORGARAN administration.

The interaction of ORGARAN with the following drugs has been studied. All effects on kinetic parameters mentioned below are considered of no clinical relevance. No clinically relevant effects have been observed on biochemical, haematological and urinary parameters.

Aspirin: no effects on hemostasis.
Acenocoumarol: slight decrease in anti-Xa clearance.
Cloxacillin: slight increase in elimination half-life of anti-Xa activity.
Ticarcillin: slight increase in anti-Xa clearance.
Digoxin: slight increase in anti-Xa clearance; slight decrease in digoxin area under the curve of plasma concentration versus time.
Chlorthalidone: slight decrease in anti-Xa clearance and central volume of distribution.
Pentobarbital: decrease of anti-IIa clearance.
Antipyrine: no significant effect on cytochrome P450 system.

Since most patients treated with ORGARAN are severely ill, often with multiple disorders, many receive a wide variety of co-medications. Many patients have received concomitant antithrombotics, the two most important of which are oral anticoagulants and thrombolytics. Such patients have been treated on average with 4 to 5 drugs other than antithrombotics. Most were antibiotics, antihypertensives, diuretics, antidiabetics, cardiac stimulants and analgesics. Anticancer or immuno-suppressive drugs have also been used frequently. Despite this variety there is no evidence of any direct interaction with ORGARAN. Occasionally it has been considered by the investigators that some drugs contribute independently to the suppression of, and possibly to delay in recovery of, the platelet count.

ORGARAN is intended primarily for subcutaneous use. When administered as an intravenous bolus, it should be given separately and not mixed with other drugs. However, ORGARAN is compatible with, and therefore, can be added to, the following infusions: normal saline, dextrose/saline, Ringer's or Lactated Ringer's and mannitol. In these solutions it remains stable for up to 48 hours at room temperature.

There is no antidote for ORGARAN overdose. Protamine is not a neutralising agent for the activity of ORGARAN. In cases of surgically uncontrollable severe bleeding, plasmapheresis has been used to reduce the circulating levels of ORGARAN, see Overdose: Symptoms and Treatment.

ADVERSE EFFECTS: Bleeding: As with any antithrombotic treatment, haemorrhagic manifestations can occur. Injection site hematomas are a common side effect with ORGARAN (danaparoid sodium) occurring at a frequency of 5% or less.

Whereas bleeding is an inherent risk with all antithrombotic therapy, no increased risk of bleeding was found during the operative and postoperative periods (based on volume of blood loss and the number of units of packed red blood cells transfused) when danaparoid 750 anti-Xa units s.c. b.i.d. administered before and after surgery was compared with placebo or active treatments (such as unfractionated heparin, warfarin and dextran). Plasma anti-Xa concentrations have not correlated with bleeding complications during danaparoid therapy, although haemorrhage has been more frequent with higher doses such as those used with HIT patients. Until further data are available, midinterval anti-Xa concentrations greater than 0.5 units/mL should be avoided during prophylaxis of thromboembolism. Risk factors associated with bleeding on therapy with heparins and heparinoids include a serious concurrent illness, surgical and accidental trauma, chronic heavy alcohol consumption, use of platelet inhibiting drugs other than aspirin or NSAIDs and severe renal failure. Bleeding may range from minor local hematomas to major haemorrhage. The early signs of bleeding may include epistaxis, hematuria, or melena, although these can also occur after severe bleeding has started. Bleeding may occur at any site and may be difficult to detect; such as retroperitoneal bleeding.

There have been cases of intra-spinal hematomas with the concurrent use of low molecular weight heparins and spinal/epidural anesthesia especially if the spinal tap has been traumatic. It can result in transient or permanent paralysis (incidence of 1:45 000). See also Warnings.

Liver: Changes in liver transaminases (AST, ALT and alkaline phosphatase) have been observed with ORGARAN. No clinical significance has been demonstrated because the patients involved were severely ill. In general there is no concordance in the changes in plasma enzyme levels suggesting a specific effect on the liver or any other source of these enzymes (muscle [cardiac, skeletal, uterine etc.], erythrocyte or kidney). Nevertheless, transient elevations of transaminases (AST and ALT) are a consistent finding with all members of the LMWH class, as well as with unfractionated heparin. The mechanism associated with the increased levels of transaminases has not been elucidated and no consistent irreversible liver damage has been observed.

Hypersensitivity: Thrombocytopenia, skin rash, and allergic reactions are rare, but occur with all LMW heparins and heparinoids. ORGARAN should be discontinued in patients showing local or systemic allergic responses. Occasionally in patients with injection site reactions to heparin these recur with ORGARAN, but with decreasing severity and may then disappear despite continued ORGARAN administration. If antibody-induced thrombocytopenia occurs, the use of ORGARAN should be stopped and the cause determined. If due to ORGARAN, then alternative treatment should be considered. Anaphylactoid reactions to unfractionated heparin and the LMW heparins have been rarely observed. Heparin, ancrod and warfarin-induced necrosis has occurred with LMWH's but has not been observed with ORGARAN.

Skeletal: No osteoporosis was observed in rats or dogs after 6 months of treatment with high i.v. doses of ORGARAN. Similarly, no osteopenic effects have been reported even in patients treated for over 3 months, including 12 pregnancies (particularly vulnerable to this side effect of heparin). However since this symptom has been reported as an adverse effect after long term treatment with unfractionated heparin at high doses, the risk of osteoporosis cannot be excluded.

Lipid Metabolism: Compared to unfractionated heparin, ORGARAN induces a smaller release of lipoprotein lipase and hepatic triglyceride lipase. The total lipase release by ORGARAN is less than 20% that of equivalent antithrombotic doses of unfractionated heparin. The lipoprotein lipase response is reduced by half and the hepatic triglyceride lipase response is reduced even further.

Table 1 lists adverse events observed in clinical trials, in which ORGARAN was given for DVT and PE Prophylaxis in Orthopedic Hip Surgery (daily dosage range: 500 U s.c. once a day—continuous i.v. infusion of 183 U/hour), DVT and PE Prophylaxis (without Orthopedic Hip Surgery) and Treatment (daily dosage range: 375 U s.c. once a day to 2000 U b.i.d.), Management of Acute or Progressing Ischemic Stroke (daily dosage range: 625 U i.v. to 9600 U/day [given as 2400 U 4 hours after bolus, 4800 U after 12 hours, 2400 U after 8 hours]), Haemodialysis (daily dosage range: 500 U to 6000 U i.v. bolus), Cardiac Catheterization (daily dosage range: 3200 U intra-arterially) or for other Clinical Pharmacology studies (daily dosage range: 100 U to 6400 U i.v.). It should be noted that placebo was only used for a limited number of clinical situations, and that the ratio of peri-operative to medical uses was much higher in the ORGARAN treated patients. This probably explains most of the differences in frequency of the events listed.

These adverse events are listed irrespective of causality by danaparoid, the disease state being treated, other concomitant diseases, concomitant medications or other unknown reasons.

In addition to the adverse effects listed in Table 1, other adverse effects observed in surgery, non-surgery and miscellaneous patients were: bruise, haematoma, haemorrhage, urine abnormal, haematuria, urinary tract bleed (microscopic), atrial fibrillation, partial loss of consciousness, urinary incontinence, involuntary muscle contractions, tremor, decreased arterial pressure, restlessness, apnea, fatigue, urinary tract bleeding, hypotension, increased alkaline phosphate, peripheral edema, confusion, insomnia, asthma, thrombocytopenia, sepsis, cerebral infarction, cerebral hemorrhage, thrombosis venous deep, hemiparesis. These events are listed regardless of causality and have not necessarily been attributed to ORGARAN.

OVERDOSE:

Symptoms: Haemorrhage is the major clinical sign of overdosage.

Table 1: ORGARAN-DVT

Incidence of Adverse Experiences (>1%) by Body System and Treatment

Body System Adverse Experience	ORGARAN n=4478 (%)	Placebo n=310 (%)
Body as a Whole		
Fever	212 (4.7)	1 (0.3)
Infection	68 (1.5)	3 (1.0)
Injection site pain	351 (7.8)	53 (17.1)
Pain	218 (4.9)	0 (0.0)
Pyrexia	78 (1.7)	0 (0.0)
Digestive System		
Constipation	86 (1.9)	0 (0.0)
Nausea	116 (2.6)	3 (1.0)
Vomiting	41 (0.9)	3 (1.0)
Hemic and Lymphatic System		
Anemia	15 (0.3)	3 (1.0)
Leukocytosis	44 (1.0)	2 (0.6)
Metabolic and Nutritional Disorders		
Hypoproteinemia	42 (0.9)	4 (1.3)
Respiratory System		
Pneumonia	46 (1.0)	2 (0.6)
Skin and Appendages		
Rash	45 (1.0)	0 (0.0)
Urogenital System		
Urinary Retention	46 (1.0)	0 (0.0)
Urinary Tract Infection	105 (2.3)	3 (1.7)

Notes: A patient may have been counted in more than one body system and in more than one adverse experience within a body system. This table does not include adverse experiences with a COSTART term of "Death". Those adverse experiences with an incidence of <1% are not listed in this table.

Treatment: In case of accidental overdosage, the routine hematological count and other coagulation parameters should be measured. Minor bleeding rarely requires specific therapy, and reducing or delaying subsequent doses of ORGARAN (danaparoid sodium) is usually sufficient. ORGARAN should be discontinued or temporarily interrupted (with subsequent continuance at a lower dose) in cases of major bleeding. Transfusion with fresh frozen plasma, or if bleeding is uncontrollable, plasmapheresis or surgery should be considered. Protamine is not a neutralizing agent for the activity of ORGARAN.

For management of a suspected drug overdose, CPhA recommends that you contact your **regional Poison Control Centre**. See the *CPS* Directory section for a list of Poison Control Centres.

DOSAGE: ORGARAN (danaparoid sodium) is expressed in U (anti-Xa units)/mL as opposed to IU/mL (as for unfractionated heparin and most of the LMW heparins). These units of measurement are not interchangeable and there is no conversion factor to convert from one to the other.

Prophylaxis of Deep Vein Thrombosis following Orthopedic, Major Abdominal Surgery and Thoracic Surgery: In general, ORGARAN is administered by subcutaneous injection at a dose of 750 anti-factor Xa units, twice daily up to 14 days for DVT prophylaxis. In surgical patients it is recommended to start prophylaxis preoperatively and to give the last preoperative dose 1 to 4 hours before surgery.

Prophylaxis of Deep Vein Thrombosis in Non-haemorrhagic Stroke Patients: In nonhaemorrhagic stroke patients, the first dose of ORGARAN can be given as an intravenous bolus injection of up to 1000 anti-Xa units, followed by 750 anti-Xa units, subcutaneously, twice daily for 7 to 14 days. In patients with normal renal function, pre-injection levels of anti-Xa activity range between 0.05 to 0.15 U/mL. At the time of maximum pharmacodynamic effect (4 to 5 hours post-injection), the levels range up to 0.4 U/mL.

The prophylactic treatment of patients with ORGARAN does not preclude the use of other modalities of prophylaxis (see Precautions, Drug Interactions).

Plasma anti-Xa activity is linearly related to the dose of ORGARAN given. If it is necessary to monitor anticoagulant activity, e.g., if the patient is very small or very large (outside the range of 55 to 90 kg) or in patients with acute renal failure, and for individual dose setting, a functional anti-factor Xa activity assay using a chromogenic peptide substrate should be used. For the results of this assay ORGARAN should be used to construct the standard curve.

In patients with severely impaired renal function (creatinine levels ≥220 μmol) the second and subsequent doses of ORGARAN may have to be reduced because the half-life of plasma anti-factor Xa activity may be prolonged. The dosage may require adjustments in order to keep the anti-Xa levels similar to those in normal patients. ORGARAN should be used with caution and the plasma anti-Xa activity monitored in case of accumulation. At steady state (3 to 4 days after initiation of therapy), consistent plasma levels of >0.5 anti-Xa units are indicative of accumulation and, therefore, suggest that dosage should be decreased or temporarily withdrawn.

Geriatrics: Clearance of anti-factor Xa has not been shown to be markedly reduced in the elderly and the usual dosage is recommended.

SUPPLIED: Each ampoule of sterile, isotonic solution contains: 0.6 mL of danaparoid sodium (750 anti-factor Xa units), sodium sulphite 0.9 mg, sodium chloride to isotonic, hydrochloric acid to pH 7.0 and water for injection to 0.6 mL. The anti-Xa unit is derived from the international heparin standard in an antithrombin-III containing buffer system. It is suitable for subcutaneous and intravenous injection. ORGARAN is intended primarily for subcutaneous use, but in cases where an immediate effect is required it may be given by the intravenous route. Glass ampoules of 1 mL, boxes of 10. Store at 2-30°C. Protect from light.

Orgaran® (HIT) Ⓟ

danaparoid sodium

Anticoagulant—Antithrombotic (Heparinoid)-Heparin-Induced Thrombocytopenia (HIT)

Schering-Plough

PHARMACOLOGY: ORGARAN (danaparoid sodium) is a mixture of non-heparin low molecular weight sulfated glycosaminoglycuronans derived from porcine intestinal mucosa. Its average molecular weight is 4000 to 8000 D and the molecular weights of the fractions range from <2000 to >10 000 D. ORGARAN consists of heparan sulfate with low affinity for antithrombin (AT) (about 80%), heparan sulfate with high affinity for AT (about 4%), dermatan sulfate (8 to 16%) and chondroitin sulfate (<8.5%). ORGARAN is devoid of heparin or heparin fragments. It has been shown both in animal models and in human studies to possess antithrombotic action.

Compared to heparin, ORGARAN has a much higher anti-factor Xa/anti-IIa ratio (more than 20:1). Its anti-Xa activity is 11 to 17 U/mg and its anti-IIa activity ≤0.5 U/mg. ORGARAN exerts a stronger catalytic effect on the inactivation of factor Xa than on the inactivation of thrombin. The anti-Xa activity is mediated by AT and is not inactivated by endogenous heparin neutralizing factors. The antithrombin activity is mediated by both AT and heparin cofactor II.

LMW heparins and heparinoids are not measured directly in the bloodstream; instead the effect on clotting mechanisms is measured. ORGARAN inhibits thrombus formation with approximately the same potency as heparin in animal models but shows greater efficacy at inhibiting extension of preformed thrombi. The APTT may not be significantly prolonged relative to unfractionated heparin. In clinical trials, ORGARAN showed improved antithrombotic activity when compared to heparin. Both of the heparan sulfate fractions, the high- and low-affinity for AT, contribute to the antithrombotic activity. ORGARAN has minimal or no effect on platelet function. It produces less bleeding-enhancing activity than heparin in experimental models at equipotent antithrombotic doses. ORGARAN does not inhibit platelet deposition at therapeutic doses and has only minimal effects on platelet degranulation during hemostatic plug formation. In experimental models, the antithrombotic activity of ORGARAN is more persistent and the hemorrhagic effects less persistent than those of heparin.

Pharmacokinetics: The absolute bioavailability of danaparoid sodium after subcutaneous administration approaches 100% and the time to reach peak plasma anti-Xa activity levels is approximately 4 to 5 hours.

The half-lives of elimination of anti-Xa and thrombin generation inhibiting activities are approximately 25 hours and 7 hours respectively, after both subcutaneous and intravenous administration. Steady-state levels of plasma anti-Xa activity are usually reached within 4 to 5 days of dosing. Measured by thrombin generation inhibiting activity steady-state levels are reached earlier, i.e., within 1 to 2 days.

ORGARAN is mainly eliminated by renal excretion and animal experiments indicate that the liver is not involved in its metabolism. In patients with severely impaired renal function the half-life of elimination of plasma anti-factor Xa activity may be prolonged.

INDICATIONS: ORGARAN treatment of patients with an acute episode of Heparin-Induced Thrombocytopenia (HIT), and for prophylaxis in patients with a history of HIT.

CONTRAINDICATIONS: Must not be administered by the intramuscular route or in patients with:

- history of thrombocytopenia and/or thrombosis with ORGARAN
- severe untreated hypertension
- diabetic or hemorrhagic retinopathy
- haemorrhagic stroke in the acute phase
- uncontrollable active bleeding state
- hypersensitivity to ORGARAN or any of its components including sulphite.

WARNINGS: ORGARAN (danaparoid sodium) should be used with care in patients with hepatic insufficiency, renal insufficiency, or a history of gastrointestinal ulceration.

ORGARAN should not be used in the following cases unless, in the opinion of the physician, the potential benefits outweigh the potential risks:

- patients with active gastric or duodenal ulcer (unless this is the reason for surgery)
- patients with severe haemorrhagic diathesis (unless no alternative antithrombotic treatment is available)
- patients with other conditions or diseases involving an increased risk of haemorrhage or haemorrhagic cerebrovascular accident (except if there are systemic emboli)
- acute or subacute bacterial endocarditis
- major blood clotting disorders
- surgery involving brain, spinal cord, eyes or ears.

Determination of anti-factor Xa levels in plasma is the only method available for monitoring danaparoid sodium activity. Anticoagulant activity is characterized by a very flat dose response curve in clotting assays such as prothrombin time, activated partial thromboplastin time, kaolin cephalin clotting time and thrombin clotting time, therefore, these routine clotting assays are unsuitable for monitoring its anticoagulant activity.

Anti-Xa units of ORGARAN have a different relationship to clinical efficacy than those of heparin and low molecular weight heparins. The plasma anti-Xa activity induced by ORGARAN is not neutralized by circulating proteins such as PF4 and histidine rich glycoprotein. Also, ORGARAN has been shown to induce three major biochemical responses in the circulation: anti-Xa activity, antithrombin activity and thrombin generation inhibitory activity, all of which have different half-lives following i.v. injection (25 hours, 4 hours, and 7 hours, respectively). Therefore, at different times after the injection of ORGARAN, different ratios of the various activities will be found and these will have a bearing on the clinical efficacy and safety of ORGARAN. Thus, there is no clear relationship between anti-Xa units and efficacy.

There is a better relationship to clinical efficacy with the actual dose of ORGARAN than with the plasma anti-Xa activity since a single dose can result in a range of plasma anti-Xa activity levels. This variation is caused by factors such as time of blood sampling, body weight, body mass index, renal function and other (unknown) factors.

Protamine is not a neutralizing agent for the activity of ORGARAN. However, in emergency, plasmapheresis has been shown to effectively reduce the plasma anti-Xa levels.

There have been cases of intraspinal hematomas with the concurrent use of low molecular weight heparins and spinal/epidural anesthesia resulting in transient or permanent paralysis. The risk of these events may be higher with the prolonged use of post-operative indwelling epidural catheters or by the concomitant use of drugs affecting haemostasis: nonsteroidal anti-inflammatory drugs (NSAIDs), platelet inhibitors, or other drugs affecting coagulation. The risk is also increased by traumatic or repeated epidural or spinal procedure. Although these effects have until now not been documented with the concomitant use of ORGARAN and spinal/epidural anesthesia, the potential risk cannot be ruled out. Therefore, ORGARAN should only be used concurrently with spinal/epidural anesthesia when the therapeutic benefits to the patients outweigh the possible risks. When used concurrently, no spinal invasion should be performed for 12 hours following the last dose of ORGARAN, and the next dose should be held until at least 2 hours after the anesthesia procedure. The same rules apply to the withdrawal or manipulation of the catheter. Careful vigilance for neurological signs is recommended with rapid diagnosis and treatment, if signs occur (see also Adverse Effects).

The dose of ORGARAN for DVT prophylaxis in HIT patients needs to be individualized and possibly decreased for those with moderate to severe renal failure. ORGARAN should be carefully monitored in patients with severely impaired renal function because the main route of elimination is via the kidney. The half-life for anti-Xa activity in patients with impaired renal function is longer than for people with normal renal function (29 to 35 hours in patients with renal impairment vs 25 hours in normal patients). In studies with renal failure patients, it was observed that the individual pharmacokinetics of plasma anti-Xa effect is not readily predictable and may show widely different patterns of inter-patient variability. For patients presenting with HIT who have to undergo renal haemodialysis or haemofiltration a specially designed dosage schedule is available (see Dosage). In patients undergoing repeated dialysis procedures, the predialysis bolus is suitably adjusted to prevent accumulation of the plasma anti-Xa activity. In patients undergoing chronic renal hemodialysis there is no need for additional DVT prophylactic dosing, since the drug's antithrombotic effect persists between dialyses.

Except under special circumstances ORGARAN should not be used when abortion is imminent or threatened. It may be used in such cases only when, in the opinion of the physician, the increased risk of bleeding is outweighed by the risk of thrombosis and thrombo-embolism.

ORGARAN contains sodium sulphite, which may cause allergic reactions including anaphylactic symptoms and life-threatening or less severe asthmatic episodes in certain susceptible people. The overall prevalence of sulfite sensitivity in the general population is unknown. Sulfite sensitivity is seen more frequently in asthmatics than in non-asthmatics.

Patients with Prosthetic Heart Valves: ORGARAN should not be used to prevent thromboembolism in patients with prosthetic heart valves because there is inadequate data to assess the safety and effectiveness in these patients. Adequate studies have not been completed to establish the conditions of use (e.g., the dosage). There have been cases of thrombosis in aortic and mitral prosthetic valves, some of which have resulted in death (see also Pregnancy).

Pregnancy: Animal studies have not demonstrated any teratogenic effects or placental transfer of ORGARAN. The use of ORGARAN in pregnancy has been studied in a small number of subjects. Observations in 23 pregnant women (13 in the first, 4 in the second and 6 in the third trimester), of whom 13 had HIT and the remainder other types of heparin intolerance, have so far given no indication that the use of ORGARAN during pregnancy leads to fetal abnormalities or to exacerbation of bleeding in mother or infant during delivery. In the few cases in which umbilical cord blood was tested for the presence of anti-Xa activity, no anti-Xa activity was found.

There has been no experience with ORGARAN during human lactation. Mothers receiving ORGARAN should avoid breast-feeding. Based on the paucity of data, it is advised, in general, that ORGARAN should not be used during pregnancy and lactation in women with HIT unless no alternative antithrombotic treatment is available and the therapeutic benefits to the patients outweigh the possible risks.

ORGARAN should not be used to prevent thromboembolism in pregnant women with prosthetic heart valves, **unless the patient has HIT**. There has been very limited use of ORGARAN in this patient population for the management of HIT Type II. In patients treated with LMW heparins, clots have developed that resulted in blockage of the valve and death. There is inadequate data to ascertain the safety, effectiveness or dosage in pregnant women with prosthetic heart valves.

Lactation: See Pregnancy.

Children: Pediatric experience with ORGARAN is very limited. The use of ORGARAN should take place in consultation with a coagulation expert, and has to be based on plasma anti-Xa levels (see Dosage).

Knee Surgery: The risk of bleeding in knee surgery patients receiving LMW heparins or heparinoids such as ORGARAN may be greater than in other orthopedic surgical procedures. It should be noted that hemarthrosis is a serious complication of knee surgery. The physician should weigh the potential risks with the potential benefits to the patient in determining whether to administer a low molecular weight heparin or heparinoid in this patient population.

PRECAUTIONS: Clinical Diagnosis of HIT: HIT can present in various ways some of which are common to other disorders. The most compelling diagnosis should be the clinical one. The following factors have all been recognized as possible or confirmatory diagnostic features of HIT:

- development of thrombocytopenia or platelet count drop of >40% within 5 to 15 days of starting heparin use;
- development of heparin resistance, i.e., the need for increasing doses to prevent extension of, or new, thromboses or to maintain the desired APTT;
- exclusion of other causes for this (extent of) platelet count reduction, e.g., surgery, drugs, sepsis, DIC;
- platelet count rises after stopping all heparin use (including small flush doses to maintain the patency of intravascular catheters etc., which are often ignored or overlooked). The rise may be slow or delayed if other reasons for platelet count suppression are present with HIT;
- observation of an (inadvertent) rechallenge platelet count reduction when heparin is reintroduced (especially following repeated dialyses);
- a new acute thromboembolic event (which may show as a white, platelet-rich clot at embolectomy) has occurred, either within the vascular system or in an artificial system, e.g., graft or dialyser.

HIT can also present in other clinical guises, e.g., heparin-induced skin necrosis, transient global amnesia, acute systemic reactions to an injection, etc. The occurrence of these or the last 2 points above can be considered as clinical confirmation of HIT.

The initial diagnosis of HIT, based upon clinical observations, may be augmented by additional laboratory investigations such as immediately repeating the platelet count, examining a blood film for platelet clumping, or identifying platelet-derived microparticles using flow cytometry. Although used in the past, the detection of high levels of immunoglobulins on the platelet surface is both insensitive and nonspecific for the diagnosis of HIT. Whenever possible, attempts should be made to detect the heparin-induced antibody (or its equivalent if a chemically related antithrombotic glycosaminoglycuronan (GAG) has been used). A number of tests are available for this. All have a very high positive predictive value, but their sensitivity for the antibody, and hence the level of false negative tests, varies. These tests are the following, listed in order of their diagnostic accuracy:

a. SRA (Serotonin Release Test/Assay): Although generally regarded as the "golden standard" it does not lend itself to routine use since it depends upon the release of ^{14}C-labeled serotonin from preloaded platelets, and it requires a license to use radioactive isotopes.
b. HIPA (Heparin-induced Platelet Activation) Test: It is a more sensitive (lower detection limit for the antibody) modification of the routine platelet aggregation test (see PAT below). The HIPA test compares favorably with the SRA. It should be noted that in the USA some investigators use the abbreviation HIPA when they are actually referring to the PAT.
c. ELISA (Enzyme-linked Immunosorbant Assay): Available in kit form and is relatively simple to perform in any laboratory. It is sensitive and able to distinguish IgG, IgM and IgA antibodies and hence to provide further insight into the pathophysiology of HIT. However, it is based upon an initial binding step involving PF4, a protein derived from the platelet, which increases the specificity of the test. This protein binds strongly to heparin (and in vivo this complex is the target of the antibody responsible for the clinical picture of HIT), but has limited or no binding to LMWHs or ORGARAN, respectively.
d. PAT (Platelet Aggregation Test): Although less sensitive than the other methods for detecting the heparin-induced antibody, it is the most widely used test. Unlike the SRA, HIPA and ELISA tests it does not require special reagents or equipment.

In some patients, even if available, a test on the first plasma sample may not be diagnostic because either interfering levels of heparin are present or the antibody concentration is too low or both. If the antibody titre is too low, this will produce false negatives with the less sensitive functional tests. Therefore, patients with clinically suspected, serologically negative HIT should have a repeat blood sample drawn 24 hours later for a retest. Interference from other plasma proteins will affect all tests particularly the ELISA. This can usually be overcome by preheating the serum to 60°C for 30 minutes. The antibody may not be induced by the usual heparin: PF4 complex but by interaction of heparin with other proteins (e.g., IL-8 or NAP2) which may produce false negative results.

In stroke patients, intracranial/intracerebral hemorrhage (hemorrhagic stroke) should be excluded by CT scan or MRI prior to the administration of ORGARAN.

Biochemical Monitoring: Danaparoid has only a moderate prolonging effect on clotting time assays such as APTT or thrombin time. For laboratory monitoring of effect, plasma anti-Xa activity using amidolytic methods are recommended. For all assay methods, ORGARAN should be used as the calibrator for the reference standard. Dose increases aimed at prolonging APTT to the same extent as with unfractionated heparin could cause overdose and bleeding.

ORGARAN is administered subcutaneously or intravenously. With subcutaneous administration, the individual patient's antifactor Xa activity level will not remain within the range that would be expected with unfractionated heparin by continuous i.v. infusion throughout the entire dosing interval. The peak plasma antifactor Xa level occurs 4 hours after subcutaneous administration. Administration of single doses of up to 3200 U of ORGARAN produce levels of less than 0.5 U/mL anti-Xa activity. Steady-state plasma anti-Xa levels are reached at day 4 to 5, but can be reached earlier with the s.c. dosing schedule if an i.v. bolus is given as a loading dose. ORGARAN administered as an i.v. bolus dose of 4000 to 4800 U produces mean anti-Xa levels of greater than 0.5 U/mL. ORGARAN should be administered as directed in Dosage.

Patient Monitoring: As with all antithrombotic agents, there is a risk of systemic bleeding with ORGARAN administration.

After treatment is initiated, patients should be carefully monitored for bleeding complications. This may be done by regular physical examination of patients, close observation of the surgical drain and periodic measurements of haemoglobin, and anti-factor Xa determinations. Bleeding complications may be considered major if haemoglobin is decreased by 2 g/dL or if a transfusion of 2 or more U has been required. With normal prophylactic doses, ORGARAN does not modify global clotting tests of activated partial thromboplastin time (APTT), prothrombin time (PT) and thrombin clotting time (TT). Therefore, treatment cannot be monitored with these tests.

Measurement of the Quick, INR, PT may not be reliable within the first 5 hours of a ORGARAN injection. Since the INR depends on PT and/or TT, this cannot be measured accurately within the first 5 hours of the overlap of OAC's and danaparoid.

ORGARAN is administered subcutaneously or intravenously. Following subcutaneous administration, the individual patient's anti-factor Xa activity level will not remain within the range that would be expected with unfractionated heparin by continuous i.v. infusion throughout the entire dosing interval. Mean plasma anti-Xa levels, measured 10 minutes after a single i.v. injection of 1500 to 1600 U, 3000 to 3200 U or 6400 U were as follows: 0.4, 0.9 and 1.6 anti-Xa U/mL, respectively. When ORGARAN was administered at steady state in doses of 800, 1600, 2400 and 3200 U, anti-Xa levels 5 minutes after injection were found to be 0.3, 0.58, 1.07 and 1.14 U/mL, respectively. Pharmacokinetic analysis shows linearity of the kinetics of anti-Xa effect after multiple i.v. bolus injections (see also Biochemical Monitoring above). ORGARAN should be administered as directed in the Dosage section.

Platelets: Platelet counts should be determined prior to commencement of therapy with ORGARAN and, subsequently, every other day during the first week, twice a week during the 2 weeks thereafter, and after 3 weeks once a week.

Caution is recommended when administering ORGARAN to patients with congenital or drug induced (other than heparin) thrombocytopenia, or platelet defects.

Cross-reactivity in Heparin-induced Thrombocytopenia Patients: The clinical implications of serological cross-reactivity testing in HIT patients are unclear. ORGARAN has been used as an alternative anticoagulant in patients who had developed thrombocytopenia with heparin. In HIT patients tested for initial therapy, the cross-reactivity with ORGARAN (<10%) was lower than with LMW heparins (>90%).

Repeated use of ORGARAN in 34 patients on 2 or more well-separated occasions has not led to sensitization during the repeat uses. If HIT is suspected or confirmed, all sources of heparin or LMWH, if the causative agent, must be eliminated.

Although the most certain test for HIT is a positive rechallenge platelet thrombocytopenia, the danger of inducing a serious thromboembolic event prohibits deliberate use in that manner. Reliance upon laboratory demonstration of heparin-induced platelet hypersensitivity or direct assay of the antibody with ORGARAN is necessary. Testing for cross-reactivity with ORGARAN is strongly advised if clinical suspicion of cross-reactivity arises. If confirmed, then danaparoid should never again be used in that patient.

Apart from problems of interference with detection of the heparin-induced antibody, inherent, to some extent, in all of the serological tests, residual heparin in the plasma sample of a patient with suspected HIT may cause confusion. This is because the "blanks/controls" will also react positive during cross-reactivity testing. There are ways of absorbing out this heparin, but the specific antibody can also be lost by this procedure, thereby reducing the sensitivity of the test.

Cross-reactivity testing of the heparin-induced antibody with alternative GAGs should be performed whenever the tests discussed above are available. However, the ELISA test is possibly less reliable in this respect because if the compound being tested binds poorly or not at all to PF4, then cross-reactivity testing may be impaired. The clinical implications of serological cross-reactivity in HIT patients are unclear. ORGARAN has been successfully used as an alternative anticoagulant in HIT patients with positive serological cross-reactivity testing.

The following salient points should be considered when evaluating platelet sensitivity testing in HIT patients but are not the only ones: 1. A negative platelet test in an acutely thrombocytopenic patient does not rule out a positive in vivo reaction. 2. A positive cross-reactivity test on a pretreatment blood sample, should not preclude careful use of ORGARAN if other heparin alternatives are unavailable. Accordingly, frequent examination for signs of clinical cross-reactivity should be instituted. 3. Samples taken a few months, or later, after a thrombocytopenic reaction may test negative for cross-reactivity because the antibody has disappeared. However, commencement of ORGARAN treatment may induce the production of cross-reaction antibody, with the accompanying risk of thrombocytopenia. 4. Use of a sensitizing agent that resulted in a positive HIT test in the past is not recommended even for a single occasion. 5. If clinical cross-reactivity with ORGARAN is suspected it should be immediately discontinued, because a fatal outcome with ORGARAN has been reported.

Antithrombotic Treatment Initiation: Due to limitations with laboratory testing and its interpretation, it is unnecessary to await a negative result before beginning ORGARAN treatment. However, careful clinical and platelet count monitoring (see above) is necessary to detect the earliest signs of clinical cross-reactivity. Treatment should be changed immediately if cross-reactivity is suspected. Cross-reactivity may manifest clinically as renewed or unresponsive platelet count reduction, a new or extension of a pre-existing thrombotic event, skin necrosis and rarely bleeding. However, although important to stop ORGARAN immediately, serological confirmation must be performed to help put into perspective other possible causes of these events. For example, sepsis, DIC, other drugs or diseases are associated with thrombocytopenia. Hemostatic factor deficiency, inappropriately low dose of ORGARAN, heparin or warfarin coadministration, anti-phospholipid syndrome/SLE may result in thrombotic events. Warfarin or heparin coadministration may cause skin necrosis. Inappropriately high doses of ORGARAN, warfarin or heparin coadministration may lead to bleeding. If cross-reactivity testing ORGARAN is negative and these other possibilities are considered to be the cause of the problem then ORGARAN can be restarted. Inappropriate dosing with danaparoid has successfully responded to appropriate dosage adjustment.

Selection of General Surgery Patients: Risk factors associated with postoperative venous thromboembolism following general surgery include history of venous thromboembolism, varicose veins, obesity, heart failure, malignancy, previous long bone fracture of a lower limb, bed rest for more than 5 days prior to surgery, predicted duration of surgery of more than 30 minutes, age 60 years or above.

Geriatrics: Age is highly correlated to risk of thrombosis. No increased bleeding tendency has been observed in the clinical studies with ORGARAN in elderly patients with normal kidney and liver function. No dose reduction should be necessary unless kidney or liver function is severely impaired.

Drug Interactions: In clinical studies no clinically significant interactions of ORGARAN with other medications have been found. In general, combination with antithrombotics that act by other mechanisms such as oral anticoagulants or ASA would be additive. ORGARAN may be used together with oral anticoagulants or drugs which interfere with platelet function, such as aspirin and non-steroidal anti-inflammatory drugs, but caution remains necessary. Monitoring of anticoagulant activity of oral anticoagulants by prothrombin time and Thrombotest is unreliable within 5 hours after ORGARAN administration.

The interaction of ORGARAN with the following drugs has been studied. All effects on kinetic parameters mentioned below are considered of no clinical relevance. No clinically relevant effects have been observed on biochemical, hematological and urinary parameters.

Aspirin: no effects on hemostasis.
Acenocoumarol: slight decrease in anti-Xa clearance.
Cloxacillin: slight increase in elimination half-life of anti-Xa activity.
Ticarcillin: slight increase in anti-Xa clearance.
Digoxin: slight increase in anti-Xa clearance; slight decrease in digoxin AUC of plasma concentration vs time.
Chlorthalidone: slight decrease in anti-Xa clearance and central volume of distribution.
Pentobarbital: decrease of anti-IIa clearance.
Antipyrine: no significant effect on cytochrome P450 system.

Since most patients treated with ORGARAN are severely ill, often with multiple disorders, many receive a wide variety of comedications. Many patients have received concomitant antithrombotics, the two most important of which are oral anticoagulants and thrombolytics. Such patients have been treated on average with 4 to 5 drugs other than antithrombotics. Most were antibiotics, antihypertensives, diuretics, antidiabetics, cardiac stimulants and analgesics. Anticancer or immunosuppressive drugs have also been used frequently and have been associated with delayed platelet count recovery. Despite this variety there is no evidence of any direct interaction with ORGARAN. Occasionally it has been considered by the investigators that some drugs contribute independently to the suppression of, and possibly to delay in recovery of, the platelet count.

ORGARAN is intended primarily for subcutaneous and intravenous use. When administered as an intravenous bolus or infusion, it should be given separately and not mixed with other drugs. However, ORGARAN is compatible with, and therefore, can be added to, the following infusions: normal saline, dextrose/saline, Ringer's or Lactated Ringer's and mannitol. In these solutions it remains stable for up to 48 hours at room temperature.

There is no antidote for ORGARAN overdose. Protamine is not a neutralizing agent for the activity of ORGARAN . In cases of surgically uncontrollable severe bleeding, plasmapheresis has been used to reduce the circulating levels of ORGARAN (see Overdose: Symptoms and Treatment).

ADVERSE EFFECTS: Adverse reactions experienced in HIT patients have not differed from those of non-HIT patients receiving danaparoid.

Bleeding: As with any antithrombotic treatment, haemorrhagic manifestations can occur. Injection site hematomas are a common side effect with ORGARAN occurring at a frequency of 5% or less.

Whereas bleeding is an inherent risk with all antithrombotic therapy, no increased risk of bleeding was found during the operative and postoperative periods (based on volume of blood loss and the number of units of packed red blood cells transfused) when danaparoid 750 anti-Xa units s.c. b.i.d. administered before and after surgery was compared with placebo or active treatments (such as unfractionated heparin, warfarin and dextran). Plasma anti-Xa activity levels have not correlated with bleeding complications during danaparoid therapy, although hemorrhage has been more frequent with higher doses such as those used with HIT patients. Until further data are available, midinterval anti-Xa concentrations greater than 0.5 U/mL should be avoided during postoperative prophylaxis of thromboembolism. Risk factors associated with bleeding on therapy with heparins and heparinoids include a serious concurrent illness, surgical and accidental trauma, chronic heavy alcohol consumption, use of platelet-inhibiting drugs other than aspirin or NSAIDs and severe renal failure. Bleeding may range from minor local hematomas to major haemorrhage. The early signs of bleeding may include epistaxis, hematuria, or melena, although these can also occur after severe bleeding has started. Bleeding may occur at any site and may be difficult to detect; such as retroperitoneal bleeding.

There have been cases of intraspinal hematomas with the concurrent use of low molecular weight heparins and spinal/epidural anesthesia especially if the spinal tap has been traumatic. It can result in transient or permanent paralysis (incidence of 1:45 000) (see also Warnings).

Liver: Changes in plasma transaminases (AST, ALT and alkaline phosphatase) have been observed with ORGARAN. No clinical significance has been demonstrated because the patients involved were severely ill. In general there is no concordance in the changes in plasma enzyme levels suggesting a specific effect on the liver or any other source of these enzymes (muscle [cardiac, skeletal, uterine, etc.], erythrocyte or kidney). Nevertheless, transient elevations of transaminases (AST and ALT) are a consistent finding with all members of the LMWH class, as well as with unfractionated heparin. The mechanism associated with the increased levels of transaminases has not been elucidated and no consistent irreversible liver damage has been observed.

Hypersensitivity: Thrombocytopenia, skin rash, and allergic reactions are rare, but occur with all LMW heparins and heparinoids. ORGARAN should be discontinued in patients showing primary local or systemic allergic responses. Occasionally in patients with injection site reactions to heparin these recur with ORGARAN, but with decreasing severity and may then disappear despite continued ORGARAN administration. If antibody-induced thrombocytopenia occurs, the use of ORGARAN should be stopped and the cause determined. If due to ORGARAN , then alternative treatment should be considered. Anaphylactoid reactions to unfractionated heparin and the low molecular weight heparins have been rarely observed. Heparin, ancrod and warfarin-induced necrosis has occurred with LMWH's but has not been observed with ORGARAN.

Skeletal: No osteoporosis was observed in rats or dogs after 6 months of treatment with high i.v. doses of danaparoid. Similarly, no osteopenic effects have been reported, even in patients treated for over 3 months, including 12 pregnancies (particularly vulnerable to this side effect of heparin). However, since this symptom has been reported as an adverse effect after long-term treatment with unfractionated heparin at high doses, the risk of osteoporosis cannot be excluded.

Lipid Metabolism: Compared to unfractionated heparin, ORGARAN induces a smaller release of lipoprotein lipase and hepatic triglyceride lipase. The total lipase release by ORGARAN is less than 20% that of equivalent antithrombotic doses of unfractionated heparin. The lipoprotein lipase response is reduced by half and the hepatic triglyceride lipase response is reduced even further.

Table 1 lists adverse events observed in clinical trials, in which ORGARAN was given for DVT and PE Prophylaxis in Orthopedic Hip Surgery [daily dosage range: 500 U s.c. daily—continuous i.v. infusion of 183 U/h], DVT and PE Prophylaxis (without Orthopedic Hip Surgery) and Treatment [daily dosage range: 375 U s.c. daily to 2000 U b.i.d.], Management of Acute or Progressing Ischemic Stroke [daily dosage range: 625 U i.v. to 9600 U/day (given as 2400 U 4 hours after bolus, 4800 U after 12 hours, 2400 U after 8 hours)], Hemodialysis [daily dosage range: 500 to 6000 U i.v. bolus], Cardiac Catheterization [daily dosage range: 3200 U intra-arterially] or for other Clinical Pharmacology studies [daily dosage range: 100 to 6400 U i.v.]. It should be noted that placebo was only used for a limited number of clinical situations, and that the ratio of perioperative to medical uses was much higher in the ORGARAN-treated patients. This probably explains most of the differences in frequency of the events listed.

These adverse events are listed irrespective of causality by danaparoid, the disease state being treated, other concomitant diseases, concomitant medications or other unknown reasons.

Table 1: ORGARAN (HIT)

Incidence of Adverse Experiences (>1%) by Body System and Treatment

Body System Adverse Experience	ORGARAN n=4478 (%)	Placebo n=310 (%)
Body as a Whole		
Fever	212 (4.7)	1 (0.3)
Infection	68 (1.5)	3 (1.0)
Injection Site Pain	351 (7.8)	53 (17.1)
Pain	218 (4.9)	0 (0.0)
Pyrexia	78 (1.7)	0 (0.0)
Digestive		
Constipation	86 (1.9)	0 (0.0)
Nausea	116 (2.6)	3 (1.0)
Vomiting	41 (0.9)	3 (1.0)
Hemic and Lymphatic		
Anemia	15 (0.3)	3 (1.0)
Leukocytosis	44 (1.0)	2 (0.6)
Metabolic and Nutritional		
Hypoproteinemia	42 (0.9)	4 (1.3)
Respiratory		
Pneumonia	46 (1.0)	2 (0.6)
Skin and Appendages		
Rash	45 (1.0)	0 (0.0)
Urogenital		
Urinary Retention	46 (1.0)	0 (0.0)
Urinary Tract Infection	105 (2.3)	3 (1.7)

Notes: A patient may have been counted in more than one body system and in more than one adverse experience within a body system.
Table 1 does not include adverse experiences with a COSTART term of "Death". Those adverse experiences with an incidence of <1% are not listed in this table.

In addition to the adverse effects listed in Table 1, other events have been observed in surgery, nonsurgery and miscellaneous patients. Some examples were: bruise, haematoma, haemorrhage, urine abnormal, haematuria, urinary tract bleed (microscopic), atrial fibrillation, partial loss of consciousness, urinary incontinence, involuntary muscle contractions, tremor, decreased arterial pressure, restlessness, apnea, fatigue, urinary tract bleeding, hypotension, increased alkaline phosphate, peripheral edema, confusion, insomnia, asthma, thrombocytopenia, sepsis, cerebral infarction, cerebral hemorrhage, thrombosis venous deep, hemiparesis. These events are listed regardless of causality and have not necessarily been attributed to ORGARAN.

OVERDOSE:

Symptoms: Hemorrhage is the major clinical sign of overdosage.

Treatment: In case of accidental overdosage, the routine hematological count and other coagulation parameters should be measured. Minor bleeding rarely requires specific therapy, and reducing or delaying subsequent doses of ORGARAN (danaparoid sodium) is usually sufficient. ORGARAN should be discontinued or temporarily interrupted (with subsequent continuance at a lower dose) in cases of major bleeding. Transfusion with fresh frozen plasma, or if bleeding is uncontrollable, plasmapheresis or surgery should be considered. Protamine is not a neutralizing agent for the activity of ORGARAN.

For management of a suspected drug overdose, CPhA recommends that you contact your **regional Poison Control Centre**. See the *CPS* Directory section for a list of Poison Control Centres.

DOSAGE: ORGARAN is expressed in U (anti-Xa units)/mL as opposed to IU/mL (as for unfractionated heparin and most of the low molecular weight heparins). These units of measurement are not interchangeable and there is no conversion factor to convert from one to the other.

Plasma anti-Xa activity is linearly related to the dose of ORGARAN given. If it is necessary to monitor anticoagulant activity, e.g., if the patient is very small or very large (outside the range of 55 to 90 kg) or in patients with acute renal failure, and for individual dose setting, a functional anti-factor Xa activity assay using a chromogenic peptide substrate should be used. For the results of this assay ORGARAN must be used to construct the standard curve.

In patients with severely impaired renal function (C_R levels ≥220 µmol) the second and subsequent doses of ORGARAN may have to be reduced because the half-life of plasma anti-factor Xa activity may be prolonged. The dosage may require adjustments in order to keep the anti-Xa levels similar to those in normal patients. ORGARAN should be used with caution and the plasma anti-Xa activity monitored in case of accumulation. At steady state (3 to 4 days after initiation of therapy), consistent plasma levels of >0.5 anti-Xa U are indicative of accumulation and, therefore, suggest that dosage should be decreased or temporarily withdrawn.

In patients with end-stage renal failure requiring hemodialysis, pre-dialysis doses for the third and subsequent procedures are reduced according to a recommended schedule (see Table 2) to avoid accumulation. To achieve this regular pre-dialysis monitoring or the plasma anti-Xa activity is recommended. For dosing in children during renal dialysis see below under "Pediatric Treatment".

Treatment or Prevention in Current or Past Episodes of HIT, with or without Thrombotic Events: If HIT is suspected or confirmed, all heparin must be discontinued immediately (including flush doses to maintain patency of vascular access and lines) and the need for further anticoagulation assessed.

Although the predictive value of in vitro cross-reactivity to HIT-associated antibodies has been queried, it is currently recommended that cross-reactivity should be excluded, when possible, before initiation of ORGARAN therapy.

HIT is such a serious side effect of heparin and the LMWH because it presents a very high risk for thrombo-embolic events which may be fatal. Hence, treatment of patients with current HIT, i.e., with circulating antibody, requires augmentation of the usual doses used to prophylax such patients when they do not have HIT. The antibody usually circulates for up to 3 months after heparin is discontinued. Therefore, in patients who have not had serological confirmation of their HIT this is a safe limit for considering HIT as current. Past HIT patients, i.e., those beyond this 3-month interval since heparin discontinuation, can be considered free of antibody and hence their risk for thrombosis is no different from other patients who have not had HIT. It must be noted that for patients who have had a prior incidence of thrombosis, the risk of developing another thrombotic event is greater. Therefore, an increased dose of ORGARAN may be required. Since the dosing schedules for ORGARAN in current HIT patients have been shown to be safe, as well as efficacious, then the same dosing regimens can be used for past HIT patients requiring similar prophylaxis or treatment of thromboembolism.

Recommended dosage regimens of ORGARAN in patients with HIT are presented in Table 2; recommendations take into account underlying diseases and coexistent hemostatic disorders.

Table 2: ORGARAN (HIT)

Recommended ORGARAN Dosage Regimens for Adults with Heparin-induced Thrombocytopenia (HIT) Who Require Further Anticoagulation

Reason for Further Anti-coagulation	Patient Characteristics/ Type of Procedure	Body Weight (kg)	Dosage (antifactor Xa U) [Duration]	Expected Plasma Antifactor Xa Levels (U/L)
DVT Prophylaxis	Current HIT	≤90	750 b.i.d. or t.i.d. s.c. [7–10 days]. For rapid attainment of prophylaxis levels, an initial i.v. bolus of 1250 can be given.	200 (on day 1), 200–400 (day 5,6h after morning dose). Plasma levels of 400 should not be exceeded. Steady state is expected after 4–5 days of therapy.
		>90	1250 b.i.d. or t.i.d. s.c. [7–10 days]. For rapid attainment of prophylaxis levels, an initial i.v. bolus of 1250 can be given.	
	Past HIT (>3 months)	≤90	750 b.i.d. or t.i.d. s.c. [7–10 days]	200 (on day 1), 150–400 (day 5, 6h after morning dose)
		>90	1250 b.i.d. or 750 t.i.d. s.c. [7–10 days]	
Established DVT or Pulmonary Embolism	Thrombosis <5 days old	55–90	2250–2500 i.v. bolus[a] then 400/h [4 h] then 300/h [4 h] then 150–200/h [5–7 days] (or maintenance of 2000 s.c. b.i.d. for 4–7 days).	500–700 (5–10 min after bolus), <1000 (during adjustment phase), 500–800 (during maintenance) 400–800 for s.c. administration
		≤55	1250–1500 iv bolus then 400/h [4 h] then 300/h [4 h] then 150–200/h [5–7 days] or maintenance of 1500 s.c. b.i.d. (for 4–7 days).	
		>90	3750 i.v. bolus then 400/h [4 h] then 300/h [4 h] then 150–200/h [5–7 days] or maintain with 1750 s.c. t.i.d. (for 4–7 days).	
	Thrombosis ≥5 days old	≤90	1250 i.v. bolus then 750 s.c. b.i.d. or t.i.d.	500–700 (5–10 mins after i.v. bolus) 300–500 (day 2–3). Plasma levels should not exceed 500 for s.c. doses. Steady state is expected after 2–3 days of therapy.
		>90	1250 i.v. bolus then 750 s.c. t.i.d. or 1250 s.c. b.i.d. or t.i.d.	
Surgical Thrombo-prophylaxis	Nonvascular surgery	≤90	750 s.c. [1–4 h before surgery] repeated ≥6 h postoperatively then 750 b.i.d. s.c. [7–10 days] (starting the day after surgery)	150–350 (on day 4–5; 6 h after morning dose). Plasma levels should not exceed 350.
		>90	750 s.c. [1–4 h before surgery] repeated ≥6 h postoperatively then 1250 b.i.d. s.c. or 750 t.i.d. s.c. [7–10 days] (starting the day after surgery)	
	Embolectomy	55–90	2250–2500 i.v. bolus before surgery then 1250 b.i.d. s.c. ≥6 h postoperatively. Patients may receive 750 b.i.d. s.c. or t.i.d. or oral anticoagulants after several days of i.v. therapy.	500–700 (5–10 min after bolus), 250–350 (on day 2–3 if started on s.c. administration postoperatively), 500–800 (on day 2–3 if started on infusion)
		>90	2250–2500 i.v. bolus before surgery then 150–200/h [5–7 days] ≥6 h postoperatively. Patients may receive 750 b.i.d. s.c. or t.i.d. or oral anticoagulants after several days of i.v. therapy.	
Cardiac Procedures	Cardiac catheterization	<90	2500 i.v. bolus before procedure	NS
		>90	3750 i.v. bolus before procedure	
	Percutaneous transluminal coronary angioplasty		2500 i.v. bolus before procedure then 150–200/h immediately postoperatively [1–2 days]. Patients may receive 750 b.i.d. or t.i.d. s.c. or oral anticoagulants after several days of i.v. therapy.	500–700 (5–10 min after bolus), 500–800 (during infusion)
	Intra-aortic balloon pump catheterization	<90	2500 i.v. bolus before procedure then 150–200/h postoperatively. If the patient has no other thrombotic complications, ORGARAN can be given 1250 i.v. bolus (if parenteral anticoagulants were stopped >24 h previously) then 750 b.i.d. or t.i.d. or 1250 b.i.d. s.c. otherwise omit bolus.	500–700 (5–10 min after bolus), 500–800 (during infusion) 300–500 (6 h after the previous s.c. injection of ORGARAN)
		>90	3750 i.v. bolus before procedure then 150–200/h postoperatively. If the patient has no other thrombotic complications, ORGARAN can be given 1250 i.v. bolus (if parenteral anticoagulants were stopped >24 h previously) then 750 b.i.d. or t.i.d. or 1250 b.i.d. s.c. otherwise omit bolus.	
Peripheral Vascular Bypass			2250–2500 i.v. bolus before surgery then 150–200/h ≥6 h postoperatively [5–7 days]. Patients may receive 750 b.i.d. or t.i.d. s.c. or oral anticoagulants after several days of i.v. therapy	500–700 (5–10 min after bolus), 500–800 (during infusion)
Cardiopul-monary Bypass			125/kg body weight i.v. bolus after thoracotomy then 3/mL as priming fluid then 7/kg/h (started at the time of bypass hook-up and stopped 45 min before expected end of bypass). Maintenance of 1250 s.c. b.i.d. or 750 s.c. t.i.d. or infusion of 150–200 U/h (starting 6 h after procedure.	1500–2000 during bypass procedure
Hemodialysis	Dialysis every other day or less frequently		3750 i.v. bolus before first 2 hemodialyses then 3000 i.v. bolus (if plasma antifactor Xa levels <300 U/L) or 2500 i.v. bolus (if plasma antifactor Xa levels 300–350) or 2000 i.v. bolus (if plasma antifactor Xa levels 350–400)[a]	500–800
		<55	2500 i.v. bolus before first 2 hemodialyses then 2000 i.v. bolus (if plasma antifactor Xa levels <300 U/L) or 1500 i.v. bolus (if plasma antifactor Xa levels 300–350) or 1500 i.v. bolus (if plasma antifactor Xa levels 350–400)[a]	
	Daily dialysis		3750 i.v. bolus before first dialysis then 2500 before second dialysis	500–800
		<55	2500 i.v. bolus before first dialysis then 2000 before second dialysis	

(cont'd)

Table 2: ORGARAN (HIT) *(cont'd)*

Recommended ORGARAN Dosage Regimens for Adults with Heparin-induced Thrombocytopenia (HIT) Who Require Further Anticoagulation

Reason for Further Anti-coagulation	Patient Characteristics/ Type of Procedure	Body Weight (kg)	Dosage (antifactor Xa U) [Duration]	Expected Plasma Antifactor Xa Levels (U/L)
Hemofiltration		55–90	2500 i.v. bolus then 600/h [4 h] then 400/h [4 h] then 200–600/h to maintain plasma antifactor Xa levels of 500–1000 U/L	500–1000
		<55	2000 i.v. bolus then 400/h [4 h] then 150–400/h to maintain plasma antifactor Xa levels of 500–1000 U/L	

[a] If plasma antifactor Xa levels are >400 U/:, ORGARAN should not be given before dialysis. However, if fibrin threads appear in the bubble chamber, 1500 antifactor Xa U may be given.

Legend: b.i.d.=twice daily; DVT=Deep Vein Thrombosis; i.v.=intravenous; s.c.=subcutaneous; t.i.d.=3 times daily.

Conversion to Oral Anticoagulant Use (OAC): Recent observations suggest that starting OACs too early in patients with HIT may lead to skin necrosis or thrombotic events, probably due to precipitate reductions in Protein C levels, unless a parenteral anticoagulant is administered at the same time. Thus, OAC therapy should not be initiated until there is adequate antithrombotic control with the parenteral drug used to replace heparin.

1. After ORGARAN 750 U b.i.d. s.c., OACs can be started before ORGARAN is withdrawn to allow the Quick, INR, PT, etc. to reach therapeutic levels. This may take up to 5 days, but since after discontinuation of ORGARAN its effect on plasma anti-Xa continues for 24 hours or more, then the patient should be adequately protected for a slightly longer transition period. Measurement of these parameters may not be reliable within 5 hours of an ORGARAN injection.

2. After ORGARAN 1250 b.i.d. s.c., OACs can be started but the ORGARAN dose should be reduced to 750 U b.i.d. s.c. and the directions followed as in 1 above.

3. OACs can be given with the i.v. infusion (maximum rate 300 U/h) which can then be stopped when the required INR is reached (maximum 3.0). However, if a bleeding risk is present then either the Organ regimen should be changed to 1250 U b.i.d., s.c. and the procedure followed as in 2 above, or the infusion rate should be reduced to 75 U/h with a delay of 24 hours before starting OACs.

4. In HIT patients for whom conversion to OACs is contraindicated (i.e., pregnant patients and patients on renal dialysis), ORGARAN has been used chronically for as long as required. It has been used at doses proposed in Table 2, in pregnant patients for up to 26 weeks and in renal dialysis patients for up to 4.5 years, without reports of adverse reactions that differed in either frequency or severity from those reported with short-term use.

Elderly: Clearance of anti-factor Xa has not been shown to be markedly reduced in the elderly and the usual dosage is recommended.

Pediatric Treatment: Acute Thrombosis (arterial and/or venous): 30 U/kg i.v. bolus injection, then 1.2 to 4 U kg/h. The expected plasma anti-Xa levels after the i.v. bolus should be 400 to 700 U/L. At steady state 400 to 600 U/L (or 500 to 800 U/L for higher doses).

Prophylaxis: 10 U/kg b.i.d. s.c.

Renal Dialysis (for the first 2 dialyses): <10 years old: 30 U/kg+1000 U; 10 to 17 years: 30 U/kg+1500 U. (3rd and subsequent dialyses): If predialysis plasma anti-Xa level >500 U/L, then no ORGARAN required for next dialysis. If 300 to 500 U/L then reduce the total dose by 250 U. If <300 U/L then give previous dialysis dose.

Flush Doses for Catheter Patency: ORGARAN can be used intermittently to maintain the patency of i.v. lines/catheters, and/or access ports thereof, if saline flushes do not work adequately. For this purpose, 1 ampul of 750 U (0.6 mL) can be diluted in 50 mL saline and 5 to 10 mL used to flush each line/port, etc. as required.

The prophylactic treatment of patients with ORGARAN does not preclude the use of other modalities of prophylaxis (see Precautions, Drug Interactions).

For information on monitoring of patients, please refer to Precautions, Biochemical Monitoring and Clinical Monitoring.

SUPPLIED: Each ampoule of sterile, isotonic solution contains: 0.6 mL of danaparoid sodium (750 anti-Xa units), sodium sulphite 0.9 mg, sodium chloride to isotonic, hydrochloric acid to pH 7.0 and water for injection to 0.6 mL. The anti-Xa unit is derived from the international heparin standard in an antithrombin-III containing buffer system. It is suitable for subcutaneous and intravenous injection. ORGARAN is intended primarily for subcutaneous use, but in cases where an immediate effect is required it may be given by the intravenous route. Glass ampoules of 1 mL, boxes of 10. Store at 2-30°C. Protect from light.

ORO-Clense Pr
chlorhexidine gluconate
Antigingivitis Oral Rinse

Germiphene

Date of Preparation: January 22, 1996

PHARMACOLOGY: ORO-Clense (0.12% Chlorhexidine Gluconate Oral Rinse) provides antimicrobial activity during oral rinsing which is maintained between rinsings. Microbiologic sampling of plaque has shown a general reduction of both aerobic and anaerobic bacterial counts through six months clinical use of 0.12% chlorhexidine gluconate oral rinse. Rinsing with 0.12% chlorhexidine gluconate oral rinse inhibits the buildup and maturation of plaque by reducing certain microbes regarded as gingival pathogens, thereby reducing gingivitis. 0.12% chlorhexidine gluconate oral rinse provides antimicrobial activity during rinsing and for several hours thereafter. No significant changes in bacterial sensitivity, overgrowth of potentially opportunistic organisms or other adverse changes in the oral microbial flora were observed following the use of 0.12% chlorhexidine gluconate oral rinse for six months. Three months after discontinued use, the number of bacteria in plaque had returned to pretreatment levels and sensitivity of plaque bacteria to chlorhexidine gluconate remained unchanged.

Pharmacokinetics: Studies conducted with human subjects and animals demonstrate that any ingested chlorhexidine gluconate is poorly absorbed in the gastrointestinal tract. Excretion of chlorhexidine gluconate occurred primarily through the feces (approximately 90%). Less than 1% of the chlorhexidine gluconate ingested by these subjects was excreted in the urine.

INDICATIONS: ORO-Clense (0.12% Chlorhexidine Gluconate Oral Rinse) is indicated for use as part of a professional program for the treatment of moderate to severe gingivitis, and for management of associated gingival bleeding and inflammation according to the recommended dosage and frequency under supervision of a dentist. For patients having coexisting gingivitis and periodontitis, see Precautions.

CONTRAINDICATIONS: ORO-Clense (0.12% Chlorhexidine Gluconate Oral Rinse) should not be used by persons who are known to be hypersensitive to chlorhexidine gluconate, chlorhexidine compounds, or other ingredients.

WARNINGS: *Pregnancy:* Reproduction and fertility studies with chlorhexidine gluconate have been conducted. No evidence of impaired fertility was observed in male and female rats at doses up to 100 mg/kg/day. No evidence of harm to the fetus was observed in rats and rabbits at doses up to 300 mg/kg/day and 40 mg/kg/day, respectively. These doses are approximately 100, 300, and 40 times that which would result from a person ingesting 30 mL (2 capfuls) of 0.12% chlorhexidine gluconate per day. Reproduction and fertility studies with chlorhexidine gluconate in pregnant women have not been conducted, so the benefits of using ORO-Clense (0.12% Chlorhexidine Gluconate Oral Rinse) should be weighed against possible risk to the fetus.

Lactation: It is not known whether chlorhexidine gluconate is excreted in human milk. In parturition and lactation studies with rats, no evidence of impaired parturition or of toxic effects to suckling pups was observed when chlorhexidine gluconate was administered at doses over 100 times greater than ingesting the recommended daily dose for rinsing. As many drugs are excreted in human milk, caution should be exercised and the benefits of use weighed against possible risk to the infant being nursed.

Children: Clinical effectiveness and safety of ORO-Clense (0.12% Chlorhexidine Gluconate Oral Rinse) have not been determined in children. The benefits of its use should be weighed against the possible risks.

PRECAUTIONS: 0.12% Chlorhexidine Gluconate Oral Rinse can cause staining of tooth surfaces, restorations, and the dorsum of the tongue in some patients especially with prolonged use and in patients who have heavier accumulations of plaque. Staining does not affect the health of oral tissues, and can be removed from most tooth surfaces by professional dental prophylaxis. Discretion should be used in prescribing 0.12% Chlorhexidine Gluconate Oral Rinse for patients who have exposed root surfaces or anterior facial restorations with rough surfaces or margins, as stains on this area may be difficult to remove and may require restoration replacement in rare instances. If natural stains cannot be removed from these surfaces by a dental prophylaxis, patients should be excluded from treatment if the risk of permanent discolouration is unacceptable.

Use of a 0.12% Chlorhexidine Gluconate Oral Rinse may cause an alteration in taste perception in some patients.

For patients having coexisting gingivitis and periodontitis, the absence of gingival inflammation following treatment with 0.12% Chlorhexidine Gluconate Oral Rinse may not be indicative of the absence of underlying periodontitis. Appropriate treatment of periodontitis is therefore indicated.

For maximum effectiveness the patient should avoid rinsing their mouth, eating, or drinking for about 30 minutes after using 0.12% chlorhexidine gluconate.

ADVERSE EFFECTS: Common side effects occurring from the use of 0.12% Chlorhexidine Gluconate Oral Rinse are staining of teeth and other oral surfaces, a slight and temporary alteration in taste perception, and an increase in supra gingival calculus formation (see Precautions). Epithelial irritation and superficial desquamation of the oral mucosa have been noted in studies of children using 0.12% chlorhexidine gluconate which were reversible upon discontinuation. Parotitis and inflammation of the salivary glands have been reported in some patients using chlorhexidine gluconate oral rinses.

OVERDOSE:

Symptoms: Ingestion of 30 to 60 mL of ORO-Clense (0.12% Chlorhexidine Gluconate Oral Rinse) by a small child may result in gastric distress, including nausea, and/or signs of alcohol intoxication.

Treatment: Medical attention should be sought if more than 100 mL is ingested or if signs of alcohol intoxication develop.

For management of a suspected drug overdose, CPhA recommends that you contact your **regional Poison Control Centre**. See the *CPS* Directory section for a list of Poison Control Centres.

DOSAGE: Use of ORO-Clense (0.12% Chlorhexidine Gluconate Oral Rinse) should begin immediately following professional dental prophylaxis. Patients should be re-examined at intervals of not more than six months and given a thorough prophylaxis. Patient referral for periodontal consultation should be done as necessary.

Rinse with 15 mL of solution for 30 (thirty) seconds, then expectorate. Use twice daily, after breakfast and before bedtime, or as prescribed. ORO-Clense is not intended for ingestion and should be expectorated after rinsing.

Do not swallow.

Note: Wait 30 minutes after brushing with conventional toothpastes before using ORO-Clense. Do not rinse the mouth, eat or drink for 30 minutes after using ORO-Clense.

The suggested initial therapy is 3 months, at which time patients should be recalled for evaluation. At the time of the recall visit, the dental professional should: Evaluate progress, remove any stain, and reinforce proper home care techniques. Discontinue use of ORO-Clense if gingival inflammation and bleeding is controlled. Recall the patient in three months to assess gingival health. Continue use of ORO-Clense for an additional 3 months if gingival inflammation and bleeding persists. Schedule a three-month recall for evaluation. Evaluate for evidence of epithelial irritation, desquamation and Parotitis.

The following generally accepted grading scheme may be of use in evaluation the severity of gingivitis (see Table 1).

Table 1: ORO-Clense

Loe and Silness: Gingival Index (GI)

Grade	Description
1	Normal gingival, no inflammation, no colouration, no bleeding
2	Mild inflammation, slight colour change, mild alteration of gingival surface, no bleeding
3	Moderate inflammation, erythema, swelling, bleeding on probing or when pressure applied
4	Severe inflammation, severe erythema and swelling, tendency toward spontaneous hemorrhage, some ulceration

SUPPLIED: A near neutral (pH range 5 to 7), green coloured, spearmint flavored liquid containing: 0.12% chlorhexidine gluconate. Nonmedicinal ingredients: ethanol, FD&C Blue 1, FD&C Yellow 5, flavour, glycerin, methyl and propyl parabens, polysorbate 60, purified water, sodium cyclamate and sorbitol solution. White containers of 227 mL, 480 mL, and 4 L. Store between 15 and 25°C.

Ortho® 1/35 Pr
norethindrone—ethinyl estradiol
Oral Contraceptive

Janssen-Ortho

Ortho® 0.5/35 Pr
norethindrone—ethinyl estradiol
Oral Contraceptive

Janssen-Ortho

Ortho® 7/7/7 Pr
norethindrone—ethinyl estradiol
Oral Contraceptive

Janssen-Ortho

Date of Preparation: October 1993
Date of Revision: May 3, 2010

INDICATIONS AND CLINICAL USE: ORTHO 1/35, ORTHO 0.5/35 and ORTHO 7/7/7 Tablets are indicated for conception control.

CONTRAINDICATIONS:

- History of or actual thrombophlebitis or thromboembolic disorders.
- Known thrombophilic conditions.
- History of or actual cerebrovascular disorders including transient ischemic attack.
- History of or actual myocardial infarction or coronary arterial disease including angina pectoris.
- Active liver disease or history of or actual benign or malignant liver tumours.
- Known or suspected carcinoma of the breast.
- Carcinoma of the endometrium or other known or suspected estrogen-dependent neoplasia.
- Undiagnosed abnormal vaginal bleeding.
- Steroid-dependent jaundice, cholestatic jaundice or history of jaundice in pregnancy.
- Any ocular lesion arising from ophthalmic vascular disease, such as partial or complete loss of vision or defect in visual fields.
- When pregnancy is suspected or diagnosed.
- Current or history of migraine with focal aura.

- Valvular heart disease with complications.
- Presence of severe or multiple risk factor(s) for arterial or venous thrombosis:
  - severe hypertension (persistent values of ≥160/100 mmHg),
  - hereditary or acquired predisposition for venous or arterial thrombosis, such as Factor V Leiden mutation and activated protein C (APC-) resistance, antithrombin-III-deficiency, protein C deficiency, protein S deficiency, hyperhomocysteinemia (e.g., due to MTHFR C677T, A1298 mutations), prothrombin mutation G20210A, and antiphospholipid-antibodies (anticardiolipin antibodies, lupus anticoagulant),
  - heavy smoking (>15 cigarettes per day) and over age 35,
  - diabetes mellitus with vascular involvement,
  - major surgery associated with an increased risk of postoperative thromboembolism,
  - prolonged immobilization.
- Hypersensitivity to this drug or to any ingredient in the formulation or component of the container. For a complete listing, see Dosage Forms, Composition and Packaging.

WARNINGS AND PRECAUTIONS:

Serious Warnings and Precautions
Cigarette smoking increases the risk of serious adverse effects on the heart and blood vessels. This risk increases with age and becomes significant in oral contraceptive users older than 35 years of age. Women should be counselled not to smoke (see Cardiovascular).

Patients should be counselled that birth control pills **DO NOT PROTECT** against sexually transmitted infections (STIs) including HIV/AIDS. For protection against STIs, patients should be counselled to use latex or polyurethane condoms **IN COMBINATION WITH** birth control pills.

General: Discontinue Medication at the Earliest Manifestation of the Following:

A. **Thromboembolic and Cardiovascular Disorders** such as thrombophlebitis, pulmonary embolism, cerebrovascular disorders, myocardial ischemia, mesenteric thrombosis, and retinal thrombosis.
B. **Conditions that Predispose to Venous Stasis and to Vascular Thrombosis** (e.g. immobilization after accidents or confinement to bed during long-term illness). Other non-hormonal methods of contraception should be used until regular activities are resumed. For use of oral contraceptives when surgery is contemplated, see Peri-Operative Considerations.
C. **Visual Defects—Partial or Complete**
D. **Papilledema or Ophthalmic Vascular Lesions**
E. **Severe Headache of Unknown Etiology or Worsening of Pre-existing Migraine Headache**
F. **Increase in Epileptic Seizures**

The following information is provided from studies of combination oral contraceptives (COCs).

The use of combination hormonal contraceptives is associated with increased risks of several serious conditions including myocardial infarction, thromboembolism, stroke, hepatic neoplasia and gallbladder disease, although the risk of serious morbidity and mortality is small in healthy women without underlying risk factors. The risk of morbidity and mortality increases significantly if associated with the presence of other risk factors such as hypertension, hyperlipidemias, obesity and diabetes.

The information contained in this section is principally from studies carried out in women who used combination oral contraceptives with higher formulations of estrogens and progestogens than those in common use today. The effect of long-term use of combination hormonal contraceptives with lower doses of both estrogen and progestogen administered orally remains to be determined.

Carcinogenesis and Mutagenesis: Breast Cancer: Increasing age and a strong family history are the most significant risk factors for the development of breast cancer. Other established risk factors include obesity, nulliparity and late age for first full-term pregnancy. The identified groups of women that may be at increased risk of developing breast cancer before menopause are long-term users of oral contraceptives (more than eight years) and starters at an early age. In a few women, the use of oral contraceptives may accelerate the growth of an existing but undiagnosed breast cancer. Since any potential increased risk related to oral contraceptive use is small, there is no reason to change prescribing habits at present.

Women receiving oral contraceptives should be instructed in self-examination of their breasts. Their physicians should be notified whenever any masses are detected. A yearly clinical breast examination is also recommended because, if a breast cancer should develop, drugs that contain estrogen may cause a rapid progression.

Cervical Cancer: The most important risk factor for cervical cancer is persistent human papillomavirus infection. Some epidemiological studies have indicated that long-term use of COCs may further contribute to this increased risk but there continues to be controversy about the extent to which this finding is attributable to confounding effects, e.g. cervical screening and sexual behaviour including use of barrier contraceptives.

Hepatocellular Carcinoma: Hepatocellular carcinoma may be associated with oral contraceptives. The risk appears to increase with duration of hormonal contraceptive use. However, the attributable risk (the excess incidence) of liver cancers in oral contraceptive users is extremely small.

Cardiovascular: Predisposing Factors for Coronary Artery Disease: Cigarette smoking increases the risk of serious cardiovascular side effects and mortality. Birth control pills increase this risk, especially with increasing age. Convincing data are available to support an upper age limit of 35 years for oral contraceptive use by women who smoke.

Other women who are independently at high risk for cardiovascular disease include those with diabetes, hypertension, abnormal lipid profile, or a family history of these. Whether oral contraceptives accentuate this risk is unclear.

In low-risk, non-smoking women of any age, the benefits of oral contraceptive use outweigh the possible cardiovascular risks associated with low-dose formulations. Consequently, oral contraceptives may be prescribed for these women up to the age of menopause.

Hypertension: Patients with essential hypertension whose blood pressure is well-controlled may be given oral contraceptives but only under close supervision. If a persistent and significant elevation of blood pressure in previously normotensive or hypertensive subjects occurs at any time during the administration of the drug, cessation of medication is necessary and an alternative method of contraception should be prescribed (see Contraindications).

Endocrine and Metabolism: Diabetes: Current low-dose oral contraceptives exert minimal impact on glucose metabolism. Diabetic patients, or those with a family history of diabetes, should be observed closely to detect any worsening of carbohydrate metabolism. Patients predisposed to diabetes who can be kept under close supervision may be given oral contraceptives. Young diabetic patients whose disease is of recent origin, well-controlled, and not associated with hypertension or other signs of vascular disease such as ocular fundal changes, should be monitored more frequently while using oral contraceptives.

Lipid and Other Metabolic Effects: A small proportion of women will have adverse lipid changes while on oral contraceptives. Alternative contraception should be used in women with uncontrolled dyslipidemias. Elevations of plasma triglycerides may lead to pancreatitis and other complications.

Gastrointestinal: Published epidemiological studies suggest a possible modest association of COC use and the development of Crohn's disease and ulcerative colitis, although this has not been firmly established.

Genitourinary: Vaginal Bleeding: Persistent irregular vaginal bleeding requires assessment to exclude underlying pathology.

Fibroids: Patients with fibroids (leiomyomata) should be carefully observed. Sudden enlargement, pain, or tenderness requires discontinuation of the use of oral contraceptives.

Hematologic: Epidemiological studies have shown that the incidence of venous thromboembolism (VTE) in users of oral contraceptives with low estrogen content (<50 µg ethinyl estradiol) ranges from about 20 to 40 cases per 100 000 women-years, but this risk estimate varies according to the progestogen. This compares with 5 to 10 cases per 100 000 women-years for non-users. The use of any combined oral contraceptive carries an increased risk of VTE compared with no use. The excess risk of VTE is highest during the first year a woman ever uses a combined oral contraceptive. The increased risk is less than the risk of VTE associated with pregnancy, which is estimated as 60 cases per 100 000 pregnancies. VTE is fatal in 1-2% of cases.

Other Risk Factors for Venous Thromboembolism: Other generalized risk factors for venous thromboembolism include but are not limited to a personal history, a family history (the occurrence of VTE in a direct relative at a relatively early age may indicate genetic predisposition), obesity (body mass index >30 kg/m^2) and systemic lupus erythematosus. The risk of VTE also increases with age and smoking. The risk of VTE is temporarily increased with prolonged immobilization, major surgery, or trauma. Also, patients with varicose veins and leg cast should be closely supervised.

If a hereditary or acquired predisposition for venous thromboembolism is suspected, the woman should be referred to a specialist for advice before deciding on any COC use.

Post-partum Period: Since the immediate postpartum period is associated with an increased risk of thromboembolism, hormonal contraceptives should be started no earlier than four weeks after delivery in women who elect not to breast-feed.

Post-abortion/Post-miscarriage: After an abortion or miscarriage that occurs at or after 20 weeks gestation, hormonal contraceptives may be started either on Day 21 post-abortion or on the first day of the first spontaneous menstruation, whichever comes first (see Dosage and Administration).

Hepatic/Biliary/Pancreatic: Acute or chronic disturbances of liver function may necessitate the discontinuation of COC use until markers of liver function return to normal.

Jaundice: Patients who have had jaundice, including a history of cholestatic jaundice during pregnancy, should be given oral contraceptives with great care and under close observation.

The development of severe generalized pruritus or icterus requires that the medication be withdrawn until the problem is resolved.

If a patient develops jaundice that proves to be cholestatic in type, the use of oral contraceptives should not be resumed. In patients taking oral contraceptives, changes in the composition of the bile may occur and an increased incidence of gallstones has been reported.

Gallbladder Disease: Patients taking oral contraceptives have a greater risk of developing gallbladder disease requiring surgery.

Hepatic Nodules: Hepatic nodules (adenoma and focal nodular hyperplasia) have been reported, particularly in long-term users of oral contraceptives. Although these lesions are extremely rare, they have caused fatal intra-abdominal hemorrhage and should be considered in women with an abdominal mass, acute abdominal pain, or evidence of intra-abdominal bleeding.

Immune: Angioedema: Exogenous estrogens may induce or exacerbate symptoms of angioedema, in particular in women with hereditary angioedema.

Neurologic: Migraine and Headache: The onset or exacerbation of migraine or the development of headache of a new pattern that is recurrent, persistent or severe requires discontinuation of oral contraceptives and evaluation of the cause. Women with migraine headaches, particularly those with aura, who take oral contraceptives may be at increased risk of stroke (see Contraindications).

Ophthalmologic: Ocular Lesions: There have been clinical case reports of retinal thrombosis associated with the use of oral contraceptives. Oral contraceptives should be discontinued if there is unexplained partial or complete loss of vision; onset of proptosis or diplopia; papilledema; or retinal vascular lesions. Appropriate diagnostic and therapeutic measures should be undertaken immediately.

Ocular Disease: Patients who are pregnant or are taking oral contraceptives may experience corneal edema that may cause visual disturbances and changes in tolerance to contact lenses, especially of the rigid type. Soft contact lenses usually do not cause disturbances. If visual changes or alterations in tolerance to contact lenses occur, temporary or permanent cessation of wear may be advised.

Peri-Operative Considerations: Thromboembolic Complications—Post-surgery: A two- to four-fold increase in relative risk of postoperative thromboembolic complications has been reported with the use of hormonal contraceptives. The relative risk of venous thrombosis in women who have predisposing conditions is twice that of women without such medical conditions.

Hormonal contraceptives should be discontinued and an alternative method substituted at least four weeks prior to elective surgery of a type associated with an increase in risk of thromboembolism and during prolonged immobilization. Hormonal contraceptives should not be resumed until the first menstrual period after hospital discharge following surgery or following prolonged immobilization.

Psychiatric: Emotional Disorders: Patients with a history of emotional disturbances, especially the depressive type, may be more prone to have a recurrence of depression while taking oral contraceptives. In cases of a serious recurrence, a trial of an alternative method of contraception should be made which may help to clarify the possible relationship. Women with premenstrual syndrome (PMS) may have a varied response to oral contraceptives, ranging from symptomatic improvement to worsening of the condition.

Renal: Fluid Retention: Hormonal contraceptives may cause some degree of fluid retention. They should be prescribed with caution, and only with careful monitoring in patients with conditions which might be aggravated by fluid retention.

Sexual Function/Reproduction: Return to Fertility: After discontinuing oral contraceptive therapy, the patient should delay pregnancy until at least one normal spontaneous menstrual cycle has occurred in order to date the pregnancy. An alternative contraceptive method should be used during this time.

Amenorrhea: In the event of amenorrhea, pregnancy should be ruled out.

In some women, withdrawal bleeding may not occur during the tablet-free interval. If the COC has been taken according to directions, it is unlikely that the woman is pregnant. However, if the COC has not been taken according to directions prior to the first missed withdrawal bleed, or if two withdrawal bleeds are missed, pregnancy must be ruled out before COC use is continued.

Women having a history of oligomenorrhea, secondary amenorrhea, or irregular cycles may remain anovulatory or become amenorrheic following discontinuation of estrogen-progestin combination therapy.

Amenorrhea, especially if associated with breast secretion, that continues for six months or more after withdrawal, warrants a careful assessment of hypothalamic-pituitary function.

Reduced Efficacy: The efficacy of COCs may be reduced in the event of missed tablets, vomiting, diarrhea or concomitant medication (see Drug Interactions).

Skin: Chloasma may occasionally occur with use of COCs, especially in women with a history of chloasma gravidarum. Women with a tendency to chloasma should avoid exposure to the sun or ultraviolet radiation while taking COCs.

Special Populations: Pregnant Women: Oral contraceptives should not be taken by pregnant women. If pregnancy occurs during treatment with ORTHO 1/35, ORTHO 0.5/35 or ORTHO 7/7/7, further pill use should be stopped. However, if conception accidentally occurs while taking the pill, there is no conclusive evidence that the estrogen and progestin contained in the oral contraceptive will damage the developing child.

Nursing Women: In breast-feeding women, the use of oral contraceptives results in the hormonal components being excreted in breast milk and may reduce its quantity and quality. Published studies of related progestins have indicated that during lactation, small amounts of the daily maternal dose of the progestin and 0.02% of the daily maternal dose of ethinyl estradiol could be transferred to the newborn via milk. Adverse effects on the child have been reported, including jaundice and breast enlargement. The nursing mother should be advised not to use oral contraceptives but to use other forms of contraception until she has completely weaned her child.

Pediatrics: The safety and efficacy of ORTHO 1/35, ORTHO 0.5/35 and ORTHO 7/7/7 has been established in women of reproductive age. Use of these products before menarche is not indicated.

Geriatrics: ORTHO 1/35, ORTHO 0.5/35 and ORTHO 7/7/7 are not indicated for use in postmenopausal women.

Monitoring and Laboratory Tests: Physical Examination and Follow-up: Before oral contraceptives are used, a thorough history and physical examination should be performed, including a blood pressure determination and the family case history carefully noted. In addition, disturbances of the clotting system should be evaluated if a first-degree family member has suffered from thromboembolic disease or event (e.g. deep vein thrombosis, stroke, myocardial infarction) at a young age. Breasts, liver, extremities and pelvic organs should be examined and a Papanicolaou (PAP) smear should be taken if the patient has been sexually active.

The first follow-up visit should be done three months after oral contraceptives are prescribed. Thereafter, examinations should be performed at least once a year, or more frequently if indicated. At each annual visit, examination should include those procedures that were done at the initial visit as outlined above or per recommendations of the Canadian Task Force on the Periodic Health Examination.

Tissue Specimens: Pathologists should be advised of oral contraceptive therapy when specimens obtained from surgical procedures and Pap smears are submitted for examination.

ADVERSE REACTIONS: Adverse Drug Reaction Overview: An increased risk of the following serious adverse reactions has been associated with the use of oral contraceptives: thrombophlebitis and venous thrombosis with or without embolism, arterial thromboembolism, pulmonary embolism, mesenteric thrombosis, neuro-ocular lesions (e.g. retinal thrombosis), myocardial infarction, cerebral thrombosis, cerebral hemorrhage, hypertension, benign hepatic tumours, gallbladder disease.

The following adverse reactions also have been reported in patients receiving oral contraceptives. Nausea and vomiting, usually the most common adverse reaction, occurs in approximately 10 per cent or less patients during the first cycle. Other reactions, as a general rule, are seen less frequently or only occasionally, as follows:

Cardiovascular System: edema, slight rise of blood pressure.

Genital Tract: breakthrough bleeding, spotting, change in menstrual flow, dysmenorrhea, amenorrhea during and after treatment, vaginal candidiasis, premenstrual-like syndrome, temporary infertility after discontinuance of treatment, vaginitis, endocervical hyperplasias, increase in cervical erosion and secretion, vaginal discharge.

Neoplasms: malignant hepatic tumors, cervical cancer, increase in size of uterine leiomyomata, breast cancer.

Breast: pain, tenderness, enlargement, and secretion, possible diminution in lactation when given immediately postpartum.

Skin and Subcutaneous Tissue: chloasma or melasma which may persist, rash (allergic), hirsutism, loss of scalp hair, erythema multiforme, erythema nodosum, Raynaud's phenomenon, hemorrhagic eruption, porphyria, acne, seborrhea, pemphigoid (herpes gestationis), urticaria, angioedema.

CNS: migraine, mental depression, headache, nervousness, dizziness, changes in libido, chorea.

Metabolic: reduced tolerance to carbohydrates, change in weight (increase or decrease), changes in appetite.

Gastrointestinal Tract: gastrointestinal symptoms (such as abdominal cramps, diarrhea and bloating), colitis, pancreatitis, abdominal pain.

Hepatobiliary: cholestatic jaundice, Budd-Chiari syndrome.

Eyes: intolerance to contact lenses, change in corneal curvature (steepening), cataracts, optic neuritis.
Urinary: impaired renal function, hemolytic uremic syndrome, cystitis-like syndrome.
Others: rhinitis, auditory disturbances, hypersensitivity, fluid retention.

DRUG INTERACTIONS: Overview: The concurrent administration of oral contraceptives with other drugs may result in an altered response to either agent (Table 1 and Table 2). Reduced effectiveness of the oral contraceptive, should it occur, is more likely with the low-dose formulations.

It is important to ascertain all drugs that a patient is taking, both prescription and non-prescription, including herbal preparations/remedies, before oral contraceptives are prescribed.

Drug-Drug Interactions: Changes in Contraceptive Effectiveness Associated with Co-administration of Other Drugs: If a woman on hormonal contraceptives takes a drug or herbal product that induces enzymes, including CYP3A4, that metabolize contraceptive hormones, she should be counselled to use additional contraception or a different method of contraception. Drugs or herbal products that induce such enzymes may decrease the plasma concentrations of contraceptive hormones, and may decrease the effectiveness of hormonal contraceptives or increase breakthrough bleeding. Some drugs or herbal products that may decrease the effectiveness of hormonal contraceptives include:*

- modafinil
- oxcarbazepine
- St. John's wort
- topiramate

HIV protease inhibitors and non-nucleoside reverse transcriptase inhibitors: Significant changes (increase or decrease) in the plasma levels of the estrogen and progestin have been noted in some cases of co-administration of HIV protease inhibitors and non-nucleoside reverse transcriptase inhibitors.

Antibiotics: There have been reports of pregnancy while taking hormonal contraceptives and antibiotics, but clinical pharmacokinetic studies have not shown consistent effects of antibiotics on plasma concentrations of synthetic steroids.

Increase in Plasma Hormone Levels Associated with Co-administered Drugs: Some drugs and grapefruit juice may increase the plasma levels of ethinyl estradiol if co-administered. Examples include:

- acetaminophen
- ascorbic acid
- CYP3A4 inhibitors (including itraconazole, ketoconazole, voriconazole and fluconazole)
- grapefruit juice
- HMG-CoA reductase inhibitors (including atorvastatin and rosuvastatin)

Changes in Plasma Levels of Co-administered Drugs: Combination hormonal contraceptives may also affect the pharmacokinetics of some other drugs if used concomitantly. Examples of drugs whose plasma levels may be increased (due to CYP inhibition) include:†

- omeprazole
- voriconazole

Examples of drugs whose plasma levels may be decreased (due to induction of glucuronidation) include:†

- morphine
- salicyclic acid
- temazepam

Combined hormonal contraceptives have been shown to significantly decrease plasma concentrations of lamotrigine when co-administered, likely due to induction of lamotrigine glucuronidation. This may reduce seizure control; therefore, dosage adjustments of lamotrigine may be necessary.

Physicians are advised to consult the labelling of concurrently used drugs to obtain further information about interactions with hormonal contraceptives or the potential for enzyme alterations.

Refer to Oral Contraceptives 1994 (Chapter 8), Health Canada, for other possible drug interactions with OCs.

Table 1: Ortho 1/35, 0.5/35, 7/7/7 Tablets
Drugs That May Decrease the Efficacy of Oral Contraceptives

Class of Compound	Drug	Proposed Mechanism	Suggested Management
Anticonvulsants	Carbamazepine Ethosuximide Phenobarbital Phenytoin Primidone	Induction of hepatic microsomal enzymes. Rapid metabolism of estrogen and increased binding of progestin and ethinyl estradiol to SHBG.	Use higher dose OCs (50 µg ethinyl estradiol), another drug or another method.
Antibiotics	Ampicillin Cotrimoxazole Penicillin	Enterohepatic circulation disturbance, intestinal hurry.	For short course, use additional method or use another drug. For long course, use another method.
	Rifampin	Increased metabolism of progestins. Suspected acceleration of estrogen metabolism.	Use another method.
	Chloramphenicol Metronidazole Neomycin Nitrofurantoin Sulfonamides Tetracyclines	Induction of hepatic microsomal enzymes. Also disturbance of enterohepatic circulation.	For short course, use additional method or use another drug. For long course, use another method.
	Troleandomycin	May retard metabolism of OCs, increasing the risk of cholestatic jaundice.	
Antifungals	Griseofulvin	Stimulation of hepatic metabolism of contraceptive steroids may occur.	Use another method.
Cholesterol Lowering Agents	Cholestyramine	May result in hastened elimination and impaired enterohepatic circulation.	
Sedatives and Hypnotics	Benzodiazepines Barbiturates Chloral Hydrate Glutethimide Meprobamate	Induction of hepatic microsomal enzymes.	For short course, use additional method or another drug. For long course, use another method or higher dose OCs.
Antacids		Decreased intestinal absorption of progestins.	Dose two hours apart.
Other Drugs	Phenylbutazone Antihistamines Analgesics Antimigraine preparations Vitamin E	Reduced OC efficacy has been reported. Remains to be confirmed.	
	Bosentan	Induction of hepatic microsomal enzymes.	Consider switching to a non-hormonal contraceptive method or adding a barrier method to oral contraceptive therapy.

* Additional drugs are listed in Table 1.
† Additional drugs are listed in Table 2.

(cont'd)

Table 1: Ortho 1/35, 0.5/35, 7/7/7 Tablets *(cont'd)*

Table 2: Ortho 1/35, 0.5/35, 7/7/7 Tablets
Modification of Other Drug Action by Oral Contraceptives

Class of Compound	Drug	Modification of Drug Action	Suggested Management
Alcohol		Possible increased levels of ethanol or acetaldehyde.	Use with caution.
Alpha-II Adrenoreceptor Agents	Clonidine	Sedation effect increased.	Use with caution.
Anticoagulants	All	OCs increase clotting factors, decrease efficacy. However, OCs may potentiate action in some patients.	Use another method.
Anticonvulsants	All	Fluid retention may increase risk of seizures.	Use another method.
	Lamotrigine	Significantly decreased lamotrigine levels (due to induction of lamotrigine glucuronidation) may lead to breakthrough seizures.	Adjust dose of drug if necessary.
Antidiabetic Drugs	Oral Hypoglycemics and Insulin	OCs may impair glucose tolerance and increase blood glucose.	Use low-dose estrogen and progestin OC or another method. Monitor blood glucose.
Antihypertensive Agents	Guanethidine and Methyldopa	Estrogen component causes sodium retention, progestin has no effect.	Use low-dose estrogen OC or use another method.
	Beta Blockers	Increased drug effect (decreased metabolism).	Adjust dose of drug if necessary. Monitor cardiovascular status.
Antipyretics	Acetaminophen	Increased metabolism and renal clearance.	Dose of drug may have to be increased.
	Antipyrine	Impaired metabolism.	Decrease dose of drug.
	ASA	Effects of ASA may be decreased by the short-term use of OCs.	Patients on chronic ASA therapy may require an increase in ASA dosage.
Aminocaproic Acid		Theoretically, a hypercoagulable state may occur because OCs augment clotting factors.	Avoid concomitant use.
Betamimetic Agents	Isoproterenol	Estrogen causes decreased response to these drugs.	Adjust dose of drug as necessary. Discontinuing OCs can result in excessive drug activity.
Caffeine		The actions of caffeine may be enhanced as OCs may impair the hepatic metabolism of caffeine.	Use with caution..
Corticosteroids	Prednisone Prednisolone	Markedly increased serum levels.	Possible need for decrease in dose.
Cyclosporine		May lead to an increase in cyclosporine levels and hepatotoxicity.	Monitor hepatic function. The cyclosporine dose may have to be decreased.
Folic Acid		OCs have been reported to impair folate metabolism.	May need to increase dietary intake, or supplement.
Meperidine		Possible increased analgesia and CNS depression due to decreased metabolism of meperidine.	Use combination with caution.
Phenothiazine Tranquilizers	All Phenothiazines, Reserpine and similar drugs	Estrogen potentiates the hyperprolactinemia effect of these drugs.	Use other drugs or lower dose OCs. If galactorrhea or hyperprolactinemia occurs, use other method.

(cont'd)

Table 2: Ortho 1/35, 0.5/35, 7/7/7 Tablets (cont'd)

Modification of Other Drug Action by Oral Contraceptives

Class of Compound	Drug	Modification of Drug Action	Suggested Management
Sedatives and Hypnotics	Chlordiazepoxide Lorazepam Oxazepam Diazepam	Increased effect (increased metabolism).	Use with caution.
Theophylline	All	Decreased oxidation, leading to possible toxicity.	Use with caution. Monitor theophylline levels.
Tricyclic Antidepressants	Clomipramine (possibly others)	Increased side effects; i.e. depression.	Use with caution.
Vitamin B_{12}		OCs have been reported to reduce serum levels of Vitamin B_{12}.	May need to increase dietary intake, or supplement.

Drug-Food Interactions: Interactions with food have not been established.

Drug-Herb Interactions: Herbal products containing St. John's wort (hypericum perforatum) may induce hepatic enzymes (cytochrome P450) and p-glycoprotein transporter and may reduce the effectiveness of contraceptive steroids. This may also result in breakthrough bleeding.

Drug-Laboratory Test Interactions: Results of laboratory tests should be interpreted in light of the fact that the patient is on oral contraceptives. The following laboratory tests are modified.

A. **Liver Function Tests:** Bromsulphthalein Retention Test (BSP): moderate increase. AST and GGT: minor increase. Alkaline Phosphatase: variable increase. Serum Bilirubin: increased, particularly in conditions predisposing to or associated with hyperbilirubinemia.

B. **Coagulation Tests:** Factors II, VII, IX, X, XII and XIII : increased. Factor VIII: mild increase. Platelet Aggregation and Adhesiveness: mild increase in response to common aggregating agents. Fibrinogen: increased. Plasminogen: mild increase. Antithrombin III: mild decrease. Prothrombin Time: increased.

C. **Thyroid Function Tests:** Protein-bound Iodine (PBI): increased. Total Serum Thyroxine (T_4): increased. Thyroid Stimulating Hormone (TSH): unchanged. T_3 resin-uptake: decreased.

D. **Adrenocortical Function Tests:** Plasma Cortisol: increased.

E. **Miscellaneous Tests:** Serum Folate: occasionally decreased. Glucose Tolerance Test: variable increase with return to normal after 6 to 12 months. Insulin Response: mild to moderate increase. c-Peptide Response: mild to moderate increase.

Lipoproteins: Small changes of unproven clinical significance may occur in lipoprotein cholesterol fractions.

Gonadotropins: LH and FSH levels are suppressed by the use of oral contraceptives. Wait at least two weeks after discontinuing the use of oral contraceptives before measurements are made.

Non-Contraceptive Benefits of Oral Contraceptives: Several health advantages other than contraception have been reported.

1. Combination oral contraceptives reduce the incidence of cancer of the endometrium and ovaries.
2. Oral contraceptives reduce the likelihood of developing benign breast disease and, as a result, decrease the incidence of breast biopsies.
3. Oral contraceptives reduce the likelihood of development of functional ovarian cysts.
4. Pill users have less menstrual blood loss and have more regular cycles, thereby reducing the chance of developing iron-deficiency anemia.
5. The use of oral contraceptives may decrease the severity of dysmenorrhea and premenstrual syndrome, and may improve acne vulgaris, hirsutism, and other androgen-mediated disorders.
6. Oral contraceptives decrease the incidence of acute pelvic inflammatory disease and, thereby, reduce as well the incidence of ectopic pregnancy.
7. Oral contraceptives have potential beneficial effects on endometriosis.

DOSAGE AND ADMINISTRATION: Information to Patients on How to Take the Birth Control Pill:

1. **Read these directions**
   - before you start taking your pills, and
   - any time you are not sure what to do.
2. **Look at your pill pack** to see if it has 21 or 28 pills:
   - **21-Pill Pack:** 21 active pills (with hormones) taken daily for three weeks, and then no pills taken for one week or
   - **28-Pill Pack:** 21 active pills (with hormones) taken daily for three weeks, and then seven "reminder" pills (no hormones) taken daily for one week.

   Also check the pill pack for instructions on 1) where to start and 2) direction to take pills (see package insert for illustrations).
3. You may wish to use a second method of birth control (e.g. latex condoms and spermicidal foam or gel) for the first seven days of the first cycle of pill use. This will provide a back-up in case pills are forgotten while you are getting used to taking them.
4. **When receiving any medical treatment, be sure to tell your doctor that you are using birth control pills.**
5. **Many women have spotting or light bleeding, or may feel sick to their stomach during the first three months on the pill.** If you do feel sick, do not stop taking the pill. The problem will usually go away. If it does not go away, check with your doctor or clinic.
6. **Missing pills also can cause some spotting or light bleeding,** even if you make up the missed pills. You also could feel a little sick to your stomach on the days you take two pills to make up for missed pills.
7. **If you miss pills at any time, you could get pregnant. The greatest risks for pregnancy are:**
   - when you start a pack late, or
   - when you miss pills at the beginning or at the very end of the pack.
8. **Always be sure you have ready:**
   - **Another kind of birth control** (such as latex condoms and spermicidal foam or gel) to use as a back-up in case you miss pills, and
   - **An extra, full pack of pills.**
9. **If you experience vomiting or diarrhea, or if you take certain medicines,** such as antibiotics, your pills may not work as well. Use a back-up method, such as latex condoms and spermicidal foam or gel, until you can check with your doctor or clinic.
10. **If you forget more than one pill two months in a row,** talk to your doctor or clinic about how to make pill-taking easier or about using another method of birth control.
11. **If your questions are not answered here, call your doctor or clinic.**

When to Start the First Pack of Pills: Be sure to read these instructions:

- before you start taking your pills, and
- any time you are not sure what to do.

Decide with your doctor or clinic what is the best day for you to start taking your first pack of pills. Your pills may be either a 21-day or a 28-day type.

Directions for 21-Day and 28-Day Pill Packs:

1. **The first day of your menstrual period (bleeding) is day 1 of your cycle.** The pills may be started up to Day 6 of your cycle. Your starting day will be chosen in discussion with your doctor. You will **always** begin taking your pills on this day of the week. Your doctor may advise you to start taking the pills on Day 1, on Day 5, or on the first Sunday after your period begins. If your period starts on Sunday, start that same day.
2. **If you are using a: 21-Day Pill Pack:** With this type of birth control pill, you are on pills for 21 days and off pills for seven days. You must not be off the pills for more than seven days in a row.

   Take one pill at approximately the same time every day for 21 days. **Then do not take a pill for seven days.** Start a new pack on the eighth day. You will probably have a period during the seven days off the pill. (This bleeding may be lighter and shorter than your usual period.)

   28-Day Pill Pack: With this type of birth control pill, you take 21 pills that contain hormones and seven pills that contain no hormones.

   Take one pill at approximately the same time every day for 28 days. Begin a new pack the next day, **not missing any days on the pills**. Your period should occur during the last seven days of using that pill pack.

Instructions for Using Your Discreet Package for Both 21-Day and 28-Day Packs: Follow these instructions carefully: (See package insert for illustrations.)

1. **For Day 1 start:** Label the DISCREET Package by selecting the day label that starts with Day 1 of your menstrual period (the first day of menstruation is Day 1). For example, if your first day of menstruation is Tuesday, attach the day label that begins with **TUE** in the space provided.

   or

   For Day 5 start: Label the DISCREET Package by selecting the day label that starts with the day that is 5 days after your period begins. (Count 5 days **including** the first day of menstruation.) For example, if your first day of menstruation is Saturday, place the day label that starts with **WED** in the space provided.

   or

   For Sunday start: No day label is required. The DISCREET Package is printed for a Sunday start. (The first Sunday **after** your period begins, or, if your period starts on Sunday, start that **same day**).
2. Place the day label in the space where you see the words "Place day label here". Having the DISCREET Package labelled with the days of the week will help remind you to take your pill every day.
3. To begin taking your pills, start with the pill inside the red circle (where you see the word **START**). This pill should correspond to the day of the week that you are taking your first pill. To remove the pill, push through the back of the DISCREET Package.
4. On the following day, take the next pill in the same row, always proceeding from left to right (→). Each row will always begin on the same day of the week.

What to Do During the Month:

1. **Take a pill at approximately the same time every day until the pack is empty.**
   - Try to associate taking your pill with some regular activity such as eating a meal or going to bed.
   - Do not skip pills even if you have bleeding between monthly periods or feel sick to your stomach (nausea).
   - Do not skip pills even if you do not have sex very often.
2. **When you finish a pack**
   - **21 Pills**

     Wait seven days to start the next pack. You will have your period during that week.
   - **28 Pills**

     Start the next pack **on the next day**. Take one pill every day. Do not wait any days between packs.

What to do if You Miss Pills: Table 3 outlines the actions you should take if you miss one or more of your birth control pills. Match the number of pills missed with the appropriate starting time for your type of pill pack.

Table 3: Ortho 1/35, 0.5/35, 7/7/7 Tablets

What to Do if You Miss Pills

Sunday Start	Other Than Sunday Start
Miss one pill	**Miss one pill**
Take it as soon as you remember and take the next pill at the usual time. This means that you might take two pills in one day.	Take it as soon as you remember, and take the next pill at the usual time. This means that you might take two pills in one day.
Miss two pills in a row	**Miss two pills in a row**
First Two Weeks: 1. Take two pills the day you remember and two pills the next day. 2. Then take one pill a day until you finish the pack. 3. Use a back-up method of birth control if you have sex in the seven days after you miss the pills. **Third Week:** 1. Keep taking one pill a day until Sunday. 2. On Sunday, safely discard the rest of the pack and start a new pack that day. 3. Use a back-up method of birth control if you have sex in the seven days after you miss the pills. 4. You may not have a period this month. **If you miss two periods in a row, call your doctor or clinic.**	**First Two Weeks:** 1. Take two pills the day you remember and two pills the next day. 2. Then take one pill a day until you finish the pack. 3. Use a back-up method of birth control if you have sex in the seven days after you miss the pills. **Third Week:** 1. Safely dispose of the rest of the pill pack and start a new pack that same day. 2. Use a back-up method of birth control if you have sex in the seven days after you miss the pills. 3. You may not have a period this month. **If you miss two periods in a row, call your doctor or clinic.**
Miss three or more pills in a row	**Miss three or more pills in a row**
Any Time in the Cycle: 1. Keep taking one pill a day until Sunday. 2. On Sunday, safely discard the rest of the pack and start a new pack that day. 3. Use a back-up method of birth control if you have sex in the seven days after you miss the pills. 4. You may not have a period this month. **If you miss two periods in a row, call your doctor or clinic.**	**Any Time in the Cycle:** 1. Safely dispose of the rest of the pill pack and start a new pack that same day. 2. Use a back-up method of birth control if you have sex in the seven days after you miss the pills. 3. You may not have a period this month. **If you miss two periods in a row, call your doctor or clinic.**

Note: 28-Day Pack: If you forget any of the seven "reminder" pills (without hormones) in Week 4, just safely dispose of the pills you missed. Then keep taking one pill each day until the pack is empty. You do not need to use a back-up method.

Always be sure you have on hand:

- a back-up method of birth control (such as latex condoms and spermicidal foam or gel) in case you miss pills, and
- an extra, full pack of pills.

If you forget more than one pill two months in a row, talk to your doctor or clinic about ways to make pill-taking easier or about using another method of birth control.

OVERDOSAGE:

Treatment of Overdose or Accidental Ingestion: In case of overdose or accidental ingestion by children, the physician should observe the patient closely, although generally no treatment is required. Gastric lavage may be utilized if considered necessary. Overdosage may cause nausea and vomiting and withdrawal bleeding may occur in females. There are no antidotes and treatment should be symptomatic.

For management of a suspected drug overdose, contact your regional Poison Control Centre. See the *CPS* Directory section for a list of Poison Control Centres.

ACTION AND CLINICAL PHARMACOLOGY: The primary mechanism of action of ORTHO 1/35, ORTHO 0.5/35 and ORTHO 7/7/7 Tablets is an inhibition of ovulation. Additionally, other effects caused by the treatment (for example, alteration of the endometrium and the thickening of the cervical mucus) appear to interfere with implantation and conception.

STORAGE AND STABILITY: Store between 15-30°C. Leave contents in protective packaging until time of use.

INFORMATION FOR THE PATIENT: Published in e-CPS, available by subscription at www.e-cps.ca.

DOSAGE FORMS, COMPOSITION AND PACKAGING: Ortho 1/35: Each peach tablet, unscored with "C135" engraved on each side, contains: norethindrone 1 mg and ethinyl estradiol 35 µg. Nonmedicinal ingredients: lactose, magnesium stearate, red ferric oxide, yellow ferric oxide and starch. In the 28-day regimen the green tablets, engraved on each side with "C-C", contain inert ingredients. Nonmedicinal ingredients: D&C Yellow No. 10 Lake, FD&C Blue No. 2 Lake, lactose, magnesium stearate, microcrystalline cellulose and starch. Available in 21-day or 28-day DISCREET Tablet Dispenser Units.

Ortho 0.5/35: Each white tablet, unscored with "C535" engraved on each side, contains: norethindrone 0.5 mg and ethinyl estradiol 35 µg. Nonmedicinal ingredients: lactose, magnesium stearate and starch. In the 28-day regimen the green tablets, engraved on each side with "C-C", contain inert ingredients. Nonmedicinal ingredients: D&C Yellow No. 10 Lake, FD&C Blue No. 2 Lake, lactose, magnesium stearate, microcrystalline cellulose and starch. Available in 21-day or 28-day DISCREET Tablet Dispenser Units.

Ortho 7/7/7: Each white tablet, unscored with "C535" engraved on each side, contains: norethindrone 0.5 mg and ethinyl estradiol 35 µg. Each light peach unscored tablet, engraved on each side with "C735", contains: norethindrone 0.75 mg and ethinyl estradiol 35 µg. Each dark peach unscored tablet, engraved on each side with "C135", contains: norethindrone 1 mg and ethinyl estradiol 35 µg. Nonmedicinal ingredients: The white, light peach and dark peach tablets contain lactose, magnesium stearate and starch. The light and dark peach tablets also contain red ferric oxide and yellow ferric oxide. In the 28-day regimen the green tablets, engraved on each side with "C-C" contain inert ingredients. Nonmedicinal ingredients: D&C Yellow No. 10 Lake, FD&C Blue No. 2 Lake, lactose, magnesium stearate, microcrystalline cellulose and starch. Available in 21-day or 28-day DISCREET Tablet Dispenser Units.

(Shown in Product Identification Section)

Ortho-Cept® ℞

desogestrel—ethinyl estradiol

Oral Contraceptive

Janssen-Ortho

Date of Preparation: July 13, 1993
Date of Revision: October 27, 2009

PHARMACOLOGY: The primary mechanism of action of Ortho-Cept tablets is an inhibition of ovulation. Additionally, other effects caused by the treatment (e.g., alteration of the endometrium and the thickening of the cervical mucus), appear to interfere with implantation and conception.

INDICATIONS: Conception control.

CONTRAINDICATIONS: History of/or actual thrombophlebitis or thromboembolic disorders. History of/or actual cerebrovascular disorders. History of/or actual myocardial infarction or coronary arterial disease. Active liver disease or history of/or actual benign or malignant liver tumors. Known or suspected carcinoma of the breast. Known or suspected estrogen-dependent neoplasia. Undiagnosed abnormal vaginal bleeding. Any ocular lesion arising from ophthalmic vascular disease, such as partial or complete loss of vision or defect in visual fields. When pregnancy is suspected or diagnosed. Valvular heart disease with complications. Severe hypertension. Diabetes with vascular involvement. Cholestatic jaundice or history of jaundice of pregnancy. Migraine with focal aura. Prolonged immobilization. Hypersensitivity to any component of this product.

WARNINGS: Predisposing Factors for Coronary Artery Disease: Cigarette smoking increases the risk of serious cardiovascular side effects and mortality. Birth control pills increase this risk, especially with increasing age. Convincing data are available to support an upper age limit of 35 years for oral contraceptive use by women who smoke.

Other women who are independently at high risk for cardiovascular disease include those with diabetes, hypertension, abnormal lipid profile, or a family history of these. Whether oral contraceptives accentuate this risk is unclear.

In low-risk, non-smoking women of any age, the benefits of oral contraceptive use outweigh the possible cardiovascular risks associated with low-dose formulations. Consequently, oral contraceptives may be prescribed for these women up to the age of menopause.

> Cigarette smoking increases the risk of serious adverse effects on the heart and blood vessels. This risk increases with age and becomes significant in oral contraceptive users older than 35 years of age. Women should be counselled not to smoke.

Thromboembolic Disease: An increased risk of venous thromboembolic disease associated with the use of oral contraceptives is well established. This risk is smaller than that associated with pregnancy, which has been estimated at 60 per 100 000. Data from some case control and cohort studies report that third generation oral contraceptives containing desogestrel (such as Ortho-Cept tablets) are associated with a 2-fold increase in the risk of venous thromboembolic disease as compared to second generation pills containing other progestins. However, it is not known to what degree methodological limitations inherent to these studies may have affected the observed difference in risk.

The incidence of venous thromboembolism in non-users of oral contraceptives is estimated to be 4 events per 100 000 woman-years, and increases to 10 to 15 events per 100 000 woman-years with the use of second generation oral contraceptives. The findings of the studies mentioned above could translate into an additional 4 to 15 events per 100 000 woman-years (to a total of 14 to 30 events per 100 000 woman-years) with the use of third generation oral contraceptives. It should be noted, however, that the incidence of venous thromboembolism in oral contraceptive users overall is rare.

Discontinue medication at the earliest manifestation of:

A. Thromboembolic and cardiovascular disorders such as: thrombophlebitis, pulmonary embolism, cerebrovascular disorders, myocardial ischemia, mesenteric thrombosis and retinal thrombosis.
B. Conditions that predispose to venous stasis and to vascular thrombosis (e.g., immobilization after accidents or confinement to bed during long-term illness). Other non-hormonal methods of contraception should be used until regular activities are resumed. For use of oral contraceptives when surgery is contemplated, see Precautions.
C. Visual defects, partial or complete.
D. Papilledema, or ophthalmic vascular lesions.
E. Severe headache of unknown etiology or worsening of pre-existing migraine headache.

PRECAUTIONS: Physical Examination and Follow-up: Before oral contraceptives are used, a thorough history and physical examination should be performed, including a blood pressure determination. Breasts, liver, extremities and pelvic organs should be examined. A Papanicolaou smear should be taken if the patient has been sexually active.

The first follow-up visit should be 3 months after oral contraceptives are prescribed. Thereafter, examinations should be performed at least once a year, or more frequently if indicated. At each annual visit, examination should include those procedures that were done at the initial visit as outlined above or per recommendations of the Canadian Workshop on Screening for Cancer of the Cervix. Their suggestion was that, for women who had 2 consecutive negative Pap smears, screening could be continued every 3 years up to the age of 69.

Pregnancy: Oral contraceptives should not be taken by pregnant women. However, if conception accidentally occurs while taking the pill, there is no conclusive evidence that the estrogen and progestin contained in the oral contraceptive will damage the developing child.

Lactation: In breast-feeding women, the use of oral contraceptives results in the hormonal components being excreted in breast milk and may reduce its quantity and quality. If the use of oral contraceptives is initiated after the establishment of lactation, there does not appear to be any effect on the quantity and quality of the milk. There is no evidence that low-dose oral contraceptives are harmful to the nursing infant.

Hepatic Function: Patients who have had jaundice, including a history of cholestatic jaundice during pregnancy, should be given oral contraceptives with great care and under close observation.

The development of severe generalized pruritus or icterus requires that the medication be withdrawn until the problem is resolved.

If a patient develops jaundice that proves to be cholestatic in type, the use of oral contraceptives should not be resumed. In patients taking oral contraceptives, changes in the composition of the bile may occur and an increased incidence of gallstones has been reported.

Hepatic nodules (adenoma and focal nodular hyperplasia) have been reported, particularly in long-term users of oral contraceptives. Although these lesions are extremely rare, they have caused fatal intra-abdominal hemorrhage and should be considered in women with an abdominal mass, acute abdominal pain or evidence of intra-abdominal bleeding.

Hypertension: Patients with essential hypertension whose blood pressure is well-controlled may be given oral contraceptives but only under close supervision. If a significant elevation of blood pressure in previously normotensive or hypertensive subjects occurs at any time during the administration of the drug, cessation of medication is necessary.

Migraine and Headache: The onset or exacerbation of migraine or the development of headache of a new pattern that is recurrent, persistent or severe, requires discontinuation of oral contraceptives and evaluation of the cause.

Diabetes: Current low-dose oral contraceptives exert minimal impact on glucose metabolism. Diabetic patients, or those with a family history of diabetes, should be observed closely to detect any worsening of carbohydrate metabolism. Patients predisposed to diabetes who can be kept under close supervision may be given oral contraceptives. Young diabetic patients whose disease is of recent origin, well-controlled and not associated with hypertension or other signs of vascular disease such as ocular fundal changes, should be monitored more frequently while using oral contraceptives.

Ocular Disease: Patients who are pregnant or are taking oral contraceptives, may experience corneal edema that may cause visual disturbances and changes in tolerance to contact lenses, especially of the rigid type. Soft contact lenses usually do not cause disturbances. If visual changes or alterations in tolerance to contact lenses occur, temporary or permanent cessation of wear may be advised.

Breasts: Increasing age and a strong family history are the most significant risk factors for the development of breast cancer. Other established risk factors include obesity, nulliparity and late age for first full-term pregnancy. The identified groups of women that may be at increased risk of developing breast cancer before menopause are long-term users of oral contraceptives (more than 8 years) and starters at an early age. In a few women, the use of oral contraceptives may accelerate the growth of an existing but undiagnosed breast cancer. Since any potential increased risk related to oral contraceptive use is small, there is no reason to change prescribing habits at present.

Women receiving oral contraceptives should be instructed in self-examination of their breasts. Their physicians should be notified whenever any masses are detected. A yearly clinical breast examination is also recommended because, if a breast cancer should develop, drugs that contain estrogen may cause a rapid progression.

Vaginal Bleeding: Persistent irregular vaginal bleeding requires assessment to exclude underlying pathology.

Fibroids: Patients with fibroids (leiomyomata) should be carefully observed. Sudden enlargement, pain or tenderness require discontinuation of the use of oral contraceptives.

Emotional Disorders: Patients with a history of emotional disturbances, especially the depressive type, may be more prone to have a recurrence of depression while taking oral contraceptives. In cases of a serious recurrence, a trial of an alternative method of contraception should be made which may help to clarify the possible relationship. Women with premenstrual syndrome (PMS) may have a varied response to oral contraceptives, ranging from symptomatic improvement to worsening of the condition.

Laboratory Tests: Results of laboratory tests should be interpreted in light of the fact that the patient is on oral contraceptives. The following laboratory tests are modified.

A. Liver Function Tests: Bromsulphthalein Retention Test (BSP): moderate increase; AST and GGT: minor increase; alkaline phosphatase: variable increase; serum bilirubin: increased, particularly in conditions predisposing to, or associated with, hyperbilirubinemia.
B. Coagulation Tests: Factors II, VII, IX, X, XII and XIII: increased; Factor VIII: mild increase; platelet aggregation and adhesiveness: mild increase in response to common aggregating agents; fibrinogen: increased; plasminogen: mild increase; antithrombin III: mild decrease; prothrombin time: increased.
C. Thyroid Function Tests: Protein-bound Iodine (PBI): increased; Total Serum Thyroxine (T_4): increased; Thyroid Stimulating Hormone (TSH): unchanged; Free T_3 resin-uptake: decreased.
D. Adrenocortical Function Tests: plasma cortisol: increased.
E. Miscellaneous Tests: serum folate: occasionally decreased; glucose tolerance test: variable increase with return to normal after 6 to 12 months; insulin response: mild to moderate increase; C-peptide response: mild to moderate increase.

Tissue Specimens: Pathologists should be advised of oral contraceptive therapy when specimens obtained from surgical procedures and Pap smears are submitted for examination.

Return to Fertility: After discontinuing oral contraceptive therapy, the patient should delay pregnancy until at least 1 normal spontaneous cycle has occurred in order to date the pregnancy. An alternative contraceptive method should be used during this time.

Amenorrhea: Women having a history of oligomenorrhea, secondary amenorrhea or irregular cycles may remain anovulatory or become amenorrheic following discontinuation of estrogen-progestin combination therapy.

Amenorrhea, especially if associated with breast secretion, that continues for 6 months or more after withdrawal, warrants a careful assessment of hypothalamic-pituitary function.

Thromboembolic Complications—Post-surgery: There is an increased risk of thromboembolic complications in oral contraceptive users after major surgery. If feasible, oral contraceptives should be discontinued and an alternative method substituted at least 1 month prior to **major** elective surgery. Oral contraceptive use should not be resumed until the first menstrual period after hospital discharge following surgery.

__Drug Interactions:__ The concurrent administration of oral contraceptives with other drugs may result in an altered response to either agent (see Table 1 and Table 2). Reduced effectiveness of the oral contraceptive, should it occur, is more likely with the low-dose formulations. It is important to ascertain all drugs that a patient is taking, both prescription and non-prescription, before oral contraceptives are prescribed.

Changes in Contraceptive Effectiveness Associated With Co-Administration of Other Drugs: If a woman on hormonal contraceptives takes a drug or herbal product that induces enzymes, including CYP3A4, that metabolize contraceptive hormones, she should be counselled to use additional contraception or a different method of contraception. Drugs or herbal products that induce such enzymes may decrease the plasma concentrations of contraceptive hormones, and may decrease the effectiveness of hormonal contraceptives or increase breakthrough bleeding. Some drugs or herbal products that may decrease the effectiveness of hormonal contraceptives include*: oxcarbazepine, St. John's wort, topiramate.

HIV protease inhibitors: Significant changes (increase or decrease) in the plasma levels of the estrogen and progestin have been noted in some cases of co-administration of HIV protease inhibitors.

Antibiotics: There have been reports of pregnancy while taking hormonal contraceptives and antibiotics, but clinical pharmacokinetic studies have not shown consistent effects of antibiotics on plasma concentrations of synthetic steroids.

Increase in Plasma Hormone Levels Associated With Co-Administered Drugs: Some drugs may increase the plasma levels of ethinyl estradiol if co-administered. Examples include: acetaminophen, ascorbic acid, CYP3A4 inhibitors (including itraconazole and ketoconazole), HMG-CoA reductase inhibitors (including atorvastatin).

Changes in Plasma Levels of Co-Administered Drugs: Combination hormonal contraceptives may also affect the pharmacokinetics of some other drugs if used concomitantly. Examples of drugs whose plasma levels may be decreased (due to induction of glucuronidation) include†: morphine, salicyclic acid, temazepam.

Physicians are advised to consult the labelling of concurrently-used drugs to obtain further information about interactions with hormonal contraceptives or the potential for enzyme alterations.

Refer to Oral Contraceptives 1994 (Chapter 8), Health Canada, for possible drug interactions with OCs.

Table 1: Ortho-Cept

Drugs That May Decrease the Efficacy of Oral Contraceptives

Class of Compound	Drug	Proposed Mechanism	Suggested Management
Anticonvulsants	Carbamazepine Ethosuximide Phenobarbital Phenytoin Primidone	Induction of hepatic microsomal enzymes: Rapid metabolism of estrogen and increased binding of progestin and ethinyl estradiol to SHBG.	Use higher dose OCs (50 µg ethinyl estradiol), another drug or another method.

* Additional drugs are listed in Table I.
† Additional drugs are listed in Table II.

(cont'd)

Table 1: Ortho-Cept *(cont'd)*

Drugs That May Decrease the Efficacy of Oral Contraceptives

Class of Compound	Drug	Proposed Mechanism	Suggested Management
Antibiotics	Ampicillin Cotrimoxazole Penicillin	Enterohepatic circulation disturbance, intestinal hurry.	For short course, use additional method or use another drug. For long course, use another method.
	Rifampin	Increased metabolism of progestins. Suspected acceleration of estrogen metabolism.	Use another method.
	Chloramphenicol Metronidazole Neomycin Nitrofurantoin Sulfonamides Tetracyclines	Induction of hepatic microsomal enzymes. Also disturbance of enterohepatic circulation.	For short course, use additional method or use another drug. For long course, use another method.
	Troleandomycin	May retard metabolism of OCs, increasing the risk of cholestatic jaundice.	
Antifungals	Griseofulvin	Stimulation of hepatic metabolism of contraceptive steroids may occur.	Use another method.
Sedatives and Hypnotics	Benzodiazepines Barbiturates Chloral Hydrate Glutethimide Meprobamate	Induction of hepatic microsomal enzymes.	For short course, use additional method or another drug. For long course, use another method or higher dose OCs.
Antacids		Decreased intestinal absorption of progestins.	Dose two hours apart.
Other Drugs	Phenylbutazone Antihistamines Analgesics Antimigraine preparations Vitamin E	Reduced OC efficacy has been reported. Remains to be confirmed.	
	Bosentan	Induction of hepatic microsomal enzymes	Consider switching to a non-hormonal contraceptive method or adding a barrier method to oral contraceptive therapy.

Table 2: Ortho-Cept

Modification of Other Drug Action by Oral Contraceptives

Class of Compound	Drug	Modification of Drug Action	Suggested Management
Alcohol		Possible increased levels of ethanol or acetaldehyde.	Use with caution.
Alpha-II Adrenoreceptor Agents	Clonidine	Sedation effect increased.	Use with caution.
Anticoagulants	All	OCs increase clotting factors, decrease efficacy. However, OCs may potentiate action in some patients.	Use another method.
Anticonvulsants	All	Fluid retention may increase risk of seizures.	Use another method.
	Lamotrigine	Significantly decreased lamotrigine levels (due to induction of lamotrigine glucuronidation) may lead to breakthrough seizures.	Adjust dose of drug if necessary.
Antidiabetic Drugs	Oral hypoglycemics and insulin	OCs may impair glucose tolerance and increase blood glucose.	Use low-dose estrogen and progestin OC or another method. Monitor blood glucose.
Antihypertensive Agents	Guanethidine and methyldopa	Estrogen component causes sodium retention, progestin has no effect.	Use low-dose estrogen OC or use another method.
	Beta-blockers	Increased drug effect (decreased metabolism).	Adjust dose of drug if necessary. Monitor cardiovascular status.
Antipyretics	Acetaminophen	Increased metabolism and renal clearance.	Dose of drug may have to be increased.
	Antipyrine	Impaired metabolism.	Decrease dose of drug.
	ASA	Effects of ASA may be decreased by the short-term use of OCs.	Patients on chronic ASA therapy may require an increase in ASA dosage.

(cont'd)

Table 2: Ortho-Cept *(cont'd)*

Modification of Other Drug Action by Oral Contraceptives

Class of Compound	Drug	Modification of Drug Action	Suggested Management
Aminocaproic Acid		Theoretically, a hypercoagulable state may occur because OCs augment clotting factors.	Avoid concomitant use.
Betamimetic Agents	Isoproterenol	Estrogen causes decreased response to these drugs.	Adjust dose of drug as necessary. Discontinuing OCs can result in excessive drug activity.
Caffeine		The actions of caffeine may be enhanced as OCs may impair the hepatic metabolism of caffeine.	Use with caution.
Corticosteroids	Prednisone Prednisolone	Markedly increased serum levels.	Possible need for decrease in dose.
Cyclosporine		May lead to an increase in cyclosporine levels and hepatotoxicity.	Monitor hepatic function. The cyclosporine dose may have to be decreased.
Folic Acid		OCs have been reported to impair folate metabolism.	May need to increase dietary intake or supplement.
Meperidine		Possible increased analgesia and CNS depression due to decreased metabolism of meperidine.	Use combination with caution.
Phenothiazine Tranquilizers	All phenothiazines, reserpine and similar drugs	Estrogen potentiates the hyperprolactinemia effect of these drugs.	Use other drugs or lower dose OCs. If galactorrhea or hyperprolactinemia occurs, use other method.
Sedatives and Hypnotics	Chlordiazepoxide Lorazepam Oxazepam Diazepam	Increased effect (increased metabolism).	Use with caution.
Theophylline	All	Decreased oxidation, leading to possible toxicity.	Use with caution. Monitor theophylline levels.
Tricyclic Antidepressants	Clomipramine (possibly others)	Increased side effects; i.e., depression.	Use with caution.
Vitamin B_{12}		OCs have been reported to reduce serum levels of Vitamin B_{12}.	May need to increase dietary intake, or supplement.

Non-contraceptive Benefits of Oral Contraceptives: Several health advantages other than contraception have been reported.

1. Combination oral contraceptives reduce the incidence of cancer of the endometrium and ovaries.
2. Oral contraceptives reduce the likelihood of developing benign breast disease and, as a result, decrease the incidence of breast biopsies.
3. Oral contraceptives reduce the likelihood of development of functional ovarian cysts.
4. Pill users have less menstrual blood loss and have more regular cycles, thereby reducing the chance of developing iron-deficiency anemia.
5. The use of oral contraceptives may decrease the severity of dysmenorrhea and premenstrual syndrome, and may improve acne vulgaris, hirsutism and other androgen-mediated disorders.
6. Oral contraceptives decrease the incidence of acute pelvic inflammatory disease and, thereby, reduce as well the incidence of ectopic pregnancy.
7. Oral contraceptives have potential beneficial effects on endometriosis.

Oral contraceptives **do not protect** against sexually transmitted diseases (STDs) including HIV/AIDS. For protection against STDs, it is advisable to use latex condoms **in combination with** oral contraceptives.

ADVERSE EFFECTS: An increased risk of the following serious adverse reactions has been associated with the use of oral contraceptives: thrombophlebitis and venous thrombosis with or without embolism, arterial thromboembolism, pulmonary embolism, mesenteric thrombosis, neuro-ocular lesions (e.g., retinal thrombosis), myocardial infarction, cerebral thrombosis, cerebral hemorrhage, hypertension, benign hepatic tumors, gallbladder disease.

The following adverse reactions also have been reported in patients receiving oral contraceptives. Nausea and vomiting, usually the most common adverse reaction, occurs in approximately 10% or less of patients during the first cycle. Other reactions, as a general rule, are seen less frequently or only occasionally, as follows: gastrointestinal symptoms (such as abdominal cramps and bloating), breakthrough bleeding, spotting, change in menstrual flow, dysmenorrhea, amenorrhea during and after treatment, temporary infertility after discontinuance of treatment, edema, chloasma or melasma which may persist, breast changes (tenderness, enlargement and secretion), change in weight (increase or decrease), endocervical hyperplasias, possible diminution in lactation when given immediately postpartum, cholestatic jaundice, migraine, increase in size of uterine leiomyomata, rash (allergic), depression, reduced tolerance to carbohydrates, vaginal candidiasis, premenstrual-like syndrome, intolerance to contact lenses, change in corneal curvature (steepening), cataracts, optic neuritis, retinal thrombosis, changes in libido, chorea, changes in appetite, cystitis-like syndrome, rhinitis, headache, nervousness, dizziness, hirsutism, loss of scalp hair, erythema multiforme, erythema nodosum, hemorrhagic eruption, vaginitis, porphyria, impaired renal function, Raynaud's phenomenon, auditory disturbances, hemolytic uremic syndrome, pancreatitis, change in cervical erosion and secretion, acne, colitis, Budd-Chiari Syndrome.

OVERDOSE:

Treatment: In case of overdose or accidental ingestion by children, the physician should observe the patient closely although generally no treatment is required. Gastric lavage may be utilized if considered necessary. Overdosage may cause nausea and vomiting and withdrawal bleeding may occur in females. There are no antidotes and treatment should be symptomatic.

For management of a suspected drug overdose, CPhA recommends that you contact your **regional Poison Control Centre**. See the *CPS* Directory section for a list of Poison Control Centres.

DOSAGE: **Information for the Patient on How to Take the Birth Control Pill:**

1. **Read these directions:**
   - before you start taking your pills, and
   - any time you are not sure what to do.
2. **Look at your pill pack:**

• **28-Pill Pack:** 21 active pills (with hormones) taken daily for 3 weeks, and then 7 "reminder" pills (no hormones) taken daily for 1 week.
Also check the pill pack for instructions on (1) where to start and (2) directions to take pills (see package insert for illustrations).
3. You may wish to use a second method of birth control (e.g., latex condoms and spermicidal foam or gel) for the first 7 days of the first cycle of pill use. This will provide a back-up in case pills are forgotten while you are getting used to taking them.
4. **When receiving any medical treatment, be sure to tell your doctor that you are using birth control pills.**
5. **Many women have spotting or light bleeding, or may feel sick to their stomach during the first 3 months on the pill.** If you do feel sick, do not stop taking the pill. The problem will usually go away. If it does not go away, check with your doctor or clinic.
6. **Missing pills also can cause some spotting or light bleeding**, even if you make up the missed pills. You also could feel a little sick to your stomach on the days you take 2 pills to make up for missed pills.
7. **If you miss pills at any time, you could get pregnant. The greatest risks for pregnancy are:**
   • when you start a pack late, or
   • when you miss pills at the beginning or at the very end of the pack.
8. **Always be sure you have ready:**
   • **another kind of birth control** (such as latex condoms and spermicidal foam or gel) to use as a back-up in case you miss pills, and
   • **an extra, full pack of pills.**
9. **If you experience vomiting or diarrhea, or if you take certain medicines**, such as antibiotics, your pills may not work as well. Use a back-up method, such as latex condoms and spermicidal foam or gel, until you can check with your doctor or clinic.
10. **If you forget more than 1 pill 2 months in a row**, talk to your doctor or clinic about how to make pill-taking easier or about using another method of birth control.
11. **If your questions are not answered here, call your doctor or clinic.**

When to start the first pack of pills: Be sure to read these instructions:
• before you start taking your pills, and
• any time you are not sure what to do.
Decide with your doctor or clinic what is the best day for you to start taking your first pack of pills.

A. 28-Day Combination: With this type of birth control pill, you take 21 pills which contain hormones and 7 pills which contain no hormones.
1. **The first day of your menstrual period (bleeding) is Day 1 of your cycle.** The pills may be started up to Day 6 of your cycle. Your starting day will be chosen in discussion with your doctor. You will **always** begin taking your pill on this day of the week. Your doctor may advise you to start taking the pills on Day 1, on Day 5, or on the first Sunday after your period begins. If your period starts on Sunday, start that same day.
2. Take 1 pill at approximately the same time every day for 28 days. Begin a new pack the next day, **not missing any days on the pills**. Your period should occur during the last 7 days of using that pill pack.

Instructions for Using Your DIALPAK Tablet Dispenser: Follow these instructions carefully: 28 Day Regimen: (see package insert for illustrations): **Always complete the orange tablets before taking the green tablets.**

Please make sure that your DIALPAK Tablet Dispenser is aligned such that the Black Day Arrow in the center of the plastic points to the Black Day Arrow at the top of the package (towards the cover) as shown in the diagram. To align the Black Day Arrows, turn the ribbed outer ring to the right. The Black Day Arrows should be pointing at the first orange tablet to the left of the green tablets.

Your starting day will be chosen in discussion with your doctor. You should **always** begin taking your tablets on this day of the week. To set the package to the day you and your doctor selected, a calendar label is enclosed. To put the label in place, identify your correct starting day, locate that day on the label, line that day up with the pill to which the Black Day Arrow is pointing, remove the label from the backing and press the label over the printed calendar on the center of the plastic. The first orange tablet you will take is to the left of the green tablets and between the Black Day Arrows. Push down on your first orange tablet with your thumb or forefinger. The tablet will come out through a hole in the back of the package. To take your second and subsequent tablets, turn the ribbed outer ring to the right. Take 1 tablet every day, first completing all 21 orange tablets, and finally the 7 green tablets. Begin your next package the very next day, your chosen starting day, whether you have finished menstruating or not. Always remember to set the starting day of each new package to the day chosen by you and your doctor.

What to do during the month:
1. **Take a pill at approximately the same time every day until the pack is empty.**
   • Try to associate taking your pill with some regular activity such as eating a meal or going to bed.
   • Do not skip pills even if you have bleeding between monthly periods or feel sick to your stomach (nausea).
   • Do not skip pills even if you do not have sex very often.
2. **When you finish a pack:**
   • **28 pills:** Start the next pack **on the next day**. Take 1 pill every day. Do not wait any days between packs.

What to do if you miss pills: Table 3 outlines the actions you should take if you miss 1 or more of your birth control pills. Match the number of pills missed with the appropriate starting time for your type of pill pack.

Note: 28-Day Pack: If you forget any of the 7 "reminder" pills (without hormones) in Week 4, just safely dispose of the pills you missed. Then keep taking 1 pill each day until the pack is empty. You do not need to use a back-up method.

Always be sure you have on hand:
• a back-up method of birth control (such as latex condoms and spermicidal foam or gel) in case you miss pills, and
• an extra, full pack of pills.

If you forget more than 1 pill 2 months in a row, talk to your doctor or clinic about ways to make pill-taking easier or about using another method of birth control.

Table 3: Ortho-Cept

What to Do if You Miss Pills

Sunday Start	Other Than Sunday Start
Miss 1 pill	**Miss 1 pill**
Take it as soon as you remember, and take the next pill at the usual time. This means that you might take 2 pills in one day.	Take it as soon as you remember, and take the next pill at the usual time. This means that you might take 2 pills in one day.
Miss 2 pills in a row	**Miss 2 pills in a row**
First 2 Weeks: 1. Take 2 pills the day you remember and 2 pills the next day. 2. Then take 1 pill a day until you finish the pack. 3. Use a back-up method of birth control if you have sex in the 7 days after you miss the pills. **Third Week:** 1. Keep taking 1 pill a day until Sunday. 2. On Sunday, safely discard the rest of the pack and start a new pack that day. 3. Use a back-up method of birth control if you have sex in the 7 days after you miss the pills. 4. You may not have a period this month. **If you miss 2 periods in a row, call your doctor or clinic.**	**First 2 Weeks:** 1. Take 2 pills the day you remember and 2 pills the next day. 2. Then take 1 pill a day until you finish the pack. 3. Use a back-up method of birth control if you have sex in the 7 days after you miss the pills. **Third Week:** 1. Safely dispose of the rest of the pill pack and start a new pack that same day. 2. Use a back-up method of birth control if you have sex in the 7 days after you miss the pills. 3. You may not have a period this month. **If you miss 2 periods in a row, call your doctor or clinic.**
Miss 3 or more pills in a row	**Miss 3 or more pills in a row**

(cont'd)

Table 3: Ortho-Cept *(cont'd)*

What to Do if You Miss Pills

Sunday Start	Other Than Sunday Start
Anytime in the Cycle: 1. Keep taking 1 pill a day until Sunday. 2. On Sunday, safely discard the rest of the pack and start a new pack that day. 3. Use a back-up method of birth control if you have sex in the 7 days after you miss the pills. 4. You may not have a period this month. **If you miss 2 periods in a row, call your doctor or clinic.**	**Anytime in the Cycle:** 1. Safely dispose of the rest of the pill pack and start a new pack that same day. 2. Use a back-up method of birth control if you have sex in the 7 days after you miss the pills. 3. You may not have a period this month. **If you miss 2 periods in a row, call your doctor or clinic.**

INFORMATION FOR THE PATIENT: Published in e-CPS, available by subscription at www.e-cps.ca.

SUPPLIED: Each orange tablet, unscored with D 150 engraved on each side, contains: desogestrel 0.15 mg and ethinyl estradiol 0.03 mg. The green tablet, engraved with ORTHO P on each side, contains: inert ingredients. Nonmedicinal ingredients: Orange tablets: colloidal silicon dioxide, hydroxypropyl methylcellulose, iron oxide (red and yellow), lactose, polyethylene glycol, povidone, starch, stearic acid, talc, titanium dioxide and vitamin E; Green tablets: hydroxypropyl methylcellulose, indigotin blue or FD&C Blue No. 1, iron oxide (red and yellow), lactose, magnesium stearate, polyethylene glycol, starch, talc and titanium dioxide. 28-Day DIALPAK Tablet Dispenser (21 active and 7 inert tablets). Store between 15 and 30°C. Leave contents in protective packaging until time of use.

(Shown in Product Identification Section)

OrthoVisc

sodium hyaluronate

Synovial Fluid Replacement/Replenishment

Helix Biopharma

DESCRIPTION: Sodium hyaluronate is a high molecular weight polysaccharide composed of sodium glucuronate and N-acetylglucosamine. Sodium hyaluronate is ubiquitously distributed throughout the tissues of the body and is present in high concentrations in such tissues as vitreous humor, synovial fluid, umbilical cord and dermis. Sodium hyaluronate functions as a tissue lubricant and is thought to play an important role in modulating the interactions between adjacent tissues. It can also act as a viscoelastic support maintaining a separation between tissues. Different sodium hyaluronate preparations may have different molecular weights, but are thought to have the same chemical structure. The sodium hyaluronate in OrthoVisc has an average molecular weight greater than one million. OrthoVisc is non-inflammatory, is non-pyrogenic and is well tolerated. Sodium hyaluronate has been shown to be non-antigenic. OrthoVisc does not interfere with normal wound healing processes.

INDICATIONS: OrthoVisc is indicated for the symptomatic treatment of osteoarthritis of the knee.

CONTRAINDICATIONS: At the present time there are no known contraindications to the use of OrthoVisc when used in the symptomatic treatment of joint disease.

OrthoVisc may contain trace quantities of gram positive bacterial proteins and is contraindicated for patients with a history of such allergies. There are minimal risks associated with the procedure of injecting substances into joints in general; primarily infection and bleeding. Pre-existing infections of the skin in the region of the intended injection or known systemic bleeding disorders may constitute relative or absolute contraindications.

PRECAUTIONS: Those precautions normally considered during injection of substances into joints are recommended. Only individuals familiar with accepted injection techniques for delivering agents to joint spaces should inject sodium hyaluronate for this application. An excess quantity of sodium hyaluronate is not to be used and the patient should be monitored closely. If pain increases during the injection procedure, the injection should be stopped and the needle withdrawn. The space should not be overfilled.

ADVERSE EFFECTS: Sodium hyaluronate is a natural component of the tissues in the body. OrthoVisc is thoroughly tested to determine that each batch is non-inflammatory. Adverse events reported in clinical trials have included mild or moderate reactions at the site of the injection. Based upon clinical studies, these reactions have occurred with a similar incidence in patients treated with saline injections. There is no evidence which attributes reactions to be specifically related to the product.

OVERDOSE:

For management of a suspected drug overdose, CPhA recommends that you contact your **regional Poison Control Centre**. See the *CPS* Directory section for a list of Poison Control Centres.

DOSAGE: OrthoVisc is injected by intra-articular injection one week apart for a total of three injections. The required amount of OrthoVisc is slowly infused through a sterile hypodermic needle of suitable gauge into the selected joint space. A plastic-hubbed needle is recommended.

The volume will vary depending upon the size of the joint space, not to exceed 2 mL for the knee.

Do not overfill the joint space.

SUPPLIED: Each mL of sterile viscoelastic preparation contains: sodium hyaluronate 15 mg adjusted to 20 000-70 000 centistokes, sodium chloride 9 mg and sterile water for injection USP q.s. Osmolality: approximately 340 mOsm. Disposable glass syringes delivering 2 mL, appropriate for the knee, of sodium hyaluronate dissolved in physiological saline. Contents of unopened and undamaged syringe are sterile. Refrigerated OrthoVisc should be allowed to reach room temperature, approximately 20 to 45 minutes, prior to use. For intra-articular use. Store between 2 and 25°C. Protect from freezing.

Osmitrol®

mannitol

Osmotic Diuretic

Baxter

SUPPLIED: Each mL of aqueous solution contains: mannitol 10% or 20% (see Table 1). Do not store above 30°C. Protect from freezing.

Table 1: Osmitrol

Viaflex Plus Plastic (polyvinyl chloride) Containers

Total Volume (mL)	Total Mannitol Content (g)	Mannitol Concentration (g/mL)
250	50	0.2
500	100	0.2
1000	100	0.1

Osmopak Plus

magnesium sulfate—benzocaine
Drawing Salve

Rougier Pharma

SUPPLIED: Each g of thick turquoise ointment with a characteristic aromatic odor, contains: magnesium sulfate equivalent to the hepta-hydrated form 60% and benzocaine 0.5% in a water miscible base. Nonmedicinal ingredients: FD&C Green #3, fir oil, hydroxyethylcellulose, lavender extract, methyl salicylate, propylene glycol and purified water. Jars of 50 g.

Ovidrel™ Ⓟ

choriogonadotropin alpha
Gonadotropin

EMD Canada

Date of Preparation: November 24, 2004

PHARMACOLOGY: Ovidrel (choriogonadotropin alpha) is a sterile solution or sterile lyophilised powder for injection preparation of choriogonadotropin alpha (recombinant human Chorionic Gonadotrophin, r-hCG). The drug substance is produced by recombinant DNA techniques. Choriogonadotropin alpha is a water soluble glycoprotein consisting of two non-covalently linked subunits—designated α and β—consisting of 92 and 145 amino acid residues, respectively, with carbohydrate moieties linked to ASN-52 and ASN-78 (on alpha subunit) and ASN-13, ASN-30, SER-121, SER-127, SER-132 and SER-138 (on beta subunit). The primary structure of the α-chain of r-hCG is identical to that of the α-chain of hCG, FSH and LH. The glycoform pattern of the α-subunit of r-hCG is closely comparable to urinary derived hCG (u-hCG), the differences mainly being due to the branching and salicylation extent of the oligosaccharides. The β-chain has both O- and N-glycosylation sites and its structure and glycosylation pattern are also very similar to that of u-hCG.

The production process involves expansion of genetically modified Chinese Hamster Ovary (CHO) cells from an extensively characterized cell bank into large scale cell culture processing. Choriogonadotropin alpha is secreted by CHO cells directly into the cell culture medium, which is then purified using a series of chromatographic steps. This process yields a product with a high level of purity and consistent product characteristics including glycoforms and biological activity. The biological activity of choriogonadotropin alpha is determined using the seminal vesicle weight gain test in male rats described in the "Chorionic Gonadotrophins" monograph of the European Pharmacopoeia. The in vivo biological activity of choriogonadotropin alpha has been calibrated against the third international reference preparation IS75/587 for chorionic gonadotrophin.

The physicochemical, immunological, and biological activities of recombinant hCG are comparable to those of placental and human pregnancy urine-derived hCG. Choriogonadotropin alpha stimulates late follicular maturation and resumption of oocyte meiosis, and initiates rupture of the pre-ovulatory ovarian follicle. Choriogonadotropin alpha, the active component of Ovidrel, is an analogue of Luteinizing Hormone (LH) and binds to the LH/hCG receptor of the granulosa and theca cells of the ovary to effect these changes in the absence of an endogenous LH surge. In pregnancy, hCG, secreted by the placenta, maintains the viability of the corpus luteum to provide the continued secretion of estrogen and progesterone necessary to support the first trimester of pregnancy. Ovidrel is administered when monitoring of the patient indicates that sufficient follicular development has occurred in response to follicle stimulating agent treatment for ovulation induction.

INDICATIONS: Ovidrel (choriogonadotropin alpha) is indicated for the induction of ovulation (OI) and pregnancy in patients undergoing fertility treatment in whom the cause of infertility is functional and not due to primary ovarian failure.

Selection of Patients:

1. Before treatment with gonadotrophins is instituted, a thorough gynecologic and endocrinologic evaluation must be performed. This should include an assessment of pelvic anatomy. Patients with tubal obstruction should receive Ovidrel only if enrolled in an in vitro fertilization program.
2. Primary ovarian failure should be excluded by the determination of gonadotrophin levels.
3. Appropriate evaluation should be performed to exclude pregnancy.
4. Women in later reproductive life have a greater predisposition to endometrial carcinoma as well as a higher incidence of anovulatory disorders. A thorough diagnostic evaluation should always be performed in patients who demonstrate abnormal uterine bleeding or other signs of endometrial abnormalities before starting follicle stimulating agent and Ovidrel therapy.
5. Evaluation of the partner's fertility potential should be included in the initial evaluation.

CONTRAINDICATIONS: Ovidrel (choriogonadotropin alpha) is contraindicated in women who exhibit:

1. Prior hypersensitivity to hCG preparations or one of their excipients.
2. Primary ovarian failure.
3. Uncontrolled thyroid or adrenal dysfunction.
4. An uncontrolled organic intracranial lesion such as a pituitary tumor.
5. Abnormal uterine bleeding of undetermined origin (see Indications, Selection of Patients).
6. Ovarian cyst or enlargement of undetermined origin (see Indications, Selection of Patients).
7. Sex hormone-dependent tumors of the reproductive organs and breasts.
8. Pregnancy.

WARNINGS: Gonadotrophins, including Ovidrel (choriogonadotropin alpha), should only be used by physicians who are thoroughly familiar with infertility problems and their management. Like other hCG products, Ovidrel is a potent gonadotrophic substance capable of causing Ovarian Hyperstimulation Syndrome (OHSS) in women with or without pulmonary or vascular complications. Gonadotrophin therapy requires a certain time commitment by physicians and supportive health professionals, and requires the availability of appropriate monitoring facilities (see Precautions, Laboratory Tests). Safe and effective induction of ovulation and use of Ovidrel in women requires monitoring of ovarian response with serum estradiol and transvaginal ultrasound on a regular basis.

Overstimulation of the Ovary Following hCG Therapy: Ovarian Enlargement: Mild to moderate uncomplicated ovarian enlargement which may be accompanied by abdominal distention and/or abdominal pain may occur in patients treated with follicle stimulating agents and hCG, and generally regresses without treatment within two or three weeks. Careful monitoring of ovarian response can further minimize the risk of overstimulation. If the ovaries are abnormally enlarged on the last day of follicle stimulating agent therapy, choriogonadotropin alpha may be withheld in this course of therapy. This will reduce the risk of development of Ovarian Hyperstimulation Syndrome.

Ovarian Hyperstimulation Syndrome (OHSS): OHSS is a medical event distinct from uncomplicated ovarian enlargement. Severe OHSS may progress rapidly (within 24 hours to several days) to become a serious medical event. It is characterized by an apparent dramatic increase in vascular permeability which can result in a rapid accumulation of fluid in the peritoneal cavity, thorax, and potentially, the pericardium. The early warning signs of development of OHSS are severe pelvic pain, nausea, vomiting, and weight gain. The following symptomatology has been seen with cases of OHSS: abdominal pain, abdominal distention, gastrointestinal symptoms including nausea, vomiting and diarrhea, severe ovarian enlargement, weight gain, dyspnea, and oliguria. Clinical evaluation may reveal hypovolemia, hemoconcentration, electrolyte imbalances, ascites, hemoperitoneum, pleural effusions, hydrothorax, acute pulmonary distress, and thromboembolic events (see Pulmonary and Vascular Complications). Transient liver function test abnormalities suggestive of hepatic dysfunction, which may be accompanied by morphologic changes on liver biopsy, have been reported in association with Ovarian Hyperstimulation Syndrome (OHSS).

OHSS occurred in 3 of 99 (3.0%) patients treated with Ovidrel 250 µg in an ovulation induction trial, and in 4 of 236 (1.7 %) patients treated with Ovidrel 250 µg in other clinical studies. OHSS occurred in 8 of 89 (9.0%) patients who received Ovidrel 500 µg. Two patients treated with Ovidrel 500 µg developed severe OHSS.

OHSS may be more severe and more protracted if pregnancy occurs. OHSS develops rapidly; therefore, patients should be followed for at least two weeks after hCG administration. Most often, OHSS occurs after treatment has been discontinued and reaches its maximum at about seven to ten days following hCG treatment. Usually, OHSS resolves spontaneously with the onset of menses. If there is evidence that OHSS may be developing prior to hCG administration (see Precautions, Laboratory Tests), the hCG should be withheld. If severe OHSS occurs, treatment with gonadotrophins must be stopped and the patient should be hospitalized. A physician experienced in the management of this syndrome, or who is experienced in the management of fluid and electrolyte imbalances should be consulted.

Pulmonary and Vascular Complications: As with other hCG products, a potential for the occurrence of arterial thromboembolism exists.

Reproductive Complications: As with other hCG products, reports of multiple births have been associated with Ovidrel treatment when used in combination with follicle stimulating agents. The risk of multiple births correlates to the number of embryos transferred or mature follicles that develop for ovulation induction. In the ovulation induction clinical trial, 2 of 15 live deliveries (13.3%) were associated with multiple births in women receiving Ovidrel. Multiple births occurred in 17 of 55 live deliveries (30.9 %) experienced by women receiving Ovidrel 250 µg in other clinical studies. The patient should be advised of the potential risk of multiple births before starting treatment with follicle stimulating agents and Ovidrel.

PRECAUTIONS: General: Careful attention should be given to the diagnosis of infertility in candidates for hCG therapy (see Indications, Selection of Patients). After the exclusion of pre-existing conditions, elevations in ALT were found in 10 (3%) of 335 patients receiving Ovidrel (chorigonadotrophin alpha) 250 µg, 9 (10%) of 89 patients receiving Ovidrel 500 µg and in 16 (4.8%) of 328 patients receiving urinary-derived hCG. The elevations ranged up to 1.2 times the upper limit of normal. The clinical significance of these findings is not known.

Information to Be Provided to the Patient: Prior to therapy with hCG, patients should be informed of the duration of treatment and monitoring of their condition that will be required. The risks of Ovarian Hyperstimulation Syndrome and multiple births in women (see Warnings) and other possible adverse reactions (see Adverse Effects) should also be discussed.

Laboratory Tests: In most instances, treatment of women with follicle stimulating agents results only in follicular recruitment and development. In the absence of an endogenous LH surge, hCG is given when monitoring of the patient indicates that sufficient follicular development has occurred. This may be estimated by ultrasound alone or in combination with measurement of serum estradiol levels. The combination of both ultrasound and serum estradiol measurement are useful for monitoring the development of follicles, for timing of the ovulatory trigger, as well as for detecting ovarian enlargement and minimizing the risk of the Ovarian Hyperstimulation Syndrome and multiple gestation. It is recommended that the number of growing follicles be confirmed using ultrasonography because serum estrogen levels do not give an indication of the size or number of follicles.

Human chorionic gonadotrophins can cross-react in the radioimmunoassay of gonadotrophins, especially luteinizing hormone. Each individual laboratory should establish the degree of cross-reactivity with their gonadotrophin assay. Physicians should make the laboratory aware of patients on hCG if gonadotrophin levels are requested.

The clinical confirmation of ovulation, with the exception of pregnancy, is obtained by direct and indirect indices of progesterone production. The indices most generally used are as follows: a rise in basal body temperature, increase in serum progesterone and menstruation following a shift in basal body temperature.

When used in conjunction with the indices of progesterone production, sonographic visualization of the ovaries will assist in determining if ovulation has occurred. Sonographic evidence of ovulation may include the following: fluid in the cul-de-sac, ovarian stigmata suggestive of a corpus luteum, collapsed follicle.

Accurate interpretation of the indices of ovulation require a physician who is experienced in the interpretation of these tests.

Carcinogenesis, Mutagenesis, Impairment of Fertility: Long-term studies to evaluate the carcinogenic potential of Ovidrel in animals have not been performed. In-vitro genotoxicity testing of Ovidrel in bacteria and mammalian cell lines, chromosome aberration assay in human lymphocytes and in-vivo mouse micronucleus have shown no indication of genetic defects.

Pregnancy: No clinical data on exposed pregnancies are available. No reproduction studies with choriogonadotropin alpha in animals were performed. The potential risk for humans is unknown.

Lactation: It is not known whether this drug is excreted in human milk. Because many drugs are excreted in human milk, caution should be exercised if hCG is administered to a nursing woman.

Pediatrics: Ovidrel is only intended for use in female patients of reproductive age, therefore, safety and effectiveness in pediatric patients has not been established.

Geriatrics: Ovidrel is only intended for use in female patients of reproductive age, therefore, safety and effectiveness in geriatric patients has not been established.

Drug Interactions: No clinically significant drug interactions have been reported during hCG therapy. Following administration, Ovidrel may interfere for up to ten days with the immunological determination of serum/urinary hCG, leading to a false positive pregnancy test.

ADVERSE EFFECTS: The safety of Ovidrel (choriogonadotropin alpha) was examined in four clinical studies that treated 752 patients of whom 335 received Ovidrel 250 µg following follicular recruitment with gonadotrophins. When patients enrolled in four clinical studies (1 in ovulation induction and 3 in assisted reproductive technologies) were injected subcutaneously with either Ovidrel or an approved urinary-derived hCG, 14.6 % (49 of 335 patients) in the Ovidrel 250 µg group experienced application site disorders compared to 28% (92 of 328 patients) in the approved u-hCG group. Adverse events reported for Ovidrel 250 µg occurring in at least 2% of patients (regardless of causality) are listed in Table 1 for the single OI study.

Table 1: Ovidrel

Incidence of Adverse Events of r-hCG in Ovulation Induction (Study 8209)

Body System Preferred Term	Ovidrel 250 µg (n=99) Incidence Rate % (n)
At Least One Adverse Event	26.2% (26)
Application Site Disorders	**16.2% (16)**
Injection Site Pain	8.1% (8)
Injection Site Bruising	3.0% (3)
Injection Site Inflammation	2.0% (2)
Injection Site Reaction	3.0% (3)
Gastro-intestinal System Disorders	**4.0% (4)**
Abdominal Pain	3.0% (3)
Reproductive Disorders, Female	**7.1% (7)**
Ovarian Cyst	3.0% (3)
Ovarian Hyperstimulation	3.0% (3)

Additional adverse events not listed in Table 1 that occurred in less than 2% of patients treated with Ovidrel 250 µg, whether or not considered causally related to Ovidrel, included: breast pain, flatulence, abdominal enlargement, pharyngitis, upper respiratory tract infection, hyperglycemia and pruritis.

In three studies involving 236 patients treated with Ovidrel 250 µg and undergoing assisted reproductive technologies (Studies 7648, 7927 and 9073—Chang, 2001), at least one adverse event was observed in 78 patients (33.1%). Application site disorders occurred in 14.0% of patients, which included injection site pain in 7.6% and injection site bruising in 4.7% of subjects. Twenty patients (8.5%) experienced gastro-intestinal system disorders, and these events included abdominal pain (4.2%), nausea (3.4%) and vomiting (2.5%). Post-operative pain was noted by 4.7% of patients participating in the studies. Adverse events that occurred in less than 2% of patients treated with Ovidrel 250 µg, whether or not considered causally related to Ovidrel, included: injection site inflammation and reaction, flatulence, diarrhea, hiccup, ectopic pregnancy, breast pain, intermenstrual bleeding, vaginal hemorrhage, vaginal discharge, cervical lesion, ovarian hyperstimulation, uterine disorders, vaginitis, vaginal discomfort, body pain, back pain, fever, dizziness, headache, hot flashes, malaise, paraesthesia, rash, emotional lability, insomnia, upper respiratory tract infection, cough, dysuria, urinary tract infection, urinary incontinence, albuminuria, cardiac arrhythmia, genital moniliasis, genital herpes, leukocytosis, heart murmur and cervical carcinoma.

The following medical events have been reported subsequent to pregnancies resulting from hCG therapy in controlled clinical studies: spontaneous abortion, ectopic pregnancy, premature labor, postpartum fever, congenital abnormalities.

Of 125 clinical pregnancies reported following treatment with FSH and Ovidrel 250 µg or 500 µg, three were associated with a congenital anomaly of the fetus or newborn. Among patients receiving Ovidrel 250 µg, cranial malformation was detected in the fetus of one woman and a chromosomal abnormality (47, XXX) in another. These events were judged by the investigators to be of unlikely or unknown relation to treatment. These three events represent an incidence of major congenital malformations of

2.4%, which is consistent with the reported rate for pregnancies resulting from natural or assisted conception. In a woman who received Ovidrel 500 µg, one birth in a set of triplets was associated with Down's syndrome and atrial septal defect. This event was considered to be unrelated to the study drug.

The following adverse reactions have been previously reported during gonadotrophin or menotropin therapy: pulmonary and vascular complications (see Warnings), adnexal torsion (as a complication of ovarian enlargement), mild to moderate ovarian enlargement, hemoperitoneum.

There have been infrequent reports of ovarian neoplasms, both benign and malignant, in women who have undergone multiple drug regimens for ovulation induction; however, a causal relationship has not been established. During Ovidrel therapy, a minor thyroid stimulation is possible, of which the clinical relevance is unknown.

OVERDOSE:

Symptoms: No case of overdosage has been reported. Nevertheless, there is a possibility that Ovarian Hyperstimulation Syndrome (OHSS) may result from an overdosage of Ovidrel (choriogonadotropin alpha) (see Warnings).

For management of a suspected drug overdose, CPhA recommends that you contact your **regional Poison Control Centre**. See the *CPS* Directory section for a list of Poison Control Centres.

DOSAGE: Ovidrel (choriogonadotropin alpha) should not be administered until adequate follicular development is indicated by serum estradiol and/or vaginal ultrasonography.

Ovidrel 250 µg should be administered subcutaneously one day following the last dose of the follicle stimulating agent. Ovidrel administration should be withheld in situations where there is an excessive ovarian response, as evidenced by multiple follicular development, clinically significant ovarian enlargement or excessive estradiol production.

Reconstituted Solutions: Solution for Injection: The solution in the pre-filled syringe is ready for use. Single use only.

Lyophilised Powder in vials: Ovidrel is for single use only. One vial of Ovidrel can be reconstituted with 1 mL of the diluent provided. Any unused product or waste material should be disposed of in accordance with local requirements.

Parenteral Products: The pre-filled syringe solution or reconstituted lyophilised powder should not be administered if it contains particles or is not clear. Administration by the subcutaneous route.

In the absence of compatibility studies, this medicinal product should not be mixed with other medicinal products.

INFORMATION FOR THE PATIENT: Published in e-CPS, available by subscription at www.e-cps.ca.

SUPPLIED: Pre-filled Syringes: Each pre-filled syringe of sterile solution contains: 250 µg of choriogonadotropin alpha, 27.3 mg of mannitol, 0.49 mg of phosphoric acid, 0.1 mg of L-methionine, 0.05 mg of Poloxamer 188, sodium hydroxide (for pH adjustment) and water for injection to 0.5 mL. Packages of 1 ready-to-use pre-filled syringe.

Vials: Each vial of sterile, lyophilised powder contains: 285 µg of choriogonadotropin alpha, 30 mg of sucrose, 0.98 mg of phosphoric acid, and sodium hydroxide (for pH adjustment) which, when reconstituted with the diluent, will deliver 250 µg of recombinant human Chorionic Gonadotrophin. Packages of 1 vial of 250 µg Ovidrel and 1 vial or ampoule of 1 mL Sterile Water for Injection, USP/Ph.Eur. Packages of 10 vials of 250 µg Ovidrel and 10 vials or ampoules of 1 mL Sterile Water for Injection, USP/Ph.Eur.

Refer to the date indicated on the labels for the expiry date. Do not freeze. Store in the original package. Protect from light. Syringes of solution are stored at 2-8°C (in a refrigerator). Patient can either store the product at 25°C (room temperature) for up to 30 days or continue to refrigerate it until the expiration date. Lyophilised vials are stable when stored at or below room temperature (25°C).

Ovol® Preparations

simethicone

Antiflatulent

Church & Dwight

INDICATIONS: Specifically for symptomatic treatment of gastrointestinal discomfort due to entrapped gas. Relief of infant's symptoms of excess gas associated with colic.

CONTRAINDICATIONS: No data supplied by the manufacturer.

WARNINGS: Do not take for more than two weeks, nor if symptoms recur, unless directed by a physician.

Do not use in children under two years of age except on the advice of a physician.

PRECAUTIONS: No data supplied by the manufacturer.

ADVERSE EFFECTS: No data supplied by the manufacturer.

OVERDOSE:

Treatment: Symptomatic.

For management of a suspected drug overdose, CPhA recommends that you contact your **regional Poison Control Centre**. See the *CPS* Directory section for a list of Poison Control Centres.

DOSAGE: Drops: Infants, 0.25 to 0.50 mL with or after each meal. May be added to formula or given directly from dropper. Maximum: 1.5 mL/24 hours.

Softgel Capsules (180 mg): Caution: Not for children under 12 years of age. Adults: 180 mg (swallow 1 softgel after meals or at bedtime. Maximum 3 softgels/24 hours).

Tablets: Adults: 80 mg (1 or 2 tablets, 4 times daily); 180 mg (1 tablet, maximum 3 tablets/24 hours).

SUPPLIED: Drops: Each mL of white, opaque, peppermint flavored suspension with a milky appearance contains: simethicone 40 mg. Nonmedicinal ingredients: aluminum magnesium silicate, cellulose, citric acid, flavor, hydrogen peroxide, parabens, polyoxyl 8 stearate, purified water and sucrose. pH: 5.9 to 7.5. Energy: 1.2 kJ (0.3 kcal). Sodium: <1 mmol (0.8 mg). Alcohol-, gluten- and tartrazine-free. Dropper bottles of 15 and 30 mL.

Softgel Capsules: Ovol-180 Ultra Strength: Each softgel capsule contains: simethicone 180 mg. Nonmedicinal ingredients: D&C Red No. 33, FD&C Blue No. 1, gelatin, glycerin, lecithin, methylparaben and propylparaben. Gluten-, lactose- and sucrose-free. Push-through packages of 8 and 32.

Tablets: Ovol-80: Each white, round, flat, peppermint-flavored chewable tablet with beveled edges, quadrisected on both sides, contains: simethicone 80 mg. Nonmedicinal ingredients: cellulose, flavor, gelatin, magnesium stearate, silicon dioxide, sucrose and talc. Energy: 13.4 kJ (3.2 kcal). Sodium: <1 mmol (0.2 mg). Alcohol-, gluten- and tartrazine-free. Push-through packages of 10 and 50.

Ovol-180 Ultra Strength: Each white, round, flat, cherry-flavored chewable tablet with beveled edges, bisected on one side, engraved Ovol-180 on the other, contains: simethicone 180 mg. Nonmedicinal ingredients: aluminum hydroxide, calcium cyclamate, cellulose, citric acid, flavor, gelatin, magnesium stearate, silicon dioxide, sucrose and talc. Energy: 10.3 kJ (2.46 kcal). Sodium: <1 mmol (0.2 mg). Alcohol-, gluten- and tartrazine-free. Push-through packages of 16 and 32.

Ovral® 21 Ⓟ

norgestrel—ethinyl estradiol

Oral Contraceptive

Pfizer

SUPPLIED: Each white tablet engraved with W on one face and a "23" on the other face, contains: 250 µg of d-norgestrel (as 500 µg of the dl-racemate) and 50 µg of ethinyl estradiol. Energy: 1.59 kJ (0.38 kcal). Nonmedicinal ingredients: lactose, magnesium stearate, microcrystalline cellulose and polacrillin potassium. Gluten- and tartrazine-free. Blister packages of 21 tablets. Store at 15-30°C. Protect from light once opened using the protective covering provided. Keep out of reach of children.

(Shown in Product Identification Section)

Oxazepam Ⓝ

CPhA Monograph

see *Benzodiazepines*

Oxeze® Turbuhaler® Ⓟ

formoterol fumarate dihydrate

Bronchodilator

AstraZeneca

Date of Preparation: February 2, 2000
Date of Revision: February 9, 2009

SUMMARY PRODUCT INFORMATION:

Route of Administration	Dosage Form/ Strength	Clinically Relevant Nonmedicinal Ingredients
Oral Inhalation	Turbuhaler/ 6 µg/metered dose formoterol fumarate dihydrate 12 µg/metered dose formoterol fumarate dihydrate	Lactose monohydrate (which may contain milk protein residue) For a complete listing see Dosage Forms, Composition and Packaging.

INDICATIONS AND CLINICAL USE: OXEZE TURBUHALER (formoterol fumarate dihydrate) is indicated for the treatment and prevention of symptoms of reversible obstructive airways disease including asthma in patients* 6 years of age and older (this includes patients on concomitant inhaled corticosteroid therapy:)

*This includes patients on concomitant inhaled corticosteroid therapy:

- requiring long-term twice daily maintenance treatment of asthma
- requiring occasional use of a bronchodilator
- experiencing acute bronchoconstriction
- with nocturnal asthma
- with exercise-induced bronchoconstriction.

Corticosteroids should not be stopped because formoterol is prescribed.

OXEZE TURBUHALER should not be used in patients whose asthma can be managed by only occasional use of inhaled short-acting beta$_2$-agonists.

When treating asthma patients, OXEZE TURBUHALER should be used only as additional therapy for patients whose conditions are not adequately controlled using low-to-medium dose inhaled corticosteroids or whose disease severity clearly warrants the initiation of treatment with two maintenance therapies, i.e. OXEZE TURBUHALER in addition to an inhaled corticosteroid (see Warnings and Precautions).

CONTRAINDICATIONS: OXEZE TURBUHALER (formoterol fumarate dihydrate) is contraindicated when there is known hypersensitivity to formoterol or inhaled lactose. Like other sympathomimetic amines, OXEZE TURBUHALER should not be used in patients with tachyarrhythmias.

WARNINGS AND PRECAUTIONS:

Serious Warnings and Precautions

- Data from a large placebo-controlled US study (Salmeterol Multi-center Asthma Research Trial) comparing the safety of the long-acting beta$_2$-adrenergic agonist salmeterol to that of a placebo added to the original asthma therapy showed an increase in asthma-related deaths in patients receiving salmeterol. Although the trial results were specific to salmeterol, one of the conclusions derived from this study is that long-acting beta$_2$-adrenergic agonists may increase the risk of asthma exacerbation and possibly asthma-related death.
- Although available data for formoterol fumarate dihydrate do not suggest increased risk, it can not be excluded that the findings with salmeterol may apply to all long-acting beta$_2$-adrenergic agonists including formoterol fumarate dihydrate, the active ingredient in OXEZE TURBUHALER.
- When treating asthma patients, OXEZE TURBUHALER should be used only as additional therapy for patients whose conditions are not adequately controlled using low-to-medium dose inhaled corticosteroids or whose disease severity clearly warrants the initiation of treatment with two maintenance therapies, i.e. OXEZE TURBUHALER in addition to an inhaled corticosteroid.

General: OXEZE TURBUHALER (formoterol fumarate dihydrate) should be used as an additional therapy to low-to-medium dose inhaled corticosteroids. Do not use OXEZE TURBUHALER as monotherapy in asthma patients or as a substitute for oral or inhaled corticosteroids.

Patients who require therapy with OXEZE TURBUHALER should also receive optimal anti-inflammatory therapy with corticosteroids. Patients must be advised to continue taking their anti-inflammatory therapy after the introduction of OXEZE TURBUHALER even when symptoms decrease. Any change in corticosteroid dosage should be made **only** after clinical evaluation.

Use of Anti-Inflammatory Agents: Patients should be receiving optimal anti-inflammatory therapy with corticosteroids before starting maintenance treatment with OXEZE TURBUHALER. Formoterol is not a substitute for inhaled or oral corticosteroids; its use is complementary to them. Corticosteroids should not be stopped when OXEZE TURBUHALER is initiated. Patients must be advised not to stop or reduce corticosteroid therapy without medical advice.

Treatment of Acute Symptoms: OXEZE TURBUHALER can be used to treat acute symptoms, however, medical attention should be sought if patients find that relief bronchodilator treatment becomes less effective or that they need more inhalations than usual (see Dosage and Administration).

OXEZE TURBUHALER and the Management of Asthma: OXEZE TURBUHALER may be used as a regular twice daily maintenance regimen and/or as needed to treat asthma. The management of asthma should normally follow a stepwise programme, as advised in asthma management guidelines, with patient response monitored clinically and by lung function tests. When used as regular, twice daily maintenance treatment, OXEZE TURBUHALER should not be used without adequate anti-inflammatory therapy. Consideration should be given to the following in the management of asthma with OXEZE TURBUHALER:

- Oral or inhaled corticosteroids, or other anti-inflammatory medications should not be stopped.
- Adequate education should be provided to the patient regarding the use of long-acting β_2-agonists and the acute treatment of asthma, with close follow-up to ensure compliance.

Increasing use of OXEZE TURBUHALER or other fast-acting bronchodilators to control symptoms indicates deterioration of asthma control and the need to reassess the patient's therapy.

Sudden or progressive deterioration in asthma control is potentially life-threatening; the treatment plan must be re-evaluated, and consideration be given to increasing corticosteroid therapy. In patients at risk, daily peak flow monitoring with precise instructions for acceptable variation limits should be considered.

Watch for Increased Need for Rescue Medication: Fast-acting, inhaled bronchodilators (e.g., formoterol, terbutaline, salbutamol) may be used for relief of breakthrough symptoms. Asthma may deteriorate acutely over a period of hours or slowly over several days or longer. **The total maximum daily dose of OXEZE TURBUHALER should not be exceeded.** Should symptoms persist, or treatment with fast-acting inhaled β_2-agonist become less effective or a patient needs more inhalations than usual, this indicates a worsening of the underlying condition and warrants reassessment of the treatment regimen and consideration given to increasing corticosteroid therapy. Patients requiring increasing doses or inhalations of fast-acting β_2-agonists for relief of symptoms should be advised to consult a physician for re-evaluation. In the case of acutely or rapidly worsening dyspnea, a doctor should be consulted immediately.

Do Not Exceed Recommended Dosage: OXEZE TURBUHALER should **not** be used at higher doses than recommended. Fatalities have been reported in association with excessive use of inhaled sympathomimetic drugs (see below).

Cardiovascular: Potentially serious ECG changes (such as increased QTc interval) and hypokalemia may result from β_2-agonist therapy. Although clinically not significant, a small increase in QTc interval and/or decrease in serum potassium has been reported at therapeutic doses of formoterol. Particular caution is advised in severe asthma as these effects may be potentiated by hypoxia and concomitant treatment with xanthine derivatives, steroids and diuretics. Hypokalemia will increase the susceptibility of digitalis patients to cardiac arrhythmias (see Warnings and Precautions). It is recommended that serum potassium levels be monitored in such situations. Therefore, OXEZE TURBUHALER, like all sympathomimetic amines, should be used with caution in patients with cardiovascular disorders, arrhythmias and hypertension.

Usually no effect on the cardiovascular or central nervous system is seen after the administration of formoterol at recommended doses, but the cardiovascular and central nervous system effects seen with all sympathomimetic drugs (e.g., increased heart rate, cardiac contractility, tremor) can occur while using formoterol. Special care and supervision, with particular emphasis on dosage limits, is required in patients receiving OXEZE TURBUHALER when the following conditions may exist: ischemic heart disease, cardiac arrhythmias, especially third degree atrioventricular block, severe cardiac decompensation, severe hypertension, hypertrophic obstructive cardiomyopathy, thyrotoxicosis or severe heart failure.

Use with caution in patients with idiopathic hypertrophic subvalvular aortic stenosis, in whom an increase in the pressure gradient between the left ventricle and the aorta may occur, causing increased strain on the left ventricle.

Caution should be observed when treating patients with known or suspected prolongation of the QTc-interval. Formoterol itself may induce prolongation of the QTc-interval.

Endocrine and Metabolism: Sympathomimetic bronchodilators should be administered cautiously to patients who are unusually responsive to sympathomimetic amines, e.g., in patients with hyperthyroidism not yet under adequate control. Since β_2-agonists may increase the blood glucose level, additional blood glucose controls are recommended when asthmatic patients with concomitant diabetes are started on OXEZE TURBUHALER.

Respiratory: Paradoxical Bronchospasm: As with other inhaled asthma medication, the potential for paradoxical bronchospasm should be kept in mind. If it occurs, treatment with OXEZE TURBUHALER should be discontinued immediately and alternative therapy instituted.

Sensitivity/Resistance: Immediate Hypersensitivity Reactions: Immediate hypersensitivity reactions may occur after administration of OXEZE TURBUHALER. OXEZE TURBUHALER contains lactose (600 µg per metered dose) and is contraindicated in patients with hypersensitivity to inhaled lactose or formoterol. The amount of lactose in OXEZE TURBUHALER does not normally cause problems in lactose intolerant people (see Contraindications).

Special Populations: Pregnant Women: The safety of formoterol during pregnancy has not yet been established. OXEZE TURBUHALER should be used during pregnancy only if the potential benefit justifies the potential risk to the fetus.

There are no well-controlled human studies that have investigated the effects of formoterol on preterm labour or labour at term. Because of the potential for β-agonist interference with uterine contractility, use of β_2-agonists, such as OXEZE TURBUHALER, during labour should be restricted to those patients in whom the benefits clearly outweigh the risks.

Nursing Women: Formoterol was found to be excreted in the milk of lactating rats after oral administration. Since there is no experience in the use of OXEZE TURBUHALER in nursing mothers, its use in such circumstances should only be considered if the expected benefit to the mother is greater than the risk to the infant.

Pediatrics: OXEZE TURBUHALER is not currently recommended for on-demand use in children younger than 12 years of age. For long-term maintenance therapy and prevention of exercise-induced bronchoconstriction, OXEZE TURBUHALER is not recommended for children younger than 6 years of age due to limited clinical data in this age group.

In children and adolescents the severity of asthma may be variable with age and periodic reassessment should be considered to determine if continued therapy with OXEZE TURBUHALER is still indicated. Compliance, especially neglect of anti-inflammatory therapy and overuse of rescue medication, should be carefully followed in this age group.

Geriatrics: No adjustment of dose should be required in the elderly, or in patients with renal or hepatic impairment, at the recommended normal doses. (See also Warnings and Precautions for patients with cardiovascular disorders.)

ADVERSE REACTIONS: Adverse Drug Reaction Overview: OXEZE TURBUHALER (formoterol fumarate dihydrate) has been used by more than 29 000 patients in clinical trials. The total post marketing exposure to OXEZE TURBUHALER is more than 2.4 million treatment-years. The most commonly reported adverse symptoms, which constitute the majority of the reports, are listed as adverse side effects of β_2-agonist therapy. There has been no indication of any particularly serious or unanticipated drug related reactions. The frequencies listed below are from the combined clinical trial and post marketing experience. Pharmacologically predictable side-effects of β_2-agonist therapy, such as tremor and palpitations, may occur but tend to be transient and reduced with regular therapy. As with other inhalation therapy, paradoxical bronchospasm may occur in very rare cases. The following adverse reactions can be classified as common (i.e. frequency ≥1% and <10%): tremor, palpitations and headache; uncommon (frequency ≥0.1% and <1%): muscle cramps, tachycardia, agitation, restlessness and sleep disturbances; rare (frequency ≥0.01% and <0.1%): cardiac arrythmias (e.g., atrial fibrillation, supraventricular tachycardia, extrasystoles), hypersensitivity reaction (e.g., bronchospasm, exanthema, urticaria, pruritus), hypokalemia; very rare: (frequency <0.01%) angina pectoris, hyperglycemia, taste disturbance, dizziness, and variations in blood pressure.

Clinical Trial Adverse Drug Reactions: The incidence of adverse events, irrespective of causality towards the drug, from four controlled trials (duration 1, 3, 3 and 6 months, respectively) with OXEZE TURBUHALER is presented in Table 1.

Table 1: OXEZE TURBUHALER

Incidence of Adverse Events (irrespective of causality) with Frequency Higher than Placebo in Four Controlled Trials of Duration 1, 3, 3 and 6 Months Respectively

	OXEZE TURBUHALER			Placebo TURBUHALER
	Total	6 µg b.i.d.	12 µg b.i.d.	
	No. (%)	No. (%)	No. (%)	No. (%)
Total Number of Evaluable Patients	359	190	169	412
Headache	66 (18%)	15 (8%)	51 (30%)	84 (20%)
Tremor	11 (3%)	4 (2%)	7 (4%)	2 (0%)
Pharynx Disorder	18 (5%)	3 (2%)	15 (9%)	10 (2%)
Cramps	10 (3%)	3 (2%)	7 (4%)	3 (1%)

DRUG INTERACTIONS: Beta-Receptor Blocking Agents: Beta-receptor blocking agents, especially non-selective ones, may partly or totally inhibit the effect of beta-stimulants.

Should a patient treated with OXEZE TURBUHALER (formoterol fumarate dihydrate) also require concomitant treatment with a beta-blocker, it is recommended that a beta-blocker (e.g., metoprolol) with less predominant β_2-blocking effects be considered. If concomitant treatment is necessary, patients should be monitored carefully for possible deterioration in pulmonary function and the need to adjust the dosage of either drug.

Xanthine Derivatives, Steroids and Diuretics: Concomitant treatment with xanthine derivatives, steroids or diuretics may potentiate a possible hypokalemic effect of β_2-agonists. Hypokalemia may increase the disposition towards arrhythmias in patients who are treated with digitalis glycosides.

Other Drugs: Concomitant treatment with quinidine, disopyramide, procainamide, phenothiazines, antihistamines (terfenadine), monoamine oxidase inhibitors and tricyclic antidepressants can prolong the QTc-interval and increase the risk of ventricular arrhythmias.

L-Dopa, L-thyroxine, oxytocin and alcohol can impair cardiac tolerance towards β_2-sympathomimetics.

Concomitant treatment with monoamine oxidase inhibitors including agents with similar properties such as furazolidone and procarbazine may precipitate hypertensive reactions.

There is elevated risk of arrhythmias in patients receiving concomitant anesthesia with halogenated hydrocarbons.

DOSAGE AND ADMINISTRATION: Dosing Considerations: When treating asthma patients, OXEZE TURBUHALER (formoterol fumarate dihydrate) should be used only as additional therapy for patients whose conditions are not adequately controlled using low-to-medium dose inhaled corticosteroids or whose disease severity clearly warrants the initiation of treatment with two maintenance therapies, i.e. OXEZE TURBUHALER in addition to an inhaled corticosteroid (see Warnings and Precautions).

OXEZE TURBUHALER SHOULD NOT BE USED AT HIGHER DOSES THAN RECOMMENDED. Asthma may deteriorate acutely over a period of hours or chronically over several days or longer. If the patient's fast-acting inhaled β_2-agonist becomes less effective or a patient needs more inhalations than usual, this may be a marker of destabilization of asthma. In this setting, the patient requires immediate reassessment of the treatment regimen. Increasing the daily dosage of OXEZE TURBUHALER in this situation is not appropriate (see Warnings and Precautions).

Bronchodilators should not be the only or the main treatment in patients with moderate to severe or unstable asthma. Patients with severe asthma may require regular medical assessment. These patients will require high dose inhaled or oral corticosteroid therapy. Sudden worsening of symptoms may require increased corticosteroid dosage which should be administered under medical supervision.

Recommended Dose and Dosage Adjustment: Since there may be serious adverse effects associated with excessive dosing, the dosage should not be increased beyond the maximum recommended dose. Dosage should be individualized and patient response should be monitored by the prescribing physician on an ongoing basis.

1. **Long-Term Twice Daily Maintenance Therapy**
   As a twice daily regular treatment, OXEZE TURBUHALER provides 24-hour bronchodilation and can replace regular use of a fast-acting, short duration inhaled bronchodilator (e.g., salbutamol or terbutaline), when used concurrently with corticosteroid therapy.
   The dose of OXEZE TURBUHALER should be individualized to the patient's needs and should be the lowest possible dose that keeps the patient symptom free or fulfills the therapeutic objective.

Adults: The normal dose is 6 or 12 µg from OXEZE TURBUHALER, twice daily, at 12 hour intervals. Some patients may need 24 µg twice daily. In adults, the maximum recommended daily dose is 48 µg.

Children (6-16 years): The usual dose is 6 or 12 µg, twice daily, at 12 hour intervals. In children, the maximum recommended daily dose is 24 µg.

On Demand Treatment:

2. **Relief of Acute Bronchoconstriction in Patients Who are on Maintenance Treatment with OXEZE TURBUHALER**
   Adults and Adolescent Children (12-16 years): The usual dose is 6 or 12 µg as needed.
3. **For relief of acute bronchoconstriction and prevention of bronchospasm for patients who remain symptomatic on inhaled corticosteroids:**
   Adults and Adolescent Children (12-16 years): The usual dose is 6 or 12 µg as needed.
4. **Prevention of Exercise-Induced Bronchoconstriction**
   Adults and Children 6 Years of Age and Older: 6 or 12 µg before exercise.
   When OXEZE TURBUHALER is used on demand, the maximum dose during a 24 hour period should not normally exceed 72 µg in adults and 48 µg in adolescent children. Prolonged use (more than 3 consecutive days) of more than 48 µg may be a sign of sub-optimal asthma control and treatment should be reassessed.
   In children and adolescents, the severity of asthma may be variable with age and periodic reassessment should be considered to identify the lowest dose required to maintain control and to determine if continued maintenance therapy with OXEZE TURBUHALER is still indicated (see Warnings and Precautions).
   OXEZE TURBUHALER is available in two strengths, 6 or 12 µg per inhalation. Use of the higher strength is recommended for patients requiring 12 µg or more, twice daily. OXEZE TURBUHALER is not currently recommended for on-demand use in children younger than 12 years of age. For long-term maintenance therapy and prevention of exercise-induced bronchoconstriction, OXEZE TURBUHALER is not recommended for children younger than 6 years of age due to limited clinical data in this age group.
   It is important to instruct patients to avoid exhaling into the device and to always replace the cover after using OXEZE TURBUHALER.
   Note: The medication from OXEZE TURBUHALER is delivered to the lungs as the patient inhales and, therefore, it is important to instruct the patient to breathe in forcefully and deeply through the mouthpiece. The patient may not taste or feel any medication when using OXEZE TURBUHALER due to the small amount of drug dispensed.

Missed Dose: If a dose of twice daily maintenance treatment of OXEZE TURBUHALER is missed, it should be taken as soon as possible within 6 hours of the missed dose; the patient should then resume their regular schedule. If more than 6 hours have passed, the missed dose should not be taken. Patients should be advised to take their next scheduled dose on time.

A double dose of OXEZE TURBUHALER should never be taken to make up for missed doses.

OVERDOSAGE:

There is limited clinical experience on the management of overdose. An overdose would likely lead to effects that are typical of β_2-adrenergic agonists: tremor, headache, palpitations. Metabolic acidosis and hypertension may also occur. Symptoms reported from isolated cases are tachycardia, hyperglycaemia, hypokalaemia, prolonged QTc-interval, arrhythmia, nausea and vomiting. Supportive and symptomatic treatment may be indicated.

For management of a suspected drug overdose, CPhA recommends that you contact your **regional Poison Control Centre**. See the *CPS* Directory section for a list of Poison Control Centres.

ACTION AND CLINICAL PHARMACOLOGY: Mechanism of Action: The active ingredient in OXEZE TURBUHALER (formoterol fumarate dihydrate), formoterol, produces bronchodilation by stimulation of the β_2-adrenergic receptors in bronchial smooth muscle, thereby causing relaxation of smooth muscle fibres.

Pharmacodynamics: Following inhalation from OXEZE TURBUHALER (formoterol fumarate dihydrate), a marked improvement in pulmonary function is observed within 1-3 minutes. This fast onset of action is similar to that seen with short-acting bronchodilators (e.g., terbutaline, salbutamol). Approximately 80% of peak effect is attained within 15 minutes of administration. In addition, formoterol has a mean duration of bronchodilator effect of 12 hours after a single dose, much like other long-acting β_2-agonists.

Pharmacokinetics: Absorption: Inhaled formoterol is rapidly absorbed. Peak plasma concentration is reached about 15 minutes after inhalation.

In studies the mean lung deposition of formoterol after inhalation via TURBUHALER ranged from 21-37% of the metered dose. The total systemic availability for the higher lung deposition was approximately 46% of the metered dose.

Distribution: Plasma protein binding is approximately 50%.

Metabolism: Formoterol is metabolized via direct glucuronidation and O-demethylation. The enzyme responsible for O-demethylation has not been identified. Total plasma clearance and volume of distribution has not been determined.

Excretion: The major part of the dose of formoterol is eliminated via metabolism. After inhalation 6-10% of the metered dose of formoterol is excreted unmetabolized in the urine. About 20% of an intravenous dose is excreted unchanged in the urine. The terminal half-life after inhalation is estimated to be 8 hours.

STORAGE AND STABILITY: OXEZE TURBUHALER (formoterol fumarate dihydrate) should be stored at room temperature between 15°C and 30°C with the cover tightened, away from moisture.

SPECIAL HANDLING INSTRUCTIONS: OXEZE TURBUHALER (formoterol fumarate dihydrate) cannot be refilled and should be discarded when empty.

INFORMATION FOR THE PATIENT: Published in e-CPS, available by subscription at www.e-cps.ca.

DOSAGE FORMS, COMPOSITION AND PACKAGING: 6 µg/metered dose: Each inhalation contains: a white to off-white or slightly yellow nonhygroscopic crystalline powder of formoterol fumarate dihydrate 6 µg. Nonmedicinal ingredients: lactose monohydrate (which may contain milk protein residue) 600 µg/metered dose (this amount does not normally cause problems in lactose-intolerant people). Turbuhaler of 60 doses with a light greenish-blue turning grip.

12 µg/metered dose: Each inhalation contains: a white to off-white or slightly yellow nonhygroscopic crystalline powder of formoterol fumarate dihydrate 12 µg. Nonmedicinal ingredients: lactose monohydrate (which may contain milk protein residue) 600 µg/metered dose (this amount does not normally cause problems in lactose-intolerant people). Turbuhaler of 60 doses with a dark greenish-blue turning grip.

(Shown in Product Identification Section)

Oxtriphylline P

CPhA Monograph

see *Theophyllines*

Oxycodone Ⓝ

CPhA Monograph

see *Opioids*

OxyContin® Ⓝ

oxycodone HCl

Opioid Analgesic

Purdue Pharma

Oxy·IR® Ⓝ

oxycodone HCl

Opioid Analgesic

Purdue Pharma

Date of Preparation: December 18, 1995
Date of Revision: August 25, 2009

PHARMACOLOGY: Oxycodone is a semi-synthetic opioid analgesic which exerts an agonist effect at specific, saturable opioid receptors in the CNS and other tissues. In man, oxycodone produces a variety of effects including analgesia, constipation from decreased gastrointestinal motility, suppression of the cough reflex, respiratory depression from reduced responsiveness of the respiratory center to CO_2, nausea and vomiting via stimulation of the chemoreceptor trigger zone, changes in mood including euphoria and dysphoria, sedation, mental clouding, and alterations of the endocrine and autonomic nervous systems.

Oxycodone retains at least one-half of its analgesic activity when administered orally and with acute dosing is approximately twice as potent as orally administered morphine.

Studies with OxyContin (oxycodone hydrochloride controlled release tablets) and Oxy•IR (oxycodone hydrochloride tablets) in normal volunteers and patients demonstrate a consistent relationship between oxycodone dosage and plasma oxycodone concentrations as well as between concentration and pharmacodynamic effects. In a single dose analgesic assay, the peak effect of OxyContin (20 and 30 mg) was greater than that of 10 mg OxyContin and was equivalent to that of two tablets of oxycodone (5 mg) plus acetaminophen (325 mg), or 15 mg of immediate release oxycodone but with a longer duration of action. In patients with pain due to osteoarthritis, OxyContin q12h was more effective than placebo in decreasing pain and in improving quality of life, mood and sleep. In patients with cancer pain, OxyContin administered q12h produced equivalent analgesia to Oxy•IR administered four times per day. In patients with low back pain, OxyContin q12h was equally effective as Oxy•IR given four times per day. Titration to analgesic effect was achieved as easily with OxyContin as with Oxy•IR.

There is no intrinsic limit to the analgesic effect of oxycodone; like morphine, adequate doses will relieve even the most severe pain. Clinically however, dosage limitations are imposed by the adverse effects, primarily respiratory depression, nausea and vomiting, which can result from high doses.

Pharmacokinetics: After oral administration, oxycodone is absorbed from the gastrointestinal tract and has a relatively high bioavailability of approximately 60-87%. Unlike morphine, oxycodone does not undergo high first pass metabolism, possibly due to the protective effect of a methoxy group in the 3 position which is a site of morphine glucuronidation. Oxycodone is metabolized in the liver to noroxycodone, oxymorphone, noroxymorphone and their glucuronides. The formation of oxymorphone and noroxycodone is mediated by cytochrome P450 2D6 and its cytochrome P450 3A4, respectively. In addition, noroxymorphone formation is mediated by both cytochrome P450 2D6 and cytochrome P450 3A4. Therefore, the rate of formation of these metabolites can, in theory, be affected by other drugs (see Precautions, Drug Interactions).

The in vitro drug-drug interaction studies with noroxymorphone using human liver microsomes resulted in no significant inhibition of CYP2D6 and CYP3A4 activities, which suggest that noroxymorphone may not alter the metabolism of other drugs that are metabolized by CYP2D6 and CYP3A4. Noroxymorphone has been shown to bind to μ-opioid receptor. Although oxymorphone has been shown to be active, the analgesic effects of the metabolites are thought to be clinically insignificant.

Oxymorphone is known to possess analgesic activity but concentrations in the plasma are very low and not as closely correlated to opioid effects as oxycodone concentrations. Although the AUC ratio of noroxycodone to oxycodone is about 0.6 following oral dosing, noroxycodone is reported to be a considerably weaker analgesic than oxycodone and is unlikely to contribute significantly to the analgesic effect of oxycodone. The analgesic activity profile of other metabolites is not known. The terminal elimination half-life after immediate release tablets is approximately 4 hours. The majority of metabolites and unchanged drug (conjugated 2.2%, unconjugated 5.5%) are excreted in the urine and feces.

Pharmacokinetic studies of OxyContin in normal volunteers demonstrate that both AUC and C_{max} increase in a dose proportional manner and that the six tablet strengths are bioequivalent. In single dose studies, OxyContin was absorbed to an equivalent extent as immediate release oxycodone but with a reduced maximum concentration (C_{max} ratio approximately 50%), a prolonged (2.4×) time to maximum concentration (t_{max} approximately 2.8 hours), with a biphasic absorption pattern, with two apparent absorption half-times of 0.6 and 6.9 hours, which describe the initial release of oxycodone from the tablet, followed by a prolonged release. Release in vitro is pH-independent. OxyContin tablets 15 mg, 30 mg and 60 mg are proportionally bioequivalent to OxyContin tablets 40 mg in terms of AUC_t, AUC_{INF} and C_{max} of oxycodone, and mean half-life values and median t_{max} values were all similar.

In steady state pharmacokinetic studies of OxyContin q12h, maximum plasma concentrations (C_{max}) of oxycodone were equivalent to those obtained with q6h administration of oral immediate release preparations and were achieved approximately 3 hours after administration of OxyContin. Steady-state was achieved within 24-36 hours of initiation of dosing. The absorption of oxycodone from OxyContin tablets is not significantly influenced when administered in the presence of food.

Following absorption, oxycodone is distributed throughout the entire body. Approximately 45% is bound to plasma protein.

Female subjects have, on average, plasma oxycodone concentrations up to 25% higher than males on a body weight adjusted basis. Plasma concentrations of oxycodone are increased by approximately 15% in elderly subjects receiving OxyContin; by 50-60% in patients with moderate degrees of renal impairment; and by approximately two-fold in patients with hepatic cirrhosis.

INDICATIONS: OxyContin (oxycodone hydrochloride controlled release tablets) are indicated for relief of moderate to severe pain requiring the continuous use of an opioid analgesic preparation for several days or more.

Oxy•IR (oxycodone hydrochloride tablets) are indicated for relief of moderate to severe pain.

CONTRAINDICATIONS: OxyContin (oxycodone hydrochloride controlled release tablets) and Oxy•IR (oxycodone hydrochloride tablets) should not be given to patients with: hypersensitivity to opioid analgesics; acute asthma or other obstructive airway disease and acute respiratory depression with hypoxia; elevated carbon dioxide levels in the blood; cor pulmonale; acute alcoholism; delirium tremens; severe CNS depression; convulsive disorders; increased cerebrospinal or intracranial pressure; head injury; suspected surgical abdomen (e.g., paralytic ileus); concomitant MAO inhibitors (or within 14 days of such therapy).

WARNINGS: OxyContin (oxycodone hydrochloride controlled release tablets) should be swallowed whole. Taking broken, chewed, dissolved or crushed OxyContin tablets could lead to the rapid release and absorption of a potentially fatal dose of oxycodone.

OxyContin 60 mg and 80 mg tablets, or a single dose greater than 40 mg, are for use in opioid tolerant patients only (see also Dosage). A single dose greater than 40 mg, or total daily doses greater than 80 mg, may cause fatal respiratory depression when administered to patients who are not tolerant to the respiratory depressant effects of opioids (see Precautions, Drug Interactions).

Patients should be instructed not to give OxyContin or Oxy•IR (oxycodone hydrochloride tablets) to anyone other than the patient for whom it was prescribed, as such inappropriate use may have severe medical consequences, including death.

Patients should be cautioned not to consume alcohol while taking OxyContin or Oxy•IR, as it may increase the chance of experiencing dangerous side effects.

Abuse of Opioid Formulations: OxyContin consists of a dual polymer matrix intended for oral use only. Abuse can lead to overdose and death. This risk is increased when the tablets are crushed, broken, dissolved or chewed, and with concurrent consumption of alcohol or other CNS depressants. With parenteral abuse, the tablet excipients, especially talc, can be expected to result in local tissue necrosis, infection, pulmonary granulomas, and increased risk of endocarditis and valvular heart injury.

Drug Dependence: As with other opioids, tolerance and physical dependence may develop upon repeated administration of oxycodone and there is a potential for development of psychological dependence. OxyContin tablets and Oxy•IR should therefore be prescribed and handled with the degree of caution appropriate to the use of a drug with abuse potential. Drug abuse is usually not a problem in patients with pain in whom oxycodone is appropriately indicated. Withdrawal symptoms may occur following abrupt discontinuation of therapy or upon administration of an opioid antagonist.

Therefore, patients on prolonged therapy should be withdrawn gradually from the drug if it is no longer required for pain control.

Use in Drug and Alcohol Addiction: OxyContin/Oxy•IR are opioids with no approved use in the management of addictive disorders. Their proper usage in individuals with drug or alcohol dependence, either active or in remission is for the management of pain requiring opioid analgesia.

CNS Depression: Oxycodone should be used with caution and in reduced dosage during concomitant administration of other opioid analgesics, general anaesthetics, phenothiazines and other tranquilizers, sedative-hypnotics, tricyclic antidepressants and other CNS depressants, including alcohol. Respiratory depression, hypotension and profound sedation or coma may result.

Severe pain antagonizes the subjective and respiratory depressant actions of opioid analgesics. Should pain suddenly subside, these effects may rapidly become manifest. Patients who are scheduled for cordotomy or other interruption of pain transmission pathways should not receive OxyContin or Oxy•IR within 24 hours of the procedure.

Pregnancy: While animal reproduction studies have revealed no evidence of harm to the fetus due to oxycodone, safe use in pregnancy has not been established. OxyContin or Oxy•IR should be given to pregnant patients only when the anticipated benefits outweigh the potential risks to the fetus and should be avoided to the extent possible in patients who are pregnant.

PRECAUTIONS: Respiratory Depression: Oxycodone should be used with extreme caution in patients with substantially decreased respiratory reserve, pre-existing respiratory depression, hypoxia or hypercapnia. Such patients are often less sensitive to the stimulatory effects of carbon dioxide (CO_2) on the respiratory centre and the respiratory depressant effects of oxycodone may reduce respiratory drive to the point of apnea.

Head Injury: The respiratory depressant effects of oxycodone, and the capacity to elevate cerebrospinal fluid pressure, may be greatly increased in the presence of an already elevated intracranial pressure produced by trauma. Also, oxycodone may produce confusion, miosis, vomiting and other side effects which obscure the clinical course of patients with head injury. In such patients, oxycodone must be used with extreme caution and only if it is judged essential.

Hypotension: Oxycodone administration may result in severe hypotension in patients whose ability to maintain adequate blood pressure is compromised by reduced blood volume, or concurrent administration of such drugs as phenothiazines or certain anaesthetics.

Acute Abdominal Conditions: Oxycodone and other morphine-like opioids have been shown to decrease bowel motility. Oxycodone may obscure the diagnosis or clinical course of patients with acute abdominal conditions.

Special Risk Groups: Oxycodone should be administered with caution, and in reduced dosages, to debilitated patients, to patients with severely reduced hepatic or renal function, and in patients with Addison's disease, hypothyroidism, toxic psychosis, pancreatitis, prostatic hypertrophy or urethral stricture.

Ambulatory Surgery and Post-Operative Use: OxyContin is not indicated for pre-emptive analgesia (administration pre-operatively for the management of post-operative pain).

OxyContin is not indicated for pain in the postoperative period if the pain is mild or not expected to persist for an extended period of time. Physicians should individualize treatment, moving from parenteral to oral analgesics as appropriate.

Patients who are already receiving OxyContin tablets as part of ongoing analgesic therapy may be continued on the drug if appropriate dosage adjustments are made considering the procedure, other drugs given including perioperative medications (see Precautions, Drug Interactions, Mixed agonist/antagonist opioid analgesics) and the temporary changes in physiology caused by the surgical intervention (see Dosage and Precautions, Drug Interactions).

Oxycodone and other morphine-like opioids have been shown to decrease bowel motility. Ileus is a common post-operative complication, especially after intra-abdominal surgery with opioid analgesia. Caution should be taken to monitor for decreased bowel motility in post-operative patients receiving opioids. Standard supportive therapy should be implemented.

OxyContin should not be used in the early post-operative period (12-24 hours post-surgery) unless the patient is ambulatory and gastrointestinal function is normal (see also Precautions, Drug Interactions, Mixed agonist/antagonist opioid analgesics).

Oxy•IR should be used with caution pre-operatively and within the first 12-24 hours post-operatively.

Labor/Delivery: In view of the potential for opioids to cross the placental barrier and to be excreted in breast milk, oxycodone use should be avoided to the extent possible in nursing mothers. Physical dependence or respiratory depression may occur in the infant if opioids are administered during labour.

Lactation: See Labor/Delivery.

Occupational Hazards: Driving and Operating Dangerous Machinery: Oxycodone may impair the mental and/or physical abilities needed for certain potentially hazardous activities such as driving a car or operating machinery. Patients should be cautioned accordingly. Patients should also be cautioned about the combined effects of oxycodone with other CNS depressants, including other opioids, phenothiazines, sedative/hypnotics and alcohol.

Drug Interactions: CNS Depressants, such as other opioids, anaesthetics, sedatives, hypnotics, antidepressants, sleeping aids, phenothiazines, neuroleptics, chloral hydrate and glutethimide may enhance the depressant effects of oxycodone (see Precautions, Ambulatory Surgery and Post-Operative Use). Oxycodone should be used with caution and started in a reduced dosage (1/3 to 1/2 of the usual dosage) in patients who are currently receiving other central nervous system depressants. Monoamine oxidase inhibitors (including procarbazine hydrochloride), pyrazolidone, antihistamines, beta-blockers and alcohol may also enhance the depressant effect of oxycodone.

Oxycodone is metabolized in part by cytochrome P450 2D6 and cytochrome P450 3A4 and in theory, can be affected by other drugs. While these pathways may be blocked by a variety of drugs, such blockage has not yet been shown to be of clinical significance with this agent.

"In Vitro" Dissolution Studies of Interaction with Alcohol: Increasing concentrations of alcohol in the dissolution medium, resulted in a slight decrease in the rate of release of oxycodone from OxyContin tablets.

Mixed agonist/antagonist opioid analgesics (i.e., pentazocine, nalbuphine, butorphanol, and buprenorphine) should be administered with caution to a patient who has received or is receiving a course of therapy with a pure opioid agonist analgesic such as oxycodone. In this situation, mixed agonist/antagonist analgesics may reduce the analgesic effect of oxycodone and/or may precipitate withdrawal symptoms in these patients.

ADVERSE EFFECTS: Adverse effects of OxyContin (oxycodone hydrochloride controlled release tablets) and Oxy•IR (oxycodone hydrochloride tablets) are similar to those of other opioid analgesics, and represent an extension of pharmacological effects of the drug class. The major hazards of opioids include respiratory and central nervous system depression and to a lesser degree, circulatory depression, respiratory arrest, shock and cardiac arrest.

The most frequently observed adverse effects of OxyContin and Oxy•IR are asthenia, constipation, dizziness, dry mouth, headache, nausea, pruritus, somnolence, sweating and vomiting.

Sedation: Sedation is a common side effect of opioid analgesics, especially in opioid naive individuals. Sedation may also occur partly because patients often recuperate from prolonged fatigue after the relief of persistent pain. Most patients develop tolerance to the sedative effects of opioids within three to five days and, if the sedation is not severe, will not require any treatment except reassurance. If excessive sedation persists beyond a few days, the dose of the opioid should be reduced and alternate causes investigated. Some of these are: concurrent CNS depressant medication, hepatic or renal dysfunction, brain metastases, hypercalcemia and respiratory failure. If it is necessary to reduce the dose, it can be carefully increased again after three or four days if it is obvious that the pain is not being well controlled. Dizziness and unsteadiness may be caused by postural hypotension, particularly in elderly or debilitated patients, and may be alleviated if the patient lies down.

Nausea and Vomiting: Nausea is a common side effect on initiation of therapy with opioid analgesics and is thought to occur by activation of the chemoreceptor trigger zone, stimulation of the vestibular apparatus and through delayed gastric emptying. The prevalence of nausea declines following continued treatment with opioid analgesics. When instituting therapy with an opioid for chronic pain, the routine prescription of an antiemetic should be considered. In the cancer patient, investigation of nausea should include such causes as constipation, bowel obstruction, uremia, hypercalcemia, hepatomegaly, tumor invasion of celiac plexus and concurrent use of drugs with emetogenic properties. Persistent nausea which does not respond to dosage reduction may be caused by opioid-induced gastric stasis and may be accompanied by other symptoms including anorexia, early satiety, vomiting and abdominal fullness. These symptoms respond to chronic treatment with gastrointestinal prokinetic agents.

Constipation: Practically all patients become constipated while taking opioids on a persistent basis. In some patients, particularly the elderly or bedridden, fecal impaction may result. It is essential to caution the patients in this regard and to institute an appropriate regimen of bowel management at the start of prolonged opioid therapy. Stimulant laxatives, stool softeners, and other appropriate measures should be used as required.

The following adverse effects occur less frequently with opioid analgesics and include those reported in OxyContin and Oxy•IR clinical trials, whether related or not to oxycodone.

No deaths were reported during treatment. No serious adverse events related to treatment were reported.
Adverse events reported in the pivotal trials are summarized in Table 1 and Table 2.

Table 1: OXYTROL

Number (%) of Adverse Events Occurring in >2% of Oxytrol-treated Patients and Greater in Oxytrol Group Than in Placebo Group (Study 1)

	Placebo (N=132)		OXYTROL (3.9 mg/day) (N=125)	
Adverse Event[a]	**N**	**%**	**N**	**%**
Application Site Pruritus	8	6.1	21	16.8
Dry Mouth	11	8.3	12	9.6
Application Site Erythema	3	2.3	7	5.6
Application Site Vesicles	0	0.0	4	3.2
Diarrhea	3	2.3	4	3.2
Dysuria	0	0.0	3	2.4

[a] Includes adverse events judged by the investigator as possibly, probably or definitely treatment-related.

Table 2: OXYTROL

Number (%) of Adverse Events Occurring in >2% of Oxytrol-treated Patients and Greater in Oxytrol Group Than in Placebo Group (Study 2)

	Placebo (N=117)		OXYTROL (3.9 mg/day) (N=121)	
Adverse Event[a]	**N**	**%**	**N**	**%**
Application Site Pruritus	5	4.3	17	14.0
Application Site Erythema	2	1.7	10	8.3
Dry Mouth	2	1.7	5	4.1
Constipation	0	0.0	4	3.3
Application Site Rash	1	0.9	4	3.3
Application Site Macules	0	0.0	3	2.5
Abnormal Vision	0	0.0	3	2.5

[a] Includes adverse events judged by the investigator as possibly, probably or definitely treatment-related.

Other adverse events reported by >1% of OXYTROL-treated patients, and judged by the investigator to be possibly, probably or definitely related to treatment include: abdominal pain, nausea, flatulence, fatigue, somnolence, headache, flushing, rash, application site burning and back pain.

Most treatment-related adverse events were described as mild or moderate in intensity. Severe application site reactions were reported by 6.4% of OXYTROL-treated patients in Study 1 and by 5.0% of OXYTROL-treated patients in Study 2.

Treatment-related adverse events that resulted in discontinuation were reported by 11.2% of OXYTROL-treated patients in Study 1 and 10.7% of OXYTROL-treated patients in Study 2. Most of these were secondary to application site reaction. In the two pivotal studies, no patient discontinued OXYTROL treatment due to dry mouth.

In the open-label extension, the most common treatment-related adverse events were: application site pruritus, application site erythema and dry mouth.

OVERDOSE:

Symptoms: Overdosage using OXYTROL (oxybutynin transdermal system) is unlikely. Each 39 cm^2 system contains 36 mg oxybutynin and delivers 3.9 mg/day when attached to the skin. Thus, 36 mg oxybutynin would be the maximum dose possible if a system were inadvertently taken internally. In terms of transdermal application, if an entire box of 24 systems were applied simultaneously and worn for 24 hours, the resulting dose would be 93.6 mg.

Case reports of oral overdose with oxybutynin chloride indicate that doses of this magnitude should resolve with withdrawal of exposure and supportive care. Overdose with oral oxybutynin chloride has been associated with anticholinergic effects including central nervous system excitation, flushing, fever, dehydration, cardiac arrhythmia, vomiting, and urinary retention. Ingestion of 100 mg oral oxybutynin chloride in association with alcohol has been reported in a 13-year-old boy who experienced memory loss, and a 34-year-old woman who developed stupor, following by disorientation and agitation on awakening, dilated pupils, dry skin, cardiac arrhythmia, and retention of urine. Both patients recovered fully with symptomatic treatment.

Treatment: In the event of a possible overdose, the transdermal system(s) should be removed immediately and medical attention sought. Plasma concentrations of oxybutynin and N-desethyloxybutynin decline within 1 to 2 hours after removal of transdermal system(s). If an overdose is suspected, patients should be monitored until symptoms resolve.

For management of a suspected drug overdose, CPhA recommends that you contact your **regional Poison Control Centre**. See the *CPS* Directory section for a list of Poison Control Centres.

DOSAGE: OXYTROL (oxybutynin transdermal system) is designed to deliver oxybutynin continuously and consistently over a 3 to 4-day time interval after application to intact skin. The OXYTROL system has a nominal in vivo delivery rate of 3.9 mg oxybutynin per day through skin of average permeability (interindividual variation in skin permeability is approximately 20%) and contains 36 mg of oxybutynin. OXYTROL adheres well to the skin when applied according to instructions (see Administration below).

Adults: The recommended starting dose is one 3.9 mg/day system applied twice weekly (every 3 to 4 days).

Administration: OXYTROL should be applied to dry, intact skin on the abdomen, hip or buttock. Apply immediately after removal from the protective pouch. A new application site should be selected with each new OXYTROL system to avoid re-application to the same site within 7 days.

INFORMATION FOR THE PATIENT: Published in e-CPS, available by subscription at www.e-cps.ca.

SUPPLIED: OXYTROL is a matrix-type transdermal system composed of 3 layers. Layer 1 (Backing Film) is a thin flexible polyester/ethylene-vinyl acetate film that provides the matrix system with occlusivity and physical integrity and protects the adhesive/drug layer. Layer 2 (Adhesive/Drug Layer) is a cast film of acrylic adhesive containing oxybutynin and triacetin USP. Layer 3 (Release Liner) is two overlapped siliconized polyester strips that are peeled off and discarded by the patient prior to applying the matrix system.

Each 39 cm^2 system imprinted with "OXYTROL 3.9" contains: 36 mg oxybutynin for nominal delivery of 3.9 mg oxybutynin per day when dosed in a twice weekly regimen. Patient Calendar Boxes of 8 systems and 24 systems. Boxes of 8 systems for use as physician samples. Store at room temperature at 15 to 30°C. Protect from moisture and humidity. Do not store outside the sealed pouch. Apply immediately after removal from protective pouch. Discard used OXYTROL in household trash in a manner that prevents accidental application or ingestion by children, pets, or others.

Ozonol® Antibiotic Plus

polymyxin B sulfate—bacitracin—lidocaine HCl

Topical First Aid

Bayer Consumer Care

Ozonol® Ointment

phenol—zinc oxide

Topical First Aid

Bayer Consumer Care

SUPPLIED: Antibiotic Plus: Each g contains: polymyxin B (as sulfate) 10 000 units, bacitracin 500 units and lidocaine hydrochloride 40 mg. Nonmedicinal ingredients: white petrolatum. Tubes of 15 and 30 g.

Ointment: Each g contains: phenol 0.18% and zinc oxide 3.72%. Nonmedicinal ingredients: aluminum potassium sulfate, camphor oil, ichthammol, lanolin, mineral oil, origanum oil, petrolatum yellow, sodium bicarbonate, thymol iodide and yellow beeswax. Tubes of 30 and 60 g.

P

Paclitaxel for Injection Ⓟ

paclitaxel

Antineoplastic

Hospira

SUPPLIED: Each mL of solution contains: paclitaxel 6 mg, Cremophor EL (polyethoxylated castor oil) 527 mg, citric acid (anhydrous) 2 mg and absolute alcohol 46.5% v/v. Single dose vials of 5 mL. Multi-dose vials of 16.7 and 50 mL. Single pack cartons. Store at room temperature (15-25°C). Retain in the original package and protect from light. Once punctured, the 16.7 mL, 25 mL and 50 mL vials of Paclitaxel for Injection are stable for 28 days at room temperature (15-25°C). These presentations are labeled as multi-dose vials. Unused portions of the 5 mL single dose format should be discarded. Solutions for infusion prepared as recommended may be stored at room temperature (15-25°C) only if necessary. However, the infusion should be initiated within 24 hours of reconstitution.

If unopened vials are refrigerated, a precipitate may form which redissolves with little or no agitation upon reaching room temperature. Product quality is not affected. If the solution remains cloudy or if an insoluble precipitate is noted, the vial should be discarded.

Palafer®

ferrous fumarate

Anemia Therapy

GlaxoSmithKline Consumer Healthcare

INDICATIONS: Increased iron requirements as in childhood, adolescence, and pregnancy; blood losses, overt or occult. Characterized microcytic hypochromic anemia; faulty iron absorption following gastrectomy; iron loss due to menstruation, sub-clinical iron deficiencies in adolescent girls due to precarious iron balance, and geriatrics.

CONTRAINDICATIONS: Hemosiderosis, hemochromatosis. Iron compounds are also contraindicated in the treatment of hemolytic anemias unless an iron-deficient state also exists, since storage of iron with a possible exogenous hemosiderosis can result.

PRECAUTIONS: Where anemia exists, its nature should be established and underlying causes determined.

Prolonged administration of iron should be avoided, except in patients with continued bleeding or repeated pregnancies. In infants, large chronic doses of iron may so interfere with the assimilation of phosphorus as to cause severe rickets.

Orally administered iron salts may aggravate existing disorders, such as peptic ulcer, regional enteritis and ulcerative colitis. They may not be absorbed in patients with steatorrhea and those who have had a partial gastrectomy.

Before initiating parenteral iron therapy, it is advisable to give test doses to help detect sensitivity. Iron overload can occur in patients given an excess of parenteral iron, as well as those with hemoglobinopathies or other refractory anemias which might be erroneously diagnosed as iron-deficiency anemia.

Do not administer oral iron preparations concomitantly with parenteral iron.

Iron binds with tetracyclines in equal molecular ratio thus preventing absorption of tetracyclines.

Warn patients that iron is toxic when overdoses are ingested by children. Severe reactions, including fatalities, have resulted.

Concomitant administration of antacids containing aluminum and magnesium salts may impair the absorption of iron.

ADVERSE EFFECTS: Oral ingestion of iron preparations may be associated with gastrointestinal discomfort (such as nausea) and dose-related bowel effects (such as constipation or diarrhea). Untoward effects usually subside with continuation of therapy or by iron ingestion with or after meals.

There is a possibility that liquid dosage forms of iron may stain teeth. To reduce this possibility, mix each dose with water or fruit juice. If staining occurs, remove by brushing with baking soda (sodium bicarbonate).

Parenteral iron administration can cause nausea, vomiting and such acute allergic reactions as chills and fever, arthralgia, urticaria and asthma. Occasional pain and staining of the skin at the site of injection may occur. Severe anaphylactoid reactions with some deaths have been reported in the literature. Although i.m. administration of iron dextran injections has caused sarcoma in laboratory animals, induced malignancy in man has never been observed.

OVERDOSE:

Iron poisoning is rare in adults but serious acute poisoning in children can result from ingestion of doses in excess of 1 g. Doses of 1 g should be considered as toxic in children and therapy instituted as soon as possible. Serum iron levels above 500 µg/100 mL can be taken as presumptive evidence of poisoning; severe poisoning is usually associated with levels well above 1000 µg/100 mL.

Symptoms: Symptoms may occur within about 30 minutes or may be delayed several hours. They are largely those of gastrointestinal irritation and necrosis with vomiting, diarrhea, tarry stools, hematemesis, fast and weak pulse, lethargy, low blood pressure, coma and signs of peripheral circulatory collapse. There may be a transient period of apparent recovery after 4 to 6 hours, followed by a second crisis characterized by cyanosis, pulmonary edema, circulatory collapse, convulsion and coma may then occur followed by death in 12 to 48 hours.

Treatment: Milk should be given immediately and vomiting induced. Eggs and milk should then be fed (to form iron-protein complexes) until it is possible to perform gastric lavage with 1% sodium bicarbonate solution (to convert the iron to a less soluble form). Gastric lavage should not be performed after the first hour of iron ingestion because of the danger of perforation due to gastric necrosis. If an iron-chelating agent such as deferoxamine mesylate is available, it should be utilized. BAL (dimercaprol) should not be used because it may form a toxic complex. Measures to combat shock, dehydration, blood loss and respiratory failure may be necessary.

> For management of a suspected drug overdose, CPhA recommends that you contact your **regional Poison Control Centre**. See the *CPS* Directory section for a list of Poison Control Centres.

DOSAGE: Capsules: Adults and children over 12 years: 1 capsule daily on an empty stomach, preferably at bedtime. Ferrous fumarate is well tolerated by most patients, however, for patients sensitive to any form of iron: 1 capsule twice a day with meals is recommended. Characterized iron deficiency anemia: 24 weeks minimum. In pregnancy, 1 capsule daily throughout gestation. Iron supplementation in clinical cases: 12 weeks minimum.

Suspension: Children 0 to 2 years: Preventive: 0 to 6 months: 0.25 mL once daily (5 mg/day of elemental iron). 6 months to 2 years: 0.75 mL once daily (15 mg/day elemental iron).

Therapeutic: 0 to 6 months: 0.25 mL t.i.d. (15 mg/day of elemental iron). 6 months to 2 years: 0.75 mL t.i.d. (45 mg/day of elemental iron).

Children 2 to 6 years: 2.5 mL (½ teaspoonful) daily at bedtime. 6 years of age and over: 5 mL (1 teaspoonful) daily at bedtime. Administer between meals with water or fruit juice.

SUPPLIED: Capsules: Each scarlet capsule, printed "PALAFER" in white ink on the body and cap, contains: ferrous fumarate M.D.I. (micro dispersible form) 300 mg representing 100 mg of elemental iron. Nonmedicinal ingredients: D&C yellow No. 10, FD&C red No. 2, FD&C red No. 3, FD&C yellow No. 6, gelatin, lactose, povidone, sucrose, talc, titanium dioxide, silicon dioxide and sodium lauryl sulphate. Energy: 4.34 kJ (1.03 kcal); 0.25 g carbohydrates. Cartons of 30 and bottles of 500.

Suspension: Each 5 mL of brown-colored suspension contains: ferrous fumarate 300 mg equivalent to 100 mg elemental iron. Nonmedicinal ingredients: artificial cherry flavor, caramel, carrageenan, glycerin, methylparaben, propylparaben, sorbitol solution, sucrose and water. Energy: 61.1 kJ (14.6 kcal)/5 mL; 3.3 g carbohydrates per 5 mL. Bottles of 100 mL.

Palafer® CF

ascorbic acid—ferrous fumarate—folic acid

Prenatal Supplement

GlaxoSmithKline Consumer Healthcare

INDICATIONS: For the treatment of hypochromic anemia and avitaminosis C and to prevent megaloblastic anemia of pregnancy due to folic acid depletion.

CONTRAINDICATIONS: Hemosiderosis, hemochromatosis. Iron compounds are also contraindicated in the treatment of hemolytic anemias unless an iron-deficient state also exists, since storage of iron with a possible exogenous hemosiderosis can result.

WARNINGS: No data supplied by the manufacturer.

PRECAUTIONS: Where anemia exists, its nature should be established and underlying causes determined.

Prolonged administration of iron should be avoided except in patients with continued bleeding or repeated pregnancies. In infants, large chronic doses of iron may so interfere with the assimilation of phosphorus as to cause severe rickets.

Orally administered iron salts may aggravate existing disorders, such as peptic ulcer, regional enteritis and ulcerative colitis. They may not be absorbed in patients with steatorrhea and those who have had a partial gastrectomy.

Before initiating parenteral iron therapy, it is advisable to give test doses to help detect sensitivity. Iron overload can occur in patients given an excess of parenteral iron, as well as those with hemoglobinopathies or other refractory anemias which might be erroneously diagnosed as iron-deficiency anemia. Do not administer oral iron preparations concomitantly with parenteral iron.

Iron binds with tetracyclines in equal molecular ratio thus preventing absorption of tetracyclines.

Warn patients that iron is toxic when overdoses are ingested by children. Severe reactions, including fatalities, have resulted.

Concomitant administration of antacids containing aluminum and magnesium salts may impair the absorption of iron.

ADVERSE EFFECTS: Oral ingestion of iron preparations may be associated with gastrointestinal discomfort (such as nausea) and dose-related bowel effects (such as constipation or diarrhea). Untoward effects usually subside with continuation of therapy or by iron ingestion with or after meals.

Parenteral iron administration can cause nausea, vomiting, and such acute allergic reactions as chills and fever, arthralgia, urticaria, and asthma. Occasional pain and staining of the skin at the site of injection may occur. Severe anaphylactoid reactions with some deaths have been reported in the literature. Although i.m. administration of iron dextran injections have caused sarcoma in laboratory animals, induced malignancy in man has never been observed.

OVERDOSE:

Iron poisoning is rare in adults but serious acute poisoning in children can result from ingestion of doses in excess of 1 g. Doses of 1 g should be considered as toxic in children and therapy instituted as soon as possible. Serum iron levels above 500 µg/100 mL can be taken as presumptive evidence of poisoning; severe poisoning is usually associated with levels well above 1000 µg/100 mL.

Symptoms: Symptoms may occur within about 30 minutes or may be delayed several hours. They are largely those of gastrointestinal irritation and necrosis with vomiting, diarrhea, tarry stools, hematemesis, fast and weak pulse, lethargy, low blood pressure, coma and signs of peripheral circulatory collapse. There may be a transient period of apparent recovery after 4 to 6 hours followed by a second crisis characterized by cyanosis, pulmonary edema, circulatory collapse, convulsion, and coma may then occur followed by death in 12 to 48 hours.

Treatment: Milk should be given immediately and vomiting induced. Eggs and milk should then be fed (to form iron-protein complexes) until it is possible to perform gastric lavage with 1% sodium bicarbonate solution (to convert the iron to a less soluble form). Gastric lavage should not be performed after the first hour of iron ingestion, because of the danger of perforation due to gastric necrosis. If an iron-chelating agent such as deferoxamine mesylate is available, it should be utilized. BAL (dimercaprol) should not be used because it may form a toxic complex. Measures to combat shock, dehydration, blood loss and respiratory failure may be necessary.

> For management of a suspected drug overdose, CPhA recommends that you contact your **regional Poison Control Centre**. See the *CPS* Directory section for a list of Poison Control Centres.

DOSAGE: One capsule daily on an empty stomach, preferably at bedtime, or as prescribed. Prophylactic administration of Palafer CF should be discontinued at term. Iron therapy alone should be administered after parturition.

SUPPLIED: Each pink and scarlet capsule, printed PALAFER CF in white ink on the body and cap, contains: microdispersed ferrous fumarate 300 mg (representing 100 mg of elemental iron), ascorbic acid 200 mg, and folic acid 0.5 mg. Nonmedicinal ingredients: D&C Yellow No. 10, FD&C Blue No. 1, FD&C Red No. 2, FD&C Red No. 3, FD&C Yellow No. 6, gelatin, lactose, magnesium stearate, povidone, silicon dioxide, sodium lauryl sulphate, sucrose, talc and titanium dioxide. Energy: 7.07 kJ (1.69 kcal per capsule); 0.41 g carbohydrates per capsule. Cartons of 30.

Pamidronate Disodium for Injection Ⓟ

pamidronate disodium

Bone Metabolism Regulator

Hospira

SUPPLIED: 3 mg/mL: Each mL of solution contains: pamidronate disodium 3 mg (formed from 2.53 mg pamidronic acid and 0.86 mg sodium hydroxide). Nonmedicinal ingredients: mannitol 47 mg and water for injection. May contain sodium hydroxide and phosphoric acid as pH adjusters. Preservative-free. Single use vials of 10 mL.

6 mg/mL: Each mL of solution contains: pamidronate disodium 6 mg (formed from 5.05 mg pamidronic acid and 1.72 mg sodium hydroxide). Nonmedicinal ingredients: mannitol 40 mg and water for injection. May contain sodium hydroxide and phosphoric acid as pH adjusters. Preservative-free. Single use vials of 10 mL.

9 mg/mL: Each mL of solution contains: pamidronate disodium 9 mg (formed from 7.58 mg pamidronic acid and 2.58 mg sodium hydroxide). Nonmedicinal ingredients: mannitol 37.5 mg and water for injection. May contain sodium hydroxide and phosphoric acid as pH adjusters. Preservative-free. Single use vials of 10 mL.

Store between 15 and 25°C. Do not freeze. Must be diluted before use. Discard unused portion.

Pamidronate Disodium for Injection Ⓟ

pamidronate disodium

Bone Metabolism Regulator

Sandoz

SUPPLIED: 3 mg/mL: Each mL of sterile concentrate for infusion contains: pamidronate disodium 3 mg (formed from 2.947 mg monosodium pamidronate and 5.8 mg sodium hydroxide). Nonmedicinal ingredients: mannitol, phosphoric acid to adjust pH and water for injection. Preservative-free. Single use vials of 10 mL, boxes of 1. Store between 15 and 30°C. Protect from heat. Discard unused portion.

6 mg/mL: Each mL of sterile concentrate for infusion contains: pamidronate disodium 6 mg (formed from 5.894 mg monosodium pamidronate and 11.6 mg sodium hydroxide). Nonmedicinal ingredients: mannitol, phosphoric acid to adjust pH and water for injection. Preservative-free. Single use vials of 10 mL, boxes of 1. Store between 15 and 30°C. Protect from heat. Discard unused portion.
9 mg/mL: Each mL of sterile concentrate for infusion contains: pamidronate disodium 9 mg (formed from 8.84 mg monosodium pamidronate and 17.4 mg sodium hydroxide). Nonmedicinal ingredients: mannitol, phosphoric acid to adjust pH and water for injection. Preservative-free. Single use vials of 10 mL, boxes of 1. Store between 15 and 30°C. Protect from heat. Discard unused portion.

Pamprin® Extra Strength Multi-Symptom
pamabrom—pyrilamine maleate—acetaminophen
Diuretic—Antihistamine—Analgesic

Chattem

Pamprin® Extra Strength PMS
pamabrom—pyrilamine maleate—acetaminophen
Diuretic—Antihistamine—Analgesic

Chattem

Pamprin® Ultra Strength Ibuprofen Formula
ibuprofen
Analgesic

Chattem

SUPPLIED: Pamprin Extra Strength Multi-Symptom: Each white, capsule-shaped tablet, with PAMPRIN embossed on one side, contains: pamabrom 25 mg, pyrilamine maleate 15 mg and acetaminophen 500 mg. Gluten-, lactose-, sodium- and tartrazine-free. Child-resistant bottles of 16 and 32.
Pamprin Extra Strength PMS: Each white, capsule-shaped tablet, with Pamprin PMS embossed on one side, contains: pamabrom 25 mg, pyrilamine maleate 15 mg and acetaminophen 500 mg. Gluten-, lactose-, sodium- and tartrazine-free. Child-resistant bottles of 16 and 32.
Pamprin Ultra Strength Ibuprofen Formula: Each brown caplet, with IBU 400 embossed on one side, contains: ibuprofen 400 mg. Gluten-, lactose-, sodium- and tartrazine-free. Child-resistant bottles of 16.

Pancrease® MT
pancrelipase
Digestant

Janssen-Ortho

DESCRIPTION: Pancrease MT capsules contain enteric-coated microtablets of pure porcine pancreatic enzyme concentrate—predominantly steapsin (pancreatic lipase), amylase and protease—isolated by a patented process that ensures high enzyme purity and activity.

PHARMACOLOGY: The enteric-coated microtablets resist gastric inactivation and deliver predictable, high levels of biologically active pancreatic enzymes (lipase, amylase, and protease) into the duodenum. The enzymes catalyze the hydrolysis of fats into glycerol and fatty acids, proteins into proteoses and derived substances, and starch into dextrins and sugars.
Pharmacokinetics: Absorption: The intestinal bioavailability of Pancrease MT 16 capsules was determined, in vitro, under simulated physiological conditions. The capsules were placed into a test tube containing an incubation medium consisting of 2 g NaCl, 9.2 g NaH_2PO_4 and distilled water (total volume: 1L). Employing a disintegration tester, the contents of the test tube were shaken at a constant speed of 30 rpm at an incubation temperature of 37°C. The pH of the mixture was adjusted by adding 4N HCl or 4N NaOH.

To simulate the acidic conditions of the stomach during a meal, a pH of 4.0 was initially established and gradually reduced in increments of 0.5 at 30 minute intervals to a pH of 2.5. To simulate the relative alkalinity of the intestine, the preparation was then transferred to a buffer where a pH of 6.6 was maintained. While the preparation was exposed to the buffer, release of pancreatic lipase, the marker enzyme, was measured as a function of time. The lipase content of the incubation medium was determined every 15 minutes for 120 minutes. More than 90% of the enzyme activity of the Pancrease MT capsules was released at 15 minutes with peak levels (97%) occurring at 30 minutes. The results demonstrate that Pancrease MT capsules are nearly 100% bioavailable and rapidly release high levels of pancreatic enzymes.
Excretion: Unused enzymes in the capsules are excreted in the feces. Digested enzymes are absorbed and are subsequently excreted in the urine.

INDICATIONS: For the treatment of steatorrhea secondary to pancreatic insufficiency in disorders such as cystic fibrosis or chronic pancreatitis.

CONTRAINDICATIONS: In patients known to be hypersensitive to pork protein and in patients with acute pancreatitis or with acute exacerbations of chronic pancreatic diseases.

WARNINGS: Should hypersensitivity occur, discontinue medication and treat the patient symptomatically.

Cases of fibrotic stricture formation in the ascending colon have been reported in cystic fibrosis patients with the use of high potency enzyme supplements in high doses (6 500 to 50 000 BP lipase units*/kg/meal). If symptoms suggestive of gastrointestinal obstruction occur the possibility of bowel strictures should be considered.

PRECAUTIONS: To protect the enteric coating, the microtablets should not be crushed or chewed. Where swallowing of capsules is difficult, they may be opened and the contents may be shaken onto a small quantity of a soft food which does not require chewing (e.g., applesauce, dessert gelatin, etc.), and swallowed immediately. Contact of the microtablets with foods having a pH greater than 7.3 (e.g., milk, custard, ice cream and many other dairy products) can dissolve the protective enteric coating and destroy enzyme activity.

To avoid irritation of the mouth, lips and tongue, opened capsules should be swallowed immediately before regular feedings or meals to minimize the likelihood that the microtablets are retained in the mouth. Proteolytic enzymes present in pancrelipase, when retained in the mouth, may begin to digest the mucous membranes and cause ulcerations.

Any change in pancreatic enzyme replacement therapy (e.g., dose or brand of medication) should be made cautiously and only under medical supervision.
Pregnancy: Teratology studies in rats (single dose level of 329 mg/kg/day) and rabbits (up to 259 mg/kg/day) did not indicate any embryo/fetal toxicity or teratogenic effects. No fertility or peri-/postnatal studies have been performed in animals.

No adequate, well-controlled studies have been conducted in pregnant women. Pancrease MT capsules should be used in pregnancy only if the potential benefit justifies the potential risk to the fetus.
Lactation: Pancreatic enzymes act locally in the gastrointestinal tract and are not likely to be systemically absorbed. Some of the constituent amino and nucleic acids are likely to be absorbed along with dietary proteins. The possibility of the protein constituents appearing in the breast milk cannot be excluded.

ADVERSE EFFECTS: Clinical evidence indicates that Pancrease MT pancrelipase capsules are well tolerated. Postmarketing, the most frequently reported adverse effects are gastrointestinal in nature and include diarrhea, abdominal pain, intestinal obstruction, vomiting, intestinal stenosis, and constipation. Frequently reported adverse events in other body systems include dermatitis.

* 1 BP lipase unit is approximately equal to 1 USP lipase unit.

Extremely high doses of exogenous pancreatic enzymes have been associated with hyperuricemia and hyperuricosuria when the preparations given were pancrelipase in powdered or capsule form or pancreatin in tablet form.

Cases of fibrosing colonopathy have been reported in cystic fibrosis patients (see Warnings).

OVERDOSE:

Symptoms: There have been no reports of accidental or purposeful overdosage with pancrelipase capsules. Pancrelipase microtablets are classified as nontoxic by the Poisindex Information System, and serious toxicity from overdose is unlikely.

Treatment: Should toxicity occur, treat symptomatically.

> For management of a suspected drug overdose, CPhA recommends that you contact your **regional Poison Control Centre**. See the *CPS* Directory section for a list of Poison Control Centres.

DOSAGE: General Guidelines: Patients with pancreatic insufficiency should consume a high-calorie, unrestricted fat diet appropriate for their age and clinical status. A nutritional assessment should be performed regularly as a component of routine care, and additionally when the dosage of pancreatic enzyme replacement is changed.

Dosage should be adjusted according to the severity of the exocrine pancreatic enzyme deficiency. The number of capsules or capsule strength given with meals and/or snacks should be estimated by assessing which dose minimizes steatorrhea and maintains good nutritional status. In some patients with pancreatic enzyme deficiency, satisfactory responses have been achieved with dosages (expressed in USP units of lipase) similar to the ones stated below. However, dosages should be adjusted according to the response of the patients. Dosage should be adjusted based on 3-day fecal fat studies.

Dose increases, if required, should be made slowly, with careful monitoring of response and symptomatology. It is important to ensure adequate hydration of patients at all times while administering Pancrease MT capsules.

There is considerable variation among individuals in response to enzymes with respect to control of steatorrhea; therefore, a range of doses is suggested.
Infants (up to 12 months): Fat Consumption Scheme: 2 000 to 4 000 USP lipase units per 120 mL of formula or per breast-feeding. This provides approximately 450 to 900 lipase units per g of fat ingested (based on 4.5 g of fat per 120 mL standard cow's milk-based formula). Higher doses are used in infants because, on average, infants ingest 5 g of fat/kg of body weight/day, whereas adults tend to ingest about 2 g of fat/kg/day.
Children (over 12 months) and Adults: Weight-based Scheme: Less than 4 years: Begin with 1 000 USP lipase units/kg/meal to a maximum of 2 500 lipase units/kg/meal. Over 4 years and Adults: Begin with 400 USP lipase units/kg/meal to a maximum of 2 500 lipase units/kg/meal.

Enzyme doses, expressed as lipase units/kg/meal, should be decreased in older patients, since they weigh more but tend to ingest less fat per kg. Usually, half the mealtime dose is given with a snack. The total daily dose should reflect approximately 3 meals and 2 snacks per day.

If doses greater than 2 500 lipase units/kg/meal (4 000 lipase units/g fat/day) are required to control malabsorption, further investigation is warranted to rule out other causes of malabsorption. Doses greater than 2 500 units/kg/meal should be used with caution and only if they are documented to be effective by 3-day fecal fat studies. It is unknown whether doses above 2 500 lipase units/kg/meal are safe.

Doses above the recommended dosing range have been associated with colonic strictures, particularly in children. Patients currently on higher doses (>2 500 lipase units/kg/meal or 4 000 lipase units/g fat/day) should be re-evaluated and the dosage either immediately decreased or titrated downward to the lowest effective clinical dose as assessed by 3-day fecal fat excretion.

SUPPLIED: Physical and Chemical Properties: Macroscopic Appearance: Pancrelipase, the enzyme component of Pancrease MT capsules, is a light beige granulate containing some lighter off-white particles.
Pancrease MT 4: Each yellow opaque, clear hard gelatin capsule, imprinted "PANCREASE MT 4" on clear cap, and "McNEIL" on body, contains: lipase 4 000 USP units, amylase 12 000 USP units and protease 12 000 USP units. Capsules are filled with off-white microtablets. Nonmedicinal ingredients: cellulose, crospovidone, gelatin, iron oxide, magnesium stearate, methacrylic acid copolymer, polydimethylsiloxane, polysorbate 80, sodium lauryl sulfate, silicon dioxide, talc, titanium dioxide, triethylcitrate, wax and other trace ingredients. Bottles of 100.
Pancrease MT 10: Each pink opaque, clear hard gelatin capsule, imprinted "PANCREASE MT 10" on clear cap, and "McNEIL" on body, contains: lipase 10 000 USP units, amylase 30 000 USP units and protease 30 000 USP units. Capsules are filled with off-white microtablets. Nonmedicinal ingredients: cellulose, crospovidone, gelatin, iron oxide, magnesium stearate, methacrylic acid copolymer, polydimethylsiloxane, polysorbate 80, sodium lauryl sulfate, silicon dioxide, talc, titanium dioxide, triethylcitrate, wax and other trace ingredients. Bottles of 100.
Pancrease MT 16: Each salmon opaque, clear hard gelatin capsule, imprinted "PANCREASE MT 16" on clear cap, and "McNEIL" on body, contains: lipase 16 000 USP units, amylase 48 000 USP units and protease 48 000 USP units. Capsules are filled with off-white microtablets. Nonmedicinal ingredients: cellulose, crospovidone, gelatin, iron oxide, magnesium stearate, methacrylic acid copolymer, polydimethylsiloxane, polysorbate 80, sodium lauryl sulfate, silicon dioxide, talc, titanium dioxide, triethylcitrate, wax and other trace ingredients. Bottles of 100.

Keep bottles tightly closed. Store between 10 to 25°C in a dry place. Do not refrigerate. Dispense in tight container.

(Shown in Product Identification Section)

Pancuronium Bromide Injection ℞
pancuronium bromide
Nondepolarizing Neuromuscular Blocking Agent

Sandoz

SUPPLIED: 1 mg/mL: Each mL of solution contains: pancuronium bromide 1 mg. Nonmedicinal ingredients: acetic acid to adjust pH to 4.0, sodium acetate, sodium chloride and water for injection. Single use vials of 5 mL, boxes of 5. Discard unused portion. Store between 2 and 8°C.
2 mg/mL: Each mL of solution contains: pancuronium bromide 2 mg. Nonmedicinal ingredients: acetic acid to adjust pH to 4.0, sodium acetate, sodium chloride and water for injection. Single use vials of 2 mL, boxes of 10. Single use vials of 5 mL, boxes of 5. Discard unused portion. Store between 2 and 8°C.

Panoxyl® 5%
benzoyl peroxide
Acne Vulgaris Therapy

Stiefel, a GSK company

Panoxyl® 10% and 20% ℞
benzoyl peroxide
Acne Vulgaris Therapy

Stiefel, a GSK company

SUPPLIED: Bars: Each g contains: benzoyl peroxide USP 5% or 10%. Nonmedicinal ingredients: colloidal silicon dioxide, purified water and tensianol base KS-1. Bars of 100 g with plastic storage tray.
Gel: Each g of gel contains: benzoyl peroxide USP 5%, 10% or 20% in an alcohol gel base containing polyoxyethylene lauryl ether. Nonmedicinal ingredients: citric acid anhydrous, ethoxylated lauryl alcohol, ethyl alcohol 95 O.P., hydroxylpropyl methyl cellulose, magnesium aluminum silicate and purified water USP. Plastic tubes of 60 g. Store between 15-30°C.

Panoxyl® 5% Wash
benzoyl peroxide
Acne Therapy

Stiefel, a GSK company

SUPPLIED: Each mL contains: benzoyl peroxide USP 5% in a lathering base of soapless cleansers (Benoxyl formulation). Nonmedicinal ingredients: citric acid, ethoxylated lauryl alcohol, hydroxypropyl methylcellulose, imidurea, magnesium aluminum silicate, purified water, sodium alkyl aryl polyethylene sulfate, sodium dialkyl octyl sulfate succinate and sodium lauryl sulfoacetate. Plastic flip top bottles of 175 mL. Keep from heat.

Panoxyl® Antibacterial Acne Creamy Wash
benzoyl peroxide
Acne Therapy

Stiefel, a GSK company

SUPPLIED: Each g contains: benzoyl peroxide 4%. Nonmedicinal ingredients: dimethyl isosorbide, glycolic acid, imidurea, methylparaben, nalidone, purified water, sodium hydroxide and tensianol soap base KS-1. Plastic tubes of 120 g.

Panoxyl® Aquagel 2.5% and 5%
benzoyl peroxide
Acne Therapy

Stiefel, a GSK company

SUPPLIED: Each g of gel contains: benzoyl peroxide USP 2.5% or 5% in an aqueous gel base (H_2Oxyl formulation). Nonmedicinal ingredients: carbomer 940, imidurea, polyoxyethylene lauryl ether, purified water and sodium hydroxide. Plastic tubes of 60 g. Keep from heat.

Panoxyl® Clear Acne Cleansing Gel
salicylic acid—triclosan
Acne Vulgaris Therapy

Stiefel, a GSK company

SUPPLIED: Each g contains: a two in one combination of 2% salicylic acid and 0.5% triclosan. Nonmedicinal ingredients: cocobetaine, cocamidopropylbetaine, glycerin, methylparaben, purified water, sodium laureth sulfate, sodium metabisulfite, tetrasodium EDTA. Plastic tubes of 120 g.

PANTO® IV Ⓟ
pantoprazole sodium
H+, K+-ATPase Inhibitor

Nycomed

Date of Revision: May 16, 2008

SUMMARY PRODUCT INFORMATION:

Route of Administration	Dosage Form/Strength	Clinically Relevant Nonmedicinal Ingredients
Intravenous	Lyophilized powder for injection/40 mg	None For a complete listing see Dosage Forms, Composition and Packaging.

INDICATIONS AND CLINICAL USE: PANTO IV (pantoprazole sodium for injection) is indicated for the short-term treatment (up to 7 days) of conditions where a rapid reduction of gastric acid secretion is required, such as the following:

- Reflux esophagitis, in hospitalized patients who cannot tolerate oral medication
- Pathological hypersecretion associated with Zollinger-Ellison Syndrome, in hospitalized patients who cannot tolerate oral medication

Geriatrics (>65 years of age): No dosage adjustment is recommended based on age. The daily dose used in elderly patients, as a rule, should not exceed the recommended dosage regimens.
Pediatrics: The safety and effectiveness of pantoprazole sodium in children have not yet been established.

CONTRAINDICATIONS: PANTO IV (pantoprazole sodium for injection) is contraindicated in patients with a history of hypersensitivity to pantoprazole sodium or to any ingredient in the formulation. For a complete listing of ingredients, see Dosage Forms, Composition and Packaging.

Pantoprazole, like all PPIs, should not be concurrently administered with atazanavir. See Drug Interactions.

WARNINGS AND PRECAUTIONS: General: In the presence of any alarm symptom (e.g. significant unintentional weight loss, recurrent vomiting, dysphagia, haematemesis, anaemia, or melaena) and when gastric ulcer is suspected, the possibility of malignancy should be excluded before therapy with PANTO IV (pantoprazole sodium for injection) is instituted since treatment with pantoprazole sodium may alleviate symptoms and delay diagnosis.

Further investigation should be considered if symptoms persist despite adequate treatment.

As with any other intravenous product containing edetate disodium (the salt form of EDTA), which is a potent chelator of metal ions including zinc, zinc supplementation should be considered in patients treated with PANTO IV who are prone to zinc deficiency. Caution should be used when other EDTA containing products are also co-administered intravenously.

Carcinogenesis and Mutagenesis: Effects of long-term treatment include hypergastrinemia, possible enterochromaffin-like (ECL) cell hyperplasia and carcinoid formation in the stomach, adenomas and carcinomas in the liver and neoplastic changes in the thyroid.

In the rat, the mechanism leading to the formation of gastric carcinoids is considered to be due to the elevated gastrin level occurring during chronic treatment. Similar observations have also been made after administration of other acid secretion inhibitors.

Short-term and long-term treatment with pantoprazole sodium in a limited number of patients up to 6 years have not resulted in any significant pathological changes in gastric oxyntic exocrine cells.

Hepatic/Biliary/Pancreatic: The daily dose in patients with severe liver disease should, as a rule, not exceed 20 mg pantoprazole. In severe hepatically impaired patients with Zollinger-Ellison syndrome,doses of pantoprazole should be adjusted according to acid output measurements, and kept at a minimum effective dose. See Action and Clinical Pharmacology, Special Populations and Conditions.

Renal: The daily dose used in renal insufficient patients, as a rule, should not exceed the recommended dosage regimens. See Action and Clinical Pharmacology, Special Populations and Conditions.

Special Populations: Pregnant Women: There are no adequate or well-controlled studies in pregnant women. PANTO IV should not be administered to pregnant women unless the expected benefits outweigh the potential risks to the fetus.

Nursing Women: Limited data is available around pantoprazole use in nursing women. Pantoprazole excretion in human milk has been detected in a study of a single nursing mother after a single 40 mg oral dose. The clinical relevance of this finding is not known. Pantoprazole sodium should not be given to nursing mothers unless its use is believed to outweigh the potential risks to the infant.

Pediatrics: The safety and effectiveness of pantoprazole sodium in children have not yet been established.

Geriatrics (>65 years of age): No dose adjustment is recommended based on age. The daily dose used in elderly patients, as a rule, should not exceed the recommended dosage regimens.

Monitoring and Laboratory Tests: Critically ill patients should be monitored carefully for any unexpected side effects.

ADVERSE EFFECTS: Adverse Drug Reaction Overview: Pantoprazole sodium is well tolerated. Most adverse events have been mild and transient showing no consistent relationship with treatment.

In four controlled clinical trials involving 407 reflux esophagitis patients receiving pantoprazole sodium i.v. therapy (40 mg daily for 5-7 days, followed by oral administration up to a maximum of 7 weeks), the following adverse events were reported with a >1% frequency during the i.v. administration phase, and relation to drug administration could not be ruled out (see Table 1).

Table 1: PANTO IV

Adverse Reactions [>1% frequency; relation to administration of pantoprazole sodium i.v. 40 mg daily (5–7 days) could not be ruled out] Reported in 4 Controlled Clinical Trials (n=407)

Gastrointestinal Disorders	
General complaints like abdominal pain, cramps, bloating and discomfort	1.97%
Constipation	1.22%
Diarrhea	1.97%
Loose/soft/mushy stools	1.72%
Nausea/nauseated	1.72%
Vomiting/retching	1.97%
Nervous System Disorders	
Headache/headache dull	3.2%
General Disorders and Administration Site Conditions	
Injection site reactions (inflammation, bruises)	1.22%
Skin and Subcutaneous Tissue Disorders	
Allergic skin reactions including pruritus and exanthema	1.22%

In two pantoprazole sodium i.v. studies in patients with Zollinger-Ellison syndrome, the following adverse events were reported most frequently and relation to drug administration (divided doses between 160-240 mg) could not be ruled out: abdominal pain, cough increased, constipation, diarrhea, headache, injection site reactions, tachycardia, taste perversion, and twitching.

In one tolerability study (n=61) comparing 40 mg pantoprazole sodium i.v. without EDTA to 40 mg pantoprazole sodium i.v. with EDTA in healthy volunteers, the following treatment emergent adverse events were reported most frequently (i.e.≥1% and <10%) in the EDTA group: abdominal pain, chest pain, face edema, headache, pain, vasodilation, nausea, vomiting, peripheral edema, dizziness, pruritus, rash, increased triglycerides, increased glucose, decreased hematocrit, decreased neutrophils, and creatinine clearance decreased. Increased potassium, decreased potassium, and increased ALT were reported in the non-EDTA group only. Constipation was reported at a frequency of ≥10%. Increased triglycerides was reported at a frequency of ≥ 10% in the non-EDTA group only. All of the adverse events were mild or moderate and no significant differences were seen between treatment groups. The EDTA formulation was well tolerated and has a similar tolerability profile to the non-EDTA formulation.

Eight subjects experienced increases in serum eosinophils (3 subjects in the non-EDTA group, 5 in the EDTA group) all of whom were noted to have elevated eosinophils before administration of the first dose. Of these 8 subjects, during the course of the study, serum eosinophils decreased in 3 subjects (all in the EDTA group), stayed approximately the same in 2 subjects (1EDTA, 1 non-EDTA), and increased slightly in 3 subjects (1 EDTA, and 2 non-EDTA).

Post-Market Adverse Drug Reactions: Spontaneous adverse events reported during postmarketing use of intravenous pantoprazole sodium (estimate of over 5 million patients with intravenous administration) are described below. As the events were reported spontaneously, no exact incidences can be provided, yet, most of them occurred very rarely. The following events were reported in postmarketing use, and causal relation to intravenous pantoprazole sodium treatment could not be ruled out:
Gastrointestinal Disorders: dry mouth.
Nervous System Disorders: dizziness, disturbance in vision (blurred vision).
Skin and Subcutaneous Tissue Disorders: urticaria, angioedema, skin rash, photosensitivity, severe skin reactions such as Stevens-Johnson syndrome, erythema multiforme, toxic epidermal necrolysis.
Hepatobiliary Disorders: increased liver enzymes (transaminases, GGT), severe hepatocellular damage leading to jaundice with or without hepatic failure.
Musculoskeletal, Connective Tissue and Bone Disorders: myalgia, arthralgia, rhabdomyolysis.
General Disorders: increased body temperature, peripheral edema.
Metabolic Disorders: elevated triglycerides.
Immune System Disorders: anaphylactic reactions including anaphylactic shock.
Psychiatric Disorders: depression, hallucination, disorientation, confusion especially in pre-disposed patients, as well as the aggravation of these symptoms in the case of pre-existence.
Renal and Urinary Disorders: interstitial nephritis.
Hematologic and Lymphatic System: leukopenia, thrombocytopenia.
General Disorders and Administration Site Conditions: injection site thrombophlebitis.
In addition, the following spontaneous post-marketing adverse events have been reported: nausea, pancreatitis, increased salivation, hypokinesia, tinnitus, speech disorder, elevated creatine phosphokinase, confusion, pancytopenia, anterior ischemic optic neuropathy.

DRUG INTERACTIONS: Overview: Pantoprazole undergoes extensive hepatic metabolism via cytochrome P450-mediated oxidation followed by sulphate conjugation via a Phase II reaction (non-saturable, non-cytochrome P450 dependent). No induction of the CYP 450 system by pantoprazole was observed during chronic administration with antipyrine as a marker. Because of the profound and long lasting inhibition of gastric acid secretion, pantoprazole sodium may interfere with the absorption of drugs where gastric pH is an important determinant of their bioavailability (e.g., ketoconazole).

It has been shown that co-administration of atazanavir 300 mg/ritonavir 100 mg with omeprazole (40 mg once daily) or atazanavir 400 mg with lansoprazole (60 mg single dose) to healthy volunteers resulted in a substantial reduction in the bioavailability of atazanavir. The absorption of atazanavir is pH dependent. Therefore all PPIs, including pantoprazol, should not be co-administered with atazanavir. See Contraindications.

Drug-Drug Interactions: Pantoprazole sodium does not interact with carbamazepine, caffeine, diclofenac, naproxen, piroxicam, ethanol, glibenclamide, metoprolol, antipyrine, diazepam, phenytoin, nifedipine, theophylline, digoxin, oral contraceptives, or cyclosporine. Concomitant use of antacids does not affect the pharmacokinetics of pantoprazole sodium.

Clinical studies have shown that there is no pharmacokinetic interaction between pantoprazole sodium and the following antibiotic combinations: metronidazole plus clarithromycin, metronidazole plus amoxicillin, amoxicillin plus clarithromycin.

Although no interaction during concomitant administration of warfarin has been observed in clinical pharmacokinetic studies, a few isolated cases of changes in INR have been reported during concomitant treatment in the post-marketing period. Therefore, in patients being treated with coumarin anticoagulants, monitoring of prothrombin time/INR is recommended after initiation, termination or during irregular use of pantoprazole.

Drug-Food Interactions: Consumption of food does not affect the pharmacokinetics (AUC and C_{max}) of pantoprazole sodium.

Drug-Laboratory Test Interactions: There have been reports of false-positive results in urine screening tests for tetrahydrocannabinol (THC) in patients receiving most proton pump inhibitors, including pantoprazole. To some extent, a cross-reactivity of proton pump inhibitors to the THC assay in the OnTrak TesTcard 9 has been seen, though this may not be limited to this screening test. In order to verify positive urine screening results, a confirmatory method should be considered.

DOSAGE AND ADMINISTRATION:

Dosing Considerations: Patients should be switched to PANTOLOC (pantoprazole sodium) tablet when feasible. In switching, the same dose mg per mg should be administered. Daily doses of up to 272 mg pantoprazole i.v. were administered and were well tolerated. PANTO IV has been administered for up to 7 days in clinical trials. Tolerance effects are not associated with the use of PANTO IV as demonstrated in clinical trials.

Recommended Dose and Dosage Adjustment: Reflux Esophagitis: The recommended adult dose of PANTO IV (pantoprazole sodium for injection) in patients with reflux esophagitis is 40 mg pantoprazole per day, administered either by slow intravenous injection over 2 to 5 minutes, or by intravenous infusion over 15 minutes.

Pathological Hypersecretion Associated with Zollinger-Ellison Syndrome: For patients with pathological hypersecretion associated with Zollinger-Ellison syndrome, the recommended adult dose is 80 mg every 12 hours, administered by intravenous infusion over 15 minutes. Doses of 120 mg twice daily and 80 mg three times per day were also used to control acid output to below 10 mEq/h.

Administration: When preparing the intravenous infusion, polyvinyl chloride (PVC) and copolymer of ethylene and propylene (PAB) infusion bags, can be used.

40 mg intravenous injection: Inject 10 mL of physiological sodium chloride solution into the vial containing the dry substance. The resulting potency of the solution is 4 mg/mL of pantoprazole, and can be administered by slow injection over 2 to 5 minutes.

After preparation, the reconstituted (ready-to-use) solution for intravenous injection must be used within 24 hours of initial puncture of the stopper.

Reconstitution Medium	Administer within:
0.9% Sodium Chloride Injection, USP	24 hours

40 mg intravenous infusion: Prepare the 40 mg intravenous injection as described above. The ready-to-use solution should then be further diluted with 90 mL 0.9% Sodium Chloride Injection USP, or 90 mL of 5% Dextrose Injection. The resulting potency of the diluted solution is 0.4 mg/mL of pantoprazole, and can be administered by infusion over 15 minutes.

80 mg intravenous infusion: Two vials of PANTO IV are required. Each vial should be reconstituted with 10 mL of physiological sodium chloride solution. The contents of the two vials should be further diluted together with 80 mL 0.9% Sodium Chloride Injection USP, or 80 mL 5% Dextrose Injection USP. The resulting potency of the diluted solution is 0.8 mg/mL of pantoprazole, and can be administered by infusion over 15 minutes.

When further diluting, the reconstituted solution in the vial must be diluted within 3 hours of the initial puncture of the stopper.

When further diluting with 0.9% sodium chloride injection USP for intravenous infusion, the solution must be administered within 21 hours.

When further diluting with 5% dextrose injection USP for intravenous infusion, the solution must be administered within 12 hours.

Diluent	Further dilute within:	Administer within:
0.9% Sodium Chloride Injection, USP	3 hours	21 hours following dilution
5% Dextrose Injection, USP	3 hours	12 hours following dilution

As with all parenteral admixtures, the reconstituted or further diluted solution should be examined for change in colour, precipitation, haziness or leakage. Discard unused portion.

Reconstitution: Parenteral Products: PANTO IV should not be simultaneously administered through the same line with other intravenous solutions, and it is recommended that a dedicated line or a flushed line be used for administration. When a flushed intravenous line is used, it should be flushed before and after administration of PANTO IV with either 0.9% sodium chloride injection USP, or 5% dextrose injection USP.

40 mg Intravenous Injection: 0.9% Sodium Chloride Injection USP. See Table 2.

Table 2: PANTO IV

40 mg Intravenous Injection—0.9% Sodium Chloride Injection USP

Vial Size (mL)	Volume of Diluent (mL) to be added to the vial	Approximate Available Volume (mL)	Nominal Concentration per mL
12	10	10	4 mg

For intravenous injection, a ready-to-use solution is prepared by injecting 10 mL of physiological sodium chloride solution into the vial containing the dry substance. The resulting potency is 4 mg/mL of pantoprazole.

40 mg Intravenous Infusion: Prepare as above; then, 1) 0.9% Sodium Chloride Injection USP. See Table 3.

Table 3: PANTO IV

40 mg Intravenous Infusion—0.9% Sodium Chloride Injection USP

Volume of ready-to-use solution (mL)	Volume of Diluent (mL)	Approximate Available Volume (mL)	Nominal Concentration per mL
10	90	100	0.4 mg

2) 5% Dextrose Injection, USP. See Table 4.

Table 4: PANTO IV

40 mg Intravenous Infusion—5% Dextrose Injection USP

Volume of ready-to-use solution (mL)	Volume of Diluent (mL)	Approximate Available Volume (mL)	Nominal Concentration per mL
10	90	100	0.4 mg

For intravenous infusion of 40 mg: the solution is prepared by injecting 10 mL of physiological sodium chloride solution into the vial containing the dry substance. The ready-to-use solution should then be further diluted with 90 mL of 0.9% Sodium Chloride Injection USP, or 90 mL of 5% Dextrose Injection USP.

80 mg Intravenous Infusion: Two vials of PANTO IV are required. Each vial should be reconstituted with 10 mL of physiological sodium solution.

1) 0.9% Sodium Chloride Injection, USP. See Table 5.

Table 5: PANTO IV

80 mg Intravenous Infusion—0.9% Sodium Chloride Injection USP

Volume of ready-to-use solution (mL)	Volume of Diluent (mL)	Approximate Available Volume (mL)	Nominal Concentration per mL
20	80	100	0.8 mg

2) 5% Dextrose Injection, USP. See Table 6.

Table 6: PANTO IV

80 mg Intravenous Infusion—5% Dextrose Injection USP

Volume of ready-to-use solution (mL)	Volume of Diluent (mL)	Approximate Available Volume (mL)	Nominal Concentration per mL
20	80	100	0.8 mg

For intravenous infusion of 80 mg: The two ready-to-use solutions should then be further diluted together with 80 mL 0.9% sodium chloride injection USP, or 80 mL of 5% dextrose injection USP.

OVERDOSAGE:

For management of a suspected drug overdose, CPhA recommends that you contact your **regional Poison Control Centre**. See the *CPS* Directory section for a list of Poison Control Centres.

Some reports of overdosage with pantoprazole sodium have been received. No consistent symptom profile was observed after ingestion of high doses of pantoprazole sodium. Daily doses of up to 272 mg pantoprazole sodium i.v., and single doses of 240 mg administered over 2 minutes, have been administered and were well tolerated.

Treatment of overdosage should be supportive and symptomatic. Pantoprazole is not removed by hemodialysis.

ACTION AND CLINICAL PHARMACOLOGY: Mechanism of Action: PANTO IV (pantoprazole sodium for injection) is a specific inhibitor of the gastric H^+, K^+-ATPase enzyme (the proton pump) that is responsible for acid secretion by the parietal cells of the stomach.

Pantoprazole sodium is a substituted benzimidazole that accumulates in the acidic environment of the parietal cells after absorption. Pantoprazole sodium is then converted into the active form, a cyclic sulphenamide, which binds to the H^+, K^+-ATPase, thus inhibiting both the basal and stimulated gastric acid secretion. Pantoprazole sodium exerts its effect in an acidic environment (pH <3), and it is mostly inactive at higher pH. Its pharmacological and therapeutic effect is achieved in the acid-secretory parietal cells.

In clinical studies investigating intravenous (i.v.) and oral administration, pantoprazole sodium inhibited pentagastrin-stimulated gastric acid secretion. With a daily oral dose of 40 mg, inhibition was 51% on Day 1 and 85% on Day 7. Basal 24-hour acidity was reduced by 37% and 98% on Days 1 and 7, respectively.

Fasting gastrin values increased during pantoprazole treatment, but in most cases the increase was only moderate. An extensive evaluation of clinical laboratory results has not revealed any clinically important changes during pantoprazole sodium treatment (except for gastrin which increased to 1.5-fold after 4 to 8 weeks).

Pharmacodynamics: Pantoprazole is a proton pump inhibitor. It inhibits H^+, K^+-ATPase, the enzyme responsible for gastric acid secretion in the parietal cells of the stomach, in a dose-dependent manner. The drug is a substituted benzimidazole that accumulates in the acid canaliculi of parietal cells after absorption. There, pantoprazole is converted into the active form, a cyclic sulphenamide that binds selectively to the proton translocating region of the H^+, K^+-ATPase. Pantoprazole's selectivity is due to the fact that it only exerts its maximal effect in a strongly acidic environment (pH <3).

Pantoprazole remains mostly inactive at higher pH values. As pantoprazole action is distal to the receptor levels, it can inhibit gastric acid secretion irrespective of the nature of the stimulus (acetylcholine, histamine, gastrin).

Pharmacokinetics: Absorption: Pantoprazole is absorbed rapidly following administration of a 40 mg enteric coated tablet. Its oral bioavailability compared to the i.v. dosage form is 77% and does not change upon multiple dosing. Following an oral dose of 40 mg, C_{max} is approximately 2.5 µg/mL with a t_{max} of 2 to 3 hours. The AUC is approximately 5 µg.h/mL. There is no food effect on AUC (bioavailability) and C_{max}.

Distribution: Pantoprazole is 98% bound to serum proteins. Elimination half-life, clearance and volume of distribution are independent of the dose.

Metabolism: Pantoprazole is almost completely metabolized in the liver. Pantoprazole sodium is mainly metabolized by CYP2C19 and to a minor extent CYPs 3A4. Studies with pantoprazole in humans reveal no inhibition or activation of the cytochrome P450 (CYP 450) system of the liver.

Excretion: Renal elimination represents the major route of excretion (about 82%) for the metabolites of pantoprazole, the remaining metabolites are excreted in feces. The main metabolite in both the serum and urine is desmethylpantoprazole as a sulphate conjugate. The half-life of the main metabolite (about 1.5 hours) is not much longer than that of pantoprazole (approximately 1 hour).

Pantoprazole shows linear pharmacokinetics, i.e., AUC and C_{max} increase in proportion with the dose within the dose-range of 10 to 80 mg after both i.v. and oral administration. Elimination half-life, clearance and volume of distribution are considered to be dose-independent. Following repeated i.v. or oral administration, the AUC of pantoprazole was similar to a single dose.

Special Populations and Conditions: Pediatrics: The safety and effectiveness of pantoprazole in children have not yet been established.

Geriatrics: After repeated intravenous administration in healthy elderly subjects, total serum clearance of pantoprazole sodium was similar to that observed in healthy younger subjects. No dosage adjustment is recommended based on age. The daily dose used in elderly patients, as a rule, should not exceed the recommended dosage regimens.

Hepatic Insufficiency: The half-life increased to between 7 and 9 h, the AUC increased by a factor of 5 to 7, and the C_{max} increased by a factor of 1.5 in patients with liver cirrhosis compared with healthy subjects following administration of 40 mg pantoprazole. Similarly, following administration of a 20 mg dose, the AUC increased by a factor of 5.5 and the C_{max} increased by a factor of 1.3 in patients with severe liver cirrhosis compared with healthy subjects. Considering the linear pharmacokinetics of pantoprazole, there is an increase in AUC by a factor of 2.75 in patients with severe liver cirrhosis following administration of a 20 mg dose compared to healthy volunteers following administration of a 40 mg dose. Thus, the daily dose in patients with severe liver disease should, as a rule, not exceed 20 mg pantoprazole.

In severe hepatically impaired patients with Zollinger-Ellison syndrome, doses of pantoprazole should be adjusted according to acid output measurements, and kept at a minimum effective dose.

Renal Insufficiency: In patients with severe renal impairment, pharmacokinetic parameters for pantoprazole sodium were similar to those of healthy subjects. No dosage adjustment is necessary in patients with renal impairment or in patients undergoing hemodialysis.

STORAGE AND STABILITY: Store at 15 to 30°C and protect from light.

SPECIAL HANDLING INSTRUCTIONS: None.

INFORMATION FOR THE PATIENT: Published in e-CPS, available by subscription at www.e-cps.ca.

DOSAGE FORMS, COMPOSITION AND PACKAGING: Each vial of lyophilized powder contains: pantoprazole 40 mg (pantoprazole sodium 42.3 mg). Nonmedicinal Ingredients: edetate disodium dihydrate and sodium hydroxide. Vials of 10 mL, bundles of 10.

(Shown in Product Identification Section)

Pantoloc® Ⓟ

pantoprazole sodium

H+, K+-ATPase Inhibitor

Nycomed

Date of Revision: June 13, 2008

SUMMARY PRODUCT INFORMATION:

Route of Administration	Dosage Form/ Strength	Clinically Relevant Nonmedicinal Ingredients
Oral	Enteric-coated Tablet 20 and 40 mg pantoprazole	None For a complete listing see Dosage Forms, Composition and Packaging.

Note: As with all proton pump inhibitors, when PANTOLOC (pantoprazole sodium) is prescribed in combination with clarithromycin, amoxicillin or metronidazole for the eradication of an *H. pylori* infection, the Product Monograph for the antibiotics used should be consulted and followed.

INDICATIONS AND CLINICAL USE: PANTOLOC (pantoprazole sodium) is indicated for the treatment of conditions where a reduction of gastric acid secretion is required, such as the following:

- Duodenal ulcer
- Gastric ulcer
- Reflux esophagitis
- Symptomatic gastro-esophageal reflux disease (such as, acid regurgitation and heartburn).
- Prevention of gastrointestinal lesions induced by non-steroidal anti-inflammatory drugs (NSAIDs) in patients with a need for continuous NSAID treatment, who have increased risk to develop NSAID-associated upper gastrointestinal lesions.
- *H. pylori* associated duodenal ulcer. Pantoprazole, in combination with clarithromycin and either amoxicillin or metronidazole, is indicated for the treatment of patients with an active duodenal ulcer who are *H. pylori* positive. Clinical trials using combinations of pantoprazole with appropriate antibiotics have indicated that such combinations are successful in eradicating *H. pylori*.

For the maintenance treatment of patients with reflux esophagitis and the resolution of symptoms associated with reflux esophagitis, such as heartburn with or without regurgitation, 20 or 40 mg pantoprazole once daily have been used for 3 years in controlled clinical trials. In continuous maintenance treatment 20 mg pantoprazole has been used in a limited number of patients for up to eight years.

Geriatrics (>65 years of age): No dose adjustment is recommended based on age. The daily dose used in elderly patients, as a rule, should not exceed the recommended dosage regimens.

Pediatrics: The safety and effectiveness of pantoprazole in children have not yet been established.

CONTRAINDICATIONS: Patients who are hypersensitive to this drug or to any ingredient in the formulation or component of the container. For a complete listing, see Dosage Forms, Composition and Packaging.

Pantoprazole, like all PPIs, should not be concurrently administered with atazanavir (see Drug Interactions).

WARNINGS AND PRECAUTIONS: General: In the presence of any alarm symptom (e.g. significant unintentional weight loss, recurrent vomiting, dysphagia, haematemesis, anaemia, or melaena) and when gastric ulcer is suspected, the possibility of malignancy should be excluded before therapy with PANTOLOC (pantoprazole sodium) is instituted since treatment with pantoprazole sodium may alleviate symptoms and delay diagnosis.

Further investigation should be considered if symptoms persist despite adequate treatment.

Carcinogenesis and Mutagenesis: Effects of long-term treatment include hypergastrinemia, possible enterochromaffin-like (ECL) cell hyperplasia and carcinoid formation in the stomach, adenomas and carcinomas in the liver and neoplastic changes in the thyroid.

In the rat, the mechanism leading to the formation of gastric carcinoids is considered to be due to the elevated gastrin level occurring during chronic treatment. Similar observations have also been made after administration of other acid secretion inhibitors.

Short-term and long-term treatment with pantoprazole sodium in a limited number of patients up to 6 years have not resulted in any significant pathological changes in gastric oxyntic exocrine cells.

Hepatic/Biliary/Pancreatic and Renal: The daily dose in patients with severe liver disease should, as a rule, not exceed 20 mg pantoprazole. See Action and Clinical Pharmacology, Special Populations and Conditions.

The daily dose used in renal insufficient patients, as a rule, should not exceed the recommended dosage regimens. See Action and Clinical Pharmacology, Special Populations and Conditions.

Pantoprazole should not be used in combination treatment for the eradication *H. pylori* in patients with severe hepatic or renal dysfunction since currently no data are available on the efficacy and safety of pantoprazole in combination treatment of these patients.

Special Populations: Pregnant Women: There are no adequate or well-controlled studies in pregnant women. Pantoprazole sodium should not be administered to pregnant women unless the expected benefits outweigh the potential risks to the fetus.

Nursing Women: Limited data is available around pantoprazole in nursing women. Pantoprazole excretion in human milk has been detected in a study of a single nursing mother after a single 40 mg oral dose. The clinical relevance of this finding is not known. Pantoprazole sodium should not be given to nursing mothers unless its use is believed to outweigh the potential risks to the infant.

Pediatrics: The safety and effectiveness of pantoprazole in children have not yet been established.

Geriatrics (>65 years of age): No dose adjustment is recommended based on age. The daily dose used in elderly patients, as a rule, should not exceed the recommended dosage regimens.

ADVERSE REACTIONS: Adverse Drug Reaction Overview: PANTOLOC (pantoprazole sodium) is well tolerated. Most adverse events have been mild and transient showing no consistent relationship with treatment. Adverse events have been recorded during controlled clinical investigations in over 13 000 patients exposed to pantoprazole sodium as the single therapeutic agent for treatment of conditions requiring acid suppression.

The following adverse events (the most frequently reported) have been reported in individuals receiving pantoprazole therapy (40 mg once daily) in controlled clinical trials of at least 6 months duration: headache (2.1%), diarrhea (1.6%), nausea (1.2%).

The following adverse reactions considered possibly, probably, or definitely related by the investigator have been reported in individuals receiving pantoprazole therapy (20 mg or 40 mg once daily) in long-term clinical trials (duration of at least 6 months). There were a limited number of *H. pylori* positive patients in these studies and therefore, definitive conclusions with regard to long-term consequences of *H. pylori* infection and acid suppressive treatment on gastric inflammation in this sub-group cannot be made. See Table 1.

Table 1: PANTOLOC

Adverse Drug Reactions With a Frequency of ≥1%, Related to 40 mg Pantoprazole Assessed as Possibly, Probably or Definitely Related by the Investigator

Preferred term	Number of patients	Percentage of patients
Headache	24	2.137
Diarrhea	18	1.603
Nausea	13	1.158

For long-term treatment with 20 mg, no such events were reported with a frequency of more than 1%.

Adverse drug reactions with a frequency of 0.1 to 1% related to 20 mg pantoprazole: Gastrointestinal Disorders: diarrhea, flatulence, abdominal pain, abdominal pain upper, abdominal distension, gastric polyps, loose stools, frequent bowel movements, eructation, dyspepsia, nausea, vomiting, constipation.

General Disorders: fatigue.

Hepatobiliary Disorders: alanine aminotransferase increased, aspartate aminotransferase increased, liver function tests abnormal, transaminases increased.

Laboratory Parameters: hyperglycaemia.

Nervous System Disorders: headache, dizziness, vertigo.

Skin and Subcutaneous Tissue Disorders: pruritus, rash.

Special Senses: visual disturbance.

Other: libido decreased.

Adverse drug reactions with a frequency of 0.1 to 1% related to 40 mg pantoprazole: Cardiovascular System: blood pressure increased, hypertension, ECG abnormal.

Gastrointestinal Disorders: flatulence, abdominal distension, abdominal pain, abdominal pain upper, loose stools, esophageal reflux aggravated, gastric polyps, abdominal discomfort, abdominal tenderness, constipation, eructation, vomiting, dyspepsia, gastroesophageal reflux, esophagitis.

General Disorders: fatigue, peripheral edema, pyrexia.

Hepatobiliary Disorders: alanine aminotransferase increased, aspartate aminotransferase increased, liver function tests abnormal, transaminases increased.

Laboratory Parameters: hypertriglyceridaemia.

Metabolic and Nutritional: appetite decreased, weight increase.

Nervous System Disorders: dysgeusia, dizziness, migraine, vertigo.

Respiratory System: cough.

Skin and Subcutaneous Tissue Disorders: pruritus, rash.

Special Senses: mouth dry, vision blurred.

Other: neoplasm.

The following adverse reactions considered possibly, probably, or definitely related by the investigator have been reported in individuals receiving pantoprazole therapy (20 mg or 40 mg once daily) in short-term clinical trials (duration of up to 3 months).

Adverse drug reactions with a frequency of 0.1 to 1% related to pantoprazole, 20 or 40 mg: Gastrointestinal Disorders: diarrhea, flatulence, nausea, constipation, abdominal pain.

Nervous System Disorders: headache, dizziness.

Skin and Subcutaneous Tissue Disorders: pruritus.

In addition, the following adverse events considered unrelated, or unlikely related by the investigator have been reported in individuals receiving pantoprazole therapy (20 mg or 40 mg once daily) in short-term and long-term clinical trials.

Adverse events with a frequency of ≥1%, 20 or 40 mg: influenza like illness, headache, diarrhea.

Adverse events with a frequency of 0.1 to 1%, 20 or 40 mg: bronchitis, nausea, back pain, abdominal pain upper, upper respiratory tract infection, nonaccidental injury, sinusitis, abdominal pain, dizziness, arthralgia, vomiting, pharyngitis, chest pain, gastroenteritis, dyspepsia, urinary tract infection, eructation, pyrexia, cough, depression, hypertension, pain in limb, constipation, fatigue, operation, neck pain, nasopharyngitis, alanine aminotransferase increased, hemorrhoids, pain, flatulence, viral infection, hypertriglyceridaemia, toothache, hypersensitivity, rash, abdominal pain lower, pneumonia, abdominal distension, dyspnoea, muscle cramp, rhinitis, peripheral edema, tonsillitis, angina pectoris, cholelithiasis, sinus congestion, influenza, vertigo, insomnia, infection, osteoarthritis, hypercholesterolaemia, pruritus, eczema, sleep disorder, migraine, aspartate aminotransferase increased, hyperglycemia, musculoskeletal discomfort, blood triglycerides increased, myocardial infarction, tendonitis, weight increased, rectal hemorrhage, cystitis, nasal congestion, arthritis, contusion, abdominal discomfort, enteritis.

The following Serious Adverse Events regardless of causality were reported with a frequency of <0.1% in either 20 mg or 40 mg: sepsis.

A total of 1217 patients were treated with triple combination therapy including pantoprazole sodium and two antibiotics. Adverse events noted at a frequency of greater than or equal to 1% when pantoprazole sodium was used in combination with antibiotics for the eradication of an *H. pylori* infection included the following:

In combination with clarithromycin and metronidazole (n=725):

Body as a Whole: headache (1.8%), tiredness (1.1%).

Central and Peripheral Nervous System: dizziness (1.4%).

Gastrointestinal: diarrhea (4.8%), nausea (3.7%), upper abdominal pain (1.9%), tongue pain (1.2%), loose stools (1.0%), buccal inflammation (1.0%).

Hepatobiliary: hepatic enzymes increased (1.2%).

Special Senses: bitter taste (4.0%), metallic taste (2.1%).

In combination with amoxicillin and clarithromycin (n=492):

Body as a Whole: headache (1.8%), pain (1.0%).

Skin and Appendages: exanthema (1.2%).

Gastrointestinal: diarrhea (10.0%), bitter taste (3.0%), upper abdominal pain (1.4%), nausea (1.2%).

Regardless of the combination regimen, the most frequently reported events were gastrointestinal system disorders, followed by autonomic nervous system disorders and "body as a whole", or generalized disorders.

Abnormal Hematologic and Clinical Chemistry Findings: Please refer to the Hepatobiliary Disorders and the Laboratory Parameters portions of the Adverse Reaction; Action and Clinical Pharmacology, Special Populations and Conditions; and Warnings and Precautions, Hepatic/Biliary/Pancreatic and Renal.

Post-Market Adverse Drug Reactions: The following adverse events were reported in post-marketing use and causal relation to pantoprazole sodium treatment could not be ruled out:

Skin and Subcutaneous Tissue Disorders: allergic reactions such as skin rash. Very rare cases of angioedema, severe skin reactions such as Stevens-Johnson Syndrome, erythema multiforme, toxic epidermal necrolysis, and photosensitivity. Isolated cases of alopecia, acne, maculopapular rash, urticaria, exfoliative dermatitis.

Nervous System Disorders: hypokinesia, disturbances in vision (blurred vision). Rare cases of somnolence, insomnia; in isolated cases vertigo, tremor, tinnitus, paresthesia, nervousness, photophobia.

Eye Disorders: anterior ischemic optic neuropathy.

Gastrointestinal Disorders: occasionally upper abdominal pain, flatulence; rare cases of increased appetite, dry mouth, nausea/vomiting, constipation, dyspeptic symptoms, acid eructation, pancreatitis, increased salivation.

Urogenital: isolated cases of hematuria and impotence. Interstitial nephritis.

Laboratory Parameters: in rare cases, increased liver enzymes (transaminases, γ-GT), elevated triglycerides.

Hematologic and Lymphatic System: pancytopenia, isolated cases of eosinophilia. Very rare cases of leukopenia, and thrombocytopenia.

General Disorders: speech disorder, very rare cases of peripheral edema, increased body temperature.

Hepatobiliary Disorders: very rare cases of severe hepatocellular damage leading to jaundice with or without hepatic failure.

Immune System Disorders: anaphylactic reactions including anaphylactic shock.

Musculoskeletal, Connective Tissue and Bone Disorders: elevated creatine phosphokinase, in rare cases, myalgia and arthralgia. In very rare cases rhabdomyolysis.

Psychiatric Disorders: confusion, rare cases of depression, hallucination, disorientation, confusion especially in pre-disposed patients, as well as the aggravation of these symptoms in the case of pre-existence.

Other: in isolated cases malaise.

DRUG INTERACTIONS: Overview: Pantoprazole undergoes extensive hepatic metabolism via cytochrome P450-mediated oxidation followed by sulphate conjugation via a Phase II reaction (non-saturable, non-cytochrome P450 dependent). Pharmacokinetic drug interaction studies in man did not demonstrate the inhibition of the oxidative metabolism of the drug. No induction of the CYP 450 system by pantoprazole was observed during chronic administration of pantoprazole sodium with antipyrine as a marker. Changes in absorption should be taken into account when drugs whose absorption is pH dependent, e.g., ketoconazole, are taken concomitantly.

It has been shown that co-administration of atazanavir 300 mg/ritonavir 100 mg with omeprazole (40 mg once daily) or atazanavir 400 mg with lansoprazole (60 mg single dose) to healthy volunteers resulted in a substantial reduction in the bioavailability of atazanavir. The absorption of atazanavir is pH dependent. Therefore all PPIs, including pantoprazole, should not be co-administered with atazanavir. See Contraindications.

Drug-Drug Interactions: Pantoprazole sodium does not interact with carbamazepine, caffeine, diclofenac, naproxen, piroxicam, ethanol, glibenclamide, metoprolol, antipyrine, diazepam, phenytoin, nifedipine, theophylline, digoxin, oral contraceptives, or cyclosporine. Concomitant use of antacids does not affect the pharmacokinetics of pantoprazole sodium.

Clinical studies have shown that there is no pharmacokinetic interaction between pantoprazole and the following antibiotic combinations: metronidazole plus clarithromycin, metronidazole plus amoxicillin, amoxicillin plus clarithromycin.

In a preclinical study, pantoprazole sodium in combination therapy with various antibiotics (including tetracycline, clarithromycin, and amoxicillin) was shown to have a potentiating effect on the elimination rate of *H. pylori* infection.

Although no interaction during concomitant administration of warfarin has been observed in clinical pharmacokinetic studies, a few isolated cases of changes in INR have been reported during concomitant treatment in the post-marketing period. Therefore, in patients being treated with coumarin anticoagulants, monitoring of prothrombin time/INR is recommended after initiation, termination or during irregular use of pantoprazole.

Drug-Food Interactions: Consumption of food does not affect the pharmacokinetics (AUC and C_{max}) of pantoprazole sodium.

Drug-Laboratory Test Interactions: There have been reports of false-positive results in some urine screening tests for tetrahydrocannabinol (THC) in patients receiving most proton pump inhibitors, including pantoprazole. A confirmatory method should be considered to verify positive results.

Other: Generally, daily treatment with any acid-blocking medicines over a long time (e.g. longer than 3 years) may lead to malabsorption of cyanocobalamin caused by hypo- or achlorhydria. Rare cases of cyanocobalamin deficiency under acid-blocking therapy have been reported in the literature and should be considered if respective clinical symptoms are observed.

DOSAGE AND ADMINISTRATION: Recommended Dose and Dosage Adjustment: Duodenal Ulcer: The recommended adult dose of PANTOLOC (pantoprazole sodium) for the oral treatment of duodenal ulcer is 40 mg as pantoprazole given once daily in the morning. Healing usually occurs within 2 weeks. For patients not healed after this initial course of therapy, an additional course of 2 weeks is recommended.

Gastric Ulcer: The recommended adult oral dose of pantoprazole for the oral treatment of gastric ulcer is 40 mg given once daily in the morning. Healing usually occurs within 4 weeks. For patients not healed after this initial course of therapy, an additional course of 4 weeks is recommended.

***H. pylori* Associated Duodenal Ulcer:** Pantoprazole/Clarithromycin/Metronidazole Triple Combination Therapy: The recommended dose for *H. pylori* eradication is treatment for seven days with PANTOLOC 40 mg together with clarithromycin 500 mg and metronidazole 500 mg, all twice daily.

Pantoprazole/Clarithromycin/Amoxicillin Triple Combination Therapy: The recommended dose for *H. pylori* eradication is treatment for seven days with PANTOLOC 40 mg together with clarithromycin 500 mg and amoxicillin 1000 mg, all twice daily.

Symptomatic Gastro-esophageal Reflux Disease (GERD): The recommended adult oral dose for the treatment of symptoms of GERD, including heartburn and regurgitation, is 40 mg once daily for up to 4 weeks. If significant symptom relief is not obtained in 4 weeks, further investigation is required.

Reflux Esophagitis: The recommended adult oral dose of pantoprazole is 40 mg, given once daily in the morning. In most patients, healing usually occurs within 4 weeks. For patients not healed after this initial course of therapy, an additional 4 weeks of treatment is recommended.

Both 20 mg and 40 mg once daily have been demonstrated to be effective in the maintenance of healing of reflux esophagitis. If maintenance therapy fails when using 20 mg once daily, consideration may be given to the 40 mg daily dose as maintenance therapy.

Prevention of Gastrointestinal Lesions Induced by NSAIDs: The recommended adult oral dose of pantoprazole is 20 mg, given once daily in the morning.

Missed Dose: If a dose is forgotten, the missed dose should be taken as soon as possible unless it is close to the next scheduled dose. Two doses should never be taken at one time to make up for a missed dose; patients should just return to the regular schedule.

Administration: Pantoprazole sodium is formulated as an enteric-coated tablet. A whole tablet should not be chewed or crushed, and should be swallowed with fluid in the morning either before, during, or after breakfast.

Reconstitution: Not applicable.

OVERDOSAGE:

Some reports of overdosage with pantoprazole have been received. No consistent symptom profile was observed after ingestion of high doses of pantoprazole. Daily doses of up to 272 mg pantoprazole i.v., and single doses of up to 240 mg i.v. administered over 2 minutes, have been administered and were well tolerated.

Treatment of overdosage should be supportive and symptomatic. Pantoprazole is not removed by hemodialysis.

> For management of a suspected drug overdose, CPhA recommends that you contact your **regional Poison Control Centre**. See the *CPS* Directory section for a list of Poison Control Centres.

ACTION AND CLINICAL PHARMACOLOGY: Mechanism of Action: PANTOLOC (pantoprazole sodium) is a specific inhibitor of the gastric H^+, K^+-ATPase enzyme (the proton pump) that is responsible for acid secretion by the parietal cells of the stomach.

Pantoprazole sodium is a substituted benzimidazole that accumulates in the acidic environment of the parietal cells after absorption. Pantoprazole sodium is then converted into the active form, a cyclic sulphenamide, which binds to the H^+, K^+-ATPase, thus inhibiting both the basal and stimulated gastric acid secretion. Pantoprazole sodium exerts its effect in an acidic environment (pH <3), and it is mostly inactive at higher pH. Its pharmacological and therapeutic effect is achieved in the acid-secretory parietal cells.

In clinical studies investigating intravenous (i.v.) and oral administration, pantoprazole sodium inhibited pentagastrin-stimulated gastric acid secretion. With a daily oral dose of 40 mg, inhibition was 51% on Day 1 and 85% on Day 7. Basal 24-hour acidity was reduced by 37% and 98% on Days 1 and 7, respectively.

In long-term international studies involving over 800 patients, a 2 to 3 fold mean increase from the pre-treatment fasting serum gastrin level was observed in the initial months of treatment with pantoprazole at doses of 40 mg per day during GERD maintenance studies and 40 mg or higher per day in patients with refractory GERD. Fasting serum gastrin levels generally remained at approximately 2 to 3 times baseline for up to 4 years of periodic follow-up in clinical trials.

Treatment with pantoprazole alone has a limited effect on infections of *H. pylori*, a bacterium implicated as a major pathogen in peptic ulcer disease. Approximately 90-100% of patients with duodenal ulcers, and 80% of patients with gastric ulcers, are *H. pylori* positive. Preclinical evidence suggests that there is a synergistic effect between pantoprazole sodium and selected antibiotics in eradicating *H. pylori*. In infected patients, eradication of the infection with pantoprazole sodium and appropriate antibiotic therapy leads to ulcer healing, accompanied by symptom relief and a decreased rate of ulcer recurrence.

In single dose clinical pharmacology studies, pantoprazole was administered concomitantly with combinations of amoxicillin, clarithromycin, and/or metronidazole. When a single dose of pantoprazole was administered to healthy volunteers in combination with metronidazole plus amoxicillin, with clarithromycin plus metronidazole, or with clarithromycin plus amoxicillin, lack of interaction between any of the medications was shown.

Pharmacodynamics: Pantoprazole is a proton pump inhibitor. It inhibits H^+,K^+-ATPase, the enzyme responsible for gastric acid secretion in the parietal cells of the stomach, in a dose-dependent manner. The drug is a substituted benzimidazole that accumulates in the acid canaliculi of parietal cells after absorption. There, pantoprazole is converted into the active form, a cyclic sulfenamide that binds selectively to the proton translocating region of the H^+,K^+-ATPase. Pantoprazole's selectivity is due to the fact that it only exerts its maximal effect in a strongly acidic environment (pH <3).

Pantoprazole remains mostly inactive at higher pH values. As pantoprazole action is distal to the receptor levels, it can inhibit gastric acid secretion irrespective of the nature of the stimulus (acetylcholine, histamine, gastrin).

Pharmacokinetics: Absorption: Pantoprazole is absorbed rapidly following administration of a 40 mg enteric coated tablet. Its oral bioavailability compared to the i.v. dosage form is 77% and does not change upon multiple dosing. Following an oral dose of 40 mg, C_{max} is approximately 2.5 µg/mL with a t_{max} of 2 to 3 hours. The AUC is approximately 5 µg·h/mL. There is no food effect on AUC (bioavailability) and C_{max}.

Distribution: Pantoprazole is 98% bound to serum proteins. Elimination half-life, clearance and volume of distribution are independent of the dose.

Metabolism: Pantoprazole is almost completely metabolized in the liver. Studies with pantoprazole in humans reveal no inhibition or activation of the cytochrome P450 (CYP 450) system of the liver.

Excretion: Renal elimination represents the major route of excretion (about 82%) for the metabolites of pantoprazole sodium, the remaining metabolites are excreted in feces. The main metabolite in both the serum and urine is desmethylpantoprazole as a sulphate conjugate. The half-life of the main metabolite (about 1.5 hours) is not much longer than that of pantoprazole (approximately 1 hour).

Pantoprazole shows linear pharmacokinetics, i.e., AUC and C_{max} increase in proportion with the dose within the dose-range of 10 to 80 mg after both i.v. and oral administration. Elimination half-life, clearance and volume of distribution are considered to be dose-independent. Following repeated i.v. or oral administration, the AUC of pantoprazole was similar to a single dose.

Special Populations and Conditions: Pediatrics: The safety and effectiveness of pantoprazole in children have not yet been established.

Geriatrics: An increase in AUC (35%) and C_{max} (22%) for pantoprazole occurs in elderly volunteers when compared to younger volunteers after 7 consecutive days oral dosing with pantoprazole 40 mg. After a single oral dose of pantoprazole 40 mg , an increase in AUC (43%) and C_{max} (26%) occurs in elderly volunteers when compared to younger volunteers. No dose adjustment is recommended based on age. The daily dose in elderly patients, as a rule, should not exceed the recommended dosage regimens.

Hepatic Insufficiency: The half-life increased to between 7 and 9 h, the AUC increased by a factor of 5 to 7, and the C_{max} increased by a factor of 1.5 in patients with liver cirrhosis compared with healthy subjects following administration of 40 mg pantoprazole. Similarly, following administration of a 20 mg dose, the AUC increased by a factor of 5.5 and the C_{max} increased by a factor of 1.3 in patients with severe liver cirrhosis compared with healthy subjects. Considering the linear pharmacokinetics of pantoprazole, there is an increase in AUC by a factor of 2.75 in patients with severe liver cirrhosis following administration of a 20 mg dose compared to healthy volunteers following administration of a 40 mg dose. Thus, the daily dose in patients with severe liver disease should, as a rule, not exceed 20 mg pantoprazole.

Renal Insufficiency: In patients with severe renal impairment, pharmacokinetic parameters for pantoprazole were similar to those of healthy subjects. No dosage adjustment is necessary in patients with renal impairment or in patients undergoing hemodialysis, as the difference in AUCs between patients who are dialyzed and those who are not is 4%.

STORAGE AND STABILITY: Store at 15 to 30°C in the recommended packaging.

SPECIAL HANDLING INSTRUCTIONS: None.

INFORMATION FOR THE PATIENT: Published in e-CPS, available by subscription at www.e-cps.ca.

DOSAGE FORMS, COMPOSITION AND PACKAGING: 20 mg: Each enteric-coated, yellow, oval, biconvex tablet, marked P20 on one side, contains: pantoprazole 20 mg (pantoprazole sodium sesquihydrate 22.6 mg). Nonmedicinal ingredients: anhydrous sodium carbonate, calcium stearate, crospovidone, ferric oxide, mannitol, methylhydroxypropyl cellulose, poly (ethylacrylate, methacrylic acid), polysorbate 80, polyvidone, propylene glycol, sodium lauryl sulfate, titanium dioxide and triethyl citrate. Bottles of 100.

40 mg: Each enteric-coated, yellow, oval, biconvex tablet, marked P40 on one side, contains: pantoprazole 40 mg (pantoprazole sodium sesquihydrate 45.1 mg). Nonmedicinal ingredients: anhydrous sodium carbonate, calcium stearate, crospovidone, ferric oxide, mannitol, methylhydroxypropyl cellulose, poly (ethylacrylate, methacrylic acid), polysorbate 80, polyvidone, propylene glycol, sodium lauryl sulfate, titanium dioxide and triethyl citrate. Bottles of 100.

(Shown in Product Identification Section)

Pantoprazole Sodium for Injection

pantoprazole sodium

H^+, K^+-ATPase Inhibitor

Sandoz

SUPPLIED: Each vial of lyophilized powder contains: pantoprazole 40 mg (as pantoprazole sodium sesquihydrate 45.11 mg). Nonmedicinal ingredients: none. Vials of 15 mL, boxes of 10. Store between 15 and 30°C and protect from light.

Pantothenic Acid

Vitamin

CPhA Monograph

Date of Revision: October 2010

> This monograph has been compiled by CPhA and reviewed by experts. It may contain information different from that found in Health Canada-approved Product Monographs. The reader is referred to the *CPS* Editorial Policy for more information.

SUMMARY PRODUCT INFORMATION:

Route of Administration	Dosage Form	Strength
Oral	Capsule, tablet	100 mg, 250 mg, 500 mg, 1000 mg
	Solution	100 mg/mL

PHARMACOLOGY: Pantothenic acid, or vitamin B_5, is a water-soluble, B complex vitamin. It is a component of coenzyme A and is essential for acetylation reactions in gluconeogenesis, carbohydrate and lipid metabolism, and in the synthesis of steroid hormones, porphyrins, acetylcholine and other compounds.

Pantothenic acid is a required nutrient, but is so widely distributed that deficiency in humans is rare. Deficiency may occur in persons with severe malnutrition and is usually found in association with other deficiency states. Requirements may be increased in malabsorption syndromes such as tropical sprue, celiac disease and enteritis.

Food sources of pantothenic acid include organ meats (e.g., liver, kidney), egg yolk, broccoli, milk, yeast, avocado, chicken, beef, tomato products, oat cereals and whole grains. Processing of foods (e.g., refining grains, canning or freezing) lowers their pantothenic acid content.

Only the dextrorotatory isomer of pantothenic acid has vitamin activity.

Pharmacokinetics: Pantothenic acid is readily absorbed from the gastrointestinal tract. It is widely distributed to all body tissues and is not metabolized. About 70% of a dose is excreted unchanged in the urine with the remainder being excreted in the feces. Normal serum concentrations of pantothenic acid are 100 µg/mL or higher.

INDICATIONS: Pantothenic acid is classified by Health Canada as a natural health product (NHP). It is recommended for prevention of deficiency.

CONTRAINDICATIONS: Patients hypersensitive to any component of pantothenic acid formulations.

WARNINGS: See Precautions.

PRECAUTIONS: *Pregnancy:* The adequate intake for pantothenic acid is increased in pregnancy (see Table 1). It is not known whether large amounts of pantothenic acid can cause fetal harm.

Lactation: The adequate intake for pantothenic acid is increased during breastfeeding. No data are available on the effects of large amounts of pantothenic acid on nursing infants.

ADVERSE EFFECTS: Pantothenic acid is usually nontoxic, even in large doses.

OVERDOSE:

> For management of a suspected drug overdose, CPhA recommends that you contact your **regional Poison Control Centre**. See the *CPS* Directory section for a list of Poison Control Centres.

DOSAGE: To prevent nutrient deficiency, adequate dietary intake is preferred over supplementation whenever possible. Food sources include organ meats (e.g., liver, kidney), egg yolk, broccoli, milk, yeast, avocado, chicken, beef, tomato products, oat cereals and whole grains. For Adequate Intakes (AI) of pantothenic acid for adults and children, see Table 1.

To treat deficiency, dosage must be individualized, based on the severity of the deficiency. Calcium pantothenate 10 mg is equivalent to 9.2 mg pantothenic acid.

Table 1: Pantothenic Acid

Daily Adequate Intake

Age or Life Stage		Daily Adequate Intake (AI)
Infants	0–6 mo	1.7 mg
	7–12 mo	1.8 mg
Children	1–3 y	2 mg
	4–8 y	3 mg
	9–13 y	4 mg
Adults	14 y and older	5 mg
Pregnancy		6 mg
Breastfeeding		7 mg

Papaverine HCl Injection USP

papaverine HCl

Smooth Muscle Relaxant

Sandoz

SUPPLIED: Each mL contains: papaverine HCl 32.5 mg, dextrose anhydrous for tonicity and water for injection. Product contains a saturated solution. Single use vials of 2 mL, boxes of 10. Store between 15 and 30°C. Protect from light. Discard unused portion. Crystallization may occur at low temperatures; in such cases, warm the vial and shake until complete dissolution of crystals.

Paricalcitol ℞

CPhA Monograph

see *Vitamin D*

Pariet™ ℞

rabeprazole sodium

H+, K+-ATPase Inhibitor

Janssen-Ortho

Date of Preparation: May 15, 2001
Date of Revision: April 20, 2009

Note: When used in combination with amoxicillin and clarithromycin, the Product Monographs for those agents must be consulted and followed.

SUMMARY PRODUCT INFORMATION:

Route of Administration	Dosage Form/Strength	Clinically Relevant Nonmedicinal Ingredients
Oral	Tablet 10 mg, 20 mg	None For a complete listing see Dosage Forms, Composition and Packaging.

INDICATIONS AND CLINICAL USE: PARIET (rabeprazole sodium) is indicated for: Treatment of conditions where a reduction of gastric acid secretion is required, such as:

1. Symptomatic relief and healing of erosive or ulcerative gastroesophageal reflux disease (GERD).
2. Long-term maintenance of healing of erosive or ulcerative gastroesophageal reflux disease (GERD).
3. Treatment of symptoms (i.e. heartburn and regurgitation) in symptomatic gastroesophageal reflux disease (GERD), also called non-erosive reflux disease (NERD).
4. Symptomatic relief and healing of duodenal ulcers.
5. Symptomatic relief and healing of gastric ulcers.
6. Long-term treatment of pathological hypersecretory conditions, including Zollinger-Ellison syndrome.
7. Eradication of *H. pylori* associated with duodenal ulcer disease (active or history within the past 5 years). Eradication of *H. pylori* has been shown to reduce the risk of duodenal ulcer recurrence. Clinical trials using combinations of rabeprazole with appropriate antibiotics have indicated that such combinations are successful in eradicating *H. pylori*. Presented in Table 1 are the data from a U.S. multicentre study (Study 604) comparing rabeprazole, amoxicillin, and clarithromycin (RAC) for 3, 7 or 10 days versus omeprazole, amoxicillin and clarithromycin (OAC) for 10 days. In a European multicentre study (Study 603), RAC was compared to OAC for 7 days.

Geriatrics: See Warnings and Precautions, Special Populations.

Pediatrics (<18 years of age): The safety and efficacy of rabeprazole have not been established in children under the age of 18 years.

CONTRAINDICATIONS:

- Patients who are hypersensitive to rabeprazole, substituted benzimidazoles or to any ingredient in the formulation or component of the container. For a complete listing, see Dosage Forms, Composition and Packaging.
- Amoxicillin is contraindicated in patients with a known hypersensitivity to any penicillin. (Please refer to the amoxicillin Product Monograph before prescribing.)
- Clarithromycin is contraindicated in patients with known hypersensitivity to clarithromycin, erythromycin or other macrolide antibacterial agents. Clarithromycin is also contraindicated in patients receiving concurrent therapy with astemizole, terfenadine, cisapride or pimozide. (Please refer to the clarithromycin tablets Product Monograph before prescribing.)

WARNINGS AND PRECAUTIONS: When gastric ulcer is suspected, the possibility of malignancy should be excluded before therapy with PARIET is instituted, as treatment with rabeprazole may alleviate symptoms and delay diagnosis.

General: Symptomatic response to therapy with PARIET (rabeprazole sodium) does not preclude the presence of gastric malignancy.

Steady state interactions of rabeprazole and warfarin have not been adequately evaluated in patients. There have been reports of increased INR and prothrombin time in patients receiving proton pump inhibitors, including rabeprazole, and warfarin concomitantly. Increases in INR and prothrombin time may lead to abnormal bleeding and even death. Patients treated with a proton pump inhibitor and warfarin concomitantly may need to be monitored for increases in INR and prothrombin time.

Table 1: PARIET

***H. pylori* Eradication[a] Rates with Rabeprazole or Omeprazole Plus Amoxicillin and Clarithromycin in Patients with Duodenal Ulcer Disease**

	Proton Pump Inhibitor in Treatment	Treatment Time	% of Patients Cured [95% Confidence Interval of the difference RAC-OAC] (Number of patients)	
			Per-protocol[b]	Intent-to-treat[c]
Study 604 North America	Rabeprazole	3 days	30% [−61%, −43%] (n=167)	27% [−55%, −37%] (n=187)
	Rabeprazole	7 days	84%[d] [−5%, +11%] (n=166)	77%[d] [−4%, +12%] (n=194)
	Rabeprazole	10 days	86%[d] [−3%, +12%] (n=171)	78%[d] [−4%, +13%] (n=196)
	Omeprazole	10 days	82% (n=179)	73% (n=206)
Study 603 Europe	Rabeprazole	7 days	94% [−0.7%, +20%] (n=65)	84% [+0.5%, +24.5%] (n=83)
	Omeprazole	7 days	84% (n=63)	72% (n=85)

a In Study 604, *H. pylori* eradication was assessed at 6 weeks but not more than 10 weeks by ^{13}C-UBT. In Study 603, successful eradication of *H. pylori* was defined as a negative ^{13}C-UBT at week 5 and week 13 post-treatment assessments.
b Patients were included in the analysis if they had *H. pylori* infection documented at baseline, defined as a positive ^{13}C-UBT plus rapid urease test or culture and were not protocol violators. Patients who dropped out of the study due to an adverse event related to the study drug were included in the evaluable analysis as failures of therapy.
c Patients were included in the analysis if they had documented *H. pylori* infection at baseline defined as a positive ^{13}C-UBT plus rapid urease test or culture, and took at least one dose of study medication.
d Equivalent to OAC; two-sided 95% confidence interval on the difference between regimens is within [−15%,+15%].

As demonstrated with other PPI's, prolonged use may impair the absorption of protein-bound Vitamin B_{12} and may contribute to the development of Vitamin B_{12} deficiency.

Information to Be Provided to the Patient: PARIET tablets can be taken with or without meals. Patients should be advised that PARIET tablets should be swallowed whole, not chewed or crushed.

Hepatic/Biliary/Pancreatic: For patients with severe liver disease, dosage adjustment should be considered.

Renal: No dosage adjustment is necessary in patients with renal insufficiency.

Special Populations: Pregnant Women: The safety of PARIET treatment in pregnancy has not been established. PARIET tablets should not be administered to pregnant women unless the expected benefits outweigh the potential risks to the fetus.

Nursing Women: It is not known whether rabeprazole is excreted in human milk. PARIET tablets should not be given to nursing mothers unless the expected benefits outweigh the potential risks to the infant.

Pediatrics (<18 years of age): The safety and efficacy of rabeprazole have not been established in children under the age of 18 years.

Geriatrics: Ulcer healing rates in elderly patients are similar to those in younger patients. Adverse events and laboratory test abnormalities in elderly patients occurred at rates similar to those in younger patients. No dose adjustment is required in elderly patients.

ADVERSE REACTIONS: Adverse Drug Reaction Overview: Worldwide, over 3094 patients have been treated with PARIET (rabeprazole sodium) in Phase II-III clinical trials involving various dosages and durations of treatment. In general, rabeprazole treatment has been well tolerated in both short-term and long-term trials.

Clinical Trial Adverse Drug Reactions: Because clinical trials are conducted under very specific conditions the adverse reaction rates observed in the clinical trials may not reflect the rates observed in practice and should not be compared to the rates in the clinical trials of another drug. Adverse drug reaction information from clinical trials is useful for identifying drug-related adverse events and for approximating rates.

Incidence in North American and European Clinical Trials: The following adverse events were reported by the treating physicians to have a possible or probable relationship to drug in at least 1% of patients treated with rabeprazole sodium compared to patients who received placebo: see Table 2.

Table 2: PARIET

Incidence of Possibly- or Probably-related Adverse Events in Short-term and Long-term Controlled North American and European Studies

	PARIET (n=1746) %	Placebo (n=388) %
Body as a Whole		
Headache	2.8	2.8
Digestive System		
Diarrhea	2.6	2.3

Less Common Clinical Trial Adverse Drug Reactions (<1%): In short- and long-term studies, the following adverse events were reported in <1% of the patients treated with PARIET without regard to causality:

Body as a Whole: enlarged abdomen, abscess, ascites, carcinoma, substernal chest pain, asthenia, allergic reaction, fever, chills, cellulitis, cyst, hangover effect, hernia, injection site hemorrhage, injection site pain, injection site reaction, malaise, moniliasis, mucous membrane disorder, neck pain, neck rigidity, neoplasm, overdose, pelvic pain, photosensitivity, suicide attempt.

Cardiovascular System: angina pectoris, arrhythmia, bradycardia, bundle branch block, cardiovascular disorder, coronary artery disorder, abnormal electrocardiogram, embolus, hypertension, increased capillary fragility, migraine, myocardial infarction, palpitation, sinus bradycardia, supraventricular tachycardia, syncope, tachycardia, thrombophlebitis, thrombosis, varicose vein, vascular disorder, ventricular extrasystoles, QTc prolongation, ventricular tachycardia.

Digestive System: abdominal pain, abnormal stools, anorexia, bloody diarrhea, cholangitis, cholecystitis, cholelithiasis, cirrhosis of liver, colitis, constipation, diarrhea, duodenal ulcer, duodenitis, dry mouth, dyspepsia, dysphagia, esophageal stenosis, esophagitis, eructation, flatulence, gastritis, gastrointestinal hemorrhage, gastroenteritis, gastrointestinal carcinoma, gingivitis, glossitis, hepatic encephalopathy, hepatitis, hepatoma, increased appetite, melena, mouth ulceration, nausea and vomiting, pancreas disorder, pancreatitis, periodontal abscess, proctitis, rectal disorder, rectal hemorrhage, salivary gland enlargement, stomach ulcer, stomatitis, tooth caries, tooth disorder, ulcer ileum, ulcerative colitis, ulcerative stomatitis.

Endocrine System: diabetes mellitus, hyperthyroidism, hypothyroidism.

Hemic and Lymphatic System: anemia, ecchymosis, hypochromic anemia, lymphadenopathy.

Metabolic and Nutritional Disorders: dehydration, edema, face edema, gout, iron deficiency anemia, liver fatty deposit, peripheral edema, thirst, weight gain, weight loss.

Musculoskeletal System: arthritis, arthrosis, bone pain, bursitis, joint disorder, leg cramps, myalgia, rheumatoid arthritis, tendon disorder.

Nervous System: abnormal dreams, acute brain syndrome, addiction, agitation, amnesia, anxiety, cerebral hemorrhage, confusion, convulsion, dementia, depression, dizziness, extrapyramidal syndrome, hyperkinesia, hypertonia, insomnia, libido decreased, nervousness, neuralgia, neuropathy, paresthesia, sleep disorder, somnolence, tremor, twitching, vasodilatation, vertigo.
Respiratory System: apnea, asthma, carcinoma of lung, dyspnea, epistaxis, hiccup, hyperventilation, hypoventilation, hypoxia, laryngitis, lung disorder, pneumonia, pulmonary embolus, respiratory disorder, voice alteration.
Skin and Appendages: acne, alopecia, contact dermatitis, dry skin, fungal dermatitis, herpes simplex, herpes zoster, nail disorder, pruritus, psoriasis, rash, seborrhea, benign skin neoplasm, skin carcinoma, skin discoloration, skin hypertrophy, skin melanoma, skin nodule, sweating, urticaria.
Special Senses: abnormal vision, amblyopia, blepharitis, blurry vision, cataract, conjunctivitis, corneal opacity, deafness, diplopia, dry eyes, ear disorder, ear pain, eye disorder, eye hemorrhage, eye pain, glaucoma, lacrimation disorder, otitis externa, otitis media, retinal degeneration, retinal disorder, strabismus, taste perversion, tinnitus, vestibular disorder, vitreous disorder.
Urogenital System: breast enlargement, breast neoplasm, breast pain, cystitis, dysmenorrhea, dysuria, hematuria, impotence, kidney calculus, leukorrhea, mastitis, menorrhagia, menstrual disorder, metrorrhagia, orchitis, polycystic kidney, polyuria, prostatic disorder, urinary frequency, urinary incontinence, urinary tract disorder, uterine hemorrhage, vaginal hemorrhage, vaginitis.
Monitoring and Laboratory Tests: An extensive evaluation of laboratory analyses has not revealed any significant and/or clinically relevant changes during PARIET treatment. The following changes in laboratory parameters were reported as adverse events: abnormal platelets, albuminuria, increased creatine phosphokinase, abnormal erythrocytes, hypercholesteremia, hyperglycemia, hyperlipemia, hypokalemia, hyponatremia, leukocytosis, leukorrhea, abnormal liver function tests, prostatic specific antigen increase, urine abnormality, abnormal WBC.

In controlled clinical studies, 3/1456 (0.2%) patients treated with rabeprazole and 2/237 (0.8%) patients treated with placebo developed treatment-emergent abnormalities (which were either new on study or present at study entry with an increase of 1.25×baseline value) in AST, ALT, or both. None of the three rabeprazole patients experienced chills, fever, right upper quadrant pain, nausea or jaundice.
Combination Treatment with Amoxicillin and Clarithromycin: In clinical trials using combination therapy with rabeprazole plus amoxicillin and clarithromycin (RAC), no adverse events unique to this drug combination were observed. In the U. S. multicentre Study 604, the most frequently reported drug-related adverse events for patients who received the triple therapy for 7 or 10 days were diarrhea (8% and 7%) and taste perversion (6% and 10%), respectively. In the European multicentre Study 603, the most frequently occurring adverse events were diarrhea (13%) and taste perversion (14%) in patients receiving RAC therapy for 7 days.

No clinically significant laboratory abnormalities particular to the drug combinations were observed. When rabeprazole sodium is used in combination with amoxicillin and clarithromycin, the Product Monographs for those agents must be consulted and followed.
Post-market Adverse Drug Reactions: Additional adverse events reported from worldwide marketing experience with rabeprazole sodium are: sudden death, coma and hyperammonemia, jaundice, rhabdomyolysis, disorientation and delirium, anaphylaxis, angioedema, bullous and other drug eruptions of the skin, interstitial pneumonia, TSH elevations, myalgia and arthralgia. In most instances, the relationship to rabeprazole sodium was unclear. There have also been rare reports of increased hepatic enzymes and rare reports of hepatitis. Rare reports of hepatic encephalopathy have been received in patients with underlying cirrhosis. In addition, agranulocytosis, hemolytic anemia, leukopenia, pancytopenia, thrombocytopenia, neutropenia and acute systemic allergic reactions (facial swelling, hypotension, dyspnea) have been reported. There have been very rare reports of interstitial nephritis, gynecomastia, erythema multiforme, toxic epidermal necrolysis and Stevens-Johnson syndrome.
DRUG INTERACTIONS: Rabeprazole is metabolized by the cytochrome P450 (CYP450) drug metabolizing system. Studies in healthy subjects have shown that rabeprazole does not have clinically significant interactions with other drugs metabolized by the CYP450 system, such as warfarin, phenytoin, theophylline or diazepam. Steady state interactions of rabeprazole and other drugs metabolized by this enzyme system have not been studied in patients. Studies with rabeprazole in humans reveal no inhibition or activation of the CYP450 system of the liver. There have been reports of increased INR and prothrombin time in patients receiving proton pump inhibitors, including rabeprazole, and warfarin concomitantly. Increases in INR and prothrombin time may lead to abnormal bleeding and even death. In vitro incubations employing human liver microsomes indicated that the degree of inhibition of cyclosporin metabolism by rabeprazole and omeprazole is similar at equivalent concentrations.

Rabeprazole produces sustained inhibition of gastric acid secretion. An interaction with compounds whose absorption depends on gastric pH may occur due to the magnitude of acid suppression seen with rabeprazole: consequently, the co-administration of ketoconazole and rabeprazole decreases the absorption of ketoconazole, thereby decreasing plasma levels, whereas the concomitant use of digoxin results in an increase in digoxin plasma levels. Therefore, patients may need to be monitored when such drugs are taken concomitantly with rabeprazole.

Co-administration of atazanavir 300 mg/ritonavir 100 mg with omeprazole (40 mg once daily) or atazanavir 400 mg with lansoprazole (60 mg once daily) to healthy volunteers resulted in a substantial reduction in atazanavir exposure. The absorption of atazanavir is pH dependent. Although not studied, similar results are expected with other proton pump inhibitors. Therefore PPIs, including rabeprazole, should not be co-administered with atazanavir.
Combination Therapy with Clarithromycin: Combination therapy consisting of rabeprazole, amoxicillin and clarithromycin resulted in increases in plasma levels of rabeprazole and 14-hydroxyclarithromycin. (See Action and Clinical Pharmacology, Special Populations and Conditions, Combination Therapy with Antimicrobials.)
Drug-Food Interactions: Taking rabeprazole with food or antacids produced no clinically relevant changes in plasma rabeprazole concentrations.

DOSAGE AND ADMINISTRATION: Recommended Dose and Dosage Adjustment: Symptomatic Relief and Healing of Erosive or Ulcerative Gastroesophageal Reflux Disease (GERD): The recommended adult oral dose is 20 mg once daily. In most patients, healing occurs in four weeks. For patients not healed after this initial course, an additional four weeks of treatment is recommended. Symptom relief is usually rapid. If symptom relief is not achieved after four weeks, further investigation is recommended (see Indications and Clinical Use).
Long-term Maintenance of Healing of Erosive or Ulcerative Gastroesophageal Reflux Disease (GERD Maintenance): 10 mg once daily has been demonstrated to be effective versus placebo in the maintenance of healing of GERD. The maximum recommended adult oral dose is 20 mg once daily (see Indications and Clinical Use).
Treatment of Symptoms (i.e. Heartburn and Regurgitation) of Symptomatic Gastroesophageal Reflux Disease (GERD) or Non-Erosive Reflux Disease (NERD): The recommended adult oral dose is 10 mg once daily to a maximum of 20 mg once daily in patients with NERD. If symptom control is not achieved after four weeks, further investigation is recommended (see Indications and Clinical Use).
Symptomatic Relief and Healing of Duodenal Ulcers: The recommended adult oral dose is 20 mg once daily for up to four weeks (see Indications and Clinical Use). Most patients with duodenal ulcer heal within four weeks but a few patients may require additional therapy to achieve healing. Symptom relief is usually rapid with improvement achieved after two weeks for most patients.
Symptomatic Relief and Healing of Gastric Ulcers: The recommended adult oral dose is 20 mg once daily for up to six weeks (see Indications and Clinical Use). Most patients with gastric ulcer heal within six weeks, but a few patients may require additional therapy to achieve healing. Symptom relief is usually rapid with improvement achieved after three weeks for most patients.
Eradication of *H. pylori* Associated with Duodenal Ulcer Disease—Triple Therapy: PARIET 20 mg: twice daily for 7 days. Amoxicillin 1000 mg: twice daily for 7 days. Clarithromycin 500 mg: twice daily for 7 days.

All three medications should be taken twice daily with the morning and evening meals.

In patients who fail therapy, susceptibility testing should be done. If resistance to clarithromycin is demonstrated or susceptibility testing is not possible, alternative antimicrobial therapy should be instituted.
Long-term Treatment of Pathological Hypersecretory Conditions Including Zollinger-Ellison Syndrome: The PARIET dosage in patients with pathologic hypersecretory conditions varies with the individual patient. The recommended adult oral starting dose is 60 mg once a day. Doses should be adjusted to individual patient needs and should continue for as long as clinically indicated. Some patients may require divided doses. Doses up to 100 mg QD and 60 mg BID have been administered. Some patients with Zollinger-Ellison syndrome have been treated continuously with PARIET tablets for up to one year.

No dosage adjustment is necessary in patients with renal insufficiency or in elderly patients. For patients with severe liver disease, dosage adjustment should be considered.
Administration: PARIET tablets can be taken with meals or on an empty stomach. PARIET tablets are enteric-coated and therefore should be swallowed whole with a beverage (not chewed or crushed).

OVERDOSAGE:
Because strategies for the management of overdose are continually evolving, it is advisable to contact a Poison Control Centre to determine the latest recommendations for the management of an overdose of any drug.

There has been no experience with large overdoses of rabeprazole although seven reports of accidental overdosage with rabeprazole have been received. The maximum established exposure has not exceeded 60 mg twice daily or 160 mg once daily. Effects are generally minimal, representative of the known adverse event profile, and reversible without any further medical intervention. No specific antidote for rabeprazole is known; in the event of overdosage, treatment should be symptomatic and supportive. Rabeprazole is extensively protein-bound and is not readily dialyzable.

For management of a suspected drug overdose, CPhA recommends that you contact your **regional Poison Control Centre**. See the *CPS* Directory section for a list of Poison Control Centres.

ACTION AND CLINICAL PHARMACOLOGY: PARIET (rabeprazole sodium) is an antisecretory compound (substituted benzimidazole proton pump inhibitor) that suppresses gastric acid secretion by inhibiting the gastric H^+, K^+-ATPase at the secretory surface of the gastric parietal cell. Because this enzyme is regarded as the acid (proton) pump within the parietal cell, PARIET has been characterized as a gastric proton pump inhibitor. PARIET blocks the final step of gastric acid secretion and produces dose-related sustained inhibition of both basal and stimulated gastric acid secretion.
Pharmacodynamics: Antisecretory Activity: The antisecretory effect begins within one hour after oral administration of PARIET tablets (20 mg), and reaches its maximum within two to four hours. The median inhibitory effect of PARIET on 24-hour gastric acidity is 88% of maximal after the first dose and the inhibition of acid secretion increases with repeated once-daily dosing to steady-state within seven days. PARIET 20 mg, versus placebo, inhibits basal and pentagastrin-induced acid secretion by 86% and 95%, respectively. At this dosage, it also increases the percentage of time (from 10% to 65%) within a 24-hour period that the gastric pH>3 (see Table 3). This relatively prolonged pharmacodynamic action compared to the short pharmacokinetic half-life (approximately one hour) reflects the sustained inactivation of the H^+, K^+-ATPase.

Table 3: PARIET

Gastric Acid Parameters—PARIET versus Placebo After 7 Days of Once-daily Dosing

Parameter	PARIET (20 mg q.d.)	Placebo
Basal Acid Output (mmol/h)	0.4[a]	2.8
Stimulated Acid Output (mmol/h)	0.6[a]	13.3
% Time Gastric pH>3	65[a]	10

[a] (p<0.01 versus placebo).

The ability of PARIET to cause a dose-related decrease in mean intragastric acidity is illustrated in Table 4.

Table 4: PARIET

Mean AUC Acidity for Three PARIET Doses versus Placebo

Parameter	PARIET (mg q.d.) 10	20	40	Placebo
Mean AUC_{0-24} acidity (mmol·h/L)	156[a]	131[a]	86[a]	678

[a] (p<0.001 versus placebo).

The decrease in gastric acidity and the increase in gastric pH observed with 20 mg PARIET were compared to the same parameters with 20 mg omeprazole and placebo, as illustrated in Table 5.

Table 5: PARIET

Gastric Acid Parameters—PARIET versus Omeprazole and Placebo on Day 1 and Day 8 of Multiple Once-daily Dosing

	PARIET 20 mg q.d.		Omeprazole 20 mg q.d.		Placebo	
Parameter	Day 1	Day 8	Day 1	Day 8	Day 1	Day 8
Mean AUC_{0-24} Acidity	340.8[b,c]	176.9[b,d]	577.1[b]	271.2[b]	925.5	862.4
Median trough pH (23-h)[a]	3.77	3.51	1.43	3.21	1.27	1.38
% Time Gastric pH>3[e]	54.6[b,c]	68.7[b,d]	36.7[b]	59.4[b]	19.1	21.7
% Time Gastric pH>4[e]	44.1[b,c]	60.3[b,d]	24.7[b]	51.4[b]	7.6	11.0

[a] No inferential statistics conducted for this parameter.
[b] (p<0.001) versus placebo.
[c] (p<0.001) versus omeprazole 20 mg q.d.
[d] (p<0.05) versus omeprazole 20 mg q.d.
[e] Gastric pH was measured every hour over a 24-hour period.

Effects on Esophageal Acid Exposure: In patients with gastroesophageal reflux disease (GERD) and moderate to severe esophageal acid exposure, PARIET doses of 20 or 40 mg/day normalized 24-hour esophageal acid exposure. After seven days' treatment, the percentage of time that the esophageal pH <4 was 5.1% at the 20 mg dose and 2.0% at the 40 mg dose, from baselines of 24.7% and 23.7%, respectively. Normalization of 24-hour intraesophageal acid exposure was correlated to gastric pH >4 for at least 35% of the 24-hour period; this level was achieved in 90% of subjects receiving a 20 mg PARIET dose and in 100% of subjects receiving a 40 mg PARIET dose. With PARIET doses of 20 or 40 mg/day, effects on gastric and esophageal pH were significant and substantial after one day of treatment and more pronounced after seven days of treatment.
Effects on Serum Gastrin: In patients given daily doses of PARIET tablets for up to eight weeks to treat ulcerative or erosive esophagitis and in patients treated for up to 52 weeks to prevent recurrence of disease, there was a dose-related increase in the median fasting gastrin level. The group median values stayed within the normal range. These data are indicative of dose-dependent inhibition on gastric acid secretion by PARIET.
Effects on Enterochromaffin-like (ECL) Cells: Increased serum gastrin secondary to antisecretory agents stimulates proliferation of gastric ECL cells which, over time, may result in ECL cell hyperplasia in laboratory rats and mice and gastric carcinoids in laboratory rats. During life-time exposure of rats with doses of rabeprazole up to 120 mg/kg/day [60 times the exposure on a body surface (mg/m^2) basis in patients given the recommended 20 mg/day (12.3 mg/m^2) dose], ECL cell hyperplasia was observed in both male and female rats, while gastric carcinoids were observed in female Sprague Dawley rats only. ECL cell hyperplasia was observed with rabeprazole in both male and female rats and mice.

Human gastric biopsy specimens from the antrum and the fundus from 330 patients receiving rabeprazole treatment for up to 8 weeks detected no consistent pattern of changes in ECL cell histology. Histological findings from 61 patients receiving rabeprazole also showed no consistent pattern of changes in degree of gastritis. No chronic atrophic gastritis was found in these patients either at baseline or endpoint assessment. There was no consistent change in the incidence of intestinal metaplasia or distribution of *H. pylori* infection.

In over 400 patients undergoing PARIET treatment (10 or 20 mg/day) for up to one year, the incidence of ECL cell hyperplasia was low and comparable to that observed with omeprazole (20 mg/day); no patient demonstrated the adenomatoid changes or carcinoid tumour as observed in rats.

Endocrine Effects: Studies in humans for up to one year have revealed no clinically significant effects on the endocrine system. In healthy male volunteers treated with PARIET tablets for 13 days, no clinically relevant changes have been detected in the following endocrine parameters examined: 17 β-estradiol, thyroid-stimulating hormone, tri-iodothyronine, thyroxine, thyroxine-binding protein, parathyroid hormone, insulin, glucagon, renin, aldosterone, follicle-stimulating hormone, luteotrophic hormone, prolactin, somatotrophic hormone, dehydroepiandrosterone, cortisol-binding globulin, urinary 6β-hydroxycortisol, and testosterone.
Other Effects: In humans treated with PARIET for up to one year, no systemic effects have been observed on the central nervous system, lymphoid, hematopoietic, renal, hepatic, cardiovascular, ocular, or respiratory systems.
Microbiology: Rabeprazole sodium, amoxicillin and clarithromycin triple therapy has been shown to be active against most strains of *H. pylori* in vitro and in clinical infections as described in Indications and Clinical Use.
Pharmacokinetics: PARIET tablets are enteric-coated. Absorption is rapid following ingestion. After oral administration of 20 mg rabeprazole sodium, peak plasma concentrations (C_{max}) are reached at an average of 1.6-5.0 hours; bioavailability compared to intravenous administration is 52%. Rabeprazole does not accumulate and its pharmacokinetics are not altered by multiple dosing. The plasma half-life is approximately one hour.
Absorption: Following oral administration, rabeprazole is rapidly absorbed and can be detected in plasma as early as 0.5 hours. The rabeprazole C_{max} and AUC are linear with doses from 10 mg to 40 mg. Taking PARIET tablets with food does not alter C_{max} or AUC relative to the fasting state; the T_{max} is increased by 1.7 hours. Antacids do not significantly affect the absorption of rabeprazole sodium. Administration of rabeprazole sodium with a high fat meal may delay its absorption by approximately 4 hours or longer; however, the C_{max} and the extent of absorption (AUC) are not altered.
Distribution: Rabeprazole is 96.3% bound to human plasma proteins.
Metabolism: In humans the thioether and carboxylic acid are the main plasma metabolites. These metabolites were not observed to have significant antisecretory activity. The sulphone, desmethyl-thioether and mercapturic acid conjugate minor metabolites were observed at lower levels. Only the desmethyl metabolite has a small amount of antisecretory activity, but it is not present in plasma.

In vitro studies have demonstrated that rabeprazole is metabolized primarily by non-enzymatic reduction to form the thioether metabolite. Rabeprazole is also metabolized in the liver by cytochromes P450 3A (CYP3A), to a sulphone metabolite, and cytochrome P450 2C19 (CYP2C19), to desmethyl rabeprazole. CYP2C19 exhibits a known genetic polymorphism due to its deficiency in some sub-populations (e.g. 3 to 5% of Caucasians and 17 to 20% of Asians). Rabeprazole metabolism is slow in these sub-populations; therefore, they are referred to as poor metabolizers of the drug.
Excretion: Following a single 20 mg ^{14}C-labelled oral dose of rabeprazole sodium, no unchanged drug was excreted in the urine. Approximately 90% of the dose was eliminated in urine mainly as two metabolites: a mercapturic acid conjugate and a carboxylic acid; there are also two unknowns. The remainder of the dose was recovered in feces.
Special Populations and Conditions: Pediatrics: The pharmacokinetic profile of PARIET in adolescents and children under the age of 18 years has not been studied.
Geriatrics: In 20 healthy elderly subjects given a 20 mg PARIET dose once daily for seven days, AUC doubled and the C_{max} increased by 60% compared to measurements in a parallel younger control group. There was no evidence of drug accumulation (see Warnings and Precautions).
Race: See Metabolism above.
Hepatic Insufficiency: In two studies in which 23 patients with varying degrees of chronic compensated hepatic cirrhosis were given a 20 mg PARIET dose, the AUC of rabeprazole approximately doubled and the C_{max} increased by 50% compared to measurements in healthy age- and sex-matched subjects.
Renal Insufficiency: In 10 patients with stable end-stage renal failure requiring maintenance hemodialysis (creatinine clearance ≤5 mL/min/1.73 m²), the pharmacokinetics of rabeprazole (PARIET 20 mg oral dose) were comparable to those in 10 healthy volunteers.
Combination Therapy with Antimicrobials: Sixteen healthy volunteers were given 20 mg rabeprazole sodium, 1000 mg amoxicillin, 500 mg clarithromycin, or the combination of all 3 rabeprazole, amoxicillin, and clarithromycin (RAC) in a four-way crossover study. Each of the four treatments was administered for 7 days with single doses administered on days 1 and 7 and twice daily on days 2-6. The AUC and C_{max} for clarithromycin and amoxicillin were similar during combined treatment compared to monotherapy. The rabeprazole AUC and C_{max} increased by 11% and 34%, respectively, and the 14-hydroxyclarithromycin (active metabolite of clarithromycin) AUC and C_{max} increased by 42% and 46%, respectively, during the combined treatment compared to values obtained during monotherapy. This increase in exposure to rabeprazole and 14-hydroxyclarithromycin is not considered to be clinically significant.

In an open-label, randomized, four-period crossover study in 20 healthy Japanese volunteers, 16 extensive metabolizers (EM) and four poor metabolizers (PM) of CYP2C19 genotype were given 20 mg rabeprazole, 400 mg clarithromycin, 750 mg amoxicillin, or the combination of rabeprazole, amoxicillin and clarithromycin. Each of the treatments consisted of a single oral administration under fasting conditions on days 1 and 7, and twice daily administration on days 2 to 6. As illustrated in Table 6, in the EM and PM subjects, an interaction was observed for clarithromycin, 14-hydroxyclarithromycin, and rabeprazole which resulted in a higher C_{max} and AUC_{0-12} during the combination treatment compared to monotherapy. For the amoxicillin treatment, no interaction was observed in the PM subjects, and only a very slight increase in C_{max}, in EM subjects, was observed in the combination treatment when compared to monotherapy.

Table 6: PARIET

Percent (%) Increase in Pharmacokinetic Parameters (C_{max} and AUC_{0-12}) for Extensive Metabolizers (EM) and Poor Metabolizers (PM) During Combination Therapy[a] vs Monotherapy[b]

Pharmacokinetic Parameter		Active Substance: Rabeprazole	Clarithromycin	Clarithromycin M-5 metabolite (14-hydroxy-clarithromycin)	Amoxicillin
% Increase C_{max} (µg/mL)	EM	38%	11%	45%	11%
	PM	22%	24%	67%	no interaction
% Increase AUC_{0-12} (µg·h/mL)	EM	32%	11%	46%	no interaction
	PM	35%	24%	73%	no interaction

[a] Test treatment (combination therapy) consisted of clarithromycin 400 mg + amoxicillin 750 mg + rabeprazole 20 mg.
[b] Reference treatments (monotherapy): A: clarithromycin 400 mg; B: amoxicillin 750 mg; C: rabeprazole 20 mg.
Legend: EM=extensive metabolizer; PM=poor metabolizer.

STORAGE AND STABILITY: Store at room temperature (15 to 25°C) protected from moisture.

INFORMATION FOR THE PATIENT: Published in e-CPS, available by subscription at www.e-cps.ca.

DOSAGE FORMS, COMPOSITION AND PACKAGING: 10 mg: Each pink enteric-coated tablet, printed "ε 241" on one side, contains: rabeprazole sodium 10 mg. Nonmedicinal ingredients: carnauba wax, diacetylated monoglycerides, ethylcellulose, hydroxypropyl cellulose, hydroxypropyl methylcellulose phthalate, iron oxide (black, red, or yellow), low-substituted hydroxypropyl cellulose, magnesium oxide, magnesium stearate, mannitol, talc and titanium dioxide. HDPE bottles of 100.
20 mg: Each light yellow enteric-coated tablet, printed "ε 243" on one side, contains: rabeprazole sodium 20 mg. Nonmedicinal ingredients: carnauba wax, diacetylated monoglycerides, ethylcellulose, glycerine fatty acid ester, hydroxypropyl cellulose, hydroxypropyl methylcellulose phthalate, iron oxide (black, red, or yellow), low-substituted hydroxypropyl cellulose, magnesium oxide, magnesium stearate, mannitol, talc and titanium dioxide. Hospital unit-dose blister packages of 50. HDPE bottles of 100.

(Shown in Product Identification Section)

Can't find information on a particular drug? Consult the CPhA Monograph Index in the front pages of the *CPS*. The CPhA monographs are compiled by the editorial staff of the Canadian Pharmacists Association and reviewed by expert Canadian physicians and pharmacists.

Parnate® Ⓟ

tranylcypromine sulfate

Antidepressant

GlaxoSmithKline

Date of Revision: May 11, 2010

PHARMACOLOGY: PARNATE is a nonhydrazine monoamine oxidase (MAO) inhibitor with a rapid onset of activity. It increases the concentration of epinephrine, norepinephrine and serotonin in storage sites in the nervous system. In theory, the increased concentration of monoamines in the brain stem is the basis for its antidepressant activity.

PARNATE differs from other MAO inhibitors in being a reversible inhibitor. When PARNATE is withdrawn, monoamine oxidase activity is generally restored within a week, although the drug is excreted in 24 hours.

INDICATIONS: PARNATE has been used successfully to treat psychotic depressive states such as: depressive phase of manic-depressive psychosis, involutional melancholia, reactive depression and psychoneurotic depression of moderate to severe intensity.

In the psychiatric treatment of severe endogenous depression, it is impossible to predict, with presently known data, which patients will respond best to PARNATE and which to electroconvulsive therapy (ECT). The drug may be indicated in some reactive depressions in which ECT is not indicated.

PARNATE is not recommended for use in mild depressive states resulting from temporary situational difficulties.
Note: Because PARNATE is a potent agent with the capability of producing serious side effects (e.g., hypertensive crises, sometimes complicated by fatal intracranial bleeding), its use should be reserved for patients who can be closely supervised.

Before prescribing PARNATE, the physician should be thoroughly familiar with information on its dosage, side effects and contraindications, as well as the principles of MAO inhibitor therapy and the side effects of this class of drugs as reported in the literature. The physician should also be familiar with the symptomatology of mental depression and alternative methods of treatment, to aid in the careful selection of patients for PARNATE therapy.
Selecting the Patient:

1. PARNATE should be used for the symptomatic treatment of moderate to severe depression. It is not recommended for those mild depressive reactions where more conservative therapy is indicated.
2. PARNATE should be reserved for those patients who can be followed closely. Blood pressure should be recorded periodically to detect evidence of pressor response to PARNATE therapy.
3. PARNATE should not be used in patients with cerebrovascular or cardiovascular disorders (e.g., arteriosclerosis, hypertension) (see Contraindications).
4. PARNATE should not be used in patients receiving any other antidepressant medication (see Contraindications).
5. PARNATE is not recommended for patients with a history of recurring or frequent headaches, especially the tension and vascular types.
6. PARNATE should not be used alone in patients with marked psychomotor agitation, since it is recognized that antidepressant drugs can aggravate some coexisting symptoms such as agitation or anxiety.

PARNATE combined with trifluoperazine: PARNATE has been combined with trifluoperazine in the treatment of coexisting anxiety and depression. Such combined therapy has been found particularly valuable when used to treat depressed patients in whom a persistent disorder of mood is associated with anxiety, moderate agitation, inappropriate mental symptoms (such as unnatural fears or suspicions and phobias) or improper response to single-agent therapy.

Combined PARNATE-trifluoperazine therapy has been used successfully in the treatment of psychiatric conditions such as psychoneurotic depression, agitated depression, schizo-affective disorders and pseudoneurotic schizophrenia. If the patient appears to have a pure depression, PARNATE should be used alone and, similarly, if the symptoms appear to indicate a pure anxiety state, trifluoperazine should be used first. The combined therapy has frequently displayed striking effectiveness in patients who obtained little benefit from treatment with a succession of single drugs.

For comprehensive prescribing information on trifluoperazine, refer to Prescribing Information on that product.

CONTRAINDICATIONS: In patients with a previous history of hypersensitivity to PARNATE or excipients.

In patients with cerebrovascular or cardiovascular disorders or a history of recurrent or frequent headaches. PARNATE should not be administered to patients with confirmed or suspected cerebrovascular defect, hypertension or cardiovascular disease. The drug should be used with caution in individuals beyond the age of 60, because of the possibility of existing cerebral sclerosis with damaged vessels.

In patients with liver damage or blood dyscrasias. Extensive clinical use and laboratory tests have revealed no evidence of liver toxicity or blood dyscrasias due to PARNATE therapy. Because rare cases of hepatitis have been reported, it is recommended that patients with known liver damage or blood dyscrasias should not be treated with PARNATE.

In pheochromocytoma. PARNATE should not be used in the presence of known or suspected pheochromocytoma, as such tumours secrete pressor substances.

In combination with certain drugs. Because the effect of many antidepressant drugs may persist for 10 to 20 days, do not commence PARNATE therapy within less than a week of discontinuing treatment with such drugs; then, use half the normal dosage for the first week. Similarly, allow 1 week to elapse between the discontinuance of PARNATE and the administration of any other drug that is contraindicated with PARNATE such as:

1. **Other monoamine oxidase inhibitors (MAOIs)** such as isocarboxazid and phenelzine sulfate.
2. **Dibenzazepine derivatives** such as amitriptyline, nortriptyline, protriptyline, desipramine, imipramine, doxepin, perphenazine, carbamazepine, cyclobenzaprine, amoxapine, maprotiline and trimipramine, as combination with these drugs may induce hypertensive crises or severe convulsive seizures.
3. **Sympathomimetics** including amphetamines, ephedrine, methyldopa, dopamine, and levodopa; as well as tryptophan. These may result in potentiation, precipitating hypertension, severe headache, and hyperpyrexia. Cerebral (subarachnoid) hemorrhage may also occur. These compounds may be found in many herbal preparations, as well as over-the-counter drugs, such as cold, hay fever, energy-enhancing and weight-reducing preparations. The combination of MAOIs and tryptophan has been reported to cause behaviour and neurologic syndromes including disorientation, confusion, amnesia, delirium, agitation, hypomanic signs, ataxia, myoclonus, hyperreflexia, shivering, ocular oscillations and Babinski signs.
4. **SSRIs or SNRIs (e.g. venlafaxine):** There have been reports of serious, sometimes fatal reactions when MAOIs are given before, with, or shortly after discontinuation with some SSRIs or SNRIs. It is recommended that MAOIs are not used in combination with SSRIs or SNRIs. If SSRIs or SNRIs are used consecutively, a suitable washout period should be observed. The following is a guide, but prescribing information for individual products should be consulted:
   - MAOI followed by SSRI or SNRI (eg. venlafaxine)—2 weeks
   - Fluoxetine followed by MAOI—5 weeks
   - Other SSRI followed by MAOI—2 weeks
   - SNRI (eg. venlafaxine) followed by MAOI—1 week
5. **Other drugs:** dextromethorphan, buspirone HCl.

In combination with foods with a high tyramine content: Tyramine is normally metabolized by monoamine oxidase in the intestinal and hepatic cells. When monoamine oxidase is inhibited, tyramine absorbed from the gastrointestinal tract passes freely into the circulation. It releases norepinephrine from adrenergic neurones, causing exaggerated hypertensive and other effects.

When excessive amounts of tyramine are consumed in conjunction with PARNATE, or within 2 weeks of stopping treatment, a serious and sometimes fatal hypertensive reaction may occur.

Tyramine occurs naturally in some foods or may occur from the bacterial breakdown of protein in foods which are fermented, aged or spoiled.

Foods that have reliably been shown to contain a high tyramine content and may also have been reported to induce a serious hypertensive reaction when consumed with PARNATE are contraindicated.
Foods that are contraindicated in combination with PARNATE:

- All matured or aged cheeses (exceptions: fresh cottage cheese, cream cheese, ricotta and processed cheese). All non-cheese dairy products can be consumed providing they are fresh.
- All aged, cured or fermented meat, fish or poultry (note: meat, fish or poultry that has not undergone aging, curing or fermenting and that is bought fresh, stored correctly and eaten fresh is not contraindicated).
- All fermented soybean products (e.g. soy sauce, miso, fermented tofu).
- Sauerkraut.
- Fava or broad bean pods.
- Banana peel (but not the pulp).

- Concentrated yeast extracts (e.g. Marmite spread).
- All tap/draught beers (Note: some bottled beers, including non-alcoholic beer, may also pose a risk).

Patients should be advised to minimize or avoid use of all alcoholic beverages while taking PARNATE.

Patients should be advised to adhere to the following dietary guidance about eating fresh foods:

Foods may be deliberately aged as part of their processing and these are contraindicated (see list above). Foods may also naturally age over time, even if they are refrigerated. It is therefore extremely important that patients are instructed to buy and eat only fresh foods or those which have been properly frozen. They should avoid eating foods if they are unsure of their storage conditions or freshness and they should be cautious of foods of unknown age or composition even if refrigerated.

The longer food is left to deteriorate and the larger the quantity of food eaten, the greater the potential quantity of tyramine ingested. Where there is any doubt, patients should be advised to either avoid the food or consume in strict moderation if it is not otherwise contraindicated.

Patients should also be warned that tyramine levels may vary by brand or even batch and a person may absorb different amounts of tyramine from a particular food at different times. Therefore, if they have accidentally consumed a prohibited food on one occasion and not had a reaction, this does not mean that they will not have a serious hypertensive reaction if they consume the same food on a different occasion.

WARNINGS: Hypertensive Crisis: The most important adverse reaction associated with PARNATE is hypertensive crisis, which has sometimes been fatal. This response is not usually dose-related. It is associated with a distinctive reaction characterized by some or all of the following symptoms: occipital headache which may radiate frontally, palpitation, neck stiffness or soreness, nausea or vomiting, sweating (sometimes with fever and sometimes with cold, clammy skin) with early pallor followed later by flushing, and photophobia. Either tachycardia or bradycardia may be present, sometimes associated with constricting chest pain. Mydriasis may occur.

The occipital headache, together with pain and stiffness in the cervical muscles, may mimic subarachnoid hemorrhage, but can equally be associated with actual intracranial bleeding, as in other conditions where a sudden rise in blood pressure occurs. Cases of such bleeding have been reported, some of which have been fatal.

Blood pressure should be followed closely in patients taking PARNATE to detect evidence of any pressor response. It is emphasized that full reliance should not be placed on blood pressure readings, but that the patient should also be observed frequently.

Therapy should be discontinued immediately upon the occurrence of palpitation or frequent headache during PARNATE therapy. These signs may be prodromal of a hypertensive reaction. Patients should be instructed to report promptly the occurrence of headache or other symptoms.

If a hypertensive reaction occurs, PARNATE should be discontinued and therapy to lower blood pressure should be given immediate consideration. Headache tends to abate as blood pressure decreases. On the basis of present evidence, phentolamine is recommended for use in acute cases (the dosage reported for phentolamine is 5 mg i.v. administered slowly). Do not use parenteral reserpine or rauwolfia alkaloids for the treatment of a hypertensive crisis, as they may, by releasing catecholamines, exacerbate the condition. Care should be taken to administer these drugs in such a way as to avoid producing an excessive hypotensive effect. Fever should be managed by means of external cooling. Other symptomatic and supportive measures may be desirable in particular cases. Acute distress generally subsides in 24 hours or less. For milder reactions, the more moderate adrenolytic action of injectable chlorpromazine may be more appropriate.

Hypotension: which may be postural, has been observed during PARNATE therapy, particularly at doses above 30 mg daily. It is seen most commonly (but not exclusively) in patients with pre-existing hypertension. In most instances, it affects the systolic readings. Rare instances of syncope have been seen. Dosage increases should be made more gradually in patients showing a tendency toward hypotension at the starting dose. Postural hypotension can usually be relieved by having the patient lie down until blood pressure returns to normal. This side effect is usually temporary, but if it persists, PARNATE should be discontinued. Blood pressure usually returns rapidly to pretreatment levels upon discontinuation of PARNATE.

Also, when PARNATE is combined with those phenothiazine derivatives or other compounds known to cause hypotension, the possibility of additive hypotensive effects should be considered.

Potential Association with the Occurrence of Behavioral and Emotional Changes, Including Self-Harm: It is unknown whether increased risk of suicidal ideation and behavior is associated with the use of PARNATE in pediatric patients and/ or adults.

However, recent analyses of placebo-controlled clinical trial safety databases from SSRIs and other newer antidepressants suggest that use of these drugs in patients under the age of 18 may be associated with behavioral and emotional changes, including an increased risk of suicidal ideation and behavior over that of placebo. Thus, rigorous clinical monitoring for suicidal ideation or other indicators of potential for suicidal behavior is advised in **patients of all ages** given any antidepressant drug. This includes monitoring for emotional and behavioral changes.

Clinical worsening and suicide risk in adults with psychiatric disorders: Patients with depression may experience worsening of their depressive symptoms and/or the emergence of suicidal ideation and behaviours (suicidality) whether or not they are taking antidepressant medications. This risk persists until significant remission occurs. As improvement may not occur during the first few weeks or more of treatment, patients should be closely monitored for clinical worsening (including development of new symptoms) and suicidality, especially at the beginning of a course of treatment, or at the time of dose changes, either increases or decreases. It is general clinical experience with all antidepressant therapies that the risk of suicide may increase in the early stages of recovery.

Patients with a history of suicidal behaviour or thoughts, and those patients exhibiting a significant degree of suicidal ideation prior to commencement of treatment, are at a greater risk of suicidal thoughts or suicide attempts, and should receive careful monitoring during treatment.

Patients (and caregivers of patients) should be alerted about the need to monitor for any worsening of their condition (including development of new symptoms) and/or the emergence of suicidal ideation/behaviour or thoughts of harming themselves and to seek medical advice immediately if these symptoms present. It should be recognised that the onset of some neuropsychiatric symptoms could be related either to the underlying disease state or the drug therapy (see Mania and bipolar disorder below).

Consideration should be given to changing the therapeutic regimen, including possibly discontinuing the medication, in patients who experience clinical worsening (including development of new symptoms) and/or the emergence of suicidal ideation/behaviour, especially if these symptoms are severe, abrupt in onset, or were not part of the patient's presenting symptoms.

Mania and Bipolar Disorder: A major depressive episode may be the initial presentation of bipolar disorder. It is generally believed (though not established in controlled trials) that treating such an episode with an antidepressant alone can increase the likelihood of precipitation of a mixed/manic episode in patients at risk for bipolar disorder. Prior to initiating treatment with an antidepressant, patients should be adequately screened to determine if they are at risk for bipolar disorder; such screening should include a detailed psychiatric history, including a family history of suicide, bipolar disorder, and depression. As with all antidepressants, PARNATE should be used with caution in patients with a history of mania.

PRECAUTIONS: Drug Interactions: (see also Contraindications): In general, the physician should bear in mind the possibility of a lowered margin of safety when PARNATE is administered in combination with potent drugs and should adjust dosage carefully.

A marked potentiating effect has been reported on some CNS depressants such as morphine, meperidine, barbiturates and alcohol. For this reason, narcotics and barbiturates should be used conservatively with PARNATE, and patients should be warned that the drug may potentiate the effects of alcoholic beverages.

Caution should be exercised when giving PARNATE with hypotensive agents: guanethidine, as its action may be antagonized; reserpine, as hyperactivity may occur; alpha-methyldopa, since the combination may give rise to central excitation.

When PARNATE is combined with those phenothiazine derivatives or other compounds known to affect blood pressure, patients should be observed more closely because of the possibility of additive hypotensive effects.

Caution should also be exercised when giving PARNATE with antiparkinson agents, as the combination may result in potentiation, with profuse sweating, tremulousness and a rise in body temperature.

Drugs which lower the seizure threshold, including MAO inhibitors, should not be used with metrizamide. As with other MAOIs, PARNATE should be discontinued at least 48 hours before myelography and should not be resumed for at least 24 hours after the procedure.

Caution should be exercised when giving PARNATE with clomipramine hydrochloride, as this drug, in combination with a MAOI, has been reported to result in hyperpyrexia, diffuse intravascular coagulation, and status epilepticus; and pethidine, as this drug in combination with a MAOI may lead to an increase of serotonin associated effects which could cause serotonin toxicity.

PARNATE should be administered with caution to patients receiving disulfiram. In a single study, rats given high intraperitoneal doses of d- or l-isomers of PARNATE sulfate plus disulfiram experienced severe toxicity including convulsions and death. Additional studies in rats given high oral doses of racemic PARNATE sulfate and disulfiram produced no adverse interaction.

PARNATE may affect ability to drive or operate machinery.

In Angina: MAOIs may have the capacity to suppress anginal pain that would otherwise serve as a warning of myocardial ischemia.

In Depression: PARNATE may aggravate coexisting symptoms in depression, such as anxiety and agitation. In depressed patients, the possibility of suicide should always be considered and adequate precautions taken. Exclusive reliance on drug therapy to prevent suicidal attempts is unwarranted, as there may be a delay in the onset of therapeutic effect or an increase in anxiety and agitation. Also, some patients fail to respond to drug therapy or may respond only temporarily.

In Epilepsy: Because the influence of PARNATE on the convulsive threshold is variable in animal experiments, suitable precautions should be taken if epileptic patients are treated.

In Hyperthyroidism: Use PARNATE with caution in hyperthyroid patients because of their increased sensitivity to pressor amines.

In Renal Dysfunction: The usual precautions should be observed in patients with impaired renal function, since there is a possibility of cumulative effects in such patients.

Pregnancy and Lactation: PARNATE has been shown to pass through the placental barrier to the fetus of the rat and into the milk of the lactating dog. Nevertheless, as with any potent drug, the physician must assess the definite medical need when prescribing for the pregnant patient. Adequate human data on use during pregnancy or lactation and adequate animal reproduction studies are not available.

In Surgery: It is suggested that PARNATE be discontinued at least 7 days before elective surgery, to allow time for recovery of monoamine oxidase activity before anesthetic agents are given.

Drug Dependency: There have been reports of drug dependency in patients using doses of PARNATE significantly in excess of the therapeutic range. Some of these patients had a history of previous substance abuse.

ADVERSE EFFECTS: The most frequently seen side effect is insomnia, which can usually be overcome by giving the last dose of the day not later than 3 p.m., by reducing the dose, or by prescribing a mild hypnotic.

Some of the following unwanted reactions have been reported in the literature; others are possible. They are classified according to their seriousness and probable cause—an arrangement intended to help the physician view them in proper perspective.

Pharmacologic Reactions of a Serious Nature:

A. Hypertensive Crisis: see Warnings.
B. Hypotension: see Warnings.
C. Overstimulation: Overstimulation, which may include increased anxiety, agitation and manic symptoms, is usually evidence of excessive therapeutic action. Dosage should be reduced, or a phenothiazine tranquilizer should be administered concomitantly.

Hematologic or Allergic Reactions: Blood dyscrasias, including anemia, leukopenia, agranulocytosis and thrombocytopenia have been reported. Rare instances of hepatitis (e.g., one case of mild jaundice, not of the serious type associated with hydrazine MAOIs) and skin rash have been reported.

Pharmacologic Reactions of a Less Serious Nature: Patients may experience restlessness, insomnia, drowsiness, dizziness, weakness, dry mouth, nausea, abdominal pain, anorexia, diarrhea or constipation. Tachycardia, palpitation, blurred vision, headache without blood pressure elevation, chills, sweating, urinary retention, edema and impotence have each been reported in at least 1 patient.

Other Reactions: Micturition difficulty has been reported. Tinnitus, muscle spasm and tremors, paresthesia and habituation have been reported so rarely that the role of PARNATE cannot be established. Alopecia has been reported very rarely.

Drug Dependency: There have been reports of drug dependency in patients using PARNATE tablets (see Precautions). Symptoms reported after stopping PARNATE include: sleep disturbances, depression, confusion, delirium, tremor, agitation, convulsion, anxiety, hallucinations, fatigue, headache.

OVERDOSE:

Symptoms: The characteristic symptoms that may arise as a result of PARNATE overdosage are usually those which have already been described under and Adverse Effects. However, an intensification of these symptoms and sometimes severe additional manifestations may be seen, depending on the degree of overdosage and on individual susceptibility.

Some patients exhibit insomnia, restlessness and anxiety, progressing in severe cases to agitation, mental confusion and incoherence. Hypotension, dizziness, weakness and drowsiness may occur, progressing in severe cases to extreme dizziness and shock. A few patients have displayed hypertension with severe headache and other symptoms. Rare instances have been reported in which hypertension was accompanied by twitching or myoclonic fibrillation of skeletal muscles with hyperpyrexia, sometimes progressing to generalized rigidity and coma.

Treatment: Treatment normally consists of general supportive measures, close observation of vital signs and steps to counteract specific symptoms as they occur. The management of hypertensive reactions is described under Warnings. Further management should be as clinically indicated or as recommended by the national poisons centre, where available.

External cooling is recommended if hyperpyrexia occurs. Barbiturates have been reported to help myoclonic reactions, but frequency of administration should be controlled carefully because PARNATE may prolong barbiturate activity.

When hypotension requires treatment, the standard measures for managing circulatory shock should be initiated. If pressor agents are required, norepinephrine is the most suitable. The rate of infusion should be regulated by careful observation of the patient. MAOIs may sometimes increase the pressor response, as has been demonstrated with norepinephrine. Mephentermine may be required if marked refractory hypotension occurs.

Although PARNATE is rapidly excreted, its MAO inhibiting action may persist for approximately 1 week.

> For management of a suspected drug overdose, contact your regional Poison Control Centre. See the *CPS* Directory section for a list of Poison Control Centres.

DOSAGE: Dosage should be adjusted to the requirements of the individual patient. If the patient responds to therapy, the response is usually seen within 48 hours to 3 weeks after starting medication.

- Recommended starting dosage is 20 mg/day (10 mg in the morning and 10 mg in the afternoon).
- Continue this dosage for 2 to 3 weeks.
- If no signs of a response appear, increase dosage to 30 mg daily (20 mg upon arising and 10 mg in the afternoon).
- Continue this dosage for at least 1 week. If no improvement occurs, continued administration is unlikely to be beneficial. Although dosages above 30 mg/day have been used, it should be borne in mind that the incidence and severity of side effects may increase as dosage is raised. Dosage increases should be made in increments of 10 mg/day, and ordinarily at intervals of 1 to 3 weeks.
- When a satisfactory response is obtained, dosage may be reduced to a maintenance level.
- Some patients will be maintained on 20 mg/day; many will need only 10 mg daily.
- Reduction from peak to maintenance dosage may be desirable before withdrawal. If withdrawn prematurely, original symptoms will recur. No tendency to produce rebound depressions of greater intensity has been seen, although this is a theoretical possibility in patients treated at high doses. Experimental work indicates that PARNATE is rapidly excreted. Inhibition of MAO activity may, however, persist for up to 1 week.
- Combined PARNATE-trifluoperazine therapy: For those physicians wishing to combine PARNATE with trifluoperazine, the usual dosage is PARNATE 10 mg plus trifluoperazine 1 mg or 2 mg twice daily (morning and afternoon) depending on the individual patient requirements. After a satisfactory response is secured, medication can often be reduced to one dose daily, usually administered in the morning. Patients displaying marked mental disturbance, especially psychotic manifestations or severe agitation, will usually require larger initial doses of trifluoperazine.
- Children and adolescents (less than 18 years of age): PARNATE is not indicated for use in children or adolescents aged less than 18 years (see Warnings and Precautions).

Note: When ECT is being administered concurrently with PARNATE, 10 mg b.i.d. can usually be given during the series, then reduced to 10 mg daily for maintenance therapy.

INFORMATION FOR THE PATIENT: Published in e-CPS, available by subscription at www.e-cps.ca.

SUPPLIED: Each biconvex, rose-red, film-coated tablet, with PARNATE and SB monogram printed in black on one side, contains: PARNATE 10 mg. Nonmedicinal ingredients: carnauba wax, citric acid, croscarmellose sodium, D&C Red No. 7, edible black printing ink, FD&C Blue No. 2, FD&C Yellow No. 6, gelatin, hydroxypropylmethyl cellulose, lactose, magnesium stearate, microcrystalline cellulose, talc, propylene glycol 400, purified water and titanium dioxide. Bottles of 100. Store at 15-30°C.

(Shown in Product Identification Section)

Paroxetine ℞

CPhA Monograph

see *Selective Serotonin Reuptake Inhibitors*

Patanol® ℞

olopatadine HCl

Antiallergic

Alcon

Date of Preparation: September 9, 1997
Date of Revision: November 28, 2006

SUMMARY PRODUCT INFORMATION:

Route of Administration	Dosage Form/ Strength	Clinically Relevant Nonmedicinal Ingredients
Topical ophthalmic	Solution 0.1% (w/v)	Preservative: benzalkonium chloride Inactive ingredients: purified water, sodium chloride, dibasic sodium phosphate, hydrochloric acid and/or sodium hydroxide (to adjust pH)

INDICATIONS AND CLINICAL USE: PATANOL (olopatadine hydrochloride) ophthalmic solution is indicated for the treatment of allergic conjunctivitis.
Geriatrics: No overall difference in safety has been observed between elderly and younger patients.
Pediatrics (3-16 years of age): PATANOL solution administered three times a day for six weeks was shown to be safe and well-tolerated in subjects who were ages 3 years and older.
CONTRAINDICATIONS: Patients who are hypersensitive to this drug or to any ingredient in the formulation or component of the container. For a complete listing, see Dosage Forms, Composition and Packaging.
WARNINGS AND PRECAUTIONS: General: For topical use only. Not for injection. Patients should be instructed not to instill PATANOL (olopatadine hydrochloride) ophthalmic solution while wearing contact lenses, but to wait for 10 minutes after instillation before inserting contact lenses.

To prevent contaminating the dropper tip and solution, care should be taken not to touch the eyelids or surrounding areas with the dropper tip of the bottle. Keep bottle tightly closed when not in use.

Sexual Function/Reproduction: Fertility: Olopatadine administered to male and female rats at oral doses of 62 500 times the maximum recommended ocular human use level resulted in a slight decrease in the fertility index and reduced implantation rate; no effects on reproductive function were observed at doses of 7800 times the maximum recommended ocular human use level.
Special Populations: Pregnant Women: Olopatadine was found not to be teratogenic in rats and rabbits at oral doses >90 000 and >60 000 times the maximum recommended ocular human use level, respectively. There are, however, no adequate and well controlled studies in pregnant women. Because animal studies are not always predictive of human responses, this drug should be used in pregnant women only if the potential benefit to the mother justifies the potential risk to the embryo or fetus.
Nursing Women: Olopatadine has been identified in the milk of nursing rats following oral administration. Rat pups of mothers administered olopatadine orally at greater than 625 times (but not at 312 times) the maximum recommended ocular human use level demonstrated reduced body weight gain during the nursing period. It is not known whether topical ocular administration could result in sufficient systemic absorption to produce detectable quantities in human breast milk. Nevertheless, caution should be exercised when PATANOL solution is administered to a nursing mother.
Pediatrics (3-16 years of age): Safety and effectiveness in pediatric patients between the ages of 3 and 16 have been established.
Geriatrics: No overall difference in safety has been observed between elderly and younger patients.
ADVERSE REACTIONS: Adverse Drug Reaction Overview: In clinical studies of PATANOL (olopatadine hydrochloride) ophthalmic solution, ocular and nonocular adverse reactions related to therapy were reported at an incidence below 1%.
Clinical Trial Adverse Drug Reactions: Because clinical trials are conducted under very specific conditions the adverse reaction rates observed in the clinical trials may not reflect the rates observed in practice and should not be compared to the rates in the clinical trials of another drug. Adverse drug reaction information from clinical trials is useful for identifying drug-related adverse events and for approximating rates.
Less Common Clinical Trial Adverse Drug Reactions: Ocular: mild transient burning or stinging, pruritus, hyperemia, foreign body sensation, superficial keratitis, lid edema, dry eye, lid dryness, lid spasm, photophobia.
Nonocular: asthenia, headache, taste perversion.
Abnormal Hematologic and Clinical Chemistry Findings: No hematologic or clinical chemistry findings have been observed.
Post-Market Adverse Drug Reactions: Approximately 30.5 million units of PATANOL solution have been sold in 69 countries. The reporting rate of all reaction terms reported between 01 January 1997 and 31 December 2004 was 0.004%, and no single reaction term occurred with a reporting rate greater than 0.0007%.

There were no new major findings bearing on the established overall safety profile of PATANOL solution.

DRUG INTERACTIONS: Overview: No clinical interaction studies have been conducted with PATANOL (olopatadine hydrochloride) ophthalmic solution. In vitro studies have shown that olopatadine does not inhibit metabolic reactions which involve cytochrome P-450 isoenzymes 1A2, 2C8, 2C9, 2C19, 2D6, 2E1 and 3A4. Olopatadine is moderately bound to plasma proteins (approximately 55%). These results indicate that olopatadine is unlikely to result in interactions with other concomitantly administered medications. Due to the low systemic exposure following topical ocular dosing, it is unlikely that PATANOL solution would interfere with immediate hypersensitivity skin testing.
Drug-Drug Interactions: Interactions with other drugs have not been established.
Drug-Food Interactions: Interactions with food have not been established.
Drug-Herb Interactions: Interactions with herbal products have not been established.
Drug-Laboratory Test Interactions: Interactions with laboratory tests have not been established.

DOSAGE AND ADMINISTRATION: Recommended Dose and Dosage Adjustment:
The recommended dose is one to two drops in each affected eye twice daily. No dosage adjustment is required in hepatic or renal impairment.
Missed Dose: If a dose is missed, a single drop should be taken as soon as possible before reverting to regular routine. Do not use a double dose to make up for the one missed.

OVERDOSAGE:
A topical overdosage may be flushed from the eye(s) with warm tap water.

> For management of a suspected drug overdose, CPhA recommends that you contact your **regional Poison Control Centre**. See the *CPS* Directory section for a list of Poison Control Centres.

ACTION AND CLINICAL PHARMACOLOGY: Mechanism of Action: Olopatadine, a structural analog of doxepin, is a non-steroidal, non-sedating, topically effective anti-allergic molecule that exerts its effects through multiple distinct mechanisms of action. Olopatadine is a mast cell stabilizer and a potent, selective histamine H_1 antagonist that inhibits the in vivo type 1 immediate hypersensitivity reaction. Olopatadine inhibits the release of mast cell inflammatory mediators [i.e., histamine, tryptase, prostaglandin D2 and TNFα] as demonstrated in in vitro studies and confirmed in patients. Olopatadine is also an inhibitor of pro-inflammatory cytokine secretion from human conjunctival epithelial cells.
Pharmacodynamics: Effects on Cardiac Repolarization (QTc): In two placebo-controlled, two-way crossover cardiac repolarization studies, no signal of QT interval prolongation was observed relative to placebo following twice daily 5 mg oral doses for 2.5 days in 102 healthy volunteers, or following twice daily 20 mg oral doses for 13.5 days in 32 healthy volunteers. In addition, no evidence of QT interval prolongation was observed, relative to placebo, in 429 perennial allergic rhinitis patients given PATANOL (olopatadine hydrochloride) Nasal Spray, 665 µg twice daily for up to 1 year.
Pharmacokinetics: Following topical ocular administration in man, olopatadine was shown to have low systemic exposure. Two studies in normal volunteers (totalling 24 subjects) dosed bilaterally with Olopatadine 0.15% ophthalmic solution once every 12 hours for 2 weeks demonstrated plasma concentrations to be generally below the quantitation limit of the assay (<0.5 ng/mL). The half-life in plasma was 7-14 hours, and elimination was predominantly through renal excretion. Approximately 60-70% of the dose was recovered in the urine as parent drug.
Special Populations and Conditions: Pediatrics: PATANOL (olopatadine hydrochloride) ophthalmic solution administered three times a day for six weeks was shown to be safe and well tolerated in subjects who were 3 years and older.
Geriatrics: No overall differences in safety and effectiveness have been observed between elderly and younger patients.
Gender: No specific pharmacokinetic study examining the effect of gender was conducted.
Race: No specific pharmacokinetic study examining the effect of race was conducted.
Hepatic Insufficiency: No specific pharmacokinetic study examining the effect of hepatic impairment was conducted. Since metabolism of olopatadine is a minor route of elimination, no adjustment of the dosing regimen of Olopatadine Hydrochloride Ophthalmic Solution, 0.1% is warranted in patients with hepatic impairment.
Renal Insufficiency: The mean plasma C_{max} values for olopatadine following single intranasal doses of olopatadine HCl nasal spray 0.6% (665 µg/spray) were not markedly different between healthy subjects (18.1 ng/mL) and patients with mild, moderate and severe renal impairment (range 15.5 to 21.6 ng/mL). Plasma AUC was 2.5-fold higher in patients with severe impairment (creatinine clearance <30 mL/min/1.73m^2). Predicted peak steady-state plasma concentrations of olopatadine in patients with renal impairment following administration of Olopatadine Hydrochloride Ophthalmic Solution, 0.1% are at least 10-fold lower than those observed following administration of olopatadine nasal spray 0.6%, and approximately 300-fold lower than those observed following the safe and well-tolerated administration of 20 mg oral doses for 13.5 days. These findings indicate that no adjustment of the dosing regimen of Olopatadine Hydrochloride Ophthalmic Solution, 0.1% is warranted in patients with renal impairment.
STORAGE AND STABILITY: Store at 4-30°C. Discard the container at the end of treatment.
SPECIAL HANDLING INSTRUCTIONS: None.
INFORMATION FOR THE PATIENT: Published in e-CPS, available by subscription at www.e-cps.ca.
DOSAGE FORMS, COMPOSITION AND PACKAGING: Each mL of ophthalmic solution contains: olopatadine HCl 1.11 mg equivalent to olopatadine 1 mg. Nonmedicinal ingredients: benzalkonium chloride (as preservative), dibasic sodium phosphate, hydrochloric acid/sodium hydroxide (to adjust pH), purified water and sodium chloride. Plastic Drop-Tainer dispensers of 5 mL.

> The reader is invited to consult CPhA's monograph **Selective Serotonin Reuptake Inhibitors**.

Paxil® ℞

paroxetine HCl

Antidepressant—Antiobsessional—Antipanic—Anxiolytic—Social Phobia (Social Anxiety Disorder)—Post-traumatic Stress Disorder Therapy

GlaxoSmithKline

Date of Revision: May 28, 2010

SUMMARY PRODUCT INFORMATION:

Route of Administration	Dosage Form/Strength	Nonmedicinal Ingredients
Oral	Tablet 10 mg, 20 mg, 30 mg	Dibasic calcium phosphate dihydrate USP, hydroxypropyl methylcellulose, hypromellose, magnesium stearate NF, polyethelene glycols, polysorbate 80, sodium starch glycolate NF, titanium dioxide, and one or more of the following: D&C Red No. 30 aluminum lake, D&C Yellow No. 10 aluminum lake, FD&C Blue No. 2 aluminum lake, FD&C Yellow No. 6 aluminum lake.

INDICATIONS AND CLINICAL USE: Adults: Depression: PAXIL (paroxetine hydrochloride) is indicated for symptomatic relief of Major Depressive Disorder (MDD).

Clinical trials have provided evidence that continuation treatment with PAXIL in patients with moderate to moderately severe depressive disorder is effective for at least 6 months.

Obsessive-Compulsive Disorder: PAXIL is indicated for the symptomatic treatment of obsessive-compulsive disorder (OCD). The obsessions or compulsions must be experienced as intrusive, markedly distressing, time-consuming, or interfering significantly with the person's social or occupational functioning.
Panic Disorder: PAXIL is indicated for the symptomatic treatment of panic disorder, with or without agoraphobia.

Panic disorder (DSM-IV) is characterized by recurrent unexpected panic attacks, i.e., a discrete period of intense fear or discomfort in which four (or more) of the following symptoms develop abruptly and reach a peak within 10 minutes: (1) palpitations, pounding heart, or accelerated heart rate; (2) sweating; (3) trembling or shaking; (4) sensations of shortness of breath or smothering; (5) feeling of choking; (6) chest pain or discomfort; (7) nausea or abdominal distress; (8) feeling dizzy, unsteady, lightheaded, or faint; (9) derealization (feelings of unreality) or depersonalization (being detached from oneself); (10) fear of losing control; (11) fear of dying; (12) paresthesias (numbness or tingling sensations); (13) chills or hot flushes.

Social Phobia (Social Anxiety Disorder): PAXIL is indicated for the symptomatic relief of generalized social phobia (social anxiety disorder), a disorder characterized by marked and persistent fear, anxious anticipation, or avoidance of multiple social situations (e.g. interacting with strangers, attending social gatherings, dealing with authority figures) and/or performance situations (e.g. eating, writing, working while being observed, or public speaking). A diagnosis of social phobia/social anxiety disorder should not be made unless the fear, anxious anticipation, or avoidance of social and/or performance situations interferes significantly with the person's normal routine, occupational functioning, or social life, or causes marked distress.
Generalized Anxiety Disorder: PAXIL is indicated for the symptomatic relief of anxiety causing significant distress in patients with Generalized Anxiety Disorder (GAD).
Post-Traumatic Stress Disorder: PAXIL is indicated for the symptomatic treatment of post-traumatic stress disorder (PTSD).

PTSD as defined by DSM-IV requires exposure to a traumatic event that involved actual or threatened death or serious injury, or threat to the physical integrity of self or others, and a response which involves intense fear, helplessness, or horror. Symptoms that occur as a result of exposure to the traumatic event include reexperiencing of the event in the form of intrusive thoughts, flashbacks or dreams, and intense psychological distress and physiological reactivity on exposure to clues to the event; avoidance of situations reminiscent of the traumatic event, inability to recall details of the event, and/or numbing of general responsiveness manifested as diminished interest in significant activities, estrangement from others, restricted range of affect, or sense of foreshortened future; and symptoms of autonomic arousal including hypervigilance, exaggerated startle response, sleep disturbance, impaired concentration, and irritability or outbursts of anger.

A diagnosis of PTSD requires that the symptoms are present for at least one month and that they cause clinically significant distress or impairment in social, occupational, or other important areas of functioning.

Long-Term Use of PAXIL: The effectiveness of PAXIL in long-term use (i.e. more than 8 weeks for GAD and 12 weeks for other indications) has not yet been established in controlled trials for OCD, panic disorder, social phobia (social anxiety disorder), generalized anxiety disorder and post-traumatic stress disorder. Therefore, the physician who elects to use PAXIL for extended periods in these indications should periodically re-evaluate the long-term usefulness of the drug for individual patients (see Dosage and Administration, Dosing Considerations).

Geriatrics (>65 years of age): Evidence from clinical studies indicates that there are differences in the pharmacokinetic profile of paroxetine in the geriatric population relative to younger adults, which may be associated with differences in safety or effectiveness. A brief discussion can be found in the appropriate sections (see Warnings and Precautions, Special Populations, Geriatrics (≥65 years of age); Action and Clinical Pharmacology and Dosage and Administration).

Pediatrics (<18 years of age): PAXIL is not indicated for use in patients below the age of 18 years (see Warnings and Precautions, General, Potential Association with Behavioural and Emotional Changes, Including Self-Harm).

CONTRAINDICATIONS: Hypersensitivity: PAXIL is contraindicated in patients who are known to be hypersensitive to the drug or any of its components. For a complete listing, see Dosage Forms, Composition and Packaging.

Monoamine Oxidase Inhibitors: In patients receiving serotonin reuptake inhibitors (SSRIs) in combination with a MAO inhibitor, there have been reports of serious, sometimes fatal, reactions including hyperthermia, rigidity, myoclonus, autonomic instability with possible rapid fluctuations of vital signs, and mental status changes that include extreme agitation progressing to delirium and coma. These reactions have also been reported in patients who have recently discontinued SSRI treatment and have begun treatment on a MAO inhibitor. Some cases presented with features resembling serotonin syndrome or neuroleptic malignant syndrome (see Warnings and Precautions, Serotonin Syndrome/Neuroleptic Malignant Syndrome). Therefore, PAXIL should not be used in combination with MAO inhibitors (including linezolid, an antibiotic which is a reversible non-selective MAO inhibitor) or within a minimum of 2 weeks of terminating treatment with MAO inhibitors. Treatment with PAXIL should then be initiated cautiously and dosage increased gradually until optimal response is reached. MAO inhibitors should not be introduced within 2 weeks of cessation of therapy with PAXIL.

Thioridazine: Thioridazine administration alone produces prolongation of the QTc interval, which is associated with serious ventricular arrhythmias, such as torsade de pointes-type arrhythmias, and sudden death. This effect appears to be dose-related. An in vivo study suggests that drugs which inhibit P450 2D6, including certain SSRIs such as paroxetine, fluoxetine and fluvoxamine, will elevate plasma levels of thioridazine. Therefore, PAXIL should not be used in combination with thioridazine or within a minimum of 2 weeks of terminating treatment with thioridazine. At least 2 weeks should be allowed after discontinuing PAXIL therapy before initiating treatment with thioridazine.

Pimozide: The concomitant use of PAXIL and pimozide is contraindicated as PAXIL has been shown to increase plasma pimozide levels. Elevation of pimozide blood concentration may result in QT interval prolongation and severe arrhythmias including torsade de pointes (see Drug Interactions).

WARNINGS AND PRECAUTIONS: General: Potential Association with Behavioural and Emotional Changes, Including Self-Harm: Pediatrics: Placebo-Controlled Clinical Trial Data:

- **Recent analyses of placebo-controlled clinical trial safety databases from SSRIs and other newer antidepressants suggests that use of these drugs in patients under the age of 18 may be associated with behavioural and emotional changes, including an increased risk of suicidal ideation and behaviour over that of placebo.**
- **The small denominators in the clinical trial database, as well as the variability in placebo rates, preclude reliable conclusions on the relative safety profiles among these drugs.**

Adult and Pediatrics: Additional Data:

- **There are clinical trial and post-marketing reports with SSRIs and other newer antidepressants, in both pediatrics and adults, of severe agitation-type adverse events coupled with self-harm or harm to others. The agitation-type events include: akathisia, agitation, disinhibition, emotional lability, hostility, aggression, depersonalization. In some cases, the events occurred within several weeks of starting treatment.**

Rigorous clinical monitoring for suicidal ideation or other indicators of potential for suicidal behaviour is advised in patients of all ages. This includes monitoring for agitation-type emotional and behavioural changes.

Discontinuation Symptoms: Patients currently taking PAXIL should not be discontinued abruptly, due to risk of discontinuation symptoms. At the time that a medical decision is made to discontinue an SSRI or other newer antidepressant drug, a gradual reduction in the dose rather than an abrupt cessation is recommended.

Discontinuation of Treatment with PAXIL: When discontinuing treatment, regardless of the indication for which PAXIL is being prescribed, patients should be monitored for symptoms which may be associated with discontinuation (e.g. dizziness, sleep disturbances including abnormal dreams, sensory disturbances (including paresthesias, electric shock sensations and tinnitus), agitation, anxiety, headache, tremor, confusion, diarrhea, nausea, vomiting and sweating or other symptoms which may be of clinical significance [see Adverse Reactions, Adverse Events following Discontinuation of Treatment (or Dose Reduction, Post-Marketing)]. A gradual reduction in the dose rather than abrupt cessation is recommended whenever possible. If intolerable symptoms occur following a decrease in the dose or upon discontinuation of treatment, dose titration should be managed on the basis of the patient's clinical response (see Adverse Reactions and Dosage and Administration).

PAXIL Treatment During Pregnancy Effects on Newborns: Epidemiological studies of pregnancy outcomes following maternal exposure to antidepressants in the first trimester have reported an increase in the risk of congenital malformations, particularly cardiovascular (e.g. ventricular and atrial septal defects), associated with the use of paroxetine. If a patient becomes pregnant while taking PAXIL, consideration should be given to switching to other treatment options. Treatment with PAXIL should only be continued for an individual pregnant patient, if the potential benefits outweigh the potential risks. Initiation of paroxetine, for women who intend to become pregnant, or are in their first trimester of pregnancy, should be considered only after other treatment options have been evaluated (see Warnings and Precautions, Special Populations)

Post-marketing reports indicate that some neonates exposed to PAXIL, SSRIs (Selective Serotonin Reuptake Inhibitors), or other newer antidepressants late in the third trimester have developed complications requiring prolonged hospitalization, respiratory support, and tube feeding. Such complications can arise immediately upon delivery. When treating a pregnant woman with PAXIL during the third trimester, the physician should carefully consider the potential risks and benefits of treatment (see Warnings and Precautions, Special Populations; Dosage and Administration, Special Patient Populations, Treatment of Pregnant Women).

Potential for Reduced Efficacy of Tamoxifen with Concomitant SSRI use, Including PAXIL: The antitumor agent tamoxifen is a pro-drug requiring metabolic activation by CYP2D6. Inhibition of CYP2D6 can lead to reduced plasma concentrations of a primary active metabolite (endoxifen). Chronic use of CYP2D6 inhibitors, including certain SSRIs, together with tamoxifen can lead to persistent reduction in levels of endoxifen (see also Drug Interactions, Tamoxifen). The clinical significance of this in terms of efficacy of tamoxifen is unclear.

Psychomotor Impairment: Although paroxetine did not cause sedation or interfere with psychomotor performance in placebo-controlled studies in normal subjects, patients should be advised to avoid driving a car or operating hazardous machinery until they are reasonably certain that PAXIL does not affect them adversely.

Bone Fracture Risk: Epidemiological studies show an increased risk of bone fractures following exposure to some antidepressants, including SSRIs. The risks appear to be greater at the initial stages of treatment, but significant increased risks were also observed at later stages of treatment. The possibility of fracture should be considered in the care of patients treated with PAXIL. Elderly patients and patients with important risk factors for bone fractures should be advised of possible adverse events which increase the risk of falls, such as dizziness and orthostatic hypotension, especially at the early stages of treatment but also soon after withdrawal. Preliminary data from observational studies show association of SSRIs and low bone mineral density in older men and women. Until further information becomes available, a possible effect on bone mineral density with long term treatment with SSRIs, including PAXIL, cannot be excluded, and may be a potential concern for patients with osteoporosis or major risk factors for bone fractures.

The following additional precautions are listed alphabetically.

Cardiovascular: PAXIL has not been evaluated or used to any appreciable extent in patients with a recent history of myocardial infarction or unstable heart disease. The usual precautions should be observed in patients with cardiac conditions.

Concomitant Illnesses: Clinical experience with PAXIL in patients with certain concomitant systemic illnesses is limited. Caution is advisable in using PAXIL in patients with diseases or conditions that could affect metabolism or hemodynamic responses.

Dependence Liability: PAXIL has not been systematically studied, in animals or humans, for its potential for abuse, tolerance, or physical dependence. Physicians should carefully evaluate patients for history of drug abuse and follow such patients closely, observing them for signs of misuse or abuse of PAXIL.

Endocrine and Metabolism: Serum Cholesterol Elevation: Several public domain studies have shown increased LDL-cholesterol levels of ~10% in volunteers and patients taking paroxetine for 8 to 12 weeks, which generally normalized after paroxetine discontinuation. In addition, of the patients in placebo-controlled clinical trials for whom baseline and on-treatment measurements were taken, total serum levels of cholesterol showed a mean increase of ~1.5 mg/dL in n=653 paroxetine-treated patients, compared to a mean decrease of ~5.0 mg/dL in placebo-treated patients (n=379). Increases from baseline of 45 mg/dL or greater were recorded in 6.6% of paroxetine-treated patients compared to 2.6% of placebo-treated patients (see Monitoring and Laboratory Tests, Serum Cholesterol Elevation).

These data should be taken into consideration when treating patients with underlying cardiac risk factors.

Hematologic: Abnormal Bleeding: There have been several reports of abnormal bleeding (mostly ecchymosis) associated with paroxetine treatment, including a report of impaired platelet aggregation. While a causal relationship to paroxetine is unclear, impaired platelet aggregation may result from platelet serotonin depletion and contribute to such occurrences.

Skin and mucous membrane bleedings (including upper gastrointestinal bleeding) have been reported following treatment with paroxetine. Paroxetine should therefore be used with caution in patients concomitantly treated with drugs that give an increased risk for bleeding (e.g. anticoagulants, nonsteroidal anti-inflammatories and ASA) and in patients with a known tendency for bleeding or those with predisposing conditions.

Hepatic/Biliary/Pancreatic: Hepatic Impairment: Pharmacokinetic studies of PAXIL in subjects with clinically significant hepatic impairment suggest that prolongation of the elimination half-life and increased plasma levels can be expected in this patient group. PAXIL should be used with caution and dosages restricted to the lower end of the range in patients with clinically significant hepatic impairment (see Dosage and Administration, Special Patient Populations and Actions and Clinical Pharmacology, Hepatic Insufficiency).

Neurologic: Epilepsy: As with other antidepressants, PAXIL should be used with caution in patients with epilepsy.

Seizures: During clinical trials, the overall incidence of seizures was 0.15% in patients treated with PAXIL. However, patients with a history of convulsive disorders were excluded from these studies. Caution is recommended when the drug is administered to patients with a history of seizures. The drug should be discontinued in any patient who develops seizures.

Serotonin Syndrome/Neuroleptic Malignant Syndrome: On rare occasions serotonin syndrome or neuroleptic malignant syndrome-like events have occured in association with treatment of PAXIL, particularly when given in combination with other serotonergic and/or neuroleptic/antipsychotic drugs. As these syndromes may result in potentially life-threatening conditions, treatment with PAXIL should be discontinued if patients develop a combination of symptoms possibly including hyperthermia, rigidity, myoclonus, autonomic instability with possible rapid fluctuations of vital signs, mental status changes including confusion, irritability, extreme agitation progressing to delirium and coma, and supportive symptomatic treatment should be initiated. Due to the risk of serotonergic syndrome or neuroleptic malignant syndrome PAXIL should not be used in combination with MAO inhibitors or serotonin-precursors (such as L-tryptophan, oxitriptan) and should be used with caution in patients receiving other serotonergic drugs (e.g., triptans, lithium, tramadol, St. John's wort, most tricyclic antidepressants) or neuroleptics/antipsychotics (see Contraindications and Drug Interactions).

Ophthalmologic: Glaucoma: As with other SSRIs, PAXIL can cause mydriasis and should be used with caution in patients with narrow angle glaucoma.

Psychiatric: Suicide: The possibility of a suicide attempt is inherent in depression and may persist until remission occurs. Patients with depression may experience worsening of their depressive symptoms and/or the emergence of suicidal ideation and behaviours (suicidality) whether or not they are taking antidepressant medications. Notwithstanding, high risk patients should be closely supervised throughout therapy with appropriate consideration to the possible need for hospitalization. In order to minimize the opportunity for overdosage, prescriptions for PAXIL should be written for the smallest quantity of drug consistent with good patient management.

Because of the well established comorbidity between depression and other psychiatric disorders, the same precautions observed when treating patients with depression should be observed when treating patients with other psychiatric disorders (see **Warnings and Precautions, Potential Association with Behavioural and Emotional Changes, Including Self-Harm**).

Activation of Mania/Hypomania: During clinical testing in a patient population comprised primarily of unipolar depressed patients, approximately 1% of PAXIL-treated patients experienced manic reactions. When bipolar patients were considered as a sub-group the incidence of mania was 2%. As with all drugs effective in the treatment of depression, PAXIL should be used with caution in patients with a history of mania.

A major depressive episode may be the initial presentation of bipolar disorder. Patients with bipolar disorder may be at an increased risk of experiencing manic episodes when treated with antidepressants alone. Therefore, the decision to initiate symptomatic treatment of depression should only be made after patients have been adequately assessed to determine if they are at risk for bipolar disorder.

Electroconvulsive Therapy (ECT): The efficacy and safety of the concurrent use of PAXIL and ECT have not been studied.

Renal: Hyponatremia: Several cases of hyponatremia have been reported. The hyponatremia appeared to be reversible when PAXIL was discontinued. The majority of these occurrences have been in elderly individuals, some in patients taking diuretics or who were otherwise volume depleted.

Renal Impairment: Since PAXIL is extensively metabolized by the liver, excretion of unchanged drug in urine is a minor route of elimination. However, single dose pharmacokinetic studies in subjects with clinically significant renal impairment suggest that plasma levels of paroxetine are elevated in such subjects. Paroxetine should therefore be used with caution and the dosage restricted to the lower end of the range in patients with clinically significant renal impairment (see Dosage and Administration, Special Patient Populations and Actions and Clinical Pharmacology, Renal Insufficiency).

Special Populations: Pregnant Women and Newborns: Risk of Cardiovascular Malformations Following First Trimester Exposure to SSRIs: Epidemiological studies of pregnancy outcomes following maternal exposure to antidepressants in the first trimester have reported an increase in the risk of congenital malformations, particularly cardiovascular (e.g. ventricular and atrial septal defects), associated with the use of paroxetine. The data suggest that the risk of having an infant with a cardiovascular defect following maternal paroxetine exposure is approximately 1/50 (2%), compared with an expected rate for such defects of approximately 1/100 (1%) infants in the general population. In general, septal defects range from those that are symptomatic and may require surgery, to those that are asymptomatic and may resolve spontaneously. Information about the severity of the septal defects reported in the studies is not available.

While on PAXIL: Pregnancy, or intent to become pregnant: If a patient becomes pregnant while taking PAXIL, or intends to become pregnant, she should be informed of the current estimate of increased risk to the fetus with PAXIL over other antidepressants. Examinations of additional databases, as well as updated analyses, may result in changes to the current risk estimates. Consideration should be given to switching to other treatment options, including another antidepressant or non-pharmaceutical treatment such as cognitive behavioural therapy. Treatment with PAXIL should only be continued for an individual patient, if the potential benefits outweigh the potential risks.

Due to the potential for discontinuation symptoms, if a decision is taken to discontinue PAXIL treatment, a gradual reduction in the dose rather than an abrupt cessation is recommended (see Warnings and Precautions, Discontinuation of Treatment with PAXIL; Adverse Reactions, Adverse Events following Discontinuation of Treatment (or Dose Reduction) and Dosage and Administration, Discontinuation of Treatment).

Initiation of Paroxetine: For women who intend to become pregnant, or are in their first trimester of pregnancy, initiation of paroxetine should be considered only after other treatment options have been evaluated.

Complications Following Late Third Trimester Exposure to SSRIs: Post-marketing reports indicate that some neonates exposed to PAXIL, SSRIs (Selective Serotonin Reuptake Inhibitors), or other newer antidepressants late in the third trimester have developed complications requiring prolonged hospitalization, respiratory support, and tube feeding. Such complications can arise immediately upon delivery. Reported clinical findings have included respiratory distress, cyanosis, apnea, seizures, temperature instability, feeding difficulty, vomiting, hypoglycemia, hypotonia, hypertonia, hyperreflexia, tremor, jitteriness, irritability, and constant crying. These features are consistent with either a direct toxic effect of SSRIs and other newer antidepressants, or, possibly, a drug discontinuation syndrome. It should be noted that, in some cases, the clinical picture is consistent with serotonin syndrome (see Warnings and Precautions, Neurologic, Serotonin Syndrome/Neuroleptic Malignant Syndrome). When treating a pregnant woman with PAXIL during the third trimester, the physician should carefully consider the potential risks and benefits of treatment (see Dosage and Administration, Special Patient Populations, Treatment of Pregnant Women).

Risk of PPHN and Exposure to SSRIs (including paroxetine): Epidemiological studies on persistent pulmonary hypertension of the newborn (PPHN) have shown that the use of SSRIs (including PAXIL) in pregnancy, particularly use in late pregnancy, was associated with an increased risk of PPHN. PPHN occurs in 1-2 per 1 000 live births in the general population and is associated with substantial neonatal morbidity and mortality. In a retrospective case-control study of 377 women whose infants were born with PPHN and 836 women whose infants were born healthy, the risk for developing PPHN was approximately six-fold higher for infants exposed to SSRIs after the 20th week of gestation compared to infants who had not been exposed to antidepressants during pregnancy (Odds Ratio 6.1, 95% CI 2.2-16.8). A study using data from the Swedish Medical Birth Register for 831,324 infants born in 1997-2005 found an increased risk of PPHN of approximately 2-fold associated with patient-reported maternal use of SSRIs in the first trimester of pregnancy (Risk Ratio 2.4, 95% CI 1.2-4.3), and an increased risk of PPHN of approximately 4-fold associated with a combination of patient-reported maternal use of SSRIs in the first trimester and an antenatal SSRI prescription in later pregnancy (Risk Ratio 3.6, 95% CI 1.2-8.3).

Nursing Women: The concentrations of paroxetine detected in the breast milk of lactating women are similar to those in the mother's plasma. Lactating women should not nurse their infants while receiving paroxetine unless in the opinion of the treating physician, breast feeding is necessary, in which case the infant should be closely monitored.

Pediatrics (<18 years of age): PAXIL is not indicated for use in patients below the age of 18 years (see Warnings and Precautions, Potential Association with Behavioural and Emotional Changes, Including Self-Harm). See also Indications, Pediatrics (<18 years of age) and Dosage and Administration, Special Patient Populations, Pediatrics).

Controlled clinical studies in depression failed to demonstrate efficacy and do not support the use of paroxetine in the treatment of children under the age of 18 years with depression. Moreover, a higher incidence of adverse events related to behavioural and emotional changes, including self harm, was reported with paroxetine treatment compared to placebo during controlled clinical trials in depression, OCD and social anxiety disorder (see Adverse Drug Reactions, Clinical Trial Adverse Drug Reactions, Pediatrics).

Geriatrics (≥65 years of age): Administration of PAXIL to the elderly is associated with increased plasma levels and prolongation of the elimination half-life relative to younger adults (see Action and Clinical Pharmacology). Elderly patients should be initiated and maintained at the lowest daily dose of paroxetine which is associated with clinical efficacy (see Dosage and Administration).

Evaluation of approximately 800 elderly patients (≥65 years) treated with PAXIL (10-40 mg daily) in worldwide premarketing clinical trials revealed no unusual pattern of adverse events relative to the clinical experience in younger patients. However, it is not possible to rule out potential age-related differences in safety and effectiveness during chronic use, particularly in elderly patients who have concomitant systemic illnesses or who are receiving concomitant drugs.

Monitoring and Laboratory Tests: Serum Cholesterol Elevation: Of the patients in placebo-controlled clinical trials for whom baseline and on-treatment measurements were taken, increases from baseline of 45 mg/dL or greater were recorded in 6.6% of paroxetine-treated patients compared to 2.6% of placebo-treated patients (see Adverse Reactions, Laboratory Changes—Cholesterol and Warnings and Precautions, Endocrine and Metabolism).

These data should be taken into consideration when treating patients with underlying cardiac risk factors.

ADVERSE REACTIONS: Adverse Drug Reaction Overview: Commonly Observed Adverse Events: The most commonly observed adverse experiences associated with the use of PAXIL in clinical trials and not seen at an equivalent incidence among placebo-treated patients were: nausea, somnolence, sweating, tremor, asthenia, dizziness, dry mouth, insomnia, constipation, diarrhea, decreased appetite and male sexual dysfunction (see Table 1 and Table 2).

Adverse Events Leading to Discontinuation of Treatment: Twenty-one percent of over 4000 patients who received PAXIL in worldwide clinical trials in depression discontinued treatment due to an adverse experience. In obsessive-compulsive disorder, panic disorder, social phobia (social anxiety disorder), generalized anxiety disorder and post-traumatic stress disorder studies, 11.8% (64/542), 9.4 % (44/469), 16.1% (84/522) 10.7% (79/735) and 11.7% (79/676), respectively, of patients treated with PAXIL discontinued treatment because of adverse events. The most common events leading to discontinuation (reported by 1% or more of subjects) included: asthenia, headache, nausea, somnolence, insomnia, agitation, tremor, dizziness, constipation, impotence, abnormal ejaculation, sweating and diarrhea.

Adverse Events following Discontinuation of Treatment (or Dose Reduction): Clinical Trials: The following adverse events have been reported at an incidence of 2% or greater for PAXIL and were at least twice that reported for placebo: abnormal dreams (2.3% vs 0.5%), paresthesias (2.0% vs 0.4%), and dizziness (7.1% vs 1.5%).

The majority of these events were mild to moderate, self-limiting and did not requiremedical intervention. These adverse events were noted in GAD and PTSD clinical trials employing a taper phase regimen for discontinuation of treatment. This regimen involved an incremental decrease in the daily dose by 10 mg/day at weekly intervals. When a daily dose of 20 mg/day was reached, patients were continued on this dose for 1 week before treatment was stopped.

Post-Marketing: There have been spontaneous reports of adverse events upon the discontinuation of PAXIL (particularly when abrupt), including but not limited to the following: dizziness, sensory disturbances (including paresthesias, electric shock sensations and tinnitus), agitation/restlessness, anxiety, nausea, tremor, confusion, diarrhea, vomiting, sweating, headache, and sleep disturbances (abnormal dreams). Generally these symptoms are mild to moderate, however, in some patients they may be severe in intensity. They usually occur within the first few days of discontinuing treatment, but there have been very rare reports of such symptoms in patients who have inadvertently missed a dose. Generally these symptoms are self-limiting and usually resolve within 2 weeks, though in some individuals they may be prolonged (2-3 months or more). Symptoms associated with discontinuation have been reported for other selective serotonin reuptake inhibitors.

Patients should be monitored for these or any other symptoms when discontinuing treatment, regardless of the indication for which PAXIL is being prescribed. If intolerable symptoms occur following a decrease in the dose or upon discontinuation of treatment, dose titration should be managed on the basis of the patient's clinical response (see Warnings and Precautions and Dosage and Administration).

Clinical Trial Adverse Drug Reactions: Because clinical trials are conducted under very specific conditions the adverse reaction rates observed in the clinical trials may not reflect the rates observed in practice and should not be compared to the rates in the clinical trials of another drug. Adverse drug reaction information from clinical trials is useful for identifying drug-related adverse events and for approximating rates.

Incidence in Controlled Clinical Trials: Adults: Multiple doses of PAXIL were administered to 4126 subjects in clinical trials for depression, 542 subjects in clinical trials for OCD, 469 subjects in clinical trials for panic disorder, 522 subjects in clinical trials for social phobia (social anxiety disorder), 735 subjects in clinical trials for generalized anxiety disorder and 676 subjects in clinical trials for post-traumatic stress disorder. Untoward experiences associated with this exposure were recorded by clinical investigators using descriptive terminology of their own choosing.

Consequently, it is not possible to provide a meaningful estimate of the proportion of individuals experiencing adverse experiences without first grouping similar types of untoward experiences into a limited (i.e., reduced) number of standardized experience categories.

Table 1 lists adverse experiences that occurred at an incidence of 1% or higher in short term (6-week) flexible dose (20-50 mg/day) placebo-controlled trials in depression. (An additional 460 patients participated in a fixed-dose placebo-controlled study).

Table 2 enumerates adverse events that occurred at a frequency of 2% or more among patients on PAXIL who participated in placebo-controlled OCD trials of 12-weeks duration in which patients were dosed in the range of 20-60 mg/day, in placebo-controlled panic disorder trials of 10-12-weeks duration in which patients were dosed in the range of 10-60 mg/day, in placebo-controlled social phobia (social anxiety disorder) trials of 12 weeks duration in which patients were dosed in a range of 20-50 mg/day, in placebo-controlled generalized anxiety disorder trials of 8 weeks in which patients were dosed in a range from 10-50 mg/day and in placebo-controlled post-traumatic stress disorder trials of 12 weeks in which patients were dosed in a range from 20-50 mg/day.

The prescriber should be aware that these figures cannot be used to predict the incidence of side effects in the course of usual medical practice where patient characteristics and other factors differ from those which prevailed in the clinical trials. Similarly the cited incidences cannot be compared with figures obtained from other clinical investigations involving different treatments, uses and investigators. The cited frequencies do however provide the prescribing physician with some basis for estimating the relative contribution of drug and non-drug factors to the side effect incidence rate in the population studied. Reported adverse experiences were classified using a COSTART-based Dictionary terminology for the depression trials and an ADECS (a modified COSTART dictionary) for OCD and panic disorder trials.

Table 1: PAXIL

Treatment-Emergent Adverse Events in Short Term Flexible Dose Placebo-Controlled Clinical Trials in Depression[a]

Body System	Preferred Term	Paroxetine (n=421) (%)	Placebo (n=421) (%)
Body as a Whole	Headache	17.6	17.3
	Asthenia	15.0	5.9
	Abdominal Pain	3.1	4.0
	Fever	1.7	1.7
	Chest Pain	1.4	2.1
	Trauma	1.4	0.5
	Back Pain	1.2	2.4
Cardiovascular	Palpitation	2.9	1.4
	Vasodilation	2.6	0.7
	Postural Hypotension	1.2	0.5
Dermatological	Sweating	11.2	2.4
	Rash	1.7	0.7
Gastrointestinal	Nausea	25.7	9.3
	Dry Mouth	18.1	12.1
	Constipation	13.8	8.6
	Diarrhea	11.6	7.6
	Decreased Appetite	6.4	1.9
	Flatulence	4.0	1.7
	Vomiting	2.4	1.7
	Oropharynx Disorder[d]	2.1	0.0
	Dyspepsia	1.9	1.0
	Increased Appetite	1.4	0.5
Musculoskeletal	Myopathy	2.4	1.4
	Myalgia	1.7	0.7
	Myasthenia	1.4	0.2
Nervous System	Somnolence	23.3	9.0
	Dizziness	13.3	5.5
	Insomnia	13.3	6.2
	Tremor	8.3	1.9
	Nervousness	5.2	2.6
	Anxiety	5.0	2.9
	Paresthesia	3.8	1.7
	Libido Decreased	3.3	0.0
	Agitation	2.1	1.9
	Drugged Feeling	1.7	0.7
	Myoclonus	1.4	0.7
	CNS Stimulation	1.2	3.6
	Confusion	1.2	0.2
Respiration	Respiratory Disorder[e]	5.9	6.4
	Yawn	3.8	0.0
	Pharyngitis	2.1	2.9
Special Senses	Blurred Vision	3.6	1.4
	Taste Perversion	2.4	0.2
Urogenital System	[b]Abnormal Ejaculation[c]	12.9	0.0
	[b]Male Genital Disorders[f]	8.0	0.0
	Urinary Frequency	3.1	0.7
	Urination Impaired[g]	2.9	0.2
	[b]Impotence	2.5	0.5
	[b]Female Genital Disorders[h]	1.8	0.0

[a] Events reported by at least 1% of patients treated with Paxil are included.
[b] Percentage corrected for gender. Placebo: male, n=206; female, n=215. Paroxetine: male, n=201; female, n=220.
[c] Primarily ejaculatory delay. In a trial of fixed doses of paroxetine, the incidence of ejaculatory disturbance in males with 20 mg/day of paroxetine was 6.5% (3/46) vs 0% (0/23) in the placebo group.
[d] Includes mostly lump in throat and tightness in throat.
[e] Includes mostly cold symptoms or URI.
[f] Includes anorgasmia, erectile difficulties, delayed ejaculation/orgasm, sexual dysfunction and impotence.
[g] Includes difficulty with micturition and urinary hesitancy.
[h] Includes anorgasmia and difficulty reaching climax/orgasm.

Table 2: PAXIL

Treatment-Emergent Adverse Experience Incidence in Placebo-Controlled Clinical Trials for Obsessive-Compulsive Disorder, Panic Disorder, Social Phobia (Social Anxiety Disorder), Generalized Anxiety Disorder and Post-Traumatic Stress Disorder[a]

		Obsessive-Compulsive Disorder		Panic Disorder		Social Phobia (Social Anxiety Disorder)		Generalized Anxiety Disorder		Post-Traumatic Stress Disorder	
Body System	**Preferred Term**	**PAXIL (n=542) (%)**	**Placebo (n=265) (%)**	**PAXIL (n=469) (%)**	**Placebo (n=324) (%)**	**PAXIL (n=425) (%)**	**Placebo (n=339) (%)**	**PAXIL (n=735) (%)**	**Placebo (n=529) (%)**	**PAXIL (n=676) (%)**	**Placebo (n=504) (%)**
Body as a Whole	Headache	25.3	29.1	25.4	25.3	22.4	21.8	16.9	14.0	18.9	19.2
	Asthenia	21.8	13.6	13.6	4.6	22.4	13.6	14.3	6.4	11.8	4.2
	Infection	5.4	4.9	5.3	6.8	3.8	5.9	5.6	3.4	4.9	3.8
	Abdominal Pain	4.8	4.9	4.3	3.1	2.1	4.7	4.5	3.6	4.3	3.2
	Chest Pain	2.8	1.9	2.3	3.1	0.7	0.3	1.0	0.6	1.2	0.8
	Back Pain	2.4	4.9	3.2	2.2	1.6	4.1	2.3	3.6	3.4	3.4
	Chills	2.0	0.8	2.3	0.6	0.2	0.3	1.0	0.0	0.1	0.4
	Trauma	3.1	3.8	3.6	3.7	2.6	0.9	2.6	3.4	5.8	5.2
Cardiovascular	Vasodilation	3.9	1.1	2.1	2.8	1.4	0.6	2.7	0.8	2.2	1.2
	Palpitation	2.0	0.4	2.3	2.5	1.2	1.8	1.1	1.1	1.0	0.8
Dermatologic	Sweating	8.9	3.0	14.3	5.9	9.2	2.1	6.3	1.5	4.6	1.4
	Rash	3.1	1.9	2.3	1.5	0.7	0.3	1.5	0.9	1.5	2.0
Gastrointestinal	Nausea	23.2	9.8	22.8	17.3	24.7	6.5	20.1	5.3	19.2	8.3
	Dry Mouth	18.1	8.7	18.1	10.8	8.9	2.9	10.9	4.7	10.1	4.8
	Constipation	15.7	6.4	7.9	5.2	5.4	1.8	10.5	1.7	5.5	3.[illegible]
	Diarrhea	10.3	9.8	11.7	6.5	8.5	5.9	9.1	6.6	10.5	5.[illegible]
	Decreased Appetite	9.0	3.4	7.0	2.8	7.8	1.5	5.2	1.1	5.9	2.5
	Dyspepsia	3.9	6.8	3.8	6.8	4.0	2.4	4.5	4.9	4.6	3.1
	Flatulence	3.0	4.2	1.7	2.8	4.0	2.4	1.4	2.1	1.0	1.0
	Increased Appetite	4.2	3.0	2.1	0.6	1.2	1.8	0.4	1.1	1.5	1.0
	Vomiting	2.2	3.4	1.9	1.5	2.4	0.6	2.7	2.5	3.0	2.0
Musculoskeletal	Myalgia	3.1	3.8	2.3	3.4	4.0	2.7	2.9	2.6	1.8	1.8
Nervous System	Somnolence	24.4	7.2	18.8	10.8	21.6	5.3	15.4	4.5	16.0	4.6
	Insomnia	23.8	13.2	17.9	10.2	20.9	15.9	10.7	7.9	11.8	1[illegible].3
	Dizziness	12.4	6.0	14.1	9.9	11.3	7.1	6.1	4.5	6.1	[illegible].6
	Tremor	10.5	1.1	8.5	1.2	8.7	1.2	4.6	0.8	4.3	[illegible].4
	Nervousness	8.5	8.3	7.9	8.3	7.5	6.5	3.9	2.8	3.0	[illegible].4
	Libido Decreased	7.2	3.8	8.5	1.2	11.5	0.9	9.4	1.5	5.2	[illegible].8
	Anxiety	4.1	6.8	4.5	4.0	4.7	4.1	1.6	0.9	3.8	4.0
	Abnormal Dreams	3.9	1.1	2.8	3.4	1.9	1.5	0.5	1.1	2.5	1.6
	Myoclonus	3.3	0.4	3.2	1.5	2.1	0.9	1.6	0.6	1.0	0.6
	Concentration Impaired	2.8	1.5	1.1	0.9	3.5	0.6	1.1	0.6	1.5	1.0
	Depersonalization	2.6	0.4	1.7	2.2	0.7	0.9	0.7	0.0	0.9	0.2
	Amnesia	2.2	1.1	0.6	0.0	0.5	0.3	0.4	0.6	1.3	1.0
	Hyperkinesia	2.2	1.5	0.9	0.9	1.2	0.0	0.8	0.0	1.3	0.2
	Agitation	1.7	2.3	4.7	3.7	2.6	0.9	1.8	1.1	1.9	3.2
Respiratory System	Pharyngitis	3.7	4.9	3.2	3.1	3.8	2.1	2.3	2.1	2.4	2.2
	Rhinitis	1.5	3.4	2.6	0.3	1.2	3.2	1.5	1.1	1.0	2.0
	Sinusitis	1.5	4.9	5.8	4.6	2.1	2.4	3.5	3.4	3.8	4.4
	Yawn	1.7	0.4	1.9	0.0	4.9	0.3	4.2	0.2	2.1	0.2
	Cough Increased	1.1	1.9	2.3	1.5	0.7	0.9	0.8	0.8	1.2	0.6
	Respiratory Disorder[a]	—	—	—	—	—	—	6.8	5.1	3.3	1.0
Special Senses	Abnormal Vision	3.7	2.3	3.0	2.8	4.0	0.3	2.2	0.6	0.3	0.0
	Taste Perversion	2.0	0.0	1.1	0.6	0.7	0.6	0.7	0.8	0.7	0.8

(cont'd)

Table 2: PAXIL *(cont'd)*

Treatment-Emergent Adverse Experience Incidence in Placebo-Controlled Clinical Trials for Obsessive-Compulsive Disorder, Panic Disorder, Social Phobia (Social Anxiety Disorder), Generalized Anxiety Disorder and Post-Traumatic Stress Disorder[a]

		Obsessive-Compulsive Disorder		Panic Disorder		Social Phobia (Social Anxiety Disorder)		Generalized Anxiety Disorder		Post-Traumatic Stress Disorder	
Body System	**Preferred Term**	**PAXIL (n=542) (%)**	**Placebo (n=265) (%)**	**PAXIL (n=469) (%)**	**Placebo (n=324) (%)**	**PAXIL (n=425) (%)**	**Placebo (n=339) (%)**	**PAXIL (n=735) (%)**	**Placebo (n=529) (%)**	**PAXIL (n=676) (%)**	**Placebo (n=504) (%)**
Urogenital System	Abnormal Ejaculation[b]	23.3	1.3	20.5	0.9	27.6	1.1	24.7	2.0	12.6	1.6
	Dysmenorrhea[b]	1.4	1.9	2.0	2.3	4.6	4.4	1.3	1.2	1.6	1.3
	Impotence[b]	8.2	1.3	5.4	0.0	5.3	1.1	4.2	3.0	9.2	0.5
	Female Genital Disorder[b,c]	3.3	0.0	8.9	0.5	8.6	0.6	4.4	0.6	4.8	0.6
	Urinary Frequency	3.3	1.1	2.1	0.3	1.6	1.8	1.0	0.6	1.0	0.2
	Urination Impaired	3.3	0.4	0.4	0.3	1.9	0.0	1.0	0.0	0.6	0.0
	Urinary Tract Infection	1.5	1.1	2.1	1.2	0.2	1.2	1.2	1.1	0.6	0.8

[a] Events reported by at least 2% of either OCD, Panic Disorder, Social Phobia (Social Anxiety Disorder), Generalized Anxiety Disorder or Post-traumatic Stress Disorder Paxil-treated patients are included, except the following events which had an incidence on placebo ≥Paxil: [OCD]: depression, paresthesia, and respiratory disorder. [Panic Disorder]: flu syndrome, depression, paresthesia, respiratory disorder. [Social Phobia (Social Anxiety Disorder)]: depression, respiratory disorder. [Generalized Anxiety Disorder]: not applicable. [Stress Disorder]: depression, respiratory disorder.

[b] Incidence is gender-corrected.
OCD: Placebo: male, n=158; female, n=107.
Paroxetine: male, n=330; female, n=212.
Panic Disorder: Placebo: male, n=111; female, n=213.
Paroxetine: male, n=166; female, n=303.
Social Phobia (Social Anxiety Disorder): Placebo: male, n=180; female, n=159.
Paroxetine: male, n=228; female, n=197.
Generalized Anxiety Disorder: Placebo: male, n=197; female, n=332.
Paroxetine: male, n=283; female, n=452.
Post-Traumatic Stress Disorder: Placebo: male, n=190; female, n=314.
Paroxetine: male, n=238; female, n=438.

[c] Includes anorgasmia and difficulty reaching climax/orgasm.

Male and Female Sexual Dysfunction with SSRIs: Although changes in sexual desire, sexual performance and sexual satisfaction often occur as manifestations of a psychiatric disorder, they may also be a consequence of pharmacologic treatment. In particular, some evidence suggests that selective serotonin reuptake inhibitors (SSRIs) can cause such untoward sexual experiences.

Reliable estimates of the incidence and severity of untoward experiences involving sexual desire, performance and satisfaction are difficult to obtain, however, in part because patients and physicians may be reluctant to discuss them. Accordingly, estimates of the incidence of untoward sexual experience and performance cited in product labeling are likely to underestimate their actual incidence.

In placebo-controlled clinical trials involving more than 3200 patients, the ranges for the reported incidence of sexual side effects in males and females with major depressive disorder, OCD, panic disorder, social anxiety disorder, GAD and PTSD are displayed in Table 3.

Table 3: PAXIL

Incidence of Sexual Adverse Events in Controlled Clinical Trials

	PAXIL	Placebo
n (males)	**1446**	**1042**
Decreased Libido	6–15%	0–5%
Ejaculatory Disturbance	13–28%	0–2%
Impotence	2–9%	0–3%
n (females)	**1822**	**1340**
Decreased Libido	0–9%	0–2%
Orgasmic Disturbance	2–9%	0–1%

There are no adequate and well-controlled studies examining sexual dysfunction with paroxetine treatment.

Paroxetine treatment has been associated with several cases of priapism. In those cases with a known outcome, patients recovered without sequelae.

While it is difficult to know the precise risk of sexual dysfunction associated with the use of SSRIs, physicians should routinely inquire about such possible side effects.

Laboratory Changes—Cholesterol: Clinically and statistically relevant increases in cholesterol levels have been noted in studies using paroxetine (see Warnings and Precautions, Endocrine and Metabolism).

Of the patients in placebo-controlled clinical trials for whom baseline and on-treatment measurements were taken, total serum levels of cholesterol showed a mean increase of ~1.5 mg/dL in n=653 paroxetine-treated patients, compared to a mean decrease of ~5.0 mg/dL in placebo-treated patients (n=379). Increases from baseline of 45 mg/dL or greater were recorded in 6.6% of paroxetine-treated patients compared to 2.6% of placebo-treated patients.

Pediatrics: In placebo-controlled clinical trials conducted with pediatric patients aged 7 to 18 years with depression, OCD and Social Anxiety Disorder (involving 633 patients treated with paroxetine and 542 patients treated with placebo), the following adverse events were reported in at least 2% of pediatric patients treated with PAXIL and occurred at a rate at least twice that for pediatric patients receiving placebo: emotional lability (including self-harm, suicidal thoughts, attempted suicide, crying, and mood fluctuations), hostility, (predominantly aggression, oppositional behaviour and anger) decreased appetite, tremor, sweating, hyperkinesia, and agitation.

In the pediatric clinical trials in depression, OCD and Social Anxiety Disorder that included a taper phase regimen (307 patients aged 7 to 18 years treated with paroxetine and 291 patients treated with placebo), events reported upon discontinuation of treatment, which occurred in at least 2% of patients who received PAXIL and which occurred at a rate at least twice that of placebo, were: emotional lability (including suicidal ideation, suicide attempt, mood changes, and tearfulness), nervousness, dizziness, nausea, and abdominal pain (see Warnings and Precautions, Discontinuation of Treatment with PAXIL).

Other Events Observed During the Clinical Development of Paroxetine: In the tabulations which follow, a COSTART or modified COSTART-based Dictionary terminology has been used to classify reported adverse experiences. The frequencies presented therefore represent the portion of the 4126, 542, 469, 522, 735 and 676 PAXIL-exposed individuals in depression, OCD, panic, social phobia (social anxiety disorder), generalized anxiety disorder and post-traumatic stress disorder trials, respectively, who experienced an event of the type cited on at least one occasion while receiving PAXIL. Experiences are further classified within body system categories and enumerated in order of decreasing frequency using the following definitions: frequent experiences are defined as those occurring on one or more occasion in at least 1/100 patients; infrequent adverse experiences are those occurring in less than 1/100 but at least 1/1000 patients; rare experiences are those occurring in less than 1/1000 patients.

All adverse experiences are included except those already listed in Table 1 and Table 2, those reported in terms so general as to be uninformative and those experiences for which the drug cause was remote. It is important to emphasize that although the experiences reported did occur during treatment with PAXIL, they were not necessarily caused by it.

Body as a Whole: Frequent: malaise, pain. Infrequent: allergic reaction, chills, face edema, infection, moniliasis, neck pain, overdose. Rare: abnormal laboratory value, abscess, adrenergic syndrome, cellulitis, chills and fever, cyst, hernia, intentional overdose, neck rigidity, pelvic pain, peritonitis, substernal chest pain, sepsis, ulcer.

Cardiovascular System: Frequent: hypertension, syncope, tachycardia. Infrequent: bradycardia, conduction abnormalities, electrocardiogram abnormal, hypotension, migraine, ventricular extrasystoles. Rare: angina pectoris, arrhythmia, atrial arrhythmia, atrial fibrillation, bundle branch block, cardiac disorder, cerebral ischemia, cerebrovascular accident, cerebrovascular disorder, congestive heart failure, extrasystoles, low cardiac output, myocardial infarct, myocardial ischemia, pallor, phlebitis, pulmonary embolus, supraventricular extrasystoles, thrombosis, varicose vein, vascular disorder, vascular headache.

Dermatological: Frequent: pruritus. Infrequent: acne, alopecia, dry skin, ecchymosis, eczema, furunculosis, herpes simplex, urticaria. Rare: angioedema, contact dermatitis, erythema nodosum, exfoliative dermatitis, herpes zoster, maculopapular rash, photosensitivity, skin discolouration, skin ulcer, skin hypertrophy, sweating decreased.

Endocrine: Rare: diabetes mellitus, fertility decreased female, goiter, hyperthyroidism, hypothyroidism, thyroiditis.

Gastrointestinal: Frequent: nausea and vomiting. Infrequent: bruxism, buccal cavity disorders, dysphagia, eructation, gastroenteritis, gastrointestinal flu, glossitis, increased salivation, liver function tests abnormal, mouth ulceration, vomiting and diarrhea, rectal hemorrhage. Rare: aphthous stomatitis, bloody diarrhea, bulimia, cardiospasm, colitis, duodenitis, esophagitis, fecal impaction, fecal incontinence, gastritis, gingivitis, hematemesis, hepatitis, ileitis, ileus, jaundice, melena, peptic ulcer, salivary gland enlargement, sialadenitis, stomach ulcer, stomatitis, tongue edema, tooth caries.

Hematologic and Lymphatic: Infrequent: anemia, leukopenia, lymphadenopathy, purpura, WBC abnormality. Rare: abnormal bleeding, predominately of the skin and mucous membranes (mostly ecchymosis), bleeding time increased, eosinophilia, iron deficiency anemia, leukocytosis, lymphedema, lymphocytosis, microcytic anemia, monocytosis, normocytic anemia, thrombocytopenia.

Metabolic and Nutritional: Frequent: weight gain, weight loss, increases in cholesterol levels. Infrequent: edema, hyperglycemia, peripheral edema, thirst. Rare: alkaline phosphatase increased, bilirubinemia, cachexia, dehydration, gout, hypocalcemia, hypoglycemia, hypokalemia, hyponatremia (predominantly in the elderly) which is sometimes due to syndrome of inappropriate antidiuretic hormone secretion (SIADH), non-protein nitrogen (NPN) increased, obesity, AST increased, ALT increased.

Musculoskeletal: Infrequent: arthralgia, arthritis, traumatic fracture. Rare: arthrosis, bone disorder, bursitis, cartilage disorder, myositis, osteoporosis, tetany.

Nervous System: Frequent: CNS stimulation, concentration impaired, depression, emotional lability, vertigo. Infrequent: akinesia, alcohol abuse, amnesia, ataxia, convulsion, depersonalization, hallucinations, hyperkinesia, hypertonia, incoordination, lack of emotion, manic reaction, paranoid reaction, thinking abnormal, hypesthesia. Rare: abnormal electroencephalogram, abnormal gait, antisocial reaction, brain edema, choreoathetosis, circumoral paraesthesia, confusion, delirium, delusions, diplopia, drug dependence, dysarthria, dyskinesia, dystonia, euphoria, fasciculations, grand mal convulsion, hostility, hyperalgesia, hypokinesia, hysteria, libido increased, manic depressive reaction, meningitis, myelitis, neuralgia, neuropathy, nystagmus, psychosis, psychotic depression, reflexes increased, stupor, torticollis, withdrawal syndrome.

Respiratory System: Frequent: cough increased, rhinitis. Infrequent: asthma, bronchitis, dyspnea, epistaxis, hyperventilation, pneumonia, respiratory flu, sinusitis. Rare: hiccup, lung fibrosis, sputum increased, stridor, trachea disorder, voice alteration.

Special Senses: Infrequent: abnormality of accommodation, conjunctivitis, ear pain, eye pain, mydriasis, otitis media, tinnitus. Rare: amblyopia, cataract specified, conjunctival edema, corneal lesion, corneal ulcer, exophthalmos, eye hemorrhage, acute glaucoma, hyperacusis, otitis externa, photophobia, retinal hemorrhage, taste loss, anisocoria, deafness, keratoconjunctivitis.

Urogenital System: Infrequent: abortion*, amenorrhea*, breast pain*, cystitis, dysmenorrhea*, dysuria, menorrhagia*, nocturia, polyuria, urinary incontinence, urinary retention, urinary tract infection, urinary urgency, vaginitis*. Rare: Breast atrophy*, cervix disorder*, endometrial disorder*, female lactation*, hematuria, kidney calculus, kidney function abnormal, kidney pain, mastitis*, nephritis, oliguria, salpingitis*, spermatogenesis arrest* urethritis, urinary casts, urine abnormality, uterine neoplasm*, vaginal moniliasis*.

Post-Market Adverse Drug Reactions: Adverse events not listed above which have been reported since market introduction in patients taking PAXIL include acute pancreatitis, hepatic events such as elevation of hepatic enzymes, and hepatitis, sometimes associated with jaundice, and/or liver failure (in very rare circumstances, with fatal outcomes), Guillain-Barré syndrome, toxic epidermal necrolysis, priapism, thrombocytopenia, aggravated hypertension, syndrome of inappropriate ADH secretion, symptoms suggestive of hyperprolactinemia and galactorrhea, blurred vision; extrapyramidal symptoms which have included akathisia, (characterized by an inner sense of restlessness and psychomotor agitation such as an inability to sit or stand still usually associated with subjective distress), bradykinesia, cogwheel rigidity, dystonia, hypertonia, oculogyric crisis which has been associated with concomitant use of pimozide, tremor and trismus, abnormal dreams (including nightmares), restless legs syndrome (RLS), neuroleptic malignant syndrome-like events and serotonin syndrome (see Warnings and Precautions, Neurologic, Serotonin Syndrome/Neuroleptic Malignant Syndrome), persistent pulmonary hypertension (PPHN; see also Warnings and Precautions, Pregnant Women and Newborns, Risk of PPHN and Exposure to SSRIs (including paroxetine)). There has been

* Incidence corrected for gender.

a case report of an elevated phenytoin level after 4 weeks of PAXIL and phenytoin co-administration. There has been a case report of severe hypotension when PAXIL was added to chronic metoprolol treatment. The causal relationship between PAXIL and the emergence of these events has not been established.

There have been spontaneous reports of adverse events upon the discontinuation of PAXIL and other selective serotonin reuptake inhibitors (particularly when abrupt) (see Warnings and Precautions, General, Discontinuation of Treatment with PAXIL and Adverse Reactions, Adverse Events following Discontinuation of Treatment (or Dose Reduction)).

DRUG INTERACTIONS:

Serious Drug Interactions
- **Monoamine Oxidase Inhibitors: See Contraindications.**
- **Thioridazine: See Contraindications.**
- **Pimozide: See Contraindications.**

Overview: Like some other selective serotonin re-uptake inhibitors, paroxetine inhibits the specific hepatic cytochrome P450 isozyme CYP2D6 which is responsible for the metabolism of debrisoquine and sparteine. Poor metabolizers of debrisoquine/sparteine represent approximately 5-10% of Caucasians. The median C_{min} (ss) for PAXIL (20 mg daily) at steady state in poor metabolizers (n=8) was almost triple that reported for extensive metabolizers (n=9). Although the full clinical significance of this effect has not been established, inhibition of CYP2D6 can lead to elevated plasma levels of co-administered drugs which are metabolized by this isozyme. Consideration should be given to decreasing the dose of the CYP2D6 metabolized drug or paroxetine and/or monitoring of drug plasma levels, especially when PAXIL is co-administered with drugs with a narrow therapeutic index.

PAXIL coadministration has been associated with elevated levels of the anticholinergic procyclidine, certain neuroleptics/antipsychotics (e.g., perphenazine, risperidone), tricyclic antidepressants (e.g., desipramine), atomoxetine, type 1C antiarrhythmics (e.g., propafenone), and theophylline.

Co-administration of phenobarbitol or phenytoin with PAXIL has been associated with decreased levels of PAXIL. When co-administered with cimetidine, PAXIL levels were elevated.

The concomitant use of PAXIL and alcohol has not been studied.

Drug-Drug Interactions: Monoamine Oxidase Inhibitors: Combined use of PAXIL and monoamine oxidase inhibitors (including linezolid, an antibiotic which is a reversible non-selective MAO inhibitor) is contraindicated due to the potential for serious reactions with features resembling serotonin syndrome or neuroleptic malignant syndrome (see Contraindications and Warnings and Precautions, Serotonin Syndrome/Neuroleptic Malignant Syndrome).

Thioridazine: Combined use of PAXIL and thioridazine is contraindicated due to a potential for elevated thioridazine plasma levels. Thioridazine treatment alone produces prolongation of the QTc interval, which is associated with serious ventricular arrhythmias, such as torsade de pointes-type arrhythmias, and sudden death (see Contraindications).

Pimozide: In an open label study of healthy volunteers, co-administration of a single dose of 2 mg pimozide, under steady state conditions of PAXIL (titrated to 60 mg daily) was associated with mean increases in pimozide AUC of 151% and C_{max} of 62%, compared to pimozide administered alone. This is likely explained by the known CYP2D6 inhibitory properties of paroxetine. Due to the narrow therapeutic index of pimozide, and its known ability to prolong the QT interval, and produce severe cardiac arrhythmias including torsade de pointes, concomitant use of pimozide and PAXIL is contraindicated (see Contraindications).

Drugs Metabolized by Cytochrome P450 (CYP2D6): In two studies, daily dosing of PAXIL (20 mg qd) under steady state conditions increased the following mean pharmacokinetic parameters for a single (100 mg) dose of desipramine in extensive metabolizers: C_{max} (2 fold), AUC (6 fold), and T½ (3-5 fold). Concomitant steady-state PAXIL treatment did not result in any further impairment of desipramine elimination in poor metabolizers. Insufficient information is available to provide recommendations on the necessary dosage adjustments for tricyclic antidepressants or PAXIL, if these drugs are to be used in combination. Plasma tricyclic antidepressant concentrations may need to be monitored in such instances.

Concomitant use of PAXIL with other drugs metabolized by CYP2D6 has not been formally studied but may require lower doses than usually prescribed for either PAXIL or the other drug. Drugs metabolized by CYP2D6 include certain tricyclic antidepressants (e.g. nortriptyline, amitriptyline, imipramine and desipramine), selective serotonin reuptake inhibitors (e.g. fluoxetine), phenothiazine neuroleptics (e.g. perphenazine), risperidone, atomoxetine, Type IC antiarrhythmics (e.g. propafenone and flecainide), and metoprolol. Due to the risk of serious ventricular arrhythmias and sudden death potentially associated with elevated plasma levels of thioridazine, PAXIL and thioridazine should not be co-administered (see Contraindications).

Fosamprenavir/Ritonavir: Co-administration of fosamprenavir/ritonavir with paroxetine significantly decreased plasma levels of paroxetine (by ~60% in one study). Any dose adjustment should be guided by clinical effect (tolerability and efficacy).

Tamoxifen: Tamoxifen is a pro-drug requiring metabolic activation by CYP2D6. Inhibition of CYP2D6 by paroxetine and other antidepressants can lead to reduced plasma concentrations of an active metabolite and hence potential for reduced efficacy of tamoxifen (see Warnings and Precautions, Potential for Reduced Efficacy of Tamoxifen with Concomitant SSRI use, Including PAXIL).

Drugs Metabolized by Cytochrome P450 (CYP3A4): An in vivo interaction study involving the co-administration under steady state conditions of PAXIL and terfenadine, a substrate for CYP3A4, revealed no effect of PAXIL on terfenadine pharmacokinetics. In addition, in vitro studies have shown ketoconazole, a potent inhibitor of CYP3A4 activity, to be at least 100 times more potent than paroxetine as an inhibitor of the metabolism of several substrates for this enzyme, including terfenadine, astemizole, cisapride, triazolam and cyclosporin. Based on the assumption that the relationship between paroxetine's in vitro Ki and its lack of effect on terfenadine's in vivo clearance predicts its effect on other CYP3A4 substrates, paroxetine's extent of inhibition of CYP3A4 activity would not be expected to be of clinical significance.

Microsomal Enzyme Inhibition/Induction: The metabolism and pharmacokinetics of PAXIL may be affected by the induction or inhibition of drug metabolizing enzymes.

Drugs Highly Bound to Plasma Protein: Paroxetine is highly bound to plasma protein, therefore administration of PAXIL to a patient taking another drug that is highly protein bound may cause increased free concentrations of the other drug, potentially resulting in adverse events. Conversely, adverse effects could result from displacement of paroxetine by other highly bound drugs.

Alcohol: The concomitant use of PAXIL and alcohol has not been studied and is not recommended. Patients should be advised to avoid alcohol while taking PAXIL.

Anticholinergic Drugs: PAXIL has been reported to increase significantly the systemic bioavailability of procyclidine. Steady state plasma levels of procyclidine (5 mg daily) were elevated by about 40% when 30 mg paroxetine was co-administered to steady-state. If anticholinergic effects are seen, the dose of procyclidine should be reduced.

Antiretroviral: Co-administration of fosamprenavir/ritonavir with paroxetine significantly decreased plasma levels of paroxetine (by ~60% in one study). Any dose adjustment should be guided by clinical effect (tolerability and efficacy).

Phenobarbital: Chronic daily dosing with phenobarbital (100 mg qid for 14 days) decreased the systemic availability of a single 30 mg dose of paroxetine in some subjects. The AUC and T½ of PAXIL were reduced by an average of 25% and 38% respectively compared to PAXIL administered alone. The effect of PAXIL on phenobarbital pharmacokinetics was not studied. No initial PAXIL dosage adjustment is considered necessary when co-administered with phenobarbital; any subsequent adjustment should be guided by clinical effect.

Anticonvulsants: In a limited number of patients with epilepsy on long-term treatment with anticonvulsants (carbamazepine 600-900 mg/day, n=6; phenytoin 250-400 mg/day, n=6; sodium valproate 300-2500 mg/day, n=8) the co-administration of PAXIL (30 mg/day for 10 days) had no significant effect on the plasma concentrations of these anticonvulsants. In healthy volunteers, co-administration of paroxetine with phenytoin has been associated with decreased plasma levels of paroxetine and an increased incidence of adverse experiences. However, no initial dosage adjustment of PAXIL is considered necessary when the drug is to be co-administered with known drug metabolizing enzyme inducers (e.g. carbamazepine, phenytoin, sodium valproate) and any subsequent dosage adjustment should be guided by clinical effect. Co-administration of PAXIL with anticonvulsants may be associated with an increased incidence of adverse experiences.

Antipsychotic Drugs/Neuroleptic Malignant Syndrome: As with other SSRIs, PAXIL should be used with caution in patients already receiving antipsychotics/ neuroleptics, since symptoms suggestive of Neuroleptic Malignant Syndrome cases have been reported with this combination (see Warnings and Precautions, Serotonin Syndrome/Neuroleptic Malignant Syndrome).

Serotonergic Drugs: Based on the mechanism of action of paroxetine and the potential for serotonin syndrome, caution is advised when PAXIL is coadministered with other drugs or agents that may affect the serotonergic neurotransmitter systems, such as tryptophan, triptans, serotonin reuptake inhibitors, lithium, fentanyl, tramadol, or St. John's wort (see Warnings and Precautions, Serotonin Syndrome/Neuroleptic Malignant Syndrome). Concomitant use of PAXIL and MAO inhibitors (including linezolid, an antibiotic which is a reversible non-selective MAO inhibitor) is contraindicated (see Contraindications).

Lithium: In a study of depressed patients stabilized on lithium, no pharmacokinetic interaction between paroxetine and lithium was observed. However, due to the potential for serotonin syndrome, caution is advised when PAXIL is coadministered with lithium.

Triptans: There have been rare postmarketing reports describing patients with weakness, hyperreflexia, and incoordination following the use of a selective serotonin reuptake inhibitor (SSRI) and the $5HT_1$ agonist, sumatriptan. If concomitant treatment with triptan and an SSRI (e.g., fluoxetine, fluvoxamine, paroxetine, sertraline) is clinically warranted, appropriate observation of the patient is advised. The possibility of such interactions should also be considered if other $5HT_1$ agonists are to be used in combination with SSRIs (see Warnings and Precautions, Serotonin Syndrome/Neuroleptic Malignant Syndrome).

Tryptophan: Tryptophan can be metabolized to serotonin. As with other serotonin reuptake inhibitors, the use of PAXIL together with tryptophan may result in adverse reactions consisting primarily of headache, nausea, sweating and dizziness as well as serotonin syndrome. Consequently, concomitant use of PAXIL with tryptophan is not recommended (see Warnings and Precautions, Serotonin Syndrome/Neuroleptic Malignant Syndrome).

CNS Drugs: Experience in a limited number of healthy subjects has shown that PAXIL does not increase the sedation and drowsiness associated with haloperidol, amylbarbitone or oxazepam, when given in combination. Since the effects of concomitant administration of PAXIL with neuroleptics have not been studied, the use of PAXIL with these drugs should be approached with caution.

Diazepam: A multiple dose study of the interaction between PAXIL and diazepam showed no alteration in the pharmacokinetics of PAXIL that would warrant changes in the dose of PAXIL for patients receiving both drugs. The effects of PAXIL on the pharmacokinetics of diazepam were not evaluated.

Cardiovascular Drugs: Multiple dose treatment with PAXIL 30 mg/day has little or no effect on the steady-state pharmacokinetics of digoxin (0.25 mg qd) or propanolol (80 mg bid).

Theophylline: Reports of elevated theophylline levels associated with PAXIL treatment have been reported. While this interaction has not been formally studied, it is recommended that theophylline levels be monitored when these drugs are concurrently administered.

Cimetidine: Steady state levels of PAXIL (30 mg daily) were elevated by about 50% when cimetidine (300 mg tid), a known drug metabolizing enzyme inhibitor, was co-administered to steady-state. Consideration should be given to using doses of PAXIL towards the lower end of the range when co-administered with known drug metabolizing enzyme inhibitors.

Drug-Food Interactions: The absorption and pharmacokinetics of PAXIL are not affected by food or antacids.

Drug-Herb Interactions: St. John's wort: In common with other SSRI's, pharmakodynamic interactions between paroxetine and the herbal remedy St. John's wort may occur and may result in an increase in undesirable effects.

Drug-Laboratory Test Interactions: Interactions with laboratory tests have not been established.

DOSAGE AND ADMINISTRATION: Dosing Considerations: General: PAXIL is not indicated for use in children under 18 years of age (see Warnings and Precautions, Potential Association with Behavioural and Emotional Changes, Including Self-Harm).

Lower initial doses of PAXIL are recommended for elderly and debilitated patients, and patients with renal or hepatic impairment (see Dosage and Administration, Special Patient Populations).

PAXIL should be administered once daily in the morning and may be taken with or without food. The tablet should be swallowed rather than chewed.

Dose Adjustments: Based on pharmacokinetic parameters, steady-state paroxetine plasma levels are achieved over a 7-14 day interval. Hence, dosage adjustments in 10 mg increments should be made at 1-2 week intervals or according to clinician judgment.

Maintenance: During long term therapy for any indication, the dosage should be maintained at the lowest effective level.

There is no body of evidence available to answer the question of how long a patient should continue to be treated with PAXIL. It is generally agreed that acute episodes of depression require several months or longer of sustained pharmacologic therapy. Whether the dose of an antidepressant needed to induce remission is identical to the dose needed to maintain and/or sustain euthymia is unknown.

Systematic evaluation of the efficacy of paroxetine hydrochloride has shown that efficacy is maintained for at least 6 months with doses that averaged about 30 mg.

Discontinuation of Treatment: Symptoms associated with the discontinuation of PAXIL have been reported in clinical trials and post marketing. Patients should be monitored for these and other symptoms when discontinuing treatment, regardless of the indication for which PAXIL is being prescribed (see Warnings and Precautions, Discontinuation of Treatment with PAXIL and Adverse Reactions, Adverse Events following Discontinuation of Treatment (or Dose Reduction)).

A gradual reduction in the dose rather than abrupt cessation is recommended whenever possible. If intolerable symptoms occur following a decrease in the dose or upon discontinuation of treatment, dose titration should be managed on the basis of the patient's clinical response (see Adverse Reactions).

Adults: Depression: Usual Adult Dose: The administration of PAXIL should be initiated at 20 mg daily. For most patients, 20 mg daily will also be the optimum dose. The therapeutic response may be delayed until the third or fourth week of treatment.

Dose Range: For those patients who do not respond adequately to the 20 mg daily dose, a gradual increase in dosage up to 40 mg daily may be considered. The maximum recommended daily dose is 50 mg.

Obsessive-Compulsive Disorder: Usual Adult Dose: The administration of PAXIL should be initiated at 20 mg daily. The recommended dose of PAXIL in the treatment of OCD is 40 mg daily.

Dose Range: For those patients who do not respond adequately to the 40 mg daily dose, a gradual increase in dosage may be considered. The maximum recommended daily dose is 60 mg.

Panic Disorder: Usual Adult Dose: The recommended starting dose of PAXIL in the treatment of panic disorder is 10 mg/day. The recommended dose of PAXIL in the treatment of panic disorder is 40 mg daily.

Dose Range: For those patients who do not respond adequately to the 40 mg daily dose, a gradual increase in dosage may be considered. The maximum recommended daily dose is 60 mg.

Social Phobia (Social Anxiety Disorder): Usual Adult Dose: The recommended initial dosage is 20 mg/day. No clear dose-relationship has been demonstrated over a 20 to 60 mg/day dose range.

Dose Range: Some patients not responding adequately to a 20 mg dosage may benefit from gradual dosage increases, in 10 mg/day increments, up to a maximum of 50 mg/day.

Generalized Anxiety Disorder: Usual Adult Dose: The recommended initial dosage is 20 mg/day.

Dose Range: Some patients not responding adequately to a 20 mg dosage may benefit from gradual dosage increases, in 10 mg/day increments, up to a maximum of 50 mg/day.

Post-Traumatic Stress Disorder: Usual Adult Dose: The recommended starting dosage is 20 mg/day.

Dose Range: Some patients not responding adequately to a 20 mg/day dosage may benefit from gradual dosage increases, in 10 mg/day increments, up to a maximum of 50 mg/day.

Special Patient Populations: Treatment of Pregnant Women: Epidemiological studies of pregnancy outcomes following maternal exposure to antidepressants in the first trimester have reported an increase in the risk of congenital malformations, particularly cardiovascular (e.g. ventricular and atrial septal defects), associated with the use of paroxetine. If a patient becomes pregnant while taking PAXIL, she should be informed of the current estimate of risk to the fetus (see Warnings and Precautions, Special Populations) and consideration should be given to switching to other treatment options. Treatment with PAXIL should only be continued for an individual patient, if the potential benefits outweigh the potential risks. For women who intend to become pregnant, or are in their first trimester of pregnancy, initiation of paroxetine should be considered only after other treatment options have been evaluated (see Warnings and Precautions, Special Populations for more details).

Post-marketing reports indicate that some neonates exposed to PAXIL, SSRIs, or other newer antidepressants late in the third trimester have developed complications requiring prolonged hospitalization, respiratory support, and tube feeding (see Warnings and Precautions, Special Populations). When treating pregnant women with PAXIL during the third trimester, the physician should carefully consider the potential risks and benefits of treatment. The physician may consider tapering PAXIL in the third trimester.

Geriatrics (>65 years): Administration of PAXIL to the elderly is associated with increased plasma levels and prolongation of the elimination half-life relative to younger adults (see Action and Clinical Pharmacology). The recommended initial dose is 10 mg/day for elderly and/or debilitated patients. The dose may be increased if indicated up to a maximum of 40 mg daily.

Pediatrics: PAXIL is not indicated for use in children under 18 years of age (see Indications and Clinical Use and Warnings and Precautions, Potential Association with Behavioural and Emotional Changes, Including Self-Harm).

Renal/Hepatic Impairment: PAXIL should be used with caution in patients with renal or hepatic impairment. The recommended initial dose is 10 mg/day in patients with clinically significant renal or hepatic impairment. A maximum dose of 40 mg should not be exceeded (see Warnings and Precautions and Action and Clinical Pharmacology).

OVERDOSAGE:

The largest known ingestion from which a patient has recovered is 2000 mg. The smallest known dose of paroxetine alone associated with a fatal outcome is approximately 400 mg.

Symptoms of Overdosage: The most commonly reported adverse events subsequent to paroxetine-only overdose include: somnolence, nausea, tremor, dizziness, vomiting, diarrhea, agitation, aggression, anxiety, confused state, headache, fatigue, insomnia, tachycardia, hyperhydrosis, mydriasis, convulsion, paraethesia, serotonin syndrome, fever, blood pressure changes, involuntary muscle contraction and loss of consciousness. It should be noted that in some cases, patients may have consumed alcohol in addition to taking an overdose of paroxetine. **Some of these symptoms may also be seen with clinical use.**

Events such as coma and ECG changes have also been reported.

Treatment of Overdosage: The physician should consider contacting a poison control centre for additional information on the treatment of any overdose.

No specific antidote is known. Treatment should consist of those general measures employed in the management of overdose with any antidepressant. Establish and maintain an airway; ensure adequate oxygenation and ventilation.

Induction of emesis is not recommended. Due to the large volume of distribution of PAXIL, forced diuresis, dialysis, hemoperfusion and exchange transfusion are unlikely to be of benefit.

Supportive care with frequent monitoring of vital signs and careful observation is indicated. An ECG should be taken and monitoring of cardiac function instituted if there is any evidence of abnormality. Patient management should be as clinically indicated, or as recommended by the national poisons centre, where available.

In managing overdosage, consider the possibility of multiple drug involvement.

A specific caution involves patients taking or recently having taken PAXIL who might ingest, by accident or intent, excessive quantities of a tricyclic antidepressant. In such a case, accumulation of the parent tricyclic and its active metabolite may increase the possibility of clinically significant sequelae and extend the time needed for close medical observation.

For management of a suspected drug overdose, contact your regional Poison Control Centre. See the *CPS* Directory section for a list of Poison Control Centres.

ACTION AND CLINICAL PHARMACOLOGY: Mechanism of Action: Paroxetine is a potent and selective serotonin (5-hydroxytryptamine, 5-HT) reuptake inhibitor (SSRI). This activity of the drug on brain neurons is thought to be responsible for its antidepressant and anxiolytic action in the treatment of depression, obsessive-compulsive disorder (OCD), panic disorder, social phobia (social anxiety disorder), generalized anxiety disorder (GAD) and post-traumatic stress disorder (PTSD). Paroxetine is a phenylpiperidine derivative which is chemically unrelated to the tricyclic or tetracyclic antidepressants. In receptor binding studies, paroxetine did not exhibit significant affinity for the adrenergic (α_1, α_2, β), dopaminergic, serotonergic ($5HT_1$, $5HT_2$), or histaminergic receptors of rat brain membrane. A weak affinity for the muscarinic acetylcholine receptor was evident. The predominant metabolites of paroxetine are essentially inactive as 5-HT reuptake inhibitors.

Pharmacokinetics: No clear dose relationship has been demonstrated for the antidepressant effects of paroxetine at doses above 20 mg/day. The results of fixed-dose studies comparing paroxetine and placebo in the treatment of depression, panic disorder, generalized anxiety disorder and post-traumatic stress disorder revealed a dose dependency for some adverse events.

Absorption: Paroxetine is well absorbed after oral administration. In healthy volunteers, the absorption of a single 30 mg oral dose of paroxetine was not appreciably affected by the presence or absence of food.

Both the rate of absorption and the terminal elimination half-life appear to be independent of dose. Steady-state plasma concentrations of paroxetine are generally achieved in 7 to 14 days. No correlation has been established between paroxetine plasma concentrations and therapeutic efficacy or the incidence of adverse reactions.

In healthy young volunteers receiving a 20 mg daily dose of paroxetine for 15 days, the mean maximal plasma concentration was 41 ng/mL at steady state (see Table 4). Peak plasma levels generally occurred within 3 to 7 hours.

Distribution: Owing to the extensive distribution of paroxetine into the tissues, less than 1% of the total drug in the body is believed to reside in the systemic circulation.

At therapeutic concentrations, the plasma protein binding of paroxetine is approximately 95%.

Metabolism: Paroxetine is subject to a biphasic process of metabolic elimination which involves presystemic (first-pass) and systemic pathways. First-pass metabolism is extensive, but may be partially saturable, accounting for the increased bioavailability observed with multiple dosing. The metabolism of paroxetine is accomplished in part by cytochrome P450 ($2D_6$). Saturation of this enzyme at clinical doses appears to account for the nonlinearity of paroxetine kinetics with increasing dose and increasing duration of treatment. The role of this enzyme in paroxetine metabolism also suggests potential drug-drug interactions (see Drug Interactions). The majority of the dose appears to be oxidized to a catechol intermediate which is converted to highly polar glucuronide and sulphate metabolites through methylation and conjugation reactions. The glucuronide and sulphate conjugates of paroxetine are about >10 000 and 3000 times less potent, respectively, than the parent compound as inhibitors of 5-HT reuptake in rat brain synaptosomes.

Excretion: Following the single or multiple dose administration of paroxetine at doses of 20 to 50 mg, the mean elimination half-life value for healthy subjects appears to be about 24 hours, although a range of 3 to 65 hours has been reported.

Approximately 64% of an administered dose of paroxetine is eliminated by the kidneys and 36% in the faeces. Less than 2% of the dose is recovered in the form of the parent compound.

Special Populations and Conditions: Geriatrics: In elderly subjects, increased steady-state plasma concentrations and prolongation of the elimination half-life were observed relative to younger adult controls (Table 4). Elderly patients should, therefore, be initiated and maintained at the lowest daily dosage of paroxetine which is associated with clinical efficacy (see Dosage and Administration).

Hepatic Insufficiency: The results from a multiple dose pharmacokinetic study in subjects with severe hepatic dysfunction suggest that the clearance of paroxetine is markedly reduced in this patient group (see Table 4). As the elimination of paroxetine is dependent upon extensive hepatic metabolism, its use in patients with hepatic impairment should be undertaken with caution. (see Dosage and Administration, Special Patient Populations).

Renal Insufficiency: In a single dose pharmacokinetic study in patients with mild to severe renal impairment, plasma levels of paroxetine tended to increase with deteriorating renal function (see Table 5). As multiple-dose pharmacokinetic studies have not been performed in patients with renal disease, paroxetine should be used with caution in such patients (see Dosage and Administration, Special Patient Populations).

Table 4: PAXIL

Steady-state Pharmacokinetics of Paroxetine after Doses of 20 mg Daily (mean and range)

	Young Healthy Subjects (n=22)	Elderly Healthy Subjects (n=22)	Hepatically[a] Impaired Subjects (n=10)
$C_{max(ss)}$ (ng/mL)	41 (12–90)	87 (18–154)	87 (11–147)
$T_{max(ss)}$ (hours)	5.0 (3–7)	5.0 (1–10)	6.4 (2–11)
$C_{min(ss)}$ (ng/mL)	21 (4–51)	58 (9–127)	66 (7–128)
$AUC_{(ss)}$ (ng·h/mL)	660 (179–1436)	1580 (221–3286)	1720 (194–3283)
$T_{½}$(hours)	19 (8–43)	31 (13–92)	66 (17–152)

[a] Galactose elimination capacity 30 to 70% of normal.

Legend: C_{max}=maximum plasma concentration; T_{max}=time to reach C_{max}; $AUC_{(ss)}$=area under the plasma concentration time curve between dosing intervals (i.e., 24 hours) at steady state; $T_{½}$=terminal elimination half-life; $_{ss}$=steady state.

A wide range of interindividual variation is observed for the pharmacokinetic parameters.

STORAGE AND STABILITY: Store at 15-30°C.

INFORMATION FOR THE PATIENT: Published in e-CPS, available by subscription at www.e-cps.ca.

DOSAGE FORMS, COMPOSITION AND PACKAGING: 10 mg: Each yellow, bisected, film-coated, oval, biconvex tablet, with the product name engraved on one side and strength engraved on the other side, contains: paroxetine HCl USP equivalent to paroxetine free base 10 mg. Nonmedicinal ingredients: dibasic calcium phosphate dihydrate, hydroxypropyl methylcellulose, hypromellose, magnesium stearate, polyethylene glycols, polysorbate 80, sodium starch glycolate and titanium dioxide. Bottles of 30.

Table 5: PAXIL

Pharmacokinetics of Paroxetine after a Single 30 mg Dose in Normal Subjects and Those with Renal Impairment

	[a]Renally Impaired Severe (n=6)	[b]Renally Impaired Moderate (n=6)	[c]Healthy Young Subjects (n=6)
C_{max} (ng/mL)	46.2 (35.9–56.7)	36 (3.6–59.4)	19.8 (1.4–54.8)
T_{max} (hours)	6.5 (4.0–11.0)	4.8 (1.5–9.0)	4.3 (1–7)
AUC_{∞} (ng·h/mL)	2046 (605–3695)	1053 (48–2087)	574 (21–2196)
$T_{½}$ (hours)	29.7 (10.9–54.8)	18.3 (11.2–32.0)	17.3 (9.6–25.1)

[a] Creatinine clearance=13–27 mL/min.
[b] Creatinine clearance=32–46 mL/min.
[c] Creatinine clearance >100 mL/min.

Legend: C_{max}=maximum plasma concentration; T_{max}=time to reach C_{max}; AUC_{∞}=area under the plasma concentration time curve at infinity; $T_{½}$=terminal elimination half-life.

20 mg: Each pink, bisected, film-coated, oval, biconvex tablet, with the product name engraved on one side and strength engraved on the other side, contains: paroxetine HCl USP equivalent to paroxetine free base 20 mg. Nonmedicinal ingredients: dibasic calcium phosphate dihydrate, hydroxypropyl methylcellulose, hypromellose, magnesium stearate, polyethylene glycols, polysorbate 80, sodium starch glycolate and titanium dioxide. Bottles of 100 and 500.

30 mg: Each blue, film-coated, oval, biconvex tablet, with the product name engraved on one side and strength engraved on the other side, contains: paroxetine HCl USP equivalent to paroxetine free base 30 mg. Nonmedicinal ingredients: dibasic calcium phosphate dihydrate, hydroxypropyl methylcellulose, hypromellose, magnesium stearate, polyethylene glycols, polysorbate 80, sodium starch glycolate and titanium dioxide. Bottles of 30.

The 10, 20 and 30 mg tablets also contain one or more of the following: D&C Red No. 30 Aluminum Lake, D&C Yellow No. 10 Aluminum Lake, FD&C Blue No. 2 Aluminum Lake and FD&C Yellow No. 6 Aluminum Lake.

(Shown in Product Identification Section)

The reader is invited to consult CPhA's monograph **Selective Serotonin Reuptake Inhibitors**.

Paxil CR®

paroxetine HCl

Selective Serotonin Reuptake Inhibitor

GlaxoSmithKline

Date of Revision: May 28, 2010

SUMMARY PRODUCT INFORMATION:

Route of Administration	Dosage Form/Strength	Nonmedicinal Ingredients
Oral	12.5 mg and 25 mg controlled release tablets	This product contains lactose monohydrate. Nonmedicinal ingredients are: colloidal silicon dioxide, glyceryl behenate, hydroxypropyl methylcellulose, magnesium stearate, methacrylic acid copolymer type C, polyethylene glycol, polysorbate 80, polyvinylpyrrolidone, sodium lauryl sulphate, talc, titanium dioxide, triethyl citrate. PAXIL CR 12.5 mg tablets also contain D&C yellow No. 10 aluminium lake, FD&C yellow No. 6 aluminium lake, and yellow ferric oxide. PAXIL CR 25 mg tablets also contains D&C red No. 30 aluminium lake and red ferric oxide. PAXIL CR 37.5 mg tablets also contain FD&C blue No. 2 and yellow ferric oxide.

INDICATIONS AND CLINICAL USE: Adults: Depression: PAXIL CR (paroxetine hydrochloride) is indicated for symptomatic relief of Major Depressive Disorder.

PAXIL CR has not been systematically evaluated beyond 12 weeks in controlled clinical trials; however, the effectiveness of immediate release paroxetine hydrochloride in maintaining a response in depression for at least 6 months has been demonstrated in a placebo controlled trial. The physician who elects to use PAXIL CR for extended periods should periodically re-evaluate the long-term usefulness of the drug for the individual patient.

Panic Disorder: PAXIL CR is indicated for the symptomatic treatment of panic disorder, with or without agoraphobia.

Panic disorder (DSM-IV) is characterized by recurrent unexpected panic attacks, i.e., a discrete period of intense fear or discomfort in which four (or more) of the following symptoms develop abruptly and reach a peak within 10 minutes: (1) palpitations, pounding heart, or accelerated heart rate; (2) sweating; (3) trembling or shaking; (4) sensations of shortness of breath or smothering; (5) feeling of choking; (6) chest pain or discomfort; (7) nausea or abdominal distress; (8) feeling dizzy, unsteady, lightheaded, or faint; (9) derealization (feelings of unreality) or depersonalization (being detached from oneself); (10) fear of losing control; (11) fear of dying; (12) paresthesias (numbness or tingling sensations); (13) chills or hot flushes.

Social Phobia (Social Anxiety Disorder): PAXIL CR is indicated for the symptomatic relief of generalized social phobia (social anxiety disorder), a disorder characterized by marked and persistent fear, anxious anticipation, or avoidance of multiple social situations (e.g. interacting with strangers, attending social gatherings, dealing with authority figures) and/or performance situations (e.g. eating, writing, working while being observed, or public speaking). A diagnosis of social phobia/social anxiety disorder should not be made unless the fear, anxious anticipation, or avoidance of social and/or performance situations interferes significantly with the person's normal routine, occupational functioning, or social life, or causes marked distress.

Premenstrual Dysphoric Disorder: PAXIL CR is indicated for the symptomatic treatment of premenstrual dysphoric disorder (PMDD). The efficacy of PAXIL CR in the treatment of PMDD was established in 3 placebo-controlled trials.

The essential features of PMDD, according to DSM-IV, include markedly depressed mood, anxiety or tension, affective lability, and persistent anger or irritability. Other features include decreased interest in usual activities, difficulty concentrating, lack of energy, change in appetite or sleep, and feeling out of control. Physical symptoms associated with PMDD include breast tenderness, headache, joint and muscle pain, bloating, and weight gain. These symptoms occur regularly, in most menstrual cycles, during the luteal phase and remit within a few days following the onset of menses; the disturbance markedly interferes with work or school or with usual social activities and relationships with others. Typically, the symptoms are comparable in severity (but not duration) to those of a major depressive episode. The presence of the cyclical pattern of symptoms must be confirmed by at least two consecutive months of prospective daily symptom ratings. It is estimated that at least 75% of women report minor or isolated premenstrual changes; however, only 3 to 5% of women experience symptoms that may meet the criteria for PMDD. In making the diagnosis, care should be taken to rule out other cyclical mood disorders that may be exacerbated by treatment with an antidepressant.

Long-term Use of PAXIL CR: The effectiveness of PAXIL CR in long-term use (i.e. more than 12 weeks for depression, panic disorder and social phobia and more than 3 menstrual cycles for premenstrual dysmorphic disorder) has not yet been established in controlled trials for depression, panic disorder, social phobia or premenstrual dysmorphic disorder. The physician who elects to use PAXIL CR for extended periods in these indications should periodically re-evaluate the long-term usefulness of the drug for individual patients (see Dosage and Administration).
Geriatrics (>65 years of age): Evidence from clinical studies indicates that there are differences in the pharmacokinetic profile of paroxetine in the geriatric population relative to younger adults, which may be associated with differences in safety or effectiveness. A brief discussion can be found in the appropriate sections (see Warnings and Precautions, Special Populations, Geriatrics (≥65 years of age); Action and Clinical Pharmacology and Dosage and Administration).
Pediatrics (<18 years of age): PAXIL CR is not indicated for use in patients below the age of 18 years (see Warnings and Precautions, General, Potential Association with Behavioural and Emotional Changes, Including Self-harm).

CONTRAINDICATIONS: Hypersensitivity: PAXIL CR (paroxetine hydrochloride) is contraindicated in patients who are known to be hypersensitive to the drug or any of its components. For a complete listing, see Dosage Forms, Composition and Packaging.
Monoamine Oxidase Inhibitors: In patients receiving serotonin reuptake inhibitors (SSRIs) in combination with a MAO inhibitor, there have been reports of serious, sometimes fatal, reactions including hyperthermia, rigidity, myoclonus, autonomic instability with possible rapid fluctuations of vital signs, and mental status changes that include extreme agitation progressing to delirium and coma. These reactions have also been reported in patients who have recently discontinued SSRI treatment and have begun treatment on a MAO inhibitor. Some cases presented with features resembling serotonin syndrome or neuroleptic malignant syndrome (see Warnings and Precautions, Neurologic, Serotonin Syndrome/Neuroleptic Malignant Syndrome). Therefore, PAXIL CR should not be used in combination with MAO inhibitors (including linezolid, an antibiotic which is a reversible non-selective MAO inhibitor) or within a minimum of 2 weeks of terminating treatment with MAO inhibitors. Treatment with PAXIL CR should then be initiated cautiously and dosage increased gradually until optimal response is reached. MAO inhibitors should not be introduced within 2 weeks of cessation of therapy with PAXIL CR.
Thioridazine: Thioridazine administration alone produces prolongation of the QTc interval, which is associated with serious ventricular arrhythmias, such as torsades de pointes-type arrhythmias, and sudden death. This effect appears to be dose-related. An in vivo study suggests that drugs which inhibit P450 2D6, including certain SSRI's such as paroxetine, fluoxetine and fluvoxamine, will elevate plasma levels of thioridazine. Therefore, PAXIL CR should not be used in combination with thioridazine or within a minimum of 2 weeks of terminating treatment with thioridazine. At least 2 weeks should be allowed after discontinuing PAXIL CR therapy before initiating treatment with thioridazine.
Pimozide: The concomitant use of PAXIL CR and pimozide is contraindicated as paroxetine has been shown to increase plasma pimozide levels. Elevation of pimozide blood concentration may result in QT interval prolongation and severe arrhythmias including torsade de pointes (see Drug Interactions).

WARNINGS AND PRECAUTIONS: General: Potential Association with Behavioural and Emotional Changes, Including Self-harm: Pediatrics: Placebo-Controlled Trial Data:

- **Recent analyses of placebo-controlled clinical trial safety databases from SSRIs and other newer antidepressants suggests that use of these drugs in patients under the age of 18 may be associated with behavioural and emotional changes, including an increased risk of suicidal ideation and behaviour over that of placebo.**
- **The small denominators in the clinical trial database, as well as the variability in placebo rates, preclude reliable conclusions on the relative safety profiles among these drugs.**

Adult and Pediatrics: Additional Data:

- **There are clinical trial and post-marketing reports with SSRIs and other newer antidepressants, in both pediatrics and adults, of severe agitation-type adverse events coupled with self-harm or harm to others. The agitation-type events include: akathisia, agitation, disinhibition, emotional lability, hostility, aggression, depersonalization. In some cases, the events occurred within several weeks of starting treatment.**

Rigorous clinical monitoring for suicidal ideation or other indicators of potential for suicidal behaviour is advised in patients of all ages. This includes monitoring for agitation-type emotional and behavioural changes.
Discontinuation Symptoms: Patients currently taking PAXIL CR should not be discontinued abruptly, due to risk of discontinuation symptoms. At the time that a medical decision is made to discontinue an SSRI or other newer antidepressant drug, a gradual reduction in the dose rather than an abrupt cessation is recommended.
Discontinuation of Treatment with PAXIL CR: When discontinuing treatment, patients should be monitored for symptoms which may be associated with discontinuation [e.g. dizziness, sleep disturbances including abnormal dreams, sensory disturbances (including paresthesias, electric shock sensations and tinnitus), agitation, anxiety, headache, tremor, confusion, diarrhea, nausea, vomiting and sweating] or other symptoms which may be of clinical significance [see Adverse Reactions, Adverse Events following Discontinuation of Treatment (or Dose Reduction), Post-Marketing]. A gradual reduction in the dose rather than abrupt cessation is recommended whenever possible. If intolerable symptoms occur following a decrease in the dose or upon discontinuation of treatment, dose titration should be managed on the basis of the patient's clinical response. (See Adverse Reactions and Dosage and Administration.)
PAXIL CR Treatment During Pregnancy Effects on Newborns: Epidemiological studies of pregnancy outcomes following maternal exposure to antidepressants in the first trimester have reported an increase in the risk of congenital malformations, particularly cardiovascular (e.g. ventricular and atrial septal defects), associated with the use of paroxetine. If a patient becomes pregnant while taking PAXIL CR, consideration should be given to switching to other treatment options. Treatment with PAXIL CR should only be continued for an individual pregnant patient, if the potential benefits outweigh the potential risks. Initiation of paroxetine, for women who intend to become pregnant, or are in their first trimester of pregnancy, should be considered only after other treatment options have been evaluated (see Warnings and Precautions, Special Populations).

Post-marketing reports indicate that some neonates exposed to PAXIL CR, SSRIs (Selective Serotonin Reuptake Inhibitors), or other newer antidepressants late in the third trimester have developed complications requiring prolonged hospitalization, respiratory support, and tube feeding. Such complications can arise immediately upon delivery. When treating a pregnant woman with PAXIL CR during the third trimester, the physician should carefully consider the potential risks and benefits of treatment (see Warnings and Precautions, Special Populations and Dosage and Administration, Special Patient Populations, Treatment of Pregnant Women during the third trimester).
Potential for Reduced Efficacy of Tamoxifen with Concomitant SSRI use, Including PAXIL CR: The antitumor agent tamoxifen is a pro-drug requiring metabolic activation by CYP2D6. Inhibition of CYP2D6 can lead to reduced plasma concentrations of a primary active metabolite (endoxifen). Chronic use of CYP2D6 inhibitors, including certain SSRIs, together with tamoxifen can lead to persistent reduction in levels of endoxifen (see also Drug Interactions, Tamoxifen). The clinical significance of this in terms of efficacy of tamoxifen is unclear.
Psychomotor Impairment: Although paroxetine did not cause sedation or interfere with psychomotor performance in placebo-controlled studies in normal subjects, patients should be advised to avoid driving a car or operating hazardous machinery until they are reasonably certain that PAXIL CR does not affect them adversely.
Bone Fracture Risk: Epidemiological studies show an increased risk of bone fractures following exposure to some antidepressants, including SSRIs. The risks appear to be greater at the initial stages of treatment, but significant increased risks were also observed at later stages of treatment. The possibility of fracture should be considered in the care of patients treated with PAXIL CR. Elderly patients and patients with important risk factors for bone fractures should be advised of possible adverse events which increase the risk of falls, such as dizziness and orthostatic hypotension, especially at the early stages of treatment but also soon after withdrawal. Preliminary data from observational studies show association of SSRIs and low bone mineral density in older men and women. Until further information becomes available, a possible effect on bone mineral density with long term treatment with SSRIs, including PAXIL CR, cannot be excluded, and may be a potential concern for patients with osteoporosis or major risk factors for bone fractures.

The following additional precautions are listed alphabetically.
Cardiovascular: PAXIL CR or PAXIL IR have not been evaluated or used to any appreciable extent in patients with a recent history of myocardial infarction or unstable heart disease. The usual precautions should be observed in patients with cardiac conditions.
Concomitant Illnesses: Clinical experience with PAXIL CR or PAXIL IR in patients with certain concomitant systemic illnesses is limited. Caution is advisable in using PAXIL CR in patients with diseases or conditions that could affect metabolism or hemodynamic responses.
Dependence/Tolerance: PAXIL CR or PAXIL IR have not been systematically studied, in animals or humans, for its potential for abuse, tolerance, or physical dependence. Physicians should carefully evaluate patients for history of drug abuse and follow such patients closely, observing them for signs of misuse or abuse of PAXIL CR.
Endocrine and Metabolism: Serum Cholesterol Elevation: Several public domain studies have shown increased LDL-cholesterol levels of ~10% in volunteers and patients taking paroxetine for 8 to 12 weeks, which generally normalized after paroxetine discontinuation. In addition, of the patients in placebo-controlled clinical trials for whom baseline and on-treatment measurements were taken, total serum levels of cholesterol showed a mean increase of ~1.5 mg/dL in n=653 paroxetine-treated patients, compared to a mean decrease of ~5.0 mg/dL in placebo-treated patients (n=379). Increases from baseline of 45 mg/dL or greater were recorded in 6.6% of paroxetine-treated patients compared to 2.6% of placebo-treated patients (see Monitoring and Laboratory Tests, Serum Cholesterol Elevation).

These data should be taken into consideration when treating patients with underlying cardiac risk factors.
Hematologic: Abnormal Bleeding: There have been several reports of abnormal bleeding (mostly ecchymosis) associated with paroxetine IR treatment, including a report of impaired platelet aggregation. While a causal relationship to paroxetine is unclear, impaired platelet aggregation may result from platelet serotonin depletion and contribute to such occurrences.

Skin and mucous membrane bleedings (including upper gastrointestinal bleeding) have been reported following treatment with paroxetine IR. Paroxetine CR should therefore be used with caution in patients concomitantly treated with drugs that give an increased risk for bleeding (e.g. anticoagulants, nonsteroidal anti-inflammatories and ASA) and in patients with a known tendency for bleeding or those with predisposing conditions.
Hepatic/Biliary/Pancreatic: Hepatic Impairment: Pharmacokinetic studies of PAXIL IR in subjects with clinically significant hepatic impairment suggest that prolongation of the elimination half-life and increased plasma levels can be expected in this patient group. PAXIL CR should be used with caution and dosages restricted to the lower end of the range in patients with clinically significant hepatic impairment (see Dosage and Administration, Special Patient Populations and Actions and Clinical Pharmacology, Hepatic Insufficiency).
Neurologic: Epilepsy: As with other antidepressants, PAXIL CR should be used with caution in patients with epilepsy.
Seizures: During clinical trials, the overall incidence of seizures was 0.15% in patients treated with PAXIL IR. However, patients with a history of convulsive disorders were excluded from these studies. Caution is recommended when the drug is administered to patients with a history of seizures. The drug should be discontinued in any patient who develops seizures.
Serotonin Syndrome/Neuroleptic Malignant Syndrome: On rare occasions serotonin syndrome or neuroleptic malignant syndrome-like events have occurred in association with treatment of PAXIL CR, particularly when given in combination with other serotonergic and/or neuroleptic/antipsychotic drugs. As these syndromes may result in potentially life-threatening conditions, treatment with PAXIL CR should be discontinued if patients develop a combination of symptoms possibly including hyperthermia, rigidity, myoclonus, autonomic instability with possible rapid fluctuations of vital signs, mental status changes including confusion, irritability, extreme agitation progressing to delirium and coma, and supportive symptomatic treatment should be initiated. Due to the risk of serotonergic syndrome or neuroleptic malignant syndrome PAXIL CR should not be used in combination with MAO inhibitors or serotonin-precursors (such as L-tryptophan, oxitriptan) and should be used with caution in patients receiving other serotonergic drugs (e.g., triptans, lithium, tramadol, St. John's wort, most tricyclic antidepressants) or neuroleptics/antipsychotics (see Contraindications and Drug Interactions).
Ophthalmologic: Glaucoma: As with other SSRIs, PAXIL CR can cause mydriasis and should be used with caution in patients with narrow angle glaucoma.
Psychiatric: Suicide: The possibility of a suicide attempt is inherent in depression and may persist until remission occurs. Patients with depression may experience worsening of their depressive symptoms and/or the emergence of suicidal ideation and behaviours (suicidality) whether or not they are taking antidepressant medications. Notwithstanding, high risk patients should be closely supervised throughout therapy with appropriate consideration to the possible need for hospitalization. In order to minimize the opportunity for overdosage, prescriptions for PAXIL CR should be written for the smallest quantity of drug consistent with good patient management.

Because of the well established comorbidity between depression and other psychiatric disorders, the same precautions observed when treating patients with depression should be observed when treating patients with other psychiatric disorders (see **Warnings and Precautions,** Potential Association with Behavioural and Emotional Changes, Including Self-harm).
Activation of Mania/Hypomania: During clinical testing in a patient population comprised primarily of unipolar depressed patients, approximately 1% of PAXIL IR-treated patients experienced manic reactions. When bipolar patients were considered as a sub-group the incidence of mania was 2%. As with all drugs effective in the treatment of depression, PAXIL CR should be used with caution in patients with a history of mania.

A major depressive episode may be the initial presentation of bipolar disorder. Patients with bipolar disorder may be at an increased risk of experiencing manic episodes when treated with antidepressants alone. Therefore, the decision to initiate symptomatic treatment of depression should only be made after patients have been adequately assessed to determine if they are at risk for bipolar disorder.
Electroconvulsive Therapy (ECT): The efficacy and safety of the concurrent use of PAXIL CR and ECT have not been studied.
Renal: Hyponatremia: Several cases of hyponatremia have been reported. The hyponatremia appeared to be reversible when PAXIL IR was discontinued. The majority of these occurrences have been in elderly individuals, some in patients taking diuretics or who were otherwise volume depleted.
Renal Impairment: Since PAXIL CR is extensively metabolized by the liver, excretion of unchanged drug in urine is a minor route of elimination. However, single dose pharmacokinetic studies in subjects with clinically significant renal impairment suggest that plasma levels of paroxetine are elevated in such subjects. Paroxetine should therefore be used with caution and the dosage restricted to the lower end of the range in patients with clinically significant renal impairment (see Dosage and Administration, Special Patient Populations and Actions and Clinical Pharmacology, Renal Insufficiency).
Special Populations: Pregnant Women and Newborns: Risk of Cardiovascular Malformations Following First Trimester Exposure to SSRIs: Epidemiological studies of pregnancy outcomes following maternal exposure to antidepressants in the first trimester have reported an increase in the risk of congenital malformations, particularly cardiovascular (e.g. ventricular and atrial septal defects), associated with the use of paroxetine. The data suggest that the risk of having an infant with a cardiovascular defect following maternal paroxetine exposure is approximately 1/50 (2%), compared with an expected rate for such defects of approximately 1/100 (1%) infants in the general population. In general, septal defects range from those that are symptomatic and may require surgery, to those that are asymptomatic and may resolve spontaneously. Information about the severity of the septal defects reported in the studies is not available.
While on PAXIL CR: Pregnancy, or intent to become pregnant: If a patient becomes pregnant while taking PAXIL CR, or intends to become pregnant, she should be informed of the current estimate of increased risk to the fetus with PAXIL CR over other antidepressants. Examinations of additional databases, as well as updated analyses, may result in changes to the current risk estimates. Consideration should be given to switching to other treatment options, including another antidepressant or non-pharmaceutical treatment such as cognitive behavioural therapy. Treatment with PAXIL CR should only be continued for an individual patient, if the potential benefits outweigh the potential risks.

Due to the potential for discontinuation symptoms, if a decision is taken to discontinue PAXIL CR treatment, a gradual reduction in the dose rather than an abrupt cessation is recommended (see Warnings and Precautions, Discontinuation of Treatment with PAXIL CR, Adverse Reactions, Adverse Events following Discontinuation of Treatment (or Dose Reduction) and Dosage and Administration, Discontinuation of Treatment with PAXIL CR).
Initiation of Paroxetine: For women who intend to become pregnant, or are in their first trimester of pregnancy, initiation of paroxetine should be considered only after other treatment options have been evaluated.
Complications Following Late Third Trimester Exposure to SSRIs: Post-marketing reports indicate that some neonates exposed to PAXIL CR, SSRIs (Selective Serotonin Reuptake Inhibitors), or other newer antidepressants late in the third trimester have developed complications requiring prolonged hospitalization, respiratory support, and tube feeding. Such complications can arise immediately upon delivery. Reported clinical findings have included respiratory distress, cyanosis, apnea, seizures, temperature instability, feeding difficulty, vomiting, hypoglycemia, hypotonia, hypertonia, hyperreflexia, tremor, jitteriness, irritability, and constant crying. These features are consistent with either a direct toxic effect of SSRIs and other newer antidepressants, or, possibly, a drug discontinuation syndrome. It should be noted that, in some cases, the clinical picture is consistent with serotonin syndrome (see Warnings and Precautions, Neurologic, Serotonin Syndrome/Neuroleptic Malignant Syndrome). When treating a pregnant woman with PAXIL CR during the third trimester, the physician should carefully consider the potential risks and benefits of treatment (see Dosage and Administration, Special Patient Populations, Treatment of Pregnant Women during the third trimester).

There have been post-marketing reports of premature birth in pregnant women exposed to paroxetine or other SSRIs. The causal relationship between PAXIL CR and the emergence of these events has not been established.
Risk of PPHN and Exposure to SSRIs (including paroxetine): Epidemiological studies on persistent pulmonary hypertension of the newborn (PPHN) have shown that the use of SSRIs (including PAXIL CR) in pregnancy, particularly use in late pregnancy, was associated with an increased risk of PPHN. PPHN occurs in 1-2 per 1 000 live births in the general population and is associated with substantial neonatal morbidity and mortality. In a retrospective case-control study of 377 women whose infants were born with PPHN and 836 women whose infants were born healthy, the risk for developing PPHN was approximately six-fold higher for infants exposed to SSRIs after the 20th week of gestation compared to infants who had not been exposed to antidepressants during pregnancy (Odds Ratio 6.1, 95% CI 2.2-16.8). A study using data from the Swedish Medical Birth Register for 831 324 infants born in 1997-2005 found an increased risk of PPHN of approximately 2-fold associated with patient-reported maternal use of SSRIs in the first trimester of pregnancy (Risk Ratio 2.4, 95% CI 1.2-4.3), and an increased risk of PPHN of approximately 4-fold associated with a combination of patient-reported maternal use of SSRIs in the first trimester and an antenatal SSRI prescription in later pregnancy (Risk Ratio 3.6, 95% CI 1.2-8.3).

Nursing Women: The concentrations of paroxetine detected in the breast milk of lactating women are similar to those in the mother's plasma. Lactating women should not nurse their infants while receiving paroxetine unless in the opinion of the treating physician, breast feeding is necessary, in which case the infant should be closely monitored.

Pediatrics (<18 years of age): PAXIL CR is not indicated for use in patients below the age of 18 years (see Warnings and Precautions, Potential Association with Behavioural and Emotional Changes, Including Self-harm). See also Indications, Pediatrics (<18 years of age) and Dosage and Administration, Special Patient Populations, Pediatrics).

Controlled clinical studies in depression failed to demonstrate efficacy and do not support the use of paroxetine in the treatment of children under the age of 18 years with depression. Moreover, a higher incidence of adverse events related to behavioural and emotional changes, including self harm, was reported with paroxetine treatment compared to placebo during controlled clinical trials in depression, OCD and social anxiety disorder (see Adverse Reactions, Clinical Trial Adverse Drug Reactions, Pediatrics).

Geriatrics (≥65 years of age): Administration of PAXIL CR to the elderly is associated with increased plasma levels and prolongation of the elimination half-life relative to younger adult (see Action and Clinical Pharmacology). Elderly patients should be initiated and maintained at the lowest daily dose of paroxetine which is associated with clinical efficacy (see Dosage and Administration).

Evaluation of approximately 800 elderly patients (≥65 years) treated with PAXIL IR (10-40 mg daily) in worldwide premarketing clinical trials revealed no unusual pattern of adverse events relative to the clinical experience in younger patients.

In a controlled study focusing specifically on elderly patients with depression, PAXIL CR (12.5-50 mg daily) was demonstrated to be safe and effective in the treatment of elderly patients (>60 years of age) with depression (see Adverse Reactions, Table 3). However, it is not possible to rule out potential age-related differences in safety and effectiveness during chronic use, particularly in elderly patients who have concomitant systemic illnesses or who are receiving concomitant drugs.

Monitoring and Laboratory Tests: Serum Cholesterol Elevation: Of the patients in placebo-controlled clinical trials for whom baseline and on-treatment measurements were taken, increases from baseline of 45 mg/dL or greater were recorded in 6.6% of paroxetine-treated patients compared to 2.6% of placebo-treated patients (see Adverse Reactions, Laboratory Changes—Cholesterol and Warnings and Precautions, Endocrine and Metabolism).

These data should be taken into consideration when treating patients with underlying cardiac risk factors.

ADVERSE REACTIONS: Adverse Drug Reaction Overview: Commonly Observed Adverse Events: Depression: The most commonly observed adverse events associated with the use of PAXIL CR in a pool of two trials (incidence of 5.0% or greater and incidence for PAXIL CR at least twice that for placebo, derived from Table 2) were: abnormal ejaculation, abnormal vision, constipation, decreased libido, diarrhea, dizziness, female genital disorders, nausea, somnolence, sweating, trauma, tremor, and yawning. Using the same criteria, the adverse events associated with the use of PAXIL CR in a study of elderly patients with depression were: abnormal ejaculation, constipation, decreased appetite, dry mouth, impotence, infection, libido decreased, sweating, and tremor.

Panic Disorder: In the pool of panic disorder studies, the adverse events meeting these criteria were: abnormal ejaculation, somnolence, impotence, libido decreased, tremor, sweating, and female genital disorders (generally anorgasmia or difficulty achieving orgasm).

Social Anxiety Disorder: The most commonly observed adverse events associated with the use of PAXIL CR (incidence of 5.0% or greater and incidence for PAXIL CR at least twice that for placebo, derived from Table 5) in the social phobia (social anxiety disorder) study were nausea, asthenia, abnormal ejaculation, sweating, somnolence, impotence, insomnia, and libido decreased.

Premenstrual Dysphoric Disorder: The most commonly observed adverse events associated with the use of PAXIL CR, either during continuous dosing or luteal phase dosing (incidence of 5.0% or greater and incidence for PAXIL CR at least twice that for placebo, derived from Table 6) were: nausea, asthenia, libido decreased, somnolence, insomnia, female genital disorders, sweating, dizziness, diarrhea and constipation.

In the luteal phase dosing PMDD trial, which employed dosing of 12.5 mg/day or 25 mg/day of PAXIL CR limited to the 2 weeks prior to the onset of menses over 3 consecutive menstrual cycles, adverse events were evaluated during the first 14 days of each off-drug phase. When the 3 off-drug phases were combined, the following adverse events were reported at an incidence of 2% or greater for PAXIL CR and were at least twice the rate of that reported for placebo: infection (5.3% versus 2.5%), depression (2.8% versus 0.8%), insomnia (2.4% versus 0.8%), sinusitis (2.4% versus 0%), and asthenia (2.0% versus 0.8%).

Adverse Events Leading to Discontinuation of Treatment: The information included under the "Adverse Events Leading to Discontinuation of Treatment" subsection of Adverse Reactions is based on data from seven short-term placebo-controlled clinical trials. Three of these studies were conducted in patients with depression, three studies were done in patients with panic disorder, and one study was conducted in patients with social anxiety disorder. Two of the studies in depression, which enrolled patients in the age range 18 to 65 years, are pooled. Information from a third study of depression, which focussed on elderly patients (ages 60 to 88), is presented separately as is the information from the panic disorder studies and the information from the social anxiety disorder study. Information on additional adverse events associated with PAXIL CR and the immediate-release formulation of paroxetine hydrochloride is included in a separate subsection (see Other Events Observed During the Clinical Development of Paroxetine).

Depression: Ten percent (21/212) of PAXIL CR patients discontinued treatment due to an adverse event in a pool of two studies of patients with depression. The most common events (≥1%) associated with discontinuation and considered to be drug related (i.e., those events associated with dropout at a rate approximately twice or greater for PAXIL CR compared to placebo) included the following:

	PAXIL CR (n=212)	Placebo (n=211)
Nausea	3.7%	0.5%
Asthenia	1.9%	0.5%
Dizziness	1.4%	0.0%
Somnolence	1.4%	0.0%

In a placebo-controlled study of elderly patients with depression, 13% (13/104) of PAXIL CR patients discontinued due to an adverse event. Events meeting the above criteria included the following:

	PAXIL CR (n=104)	Placebo (n=109)
Nausea	2.9%	0.0%
Headache	1.9%	0.9%
Depression	1.9%	0.0%
LFT's abnormal	1.9%	0.0%

Panic Disorder: Eleven percent (50/444) of PAXIL CR patients in panic disorder studies discontinued treatment due to an adverse event. Events meeting the above criteria included the following:

	PAXIL CR (n=444)	Placebo (n=445)
Nausea	2.9%	0.4%
Insomnia	1.8%	0.0%
Headache	1.4%	0.2%
Asthenia	1.1%	0.0%

Social Anxiety Disorder: Three percent (5/186) of patients treated with PAXIL CR in the social anxiety disorder study discontinued treatment due to an adverse event. Events meeting the above criteria included the following:

	PAXIL CR (n=186)	Placebo (n=184)
Nausea	2.2%	0.5%
Headache	1.6%	0.5%
Diarrhea	1.1%	0.5%

Premenstrual Dysphoric Disorder: Thirteen percent (88/681) of patients treated with PAXIL CR in PMDD studies of continuous dosing discontinued treatment due to an adverse event. Nine percent (34/366) of patients treated with PAXIL CR in PMDD studies of luteal phase dosing discontinued treatment due to an adverse event.

The most common events (>1%) associated with discontinuation and considered to be drug related (i.e., those events associated with dropout at a rate approximately twice or greater for PAXIL CR compared to placebo) included the following: see Table 1.

Table 1: PAXIL CR

Most Common Events (>1%) Associated with Discontinuation and Considered to Be Drug Related

	Continuous Dosing			Intermittent Dosing		
	PAXIL CR 25 mg (n=348)	PAXIL CR 12.5 mg (n=333)	Placebo (n=349)	PAXIL CR 25 mg (n=116)	PAXIL CR 12.5 mg (n=130)	Placebo (n=120)
Total	15%	9.9%	6.3%	5.2%	5.4%	0.0%
Nausea[a]	6.0%	2.4%	0.9%	3.4%	2.3%	0.0%
Asthenia	4.9%	3.0%	1.4%	0.9%	1.5%	0.0%
Somnolence[a]	4.3%	1.8%	0.3%	—	—	—
Insomnia	2.3%	1.5%	0.0%	1.7%	3.1%	0.0%
Concentration Impaired[a]	2.0%	0.6%	0.3%	—	—	—
Dry Mouth[a]	2.0%	0.6%	0.3%	—	—	—
Dizziness[a]	1.7%	0.6%	0.6%	2.6%	0.8%	0.0%
Decreased Appetite[a]	1.4%	0.6%	0.0%	—	—	—
Sweating[a]	1.4%	0.0%	0.3%	—	—	—
Tremor[a]	1.4%	0.3%	0.0%	1.7%	0.8%	0.0%
Yawn[a]	1.1%	0.0%	0.0%	—	—	—
Diarrhea	0.9%	1.2%	0.0%	—	—	—

[a] Events considered to be dose dependent are defined as events having an incidence rate with 25 mg of PAXIL CR that was at least twice that with 12.5 mg of PAXIL CR (as well as the placebo group).

Adverse Events following Discontinuation of Treatment (or Dose Reduction): Clinical Trials: Adverse events while discontinuing therapy with PAXIL CR were not systematically evaluated in most clinical trials; however, in one placebo-controlled clinical trial in social anxiety disorder involving 370 patients (186 on PAXIL CR and 184 on placebo), utilizing daily doses of PAXIL CR up to 37.5 mg/day, spontaneously reported adverse events while discontinuing therapy with PAXIL CR were evaluated. Patients receiving 37.5 mg/day underwent an incremental decrease in the daily dose by 12.5 mg/day to a dose of 25 mg/day for 1 week before treatment was stopped. For patients receiving 25 mg/day or 12.5 mg/day, treatment was stopped without an incremental decrease in dose. With this regimen, the following adverse events were reported at an incidence of 2% or greater for PAXIL CR and were at least twice that reported for placebo: dizziness (13.9% versus 2.2%), insomnia (4.4% versus 2.2%), paresthesia (4.4% versus 0%) vertigo (3.3% versus 0%), and additional symptoms described by the investigator as associated with tapering or discontinuing PAXIL CR including electric shock sensations (5.6% versus 0.6%). These events were reported as serious in 1.7% (3/180) of patients who discontinued therapy with PAXIL CR.

The following adverse events have been reported at an incidence of 2% or greater for PAXIL IR and were at least twice that reported for placebo: abnormal dreams (2.3% vs 0.5%), paresthesias (2.0% vs 0.4%), and dizziness (7.1% vs 1.5%). The majority of these events were mild to moderate, self-limiting and did not require medical intervention. These adverse events were noted in GAD and PTSD clinical trials employing a taper phase regimen for discontinuation of treatment. This regimen involved an incremental decrease in the daily dose by 10 mg/day at weekly intervals. When a daily dose of 20 mg/day was reached, patients were continued on this dose for 1 week before treatment was stopped.

Post-Marketing: There have been spontaneous reports of adverse events upon the discontinuation of PAXIL and PAXIL CR (particularly when abrupt), including but not limited to the following: dizziness, sensory disturbances (including paresthesias, electric shock sensations and tinnitus), agitation/restlessness, anxiety, nausea, tremor, confusion, diarrhea, vomiting, sweating, headache, and sleep disturbances (abnormal dreams). Generally these symptoms are mild to moderate; however, in some patients they may be severe in intensity. They usually occur within the first few days of discontinuing treatment, but there have been very rare reports of such symptoms in patients who have inadvertently missed a dose. Generally these symptoms are self-limiting and usually resolve within 2 weeks, though in some individuals they may be prolonged (2-3 months or more). Symptoms associated with discontinuation have been reported for other selective serotonin reuptake inhibitors.

Patients should be monitored for these or any other symptoms when discontinuing treatment. If intolerable symptoms occur following a decrease in the dose or upon discontinuation of treatment, dose titration should be managed on the basis of the patient's clinical response (see Warnings and Precautions and Dosage and Administration).

Clinical Trial Adverse Drug Reactions: Because clinical trials are conducted under very specific conditions the adverse reaction rates observed in the clinical trials may not reflect the rates observed in practice and should not be compared to the rates in the clinical trials of another drug. Adverse drug reaction information from clinical trials is useful for identifying drug-related adverse events and for approximating rates.

Incidence in Controlled Clinical Trials: Adults: Table 2 enumerates adverse events that occurred at an incidence of 1% or more among PAXIL CR-treated patients, aged 18-65, who participated in two short-term (12-week) placebo-controlled trials in depression in which patients were dosed in a range of 25 to 62.5 mg/day. Table 3 enumerates adverse events reported at an incidence of 5% or greater among elderly PAXIL CR-treated patients (ages 60-88) who participated in a short-term (12-week) placebo-controlled trial in depression in which patients were dosed in a range of 12.5 to 50 mg/day. Table 4 enumerates adverse events reported at an incidence of 1% or greater among PAXIL CR-treated patients (ages 19-72) who participated in short-term (10-week) placebo-controlled trials in panic disorder in which patients were dosed in a range of 12.5 to 75 mg/day. Table 5 enumerates adverse events reported at an incidence of 1% or greater among adult patients treated with PAXIL CR who participated in a short-term (12-week) double-blind, placebo-controlled trial in Table 6 social anxiety disorder in which patients were dosed at a range of 12.5 to 37.5 mg/day enumerates adverse events that occurred at an incidence of 1% or more among PAXIL CR-treated patients who participated in three 12-week placebo-controlled trials in PMDD in which patients were dosed at 12.5 mg/day or

25 mg/day and in one 12-week placebo-controlled trial in which patients were dosed for 2 weeks prior to the onset of menses (luteal phase dosing) at 12.5 mg/day or 25 mg/day. Reported adverse events were classified using a standard COSTART-based Dictionary terminology.

The prescriber should be aware that these figures cannot be used to predict the incidence of side effects in the course of usual medical practice where patient characteristics and other factors differ from those which prevailed in the clinical trials. Similarly, the cited frequencies cannot be compared with figures obtained from other clinical investigations involving different treatments, uses and investigators. The cited figures, however, do provide the prescribing physician with some basis for estimating the relative contribution of drug and nondrug factors to the side effect incidence rate in the population studied.

Table 2: PAXIL CR

Treatment-Emergent Adverse Events Occurring In ≥1% of PAXIL CR Patients in a Pool of Two Studies in Depression[a,b]

Body System/Adverse Event	% Reporting Event	
	PAXIL CR (n=212)	Placebo (n=211)
Body as a Whole		
Headache	27%	20%
Asthenia	14%	9%
Infection[c]	8%	5%
Abdominal Pain	7%	4%
Back Pain	5%	3%
Trauma[d]	5%	1%
Pain[e]	3%	1%
Allergic Reaction[f]	2%	1%
Cardiovascular System		
Tachycardia	1%	0%
Vasodilatation[g]	2%	0%
Digestive System		
Nausea	22%	10%
Diarrhea	18%	7%
Dry Mouth	15%	8%
Constipation	10%	4%
Flatulence	6%	4%
Decreased Appetite	4%	2%
Vomiting	2%	1%
Nervous System		
Somnolence	22%	8%
Insomnia	17%	9%
Dizziness	14%	4%
Libido Decreased	7%	3%
Tremor	7%	1%
Hypertonia	3%	1%
Paresthesia	3%	1%
Agitation	2%	1%
Confusion	1%	0%
Respiratory System		
Yawn	5%	0%
Rhinitis	4%	1%
Cough Increased	2%	1%
Bronchitis	1%	0%
Skin and Appendages		
Sweating	6%	2%
Photosensitivity	2%	0%
Special Senses		
Abnormal Vision[h]	5%	1%

(cont'd)

Table 2: PAXIL CR *(cont'd)*

Treatment-Emergent Adverse Events Occurring In ≥1% of PAXIL CR Patients in a Pool of Two Studies in Depression[a,b]

Body System/Adverse Event	% Reporting Event	
	PAXIL CR (n=212)	Placebo (n=211)
Taste Perversion	2%	0%
Urogenital System		
Abnormal Ejaculation[i,j]	26%	1%
Female Genital Disorder[i,k]	10%	<1%
Impotence[i]	5%	3%
Urinary Tract Infection	3%	1%
Menstrual Disorder[i]	2%	<1%
Vaginitis[i]	2%	0%

a Adverse events for which the PAXIL CR (paroxetine hydrochloride) reporting incidence was less than or equal to the placebo incidence are not included. These events are: abnormal dreams, anxiety, arthralgia, depersonalization, dysmenorrhea, dyspepsia, hyperkinesia, increased appetite, myalgia, nervousness, pharyngitis, purpura, rash, respiratory disorder, sinusitis, urinary frequency, and weight gain.
b <1% means greater than zero and less than 1%.
c Mostly flu.
d A wide variety of injuries with no obvious pattern.
e Pain in a variety of locations with no obvious pattern.
f Most frequently seasonal allergic symptoms.
g Usually flushing.
h Mostly blurred vision.
i Based on the number of males or females.
j Mostly anorgasmia or delayed ejaculation.
k Mostly anorgasmia or delayed orgasm.

Table 3: PAXIL CR

Treatment-Emergent Adverse Events Occurring in ≥5% of PAXIL CR Patients in a Study of Elderly Patients with Depression[a,b]

Body System/Adverse Event	% Reporting Event	
	PAXIL CR (n=104)	Placebo (n=109)
Body as a Whole		
Headache	17%	13%
Asthenia	15%	14%
Trauma	8%	5%
Infection	6%	2%
Digestive System		
Dry Mouth	18%	7%
Diarrhea	15%	9%
Constipation	13%	5%
Dyspepsia	13%	10%
Decreased Appetite	12%	5%
Flatulence	8%	7%
Nervous System		
Somnolence	21%	12%
Insomnia	10%	8%
Dizziness	9%	5%
Libido Decreased	8%	<1%
Tremor	7%	0%
Skin and Appendages		
Sweating	10%	<1%
Urogenital System		
Abnormal Ejaculation[c,d]	17%	3%
Impotence[c]	9%	3%

a Adverse events for which the PAXIL CR (paroxetine hydrochloride) reporting incidence was less than or equal to the placebo incidence are not included. These events are nausea and respiratory disorder.
b <1% means greater than zero and less than 1%.
c Based on the number of males.
d Mostly anorgasmia or delayed ejaculation.

Table 4: PAXIL CR

Treatment-Emergent Adverse Events Occurring in ≥1% of PAXIL CR Patients in a Pool of Three Panic Disorder Studies[a,b]

Body System/Adverse Event	% Reporting Event PAXIL CR (n=444)	% Reporting Event Placebo (n=445)
Body as a Whole		
Asthenia	15%	10%
Abdominal Pain	6%	4%
Trauma[c]	5%	4%
Cardiovascular System		
Vasodilation[d]	3%	2%
Digestive System		
Nausea	23%	17%
Dry Mouth	13%	9%
Diarrhea	12%	9%
Constipation	9%	6%
Decreased Appetite	8%	6%
Metabolic/Nutritional Disorders		
Weight Loss	1%	0%
Musculoskeletal System		
Myalgia	5%	3%
Nervous System		
Insomnia	20%	11%
Somnolence	20%	9%
Libido Decreased	9%	4%
Nervousness	8%	7%
Tremor	8%	2%
Anxiety	5%	4%
Agitation	3%	2%
Hypertonia[e]	2%	<1%
Myoclonus	2%	<1%
Respiratory System		
Sinusitis	8%	5%
Yawn	3%	0%
Skin and Appendages		
Sweating	7%	2%
Special Senses		
Abnormal Vision[f]	3%	<1%
Urogenital System		
Abnormal Ejaculation[g,h]	27%	3%
Impotence[g]	10%	1%
Female Genital Disorders[i,j]	7%	1%
Urinary Frequency	2%	<1%
Urination Impaired	2%	<1%
Vaginitis[i]	1%	<1%

[a] Adverse events for which the PAXIL CR reporting rate was less than or equal to the placebo rate are not included. These events are: abnormal dreams, allergic reaction, back pain, bronchitis, chest pain, concentration impaired, confusion, cough increased, depression, dizziness, dysmenorrhea, dyspepsia, fever, flatulence, headache, increased appetite, infection, menstrual disorder, migraine, pain, paresthesia, pharyngitis, respiratory disorder, rhinitis, tachycardia, taste perversion, thinking abnormal, urinary tract infection, and vomiting.
[b] <1% means greater than zero and less than 1%.
[c] Various physical injuries.
[d] Mostly flushing.
[e] Mostly muscle tightness or stiffness.
[f] Mostly blurred vision.
[g] Based on the number of male patients.
[h] Mostly anorgasmia or delayed ejaculation.
[i] Based on the number of female patients.
[j] Mostly anorgasmia or difficulty achieving.

Table 5: PAXIL CR

Treatment-Emergent Adverse Effects Occurring in ≥1% of Patients Treated with PAXIL CR in a Social Phobia (social Anxiety Disorder) Study[a,b]

Body System/Adverse Event	% Reporting Event PAXIL CR (n=186)	% Reporting Event Placebo (n=184)
Body as a Whole		
Headache	23%	17%
Asthenia	18%	7%
Abdominal Pain	5%	4%
Back Pain	4%	1%
Trauma[c]	3%	<1%
Allergic Reaction[d]	2%	<1%
Chest Pain	1%	<1%
Cardiovascular System		
Hypertension	2%	0%
Migraine	2%	1%
Tachycardia	2%	1%
Digestive System		
Nausea	22%	6%
Diarrhea	9%	8%
Constipation	5%	2%
Dry Mouth	3%	2%
Dyspepsia	2%	<1%
Decreased Appetite	1%	<1%
Tooth Disorder	1%	0%
Metabolic/Nutritional Disorders		
Weight Gain	3%	1%
Weight Loss	1%	0%
Nervous System		
Insomnia	9%	4%
Somnolence	9%	4%
Libido Decreased	8%	1%
Dizziness	7%	4%
Tremor	4%	2%
Anxiety	2%	1%
Concentration Impaired	2%	0%
Depression	2%	1%
Myoclonus	1%	<1%
Paresthesia	1%	<1%
Respiratory System		
Yawn	2%	0%
Skin and Appendages		
Sweating	14%	3%
Eczema	1%	0%
Special Senses		
Abnormal Vision[e]	2%	0%
Abnormality of Accommodation	2%	0%
Urogenital System		
Abnormal Ejaculation[f,g]	15%	1%
Impotence[f]	9%	0%

(cont'd)

Table 5: PAXIL CR *(cont'd)*

Treatment-Emergent Adverse Effects Occurring in ≥1% of Patients Treated with PAXIL CR in a Social Phobia (social Anxiety Disorder) Study[a,b]

Body System/Adverse Event	% Reporting Event	
	PAXIL CR (n=186)	Placebo (n=184)
Female Genital Disorders[h,i]	3%	0%

[a] Adverse events for which the PAXIL CR reporting rate was less than or equal to the placebo rate are not included. These events are: dysmenorrhea, flatulence, gastroenteritis, hypertonia, infection, pain, pharyngitis, rash, respiratory disorder, rhinitis, and vomiting.
[b] <1% means greater than zero and less than 1%.
[c] Various physical injuries.
[d] Most frequently seasonal allergic symptoms.
[e] Mostly blurred vision.
[f] Based on the number of male patients.
[g] Mostly anorgasmia or delayed ejaculation.
[h] Based on the number of female patients.
[i] Mostly anorgasmia or difficulty achieving orgasm.

Table 6: PAXIL CR

Treatment-Emergent Adverse Events Occurring in >1% of PAXIL CR Patients in a Pool of Three Premenstrual Dysphoric Disorder Studies[a,b] or in 1 Premenstrual Dysphoric Disorder Study with Luteal Phase Dosing

Body System/ Adverse Event	% Reporting Event Continuous Dosing		% Reporting Event Luteal Phase Dosing	
	PAXIL CR (n=681)	Placebo (n=349)	PAXIL CR (n=246)	Placebo (n=120)
Body as a Whole				
Asthenia	17%	6%	15%	4%
Headache	15%	12%	—	—
Infection	6%	4%	—	—
Abdominal Pain	—	—	3%	0%
Cardiovascular System				
Migraine	1%	<1%	—	—
Digestive System				
Nausea	17%	7%	18%	2%
Diarrhea	6%	2%	6%	0%
Constipation	5%	1%	2%	<1%
Dry Mouth	4%	2%	2%	<1%
Increased Appetite	3%	<1%	—	—
Decreased Appetite	2%	<1%	2%	0%
Dyspepsia	2%	1%	2%	2%
Gingivitis	—	—	1%	0%
Metabolic and Nutritional Disorders				
Generalized Edema	—	—	1%	<1%
Weight Gain	—	—	1%	<1%
Musculoskeletal System				
Arthralgia	2%	1%	—	—
Nervous System				
Libido Decreased	12%	5%	9%	6%
Somnolence	9%	2%	3%	<1%
Insomnia	8%	2%	7%	3%
Dizziness	7%	3%	6%	3%
Tremor	4%	<1%	5%	0%
Concentration Impaired	3%	<1%	1%	0%
Nervousness	2%	<1%	3%	2%
Anxiety	2%	1%	—	—
Lack of Emotion	2%	<1%	—	—
Depression	—	—	2%	<1%
Vertigo	—	—	2%	<1%
Abnormal Dreams	1%	<1%	—	—

(cont'd)

Table 6: PAXIL CR *(cont'd)*

Treatment-Emergent Adverse Events Occurring in >1% of PAXIL CR Patients in a Pool of Three Premenstrual Dysphoric Disorder Studies[a,b] or in 1 Premenstrual Dysphoric Disorder Study with Luteal Phase Dosing

Body System/ Adverse Event	% Reporting Event Continuous Dosing		% Reporting Event Luteal Phase Dosing	
	PAXIL CR (n=681)	Placebo (n=349)	PAXIL CR (n=246)	Placebo (n=120)
Amnesia	—	—	1%	0%
Respiratory System				
Sinusitis	—	—	4%	2%
Yawn	2%	<1%	—	—
Bronchitis	—	—	2%	0%
Cough Increased	1%	<1%	—	—
Skin and Appendages				
Sweating	7%	<1%	6%	<1%
Special Senses				
Abnormal Vision	—	—	1%	0%
Urogenital System				
Female Genital Disorders[c]	8%	1%	2%	0%
Menorrhagia	1%	<1%	—	—
Vaginal Moniliasis	1%	<1%	—	—
Menstrual Disorder	—	—	1%	0%

[a] Adverse events for which the PAXIL CR reporting rate was less than or equal to the placebo rate are not included. These events are: abdominal pain, back pain, pain, trauma, weight gain, myalgia, pharyngitis, respiratory disorder, rhinitis, sinusitis, pruritus, dysmenorrhea, menstrual disorder, urinary tract infection, vomiting.
[b] <1% means greater than zero and less than 1%.
[c] Mostly anorgasmia or difficulty achieving orgasm.

Dose Dependency of Adverse Events: Table 7 shows results in PMDD trials of common adverse events, defined as events with an incidence of 1% with 25 mg of PAXIL CR that was at least twice that with 12.5 mg of PAXIL CR and with placebo.

Table 7: PAXIL CR

Incidence of Common Adverse Events in Placebo, 12.5 mg and 25 mg of PAXIL CR in a Pool of 3 Fixed-dose Continuous Dosing PMDD Trials

	PAXIL CR 25 mg (n=348)	PAXIL CR 12.5 mg (n=333)	Placebo (n=349)
Common Adverse Event			
Sweating	8.9%	4.2%	0.9%
Tremor	6.0%	1.5%	0.3%
Concentration Impaired	4.3%	1.5%	0.6%
Yawn	3.2%	0.9%	0.3%
Paresthesia	1.4%	0.3%	0.3%
Hyperkinesia	1.1%	0.3%	0.0%
Vaginitis	1.1%	0.3%	0.3%

A comparison of adverse event rates in a fixed-dose study comparing immediate-release paroxetine with placebo in the treatment of depression revealed a clear dose dependency for some of the more common adverse events associated with the use of immediate-release paroxetine.

Male and Female Sexual Dysfunction with SSRIs: Although changes in sexual desire, sexual performance and sexual satisfaction often occur as manifestations of a psychiatric disorder, they may also be a consequence of pharmacologic treatment. In particular, some evidence suggests that selective serotonin reuptake inhibitors (SSRIs) can cause such untoward sexual experiences.

Reliable estimates of the incidence and severity of untoward experiences involving sexual desire, performance and satisfaction are difficult to obtain, however, in part because patients and physicians may be reluctant to discuss them. Accordingly, estimates of the incidence of untoward sexual experience and performance, cited in product labeling, are likely to underestimate their actual incidence.

The percentage of patients reporting symptoms of sexual dysfunction in the pool of two placebo-controlled trials in non-elderly patients with depression, in the pool of three placebo-controlled trials in patients with panic disorder, in the placebo-controlled trial in patients with social anxiety disorder, and in the luteal phase dosing and in the pool of 3 placebo-controlled trials in female patients with PMDD are as follows: See Table 8.

There are no adequate, controlled studies examining sexual dysfunction with paroxetine treatment.

Paroxetine treatment has been associated with several cases of priapism. In those cases with a known outcome, patients recovered without sequelae.

While it is difficult to know the precise risk of sexual dysfunction associated with the use of SSRIs, physicians should routinely inquire about such possible side effects.

Laboratory Changes—Cholesterol: Clinically and statistically relevant increases in cholesterol levels have been noted in studies using paroxetine (see Warnings and Precautions, Endocrine and Metabolism).

Of the patients in placebo-controlled clinical trials for whom baseline and on-treatment measurements were taken, total serum levels of cholesterol showed a mean increase of ~1.5 mg/dL in n=653 paroxetine-treated patients, compared to a mean decrease of ~5.0 mg/dL in placebo-treated patients (n=379). Increases from baseline of 45 mg/dL or greater were recorded in 6.6% of paroxetine-treated patients compared to 2.6% of placebo-treated patients.

Pediatrics: In placebo-controlled clinical trials conducted with pediatric patients aged 7 to 18 years with depression, OCD and Social Anxiety Disorder (involving 633 patients treated with paroxetine and 542 patients treated with placebo), the following adverse events were reported in at least 2% of pediatric patients treated with PAXIL IR and occurred at a rate at least twice that

Table 8: PAXIL CR

The Percentage of Patients Reporting Symptoms of Sexual Dysfunction

	Depression		Panic Disorder		Social Anxiety Disorder		PMDD Continuous Dosing		PMDD Luteal Phase Dosing	
	PAXIL CR	Placebo	PAXIL CR	Placebo	PAXIL CR	Placebo	PAXIL CR	Placebo	PAXIL CR	Placebo
n (males)	**78**	**78**	**162**	**194**	**88**	**97**	**n/a**	**n/a**	**n/a**	**n/a**
Decreased Libido	10%	5%	9%	6%	13%	1%	n/a	n/a	n/a	n/a
Ejaculatory Disturbance	26%	1%	27%	3%	15%	1%	n/a	n/a	n/a	n/a
Impotence	5%	3%	10%	1%	9%	0%	n/a	n/a	n/a	n/a
n (females)	**134**	**133**	**282**	**251**	**98**	**87**	**681**	**349**	**246**	**120**
Decreased Libido	4%	2%	8%	2%	4%	1%	12%	5%	9%	6%
Orgasmic Disturbance	10%	<1%	7%	1%	3%	0%	8%	1%	2%	0%

for pediatric patients receiving placebo: emotional lability (including self-harm, suicidal thoughts, attempted suicide, crying, and mood fluctuations), hostility, (predominantly aggression, oppositional behaviour and anger) decreased appetite, tremor, sweating, hyperkinesia, and agitation.

In the pediatric clinical trials in depression, OCD and Social Anxiety Disorder that included a taper phase regimen (307 patients aged 7 to 18 years treated with paroxetine and 291 patients treated with placebo), events reported upon discontinuation of treatment, which occurred in at least 2% of patients who received PAXIL IR and which occurred at a rate at least twice that of placebo, were: emotional lability (including suicidal ideation, suicide attempt, mood changes, and tearfulness), nervousness, dizziness, nausea, and abdominal pain (see Warnings and Precautions, Discontinuation of Treatment with PAXIL CR).

Other Events Observed During the Clinical Development of Paroxetine: The following adverse events were reported during the clinical development of PAXIL CR tablets and/or the clinical development of the immediate-release formulation of paroxetine.

Adverse events for which frequencies are provided below occurred in clinical trials with the controlled release formulation of paroxetine. During its premarketing assessment in depression, panic disorder, social anxiety disorder, and PMDD, multiple doses of PAXIL CR were administered to 1627 patients in phase 3 double-blind, controlled, outpatient studies. Untoward events associated with this exposure were recorded by clinical investigators using terminology of their own choosing. Consequently, it is not possible to provide a meaningful estimate of the proportion of individuals experiencing adverse events without first grouping similar types of untoward events into a smaller number of standardized event categories.

In the tabulations that follow, reported adverse events were classified using a COSTART-based dictionary. The frequencies presented, therefore, represent the proportion of the 1627 patients exposed to PAXIL CR controlled release who experienced an event of the type cited on at least one occasion while receiving PAXIL CR. All reported events are included except those already listed in Table 2, Table 3, Table 4, Table 5 or Table 6 and those events where a drug cause was remote. If the COSTART term for an event was so general as to be uninformative, it was deleted or, when possible, replaced with a more informative term. It is important to emphasize that although the events reported occurred during treatment with paroxetine, they were not necessarily caused by it.

Events are further categorized by body system and listed in order of decreasing frequency according to the following definitions: frequent adverse events are those occurring on one or more occasions in at least 1/100 patients (only those not already listed in the tabulated results from placebo-controlled trials appear in this listing); infrequent adverse events are those occurring in 1/100 to 1/1000 patients; rare events are those occurring in fewer than 1/1000 patients.

Adverse events for which frequencies are not provided occurred during the premarketing assessment of immediate-release paroxetine in phase 2 and 3 studies of depression, obsessive compulsive disorder, panic disorder, social anxiety disorder, generalized anxiety disorder, and posttraumatic stress disorder. The conditions and duration of exposure to immediate-release paroxetine varied greatly and included (in overlapping categories) open and double-blind studies, uncontrolled and controlled studies, inpatient and outpatient studies, and fixed-dose and titration studies. Only those events not previously listed for controlled release paroxetine are included. The extent to which these events may be associated with PAXIL CR is unknown.

Events are listed alphabetically within the respective body system. Events of major clinical importance are also described in Warnings and Precautions.

Body as a Whole: Infrequent were, chills, face edema, fever, flu syndrome, malaise; rare were abscess, anaphylactoid reaction, anticholinergic syndrome, hypothermia; also observed were adrenergic syndrome, neck rigidity, sepsis.

Cardiovascular System: Infrequent were angina pectoris, bradycardia, bundle branch block, hematoma, hypertension, hypotension, palpitation, postural hypotension, supraventricular tachycardia, syncope; rare was bundle branch block; also observed were arrhythmia nodal, atrial fibrillation, cerebrovascular accident, congestive heart failure, low cardiac output, myocardial infarct, myocardial ischemia, pallor, phlebitis, pulmonary embolus, supraventricular extrasystoles, thrombophlebitis, thrombosis, vascular headache, ventricular extrasystoles.

Digestive System: Infrequent were bruxism, dysphagia, eructation, gastritis, gastroenteritis, gastroesophageal reflux, gingivitis, hemorrhoids, liver function tests abnormal, melena, pancreatitis, rectal hemorrhage, toothache, ulcerative stomatitis; rare were colitis, glossitis, gum hyperplasia, hepatosplenomegaly, increased salivation, intestinal obstruction, peptic ulcer, stomach ulcer, throat tightness; also observed were aphthous stomatitis, bloody diarrhea, bulimia, cardiospasm, cholelithiasis, duodenitis, enteritis, esophagitis, fecal impactions, fecal incontinence, gum hemorrhage, hematemesis, hepatitis, ileitis, ileus, jaundice, mouth ulceration, salivary gland enlargement, sialadenitis, stomatitis, tongue discoloration, tongue edema.

Endocrine System: Infrequent were, ovarian cyst, testes pain; rare were diabetes mellitus, hyperthyroidism; also observed were, goiter, hypothyroidism, thyroiditis.

Hemic and Lymphatic System: Infrequent were anemia, eosinophilia, hypochromic anemia, leukocytosis, leukopenia, lymphadenopathy, purpura; rare was thrombocytopenia; also observed were anisocytosis, basophilia, bleeding time increased, lymphedema, lymphocytosis, lymphopenia, microcytic anemia, monocytosis, normocytic anemia, thrombocythemia.

Metabolic and Nutritional Disorders: Frequent were increases in cholesterol levels. Infrequent were generalized edema, hyperglycemia, hyperkalemia, hypokalemia, peripheral edema, AST increased, ALT increased, thirst; rare were billirubinemia, dehydration, hyperkalemia, obesity; also observed were alkaline phosphatase increased, BUN increased, creatinine phosphokinase increased, gamma globulins increased, gout, hypercalcemia, hyperphosphatemia, hypocalcemia, hypoglycemia, hyponatremia, ketosis, lactic dehydrogenase increased, non-protein nitrogen (NPN) increased.

Musculoskeletal System: Infrequent were arthritis, bursitis, tendonitis; rare were myasthenia, myopathy, myositis; also observed were generalized spasm, osteoporosis, tenosynovitis, tetany.

Nervous System: Frequent was depression; infrequent were amnesia, convulsion, depersonalization, dystonia, emotional lability, hallucinations, hyperkinesia, hypesthesia, hypokinesia, incoordination, libido increased, neuralgia, neuropathy, nystagmus, paralysis, vertigo; rare were ataxia, coma, diplopia, dyskinesia, hostility, paranoid reaction, torticollis, withdrawal syndrome; also observed were abnormal gait, akathisia, akinesia, aphasia, choreoathetosis, circumoral paresthesia, delirium, delusions, dysarthria, euphoria, extrapyramidal syndrome, fasciculations, grand mal convulsion, hyperalgesia, irritability, manic reaction, manic-depressive reaction, meningitis, myelitis, peripheral neuritis, psychosis, psychotic depression, reflexes decreased, reflexes increased, stupor, trismus.

Respiratory System: Frequent was pharyngitis; infrequent were asthma, dyspnea, epistaxis, laryngitis, pneumonia; rare was stridor; also observed were dysphonia, emphysema, hemoptysis, hiccups, hyperventilation, lung fibrosis, pulmonary edema, respiratory flu, sputum increased.

Skin and Appendages: Frequent was rash; infrequent were acne, alopecia, dry skin, eczema, pruritus, urticaria; rare were exfoliative dermatitis, furunculosis, pustular rash, seborrhea; also observed were angioedema, ecchymosis, erythema multiforme, erythema nodosum, hirsutism, maculopapular rash, skin discoloration, skin hypertrophy, skin ulcer, sweating decreased, vesiculobullous rash.

Special Senses: Infrequent were conjunctivitis, earache, keratoconjunctivitis, mydriasis, photophobia, retinal hemorrhage, tinnitus; rare were blepharitis, visual field defect; also observed were amblyopia, anisocoria, blurred vision, cataract, conjunctival edema, corneal ulcer, deafness, exophthalmos, glaucoma, hyperacusis, night blindness, parosmia, ptosis, taste loss.

Urogenital System: Frequent was dysmennorhea*; infrequent were albuminuria, amenorrhea*, breast pain*, cystitis, dysuria, prostatitis*, urinary retention; rare were breast enlargement, breast neoplasm*, female lactation, hematuria, kidney calculus, metorrhagia, nephritis, nocturia, pregnancy and puerperal disorders*, salpingitis, urinary incontinence, uterine fibroids enlarged*; also observed were breast atrophy, ejaculatory disturbance, endometrial disorder, epididymitis, fibrocystic breast, leukorrhea, mastitis, oliguria, polyuria, pyuria, urethritis, urinary casts, urinary urgency, urolith, uterine spasm, vaginal hemorrhage.

Post-Market Adverse Drug Reactions: Adverse events not listed above which have been reported since market introduction in patients taking immediate-release paroxetine hydrochloride include acute pancreatitis, hepatic events such as elevation of hepatic enzymes, and hepatitis, sometimes associated with jaundice, and/or liver failure (in very rare circumstances, with fatal outcomes), Guillain-Barré syndrome, toxic epidermal necrolysis, priapism, thrombocytopenia, aggravated hypertension, syndrome of inappropriate ADH secretion, symptoms suggestive of hyperprolactinemia and galactorrhea, blurred vision, extrapyramidal symptoms which have included akathisia, (characterized by an inner sense of restlessness and psychomotor agitation such as an inability to sit or stand still usually associated with subjective distress), bradykinesia, cogwheel rigidity, dystonia, hypertonia, oculogyric crisis which has been associated with concomitant use of pimozide, tremor and trismus, abnormal dreams (including nightmares), restless legs syndrome (RLS), vomiting, neuroleptic malignant syndrome-like events; serotonin syndrome (see Warnings and Precautions, Neurologic, Serotonin Syndrome/Neuroleptic Malignant Syndrome), persistent pulmonary hypertension (PPHN; see also Warnings and Precautions, Pregnant Women and Newborns, Risk of PPHN and Exposure to SSRIs (including paroxetine)). There has been a case report of an elevated phenytoin level after 4 weeks of PAXIL IR and phenytoin coadministration. There has been a case report of severe hypotension when PAXIL IR was added to chronic metoprolol treatment. The causal relationship between PAXIL IR and the emergence of these events has not been established.

There have been spontaneous reports of adverse events upon the discontinuation of PAXIL CR and other selective serotonin reuptake inhibitors (particularly when abrupt) (see Warnings and Precautions, General, Discontinuation of Treatment with PAXIL CR and Adverse Reactions, Adverse Events following Discontinuation of Treatment (or Dose Reduction)).

DRUG INTERACTIONS:

Serious Drug Interactions
- **Monoamine Oxidase Inhibitors: See Contraindications**
- **Thioridazine: See Contraindications**
- **Pimozide: See Contraindications**

Overview: Like some other selective serotonin re-uptake inhibitors, paroxetine inhibits the specific hepatic cytochrome P450 isozyme CYP2D6 which is responsible for the metabolism of debrisoquine and sparteine. Poor metabolizers of debrisoquine/sparteine represent approximately 5-10% of Caucasians. The median C_{min} (ss) for PAXIL (20 mg daily) at steady state in poor metabolizers (n=8) was almost triple that reported for extensive metabolizers (n=9). Although the full clinical significance of this effect has not been established, inhibition of CYP2D6 can lead to elevated plasma levels of coadministered drugs which are metabolized by this isozyme. Consideration should be given to decreasing the dose of the CYP2D6 metabolized drug or paroxetine and/or monitoring of drug plasma levels, especially when PAXIL is coadministered with drugs with a narrow therapeutic index.

PAXIL CR coadministration has been associated with elevated levels of the anticholinergic procyclidine, certain neuroleptics/antipsychotics (e.g., perphenazine, risperidone), tricyclic antidepressants (e.g., desipramine), atomoxetine, type 1C antiarrhythmics (e.g., propafenone), and theophylline.

Coadministration of phenobarbitol or phenytoin with PAXIL CR has been associated with decreased levels of PAXIL CR or IR. When coadministered with cimetidine, PAXIL CR levels were elevated.

The concomitant use of PAXIL CR and alcohol has not been studied.

Drug-Drug Interactions: Monoamine Oxidase Inhibitors: Combined use of PAXIL CR and monoamine oxidase inhibitors (including linezolid, an antibiotic which is a reversible non-selective MAO inhibitor) is contraindicated due to the potential for serious reactions with features resembling serotonin syndrome or neuroleptic malignant syndrome (see Contraindications and Warnings and Precautions, Neurologic, Serotonin Syndrome/Neuroleptic Malignant Syndrome).

Thioridazine: Combined use of PAXIL CR and thioridazine is contraindicated due to a potential for elevated thioridazine plasma levels. Thioridazine treatment alone produces prolongation of the QTc interval, which is associated with serious ventricular arrhythmias, such as torsades de pointes-type arrhythmias, and sudden death (see Contraindications).

Pimozide: In an open label study of healthy volunteers, coadministration of a single dose of 2 mg pimozide, under steady state conditions of PAXIL (titrated to 60 mg daily) was associated with mean increases in pimozide AUC of 151% and C_{max} of 62%, compared to pimozide administered alone. This is likely explained by the known CYP2D6 inhibitory properties of paroxetine. Due to the narrow therapeutic index of pimozide and its known ability to prolong the QT interval, and produce severe cardiac arrhythmias including torsade de pointes, concomitant use of pimozide and PAXIL CR is contraindicated (see Contraindications).

Drugs Metabolized by Cytochrome P450 (CYP2D6): In two studies, daily dosing of PAXIL (20 mg qd) under steady state conditions increased the following mean pharmacokinetic parameters for a single (100 mg) dose of desipramine in extensive metabolizers: C_{max} (2 fold), AUC (6 fold), and $T_{½}$ (3-5 fold). Concomitant steady-state PAXIL treatment did not result in any further impairment of desipramine elimination in poor metabolizers. Insufficient information is available to provide recommendations on the necessary dosage adjustments for tricyclic antidepressants or PAXIL CR, if these drugs are to be used in combination. Plasma tricyclic antidepressant concentrations may need to be monitored in such instances.

Concomitant use of PAXIL CR with other drugs metabolized by CYP2D6 has not been formally studied but may require lower doses than usually prescribed for either PAXIL CR or the other drug. Drugs metabolized by CYP2D6 include certain tricyclic antidepressants (e.g. nortriptyline, amitriptyline, imipramine and desipramine), selective serotonin reuptake inhibitors (e.g. fluoxetine), phenothiazine neuroleptics (e.g. perphenazine), risperidone, atomoxetine, Type IC antiarrhythmics (e.g. propafenone and flecainide), and metoprolol. Due to the risk of serious ventricular arrhythmias and sudden death potentially associated with elevated plasma levels of thioridazine, PAXIL CR and thioridazine should not be coadministered (see Contraindications).

Fosamprenavir/Ritonavir: Coadministration of fosamprenavir/ritonavir with paroxetine significantly decreased plasma levels of paroxetine (by ~60% in one study). Any dose adjustment should be guided by clinical effect (tolerability and efficacy).

* Based on the number of men and women as appropriate.

Tamoxifen: Tamoxifen is a pro-drug requiring metabolic activation by CYP2D6. Inhibition of CYP2D6 by paroxetine and other antidepressants can lead to reduced plasma concentrations of an active metabolite and hence potential for reduced efficacy of tamoxifen (see Warnings and Precautions, Potential for Reduced Efficacy of Tamoxifen with Concomitant SSRI use, Including PAXIL CR).

Drugs Metabolized by Cytochrome P450 (CYP3A4): An in vivo interaction study involving the coadministration under steady state conditions of PAXIL and terfenadine, a substrate for CYP3A4, revealed no effect of PAXIL on terfenadine pharmacokinetics. In addition, in vitro studies have shown ketoconazole, a potent inhibitor of CYP3A4 activity, to be at least 100 times more potent than paroxetine as an inhibitor of the metabolism of several substrates for this enzyme, including terfenadine, astemizole, cisapride, triazolam and cyclosporin. Based on the assumption that the relationship between paroxetine's in vitro Ki and its lack of effect on terfenadine's in vivo clearance predicts its effect on other CYP3A4 substrates, paroxetine's extent of inhibition of CYP3A4 activity would not be expected to be of clinical significance.

Microsomal Enzyme Inhibition/Induction: The metabolism and pharmacokinetics of PAXIL CR may be affected by the induction or inhibition of drug metabolizing enzymes.

Drugs Highly Bound to Plasma Protein: Paroxetine is highly bound to plasma protein, therefore administration of PAXIL CR to a patient taking another drug that is highly protein bound may cause increased free concentrations of the other drug, potentially resulting in adverse events. Conversely, adverse effects could result from displacement of paroxetine by other highly bound drugs.

Alcohol: The concomitant use of PAXIL CR or IR and alcohol has not been studied and is not recommended. Patients should be advised to avoid alcohol while taking PAXIL CR.

Anticholinergic Drugs: PAXIL IR has been reported to increase significantly the systemic bioavailability of procyclidine. Steady state plasma levels of procyclidine (5 mg daily) were elevated by about 40% when 30 mg paroxetine was coadministered to steady-state. If anticholinergic effects are seen, the dose of procyclidine should be reduced.

Antiretroviral: Coadministration of fosamprenavir/ritonavir with paroxetine significantly decreased plasma levels of paroxetine (by ~60% in one study). Any dose adjustment should be guided by clinical effect (tolerability and efficacy).

Phenobarbital: Chronic daily dosing with phenobarbital (100 mg qid for 14 days) decreased the systemic availability of a single 30 mg dose of paroxetine in some subjects. The AUC and $T_{½}$ of PAXIL IR were reduced by an average of 25% and 38% respectively compared to PAXIL IR administered alone. The effect of PAXIL CR or IR on phenobarbital pharmacokinetics was not studied. No initial PAXIL CR or IR dosage adjustment is considered necessary when coadministered with phenobarbital; any subsequent adjustment should be guided by clinical effect.

Anticonvulsants: In a limited number of patients with epilepsy on long-term treatment with anticonvulsants (carbamazepine 600-900 mg/day, n=6; phenytoin 250-400 mg/day, n=6; sodium valproate 300-2500 mg/day, n=8) the coadministration of PAXIL IR (30 mg/day for 10 days) had no significant effect on the plasma concentrations of these anticonvulsants. In healthy volunteers, coadministration of paroxetine with phenytoin has been associated with decreased plasma levels of paroxetine and an increased incidence of adverse experiences. However, no initial dosage adjustment of PAXIL CR is considered necessary when the drug is to be coadministered with known drug metabolizing enzyme inducers (e.g. carbamazepine, phenytoin, sodium valproate) and any subsequent dosage adjustment should be guided by clinical effect. Coadministration of PAXIL CR with anticonvulsants may be associated with an increased incidence of adverse experiences.

Antipsychotic Drugs/Neuroleptic Malignant Syndrome: As with other SSRIs, PAXIL CR should be used with caution in patients already receiving antipsychotics/neuroleptics, since symptoms suggestive of Neuroleptic Malignant Syndrome cases have been reported with this combination (see Warnings and Precautions, Neurologic, Serotonin Syndrome/Neuroleptic Malignant Syndrome).

Serotonergic Drugs: Based on the mechanism of action of paroxetine and the potential for serotonin syndrome, caution is advised when PAXIL CR is coadministered with other drugs or agents that may affect the serotonergic neurotransmitter systems, such as tryptophan, triptans, serotonin reuptake inhibitors, lithium, fentanyl, tramadol, or St. John's wort (see Warnings and Precautions, Neurologic, Serotonin Syndrome/Neuroleptic Malignant Syndrome). Concomitant use of PAXIL CR and MAO inhibitors (including linezolid, an antibiotic which is a reversible non-selective MAO inhibitor) is contraindicated (see Contraindications).

Lithium: In a study of depressed patients stabilized on lithium, no pharmacokinetic interaction between paroxetine and lithium was observed. However, due to the potential for serotonin syndrome, caution is advised when PAXIL CR is coadministered with lithium.

Triptans: There have been rare postmarketing reports describing patients with weakness, hyperreflexia, and incoordination following the use of a selective serotonin reuptake inhibitor (SSRI) and the $5HT_1$ agonist, sumatriptan. If concomitant treatment with triptan and an SSRI (e.g., fluoxetine, fluvoxamine, paroxetine, sertraline) is clinically warranted, appropriate observation of the patient is advised. The possibility of such interactions should also be considered if other $5HT_1$ agonists are to be used in combination with SSRIs (see Warnings and Precautions, Neurologic, Serotonin Syndrome/Neuroleptic Malignant Syndrome).

Tryptophan: Tryptophan can be metabolized to serotonin. As with other serotonin reuptake inhibitors, the use of PAXIL CR together with tryptophan may result in adverse reactions consisting primarily of headache, nausea, sweating and dizziness as well as serotonin syndrome. Consequently, concomitant use of PAXIL CR with tryptophan is not recommended (see Warnings and Precautions, Neurologic, Serotonin Syndrome/Neuroleptic Malignant Syndrome).

CNS Drugs: Experience in a limited number of healthy subjects has shown that PAXIL IR does not increase the sedation and drowsiness associated with haloperidol, amylbarbitone or oxazepam, when given in combination. Since the effects of concomitant administration of PAXIL CR or IR with neuroleptics have not been studied, the use of PAXIL CR with these drugs should be approached with caution.

Diazepam: A multiple dose study of the interaction between PAXIL IR and diazepam showed no alteration in the pharmacokinetics of PAXIL IR that would warrant changes in the dose of PAXIL CR for patients receiving both drugs. The effects of PAXIL IR or CR on the pharmacokinetics of diazepam were not evaluated.

Cardiovascular Drugs: Multiple dose treatment with PAXIL IR 30 mg/day has little or no effect on the steady-state pharmacokinetics of digoxin (0.25 mg qd) or propanolol (80 mg bid).

Theophylline: Reports of elevated theophylline levels associated with PAXIL treatment have been reported. While this interaction has not been formally studied, it is recommended that theophylline levels be monitored when these drugs are concurrently administered.

Cimetidine: Steady state levels of PAXIL (30 mg daily) were elevated by about 50% when cimetidine (300 mg tid), a known drug metabolizing enzyme inhibitor, was coadministered to steady-state. Consideration should be given to using doses of PAXIL CR towards the lower end of the range when coadministered with known drug metabolizing enzyme inhibitors.

Drug-Food Interactions: At steady state, the bioavailability of 25 mg PAXIL CR is not affected by food.

Drug-Herb Interactions: St. John's wort: In common with other SSRIs, pharmakodynamic interactions between paroxetine and the herbal remedy St. John's wort may occur and may result in an increase in undesirable effects.

Drug-Laboratory Test Interactions: Interactions with laboratory tests have not been established.

DOSAGE AND ADMINISTRATION:

Dosing Considerations: General: PAXIL CR is not indicated for use in children under 18 years of age (see Warnings and Precautions, Potential Association with Behavioural and Emotional Changes, Including Self-harm).

Lower initial doses of PAXIL CR are recommended for elderly and debilitated patients, and patients with renal or hepatic impairment (see Dosage and Administration, Special Patient Populations).

PAXIL CR should be administered as a single daily dose, usually in the morning, with or without food. Patients should be cautioned that the PAXIL CR tablet should not be chewed or crushed, and should be swallowed whole.

Discontinuation of Treatment with PAXIL CR: Symptoms associated with the discontinuation of PAXIL IR and PAXIL CR have been reported in clinical trials and post marketing. Patients should be monitored for these and other symptoms when discontinuing treatment, regardless of the indication for which PAXIL CR is being prescribed (see Warnings and Precautions, Discontinuation of Treatment with PAXIL CR and Adverse Reactions, Adverse Events following Discontinuation of Treatment (or Dose Reduction)).

A gradual reduction in the dose rather than abrupt cessation is recommended whenever possible. If intolerable symptoms occur following a decrease in the dose or upon discontinuation of treatment, dose titration should be managed on the basis of the patient's clinical response (see Adverse Reactions).

Adults: Depression: Usual Initial Dosage: The recommended initial dose is 25 mg/day. Patients were dosed in a range of 25 mg to 62.5 mg/day in the clinical trials demonstrating the effectiveness of PAXIL CR in the treatment of depression. As with all drugs effective in the treatment of depression, the full effect may be delayed. Some patients not responding to a 25 mg dose may benefit from dose increases, in 12.5 mg/day increments, up to a maximum of 62.5 mg/day. Dose changes should occur at intervals of at least 1 week.

Maintenance Therapy: There is no body of evidence available to answer the question of how long a patient should continue to be treated with PAXIL CR for the symptoms of panic and depression. It is generally agreed that acute episodes of depression require several months or longer of sustained pharmacologic therapy. Whether the dose of an antidepressant needed to induce remission is identical to the dose needed to maintain and/or sustain euthymia is unknown.

Systematic evaluation of the efficacy of PAXIL IR has shown that efficacy is maintained for at least 6 months with doses that averaged about 30 mg, which corresponds to a 37.5 mg dose of PAXIL CR, based on relative bioavailability considerations.

Panic Disorder: Usual Initial Dosage: Patients should be started on 12.5 mg/day. Dose changes should occur in 12.5 mg/day increments and at intervals of at least 1 week. Patients were dosed in a range of 12.5 to 75 mg/day in the clinical trials demonstrating the effectiveness of PAXIL CR. The maximum dosage should not exceed 75 mg/day.

Maintenance Therapy: Panic disorder is a chronic condition, and it is reasonable to consider continuation of treatment for a responding patient. Dosage adjustments should be made to maintain the patient on the lowest effective dosage, and patients should be periodically reassessed to determine the need for continued treatment.

Social Phobia (Social Anxiety Disorder): Usual Initial Dosage: The recommended initial dose is 12.5 mg/day. In the clinical trial demonstrating the effectiveness of PAXIL CR in the treatment of social anxiety disorder, patients were dosed in a range of 12.5 mg to 37.5 mg/day. Some patients not responding to a 12.5 mg dose may benefit from dose increases, in 12.5 mg/day increments, up to a maximum of 37.5 mg/day. Dose changes should occur at intervals of at least 1 week.

Maintenance Therapy: There is no body of evidence available to answer the question of how long the patient treated with PAXIL CR should remain on it. Although the efficacy of PAXIL CR beyond 12 weeks of dosing has not been demonstrated in controlled clinical trials, social anxiety disorder is recognized as a chronic condition, and it is reasonable to consider continuation of treatment for a responding patient. Dosage adjustments should be made to maintain the patient on the lowest effective dosage, and patients should be periodically reassessed to determine the need for continued treatment.

Premenstrual Dysphoric Disorder: Usual Initial Dosage: In clinical trials, both 12.5 mg/day and 25 mg/day were shown to be effective with continuous dosing, or intermittent luteal phase dosing.

The recommended dose is 12.5 mg/day limited to the luteal phase of the menstrual cycle, starting 14 days prior to the expected onset of menses, and terminating on the first day of menses. Some patients not responding to a 12.5 mg dose may benefit from a dose increase to 25 mg/day. Dose changes should occur at intervals of at least 1 week. Continuous dosing of PAXIL CR, administered daily throughout the menstrual cycle may be considered if efficacy with luteal phase dosing is sub-optimal. Dose changes should occur at intervals of at least 1 week.

Maintenance/Continuation Therapy: The effectiveness of PAXIL CR in long-term use, that is, for more than 3 menstrual cycles has not been evaluated in controlled trials. Therefore, the physician who elects to use PAXIL CR for extended periods should periodically reevaluate the long-term usefulness of the drug for the individual patient.

Special Patient Populations: Treatment of Pregnant Women: Epidemiological studies of pregnancy outcomes following maternal exposure to antidepressants in the first trimester have reported an increase in the risk of congenital malformations, particularly cardiovascular (e.g. ventricular and atrial septal defects), associated with the use of paroxetine. If a patient becomes pregnant while taking PAXIL CR, she should be informed of the current estimate of risk to the fetus (see Warnings and Precautions, Special Populations) and consideration should be given to switching to other treatment options. Treatment with PAXIL CR should only be continued for an individual patient, if the potential benefits outweigh the potential risks. For women who intend to become pregnant, or are in their first trimester of pregnancy, initiation of paroxetine should be considered only after other treatment options have been evaluated (see Warnings and Precautions, Special Populations for more details).

Post-marketing reports indicate that some neonates exposed to PAXIL CR, SSRIs, or other newer antidepressants late in the third trimester have developed complications requiring prolonged hospitalization, respiratory support, and tube feeding (see Warnings and Precautions, Special Populations). When treating pregnant women with PAXIL CR during the third trimester, the physician should carefully consider the potential risks and benefits of treatment. The physician may consider tapering PAXIL CR in the third trimester.

Geriatrics (>65 years) or Debilitated: Administration of PAXIL CR to the elderly is associated with increased plasma levels and prolongation of the elimination half-life relative to younger adults. (See Action and Clinical Pharmacology.) The recommended initial dose of PAXIL CR is 12.5 mg/day for elderly patients and debilitated patients. The dose may be increased if indicated up to a maximum of 50 mg/day.

Pediatrics: PAXIL CR is not indicated for use in children under 18 years of age (see Indications and Clinical Use and Warnings and Precautions, Potential Association with Behavioural and Emotional Changes, Including Self-harm).

Renal/Hepatic Impairment: PAXIL CR should be used with caution in patients with renal or hepatic impairment. The recommended initial dose is 12.5 mg/day in patients with clinically significant renal or hepatic impairment. A maximum dose of 50 mg/day should not be exceeded (see Warnings and Precautions and Action and Clinical Pharmacology).

OVERDOSAGE:

The largest known ingestion from which a patient has recovered is 2000 mg. The smallest known dose of paroxetine alone associated with a fatal outcome is approximately 400 mg.

Symptoms of Overdosage: The most commonly reported adverse events subsequent to paroxetine-only overdose include: somnolence, nausea, tremor, dizziness, vomiting, diarrhea, agitation, aggression, anxiety, confused state, headache, fatigue, insomnia, tachycardia, hyperhydrosis, mydriasis, convulsion, paraethesia, serotonin syndrome, fever, blood pressure changes, involuntary muscle contraction and loss of consciousness. It should be noted that in some cases, patients may have consumed alcohol in addition to taking an overdose of paroxetine. **Some of these symptoms may also be seen with clinical use.**

Events such as coma and ECG changes have also been reported.

Treatment of Overdosage: The physician should consider contacting a poison control centre for additional information on the treatment of any overdose.

No specific antidote is known. Treatment should consist of those general measures employed in the management of overdose with any antidepressant. Establish and maintain an airway; ensure adequate oxygenation and ventilation.

Induction of emesis is not recommended. Due to the large volume of distribution of PAXIL CR, forced diuresis, dialysis, hemoperfusion and exchange transfusion are unlikely to be of benefit.

Supportive care with frequent monitoring of vital signs and careful observation is indicated. An ECG should be taken and monitoring of cardiac function instituted if there is any evidence of abnormality. Patient management should be as clinically indicated, or as recommended by the national poisons centre, where available.

In managing overdosage, consider the possibility of multiple drug involvement.

A specific caution involves patients taking or recently having taken PAXIL CR who might ingest, by accident or intent, excessive quantities of a tricyclic antidepressant. In such a case, accumulation of the parent tricyclic and its active metabolite may increase the possibility of clinically significant sequelae and extend the time needed for close medical observation.

> For management of a suspected drug overdose, contact your regional Poison Control Centre. See the *CPS* Directory section for a list of Poison Control Centres.

ACTION AND CLINICAL PHARMACOLOGY: Mechanism of Action: Paroxetine is a potent and selective serotonin (5-hydroxytryptamine, 5-HT) reuptake inhibitor (SSRI). This activity of the drug on brain neurons is thought to be responsible for its antidepressant and anxiolytic action in the treatment of depression, panic disorder and social anxiety disorder.

Paroxetine is a phenylpiperidine derivative which is chemically unrelated to the tricyclic or tetracyclic antidepressants. In receptor binding studies, paroxetine did not exhibit significant affinity for the adrenergic (α1, α2, β), dopaminergic, serotonergic ($5HT_1$, $5HT_2$), or histaminergic receptors of rat brain membrane. A weak affinity for the muscarinic acetylcholine receptor was evident. The predominant metabolites of paroxetine are essentially inactive as 5-HT reuptake inhibitors.

Pharmacokinetics: PAXIL CR tablets contain a degradable polymeric matrix (Geomatrix, a trademark of Jago Pharma, Muttenz, Switzerland) designed to control the dissolution rate of paroxetine over a period of approximately 4 to 5 hours. In addition to controlling the rate of drug release in vivo, an enteric coat delays the start of drug release until PAXIL CR tablets have left the stomach.

Absorption: Paroxetine hydrochloride is completely absorbed after oral dosing of a solution of the hydrochloride salt. In a study in which normal male and female subjects (n=23) received single oral doses of PAXIL CR at four dosage strengths (12.5 mg, 25 mg, 37.5 mg and 50 mg), paroxetine C_{max} and AUC_{0-inf} increased disproportionately with dose (as seen also with immediate-release formulations). Mean C_{max} and AUC_{0-inf} values at these doses were 2.0, 5.5, 9.0, and 12.5 ng/mL, and 121, 261, 338, and 540 ng/h/mL, respectively. T_{max} was observed typically between 6 and 10 hours post-dose, reflecting a reduction in absorption rate compared with immediate-release formulations (IR). The mean elimination half-life of paroxetine was 15 to 20 hours throughout this range of single PAXIL CR doses. The bioavailability of 25 mg PAXIL CR is not affected by food.

During repeated administration of PAXIL CR (25 mg once daily), steady state was reached within two weeks (i.e., comparable to immediate-release formulations). In a repeat-dose study in which normal male and female subjects (n=23) received PAXIL CR (25 mg daily), mean steady state C_{max}, C_{min} and AUC_{0-24} values were 30 ng/mL, 20 ng/mL and 550 ng·h/mL, respectively.

Based on studies using IR formulations, steady-state drug exposure based on AUC_{0-24} was several-fold greater than would have been predicted from single-dose data. The excess accumulation is a consequence of the fact that one of the enzymes that metabolizes paroxetine is readily saturable.

In steady-state dose proportionality studies involving elderly and nonelderly patients, at doses of the IR formulation of 20 to 40 mg daily for the elderly and 20 to 50 mg daily for the nonelderly, some nonlinearity was observed in both populations, again reflecting a saturable metabolic pathway. In comparison to C_{min} values after 20 mg daily, values after 40 mg daily were only about 2 to 3 times greater than doubled.

In healthy young volunteers receiving a 20 mg daily dose of paroxetine IR for 15 days, the mean maximal plasma concentration was 41 ng/mL at steady state (see Table 9). Peak plasma levels generally occurred within 3 to 7 hours.

Distribution: At therapeutic concentrations, the plasma protein binding of paroxetine is approximately 95%.

Metabolism: Paroxetine is subject to a biphasic process of metabolic elimination which involves presystemic (first-pass) and systemic pathways. First-pass metabolism is extensive, but may be partially saturable, accounting for the increased bioavailability observed with multiple dosing. The metabolism of paroxetine is accomplished in part by cytochrome P450 (IID_6). Saturation of this enzyme at clinical doses appears to account for the nonlinearity of paroxetine kinetics with increasing dose and increasing duration of treatment. The role of this enzyme in paroxetine metabolism also suggests potential drug-drug interactions (see Drug Interactions). The majority of the dose appears to be oxidized to a catechol intermediate which is converted to highly polar glucuronide and sulphate metabolites through methylation and conjugation reactions. The glucuronide and sulphate conjugates of paroxetine are about >10 000 and 3000 times less potent, respectively, than the parent compound as inhibitors of 5-HT reuptake in rat brain synaptosomes.

Excretion: Approximately 64% of an administered dose of paroxetine is eliminated by the kidneys and 36% in the faeces. Less than 2% of the dose is recovered in the form of the parent compound.

Special Populations and Conditions: Geriatrics: In elderly subjects, increased steady-state plasma concentrations and prolongation of the elimination half-life were observed relative to younger adult controls (Table 9). Elderly patients should, therefore, be initiated and maintained at the lowest daily dosage of paroxetine which is associated with clinical efficacy (see Dosage and Administration).

Hepatic Insufficiency: The results from a multiple dose pharmacokinetic study with paroxetine IR, in subjects with severe hepatic dysfunction, suggest that the clearance of paroxetine is markedly reduced in this patient group (see Table 9). As the elimination of paroxetine is dependent upon extensive hepatic metabolism, its use in patients with hepatic impairment should be undertaken with caution (see Dosage and Administration, Special Patient Populations).

Renal Insufficiency: In a single dose pharmacokinetic study in patients with mild to severe renal impairment, plasma levels of paroxetine tended to increase with deteriorating renal function (see Table 10).

As multiple-dose pharmacokinetic studies have not been performed in patients with renal disease, paroxetine should be used with caution in such patients (see Dosage and Administration, Special Patient Populations).

Table 9: PAXIL CR

Steady State Pharmacokinetics of Paroxetine IR After Doses of 20 mg Daily (mean and range)

	Young Healthy Subjects [n=22]	Elderly Healthy Subjects [n=22]	Hepatically[a] Impaired Subjects [n=10]
$C_{max\ (ss)}$ (ng/mL)	41 (12–90)	87 (18–154)	87 (11–147)
$T_{max\ (ss)}$ (hours)	5.0 (3–7)	5.0 (1–10)	6.4 (2–11)
$C_{min\ (ss)}$ (ng/mL)	21 (4–51)	58 (9–127)	66 (7–128)
$AUC_{(ss)}$ (ng·h/mL)	660 (179–1436)	1580 (221–3286)	1720 (194–3283)
$T_{½}$ (hour)	19 (8–43)	31 (13–92)	66 (17–152)

[a] Galactose elimination capacity 30-70% of normal.

Legend: C_{max}=maximum plasma concentration; T_{max}=time to reach C_{max}; AUC=area under the plasma concentration time curve between dosing intervals (i.e. 24 hrs) at steady-state; $T_{½}$=terminal elimination half-life; ss=steady state.

Table 10: PAXIL CR

Pharmacokinetics of Paroxetine IR After a Single 30 mg Dose in Normal Subjects and Those with Renal Impairment

	[a]Renally Impaired Subjects Severe [n=6]	[b]Renally Impaired Subjects Moderate [n=6]	[c]Healthy Young Subjects [n=6]
C_{max} (ng/mL)	46.2 (35.9–56.7)	36 (3.6–59.4)	19.8 (1.4–54.8)
T_{max} (hour)	6.5 (4.0–11.0)	4.8 (1.5–9.0)	4.3 (1–7)
AUC_{∞} (ng·h/mL)	2046 (605–3695)	1053 (48–2087)	574 (21–2196)
$T_{½}$ (hour)	29.7 (10.9–54.8)	18.3 (11.2–32.0)	17.3 (9.6–25.1)

[a] Creatinine clearance=13-27 mL/min.

[b] Creatinine clearance=32-46 mL/min.

[c] Creatinine clearance >100 mL/min.

Legend: C_{max}=maximum plasma concentration; T_{max}=time to reach C_{max}; AUC_{∞}=area under the plasma concentration time curve at infinity; $T_{½}$=terminal elimination half-life.

STORAGE AND STABILITY: Store between 15 and 25°C.

INFORMATION FOR THE PATIENT: Published in e-CPS, available by subscription at www.e-cps.ca.

DOSAGE FORMS, COMPOSITION AND PACKAGING: 12.5 mg: Each yellow, round and biconvex, enteric, film-coated, controlled-release tablet, with GSK engraved on one side and strength engraved on the other side, contains: paroxetine HCl equivalent to paroxetine 12.5 mg. Nonmedicinal ingredients: colloidal silicon dioxide, D&C Yellow No. 10 Aluminum Lake, FD&C Yellow No. 6 Aluminum Lake, glyceryl behenate, hydroxypropyl methylcellulose, lactose monohydrate, magnesium stearate, methacrylic acid copolymer type C, polyethylene glycol, polysorbate 80, polyvinylpyrrolidone, sodium lauryl sulphate, talc, titanium dioxide, triethyl citrate and yellow ferric oxide. Bottles of 30.

25 mg: Each pink, round and biconvex, enteric, film-coated, controlled-release tablet, with GSK engraved on one side and strength engraved on the other side, contains: paroxetine HCl equivalent to paroxetine 25 mg. Nonmedicinal ingredients: colloidal silicon dioxide, D&C Red No. 30 Aluminum Lake, glyceryl behenate, hydroxypropyl methylcellulose, lactose monohydrate, magnesium stearate, methacrylic acid copolymer type C, polyethylene glycol, polysorbate 80, polyvinylpyrrolidone, red ferric oxide, sodium lauryl sulphate, talc, titanium dioxide and triethyl citrate. Bottles of 30.

(Shown in Product Identification Section)

Pediacel®

diphtheria and tetanus toxoids and acellular pertussis vaccine adsorbed combined with inactivated poliomyelitis vaccine and Haemophilus b conjugate vaccine (tetanus protein-conjugate)

Active Immunizing Agent

sanofi pasteur

Date of Revision: January 2009

SUMMARY PRODUCT INFORMATION:

Route of Administration	Dosage Form/ Strength	Clinically Relevant Nonmedicinal Ingredients
Intramuscular injection	Suspension for injection: Each 0.5 mL dose is formulated to contain: Diphtheria toxoid, tetanus toxoid, acellular pertussis [pertussis toxoid (PT), filamentous haemagglutinin (FHA), pertactin (PRN), fimbriae types 2 and 3 (FIM)], inactivated poliomyelitis vaccine [type 1 (Mahoney), type 2 (MEF1), type 3 (Saukett)] and purified polyribosylribitol phosphate capsular polysaccharide (PRP) of *H. influenzae* type b covalently bound to tetanus protein	Excipients: aluminum phosphate (adjuvant), 2-phenoxyethanol, polysorbate 80. Manufacturing process residuals: bovine serum albumin, neomycin, polymyxin B and trace amounts of streptomycin, formaldehyde and glutaraldehyde. For a complete listing see Dosage Forms, Composition and Packaging.

DESCRIPTION: PEDIACEL [Diphtheria and Tetanus Toxoids and Acellular Pertussis Vaccine Adsorbed Combined with Inactivated Poliomyelitis Vaccine and Haemophilus b Conjugate Vaccine (Tetanus Protein-Conjugate)] is a sterile, uniform, cloudy, white to off-white suspension of diphtheria and tetanus toxoids and acellular pertussis vaccine adsorbed separately on aluminum phosphate combined with inactivated poliomyelitis vaccine (vero cell origin) types 1, 2 and 3 (IPV), and *H. influenzae* type b capsular polysaccharide (polyribosylribitol phosphate, PRP) covalently bound to tetanus protein, and suspended in water for injection. The acellular pertussis vaccine is composed of 5 purified pertussis antigens (PT, FHA, PRN and FIM).

INDICATIONS AND CLINICAL USE: PEDIACEL is indicated for primary immunization of infants from the age of 2 months and in children up to 6 years of age (prior to their 7th birthday) against diphtheria, tetanus, pertussis (whooping cough), poliomyelitis and invasive *H. influenzae* type b disease. (See Dosage and Administration.)

Currently, Haemophilus b conjugate vaccines are not recommended for infants younger than 2 months of age.

According to the National Advisory Committee on Immunization (NACI), children who have had pertussis, tetanus, diphtheria or *H. influenzae* type b (Hib) invasive disease should still be immunized since these clinical infections do not always confer immunity. For persons who have been exposed to invasive Hib and who are incompletely immunized, refer to the guidelines in the Canadian Immunization Guide.

NACI recommends that Human Immunodeficiency Virus (HIV)-infected persons, both asymptomatic and symptomatic, should be immunized against diphtheria, tetanus, pertussis, poliomyelitis and *H. influenzae* type b, according to standard schedules.

PEDIACEL is not to be used for the treatment of diseases caused by *C. diphtheriae*, *C. tetani*, *B. pertussis*, poliovirus or *H. influenzae* type b infections.

Pediatrics: PEDIACEL is not indicated for persons less than 2 months or to persons 7 years of age or older.

Geriatrics: PEDIACEL is not indicated for use in adult and elderly populations.

CONTRAINDICATIONS: Hypersensitivity: NACI recommends that known systemic hypersensitivity reaction to any component of PEDIACEL or a life-threatening reaction after previous administration of the vaccine or a vaccine containing one or more of the same components are contraindications to vaccination. (See Summary Product Information.) Because of uncertainty as to which component of the vaccine may be responsible, none of the components should be administered. Alternatively, such persons may be referred to an allergist for evaluation if further immunizations are considered.

Acute Neurological Disorders: According to the Advisory Committee on Immunization Practices (ACIP), the following events are contraindications to administration of any pertussis-containing vaccine, including PEDIACEL:

Encephalopathy (e.g., coma, decreased level of consciousness, prolonged seizures) within 7 days of a previous dose of a pertussis-containing vaccine that is not attributable to another identifiable cause.

Progressive neurologic disorder, including infantile spasms, uncontrolled epilepsy, progressive encephalopathy. Pertussis vaccine should not be administered to persons with such conditions until a treatment regimen has been established and the condition has stabilized.

WARNINGS AND PRECAUTIONS: General: Before administration of PEDIACEL, health-care providers should inform the parent or guardian of the recipient to be immunized of the benefits and risks of immunization, inquire about the recent health status of the recipient, review the recipient's history concerning possible hypersensitivity to the vaccine or similar vaccine, previous immunization history, the presence of any contraindications to immunization and comply with any local requirements with respect to information to be provided to the parent or guardian before immunization and the importance of completing the immunization series.

It is extremely important that the parent or guardian be questioned concerning any symptoms and/or signs of an adverse reaction after a previous dose of vaccine. (See Contraindications and Adverse Reactions.)

NACI states that the rates and severity of adverse events in recipients of tetanus toxoid are influenced by the number of prior doses and level of pre-existing antitoxins.

As with any vaccine, PEDIACEL may not protect 100% of vaccinated individuals.

Vaccines that contain Hib antigen do not provide protection against infections with other types of *H. influenzae*, or against meningitis of other origin.

Under no circumstances can the tetanus protein contained in conjugate vaccines containing tetanus toxoid as protein carrier be used to replace the usual tetanus vaccination.

Sudden infant death syndrome (SIDS) has occurred in infants following administration of DTaP vaccines. By chance alone, some cases of SIDS can be expected to follow receipt of PEDIACEL.

Administration Route—Related Precautions: Do not administer PEDIACEL by intravascular injection; ensure that the needle does not penetrate a blood vessel.

Intradermal or subcutaneous routes of administration are not to be utilized.

PEDIACEL should not be administered into the buttocks.

Granuloma or sterile abscess at the injection site has been reported with a product containing the same antigens.

Febrile or Acute Disease: ACIP recommends that vaccination should be postponed in cases of acute or febrile disease. However, a disease with low-grade fever should not usually be a reason to postpone vaccination.

If any of the following events occur within the specified period after administration of a whole-cell pertussis vaccine or a vaccine containing an acellular pertussis component, the decision to administer PEDIACEL should be based on careful consideration of potential benefits and possible risks: temperature of ≥40.5°C within 48 hours, not attributable to another identifiable cause; collapse or shock-like state (hypotonic-hyporesponsive episode) within 48 hours; persistent crying lasting ≥3 hours within 48 hours; convulsions with or without fever within 3 days.

Hematologic: Because any intramuscular injection can cause an injection site hematoma in persons with any bleeding disorders, such as hemophilia or thrombocytopenia, or in persons on anticoagulant therapy, intramuscular injections with PEDIACEL should not be administered to such persons unless the potential benefits outweigh the risk of administration. If the decision is made to administer any product by intramuscular injection to such persons, it should be given with caution, with steps taken to avoid the risk of hematoma formation following injection.

Immune: The possibility of allergic reactions in persons sensitive to components of the vaccine should be evaluated. Hypersensitivity reactions may occur following the use of PEDIACEL even in persons with no prior history of hypersensitivity to the product components. Cases of allergic or anaphylactic reaction have been reported after receiving some preparations containing diphtheria and tetanus toxoids and/or pertussis antigens.

As recommended by NACI and as with all other products, epinephrine hydrochloride solution (1:1000) and other appropriate agents should be available for immediate use in case an anaphylactic or acute hypersensitivity reaction occurs. Health-care providers should be familiar with current recommendations for the initial management of anaphylaxis in non-hospital settings, including proper airway management. For instructions on recognition and treatment of anaphylactic reactions see the current edition of the Canadian Immunization Guide or visit the Health Canada website.

According to NACI, immunocompromised persons (whether from disease or treatment) may not obtain the expected immune response. If possible, consideration should be given to delaying vaccination until after the completion of any immunosuppressive treatment. Nevertheless, vaccination of persons with chronic immunodeficiency such as HIV infection is recommended even if the antibody response might be limited.

Neurologic: A review by the IOM found evidence for a causal relation between tetanus toxoid and both brachial neuritis and Guillain-Barré syndrome (GBS). ACIP recommends that if GBS occurred within 6 weeks of receipt of prior vaccine containing tetanus toxoid, the decision to give PEDIACEL or any vaccine containing tetanus toxoid should be based on careful consideration of potential benefits and possible risks.

A few cases of demyelinating diseases of the central nervous system, peripheral mononeuropathies, and cranial mononeuropathies have been reported following vaccines containing tetanus and/or diphtheria toxoids, although the IOM concluded that the evidence is inadequate to accept or reject a causal relation between these conditions and vaccination.

ACIP recommends for infants or children at higher risk for seizures than the general population, an appropriate antipyretic may be administered (in the dosage recommended in its prescribing information) at the time of vaccination with a vaccine containing an acellular pertussis component (including PEDIACEL) and for the following 24 hours, to reduce the possibility of post-vaccination fever.

Hypotonic-hyporesponsive episodes (HHEs) rarely follow vaccination with whole-cell pertussis containing DTP vaccines and occur even less commonly after acellular pertussis-containing DTP vaccines and DT vaccines. The NACI states that a history of HHEs is not a contraindication to the use of acellular pertussis vaccines but recommends caution in these cases.

Pregnant Women: The vaccine should not be administered to pregnant women.

Nursing Women: The vaccine should not be administered to nursing women.

ADVERSE REACTIONS: Clinical Trial Adverse Drug Reactions: Because clinical trials are conducted under widely varying conditions, adverse reaction rates observed in the clinical trials of a vaccine cannot be directly compared to rates in the clinical trials of another vaccine and may not reflect rates observed in practice. The adverse reaction information from clinical trials does, however, provide a basis for identifying the adverse events that appear to be related to vaccine use and for approximating rates of those events.

In a randomized, controlled clinical trial conducted in Canada, 339 infants were immunized with PEDIACEL at 2, 4 and 6 months of age. In addition, 301 of these children were immunized as toddlers at 18 months. Injection site reactions were generally mild. Up to one third of children receiving PEDIACEL experienced some degree of redness, swelling or tenderness around the injection site. Solicited injection site reaction rates are shown in Table 1.

Table 1: PEDIACEL

Frequency (%) of Solicited Reactions Observed Within 24 Hours Following a Single Dose with PEDIACEL Administered at 2, 4, 6 and 18 Months of Age

Solicited Reactions	2 months (N=336)	4 months (N=331)	6 months (N=330)	18 months (N=300)
Injection Site Reactions				
Redness	6.8	12.7	9.7	19.7
Swelling	12.5	10.3	9.7	13.7
Tenderness	22.6	22.1	14.8	33.0
Systemic Reactions				
Fever ≥38.0°C	13.4	19.6	15.9	19.5
Crying	27.7	34.7	23.0	17.0
Eating Less	29.2	19.3	15.2	13.3
Diarrhea	9.2	4.8	7.0	7.0
Vomiting	6.8	5.7	3.3	4.0
Fussiness	42.3	46.8	38.2	27.7
Less Active	44.9	29.9	13.9	12.0

Data from Post-Marketing Experience: The following additional adverse events have been spontaneously reported during the post-marketing use of PEDIACEL worldwide. Because these events are reported voluntarily from a population of uncertain size, it is not always possible to reliably estimate their frequency or establish a causal relationship to vaccine exposure. Decisions to include these events in labelling were based on one or more of the following factors: 1) severity of the event, 2) frequency of reporting, or 3) strength of causal connection to PEDIACEL.

Immune System Disorders: hypersensitivity, anaphylactic reaction (such as urticaria, angiodema).

Psychiatric Disorders: screaming.

Nervous System Disorders: convulsion (with or without fever), prolonged or unusual high-pitched crying, hypotonic hyporesponsive episode (infant appears pale, hypotonic [limp] and unresponsive to parents). To date, this condition has not been associated with any permanent sequelae.

Vascular Disorders: Edematous reactions affecting one or both lower limbs have occurred following vaccination with *H. influenza* type b containing vaccines. When this reaction occurs, it does so mainly after primary injections and is observed within the first few hours following vaccination. Associated symptoms may include cyanosis, redness, transient purpura and severe crying. All events resolved spontaneously without sequelae within 24 hours.

Skin and Subcutaneous Tissue Disorders: erythema, rash.

Musculoskeletal, Connective Tissue and Bone Disorders: pain in vaccinated limb.

General Disorders and Administration Site Conditions: high fever (>40.5°C), injection site mass, pallor, somnolence, asthenia, irritability and listlessness.

Large injection site reactions (>50 mm) including extensive limb swelling which may extend from the injection site beyond one or both joints, have been reported in children following PEDIACEL administration. These reactions start within 24-72 hours after vaccination, may be associated with erythema, warmth, tenderness or pain at the injection site and resolve spontaneously within 3 to 5 days. The risk appeared to be dependent on the number of prior doses of acellular pertussis containing vaccine, with a greater risk following the 4th and 5th doses.

Physicians, nurses and pharmacists should report any adverse occurrences temporally related to the administration of the product in accordance with local requirements and to the Global Pharmacovigilance Department, Sanofi Pasteur Limited, 1755 Steeles Avenue West, Toronto, ON, M2R 3T4 Canada. 1-888-621-1146 (phone) or 416-667-2435 (fax).

DRUG INTERACTIONS: Vaccine-Drug Interactions: Immunosuppressive treatments may interfere with the development of the expected immune response. (See Warnings and Precautions.)

Concomitant Vaccine Administration: NACI states that administering the most widely used live and inactivated vaccines during the same patient visit has produced seroconversion rates and rates of adverse reactions similar to those observed when the vaccines are administered separately. NACI recommends that vaccines administered simultaneously should be given using separate syringes at separate sites. Simultaneous administration is suggested, particularly when there is concern that a person may not return for subsequent vaccination.

PEDIACEL should not be mixed in the same syringe with other parenterals.

Vaccine-Laboratory Test Interactions: Antigenuria has been detected in some instances following administration of a vaccine containing Hib antigen. Therefore, urine antigen detection may not have definite diagnostic value in suspected *H. influenzae* type b disease within two weeks of immunization.

DOSAGE AND ADMINISTRATION: Recommended Dose: For routine immunization, PEDIACEL is recommended as a 4-dose series, with a single dose of 0.5 mL of PEDIACEL at 2, 4, 6 and 18 months of age.

If for any reason this schedule is delayed, it is recommended that 3 doses be administered with an interval of 2 months between each dose followed by a fourth dose approximately 6 to 12 months after the third dose.

Whenever feasible, PEDIACEL should be used for all 4 doses in the vaccination series as there are no clinical data to support the use of PEDIACEL with any other licensed acellular pertussis combination vaccine in a mixed sequence. For situations where a different brand of DTaP or DTaP-IPV or DTaP-IPV/Hib vaccine was originally used, or where the brand is unknown, please refer to the latest edition of the Canadian Immunization Guide.

NACI recommends that premature infants whose clinical condition is satisfactory should be immunized with full doses of vaccine at the same chronological age and according to the same schedule as full-term infants, regardless of birth weight.

Fractional doses (doses <0.5 mL) should not be given. The effect of fractional doses on the safety and efficacy has not been determined.

In compliance with NACI's recommended immunization schedule, the childhood immunization series should be completed with a single 0.5 mL dose of Sanofi Pasteur Limited's QUADRACEL [Diphtheria and Tetanus Toxoids and Acellular Pertussis Vaccine Adsorbed Combined with Inactivated Poliomyelitis Vaccine] between 4 and 6 years of age (i.e., at the time of school entry). Alternatively, ADACEL [Tetanus Toxoid, Reduced Diphtheria Toxoid and Acellular Pertussis Vaccine Adsorbed] and IPV may be administered at separate sites for this booster at 4 to 6 years of age. This booster dose is unnecessary if the fourth dose of PEDIACEL was administered after the child's fourth birthday.

A subsequent booster should be administered 10 years later, during adolescence with ADACEL or Td Adsorbed. Thereafter, routine booster immunizations should be with Td at intervals of 10 years.

PEDIACEL should not be administered to persons less than 2 months or to persons 7 years of age or older. (See Indications and Clinical Use.)

Administration: Inspect for extraneous particulate matter and/or discolouration before use. If these conditions exist, the product should not be administered.

Shake the vial well until a uniform, cloudy, suspension results. Cleanse the vial stopper with a suitable germicide prior to withdrawing the dose. Do not remove either the stopper or the metal seal holding it in place.

Aseptic technique must be used. Use a separate, sterile syringe and needle, or a sterile disposable unit, for each individual patient to prevent disease transmission. Needles should not be recapped but should be disposed of according to biohazard waste guidelines.

Before injection, the skin over the site to be injected should be cleansed with a suitable germicide. Administer the total volume of 0.5 mL **intramuscularly** (I.M.). In infants younger than 1 year, the anterolateral aspect of the thigh provides the largest muscle and is the preferred site of injection. In older children, the deltoid muscle is usually large enough for injection.

Give the patient a permanent personal immunization record. In addition, it is essential that the physician or nurse record the immunization history in the permanent medical record of each patient. This permanent office record should contain the name of the vaccine, date given, dose, manufacturer and lot number.

ACTION AND CLINICAL PHARMACOLOGY: Diphtheria and Tetanus: Strains of *C. diphtheriae* that produce diphtheria toxin can cause severe or fatal illness characterized by membranous inflammation of the upper respiratory tract and toxin-induced damage to the myocardium and nervous system. Protection against disease attributable to *C. diphtheriae* is due to the development of neutralizing antibodies to diphtheria toxin. ACIP states that a serum diphtheria antitoxin level of 0.01 IU/mL is considered the lowest level giving some degree of protection. Antitoxin levels of at least 0.1 IU/mL are generally regarded as protective. Levels of 1.0 IU/mL have been associated with long-term protection.

Tetanus is an acute and often fatal disease caused by an extremely potent neurotoxin produced by *C. tetani*. The toxin causes neuromuscular dysfunction, with rigidity and spasms of skeletal muscles. Protection against disease attributable to *C. tetani* is due to the development of neutralizing antibodies to tetanus toxin. ACIP states that a serum tetanus antitoxin level of at least 0.01 IU/mL, measured by neutralization assay, is considered the minimum protective level. A tetanus antitoxin level of at least 0.1 IU/mL as measured by the ELISA used in clinical studies of PEDIACEL is considered protective for tetanus. Levels of 1.0 IU/mL have been associated with long-term protection.

In a clinical trial in Canada, after 4 doses of PEDIACEL, 100% (N=300) of immunized children achieved serum diphtheria and tetanus antitoxin levels of at least 0.01 IU/mL and 100% of these children achieved serum antitoxin levels of at least 0.1 IU/mL for diphtheria and tetanus. After completion of the childhood immunization series, circulating antibodies to diphtheria and tetanus toxoids gradually decline but are thought to persist at protective levels for up to 10 years. NACI recommends diphtheria and tetanus toxoids boosters every 10 years.

Pertussis: Pertussis (whooping cough) is a respiratory disease caused by *B. pertussis*. This Gram-negative coccobacillus produces a variety of biologically active components, though their role in either the pathogenesis of, or immunity to, pertussis has not been clearly defined. The mechanism of protection from *B. pertussis* disease is not well understood. However, in a clinical trial in Sweden (Sweden I Efficacy Trial), pertussis components in PEDIACEL (i.e., PT, FHA, PRN and FIM) have been shown to prevent pertussis in infants with a protective efficacy of 85.2% using the World Health Organization (WHO) case definition (≥21 consecutive days of paroxysmal cough with culture or serologic confirmation or epidemiological link to a confirmed case). In the same study, the protective efficacy against mild disease was 77.9%.

Minimum serum antibody levels to specific pertussis vaccine components that confer protection against the development of clinical pertussis have not been identified. Nevertheless, a number of studies have demonstrated a correlation between the presence of serum antibody responses to pertussis vaccine components and protection against clinical disease. In a controlled clinical trial in Sweden (Sweden II Trial), the efficacy of a DTaP vaccine with the same formulation in pertussis antigens as PEDIACEL was demonstrated to provide a two-fold to three-fold higher protection against pertussis with any cough compared to the three pertussis antigens vaccine. The observed difference supports the role of fimbriae types 2 and 3 in the protection against colonization of *B. pertussis* and mild disease.

PEDIACEL is a fully liquid version of PENTACEL [Haemophilus b Conjugate Vaccine (Tetanus Protein-Conjugate) Reconstituted with Diphtheria and Tetanus Toxoids and Acellular Pertussis Vaccine Adsorbed Combined with Inactivated Poliomyelitis Vaccine] with both vaccines containing similar antigens. PENTACEL has been used in the prevention and control of pertussis in Canada since it was introduced in 1997-1998. Over 13 million doses of PENTACEL have been administered to Canadian children (at 2, 4, 6 and 18 months of age) since 1997.

In a recent publication, Bettinger et al reviewed pertussis cases during 1991-2004 using surveillance data from the Canadian Immunization Monitoring Program, Active (IMPACT), an active surveillance network based in 12 pediatric tertiary-care hospitals across Canada. Overall, the data show declining rates of pertussis during the years in which PENTACEL has been used (1999-2004) compared to the period when whole-cell pertussis vaccine was used (1991-1996). Among children 1-4 years of age, incidence of pertussis declined 85%. Data from the Northwest Territories, Newfoundland and Labrador and British Columbia support national and IMPACT data demonstrating a progressive decline of pertussis cases among infants and children through 9 years of age.

Poliomyelitis: Inactivated poliomyelitis vaccine induces the production of detectable levels of neutralizing antibodies against each type of poliovirus. The detection of type-specific neutralizing antibodies has been correlated with protection. A clinical study of PEDIACEL in 300 Canadian infants showed that, after 4 doses, more than 99.7% of vaccinated children achieved protective antibody levels (titres ≥1:8) to poliovirus types 1, 2 and 3 following the primary series.

***H. influenzae* Type b:** The response to a Haemophilus b conjugate vaccine is typical of a T-dependent immune response with induction of immunological priming and memory. Bactericidal activity against Hib is demonstrated in serum after immunization and correlates with the anti-PRP antibody response induced by Hib conjugate vaccine. In children aged ≥24 months, antibody titres to *H. influenzae* capsular polysaccharide (anti-PRP) of ≥0.15 µg/mL following vaccination with unconjugated PRP vaccine correlated with protection against invasive *H. influenzae* type b disease immediately after immunization, whereas titres ≥1.0 µg/mL correlated with protection for at least 1 year. Although the relevance of the 0.15 µg/mL and 1.0 µg/mL thresholds to clinical protection after immunization with conjugate vaccines is not known, these levels have been used to gauge antibody response to vaccination. In a clinical study of PEDIACEL in 300 infants in Canada after 4 doses, 100% of vaccinated children achieved protective antibody titres ≥0.15 µg/mL, and 99.0% achieved protective antibody levels ≥1.0 µg/mL.

Duration of Effect: To ensure optimal protection during childhood, 4 consecutive doses should be given at 2, 4, 6 and 18 months of age. A booster with a vaccine containing diphtheria, tetanus, acellular pertussis with or without IPV is required at 4 to 6 years.

STORAGE AND STABILITY: Store at 2 to 8°C. Do not freeze. Discard product if exposed to freezing. Do not use after expiration date.

INFORMATION FOR THE PATIENT: Published in e-CPS, available by subscription at www.e-cps.ca.

DOSAGE FORMS, COMPOSITION AND PACKAGING: PEDIACEL is supplied as a sterile, uniform, cloudy, white to off-white suspension in a vial. Each single dose (0.5 mL) contains: diphtheria toxoid 15 Lf; tetanus toxoid 5 Lf; acellular pertussis: pertussis toxoid (PT) 20 µg, filamentous haemagglutinin (FHA) 20 µg, pertactin (PRN) 3 µg, fimbriae types 2 and 3 (FIM) 5 µg; inactivated poliomyelitis vaccine: type 1 (Mahoney) 40 D-antigen units, type 2 (MEF1) 8 D-antigen units, type 3 (Saukett) 32 D-antigen units; purified polyribosylribitol phosphate capsular polysaccharide (PRP) of *H. influenzae* type b covalently bound to 20 µg of tetanus protein 10 µg. Excipients: aluminum phosphate (adjuvant) 1.5 mg, 2-phenoxyethanol 0.6% v/v, polysorbate 80 ≤0.1% w/v (by calculation). Manufacturing Process Residuals: bovine serum albumin, neomycin, polymyxin B, streptomycin, formaldehyde and glutaraldehyde are present in trace amounts. The container closure system does not contain latex (natural rubber). Single dose Type 1 glass vials of 0.5 mL, packages of 1 and 5.

Pediapred® ℞

prednisolone sodium phosphate

Glucocorticoid—Anti-inflammatory

sanofi-aventis

SUPPLIED: Each 5 mL of dye-free, colorless to light straw-colored, raspberry-flavored solution contains: prednisolone base 5 mg (as prednisolone sodium phosphate USP) in a palatable, aqueous vehicle. Nonmedicinal ingredients: disodium edetate, flavor raspberry, methylparaben, purified water, sodium phosphate and sorbitol. Bottles of 120 mL. Store at 15 to 30°C. Do not refrigerate. Keep cap tightly closed.

Pediatric Electrolyte

electrolytes

Electrolyte Solution

PendoPharm

SUPPLIED: Solutions: Apple Flavor: Contains: acesulfame potassium, artificial apple flavor, benzoic acid (237 mL format), caramel color, citric acid, dextrose, fructose, potassium citrate, sodium chloride, sodium citrate, sucralose and water. Plastic bottles of 237 and 1000 mL.

Cherry Flavor: Contains: acesulfame potassium, benzoic acid (237 mL format), citric acid, dextrose, fructose, natural and artificial cherry flavors (FD&C Red No. 40), potassium citrate, sodium chloride, sodium citrate, sucralose and water. Plastic bottles of 237 and 1000 mL.

Fruit Flavor: Contains: acesulfame potassium, benzoic acid (237 mL format), citric acid, dextrose, FD&C Yellow No. 6, fructose, natural and artificial fruit flavor, potassium citrate, sodium chloride, sodium citrate, sucralose and water. Plastic bottles of 237 and 1000 mL.

Grape Flavor: Contains: acesulfame potassium, artificial grape flavor, benzoic acid (237 mL format), citric acid, dextrose, FD&C Blue No. 1, FD&C Red No. 40, fructose, potassium citrate, sodium chloride, sodium citrate, sucralose and water. Plastic bottles of 237 and 1000 mL.

Unflavored: Contains: benzoic acid (237 mL format), citric acid, dextrose, potassium citrate, sodium chloride, sodium citrate and water. Plastic bottles of 237 and 1000 mL.

Do not freeze. Protect from heat. Discard unused portion of opened 237 mL bottle. After opening 1 L Pediatric Electrolyte, replace cap, refrigerate and use within 48 hours.

Freezer Pops: Cherry Flavor: Contains: acesulfame potassium, benzoic acid (a preservative), citric acid, cornstarch, dextrose, ethyl acetate, FD&C Red No. 40, maltodextrin, natural and artificial cherry flavors, potassium citrate, sodium carboxymethylcellulose, sodium chloride, sodium citrate, sucralose, sulfites and water. Boxes of 16 pops of 62.5 mL each.

Grape Flavor: Contains: acesulfame potassium, acetic acid, benzoic acid (a preservative), citric acid, cornstarch, dextrose, EDTA calcium, ethyl acetate, FD&C Red No. 40, FD&C Blue No. 1, maltodextrin, natural and artificial grape flavor, potassium citrate, sodium ascorbate, sodium carboxymethylcellulose, sodium chloride, sodium citrate, sucralose and water. Boxes of 16 pops of 62.5 mL each.

Orange Flavor: Contains: acesulfame potassium, benzoic acid (a preservative), citric acid, cornstarch, dextrose, FD&C Red No. 40, FD&C Yellow No. 6, maltodextrin, natural and artificial orange flavors, potassium citrate, sodium carboxymethylcellulose, sodium chloride, sodium citrate, sucralose, tocopherol and water. Boxes of 16 pops of 62.5 mL each.

Wild Berry Flavor: Contains: acesulfame potassium, acetic acid, benzoic acid (a preservative), citric acid, cornstarch, dextrose, FD&C Blue No. 1, maltodextrin, natural and artificial wild berry flavor, potassium citrate, sodium carboxymethylcellulose, sodium chloride, sodium citrate, sucralose, triacetin and water. Boxes of 16 pops of 62.5 mL each.

Pediatrix

acetaminophen

Antipyretic—Analgesic

Rougier Pharma

SUPPLIED: Drops: Each mL of red clear solution contains: acetaminophen 80 mg. Nonmedicinal ingredients: artificial coloring and flavorings, citric acid, glycerin, methylparaben, polyethylene glycol, propylene glycol, propylparaben, purified water, sodium cyclamate and sodium phosphate dibasic. Alcohol-, gluten-, lactose-, sucrose- and tartrazine-free. Plastic bottles of 24 mL (child resistant cap) with a calibrated dropper. Concentrated, for dropper dosage only.

Oral Solution: Each 5 mL of red clear solution contains: acetaminophen 160 mg. Nonmedicinal ingredients: artificial coloring and flavoring, citric acid, FD&C Yellow #6, glycerin, methylparaben, polyethylene glycol, propylene glycol, propylparaben, purified water, sodium cyclamate, sodium phosphate dibasic and sorbitol. Alcohol-, gluten-, lactose-, sucrose- and tartrazine-free. Amber plastic bottles of 100 mL (child resistant closure) and 500 mL (for pharmacists and hospitals only). All bottles are safety sealed.

Store between 15 and 30°C.

Pegalax™

polyethylene glycol

Laxative

Medical Futures

SUMMARY PRODUCT INFORMATION:

Route of Administration	Dosage Form/ Strength	Clinically Relevant Nonmedicinal Ingredients
Oral	Powder for oral solution/100% w/w	None

INDICATIONS AND CLINICAL USE: Pegalax is indicated for the treatment of occasional constipation and irregularity. This product should be used for 7 days or less or as directed by a physician.

CONTRAINDICATIONS: Pegalax is contraindicated in patients with known or suspected bowel obstruction and patients known to be allergic to polyethylene glycol.

WARNINGS AND PRECAUTIONS: This product should be used for one week or less.

Overuse or extended use of any laxative may cause dependence for bowel function.

A laxative should not be taken within two hours of another medicine because the desired effect of the other medicine may be reduced.

Patients should be instructed to consult their physician if unusual cramps, bloating or diarrhea occur.

Patients with symptoms suggestive of bowel obstruction, appendicitis, or inflamed bowel (fever, nausea, vomiting, abdominal pain or bloating) should be evaluated to rule out these conditions before initiating Pegalax therapy.

Patients presenting with complaints of constipation should have a thorough medical history and physical examination to detect associated metabolic, endocrine and neurogenic conditions, and medications. A diagnostic evaluation should include a structural examination of the colon. Patients should be educated about good defecatory and eating habits (such as high fiber diets) and lifestyle changes (adequate dietary fiber and fluid intake, regular exercise) which may produce more regular bowel habits.

Carcinogenesis and Mutagenesis: Long term carcinogenicity studies, genetic toxicity studies and reproductive toxicity studies in animals have not been performed with Pegalax.

Special Populations: Pregnant Women: Category C. Animal reproductive studies have not been performed with Pegalax. It is also not known whether Pegalax can cause fetal harm when administered to a pregnant woman, or can affect reproductive capacity. The use of Pegalax should be avoided in women who are pregnant unless clearly needed and directed by a physician.

Nursing Women: It is unknown if Pegalax is excreted in human milk. Because many drugs are excreted in human milk, precaution should be exercised. The use of Pegalax should be avoided in nursing women unless clearly needed and directed by a physician.

Pediatrics: Safety and effectiveness in pediatric patients has not been established. Pegalax should not be used in children under 18 years of age.

Geriatrics: There is no evidence for special considerations when Pegalax is administered to elderly patients. In geriatric nursing home patients a higher incidence of diarrhea occurred at the recommended 17 g dose. If diarrhea occurs Pegalax should be discontinued.

Monitoring and Laboratory Tests: No clinically significant effects on laboratory tests have been demonstrated.

ADVERSE REACTIONS: Nausea, abdominal bloating, cramping and flatulence may occur. High doses may produce diarrhea and excessive stool frequency, particularly in elderly nursing home patients.

Patients taking other medications containing polyethylene glycol have occasionally developed urticaria suggestive of an allergic reaction.

DRUG INTERACTIONS: Drug-Drug Interactions: A laxative should not be taken within two hours of another medicine because the desired effect of the other medicine may be reduced.

DOSAGE AND ADMINISTRATION: Recommended Dose and Dosage Adjustment: The usual dose is 17 g (1 sachet) of Pegalax per day.

Treatment for two to four days (48 to 96 hours) may be required to produce a bowel movement.

Pegalax should be used once a day only.

Administration: Oral.

Reconstitution: Oral Solutions: The usual daily dose of Pegalax powder (17 g) should be stirred in 250 mL or 8 ounces of water, juice, soda, coffee or tea until completely dissolved.

The solution should be drunk immediately.

OVERDOSAGE:

There have been no reports of accidental over dosage. In the event of over dosage diarrhea would be the expected major event. If an overdose of drug occurred without concomitant ingestion of fluid, dehydration due to diarrhea may result. Medication should be terminated and free water administered.

For management of a suspected drug overdose, contact your **regional Poison Control Centre**. See the *CPS* Directory section for a list of Poison Control Centres.

ACTION AND CLINICAL PHARMACOLOGY: Mechanism of Action: Pegalax (polyethylene glycol 3350, powder for oral solution) is a synthetic polyglycol having an average molecular weight of 3350. The actual molecular weight is not less than 90.0 percent and not greater than 110.0 percent of the nominal value. The chemical formula is HO(C2H4O)nH in which n represents the average number of oxyethylene groups. Below 55°C it is a free flowing white powder freely soluble in water. Pegalax is an osmotic agent for the treatment of constipation.

Pegalax softens the stool and increases the frequency of bowel movements by retaining water in the stool.

Pharmacology: Pegalax is an osmotic agent which causes water to be retained with the stool. Essentially, complete recovery of Pegalax was shown in normal subjects without constipation. Attempts at recovery of Pegalax in constipated patients resulted in incomplete and highly variable recovery. An in-vitro study showed indirectly that Pegalax was not fermented into hydrogen or methane by the colonic microflora in human feces. Pegalax appears to have no effect on the active absorption or secretion of glucose or electrolytes. There is no evidence of tachyphylaxis.

Pharmacodynamics: Pharmacotherapeutic group: A06A D15.

Polyethylene glycol 3350 exerts an osmotic action in the gut, which induces a laxative effect. PEG 3350 increases the stool volume, which triggers colon motility via neuromuscular pathways. The physiological consequence is a propulsive colonic transportation of the softened stools.

Pharmacokinetics: Polyethylene glycol 3350 is unchanged along the gut. It is virtually unabsorbed from the gastro-intestinal tract. Any PEG 3350 that is absorbed is excreted via the urine.

STORAGE AND STABILITY: Store at 15-30°C, in a dry area.

Keep out of reach of children.

Shelf life period: 2 years.

DOSAGE FORMS, COMPOSITION AND PACKAGING: Each sachet of white powder for oral solution contains: 100% of polyethylene glycol 3350. Powder sachets of laminated low density polyethylene/aluminium/low density polyethylene/paper of 17 g, cardboard cartons of 4 and 14 sachets. Each carton box is supplied with a label.

Pegasys® ℞

peginterferon alfa-2a

Biological Response Modifier

Roche

Date of Revision: March 10, 2010

SUMMARY PRODUCT INFORMATION:

Route of Administration	Dosage Form/ Strength	Clinically Relevant Nonmedicinal Ingredients
Subcutaneous	Solution in vial: 180 µg/1.0 mL	Benzyl alcohol For a complete listing see Dosage Forms, Composition and Packaging.
	Solution in pre-filled syringe: 180 µg/0.5 mL	Benzyl alcohol For a complete listing see Dosage Forms, Composition and Packaging.

DESCRIPTION: PEGASYS: Peginterferon alfa-2a is a covalent conjugate of recombinant alfa-2a interferon (approximate molecular weight [MW] 20 kD) with a single branched bis-monomethoxy polyethylene glycol (PEG) chain (approximate MW 40 kD). Interferon alfa-2a is produced biosynthetically using recombinant DNA technology, and is the product of a cloned human leukocyte interferon gene inserted into and expressed in *E. coli*.

INDICATIONS AND CLINICAL USE: Chronic Hepatitis C (CHC): PEGASYS (peginterferon alfa-2a) is indicated for the treatment of chronic hepatitis C in:

- Adult patients without cirrhosis
- Adult patients with compensated cirrhosis,

including HCV/HIV co-infection patients with stable HIV disease with or without antiretroviral therapy.

Chronic Hepatitis B (CHB): PEGASYS is indicated for the treatment of both HBeAg-positive and HBeAg-negative chronic hepatitis B in:

- Patients with compensated liver disease, liver inflammation and evidence of viral replication (both cirrhotic and non-cirrhotic disease).

CONTRAINDICATIONS: PEGASYS (peginterferon alfa-2a) is contraindicated in:

- Patients with known hypersensitivity to alpha interferons, to *E. coli* derived products, to polyethyleneglycol or to any component of the product (see Dosage Forms, Composition and Packaging),
- Patients with autoimmune hepatitis,
- Patients with decompensated cirrhosis,
- HIV-HCV patients with cirrhosis and a base-line Child-Pugh score ≥6 (see Warnings and Precautions, Hepatic/Biliary/Pancreas and Dosage and Administration, Special Populations).
- Neonates and infants because PEGASYS contains benzyl alcohol. There have been rare reports of death in neonates and infants associated with excessive exposure to benzyl alcohol. The amount of benzyl alcohol at which toxicity or adverse effects may occur in neonates or infants is not known.

WARNINGS AND PRECAUTIONS:

> **Serious Warnings and Precautions**
> **Alpha interferons, including PEGASYS (peginterferon alfa-2a), cause or aggravate fatal or life-threatening neuropsychiatric, autoimmune, ischemic, and infectious disorders. Patients should be monitored closely with periodic clinical and laboratory evaluations. Patients with persistently severe or worsening signs or symptoms of these conditions should be withdrawn from therapy. In many cases, but not all cases, these disorders resolve after stopping interferon therapy (see Warnings and Precautions).**

General: The safety and efficacy of PEGASYS have not been established in patients who have failed other alpha interferon treatments.

Treatment with PEGASYS should be administered under the guidance of a qualified physician and may lead to moderate to severe adverse experiences requiring dose reduction, temporary dose cessation or discontinuation of therapy.

Patients should be informed regarding the potential benefits and risks attendant to the use of PEGASYS. If home use is determined to be desirable by the physician, instructions on appropriate use should be given, including review of the contents of the Consumer Information, which does not disclose all possible adverse effects of PEGASYS (see Information for the Patient).

If home use is prescribed, patients should be thoroughly instructed in the importance of proper disposal of, and cautioned against, reuse of any needles and syringes.

Patients should be cautioned not to change to other pegylated interferons or switch to other alpha interferons without a medical consultation; changing from one interferon to another may require dosage change or adjustment.

Patients who develop dizziness, confusion, somnolence, or fatigue should be cautioned to avoid driving or operating machinery.

Cardiovascular: Cardiovascular events such as hypertension, supraventricular arrhythmias, congestive heart failure, chest pain and myocardial infarction have been associated with interferon therapies, including PEGASYS. Therefore, PEGASYS should be administered with caution to patients with pre existing cardiac disease. Patients should be assessed before initiation of therapy and should be appropriately monitored during therapy. It is recommended that patients who have pre existing cardiac abnormalities have an electrocardiogram prior to initiation of PEGASYS. As with other alpha interferons, treatment with PEGASYS is not recommended in patients with pre existing severe, unstable or uncontrolled cardiac disease; if there is any deterioration of cardiovascular status, PEGASYS therapy should be suspended or discontinued.

Cerebrovascular: Ischemic and hemorrhagic cerebrovascular events have been observed in patients treated with interferon alfa-based therapies, including PEGASYS. Events occurred in patients with few or no reported risk factors for stroke, including patients less than 45 years of age. Because these are spontaneous reports, estimates of frequency cannot be made and a causal relationship between interferon alfa-based therapies and these events is difficult to establish.

Endocrine and Metabolism: Endocrine: As with other interferons, PEGASYS may cause or aggravate hypothyroidism and hyperthyroidism. Hypoglycemia, hyperglycemia, and diabetes mellitus have been observed in patients treated with PEGASYS. Patients with these conditions at baseline who cannot be effectively controlled by medication should not be started on PEGASYS therapy. Patients who develop these conditions during treatment and cannot be controlled with medication should not continue PEGASYS therapy.

Gastrointestinal: Colitis: Hemorrhagic/ischemic colitis, sometimes fatal, has been observed within 12 weeks of starting alpha interferon treatment. Abdominal pain, bloody diarrhea, and fever are the typical manifestations of colitis. PEGASYS treatment should be discontinued immediately if these symptoms develop. The colitis usually resolves within 1 to 3 weeks following discontinuation of alpha interferon. Ulcerative colitis has also been observed in patients treated with alpha interferon.

Hematologic: Alpha interferons, including PEGASYS, may suppress bone marrow function which may result in severe cytopenias. Very rarely alpha interferons may be associated with pancytopenia including aplastic anemia. Therefore, caution should be exercised when administering PEGASYS in combination with other potentially myelosuppressive agents. It is advised that complete blood counts (CBC) be obtained pre treatment and monitored routinely during therapy (see Warnings and Precautions, Monitoring and Laboratory Tests).

PEGASYS should be used with caution in patients with baseline absolute neutrophil counts (ANC) <1.5×10⁹/L, with baseline platelets <90×10⁹/L or baseline hemoglobin <100 g/L. PEGASYS should be discontinued, at least temporarily, in patients who develop severe decreases in ANC (<0.5×10⁹/L) and/or platelet (<25×10⁹/L) counts (see Dosage and Administration, Recommended Dose and Dosage Adjustment).

Hepatic/Biliary/Pancreas: Hepatic: In patients who develop evidence of hepatic decompensation during treatment, PEGASYS treatment should be discontinued. HIV-HCV co-infected patients with advanced cirrhosis receiving concomitant HAART may be at an increased risk of hepatic decompensation and possibly death when treated with ribavirin in combination with alpha interferons, including PEGASYS. During treatment, co-infected patients should be closely monitored, periodically assessing their clinical status and hepatic function and should be immediately discontinued if they decompensate (Child-Pugh score ≥6) (see Dosage and Administration).

CHC: As with other alpha interferons, increases in ALT levels above baseline have been observed in patients treated with PEGASYS, including those patients who exhibit a virological response.

When the increase in ALT levels is progressive despite dose reduction or is accompanied by increased bilirubin, therapy should be discontinued (see Dosage and Administration).

CHB: Unlike CHC, disease exacerbations during therapy are not uncommon and are characterized by transient and potentially significant increases in serum ALT. Transient ALT elevations are common during CHB therapy with PEGASYS. Flares have been accompanied by elevations of total bilirubin and alkaline phosphatase and less commonly with prolongation of PT and reduced albumin levels. In clinical trials with PEGASYS in HBV, marked transaminase flares have been accompanied by mild changes in other measures of hepatic function and without evidence of hepatic decompensation. In approximately half the case of flares exceeding 10 times the upper limit of normal, PEGASYS dosing was reduced or withheld until the transaminase elevations subsided, while in the rest therapy was continued unchanged. More frequent monitoring of hepatic function was recommended in all instances (see Adverse Reactions and Dosage and Administration).

Pancreatitis: Pancreatitis, sometimes fatal, has occurred during alpha interferon treatment. PEGASYS treatment should be suspended if symptoms or signs suggestive of pancreatitis are observed. PEGASYS should be discontinued in patients diagnosed with pancreatitis.

Hydration: Adequate hydration must be maintained in patients undergoing therapy with PEGASYS, since hypotension related to fluid depletion has been seen in some patients treated with alpha interferons. Fluid replacement may be necessary.

Hypersensitivity: Serious, acute hypersensitivity reactions (e.g. urticaria, angioedema, bronchoconstriction, anaphylaxis) have been rarely observed during alpha interferon therapy and cutaneous eruptions (Stevens-Johnson syndrome, toxic epidermal necrolysis) have been very rarely reported. If such a reaction develops during treatment with PEGASYS, treatment should be discontinued and appropriate medical therapy should be instituted immediately. Transient rashes do not necessitate interruption of treatment.

Immune: Exacerbation of autoimmune disease including myositis, hepatitis, immune thrombocytopenic purpura (ITP), rheumatoid arthritis, interstitial nephritis, thyroiditis and systemic lupus erythematosus has been reported in patients receiving alpha interferon therapy. PEGASYS should be used with extreme caution in patients with autoimmune disorders. Use of alpha interferons has been associated with exacerbation or provocation of psoriasis. PEGASYS must be used with caution in patients with psoriasis; in case of appearance or worsening of psoriatic lesions, discontinuation of therapy should be considered.

Infections: While fever may be associated with the flu-like syndrome reported commonly during interferon therapy, other causes of persistent fever must be ruled out, particularly in patients with neutropenia. Serious infections (bacterial, viral, fungal) have been reported during treatment with alpha interferons including PEGASYS. Appropriate anti-infective therapy should be started immediately and discontinuation of therapy should be considered.

Ophthalmologic: As with other interferons, retinopathy including retinal hemorrhages, cotton wool spots, papilledema, retinal artery or vein obstruction and serous retinal detachment have been reported in rare instances after treatment with PEGASYS. As with other interferons, decrease or loss of vision, macular edema and optic neuritis may be induced or aggravated by PEGASYS treatment. All patients should receive an eye examination at baseline. Patients with preexisting ophthalmologic disorders (e.g. diabetic or hypertensive retinopathy) should receive periodic ophthalmologic exams during PEGASYS treatment. Any patient complaining of decreased or loss of vision must have a prompt and complete eye examination. PEGASYS treatment should be discontinued in patients who develop new or worsening ophthalmologic disorders.

Psychiatric: Severe psychiatric adverse reactions may manifest in patients receiving therapy with interferons, including PEGASYS. Depression, suicidal ideation, and suicidal attempt may occur in patients with and without previous psychiatric illness. Other CNS effects including aggressive behavior, confusion and other alterations of mental status have been observed with alpha interferon. PEGASYS should be used with extreme caution in patients who report a history of depression and physicians should monitor all patients for evidence of depression. Physicians should inform patients of the possible development of depression prior to initiation of PEGASYS therapy, and patients should report any sign or symptom of depression immediately. If severe symptoms persist, therapy should be stopped and psychiatric intervention sought (see Adverse Reactions).

Renal: Renal impairment is associated with decreased total apparent clearance and prolonged half life. In subjects with a creatinine clearance between 0.33 and 0.67 mL/sec, the average total apparent clearance is reduced by approximately 30% compared with subjects with normal renal function following single doses of PEGASYS. There is no information available following multiple doses of drug, in patients with creatinine clearance <0.83 mL/sec. As with all patients treated with PEGASYS, patients with renal impairment may require dose modification for moderate to severe adverse reactions (clinical and/or laboratory) occurring during therapy (see Dosage and Administration, Recommended Dose and Dosage Adjustment, Dose Adjustments and Action and Clinical Pharmacology, Pharmacokinetics of PEGASYS in Special Populations and Conditions).

Respiratory: As with other alpha interferons, pulmonary symptoms, including dyspnea, pulmonary infiltrates, pneumonia, and pneumonitis, including fatality, have been reported during therapy with PEGASYS. Any patient developing fever, cough, and dyspnea or other respiratory symptoms must have a chest X ray taken. If there is evidence of persistent or unexplained pulmonary infiltrates or pulmonary function impairment, treatment should be discontinued.

Sexual Function/Reproduction: Peginterferon alfa-2a has not been studied for its teratogenic effect. Treatment with interferon alfa-2a resulted in a statistically significant increase in abortifacient activity in rhesus monkeys; no teratogenic effects were seen in the offspring delivered at term (see Special Populations, Pregnant Women).

Transplantation: The safety and efficacy of PEGASYS treatment have not been established in patients with liver or other transplantations. As with other alpha interferons, liver and renal graft rejections have been reported on PEGASYS, alone or in combination with COPEGUS.

Special Populations: Pregnant Women: The safety of PEGASYS during pregnancy has not been established. Therefore, PEGASYS should be used during pregnancy only if the potential benefit justifies the potential risk to the fetus.

As with other alpha interferons, women of childbearing potential receiving PEGASYS therapy should be advised to use effective contraception during therapy (see Sexual Function/Reproduction).

Nursing Women: It is not known whether PEGASYS or its components are excreted in human milk. The effect of orally ingested PEGASYS from breast milk on the nursing infant has not been evaluated. Because of the potential for adverse reactions from the drug in nursing infants, a decision should be made to discontinue nursing or PEGASYS, based on the importance of the therapy to the mother.

Pediatrics (<18 years of age): Safety and effectiveness have not been established in patients below the age of 18. In addition, PEGASYS injection solutions contain benzyl alcohol. Therefore, PEGASYS should not be used in neonates or infants (see Contraindications).

Monitoring and Laboratory Tests: Before beginning PEGASYS therapy, standard hematological and biochemical profiles should be obtained for all patients. After initiation of therapy, hematological tests should be performed at 2 weeks and biochemical tests should be performed at 4 weeks. Additional testing should be performed periodically during therapy.

The enrolment criteria used for the clinical studies of PEGASYS may be considered as a guideline to acceptable baseline values for initiation of treatment: platelet count ≥90×10⁹/L (75×10⁹/L in patients with cirrhosis or transition to cirrhosis); ANC ≥1.5×10⁹/L; serum creatinine concentration <1.5×upper limit of normal; TSH and T_4 within normal limits or adequately controlled thyroid function; HIV-HCV co-infection: CD4+ ≥200/µL or CD4+ ≥100/µ-<200/µL and HIV-1 RNA <5000 copies/mL using Amplicor HIV-1 Monitor Test, v 1.5.

PEGASYS treatment was associated with decreases in both total white blood cell (WBC) count and ANC, usually starting within the first 2 weeks of treatment (see Adverse Reactions). In clinical studies, progressive decreases thereafter were infrequent. Dose reduction is recommended when ANC decreases to levels below 0.75×10⁹/L (see Dosage and Administration, Recommended Dose and Dosage Adjustment, Dose Adjustments). For patients with ANC values below 0.5×10⁹/L treatment should be suspended until ANC values return to more than 1.0×10⁹/L. In clinical trials with PEGASYS, the decrease in ANC was reversible upon dose reduction or cessation of therapy.

PEGASYS treatment was associated with decreases in platelet count, which returned to pre treatment (baseline) levels during the post treatment observation period (see Adverse Reactions). Dose reduction is recommended when platelet count decreases to levels below 50×10⁹, and discontinuation of therapy is recommended when platelet count decreases to levels below 25×10⁹/L (see Dosage and Administration, Recommended Dose and Dosage Adjustment, Dose Adjustments).

ADVERSE REACTIONS: Adverse Drug Reaction Overview: The frequency and severity of the most commonly reported adverse reactions are similar in patients treated with PEGASYS (peginterferon alfa-2a) and interferon alfa-2a.

The most frequently reported adverse reactions with 180 µg PEGASYS were mostly mild to moderate in severity and were manageable without the need for modification of dosage or discontinuation of therapy.

Clinical Trial Adverse Drug Reactions: Chronic Hepatitis C Mono-infection: In mono-infection clinical trials, the incidence of withdrawal from treatment for all patients due to adverse events and laboratory abnormalities was 10%, 9% and 13% for interferon alfa-2a (IFN), PEGASYS or for PEGASYS RBV (peginterferon alfa-2a and ribavirin) combination therapy, respectively. Only 1% or 3% of patients required discontinuation of either PEGASYS or PEGASYS RBV combination therapy for laboratory abnormalities. The withdrawal rates for patients with cirrhosis were similar to those of the overall population.

HIV-HCV Co-infection : In HIV-HCV co-infected patients, the clinical adverse events reported on PEGASYS, PEGASYS RBV and interferon alfa-2a plus ribavirin were similar to that observed in HCV mono-infected patients.

In the co-infection study, the incidence of withdrawal from treatment for clinical adverse events, laboratory abnormalities or AIDS-defining events was 16% for PEGASYS monotherapy and 15% for both PEGASYS RBV and interferon alfa-2a plus ribavirin given for 48 weeks. Respectively, 4%, 3% or 1% of patients required discontinuation of PEGASYS or PEGASYS RBV or interferon alfa-2a plus ribavirin for laboratory abnormalities. In PEGASYS RBV combination therapy, the PEGASYS dose modification occurred in 39%, and the COPEGUS dose modification occurred in 37%, of the co-infected patients. In interferon alfa-2a plus ribavirin therapy, the interferon alfa-2a dose modification occurred in 16%, and the COPEGUS dose modification occurred in 28%, of the co-infected patients. In PEGASYS monotherapy, PEGASYS dose modification occurred in 38% of the co-infected patients. Serious adverse events were reported in 21%, 17% and 15% of those receiving PEGASYS monotherapy, PEGASYS RBV or interferon alfa-2a plus ribavirin, respectively.

Limited safety data (N=31) is available in co-infected patients with CD4+ cell counts <200/µL treated with PEGASYS and PEGASYS RBV. PEGASYS containing treatment was associated with an on-treatment reduction in absolute CD4+ cell count without a reduction in CD4+ cell percentage. CD4+ cell count indices returned to baseline values during the follow-up period of the study. PEGASYS containing treatment had no apparent negative impact on the control of HIV viremia during therapy or follow-up.

Chronic Hepatitis B: In clinical trials of 48 week treatment and 24 weeks follow-up, the safety profile for PEGASYS in chronic hepatitis B (CHB) was similar to that seen in chronic hepatitis C (see Table 1). 88% of PEGASYS-treated patients experienced adverse events, as compared to 53% of patients in the lamivudine comparator group, while 6% of the PEGASYS treated and 4% of the lamivudine treated patients experienced serious adverse events during the studies. Five percent of patients withdrew from PEGASYS treatment due to adverse events or laboratory abnormalities, while less than 1% withdrew from lamivudine treatment for safety reasons. The withdrawal rates for patients with cirrhosis were similar to those of the overall population in each treatment group. The addition of lamivudine had no effect on the safety profile of PEGASYS.

Because clinical trials are conducted under very specific conditions the adverse drug reaction rates observed in the clinical trials may not reflect the rates observed in practice and should not be compared to the rates in the clinical trials of another drug. Adverse drug reaction information from clinical trials is useful for identifying drug-related adverse events and for approximating rates.

Table 1: PEGASYS

Adverse Reactions (≥10% of Incidence in Any Treatment Group)

	HBV		HCV						HIV-HCV			
	PEGASYS 180 µg[a] N=448		Interferon alfa 2a 3 MIU N=323		Interferon alfa 2a 6/3 MIU N=261		PEGASYS 180 µg N=827		INF alfa-2a 3 MIU + ribavirin 800 mg N=285		PEGASYS 180 µg N=286	
	N	(%)	N	(%)	N	(%)	N	(%)	N	(%)	N	(%)
Gastrointestinal												
Nausea	29	(6)	101	(31)	80	(31)	199	(24)	54	(19)	54	(19)
Diarrhea	28	(6)	44	(14)	48	(18)	132	(16)	29	(10)	35	(12)
Abdominal pain	19	(4)	50	(15)	35	(13)	120	(15)	17	(6)	18	(6)
Nausea and vomiting	9	(2)	19	(6)	25	(10)	43	(5)	22	(8)	18	(6)
General												
Fatigue	93	(21)	147	(46)	152	(58)	405	(49)	102	(36)	104	(36)
Rigors	28	(6)	134	(41)	112	(43)	219	(30)	49	(17)	41	(14)
Pyrexia	233	(52)	94	(29)	141	(54)	249	(35)	92	(32)	101	(35)
Injection site reaction	33	(7)	71	(22)	40	(15)	178	(22)	24	(8)	23	(8)
Pain	6	(1)	46	(14)	27	(10)	89	(11)	11	(4)	14	(5)
Asthenia	50	(11)	27	(8)	9	(3)	56	(7)	65	(23)	56	(20)
Metabolic and Nutritional												
Anorexia	59	(13)	37	(11)	61	(23)	131	(16)	71	(25)	59	(21)
Weight decreased	18	(4)	11	(3)	7	(3)	44	(5)	36	(13)	44	(15)
Musculoskeletal, Connective Tissue and Bone												
Myalgia	114	(25)	115	(36)	108	(41)	307	(37)	77	(27)	82	(29)
Arthralgia	43	(10)	87	(27)	82	(31)	211	(26)	36	(13)	43	(15)
Back pain	8	(2)	31	(10)	27	(10)	67	(8)	8	(3)	18	(6)
Neurological												
Headache	103	(23)	174	(54)	165	(63)	428	(52)	97	(34)	84	(29)
Insomnia	25	(6)	78	(24)	57	(22)	167	(20)	66	(23)	46	(16)
Dizziness (excluding vertigo)	28	(6)	33	(10)	39	(15)	120	(15)	26	(9)	7	(2)
Concentration impairment	9	(2)	31	(10)	26	(10)	76	(9)	7	(2)	7	(2)
Psychiatric												
Depression	17	(4)	51	(16)	57	(22)	148	(18)	57	(20)	45	(16)
Irritability	14	(3)	67	(21)	29	(11)	141	(17)	48	(17)	45	(16)
Skin and Subcutaneous Tissue												
Alopecia	78	(17)	78	(24)	92	(35)	187	(23)	13	(5)	19	(7)
Pruritus	25	(6)	20	(6)	24	(9)	104	(13)	11	(4)	12	(4)

[a] In clinical trials, 450 patients received PEGASYS in combination with lamivudine. The addition of lamivudine had no effect on the safety profile of PEGASYS.

Table 2: PEGASYS

Adverse Reactions Reported in ≥1% to <10% on PEGASYS RBV Combination or PEGASYS Monotherapy in Patients in Clinical Trials Were:

	Any Treatment Group		HIV-HCV Only
Body System	**Common ≥5% to <10%**	**Common ≥1% to <5%**	**Other Adverse Reactions ≥1% to ≤3%**
Blood and Lymphatic System Disorders		lymphadenopathy, thrombocytopenia	
Cardiac Disorders		palpitation,oedema peripheral, tachycardia	

(cont'd)

Table 2: PEGASYS *(cont'd)*

Adverse Reactions Reported in ≥1% to <10% on PEGASYS RBV Combination or PEGASYS Monotherapy in Patients in Clinical Trials Were:

	Any Treatment Group		HIV-HCV Only
Body System	**Common ≥5% to <10%**	**Common ≥1% to <5%**	**Other Adverse Reactions ≥1% to ≤3%**
Ear and Labyrinth Disorders		vertigo, earache, tinnitus	
Endocrine Disorders		hypothyroidism, hyperthyroidism	
Eye Disorders		vision blurred, eye inflammation, xerophthalmia, eye pain	
Gastrointestinal Disorders	dry mouth, dyspepsia	mouth ulceration, flatulence, gingival bleeding, stomatitis, constipation, dysphagia, glossitis	cheilitis
General Disorders and Administration Site Conditions	malaise	lethargy, chest pain, hot flushes, thirst, influenza-like illness	
Infections and Infestations		herpes simplex, URI infection bronchitis, oral candidiasis	influenza, pneumonia
Injury and Poisoning		substance abuse	
Metabolism and Nutrition Disorders		dehydration	hyperlactacidemia/ lactic acidosis
Musculoskeletal, Connective Tissue and Bone Disorders	back pain	muscle cramps, neck pain, musculoskeletal pain, bone pain, arthritis, muscle weakness	
Nervous System Disorders	memory impairment	taste disturbance, weakness, paraesthesia, hypoaesthesia, tremor, migraine, somnolence, hyperaesthesia, nightmares, syncope	
Psychiatric Disorders	anxiety, mood alteration, emotional disorders	nervousness, libido decreased, aggression, suicidal ideation, confusional state	affect lability, apathy
Renal and Urinary Disorders			chromaturia
Reproductive System and Breast Disorders		impotence	
Respiratory, Thoracic and Mediastinal Disorders	dyspnoea, cough	sore throat, pharyngolaryngeal pain, dyspnoea exertional, epistaxis, nasopharyngitis, sinus congestion, rhinitis, nasal congestion	
Skin and Subcutaneous Tissue Disorders	rash, sweating increased	eczema, night sweats, psoriasis, photosensitivity reaction, urticaria, skin disorder	acquired lipodystrophy
Vascular Disorders		flushing, hypertension	

As with other alpha interferon therapies, uncommon to rare cases (<1%) of the following serious adverse events have been reported in patients receiving PEGASYS RBV combination or PEGASYS monotherapy during clinical trials:

Blood and the Lymphatic System Disorders: thrombotic thrombocytopenic purpura (TTP).
Cardiac Disorders: arrhythmia, atrial fibrillation, pericarditis.
Eye Disorders: corneal ulcer.
Gastrointestinal Disorders: peptic ulcer, gastrointestinal bleeding, pancreatitis, abdominal distention.
Immune System Disorders: autoimmune phenomena (e.g. ITP, thyroiditis, psoriasis, rheumatoid arthritis, SLE), sarcoidosis.
Infections and Infestations: skin infection, otitis externa, endocarditis.
Hepato-Biliary: hepatic dysfunction, fatty liver, cholangitis, malignant hepatic neoplasm.
Nervous System Disorders: myositis, peripheral neuropathy*, coma.
Psychiatric Disorders: suicide, panic attack, psychotic disorder, hallucination.
Respiratory, Thoracic and Mediastinal Disorders: interstitial pneumonitis with fatal outcome, pulmonary embolism.
Vascular Disorders: cerebral hemorrhage.

Rarely, alpha interferon including PEGASYS RBV or PEGASYS monotherapy may be associated with pancytopenia, and very rarely, aplastic anemia has been reported.

Uncommon to very rare cases of hearing impairment (deafness) have been reported.

The adverse reactions observed with other alpha interferons may be expected with PEGASYS, including colitis and pancreatitis.

Abnormal Hematologic and Clinical Chemistry Findings: Hematology: As with other interferons, treatment with 180 µg PEGASYS and PEGASYS RBV combination therapy was associated with decreases in hematological values, which generally improved with dosage modification and returned to pretreatment levels within 4 to 8 weeks upon cessation of therapy (see Warnings and Precautions and Dosage and Administration).

Although hematological toxicities of neutropenia, thrombocytopenia and anemia occurred more frequently in HIV-HCV patients, the majority could be managed by dose modification and the use of growth factors and infrequently required premature discontinuation of treatment.

Hemoglobin and Hematocrit: Treatment with 180 mcg PEGASYS and 3 MIU and 6/3 MIU interferon alfa-2a for HCV were associated with small gradual decreases in hemoglobin and hematocrit. Less than 1% of all patients treated with PEGASYS including those with cirrhosis, required dose modification for anemia (hemoglobin <100 g/L). No patients receiving interferon alfa-2a required anemia-related dose modifications, due to drops in hemoglobin levels. Anemia due to hemolysis is the most significant toxicity of ribavirin therapy. Anemia (hemoglobin <100 g/L) was observed in 13% of PEGASYS RBV combination-treated patients in clinical trials. The maximum drop in hemoglobin occurred during the first 8 weeks of initiation of ribavirin therapy (see Dosage and Administration, Recommended Dose and Dosage Adjustment, Dose Adjustments).

Approximately 10% of patients on PEGASYS RBV combination therapy required COPEGUS dose modification for anemia. Patients receiving 800 mg of COPEGUS for 24 weeks had the lowest frequency of decrease in hemoglobin levels to <100 g/L; hemoglobin levels did not fall to <85 g/L in any of these patients.

* In protocol NR15961(HIV-HCV) the frequency was reported as 2% in the PEGASYS monotherapy arm.

Anemia (hemoglobin <100 g/L) was reported in 8% and 14% of HIV-HCV co-infected patients treated with PEGASYS monotherapy or PEGASYS RBV combination therapy, respectively.

White Blood Cells: Treatment with PEGASYS for HCV was associated with decreases in values for both total WBC and ANC. Transient decreases in ANC to levels below 0.5×10^9/L at some time during therapy, were observed in 3.8% and 5% of patients treated with PEGASYS and PEGASYS RBV versus 1.2% and 1.5% of patients treated with 3 MIU and 6/3 MIU interferon alfa-2a, respectively.

In HIV-HCV co-infected patients, 13% and 11% of those receiving PEGASYS monotherapy and PEGASYS RBV combination therapy, respectively, had decreases in ANC levels below 0.5×10^9/L.

Platelet Count: Treatment with PEGASYS was associated with decreases in values for platelet counts. In HCV clinical trials for chronic hepatitis C, approximately 5% of patients had decreases in platelet counts to levels below 50×10^9/L versus 2.5% and 1.5% of patients in the 3 MIU and 3/6 MIU interferon alfa-2a treatment groups, respectively. Most of these patients were cirrhotic at baseline and/or entered the study with a baseline platelet count as low as 75×10^9/L.

In HIV-HCV patients, 10% and 8% of those receiving PEGASYS monotherapy and PEGASYS RBV combination therapy, respectively, had decreases in platelets below 50×10^9/L.

In clinical trials for hepatitis B, 14% of patients had decreases in platelet counts to below 50×10^9/L, mostly in patients who entered the study with low baseline platelet counts.

Clinical Chemistry: ALT: In clinical trials in CHB, 25% and 27% of patients experienced ALT elevations of 5 to 10×the ULN and 12% and 18% exhibited elevations of >10×ULN during treatment of HBeAg negative and HBeAg positive disease respectively. Overall, 11% of patients had dose modifications due to ALT flares and <1% of patients were withdrawn from treatment for this reason. ALT flares of 5-10×ULN occurred in 13% and 16% of patients, while ALT flares of >10×ULN occurred in 7% and 12% of patients in the HBeAG negative and HBeAG positive patients respectively, after discontinuation of PEGASYS therapy (see Warnings and Precautions and Dosage and Administration).

Thyroid Function: PEGASYS treatment was associated with clinically significant abnormalities in thyroid laboratory values requiring clinical intervention (see Warnings and Precautions, Monitoring and Laboratory Tests). The frequencies observed with PEGASYS were similar to those observed with other interferons.

Triglycerides: Triglyceride levels are found to be elevated in patients receiving alpha interferon therapy, including PEGASYS.

For a full listing of PEGASYS RBV combination adverse reactions, please refer to the current PEGASYS RBV product monograph.

Post-Market Adverse Drug Reactions: During the post-marketing period, erythema multiforme, Stevens-Johnson Syndrome, toxic epidermal necrolysis, pure red cell aplasia (PRCA) and homicidal ideation have been reported very rarely with PEGASYS RBV combination therapy.

Dehydration has been reported rarely with PEGASYS RBV combination therapy.

As with other alpha interferons, serous retinal detachment has been reported with PEGASYS RBV combination therapy.

As with other alpha interferons, liver and renal graft rejections have been reported on PEGASYS, alone or in combination with COPEGUS.

DRUG INTERACTIONS: Overview: No pharmacokinetic interactions between PEGASYS (peginterferon alfa-2a) and ribavirin have been observed in HCV clinical trials in which PEGASYS was used in combination with ribavirin. Similarly, lamivudine had no effect on PEGASYS pharmacokinetics in HBV clinical trials in which PEGASYS was used in combination with lamivudine.

Treatment with 180 µg PEGASYS once weekly for 4 weeks had no effect on the pharmacokinetic profiles of tolbutamide (CYP 2C9), mephenytoin (CYP 2C19), debrisoquine (CYP 2D6), and dapsone (CYP 3A4) in healthy male subjects.

Drug-Drug Interactions: See Table 3.

Table 3: PEGASYS

Established or Potential Drug-Drug Interactions

Proper Name	Ref	Effect	Clinical Comment
Peginterferon alfa-2a and Methadone	CT	In a pharmacokinetic study of 24 HCV patients concomitantly receiving methadone maintenance therapy (median dose 95 mg; range 30 mg to 150 mg), treatment with PEGASYS 180 µg sc once weekly for 4 weeks was associated with mean methadone levels that were 10% to 15% higher than at baseline.	The clinical significance of this finding is unknown; nonetheless, patients should be monitored for the signs and symptoms of methadone toxicity.
Peginterferon alfa-2a and Theophylline	T	PEGASYS is a modest inhibitor of cytochrome P450 1A2: a 25% increase in theophylline's AUC was observed in the same study. Comparable effects on the pharmacokinetics of theophylline have been seen after treatment with standard alpha interferons. Alpha interferons have been shown to affect the oxidative metabolism of some drugs by reducing the activity of hepatic microsomal cytochrome P450 enzymes.	Theophylline serum concentrations should be monitored and appropriate dose adjustments of theophylline made for patients taking theophylline and PEGASYS concomitantly.

Legend: C=case study; CT=clinical trial; T=theoretical.

Peginterferon alfa-2a and Telbivudine: A non-Roche sponsored pilot clinical trial in Hepatitis B investigating the combination of telbivudine 600 mg daily, with pegylated interferon alfa -2a, 180 µg once weekly by subcutaneous administration, indicated that this combination is associated with an increased risk for developing **serious peripheral neuropathy** at a rate of 10%. An increased risk can not be ruled out for combination treatment with other interferon products (pegylated or standard). The benefit of telbivudine in combination with interferon alfa (pegylated or standard) is not currently established in patients. It is not recommended that telbivudine be given in combination with PEGASYS.

Drug-Herb Interactions: Pulmonary symptoms have been reported more frequently when sho-saiko-to, a Chinese herbal medicine, also known as Xiao-Chai-Hu was given with interferon alfa-2a. This herb should not be taken by patients receiving interferon.

DOSAGE AND ADMINISTRATION:

Dosing Considerations: Treatment should be individualized to the patient depending on response to therapy and tolerability of the regimen.

Recommended Dose and Dosage Adjustment: Recommended Dose: Chronic Hepatitis C Mono-infection: The recommended dose of PEGASYS (peginterferon alfa-2a) is 180 µg once-weekly for 48 weeks by subcutaneous administration in the abdomen or thigh.

HIV-HCV Co-infection: The recommended dosage of PEGASYS is 180 µg once weekly subcutaneously for 48 weeks, regardless of genotype. The safety and efficacy of a duration of therapy less than 48 weeks has not been studied.

Early Predictability of Response: After 12 weeks of treatment, virologic response should be assessed. Treatment discontinuation should be considered in any HCV (including HIV-HCV) patient who has not achieved viral clearance or an HCV-RNA reduction from baseline of at least 99% by week 12.

Chronic Hepatitis B: The recommended dose of PEGASYS (peginterferon alfa-2a) is 180 µg once-weekly for 48 weeks by subcutaneous administration in the abdomen or thigh.

Dose Adjustments: General: When dose modification is required for moderate to severe adverse reactions (clinical and/or laboratory), initial dose reduction to 135 µg is generally adequate. However, in some cases, dose reduction to 90 µg is necessary. Following improvement of the adverse reaction, dose increases to or toward the original dose may be considered (see Warnings and Precautions and Adverse Reactions).

Hematological: Dose reduction to 135 µg PEGASYS is recommended if the ANC is less than 7.5×10^9/L. For patients with ANC values below 0.5×10^9/L, treatment should be suspended until ANC values return to over 1.0×10^9/L. Therapy should initially be reinstituted at 90 µg PEGASYS, and the ANC monitored.

Dose reduction to 90 µg PEGASYS is recommended if the platelet count is less than 50×10^9/L. Cessation of therapy is recommended when platelet count decreases to levels below 25×10^9/L.

Liver Function: Fluctuations in abnormalities of liver function tests are common in patients with chronic hepatitis C. However, as with other alpha interferons, increases in ALT levels above baseline have been observed in patients treated with PEGASYS, including patients with a virological response.

For CHC patients, the dose should be reduced initially to 90 µg in the presence of progressive ALT increases above baseline values. When increase in ALT levels is progressive despite dose reduction, or is accompanied by increased bilirubin or evidence of hepatic decompensation, therapy should be discontinued.

For CHB patients, transient flares of ALT levels sometimes exceeding 10 times the upper limit of normal are not uncommon, and may reflect immune clearance. Consideration should be given to continuing treatment with more frequent monitoring of liver function during ALT flares. If the PEGASYS dose is reduced or withheld, therapy can be restored once the flare is subsiding (see Warnings and Precautions).

Special Populations: Renal Impairment: No dose adjustments in the recommended starting dose of PEGASYS 180 µg once weekly is required in patients with creatinine clearance >0.33 mL/sec. In patients with impaired renal function, signs and symptoms of interferon toxicity should be closely monitored.

In subjects with end-stage renal disease requiring hemodialysis, a starting dose of 135 µg should be used. Regardless of the starting dose or degree of renal impairment, patients should be monitored and appropriate dose reductions of PEGASYS during the course of therapy should be made in the event of adverse reactions (see Warnings and Precautions and Action and Clinical Pharmacology, Pharmacokinetics, Special Populations and Conditions).

Geriatrics: No special dosage modification is required for geriatric patients with normal renal function, based upon pharmacokinetic, pharmacodynamic, tolerability, and safety data from clinical trials.

Hepatic Impairment: PEGASYS has been shown to be effective and safe in patients with compensated cirrhosis (e.g. Child-Pugh A). PEGASYS has not been studied in patients with decompensated liver disease (e.g. Child-Pugh B/C or bleeding esophageal varices) (see Contraindications and Warnings and Precautions).

The Child-Pugh classification divides patients into groups A, B, and C, or "Mild", "Moderate" and "Severe" corresponding to scores of 5-6, 7-9 and 10-15, respectively.

Table 4: PEGASYS

Modified Assessment

Assessment	Degree of Abnormality	Score
Encephalopathy	None	1
	Grade 1-2	2
	Grade 3-4[a]	3
Ascites	Absent	1
	Slight	2
	Moderate	3
S-Bilirubin (mg/dL)	<2	1
	2–3	2
	>3	3
(SI=µmol/L)	<34	1
	34–51	2
	>51	3
S-Albumin (g/L)	>35	1
	35–28	2
	<28	3
INR	<1,7	1
	1,7–2,3	2
	>2,3	3

[a] Grading according to Trey, Burns and Saunders (1966).

Missed Dose: If the PEGASYS dose is missed and remembered within 2 days of the scheduled dose, the PEGASYS dose should be administered as soon as possible. The next scheduled PEGASYS dose should be given on the usual day. If more than 2 days have elapsed, the dosage schedule should be based on the clinical judgment of the physician.

Administration: PEGASYS (peginterferon alfa-2a) is administered subcutaneously in the abdomen or thigh once weekly (see Dosage and Administration). Visually inspect the solution prior to administration. Do not use if discoloured or if particles are present.

OVERDOSAGE:

There is limited experience with overdosage. The maximum dose received by any patient was 7 times the intended dose of PEGASYS (peginterferon alfa-2a), (180 µg/day for 7 days). There were no serious reactions attributed to overdosages. Weekly doses of up to 630 µg have been administered to patients with cancer. Dose limiting toxicities were fatigue, elevated liver enzymes, neutropenia and thrombocytopenia. There is no specific antidote for PEGASYS. Hemodialysis and peritoneal dialysis are not effective.

For management of a suspected drug overdose, CPhA recommends that you contact your **regional Poison Control Centre**. See the *CPS* Directory section for a list of Poison Control Centres.

ACTION AND CLINICAL PHARMACOLOGY: Mechanism of Action: PEGASYS (peginterferon alfa-2a) possesses the in vitro antiviral and antiproliferative activities of interferon alfa-2a. Interferons bind to specific receptors on the cell surface initiating a complex intracellular signalling pathway and rapid activation of gene transcription. Interferon-stimulated genes modulate many biological effects including the inhibition of viral replication in infected cells, inhibition of cell proliferation, and immunomodulation. The clinical relevance of these in vitro activities is not known.

Pharmacodynamics: HCV RNA levels decline in a biphasic manner in responding patients with hepatitis C with and without compensated cirrhosis who have received treatment with 180 µg PEGASYS. The first phase of decline occurs within 24 to 36 hours after the first PEGASYS dose in sustained responders and in some patients that do not achieve a sustained virological response. In those individuals who are sustained responders, the second phase of decline occurs over the next 4 to 16 weeks. Treatment with 180 µg PEGASYS per week enhances the virion clearance and improves the virological end of treatment responses compared to treatment with interferon alfa-2a.

PEGASYS stimulates the production of effector proteins such as serum neopterin, 2',5'-oligoadenylate synthetase (2',5'-OAS), raises body temperature and causes reversible decreases in leukocyte and platelet counts. The stimulation of 2',5'-OAS is maximal after single doses of 135 to 180 µg PEGASYS and stays maximal throughout the one week dosing interval. The magnitude and duration of 2',5'-OAS activity induced by PEGASYS were reduced in subjects older than 62 years and in subjects with significant renal impairment (creatinine clearances of 0.33 to 0.67 mL/sec) compared to that seen in healthy subjects. The correlation between the in vitro and in vivo pharmacology and pharmacodynamic and clinical effects is unknown.

Pharmacokinetics: The structure of the PEG moiety directly affects the clinical pharmacology of PEGASYS. Specifically, the size, branching and location of attachment of the 40 kD PEG moiety contribute to defining the absorption, distribution and elimination characteristics of PEGASYS. The pharmacokinetics of PEGASYS were studied in healthy volunteers and hepatitis C virus (HCV) -infected patients. The results for patients with chronic hepatitis B were similar to those for patients with chronic hepatitis C.

Absorption: The absorption of PEGASYS is sustained with peak serum concentrations reached 72 to 96 hours after dosing. Serum concentrations are measurable within 3 to 6 hours of a single dose. Dose proportional increases in AUC and C_{max} are seen in patients that received once weekly doses of PEGASYS.

The absolute bioavailability of PEGASYS following sc administration in the abdomen is 84% and is similar to that seen with interferon alfa-2a.

Distribution: The volume of distribution at steady-state (V_{ss}) of 6 to 14 liters after intravenous dosing suggests that the drug is found mainly in the bloodstream and extracellular fluid.

Metabolism: The metabolic profile of PEGASYS is not fully characterized.

Excretion: The systemic clearance of PEGASYS is about 100 mL/h, which is 100-fold lower than that of interferon alfa-2a. After an intravenous dose, the terminal half-life of PEGASYS in healthy subjects is about 60 hours compared to 3 to 4 hours for standard interferon. The terminal half-life after subcutaneous administration in patients is longer with a mean value of 160 hours (84 to 353 hours). The terminal half-life after subcutaneous dosing may be reflecting the sustained absorption of PEGASYS and not the elimination of the drug.

The kidneys eliminate less than 10% of a dose as the intact peginterferon alfa-2a. The rest is broken down metabolically.

Steady state serum levels are reached within 5 to 8 weeks of once-weekly dosing. Once steady state has been achieved, there is no accumulation of peginterferon alfa-2a. The peak to trough ratio after 48 weeks of treatment is about 1.5 to 2.0. Peginterferon alfa-2a serum concentrations are sustained throughout the 1 week dosing interval (168 hours) [Table 5 and Figure 1].

Table 5: PEGASYS

Pharmacokinetic Parameters of PEGASYS After Single and Multiple Dose of 180 µg

	Healthy Subjects 180 µg sc (N=50)	CHC Patients 180 µg sc (N=16)	
PEGASYS Pharmacokinetic Parameter	**Single Dose Mean±SD [Range]**	**Single Dose Mean±SD [Range]**	**Week 48 Dose Mean±SD [Range]**
C_{max} (ng/mL)	14±5 [6–26]	15±4 [7–23]	26±9 [10–40]
T_{max} (h)	92±27 [48–168]	80±28 [23–119]	45±36 [0–97]
AUC_{1-168h} (ng·h/mL)	1725±586 [524–3013]	1820±586 [846–2609]	3334±994 [1265–4824]
Clearance/F (mL/h)	94±56 [34–337]	83±50 [33–186]	60±25 [37–142]
Week 48 trough concentration (ng/mL)	Not applicable	Not applicable	16±6 [4–28]
Peak to trough ratio for week 48	Not applicable	Not applicable	1.7±0.4 [1.1–2.5]
Accumulation ($AUC_{Week\ 48}/AUC_{Single\ Dose}$)	Not applicable	Not applicable	2.3±1.0 [1.1–4.0]

Figure 1: PEGASYS

Mean Steady-State PEGASYS Concentrations in Patients with CHC

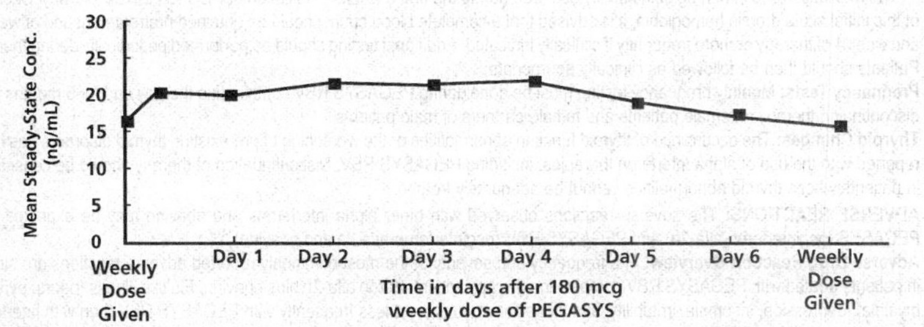

Special Populations and Conditions: Pediatrics (<18 years of age): The pharmacokinetics of PEGASYS have not been adequately studied in pediatric patients.

Geriatrics: In subjects older than 62 years, the AUC was modestly increased (1663 vs 1295 ng·h/mL, older than 62 years vs younger, respectively), but peak concentrations (9.1 vs 10.3 ng/mL) were similar in the two age groups (see Dosage and Administration).

Gender: The pharmacokinetics of PEGASYS after single subcutaneous injections were comparable between male and female healthy subjects.

Hepatic Insufficiency: The pharmacokinetics of PEGASYS were similar between healthy subjects and patients with chronic hepatitis B or chronic hepatitis C. Comparable pharmacokinetic profiles were seen in cirrhotic patients with compensated liver disease and patients without cirrhosis.

Renal Insufficiency: Renal impairment is associated with decreased total apparent clearance and prolonged half-life. In subjects with a creatinine clearance between 0.33 and 0.67 mL/sec, the average total apparent clearance is reduced by approximately 30% compared with subjects with normal renal function following single doses of PEGASYS.

In subjects with end-stage renal disease undergoing hemodialysis, there is a 25% to 45% reduction in the clearance of peginterferon alfa-2a and doses of 135 µg provide exposure similar to those observed in subjects with normal renal function receiving 180 µg doses. Regardless of the starting dose or degree of renal impairment, patients should be monitored and appropriate dose reductions of PEGASYS during the course of therapy should be made in the event of adverse reactions (see Warnings and Precautions and Dosage and Administration, Recommended Dose and Dosage Adjustment, Dose Adjustments).

STORAGE AND STABILITY: Stability and Storage Recommendations: Store in refrigerator at 2 to 8°C. Protect from light. Do not freeze or shake. Do not use PEGASYS (peginterferon alfa-2a) beyond the date of expiry.

Parenteral drug products such as PEGASYS should be inspected visually for particulate matter and discolouration before administration. Do not use PEGASYS if it contains particulate matter or it appears discoloured.

SPECIAL HANDLING INSTRUCTIONS: PEGASYS (peginterferon alfa-2a): Disposal of syringes/sharps: The following points should be strictly adhered to regarding the use and disposal of syringes and other medicinal sharps:

- Needles and syringes should never be reused.
- Place all used needles and syringes into a sharps container (puncture-proof disposable container).
- Keep this container out of the reach of children.
- Placing used sharps containers in the household waste should be avoided.
- Dispose of the full container according to local requirements or as instructed by your healthcare provider

For home use, a puncture resistant container for the disposal of used syringes and needles should be supplied to the patients.

Disposal of unused/expired medicines: The release of pharmaceuticals in the environment should be minimized. Medicines should not be disposed of via wastewater and disposal through household waste should be avoided. Use established "collection systems" if available in your location.

INFORMATION FOR THE PATIENT: Published in e-CPS, available by subscription at www.e-cps.ca.

DOSAGE FORMS, COMPOSITION AND PACKAGING: Pre-Filled Syringes: Each 0.5 mL of sterile, ready to use solution for subcutaneous injection contains: peginterferon alfa-2a 180 µg (expressed as the amount of interferon alfa-2a), sodium chloride 4 mg, 80 polysorbate 0.025 mg, benzyl alcohol 5 mg, sodium acetate trihydrate 1.3085 mg, acetic acid 0.0231 mg and water for injection. Single use, graduated, clear glass pre-filled syringes, packages of 1 and 4.

Single-Use Vials: Each mL of sterile, ready to use solution for subcutaneous injection contains: peginterferon alfa-2a 180 µg (expressed as the amount of interferon alfa-2a), sodium chloride 8 mg, 80 polysorbate 0.05 mg, benzyl alcohol 10 mg, sodium acetate trihydrate 2.617 mg, acetic acid 0.0462 mg and water for injection. Single-use, clear glass vials of 1 mL, packages of 1 and 4.

Pegasys RBV® (Pegasys® and Copegus®) Ⓟ

peginterferon alfa-2a—ribavirin

Biological Response Modifier—Antiviral Agent

Roche

Date of Revision: March 10, 2010

SUMMARY PRODUCT INFORMATION:

Route of Administration	Dosage Form/ Strength	Clinically Relevant Nonmedicinal Ingredients
Subcutaneous	Solution in vial: 180 µg/1.0 mL	Benzyl alcohol For a complete listing see Dosage Forms, Composition and Packaging.
	Solution in pre-filled syringe: 180 µg/0.5 mL	Benzyl alcohol For a complete listing see Dosage Forms, Composition and Packaging.
Oral	Tablet/200 mg	None For a complete listing see Dosage Forms, Composition and Packaging.

DESCRIPTION: PEGASYS RBV (peginterferon alfa-2a and ribavirin) is a combination of PEGASYS (peginterferon alfa-2a) and COPEGUS (ribavirin) tablets.

PEGASYS: Peginterferon alfa-2a is a covalent conjugate of recombinant alfa-2a interferon (approximate molecular weight [MW] 20 kD) with a single branched bis-monomethoxy polyethylene glycol (PEG) chain (approximate MW 40 kD). Interferon alfa-2a is produced biosynthetically using recombinant DNA technology, and is the product of a cloned human leukocyte interferon gene inserted into and expressed in *E. coli*.

COPEGUS: Ribavirin, a synthetic nucleoside analog, has shown in vitro activity against some RNA and DNA viruses, as well as immunomodulatory activity.

INDICATIONS AND CLINICAL USE: PEGASYS RBV (peginterferon alfa-2a and ribavirin) is indicated for the treatment of chronic Hepatitis C in:

- Adult patients without cirrhosis
- Adult patients with compensated cirrhosis,

including HCV/HIV co-infection patients with stable HIV disease with or without antiretroviral therapy.

CONTRAINDICATIONS: PEGASYS RBV (peginterferon alfa-2a and ribavirin) is contraindicated in:

- Women who are pregnant or by men whose female partners are pregnant. PEGASYS RBV should not be initiated until a report of a negative pregnancy test has been obtained immediately prior to initiation of therapy. Women of childbearing potential and their male partners must not receive PEGASYS RBV therapy unless they are using effective contraception (two reliable forms, one for each partner) during treatment with PEGASYS RBV and for the 6-month post-therapy period.
- Patients who are hypersensitive to alpha interferons, *E. coli*-derived products, polyethylene glycol, ribavirin and/or any ingredient in the formulation or component of PEGASYS or COPEGUS (see Dosage Forms, Composition and Packaging).
- Patients with autoimmune hepatitis and patients with decompensated cirrhosis.
- HIV-HCV patients with cirrhosis and a base-line Child-Pugh score ≥6 (see Warnings and Precautions, Hepatic/Biliary/Pancreatic and Dosage and Administration, Special Populations).
- Patients with a history of autoimmune disease.
- Patients with hemoglobinopathies (e.g. thalassemia, sickle-cell anemia).
- Neonates and infants because the PEGASYS component contains benzyl alcohol. There have been rare reports of death in neonates and infants associated with excessive exposure to benzyl alcohol. The amount of benzyl alcohol at which toxicity or adverse effects may occur in neonates or infants is not known.
- Patients who have a pre-existing severe psychiatric condition or a history of a severe psychiatric disorder, who have pre-existing thyroid abnormalities for which thyroid function cannot be maintained in the normal range by medication, and in women who are breast feeding.

WARNINGS AND PRECAUTIONS:

> **Serious Warnings and Precautions**
> **Alpha interferons, including PEGASYS (peginterferon alfa-2a), cause or aggravate fatal or life-threatening neuropsychiatric, autoimmune, ischemic, and infectious disorders. Patients should be monitored closely with periodic clinical and laboratory evaluations. Patients with persistently severe or worsening signs or symptoms of these conditions should be withdrawn from therapy. In many cases, but not all cases, these disorders resolve after stopping interferon therapy (see Warnings and Precautions).**

General: Ribavirins, including the COPEGUS component of PEGASYS RBV (peginterferon alfa-2a and ribavirin) may cause birth defects and/or death of the exposed fetus. COPEGUS (ribavirin) must not be used by women who are pregnant or by men whose female partners are pregnant.

Treatment with PEGASYS RBV should be administered under the guidance of a qualified physician and may lead to moderate to severe adverse experiences requiring dose reduction, temporary dose cessation or discontinuation of therapy.

Based on results of clinical trials, the use of ribavirin as monotherapy is not effective and COPEGUS must not be used alone.

The safety and efficacy of PEGASYS RBV have not been established in patients who have failed other alpha interferon treatments.

Patients should be informed regarding the potential benefits and risks attendant to the use of PEGASYS RBV. If home use is determined to be desirable by the physician, instructions on appropriate use should be given, including review of the contents of the Consumer Information, which does not disclose all possible adverse effects of PEGASYS RBV (see Information for the Patient).

If home use is prescribed, patients should be thoroughly instructed in the importance of proper disposal of, and cautioned against, reuse of any needles and syringes.

Patients should be cautioned not to change to other pegylated interferons or switch to other alpha interferons without a medical consultation; changing from one interferon to another may require dosage change or adjustment.

Patients who develop dizziness, confusion, somnolence, or fatigue should be cautioned to avoid driving or operating machinery.

Cardiovascular: Because cardiac disease may be worsened by ribavirin-induced anemia, patients with a history of significant or unstable cardiac disease in the previous six months should not use the COPEGUS component of PEGASYS RBV. Cardiovascular events such as hypertension, supraventricular arrhythmias, congestive heart failure, chest pain and myocardial infarction have been associated with interferon therapies, including PEGASYS. Therefore, PEGASYS RBV should be administered with caution to patients with pre-existing cardiac disease. Patients should be assessed before initiation of therapy and should be appropriately monitored during therapy. It is recommended that patients who have pre existing cardiac abnormalities have an electrocardiogram prior to initiation of PEGASYS RBV treatment and during the course of treatment. PEGASYS RBV should not be used in patients with pre existing severe, unstable or uncontrolled cardiac disease; if there is any deterioration of cardiovascular status, PEGASYS RBV therapy should be suspended or discontinued (see Warnings and Precautions, Hematologic).

Cerebrovascular: Ischemic and hemorrhagic cerebrovascular events have been observed in patients treated with interferon alfa-based therapies, including PEGASYS. Events occurred in patients with few or no reported risk factors for stroke, including patients less than 45 years of age. Because these are spontaneous reports, estimates of frequency cannot be made and a causal relationship between interferon alfa-based therapies and these events is difficult to establish.

Endocrine and Metabolism: Endocrine: As with other interferons, PEGASYS may cause or aggravate hypothyroidism and hyperthyroidism. Hypoglycemia, hyperglycemia, and diabetes mellitus have been observed in patients treated with PEGASYS RBV. Patients with these conditions at baseline who cannot be effectively controlled by medication should not be started on PEGASYS RBV therapy. Patients who develop these conditions during treatment and cannot be controlled with medication should not continue PEGASYS RBV therapy.

Gastrointestinal: Colitis: Hemorrhagic/ischemic colitis, sometimes fatal, has been observed within 12 weeks of starting alpha interferon treatment. Abdominal pain, bloody diarrhea, and fever are the typical manifestations of colitis. PEGASYS RBV treatment should be discontinued immediately if these symptoms develop. The colitis usually resolves within 1 to 3 weeks following discontinuation of alpha interferon. Ulcerative colitis has also been observed in patients treated with alpha interferon.

Hematologic: Alpha interferons, including PEGASYS, may suppress bone marrow function which may result in severe cytopenias. Very rarely alpha interferons may be associated with pancytopenia including aplastic anemia. On the other hand, the primary toxicity of the COPEGUS component is hemolytic anemia (hemoglobin <100 g/L), which was observed in approximately 13% of PEGASYS RBV treated patients in clinical trials. The anemia associated with COPEGUS occurs within 1 to 2 weeks of initiation of therapy. Because the initial acute drop in hemoglobin may be significant, it is advised that complete blood counts (CBC) should be obtained pretreatment and at week 2 and week 4 of therapy, or more frequently if clinically indicated. Patients should then be followed as clinically appropriate.

Extreme caution should be exercised when administering PEGASYS RBV in combination with other potentially myelosuppressive agents (see Warnings and Precautions, Monitoring and Laboratory Tests).

PEGASYS RBV should be used with caution in patients with baseline absolute neutrophil counts (ANC) $<1.5\times10^9$/L, with baseline platelets $<90\times10^9$/L or baseline hemoglobin <100 g/L. PEGASYS RBV should be discontinued, at least temporarily, in patients who develop severe decreases in ANC ($<0.5\times10^9$/L) and/or platelet ($<25\times10^9$/L) counts (see Dosage and Administration, Recommended Dose and Dosage Adjustment, Dose Adjustments).

If there is any deterioration of hemoglobin blood concentration, COPEGUS should be suspended or discontinued (see Dosage and Administration, Recommended Dose and Dosage Adjustment, Dose Adjustments). Although ribavirin has no direct cardiovascular effects, the anemia associated with PEGASYS RBV combination therapy may result in deterioration of cardiac function and/or exacerbation of the symptoms of cardiovascular disease. If there is any deterioration of cardiovascular status, COPEGUS therapy should be suspended or discontinued (see Warnings and Precaution, Cardiovascular and Dosage and Administration).

Pancytopenia (marked decreases in RBCs, neutrophils and platelets) and bone marrow suppression have been reported in the literature to occur within 3 to 7 weeks after the concomitant administration of ribavirin and azathioprine. This myelotoxicity was reversible within 4 to 6 weeks upon withdrawal of HCV antiviral therapy and concomitant azathioprine and did not recur upon reintroduction of either treatment alone (see Drug Interactions).

Hepatic/Biliary/Pancreatic: Hepatic: In patients who develop evidence of hepatic decompensation during treatment, PEGASYS RBV treatment should be discontinued. HIV-HCV co-infected patients with advanced cirrhosis receiving concomitant HAART may be at an increased risk of hepatic decompensation and possibly death when treated with ribavirin in combination with alpha interferons, including PEGASYS RBV. During treatment, co-infected patients should be closely monitored, periodically assessing their clinical status and hepatic function and should be immediately discontinued if they decompensate (Child-Pugh score ≥6) (see Dosage and Administration).

As with other alpha interferons, increases in ALT levels above baseline have been observed in patients treated with PEGASYS RBV, including those patients who exhibit a virological response. When the increase in ALT levels is progressive despite dose reduction or is accompanied by increased bilirubin, therapy should be discontinued (see Dosage and Administration).

Pancreatitis: Pancreatitis, sometimes fatal, has occurred during alpha interferon treatment. PEGASYS RBV treatment should be suspended if symptoms or signs suggestive of pancreatitis are observed. PEGASYS RBV should be discontinued in patients diagnosed with pancreatitis.

HBV : The safety and efficacy of PEGASYS RBV treatment has not been established for patients with hepatitis B virus (HBV).

Hydration: Adequate hydration must be maintained in patients undergoing therapy with PEGASYS RBV, since hypotension related to fluid depletion has been seen in some patients treated with alpha interferons. Fluid replacement may be necessary.

Hypersensitivity: Serious, acute hypersensitivity reactions (e.g. urticaria, angioedema, bronchoconstriction, anaphylaxis) have been rarely observed during alpha interferon therapy and cutaneous eruptions (Stevens-Johnson syndrome, toxic epidermal necrolysis) have been very rarely reported. If such a reaction develops during treatment with PEGASYS RBV, treatment should be discontinued and appropriate medical therapy should be instituted immediately. Transient rashes do not necessitate interruption of treatment.

Immune: Exacerbation of autoimmune disease including myositis, hepatitis, immune thrombocytopenic purpura (ITP), rheumatoid arthritis, interstitial nephritis, thyroiditis and systemic lupus erythematosus has been reported in patients receiving alpha interferon therapy; PEGASYS RBV is contraindicated in patients with a history of autoimmune disease. In case of appearance of psoriatic lesions and sarcoidosis, discontinuation of therapy should be considered.

Infections: While fever may be associated with the flu-like syndrome reported commonly during interferon therapy, other causes of persistent fever must be ruled out, particularly in patients with neutropenia. Serious infections (bacterial, viral, fungal) have been reported during treatment with alpha interferons including PEGASYS. Appropriate anti-infective therapy should be started immediately and discontinuation of therapy should be considered.

Ophthalmologic: As with other interferons, retinopathy including retinal hemorrhages, cotton wool spots, papilledema, retinal artery or vein obstruction and serous retinal detachment, have been reported in rare instances after treatment with PEGASYS RBV. As with other interferons, decrease or loss of vision, macular edema and optic neuritis may be induced or aggravated by PEGASYS RBV treatment. All patients should receive an eye examination at baseline. Patients with preexisting ophthalmologic disorders (e.g. diabetic or hypertensive retinopathy) should receive periodic ophthalmologic exams during PEGASYS RBV treatment. Any patient complaining of loss of visual acuity or visual field must have a prompt and complete eye examination. PEGASYS RBV treatment should be discontinued in patients who develop new or worsening ophthalmologic disorders.

Psychiatric: Severe psychiatric adverse reactions may manifest in patients receiving therapy with interferons, including PEGASYS. Depression, suicidal ideation, and suicidal attempt may occur in patients with and without previous psychiatric illness. Other CNS effects including aggressive behavior, confusion and other alterations of mental status have been observed with alpha interferons. PEGASYS RBV should be used with extreme caution in patients who report a history of depression and physicians should monitor all patients for evidence of depression. Physicians should inform patients of the possible development of depression prior to initiation of PEGASYS RBV therapy, and patients should report any sign or symptom of depression immediately. If severe symptoms persist, therapy should be stopped and psychiatric intervention sought (see Adverse Reactions and Dosage and Administration, Recommended Dose and Dosage Adjustment, Dose Adjustments).

Renal: PEGASYS RBV therapy should not be initiated in patients with renal impairment, whether or not on hemodialysis, or continued if renal impairment occurs while on treatment, unless it is considered to be essential. It is recommended that renal function be evaluated in all patients prior to initiation of PEGASYS RBV therapy, preferably by estimating the patient's creatinine clearance. PEGASYS RBV should not be administered to patients with serum creatinine >177 µmol/L or with creatinine clearance <0.83 mL/sec as substantial increases in ribavirin plasma concentrations are seen at the recommended dosing regimen. There are insufficient data on the safety and efficacy in such patients to support recommendations for dose adjustments. Therefore, PEGASYS RBV must be administered with extreme caution and corrective action including drug discontinuation must be considered if adverse events develop (see Dosage and Administration, Recommended Dose and Dosage Adjustment, Dose Adjustments and Action and Clinical Pharmacology, Pharmacokinetics of PEGASYS RBV in Special Populations).

Respiratory: As with other alpha interferons, pulmonary symptoms, including dyspnea, pulmonary infiltrates, pneumonia, and pneumonitis, including fatality, have been reported during therapy with PEGASYS RBV. Any patient developing fever, cough, and dyspnea or other respiratory symptoms must have a chest X-ray taken. If there is evidence of persistent or unexplained pulmonary infiltrates or pulmonary function impairment, treatment should be discontinued. PEGASYS RBV should not be administered to patients with chronic obstructive pulmonary disease (COPD).

Sexual Function/Reproduction: Reproduction: Ribavirin accumulates intracellularly and is cleared from the body very slowly. It is not known whether ribavirin contained in sperm will exert a potential teratogenic effect upon fertilization of the ova. Therefore, men must be instructed to use a condom to minimize delivery of ribavirin to their female partners. Male patients and their female partners of childbearing age must practice effective contraception (two reliable forms, one for each partner) during ribavirin therapy and for 6 months (based on the half-life of ribavirin of 12 days when the drug is administered at multiple doses) after treatment has stopped (see Pharmacokinetics of COPEGUS).

Evaluation of experimental animal studies showed reproductive toxicity. Significant teratogenic and/or embryocidal potential have been demonstrated for ribavirin in all animal species in which adequate studies have been conducted, occurring at doses well below the recommended human dose. Malformations of the skull, palate, eye, jaw, limbs, skeleton and gastrointestinal tract were noted. The incidence and severity of teratogenic effects increased with escalation of the ribavirin dose. Survival of fetuses and offspring was reduced.

Peginterferon alfa-2a has not been studied for its teratogenic effect. Treatment with interferon alfa-2a resulted in a statistically significant increase in abortifacient activity in rhesus monkeys; no teratogenic effects were seen in the offspring delivered at term (see Special Populations, Pregnant Women).

Transplantation: Organ Transplant Recipients: The safety and efficacy of PEGASYS RBV treatment have not been established in patients with liver or other transplantations. As with other alpha interferons, liver and renal graft rejections have been reported on PEGASYS, alone or in combination with COPEGUS.

Special Populations: Pregnant Women: Ribavirins, including the COPEGUS component of PEGASYS RBV may cause birth defects and/or death of the exposed fetus. COPEGUS must not be used by women who are pregnant or by men whose female partners are pregnant.

PEGASYS RBV therapy must not be initiated until a report of a negative pregnancy test has been obtained immediately prior to initiation of therapy. Females of childbearing potential and males with female partners receiving PEGASYS RBV must be advised of the teratogenic/embryocidal risks and must be instructed to use two forms of effective contraception (two reliable forms, one for each partner) during treatment and for 6 months after treatment has concluded. Routine monthly pregnancy tests must be performed during this time (see Contraindications). Patients should be advised to notify the physician immediately in the event of a pregnancy. If pregnancy does occur during treatment or within six months from stopping treatment, the patient must be advised of the significant teratogenic risk of ribavirin to the fetus (see Sexual Function/Reproduction, Reproduction).

As with other alpha interferons, women of childbearing potential receiving PEGASYS therapy should be advised to use effective contraception during therapy (see Sexual Function/Reproduction, Reproduction).

Nursing Women: It is not known whether the components of PEGASYS RBV are excreted in human milk. Because many drugs are excreted in human milk and to avoid any potential for serious adverse reactions in nursing infants from PEGASYS RBV, nursing must be discontinued prior to the start of PEGASYS RBV therapy.

Pediatrics (<18 years of age): Safety and effectiveness of PEGASYS RBV have not been established in patients below the age of 18. Therefore, PEGASYS RBV is not recommended for use in children and adolescents under the age of 18 years (also see Contraindications).

Monitoring and Laboratory Tests: Before beginning PEGASYS RBV combination therapy, standard hematological and biochemical profiles should be obtained for all patients. After initiation of therapy, hematological tests should be performed at 2 and 4 weeks and biochemical tests should be performed at 4 weeks. Additional testing should be performed periodically during therapy.

The enrolment criteria used for the clinical studies of PEGASYS RBV may be considered as a guideline to acceptable baseline values for initiation of treatment: platelet count $\geq90\times10^9$/L (75×10^9/L in patients with cirrhosis or transition to cirrhosis); ANC $\geq1.5\times10^9$/L; serum creatinine concentration <1.5×upper limit of normal; TSH and T4 within normal limits or adequately controlled thyroid function; HIV-HCV co-infection: CD4+ ≥200/µL or CD4+ ≥100/µL-<200/µl and HIV-1 RNA <5000 copies/mL using Amplicor HIV-1 Monitor Test, v 1.5.

PEGASYS RBV treatment was associated with decreases in both total white blood cell (WBC) count and ANC, usually starting within the first 2 weeks of treatment (see Adverse Reactions). In clinical studies, progressive decreases thereafter were infrequent. PEGASYS dose reduction is recommended when ANC decreases to levels below 0.75×10^9/L (see Dosage and Administration, Recommended Dose and Dosage Adjustment, Dose Adjustments). For patients with ANC values below 0.5×10^9/L treatment should be suspended until ANC values return to more than 1.0×10^9/L. In clinical trials with PEGASYS RBV, the decrease in ANC was reversible upon dose reduction of PEGASYS or cessation of therapy.

PEGASYS RBV treatment was associated with decreases in platelet count, which returned to pre-treatment (baseline) levels during the post-treatment observation period (see Adverse Reactions). PEGASYS dose reduction is recommended when platelet count decreases to levels below 50×10^9/L, and discontinuation of therapy is recommended when platelet count decreases to levels below 25×10^9/L (see Dosage and Administration, Recommended Dose and Dosage Adjustment, Dose Adjustments).

The maximum drop in hemoglobin usually occurred during the first 8 weeks of initiation of PEGASYS RBV therapy. Because of this initial acute drop in hemoglobin, it is advised that a complete blood count should be obtained pretreatment and at week 2 and week 4 of therapy or more frequently if clinically indicated. Additional testing should be performed periodically during therapy. Patients should then be followed as clinically appropriate.

Pregnancy Tests: Monthly pregnancy testing must be done during PEGASYS RBV combination therapy and for 6 months after discontinuing therapy in female patients and female partners of male patients.

Thyroid Changes: The occurrence of thyroid function abnormalities or the worsening of pre-existing thyroid disorders has been reported with the use of alpha interferon therapies, including PEGASYS RBV. Discontinuation of therapy should be considered in patients whose thyroid abnormalities cannot be adequately treated.

ADVERSE REACTIONS: The adverse reactions observed with other alpha interferons and ribavirin may be expected with PEGASYS (peginterferon alfa-2a) and PEGASYS RBV (peginterferon alfa-2a and ribavirin).

Adverse Drug Reaction Overview: The frequency and severity of the most commonly reported adverse reactions are similar in patients treated with PEGASYS RBV combination therapy and interferon alfa-2b plus ribavirin. Flu like illness (rigors, pyrexia, myalgia), depression, insomnia, irritability, and alopecia were reported less frequently with PEGASYS RBV than with interferon alfa-2b plus ribavirin (>5% difference between treatment groups). The most frequently reported adverse reactions with PEGASYS RBV combination therapy were mostly mild to moderate in severity and were manageable without the need for discontinuation of therapy.

Clinical Trial Adverse Drug Reactions: Chronic Hepatitis C Mono-infection: In mono-infected clinical trials, the incidence of withdrawal from treatment for all patients due to adverse events and laboratory abnormalities was 9% for PEGASYS monotherapy and 13% for PEGASYS RBV combination therapy. Respectively, only 1% or 3% of patients required discontinuation of either PEGASYS or PEGASYS RBV combination therapy due to laboratory abnormalities. Treatment-limiting events including serious and severe adverse events and adverse events and laboratory abnormalities leading to premature withdrawal or requiring dose modification with the combination treatment occurred with the lowest frequency in patients receiving 24 weeks of treatment and the 800 mg dose of COPEGUS.

HIV-HCV Co-infection: In HIV-HCV co-infected patients, the clinical adverse events reported on PEGASYS, PEGASYS RBV and interferon alfa-2a plus ribavirin were similar to that observed in HCV mono-infected patients.

In the co-infection study, the incidence of withdrawal from treatment for clinical adverse events, laboratory abnormalities or AIDS-defining events was 16% for PEGASYS monotherapy and 15% for both PEGASYS RBV and interferon alfa-2a plus ribavirin given for 48 weeks. Respectively, 4%, 3% or 1% of patients required discontinuation of PEGASYS or PEGASYS RBV or interferon alfa-2a plus ribavirin for laboratory abnormalities. In PEGASYS RBV combination therapy, the PEGASYS dose modification occurred in 39%, and the COPEGUS dose modification occurred in 37%, of the co-infected patients. In interferon alfa-2a plus ribavirin therapy, the interferon alfa-2a dose modification occurred in 16%, and the COPEGUS dose modification occurred in 28%, of the co-infected patients. In PEGASYS monotherapy, PEGASYS dose modification occurred in 38% of the co-infected patients. Serious adverse events were reported in 21%, 17% and 15% of those receiving PEGASYS monotherapy, PEGASYS RBV or interferon alfa-2a plus ribavirin, respectively.

Limited safety data (N=31) is available in co-infected patients with CD4+ cell counts <200/µL treated with PEGASYS and PEGASYS RBV. PEGASYS containing treatment was associated with an on-treatment reduction in absolute CD4+ cell count without a reduction in CD4+ cell percentage. CD4+ cell count indices returned to baseline values during the follow-up period of the study. PEGASYS containing treatment had no apparent negative impact on the control of HIV viremia during therapy or follow-up.

Because clinical trials are conducted under very specific conditions the adverse drug reaction rates observed in the clinical trials may not reflect the rates observed in practice and should not be compared to the rates in the clinical trials of another drug. Adverse drug reaction information from clinical trials is useful for identifying drug-related adverse events and for approximating rates. See Table 1 and Table 2.

Table 1: PEGASYS RBV

Adverse Reactions (≥5% of Incidence in Any Treatment Group)

	HCV			HIV-HCV	
Body System	**Interferon alfa-2b 3MIU + 1000 or 1200 mg Ribavirin 48 Weeks N=443[a] %**	**PEGASYS 180 µg + 1000 or 1200 mg Ribavirin 48 Weeks N=887[b] %**	**PEGASYS 180 µg + 800 mg Ribavirin 24 Weeks N=207[c] %**	**INF alfa-2a 3MIU + Ribavirin 800 mg 48 Weeks N=285[d] %**	**PEGASYS 180 µg + 800 mg Ribavirin 48 Weeks N=288[d] %**
Endocrine Disorders					
Hypothyroidism	5	4	2	1	<1
Gastrointestinal					
Nausea	28	28	29	19	24
Diarrhea	10	14	15	10	16
Abdominal pain	9	10	9	7	7
Dry mouth	7	6	8	2	5
Nausea and vomiting	6	7	8	8	8
Dyspepsia	5	6	2	6	4
General					
Fatigue	53	49	45	36	40
Pyrexia	54	39	37	32	41
Rigors	34	25	30	17	16
Injection site reaction	16	21	28	8	10
Asthenia	16	15	18	23	26
Pain	9	10	9	4	6
Malaise	3	4	3	7	6
Metabolic and Nutritional					
Anorexia	26	27	20	25	23
Weight decrease	10	7	2	13	16
Appetite decrease	—	—	—	9	7
Musculoskeletal, Connective Tissue and Bone					
Myalgia	49	38	42	27	32
Arthralgia	23	22	20	13	16
Back pain	5	5	3	3	3
Neurological					
Headache	49	47	48	34	35
Insomnia	37	32	30	23	19
Dizziness (excluding vertigo)	14	15	13	9	7
Concentration impairment	13	10	8	2	2
Memory impairment	5	5	4	<1	1
Psychiatric					
Depression	28	21	17	20	22
Irritability	27	24	28	17	15
Anxiety	12	8	8	7	8
Mood alteration	6	6	8	2	<1
Emotional disorders	4	5	5	1	<1
Libido decreased	3	3	5	1	2
Nervousness	5	3	—	1	1
Respiratory, Thoracic and Mediastinal					
Dyspnea	14	13	11	3	7
Cough	7	13	8	2	3
Dyspnea (exertional)	7	4	3	2	3
Skin and Subcutaneous Tissue					
Alopecia	33	24	25	5	10
Pruritus	18	21	25	3	4
Dermatitis	13	16	15	<1	1
Dry skin	13	12	13	4	4
Rash	5	9	7	5	5
Sweating increased	5	5	2	2	5

[a] Data from study 1.
[b] Pooled data from studies 1 and 2.
[c] Data from study 2.
[d] Data from study 3.

Table 2: PEGASYS RBV

Adverse Reactions Reported in ≥1% to <5% on PEGASYS RBV Combination or PEGASYS Monotherapy in Patients in Clinical Trials Were:

Body System	**Any Treatment Group Common ≥1% to <5%**	**HIV-HCV Only Other Adverse Reactions ≥1% to ≤3%**
Blood and Lymphatic System Disorders	lymphadenopathy, thrombocytopenia	
Cardiac Disorders	palpitations, oedema peripheral, tachycardia	
Ear and Labyrinth Disorders	vertigo, earache, tinnitus	
Endocrine Disorders	hyperthyroidism	
Eye Disorders	vision blurred, eye inflammation, xerophthalmia, eye pain	
Gastrointestinal Disorders	mouth ulceration, flatulence, gingival bleeding, stomatitis, constipation, dysphagia, glossitis	cheilitis
General Disorders and Administration Site Conditions	lethargy, chest pain, hot flushes, thirst, influenza-like illness	
Infections and Infestations	herpes simplex, URI infection, bronchitis, oral candidiasis	influenza, pneumonia
Injury and Poisoning	substance abuse	
Metabolism and Nutrition Disorders	dehydration	hyperlactacidemia/lactic acidosis
Musculoskeletal, Connective Tissue and Bone Disorders	muscle cramps, neck pain, musculoskeletal pain, bone pain, arthritis, muscle weakness	
Nervous System Disorders	taste disturbance, weakness, paraesthesia, hypoaesthesia, tremor, migraine, somnolence, hyperaesthesia, nightmares, syncope	
Psychiatric Disorders	aggression, suicidal ideation, confusional state	affect lability, apathy
Renal and Urinary Disorders		chromaturia
Reproductive System and Breast Disorders	impotence	
Respiratory, Thoracic and Mediastinal Disorders	sore throat, pharyngolaryngeal pain, epistaxis, nasopharyngitis, sinus congestion, rhinitis, nasal congestion	
Skin and Subcutaneous Tissue Disorders	eczema, night sweats, psoriasis, photosensitivity reaction, urticaria, skin disorder	acquired lipodystrophy
Vascular Disorders	flushing, hypertension	

As with other alpha interferon therapies, uncommon to rare cases (<1%) of the following **serious** adverse events have been reported in patients receiving PEGASYS RBV combination or PEGASYS monotherapy during clinical trials:

Blood and the Lymphatic System Disorders: thrombotic thrombocytopenic purpura (TTP).
Cardiac Disorders: arrhythmia, atrial fibrillation, pericarditis.
Eye Disorders: corneal ulcer.
Gastrointestinal Disorders: peptic ulcer, gastrointestinal bleeding, pancreatitis, abdominal distention.
Immune System Disorders: autoimmune phenomena (e.g. ITP, thyroiditis, psoriasis, rheumatoid arthritis, SLE), sarcoidosis.
Infections and Infestations: skin infection, otitis externa, endocarditis.
Hepatobiliary: hepatic dysfunction, fatty liver, cholangitis, malignant hepatic neoplasm.

Nervous System Disorders: myositis, peripheral neuropathy*, coma.
Psychiatric Disorders: suicide, panic attack, psychotic disorder, hallucination.
Respiratory, Thoracic and Mediastinal Disorders: interstitial pneumonitis with fatal outcome, pulmonary embolism.
Vascular Disorders: cerebral hemorrhage.

Rarely, alpha interferon including PEGASYS RBV or PEGASYS monotherapy may be associated with pancytopenia, and very rarely, aplastic anemia has been reported.

Uncommon to very rare cases of hearing impairment (deafness) have been reported.

Abnormal Hematologic and Clinical Chemistry Findings: Hematology: As with other interferon therapies, treatment with PEGASYS monotherapy and PEGASYS RBV combination therapy was associated with decreases in hematological values, which generally improved with dosage modification and returned to pretreatment levels within 4 to 8 weeks upon cessation of therapy (see Warnings and Precautions and Dosage and Administration).

Although hematological toxicities of neutropenia, thrombocytopenia and anemia occurred more frequently in HIV-HCV patients, the majority could be managed by dose modification and the use of growth factors and infrequently required premature discontinuation of treatment.

Hemoglobin: Treatment with PEGASYS monotherapy for HCV was associated with small gradual decrease in hemoglobin and hematocrit. Less than 1% of all patients treated with PEGASYS, including those with cirrhosis, required dose modification for anemia (<100 g/L). No patients receiving interferon alfa-2a required anemia-related dose modifications, due to drops in hemoglobin levels. Anemia due to hemolysis is the most significant toxicity of ribavirin therapy. Anemia (hemoglobin <100 g/L) was observed in 13% of PEGASYS RBV combination-treated patients in HCV clinical trials. The maximum drop in hemoglobin occurred during the first 8 weeks of initiation of ribavirin therapy (see Dosage and Administration, Recommended Dose and Dosage Adjustment, Dose Adjustments).

Approximately 10% of patients on PEGASYS RBV combination therapy required COPEGUS dose modification for anemia. Patients receiving 800 mg of COPEGUS for 24 weeks had the lowest frequency of decrease in hemoglobin levels to <100 g/L; hemoglobin levels did not fall to <85 g/L in any of these patients.

Anemia (hemoglobin <100g/L) was reported in 8% and 14% of HIV-HCV co-infected patients treated with PEGASYS monotherapy or PEGASYS RBV combination therapy, respectively.

White Blood Cells: Treatment with PEGASYS for HCV was associated with decreases in values for both total WBC and ANC. Approximately 4% and 5% of patients on PEGASYS monotherapy or PEGASYS RBV combination therapy, respectively, had transient decreases in ANC to levels below 0.5×10^9/L at some time during therapy.

In HIV-HCV co-infected patients, 13% and 11% of those receiving PEGASYS monotherapy and PEGASYS RBV combination therapy, respectively, had decreases in ANC levels below 0.5×10^9/L.

Platelet Count: Treatment with PEGASYS was associated with decreases in values for platelet counts. In HCV clinical trials, approximately 5% of patients had decreases in platelet counts to levels below 50×10^9/L. Most of these patients were cirrhotic at baseline and/or entered the study with a baseline platelet count as low as 75×10^9/L.

Table 3: PEGASYS RBV

Laboratory Test Values

	Interferon alfa-2b 3MIU + 1000 or 1200 mg Ribavirin 48 Weeks N=443[a] %	Peginterferon alfa-2a 180 µg + 1000 or 1200 mg Ribavirin 48 Weeks N=887[b] %	Peginterferon alfa-2a 180 µg + 800 mg Ribavirin 24 Weeks N=207[c] %
Hemoglobin level (<100 g/L)	10.8	13	3.4
ANC (<0.5×10^9/L)	1.1	5	3.4
Platelet counts (<50×10^9/L)	0.2	5	3.9

[a] Data from study 1.
[b] Pooled data from studies 1 and 2.
[c] Data from study 2.

In HIV-HCV patients, 10% and 8% of those receiving PEGASYS monotherapy and PEGASYS RBV combination therapy, respectively, had decreases in platelets below 50×10^9/L.

Clinical Chemistry: Thyroid Function: PEGASYS treatments was associated with clinically significant abnormalities in thyroid laboratory values requiring clinical intervention (see Warnings and Precautions, Monitoring and Laboratory Tests). The frequencies observed with PEGASYS treatments were similar to those observed with other interferons.

Triglycerides: Triglyceride levels are found to be elevated in patients receiving alpha interferon therapy, including PEGASYS.

For a full listing of PEGASYS monotherapy adverse reactions, please refer to the current PEGASYS product monograph.

Post-Market Adverse Drug Reactions: During the post-marketing period, erythema multiforme, Stevens-Johnson Syndrome and toxic epidermal necrolysis, pure red cell aplasia (PRCA) and homicidal ideation have been reported very rarely with PEGASYS RBV combination therapy.

Dehydration has been reported rarely with PEGASYS RBV combination therapy.

As with other alpha interferons, serous retinal detachment has been reported with PEGASYS RBV combination therapy.

As with other alpha interferons, liver and renal graft rejections have been reported on PEGASYS, alone or in combination with COPEGUS.

DRUG INTERACTIONS: Overview: PEGASYS RBV (peginterferon alfa-2a and ribavirin): No pharmacokinetic interactions between PEGASYS (peginterferon alfa-2a) and COPEGUS (ribavirin) have been observed in HCV clinical trials in which PEGASYS was used in combination with ribavirin.

PEGASYS: Treatment with 180 µg PEGASYS once weekly for 4 weeks had no effect on the pharmacokinetic profiles of tolbutamide (CYP 2C9), mephenytoin (CYP 2C19), debrisoquine (CYP 2D6), and dapsone (CYP 3A4) in healthy male subjects.

COPEGUS: Results of in vitro studies using both human and rat liver microsome preparations indicated no cytochrome P450 enzyme mediated metabolism of ribavirin. Ribavirin does not inhibit cytochrome P450 enzymes. There is no evidence from toxicity studies that ribavirin induces liver enzymes. Therefore, there is a minimal potential for P450 enzyme-based interactions.

The bioavailability of ribavirin 600 mg was decreased by coadministration with an antacid containing magnesium, aluminium and methicone; AUC_{tf} decreased 14%. It is possible that the decreased bioavailability in this study was due to delayed transit of ribavirin or modified pH. This interaction is not considered to be clinically relevant.

Any potential for interactions may persist for up to 2 months (5 half-lives for ribavirin) after cessation of ribavirin therapy due to the long half-life.

Drug-Drug Interactions: See Table 4.

Table 4: PEGASYS RBV

Established or Potential Drug-Drug Interactions

Proper Name	Ref	Effect	Clinical Comment
Peginterferon alfa-2a and Methadone	CT	In a pharmacokinetic study of 24 HCV patients concomitantly receiving methadone maintenance therapy (median dose 95 mg; range 30 mg to 150 mg), treatment with PEGASYS 180 µg sc once weekly for 4 weeks was associated with mean methadone levels that were 10% to 15% higher than at baseline.	The clinical significance of this finding is unknown; nonetheless, patients should be monitored for the signs and symptoms of methadone toxicity.

* In protocol NR15961 (HIV-HCV) the frequency was reported as 2% in the PEGASYS monotherapy arm.

(cont'd)

Table 4: PEGASYS RBV *(cont'd)*

Established or Potential Drug-Drug Interactions

Proper Name	Ref	Effect	Clinical Comment
Peginterferon alfa-2a and Theophylline	T	PEGASYS is a modest inhibitor of cytochrome P450 1A2: a 25% increase in theophylline's AUC was observed in the same study. Comparable effects on the pharmacokinetics of theophylline have been seen after treatment with standard alpha interferons. Alpha interferons have been shown to affect the oxidative metabolism of some drugs by reducing the activity of hepatic microsomal cytochrome P450 enzymes.	Theophylline serum concentrations should be monitored and appropriate dose adjustments of theophylline made for patients taking theophylline and PEGASYS concomitantly.
Ribavirin and Didanosine	CT	Ribavirin potentiated the antiretroviral effect of didanosine (ddI) in vitro and in animals by increasing the formation of the active triphosphate anabolite (ddATP). This observation also raised the possibility that concomitant administration of ribavirin and ddI might increase the risk of adverse reactions related to ddI (such as peripheral neuropathy, pancreatitis, and hepatic steatosis with lactic acidosis). While the clinical significance of these findings is unknown, one study of concomitant ribavirin and ddI in patients with HIV disease did not result in further reductions in viraemia or an increase in adverse reactions. Plasma pharmacokinetics of ddI were not significantly affected by concomitant ribavirin in this study, although intracellular ddATP was not measured. Exposure to didanosine or its active metabolite (dideoxyadenosine 5'-triphosphate) is increased when didanosine is coadministered with ribavirin.	Coadministration of ribavirin and didanosine is not recommended. Reports of fatal hepatic failure, as well as, peripheral neuropathy, pancreatitis, and symptomatic hyperlactatemia/lactic acidosis have been reported.
Ribavirin and Lamivudine, Stavudine, Zidovudine	T	Ribavirin was shown in-vitro to inhibit phosphorylation of zidovudine and stavudine. The clinical significance of these findings is unknown. However, these in-vitro findings raise the possibility that concurrent use of ribavirin with either zidovudine or stavudine might lead to increased HIV plasma viremia.	Therefore, it is recommended that plasma HIV RNA levels be closely monitored in patients treated with ribavirin concurrently with either of these two agents. If HIV RNA levels increase, the use of ribavirin concomitantly with reverse transcriptase inhibitors must be reviewed.
	CT	No evidence of drug interaction was observed in 47 HIV-HCV co-infected patients who completed a 12 week pharmacokinetic substudy to examine the effect of ribavirin on the intracellular phosphorylation of some nucleoside reverse transcriptase inhibitors (lamivudine, zidovudine, or stavudine).	Plasma exposure of ribavirin did not appear to be affected by concomitant administration of NRTIs.

Legend: C=case study; CT=clinical trial; T=theoretical.

Peginterferon alfa-2a and Telbivudine: A non-Roche sponsored pilot clinical trial in Hepatitis B investigating the combination of telbivudine 600 mg daily, with pegylated interferon alfa -2a, 180 µg once weekly by subcutaneous administration, indicated that this combination is associated with an increased risk for developing **serious peripheral neuropathy** at a rate of 10%. An increased risk can not be ruled out for combination treatment with other interferon products (pegylated or standard). The benefit of telbivudine in combination with interferon alfa (pegylated or standard) is not currently established in patients. It is not recommended that telbivudine be given in combination with PEGASYS.

Azathioprine: Ribavirin, by having an inhibitory effect on inosine monophosphate dehydrogenase, may interfere with azathioprine metabolism possibly leading to an accumulation of 6-methylthioinosine monophosphate (6-MTIMP), which has been associated with myelotoxicity in patients treated with azathioprine.

In individual cases where the benefit of administering ribavirin concomitantly with azathioprine warrants the potential risk, it is recommended that close hematologic monitoring be done during concomitant azathioprine use to identify signs of myelotoxicity, at which time treatment with these drugs should be stopped (see Warnings and Precautions, Hematologic).

Drug-Herb Interactions: Pulmonary symptoms have been reported more frequently when sho-saiko-to, a Chinese herbal medicine, also known as Xiao-Chai-Hu was given with interferon alfa-2a. This herb should not be taken by patients receiving interferon.

DOSAGE AND ADMINISTRATION: Dosing Considerations: Treatment should be individualized to the patient depending on baseline disease characteristics, response to therapy, and tolerability of the regimen.

Recommended Dose and Dosage Adjustment: Recommended Dose: Chronic Hepatitis C Mono-infection: See Table 5.

Table 5: PEGASYS RBV

Dosing Recommendations

Genotype	PEGASYS Dose	COPEGUS Dose (Take with Food)	Duration
Genotype 1, 4	180 µg	<75 kg=1000 mg ≥75 kg=1200 mg	48 weeks 48 weeks
Genotype 2, 3	180 µg	800 mg (regardless of weight)	24 weeks

PEGASYS (peginterferon alfa-2a): The recommended dose of PEGASYS is 180 µg administered subcutaneously in the abdomen or thigh once-weekly for 48 weeks for Genotype 1, 4 patients and for 24 weeks for Genotype 2, 3 patients.

The recommended duration of PEGASYS RBV treatment for patients previously untreated with interferon alfa-2a is 24 to 48 weeks. The duration of treatment should be individualized to the patient depending on baseline disease characteristics, response to therapy, and tolerability of the regimen.

A treatment duration of 24 weeks is recommended for Genotype 2, 3 patients and a treatment duration of 48 weeks is recommended for Genotype 1, 4 patients.

COPEGUS (ribavirin): The daily dose of COPEGUS is 1000 mg to 1200 mg for 48 weeks for Genotype 1, 4 patients and 800 mg for 24 weeks for Genotype 2, 3 patients administered orally in two divided doses. The dose should be individualized to the patient depending on baseline disease characteristics (eg, genotype as indicated), response to therapy, and tolerability of the regimen (see Table 5). In the pivotal clinical trials, patients were instructed to take COPEGUS with food; therefore, patients are advised to take COPEGUS with food.

HIV-HCV Co-infection: See Table 6.

Table 6: PEGASYS RBV

PEGASYS RBV Dosing Recommendations

Genotype	PEGASYS Dose	COPEGUS Dose (Take with Food)	Duration
Genotype 1, 2, 3, 4	180 µg	800 mg (regardless of weight)	48 weeks

The recommended dosage of PEGASYS in combination with 800 mg daily COPEGUS (ribavirin) is 180 µg once weekly subcutaneously for 48 weeks, regardless of genotype. The safety and efficacy of combination therapy with COPEGUS doses greater than 800 mg daily or a duration of therapy less than 48 weeks has not been studied.

Early Predictability of Response: After 12 weeks of treatment, virologic response should be assessed. Treatment discontinuation should be considered in any HCV (including HIV-HCV) patient who has not achieved viral clearance or an HCV-RNA reduction from baseline of at least 99% by week 12.

Dose Adjustments: PEGASYS: General: When dose modification is required for moderate to severe adverse reactions (clinical and/or laboratory), initial dose reduction to 135 µg is generally adequate. However, in some cases, dose reduction to 90 µg is necessary. Following improvement of the adverse reaction, dose increases to or toward the original dose may be considered (see Warnings and Precautions and Adverse Reactions).

Hematological: Dose reduction to 135 µg PEGASYS is recommended if the ANC is less than 0.75×10^9/L. For patients with ANC values below 0.5×10^9/L, treatment should be suspended until ANC values return to over 1.0×10^9/L. Therapy should initially be reinstituted at 90 µg PEGASYS, and the ANC monitored.

Dose reduction to 90 µg PEGASYS is recommended if the platelet count is less than 50×10^9/L. Cessation of therapy is recommended when platelet count decreases to levels below 25×10^9/L.

COPEGUS: See Table 7.

Table 7: PEGASYS RBV

COPEGUS Dosage Modification Guidelines for Management of Treatment Emergent Anemia

Laboratory Values	Reduce COPEGUS Dose to 600 mg/day[a] Only if:	Discontinue COPEGUS if[b]:
Hemoglobin: Patients with no cardiac disease	<100 g/L	<85 g/L
Hemoglobin: Patients with history of stable cardiac disease	>20 g/L decrease in hemoglobin during any 4 week period during treatment (permanent dose reduction)	<120 g/L after 4 weeks of dose reduction

[a] Patients whose dose of COPEGUS is reduced to 600 mg daily receive one 200 mg tablet in the morning and two 200 mg tablets in the evening.

[b] If the abnormality is reversed, COPEGUS may be restarted at 600 mg daily, and further increased to 800 mg daily at the discretion of the treating physician. However, a return to higher doses is not recommended.

In case of intolerance to COPEGUS, PEGASYS monotherapy may be continued.

Liver Function: PEGASYS: Fluctuations in abnormalities of liver function tests are common in patients with chronic hepatitis. However, as with other alpha interferons, increases in ALT levels above baseline have been observed in patients treated with PEGASYS, including patients with a virological response.

The dose should be reduced initially to 90 µg in the presence of progressive ALT increases above baseline values. When increase in ALT levels is progressive despite dose reduction, or is accompanied by increased bilirubin or evidence of hepatic decompensation, therapy should be discontinued.

Depression: PEGASYS RBV should be used with extreme caution in patients who report a history of depression and physicians should monitor all patients for evidence of depression. For mild depression, no dose adjustment is necessary. For moderate depression, an initial dose reduction to 135 µg is recommended; however, dose reduction to 90 µg may be needed. Patients should be closely monitored. The frequency and nature of the monitoring should be based on the clinical judgment of the physician. If severe symptoms persist, therapy should be stopped and psychiatric intervention sought (see Warnings and Precautions).

Special Populations: Geriatric Use: PEGASYS: No special dosage modification is required for geriatric patients with normal renal function, based upon pharmacokinetic, pharmacodynamic, tolerability, and safety data from clinical trials.

COPEGUS: There does not appear to be a significant age-related effect on the pharmacokinetics of ribavirin. However, as in younger patients, renal function must be determined prior to administration of COPEGUS.

Hepatic Impairment: PEGASYS RBV has been shown to be effective and safe in patients with compensated cirrhosis (e.g. Child-Pugh A). PEGASYS RBV has not been studied in patients with decompensated liver disease (e.g. Child-Pugh B/C or bleeding esophageal varices) (see Contraindications and Warnings and Precautions).

The Child-Pugh classification divides patients into groups A, B, and C, or "Mild", "Moderate" and "Severe" corresponding to scores of 5-6, 7-9 and 10-15, respectively.

Table 8: PEGASYS RBV

Modified Assessment

Assessment	Degree of Abnormality	Score
Encephalopathy	None	1
	Grade 1-2	2
	Grade 3-4[a]	3
Ascites	Absent	1
	Slight	2
	Moderate	3
S-Bilirubin (mg/dL)	<2	1
	2–3	2
	>3	3
(SI unit=µmol/L)	<34	1
	34–51	2
	>51	3
S-Albumin (g/L)	>35	1
	35–28	2
	<28	3
INR	<1.7	1
	1.7–2.3	2
	>2.3	3

[a] Grading according to Trey, Burns and Saunders (1966).

COPEGUS: No pharmacokinetic interaction appears between ribavirin and hepatic function. Therefore, no dose adjustment of COPEGUS is required in patients with hepatic impairment.

Renal Impairment: PEGASYS: No dose adjustments in the recommended starting dose of PEGASYS 180 µg once weekly is required in patients with creatinine clearance >0.33 mL/sec. In patients with impaired renal function, signs and symptoms of interferon toxicity should be closely monitored.

In subjects with end-stage renal disease requiring hemodialysis, a starting dose of 135 µg should be used. Regardless of the starting dose or degree of renal impairment, patients should be monitored and appropriate dose reductions of PEGASYS during the course of therapy should be made in the event of adverse reactions.

COPEGUS: The pharmacokinetics of ribavirin are altered in patients with renal dysfunction due to reduction of apparent clearance in these patients. Therefore, it is recommended that renal function be evaluated in all patients prior to initiation of COPEGUS, preferably by estimating the patient's creatinine clearance. Substantial increases in ribavirin plasma concentrations are seen at the recommended dosing regimen in patients with serum creatinine >177 µmol/L or with creatinine clearance <0.83 mL/sec. There are insufficient data on the safety and efficacy in these patients and therefore, drug discontinuation, must be considered if adverse events develop (see Warnings and Precautions and Action and Pharmacology, Pharmacokinetics of PEGASYS RBV in Special Populations).

Missed Dose: PEGASYS: If the PEGASYS dose is missed and remembered within 2 days of the scheduled dose, the PEGASYS dose should be administered as soon as possible. The next scheduled PEGASYS dose should be given on the usual day. If more than 2 days have elapsed, the dosage schedule should be based on the clinical judgement of the physician.

COPEGUS: If a COPEGUS dose is missed but remembered within the same day, it should be taken as soon as possible. If an entire day has passed, the next dose should be taken based on the clinical judgement of the physician. Two doses should not be taken at the same time.

Administration: PEGASYS is administered subcutaneously in the abdomen or thigh once-weekly (see Dosage and Administration). Visually inspect the solution prior to administration. Do not use if discoloured or if particles are present.

COPEGUS is administered orally in two divided doses. In the pivotal clinical trials, patients were instructed to take COPEGUS with food; therefore, patients are advised to take COPEGUS with food (see Dosage and Administration).

OVERDOSAGE:

PEGASYS RBV (peginterferon alfa-2a and ribavirin): There is limited experience with overdosage with PEGASYS (peginterferon alfa-2a). The maximum dose received by any patient was 7 times the intended dose of PEGASYS (180 µg/day for 7 days). There were no serious reactions attributed to overdosages. Weekly doses of up to 630 µg have been administered to patients with cancer. Dose-limiting toxicities were fatigue, elevated liver enzymes, neutropenia and thrombocytopenia. There is no specific antidote for PEGASYS. Hemodialysis and peritoneal dialysis are not effective.

No cases of overdose with COPEGUS (ribavirin) have been reported in clinical trials. Absorption of ribavirin is generally complete after one hour. Hypocalcemia and hypomagnesemia have been observed in persons administered dosages greater than four times the maximal recommended dosages. In many of these cases ribavirin was administered intravenously. Treatment of overdose with ribavirin should consist of general supportive measures including monitoring of vital signs and observation of clinical status of the patient. There is no specific antidote for overdose with ribavirin. Ribavirin concentration is essentially unchanged by hemodialysis.

> For management of a suspected drug overdose, CPhA recommends that you contact your **regional Poison Control Centre**. See the *CPS* Directory section for a list of Poison Control Centres.

ACTION AND CLINICAL PHARMACOLOGY: PEGASYS RBV (peginterferon alfa-2a and ribavirin): Mechanism of Action: PEGASYS: Peginterferon alfa-2a possesses the in vitro antiviral and antiproliferative activities of interferon alfa-2a. Interferons bind to specific receptors on the cell surface initiating a complex intracellular signalling pathway and rapid activation of gene transcription. Interferon-stimulated genes modulate many biological effects including the inhibition of viral replication in infected cells, inhibition of cell proliferation, and immunomodulation. The clinical relevance of these in vitro activities is not known.

COPEGUS: The mechanism by which ribavirin in combination with peginterferon alfa-2a exerts its effects against hepatitis C virus (HCV) is unknown, although it is likely to involve both direct antiviral and immunomodulatory activities. More than additive inhibition of HCV subgenomic RNA replication in human liver cells has been seen in combination with PEGASYS.

Pharmacodynamics of PEGASYS: HCV RNA levels decline in a biphasic manner in responding patients with hepatitis C with and without compensated cirrhosis who have received treatment with 180 µg PEGASYS. The first phase of decline occurs within 24 to 36 hours after the first dose of PEGASYS and the second phase of decline occurs over the next 4 to 16 weeks in patients who achieve a sustained response. Treatment with 180 µg PEGASYS per week enhances the virion clearance and improves the virological end of treatment responses compared to treatment with interferon alfa-2a.

PEGASYS stimulates the production of effector proteins such as serum neopterin and 2', 5'-oligoadenylate synthetase (2', 5'-OAS) raises body temperature and causes reversible decreases in leukocyte and platelet counts. The stimulation of 2', 5'-OAS is maximal after single doses of 135 to 180 µg PEGASYS and stays maximal throughout the one week dosing interval. The magnitude and duration of 2',5'-OAS activity induced by PEGASYS were reduced in subjects older than 62 years and in subjects with significant renal impairment (creatinine clearances of 0.33 to 0.67 mL/sec) compared to that seen in healthy subjects. The correlation between the in vitro and in vivo pharmacology and pharmacodynamic and clinical effects is unknown.

Pharmacokinetics: PEGASYS: The structure of the PEG moiety directly affects the clinical pharmacology of PEGASYS. Specifically, the size, branching and location of attachment of the 40 kD PEG moiety contribute to defining the absorption, distribution and elimination characteristics of PEGASYS. The pharmacokinetics of PEGASYS were studied in healthy volunteers and hepatitis C virus (HCV)-infected patients.

Absorption: The absorption of PEGASYS is sustained with peak serum concentrations reached 72 to 96 hours after dosing. Serum concentrations are measurable within 3 to 6 hours of a single dose. Dose proportional increases in AUC and C_{max} are seen in patients that received once weekly doses of PEGASYS.

The absolute bioavailability of PEGASYS following sc administration in the abdomen is 84% and is similar to that seen with interferon alfa-2a.

Distribution: The volume of distribution at steady-state (Vss) of 6 to 14 liters after intravenous dosing suggests that the drug is found mainly in the bloodstream and extracellular fluid.

Metabolism: The metabolic profile of PEGASYS is not fully characterized.

Excretion: The systemic clearance of PEGASYS is about 100 mL/h, which is 100-fold lower than that of interferon alfa-2a. After an intravenous dose, the terminal half-life of PEGASYS in healthy subjects is about 60 hours compared to 3 to 4 hours for standard interferon. The terminal half-life after subcutaneous administration in patients is longer with a mean value of 160 hours (84 to 353 hours). The terminal half-life after subcutaneous dosing may be reflecting the sustained absorption of PEGASYS and not the elimination of the drug.

The kidneys eliminate less than 10% of a dose as the intact peginterferon alfa-2a. The rest is broken down metabolically.

Steady state serum levels are reached within 5 to 8 weeks of once-weekly dosing. Once steady state has been achieved, there is no accumulation of peginterferon alfa-2a. The peak to trough ratio after 48 weeks of treatment is about 1.5 to 2.0. Peginterferon alfa-2a serum concentrations are sustained throughout the 1 week dosing interval (168 hours) [see Table 9 and Figure 1].

Table 9: PEGASYS RBV

Pharmacokinetic Parameters of PEGASYS After Single and Multiple Dose of 180 µg

PEGASYS Pharmacokinetic Parameter	Healthy Subjects 180 µg sc (N=50)	CHC Patients 180 µg sc (N=16)	
	Single Dose Mean±SD [Range]	Single Dose Mean±SD [Range]	Week 48 Dose Mean±SD [Range]
C_{max} (ng/mL)	14±5 [6–26]	15±4 [7–23]	26±9 [10–40]
T_{max} (h)	92±27 [48–168]	80±28 [23–119]	45±36 [0–97]
$AUC_{1\text{-}168h}$ (ng·h/mL)	1725±586 [524–3013]	1820±586 [846–2609]	3334±994 [1265–4824]
Clearance/F (mL/h)	94±56 [34–337]	83±50 [33–186]	60±25 [37–142]
Week 48 trough concentration (ng/mL)	Not applicable	Not applicable	16±6 [4–28]
Peak to trough ratio for week 48	Not applicable	Not applicable	1.7±0.4 [1.1–2.5]
Accumulation ($AUC_{Week\ 48}/AUC_{Single\ Dose}$)	Not applicable	Not applicable	2.3±1.0 [1.1–4.0]

Figure 1: PEGASYS RBV

Mean Steady-state PEGASYS Concentrations in Patients with CHC Following 180 µg Peginterferon alfa-2a in Combination Therapy

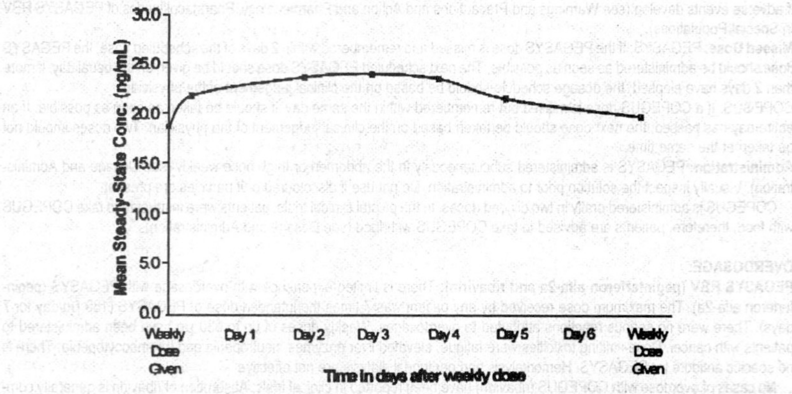

COPEGUS: Absorption: Orally administrated ribavirin is absorbed rapidly, reaching maximal plasma concentrations between 1 and 2 hours. The $AUC_{0\text{-}192h}$ and C_{max} following a single oral dose of 600 mg of ribavirin ranged from 14 to 20 mg·h/mL and from 650 to 770 ng/mL, respectively. Intersubject variability was high, with values of approximately 30% for $AUC_{0\text{-}192h}$ and 40% for C_{max}. Absorption is extensive with about 10% to 15% of a radiolabelled dose excreted in the feces. However, the absolute bioavailability is between 33% to 65%, probably due to high first-pass metabolism. Ribavirin is absorbed from the gastrointestinal tract via an active sodium dependent nucleoside transport process. Since this process is saturable, less than proportional increases in C_{max} were observed for doses above 800 mg. However, the exposure as measured by $AUC_{0\text{-}192h}$ was proportional up to a 2400 mg dose.

Bioavailability of a single oral dose of ribavirin was increased by coadministration with a high-fat meal. The absorption was slowed (T_{max} was doubled) and the $AUC_{0\text{-}192h}$ and C_{max} increased by 42% and 66%, respectively, when the ribavirin film-coated tablet was taken with a high-fat meal compared with fasting conditions.

Distribution: Ribavirin partitions into all cells rapidly and extensively and a very large steady-state volume of distribution of about 850 liters after intravenous dosing. This distribution is facilitated by the sodium independent es nucleoside transporter that is present in all types of cells and thus ribavirin accumulates in erythrocytes, ova and spermatozoa. Ribavirin sequesters in erythrocytes extensively with a ratio of 60:1 between whole blood and plasma concentrations. Ribavirin does not bind to plasma proteins.

Metabolism: Ribavirin is metabolized via two major pathways:

- A reversible phosphorylation in nucleated cells forming mono-, di-, and tri-phosphate metabolites and
- Deribosylation and amide hydrolysis forming the triazole carboxylic acid metabolite. The triazole carboxylic acid and triazole carboxamide were the principal metabolites. The cytochrome P450 enzyme system is not involved in the metabolism of ribavirin.

Excretion: Both renal excretion and metabolism are major routes of elimination of ribavirin in humans and animals. Total body clearance after intravenous dosing was about 20 L/h to 25 L/h, with about 30% accounted for by renal clearance. In humans, about 61% of the radioactivity of a 600-mg oral dose was eliminated in the urine within 336 hours, of which unchanged ribavirin accounted for 17%.

Due to extensive distribution, the terminal half-life of a single oral or intravenous dose is about 120 to 170 hours. This half-life is further prolonged to 270 to 300 hours following multiple doses. Extensive accumulation of ribavirin is seen after multiple dosing (BID) such that the AUC at steady state was sixfold higher than that of a single dose.

Pharmacokinetics Analysis of PEGASYS RBV: No pharmacokinetic interactions between PEGASYS and COPEGUS have been observed in clinical trials in which PEGASYS is used in combination with COPEGUS. Results from a pharmacokinetic substudy of a pivotal phase III trial demonstrated no pharmacokinetic interaction between peginterferon alfa-2a and ribavirin.

Special Populations and Conditions: Pediatrics (<18 years of age): PEGASYS: The pharmacokinetics of PEGASYS have not been adequately studied in pediatric patients.

COPEGUS: Pharmacokinetic evaluations in pediatric patients have not been performed.

Geriatrics: PEGASYS: In subjects older than 62 years, the AUC was modestly increased (1663 vs 1295 ng·h/mL, older than 62 years vs younger, respectively), but peak concentrations (9.1 vs 10.3 ng/mL) were similar in the two age groups (see Dosage and Administration).

COPEGUS: Specific pharmacokinetic evaluations for elderly patients have not been performed. However, in a published population pharmacokinetic study, age was not a key factor in the kinetics of ribavirin; renal function is the determining factor.

Gender: PEGASYS: The pharmacokinetics of PEGASYS after single subcutaneous injections were comparable between male and female healthy subjects.

COPEGUS: No clinically significant differences in the pharmacokinetics of ribavirin were observed between male and female subjects in a population pharmacokinetic analysis of 3600 sparsely collected serum concentration data from 138 patients.

Race: COPEGUS: A pharmacokinetic study in 42 subjects demonstrated there is no clinically significant difference in ribavirin pharmacokinetics among Black (n=14), Hispanic (n=13) and Caucasian (n=15) subjects.

Hepatic Insufficiency: PEGASYS: The pharmacokinetics of PEGASYS were similar between healthy subjects and patients with hepatitis C. Comparable pharmacokinetic profiles were seen in cirrhotic patients with compensated liver disease and patients without cirrhosis.

COPEGUS: Single-dose pharmacokinetics of ribavirin in patients with mild, moderate or severe hepatic dysfunction are similar to those of normal controls.

Renal Insufficiency: PEGASYS: Renal impairment is associated with decreased total apparent clearance and prolonged half-life. In subjects with a creatinine clearance between 0.33 and 0.67 mL/sec, the average total apparent clearance is reduced by approximately 30% compared with subjects with normal renal function following single doses of PEGASYS. Adverse events and laboratory abnormalities that occurred during the study were those expected following interferon administration and occurred with only slightly greater frequency in subjects with renal impairment (see Warnings and Precautions).

In subjects with end-stage renal disease undergoing hemodialysis, there is a 25% to 45% reduction in the clearance of peginterferon alfa-2a and doses of 135 µg provide exposure similar to those observed in subjects with normal renal function receiving 180 µg doses. Regardless of the starting dose or degree of renal impairment, patients should be monitored and appropriate dose reductions of PEGASYS during the course of therapy should be made in the event of adverse reactions (see Warnings and Precautions and Dosage and Administration, Recommended Dose and Dosage Adjustment, Dose Adjustments).

COPEGUS: Single-dose ribavirin pharmacokinetics were altered (increased AUC_{tf} and C_{max}) in patients with renal dysfunction compared with control subjects whose creatinine clearance was greater than 1.50 mL/sec. The oral clearance of ribavirin is substantially reduced in patients with serum creatinine >177 µmol/L or creatinine clearance <0.83 mL/sec. There are insufficient data on the safety and efficacy of ribavirin in these patients and therefore, COPEGUS must be administered with extreme caution and corrective action including drug discontinuation must be considered if adverse events develop (see Warnings and Precautions and Dosage and Administration, Recommended Dose and Dosage Adjustment, Dose Adjustments). Plasma concentrations of ribavirin are essentially unchanged by hemodialysis.

STORAGE AND STABILITY: Stability and Storage Recommendations: Store PEGASYS RBV (peginterferon alfa-2a and ribavirin) packages in the refrigerator at 2 to 8°C. Protect from light. Do not freeze or shake. Do not use PEGASYS RBV beyond the date of expiry.

If Package Components are Separated: Store PEGASYS vials or pre-filled syringes in the refrigerator at 2 to 8°C. Protect from light. Do not freeze or shake. Do not use PEGASYS beyond the date of expiry.

Parenteral drug products such as PEGASYS should be inspected visually for particulate matter and discolouration before administration. Do not use PEGASYS if it contains particulate matter or it appears discoloured. Store COPEGUS below 30°C or under refrigeration. Keep bottle tightly closed.

SPECIAL HANDLING INSTRUCTIONS: PEGASYS RBV (peginterferon alfa-2a and ribavirin): Disposal of Syringes/Sharps: The following points should be strictly adhered to regarding the use and disposal of syringes and other medicinal sharps:

- Needles and syringes should never be reused.
- Place all used needles and syringes into a sharps container (puncture-proof disposable container).
- Keep this container out of the reach of children.
- Placing used sharps containers in the household waste should be avoided.
- Dispose of the full container according to local requirements or as instructed by your healthcare provider.

For home use, a puncture resistant container for the disposal of used syringes and needles should be supplied to the patients.

Disposal of Unused/Expired Medicines: The release of pharmaceuticals in the environment should be minimized. Medicines should not be disposed of via wastewater and disposal through household waste should be avoided. Use established "collection systems" if available in your location.

INFORMATION FOR THE PATIENT: Published in e-CPS, available by subscription at www.e-cps.ca.

DOSAGE FORMS, COMPOSITION AND PACKAGING: PEGASYS Pre-filled Syringes: Each 0.5 mL of sterile, ready to-use solution contains: peginterferon alfa-2a 180 µg (expressed as the amount of interferon alfa-2a), sodium chloride 4 mg, polysorbate 80 0.025 mg, benzyl alcohol 5 mg, sodium acetate trihydrate 1.3085 mg, acetic acid 0.0231 mg and water for injection. Single-use, graduated, clear glass pre-filled syringes of 0.5 mL.

PEGASYS Vials: Each mL contains: peginterferon alfa-2a 180 µg (expressed as the amount of interferon alfa-2a), sodium chloride 8.0 mg, polysorbate 80 0.05 mg, benzyl alcohol 10.0 mg, sodium acetate trihydrate 2.617 mg, acetic acid 0.0462 mg and water for injection. Single-use, clear glass vials of 1 mL.

COPEGUS Tablets: Each light pink to pink, flat, oval, film-coated tablet, with RIB and 200 engraved on one side and ROCHE on the other side contains: ribavirin 200 mg. Nonmedicinal ingredients: ethyl cellulose, hydroxypropyl methylcellulose, iron oxide red, iron oxide yellow, magnesium stearate, maize starch, microcrystalline cellulose, pregelatinized starch, sodium starch glycolate, talc, titanium dioxide and triacetin.

PEGASYS RBV: PEGASYS Pre-filled Syringes (PFS) and COPEGUS: Cartons containing: 1 PFS of PEGASYS 180 µg/0.5 mL and 1 injection needle (27 gauge×½ inch); 1 bottle of COPEGUS containing 28 tablets; 1 alcohol swab. Cartons containing 1 PFS of PEGASYS 180 µg/0.5 mL and 1 injection needle (27 gauge×½ inch); 1 bottle of COPEGUS containing 35 tablets; 1 alcohol swab. Cartons containing 1 PFS of PEGASYS 180 µg/0.5 mL and 1 injection needle (27 gauge×½ inch); 1 bottle of COPEGUS containing 42 tablets; 1 alcohol swab. Cartons containing 4 PFS of PEGASYS 180 µg/0.5 mL and 4 injection needles (27 gauge×½ inch); 1 bottle of COPEGUS containing 112 tablets; 4 alcohol swabs. Cartons containing 4 PFS of PEGASYS 180 µg/0.5 mL and 4 injection needles (27 gauge×½ inch); 1 bottle of COPEGUS containing 140 tablets; 4 alcohol swabs. Cartons containing 4 PFS of PEGASYS 180 µg/0.5 mL and 4 injection needles (27 gauge× ½ inch); 1 bottle of COPEGUS containing 168 tablets; 4 alcohol swabs. Cartons containing 4 PFS of PEGASYS 180 µg/0.5 mL and 4 injection needles (27 gauge× ½ inch); 1 bottle of COPEGUS containing 168 tablets + 1 bottle of COPEGUS containing 28 tablets; 4 alcohol swabs.

PEGASYS RBV: PEGASYS Vials and COPEGUS: Cartons containing 1 vial of PEGASYS 180 µg/mL; 1 bottle of COPEGUS containing 42 tablets; 2 alcohol swabs. Cartons containing 4 vials of PEGASYS 180 µg/mL; 1 bottle of COPEGUS containing 112 tablets; 8 alcohol swabs. Cartons containing 4 vials of PEGASYS 180 µg/mL; 1 bottle of COPEGUS containing 140 tablets; 8 alcohol swabs. Cartons containing 4 vials of PEGASYS 180 µg/mL; 1 bottle of COPEGUS containing 168 tablets; 8 alcohol swabs.

Pegetron® Pr

ribavirin—peginterferon alfa-2b

Antiviral Agent—Biological Response Modifier

Schering-Plough

Date of Revision: July 28, 2010

SUMMARY PRODUCT INFORMATION:

Route of Administration	Dosage Form/ Strength	Clinically Relevant Nonmedicinal Ingredients
Ribavirin: oral	Capsules/ 200 mg	Lactose monohydrate For a complete listing see Dosage Forms, Composition and Packaging.
Peginterferon alfa-2b: subcutaneous	Powder for Solution in Vial/ 50 µg/0.5 mL, 150 µg/0.5 mL	None For a complete listing see Dosage Forms, Composition and Packaging.
	Powder for Solution in REDIPEN Single Dose Delivery System/ 80 µg/0.5 mL, 100 µg/0.5 mL, 120 µg/0.5 mL, 150 µg/0.5 mL	

DESCRIPTION: PEGETRON product is a combination of ribavirin and peginterferon alfa-2b, specifically PEGETRON (ribavirin) Capsules and PEGETRON (peginterferon alfa-2b) Powder for Solution.

PEGETRON (ribavirin) Capsules: Ribavirin is a synthetic nucleoside analog, which has shown in vitro activity against some, but not all, RNA and DNA viruses.

PEGETRON (peginterferon alfa-2b) Powder for Solution: Peginterferon alfa-2b is a covalent conjugate of recombinant interferon alfa-2b with monomethoxy polyethylene glycol (PEG, with an average molecular weight of 12 000 daltons). The average molecular weight of the conjugated molecule is approximately 31 000 daltons.

INDICATIONS AND CLINICAL USE: PEGETRON (ribavirin plus peginterferon alfa-2b) is indicated for:

- Treatment of adult patients (≥18 years of age) with chronic hepatitis C who have compensated liver disease and are positive for HCV-RNA, including patients who have not received previous treatment or who failed prior treatment with interferon alpha (pegylated or non-pegylated) and ribavirin combination therapy.

Retreatment should be considered in the context of each patient's characteristics and assessment of individual benefit/risk.

- Patients with the following characteristics are more likely to benefit from retreatment after failing a course of combination therapy: previous relapse, previously treated with interferon therapy (non-pegylated), lower fibrosis score, lower baseline viral load, or infection with HCV genotype 2 or 3.
- Patients with the following characteristics are less likely to benefit from retreatment after failing a course of combination therapy: previous non-response, previously treated with pegylated interferon therapy, significant bridging fibrosis or cirrhosis, or infection with HCV genotype 1.

CONTRAINDICATIONS:

- PEGETRON is contraindicated in patients with a hypersensitivity to any interferons and/or ribavirin or any component of the injection and/or capsule. For a complete listing, see Dosage Forms, Composition and Packaging.
- PEGETRON must not be used by pregnant women or by men whose female partners are pregnant. Extreme care must be taken to avoid pregnancy in female patients and in female partners of male patients taking PEGETRON therapy. PEGETRON therapy must not be initiated until a report of a negative pregnancy test has been obtained immediately prior to initiation of therapy. Women of childbearing potential and their male partners must not receive PEGETRON therapy unless they are using effective contraception (two reliable forms, one for each partner) during treatment with PEGETRON and for the 6-month post-therapy period (i.e., 15 half-lives for ribavirin clearance from the body). Significant teratogenic and/or embryocidal effects have been demonstrated for ribavirin in all animal species in which adequate studies have been conducted. These effects occurred at doses as low as one twentieth of the recommended human dose of PEGETRON (ribavirin) Capsules (see Warnings and Precautions).
- Patients with autoimmune hepatitis or a history of autoimmune disease must not be treated with PEGETRON therapy.
- PEGETRON is contraindicated in patients who have pre-existing severe psychiatric condition or a history of severe psychiatric disorder.
- PEGETRON is contraindicated in patients who have pre-existing thyroid abnormalities for which thyroid function cannot be maintained in the normal range by medication.
- Patients with severe renal dysfunction (creatinine clearance <50 mL/min) must not be treated with PEGETRON.
- Patients with decompensated liver disease should not be treated with PEGETRON.
- PEGETRON is contraindicated in patients who have epilepsy.

WARNINGS AND PRECAUTIONS:

Serious Warnings and Precautions

Alpha interferons, including PEGETRON, cause or aggravate fatal or life-threatening neuropsychiatric, autoimmune, ischemic, and infectious disorders. Patients should be monitored closely with periodic clinical and laboratory evaluations. Patients with persistently severe or worsening signs or symptoms of these conditions should be withdrawn from therapy. In many cases, but not all cases, these disorders resolve after stopping interferon therapy.

Life-threatening or fatal psychiatric effects, particularly severe depression, suicidal behavior (suicidal ideation, attempted suicide and suicide), psychosis including hallucinations, and aggressive behavior, sometimes directed towards others, have occurred in patients with and without previous psychiatric disorders during ribavirin plus peginterferon alfa-2b or ribavirin plus interferon alfa-2b treatment and follow-up (see Adverse Reactions). Other Central Nervous System (CNS) effects including confusion and alterations of mental status have been observed with alpha interferons, including peginterferon alfa-2b.

PEGETRON therapy should be used with extreme caution in patients with a history of pre-existing psychiatric disorders who report a history of severe depression. If patients develop psychiatric or CNS problems, including clinical depression, it is recommended that the patients be carefully monitored during treatment and in the 6 month follow-up period, due to the potential seriousness of these undesirable effects. If such symptoms appear, the potential seriousness of these undesirable effects must be borne in mind by the prescribing physician. If symptoms persist or worsen, discontinue PEGETRON therapy.

General: PEGETRON therapy should not be used in patients with severe, debilitating medical conditions.

Based on results of clinical trials, the use of PEGETRON (ribavirin) Capsules as monotherapy is not effective and PEGETRON (ribavirin) Capsules must not be used alone. The safety and efficacy of ribavirin has only been established in combination with peginterferon alfa-2b (PEGETRON).

PEGETRON may cause moderate to severe adverse experiences requiring dose reduction or temporary interruption of PEGETRON (peginterferon alfa-2b) Powder for Solution or PEGETRON (ribavirin) Capsules therapy, or temporary cessation of both drugs. Generally, medical management of these adverse experiences is accomplished with these modifications. Occasionally, discontinuation from further therapy is required. More stringent dose-modification guidelines are recommended for cardiac patients (see Dosage and Administration).

Carcinogenesis and Mutagenesis: Conventional carcinogenicity studies in rodents with low exposures compared to human exposure under therapeutic conditions (factor 0.1 in rats and 1 in mice) did not reveal tumorigenicity of ribavirin. In addition, in a 26 week carcinogenicity study using the heterozygous p53 (+/-) mouse model, ribavirin did not produce tumors at the maximally tolerated dose of 300 mg/kg (plasma exposure factor approximately 2.5 compared to human exposure). Ribavirin was non-carcinogenic when administered for 2 years to rats at doses up to 40 mg/kg (estimated human equivalent of 5.71 mg/kg based on body surface area adjustment for a 60 kg adult). While these studies do not suggest a carcinogenic potential of PEGETRON (ribavirin) Capsules in humans, this dose was less than the maximum tolerated dose, and therefore the 2-year study was not adequate to fully characterize the carcinogenic potential of ribavirin. Ribavirin should be considered a potential carcinogen.

Ribavirin is genotoxic and mutagenic in some in vivo and in vitro genotoxicity assays. Studies indicated that ribavirin was not oncogenic in mice at oral gavage doses up to 75 mg/kg/day, or in rats at oral gavage doses up to 40 mg/kg/day.

Cardiovascular: Chest pain, hypertension, cardiac arrhythmia, cardiac ischemia, and myocardial infarction have been reported in patients with and without a history of cardiac disorder or abnormality in association with the use of alpha interferon therapies including peginterferon alfa-2b (see Adverse Reactions). PEGETRON should not be administered to patients with a history of severe pre-existing cardiac disease including unstable or uncontrolled cardiac disease in the previous 6 months. As with other alpha interferons, patients with a history of congestive heart failure, myocardial infarction and/or previous or current arrhythmic disorders receiving PEGETRON therapy require close monitoring. It is recommended that patients who have preexisting cardiac abnormalities have electrocardiograms taken prior to and during the course of treatment. Cardiac arrhythmias (primarily supraventricular) usually respond to conventional therapy but may require discontinuation of PEGETRON therapy. Cardiomyopathy, that may be reversible upon discontinuation of alpha interferon therapy, has been reported rarely in patients without prior evidence of cardiac disease.

A case of deep vein thrombosis has been reported from a clinical trial of retreatment of patients who failed previous treatment with interferon and ribavirin combination therapy.

Hydration: Adequate hydration must be maintained in patients undergoing therapy with PEGETRON since hypotension related to fluid depletion has been seen in some patients treated with alpha interferons, including peginterferon alfa-2b. Fluid replacement may be necessary.

Cerebrovascular Disorders: Ischemic and hemorrhagic cerebrovascular events have been observed in patients treated with interferon alfa-based therapies, including peginterferon alfa-2b. Events occurred in patients with few or no reported risk factors for stroke, including patients less than 45 years of age. Because these are spontaneous reports, estimates of frequency cannot be made and a causal relationship between interferon alfa-based therapies and these events is difficult to establish.

Dental and Periodontal Disorders: Dental and periodontal disorders have been reported in patients receiving ribavirin and peginterferon combination therapy. In addition, dry mouth could have a damaging effect on teeth and mucous membranes of the mouth during long-term treatment with the combination of ribavirin and peginterferon alfa-2b. Patients should brush their teeth thoroughly twice daily and have regular dental examinations. In addition some patients may experience vomiting. If this reaction occurs, they should be advised to rinse out their mouth thoroughly afterwards.

Ear/Nose/Throat: Hearing disorder and hearing loss have been reported with the use of alpha interferons, including peginterferon alfa-2b therapy.

Endocrine and Metabolism: Diabetes Mellitus and Hyperglycemia: As with other alpha interferons, diabetes mellitus and hyperglycemia have been observed in patients treated with peginterferon alfa-2b therapy. Symptomatic patients should have their blood glucose measured and followed up accordingly. Patients with diabetes mellitus may require adjustment of their anti-diabetic regimen.

Thyroid Changes: Infrequently, patients treated for chronic hepatitis C with alpha interferons, including peginterferon alfa-2b, have developed thyroid abnormalities, either hypothyroidism or hyperthyroidism. After discontinuation of therapy, thyroid dysfunction may or may not be reversed. Determine thyroid-stimulating hormone (TSH) levels if, during the course of therapy, a patient develops symptoms consistent with possible thyroid dysfunction. In the presence of thyroid dysfunction, PEGETRON treatment may be initiated or continued only if TSH levels can be maintained in the normal range by medication.

Hypertriglyceridemia: Hypertriglyceridemia and aggravation of hypertriglyceridemia, sometimes severe, have been observed with peginterferon alfa-2b therapy. Monitoring of lipid levels is, therefore, recommended.

Gastrointestinal: Colitis: As seen with other alpha interferons, ulcerative and ischemic colitis, sometimes serious, have been observed within 12 weeks of starting peginterferon alfa-2b therapy. PEGETRON should be discontinued immediately if symptoms of colitis develop (typical manifestations include abdominal pain, bloody diarrhea and fever). The colitis usually resolves within 1 to 3 weeks of discontinuation of alpha interferon.

Hematologic: Anemia: Hemolytic anemia (hemoglobin levels to <10 g/dL) was observed in up to 28% of patients treated with ribavirin in combination with peginterferon alfa-2b in clinical trials. Anemia occurred within 1-4 weeks of initiation of PEGETRON (ribavirin) Capsules therapy. Because of this initial acute drop in hemoglobin, it is advised that complete blood counts (CBC) should be obtained pretreatment and at Week 2 and Week 4 of therapy or more frequently if clinically indicated. Patients should then be followed as clinically appropriate.

Although ribavirin has no direct cardiovascular effects, anemia associated with ribavirin may result in deterioration of cardiac function and/or exacerbation of the symptoms of coronary disease. Patients should be assessed before initiation of therapy and should be appropriately monitored during therapy. If there is any deterioration of cardiovascular status, therapy should be suspended or discontinued (see Dosage and Administration). Because cardiac disease may be worsened by drug-induced anemia, patients with a history of significant or unstable cardiac disease should not be treated with PEGETRON.

PEGETRON therapy should not be used in patients with hemoglobinopathies (e.g., thalassemia, sickle-cell anemia).

Hepatic/Biliary/Pancreatic: Hepatic Function: Any patient developing liver function abnormalities or hepatopathy during treatment should be monitored closely. As with treatment with any interferon, discontinue treatment with PEGETRON in patients who develop prolongation of coagulation markers or other markers of hepatic function, which might indicate liver decompensation (see Dosage and Administration). The safety and efficacy of peginterferon alfa-2b have not been evaluated in patients with severe hepatic dysfunction. Therefore, PEGETRON must not be used for these patients. PEGETRON therapy should be discontinued for any patient developing signs and symptoms of liver failure. Patients should be tested for the presence of hepatitis C virus (HCV) antibodies. Other causes of chronic hepatitis including autoimmune hepatitis should be excluded.

There is limited data available for the use of PEGETRON in patients with mild and moderate hepatic dysfunction. In a single dose, parallel group, Phase I study in a limited number of patients (n=5 to 7 subjects per group) with various degrees of hepatic dysfunction (mild, moderate and severe) C_{max} increased with increasing severity of liver dysfunction ($P < 0.05$). While there were no statistically significant differences detected with AUC_t, the limited size of the study population does not permit any generalizations to be made.

Pancreatitis: Pancreatitis, sometimes life-threatening, has occurred in patients treated with alpha interferons, including peginterferon alfa-2b. PEGETRON therapy should be suspended if symptoms or signs of pancreatitis are observed. PEGETRON should be discontinued in patients diagnosed with pancreatitis.

Immune: Acute Hypersensitivity: Acute hypersensitivity reactions, (e.g., angioedema, bronchoconstriction and anaphylaxis), have been observed rarely during alpha interferon therapy. If such a reaction develops during treatment with PEGETRON, discontinue treatment and institute appropriate medical therapy immediately. As with other alpha interferons, urticaria has been observed rarely during peginterferon alfa-2b therapy. Transient rashes do not necessitate interruption of treatment.

Bone Marrow Toxicity: Alpha interferons, including peginterferon alfa-2b, may suppress bone marrow function which may result in severe cytopenias. As with other alpha interferons, peginterferon alfa-2b may be very rarely associated with aplastic anemia. PEGETRON dosing should be reduced or discontinued in patients developing decreases in neutrophil or platelet counts (see Dosage and Administration, Dose Modification).

Immunological Effects: A number of immune-mediated dermatological reactions associated with the use of alpha interferons have been reported ranging from erythema multiforme to more severe but very rare occurrences of Stevens-Johnson syndrome and toxic epidermal necrolysis.

Autoimmune Disease: As with other alpha interferons, the development of autoantibodies has been reported during treatment with peginterferon alfa-2b. Clinical manifestations of autoimmune disease during interferon therapy may occur more frequently in patients predisposed to the development of autoimmune disorders.

Fever: While fever may be associated with the "flu-like" syndrome reported commonly during interferon therapy, other causes of persistent fever must be ruled out.

Neurologic: More significant obtundation and coma, including cases of encephalopathy, have been observed in some patients, usually elderly, treated at higher doses. While these effects are generally reversible upon discontinuation of therapy, in a few patients full resolution took up to three weeks. Very rarely, seizures have occurred with high doses of peginterferon alfa-2b.

Effects on Ability to Drive and Use Machines: Patients who develop fatigue, somnolence or confusion during treatment with PEGETRON therapy are cautioned to avoid driving or operating machinery.

Ophthalmologic: Ocular Changes: As with other alpha interferons, ophthalmologic disorders, including retinopathies (including macular edema), retinal hemorrhages, retinal artery or vein obstruction, serous retinal detachment, cotton wool spots, loss of visual acuity or visual field, optic neuritis, and papilledema have been reported in rare instances after treatment with peginterferon alfa-2b (see Adverse Reactions). These events have been reported after treatment for several months, but also have been reported after shorter treatment periods. All patients should have a baseline eye examination. Any patient complaining of ocular symptoms, including loss of visual acuity or visual field must have a prompt and complete eye examination. Because these ocular events may occur in conjunction with other disease states, periodic ocular examinations during PEGETRON therapy are recommended in patients with disorders that may be associated with retinopathy, such as diabetes mellitus or hypertension. Discontinuation of PEGETRON therapy should be considered in patients who develop new or worsening ophthalmological disorders.

Renal: Renal Function: It is recommended that renal function be evaluated in all patients prior to initiation of PEGETRON therapy and that patients be monitored closely during treatment (see Dosage and Administration). Increases in serum creatinine levels have been observed in patients with renal insufficiency treated with interferons, including PEGETRON. Patients with impairment of renal function should be closely monitored for signs and symptoms of toxicity, including increases in serum creatinine, and, should have their weekly dose of peginterferon alfa-2b reduced if medically appropriate (see Dosage and Administration). Patients with impaired renal function and/or those over the age of 50 should be more carefully monitored with respect to the development of anemia. Patients with severe renal dysfunction (creatinine clearance <50 mL/min) must not be treated with PEGETRON, as the clearance of peginterferon alfa-2b is reduced in patients with significant renal impairment (see Action and Clinical Pharmacology and Contraindications). If serum creatinine rises to >2 mg/dL, PEGETRON must be discontinued.

The pharmacokinetics of ribavirin were assessed, in a limited number of subjects (n=6 per group), after administration of a single oral dose (400 mg) of ribavirin to subjects with varying degrees of renal function. Both C_{max} and AUC_f of ribavirin appeared to increase with increasing severity of renal dysfunction. Due to the limited size of the study groups, no dosing recommendations can be made and, therefore, the use of PEGETRON in the presence of moderate to severe renal dysfunction cannot be recommended.

Respiratory: Pulmonary Changes: As with other alpha interferons, pulmonary infiltrates, pneumonitis, pulmonary hypertension, and pneumonia, occasionally resulting in fatality, have been observed rarely in peginterferon alfa-2b treated patients. Any patient developing fever, cough, dyspnea or other respiratory symptoms must have a chest X-ray taken. If the chest X-ray shows pulmonary infiltrates or there is evidence of pulmonary function impairment, the patient is to be monitored closely. If appropriate, discontinue PEGETRON therapy. Prompt discontinuation of therapy and treatment with corticosteroids appear to be associated with resolution of pulmonary adverse events (AEs). These symptoms have been reported more frequently when Shosaikoto (also known as Xiao-Chai-Hu-Tang), a Chinese herbal medication, has been administered concomitantly with alpha interferons. PEGETRON should not be administered to patients with chronic obstructive pulmonary disease (COPD).

Sexual Function/Reproduction: Effects on Fertility: No reproductive toxicology studies have been performed using peginterferon alfa-2b in combination with ribavirin. However, evidence provided below for interferon and ribavirin when administered alone indicate that both agents have adverse effects on reproduction. It should be assumed that the effects produced by either agent alone will also be caused by the combination of the two agents.

Interferons, including peginterferon alfa-2b, may impair fertility. In studies of interferon administration in non-human primates, menstrual cycle abnormalities have been observed. Decreases in serum estradiol and progesterone concentrations have been reported in women treated with human leukocyte interferon. The effects of interferon on male fertility have not been studied. Therefore, a possible effect on male fertility should be considered. The genotoxicity of peginterferon alfa-2b was evaluated in bacterial (Ames) and mammalian cell clastogenicity (HPBL) assays, and was negative in both assays.

PEGETRON therapy should be used with caution in fertile men. In studies in mice to evaluate the time course and reversibility of ribavirin-induced testicular degeneration at doses of 15 to 150 mg/kg/day (estimated human equivalent of 1.25-12.5 mg/kg/day, based on body surface area adjustment for a 60 kg adult; 0.2-0.8 times the maximum human 24-hour dose of ribavirin) administered for 3 or 6 months, abnormalities in sperm occurred. Upon cessation of treatment, essentially total recovery from ribavirin-induced testicular toxicity was apparent within one or two spermatogenesis cycles.

Skin: Psoriatic Disease and Sarcoidosis: Use of alpha interferons, including peginterferon alfa-2b, has been associated with exacerbating pre-existing psoriatic disease and sarcoidosis. Use of PEGETRON in patients with psoriasis or sarcoidosis is recommended only if the potential benefit justifies the potential risk.

Special Populations: Pregnant Women: (See Contraindications.) PEGETRON **must not** be used during pregnancy. Interferon alfa-2b has been shown to have abortifacient effects in Macaca mulatta (rhesus monkeys) at 15 and 30 million IU/kg (estimated human equivalent of 5 and 10 million IU/kg, based on body surface area adjustment for a 60 kg adult). This same effect is expected with peginterferon alfa-2b. High doses of other forms of interferon alpha and beta are known to produce dose-related anovulatory and abortifacient effects in rhesus monkeys.

Significant teratogenic and/or embryocidal potential have been demonstrated for ribavirin in all animal species in which adequate studies have been conducted, occurring at doses as low as one twentieth of the recommended human dose. Malformations of the skull, palate, eye, jaw, limbs, skeleton and gastrointestinal tract were noted. The incidence and severity of teratogenic effects increased with escalation of the ribavirin dose. Survival of fetuses and offspring was reduced. In conventional embryotoxicity/teratogenicity studies in rats and rabbits, observed no effect dose levels were well below those for proposed clinical use (0.3 mg/kg/day for both the rat and rabbit; approximately 0.06 times the recommended human 24-hour dose of ribavirin). No maternal toxicity or effects on offspring were observed in a peri/postnatal toxicity study in rats dosed orally at up to 1 mg/kg/day (estimated human equivalent dose of 0.17 mg/kg based on body surface area adjustment for a 60 kg adult; approximately 0.01 times the maximum recommended human 24-hour dose of ribavirin).

Treatment and Post-Treatment: Potential Risk to the Fetus: Because of the potential human teratogenic effects of PEGETRON (ribavirin) Capsules, male patients must be advised to take every precaution to avoid risk of pregnancy for their female partners during treatment with PEGETRON and for six months after treatment has been concluded (i.e., 15 half-lives for ribavirin clearance from the body). Ribavirin accumulates intracellularly and is cleared from the body very slowly. In animal studies, ribavirin produced changes in sperm at doses below the clinical dose. It is unknown whether the ribavirin that is contained in sperm will exert its known teratogenic effects upon fertilization of the ova. In a study in rats, it was concluded that dominant lethality was not induced by ribavirin at doses up to 200 mg/kg for 5 days (estimated human equivalent doses of 7.14-28.6 mg/kg, based on body surface area adjustment for a 60 kg adult; up to 1.7 times the maximum recommended human dose of ribavirin).

Women of childbearing potential and their male partners must not receive PEGETRON therapy unless the patient and his/her partner are using effective contraceptive (two reliable forms, one for each partner) during the therapy period. In addition, effective contraception should be utilized for six months post-therapy based on a multiple dose half-life ($t_{1/2}$) of ribavirin of 12 days.

Male patients and their female partners must practice effective contraception (two reliable forms, one for each partner) during treatment with PEGETRON and for the 6-month post-therapy period (e.g., 15 half-lives for ribavirin clearance from the body).

If pregnancy occurs in a patient or partner of a patient during treatment or during the six months after treatment cessation, the patient must be advised of the significant teratogenic risk of PEGETRON (ribavirin) Capsules to the fetus and physicians should report such cases by calling Schering-Plough Canada Inc., Medical Information Department at 1-800-463-5442.

Nursing Women: It is not known whether interferon alfa-2b, peginterferon alfa-2b and/or ribavirin are excreted in human milk. Because of the potential for serious adverse reactions from PEGETRON in nursing infants, nursing must be discontinued prior to the start of PEGETRON therapy.

Pediatrics (<18 years of age): Safety and effectiveness of PEGETRON in these patients have not been evaluated (see Indications and Clinical Use). PEGETRON is not recommended for use in children and adolescents under the age of 18 years.

HCV/HIV/HBV Co-Infection: The safety and efficacy of PEGETRON treatment have not been established for hepatitis C patients co-infected with human immunodeficiency virus (HIV) or hepatitis B virus (HBV).

Transplantation: The safety and efficacy of PEGETRON treatment have not been established for patients with liver or other organ transplants. Preliminary data indicates that interferon alpha therapy may be associated with an increased rate of kidney graft rejection. Liver graft rejection has also been reported but a causal association with interferon alpha therapy has not been established.

Monitoring and Laboratory Tests: Standard hematologic tests, blood chemistry and a test of thyroid function must be conducted in all patients prior to initiating therapy. Acceptable baseline values that may be considered as a guideline prior to initiation of PEGETRON therapy are:

- Hemoglobin: ≥12 g/dL (females), ≥13 g/dL (males)
- Platelets: $\geq 100 \times 10^9$/L
- Neutrophil Count: $\geq 1.5 \times 10^9$/L
- TSH Levels: must be within normal limits

Laboratory evaluations are to be conducted at weeks 2 and 4 of therapy, and periodically thereafter as clinically appropriate.

Uric acid may increase due to hemolysis with PEGETRON (ribavirin) Capsules use; therefore, the potential for development of gout must be carefully monitored in predisposed patients.

ADVERSE REACTIONS: Adverse Drug Reaction Overview: Potentially serious adverse reactions have been reported with PEGETRON in controlled clinical trials (see Adverse Reactions, General Safety Information).

The most frequently reported adverse reactions (≥25%) with PEGETRON were fatigue, fever, headache, rigors, myalgia, insomnia, injection site inflammation, injection site reaction, "flu-like" symptoms, weight decreased, anorexia, nausea, arthralgia, myalgia, depression, irritability, dyspnea, alopecia, pruritus, anemia, and neutropenia. The most frequently reported adverse reactions were mostly mild to moderate in severity and were manageable without the need for modification of doses or discontinuation of therapy.

Clinical Trial Adverse Drug Reactions: Because clinical trials are conducted under very specific conditions the adverse reaction rates observed in the clinical trials may not reflect the rates observed in practice and should not be compared to the rates in the clinical trials of another drug. Adverse drug reaction information from clinical trials is useful for identifying drug-related adverse events and for approximating rates.

The safety of PEGETRON was evaluated in two controlled clinical trials of over 3500 HCV-infected naïve adult patients treated with ribavirin plus peginterferon alfa-2b for up to 48 weeks. Additionally, the safety of PEGETRON was evaluated in one controlled clinical trial of over 2200 HCV-infected adults who had failed previous treatment combination alpha interferon/ribavirin and who were subsequently treated with peginterferon alfa-2b for up to 48 weeks.

Study 1: ribavirin plus peginterferon alfa-2b vs ribavirin plus interferon alfa-2b in naïve patients: A PEGETRON randomized study compared treatment with two peginterferon alfa-2b/ribavirin regimens [peginterferon alfa-2b 1.5 µg/kg subcutaneously once weekly/ribavirin Capsules 800 mg p.o. daily (in divided doses); peginterferon alfa-2b 1.5 µg/kg subcutaneously once weekly for 4 weeks then 0.5 µg/kg subcutaneously once weekly for 44 weeks/ribavirin 1000/1200 mg p.o. daily (in divided doses)] with INTRON A (interferon alfa-2b) [3 MIU subcutaneously thrice weekly/ribavirin 1000/1200 mg p.o. daily (in divided doses)] in 1530 adults. Interferon-naïve patients were treated for 48 weeks and followed for 24 weeks post-treatment.

The most common adverse events that occurred with ≥10% incidence are provided in Table 1 by treatment group.

Table 1: PEGETRON

Adverse Events Reported in Study 1 (10% of patients in any treatment group)

	% of Patients			
	PEGETRON			Interferon alfa-2b+Ribavirin
	PEG2b 1.5/R			
	800 mg N=511	>10.6 mg/kg N=188	PEG2b 0.5/R N=514	I/R N=505
Application Site Disorder				
Injection Site Inflammation	25	20	27	18
Injection Site Reaction	58	54	59	36
Autonomic Nervous System				
Mouth Dry	12	11	8	8
Sweating Increased	11	7	9	7
Body as a Whole				
Asthenia	18	28	16	18
Fatigue	64	56	62	60
Fever	46	41	44	33
Headache	62	59	58	58
Flu-like Symptoms	24	21	27	23
Rigors	48	43	45	41
RUQ[a] Pain	12	10	7	6
Weight Decrease	29	30	17	20
Central Nervous System				
Dizziness	21	18	19	17
Gastrointestinal System				
Abdominal Pain	13	15	12	13
Anorexia	32	35	29	27
Diarrhea	22	22	16	17
Nausea	43	43	36	33
Vomiting	14	16	14	12
Musculoskeletal				
Arthralgia	34	32	34	28
Musculoskeletal Pain	21	19	17	19
Myalgia	56	51	48	50
Psychiatric				
Anxiety	15	16	15	15
Concentration Impaired	17	19	16	21
Depression	31	34	29	34
Emotional Lability	11	11	11	10
Insomnia	40	38	40	41
Irritability	35	32	34	34
Resistance Mechanism				
Infection Viral	12	15	10	12
Respiratory System				
Coughing	17	19	15	13
Dyspnea	26	27	23	24
Pharyngitis	12	16	11	13
Rhinitis	8	10	8	6
Skin and Appendages				
Alopecia	36	45	29	32
Pruritus	29	28	26	28
Rash	24	23	22	23

(cont'd)

Table 1: PEGETRON *(cont'd)*

Adverse Events Reported in Study 1 (10% of patients in any treatment group)

	% of Patients			
	PEGETRON			Interferon alfa-2b+Ribavirin
	PEG2b 1.5/R			
	800 mg N=511	>10.6 mg/kg N=188	PEG2b 0.5/R N=514	I/R N=505
Skin Dry	24	26	18	23

[a] Right Upper Quadrant.
Legend: PEG2b=peginterferon alfa-2b; R=ribavirin; I=interferon alfa-2b.

Adverse events reported between 5 and 10% in the treatment group receiving the recommended dose of PEGETRON were chest pain, right upper quadrant (RUQ) pain, paresthesia, hypothyroidism, constipation, dyspepsia, tachycardia, agitation, nervousness, menorrhagia, menstrual disorder, nonproductive cough, rhinitis, taste perversion, and blurred vision.

Adverse events reported between 2 and 5% in the treatment group receiving the recommended dose of PEGETRON were injection site pain, flushing, hypotension, lacrimal gland disorder, erythema, malaise, hypertension, syncope, confusion, hyperesthesia, hypoesthesia, hypertonia, decreased libido, tremor, vertigo, hyperthyroidism, flatulence, gingival bleeding, glossitis, loose stools, stomatitis, ulcerative stomatitis, hearing impairment/loss, tinnitus, palpitation, thirst, thrombocytopenia, aggressive behavior, somnolence, herpes simplex, fungal infection, amenorrhea, prostatitis, otitis media, bronchitis, nasal congestion, respiratory disorder, rhinorrhea, sinusitis, eczema, abnormal hair texture, photosensitivity reaction, erythematous rash, maculopapular rash, migraine, conjunctivitis, neutropenia, thyroid disorders, eye pain, apathy, and lymphadenopathy.

Study 2 (IDEAL): ribavirin plus peginterferon alfa-2b vs ribavirin plus peginterferon in naïve patients: This PEGETRON study with 3070 adults compared two peginterferon alfa-2b (1.5 µg/kg/week and 1 µg/kg/week) doses in combination with ribavirin (800-1400 mg/day) and included a third treatment group in which patients received peginterferon alfa-2a (180 µg/week)/ribavirin (1000-1200 mg/day).

Table 2: PEGETRON

Adverse Reactions Reported in Study 2 Occurring in ≥1% of Patients in either PEG2b Arm

	Number (%) of Patients		
SOC/Adverse Reactions	PEG2b 1.5/R n=1019	PEG2b 1.0/R n=1016	PEG2a/R n=1035
Blood and Lymphatic System Disorders	499 (49)	413 (41)	540 (52)
Anemia	343 (34)	293 (29)	348 (34)
Neutropenia	263 (26)	188 (19)	325 (31)
Leukopenia	95 (9)	69 (7)	106 (10)
Thrombocytopenia	28 (3)	23 (2)	66 (6)
Hemolytic anemia	16 (2)	8 (<1)	3 (<1)
Cardiac Disorders	23 (2)	34 (3)	29 (3)
Palpitations	9 (<1)	23 (2)	16 (2)
Ear and Labyrinth Disorders	46 (5)	46 (5)	43 (4)
Tinnitus	19 (2)	13 (1)	9 (<1)
Endocrine Disorders	61 (6)	55 (5)	61 (6)
Hypothyroidism	54 (5)	38 (4)	46 (4)
Hyperthyroidism	13 (1)	22 (2)	21 (2)
Eye Disorders	133 (13)	113 (11)	146 (14)
Vision blurred	38 (4)	54 (5)	64 (6)
Dry eye	30 (3)	17 (2)	35 (3)
Eye pain	11 (1)	5 (<1)	13 (1)
Photophobia	14 (1)	7 (<1)	5 (<1)
Retinal exudates	12 (1)	4 (<1)	8 (<1)
Visual disturbance	11 (1)	9 (<1)	12 (1)
Gastrointestinal Disorders	630 (62)	583 (57)	577 (56)
Nausea	412 (40)	357 (35)	351 (34)
Diarrhea	154 (15)	162 (16)	147 (14)
Vomiting	121 (12	100 (10)	87 (8)
Constipation	51 (5)	59 (6)	51 (5)
Dry mouth	53 (5)	50 (5)	45 (4)
Abdominal pain	38 (4)	31 (3)	37 (4)
Dyspepsia	45 (4)	42 (4)	55 (5)
Abdominal pain upper	32 (3)	32 (3)	36 (3)
Stomatitis	28 (3)	33 (3)	25 (2)

(cont'd)

Table 2: PEGETRON *(cont'd)*

Adverse Reactions Reported in Study 2 Occurring in ≥1% of Patients in either PEG2b Arm

	Number (%) of Patients		
SOC/Adverse Reactions	PEG2b 1.5/R n=1019	PEG2b 1.0/R n=1016	PEG2a/R n=1035
Gastroesophageal reflux disease	23 (2)	25 (2)	33 (3)
Mouth ulceration	17 (2)	21 (2)	21 (2)
Abdominal distension	13 (1)	11 (1)	15 (1)
Aphthous stomatitis	12 (1)	10 (1)	12 (1)
Abdominal discomfort	6 (<1)	10 (1)	3 (<1)
Cheilitis	14 (1)	6 (<1)	5 (<1)
Glossodynia	14 (1)	14 (1)	11 (1)
Stomach discomfort	15 (1)	14 (1)	12 (1)
Flatulence	8 (<1)	10 (1)	5 (<1)
Gingival bleeding	10 (1)	6 (<1)	3 (<1)
General Disorders and Administration Site Conditions	917 (90)	933 (92)	892 (86)
Fatigue	663 (65)	665 (65)	649 (63)
Chills	397 (39)	362 (36)	241 (23)
Pyrexia	352 (35)	323 (32)	219 (21)
Irritability	251 (25)	259 (25)	262 (25)
Influenza like illness	164 (16)	152 (15)	157 (15)
Injection site erythema	166 (16)	178 (18)	123 (12)
Pain	120 (12)	133 (13)	90 (9)
Injection site reaction	101 (10)	112 (11)	57 (6)
Asthenia	50 (5)	43 (4)	41 (4)
Chest pain	39 (4)	31 (3)	27 (3)
Injection site rash	41 (4)	38 (4)	20 (2)
Injection site pruritus	29 (3)	19 (2)	13 (1)
Chest discomfort	16 (2)	22 (2)	12 (1)
Feeling abnormal	19 (2)	10 (1)	12 (1)
Malaise	21 (2)	18 (2)	20 (2)
Injection site irritation	12 (1)	10 (1)	7 (<1)
Injection site pain	12 (1)	13 (1)	8 (<1)
Edema peripheral	5 (<1)	11 (1)	11 (1)
Temperature intolerance	6 (<1)	10 (1)	3 (<1)
Infections and Infestations	162 (16)	152 (15)	197 (19)
Sinusitis	30 (3)	11 (1)	27 (3)
Influenza	20 (2)	19 (2)	14 (1)
Bronchitis	14 (1)	11 (1)	21 (2)
Cellulitis	7 (<1)	10 (1)	9 (<1)
Oral herpes	14 (1)	20 (2)	19 (2)
Upper respiratory tract infection	7 (<1)	19 (2)	19 (2)
Investigations	225 (22)	183 (18)	189 (18)
Weight decreased	135 (13)	100 (10)	100 (10)
Hemoglobin decreased	21 (2)	19 (2)	21 (2)
Blood amylase increased	7 (<1)	12 (1)	5 (<1)
Blood thyroid stimulating hormone increased	12 (1)	13 (1)	11 (1)
Neutrophil count decreased	13 (1)	7 (<1)	13 (1)
Platelet count decreased	12 (1)	9 (<1)	15 (1)
Metabolism and Nutrition Disorders	340 (33)	284 (28)	252 (24)
Decreased appetite	182 (18)	156 (15)	141 (14)

(cont'd)

Table 2: PEGETRON *(cont'd)*

Adverse Reactions Reported in Study 2 Occurring in ≥1% of Patients in either PEG2b Arm

SOC/Adverse Reactions	Number (%) of Patients		
	PEG2b 1.5/R n=1019	PEG2b 1.0/R n=1016	PEG2a/R n=1035
Anorexia	121 (12)	95 (9)	75 (7)
Hyperuricemia	14 (1)	17 (2)	17 (2)
Dehydration	11 (1)	6 (<1)	7 (<1)
Musculoskeletal Pain	473 (46)	505 (50)	467 (45)
Myalgia	271 (27)	264 (26)	226 (22)
Arthralgia	218 (21)	219 (22)	228 (22)
Back pain	59 (6)	65 (6)	72 (7)
Muscle spasms	46 (5)	39 (4)	54 (5)
Pain in extremity	35 (3)	40 (4)	39 (4)
Neck pain	9 (<1)	10 (1)	10 (1)
Musculoskeletal pain	8 (<1)	10 (1)	15 (1)
Nervous System Disorders	664 (65)	626 (62)	601 (58)
Headache	501 (49)	474 (47)	426 (41)
Dizziness	155 (15)	139 (14)	136 (13)
Dysgeusia	79 (8)	69 (7)	66 (6)
Disturbance in attention	71 (7)	51 (5)	71 (7)
Hypoesthesia	28 (3)	25 (2)	26 (3)
Memory impairment	27 (3)	37 (4)	33 (3)
Amnesia	16 (2)	29 (3)	18 (2)
Hyperesthesia	17 (2)	10 (1)	3 (<1)
Migraine	17 (2)	15 (1)	13 (1)
Paresthesia	25 (2)	24 (2)	17 (2)
Sinus headache	17 (2)	6 (<1)	5 (<1)
Tremor	20 (2)	10 (1)	21 (2)
Poor quality of sleep	9 (<1)	14 (1)	12 (1)
Syncope	14 (1)	12 (1)	12 (1)
Somnolence	8 (<1)	11 (1)	7 (<1)
Lethargy	5 (<1)	10 (1)	5 (<1)
Psychiatric Disorders	588 (58)	561 (55)	587 (57)
Insomnia	384 (38)	377 (37)	417 (40)
Depression	254 (25)	192 (19)	209 (20)
Anxiety	107 (11)	111 (11)	105 (10)
Affect lability	31 (3)	23 (2)	21 (2)
Agitation	17 (2)	15 (1)	16 (2)
Anger	25 (2)	20 (2)	10 (1)
Crying	16 (2)	12 (1)	4 (<1)
Libido decreased	24 (2)	11 (1)	13 (1)
Mood swings	18 (2)	19 (2)	16 (2)
Restlessness	14 (1)	16 (2)	6 (<1)
Confusional state	10 (1)	8 (<1)	5 (<1)
Mood altered	9 (<1)	12 (1)	11 (1)
Nervousness	6 (<1)	10 (1)	8 (<1)
Renal and Urinary Disorders	34 (3)	32 (3)	24 (2)
Pollakiuria	14 (1)	15 (1)	10 (1)
Reproductive System and Breast Disorders	38 (4)	38 (4)	50 (5)
Erectile Dysfunction	13 (1)	15 (1)	18 (2)

(cont'd)

Table 2: PEGETRON *(cont'd)*

Adverse Reactions Reported in Study 2 Occurring in ≥1% of Patients in either PEG2b Arm

SOC/Adverse Reactions	Number (%) of Patients		
	PEG2b 1.5/R n=1019	PEG2b 1.0/R n=1016	PEG2a/R n=1035
Respiratory, Thoracic and Mediastinal Disorders	383 (38)	391 (38)	411 (40)
Dyspnea	170 (17)	160 (16)	165 (16)
Cough	139 (14)	155 (15)	172 (17)
Dyspnea exertional	55 (5)	54 (5)	72 (7)
Pharyngolaryngeal pain	32 (3)	39 (4)	37 (4)
Respiratory tract congestion	26 (3)	18 (2)	17 (2)
Epistaxis	21 (2)	24 (2)	29 (3)
Nasal congestion	18 (2)	20 (2)	28 (3)
Productive cough	23 (2)	7 (<1)	8 (<1)
Sinus congestion	23 (2)	24 (2)	30 (3)
Increased upper airway secretion	13 (1)	6 (<1)	5 (<1)
Nasal dryness	10 (1)	8 (<1)	8 (<1)
Postnasal drip	11 (1)	12 (1)	5 (<1)
Rhinorrhea	7 (<1)	10 (1)	9 (<1)
Skin and Subcutaneous Tissue Disorders	592 (58)	547 (54)	617 (60)
Alopecia	232 (23)	205 (20)	176 (17)
Rash	212 (21)	205 (20)	274 (26)
Pruritus	156 (15)	133 (13)	173 (17)
Dry skin	117 (11)	110 (11)	128 (12)
Rash generalized	42 (4)	25 (2)	36 (3)
Rash pruritic	38 (4)	27 (3)	38 (4)
Hyperhidrosis	30 (3)	31 (3)	33 (3)
Dermatitis	23 (2)	16 (2)	20 (2)
Erythema	16 (2)	17 (2)	9 (<1)
Pruritus generalized	25 (2)	20 (2)	24 (2)
Eczema	14 (1)	10 (1)	4 (<1)
Night sweats	13 (1)	21 (2)	16 (2)
Psoriasis	9 (<1)	11 (1)	13 (1)
Rash erythematous	12 (1)	5 (<1)	13 (1)
Rash papular	12 (1)	6 (<1)	16 (2)
Skin exfoliation	3 (<1)	10 (1)	7 (<1)
Vascular Disorders	45 (4)	47 (5)	47 (5)
Hot flush	19 (2)	12 (1)	17 (2)
Hypertension	12 (1)	18 (2)	18 (2)

Legend: SOC=System Organ Class; PEG2b=peginterferon alfa-2b; R=ribavirin; PEG2a=peginterferon alfa-2a.

Study 3 (EPIC): retreatment of prior treatment failures (relapser and non-responder patients): In a single-arm trial, adult patients with moderate to severe fibrosis who failed previous treatment with combination of alpha interferon (pegylated or non-pegylated) and ribavirin, including non-responders and relapsers, were subsequently retreated with peginterferon alfa-2b, 1.5 µg/kg subcutaneously, once weekly, in combination with body weight-adjusted ribavirin (800-1400 mg/day, p.o.). Prior non-responders (n=1401) were defined as patients who were HCV-RNA positive at the end of a minimum 12 weeks of treatment and prior relapsers (n=647) were defined as patients who were HCV-RNA negative at the end of a minimum 12 weeks of treatment and subsequently relapsed after post-treatment follow-up.

A total of 2312 patients were eligible for safety analysis, while 2293 patients were included in efficacy analysis. 943 patients (41%) completed dosing of combination therapy and were treated for 48 weeks. 1061 patients (46%) were identified as virologic treatment failures after 12 weeks of treatment, were discontinued from the study by Treatment Week 18 and were eligible for other studies; 308 patients (13%) were discontinued from the study due to other reasons.

There was a trend of increasing incidence with increasing dose of ribavirin for diarrhea, dry mouth, injection site erythema, anxiety, and exertional dyspnea. The following AEs were more common (≥5% difference) with the 1400 mg ribavirin dose than with the lower doses: thrombocytopenia, decrease hemoglobin, decreased neutrophil count, nausea, vomiting, chills, fatigue, irritability, pain, headache, and dyspnea. There is a tendency of increased Serious Adverse Events and discontinuation of treatment due to AEs with increasing ribavirin dose. Dose modification due to AEs occurred more often in 1400 mg/day group.

Less Common Clinical Trial Adverse Drug Reactions (<1%) (IDEAL and EPIC): Some Adverse Drug Reactions (ADRs) were only reported in a single trial. Some ADRs with an incidence of ≥1% for the EPIC trial but were <1% in the IDEAL trial are also reported in Table 3.

Table 3: PEGETRON

Adverse Reactions Reported in Study 3 Occurring in ≥1% of Patients

SOC/Adverse Reactions	Number (%) of Patients[a] PEG2b 1.5/R n=2312
Blood and Lymphatic System Disorders	**738 (32)**
Neutropenia	459 (20)
Anemia	368 (16)
Leukopenia	239 (10)
Thrombocytopenia	127 (7)
Lymphopenia	25 (1)
Ear and Labyrinth Disorders	**90 (4)**
Vertigo	46 (2)
Endocrine Disorders	**54 (2)**
Hypothyroidism	46 (2)
Eye Disorders	**172 (7)**
Dry eye	44 (2)
Vision blurred	40 (2)
Gastrointestinal Disorders	**1097 (47)**
Nausea	560 (24)
Diarrhea	281 (12)
Vomiting	178 (8)
Dry mouth	132 (6)
Abdominal pain upper	114 (5)
Dyspepsia	95 (4)
Constipation	58 (3)
Stomatitis	33 (1)
Aphthous stomatitis	28 (1)
Gastroesophageal reflux disease	27 (1)
Gastritis	24 (1)
Mouth ulceration	24 (1)
General Disorders and Administration Site Conditions	**1972 (85)**
Pyrexia	887 (38)
Fatigue	747 (32)
Chills	505 (22)
Asthenia	492 (21)
Influenza like illness	491 (21)
Irritability	394 (17)
Injection site erythema	236 (10)
Injection site reaction	120 (5)
Malaise	92 (4)
Pain	85 (4)
Chest pain	44 (2)
Injection site pruritus	29 (1)
Injection site irritation	28 (1)
Injection site rash	25 (1)
Hepatobiliary Disorders	**63 (3)**
Hyperbilirubinemia	42 (2)
Infections and Infestations	**311 (13)**
Oral herpes	50 (2)
Influenza	39 (2)

(cont'd)

Table 3: PEGETRON *(cont'd)*

Adverse Reactions Reported in Study 3 Occurring in ≥1% of Patients

SOC/Adverse Reactions	Number (%) of Patients[a] PEG2b 1.5/R n=2312
Nasopharyngitis	25 (1)
Investigations	**366 (16)**
Weight decreased	151 (7)
Hemoglobin decreased	82 (4)
Neutrophil count decreased	59 (3)
Platelet count decreased	45 (2)
White blood cell count decreased	42 (2)
Blood bilirubin increased	27 (1)
Blood uric acid increased	23 (1)
Metabolism and Nutrition Disorders	**561 (24)**
Anorexia	284 (12)
Decreased appetite	195 (8)
Hyperuricemia	37 (2)
Musculoskeletal and Connective Tissue Disorders	**1071 (46)**
Myalgia	705 (30)
Arthralgia	371 (16)
Back pain	109 (5)
Pain in extremity	62 (3)
Muscle spasms	53 (2)
Musculoskeletal pain	36 (2)
Bone pain	28 (1)
Nervous System Disorders	**1167 (50)**
Headache	907 (39)
Dizziness	223 (10)
Disturbance in attention	109 (5)
Lethargy	73 (3)
Dysgeusia	68 (3)
Memory impairment	38 (2)
Paresthesia	35 (2)
Tremor	31 (1)
Hypoesthesia	24 (1)
Psychiatric Disorders	**924 (40)**
Insomnia	487 (21)
Depression	272 (12)
Anxiety	182 (8)
Sleep disorder	56 (2)
Depressed mood	34 (1)
Affect lability	33 (1)
Libido decreased	33 (1)
Mood altered	33 (1)
Mood swings	33 (1)
Aggression	29 (1)
Nervousness	23 (1)
Respiratory, Thoracic and Mediastinal Disorders	**699 (30)**
Cough	325 (14)
Dyspnea	238 (10)

(cont'd)

Table 3: PEGETRON *(cont'd)*

Adverse Reactions Reported in Study 3 Occurring in ≥1% of Patients

	Number (%) of Patients[a]
SOC/Adverse Reactions	**PEG2b 1.5/R n=2312**
Dyspnea exertional	81 (4)
Epistaxis	57 (2)
Pharyngolaryngeal pain	57 (2)
Nasal congestion	31 (1)
Skin and Subcutaneous Tissue Disorders	**1012 (44)**
Alopecia	388 (17)
Pruritus	338 (15)
Rash	213 (9)
Dry skin	192 (8)
Erythema	73 (3)
Hyperhidrosis	56 (2)
Eczema	36 (2)
Vascular Disorders	**73 (3)**
Hypertension	29 (1)

[a] Includes all METAVIR scores (F1-F4) and missing METAVIR scores.
Legend: SOC=System Organ Class; PEG2b=peginterferon alfa-2b; R=ribavirin.

Blood and Lymphatic System Disorders: lymphadenopathy, pancytopenia.
Cardiac Disorders: tachycardia, cardiomyopathy, myocardial infarction, pericarditis.
Ear and Labyrinth Disorders: ear pain, vertigo.
Eye Disorders: abnormal sensation in eye, eye irritation, retinopathy, visual acuity reduced.
Gastrointestinal Disorders: gingival pain, hemorrhoids, oral pain, rectal hemorrhage, toothache, abdominal pain lower, glossitis, oral disorder, rectal hemorrhage, retching, tongue ulceration colitis ischemic, gingivitis, pancreatitis.
General Disorders and Administration Site Conditions: feeling hot, injection site bruising, injection site dryness, thirst, feeling jittery, injection site hemorrhage, face edema, injection site inflammation, injection site necrosis, non-cardiac chest pain, edema.
Hepatobiliary Disorders: hepatic pain, hyperbilirubinemia.
Immune System Disorders: drug hypersensitivity, sarcoidosis.
Infections and Infestations: candidiasis, nasopharyngitis, oral candidiasis, urinary tract infection, onychomycosis, ear infection, sinusitis, infection bacterial including sepsis, fungal infection, furuncle, herpes simplex, injection site infection, lower respiratory tract infection, otitis media, respiratory tract infection, rhinitis, upper respiratory tract infection.
Injury, Poisoning and Procedural Complications: contusion, overdose.
Investigations: blood pressure increased, blood thyroid stimulating hormone decreased, blood triglycerides increased, blood uric acid increased, heart rate increased, blood glucose increased, hematocrit decreased, blood alkaline phosphatase increased, white blood cell count decreased.
Metabolism and Nutrition Disorders: hyperglycemia, hypertriglyceridemia, diabetes mellitus, increased appetite, diabetic ketoacidosis, hypercalcemia.
Musculoskeletal and Connective Tissue Disorders: flank pain, joint stiffness, muscle tightness, muscle weakness, bone pain, arthritis, rheumatoid arthritis.
Nervous System Disorders: parosmia, restless leg syndrome, hypogeusia, neuralgia, neuropathy, neuropathy peripheral.
Psychiatric Disorders: apathy, depressed mood, suicidal ideation, tearfulness, stress, abnormal behavior, abnormal dreams, psychosis, aggression, bipolar disorder, hallucination, homicidal ideation, panic attack, sleep disorder, suicide attempt.
Renal and Urinary Disorders: dysuria, micturition frequency decreased, micturition urgency, polyuria renal failure, urine abnormality.
Reproductive System and Breast Disorders: menorrhagia, amenorrhea, menstrual disorder, menstruation irregular, breast pain, prostatitis, sexual dysfunction.
Respiratory, Thoracic and Mediastinal Disorders: dysphonia, paranasal sinus hypersecretion, wheezing, dry throat, nasal ulcer.
Skin and Subcutaneous Tissue Disorders: increased tendency to bruise, skin discoloration, skin lesions, rash macular, rash maculo-papular, hair texture abnormal, photosensitivity reaction, skin ulcer, urticaria, pain of skin, cutaneous sarcoidosis, erythema multiforme, nail disorder.
Vascular Disorders: pallor, flushing, hypotension, vasculitis, deep vein thrombosis.
General Safety Information: In clinical trials, approximately 1.2% of patients treated with PEGETRON reported life-threatening psychiatric events during treatment. These events included suicide, attempted suicide, suicidal ideation, psychosis including hallucinations, bipolar disorders and aggressive behavior, sometimes directed towards others (see Warnings and Precautions).

As with other alpha interferons, ophthalmological disorders including retinopathies (including macular edema), retinal hemorrhages, retinal artery or vein obstruction, cotton wool spots, loss of visual acuity or visual field, optic neuritis, and papilledema have been rarely reported during therapy with peginterferon alfa-2b (see Warnings and Precautions).

Adverse reactions of the cardiovascular system (CVS), particularly arrhythmia, appeared to be correlated mostly with pre-existing CVS disease and prior cardiotoxic therapy. Cardiomyopathy was also observed in patients treated with peginterferon alfa and has been reported more frequently in patients with known risk factors for cardiovascular diseases. There are limited data to assess the reversibility of cardiomyopathy reported with the use of peginterferon alfa; however cases of reversible cardiomyopathy have been reported with the use of interferon alfa.

As with other alpha interferons, seizures, pancreatitis, hypertriglyceridemia, arrhythmia, diabetes, peripheral neuropathy, colitis (including ischemic and ulcerative), aplastic anemia, hypertension, cardiac ischemia, myocardial infarction, cerebrovascular ischemia, cerebrovascular hemorrhage, encephalopathy (see Warnings and Precautions), sarcoidosis or exacerbation of sarcoidosis, erythema multiforme, Stevens-Johnson syndrome, toxic epidermal necrolysis, injection site necrosis, rhabdomyolysis, myositis, renal failure and renal insufficiency have been rarely or very rarely reported during therapy with peginterferon alfa-2b.

Very rarely, alpha interferons, including peginterferon alfa-2b used alone or in combination with ribavirin, may be associated with pure red cell aplasia (PRCA).

Alpha interferons have been associated with altered lipid metabolism (including hypercholesterolemia and hyperlipemia) and pulmonary hypertension.

Adequate hydration must be maintained in patients undergoing peginterferon alfa-2b therapy since hypotension related to fluid depletion has been seen in some patients treated with alpha interferons. Fluid replacement may be necessary.

Abnormal Hematologic and Clinical Chemistry Findings from Studies 1 and 2: Hemoglobin levels dropped below 10 g/dL in up to 14% of patients treated with PEGETRON. Most cases of anemia, neutropenia and thrombocytopenia were mild (WHO grades 1 or 2). Some cases of more severe neutropenia in patients treated with the recommended doses of PEGETRON were reported (WHO grade 3 [21%] and grade 4 [7%]).

In addition, patients receiving peginterferon alfa-2b (1.5 µg/kg)/ribavirin, in the IDEAL study (study 2), had decreases in hemoglobin levels to between 8.5 to <10 g/dL (28%) and to <8.5 g/dL (3%). WHO grades 3 and 4 leukopenia was also reported in 7% and 0.3% of this treatment group.

An increase in uric acid and indirect bilirubin values associated with hemolysis was observed in some patients treated with PEGETRON, but values returned to baseline levels by four weeks after the end of therapy. Among those patients with elevated uric acid levels, very few patients treated with PEGETRON developed clinical gout, none of which required treatment modification or discontinuation from the clinical trials.

Post-Market Adverse Drug Reactions: Very rarely, post-marketing reports of pancreatitis, seizures, ulcerative and ischemic colitis, rhabdomyolysis, myositis, stomatitis, vertigo, renal insufficiency, renal failure, injection site necrosis, erythema multiforme, Stevens-Johnson syndrome, toxic epidermal necrolysis, cerebrovascular ischemia, cerebrovascular hemorrhage, hearing impairment, hearing loss, cardiac ischemia, and myocardial infarction have been received.

A wide variety of autoimmune and immune-mediated disorders have been reported with alpha interferons including idiopathic thrombocytopenic purpura, thrombotic thrombocytopenic purpura, rheumatoid arthritis, systemic lupus erythematosus, vasculitis and Vogt-Koyanagi-Harada syndrome.

Very rare cases of PRCA were reported in patients receiving both anti-hepatitis C therapy and erythropoietin (EPO) stimulating agents. The potential for an increased risk of PRCA and development of anti-EPO antibodies should therefore be kept in mind when considering EPO stimulating agents use for hepatitis C treatment induced-anemia.

Cases of acute hypersensitivity reactions, including anaphylaxis, urticaria and angioedema have been reported.

Other adverse events reported with peginterferon alfa-2b alone or in combination with ribavirin include: abdominal pain, anxiety, asthenic conditions (including asthenia, malaise and fatigue), bacterial infection (including sepsis), chest pain, cough, dehydration, dyspnea, dry skin, emotional lability, facial palsy, fungal infection, hypertension, hyperthyroidism, hypotension, hypothyroidism, irritability, migraine headache, palpitations, paresthesia, peripheral neuropathy, pruritus, rash, and serous retinal detachment.

DRUG INTERACTIONS: Overview: Results of in vitro studies using both human and rat liver microsome preparations indicated no cytochrome P450 enzyme-mediated metabolism of ribavirin. Ribavirin does not inhibit cytochrome P450 enzymes. There is no evidence from toxicity studies that ribavirin induces liver enzymes. Therefore there is minimal potential for P450 enzyme-based interactions.

Results of a single dose study with peginterferon alfa-2b demonstrated no effect on the activity of cytochrome P450 isoenzymes CYP1A2, CYP2C8/9, CYP2D6, and CYP3A4 or hepatic N-acetyl transferase. The literature, however, reports up to a 50% reduction in clearance of CYP1A2 substrates (e.g., theophylline) when administered with other forms of interferon alpha and therefore caution should be exercised when PEGETRON (peginterferon alfa-2b) Powder for Solution is used with medications metabolized by CYP1A2.

A multi-dose probe study assessing P450 substrates was performed in 26 subjects with chronic hepatitis C, who received a once-weekly peginterferon alfa-2b (1.5 µg/kg) for 4 weeks. There was no inhibition of CYP1A2, 3A4 or N-acetyltransferase. There was a 27% increase in activity of CYP2C8/9 and a 69% increase in CYP2D6. Caution should be used when administering peginterferon alfa-2b with medications metabolized by CYP2C8/9 and CYP2D6.

No pharmacokinetic interactions were noted between PEGETRON (peginterferon alfa-2b) Powder for Solution and PEGETRON (ribavirin) Capsules in a multiple-dose pharmacokinetic study.

Drug-Drug Interactions: Ribavirin was shown in vitro to inhibit phosphorylation of the nucleoside analog reverse transcriptase inhibitors (NRTIs) zidovudine and stavudine. The clinical significance of these findings is unknown. However, these in vitro findings raise the possibility that concurrent use of PEGETRON (ribavirin) Capsules with either zidovudine or stavudine might lead to increased HIV plasma viremia. Therefore, it is recommended that plasma HIV-RNA levels be closely monitored in patients treated with PEGETRON (ribavirin) Capsules concurrently with either of these two agents. If HIV-RNA levels increase, the use of PEGETRON (ribavirin) Capsules concomitantly with NRTIs must be reviewed.

Use of nucleoside analogs, alone or in combination with other nucleosides, has resulted in lactic acidosis. Pharmacologically, ribavirin increases phosphorylated metabolites of purine nucleosides in vitro. This activity could potentiate the risk of lactic acidosis induced by purine nucleoside analogues (e.g., didanosine or abacavir). Co-administration of ribavirin and didanosine is not recommended. Reports of mitochondrial toxicity in particular lactic acidosis and pancreatitis, of which some fatal, have been reported.

An increased risk of developing peripheral neuropathy cannot be ruled out for treatments combining telbivudine with any alfa (standard or pegylated types) and beta interferon products. This risk might occur when the drug is used with interferon products other than pegylated interferon alfa-2a. Development of peripheral neuropathy was reported in a small clinical trial in Hepatitis B investigating the use of both 600 mg daily of telbivudine and 180 µg once weekly by subcutaneous administration of pegylated interferon alfa-2a. The safety and efficacy of telbivudine in combination with interferon alfa-2b has not been established in patients with Hepatitis B; therefore, telbivudine in combination with alpha interferons is not recommended.

There are limited data regarding the efficacy and safety of combining PEGETRON with Highly Active Anti-Retroviral Therapy (HAART) for HIV-HCV co-infected patients. Patients coinfected with HIV and who are receiving HAART may be at increased risk of developing lactic acidosis. Caution should be used when treating HIV-HCV co-infected subjects with PEGETRON in combination with HAART.

Any potential for interactions may persist for up to two months (5 half-lives for PEGETRON (ribavirin) Capsules) after cessation of PEGETRON therapy due to the long half-life of PEGETRON (ribavirin) Capsules.

There is no evidence that ribavirin interacts with non-nucleoside reverse transcriptase inhibitors (NNRTIs) protease inhibitors.

Antacid: The bioavailability of ribavirin (600 mg) was decreased by co-administration with an antacid containing magnesium aluminum and simethicone; AUC_{tf} decreased 14%. This interaction is not considered to be clinically relevant.

Drug-Food Interactions: Interactions with food have not been established.

Drug-Herb Interactions: As with other alpha interferons, pulmonary infiltrates, pneumonitis, and pneumonia, occasionally resulting in fatality, have been observed rarely in peginterferon alfa-2b treated patients. These symptoms have been reported more frequently when Shosaikoto (also known as Xiao-Chai-Hu-Tang), a Chinese herbal medication, has been administered concomitantly with alpha interferons.

Drug-Laboratory Test Interactions: Interactions with laboratory tests have not been established.

DOSAGE AND ADMINISTRATION: Recommended Dose and Dosage Adjustment: PEGETRON (peginterferon alfa-2b) Powder for Solution is administered subcutaneously using either the plastic disposable syringes or the REDIPEN Single Dose Delivery System with the disposable needles supplied. PEGETRON (ribavirin) Capsules are for oral administration only.

PEGETRON treatment should be initiated only by a physician experienced in the treatment of patients with hepatitis C.

Recommended Dose: Based on the results of the clinical trial, the recommended dose of PEGETRON (peginterferon alfa-2b) Powder for Solution is 1.5 µg/kg/week subcutaneously in combination with PEGETRON (ribavirin) Capsules. PEGETRON (peginterferon alfa-2b) Powder for Solution should be administered once a week. The dose of PEGETRON (ribavirin) Capsules to be used in combination with PEGETRON (peginterferon alfa-2b) Powder for Solution is based on patient body weight. PEGETRON (ribavirin) Capsules are taken daily. PEGETRON (ribavirin) Capsules are to be administered orally each day in two divided doses with food (morning and evening).

Recommended Dose for Treatment Naïve Patients Infected with HCV Genotype 1: PEGETRON (peginterferon alfa-2b) Powder for Solution: 1.5 µg/kg/week.
PEGETRON (ribavirin) Capsules: 800-1400 mg daily based upon patient weight.

Table 4: PEGETRON

PEGETRON Dosing Recommendations for Treatment Naïve Patients Infected with HCV Genotype 1[a]

	PEG2b Powder for Solution		ribavirin Capsules	
Patient Weight (kg)	**Weekly Dose (µg/kg)**	**Vial or REDIPEN Size (µg/0.5 mL)[b]**	**Daily Dose (mg)**	**Number of Capsules (200 mg)**
<40	1.5	50	800	2×200 mg capsules A.M. 2×200 mg capsules P.M.
40 to 50	1.5	80	800	2×200 mg capsules A.M. 2×200 mg capsules P.M.
51 to 65	1.5	100	800	2×200 mg capsules A.M. 2×200 mg capsules P.M.

(cont'd)

Table 4: PEGETRON *(cont'd)*

PEGETRON Dosing Recommendations for Treatment Naïve Patients Infected with HCV Genotype 1[a]

Patient Weight (kg)	PEG2b Powder for Solution: Weekly Dose (µg/kg)	PEG2b Powder for Solution: Vial or REDIPEN Size (µg/0.5 mL)[b]	ribavirin Capsules: Daily Dose (mg)	ribavirin Capsules: Number of Capsules (200 mg)
66 to 80	1.5	120	1000	2×200 mg capsules A.M. 3×200 mg capsules P.M.
81 to 105	1.5	150	1200	3×200 mg capsules A.M. 3×200 mg capsules P.M.
>105	1.5	[c]	1400	3×200 mg capsules A.M. 4×200 mg capsules P.M.

[a] The daily dose for PEGETRON (ribavirin) Capsules approximately falls within 13±2 mg/kg/day.
[b] When reconstituted as instructed.
[c] Should be calculated based on the body weight of an individual patient.
Legend: PEG2b = peginterferon alfa-2b.

Recommended Dose for Treatment Naïve Patients Infected with HCV non-Genotypes 1: PEGETRON (peginterferon alfa-2b) Powder for Solution: 1.5 µg/kg/week.
PEGETRON (ribavirin) Capsules: 800-1200 mg daily based upon patient weight

Table 5: PEGETRON

Dosing Recommendations for Treatment Naïve Patients Infected with HCV non-Genotypes 1[a]

Patient Weight (kg)	PEG2b Powder for Solution: Weekly Dose (µg/kg)	PEG2b Powder for Solution: Vial or REDIPEN Size (µg/0.5 mL)[b]	ribavirin Capsules: Daily Dose (mg)	ribavirin Capsules: Number of Capsules (200 mg)
<40	1.5	50	800	2×200 mg capsules A.M. 2×200 mg capsules P.M.
40 to 50	1.5	80	800	2×200 mg capsules A.M. 2×200 mg capsules P.M.
51 to 65	1.5	100	800	2×200 mg capsules A.M. 2×200 mg capsules P.M.
66 to 85	1.5	120	1000	2×200 mg capsules A.M. 3×200 mg capsules P.M.
>85	1.5	150	1200	3×200 mg capsules A.M. 3×200 mg capsules P.M.

[a] The daily dose for PEGETRON (ribavirin) Capsules approximately falls within 13±2 mg/kg/day.
[b] When reconstituted as instructed.
Legend: PEG2b = peginterferon alfa-2b.

Recommended Dose for Retreatment of Prior Treatment Failures (Relapser and Non-responder Patients) Infected with Any HCV Genotypes: PEGETRON (peginterferon alfa-2b) Powder for Solution: 1.5 µg/kg/week.
PEGETRON (ribavirin) Capsules: 800-1400 mg daily based upon patient weight.

Table 6: PEGETRON

Dosing Recommendations for Retreatment of Prior Treatment Failures (Relapser and Non-responder Patients) Infected with Any HCV Genotypes[a]

Patient Weight (kg)	PEG2b Powder for Solution: Weekly Dose (µg/kg)	PEG2b Powder for Solution: Vial or REDIPEN Size (µg/0.5 mL)[b]	ribavirin Capsules: Daily Dose (mg)	ribavirin Capsules: Number of Capsules (200 mg)
<40	1.5	50	800	2×200 mg capsules A.M. 2×200 mg capsules P.M.
40 to 50	1.5	80	800	2×200 mg capsules A.M. 2×200 mg capsules P.M.
51 to 65	1.5	100	800	2×200 mg capsules A.M. 2×200 mg capsules P.M.
66 to 85	1.5	120	1000	2×200 mg capsules A.M. 3×200 mg capsules P.M.
86 to 105	1.5	150	1200	3×200 mg capsules A.M. 3×200 mg capsules P.M.
>105	1.5	[c]	1400	3×200 mg capsules A.M. 4×200 mg capsules P.M.

[a] The daily dose for PEGETRON (ribavirin) Capsules approximately falls within 13 ± 2 mg/kg/day.
[b] When reconstituted as instructed.
[c] Should be calculated based on the body weight of an individual patient.
Legend: PEG2b = peginterferon alfa-2b.

Duration of Treatment: Naïve Patients: The recommended duration of treatment is 48 weeks. Duration should be individualized in accordance with the baseline characteristics of the disease, response to therapy, and tolerance of the regimen. Virological response by week 12 has been shown to be predictive for sustained response. After 12 weeks of treatment with no virologic response (HCV-RNA positive and <2 $\log_{10}$ decrease from baseline) for an adult genotype 1 patient, discontinuation of treatment should be considered. After 24 weeks of treatment, virologic response (HCV-RNA below lower limit of detection) should be assessed. If a virologic response has not occurred by 24 weeks of treatment, PEGETRON should be discontinued, as a virologic response is unlikely to occur after this time.

Therapeutic Milestones: Futility Rule at Week 12: If chronic hepatitis C genotype 1 adult patient fails to demonstrate an early virologic response (EVR), defined as either detectable HCV-RNA with at least a 2 $\log_{10}$ reduction from baseline in viral titer or undetectable HCV-RNA, at the end of 12 weeks of therapy, with peginterferon alfa-2b in combination with ribavirin, consideration should be given to treatment withdrawal.
Futility Rule at Week 24: Those chronic hepatitis C genotype 1 adult patients who had detectable HCV-RNA with at least a 2 log10 reduction in viral titer from baseline after 12 weeks of treatment, who fail to achieve undetectable HCV-RNA after 24 weeks of therapy, warrant withdrawal of treatment.
Retreatment of Prior Treatment Failures (Relapser and Non-responder Patients): All patients, irrespective of genotype, who have demonstrated serum HCV-RNA below the limits of detection at Week 12, should receive 48 weeks of therapy. Retreated patients who fail to achieve undetectable HCV-RNA at Week 12 of therapy are highly unlikely to become sustained virological responders after 48 weeks of therapy and discontinuation of therapy should be considered.
Dose Modification: In general, the dosage may be adjusted according to the patient's tolerance to the medication. If severe adverse reactions or laboratory abnormalities develop during the course of treatment, the dosage should be modified or therapy should be temporarily discontinued until the adverse reactions abate. If persistent or recurrent intolerance develops despite adequate dosage adjustment, or if the disease progresses rapidly, treatment with PEGETRON should be discontinued.
Dose Modification for Naïve Patients Infected with HCV Genotype 1: It is recommended that a patient whose hemoglobin level falls below 10 g/dL have his/her PEGETRON (ribavirin) Capsules dose reduced (see Table 7). A patient whose hemoglobin level falls below 8.5 g/dL should be permanently discontinued from PEGETRON therapy.

Table 7: PEGETRON

PEGETRON (ribavirin) Capsules Dose Reduction for Naïve Patients Infected with HCV Genotype 1

Starting Dose (mg)	Dose after 1st dose reduction (mg)	Dose after 2nd dose reduction, if required (mg)
800	600	400
1000	800	600
1200	1000	800
1400	1000	800

For patients with a history of stable cardiovascular disease, a PEGETRON (ribavirin) Capsule dose reduction is required if the hemoglobin decreases by ≥2 g/dL during any 4 week period. In addition, for these cardiac history patients, if the hemoglobin remains <12 g/dL after 4 weeks on a reduced dose, the patient should discontinue PEGETRON therapy.

It is recommended that a patient whose neutrophil count falls below 0.75×10^9/L, have his/her PEGETRON (peginterferon alfa-2b) Powder for Solution dose reduced (see Table 8). A patient whose neutrophil count falls below 0.5×10^9/L should be permanently discontinued from PEGETRON therapy.

Table 8: PEGETRON

PEGETRON (peginterferon alfa-2b) Powder for Solution Dose Reduction for Naïve Patients Infected with HCV Genotype 1

Starting dose (µg/kg/week)	Dose after 1st dose reduction (µg/kg/week)	Dose after 2nd dose reduction, if required (µg/kg/week)
1.5	1	0.5

The following guidelines for dose modification were developed in clinical trials based on laboratory values:

Table 9: PEGETRON

Dose Modification for Naïve Patients Infected with HCV Genotype 1

	Reduce only (ribavirin) dose, if[a]:	Reduce only PEG2b, if[b]:	Discontinue combination therapy if:
Hemoglobin	<10 g/dL	—	<8.5 g/dL
Hemoglobin in patients with history of stable cardiac disease	≥2 g/dL decrease in hemoglobin during any 4-week period during treatment (permanent dose reduction)		<12 g/dL after 4 weeks of dose reduction
White blood cell count	—	$<1.5 \times 10^9$/L	$<1.0 \times 10^9$/L
Neutrophil count	—	$<0.75 \times 10^9$/L	$<0.5 \times 10^9$/L
Platelet count	—	$<50 \times 10^9$/L	$<25 \times 10^9$/L
Bilirubin-direct	—		2.5×upper limit of normal
Bilirubin-indirect	>5 mg/dL		>4 mg/dL (for >4 weeks)
Creatinine	—	—	>2.0 mg/dL
ALT/AST	—	—	2×baseline and >10×upper limit of normal

[a] **Ribavirin dose reduction:** 1st dose reduction of ribavirin for adult patients is by 200 mg/day except in patients receiving the 1400 mg; it is by 400 mg/day. If needed, 2nd dose reduction of ribavirin is by an additional 200 mg/day.
[b] **Peginterferon alfa-2b dose reduction:** dose reduction of peginterferon alfa-2b should be implemented in increments of 0.5 µg/kg/week.
Legend: PEG2b = peginterferon alfa-2b.

Dose Modification for Naïve Patients Infected with HCV non-Genotypes 1: For patients with a history of stable cardiovascular disease, a PEGETRON (ribavirin) Capsules dose reduction to 600 mg/day (1x200 mg capsule in AM and 2x200 mg capsules in PM) is required if the hemoglobin decreases by >2 g/dL during any 4 week period. In addition, for these cardiac history patients, if the hemoglobin remains <12 g/dL after 4 weeks on a reduced dose, the patient should discontinue PEGETRON therapy.

It is recommended that a patient whose hemoglobin level falls below 10 g/dL have his/her PEGETRON (ribavirin) Capsules dose reduced to 600 mg daily. A patient whose hemoglobin level falls below 8.5 g/dL should be permanently discontinued from PEGETRON therapy.

It is recommended that a patient whose neutrophil count falls below 0.75×10^9/L, have his/her PEGETRON (peginterferon alfa-2b) Powder for Solution dose reduced to 0.75 µg/kg/week. A patient whose neutrophil count falls below 0.5×10^9/L should be permanently discontinued from PEGETRON therapy.

The following guidelines for dose modification were used in clinical trials: See Table 10.

Dose Modification for Retreatment of Prior Treatment Failures (Relapser and Non-responder Patients) Infected with Any HCV Genotypes: It is recommended that a patient whose hemoglobin level falls below 10 g/dL have his/her PEGETRON (ribavirin) Capsules dose reduced (see Table 11). A patient whose hemoglobin level falls below 8.5 g/dL should be permanently discontinued from PEGETRON therapy.

Table 10: PEGETRON

Dose Modification for Naïve Patients Infected with HCV non-Genotypes 1

	Reduce only PEGETRON (ribavirin) Capsules dose to 600 mg/day[a], if:	Reduce only PEG2b Powder for Solution to one-half dose if:	Permanent Discontinuation of PEGETRON therapy if:
Hemoglobin	<10 g/dL	—	<8.5 g/dL
Hemoglobin in patients with history of stable cardiac disease	≥2 g/dL decrease in hemoglobin during any 4-week period during treatment (permanent dose reduction)		<12 g/dL after 4 weeks of dose reduction
White blood cell count	—	<1.5×10^9/L	<1.0×10^9/L
Neutrophil count	—	<0.75×10^9/L	<0.5×10^9/L
Platelet count	—	<80×10^9/L	<50×10^9/L
Bilirubin-direct	—	—	2.5×upper limit of normal
Bilirubin-indirect	>5 mg/dL	—	>4 mg/dL (for >4 weeks)
Creatinine	—	—	>2.0 mg/dL
ALT/AST	—	—	2×baseline **and** >10×upper limit of normal

[a] Patients whose dose of PEGETRON (ribavirin) Capsules is reduced to 600 mg daily receive one 200 mg capsule in the morning and two 200 mg capsules in the evening.

Legend: PEG2b = peginterferon alfa-2b.

Table 11: PEGETRON

Dose Modification for Retreatment of Prior Treatment Failures (Relapser and Non-responder Patients) Infected with Any HCV Genotypes

Starting Dose (mg)	Dose after 1st dose reduction (mg)	Dose after 2nd dose reduction, if required (mg)
800	600	400
1000	800	600
1200	800	600
1400	1000	800

For patients with a history of stable cardiovascular disease, a PEGETRON (ribavirin) Capsule dose reduction is required if the hemoglobin decreases by ≥2 g/dL during any 4 week period. In addition, for these cardiac history patients, if the hemoglobin remains <12 g/dL after 4 weeks on a reduced dose, the patient should discontinue PEGETRON therapy.

It is recommended that a patient whose neutrophil count falls below 0.75×10^9/L, have his/her PEGETRON (peginterferon alfa-2b) Powder for Solution dose reduced (see Table 12). A patient whose neutrophil count falls below 0.5×10^9/L should be permanently discontinued from PEGETRON therapy.

Table 12: PEGETRON

PEGETRON (peginterferon alfa-2b) Powder for Solution Dose Reduction for Retreatment of Prior Treatment Failures (Relapser and Non-responder Patients) Infected with All HCV Genotypes

Starting dose (µg/kg/week)	Dose after 1st dose reduction (µg/kg/week)	Dose after 2nd dose reduction, if required (µg/kg/week)
1.5	1	0.5

The following guidelines for dose modification were used in clinical trials:

Table 13: PEGETRON

Dose Modification for Retreatment of Prior Treatment Failures (Relapser and Non-responder Patients) Infected with Any HCV Genotypes

	Reduce only (ribavirin) dose, if[a]:	Reduce only PEG2b if[b]:	Discontinue combination therapy if:
Hemoglobin	<10 g/dL	—	<8.5 g/dL
Hemoglobin in patients with history of stable cardiac disease	≥2 g/dL decrease in hemoglobin during any 4-week period during treatment (permanent dose reduction)		<12 g/dL after 4 weeks of dose reduction
White blood cell count	—	<1.5×10^9/L	<1.0×10^9/L
Neutrophil count	—	<0.75×10^9/L	<0.5×10^9/L
Platelet count	—	<50×10^9/L	<25×10^9/L
Bilirubin-direct	—	—	2.5×upper limit of normal
Bilirubin-indirect	>5 mg/dL	—	>4 mg/dL (for >4 weeks)
Creatinine	—	—	>2.0 mg/dL
ALT/AST	—	—	2×baseline AND >10×upper limit of normal

[a] **Ribavirin dose reduction:** 1st dose reduction of ribavirin for adult patients is by 200 or 400 mg/day depending on starting dose (see Table 11).

[b] **Peginterferon alfa-2b dose reduction:** dose reduction of peginterferon alfa-2b should be implemented in increments of 0.5 µg/kg/week.

Legend: PEG2b = peginterferon alfa-2b.

Concomitant Therapy: Acetaminophen has been used successfully to alleviate the symptoms of fever and headache, which can occur with peginterferon alfa-2b therapy. The recommended acetaminophen dosage is 500 mg to 1 g given 30 minutes before administration of PEGETRON (peginterferon alfa-2b) Powder for Solution. The maximum dosage of acetaminophen to be given is 1 g four times daily. In order to properly assess the source of fever, adjunctive acetaminophen should be limited to a maximum of 5 consecutive days unless otherwise specified by the prescribing physician.

Reconstitution: To Reconstitute the PEGETRON (peginterferon alfa-2b) Powder for Solution in Vials: Each vial of PEGETRON (peginterferon alfa-2b) Powder for Solution must be reconstituted with 0.7 mL of the accompanying Sterile Water for Injection to give a final volume of 0.74 mL for administration of up to 0.5 mL of solution. The reconstituted solutions will have concentrations of 100 and 300 µg/mL respectively.

To reconstitute use a sterilized syringe and injection needle, inject 0.7 mL of diluent **slowly**, into the vial of PEGETRON (peginterferon alfa-2b) Powder for Solution aiming the stream of liquid at the glass wall of the vial. It is best not to aim the stream directly at the white solid or powder, or to inject the liquid quickly, as this causes a greater amount of bubbles. The solution may appear cloudy or bubbly for a few minutes. Swirl the vial gently to complete dissolution of the powder. **Do not shake**, but gently turn the vial upside down. The contents should now be completely dissolved. Once the solution has settled and all bubbles have risen to the top of the solution, you should have a clear solution with a small ring of tiny bubbles around the top. The appropriate dose can now be withdrawn with a sterilized injection syringe and injected.

A small volume is lost during preparation of PEGETRON (peginterferon alfa-2b) solution when the dose is measured and injected. Thus, each unit contains an excess amount of diluent and PEGETRON (peginterferon alfa-2b) Powder for Solution to ensure delivery of the labeled dose in 0.5 mL of PEGETRON (peginterferon alfa-2b) Injection. **The labeled strength will be contained in 0.5 mL of the reconstituted solution.** The reconstituted solution for each of the available strengths will have a concentration of 50 µg/0.5 mL or 150 µg/0.5 mL.

As for all parenteral medicinal products, inspect visually the reconstituted solution prior to administration. Do not use if discoloration is present. Discard any unused solution. PEGETRON (peginterferon alfa-2b) Powder for Solution must not be mixed with other injectable products.

Incompatibilities: PEGETRON (peginterferon alfa-2b) Powder for Solution should only be reconstituted with Sterile Water for Injection and must not be mixed with other medicinal products.

PEGETRON (peginterferon alfa-2b) Powder for Solution vials are single dose vials. Once reconstituted, use immediately (see Storage of PEGETRON (peginterferon alfa-2b) Powder for Solution).

To Reconstitute the PEGETRON (peginterferon alfa-2b) Powder for Solution in REDIPEN Delivery System: Before you inject PEGETRON (peginterferon alfa-2b) Powder for Solution using the REDIPEN Single Dose Delivery System, the two cartridges must be activated, as directed, to mix (reconstitute) the powder with the sterile diluent to form a solution. The powder must be completely dissolved. The appropriate PEGETRON dose should be properly dialed and injected subcutaneously.

As for all parenteral medicinal products, inspect visually the reconstituted solution prior to administration. Do not use if discoloration is present.

PEGETRON should be administered at room temperature.

OVERDOSAGE:

Distinction between the therapeutic dose of peginterferon alfa-2b and overdose has not been clearly defined. Symptoms of overdose may include amplification of the adverse effects, notably "flu-like" symptoms, leukopenia or thrombocytopenia and increased serum liver enzyme levels. The severity of the adverse reactions can be ameliorated by adjusting the dose level and schedule, or in some cases termination of peginterferon alfa-2b therapy. Cardiovascular side effects such as hypotension and arrhythmia may require supportive therapy.

There is limited experience with overdosage. The primary effects of overdose were an increased incidence and severity of adverse events reported at the therapeutic doses of PEGETRON. Serious adverse events reported in cases of PEGETRON overdose include affect lability, anemia, anxiety, ataxia, bursitis, dehydration, depression, fatigue, hallucination, hallucination auditory, hyperesthesia, hypothyroidism, mental disorder, myalgia, nausea, non-accidental overdose, neutropenia, paranoia, pneumonia, pyrexia, suicidal ideation, suicide attempt, thyroid disorder, urinary tract infection, and vomiting. In cases of overdoses, symptomatic treatment and close observation of the patient are recommended (see Dosage and Administration, Dose Modification).

In ribavirin plus interferon alfa-2b clinical trials, the maximum overdose reported was 10 g of ribavirin capsules (50×200 mg capsules) taken with a dose of 39 million units of interferon alfa-2b (13 subcutaneous injections of 3 million IU each). The patient was observed for two days in the emergency room during which time no adverse event from the overdose was noted.

Absorption of ribavirin is generally complete after one hour. Treatment of overdose with ribavirin consists of general supportive measures including monitoring of vital signs and observation of clinical status of the patient. There is no specific antidote for overdose with ribavirin. Although no data currently exists, administration of activated charcoal may be used to aid in the removal of unabsorbed drug. Ribavirin concentration is essentially unchanged by hemodialysis.

> For management of a suspected drug overdose, contact your regional Poison Control Centre. See the *CPS* Directory section for a list of Poison Control Centres.

ACTION AND CLINICAL PHARMACOLOGY: Mechanism of Action: PEGETRON (ribavirin) Capsules: The mechanism by which ribavirin exerts its effects against HCV is unknown. At physiologic concentrations, neither ribavirin nor its intracellular nucleotide metabolites have been shown to inhibit HCV-specific enzymes or HCV replication. Oral formulations of ribavirin monotherapy have been investigated as therapy for chronic hepatitis C in several clinical studies showing that ribavirin monotherapy had no effect on eliminating serum HCV or improving hepatic histology after 6 to 12 months of therapy and 6 months of follow up. However, when used in combination with peginterferon alfa-2b in the treatment of chronic hepatitis C, ribavirin has been shown to increase the efficacy of peginterferon alfa-2b used alone, as measured by reduction of viral load.

PEGETRON (peginterferon alfa-2b) Powder for Solution: For information on the mechanism of action of peginterferon alfa-2b, refer to the product monograph for UNITRON PEG (peginterferon alfa-2b) Powder for Solution.

PEGETRON (ribavirin plus peginterferon alfa-2b): The mechanism of inhibition of HCV RNA by PEGETRON therapy has not been established.

Pharmacokinetics: PEGETRON (ribavirin) Capsules: Ribavirin is rapidly and extensively absorbed following oral administration. However, due to first-pass metabolism, absolute bioavailability is approximately 33%-64%. There is a linear relationship between dose and AUC_{tf} following single doses of 200-1200 mg ribavirin. Volume of distribution is approximately 5000 L. Based upon C_{max} from single dose to 6 weeks, accumulation of ribavirin in plasma is approximately 4.7 fold, although steady state may not have been achieved at 6 weeks. Following oral dosing with 600 mg ribavirin BID, mean plasma concentrations of 2200 (37%) ng/mL were achieved. Upon discontinuation of dosing, the mean half-life was 298 (30%) hours, which probably reflects slow elimination from non-plasma compartments.

Ribavirin has been shown to produce high inter- and intra-subject pharmacokinetic variability following single oral doses (intra-subject variability of approximately 30% for both AUC and C_{max}). This may be due to extensive first pass metabolism and transfer within and beyond the blood compartment.

Ribavirin transport into non-plasma compartments has been most extensively studied in red cells, and has been identified to be primarily via an e_s-type equilibrative nucleoside transporter. This type of transporter is present on virtually all cell types and may account for the high volume of distribution of ribavirin. The ratio of whole blood:plasma ribavirin concentrations is approximately 60:1; the excess of ribavirin in whole blood exists as ribavirin nucleotides sequestered in erythrocytes.

Ribavirin has two pathways of metabolism: (i) a reversible phosphorylation pathway in nucleated cells; and (ii) a degradative pathway involving deribosylation and amide hydrolysis to yield a triazole carboxamide metabolite. Ribavirin and its triazole carboxylic acid metabolites are excreted renally. Following oral administration of 600 mg of ^{14}C-ribavirin, approximately 61% and 12% of the radioactivity was eliminated in the urine and feces, respectively, in 336 hours. Unchanged ribavirin accounted for 17% of the administered dose.

Effect of Food on Absorption of Ribavirin: Both AUC_t (AUC from time zero to last measurable concentration) and C_{max} increased by 70% when ribavirin was administered with a high fat meal (841 kcal, 53.8 g fat, 31.6 g protein, and 57.4 g carbohydrate) in a single-dose pharmacokinetic study. It is possible that the increased bioavailability in this study was due to delayed transit of ribavirin or modified pH. The clinical relevance of results from this single dose study is unknown. In the pivotal clinical efficacy trial, patients were instructed to take ribavirin with food to achieve the maximal plasma concentration of ribavirin.

PEGETRON (peginterferon alfa-2b) Powder for Solution: Peginterferon alfa-2b is a well-characterized polyethylene glycol-modified ("pegylated") derivative of interferon alfa-2b and is predominantly composed of monopegylated species with small amounts of dipegylated and free interferon alfa-2b. The plasma half-life of peginterferon alfa-2b is prolonged compared with non-pegylated interferon alfa-2b. Peginterferon alfa-2b has a potential to depegylate to free interferon alfa-2b. The biologic activity of the pegylated isomers is qualitatively similar to, but lower than that of free interferon alfa-2b.

Following subcutaneous administration, maximal serum concentrations occur between 15-44 hours post-dose, and are sustained for up to 48-72 hours post-dose. Peginterferon alfa-2b C_{max} and AUC measurements increase in a dose-related manner. Mean apparent volume of distribution is 0.99 L/kg.

Upon multiple dosing, there is an accumulation of immunoreactive interferons. There is, however, only a modest increase in biologic activity as measured by a bioassay.

Mean peginterferon alfa-2b elimination half-life is approximately 40 hours, with apparent clearance of 22.0 mL/hr×kg. The mechanisms involved in clearance of interferons in man have not yet been fully elucidated. Based on a retrospective regression analysis of UNITRON PEG CI/F and creatinine clearance, from an expanded database, it is estimated that renal clearance of UNITRON PEG may account for approximately 30% of the apparent clearance.

Pharmacokinetic Analysis of Combined Ribavirin and Peginterferon alfa-2b Administration: A ribavirin population pharmacokinetic analysis was conducted upon serum samples obtained at weeks 12, 24 and 48 during treatment with PEGETRON. Based upon pharmacokinetic modeling, the recommended dose of 800/1000/1200 mg/day based on body weights of <65/65-85/>85 kg (in combination with peginterferon alfa-2b 1.5 µg/kg), showed an overall 6.3% improved sustained response* rate relative to a fixed dose of 800 mg/day. The improved sustained response rate was larger (+7.4%) in the patients with HCV Genotype 1 compared to patients with HCV Genotype non-1 (3.8%).

The toxicity rate, defined as the percentage of patients with hemoglobin below 10.5 mg/dL at week four of treatment was only minimally increased by 2.5% relative to a fixed dose of 800 mg/day. This increase in toxicity was considered mild and clinically manageable.

Peginterferon alfa-2b trough concentrations were obtained at weeks 12, 24 and 48 during treatment with PEGETRON. The observed concentrations and the trend toward accumulation was similar to that observed previously with peginterferon alfa-2b monotherapy for chronic hepatitis C, supporting the lack of pharmacokinetic interaction between peginterferon alfa-2b and ribavirin.

Special Populations and Conditions: Pediatrics: Specific pharmacokinetic evaluations in patients under 18 years of age were not performed. Safety and effectiveness of PEGETRON in these patients have not been evaluated.

PEGETRON is indicated for the treatment of chronic hepatitis C only in patients 18 years of age or older.

Geriatrics (≥65 years of age): In a single dose study using a subcutaneous dose of 1.0 µg/kg, the pharmacokinetics of peginterferon alfa-2b were not affected by age. The study was not powered to detect specified differences between the age groups (20-45 years and 65-80 years). There does not appear to be a significant age-related effect on the pharmacokinetics of ribavirin. However, as in younger patients, renal function must be determined prior to the administration of PEGETRON therapy.

Hepatic Insufficiency:

- PEGETRON (ribavirin) Capsules: Single-dose pharmacokinetics of ribavirin in patients with mild, moderate or severe hepatic dysfunction (Child-Pugh classification A, B or C) showed a similar extent of absorption to that of normal controls.
- PEGETRON (peginterferon alfa-2b) Powder for Solution: The pharmacokinetics of peginterferon alfa-2b have not been evaluated in patients with severe hepatic dysfunction. Therefore, PEGETRON must not be used in these patients.

Renal Insufficiency:

- PEGETRON (ribavirin) Capsules: Single-dose ribavirin pharmacokinetics were altered (increased AUC_{tf} and C_{max}) in patients with renal dysfunction compared with control subjects (creatinine clearance >90 mL/minute). This appears to be due to reduction of apparent clearance in these patients.
- PEGETRON (peginterferon alfa-2b) Powder for Solution: Renal clearance appears to account for 30% of total clearance of peginterferon alfa-2b. In a single dose study (1.0 µg/kg) in patients with impaired renal function, C_{max}, AUC, and half-life increased in relation to the degree of renal impairment (see Contraindications and Warnings and Precautions). Because of marked intra-subject variability in interferon pharmacokinetics, it is recommended that patients be monitored closely during treatment with PEGETRON (see Warnings and Precautions).

Patients with severe renal dysfunction (creatinine clearance <50 mL/min) must not be treated with PEGETRON (see Contraindications).

STORAGE AND STABILITY: Storage of PEGETRON Packages: Store the PEGETRON (ribavirin) Capsules plus PEGETRON (peginterferon alfa-2b) Powder for Solution package refrigerated between 2 and 8°C.

Storage of PEGETRON (ribavirin) Capsules: When separated, PEGETRON (ribavirin) Capsules should be stored in the refrigerator between 2 and 8°C or at room temperature between 15 and 30°C.

Storage of PEGETRON (peginterferon alfa-2b) Powder for Solution: When separated and before reconstitution, the individual carton of PEGETRON (peginterferon alfa-2b) Powder for Solution should be stored in the refrigerator at 2 to 8°C. After reconstitution with Sterile Water for Injection, the reconstituted product is to be used immediately. Since no preservative is present, it is recommended that administration of the solution occur as soon as possible and within 3 hours of reconstitution. For reconstitution under controlled and validated aseptic conditions such as a hospital pharmacy, the chemical and physical in-use stability for the reconstituted solution has been demonstrated for 24 hours at 2-8°C. Discard any unused portion.

Do not use past expiry date on the label.

Storage for PEGETRON REDIPEN Delivery System: When separated and before reconstitution, store the individual carton of PEGETRON REDIPEN at 2 to 8°C. Once reconstituted PEGETRON REDIPEN should be used immediately but may be stored at 2-8°C for up to 24 hours. Do not freeze.

Do not use past expiry date on the label.

INFORMATION FOR THE PATIENT: Published in e-CPS, available by subscription at www.e-cps.ca.

DOSAGE FORMS, COMPOSITION AND PACKAGING: Please refer to Dosage and Administration for recommended dosing.

Capsules: Each opaque, white, hard gelatin capsule filled with a white powder and printed with the Schering-Plough logo and "200 mg" in blue ink, contains: ribavirin 200 mg. Nonmedicinal ingredients: croscarmellose sodium, lactose monohydrate, magnesium stearate and microcrystalline cellulose; capsule shell: gelatin, silicon dioxide, sodium lauryl sulfate and titanium dioxide.

Powder for Solution in Vials: Each single-dose vial of lyophilized powder contains: peginterferon alfa-2b 74 or 222 µg and delivers either 50 or 150 µg in each 0.5 mL of reconstituted solution. Nonmedicinal ingredients: polysorbate 80, sodium phosphate dibasic anhydrous, sodium phosphate monobasic dihydrate and sucrose. Each vial of diluent contains 1 mL of Sterile Water for Injection.

Powder for Solution in REDIPEN Delivery System: Pegetron REDIPEN Single Dose Delivery System consists of a dual-chamber glass cartridge with a sterile active chamber containing PEGETRON as a white to off-white lyophilized powder and a diluent chamber containing Sterile Water for Injection. The cartridge is provided in a pen device for reconstitution, dose preparation and subcutaneous administration, to deliver doses of 80, 100, 120 or 150 µg in 0.5 mL of reconstituted solution. Each REDIPEN contains 108, 135, 162 or 202.5 µg of peginterferon alfa-2b. Following reconstitution of the powder with the diluent contained within the cartridge, each REDIPEN gives a final volume of 0.675 mL for administration of up to 0.5 mL. The reconstituted solution contains 160, 200, 240, 300 µg/mL respectively. Nonmedicinal ingredients: sodium phosphate dibasic anhydrous, sodium phosphate monobasic dihydrate, sucrose and polysorbate 80.

PEGETRON is available in the following package presentations, which provide sufficient ribavirin and peginterferon alfa-2b for two weeks of PEGETRON therapy:

Deliverable Dose 50 µg/0.5 mL:

1. A box containing 2 vials of PEGETRON (peginterferon alfa-2b) Powder for Solution, 50 µg/vial, with 2 vials of diluent containing 1 mL of Sterile Water for Injection, 4 syringes and 4 alcohol swabs; plus two boxes of 28 PEGETRON (ribavirin) Capsules each for a total of 56 PEGETRON (ribavirin) Capsules.

Deliverable Dose 80 µg/0.5 mL:

1. A box containing 2 PEGETRON (peginterferon alfa-2b) REDIPEN Single Dose Delivery Systems, 80 µg/REDIPEN, with two 30-gauge needles (0.3×8 mm), 4 alcohol swabs and two pen holders; plus two boxes of 28 PEGETRON (ribavirin) Capsules each for a total of 56 PEGETRON (ribavirin) Capsules.

Deliverable Dose 100 µg/0.5 mL:

1. A box containing 2 PEGETRON (peginterferon alfa-2b) REDIPEN Single Dose Delivery Systems, 100 µg/REDIPEN, with two 30-gauge needles (0.3x8 mm), 4 alcohol swabs and two pen holders; plus two boxes of 28 PEGETRON (ribavirin) Capsules each for a total of 56 PEGETRON (ribavirin) Capsules.

Deliverable Dose 120 µg/0.5 mL:

1. A box containing 2 PEGETRON (peginterferon alfa-2b) REDIPEN Single Dose Delivery Systems, 120 µg/REDIPEN, with two 30-gauge needles (0.3x8 mm), 4 alcohol swabs and two pen holders; plus two boxes of 35 PEGETRON (ribavirin) Capsules each for a total of 70 PEGETRON (ribavirin) Capsules.

Deliverable Dose 150 µg/0.5 mL:

1. A box containing 2 vials of PEGETRON (peginterferon alfa-2b) Powder for Solution, 150 µg/vial, with 2 vials of diluent containing 1 mL of Sterile Water for Injection, 4 syringes and 4 alcohol swabs; plus two boxes of 42 PEGETRON (ribavirin) Capsules each for a total of 84 PEGETRON (ribavirin) Capsules.
2. A box containing 2 PEGETRON (peginterferon alfa-2b) REDIPEN Single Dose Delivery Systems, 150 µg/REDIPEN, with two 30-gauge needles (0.3x8 mm), 4 alcohol swabs and two pen holders; plus two boxes of 42 PEGETRON (ribavirin) Capsules each for a total of 84 PEGETRON (ribavirin) Capsules.
3. A box containing 2 vials of PEGETRON (peginterferon alfa-2b) Powder for Solution, 150 µg/vial, with 2 vials of diluent containing 1 mL of Sterile Water for Injection, 4 syringes and 4 alcohol swabs; plus two boxes of 49 PEGETRON (ribavirin) Capsules each for a total of 98 PEGETRON (ribavirin) Capsules.
4. A box containing 2 PEGETRON (peginterferon alfa-2b) REDIPEN Single Dose Delivery Systems, 150 µg/REDIPEN, with two 30-gauge needles (0.3x8 mm), 4 alcohol swabs and two pen holders; plus two boxes of 49 PEGETRON (ribavirin) Capsules each for a total of 98 PEGETRON (ribavirin) Capsules.

(Shown in Product Identification Section)

* Sustained response was assessed by the response rate 24 weeks after the cessation of treatment.

PegLyte™

polyethylene glycol—electrolytes

Gastrointestinal Lavage

PendoPharm

SUPPLIED: 4 L Bottles: Each disposable 4 L jug contains: 238.18 g polyethylene glycol 3350, sodium chloride 5.85 g, potassium chloride 3.05 g, sodium bicarbonate 6.76 g and sodium sulfate 22.96 g. Peglyte also contains sodium saccharin, pineapple artificial flavour and tutti-frutti artificial flavour.

4 × 1 L Sachets: Each 1 L sachet contains: 59.55 g polyethylene glycol 3350, sodium sulfate 5.74 g, sodium bicarbonate 1.69 g, sodium chloride 1.46 g and potassium chloride 0.76 g. Peglyte also contains sodium saccharin, pineapple artificial flavour and tutti-frutti artificial flavour.

After reconstitution of water-soluble components each PegLyte preparation delivers the following, in g/L: polyethylene glycol 3350 59.5, sodium chloride 1.46, potassium chloride 0.76, sodium bicarbonate 1.69, sodium sulfate (anhydrous) 5.74. The reconstituted solution is isosmotic.

Reconstituted solution should be used within 48 hours after mixing if stored at room temperature. If kept refrigerated (2-8°C) use within 30 days. Discard unused portion.

Penicillin G 🄿

penicillin G benzathine

penicillin G sodium

Antibiotic

CPhA Monograph

Penicillin V 🄿

penicillin V potassium

Antibiotic

CPhA Monograph

Date of Revision: October 2009

This monograph has been compiled by CPhA and reviewed by experts. It may contain information different from that found in Health Canada-approved Product Monographs. The reader is referred to the *CPS* Editorial Policy for more information.

SUMMARY PRODUCT INFORMATION:

Drug	Route of Administration	Dosage Form	Strength
Penicillin V Potassium	Oral	Suspension	25 mg/mL, 60 mg/mL
		Tablet	300 mg
Penicillin G Sodium	Injectable (IM, IV)	Powder	1, 5, 10 million units/vial
Penicillin G Benzathine	Injectable (IM)	Suspension	600 000 units/mL (available in 2 mL vials)

PHARMACOLOGY: Penicillins G and V, known as the natural penicillins, are bactericidal against susceptible organisms. Penicillins interfere with the synthesis of cell wall mucopeptides, resulting in the formation of defective cell walls that will lyse and eventually result in death of the organism.

The spectra of activity of penicillins G and V are similar. Penicillin G is more active against gram-negative organisms (e.g., Neisseria) and some anaerobes than is penicillin V. Penicillin G can be given parenterally, enabling the attainment of high serum concentrations, and is used for the treatment of serious infections involving penicillin-susceptible bacteria. Penicillin V is more resistant to hydrolysis by acidic gastric secretions and is absorbed orally to a much greater extent than penicillin. Currently, only penicillin V is available orally, for the treatment of penicillin-susceptible infections of mild to moderate severity, in which the oral route of administration is desirable.

The in vitro spectrum of activity of the natural penicillins is as follows: Gram-positive aerobic bacteria: non-β-lactamase-producing staphylococci, streptococci Groups A, B, C, G, H, K, L and M, *S. pneumoniae* (increasingly not susceptible), nonenterococcal group D streptococci, viridans streptococci and some strains of enterococci, *C. diphtheriae*, *L. monocytogenes*, *B. anthracis* and *E. rhusiopathiae*.

Gram-negative aerobic bacteria: non-β-lactamase-producing *N. gonorrhoeae*, *N. meningitidis*, *E. corrodens*, *P. multocida*.

Gram-positive anaerobic bacteria: *A. israelii*, *C. tetani*, *C. perfringens*, *C. botulinum*, Eubacterium, Lactobacillus, Peptococcus, Peptostreptococcus, Propionibacterium.

Gram-negative anaerobic bacteria: Fusobacterium; most Bacteroides species are resistant.

Spirochetes: *T. pallidum*, *B. recurrentis*, *B. burgdorferi*, Leptospira.

Pharmacokinetics: After oral administration, penicillin is absorbed mainly from the duodenum and upper jejunum. The extent of absorption depends on the presence of food in the gastrointestinal tract, gastric and intestinal pH and the relative acid-stability of the penicillin derivative. Both natural penicillins are hydrolyzed in the presence of acidic gastric secretions. Penicillin V is more stable than penicillin G in the presence of gastric acid and although it may be taken with meals, higher serum levels are achieved if it is taken on an empty stomach.

Peak serum levels are reached within 30 to 60 minutes. The oral form of penicillin V benzathine (oral solution) reaches a lower peak level when compared with other forms of oral penicillin but levels are sustained for a longer period of time.

Aqueous penicillin G may be administered im or iv. Following im injection peak levels are attained within 15 to 30 minutes.

Repository preparations of penicillin G benzathine are intended for deep im injection and provide a tissue depot from which absorption takes place over several hours to several days.

The natural penicillins are readily distributed into ascitic, synovial, pleural and pericardial fluids. Distribution into tissues varies widely, with highest amounts in the kidney and lower concentrations in the liver, lungs, skin, intestines and muscle. Small amounts are found in all other body tissues and in the CSF. When the meninges are inflamed, the CSF concentration is about 5% of the serum concentration and can be therapeutic against sensitive organisms. Penicillins readily cross the placenta and are distributed into breast milk.

Penicillin V is more highly protein bound (75 to 89%) than penicillin G (45 to 68%).

In patients with normal kidney function, penicillin is excreted rapidly by filtration and active tubular secretion. The elimination half-life is about 30 minutes. In neonates and young infants and in individuals with impaired kidney function, excretion is considerably delayed, occasionally necessitating longer dosing intervals and smaller doses.

Penicillin G is removed by hemodialysis but only minimally removed by peritoneal dialysis. It is not known whether penicillin V is dialyzable.

INDICATIONS: Penicillin is considered the drug of choice for the following infections: actinomycosis, streptococcal pharyngitis, erysipelas, erysipeloid, leptospirosis, trench mouth, syphilis, bejel, pinta, yaws, clostridial and streptococcal necrotizing infections, *P. multocida* infections, leptospirosis, rat-bite fever and the prophylaxis of rheumatic fever.

Penicillin G is indicated for the treatment of infections due to susceptible organisms of moderate to severe infections. Penicillin V is indicated for treatment of mild to moderately severe infections. Penicillin G benzathine is used for moderately severe infections that respond to low levels of penicillin.

Both penicillin G and penicillin V are indicated for the treatment of: actinomycosis caused by Actinomyces species; anthrax caused by *B. anthracis*; bronchitis, acute otitis media, pharyngitis, sinusitis, skin and soft tissue infections caused by susceptible organisms; erysipelas caused by susceptible strains of group A streptococci; erysipeloid (including endocarditis and septicemia) caused by *E. rhusiopathiae*; acute, necrotizing, ulcerative gingivitis (Vincent's angina or "trench mouth") caused by anaerobes and spirochetes; *P. multocida* infections; rat-bite fever caused by *S. moniliformis* or *S. minor*; scarlet fever caused by group A streptococci; Lyme disease caused by *B. burgdorferi*.

Penicillin V is indicated for the prophylaxis of rheumatic fever caused by group A streptococci. Penicillin V is also used to reduce the incidence of *S. pneumoniae* septicemia in children >5 years with sickle cell anemia.

Parenteral penicillin G is indicated for the treatment of bone and joint infections, bacterial endocarditis, intra-abdominal infections, meningitis, pericarditis, pneumonia and septicemia caused by susceptible organisms; listeriosis caused by *L. monocytogenes*; tetanus; yaws caused by *T. pallidum pertenue*; tertiary and neurosyphilis; gas gangrene caused by Clostridium species; leptospirosis caused by Leptospira species; diphtheria caused by *C. diphtheriae*, as an adjunct to antitoxin.

Penicillin G benzathine is used for the treatment of bejel caused by *T. pallidum endemicum*, pinta caused by *T. carateum* and yaws caused by *T. pertenue*. Penicillin G benzathine is also used for the treatment of pharyngitis and early or late benign syphilis (not neurosyphilis) and in the prophylaxis of diphtheria and recurrent rheumatic fever.

CONTRAINDICATIONS: A clear history of penicillin allergy; infections caused by beta-lactamase producing organisms.

Oral penicillin should not be used as adjunctive prophylaxis for genitourinary instrumentation or surgery, lower intestinal tract surgery, sigmoidoscopy or childbirth, or for the active treatment of syphilis, meningitis, bacterial endocarditis, diphtheria, gas gangrene or other severe infections due to penicillin-susceptible microorganisms.

Severe pneumonia, empyema, bacteremia, pericarditis, meningitis and septic arthritis should not be treated with oral penicillin during the acute stage.

Topical application of penicillin is contraindicated since sensitization is a frequent complication.

WARNINGS: Serious and occasionally fatal hypersensitivity reactions have been reported in patients receiving penicillin therapy. Although anaphylaxis is more frequent following parenteral therapy, it has occurred in patients receiving oral penicillin (see Overdose, Symptoms and Treatment).

Cross-sensitivity between penicillins and cephalosporins is estimated to be very low. According to current opinion, the true incidence of cross-sensitivity is about 1%. The beta-lactam subunit is not considered the primary allergenic determinant; rather, the side chain predicts cross-reactivity [*Pediatrics* 2005;115(4):1048-57]. Therefore the likelihood of a cross-reaction with a cephalosporin varies and is expected to be highest with first-generation cephalosporins. After thorough investigation into the nature of the allergy, a penicillin should only be considered in a cephalosporin-allergic patient provided there is no history of an immediate-sensitivity reaction. Although the risk of cross-reaction is predicted to be low the patient should be monitored for signs of a sensitivity reaction.

The use of antibacterial agents can result in overgrowth of nonsusceptible organisms, such as *C. difficile* or *C. albicans*. The possibility of C. difficile infection should be considered in patients presenting with diarrhea during or following therapy with penicillin.

Extreme care must be taken not to inject penicillin G benzathine intravenously, intra-arterially or near a peripheral nerve or vessel as severe and/or permanent neurovascular damage may occur. Injections should be discontinued if sudden severe pain occurs at the injection site.

PRECAUTIONS: Oral administration should not be relied upon in patients with severe illness, or with nausea, vomiting, gastric dilatation, cardiospasm or intestinal hypermotility.

Occasionally, certain patients will not absorb therapeutic amounts of orally administered penicillin.

In streptococcal infections, therapy should be given for a minimum of 10 days. Cultures should be taken following treatment to ensure eradication of streptococci.

Patients with impaired renal function (ClCr <50 mL/min) require modification of dose and interval.

The passage of any penicillin from blood into brain is facilitated by inflamed meninges and during cardiopulmonary bypass. In the presence of such factors, particularly in renal failure when high serum concentrations can be attained, CNS adverse effects including myoclonia, seizures and depressed consciousness can be expected.

Drug Interactions: Aminoglycosides: A synergistic bactericidal effect occurs in vitro against some strains of enterococci and against viridans streptococci when penicillin G is used in conjunction with aminoglycosides. This effect is used therapeutically to treat bacterial endocarditis.

Bacteriostatic Antibiotics (e.g., chloramphenicol, erythromycin, tetracycline): May decrease the effectiveness of penicillin.

Methotrexate: Increased serum levels of methotrexate through competitive inhibition of renal tubular secretion. If possible, consider alternate antibiotic therapy. If penicillin is necessary monitor for toxicity of methotrexate and modify dose or discontinue methotrexate as appropriate.

Oral Contraceptives: Whether penicillins decrease the effectiveness of oral contraceptives is controversial. Some clinicians recommend adding an alternative method of contraception for the duration of the cycle when a penicillin is taken.

Probenecid: Decreases renal tubular secretion of penicillin leading to higher and more prolonged serum concentrations, higher CSF concentrations and an increased risk of toxicity. Alternatively, it has been used therapeutically in select cases to increase penicillin serum levels.

Pregnancy: Usual doses appear to be safe in pregnant women.

Lactation: Penicillin does not appear in breast milk in sufficient quantities to treat infections in the infant but does appear in trace quantities which could lead to allergic sensitization or disruption of the gastrointestinal flora.

ADVERSE EFFECTS: Central Nervous System: Usually associated with administration of large parenteral dosages to patients with impaired renal function; manifested as hallucinations, confusion, lethargy, dysphasia, twitching, hyperreflexia, asterixis, localized or generalized seizures, coma or fatal encephalopathy.

Gastrointestinal: nausea, vomiting, epigastric distress, diarrhea, black hairy tongue, antibiotic associated pseudomembranous colitis.

Hepatic: Hepatotoxicity may be associated with hypersensitivity.

Hematologic: eosinophilia (hypersensitivity), hemolytic anemia, transient neutropenia, leukopenia, thrombocytopenia and thrombocytopenic purpura. These reactions are more common with larger parenteral doses of penicillin.

Hypersensitivity: Hypersensitivity reactions are usually more severe following parenteral administration, however all degrees of hypersensitivity including fatal anaphylaxis have followed even oral administration of the drug. The most common manifestations of hypersensitivity are: skin eruptions (from mild rash to exfoliative dermatitis) with an overall incidence of approximately 2%, urticaria, chills, fever, edema, eosinophilia and anaphylaxis (overall incidence about 0.05%). A serum sickness-like reaction has been reported, characterized by fever, malaise, urticaria, arthralgia, myalgia, lymphadenopathy and splenomegaly.

Renal: Rarely, acute interstitial nephritis (fever, proteinuria and hematuria); high doses of parenterally administered penicillin sodium may result in electrolyte disturbances, especially in patients with poor renal function.

Miscellaneous: Jarisch-Herxheimer Reaction: Frequently occurs 2 to 12 hours after penicillin is started to treat syphilis or other spirochetal infections and is thought to result from the phagocytized organism's release of endotoxins and/or other pyrogens. The reaction is characterized by headache, fever, chills, sweating, sore throat, myalgia, arthralgia, malaise, tachycardia, hypertension followed by hypotension. The reaction usually subsides within 24 hours.

OVERDOSE:

Symptoms: Hypersensitivity reactions including anaphylaxis may occur with any dosage. Oral ingestion of excessive amounts may cause nausea, vomiting, diarrhea, abdominal pain. Parenteral administration of high doses may lead to cardiovascular or electrolyte abnormalities or neurological effects such as drowsiness, seizures or coma.

Treatment: Following oral ingestion of large amounts of penicillin administration of activated charcoal with a cathartic may be of benefit. Patients must be observed for signs of a hypersensitivity reaction (see below). If seizures, cardiac arrhythmias or fluid or electrolyte disturbances occur following parenteral administration, appropriate measures must be taken. Dialysis may be helpful in removing Penicillin G.

Anaphylaxis: Mild cases involving only urticaria may be managed with antihistamine therapy. Severe anaphylaxis may require oxygen supplementation, airway management, epinephrine administration, ECG monitoring and iv fluids.

For management of a suspected drug overdose, CPhA recommends that you contact your **regional Poison Control Centre**. See the *CPS* Directory section for a list of Poison Control Centres.

DOSAGE: Oral therapy is generally used for the treatment of mild to moderately severe infections. Maximal absorption of both natural penicillins occurs on an empty stomach (1 hour before or 2 hours after meals); however, penicillin V may be taken with or without food without loss of clinical effectiveness. Parenteral (IV) administration is required for the treatment of severe infections including meningitis, endocarditis, syphilis and clostridial infections.

Dosage must be individualized according to the causative organism, severity of the infection and host factors such as age and renal function.

Penicillin V 500 000 units is equivalent to 300 mg.

Penicillin G 500 000 units is equivalent to 312 mg.

Usual therapeutic dosages are as follows:

Oral: Penicillin V: Adults and Children >12 Years: 1-4 g daily in 3 to 4 divided doses. Children <12 Years: 25-100 mg/kg/day in 3 to 4 divided doses, maximum 3 g/day. Treatment of Group A beta-hemolytic streptococcal infections may be dosed every 12 hours for adults and children.

Rheumatic Fever Prophylaxis: Prevention of recurrent Group A beta-hemolytic streptococcal infections in patients who have had rheumatic fever and/or chorea: penicillin V 250-300 mg orally twice daily.

Parenteral: Aqueous Penicillin G IM/IV: Adults and Children >12 Years: Dosage may range from 1 million units daily im to 24 million units daily iv in 4 to 6 divided doses. Intermittent iv infusions should be given over 1 to 2 hours.

Children 1 Month to 12 Years: 50 000 to 250 000 units/kg/day in 4 divided doses. Higher doses such as 250 000 to 400 000 units/kg/day (up to a maximum of 24 million units/day) in divided doses every 4 to 6 hours may be required to treat more severe infections. IV infusion should be given over 15 to 30 minutes.

Table 1: Penicillin G

Dose in Renal Impairment

Creatinine Clearance	Dose Adjustment
>50 mL/min	Usual dose
10–50 mL/min	75% of usual dose
<10 mL/min	20–50% of usual dose

Penicillin G Benzathine IM: Administer by deep im injection. Adults and Children >27 kg: 1.2 million units as a single dose. Children ≤27 kg: 600 000 units as a single dose. The treatment for primary, secondary and early latent syphilis in adults is one dose of penicillin G benzathine 2.4 million units im. Late latent and tertiary syphilis is treated with 2.4 million units im once weekly for 3 weeks.

Rheumatic Fever Prophylaxis: Adults and Children >27 kg: penicillin G benzathine 1.2 million units im every 4 weeks. Children ≤27 kg: 600 000 units every 4 weeks.

Penlac™ Ⓟ

ciclopirox

Topical Antifungal

sanofi-aventis

Date of Revision: December 4, 2007

PHARMACOLOGY: Ciclopirox free acid is an antimycotic agent that inhibits the growth of a number of fungi in vitro including *T. mentagrophytes, T. rubrum, M. canis, E. floccosum, C. albicans, C. tropicalis* and *C. pseudotropicalis*.

The mechanism of action of ciclopirox has been investigated using various in vitro and in vivo infection models. One in vitro study suggested that ciclopirox acts by chelation of polyvalent cations (Fe^{+3} or Al^{+3}) resulting in the inhibition of the metal-dependent enzymes that are responsible for the degradation of peroxides within the fungal cell. The clinical significance of this observation is not known.

Pharmacokinetics: As demonstrated in pharmacokinetic studies in animals and man, ciclopirox olamine is rapidly absorbed after oral administration and completely eliminated in all species via feces and urine. Most of the compound is excreted either unchanged or as glucuronide. After oral administration of 10 mg of radiolabelled drug (^{14}C-ciclopirox) to healthy volunteers, approximately 96% of the radioactivity was excreted renally within 12 hours of administration. Ninety-four percent of the renally excreted radioactivity was in the form of glucuronides. Thus, glucuronidation is the main metabolic pathway of this compound.

Systemic absorption of ciclopirox was determined in 5 patients with dermatophytic onychomycoses after application of PENLAC (Ciclopirox Topical Solution, 8% w/w) NAIL LACQUER, to all 20 digits and adjacent 5 mm of skin once daily for six months. Random serum concentrations and 24 hour urinary excretion of ciclopirox were determined at two weeks and at 1, 2, 4 and 6 months after initiation of treatment and 4 weeks post-treatment. In this study, ciclopirox serum levels ranged from 12-80 ng/mL. Based on urinary data, mean absorption of ciclopirox from the dosage form was <5% of the applied dose. One month after cessation of treatment, serum and urine levels of ciclopirox were below the limit of detection.

In two vehicle-controlled trials, patients applied PENLAC to all toenails and affected fingernails. Out of a total of 66 randomly selected patients on active treatment, 24 had detectable serum ciclopirox concentrations at some point during the dosing interval (range 10.0-24.6 ng/mL). It should be noted that eleven of these 24 patients took concomitant medication containing ciclopirox as ciclopirox olamine (Loprox Cream).

The penetration of PENLAC was evaluated in an in vitro investigation. Radiolabelled ciclopirox applied once to onychomycotic toenails that were avulsed demonstrated penetration up to a depth of approximately 0.4 mm. Nail plate concentrations decreased as a function of nail depth. The clinical significance of these findings in nail plates is unknown. Nail bed concentrations were not determined.

INDICATIONS: Please read this entire section carefully to fully understand the indication for this product.

Topical treatment with PENLAC (Ciclopirox Topical Solution, 8% w/w) NAIL LACQUER is indicated as part of a comprehensive nail management program in immunocompetent patients with mild to moderate onychomycosis (due to *T. rubrum*) of fingernails and toenails without lunula involvement. The comprehensive management program includes frequent removal of unattached, infected nails (e.g., monthly) by a health care professional with special competence in the diagnosis and treatment of nail disorders, including minor nail procedures. PENLAC should therefore be used only under medical supervision. The safety and efficacy of daily use for longer than 48 weeks have not been established. (See Precautions.)

Pivotal Clinical Trial Data: PENLAC was used to treat onychomycosis of the great toenail (without lunula involvement) in two double-blind, placebo-controlled pivotal studies (see Table 1). Patients were treated once daily for up to 48 weeks in conjunction with monthly removal of the unattached, infected toenail by the investigator. At baseline, patients had 20-65% involvement of the target nail plate.

Table 1: PENLAC

Endpoint ITT Population

	Study 312[d]		Study 313[d]	
Efficacy Variable	Ciclopirox	Placebo	Ciclopirox	Placebo
Treatment Success[a]	8/107 (8%)	1/107 (1%)	13/115 (11%)	1/115 (1%)
Treatment Cure[b]	6/110 (6%)[e]	1/109 (1%)	10/118 (9%)	0/117 (0%)

(cont'd)

Table 1: PENLAC *(cont'd)*

Endpoint ITT Population

Efficacy Variable	Study 312[d]		Study 313[d]	
	Ciclopirox	Placebo	Ciclopirox	Placebo
Mycological Cure[c]	30/105 (29%)	14/105 (13%)	39/113 (35%)	10/114 (9%)

[a] Treatment Success: negative culture, negative KOH, ≤10% involvement target nail.
[b] Treatment Cure: negative culture & KOH, Global Evaluation Score=Cleared.
[c] Mycological Cure: negative culture, negative KOH.
[d] Denominators differ across variables because of missing data.
[e] p=0.055. All other values statistically significant (CMH ≤0.02, stratified by centre).

Post-treatment efficacy assessments were scheduled only for patients who achieved treatment cure. Some data on the post-treatment efficacy of the product are available for 12 patients. Twelve weeks after stopping ciclopirox treatment, 3/6 patients maintained treatment success, and 6/9 patients maintained negative mycology reports.

CONTRAINDICATIONS: PENLAC (Ciclopirox Topical Solution, 8% w/w) NAIL LACQUER is contraindicated in individuals who have shown hypersensitivity to any of its components.

WARNINGS: PENLAC (Ciclopirox Topical Solution, 8% w/w) NAIL LACQUER is not for ophthalmic, oral, or intravaginal use. For use on nails and immediately adjacent skin only.

PRECAUTIONS: No studies have been conducted to determine whether ciclopirox might reduce the effectiveness of systemic antifungal agents for onychomycosis. Therefore, the concomitant use of PENLAC (Ciclopirox Topical Solution, 8% w/w) NAIL LACQUER and systemic antifungal agents for onychomycosis, is not recommended. (See Indications.)

The effectiveness and safety in the following populations have not been studied, as the clinical trials with PENLAC excluded patients who: were pregnant or nursing, planned to become pregnant, had a history of immunosuppression (e.g., extensive, persistent, or unusual distribution of dermatomycoses, extensive seborrheic dermatitis, recent or recurring herpes zoster, or persistent herpes simplex), were HIV seropositive, received organ transplant, required medication to control epilepsy, were insulin dependent diabetics or had diabetic neuropathy. Patients with severe plantar (moccasin) tinea pedis were also excluded.

So far there is no relevant clinical experience with patients with insulin dependent diabetes or who have diabetic neuropathy. The risk of removal of the unattached, infected nail, by the health care professional and trimming by the patient should be carefully considered before prescribing to patients with a history of insulin dependent diabetes mellitus or diabetic neuropathy.

If a reaction suggesting sensitivity or chemical irritation should occur with the use of PENLAC, treatment should be discontinued and appropriate therapy instituted.

Pregnancy: Teratology studies in mice, rats, rabbits, and monkeys at oral doses of up to 77, 23, 23, or 38.5 mg, respectively, of ciclopirox as ciclopirox olamine/kg/day, or in rats and rabbits receiving topical doses of up to 92.4 and 77 mg/kg/day, respectively, did not indicate any significant fetal malformations.

Teratology studies with ciclopirox free acid were performed in rats with oral doses of 20, 50, or 125 mg/kg/day and in rabbits with oral doses of 12.5, 32, or 80 mg/kg/day; no significant fetal malformations were noted.

There are no adequate or well-controlled studies of topically applied ciclopirox in pregnant women. PENLAC should be used during pregnancy only if the potential benefit justifies the potential risk to the fetus.

Lactation: It is not known whether this drug is excreted in human milk. Since many drugs are excreted in human milk, caution should be exercised when PENLAC is administered to a nursing woman.

Pediatrics: Safety and effectiveness in pediatric patients have not been established.

Geriatrics: Vehicle-controlled clinical trials of PENLAC conducted in the US did not include sufficient numbers of patients aged 65 and over to determine whether they respond differently from younger patients. Other reported clinical experience has not identified differences in responses between elderly and younger patients.

Information to Be Provided to the Patient: **Patients should be provided with instructions regarding the use of PENLAC (see Information for the Patient).**

The patient should be told:

1. To avoid contact with the eyes and mucous membranes. Contact with skin other than skin immediately surrounding the treated nail(s) should be avoided. PENLAC is for external use only.
2. To apply PENLAC evenly over the entire nail plate and 5 mm of surrounding skin. If possible, PENLAC should be applied to the nail bed, hyponychium, and the under surface of the nail plate when it is free of the nail bed (e.g., onycholysis). Contact with the surrounding skin may produce mild, transient irritation (redness).
3. To file and trim nails on a weekly basis during treatment with PENLAC.
4. That removal of the unattached, infected nail, as frequently as monthly, by a health care professional is needed with use of this medication.
5. To inform a health care professional if they have diabetes or problems with numbness in the toes or fingers for consideration of the appropriate nail management program.
6. To inform a health care professional if the area of application shows signs of increased irritation (redness, itching, burning, blistering, swelling, oozing).
7. That up to 48 weeks of daily application with PENLAC and professional removal of the unattached, infected nail, as frequently as monthly, are considered the full treatment needed to achieve a clear or almost clear nail (defined as 10% or less residual nail involvement).
8. That six months of therapy with professional removal of the unattached, infected nail may be required before initial improvement of symptoms is noticed.
9. That a completely clear nail may not be achieved with use of this medication. In clinical studies less than 12% of patients were able to achieve either a completely clear or almost clear toenail.
10. That he/she should not use nail polish or other nail cosmetic products on the treated nails.
11. To not use the medication for any disorder other than that for which it is prescribed.
12. To avoid use near heat or open flame, because product is flammable.

ADVERSE EFFECTS: In the vehicle-controlled clinical trials conducted in the US, 9% (30/327) of patients treated with PENLAC (Ciclopirox Topical Solution, 8% w/w) NAIL LACQUER and 7% (23/328) of patients treated with vehicle reported treatment-emergent adverse events (TEAE) considered by the investigator to be causally related to the test material. With the exception of Skin and Appendages, the incidence of these adverse events, within each body system, was similar between the treatment groups and was less than 1%. For Skin and Appendages, 8% (27/327) and 4% (14/328) of patients in the ciclopirox and vehicle groups, respectively, reported at least one adverse event.

Periungual erythema and erythema of the proximal nail fold were the most common TEAEs causally related to study drug. These events (coded as "rash") were reported in 5% (16/327) of patients treated with PENLAC and 1% (3/328) of patients treated with vehicle.

Other TEAEs thought to be causally related to study material in the US vehicle-controlled studies included nail disorders such as shape change, irritation, ingrown toenail, and discoloration. The incidence of nail disorders was similar between the treatment groups (2% [6/327] in the PENLAC group and 2% [7/328] in the vehicle group).

Application site reactions and/or burning sensation of the skin were considered causally related to study drug in 1% of both PENLAC- and vehicle-treated patients (3/327 and 4/328, respectively).

Table 2 summarizes the most common TEAEs considered causally related to study drug, as reported in the US Phase II/III vehicle-controlled trials.

Use of PENLAC for 48 additional weeks was evaluated in an open-label extension study conducted in patients previously treated in the vehicle-controlled studies. Three percent (9/281) of patients treated with PENLAC experienced at least one TEAE that the investigator thought was causally related to the test material. Mild rash in the form of periungual erythema (1% [2/281]) and nail disorders (1% [4/281]) were the most frequently reported. The remainder of TEAEs considered causally related to study drug occurred at an incidence of <1%.

In controlled and open-label clinical trials conducted with ciclopirox nail lacquer, 8% outside of the US, adverse events reported were consistent with those seen in the US studies.

Postmarketing Experience: Contact dermatitis has been reported as an adverse reaction in post-marketing surveillance of ciclopirox-containing products, including ciclopirox nail lacquer, 8%.

Table 2: PENLAC

Most Common TEAEs Considered Causally Related to Study Drug

Body System TEAE	PENLAC n (%)	Vehicle n (%)
No. of Patients Treated	327 (100.0)	328 (100.0)
Patients with Related TEAEs	30 (9.2)	23 (7.0)
Skin and Appendages	27 (8.3)	14 (4.3)
Periungual erythema/erythema of proximal nail fold	16 (4.9)	3 (0.9)
Nail Disorders[a]	6 (1.8)	7 (2.1)
Application Site Reaction/Burning Sensation	3 (0.9)	4 (1.2)
Other[b]	2 (0.6)	0 (0.0)
All other Body Systems	0–1 (0.0–0.3)	0–3 (0–0.9)

[a] Nail disorders such as shape change, irritation, ingrown toenail and discolouration.
[b] Other: Dry skin, pruritus.

OVERDOSE:
The likelihood of overdosage from topical administration of ciclopirox nail lacquer, 8% is extremely low.

In a test of acute oral toxicity in the rat, the LD50 was greater than 10 mL/kg of ciclopirox nail lacquer, 8%. This would be equivalent to 600 mL for an adult person weighing 60 kg or more than 1000 vials of 3 mL. Furthermore, overdosage by oral ingestion of nail lacquer would be unlikely because of its unpalatable taste.

For management of a suspected drug overdose, CPhA recommends that you contact your **regional Poison Control Centre**. See the *CPS* Directory section for a list of Poison Control Centres.

DOSAGE: PENLAC (Ciclopirox Topical Solution, 8% w/w) NAIL LACQUER should be used as a component of a comprehensive management program for onychomycosis. Removal of the unattached, infected nail—as frequently as monthly—by a health care professional, weekly trimming by the patient, and daily application of the medication are all integral parts of this therapy. Careful consideration of the appropriate nail management program should be given to patients with diabetes. (See Precautions.)

Nail Care By Health Care Professionals: Removal of the unattached, infected nail—as frequently as monthly—trimming of onycholytic nail, and filing of excess horny material should be performed by professionals trained in the treatment of nail disorders.

Nail Care By Patient: Patients should file away (with emery board) loose nail material and trim nails, as required, or as directed by the health care professional, every seven days after PENLAC is removed with isopropyl alcohol.

PENLAC should be applied once daily (preferably at bedtime or eight hours before washing) to all affected nails with the applicator brush provided.

PENLAC should be applied evenly over the entire nail plate.

If possible, PENLAC should be applied to the nail bed, hyponychium, and the under surface of the nail plate when it is free of the nail bed (e.g., onycholysis).

PENLAC should not be removed on a daily basis. Daily applications should be made over the previous coat and removed with isopropyl alcohol every seven days. This cycle should be repeated throughout the duration of therapy.

INFORMATION FOR THE PATIENT: Published in e-CPS, available by subscription at www.e-cps.ca.

SUPPLIED: Each g of clear, colourless to slightly yellowish solution for topical application to fingernails, toenails and immediately adjacent skin only, contains: ciclopirox 80 mg in a solution base consisting of ethyl acetate, isopropyl alcohol, and butyl monoester of poly[methylvinyl ether/maleic acid] in isopropyl alcohol. Ethyl acetate and isopropyl alcohol are solvents that vaporize after application. Glass bottles of 3, 6 and 12 g with screw caps which are fitted with brushes. Store at room temperature between 15 and 30°C. To protect from light, replace the bottle into the carton after each use. **Caution:** Flammable. Keep away from heat and flame.

Pennsaid® Ⓟ

diclofenac sodium

Topical Anti-inflammatory—Analgesic

Paladin

Date of Revision: April 14, 2009

PHARMACOLOGY: Diclofenac sodium is a non-steroidal anti-inflammatory drug (NSAID) of the arylacanoic acid group, with analgesic and anti-inflammatory properties. The mode of action of diclofenac sodium is not fully known, but it is considered to be primarily through its inhibitory effects on prostaglandin synthesis by interfering with the action of prostaglandin synthetase/cyclo-oxygenase, isoforms 1 and 2 (COX-1 and COX-2). It does not act through the pituitary-adrenal axis. Diclofenac sodium does not alter the course of the underlying disease in patients with osteoarthritis; it has been found to relieve pain, reduce swelling and tenderness, and increase mobility.

In an 84-day (12-week), double-blind, vehicle-controlled clinical trial in patients with osteoarthritis of the knee, the efficacy of PENNSAID was demonstrated by three primary variables—pain and physical function, as measured with the WOMAC LK3.1 Osteoarthritis Index—plus Patient Global Assessment. Efficacy was confirmed by the secondary variable, stiffness, as measured by WOMAC LK3.1 Osteoarthritis Index. For all treated patients (ALL), descriptive statistical analysis revealed that the PENNSAID group showed greater improvement in scores than the vehicle-control group for all variables. Based on ANCOVA, using baseline score as a covariate, PENNSAID was found to be statistically significantly (p<0.05) more effective than vehicle-control for all variables (see Table 1).

Table 1: PENNSAID

Efficacy Data for 84-day Vehicle-Controlled Study

Improvement in Score of:	All			
	N	Mean Baseline Score (S.D.)	Mean Change in Score[a] (S.D.)	p value[b] PENNSAID >C
Pain				
PENNSAID	164	42.0 (11.7)	−15.3 (15.2)	p=0.0024
Vehicle-control (C)	162	41.3 (11.6)	−10.3 (13.9)	
Physical Function				

(cont'd)

Table 1: PENNSAID *(cont'd)*

Efficacy Data for 84-day Vehicle-Controlled Study

Improvement in Score of:	All			
	N	Mean Baseline Score (S.D.)	Mean Change in Score[a] (S.D.)	p value[b] PENNSAID >C
PENNSAID	164	42.0 (11.7)	−15.3 (15.2)	p=0.0024
Vehicle-control (C)	162	41.3 (11.6)	−10.3 (13.9)	
Patient Global Assessment				
PENNSAID	164	3.1 (0.7)	−1.3 (1.2)	p=0.0052
Vehicle-control (C)	162	3.1 (0.7)	−1.0 (1.1)	
Stiffness				
PENNSAID	164	5.2 (1.5)	−1.8 (2.1)	p=0.0086
Vehicle-control (C)	162	5.2 (1.5)	−1.3 (2.0)	

[a] Final—Baseline; WOMAC LK3.1.
[b] ANCOVA (baseline score as a covariate).

In a 42-day (6-week), double-blind, vehicle-controlled clinical trial in patients with osteoarthritis of the knee, the efficacy of PENNSAID was demonstrated by three primary variables—pain and physical function, as measured with the WOMAC LK3.1 Osteoarthritis Index—plus Patient Global Assessment. Efficacy was confirmed by the secondary variable, stiffness, as measured by WOMAC LK3.1 Osteoarthritis Index. For all treated patients (ALL), descriptive statistical analysis revealed that the PENNSAID group showed greater improvement in scores than the vehicle-control group for all variables. Based on ANCOVA, using baseline score as a covariate, PENNSAID was found to be statistically significantly ($p<0.05$) more effective than the vehicle-control for all variables (see Table 2).

Table 2: PENNSAID

Efficacy Data for 42-day Vehicle-Controlled Study

Improvement in Score of:	All			
	N	Mean Baseline Score (S.D.)	Mean Change in Score[a] (S.D.)	p value[b] PENNSAID >C
Pain				
PENNSAID	107	13.0 (3.2)	−5.3 (5.0)	p=0.0040
Vehicle-control (C)	109	12.8 (3.1)	−3.4 (4.3)	
Physical Function				
PENNSAID	107	40.7 (12.0)	−13.0 (16.2)	p=0.0041
Vehicle-control (C)	109	40.4 (11.2)	−7.3 (13.4)	
Patient Global Assessment				
PENNSAID	107	3.1 (0.8)	−1.2 (1.3)	p=0.0004
Vehicle-control (C)	109	3.2 (0.8)	−0.7 (1.2)	
Stiffness				
PENNSAID	107	5.2 (1.5)	−1.7 (2.1)	p=0.0023
Vehicle-control (C)	109	5.2 (1.5)	−1.0 (1.9)	

[a] Final—Baseline; WOMAC LK3.1.
[b] ANCOVA (baseline score as a covariate).

In a 28-day (4-week), double-blind, vehicle- and placebo-controlled clinical trial in patients with osteoarthritis of the knee, the efficacy of PENNSAID was demonstrated by the primary variable—pain, as measured with the WOMAC LK3.0 Osteoarthritis Index. Efficacy was confirmed by three secondary variables—physical function and stiffness, as measured by the WOMAC LK3.0 Osteoarthritis Index—plus Patient Global Assessment. For all treated patients (ALL) descriptive statistical analysis revealed that the PENNSAID group showed greater improvement in scores than the vehicle-control and placebo groups for all WOMAC variables and for the Patient Global Assessment. Based on ANOVA (contrast analysis between least squares means) PENNSAID was found to be statistically significantly ($p<0.05$) more effective than vehicle-control and placebo for all variables (see Table 3).

Table 3: PENNSAID

Efficacy Data for 28-day Vehicle- and Placebo-Controlled Study

Improvement in Score of:	All			
	N	Mean Baseline Score (S.D.)	Mean Change in Score[b] (S.D.)	p value[a]
Pain				
PENNSAID	84	9.2 (0.4)	−3.9 (4.4)	
Vehicle-control (C)	80	9.2 (0.4)	−2.3 (3.4)	PENNSAID >C; p=0.008
Placebo (P)	84	9.6 (0.4)	−2.7 (4.0)	PENNSAID >P; p=0.034
Physical Function				
PENNSAID	84	29.5 (13.7)	−11.5 (14.5)	
Vehicle-control (C)	80	30.5 (11.8)	−5.6 (11.1)	PENNSAID >C; p=0.002
Placebo (P)	84	30.9 (13.1)	−7.2 (12.3)	PENNSAID >P; p=0.017

(cont'd)

Table 3: PENNSAID *(cont'd)*

Efficacy Data for 28-day Vehicle- and Placebo-Controlled Study

Improvement in Score of:	All			
	N	Mean Baseline Score (S.D.)	Mean Change in Score[b] (S.D.)	p value[a]
Patient Global Assessment[c]				
PENNSAID	82	NA[d]	6.6 (3.1)	
Vehicle-control (C)	76	NA[d]	7.7 (3.5)	PENNSAID >C; p=0.040
Placebo (P)	83	NA[d]	7.8 (3.0)	PENNSAID >P; p=0.024
Stiffness				
PENNSAID	84	3.7 (1.7)	−1.5 (1.8)	
Vehicle-control (C)	80	3.5 (1.7)	−0.7 (2.0)	PENNSAID >C; p=0.011
Placebo (P)	84	3.7 (1.8)	−0.7 (1.9)	PENNSAID >P; p=0.006

[a] ANOVA (contrast analysis between least squares means).
[b] Final—Baseline; WOMAC LK3.0.
[c] Sum of weekly scores; some patients had no Patient Global Assessment data.
[d] NA=Not applicable.

Vehicle-control (C) and Placebo (P) were not statistically significantly different for any of the efficacy variables—pain (p=0.557); physical function (p=0.412); Patient Global Assessment (p=0.882); stiffness (p=0.873).

The efficacy of PENNSAID (50 drops, 3 times a day) versus oral diclofenac (50 mg, 3 times a day) in relieving symptoms of primary osteoarthritis (OA) of the knee was assessed in an 84-day, randomized, double blind, double-dummy clinical study. The three primary efficacy variables were change from baseline to final assessment in (1) WOMAC Index VA3.1 pain subscale score, (2) WOMAC Index VA3.1 physical function subscale score and (3) Patient Global Assessment score. The primary efficacy results on the Per Protocol (PP) dataset are summarized in Table 4. Efficacy was also supported by secondary efficacy variable, stiffness, as measured by WOMAC Index VA3.1.

Table 4: PENNSAID

Efficacy Data for 84-day Study Comparing PENNSAID (50 drops tid) and Oral Diclofenac (50 mg tid) (data normalized to 100 mm) VAS)

	WOMAC Pain	WOMAC Physical Function	Patient Global Assessment	Stiffness
PENNSAID				
N	237	237	234	237
Mean Change (SD)	−25.4 (24.0)	−22.4 (23.3)	−29.5 (30.9)	−24.1 (29.5)
Oral Diclofenac				
N	255	255	251	255
Mean Change (SD)	−28.0 (25.3)	−26.6 (25.3)	−33.8 (30.7)	−27.3 (30.5)
Absolute Difference of Means (95% CI)				
	2.7 (−1.7 to 7.0)	4.2 (−0.1 to 8.5)	4.3 (−1.2 to 9.8)	3.2 (−2.2 to 8.5)

INDICATIONS: PENNSAID is indicated for treatment of the symptoms associated with osteoarthritis of the knee(s) only, for a treatment regimen of not more than three months duration, whether continuous or intermittent.

CONTRAINDICATIONS: Active peptic ulcer, a history of recurrent ulceration or active inflammatory disease of the gastrointestinal system.

Known or suspected hypersensitivity to diclofenac sodium or other non-steroidal anti-inflammatory drugs. The potential for cross-reactivity between different NSAIDs must be kept in mind.

PENNSAID should not be used in patients with the complete or partial syndrome of ASA intolerance (rhinosinusitis, urticaria/angioedema, nasal polyps and asthma), in whom asthma, anaphylaxis, urticaria, rhinitis or other allergic manifestations are precipitated by ASA or other non-steroidal anti-inflammatory agents. Fatal anaphylactoid reactions have occurred in such individuals. As well, individuals with the above medical problems are at risk of a severe reaction even if they have taken NSAIDs in the past without any adverse effects.

Significant hepatic impairment or active liver disease.

Severely impaired or deteriorating renal function (creatinine clearance <30 mL/min). Individuals with lesser degrees of renal impairment are at risk of deterioration of their renal function when prescribed NSAIDs and must be monitored.

PENNSAID is not recommended for use with other NSAIDs because of the absence of any evidence demonstrating synergistic benefits and the potential for additive side effects.

PENNSAID contains 45% dimethyl sulfoxide (DMSO), propylene glycol, glycerine and alcohol and should not be used by patients with allergy to any of these substances. Because the long-term safety of PENNSAID is unknown, PENNSAID should not be used for a treatment regimen of longer duration than 3 months.

PENNSAID should not be used in children and pregnant and lactating women as its safety in these groups has not been established.

WARNINGS: Gastrointestinal System (GI): In clinical studies, PENNSAID has not been associated with serious GI toxicity, such as peptic ulceration, perforation and GI bleeding.

Serious GI toxicity, such as peptic ulceration, perforation and gastrointestinal bleeding, sometimes severe and occasionally fatal, can occur at any time, with or without symptoms, in patients treated with NSAIDs, including diclofenac sodium.

Gastrointestinal symptoms, such as dyspepsia, are common, usually developing early in therapy. Physicians should remain alert for the signs and symptoms of ulceration and bleeding in patients treated with NSAIDs, even in the absence of previous GI tract symptoms.

In patients observed in clinical trials of NSAIDs given orally, symptomatic upper GI ulcers, gross bleeding, or perforation appear to occur in approximately 1% of patients treated for 3-6 months and in about 2-4% of patients treated for one year. The incidence of these complications is related to dose, past history of known ulcer disease, and advanced age.

PENNSAID should be given under close medical supervision to patients with a history of ulcer of the gastrointestinal tract, or inflammatory disease of the gastrointestinal tract, such as ulcerative colitis or Crohn's disease. In these cases the physician must weigh the benefits of treatment against the possible hazards.

Physicians should inform patients about the signs and/or symptoms of serious GI toxicity and instruct them to contact a physician immediately if they experience persistent dyspepsia or other symptoms or signs suggestive of gastrointestinal ulceration or bleeding.

Because serious GI tract ulceration and bleeding can occur without warning symptoms, physicians should follow patients and watch for the signs and symptoms of ulceration and bleeding and should inform the patients of the importance of this follow-up.

If ulceration is suspected or confirmed, or if GI bleeding occurs, PENNSAID should be discontinued immediately, appropriate treatment instituted and the patient monitored closely.

No studies, to date, have identified any group of patients not at risk of developing ulceration and bleeding. The major risk factors are a prior history of serious GI events and increasing age. Possible risk factors include *H. pylori* infection, excess alcohol intake, smoking, concomitant oral steroids, anticoagulants, anti-platelet agents (including ASA) and selective serotonin reuptake inhibitors (SSRIs).

Geriatrics: Patients older than 65 years and frail or debilitated patients are most susceptible to a variety of adverse reactions from non-steroidal anti-inflammatory drugs (NSAIDs); the incidence of these adverse reactions increases with dose and duration of treatment. In addition, these patients are less tolerant to ulceration and bleeding. Most reports of fatal GI events are in this population. Older patients are also at risk of lower esophageal ulceration and bleeding.

For such patients, consideration should be given to a starting dose lower than the one usually recommended, with individual adjustment when necessary and under close supervision. See Precautions for further advice.

Cross-Sensitivity: Patients sensitive to any one of the NSAIDs may be sensitive to any of the other NSAIDs also.

Aseptic Meningitis: In rare cases, with some NSAIDs, the symptoms of aseptic meningitis (stiff neck, severe headaches, nausea and vomiting, fever or clouding of consciousness) have been observed. Patients with autoimmune disorders (systemic lupus erythematosus, mixed connective tissue diseases, etc.) seem to be pre-disposed. Therefore, in such patients, the physician must be vigilant to the development of this complication.

Pregnancy: See Contraindications.

Labor: See Contraindications.

Lactation: See Contraindications.

Children: See Contraindications.

Dermatological: PENNSAID should not be used under occlusive dressings. Do not apply PENNSAID to open, abraded or infected skin. Avoid contact with the eyes or mucous membranes.

Hypersensitivity: Dimethyl sulfoxide may initiate the liberation of histamine and occasional hypersensitivity reactions have occurred with topical administration. If anaphylactoid symptoms develop, appropriate therapy should be instituted and further use of PENNSAID immediately discontinued.

PRECAUTIONS: Gastrointestinal System: There is no definitive evidence that the concomitant administration of histamine H_2-receptor antagonists and/or antacids will either prevent the occurrence of gastrointestinal side effects or allow the continuation of PENNSAID therapy when, and if, these adverse reactions appear.

Renal Function: In clinical studies with PENNSAID, increase in urea or creatinine, or any other renal toxicity has not been observed.

Long-term administration of NSAIDs to animals has resulted in renal papillary necrosis and other abnormal renal pathology. In humans, there have been reports of acute interstitial nephritis with hematuria, proteinuria, and occasionally nephrotic syndrome.

A second form of renal toxicity has been seen in patients with prerenal conditions leading to reduction in renal blood flow or blood volume, where the renal prostaglandins have a supportive role in the maintenance of renal perfusion. In these patients, administration of an NSAID may cause a dose-dependent reduction in prostaglandin formation and may precipitate overt renal decompensation. Patients at greatest risk of this reaction are those with impaired renal function, heart failure, liver dysfunction, those taking diuretics, and the elderly. Discontinuation of NSAID therapy is usually followed by recovery to the pretreatment state.

Diclofenac sodium and its metabolites are eliminated primarily (60%) by the kidneys; therefore, PENNSAID should be used with great caution in patients with impaired renal function. In these cases, utilization of lower doses of PENNSAID should be considered and patients carefully monitored.

Genitourinary Tract: Some NSAIDs are known to cause persistent urinary symptoms (bladder pain, dysuria, urinary frequency), hematuria or cystitis. The onset of these symptoms may occur at any time after the initiation of therapy with an NSAID. Some cases have become severe on continued treatment. Should urinary symptoms occur, treatment with PENNSAID must be stopped immediately to obtain recovery. This should be done before any urological investigation or treatment is carried out.

Hepatic Function: As with other NSAIDs, borderline elevations of liver function tests may occur in up to 15% of patients. These abnormalities may progress, may remain essentially unchanged, or may be transient with continued therapy. A patient with symptoms and/or signs suggesting liver dysfunction, or in whom an abnormal liver test has occurred, should be evaluated for evidence of the development of more severe hepatic reaction, while on therapy with PENNSAID. Severe hepatic reactions including jaundice and cases of fatal hepatitis have been reported with NSAIDs.

Although such reactions are rare, if abnormal liver tests persist or worsen, if clinical signs and symptoms consistent with liver disease develop, or if systemic manifestations occur (e.g. eosinophilia, rash, etc.), this drug should be discontinued.

Toxicity studies in animals with high doses of DMSO have shown occasional, transient elevation of liver function tests.

In two clinical trials with PENNSAID, a mild elevation of AST was seen in 4 of 117 (3.4%) patients using PENNSAID, 2 of 109 (1.8%) using vehicle-control (both of these solutions contained DMSO 45.5%) and 1 of 110 (0.9%) using Placebo. A mild elevation of ALT was seen in 4 of 117 (3.4%) patients using PENNSAID, 6 of 111 (5.4%) using vehicle-control and 2 of 108 (1.9%) using placebo. In most cases the increase was minimal and in two patients (one treated with PENNSAID, one treated with vehicle-control) the increase was 2.5 times normal. If there is a need to prescribe this drug in the presence of impaired liver function, it must be done under strict observation.

Caution is called for when using diclofenac sodium in patients with hepatic porphyria, since diclofenac sodium may trigger an attack.

Fluid and Electrolyte Balance: In clinical studies with PENNSAID, fluid or electrolyte abnormalities have not been observed.

Fluid retention and edema have been observed in patients treated with diclofenac sodium. Therefore, as with many other NSAIDs, the possibility of precipitating congestive heart failure in elderly patients or those with compromised cardiac function should be borne in mind. PENNSAID should be used with caution in patients with heart failure, hypertension or other conditions predisposing to fluid retention.

With NSAID treatment, there is a potential risk of hyperkalemia, particularly in patients with conditions such as diabetes mellitus or renal failure; elderly patients; or in patients receiving concomitant therapy with β-adrenergic blockers, angiotensin-converting enzyme inhibitors, angiotensin-II receptor antagonists or some diuretics. Patients at risk should be monitored periodically.

Hematology: In clinical studies with PENNSAID, abnormal hemoglobin, WBC or platelet counts have not been observed. Platelet function during treatment with PENNSAID has not been studied.

The effect of PENNSAID on platelet function was studied in 10 healthy patients randomly selected to participate in a sub-study of multiple-dose pharmacokinetic study where 40 drops of PENNSAID were applied to each knee four times a day for 7 days. Following 7-day treatment with PENNSAID, the mean change in % aggregation for ADP-collagen-, epinephrine- and arachidonic acid-induced aggregation was 1.31%, −0.19%, 9.85% and −0.95%, respectively. These results indicate that there was no marked effect on platelet aggregation after application of the maximum clinical dose for 7 days.

Drugs inhibiting prostaglandin biosynthesis do interfere with platelet function to varying degrees; therefore, patients who may be adversely affected by such an action should be carefully observed when PENNSAID is administered.

Blood dyscrasias (such as neutropenia, leukopenia, thrombocytopenia, aplastic anemia and agranulocytosis) associated with the use of NSAIDs are rare, but could occur with severe consequences. Patients on long-term diclofenac sodium treatment should have their hemopoietic system evaluated periodically.

Infection: In common with other NSAIDs, diclofenac sodium may mask the usual signs of infection (i.e. fever).

Ophthalmology: Blurred and/or diminished vision has been reported with the use of NSAIDs. Changes in the refractive index and lens opacities have been seen in non-primate animals with chronic administration of dimethyl sulfoxide, in doses far in excess of those used in humans. If ophthalmological symptoms develop, PENNSAID should be discontinued and an ophthalmologic examination performed.

Central Nervous System: Some patients may experience drowsiness, dizziness, vertigo, insomnia or depression with the use of PENNSAID. If patients experience these side effects, they should exercise caution in carrying out activities that require alertness.

Hypersensitivity Reactions: Dimethyl sulfoxide may initiate the liberation of histamine and occasional hypersensitivity reactions have occurred with topical administration. If anaphylactoid symptoms develop, appropriate therapy should be instituted and further use of PENNSAID immediately discontinued.

As with other NSAIDs, allergic reactions, including anaphylactic/anaphylactoid reactions, can occur without prior exposure to drug. Careful questioning for patient history of asthma, nasal polyps, urticaria, and hypotension associated with NSAIDs is important before starting therapy. Because hypersensitivity reactions may occur even at a low systemic level, the possibility of such adverse effects with PENNSAID cannot be completely excluded.

In rare cases, serious skin reactions such as Stevens-Johnson syndrome, toxic epidermal necrolysis, exfoliative dermatitis and erythema multiforme have been associated with the use of some NSAIDs. Because the rate of these reactions is low, they have usually been noted during post-marketing surveillance in patients taking other medications also associated with the potential development of these serious skin reactions. Thus causality is not clear. These reactions are potentially life-threatening, but may be reversible if the causative agent is discontinued and appropriate treatment instituted. Patients should be advised that if they experience a generalized skin rash they should discontinue PENNSAID and contact their physician for assessment and advice, including which additional therapies to discontinue.

Information to Be Provided to the Patients: PENNSAID should not be used under occlusive dressings.

Do not apply PENNSAID to open, abraded or infected skin.

Do not apply any other medication to treated area.

Avoid contact with the eyes or mucous membranes.

Avoid contact of synthetic fibres with skin wetted with DMSO.

See Information for the Patient.

Drug Interactions: Acetylsalicylic Acid (ASA) or Other NSAIDs: The use of PENNSAID in addition to any other NSAID, including those over-the-counter ones (such as ASA and ibuprofen) is not recommended due to the possibility of additive side effects. Low dose ASA (≤325 mg/day) for cardiovascular prophylaxis, is permitted.

Digoxin: Diclofenac sodium may increase the plasma concentration of digoxin. Dosage adjustment of digoxin may be required.

Anticoagulants, Heparin, Thrombolytic Agents and Other Platelet Aggregation Inhibitors: Numerous studies have shown that the concomitant use of NSAIDs and anticoagulants increases the risk of GI adverse events such as ulceration and bleeding.

Because prostaglandins play an important role in hemostasis, and NSAIDs affect platelet function, concurrent therapy of PENNSAID with warfarin requires close monitoring to be certain that no change in anticoagulant dosage is necessary.

Oral Hypoglycemics: Pharmacodynamic studies have shown no potentiation of effect with concurrent administration with diclofenac sodium; however, there are isolated reports of both hypoglycemic and hyperglycemic effects in the presence of diclofenac sodium, which necessitated changes in the dosage of hypoglycemic agents.

Diuretics: NSAIDs have been reported to decrease the activity of diuretics. Concomitant treatment with potassium-sparing diuretics may be associated with increased serum potassium, thus making it necessary to monitor levels.

Antihypertensives: Like other NSAIDs, diclofenac sodium can reduce the antihypertensive effects of propranolol and other beta-blockers, as well as other antihypertensive agents.

Glucocorticoids: Numerous studies have shown that concomitant use of NSAIDs and oral glucocorticoids increases the risk of GI side effects such as ulceration and bleeding. This is especially the case in older (>65 years of age) individuals.

Methotrexate: Caution should be exercised when NSAIDs are administered less than 24 hours before or after treatment with methotrexate. Elevated blood concentrations of methotrexate may occur, increasing its toxicity.

Acetaminophen: There may be an increased risk of adverse renal effects when administered concomitantly with NSAIDs.

Alcohol: There may be an increased risk of GI side effects, including ulceration or hemorrhage, when taken concomitantly with NSAIDs.

Cyclosporine: The nephrotoxicity of cyclosporine may be increased because of the effects of NSAIDs on renal prostaglandins.

Lithium: Lithium plasma concentrations will increase when administered concomitantly with diclofenac sodium (which affects lithium renal clearance). Dosage adjustment of lithium may be required.

Probenecid: May decrease the excretion and increase serum concentration of NSAIDs, possibly enhancing effectiveness and/or increasing the potential for toxicity. Concurrent therapy of NSAIDs with probenecid requires close monitoring of dosage.

Quinolone Antibacterials: There have been isolated reports of convulsions, which may have been due to concomitant use of quinolones and NSAIDs.

Clinical Laboratory Tests: Diclofenac sodium increases platelet aggregation time but does not affect bleeding time, plasma thrombin clotting time, plasma fibrinogen, or factors V and VII to XII. Statistically significant changes in prothrombin and partial thromboplastin times have been reported in normal volunteers. The mean changes were observed to be less than 1 second in both instances, and are unlikely to be clinically important.

Persistently abnormal or worsening renal, hepatic or hematological test values should be followed up carefully since they may be related to therapy.

ADVERSE EFFECTS: Adverse reaction reporting is based on double-blind, controlled clinical studies in which 446 patients were exposed to PENNSAID. Mean drop-out rates were: PENNSAID, 22.0%; vehicle-control (C), 28.3%; diclofenac control, 19.2%; placebo, 20.6%.

Application-site, dermatological reactions are the most commonly seen adverse events with PENNSAID (see Table 5).

The most common adverse reactions encountered with oral NSAIDs are gastrointestinal, of which peptic ulcer, with or without bleeding, is the most severe. Fatalities have occurred, particularly in the elderly. The most severe, albeit rare, dermatological reactions observed were erythema multiforme (Stevens-Johnson syndrome and Lyell's syndrome).

Table 5 lists all adverse events, regardless of causality, occurring in ≥2% of patients receiving PENNSAID from five controlled studies conducted in patients with osteoarthritis that included a vehicle-control, active-control and/or placebo-control group.

Table 5: PENNSAID

Adverse Events Occurring in ≥2% of PENNSAID Patients in Five Vehicle-Controlled Studies

Adverse Event	PENNSAID (n=446) (%)	Control-DMSO[a] (n=442) (%)	Control-diclofenac[b] (n=52) (%)	Placebo[c] (n=175) (%)
Gastrointestinal				
Dyspepsia	4.48	3.85	9.62	4
Nausea	2.02	2.26	3.85	1.71
Central and Peripheral Nervous System				
Paresthesia	2.02	1.58	0	1.14
Paresthesia (Application Site)	7.85	9.05	7.69	10.29
Skin and Appendages				
Application Site Reaction	2.47	1.13	5.77	1.71
Dry Skin (Application Site)	41.93	23.3	23.08	6.86
Pruritus (Application Site)	2.91	4.52	3.85	4
Rash	2.02	1.81	3.85	2.86
Rash (Application Site)	9.64	4.98	7.69	2.86
Special Senses				
Taste Perversion	3.81	3.62	0	4.57
Respiratory				
Pharyngitis	5.38	2.71	5.77	6.86
Musculoskeletal				
Arthralgia	16.82	16.52	40.38	37.14
Arthrosis	4.04	3.85	3.85	12
Joint Disorder	4.71	5.43	7.69	15.43
Body as a Whole				
Abdominal Pain	3.14	1.58	0	5.14

(cont'd)

Table 5: PENNSAID *(cont'd)*

Adverse Events Occurring in ≥2% of PENNSAID Patients in Five Vehicle-Controlled Studies

Adverse Event	PENNSAID (n=446) (%)	Control-DMSO[a] (n=442) (%)	Control-diclofenac[b] (n=52) (%)	Placebo[c] (n=175) (%)
Back Pain	6.5	5.66	15.38	7.43
Flu Syndrome	4.04	4.07	0	4.57
Headache	12.11	13.12	32.69	26.86
Infection	3.14	2.71	11.54	4.57
Pain	6.05	6.33	17.31	10.86

[a] Contains the full carrier with DMSO, no diclofenac sodium.
[b] Contains negligible DMSO with the full dose of diclofenac sodium.
[c] Contains negligible DMSO with no diclofenac sodium.

The following spontaneous adverse events occurred in 0.2 to 1.8% of patients treated with PENNSAID regardless of causality:
Gastrointestinal: colitis, constipation, diarrhea, dry mouth, flatulence, gastritis, gastroenteritis, gingivitis, periodontal abscess, rectal disorder, thirst, tooth caries, vomiting.
Central and Peripheral Nervous System: aphasia, confusion, dizziness, depression, dysthymia, hypertonia, insomnia, nervousness, neuritis, sleep disorder, speech disorder, thinking abnormal, vertigo.
Skin and Appendages: acne, acne (application site), contact dermatitis, dry skin, furunculosis, hair disorder, maculopapular rash, nail disorder, pruritus, pustular rash, skin nodule, urticaria, vesiculobullous rash.
Cardiovascular: arrhythmia, arteriosclerosis, bradycardia, cardiovascular disorder, hypertension, myocardial infarction, migraine, palpitation, vasodilation, vasodilation (application site).
Special Senses: amblyopia, cataract, ear pain, eye pain, lacrimation disorder.
Hemic and Lymphatic: ecchymosis.
Urogenital: dysmenorrhea, prostatic specific antigen increase, testis disorder, vaginal hemorrhage.
Metabolic and Nutritional: edema, gout, hypercholesterolemia, peripheral edema.
Respiratory: asthma, bronchitis, congestion, cough increased, dyspnea, epistaxis, rhinitis, sinusitis.
Musculoskeletal: abnormal gait, arthritis, bone pain, leg cramps, myasthenia.
Body as a Whole: accidental injury, allergic reaction, asthenia, body odour, carcinoma, chest pain, chills, face edema, fever, halitosis, hernia, malaise, neck pain, neck rigidity.

In a controlled clinical trial conducted to assess the alternative dose regimen of 50 drops t.i.d, a total of 311 patients received at least one dose of PENNSAID for mean treatment duration of 66 days. The safety profile observed in this study was consistent with that reported in previous studies, the primary adverse events experiences by PENNSAID patients being application-site reactions.

In a long-term, uncontrolled clinical trial (approximately 800 patients were treated with PENNSAID for one year or longer), the adverse event profile was similar to that observed in the controlled clinical trials.
Post-Market Adverse Drug Reactions: In post-marketing surveillance for PENNSAID, the following adverse reactions have been reported:
Body as a Whole: abdominal pain, accidental injury, allergic reaction, asthenia, back pain, body odor, chest pain, edema, face edema, halitosis, headache, lack of drug effect, neck rigidity, pain.
Cardiovascular: cardiovascular disorder, palpitation.
Digestive: diarrhea, dry mouth, dyspepsia, mouth ulceration, nausea, rectal hemorrhage, ulcerative stomatitis.
Metabolic and Nutritional: creatinine increased.
Musculoskeletal: leg cramps, myalgia.
Nervous: depression, dizziness, drowsiness, paresthesia, paresthesia, app. site.
Respiratory: asthma, dyspnea, laryngismus, laryngitis, pharyngitis.
Skin and Appendages: At the application site: contact dermatitis, contact dermatitis with vesicles, dry skin, pruritus, rash. Other skin adverse reaction: rash, skin discoloration, urticaria.
Special Senses: abnormal vision, blurred vision, cataract, ear pain, eye disorder, eye pain, taste perversion.

OVERDOSE:

Treatment: In the event of ingestion of PENNSAID (1.5% w/w diclofenac sodium in 45% dimethyl sulfoxide), there is no specific antidote. An entire 60 mL bottle of PENNSAID contains approximately 960 mg of diclofenac sodium. Systemic absorption should be prevented as soon as possible by the induction of vomiting, gastric lavage or treatment with activated charcoal. Supportive and symptomatic treatment should be given for complications such as hypotension, renal failure, convulsions, gastrointestinal irritation and respiratory depression. Measures to accelerate elimination (forced diuresis, hemoperfusion, dialysis) may be considered, but may be of limited use because of the high protein binding and extensive metabolism of diclofenac.

A 60 mL bottle of PENNSAID contains approximately 29 g of DMSO, well below any toxic level. (The oral LD_{50} for monkeys is >4 g/kg. The dermal LD_{50} of DMSO for monkeys is >11 g/kg). Acute toxicity through inhalation of high vapour concentrations of DMSO, through the use or abuse of PENNSAID, is remote. In the event that exposure should occur, it may lead to irritation of the mucous membranes of the upper respiratory tract, wheezing, nausea or vomiting. Treatment includes administration of oxygen or other symptomatic measures as necessary.

In the event of topical application of an excessive dose, wash the area with soap and water as soon as possible. Local irritation may occur. Treatment includes symptomatic measures as necessary.

> For management of a suspected drug overdose, CPhA recommends that you contact your **regional Poison Control Centre**. See the *CPS* Directory section for a list of Poison Control Centres.

DOSAGE: Table 6 summarizes the recommended dosage and administration of PENNSAID.

Table 6: PENNSAID

Dosage and Administration of PENNSAID (1.5% w/w diclofenac sodium solution)

Medical Condition	Population (age group)	Dose	Route of Administration	Maximum Duration of Treatment (days)
Osteoarthritis of the knee(s)	Adults (≥18 years old)	50 drops per knee, 3 times a day, or 40 drops per knee, 4 times a day	Topical	3 months

The following treatment regimen is recommended for patients:
- PENNSAID is intended for external use only.
- Apply PENNSAID to clean, dry skin; do not use under bandages or dressings.
- Dispense 10 drops of PENNSAID into the hand, or directly onto the knee.
- Spread PENNSAID evenly around front, back and sides of the knee.
- Repeat this procedure until 40 drops or 50 drops (depending on the recommended dose) have been applied and the knee is completely covered.
- To treat the other knee, repeat the procedure.
- Allow several minutes for PENNSAID to dry.
- Avoid contact with the eyes or mucous membranes.
- After application, wash the hands.
- Follow the same procedure 3 times (for 50 drops) or 4 times (for 40 drops), spaced evenly throughout the day. PENNSAID treatment has no relationship to food intake.
- There is no need to adjust the dosage of PENNSAID for elderly or debilitated patients.
- PENNSAID is not indicated for pediatric patients.
- PENNSAID is indicated for a treatment regimen of not more than three months duration, whether continuous or intermittent.
- PENNSAID therapy should be discontinued if the application site displays signs of significant skin reaction, including swelling, urticaria or vesiculobullous rash.

INFORMATION FOR THE PATIENT: Published in e-CPS, available by subscription at www.e-cps.ca.

SUPPLIED: Each bottle of clear, odorless liquid contains: diclofenac sodium 1.5% w/w in a solution base consisting of dimethyl sulfoxide, glycerine, propylene glycol, ethanol and purified water. Low-density polyethylene bottles of 15 mL and packages of 2×60 mL. High-density polyethylene bottles of 15 mL and packages of 2×60 mL. All have a plastic dropper cap. Store at room temperature (15-25°C).

Penta/3b®
vitamin B complex
Intensive Vitamin Therapy

Sandoz

Penta/3b® Plus
multiple vitamins
Intensive Vitamin Therapy

Sandoz

Penta/3b®+C
ascorbic acid—vitamin B complex
Intensive Vitamin Therapy

Sandoz

SUPPLIED: Penta/3b: Each round, biconvex, film-coated, dark red tablet contains: vitamin B_1 (thiamine hydrochloride) 250 mg, vitamin B_6 (pyridoxine hydrochloride) 125 mg and vitamin B_{12} (cyanocobalamin) 250 µg. Bottles of 50 and 300.
Penta/3b Plus: Each scarlet red decavitamin capsule, imprinted with "DIN" over "01980610" on one side and "Sabex®" on the other side, contains: vitamin B_1 (thiamine hydrochloride) 250 mg, vitamin B_2 (riboflavin) 2 mg, vitamin B_6 (pyridoxine hydrochloride) 125 mg, niacinamide 20 mg, folic acid 0.1 mg, vitamin B_{12} (cyanocobalamin) 250 µg, vitamin C (ascorbic acid) 75 mg, vitamin D (as ergocalciferol) 400 IU, vitamin E (as dl-alpha-tocopheryl acetate) 15 mg, vitamin A (as palmitate) 4000 IU, and pantothenic acid (as calcium pantothenate) 9 mg. Bottles of 50.
Penta/3b+C: Each round, biconvex, film-coated, yellow tablet contains: vitamin B_1 (thiamine hydrochloride) 250 mg, vitamin B_6 (pyridoxine hydrochloride) 125 mg, vitamin B_{12} (cyanocobalamin) 250 µg and vitamin C (ascorbic acid) 250 mg. Bottles of 50.

Pentamycetin®
chloramphenicol
Antibiotic

Sandoz

Pentamycetin®/HC
chloramphenicol—hydrocortisone acetate
Antibiotic—Corticosteroid

Sandoz

SUPPLIED: Pentamycetin: Ophthalmic Ointment 1%: Each g contains: chloramphenicol 10 mg in a sterile petrolatum base. Tubes of 3.5 g. Store between 15 and 30°C. Protect from freezing.
Ophthalmic Solution: 0.25%: Each mL contains: chloramphenicol 2.5 mg and chlorobutanol 0.5% (as preservative) in a sterile buffered solution. Plastic dropper bottles of 10 mL. Refrigerate until dispensed. After dispensing, the solution may be kept at room temperature for 21 days; after that period, discard unused portion. Protect from freezing.
0.5%: Each mL contains: chloramphenicol 5 mg and chlorobutanol 0.5% (as preservative) in a sterile buffered solution. Plastic dropper bottles of 10 mL. Refrigerate until dispensed. After dispensing, the solution may be kept at room temperature for 21 days; after that period, discard unused portion. Protect from freezing.
Pentamycetin/HC: Eye and Ear Ointment: Each g contains: chloramphenicol 10 mg and hydrocortisone acetate 10 mg in a sterile petrolatum base. Tubes of 3.5 g. Store between 15 and 30°C. Protect from freezing.
Eye and Ear Suspension: Each mL contains: chloramphenicol 2 mg and hydrocortisone acetate 10 mg in a sterile buffered vehicle. Plastic dropper bottles of 5 mL. Refrigerate until dispensed. After dispensing, the suspension may be kept at room temperature for 21 days; after that period, discard unused portion. Protect from freezing. Shake well before each use.

Pentasa®
5-ASA
Gastrointestinal Anti-inflammatory

Ferring

Date of Preparation: August 15, 1994
Date of Revision: January 17, 2006

PHARMACOLOGY: PENTASA (5-aminosalicylic acid or 5-ASA) is an ethylcellulose-coated, extended-release formulation of 5-ASA, an aminosalicylate, gastrointestinal anti-inflammatory agent. Aminosalicylates are considered to be first line therapy for inflammatory bowel diseases. 5-ASA is known to be therapeutically active in Crohn's Disease and ulcerative colitis.

5-ASA has in vitro and in vivo pharmacologic effects that decrease leukotriene production, scavenge for free radicals and inhibit leukocyte chemotaxis. While the exact mode of action is currently unknown, any of these biochemical mechanisms may play a role in the clinical effectiveness of 5-ASA.

Regardless of its mode of action, 5-ASA appears to exert its therapeutic effect by topical action on the affected areas of inflammation. The oral dosage form of PENTASA extended-release tablets allows a very predictable, uniform, and continuous release of drug in the small (duodenum, jejunum and ileum) and large bowel (colon), at all enteral pH conditions, which is not significantly compromised by diarrhoea or increased bowel acidity, conditions which accompany active inflammatory bowel disease. The PENTASA dosage forms designed for rectal administration, enemas and suppositories, are well suited to deliver the active ingredient, 5-ASA, directly to affected areas along the mucosal lumen of the rectum, sigmoid and distal large bowel.

Based on urinary excretion data, 20% to 30% of 5-ASA in PENTASA extended-release tablets is absorbed. It is rapidly acetylated to N-acetyl-5-ASA. Plasma 5-ASA concentration peaks at approximately 1 µg/mL three hours after a 1 g dose of PENTASA, and declines rapidly in a biphasic manner. N-acetyl-5-ASA peaks at approximately 1.8 µg/mL and its concentration also follows a biphasic decline. Pharmacological activities of N-acetyl-5-ASA are unknown and other metabolites have not been identified.

Under steady-state conditions, 15% of the 2 g daily dose was recovered in the urine (mostly as the acetylated metabolite) after administration of PENTASA (5-ASA) enema, with 10% urinary recovery observed after administration of PENTASA suppositories. Maximum plasma concentrations of 5-ASA and of N-acetyl-5-ASA (approximately 0.7 µg/mL and 1.2 µg/mL respectively for the enema; 0.3 µg/mL and 0.8 µg/mL respectively for the suppositories) were reached 2 hours following administration of the enema and 5 to 6 hours following administration of the suppositories. About 130 mg of free 5-ASA was recovered in the faeces following a single 1 g dose of PENTASA (2×500 mg tablets). Elimination of free 5-ASA and salicylates in faeces increased proportionately with dose. N-acetyl-5-ASA was the primary compound excreted in the urine (19%-30% of dose).

Local availability, as shown by recovery of free 5-ASA in the faeces, was higher for both the enema (mean 30%) and the suppositories (mean 45%) than for the oral dosage forms of 5-ASA.

Scintigraphic studies have shown that in the stomach, PENTASA tablets disintegrate immediately into discrete microgranules which are spread throughout the entire gastrointestinal tract. The microgranules are emptied from the stomach within 17+5 minutes under fasted conditions and within about 30 minutes when a breakfast meal is served 5 minutes post-dose. Therefore the residence time in the stomach is not affected by simultaneous food intake. The transit time through the small intestine has been shown to be 213+45 minutes after which the microgranules arrive in the caecum. The small intestinal transit is not affected by food intake since no statistically significant difference could be detected between fasted and fed conditions. The small intestinal transit time was 3.7 hours in fasted subjects and 3.1 hours in a fasted subject that had a breakfast meal 5 minutes post-dose. The microgranules reside in the colon for about 8 hours. The independence of food intake and intestinal transit has also been shown in another study, where the gastric emptying and small intestinal transit of 5-ASA microgranules occurred within the digestive period and synchronous with the meal.

Coadministration of 5-ASA tablets and a high-fat meal was found to inhibit 5-ASA and N-acetyl-5-ASA systemic absorption. Bioavailability of 5-ASA decreased by about 70% and peak concentration decreased by about 60% as compared to the fasting state. N-acetyl-5-ASA pharmacokinetics were affected to a lesser extent, i.e., a 24% decrease in bioavailability and peak concentration. When food was present, less free 5-ASA was eliminated in the feces (33%), although 15.2% more salicylates were eliminated in the feces than under fasting conditions. The same effect was observed after administration of 5-ASA in a suspension, indicating that the interaction involves 5-ASA, not the PENTASA delivery system.

INDICATIONS: PENTASA (5-ASA) extended-release tablets are indicated for the treatment of mild to moderate active ulcerative colitis and for long-term maintenance therapy in order to maintain remission and prevent relapse of active disease. PENTASA (5-ASA) extended-release tablets are also indicated for the management of mild to moderate Crohn's Disease, and as maintenance therapy for patients with Crohn's Disease in remission induced by surgery or medication.

PENTASA (5-ASA) rectal suspension is indicated for the treatment of acute distal ulcerative colitis extending to the splenic flexure and for long-term maintenance therapy in order to maintain remission and prevent relapse of active disease. Clinical experience has shown that topical PENTASA (i.e. enemas/suppositories) is superior to oral PENTASA (i.e tablets) with regard to therapeutic efficacy in distal ulcerative colitis.

PENTASA (5-ASA) suppositories are indicated for the treatment of acute ulcerative proctitis and for long-term maintenance therapy in order to maintain remission and prevent relapse of active disease.

CONTRAINDICATIONS: In patients with existing gastric or duodenal ulcer. In patients with urinary tract obstruction, renal parenchymal disease or severe renal impairment. Very rarely, 5-ASA may induce nephrotoxicity which would be additive in these patients. Renal function should be determined prior to beginning therapy (e.g., serum creatinine), and the benefits of therapy versus the increased risk of nephrotoxicity carefully assessed. See Warnings; patients who have demonstrated hypersensitivity to derivatives of salicylate.

WARNINGS: Impaired Renal or Hepatic Function: Caution should be exercised if PENTASA (5-ASA) is administered to patients with impaired renal or hepatic function. Rare reports of Nephrotic Syndrome and interstitial nephritis associated with 5-ASA therapy have been described in the literature. Animal studies have demonstrated a dose-dependent nephrotoxicity.

Patients with pre-existing renal disease, increased BUN or serum creatinine, or proteinuria should be carefully monitored. 5-ASA-induced nephrotoxicity should be suspected in patients developing renal dysfunction during therapy. The concurrent use of other known nephrotoxic agents, such as NSAIDs and azathioprine, may increase the risk of renal reactions. Renal function should be determined prior to beginning therapy (e.g. serum creatinine) and should be frequently monitored, especially during the initial phase of treatment.

Cardiac Hypersensitivity Reactions and Myelosuppression: 5-ASA-induced cardiac hypersensitivity reactions (myocarditis and pericarditis) and serious myelosuppression have been reported rarely. Concomitant treatment with mesalazine can increase the risk of myelosuppression in patients receiving azathioprine or 6-mercaptopurine. Treatment should be discontinued on suspicion or upon evidence of these adverse reactions.

Pregnancy: PENTASA should be used during pregnancy only if clearly needed. 5-ASA is known to cross the placental barrier. However no teratogenic effects have been observed in animal studies.

Blood disorders (leukopenia, thrombocytopenia, anemia) have been reported in newborns of mothers being treated with PENTASA.

Lactation: Caution should be exercised when PENTASA is administered to a nursing woman. 5-ASA is excreted in breast milk. The concentration of 5-ASA is much lower than in maternal blood, but the metabolite N-acetyl-5-ASA appears in similar concentrations. There is limited experience of the use of oral mesalazine in lactating women. No controlled studies with PENTASA during breast-feeding have been carried out. Hypersensitivity reactions like diarrhea in the infants cannot be excluded.

Children: The safety and efficacy of PENTASA have not been established in children under 12 years of age. The potential benefits of therapy should be weighed against the possible risks.

PRECAUTIONS: General: 5-ASA has been associated with the production of an acute intolerance syndrome which may be difficult to distinguish from a flare-up of inflammatory bowel disease. Symptoms include cramping, acute abdominal pain and bloody diarrhea, sometimes fever, headache and rash. If acute intolerance syndrome is suspected, prompt withdrawal is required. If a rechallenge is performed later in order to validate the hypersensitivity, it should be carried out under close medical supervision at reduced dose and only if clearly needed.

In ulcerative colitis studies, most patients who were intolerant or hypersensitive to sulfasalazine were able to take PENTASA (5-ASA) without evidence of allergic reaction (e.g., rash, fever, pruritus) or intolerance. Nevertheless, since rash is more often seen in PENTASA-treated patients than in placebo-treated patients (1.6% vs 0.6%), caution should be exercised when PENTASA is used in patients known to be allergic to sulfasalazine. These patients should be instructed to discontinue therapy if signs of rash or fever become apparent.

Semen abnormalities and infertility in men, which are associated with sulfasalazine, have not been reported with PENTASA during controlled clinical trials. Semen quality significantly improved when patients were transferred from sulfasalazine to PENTASA.

Drug Interactions: A potential risk of myelosuppression, particularly leucopenia when aminosalicylates are coadministered with azathioprine or 6-mercaptopurine.

A potential risk of renal failure when aminosalicylates are coadministered with other nephrotoxic agents such as NSAIDs and azathioprine.

ADVERSE EFFECTS: The most frequent adverse reactions seen in clinical trials are diarrhea (3%), nausea (3%), abdominal pain (3%), headache (3%), vomiting (1%) and rash (1%). See Table 1 for typical expected reactions to therapy with PENTASA.

Table 1: PENTASA

Frequency of Expected Adverse Effects, Based on Clinical Trials Reports and Reports from Post-marketing Surveillance

Frequency of Adverse Effect	Organ System Affected	Symptom
Common (≥1% and <10%)	Nervous System Disorders Gastrointestinal Disorders	Headache Diarrhea Abdominal pain Nausea Vomiting
	Skin and Subcutaneous Tissue Disorders	Rash including urticaria Exanthema
Rare (≥0.01% and <0.1%)	Cardiac Disorders	Myocarditis Pericarditis
	Gastrointestinal Disorders	Increased amylase Pancreatitis
Very rare (<0.01%)	Skin and Subcutaneous Tissue Disorders	Reversible alopecia
	Hepato-biliary Disorders	Increased liver enzymes and bilirubin, hepatotoxicity (incl. hepatitis, cirrhosis, hepatic failure)
	Renal and Urinary Disorders	Nephropathy including interstitial nephritis Nephrotic syndrome, urine discolouration
	Respiratory, Thoracic and Mediastinal Disorders	Allergic lung reactions (incl. dyspnea, coughing, allergic alveolitis, pulmonary eosinophilia, pulmonary infiltration, pneumonitis)
	Musculoskeletal, Connective Tissue and Bone Disorders	Myalgia Arthralgia Isolated reports of lupus-erythematosus-like reactions
	Blood and Lymphatic System Disorders	Eosinophilia (as part of an allergic reaction), anemia, aplastic anemia, leukopenia (incl. sgranulocytopenia), thrombocytopenia, agranulocytosis, pancytopenia
	Nervous System Disorders	Peripheral neuropathy

The mechanism of 5-ASA-induced myocarditis and pericarditis, pancreatitis, nephritis and hepatitis is unknown, but may be of allergic origin. It is important to note that several of these disorders may also be attributable to the underlying inflammatory bowel disease itself.

Following rectal administration, local reactions such as pruritus, rectal discomfort and urgency may occur.

The following events have been reported infrequently during trials and represent sporadic, idiosyncratic or hypersensitivity reactions, to be expected rarely.

Gastrointestinal: abdominal distention, anorexia, duodenal ulcer, eructation, esophageal ulcer, fecal incontinence, bloody stools or diarrhea, intestinal obstruction, melena, dysphagia, mouth ulcer, oral moniliasis, pancreatitis, rectal bleeding, rectal urgency, thirst.

Diarrhea is a commonly reported adverse event (about 3% frequency in clinical trials; somewhat less from spontaneous post-market surveillance reports), which is not dose-related. Diarrhea is also a symptom of the underlying disease, and may indeed be indicative of inadequate dosage with PENTASA in some patients. Rarely 5-ASA may exacerbate the inflammatory bowel disease itself.

It may be noted that melena has been reported as an adverse event rarely during 5-ASA therapy, but it has not been definitely linked to treatment. Gastrointestinal bleeding has been assumed from observations of bloody diarrhea or stools. Again, blood in fecal matter may be a symptom of the underlying disease and has not been definitely linked to treatment.

Dermatological: acne, alopecia, dry skin, eczema, erythema nodosum, erythematous rash, hirsutism, nail disorder, photosensitivity, pruritus, skin discoloration, sweating.

Reversible alopecia has been reported in 5-ASA-treated patients, as well as in placebo-treated patients, indicating that hair loss could be part of the underlying disease. Two cases of alopecia in patients on treatment with 5-ASA at a dose of 4 g/day were confirmed by positive rechallenge. In one of the cases, the hair loss improved after dosage reduction to 2 g/day. However, the available data are insufficient to establish a dose relationship with 5-ASA treatment generally.

Three cases of erythema nodosum have been reported in connection with PENTASA therapy. The causality was assessed as probable (1 case), possible (1 case) and not related (1 case) due to negative dechallenge. Erythema nodosum is a well-known extra-intestinal manifestation of inflammatory bowel disease.

Nervous System: anxiety, abnormal dreams, dizziness, insomnia, somnolence, paresthesia.

Cardiovascular: postural hypotension, tachycardia.

Respiratory: dyspnea, increased coughing, pharyngitis.

Metabolic: alkaline phosphatase increase, amylase increase, C reactive protein increase, creatinine increase, GGTP increase, LDH increase, proteinuria, AST increase, ALT increase, weight decrease, weight increase.

Rise in liver enzymes by 3 to 5 times the normal range may be expected in a small percentage of patients treated with PENTASA. This variable and transient occurrence is difficult to relate definitely to drug treatment due to the concomitant drug therapy usual with patients, and due to enzyme fluctuations caused by the disease itself. In many cases, the enzyme increases resolve without drug discontinuation or reduction. In most cases, enzyme abnormalities are reversed on discontinuation of therapy. Rarely, increase in liver enzymes is indicative of developing hepatitis.

Similarly, increases in serum amylase and lipase levels by 3 to 5 times the normal range may occur, and are usually reversible upon dosage reduction or discontinuation. Very rarely, patients develop pancreatitis.

Weight loss is an expected consequence of inflammatory bowel disease. Weight gain is usually indicative of a positive clinical response to PENTASA therapy.

Renal/Genitourinary: albuminuria, urinary frequency, urinary infection, urination disorder, vaginitis, isolated cases of nephrotic syndrome and interstitial nephritis.

Other: anemia, appetite decrease, arthralgia, breast pain, chest pain/pressure, chills, conjunctivitis, dry eyes, eye pain, ecchymosis, edema, eosinophilia, ESR increase, fatigue, fever, flu syndrome, leg cramps, malaise, menorrhagia, myalgia, scotoma, sore throat.

OVERDOSE:

Symptoms: There is no clinical experience with PENTASA (5-ASA) overdosage. Single oral doses of 5-ASA up to 5 g/kg in pigs and a single i.v. dose of 5-ASA at 920 mg/kg in rats were not lethal.

Treatment: In cases of suspected overdose, symptomatic treatment at hospital is required. Fluid and electrolyte, as well as acid/base imbalances, should be corrected by the administration of appropriate i.v. therapy. Close monitoring of renal function is required in order to maintain adequate renal function. No cases of overdose have been reported.

For management of a suspected drug overdose, CPhA recommends that you contact your **regional Poison Control Centre**. See the *CPS* Directory section for a list of Poison Control Centres.

DOSAGE: Extended-release Tablets 500 mg: Management of mild to moderate active ulcerative colitis and maintenance therapy: Therapy should be initiated at 0.5 g 4 times daily (2 g daily dose). The dose may be increased to 1 g 4 times daily (4 g daily dose) if additional therapeutic benefit is needed.

Management of mild to moderate Crohn's disease: The optimal dose is 1 g 4 times daily (4 g daily dose). For patients with Crohn's disease in remission, a dose of 0.75 g 4 times daily (3 g daily dose) is recommended.

PENTASA extended-release tablets should not be chewed, broken or crushed but should be swallowed whole.

PENTASA extended-release tablets may be taken before meals without affecting drug bioavailability. Taking PENTASA with food may be helpful in alleviating gastrointestinal pain and nausea if these symptoms have been reported after taking the product on an empty stomach.

Rectal Suspension: The recommended dose ranges from 1 to 4 g of 5-ASA, depending on disease activity. PENTASA may be self-administered once daily at bedtime. Dosage may be adjusted according to the individual patient's needs consistent with therapeutic goals. Prolonged retention is expected to achieve the best therapeutic response.

Suppositories: The usual dose of PENTASA suppositories is 1 suppository containing 1 g of 5-ASA, self-administered once daily at bedtime. Prolonged retention is expected to achieve the best therapeutic response. The frequency of dosage may be adjusted according to the individual patient's needs consistent with therapeutic goals.

INFORMATION FOR THE PATIENT: Published in e-CPS, available by subscription at www.e-cps.ca.

SUPPLIED: Extended-release Tablets: Each round, flat, speckled beige, extended-release tablet with beveled edges, one face debossed with "PENTASA", other face scored, debossed with "500" above scoreline and with "mg" below scoreline, contains: 5-ASA 500 mg. Nonmedicinal ingredients: cellulose, ethylcellulose, magnesium stearate, povidone and talc. Gluten-free. Bottles of 240. Store at room temperature (15 to 30°C).

Rectal Suspension: Each unit dose (100 mL) of rectal suspension enema contains: 5-ASA 1 g or 4 g. Nonmedicinal ingredients: hydrochloric acid (to adjust the pH to 4.8), purified water, sodium acetate, sodium edetate, sodium metabisulfite. Cartons of 7 enemas together with 7 hygienic bags. Store at controlled room temperature, preferably below 25°C. Dispense in the respective carton.

Suppositories: Each suppository contains: 5-ASA 1 g. Nonmedicinal ingredients: magnesium stearate, polyethylene glycol, povidone, talc. Cartons of 30 suppositories in individual foil pouches with finger protectors. Store at controlled temperature, preferably below 25°C. Dispense in the respective carton.

Pentaspan®

pentastarch

Plasma Volume Expander

Bristol-Myers Squibb

Date of Preparation: November 19, 2001
Date of Revision: June 19, 2007

PHARMACOLOGY: The colloidal properties of pentastarch render it useful as a plasma volume expander. I.V. infusion of pentastarch results in expansion of the plasma volume in excess of the volume infused. This expansion persists for approximately 18 to 24 hours and is expected to improve the hemodynamic status for 12 to 18 hours.

Pentastarch molecules below 50 000 molecular weight are rapidly eliminated by renal excretion. A single dose of approximately 500 mL of pentastarch results in elimination in the urine of approximately 70% of the dose within 24 hours, and approximately 80% of the dose within 1 week. The remaining percentage of the administered dose is presumed to be eliminated at a slower rate. Although this process is variable, it generally results in an intravascular pentastarch concentration below the level of detection by 1 week. The hydroxyethyl group is not cleaved, but remains intact and attached to glucose units when excreted.

INDICATIONS: When plasma volume expansion is desired as an adjunct in the management of shock due to hemorrhage, surgery, sepsis, burns or other trauma. It is not a substitute for red blood cells or coagulation factors in plasma.

CONTRAINDICATIONS: In patients with known hypersensitivity to hydroxyethyl starch, or with bleeding disorders, or with congestive heart failure where volume overload is a potential problem. Pentastarch should not be used in renal disease with oliguria or anuria not related to hypovolemia.

WARNINGS: General: Administration of large volumes of pentastarch will decrease hemoglobin concentration and dilute plasma proteins excessively. Administration should be kept below the recommended ceiling of 2000 mL in 24 hours (see Dosage).

As with other plasma volume expanders, large volumes of pentastarch will alter the coagulation mechanisms, inasmuch as a prolongation of prothrombin, partial thromboplastin and clotting times will occur. The physician should also be alert to the possibility of transient prolongation of bleeding time.

Hypersensitivity has been seen (wheezing, urticaria and hypotension). Anaphylactic/anaphylactoid reactions have been reported with pentastarch; a causal relationship has not been established. If hypersensitivity effects occur, discontinue the drug and, if necessary, administer appropriate therapy.

Pregnancy: Pentastarch has been shown to be embryocidal in New Zealand rabbits and in Swiss mice when given in doses 5 times the human dose. There are no adequate and well-controlled clinical studies using pentastarch in pregnant women. Pentastarch should not be used during pregnancy unless potential benefits justify the potential risk to the fetus.

Lactation: It is not known whether pentastarch is excreted in human milk. Because many drugs are excreted in human milk, caution should be exercised when pentastarch is administered to a nursing woman.

Children: The safety and effectiveness of pentastarch in children have not been established.

PRECAUTIONS: Pentastarch, like all plasma volume expanders, is not a substitute for red blood cells or coagulation factors in plasma.

The possibility of circulatory overload should be kept in mind.

Caution should be used when the risk of pulmonary edema and/or congestive heart failure is increased. Special care should be exercised in patients who have impaired renal clearance since this is the principal route by which pentastarch is eliminated.

The serum chemistries of 16 normal volunteers who were given pentastarch in doses of 500 to 2000 mL (2×1000 mL infusions on separate days) were essentially unchanged from pre- to 7 days post infusion, except for dilutional effects. There were no clinically significant abnormal values except for one creatinine phosphokinase level following an episode of venospasm. However, indirect bilirubin levels of 8.3 mg/L (normal 0 to 7 mg/L) have been reported in 2 out of 20 normal subjects who received multiple infusions of a 6% hetastarch product. Total bilirubin was within normal limits at all times; indirect bilirubin returned to normal by 96 hours following the final infusion. The significance, if any, of these elevations is not known; however, caution should be observed before administering pentastarch to patients with a history of liver disease.

Caution should be exercised when administering pentastarch to patients allergic to corn because such patients can also be allergic to pentastarch.

Elevated serum amylase levels may be observed temporarily following administration of pentastarch although no association with pancreatitis has been demonstrated. A 6% hetastarch injection product has not been shown to increase serum lipase. Similar effects may be expected with pentastarch.

ADVERSE EFFECTS: Coagulation disorders or hemorrhage have been reported in association with the use of pentastarch as a plasma volume expander. Headache, diarrhea, nausea, weakness, temporary weight gain, insomnia, fatigue, fever, edema, paresthesia, acne, malaise, shakiness, dizziness, chest pain, chills, nasal congestion, anxiety and increased heart rate have also been reported in clinical studies involving pentastarch.

It is uncertain whether any of these adverse experiences are attributable to the drug, medical procedures, concurrent adjunctive medication, or a combination of these factors.

Hypersensitivity has been seen (wheezing, urticaria and hypotension). Anaphylactic/anaphylactoid reactions have been reported with pentastarch (see Warnings).

OVERDOSE:

Treatment: The treatment of overdosage would be essentially symptomatic and supportive.

> For management of a suspected drug overdose, CPhA recommends that you contact your **regional Poison Control Centre**. See the *CPS* Directory section for a list of Poison Control Centres.

DOSAGE: Pentastarch is administered by i.v. infusion only. Total dosage and rate of infusion depend upon the amount of blood or plasma lost. In adults, the amount usually administered is 500 to 2000 mL. Total dosage does not usually exceed 2000 mL/day or approximately 28 mL/kg of body weight for the typical 70 kg patient. In acute hemorrhagic shock, an administration rate approaching 20 mL/kg/hour may be used. Use beyond 72 hours has not been studied.

Parenteral drug products should be inspected for particulate matter and discoloration prior to administration whenever solution and container permit.

The solution is intended for i.v. administration using sterile equipment. It is recommended that i.v. administration apparatus be replaced at least once every 24 hours.

Special Instructions: Caution: Before administering to patient, review these directions: Visual Checking: 1. Do not remove the plastic infusion container from its overwrap until immediately before use. 2. While the overwrap is intact, identify the solution (Pentaspan), lot number and expiration date. 3. Check that the solution is clear. 4. Inspect the intact unit for signs of obvious damage. If present, the unit should not be used.

Removal of Overwrap: A peelable area is located in the lower right hand corner of the unit (the label facing upward and the port facing downward). Pull apart the two edges. You can also tear at any notch located at either end of the unit. After removing overwrap, check for minute leaks by squeezing container firmly. If leaks are found, discard unit as sterility may be impaired.

Preparation for Administration (Use aseptic technique): 1. Close flow control clamp of administration set. 2. Twist off plug from port designated "Infusion Set Port". 3. Insert spike of infusion set into port with a twisting motion until the set is firmly sealed. 4. Suspend container from hanger. 5. Follow manufacturer's recommended procedures for the administration set. 6. Discontinue administration and notify physician immediately if patient exhibits signs of adverse reactions.

SUPPLIED: Each 100 mL of sterile, clear, pale yellow to amber-colored, nonpyrogenic solution contains: pentastarch 10 g, sodium chloride USP 0.9 g and water for injection USP qs. pH adjusted with sodium hydroxide to approximately 5.0. Approximate concentration of electrolytes (mEq/L): sodium 154, chloride 154. Calculated osmolality: approximately 326 mOsm/kg. Plastic, intravenous infusion bags of 250 and 500 mL. Exposure of pharmaceutical products to heat should be minimized. Avoid excessive heat. Protect from freezing. Store at room temperature (15 to 25°C).

Pentazocine Ⓝ

CPhA Monograph

see *Opioids*

Pentobarbital Ⓒ

CPhA Monograph

see *Barbiturates*

Pentothal® Ⓒ

thiopental sodium

I.V. Anesthetic

Hospira

Date of Preparation: March 31, 1997
Date of Revision: June 30, 2003

INDICATIONS: PENTOTHAL (Thiopental Sodium for Injection USP) is indicated as the sole anesthetic agent for brief (15-minute) procedures; for induction of anesthesia prior to administration of other anesthetic agents; to supplement regional anesthesia; to provide hypnosis during balanced anesthesia with other agents for analgesia or muscle relaxation; for the control of convulsive states during or following inhalation anesthesia, local anesthesia, or other causes; in neurosurgical patients with increased intracranial pressure, if adequate ventilation is provided; and for narcoanalysis and narcosynthesis in psychiatric disorders.

CONTRAINDICATIONS: Absolute Contraindications: Absence of suitable veins for i.v. administration; hypersensitivity (allergy) to barbiturates; variegate porphyria (South African) or acute intermittent porphyria; patients with severe respiratory embarrassment; status asthmaticus and; inflammatory conditions of the mouth, jaw, and neck.

Relative Contraindications: Severe cardiovascular disease; hypotension or shock; and conditions in which the hypnotic effect may be prolonged or potentiated-excessive premedication, Addison's disease, hepatic or renal dysfunction, myxedema, increased blood urea, severe anemia, asthma and myasthenia gravis.

Diluents in PENTOTHAL (Thiopental Sodium for Injection USP) Ready-to-Mix LifeShield Syringes should not be used for fluid replacement. Do not use unless diluent is clear and the syringe package is undamaged.

WARNINGS: Keep resuscitative and endotracheal intubation equipment and oxygen readily available. Maintain patency of the airway at all times.

This drug should be administered only by persons qualified in the use of i.v. anesthetics.

Avoid extravasation or intra-arterial injection.

May be habit forming.

I.V. administration of Sterile Water for Injection USP, without a solute, may result in hemolysis.

Use aseptic technique for preparing PENTOTHAL (Thiopental Sodium for Injection USP) solutions.

Administer only clear, reconstituted solutions.

Use within 24 hours after reconstitution. Discard unused portions.

PRECAUTIONS: General: A person competent in anesthesia management should be in constant attendance and adequate facilities for support of respiration and circulation should be available when PENTOTHAL (Thiopental Sodium for Injection USP) is being used.

Observe aseptic precautions at all times in preparation and handling of Thiopental Sodium for Injection USP solutions.

If used in conditions involving relative contraindications, reduce dosage and administer slowly.

Thiopental Sodium for Injection USP should be administered with caution to patients with pre-existing hypotension or in conditions where the hypnotic effect may be prolonged or intensified, such as in the presence of liver disease and renal disease.

Care should be taken in administering the drug to patients with advanced cardiac disease, increased intracranial pressure, ophtalmoplegia, asthma, myasthenia gravis and endocrine insufficiency (pituitary, thyroid, adrenal, pancreas).

<u>*Drug Interactions:*</u> The following drug interactions have been reported with thiopental (see Table 1).

Table 1: PENTOTHAL

Drug Interactions

Drug	Effect
Probenecid	Prolonged action of thiopental
Diazoxide	Hypotension
Opioid analgesics	Decreased antinociceptive action
Aminophylline	Thiopental antagonism
Midazolam	Synergism
Sulfisoxazole (i.v.)	Reduced thiopental dosage requirements

Pregnancy: It is not known whether Thiopental Sodium for Injection USP can cause fetal harm when administered to a pregnant woman or can affect reproductive capacity. Thiopental Sodium for Injection USP should be given to a pregnant woman only if clearly needed.

Lactation: Thiopental sodium readily crosses the placenta barrier and small amounts may appear in the milk of nursing mothers following administration of large doses.

ADVERSE EFFECTS: Adverse reactions include respiratory depression, myocardial depression, cardiac arrhythmias, prolonged somnolence and recovery, hypotension, tachycardia, sneezing, coughing, bronchospasm, laryngospasm and shivering. Anaphylactic and anaphylactoid reactions to PENTOTHAL(Thiopental Sodium for Injection USP) have been reported. Symptoms, e.g., urticaria, bronchospasm, vasodilation and edema should be managed by conventional means.

Hypersensitivity reactions to barbiturates, including thiopental sodium have been reported.

Rarely, immune hemolytic anemia with renal failure and radial nerve palsy have been reported.

Reactions which may occur because of the diluents, technique of preparation or mixing, or administration of reconstituted solutions of Thiopental Sodium for Injection USP include febrile response or infection at the site of injection, venous thrombosis or phlebitis extending from the site of injection and extravasation.

If an adverse reaction does occur, discontinue the injection, evaluate the patient, institute appropriate therapeutic countermeasures and save the remainder of unused solution (or the used container or syringe) for examination if deemed necessary.

OVERDOSE:

Symptoms: Overdosage may occur from too rapid or repeated injections. Too rapid injection may be followed by an alarming fall in blood pressure even to shock levels. Apnea, occasional laryngospasm, coughing and other respiratory difficulties with excessive or too rapid injections may occur. In the event of suspected or apparent overdosage, the drug should be discontinued, a patent airway established (intubate if necessary) or maintained, and oxygen should be administered, with assisted ventilation if necessary. The lethal dose of barbiturates varies and cannot be stated with certainty. Lethal blood level may be as low as 1 mg/100 mL for short-acting barbiturates; less if other depressant drugs or alcohol are also present.

Cardiovascular collapse may also follow too rapid injection or overdosage. Treatment should be directed toward supporting the blood pressure and using volume expansion and/or vasopressor agents as appropriate.

Treatment: It is generally agreed that respiratory depression or arrest, due to unusual sensitivity to thiopental sodium or overdosage, is easily managed if there is no concomitant respiratory obstruction. If the airway is patent, any method of ventilating the lungs (that prevents hypoxia) should be successful in maintaining other vital functions. Since depression of respiratory activity is one of the characteristic actions of the drug, it is important to observe respiration closely.

Should laryngospasm occur, it may be relieved by one of the usual methods, such as the use of a relaxant drug or positive pressure oxygen. Endotracheal intubation may be indicated in difficult cases.

For management of a suspected drug overdose, CPhA recommends that you contact your **regional Poison Control Centre**. See the *CPS* Directory section for a list of Poison Control Centres.

DOSAGE: PENTOTHAL (Thiopental Sodium for Injection USP) is administered by i.v. route only. Individual response to the drug is so varied that there can be no fixed dosage. The drug should be titrated against patient requirements as governed by age, sex and body weight. Younger patients require relatively larger doses than middle-aged and elderly persons: the latter metabolize the drug more slowly. Prepuberty requirements are the same for both sexes, but adult females require less than adult males. Dose is usually proportional to body weight and obese patients require a larger dose than relatively lean persons of the same weight.

Reconstituted solutions of thiopental sodium should be inspected visually for particular matter and discoloration, whenever solution and container permit.

Premedication: Premedication usually consists of atropine or scopolamine to suppress vagal reflexes and inhibit secretions. In addition, a barbiturate or an opiate is often given. Pentobarbital Sodium Injection USP (Nembutal) is suggested because it provides a preliminary indication of how the patient will react to barbiturate anesthesia. Ideally, the peak effect of these medications should be reached shortly before the time of induction.

Test Dose: It is advisable to inject a small "test" dose of 25 to 75 mg: (1 to 3 mL of a 2.5% solution) of (Thiopental Sodium for Injection USP) to assess tolerance or unusual sensitivity to Thiopental Sodium for Injection USP, and pause to observe patient reaction for at least 60 seconds. If unexpectedly deep anesthesia develops or if respiratory depression occurs, consider these possibilities: the patient may be unusually sensitive to Thiopental Sodium for Injection USP, the solution may be more concentrated than had been assumed, or the patient may have received too much premedication.

Anesthesia: Moderately slow induction can usually be accomplished in the "average" adult by injection of 50 to 75 mg (2 to 3 mL of a 2.5% solution) at intervals of 20 to 40 seconds, depending on the reaction of the patient. Once anesthesia is established, additional injections of 25 to 50 mg can be given whenever the patient moves.

Slow injection is recommended to minimize respiratory depression and the possibility of overdosage. The smallest dose consistent with attaining the surgical objective is the desired goal. Momentary apnea following each injection is typical, and progressive decrease in the amplitude of respiration appears with increasing dosage. Pulse remains normal or increases slightly and returns to normal. Blood pressure usually falls slightly and returns toward normal. Muscles usually relax about 30 seconds after unconsciousness is attained, but this may be masked if a skeletal muscle relaxant is used. The tone of jaw muscles is a fairly reliable index. The pupils may dilate but later contract: sensitivity to light is not usually lost until a level of anesthesia deep enough to permit surgery is attained. Nystagmus and divergent strabismus are characteristic during early stages, but at the level of surgical anesthesia, the eyes are central and fixed. Corneal and conjunctival reflexes disappear during surgical anesthesia.

When (Thiopental Sodium for Injection USP) is used for induction in balanced anesthesia with a skeletal muscle relaxant and an inhalation agent, the total dose of Thiopental Sodium for Injection USP can be estimated and then injected in two to four fractional doses. With this technique, brief periods of apnea may occur which may require assisted or controlled pulmonary ventilation. As an initial dose, 210 to 280 mg (3 to 4 mg/kg) of Thiopental Sodium for Injection USP is usually required for rapid induction in the average adult (70 kg).

When Thiopental Sodium for Injection USP is used as the sole anesthetic agent, the desired level of anesthesia can be maintained by injection of small, repeated doses as needed or by using a continuous intravenous drip in a 0.2% or 0.4% concentration. (Sterile Water should not be used as the diluent in these concentrations, since hemolysis will occur. Solutions may be prepared with 5% Dextrose in water, Sodium Chloride Injection or Normosol-R.) With continuous drip, the depth of anesthesia is controlled by adjusting the rate of infusion.

Convulsive States: For the control of convulsive states following anesthesia (inhalation or local) or other causes, 75 to 125 mg (3 to 5 mL of a 2.5% solution) should be given as soon as possible after the convulsion begins. Convulsions following the use of a local anesthetic may require 125 to 250 mg of Thiopental Sodium for Injection USP, given over a ten-minute period. If the convulsion is caused by a local anesthetic, the required dose of Thiopental Sodium for Injection USP will depend upon the amount of local anesthetic given and its convulsant properties.

Neurosurgical Patients with Increased Intracranial Pressure: In neurosurgical patients, intermittent bolus injections of 1.5 to 3.5 mg/kg of body weight may be given to reduce intraoperative elevations of intracranial pressure, if adequate ventilation is provided.

Psychiatric Disorders: For narcoanalysis and narcosynthesis in psychiatric disorders, premedication with an anticholinergic agent may precede administration of Thiopental Sodium for Injection USP. After a test dose, Thiopental Sodium for Injection USP is injected at a slow rate of 100 mg/min (4 mL/min of a 2.5% solution) with the patient counting backwards from 100. Shortly after counting, the patient becomes confused but before actual sleep is produced, the injection is discontinued. Allow the patient to return to a semidrowsy state where conversation is coherent. Alternatively, Thiopental Sodium for Injection USP may be administered by rapid i.v. drip using a 0.2% concentration in 5 % Dextrose in water. At this concentration, the rate of administration should not exceed 50 mL/min.

Management of Some Complications: Respiratory depression (hypoventilation, apnea), which may result from either unusual responsiveness to PENTOTHAL (Thiopental Sodium for Injection USP) or overdosage, is managed as stated above. Thiopental Sodium for Injection USP should be considered to have the same potential for producing respiratory depression as an inhalation agent, and patency of the airway must be protected at all times.

Laryngospasm may occur with light Thiopental Sodium for Injection USP narcosis at intubation, or in the absence of intubation if foreign matter or secretions in the respiratory tract create irritation. Laryngeal and bronchial vagal reflexes can be suppressed, and secretions minimized by giving atropine or scopolamine premedication and a barbiturate or opiate. Use of a skeletal muscle relaxant or positive pressure oxygen will usually relieve laryngospasm. Tracheotomy may be indicated in difficult cases.

Myocardial depression, proportional to the amount of drug in direct contact with the heart, can occur and may cause hypotension, particularly in patients with an unhealthy myocardium. Arrhythmias may appear if P_{CO_2} is elevated, but they are uncommon with adequate ventilation. Management of myocardial depression is the same as for overdosage. Thiopental does not sensitize the heart to epinephrine or other sympathomimetic amines.

Extravascular infiltration should be avoided. Care should be taken to insure that the needle is within the lumen of the vein before injection of Thiopental Sodium for Injection USP. Extravascular injection may cause chemical irritation of the tissues varying from slight tenderness to venospasm, extensive necrosis and sloughing. This is due primarily to the high alkalinity (pH 10 to 11) of clinical concentrations of the drug. If extravasation occurs, the local irritant effects can be reduced by injection of 1 % procaine locally to relieve pain and enhance vasodilatation. Local application of heat also may help to increase local circulation and removal of the infiltrate.

Intra-arterial injection can occur inadvertently, especially if an aberrant superficial artery is present at the medial aspect of the antecubital fossa. The area selected for i.v. injection of the drug should be palpated for detection of an underlying pulsating vessel. Accidental intra-arterial injection can cause arteriospasm and severe pain along the course of the artery with blanching of the arm and fingers. Appropriate corrective measures should be instituted promptly to avoid possible development of gangrene. Any patient complaint of pain warrants stopping the injection. Methods suggested for dealing with this complication vary with the severity of symptoms. The following have been suggested: Dilute the injected PENTOTHAL by removing the tourniquet and any restrictive garments; leave the needle in place, if possible; inject the artery with a dilute solution of papaverine, 40 to 80 mg, or 10 mL of 1% procaine, to inhibit smooth muscle spasm; if necessary, perform sympathetic block of the brachial plexus and/or stellate ganglion to relieve pain and assist in opening collateral circulation (papaverine can be injected into subclavian artery, if desired); unless otherwise contraindicated, institute immediate heparinization to prevent thrombus formation; consider local infiltration of an alpha-adrenergic blocking agent such as phentolamine into the vasospastic area; and provide additional symptomatic treatment as required.

Shivering after Thiopental Sodium for Injection USP anesthesia, manifested by twitching face muscles and occasional progression to tremors of the arms, head, shoulders and body, is a thermal reaction due to increased sensitivity to cold. Shivering appears if the room environment is cold and if a large ventilatory heat loss has been sustained with balanced inhalation anesthesia employing nitrous oxide. Treatment consists of warming the patient with blankets, maintaining room temperature near 22°C, and administration of chlorpromazine or methylphenidate.

Reconstitution of Solutions: PENTOTHAL (Thiopental Sodium for Injection USP) is supplied as a sterile, yellowish, hygroscopic powder stabilized with anhydrous sodium carbonate as a buffer.

The diluent (0.9% Sodium Chloride Injection, USP) in PENTOTHAL Ready-to-Mix Lifeshield Syringes is supplied in a separate container to allow for mixing with the PENTOTHAL in the powder vial to permit immediate i.v. injection of reconstituted solution into a vein or attachment to a standard stopcock assembly.

Since PENTOTHAL contains no added bacteriostatic agent, extreme care in preparation and handling should be exercised at all times to prevent the introduction of microbial contaminants. Solutions should be **freshly prepared** and used promptly. Reconstituted solutions of Thiopental Sodium for Injection USP may be kept, tightly stoppered, under refrigeration up to 24 hours, unused portions should be discarded after 24 hours. Sterilization by heating should not be attempted.

Directions for Preparing the PENTOTHAL (Thiopental Sodium for Injection USP) solutions, excluding Ready-to-Mix Lifeshield Syringes: Solutions should be prepared **aseptically** with 1 of the 3 following diluents: Sterile Water for Injection, USP, sodium chloride injection, USP, or 5% dextrose injection, USP. Clinical concentrations used for intermittent i.v. administration vary between 2 and 5%. A 2 or 2.5% solution is most commonly used. A 3.4% concentration in sterile water for injection is isotonic; concentrations less than 2% in this diluent are not used because they cause hemolysis. For continuous i.v. drip administration, concentrations of 0.2 or 0.4% are used. Solutions may be prepared by adding Pentothal to 5% dextrose injection, USP, sodium chloride injection, USP, or Normosol R pH 7.4. Calculations for various concentrations of PENTOTHAL are listed in Table 2.

Table 2: PENTOTHAL

Calculations For Various Concentrations

Concentration Desired		Amounts to Use: PENTOTHAL	Diluent
%	**mg/mL**	**g**	**mL**
0.2	2	1	500
0.4	4	1	250
		2	500
2.0	20	1	50
		5	250
		10	500
2.5	25	0.5	20
		1	40
		5	200
5	50	1	20
		5	100

Directions for Preparing the PENTOTHAL (Thiopental Sodium for Injection USP) Ready-to-Mix Lifeshield Syringes: Use aseptic technique: Do not assemble until ready to use.

1. Remove piercing pin from pouch. Remove cover from piercing pin. Remove fliptop from diluent vial. Swab stopper. While holding the diluent vial on a flat surface, insert the piercing pin into the target area of the stopper with a downward twisting motion.
2. Remove purple caps from powder vial and phlange end of injector. Insert powder vial into injector and rotate clockwise approximately three turns.
3. Remove covers from luer ends of piercing pin and injector. Push piercing pin onto luer end of injector and turn clockwise until secure.
4. Position syringe upright and transfer diluent into powder vial by slowly pulling back on powder vial. **Do not displace air into the diluent vial by pushing on the powder vial, as this may cause leakage through the vent in the piercing pin.**
5. When all of the diluent has been transferred, remove piercing pin and empty diluent vial together and discard. Replace luer end cover of injector. Shake until powder is completely dissolved.
6. **Use reconstituted solution only if it is clear, free from precipitate and not discolored.**

For intravenous use. Medication, fluid path and needle are sterile if caps and protective covers are undisturbed and package is intact. Component exteriors are not sterile. Single-dose unit. Discard unused portion.

Compatibility: **Any solution of thiopental sodium for injection usp with a visible precipitate should be discarded.** The stability of Thiopental Sodium for Injection USP solutions depends upon several factors, including the diluent, temperature of storage and the amount of carbon dioxide from room air that gains access to the solution. Any factor or condition which tends to lower pH (increased acidity) of Thiopental Sodium for Injection USP solutions will increase the likelihood of precipitation of thiopental acid. Such factors include the use of diluents which are too acidic and the absorption of carbon dioxide, which can combine with water to form carbonic acid.

Solutions of succinylcholine, tubocurarine or other drugs which have an acid pH should not be mixed with Thiopental Sodium for Injection USP solutions. The most stable solutions are those reconstituted in water or isotonic saline, kept under refrigeration and tightly stoppered.

SUPPLIED: Combination Kits: 500 mg/vial: Each kit contains: one 500 mg thiopental sodium vial with sodium carbonate as buffer and one 20 mL vial of water for injection to provide 2.5% solution after reconstitution. Packages of 25 kits. Store between 15 and 25°C. Protect from freezing. Avoid excessive heat (above 38°C).

1 g/vial: Each kit contains: one 1 g thiopental sodium vial with sodium carbonate as buffer and one 50 mL vial of water for injection to provide a 2% solution after reconstitution. To obtain a 2.5% solution after reconstitution, use only 40 mL of water for injection. Packages of 25 kits. Store between 15 and 25°C. Protect from freezing. Avoid excessive heat (above 38°C).

Vials: 500 mg: Each vial of sterile, yellowish, hydroscopic powder for injection, stabilized with anydrous sodium carbonate as a buffer, contains: thiopental sodium 500 mg. Packages of 25 vials. Store at controlled room temperature (15 to 25°C).

1 g: Each vial of sterile, yellowish, hydroscopic powder for injection, stabilized with anydrous sodium carbonate as buffer, contains: thiopental sodium 1 g. Packages of 25 vials. Store at controlled room temperature (15 to 25°C).

Ready to Mix Syringes: Each single dose unit contains: thiopental sodium powder 500 mg accompanied with 20 mL of diluent, providing a reconstituted concentration of 2.5%. Store at controlled room temperature (15 to 30°C). Protect from freezing. Avoid excessive heat and high temperatures (above 38°C).

Pepcid AC®

famotidine

Histamine H2-Receptor Antagonist

Johnson & Johnson • Merck

PHARMACOLOGY: Famotidine is a competitive inhibitor of histamine H_2-receptors. The primary clinically important pharmacologic activity of famotidine is inhibition of gastric juice secretion. Famotidine reduces the acid and pepsin content, as well as the volume, of basal, nocturnal, and stimulated gastric secretion.

Pharmacokinetics: Famotidine is incompletely absorbed. The bioavailability of oral doses is 40 to 45%. The bioavailability of the 10 mg chewable tablet was found to be equivalent to the 10 mg film-coated tablet. Bioavailability may be slightly increased by food; however, this effect is of no clinical significance. Bioavailability of Pepcid AC at recommended doses is not affected by customary doses of antacids. Famotidine undergoes minimal first-pass metabolism. After oral doses, peak plasma levels occur in 1 to 3 hours.

C_{max} values of 41 ng/mL and 40 ng/mL for the 10 mg film-coated and chewable tablet, respectively, were found in 1 bioequivalence study. Plasma levels after multiple doses are similar to those after single doses. Fifteen to 20% of famotidine in plasma is protein bound. Famotidine has an elimination half-life of 2.5 to 3.5 hours. Famotidine is eliminated by renal (65 to 70%) and metabolic (30 to 35%) routes. Renal clearance is 250 to 450 mL/min, indicating some tubular excretion.

Twenty-five to 30% of an oral dose and 65 to 70% of an i.v. dose are recovered in the urine as unchanged compound. The only metabolite identified in man is the S-oxide. There is a close relationship between creatinine clearance values and the elimination half-life of famotidine. In patients with severe renal insufficiency, i.e., creatinine clearance less than 10 mL/min, elimination half-life of famotidine may exceed 20 hours (see Dosage). In elderly patients, there are no clinically significant age-related changes in the pharmacokinetics of famotidine.

INDICATIONS: The treatment of the following conditions where a controlled reduction of gastric secretion is required, such as acid indigestion, heartburn, sour or upset stomach. It is also indicated for the prevention of these symptoms when associated with the consumption of food and/or beverage including nocturnal symptoms associated with the evening meal and expected to cause sleep disturbance.

CONTRAINDICATIONS: Hypersensitivity to any component of this medication.

Cross-sensitivity in this class of compounds has been observed. Therefore, famotidine should not be administered to patients with a history of hypersensitivity to other H_2-receptor antagonists.

WARNINGS: No data supplied by the manufacturer.

PRECAUTIONS: General: In clinical trials, patients with other underlying acid gastrointestinal diseases (e.g., duodenal ulcer, gastric ulcer) did not experience complications; in general, they did not exhibit a clinically significant deterioration in their condition. However, if patients have difficulty swallowing or if abdominal discomfort persists, the underlying cause should be determined. Symptomatic response to therapy with famotidine does not preclude the presence of gastric malignancy.

Patients with severe kidney disease, previous history of ulcer disease complications, severe coexisting illness, those who are experiencing unintended weight loss in association with dyspeptic symptoms, and those who are middle-aged or older with new or recently changed dyspeptic symptoms should consult a physician before commencing therapy with famotidine.

Patients consuming NSAIDs may have dyspepsia as a side effect of these medicines and should consult a physician or a pharmacist before taking famotidine.

Therapy should not exceed 2 weeks of continuous treatment without medical consultation.

Drug Interactions: Studies with famotidine in man, in animal models, and in vitro have shown no significant interference with the disposition of compounds metabolized by the hepatic microsomal enzymes, e.g., cytochrome P450 system. Compounds tested in man have included warfarin, theophylline, phenytoin, diazepam, aminopyrine and antipyrine. Indocyanine green as an index of hepatic blood flow and/or hepatic drug extraction has been tested and no significant effects have been found.

Concomitant use of aluminum hydroxide/magnesium hydroxide at commonly used doses, does not influence the pharmacodynamics or bioavailability of Pepcid AC. Famotidine does not affect gastric alcohol dehydrogenase and, consequently, blood ethanol levels.

Pregnancy: Reproductive studies have been performed in rats and rabbits at oral doses of up to 2000 and 500 mg/kg/day, respectively (approximately 2500 and 625 times the maximum recommended prescription human dose [80 mg], respectively), and have revealed no evidence of impaired fertility or harm to the fetus due to famotidine. There are, however, no adequate or well-controlled studies in pregnant women.

Since the safe use of famotidine in pregnant women has not been established, pregnant women should not use famotidine unless directed otherwise by a physician.

Lactation: Famotidine is detectable in human milk. Nursing mothers should either stop this drug or should stop nursing.

Children: Safety and effectiveness in children have not been established. Pepcid AC should not be administered to children under 12 years of age.

Geriatrics: No dosage adjustment is required based on age (see Pharmacology, Pharmacokinetics).

ADVERSE EFFECTS: Famotidine has been demonstrated to be generally well tolerated. Adverse reactions reported in ≥1% of patients were headache and dizziness. These occurred with comparable frequency in patients treated with placebo.

Laboratory parameters may be affected during treatment with famotidine, but the changes are usually not considered serious. Among the laboratory changes that were reported during clinical trials were increases in AST, ALT, and WBC count, and decreases in hemoglobin and hematocrit. These changes were rarely of clinical significance.

No famotidine-treated patients/subjects had to be discontinued from therapy because of laboratory adverse experiences.

During marketed use of prescription doses, which are higher than those recommended for nonprescription use, the following adverse reactions have been reported; urticaria, liver enzyme abnormalities, cholestatic jaundice, anaphylaxis, angioedema. Toxic epidermal necrolysis has been reported very rarely with H_2-receptor antagonists.

The following adverse reactions have been reported; however, a causal relationship to therapy with famotidine has not been established: agitation, confusion, hallucinations, grand mal seizures, rare cases of impotence, thrombocytopenia, pancytopenia, leukopenia and agranulocytosis.

Gynecomastia has been reported rarely. In most cases that were followed up, it was reversible after discontinuing treatment.

OVERDOSE:

There is no experience to date with deliberate overdosage. Doses of up to 800 mg/day have been employed in patients with pathological hypersecretory conditions with no serious adverse effects.

Treatment: In the event of overdosage, treatment should be symptomatic and supportive. Unabsorbed material should be removed from the gastrointestinal tract, the patient should be monitored, and supportive therapy should be employed.

The oral LD_{50} of famotidine in male and female rats and mice was >5000 mg/kg.

> For management of a suspected drug overdose, CPhA recommends that you contact your **regional Poison Control Centre**. See the *CPS* Directory section for a list of Poison Control Centres.

DOSAGE: Adults and children 12 years of age or older: 10 mg, as required to relieve symptoms.

For prevention of acid-related symptoms associated with the consumption of food and/or beverage: 10 mg 10 to 15 minutes before eating. Repeat if symptoms return, up to a maximum of 20 mg in a 24-hour period.

Therapy should not exceed 2 weeks of continuous treatment without medical consultation.

Concomitant Use with Antacids: Antacids may be given concomitantly if needed.

INFORMATION FOR THE PATIENT: Published in e-CPS, available by subscription at www.e-cps.ca.

SUPPLIED: Each rounded-square, pale rose (pink) colored, film-coated tablet, with Pepcid AC embossed on one side, contains: famotidine 10 mg. Nonmedicinal ingredients: hydroxypropyl cellulose, hypromellose, magnesium stearate, microcrystalline cellulose, red ferric oxide, starch, talc and titanium dioxide. Boxes of 6, 18, 30 and 60 individually packaged in blisters. Store at room temperature (15 to 30°C). Protect from moisture.

Pepcid® AC, Maximum Strength

famotidine

Histamine H2-Receptor Antagonist

Johnson & Johnson • Merck

Date of Preparation: September 4, 1986
Date of Revision: November 16, 2005

PHARMACOLOGY: PEPCID (famotidine) is a competitive inhibitor of histamine H_2-receptors. The primary clinically important pharmacologic activity of MAXIMUM STRENGTH PEPCID AC is inhibition of gastric juice secretion. MAXIMUM STRENGTH PEPCID AC reduces the acid and pepsin content, as well as the volume, of basal, nocturnal, and stimulated gastric secretion.

Pharmacokinetics: Famotidine exhibits a linear pharmacokinetic profile for AUC and gastric pH in the 5- to 40-mg range. In this same range, associations have been demonstrated between mean plasma famotidine concentrations and mean inhibition of meal stimulated acid secretion. However "area under the gastric pH-time curve" has not been shown to be directly associated or correlated with heartburn relief.

Clinical studies have demonstrated that: MAXIMUM STRENGTH PEPCID AC famotidine 20 mg prevents heartburn in patients with moderate to severe symptoms when taken before a meal. A dose response is demonstrated between 10 mg famotidine and 20 mg famotidine in successfully preventing acid-related symptoms and effectively relieving heartburn.

INDICATIONS: MAXIMUM STRENGTH PEPCID AC 20 mg is indicated in the treatment of conditions where a controlled reduction of gastric secretion is required, such as heartburn, acid indigestion, sour or upset stomach. MAXIMUM STRENGTH PEPCID AC is also indicated for the prevention of these symptoms when associated with the consumption of food and/or beverage including nocturnal symptoms associated with the evening meal and expected to cause sleep disturbance

CONTRAINDICATIONS: Hypersensitivity to any component of this medication. Cross sensitivity in this class of compounds has been observed. Therefore, MAXIMUM STRENGTH PEPCID AC should not be administered to patients with a history of hypersensitivity to other histamine H_2 receptor antagonists (H2RAs).

WARNINGS: No data supplied by the manufacturer.

PRECAUTIONS: General: In clinical trials, patients with other underlying acid gastrointestinal diseases (e.g. duodenal ulcer, gastric ulcer) did not experience complications; in general, they did not exhibit a clinically significant deterioration in their condition. However, if patients have difficulty swallowing, pain on swallowing, unexpected weight loss, vomiting of blood or passage of blood in the stools or if abdominal discomfort persists, the underlying cause should be determined. Symptomatic response to therapy with MAXIMUM STRENGTH PEPCID AC (famotidine) does not preclude the presence of gastric malignancy.

Patients with severe kidney disease, previous history of ulcer disease complications, severe coexisting illness, those who are experiencing unintended weight loss in association with dyspeptic symptoms, and those who are middle aged or older with new or recently changed dyspeptic symptoms should consult a physician before commencing therapy with MAXIMUM STRENGTH PEPCID AC.

Patients consuming nonsteroidal anti inflammatory drugs may have dyspepsia as a side effect of these medicines and should consult a physician or a pharmacist before taking MAXIMUM STRENGTH PEPCID AC.

Further medical evaluation is required if therapy exceeds two weeks of continuous treatment, if two 14 day courses of treatment are needed at intervals of less than 6 weeks, or if heartburn is frequent (>3 times per week) and/or severe.

Patients with Moderate or Severe Renal Insufficiency: Since CNS adverse effects have been reported in patients with moderate and severe renal insufficiency, longer intervals between doses or lower doses may need to be used in patients with moderate (creatinine clearance 30-50 mL/min) or severe (creatinine clearance <30 mL/min) renal insufficiency to adjust for the longer elimination half-life of famotidine (see Dosage).

Drug Interactions: Studies with famotidine in man, in animal models, and in vitro have shown no significant interference with the disposition of compounds metabolized by the hepatic microsomal enzymes, e.g., cytochrome P450 system. Compounds tested in man have included warfarin, theophylline, phenytoin, diazepam, aminopyrine and antipyrine. Indocyanine green as an index of hepatic blood flow and/or hepatic drug extraction has been tested and no significant effects have been found.

Concomitant use of aluminum hydroxide/magnesium hydroxide at commonly used doses, does not influence the pharmacodynamics or bioavailability of MAXIMUM STRENGTH PEPCID AC. Famotidine does not affect gastric alcohol dehydrogenase and, consequently, blood ethanol levels.

Pregnancy: Reproductive studies have been performed in rats and rabbits at oral doses of up to 2000 and 500 mg/kg/day, respectively (approximately 2500 and 625 times the maximum recommended prescription human dose [80 mg], respectively), and have revealed no evidence of impaired fertility or harm to the fetus due to famotidine. There are, however, no adequate or well controlled studies in pregnant women.

Since the safe use of MAXIMUM STRENGTH PEPCID AC in pregnant women has not been established, pregnant women should not use MAXIMUM STRENGTH PEPCID AC unless directed otherwise by a physician.

Lactation: Famotidine is detectable in human milk. Nursing mothers should either stop this drug or should stop nursing.

Children: Safety and effectiveness in children have not been established. MAXIMUM STRENGTH PEPCID AC should not be administered to children under 12 years of age.

Geriatrics: No dosage adjustment is required based on age. This drug is known to be substantially excreted by the kidney, and the risk of toxic reactions to this drug may be greater in patients with impaired renal function. Because elderly patients are more likely to have decreased renal function, care should be taken in dose selection, and it may be useful to monitor renal function (see Precautions, Patients with Moderate or Severe Renal Insufficiency and Dosage, Dosage Adjustment for Patients with Moderate or Severe Renal Insufficiency).

ADVERSE EFFECTS: MAXIMUM STRENGTH PEPCID AC 20 mg (famotidine) has been demonstrated to be generally well tolerated. The following adverse reactions have been reported in ≥1% of patients using MAXIMUM STRENGTH PEPCID AC in controlled clinical trials (prevention or treatment): headache (6.9%), diarrhea (2.9%), upper respiratory infection (2.9%), vomiting (2.4%), constipation (2.0%), nausea (2.0%), pharyngitis (2.0%), flu-like illness (1.6%), back pain (1.2%) and rash (1.2%). These occurred with comparable frequency across treatment groups and control groups.

Other reactions reported in patients using MAXIMUM STRENGTH PEPCID AC in controlled clinical trials at rates <1%. These observations are listed.

Body as Whole/Site Unspecified 1.0%: asthenia/fatigue 0.1%; pain–abdominal 0.3%; pain–chest 0.1%. Each of the following at <0.1%: fever, infection-viral, pain-pelvic.

Cardiovascular System 0.2%: Each of the following at <0.1%: extravasation, premature atrial contraction, premature ventricular contraction.

Digestive System 1.7%: dyspepsia 0.1%. Each of the following at <0.1% : erosive esophagitis, esophagitis, gingivitis and glossodynia.

Musculoskeletal System 0.5%: myalgia 0.1%; pain–shoulder 0.1%. Each of the following at <0.1%: pain–foot, pain–knee, pain–neck.

Nervous System and Psychiatric 2.4%: anxiety 0.1%; dizziness 0.1%. Each of the following at <0.1%: agitation, migraine.

Respiratory System 1.3%: sinusitis 0.1%. Each of the following at <0.1%: bronchitis, congestion-nasal, cough, dry throat, influenza, sinus disorder, sneezing, wheezing.

Skin and Skin Appendages 0.4%: Each of the following at <0.1% edema–angioneurotic, infection–skin, laceration, measles.

Special Senses 0.2%: Each of the following at <0.1%: eustachian tube disorder, hemorrhage–corneal, pain–ear.

Urogenital System 0.4%: mass, breast 0.1%. Each of the following at <0.1%: benign prostatic hypertrophy, dysuria, hematuria, impotence, menstruation disorder, urinary frequency.

Laboratory parameters may be affected during treatment with PEPCID famotidine, but the changes are usually not considered serious. Among the laboratory changes reported during clinical trials were increases in AST, ALT, BUN, WBC count and serum creatinine, and decreases in hemoglobin and hematocrit. These changes were rarely of clinical significance.

No famotidine treated patients/subjects had to be discontinued from therapy because of laboratory adverse experiences.

During marketed use of prescription doses of famotidine, the following adverse reactions have been reported; urticaria, liver enzymes abnormalities, cholestatic jaundice, anaphylaxis, angioedema. Toxic epidermal necrolysis has been reported very rarely with H_2-receptor antagonists. As with other H_2-receptor antagonists, cases of bradycardia, A-V block and other arrhythmia have been reported rarely in patients treated with famotidine.

The following adverse reactions have been reported; however, a causal relationship to therapy with PEPCID famotidine has not been established: agitation, confusion, hallucinations, depression, disorientation, mental disorder, insomnia, psychotic disorder, pruritus, alopecia, photosensitivity, Steven-Johnson syndrome, hypotrichosis, neutropenia, anaemia, paraesthesia, dysgeusia, convulsions, syncope, grand mal seizures, rare cases of impotence, thrombocytopenia, pancytopenia, leukopenia, bone marrow depression and agranulocytosis.

Gynecomastia has been reported rarely. In most cases that were followed up, it was reversible after discontinuing treatment.

OVERDOSE:

Symptoms: Doses of up to 800 mg/day have been employed in patients with pathological hypersecretory conditions with no serious adverse effects. In the event of overdosage, treatment should be symptomatic and supportive. Unabsorbed material should be removed from the gastrointestinal tract, the patient should be monitored, and supportive therapy should be employed.

The oral LD50 of famotidine in male and female rats and mice was >5000 mg/kg.

Intentional exposure is defined as a purposeful action in patients who use a substance inappropriately for self-destructive or manipulative reasons, including suicides, suicide gestures, and attempts. The inappropriate use of famotidine (single agent) or with other agents for suicide attempts is very uncommon. There have been no reports that identified an overdose fatality with famotidine (single agent) or taken with other agents. For all overdose exposures, the duration of clinical effects, considered moderate or major, resolved in ≤3 days, the large majority and single-agent famotidine exposures resolved in ≤24 hours.

According to data from the Toxic Exposure Surveillance System (TESS) of the American Association of Poison Control Centers (AAPCC), of the single-agent famotidine exposures, the most common cardiovascular symptom was tachycardia (0.3%). For neurological symptoms, the proportions of subjects who experienced drowsiness/lethargy was 1.5%; headache, 0.6%; dizziness/vertigo, 1.0%; and agitated/irritable, 0.5%. Abdominal pain (1.9%), nausea (1.2%), vomiting (1.6%), and diarrhea (1.0%) were observed as gastrointestinal side effects. It is not known the extent to which the use of an emetic in hospital emergency rooms may have contributed to the occurrence of the symptoms nausea and vomiting.

Treatment: See Symptoms.

For management of a suspected drug overdose, CPhA recommends that you contact your **regional Poison Control Centre**. See the *CPS* Directory section for a list of Poison Control Centres.

DOSAGE: Adults and Children 12 Years of Age or Older: The patient should take one tablet for relief of heartburn, acid indigestion and sour or upset stomach. To prevent these symptoms, one tablet should be taken 10-15 minutes before a meal. The patient should not take more than 1 tablet at a time and the patient should not take more than two tablets in 24 hours. Therapy should not exceed two weeks of continuous treatment without medical consultation.

Concomitant Use with Other Medications: Antacids may be given concomitantly if needed. It is not appropriate to use this product and other H2RAs concomitantly.

Dosage Adjustment for Patients with Moderate or Severe Renal Insufficiency: In patients with moderate (creatinine clearance 30-50 mL/min) or severe (creatinine clearance <30 mL/min) renal insufficiency, the elimination half life of PEPCID famotidine is increased. For patients with severe renal insufficiency, it may exceed 20 hours, reaching approximately 24 hours in anuric patients. Since CNS adverse reactions have been reported in patients with moderate and severe renal insufficiency, to avoid excess accumulation of the drug in patients with moderate or severe renal insufficiency, the dose of PEPCID famotidine may be reduced to half the dose or the dosing interval may be prolonged to 36-48 hours as indicated by the patient's clinical response.

INFORMATION FOR THE PATIENT: Published in e-CPS, available by subscription at www.e-cps.ca.

SUPPLIED: Each white, "D" shaped, film-coated tablet, PAC20 debossed one side and blank on the other contains: famotidine 20 mg. Nonmedicinal ingredients: carnauba wax, hydroxypropyl cellulose, hypromellose, magnesium stearate, microcrystalline cellulose, starch, talc and titanium dioxide. Boxes of 5 and 25, packaged in blisters. Pouches of 1 tablet. Store at room temperature (15-30°C). Protect from moisture.

Pepcid® Complete

famotidine—calcium carbonate—magnesium hydroxide

Histamine H2-Receptor Antagonist—Antacid

Johnson & Johnson • Merck

PHARMACOLOGY: Heartburn is a common symptom for which a variety of treatments exist. Single doses of antacid alone and histamine H_2-receptor antagonists (acid reducers) alone have been shown to relieve heartburn more effectively than placebo. Although both agents are believed to act by reducing intraluminal acidity, their mechanisms of action and pharmacodynamic profiles differ substantially.

Antacids are believed to provide a fast onset of action by neutralizing intraluminal acid on contact but their duration of action is limited by physiologic clearing mechanisms. Histamine H_2-receptor antagonists inhibit gastric juice secretion, reducing acid and pepsin content, as well as the volume, of basal, nocturnal and stimulated gastric secretion. These acid reducers are believed to require a longer time to onset of effect than antacids but these antagonists have an appreciably longer duration of action.

Pepcid Complete contains both antacids (calcium carbonate and magnesium hydroxide) and an acid reducer, famotidine (an H_2-receptor antagonist).

In a clinical study to determine the pharmacodynamic profile of Pepcid Complete, esophageal and gastric pH were measured following administration of either Pepcid Complete, famotidine 10 mg, antacid (calcium carbonate/magnesium hydroxide 21 mEq) or placebo.

Figure 1 displays gastric pH by treatment from 2 hours prior to dosing to 12 hours postdose. During 5- to 9-hours postdose, the mean intragastric pH was significantly greater with Pepcid Complete and famotidine treatments than with the antacid (calcium carbonate/magnesium hydroxide 21 mEq) and placebo. The mean intragastric pH for the antacid and placebo treatments were similar during the 5 to 9 hour postdose period. These results demonstrate the longer duration of effect on gastric pH of the acid reducer and Pepcid Complete over the antacid.

Figure 1: Pepcid Complete

Gastric pH Means at 30-minute Time Intervals Relative to Dosing (n=23)

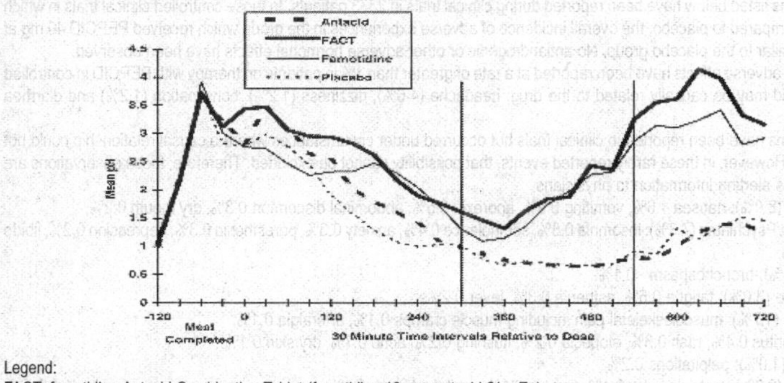

Legend:
FACT=famotidine Antacid Combination Tablet (famotidine 10 mg, antacid 21 mEq).
Famotidine=famotidine 10 mg film-coated tablet.
Antacid=calcium carbonate/magnesium hydroxide 21 mEq.

Figure 2 displays mean esophageal pH by treatment from 15 minutes prior to dosing to 60 minutes postdose. Compared to famotidine and placebo, mean intraesophageal pH was significantly greater in the Pepcid Complete and antacid groups during the first hour. These results demonstrate that Pepcid Complete and the antacid have a faster onset of effect on esophageal pH than the acid reducer (famotidine 10 mg).

This study shows that the pharmacodynamic profile of Pepcid Complete reflects the action of both the antacid and acid reducer components. The Pepcid Complete combination tablet has a faster onset of effect on esophageal pH than the acid reducer and a longer duration of effect on gastric pH than the antacid.

Figure 2: Pepcid Complete

Esophageal pH Means at 1-minute Time Intervals Relative to Dose: 0 to 60 Minutes Postdose (n=23)

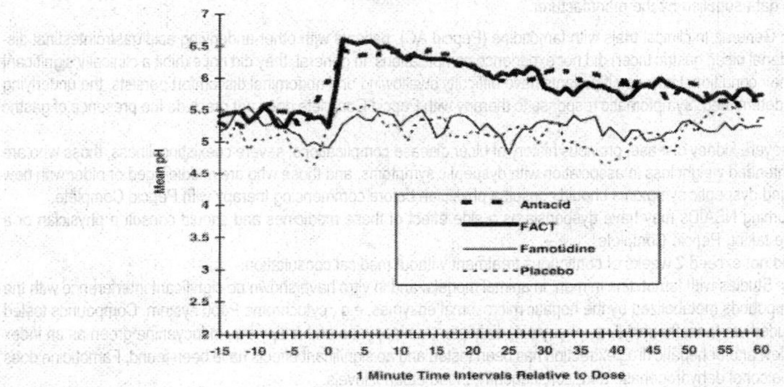

Legend:
FACT=famotidine Antacid Combination Tablet (famotidine 10 mg, antacid 21 mEq).
Famotidine=famotidine 10 mg film-coated tablet.
Antacid=calcium carbonate/magnesium hydroxide 21 mEq.

These results are consistent with clinical data, obtained from 3 studies, demonstrating the onset and duration benefits of Pepcid Complete in heartburn relief. According to the data, Pepcid Complete relieved heartburn significantly longer than the antacid and significantly faster than the acid reducer.

In a double-blind, randomized, parallel-group, multiple-dose study comparing Pepcid Complete to famotidine 10 mg, antacid (calcium carbonate/magnesium hydroxide 21 mEq) and placebo in patients with frequent heartburn, the adequacy of relief was assessed at 15-minute intervals for the first hour post-dose, then hourly for 8 hours postdose. Table 1 shows the number of heartburn episodes each patient recorded with adequate relief first occurring at each time point within 2 hours. Heartburn treated with Pepcid Complete was statistically more likely to achieve adequate relief at an earlier time point than episodes treated with the acid reducer, famotidine 10 mg (p=0.011). Heartburn episodes for Pepcid Complete patients were also more likely to achieve adequate relief at an earlier time point than episodes for the antacid (calcium carbonate/magnesium hydroxide 21 mEq) and placebo patients, respectively (p=0.042 and p<0.001).

Results presented in Table 2 show that, in this same study, Pepcid Complete produces a statistically longer duration of adequate relief than the antacid. The proportion of episodes relieved for at least 7 hours was greater with Pepcid Complete than antacid (p=0.001) and placebo (p<0.001).

Table 1: Pepcid Complete

Onset Data-Number (Cumulative %) of Heartburn Episodes Adequately Relieved (N=1231)

	FACT n=305 Tot Eps[a]=1205		Famotidine 10 mg FCT n=311 Tot Eps=1229		Antacid 21 mEq n=308 Tot Eps=1212		Placebo n=307 Tot Eps=1217	
Relief at:	n	cum %[b]	n	cum %[b]	n	cum %[b]	n	cum %[b]
15 minutes	322	27.0	249	20.3	301	25.1	191	15.7
30 minutes	222	45.3	215	37.8	190	40.9	210	33.0
45 minutes	234	64.6	257	58.6	200	57.4	262	54.4
60 minutes	172	78.8	190	73.9	159	70.5	203	71.2
120 minutes	77	85.3	94	81.5	102	78.8	77	77.5
>120 minutes	178	100.0	224	100.0	260	100.0	274	100.0

[a] Eps=Episodes.
[b] Cumulative percentages are based on the number of episodes within each patient.

Legend:
FACT=Famotidine Antacid Combination Tablet.
FCT=Film-coated Tablet.
Antacid=calcium carbonate/magnesium hydroxide 21 mEq.

Table 2: Pepcid Complete

Duration Data-Number (Cumulative %) of Heartburn Episodes Adequately Relieved (N=1231)

	FACT n=305 Tot Eps[a]=1205		Famotidine 10 mg FCT n=311 Tot Eps=1229		Antacid 21 mEq n=308 Tot Eps=1212		Placebo n=307 Tot Eps=1217	
Adequate Relief for:	n	cum %[b]	n	cum %[b]	n	cum %[b]	n	cum %[b]
≥7 hours	845	70.4	842	68.3	741	61.3	718	59.0
6 hours	20	72.0	19	69.8	14	62.4	22	60.8
5 hours	28	74.3	29	72.2	30	64.9	43	64.3
4 hours	26	76.5	31	74.7	41	68.2	48	68.2
<4 hours	152	89.0	142	86.2	180	83.2	182	83.2
No onset	134	100.0	166	100.0	206	100.0	204	100.0

[a] Eps=Episodes.
[b] Cumulative percentages are based on the number of episodes within each patient.

Legend:
FACT=Famotidine Antacid Combination Tablet.
FCT=Film-coated Tablet.
Antacid=calcium carbonate/magnesium hydroxide 21 mEq.

INDICATIONS: The treatment of the following conditions where neutralization of gastric acid and a controlled reduction of gastric secretion is required, such as acid indigestion, heartburn, sour or upset stomach. Pepcid Complete is also indicated for the prevention of these symptoms when associated with the consumption of food and/or beverage. Pepcid Complete relieves and prevents daytime heartburn symptoms and relieves heartburn during the night.

CONTRAINDICATIONS: In individuals with a hypersensitivity to any component of this medication. Cross-sensitivity has been observed between H_2-receptor antagonists. Therefore, Pepcid Complete should not be taken by individuals with a history of hypersensitivity to other drugs in this class of compounds.

WARNINGS: No data supplied by the manufacturer.

PRECAUTIONS: General: In clinical trials with famotidine (Pepcid AC), patients with other underlying acid gastrointestinal diseases (e.g., duodenal ulcer, gastric ulcer) did not experience complications; in general, they did not exhibit a clinically significant deterioration in their condition. However, if patients have difficulty swallowing or if abdominal discomfort persists, the underlying cause should be determined. Symptomatic response to therapy with Pepcid Complete does not preclude the presence of gastric malignancy.

Patients with severe kidney disease, previous history of ulcer disease complications, severe coexisting illness, those who are experiencing unintended weight loss in association with dyspeptic symptoms, and those who are middle-aged or older with new or recently changed dyspeptic symptoms should consult a physician before commencing therapy with Pepcid Complete.

Patients consuming NSAIDs may have dyspepsia as a side effect of these medicines and should consult a physician or a pharmacist before taking Pepcid Complete.

Therapy should not exceed 2 weeks of continuous treatment without medical consultation.

Drug Interactions: Studies with famotidine in man, in animal models, and in vitro have shown no significant interference with the disposition of compounds metabolized by the hepatic microsomal enzymes, e.g., cytochrome P450 system. Compounds tested in man have included warfarin, theophylline, phenytoin, diazepam, aminopyrine and antipyrine. Indocyanine green as an index of hepatic blood flow and/or hepatic drug extraction has been tested and no significant effects have been found. Famotidine does not affect gastric alcohol dehydrogenase and, consequently, blood ethanol levels.

Concomitant administration of antacids can reduce the absorption of a variety of drugs, such as tetracyclines, phenothiazines, benzodiazepines, and iron. Given the known drug-interaction profiles of the Pepcid Complete components, no studies were conducted with Pepcid Complete to directly characterize any potential interactions. Patients taking a prescription drug should check with their pharmacist or physician before taking Pepcid Complete. Most interactions can be avoided by taking Pepcid Complete 2 hours before or after ingestion of other drugs.

Pregnancy: Reproductive studies with famotidine have been performed in rats and rabbits at oral doses of up to 2000 and 500 mg/kg/day, respectively (approximately 2500 and 625 times the maximum recommended human prescription dose [80 mg] of famotidine, respectively), and have revealed no evidence of impaired fertility or harm to the fetus due to famotidine. There are, however, no adequate or well-controlled studies in pregnant women with famotidine.

Since the safe use of Pepcid Complete in pregnant women has not been established, pregnant women should not use Pepcid Complete unless directed otherwise by a physician.

Lactation: Famotidine is detectable in human milk. Nursing mothers should either stop Pepcid Complete or should stop nursing.

Children: Safety and effectiveness in children have not been established. Pepcid Complete should not be administered to children under 12 years of age.

Geriatrics: No dosage adjustment is required based on age.

ADVERSE EFFECTS: Pepcid Complete has been demonstrated to be generally well tolerated. In primary studies (comparing Pepcid Complete, antacid 21.5 mEq, famotidine 10 mg and placebo), Pepcid Complete and the antacid groups (calcium carbonate/magnesium hydroxide 21 mEq) had similar proportions of patients with adverse experiences. The most common adverse experience was headache, occurring in 2.6% of patients receiving Pepcid Complete.

Changes in laboratory parameters have been observed with famotidine 10 mg.

Among the laboratory changes that were reported during clinical trials with Pepcid AC were increases in AST, ALT, and WBC count, and decreases in hemoglobin and hematocrit. These changes were rarely of clinical significance. No famotidine-treated patients/subjects had to be discontinued from therapy because of laboratory adverse experiences.

During marketed use of prescription doses of famotidine, which are higher than those recommended for nonprescription use, the following adverse reactions have been reported; urticaria, liver enzymes abnormalities, cholestatic jaundice, anaphylaxis, angioedema. Toxic epidermal necrolysis has been reported very rarely with H_2-receptor antagonists.

The following adverse reactions have been reported; however, a causal relationship to therapy with Pepcid has not been established: agitation, confusion, hallucinations, grand mal seizures, rare cases of impotence, thrombocytopenia, pancytopenia, leukopenia and agranulocytosis.

Gynecomastia has been reported rarely. In most cases that were followed up, it was reversible after discontinuing treatment.

OVERDOSE:
There is no experience to date with deliberate overdosage. Doses of up to 800 mg/day of famotidine have been employed in patients with pathological hypersecretory conditions with no serious adverse effects.

Treatment: In the event of overdosage, treatment should be symptomatic and supportive. Unabsorbed material should be removed from the gastrointestinal tract, the patient should be monitored, and supportive therapy should be employed.

The oral LD_{50} of famotidine in male and female rats and mice was >5000 mg/kg.

For management of a suspected drug overdose, CPhA recommends that you contact your **regional Poison Control Centre**. See the *CPS* Directory section for a list of Poison Control Centres.

DOSAGE: **Heartburn or Acid Indigestion** Adults and children 12 years and older: For fast, long-lasting and effective relief of symptoms: 1 tablet. If symptoms return, another tablet may be taken. For prevention of acid-related symptoms brought on by consuming food and/or beverage: 1 tablet 1 hour before eating. Maximum 2 tablets in 24 hours.

If symptoms persist for more than 2 consecutive weeks, a physician should be consulted. Individuals with kidney disease should not take this product except on the advice of a physician. This product should not be taken within 2 hours of another medicine because the effectiveness of the other medicine may be altered.

INFORMATION FOR THE PATIENT: Published in e-CPS, available by subscription at www.e-cps.ca.

SUPPLIED: Berry Flavour: Each chewable, berry flavoured, round, flat, purple coloured tablet, embossed with "P", contains: famotidine 10 mg, calcium carbonate 800 mg and magnesium hydroxide 165 mg. Nonmedicinal ingredients: cellulose acetate, D&C Red No. 7, dextrates, FD&C Blue No. 1, FD&C Red No. 40, flavours, hydroxypropyl cellulose, hypromellose, lactose, magnesium stearate, pregelatinized starch, sodium lauryl sulfate and sugar. Bottles of 25 and 50. Cartons of 5. Store at 15 to 25°C. Protect from moisture.

Mint Flavour: Each chewable, mint flavoured, round, flat, rose (pink) coloured tablet, embossed with "P", contains: famotidine 10 mg, calcium carbonate 800 mg and magnesium hydroxide 165 mg. Nonmedicinal ingredients: cellulose acetate, dextrates, flavours, hydroxypropyl cellulose, hypromellose, lactose, magnesium stearate, pregelatinized starch, red ferric oxide, sodium lauryl sulfate and sugar. Blisters of 5, 25 and 50. Bottles of 25 and 50. Cartons of 5. Store at 15 to 25°C. Protect from moisture.

Each chewable tablet, mint and berry flavoured, provides 320 mg of elemental calcium and 69 mg of elemental magnesium. Low sodium.

Pepcid® Tablets ℞

famotidine

Histamine H2-Receptor Antagonist

Merck Frosst

Date of Revision: March 30, 2010

PHARMACOLOGY: PEPCID (famotidine) is a competitive inhibitor of histamine H_2-receptors. The primary clinically important pharmacologic activity of PEPCID is inhibition of gastric juice secretion. PEPCID reduces the acid and pepsin content, as well as the volume, of basal, nocturnal, and stimulated gastric secretion.

In both normal volunteers and hypersecretors, PEPCID (famotidine) inhibited basal nocturnal and daytime gastric secretion, as well as secretion stimulated by a variety of stimuli, such as pentagastrin and food.

After oral administration, the onset of the antisecretory effect occurred within one hour; the maximum effect was dose-dependent, occurring within one to three hours. Duration of inhibition of secretion was 10 to 12 hours. After intravenous administration, the maximum effect was achieved within 30 minutes. Single intravenous doses of 10 and 20 mg inhibited basal nocturnal secretion for a period of 10-12 hours. The 20 mg dose was associated with the longest duration of action in most subjects. Single oral doses of 20 and 40 mg inhibited basal nocturnal acid secretion in all subjects; mean gastric acid secretion was inhibited by 86% and 94%, respectively, for a period of at least 10 hours. Similar doses given in the morning suppressed food-stimulated acid secretion in all subjects, with mean suppression of 76% and 84%, respectively, 3 to 5 hours after drug, and of 25% and 30%, respectively, 8 to 10 hours after drug; however, in some subjects who received the 20 mg dose, the antisecretory effect was dissipated earlier, within 6-8 hours. There was no cumulative effect with repeated doses. The basal nocturnal intragastric pH was raised by evening doses of 20 and 40 mg of PEPCID to mean values of 5.0 and 6.4, respectively. When PEPCID was given in the morning, the basal daytime interdigestive pH at 3 and 8 hours after 20 or 40 mg of PEPCID was raised to about 5.0.

Fasting and postprandial serum gastrin levels may be slightly elevated during periods of drug antisecretory effect, and with chronic therapy an increase in gastric bacterial flora may occur. Gastric emptying and exocrine pancreatic function are not affected by PEPCID.

The presence of gastroesophageal reflux disease appears to correlate best with the percentage of time over 24 hours during which the esophagus is exposed to acid. In gastroesophageal reflux disease patients, 20 mg twice a day and 40 mg twice a day of PEPCID reduced intraesophageal acid exposure into the normal range as measured by 24-hour intraesophageal pH monitoring. In clinical studies of gastroesophageal reflux disease patients with endoscopically verified erosive or ulcerative esophagitis, 40 mg twice a day was more effective than 20 mg twice a day in healing esophageal lesions. Both dosage regimens were superior to placebo.

In patients treated for six months with PEPCID, relapse of esophageal erosion or ulceration was significantly less than in patients treated with placebo. PEPCID was also shown to be superior to placebo in preventing symptomatic deterioration.

Other Effects: Systemic pharmacologic effects of PEPCID in the CNS, cardiovascular, respiratory or endocrine systems have not been found to date. Serum prolactin levels do not rise after intravenous bolus doses of 20 mg of famotidine and no antiandrogenic effects have been detected.

Pharmacokinetics: PEPCID is incompletely absorbed. The mean bioavailability of oral doses is 40-45%. Bioavailability may be slightly increased by food, or slightly decreased by antacids; however, these effects are of no clinical consequence. PEPCID undergoes minimal first-pass metabolism. After oral doses, peak plasma levels occur in 1-3 hours. Plasma levels after multiple doses are similar to those after single doses. Fifteen to 20% of PEPCID in plasma is protein bound. PEPCID has an elimination half-life of 2.5-3.5 hours. PEPCID is eliminated by renal (65-70%) and metabolic (30-35%) routes. Renal clearance is 250-450 mL/min., indicating some tubular excretion.

Twenty-five to 30% of an oral dose and 65-70% of an intravenous dose are recovered in the urine as unchanged compound. The only metabolite identified in man is the S-oxide. There is a close relationship between creatinine clearance values and the elimination half-life of PEPCID. In patients with severe renal insufficiency, i.e., creatinine clearance less than 30 mL/min., elimination half-life of famotidine may exceed 20 hours and adjustment of dosing intervals in moderate and severe renal insufficiency may be necessary (see Precautions and Dosage). Iln elderly patients, there are no clinically significant age-related changes in the pharmacokinetics of PEPCID. However, in elderly patients with decreased renal function, the clearance of the drug may be decreased (see Precautions, Geriatrics).

INDICATIONS: PEPCID (famotidine) is indicated in the treatment of the following conditions where a controlled reduction of gastric secretion is required: treatment of acute duodenal ulcer; prophylactic use in duodenal ulcer; treatment of acute benign gastric ulcer; treatment of pathological hypersecretory conditions (e.g., Zollinger-Ellison syndrome); treatment of gastroesophageal reflux disease (GERD); maintenance of remission of patients with GERD.

CONTRAINDICATIONS: Hypersensitivity to any component of this medication. Cross sensitivity in this class of compounds has been observed. Therefore, PEPCID (famotidine) should not be administered to patients with a history of hypersensitivity to other H_2-receptor antagonists.

WARNINGS: No data supplied by the manufacturer.

PRECAUTIONS: Patients with Moderate or Severe Renal Insufficiency: Since CNS adverse effects have been reported in patients with moderate and severe renal insufficiency, longer intervals between doses or lower doses may need to be used in patients with moderate (creatinine clearance 30-50 mL/min) or severe (creatinine clearance <30 mL/min) renal insufficiency to adjust for the longer elimination half-life of famotidine (see Pharmacology, Pharmacokinetics and Dosage).

Drug Interactions: Studies with famotidine in man, in animal models, and in vitro have shown no significant interference with the disposition of compounds metabolized by the hepatic microsomal enzymes, e.g., cytochrome P450 system. Compounds tested in man have included warfarin, theophylline, phenytoin, diazepam, aminopyrine and antipyrine. Indocyanine green as an index of hepatic blood flow and/or hepatic drug extraction has been tested and no significant effects have been found. In addition, studies with famotidine have shown no augmentation of expected blood alcohol levels resulting from alcohol ingestion.

Use in Gastric Ulcer: Gastric malignancy should be excluded prior to initiation of therapy of gastric ulcer with PEPCID. Symptomatic response of gastric ulcer to therapy with PEPCID does not preclude the presence of gastric malignancy.

Pregnancy: Reproductive studies have been performed in rats and rabbits at oral doses of up to 2000 and 500 mg/kg/day, respectively (approximately 2500 and 625 times the maximum recommended human dose, respectively), and have revealed no evidence of impaired fertility or harm to the fetus due to PEPCID. There are, however, no adequate or well-controlled studies in pregnant women.

Since the safe use of PEPCID in pregnant women has not been established, the benefits of treatment with PEPCID should be weighed against potential risks.

Lactation: Famotidine is detectable in human milk. Nursing mothers should either stop this drug or should stop nursing.

Children: Safety and effectiveness in children have not been established.

Geriatrics: No dosage adjustment is required based on age (see Pharmacology, Pharmacokinetics). This drug is known to be substantially excreted by the kidney, and the risk of toxic reactions to this drug may be greater in patients with impaired renal function. Because elderly patients are more likely to have decreased renal function, care should be taken in dose selection, and it may be useful to monitor renal function. Dosage adjustment in the case of moderate or severe renal impairment is necessary (see Precautions, Patients with Moderate or Severe Renal Insufficiency and Dosage, Dosage Adjustment for Patients with Moderate or Severe Renal Insufficiency).

Occupational Hazards: Driving and Operating Machinery: PEPCID may cause certain side effects such as dizziness, confusion, or hallucinations and, therefore, patients should know how they react to PEPCID before they operate an automobile or machinery or engage in activities requiring mental alertness and coordination (see Adverse Effects).

ADVERSE EFFECTS: PEPCID (famotidine) is usually well tolerated; most adverse reactions have been mild and transient. The adverse reactions listed below have been reported during clinical trials in 2333 patients. In those controlled clinical trials in which PEPCID was compared to placebo, the overall incidence of adverse experiences in the group which received PEPCID 40 mg at bedtime was similar to the placebo group. No antiandrogenic or other adverse hormonal effects have been observed.

The following adverse effects have been reported at a rate of greater than 1% in patients on therapy with PEPCID in controlled clinical trials, and may be causally related to the drug: headache (4.6%), dizziness (1.2%), constipation (1.2%) and diarrhea (1.6%).

Other reactions have been reported in clinical trials but occurred under circumstances where a causal relationship could not be established. However, in these rarely reported events, that possibility cannot be excluded. Therefore, these observations are listed to serve as alerting information to physicians.

Gastrointestinal (8.0%): nausea 1.6%, vomiting 0.9%, anorexia 0.5%, abdominal discomfort 0.3%, dry mouth 0.2%.
Nervous System/Psychiatric (7.3%): insomnia 0.6%, somnolence 0.4%, anxiety 0.3%, paresthesia 0.3%, depression 0.2%, libido decreased 0.1%.
Respiratory (4.4%): bronchospasm <0.1%.
Body as a Whole (3.0%): fatigue 0.6%, asthenia 0.3%, fever 0.2%.
Musculoskeletal (1.7%): musculoskeletal pain including muscle cramps 0.1%, arthralgia 0.1%.
Skin (1.7%): pruritus 0.4%, rash 0.3%, alopecia 0.2%, flushing 0.2%, acne 0.1%, dry skin 0.1%.
Cardiovascular (1.0%): palpitations 0.2%.
Special Senses (0.9%): taste disorder 0.1%, tinnitus 0.1%, orbital edema <0.1%.
Urogenital (0.9%).

The following additional adverse reactions have been reported since the drug was marketed: urticaria, alopecia, liver enzymes abnormalities, hepatitis, cholestatic jaundice, anaphylaxis, angioedema. Interstitial pneumonia and Stevens-Johnson syndrome/toxic epidermal necrolysis has been reported very rarely. Convulsions, in patients with impaired renal function, have been reported very rarely. As with other H_2-receptor antagonists, cases of bradycardia, A-V block and other arrhythmias have been reported rarely in patients treated with famotidine.

The following adverse reactions have been reported; however, a causal relationship to therapy with PEPCID has not been established: agitation, confusion, hallucinations, grand mal seizures, rare cases of impotence, thrombocytopenia, pancytopenia, leukopenia, neutropenia, and agranulocytosis.

Gynecomastia has been reported rarely. In most cases that were followed up, it was reversible after discontinuing treatment.

Laboratory Abnormalities: Laboratory parameters may be affected during treatment with PEPCID, but the changes are usually not considered serious. Among the laboratory changes that were reported during clinical trials were increases in AST, ALT, BUN, and serum creatinine. These changes were rarely of clinical significance.

Only three patients had to be discontinued from therapy because of laboratory adverse experiences, however laboratory abnormalities were present at baseline.

OVERDOSE:

Symptoms: The adverse reactions in overdose cases are similar to the adverse reactions encountered in normal clinical experience (see Adverse Effects). Doses of up to 800 mg/day have been employed in patients with pathological hypersecretory conditions with no serious adverse effects.

Treatment: In the event of overdosage, treatment should be symptomatic and supportive. Unabsorbed material should be removed from the gastrointestinal tract, the patient should be monitored, and supportive therapy should be employed.

The oral LD_{50} of famotidine in male and female rats and mice was >5000 mg/kg.

For management of a suspected drug overdose, contact your regional Poison Control Centre. See the *CPS* Directory section for a list of Poison Control Centres.

DOSAGE: Duodenal Ulcer: Acute Therapy: The recommended adult oral dosage of PEPCID (famotidine) for acute duodenal ulcer is 40 mg once a day at bedtime. Treatment should be given for 4-8 weeks, but the duration of treatment may be shortened if healing can be documented. Healing occurs within 4 weeks in most cases of duodenal ulcer.

Maintenance Therapy: For the prevention of recurrence of duodenal ulcer, it is recommended that therapy with PEPCID be continued with a dose of 20 mg once a day at bedtime, for a duration of up to 6-12 months depending on the severity of the condition.

Benign Gastric Ulcer: Acute Therapy: The recommended adult oral dosage for acute benign gastric ulcer is 40 mg once a day at bedtime. Treatment should be given for 4 to 8 weeks, but the duration of treatment may be shortened if healing can be documented.

Pathological Hypersecretory Conditions (such as Zollinger-Ellison syndrome): The dosage of PEPCID in patients with pathological hypersecretory conditions varies with the individual patient. The recommended adult oral starting dose for pathological hypersecretory conditions is 20 mg every six hours. In some patients, a higher starting dose may be required. Doses should be adjusted to individual patient needs and should continue as long as clinically indicated. Doses up to 800 mg/day have been administered to some patients with severe Zollinger-Ellison syndrome.

Gastroesophageal Reflux Disease: The recommended dosage for the symptomatic relief of gastroesophageal reflux disease is 20 mg of famotidine twice a day.

For the treatment of esophageal erosion or ulceration associated with gastroesophageal reflux disease, the recommended dosage is 40 mg of famotidine twice a day.

For the maintenance of remission of patients with GERD, the recommended dosage is 20 mg of famotidine twice a day.

Concomitant Use with Antacids: Antacids may be given concomitantly if needed.

Dosage Adjustment for Patients with Moderate or Severe Renal Insufficiency: In patients with moderate (creatinine clearance 30-50 mL/min) or severe (creatinine clearance <30 mL/min) renal insufficiency, the elimination half-life of PEPCID is increased. For patients with severe renal insufficiency, it may exceed 20 hours, reaching approximately 24 hours in anuric patients. Since CNS adverse reactions have been reported in patients with moderate and severe renal insufficiency, to avoid excess accumulation of the drug in patients with moderate or severe renal insufficiency, the dose of PEPCID may be reduced to half the dose or the dosing interval may be prolonged to 36-48 hours as indicated by the patient's clinical response.

INFORMATION FOR THE PATIENT: Published in e-CPS, available by subscription at www.e-cps.ca.

SUPPLIED: 20 mg: Each beige, rounded-square shaped coated tablet, with MSD 963 engraved on one side and plain on the other side, contains: famotidine 20 mg. Nonmedicinal ingredients: hydroxypropyl cellulose, hydroxypropyl methylcellulose, magnesium stearate, microcrystalline cellulose, red ferric oxide, starch pregelatinized, talc, titanium dioxide and yellow ferric oxide. Blisters of 28. Store at 15-30°C in a tightly closed container. Protect from light.

40 mg: Each tan, rounded-square shaped coated tablet, with MSD 964 engraved on one side and plain on the other side, contains: famotidine 40 mg. Nonmedicinal ingredients: hydroxypropyl cellulose, hydroxypropyl methylcellulose, magnesium stearate, microcrystalline cellulose, red ferric oxide, starch pregelatinized, talc, titanium dioxide and yellow ferric oxide. Blisters of 28. Store at 15-30°C in a tightly closed container. Protect from light.

(Shown in Product Identification Section)

Pepto-Bismol® Caplets

bismuth subsalicylate

Heartburn Relief—Indigestion Relief—Upset Stomach Relief—Nausea Relief—Diarrhea Relief

Procter & Gamble

Pepto-Bismol® Liquid

bismuth subsalicylate

Heartburn Relief—Indigestion Relief—Upset Stomach Relief—Nausea Relief—Diarrhea Relief

Procter & Gamble

SUPPLIED: Caplets: Each swallowable caplet contains: bismuth subsalicylate 262 mg. Nonmedicinal ingredients: calcium carbonate, magnesium stearate, mannitol, microcrystalline cellulose, polysorbate 80, PVP, Red 27 Lake, silica and sodium carboxymethyl starch. Cartons of 24.

Liquid: Original: Each mL contains: bismuth subsalicylate 17.6 mg. Nonmedicinal ingredients: benzoic acid, flavour, magnesium aluminum silicate, methylcellulose, Red 22, Red 28, sodium saccharin, salicylic acid, sodium salicylate, sorbic acid and water. Bottles of 115, 230, 350 and 480 mL, or twin packs of 2×480 mL bottles.

Cherry-Flavoured: Each mL contains: bismuth subsalicylate 17.6 mg. Nonmedicinal ingredients: benzoic acid, flavour, magnesium aluminum silicate, methylcellulose, Red 22, Red 28, sodium saccharin, salicylic acid, sodium salicylate, sorbic acid, sucralose and water. Bottles of 230 and 480 mL.

Liquid Extra Strength: Original: Each mL contains: bismuth subsalicylate 35.2 mg. Nonmedicinal ingredients: benzoic acid, flavour, magnesium aluminum silicate, methylcellulose, Red 22, Red 28, sodium saccharin, salicylic acid, sodium salicylate, sorbic acid and water. Bottles of 350 mL.

Cherry-Flavoured: Each mL contains: bismuth subsalicylate 35.2 mg. Nonmedicinal ingredients: benzoic acid, flavour, magnesium aluminum silicate, methylcellulose, Red 22, Red 28, sodium saccharin, salicylic acid, sodium salicylate, sorbic acid, sucralose and water. Bottles of 350 mL.

Pepto-Bismol® Chewable Tablets

bismuth subsalicylate—calcium carbonate

Heartburn Relief—Indigestion Relief—Upset Stomach Relief—Nausea Relief—Diarrhea Relief

Procter & Gamble

SUPPLIED: Original: Each tablet contains: bismuth subsalicylate 262 mg and calcium carbonate 350 mg. Nonmedicinal ingredients: flavour, magnesium stearate, mannitol, PVP, Red 27 Lake, sodium saccharin and talc. Cartons of 48. Bottles of 24.

Cherry-Flavoured: Each cherry-flavoured tablet contains: bismuth subsalicylate 262 mg and calcium carbonate 350 mg. Nonmedicinal ingredients: adipic acid, flavour, magnesium stearate, mannitol, PVP, Red 27 Lake, Red 40, sodium saccharin and talc. Cartons of 48.

Pepto-Bismol® with InstaCool™

bismuth subsalicylate

Heartburn Relief—Indigestion Relief—Upset Stomach Relief—Nausea Relief—Diarrhea Relief

Procter & Gamble

SUPPLIED: Each peppermint flavoured chewable tablet contains: bismuth subsalicylate 262 mg. Nonmedicinal ingredients: calcium carbonate, magnesium stearate, mannitol, peppermint flavour, PVP, Red 27 Lake, sodium saccharin and talc. Cartons of 18 bottles.

Percocet® Ⓝ

oxycodone HCl—acetaminophen

Opioid Analgesic

Bristol-Myers Squibb

Percocet®-Demi Ⓝ

oxycodone HCl—acetaminophen

Opioid Analgesic

Bristol-Myers Squibb

Date of Preparation: December 31, 1977
Date of Revision: November 5, 2001

PHARMACOLOGY: The principal ingredient, oxycodone, is a semisynthetic opioid analgesic with multiple actions qualitatively similar to those of morphine; the most prominent of these involve the CNS and organs composed of smooth muscle. The principal actions of therapeutic value of the oxycodone in Percocet are analgesia and sedation.

Oxycodone is similar to codeine and methadone in that it retains at least one half of its analgesic activity when administered orally. It has been suggested that less rapid biotransformation in the liver may be due to the protective effect of a methoxy group in the 3-position, the site of glucuronide conjugation in morphine.

Percocet also contains the non-opioid, antipyretic analgesic, acetaminophen; the latter exerts its effects by a mechanism similar to that of the salicylates but, unlike the salicylates, does not have anti-inflammatory or uricosuric properties. Acetaminophen is rapidly and almost completely absorbed from the gastrointestinal tract, peak plasma levels being obtained within 10 minutes to 1 hour.

INDICATIONS: The relief of moderate to moderately severe pain, including conditions accompanied by fever.

CONTRAINDICATIONS: Status asthmaticus, pre-existing respiratory depression or convulsive states, hypersensitivity to oxycodone or acetaminophen.

WARNINGS: Drug Dependence: Oxycodone can produce drug dependence of the morphine type and, therefore, has the potential of being abused. Psychic dependence, physical dependence and tolerance may develop upon repeated administration of Percocet, and it should be prescribed and administered with the same degree of caution appropriate to the use of other oral medication containing opioids.

Occupational Hazards: Oxycodone may impair the mental and/or physical abilities required for the performance of potentially hazardous tasks such as driving a car or operating machinery. The patient using Percocet should be cautioned accordingly.

Interaction with other CNS depressants: Patients receiving other opioid analgesics, general anesthetics, monoamine oxidase inhibitors, tricyclic antidepressants, phenothiazines, other tranquilizers, sedative-hypnotics or other CNS depressants (including alcohol), concomitantly with Percocet may exhibit an additive CNS depression. When such combined therapy is contemplated, the dose of one or both agents should be reduced.

Pregnancy: Safe use in pregnancy has not been established relative to possible adverse effects on fetal development. Therefore, Percocet should not be given to pregnant women unless, in the judgment of the physician, the potential benefits outweigh the possible hazards. The administration of Percocet to obstetrical patients in labor may be associated with respiratory depression of the newborn.

Children: The more potent formula, Percocet, should not be administered to infants or children. However, Percocet-Demi, containing half the amount of oxycodone, can be considered for children of 6 years of age or older.

PRECAUTIONS: Head Injury and Increased Intracranial Pressure: The respiratory depressant effects of opioids and their capacity to elevate cerebrospinal fluid pressure may be markedly exaggerated in the presence of head injury, other intracranial lesions or a pre-existing elevated intracranial pressure. Furthermore, opioids may produce adverse reactions which can obscure the clinical course of patients with head injuries.

Acute Abdominal Conditions: The administration of Percocet or other opioids may obscure the diagnosis or clinical course in patients with acute abdominal conditions.

Special Risk Patients: Percocet should be given with caution to certain patients such as the elderly or debilitated, because of the danger of cardiac or respiratory depression, as well as to those patients with hemorrhage, severe impairment of hepatic, respiratory or renal function, hypothyroidism, Addison's disease, prostatic hypertrophy or urethral stricture.

Headache: Because headache often involves a significant psychological component, an opioid analgesic should only be employed for the treatment of headache when no other treatment is effective, in order to minimize the risk of psychological and physical dependence.

Drug Interactions: The CNS depressant effects of Percocet may be additive with those of other CNS depressants (see Warnings).

Other: Patients should be instructed to store Percocet as for any medication, safely out of the reach of children.

ADVERSE EFFECTS: The most frequently observed adverse reactions include: light-headedness, dizziness, sedation, nausea, and vomiting. These effects seem to be more prominent in ambulatory than in nonambulatory patients, and some of these adverse reactions may be alleviated if the patient lies down.

Other adverse reactions include: euphoria, dysphoria, constipation and pruritus.

OVERDOSE:

Symptoms: Serious overdose is characterized by respiratory depression (a decrease in respiratory rate and/or tidal volume, Cheyne-Stokes respiration, cyanosis), extreme somnolence progressing to stupor or coma, skeletal muscle flaccidity, cold and clammy skin and sometimes bradycardia and hypotension. In severe overdose, apnea, circulatory collapse, cardiac arrest, and death may occur. The ingestion of very large amounts of Percocet may, in addition, result in acute acetaminophen intoxication, characterized by anorexia, nausea, vomiting and sweating within 2 or 3 hours of ingestion, and possibly cyanosis with methemoglobinemia. Within 48 hours, liver function tests rise abnormally, and the liver becomes enlarged and tender. Within 3 to 5 days, jaundice, coagulation defects, myocardiopathy, encephalopathy and renal failure occur, followed by death due to hepatic necrosis. The ingestion of 10 g of acetaminophen is considered to result in intoxication, with the possibility of a fatal outcome if the amount exceeds 15 g. Hepatotoxicity occurs when plasma levels of 300 µg/mL are observed within 4 hours of ingestion.

Treatment: Primary attention should be given to the re-establishment of adequate respiratory exchange through provision of a patent airway and the institution of assisted or controlled ventilation. The opioid antagonist naloxone is a specific antidote against respiratory depression which may result from overdosage or unusual sensitivity to opioids, including oxycodone. Therefore, an appropriate dose of this antagonist should be administered, preferably by the i.v. route, simultaneously with efforts at respiratory resuscitation. Since the duration of action of oxycodone may exceed that of the antagonist, the patient should be kept under continued surveillance and repeat doses of the antagonist should be administered as needed to maintain adequate respiration. The instructions contained in the package insert provided by the manufacturer should be carefully observed.

An antagonist should not be administered in the absence of clinically significant respiratory or cardiovascular depression.

Oxygen, i.v. fluids, vasopressors and other supportive measures should be employed as indicated.

Gastric emptying by emesis or lavage may be useful in removing unabsorbed drug and should be carried out at an early stage of treatment. Plasma levels of acetaminophen should be determined. If hemodialysis is carried out within 10 hours of ingestion, it may be of some value.

The drug PARVOLEX (N-acetylcysteine, Bioniche) is a specific antidote for acetaminophen intoxication. For directions for use, refer to the manufacturer's Product Monograph or the CPS.

For management of a suspected drug overdose, CPhA recommends that you contact your **regional Poison Control Centre**. See the *CPS* Directory section for a list of Poison Control Centres.

DOSAGE: Dosage should be adjusted according to the severity of the pain and the patient's response. It may occasionally be necessary to exceed the usual dosage recommended below in cases of more severe pain or in those patients who have become tolerant to the analgesic effect of opioids.

Percocet: Adults: 1 tablet every 6 hours as needed for pain.

Percocet-Demi: Adults: 1 or 2 tablets every 6 hours. Children: 12 years and older: one half tablet every 6 hours. Children: 6 to 12 years: quarter of a tablet every 6 hours. Not indicated for children under 6 years of age.

SUPPLIED: Percocet: Each white to off-white biconvex tablet, one side embossed with "PERCOCET" and the other side bisected contains: oxycodone HCl 5 mg and acetaminophen 325 mg. Nonmedicinal ingredients: cornstarch, microcrystalline cellulose, povidone, pregelatinized starch, silicon dioxide (colloidal) and stearic acid. Lactose-, sodium- and tartrazine-free. Bottles of 100 and 500. Store at room temperature (15 to 30°C).

Percocet-Demi: Each blue-colored biconvex tablet, one side quadrisected and embossed with "PERCOCET-DEMI" and the other side blank contains: 2.5 mg oxycodone HCl and acetaminophen 325 mg. Nonmedicinal ingredients: cornstarch, microcrystalline cellulose, FD&C Blue No. 2 Lake, povidone, pregelatinized starch, silicon dioxide (colloidal) and stearic acid. Lactose-, sodium- and tartrazine-free. Bottles of 100. Store at room temperature (15 to 30°C).

(Shown in Product Identification Section)

Perindopril

CPhA Monograph

see *ACE Inhibitors*

Periostat™

doxycycline hyclate

Collagenase Inhibitor for Periodontal Use

Pharmascience

PHARMACOLOGY: Periostat contains doxycycline hyclate which is a semi-synthetic tetracycline. Doxycycline is an inhibitor of collagenase activity. Studies have shown that doxycycline reduces the elevated collagenase activity in the gingival crevicular fluid of patients with chronic adult periodontitis, in an action unrelated to its antibacterial mode of action. The clinical significance of these findings is not known.

INDICATIONS: Periostat is indicated for use as an adjunct to scaling and root planing to promote attachment level gain and to reduce pocket depth in patients with adult periodontitis.

CONTRAINDICATIONS: This drug is contraindicated in persons who have shown hypersensitivity to any of the tetracyclines, and in patients with myasthenia gravis. Periostat should not be used during tooth development (second half of pregnancy, infancy and in childhood).

WARNINGS: The use of drugs of the tetracycline class during tooth development (last half of pregnancy, infancy and childhood to the age of 8 years) may cause permanent discoloration of the teeth (yellow-gray-brown). This adverse reaction is more common during long-term use of the drugs but has been observed following repeated short-term courses. Enamel hypoplasia has also been reported. Tetracyclines drugs, therefore, should not be used in this age group and in pregnant or nursing mothers unless the potential benefits may be acceptable despite the potential risks.

Doxycycline can cause fetal harm when administered to a pregnant woman. Results of animals studies indicate that tetracyclines cross the placenta, are found in fetal tissues, and can have toxic effects on the developing fetus (often related to retardation of skeletal development). Evidence of embryotoxicity has also been noted in animals treated early in pregnancy. If any tetracyclines are used during pregnancy, or if the patient becomes pregnant while taking this drug, the patient should be apprised of the potential hazard to the fetus.

Photosensititvity manifested by an exaggerated sunburn reaction has been observed in some individuals taking tetracyclines. Patients apt to be exposed to direct sunlight or ultraviolet light should be advised that this reaction can occur with tetracycline drugs, and treatment should be discontinued at the first evidence of skin erythema.

Pregnancy: Teratogenic Effects: Pregnancy Category D. Results from animal studies indicate that doxycycline crosses the placenta and is found in fetal tissues.

PRECAUTIONS: Although not seen in clinical trials, overgrowth by opportunistic microorganisms, as with other antimicrobials, may occur. Exceeding the recommended dose of Periostat may result in the following:

The use may increase the incidence of vaginal candidiasis.

Periostat should be used with caution in patients with a history or predisposition to oral candidiasis. The safety and effectiveness of Periostat has not been established for the treatment of periodontitis in patients with coexistent oral candidiasis.

If superinfection is suspected, Periostat treatment should be discontinued and appropriate measures should be taken.

Laboratory Tests: In long-term therapy, periodic laboratory evaluations of organ systems, including hematopoietic, renal, and hepatic studies should be performed.

Drug Interactions: Because tetracyclines have been shown to depress plasma prothrombin activity, patients who are on anticoagulant therapy may require downward adjustment of their anticoagulant dosage.

Since bacterial antibiotics, such as the tetracycline class of antibiotics, may interfere with the bactericidal action of members of the β-lactam (e.g. penicillin) class of antibiotics, it is not advisable to administer these antibiotics concomitantly.

Absorption of doxycycline is impaired by antacids containing aluminum, calcium, or magnesium, and iron-containing preparations. Absorption is also impaired by bismuth subsalicylate.

Barbiturates, carbamazepine, and phenytoin decrease the half-life of doxycycline.

The concurrent use of tetracycline and Penthrane (methoxy-fluorane) has been reported to result in fatal renal toxicity.

Concurrent use of doxycycline may render oral contraceptives less effective.

Drug/Laboratory Test Interactions: False elevations of urinary catecholamine levels may occur due to interference with the fluorescence test.

ADVERSE EFFECTS: Adverse Reactions in Clinical Trials of Periostat: In clinical trials of adult patients with periodontal disease 213 patients received Periostat 20 mg BID over a 9-12 month period. The most frequent adverse reactions occurring in studies involving treatment with Periostat or placebo are listed in Table 1.

Table 1: Periostat

Adverse Reactions

Incidence (%) of Adverse Reactions in Periostat Clinical Trials		
	Periostat 20 mg BID (n=213)	**Placebo (n=215)**
Headache	55 (26%)	56 (26%)
Common Cold	47 (22%)	46 (21%)
Flu Symptoms	24 (11%)	40 (19%)
Tooth Ache	14 (7%)	28 (13%)
Periodontal Abcess	8 (4%)	21 (10%)
Tooth Disorder	13 (6%)	19 (9%)
Nausea	17 (8%)	12 (6%)
Sinusitis	7 (3%)	18 (8%)
Injury	11 (5%)	18 (8%)
Dyspepsia	13 (6%)	5 (2%)
Sore Throat	11 (5%)	13 (6%)
Joint Pain	12 (6%)	8 (4%)
Diarrhea	12 (6%)	8 (4%)
Sinus Congestion	11 (5%)	11 (5%)
Coughing	9 (4%)	11 (5%)
Sinus Headache	8 (4%)	8 (4%)
Rash	8 (4%)	6 (3%)
Back Pain	7 (3%)	8 (4%)
Back Ache	4 (2%)	9 (4%)
Menstrual Cramp	9 (4%)	5 (2%)
Acid Indigestion	8 (4%)	7 (3%)
Pain	8 (4%)	5 (2%)
Infection	4 (2%)	6 (3%)
Gum Pain	1 (%)	6 (3%)
Bronchitis	7 (3%)	5 (2%)
Muscle Pain	2 (1%)	6 (3%)

(cont'd)

Note: Percentages are based on total number of study participants in each treatment group.

OVERDOSE:

Treatment: In case of overdosage, discontinue medication, treat symptomatically and institute supportive measures. Dialysis does not alter serum half-life and thus would not be of benefit in treating cases of overdose.

For management of a suspected drug overdose, CPhA recommends that you contact your **regional Poison Control Centre**. See the *CPS* Directory section for a list of Poison Control Centres.

DOSAGE: The dosage of Periostat differs from that of doxycycline used to treat infections. Exceeding the recommended dosage may result in an increased incidence of side effects including the development of resistant microorganisms.

Periostat 20 mg twice daily as an adjunct following scaling and root planing may be administered for up to 9 months. Safety beyond 12 months and efficacy beyond 9 months have not been established.

Periostat should be administered at least one hour prior to morning and evening meals. Administration of adequate amounts of fluid along with the capsules is recommended to wash down the drug and reduce the risk of esophageal irritation and ulceration.

SUPPLIED: Each white capsule, imprinted with TM Periostat 20 mg contains: doxycycline hyclate equivalent to doxycycline 20 mg. Bottles of 100. Store at controlled room temperature between 15 and 30°C and dispense in tight, light-resistant containers, protected from excessive humidity.

Persantine®

dipyridamole

Coronary Vasodilator—Inhibitor of Platelet Adhesion and Aggregation

Boehringer Ingelheim

Date of Preparation: March 15, 1995

Date of Revision: May 20, 2005

SUMMARY PRODUCT INFORMATION:

Route of Administration	Dosage Form/Strength	Clinically Relevant Nonmedicinal Ingredients
Oral	Tablet 50 mg , 75 mg	Acacia, calcium hydrogen phosphate, carnauba wax, colloidal silica, FDC yellow, magnesium stearate, polyethylene glycol, starch, sucrose, talc, titanium dioxide, white wax, and red iron oxide (50 mg tablet only).
I.V. (intravenous)	10 mL ampoules, 5 mg/mL	Tartaric acid, polyethylene glycol, hydrochloric acid and sterile water for injection.

INDICATIONS AND CLINICAL USE: Thromboembolic Disease: Persantine (dipyridamole) tablets are indicated for:

- The prevention of post-operative thromboembolic complications associated with prosthetic heart valve.

Myocardial Perfusion Imaging: Persantine (dipyridamole) ampoules can be used to:
- Induce pharmacologic vasodilation for myocardial perfusion imaging.

CONTRAINDICATIONS:
- Patients who are hypersensitive to this drug or to any ingredient in the formulation or component of the container. For a complete listing, see Dosage Forms, Composition and Packaging.
- Intravenous administration of Persantine is not recommended in states of shock or collapse.

WARNINGS AND PRECAUTIONS: General: Rare serious adverse reactions associated with the administration of intravenous Persantine for myocardial imaging have been reported. These have included fatal and non-fatal myocardial infarction, ventricular fibrillation, symptomatic ventricular tachycardia, stroke and transient cerebral ischemia.

Cardiovascular: Since excessive doses of dipyridamole (intravenous or oral) or intravenous doses given too rapidly can produce peripheral vasodilation, Persantine should be used with caution in patients with hypotension, coronary artery disease, including rapidly worsening angina, left ventricular outflow obstruction, (including subvalvular aortic stenosis), or hemodynamic instability. In rare cases, such patients may be at risk for developing myocardial ischemia and infarction.

Clinical experience suggests that patients being treated with oral dipyridamole who also require pharmacological stress testing with intravenous dipyridamole, should discontinue drugs containing oral dipyridamole for twenty-four hours prior to stress testing. Failure to do so may impair the sensitivity of the test.

An intravenous bolus of Persantine (40-50 mg over 4 minutes) can result in chest pain in patients with coronary artery disease. Rarely, hypotension or ventricular arrhythmias occur with a rapid, i.v. bolus. The infusion rate should be monitored to minimize this risk. The symptoms can generally be reversed with an intravenous injection of 50-250 mg of aminophylline over several minutes.

Intravenous Persantine (dipyridamole) as an adjunct to myocardial perfusion imaging should be used with caution in patients with unstable angina; as such patients may be at risk for severe myocardial infarction.

As with exercise induced stress, the use of intravenous Persantine as an adjunct to myocardial perfusion imaging may occasionally precipitate cardiac arrhythmias in patients with severe heart disease. Scanning should therefore be performed with constant monitoring of the patient's ECG. Parenteral aminophylline should be readily available and should be administered as a slow intravenous injection of 50-250 mg in the event of occurrences such as chest pain, bronchospasm, severe nausea/vomiting, hypotension, severe headache.

In the case of severe hypotension, the patient should be placed in a supine position with the head tilted down if necessary, before administration of parenteral aminophylline. If 250 mg of aminophylline does not relieve chest pain symptoms within a few minutes, sublingual nitroglycerin may be administered. If chest pain continues despite use of aminophylline and nitroglycerin, the possibility of myocardial infarction should be considered. If the clinical condition of a patient with an adverse event permits a one minute delay in the administration of parenteral aminophylline, thallium-201 may be injected and allowed to circulate for one minute before the injection of aminophylline. This will allow initial thallium perfusion imaging to be performed before reversal of the pharmacologic effects of Persantine on the coronary circulation.

Hepatic/Biliary/Pancreatic: A small number of cases have been reported in which unconjugated dipyridamole was shown to be incorporated into gallstones to a variable extent (up to 70% by dry weight of stone). These patients were all elderly, had evidence of ascending cholangitis and had been treated with oral dipyridamole for a number of years. There is no evidence that dipyridamole was the initiating factor in causing gallstones to form in these patients. It is possible that bacterial deglucuronidation of conjugated dipyridamole in bile may be the mechanism responsible for the presence of dipyridamole in gallstones.

Respiratory: Patients with a history or presence of bronchial hyperreactivity may be at risk of developing bronchospasm during the use of intravenous Persantine as an adjunct to myocardial perfusion imaging. Although the actual overall incidence of this occurrence is small (~0.2%), the clinical information to be gained through the use of intravenous Persantine should be weighed against the potential risk to the patient.

Special Populations: Pregnant Women: Reproductive studies have been performed in mice, rats, and rabbits at doses of up to 125 mg/kg and have not revealed evidence of impaired embryonic development attributable to dipyridamole. However, there have not been adequate, well controlled studies in pregnant women and the drug should be used during pregnancy only if the expected benefits outweigh the potential risks.

Nursing Women: Dipyridamole is excreted in human milk. Caution should therefore be used when this drug is administered to nursing mothers.

Pediatrics: The safety and effectiveness of Persantine have not been established in the pediatric population.

ADVERSE REACTIONS: Parenteral Administration (i.v. infusion): Adverse Drug Reaction Overview: Serious adverse events (fatal and non-fatal myocardial infarction, severe ventricular arrhythmias, and serious CNS abnormalities) associated with the intravenous administration of Persantine for myocardial imaging are described in Warnings and Precautions.

Clinical Trial Adverse Drug Reactions: Because clinical trials are conducted under very specific conditions the adverse reaction rates observed in the clinical trials may not reflect the rates observed in practice and should not be compared to the rates in the clinical trials of another drug. Adverse drug reaction information from clinical trials is useful for identifying drug-related adverse events and for approximating rates.

When intravenous Persantine was used as an adjunct to myocardial perfusion imaging in a study of 3911 patients, the following events occurred in greater than 1% of the patients (see Table 1).

Table 1: Persantine

Adverse Effects—I.V. Use

Event Description	Incidence (%) of Occurrence in 3911 Patients
Chest Pain/Angina Pectoris	19.7
Headache	12.2
Dizziness	11.8
Electrocardiographic Abnormalities/ST-T Changes	7.5
Electrocardiographic Abnormalities/Extrasystoles	5.2
Hypotension	4.6
Nausea	4.6
Flushing	3.4
Electrocardiographic Abnormalities/Tachycardia	3.2
Dyspnea	2.6
Pain Unspecified	2.6
Blood Pressure Lability	1.6
Hypertension	1.5
Paresthesia	1.3
Fatigue	1.2

Less Common Clinical Trial Adverse Drug Reactions (<1%): Cardiovascular: electrocardiographic abnormalities unspecified, arrhythmia unspecified, palpitation, ventricular tachycardia, bradycardia, myocardial infarction, AV block, syncope, orthostatic hypotension, atrial fibrillation, supraventricular tachycardia, ventricular arrhythmia unspecified, heart block unspecified, cardiomyopathy, and edema.

Central and Peripheral Nervous System: hypoaesthesia, hypertonia, nervousness/anxiety, tremor, abnormal coordination, somnolence, dysphonia, migraine, vertigo.

Respiratory: pharyngitis, bronchospasm, hyperventilation, rhinitis, coughing, pleural pain.

Gastrointestinal: dyspepsia, dry mouth, abdominal pain, flatulence, vomiting, eructation, dysphagia, tenesmus, increased appetite.

Other: myalgia, back pain, injection site reaction unspecified, diaphoresis, asthenia, malaise, arthralgia, injection site pain, rigor, earache, tinnitus, vision abnormalities unspecified, dysgeusia, thirst, depersonalization, eye pain, renal pain, perineal pain, breast pain, intermittent claudication, leg cramping.

Post-market Adverse Drug Reactions: When using Persantine as an adjunct to myocardial imaging, the following adverse events have been reported: cardiac death, cardiac arrest, myocardial infraction (rarely fatal), arrhythmias (e.g. sinus node arrest), tachycardia, fibrillation, and cerebrovascular events (e.g. stroke, TIA, seizures). Persantine may cause severe hypotension and hot flushes. Diarrhoea has been observed.

Hypersensitivity reactions such as rash, urticaria, angio-oedema, laryngospasm, severe bronchospasm and very rarely anaphylactoid reactions have been reported.

Oral Administration: Adverse reactions at therapeutic doses are usually minimal and transient. Occasionally diarrhoea, vomiting, headache, dizziness, nausea, flushing, syncope or weakness, myalgia, and skin rash have occurred during initiation of therapy. Mild occasional gastric distress can be avoided by administration of the tablets with a glass of milk. Gastric irritation, emesis and abdominal cramping may occur at high dosage levels. Rare cases of what appears to be an aggravation of angina pectoris have been reported, usually at the initiation of therapy.

On those uncommon occasions when adverse reactions have been persistent or intolerable to the patient, withdrawal of the medication has been followed promptly by cessation of the undesirable symptoms.

When Persantine (dipyridamole) is used in combination with ASA, the only side effect clearly attributable to Persantine is headache. This symptom shows an increase of 5.5% in the combination treated group over that occurring in a group of patients treated with ASA alone. Other adverse reactions which occur during combination therapy are similar to those mentioned above, together with the well documented side effects of ASA therapy, notably gastric distress and gastrointestinal bleeding.

At the higher doses of Persantine there may be an increase in the incidence of adverse reactions.

In very rare cases, increased bleeding during or after surgery has been reported.

Post-market Adverse Drug Reactions: As a result of its vasodilator properties, Persantine may cause hypotension, hot flushes, and tachycardia. Worsening of symptoms of coronary heart disease has been observed.

Hypersensitivity reactions such as rash, urticaria, severe bronchospasm and angio-oedema have been reported.

Dipyridamole has been shown to be incorporated into gallstones (see Warnings and Precautions).

Isolated cases of thrombocytopenia have been reported in conjunction with treatment with Persantine.

DRUG INTERACTIONS: Drug-Drug Interactions: See Table 2.

Table 2: Persantine

Established or Potential Drug-Drug Interactions

Persantine	Effect	Clinical Comment
Persantine–Adenosine	Dipyridamole increases plasma levels and cardiovascular effects of adenosine.	Adjustment of adenosine dosage should be considered.
Persantine Ampoules–Theophylline, Aminophylline	The use of oral maintenance xanthines (e.g., theophylline, aminophylline) may abolish the coronary vasodilation produced by intravenous dipyridamole administration.	This could lead to false negative imaging results.
Persantine ampoules–Oral Dipyridamole	In patients already receiving oral dipyridamole, clinical experience suggests that the sensitivity of the intravenous dipyridamole testing may be impaired.	Oral dipyridamole treatment should be discontinued for 24-hours prior to testing.
Persantine–Anticoagulants, Thrombolytics	The combined use of such agents may result in an increased risk of hemorrhage.	Caution is necessary when dipyridamole is used concurrently with anticoagulants or thrombolytics.
Persantine–ASA	The addition of dipyridamole to acetylsalicylic acid does not increase the incidence of bleeding events.	
Persantine–Warfarin	When dipyridamole was administered concomitantly with warfarin, bleeding was no greater in frequency or severity than that observed when warfarin was administered alone.	
Persantine–Blood Pressure Lowering Drugs	Dipyridamole may increase the hypotensive effect of blood pressure lowering drugs.	
Persantine–Cholinesterase Inhibitors	Dipyridamole may counteract the anticholinesterase effect of cholinesterase inhibitors.	In patients with myasthenia gravis, readjustment of therapy may be necessary during treatment with dipyridamole.

Drug-Food Interactions: Xanthine derivatives (e.g., found in coffee, tea) may weaken the effect of Persantine and therefore should be avoided 24 hours before myocardial imaging with Persantine.

DOSAGE AND ADMINISTRATION: Dosing Considerations: Oral Administration: Thromboembolic Disease: Recommended Dose and Dosage Adjustment: The recommended oral dose is 100 mg q.i.d., one hour before meals. The maximum daily dose is 600 mg. A lower dose of 100 mg of Persantine (dipyridamole) daily together with 1 g ASA daily, prolongs platelet survival to the same extent.

Parenteral Administration: Myocardial Perfusion Imaging: Recommended Dose and Dosage Adjustment: The dose of intravenous Persantine used as an adjunct to myocardial perfusion imaging should be adjusted according to the weight of the patient.

Immediately prior to infusion, Persantine i.v. should be diluted at least 1:2 with Dextrose Injection, USP 5%. The recommended dose is 0.142 mg/kg/min., infused over 4 minutes.

A total dose of greater than 60 mg is not recommended for use in any patient. The imaging agent should be injected within 5 minutes following the 4 minute infusion of Persantine. Do not mix i.v. Persantine with other drugs in the same syringe or infusion container. Infusion of undiluted Persantine may cause local irritation.

As with all parenteral drug products, intravenous admixtures should be inspected visually for clarity, particulate matter, precipitate, discolouration and leakage prior to administration, whenever solution and container permit. Solutions showing haziness, particulate matter, precipitate, discolouration or leakage should not be used. Discard unused portion.

OVERDOSAGE:

Hypotension, if it occurs, is likely to be of short duration but vasopressor substances may be used if necessary. Symptoms such as feeling warm, flushes, sweating, accelerated pulse, restlessness, feeling of weakness and dizziness, and anginal complaints may occur. A drop in blood pressure and tachycardia might be observed.

Oral Administration: Symptomatic therapy is recommended. A gastric decontamination procedure should be considered. Administration of xanthine derivatives (e.g. aminophylline) may reverse the haemodynamic effects of dipyridamole overdose. Due to its wide distribution to tissues and its predominantly hepatic elimination, dipyridamole is not likely to be accessible to enhanced removal procedures.

Parenteral Administration (I.V. Infusion): No cases of overdose in humans have been reported in this indication. Signs and symptoms as described under Side Effects are expected to occur. Aminophylline, as described in Warnings and Precautions may be administered. Due to its wide distribution to tissue and its predominantly hepatic elimination, dipyridamole is not likely to be accessible to enhanced removal procedures.

> For management of a suspected drug overdose, CPhA recommends that you contact your **regional Poison Control Centre**. See the *CPS* Directory section for a list of Poison Control Centres.

ACTION AND CLINICAL PHARMACOLOGY: Mechanism of Action: Persantine (dipyridamole) normalizes increased platelet adhesiveness and tendency to aggregate (Hellem's Method). Persantine has been found to lengthen abnormally shortened platelet survival time in a dose-dependent manner; 400 mg/day or 100 mg/day plus 1 g ASA.

It is believed that platelet reactivity and interaction with prosthetic cardiac valve surfaces, resulting in abnormal shortened platelet survival time is a significant factor in connection with prosthetic heart valve replacement.

In a controlled clinical trial involving patients who had undergone surgical placement of prosthetic heart valves (mitral and/or aortic valve replacement), Persantine, in combination with anticoagulants, significantly decreased the incidence of post-operative thromboembolic events, without increasing hemorrhagic complications. The incidence of thromboembolic events in patients receiving dipyridamole in a dose of 400 mg/day in combination with anticoagulants was 1.3% compared to 14.3% to the control group treated with anticoagulant alone.

In vitro dipyridamole potentiates the aggregation-inhibiting effects of adenosine and prostaglandin E_1, inhibits platelet uptake of adenosine, serotonin and glucose, and increases platelet cyclic AMP levels. At higher concentrations dipyridamole inhibits platelet aggregation induced by ADP or collagen.

Myocardial blood flow increases in a dose-dependent fashion after i.v. or oral dipyridamole, with flows 170% or more above normal. Maximal increases are achieved at about 2.0 µg/mL with 0.8 µg/mL being the threshold serum level. Single oral doses of 150 mg dipyridamole produce the maximal response. At normal therapeutic doses, no significant alterations of peripheral blood flow, systemic blood pressure, or heart rate have been observed.

Pharmacodynamics: Persantine is a coronary vasodilator in man. The mechanism of vasodilation has not been fully elucidated, but may result from inhibition of uptake of adenosine, an important mediator of coronary vasodilation. The vasodilatory effects of Persantine are abolished by administration of the adenosine receptor antagonist theophylline.

How Persantine-induced vasodilation leads to abnormalities in thallium distribution (when administered intravenously for myocardial perfusion imaging) and ventricular function is also uncertain, but presumably represents a "steal" phenomenon. In this situation, relatively intact vessels dilate, and sustain enhanced flow, leaving reduced pressure and flow across areas of hemodynamically important coronary vascular constriction.

Pharmacokinetics: Absorption: Dipyridamole is readily absorbed from the gastrointestinal tract, reaching peak plasma levels in man 1-3 hours following oral administration. Peak plasma levels are dose-dependent and range from about 0.5 µg/mL after a 25 mg dose to 1.6 µg/mL after a 75 mg dose. Blood levels are quite variable, possibly depending on food intake and gastrointestinal peristalsis. Ingestion on an empty stomach may result in higher blood levels.

Distribution: Following intravenous administration, the distribution half-life in man is about 25 minutes and after oral administration about 3 hours. When plasma levels of drug are followed for up to 60 hours after i.v. or oral administration of 20 to 50 mg, plasma levels decline tri-exponentially with half-lives of 5 minutes (i.v. only), 53 minutes and about 10-12 hours. The volume of distribution is about 140 L with about 92-99% binding to plasma proteins, primarily alpha1-acid glycoprotein.

STORAGE AND STABILITY: The Persantine Tablets should be stored at room temperature (15-30°C).

The Persantine Ampoule should be stored at room temperature (15-30°C).

SPECIAL HANDLING INSTRUCTIONS: Protect Persantine ampoules from direct light, and avoid freezing.

INFORMATION FOR THE PATIENT: Published in e-CPS, available by subscription at www.e-cps.ca.

DOSAGE FORMS, COMPOSITION AND PACKAGING: Parenteral: Each mL contains: dipyridamole 5 mg. Nonmedicinal ingredients: hydrochloric acid, polyethylene glycol, tartaric acid and sterile water for injection (SWFI). Ampuls of 10 mL, packages of 5.

Tablets: 50 mg: Each coral-red, round, sugar-coated tablet, imprinted with the Ingelheim tower on one side contains: dipyridamole 50 mg. Nonmedicinal ingredients: acacia, calcium hydrogen phosphate, carnauba wax, colloidal silica, FD&C Yellow No. 6, magnesium stearate, maize starch, polyethylene glycol, red iron oxide, sucrose, talc, titanium dioxide and white wax. Bottles of 100.

75 mg: Each reddish-orange, round, sugar-coated tablet, imprinted with the Ingelheim tower on one side contains: dipyridamole 75 mg. Nonmedicinal ingredients: acacia, calcium hydrogen phosphate, carnauba wax, colloidal silica, FD&C Yellow No. 6, magnesium stearate, maize starch, methyl and propyl parabens, polyethylene glycol, sucrose, talc, titanium dioxide and white wax. Bottles of 100.

Pethidine Ⓝ

CPhA Monograph

see *Opioids*

Pharmorubicin® PFS® Ⓟ

epirubicin HCl

Antineoplastic

Pfizer

Date of Preparation: September 5, 2003
Date of Revision: October 1, 2009

Caution: PHARMORUBICIN PFS (epirubicin hydrochloride injection) is a potent drug and should be used only by physicians experienced with cancer chemotherapeutic drugs (see Warnings and Precautions). Blood counts and hepatic function tests should be performed regularly. Irreversible cardiac toxicity may occur as the cumulative dose approaches 1000 mg/m². Cardiac monitoring is advised in those patients who have received mediastinal radiotherapy, other anthracycline or anthracene therapy, with pre-existing cardiac disease, or received prior epirubicin cumulative doses exceeding 650 mg/m².

Secondary acute myeloid leukemia (AML) with or without a preleukemic phase (Myelodysplastic Syndrome or MDS) has been reported in patients treated with epirubicin-containing regimens. The cumulative risk of developing treatment-related AML/MDS in 7110 patients with early breast cancer who received adjuvant treatment with epirubicin-containing regimens was estimated as 0.27% at 3 years, 0.46% at 5 years, and 0.55% at 8 years.

SUMMARY PRODUCT INFORMATION:

Route of Administration	Dosage Form/ Strength	Clinically Relevant Nonmedicinal Ingredients
Intravenous	Sterile solution for injection/2 mg/mL	Not applicable. For a complete listing see Dosage Forms, Composition and Packaging.

INDICATIONS AND CLINICAL USE: PHARMORUBICIN PFS (epirubicin hydrochloride injection) has been used successfully as a single agent and in combination with other chemotherapeutic agents to produce regression in a variety of tumour types such as lymphoma, lung, cancer of the breast, ovary and stomach.

PHARMORUBICIN PFS is recommended for the treatment of metastatic breast cancer.

PHARMORUBICIN PFS may also be used as a component in the adjuvant treatment of early stage breast cancer for pre- and peri- menopausal women.

PHARMORUBICIN PFS is also recommended in small cell lung cancer (both limited and extensive disease) advanced non-small cell lung cancer, non-Hodgkin's lymphoma, Hodgkin's disease, Stage III and IV (FIGO) ovarian carcinoma and metastatic and locally unresectable gastric carcinoma.

CONTRAINDICATIONS:

- hypersensitivity to epirubicin or any other component of the product, or other anthracyclines or anthracenediones such as doxorubicin hydrochloride, daunorubicin hydrochloride, mitoxantrone or mitomycin C.
- marked persistent myelosuppression induced by prior treatment with other antitumour agents or by radiotherapy
- severe hepatic impairment
- severe myocardial insufficiency
- recent myocardial infarction
- severe arrhythmias
- history of severe cardiac disease
- previous treatments with maximum cumulative doses of epirubicin and/or other anthracyclines and anthracenediones (see Warnings and Precautions).

WARNINGS AND PRECAUTIONS: Cardiac Function: Cardiotoxicity is a risk of anthracycline treatment that may be manifested by early (i.e., acute) or late (i.e., delayed) events.

Early (i.e., Acute) Events: Early cardiotoxicity of epirubicin consists mainly of sinus tachycardia and/or ECG abnormalities such as non-specific ST-T wave changes. Tachyarrhythmias, including premature ventricular contractions, ventricular tachycardia, and bradycardia, as well as atrioventricular and bundle-branch block have also been reported. These effects do not usually predict subsequent development of delayed cardiotoxicity, are rarely of clinical importance, and are generally not a consideration for the discontinuation of epirubicin treatment.

Late (i.e., Delayed) Events: Delayed cardiotoxicity usually develops late in the course of therapy with epirubicin or within 2 to 3 months after treatment termination, but later events several months to years after completion of treatment have also been reported. Delayed cardiomyopathy is manifested by reduced left ventricular ejection fraction (LVEF) and/or signs and symptoms of congestive heart failure (CHF) such as dyspnea, pulmonary edema, dependent edema, cardiomegaly and hepatomegaly, oliguria, ascites, pleural effusion, and gallop rhythm. Life-threatening CHF is the most severe form of anthracycline-induced cardiomyopathy and represents the cumulative dose-limiting toxicity of the drug.

Cardiac function should be assessed before patients undergo treatment with epirubicin and must be monitored throughout therapy to minimize the risk of incurring severe cardiac impairment. The risk may be decreased through regular monitoring of LVEF during the course of treatment with prompt discontinuation of epirubicin at the first sign of impaired function. The appropriate quantitative method for repeated assessment of cardiac function (evaluation of LVEF) includes multi-gated radionuclide angiography (MUGA) or echocardiography (ECHO). A baseline cardiac evaluation with an ECG and either a MUGA scan or an ECHO is recommended, especially in patients with risk factors for increased cardiotoxicity. Repeated MUGA or ECHO determinations of LVEF should be performed, particularly with higher, cumulative anthracycline doses. The technique used for assessment should be consistent throughout follow-up.

Congestive heart failure and/or cardiomyopathy may be encountered several weeks after discontinuation of PHARMORUBICIN PFS therapy.

Given the risk of cardiomyopathy, a cumulative dose of 900 to 1000 mg/m² epirubicin should generally not be exceeded. Risk factors for cardiac toxicity include active or dormant cardiovascular disease, prior or concomitant radiotherapy to the mediastinal/pericardial area, previous therapy with other anthracyclines or anthracenediones, and concomitant use of other drugs with the ability to suppress cardiac contractility or cardiotoxic drugs. Anthracyclines including epirubicin should not be administered in combination with other cardiotoxic agents unless the patient's cardiac function is closely monitored.

Patients receiving anthracyclines after stopping treatment with other cardiotoxic agents, especially those with long half-lives such as trastuzumab, may also be at an increased risk of developing cardiotoxicity. The half-life of trastuzumab is approximately 28.5 days and may persist in the circulation for up to 24 weeks. Therefore, physicians should avoid anthracycline-based therapy for up to 24 weeks after stopping trastuzumab when possible. If anthracyclines are used before this time, careful monitoring of cardiac function is recommended.

Cardiac function monitoring must be particularly strict in patients receiving high cumulative doses and in those with risk factors. While cardiotoxicity with epirubicin may occur at lower cumulative doses whether or not cardiac risk factors are present, it may be more likely to occur at lower cumulative doses in patients with these risk factors.

Available evidence appears to indicate that cardiotoxicity is cumulative across members of the anthracycline and anthracene class of drugs. Patients who have previously received other anthracyclines and anthracenes are at particular risk for possible cardiotoxic effects of PHARMORUBICIN PFS at a lower total dose than previously untreated patients and, therefore, should be carefully monitored. The total dose of PHARMORUBICIN administered to a patient should take into account: prior or concomitant therapy with related compounds such as doxorubicin and daunorubicin or anthracene derivatives; and/or radiotherapy to the mediastinal area.

Anthracycline-induced cardiac failure is often resistant to currently available therapeutic and physical measures used for the treatment of cardiac failure. Early clinical diagnosis of drug-induced heart failure is essential. Treatment measures include digitalis, diuretics, peripheral vasodilators, low salt diet, and bed rest. Severe cardiac toxicity may occur precipitously without antecedent EKG changes. An EKG, echocardiogram or radionuclide angiography (MUGA) performed at baseline and prior to each dose or course after a cumulative dose of 650 mg/m² is suggested. Transient EKG changes consisting of T-wave flattening, S-T depression and arrhythmias occurring up to two weeks after a dose or course of PHARMORUBICIN PFS are presently not considered indications for suspension of PHARMORUBICIN PFS therapy.

PHARMORUBICIN PFS cardiomyopathy has been reported to be associated with a reduction of the ejection fraction as determined by radionuclide scan or echocardiography. None of these tests have yet consistently identified those individual patients that are approaching their maximally tolerated cumulative dose of PHARMORUBICIN PFS. If test results indicate a change in cardiac status associated with PHARMORUBICIN PFS therapy, the benefit of continued therapy must be carefully weighed against the risk of producing irreversible cardiac damage.

Hematologic Toxicity: Careful hematologic monitoring is required since bone marrow depression, primarily of leukocytes may occur. Hematologic profiles should be assessed before and during each cycle of therapy with epirubicin, including differential white blood cell counts (WBC).

With the recommended dosage schedule (see Dosage and Administration) leukopenia is transient, reaching its nadir 10-14 days after treatment, with recovery usually occurring by the 21st day. White blood cell counts as low as 1000/mm³ are to be expected during treatment with PHARMORUBICIN PFS.

Red blood cell and platelet levels should be monitored since they may also be depressed. Haematologic toxicity may require dose reduction or delay or suspension of PHARMORUBICIN PFS therapy. Persistent myelosuppression may result in infection or haemorrhage.

PHARMORUBICIN PFS may potentiate the toxicity of other anticancer therapies as well as radiation induced toxicity to the myocardium, mucosa and skin. Patients should recover from acute toxicities (such as stomatitis, neutropenia, thrombocytopenia and generalized infections) of prior cytotoxic treatment before beginning treatment with PHARMORUBICIN PFS.

While treatment with high doses of epirubicin (e.g., ≥90 mg/m² every 3 to 4 weeks) causes adverse events generally similar to those seen at standard doses (<90 mg/m² every 3 to 4 weeks), the severity of the neutropenia and stomatitis/mucositis may be increased. Treatment with high doses of the drug does require special attention for possible clinical complications due to profound myelosuppression.

Immunosuppressant Effects/Increased Susceptibility to Infections : Administration of live or live-attenuated vaccines in patients immunocompromised by chemotherapeutic agents including epirubicin, may result in serious or fatal infections. Vaccination with a live vaccine should be avoided in patients receiving epirubicin. Killed or inactivated vaccines may be administered; however, the response to such vaccines may be diminished.

Liver Function: Epirubicin is extensively metabolized by the liver and its major route of elimination is the hepatobiliary system. Serum total bilirubin and AST levels should be evaluated before and during treatment with epirubicin. Patients with elevated bilirubin or AST may experience slower clearance of drug with an increase in overall toxicity. Lower doses are recommended in these patients (see Dosage and Administration). Patients with severe hepatic impairment should not receive epirubicin (see Contraindications).

Renal Function: Serum creatinine should be assessed before and during therapy. Dosage adjustment is necessary in patients with serum creatinine >5 mg/dL (see Dosage and Administration).

Secondary Leukemia: The occurrence of secondary acute myeloid leukemia (AML) with or without a preleukemic phase (myelodysplastic syndrome or MDS) has been reported in patients treated with epirubicin-containing regimens. Such cases could have a short (1-3 years) latency period (see below and in Table 2 under Adverse Effects).

The quantified risk of developing acute myeloid leukemia (AML), including myelodysplastic syndrome (MDS), following epirubicin or epirubicin-containing therapy, has been estimated by analyzing data collected prospectively from 19 randomized trials for the adjuvant treatment of early breast cancer, that were either company-sponsored or conducted by independent institutions (including the National Institute of Canada's MA.5 trial). As of 31 December 2001, 28 (0.39%) of the 7,110 evaluable patients treated with epirubicin, had presented with either AML or MDS. An additional 4 patients were diagnosed with other types of leukemia: 3 with acute lymphoblastic leukemia (ALL), and 1 with chronic lymphocytic leukemia (CLL). The time elapsed from the start of adjuvant treatment to the diagnosis of AML/MDS ranged from 8 to 126 months, with a median of 33 months. Of the 23 cases of AML/MDS for whom cytogenetic information was available, in 12 there was evidence of balanced chromosome translocations, and in 7 these translocations involved chromosome 11 or 21. Therapy-induced leukemia secondary to topoisomerase inhibitors generally has a short induction period (6 months to 5 years) and is known to be associated with translocations involving chromosome 11 or 21.

In this most recent analysis, the cumulative risk of developing AML/MDS in the 7,110 patients treated with epirubicin was 0.27% (95% confidence interval 0.14%, 0.40%) at 3 years, 0.46% (95% confidence interval 0.28%, 0.65%) at 5 years, and 0.55% (95% confidence interval, 0.33%, 0.78%) at 8 years. AML/MDS rates increased with epirubicin dose per cycle, and cumulative dose. For instance, in the MA.5 trial, in patients that received intensive doses of epirubicin (120 mg/m^2), the incidence of AML/MDS was 1.1% at 5 years with no additional cases observed during the second 5 years (years 6-10) of follow-up.

Since the completion of these analyses, in the period up to and including September 2003, further spontaneous, literature and study reports of AML/MDS have been received.

In addition, in 10 trials for the treatment of advanced breast cancer (3061 patients, follow-up until March 1999), two cases of AML occurred. However, due to the small number of cases and the limited follow-up as a result of the natural history of advanced breast cancer in these patients, risk estimates could not be made for this patient population.

General: PHARMORUBICIN PFS must not be administered by intramuscular or subcutaneous injection.

Severe local tissue necrosis can occur if PHARMORUBICIN PFS is extravasated during intravenous administration. Extravasation may occur with or without an accompanying stinging or burning sensation even if blood returns well on aspiration of the infusion needle (see Dosage and Administration). If signs or symptoms of extravasation occur the injection or infusion should be terminated immediately and restarted in another vein.

As with other cytotoxic agents, thrombophlebitis and thromboembolic phenomena, including pulmonary embolism (in some cases fatal) have been coincidentally reported with the use of epirubicin.

PHARMORUBICIN PFS is mutagenic, clastogenic, and carcinogenic in animals and has been associated with an increased risk of secondary leukemia (AML) in clinical trials of adjuvant treatment of breast cancer (see Adverse Reactions). In addition, epirubicin could induce chromosomal damage in human spermatozoa. Men undergoing treatment with epirubicin should use effective contraceptive methods.

Epirubicin may cause amenorrhea or premature menopause in premenopausal women.

PHARMORUBICIN PFS imparts a red colouration to the urine for 1 or 2 days after administration. Patients should be advised to expect this during active therapy.

Pregnant Women: There is no conclusive information about epirubicin adversely affecting human fertility, or causing teratogenesis; however, at high doses PHARMORUBICIN PFS is embryotoxic and teratogenic in rats and embryotoxic and abortifacient in rabbits. There are no studies in pregnant women. Therefore, women of childbearing potential should be advised to avoid pregnancy.

Epirubicin should be used during pregnancy only if the potential benefit justifies the potential risk to the fetus. If PHARMORUBICIN PFS is to be used during pregnancy, or if the patient becomes pregnant during therapy, the patient should be informed of the potential hazard to the fetus.

Nursing Women: Mothers should be advised not to breast-feed while undergoing chemotherapy with epirubicin.

Monitoring and Laboratory Tests: Initial treatment with PHARMORUBICIN PFS requires close observation of the patient and extensive laboratory monitoring. Like other cytotoxic drugs, PHARMORUBICIN PFS may induce hyperuricemia secondary to rapid lysis of neoplastic cells. The physician should monitor the patient's serum chemistry and blood uric acid level and be prepared to institute appropriate measures that might be necessary to control this problem. Hydration, urine alkalinization, and prophylaxis with allopurinol to prevent hyperuricemia may minimize potential complications of tumor-lysis syndrome.

PHARMORUBICIN PFS is not an anti-microbial agent.

Information to Be Provided to the Patient: Patients should be counseled about the known adverse effects that they could experience during chemotherapy with PHARMORUBICIN PFS, including cardiotoxicity, myelosuppression and risk of infection, thrombocytopenia, anemia, nausea, vomiting, and stomatitis.

Physicians should also clearly lay out early on the risks and benefits of the various chemotherapeutic options available, thus enabling the patient to make an informed treatment choice. Patients should be aware that higher dose regimens may have a greater toxicity that includes secondary leukemia. Wherever possible, the physician should discuss the information presented in the Information for the Patient section.

ADVERSE REACTIONS: Dose limiting toxicities are myelosuppression and cardiotoxicity (see Warnings and Precautions). Other reactions reported are:

Cutaneous: Reversible partial or complete alopecia occurs in most patients. Alopecia and lack of beard growth in males are usually reversible. Recall of skin reaction associated with prior radiotherapy may occur with PHARMORUBICIN PFS (epirubicin hydrochloride injection) administration. Local toxicity, rash/itch and skin changes may also occur.

Gastrointestinal: Acute nausea and vomiting occurs frequently in most patients. This may be alleviated by antiemetic therapy. Mucositis (stomatitis and esophagitis) has been reported to occur 5-10 days after administration. This may lead to ulceration and represents a site of origin for severe infections. Diarrhea has been reported. Most patients recover from this adverse event by the third week of therapy.

Local: Severe cellulitis, vesication, local pain and tissue necrosis can occur if PHARMORUBICIN PFS is extravasated during administration (see Dosage and Administration). Erythematous streaking and/or transient urticaria along the vein proximal to the site of administration may occur. Venous sclerosis may result from injection into small veins or repeated injection into the same vein. Following the recommended administration procedures may minimize the risk of phlebitis/thrombophlebitis at the injection site (see Special Handling Instructions).

Haematological: A dose-dependent, reversible leukopenia and/or granulocytopenia (neutropenia) are the predominant manifestations of epirubicin bone marrow/haematologic toxicity and represents the acute dose-limiting toxicity of this drug. Leukopenia and neutropenia are usually more severe after administration of high-dose regimens; under these conditions appropriate bone marrow support e.g., peripheral blood progenitor cells and/or colony-stimulating factors) may be required. Thrombocytopenia and anemia may also occur. Clinical consequences of severe myelosuppression include fever, infection, sepsis/septicemia, septic shock, hemorrhage, tissue hypoxia, or death.

Secondary Leukemia: See Warnings and Precautions.

Body as a Whole: Phlebitis, fever and malaise/asthenia have been reported following administration of PHARMORUBICIN PFS.

Drug-related adverse events also occurred in the following systems:

Endocrine: amenorrhea and hot flashes.

Cardiovascular: asymptomatic drops in left ventricular ejection fraction and congestive heart failure.

Ocular: conjunctivitis, keratitis.

Other: infection, acute lymphocytic leukemia, acute myelogenous leukemia.

Adverse Reactions in Early Breast Cancer Adjuvant Treatment: On-Study Events: Integrated safety data are available from two studies (Studies MA.5 and GFEA-05 [FASG-05]) evaluating epirubicin-containing combination regimens in patients with early breast cancer. Of the 1260 patients treated in these studies, 620 patients received the higher-dose epirubicin regimen (FEC-100/CEF-120), 280 patients received the lower-dose epirubicin regimen (FEC-50), and 360 patients received CMF. Serotonin-specific anti-emetic therapy and colony-stimulating factors were not used in these trials. Clinically relevant acute adverse events are summarized inTable 1.

Delayed Events: Table 2 describes the incidence of delayed adverse events in patients participating in the MA.5 and GFEA-05 (FASG-05) trials.

Within the first 5 year follow-up period, two cases of acute lymphoid leukemia (ALL) were also observed in patients receiving epirubicin. However, an association between anthracyclines such as epirubicin and ALL has not been clearly established.

Over the 10 year follow-up period for study GFEA-05 (FASG-05), the overall incidence of cardiac events in patients treated with FEC-100 remained similar to that reported in patients receiving FEC-50. There were, however, two new cases of decreased left ventricular ejection fraction reported in FEC-100 treated patients. Therefore, the incidence of decreased left ventricular ejection fraction was 1.1 % (3/280) in the FEC-50 group and 3% (8/266) in the FEC-100 group. No new cases of delayed CHF were reported. Thus the frequency of CHF remains at 0.4% (1/280) in the FEC-50 and at 1.1% (3/266) in the FEC-100 group. In a subset of patients from this study who were without disease at median follow up time of 102 months, a subsequent analysis of long term cardiac function identified 2 patients with CHF amongst the 85 FEC-100 patients evaluated. Cardiac function was not monitored after 5 years in MA.5 study.

No new cases of secondary leukemia were reported in the 10 year follow up for both MA.5 and GFEA-05 (FASG-05) trials.

Post-Market Adverse Drug Reactions: Gastrointestinal: pain or burning sensation, erythema, erosions, ulcerations, bleeding, dehydration, hyperpigmentation of the oral mucosa.

Table 1: PHARMORUBICIN PFS

Clinically Relevant Acute Adverse Events in Patients with Early Breast Cancer

	% of Patients					
	FEC-100/CEF-120 (N=620)		FEC-50 (N=280)		CMF (N=360)	
Event	**Grades 1-4**	**Grades 3/4**	**Grades 1-4**	**Grades 3/4**	**Grades 1-4**	**Grades 3/4**
Hematologic						
Leukopenia	80.3	58.6	49.6	1.5	98.1	60.3
Neutropenia	80.3	67.2	53.9	10.5	95.8	78.1
Anemia	72.2	5.8	12.9	0	70.9	0.9
Thrombocytopenia	48.8	5.4	4.6	0	51.4	3.6
Endocrine						
Amenorrhea	71.8	0	69.3	0	67.7	0
Hot Flashes	38.9	4.0	5.4	0	69.1	6.4
Body as a Whole						
Lethargy	45.8	1.9	1.1	0	72.7	0.3
Fever	5.2	0	1.4	0	4.5	0
Gastrointestinal						
Nausea/Vomiting	92.4	25.0	83.2	22.1	85.0	6.4
Mucositis	58.5	8.9	9.3	0	52.9	1.9
Diarrhea	24.8	0.8	7.1	0	50.7	2.8
Anorexia	2.9	0	1.8	0	5.8	0.3
Infection						
Infection	21.5	1.6	15.0	0	25.9	0.6
Febrile Neutropenia	NA	6.1	0	0	NA	1.1
Ocular						
Conjunctivitis/Keratitis	14.8	0	1.1	0	38.4	0
Skin						
Alopecia	95.5	56.6	69.6	19.3	84.4	6.7
Local Toxicity	19.5	0.3	2.5	0.4	8.1	0
Rash/Itch	8.9	0.3	1.4	0	14.2	0
Skin Changes	4.7	0	0.7	0	7.2	0

Grade 1 or 2 changes in transaminase levels were observed but were more frequently seen with CMF than with CEF.
Legend: FEC & CEF=cyclophosphamide+epirubicin+fluorouracil; CMF=cyclophosphamide+methotrexate+flurouracil; NA=not available.

Table 2: PHARMORUBICIN PFS

Long-term Adverse Events in Patients with Early Breast Cancer (5-year follow-up data)[a]

	% of Patients		
Event	**FEC-100/CEF-120 (N=620)**	**FEC-50 (N=280)**	**CMF (N=360)**
Cardiac Toxicity			
Asymptomatic drops in LVEF	1.8	1.4	0.8
CHF	1.5	0.4	0.3
AML/MDS			
AML	0.8	0	0.3
MDS	0	0	0

[a] In study MA.5 cardiac function was not monitored after 5 years. In study GFEA-05 (FASG-05) monitoring of cardiac function was optional.

Cutaneous: flushes, skin and nail hyperpigmentation, photosensitivity, hypersensitivity to irradiated skin (radiation-recall reaction).

Hypersensitivity Reactions: urticaria, anaphylaxis, fever, chills, shock.

Vascular: phlebitis, thrombophlebitis.

Urological: red colouration of urine for 1 to 2 days after administration.

DRUG INTERACTIONS: Epirubicin is mainly used in combination with other cytotoxic drugs. Additive toxicity may occur especially with regard to bone marrow/haematologic and gastro-intestinal effects (see Warnings and Precautions). The use of epirubicin in combination chemotherapy with other potentially cardiotoxic drugs, as well as the concomitant use of other cardioactive compounds (e.g., calcium channel blockers), requires monitoring of cardiac function throughout treatment.

Cimetidine increased the AUC of epirubicin by 50% when given for seven days, starting five days before chemotherapy. Cimetidine should be stopped prior to treatment with epirubicin.

DOSAGE AND ADMINISTRATION: Refer to Special Handling Instructions.

Dosage: A variety of dose schedules have been used. The following recommendations are for use as a single agent or in combination with other chemotherapeutic agents.

Dosage is usually calculated on the basis of body surface area. The lower dose should be given to patients with inadequate marrow reserves due to prior therapy or neoplastic marrow infiltration. Standard starting doses and regimens have been used in the elderly.

Hepatic Dysfunction: As PHARMORUBICIN PFS is extensively metabolized by the liver and excreted primarily by the biliary system, its dosage must be reduced in patients with impaired liver function indicated by elevated bilirubin or serum AST values as follows: Serum bilirubin 21-51 µmol/L or AST 2 to 4 times upper limit of normal—give ½ of recommended starting dose; Serum bilirubin >51 µmol/L or AST >4 times upper limit of normal—give ¼ of recommended starting dose. Patients with severe hepatic impairment should not receive epirubicin (see Contraindications).

Renal Dysfunction: While no specific dose recommendation can be made based on the limited available data in patients with renal impairment, lower starting doses are necessary in patients with severe renal impairment (serum creatinine >5 mg/dL).

Other Special Populations: Lower starting doses or longer intervals between cycles may need to be considered for heavily pretreated patients or patients with neoplastic bone marrow infiltration (see Warnings and Precautions). Standard starting doses and regimens have been used in the elderly.

Carcinoma of the Breast: Early Breast Cancer-Adjuvant Treatment: Breast cancer has been managed using epirubicin in combination with various chemotherapeutic agents. The recommended adjuvant treatment of early breast cancer should employ a cyclophosphamide, epirubicin, and 5-fluorouracil combination regimen (CEF 120) in a cycle to be repeated every 4 weeks for 6 cycles as follows:

- cyclophosphamide 75 mg/m² p.o. on days 1 to14,
- epirubicin 60 mg/m² i.v. on days 1 and 8, and
- 5-fluorouracil 500 mg/m² i.v. days 1 and 8.

Metastatic Breast Cancer: Single Agent: The most commonly used dosage schedule of PHARMORUBICIN PFS (epirubicin hydrochloride injection) in metastatic breast cancer, when employed as a single agent for adults, is 75-90 mg/m² administered at 21-day intervals. The recommended single dose may be divided over 2 successive days. An alternative weekly dosage schedule of 12.5 to 25 mg/m² has been used and has been reported to produce less clinical toxicity than higher doses given every three weeks.

Combination Therapy: In metastatic breast cancer, epirubicin can be used in combination with cyclophosphamide and 5-fluorouracil (FEC), at a dose of 50 mg/m².

Small Cell Lung Cancer: Single Agent: PHARMORUBICIN PFS, as a single agent, can be used at 90-120 mg/m² administered every 3 weeks.

Combination Therapy: Epirubicin has been used in several different combinations with other antineoplastic agents at doses ranging from 50-90 mg/m². The following combinations have proven effective: Epirubicin in combination with either cisplatin or ifosfamide; epirubicin with cyclophosphamide and vincristine (CEV); epirubicin with cyclophosphamide and etoposide (CEVP-16) and epirubicin with cisplatin and etoposide.

Non-small Cell Lung Cancer: Single Agent: PHARMORUBICIN PFS, as a single agent, can be used at doses of 120-150 mg/m² administered day 1, every 3-4 weeks.

Combination Therapy: Epirubicin, in combination with etoposide, cisplatinum, mitomycin, vindesine and vinblastine, can be used at doses of 90-120 mg/m² administered day 1, every 3-4 weeks.

Non-Hodgkin's Lymphoma: Single Agent: PHARMORUBICIN PFS, as a single agent, can be used at doses of 75 to 90 mg/m² at 21-day intervals.

Combination Therapy: Epirubicin at doses of 60-75 mg/m² can be used in combination with cyclophosphamide, vincristine and prednisone with or without bleomycin (replacing doxorubicin in the CHOP, CHOP-Bleo or BACOP regimens) for the treatment of newly diagnosed non-Hodgkin's lymphoma.

Hodgkin's Disease: Combination Therapy: Epirubicin, in combination with bleomycin, vinblastine and dacarbazine, can be used at 35 mg/m² every 2 weeks or 70 mg/m² every 3-4 weeks (replacing doxorubicin in the ABVD regimen).

Ovarian Cancer: Single Agent: In patients with prior therapy, epirubicin can be used as single agent at doses of 50-90 mg/m² at 3-4 week intervals.

Combination Therapy: In patients with prior therapy epirubicin can be used in combination at doses of 50-90 mg/m² at 3-4 week intervals. Epirubicin at doses of 50-90 mg/m² in combination with cisplatin and cyclophosphamide can be used for initial therapy of ovarian cancer repeated at 3-4 week intervals.

Gastric Cancer: Single Agent: Epirubicin, as a single agent, can be used for the treatment of locally unresectable or metastatic gastric carcinoma at doses of 75-100 mg/m².

Combination Therapy: Epirubicin, at a dose of 80 mg/m² can be used in combination with fluorouracil for the treatment of locally unresectable or metastatic gastric carcinoma.

Administration: Care in the administration of PHARMORUBICIN PFS will reduce the chance of perivenous infiltration. It may also decrease the chance of local reactions such as urticaria and erythematous streaking. On intravenous administration of PHARMORUBICIN PFS extravasation may occur with or without an accompanying stinging or burning sensation even if blood returns well on aspiration of the infusion needle. If any signs or symptoms of extravasation have occurred the injection or infusion should be immediately terminated and restarted in another vein. If it is known or suspected that subcutaneous extravasation has occurred, the following steps are recommended:

1. Attempt aspiration of the infiltrated PHARMORUBICIN PFS solution.
2. Local intermittent application of ice for up to 3 days.
3. Elevation of the affected limb.
4. Close observation of the lesion.
5. Consultation with a plastic surgeon familiar with drug extravasation if local pain persists or skin changes progress after 3 to 4 days. If ulceration begins, early wide excision of the involved area should be considered.

PHARMORUBICIN PFS should be slowly administered into the tubing of a freely running intravenous infusion of Sodium Chloride Solution USP (0.9%) or 5% Dextrose Solution USP. The tubing should be attached to a Butterfly needle or other suitable device and inserted preferably into a large vein. If possible, avoid veins over joints or in extremities with compromised venous or lymphatic drainage. To minimize the risk of thrombosis or perivenous extravasation, the usual infusion times range between 3 and 20 minutes depending upon dosage and volume of the infusion solution. The infusion time should be not less than 3 to 5 minutes. A direct push injection is not recommended due to the risk of extravasation, which may occur even in the presence of adequate blood return upon needle aspiration (see Warnings and Precautions). Local erythematous streaking along the vein as well as facial flushing may be indicative of too rapid administration. A burning or stinging may be indicative of perivenous infiltration and the infusion should be immediately terminated and restarted in another vein. Perivenous infiltration may occur painlessly.

Unless specific compatibility data are available, mixing PHARMORUBICIN PFS with other drugs is not recommended.

PHARMORUBICIN PFS has been used concurrently with other approved chemotherapeutic agents. Evidence is available that combination chemotherapy is superior to single agents. The benefits and risks of such therapy continue to be elucidated.

For Safe Preparation and Handling of PHARMORUBICIN PFS refer to "Special Handling Instructions".

OVERDOSAGE:

Acute overdosage with PHARMORUBICIN PFS (epirubicin hydrochloride injection) may cause an acute myocardial dysfunction within 24 hours. Pronounced mucositis, leukopenia and thrombocytopenia could be observed within 7-14 days. Treatment of acute overdosage consists of hospitalization of the severely myelosuppressed patient, platelet and granulocyte transfusions, antibiotics, and symptomatic treatment of mucositis.

For management of a suspected drug overdose, CPhA recommends that you contact your **regional Poison Control Centre**. See the *CPS* Directory section for a list of Poison Control Centres.

ACTION AND CLINICAL PHARMACOLOGY: The mechanism of action of epirubicin, although not completely elucidated, appears to be related to its ability to bind to nucleic acids by intercalation of the planar anthracycline nucleus with the DNA double helix.

Binding to cell membranes as well as to plasma proteins may also be involved. Cell culture studies have demonstrated rapid cell penetration and perinucleolar chromatin binding, rapid inhibition of mitotic activity, mutagenesis and chromosomal aberrations.

Animal studies have shown activity in a wide spectrum of experimental tumours, immunosuppression, mutagenic and carcinogenic properties in rodents, and a variety of toxic effects, including myelosuppression in all species and atrophy of the seminiferous tubules of testes in rats and dogs.

Data from different animal species and in vitro models have shown that epirubicin is less toxic, and in particular less cardiotoxic than doxorubicin.

At equally effective doses, epirubicin produces less severe non-haematologic side effects such as vomiting and mucositis, than doxorubicin.

Early Stage Breast Cancer Studies: Two randomized, open-label, multi center studies evaluated PHARMORUBICIN 100 to 120 mg/m² in combination with cyclophosphamide and fluorouracil in adjuvant treatment of axillary-node-positive breast cancer with no evidence of distant metastatic disease (see Adverse Reactions).

Study MA.5 evaluated 120 mg/m² doses of epirubicin per course in combination with cyclophosphamide and fluorouracil (CEF-120 regimen) versus a CMF (methotrexate) regimen in pre- and peri-menopausal women.

Study GFEA-05 (FASG-05) evaluated 100 mg/m² doses of epirubicin per course in combination with fluorouracil and cyclophosphamide (FEC-100) or lower-dose FEC-50 in pre- and post-menopausal women.

In the pivotal trial MA.5, the Cox proportional model showed that node number is a significant (p=0.0001) outcome predictor overall (conditional risk ratio of 1.7 for ≥4 versus <3 involved nodes). Non-significant trends indicate that the CEF treatment may show superiority over CMF in patients with ≥4 nodes than those with <3. The trial was insufficiently powered to demonstrate a subset difference; it must be borne in mind that the majority of patients (61%) in both treatments had 1-3 positive nodes, yet CEF-120 still produced overall advantages in relapse free survival (RFS) and overall survival (OS) (see below). Nonetheless, CEF versus CMF RFS in the <3 node group was 68 vs. 62%, while in the ≥4 node group the values were 52 vs. 39%.

In the supporting trial GFEA-05 (FASG-05), similar improvements in RFS and OS were observed in both pre- and post-menopausal women treated with FEC-100 compared to FEC-50.

The median follow-up time in the MA.5 study was 8.8 years (range: 0.2 to 12.1 years) and 8.7 years (range: 0.7 to 12.1 years) for the CEF and CMF treatment groups, respectively. In MA.5, the CEF-120 therapy demonstrated superior RFS to CMF, both over the 5- and 10-year follow-up. The overall reduction in risk of relapse was 24% over 5 years and 22% over 10 years. The 5- and 10-year OS were also greater for the epirubicin-containing CEF-120 regimen than for the CMF regimen. The overall relative reduction in the risk of death was 29% over 5 years and 18% over 10 years.

Pharmacokinetics: Pharmacokinetic studies show an initial rapid elimination of the parent compound from plasma. The terminal half-life of elimination of the parent drug from plasma approximates 30-40 hours in humans. Urinary excretion accounts for approximately 9-10% of the administered dose in 48 hours. Biliary excretion represents the major route of elimination, about 40% of the administered dose being recovered in the bile in 72 hours. The major metabolites that have been identified are epirubicinol (13-OH epirubicin) and glucuronides of epirubicin and epirubicinol.

The 4'-O-glucuronidation distinguishes epirubicin from doxorubicin and may account for the faster elimination of epirubicin and its reduced toxicity. Plasma levels of the main metabolite, the 13-OH derivative (epirubicinol) are consistently lower and virtually parallel to those of the unchanged drug.

Impairment of hepatic function results in higher plasma levels.

Distribution studies in the rat have shown that epirubicin does not appear to cross the blood-brain barrier.

STORAGE AND STABILITY: PHARMORUBICIN PFS (epirubicin hydrochloride injection) should be stored under refrigeration (2-8°C), and retained in original carton until time of use. Unused solution should be discarded.

Dispensing from the Pharmacy Bulk Vial should be completed within eight hours of initial entry because of the potential for microbial contamination.

Incompatibility: Unless specific compatibility data are available, PHARMORUBICIN PFS should not be mixed with other drugs.

Contact with any solution of an alkaline pH should be avoided, as it will result in hydrolysis of the drug. Epirubicin should also not be mixed with heparin due to chemical incompatibility that may lead to precipitation.

SPECIAL HANDLING INSTRUCTIONS: Preparation and Handling:

1. Personnel should be trained in good technique for reconstitution and handling. Pregnant staff should be excluded from working with this drug.
2. Preparation of antineoplastic solutions should be done in a vertical laminar flow hood (Biological Safety Cabinet-Class II) and the work surface should be protected by disposable, plastic-backed absorbent paper.
3. Personnel handling epirubicin solutions should wear PVC gloves, safety glasses and protective clothing such as disposable gowns and masks. If epirubicin solutions contact the skin or mucosa, the area should be washed with soap and water or sodium bicarbonate immediately. Do not abrade the skin by using a scrub brush and always wash hands after removing gloves.
4. In case of contact with the eye(s), hold back the eyelid of the affected eye(s) and flush with copious amounts of water for at least 15 minutes, proceed to a physician for medical evaluation.
5. Personnel regularly involved in the preparation and handling of antineoplastics should have blood examinations on a regular basis.
6. Directions for Dispensing from Pharmacy Bulk Vial:

   The use of Pharmacy Bulk Vials is restricted to hospitals with a recognized intravenous admixture program. The Pharmacy Bulk Vial is intended for single puncture, multiple dispensing and for intravenous use only.

   Entry into the vial must be made with a sterile dispensing device such as the Econ-O-Set Sterile Transfer System. Multiple use of a syringe with needle is not recommended since it may cause leakage as well as increasing the potential for microbial and particulate contamination.

   Swab the vial stopper with an antiseptic solution. Following carefully the manufacturer's instructions, insert the device into the vial. Withdraw contents of vial into syringes, using aseptic technique. Discard any unused portion within eight hours of initial entry.

Disposal:

1. Avoid contact with skin and inhalation of airborne particles by use of PVC gloves and disposable gowns and masks.
2. All needles, syringes, vials and other materials which have come in contact with epirubicin should be segregated in plastic bags, sealed, and marked as hazardous waste. Incinerate at 1000°C or higher. Sealed containers may explode if a tight seal exists.
3. If incineration is not available, epirubicin hydrochloride may be detoxified by adding sodium hypochlorite solution (household bleach) to the vial, in sufficient quantity to decolourize the epirubicin, care being taken to vent the vial to avoid a pressure build-up of the chlorine gas which is generated. Dispose of detoxified vials in a safe manner.

Needles, Syringes, Disposable and Nondisposable Equipment: Rinse equipment with an appropriate quantity of sodium hypochlorite solution. Discard the solution and disposable equipment in a safe manner. Thoroughly wash non-disposable equipment in soap and water.

Spillage/Contamination: Wear gloves, mask, protective clothing. Treat spilled liquid with sodium hypochlorite solution. Carefully absorb solution with gauze pads or towels, wash area with water and absorb with gauze or towels again and place in polyethylene bag; seal, double bag and mark as hazardous waste. Disposal of waste by incineration or by other methods approved for hazardous materials. Personnel involved in clean-up should wash with soap and water.

INFORMATION FOR THE PATIENT: Published in e-CPS, available by subscription at www.e-cps.ca.

DOSAGE FORMS, COMPOSITION AND PACKAGING: Each mL of sterile, ready-to-use, red-orange, isotonic, non-preserved solution contains: epirubicin HCl 2 mg, sodium chloride USP 9 mg and water for injection q.s. Also contains hydrochloric acid for pH adjustment. Single glass and polypropylene vials of 5, 25 and 100 mL.

Phenobarbital ©

CPhA Monograph

see *Barbiturates*

Phenobarbital Sodium Injection USP ©

phenobarbital sodium

Anticonvulsant—Hypnotic—Sedative (Barbiturate)

Sandoz

Date of Preparation: December 11, 2007
Date of Revision: November 18, 2008

PHARMACOLOGY: Phenobarbital, like many other barbiturates, is a nonselective central nervous system (CNS) depressant, capable of producing all degrees of depression from mild sedation and hypnosis to general anesthesia, deep coma and death. The extent of CNS depression varies with the route of administration, dose and pharmacokinetic characteristics of the particular barbiturates. Patient specific factors such as age, physical or emotional state and the concomitant use of other drugs will also affect response.

The mechanism of action of phenobarbital is not completely known. Phenobarbital may act by enhancing and/or mimicking the synaptic action of gamma-aminobutyric acid (GABA), an inhibitory neurotransmitter. The sedative-hypnotic action of phenobarbital may be due to an inhibition of conduction in the reticular formation resulting in a decrease in the number of impulses reaching the cerebral cortex.

Anticonvulsant activity may result from a reduction in CNS synaptic transmission and an increase in the threshold for electrical stimulation of the motor cortex. Phenobarbital is the only barbiturate with anticonvulsant activity at subhypnotic doses.

The therapeutic index of barbiturates, such as phenobarbital, is narrow. Therefore, the use of phenobarbital is almost always accompanied by some degree of impairment of cognitive function. Supratherapeutic doses lead to marked mental and motor impairment. In some patients (especially children and the elderly), drowsiness may be paradoxically preceded by transient euphoria, elation, excitement and confusion.

Pharmacokinetics: The pharmacokinetics of phenobarbital as well as other common barbiturates are shown in Table 1. After oral administration, absorption is usually rapid and relatively complete. The sodium salts undergo rapid dissolution and are absorbed more quickly than their corresponding free acids. The rate of absorption is increased when the barbiturate is formulated as a liquid, when the stomach is empty and when alcohol is ingested concurrently. The onset of action following rectal administration is similar to that following oral administration. After IV administration, the onset of action is immediate for amobarbital and pentobarbital and within 5 minutes for phenobarbital. The onset of action following IM administration is slightly faster than when the drugs are administered orally or rectally.

Once absorbed, phenobarbital is rapidly distributed to all tissues and fluids. High concentrations appear in the brain, liver and kidneys. Secobarbital has the highest degree of lipid solubility and thus the fastest distribution, phenobarbital is the least lipid soluble and has the slowest distribution. Phenobarbital readily cross the placenta and is excreted into breast milk. If administered IV, fetal blood concentrations are approximately equal to maternal serum concentration; if administered orally, fetal concentrations are less than maternal levels.

Barbiturates are slowly metabolized and/or conjugated in the liver and then excreted renally. Amobarbital, pentobarbital and secobarbital are almost completely metabolized. Due to its lower lipid solubility, phenobarbital is not metabolized as extensively and almost 25% is excreted unchanged in the urine. One of the metabolites of primidone is phenobarbital.

Metabolic elimination is influenced by age (being slower in the elderly and infants), chronic liver disease and other drugs.

Table 1: Phenobarbital Sodium Injection USP

Barbiturates Pharmacokinetics

Drug	Onset of Action (minutes)	Half-life (hours)	Duration of Action (hours)
Amobarbital[a]	45 to 60	8 to 42	6 to 8
Butalbital[a]	15 to 60	35	4 to 6
Pentobarbital[a]	10 to 15	15 to 48	3 to 4
Phenobarbital[a]	60	80 to 120	10 to 12
Primidone	N/A	10 to 12	10 to 12
Secobarbital[a]	10 to 15	15 to 40	3 to 4
Thiopental[b]	1	8 to 10	10 to 30 minutes

[a] Oral administration.
[b] Intravenous administration.

INDICATIONS: The use of barbiturates as sedative/hypnotics has largely been replaced by less toxic agents such as benzodiazepines. Barbiturates have been used parenterally in the management of status epilepticus or acute seizure episodes that are secondary to meningitis or other causes.

Phenobarbital is indicated for the control of generalized tonic-clonic and complex partial seizures.

CONTRAINDICATIONS: Phenobarbital should not to be administered to patients who are known to be hypersensitive to barbituric acid derivatives, or patients with porphyria, severe respiratory depression or pulmonary insufficiency, renal impairment, hepatic impairment, sleep apnea, suicidal potential, alcoholism, drug dependence or in the presence of uncontrolled pain (paradoxical excitement may be produced). With the exception of phenobarbital, barbiturates should be avoided in older individuals.

WARNINGS: See Precautions.

PRECAUTIONS: Prolonged use of phenobarbital, even in therapeutic dosages, may result in psychologic and physiologic dependence. Patients may escalate dosage without medical advice. Withdrawal symptoms may occur following abrupt termination of hypnotic doses causing nightmares or insomnia, sweating, irritability, tremor, weight loss, anorexia or after chronic use of large doses, resulting in delirium, seizures, or death. Withdrawal should be cautious and gradual.

Rarely, rickets and osteomalacia have been reported following prolonged usage of phenobarbital due to increased metabolism of vitamin D.

Phenobarbital should be used with caution in patients with impaired liver function or in patients with a history of drug dependence or abuse. Caution is essential when the drug is administered in the presence of any respiratory difficulty. Special care should be taken when phenobarbital is administered to patients in whom the hypnotic effect may be prolonged or intensified, as in those suffering from shock, hepatic dysfunction, uremia, or after recent administration of other respiratory depressants.

Since phenobarbital is a potent CNS depressant, IV administration should not be attempted without adequate provisions for supporting respiration and circulation. Rapid injection can cause cardiovascular collapse. Slow administration will usually prevent this occurrence but may cause apnea, laryngospasm, coughing, or other respiratory difficulties. IM injection should not exceed a volume of 5 mL at any one site because of possible tissue damage.

Phenobarbital solutions are highly alkaline. Extreme care should be exercised to avoid extravasation or intra-arterial injection. Extravascular injection may cause local tissue damage with subsequent necrosis. The consequences of intra-arterial injection may vary from transient pain along the course of the artery to gangrene of the limb. Signs of accidental injection by this route include, in addition to pain, delayed onset of hypnosis, pallor and cyanosis of the extremity and patchy discolouration of the skin. Any complaint of pain in the limb warrants stopping the injection.

Hypotension may result from IV administration of the drug, particularly in patients with hypertension. Slow administration will usually prevent this occurrence.

Solutions that appear cloudy or in which a precipitate has formed should not be used.

Occupational Hazards: Phenobarbital may impair the mental and/or physical abilities required for the performance of potentially hazardous tasks such as driving a vehicle or operating machinery. The concomitant use of alcohol or other CNS depressants may have an additive effect. Patients should be warned accordingly. The incidence of fractures due to falls may be increased, particularly in the elderly. Following use of phenobarbital in office procedures, warn patients against operating motor vehicles for the remainder of the day.

Drug Interactions: Most drug interactions have been documented with phenobarbital, however they are likely applicable to other barbiturates as well. The barbiturates are inducers of cytochrome P450 isoenzymes CYP1A2, CYP2C9, CYP2C19 and CYP3A4, and are capable of increasing the clearance of many hepatically metabolized drugs. This can result in two concerns: i) decrease in or loss of effectiveness of other drug(s) during phenobarbital use; ii) increase in effect or frank toxicity of the other drug(s) on discontinuation of phenobarbital.

When adding or deleting any barbiturate to or from the patient's therapeutic regimen, pharmacotherapy must be monitored closely as dosage adjustment may be necessary.

Anticoagulants, Oral: Metabolism of coumarin anticoagulants may be accelerated, resulting in decreased anticoagulant response. Correspondingly, if phenobarbital is discontinued from a stabilized regimen, the hypoprothrombinemic response may be greatly increased, potentially resulting in hemorrhagic complications. Prothrombin times should be monitored closely when barbiturates are added to or deleted from a regimen that includes oral anticoagulants.

Anticonvulsants: Phenytoin: When phenobarbital is used with phenytoin, concentrations of either or both drugs may be increased, decreased or unchanged. While phenobarbital may induce the metabolism of phenytoin, it may also decrease it because both drugs compete for the same metabolic pathway. Plasma concentrations of both drugs should be monitored when any change in the therapeutic regimen occurs.

Valproic Acid: Concomitant administration of valproic acid and phenobarbital usually results in increased levels of phenobarbital and resultant oversedation. There have been case reports of progression of CNS depression to coma. Plasma concentrations of both drugs should be monitored when any change in the therapeutic regimen occurs.

Carbamazepine: When phenobarbital and carbamazepine are used together, the metabolism of carbamazepine is usually accelerated and plasma concentrations may be decreased. The clinical significance of this interaction is not known. Plasma concentrations of both drugs should be monitored when any change in the therapeutic regimen occurs.

Antidepressants, MAO Inhibitors: MAO inhibitors may inhibit phenobarbital metabolism, resulting in increased CNS depressant effects. A reduction in phenobarbital dosage may be required.

Antidepressants, Tricyclic: Phenobarbital may increase metabolism of tricyclic antidepressants resulting in lack of effect. Plasma tricyclic concentrations should be monitored if possible, especially if the patient is not responding to standard dosages of antidepressant. The use of both drugs concomitantly may result in additive respiratory depressant effects.

CNS Depressants: Alcohol, benzodiazepines and other CNS depressants used concurrently with phenobarbital may result in excessive CNS depression.

Corticosteroids: Phenobarbital may increase the metabolism of corticosteroids. There have been several reports of exacerbation of asthma and other conditions when phenobarbital was added to regimens containing corticosteroids.

Contraceptives, Oral: Phenobarbital may accelerate the metabolism of both the estrogenic and progestagenic components of the contraceptive, resulting in decreased effectiveness, which may or may not be signalled by breakthrough bleeding. There have been reports of pregnancy resulting from this combination. If phenobarbital is necessary it would be advisable to use some other form of contraception.

Miscellaneous: Phenobarbital has been reported to increase the metabolism and correspondingly reduce the effectiveness of the following: griseofulvin, digitoxin and doxycycline. When ketamine is used for anesthesia following preoperative administration of phenobarbital, profound respiratory depression may result.

Pregnancy: Phenobarbital readily crosses the placental barrier.

Phenobarbital and Primidone: The great majority of mothers on antiepileptic medication deliver normal infants. It is important to note that antiepileptic drugs should not be discontinued in patients in whom the drug is administered to prevent major seizures because of the strong possibility of precipitating status epilepticus with attendant hypoxia and threat to life. In individual cases where the severity and frequency of the seizure disorder are such that the removal of medication does not pose a serious threat to the patient, discontinuation of the drug may be considered prior to and during pregnancy, although it cannot be said with any confidence that even minor seizures do not pose some hazard to the developing embryo or fetus.

In addition to reports of increased incidence of congenital malformations such as cleft lip/palate and heart malformations in children of women receiving phenobarbital and other antiepileptic drugs, there have been reports of fetal hydantoin syndrome. This consists of prenatal growth deficiency, microcephaly and mental deficiency in children born to mothers who have received phenobarbital, phenytoin, alcohol or trimethadione. However, these features are all interrelated and are frequently associated with intrauterine growth retardation from other causes.

The prescribing physician should weigh these considerations in treating or counseling epileptic women of childbearing potential.

The serum level of anticonvulsants may decline during pregnancy requiring adjustments in dosage. Postpartum restoration of the original dosage will probably be indicated.

Neonatal coagulation defects have been reported within the first 24 hours in babies born to epileptic mothers receiving phenobarbital, primidone and/or phenytoin. Vitamin K has been shown to prevent or correct this defect and has been recommended to be given to the mother before delivery and to the neonate after birth.

Phenobarbital withdrawal has occurred in newborns who were exposed to the drug in utero and may be characterized by hypotonia, irritability and vomiting.

Lactation: Breast milk concentrations of barbiturates are 35 to 50% of maternal serum concentrations. Phenobarbital is eliminated slowly in neonates and may accumulate. Breastfed infants should be observed for excessive drowsiness, feeding problems, rash or other adverse effects. If any of these occur, breastfeeding should be discontinued. When breastfeeding is discontinued there is a potential for withdrawal symptoms in infants.

ADVERSE EFFECTS: CNS: Drowsiness is frequent, especially at initiation of therapy. Mild impairment of concentration, judgment, memory, and fine motor skills may occur. Disturbances of sleep, dizziness, vertigo, headache and depression may occur. Patients with uncontrolled pain may experience paradoxical euphoria, elation, excitement and confusion. In children, hyperactivity is not uncommon; behavioural disturbances and cognitive impairment may occur. Geriatric patients may experience excitation, confusion or depression.

Cardiovascular: Hypotension may be observed with IV administration and is generally related to the rate of administration (see Precautions).

Gastrointestinal: nausea, vomiting, diarrhea and constipation.

Hematologic: megaloblastic anemia (responds to folic acid therapy). Agranulocytosis and thrombocytopenia are rare.

Hypersensitivity: Facial edema, skin rash (1 to 2%) may be purpuric, vesicular or erythematous. Exfoliative dermatitis and erythema multiforme are rare. Hypersensitivity reactions have a greater tendency to occur in patients with a history of asthma, urticaria or angioedema.

Metabolic: Phenobarbital may increase vitamin D requirements, possibly by increasing vitamin D metabolism via enzyme induction. Rarely, rickets and osteomalacia have been reported following prolonged use of phenobarbital.

Respiratory: respiratory depression (see Precautions).

Hepatic: Severe allergic reactions may result in jaundice due to degenerative changes in the liver. Toxic hepatitis is rare.

Miscellaneous: exacerbation of porphyria, pain at the injection site, withdrawal (see Precautions).

OVERDOSE:

Symptoms: Acute overdosage with phenobarbital primarily affects the CNS and the cardiovascular system. Mild overdose resembles alcohol intoxication. Drowsiness, confusion, stupor, respiratory depression, ataxia, sluggish or absent reflexes, early hypothermia, late fever, cardiovascular depression with hypotension, renal failure, cardiac arrhythmias, pulmonary edema, aspiration pneumonia, bullae over pressure points and decreased gastrointestinal motility are all possible symptoms. Severe overdose may progress to shock, coma and death.

Doses that result in toxicity vary widely among patients. The lethal dose of phenobarbital is believed to be 5 g.

Chronic ingestion of phenobarbital results in the development of tolerance and large doses can be ingested without overt toxicity. Serious toxicity can result at lower phenobarbital levels if combined with alcohol or other CNS depressant drugs.

Treatment: Patients who have ingested phenobarbital in overdose often require respiratory and hemodynamic support. This may include intubation, ventilation, boluses of isotonic IV fluids, and inotrope infusions. Once a patient's airway is protected, activated charcoal should be administered to minimize absorption of orally administered phenobarbital. Administering multiple doses of activated charcoal enhances the clearance of phenobarbital, though there is no evidence that it actually improves clinical outcomes such as duration of intubation. In patients with normal renal and cardiac function, urinary alkalinization also enhances phenobarbital clearance. Likewise, urinary alkalinization has not actually been shown to improve clinical outcomes.

For management of a suspected drug overdose, contact your regional Poison Control Centre. See the *CPS* Directory section for a list of Poison Control Centres.

DOSAGE: The general use of phenobarbital as a sedative or hypnotic has for the most part, been supplanted by other less toxic drugs (i.e. benzodiazepines). Decreased dosage is recommended in older individuals and in patients with decreased renal or hepatic function. The phenobarbital can be given by deep IM or slow IV injection.

Preoperative: For intramuscular or slow intravenous injection.
Adults: 130 to 200 mg 1 to 2 hours prior to surgery.
Children: 1 to 3 mg/kg 1 to 2 hours prior to surgery.
Anticonvulsant: For intramuscular or slow intravenous injection.
Adults: 100 to 320 mg IV with additional doses if necessary to a maximum daily dose of 600 mg.
Children: Initial Loading Dose: 10-20 mg/day, maximum 125 mg/m² daily.
Maintenance Dose: 1 to 6 mg/kg/day.
Status Epilepticus: For slow intravenous injection.
Adults: 20 mg/kg IV at a rate of 50-75 mg/min [Barbiturates [product monograph]. In: Compendium of pharmaceuticals and specialties: the Canadian drug reference for health professionals. Ottawa (ON): CPhA; 2008. p. 302-3].
Children: 20 mg/kg IV over 20 minutes [Barbiturates [product monograph]. In: Compendium of pharmaceuticals and specialties: the Canadian drug reference for health professionals. Ottawa (ON): CPhA; 2008. p. 302-3].
Not for use in newborns.

SUPPLIED: 30 mg/mL: Each mL of sterile injection solution contains: phenobarbital sodium 30 mg. Nonmedicinal ingredients: benzyl alcohol (as a preservative), hydrochloric acid to adjust pH, propylene glycol and water for injection. Ampoules of 1 mL, boxes of 10. Store between 15 and 25°C. Protect from light. Protect from freezing. Do not use if precipitate is present.
120 mg/mL: Each mL of sterile injection solution contains: phenobarbital sodium 120 mg. Nonmedicinal ingredients: benzyl alcohol (as a preservative), hydrochloric acid to adjust pH, propylene glycol and water for injection. Ampoules of 1 mL, boxes of 10. Store between 15 and 25°C. Protect from light. Protect from freezing. Do not use if precipitate is present.

Phenytoin Pr

phenytoin
phenytoin sodium

Antiepileptic

CPhA Monograph

Date of Revision: November 2005

This monograph has been compiled by CPhA and reviewed by experts. It may contain information different from that found in Health Canada-approved Product Monographs. The reader is referred to the *CPS* Editorial Policy for more information.

PHARMACOLOGY: Phenytoin (also known as diphenylhydantoin) is an antiepileptic drug that elevates the seizure threshold in the motor cortex by limiting the post-tetanic potentiation (PTP) of synaptic transmission. It exerts this effect by preventing the excessive accumulation of intracellular sodium during tetanic stimulation by either reducing the passive influx of sodium or increasing the efficiency of the sodium pump. By limiting PTP, phenytoin prevents the spread of seizure activity to adjacent cortical areas.

Phenytoin also possesses antiarrhythmic activity similar to that of quinidine and procainamide. It increases the conduction velocity of the AV node and Purkinje fibres especially when conduction has been depressed by digitalis glycosides. Phenytoin decreases the automaticity of cardiac tissue by prolonging the effective refractory period. It also decreases the force of cardiac contraction. It may produce hypotension following i.v. administration.

Phenytoin is also available parenterally as the prodrug, fosphenytoin. For information on fosphenytoin, consult the product monograph.

Pharmacokinetics: Following oral administration, phenytoin is slowly absorbed from the gastrointestinal tract. Absorption may be variable and sometimes incomplete. Dissolution is the rate-limiting step.

Phenytoin is slowly and erratically absorbed following i.m. administration due to precipitation of the drug at the injection site. Following absorption, the drug is rapidly distributed to all tissues. Peak serum drug concentrations are achieved between 3 and 12 hours after administration of an oral dose.

The plasma half-life in man after oral phenytoin administration averages 22 hours, with a range of 7 to 42 hours. Time to steady state is highly variable, ranging from 1 to 5 weeks. Therapeutic drug concentrations can be obtained in 1 to 2 hours when the drug is administered i.v. The clinically effective serum trough concentration is usually 40 to 80 µmol/L.

Phenytoin is greater than 90% protein bound. Free fraction may increase in patients with renal or hepatic failure and/or hypoalbuminemia. These patients are predisposed to toxicity, and free/unbound phenytoin levels may be helpful in their management. If free phenytoin levels are not readily available, the following equation can be used to correct for the presence of hypoalbuminemia in patients with creatinine clearance >0.17 mL/s:

$$C_{norm} = \frac{C_{obs}}{(0.02)(Alb) + 0.1}$$

where C_{norm} = approximate phenytoin level adjusted for low albumin

C_{obs} = measured total phenytoin level

Alb = patient's albumin level (g/L).

Phenytoin is metabolized by the hepatic microsomal isoenzyme CYP2C9 to an inactive metabolite 5-(p-hydroxyphenyl)-5-phenylhydantoin (HPPH), which undergoes enterohepatic circulation. Approximately 60 to 75% of the daily dose of the drug is excreted in the urine as the glucuronide. Other minor metabolites also appear in the urine. In therapeutic doses, approximately 1% is excreted unchanged in the urine; in toxic doses, up to 10% of the ingested drug may be excreted unchanged by the kidneys.

Phenytoin kinetics are nonlinear and saturable, resulting in highly variable concentrations with even minor dosage changes. The steady-state plasma concentration may double or triple from as little as a 10% increase in dose, possibly resulting in toxicity.

INDICATIONS: Phenytoin is used in the management of generalized tonic-clonic and simple or complex partial seizures, in the treatment and prevention of seizures during or following neurosurgery, and in the management of status epilepticus.

Phenytoin has also been used in the management of neuropathic pain and dermatologic conditions such as decubitus ulcers and epidermolysis bullosa.

CONTRAINDICATIONS: Known hypersensitivity to hydantoin products. Because of its effect on ventricular automaticity, i.v. phenytoin is contraindicated in sinus bradycardia, sinoatrial block, second- and third-degree AV block without a functioning pacemaker, patients with Adams-Stokes syndrome.

WARNINGS: When used i.v., phenytoin must be administered slowly. I.V. administration should not exceed 50 mg/min in adults. In neonates, the drug should be administered at a rate not exceeding 1 to 3 mg/kg/min. The response to phenytoin may be significantly altered by the concomitant use of other drugs (see Precautions, Drug Interactions).

Abrupt withdrawal of phenytoin in epileptic patients may precipitate seizures. When the need for dosage reduction, discontinuation, or substitution of other antiepileptic medication arises, this should be done gradually. However, in the event of an allergic or hypersensitivity reaction, rapid initiation of alternative therapy may be necessary. In this case, alternative therapy should be an antiepileptic drug not belonging to the hydantoin chemical class. In addition, caution should be exercised if using structurally similar compounds (e.g., barbiturates, ethosuximide, methsuximide) in patients who have previously experienced phenytoin hypersensitivity.

Severe cardiotoxic reactions and fatalities have been reported with atrial and ventricular conduction depression and ventricular fibrillation. Severe complications are most commonly encountered in elderly or gravely ill patients.

Phenytoin should be used with caution in patients with hypotension and severe myocardial insufficiency.

Hypotension is associated with rapid i.v. administration (see Dosage).

The i.m. route is not recommended since absorption of the drug may be erratic and because it may cause pain, necrosis and abscess formation.

An uncommon but serious reaction known as anticonvulsant hypersensitivity syndrome (AHS) has been associated with the use of aromatic antiepileptic drugs such as phenytoin, phenobarbital, lamotrigine and carbamazepine. AHS typically occurs within 1 to 3 months following initiation of therapy, is more common in Blacks, and is reported to be associated with an inborn error of metabolism leading to an accumulation of intermediary aromatic hydrocarbon metabolites, which may stimulate an immune reaction. Manifestations include lymphadenopathy, fever, rash, hepatitis and various dermatologic sequelae including toxic epidermal necrolysis and Stevens-Johnson syndrome. Other possible effects include rhabdomyolysis, interstitial nephritis, hemolysis and acute renal failure. Management of AHS involves discontinuation of the offending drug and supportive treatment. Because of the proposed genetic etiology and a high degree of cross-reactivity, aromatic antiepileptic drugs should be avoided in patients who have experienced AHS, and in their first-degree relatives.

Acute alcohol intake may increase phenytoin serum levels while chronic use may decrease serum levels.

Occupational Hazards: Phenytoin may impair mental and/or physical abilities required for performance of hazardous tasks such as operating machinery or driving a motor vehicle.

Pregnancy: The majority of mothers on antiepileptic medication deliver normal infants. It is important to note that AEDs should not be discontinued in patients in whom the drug is administered to prevent major seizures because of the strong possibility of precipitating status epilepticus with attendant hypoxia and threat to life. In individual cases where the severity and frequency of the seizure disorder are such that the removal of medication does not pose a serious threat to the patient, discontinuation of the drug may be considered prior to and during pregnancy, although it cannot be said with any confidence that even minor seizures do not pose some hazard to the developing embryo or fetus. The prescribing physician should weigh these considerations in treating or counseling epileptic women of childbearing potential.

In addition to reports of increased incidence of congenital malformations, such as cleft lip/palate and heart malformations in children of women receiving phenytoin and other AEDs, there have been reports of fetal hydantoin syndrome. This consists of prenatal growth deficiency, microcephaly and mental deficiency in children born to mothers who have received phenytoin, barbiturates or alcohol. However, these features are all interrelated and are frequently associated with intrauterine growth retardation from other causes.

Phenytoin causes decreased folic acid levels, which may contribute to the risk of congenital malformations. Folic acid supplementation should begin several months prior to conception and continue for the first trimester of pregnancy, as for any woman who could become pregnant.

There have been isolated reports of malignancies, including neuroblastoma, in children whose mothers received phenytoin during pregnancy.

An increase in seizure frequency during pregnancy occurs in a high proportion of patients, because of altered phenytoin absorption or metabolism. Periodic measurement of serum phenytoin levels is particularly valuable in the management of a pregnant epileptic patient as a guide to appropriate dosage adjustment; however, restoration of the original dosage will probably be indicated postpartum.

Neonatal coagulation defects have been reported within the first 24 hours in babies born to epileptic mothers receiving phenobarbital and/or phenytoin. Vitamin K has been shown to prevent or correct this defect and has been recommended to be given to the mother before delivery and to the neonate after birth.

PRECAUTIONS: Anticonvulsant hypersensitivity syndrome: see Warnings.

The liver is the chief site of biotransformation of phenytoin; patients with impaired liver function, elderly patients, or those who are gravely ill may be particularly susceptible to toxicity.

A small percentage of individuals who have been treated with phenytoin have been shown to metabolize the drug slowly. Slow metabolism may be due to limited enzyme availability and lack of induction; it appears to be genetically determined.

Phenytoin should be discontinued if a skin rash appears (see Warnings). If the rash is exfoliative, purpuric, or bullous or if lupus erythematosus, Stevens-Johnson syndrome or toxic epidermal necrolysis is suspected, use of this drug should not be resumed and alternative therapy should be considered (see Adverse Effects). If the rash is of a milder type (measles-like or scarlatiniform), therapy may be resumed after the rash has completely disappeared. If the rash recurs upon reinstitution of therapy, further phenytoin therapy is contraindicated. Patients should be instructed to call their physician if skin rash develops.

The importance of good dental hygiene should be stressed in order to minimize the development of gingival hyperplasia and its potential complications (e.g., halitosis, gingivitis/periodontitis).

Hyperglycemia, resulting from the drug's inhibitory effects on insulin release, has been reported. Phenytoin may also raise the serum glucose level in diabetic patients.

Phenytoin, like some other AEDs, is associated with adverse effects on bone (see Adverse Effects). There is no consensus on how best to detect or prevent this problem. Some clinicians recommend screening all adults who are or will be prescribed long-term AEDs with measurements of baseline fasting serum calcium, phosphate and alkaline phosphatase and analysis of bone mineral density (BMD). In children, the same screening protocol has been suggested but with measurement of the serum intact parathyroid hormone level replacing the measurement of BMD. Others suggest limiting screening to measurements of 25-hydroxyvitamin D levels in those individuals at higher risk of bone-related adverse effects, and prophylactically supplementing other patients with calcium and vitamin D to ensure they receive the appropriate amounts.

Phenytoin is not indicated for seizures that are due to hypoglycemia or other metabolic causes.

Phenytoin is not effective for and may worsen absence (petit mal) seizures. If both tonic-clonic (grand mal) and absence (petit mal) seizures are present, combined drug therapy is needed.

Phenytoin may exacerbate porphyria, and should be used with caution in patients with this condition.

Each injection of i.v. phenytoin sodium should be followed by an injection of sterile saline through the same needle or i.v. catheter to avoid local venous irritation due to the alkalinity of the solution. Continuous infusion should be avoided.

Soft tissue irritation and inflammation have occurred at the site of injection with and without extravasation of i.v. phenytoin. Soft tissue irritation varying from slight tenderness to extensive necrosis and sloughing has been noted. Subcutaneous or perivascular injection should be avoided.

Serum levels of phenytoin sustained above the optimal range may produce confusional states referred to as delirium, psychosis, or encephalopathy, or rarely, irreversible cerebellar dysfunction. Accordingly, at the first sign of acute toxicity, plasma level determinations are recommended. Dose reduction of phenytoin therapy is indicated if plasma levels are excessive; if symptoms persist, termination is recommended (see Warnings).

Patients should be cautioned about the use of other drugs or alcoholic beverages without first seeking the physician's advice.

Patients should carry identification (e.g., bracelet, wallet card) indicating phenytoin usage and epilepsy.

Do not use capsules that are discolored.

Drug Interactions: There are many drugs that may increase or decrease phenytoin levels or that phenytoin may affect. The most commonly occurring drug interactions are listed below.

When adding or deleting phenytoin from a patient's therapeutic regimen, pharmacotherapy must be monitored closely as dosage adjustment may be necessary. Serum level determinations of each drug are especially helpful when possible drug interactions are suspected.

Drugs that may increase phenytoin serum levels include: amiodarone, chloramphenicol, cimetidine, ciprofloxacin, erythromycin, fluconazole, fluoxetine, isoniazid, ketoconazole, methylphenidate, norfloxacin, omeprazole, phenylbutazone, salicylates, sulfonamides, trazodone, warfarin and acute alcohol ingestion.

Drugs that may decrease phenytoin levels include: carbamazepine, chronic alcohol abuse, diazoxide, rifampin and theophylline.

Drugs that may either increase or decrease phenytoin serum levels include: phenobarbital, valproic acid and sodium valproate. Similarly, the effect of phenytoin on phenobarbital, valproic acid and sodium valproate serum levels is unpredictable.

Drugs whose efficacy may be impaired by phenytoin include: corticosteroids, diazoxide, digitalis glycosides, doxycycline, estrogens, furosemide, itraconazole, levodopa, methadone, oral contraceptives, quinidine, theophylline, vitamin D and warfarin.

Phenytoin is an inducer of CYP1A2, 2C9, 2D6, 3A4 and 2B6, and may interact with drugs metabolized by these enzymes.

Administration of phenytoin with sulcralfate, enteral feeds, antacids or calcium preparations should be separated by at least 3 hours to prevent a decrease in phenytoin absorption. Dosage adjustments may also be necessary.

Concurrent use of i.v. phenytoin with lidocaine or propranolol may produce additive cardiac depressant effects.

Although not a true drug interaction, tricyclic antidepressants may precipitate seizures in susceptible patients and phenytoin dosage may need to be adjusted.

Drug-Laboratory Test Interactions: Phenytoin may produce lower than normal values for dexamethasone or metyrapone tests. Phenytoin may cause increased serum levels of glucose and alkaline phosphatase. Like other inducers of hepatic microsomal enzymes, phenytoin administration will increase serum levels of gamma-glutamyl transferase (GGT).

Drug-Food Interactions: The presence of food may affect phenytoin absorption, but may also reduce its gastrointestinal side effects. Taking phenytoin with food on a consistent basis should minimize any food-associated fluctuations in bioavailability.

Phenytoin bioavailability can be significantly reduced in the presence of enteral nutrition products. Tube feeds should be held for 2 hours before and after phenytoin doses. See Dosage, Antiepileptic Dosage: Oral.

Pregnancy: See Warnings.

Lactation: If maternal levels are kept within therapeutic range, there is little risk of drug accumulation in the infant. Phenytoin is generally considered compatible with breast-feeding.

Children: AEDs, including phenytoin, may have adverse effects on behavior and cognition in children. Effects of phenytoin on behavior may include unsteadiness, involuntary movements, tiredness and alteration of emotional state. Effects of phenytoin on cognition may include deficits on neuropsychologic tests; impaired attention, problem-solving and visuomotor skills. Children treated with phenytoin and/or other antiepileptics should be closely monitored by clinicians, parents and teachers for changes in cognitive function, mood and behavior. If significant changes occur and another explanation is not obvious, the possibility that the antiepileptic is responsible should be considered. Dosage reduction or substitution of another AED may be necessary.

ADVERSE EFFECTS: Bone: Phenytoin and other AEDs have been associated with adverse effects on bone, ranging from biochemical abnormalities to rickets and osteomalacia. These effects are thought to be secondary to phenytoin-induced vitamin D deficiency. Subclinical disease may consist of decreased serum calcium or 25-hydroxyvitamin D, increased serum parathyroid hormone levels, decreased bone density or abnormal bone biopsy findings (increased osteoid). These effects may occur early in therapy. Rickets and osteomalacia are most often seen in non-ambulatory patients, likely because of coexisting risk factors for these conditions (e.g., insufficient intake of calcium or vitamin D, infrequent exposure to sunlight, inadequate physical activity). In addition, long-term AED therapy likely increases the risk of fractures, especially of the hip.

If adverse effects on bone are identified (see Precautions), many clinicians recommend treatment with calcium and vitamin D (cholecalciferol or ergocalciferol). Though the optimum treatment regimen has not been defined, it would seem prudent to start with amounts sufficient to attain the Dietary Reference Intake, and then modify the dose of calcium and vitamin D based on the degree of improvement of identified abnormalities in response to treatment.

Cardiovascular: Severe cardiotoxic reactions and fatalities have been reported with atrial and ventricular conduction depression and ventricular fibrillation. Severe complications are most commonly encountered in elderly or gravely ill patients.

The most notable signs of toxicity associated with the i.v. use of phenytoin are cardiovascular collapse and/or CNS depression. Hypotension does occur when the drug is administered rapidly by the i.v. route. The rate of administration is very important; it should not exceed 50 mg/min in adults, and 1 to 3 mg/kg/min in neonates. In geriatric patients with heart disease, it has been recommended that phenytoin be given at a rate of 50 mg over 2 to 3 minutes. At this rate, toxicity should be minimized.

Central Nervous System: nystagmus, ataxia, slurred speech, decreased coordination and mental confusion. These are usually related to increased drug serum concentrations. Dizziness, insomnia, transient nervousness, motor twitching and headache have also been observed. There have also been rare reports of phenytoin induced dyskinesias, including chorea, dystonia and tremor, similar to those induced by phenothiazine and other antipsychotic drugs.

A predominantly sensory peripheral polyneuropathy has been observed in patients receiving long-term phenytoin therapy.

Connective Tissue: gingival hyperplasia, which is especially frequent in children, coarsening of the facial features, enlargement of the lips, systemic lupus erythematosus, hypertrichosis and Peyronie's disease.

Dermatologic: scarlatiniform or morbilliform rashes sometimes accompanied by fever. Other more serious reactions which may be fatal have included bullous, exfoliative or purpuric dermatitis, lupus erythematosus, Stevens-Johnson syndrome and toxic epidermal necrolysis (see Warnings and Precautions).

Gastrointestinal: nausea, vomiting, and constipation.

Hematologic: thrombocytopenia, leukopenia, granulocytopenia, agranulocytosis, and pancytopenia with or without bone marrow suppression. Some reactions have been fatal. While macrocytosis and megaloblastic anemia have occurred, these conditions usually respond to folic acid therapy. Lymphadenopathy including benign lymph node hyperplasia, pseudolymphoma, lymphoma, and Hodgkin's disease have been reported (see Warnings).

Injection Site: Local irritation, inflammation, tenderness, necrosis, and sloughing have been reported with or without extravasation of i.v. phenytoin.

Other: Periarteritis nodosa, toxic hepatitis, liver damage, and immunoglobulin abnormalities may occur.

OVERDOSE:

Symptoms: Symptoms may include nausea and vomiting, nystagmus and neurologic symptoms such as ataxia, tremor, hyperreflexia, slurred speech. Other neurologic symptoms may include hallucinations, opisthotonos (spastic state in which head, spine and heels are arched backward), choreoathetoid movements, and rarely seizures or coma. Seizures may occur in patients with or without pre-existing seizure disorder. Agitation and combativeness may alternate with periods of CNS depression. Respiratory depression occurs rarely, in severe cases.

Rapid i.v. injection may lead to hypotension, arrhythmias, seizures and cardiorespiratory arrest. These effects are generally not associated with oral overdose of phenytoin alone.

Death from phenytoin overdose is rare and usually associated with multiple drug ingestion or lack of adequate supportive care.

In overdose, phenytoin serum concentrations may not correlate well with clinical presentation. Therapeutic phenytoin levels range from 40 to 80 µmol/L. Mild to moderate neurologic toxicity is associated with levels of 80 to 160 µmol/L. At levels above 160 µmol/L, severe neurologic toxicity may occur. Patients with reduced protein binding may be at increased risk of toxicity due to higher free phenytoin levels.

Treatment: Respiratory and circulatory function should be carefully monitored and appropriate supportive measures employed. In addition, ECG, phenytoin serum levels and blood glucose should be monitored. Agitation and seizures may be managed with i.v. diazepam. Activated charcoal should be considered even if significant time has elapsed since ingestion. Studies have shown that multiple dose activated charcoal (MDAC) substantially increases phenytoin's rate of elimination, though it has not been demonstrated that this results in improved clinical outcomes. MDAC may be helpful even in cases of parenteral exposure. Forced diuresis, hemodialysis, peritoneal dialysis, charcoal hemoperfusion, exchange transfusion and plasmapheresis do not appear to enhance elimination significantly.

In acute overdose, the possibility of ingestion of other CNS depressants, including alcohol, should be considered.

> For management of a suspected drug overdose, CPhA recommends that you contact your **regional Poison Control Centre**. See the *CPS* Directory section for a list of Poison Control Centres.

DOSAGE: Dosage should be individualized to provide maximum benefit with minimum adverse effects. In many cases, serum concentration determinations will be necessary for optimal dosage adjustments; the clinically effective serum concentration is usually in the range of 40 to 80 µmol/L. Serum level determinations are especially helpful when toxicity, drug interactions or poor adherence to prescribed therapy is suspected. Dosage adjustments should not be made solely on the basis of serum levels, but should be based chiefly upon careful consideration of the patient's clinical response.

If dosage adjustment is required, phenytoin's nonlinear pharmacokinetics must be taken into consideration. Maintenance doses should generally only be increased in small increments, often by no more than 10% of the total daily dose. Some experts suggest that, in adults, if the steady-state serum level is less than 28 µmol/L, the dose should be increased by 100 mg/day. If the concentration is between 28 and 48 µmol/L, the dose can be increased by 50 mg/day. If the concentration is greater than 48 µmol/L, the dose should be increased by 30 mg/day or less. The time required to reach steady-state after each dosage adjustment may be prolonged (e.g., several weeks), and must be taken into account in order to avoid premature and unnecessary modifications which might result in toxicity or loss of seizure control (see Pharmacokinetics).

Both phenytoin acid and its sodium salt may be administered orally. Phenytoin sodium may also be administered i.v. Phenytoin sodium 100 mg is approximately equivalent to phenytoin acid 92 mg. This should be taken into consideration when a patient is switched from one form to the other.

Antiepileptic Dosage: Oral: In most adults, phenytoin may be administered in a once-daily dose using the extended-release capsules. The suspension and chewable tablets are not recommended for once-daily dosing. When using the suspension, it is important to shake the suspension well before measuring and to measure the dose accurately using a calibrated measuring device. Otherwise, clinically significant variations in dose may occur.

The suspension may be administered through a nasogastric tube. If this is necessary, the suspension should be diluted (e.g., 2- to 3-fold) with a compatible diluent (e.g., sterile water) prior to administration, and the tube should be flushed with at least 20 mL of diluent before and after administration. Enteral feeds should be stopped 2 hours before and resumed 2 hours after phenytoin doses, to minimize reduction of phenytoin bioavailability.

Adults: The usual starting dose of phenytoin is 5 mg/kg/day. The dose should be adjusted, if necessary, as described above.

Some clinicians have advocated the use of oral loading doses in adults who require rapid attainment of steady-state levels and where i.v. administration is not desirable or feasible. Approximately 18 mg/kg is administered in divided doses over 4 hours. For example, a 1 g dose would be divided into 3 doses (400 mg, 300 mg, 300 mg) which would be administered every 2 hours. Normal maintenance dose is then instituted 24 hours after completion of the loading dose. This should generally only be performed in a clinic or hospital setting where the patient can be closely monitored for adverse effects, and should be used in patients with normal renal and hepatic function.

Children: Initially, 5 mg/kg/day in 2 or 3 equally divided doses with subsequent dosage individualization. The usual maintenance dose varies from 4 to 8 mg/kg/day.

Parenteral: Whenever parenteral administration of phenytoin is necessary, the use of the prodrug fosphenytoin should be considered. For specific information on fosphenytoin, please consult the product monograph.

I.M. injection of phenytoin is not recommended (see Warnings).

Parenteral phenytoin should be injected slowly and directly into a large vein through a large-gauge needle or i.v. catheter or administered as an intermittent infusion. The patency of the vein and position of the venous catheter must be ascertained prior to injection, since extravasation of phenytoin can cause serious tissue damage (see Precautions and Adverse Effects). Each injection should be followed by an injection of sterile saline through the same needle or catheter to avoid local venous irritation due to the alkalinity of phenytoin solution. If given as an intermittent infusion, phenytoin should be administered under close observation immediately after preparation. Many clinicians recommend the use of a 0.22 µm in-line filter during infusion. Phenytoin is not compatible with solutions containing dextrose.

Do not exceed an injection rate of 50 mg/min in adults or 1 to 3 mg/kg/min (maximum 50 mg/min) in children. In geriatric patients, or patients with cardiovascular disease, a maximum rate of 25 mg/min has been advocated by some experts (see Warnings and Overdose). Many clinicians recommend continuous monitoring of ECG and blood pressure during injection. The patient should be observed for signs of respiratory depression.

Adults: When rapid attainment of therapeutic serum concentrations is desired, an i.v. loading dose may be administered. The usual dose is 15 to 20 mg/kg i.v. given at a rate of 25 to 50 mg/min (see above).

Generalized Convulsive Status Epilepticus (GCSE): Adults: 15 to 20 mg/kg administered at a rate of 25 to 50 mg/min. If seizures are not controlled, additional doses of 5 to 10 mg/kg (max 30 mg/kg) may be given.

Children: Children in GCSE not currently on phenytoin should receive 20 mg/kg i.v. initially, administered at a rate of 1 mg/kg/min (children <50 kg) or 50 mg/min (children ≥50 kg). If the seizure continues, additional 5 mg/kg doses may be given. A maximum of 30 mg/kg (up to 1000 mg) can be given in total.

Children in GCSE already on phenytoin may receive an initial booster dose of 5 mg/kg, pending serum level determinations.

Phillips'® Preparations
magnesium hydroxide
Antacid—Laxative

Bayer Consumer Care

SUPPLIED: Phillips' Milk of Magnesia: Fresh Mint: Each mL contains: magnesium hydroxide 80 mg. Nonmedicinal ingredients: mineral oil, peppermint flavor, sodium hypochlorite solution, sodium saccharin and water. Bottles of 350 mL.
Original: Each mL contains: magnesium hydroxide 80 mg. Nonmedicinal ingredients: sodium hypochlorite and water. Bottles of 350 and 769 mL.
Wild Cherry: Each mL contains: magnesium hydroxide 80 mg. Nonmedicinal ingredients: carboxymethylcellulose sodium, cherry flavor, citric acid, D&C Red #28, ethanol, glycerin, microcrystalline cellulose, sodium citrate, sodium hypochlorite, sucrose, water and xanthan gum. Bottles of 350 and 769 mL.
Phillips' Magnesia Tablets: Each tablet contains: magnesium hydroxide 311 mg. Nonmedicinal ingredients: dextrates, magnesium stearate, maltodextrin, peppermint oil, silicon dioxide, starch and sucrose. Packages of 100.

pHisoHex® Ⓟ
hexachlorophene
Antibacterial—Skin Cleanser

sanofi-aventis

SUPPLIED: Each mL of white to slightly off-white emulsion contains: hexachlorophene 3%. Nonmedicinal ingredients: lanolin cholesterols, lauryl myristyl diethanolamide, methylcellulose, petrolatum (white), polyethylene glycol 400, polyethylene glycol 400 monostearate, purified water, sodium benzoate and sodium octylphenoxyethoxyethyl ether sulfonate. Bottles of 150 mL, 450 mL and 3.75 L.

Phoslax™
sodium phosphates
Laxative

Odan

SUPPLIED: Each clear, colorless teaspoonful (5 mL) contains: monobasic sodium phosphate USP 2.4 g and dibasic sodium phosphate USP 0.9 g. Nonmedicinal ingredients: glycerin, grape flavour, purified water, sodium benzoate and sodium saccharin. Plastic bottles of 50 mL. Store at room temperature (15 to 30°C).

PhosLo® Ⓟ
calcium acetate
Phosphate Binder

Fresenius Medical Care

Date of Preparation: October 2007

PHARMACOLOGY: When taken with meals, PhosLo (calcium acetate) combines with dietary phosphate to form insoluble calcium phosphate, which is excreted in the feces. PhosLo is highly soluble at neutral pH, making the calcium readily available for binding to phosphate in the proximal small intestine. Calcium acetate is a more efficient phosphate binder than other calcium salts. When phosphate binding in the proximal small intestinal lumen occurs, the calcium available for absorption decreases, thus reducing the risk of hypercalcemia in these patients.

The absorption of phosphorus plays a critical role in the development of metabolic bone diseases in patients with chronic renal failure. The retention of phosphate plays a pivotal role in causing secondary hyperparathyroidism associated with osteodystrophy and soft tissue calcification. The majority of patients with advanced renal insufficiency (glomerular filtration rate less than 30 mL/min) exhibit phosphate retention with hyperphosphatemia.

The rate of removal of phosphate by dietary manipulation or by dialysis is insufficient to prevent hyperphosphatemia in most dialysis patients. Dialysis patients absorb 40% to 80% of dietary phosphorus. Therefore, the fraction of dietary phosphate absorbed from the diet needs to be reduced. Phosphate binders in most renal failure patients on maintenance dialysis are effective in accomplishing that.

INDICATIONS: PhosLo (calcium acetate) is indicated for the control of hyperphosphatemia in end stage renal failure.

CONTRAINDICATIONS: PhosLo (calcium acetate) is contraindicated in patients with hypercalcemia.

WARNINGS: PhosLo (calcium acetate) should not be given concurrently with calcium supplements because patients with end stage renal failure may develop hypercalcemia.

Progressive hypercalcemia due to overdose of calcium salts administered to patients with chronic renal impairment may be sufficiently severe to require emergency measures. Chronic hypercalcemia may lead to vascular calcification and other soft tissue calcifications. The serum calcium concentration should be monitored twice weekly during the early dose adjustment period and regularly thereafter. **The serum calcium times phosphate (CaXP) product should not be allowed to exceed 5.33 mmol²/L².** Radiographic evaluation of the suspect anatomical region may be helpful in early detection of soft tissue calcification.

PRECAUTIONS: General: Excessive dosage of PhosLo (calcium acetate) could induce hypercalcemia; therefore, early in the treatment during dosage adjustment, serum calcium should be determined twice weekly, and monitored regularly thereafter. Should hypercalcemia develop, the dosage should be reduced or the treatment discontinued immediately depending on the severity of hypercalcemia. Calcium salts should not be given to patients on digitalis because hypercalemia may precipitate cardiac arrhythmias. Therapy with phosphate binders should always be started at low doses and should not be increased without careful monitoring of serum calcium. An estimate of daily dietary calcium intake should be made initially and the intake adjusted as needed. Serum phosphorous should also be determined periodically.

Pregnancy: The safety and efficacy of PhosLo (calcium acetate) in pregnant women has not been established; therefore, PhosLo (calcium acetate) should be prescribed during pregnancy only if the benefits outweigh potential risks. Animal reproduction studies have not been conducted with PhosLo (calcium acetate), nor is it known whether PhosLo (calcium acetate) can cause fetal harm when administered to pregnant women or whether it can affect reproductive capacity.

Children: The safety and efficacy of PhosLo (calcium acetate) in children have not been established.

Drug Interactions: PhosLo (calcium acetate) may decrease the bioavailability of tetracyclines. PhosLo (calcium acetate) should not be taken with non-prescription antacids because these drugs contain calcium.

Information to Be Provided to the Patient: The patient should be informed about compliance with dosage instructions, adherence to instructions about diet and avoidance of the use of non-prescription antacids. Patients should be informed about the symptoms of hypercalcemia (see Adverse Effects).

ADVERSE EFFECTS: The most frequent adverse reaction to PhosLo (calcium acetate) was hypercalcemia, which occurred in 15% of the patients in clinical studies. Mild hypercalcemia (Ca >2.63 mmol/L) may be asymptomatic or manifest itself as constipation, anorexia, nausea and vomiting. More severe hypercalcemia (Ca >3 mmol/L) is associated with confusion, delirium, stupor and coma. The serum calcium concentration should be monitored, and the dose should be adjusted accordingly. Decreasing dialysate calcium concentration could reduce the incidence and severity of hypercalcemia induced by PhosLo (calcium acetate).

In clinical studies, 7% of patients experienced nausea (including vomiting) and gastrointestinal disturbance during PhosLo (calcium acetate) therapy. Frequently this was a consequence of hypercalcemia.

The long-term effect of PhosLo (calcium acetate) on the progression of vascular or soft tissue calcification has not been determined.

OVERDOSE:

Symptoms: Administration of PhosLo (calcium acetate) in excess of the appropriate daily dosage can cause severe hypercalcemia (see Adverse Effects).

Treatment: Mild hypercalcemia is easily controlled by reducing the PhosLo (calcium acetate) dose or temporarily discontinuing therapy. Severe hypercalcemia can be treated by acute hemodialysis and discontinuing PhosLo (calcium acetate) therapy.

> For management of a suspected drug overdose, CPhA recommends that you contact your **regional Poison Control Centre**. See the *CPS* Directory section for a list of Poison Control Centres.

DOSAGE: The recommended initial dose of PhosLo (calcium acetate) for the adult dialysis patient is 2 tablets with each meal. The dosage may be increased gradually to bring the serum phosphate value below 1.94 mmol/L, as long as hypercalcemia does not develop. Most patients require 3-4 tablets with each meal. Tablets should be swallowed whole and not chewed.

SUPPLIED: Each white, round tablet, stamped "BRA200", contains: 667 mg calcium acetate USP equal to 169 mg calcium. Nonmedicinal ingredients: polyethylene glycol 8000 NF. Bottles of 200. Tablets should be swallowed whole and not chewed. Store at controlled room temperature (15-30°C).

(Shown in Product Identification Section)

Phosphate-Novartis
sodium acid phosphate
Hypercalciuria—Electrolyte Replenisher

Novartis Pharmaceuticals

INDICATIONS: Hypercalciuria, electrolyte replenisher.

CONTRAINDICATIONS: Do not use this medication if hyperphosphatemia is present or in the presence of severe impairment of renal function (less than 30% of normal).

WARNINGS: Use carefully in patients with cardiac disease treated with digitalis and in conditions where high potassium concentration may be encountered such as: adrenal insufficiency, acute dehydration, severe renal insufficiency, in conditions such as in severe burns, where high tissue breakdown is expected.

Because of the sodium content of this product, use carefully in the presence of cardiac failure, liver cirrhosis or severe hepatic disease, edema, hypernatremia, hypertension and toxemia of pregnancy.

PRECAUTIONS: High phosphate intake may result in high serum concentrations which may be associated with an increase in extraskeletal calcification. If long-term therapy is prescribed, the following patient monitoring may be warranted: evaluation of renal function, and serum determination of the following ions: calcium, phosphorus, potassium, sodium.

Pregnancy: No well-controlled studies have been conducted in humans or in animals to determine the effect of phosphate during pregnancy. Nevertheless, the benefit of treatment should be considered in relation to the risks before instituting treatment in a pregnant woman.

Lactation: It is not known if phosphates are excreted in breast milk. However, problems in nursing infants have not been documented.

Drug Interactions: Concurrent use of sodium phosphates with glucocorticoids and related compounds may result in hypernatremia.

Androgens and anabolic steroids may increase the risk of edema.

Oxalates and phytates in food, and aluminum and/or magnesium antacids may bind phosphates and prevent absorption.

Calcium containing drugs (e.g. dietary supplement and antacids) may increase the risk of calcium deposition in soft tissues.

Drugs containing potassium and ACE inhibitors may produce hyperkalemia.

Thiazide diuretics taken with phosphates may cause or worsen renal damage.

Iron supplements will form insoluble complex with phosphates resulting in a decreased absorption of iron.

Phosphates by producing marked acidification of urine may accelerate excretion of mexiletine and decrease salicylate excretion. Potassium content in this drug may enhance quinidine's effects.

Vitamin D enhances phosphate absorption and may increase potential for hyperphosphatemia if taken with high doses of phosphate.

ADVERSE EFFECTS: The following reactions have been reported: nausea, vomiting, stomach pain, laxative effect or diarrhea, and less frequently: fluid retention associated with swelling of feet and/or weight gain, hyperkalemia associated with confusion; tiredness or weakness; irregular or slow heartbeat; numbness or tingling around lips, hands or feet; unexplained anxiety; breathing problems, hypernatremia associated with confusion; convulsions; decrease in urine volume or in frequency of urination; fast heartbeat; headache or dizziness; increased thirst; hyperphosphatemia or hypocalcemic tetany associated with muscle cramps; numbness, tingling, pain, or weakness in hands or feet; shortness of breath or troubled breathing.

OVERDOSE:

Treatment: Withhold further administration of phosphates. Correct deficient serum electrolyte concentrations (such as that of calcium). Implement general supportive measures.

> For management of a suspected drug overdose, CPhA recommends that you contact your **regional Poison Control Centre**. See the *CPS* Directory section for a list of Poison Control Centres.

DOSAGE: Adults: Usual dosage for hypercalciuria and as an electrolyte replenisher: 1 tablet 2 times a day with meals. Adjust dose according to patient response.

Children: Half of the adult dose.

Take tablets only when dissolved in water. Use preferably 250 mL of diluent. Use only on the advice of a physician.

Do not take if renal function is impaired or if sodium (table salt) restriction has been prescribed.

SUPPLIED: Each white, round, flat tablet, approximately 25 mm in diameter with a coarse surface, contains: phosphorus 500 mg (16.1 mmol) from anhydrous sodium acid phosphate 1 936 mg. Also contains potassium bicarbonate and sodium bicarbonate providing 123 mg (3.1 mmol) potassium and 469 mg (20.4 mmol) sodium, citric acid anhydrous, orange flavor, polyethylene glycol, saccharin sodium and sucrose. Energy: 3.29 kcal. Lactose-, paraben-, starch-, sulfite- and tartrazine-free. Tubes of 20. Store at 15 to 30°C, protect from heat and humidity.

(Shown in Product Identification Section)

Phosphates Solution
sodium phosphates
Laxative

PendoPharm

SUPPLIED: Each 5 mL of solution contains: monobasic sodium phosphate monohydrate 2.4 g and dibasic sodium phosphate heptahydrate 0.9 g. Nonmedicinal ingredients: glycerin, natural ginger-lemon flavor, purified water, sodium benzoate and sodium saccharin. White opaque bottles of 45 mL.

Photofrin®
porfimer sodium
Antineoplastic Photosensitizing Agent

Axcan Pharma

> Caution: PHOTOFRIN is an injectable photosensitizing drug for use in photodynamic therapy (PDT) for treatment of cancer and pre-malignant conditions (e.g., high-grade dysplasia in Barrett's esophagus). Photodynamic therapy is a photochemical process requiring specific lasers and fiber optics. Photodynamic therapy with PHOTOFRIN should only be applied by physicians trained in the endoscopic use of PDT with PHOTOFRIN and only in those facilities properly equipped for the procedure. PHOTOFRIN may cause residual photosensitivity for 30 days or more resulting in erythema and blistering of the skin when it is exposed to direct sunlight or brightly focused indoor light (e.g., from examination lamps, operating room lamps, floodlights, halogen lamps, etc.).

PHARMACOLOGY: Pharmacodynamics: The cytotoxic and antitumor actions of PHOTOFRIN (porfimer sodium) are light and oxygen dependent. Photodynamic therapy (PDT) with PHOTOFRIN is a 2-stage process. The first stage is the i.v. injection of PHOTOFRIN. Clearance from a variety of tissues occurs over 40-72 hours; but tumor, skin, and organs of the reticuloendothelial system (including liver and spleen) retain PHOTOFRIN for a longer period. Illumination with 630 nm wavelength laser light constitutes the second and final stage of therapy. Tumor selectivity in treatment occurs through a combination of selective retention of PHOTOFRIN and selective delivery of light. Photodynamic therapy-induced cytotoxicity may be due to free radical (superoxide or hydroxyl) generation and the production of singlet oxygen via energy transfer from light to triplet oxygen. Tumor death also occurs through ischemic necrosis secondary to vascular occlusion that appears to be partly mediated by thromboxane A_2 release. The laser treatment induces a photochemical, not a thermal effect. The necrotic reaction and associated inflammatory responses may evolve over several days.

Pharmacokinetics: A pharmacokinetic study was performed on 12 lung cancer patients given 2 mg/kg of PHOTOFRIN via the i.v. route. Samples of plasma were obtained up to 56 days post-injection. PHOTOFRIN was slowly cleared from the body with a mean apparent elimination half-life of 21.5 days (range 11-28 days).

The pharmacokinetics of PHOTOFRIN was also studied in 24 healthy subjects (12 men and 12 women) who received a single dose of 2 mg/kg PHOTOFRIN given via the i.v. route. Serum samples were collected out to 36 days after injection. The serum decay was bi-exponential, with a slow distribution phase and a very long elimination phase that started approximately 24 hours after injection. The elimination half-life was 415 hours (17 days). C_{max} was determined to be 40 µg/mL, and $AUC_{(inf)}$ was 2400 µg.h/mL. Gender had no effect on pharmacokinetic parameters except for t_{max}, which was approximately 1.5 hours in women and 0.17 hours in men. At the time of intended photoactivation 40 to 50 hours after injection, the pharmacokinetic profiles of PHOTOFRIN in men and women were very similar.

No special precautions in renally impaired patients are necessary because excretion is primarily via the fecal route. The influence of impaired hepatic function on porfimer sodium disposition has not been evaluated.

PHOTOFRIN was approximately 90% protein bound in human serum, studied in vitro. The binding was independent of concentration over the concentration range of 20 to 100 µg/mL.

Clinical Studies: Papillary Bladder Cancer: A Phase III, multicentre, randomized, open-label study was performed in patients with superficial papillary transitional cell carcinoma of the urinary bladder, stage TaG1 with frequently recurring disease or stages TaG2, T1G1-3. Following transurethral resection, patients were randomized to either single doses of PHOTOFRIN plus light or an observation control arm and the time to tumor recurrence was compared between groups. Efficacy analysis was performed on 30 patients. The median follow-up time for all randomized patients was 456 days. In the PHOTOFRIN group, 9 of 17 patients (53%) recurred compared with 10 of 13 patients (77%) in the observation group. The median time to tumor recurrence for patients who received PHOTOFRIN was 379 days versus 93 days for the observed group.

Esophageal Cancer: A Phase III, multicentre, randomized, open-label clinical trial was conducted comparing PDT with PHOTOFRIN and controlled uniform laser light versus thermal ablation therapy using the Nd:YAG laser for the removal of tumor mass and subsequent local palliation of dysphagia in 236 patients with partially obstructing esophageal carcinoma. Each course of PDT with PHOTOFRIN consisted of 1 injection of the drug followed by up to 2 laser light applications. A maximum of 3 courses of PDT with PHOTOFRIN was allowed. Repeat Nd:YAG laser sessions were given until maximal anticipated tumor debulking and palliation of dysphagia were achieved. Thus, a course of Nd:YAG laser therapy consisted of multiple laser application sessions. An unlimited number of Nd:YAG courses was permitted. Efficacy results after 1 course of therapy, based on all 236 randomized patients, are provided in Table 1. Based on all courses, 9 PDT-treated patients and 2 Nd:YAG-treated patients had no visible evidence of tumor and were considered to be in complete response (CR). In 6 PDT-treated patients and 2 Nd:YAG-treated patients, CR was verified by pathology.

Table 1: PHOTOFRIN

Course 1 Efficacy Results in Patients with Partially Obstructing Esophageal Cancer

	Month 1 Improvement in Dysphagia (% of Pts)	Month 1 Objective Tumor Response Rate (% of Pts)	Median TPF[a] (Days)	Mean No. of Treatment Endoscopies Per Patient[b]
PHOTOFRIN PDT (n=118)	35%	32%* (CR 2%, PR[c] 30%)	34	2.1
Nd:YAG (n=118)	29%	20% (CR 0%, PR 20%)	42	2.8

[a] Time to palliation failure.
[b] Treatments not compared statistically.
[c] Partial response, based on change in smallest esophageal luminal diameter.
Legend:
* Statistically significant difference between PDT and Nd:YAG (p <0.05).

In addition, PDT with PHOTOFRIN was utilized in a Phase III, multicentre, single-arm study in 19 patients with completely obstructing esophageal carcinoma using the same schedule as above. Based on Month 1 assessments for Course 1 for all 19 patients enrolled, 42% of patients showed improvement in dysphagia grade, 32% of patients achieved partial objective tumor responses (PR), and median time to palliation failure was 30 days. Based on all courses, 3 patients achieved a complete tumor response; one of these was verified by pathology.

Endobronchial Cancer: Two randomized multicenter Phase III studies were conducted to compare the safety and efficacy of PHOTOFRIN PDT versus Nd:YAG laser therapy for reduction of obstruction and palliation of symptomatic patients with partially or completely obstructing endobronchial nonsmall cell lung cancer. Assessments were made at 1 week and at monthly intervals after treatment. Table 2 shows the results from all randomized patients in the two studies combined. Objective tumor response rates (CR+PR), which demonstrate reduction of obstruction, were 59% for PDT and 58% for Nd:YAG at Week 1. The response rates at 1 month were 55% for PDT and 29% for Nd:YAG. These reductions in endobronchial obstruction resulted in improvements in atelectasis and pulmonary symptoms in many patients (Table 2 and Table 3).

Table 2: PHOTOFRIN

Efficacy Results from Studies in Late-stage Obstructing Endobronchial Cancer—All Randomized Patients[a]

Efficacy Parameter (% of Patients)	PDT N=102	Nd:YAG N=109
Objective Tumor Response[b]		
Week 1	59%	58%
Month 1	55%	29%
Symptom Improvement[c]		
Week 1	58%	51%
Month 1	54%	35%
Atelectasis Improvement[d]	n=60	n=71
Any Time in Course 1	50%	34%

a Statistical comparisons were precluded by the amount of missing data at Month 1 (e.g., for tumor response PDT 32%, Nd:YAG 46%).
b CR+PR, CR=complete response (absence of bronchoscopically visible tumor), PR=partial response (increase of ≥50% in the smallest luminal diameter); for completely obstructing tumors, any appearance of a lumen).
c Individual symptoms were evaluated using 5- or 6-grade severity scales. A change of at least 1 grade on at least 1 symptom was counted as improvement. Clinically significant improvements for specific symptoms are summarized in Table 3.
d In patients with atelectasis at baseline.

Patient symptoms were evaluated using a 5- or 6-grade pulmonary symptom severity rating scale for dyspnea, cough, and hemoptysis. Patients with moderate to severe symptoms are those most in need of palliation. Improvements of 2 or more grades are considered to be clinically significant. Table 3 shows the percentages of patients with moderate to severe symptoms at baseline who demonstrated at least a 2-grade improvement at any time during the interval evaluated.

Table 3: PHOTOFRIN

Efficacy Results from Studies in Late-stage Obstructing Endobronchial Cancer—Clinically Significant Improvements in Patients with Moderate to Severe Symptoms at Baseline[a]

Clinically Significant Symptom Improvement[b] (% of Patients)	PDT	Nd:YAG
Any Symptom	n=89	n=89
Week 1	25%	29%
Month 1	35%	17%
Dyspnea	n=60	n=68
Week 1	15%	18%
Month 1	20%	7%
Cough	n=63	n=65
Week 1	6%	9%
Month 1	13%	5%
Hemoptysis	n=24	n=31
Week 1	58%	29%
Month 1	71%	32%

a Statistical comparisons were precluded by the amount of missing data at Month 1.
b Dyspnea was graded on a 6-point severity rating scale; cough and hemoptysis on 5-point scales. Clinically significant improvement was defined as a change of at least 2 grades from baseline.

In a separate retrospective analysis, patients were individually evaluated to identify those patients whose benefit to risk ratio was most favorable, i.e., those who obtained clinically important benefit with minimal adverse reactions. Clinically important benefit was defined as one of the following:

1. a substantial improvement in pulmonary symptoms at Month 1 or later (dyspnea ≥2 grades, hemoptysis ≥3 grades, cough ≥3 grades or increase in FEV_1 ≥40%); 2. a moderate improvement in symptoms at Month 2 or later (dyspnea ≥1 grade, cough 2 grades, hemoptysis 2 grades or increase in FEV_1 ≥20%); or 3. a durable objective tumor response (CR or PR maintained to Month 2 or longer).

Thirty-six of the 99 PDT-treated patients (36%) and 23 of the 99 Nd:YAG-treated patients (23%) received clinically important benefit with only minimal or moderate toxicities of short duration. Thirty-four of 99 PDT-treated patients demonstrated improvements in 2 or more efficacy endpoints (dyspnea, cough, hemoptysis, sputum, atelectasis, pulmonary function tests of FEV1 or FVC, Karnofsky Performance Score or tumor response) and 29 patients had improvements in 3 or more. The median duration of documented benefit in the 36 patients was 63 days.

PHOTOFRIN PDT was also evaluated in the treatment of superficial endobronchial tumors in 100 inoperable patients in 3 non-comparative studies. These patients had either carcinoma in situ or microinvasive tumors. Microinvasive lung cancer is defined histologically as disease which invades beyond the basement membrane but not through or into the cartilage. For 24 of the 100 patients, it was clearly documented that surgery and radiotherapy were not indicated. These 24 patients were all inoperable for medical or technical reasons. Radiotherapy was not indicated due to prior high-dose radiotherapy (9 patients), poor pulmonary function (7 patients), multifocal multilobar disease (8 patients), and poor medical condition (1 patient). As shown in Table 4, the tumor response rate (biopsy proven at any time after treatment) was 92%, median time to tumor recurrence was more than 2.7 years, median survival was 3.4 years and disease-specific survival was >3.5 years. The results from the whole population were comparable to those in the subset and in the remaining patients.

High-Grade Dysplasia associated with Barrett's Esophagus: A multicentre, partially blinded, randomized, controlled study was conducted in North America and Europe to assess the efficacy of PDT with PHOTOFRIN for injection plus omeprazole (PHOTOFRIN PDT+OM) in producing complete ablation of HGD in patients with BE as compared to patients receiving omeprazole alone (OM Only). Omeprazole was administered as 20 mg twice daily. Patients were centrally randomized in a 2:1 design to receive PHOTOFRIN PDT plus omeprazole or omeprazole alone. All patients underwent rigorous systematic quarterly endoscopic biopsy surveillance. Four-quadrant jumbo biopsies at every 2 cm of the entire Barrett's mucosa were obtained at each follow-up visit. All histological assessments were carried out at a central pathology laboratory and read by pathologists blinded to the treatment administered. The main efficacy endpoint was the complete response rate (CR3 responders) defined as the complete ablation of HGD at any one of the endoscopic assessment time points. The secondary efficacy endpoints were the quality of the complete response defined as CR2 responders (complete ablation of all grades of dysplasia) and CR1 responders (complete replacement of all Barrett's metaplasia and dysplasia with normal squamous cell epithelium), Duration of Response (CR), Time to Progression to Cancer (TTP), Time to Treatment Failure (TTF), and Survival time. A total of 208 patients who had biopsy-proven HGD in BE and no esophageal invasive cancer or history of cancer participated in the study. The mean age was 66.13 years (38.4 to 88.5 years) in the PHOTOFRIN PDT+OM group, and 67.27 (36.1 to 87.6) in the OM Only group. The patients in both treatment groups were predominantly male (85%), Caucasian (99%), and former smokers (64%).

Table 4: PHOTOFRIN

Overall Efficacy Results in Patients with Superficial Endobronchial Tumors

Efficacy Parameter	PHOTOFRIN PDT N=24	N=100
Complete Tumor Response, Biopsy-proven		
Number of Patients (%)	22 (92%)	79 (79%)
Time to Tumor Recurrence in Patients with Complete Response		
Number of Patients (%) with Recurrences	10 (46%)	33 (42%)
Median Time to Tumor Recurrence	2.7 years	2.8 years
[95% Confidence Interval]	[1.0;—[a]]	[1.5;—[a]]
Survival		
Number of Patients (%) who Died of Any Cause	9 (38%)	44 (44%)
Median Survival	3.4 years	3.5 years
[95% Confidence Interval]	[2.9;—[a]]	[2.9; 6.1]
Disease-specific Survival		
Number of Patients (%) who Died of Lung Cancer	7 (29%)	31 (31%)
Median Disease-Specific Survival	>3.5 years	5.7 years
[95% Confidence Interval]	[3.2;—[a]]	[3.5;—[a]]

a The upper limit of the confidence interval could not be estimated due to an insufficient number of patients whose tumors recurred (Time to Tumor Recurrence) or who died (Survival).

Table 5 presents the overall clinical response for both treatment groups in the ITT population whose response was at CR3 or better at any one of the evaluation time points.

Table 5: PHOTOFRIN

Complete Response Rates (ITT Population)

Responders		Treatment Groups PHOTOFRIN PDT+OM		OM Only		
Follow-up Period		6-month	24-month	6-month	24-month	p value[a]
Numbers of patients	N	138	138	70	70	
CR3 or better[b]	n	99	106	22	27	
	Proportion 95% CI	0.717 (0.642, 0.739)	0.768 (0.698, 0.839)	0.314 (0.206, 0.423)	0.386 (0.272, 0.500)	<0.0001

a Fisher's Exact test.
b CR3 or better: Ablation of all areas of HGD.
Note: Six patients in the PHOTOFRIN PDT+OM group and three patients in the OM Only group without post-baseline biopsy are considered as non-responders.

Table 6: PHOTOFRIN

Proportion of patients responding to treatment, progressing to cancer, and developing esophageal stricture per response category after a minimum of 6 and 24 months of follow-up (ITT population)

Response Category	Outcome Parameters	Statistics	Treatment Groups PHOTOFRIN PDT+OM N=138 6-month Follow-up	24-month Follow-up	OM Only N=70 6-month Follow-up	24-month Follow-up
Overall	CR3 or better responders[a]	n (%)	99 (72)	106 (77)	22 (31)	27 (39)
	Cancer rate	n (%)	14 (10)	18 (13)	13 (19)	20 (28)
	Esophageal strictures[b]	n (%)	48 (35)	49 (37)	0	0
CR3 or better responders	CR3 or better responders[a]	n (%)	99 (72)	106 (77)	22 (31)	27 (39)
	Cancer rate	n (%)	4 (4)	6 (6)	0	1 (4)
	Esophageal strictures[b]	n (%)	28 (28)	39 (37)	0	0

(cont'd)

Table 6: PHOTOFRIN *(cont'd)*

Proportion of patients responding to treatment, progressing to cancer, and developing esophageal stricture per response category after a minimum of 6 and 24 months of follow-up (ITT population)

Response Category	Outcome Parameters	Statistics	Treatment Groups: PHOTOFRIN PDT+OM N=138 6-month Follow-up	PHOTOFRIN PDT+OM N=138 24-month Follow-up	OM Only N=70 6-month Follow-up	OM Only N=70 24-month Follow-up
Non-responders	CR3 or better responders[a]	n (%)	39 (28)	32 (23)	48 (69)	43 (61)
	Cancer rate	n (%)	10 (26)	12 (38)	13 (27)	19 (44)
	Esophageal stricture[b]	n (%)	20 (51)	10 (31)	0	0

[a] Complete ablation of high-grade dysplasia.
[b] Defined as dilated esophageal narrowing.

The proportion of responders was significantly higher in the PHOTOFRIN PDT+OM group as compared to the proportion of responders observed in the OM Only group (77% versus 39%, respectively; p<0.0001).

The quality of response in the PHOTOFRIN PDT+OM group was significantly better than that measured in the OM Only group at all response levels. Seventy-two (52.2%) patients in the PHOTOFRIN PDT+OM group achieved a CR1 response as compared to five (7.1%) patients in the OM Only group. Eighty-one (58.7%) patients in the PHOTOFRIN PDT+OM group achieved a CR2 or better response as compared to ten (14.3%) patients in the OM Only group. The rate of patients who progressed to cancer in the PHOTOFRIN PDT+OM group was statistically lower than that in the OM only group (p=0.0060). By the end of the minimum 2-year follow-up, 18 (13%) of patients in the PHOTOFRIN PDT+OM group had progressed to cancer in contrast with 20 patients (28%) in the OM Only group. By the end of the 24-month follow-up period, patients in the PHOTOFRIN PDT+OM group experienced a significant delay in the TTP compared to those in the OM Only group (p=0.0014). Figure 1 shows a comparison of TTP between the two treatment groups. The TTP for the OM Only group started to differ significantly from that for the PHOTOFRIN PDT+OM group at the 90-day time point. A further, more pronounced disparity in TTP occurred at the 650-day time point.

Figure 1: PHOTOFRIN

Time to Progression to Cancer

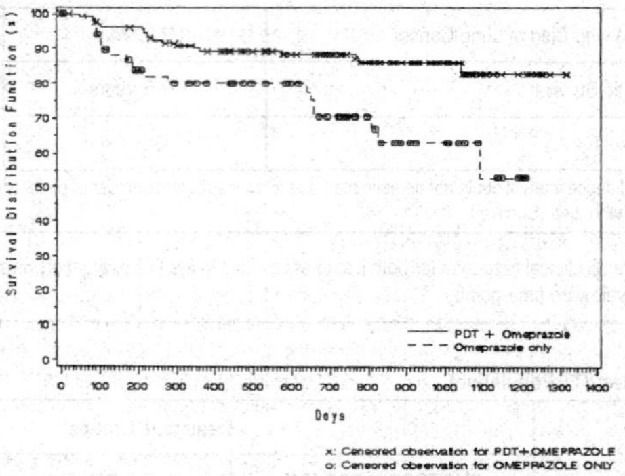

INDICATIONS: Papillary Bladder Cancer: Photodynamic therapy with PHOTOFRIN is indicated following transurethral resection in patients with recurring superficial papillary bladder cancer as second-line treatment for those who have failed a standard intravesical therapy.

Esophageal Cancer: Photodynamic therapy with PHOTOFRIN is indicated for the reduction of obstruction and palliation of dysphagia in patients with completely or partially obstructing esophageal cancer.

Endobronchial Cancer: Photodynamic therapy with PHOTOFRIN is indicated for: reduction of obstruction and palliation of symptoms in patients with completely or partially obstructing endobronchial nonsmall cell lung cancer, and treatment of superficial endobronchial nonsmall cell lung cancer (carcinoma in situ or microinvasive tumors) in patients for whom surgery and radiotherapy are not indicated.

High-Grade Dysplasia associated with Barrett's Esophagus: Photodynamic therapy with PHOTOFRIN is indicated for ablation of high-grade dysplasia (HGD) in Barrett's esophagus (BE) in patients who refuse esophagectomy and are in overall good health. PDT with PHOTOFRIN reduces the risk of progression to esophageal cancer. Rigorous endoscopic surveillance is recommended every three months (until four consecutive negative evaluations have been recorded; further follow-up may be scheduled every 6 to 12 months, as per judgment of physicians) to ensure the detection and biopsy of cancer at an early stage. Ablation of HGD in BE with PDT was better achieved in patients having a single focus HGD and in those taking omeprazole for at least three months prior to PDT treatment.

CONTRAINDICATIONS: Photodynamic therapy (PDT) with PHOTOFRIN (porfimer sodium) is contraindicated in patients with porphyria or in patients with known allergies to porphyrins.

Photodynamic therapy is contraindicated in patients with tumors eroding into a major blood vessel.

Photodynamic therapy is contraindicated in patients with an existing tracheoesophageal or bronchoesophageal fistula.

Papillary Bladder Cancer: Patients with prior total bladder irradiation, or with a functional bladder capacity less than 200 mL, must not be treated with PDT to the bladder; there is the possibility of irreversible bladder contracture from increased fibrosis.

Patients with coexisting bladder tumors of stage greater than T1, who have invasive cancer, must not receive PDT.

Endobronchial Cancer: Photodynamic Therapy is not suitable for emergency treatment of patients with severe acute respiratory distress caused by an obstructing endobronchial lesion because 40 to 50 hours are required between injection with PHOTOFRIN and laser light treatment.

High-Grade Dysplasia associated with Barrett's Esophagus: PDT is not suitable for patients with esophageal or gastric varices or patients with esophageal ulcers >1 cm in diameter.

WARNINGS: Following injection with PHOTOFRIN precautions must be taken to avoid exposure of skin and eyes to direct sunlight or bright indoor light (see Precautions, General Precautions and Information for the Patient).

Esophageal Cancer: If the esophageal tumor is eroding into the trachea or bronchial tree, the likelihood of tracheoesophageal or bronchoesophageal fistula resulting from treatment is sufficiently high that PDT is not recommended.

Patients with esophageal varices should be treated with extreme caution. Light should not be given directly to the variceal area because of the high risk of bleeding.

Endobronchial Cancer: Patients should be assessed for the possibility that a tumor may be eroding into a pulmonary blood vessel (see Contraindications). Patients at high risk for fatal hemoptysis include those with large, centrally located tumors, those with cavitating tumors or those with extensive tumor extrinsic to the bronchus.

If the endobronchial tumor invades deeply into the bronchial wall, the possibility exists for fistula formation upon resolution of the tumor.

Photodynamic therapy should be used with extreme caution for endobronchial tumors in locations where treatment-induced inflammation could obstruct the main airway, e.g., long or circumferential tumors of the trachea, tumors of the main carina that involve both mainstem bronchi circumferentially, or circumferential tumors in the mainstem bronchus in patients with prior pneumonectomy.

High-Grade Dysplasia associated with Barrett's Esophagus: The long-term effect with therapy of this nature is unknown. There is always a possibility of leaving cancer behind or leaving residual abnormal epithelium beneath the new squamous epithelium, facts that emphasize the risk of overlooking cancer in such patients and the need for rigorous continuing surveillance despite the endoscopic appearance of complete squamous reepithelialization. The follow-up of the pivotal study at the time of approval was a minimum of two years (ranging from 2 to 3.6 years).

PRECAUTIONS: Photosensitivity: All patients who receive PHOTOFRIN will be photosensitive for 30 days or more and must observe precautions to avoid exposure of eyes and skin to direct sunlight or brightly focused indoor light (from examination lamps, dental lamps, operating room lamps, floodlights, halogen lamps, etc.). Some patients may remain photosensitive for up to 90 days or more. **Conventional UV sunscreens are of no value in protecting against photosensitivity reactions because photoactivation is caused by visible light.** When outdoors, patients should wear protective clothing and dark sunglasses. The photosensitivity is due to residual drug which will be present in all parts of the skin. Exposure of the skin to ambient indoor light is, however, beneficial because the remaining drug will be inactivated gradually and safely through a photobleaching reaction. Therefore, patients should not stay in a darkened room during this period and should be encouraged to expose their skin to ambient indoor light. The level of photosensitivity will vary for different areas of the body, depending on the extent of previous exposure to light. Before exposing any area of skin to direct sunlight or bright indoor light, the patient should test it for residual photosensitivity. A small area of skin should be exposed to sunlight for 10 minutes. If no photosensitivity reaction (erythema, edema, blistering) occurs within 24 hours, the patient can gradually resume normal outdoor activities, initially continuing to exercise caution and gradually allowing increased exposure. If some photosensitivity reaction occurs with the limited skin test, the patient should continue precautions for another 2 weeks before retesting. The tissue around the eyes may be more sensitive, and therefore, it is not recommended that the face be used for testing. If patients travel to a different geographical area with greater sunshine, they should retest their level of photosensitivity.

Ocular Sensitivity: Ocular discomfort, commonly described as sensitivity to sun, bright lights, or car headlights, has been reported in patients who received PHOTOFRIN. For 30 days, when outdoors, patients should wear dark sunglasses which have an average white light transmittance of <4%.

Respiratory Distress: Patients with endobronchial lesions must be closely monitored between the laser light therapy and the mandatory debridement bronchoscopy for any evidence of respiratory distress. Inflammation and mucositis may result from exposure of normal tissue to too much light. Necrotic debris may also obstruct the airway. If respiratory distress occurs, the physician should be prepared to carry out immediate bronchoscopy to remove secretions and debris to open the airway.

Use Before or After Radiotherapy: If PDT is to be used before or after radiotherapy, sufficient time should be allotted between the two therapies to ensure that the inflammatory response produced by the first treatment has subsided before commencing the second treatment. The inflammatory response from PDT will depend on tumor size and extent of surrounding normal tissue that receives light. It is recommended that 2 to 4 weeks be allowed after PDT before commencing radiotherapy. Similarly, if PDT is to be given after radiotherapy, the acute inflammatory reaction from radiotherapy usually subsides within 4 weeks after completing radiotherapy, after which PDT may be given.

Chest Pain: As a result of PDT treatment in esophageal or endobronchial cancer, or HGD in BE, patients may complain of substernal chest pain because of inflammatory responses within the area of treatment. Such pain may be of sufficient intensity to warrant the short-term prescription of opiate analgesics.

Esophageal Strictures: Esophageal stenosis as a result of PDT in HGD in BE is a common side event. Esophageal stenosis includes esophageal narrowing and esophageal strictures. An esophageal narrowing was defined as a lumen narrowing without solid food dysphagia and not requiring dilation. An esophageal stricture was defined as a fixed lumen narrowing with solid food dysphagia and requiring dilation. In the pivotal study, 128 events of esophageal stenosis were reported in the PHOTOFRIN PDT+OM group (55% mild, 37% moderate, 8% severe). Esophageal strictures occurred in 36% of the patients within six months following PDT and were manageable through dilations (see Pharmacology, Clinical Studies). Multiple dilations of esophageal strictures may be required. Special care should be taken during dilation to avoid perforation of the esophagus. A high proportion of patients who developed an esophageal stricture received a nodule pre-treatment prior to developing the event (49%) was compared to patients who did not develop esophageal strictures during the study (37%). A high proportion of patients who developed an esophageal stricture had a mucosal segment treated twice (82%) as compared to patients who did not develop esophageal stricture (52%). Therefore, nodule pre-treatment and re-treating the same mucosal segment more than once may influence the risk of developing an esophageal stricture.

PDT with PHOTOFRIN should be applied by physicians trained in the endoscopic use of PDT with PHOTOFRIN and only in those facilities properly equipped for the procedure.

Others: PDT has not been studied in patients with significant cardiopulmonary symptoms. The effect on such patients is not known.

Drug Interactions: There is no clinical information concerning drug-drug interactions involving PHOTOFRIN. However, it is possible that concomitant use of other agents known to produce photosensitivity reactions (e.g., tetracyclines, sulfonamides, phenothiazines, sulfonylurea hypoglycemic agents, thiazide diuretics, griseofulvin and fluoroquinolones) would have the potential to increase the photosensitivity reaction.

Since the basic effects of PDT are thought to involve vasoconstriction and platelet activation and aggregation at the site of treatment, as well as the generation of active oxygen species, treatments which alter blood flow or availability of oxygen would be expected to affect the effectiveness of PDT. Data from animal models and in vitro tissue culture studies suggest the following: Thromboxane A_2 receptor antagonists, thromboxane synthetase inhibitors, drugs which quench active oxygen species, and compounds which react with hydroxyl radicals, including dimethyl sulfoxide (DMSO), ethanol, formate, and mannitol, have been shown to decrease the effectiveness of PDT. Steroids administered 24 to 48 hours following PDT enhanced antitumor effects, whereas steroids administered concomitantly inhibited the PDT effect. Animal or in vitro studies involving combination therapy with PDT and standard antineoplastic agents (including doxorubicin, mitomycin C, and BCG for bladder cancer, and mitomycin C in a colon cancer cell line) resulted in an increase in effectiveness compared with single therapies. Similarly, combinations of PDT with PHOTOFRIN and different photosensitizers with different biodistribution properties (including tetraphenylporphine sulfonate) resulted in enhanced tumor eradication in a murine mammary tumor model.

Pregnancy: There are no adequate and well controlled studies in pregnant women. PHOTOFRIN should be used during pregnancy only if the potential benefit justifies the potential risk to the fetus. Women of childbearing potential should practice an effective method of contraception during therapy, and have a pretreatment pregnancy test performed.

Lactation: It is unknown whether the drug is excreted in human milk. Therefore, women receiving PHOTOFRIN must not breastfeed.

Children: Safety and effectiveness in children have not been established.

Geriatrics: Approximately 70% of the patients treated with PDT using PHOTOFRIN in clinical trials were over 60 years of age. There was no apparent difference in effectiveness or safety in these patients compared to younger people. Dose modification based upon age is not required.

ADVERSE EFFECTS: The skin of all patients who receive PHOTOFRIN, will be photosensitive for 30 days or more (see Precautions). Photosensitivity reactions are avoidable through proper patient education. In clinical studies in cancer, the incidence of photosensitivity was 20%; this incidence was 68% in patients with HGD in BE. Typically these reactions were mostly mild to moderate erythema but they also included swelling, itching, burning sensations, feeling hot, or blisters. In a single study of 24 healthy subjects, some evidence of photosensitivity reactions occurred in all subjects (incidence of 100%). Other less common skin manifestations, in areas where photosensitivity reactions had occurred, were also reported such as increased hair growth, skin discoloration, skin nodules, increased wrinkles and increased skin fragility. These manifestations may be attributed to a pseudoporphyria state (temporary drug-induced cutaneous porhyria). Ocular discomfort (sensitivity to sun, bright lights or car headlights) has also been reported. The only other known systemic reaction is constipation.

The toxicities associated with PDT across all indications are primarily local, in the immediate area that received laser light, and sometimes extending into adjacent tissues. The local/regional reactions are consistent with an inflammatory reaction induced by the photodynamic effect (see below for specific reactions by indication).

A few cases of fluid imbalance have been reported following the use of PDT with PHOTOFRIN in patients with overtly disseminated intraperitoneal malignancies. Fluid imbalance is an expected PDT treatment related event.

Accelerated development of early bilateral cataracts following therapy has been reported in one patient with positive family history of cataracts.

Papillary Bladder Cancer: Patients with papillary bladder cancer may develop transient (up to several weeks) irritative bladder symptoms after PDT with PHOTOFRIN. This post-PDT response, thought to be due to inflammation, includes increased micturition frequency (60% of patients), hematuria (56%), dysuria (36%), urgency (32%) and suprapubic pain (20%). Additional common urinary symptoms observed were strangury (32%), genital edema (24%), urinary incontinence (20%) and nocturia (12%), and urinary tract infection (12%). Transient reduction in bladder capacity may occur; irreversible bladder contracture occurred in 20% of patients, a median of 99 days post PDT.

Additional adverse reactions which occurred in ≥10% of patients with papillary bladder cancer were anxiety (12%), insomnia (20%), peripheral edema (16%), nonspecific pain (12%), nausea (12%) and constipation (12%).

Esophageal Cancer: In a clinical trial involving patients with partially-obstructing esophageal cancer PDT with PHOTOFRIN was compared to thermal ablation with the Nd:YAG laser. Adverse events that occurred significantly more often in PDT-treated than in Nd:YAG-treated patients (besides photosensitivity) were fever (33% versus 10%, respectively), pleural effusion (28% versus 6%), respiratory insufficiency (10% versus 1%), anemia (26% versus 12%), and constipation (23% versus 9%). With the exception of anemia and respiratory insufficiency, these reactions were generally mild or moderate in severity and easily managed. Anemia was manageable by transfusion and was more common in patients with large tumors (>10 cm) and in tumors in the lower area of the esophagus. The etiology of respiratory insufficiency is unclear. Fever and pleural effusion, as well as pain (22% versus 20%), esophageal edema (6% versus 2%) and atrial fibrillation (8% versus 4%) are thought to be manifestations of a local/regional inflammatory reaction. Esophageal edema occurred more frequently when the tumor was located in the upper third of the esophagus; atrial fibrillation was more likely to occur when the tumor was in the middle of the esophagus.

Other adverse reactions which occurred commonly (>10% of either group of patients) in both the PDT group and the Nd:YAG laser group were insomnia (14% versus 9%), abdominal pain (19% versus 11%), hematemesis (11% versus 7%), nausea (21% versus 15%), vomiting (16% versus 8%), dyspnea (18% versus 15%), pneumonia (16% versus 13%) and chest pain (23% versus 19%). Some of these adverse events reflect symptoms of esophageal cancer or concurrent conditions such as respiratory disease, although they may have been exacerbated by either treatment.

Endobronchial Cancer: Adverse events reported in 5% or more of patients (n=99) with obstructing endobronchial nonsmall cell lung cancer were most commonly associated with the respiratory system; their relationship to therapy is unclear: dyspnea (32%), coughing (17%), pneumonia (13%), nonfatal hemoptysis (12%), bronchitis (11%), fatal massive hemoptysis (10%), increased sputum (9%) and respiratory insufficiency (7%). Other frequent events were photosensitivity reaction (20%), fever (15%), chest pain (9%), insomnia (7%), anxiety (5%) and constipation (5%).

Transient inflammatory reactions occur in about 10% of patients and manifest as fever, bronchitis, chest pain and dyspnea. Most cases of bronchitis occurred within 1 week of treatment and all but one were mild or moderate in intensity. The events usually resolved within 10 days with antibiotic therapy. Treatment-related worsening of dyspnea is generally transient and self-limiting. Debridement of the treated area is mandatory to remove exudate and necrotic tissue. Life-threatening respiratory insufficiency likely due to therapy occurred in 3% of PDT-treated patients and in 2% of patients treated with the comparator, Nd:YAG thermal ablation (see Warnings and Precautions).

There was a trend toward a higher rate of fatal hemoptysis (FMH) occurring on the PDT arm (10%) versus Nd:YAG (5%), however, the rate of FMH occurring within 30 days of treatment was the same for PDT and Nd:YAG (4% total events, 3% treatment-associated events) and median survival was similar in the two groups (PDT 174 days, Nd:YAG 161 days). Patients who have received radiation therapy have a higher incidence of FMH after treatment with PDT and after other forms of local therapy than patients who have not received radiation therapy, but analyses suggest that this increased risk may be due to associated prognostic factors such as having a recurrent, centrally located tumor. The incidence of FMH in patients previously treated with radiotherapy was 21% (6/29) in the PDT group and 10% (3/29) in the Nd:YAG group. Characteristics of patients at high risk for FMH are described in Warnings.

Serious and other notable adverse events observed in less than 5% of PDT-treated patients with obstructing endobronchial cancer included pleural effusion, pulmonary thrombosis, pulmonary embolism and lung abscess. Cardiac failure, sepsis, and possible cerebrovascular accident have also been reported in 1 patient each. Their relationship to therapy is uncertain.

In patients with superficial endobronchial tumors, adverse events were similar in nature to those reported in patients with late-stage disease, but much less frequent and milder in intensity. Fifty-one of 102 patients (50%) experienced an adverse event, two-thirds of which were related to the respiratory system. A mucositis reaction occurred more frequently in patients with superficial tumors; one-fifth of the patients experienced manifestations of mucositis, such as edema, exudate, and obstruction. The obstruction (mucous plug) is easily removed with suction or forceps. Mucositis can be minimized by avoiding exposure of normal tissue to excessive light (see Precautions). Three patients experienced life-threatening dyspnea: one was given a double dose of light, one was treated concurrently in both mainstem bronchi and the other had had prior pneumonectomy and was treated in the sole remaining main airway (see Warnings). In addition, fatal massive hemoptysis occurred within 30 days of treatment in 1 patient who had received prior endobronchial brachytherapy. Stent placement was required in 3% of the patients due to endobronchial stricture.

High-Grade Dysplasia associated with Barrett's Esophagus: In a clinical trial, PDT with PHOTOFRIN plus omeprazole (PDT+OM) was compared to a control group of patients receiving omeprazole alone (OM Only) in producing complete ablation of High-Grade Dysplasia (HGD) in patients with Barrett's esophagus (BE). The majority (99%) of patients in the PHOTOFRIN PDT+OM group reported treatment emergent adverse events (regardless of association with treatment) compared to 74% of patients in the OM Only group. Adverse events that occurred significantly more often in PHOTOFRIN PDT+OM group than in the OM Only group (>10% in either group of patients) were photosensitivity reaction (68% versus 0%), esophageal narrowing/strictures (40% versus 1%), vomiting (38% versus 6%), constipation (27% versus 7%), chest pain (25% versus 12%), fever (24% versus 4%), upper or lower abdominal pain (20% versus 6%), dysphagia (19% versus 1%), nausea (14% versus 7%), dehydration (12% versus 3%), hiccups (11% versus 0%), and dyspnea (10% versus 4%). Other adverse reactions, which occurred commonly (>10% of either group of patients) in both groups, were diarrhea (16% versus 10%) and headache (11% versus 9%). Other adverse events reported included pleural effusion (6 % versus 0%) and atrial fibrillation (3% versus 1%).

Esophageal stenosis as a result of PDT in HGD in BE is a common side event. Esophageal stenosis includes esophageal narrowing, defined as a lumen narrowing without solid food dysphagia and not requiring dilation, and esophageal strictures, defined as a fixed lumen narrowing with solid food dysphagia and requiring dilation. The majority of esophageal stenosis reported in the PHOTOFRIN PDT+OM group were of mild or moderate intensity (55% mild, 37% moderate). Approximately 8% of events were of severe intensity. The majority of esophageal strictures reported in the PHOTOFRIN PDT+OM group were reported during Course 2 of treatment. All esophageal strictures were considered to be associated with treatment. Most esophageal strictures were manageable through dilations.

OVERDOSE:

There is no information on overdosage situations involving PHOTOFRIN. Higher than recommended drug doses of two 2 mg/kg doses given 2 days apart (10 patients), and three 2 mg/kg doses given within 2 weeks (1 patient), were tolerated without notable adverse reactions. Effects of overdosage on the duration of photosensitivity are unknown. Laser treatment should not be given if an overdose of PHOTOFRIN is administered. In the event of an overdose, patients should protect their eyes and skin from direct sunlight or bright indoor lights for 30 days. At this time, patients should test for residual photosensitivity (see Precautions). PHOTOFRIN is not dialyzable.

Overdose of Laser Light Following PHOTOFRIN Injection: Papillary Bladder Cancer: Whole bladder photoradiation at light levels exceeding the recommended dose may significantly increase adverse urinary symptoms seen after PDT treatment, and may create irreversible bladder contracture in some patients.

Esophageal Cancer: There is no information on overdose of laser light following PHOTOFRIN injection in patients with esophageal carcinoma.

Endobronchial Cancer: Light doses of 2 to 3 times the recommended dose have been administered to a few patients with superficial endobronchial tumors. One patient experienced life-threatening dyspnea and the others had no notable complications. Increased symptoms and damage to normal tissue might be expected following an overdose of light.

High-Grade Dysplasia associated with Barrett's Esophagus:

There is no information on overdose of laser light following PHOTOFRIN injection in patients with Barrett's esophagus.

For management of a suspected drug overdose, CPhA recommends that you contact your **regional Poison Control Centre**. See the *CPS* Directory section for a list of Poison Control Centres.

DOSAGE: Photodynamic therapy (PDT) with PHOTOFRIN is a 2-stage process requiring administration of both drug and light. Physicians should be trained in the safe and efficacious treatment of papillary bladder, esophageal or endobronchial cancer, or HGD in BE using photodynamic therapy with PHOTOFRIN and associated light delivery devices. The first stage of PDT is the i.v. injection of PHOTOFRIN at 2 mg/kg. The second stage of therapy is illumination with laser light 40 to 50 hours following injection with PHOTOFRIN. In patients with bladder cancer, no further doses of drug or light should be administered due to increased risk of bladder contracture; patients with esophageal cancer, endobronchial cancer, or HGD in BE may receive a second laser light application 96 to 120 hours after drug administration. If needed, up to 1 or 2 more courses of drug and light may be given, with each injection separated by a minimum of 30 days, except for HGD in BE where each injection should be separated by a minimum of 90 days.

PHOTOFRIN Administration: PHOTOFRIN should be reconstituted according to the directions given under Reconstitution and administered as a single slow i.v. injection over 3 to 5 minutes at 2 mg/kg body weight. As with all i.v. injections, care should be taken to prevent extravasation at the injection site. If extravasation occurs, the area should be protected from light for a minimum of 30 days. There is no known benefit from injecting the extravasation site with another substance.

Photoactivation of PHOTOFRIN: Uniform and complete light delivery to the tumor mass is essential for activation of PHOTOFRIN. Light from a laser is delivered to the tumor or Barrett's segment via Optiguide Fiber Optic Diffusers, designed specifically for use in photodynamic therapy. While there are numerous lasers available for medical applications, the use of the Optiguide Fiber Optics for photoactivation of PHOTOFRIN requires a continuous output laser operating at a wavelength of 630±3 nm, and producing a stable power output. The choice of the type and size of the fiber optic diffuser tip will depend on the indication, tumor or Barrett's segment location and size.

Photoactivation of PHOTOFRIN is controlled by the total energy delivered to the tumor or Barrett's segment site. This is determined by the power delivered from the Optiguide Fiber Optic to the treatment site and the total treatment time.

The Optiguide Package Insert provides details relating to the assembly, function and operation of the fiber optic light delivery system, including accepted laser light sources, and should be used in conjunction with the information presented for each indication below.

Superficial Papillary Bladder Cancer: Whole bladder treatment will require a total light delivery of 15 joules/cm², using the spherical cavity diffuser. Approximately 40 to 50 hours after injection with PHOTOFRIN, the patient should be anesthetized and the bladder distended with a volume of saline or water sufficient to smooth mucosal folds, without compromising circulation. This "treatment volume" should be within 50 to 75% of the bladder's functional capacity, as measured by cystometrography.

Referring to the Optiguide Package Insert, attach the Optiguide Model DSPH spherical cavity diffuser to an acceptable laser light source. To minimize the treatment time and thus the period of bladder distention, the total power output at the fiber optic tip should be at least 1.25 watts but less than the maximum power specification for the fiber optic.

The cystocope should be positioned securely at the bladder neck using clamps and metal rods, a gooseneck or similar stationary apparatus, and should not be moved once it is secured. The patient is placed in Trendelenberg position which relaxes the abdominal wall to facilitate centering the treatment tip. By adjusting the position of the patient, the cystoscope is aimed at the point where the posterior wall meets the dome, which is the maximum distance from the bladder neck. The trigone should not be visible. Correct placement of the fiber tip in the center of the bladder is essential to ensure uniform irradiation of the bladder, as areas which receive excessive amounts of light may result in pain or sensitivity post-treatment. Correct placement can be achieved by one of two methods:

a. Ultrasound Imaging: Ultrasound imaging is recommended to verify the mid-bladder placement of the fiber tip, as well as to monitor the bladder volume during treatment: (1) after the bladder is filled, an initial examination of the bladder is made in cross-sectional and longitudinal planes using an ultrasound apparatus. (2) The probe is then placed in the longitudinal position in the midline of the abdomen just above the symphysis pubis. Once the bladder filling has begun, the fluid can be easily detected as a black or clear space in the ultrasound image. The probe may have to be moved side to side (right to left or left to right) to locate the optimum long axis of the bladder once the bladder is filled. (3) Once the bladder has been filled, the cystocope can easily be imaged by ultrasound. (4) Centering of the cystoscope and laser fiber should be done using the linear distance calipers on the ultrasound equipment.

b. Sounding: To determine the midpoint of the bladder by sounding, a urethral catheter with one end plugged to prevent leakage is directed to the dome. The maximum distance is measured from the bladder neck to the point where the posterior bladder wall meets the dome. The spherical diffuser tip is passed through the port of the cystocope to the midpoint of the neck-dome measurement. Once the spherical diffuser tip is situated at the midpoint of the bladder, the catheter should be withdrawn.

Calculation of Treatment Time: The surface area of the bladder wall and the subsequent treatment time required to deliver a total light dose of 15 joules/cm² should be calculated knowing the bladder treatment volume (i.e., the volume instilled to distend the bladder) and the laser power output from the fiber optic tip, using the following equation:

$$\text{Light dose (J/cm}^2\text{)} = \frac{\text{Power output from diffuser (W)} \times \text{Treatment time (sec)}}{\text{Bladder surface area (cm}^2\text{)}}$$

where:

Light dose=15 joules/cm²

Bladder surface area=4.83×(bladder treatment volume)$^{2/3}$

Urine production or irrigant leakage during treatment can change the bladder surface area and therefore the power density and the delivered light dose. The bladder volume, power output at the fiber tip and positioning of the fiber tip should be checked at the beginning, middle (particularly if the total treatment time is to exceed 45 minutes) and end, and at any time that bleeding is observed or significant changes in bladder volume, fiber power output or fiber tip position are suspected. Whenever treatment is interrupted, "pause" the laser output, ensuring that the original laser settings and elapsed treatment time are retained. If the bladder appears to be filling during the procedure, sufficient urine should be evacuated to restore the original volume. By the end of the procedure, the cumulative laser light dose should total 15±1 joules/cm².

The patient should remain under observation for 24 hours post-cystoscopy or until the physician determines that he or she may be safely discharged.

No further courses of treatment with PHOTOFRIN or light should be used to treat superficial papillary bladder cancer, due to increased risk of bladder contracture.

Esophageal or Endobronchial Cancers: Approximately 40 to 50 hours after PHOTOFRIN administration, light should be delivered to the tumor by Optiguide Fiber Optic Diffusers passed through the operating channel of the endoscope/bronchoscope.

Light Doses: Photoactivation of PHOTOFRIN is controlled by the total light energy (light dose) delivered to the tumor site and depends on the indication, as follows: For endobronchial (obstructing or superficial) tumors: 200 joules/cm of tumor length. For esophageal tumors: 300 joules/cm of tumor length.

The cylindrical diffuser uniformly distributes laser light radially in a cylindrical pattern over the entire length of the fiber optic tip. The following light dosimetry equation applies.

$$\text{Light dose (J/cm)} = \frac{\text{Total power output from diffuser (W)} \times \text{Treatment time (sec)}}{\text{Diffuser length (cm)}}$$

It is recommended that the total power output from the diffuser, as measured by a suitable integrating sphere power meter, be set to [400 mW/cm×cm diffuser length] which will deliver the appropriate dose using exposure times of either 8 minutes, 20 seconds (endobronchial tumors, 200 J/cm) or 12 minutes, 30 seconds (esophageal tumors, 300 J/cm).

Optiguide cylindrical diffusers are available in several lengths (refer to Optiguide Package Insert) and the diffuser tip length should be chosen to match the length of the tumor. Tumors that differ from available diffuser lengths may require multiple use of a single diffuser or the use of 2 or more diffusers of differing lengths. Diffuser length should be sized to avoid exposure of non-malignant tissue to light and to prevent overlapping of previously treated malignant tissue. Diffusers or combinations of diffusers should be selected to minimize patient treatment time.

Examples of diffuser lengths/tumor sizes follow: See Table 7.

Table 7: PHOTOFRIN

Examples of Use of Optiguide Cylindrical Diffusers

Optiguide			Fiber Optic Power Output (mW)	Esophageal Cancer (300 J/cm)		Endobronchial Cancer (200 J/cm)[a]	
Tumor Length (cm)	**Diffuser Length (cm)**	**Segment Number**		**Min:Sec per Segment**	**Total Time (min:sec)**	**Min:Sec per Segment**	**Total Time (min:sec)**
1.0	1.0	1	400	12:30	12:30	8:20	8:20
2.0	2.0	1	800	12:30	12:30	8:20	8:20
3.0	1.5	1	600	12:30	25:00	8:20	16:40
	1.5	2	600	12:30		8:20	
5.0	5.0	1	2000	12:30	12:30	8:20	8:20

(cont'd)

Table 7: PHOTOFRIN *(cont'd)*

Examples of Use of Optiguide Cylindrical Diffusers

Optiguide			Fiber Optic Power Output (mW)	Esophageal Cancer (300 J/cm)		Endobronchial Cancer (200 J/cm)[a]	
Tumor Length (cm)	Diffuser Length (cm)	Segment Number		Min:Sec per Segment	Total Time (min:sec)	Min:Sec per Segment	Total Time (min:sec)
7.0	5.0	1	2000	12:30	25:00	8:20	16:40
	2.0	2	800	12:30		8:20	

[a] For superficial or obstructing tumors.

The cylindrical diffusers may be used either interstitially or intraluminally. For non-circumferential endobronchial tumors that are soft enough to penetrate, interstitial fiber placement is preferred to intraluminal activation, since this method produces better efficacy and results in less exposure of normal bronchial mucosa to the light. When the interstitial technique is used, up to 90% of the length of the diffuser should be inserted into the tumor mass.

Debridement and Retreatment: In patients with endobronchial tumors, gentle debridement is mandatory to remove necrotic tumor debris and clear secretions or mucous plugs, thereby preventing dyspnea, obstruction, atelectasis and infection. For esophageal cancer, debridement is optional since the residua will be removed naturally by peristaltic action. Debridement of residua should be performed 2 days after light treatment. Vigorous debridement may cause tumor bleeding. Debridement should be discontinued if the volume of bleeding increases, as this may indicate that debridement has gone beyond the zone of PDT treatment effect. Patients with residual tumor may be retreated with laser light at the time of debridement at the same dose as used in the initial treatment. The second light dose is administered 96 to 120 hours after the PHOTOFRIN injection.

Patients may receive a second course of PDT a minimum of 30 days after the initial therapy; up to 3 courses of PDT (each injection separated by a minimum of 30 days) can be given. Before each course of treatment, patients should be evaluated for the presence of a tracheoesophageal or bronchoesophageal fistula or the possibility that the tumor may be eroding into a major blood vessel (see Contraindications).

High-Grade Dysplasia in Barrett's Esophagus: Approximately 40-50 hours after PHOTOFRIN administration, light should be delivered by a fiber optic diffuser passed through the central channel of a centering balloon. The choice of fiber optic/balloon diffuser combination will depend on the length of esophagus to be treated (see Table 8).

Table 8: PHOTOFRIN

Fiber Optic Diffuser/Balloon Combination[a]

Treated Barrett's Mucosa Length (cm)	Fiber Optic Diffuser Size (cm)	Balloon Window Size (cm)
6–7	9	7
4–5	7	5
1–3	5	3

[a] Whenever possible, the BE segment selected for treatment should include normal tissue margins of a few millimetres at the proximal and distal ends.

Light Doses: Photoactivation is controlled by the total light dose delivered. The objective is to expose and treat all areas of HGD and the entire length of BE. The light dose administered will be 130 J/cm of diffuser length using a centering balloon. Based on preclinical studies, acceptable light intensity for the balloon/diffuser combinations range from 175-270 mW/cm of diffuser.

To calculate the light dose, the following specific light dosimetry equation applies for all fiber optic diffusers:

$$\text{Light dose (J/cm)} = \frac{\text{Power output from diffuser (W)} \times \text{Treatment time (sec)}}{\text{Diffuser length (cm)}}$$

Table 9 provides the settings that will be used to deliver the dose within the shortest time (light intensity of 270 mW/cm). A second option (light intensity of 200 mW/cm) has also been included where necessary to accommodate lasers with a total capacity that dose not exceed 2.5 W.

Table 9: PHOTOFRIN

Fiber Optic Power Outputs and Treatment Times Required to Deliver 130 J/cm of Diffuser Length Using the Balloon for Areas with HGD

Balloon Window Length (cm)	Diffuser Length (cm)	Light Intensity (mW/cm)	Required Power Output from Diffuser[a] (W)	Treatment Time (sec)	Treatment Time (min:sec)
3	5	270	1.35	480	8:00
5	7	270	1.90	480	8:00
		200	1:40	650	10:50
7	9	270	2:44	480	8:00
		200	1:80	650	10:50

[a] As measured by immersing the diffuser into the cuvet in the power meter and slowly increasing the laser power. Note: No more than 1.5 times the required diffuser power output should be needed from the laser. If more than this is required, the system should be checked.

Omeprazole administration: As an adjunctive treatment in BE with HGD, omeprazole should be administered at a minimum of 20 mg twice daily or higher if judged necessary by the attending physician, beginning at least two days before the PHOTOFRIN injection. For additional information, please refer to the Product Monograph for omeprazole.

Pre-treatment of Nodules and Post-treatment of Skip Areas: Short fiber optic diffusers (≤2.5 cm) are to be used to pretreat nodules with 50 J/cm diffuser length prior to regular balloon treatment in the first laser light session or for the retreatment of "skip" areas after the first light session. For this treatment, the fiber optic diffuser is used without a balloon, and a light intensity of 400 mW/cm should be used. Table 10 lists appropriate fiber optic power outputs and treatment times using a light intensity of 400 mW/cm.

Nodules are to be pre-treated at a light dose of 50 J/cm of diffuser length with a short (≤2.5 cm) fiber optic diffuser placed directly against the nodule followed by standard balloon application as described above.

First Treatment Course: A maximum of 7 cm of Barrett's mucosa is treated at the first light session using an appropriate size of centering balloon and fiber optic diffuser (Table 8). Whenever possible, the segment selected for the first light application should contain all the areas of HGD. Also, whenever possible, the BE segment selected for the first light application should include normal tissue margin of a few millimeters at the proximal and distal ends.

Repeat Light Application (Treatment of Skip Areas): A second laser light application may be given to a previously treated segment that shows a 'skip' area, (i.e., an area that does not show sufficient mucosal response) using a short, ≤2.5 cm fiber optic diffuser at the light dose of 50 J/cm of the diffuser length (see Table 10).

Table 10: PHOTOFRIN

Short Fiber Optic Diffusers to be Used Without A Centering Balloon to Deliver 50 J/cm of Diffuser Length at a Light Intensity of 400 mW/cm for Nodules and Skipped Areas

Diffuser Length (cm)	Required Power Output From Diffuser[a] (W)	Treatment Time (sec)	Treatment Time (min:sec)
1.0	0.4	125	2:05
1.5	0.6	125	2:05
2.0	0.8	125	2:05
2.5	1.0	125	2:05

[a] As measured by immersing the diffuser into the cuvet in the power meter and slowly increasing the laser power.
Note: No more than 1.5 times the required diffuser power output should be needed from the laser. If more than this is required, the system should be checked.

The treatment regimen is summarized in Table 11. Patients with BE >7 cm, should have the remaining untreated length of Barrett's epithelium treated with a second PDT course at least 90 days later.

Table 11: PHOTOFRIN

High-Grade Dysplasia in Barrett's Esophagus of ≤7 cm

Procedure	Study Day	Light Delivery Devices	Treatment Intent
PHOTOFRIN Injection	Day 1	NA	Uptake of photosensitizer
Laser Light Application	Day 3[a]	3, 5 or 7 cm balloon (130 J/cm)	Photoactivation
Laser Light Application (Optional)	Day 5	short (≤2.5 cm) fiber optic diffuser (50 J/cm)	Treatment of "skip" areas only

[a] Discrete nodules will receive an initial light application of 50 J/cm (using a short diffuser) before the balloon light application.

Additional Treatment Courses: Patients may receive a second course of PDT a minimum of 90 days after the initial therapy; up to three courses of PDT (each injection separated by a minimum of 90 days) can be given to a previously treated segment which still shows HGD, low-grade dysplasia (LGD) or Barrett's metaplasia, or to a new segment if the initial Barrett's segment was >7 cm in length. Both residual and additional segments may be treated in the same light session(s) provided that the total length of the segments treated with the balloon/diffuser combination is not greater than 7 cm. In the case of a previously treated esophageal segment, if it has not sufficiently healed and/or histological assessment of biopsies is not clear, the subsequent course of PDT may be delayed for an additional 1-2 months.

Surveillance: PDT therapy is an adjunct to rigorous surveillance with biopsies (four quadrant jumbo biopsies every 1-2 cm) every three months (until four consecutive negative evaluations have been recorded; further follow-up may be scheduled every 6 to 12 months, as per judgment of physicians).

Reconstitution: PHOTOFRIN in the 75 mg or 15 mg vial should be reconstituted as follows with 5% Dextrose for injection, USP resulting in a final concentration of 2.5 mg porfimer sodium/mL. See Table 12.

Table 12: PHOTOFRIN

Reconstitution

Vial Size[a]	Volume of Diluent to be Added to Vial	Approximate Available Volume	Concentration
75 mg	31.8 mL	30.0 mL	2.5 mg/mL
15 mg	6.6 mL	6.0 mL	2.5 mg/mL

[a] Some excess added to allow complete recovery of vial contents.

Store reconstituted solutions at 2 to 8°C protected from light. Discard unused portion after 24 hours.

Incompatibilities: PHOTOFRIN should only be reconstituted with Dextrose 5% in water. PHOTOFRIN should not be mixed with other drugs in the same solution.

Special Instructions: Spills and Disposal: Spills of PHOTOFRIN should be wiped up with a damp cloth, at which time the wearing of rubber gloves and eye protection are recommended. Skin and eye contact should be avoided. All contaminated materials should be disposed of in a polyethylene bag in a manner consistent with local regulations.

Accidental Exposure: PHOTOFRIN is neither a primary ocular irritant nor a primary dermal irritant. Because of its potential to induce photosensitivity, PHOTOFRIN might be an eye and/or skin irritant in the presence of bright light. It is important to avoid contact with the eyes and skin during preparation and/or administration. As with therapeutic overdosage, any accidentally exposed persons must be protected from bright light.

INFORMATION FOR THE PATIENT: Published in e-CPS, available by subscription at www.e-cps.ca.

SUPPLIED: Each vial contains: porfimer sodium 15 or 75 mg as a sterile freeze-dried cake or powder. Sodium hydroxide and/or hydrochloric acid are used in the manufacturing process to adjust pH. There are no antimicrobial preservatives or formulation excipients. Store unreconstituted PHOTOFRIN for injection at 15 to 25°C.

Phytonadione

CPhA Monograph

see *Vitamin K*

Pico-Salax®

picosulfate sodium—magnesium oxide—citric acid

Purgative

Ferring

PHARMACOLOGY: The active components of PICO-SALAX are sodium picosulfate and magnesium citrate.

Picosulfate is a stimulant cathartic active locally in the colon.

Magnesium citrate (magnesium oxide and citric acid) acts as an osmotic laxative by retaining moisture in the colon. The action is of a powerful "washing out" effect combined with peristaltic stimulation to clear the bowel prior to radiography, colonoscopy or surgery. Full doses of the saline cathartics (15 g of magnesium sulfate or its equivalent) produces a semi-fluid of watery evacuation within 3-6 hours or less.

The product is not intended for use as a routine laxative.

Systemic Effects: Some absorption of the component ions of the saline cathartics does occur, and in certain instances they may produce systemic toxicity. This is especially true for magnesium salts, since 20% or more of the administered cation is absorbed. If renal function is normal, the absorbed magnesium is rapidly excreted. However, if a magnesium cation is given to an individual with impaired renal function, the accumulation of magnesium ion in the body fluids may be sufficient to cause magnesium intoxication.

In most instances, salts that gain access to the systemic circulation are rapidly excreted by the kidneys.

INDICATIONS: PICO-SALAX is used for clearance of the bowel prior to x-ray examination, endoscopy or surgery.

CONTRAINDICATIONS: Hypersensitivity to any of the ingredients of the product, congestive cardiac failure, gastric retention, gastrointestinal ulceration, toxic colitis, toxic megacolon, ileus, nausea and vomiting, acute surgical abdominal conditions such as acute appendicitis and known or suspected gastrointestinal obstruction or perforation.

In patients with severely reduced renal function, accumulation of magnesium in plasma may occur. Another preparation should be used in such cases.

WARNINGS: See Precautions.

PRECAUTIONS: Recent gastrointestinal surgery. Care should also be taken in patients with renal impairment, heart disease or inflammatory bowel disease.

Use with caution in patients on drugs that might affect water and/or electrolyte balance e.g. diuretics, corticosteroids, lithium (see Drug Interactions and Adverse Effects).

Patients should avoid taking oral iron preparations for a week before colonoscopy. Constipating drugs (i.e. cholinergics, opioids) should be suspended for a few days before the procedure, after consulting with your doctor.

PICO-SALAX may modify the absorption of regularly prescribed oral medication and should be used with caution e.g. there have been isolated reports of seizures in patients on antiepileptics, with previously controlled epilepsy (see Drug Interactions and Adverse Effects).

An inadequate oral intake of water and electrolytes could create clinically significant, deficiencies, particularly in less fit patients. In this regard, the elderly, debilitated individuals and patients at risk of hypokalaemia may need particular attention. Prompt corrective action should be taken to restore fluid/electrolyte balance in patients with signs or symptoms of hyponatraemia.

The period of bowel cleansing should not exceed 24 hours because longer preparation may increase the risk of water and electrolyte imbalance.

Pregnancy: Reproduction studies with sodium picosulfate performed in animals have revealed no evidence of a harmful action on the fetus. However, clinical experience of the use of PICO-SALAX during pregnancy is limited and caution should be observed, particularly during the first trimester.

Lactation: Neither sodium picosulfate nor magnesium citrate have been shown to be excreted in breast milk.

Drug Interactions: As a purgative, PICO-SALAX increases the gastrointestinal transit rate. The absorption of other orally administered medicines (e.g. antiepileptics, contraceptives, antidiabetics, antibiotics) may therefore be modified during the treatment period (see above).

The efficacy of PICO-SALAX is lowered by bulk-forming laxatives.

Care should be taken with patients already receiving drugs which may be associated with hypokalaemia (such as diuretics or corticosteroids, or drugs where hypokalaemia is a particular risk i.e. cardiac glycosides). Caution is also advised when PICO-SALAX is used in patients on nonsteroidal anti-inflammatory drugs (NSAIDs) or drugs known to induce Antidiuretic Hormone Secretion (SIADH) e.g. tricyclic antidepressants, selective serotonin re-uptake inhibitors, antipsychotic drugs and carbamazepine as these drugs may increase the risk of water retention and/or electrolyte imbalance.

ADVERSE EFFECTS: Adverse reactions to PICO-SALAX are very rare (<1 in 10 000) and are presented below by System Organ Class and Preferred term.

Immune System Disorders: anaphylactoid reaction, hypersensitivity.

Metabolism and Nutrition Disorders: hyponatraemia.

Nervous System Disorders: epilepsy, grand mal convulsion, convulsions, confusional state, headache.

Gastrointestinal Disorders: vomiting, diarrhoea, abdominal pain, nausea, proctalgia.

Skin and Subcutaneous Tissue Disorders: rash (including erythematous and maculo-papular rash), urticaria, pruritus, purpura.

General Disorders: Drug interaction: Hyponatraemia has been reported with or without associated convulsions. In epileptic patients, there have been isolated reports of seizure/grand mal convulsion without associated hyponatraemia (see Precautions). There have been isolated reports of anaphylactoid reaction (see Contraindications). Isolated cases of mild ulcers in the small bowel have also been reported.

OVERDOSE:

For management of a suspected drug overdose, CPhA recommends that you contact your **regional Poison Control Centre**. See the *CPS* Directory section for a list of Poison Control Centres.

DOSAGE: Two doses are normally taken 6 to 8 hours apart on the day **before** the hospital procedure. Drink plenty of clear fluids during use.

Adults: Mix and dissolve the contents of one sachet in a cup of cold water. Stir for 2-3 minutes and drink the solution. If it becomes hot, wait until it cools before you drink it.

First dose: 1 sachet before 8 am on the day **before** the procedure.

Second dose: 1 sachet between 2 pm and 4 pm on the day **before** the procedure.

Children (1 to 6 years old): ¼ sachet morning, ¼ sachet afternoon.

Children (6 to 12 years old): ½ sachet morning, ½ sachet afternoon.

In order to replace fluid lost from the body, it is important to drink plenty of clear fluids throughout the treatment with PICO-SALAX until the bowel movements have ceased. In general, patients should drink about 250 mL of water or clear fluid **every hour** while they feel the effects of PICO-SALAX.

INFORMATION FOR THE PATIENT: Published in e-CPS, available by subscription at www.e-cps.ca.

SUPPLIED: Each sachet contains: sodium picosulfate 10 mg, magnesium oxide 3.5 g and citric acid 12 g. Nonmedicinal ingredients: orange flavor, potassium bicarbonate and saccharin sodium. Cartons of 1 or 2.

Pilopine HS® ℞

pilocarpine HCl

Topical Miotic

Alcon

SUPPLIED: Each tube of gel contains: pilocarpine HCl 4%. Preserved with benzalkonium chloride 0.008%. Nonmedicinal ingredients: carbomer 940, edetate disodium, hydrochloric acid, purified water and sodium hydroxide. Tubes of 5 g.

Pioglitazone Hydrochloride Tablets ℞

pioglitazone HCl

Antidiabetic Agent—Insulin Resistance Reducing Agent

Accord Healthcare

SUPPLIED: 30 mg: Each white to off-white, round, flat, uncoated tablet with bevelled edges, debossed with 'PIO' on one side and "30" on other side, contains: pioglitazone hydrochloride 30 mg. Nonmedicinal ingredients: carboxymethylcellulose calcium, hydroxypropylcellulose, lactose monohydrate and magnesium stearate. Bottles of 30, 90 and 500. Store at controlled room temperature (15-30°C). Keep container tightly closed and protect from moisture and humidity.

45 mg: Each white to off-white, round, flat, uncoated tablet with bevelled edges, debossed with 'PIO' on one side and "45" on other side, contains: pioglitazone hydrochloride 45 mg. Nonmedicinal ingredients: carboxymethylcellulose calcium, hydroxypropylcellulose, lactose monohydrate and magnesium stearate. Bottles of 30, 90 and 500. Store at controlled room temperature (15-30°C). Keep container tightly closed and protect from moisture and humidity.

Piperacillin for Injection ℞

piperacillin sodium

Antibiotic

Hospira

SUPPLIED: 2 g: Each vial of sterile lyophilized powder contains: piperacillin sodium equivalent to 2 g of piperacillin. Nonmedicinal ingredients: none. Preservative-free. Single use vials, cartons of 10. Store between 15 and 30°C, protected from light. Discard unused portion.

3 g: Each vial of sterile lyophilized powder contains: piperacillin sodium equivalent to 3 g of piperacillin. Nonmedicinal ingredients: none. Preservative-free. Single use vials, cartons of 10. Boxes of 10. Store between 15 and 30°C, protected from light. Discard unused portion.

4 g: Each vial of sterile lyophilized powder contains: piperacillin sodium equivalent to 4 g of piperacillin. Nonmedicinal ingredients: none. Preservative-free. Single use vials, cartons of 4. Boxes of 4. Store between 15 and 30°C, protected from light. Discard unused portion.

Piperacillin Sodium/Tazobactam Sodium Powder for Injection ℞

piperacillin sodium—tazobactam sodium

Antibiotic—Beta-lactamase Inhibitor

Sandoz

SUMMARY PRODUCT INFORMATION:

Route of Administration	Dosage Form/ Strength	Clinically Relevant Nonmedicinal Ingredients
Intravenous Infusion	Powder for Injection Piperacillin 2 g (as piperacillin sodium) and Tazobactam 0.25 g (as tazobactam sodium) per vial Piperacillin 3 g (as piperacillin sodium) and Tazobactam 0.375 g (as tazobactam sodium) per vial Piperacillin 4 g (as piperacillin sodium) and Tazobactam 0.5 g (as tazobactam sodium) per vial Piperacillin 12 g (as piperacillin sodium) and Tazobactam 1.5 g (as tazobactam sodium) per vial	No nonmedicinal ingredients are used in the formulation.

INDICATIONS AND CLINICAL USE: Piperacillin Sodium/Tazobactam Sodium Powder for Injection (sterile piperacillin sodium/tazobactam sodium) is indicated for the treatment of patients with systemic and/or local bacterial infections, caused by piperacillin resistant, piperacillin/tazobactam susceptible, β-lactamase producing strains of the designated microorganisms in the specified conditions listed below:

Intra-Abdominal Infections: Appendicitis (complicated by rupture or abscess) and peritonitis caused by piperacillin resistant, β-lactamase producing strains of *E. coli* or members of the *B. fragilis* group.

Skin and Skin Structure Infections: Uncomplicated and complicated skin and skin structure infections, including cellulitis, cutaneous abscess, acute ischemic/diabetic foot infections caused by piperacillin resistant β-lactamase producing strains of *S. aureus* (not methicillin-resistant strains).

Gynecological Infections: Postpartum endometritis or pelvic inflammatory disease caused by piperacillin resistant, β-lactamase producing strains of *E. coli*.

Community-Acquired Lower Respiratory Tract Infections: Community-acquired pneumonia (moderate severity only) caused by piperacillin resistant, β-lactamase producing strains of *H. influenzae*.

Nosocomial Pneumonia: Nosocomial pneumonia (moderate to severe) caused by piperacillin-resistant, β-lactamase producing strains of *S. aureus* and by piperacillin/tazobactam-susceptible *A. baumannii*, *H. influenzae*, *K. pneumoniae*, and *P. aeruginosa* (Nosocomial pneumonia caused by *P. aeruginosa* should be treated in combination with an aminoglycoside) (see Drug Interactions and Dosage and Administration).

While Piperacillin Sodium/Tazobactam Sodium Powder for Injection is indicated only for the conditions listed above, infections caused by piperacillin susceptible organisms are also amenable to Piperacillin Sodium/Tazobactam Sodium Powder for Injection treatment due to its piperacillin content. The tazobactam component of this combination product does not decrease the activity of the piperacillin component against piperacillin susceptible organisms. Therefore, the treatment of polymicrobial infections caused by piperacillin susceptible organisms and β-lactamase producing organisms susceptible to Piperacillin Sodium/Tazobactam Sodium Powder for Injection should not require the addition of another antibiotic.

Piperacillin Sodium/Tazobactam Sodium Powder for Injection may be useful as presumptive therapy in the indicated conditions prior to identification of causative organisms because of its broad spectrum of bactericidal activity against gram-positive and gram-negative aerobic and anaerobic organisms.

Appropriate cultures should usually be performed before initiating antimicrobial treatment in order to isolate and identify the organisms causing infection and to determine their susceptibility to Piperacillin Sodium/Tazobactam Sodium Powder for Injection. Antimicrobial therapy should be adjusted, if appropriate, once results of culture(s) and antimicrobial susceptibility testing are known.

CONTRAINDICATIONS: The use of Piperacillin Sodium/Tazobactam Sodium Powder for Injection (sterile piperacillin sodium/tazobactam sodium) is contraindicated in:

- patients with a history of allergic reactions to any of the penicillins and/or cephalosporins or β-lactamase inhibitors.

WARNINGS AND PRECAUTIONS: Warnings: Serious and occasionally fatal hypersensitivity (anaphylactic/anaphylactoid [including shock]) reactions have been reported in individuals receiving therapy with penicillins. These reactions are more apt to occur in individuals with a history of sensitivity to multiple allergens. There have been reports of individuals with a history of penicillin hypersensitivity who have experienced severe hypersensitivity reactions when treated with cephalosporins. Before initiating therapy with Piperacillin Sodium/Tazobactam Sodium, careful inquiry should be made concerning previous hypersensitivity reactions to penicillins, cephalosporins, or other allergens. If an allergic reaction occurs during therapy with Piperacillin Sodium/Tazobactam Sodium, the antibiotic should be discontinued and appropriate therapy instituted. Serious anaphylactoid reactions require immediate emergency treatment with epinephrine, oxygen and intravenous steroids and airway management, including intubation, should also be administered as indicated.

C. difficile-associated disease (CDAD) has been reported with use of many antibacterial agents, including piperacillin/tazobactam. CDAD may range in severity from mild diarrhea to fatal colitis. It is important to consider this diagnosis in patients who present with diarrhea, or symptoms of colitis, pseudomembranous colitis, toxic megacolon, or perforation of colon subsequent to the administration of any antibacterial agent. CDAD has been reported to occur over 2 months after the administration of antibacterial agents.

Treatment with antibacterial agents may alter the normal flora of the colon and may permit overgrowth of *C. difficile*. *C. difficile* produces toxins A and B, which contribute to the development of CDAD. CDAD may cause significant morbidity and mortality. CDAD can be refractory to antimicrobial therapy.

If the diagnosis of CDAD is suspected or confirmed, appropriate therapeutic measures should be initiated. Mild cases of CDAD usually respond to discontinuation of antibacterial agents not directed against *C. difficile*. In moderate to severe cases, consideration should be given to management with fluids and electrolytes, protein supplementation, and treatment with an antibacterial agent clinically effective against *C. difficile*. Surgical evaluation should be instituted as clinically indicated, as surgical intervention may be required in certain severe cases (see Adverse Reactions).

Precautions: General: Bleeding manifestations or significant leukopenia following prolonged administration have occurred in some patients receiving β-lactam antibiotics, including piperacillin. These reactions have sometimes been associated with abnormalities of coagulation tests such as clotting time, platelet aggregation and prothrombin time and are more likely to occur in patients with renal failure. If bleeding manifestations occur, the antibiotic should be discontinued and appropriate therapy instituted.

The possibility of the emergence of resistant organisms that might cause superinfections should be kept in mind. If this occurs, appropriate measures should be taken.

As with other penicillins, patients may experience neuromuscular excitability or convulsions if higher than recommended doses are given intravenously (particularly in the presence of renal failure).

Piperacillin Sodium/Tazobactam Sodium Powder for Injection contains a total of 2.35 mEq (54 mg) of sodium (Na^+) per gram of piperacillin in the combination product. This should be considered when treating patients requiring restricted salt intake. Periodic electrolyte determinations should be performed in patients with low potassium reserves, and the possibility of hypokalemia should be kept in mind with patients who have potentially low potassium reserves and who are receiving cytotoxic therapy or diuretics.

Leukopenia and neutropenia may occur, especially during prolonged therapy. Therefore, periodic assessment of hematopoietic function should be performed.

As with other semisynthetic penicillins, piperacillin therapy has been associated with an increased incidence of fever and rash in cystic fibrosis patients.

In patients with creatinine clearance <40 mL/min and dialysis patients [hemodialysis and chronic ambulatory peritoneal dialysis (CAPD)], the intravenous dose should be adjusted to the degree of renal function impairment (see Dosage and Administration).

Because of chemical instability, piperacillin/tazobactam should not be used for intravenous administration with solutions containing **only** sodium bicarbonate (see Dosage and Administration, Incompatibilities).

Piperacillin/tazobactam should not be added to blood products or albumin hydrolysates.

Special Populations: Pregnant Women: Obstetrics and Teratology: Reproduction studies have been performed in rats and have revealed no evidence of impaired fertility due to piperacillin/tazobactam administered up to a dose which is similar to the maximum recommended human daily dose based on body-surface area (mg/m^2). Teratology studies have been performed in mice and rats and have revealed no evidence of harm to the fetus due to piperacillin/tazobactam at doses 1-2 and 2-3 times the human dose of piperacillin and tazobactam, respectively, based on body-surface area (mg/m^2).

Piperacillin: Reproduction and teratology studies have been performed in mice and rats and have revealed no evidence of impaired fertility or harm to the fetus due to piperacillin administered up to a dose which is half (mice) or similar (rats) to the human dose based on body-surface area (mg/m^2).

Tazobactam: Reproduction studies have been performed in rats and have revealed no evidence of impaired fertility due to tazobactam administered up to a dose 3 times the human dose based on body-surface area (mg/m^2). Teratology studies have been performed in mice and rats and have revealed no evidence of harm to the fetus due to tazobactam up to a dose which is 6 (mice) and 14 (rats) times the human dose based on body-surface area (mg/m^2). In rats, tazobactam crosses the placenta. Concentrations in the fetus are less than or equal to 10% of that found in maternal plasma.

There are no adequate and well-controlled studies with the piperacillin/tazobactam combination or with piperacillin or tazobactam alone in pregnant women. Piperacillin and tazobactam cross the placenta. Because animal reproduction studies are not always predictive of human response pregnant women should be treated with piperacillin/tazobactam only if the expected benefit outweighs the possible risks to the pregnant woman and fetus.

Nursing Women: Caution should be exercised when piperacillin/tazobactam is administered to nursing mothers. Piperacillin is excreted in low concentrations in human milk; tazobactam concentrations in milk have not been studied. Women who are breast-feeding should be treated only if the expected benefit outweighs the possible risks to the woman and child.

Pediatrics: Safety and efficacy in children below the age of 12 have not been established.

Geriatrics: Patients over 65 years of age are not at an increased risk of developing adverse effects solely because of age. However, dosage should be adjusted in the presence of renal insufficiency (see Dosage and Administration).

In general, dose selection for an elderly patient should be approached with caution, usually starting at the low end of the dosing range, reflecting the greater frequency of decreased hepatic, renal, or cardiac function, and of concomitant disease or other drug therapy.

Piperacillin Sodium/Tazobactam Sodium Powder for Injection contains 54 mg (2.35 mEq) of sodium per gram of piperacillin in the combination product. At the usual recommended doses, patients would receive between 648 and 864 mg/day (28.2 and 37.6 mEq) of sodium. The geriatric population may respond with a blunted natriuresis to salt loading. This may be clinically important with regard to diseases such as congestive heart failure.

Piperacillin/tazobactam is known to be substantially excreted by the kidney, and the risk of toxic reactions to this drug may be greater in patients with impaired renal function. Elderly patients are more likely to have decreased renal function and therefore care should be taken in dose selection. It may be useful to monitor renal function.

ADVERSE REACTIONS: Clinical Trial Adverse Drug Reactions: During the clinical investigations, 2621 patients worldwide were treated with piperacillin/tazobactam in phase 3 trials.

In the key North American clinical trials (n=830 patients), 90% of the adverse events reported were mild to moderate in severity and transient in nature. However, in 3.2% of the patients treated worldwide, piperacillin/tazobactam was discontinued because of adverse events primarily involving the skin (1.3%), including rash and pruritus; the gastrointestinal system (0.9%), including diarrhea, nausea, and vomiting; and allergic reactions (0.5%).

Adverse local reactions that were reported, irrespective of relationship to therapy with piperacillin/tazobactam, were phlebitis (1.3%), injection site reaction (0.5%), pain (0.2%), inflammation (0.2%), thrombophlebitis (0.2%), and edema (0.1%).

Based on patients from the North American trials (n=1063), the events with the highest incidence in patients, irrespective of relationship to piperacillin/tazobactam therapy, were diarrhea (11.3%); headache (7.7%); constipation (7.7%); nausea (6.9%); insomnia (6.6%); rash (4.2%), including maculopapular, bullous, urticarial, and eczematoid; vomiting (3.3%); dyspepsia (3.3%); pruritus (3.1%); stool changes (2.4%); fever (2.4%); agitation (2.1%); pain (1.7%); moniliasis (1.6%); hypertension (1.6%); dizziness (1.4%); abdominal pain (1.3%); chest pain (1.3%); edema (1.2%); anxiety (1.2%); rhinitis (1.2%); and dyspnea (1.1%).

Additional adverse systemic clinical events reported in 1.0% or less of the patients are listed below within each body system:

Autonomic Nervous System: hypotension, ileus, syncope.

Body as a Whole: rigors, back pain, malaise, candidal superinfection.

Cardiovascular: tachycardia, including supraventricular and ventricular; bradycardia; arrhythmia, including atrial fibrillation, ventricular fibrillation, cardiac arrest, cardiac failure, circulatory failure, myocardial infarction.

Central Nervous System: tremor, convulsions, vertigo.

Gastrointestinal: melena, flatulence, hemorrhage, gastritis, hiccough, ulcerative stomatitis, jaundice.

Pseudomembranous colitis was reported in one patient during the clinical trials. The onset of pseudomembranous colitis symptoms may occur during or over 2 months after the administration of antibacterial treatment (see Warnings).

Hearing: tinnitus.

Hypersensitivity: anaphylaxis (including shock). Incidence of rash and fever is higher in patients with cystic fibrosis.

Metabolic and Nutritional: symptomatic hypoglycemia, thirst.

Musculoskeletal: myalgia, arthralgia.

Platelet, Bleeding, Clotting: mesenteric embolism, purpura, epistaxis, pulmonary embolism (see Precautions, General).

Psychiatric: confusion, hallucination, depression.

Reproductive, Female: leukorrhea, vaginitis.

Respiratory: pharyngitis, pulmonary edema, bronchospasm, coughing.

Skin and Appendages: genital pruritus, diaphoresis, toxic epidermal necrolysis.

Special Senses: taste perversion.

Urinary: retention, dysuria, oliguria, hematuria, incontinence.

Vision: photophobia.

Vascular (extracardiac): flushing.

Nosocomial Pneumonia Trials: In a completed study of nosocomial pneumonia, 222 patients were treated with piperacillin/tazobactam in a dosing regimen of **4.5 g every 6 hours in combination with an aminoglycoside and 215 patients were treated with a comparator in combination with an aminoglycoside**. In this trial, treatment-emergent adverse events were reported by 402 patients, 204 (91.9%) in the piperacillin/tazobactam group and 198 (92.1%) in the comparator group. Twenty-five (25, 11.0%) patients in the piperacillin/tazobactam group and 14 (6.5%) in the comparator group (p >0.05) discontinued treatment due to an adverse event.

In this study of piperacillin/tazobactam in combination with an aminoglycoside, adverse events that occurred in more than 1% of patients and were considered by the investigator to be drug-related were: diarrhea (17.6%), fever (2.7%), vomiting (2.7%), urinary tract infection (2.7%), rash (2.3%), abdominal pain (1.8%), generalized edema (1.8%), moniliasis (1.8%), nausea (1.8%), oral moniliasis (1.8%), BUN increased (1.8%), creatinine increased (1.8%), peripheral edema (1.8%), abdomen enlarged (1.4%), headache (1.4%), constipation (1.4%), liver function tests abnormal (1.4%), thrombocythemia (1.4%), excoriations (1.4%), and sweating (1.4%).

Drug-related adverse events reported in 1% or less of patients in the nosocomial pneumonia study of piperacillin/tazobactam with an aminoglycoside were: acidosis, acute kidney failure, agitation, alkaline phosphatase increased, anemia, asthenia, atrial fibrillation, chest pain, CNS depression, colitis, confusion, convulsion, cough increased, thrombocytopenia, dehydration, depression, diplopia, drug level decreased, dry mouth, dyspepsia, dysphagia, dyspnea, dysuria, eosinophilia, fungal dermatitis, gastritis, glossitis, grand mal convulsion, hematuria, hyperglycemia, hypernatremia, hypertension, hypertonia, hyperventilation, hypochromic anemia, hypoglycemia, hypokalemia, hyponatremia, hypophosphatemia, hypoxia, ileus, injection site edema, injection site pain, injection site reaction, kidney function abnormal, leukocytosis, leukopenia, local reaction to procedure, melena, pain, prothrombin decreased, pruritus, respiratory disorder, AST increased, ALT increased, sinus bradycardia, somnolence, stomatitis, stupor, tremor, tachycardia, ventricular extrasystoles, and ventricular tachycardia.

Post-Market Adverse Drug Reactions: Additional adverse events reported from worldwide marketing experience with piperacillin/tazobactam occurring under circumstances where causal relationship to piperacillin/tazobactam is uncertain:

Gastrointestinal: hepatitis, cholestatic jaundice.

Hematologic: hemolytic anemia, anemia, thrombocytosis, agranulocytosis, pancytopenia.

Immune: hypersensitivity reactions, anaphylactic/anaphylactoid reactions (including shock).

Infections: candidial superinfections.

Renal: interstitial nephritis, renal failure.

Skin and Appendages: erythema multiforme, Stevens-Johnson syndrome, toxic epidermal necrolysis.

Abnormal Hematologic and Clinical Chemistry Findings: Changes in laboratory parameters, without regard to drug relationship, were reported in all studies, including studies of nosocomial pneumonia in which a higher dose of piperacillin/tazobactam was used in combination with an aminoglycoside. The changes in laboratory parameters include:

Hematologic: agranulocytosis, pancytopenia, anemia, decreases in hemoglobin and hematocrit, thrombocytopenia, increases in platelet count, eosinophilia, leukopenia, neutropenia. The leukopenia/neutropenia associated with piperacillin/tazobactam administration appears to be reversible and most frequently associated with prolonged administration, i.e. ≥21 days of therapy. These patients were withdrawn from therapy; some had accompanying systemic symptoms (e.g., fever, rigors, chills).

Coagulation: positive direct Coombs test, prolonged prothrombin time, prolonged partial thromboplastin time, bleeding time prolonged.

Hepatic: transient elevations of AST, ALT, alkaline phosphatase, bilirubin, gamma-glutamyltransferase increased.

Renal: increases in serum creatinine, blood urea nitrogen, renal failure.

Urinalysis: proteinuria, hematuria, pyuria.

Additional laboratory events include abnormalities in electrolytes (i.e., increases and decreases in sodium, potassium, and calcium), hyperglycemia, decreases in total protein or albumin. In individuals with liver disease or those receiving cytotoxic therapy or diuretics, piperacillin/tazobactam has been reported rarely to produce a decrease in serum potassium levels at high doses of piperacillin.

The following adverse reactions have also been reported for sterile piperacillin sodium:

Skin and Appendages: erythema multiforme and Stevens-Johnson syndrome, rarely reported.

Gastrointestinal: cholestatic hepatitis.

Renal: rarely, interstitial nephritis.

Skeletal: Prolonged muscle relaxation (see Drug Interactions).

DRUG INTERACTIONS: Drug-Drug Interactions: Aminoglycosides: The mixing of beta-lactam antibiotics with aminoglycosides in vitro can result in substantial inactivation of the aminoglycoside. However, amikacin and gentamicin were determined to be compatible in vitro with Piperacillin Sodium/Tazobactam Sodium Powder for Injection in certain diluents at specific concentrations for a simultaneous Y-site infusion (see Dosage and Administration).

The inactivation of aminoglycosides in the presence of penicillin-class drugs has been recognized. It has been postulated that penicillin-aminoglycoside complexes form; these complexes are microbiologically inactive and of unknown toxicity. Sequential administration of piperacillin/tazobactam with tobramycin to patients with normal renal function and mild to moderate renal impairment has been shown to modestly decrease serum concentrations of tobramycin but does not significantly affect tobramycin pharmacokinetics. When aminoglycosides are administered in combination with piperacillin to patients with end-stage renal disease requiring hemodialysis, the concentrations of the aminoglycosides (especially tobramycin) may be significantly altered and should be monitored. Since aminoglycosides are not equally susceptible to inactivation by piperacillin, consideration should be given to the choice of the aminoglycoside when administered in combination with piperacillin to these patients.

Probenecid: Concomitant administration of piperacillin/tazobactam and probenecid results in prolonged half-life of piperacillin (21%), and tazobactam (71%) and lower renal clearance for both piperacillin and tazobactam; however, peak plasma concentrations of either drug are unaffected.

Vancomycin: No pharmacokinetic interactions are found between piperacillin/tazobactam and vancomycin.

Heparin: Coagulation parameters should be tested more frequently and monitored regularly, during simultaneous administration of high doses of heparin, oral anticoagulants and other drugs that may affect the blood coagulation system and/or the thrombocyte function.

Vecuronium: Piperacillin used concomitantly with vecuronium has been implicated in the prolongation of the neuromuscular blockade of vecuronium. Piperacillin/tazobactam could produce the same phenomenon if given along with vecuronium. Due to their similar mechanism of action, it is expected that the neuromuscular blockade produced by any of the non-depolarizing muscle relaxants could be prolonged in the presence of piperacillin (see package insert for vecuronium bromide).

Methotrexate: Piperacillin may reduce the excretion of methotrexate; therefore, serum levels of methotrexate should be monitored in patients to avoid drug toxicity.

Where piperacillin/tazobactam is administered concurrently with another antibiotic the drugs should **not** be mixed in the same solution but must be administered separately.

Drug-Laboratory Test Interactions: As with other penicillins, the administration of piperacillin/tazobactam may result in a false-positive reaction for glucose in the urine using a copper-reduction method (CLINITEST). It is recommended that glucose tests based on enzymatic glucose oxidase reactions (such as DIASTIX or TES-TAPE) be used.

There have been reports of positive test results using the Bio-Rad Laboratories Platelia Aspergillus EIA test in patients receiving piperacillin/tazobactam injection who were subsequently found to be free of Aspergillus infection. Cross-reactions with non-Aspergillus polysaccharides and polyfuranoses with Bio-Rad Laboratories Platelia Aspergillus EIA test have been reported. Therefore, positive test results in patients receiving piperacillin/tazobactam should be interpreted cautiously and confirmed by other diagnostic methods.

DOSAGE AND ADMINISTRATION: Dosage: The usual total daily dose of Piperacillin Sodium/Tazobactam Sodium Powder for Injection for adults is 12 g/1.5 g, given as 3 g/0.375 g every six hours.

Clinical trial data in the treatment of intra-abdominal infections support the efficacy of 4 g/0.5 g given every eight hours.

Initial presumptive treatment of patients with nosocomial pneumonia should start with Piperacillin Sodium/Tazobactam Sodium Powder for Injection at a dosage of 4.5 g every six hours plus an aminoglycoside, totalling 18.0 g (16.0 g piperacillin sodium/2.0 g tazobactam sodium). Treatment with the aminoglycoside should be continued in patients from whom *P. aeruginosa* is isolated. If *P. aeruginosa* is not isolated, the aminoglycoside may be discontinued at the discretion of the treating physician.

Due to the in vitro inactivation of the aminoglycoside by beta-lactam antibiotics, Piperacillin Sodium/Tazobactam Sodium Powder for Injection and the aminoglycoside should be reconstituted and diluted separately when concomitant therapy with aminoglycosides is indicated (see Drug Interactions).

When concomitant therapy with an aminoglycoside is indicated, Piperacillin Sodium/Tazobactam Sodium Powder for Injection and the aminoglycoside should be administered separately.

In certain circumstances where co-administration is preferred, compatibility for simultaneous co-administration via Y-site infusion has been established for Piperacillin Sodium/Tazobactam Sodium Powder for Injection supplied in vials with the following aminoglycosides under the following conditions:

The following compatibility information only applies to Piperacillin Sodium/Tazobactam Sodium Powder for Injection.

Table 1: Piperacillin/Tazobactam for Injection

Compatibility Information

Aminoglycoside	Piperacillin/ Tazobactam (grams) dose	Piperacillin/ Tazobactam Diluent Volume (mL)	Aminoglycoside Concentration Range[a] (mg/mL)	Acceptable Diluents
Amikacin	2.25, 3.375, 4.5	50, 100, 150	1.75–7.5	0.9% sodium chloride or 5% dextrose

(cont'd)

Table 1: Piperacillin/Tazobactam for Injection *(cont'd)*
Compatibility Information

Aminoglycoside	Piperacillin/ Tazobactam (grams) dose	Piperacillin/ Tazobactam Diluent Volume (mL)	Aminoglycoside Concentration Range[a] (mg/mL)	Acceptable Diluents
Gentamicin	2.25, 3.375, 4.5	100, 150	0.7–3.32	0.9% sodium chloride

[a] The dose of aminoglycoside should be based on patient weight, status of infection (serious or life threatening) and renal function (creatinine clearance).

Piperacillin/tazobactam is not compatible with tobramycin for simultaneous coadministration via Y-site infusion. Compatibility of piperacillin/tazobactam with other aminoglycosides has not been established. Only the concentration and diluents of amikacin or gentamicin with the dosages of Piperacillin Sodium/Tazobactam Sodium Powder for Injection listed in Table 1 have been established as compatible for co-administration via Y-site infusion. Simultaneous administration via Y-site infusion in any manner other than listed above may result in inactivation of the aminoglycoside by piperacillin/tazobactam.

Renal Insufficiency: In patients with renal insufficiency, the intravenous dose should be adjusted to the degree of actual renal function impairment. In patients with nosocomial pneumonia receiving concomitant aminoglycoside therapy, the aminoglycoside dosage should be adjusted according to the recommendations of the aminoglycoside used. The recommended daily doses of Piperacillin Sodium/Tazobactam Sodium Powder for Injection for patients with renal insufficiency are as follows: See Table 2.

Table 2: Piperacillin/Tazobactam for Injection
Recommended Dosing of Piperacillin Sodium/Tazobactam Sodium Powder for Injection in Patients with Normal Renal Function and Renal Insufficiency (As total grams piperacillin/tazobactam)

Renal Function (Creatinine Clearance, mL/min)	All Indications (except Nosocomial Pneumonia)	Nosocomial Pneumonia
>40 mL/min	3.375 q6h	4.5 q6h
20–40 mL/min[a]	2.25 q6h	3.375 q6h
<20 mL/min[a]	2.25 q8h	2.25 q6h
Hemodialysis[b]	2.25 q12h	2.25 q8h
CAPD	2.25 q12h	2.25 q8h

[a] Creatinine clearance for patients not receiving hemodialysis.
[b] 0.75 g should be administered following each hemodialysis session on hemodialysis days.

For patients on hemodialysis, the maximum dose is 2.25 g piperacillin/tazobactam given every twelve hours for all indications other than nosocomial pneumonia and 2.25 g every eight hours for nosocomial pneumonia. In addition, because hemodialysis removes 30% to 40% of piperacillin/tazobactam dose in four hours, one additional dose of 0.75 g piperacillin/tazobactam should be administered following each dialysis period. For patients with renal failure, measurement of serum levels of piperacillin/tazobactam will provide additional guidance for adjusting dosage.

Dosage adjustment is based on pharmacokinetic data. Clinical studies with piperacillin/tazobactam have not been performed in patients with impaired renal function.

Duration of Therapy: The usual duration of Piperacillin Sodium/Tazobactam Sodium Powder for Injection treatment is from seven to ten days. However, the recommended duration of Piperacillin Sodium/Tazobactam Sodium Powder for Injection treatment of nosocomial pneumonia is 7 to 14 days. In all conditions, the duration should be guided by the severity of the infection and the patient's clinical and bacteriological progress.

Administration: Piperacillin Sodium/Tazobactam Sodium Powder for Injection should be administered by intravenous infusion over 30 minutes.

Reconstitution for Single Dose Vial: Reconstitute Piperacillin Sodium/Tazobactam Sodium Powder for Injection with at least 5 mL of a suitable diluent per gram of piperacillin from the list of diluents provided below. Swirl until dissolved. It should be further diluted to the desired final volume with an acceptable diluent.

Table 3: Piperacillin/Tazobactam for Injection
Reconstitution for Single Dose Vial

Vial Size (piperacillin/tazobactam)	Volume of Diluent to be Added to Vial	Approximate Available Volume	Nominal Concentration per mL
2.25 g (2 g/0.25 g)	10 mL	11.60 mL	0.194 g/mL (0.172 g/mL/0.022 g/mL)
3.375 g (3 g/0.375 g)	15 mL	17.36 mL	0.194 g/mL (0.172 g/mL/0.022 g/mL)
4.50 g (4 g/0.50 g)	20 mL	23.15 mL	0.194 g/mL (0. 172 g/mL/0.022 g/mL)

Table 4: Piperacillin/Tazobactam for Injection
Reconstitution

Reconstitute Piperacillin Sodium /Tazobactam Sodium Powder for Injection per gram of piperacillin with 5 mL of a **Compatible Reconstitution Diluent** (listed below)	**Further dilute** the reconstituted Piperacillin Sodium/Tazobactam Sodium Powder for Injection with 50 mL to 150 mL of a **Compatible Intravenous Solution** (listed below)
0.9% Sodium Chloride Injection Sterile Water for Injection 5% Dextrose Injection	0.9% Sodium Chloride Injection Sterile Water for Injection[a] 6% Dextran in Saline 5% Dextrose Injection Lactated Ringer's Injection
Bacteriostatic Water/Parabens Bacteriostatic Saline/Benzyl Alcohol Bacteriostatic Water/Benzyl Alcohol	0.9% Sodium Chloride Injection

[a] Maximum recommended volume per dose of Sterile Water for Injection is 50 mL.
Lactated Ringer's Injection is compatible with Piperacillin Sodium/Tazobactam Sodium Powder for Injection.

Reconstitution for Pharmacy Bulk Vial: Reconstitute the pharmacy bulk vial with exactly 51 mL of a compatible reconstitution diluent, listed in Table 5, to a concentration of 200 mg/mL of piperacillin and 25 mg/mL of tazobactam. Swirl well until dissolved. It should be further diluted to the desired final volume with an acceptable diluent.

Table 5: Piperacillin/Tazobactam for Injection
Reconstitution for Pharmacy Bulk Vial

Reconstitute Piperacillin Sodium/Tazobactam Sodium Powder for Injection per pharmacy bulk vial with 51 mL of a **Compatible Reconstitution Diluent** (listed below)	**Further dilute** the reconstituted Piperacillin Sodium/Tazobactam Sodium Powder for Injection with 50 mL to 150 mL of a **Compatible Intravenous Solution** (listed below)
Sodium Chloride for Injection 0.9% Sterile Water for Injection Dextrose Injection 5%	Sodium Chloride for Injection 0.9% Sterile Water for Injection[a] Dextran in Saline 6% Dextrose Injection 5% Lactated Ringer's Injection
Bacteriostatic Water/Parabens Bacteriostatic Saline/Benzyl Alcohol Bacteriostatic Water/Benzyl Alcohol	Sodium Chloride for Injection 0.9%

[a] Maximum recommended volume per dose of Sterile Water for Injection is 50 mL.
Lactated Ringer's Injection is compatible with Piperacillin Sodium/Tazobactam Sodium Powder for Injection.

Intermittent Intravenous Infusion: Reconstitute as previously described, with 5 mL of an acceptable diluent per 1 gram of piperacillin and then further dilute in the desired volume (at least 50 mL). This diluted solution must be used immediately. Administer by infusion over a period of at least 30 minutes. During the infusion it is desirable to discontinue the primary infusion solution.

Stability of Piperacillin Sodium/Tazobactam Sodium Powder for Injection Following Reconstitution: Piperacillin Sodium/Tazobactam Sodium Powder for Injection is stable in glass and plastic containers (plastic syringes, IV bags and tubing) when reconstituted with acceptable diluents.

Stability studies of Piperacillin Sodium/Tazobactam Sodium Powder for Injection in glass vials have demonstrated chemical stability [potency, pH of reconstituted solution, appearance, and clarity of solution] for up to 24 hours at room temperature (between 20 and 25°C) and up to 48 hours at refrigerated temperatures (between 2 and 8°C). Discard unused portions after storage for 24 hours at room temperature or 48 hours when refrigerated.

Stability studies of Piperacillin Sodium/Tazobactam Sodium Powder for Injection in glass vials have demonstrated chemical stability with Lactated Ringer's Injection [potency, pH of reconstituted solution, appearance, and clarity of solution] for up to 24 hours at room temperature (between 20 and 25°C) and up to 72 hours at refrigerated temperatures (between 2 and 8°C). Discard unused portions.

Due to microbial considerations, intravenous admixtures are usually recommended for use within a maximum of 24 hours at room temperature or 72 hours when refrigerated (2-8°C).

Stability studies of Piperacillin Sodium/Tazobactam Sodium Powder for Injection in PVC IV bags have demonstrated chemical stability (potency, appearance, and clarity of solution) for up to 24 hours at room temperature and up to 72 hours at refrigerated temperature. Piperacillin Sodium/Tazobactam Sodium Powder for Injection contains no preservatives. Appropriate consideration of aseptic technique should be used.

Directions for Dispensing From Pharmacy Bulk Vial: The use of pharmacy bulk vial is restricted to hospitals with a recognized intravenous admixture program. The pharmacy bulk vial is intended for single puncture, multiple dispensing.

As with all parenteral drug products, intravenous admixtures should be inspected visually for clarity, particulate matter, precipitate, discoloration and leakage prior to administration, whenever solution and container permit. Solutions showing haziness, particulate matter, precipitate, discoloration or leakage should not be used. Discard unused portion.

Incompatibilities: Not to be added to blood products or albumin hydrolysates.

Because of chemical instability, Piperacillin Sodium/Tazobactam Sodium Powder for Injection should not be used for intravenous administration with solutions containing sodium bicarbonate alone. It may be used with intravenous admixtures containing other ingredients as well as sodium bicarbonate for up to 24 hours at room temperature and 48 hours refrigerated.

Solutions containing Piperacillin Sodium/Tazobactam Sodium Powder for Injection and protein hydrolysates or amino acids should be used within 12 hours if stored at room temperature and 24 hours if refrigerated.

Piperacillin Sodium/Tazobactam Sodium Powder for Injection should not be mixed with other drugs in a syringe or infusion bottle since compatibility has not been established.

OVERDOSAGE:

Symptoms: There have been post-marketing reports of overdose with piperacillin/tazobactam. The majority of those events experienced including nausea, vomiting, and diarrhea have also been reported with the usual recommended dosages. Patients may experience neuromuscular excitability or convulsions if higher than recommended doses are given intravenously (particularly in the presence of renal failure).

Treatment: Treatment should be supportive and symptomatic according to the patient's clinical presentation.

Excessive serum levels of either tazobactam or piperacillin may be reduced by hemodialysis, although no specific antidote is known. As with other penicillins, neuromuscular excitability or convulsions have occurred following large intravenous doses, primarily in patients with impaired renal function.

In the case of motor excitability or convulsions, general supportive measures, including administration of anticonvulsive agents (e.g. diazepam or barbiturates) may be considered.

For management of a suspected drug overdose, CPhA recommends that you contact your **regional Poison Control Centre**. See the *CPS* Directory section for a list of Poison Control Centres.

ACTION AND CLINICAL PHARMACOLOGY: Piperacillin Sodium/Tazobactam Sodium Powder for Injection (sterile piperacillin sodium/tazobactam sodium) is an injectable antibacterial combination consisting of the semisynthetic antibiotic piperacillin sodium and the β-lactamase inhibitor tazobactam sodium for intravenous administration.

Mechanism of Action: Piperacillin sodium exerts bactericidal activity by inhibiting septum formation and cell wall synthesis. In vitro, piperacillin is active against a variety of gram-positive and gram-negative aerobic and anaerobic bacteria. Tazobactam sodium is a β-lactamase inhibitor. Tazobactam, in combination with piperacillin enhances and extends the antibiotic spectrum of piperacillin to include β-lactamase producing bacteria normally resistant to piperacillin.

Piperacillin is metabolized to a minor microbiologically active desethyl metabolite. Tazobactam is metabolized to a single metabolite which lacks pharmacological and antibacterial activities.

Both tazobactam and piperacillin are eliminated by the kidney via glomerular filtration and tubular secretion. Tazobactam and its metabolite are eliminated primarily by renal excretion with 80% of the dose as unchanged drug and the remainder as the single metabolite. Piperacillin is excreted rapidly as unchanged drug, with 68% of the dose in the urine. Piperacillin, tazobactam and desethyl piperacillin are also secreted into the bile.

Tazobactam and piperacillin are widely distributed into tissues and body fluids including, but not limited to, intestinal mucosa, gallbladder, lung, female reproductive tissues (uterus, ovary and fallopian tube), interstitial fluid and bile. Mean tissue concentrations were generally 50-100% of those in plasma. Distribution of tazobactam and piperacillin into cerebrospinal fluid is low in subjects with non-inflamed meninges, as with other penicillins.

In subjects with renal impairment, the half-lives of tazobactam and piperacillin, after single doses, increase with decreasing creatinine clearance. At creatinine clearance below 20 mL/min., the increase in half-life is four-fold for tazobactam and two-fold for piperacillin compared to subjects with normal renal function. Dosage adjustments for Piperacillin Sodium/Tazobactam Sodium Powder for Injection are recommended when creatinine clearance is below 40 mL/min in patients receiving the recommended daily dose of Piperacillin Sodium/Tazobactam Sodium Powder for Injection (see Dosage and Administration).

Hemodialysis removes 30-40% of a piperacillin/ tazobactam dose with an additional 5% of the tazobactam dose removed as the tazobactam metabolite. Peritoneal dialysis removes approximately 21% and 6% of the tazobactam and piperacillin doses, respectively, with up to 16% of the tazobactam dose removed as the tazobactam metabolite. For dosage recommendations for patients undergoing hemodialysis, see Dosage and Administration.

Tazobactam and piperacillin half-lives increase by approximately 18% and 25% respectively, in patients with hepatic cirrhosis compared to healthy subjects. However, dosage adjustment of Piperacillin Sodium/Tazobactam Sodium Powder for Injection due to hepatic cirrhosis is not necessary.

STORAGE AND STABILITY: Piperacillin Sodium/Tazobactam Sodium Powder for Injection vials should be stored between 15 and 30°C.

For single dose vial and pharmacy bulk vial, discard unused portions.

DOSAGE FORMS, COMPOSITION AND PACKAGING: 2.25 g: Each vial of white to off-white sterile, cryodesiccated powder contains: tazobactam sodium equivalent to 0.25 g of tazobactam and piperacillin sodium equivalent to 2 g of piperacillin. Sodium: 4.69 mEq (108 mg). Glass vials with rubber stoppers and flip-top bordered caps of 30 mL, boxes of 10.

3.375 g: Each vial of white to off-white sterile, cryodesiccated powder contains: tazobactam sodium equivalent to 0.375 g of tazobactam and piperacillin sodium equivalent to 3 g of piperacillin. Sodium: 7.03 mEq (162 mg). Glass vials with rubber stoppers and flip-top bordered caps of 30 mL, boxes of 10.

4.5 g: Each vial of white to off-white sterile, cryodesiccated powder contains: tazobactam sodium equivalent to 0.5 g of tazobactam and piperacillin sodium equivalent to 4 g of piperacillin. Sodium: 9.37 mEq (216 mg). Glass vials with rubber stoppers and flip-top bordered caps of 50 mL, boxes of 10.

13.5 g: Each pharmacy bulk vial of white to off-white sterile, cryodesiccated powder contains: tazobactam sodium equivalent to 1.5 g of tazobactam and piperacillin sodium equivalent to 12 g of piperacillin. Sodium: 28.17 mEq (648 mg). Glass vials with rubber stoppers and flip-top bordered caps of 100 mL, boxes of 1.

Piportil® L4 Ⓟ

pipotiazine palmitate

Antipsychotic

sanofi-aventis

Date of Revision: March 5, 2010

PHARMACOLOGY: Piportil L4 (pipotiazine palmitate) is the palmitic ester of pipotiazine, a piperidine phenothiazine with antipsychotic properties and weak sedative activity. The esterification of pipotiazine is responsible for its prolonged duration of action. The onset of action appears usually within the first 2 to 3 days after injection and the effects of the drug on psychotic symptoms are significant within 1 week. Improvement in symptomatology lasts from 3 to 6 weeks, but adequate control may frequently be maintained with one injection every 4 weeks. However, in view of the variations in individual response, careful supervision is required throughout treatment.

Piportil L4 has actions similar to those of other phenothiazines. Among the different phenothiazine derivatives, Piportil L4 appears to be less sedating and to have a weak propensity for causing hypotension or potentiating the effects of CNS depressants and anesthetics. However, it produces a high incidence of extrapyramidal reactions.

INDICATIONS: Piportil L4 (pipotiazine palmitate) is indicated in the maintenance treatment of chronic non-agitated schizophrenic patients.

CONTRAINDICATIONS: Piportil L4 (pipotiazine palmitate) should not be administered in the presence of circulatory collapse, altered states of consciousness or comatose states, particularly when these are due to intoxication with central depressant drugs, e.g., alcohol, hypnotics, narcotics. In severely depressed patients, in the presence of blood dyscrasias, liver disease, renal insufficiency, pheochromocytoma, or in patients with severe cardiovascular disorders or a history of hypersensitivity to phenothiazine derivatives.

Pipotiazine palmitate is not indicated for the management of psychoneurotic patients or geriatric patients with confusion and/or agitation.

As with other phenothiazines, pipotiazine is contraindicated in patients with suspected or established subcortical brain damage, with or without hypothalamic damage, since a hyperthermic reaction with temperatures above 40°C may occur, sometimes not until 14 to 16 hours after drug administration.

Phenothiazine compounds should not be used in patients receiving large doses of hypnotics, due to the possibility of potentiation.

Children: The safety and efficacy of pipotiazine palmitate in children have not been established. Therefore, Piportil L4 is not indicated for use in children.

WARNINGS: Elderly Patients with Dementia: Analyses of thirteen placebo-controlled trials with various atypical antipsychotics (modal duration of 10 weeks) in elderly patients with dementia showed a mean 1.6 fold increase in the death rate in the drug-treated patients. Although the causes of death were varied, most of the deaths appeared to be either cardiovascular (e.g., heart failure, sudden death) or infectious (e.g., pneumonia) in nature. Observational studies suggest that, similar to atypical antipsychotic drugs, treatment with conventional antipsychotic drugs may increase mortality. The extent to which the findings of increased mortality in observational studies may be attributed to the antipsychotic drug as opposed to some characteristic(s) of the patients is not clear. Piportil L4 is not indicated for the treatment of patients with dementia (see Precautions, Mortality in Geriatric Patients with Dementia-Related Psychosis).

Severe adverse reactions requiring immediate medical attention may occur and are difficult to predict. Therefore, Piportil L4 (pipotiazine palmitate) should be administered under the supervision of physicians experienced in the use of psychotropic drugs and facilities should be readily available to cope with any emergency situation.

Occupational Hazards: The use of this drug may impair the mental and physical abilities required for the performance of potentially hazardous tasks, such as driving a car or operating machinery.

Potentiation of the effects of alcohol may also occur.

As with other neuroleptics, very rare cases of QT interval prolongation have been reported with Piportil L4. Neuroleptic phenothiazines may potentiate QT interval prolongation, which increases the risk of onset of serious ventricular arrhythmias of the torsade de pointes type, which is potentially fatal (sudden death). QT prolongation is exacerbated, in particular, in the presence of bradycardia, hypokalemia, and congenital or acquired (i.e., drug induced) QT prolongation. If the clinical situation permits, medical and laboratory evaluations should be performed to rule out possible risk factors before initiating treatment with a neuroleptic agent and as deemed necessary during treatment (see also Precautions and Adverse Effects).

Tardive Dyskinesia: As with all antipsychotic agents, tardive dyskinesia may appear in some patients on long-term therapy or after drug discontinuation. The syndrome is mainly characterized by rhythmical involuntary movements of the tongue, face, mouth or jaw. The manifestations may be permanent in some patients. The syndrome may be masked when treatment is reinstituted, when the dosage is increased or when a switch is made to a different antipsychotic drug. Piportil L4 should be prescribed in a manner that is most likely to minimize the risk of tardive dyskinesia. The lowest effective dose and the shortest duration of treatment should be used, and treatment should be discontinued at the earliest opportunity, or if a satisfactory response cannot be obtained. If the signs and symptoms of tardive dyskinesia appear during treatment, discontinuation of Piportil L4 should be considered.

Neuroleptic Malignant Syndrome (NMS): NMS may occur in patients receiving antipsychotic drugs. NMS is characterized by hyperthermia, muscle rigidity, altered conciousness and signs of autonomic instability including irregular blood pressure, tachycardia, cardiac arrhythmias and diaphoresis. Additional signs may include elevated serum creatine kinase, myoglobinuria (rhabdomyolysis), acute renal failure and leukocytosis. Hyperthermia is often an early sign of this syndrome. Antipsychotic treatment should be withdrawn immediately and appropriate supportive therapy and careful monitoring instituted.

As with other psychotropic drugs, rare cases of priapism have been reported. This reaction did not appear to be dose-dependent and did not correlate with the duration of treatment. The most likely mechanism of action of priapism is a relative decrease in sympathetic tone.

Elderly patients with dementia treated with certain atypical antipsychotic drugs are at an increased risk of Cerebrovascular Adverse Events (CVAEs) such as stroke and transient ischemic attacks, as well as death, compared to placebo. The mechanism of this increased risk is not known. As an increase in the risk with other antipsychotic drugs cannot be excluded, Piportil L4 should be used with caution in the elderly with dementia.

Cases of venous thromboembolism, sometimes fatal, have been reported with antipsychotic drugs. Therefore Piportil L4 should be used with caution in patients with risk factors for thromboembolism (see also Adverse Effects).

Pregnancy: Since the safety of Piportil L4 during pregnancy has not been established, the drug should not be used in women of childbearing potential unless, in the opinion of the physician, the expected benefit to the patient outweighs the possible risk to the fetus.

PRECAUTIONS: Phenothiazines, particularly those that are long acting, should be used with caution in patients with a history of convulsive disorders; treatment should not be initiated unless such patients are receiving appropriate anticonvulsive medication.

The increased incidence of seizures, which occasionally occur in epileptics started on antipsychotic medication, may be controlled by increasing the dosage of their anticonvulsant. Patients with a familial history of seizures or febrile convulsions are more likely to develop seizures than those who have no such history.

Hypotensive phenomena may develop in phenothiazine treated patients who are undergoing surgery. Careful observation is necessary and dosages of anesthetics or CNS depressants may have to be reduced. Antipsychotic agents should be temporarily discontinued in patients receiving spinal or epidural anesthesia, if possible, to allow time for the residual drug to be metabolized.

Particularly during the first 2 or 3 months of therapy, it is advisable to perform periodic liver function tests and blood counts as cholestatic jaundice and blood dyscrasias may occur, necessitating discontinuation of treatment. During long-term therapy renal function should be monitored and, if BUN becomes abnormal, treatment should be discontinued.

The effects of anticholinergic drugs may be potentiated by pipotiazine. Paralytic ileus, even resulting in death, may occur, especially in the elderly. Caution should be observed if constipation develops.

Retinal changes, lenticular and corneal deposits and abnormal skin pigmentation have been observed with other phenothiazines and may occur after prolonged therapy. The possibility of persistent tardive dyskinesia should also be borne in mind where patients are under long-term treatment.

Patients receiving pipotiazine should be cautioned against exposure to extreme heat or organophosporus insecticides.

False positive or negative pregnancy tests have occurred in patients receiving phenothiazine therapy.

Hypotension and ECG changes, particularly nonspecific and usually reversible Q and T wave distortions, have been associated with the administration of phenothiazines. Therefore, pipotiazine palmitate should be used with caution in patients with compensated cardiovascular and cerebrovascular disorders.

Neuroleptic phenothiazines may potentiate QT interval prolongation. QT prolongation is exacerbated, in particular, in the presence of bradycardia, hypokalemia, and congenital or acquired (i.e., drug induced) QT prolongation (see Warnings and Adverse Effects).

The antiemetic effects of most phenothiazines can obscure toxic signs due to overdosage of other drugs or they may mask the symptoms of diseases such as brain tumors or intestinal obstruction.

Unexpected, sudden deaths have occurred in hospitalized patients treated with phenothiazines. Previous brain damage or seizures may predispose. High doses should be avoided in known seizure patients. Sudden exacerbations of psychotic behavior patterns occurred in several patients shortly before death. Acute fulminating pneumonia or pneumonitis and aspiration of gastric contents also were observed. Therefore, the physician also should keep in mind the possible development of "silent pneumonias".

Neuroleptic drugs elevate prolactin levels; the elevation persists during chronic administration. Tissue culture experiments indicate that approximately one third of human breast cancers are prolactin-dependent in vitro, a factor of potential importance if the prescription of these drugs is contemplated in a patient with a previously detected breast cancer. Although disturbances such as galactorrhea, amenorrhea, gynecomastia and impotence have been reported, the clinical significance of elevated serum prolactin levels is unknown for most patients. An increase in mammary neoplasms has been found in rodents after chronic administration of neuroleptic drugs. Neither clinical studies, nor epidemiologic studies conducted to date, however, have shown an association between chronic administration of these drugs and mammary tumorogenesis; the available evidence is considered too limited to be conclusive at this time.

Withdrawal Emergent Neurological Signs: Abrupt withdrawal after short-term administration of antipsychotic drugs does not generally pose problems. However, transient dyskinetic signs are experienced by some patients on maintenance therapy after abrupt withdrawal. The signs are very similar to those described under Tardive Dyskinesia, except for duration. Although it is not known whether gradual withdrawal of antipsychotic drugs will decrease the incidence of withdrawal emergent neurological signs, gradual withdrawal would appear to be advisable.

Geriatrics: The incidence of adverse reactions may be greater in patients over 55 years of age, since the half-lives of antipsychotic drugs are often prolonged. To minimize this possibility, the maintenance dosage should be reduced to the lowest effective level as soon as possible after initial titration and periodically reviewed.

Since psychiatric syndromes in the elderly can be caused by drugs or organic disease, withdrawal of the precipitating drug or treatment of the medical condition should supersede initiation of antipsychotic medication. These agents should not be used for non-psychiatric conditions for which other drugs are available, since the elderly are especially prone to develop adverse effects from antipsychotic drugs.

Mortality in Geriatric Patients with Dementia-Related Psychosis: In elderly patients with dementia-related psychosis, the efficacy and safety of Piportil L4 has not been studied. Observational studies suggest that elderly patients with dementia-related psychosis treated with antipsychotic drugs are at an increased risk of death. Piportil L4 is not indicated for the treatment of patients with dementia-related psychosis.

Cerebrovascular Adverse Events (CVAEs) Including Stroke in Elderly Patients with Dementia: An increased risk of cerebrovascular adverse events has been seen in the dementia population in clinical trials with some atypical antipsychotics. The mechanism for this increased risk is not known. There is insufficient data to know if there is an increased risk of cerebrovascular events associated with Piportil L4. An increased risk however cannot be excluded. Piportil L4 is not indicated in elderly patients with dementia.

Vascular Disease: Piportil L4 should be used with caution in patients with risk factors for stroke or with a history of stroke.

Hyperglycaemia or intolerance to glucose has been reported in patients treated with Piportil L4. Patients with an established diagnosis of diabetes mellitus or with risk factors for the development of diabetes who are started on Piportil L4, should get appropriate glycaemic monitoring during treatment (see Adverse Effects).

ADVERSE EFFECTS: Neurological: The side effects most frequently reported are extrapyramidal reactions including tremor, rigidity, akathisia, dystonia, dyskinesia, oculogyric crises, opisthotonos, hyperreflexia and sialorrhea which tend to occur in the first few days after an injection of Piportil L4 (pipotiazine palmitate). Piportil L4 tends to produce a higher incidence of extrapyramidal reactions than some other phenothiazine derivatives. Extrapyramidal reactions may be alarming, and the patient should be forewarned and reassured. These reactions may tend to subside as treatment is continued but are often dose-related and may respond to a reduction of the dose. Anti-parkinsonian medication may be required to control serious reactions or, if intractable, the drug may have to be withdrawn. The information available tends to indicate that persistent tardive dyskinesia results from heavy drug overloading of the extrapyramidal system. Therefore, caution should be exercised to avoid overdosing of Piportil L4 and the optimum dosage should not be exceeded since this will tend to elicit marked extrapyramidal reactions.

Persistent Tardive Dyskinesia: As with other antipsychotic agents, tardive dyskinesia may occur in patients on long-term therapy or may be observed after drug therapy has been discontinued. The risk seems to be greater in elderly patients on high doses, especially females. The symptoms are persistent and in some patients appear to be irreversible. The syndrome is characterized by rhythmical involuntary movements of the tongue, face, mouth or jaw, e.g., protrusion of tongue, puffing of cheeks, puckering of mouth, chewing movements. Sometimes, these may be accompanied by involuntary movements of the extremities.

There is no known effective treatment for tardive dyskinesia; antiparkinsonian agents usually do not alleviate the symptoms of this syndrome. It is suggested that all antipsychotic agents be discontinued if these symptoms appear. Should it be necessary to reinstitute treatment, or increase the dosage of the agent, or switch to a different antipsychotic agent, the syndrome may be masked. It has been reported that fine vermicular movements of the tongue may be an early sign of the syndrome and if the medication is stopped at that time, the syndrome may not develop. The physician may be able to reduce the risk of this syndrome by minimizing the unnecessary use of neuroleptic drugs and reducing the dose or discontinuing the drug, if possible, when manifestations of this syndrome are recognized, particularly in patients over the age of 50.

Behavioral: Sleep disturbances, drowsiness, fatigue, insomnia, and depression have been reported and may, in severe cases, necessitate reduction in dosage. As with other phenothiazine derivatives, reactivation or aggravation of psychotic processes may be encountered.

Paradoxical effects such as agitation, anxiety, restlessness, excitement and bizarre dreams, have been observed in some patients.

Autonomic Nervous System: Dry mouth, nausea and constipation were most frequently seen during Piportil L4 therapy. Tachycardia, hypotension, syncope, dizziness, blurred vision, vomiting, sweating, nasal congestion, and urinary incontinence have also been observed.

Patients with pheochromocytoma, cerebral vascular or renal insufficiency, or a severe cardiac reserve deficiency such as mitral insufficiency appear to be particularly prone to hypotensive reactions with phenothiazine compounds, and should therefore be observed closely when the drug is administered. Should hypotension occur in patients receiving Piportil L4 and a vasopressor agent be required, i.v. norepinephrine or phenylephrine should be used, and not epinephrine, since phenothiazine derivatives can reverse the pressor effect of the latter drug.

Other autonomic reactions which have occurred with phenothiazines are salivation, polyuria, glaucoma, bladder paralysis, adynamic ileus, and fecal compaction.

Metabolic and Endocrine: Anorexia, menstrual irregularities, impotence, and increased thirst have been reported with Piportil L4.

Weight changes, increased appetite, peripheral edema, galactorrhea, gynecomastia and changes in libido have also occurred in patients receiving phenothiazine therapy.

Allergic or Toxic: Pruritus, dermatitis and rash have been observed with Piportil L4. Other allergic reactions reported with phenothiazine derivatives are erythema, urticaria, seborrhea, eczema, exfoliative dermatitis, and photosensitivity. The possibility of an anaphylactoid reaction should be borne in mind.

Blood dyscrasias including leukopenia, agranulocytosis, pancytopenia, thrombocytopenic or nonthrombocytopenic purpura, eosinophilia, and anemia, have been associated with phenothiazine therapy. Routine blood counts are therefore advisable during prolonged therapy. If any soreness of the mouth, gums or throat or any symptoms of upper respiratory infection occur and confirmatory leukocyte count indicates cellular depression, therapy should be discontinued and other appropriate measures instituted immediately.

Cholestatic jaundice and biliary stasis may be encountered, particularly during the first months of therapy, and require immediate discontinuation of treatment.

Miscellaneous: The following adverse reactions have been reported in patients receiving phenothiazine derivatives: headache, asthma, laryngeal, cerebral and angioneurotic edema, altered cerebrospinal fluid proteins, systemic lupus erythematosus-like syndrome, hyperpyrexia, ECG and EEG changes and hypotension severe enough to cause fatal cardiac arrest. Skin pigmentation, epithelial keratopathy, lenticular and corneal deposits have been associated with long-term administration.

Very rare cases of QT interval prolongation have been reported. There have been isolated reports of sudden death, with possible causes of cardiac origin (see Warnings and Precautions) as well as cases of unexplained sudden death have been reported in patients receiving neuroleptic phenothiazines.

Cases of venous thromboembolism, including cases of pulmonary embolism, sometimes fatal, and cases of deep vein thrombosis have been reported with antipsychotic drugs (see also Warnings).

Sudden, unexpected and unexplained deaths have been reported in hospitalized psychotic patients receiving phenothiazines. Previous brain damage or seizures may be predisposing factors; high doses should be avoided in known seizure patients. Several patients have shown flare-ups of psychotic behaviour patterns shortly before death. Autopsy findings have usually revealed acute fulminating pneumonia or pneumonitis, aspiration of gastric contents or intramyocardial lesions.

Potentiation of CNS depressants (barbiturates, narcotics, analgesics, alcohol, antihistamines), may occur. Local tolerance to pipotiazine is good and reactions at the site of injection are seldom seen.

Hyperglycaemia or intolerance to glucose has been reported in patients treated with Piportil L4 (see Precautions).

OVERDOSE:

Symptoms: In case of overdosage, severe extrapyramidal manifestations, hypotension, lethargy and sedation are most likely to be observed. Initial hospitalization may be required and close medical supervision should be maintained until symptoms are well under control.

Treatment: Treatment is essentially symptomatic and supportive. Severe extrapyramidal reactions may be treated with an appropriate antiparkinsonian agent. Maintain an adequate airway and, in cases of severe hypotension, administer i.v. norepinephrine or phenylephrine (not epinephrine as it may further depress the blood pressure).

When a sufficient amount of time has elapsed or when the patient shows signs of relapse, treatment may be resumed at a lower dosage.

For management of a suspected drug overdose, contact your regional Poison Control Centre. See the *CPS* Directory section for a list of Poison Control Centres.

DOSAGE: Piportil L4 (pipotiazine palmitate) is to be administered as an i.m. injection only. Piportil L4, as a long-acting depot phenothiazine, it has been found useful in the maintenance therapy of non-agitated, chronic schizophrenic patients stabilized with shorter acting neuroleptics who might benefit from a transfer to a long-acting injectable drug.

The changeover to Piportil L4 should aim at maintaining a clinical outcome similar to or better than that obtained with the previously used antipsychotic agent in patients who cannot be relied upon to take oral medication regularly. In those patients who might benefit from a long-acting neuroleptic, it is suggested to discontinue the previous antipsychotic medication prior to the changeover of drugs.

The initial dose and the interval between injections should be selected on an individual basis, considering such factors as age, physical condition, symptoms and severity of illness, and previous drug history. Depending on the previous drug history or other individual factors, an initial dose of 50 to 100 mg may be administered. If necessary, further symptom control can usually be obtained by increasing the dose by increments of 25 mg every 2 or 3 weeks. The optimal dose and the interval between injections must be determined in accordance with the patient's response. A single injection of Piportil L4 may effectively control the schizophrenic symptoms for 3 to 6 weeks. However, it is frequently possible to achieve adequate control with a dosage between 75 and 150 mg administered every 4 weeks. Some patients may not require more than 25 to 50 mg every 4 weeks, while in others, doses of up to 250 mg may be needed.

Lower doses should be used in patients over the age of 50 when initiating therapy with Piportil L4.

The dosage should not be increased in order to prolong the interval between injections. Some patients may benefit from the use of lower doses administered every 3 weeks. Regular and continuous supervision is considered essential in order to maintain the patient on the lowest effective individual dose and to make any additional adjustments in the dosage which may be required to avoid overdosage and troublesome adverse effects.

Although the incidence of extrapyramidal reactions is high, antiparkinsonian medication should be prescribed only to treat emergent symptoms that may occur. They should not be used prophylactically against such reactions.

A dry syringe and a needle of at least 21 gauge should be used to inject Piportil L4. Use of a wet needle or syringe may cause the solution to become cloudy.

INFORMATION FOR THE PATIENT: Published in e-CPS, available by subscription at www.e-cps.ca.

SUPPLIED: 25 mg/mL: Each mL contains: pipotiazine palmitate 25 mg. Nonmedicinal ingredients: sesame oil. Ampuls of 1 mL, boxes of 5. Store at room temperature (15 to 30°C) and protect from light.

50 mg/mL: Each mL contains: pipotiazine palmitate 50 mg. Nonmedicinal ingredients: sesame oil. Ampuls of 1 mL, boxes of 5. Ampuls of 2 mL, boxes of 5. Store at room temperature (15 to 30°C) and protect from light.

Pizotifen ℞
Serotonin Antagonist

CPhA Monograph

Date of Preparation: November 2007

This monograph has been compiled by CPhA and reviewed by experts. It may contain information different from that found in Health Canada-approved Product Monographs. The reader is referred to the *CPS* Editorial Policy for more information.

SUMMARY PRODUCT INFORMATION:

Route of Administration	Dosage Form	Strength
Oral	Tablet	0.5 mg, 1 mg

INDICATIONS AND CLINICAL USE: Pizotifen (also known as pizotyline) is used for the prevention of migraine headaches. Prophylaxis for migraine headaches is generally recommended for patients experiencing three or more attacks per month that fail to respond adequately to symptomatic treatment and interfere with the patient's quality of life.

Pizotifen is not effective treatment for acute migraine or tension headaches.

Pediatrics: Although there is a lack of evidence of efficacy in the pediatric population, pizotifen is sometimes used for migraine headache prophylaxis in children.

Pizotifen may be effective in reducing the frequency and severity of abdominal migraine. Children with abdominal migraine experience episodes of midline abdominal pain lasting 1 to 72 hours that can be accompanied by anorexia, nausea, vomiting and pallor. Less commonly, flushing rather than pallor is the predominant vasomotor symptom. Children with abdominal migraine often develop migraine headache later in life.

CONTRAINDICATIONS: According to the manufacturer's product monograph, pizotifen is contraindicated in:

- Patients who are hypersensitive to pizotifen prior to any ingredient in the formulation or component of the container.
- Patients taking monoamine oxidase (MAO) inhibitors.
- Patients with a pyloroduodenal obstruction and/or stenosing pyloric ulcer.

WARNINGS AND PRECAUTIONS: Endocrine and Metabolism: Pizotifen-associated weight gain may contribute to or exacerbate other conditions associated with overweight such as obesity, diabetes mellitus or metabolic syndrome.

Genitourinary: The anticholinergic effects of pizotifen may exacerbate urinary symptoms in patients with conditions such as prostatic hyperplasia.

Ophthalmologic: Pizotifen's anticholinergic action warrants caution in patients with angle closure glaucoma.

Other: Exercise caution in patients with a history of hypersensitivity or intolerance to tricyclic antidepressants (TCAs), phenothiazines or cyproheptadine.

Special Populations: Pregnant Women: There is little published information on the use of pizotifen in pregnant women. In general, migraine prophylaxis during pregnancy should be considered only when migraine is associated with severe disabling attacks accompanied by nausea, vomiting and dehydration. Like other medications used for headache prophylaxis, pizotifen should be used in pregnancy only when the potential benefits of therapy outweigh the possible risks to mother and fetus.

Nursing Women: Distribution into milk has been demonstrated in animal studies. Because there is little published information on the potential effects of pizotifen on nursing infants, women taking pizotifen should probably not breastfeed while taking the drug.

Monitoring and Laboratory Tests: To assess the clinical benefit of therapy and ongoing need for the drug, frequent monitoring of headache frequency, duration and severity is recommended throughout the treatment period.

Occupational Hazards: Pizotifen's sedative effects may decrease alertness. Activities such as driving a vehicle or operating dangerous machinery should be suspended until the degree of sedative effect on the patient is known.

ADVERSE REACTIONS: More Common Adverse Drug Reactions (≥ 1%) : See Table 1.

Table 1: Pizotifen

More Common Adverse Drug Reactions (≥ 1%)

Body System	Effect	Clinical Comment
Endocrine and Metabolism	Weight gain	Estimated frequency: 4–60%. Average weight gain is between 1–3 kg and is associated with increased appetite. Excessive weight gain may be managed with appropriate dietary recommendations. Body weight usually stabilizes with continued therapy.
Central Nervous System	Drowsiness	Estimated frequency: 4–30%. As the trial period progresses, sedative effects often diminish. Gradual titration of the dose may mitigate the early sedative effects.
Gastrointestinal	Constipation, diarrhea, dry mouth, and nausea	Estimated frequency: 2–12%.
Musculoskeletal	Muscle pain or cramps	Estimated frequency: 6%

Less Common Adverse Drug Reactions (<1%): Cardiovascular: Edema, hypotension and tachycardia may occur occasionally.

Theoretically, pizotifen's tricyclic configuration may confer similar cardiovascular risks to those associated with tricyclic antidepressants, such as a dose-related increased incidence of sudden cardiac death.

Central Nervous System: Infrequently, depression, dizziness, headache, nervousness and weakness have occurred. CNS stimulation may occur in children. "Heaviness in the legs" and tingling/coldness in extremities have also been reported.

Allergic/Dermatologic: Facial flushing occurs rarely.

Hepatic/Biliary/Pancreatic: One case report suggested pizotifen as the possible cause of cholestatic hepatotoxicity.

Ophthalmologic: Blurred vision, thought to be related to pizotifen's anticholinergic effects, occasionally occurs.

Sexual Function/Reproduction: Erectile dysfunction is a rare adverse effect.

DRUG INTERACTIONS: Drug-Drug Interactions: See Table 2.

Table 2: Pizotifen

Drug-Drug Interactions

Interacting Drug	Effect	Clinical Comment
CNS depressants	Additive sedative effects	Use caution when combining pizotifen with other CNS depressants to avoid excessive sedation/impairment
Anticholinergics	Additive anticholinergic effects	Use caution when combining pizotifen with other drugs possessing anticholinergic properties.

Drug-Laboratory Interactions: Theoretically, pizotifen's antihistaminic action may suppress the cutaneous histamine response to allergen extracts applied in an allergy skin test. Therapy should be temporarily discontinued several days before scheduled skin testing.

DOSAGE AND ADMINISTRATION: Recommended Dose and Dosage Adjustment: Adults: See Table 3.

Table 3: Pizotifen

Dose in Adult Patients

Indication	Initial Dose	Dose Titration	Usual Dose	Maximum Dose	Duration of Therapy	Clinical Comment
Migraine headache prophylaxis	0.5 mg at bedtime	Gradually increase to 1.5 mg/day in 3 divided doses.	Usual dose: 1.5 mg/day. Doses higher than 1.5 mg/day have not been shown to increase efficacy.	Maximum dose: 6 mg/day. A single dose should **not** exceed 3 mg.	A 4-wk trial to determine efficacy has been suggested; however, clinical benefit may take as long as 2–3 months to manifest. After several months of treatment, reassess the need to continue therapy. If pizotifen is to be discontinued, gradually reduce the dose over a 2-wk period to avoid rebound headache. If signs and symptoms reappear, prophylactic therapy may be reinstituted.	Giving a larger portion of the daily dose in the evening may help reduce daytime sedation and mitigate increased appetite/weight gain.

Pediatrics: See Table 4.

Table 4: Pizotifen
Dose in Pediatric Patients

Indication	Initial Dose	Dose Titration	Maximum Dose	Duration of Therapy	Clinical Comment
Migraine headache prophylaxis	0.5 mg at bedtime	Gradually increase as needed up to 1.5 mg/day taken in three divided doses	Maximum dose: 1.5 mg/day. A single nighttime dose should be ≤1 mg.	A 4-wk trial to determine efficacy has been suggested; however, clinical benefit may take as long as 2–3 months to manifest. After several months of treatment, reassess the need to continue therapy. If pizotifen is to be discontinued, gradually reduce the dose over a 2-wk period to avoid rebound headache. If signs and symptoms reappear, prophylactic therapy may be reinstituted.	Pizotifen lacks evidence of clinical efficacy in children. Other prophylactic therapy may be preferable initial choices.

Dose in Adult Patients with Renal Impairment: Use with caution; no data.
Hepatic Impairment: Use with caution; no data.

OVERDOSAGE:

For management of a suspected drug overdose, CPhA recommends that you contact your **regional Poison Control Centre**. See the *CPS* Directory section for a list of Poison Control Centres.

ACTION AND CLINICAL PHARMACOLOGY: Mechanism of Action: Pizotifen is classified as a benzocycloheptathiophene derivative with a tricyclic configuration resembling that of amitriptyline and cyproheptadine. Its exact mechanism of action has not been determined but serotonin (5-HT) antagonism and antihistaminic properties are thought to be responsible for its clinical effects. Inhibition of serotonin activity is achieved by binding to and blocking 5-HT receptors, primarily the 5-HT_2-receptor for which pizotifen exhibits a particularly high affinity. Calcium channel blocking activity has also been suggested as a possible mechanism of action in migraine prophylaxis. Antagonism of the H_1-receptor in combination with antibradykinin and peripheral anticholinergic action is thought to be the cause of sedation, increased appetite and weight gain.
Pharmacokinetics: Adults: Absorption: Pizotifen is well absorbed from the gastrointestinal tract, reaching peak plasma concentrations within 5-7 hours after a single oral dose. Absorption is unaffected by concomitant food intake.
Distribution: Pizotifen is over 90% bound to plasma proteins.
Metabolism: Extensive hepatic metabolism converts pizotifen primarily to an N-glucuronide conjugate as well as other minor metabolites.
Excretion: Over 50% of the drug and its metabolites are excreted in the urine. A significant proportion is excreted in the feces. Pizotifen's biological half-life is approximately 26 hours.
STORAGE AND STABILITY: Protect pizotifen preparations from exposure to light.

Plan B®
levonorgestrel
Emergency Contraception

Paladin

Date of Revision: June 10, 2010

SUMMARY PRODUCT INFORMATION:

Route of Administration	Dosage Form/ Strength	Clinically Relevant Nonmedicinal Ingredients
Oral	Tablet 0.75 mg	Lactose monohydrate For a complete listing see Dosage Forms, Composition and Packaging.

INDICATIONS AND CLINICAL USE: Plan B (levonorgestrel 0.75 mg tablets) is an emergency contraceptive that can prevent pregnancy if two tablets are taken together within 72 hours (three days) following unprotected intercourse or a contraceptive accident.

As an emergency contraceptive, Plan B is indicated following any unprotected act of sexual intercourse, including:
- when no contraceptive has been used
- when a contraceptive method may have failed, including:
  - condom rupture, slippage, or misuse
  - diaphragm or cap dislodgment, breakage or early removal
  - failed coitus interruptus
  - miscalculation of periodic abstinence method
  - IUD expulsion
  - missed oral contraceptive
  - a delay in starting a new packet of oral contraceptives
  - a delay in getting a scheduled contraceptive injection
- in cases of sexual assault

Treatment should not be delayed as efficacy may decline with an increased interval between intercourse and the start of treatment. Efficacy is greatest when treatment is taken within 24 hours of unprotected intercourse, decreasing somewhat during each subsequent 24 hour period.

The pregnancy rate of Plan B (levonorgestrel 0.75 mg tablets) is calculated for a single use. If Plan B is used on more than one occasion, the cumulative pregnancy rate will be higher. Plan B is not recommended for routine use as a contraceptive.

Plan B will not prevent pregnancy from future acts of unprotected intercourse. Following use of this product, the woman should either abstain or use an alternative contraceptive method until her next menstrual cycle.
Note to Pharmacist: If you determine that a woman is a repeat user of Emergency Contraception (defined as use more than once a month on a regular basis) or that Plan B has been used within the past cycle, you should consider discussing other, more effective contraceptive methods with the woman, as well as encouraging her to see her physician or other health professional for contraceptive counseling services and advise on other methods of contraception and prevention of sexually transmitted infections. Plan B should still be dispensed, if indicated.
Geriatrics: Plan B has not been studied in this population.
Pediatrics: Plan B has not been studied in this population.

CONTRAINDICATIONS:
- Patients who are hypersensitive to this drug or to any ingredient in the formulation or component of the container. For a complete listing, see Dosage Forms, Composition and Packaging.
- Women with known or suspected pregnancy. The method is not to be used by a woman who is pregnant due to a previous act of intercourse.
- Patients with undiagnosed abnormal vaginal bleeding.

Progestin-only oral contraceptives are used as a routine method of birth control over longer periods of time, and are contraindicated in some conditions (acute liver disease or history of or actual benign or malignant liver tumours, known or suspected carcinoma of the breast, and undiagnosed abnormal vaginal bleeding). It is not known whether these same conditions apply to the Plan B regimen consisting of the emergency use of two progestin pills, but these risks should be considered if Plan B needs to be administered several times.

WARNINGS AND PRECAUTIONS: General: Plan B is not an abortifacient. Patients should be advised that Plan B provides no protection against HIV infection (AIDS) and other sexually transmitted diseases.

The use of cyclic combination oral contraceptives containing estrogen and progestin is associated with increased risks of several serious conditions, including thromboembolic and cardiovascular disorders (e.g. thrombophlebitis, pulmonary embolism, cerebrovascular disorders, myocardial ischemia, mesenteric thrombosis, retinal thrombosis), hepatic neoplasia and gallbladder disease. These conditions have not been associated with the routine use of progestin-only oral contraceptives, but whether short-term (single dose) use of high-dose progestin-only contraceptives would accentuate the risk is unknown. Plan B does not contain estrogen. Controlled clinical trials using Plan B and post-market experience with levonorgestrel for postcoital and emergency contraception have not so far identified any serious adverse events.

Plan B **is not recommended for routine use as a contraceptive**. The pregnancy rate of Plan B (levonorgestrel 0.75 mg tablets) is calculated for a single use. If Plan B is used on more than one occasion, the cumulative pregnancy rate will be higher.
Migraine and Headache: During the use of Plan B, the onset or exacerbation of migraine or the development of a new pattern that is recurrent, persistent or severe requires evaluation of the cause and may require re-evaluation of a future use of emergency contraceptive pills.
Cardiovascular: Hypertension: Patients with essential hypertension whose blood pressure is well controlled may be given combined oral contraceptives containing estrogen and progestin, but only under close supervision. Progestin-only oral contraceptives are not contraindicated for such patients.
Endocrine and Metabolism: Diabetes: The effects of Plan B on carbohydrate metabolism are unknown. Some users of progestin-only oral contraceptives experience slight deterioration in glucose tolerance, with increases in plasma insulin; however, women with diabetes mellitus who use progestin-only oral contraceptives do not generally experience changes in their insulin requirements. Nevertheless, diabetic women should be monitored while taking Plan B.
Hepatic/Biliary/Pancreatic: Following a single oral dose of 0.75 mg, levonorgestrel does not appear to be significantly metabolized by the liver. The risks of Plan B to women with a history of liver disease are unknown. Women with a history of liver disease should be given Plan B under medical supervision especially if the method needs to be administered more than once.
Sexual Function/Reproduction: Effects on Menses: Menstrual bleeding patterns are often irregular among women using progestin-only oral contraceptives and in clinical studies of levonorgestrel for postcoital and emergency contraceptive use. Some women may experience spotting a few days after taking Plan B. At the time of expected menses, approximately 77% of women using Plan B had vaginal bleeding similar to their normal menses, 11-12% bled more than usual and 11% bled less than usual. The majority of women (78%) had their next menstrual period at the expected time or within ±5 days, while only 4.5% had a delay of more than 7 days beyond the anticipated onset of menses. **If there is a delay in the onset of menses beyond 1 week, the possibility of pregnancy should be considered.**
Ectopic Pregnancy: Ectopic pregnancies account for approximately 2% of reported pregnancies (19.7 per 1000 reported pregnancies). **Up to 10% of pregnancies reported in clinical studies of routine use of progestin-only oral contraceptives are ectopic.** However, there appears to be no increase in the rate of ectopic pregnancy after use of levonorgestrel for emergency contraception. A history of ectopic pregnancy need not be considered a contraindication to use of this emergency contraceptive method. However, physicians should be alert to the possibility of an ectopic pregnancy in women who become pregnant or complain of lower abdominal pain after taking Plan B.
Suspected Pregnancy: A pregnancy test is warranted if pregnancy is suspected. Women should be counseled to abstain from sexual intercourse or use an alternative contraceptive method until the onset of their next menstrual period. If a normal menstrual period is delayed beyond 1 week, the patient's pregnancy status should be confirmed with a pregnancy test and follow-up with a health professional. Counseling on routine contraception for future use should be provided as appropriate.
Special Populations: Pregnant Women: Plan B is not an abortifacient and should not be taken by pregnant women, as it will not be effective. Studies involving women who have taken combined oral contraceptives containing levonorgestrel inadvertently during early pregnancy do not suggest that these drugs have an adverse effect on the fetus and there is no evidence that Plan B (levonorgestrel 0.75 mg tablets) taken as an emergency contraceptive would have an adverse effect on an established pregnancy. However, there are insufficient data to rule out the possibility of adverse effects on the fetus if Plan B is used after a woman is already pregnant or in cases of method failure.
Nursing Women: Administration of combined oral contraceptives and progestin-only contraceptives to breastfeeding women has been reviewed in the literature. Seven studies were reviewed that analyzed the transmission of progestins in breast milk. Data were obtained as early as one week post-partum up to approximately six months post-partum. Very small amounts of progestin have been measured in the milk of breastfeeding mothers who are taking progestin-only contraceptives. Levonorgestrel is transferred from maternal breast milk to infants, with infant plasma levels approximately 40% of those in breast milk and approximately 1% to 6% of maternal plasma. No adverse effects due to progestin-only oral contraceptives have been found on breastfeeding performance, either in the quality or quantity of the milk, or on the health, growth, or development of the infant.
Pediatrics: No data is available.
Geriatrics: No data is available.

ADVERSE REACTIONS: Adverse Drug Reaction Overview: There are in general no serious adverse drug reactions to report following the use of Plan B, either in clinical trials or post-market surveillance. Most commonly observed adverse drug reactions are presented in the following sections.
Clinical Trial Adverse Drug Reactions: Because clinical trials are conducted under very specific conditions the adverse reaction rates observed in the clinical trials may not reflect the rates observed in practice and should not be compared to the rates in the clinical trials of another drug. Adverse drug reaction information from clinical trials is useful for identifying drug-related adverse events and for approximating rates.
Plan B Divided Dose Regimen: The most common adverse events reported in the Pivotal Study (Study 92908) of Plan B (levonorgestrel 0.75 mg tablet) when administered as two doses of 0.75 mg at a 12-hour interval included: nausea 23%; abdominal pain 18%; fatigue 17%; headache 17%; vomiting 6%; intermenstrual bleeding and altered menstrual cycles: Some women may experience spotting a few days after taking Plan B. The majority of women (58%) will have their next menstrual period at about the expected time or a few days early or late; if there is a delay in the onset of menses of more than one week, the possibility of pregnancy should be excluded. Women who take Plan B frequently are likely to experience disruptions of the menstrual cycle. Other: breast tenderness, dizziness and diarrhea have been reported in women using Plan B and may be drug related.

In this comparative clinical study involving 1955 evaluable women, the incidence of nausea and vomiting, were significantly (P<0.01) less for women using Plan B than for women receiving the Yuzpe regimen. Adverse events reported in the other controlled clinical trial of the Plan B regimen by Ho and Kwan were consistent with those in the Pivotal Study (Study 92908) (see Table 1).

In the combined controlled clinical trials, the proportion of women receiving levonorgestrel who reported nausea was less than half of the proportion in the Yuzpe group (see Table 2). The proportion that reported vomiting in the levonorgestrel group was only one-fourth that in the Yuzpe group.

The Plan B OTC Label Comprehension Study 18 was conducted to evaluate whether Plan B can be used safely and effectively without oversight by a licensed medical practitioner. A total of 540 women used the study product. No serious adverse events were reported. The findings of the study, compared to those of the Pivotal study, indicate that the pattern of adverse events does not change when the product is provided in a non-prescription setting (see Table 3).
Plan B Single Dose Administration : In a double-blind pivotal trial, the safety profile of levonorgestrel was compared following the administration of a single dose of 1.5 mg or two doses of 0.75 mg at a 12-hour interval (Study 97902). A total of 2756 women used the study product. There was no statistically significant difference in the incidence of the adverse events between the two levonorgestrel groups (see Table 4).
Less Common Clinical Trial Adverse Drug Reactions (<1%): Body as a Whole: back muscular pain, influenza, light headedness, numbness in lower extremities, migraine NOS, redness arms, redness of the chest, tiredness.
Cardiovascular: palpitations.
Ear and Nose: otitis.
Gastrointestinal: acute appendicitis, air in stomach, constipation, polydipsia.
Hematology: high platelets counts, low haemoglobin (anaemia hypochromic).
Immunology: acute tonsillitis, otitis, pharyngitis.
Metabolic: blood glucose increased.

Musculoskeletal: muscle twitching, leg cramps.
Psychiatric: weeping.
Reproductive: corpus luteum cyst or haematoma, ectopic pregnancy termination, late menses, vaginal mycosis.
Respiratory: coughing, rhinitis, sinusitis NOS.
Skin and Appendages: acne, acne aggravated, chapped lips, rash.
Urinary: blood in urine, cystitis, ketone positive in urine, urinary protein increased, white blood cells positive in urine.
Post-Market Adverse Drug Reactions: Data were compiled from a number of sources in order to provide an assessment of the post-marketing safety profile of levonorgestrel 0.75 mg tablets; the results yielded very low numbers of adverse events. There were no signals in the reporting that identified any concerns. When the total adverse events were compared to the estimated sales and usage, the percentages were extremely low. The most common adverse events were consistent with those reported in clinical studies and published data.

Table 1: Plan B

Frequency of Adverse Experiences by Body System Reported in ≥1% of Subjects for Emergency Contraception: Subjects in Controlled Clinical Trials (June 1998)

	(WHO/HRP 1998—Study 92908)		Ho and Kwan, 1993	
Body System/ Preferred Term	**Levonorgestrel N=977 (%)**	**Yuzpe N=979 (%)**	**Levonorgestrel N=410 (%)**	**Yuzpe N=424 (%)**
Body, Whole				
Abdominal Pain	172 (17.6)	205 (20.9)	—	—
Fatigue	165 (16.9)	279 (28.5)	98 (23.9)[a]	156 (36.8)
Flu Syndrome	10 (1.0)	9 (0.9)	—	—
Digestive				
Diarrhea	49 (5.0)	64 (6.5)	—	—
Nausea	226 (23.1)[a]	494 (50.5)	66 (16.1)[a]	197 (46.5)
Vomiting	55 (5.6)[a]	184 (18.8)	11 (2.7)[a]	95 (22.4)
Nervous				
Dizziness	109 (11.2)	163 (16.6)	76 (18.5)	98 (23.1)
Headache	164 (16.8)	198 (20.2)	—	—
Urogenital				
Breast Tenderness	105 (10.7)	118 (12.1)	65 (15.9)	88 (20.8)
Bleeding More	133 (15.6)	116 (11.8)	—	—
Vaginal Hemorrhage	10 (1.0)	12 (1.2)	14 (3.4)	18 (4.2)

[a] Significantly different, P<0.001.

Table 2: Plan B

Frequency of Adverse Experiences by Body System Reported in ≥1% of Subjects for Emergency Contraception: Subjects in Controlled Clinical Trials (Pooled), March 1999

Body System/ Preferred Term	**Levonorgestrel N=1387 (%)**	**Yuzpe N=1403 (%)**
Body, Whole		
Fatigue	263 (19.0)[a]	435 (31.0)
Digestive		
Nausea	292 (21.1)[a]	691 (49.3)
Vomiting	66 (4.8)[a]	279 (19.9)
Nervous		
Dizziness	185 (13.3)[a]	261 (18.7)
Urogenital		
Breast Tenderness	170 (12.3)	206 (14.7)
Spotting/Bleeding	24 (1.7)	30 (2.1)

[a] Significantly different, P<0.001.

Table 3: Plan B

Adverse Events in OTC Actual Use Study and WHO Pivotal Clinical Trial

	% Subjects Reporting Adverse Events	
Adverse Event	**OTC Actual Use Study WCC/FHI 2002 N=540**	**WHO/HRP 1998 Study 92908 N=979**
Abdominal Pain	14.3	17.6
Asthenia (Fatigue)	8.0	16.9
Headache	11.3	5.6
Nausea	12.4	23.1
Vomiting	1.2	5.6
Metrorrhagia	4.3	—
Dizziness	3.7	11.2
All Other	29.6	13.5

(cont'd)

Table 3: Plan B *(cont'd)*

Table 4: Plan B

Frequency of Adverse Experiences by Body System Reported in ≥1% of Subjects for Emergency Contraception: Subjects in Study 97902

	Levonorgestrel One Dose of 1.5 mg N=1379 (%)	**Levonorgestrel Two Tablets of 0.75 mg Administered at a 12-hour Interval N=1377 (%)**
Lower Abdominal Pain	183 (13.3)	198 (14.4)
Fatigue	184 (13.3)	182 (13.2)
Diarrhea	53 (3.8)	44 (3.2)
Nausea	189 (13.7)	199 (14.5)
Vomiting	19 (1.4)	19 (1.4)
Dizziness	132 (9.6)	126 (9.2)
Headache	142 (10.3)	130 (9.4)
Breast Tenderness	113 (8.2)	115 (8.4)
Bleeding More	426 (30.9)	426 (30.9)
Delay of Menses More Than 7 Days[a]	61 (4.5)	61 (4.5)

[a] The denominator for "Delay of menses more than 7 days" is 1359 and 1353, compared to 1379 and 1377 for the other adverse experiences listed in the table.

DRUG INTERACTIONS: Overview: There are no published drug interaction studies of levonorgestrel. Contraceptive steroids are known to be sensitive to anticonvulsants, griseofulvin, rifampicin, and certain other antibiotics (decreased efficacy) and acetaminophen. As the efficacy of Plan B may be decreased in cases of concomitant intake of these drugs, it is recommended that patients perform a pregnancy test if menses is delayed beyond 1 week.
Drug-Drug Interactions: Anticonvulsant Drugs: There was a marked decrease in the AUC of levonorgestrel following 12 weeks of treatment with phenytoin and carbamazepine (42% and 40%, respectively). In contrast, sodium valproate had no detectable effect. These results are consistent with the known effects of the drugs on liver enzyme induction. A number of reports exist in the literature on oral contraceptive failures in women using certain anticonvulsants, most commonly phenytoin, primidone and phenobarbital.
Antibiotics: (See below for rifampicin and rifabutin.) No consistent effect has been found in formal pharmacokinetic studies of a number of antibiotics (including ampicillin, clotrimoxazole, tetracycline, the quinolone temafloxacin, and the macrolide clarithromycin) on plasma concentrations of steroids, in particular ethinyl estradiol. It is impossible at the present time to evaluate fully the potential impact of antibiotics on efficacy based on the literature.
Rifampicin/Rifabutin: Rifampicin is a potent enzyme inducer and, as with anticonvulsant drugs, there is a molecular basis for expecting an interaction with contraceptive steroid efficacy. Oral contraceptive failures, menstrual abnormalities, and low progestin levels have been shown in subjects being treated simultaneously with oral contraceptives and rifampicin. The metabolism of levonorgestrel is enhanced by the concomitant use of rifabutin.
Acetaminophen: Paracetamol is metabolized primarily by conjugation with sulfuric and glucuronic acids and hence has the potential for interfering with ethinyl estradiol metabolism. However, a similar effect on levonorgestrel was not shown in the same study.
Drug-Food Interactions: No formal pharmacokinetic studies of the effect of food have been performed. Efficacy is presumed to be independent of the timing of meals since no instruction on timing of dosing relative to meals was provided to the participants in the primary clinical trials supporting the indication.
Drug-Herb Interactions: The concomitant use of Hypericum perforatum (St. John's wort) can decrease the efficacy of Plan B. Interactions with other herbal products have not been established.
Drug-Laboratory Test Interactions: Use of oral contraceptives can modify the results of laboratory tests. Lab tests should therefore be done prior to dosing or more than 3 days after dosing to avoid misinterpretation of the results. Pathologists should be advised about oral contraceptive therapy when specimens obtained from Pap smears are submitted for examination.

DOSAGE AND ADMINISTRATION: Dosing Considerations: Plan B can be administered at any time during the menstrual cycle.
Recommended Dose and Dosage Adjustment: Two tablets of Plan B (levonorgestrel 0.75 mg) should be taken at the same time, orally, as soon as possible but within 72 hours after unprotected intercourse. The total dosage for one complete regimen of Plan B consists in a single dose of 1.50 mg levonorgestrel.

The patient should be instructed to contact her health care provider if she vomits in the first two hours after taking the dose of medication. An additional dose may be administered, based on the judgment of the health care provider. In clinical studies, of the 55 women who vomited as a result of taking Plan B, 40 took a replacement dose. Statistical analysis showed that the replacement dose did not increase efficacy significantly. If vomiting occurs as a result of taking Plan B, it is possible that sufficient quantities of the hormone have been absorbed, as the maximum blood level after oral consumption is reached in about 1.6 hours. If vomiting occurs, for other reasons (such as the flu), or if the pills are visible in the emesis, a replacement dose may be warranted.

The patient should be counselled to abstain of or use an alternative method of contraception (e.g., diaphragm or condom) until the next menstrual cycle. Most patients will have their next menstrual period at the expected time or within a week of the expected time. If a normal period is delayed beyond 1 week, the patient's pregnancy status should be confirmed with a pregnancy test and follow-up with a health professional.

OVERDOSAGE:
There are no data on overdosage of Plan B; however, it is anticipated that the incidence and severity of nausea and vomiting and of menstrual cycle disturbances may be increased. In case of overdose or accidental ingestion by children, treatment is generally not required, but the patient should be closely observed by the physician and gastric lavage may be employed if considered necessary.

For management of a suspected drug overdose, CPhA recommends that you contact your **regional Poison Control Centre**. See the *CPS* Directory section for a list of Poison Control Centres.

Table 5: Plan B

Summary of Pharmacokinetic Parameter Values for Studies

Study	N	Dose	Mean (±S.D.) C_{max} (ng/mL)	T_{max} (h)	T_{α} (h)	T_{β} (h)	Vd (L)	CL (L/h)	$AUC_{0-\infty}$ (ng/mL/h)
WCC-Sponsored Study of Proposed Commercial Formulation									
WCC-PK 001	16	0.75 mg	14.1±7.7	1.6±0.7	—	24.4±5.3	260	7.7±2.7	123.1±50.1
Other Studies Performed with Gedeon Richter Formulation									
He 1990	10	0.75 mg	11.2±3.4	1.9±0.6	1.3±0.6	13.3±3.7	115±41	6.1±1.9	124±43
Landgren 1989	10	0.75 mg	16	—	—	14.5	—	—	—
Shi 1988	6	0.75 mg	9.0±2.2	2±4	—	8.9±1.9	88.6±25.6	7.2±2.7	116±41

ACTION AND CLINICAL PHARMACOLOGY: Mechanism of Action: Emergency contraceptives are intended to be used after known or suspected contraceptive failure or unprotected intercourse. They are not effective if a woman is already pregnant. Plan B (levonorgestrel) is believed to act as an emergency contraceptive principally by preventing ovulation or by inhibiting fertilization (by altering tubal transport of sperm and/or ova). It may also prevent implantation (by altering the endometrium). It is not effective once the process of implantation has begun.

Pharmacokinetics: Absorption and Distribution: The absolute bioavailability of Plan B in humans has not been specifically investigated. However, levonorgestrel is reported in the literature to be rapidly and completely absorbed following oral administration and does not undergo first pass metabolism.

Single Dose Studies: In WCC-PK 001, investigators administered single doses of 0.75 mg tablets to 16 healthy young women. The same subjects received levonorgestrel 0.75 mg as an oral suspension, prepared immediately prior to dosing. The rate and extent of absorption following administration of the suspension were lower than those measured following administration of the tablet (mean C_{max} of 7.52±4.14 ng/mL occurring on average 2.8±1.1 hours post-dose for the suspension versus 14.1±7.7 ng/mL and 1.6±0.7 hours post-dose for the tablets). This pattern was observed in 14 of 16 subjects. (The lower bioavailability of the oral suspension is attributed to the larger particle size in the micronized drug substance as compared with that in the tablet.)

The volume of distribution (Vd) was estimated to be 260.0 L. Serum levels declined with a mean terminal half-life of 24.4±5.3 hours following administration as a tablet and 27.3±6.3 hours following administration as a suspension.

Results for the three published studies were similar to one another and also to results for the tablet in the WCC-sponsored study (see Table 5). Reported half-lives were shorter in the published single dose studies, approximately 13 to 14 hours. The duration of sampling was shorter.

Multiple Dose Study: One study, also provided results for seven-day dosing of six healthy young women. Serum levels on Day 7 were found to be somewhat lower than Day 1 levels (mean C_{max} value of 9.0 ng/mL for Day 1; 5.3 ng/mL mean C_{max} for Day 7 corrected values), and a longer half-life was reported (mean 12.6 hours on Day 7). Steady state was obtained on the fourth day, with no unanticipated accumulation.

Orally administered levonorgestrel is found in breast milk at levels approximating a plasma/milk ratio of 100:15.

Metabolism: Following a single oral dosage, levonorgestrel does not appear to be extensively metabolized by the liver. The primary metabolites are 3a,5b- and 3a,5a-tetrahydrolevonorgestrel with 16b-hydroxynorgestrel also identified. Together, these account for less than 10% of parent plasma levels. Urinary metabolites hydroxylated at the 2a and 16b positions have also been identified. Small amounts of the metabolites are present in plasma as sulfate and glucuronide conjugates.

Special Populations and Conditions: Age Effects: Due to the age range of women participating in these studies (19-44 years), and given that the target population for levonorgestrel emergency contraception is comparable, age effects have not been evaluated.

Race: Pharmacokinetic parameters have been summarized separately by ethnicity (see Table 6). Ethnicity was not stated in the three published studies. Two studies were conducted in China, and presumably, all 16 subjects were Chinese. Similarly, the ten subjects participating in Sweden are all assumed to be Caucasian. There is a suggestion of lower concentrations in Asian subjects. These observations should be interpreted with caution, however, as in the U.S.-based study, there was only one Asian subject, and the assay methodology in the other studies differed.

Table 6: Plan B

Summary of Levonorgestrel 0.75 mg Single Dose Tablet Pharmacokinetic Parameter Values by Ethnicity

Parameters	WCC-PK 001 Caucasian (U.S.) (N=9)	WCC-PK 001 Black (U.S.) (N=6)	WCC-PK 001 Asian/Pacific Islander (U.S.) (N=1)	Landgren, 1989 — (Sweden) (N=10)	He, 1990 — (China) (N=10)	Shi, 1988 — (China) (N=6)
C_{max} (ng/mL)	15.9	12.2	9.4	16	11.2±3.4	9.0±2.2
T_{max} (h)	1.8	1.4	1.3	—	1.9±0.6	2-4
$AUC_{0-\infty}$ (ng/mL/h)	131.5	120.7	62.5	—	124±43	116±41
Half life (h)	24.6	24.5	22.9	14.5	13.3±3.7	8.9±1.9
CL (L/h)	6.4	7.2	12	—	6.1±1.9	7.2±2.7

Hepatic and Renal Insufficiency: No formal pharmacokinetic studies have been conducted in patients with renal or hepatic impairment. Since the product is administered as a single course of treatment there is no concern about the potential accumulation that might occur with chronic dosing in patients with hepatic or renal impairment.

STORAGE AND STABILITY: Store Plan B tablets between 15 and 30°C. Protect from high humidity.

INFORMATION FOR THE PATIENT: Published in e-CPS, available by subscription at www.e-cps.ca.

DOSAGE FORMS, COMPOSITION AND PACKAGING: Each almost white, flat, rimmed tablet of about 6 mm diameter with an impressed mark of "INOR" on one side, contains: levonorgestrel 0.75 mg [18,19-Dinorpregn-4-en-20-yn-3-one,13-ethyl-17-hydroxy-(17α)-(-)-], a totally synthetic progestogen. Nonmedicinal ingredients: colloidal silicon dioxide, cornstarch, lactose monohydrate, magnesium stearate, potato starch and talc. PVC/aluminum foil blister packages of two tablets each, which are permanently sealed in a double-layer, four-panel outer package.

(Shown in Product Identification Section)

Plaquenil® Pr

hydroxychloroquine sulfate

Anti-inflammatory—Antimalarial

sanofi-aventis

Date of Revision: October 25, 2006

PHARMACOLOGY: Hydroxychloroquine has been beneficial for a high percentage of patients with rheumatoid arthritis and lupus erythematosus, especially chronic discoid lupus. The exact mode of action in controlling these diseases is unknown. The action of this compound against malarial parasites is similar to that of chloroquine phosphate.

INDICATIONS: For the treatment of rheumatoid arthritis, and discoid and systemic lupus erythematosus, in patients who have not responded satisfactorily to drugs with less potential for serious side effects.

It is also indicated for the suppressive treatment and treatment of acute attacks of malaria due to *P. vivax*, *P. malariae*, *P. ovale*, and susceptible strains of *P. falciparum*. It is not active against the exo-erythrocytic forms of *P. vivax*, *P. malariae* and *P. ovale* and therefore will neither prevent infection due to these organisms when given prophylactically, nor prevent relapse of infection due to these organisms. It is highly effective as a suppressive agent in patients with vivax or malariae malaria in terminating acute attacks and significantly lengthening the interval between treatment and relapse. In patients with falciparum malaria, it abolishes the acute attack and effects complete cure of the infection, unless due to a resistant strain of *P. falciparum*.

CONTRAINDICATIONS: Pre-existing retinopathy of the eye, patients with known hypersensitivity to 4-aminoquinoline compounds and use in children below 6 years of age (200 mg tablets not adapted for weight <35 kg).

WARNINGS: Ophthalmic: Irreversible retinal damage has been observed in some patients who had received long-term or high-dosage 4-aminoquinoline therapy for discoid and systemic lupus erythematosus, or rheumatoid arthritis. Before starting a long term treatment, both eyes should be examined by careful ophthalmoscopy for visual acuity, central visual field and color vision, and fundoscopy. Then, the examination should be repeated at least annually.

Retinal toxicity is largely dose-related. The risk of retinal damages is small with daily doses of up to 6.5 mg/kg ideal (lean) body weight. Exceeding the recommended daily dose sharply increase the risk of retinal toxicity.

This examination should be more frequent and adapted to the patient, in the following situations:

- daily doses exceeding 6.5 mg/kg ideal (lean) body weight. Absolute body weight used as a guide to dosage, could result in an overdosage in the obese;
- renal insufficiency;
- cumulative dose more than 200 g;
- elderly;
- impaired visual acuity.

If there is any indication of abnormality in the visual acuity, visual field, or retinal macular areas (such as pigmentary changes, loss of foveal reflex), or any visual symptoms (such as light flashes and streaks) that are not fully explainable by difficulties of accommodation or coroneal opacities, the drug should be stopped immediately. The patient should be closely observed for possible progression of the abnormality. Retinal changes (and visual disturbances) may progress even after cessation of the therapy.

Anti-inflammatory: Dermatological reactions to Plaquenil (hydroxychloroquine sulfate) may occur. It is not recommended for the treatment of psoriasis or porphyria as these conditions may be exacerbated by its use. The preparation should only be used in these conditions, when in the judgment of the physician, the benefit outweighs the risk in those patients.

All patients on long-term therapy with this preparation should be questioned and examined periodically. Including the testing of knee and ankle reflexes, to detect any evidence of muscular weakness. If weakness occurs, discontinue the drug.

Malaria: Plaquenil is not effective against chloroquine-resistant strains of *P. falciparum* and is not active against the exo-erythrocytic forms of *P. vivax*, *P. ovale* and *P. malariae* and therefore will neither prevent infection due to these organisms when given prophylactically, nor prevent relapse of infection due to these organisms.

Pregnancy: Hydroxychloroquine crosses the placenta. Data are limited regarding the use of hydroxychloroquine during pregnancy. Plaquenil should be avoided in pregnancy except when, in the judgment of the physician, the potential benefits outweigh the potential hazards. It should be noted that the 4-aminoquinolines in therapeutic doses have been associated with central nervous system damage, including ototoxicity (auditory and vestibular toxicity, congenital deafness), retinal hemorrhages and abnormal retinal pigmentation to the foetus.

Lactation: Careful consideration should be given to using hydroxychloroquine during lactation, since it has been known to be excreted in small amounts in human breast milk and it is known that infants are extremely sensitive to the toxic effects of 4-aminoquinolines.

Children: Safety and efficacy has not been established in rheumatoid arthritis or systemic lupus erythematosus in children. Children are especially sensitive to the 4-aminoquinoline compounds. The most reported fatalities follow the accidental ingestion of chloroquine, sometimes in small doses. Patients should be strongly warned to keep these drugs out of the reach of children.

PRECAUTIONS: Observe caution in patients with hepatic or renal disease, in whom a reduction in dosage may be necessary, as well as in those taking medicines known to affect these organs.

Observe caution also in patients with gastrointestinal, neurological, or blood disorders, in those with a sensitivity to quinine, and in glucose-6-phosphate dehydrogenase deficiency, porphyria and psoriasis.

Methods recommended for early diagnosis of retinopathy consist of (1) funduscopic examination of the macula for fine pigmentary disturbances or loss of the foveal reflex and (2) examination of the central visual field with a small red test object for pericentral or paracentral scotoma or determination of retinal thresholds to red. Any unexplained visual symptoms, such as light flashes or streaks also should be regarded with suspicion as possible manifestations of retinopathy.

If serious toxic symptoms occur from overdosage or sensitivity, it has been suggested that ammonium chloride (8 g daily in divided doses for adults) 3 or 4 days a week be administered for several months after therapy has been stopped, as acidification of the urine increases renal excretion of the 4-aminoquinoline compounds by 20 to 90%. However, caution must be exercised in patients with impaired renal function and/or metabolic acidosis. Although the risk of bone marrow depression is low, periodic blood counts should be obtained in patients requiring prolonged therapy. If any severe blood disorder appears that is not attributable to the disease under treatment, the drug should be discontinued.

Drug Interactions: Concomitant hydroxychloroquine and digoxin therapy may result in increased serum digoxin levels; serum digoxin levels should be closely monitored in patients receiving combined therapy.

As hydroxychloroquine may enhance the effects of a hypoglycemic treatment, a decrease in doses of insulin or antidiabetic drugs may be required.

Occupational Hazards: Effects on Ability to Drive and Use Machinery: Patients should be warned about driving and operating machinery since hydroxychloroquine can impair accommodation and cause blurring of vision. If the condition is not self-limiting, dosage may need to be temporarily reduced.

ADVERSE EFFECTS: Retinopathy with changes in pigmentation and visual field defects, can occur following hydroxychloroquine administration, but is rare. In its early form, it appears reversible upon discontinuation of the drug. If allowed to develop however, there may be a risk of progression even after treatment withdrawal.

Patients with retinal changes may be asymptomatic initially, or may have scotomatous vision with paracentral, pericentral ring types, temporal scotomas, abnormal colour visions, reduction in visual acuity, night blindness, difficulty reading and skipping words.

Corneal changes including edema and opacities have been reported. They are either symptomless or may cause disturbances such as halos around lights especially at night, blurring of vision or photophobia. They may be transient or are reversible upon discontinuation of therapy.

Blurring of vision due to a disturbance of accommodation which is dose dependent and reversible may also occur.

Skin rashes sometimes occur; pruritus, pigmentary changes in skin and mucous membranes, bleaching of hair, and alopecia have also been reported. These usually resolve readily upon cessation of therapy.

Bullous eruptions including (urticarial, morbilliform, lichenoid, maculopapular, purpuric, erythema annulare centrifugum) and very rare cases of erythema multiforme, Stevens-Johnson syndrome, photosensitivity and isolated cases of exfoliative dermatitis have been reported.

Very rare cases of acute generalized exanthematous pustulosis (AGEP) has to be distinguished from psoriasis, although hydroxychloroquine may precipitate attacks of psoriasis. It may be associated with fever and hyperleukocytosis. Outcome is usually favorable after discontinuation of drug.

Other adverse reactions include gastrointestinal disturbances such as nausea, diarrhea, anorexia, abdominal pain and, rarely, vomiting may occur. These symptoms usually resolve immediately upon reducing the dose or upon stopping the treatment.

Less frequently, dizziness, vertigo, tinnitus, hearing loss including very rare cases of irreversible hearing loss, headache, nervousness, emotional lability, psychosis and convulsions have been reported with this class of drugs.

Skeletal muscle palsies or skeletal muscle myopathy or neuromyopathy leading to progressive weakness and atrophy of proximal muscle groups which may be associated with mild sensory changes, depression of tendon reflexes and abnormal nerve conduction have been noted. Myopathy may be reversible after drug discontinuation, but recovery may take many months.

Rarely, there have been reports of cardiomyopathy.

Chronic toxicity should be suspected when conduction disorders (bundle branch block/atrioventricular heart block) as well as biventricular hypertrophy are found. Drug discontinuation may lead to recovery.

Rarely, there have been reports of bone marrow depression.

Blood disorders such as anemia, aplastic anemia, agranulocytosis, decrease in white blood cells and thrombocytopenia have been reported.

Hydroxychloroquine may exacerbate porphyria.

Isolated cases of abnormal liver function tests have been reported and few cases of fulminant hepatic failure have been published.

Urticaria, angioedema and bronchospasm have been reported.

OVERDOSE:

Overdosage with the 4-aminoquinolines is dangerous particularly in infants, as little as 1-2 g having proved fatal.

Symptoms: The 4-aminoquinoline compounds are very rapidly and completely absorbed following ingestion and in accidental overdosage toxic symptoms may occur within 30 minutes. These consist of headache, drowsiness, visual disturbances, cardiovascular collapse, hypokalemia and convulsions, followed by sudden and early respiratory and cardiac arrest. The ECG may reveal atrial standstill, nodal rhythm, prolonged intraventricular conduction time, and progressive bradycardia leading to ventricular fibrillation and/or arrest.

Treatment: Treatment is symptomatic and must be prompt with immediate evacuation of the stomach by emesis (at home, before transportation to the hospital), or gastric lavage until the stomach is completely emptied. If finely powdered activated charcoal is introduced by the stomach tube, after lavage and within 30 minutes after ingestion of the tablets, it may inhibit further intestinal absorption of the drug. To be effective, the dose of activated charcoal should be at least five times the estimated dose of ingested hydroxychloroquine. Convulsions, if present, should be controlled before attempting gastric lavage. If due to cerebral stimulation, cautious administration of an ultrashort-acting barbiturate may be tried but, if due to anoxia, convulsions should be corrected by oxygen administration, artificial respiration or, in shock with hypotension, by vasopressor therapy. Because of the importance of supporting respiration, tracheal intubation or tracheostomy, followed by gastric lavage, has also been advised. Exchange transfusions have been used to reduce the level of 4-aminoquiolines in the blood.

Consideration should be given to administering diazepam parenterally, since studies have reported it beneficial in reversing chloroquine cardiotoxicity.

A patient who survives the acute phase and is asymptomatic should be closely observed for at least 6 hours. Fluids may be forced, and sufficient ammonium chloride may be administered for a few days to acidify the urine to help promote urinary excretion.

For management of a suspected drug overdose, CPhA recommends that you contact your **regional Poison Control Centre**. See the *CPS* Directory section for a list of Poison Control Centres.

DOSAGE: Absolute body weight used as a guide to dosage, could result in an overdosage; daily doses should not exceed 6.5 mg/kg ideal (lean) body weight. Exceeding the recommended daily dose sharply increase the risk of retinal toxicity.

The dosages cited below are stated in terms of hydroxychloroquine sulfate. One 200 mg tablet is equivalent to 155 mg base. Each dose should be taken with a meal or a glass of milk.

Rheumatoid Arthritis: The compound is cumulative in action and will require several weeks to exert its beneficial therapeutic effects, whereas minor side effects may occur somewhat early. Several months of therapy may be required before maximum effects can be obtained. If objective improvement (such as reduced joint swelling, increased mobility) does not occur within 6 months, the drug should be stopped. Safe use of the drug in the treatment of juvenile rheumatoid arthritis has not been established.

Initial Dosage: Adults: 400 to 600 mg daily. In a few patients, the side effects may require temporary reduction of the initial dosage. Generally, after 5 to 10 days the dose may be gradually increased to the optimum response level, frequently, without return of side effects.

Maintenance Dosage: When a good response is obtained (usually in 4 to 12 weeks), the dosage is reduced by 50% and continued at an acceptable maintenance level of 200 to 400 mg daily. The incidence of retinopathy has been reported to be higher when the maintenance dose is exceeded.

If a relapse occurs after medication is withdrawn, therapy may be resumed or continued on an intermittent schedule if there are no ocular contraindications.

Use in Combination Therapy: Hydroxychloroquine may be used safely and effectively in combination with corticosteroids, salicylates, NSAIDs, and methotrexate and other second line therapeutic agents. Corticosteroids and salicylates can generally be decreased gradually in dosage or eliminated after the drug has been used for several weeks. When gradual reduction of steroid dosage is suggested, it may be done by reducing, every 4 to 5 days, the dose of cortisone by no more than 5 to 15 mg; of hydrocortisone from 5 to 10 mg; of prednisolone and prednisone from 1 to 2.5 mg; of methylprednisolone and triamcinolone from 1 to 2 mg and dexamethasone from 0.25 to 0.5 mg. Regimens of treatment using other agents than steroids and NSAIDs are under development. No definitive dose combinations have been established.

Lupus Erythematosus: Initially, the average **adult** dose is 400 mg once or twice daily. This may be continued for several weeks or months, depending upon the response of the patient. For prolonged maintenance therapy, a smaller dose, from 200 to 400 mg daily will suffice. The incidence of retinopathy has been reported to be higher when this maintenance dose is exceeded.

Malaria: Suppression: **In adults**, 400 mg on exactly the same day of each week. **In infants and children**, the weekly suppressive dose is 5 mg base/kg, but should not exceed the adult dose regardless of body weight.

Suppressive therapy should begin 2 weeks before exposure. When not administered before exposure, give an initial loading dose of 800 mg to adults, or 10 mg base/kg to children in 2 divided doses, 6 hours apart. The suppressive therapy should be continued for 8 weeks after leaving the endemic area.

Treatment of the Acute Attack: **In adults**, an initial loading dose of 800 mg followed by 400 mg in six to eight hours. This is followed by 400 mg on each of the next two days for a total of 2 g of hydroxychloroquine sulfate or 1.55 g base. Alternatively, the administration of a single dose of 800 mg has also proved effective. The dosage for adults may also be calculated by body weight.

For Infants and Children: Dosage calculated by body weight is preferred. A total dose representing 25 mg of base/kg is administered over 3 days as follows:

First dose: 10 mg base/kg (not to exceed 620 mg base).

Second dose: 5 mg base/kg 6 hours after the first dose (not to exceed 310 mg base).

Third dose: 5 mg base/kg 18 hours after the second dose.

Fourth dose: 5 mg base/kg 24 hours after the third dose.

For radical cure of vivax and malariae malaria, concomitant therapy with an 8-aminoquinoline compound is necessary.

INFORMATION FOR THE PATIENT: Published in e-CPS, available by subscription at www.e-cps.ca.

SUPPLIED: Each white to off-white, film-coated, peanut-shaped tablet, with PLAQUENIL in black on one side, contains: hydroxychloroquine sulfate 200 mg (equivalent to 155 mg of base). Nonmedicinal ingredients: black ink, calcium hydrogenophosphate, carnauba wax, corn starch, magnesium stearate, Opadry White YS-1-7443 and polyethylene glycol 400. Bottles of 100. Store at room temperature (15-30°C). Keep in a safe place out of reach of children.

(Shown in Product Identification Section)

Plasbumin®-5

albumin (human)

Plasma Substitute/Blood Derivative

Talecris

Date of Revision: January 19, 2009

SUMMARY PRODUCT INFORMATION:

Route of Administration	Dosage Form/ Strength	Clinically Relevant Nonmedicinal Ingredients
Intravenous injection	Intravenous solution, 5%	For a complete listing see Dosage Forms, Composition and Packaging section.

DESCRIPTION: PLASBUMIN-5 (Albumin [Human] 5%, USP) is a 5% sterile solution of albumin in an aqueous diluent. The preparation is stabilized with 0.004 M sodium caprylate and 0.004 M acetyltryptophan and buffered with sodium carbonate. The approximate sodium content of the product is 145 mEq/L. It contains no preservative. PLASBUMIN-5 must be administered intravenously.

PLASBUMIN-5 is made from pooled human venous plasma using the Cohn cold ethanol fractionation process. It is prepared in accordance with the applicable requirements established by the U.S. Food and Drug Administration.

INDICATIONS AND CLINICAL USE: The oncotic and colloid properties of PLASBUMIN-5 are used to restore and maintain circulating blood volume, when needed, and when the use of a colloid is appropriate. The choice of PLASBUMIN-5 over artificial colloid or crystalloid solutions will depend on the clinical situation of the individual patient, according to current therapeutic guidelines and recommendations.

PLASBUMIN-5 is primarily used in the treatment of shock associated with hemorrhage, surgery, trauma, burns, and bacteremia.

Emergency Treatment of Hypovolemic Shock: PLASBUMIN-5 is iso-oncotic with normal plasma and on intravenous infusion will expand the circulating blood volume by an amount approximately equal to the volume infused. In conditions associated mainly with a volume deficit, albumin is best administered as a 5% solution (PLASBUMIN-5); but where there is an oncotic deficit, PLASBUMIN-25 may be preferred. This is also an important consideration where the treatment of the shock state has been delayed. If PLASBUMIN-25 is used, appropriate additional crystalloid should be administered.

Crystalloid solutions in volumes several times greater than that of PLASBUMIN-5 may be effective in treating shock in younger individuals who have no preexisting illness at the time of the incident. Older patients, especially those with preexisting debilitating conditions, or those in whom the shock is caused by a medical disorder, or where the state of shock has existed for some time before active therapy could be instituted, may not tolerate hypoalbuminemia as well.

Removal of ascitic fluid from a patient with cirrhosis may cause changes in cardiovascular function and even result in hypovolemic shock. In such circumstances, the use of albumin infusion may be required to support the blood volume.

Burn Therapy: An optimal therapeutic regimen with respect to the administration of colloids, crystalloids, and water following extensive burns has not been established. During the first 24 hours after sustaining thermal injury, large volumes of crystalloids are infused to restore the depleted extracellular fluid volume. Beyond 24 hours PLASBUMIN-25 may be preferred for this purpose.

Cardiopulmonary Bypass: With the relatively small priming volume required with modern pumps, preoperative dilution of the blood using albumin and crystalloid has been shown to be safe and well-tolerated. Although the limit to which the hematocrit and plasma protein concentration can be safely lowered has not been defined, it is common practice to adjust the albumin and crystalloid pump prime to achieve a hematocrit of 20% and a plasma albumin concentration of 2.5 g per 100 mL in the patient.

Acute Liver Failure: In the uncommon situation of rapid loss of liver function, with or without coma, administration of albumin may serve the double purpose of supporting the colloid osmotic pressure of the plasma as well as binding excess plasma bilirubin.

Sequestration of Protein Rich Fluids: This occurs in such conditions as acute peritonitis, pancreatitis, mediastinitis, and extensive cellulitis. The magnitude of loss into the third space may require treatment of reduced volume or oncotic activity with an infusion of albumin.

Situations in Which Albumin Administration is Not Warranted: In chronic nephrosis, infused albumin is promptly excreted by the kidneys with no relief of the chronic edema or effect on the underlying renal lesion. It is of occasional use in the rapid "priming" diuresis of nephrosis. Similarly, in hypoproteinemic states associated with chronic cirrhosis, malabsorption, protein losing enteropathies, pancreatic insufficiency, and undernutrition, the infusion of albumin as a source of protein nutrition is not justified.

CONTRAINDICATIONS:

- PLASBUMIN-5 should not be given to patients who are hypersensitive to albumin or to any ingredient in the formulation or component of the container. For a complete listing, see Dosage Forms, Composition and Packaging.
- PLASBUMIN-5 should not be given to patients at special risk of developing circulatory overload (i.e., those with a history of congestive cardiac failure, renal insufficiency or stabilized chronic anemia).

WARNINGS AND PRECAUTIONS: General: PLASBUMIN-5 is made from human plasma. Products made from human plasma may contain infectious agents, such as viruses, that can cause disease. The risk that such products will transmit an infectious agent has been reduced by screening plasma donors for prior exposure to certain viruses, by testing for the presence of certain current virus infections, and by inactivating and/or removing certain viruses. Despite these measures, such products can still potentially transmit disease. There is also the possibility that unknown infectious agents may be present in such products. Individuals who receive infusions of blood or plasma products may develop signs and/or symptoms of some viral infections, particularly hepatitis C. All infections thought by a physician possibly to have been transmitted by this product should be reported by the physician or other healthcare provider to Talecris Biotherapeutics Ltd. [1-866-482-5226].

Albumin is a derivative of human blood. Based on effective donor screening and product manufacturing processes, it carries an extremely remote risk for transmission of viral diseases. A theoretical risk for transmission of Creutzfeldt-Jakob Disease (CJD), including variant Creutzfeldt-Jakob disease (vCJD), also is considered extremely remote. No cases of transmission of viral diseases or CJD, including vCJD, have ever been identified for albumin.

The physician should discuss the risks and benefits of this product with the patient, before prescribing or administering to the patient.

PLASBUMIN-5 must not be diluted with sterile water for injection as this may cause hemolysis and acute renal failure in recipients (see Dosage and Administration).

Blood coagulation parameters, the hematocrit and serum electrolytes should be monitored when a large volume of PLASBUMIN-5 solution is administered.

Patients should always be monitored carefully in order to guard against the possibility of circulatory overload. PLASBUMIN-5 is iso-oncotic with normal plasma and will not tend to aggravate tissue dehydration. Appropriate additional crystalloids should be administered, if required by the patient, to maintain normal fluid balance.

PLASBUMIN-5 is not tested for aluminum content and may contain more than 200 µg/L of aluminum. It should, therefore, not be used to treat infants or patients on hemodialysis.

In hemorrhage the administration of albumin should be supplemented by the transfusion of whole blood to treat the relative anemia associated with hemodilution. When circulating blood volume has been reduced, hemodilution following the administration of albumin persists for many hours. In patients with a normal blood volume, hemodilution lasts for a much shorter period.

The rapid rise in blood pressure which may follow the administration of a colloid with positive oncotic activity necessitates careful observation to detect and treat severed blood vessels which may not have bled at the lower blood pressure.

Special Populations: Pregnant and Nursing Women: Animal reproduction studies have not been conducted with PLASBUMIN-5. It is not known whether it can cause harm to the fetus or nursing child. PLASBUMIN-5 should be given to a pregnant or nursing woman only if the benefit outweighs any potential risk.

Pediatrics: The use of PLASBUMIN-5 in children has not been associated with any special or specific hazard, if the dose is appropriate for the child's body weight. However, its use should be carefully evaluated for risk and benefit in pediatric treatment and PLASBUMIN-5 should not be used in neonates and infants (see Warnings and Precautions, General).

ADVERSE REACTIONS: Adverse Drug Reaction Overview: Adverse reactions to albumin are rare. Such reactions may be allergic in nature or due to high plasma protein levels from excessive albumin administration. Allergic manifestations include urticaria, chills, fever, and changes in respiration, pulse and blood pressure. The possibility of an anaphylactic reaction occurring in association with albumin is considered extremely rare. In the case of an anaphylactic reaction, discontinue infusion and treat appropriately.

The Cochrane Injuries Group published a meta-analysis (July 1998) in which an increase in mortality was reported in albumin–treated patients compared to patients who had received crystalloids or no treatment. However, the analysis was criticized by many authors, due to substantial methodological concerns.

In 2001, Wilkes et. al. published a revised meta-analysis, which showed no evidence of excess albumin-associated mortality, but suggested that albumin might actually reduce mortality.

The Saline versus Albumin Fluid Evaluation (SAFE) Study reported in the New England Journal of Medicine in May 2004, involving nearly 7000 critically ill patients, addressed one of the most fundamental and contentious issues in critical care: the value of colloids as opposed to crystalloids in the resuscitation of seriously ill patients. Based on these results, the administration of albumin appears to be safe for up to 28 days in a heterogeneous population of critically ill patients, and may be beneficial in patients with severe sepsis. A greater number of patients with trauma involving brain injury died among those randomly assigned to albumin as opposed to saline (59 of 241 in the albumin group compared to 38 of 251 in the saline group with a relative risk of 1.62 and p=0.009). However, the overall number of these patients was relatively small. The study had insufficient power to detect differences in mortality among the predefined subgroups and the authors warn that the observed difference should be interpreted with caution.

A second review by the Albumin Reviewers of the Cochrane Collaboration, published in October 2004, included the results of the SAFE study and concluded that "there is no evidence that albumin reduces mortality when compared with cheaper alternatives, such as saline", for patients with hypovolemia or in critically ill patients with burns and hypoalbuminemia.

DRUG INTERACTIONS: Drug-Drug Interactions: PLASBUMIN-5 is compatible with the standard isotonic carbohydrate and electrolyte solutions intended for intravenous use. It should not be mixed with protein hydrolysates, amino acid solutions or solutions containing alcohol. It should also not be mixed with whole blood, packed red cells, and other medicinal products. Specialized references (e.g. Trissel's Handbook of Injectable Drugs) should be consulted for specific compatibility information.

DOSAGE AND ADMINISTRATION: Recommended Dose and Dosage Adjustment: The volume administered should be adapted to the response of the individual patient. The infusion rate must be adjusted to individual requirements, based on initial assessment and monitoring of the patient's status. It should normally not exceed 5 mL/minute.

Hypovolemic Shock: The volume infused should be related to the estimated volume deficit and the speed of administration adapted to the response of the patient.

Burn Therapy: After a burn injury (usually beyond 24 hours) there is a close correlation between the amount of albumin infused and the resultant increase in plasma colloid osmotic pressure. The aim should be to maintain the plasma albumin concentration in the region of 2.5 g±0.5 g per 100 mL with a plasma oncotic pressure of 20 mmHg (equivalent to a total plasma protein concentration of 5.2 g per 100 mL). This is best achieved by the intravenous administration of PLASBUMIN, usually as PLASBUMIN-25. The duration of therapy is decided by the loss of protein from burned areas and in the urine. In addition, oral or parenteral feeding with amino acids should be initiated, as the long-term administration of albumin should not be considered as a source of nutrition.

Cardiopulmonary Bypass: See Indications and Clinical Use, Cardiopulmonary Bypass.

Acute Liver Failure: See Indications and Clinical Use, Acute Liver Failure.

Sequestration of Protein Rich Fluids: See Indications and Clinical Use, Sequestration of Protein Rich Fluids.

Administration: PLASBUMIN-5 should always be administered by intravenous infusion. The choice between the use of PLASBUMIN-5 and PLASBUMIN-25 depends upon whether or not the patient requires primarily a higher colloid osmotic activity (PLASBUMIN-25). Albumin solutions must not be diluted with sterile water for injection to avoid hemolysis and acute renal failure in recipients (see Drug Interactions).

Remove seal to expose stopper. Always swab stopper top immediately with a suitable antiseptic prior to entering vial.

Parenteral drug products should be inspected visually for particulate matter and discoloration prior to administration, whenever solution and container permit.

Dispensing pins or 16 gauge needles should only be used with 20 mL vial sizes and larger. Needles or dispensing pins should only be inserted within the stopper area delineated by the raised ring. The stopper should be penetrated perpendicular to the plane of the stopper within the ring.

Solutions which have been frozen should not be used. Do not use if turbid. Do not begin administration more than 4 hours after the container has been entered. Partially used vials must be discarded. Vials which are cracked or which have been previously entered or damaged should not be used, as this may have allowed the entry of microorganisms. PLASBUMIN-5 contains no preservative.

There exists a risk of potentially fatal hymolysis and acute renal failure from the use of sterile water for injection as a diluent for PLASBUMIN-5. Acceptable diluents include 0.9% sodium chloride or 5% dextrose in water.

OVERDOSAGE:

To date, there have been no reported cases of overdose for PLASBUMIN-5. No data are available in regard to overdosage in humans; however, because PLASBUMIN-5 is hyperoncotic, patients should be monitored against the possibility of circulatory overload. If overdose occurs, provide standard supportive treatment as necessary.

Hypervolemia may occur if the dosage and rate of infusion are too high. If hypervolemia is suspected, the infusion should be stopped immediately and the patient's hemodynamic parameters should be carefully monitored.

> For management of a suspected drug overdose, CPhA recommends that you contact your **regional Poison Control Centre**. See the *CPS* Directory section for a list of Poison Control Centres.

ACTION AND CLINICAL PHARMACOLOGY: Mechanism of Action: PLASBUMIN-5 is oncotically (colloid osmotic) equivalent volume for volume to normal human plasma.

When administered intravenously to an adequately hydrated subject, the oncotic effect of PLASBUMIN-5 is to expand the circulating blood volume by an amount approximately equal to the volume infused.

Albumin is a transport protein that binds to many substances, including drugs and bilirubin. This could be of importance in acute liver failure where albumin might serve the dual role of supporting plasma oncotic pressure, as well as binding excessive plasma bilirubin.

STORAGE AND STABILITY: Store at room temperature not exceeding 30°C. Do not freeze. Do not use after expiration date.

The product should be used within 4 hours after the container has been entered.

INFORMATION FOR THE PATIENT: Published in e-CPS, available by subscription at www.e-cps.ca.

DOSAGE FORMS, COMPOSITION AND PACKAGING: Each vial of sterile, aqueous solution for i.v. administration contains albumin (human) 5%, USP: 2.5 g (in 50 mL) and 12.5 g (in 250 mL). Also contains sodium caprylate 0.004 M, and acetyltryptophan 0.004 M and is buffered with sodium carbonate. Preservative-free. Approximate sodium content: 145 mEq/L. Rubber-stoppered vials of 50 (pediatric size) and 250 mL.

A sterile filter needle is provided with the 50 mL size of PLASBUMIN-5. The filter needle is to be used to facilitate the administration of albumin to patients in a pediatric setting.

Plasbumin®-25

albumin (human)

Plasma Substitute/Blood Derivative

Talecris

Date of Revision: January 19, 2009

SUMMARY PRODUCT INFORMATION:

Route of Administration	Dosage Form/ Strength	Clinically Relevant Nonmedicinal Ingredients
Intravenous injection	Intravenous solution, 25%	For a complete listing see Dosage Forms, Composition and Packaging.

DESCRIPTION: PLASBUMIN-25 (Albumin [Human] 25%, USP) is a 25% sterile solution of albumin in an aqueous diluent. The preparation is stabilized with 0.02 M sodium caprylate and 0.02 M acetyltryptophan and buffered with sodium carbonate. The approximate sodium content of the product is 145 mEq/L. It contains no preservative. PLASBUMIN-25 must be administered intravenously.

PLASBUMIN-25 is made from pooled human venous plasma using the Cohn cold ethanol fractionation process. Part of the fractionation may be performed by another licensed manufacturer. It is prepared in accordance with the applicable requirements established by the U.S. Food and Drug Administration.

INDICATIONS AND CLINICAL USE: The oncotic and colloid properties of PLASBUMIN-25 are used to restore and maintain circulating blood volume, when needed, and when the use of a colloid is appropriate. The choice of PLASBUMIN-25 over artificial colloid or crystalloid solutions will depend on the clinical situation of the individual patient, according to current therapeutic guidelines and recommendations.

Emergency Treatment of Hypovolemic Shock: PLASBUMIN-25 is hyperoncotic and on intravenous infusion will expand the plasma volume by an additional amount three to four times the volume actually administered, by withdrawing fluid from the interstitial spaces, provided the patient is normally hydrated interstitially or there is interstitial edema. If the patient is dehydrated, additional crystalloids must be given or alternatively, PLASBUMIN-5 should be used. The patient's hemodynamic response should be monitored and the usual precautions against circulatory overload observed. The total dose should not exceed the level of albumin found in the normal individual, i.e., about 2 g per kg body weight in the absence of active bleeding. Although PLASBUMIN-5 is to be preferred for the usual volume deficits, PLASBUMIN-25 with appropriate crystalloids may offer therapeutic advantages in oncotic deficits or in long-standing shock where treatment has been delayed.

Removal of ascitic fluid from a patient with cirrhosis may cause changes in cardiovascular function and even result in hypovolemic shock. In such circumstances, the use of an albumin infusion may be required to support the blood volume.

Burn Therapy: An optimal therapeutic regimen with respect to the administration of colloids, crystalloids, and water following extensive burns has not been established. During the first 24 hours after sustaining thermal injury, large volumes of crystalloids are infused to restore the depleted extracellular fluid volume. Beyond 24 hours PLASBUMIN-25 can be used to maintain plasma colloid osmotic pressure.

Hypoproteinemia With or Without Edema: During major surgery, patients can lose over half of their circulating albumin with the attendant complications of oncotic deficit. A similar situation can occur in sepsis or intensive care patients. Treatment with PLASBUMIN-25 may be of value in such cases.

Adult Respiratory Distress Syndrome (ARDS): This is characterized by deficient oxygenation caused by pulmonary interstitial edema complicating shock and postsurgical conditions. When clinical signs are those of hypoproteinemia with a fluid volume overload, PLASBUMIN-25 together with a diuretic may play a role in therapy.

Cardiopulmonary Bypass: With the relatively small priming volume required with modern pumps, preoperative dilution of the blood using albumin and crystalloid has been shown to be safe and well-tolerated. Although the limit to which the hematocrit and plasma protein concentration can be safely lowered has not been defined, it is common practice to adjust the albumin and crystalloid pump prime to achieve a hematocrit of 20% and a plasma albumin concentration of 2.5 g per 100 mL in the patient.

Acute Liver Failure: In the uncommon situation of rapid loss of liver function with or without coma, administration of albumin may serve the double purpose of supporting the colloid osmotic pressure of the plasma as well as binding excess plasma bilirubin.

Neonatal Hemolytic Disease: The administration of PLASBUMIN-25 may be indicated prior to exchange transfusion, in order to bind free bilirubin, thus lessening the risk of kernicterus. A dosage of 1 g/kg body weight is given about 1 hour prior to exchange transfusion. Caution must be observed in hypervolemic infants (see Warnings and Precautions).

Sequestration of Protein Rich Fluids: This occurs in such conditions as acute peritonitis, pancreatitis, mediastinitis, and extensive cellulitis. The magnitude of loss into the third space may require treatment of reduced volume or oncotic activity with an infusion of albumin.

Erythrocyte Resuspension: Albumin may be required to avoid excessive hypoproteinemia, during certain types of exchange transfusion, or with the use of very large volumes of previously frozen or washed red cells. About 25 g of albumin per liter of erythrocytes is commonly used, although the requirements in preexistent hypoproteinemia or hepatic impairment can be greater. PLASBUMIN-25 is added to the isotonic suspension of washed red cells immediately prior to transfusion.

Acute Nephrosis: Certain patients may not respond to cyclophosphamide or steroid therapy. The steroids may even aggravate the underlying edema. In this situation a loop diuretic and 100 mL PLASBUMIN-25 repeated daily for 7 to 10 days may be helpful in controlling the edema and the patient may then respond to steroid treatment.

Renal Dialysis: Although not part of the regular regimen of renal dialysis, PLASBUMIN-25 may be of value in the treatment of shock or hypotension in these patients. The usual volume administered is about 100 mL, taking particular care to avoid fluid overload as these patients are often fluid overloaded and cannot tolerate substantial volumes of salt solution.

Situations in Which Albumin Administration is Not Warranted: In chronic nephrosis, infused albumin is promptly excreted by the kidneys with no relief of the chronic edema or effect on the underlying renal lesion. It is of occasional use in the rapid "priming" diuresis of nephrosis. Similarly, in hypoproteinemic states associated with chronic cirrhosis, malabsorption, protein losing enteropathies, pancreatic insufficiency, and undernutrition, the infusion of albumin as a source of protein nutrition is not justified.

CONTRAINDICATIONS:

- PLASBUMIN-25 should not be given to patients who are hypersensitive to albumin or to any ingredient in the formulation or component of the container. For a complete listing, see Dosage Forms, Composition and Packaging.
- PLASBUMIN-25 should not be given to patients at special risk of developing circulatory overload (i.e., those with a history of congestive cardiac failure, renal insufficiency or stabilized chronic anemia).

WARNINGS AND PRECAUTIONS: General: PLASBUMIN-25 is made from human plasma. Products made from human plasma may contain infectious agents, such as viruses, that can cause disease. The risk that such products will transmit an infectious agent has been reduced by screening plasma donors for prior exposure to certain viruses, by testing for the presence of certain current virus infections, and by inactivating and/or removing certain viruses. Despite these measures, such products can still potentially transmit disease. There is also the possibility that unknown infectious agents may be present in such products. Individuals who receive infusions of blood or plasma products may develop signs and/or symptoms of some viral infections, particularly hepatitis C. ALL infections thought by a physician possibly to have been transmitted by this product should be reported by the physician or other healthcare provider to Talecris Biotherapeutics Ltd. [1-866-482-5226].

Albumin is a derivative of human blood. Based on effective donor screening and product manufacturing processes, it carries an extremely remote risk for transmission of viral diseases. A theoretical risk for transmission of Creutzfeldt-Jakob Disease (CJD), including variant Creutzfeldt-Jakob disease (vCJD), also is considered extremely remote. No cases of transmission of viral diseases or CJD, including vCJD, have ever been identified for albumin.

The physician should discuss the risks and benefits of this product with the patient, before prescribing or administering to the patient.

PLASBUMIN-25 must not be diluted with sterile water for injection as this may cause hemolysis and acute renal failure in recipients (see Dosage and Administration).

Blood coagulation parameters, the hematocrit and serum electrolytes should be monitored when a large volume of PLASBUMIN-25 solution is administered.

Patients should always be monitored carefully in order to guard against the possibility of circulatory overload. PLASBUMIN-25 is hyperoncotic, therefore, in the presence of dehydration, albumin must be given with or followed by addition of fluids.

PLASBUMIN-25 is not tested for aluminum content and may contain more than 200 µg/L of aluminum. It should, therefore, not be used to treat infants or patients on hemodialysis.

In hemorrhage the administration of albumin should be supplemented by the transfusion of whole blood to treat the relative anemia associated with hemodilution. When circulating blood volume has been reduced, hemodilution following the administration of albumin persists for many hours. In patients with a normal blood volume, hemodilution lasts for a much shorter period.

The rapid rise in blood pressure which may follow the administration of a colloid with positive oncotic activity necessitates careful observation to detect and treat severed blood vessels which may not have bled at the lower blood pressure.

Special Populations: Pregnant and Nursing Women: Animal reproduction studies have not been conducted with PLASBUMIN-25. It is not known whether it can cause harm to the fetus or nursing child. PLASBUMIN-25 should be given to a pregnant or nursing woman only if the benefit outweighs any potential risk.

Pediatrics: The use of PLASBUMIN-25 in children has not been associated with any special or specific hazard, if the dose is appropriate for the child's body weight. However, its use should be carefully evaluated for risk and benefit in pediatric treatment and PLASBUMIN-25 should not be used in neonates and infants (see Warnings and Precautions: General).

ADVERSE REACTIONS: Adverse Drug Reaction Overview: Adverse reactions to albumin are rare. Such reactions may be allergic in nature or due to high plasma protein levels from excessive albumin administration. Allergic manifestations include urticaria, chills, fever, and changes in respiration, pulse and blood pressure. The possibility of an anaphylactic reaction occurring in association with albumin is considered extremely rare. In the case of an anaphylactic reaction, discontinue infusion and treat appropriately.

The Cochrane Injuries Group published a meta-analysis (July 1998) in which an increase in mortality was reported in albumin-treated patients compared to patients who had received crystalloids or no treatment. However, the analysis was criticized by many authors, due to substantial methodological concerns.

In 2001, Wilkes et. al. published a revised meta-analysis, which showed no evidence of excess albumin-associated mortality, but suggested that albumin might actually reduce mortality.

The Saline versus Albumin Fluid Evaluation (SAFE) Study reported in the New England Journal of Medicine in May 2004, involving nearly 7000 critically ill patients, addressed one of the most fundamental and contentious issues in critical care: the value of colloids as opposed to crystalloids in the resuscitation of seriously ill patients. Based on these results, the administration of albumin appears to be safe for up to 28 days in a heterogeneous population of critically ill patients, and may be beneficial in patients with severe sepsis. A greater number of patients with trauma involving brain injury died among those randomly assigned to albumin as opposed to saline (59 of 241 in the albumin group compared to 38 of 251 in the saline group with a relative risk of 1.62 and p=0.009). However, the overall number of these patients was relatively small. The study had insufficient power to detect differences in mortality among the predefined subgroups and the authors warn that the observed difference should be interpreted with caution.

A second review by the Albumin Reviewers of the Cochrane Collaboration, published in October 2004, included the results of the SAFE study and concluded that "there is no evidence that albumin reduces mortality when compared with cheaper alternatives, such as saline", for patients with hypovolemia or in critically ill patients with burns and hypoalbuminemia.

DRUG INTERACTIONS: Drug-Drug Interactions: PLASBUMIN-25 is compatible with the standard isotonic carbohydrate and electrolyte solutions intended for intravenous use. It should not be mixed with protein hydrolysates, amino acid solutions or solutions containing alcohol. It should also not be mixed with whole blood, packed red cells, and other medicinal products. Specialized references (e.g. Trissel's Handbook of Injectable Drugs) should be consulted for specific compatibility information.

DOSAGE AND ADMINISTRATION: Recommended Dose and Dosage Adjustment: The infusion rate must be adjusted to individual requirements, based on initial assessment and monitoring of the patient's status. It should normally not exceed 1 to 2 mL/minute.

Hypovolemic Shock: For treatment of hypovolemic shock, the volume administered and the speed of infusion should be adapted to the response of the individual patient.

Burn Therapy: After a burn injury (usually beyond 24 hours) there is a close correlation between the amount of albumin infused and the resultant increase in plasma colloid osmotic pressure. The aim should be to maintain the plasma albumin concentration in the region of 2.5 g±0.5 g per 100 mL with a plasma oncotic pressure of 20 mmHg (equivalent to a total plasma protein concentration of 5.2 g per 100 mL). This is best achieved by the intravenous administration of PLASBUMIN-25. The duration of therapy is decided by the loss of protein from the burned areas and in the urine. In addition, oral or parenteral feeding with amino acids should be initiated, as the long-term administration of albumin should not be considered as a source of nutrition.

Hypoproteinemia With or Without Edema: Unless the underlying pathology responsible for the hypoproteinemia can be corrected, the intravenous administration of PLASBUMIN-25 must be considered purely symptomatic or supportive (see Indications and Clinical Use, Situations in Which Albumin Administration is Not Warranted). The usual daily dose of albumin for adults is 50 to 75 g and for children 25 g. Patients with severe hypoproteinemia who continue to lose albumin may require larger quantities. Since hypoproteinemic patients usually have approximately normal blood volumes, the rate of administration of PLASBUMIN-25 should not exceed 2 mL per minute, as more rapid injection may precipitate circulatory embarrassment and pulmonary edema.

Adult Respiratory Distress Syndrome (ARDS): See Indications and Clinical Use, Adult Respiratory Distress Syndrome (ARDS).

Cardiopulmonary Bypass: See Indications and Clinical Use, Cardiopulmonary Bypass.

Acute Liver Failure: See Indications and Clinical Use, Acute Liver Failure.

Neonatal Hemolytic Disease: See Indications and Clinical Use, Neonatal Hemolytic Disease.

Sequestration of Protein Rich Fluids: See Indications and Clinical Use, Sequestration of Protein Rich Fluids.

Erythrocyte Resuspension: See Indications and Clinical Use, Erythrocyte Resuspension.

Acute Nephrosis: See Indications and Clinical Use, Acute Nephrosis.

Renal Dialysis: See Indications and Clinical Use, Renal Dialysis.

Administration: PLASBUMIN-25 should always be administered by intravenous infusion. If sodium restriction is required, PLASBUMIN-25 may be administered either undiluted or diluted in a sodium-free carbohydrate solution such as 5% dextrose in water. PLASBUMIN-25 must not be diluted with sterile water for injection to avoid hemolysis and acute renal failure in recipients (see Drug Interactions).

Remove seal to expose stopper. Always swab stopper top immediately with a suitable antiseptic prior to entering vial.

Parenteral drug products should be inspected visually for particulate matter and discoloration prior to administration, whenever solution and container permit.

Dispensing pins or 16 gauge needles should only be used with 20 mL vial sizes and larger. Needles or dispensing pins should only be inserted within the stopper area delineated by the raised ring. The stopper should be penetrated perpendicular to the plane of the stopper within the ring.

Solutions which have been frozen should not be used. Do not use if turbid. Do not begin administration more than 4 hours after the container has been entered. Partially used vials must be discarded. Vials which are cracked or which have been previously entered or damaged should not be used, as this may have allowed the entry of microorganisms. PLASBUMIN-25 contains no preservative.

There exists a risk of potentially fatal hemolysis and acute renal failure from the use of sterile water for injection as a diluent for PLASBUMIN-25. Acceptable diluents include 0.9% sodium chloride or 5% dextrose in water.

OVERDOSAGE:

To date, there have been no reported cases of overdose for PLASBUMIN-25. No data are available in regard to overdosage in humans; however, because PLASBUMIN-25 is hyperoncotic, patients should be monitored against the possibility of circulatory overload. If overdose occurs, provide standard supportive treatment as necessary.

Hypervolemia may occur if the dosage and rate of infusion are too high. If hypervolemia is suspected, the infusion should be stopped immediately and the patient's hemodynamic parameters should be carefully monitored.

For management of a suspected drug overdose, CPhA recommends that you contact your **regional Poison Control Centre**. See the *CPS* Directory section for a list of Poison Control Centres.

ACTION AND CLINICAL PHARMACOLOGY: Mechanism of Action: Each 100 mL vial of PLASBUMIN-25 supplies the oncotic (colloid osmotic) equivalent of approximately 500 mL citrated plasma.

When administered intravenously to an adequately hydrated subject, the oncotic effect of 20 mL PLASBUMIN-25 is such that it will draw approximately a further 70 mL of fluid from the extravascular tissues into the circulation within 15 minutes, thus increasing the total blood volume and reducing both hemoconcentration and whole blood viscosity. Accordingly, the main clinical indications are for hypoproteinemic states involving reduced oncotic pressure, with or without accompanying edema. PLASBUMIN-25 can also be used as a plasma volume expander.

Albumin is a transport protein that binds to many substances, including drugs and bilirubin. Infused albumin may reduce the level of free bilirubin in the blood.

This could also be of importance in acute liver failure where albumin might serve the dual role of supporting plasma oncotic pressure, as well as binding excessive plasma bilirubin.

STORAGE AND STABILITY: Store at room temperature not exceeding 30°C. Do not freeze. Do not use after expiration date. The product should be used within 4 hours after the container has been entered.

INFORMATION FOR THE PATIENT: Published in e-CPS, available by subscription at www.e-cps.ca.

DOSAGE FORMS, COMPOSITION AND PACKAGING: Each vial of sterile, aqueous solution for i.v. administration contains: 25 g albumin (human) 25%, USP. The solution also contains sodium caprylate 0.02 M and acetyltryptophan 0.02 M and is buffered with sodium carbonate. Preservative-free. Approximate sodium content: 145 mEq/L. Rubber-stoppered vials of 100 mL.

Plavix® Ⓟ

clopidogrel bisulfate

Platelet Aggregation Inhibitor

sanofi-aventis

Date of Revision: September 4, 2009

SUMMARY PRODUCT INFORMATION:

Route of Administration	Dosage Form/ Strength	All Nonmedicinal Ingredients
Oral	Tablet 75 and 300 mg	Tablet Core: mannitol, microcrystalline cellulose, polyethelene glycol 6000, low-substituted hydroxypropylcellulose, hydrogenated castor oil Coating: lactose, hypromellose, titanium dioxide, triacetin, red iron oxide Polishing: carnauba wax

INDICATIONS AND CLINICAL USE: MI, Stroke or Established Peripheral Arterial Disease: PLAVIX (clopidogrel bisulfate) is indicated for the secondary prevention of atherothrombotic events (myocardial infarction, stroke and vascular death) in patients with atherosclerosis documented by stroke, myocardial infarction, or established peripheral arterial disease.

Acute Coronary Syndrome:

- PLAVIX, in combination with acetylsalicylic acid (ASA), is indicated for the early and long-term secondary prevention of atherothrombotic events (myocardial infarction, ischemic stroke, cardiovascular death and/or refractory ischemia) in patients with acute coronary syndromes- without ST segment elevation (ie. unstable angina or non-Q-wave myocardial infarction). These benefits of PLAVIX have been shown only when these patients were concomitantly treated with ASA in addition to other standard therapies. These benefits were also seen in patients who were managed medically and those who were managed with percutaneous coronary intervention (with or without stent) or CABG (coronary artery bypass graft).
- For patients with ST-segment elevation acute myocardial infarction, PLAVIX has been shown to reduce the rate of an endpoint of all-cause mortality and the rate of a combined endpoint of death, re-infarction or stroke.

Pediatrics (<18 years of age): No data available.

CONTRAINDICATIONS:

- Patients who are hypersensitive to this drug or to any ingredient in the formulation or component of the container. For a complete listing, see Dosage Forms, Composition and Packaging.
- Active bleeding such as peptic ulcer and intracranial hemorrhage.
- Significant liver impairment or cholestatic jaundice.

WARNINGS AND PRECAUTIONS: General: As with other antiplatelet agents, when considering prescribing PLAVIX (clopidogrel bisulfate), physicians should inquire whether the patient has a history of bleeding. Clopidogrel should be used with caution in patients who may be at risk of increased bleeding from recent trauma, surgery or other pathological condition(s).

Because of the increased risk of bleeding, the concomitant administration of warfarin with clopidogrel should be undertaken with caution (see Drug Interactions).

In patients with recent transient ischaemic attack (TIA) or stroke who are at high risk of recurrent ischemic events, the combination of aspirin and PLAVIX has not been shown to be more effective than PLAVIX alone, but the combination has been shown to increase major bleeding (see Drug Interactions).

If a patient is to undergo elective surgery, consideration should be given to discontinue PLAVIX 5 to 7 days prior to surgery to allow for the reversal of the effect.

Platelet transfusion may be used to reverse the pharmacological effects of PLAVIX when quick reversal is required.

Concomitant Use of PLAVIX and Proton-Pump Inhibitors (PPI): Observational studies have reported that PPIs may reduce the inhibitory effect of clopidogrel on platelet aggregation and, thereby, the antithrombotic activity. Pending definitive data of the results of adequately designed clinical trials to characterize the clinical significance of this possible interaction, the concomitant therapy of PLAVIX and PPIs is discouraged (see Drug Interactions, Table 5; see also Action and Clinical Pharmacology, Pharmacokinetics, Pharmacogenetics).

Concomitant Use of PLAVIX and CYP2C19 Isoenzyme Inhibitors: Since clopidogrel is metabolized to its active metabolite partly by CYP2C19, use of drugs that inhibit the activity of this enzyme would be expected to result in reduced drug levels of the active metabolite of clopidogrel and a reduction in clinical efficacy. The use of drugs known to inhibit CYP2C19 should be discouraged in patients taking clopidogrel (see Drug Interactions).

Pharmacogenetics—Metabolism: Based on literature data, patients with genetically reduced CYP2C19 function have lower systemic exposure to the active metabolite of clopidogrel and diminished antiplatelet responses, and generally exhibit higher cardiovascular event rates following myocardial infarction or stent placement than do patients with normal CYP2C19 function (see Action and Clinical Pharmacology, Pharmacokinetics, Pharmacogenetics).

Gastrointestinal: Active GI Lesions: PLAVIX (clopidogrel bisulfate) prolongs bleeding time. Although PLAVIX has shown a lower incidence of gastrointestinal bleeding compared to ASA in a large controlled clinical trial (CAPRIE), PLAVIX should not be used in patients who have lesions with a propensity to bleed. In CURE, the incidence of major GI bleeding was 1.3% versus 0.7% (PLAVIX+ASA versus placebo+ASA, respectively).

In patients taking PLAVIX, drugs that might induce GI lesions should be used with caution.

Hematologic: Thrombotic Thrombocytopenic Purpura (TTP): Thrombotic thrombocytopenic purpura (TTP) has been reported rarely following the use of PLAVIX, but it can occur anytime during the first year of exposure. Few cases have been reported after more than one year of exposure. TTP is a potentially fatal condition requiring prompt treatment with plasmapheresis. It is characterized by thrombocytopenia, microangiopathic hemolytic anemia (schistocytes [fragmented RBC's] seen on peripheral smear), neurological findings, renal dysfunction, and fever.

Hepatic/Biliary/Pancreatic: Experience is limited in patients with moderate hepatic impairment who may have bleeding diatheses. As with any patient exhibiting hepatic impairment, liver function should be carefully monitored and PLAVIX should be used with caution.

In the CAPRIE study, there were 344 hepatically impaired patients (Alkaline phosphatase >300 U/L, or ALT >120 U/L, or AST >75 U/L) and 168 received clopidogrel for a mean duration of 18 months. The adverse events were more common in this population, compared to the rest of the CAPRIE population, and more common in the clopidogrel (N=168) than in the ASA (N=176) group (any bleeding disorders, N=17 vs N=14; any rash, N=11 vs N=6; diarrhea, N=8 vs N=3, respectively).

Peri-Operative Considerations: If a patient is to undergo elective surgery, consideration should be given to discontinue PLAVIX 5 to 7 days prior to surgery to allow for a reversal of its effect.

Clopidogrel should be used with caution in patients who may be at risk of increased bleeding from recent surgery.

Renal: Therapeutic experience with clopidogrel is limited in patients with severe and moderate renal impairment. Therefore, PLAVIX should be used with caution in these patients.

Special Populations: Pregnant Women: There are no adequate and well-controlled studies in pregnant women.

Reproduction studies have been performed in rats at doses up to 500 mg/kg per day and in rabbits at doses up to 300 mg/kg per day and have revealed no evidence of impaired fertility or harm to the fetus due to clopidogrel. Because animal reproduction studies are not always predictive of a human response, PLAVIX should be used during pregnancy only if the potential benefits outweigh the potential risks to the fetus.

Nursing Women: Studies in rats have shown that clopidogrel and/or its metabolites are excreted in milk. It is not known whether this drug is excreted in human milk. Therefore, clopidogrel should not be used by lactating women.

Pediatrics (<18 years of age): Safety and effectiveness in subjects below the age of 18 have not been established.

ADVERSE REACTIONS: Adverse Drug Reaction Overview: The safety profile of clopidogrel has been evaluated in clinical trials in more than 42 000 patients and further assessed during post-marketing experience.

Of the patients who participated in the CAPRIE, CURE and CLARITY double-blind international clinical trials, approximately 50% were elderly patients (>65 years) and 15% were 75 years and older. 9000 patients were treated for one year or more. In COMMIT, approximately 58% of the patients treated with PLAVIX were 60 years and older, 26% of whom were 70 years and older.

The most frequent adverse drug reactions (≥1%) with PLAVIX (with or without associated ASA) in controlled clinical trials were hemorrhage and bleeding disorders including purpura, any rash, dyspepsia, abdominal pain and diarrhea (see Clinical Trial Adverse Drug Reactions).

The most serious adverse drug reactions from controlled clinical trials rarely reported (<1%) were bleeding and clotting disorders including gastrointestinal hemorrhage, hemorrhagic ulcer and hemothorax.

Blood Disorders: agranulocytosis/granulocytopenia, aplastic anemia, neutropenia and thrombocytopenia.
Gastrointestinal System Disorders: duodenal, gastric or peptic ulcer, gastritis.
Skin Disorders: any rash and bullous eruption.

The overall incidence of study drug discontinuation because of adverse events was similar in both groups in CAPRIE (PLAVIX 11.9% and ASA 11.9%). In CURE, study drug discontinuation occurred in 5.8 % of patients with PLAVIX plus ASA and 3.9% of patients with placebo plus ASA. In CLARITY, study drug discontinuation was greater in the placebo group (8.6%) compared with the clopidogrel group (6.9%). In COMMIT, the overall incidence of discontinuations was similar between the two treatment groups (2.4% in the clopidogrel group versus 2.2% in the placebo group).

Clinical Trial Adverse Drug Reactions: Because clinical trials are conducted under very specific conditions the adverse reaction rates observed in the clinical trials may not reflect the rates observed in practice and should not be compared to the rates in the clinical trials of another drug. Adverse drug reaction information from clinical trials is useful for identifying drug-related adverse events and for approximating rates.

CAPRIE: With few exceptions (see Table 1) the overall tolerability of PLAVIX was similar regardless of age, sex and race. However, in women there was a slightly higher incidence of bleeding disorders in the clopidogrel group (11.36% vs 9.88%).

Clinically Important Adverse Events: The clinically important adverse events observed in CAPRIE were the following:

Bleeding and Clotting Disorders: One case of Henoch-Schönlein purpura (acute visceral symptoms: vomiting, diarrhea, abdominal distension, hematuria, renal colic) was reported in a patient taking PLAVIX. The patient recovered without sequellae within one month. Rare cases of platelet count ≤30 000/mm³ have been reported. The overall incidence of bleeding on clopidogrel and ASA was the same (9.3%). The incidence of severe cases was 1.4% and 1.6% in the clopidogrel and ASA groups respectively. The overall incidence of other bleeding disorders was higher in the clopidogrel group (7.3%) compared to ASA (6.5%). However, the incidence of severe events was similar in both treatment groups (0.6% vs 0.4%).

Gastrointestinal: Overall, the incidence of gastrointestinal events (e.g. abdominal pain, dyspepsia, gastritis and constipation) in patients receiving PLAVIX (clopidogrel bisulfate) was 27.1%, compared to 29.8% in those receiving ASA. The incidence of patients withdrawing from treatment because of gastrointestinal adverse reactions was 3.2% for PLAVIX and 4.0% for ASA.

Hepatic and Biliary Disorders: The overall incidence of hepatic and biliary disorders was similar in patients treated with clopidogrel (3.5%) compared to ASA (3.4%). The most frequent events were increased liver enzymes and bilirubinemia.

Skin Disorders: The incidence of skin and appendage disorders in patients receiving PLAVIX was 15.8% (0.7% serious); the corresponding rate in ASA patients was 13.1% (0.5% serious). There was no notable difference between treatment groups in the incidence of bullous eruptions (0.23% PLAVIX versus 0.16% ASA). One case of a severe bullous eruption was reported in a patient taking PLAVIX. The overall incidence of patients withdrawing from treatment because of skin and appendage disorders adverse reactions was 1.5% for PLAVIX and 0.8% for ASA.

A summary of the clinically relevant adverse effects observed in CAPRIE are presented in Table 1. In CAPRIE, patients with a known intolerance to ASA were excluded from the study.

Table 1: PLAVIX

Summary of Adverse Events Occurring in ≥1% of PLAVIX Patients in CAPRIE Trial

Adverse Event	PLAVIX (n=9599) %	ASA (n=9586) %
Body as a Whole		
Accidental/Inflicted Injury	7.9	7.3
Chest Pain	8.3	8.3
Influenza-like Symptoms	7.5	7
Fatigue	3.3	3.4
Pain	6.4	6.3
Cardiovascular		
Dependent Edema	1.2	1.3
Edema	1.0	1.2
Heart and Rhythm Disorder	4.3	5.0[a]
Hypertension	4.3	5.1
Peripheral Edema	1.2	1.6
Central Nervous System		
Dizziness	6.2	6.7
Headache	7.6	7.2
Endocrine and Metabolism		
Hypercholesterolemia	4.0	4.4
Gastrointestinal		
Any Event	27.1	29.8
Abdominal Pain	5.6	7.1[a]
Constipation	2.4	3.3[a]
Diarrhea severe[b] leading to discontinuation[b]	4.5[a] 0.2 0.4	3.4 0.1 0.3
Dyspepsia	5.2	6.1[a]
Flatulence	1.0	1.1
Nausea	3.4	3.8
Vomiting	1.3	1.4
Genitourinary		
Urinary Tract Infection	3.1	3.5
Hemorrhages or Bleeding		

(cont'd)

Table 1: PLAVIX *(cont'd)*

Summary of Adverse Events Occurring in ≥1% of PLAVIX Patients in CAPRIE Trial

Adverse Event	PLAVIX (n=9599) %	ASA (n=9586) %
Epistaxis	2.9	2.5
Hematoma	1.6	1.5
Gastrointestinal Hemorrhage requiring hospitalization	2.0 0.7	2.7[a] 1.1
Purpura (primarily bruising & ecchymosis)	5.3[a]	3.7
Musculoskeletal		
Arthralgia	6.3	6.2
Back Pain	5.8	5.3
Psychiatric Disorder		
Depression	3.6	3.9
Skin		
Any Event	15.8	13.1
Pruritus	3.3[a]	1.6
Rash severe[b] leading to discontinuation[b]	4.2[a] 0.1 0.5	3.5 0.1 0.2
Respiratory		
Bronchitis	3.7	3.7
Coughing	3.1	2.7
Dyspnea	4.5	4.7
Rhinitis	4.2	4.2
Upper Respiratory Tract Infection	8.7	8.3

[a] Statistically significant difference between treatments (p≤0.05).
[b] Patients may be included in more than 1 category.

No clinically relevant events other than those observed in CAPRIE have been reported with a frequency ≥2.5% during the CURE, CLARITY and COMMIT controlled studies.

The number of patients discontinuing due to adverse reactions in CAPRIE are shown in Table 2.

Table 2: PLAVIX

Patients Discontinued Because of Adverse Experiences in CAPRIE (number and percentage of patients)

Adverse Experience	Study Drug Permanently Discontinued	
	PLAVIX N=9599 (%)	ASA N=9586 (%)
Rash	0.90	0.41[a]
Diarrhea	0.42	0.27
Indigestion/Nausea/Vomiting	1.9	2.41[a]
Any Bleeding Disorder	1.20	1.37
Intracranial Hemorrhage	0.21	0.33
Gastrointestinal Hemorrhage	0.52	0.93[a]
Abnormal Liver Function	0.23	0.29

[a] Statistically significant, p<0.05.

CURE: In CURE, PLAVIX was given with ASA and was not associated with a significant increase in life-threatening or fatal bleeds compared to placebo given with ASA; the incidences of non-life threatening major bleeding and minor bleeding were significantly larger in the PLAVIX+ASA group. The incidence of intracranial hemorrhage was 0.1% in both groups. The principal sites for major bleeding were primarily gastrointestinal and at arterial puncture sites. In patients receiving both PLAVIX and ASA in CURE, the incidence of bleeding is described in Table 3.

Table 3: PLAVIX

Incidence of Bleeding Complications (% patients)—CURE Trial

Event	PLAVIX+ASA[a] (N=6259)	Placebo+ASA[a] (N=6303)	p-value
Life-threatening Bleeding	2.2	1.8	0.13
Fatal	0.2	0.2	
5 g/dL Hemoglobin Drop	0.9	0.9	
Requiring Surgical Intervention	0.7	0.7	
Hemorrhagic Strokes	0.1	0.1	

(cont'd)

Table 3: PLAVIX *(cont'd)*

Incidence of Bleeding Complications (% patients)—CURE Trial

Event	PLAVIX+ASA[a] (N=6259)	Placebo+ASA[a] (N=6303)	p-value
Requiring Inotropes	0.5	0.5	
Requiring Transfusions (≥4 units)	1.2	1	
Other Major Bleeding	1.6	1	0.005
Significantly Disabling	0.4	0.3	
Intraocular Bleeding with Significant Loss of Vision	0.05	0.03	
Requiring 2–3 Units of Blood	1.3	0.9	
Major Bleeding[b]	3.7[c]	2.7[d]	0.001
Minor Bleeding[e]	5.1	2.4	<0.001
Total with Bleeding Complications	8.5	5.0	<0.001

[a] Other standard therapies were used as appropriate. All patients received ASA 75–325 mg daily (mean=160 mg).
[b] Life threatening and other major bleeding necessitating transfusion of ≥2 units of blood.
[c] Major bleeding event rate for PLAVIX+ASA was dose-dependent on ASA: <100 mg=2.6%; 100-200 mg=3.5%; >200 mg=4.9%.
[d] Major bleeding event rate for placebo+ASA was dose-dependent on ASA: <100 mg=2.0%; 100-200 mg=2.3%; >200 mg=4.0%.
[e] Led to interruption of study medication.

The number of patients with bleeding that met the criteria for major bleeding established by the Thrombolysis in Myocardial Infarction (TIMI) trial was 68 (1.09%) in the clopidogrel group and 73 (1.16%) in the placebo group (relative risk, 0.94; p=0.70). The number with bleeding that met the criteria for life-threatening or severe bleeding established by the Global Utilization of Streptokinase and Tissue Plasminogen Activator for Occluded Coronary Arteries (GUST) trial was 78 in the clopidogrel group and 70 in the placebo group (relative risk, 1.12; p=0.48). Some patients had more than one bleeding episode.

Ninety-two percent (92%) of the patients in the CURE study received unfractionated or low molecular weight heparin, and the rate of bleeding in these patients was similar to the overall results.

There was no excess in major bleeds within seven days after coronary bypass graft surgery in patients who stopped therapy more than five days prior to surgery (event rate 4.4% PLAVIX+ASA; 5.3% placebo+ASA). In patients who remained on therapy within five days of bypass graft surgery, the event rate was 9.6% for PLAVIX+ASA, and 6.3% for placebo+ASA, which was not significantly different.

Other potentially serious adverse events which may be of clinical interest but were rarely reported (<1%) in patients who received PLAVIX in the CAPRIE or CURE controlled clinical trials are listed below regardless of relationship to PLAVIX. In general, the incidence of these events was similar to that in patients receiving aspirin (in CAPRIE) or placebo+aspirin (in CURE).

Body as a Whole: allergic reaction and necrosis ischemic.
Cardiovascular Disorders: edema generalized.
Gastrointestinal System Disorders: gastric ulcer perforated, gastritis hemorrhagic and upper GI ulcer hemorrhagic.
Liver and Biliary System Disorders: bilirubinemia, hepatitis infectious and liver fatty.
Platelet, Bleeding and Clotting Disorders: hemarthrosis, hematuria, hemoptysis, hemorrhage intracranial, hemorrhage retroperitoneal, hemorrhage of operative wound, ocular hemorrhage, pulmonary embolism, pulmonary hemorrhage, purpura allergic.
Red Blood Cell Disorders: anemia aplastic, anemia hypochromic.
Reproductive Disorders, Female: menorrhagia.
Respiratory System Disorders: hemothorax.
Skin and Appendage Disorders: bullous eruption, rash erythematous, rash maculopapular, urticaria.
Urinary System Disorders: abnormal renal function, acute renal failure.
White Cell and Reticuloendothelial System Disorders: agranulocytosis, granulocytopenia, leukemia.

Other clinically relevant adverse drug reactions pooled from CAPRIE and CURE studies, or observed in other studies, with an incidence >0.1% as well as serious and relevant adverse drug reactions with an incidence <0.1% are presented below:

Central and Peripheral Nervous System Disorders: Uncommon: dizziness and paraesthesia. Rare: vertigo.
Gastrointestinal System Disorders: Common: dyspepsia, abdominal pain, diarrhea. Uncommon: nausea, gastritis, flatulence, constipation, vomiting, gastric ulcer, duodenal ulcer.
Platelet Bleeding and Clotting Disorders: Uncommon: bleeding time increased, platelets decreased. Very rare: thrombotic thrombocytopenic purpura (TTP).
Skin and Appendages Disorders: Uncommon: rash, pruritus.
White Cell and RES Disorders: Uncommon: leucopenia, neutrophils decreased, eosinophilia.

CLARITY: In CLARITY, the incidence of major bleeding (defined as intracranial bleeding or bleeding associated with a fall in hemoglobin >5 g/dL) was similar between groups (1.3% versus 1.1% in the PLAVIX+aspirin and in the placebo+aspirin groups, respectively). This was consistent across subgroups of patients defined by baseline characteristics, and type of fibrinolytics or heparin therapy. The incidence of fatal bleeding (0.8% versus 0.6% in the PLAVIX+aspirin and in the placebo+aspirin groups, respectively) and intracranial hemorrhage (0.5% versus 0.7%, respectively) was low and similar in both groups.

COMMIT: The overall rate of noncerebral major bleeding or cerebral bleeding in COMMIT was low and similar in both groups as shown in Table 4.

Table 4: PLAVIX

Number (%) of Patients with Bleeding Events in COMMIT

Type of Bleeding	PLAVIX (+ aspirin) (N=22 961)	Placebo (+ aspirin) (N=22 891)	P-value
Major[a] Noncerebral or Cerebral Bleeding[b]	134 (0.6%)	125 (0.5%)	0.59
Major Noncerebral	82 (0.4%)	73 (0.3%)	0.48
Fatal	36 (0.2%)	37 (0.2%)	0.9
Hemorrhagic Stroke	55 (0.2%)	56 (0.2%)	0.91
Fatal	39 (0.2%)	41 (0.2%)	0.81
Other Noncerebral Bleeding (non-major)	831 (3.6%)	721 (3.1%)	0.005

(cont'd)

Table 4: PLAVIX *(cont'd)*

Number (%) of Patients with Bleeding Events in COMMIT

Type of Bleeding	PLAVIX (+ aspirin) (N=22 961)	Placebo (+ aspirin) (N=22 891)	P-value
Any Noncerebral Bleeding	896 (3.9%)	777 (3.4%)	0.004

[a] Major bleeds are cerebral bleeds or non-cerebral bleeds thought to have caused death or that required transfusion.
[b] The relative rate of major noncerebral or cerebral bleeding was independent of age. Event rates for PLAVIX+aspirin by age were: <60 years=0.3%, ≥60 to <70 years=0.7%, ≥70 years 0.8%. Event rates for placebo+aspirin by age were: <60 years=0.4%, ≥60 to <70 years=0.6%, ≥70 years 0.7%.

Post-Market Adverse Drug Reactions: The following additional adverse reactions were reported in marketed use, however a causal relationship with clopidogrel has not been clearly established.
Blood and Lymphatic System Disorders: Very rare: agranulocytosis, aplastic anemia/pancytopenia; cases of bleeding with fatal outcome (especially gastrointestinal, intracranial and retroperitoneal hemorrhage); serious cases of bleeding, mainly eye (conjuctival, ocular, retinal), musculoskeletal, respiratory tract and skin bleeding, epistaxis, hematuria and hemorrhage of operative wound, hematoma; thrombotic thrombocytopenic purpura (TTP). Some cases of TTP resulted in fatal outcomes (see Warnings and Precautions).
Cardiovascular Disorders: Very rare: hypotension, often related to bleeding or allergic reaction.
Gastrointestinal Disorders: Very rare: colitis (including ulcerative or lymphocytic colitis), pancreatitis, stomatitis.
General Disorders and Administration Site Conditions: Very rare: fever.
Hepato-Biliary Disorders: Very rare: hepatitis, abnormal liver function test, acute liver failure.
Immune System Disorders: Very rare: anaphylactoid reactions, serum sickness.
Musculoskeletal Connective Tissue and Bone Disorders: Very rare: arthralgia, arthritis, myalgia.
Nervous System Disorders: Very rare: taste disturbances.
Psychiatric Disorders: Very rare: confusion, hallucinations.
Renal and Urinary Disorders: Very rare: glomerulopathy, elevated blood creatinine.
Respiratory, Thoracic and Mediastinal Disorders: Very rare: bronchospasm, interstitial pneumonitis.
Skin and Subcutaneous Tissue Disorders: Very rare: maculopapular or erythematous rash, urticaria, pruritus, angioedema, bullous dermatitis (erythema multiforme), Stevens-Johnson syndrome, toxic epidermal necrolysis, eczema, lichen planus.
Vascular Disorders: Very rare: vasculitis.

DRUG INTERACTIONS: Overview: Anticoagulant Drugs: In view of the possible increased risk of bleeding, anticoagulant drugs should be used with caution as tolerance and safety of simultaneous administration with clopidogrel has not been established. Risk factors should be assessed for individual patients before using clopidogrel.

Because of the increased risk of bleeding, the concomitant administration of warfarin with clopidogrel should be undertaken with caution.

Clinically significant adverse interactions were not detected in clinical trials with PLAVIX where patients received a variety of concomitant medications including ASA, diuretics, beta-blocking agents, angiotensin converting enzyme (ACE) inhibitors, calcium channel blockers, lipid-lowering agents, coronary vasodilators, antidiabetic agents (including insulin), thrombolytics, unfractionated and/or LMW heparin, glycoprotein IIb/IIIa inhibitors, antiepileptic agents, and hormone replacement therapy (however, see Table 5 regarding ASA and glycoprotein IIb/IIIa inhibitors). A review of the clinical trial data indicates that there is no evidence of an interaction between PLAVIX and atorvastatin. In CAPRIE, patients on HMG CoA reductase inhibitors and clopidogrel experienced a higher incidence of bleeding events (primarily epistaxis). Patients on HMG CoA reductase inhibitors and ASA experienced a higher incidence of intracranial hemorrhage. There is no known pathophysiological or pharmacological explanation for this observation.

Data from studies with human liver microsomes indicated that the carboxylic acid metabolite of clopidogrel could inhibit the activity of cytochrome P450 2C9. However, in vivo, clopidogrel does not modify the pharmacokinetics of S-warfarin (typical CYP2C9 substrate). Accordingly, it is unlikely that clopidogrel may interfere with the metabolism of drugs such as phenytoin and tolbutamide and the NSAIDs, which are metabolised by cytochrome P450 2C9. Data from the CAPRIE study indicate that phenytoin and tolbutamide can be safely coadministered with clopidogrel.

No clinically significant pharmacodynamic interactions were observed when clopidogrel was coadministered in clinical studies to investigate drug interaction with atenolol, nifedipine, or both atenolol and nifedipine. The pharmacodynamic activity of PLAVIX was slightly enhanced by the coadministration of phenobarbital, however this was not considered to be clinically significant. Pharmacodynamic activity of PLAVIX was not changed with the coadministration of cimetidine. Pharmacodynamic activity of PLAVIX was not significantly influenced by the coadministration of estrogen.

Drug-Drug Interactions: The drugs listed in Table 5 are based on either drug interaction case reports or studies, or potential interactions due to the expected magnitude and seriousness of the interaction (i.e., those identified as contraindicated).

Table 5: PLAVIX

Established or Potential Drug-Drug Interactions

Agent	Ref	Effect	Clinical Comment
Inhibitors of CYP2C19 (e.g. omeprazole)	CT	Reduced drug levels of the active metabolite of clopidogrel	Since clopidogrel is metabolized to its active metabolite partly by CYP2C19, use of drugs that inhibit the activity of this enzyme would be expected to result in reduced drug levels of the active metabolite of clopidogrel and a reduction in clinical efficacy. The use of drugs known to inhibit CYP2C19 should be discouraged in patients taking clopidogrel. Inhibitors of CYP2C19 include but are not limited to: omeprazole, lansoprazole, cimetidine, ticlopidine, fluvoxamine, fluoxetine, moclobemide, felbamate, chloramphenicol, ketoconazole.
ASA	CT	Potentiated effect of ASA on collagen-induced platelet aggregation	ASA (2×500 mg once) did not modify the clopidogrel-mediated inhibition of ADP-induced platelet aggregation. Potential increased risk of gastrointestinal bleeding with concomitant administration of ASA. PLAVIX (75 mg) and ASA (75–325 mg) have been administered together for up to 1 year. In patients with recent TIA or stroke who are at high risk of recurrent ischemic events, the combination of aspirin and PLAVIX has not been shown to be more effective than PLAVIX alone, but the combination has been shown to increase major bleeding (see Drug Interactions).
Atenolol, nifedipine	CT	No effect	No clinically significant pharmacodynamic interactions observed, with atenolol, nifedipine or both atenolol and nifedipine.

(cont'd)

Table 5: PLAVIX *(cont'd)*

Established or Potential Drug-Drug Interactions

Agent	Ref	Effect	Clinical Comment
Cimetidine	CT	No effect	Pharmacodynamic activity of PLAVIX not changed with coadministration.
Digoxin, Theophylline, Antacids	CT	No effect	There was no modification of the pharmacokinetics of digoxin or theophylline with the coadministration of PLAVIX at steady state. Antacids did not modify the extent of PLAVIX absorption.
Estrogens	CT	No effect	Pharmacodynamic activity of PLAVIX not significantly influenced by coadministration.
Glycoprotein IIb/IIIa Inhibitors	T		As a pharmacodynamic interaction is possible, concomitant use should be undertaken with caution.
Injectable Anticoagulants (Heparin)	CT	No effect	Clopidogrel at steady state did not modify the effect of heparin on coagulation in healthy volunteers. Coadministration of heparin had no effect on platelet aggregation inhibition induced by PLAVIX.
NSAIDs	T	↑ occult gastrointestinal blood loss (with naproxen coadministration)	Potential increased risk of gastrointestinal bleeding with concomitant administration of NSAIDs.
Oral Anticoagulants (Warfarin)	T		Because of the increased risk of bleeding, the concomitant administration of warfarin with clopidogrel should be undertaken with caution (See Warnings and Precautions).
Phenobarbitol	CT	Slight ↑ pharmacodynamic activity of PLAVIX.	Increase not considered clinically significant.
Thrombolytics	CS		The safety of the concomitant administration of clopidogrel, rt-PA and heparin was assessed in patients with recent myocardial infarction. Based on historical data, the incidence of clinically significant bleeding was similar to that observed when rt-PA and heparin are coadministered with acetylsalicylic acid.

Legend: C=case study; CT=clinical trial; T=theoretical.

Drug-Food or Drug-Herb Interactions: There is no interaction of PLAVIX with food since administration of PLAVIX with meals did not significantly modify the bioavailability of clopidogrel. Interactions with herbal products have not been established.
Drug-Laboratory Test Interactions: None known.

DOSAGE AND ADMINISTRATION:

Recommended Dose and Dosage Adjustment: MI, Stroke or Established Peripheral Arterial Disease: The recommended dose of PLAVIX is 75 mg once daily long term with or without food.
Acute Coronary Syndrome: For patients with non-ST-segment elevation acute coronary syndrome (unstable angina/non-Q-wave MI), PLAVIX should be initiated with a 300 mg loading dose and continued long term at 75 mg once a day with ASA (80 mg-325 mg daily).

For patients with ST-segment elevation acute myocardial infarction, the recommended dose of PLAVIX is 75 mg once daily, administered in combination with aspirin, with or without thrombolytics. PLAVIX may be initiated with or without a loading dose (300 mg was used in CLARITY).

No dosage adjustment is necessary for elderly patients or patients with renal impairment (see Action and Clinical Pharmacology, Special Populations and Conditions).
Pharmacogenetics: CYP2C19 poor metaboliser status is associated with diminished response to clopidogrel. The optimal dose regimen for poor metabolisers has yet to be determined (see Action and Clinical Pharmacology, Pharmacokinetics, Pharmacogenetics).
Missed Dose: If a dose of PLAVIX is missed, it should be taken as soon as possible. However, if it is close to the time of the next dose, disregard the missed dose and return to the regular dosing schedule. Do not double doses.

OVERDOSAGE:

Overdose following clopidogrel administration may lead to prolonged bleeding time and subsequent bleeding complications. Appropriate therapy should be considered if bleeding is observed or suspected.

A single oral dose of clopidogrel at 1500 or 2000 mg/kg was lethal to mice and rats, and at 3000 mg/kg to baboons.
Treatment: No antidote to the pharmacological activity of clopidogrel has been found. Platelet transfusion may be used to reverse the pharmacological effects of PLAVIX when quick reversal is required.

For management of a suspected drug overdose, contact your **regional Poison Control Centre**. See the *CPS* Directory section for a list of Poison Control Centres.

ACTION AND CLINICAL PHARMACOLOGY: Mechanism of Action: The role of platelets in the pathophysiology of atherosclerotic disease and atherothrombotic events has been established. Long-term prophylactic use of antiplatelet drugs has shown consistent benefit in the prevention of ischemic stroke, myocardial infarction, unstable angina, peripheral arterial disease, need for vascular bypass or angioplasty, and vascular death in patients at increased risk of such outcomes, including those with established atherosclerosis or a history of atherothrombosis. PLAVIX (clopidogrel bisulfate) is a specific inhibitor of adenosine diphosphate (ADP)-induced platelet aggregation.
Pharmacodynamics: Clopidogrel is a prodrug, one of whose metabolites is an inhibitor of platelet aggregation. Clopidogrel must be metabolised by CYP450 enzymes to produce the active metabolite that inhibits platelet aggregation. The active metabolite of clopidogrel selectively inhibits the binding of adenosine diphosphate (ADP) to its platelet P2Y12 receptor and the subsequent ADP-mediated activation of the glycoprotein GPIIb/IIIa complex, thereby inhibiting platelet aggregation. Platelet aggregation induced by agonists other than ADP is also inhibited by blocking the amplification of platelet activation by released ADP. Because the active metabolite is formed by CYP450 enzymes, some of which are polymorphic or subject to inhibition by other drugs, not all patients will have adequate platelet inhibition.

Clopidogrel does not inhibit phosphodiesterase activity. Acetylsalicylic acid (ASA) inhibits the cyclooxygenase enzyme pathway preventing the production of prostaglandin and thus, the synthesis of thromboxane A2 which induces platelet aggregation. Clopidogrel acts on the ADP receptor and ASA acts on a separate receptor thereby inhibiting different pathways of platelet activation and aggregation. Therefore, there is potential for synergy between the two agents.

Clopidogrel acts by modifying irreversibly the platelet ADP receptor. Consequently, platelets exposed to clopidogrel are affected for the remainder of their lifespan (approximately 7-10 days) and recovery of normal platelet function occurs at a rate consistent with platelet turnover. Single administration is not sufficient to reach a desired therapeutic effect. Statistically significant and dose-dependent inhibition of platelet aggregation was noted 2 hours after single oral doses of clopidogrel. Repeated doses of 75 mg per day produced inhibition of ADP-induced platelet aggregation from the first day. Steady state was reached between Day 3 and Day 7. At steady state, with a dose of 75 mg per day, the average inhibition level observed was between 40% and 60%. The aggregation level and bleeding time gradually returned to baseline values within 5-7 days after treatment was discontinued. The precise correlation between inhibition of platelet aggregation, prolongation of bleeding time and prevention of atherothrombotic events has not been established. The effect of a loading dose has been clinically evaluated in the CURE study (Clopidogrel in Unstable Angina to Prevent Recurrent Ischemic Events). The benefits of clopidogrel with concomitant ASA were apparent within 24 hours after randomization in the CURE trial.
Pharmacokinetics: The main pharmacokinetic parameters for clopidogrel are presented in the table below.

	C_{max}	$t_{1/2}$ (h)	AUC $_{0-\infty}$
Single Dose Mean	2.2–2.5 ng/mL	6 h	2.7 ng·h/L

Absorption: After single and repeated oral doses of 75 mg per day, clopidogrel is rapidly absorbed. Mean peak plasma levels of unchanged clopidogrel (approximately 2.2-2.5 ng/mL after a single 75-mg oral dose) occurred approximately 45 minutes after dosing.

Absorption is at least 50%, based on urinary excretion of clopidogrel metabolites.

Administration of PLAVIX with meals did not significantly modify the bioavailability of clopidogrel as assessed by the pharmacokinetics of the main circulating metabolite.
Distribution: Clopidogrel and the main circulating (inactive) metabolite bind reversibly in vitro to human plasma proteins (98% and 94%, respectively). The binding is non saturable in vitro up to a concentration of 100 μg/mL.
Metabolism: Clopidogrel is extensively metabolized by the liver. In vitro and in vivo, clopidogrel is metabolised according to two main metabolic pathways: one mediated by esterases and leading to hydrolysis into its inactive carboxylic acid derivative (85% of circulating metabolites), and one mediated by multiple cytochromes P450. Clopidogrel is first metabolised to a 2-oxo-clopidogrel intermediate metabolite. Subsequent metabolism of the 2-oxo-clopidogrel intermediate metabolite results in formation of the active metabolite, a thiol derivative of clopidogrel. In vitro, this metabolic pathway is mediated by CYP3A4, CYP2C19, CYP1A2 and CYP2B6. The active thiol metabolite which has been isolated in vitro, binds rapidly and irreversibly to platelet receptors, thus inhibiting platelet aggregation.
Excretion: Following an oral dose of ^{14}C-labeled clopidogrel in humans, approximately 50% was excreted in the urine and approximately 46% in the feces in the 5 days after dosing. After a single, oral dose of 75 mg, clopidogrel has a half-life of approximately 6 hours. The elimination half-life of the main circulating (inactive) metabolite was 8 hours after single and repeated administration. Covalent binding to platelets accounted for 2% of the radiolabel with a half-life of 11 days.
Pharmacogenetics: Several polymorphic CYP450 enzymes activate clopidogrel. CYP2C19 is involved in the formation of both the active metabolite and the 2-oxo-clopidogrel intermediate metabolite. Clopidogrel active metabolite pharmacokinetics and antiplatelet effects, as measured by ex vivo platelet aggregation assays, differ according to CYP2C19 genotype. The CYP2C19*1 allele corresponds to fully functional metabolism while the CYP2C19*2 and CYP2C19*3 alleles correspond to reduced metabolism. The CYP2C19*2 and CYP2C19*3 alleles account for 85% of reduced function alleles in whites and 99% in Asians. Other alleles associated with reduced metabolism include CYP2C19*4, *5, *6, *7, and *8, but these are less frequent in the general population. Published frequencies for the common CYP2C19 phenotypes and genotypes are listed in Table 6.

Table 6: PLAVIX

CYP2C19 Phenotype and Genotype Frequency

	Frequency (%)		
	White (n=1356)	Black (n=966)	Chinese (n=573)
Extensive metabolism: CYP2C19*1/*1	74	66	38
Intermediate metabolism: CYP2C19*1/*2 or *1/*3	26	29	50
Poor metabolism: CYP2C19*2/*2, *2/*3 or *3/*3	2	4	14

To date, the impact of CYP2C19 genotype on the pharmacokinetics of the active metabolite of clopidogrel has been evaluated in 227 subjects from 7 reported studies. Reduced CYP2C19 metabolism in intermediate and poor metabolisers decreased the Cmax and AUC of the active metabolite by 30-50% following 300- or 600-mg loading doses and 75-mg maintenance doses. Lower active metabolite exposure results in less platelet inhibition or higher residual platelet reactivity. To date, diminished antiplatelet responses to clopidogrel have been described for intermediate and poor metabolisers in 21 reported studies involving 4520 subjects. The relative difference in antiplatelet response between genotype groups varies across studies depending on the method used to evaluate response, but is typically greater than 30%.

The association between CYP2C19 genotype and clopidogrel treatment outcome was evaluated in 2 post-hoc analyses in 1942 patients from 2 clinical trials which included a total of 17 099 patients and in 5 cohort studies (total n=6489). In the first post hoc analysis (n=465) and the cohort study by Trenk et al (n=765), cardiovascular event rates did not differ significantly by genotype. In the second post-hoc analysis (n=1477) and in 3 of the cohort studies (n=3516), patients with an impaired metabolizer status (intermediate and poor combined) had a higher rate of cardiovascular events (death, myocardial infarction, and stroke) or stent thrombosis compared to extensive metabolizers. In the fifth cohort study (n=2208), patients carrying CYP2C19 loss-of-function alleles had a higher rate of cardiovascular events than those who were not.

Pharmacogenetic testing can identify genotypes associated with variability in CYP2C19 activity.

There may be genetic variants of other CYP450 enzymes with effects on the ability to form the active metabolite of clopidogrel.
Special Populations and Conditions: Geriatrics: In elderly (≥75 years) volunteers compared to young healthy subjects, there were no differences in platelet aggregation and bleeding time (see Dosage and Administration). No dosage adjustment is needed for the elderly.
Gender: In a small study comparing men and women (N=10 males and 10 females), less inhibition of ADP-induced platelet aggregation was observed in women. In the CAPRIE study (Clopidogrel versus ASA in Patients at Risk of Ischemic Events; for details see below), the incidence of clinical outcome events was similar in men and women.
Paediatric Patients: No information available.
Renal Insufficiency: After repeated doses of 75 mg per day in subjects with moderate and severe renal impairment (creatinine clearance from 30 to 60 mL/min and from 5 to 15 mL/min, respectively), a 25% inhibition of ADP-induced platelet aggregation was observed. Although this effect was lower than that typically observed in healthy subjects, the prolongation in bleeding time was similar to healthy volunteers.

Since no differences in C_{max}, for both clopidogrel and the main circulating metabolite were observed, a compensatory phenomenon i.e. biliary excretion, which has been observed in animals, may explain the lower values of AUC observed in subjects with severe chronic renal failure (see Dosage and Administration).
Ethnicity: The prevalence of CYP2C19 alleles that result in intermediate and poor CYP2C19 metabolism differs according to ethnicity (see Action and Clinical Pharmacology, Pharmacokinetics, Pharmacogenetics). From literature, limited data in Asian populations are available to assess the clinical implication of genotyping of this CYP on clinical outcome events.

STORAGE AND STABILITY: For blisters, store between 15 and 30°C and protect from moisture. For bottles, store between 15 and 30°C.

SPECIAL HANDLING INSTRUCTIONS: None.

INFORMATION FOR THE PATIENT: Published in e-CPS, available by subscription at www.e-cps.ca.

DOSAGE FORMS, COMPOSITION AND PACKAGING: 75 mg: Each round, pink, slightly biconvex, film-coated tablet, engraved with "75" on one side and "1171" on the other side, contains: clopidogrel bisulfate 97.9 mg which is the molar equivalent of 75 mg of clopidogrel base. Nonmedicinal ingredients: hydrogenated castor oil, low substituted hydroxypropylcellulose, mannitol, microcrystalline cellulose and polyethylene glycol 6000; coating: carnauba wax, hypromellose, lactose, red iron oxide, titanium dioxide and triacetin. Energy: 2.5 kJ (0.6 kcal). Blister cards of 28, cartons of 1. Bottles of 500.
300 mg: Each oblong, pink, film-coated tablet, engraved with "300" on one side and "1332" on the other side, contains: clopidogrel bisulfate 391.5 mg which is the molar equivalent of 300 mg of clopidogrel base. Nonmedicinal ingredients: hydrogenated castor oil, low substituted hydroxypropylcellulose, mannitol, microcrystalline cellulose and polyethylene glycol 6000; coating: carnauba wax, hypromellose, lactose, red iron oxide, titanium dioxide and triacetin. Blister cards of 30 (3×10 blister-packed).

(Shown in Product Identification Section)

The reader is invited to consult CPhA's monograph **Calcium Channel Blockers**.

Plendil® ℞

felodipine

Antihypertensive

AstraZeneca

Date of Preparation: February 3, 2000
Date of Revision: June 12, 2008

PHARMACOLOGY: Felodipine is a calcium ion influx inhibitor (calcium channel blocker). Felodipine is a member of the dihydropyridine class of calcium channel blockers.

Mechanism of Action: The therapeutic effect of this group of drugs is believed to be related to their specific cellular action of selectively inhibiting transmembrane influx of calcium ions into cardiac muscle and vascular smooth muscle. The contractile processes of these tissues are dependent upon the movement of extracellular calcium into the cells through specific ion channels. Felodipine blocks transmembrane influx of calcium through the slow channel without affecting to any significant degree the transmembrane influx of sodium through the fast channel. This results in a reduction of free calcium ions available within cells of the above tissues.

Felodipine does not alter total serum calcium. In vitro studies show that the effects of felodipine on contractile mechanisms are selective, with greater effects on vascular smooth muscle than on cardiac muscle. Negative inotropic effects can be detected in vitro, but such effects have not been seen in intact animals.

The effect of felodipine on blood pressure in man is principally a consequence of a dose-related decrease in peripheral vascular resistance, with a modest reflex increase in heart rate (see Pharmacodynamics).

Pharmacokinetics: Felodipine is completely absorbed from the gastrointestinal tract after oral administration. Due to rapid biotransformation of felodipine during its first pass through the portal circulation, the systemic availability is approximately 15% and is independent of the dose in the range of 5 to 20 mg/day. The plasma protein binding of felodipine is approximately 99%. It is bound predominately to the albumin fraction.

Felodipine is extensively metabolized by the liver, predominantly by cytochrome P450 CYP 3A4. After 72 hours, approximately 70% of a given dose is excreted as metabolites in the urine and 10% is secreted in the feces. Less than 0.5% of a dose is recovered unchanged in the urine. Six metabolites, which account for 23% of the oral dose, have been identified: none has significant vasodilating activity.

Felodipine has been observed to have a mean blood clearance of 914±355 mL/min in hypertensive patients, 606±245 mL/min in elderly hypertensive patients and 1337±413 mL/min in young healthy volunteers. Its mean terminal half-life was 24.5±7.0 hours in hypertensive patients, 27.5±8.4 hours in elderly hypertensive patients and 14.1±5.6 hours in young healthy volunteers.

The extended release formulation prolongs the absorption phase of felodipine resulting in an increased time to reach peak plasma concentrations (t_{max}), and a reduced maximum plasma concentration (C_{max}). The mean t_{max} ranges from 2.5 to 5 hours. The area under the plasma concentration versus time curve and C_{max} are linearly related to the dose in the 10 to 40 mg range. Following administration of felodipine to hypertensive patients, mean C_{max} at steady state is approximately 20% higher after multiple doses than after a single dose. No increase in the AUC is found during multiple dosing. The inter-individual variation in C_{max} and AUC after repeated dosing is approximately 3-fold and indicates a need for individualized dosing.

The bioavailability of felodipine is not influenced by the presence of food in the gastrointestinal tract. However, the peak plasma concentration of felodipine (C_{max}) is significantly increased by 1.5- to 2-fold when felodipine is taken after a high fat or high carbohydrate meal versus fasting. Because the effects of felodipine on blood pressure are related to plasma levels, this increase in C_{max} may cause a clinically significant fall in blood pressure. Therefore felodipine should not be administered with meals rich in carbohydrate or fat. However, the absorption characteristics of felodipine are not affected when felodipine is administered with a light meal low in fat and carbohydrates (i.e., 2 slices of toast with cheese, 150 mL of milk with cornflakes, and 150 mL of orange juice).

Studies in healthy male volunteers showed significant alterations in the pharmacokinetics of felodipine when felodipine was administered concomitantly with grapefruit juice. Following the administration of a single dose of plain felodipine 5 mg tablets with 200 mL grapefruit juice or 200 mL water AUC and C_{max} of felodipine increased about 3-fold as compared to administration with water. When felodipine extended release tablets were administered as Plendil 10 mg with 250 mL grapefruit juice felodipine AUC and C_{max} values doubled as compared to those observed with water. When grapefruit juice was taken for up to 24 hours prior to felodipine administration, a significant pharmacokinetic interaction was observed (see Precautions, Interaction with Grapefruit Juice).

Plasma concentrations of felodipine, after a single dose and at steady state, increase with age. Mean clearance of felodipine in elderly hypertensives (mean age 74 years) was only 45% of that in young volunteers (mean age 26 years). At steady state mean AUC for young patients was 39% of that for the elderly patients.

In patients with hepatic disease, the clearance of felodipine was reduced to about 60% of that seen in normal young volunteers.

Renal impairment does not alter the plasma concentration profile of felodipine. Although higher concentrations of the metabolites are present in the plasma due to decreased urinary excretion, these are hemodynamically inactive.

Animal studies have demonstrated that felodipine crosses the blood-brain barrier and the placenta.

Pharmacodynamics: The acute hemodynamic effect of felodipine is a reduction in total peripheral resistance which leads to a decrease in blood pressure associated with a modest reflex increase in heart rate. This reflex increase in heart rate frequently occurs during the first week of therapy and generally attenuates over time. Heart rate increases of 5 to 10 beats/minute may be seen during chronic administration. The effect on the heart rate is inhibited by beta-blocking agents.

Following administration of felodipine a reduction in blood pressure generally occurs within 2 to 5 hours.

During chronic administration, substantial blood pressure control lasts for approximately 24 hours; reductions in diastolic blood pressure at trough plasma levels were 40 to 60% of those at peak plasma levels. The antihypertensive effect is dose-dependent and correlates with the plasma concentration of felodipine.

Felodipine in therapeutic doses has no effect on conduction in the conducting system of the heart and no effect on the AV nodal refractoriness. No direct additional effects to those registered after beta-blockade are observed when felodipine is given concomitantly.

Renal vascular resistance is decreased by felodipine while glomerular filtration rate remains unchanged. Mild diuresis, natriuresis and kaliuresis have been observed during the first week of therapy. No significant effects on serum electrolytes have been observed during short- and long-term therapy. No general salt and water retention occurs during long-term therapy. In clinical trials increases in norepinephrine plasma levels have been observed.

INDICATIONS: In the treatment of mild to moderate essential hypertension. Felodipine should normally be used in those patients in whom treatment with a diuretic or a beta-blocker was found ineffective or has been associated with unacceptable adverse effects.

Felodipine can be tried as an initial agent in those patients in whom the use of diuretics and/or beta-blockers is contraindicated or in patients with medical conditions in which these drugs frequently cause serious adverse effects.

Combination of felodipine with a thiazide diuretic or a beta-blocker has been found to be compatible and showed an additive antihypertensive effect. Safety and efficacy of concurrent use of felodipine with other antihypertensive agents has not been established.

CONTRAINDICATIONS: In patients with a known hypersensitivity to felodipine or any other components of the product. In patients with a known hypersensitivity to other dihydropyridines.

Pregnancy: In women of childbearing potential, in pregnancy, and during lactation. Fetal malformations and adverse effects on pregnancy have been reported in animals.

Teratogenic Effects: Studies in pregnant rabbits administered doses of 0.46, 1.2, 2.3 and 4.6 mg/kg/day (from 0.4 to 4 times the maximum recommended human dose on a mg/m² basis) showed digital anomalies consisting of reduction in size and degree of ossification of the terminal phalanges in the fetuses. The frequency and severity of the changes appeared dose-related and were noted even at the lowest dose. These changes have been shown to occur with other members of the dihydropyridine class. Similar fetal anomalies were not observed in rats given felodipine.

In a teratology study in cynomolgus monkeys, no reduction in the size of the terminal phalanges was observed but an abnormal position of the distal phalanges was noted in about 40% of the fetuses.

Nonteratogenic Effects: In a study on fertility and general reproductive performance in rats, prolongation of parturition with difficult labor and an increased frequency of fetal and early postnatal deaths were observed in the groups treated with doses of 9.6 mg/kg/day and above.

Significant enlargement of the mammary glands in excess of the normal enlargement for pregnant rabbits was found with doses greater than or equal to 1.2 mg/kg/day. This effect occurred only in pregnant rabbits and regressed during lactation. Similar changes in the mammary glands were not observed in rats or monkeys.

Lactation: See Pregnancy.

WARNINGS: Congestive Heart Failure: The safety and efficacy of felodipine in patients with heart failure have not been established. Caution should, therefore, be exercised when using felodipine in hypertensive patients with compromised ventricular function, particularly in combination with a beta-blocker. Acute hemodynamic studies in a small number of patients with New York Heart Association Class II or III heart failure treated with felodipine have not demonstrated negative inotropic effects.

Hypotension, Myocardial Ischemia: Felodipine may, occasionally, precipitate symptomatic hypotension and rarely syncope. It may lead to reflex tachycardia which, particularly in patients with severe obstructive coronary artery disease, may result in myocardial ischemia. Careful monitoring of blood pressure during the initial administration and titration of felodipine is recommended.

Care should be taken to avoid hypotension especially in patients with a history of cerebrovascular insufficiency, and in those taking medications known to lower blood pressure.

Beta-blocker Withdrawal: Felodipine gives no protection against the dangers of abrupt beta-blocker withdrawal; any such withdrawal should be a gradual reduction of the dose of beta-blockers.

Outflow Obstruction: Felodipine should be used with caution in the presence of fixed left ventricular outflow obstruction.

Dermatologic Lesions: Along with leucocytoclastic vasculitis, other dermatologic events have been observed. These include rash and flush. All cases of dermatologic lesions should be carefully diagnosed and monitored.

PRECAUTIONS: Peripheral Edema: Mild to moderate peripheral edema was the most common adverse event in the clinical trials. The incidence of peripheral edema was dose-dependent. Frequency of peripheral edema ranged from about 10% in patients under 50 years of age taking 5 mg daily to about 30% in those over 60 years of age taking 20 mg daily. This adverse effect generally occurs within 2 to 3 weeks of the initiation of treatment. Care should be taken to differentiate this peripheral edema from the effects of increasing left ventricular dysfunction.

Geriatrics: Patients over 65 years of age may have elevated plasma concentrations of felodipine and, therefore, may require lower doses of felodipine (see Pharmacology, Pharmacokinetics). These patients should have their blood pressure monitored closely during initial administration and after dosage adjustment of felodipine. A dosage of 10 mg daily should not be exceeded (see Dosage, Geriatrics).

Patients with Impaired Liver Function: Patients with impaired liver function may have elevated plasma concentrations of felodipine and, therefore, may require lower doses of felodipine (see Pharmacology, Pharmacokinetics). These patients should have their blood pressure monitored closely during initial administration and after dosage adjustment of felodipine. A dosage of 10 mg daily should not be exceeded (see Dosage, Patients with Impaired Liver Function).

Gingival Hyperplasia: Felodipine can induce gingival enlargement in patients with pronounced gingivitis and parodontitis. However, such changes may be reversed by measures of good oral hygiene and mechanical debridement of the teeth. In very rare instances, felodipine has also caused gingivitis.

Pregnancy: See Contraindications.

Lactation: See Contraindications.

Children: Felodipine is not recommended in children since the safety and efficacy in children have not been established.

Interaction with Grapefruit Juice: Published data show that through inhibition of cytochrome P450, grapefruit juice can increase plasma levels and augment pharmacodynamic effects of dihydropyridine calcium channel blockers. In view of the absolute bioavailability of felodipine, the potential for a significant increase in pharmacodynamic effects exists (see Pharmacology, Pharmacokinetics). Therefore, the consumption of grapefruit juice, prior to or during treatment with felodipine should be avoided.

Drug Interactions: As with all drugs, care should be exercised when treating patients with multiple medications. Dihydropyridine calcium channel blockers undergo biotransformation by the cytochrome P450 system, mainly via the CYP 3A4 isoenzyme. Coadministration of felodipine with other drugs which follow the same route of biotransformation may result in altered bioavailability of felodipine or these drugs. Dosages of similarly metabolized drugs, particularly those of low therapeutic ratio, and especially in patients with renal and/or hepatic impairment, may require adjustment when starting or stopping concomitantly administered felodipine to maintain optimum therapeutic blood levels.

Drugs known to be inhibitors of the cytochrome P450 system include: azole antifungals, cimetidine, cyclosporine, erythromycin, quinidine, warfarin.

Drugs known to be inducers of the cytochrome P450 system include: phenobarbital, phenytoin, rifampin.

Felodipine may increase the concentration of tacrolimus. When used together, the tacrolimus serum concentration should be followed and the tacrolimus dose may need to be adjusted.

Drugs known to be biotransformed via P450 include: benzodiazepines, flecainide, imipramine, propafenone, terfenadine, theophylline.

Cytochrome P450 Enzyme Inhibitors: Cimetidine: In healthy volunteers pharmacokinetic studies showed an approximately 50% increase in the area under the plasma concentration time curve (AUC) as well as the C_{max} of felodipine when given concomitantly with cimetidine. It is anticipated that a clinically significant interaction may occur in some hypertensive patients. Therefore, it is recommended that low doses of felodipine be used when given concomitantly with cimetidine.

Erythromycin: Concomitant treatment with erythromycin has been shown to cause an increase in felodipine plasma levels.

Cytochrome P450 Enzyme Inducers: Phenytoin, Carbamazepine and Phenobarbital: In a pharmacokinetic study maximum plasma concentrations of felodipine were considerably lower in epileptic patients on long-term anticonvulsant therapy (phenytoin, carbamazepine, phenobarbital) than in healthy volunteers. The mean area under the felodipine plasma concentration-time curve was also reduced in epileptic patients to approximately 6% of that observed in healthy volunteers. Since a clinically significant interaction may be anticipated, alternative antihypertensive therapy should be considered in these patients.

Alcohol: Alcohol can enhance the hemodynamic effects of felodipine.

Beta-adrenoceptor Blocking Agents: A pharmacokinetic study of felodipine in conjunction with metoprolol demonstrated no significant effects on the pharmacokinetics of felodipine. The AUC and C_{max} of metoprolol, however, were increased approximately 31 and 36%, respectively. In controlled clinical trials, however, beta-blockers including metoprolol were concurrently administered with felodipine and were well tolerated.

Digoxin: When given concomitantly with felodipine as conventional tablets the peak plasma concentration of digoxin was significantly increased. With the extended release formulation of felodipine there was no significant change in peak plasma levels or AUC of digoxin.

Other Concomitant Therapy: In healthy subjects there were no clinically significant interactions when felodipine was given concomitantly with indomethacin or spironolactone.

ADVERSE EFFECTS: In 861 essential hypertensive patients treated once daily with 2.5 to 10 mg felodipine as monotherapy in controlled clinical trials, the most common clinical adverse events were peripheral edema and headache.

Adverse events that occurred with an incidence of 1.5% or greater at any of the recommended doses of 2.5 to 10 mg once a day, without regard to causality, are listed by dose in Table 1. These events are reported from controlled clinical trials with patients who were randomized to either a fixed dose of felodipine or titrated from an initial dose of 2.5 or 5 mg once a day. **A dose of 20 mg once a day has been evaluated in some clinical studies. Although the antihypertensive effect of felodipine is increased at 20 mg once per day, there is a disproportionate increase in adverse events, especially those associated with vasodilatory effects** (see Dosage).

Table 1: Plendil

Percent of Patients With Adverse Events in Controlled Trials of Plendil (N=861)[a] as Monotherapy Without Regard to Causality (Incidence of Discontinuations Shown in Parentheses)

Body System Adverse Events	Placebo N=334	2.5 mg N=255	5 mg N=581	10 mg N=408
Body as a Whole				
Peripheral Edema	3.3 (0.0)	2.0 (0.0)	8.8 (2.2)	17.4 (2.5)
Asthenia	3.3 (0.0)	3.9 (0.0)	3.3 (0.0)	2.2 (0.0)

(cont'd)

Table 1: Plendil *(cont'd)*

Percent of Patients With Adverse Events in Controlled Trials of Plendil (N=861)[a] as Monotherapy Without Regard to Causality (Incidence of Discontinuations Shown in Parentheses)

Body System / Adverse Events	Placebo N=334	2.5 mg N=255	5 mg N=581	10 mg N=408
Cardiovascular				
Palpitation	2.4 (0.0)	0.4 (0.0)	1.4 (0.3)	2.5 (0.5)
Warm Sensation/Flushing	0.9 (0.3)	3.9 (0.0)	6.2 (0.9)	8.4 (1.2)
Digestive				
Nausea	1.5 (0.9)	1.2 (0.0)	1.7 (0.3)	1.0 (0.7)
Dyspepsia	1.2 (0.0)	3.9 (0.0)	0.7 (0.0)	0.5 (0.0)
Constipation	0.9 (0.0)	1.2 (0.0)	0.3 (0.0)	1.5 (0.2)
Nervous				
Headache	10.2 (0.9)	10.6 (0.4)	11.0 (1.7)	14.7 (2.0)
Dizziness	2.7 (0.3)	2.7 (0.0)	3.6 (0.5)	3.7 (0.5)
Paresthesia	1.5 (0.3)	1.6 (0.0)	1.2 (0.0)	1.2 (0.2)
Respiratory				
Upper Respiratory Infection	1.8 (0.0)	3.9 (0.0)	1.9 (0.0)	0.7 (0.0)
Cough	0.3 (0.0)	0.8 (0.0)	1.2 (0.0)	1.7 (0.0)
Skin				
Rash	0.9 (0.0)	2.0 (0.0)	0.2 (0.0)	0.2 (0.0)

[a] Some patients have been exposed to more than one dose level of Plendil.

Adverse events that occurred in 0.5 up to 1.5% of patients who received felodipine in all controlled clinical trials at the recommended dosage range of 2.5 to 10 mg once a day or during postmarketing experience are listed below. These events are listed in order of decreasing severity within each category regardless of relationship to felodipine therapy:

Body as a Whole: chest pain, facial edema, flu-like illness, fever.

Cardiovascular: tachycardia, premature beats, postural hypotension, bradycardia.

Gastrointestinal: abdominal pain, diarrhea, vomiting, dry mouth, flatulence, acid regurgitation, cholestatic hepatitis, gingival hyperplasia, salivary gland enlargement.

Metabolic: ALT increased.

Musculoskeletal: arthralgia, muscle cramps, myalgia.

Nervous/Psychiatric: insomnia, depression, anxiety disorders, irritability, nervousness, somnolence, decrease in libido, tremor, confusion.

Respiratory: dyspnea, epistaxis.

Dermatologic: pruritus, erythema multiforme, erythema nodosum, leucocytoclastic vasculitis, urticaria, photosensitivity reactions.

Special Senses: visual disturbances.

Urogenital: impotence/sexual dysfunction, urinary frequency, urinary urgency, dysuria, polyuria.

Serious adverse events reported from controlled clinical trials and during marketing experience (incidence <0.5%) were myocardial infarction, hypotension, syncope, angina pectoris, arrhythmia and anemia.

Isolated cases of angioedema have been reported. Angioedema may be accompanied by breathing difficulty.

Laboratory Tests: For the following laboratory values statistically significant decreases were observed; bilirubin, red blood count, hemoglobin, and urate. Statistically significant increases were found in erythrocyte sedimentation rate and thrombocyte count. In isolated cases, there were increased liver enzymes. None of the changes were considered to be of clinical significance.

OVERDOSE:

Symptoms: Overdosage can cause excessive peripheral vasodilation with marked hypotension and possibly bradycardia.

Treatment: In the case of known overdosage, activated charcoal may be used. If severe hypotension occurs, symptomatic treatment should be instituted. The patient should be placed supine with the legs elevated. The i.v. administration of fluids may be used to treat hypotension. Plasma volume may be increased by infusion of a plasma volume expander. When accompanied by bradycardia, atropine 0.5 to 1 mg should be administered i.v. Sympathomimetic drugs predominantly affecting the α_1-adrenoceptor may be given if the above-mentioned measures are considered insufficient. Removal of felodipine from the circulation by hemodialysis has not been established.

For management of a suspected drug overdose, CPhA recommends that you contact your **regional Poison Control Centre**. See the *CPS* Directory section for a list of Poison Control Centres.

DOSAGE: Felodipine should be swallowed whole and not crushed or chewed. The tablets should not be administered with a meal rich in carbohydrates or fat (see Pharmacology, Pharmacokinetics).

The usual recommended initial dose is 5 mg once daily (see Geriatrics, and Patients with Impaired Liver Function).

Depending on the patient's response, the dosage should be adjusted accordingly. Dose adjustment, if necessary, should be done at intervals of not less than 2 weeks.

The maintenance dosage range is 2.5 to 10 mg once daily.

In clinical trials, doses above 10 mg daily showed an increased blood pressure response but a disproportionately higher incidence of peripheral edema and other vasodilatory adverse events.

Modification of the recommended dosage is usually not required in patients with renal impairment.

Geriatrics: Patients over 65 years of age may develop elevated plasma concentrations of felodipine. A starting dose no higher than 2.5 mg once daily is recommended. A dosage of 10 mg daily should not be exceeded (see Precautions, Geriatrics).

Patients with Impaired Liver Function: Patients with impaired liver function may develop elevated plasma concentrations of felodipine. A starting dose no higher than 2.5 mg once daily is recommended. A dosage of 10 mg daily should not be exceeded (see Precautions, Patients with Impaired Liver Function).

INFORMATION FOR THE PATIENT: Published in e-CPS, available by subscription at www.e-cps.ca.

SUPPLIED: 2.5 mg: Each yellow, circular, biconvex, film-coated, extended release tablet, engraved A/FL on one side and 2.5 on the other, contains: felodipine 2.5 mg. Nonmedicinal ingredients: Tablet Core: aluminum silicate, hydroxypropyl cellulose, hydroxypropyl methylcellulose, lactose anhydrous, microcrystalline cellulose, polyoxy 40 hydrogenated castor oil, propyl gallate and sodium stearyl fumarate; Coating Layer: carnauba wax, color iron oxide yellow, color titanium dioxide, hydrogen peroxide, hydroxypropyl methylcellulose and polyethylene glycol. Compliance blister packages of 30 tablets.

5 mg: Each pink, circular, biconvex, film-coated, extended release tablet, engraved A/FM on one side and 5 on the other, contains: felodipine 5 mg. Nonmedicinal ingredients: Tablet Core: aluminum silicate, hydroxypropyl cellulose, hydroxypropyl methylcellulose, lactose anhydrous, microcrystalline cellulose, polyoxy 40 hydrogenated castor oil, propyl gallate and sodium stearyl fumarate; Coating Layer: carnauba wax, color iron oxide red-brown, color iron oxide yellow, color titanium dioxide, hydrogen peroxide, hydroxypropyl methylcellulose and polyethylene glycol. Compliance blister packages of 30 tablets.

10 mg: Each red-brown, circular, biconvex, film-coated, extended release tablet, engraved A/FE on one side and 10 on the other, contains: felodipine 10 mg. Nonmedicinal ingredients: Tablet Core: aluminum silicate, hydroxypropyl cellulose, hydroxypropyl methylcellulose, lactose anhydrous, microcrystalline cellulose, polyoxy 40 hydrogenated castor oil, propyl gallate and sodium stearyl fumarate; Coating Layer: carnauba wax, color iron oxide red-brown, color iron oxide yellow, color titanium dioxide, hydrogen peroxide, hydroxypropyl methylcellulose and polyethylene glycol. Compliance blister packages of 30 tablets.

Note: These extended release tablets must not be divided, crushed or chewed.

Store between 15 and 30°C.

(Shown in Product Identification Section)

The reader is invited to consult CPhA's monograph **Bisphosphonates: Oral**.

PMS-Alendronate FC Pr

alendronate sodium

Bone Metabolism Regulator

Pharmascience

SUPPLIED: Each white, oval-shaped, biconvex, film-coated tablet, debossed with "P" logo on one side and "70" on the other side, contains: alendronate sodium 91.37 mg, which is the molar equivalent to 70 mg of free acid. Nonmedicinal ingredients: cornstarch, hydroxypropyl methylcellulose, magnesium stearate, mannitol, microcrystalline cellulose and sodium potato starch glycolate. Blisters of 4. Bottles of 30. Store at room temperature (15-30°C).

PMS-Amiodarone Pr

amiodarone HCl

Antiarrhythmic

Pharmascience

SUPPLIED: 100 mg : Each pink, round, flat face, beveled edge tablet, debossed with "P" logo on one side and "100" on the other, contains: amiodarone HCl 100 mg. Nonmedicinal ingredients: FD&C Red No. 40 Aluminum Lake, lactose, magnesium stearate, povidone, silicon dioxide and sodium starch glycolate. Bottles of 100. Store between 15 and 30°C. Protect from light and excessive heat.

200 mg: Each pink, round, flat face, beveled edge tablet, scored on one side and debossed with "P" logo and "200" on the other, contains: amiodarone HCl 200 mg. Nonmedicinal ingredients: FD&C Red No. 40 Aluminum Lake, lactose, magnesium stearate, povidone, silicon dioxide and sodium starch glycolate. Bottles of 100. Store between 15 and 30°C. Protect from light and excessive heat.

PMS-Amlodipine Pr

amlodipine besylate

Antihypertensive—Antianginal

Pharmascience

SUPPLIED: 2.5 mg: Each white, octagonal tablet, debossed with "2.5" on one side and plain on the other side, contains: amlodipine 2.5 mg (as amlodipine besylate). Nonmedicinal ingredients: dibasic calcium phosphate, magnesium stearate, microcrystalline cellulose and sodium starch glycolate. HDPE bottles of 100. Store at 15 to 30°C, protected from light.

5 mg: Each white, octagonal tablet, debossed with a "P" logo on one side and "5" on the other side, contains: amlodipine 5 mg (as amlodipine besylate). Nonmedicinal ingredients: dibasic calcium phosphate, magnesium stearate, microcrystalline cellulose and sodium starch glycolate. Bottles of 100 and 500. Store at 15 to 30°C, protected from light.

10 mg: Each white, octagonal tablet, debossed with "10" on one side and plain on the other side, contains: amlodipine 10 mg (as amlodipine besylate). Nonmedicinal ingredients: dibasic calcium phosphate, magnesium stearate, microcrystalline cellulose and sodium starch glycolate. Bottles of 100 and 500. Store at 15 to 30°C, protected from light.

PMS-Atenolol Pr

atenolol

Beta-adrenergic Receptor Blocking Agent

Pharmascience

SUPPLIED: 25 mg: Each white, round, biconvex, film-coated tablet, debossed with a "P" logo on one side and "A 25" on the other side contains: atenolol 25 mg. Nonmedicinal ingredients: croscarmellose sodium, hydroxypropyl cellulose, hydroxypropyl methylcellulose, magnesium stearate, magnesium trisilicate, microcrystalline cellulose, polyethylene glycol, talc and titanium dioxide. Bottles of 100 and 500. Store at room temperature (15-30°C). Protect from light and moisture.

50 mg: Each white, round, biconvex, film-coated tablet, debossed with a "P" logo with deep score over "50" on one side and "ATENOLOL" on the other side contains: atenolol 50 mg. Nonmedicinal ingredients: croscarmellose sodium, hydroxypropyl cellulose, hydroxypropyl methylcellulose, magnesium stearate, magnesium trisilicate, microcrystalline cellulose, polyethylene glycol, talc and titanium dioxide. Compliance packs of 30. Bottles of 100 and 500. Store at room temperature (15-30°C). Protect from light and moisture.

100 mg: Each white, round, biconvex, film-coated tablet, debossed with a "P" logo with deep score over "100" on one side and "ATENOLOL" on the other side contains: atenolol 100 mg. Nonmedicinal ingredients: croscarmellose sodium, hydroxypropyl cellulose, hydroxypropyl methylcellulose, magnesium stearate, magnesium trisilicate, microcrystalline cellulose, polyethylene glycol, talc and titanium dioxide. Compliance packs of 30. Bottles of 100 and 500. Store at room temperature (15-30°C). Protect from light and moisture.

The reader is invited to consult CPhA's monograph **HMG-CoA Reductase Inhibitors**.

PMS-Atorvastatin Pr

atorvastatin calcium

Lipid Metabolism Regulator

Pharmascience

SUPPLIED: 10 mg: Each white, elliptical, film-coated tablet, debossed with "10" on one side and "GD" on the other side contains: atorvastatin calcium 10 mg. Nonmedicinal ingredients: calcium carbonate, candelilla wax, croscarmellose sodium, hydroxypropyl cellulose, hydroxypropyl methylcellulose, lactose, magnesium stearate, microcrystalline cellulose, polyethylene glycol, polysorbate 80, simethicone emulsion, talc and titanium dioxide. Bottles of 90 and 500. Store at controlled room temperature 15 to 30°C.

20 mg: Each white, elliptical, film-coated tablet, debossed with "20" on one side and "GD" on the other side contains: atorvastatin calcium 20 mg. Nonmedicinal ingredients: calcium carbonate, candelilla wax, croscarmellose sodium, hydroxypropyl cellulose, hydroxypropyl methylcellulose, lactose, magnesium stearate, microcrystalline cellulose, polyethylene glycol, polysorbate 80, simethicone emulsion, talc and titanium dioxide. Bottles of 90 and 500. Store at controlled room temperature 15 to 30°C.
40 mg: Each white, elliptical, film-coated tablet, debossed with "40" on one side and "GD" on the other side contains: atorvastatin 40 mg. Nonmedicinal ingredients: calcium carbonate, candelilla wax, croscarmellose sodium, hydroxypropyl cellulose, hydroxypropyl methylcellulose, lactose, magnesium stearate, microcrystalline cellulose, polyethylene glycol, polysorbate 80, simethicone emulsion, talc, and titanium dioxide. Bottles of 90 and 500. Store at controlled room temperature 15 to 30°C.
80 mg: Each white, elliptical, film-coated tablet, debossed with "80" on one side and "GD" on the other side contains: atorvastatin calcium 80 mg. Nonmedicinal ingredients: calcium carbonate, croscarmellose sodium, hydroxypropyl cellulose, hydroxypropyl methylcellulose, lactose, magnesium stearate, microcrystalline cellulose, polyethylene glycol, polysorbate 80, simethicone emulsion, talc and titanium dioxide. Bottles of 90 and 500. Store at controlled room temperature 15 to 30°C.

PMS-Azithromycin ℞
azithromycin monohydrate hemiethanolate
Antibiotic

Pharmascience

SUPPLIED: Tablets: 250 mg: Each dark pink, coated, modified capsule-shaped tablet, debossed with a "AZI" logo on one side and "250" on the other side, contains: azithromycin monohydrate hemiethanolate equivalent to azithromycin 250 mg. Nonmedicinal ingredients: colloidal silicon dioxide, croscarmellose sodium, D&C Red No. 27 Aluminum Lake, FD&C Blue No. 2 Aluminum Lake, FD&C Red No. 40 Aluminum Lake, FD&C Yellow No. 6 Aluminum Lake, hydroxypropylmethylcellulose, lactose, magnesium stearate, microcrystalline cellulose, poloxamer 188, polyethylene glycol, povidone, talc and titanium dioxide. Blisters of 6. Bottles of 100. Store between 15 and 30°C.
600 mg: Each white to off-white, coated, modified capsule-shaped tablet, debossed with a "P" logo on one side and "600" on the other side, contains: azithromycin monohydrate hemiethanolate equivalent to azithromycin 600 mg. Nonmedicinal ingredients: colloidal silicon dioxide, croscarmellose sodium, hydroxypropylmethylcellulose, lactose, magnesium stearate, microcrystalline cellulose, poloxamer 188, polyethylene glycol, polysorbate 80, povidone, talc and titanium dioxide. Bottles of 30. Store between 15 and 30°C.
Powder for suspension: The pink granulated powder forms a pink-red cherry flavoured suspension when reconstituted with water as directed in the labeling. After reconstitution, the 300 mg (15 mL) size contains a 100 mg/5 mL suspension, and the 600 mg (15 mL) and 900 mg (22.5 mL) contain a 200 mg/5 mL suspension. Nonmedicinal ingredients: artificial cherry flavour, carboxyvinyl polymer, colloidal silicon dioxide, FD&C Red No. 40 Aluminum Lake, polyethylene glycol, sodium chloride, sodium citrate dihydrate, sodium lauryl sulfate and sucrose. Store the powder between 15 and 30°C and the reconstituted suspension between 5 and 30°C. Discard unused portion after 10 days.

PMS-Carvedilol ℞
carvedilol
Congestive Heart Failure Agent

Pharmascience

SUPPLIED: 3.125 mg: Each white, oval shaped, film-coated tablet, debossed with "CV" on one side and plain on the other side, contains: carvedilol 3.125 mg. Nonmedicinal ingredients: colloidal silicon dioxide, crospovidone, hydroxypropyl methylcellulose, lactose, magnesium stearate, microcrystalline cellulose, polydextrose, polyethylene glycol, povidone, titanium dioxide and triethyl citrate. Bottles of 100. Store at room temperature, between 15 and 30°C, in tightly closed containers or dispense in a tight, light-resistant container. Protect from high humidity. Since the tablets discolour when exposed to light, they should be kept in light-resistant container.
6.25 mg: Each white, oval shaped, film-coated tablet, debossed with "CV" on one side and "6.25" on the other side, contains: carvedilol 6.25 mg. Nonmedicinal ingredients: colloidal silicon dioxide, crospovidone, hydroxypropyl methylcellulose, lactose, magnesium stearate, microcrystalline cellulose, polydextrose, polyethylene glycol, povidone, titanium dioxide and triethyl citrate. Bottles of 100. Store at room temperature, between 15 and 30°C, in tightly closed containers or dispense in a tight, light-resistant container. Protect from high humidity. Since the tablets discolour when exposed to light, they should be kept in light-resistant container.
12.5 mg: Each white, oval shaped, film-coated tablet, debossed with "CV" on one side and "12.5" on the other side, contains: carvedilol 12.5 mg. Nonmedicinal ingredients: colloidal silicon dioxide, crospovidone, hydroxypropyl methylcellulose, lactose, magnesium stearate, microcrystalline cellulose, polydextrose, polyethylene glycol, povidone, titanium dioxide and triethyl citrate. Bottles of 100. Store at room temperature, between 15 and 30°C, in tightly closed containers or dispense in a tight, light-resistant container. Protect from high humidity. Since the tablets discolour when exposed to light, they should be kept in light-resistant container.
25 mg: Each white, oval shaped, film-coated tablet, debossed with "CV" on one side and "25" on the other side, contains: carvedilol 25 mg. Nonmedicinal ingredients: colloidal silicon dioxide, crospovidone, hydroxypropyl methylcellulose, lactose, magnesium stearate, microcrystalline cellulose, polydextrose, polyethylene glycol, povidone, titanium dioxide and triethyl citrate. Bottles of 100. Store at room temperature, between 15 and 30°C, in tightly closed containers or dispense in a tight, light-resistant container. Protect from high humidity. Since the tablets discolour when exposed to light, they should be kept in light-resistant container.

PMS-Cetirizine ℞
cetirizine HCl
Histamine H1-Receptor Antagonist

Pharmascience

SUPPLIED: Each white, modified rectangle shape, biconvex, coated tablet debossed with "20" on the left and "P" on the right of a score line on one side and plain on the other side, contains: cetirizine 2.5 mg (as cetirizine hydrochloride). Nonmedicinal ingredients: corn starch, hydroxypropyl methylcellulose, lactose, magnesium stearate, polyethylene glycol, povidone and titanium dioxide. Bottles of 100. Store between 15 and 30°C.

PMS-Cholestyramine ℞
cholestyramine resin
Antihypercholesterolemic—Antidiarrheal

Pharmascience

SUPPLIED: Light Lemon-lime Flavour: Each sachet (5 g dose) of an off-white to pale yellow powder with a slight lemon-lime aroma contains: cholestyramine resin 4 g (dried basis). Nonmedicinal ingredients: aspartame, citric acid, colloidal silicon dioxide, D&C Yellow No. 10 Aluminum Lake, natural lemon-lime flavour and propylene glycol alginate. Sugar-free. Cartons of 30 sachets (30 doses). Store at room temperature (15 to 30°C). Protect from moisture.
Light Orange Flavour: Each sachet (5 g dose) of an off-white to orange powder with a slight orange aroma contains: cholestyramine resin 4 g (dried basis). Nonmedicinal ingredients: aspartame, citric acid, colloidal silicon dioxide, FD&C Yellow No. 6, natural orange flavour and propylene glycol alginate. Sugar-free. Cartons of 30 sachets (30 doses). Store at room temperature (15 to 30°C). Protect from moisture.
Regular Orange Flavour: Each sachet (9 g dose) of an off-white to yellowish powder with a slight orange aroma contains: cholestyramine resin 4 g (dried basis). Nonmedicinal ingredients: citric acid, colloidal silicon dioxide, D&C Yellow No. 10 Aluminum Lake, FD&C Yellow No. 6, natural and artificial orange flavour, propylene glycol alginate and sucrose. Energy: 77.4 kJ (18.5 kcal)/9 g. Sodium- and tartrazine-free. Cartons of 30 sachets (30 doses). Store at room temperature (15 to 30°C). Protect from moisture.

The reader is invited to consult CPhA's monograph **Selective Serotonin Reuptake Inhibitors**.

PMS-Citalopram ℞
citalopram HBr
Antidepressant

Pharmascience

SUPPLIED: 10 mg: Each white, oval, coated tablet, debossed with "10" on one side and plain on the other side, contains: citalopram 10 mg as citalopram HBr. Nonmedicinal ingredients: colloidal silicon dioxide, hydroxypropyl cellulose, hydroxypropyl methylcellulose, lactose, magnesium stearate, microcrystalline cellulose, polyethylene glycol, sodium starch glycolate and titanium dioxide. Bottles of 100. Store between 15 and 30°C and keep in a dry place.
20 mg: Each white to off-white, oval, film-coated tablet, debossed "20" on one side and scored on the other side, contains: citalopram 20 mg as citalopram HBr. Nonmedicinal ingredients: colloidal silicon dioxide, hydroxypropyl cellulose, hydroxypropyl methylcellulose, lactose, magnesium stearate, microcrystalline cellulose, polyethylene glycol, sodium starch glycolate and titanium dioxide. Bottles of 100 and 500. Blisters of 30. Store between 15 and 30°C and keep in a dry place.
40 mg: Each white to off-white, oval, film-coated tablet, debossed "40" on one side and scored on the other side, contains: citalopram 40 mg as citalopram HBr. Nonmedicinal ingredients: colloidal silicon dioxide, hydroxypropyl cellulose, hydroxypropyl methylcellulose, lactose, magnesium stearate, microcrystalline cellulose, polyethylene glycol, sodium starch glycolate and titanium dioxide. Bottles of 100. Blisters of 30. Store between 15 and 30°C and keep in a dry place.

PMS-Clonazepam ℞
clonazepam
Anticonvulsant

Pharmascience

SUPPLIED: PMS-Clonazepam: 0.25 mg: Each round, blue, biconvex tablet, debossed "CLONAZEPAM" on one side and plain on the other side, contains: clonazepam 250 µg. Nonmedicinal ingredients: cornstarch, FD&C Blue No. 1 Aluminum Lake, lactose, magnesium stearate and microcrystalline cellulose. Bottles of 100. Store between 15 and 30°C. Keep in tightly closed, light-resistant container.
0.5 mg: Each round, orange, biplane, beveled-edge tablet, debossed "CLONAZEPAM" on one side and "pms" score "0.5" on the other side, contains: clonazepam 500 µg. Nonmedicinal ingredients: cornstarch, FD&C Yellow No. 6 Aluminum Lake, lactose, magnesium stearate and microcrystalline cellulose. Bottles of 100 and 500. Store between 15 and 30°C. Keep in tightly closed, light-resistant container.
1 mg: Each round, pink, biconvex tablet, debossed "CLONAZEPAM" on one side and "1.0" on the other side, contains: clonazepam 1 mg. Nonmedicinal ingredients: cornstarch, FD&C Red No. 40 Aluminum Lake, lactose, magnesium stearate and microcrystalline cellulose. Bottles of 100, 500 and 1000. Store between 15 and 30°C. Keep in tightly closed, light-resistant container.
2 mg: Each round, white, biplane, beveled-edge tablet, debossed "CLONAZEPAM" on one side and "2.0" under the score line on the other side, contains: clonazepam 2 mg. Nonmedicinal ingredients: cornstarch, lactose, magnesium stearate and microcrystalline cellulose. Bottles of 100, 500 and 1000. Store between 15 and 30°C. Keep in tightly closed, light-resistant container.
PMS-Clonazepam-R: Each round, orange, biplane, beveled-edge tablet, debossed "CLONAZEPAM" on one side and "0.5" under the score line on the other side, contains: clonazepam 500 µg. Nonmedicinal ingredients: cornstarch, FD&C Yellow No. 6 Aluminum Lake, lactose, magnesium stearate and microcrystalline cellulose. Bottles of 100 and 500. Store between 15 and 30°C. Keep in tightly closed, light-resistant container.

PMS-Desmopressin ℞
desmopressin acetate
Antidiuretic

Pharmascience

SUPPLIED: 0.1 mg: Each white, oval-shaped tablet with "0.1" debossed on one side and scored on the other side, contains: desmopressin acetate trihydrate 0.1 mg. Nonmedicinal ingredients: lactose, magnesium stearate, microcrystalline cellulose and sodium starch glycolate. Bottles of 100. Store at room temperature (15-30°C). Avoid humidity and light exposure.
0.2 mg: Each white, round tablet with "0.2" debossed on one side and scored on the other side, contains: desmopressin acetate trihydrate 0.2 mg. Nonmedicinal ingredients: lactose, magnesium stearate, microcrystalline cellulose and sodium starch glycolate. Bottles of 100. Store at room temperature (15-30°C). Avoid humidity and light exposure.

The reader is invited to consult CPhA's monograph **Corticosteroids: Topical**.

PMS-Desonide ℞
desonide
Topical Corticosteroid

Pharmascience

SUPPLIED: Cream: Each tube contains: desonide 0.05%. Nonmedicinal ingredients: aluminum acetate, cetyl stearyl alcohol, glycerin, methylparaben, mineral oil, purified water, sodium lauryl sulfate, wax and white petrolatum. Tubes of 15, 60 and 454 g.
Ointment: Each tube contains: desonide 0.05%. Nonmedicinal ingredients: white petrolatum. Tubes of 60 g.

PMS-Dexamethasone Elixir/Tablets ℞
dexamethasone
Corticosteroid

Pharmascience

PMS-Dexamethasone Injection ℞
dexamethasone sodium phosphate
Corticosteroid

Pharmascience

SUPPLIED: Elixir: Each 5 mL of clear, red, raspberry-flavored elixir, contains: dexamethasone 0.5 mg. Nonmedicinal ingredients: alcohol, artificial raspberry flavor, benzoic acid, citric acid, FD&C Red No. 40, methylparaben, propylparaben, propylene glycol and sucrose. Bottles of 100 mL. Store at 15 to 30°C. Protect from light.
Tablets: 0.5 mg: Each cream colored, pentagonal, flat, beveled-edge tablet, debossed with a "P" logo over a score line and "084" under it on one side, and plain on the other side, contains: dexamethasone 0.5 mg. Nonmedicinal ingredients: croscarmellose sodium, D&C Yellow No. 10 Aluminum Lake, lactose, magnesium stearate, microcrystalline cellulose and stearic acid. Bottles of 100. Store at 15 to 30°C. Protect from light.
0.75 mg: Each blue, pentagonal, flat, beveled-edge tablet, debossed with a "P" logo over a score line and "085" under it on one side, and plain on the other side, contains: dexamethasone 0.75 mg. Nonmedicinal ingredients: croscarmellose sodium, D&C Yellow No. 10 Aluminum Lake, FD&C Blue No. 1 Aluminum Lake, lactose, magnesium stearate, microcrystalline cellulose and stearic acid. Bottles of 100. Store at 15 to 30°C. Protect from light.
2 mg: Each white, pentagonal, flat, beveled-edge tablet, debossed with a "P" logo over a score line and "086" under it on one side, and plain on the other side, contains: dexamethasone 2 mg. Nonmedicinal ingredients: croscarmellose sodium, lactose, magnesium stearate, microcrystalline cellulose and stearic acid. Bottles of 100. Store at 15 to 30°C. Protect from light.
4 mg: Each white, pentagonal, flat, beveled-edge tablet, debossed with a "P" logo over a score line and "087" under it on one side, and plain on the other side, contains: dexamethasone 4 mg. Nonmedicinal ingredients: croscarmellose sodium, lactose, magnesium stearate, microcrystalline cellulose and stearic acid. Bottles of 100. Store at 15 to 30°C. Protect from light.
Injection: Each mL of clear, colorless to light yellow, aqueous solution contains: dexamethasone sodium phosphate 10 mg. Nonmedicinal ingredients: benzyl alcohol, sodium citrate, sodium sulfite and water. Vials of 10 mL. Store at 15 to 30°C, do not freeze. Protect from light.

PMS-Finasteride ℞
finasteride
Type II 5 Alpha-reductase Inhibitor

Pharmascience

SUPPLIED: 1 mg: Each tan-colored, round, biconvex, film-coated tablet, debossed with "FS" on one side and "1" on the other side contains: finasteride 1 mg. Nonmedicinal ingredients: docusate sodium, hydroxypropylcellulose, hypromellose, iron oxide red, lactose, magnesium stearate, microcrystalline cellulose, pregelatinized starch, sodium starch glycolate, talc, titanium dioxide and yellow iron oxide. Blisters of 10. Bottles of 100. Store at room temperature 15-30°C and protect from light to prevent discoloration. Crushed or broken finasteride tablets should not be handled by women when they are or may potentially be pregnant.
5 mg: Each blue, round, biconvex, film-coated tablet, debossed with "FS" on one side and "5" on the other side contains: finasteride 5 mg. Nonmedicinal ingredients: docusate sodium, FD&C Blue No. 2 Aluminum Lake, hydroxypropyl cellulose, hypromellose, lactose, magnesium stearate, microcrystalline cellulose (Avicel PH 102), pregelatinized starch, sodium starch glycolate, talc, titanium dioxide and yellow iron oxide. Blisters of 10. Bottles of 100. Store at room temperature (15-30°C) and protect from light to prevent discoloration. Crushed or broken finasteride tablets should not be handled by women when they are or may potentially be pregnant.

The reader is invited to consult CPhA's monograph **Selective Serotonin Reuptake Inhibitors**.

PMS-Fluoxetine ℞
fluoxetine HCl
Antidepressant—Antiobsessional—Antibulimic

Pharmascience

SUPPLIED: 10 mg: Each hard gelatin capsule with an opaque green cap and opaque grey body, both printed in black ink "P10" contains: fluoxetine HCl equivalent to fluoxetine 10 mg (32.3 μmol). Nonmedicinal ingredients: colloidal silicone dioxide and cornstarch; capsule shell: D&C Yellow No. 10, FD&C Blue No. 1, FD&C Yellow No. 6, gelatin, iron oxide black and titanium dioxide. Bottles of 100. Store at 15 to 30°C. Keep tightly closed.
20 mg: Each hard gelatin capsule with an opaque green cap and opaque ivory body, both printed in black ink "P20" contains: fluoxetine HCl equivalent to fluoxetine 20 mg (64.7 μmol). Nonmedicinal ingredients: colloidal silicone dioxide and cornstarch; capsule shell: D&C Yellow No. 10, FD&C Blue No. 1, FD&C Yellow No. 6, gelatin and titanium dioxide. Bottles of 100 and 500. Store at 15 to 30°C. Keep tightly closed.

PMS-Gabapentin ℞
gabapentin
Antiepileptic

Pharmascience

SUPPLIED: 100 mg: Each hard gelatin capsule, with white opaque body and cap ink-printed in blue with "Gabapentin/100 mg" on the cap, contains: gabapentin 100 mg. Nonmedicinal ingredients: cornstarch, lactose and talc; shell: gelatin and titanium dioxide. Bottles of 100 and 500. Store at room temperature, between 15 and 30°C.
300 mg: Each hard gelatin capsule, with yellow opaque body and cap ink-printed in blue with "Gabapentin/300 mg" on the cap, contains: gabapentin 300 mg. Nonmedicinal ingredients: cornstarch, lactose and talc; shell: gelatin, titanium dioxide and yellow iron oxide. Bottles of 100 and 500. Store at room temperature, between 15 and 30°C.
400 mg: Each hard gelatin capsule, with orange opaque body and cap ink-printed in blue with "Gabapentin/400 mg" on the cap, contains: gabapentin 400 mg. Nonmedicinal ingredients: cornstarch, lactose and talc; shell: gelatin, titanium dioxide, red iron oxide and yellow iron oxide. Bottles of 100 and 500. Store at room temperature, between 15 and 30°C.
600 mg: Each white to off-white, film-coated, elliptical-shaped tablet, debossed with "G" over "600" on one side and plain on the other side, contains: gabapentin 600 mg. Nonmedicinal ingredients: copovidone, hydroxypropyl cellulose, hydroxypropyl methylcellulose, magnesium stearate, microcrystalline cellulose, polyethylene glycol, sodium starch glycolate and talc. Bottles of 100. Store at room temperature, between 15 and 30°C.
800 mg: Each white to off-white, film-coated, elliptical-shaped tablet, debossed with "G" over "800" on one side and "P" on the other side, contains: gabapentin 800 mg. Nonmedicinal ingredients: copovidone, hydroxypropyl cellulose, hydroxypropyl methylcellulose, magnesium stearate, microcrystalline cellulose, polyethylene glycol, sodium starch glycolate and talc. Bottles of 100. Store at room temperature, between 15 and 30°C.

PMS-Hydrocodone Ⓝ
hydrocodone bitartrate
Antitussive

Pharmascience

SUPPLIED: Each mL of red-cherry-flavored syrup contains: hydrocodone bitartrate 1 mg. Nonmedicinal ingredients: artificial cherry flavor, caramel colour, FD&C Red No. 2 Aluminum Lake, methylparaben, propylparaben, purified water, sorbitol and sucrose. Bottles of 500 mL. Keep out of reach of children. Store at 15 to 30°C. Dispense syrup in a tight, light resistant container.

PMS-Hydromorphone Ⓝ
hydromorphone HCl
Analgesic—Narcotic

Pharmascience

SUPPLIED: Suppositories: Each suppository contains: hydromorphone HCl 3 mg. Nonmedicinal ingredients: Wecobee. Boxes of 10. Store between 15 to 30°C. Protect from light.
Syrup: Each mL of syrup contains: hydromorphone HCl 1 mg. Nonmedicinal ingredients: dextrose, glycerine, propylene glycol and sodium benzoate. Bottles of 500 mL. Store between 15 to 30°C. Protect from light.
Tablets: 1 mg: Each pale green, round, biconvex tablet, debossed "1" in the centre of the score line on one side and "PMS" on the other side, contains: hydromorphone HCl 1 mg. Nonmedicinal ingredients: D&C Yellow No. 10 Aluminum Lake, FD&C Blue No. 1 Aluminum Lake, FD&C Yellow No. 6 Aluminum Lake, lactose, magnesium stearate and microcrystalline cellulose. Bottles of 100. Control packs of 25 (4×25). Store at 15 to 30°C. Protect from light.
2 mg: Each pale orange, round, biconvex tablet, debossed "2" in the centre of the score line on one side and "PMS" on the other side, contains: hydromorphone HCl 2 mg. Nonmedicinal ingredients: D&C Yellow No. 10 Aluminum Lake, FD&C Yellow No. 6 Aluminum Lake, lactose, magnesium stearate and microcrystalline cellulose. Bottles of 100. Control packs of 25 (4×25). Store at 15 to 30°C. Protect from light.
4 mg: Each yellow, round, biconvex tablet, debossed "4" in the centre of the score line on one side and "PMS" on the other side, contains: hydromorphone HCl 4 mg. Nonmedicinal ingredients: D&C Yellow No. 10 Aluminum Lake, FD&C Yellow No. 6 Aluminum Lake, lactose, magnesium stearate and microcrystalline cellulose. Bottles of 100. Control packs of 25 (4×25). Store at 15 to 30°C. Protect from light.
8 mg: Each white, round, biconvex tablet, debossed "8" in the centre of the score line on one side and "PMS" on the other side, contains: hydromorphone HCl 8 mg. Nonmedicinal ingredients: lactose, magnesium stearate and microcrystalline cellulose. Bottles of 100. Control packs of 25 (4×25). Store at 15 to 30°C. Protect from light.

PMS-Letrozole ℞
letrozole
Nonsteroidal Aromatase Inhibitor—Inhibitor of Estrogen Biosynthesis—Antitumour Agent

Pharmascience

SUPPLIED: Each dark yellow, slightly biconvex, bevel-edged, round tablet, debossed with "LT" on one side and "2.5" on the other side, contains: letrozole 2.5 mg. Nonmedicinal ingredients: colloidal anhydrous silica, FD&C Yellow No. 5 Aluminum Lake, hypromellose, lactose monohydrate, magnesium stearate, microcrystalline cellulose, polyethylene glycol, red iron oxide, sodium starch glycolate, titanium dioxide and yellow iron oxide. Blister packages of 30. Protect from heat (store at room temperature 15 to 30°C). Protect from moisture.

The reader is invited to consult CPhA's monograph **Fluoroquinolones**.

PMS-Levofloxacin ℞
levofloxacin
Antibacterial

Pharmascience

SUPPLIED: 250 mg: Each pink, modified rectangular-shaped, coated tablet, debossed with "P" logo on one side and "250" on the other side, contains: levofloxacin 250 mg. Nonmedicinal ingredients: colloidal silicon dioxide, copovidone, crospovidone, iron oxide red, magnesium stearate, microcrystalline cellulose, polyethylene glycol, polyvinyl alcohol, talc and titanium dioxide. Bottles of 100. Store at controlled room temperature (15-30°C) in well-closed containers.
500 mg: Each peach, modified rectangular-shaped, coated tablet, debossed with "P" logo on one side and "500" on the other side, contains: levofloxacin 500 mg. Nonmedicinal ingredients: colloidal silicon dioxide, copovidone, crospovidone, hydroxypropyl methylcellulose, iron oxide red, iron oxide yellow, magnesium stearate, microcrystalline cellulose, polydextrose, polyethylene glycol, titanium dioxide and triacetin. Bottles of 100. Store at controlled room temperature (15-30°C) in well-closed containers.
750 mg: Each white, modified rectangular-shaped, coated tablet, debossed with "P" logo on one side and "750" on the other side, contains: levofloxacin 750 mg. Nonmedicinal ingredients: colloidal silicon dioxide, copovidone, crospovidone, magnesium stearate, microcrystalline cellulose, polyethylene glycol, polyvinyl alcohol, talc and titanium dioxide. Bottles of 100. Store at controlled room temperature (15-30°C) in well-closed containers.

PMS-Lindane
lindane
Scabicide—Pediculicide

PendoPharm

SUPPLIED: Lotion: Each mL of nongreasy lotion contains: lindane USP (gamma benzene hexachloride) 1%. Nonmedicinal ingredients: butylparaben, carbomer 934P, emulsifying wax, ethylparaben, geranium fragrance, isobutylparaben, methylparaben, phenoxyethanol, propylene glycol, propylene glycol dicaprylate/dicaprate, propylparaben, stearic acid, sorbitan monolaurate, triethanolamine and water. Bottles of 50 and 500 mL.
Shampoo: Each mL contains: lindane USP (gamma benzene hexachloride) 1%. Nonmedicinal ingredients: acetone, 5-bromo-5-nitro-1,3-dioxane, citric acid, cocamide diethanolamine, polysorbate, propylene glycol, triethanolamine lauryl sulfate and water. Bottles of 50 and 500 mL.

PMS-Loxapine ℞
loxapine succinate
Antipsychotic

Pharmascience

SUPPLIED: 2.5 mg: Each round, scored, biconvex, blue, film-coated tablet, debossed with a "P" logo on one side and "L" over "2.5" on the scored side, contains: loxapine 2.5 mg as the succinate salt. Nonmedicinal ingredients: colloidal silicon dioxide, corn starch, croscarmellose sodium, FD&C Blue No. 1 Aluminum Lake, FD&C Yellow No. 6 Aluminum Lake, hydroxypropyl methylcellulose, lactose, magnesium stearate, microcrystalline cellulose, polyethylene glycol, polysorbate and titanium dioxyde. Bottles of 100. Store at room temperature (15-30°C).

5 mg: Each round, scored, biconvex, yellow, film-coated tablet, debossed with a "P" logo on one side and "L" over "5" on the scored side, contains: loxapine 5 mg as the succinate salt. Nonmedicinal ingredients: colloidal silicon dioxide, corn starch, croscarmellose sodium, D&C Yellow No. 10 Aluminum Lake, FD&C Blue No. 2 Aluminum Lake, FD&C Yellow No. 10 Aluminum Lake, hydroxypropyl methylcellulose, lactose, magnesium stearate, microcrystalline cellulose, polyethylene glycol, polysorbate and titanium dioxide. Bottles of 100 and 500. Store at room temperature (15-30°C).
10 mg: Each round, scored, biconvex, green, film-coated tablet, debossed with a "P" logo on one side and "L" over "10" on the scored side, contains: loxapine 10 mg as the succinate salt. Nonmedicinal ingredients: colloidal silicon dioxide, corn starch, croscarmellose sodium, D&C Yellow No. 10 Aluminum Lake, FD&C Blue No. 1 Aluminum Lake, FD&C Red No. 40 Aluminum Lake, hydroxypropyl methylcellulose, lactose, magnesium stearate, microcrystalline cellulose, polyethylene glycol, polysorbate and titanium dioxide. Bottles of 100 and 500. Store at room temperature (15-30°C).
25 mg: Each round, scored, biconvex, pink, film-coated tablet, debossed with a "P" logo on one side and "L" over "25" on the scored side, contains: loxapine 25 mg as the succinate salt. Nonmedicinal ingredients: colloidal silicon dioxide, corn starch, croscarmellose sodium, D&C Red No. 27 Aluminum Lake, FD&C Red No. 40 Aluminum Lake, hydroxypropyl methylcellulose, lactose, magnesium stearate, microcrystalline cellulose, polyethylene glycol, polysorbate and titanium dioxide. Bottles of 100 and 500. Store at room temperature (15-30°C).
50 mg: Each round, scored, biconvex, white, film-coated tablet, embossed with "P" logo on one side and "L" over "50" on the scored side, contains: loxapine 50 mg as the succinate salt. Nonmedicinal ingredients: colloidal silicon dioxide, corn starch, croscarmellose sodium, hydroxypropyl methylcellulose, lactose, magnesium stearate, microcrystalline cellulose, polyethylene glycol and titanium dioxide. Bottles of 100 and 500. Store at room temperature (15-30°C).

PMS-Memantine ℞
memantine HCl
N-methyl-D-aspartate (NMDA) Receptor Antagonist

Pharmascience

SUPPLIED: Each white to off-white, oblong, biconvex, scored tablet, debossed with "MT" divided by the score on one side and "10" divided by the score on the other side, contains: memantine HCl 10 mg. Nonmedicinal indredients: colloidal silicon dioxide, crospovidone, hydroxypropyl methylcellulose, lactose, magnesium stearate, microcrystalline cellulose, polyethylene glycol, polysorbate 80 and titanium dioxide. Bottles of 100. Blister packages of 30. Store in a dry place at room temperature between 15 and 30°C, protect from moisture.

PMS-Metformin ℞
metformin HCl
Antihyperglycemic

Pharmascience

SUPPLIED: 500 mg: Each white, round, biconvex coated tablet, debossed "MET" over "500" on the scored side and plain on the other side, contains: metformin HCl 500 mg. Nonmedicinal ingredients: colloidal silicon dioxide, corn starch, croscarmellose sodium, hydroxypropyl methylcellulose, magnesium stearate, microcrystalline cellulose, polyethylene glycol and povidone. Bottles of 100 and 500. Store at room temperature between 15 and 30°C.
850 mg: Each white, capsule-shaped, biconvex coated tablet, debossed "MET" on one side and "850" on the other side, contains: metformin 850 mg. Nonmedicinal ingredients: colloidal silicon dioxide, corn starch, croscarmellose sodium, hydroxypropyl methylcellulose, magnesium stearate, microcrystalline cellulose, polyethylene glycol and povidone. Bottles of 100 and 500. Store at room temperature between 15 and 30°C.

PMS-Methylphenidate Ⓒ
methylphenidate HCl
CNS Stimulant

Pharmascience

SUPPLIED: 5 mg: Each salmon, round, biconvex, scored tablet, debossed "MP" over "5" on one side and "130" on the other side, contains: methylphenidate HCl USP 5 mg. Nonmedicinal ingredients: cornstarch, dibasic calcium phosphate, FD&C Yellow No. 6 Aluminum Lake, lactose, magnesium stearate and microcrystalline cellulose. Bottles of 100 and 500. Store at controlled room temperature 15 to 30°C.
10 mg: Each blue, round, biconvex, scored tablet, debossed "MP" over "10" on one side and "110" on the other side, contains: methylphenidate HCl USP 10 mg. Nonmedicinal ingredients: cornstarch, dibasic calcium phosphate, FD&C Green No. 3, lactose, magnesium stearate and microcrystalline cellulose. Bottles of 100 and 500. Store at controlled room temperature 15 to 30°C.
20 mg: Each yellow, round, biconvex, scored tablet, debossed "MP" over "20" on one side and "123" on the other side, contains: methylphenidate HCl USP 20 mg. Nonmedicinal ingredients: cornstarch, dibasic calcium phosphate, FD&C Yellow No. 10 Aluminum Lake, lactose, magnesium stearate and microcrystalline cellulose. Bottles of 100. Store at controlled room temperature 15 to 30°C.

PMS-Metoprolol-L ℞
metoprolol tartrate
Beta-blocking Agent

Pharmascience

SUPPLIED: 25 mg: Each white, oblong, biconvex, coated, scored tablet, debossed "L/25" on one side and "MTP" on the other side, contains: metoprolol tartrate 25 mg. Nonmedicinal ingredients: colloidal silicon dioxide, hydroxypropylmethylcellulose, lactose, magnesium stearate, microcrystalline cellulose, polydextrose, polyethylene glycol, povidone, sodium starch glycolate, titanium dioxide and triethyl citrate. Bottles of 100 and 500. Store at room temperature between 15 to 30°C. Protect from light and humidity.
50 mg: Each pink, oblong, biconvex, coated, scored tablet, debossed "L/50" on one side and "MTP" on the other side, contains: metoprolol tartrate 50 mg. Nonmedicinal ingredients: colloidal silicon dioxide, D&C Red No. 30, D&C Yellow No. 10 Aluminum Lake, hydroxypropyl methylcellulose, lactose, magnesium stearate, microcrystalline cellulose, polyethylene glycol, polysorbate, povidone, sodium starch glycolate and titanium dioxide. Bottles of 100, 500 and 1000. Store at room temperature between 15 to 30°C. Protect from light and humidity.
100 mg: Each light blue, oblong, biconvex, coated, scored tablet, debossed "L/100" on one side and "MTP" on the other side, contains: metoprolol tartrate 100 mg. Nonmedicinal ingredients: colloidal silicon dioxide, FD&C Blue No. 2 Aluminum Lake, hydroxypropyl methylcellulose, lactose, magnesium stearate, microcrystalline cellulose, polyethylene glycol, polysorbate, povidone, sodium starch glycolate and titanium dioxide. Bottles of 100, 500 and 1000. Store at room temperature between 15 to 30°C. Protect from light and humidity.

PMS-Mirtazapine ℞
mirtazapine
Antidepressant

Pharmascience

SUPPLIED: 15 mg: Each yellow, oval, scored, coated tablet, debossed with the "1" on the left side of a score line and "5" on the right side and with the letters "MIR" on the other side, contains: mirtazapine 15 mg. Nonmedicinal ingredients: colloidal silicon dioxide, hydroxypropyl methylcellulose, iron oxide yellow, lactose, magnesium stearate, microcrystalline cellulose, polyethylene glycol, polysorbate, sodium starch glycolate and titanium dioxide. Bottles of 100. Store between 15 and 30°C, in a tightly closed light resistant container.
30 mg: Each red-brown, oval, coated tablet, debossed with the "3" on the left side of a score line and "0" on the right side and the letters "MIR" on the other side, contains: mirtazapine 30 mg. Nonmedicinal ingredients: colloidal silicon dioxide, iron oxide yellow, iron oxide red, lactose, magnesium stearate, microcrystalline cellulose, polyethylene glycol, polyvinyl alcohol, sodium starch glycolate, talc and titanium dioxide. Bottles of 100. Blisters of 30. Store between 15 and 30°C in a tightly closed light resistant container.

PMS-Naproxen ℞
naproxen
Anti-inflammatory

Pharmascience

PMS-Naproxen EC ℞
naproxen
Anti-inflammatory—Analgesic—Antipyretic

Pharmascience

SUPPLIED: PMS-Naproxen: Each white to off-white suppository contains: naproxen 500 mg. Nonmedicinal ingredients: wecobee. Boxes of 30. Store at room temperature (15-30°C). Protect from freezing.
PMS-Naproxen EC: 375 mg: Each white to off-white, convex, oblong, enteric-coated tablet, imprinted with the "P" logo and "375" in black ink on one side, contains: naproxen 375 mg. Nonmedicinal ingredients: black iron oxide, croscarmellose sodium, ethyl alcohol, isobutyl alcohol, magnesium stearate, methacrylic acid copolymer, polyethylene glycol 8000, polyethylene wax, polyvinyl pyrrolidone, povidone, shellac, simethicone emulsion, sodium hydroxide, talc and titanium dioxide. Bottles of 100. Store at room temperature between 15 and 30°C. Protect from moisture and light.
500 mg: Each white to off-white, convex, oblong, enteric-coated tablet, imprinted with the "P" logo and "500" in black ink on one side, contains: naproxen 500 mg. Nonmedicinal ingredients: black iron oxide, croscarmellose sodium, ethyl alcohol, isobutyl alcohol, magnesium stearate, methacrylic acid copolymer, polyethylene glycol, polyethylene wax, polyvinyl pyrrolidone, povidone, shellac, simethicone emulsion, sodium hydroxide, talc and titanium dioxide. Bottles of 100. Store at room temperature between 15 and 30°C. Protect from moisture and light.

PMS-Nizatidine ℞
nizatidine
Histamine H2-Receptor Antagonist

Pharmascience

SUPPLIED: 150 mg: Each hard gelatin capsule with opaque yellow cap ink-printed in black with "ab" and lighter yellow opaque body with "N150", contains: nizatidine 150 mg. Nonmedicinal ingredients: benzyl alcohol, carboxymethylcellulose sodium, corn starch, edetate calcium disodium, gelatin, iron oxide yellow, magnesium stearate, parabens (benzyl, propyl and methyl), silicone, sodium lauryl sulfate, sodium propionate and titanium dioxide. Bottles of 100. Store at 15-30°C.
300 mg: Each hard gelatin capsule with opaque brown cap ink-printed in black with "ab" and opaque yellow body with "N300", contains: nizatidine 300 mg. Nonmedicinal ingredients: benzyl alcohol, carboxymethylcellulose sodium, corn starch, edetate calcium disodium, gelatin, iron oxide yellow, parabens (benzyl, propyl and methyl), povidone, silicone, sodium lauryl sulfate, sodium propionate, talc and titanium dioxide. Bottles of 100. Store at 15-30°C.

PMS-Olanzapine ℞
olanzapine
Antipsychotic—Antimanic Agent

Pharmascience

PMS-Olanzapine ODT ℞
olanzapine
Antipsychotic—Antimanic Agent

Pharmascience

SUPPLIED: PMS-Olanzapine: 2.5 mg: Each white, round, biconvex, coated tablet, ink-printed in blue with "OZ 2.5" on one side and plain on the other side, contains: olanzapine 2.5 mg. Nonmedicinal ingredients: crospovidone, hydroxypropyl cellulose, hydroxypropyl methylcellulose, lactose, magnesium stearate, microcrystalline cellulose, pharmaceutical ink, polyethylene glycol and titanium dioxide. Bottles of 100. Store at 15-30°C. Protect from light and moisture.
5 mg: Each white, round, biconvex, coated tablet, ink-printed in blue with "OZ 5" on one side and plain on the other side, contains: olanzapine 5 mg. Nonmedicinal ingredients: crospovidone, hydroxypropyl cellulose, hydroxypropyl methylcellulose, lactose, magnesium stearate, microcrystalline cellulose, pharmaceutical ink, polyethylene glycol and titanium dioxide. Bottles of 100. Store at 15-30°C. Protect from light and moisture.
7.5 mg: Each white, round, biconvex, coated tablet, ink-printed in blue with "OZ 7.5" on one side and plain on the other side, contains: olanzapine 7.5 mg. Nonmedicinal ingredients: crospovidone, hydroxypropyl cellulose, hydroxypropyl methylcellulose, lactose, magnesium stearate, microcrystalline cellulose, pharmaceutical ink, polyethylene glycol and titanium dioxide. Bottles of 100. Store at 15-30°C. Protect from light and moisture.
10 mg: Each white, round, biconvex, coated tablet, ink-printed in blue with "OZ 10" on one side and plain on the other side, contains: olanzapine 10 mg. Nonmedicinal ingredients: crospovidone, hydroxypropyl cellulose, hydroxypropyl methylcellulose, lactose, magnesium stearate, microcrystalline cellulose, pharmaceutical ink, polyethylene glycol and titanium dioxide. Bottles of 100. Store at 15-30°C. Protect from light and moisture.
15 mg: Each light blue, elliptical, coated tablet, debossed with "OZ 15" on one side and plain on the other side, contains: olanzapine 15 mg. Nonmedicinal ingredients: crospovidone, FD&C Blue No. 2 Aluminum Lake, hydroxypropyl cellulose, hydroxypropyl methylcellulose, lactose, magnesium stearate, microcrystalline cellulose, polyethylene glycol and titanium dioxide. Bottles of 100. Store at 15-30°C. Protect from light and moisture.
PMS-Olanzapine ODT: 5 mg: Each yellow, round orally disintegrating tablet, convex on one side and flat faced on the other side, contains: olanzapine 5 mg. Nonmedicinal ingredients: aspartame, colloidal silicon dioxide, crospovidone, guar gum, magnesium stearate, mannitol, microcrystalline cellulose, pregelatinized starch and sodium lauryl sulphate. Blisters of 30. Store at 15-30°C. Protect from light and moisture.
10 mg: Each yellow, round orally disintegrating tablet, convex on one side and flat faced on the other side, contains: olanzapine 10 mg. Nonmedicinal ingredients: aspartame, colloidal silicon dioxide, crospovidone, guar gum, magnesium stearate, mannitol, microcrystalline cellulose, pregelatinized starch and sodium lauryl sulphate. Blisters of 30. Store at 15-30°C. Protect from light and moisture.
15 mg: Each yellow, round orally disintegrating tablet, convex on one side and flat faced on the other side, contains: olanzapine 15 mg. Nonmedicinal ingredients: aspartame, colloidal silicon dioxide, crospovidone, guar gum, magnesium stearate, mannitol, microcrystalline cellulose, pregelatinized starch and sodium lauryl sulphate. Blisters of 30. Store at 15-30°C. Protect from light and moisture.

PMS-Omeprazole ℞

omeprazole

H+, K+-ATPase Inhibitor

Pharmascience

SUPPLIED: Each pellet-filled capsule, consisting of a dark pink cap and a pink body, imprinted with "OME 20" on the cap and body, contains: omeprazole 20 mg. Nonmedicinal ingredients: carrageenan, croscarmellose sodium, dibutyl sebacate, hypromellose, hypromellose phthalate, iron oxide red, lactose, hydroxypropyl cellulose, microcrystalline cellulose, polysorbate, potassium chloride, povidone, talc, titanium dioxide and water. Bottles of 100 and 500. Store bottle tightly capped between 15 and 30°C. Protect from moisture.

PMS-Omeprazole DR ℞

omeprazole magnesium

H+, K+-ATPase Inhibitor

Pharmascience

SUPPLIED: Each red-brown, biconvex, round, coated, delayed release tablet, ink-printed in black with "P 20" on one side and nothing on the other side, contains: omeprazole magnesium 20 mg. Nonmedicinal ingredients: colloidal silicon dioxide, copovidone, croscarmellose sodium, FD&C Blue No. 1 Aluminum Lake, FD&C Red No. 40 Aluminum Lake, FD&C Yellow No. 6 Aluminum Lake, lactose, lecithin, methacrylic acid copolymer, microcrystalline cellulose, shellac, simethicone, sodium lauryl sulfate, sodium stearyl fumarate, talc, titanium dioxide, triethyl citrate and red iron oxide. Bottles of 100 and 500. Blisters of 30. Store between 15 and 30°C. Protect from moisture.

PMS-Ondansetron ℞

ondansetron HCl dihydrate

Antiemetic

Pharmascience

SUPPLIED: 4 mg: Each yellow, oval shaped, film-coated tablet, debossed with a "P" logo on one side and "4" on the other side, contains: ondansetron 4 mg as ondansetron hydrochloride dihydrate. Nonmedicinal ingredients: cornstarch, croscarmellose sodium, iron oxide yellow, lactose, magnesium stearate, microcrystalline cellulose, polyethylene glycol, polyvinyl alcohol, talc and titanium dioxide. Blisters of 10. Bottles of 100. Store between 2 and 30°C. Protect from light.

8 mg: Each yellow, oval shaped, film-coated tablet, debossed with "OD" on one side and "8" on the other side, contains: ondansetron 8 mg as ondansetron hydrochloride dihydrate. Nonmedicinal ingredients: cornstarch, croscarmellose sodium, iron oxide yellow, lactose, magnesium stearate, microcrystalline cellulose, polyethylene glycol, polyvinyl alcohol, talc and titanium dioxide. Blisters of 10. Bottles of 100. Store between 2 and 30°C. Protect from light.

PMS-Oxybutynin ℞

oxybutynin chloride

Anticholinergic—Antispasmodic

Pharmascience

SUPPLIED: Syrup: Each 5 mL of clear, green-colored, strawberry flavoured syrup contains: oxybutynin chloride 5 mg. Nonmedicinal ingredients: artificial strawberry flavour, citric acid, FD&C Green No. 3 Aluminum Lake, glycerin, sodium methylparaben, sorbitol, sucrose, sodium hydroxide and water. Bottles of 500 mL. Store at room temperature of 15 to 30°C in a tight container and protect from light.

Tablets: 2.5 mg: Each round, biconvex, white tablet, debossed with a "P" logo on one side and "2.5" on the other side, contains: oxybutynin chloride 2.5 mg. Nonmedicinal ingredients: calcium stearate, lactose and microcrystalline cellulose. Bottles of 100. Store at room temperature of 15 to 30°C in tight, light-resistant containers.

5 mg: Each round, scored, blue tablet, debossed with a "P" logo on one side and "OXY" over "5" on the other side, contains: oxybutynin chloride 5 mg. Nonmedicinal ingredients: calcium stearate, FD&C Blue No. 1 Aluminum Lake, lactose and microcrystalline cellulose. Bottles of 100 and 500. Store at room temperature of 15 to 30°C in tight, light-resistant containers.

PMS-Oxycodone Ⓝ

oxycodone HCl

Opioid Analgesic

Pharmascience

SUPPLIED: 5 mg: Each blue, round, scored tablet, debossed with "5" over "OXY" on one side and scored on the other side, contains: oxycodone 5 mg (as oxycodone hydrochloride). Nonmedicinal ingredients: croscarmellose sodium, dibasic calcium phosphate, FD&C Blue No. 1 Aluminum Lake, magnesium stearate and microcrystalline cellulose. Bottles of 100. Store between 15 and 30°C.

10 mg: Each white, round, scored tablet, debossed with "10" over "OXY" on one side and scored on the other side, contains: oxycodone 10 mg (as oxycodone hydrochloride). Nonmedicinal ingredients: croscarmellose sodium, dibasic calcium phosphate, magnesium stearate and microcrystalline cellulose. Bottles of 100. Store between 15 and 30°C.

20 mg: Each white, oval, scored tablet, debossed with "20 OXY" on one side and scored on the other side, contains: oxycodone 20 mg (as oxycodone hydrochloride). Nonmedicinal ingredients: croscarmellose sodium, dibasic calcium phosphate, magnesium stearate and microcrystalline cellulose. Bottles of 50. Store between 15 and 30°C.

PMS-Pantoprazole IV ℞

pantoprazole sodium

H+, K+-ATPase Inhibitor

Pharmascience

SUPPLIED: Each vial of white to off-white lyophilized powder contains: pantoprazole 40 mg (as pantoprazole sodium sesquihydrate). Clear glass vials of 10 mL, closed with a grey rubber stopper, an aluminum seal and a white plastic flip-off cap. Store between 15 and 30°C. Protect from light.

PMS-Pantoprazole Tablets ℞

pantoprazole sodium

H+, K+-ATPase Inhibitor

Pharmascience

SUPPLIED: Each yellow, oval, biconvex coated tablet with "PT 40" printed in black ink on one side and nothing on the other side, contains: pantoprazole 40 mg (as pantoprazole sodium). Nonmedicinal ingredients: calcium stearate, crospovidone, hydroxypropyl cellulose, hydroxypropyl methylcellulose, mannitol, methacrylic acid copolymer, pharmaceutical ink, polyethylene glycol, sodium carbonate, talc, titanium dioxide, triethyl citrate, yellow iron oxide and Zein F 4000. Bottles of 100 and 500. Store between 15 and 30°C.

The reader is invited to consult CPhA's monograph **Selective Serotonin Reuptake Inhibitors**.

PMS-Paroxetine ℞

paroxetine HCl

Antidepressant—Antiobsessional—Antibulimic—Antipanic—Anxiolytic—Post-traumatic Stress Disorder Therapy

Pharmascience

SUPPLIED: 10 mg: Each yellow, film-coated, oval, biconvex tablet, debossed with "PXT" on one side and "1" and "0" on the scored side, contains: paroxetine HCl 10 mg. Nonmedicinal ingredients: colloidal silicon dioxide, croscarmellose sodium, D&C Yellow No. 10 Lake, FD&C Yellow No. 6 Lake, hypromellose, magnesium stearate, microcrystalline cellulose, polydextrose, polyethylene glycol, titanium dioxide and triacetin. Bottles of 30 and 100. Store at room temperature (15-30°C).

20 mg: Each pink, film-coated, oval, biconvex tablet, debossed with "PXT" on one side and "2" and "0" on the scored side, contains: paroxetine HCl 20 mg. Nonmedicinal ingredients: colloidal silicon dioxide, croscarmellose sodium, D&C Red No. 30 Lake, hypromellose, magnesium stearate, microcrystalline cellulose, polydextrose, polyethylene glycol, titanium dioxide and triacetin. Bottles of 100 and 500. Blisters of 30. Store at room temperature (15-30°C).

30 mg: Each blue, film-coated, oval, biconvex tablet, debossed with "PXT" on one side and "3" and "0" on the scored side, contains: paroxetine HCl 30 mg. Nonmedicinal ingredients: colloidal silicon dioxide, croscarmellose sodium, FD&C Blue No. 2 Lake, hydroxypropyl methylcellulose, magnesium stearate, microcrystalline cellulose, polydextrose, polyethylene glycol, titanium dioxide and triacetin. Bottles of 30 and 100. Store at room temperature (15-30°C).

40 mg: Each green, film-coated, oval, biconvex tablet, debossed with "PXT" on one side and "4" and "0" on the scored side, contains: paroxetine HCl 40 mg. Nonmedicinal ingredients: colloidal silicon dioxide, croscarmellose sodium, D&C Yellow No. 10 Aluminum Lake, FD&C Blue No. 2 Aluminum Lake, magnesium stearate, microcrystalline cellulose, polyethylene glycol, polyvinyl alcohol, soy lecithin, talc and titanium dioxide. Bottles of 100. Store at room temperature (15-30°C).

PMS-Phenobarbital Ⓒ

phenobarbital

Sedative—Hypnotic—Anticonvulsant—Antihyperbilirubinemic

Pharmascience

SUPPLIED: Elixir: Each mL of clear red liquid contains: phenobarbital USP 5 mg. Nonmedicinal ingredients: alcohol, anise oil, FD&C Red No. 2, glycerin, methyl paraben, natural & artificial flavour (lemon and orange), propyl paraben, purified water, sodium chloride, sodium cyclamate and sucrose. Bottles of 100 mL. Store at room temperature. Protect from freezing.

Tablets: 15 mg: Each pink, round, scored tablet contains: phenobarbital USP 15 mg. Nonmedicinal ingredients: carboxymethylcellulose sodium, D&C Red No. 27 Lake, FD&C Red No. 40 Lake, magnesium stearate, microcrystalline cellulose and sodium lauryl sulfate. Bottles of 500.

30 mg: Each yellow, round, scored tablet contains: phenobarbital USP 30 mg. Nonmedicinal ingredients: carboxymethylcellulose sodium, cornstarch, D&C Yellow No. 10 Aluminum Lake, glyceryl behenate, microcrystalline cellulose and sodium bicarbonate. Bottles of 500.

60 mg: Each green, round, scored tablet contains: phenobarbital USP 60 mg. Nonmedicinal ingredients: carboxymethylcellulose sodium, cornstarch, D&C Yellow No. 10 Aluminum Lake, FD&C Blue No. 1 Lake, glyceryl behenate, microcrystalline cellulose, sodium bicarbonate and sodium lauryl sulfate. Bottles of 500.

100 mg: Each blue, round, scored tablet contains: phenobarbital USP 100 mg. Nonmedicinal ingredients: carboxymethylcellulose sodium, cornstarch, FD&C Blue No. 1 Lake, glyceryl behenate, microcrystalline cellulose, sodium bicarbonate and sodium lauryl sulfate. Bottles of 500.

The reader is invited to consult CPhA's monograph **HMG-CoA Reductase Inhibitors**.

PMS-Pravastatin ℞

pravastatin sodium

Lipid Metabolism Regulator

Pharmascience

SUPPLIED: 10 mg: Each pink to peach, rounded, rectangular-shaped, biconvex tablet, debossed with "P 10" on one side and with the "P" logo on the other side, contains: pravastatin sodium 10 mg. Nonmedicinal ingredients: calcium phosphate, carboxymethylcellulose sodium, colloidal silicon dioxide, iron oxide red, lactose, magnesium stearate, microcrystalline cellulose, polyethylene glycol and povidone. Bottles of 100. Blisters of 30. Store at room temperature (15-30°C).

20 mg: Each yellow, rounded, rectangular-shaped, biconvex tablet, debossed with "P 20" on one side and with the "P" logo on the other side, contains: pravastatin sodium 20 mg. Nonmedicinal ingredients: calcium phosphate, carboxymethylcellulose sodium, colloidal silicon dioxide, iron oxide yellow, lactose, magnesium stearate, microcrystalline cellulose, polyethylene glycol and povidone. Bottles of 100 and 500. Blisters of 30. Store at room temperature (15-30°C).

40 mg: Each green, rounded, rectangular-shaped, biconvex tablet, debossed with "P 40" on one side and with the "P" logo on the other side, contains: pravastatin sodium 40 mg. Nonmedicinal ingredients: calcium phosphate, carboxymethylcellulose sodium, colloidal silicon dioxide, D&C Yellow No. 10 Aluminum Lake, FD&C Blue No. 1 Aluminum Lake, lactose, magnesium stearate, microcrystalline cellulose, polyethylene glycol and povidone. Bottles of 100. Blisters of 30. Store at room temperature (15-30°C).

PMS-Quetiapine ℞

quetiapine fumarate

Antipsychotic

Pharmascience

SUPPLIED: 25 mg: Each peach, round, biconvex, coated tablet debossed with a "P" logo on one side and "25" on the other side, contains: quetiapine 25 mg (as quetiapine fumarate). Nonmedicinal ingredients: dibasic calcium phosphate, hydroxypropyl methylcellulose, lactose, magnesium stearate, microcrystalline cellulose, polyethylene glycol, povidone, red iron oxide, sodium starch glycolate, titanium dioxide and yellow iron oxide. Bottles of 100 and 500. Blisters of 60. Store between 15 and 30°C.

100 mg: Each yellow, round, biconvex, coated tablet debossed with a "P" logo on one side and "100" on the other side, contains: quetiapine 100 mg (as quetiapine fumarate). Nonmedicinal ingredients: dibasic calcium phosphate, hydroxypropyl methylcellulose, lactose, magnesium stearate, microcrystalline cellulose, polyethylene glycol, povidone, sodium starch glycolate, titanium dioxide and yellow iron oxide. Bottles of 100 and 500. Blisters of 90. Store between 15 and 30°C.

200 mg: Each white, round, biconvex, coated tablet debossed with a "P" logo on one side and "200" on the other side, contains: quetiapine 200 mg (as quetiapine fumarate). Nonmedicinal ingredients: dibasic calcium phosphate, hydroxypropyl methylcellulose, lactose, magnesium stearate, microcrystalline cellulose, polyethylene glycol, povidone, sodium starch glycolate, talc and titanium dioxide. Bottles of 100 and 500. Blisters of 90. Store between 15 and 30°C.
300 mg: Each white, capsule-shaped, biconvex, coated tablet debossed with a "P" logo on one side and "300" on the other side, contains: quetiapine 300 mg (as quetiapine fumarate). Nonmedicinal ingredients: dibasic calcium phosphate, hydroxypropyl methylcellulose, lactose, magnesium stearate, microcrystalline cellulose, polyethylene glycol, povidone, sodium starch glycolate, talc and titanium dioxide. Bottles of 100 and 500. Store between 15 and 30°C.

PMS-Rabeprazole EC

rabeprazole sodium
H+, K+-ATPase Inhibitor

Pharmascience

SUPPLIED: 10 mg: Each pink, round, biconvex, enteric-coated tablet, ink-printed in black with "RB10" on one side and plain on the other side, contains: rabeprazole sodium 10 mg. Nonmedicinal ingredients: antifoam, black iron oxide, hydroxypropyl cellulose, hydroxypropyl methylcellulose, hypromellose, industrial methylated spirit, lecithin (soya), magnesium oxide, magnesium stearate, mannitol, methacrylic acid, polyethylene glycol, red iron oxide, shellac glaze, sodium lauryl sulfate, talc, titanium dioxide, triethyl citrate and zein. Bottles of 100 and 500. Blister packages of 10. Store at room temperature (15 to 30°C) protected from moisture.
20 mg: Each yellow, round, biconvex, enteric-coated tablet, ink-printed in red with "RB20" on one side and plain on the other side, contains: rabeprazole sodium 20 mg. Nonmedicinal ingredients: ammonium hydroxide, FD&C red/allura red AC Aluminum Lake, hydroxypropyl cellulose, hydroxypropyl methylcellulose, magnesium oxide, magnesium stearate, mannitol, methacrylic acid, polyethylene glycol, propylene glycol, shellac glaze, sodium lauryl sulfate, talc, titanium dioxide, triethyl citrate, yellow iron oxide and zein. Bottles of 100 and 500. Blister packages of 10. Store at room temperature (15 to 30°C) protected from moisture.

PMS-Ranitidine

ranitidine HCl
Histamine H2-Receptor Antagonist

Pharmascience

SUPPLIED: 150 mg: Each white, round, biconvex, film-coated tablet, debossed with "RNT" on one side and "150" on the other side, contains: ranitidine HCl 150 mg. Nonmedicinal ingredients: colloidal silicon dioxide, croscarmellose sodium, magnesium stearate, microcrystalline cellulose, polyvinyl alcohol, soy lecithin, talc, titanium dioxide and xanthan gum. Bottles of 60, 100 and 500. Blisters of 60. Store at room temperature between 15 and 30°C. Protect from light.
300 mg: Each white, capsule-shaped, biconvex, film-coated tablet, debossed with "RNT" on one side and "300" on the other side, contains: ranitidine HCl 300 mg. Nonmedicinal ingredients: colloidal silicon dioxide, croscarmellose sodium, magnesium stearate, microcrystalline cellulose, polyvinyl alcohol, soy lecithin, talc, titanium dioxide and xanthan gum. Bottles of 30, 100 and 250. Blisters of 30. Store at room temperature between 15 and 30°C. Protect from light.

The reader is invited to consult CPhA's monograph **Bisphosphonates: Oral.**

PMS-Risedronate

risedronate sodium hemi-pentahydrate
Bone Metabolism Regulator

Pharmascience

SUPPLIED: Each oval, orange coated tablet, debossed with "RS" on one side and "35" on the other side contains: the equivalent of 35 mg of anhydrous risedronate sodium in the form of the hemipentahydrate with small amounts of monohydrate. Nonmedicinal ingredients: colloidal silicon dioxide, iron oxide red, iron oxide yellow No. 10, maltodextrin, mannitol, polyvinyl alcohol-polyethylene glycol graft copolymer, povidone, pregelatinized starch, sodium starch glycolate, sodium stearyl fumarate, sucrose, talc, titanium dioxide and triethyl citrate. Bottles of 30. Blister packages of 4. Store at controlled room temperature (15-30°C).

PMS-Risperidone

risperidone
Atypical Antipsychotic

Pharmascience

SUPPLIED: Oral Solution: Each mL of clear and odourless solution contains: risperidone 1 mg as risperidone tartrate. Nonmedicinal ingredients: benzoic acid, purified water, sodium hydroxide, sorbitol solution and tartaric acid. Bottles of 30 mL with child-resistant closure and calibrated syringe. Store between 15 and 30°C. Protect from light and freezing.
Tablets: 0.25 mg: Each orange, oblong, coated tablet, debossed with "R" on one side and "0.25" on the other side, contains: risperidone 0.25 mg. Nonmedicinal ingredients: colloidal silicon dioxide, cornstarch, iron oxide yellow, lactose, magnesium stearate, microcrystalline cellulose, polyethylene glycol, polyvinyl alcohol, sodium laurylsulfate, talc and titanium dioxide. Bottles of 100 and 500. Store between 15 and 30°C. Protect from light and moisture.
0.5 mg: Each brownish-red, scored, oblong, coated tablet, debossed with "R" on one side of the score and "0.5" on the other side of the tablet, contains: risperidone 0.5 mg. Nonmedicinal ingredients: colloidal silicon dioxide, cornstarch, iron oxide red, lactose, magnesium stearate, microcrystalline cellulose, polyethylene glycol, polyvinyl alcohol, sodium laurylsulfate, talc and titanium dioxide. Bottles of 100 and 500. Store between 15 and 30°C. Protect from light and moisture.
1 mg: Each white, non scored, oblong, coated tablet, debossed with "R" and "1" on one side; plain on the reverse side, contains: risperidone 1 mg. Nonmedicinal ingredients: colloidal silicon dioxide, cornstarch, hydroxypropylmethylcellulose, lactose, magnesium stearate, microcrystalline cellulose, polydextrose, polyethylene glycol, sodium laurylsulfate, titanium dioxide and triethyl citrate. Bottles of 100 and 500. Blisters of 60. Store between 15 and 30°C. Protect from light and moisture.
2 mg: Each salmon, scored, oblong, coated tablet, debossed with "R" and "2" respectively, on either side of the score, plain on the reverse side, contains: risperidone 2 mg. Nonmedicinal ingredients: colloidal silicon dioxide, cornstarch, FD&C Yellow No. 6 Aluminum Lake, lactose, magnesium stearate, microcrystalline cellulose, polyethylene glycol, polyvinyl alcohol, sodium laurylsulfate, talc and titanium dioxide. Bottles of 100 and 500. Blisters of 60. Store between 15 and 30°C. Protect from light and moisture.
3 mg: Each yellow, scored, oblong, coated tablet, debossed with "R" and "3" respectively, on either side of the score, plain on the reverse side, contains: risperidone 3 mg. Nonmedicinal ingredients: colloidal silicon dioxide, D&C Yellow No. 10 Aluminum Lake, FD&C Yellow No. 6 Aluminum Lake, lactose, magnesium stearate, microcrystalline cellulose, polyethylene glycol, polyvinyl alcohol, sodium laurylsulfate, talc and titanium dioxide. Bottles of 100 and 500. Blisters of 60. Store between 15 and 30°C. Protect from light and moisture.
4 mg: Each light green, scored, oblong, coated tablet, debossed with "R" and "4" respectively, on either side of the score, plain on the reverse side, contains: risperidone 4 mg. Nonmedicinal ingredients: colloidal silicon dioxide, cornstarch, D&C Yellow No. 10 Aluminum Lake, FD&C Blue No. 2 Aluminum Lake, lactose, magnesium stearate, microcrystalline cellulose, polyethylene glycol, polyvinyl alcohol, sodium laurylsulfate, talc and titanium dioxide. Bottles of 100. Store between 15 and 30°C. Protect from light and moisture.

PMS-Rivastigmine

rivastigmine hydrogen tartrate
Cholinesterase Inhibitor

Pharmascience

SUPPLIED: 1.5 mg: Each yellow, hard gelatin capsule, ink-printed in red with "RV" over "1.5" on the body of the capsule and nothing on the cap, contains: rivastigmine 1.5 mg (as rivastigmine hydrogen tartrate). Nonmedicinal ingredients: colloidal silicon dioxide, hydroxypropyl methylcellulose, magnesium stearate and microcrystalline cellulose; capsule: D&C Yellow No. 10, FD&C Yellow No. 6, gelatin and titanium dioxide. Blisters of 60. Bottles of 100. Store at room temperature (15-30°C).
3 mg: Each orange, hard gelatin capsule, ink-printed in red with "RV" over "3" on the body of the capsule and nothing on the cap, contains: rivastigmine 3 mg (as rivastigmine hydrogen tartrate). Nonmedicinal ingredients: colloidal silicon dioxide, hydroxypropyl methylcellulose, magnesium stearate and microcrystalline cellulose; capsule: D&C Red No. 28, FD&C Red No. 40, FD&C Yellow No. 10, gelatin and titanium dioxide. Blisters of 60. Bottles of 100. Store at room temperature (15-30°C).
4.5 mg: Each red, hard gelatin capsule, ink-printed in white with "RV" over "4.5" on the body of the capsule and nothing on the cap, contains: rivastigmine 4.5 mg (as rivastigmine hydrogen tartrate). Nonmedicinal ingredients: colloidal silicon dioxide, hydroxypropyl methylcellulose, magnesium stearate and microcrystalline cellulose; capsule: gelatin, red iron oxide, titanium dioxide and yellow iron oxide. Blisters of 60. Bottles of 100. Store at room temperature (15-30°C).
6 mg: Each orange and red, hard gelatin capsule, ink-printed in red with "RV" over "6" on the orange coloured body of the capsule and nothing on the red coloured cap, contains: rivastigmine 6 mg (as rivastigmine hydrogen tartrate). Nonmedicinal ingredients: colloidal silicon dioxide hydroxypropyl methylcellulose, magnesium stearate and microcrystalline cellulose; capsule: gelatin, red iron oxide, titanium dioxide and yellow iron oxide. Blisters of 60. Bottles of 100. Store at room temperature (15-30°C).

PMS-Ropinirole

ropinirole HCl
Antiparkinsonian Agent—Dopamine Agonist

Pharmascience

SUPPLIED: 0.25 mg: Each white, round, biconvex, coated tablet, with a pentagon debossed on one side and "R" on the other side, contains: ropinirole 0.25 mg (as ropinirole hydrochloride). Nonmedicinal ingredients: colloidal silicon dioxide, croscarmellose sodium, hydroxypropyl methylcellulose, lactose, magnesium stearate, methionine racemic, microcrystalline cellulose, polyethylene glycol and titanium dioxide. Sucrose-, tartrazine- or any other azo dyes-free. Blisters of 10. Bottles of 100. Store between 15-30°C. Protect from light and moisture.
1 mg: Each green, round, biconvex, coated tablet, with a pentagon debossed on one side and "R1" on the other side, contains: ropinirole 1 mg (as ropinirole hydrochloride). Nonmedicinal ingredients: colloidal silicon dioxide, croscarmellose sodium, FD&C Blue No. 2 Aluminum Lake, hydroxypropyl methylcellulose, iron oxide yellow, lactose, magnesium stearate, methionine racemic, microcrystalline cellulose, polyethylene glycol and titanium dioxide. Sucrose-, tartrazine- or any other azo dyes-free. Blisters of 10. Bottles of 100. Store between 15-30°C. Protect from light and moisture.
2 mg: Each pink, round, biconvex, coated tablet, with a pentagon debossed on one side and "R2" on the other side, contains: ropinirole 2 mg (as ropinirole hydrochloride). Nonmedicinal ingredients: colloidal silicon dioxide, croscarmellose sodium, FD&C Blue No. 2 Aluminum Lake, FD&C Yellow No. 6 Aluminum Lake, hydroxypropyl methylcellulose, iron oxide red, lactose, magnesium stearate, methionine racemic, microcrystalline cellulose, polyethylene glycol and titanium dioxide. Sucrose-, tartrazine- or any other azo dyes-free. Blisters of 10. Bottles of 100. Store between 15-30°C. Protect from light and moisture.
5 mg: Each blue, round, biconvex, coated tablet, with a pentagon debossed on one side and "R5" on the other side, contains: ropinirole 5 mg (as ropinirole hydrochloride). Nonmedicinal ingredients: colloidal silicon dioxide, croscarmellose sodium, FD&C Blue No. 2 Aluminum Lake, hydroxypropyl methylcellulose, lactose, magnesium stearate, methionine racemic, microcrystalline cellulose, polyethylene glycol, polysorbate 80 and titanium dioxide. Sucrose-, tartrazine- or any other azo dyes-free. Blisters of 10. Bottles of 100. Store between 15-30°C. Protect from light and moisture.

The reader is invited to consult CPhA's monograph **Selective Serotonin Reuptake Inhibitors.**

PMS-Sertraline

sertraline HCl
Antidepressant—Antipanic—Antiobsessional

Pharmascience

SUPPLIED: 25 mg: Each hard gelatin capsule, with yellow opaque body imprinted "Sertraline" over "25" and yellow opaque cap imprinted with "P", contains: sertraline HCl equivalent to sertraline 25 mg. Nonmedicinal ingredients: cornstarch, D&C Yellow No. 10, FD&C Yellow No. 6, gelatin, lactose, magnesium stearate, sodium lauryl sulfate and titanium dioxide. Bottles of 100. Store at controlled room temperature between 15 and 30°C.
50 mg: Each hard gelatin capsule, with white opaque body imprinted "Sertraline" over "50" and yellow opaque cap imprinted with "P", contains: sertraline HCl equivalent to sertraline 50 mg. Nonmedicinal ingredients: cornstarch, D&C Yellow No. 10, FD&C Yellow No. 6, gelatin, lactose, magnesium stearate, sodium lauryl sulfate and titanium dioxide. Bottles of 100 and 250. Bottles of 100. Store at controlled room temperature between 15 and 30°C.
100 mg: Each hard gelatin capsule, with orange opaque body imprinted "Sertraline" over "100" and orange opaque cap imprinted with "P", contains: sertraline HCl equivalent to sertraline 100 mg. Nonmedicinal ingredients: cornstarch, D&C Yellow No. 10, FD&C Red No. 40, gelatin, lactose, magnesium stearate, sodium lauryl sulfate and titanium dioxide. Bottles of 100 and 250. Bottles of 100. Store at controlled room temperature between 15 and 30°C.

The reader is invited to consult CPhA's monograph **HMG-CoA Reductase Inhibitors.**

PMS-Simvastatin

simvastatin
Lipid Metabolism Regulator

Pharmascience

SUPPLIED: 5 mg: Each buff, shield-shaped, film-coated tablet, debossed with a "P" logo on one side and "5" on the other, contains: simvastatin 5 mg. Nonmedicinal ingredients: ascorbic acid, butylated hydroxyanisole, citric acid, cornstarch, hydroxypropyl methylcellulose, iron oxide yellow, lactose, magnesium stearate, microcrystalline cellulose, polydextrose, polyethylene glycol, titanium dioxide and triacetin. Bottles of 100. Blisters of 30. Store at room temperature (15-30°C).
10 mg: Each pink, shield-shaped, film-coated tablet, debossed with a "P" logo on one side and "10" on the other, contains: simvastatin 10 mg. Nonmedicinal ingredients: ascorbic acid, butylated hydroxyanisole, citric acid, cornstarch, hydroxypropyl methylcellulose, iron oxide red, lactose, magnesium stearate, microcrystalline cellulose, polydextrose, polyethylene glycol, titanium dioxide and triacetin. Bottles of 100. Blisters of 30. Store at room temperature (15-30°C).
20 mg: Each tan, shield-shaped, film-coated tablet, debossed with a "P" logo on one side and "20" on the other, contains: simvastatin 20 mg. Nonmedicinal ingredients: ascorbic acid, butylated hydroxyanisole, citric acid, cornstarch, hydroxypropyl methylcellulose, iron oxide red iron oxide yellow, lactose, magnesium stearate, microcrystalline cellulose, polydextrose, polyethylene glycol, titanium dioxide and triacetin. Bottles of 100 and 500. Blisters of 30. Store at room temperature (15-30°C).

40 mg: Each pink, shield-shaped, film-coated tablet, debossed with a "P" logo on one side and "40" on the other, contains: simvastatin 40 mg. Nonmedicinal ingredients: ascorbic acid, butylated hydroxyanisole, citric acid, cornstarch, FD&C Blue No. 2 Aluminum Lake, FD&C Red No. 40 Aluminum Lake, FD&C Yellow No. 6 Aluminum Lake, hydroxypropyl methylcellulose, lactose, magnesium stearate, microcrystalline cellulose, polydextrose, polyethylene glycol, titanium dioxide and triacetin. Bottles of 100. Blisters of 30. Store at room temperature (15-30°C).

80 mg: Each pink, capsule shaped, film-coated tablet, debossed with a "P" logo on one side and "80" on the other, contains: simvastatin 80 mg. Nonmedicinal ingredients: ascorbic acid, butylated hydroxyanisole, citric acid, cornstarch, FD&C Blue No. 2 Aluminum Lake, FD&C Red No. 40 Aluminum Lake, FD&C Yellow No. 6 Aluminum Lake, hydroxypropyl methylcellulose, lactose, magnesium stearate, microcrystalline cellulose, polydextrose, polyethylene glycol, titanium dioxide and triacetin. Bottles of 100. Blisters of 30. Store at room temperature (15-30°C).

PMS-Sulfasalazine ℞
sulfasalazine
Anti-inflammatory

Pharmascience

PMS-Sulfasalazine EC ℞
sulfasalazine
Anti-inflammatory

Pharmascience

SUPPLIED: PMS-Sulfasalazine: Each dark yellow to yellowish-brown, round, biconvex tablet, scored on one side and debossed with "PMS" on the other side, contains: sulfasalazine 500 mg. Nonmedicinal ingredients: croscarmellose sodium, magnesium stearate, microcrystalline cellulose and povidone. Bottles of 500.

PMS-Sulfasalazine EC: Each dark yellow, oval, enteric-coated tablet, contains: sulfasalazine 500 mg. Nonmedicinal ingredients: croscarmellose sodium, magnesium stearate, microcrystalline cellulose and povidone; enteric coating: colloidal silicon dioxide, croscarmellose sodium, D&C Yellow No. 10 Aluminum Lake, FD&C Blue No. 2 Aluminum Lake, FD&C Red No. 40 Aluminum Lake, FD&C Yellow No. 6 Aluminum Lake, methacrylic acid copolymer, polyethylene glycol, propylene glycol, red iron oxide, sodium bicarbonate, sodium citrate dihydrate, sodium lauryl sulfate, talc, titanium dioxide and triethyl citrate. Bottles of 100 and 500.

PMS-Testosterone Ⓒ
testosterone undecanoate
Androgen

Pharmascience

Date of Preparation: February 6, 2009
Date of Revision: April 21, 2009

SUMMARY PRODUCT INFORMATION:

Route of Administration	Dosage Form/ Strength	Clinically Relevant Nonmedicinal Ingredients
Oral	Capsule 40 mg	Gelatin For a complete listing see Dosage Forms, Composition and Packaging.

INDICATIONS AND CLINICAL USE: pms-TESTOSTERONE (testosterone undecanoate capsules) is indicated for testosterone replacement therapy in adult males for conditions associated with a deficiency or absence of endogenous testosterone. pms-TESTOSTERONE should not be used to treat non-specific symptoms suggestive of hypogonadism if testosterone deficiency has not been demonstrated and if other etiologies responsible for the symptoms have not been excluded. Testosterone deficiency should be clearly demonstrated by clinical features and confirmed by two separate validated biochemical assays (morning testosterone) before initiating therapy with any testosterone replacement, including pms-TESTOSTERONE treatment.

Geriatrics (>65 years of age): There is limited pms-TESTOSTERONE use in the geriatric population.

Pediatrics (<18 years of age): pms-TESTOSTERONE is not indicated for use in children <18 years of age since safety and efficacy have not been established in this patient population (see Warnings and Precautions).

CONTRAINDICATIONS:
- pms-TESTOSTERONE (testosterone undecanoate capsules) should not be used in patients with known hypersensitivity to any of its ingredients. For a complete listing of ingredients see Dosage Forms, Composition and Packaging.
- Testosterone replacement therapies are contraindicated in men with known or suspected carcinoma of the prostate or breast.
- pms-TESTOSTERONE is not indicated for use in women.
- Contraindicated drug-drug interactions appear in the Drug Interactions section (see Drug Interactions).

WARNINGS AND PRECAUTIONS: General: There is very limited data from clinical trials with testosterone undecanoate capsules in the geriatric male (>65 years of age) to support the efficacy and safety of prolonged use. Impacts to prostate and cardiovascular event rates and patient important outcomes are unknown.

Patients with clinical or demographic characteristics that are recognized to be associated with an increased risk of prostate cancer should be evaluated for the presence of prostate cancer prior to initiation of testosterone replacement therapy.

Testosterone replacement therapy should not be used to attempt to improve body composition, bone and muscle mass, increase lean body mass and decrease total fat mass. Efficacy and safety have not been established. Serious long term deleterious health issues may arise.

Testosterone replacement therapy has not been shown to be safe and effective for the enhancement of athletic performance. Because of the potential risk of serious adverse health effects, this drug should not be used for such purpose.

If testosterone deficiency has not been established, testosterone replacement therapy should not be used for the treatment of sexual dysfunction.

Clinical studies have not established testosterone replacement therapy as a treatment for male infertility.

Carcinogenesis and Mutagenesis: Prostatic: Geriatric patients treated with testosterone products may be at an increased risk for the development of prostatic hyperplasia and prostatic carcinoma but their role in the initiation of either disease is unknown.

Breast: Patients using long-term parenteral testosterone replacement therapy may be at an increased risk for the development of breast cancer.

Skeletal: Patients with skeletal metastases are at a risk of exacerbating hypercalcemia/ hypercalciuria with concomitant testosterone replacement therapy.

Cardiovascular: Testosterone may increase blood pressure and should be used with caution in patients with hypertension.

Edema, with or without congestive heart failure, may be a serious complication in patients with pre-existing cardiac, renal, or hepatic disease. Diuretic therapy may be required, in addition to discontinuation of the drug.

Dependence/Tolerance: Testosterone undecanoate contains testosterone, a Schedule G controlled substance as defined by the Food and Drugs Act.

Endocrine and Metabolism: Testosterone products have been shown to alter glucose tolerance tests. Diabetics should be followed carefully and the insulin or oral hypoglycemic dosage adjusted accordingly (see Drug Interactions, Drug-Drug Interactions).

Hypercalciuria/hypercalcemia (caused by malignant tumors) may be exacerbated by androgen treatment. Androgens should be used with caution in cancer patients at risk of hypercalcemia (and associated hypercalciuria). Regular monitoring of serum calcium concentrations is recommended in patients at risk of hypercalciuria/hypercalcemia. Hypercalcemia may occur in immobilized patients. If any hypercalcemia occurs, the drug should be discontinued.

Genitourinary: Patients with benign prostatic hyperplasia may develop acute urethral obstruction.

Hematologic: Hemoglobin and hematocrit levels should be checked periodically (to detect polycythemia) in patients on long-term testosterone replacement therapy (see Monitoring and Laboratory Tests).

Respiratory: The treatment of hypogonadal men with testosterone products may potentiate sleep apnea, particularly for those with risk factors such as obesity or chronic lung diseases.

Sexual Function/Reproduction: Gynecomastia may develop and occasionally persist in patients being treated for hypogonadism. Priapism or excessive sexual stimulation may develop.

Oligospermia may occur after prolonged administration or excessive dosage.

Special Populations: Pregnant Women and Nursing Women: Testosterone undecanoate should not be used in pregnant or nursing women. Testosterone may cause fetal harm. Testosterone exposure during pregnancy has been reported to be associated with fetal abnormalities (see Contraindications).

Pediatrics (<18 years of age): Testosterone replacement therapy should be used cautiously in males with hypogonadism causing delayed puberty. Androgens can accelerate bone maturation without producing compensatory gain in linear growth. This adverse effect may result in compromised adult stature. The younger the child is the greater risk of compromising final mature height. The effect of androgens on bone maturation should be monitored closely by assessing bone age of the wrist and hand on a regular basis.

Geriatrics (>65 years of age): There are very limited controlled clinical study data supporting the use of testosterone in the geriatric population and virtually no controlled clinical studies on subjects 75 years and over.

Geriatric patients treated with testosterone products may be at an increased risk for the development of prostatic hyperplasia and prostatic carcinoma but their role in the initiation of either disease is unknown.

In men receiving testosterone replacement therapy, surveillance for prostate cancer should be consistent with current practices for eugonadal men.

Monitoring and Laboratory Tests: The patient should be monitored (including serum testosterone levels) on a regular basis to ensure adequate response to treatment. Good clinical judgment must be employed using serum bioavailable testosterone levels or if this is unavailable Calculated Free Testosterone Fractions since the levels have daily fluctuations with use of testosterone undecanoate. Serum Bioavailable Testosterone (Bio-T) level or Calculated Free Testosterone Fractions must be obtained about 5 hours after testosterone undecanoate capsule intake, at C_{max}, and in a non-fasted subject.

Currently there is no consensus about age specific testosterone levels. The normal serum testosterone level for young eugonadal men is generally accepted to be approximately 10.4-34.6 nmol/L (300-1000 ng/dL). It should be taken into account that physiological testosterone levels (mean and range) decrease with increasing age.

The following laboratory tests, performed routinely, are recommended to ensure that adverse experience possibly caused by or related to testosterone replacement therapy is detected and addressed:
- hemoglobin and hematocrit levels should be checked periodically (to detect polycythemia);
- liver function tests;
- prostate specific antigen (PSA), digital rectal examination (DRE), especially if the patient presents with progressive difficulty with urination or a change in voiding habits;
- lipid profile, total cholesterol, LDL, HDL, and triglycerides; serum cholesterol levels may increase and/or decrease during androgen therapy.
- diabetics should be followed carefully and the insulin or oral hypoglycemic dosage adjusted accordingly (see Drug Interactions, Drug-Drug Interactions).

ADVERSE REACTIONS: Adverse Drug Reaction Overview: Clinical Trial Adverse Drug Reactions: Because clinical trials are conducted under very specific conditions the adverse reaction rates observed in the clinical trials may not reflect the rates observed in practice and should not be compared to the rates in the clinical trials of another drug. Adverse drug reaction information from clinical trials is useful for identifying drug-related adverse events and for approximating rates.

The following adverse reactions have occurred with androgen therapy in general: fluid retention, nervousness, mood disturbance, myalgia, hypertension, pruritus, priapism, prostatic cancer, prostatic disorder, abnormal hepatic function , lipid abnormality, increased PSA, inhibition of testicular function, testicular atrophy and oligospermia, impotence, gynecomastia, epididymitis and bladder irritability, nausea, cholestatic jaundice, peliosis hepatis, polycythemia, headache, anxiety, depression, generalized paresthesia and rarely anaphylactoid reaction. In addition, the following reactions are known to occur with anabolic steroids: increased or decreased libido, flushing of the skin, acne, habituation, excitation and sleeplessness, chills, leukopenia, and bleeding in patients on concomitant anticoagulant therapy.

Post-Market Adverse Drug Reactions: In addition to those adverse events reported during clinical trials, the following adverse reactions have been identified during post-marketing use of testosterone undecanoate capsules (see Table 1) and known reactions of other testosterone preparations in general (see Table 2). Because these reactions are reported voluntarily from a population of uncertain size, it is not always possible to reliably estimate their frequency or establish a causal relationship to drug exposure.

Table 1: pms-TESTOSTERONE
Adverse Drug Reactions from Post-marketing Experience of Testosterone Undecanoate

MedDRA System Organ Class (SOC)	Adverse Drug Reaction
Blood and the Lymphatic System Disorders	Polycythemia
Endocrine Disorders	Abnormal accelerated growth
Gastrointestinal Disorders	Nausea, vomiting, diarrhea, abdominal pain, gastrointestinal bleeding
General Disorders and Administration Site Conditions	Edema, malaise, fatigue
Hepatobiliary Disorders	Hepatic neoplasms
Immune System Disorders	Allergic reaction/hypersensitivity reaction
Investigations	Weight increase, fluctuating testosterone levels, testosterone decreased, abnormal liver function tests (e.g. elevated GGTP), lipid abnormalities
Metabolism and Nutrition Disorders	Increased appetite, electrolyte changes (nitrogen, potassium, phosphorus, sodium), glucose tolerance impaired, elevated cholesterol
Musculoskeletal and Connective Tissue Disorders	Myalgia, arthralgia
Nervous System Disorders	Headache, dizziness
Psychiatric Disorders	Personality disorder, confusion, aggression, depression, anxiety, decreased libido, cognitive disturbance
Renal and Urinary Disorders	Renal disorders
Reproductive System and Breast Disorders	Prostate carcinoma, enlarged prostate (benign), free prostate-specific antigen increased, epididymitis, oligospermia, priapism, impotence, precocious puberty, gynecomastia
Skin and Subcutaneous Tissue Disorders	Pruritus, rash, urticaria, vesiculo-bullous rash, acne, alopecia, hirsutism

(cont'd)

Table 1: pms-TESTOSTERONE *(cont'd)*

Adverse Drug Reactions from Post-marketing Experience of Testosterone Undecanoate

MedDRA System Organ Class (SOC)	Adverse Drug Reaction
Vascular Disorders	Hypertension

Table 2: pms-TESTOSTERONE

Adverse Drug Reactions from Other Testosterone Preparations

MedDRA System Organ Class (SOC)	Adverse Drug Reaction
Blood and the Lymphatic System Disorders	Erythropoiesis abnormal
General Disorders and Administration Site Conditions	Application site burning, application site induration, application site rash, application site dermatitis, application site blister, application site erythema
Hepatobiliary Disorders	Peliosis hepatis
Metabolism and Nutrition Disorders	Urine calcium decrease
Nervous System Disorders	Insomnia
Psychiatric Disorders	Anger
Renal and Urinary Disorders	Dysuria, hematuria, incontinence, bladder irritability
Reproductive System and Breast Disorders	Testicular atrophy, mastodynia
Respiratory, Thoracic and Mediastinal Disorders	Dyspnea, sleep apnea
Skin and Subcutaneous Tissue Disorders	Seborrhea, male pattern baldness, hirsutism

DRUG INTERACTIONS: Drug-Drug Interactions: Insulin: In diabetic patients, the metabolic effects of Androgens may decrease blood glucose and, therefore, insulin requirements.

Propranolol: In a published pharmacokinetic study of an injectable testosterone product, administration of testosterone cypionate led to an increased clearance of propranolol in the majority of men tested. It is unknown if this would apply to testosterone undecanoate capsules.

Corticosteroids: The concurrent administration of testosterone with ACTH or corticosteroids may enhance edema formation; thus these drugs should be administered cautiously particularly in patients with cardiac, renal or hepatic disease.

Anticoagulants: Androgens may increase sensitivity to oral anticoagulants. Dosage of the anticoagulant may require reduction in order to maintain satisfactory therapeutic hypoprothrombinemia.

Cyclosporine: Testosterone replacement therapy may potentiate cyclosporine and increase risk of nephrotoxicity.

Drug-Food Interactions: Testosterone undecanoate must be taken with meal since fat enhances its absorption.

Drug-Herb Interactions: It was found that some herbal products (e.g. St. John's Wort) which are available as over-the-counter (OTC) products might interfere with steroid metabolism and therefore may decrease plasma testosterone levels.

Drug-Laboratory Test Interactions: Testosterone products may decrease levels of thyroxine-binding globulin, resulting in decreased total T_4 serum levels and increased resin uptake of T_3 and T_4. Free thyroid hormone levels remain unchanged, however, and there is no clinical evidence of thyroid dysfunction.

DOSAGE AND ADMINISTRATION: Recommended Dose and Dosage Adjustment: Usually, a daily dosage of 120-160 mg divided in two doses, taken once in the morning and once in the evening for 2-3 weeks is adequate. Subsequent dosage (40-120 mg daily) should be based on the subsequent testosterone levels and/or clinical effect obtained during therapy.

Missed Dose: Should you forget a dose, take your dose at the next scheduled time. Do not take a double dose of this medicine.

Administration: To ensure adequate absorption, testosterone undecanoate capsules must be taken with a meal and swallowed without chewing.

OVERDOSAGE:

No experience with overdosage has been reported. No specific antidote is available.

> For management of a suspected drug overdose, contact your **regional Poison Control Centre**. See the *CPS Directory* section for a list of Poison Control Centres.

ACTION AND CLINICAL PHARMACOLOGY: Mechanism of Action: Testosterone undecanoate, an orally active testosterone preparation, is a fatty acid ester of the natural androgen testosterone. Unlike other oral testosterone preparations, testosterone undecanoate is able to by-pass the liver via the lymphatic system and is therefore orally bioavailable.

Therapy with testosterone undecanoate increases plasma levels of testosterone and its active metabolites, leading to a regular therapeutic effect. In eugonadal men, peak testosterone levels are reached approximately 4-5 hours after ingestion, returning to basal levels after about 10 hours. In volunteers and hypogonadal men, 77-93% of an orally administered dose of testosterone undecanoate was excreted in the urine and faeces within 3 to 4 days.

Testosterone undecanoate dissolved in a mixture of castor oil and propylene glycol monolaurate has been found to exhibit comparable testosterone bioavailability to testosterone undecanoate in oleic acid.

Testosterone undecanoate delivers physiologic amounts of testosterone, producing circulating testosterone levels that approximate normal levels (e.g. 10.4-34.6 nmol/L [300-1000 ng/dL]) seen in young healthy men.

Pharmacodynamics: Testosterone and Hypogonadism: Testosterone and dihydrotestosterone (DHT), endogenous androgens, are responsible for normal growth and development of the male sex organs and for maintenance of secondary sex characteristics. These effects include the growth and maturation of the prostate, seminal vesicles, penis, and scrotum; the development of male hair distribution, such as facial, pubic, chest, and axillary hair; laryngeal enlargement; vocal cord thickening; alterations in body musculature; and fat distribution.

Male hypogonadism results from insufficient secretion of testosterone and is characterized by low serum testosterone concentrations. Symptoms associated with male hypogonadism include decreased sexual desire with or without impotence, fatigue and loss of energy, mood depression, regression of secondary sexual characteristics, and osteoporosis. Hypogonadism is a risk factor for osteoporosis in men

General Androgen Effects: Drugs in the androgen class also promote retention of nitrogen, sodium, potassium, phosphorus, and decreased urinary excretion of calcium.

Androgens have been reported to increase protein anabolism and decrease protein catabolism. Nitrogen balance is improved only when there is sufficient intake of calories and protein.

Androgens have been reported to stimulate the production of red blood cells by enhancing erythropoietin production.

Androgens are responsible for the growth spurt of adolescence and for the eventual termination of linear growth brought about by fusion of the epiphyseal growth centers. In children, exogenous androgens accelerate linear growth rates but may cause a disproportionate advancement in bone maturation. Use over long periods may result in fusion of the epiphyseal growth centers and termination of the growth process.

During exogenous administration of androgens, endogenous testosterone release may be inhibited through feedback inhibition of pituitary luteinizing hormone (LH). At large doses of exogenous androgens, spermatogenesis may also be suppressed through feedback inhibition of pituitary follicle-stimulating hormone (FSH).

In hypogonadal men treatment with testosterone undecanoate results in improvement of testosterone deficiency symptoms. Testosterone treatment has been reported to increase bone mineral density and lean body mass and decrease body fat with no clinical relevance. Serum cholesterol, LDL, HDL, and triglycerides levels may increase and/or decrease during androgen therapy. Hemoglobin and hematocrit increase during testosterone therapy in a dose dependant manner. In small clinical studies reported in the literature testosterone undecanoate has not been associated with increases in serum liver enzyme activities. In short term (up to 2 years) studies involving small numbers of patients testosterone undecanoate has not been shown to be associated with significant increases in PSA levels. In other trials testosterone therapy has a variable effect on PSA measurements. Clinical studies report that testosterone treatment including testosterone undecanoate may result in an increase in prostate size but this has not been associated with symptoms of prostatism. In hypogonadal diabetic patients the metabolic effects of Androgens may decrease blood glucose, and therefore insulin requirements.

Pharmacokinetics: Absorption: The active substance, testosterone undecanoate is well absorbed from the gastrointestinal tract. Both testosterone undecanoate and the newly formed 5-alpha-dihydrotestosterone undecanoate are partly absorbed via the lymphatic system, circumventing first passage through the liver. Following oral administration of testosterone undecanoate, an important part of the active substance testosterone undecanoate is co-absorbed with the lipophilic solvent from the intestine into the lymphatic system, thus partially circumventing the first-pass inactivation by the liver. Testosterone undecanoate must be taken with a normal meal or breakfast to ensure absorption. The bioavailability is about 7%.

Distribution: Administration of radioactively labelled testosterone undecanoate (^{3}H-TU) to men resulted in radioactivity in the lymph associated with unmetabolized testosterone undecanoate and 5-alpha-dihydrotestosterone undecanoate. Peak levels of radioactivity appeared in the lymph and plasma 2.5-5 hours after administration.

Metabolism: It is metabolized partly in the intestinal wall into 5-alpha-dihydrotestosterone undecanoate (DHTU) and in plasma and tissues TU is hydrolyzed to free testosterone and DHTU to DHT. Free testosterone is rapidly converted to 5-alpha-dihydrotestosterone, androstenedione and estradiol.

Excretion: The highest concentration of radioactivity in urine was found 2 hours later. During the first 24 hours approximately 40% of the administered dose was found in urine and the total recovery of the dose in urine during the first week was 45-48%.

Special Populations and Conditions: Pediatrics: Testosterone undecanoate may be used to stimulate puberty in carefully selected males with clearly delayed puberty not secondary to a pathological disorder. Androgens can accelerate bone maturation without producing compensatory gain in linear growth. The effect on bone maturation should be monitored by assessing bone age of the wrist and hand every six months. These adverse effects may result in compromised adult stature. The younger the child the greater the risk of compromising final mature height.

Geriatrics: Geriatric patients treated with androgens may be at an increased risk of developing prostatic hypertrophy and prostatic carcinoma although conclusive evidence to support this concept is lacking.

STORAGE AND STABILITY: Store between 15-30°C. Protect from light and moisture. Do not refrigerate. Keep blister in the outer carton.

SPECIAL HANDLING INSTRUCTIONS: Not applicable.

INFORMATION FOR THE PATIENT: Published in e-CPS, available by subscription at www.e-cps.ca.

DOSAGE FORMS, COMPOSITION AND PACKAGING: Each oval, orange clear, soft gelatin capsule, ink-printed in white with "P" logo and "40" on the same line, contains: testosterone undecanoate 40 mg in the presence of caprylic-capric acid tryglicerides. Nonmedicinal ingredients: capsule shell: glycerin, pork gelatin, sodium methylparaben (Nipagin m-sodium), sodium propylparaben nipasol and sorbitol special polyol. Bottles of 100 capsules. Blister packs of 10 capsules, boxes of 3, 6 or 12 blister packs.

PMS-Topiramate Pr

topiramate

Antiepileptic

Pharmascience

SUPPLIED: 25 mg: Each white, round, coated tablet, debossed with a "T" on one side and "25" on the other side, contains: topiramate 25 mg. Nonmedicinal ingredients: colloidal silicon dioxide, copovidone, hydroxypropyl methylcellulose, lactose, magnesium stearate, polydextrose (corn), polyethylene glycol, sodium starch glycolate, titanium dioxide and triethyl citrate. Bottles of 100 and 500. Store at controlled room temperature (15 to 30°C) and protect from moisture.

50 mg: Each pale yellow, round, coated tablet, debossed with a "T" on one side and "50" on the other side, contains: topiramate 50 mg. Nonmedicinal ingredients: colloidal silicon dioxide, copovidone, iron oxide yellow, lactose, magnesium stearate, polyethylene glycol, polyvinyl alcohol, sodium starch glycolate, talc and titanium dioxide. Bottles of 100. Store at controlled room temperature (15 to 30°C) and protect from moisture.

100 mg: Each yellow, round, coated tablet, debossed with a "T" on one side and "100" on the other side, contains: topiramate 100 mg. Nonmedicinal ingredients: colloidal silicon dioxide, copovidone, iron oxide yellow, lactose, magnesium stearate, polyethylene glycol, polyvinyl alcohol, sodium starch glycolate, talc and titanium dioxide. Bottles of 100 and 500. Store at controlled room temperature (15 to 30°C) and protect from moisture.

200 mg: Each salmon, round, coated tablet, debossed with a "T" on one side and "200" on the other side, contains: topiramate 200 mg. Nonmedicinal ingredients: colloidal silicon dioxide, copovidone, iron oxide red, lactose, magnesium stearate, polyethylene glycol, polyvinyl alcohol, sodium starch glycolate, talc and titanium dioxide. Bottles of 100. Store at controlled room temperature (15 to 30°C) and protect from moisture.

PMS-Trazodone Pr

trazodone HCl

Antidepressant

Pharmascience

SUPPLIED: 50 mg: Each orange, biconvex, scored tablet identified "Trazodone" and "pms/50" on opposite sides, contains: trazodone HCl 50 mg equivalent to 45.5 mg of trazodone base. Nonmedicinal ingredients: cornstarch, croscarmellose sodium, dibasic calcium phosphate, FD&C Yellow No. 6 Aluminum Lake, lactose, magnesium stearate and microcrystalline cellulose. Bottles of 100, 250 and 500. Store at room temperature (15-30°C). Protect from light.

75 mg: Each salmon, round, biconvex tablet, identified "Trazodone" and "pms" over "75" on opposite sides, contains: trazodone HCl 75 mg equivalent to 68.25 mg of trazodone base. Nonmedicinal ingredients: cornstarch, croscarmellose sodium, dibasic calcium phosphate, FD&C Yellow No. 6 Aluminum Lake, lactose, magnesium stearate and microcrystalline cellulose. Bottles of 100. Store at room temperature (15-30°C). Protect from light.

100 mg: Each white, biconvex, scored tablet identified "Trazodone" and "pms/100" on opposite sides, contains: trazodone HCl 100 mg equivalent to 91 mg of trazodone base. Nonmedicinal ingredients: cornstarch, croscarmellose sodium, dibasic calcium phosphate, lactose, magnesium stearate and microcrystalline cellulose. Bottles of 100 and 500. Store at room temperature (15-30°C). Protect from light.

PMS-Ursodiol C Pr

ursodiol

Cholestatic Liver Disease

Pharmascience

SUPPLIED: 250 mg: Each white, elliptical, biconvex, coated tablet, debossed with "250" on one side and the "P" logo on the other side, contains: ursodiol 250 mg. Nonmedicinal ingredients: hydroxypropyl methylcellulose, magnesium stearate, microcrystalline cellulose, polyethylene glycol, povidone, sodium lauryl sulfate and sodium starch glycolate. Bottles of 100 and 500. Store at controlled room temperature between 15 and 30°C in a tightly closed container.

500 mg: Each white, elliptical, biconvex, coated tablet, debossed with "500" on one side and the "P" logo on the other side, contains: ursodiol 500 mg. Nonmedicinal ingredients: hydroxypropyl methylcellulose, magnesium stearate, microcrystalline cellulose, polyethylene glycol, povidone, sodium lauryl sulfate and sodium starch glycolate. Bottles of 100. Store at controlled room temperature between 15 and 30°C in a tightly closed container.

PMS-Valacyclovir ℞
valacyclovir HCl
Antiviral Agent

Pharmascience

SUPPLIED: Each blue, coated, capsule-shaped caplet, debossed with "VC" followed by "500" on one side and nothing on the other side, contains: valacyclovir hydrochloride equivalent to 500 mg valacyclovir. Nonmedicinal ingredients: crospovidone, FD&C Blue #2 Aluminum Lake, hydroxypropyl methylcellulose, magnesium stearate, microcrystalline cellulose, polyethylene glycol 400, polysorbate 80 and titanium dioxide. Bottles of 100. Store between 15 and 30°C and protect from light.

PMS-Venlafaxine XR ℞
venlafaxine HCl
Antidepressant—Anxiolytic

Pharmascience

SUPPLIED: 37.5 mg: Each extended release, hard gelatin capsule, with a peach body printed "37.5" in red ink and a light grey cap printed "P" logo in red ink, contains: venlafaxine 37.5 mg as venlafaxine HCl. Nonmedicinal ingredients: ammonium hydroxide, black iron oxide, dibutyl sebecate, ethyl cellulose, gelatin, isopropyl alcohol, n-butyl alcohol, povidone, propylene glycol, red iron oxide, shellac glaze, simethicone, sugar spheres, titanium dioxide and yellow iron oxide. Bottles of 100 and 500. Store at room temperature (15-30°C) in a dry place.
75 mg: Each extended release, hard gelatin peach capsule printed in red ink "75" on the body and "P" logo on cap, contains: venlafaxine 75 mg as venlafaxine HCl. Nonmedicinal ingredients: ammonium hydroxide, dibutyl sebecate, ethyl cellulose, gelatin, isopropyl alcohol, n-butyl alcohol, povidone, propylene glycol, red iron oxide, shellac glaze, simethicone, sugar spheres, titanium dioxide and yellow iron oxide. Bottles of 100 and 500. Store at room temperature (15-30°C) in a dry place.
150 mg: Each extended release, hard gelatin capsule with a dark orange opaque body printed "150" in white ink and a dark orange opaque cap printed "P" logo in white ink, contains: venlafaxine 150 mg as venlafaxine HCl. Nonmedicinal ingredients: butyl alcohol, dehydrated alcohol, dibutyl sebecate, ethyl cellulose, gelatin, isopropyl alcohol, povidone, propylene glycol, red iron oxide, shellac, sodium hydroxide, sugar spheres, titanium dioxide, and yellow iron oxide. Bottles of 100 and 500. Store at room temperature (15-30°C) in a dry place.

PMS-Zopiclone ℞
zopiclone
Hypnotic

Pharmascience

SUPPLIED: 5 mg: Each white, round, biconvex, film-coated tablet, debossed "Z" over "5" on one side and plain on the other side, contains: zopiclone 5 mg. Nonmedicinal ingredients: carboxymethylcellulose sodium, cornstarch, dibasic calcium phosphate, hydroxypropyl cellulose, hydroxypropyl methylcellulose, lactose, magnesium stearate, microcrystalline cellulose, polyethylene glycol and titanium dioxide. Bottles of 100. Store in a dry place at room temperature (15-30°C). Protect from light.
7.5 mg: Each blue, oval, biconvex, film-coated tablet, debossed "7.5" score "Z" on the scored side and plain on the other side, contains: zopiclone 7.5 mg. Nonmedicinal ingredients: carboxymethylcellulose sodium, cornstarch, dibasic calcium phosphate, FD&C Blue No. 1 Aluminum Lake, FD&C Yellow No. 6 Aluminum Lake, hydroxypropyl methylcellulose, lactose, magnesium stearate, microcrystalline cellulose, polyethylene glycol, polysorbate, and titanium dioxide. Bottles of 100 and 500. Store in a dry place at room temperature (15-30°C). Protect from light.

Pneumo 23®
pneumococcal polysaccharide vaccine
Active Immunizing Agent

sanofi pasteur

Date of Revision: July 18, 2008

PHARMACOLOGY: PNEUMO 23 [Pneumococcal Polysaccharide Vaccine] is a capsular polysaccharide vaccine against disease caused by 23 of the most common serotypes of *S. pneumoniae* (pneumococcus).

S. pneumoniae causes invasive bacterial infections including primary bacterial pneumonia, meningitis, and bacteremia. Invasive disease is most common in the very young, the elderly and in certain specific groups at high risk, such as individuals with functional or anatomic asplenia and congenital or acquired immune deficiency. Given that not every case of invasive pneumococcal disease would have had cultures taken before starting antibiotics, these estimates likely represent the minimum incidence rates. Population surveillance data from 9 selected health units across Canada show that the age-specific incidence of invasive pneumococcal disease is greatest in children <5 years of age (55.3 cases per 100 000) and in persons ≥65 years of age (46.4 cases per 100 000). Ninety-four percent of cases were caused by serotypes contained in the 23-valent pneumococcal vaccine. Other Canada-wide estimates suggest that approximately 90% of cases of pneumococcal bacteremia and meningitis are caused by these 23 types. Penicillin-resistant strains generally appear in serotypes included in the vaccine and have become more common in Canada, increasing from 2.5% in 1991 to 11.3% in 1998. The six serotypes that most often cause drug-resistant invasive pneumococcal infection are included in this vaccine. The overall case fatality rate from invasive pneumococcal disease is 11% increasing to 20% for those in the ≥65 age group.

Efficacy of pneumococcal polysaccharide vaccine is in the range of 50 to 80% among the elderly and in specific patient groups such as those with diabetes mellitus, anatomic or physiologic asplenia, congestive heart failure or chronic pulmonary disease. Pneumococcal polysaccharide vaccine is not indicated for children ≤2 years of age; however, it may broaden serotype coverage for high-risk children ≥2 years of age. Although the duration of immunity is not precisely known, serotype-specific antibody levels appear to decline after 5 to 10 years, decreasing more rapidly in some groups than others.

In clinical studies involving more than 1000 volunteers, serum capsular polysaccharide antibodies start to increase 10 to 15 days following immunization with PNEUMO 23. Clinical trials with PNEUMO 23 vaccine have shown that healthy adults develop excellent antibody responses following pneumococcal vaccination: 80% or more of subjects develop at least a two-fold rise in antibody levels, inducing IgG and IgM antibodies in individuals immunized intramuscularly.

In a clinical trial conducted in The Gambia, 150 women in the third trimester of pregnancy received either PNEUMO 23 (n=75) or a control vaccine (n=75). No significant side effects were recorded among vaccinated women except soreness at the injection site. Rates of stillbirth (1 in the PNEUMO 23 group and 3 in the control vaccine group) were less than might have been expected in the community. In a clinical trial conducted in Papua New Guinea, 235 women received PNEUMO 23 at 28 to 38 weeks gestation. A control group of 202 was unimmunized. There were no excess stillbirths in the vaccinated group and no differences in mortality rates during infancy between babies of immunized and unimmunized mothers.

INDICATIONS: PNEUMO 23 [Pneumococcal Polysaccharide Vaccine] is indicated in persons two years of age or older for the prevention of invasive infection, such as bacteremia, pneumonia or meningitis, caused by the serotypes of pneumococci contained in the vaccine.

A single dose of pneumococcal polysaccharide vaccine is recommended for all individuals ≥65 years of age including those with unknown vaccination histories.

In accordance with the National Advisory Committee on Immunization (NACI), pneumococcal polysaccharide vaccine is recommended for individuals ≥5 years of age who are at high risk of invasive pneumococcal infection including:
- individuals with asplenia, splenic dysfunction or sickle cell disease
- individuals with chronic cardiorespiratory disease (except asthma)
- individuals with cirrhosis, alcoholism, chronic renal disease or nephrotic syndrome
- individuals with chronic cerebrospinal fluid leak
- individuals with diabetes mellitus
- individuals with HIV infection and other chronic conditions associated with immunosuppression (Hodgkin's disease, lymphoma, multiple myeloma, immunosuppression for organ transplantation)
- candidates for and recipients of cochlear implants

Pneumococcal polysaccharide vaccine should also be given to smokers.

Children from 2-5 years of age who have previously been immunized with a pneumococcal conjugate vaccine may receive pneumococcal polysaccharide vaccine both as a booster dose and to increase the serogroup coverage (see Dosage).

History of a confirmed or suspected pneumococcal infection is not a contraindication and should be considered according to underlying risk status. PNEUMO 23 is not recommended for prevention of recurrent upper respiratory tract infections, particularly otitis media and sinusitis.

Children who have experienced invasive pneumococcal disease should receive all recommended doses of pneumococcal vaccine appropriate for their age and underlying condition.

Revaccination should be considered in some individuals (see Dosage).

CONTRAINDICATIONS: Immunization with PNEUMO 23 [Pneumococcal Polysaccharide Vaccine] should be deferred in the presence of any acute illness, including febrile illness, to avoid superimposing adverse effects from the vaccine on the underlying illness or mistakenly identifying a manifestation of the underlying illness as a complication of vaccine use. A minor illness such as mild upper respiratory infection is not a reason to defer immunization.

Allergy to any component of PNEUMO 23, its container or an anaphylactic or other allergic reaction to a previous dose of PNEUMO 23 are contraindications to vaccination (see Supplied).

WARNINGS: PNEUMO 23 [Pneumococcal Polysaccharide Vaccine] will not immunize against types of pneumococci other than those contained in the vaccine.

In patients receiving antibiotic prophylaxis against pneumococcal infection, such prophylaxis should not be discontinued after immunization with PNEUMO 23.

Intramuscular injections should be given with care in persons suffering from coagulation disorders or on anticoagulant therapy because of the risk of hemorrhage.

PNEUMO 23 should not be administered into the buttocks due to the varying amount of fatty tissue in this region, nor by the intradermal route, since these methods of administration may induce a weaker immune response.

Where possible, the vaccine should be given at least 10 to 14 days before splenectomy or initiation of chemotherapy or immunosuppressive therapy or early in the course of HIV infection.

Immunocompromised persons (whether from disease or treatment) may not obtain the expected immune response. If possible, consideration should be given to delaying vaccination until after the completion of any immunosuppressive treatment. If PNEUMO 23 is given less than 14 days prior to splenectomy or initiation of chemotherapy, it may not elicit the expected immune response.

As with any vaccine, immunization with PNEUMO 23 may not protect 100% of susceptible individuals.

PRECAUTIONS: The possibility of allergic reactions in persons sensitive to components of the vaccine should be evaluated. Epinephrine Hydrochloride Solution (1:1000) and other appropriate agents should be available for immediate use in case an anaphylactic or acute hypersensitivity reaction occurs. Health-care providers should be familiar with current recommendations for the initial management of anaphylaxis in non-hospital settings, including proper airway management.

For instructions on recognition and treatment of anaphylactic reactions, see the current edition of the Canadian Immunization Guide or visit the Health Canada website.

Before administration, take all appropriate precautions to prevent adverse reactions. This includes a review of the patient's history concerning possible hypersensitivity to the vaccine or similar vaccine, previous immunization history, the presence of any contraindications to immunization and current health status.

Before administration of PNEUMO 23 [Pneumococcal Polysaccharide Vaccine], health-care providers should inform the patient, parent or guardian of the benefits and risks of immunization, inquire about the recent health status of the patient and comply with any local requirements regarding information to be provided to the patient before immunization.

It is extremely important that the patient, parent or guardian be questioned concerning any symptoms and/or signs of an adverse reaction after a previous dose of vaccine (see Contraindications and Adverse Effects).

Do not inject into a blood vessel.

Use a separate sterile needle and syringe, or a sterile disposable unit, for each individual dose to prevent disease transmission.

Children: PNEUMO 23 is not recommended for children <2 years of age.

Pregnancy: Animal reproductive studies have not been conducted with PNEUMO 23. Clinical trials using PNEUMO 23 have been conducted in pregnant women during the third trimester and no significant adverse events were recorded (see Pharmacology). According to the Canadian Immunization Guide, neither pregnancy nor breast-feeding is a contraindication to either the polysaccharide or the conjugate pneumococcal vaccine. The benefits versus the risks of administering PNEUMO 23 in pregnancy should carefully be evaluated.

Lactation: Breast-feeding is not a contraindication to pneumococcal polysaccharide vaccines.

Drug Interactions: PNEUMO 23 should not be mixed in the same syringe with other parenterals. If any other vaccines are administered during the same visit, they must be given at separate sites and with separate syringes.

PNEUMO 23 may be given simultaneously with influenza, meningococcal and Hib conjugate vaccines at separate sites with separate syringes.

According to the Canadian Immunization Guide, there are obvious practical advantages to giving more than one vaccine at the same time, especially in preparation for foreign travel or when there is doubt that the patient will return for further doses of vaccine. Most of the commonly used antigens can safely be given simultaneously. No increase in the frequency or severity of clinically significant side effects has been observed. The immune response to each antigen is generally adequate and comparable to that found in patients receiving these vaccines at separate times.

ADVERSE EFFECTS: Local reactions at the injection site including pain, erythema, and induration occur in approximately 60% of vaccinees. These reactions are generally mild and transient.

Very rarely, Arthus-like reactions have been reported. They resolve without after-effects and mainly occur in persons with high initial pneumococcal antibody levels.

Systemic Reactions: Fever ≥38.5°C occurs in approximately 2% of vaccinees. Febrile episodes generally occur soon after vaccination and resolve within 24 hours. Headache and/or general malaise occur in <8%.

In post-marketing surveillance, other general reactions such as lymphadenopathy, rash, urticaria, arthralgia, anaphylactoid reactions, myalgia, asthenia and fatigue have very rarely been reported. Injection site cellulitis and peripheral edema in the injected extremity have also been reported.

Very rarely, more severe systemic reactions have been reported in the literature following administration of pneumococcal polysaccharide vaccines. These include thrombocytopenia, vasculitis, generalized rash, and relapse of known underlying immune conditions. The relationship, if any, between these reactions and pneumococcal vaccine is unknown.

Physicians, nurses, and pharmacists should report any adverse occurrences temporally related to the administration of the product in accordance with local requirements and to the Global Pharmacovigilance Department, Sanofi Pasteur Limited, 1755 Steeles Avenue West, Toronto, ON, M2R 3T4, Canada. 1-888-621-1146 (phone) or 416-667-2435 (fax).

DOSAGE: The immunizing dose is a single injection of 0.5 mL given intramuscularly or subcutaneously.

When PNEUMO 23 [Pneumococcal Polysaccharide Vaccine] is administered to broaden serotype coverage following a series of pneumococcal conjugate (PCV7) vaccinations, PNEUMO 23 should be given no earlier than 8 weeks after the last dose of pneumococcal conjugate (PCV7) vaccine.

Revaccination: One injection of 0.5 mL.

According to NACI, people for whom revaccination with pneumococcal polysaccharide vaccine should be considered include those with functional or anatomic asplenia or sickle cell disease; hepatic cirrhosis; chronic renal failure or nephrotic syndrome; HIV infection; and immunosuppression related to disease or therapy. A single revaccination is recommended after 5 years in those who received their first pneumococcal vaccine at age >10 years and after 3 years in those who received their 1st pneumococcal vaccination at age ≤10 years.

Immunization Schedule in Conjunction with the Pneumococcal Conjugate Vaccine: Children who have completed the pneumococcal conjugate vaccination series (PCV7) before they are 2 years of age, and who are among the risk groups for which PNEUMO 23 is already recommended (see Indications), should receive one dose of PNEUMO 23 at 2 years of age (>8 weeks after the last dose of pneumococcal conjugate vaccine).

Inspect for extraneous particulate matter and/or discolouration before use. If these conditions exist, the product should not be administered.

For information on vaccine administration see the current edition of the Canadian Immunization Guide or visit the Health Canada website.

Before injection, the skin over the site to be injected should be cleansed with a suitable germicide.

Shake the prefilled syringe well to uniformly distribute the suspension.

Administer the vaccine **intramuscularly or subcutaneously**. The preferred site is the deltoid area.

Do not inject intravenously.

Needles should not be recapped and should be disposed of properly.

Give the patient a permanent personal immunization record. In addition, it is essential that the physician or nurse record the immunization history in the permanent medical record of each patient. This permanent office record should contain the name of the vaccine, date given, dose, manufacturer and lot number.

SUPPLIED: PNEUMO 23 [Pneumococcal Polysaccharide Vaccine] is a clear, colorless liquid prepared from purified pneumococcal capsular antigens. Each dose of 0.5 mL contains: purified *S. pneumoniae* polysaccharides, 25 µg of each of the following serotypes: 1, 2, 3, 4, 5, 6B, 7F, 8, 9N, 9V, 10A, 11A, 12F, 14, 15B, 17F, 18C, 19A, 19F, 20, 22F, 23F, 33F; phenol ≤1.25 mg (as a preservative); sodium chloride 4.150 mg, disodium phosphate 0.065 mg, monosodium phosphate 0.023 mg, water for injection q.s. 0.5 mL.

Prefilled syringes of 0.5 mL (single dose), packages of 1, 10 and 20. Store at 2 to 8°C. **Do not freeze.** Discard product if exposed to freezing.

Do not use vaccine after expiration date.

The plunger, stopper and needle shields of the syringe for this product do not contain dry natural latex rubber.

Pneumovax® 23

pneumococcal vaccine, polyvalent, MSD Std.

Active Immunizing Agent Against Infections Caused by Pneumococci

Merck Frosst

Date of Revision: July 15, 2009

SUMMARY PRODUCT INFORMATION:

Route of Administration	Dosage Form/ Strength	Clinically Relevant Nonmedicinal Ingredients
Intramuscular or subcutaneous injection	Solution Each 0.5 mL dose contains 25 µg of capsular polysaccharide from each of 23 types of pneumococci: 1, 2, 3, 4, 5, 6B, 7F, 8, 9N, 9V, 10A, 11A, 12F, 14, 15B, 17F, 18C, 19A, 19F, 20, 22F, 23F, 33F	Phenol For a complete listing see Dosage Forms, Composition and Packaging.

DESCRIPTION: PNEUMOVAX 23 (pneumococcal vaccine, polyvalent, MSD Std.), is a sterile, liquid vaccine for intramuscular or subcutaneous injection. It consists of a mixture of highly purified capsular polysaccharides from the 23 most prevalent or invasive pneumococcal types of *S. pneumoniae*, including the six serotypes that most frequently cause invasive drug-resistant pneumococcal infections among children and adults in the United States (see Dosage Forms, Composition and Packaging). The 23-valent vaccine accounts for at least 90% of pneumococcal blood isolates and at least 85% of all pneumococcal isolates from sites which are generally sterile as determined by ongoing surveillance of United States data. Canadian population based surveillance for invasive pneumococcal disease in metropolitan Toronto-Peel region found that 92% of cases were caused by serotypes contained in PNEUMOVAX 23. Similarly, the Sentinel Health Unit Surveillance System (SHUSS) study documented 94% of cases being caused by serotypes contained in PNEUMOVAX 23.

INDICATIONS AND CLINICAL USE: PNEUMOVAX 23 (pneumococcal vaccine, polyvalent, MSD Std.) is indicated for vaccination against pneumococcal disease caused by those pneumococcal types included in the vaccine. Effectiveness of the vaccine in the prevention of pneumococcal pneumonia and pneumococcal bacteremia has been demonstrated in controlled trials in South Africa, France and in case-controlled studies.

PNEUMOVAX 23 will not prevent disease caused by capsular types of pneumococcus other than those contained in the vaccine.

If it is known that a person has not received any pneumococcal vaccine or if earlier pneumococcal vaccination status is unknown, then persons in the categories listed below should be administered pneumococcal vaccine; however, if a person has received a primary dose of pneumococcal vaccine, before administering an additional dose of vaccine, please refer to the Revaccination section.

Vaccination with PNEUMOVAX 23 is recommended for selected individuals as follows:

Immunocompetent Persons:

- Routine vaccination for persons 50 years of age or older
- Persons aged ≥2 years with chronic cardiovascular disease (including congestive heart failure and cardiomyopathies), chronic pulmonary disease (including chronic obstructive pulmonary disease and emphysema), or diabetes mellitus
- Persons aged ≥2 years with alcoholism, chronic liver disease (including cirrhosis) or cerebrospinal fluid leaks
- Persons aged ≥2 years with functional or anatomic asplenia (including sickle cell disease and splenectomy)
- Persons aged ≥2 years living in special environments or social settings (including Aboriginals)
- In Canada, the National Advisory Committee on Immunization (NACI) currently recommends the vaccination of smokers with the 23-valent polysaccharide pneumococcal vaccine.

Immunocompromised Persons:

- Persons aged ≥2 years, including those with HIV infection, leukemia, lymphoma, Hodgkin's disease, multiple myeloma, generalized malignancy, chronic renal failure or nephrotic syndrome; those receiving immunosuppressive chemotherapy (including corticosteroids); and those who have received an organ or bone marrow transplant. For selected groups, see Timing of Vaccination.

According to NACI guidelines, children aged 2 years to <5 years of age who are at increased risk of invasive pneumococcal disease (IPD) should receive pneumococcal conjugate vaccine, with pneumococcal polysaccharide vaccine being used as a booster dose in this age group to increase the serotype coverage. Children at increased risk of IPD include those who attend child care centres, are Aboriginal, have sickle cell disease and other sickle cell hemoglobinopathies, have other types of functional or anatomic asplenia, HIV infection, immunocompromising conditions (e.g., primary immunodeficiencies; malignancies; conditions resulting from immunosuppressive therapy, solid organ transplantation, or use of long-term systemic corticosteroids; nephrotic syndrome), chronic medical conditions (e.g., chronic cardiac and pulmonary disease such as bronchopulmonary dysplasia, diabetes mellitus, chronic renal disease or CSF leak) and children with cochlear implants or those receiving cochlear implants. Pneumococcal polysaccharide vaccine should be given to all individuals ≥5 years of age who have not received the conjugate vaccine previously and who are at higher risk of IPD.

Timing of Vaccination: Pneumococcal vaccine should be given at least two weeks before elective splenectomy, if possible.

For planning cancer chemotherapy or other immunosuppressive therapy (e.g., for patients with Hodgkin's disease or those who undergo organ or bone marrow transplantation), pneumococcal vaccination should be administered at least two weeks prior to the initiation of immunosuppressive therapy. Vaccination during chemotherapy or radiation therapy should be avoided. Based on literature reports, pneumococcal vaccine may be given as early as several months following completion of chemotherapy or radiation therapy for neoplastic disease. In Hodgkin's disease, immune response to vaccination may be impaired for two years or longer after intense chemotherapy (with or without radiation). During the two years following the completion of chemotherapy or other immunosuppressive therapy, antibody responses improve in some patients as the interval between the end of treatment and pneumococcal vaccination increases.

Persons with asymptomatic or symptomatic HIV infection should be vaccinated as soon as possible after their diagnosis is confirmed.

Revaccination: Revaccination of immunocompetent persons previously vaccinated with 23-valent polysaccharide vaccine is not routinely recommended. However, revaccination once is recommended for persons ≥2 years of age who are at highest risk of serious pneumococcal infection and those likely to have a rapid decline in pneumococcal antibody levels, provided that at least five years have passed since receipt of a first dose of pneumococcal vaccine.

The highest risk group includes persons with functional or anatomic asplenia (e.g., sickle cell disease or splenectomy), HIV infection, leukemia, lymphoma, Hodgkin's disease, multiple myeloma, generalized malignancy, chronic renal failure, nephrotic syndrome, or other conditions associated with immunosuppression (e.g., organ or bone marrow transplantation), and those receiving immunosuppressive chemotherapy (including long-term systemic corticosteroids) (see Timing of Vaccination).

For children ≤10 years of age at the time of initial immunization and at highest risk of severe pneumococcal infection (e.g., children with functional or anatomic asplenia, including sickle cell disease or splenectomy or conditions associated with rapid antibody decline after initial vaccination including nephrotic syndrome, renal failure or renal transplantation), the United States Advisory Committee on Immunization Practices (ACIP) and NACI recommend that a single revaccination may be considered three years after the initial dose.

For children >10 years of age at the time of initial immunization and at highest risk of severe pneumococcal infection (as described above) the ACIP and NACI recommend that a single revaccination may be considered five years after the initial dose.

If prior vaccination status is unknown for patients in the high risk group, patients should be given pneumococcal vaccine.

All persons ≥65 years of age who have not received vaccine within 5 years (and were <65 years of age at the time of vaccination) should receive another dose of vaccine.

Because data are insufficient concerning the safety of pneumococcal vaccine when administered three or more times, revaccination following a second dose is not routinely recommended.

CONTRAINDICATIONS: Hypersensitivity to any component of the vaccine.

According to the Canadian National Advisory Committee on Immunization, anaphylactic reaction to polysaccharide pneumococcal vaccine is a contraindication to re-immunization with that product.

WARNINGS AND PRECAUTIONS: General: In case of severe hypersensitivity or anaphylactoid reaction to the vaccine, refer to NACI recommendations regarding the management of these reactions in the Canadian Immunization Guide.

Epinephrine injection (1:1000) must be immediately available should an acute anaphylactoid reaction occur due to any component of the vaccine.

For planning cancer chemotherapy or other immunosuppressive therapy (e.g., for patients with Hodgkin's disease or those who undergo organ or bone marrow transplantation), the timing of the vaccination is critical (see Indications and Clinical Use, Timing of Vaccination).

If the vaccine is administered to patients who are immunosuppressed due to either an underlying condition or medical treatment (e.g., immunosuppressive therapy such as cancer chemotherapy or radiation therapy), the expected serum antibody response may not be obtained and potential impairment of future immune responses to pneumococcal antigens may occur (see Indications and Clinical Use, Timing of Vaccination).

Intradermal administration may cause severe local reactions.

Caution and appropriate care should be exercised in administering PNEUMOVAX 23 (pneumococcal vaccine, polyvalent MSD Std.) to individuals with severely compromised cardiovascular and/or pulmonary function in whom a systemic reaction would pose a significant risk.

Any febrile respiratory illness or other active infection is reason for delaying use of PNEUMOVAX 23, except when, in the opinion of the physician, withholding the agent entails even greater risk.

In patients who require penicillin (or other antibiotic) prophylaxis against pneumococcal infection, such prophylaxis should not be discontinued after vaccination with PNEUMOVAX 23.

PNEUMOVAX 23 may not be effective in preventing pneumococcal meningitis in patients who have chronic cerebrospinal fluid (CSF) leakage resulting from congenital lesions, skull fractures, or neurosurgical procedures.

Routine revaccination of immunocompetent persons previously vaccinated with a 23-valent vaccine is not recommended. However, revaccination once is recommended for persons aged ≥2 years who are at highest risk for serious pneumococcal infections and those likely to have a rapid decline in pneumococcal antibody levels (see Indications and Clinical Use, Revaccination).

As with any vaccine, vaccination with PNEUMOVAX 23 may not result in complete protection in all recipients and lack of effect following PNEUMOVAX 23 vaccination has been reported through post-market surveillance.

Special Populations: Pregnant Women: Animal reproduction studies have not been conducted with PNEUMOVAX 23. It is also not known whether PNEUMOVAX 23 can cause fetal harm when administered to a pregnant woman or can affect reproduction capacity. PNEUMOVAX 23 should be given to a pregnant woman only if clearly needed.

Nursing Women: It is not known whether this vaccine is excreted in human milk. Because many drugs are excreted in human milk, caution should be exercised when PNEUMOVAX 23 is administered to a nursing woman.

Pediatrics (<2 years of age): PNEUMOVAX 23 is not recommended for use in children less than 2 years of age. Safety and effectiveness in children below the age of 2 years have not been established. Children in this age group respond poorly to the capsular types contained in this vaccine (see Actions and Clinical Pharmacology, Immunogenicity).

Geriatrics: Persons 65 years of age or older were enrolled in several clinical studies of PNEUMOVAX 23 that were conducted pre- and post-licensure. In the largest of these studies, the safety of PNEUMOVAX 23 in adults 65 years of age and older (n=629) was compared to the safety of PNEUMOVAX 23 in adults 50 to 64 years of age (n=379). The data did not suggest an increased rate of adverse reactions among subjects ≥65 years of age compared to those 50 to 64 years of age. However, since elderly individuals may not tolerate medical interventions as well as younger individuals, a higher frequency and/or a greater severity of reactions in some older individuals cannot be ruled out.

ADVERSE REACTIONS: Adverse Drug Reaction Overview: The following adverse experiences have been reported with PNEUMOVAX 23 (pneumococcal vaccine, polyvalent, MSD Std.) in clinical trials and/or post-marketing experience: Injection site reactions, consisting of pain, soreness, erythema, warmth, swelling, local induration, decreased limb mobility and peripheral edema in the injected extremity. Very rarely, cellulitis-like reactions were reported. These cellulitis-like reactions, reported in post-marketing experience, show short onset time from vaccine administration. Local reactions may be accompanied by systemic signs and symptoms including fever, leukocytosis and an increase in the laboratory value for serum C-reactive protein.

The most common adverse experiences reported in clinical trials were fever (≤38.8°C), injection site reactions including soreness, erythema, warmth, swelling and local induration.

Clinical Trial Adverse Drug Reactions: Because clinical trials are conducted under very specific conditions the adverse reaction rates observed in the clinical trials may not reflect the rates observed in practice and should not be compared to the rates in the clinical trials of another vaccine. Adverse drug reaction information from clinical trials is useful for identifying vaccine-related adverse events and for approximating rates.

In a clinical trial, an increased rate of self-limited local reactions has been observed with revaccination at 3-5 years following primary vaccination. It was reported that the overall injection-site adverse experiences rate for subjects ≥65 years of age was higher following revaccination (79.3%) than following primary vaccination (52.9%). The reported overall injection-site adverse experiences rate for re-vaccinees and primary vaccinees who were 50 to 64 years of age were similar (79.6% and 72.8% respectively). In both age groups, re-vaccinees reported a higher rate of a composite endpoint (any of the following: moderate pain, severe pain, and/or large induration at the injection site) than primary vaccinees. Among subjects ≥65 years of age, the composite endpoint was reported by 30.6% and 10.4% of revaccination and primary vaccination subjects, respectively, while among subjects 50-64 years of age, the endpoint was reported by 35.5% and 18.9% respectively. The injection site reactions occurred within the 3 day monitoring period and typically resolved by day 5. The rate of overall systemic adverse experiences was similar among both primary vaccinees and re-vaccinees within each age group. The most common systemic adverse experiences were asthenia/fatigue, myalgia and headache. Among subjects ≥65 years of age, asthenia/fatigue and myalgia were reported more frequently following revaccination than primary vaccination. The observed generally small increase (≤13%) in post-vaccination use of analgesics returned to baseline by day 5.

Other adverse experiences reported in clinical trials and/or in post-marketing experience include:

Body as a Whole: cellulitis, asthenia, fever, chills, malaise.

Digestive System: nausea, vomiting.

Hematologic/Lymphatic System: lymphadenitis, lymphadenopathy, thrombocytopenia in patients with stabilized idiopathic thrombocytopenic purpura, hemolytic anemia in patients who have had other hematologic disorders, leukocytosis.

Hypersensitivity Reactions Including: anaphylactoid reactions, serum sickness, angioneurotic edema.

Musculoskeletal System: arthralgia, arthritis, myalgia.

Nervous System: headache, paresthesia, radiculoneuropathy, Guillain-Barré syndrome, febrile convulsion.

Skin: rash, urticaria.

DRUG INTERACTIONS: Use with Other Vaccines: It is recommended that pneumococcal vaccine may be administered at the same time as influenza vaccine (by separate injection in the other arm) without an increase in side effects or decreased antibody response to either vaccine.

In contrast to pneumococcal vaccine, influenza vaccine is recommended annually, for appropriate populations.

PNEUMOVAX 23 and ZOSTAVAX (zoster vaccine live, attenuated [Oka/Merck]) should not be given concurrently because concomitant use in a clinical trial resulted in reduced immunogenicity of ZOSTAVAX. In this trial, the immunogenicity of PNEUMOVAX 23 was not affected by ZOSTAVAX.

DOSAGE AND ADMINISTRATION: Dosing Considerations: The healthcare provider should determine the current health status and previous vaccination history of the vaccinee (see Indications and Clinical Use, Revaccination).

The healthcare provider should question the patient, parent or guardian about reactions to a previous dose of PNEUMOVAX 23 (pneumococcal vaccine, polyvalent, MSD Std.) or other pneumococcal vaccine.

Recommended Dose and Dosage Adjustment: The recommended dose of PNEUMOVAX 23 is a single 0.5 mL injection given subcutaneously or intramuscularly (see Administration).

Administration: Do not inject intravenously or intradermally.

Parenteral drug products should be inspected visually for particulate matter and discolouration prior to administration, whenever solution and container permit. PNEUMOVAX 23 is a clear, colourless solution. The vaccine is used directly as supplied. No dilution or reconstitution is necessary. Phenol 0.25% has been added in the vaccine as a preservative.

It is important to use a separate sterile syringe and needle for each individual patient to prevent transmission of infectious agents from one person to another.

Withdraw 0.5 mL from the vial using a sterile needle and syringe free of preservatives, antiseptics and detergents.

Administer a single 0.5 mL dose of PNEUMOVAX 23 subcutaneously or intramuscularly (preferably in the deltoid muscle or lateral mid-thigh), with appropriate precautions to avoid intravascular administration.

OVERDOSAGE:

There are no data with regard to overdose.

> For management of a suspected drug overdose, CPhA recommends that you contact your **regional Poison Control Centre**. See the *CPS* Directory section for a list of Poison Control Centres.

ACTION AND CLINICAL PHARMACOLOGY: Infections caused by *S. pneumoniae* are a major cause of morbidity and mortality all over the world and a major cause of pneumonia, bacteremia, meningitis, and otitis media.

Strains of drug-resistant *S. pneumoniae* have become increasingly common in the United States and in other parts of the world. In some areas as many as 35% of pneumococcal isolates have been reported to be resistant to penicillin. Many penicillin-resistant pneumococci are also resistant to other antimicrobial drugs (e.g., erythromycin, trimethoprim-sulfamethoxazole and extended-spectrum cephalosporins), therefore emphasizing the importance of vaccine prophylaxis against pneumococcal disease.

According to the results of a Canadian National Survey among 1089 clinical isolates of *S. pneumoniae* obtained from 39 laboratories across Canada between October 1994 and August 1995, the prevalence of antimicrobial resistance has increased in Canada in just a few years.

Immunogenicity: It has been established that the purified pneumococcal capsular polysaccharides induce antibody production and that such antibody is effective in preventing pneumococcal disease. Clinical studies have demonstrated the immunogenicity of each of the 23 capsular types when tested in polyvalent vaccines.

Studies with 12-, 14-, and 23-valent pneumococcal vaccines in children two years of age and older and in adults of all ages showed immunogenic responses. Protective capsular type-specific antibody levels generally develop by the third week following vaccination.

Bacterial capsular polysaccharides induce antibodies primarily by T-cell-independent mechanisms. Therefore, antibody response to most pneumococcal capsular types is generally poor or inconsistent in children aged <2 years whose immune systems are immature.

Additional Relevant Information: Epidemiology: Pneumococcal infection causes approximately 40 000 deaths annually in the United States.

In Canada, population-based surveillance for invasive pneumococcal disease in metropolitan Toronto-Peel region (population 3.4 million) revealed an overall incidence of 11.8-16.1 cases per 100 000 population in 1995-1997. At least 500 000 cases of pneumococcal pneumonia are estimated to occur annually in the United States; *S. pneumoniae* accounts for approximately 25-35% of cases of community-acquired bacterial pneumonia in persons who require hospitalization.

Pneumococcal disease accounts for an estimated 50 000 cases of pneumococcal bacteremia annually in the United States. Some studies suggest the overall annual incidence of bacteremia to be approximately 15 to 30 cases/100 000 population with 50 to 83 cases/100 000 for persons 65 years of age and older and 160 cases/100 000 for children less than two years of age. The incidence of pneumococcal bacteremia is as high as 1% (940 cases/100 000 population) among persons with acquired immunodeficiency syndrome (AIDS). In the United States, the risk of acquiring bacteremia is lower among whites than among persons in some other racial/ethnic groups (i.e., blacks, Alaskan Natives, and American Indians). Despite appropriate antimicrobial therapy and intensive medical care, the overall case-fatality rate for pneumococcal bacteremia is 15%-20% among adults, and among elderly patients this rate is approximately 30-40%. An overall case-fatality rate of 36% was documented for adult inner-city residents who were hospitalized for pneumococcal bacteremia.

The SHUSS (Sentinel Health Unit Surveillance System), an active population-based surveillance for laboratory-confirmed disease conducted in nine health units within eight Canadian provinces, revealed an overall incidence of 15.1 cases of invasive pneumococcal disease per 100 000 population. The age-specific incidence was greatest in children <5 years of age (55.3 cases per 100 000) and in persons ≥65 years of age (46.4 cases per 100 000). Ninety-four percent of cases were caused by serotypes contained in the 23-valent pneumococcal vaccine.

In the United States, pneumococcal disease accounts for an estimated 3000 cases of meningitis annually. The estimated overall annual incidence of pneumococcal meningitis is approximately 1 to 2 cases per 100 000 population. The incidence of pneumococcal meningitis is highest among children 6 to 24 months and persons aged ≥65 years; rates for blacks are twice as high as those for whites or Hispanics. Recurrent pneumococcal meningitis may occur in patients who have chronic cerebrospinal fluid leakage resulting from congenital lesions, skull fractures, or neurosurgical procedures.

Invasive pneumococcal disease (e.g., bacteremia or meningitis) and pneumonia cause high morbidity and mortality in spite of effective antimicrobial control by antibiotics. These effects of pneumococcal disease appear due to irreversible physiologic damage caused by the bacteria during the first 5 days following onset of illness, and occur irrespective of antimicrobial therapy. The incidence of penicillin resistance in many areas of the world has been steadily increasing. The National Centre for Streptococcus (NCS) in Edmonton, a voluntary passive surveillance reporting system, found that 7.8% of isolates submitted between 1992 and 1995 had diminished susceptibility to penicillin. During 1996 to 1997, this proportion had increased to 10.2%. In a similar study, SHUSS identified 7.4% of isolates having diminished susceptibility to penicillin in 1996. Vaccination offers an effective means of further reducing the mortality and morbidity of this disease.

Risk Factors: In addition to the very young and persons 65 years of age or older, patients with certain chronic conditions are at increased risk of developing pneumococcal infection and severe pneumococcal illness.

Patients with chronic cardiovascular diseases (e.g., congestive heart failure or cardiomyopathy), chronic pulmonary diseases (e.g., chronic obstructive pulmonary disease or emphysema), or chronic liver diseases (e.g., cirrhosis), diabetes mellitus, alcoholism or asthma (when it occurs with chronic bronchitis, emphysema, or long-term use of systemic corticosteroids) have an increased risk of pneumococcal disease. In adults, this population is generally immunocompetent.

Patients at high risk are those who have a decreased responsiveness to polysaccharide antigen or an increased rate of decline in serum antibody concentrations as a result of: immunosuppressive conditions (congenital immunodeficiency, human immunodeficiency virus [HIV] infection, leukemia, lymphoma, multiple myeloma, Hodgkin's disease, or generalized malignancy); organ or bone marrow transplantation; therapy with alkylating agents, antimetabolites, or systemic corticosteroids; chronic renal failure or nephrotic syndrome.

Patients at the highest risk of pneumococcal infection are those with functional or anatomic asplenia (e.g., sickle cell disease or splenectomy), because this condition leads to reduced clearance of encapsulated bacteria from the bloodstream. Children who have sickle cell disease or have had a splenectomy are at increased risk for fulminant pneumococcal sepsis associated with high mortality.

STORAGE AND STABILITY: Store unopened and opened vials at 2-8°C.

All vaccines must be discarded after the expiration date.

INFORMATION FOR THE PATIENT: Published in e-CPS, available by subscription at www.e-cps.ca.

DOSAGE FORMS, COMPOSITION AND PACKAGING: Each single dose (0.5 mL) of sterile, clear, colourless liquid contains: 25 µg of capsular polysaccharide from each of the following 23 serotypes of *S. pneumoniae* (Danish nomenclature): 1, 2, 3, 4, 5, 6B*, 7F, 8, 9N, 9V*, 10A, 11A, 12F, 14*, 15B, 17F, 18C, 19A*, 19F*, 20, 22F, 23F*, 33F. Nonmedicinal ingredients: phenol 0.25% (w/w), sodium chloride 0.9% (w/w) and Water for injection to volume. The vaccine should be used directly as supplied; no dilution or reconstitution is necessary. Single-dose 3 mL Type I glass vials containing one 0.5 mL dose of liquid vaccine, cartons of 1 and 10. The container closure system is free of latex.

* These serotypes most frequently cause drug-resistant pneumococcal infections.

Podofilm® ℞

podophyllum resin

Vesicant—Wart Remover

Paladin

SUPPLIED: Each bottle contains: podophyllum resin 25% in an adherent film-forming vehicle (tincture of benzoin compound). Bottles of 25 mL. Keep away from heat, fire and flame. Close tightly immediately after use. Store at room temperature.

Pollinex®-R

modified ragweed tyrosine adsorbate

Vaccine

Nycomed

Date of Preparation: March 20, 1998
Date of Revision: April 3, 2005

PHARMACOLOGY: The exact mode of therapeutic action of POLLINEX-R (modified ragweed tyrosine adsorbate), as with other allergy vaccines, is unknown. It has been proposed that elevations of IgG blocking antibodies may interfere with the immediate hypersensitivity reaction of patients exposed to ragweed pollen. In addition, patients receiving POLLINEX-R have lesser post-seasonal increase in ragweed specific IgE antibody compared to placebo treated patients. It is possible that suppression of IgE antibody by POLLINEX-R during the ragweed season could influence the response of ragweed allergic patients to the pollen in their environment.

INDICATIONS: POLLINEX-R (modified ragweed tyrosine adsorbate) is indicated for the pre-seasonal immunotherapy of adults and children, over the age of 8 years, who have demonstrated ragweed allergic rhinitis by careful patient history and physical examination, supplemented by skin testing and/or immunological assay.

POLLINEX-R is generally not expected to completely eliminate the various allergic symptoms but should reduce their severity. POLLINEX-R should also be expected in many patients to reduce their dependence on other medication, such as antihistamines and other cough/cold over-the-counter medications that are taken during the season to alleviate rhinitis symptoms. There is also evidence that the use of more potent therapy, such as nasal and oral steroids, is reduced in patients who have received a course of POLLINEX-R.

CONTRAINDICATIONS: POLLINEX-R (modified ragweed tyrosine adsorbate) should not be administered to a patient who has experienced a previous severe anaphylactic reaction to ragweed vaccine immunotherapy.

Immunotherapy with POLLINEX-R is contraindicated in those individuals who do not exhibit skin test reactions and clinical sensitivity to ragweed.

Any injections, including immunotherapy with POLLINEX-R, should be avoided in patients with diseases characterized by a bleeding diathesis.

WARNINGS: Patients suffering from febrile conditions or an acute attack of asthma should not be given POLLINEX-R (modified ragweed tyrosine adsorbate) until twenty-four (24) hours after their condition has returned to normal. Acute immediate anaphylactic reactions characterized by difficulty in breathing, cyanosis and shock have rarely occurred with POLLINEX-R treatment, but if such should occur, standard emergency measures must be adopted with the use of a tourniquet above the injection site, epinephrine, oxygen, intravenous steroids and airway management including intubation if required. Similarly, delayed anaphylactic reaction have rarely been reported with POLLINEX-R, however, the patient should be advised to report to their physician immediately if symptoms of such a reaction should be manifested.

Recent evidence suggests that patients on beta-blockers may be more prone to anaphylaxis during immunotherapy and in such patients, anaphylaxis may be less responsive to conventional treatment.

Hence, in such patients, the need for continued immunotherapy and/or continued beta-blocker use should be carefully reviewed.

Do not administer POLLINEX-R during the ragweed season, which usually starts in mid-August through to the end of September or until the first killing frost.

As routine immunizations may exacerbate autoimmune diseases,POLLINEX-R immunotherapy should be given cautiously to such patients.

Patients with unstable asthma or steroid dependant asthma and patients with underlying cardiovascular disease are at additional risk during a systemic reaction. The risk must be weighted against the benefit.

PRECAUTIONS: All administrations of POLLINEX-R (modified ragweed tyrosine adsorbate) must be given by the subcutaneous route, by or under the supervision of a physician. Care must be taken never to inject POLLINEX-R directly into a blood vessel.

All patients should remain under observation in the doctor's office or clinic for 20 to 30 minutes after each vaccine injection and then should avoid strenuous physical exercise for at least twenty-four (24) hours.

Patients should be advised not to eat a heavy meal immediately before receiving their injection of POLLINEX-R. It is advisable to administer an antihistamine about one hour prior to an injection of POLLINEX-R. Epinephrine hydrochloride 1:1000 solution should always be kept on hand for use in the very unlikely event of a severe immediate reaction.

It is extremely important to shake the syringe containing the vaccine prior to injection, thus greatly reducing the possibility of needle blockage.

Pregnancy: Safety for the use of POLLINEX-R in pregnancy has not been established.

Lactation: Safety for the use of POLLINEX-R in nursing mothers has not been established.

Geriatrics: Safety for the use of POLLINEX-R in geriatric populations has not been established. Patients over 60 years of age may have an increased risk of impaired cardiovascular or pulmonary function.

Children: Safety for the use of POLLINEX-R in pediatric populations has not been established, POLLINEX-R should not be used to treat patients under 8 years of age.

Safety for the use of POLLINEX-R in combination with other allergens has not been established.

POLLINEX-R administration should not be instituted unless other ragweed pollen extract therapy has been discontinued.

ADVERSE EFFECTS: The following adverse reactions may occur during therapy with POLLINEX-R:

Hypersensitivity Reactions: erythema, swelling, pruritus, wheal, papule, mild hives, anaphylactoid reaction.

Other: Local reactions, such as pain accompanied by induration at the site of injection have been reported; wheezing, stuffy and/or runny nose, chest tightness.

OVERDOSE:

It is not possible to administer to a patient an overdosage of POLLINEX-R, as long as no more than 0.5 mL of the vaccine is administered starting with either syringe or vial number 1, followed in sequence by syringe or vial 2, 3 and lastly 4.

In patients with severe allergic reactions, general supportive measures (if the patient is in shock) or symptomatic therapy similar to that applied in all cases of hypersensitivity, are recommended. Agents such as pressor amines, antihistamines and corticosteroids should be readily available. POLLINEX-R is not suitable for such patients with severe allergic reactions.

> For management of a suspected drug overdose, CPhA recommends that you contact your **regional Poison Control Centre**. See the *CPS* Directory section for a list of Poison Control Centres.

DOSAGE: POLLINEX-R (modified ragweed tyrosine adsorbate) must be given prior to the ragweed season which usually starts in mid-August. The course of vaccine therapy should start toward the end of June and be given such that the last injection is received about the first week in August.

Pre-filled Syringes: The dosage regimen is outlined in Table 1. Each course of POLLINEX-R consists of a patient treatment pack of four sterile pre-filled syringes clearly labeled 1,2,3 and 4 containing the following POLLINEX-R strengths each in a volume of 0.5 mL.

Table 1: POLLINEX-R

Syringes

Syringe Number	Strength in Protein Nitrogen Units/0.5 mL	Strength in Noon Units/0.5 mL
1	105	300
2	250	700
3	700	2000
4	2150	6000

The vaccine treatment regimen consists of the administration of POLLINEX-R by subcutaneous injection. On the first occasion, the contents of No. 1 syringe are given, followed in order by syringe numbers 2, 3 and 4 at a recommended interval of approximately 7 days between injections.

The operation of the syringe is as follows:

1. Withdraw the syringe from the cold storage condition well before time of administration and allow to attain room temperature. Do not heat.
2. **Do not remove the needle guard until ready for use.**
3. Withdraw syringe plunger slightly and shake the syringe thoroughly to ensure a homogeneous suspension.
4. Release the pressure in the syringe by withdrawing the plunger slightly.
5. Shake the syringe thoroughly again, remove needle guard, then carefully express the air from the syringe with the needle held upwards, to minimize loss of contents.
6. **Slowly** inject the suspension **deep subcutaneously.**
7. **Do not inject into a blood vessel.**

Vials: Each patient treatment pack consists of four sterile vials clearly labeled 1, 2, 3 and 4 containing the following POLLINEX-R strengths each in a volume of 1.0 mL. See Table 2.

Table 2: POLLINEX-R

Vials

Vial Number	Strength in Protein Nitrogen Units/1.0 mL	Strength in Noon Units/1.0 mL
1	210	600
2	500	1400
3	1400	4000
4	4300	12 000

The vaccine treatment regimen consists of the administration of POLLINEX-R by subcutaneous injection. On the first occasion, 0.5 mL of the contents of No. 1 vial are given, followed in order by 0.5 mL of vial numbers 2, 3 and 4 at a recommended interval of approximately 7 days between injections.

Procedure:

1. Withdraw the vial from the cold storage condition well before time of administration and allow to attain room temperature. Do not heat.
2. Shake vial thoroughly to ensure a homogeneous suspension.
3. Using a sterile disposable syringe, withdraw 0.5 mL of suspension.
4. Carefully express the air from the syringe with the needle held upwards to minimize loss of contents.
5. **Slowly** inject the suspension **deep subcutaneously.**
6. **Do not inject into a blood vessel.**

SUPPLIED: POLLINEX-R (modified ragweed tyrosine adsorbate) is an aqueous extract of short ragweed pollen (Ambrosia elatior) chemically modified with glutaraldehyde adsorbed onto tyrosine and then suspended in saline.

Pre-filled Syringes: Each patient treatment package consists of 4 pre-filled sterile syringes each containing 0.5 mL of suspension. Each syringe is labeled as to syringe number and strength in total Protein Nitrogen Units (see Table 3). Contains phenol as preservative.

Table 3: POLLINEX-R

Pre-filled Syringes

Syringe Number	Dosage in Protein Nitrogen Units
1	105
2	250
3	700
4	2150

Vials: Each patient treatment package consists of 4 sterile vials each containing 1 mL of suspension. Each vial is clearly labeled as to vial number and strength in total Protein Nitrogen Units (see Table 4). Contains phenol as preservative.

Table 4: POLLINEX-R

Vials

Vial Number	Total Protein Nitrogen Units/Vial
1	210
2	500
3	1400
4	4300

Store at 2-8°C.

(Shown in Product Identification Section)

Polyderm

bacitracin zinc—polymyxin B sulfate

Antibiotic

Taro

SUPPLIED : Each g of ointment contains: bacitracin zinc 500 units and polymyxin B sulfate 10 000 units. Nonmedicinal ingredients: white petrolatum. Tubes of 15 and 30 g. Store at room temperature (15-30°C).

Polysporin® Antibiotic Cream

polymyxin B sulfate—gramicidin

Antibiotic

Johnson & Johnson

Polysporin® Antibiotic Ointment

polymyxin B sulfate—bacitracin zinc

Antibiotic

Johnson & Johnson

Polysporin® Antibiotic Plus Pain Relief Cream

polymyxin B sulfate—gramicidin—lidocaine HCl

Antibiotic—Anesthetic—Antipruritic

Johnson & Johnson

Polysporin® Complete Antibiotic Ointment

polymyxin B sulfate—bacitracin zinc—gramicidin—lidocaine

Antibiotic—Anesthetic—Antipruritic

Johnson & Johnson

Polysporin® Eye/Ear Drops

polymyxin B sulfate—gramicidin

Antibiotic

Johnson & Johnson

Polysporin® For Kids Cream

polymyxin B sulfate—gramicidin—lidocaine HCl

Antibiotic—Anesthetic—Antipruritic

Johnson & Johnson

Polysporin® Ophthalmic Ointment

polymyxin B sulfate—bacitracin zinc

Antibiotic

Johnson & Johnson

Polysporin® Plus Pain Relief Ear Drops

polymyxin B sulfate—lidocaine HCl

Antibiotic—Anesthetic—Antipruritic

Johnson & Johnson

Polysporin® Triple Antibiotic Ointment

polymyxin B sulfate—bacitracin zinc—gramicidin

Antibiotic

Johnson & Johnson

INDICATIONS: Antibiotic Ointment: For treating local infections due to susceptible organisms and amenable to local treatment; these include infected wounds, burns and skin grafts; furuncles, acne, and for eye infections such as conjunctivitis.

Triple Antibiotic Ointment: In addition to the above, for use as prophylactic therapy in the prevention of central venous catheter related infections in hemodialysis patients.

Antibiotic Cream: For infection in dermatologic disorders particularly where the lesions are moist or weeping. Prophylactically, against bacterial contamination in burns, skin grafts, incisions and other clean lesions. For abrasions, minor cuts and wounds, the cream may prevent infection and permit healing.

Antibiotic Plus Pain Relief Cream: For treatment and prevention of infection of minor burns and scalds and for relief of skin pain.

For Kids Cream: To prevent infection, aid healing and provide temporary relief of pain in minor cuts, scrapes, and burns.

Complete Antibiotic Ointment: For treatment and prevention of infection of minor cuts, nicks, scrapes, scratches and burns, and for the temporary relief of pain, discomfort and/or itching in minor cuts, nicks, scrapes, scratches and burns.

Eye/Ear Drops: For external infections of the eye and ear when due to susceptible organisms, including acute and chronic conjunctivitis, pink eye, infected sockets, corneal ulcers, keratitis, episcleritis, blepharitis, and dacryocystitis. Used in situations in which drops may be preferred to an ointment. Prophylactically it is useful following removal of foreign bodies, and before and after ophthalmic surgery, to help provide and maintain a sterile field. Also for pyogenic infections of the ear.

Ophthalmic Ointment: For treatment of superficial ocular infections involving the conjunctiva and/or cornea caused by organisms susceptible to polymyxin B sulfate and bacitracin zinc.

Plus Pain Relief Ear Drops: The prevention of exacerbations and treatment of infection due to susceptible organisms, relief of pain and itching associated with otitis externa, including "swimmer's ear", postoperative aural cavities, furunculosis.

CONTRAINDICATIONS: Hypersensitivity to any of the components.

Eye/Ear Drops: Should not be given subconjunctivally or intraocularly, nor should it be used for the irrigation of fistulous tracts in or about the eye or its socket.

WARNINGS: No data supplied by the manufacturer.

PRECAUTIONS: As with any antibiotic containing medication, prolonged use may result in the overgrowth of nonsusceptible organisms, including fungi. Should superinfection occur, the preparation should be discontinued and/or appropriate therapy instituted.

Following application to extensive areas of raw skin, the possibility of systemic absorption of the active ingredients exists.

Allergic hypersensitivity following topical application of polymyxin B and bacitracin zinc is rare but has been reported. Rarely anaphylactic reactions following topical administration of bacitracin zinc have been reported. Following significant systemic absorption, polymyxin B can intensify and prolong the respiratory depressant effects of neuromuscular blocking agents.

In case of laceration, deep wounds or serious burns, physician should be consulted.

If an adverse reaction or irritation occurs, use should be discontinued and physician should be consulted.

Polysporin topical preparations are for external use only and contact with eyes should be avoided.

Eye/ear drops: If irritation occurs or in case of serious infection or if infection has not started to clear in 2 days, use should be discontinued and physician should be consulted. Physician should be consulted prior to use if the cause of the pink eye is unclear, or if there is a marked sensation of something in the eye, sensitivity to light, continuous, abundant discharge, pain in the eye, impaired vision, severe hearing loss or fever.

Ophthalmic Ointment: If irritation occurs or in case of serious infection or if infection has not started to clear in 2 days, use should be discontinued and physician should be consulted. Physician should be consulted prior to use if there is sensitivity to light, continuous, abundant discharge, pain in the eye, impaired vision, fever or scaling around the stye.

Plus Pain Relief Ear Drops: If irritation occurs or if itch and pain has not started to clear in 2 days, use should be discontinued and physician should be consulted. Do not use with ear tubes, after ear surgery or with damaged ear drums unless directed by physician. Physician should be consulted prior to use if there is severe pain in the ear, severe hearing loss or fever.

Geriatrics: No specific information is available regarding the use of Polysporin in the elderly; however, the maximum dosage should be reduced in cases where a decrease in renal function may exist.

Pregnancy: Polysporin has been used for several years without any evidence of untoward effects in pregnancy. The clinical benefit of treatment to the patient must be balanced against any possible, but unknown hazards to the fetus.

ADVERSE EFFECTS: No data supplied by the manufacturer.

OVERDOSE:

Treatment: If toxic symptoms develop following significant systemic absorption, treatment with Polysporin should be stopped and the patient's general status, renal function and neuromuscular function should be monitored and blood levels of polymyxin B sulfate and bacitracin zinc determined.

> For management of a suspected drug overdose, CPhA recommends that you contact your **regional Poison Control Centre**. See the *CPS* Directory section for a list of Poison Control Centres.

DOSAGE: Antibiotic Ointment: Apply to affected area, 1 to 3 times daily. May be covered with a dressing or left exposed.

Triple Antibiotic Ointment (prophylactic therapy in the prevention of central venous catheter related infections in hemodialysis patients): Cleanse central venous catheter insertion site with chlorhexidine gluconate. Apply 1 cm of Polysporin Triple ointment to the catheter insertion site and apply a 2"×2" dry gauze dressing. Apply ointment at the end of each dialysis session and at dressing changes.

Antibiotic Cream: Apply to affected area, 1 to 3 times daily; rub in gently if condition permits. May be covered with a dressing or left exposed.

Antibiotic Plus Pain Relief Cream: Apply to affected area, 1 to 3 times daily. May be covered with a dressing or left exposed.

Complete Antibiotic Ointment: Apply to affected area, 1 to 3 times daily. May be covered with a dressing or left exposed.

For Kids Cream: Apply to affected area, 1 to 3 times daily. May be covered with a dressing or left exposed.

Eye/Ear Drops: 1 or 2 drops in the affected eye or ear, 4 times daily, or more frequent as required.

Ophthalmic Ointment: Apply 4 times daily or more frequently, depending on the severity of the disease.

Plus Pain Relief Ear Drops: Apply 3 or 4 drops in the affected ear 4 times daily. For infants and children, 2 or 3 drops are suggested. Solution may be applied by saturating a gauze or cotton wick which may be left in the canal for 24 to 48 hours, keeping the wick moist by adding a few drops of solution as required.

SUPPLIED: Antibiotic Ointment: Each g contains: polymyxin B (as sulfate) 10 000 units and bacitracin zinc 500 units. Nonmedicinal ingredients: butylated hydroxytoluene, cocoa butter, cotton seed oil, olive oil, petrolatum, sodium pyruvate and vitamin E (dl-alpha tocopheryl acetate). Tubes of 15 and 30 g.

Triple Antibiotic Ointment: Each g contains: polymyxin B (as sulfate) 10 000 units, bacitracin zinc 500 units and gramicidin 0.25 mg. Nonmedicinal ingredients: butylated hydroxytoluene, cocoa butter, cotton seed oil, olive oil, petrolatum, sodium pyruvate and vitamin E (dl-alpha tocopheryl acetate). Tubes of 15 and 30 g.

Antibiotic Cream: Each g contains: polymyxin B (as sulfate) 10 000 units and gramicidin 0.25 mg. Nonmedicinal ingredients: methylparaben, mineral oil, petrolatum, poloxamer, propylene glycol, water and wax. Tubes of 15 and 30 g.

Antibiotic Plus Pain Relief Cream: Each g contains: polymyxin B (as sulfate) 10 000 units, gramicidin 0.25 mg and lidocaine HCl 50 mg. Nonmedicinal ingredients: methylparaben, mineral oil, petrolatum, polysorbate, propylene glycol, water and wax. Tubes of 15 and 30 g.

Complete Antibiotic Ointment: Each g contains: polymyxin B (as sulfate) 10 000 units, bacitracin zinc 500 units, gramicidin 0.25 mg and lidocaine 50 mg. Nonmedicinal ingredients: butylated hydroxytoluene, cocoa butter, cotton seed oil, olive oil, petrolatum, sodium pyruvate and vitamin E (dl-alpha tocopheryl acetate). Tubes of 15 and 30 g.

For Kids Cream: Each g contains: polymyxin B (as sulfate) 10 000 units, gramicidin 0.25 mg and lidocaine HCl 50 mg. Nonmedicinal ingredients: methylparaben, mineral oil, petrolatum, polysorbate, propylene glycol, water and wax. Tubes of 15 and 30 g.

Eye/Ear Drops: Each mL contains: polymyxin B (as sulfate) 10 000 units and gramicidin 0.025 mg. Nonmedicinal ingredients: alcohol, benzalkonium chloride, poloxamer, propylene glycol and water. Plastic dropper bottles of 10 mL.

Ophthalmic Ointment: Each g contains: polymyxin B (as sulfate) 10 000 units and bacitracin zinc 500 units. Nonmedicinal ingredients: butylated hydroxytoluene and petrolatum. Tubes of 3.5 g.

Plus Pain Relief Ear Drops: Each mL contains: polymyxin B (as sulfate) 10 000 units, lidocaine HCl 50 mg (5%). Nonmedicinal ingredients: cupric sulfate, hydrochloric acid, propylene glycol and water. Plastic dropper bottles of 10 mL.

Store between 15 and 30°C.

Polytar®
polytar
Antidandruff

Stiefel, a GSK company

SUPPLIED: Mild: Each mL of shampoo contains: Polytar 0.5%, a blend of wood and mineral tars in a soapless lather. Nonmedicinal ingredients: citric acid monohydrate, coconut diethanolamide, collagen protein derived, fragrance, hexylene glycol, imidurea, oleth 10, oleyl alcohol, polysorbate 80, purified water USP, sodium chloride and triethanolamine lauryl sulfate. Buffered to a natural pH balance of hair. Plastic bottles of 150 and 350 mL.

Regular: Each mL of shampoo contains: Polytar 1%, a blend of wood and mineral tars in a soapless lather. Nonmedicinal ingredients: citric acid monohydrate, coconut diethanolamide, fragrance, hexylene glycol, imidurea, oleyl alcohol, polysorbate 80, purified water USP, sodium chloride and triethanolamine lauryl sulfate. Buffered to a natural pH balance of hair. Plastic bottles of 150 and 350 mL.

Polytar® AF
coal tar—pyrithione disulfide—salicylic acid—menthol
Antidandruff and Psoriasis Therapy

Stiefel, a GSK company

SUPPLIED: Each mL of shampoo contains: decolorized coal tar 0.5%, pyrithione disulfide 1% w/v, salicylic acid 2% w/v and 0.5% menthol in a soapless shampoo base with conditioners. Buffered to natural pH balance of hair. Nonmedicinal ingredients: fragrance, hexylene glycol, modified lauric diethanolamine, oleyl alcohol, polymer JR-30 M, polysorbate 80, purified water USP, triethanolamine and triethanolamine lauryl sulfate. Plastic bottles of 150 mL.

Polytopic® Cream
polymyxin B sulfate—gramicidin
Antibiotic

Sandoz

Polytopic® Ointment
polymyxin B sulfate—bacitracin
Antibiotic

Sandoz

SUPPLIED: Cream: Each g of cream contains: polymyxin B (as sulfate) 10 000 units and gramicidin 0.25 mg. Nonmedicinal ingredients: emulsifying wax, light mineral oil, methylparaben, petrolatum, poloxamer and propylene glycol. Tubes of 15 g, boxes of 1. Store between 15 and 30°C.

Ointment: Each g of ointment contains: polymyxin B (as sulfate) 10 000 units and bacitracin 500 units. Nonmedicinal ingredients: light mineral oil and petrolatum. Tubes of 15 g, boxes of 1. Tubes of 30 g, boxes of 1. Store between 15 and 30°C.

Polytrim™ Ⓟ
trimethoprim sulfate—polymyxin B sulfate
Antibacterial

Allergan

SUPPLIED: Each mL of sterile ophthalmic solution contains: trimethoprim (as sulfate) 1 mg, polymyxin B (as sulfate) 10 000 units. Nonmedicinal ingredients: benzalkonium chloride 0.004% (as preservative), sodium chloride, sodium hydroxide or sulfuric acid and water for injection. Plastic drop-dose dispensers of 10 mL. Store at 15 to 25°C. Protect from light.

Pontocaine®
tetracaine HCl
Anesthetic

Hospira

PHARMACOLOGY: Tetracaine is 2-(dimethylamino) ethyl p-(butylamino) benzoate monohydrochloride. It is a white crystalline odorless powder that is readily soluble in water, physiologic saline solution or dextrose solution. Tetracaine is a local anesthetic of the ester-linkage type, related to procaine. Tetracaine is detoxified by plasma esterases to para-aminobenzoic acid and diethylaminoethanol.

In the concentrations ordinarily employed for surface anesthesia (from 0.5 to 2%) tetracaine exhibits a higher efficiency than cocaine solutions of corresponding strength. 0.5% and 1% solutions have proved equal in anesthetic power to the 5% and 10% solutions of cocaine.

The application of tetracaine to mucous membranes is usually unattended with tissue injury, but may cause transitory smarting.

INDICATIONS: Spinal Anesthesia: Where spinal anesthesia is indicated for operations requiring 2 to 3 hours of anesthesia.

To be used only on the advice of a physician.

CONTRAINDICATIONS: In patients with known hypersensitivity to tetracaine or to drugs of a similar chemical configuration (ester-type local anesthetics), or para-aminobenzoic acid or its derivatives, or to any other ingredient in these preparations. Spinal anesthesia with tetracaine is also contraindicated in patients for whom spinal anesthesia as a technique is contraindicated.

WARNINGS: Resuscitative equipment and drugs should be immediately available whenever any local anesthetic drug is used.

Large doses of local anesthetics should not be used in patients with heart block.

Reactions resulting in fatality have occurred on rare occasions with the use of local anesthetics, such as tetracaine, even in the absence of a history of hypersensitivity.

Excessive doses may produce serious or fatal reactions.

For anesthetizing the larynx, trachea, or esophagus, the total absorbed dose of tetracaine should not usually exceed 20 mg using a 0.5% solution by direct application or a 0.5% solution nebulized for oral inhalation. Absorption may be retarded by the addition of 0.06 mL epinephrine 1:1000 to each mL of anesthetic solution. In order to avoid rapid absorption and high blood levels of the anesthetic, the solution should not be administered in a coarse stream or by forceful injection, and care should be taken in dose measurement. In every instance, the dose should be measured accurately.

Protection of the anesthetized eye from irritating chemicals, foreign bodies, and rubbing is very important. Patients should be warned not to rub an eye to which tetracaine has been applied, because inadvertent damage may be done to the anesthetized cornea and conjunctiva.

PRECAUTIONS: The safety and effectiveness of any spinal anesthetic or of local anesthetics depend upon proper dosage, correct technique, adequate precautions, and readiness for emergencies. The lowest dosage that results in effective anesthesia should be used to avoid high plasma levels and serious systemic side effects. Tolerance varies with the status of the patient; debilitated, elderly patients or acutely ill patients should be given reduced doses commensurate with their weight, age, and physical status. Reduced doses are also indicated for obstetric patients and those with increased intra-abdominal pressure.

Tetracaine should be applied more sparingly on open lesions, in cases of allergy, cardiac or hepatic disease, emaciation, hyperthyroidism and other endocrine disorders in which tolerance may be diminished.

Caution should be used in administering tetracaine to patients with abnormal or reduced levels of plasma esterases.

As is the case with all spinal anesthetics, the patient's blood pressure should be monitored during anesthesia.

Spinal anesthetics should be used with caution in patients with severe disturbances of cardiac rhythm, shock or heart block.

Tetracaine should not be used if the patient is being treated with a sulfonamide because para-aminobenzoic acid inhibits the action of sulfonamides.

Hypotension should be corrected early if it develops during saddle block for normal vaginal delivery, since hypoxic fetal bradycardia may occur. If a vasoconstrictor is given to correct hypotension, the obstetrician should be cautioned that if an oxytocic drug is employed, severe persistent hypertension and even rupture of a cerebral blood vessel may occur during the postpartum period.

Children: Safety and effectiveness of tetracaine in children have not been established.

There is no evidence from human data that tetracaine may be carcinogenic or mutagenic or that it impairs fertility.

Pregnancy: Tetracaine should be given to a pregnant woman only if clearly needed and the benefits outweigh the risks.

Lactation: It is not known whether or not tetracaine is excreted in human milk. However, it is rapidly metabolized following absorption into the plasma.

ADVERSE EFFECTS: Spinal Anesthesia: CNS: Effects are characterized by excitation or depression. The first manifestation may be nervousness, dizziness, blurred vision, or tremors, followed by drowsiness, convulsions, unconsciousness, and possibly respiratory and cardiac arrest. Because excitement may be transient or absent, the first manifestation may be drowsiness, sometimes merging into unconsciousness and respiratory and cardiac arrest. Other CNS effects may be nausea, vomiting, chills, constriction of the pupils, or tinnitus.

Cardiovascular system reactions include depression of the myocardium, blood pressure changes (usually hypotension), and cardiac arrest.

Allergic reactions which may be due to hypersensitivity, idiosyncrasy or diminished tolerance, are characterized by cutaneous lesions (e.g., urticaria), edema, and other manifestations of allergy. Detection of sensitivity by skin testing is of limited value. Severe allergic reactions including anaphylaxis have occurred rarely and are not usually dose related.

Reactions associated with spinal anesthesia techniques:

CNS: post-spinal headache, meningismus, arachnoiditis, palsies, or spinal nerve paralysis.

Cardiovascular: hypotension due to vasomotor paralysis and pooling of the blood in the venous bed.

Respiratory: respiratory impairment or paralysis due to the level of anesthesia extending to the upper thoracic and cervical segments.
Gastrointestinal: nausea and vomiting.

In spinal anesthesia, sympathetic blockade also occurs as a pharmacological action, resulting in peripheral vasodilation and often hypotension. The extent of the hypotension will usually depend on the number of dermatomes blocked. The blood pressure should therefore be monitored in the early phases of anesthesia. If hypotension occurs, it is readily controlled by vasoconstrictors administered either by i.m. or the i.v. route, the dosage of which would depend on the severity of the hypotension and the response to treatment.

Ophthalmology: Prolonged ophthalmic use of topical anesthetics has been associated with corneal epithelial erosions, retardation or prevention of healing of corneal erosions and reports of severe keratitis and permanent corneal opacification and scarring. Inadvertent damage may be done to the anesthetized cornea and conjunctiva by rubbing an eye to which topical anesthetics have been applied. Tetracaine occasionally causes transient smarting in the eye when concentrations higher than 0.5% are used. On rare occasions, local idiosyncratic reactions, including lacrimation, photophobia, and chemosis, have been observed. Although exceedingly rare with ophthalmic application of local anesthetics, systemic toxicity, usually manifested as CNS stimulation followed by CNS and cardiovascular depression, may occur.

Rhinolaryngology: Excessive doses of rapid absorption producing high blood levels can result in systemic toxic reactions which can lead to cardiac arrest and death if not promptly and correctly treated. Systemic reactions to tetracaine are characteristic of those associated with other local anesthetics and can involve the CNS and the cardiovascular system. A small number of reactions may result from hypersensitivity, idiosyncrasy or diminished tolerance to normal dosage. CNS effects are characterized by excitation or depression. The first manifestation may be nervousness, dizziness, blurred vision, or tremors, followed by drowsiness, convulsions, unconsciousness, and possibly respiratory and cardiac arrest. Because excitement may be transient or absent, the first manifestation may be drowsiness, sometimes merging into unconsciousness and respiratory and cardiac arrest. Other CNS effects may be nausea, vomiting, chills, constriction of the pupils, or tinnitus. Cardiovascular system reactions include depression of the myocardium, blood pressure changes (usually hypotension), and cardiac arrest. Allergic reactions, which may be due to hypersensitivity, idiosyncrasy or diminished tolerance, are characterized by cutaneous lesions (e.g., urticaria), edema, and other manifestations of allergy. Detection of sensibility by skin testing is of limited value. Severe allergic reactions including anaphylaxis have occurred rarely and are not usually dose related.

Treatment of Systemic Toxic Reactions: Toxic effects of local anesthetics require symptomatic treatment; there is no specific cure. The most important measure is oxygenation of the patient by maintaining an airway and supporting ventilation. Supportive treatment of the cardiovascular system includes i.v. fluids and, when appropriate, vasopressors (preferably those that stimulate the myocardium). Convulsions are usually controlled with adequate oxygenation alone but i.v. administration in small increments of a barbiturate (preferably an ultrashort-acting barbiturate such as thiopental and thiamylal) or diazepam can be utilized. I.V. barbiturates or anticonvulsant agents should only be administered by those familiar with their use and only if ventilation and oxygenation have first been assured. Muscle relaxants such as succinylcholine may also be required.

OVERDOSE:

For management of a suspected drug overdose, CPhA recommends that you contact your **regional Poison Control Centre**. See the *CPS* Directory section for a list of Poison Control Centres.

DOSAGE: **Spinal Anesthesia**: See Table 1.

Table 1: Pontocaine

Suggested Dosage for Spinal Anesthesia Using Niphanoid

Extent of Anesthesia	Dose of Niphanoid (mg)	Volume of Spinal Fluid (mL)	Site of Injection (lumbar interspace)
Perineum	5[a]	1	4th
Perineum and Lower extremities	10	2	3rd or 4th
Up to Costal Margin	15 to 20[b]	3	2nd, 3rd, or 4th

[a] For vaginal delivery (saddle block), from 2 to 5 mg in dextrose.
[b] Doses exceeding 15 mg are rarely required and should be used only in exceptional cases. Inject solution at rate of about 1 mL per 5 seconds.

When spinal fluid is added to the Niphanoid, some turbidity results, the degree depending on the pH of the spinal fluid, the temperature of the solution during mixing, as well as the amount of drug and diluent employed. This cloudiness is due to the release of the base from the hydrochloride. Liberations of base (which is completed within the spinal canal) is held to be essential for satisfactory results with any spinal anesthetic.

The specific gravity of spinal fluid at 25°/25°C varies under normal conditions from 1.0063 to 1.0075. A solution of the instantly soluble form (Niphanoid) in spinal fluid has only a slightly greater specific gravity.

For a hyperbaric solution Pontocaine Niphanoid is first dissolved in dextrose solution 10% in a ratio of 1 mL dextrose to 10 mg of the anesthetic. Further dilution is made with an equal volume of spinal fluid. The resulting solution now contains 5% dextrose with 5 mg of anesthetic agent per mL.

A hypobaric solution may be prepared by dissolving the Niphanoid in sterile water for injection, USP (1 mg/mL). The specific gravity of this solution is essentially the same as that of water, 1.000 at 25°/25°C.

Examine ampuls carefully before use. Do not use if discoloration is observed in the ampuls, or if crystals or cloudiness is observed in the reconstituted product. This formulation of sterile tetracaine hydrochloride does not contain preservatives; therefore, unused portions should be discarded and the reconstituted Niphanoid should be used immediately.

Sterilization: The drug in intact ampuls is sterile. The preferred method to destroy bacteria on the exterior of ampuls before opening is heat sterilization (autoclaving). The ampuls should be set in an upright position for autoclaving. Immersion in antiseptic solution is not recommended.

Autoclave at 15 pounds pressure, at 121°C, for 15 to 20 minutes. The crystals may lose their snow-like appearance and tend to adhere to the sides of the ampul. This effect may slightly decrease the rate at which the drug dissolves but does not interfere with its anesthetic potency.

Autoclaving increases the likelihood of crystal formation. Unused autoclaved ampuls should be discarded. In no case should unused autoclaved ampuls be placed back in stock for later use.

SUPPLIED: Spinal Anesthesia: Each ampul of dry powder contains: tetracaine HCl 20 mg. Gluten-, lactose-, preservative-, starch and sulfite-free. Ampuls of 20 mg, boxes of 10. Protect ampuls from light.

To be used only on the advice of a physician.

Portia™ 21 Pr

levonorgestrel—ethinyl estradiol

Oral Contraceptive

Apotex

Portia™ 28 Pr

levonorgestrel—ethinyl estradiol

Oral Contraceptive

Apotex

Date of Preparation: June 1, 2007
Date of Revision: February 29 2008

SUMMARY PRODUCT INFORMATION:

Route of Administration	Dosage Form/ Strength	Clinically Relevant Nonmedicinal Ingredients
Oral	Levonorgestrel and ethinyl estradiol Tablet/0.15 mg+0.03 mg	Anhydrous lactose For a complete listing see Dosage Forms, Composition and Packaging.

INDICATIONS AND CLINICAL USE: PORTIA Tablets are indicated for conception control.

CONTRAINDICATIONS:

1. Hypersensitivity to PORTIA 21 or PORTIA 28 (levonorgestrel/ethinyl estradiol tablets) or to any ingredient in the formulation or component of the container. For a complete listing, see Dosage Forms, Composition and Packaging.
2. History of or actual thrombophlebitis or thromboembolic disorders.
3. History of or actual cerebrovascular disorders.
4. History of or actual myocardial infarction or coronary arterial disease.
5. Deep vein thrombosis (current or history).
6. Thrombogenic valvulopathies and thrombogenic rhythm disorders.
7. Hereditary or acquired thrombophilias.
8. Migraine with focal neurological symptoms such as aura (current or history).
9. Acute liver disease, or history of or actual benign or malignant liver tumours.
10. Known or suspected carcinoma of the breast.
11. Carcinoma of the endometrium or other known or suspected estrogen-dependent neoplasia.
12. Undiagnosed abnormal vaginal bleeding.
13. Any ocular lesion arising from ophthalmic vascular disease, such as partial or complete loss of vision or defect in visual fields.
14. When pregnancy is suspected or diagnosed.
15. Diabetes with vascular involvement.
16. Uncontrolled hypertension.

WARNINGS AND PRECAUTIONS:

Serious Warnings and Precautions
Women using a birth control pill should be counselled that this product (as with other combined hormonal contraceptives) does not protect against HIV infection (AIDS) and other sexually transmitted diseases (STDs). For protection against STDs, it is advisable to use latex condoms in combination with this product.
Cigarette smoking increases the risk of serious adverse effects on the heart and blood vessels. This risk increases with age and becomes significant in oral contraceptive-users over 35 years of age. Women who use combination hormonal contraceptives including this product should be counselled not to smoke.

General: The following information is provided from studies of combination oral contraceptives (COC). The use of combination hormonal contraceptives is associated with increased risks of several serious conditions including myocardial infarction, thromboembolism, stroke, hepatic neoplasia and gallbladder disease, although the risk of serious morbidity and mortality is small in healthy women without underlying risk factors. The risk of morbidity and mortality increases significantly if associated with the presence of other risk factors such as hypertension, hyperlipidemias, obesity and diabetes.

The information contained in this section is principally from studies carried out in women who used combination oral contraceptives with higher formulations of estrogens and progestogens than those in common use today. The effect of long-term use of combination hormonal contraceptives with lower doses of both estrogen and progestogen administered orally remains to be determined.

Predisposing Factors for Coronary Artery Disease: Cigarette smoking increases the risk of serious cardiovascular side effects and mortality from COC use. This risk increases with age and with the extent of smoking. Convincing data are available to support an upper age limit of 35 years for oral contraceptive (OC) use by women who smoke.

Other women who are independently at high risk for cardiovascular disease include those with diabetes, hypertension, abnormal lipid profile, or a family history of these. Whether COCs accentuate this risk is unclear.

In low-risk, non-smoking women of any age, the benefits of oral contraceptive use outweigh the possible cardiovascular risks associated with low dose formulations. Consequently, oral contraceptives may be prescribed for these women up to the age of menopause.

Epidemiological studies have shown that the incidence of venous thromboembolism (VTE) in users of oral contraceptives with low estrogen content (<50 μg ethinyl estradiol) ranges from about 20 to 40 cases per 100 000 women-years, but this risk estimate varies according to the progestogen. This compares with 5 to 10 cases per 100 000 women-years for non-users.

The use of any combined oral contraceptive carries an increased risk of venous thromboembolism (VTE) compared with no use. The excess risk of VTE is highest during the first year a woman ever uses a combined oral contraceptive. The increased risk is less 100 000 pregnancies. VTE is fatal in 1-2 % of cases.

Discontinue Medication at the Earliest Manifestation of the Following:

A. **Thromboembolic and Cardiovascular Disorders** such as thrombophlebitis, pulmonary embolism, cerebrovascular disorders, myocardial ischemia, mesenteric thrombosis, and retinal thrombosis.
B. **Conditions that Predispose to Venous Stasis and to Vascular Thrombosis** (e.g. immobilization after accidents or confinement to bed during long-term illness). Other nonhormonal methods of contraception should be used until regular activities are resumed. For use of oral contraceptives when surgery is contemplated, see Warnings and Precautions.
C. **Visual Defects—Partial or Complete**
D. **Papilledema or Ophthalmic Vascular Lesions**
E. **Severe Headache of Unknown Etiology or Development of new Migraine**

Carcinogenesis and Mutagenesis: Breasts: Increasing age and a strong family history are the most significant risk factors for the development of breast cancer. Other established risk factors include obesity, nulliparity and late age for first full-term pregnancy. The identified groups of women that may be at increased risk of developing breast cancer before menopause are long-term users of oral contraceptives (more than eight years) and starters at early age. In a few women, the use of oral contraceptives may accelerate the growth of an existing but undiagnosed breast cancer. Since any potential increased risk related to oral contraceptive use is small, there is no reason to change prescribing habits at present.

Women receiving oral contraceptives should be instructed in self-examination of their breasts. Their physicians should be notified whenever any masses are detected. A yearly clinical breast examination is also recommended because, if a breast cancer should develop, drugs that contain estrogen may cause a rapid progression.

Cardiovascular: Patients with essential hypertension whose blood pressure is well controlled may be given oral contraceptives but only under close supervision. If a significant elevation of blood pressure in previously normotensive or hypertensive subjects occurs at any time during the administration of the drug, cessation of medication is necessary.

Endocrine and Metabolism: Diabetes: Current low-dose oral contraceptives exert minimal impact on glucose metabolism. Diabetic patients, or those with a family history of diabetes, should be observed closely to detect any worsening of carbohydrate metabolism. Patients predisposed to diabetes who can be kept under close supervision may be given oral contraceptives. Young diabetic patients whose disease is of recent origin, well-controlled, and not associated with hypertension or other signs of vascular disease such as ocular fundal changes, should be monitored more frequently while using oral contraceptives.

Lipid Effects: A small proportion of women will have adverse lipid changes while on OCs. Alternative contraception should be considered in women with uncontrolled dyslipidemias. Elevations of plasma triglycerides may lead to pancreatitis and other complications.

Women who are being treated for hyperlipidemias should be followed closely if they elect to use OCs.

Hepatic/Biliary/Pancreatic: Patients who have had jaundice, including a history of cholestatic jaundice during pregnancy, or a history of COC-related cholestasis, are more likely to have this condition with COC use and, they should be given COCs with great care and under close observation. If these patients receive a COC they should be carefully monitored and, if the condition recurs, the COC should be discontinued.

The development of severe generalized pruritus or icterus requires that the medication be withdrawn until the problem is resolved.

If a patient develops jaundice that proves to be cholestatic in type, the use of oral contraceptives should not be resumed. In patients taking oral contraceptives, changes in the composition of the bile may occur and an increased incidence of gallstones has been reported.

Hepatic nodules (adenoma and focal nodular hyperplasia) have been reported, particularly in long-term users of oral contraceptives. Although these lesions are extremely rare, they have caused fatal intra-abdominal hemorrhage and should be considered in women with an abdominal mass, acute abdominal pain, or evidence of intra-abdominal bleeding.

Hepatocellular carcinoma may be associated with COC use. The risk appears to increase with duration of COC use. However, the attributable risk (the excess incidence) of liver cancer in OC users is extremely small.

OC-related cholestasis has been described in women with a history of pregnancy-related cholestasis. Women with a history of cholestasis may have the condition recur with subsequent OC use.

Gastrointestinal: Diarrhea and/or vomiting may reduce hormone absorption resulting in decreased serum concentrations.

Genitourinary: Cervix: Some studies suggest that COC use may be associated with an increase in the risk of cervical intraepithelial neoplasia or invasive cervical cancer in some populations of women.

In cases of undiagnosed abnormal genital bleeding, adequate diagnostic measures are indicated.

Neurologic: The onset or exacerbation of migraine or the development of headache of a new pattern that is recurrent, persistent or severe, requires discontinuation of oral contraceptives and evaluation of the cause.

Ophthalmologic: Patients who are pregnant or are taking oral contraceptives, may experience corneal edema that may cause visual disturbances and changes in tolerance to contact lenses, especially of the rigid type. Soft contact lenses usually do not cause disturbances. If visual changes or alterations in tolerance to contact lenses occur, temporary or permanent cessation of wear may be advised.

With use of OCs, there have been reports of retinal vascular thrombosis which may lead to partial or complete loss of visions. If there are signs or symptoms such as visual changes, onset of proptosis or diplopia, papilledema, or retinal vascular lesions, the OC should be discontinued and the cause immediately evaluated.

Peri-Operative Considerations: There is an increased risk of thromboembolic complications in oral contraceptive users after major surgery. If feasible, oral contraceptives should be discontinued and an alternative method substituted at least one month prior to **major** elective surgery. Oral contraceptive use should not be resumed until the first menstrual period after hospital discharge following surgery.

Psychiatric: Patients with a history of emotional disturbances, especially the depressive type, may be more prone to have a recurrence of depression while taking oral contraceptives. In cases of a serious recurrence, a trial of an alternative method of contraception should be made which may help to clarify the possible relationship. Women with premenstrual syndrome (PMS) may have a varied response to oral contraceptives, ranging from symptomatic improvement to worsening of the condition.

Sexual Function/Reproduction: Vaginal Bleeding: Persistent irregular vaginal bleeding requires assessment to exclude underlying pathology.

In some women withdrawal bleeding may not occur during the tablet free interval. If the OC has not been taken according to directions prior to the first missed withdrawal bleed, or if two consecutive withdrawal bleeds are missed, the possibility of pregnancy should be evaluated.

Fibroids: Patients with fibroids (leiomyomata) should be carefully observed. Sudden enlargement, pain, or tenderness require discontinuation of the use of oral contraceptives.

Return to Fertility: After discontinuing oral contraceptive therapy, the patient should delay pregnancy until at least one normal spontaneous menstrual cycle has occurred in order to date the pregnancy. An alternative contraceptive method should be used during this time.

Amenorrhea: Women having a history of oligomenorrhea, secondary amenorrhea, or irregular cycles may remain anovulatory or become amenorrheic following discontinuation of estrogen-progestin combination therapy.

Amenorrhea, especially if associated with breast secretion, that continues for six months or more after withdrawal, warrants a careful assessment of hypothalamic-pituitary function.

Special Populations: Pregnant Women: Oral contraceptives should not be taken by pregnant women. However, if conception accidentally occurs while taking the pill, there is no conclusive evidence that the estrogen and progestin contained in the oral contraceptive will damage the developing child.

Nursing Women: In breast-feeding women, the use of oral contraceptives results in the hormonal components being excreted in breast milk and may reduce its quantity and quality. If the use of oral contraceptives is initiated after the establishment of lactation, there does not appear to be any effect on the quantity and quality of the milk. Some adverse effects on the child have been reported, including jaundice and breast enlargement.

The use of OCs is generally not recommended until the nursing mother has completely weaned her child.

Pediatrics: No data available.

Monitoring and Laboratory Tests: Physical Examination and Follow-up: Before oral contraceptives are used, a thorough history and physical examination should be performed, including a blood pressure determination. Breasts, liver, extremities, and pelvic organs should be examined. A Papanicolaou smear should be taken if the patient has been sexually active.

The first follow-up visit should be done three months after oral contraceptives are prescribed. Thereafter, examinations should be performed at least once a year, or more frequently if indicated. At each annual visit, examination should include those procedures that were done at the initial visit as outlined above or per recommendations of the "Canadian Task Force on the Periodic Health Examination."

ADVERSE REACTIONS: Adverse Drug Reaction Overview: An increased risk of the following serious adverse reactions has been associated with the use of COCs: thrombophlebitis; pulmonary embolism; mesenteric thrombosis; neuro-ocular lesions (e.g. retinal thrombosis); myocardial infarction; cerebral thrombosis; cerebral hemorrhage; hypertension; benign hepatic tumours; gallbladder disease, including gallstones*; stroke; transient ischemic attack; venous thrombosis; cervical intraepithelial neoplasia; cervical cancer; being diagnosed with breast cancer.

The following adverse reactions also have been reported in patients receiving COCs: Nausea and vomiting, usually the most common adverse reactions, occurs in approximately 10 percent or fewer of patients during the first cycle. Other reactions, as a general rule, are seen less frequently or only occasionally.

Other Adverse Reactions: The following adverse reactions have been reported in patients receiving COCs and are believed to be drug related: gastrointestinal symptoms (such as abdominal pain, cramps and bloating); breakthrough bleeding; spotting; change in menstrual flow; amenorrhea; dysmenorrhea; temporary infertility after discontinuance of treatment; fluid retention/edema; chloasma (melasma) which may persist; breast changes: tenderness, enlargement, and secretion; change in weight (increase or decrease); change in cervical erosion and secretion; diminution in lactation when given immediately postpartum; cholestatic jaundice; headache, including migraines; rash (allergic); mood changes, including depression; reduced tolerance to carbohydrates; vaginitis including candidiasis; change in corneal curvature (steepening); intolerance to contact lenses; retinal vascular thrombosis.

The following adverse reactions have been reported in users of COCs, and the association has been neither confirmed nor refuted: congenital anomalies; premenstrual syndrome; cataracts; optic neuritis†; changes in appetite (increase or decrease); cystitis-like syndrome; headache; nervousness; dizziness; hirsutism; loss of scalp hair; erythema multiforme; erythema nodosum; hemorrhagic eruption; vaginitis; exacerbation of porphyria; impaired renal function; hemolytic uremic syndrome; Budd-Chiari syndrome; acne; changes in libido; colitis; sickle-cell disease; cerebral-vascular disease with mitral valve prolapse; lupus-like syndromes; anaphylactic (anaphylactoid reactions, including very rare cases of urticaria, angioedema, and severe reactions with respiratory and circulatory symptoms): exacerbation of systemic lupus erythematosus; exacerbation of chorea; aggravation of varicose veins; pancreatitis; hepatic adenomas; hepatocellular carcinomas; changes in serum lipid levels, including hypertriglyceridemia; decrease in serum folate levels‡.

Clinical Trial Adverse Drug Reactions: Because clinical trials are conducted under very specific conditions the adverse reaction rates observed in the clinical trials may not reflect the rates observed in practice and should not be compared to the rates in the clinical trials of another drug. Adverse drug reaction information from clinical trials is useful for identifying drug-related adverse events and for approximating rates.

The side effects reported in clinical trials were those commonly associated with oral contraceptives and are listed by the percentage of their occurrence by cycle (Table 1). The most frequent side effects noted were spotting (8.6%), breakthrough bleeding (6.9%), simple headache (5.5%), dysmenorrhea (3.4%), GI symptoms (2.3%), acne (2.0%), nausea (1.9%), breast discomfort (1.8%), vaginal discharge (1.3%), appetite increase (1.1%), and depression (1.1%). These symptoms were usually mild and decreased with time on therapy.

The incidence of missed withdrawal bleeding (termed amenorrhea pre-treatment) is low with the use of 150 µg of levonorgestrel and 30 µg of ethinyl estradiol; 1.5% of total cycles. If one period is missed however, appropriate diagnostic procedures should be undertaken to rule out pregnancy and medication should be discontinued during this time and an alternate method of contraception employed. Prompt return to fertility has been demonstrated following discontinuation of therapy with 150 µg of levonorgestrel and 30 µg of ethinyl estradiol. Of the subjects reporting, 98.7% resumed menses within 30 days of stopping the medication, while five (1.3%) subjects resumed within 60 days.

Table 1: PORTIA

Side Effects by Percentage in Levonorgestrel and Ethinyl Estradiol Treated Patients

No. Enrolled 1084	Cycle 1	Cycle 2	Cycle 3	Cycle 6	Cycle 12	Cycle 18	Cycle 20	Total Cycles 8186
Acne	5.5	3.1	2.4	1.6	1.4	—	—	2.0
Allergic Rash	0.2	0.3	—	—	0.4	—	—	0.1
Appetite Decrease	0.7	0.3	0.3	0.6	—	—	—	0.3
Appetite Increase	2.1	1.2	1.7	1.4	0.4	—	—	1.1
Backache	2.1	1.4	1.5	0.3	0.4	—	—	1.0
Breakthrough Bleeding	10.1	8.5	7.6	5.6	4.6	2.9	2.6	6.9
Breast Discomfort	4.0	2.4	2.4	1.0	2.1	—	—	1.8
Breast Enlargement	2.0	0.7	0.7	0.5	0.4	—	—	0.6
Breast Secretion	0.2	0.2	—	0.3	—	—	—	0.1
Chloasma or Melasma	—	0.1	0.1	—	—	—	—	0.1
Depression	2.0	1.3	0.6	1.1	1.4	1.5	—	1.1
Dizziness	1.1	1.1	0.8	0.6	0.7	—	—	0.5
Dysmenorrhea	6.3	3.5	4.3	2.4	2.8	1.5	—	3.4
Dyspareunia	0.5	0.3	0.2	—	—	—	—	0.1
Edema	0.9	0.1	0.1	1.0	0.4	—	—	0.4
Fatigue	2	0.7	1.6	0.5	0.4	—	—	0.9
G.I. Symptoms	5.6	2.9	3.4	1.8	1.4	—	—	2.3
Headache Migraine	1.2	0.5	0.3	0.5	—	1.5	2.6	0.5
Headache Simple	9.6	5.4	5.8	4.8	4.6	8.8	7.9	5.5
Hirsutism	0.3	—	—	—	—	—	—	—
Itching	1.4	0.3	0.7	0.6	0.4	—	—	0.6
Leg Cramps	1.5	0.4	0.6	0.5	—	—	2.6	0.4
Libido Decrease	0.9	1.2	1.2	0.5	0.4	—	—	0.7
Libido Increase	0.6	0.1	0.2	—	—	—	—	0.2
Loss of Scalp Hair	—	0.1	0.2	—	—	—	—	—
Nausea	6.9	2.1	1.3	0.8	2.1	1.5	—	1.9
Nervousness	1.8	0.7	0.6	0.6	0.4	—	—	0.7
Spotting	16.2	10.6	8.4	7.5	5.3	4.4	2.6	8.6
Vaginal Discharge	1.8	1.1	1.9	1.9	2.1	—	—	1.3
Vomiting	1.0	0.5	0.6	0.2	—	1.5	—	0.4

DRUG INTERACTIONS: Overview: The concurrent administration of oral contraceptives with other substances may result in an altered response to either agent. Decreased ethinyl estradiol (EE) serum concentration may cause an increased incidence of breakthrough bleeding and menstrual irregularities and may possibly reduce efficacy of the COC. During concomitant use of EE containing products and substances that may lead to decreased EE serum concentration, it is recommended that a nonhormonal back-up method of birth control (such as condoms and spermicide) be used in addition to the regular intake of PORTIA. In the case of prolonged use of such substances COCs should not be considered the primary contraceptive.

After discontinuation of substances that may lead to decreased EE serum concentrations, use of a nonhormonal back-up method is recommended for at least 7 days. Longer use of a back-up method is advisable after discontinuation of substances that have lead to induction of hepatic microsomal enzymes, resulting in decreased EE serum concentrations. It may sometimes take several weeks until enzyme induction has completely subsided, depending on dosage, duration of use and rate of elimination of the inducing substance.

Reduced effectiveness of the COC, should it occur, is more likely with the low dose formulations. It is important to ascertain all drugs that a patient is taking, both prescription and non-prescription, before COCs are prescribed.

Examples of substances that may decrease serum EE concentration:

- Any substance that reduces gastrointestinal transit time.
- Hypericum perforatum, also known as St. John's Wort, possibly by induction of hepatic microsomal enzymes.
- Substances that induce hepatic microsomal enzymes, such as rifampicin, rifabutin, dexamethasone, modafinil, protease inhibitors, topiramate.

Examples of substances that may increase serum EE concentrations:

- Atorvastatin.
- Competitive inhibitors for sulfation in the gastrointestinal wall, such as ascorbic acid (vitamin C)—Sulfation of EE occurs in the gastrointestinal wall.
- Substances that inhibit cytochrome $P450_{3A4}$ isoenzymes such as indinavir, fluconazole and troleandomycin.

Troleandomycin may increase the risk of intrahepatic cholestasis during coadministration with COCs. Ethinyl estradiol may interfere with the metabolism of other drugs by inhibiting hepatic microsomal enzymes, or by inducing hepatic drug conjugation, particularly glucuronidation. Accordingly, plasma and tissue concentrations of some drugs may either be increased (e.g. cyclosporine, theophylline, corticosteroids) or decreased (e.g. lamotrigine) by ethinyl estradiol.

Drug-Drug Interactions: For possible drug interactions with COCs, see Table 2 and Table 3.

* COCs may worsen existing gallbladder disease and may accelerate the development of this disease in previously asymptomatic women.

† Optic neuritis may lead to partial or complete loss of vision.

‡ Serum folate levels may be depressed by COC therapy.

Table 2: PORTIA[a]

Drugs That May Decrease the Efficacy of Oral Contraceptives

Class of Compound	Drug	Proposed Mechanism	Suggested Management
Anticonvulsants	Carbamazepine Ethosuximide Phenobarbital Phenytoin Primidone	Induction of hepatic microsomal enzymes. Rapid metabolism of estrogen and increased binding of progestin and ethinyl estradiol to SHBG.	Use higher dose COCs (50 μg ethinyl estradiol), another drug or another method.
Antibiotics	Ampicillin Cotrimoxazole Penicillin	Enterohepatic circulation disturbance, intestinal hurry.	For short course, use additional method or use another drug. For long course, use another method.
	Rifampin	Increased metabolism of progestins. Suspected acceleration of estrogen metabolism.	Use another method.
	Chloramphenicol Metronidazole Neomycin Nitrofurantoin Sulfonamides Tetracyclines	Induction of hepatic microsomal enzymes. Also disturbances of enterohepatic circulation.	For short course, use additional method or use another drug. For long course, use another method.
	Troleandomycin	May retard metabolism of COCs, increasing the risk of cholestatic jaundice.	
Antifungals	Griseofulvin	Stimulation of hepatic metabolism of contraceptive steroids may occur.	Use another method.
Cholesterol Lowering Agents	Clofibrate	Reduces elevated serum triglycerides and cholesterol; this reduces COC efficacy.	Use another method.
Sedatives and Hypnotics	Benzodiazepines Barbiturates Chloral Hydrate Glutethimide Meprobamate	Induction of hepatic microsomal enzymes.	For short course, use additional method or another drug. For long course, use another method or higher dose COCs.
Antacids		Decreased intestinal absorption of progestins.	Dose 2 hours apart.
Other Drugs	Phenylbutazone[b] Antihistamines[b] Analgesics[b] Antimigraine preparations[b] Vitamin E	Reduced COC efficacy has been reported. Remains to be confirmed.	

[a] Adapted from Dickey, RP, ed.: Managing Contraceptive Pill Patients, 5th edition, Creative Informatics Inc., Durant, OK, 1987.

[b] Refer to Oral Contraceptives 1994, A Report by the Special Advisory Committee on Reproductive Physiology to the Drugs Directorate, Health Protection Branch, Health Canada.

Table 3: PORTIA[a]

Modification of Other Drug Action by Oral Contraceptives

Class of Compound	Drug	Modification of Drug Action	Suggested Management
Alcohol		Possible increased levels of ethanol or acetaldehyde.	Use with caution.
Alpha-II Adrenoreceptor Agents	Clonidine	Sedation effect increased.	Use with caution.
Anticoagulants	All	COCs increase clotting factors, decrease efficacy. However, COCs may potentiate action in some patients.	Use another method.
Anticonvulsants	All	Fluid retention may increase risk of seizures.	Use another method.
Antidiabetic Drugs	Oral Hypoglycemics and Insulin	COCs may impair glucose tolerance and increase blood glucose.	Use low-dose estrogen and progestin COC or another method. Monitor blood glucose.
Antihypertensive Agents	Guanethidine and Methyldopa	Estrogen component causes sodium retention, progestin has no effect.	Use low-dose estrogen COC or use another method.
	Beta-blockers	Increased drug effect (decreased metabolism).	Adjust dose of drug if necessary. Monitor cardiovascular status.
Antipyretics	Acetaminophen	Increased metabolism and renal clearance.	Dose of drug may have to be increased.
	Antipyrine	Impaired metabolism.	Decrease dose of drug.
	ASA	Effects of ASA may be decreased by the short-term use of COCs.	Patients on chronic ASA therapy may require an increase in ASA dosage.

(cont'd)

Table 3: PORTIA[a] *(cont'd)*

Modification of Other Drug Action by Oral Contraceptives

Class of Compound	Drug	Modification of Drug Action	Suggested Management
Aminocaproic Acid		Theoretically, a hypercoagulable state may occur because COCs augment clotting factors.	Avoid concomitant use.
Betamimetic Agents	Isoproterenol	Estrogen causes decreased response to these drugs.	Adjust dose of drug as necessary. Discontinuing COCs can result in excessive drug activity.
Caffeine		The actions of caffeine may be enhanced as COCs may impair the hepatic metabolism of caffeine.	Use with caution.
Cholesterol-Lowering Agents	Clofibrate	Their action may be antagonized by COCs. COCs may also increase metabolism of clofibrate.	May need to increase dose of clofibrate.
Corticosteroids	Prednisone	Markedly increased serum levels.	Possible need for decrease in dose.
Cyclosporine		May lead to an increase in cyclosporine levels and hepatotoxicity.	Monitor hepatic function. The cyclosporine dose may have to be decreased.
Folic Acid		COCs have been reported to impair folate metabolism.	May need to increase dietary intake, or supplement.
Meperidine		Possible increased analgesia and CNS depression due to decreased metabolism of meperidine.	Use combination with caution.
Phenothiazine Tranquilizers	All Phenothiazines, Reserpine and similar drugs	Estrogen potentiates the hyperprolactinemia effect of these drugs.	Use other drugs or lower dose COCs. If galactorrhea or hyperprolactinemia occurs, use other method.
Sedatives and Hypnotics	Chlordiazepoxide Lorazepam Oxazepam Diazepam	Increased effect (increased metabolism).	Use with caution.
Theophylline	All	Decreased oxidation, leading to possible toxicity.	Use with caution. Monitor theophylline levels.
Tricyclic Antidepressants	Clomipramine (possibly others)	Increased side effects: i.e., depression.	Use with caution.
Vitamin B_{12}		COCs have been reported to reduce serum levels of Vitamin B_{12}.	May need to increase dietary intake, or supplement.

[a] Adapted from Dickey, RP, ed.: Managing Contraceptive Pill Patients, 5th edition, Creative Informatics Inc., Durant, OK, 1987.

Drug-Food Interactions: The actions of caffeine may be enhanced by concomitant use of oral contraceptives. Oral contraceptives may impair the hepatic metabolism of caffeine, therefore use with caution.

The use of alcohol with oral contraceptives may possibly result in increased levels of ethanol or acetaldehyde, therefore use with caution.

Drug-Herb Interactions: The metabolism of oral contraceptives may be influenced by various drugs and herbal preparations including St. John's Wort. Of potential clinical importance are drugs and herbal supplements that are known to affect the induction of enzymes that are responsible for the degradation of contraceptive steroid hormones (e.g. St. John's Wort). Decreased effectiveness of the estrogenic component of oral contraceptives may result in spotting, breakthrough bleeding and possible pill failure. It is possible that induction of these enzymes may lead to reductions in the circulating levels of the progestational component of PORTIA Tablets. In actual practice, reduced efficacy has been associated with concomitant use of St. John's Wort.

Drug-Laboratory Test Interactions: Laboratory Test:

Liver Function Tests	
Bromsulphthalein Retention Test (BSP)	Moderate increase
AST and GGT	Minor increase
Alkaline Phosphatase	Variable increase
Serum Bilirubin	Increased, particularly in conditions predisposing to or associated with hyperbilirubinemia
Coagulation Tests	
Factors II, VII, IX, X, XII, and XIII	Increased
Factor VIII	Mild increase
Platelet aggregation and adhesiveness	Mild increase in response to common aggregating agents
Fibrinogen	Increased
Plasminogen	Mild increase
Antithrombin III	Mild increase
Prothrombin Time	Increased
Thyroid Function Tests	

Protein-bound Iodine (PBI)	Increased
Total Serum Thyroxine (T_3 and T_4)	Increased
Thyroid Stimulating Hormone (TSH)	Unchanged
Free T_3 Resin Uptake	Decreased
Adrenocortical Function Tests	
Plasma Cortisol	Increased
Cortisol Binding Globulin	Increased
Dehydroepiandrosterone sulfate (DHEAS)	Decreased
Renal Function	
Plasma Creatinine	Increased
Creatinine Clearance	Increased
Miscellaneous Tests	
Serum Folate	Occasionally decreased
Glucose Tolerance Test	Variable increase with return to normal after 6 to 12 months
Insulin Response	Mild to moderate increase
c-Peptide Response	Mild to moderate increase

Tissue Specimens: Pathologists should be advised of oral contraceptive therapy when specimens obtained from surgical procedures and Pap smears are submitted for examination.

Non-Contraceptive Benefits of Oral Contraceptives: Several health advantages other than contraception have been reported.

1. Combination oral contraceptives reduce the incidence of cancer of the endometrium and ovaries.
2. Oral contraceptives reduce the likelihood of developing benign breast disease.
3. Oral contraceptives reduce the likelihood of development of functional ovarian cysts.
4. Pill users have less menstrual blood loss and have more regular cycles, thereby reducing the chance of developing iron-deficiency anemia.
5. The use of oral contraceptives may decrease the severity of dysmenorrhea and premenstrual syndrome, and may improve acne vulgaris, hirsutism, and other androgen-mediated disorders.
6. Other non-contraceptive benefits are outlined in Oral Contraceptives 1994, Health Canada.

DOSAGE AND ADMINISTRATION:

PORTIA 21 Tablets Regimen: Each cycle consists of 21 days on medication and a 7-day interval without medication (three weeks on, one week off).

The dosage of PORTIA Tablets is one tablet daily for 21 consecutive days per menstrual cycle, according to prescribed schedule.

For the first cycle of medication, the patient is instructed to take one PORTIA Tablet daily for 21 consecutive days beginning on Day 1 of her menstrual cycle, on Day 5, or on the first Sunday after her period begins. (For the first cycle only, the first day of menstrual flow is considered Day 1.) The tablets are then discontinued for seven days (one week). Withdrawal bleeding should usually occur within three days following discontinuation of PORTIA.

The patient begins her next and all subsequent 21-day courses of PORTIA Tablets (following the same 21 days on, 7 days off) on the same day of the week that she began her first course. She begins taking her tablets seven days after discontinuation, regardless of whether or not withdrawal bleeding is still in progress.

PORTIA 28 Tablets Regimen: Each cycle consists of 21 days of white PORTIA Tablets followed by 7 days of pink inert tablets (three weeks on PORTIA, one week on inert tablets).

The dosage of PORTIA Tablets is one tablet daily for 21 consecutive days per menstrual cycle according to prescribed schedule, followed by one inert tablet daily for 7 consecutive days according to prescribed schedule.

For the first cycle of medication, the patient is instructed to take one white tablet daily for 21 consecutive days beginning on Day 1 of her menstrual cycle, on Day 5, or on the first Sunday after her period begins. (For the first cycle only, the first day of menstrual flow is considered Day 1.) One pink tablet is taken daily for the following seven consecutive days. Withdrawal bleeding should usually occur within three days following the discontinuation of white PORTIA Tablets, i.e., during the week the patient is taking the pink inert tablets. The patient begins her next and all subsequent 28-day courses of tablets on the same day of the week that she began her first course. She continues her next course of 28 tablets immediately after the last course, regardless of whether or not a period of withdrawal bleeding is still in progress. There is no need for the patient to count days between cycles because there are no "off-tablet days".

Missed Dose: The patient should be instructed to use Table 4 if she misses one or more of her birth control pills. She should be told to match the number of pills with the appropriate starting time for her type of pill.

Table 4: PORTIA

What to Do if You Miss Pills

Sunday Start	**Other than Sunday Start**
Miss 1 Pill	**Miss 1 Pill**
Take it as soon as you remember, and take the next pill at the usual time. This means that you might take 2 pills in one day.	Take it as soon as you remember, and take the next pill at the usual time. This means that you might take 2 pills in one day.
Miss 2 Pills in a Row	**Miss 2 Pills in a Row**
First 2 weeks: 1. Take 2 pills the day you remember and 2 pills the next day. 2. Then take 1 pill a day until you finish the pack. 3. Use a nonhormonal back-up method of birth control if you have sex in the 7 days after you miss the pills. **Third week:** 1. Keep taking 1 pill a day until Sunday. 2. On Sunday, safely discard the rest of the pack and start a new pack that day. 3. Use a nonhormonal back-up method of birth control if you have sex in the 7 days after you miss the pills. 4. You may not have a period this month. **If you miss 2 periods in a row, call your doctor, pharmacist or clinic.**	**First 2 weeks:** 1. Take 2 pills the day you remember and 2 pills the next day. 2. Then take 1 pill a day until you finish the pack. 3. Use a nonhormonal back-up method of birth control if you have sex in the 7 days after you miss the pills. **Third week:** 1. Safely dispose of the rest of the pill pack and start a new pack that same day. 2. Use a nonhormonal back-up method of birth control if you have sex in the 7 days after you miss the pills. 3. You may not have a period this month. **If you miss 2 periods in a row, call your doctor, pharmacist or clinic.**
Miss 3 or More Pills in a Row	**Miss 3 or More Pills in a Row**
Anytime in the cycle: 1. Keep taking 1 pill a day until Sunday. 2. On Sunday, safely discard the rest of the pack and start a new pack that day. 3. Use a nonhormonal back-up method of birth control if you have sex in the 7 days after you miss the pills. 4. You may not have a period this month. **If you miss 2 periods in a row, call your doctor, pharmacist or clinic.**	**Anytime in the cycle:** 1. Safely dispose of the rest of the pill pack and start a new pack that same day. 2. Use a nonhormonal back-up method of birth control if you have sex in the 7 days after you miss the pills. 3. You may not have a period this month. **If you miss 2 periods in a row, call your doctor, pharmacist or clinic.**

(cont'd)

Table 4: PORTIA *(cont'd)*

Contraceptive reliability may be reduced if active tablets are missed and particularly if the missed tablets extend the tablet-free interval. If active tablets were missed and intercourse took place in the week before the tablets were missed, the possibility of pregnancy should be considered.

Special Notes on Administration: It is recommended that PORTIA Tablets be taken at the same time each day, preferably after the evening meal or at bedtime.

PORTIA is effective from the first day of therapy if the tablets are begun as described under Dosage and Administration.

If PORTIA Tablets administration is initiated after Day 1 of the first menstrual cycle of medication or postpartum, contraceptive reliance should not be placed on PORTIA until after the first seven consecutive days of administration. The possibility of ovulation and conception prior to initiation of medication should be considered. Therefore, nonhormonal methods of contraception (such as condoms and spermicide) should be used for the first 7 days of tablet taking.

If spotting or breakthrough bleeding occurs, the patient is instructed to continue on the same regimen. This type of bleeding usually is transient and without significance; however, if the bleeding is persistent or prolonged, the patient is advised to consult her physician.

Advice in Case of Vomiting: If vomiting occurs within 3-4 hours after tablet-taking, absorption may not be complete. In such event, advice concerning the Management of Missed Tablet is outlined in the above chart.

The woman must take the extra active tablet(s) needed from a backup pack.

No Preceding Hormonal Contraceptive Use (in the Past Month): Tablet-taking should start on day 1 of the woman's natural cycle (i.e., the first day of her menstrual bleeding). Starting on days 2-7 (e.g., Sunday start) is allowed, but for the first 7 days of tablet-taking during the first cycle, a nonhormonal back-up method of birth control (such as condoms and spermicide) is recommended.

Changing from Another OC Pill: The woman should start PORTIA preferably on the day after the last active tablet of her previous OC, but at the latest, on the day following the usual tablet-free or inactive tablet interval of her previous OC.

Changing from a Progestin Only Method (Progestin-only Pill, Injection, Implant): The woman may switch any day from the progestin-only pill and should begin PORTIA the next day. She should start PORTIA on the day of an implant removal or, if using an injection, the day the next injection would be due. In all of these situations, the woman should be advised to use a nonhormonal back-up method for the first 7 days of tablet-taking.

Following First-trimester Abortion: The woman may start PORTIA immediately. Additional contraceptive measures are not needed.

Following Delivery or Second-trimester Abortion: Since the immediate post-partum period is associated with an increased risk of thromboembolism, COCs should be started no earlier than day 28 after delivery in the nonlactating mother or second-trimester abortion. The woman should be advised to use a nonhormonal back-up method for the first 7 days of tablet-taking. However, if intercourse has already occurred, pregnancy should be excluded before the actual start of COC use or the woman must wait for her first menstrual period.

OVERDOSAGE:

Symptoms of COC overdosage in adults and children may include nausea, vomiting, breast tenderness, dizziness, abdominal pain, drowsiness/fatigue; withdrawal bleeding may occur in females. There is no specific antidote and further treatment of overdose, if necessary, is directed to the symptoms.

> For management of a suspected drug overdose, contact your **regional Poison Control Centre**. See the *CPS* Directory section for a list of Poison Control Centres.

ACTION AND CLINICAL PHARMACOLOGY: Mechanism of Action: Although the primary mechanism of action is inhibition of ovulation, the effectiveness of PORTIA Tablets may also result from other mechanisms of action, such as hostility of the cervical mucus to sperm penetration and migration.

Pharmacodynamics: Progestogens can have, in addition to progestational activity, estrogenic, anti-estrogenic and androgenic activity. When combined with estrogen, the progestogen will markedly affect the overall biological activity by producing a synergistic, summative or diminutional effect on activity. Comparisons of progestogen potency are not considered scientifically valid because the effects of one progestogen cannot be directly compared with those of another.

A study of serum luteinizing hormone (LH), follicle stimulating hormone (FSH), progesterone and 17ß-estradiol in patients taking 150 µg d-norgestrel (as the dl-racemate) plus 30 µg ethinyl estradiol indicated reduction or abolition of the mid-cycle ovulatory peak and post-ovulatory levels commonly associated with these hormones and gonadotrophins respectively.

Endometrial biopsies taken during the course of therapy with 250 µg d-norgestrel (as the dl-racemate) plus 50 µg ethinyl estradiol revealed a histological sequence in the menstrual cycle of early glandular epithelial stimulation followed by later inhibition after the first half of the menstrual cycle.

Cervical mucus studies with 250 µg d-norgestrel (as the dl-racemate) plus 50 µg ethinyl estradiol, and 37.5 µg d-norgestrel (as the dl-racemate) revealed absence of ferning and decreased spinnbarkeit, indicative of poor conditions for sperm penetration and migration.

The results of assays for prolactin in a group of 11 normally ovulating women given 150 µg d-norgestrel (as the dl-racemate) plus 30 µg ethinyl estradiol over a continuous period of three months indicated no clinically or statistically significant elevation or depression of hormone levels during the course of active drug ingestion, nor in the first post-treatment cycle.

A human study of the metabolism of ^{14}C-labelled norgestrel, revealed that most of the urinary excretion of norgestrel occurred on the first day. There was no difference in the rate of excretion of norgestrel whether administered orally or intravenously. The amount of radioactivity in plasma fell rapidly within the first few hours and at the end of two days only small amounts were present. The foregoing and other studies with ^{14}C-labelled and unlabelled norgestrel have shown that saturation of the 4,5-double bond with and without concomitant reduction of the 3-carbonyl to a 3-hydroxyl group are important reactions during metabolism.

Pharmacokinetics: See Table 5.

Absorption: Oral contraceptive steroids are generally well absorbed from the GI tract.

Levonorgestrel is rapidly and completely absorbed after oral administration (bioavailability about 100%) and is not subject to first-pass metabolism. Ethinyl estradiol is rapidly and almost completely absorbed from the gastrointestinal tract, but due to first-pass metabolism in gut mucosa and liver, the bioavailability of ethinyl estradiol is between 38% and 48%.

Based on literature and previous studies, the following parameters were found for a single dose of levonorgestrel (0.10 mg) and ethinyl estradiol (0.02 mg): for levonorgestrel C_{max} was reported to be 2.8 ng/mL at approximately 1.6 hour; for ethinyl estradiol C_{max} was reported to be 62 ng/mL at approximately 1.5 hour. The average elimination half-life has been reported to range between 11 to 40 hours for levonorgestrel and between 6 to 20 hours for ethinyl estradiol. The intra-subject variability (CV%) for ethinyl estradiol ranged from 20-26% for C_{max}, and from 12-25% for AUC, but was less variable for levonorgestrel.

Distribution: Levonorgestrel in serum is primarily bound to SHBG. Ethinyl estradiol is about 97% bound to plasma albumin. Ethinyl estradiol does not bind to SHBG, but induces SHBG synthesis.

Metabolism: Levonorgestrel: The most important metabolic pathway occurs in the reduction of the (DELTA)4-3-oxo group and hydroxylation at positions 2α, 1β, and 16β, followed by conjugation. Most of the metabolites that circulate in the blood are sulfates of 3α,5β-tetrahydro-levonorgestrel, while excretion occurs predominantly in the form of glucuronides. Some of the parent levonorgestrel also circulates as 17β-sulfate. Metabolic clearance rates may differ among individuals by several-fold, and this may account in part for the wide variation observed in levonorgestrel concentrations among users. Levonorgestrel is not subject to first-pass metabolism.

Table 5: PORTIA

Summary of Mean Pharmacokinetic Parameters of PORTIA in Normal Volunteers

Single dose of 2 tablets	C_{max} (pg/mL)	$t_{½}$ (hours)	$AUC_{0-\infty}$ (pg·h/mL)
Ethinyl Estradiol	147.13±50.57	17.22±8.34	1650.33±599.06
Levonorgestrel	6347.68±2270.57	28.62±10.60	86 366.33±59 053.98

Ethinyl estradiol: Cytochrome P450 enzymes (CYP3A4) in the liver are responsible for the 2-hydroxylation that is the major oxidative reaction. The 2-hydroxy metabolite is further transformed by methylation and glucuronidation prior to urinary and fecal excretion. Levels of Cytochrome P450 (CYP3A) vary widely among individuals and can explain the variation in rates of ethinyl estradiol 2-hydroxylation. Ethinyl estradiol is subject to first-pass metabolism in gut mucosa and liver.

Excretion: Levonorgestrel and its metabolites are primarily excreted in the urine (40% to 68%) and about 16% to 48% are excreted in feces. Ethinyl estradiol is excreted in the urine and feces as glucuronide and sulfate conjugates, and undergoes enterohepatic circulation. The elimination half-life for levonorgestrel is approximately 36±13 hours at steady state. The elimination half-life of ethinyl estradiol is 18±4.7 hours at steady state.

Special Populations and Conditions: Pediatrics: Pharmacokinetic differences in pediatrics in comparison to adults have not been studied. This medication should not be used before menarche.

Race: Pharmacokinetic differences based on race have not been studied.

Renal Insufficiency: No studies have been conducted in women with renal insufficiency.

Genetic Polymorphism: Pharmacokinetic differences based on genetic polymorphism have not been studied.

STORAGE AND STABILITY: Store at 15-30°C.

SPECIAL HANDLING INSTRUCTIONS: PORTIA 21 and PORTIA 28 should be protected from light once opened using the protective covering provided.

Keep out of reach of children.

INFORMATION FOR THE PATIENT: Published in e-CPS, available by subscription at www.e-cps.ca.

DOSAGE FORMS, COMPOSITION AND PACKAGING: PORTIA 21: Each pink, round, film-coated, biconvex, unscored tablet, debossed with "b" on one side and "992" on the other side, contains: levonorgestrel 0.15 mg and ethinyl estradiol 0.03 mg. Nonmedicinal ingredients: anhydrous lactose, FD&C Blue no. 1, FD&C Red no 40, hypromellose, magnesium stearate, microcrystalline cellulose, polyethylene glycol, polysorbate 80 and titanium dioxide. Packs of 21 active tablets.

PORTIA 28: Each pink, round, film-coated, biconvex, unscored tablet, debossed with "b" on one side and "992" on the other side, contains: levonorgestrel 0.15 mg and ethinyl estradiol 0.03 mg. Each white, round, biconvex, unscored tablet, debossed with "b" on one side and "208" on the other side, contains: inert ingredients. Nonmedicinal ingredients: active tablet: anhydrous lactose, FD&C Blue no. 1, FD&C Red no 40, hypromellose, magnesium stearate, microcrystalline cellulose, polyethylene glycol, polysorbate 80 and titanium dioxide; inert tablet: anhydrous lactose, hypromellose, magnesium stearate and microcrystalline cellulose. Packs of 21 active tablets and 7 inert tablets.

Posanol™ Pr

posaconazole

Antifungal

Schering-Plough

Date of Preparation: June 11, 2008

SUMMARY PRODUCT INFORMATION:

Route of Administration	Dosage Form/ Strength	Clinically Relevant Nonmedicinal Ingredients
Oral	Suspension, 40 mg/mL posaconazole	For a complete listing see Dosage Forms, Composition and Packaging.

INDICATIONS AND CLINICAL USE: POSANOL (posaconazole) is indicated for:

- prophylaxis of Aspergillus and Candida infections in patients, 13 years of age and older, who are at high risk of developing these infections, such as patients with prolonged neutropenia or hematopoietic stem cell transplant (HSCT) recipients.
- treatment of invasive aspergillosis in patients 13 years of age or older with disease that is refractory to amphotericin B or itraconazole, or in patients who are intolerant of these medicinal products. Refractoriness is defined as progression of infection or failure to improve after a minimum of 7 days of prior therapeutic doses of effective antifungal therapy.
- treatment of oropharyngeal candidiasis (OPC) in patients 13 years of age or older.

Geriatrics (≥65 years of age): Limited evidence from clinical studies and experience suggests that use in the geriatric population is associated with no overall differences in safety or effectiveness.

Pediatrics (13-17 years of age): Safety and effectiveness in pediatric subjects below the age of 13 years have not been studied. A limited number of subjects between the ages of 13 and 17 have received POSANOL including 11 patients in the refractory invasive fungal infection (rIFI) studies and 12 patients in the prophylaxis studies. The safety profile in these patients <18 years appears similar to the safety profile observed in adults.

CONTRAINDICATIONS:

- Patients who are hypersensitive to this drug or to any ingredient in the formulation or component of the container. For a complete listing, see Dosage Forms, Composition and Packaging. There is no information regarding cross-sensitivity between POSANOL and other azole antifungal agents. Caution should be used when prescribing POSANOL to patients with hypersensitivity to other azoles.
- Co-administration of POSANOL and ergot alkaloids. POSANOL may increase the plasma concentrations of ergot alkaloids, which may lead to ergotism (see Drug Interactions).
- Co-administration of POSANOL and certain medicinal products metabolized through the CYP3A4 system: terfenadine*, astemizole†, cisapride‡, pimozide, and quinidine. Although not studied in vitro or in vivo, co-administration of these CYP3A4 substrates may result in increased plasma concentrations of those medicinal products, leading to potentially serious and/or life threatening adverse events, such as QT prolongation and rare occurrences of torsade de pointes (see Drug Interactions).

WARNINGS AND PRECAUTIONS:

Serious Warnings and Precautions

- **Drug Interactions (see Contraindications and Drug Interactions)**
- **Cardiovascular effects—QT interval prolongation (see Cardiovascular)**
- **Hepatic toxicity (see Hepatic/Biliary/Pancreatic)**

General: Hypersensitivity: There is no information regarding cross-sensitivity between POSANOL and other azole antifungal agents. Caution should be used when prescribing POSANOL to patients with hypersensitivity to other azoles.

This medicine contains glucose. Patients with rare glucose-galactose malabsorption should not take this medicine.

No data on the effects of POSANOL on the ability to drive and use machines are available.

* Please note that terfenadine is no longer available on the Canadian market.

† Please note that astemizole is no longer available on the Canadian market.

‡ Please note that cisapride is no longer available on the Canadian market.

Carcinogenesis and Mutagenesis: Carcinogenicity studies did not reveal special hazards for humans.

Cardiovascular: POSANOL has been associated with prolongation of the QT interval of the electrocardiogram (ECG) in some patients. Prolongation of the QT interval may increase the risk of arrhythmia.

Due to limited clinical experience, POSANOL should be administered with caution to patients with potentially proarrhythmic conditions such as congenital or acquired QT_c prolongation, congestive heart failure, bradycardia, and acute myocardial ischemia. Electrolyte disturbances, especially those involving potassium, magnesium or calcium levels, should be monitored and corrected as necessary before and during POSANOL therapy.

Caution should be exercised if POSANOL is used in patients taking other drugs that may prolong the QT interval, such as antipsychotics, tricyclic antidepressants, methadone, erythromycin, Class IA (e.g., procainamide, quinidine) and Class III (e.g., amiodarone, sotalol) antiarrhythmic agents. Drugs metabolized by the hepatic cytochrome P450 isoenzymes may be affected by POSANOL levels, with possible resulting QT effects. Such drugs include tacrolimus, HIV protease inhibitors and macrolide antibiotics. (See Contraindications, Drug Interactions and Action and Clinical Pharmacology.)

During clinical development there was a single case of torsade de pointes in a patient taking POSANOL. This report involved a seriously ill patient with multiple confounding risk factors. (See Adverse Reactions, Less Common Clinical Trial Adverse Drug Reactions (<2%).)

Dependence/Tolerance: There is no known abuse potential for POSANOL.

Hematologic: Rare cases of hemolytic uremic syndrome and thrombotic thrombocytopenic purpura have been reported primarily among patients who had been receiving concomitant cyclosporine or tacrolimus for management of transplant rejection or graft vs. host disease (GVHD).

Hepatic/Biliary/Pancreatic: Hepatic Toxicity: In clinical trials, there were infrequent cases of hepatic reactions (e.g., mild to moderate elevations in ALT (alanine aminotransferase), AST (aspartate aminotransferase), alkaline phosphatase, total bilirubin, and/or clinical hepatitis) during treatment with POSANOL. The elevations in liver function tests were generally reversible on discontinuation of therapy, and in some instances these tests normalized without drug interruption and rarely required drug discontinuation. Rarely, more severe hepatic reactions including cholestasis or hepatic failure were reported in patients with serious underlying medical conditions (e.g., hematologic malignancy) during treatment with POSANOL.

Monitoring of Hepatic Function: Liver function tests should be evaluated at the start of and during the course of POSANOL therapy. Patients who develop abnormal liver function tests during POSANOL therapy should be monitored for the development of more severe hepatic injury. Patient management should include laboratory evaluation of hepatic function (particularly liver function tests and bilirubin). Discontinuation of POSANOL should be considered if clinical signs and symptoms are consistent with development of worsening liver disease.

Special Populations: Pregnant Women: There is insufficient information on the use of POSANOL in pregnant women. The extent of exposure in pregnancy during clinical trials is very limited. There are no adequate and well-controlled studies in pregnant women. Studies in animals have shown reproductive toxicity. The potential risk to humans is unknown. Women of childbearing potential must always use adequate contraceptive measures while on treatment. POSANOL should be used in pregnancy only if the potential benefit justifies the potential risk to the fetus.

Nursing Women: POSANOL is excreted into the milk of lactating rats. The excretion of POSANOL in human breast milk has not been investigated. POSANOL should not be used by nursing mothers unless the benefit to the mother clearly outweighs the risk to the infant.

Hepatic Impairment: POSANOL should be used with caution in patients with severe hepatic impairment. Prolonged elimination half-life may lead to increased exposure.

Patients Taking Immunosuppressant: Cases of elevated cyclosporine levels resulting in rare serious adverse events, including nephrotoxicity and leukoencephalopathy, and death were reported in clinical efficacy studies. Dose reduction and more frequent clinical monitoring of cyclosporine, tacrolimus, and sirolimus should be preformed when POSANOL therapy is initiated. (See Drug Interactions.)

ADVERSE REACTIONS: Adverse Drug Reaction Overview: The safety of POSANOL therapy has been assessed in 1844 patients. This includes 605 patients in the prophylaxis studies, 796 in OPC/rOPC studies and 428 patients treated for invasive fungal infections (IFIs). POSANOL therapy was given to 171 patients for ≥6 months, with 58 patients receiving POSANOL therapy for ≥12 months. The most frequently reported adverse reactions reported across the whole population of healthy volunteers and patients were nausea (6%) and headache (6%).

Clinical Trial Adverse Drug Reactions: Because clinical trials are conducted under very specific conditions the adverse reaction rates observed in the clinical trials may not reflect the rates observed in practice and should not be compared to the rates in the clinical trials of another drug. Adverse drug reaction information from clinical trials is useful for identifying drug-related adverse events and for approximating rates.

Studies P01899 and C/I98-316: Study P01899 was a randomised, evaluator-blinded study that compared POSANOL oral suspension (200 mg three times a day) with fluconazole suspension (400 mg once daily) or itraconazole oral solution (200 mg twice a day [BID]) as prophylaxis against IFIs in neutropenic patients who were receiving cytotoxic chemotherapy for acute myelogenous leukemia or myelodysplastic syndromes. The mean duration of therapy was comparable between the two treatment groups (29 days, POSANOL; 25 days, fluconazole/itraconazole). In this study, 304 patients were randomly assigned to POSANOL therapy and 240 patients were assigned to fluconazole, and 58 were assigned to itraconazole therapy as the local standard of care.

Study C/I98-316 was a randomised, double-blind trial that compared POSANOL oral suspension (200 mg three times a day) with fluconazole capsules (400 mg once daily) as prophylaxis against IFIs in allogeneic HSCT recipients with GVHD. The mean duration of therapy was comparable between the two treatment groups (80 days, POSANOL; 77 days, fluconazole). In this study, 301 patients were randomly assigned to POSANOL therapy and 299 patients were assigned to fluconazole therapy. See Table 1.

Table 1: POSANOL

Treatment-Related Adverse Reactions Reported in POSANOL, Fluconazole and Itraconazole Subjects Reported at an Incidence of ≥1% for the Prophylaxis Studies C/I98-316 and P01899

Adverse Reactions	POSANOL n=605 (%)	Fluconazole n=539 (%)	Itraconazole n=58 (%)
Blood and Lymphatic System			
Anemia	5 (1)	2 (<1)	0
Thrombocytopenia	4 (1)	3 (1)	0
Cardiovascular			
QT/QT_c prolongation	14 (2)	6 (1)	4 (7)
Hypertension	3 (<1)	5 (1)	0
Tachycardia	4 (1)	1 (<1)	0
Bradycardia	1 (<1)	0	2 (3)
Vasculitis	0	0	1 (2)
Eye			
Vision blurred	3 (<1)	6 (1)	0
Gastrointestinal			
Nausea	44 (7)	45 (8)	8 (14)
Vomiting	27 (4)	29 (5)	6 (10)
Diarrhea	28 (5)	24 (4)	9 (16)

(cont'd)

Table 1: POSANOL *(cont'd)*

Treatment-Related Adverse Reactions Reported in POSANOL, Fluconazole and Itraconazole Subjects Reported at an Incidence of ≥1% for the Prophylaxis Studies C/I98-316 and P01899

Adverse Reactions	POSANOL n=605 (%)	Fluconazole n=539 (%)	Itraconazole n=58 (%)
Abdominal pain	13 (2)	15 (3)	1 (2)
Constipation	4 (1)	12 (2)	0
Dyspepsia	8 (1)	9 (2)	0
Loose stools	1 (<1)	5 (1)	0
Abdominal distension	4 (1)	2 (<1)	0
Gastritis	2 (<1)	3 (1)	0
Nausea aggravated	2 (<1)	1 (<1)	2 (3)
Dry mouth	3 (<1)	1 (<1)	1 (2)
Mucositis not otherwise specified	7 (1)	0	0
Stomatitis aphtous	1 (<1)	0	1 (2)
Gastric disorder	0	0	1 (2)
Rectal pain	0	0	1 (2)
General and Administration Site Conditions			
Fatigue	7 (1)	7 (1)	0
Weakness	3 (<1)	5 (1)	0
Asthenia	2 (<1)	3 (1)	0
Fever	2 (<1)	3 (1)	0
Hepatobiliary			
Bilirubinemia	15 (2)	10 (2)	3 (5)
Hepatic enzymes increased	15 (2)	10 (2)	0
ALT increased	16 (3)	8 (1)	1 (2)
Gamma glutamyl transferase (GGT) increased	14 (2)	8 (1)	1 (2)
AST increased	14 (2)	7 (1)	1 (2)
Hepatic function abnormal	2 (<1)	5 (1)	0
Jaundice	5 (1)	2 (<1)	0
Hepatocellular damage	5 (1)	0	0
Immune			
Allergic reaction	3 (<1)	3 (1)	0
Metabolism and Nutrition			
Hypokalemia	11 (2)	6 (1)	1 (2)
Anorexia	6 (1)	8 (1)	1 (2)
Hypomagnesemia	2 (<1)	6 (1)	0
Hyperkalemia	2 (<1)	4 (1)	0
Weight decrease	1 (<1)	4 (1)	0
Hyperglycemia	2 (<1)	3 (1)	0
Weight increase	1 (<1)	0	1 (2)
Musculoskeletal and Connective Tissue			
Myalgia	2 (<1)	3 (1)	0
Nervous System			
Headache	8 (1)	8 (1)	1 (2)
Dizziness	4 (1)	7 (1)	0
Taste perversion	3 (<1)	7 (1)	1 (2)
Tremor	4 (1)	6 (1)	0
Paresthesia	5 (1)	3 (1)	0
Somnolence	2 (<1)	3 (1)	0
Syncope	2 (<1)	0	1 (2)

(cont'd)

Table 1: POSANOL *(cont'd)*

Treatment-Related Adverse Reactions Reported in POSANOL, Fluconazole and Itraconazole Subjects Reported at an Incidence of ≥1% for the Prophylaxis Studies C/I98-316 and P01899

Adverse Reactions	POSANOL n=605 (%)	Fluconazole n=539 (%)	Itraconazole n=58 (%)
Renal and Urinary System			
Blood creatinine increased	6 (1)	5 (1)	0
Creatinine clearance decreased	2 (<1)	4 (1)	0
Renal insufficiency	1 (<1)	4 (1)	0
Renal function abnormal	2 (<1)	3 (1)	0
Respiratory			
Coughing	2 (<1)	2 (<1)	1 (2)
Skin and Subcutaneous Tissue			
Rash	12 (2)	10 (2)	1 (2)
Pruritus	4 (1)	5 (1)	0
Rash pruritic	3 (<1)	5 (1)	0
Rash maculopapular	5 (1)	2 (<1)	0
Sweating increased	1 (<1)	0	1 (2)
Cellulitis	0	0	1 (2)
Investigations			
Phosphatase alkaline increased	6 (1)	6 (1)	1 (2)
Drug level altered	5 (1)	2 (<1)	0
LDH increased	5 (1)	0	0

The most common treatment-related serious adverse events (1% each) in the combined prophylaxis studies were bilirubinemia, increased hepatic enzymes, hepatocellular damage, nausea, and vomiting.

Studies P01893 and P00041: Study P01893 was an open-label, randomized, parallel group, study of the safety, tolerability, efficacy, and pharmacokinetic profile of POSANOL in the treatment of immunocompromised patients with rIFI or in febrile neutropenic subjects who required empiric antifungal therapy. POSANOL oral suspension was given as follows: 200 mg administered 4 times daily, 400 mg administered 4 times daily, 800 mg administered twice daily for 2 days followed by 400 mg administered twice daily, 600 mg administered twice daily, or 800 mg administered every day, respectively, for the remainder of the study. For subjects with rIFIs, daily administration of the study drug was continued for a maximum duration of 6 months. For febrile neutropenic subjects, daily administration of the study drug was continued until after completion of the study or until the recovering absolute neutrophil count reached 500 cells/mm³. In this study, 98 patients were randomized and 93 received POSANOL therapy.

Study P00041 was an open-label, non-comparative study of the safety and efficacy of POSANOL as treatment of IFIs in patients who had disease which was refractory to amphotericin B (including liposomal formulations) or itraconazole or in patients who were intolerant of these medicinal products. Patients were administered POSANOL 800 mg/day in divided doses. In this study, 330 patients received POSANOL therapy. The median duration of POSANOL therapy was 102.5 days (1-609 days). The majority of patients were severely immunocompromised with underlying conditions such as hematologic malignancies, including bone marrow transplantation; solid organ transplantation; solid tumors and/or AIDS.

Studies C/I96-209, C/I97-331, C/I97-330 and P00298: Study C/I96-209 was a randomised, double-blind, controlled study of four different dose levels of POSANOL as compared to fluconazole in the treatment of HIV-infected patients with azole-susceptible OPC. Patients were treated with POSANOL capsules 400 mg BID for 1 day, followed by 50 mg, 100 mg, 200 mg, or 400 mg QD for 13 days, or with fluconazole 200 mg QD for 1 day, followed by 100 mg QD for 13 days. In this study, 379 patients received POSANOL therapy and 90 patients received fluconazole therapy.

Study C/I97-331 was a randomised, evaluator-blinded, controlled study in HIV-infected patients with azole-susceptible OPC. Patients were treated with POSANOL or fluconazole oral suspension (both- POSANOL and fluconazole were given as follows: 100 mg BID for 1 day followed by 100 mg once a day for 13 days). In this study, 182 patients received POSANOL therapy and 184 patients received fluconazole therapy.

Study C/I97-330 was an open-label, non-comparative study in 199 HIV-infected patients with azole-refractory OPC treated with one of two POSANOL regimens: 400 mg BID for 3 days, followed by 400 mg QD for 25 days with an option for further treatment during a 3-month maintenance period, or 400 mg BID for 28 days.

Study P00298 was an open-label, non-comparative, long-term safety study in 100 HIV-infected patients with azole-refractory OPC treated with POSANOL 400 mg BID for up to 15 months. A total of 60 of these patients had been previously treated in Study C/I97-330 and 1 patient had been previously treated in Study P00041. See Table 2.

Table 2: POSANOL

Treatment-Related Adverse Reactions Reported in POSANOL-Treated Subjects (Divided Into Subgroups Bone Marrow Transplant [BMT], Non-BMT, Non-Refractory OPC & Refractory OPC) by Body Systems Reported at an Incidence of ≥2% for the rIFI Studies (P01893 & P00041) and OPC Studies (C/I96-209, C/I97-331, C/I97-330 & P00298)

	rIFI Studies (P01893 and P00041)		OPC Studies (C/I96-209, C/I97-331, C/I97-330 and P00298)		
	POSANOL		Non-Refractory OPC		Refractory OPC
Adverse Reactions	BMT n=124 (%)	Non-BMT n=304 (%)	POSANOL n=557 (%)	Fluconazole n=262 (%)	POSANOL n=239 (%)
Blood and Lymphatic System					
Neutropenia	0	0	10 (2)	4 (2)	20 (8)
Anemia	0	4 (1)	2 (<1)	0	6 (3)
Thrombocytopenia	0	2 (1)	3 (1)	0	4 (2)
Cardiovascular					

(cont'd)

Table 2: POSANOL *(cont'd)*

Treatment-Related Adverse Reactions Reported in POSANOL-Treated Subjects (Divided Into Subgroups Bone Marrow Transplant [BMT], Non-BMT, Non-Refractory OPC & Refractory OPC) by Body Systems Reported at an Incidence of ≥2% for the rIFI Studies (P01893 & P00041) and OPC Studies (C/I96-209, C/I97-331, C/I97-330 & P00298)

	rIFI Studies (P01893 and P00041)		OPC Studies (C/I96–209, C/I97–331, C/I97–330 and P00298)		
	POSANOL		Non-Refractory OPC		Refractory OPC
Adverse Reactions	**BMT n=124 (%)**	**Non-BMT n=304 (%)**	**POSANOL n=557 (%)**	**Fluconazole n=262 (%)**	**POSANOL n=239 (%)**
QT/QT$_c$ prolongation	0	6 (2)	0	0	0
Gastrointestinal					
Nausea	10 (8)	25 (8)	27 (5)	18 (7)	20 (8)
Diarrhea	3 (2)	12 (4)	19 (3)	13 (5)	26 (11)
Vomiting	7 (6)	18 (6)	20 (4)	4 (2)	16 (7)
Abdominal pain	3 (2)	15 (5)	10 (2)	8 (3)	12 (5)
Dry mouth	0	6 (2)	7 (1)	6 (2)	5 (2)
Flatulence	0	3 (1)	6 (1)	0	11 (5)
General and Administration Site Conditions					
Fatigue	4 (3)	3 (1)	8 (1)	5 (2)	7 (3)
Asthenia	1 (1)	3 (1)	4 (1)	2 (1)	6 (3)
Fever	1 (1)	2 (1)	10 (2)	1 (<1)	6 (3)
Hepatobiliary					
ALT increased	2 (2)	9 (3)	4 (1)	3 (1)	3 (1)
AST increased	1 (1)	8 (3)	5 (1)	2 (1)	1 (<1)
Hepatic enzymes increased	2 (2)	5 (2)	1 (<1)	0	5 (2)
Hepatic function abnormal	1 (1)	2 (1)	3 (1)	4 (2)	0
Metabolism and Nutrition					
Anorexia	2 (2)	6 (2)	6 (1)	1 (<1)	7 (3)
Muscoskeletal System					
Myalgia	0	1 (<1)	1 (<1)	0	4 (2)
Nervous System					
Headache	3 (2)	17 (6)	16 (3)	5 (2)	18 (8)
Dizziness	1 (1)	6 (2)	9 (2)	5 (2)	8 (3)
Somnolence	0	3 (1)	4 (1)	5 (2)	3 (1)
Paresthesia	1 (1)	5 (2)	3 (1)	2 (1)	2 (1)
Convulsions	2 (2)	0	0	0	2 (1)
Psychiatric					
Insomnia	0	0	3 (1)	0	6 (3)
Renal and Urinary System					
Blood creatinine increased	0	5 (2)	2 (<1)	0	2 (1)
Reproductive System and Breast					
Menstrual disorder	0	2 (2)	0	0	0
Skin and Subcutaneous Tissue					
Rash	2 (2)	8 (3)	8 (1)	4 (2)	10 (4)
Pruritus	1 (1)	3 (1)	6 (1)	2 (1)	5 (2)
Investigations					
Phosphatase alkaline increased	1 (1)	5 (2)	3 (1)	3 (1)	5 (2)
Drug level altered	2 (2)	5 (2)	0	0	0

Treatment-related serious adverse events reported in 428 patients with IFIs (1% each) included altered concentration of other medicinal products, increased hepatic enzymes, nausea, rash, and vomiting.

Adverse events were reported more frequently in the pool of patients with refractory OPC. Among these highly immunocompromised patients with advanced HIV disease, serious adverse events (SAEs) were reported in 55% (132/239). The most commonly reported SAEs were fever (13%) and neutropenia (10%).

Treatment-related SAEs were reported for 14% (34/239) of these patients and included neutropenia (5%) and abdominal pain (2%). POSANOL was discontinued in two patients who developed neutropenia that was considered serious and treatment-related. All other reported treatment-related SAEs occurred in <1% of subjects on POSANOL.

Less Common Clinical Trial Adverse Drug Reactions (<2%): Benign and Malignant Neoplasms: lipoma, Kaposi's Sarcoma.

Blood and Lymphatic System: abnormal blood gases not otherwise specified (NOS), abnormal platelets, anemia aggravated, blood neutrophil count decreased, bone marrow aplasia, coagulation disorder, coagulation time increased, eosinophilia, hematoma, hemoglobin decreased, hemorrhage NOS, leukopenia, lymphadenopathy, neutropenia aggravated, neutrophilia, pancytopenia, platelet count decreased, platelet count increased, prothrombin decreased, prothrombin time prolonged, purpura, splenomegaly, white blood cell count decreased.

In addition, rare cases of hemolytic uremic syndrome and thrombotic thrombocytopenic purpura have been reported primarily among patients who had been receiving concomitant cyclosporine or tacrolimus for management of transplant rejection or GVHD.

Cardiovascular: abnormal ECG, abnormal ECG specific, aortic valve sclerosis, arrhythmia, atherosclerosis, atrial fibrillation, atrial fibrillation aggravated, atrial flutter, AV block, bradycardia, bundle branch block, cardiac failure, cardiomegaly, cardio-respiratory arrest, cerebrovascular accident NOS, deep venous thrombosis NOS, dependent edema, ejection fraction decreased, extrasystoles, flushing, hot flushes, hypotension, hypotension postural, ischemia, mitral valve disease NOS, myocardial infarction, palpitation, premature atrial contractions, premature ventricular contractions, pulmonary embolism, sinus tachycardia, sudden death, supraventricular tachycardia, tachycardia, vascular disorder, ventricular hypertrophy, ventricular tachycardia.

During clinical development there was a single case of torsade de pointes in a patient taking POSANOL. This report involved a seriously ill patient with multiple confounding, potentially contributory risk factors, such as a history of palpitations, recent cardiotoxic chemotherapy, hypokalemia, and hypomagnesemia.

Ear and Labyrinth: earache, hearing impairment, tinnitus, vertigo, vestibular disorder.

Endocrine: adrenal insufficiency, glucocorticoids decreased, gonadotropins decreased.

Eye: conjunctivitis, diplopia, dry eyes, eye irritation, eye pain, periorbital edema, photophobia, scotoma.

Gastrointestinal: abdominal distention, abdominal pain aggravated, abdominal tenderness, ascites, ascites aggravated, bowel motility decreased, cheilitis, diverticulitis aggravated, dysphagia, eructation, esophagitis, esophagus ulceration, feces malodorous, gastritis, gastroenteritis, gastroesophageal reflux, gastrointestinal tract hemorrhage, hiccup, gingivitis, glossitis, hemorrhagic diarrhea, hemorrhagic gastritis, ileus, loose stools, melena, mouth ulceration, odynophagia, pancreatic enzymes NOS increased, pancreatitis, proctalgia, retching, saliva altered, stomatitis, tenesmus, thirst, tongue discoloration, tongue disorder, tooth discoloration, vomiting aggravated.

General and Administration Site Conditions: appetite increased, death, drug interaction, edema, fall, fatigue aggravated, fistula, generalized edema, influenza-like symptoms, laboratory test abnormality, legs edema, malaise, pain, pallor, peripheral edema, rigors.

Hepatobiliary: asterixis, biliary sludge, bilirubinemia aggravated, cholestasis, hepatic failure, hepatitis, hepatitis aggravated, hepatitis cholestatic, hepatocellular damage, hepatomegaly, hepatosplenomegaly, jaundice, liver tenderness.

Immune System: allergic reaction, allergy, GVHD aggravated, hypersensitivity reaction, non-specific inflammation, sarcoidosis aggravated, Stevens-Johnson syndrome.

Infections and Infestations: catheter related infection, non herpetic cold sores, esophageal candidiasis, fungal infection, moniliasis, oral candidiasis, pneumonia, pseudomonas aeruginosa infection, sinusitis, upper respiratory tract infection, urinary tract infection.

Injury and Poisoning: drug toxicity NOS, ecchymoses, overdose NOS, skin trauma.

Metabolism and Nutrition: amylase increased, dehydration, electrolyte abnormality, hypercalcemia, hypercholesterolemia, hypercholesterolemia aggravated, hyperlipemia, hypernatremia, hyperphosphatemia, hyperproteinemia, hypertriglyceridemia, hyperuricemia, hypoalbuminemia, hypocalcemia, hyponatremia, hypophosphatemia, lipase increased, malnutrition, metabolic acidosis, metabolic disorder NOS, NPN increased, renal tubular acidosis, vitamin K deficiency.

Musculoskeletal and Connective Tissue: arthralgia, arthralgia aggravated, back pain, bone pain, chest wall pain, extremities cramps, fasciitis, flank pain, legs cramps, muscle cramps, muscle weakness, musculoskeletal pain, neck stiffness.

Nervous System: abnormal EEG, areflexia, ataxia, central nervous system (CNS) dysfunction, delirium, dysphonia, dystonia, encephalopathy, gait abnormal aggravated, headache aggravated, hemiparesis, hyperkinesia, hyperreflexia, hypoesthesia, hyporeflexia, hypotonia, impaired coginition, impaired concentration, memory impairment, meningism, meningitis, migraine, mononeuritis, neuritis, neuropathy, paraplegia, peripheral neuropathy, restless leg syndrome, sciatica, speech disorder, stupor, twitching.

Psychiatric: abnormal dreaming, altered mental status, amnesia, anxiety, anxiety aggravated, confusion, depression, depression psychotic, emotional lability, libido decreased, nightmare, psychosis, sleep disorder.

Renal and Urinary System: abnormal urine, albuminuria, BUN increased, dysuria, hematuria, micturition disorder, micturition frequency, nephritis interstitial, nocturia, renal calculus, renal failure, renal failure acute, renal insufficiency aggravated, urinary tract obstruction NOS.

Reproductive System and Breast: balanoposthitis, breast pain.

Respiratory, Thoracic and Mediastinal: atelectasis, chest pain, nonproductive cough, dry throat, dyspnea, dyspnea aggravated, epistaxis, epistaxis aggravated, interstitial pneumonia, nasal congestion, nasal irritation, pharyngitis, pneumonitis, postnasal drip, pulmonary hypertension, pulmonary infiltration, rales, respiratory disorder, rhinitis, rhinorrhea.

Surgical and Medical Procedures: cardioversion.

Skin and Subcutaneous Tissue: acne, alopecia, dermatitis, dry skin, erythema, erythematous rash, face edema, fissures, follicular rash, furunculosis, macular rash, maculopapular rash, night sweats, pruritic rash, rash aggravated, seborrhea, skin disorder, skin nodule, urticaria, vesicular rash.

Abnormal Hematologic and Clinical Chemistry Findings: In (uncontrolled) trials of patients with IFIs treated with POSANOL doses ≥800 mg/day, the incidence of clinically significant liver function test abnormalities was: ALT and AST (>3×Upper Limit Normal [ULN]) 6% and 5%, respectively; total bilirubin (>1.5×ULN) 4%; and alkaline phosphatase (>3×ULN) 4%. In healthy volunteers, elevation of hepatic enzymes did not appear to be associated with higher plasma concentrations of POSANOL. In patients, the majority of abnormal liver function tests results showed minor and transient changes and rarely led to discontinuation of therapy.

In the comparative trials of patients infected with HIV and OPC treated with POSANOL at doses up to 400 mg, the incidence of clinically significant liver function test abnormalities was as follows; ALT and AST (>3×ULN), 1% and 3%, respectively: total bilirubin (>1.5×ULN), <1%; and alkaline phosphatase (>3×ULN), 1%.

In the comparative trials of hematopoietic stem cell recipients or patients with acute myelogenous leukemia receiving POSANOL as prophylaxis at doses up to 600 mg, the incidence of clinically significant liver function test abnormalities was as follows; ALT and AST (>3×ULN), 12 % and 4 %, respectively: total bilirubin (>1.5×ULN), 8 %; and alkaline phosphatase (>3×ULN), 2%.

Post-Market Adverse Drug Reactions: The following adverse events have been reported during the post-approval use of POSANOL in the US and Europe. Because these reactions are reported voluntarily from a population of uncertain size, it is not always possible to reliably estimate their frequency. A causal relationship to POSANOL could not be excluded for these adverse events, which included:

Blood and Lymphatic System: agranulocytosis.

Hepatobiliary: cytolytic hepatitis, toxic hepatitis (including fatality).

Cardiovascular: QT prolongation, torsades de pointes.

Infections and Infestations: Trichosporon sepsis.

DRUG INTERACTIONS:

Serious Drug Interactions

Contraindicated Drugs: ergot alkaloids, terfenadine, astemizole, cisapride, pimozide and quinidine (see Contra-indications)

Drugs whose concomitant use should be avoided: cimetidine, rifabutin and phenytoin (see Table 3 and Table 4 in Drug Interactions).

Drugs whose concomitant use requires consideration of dose reduction at initiation of concomitant treatment and close therapeutic monitoring of drug levels during treatment: cyclosporine, tacrolimus and sirolimus (see Table 4 in Drug Interactions).

Drugs whose concomitant use requires consideration of dose reduction and close monitoring for adverse events during treatment: vinca alkaloids, midazolam, HMG-CoA reductase inhibitors (statins), calcium channel blockers (see Table 4 in Drug Interactions).

Overview: Effect of Other Drugs on POSANOL Pharmacokinetics: POSANOL is metabolized via UDP glucuronidation (phase 2 enzymes) and is a substrate for p-glycoprotein efflux. Therefore, inhibitors or inducers of these clearance pathways may affect POSANOL plasma concentrations. POSANOL does not have any major circulating oxidative (CYP450 mediated) metabolites and its concentrations are thus unlikely to be altered by inhibitors of CYP450 enzymes.

Effects of POSANOL on Pharmacokinetics of Other Drugs: POSANOL is an inhibitor of CYP3A4 and thus the plasma levels of medicinal products that are metabolized through this enzyme pathway may increase when administered with POSANOL.

Drug-Drug Interactions: The drugs listed in Table 3 and Table 4 are based on either drug interaction case reports or studies, or potential interactions due to the expected magnitude and seriousness of the interaction (i.e., those identified as contraindicated).

The majority of drug interaction studies were performed with the POSANOL tablet, which is 36% less bioavailable than the suspension. The majority of drug interaction studies were performed using the 200 mg QD schedule whereas the recommended dosing schedule depends on the indication and may be as high as 400mg BID (rIFIs) or 200mg TID (prophylaxis). As a result of these limitations, the maximal exposure was not studied in the majority of these drug interaction studies.

Table 3: POSANOL

Summary of the Effect of Co-administered Drugs on POSANOL in Healthy Volunteers

Co-administered Drug (Postulated Mechanism of Interaction)	Ref	Co-administered Drug Dose/Schedule	POSANOL Dose/Schedule	Effect on Bioavailability of POSANOL: Change in Mean C_{max} (ratio estimate[a]; 90% CI of the ratio estimate)	Effect on Bioavailability of POSANOL: Change in Mean AUC[b] (ratio estimate; 90% CI of the ratio estimate)	Recommendations
Rifabutin (UDP-G Induction)	clinical trial	300 mg QD[c]×17 days	200 mg (tablets) QD×10 days	↓ 43% (0.57; 0.43–0.75)	↓ 49% (0.51; 0.37–0.71)	Concomitant use of POSANOL and rifabutin should be avoided unless the benefit to the patient outweighs the risk.
Phenytoin (UDP-G Induction)	clinical trial	200 mg QD×10 days	200 mg (tablets) QD×10 days	↓ 41% (0.59; 0.44–0.79)	↓ 50% (0.50; 0.36–0.71)	Concomitant use of POSANOL and phenytoin should be avoided unless the benefit to the patient outweighs the risk.
Cimetidine (Alteration of Gastric pH)	clinical trial	400 mg BID[d]×10 days	200 mg (tablets) QD×10 days	↓ 39% (0.61; 0.53–0.70)	↓ 39% (0.61; 0.54–0.69)	Concomitant use of POSANOL and cimetidine should be avoided unless the benefit outweighs the risk.
Antacids	clinical trial			No clinically relevant effect on POSANOL bioavailability was observed when administered with an antacid.		No differences in prophylactic efficacy or safety were observed, suggesting these agents may be used concomitantly with POSANOL.
H_2 receptor antagonists (H2RA) other than cimetidine	clinical trial			No clinically relevant effect on POSANOL bioavailability was observed when administered with an H2RA other than cimetidine. The effect of other H2RA (e.g., famotidine, ranitidine) on POSANOL Cav was evaluated in a large prophylaxis study (Study P01899). The concomitant use of H2RA, other than cimetidine, did not affect POSANOL Cav.		No differences in prophylactic efficacy or safety were observed, suggesting these agents may be used concomitantly with POSANOL.
Proton pump inhibitors (PPI)	clinical trial			No clinically relevant effect on POSANOL bioavailability was observed when administered with a PPI. The effect of other PPI (e.g., omeprazole) on POSANOL Cav was evaluated in a large prophylaxis study (Study P01899). The concomitant use of PPI was associated with an approximately 29 % reduction in the mean POSANOL plasma Cav.		No differences in prophylactic efficacy or safety were observed, suggesting these agents may be used concomitantly with POSANOL.
Glipizide	clinical trial	10 mg single dose		Glipizide had no clinically significant effect on POSANOL C_{max} and AUC.		No dose adjustments required. Glucose concentrations decreased in some healthy volunteers when glipizide was co-administered with POSANOL. Glucose concentrations should be monitored in accordance with the current standard of care for patients with diabetes when POSANOL is co-administered with glipizide.
Ritonavir	clinical trial	600 mg BID		Ritonavir had no clinically significant effect on POSANOL C_{max} and AUC.		No dose adjustments required.

[a] ratio estimate=ratio of co-administered drug plus POSANOL to POSANOL alone for C_{max} or AUC.
[b] AUC=area under the plasma concentration time curve.
[c] QD=once daily.
[d] BID=twice a day.

Table 4: POSANOL

Summary of the Effect of POSANOL on Co-administered Drugs in Healthy Volunteers and Patients

Co-administered Drug (Postulated Mechanism of Interaction)	Ref	Co-administered Drug Dose/Schedule	POSANOL Dose/Schedule	Effect on Bioavailability of POSANOL: Change in Mean C_{max} (ratio estimate[a]; 90% CI of the ratio estimate)	Effect on Bioavailability of POSANOL: Change in Mean AUC[b] (ratio estimate; 90% CI of the ratio estimate)	Recommendations
Cyclosporine (inhibition of CYP3A4 by POSANOL)	clinical trial	Stable maintenance dose in heart transplant recipients	200 mg (tablets) QD[c]×10 days	↑ cyclosporine whole blood trough concentrations Cyclosporine dose reductions of up to 29% were required		When initiating treatment with POSANOL in patients already receiving cyclosporine, reduction of the cyclosporine dose should be considered (e.g., to about 3/4 of the current dose). Thereafter blood levels of cyclosporine should be monitored carefully during co-administration and upon discontinuation of POSANOL treatment, the dose of cyclosporine should be adjusted as necessary.
Tacrolimus (inhibition of CYP3A4 by POSANOL)	clinical trial	0.05 mg/kg single oral dose	400 mg (oral suspension) BID[d]×7 days	↑ 121% (2.21; 2.01–2.42)	↑ 358% (4.58; 4.03–5.19)	When initiating treatment with POSANOL in patients already receiving tacrolimus, reduction of the tacrolimus dose should be considered (e.g., to about 1/3 of the current dose). Thereafter blood levels of tacrolimus should be monitored carefully during co-administration, and upon discontinuation of POSANOL, and the dose of tacrolimus should be adjusted as necessary.
Rifabutin (inhibition of CYP3A4 by POSANOL)	clinical trial	300 mg QD×17 days	200 mg (tablets) QD×10 days	↑ 31% (1.31; 1.10–1.57)	↑ 72% (1.72; 1.51–1.95)	Concomitant use of POSANOL and rifabutin should be avoided unless the benefit to the patient outweighs the risk. If the medicinal products are co-administered, careful monitoring of full blood counts and adverse effects related to increased rifabutin levels (e.g., uveitis) is recommended.
Midazolam (inhibition of CYP3A4 by POSANOL)	clinical trial	Single 30 min IV infusion of 0.05 mg/kg	200 mg (tablets) QD×10 days	NA[f]	↑ 83% (1.83; 1.57–2.14)	Dose adjustments of benzodiazepines metabolized by CYP3A4 should be considered during co-administration with POSANOL.
Phenytoin (inhibition of CYP34A by POSANOL)	clinical trial	200 mg QD PO[e]×10 days	200 mg (tablets) QD×10 days	↑ 16% (1.16; 0.85–1.57)	↑ 16% (1.16; 0.84–1.59)	Concomitant use of POSANOL and phenytoin should be avoided unless the benefit to the patient outweighs the risk. If the medicinal products are co-administered, frequent monitoring of phenytoin concentrations should be performed and dose reduction of phenytoin should be considered.
Ergot alkaloids	theoretical	NA, since theoretical		Although not studied in vitro or in vivo, POSANOL may ↑ the plasma concentration of ergot alkaloids (ergotamine and dihydroergotamine), which may lead to ergotism.		Co-administration of POSANOL and ergot alkaloids is contraindicated (see Contraindications).

(cont'd)

Table 4: POSANOL *(cont'd)*

Summary of the Effect of POSANOL on Co-administered Drugs in Healthy Volunteers and Patients

Co-administered Drug (Postulated Mechanism of Interaction)	Ref	Co-administered Drug Dose/Schedule	POSANOL Dose/Schedule	Effect on Bioavailability of POSANOL: Change in Mean C_{max} (ratio estimate[a]; 90% CI of the ratio estimate)	Change in Mean AUC[b] (ratio estimate; 90% CI of the ratio estimate)	Recommendations
Terfenadine Astemizole Cisapride Pimozide Quinidine	theoretical	NA, since theoretical		Although not studied in vitro or in vivo, co-administration of POSANOL and certain drugs such as cisapride, pimozide, and quinidine, metabolized through the CYP3A4 system may result in ↑ plasma concentrations of these medicinal products, leading to potentially serious and/or life threatening adverse events (QT prolongation and rare occurrences of torsade de pointes).		Co-administration of these drugs with POSANOL is contraindicated (see Contraindications).
Sirolimus	theoretical	NA, since theoretical		Although not studied in vitro or in vivo, POSANOL may ↑ the plasma concentration of sirolimus.		Monitoring of sirolimus blood levels should be performed upon initiation, during co-administration, and at discontinuation of POSANOL treatment, with sirolimus doses adjusted accordingly.
Vinca alkaloids	theoretical	NA, since theoretical		Although not studied in vitro or in vivo, POSANOL may ↑ the plasma concentration of vinca alkaloids (e.g., vincristine and vinblastine), which may lead to neurotoxicity.		It is recommended that the dose adjustment of vinca alkaloids be considered.
HMG-CoA reductase inhibitors metabolized through CYP3A4	theoretical	NA, since theoretical		Although not studied in vitro or in vivo, ↑ HMG-CoA reductase inhibitor concentrations in plasma can be associated with rhabdomyolysis.		Dose adjustments of HMG-CoA reductase inhibitors metabolized by CYP3A4 should be considered during co-administration with POSANOL.
Zidovudine (AZT) Lamivudine (3TC) Ritonavir Indinavir	clinical trial	In HIV infected patients on stable doses of AZT (300 mg BID or 200 mg every 8 hours (h)), 3TC (150 mg BID), ritonavir (600 mg BID) and/or indinavir (800 mg every 8 h).	200 mg (tablets) QD[c]×10 days	POSANOL had no clinically significant effect on the C_{max} and AUC of these medicinal products.		No dose adjustments required.
Calcium channel blockers metabolized through CYP3A4	theoretical	NA, since theoretical		Although not studied in vitro or in vivo, co-administration of POSANOL with calcium channel blockers metabolized through CYP3A4 may result in significant drug interactions.		Frequent monitoring for adverse effects and toxicity related to calcium channel blockers is recommended during co-administration with POSANOL. Dose adjustment of calcium channel blockers may be required.
Digoxin	theoretical	NA, since theoretical		POSANOL may increase plasma concentration of digoxin.		Co-administration of other azoles with digoxin has been associated with increases in digoxin levels. Thus, POSANOL may increase plasma concentration of digoxin and digoxin levels should be monitored when initiated or discontinuing POSANOL treatment.

[a] ratio estimate=ratio of co-administered drug plus POSANOL to POSANOL alone for C_{max} or AUC.
[b] AUC=area under the plasma concentration time curve.
[c] QD=once daily.
[d] BID=twice a day.
[e] PO=per os.
[f] NA=Not applicable if administered as an IV.

Drug-Food Interactions: See Table 5.

Table 5: POSANOL

Established or Potential Drug-food Interactions

Proper name	Ref	Effect	Clinical comment
Caffeine	clinical trial	No clinically significant effect has been noted.	No dose adjustments required.
Food or nutritional supplement	clinical trial	The AUC of POSANOL is about 4 times greater when administered with a high-fat meal (~50 grams fat) and about 2.6 times greater when administered with a nonfat meal or nutritional supplement (14 g fat) relative to the fasted state.	Each dose of POSANOL should be administered with food or nutritional supplement (see Dosage and Administration).

Drug-Herb Interactions: Interactions with herbal products have not been studied.
Drug-Laboratory Test Interactions: Interactions with laboratory tests have not been studied.

DOSAGE AND ADMINISTRATION: Dosing Considerations:

- Each dose of POSANOL should be administered with a meal, or with a nutritional supplement in patients who cannot tolerate food to enhance the oral absorption. For patients who cannot eat a full meal or tolerate an oral nutritional supplement, alternative antifungal therapy should be considered or patients should be monitored closely for breakthrough fungal infections.
- Patients who have severe diarrhea or vomiting should be monitored closely for breakthrough fungal infections
- Co-administration of drugs that can decrease the plasma concentrations of POSANOL should generally be avoided unless the benefit outweighs the risk. If such drugs are necessary, patients should be monitored closely for breakthrough fungal infections. (See Drug Interactions.)

Recommended Dose and Dosage Adjustment: See Table 6.

Table 6: POSANOL

Recommended Dose According to Indication

Indication	Dose and Duration of Therapy
Prophylaxis of Invasive Fungal Infections (IFIs)	200 mg (5 mL) three times a day. The duration of therapy is based on recovery from neutropenia or immunosuppression. For patients with acute myelogenous leukemia (AML) or myelodysplastic syndromes (MDS), prophylaxis with POSANOL should start several days before the anticipated onset of neutropenia and continue for 7 days after the neutrophil count rises above 500 cells per mm^3.
Refractory IFIs/Intolerant Patients with IFIs	400 mg (10 mL) twice a day. In patients who cannot tolerate a meal or a nutritional supplement, POSANOL should be administered at a dose of 200 mg (5 mL) four times a day. Duration of therapy should be based on the severity of the underlying disease, recovery from immunosuppression, and clinical response.
Oropharyngeal Candidiasis (OPC)	Loading dose of 100 mg (2.5 mL) twice a day on the first day, then 100 mg (2.5 mL) once a day for 13 days.

Increasing the total daily dose above 800 mg does not further enhance the exposure to POSANOL.

Use in Renal Impairment: POSANOL is not significantly renally eliminated. No dose adjustment is required in patients with renal dysfunction. (See Action and Clinical Pharmacology.)

Use in Hepatic Impairment: There are limited pharmacokinetic data in patients with hepatic insufficiency; therefore, no recommendation for dose adjustment can be made. In the small number of subjects studied who had hepatic insufficiency, there was an increase in half-life with a decrease in hepatic function (see Action and Clinical Pharmacology). Use with caution in patients with severe hepatic impairment. (See Action and Clinical Pharmacology.)

Use in Pediatrics (13-17 years): A total of 11 patients 13-17 years of age were treated with 800 mg/day in a study for IFIs. Additionally, 12 patients 13-17 years of age received 600 mg/day for prophylaxis of IFIs (studies C/I98-316 and P01899). The safety profile in these patients <18 years of age appears similar to the safety profile observed in adults. Based on pharmacokinetic data in 10 of these pediatric patients, the pharmacokinetic profile appears to be similar to patients ≥18 years of age (see Action and Clinical Pharmacology).

Missed Dose: If a dose of this medication is missed, it should be taken as soon as possible. This will help to keep a constant amount of medication in the blood. However, if it is almost time for the next dose, it might be better to skip the missed dose and to go back to the regular dosing schedule.

Administration: Shake well before each use.

OVERDOSAGE:

During clinical trials, patients who received POSANOL doses up to 1,600 mg/day had no noted adverse reactions different from those reported with patients at the lower doses. In addition, accidental overdose was noted in one patient who took 1,200 mg BID for 3 days. No adverse reactions were noted by the investigator.

In a trial of patients with severe hemodialysis-dependent renal dysfunction (Cl_{cr} <20 mL/min), POSANOL was not removed by hemodialysis.

Activated charcoal may be used to remove unabsorbed drug.

For management of a suspected drug overdose, CPhA recommends that you contact your **regional Poison Control Centre**. See the *CPS* Directory section for a list of Poison Control Centres.

ACTION AND CLINICAL PHARMACOLOGY: Mechanism of Action: POSANOL is a potent inhibitor of the enzyme lanosterol 14α-demethylase, which catalyses an essential step in ergosterol biosynthesis. Consequently, POSANOL exhibits broad-spectrum antifungal activity against a variety of yeasts and moulds including species of Candida (including *C. albicans* isolates resistant to fluconazole, voriconazole and itraconazole, *C. krusei* and *C. glabrata* which are inherently less susceptible to fluconazole, and *C. lusitaniae* which is inherently less susceptible to amphotericin B), Aspergillus (including isolates resistant to fluconazole, voriconazole, itraconazole and amphotericin B) and organisms not previously regarded as being susceptible to azoles such as the zygomycetes (e.g., species of Absidia, Mucor, Rhizopus and Rhizomucor). In vitro POSANOL exhibited fungicidal activity against species of Aspergillus, dimorphic fungi (*B. dermatitidis, H. capsulatum, P. marneffei*, and *C. immitis*) and some species of Candida. In animal infection models POSANOL was active against a wide variety of fungal infections caused by moulds or yeasts. However, there was no consistent correlation between minimum inhibitory concentration (MIC) and efficacy.

Pharmacodynamics: A correlation between total drug exposure (AUC) and clinical outcome has been observed. For subjects with Aspergillus infections, effective drug exposure appears to be higher than that for infections caused by Candida species, although the critical AUC/MIC ratio associated with clinical success is uncertain. It is particularly important to try to ensure that maximal plasma levels are achieved in patients infected with Aspergillus (see Dosage and Administration and Action and Clinical Pharmacology, Pharmacokinetics on recommended dose regimens and the effects of food on absorption).

Pharmacokinetics: The mean pharmacokinetic parameters in healthy volunteers following administration of POSANOL 400 mg BID for 7 days are displayed in Table 7.

Dose proportional increases in plasma exposure (AUC) to POSANOL were observed following single oral doses from 50 mg to 800 mg and following multiple dose administration from 50 mg BID to 400 mg BID. No further increases in exposure were observed when the dose was increased from 400 BID to 600 mg BID in febrile neutropenic patients or those with rIFIs.

Absorption: POSANOL is absorbed with a median T_{max} of ~3 to 5 hours. Dose proportional increases in plasma exposure (AUC) to POSANOL were observed following single oral doses from 50 mg to 800 mg and following multiple-dose administration from 50 mg BID to 400 mg BID. No further increases in exposure were observed when the dose was increased from 400 mg BID to 600 mg BID in febrile neutropenic patients or those with rIFIs. Steady-state plasma concentrations are attained at 7 to 10 days following multiple-dose administration.

Table 7: POSANOL

Mean Pharmacokinetic Parameters of POSANOL in Healthy Volunteers

Population	Dose	Mean (% CV)				
		C_{max} (ng/mL)	$t_{½}$ (h)	$AUC_{(t)}$ (ng·h/mL)	Clearance (L/h)	Volume of Distribution (L)
Healthy Volunteers	400 mg BID (n=174)	2850	35	29 453	32.3	1744

Following single-dose administration of 200 mg, the mean AUC and C_{max} of POSANOL are approximately 3 times higher when administered with a nonfat meal and approximately 4 times higher when administered with a high-fat meal (~50 g fat) relative to the fasted state. Following single-dose administration of 400 mg, the mean AUC and C_{max} of POSANOL are approximately 3 times higher when administered with a liquid nutritional supplement (14 g fat) relative to the fasted state (see Table 8). In order to assure attainment of adequate plasma concentrations, it is recommended to administer POSANOL with food or a nutritional supplement. (See Dosage and Administration.)

Table 8: POSANOL

The Mean (% CV) [min-max] POSANOL Pharmacokinetic Parameters Following Single-Dose Suspension Administration of 200 mg and 400 mg Under Fed and Fasted Conditions

Dose (mg)	C_{max} (ng/mL)	T_{max}[a] (h)	AUC(I) (ng·h/mL)	CL/F (L/h)	$t_{½}$ (h)
200 mg fasted (n=20)[c]	132 (50) [45–267]	3.50 [1.5–36[b]]	4179 (31) [2705–7269]	51 (25) [28–74]	23.5 (25) [15.3–33.7]
200 mg nonfat (n=20)[c]	378 (43) [131–834]	4 [3–5]	10 753 (35) [4579–17 092]	21 (39) [12–44]	22.2 (18) [17.4–28.7]
200 mg high fat (54 g fat) (n=20)[c]	512 (34) [241–1016]	5 [4–5]	15 059 (26) [10 341–24 476]	14 (24) [8.2–19]	23.0 (19) [17.2–33.4]
400 mg fasted (n=23)[d]	121 (75) [27–366]	4 [2–12]	5258 (48) [2834–9567]	91 (40) [42–141]	27.3 (26) [16.8–38.9]
400 mg with liquid nutritional supplement (14 g fat) (n=23)[d]	355 (43) [145–720]	5 [4–8]	11 295 (40) [3865–20 592]	43 (56) [19–103]	26.0 (19) [18.2–35.0]

[a] Median [min-max].
[b] The subject with T_{max} of 36 h had relatively constant plasma levels over 36 h (1.7 ng/mL difference between 4 h and 36 h).
[c] n=15 for AUC(I), CL/F and $t_{½}$.
[d] n=10 for AUC(I), CL/F and $t_{½}$.

Distribution: POSANOL has an apparent volume of distribution of 1774 L, suggesting extensive extravascular distribution and penetration into the body tissues.

POSANOL is highly protein bound (>98%), predominantly to albumin.

Metabolism: POSANOL primarily circulates as the parent compound in plasma. Of the circulating metabolites, the majority are glucuronide conjugates formed via UDP glucuronidation (phase 2 enzymes). POSANOL does not have any major circulating oxidative (CYP450 mediated) metabolites. The excreted metabolites in urine and feces account for ~17% of the administered radiolabeled dose.

Excretion: POSANOL is eliminated with a mean half-life ($t_{½}$) of 35 hours (range 20 to 66 hours) and a total body clearance (CL/F) of 32 L/h. POSANOL is predominantly eliminated in the feces (71% of the radiolabeled dose up to 120 hours) with the major component eliminated as parent drug (66% of the radiolabeled dose). Renal clearance is a minor elimination pathway, with 13% of the radiolabeled dose excreted in urine up to 120 hours (<0.2% of the radiolabeled dose is parent drug).

Summary of Pharmacokinetic Parameters: The mean (% CV) [min-max] POSANOL average steady-state plasma concentrations (Cav) and steady-state pharmacokinetic parameters in patients following administration of 200 mg TID and 400 mg BID of the oral suspension are provided in Table 9.

Table 9: POSANOL

The Mean (% CV) [min-max] POSANOL Steady-State Pharmacokinetic Parameters in Patients Following Oral Administration of Posaconazole 200 mg TID and 400 mg BID

Dose[a]	Cav (ng/mL)	AUC[e] (ng·h/mL)	CL/F (L/h)	V/F (L)	$t_{½}$ (h)
200 mg TID[b] (n=252)	1103 (67) [21.5–3650]	ND[f]	ND[f]	ND[f]	ND[f]
200 mg TID[c] (n=215)	583 (65) [89.7–2200]	15 900 (62) [4100–56 100]	51.2 (54) [10.7–146]	2425 (39) [828–5702]	37.2 (39) [19.1–148]
400 mg BID[d] (n=23)	723 (86) [6.70–2256]	9093 (80) [1564–26 794]	76.1 (78) [14.9–256]	3088 (84) [407–13 140]	31.7 (42) [12.4–67.3]

[a] Oral suspension administration.
[b] Allogeneic hematopoietic stem cell transplant (HSCT) recipients with graft-versus-host disease.
[c] Neutropenic patients who were receiving cytotoxic chemotherapy for acute myelogenous leukemia or myelodysplastic syndromes.
[d] Febrile neutropenic patients or patients with refractory invasive fungal infections, Cav n=24.
[e] AUC (0-24 h) for 200 mg TID and AUC (0-12 h) for 400 mg BID.
[f] Not done.
Note: Cav based on observed data; other pharmacokinetic parameters based on estimates from population pharmacokinetic analyses.

The variability in average plasma posaconazole concentrations in patients was relatively higher than that in healthy subjects.

Special Populations and Conditions: Pediatrics: Mean trough plasma concentrations from 12 patients 8-17 years of age were similar to concentrations from 194 patients 18-64 years of age. No pharmacokinetic data are available from pediatric patients less than 8 years of age.

Geriatrics: The pharmacokinetics of POSANOL are comparable in young and elderly subjects (≥65 years of age). No adjustment in the dosage of POSANOL is necessary in elderly patients (≥65 years of age) based on age.

Gender: The pharmacokinetics of POSANOL are comparable in men and women. No adjustment in the dosage of POSANOL is necessary based on gender.

Race: The AUC and C_{max} of POSANOL decreased slightly in Black subjects relative to Caucasian subjects. No other races were studied.

Hepatic Insufficiency: The pharmacokinetic data in subjects with hepatic impairment was not sufficient to determine if dose adjustment is necessary in patients with hepatic dysfunction. It is recommended that POSANOL be used with caution in patients with hepatic impairment. (See Warnings and Precautions and Dosage and Administration.)

Renal Insufficiency: Following single-dose administration of 400 mg of the oral suspension, there was no significant effect of mild (Cl_{cr}: 50-80 mL/min/1.73m^2, n=6) and moderate (Cl_{cr}: 20-49 mL/min/1.73m^2, n=6) renal insufficiency on posaconazole pharmacokinetics; therefore, no dose adjustment is required in patients with mild to moderate renal impairment. In subjects with severe renal insufficiency (Cl_{cr}: <20 mL/min/1.73m^2), the mean plasma exposure (AUC) was similar to that in patients with normal renal function (Cl_{cr}: >80 mL/min/1.73m^2); however, the range of the AUC estimates was highly variable (CV=96%) in these subjects with severe renal insufficiency as compared to that in the other renal impairment groups (CV <40%). Due to the variability in exposure, patients with severe renal impairment should be monitored closely for breakthrough fungal infections. (See Dosage and Administration.)

STORAGE AND STABILITY: Store at room temperature (15 to 30°C). Do not freeze.
Do not use past expiry date on the label.

Shelf Life: After first opening the container: 4 weeks

SPECIAL HANDLING INSTRUCTIONS: The oral suspension must be shaken well before each use.

INFORMATION FOR THE PATIENT: Published in e-CPS, available by subscription at www.e-cps.ca.

DOSAGE FORMS, COMPOSITION AND PACKAGING: Each mL of white, cherry flavored immediate-release oral suspension contains: posaconazole 40 mg. Nonmedicinal ingredients: artificial cherry flavor, citric acid monohydrate, glycerin, liquid glucose, polysorbate 80, purified water, simethicone, sodium benzoate, sodium citrate dihydrate, titanium dioxide and xanthan gum. Bottles (glass amber type IV) of 123 mL (105 mL of oral suspension) closed with a plastic child-resistant cap (polypropylene) and a measuring spoon (polystyrene) with 2 graduations: 2.5 mL and 5 mL.

Potaba® Ⓟ

aminobenzoate potassium

Antifibrotic

Glenwood

INDICATIONS: Peyronie's disease. Scleroderma. Dermatomyositis. Morphea and linear scleroderma.

CONTRAINDICATIONS: Patients taking sulfonamides.

WARNINGS: *Pregnancy:* Safety for use in pregnancy has not been established.
Lactation: Safety for use during lactation has not been established.

PRECAUTIONS: Should anorexia or nausea occur, therapy is interrupted until the patient is eating normally again. This permits prompt subsidence of symptoms and also avoids the possible development of hypoglycemia. Give cautiously to patients with renal disease. If a hypersensitivity reaction should occur, aminobenzoate should be stopped.

ADVERSE EFFECTS: Anorexia, nausea, fever and rash have occurred infrequently and subside with omission of the drug. Desensitization can be accomplished and treatment resumed.

OVERDOSE:
No data supplied by the manufacturer.

For management of a suspected drug overdose, CPhA recommends that you contact your **regional Poison Control Centre**. See the *CPS* Directory section for a list of Poison Control Centres.

DOSAGE: Adults: 12 g given in 4 divided doses.

Tablets and capsules are given at the rate of 6 tablets or capsules 4 times daily, usually with meals, and at bedtime with a snack. Tablets must be crushed and taken with an adequate amount of liquid to prevent gastrointestinal upset.

Envules each contain 2 g of pure drug, and constitute the individual average dose. Six envules are given for a total of 12 g daily.

INFORMATION FOR THE PATIENT: Published in e-CPS, available by subscription at www.e-cps.ca.

SUPPLIED: Capsules: Each capsule contains: aminobenzoate potassium USP 500 mg. Nonmedicinal ingredients: magnesium stearate NF, microcrystalline cellulose NF, povidone USP, silica gel NF, sodium starch glycolate NF, stearic acid NF. Bottles of 250 and 1 000.

Powder: Each envule contains: aminobenzoate potassium USP 2 g. Nonmedicinal ingredients: magnesium stearate NF, microcrystalline cellulose NF, povidone USP, silica gel NF, sodium starch glycolate NF, stearic acid NF. Boxes of 50.

Tablets: Each tablet contains: aminobenzoate potassium USP 500 mg. Nonmedicinal ingredients: magnesium stearate NF, microcrystalline cellulose NF, povidone USP, silica gel NF, sodium starch glycolate NF, stearic acid NF. Bottles of 100 and 1 000.

Store in a cool place and in well-closed containers.

Potassium Chloride

potassium chloride

Electrolyte Replenisher

Hospira

SUPPLIED: Each mL contains: potassium 2 mEq (potassium chloride 149 mg). Nonmedicinal ingredients: hydrochloric acid and water for injection. Single-dose vials of 10 mL (20 mEq K^+) and 20 mL (40 mEq K^+) both available in trays of 25 vials, and 250 mL (500 mEq K^+) available in trays of 12 vials. Must be diluted for i.v. use. Avoid excessive heat. Protect from freezing. Store at room temperature (25°C).

Potassium Salts

potassium chloride
potassium citrate
potassium gluconate

Potassium Replacement Therapy

CPhA Monograph

Date of Revision: October 2006

This monograph has been compiled by CPhA and reviewed by experts. It may contain information different from that found in Health Canada-approved Product Monographs. The reader is referred to the *CPS* Editorial Policy for more information.

SUMMARY PRODUCT INFORMATION:

Drug	Route of Administration	Dosage Form	Strength
Potassium chloride	IV	solution	2 mEq potassium/mL (single dose vials 10, 20, 30 mL)
	Oral	capsules, microencapsulated — sustained release	8 mEq potassium/capsule
	Oral	liquid	20 mEq potassium/15 mL (500 mL)
	Oral	powder	25 mEq potassium/packet plus 25 mEq chloride/packet (30 packets)
	Oral	tablets, sustained release	20 mEq potassium/tablet
	Oral	tablets, wax matrix — slow release	8 mEq potassium/tablet
Potassium citrate	Oral	solution	10 mEq potassium/5 mL (475 mL)
	Oral	tablets, effervescent	25 mEq potassium/tablet (30 tablets)
Potassium gluconate	Oral	caplets	166 mg potassium/tablet
	Oral	solution	20 mEq potassium/15 mL (500 mL)

PHARMACOLOGY: Potassium is the principal intracellular cation of body tissues. Potassium ions are involved in a number of essential physiologic processes, such as the maintenance of intracellular acid-base balance and isotonicity. Potassium also plays an integral role in the transmission of nerve impulses, contraction of cardiac, skeletal and smooth muscle, gastric secretion, normal renal function, tissue synthesis and carbohydrate metabolism.

Hypokalemia: Potassium depletion may occur whenever the rate of loss exceeds the rate of intake. Causes of hypokalemia include: inadequate intake diuretic therapy, diabetic ketoacidosis, metabolic alkalosis, potassium-losing nephropathy, severe diarrhea, prolonged vomiting, drainage of gastrointestinal fluids, hyperaldosteronism, hepatic cirrhosis with ascites, Bartter's syndrome and long-term corticosteroid therapy. The need for potassium supplementation in patients taking potassium-depleting medications may sometimes be avoided by increasing dietary intake of potassium. Potassium is found in foods such as green leafy vegetables, fruit (e.g., bananas, oranges), potatoes, lean meat, whole grains and milk.

Potassium deficiency is often asymptomatic, especially if mild. However, symptoms may include vomiting, abdominal distention, paralytic ileus, acute muscular weakness, paralysis, paresthesia, polydipsia and an inability to concentrate urine, hypotension, cardiac arrhythmias, and coma. Hypokalemia may also potentiate digoxin cardiotoxicity.

Hyperkalemia: Manifestations of hyperkalemia include ECG changes which ultimately may progress to complete heart block, ventricular arrhythmias or cardiac arrest. Symptoms of hyperkalemia may or may not be present and can include weakness, parasthesias of the extremities, listlessness, confusion, cold skin, gray pallor, peripheral vascular collapse, hypotension and muscular or respiratory paralysis (see Overdose).

Pharmacokinetics: Potassium is readily absorbed from the gastrointestinal tract. Potassium is actively transported into cells from the extracellular fluid. Dextrose, insulin and bicarbonate facilitate movement of potassium into cells. Normal adult values for serum potassium range from 3.5 to 5 mmol/L. Serum potassium concentrations may not be an accurate indicator of total body stores, as intracellular potassium accounts for 98% of total body amount. Excretion is mainly in the urine (85 to 90%) and closely follows potassium intake. Potassium is readily removed by peritoneal dialysis or hemodialysis.

Slow-Release Preparations: Expanded controlled-release matrix may be seen in stools; this is not an indication of poor bioavailability.

INDICATIONS: Potassium is indicated for:

- prevention of potassium depletion when dietary intake of potassium is inadequate
- treatment of potassium depletion in patients with hypokalemia
- treatment of chronic digitalis intoxication associated with hypokalemia
- treatment of hypokalemic familial periodic paralysis

CONTRAINDICATIONS: In hyperkalemia; renal impairment with oliguria, anuria or azotemia; ventricular fibrillation; untreated Addison's disease; salt-losing adrenal hyperplasia; in extensive tissue breakdown as in severe burns, crush syndrome, acute dehydration and heat cramps; severe hemolytic syndrome; increased sensitivity to potassium administration (e.g., in congenital paramyotonia or adynamia episodica hereditaria); hyporeninemic hypoaldosteronism or hyperadrenalism associated with adrenogenital syndrome.

All solid dosage forms of potassium supplements are contraindicated in any patient in whom there is cause for arrest or delay in tablet passage through the gastrointestinal tract. In these instances, potassium supplementation should be with a liquid preparation.

Slow-release potassium chloride preparations have produced esophageal ulceration in certain cardiac patients with esophageal compression due to an enlarged left atrium. The administration of these preparations is contraindicated in such patients as well as in patients with dysphagia.

WARNINGS: In patients with impaired mechanisms for excreting potassium, e.g., renal function impairment, administration of potassium salts can produce hyperkalemia and cardiac arrest. This is of particular concern in patients receiving i.v. potassium but may also occur in patients taking oral potassium. Potentially fatal hyperkalemia can develop rapidly and may be asymptomatic. Careful monitoring of the serum potassium concentration and appropriate dosage adjustment is required.

The concomitant use of potassium supplements with drugs that increase serum potassium may result in severe hyperkalemia (see Precautions, Drug Interactions).

Slow-release preparations should be avoided in patients at high risk for potassium chloride-induced gastrointestinal lesions, i.e., patients with cardiomegaly, esophageal stricture or compression, dysphagia, recent gastric surgery, delayed intestinal transit, ulcerative bowel disease or diverticulitis. Wax-matrix or extended-release tablets should be discontinued immediately if abdominal pain, distension, severe vomiting or gastrointestinal bleeding occur. Enteric-coated tablets have an unacceptably high rate of gastrointestinal adverse effects (40 to 50 incidents per 100 000 patient years) and should not be used.

Administration of undiluted potassium injection can be fatal. Parenteral potassium chloride solutions must be well diluted, thoroughly mixed and administered by slow i.v. infusion. Pain at the injection site and phlebitis may occur. Extravasation is to be avoided.

PRECAUTIONS: The treatment of potassium depletion, particularly in the presence of cardiac disease, renal disease or acidosis, requires careful attention to acid-base balance and appropriate monitoring of serum electrolytes, ECG and the patient's clinical status.

Use potassium with caution in diseases associated with heart block since increased serum potassium may increase the degree of block.

Potassium balance is markedly altered in patients with diabetic ketoacidosis. Generally, total potassium is depleted and patients present with potassium deficits of 3 to 5 mmol/kg or greater; however the serum potassium concentration may be high, normal or low depending on the degree of acidosis and volume depletion. Following insulin administration, monitor serum potassium concentrations closely as hyperkalemia can be rapidly converted to hypokalemia.

The presence of hypomagnesemia can make it more difficult to correct a coexisting hypokalemia. Therefore, hypomagnesemia should be corrected at the same time as hypokalemia.

The use of salt substitutes containing potassium chloride can lead to hyperkalemia in patients with renal impairment.

Pregnant women: Exogenous potassium may be indicated in pregnant women with low potassium levels. Appropriate monitoring of potassium serum levels is recommended, as high or low potassium levels can be detrimental to both maternal and fetal cardiac function.

Nursing women: If maternal serum potassium levels are maintained in the physiologic range, potassium supplementation is considered compatible with breast-feeding.

Drug Interactions: Extreme caution is advised if potassium salts are used concomitantly with angiotensin converting enzyme (ACE) inhibitors or potassium-sparing diuretics, i.e., amiloride, spironolactone or triamterene because of the potential for severe hyperkalemia. Closely monitor potassium levels and renal function.

ADVERSE EFFECTS: Nausea, vomiting, diarrhea, unpleasant taste (liquids) and abdominal cramps have been reported. Injection site pain or phlebitis can occur with i.v. administration of solutions of potassium salts. This is more common if the concentration of potassium is above 30 mmol/L. Severe adverse effects reported with potassium preparations have included hyperkalemia and arrhythmias (see Overdose); intestinal, esophageal and gastric ulceration (see Warnings).

OVERDOSE:

Signs and Symptoms: If excretory mechanisms are impaired or if potassium is administered too rapidly i.v., potentially fatal hyperkalemia can result. Paresthesia of the extremities, listlessness, mental confusion, gastrointestinal symptoms, weakness, heaviness of legs, paralysis, hypotension, cardiac arrhythmias, heart block and cardiac arrest may occur. Frequently, hyperkalemia is asymptomatic and may be manifested only by increased serum potassium concentration and characteristic ECG changes.

Progressive ECG changes occur with increasing serum potassium levels and indicate the need for immediate treatment. ECG changes include increased amplitude and peaking of the T waves, depression of the ST segment, reduction in the amplitude of the R wave, widening of the QRS complex, prolongation of the PR interval, and a decrease in the amplitude and ultimately disappearance of the P wave. Widening of the QRS complex is one of the most ominous signs and indicates the need for aggressive treatment. The terminal event is usually asystole or ventricular fibrillation.

Recommended Management: Discontinue administration of potassium-rich foods, medications and i.v. solutions containing potassium, or medications that can induce hyperkalemia.

In patients with severe hyperkalemia (e.g., serum potassium exceeds 7 mmol/L) or if any ECG manifestations of hyperkalemia exist, immediate treatment is required. The plasma potassium concentration and ECG must be monitored, as well as serum electrolytes, creatinine, glucose and arterial blood gases. I.V. calcium may be administered to antagonize the cardiotoxic effects of potassium. The usual dose of calcium is 10 to 20 mL of calcium gluconate 10% i.v. over 2 to 5 min. This may be repeated once after 5 to 10 min if the ECG does not improve. The ECG should be monitored continuously during administration of i.v. calcium. The use of i.v. calcium is not recommended in patients receiving digoxin. To promote a shift of potassium from the extracellular to the intracellular compartment, agents such as dextrose and insulin or sodium bicarbonate may be used. 300 to 500 mL of dextrose 10% containing 10 to 20 units of regular insulin per litre may be infused over a 1-hour period. Alternately, give 25 g of dextrose i.v. (e.g., 50 mL of a dextrose 50% prefilled syringe) accompanied by 5 to 10 units of regular insulin i.v. over 5 minutes. To correct acidosis and to promote intracellular potassium shift, sodium bicarbonate 50 mmol (e.g., 50 mL of a sodium bicarbonate 8.4% prefilled syringe) may be given i.v. over 5 minutes and repeated every 5 to 10 minutes as necessary. Bicarbonate must be used with caution in patients at risk for fluid overload.

When ECG approaches normal, measures to reduce total body stores of potassium such as cation exchange resins (e.g., sodium or calcium polystyrene sulfonate) may be employed. Hemodialysis or peritoneal dialysis should be considered if the above measures fail or the patient is in renal failure. However, peritoneal dialysis is only 15 to 20% as effective as hemodialysis.

In treating hyperkalemia in patients receiving digoxin, lowering the serum potassium concentration too rapidly can produce digoxin toxicity.

For management of a suspected drug overdose, CPhA recommends that you contact your **regional Poison Control Centre**. See the *CPS* Directory section for a list of Poison Control Centres.

DOSAGE: The usual dietary intake of potassium by the average adult is 40 to 80 mmol/day. For information on food sources of potassium, see Pharmacology.

Potassium depletion sufficient to cause hypokalemia usually requires the loss of ≥200 mmol of potassium from the total body store.

Dosage must be individualized according to the patient's needs. Whenever possible, potassium supplementation should be given orally (or via nasogastric tube). Dosage must be reduced in patients with renal failure and administered with great caution, if at all.

Table 1 lists the elemental potassium content of the various salts.

Table 1: Potassium Salts

Elemental Potassium Content

Potassium Salt	% elemental K^+	Elemental K^+/g (mmol)[a]
Potassium acetate	40	10.2
Potassium chloride	52	13.4
Potassium citrate	36	9.3
Potassium gluconate	17	4.3

[a] 1 g elemental K^+ = 25.6 mEq = 25.6 mmol.

Potassium chloride is generally the salt of choice in treating hypokalemia, as hypochloremia is usually an accompanying factor. However, metabolic acidosis may rarely coincide with hypokalemia, in which case an alkalinizing salt may be preferable, e.g., citrate or gluconate.

Oral: Adults: Tablets should be administered whole with a full glass of water, and should not be broken or chewed. Oral liquids, soluble powders and effervescent tablets should be mixed or dissolved completely in 100 to 200 mL of cold water, juice or other liquid and drunk slowly. Administer with or after meals in 2 or 3 divided doses per day to minimize gastric irritation and prevent too rapid absorption.

Prevention of Hypokalemia: 20 to 40 mmol/day.

Treatment of Depletion: 40 to a maximum of 100 mmol/day. In general, a daily dose exceeding 60 mmol should not be required.

Parenteral: For i.v. administration only; **dilute concentrated solutions before infusing**. The dose and rate of infusion are dependent on the individual patient's condition.

Adults: Generally, potassium concentrations in peripheral i.v. solutions should not exceed 40 mmol/L. Higher concentrations (e.g., 60 mmol/L) may be needed in cases of severe hypokalemia or fluid restriction and should be administered via a central line. Care must be taken to avoid extravasation.

In patients whose serum potassium concentration is above 2.5 mmol/L, the rate of infusion should not exceed 10 mmol/hour. The total dose should not exceed 200 mmol/24 hours.

For urgent treatment (serum potassium concentration <2 mmol/L with ECG changes or paralysis), infuse potassium at a rate of 40 mmol/hour, up to a maximum of 400 mmol/24-hour period. If doses greater than 20 mmol/hour are used, an infusion pump, ECG and frequent serum potassium monitoring are essential. In critical states, potassium may be infused in saline (unless saline is contraindicated) rather than in dextrose solutions, as the latter may decrease serum potassium concentrations by producing an intracellular shift.

Children: 2 to 3 mmol/kg/day or 40 mmol/m²/day with serum level monitoring.

Pradax™ 🅿

dabigatran etexilate mesilate

Anticoagulant

Boehringer Ingelheim

Date of Revision: July 31, 2009

SUMMARY PRODUCT INFORMATION:

Route of Administration	Dosage Form/ Strength	Clinically Relevant Nonmedicinal Ingredients
Oral	Capsules 75 mg, 110 mg	Tartaric acid, acacia, hypromellose, dimeticone, talc, hydroxypropyl cellulose For a complete listing see Dosage Forms, Composition and Packaging.

INDICATIONS AND CLINICAL USE: PRADAX (dabigatran etexilate) is indicated for the prevention of venous thromboembolic events (VTE) in patients who have undergone elective total hip replacement or total knee replacement surgery.

Geriatrics (>65 years of age): Clinical studies have been conducted in a patient population with a mean age >65 years (see Warnings and Precautions, Geriatrics (>65 years of age), and Renal; Dosage and Administration, Renal Impairment, and Elderly).

Pediatrics (<18 years of age): The safety and efficacy of PRADAX have not been established in children less than 18 years of age, therefore PRADAX is not recommended in this patient population.

CONTRAINDICATIONS:

- Severe renal impairment (CrCL <30 mL/min)
- Haemorrhagic manifestations, bleeding diathesis, or patients with spontaneous or pharmacological impairment of haemostasis
- Lesions at risk of clinically significant bleeding, e.g. cerebral infarction (hemorrhagic or ischemic) within the last 6 months
- Concomitant treatment with strong P-glycoprotein inhibitors, e.g. quinidine (see Drug Interactions)
- Known hypersensitivity to dabigatran or dabigatran etexilate or to any ingredient in the formulation or component of the container. For a complete listing, see the Dosage Forms, Composition and Packaging.

WARNINGS AND PRECAUTIONS: The following Warnings and Precautions are listed in alphabetical order.

Hematologic: As with all anticoagulants, bleeding may occur. Should severe bleeding occur, treatment with PRADAX must be discontinued and the source of bleeding investigated promptly.

Treatment that should NOT be administered concomitantly with PRADAX due to increase in bleeding risk, includes: unfractionated heparin and heparin derivatives, low molecular weight heparins (LMWH), fondaparinux, bivalirudin, thrombolytic agents, GPIIb/IIIa receptor antagonists, clopidogrel, ticlopidine, sulfinpyrazone, and vitamin K antagonists, such as warfarin. Unfractionated heparin can be administered at doses necessary to maintain a patent central venous or arterial catheter.

Acetylsalicylic acid (ASA) at doses of 81 to 325 mg daily has been shown to increase risk of bleeding when given concomitantly with PRADAX at doses above those currently recommended, i.e. above 220 mg daily. Co-administration of low-dose ASA, i.e. ≤160 mg daily with PRADAX has not been adequately studied and is not recommended.

Close observation, e.g. looking for signs of bleeding or anemia is required in the following situations that may increase the hemorrhagic risk:

- Recent events, including: biopsy or major trauma; cerebral, spinal or ophthalmic surgery
- Concomitant use of NSAIDs should be undertaken with caution
- Diseases associated with an increased risk of bleeding, such as congenital or acquired coagulation disorders, thrombocytopenia or functional platelet defects, active ulcerative gastrointestinal disease, history of intracranial hemorrhage or hemorrhagic infarction, bacterial endocarditis
- The concomitant administration of a strong P-gp inhibitor (e.g. verapamil) with PRADAX may elevate dabigatran plasma concentrations resulting in an increased bleeding risk. Treatment initiation with verapamil should be avoided in patients who are already treated with PRADAX. Simultaneous initiation of treatment with PRADAX and verapamil should also be avoided (see Drug Interactions, P-glycoprotein Inhibitors).

Hepatic/Biliary/Pancreatic: Patients with moderate or severe hepatic impairment (Child-Pugh classification B and C), or with elevated liver enzymes >2 ULN were excluded from clinical trials. Therefore, PRADAX is not recommended in these patients.

Peri-Operative Spinal/Epidural Anaesthesia, Lumbar Puncture: In patients treated with dabigatran etexilate for VTE prevention following major orthopedic surgery and who undergo spinal or epidural anesthesia, or in whom lumbar puncture is performed in follow-up to surgery, the formation of spinal or epidural hematomas that may result in long-term or permanent paralysis cannot be excluded.

In the case of these peri-spinal procedures, administration of the first dose of PRADAX should occur after hemostasis has been obtained and no sooner than 2 hours following puncture or removal of catheters related to these procedures.

The risk of these rare events may be higher with post-operative use of indwelling epidural catheters or the concomitant use of other products affecting hemostasis. Accordingly, the use of PRADAX is not recommended in patients undergoing anesthesia with post-operative indwelling epidural catheters.

Renal: Following oral dosing with dabigatran etexilate, there is a direct correlation of systemic exposure to dabigatran with degree of renal impairment. Severe renal insufficiency (CrCl <30 mL/min) has been shown to increase exposure to dabigatran six-fold (see Contraindications), while moderate renal impairment (CrCL 30-50 mL/min) increased exposure 2.7-fold. While the standard dose of PRADAX is 220 mg daily for patients with intact renal function, for patients with moderate renal impairment (CrCL 30-50 mL/min), the recommended daily dose is 150 mg daily (see Dosage and Administration, Renal Impairment). PRADAX is contraindicated in cases of severe renal impairment (CrCL <30 mL/min). Patients who develop acute renal failure while on PRADAX should discontinue such treatment.

As dose selection of PRADAX is based on renal function, creatinine clearance should be evaluated before initiating treatment, and during treatment as appropriate (see Dosage and Administration, Renal Impairment).

Special Populations: Pregnant Women: Since there are no studies of PRADAX in pregnant women, the potential risk in these patients is unknown. Animal reproductive studies did not show any adverse effects on fertility or postnatal development of the neonate.

Women of child-bearing potential should avoid pregnancy during treatment with PRADAX and when pregnant, women should not be treated with PRADAX unless the expected benefit is greater than the risk.

Nursing Women: Breast-feeding during treatment with PRADAX is not recommended. There are no clinical data available on the excretion of dabigatran into breast milk.

Pediatrics (<18 years of age): The safety and efficacy of PRADAX have not been established in children less than 18 years of age, therefore PRADAX is not recommended in this patient population.

Geriatrics (>65 years of age): In general, patients should be treated with a standard dose of 220 mg PRADAX daily. In patients >75 years of age, PRADAX should be used with caution, and a dose of 150 mg daily should be considered since age-related decrease of renal function is frequently encountered (see Warnings and Precautions, Renal). Regardless of age, in patients with moderate renal impairment (CrCL 30-50 mL/min), because of an increased risk of bleeding, the recommended dose of PRADAX is 150 mg daily (see Dosage and Administration, Renal Impairment).

Patients of Low Body Weight (<50 kg): Since limited data are available in these patients, PRADAX should be used with caution.

Monitoring and Laboratory Tests: At recommended doses of PRADAX, dabigatran prolongs the activated partial thromboplastin time (aPTT). In patients who are bleeding due to excess activity of dabigatran, the aPTT test would be expected to be elevated. Both thrombin time (TT) and ecarin clotting time (ECT) may be helpful in assessing anticoagulant activity of dabigatran, if necessary (see Action and Clinical Pharmacology, Pharmacodynamics). In the therapeutic range, aPTT is less sensitive to anticoagulant activity than either TT or ECT and should not be relied upon (see Drug Interactions, Drug-Laboratory Test Interactions).

ADVERSE REACTIONS: A total of 10 084 patients were exposed to at least one dose of study medication in four active-controlled clinical trials conducted to evaluate the safety and effectiveness of dabigatran etexilate in the prevention of venous thromboembolic events (VTE) following major elective orthopedic surgery. Of these, 5419 were treated with 150 mg or 220 mg daily of PRADAX, while 389 received doses of less than 150 mg daily, and 1168 received doses in excess of 220 mg daily.

The adverse reactions that can with reasonable certainty be attributed to dabigatran are those of bleeding or signs of bleeding, e.g. wound bleeding and anemia. See Table 1 and Table 2.

Although rare in frequency in clinical trials, major or severe bleeding may occur and, regardless of location, may lead to disabling, life-threatening or even fatal outcomes.

Table 1: PRADAX

Number (%) of Patients Experiencing Bleeding Events During the Treatment Period in the VTE Prevention in the REMODEL and RENOVATE Trials, According to Dose

	Dabigatran Etexilate 150 mg N (%)	Dabigatran Etexilate 220 mg N (%)	Enoxaparin 40 mg QD N (%)
Treated	1866 (100.0)	1825 (100.0)	1848 (100.0)
Major bleeding[a]	24 (1.3)	33 (1.8)	27 (1.5)
Any bleeding	258 (13.8)	251 (13.8)	247 (13.4)

[a] Major Bleeding: Major bleeding was defined as clinically overt bleeding associated with ≥20 g/L fall in hemoglobin; clinically overt bleeding leading to transfusion of ≥2 units packed cells or whole blood; fatal, retroperitoneal, intracranial, intraocular or intraspinal bleeding; bleeding warranting treatment cessation or leading to reoperation. Major bleeding included those events occurring at the surgical site.

Table 2: PRADAX

Number (%) of Patients Experiencing Bleeding Events During the Treatment Period in the VTE Prevention in the REMOBILIZE Trial, According to Dose

	Dabigatran Etexilate 150 mg N (%)	Dabigatran Etexilate 220 mg N (%)	Enoxaparin 30 mg BID N (%)
Treated	871 (100.0)	857 (100.0)	868 (100.0)
Major bleeding[a]	5 (0.6)	5 (0.6)	12 (1.4)
Any bleeding	72 (8.3)	74 (8.6)	84 (9.7)

[a] Major Bleeding: Major bleeding was defined as clinically overt bleeding associated with ≥20 g/L fall in hemoglobin; clinically overt bleeding leading to transfusion of ≥2 units packed cells or whole blood; fatal, retroperitoneal, intracranial, intraocular or intraspinal bleeding; bleeding warranting treatment cessation or leading to reoperation. Major bleeding included those events occurring at the surgical site.

There were no documented cases of hypersensitivity following oral administration of dabigatran etexilate.

Clinical Trial Adverse Drug Reactions: Because clinical trials are conducted under very specific conditions the adverse reaction rates observed in the clinical trials may not reflect the rates observed in practice and should not be compared to the rates in the clinical trials of another drug. Adverse drug reaction information from clinical trials is useful for identifying drug-related adverse events and for approximating rates. See Table 3.

Table 3: PRADAX

Common Adverse Reactions Observed in ≥1% of Dabigatran-Treated Patients in Active-Controlled VTE Prevention Trials

	Dabigatran Etexilate 150 mg N (%)	Dabigatran Etexilate 220 mg N (%)	Enoxaparin N (%)
	2737 (100)	2682 (100)	3108 (100)
Blood and Lymphatic System			
Anemia	110 (4.0)	117 (4.4)	141 (4.5)
Gastrointestinal hemorrhage	33 (1.2)	17 (0.6)	20 (0.6)
Hematuria	34 (1.2)	31 (1.2)	25 (0.8)
Vascular Disorders			
Hematoma	38 (1.4)	37 (1.4)	55 (1.8)
Wound hemorrhage	35 (1.3)	28 (1.0)	31 (1.0)
Investigations			
Hemoglobin decreased	45 (1.6)	35 (1.3)	74 (2.4)
Injury, Poisoning and Procedural Complications			
Wound secretion	130 (4.7)	130 (4.8)	93 (3.0)
Post-procedural hematoma	66 (2.4)	45 (1.7)	78 (2.5)
Post-procedural hemorrhage	28 (1.5)	43 (2.4)	32 (1.7)
Anemia post-operative	37 (1.4)	54 (2.0)	56 (1.8)
Traumatic hematoma	37 (1.4)	41 (1.5)	51 (1.6)
Post-procedural discharge	31 (1.1)	34 (1.3)	31 (1.0)
Laboratory Investigations			
ALT ≥3×ULN	68 (2.5)	58 (2.2)	95 (3.5)[a]

[a] Based on N=2716.

Less Common Clinical Trial Adverse Drug Reactions (<1%): Observed with exposure to dabigatran 150 mg and 220 mg during active-controlled venothromboembolic prevention trials in the context of major orthopedic surgery:

Blood and Lymphatic System: thrombocytopenia.

Gastrointestinal Disorders: hemorrhoidal haemorrhage, rectal hemorrhage.

General: bloody discharge, catheter site hemorrhage.

Hepatobiliary Disorders: alanine aminotransferase increased, aspartate aminotransferase increased, hepatic enzyme increased, hepatic function abnormal/liver function test abnormal, transaminases increased.

Injury, Poisoning and Procedural Complications: incision site hemorrhage.

Investigations: occult blood positive, blood urine present, hematocrit decrease.

Musculoskeletal and Cumulative Tissue Disorders: hemarthrosis.

Respiratory and Thoracic System: epistaxis.
Skin and Sub-Cutaneous Tissue: ecchymosis.
Surgical and Medical Procedures: post-procedural drainage, wound drainage.
Vascular Disorders: hemorrhage.

DRUG INTERACTIONS: Based on in vitro evaluation, neither dabigatran etexilate or its active moiety, dabigatran, were shown to be metabolised by the human cytochrome P450 system, nor did they exhibit effects on human CYP P450 isozymes.

Concomitant use of PRADAX with treatment that acts on hemostasis or coagulation increases bleeding risk (see Warnings and Precautions, Hematologic). Co-administration of PRADAX with other anticoagulants or antithrombotic therapy has not been adequately studied and is not recommended.

Drug-Drug Interactions: Transporter Interactions: Dabigatran etexilate, but not dabigatran, is a substrate with moderate affinity for the efflux P-glycoprotein (P-gp) transporter. Therefore potent P-glycoprotein inducers or inhibitors may be expected to impact exposure to dabigatran.

P-glycoprotein Inhibitors: Potent P-gp inhibitors like verapamil, clarithromycin and amiodarone may be expected to increase systemic exposure to dabigatran, see Table 4. The P- glycoprotein inhibitor, quinidine, is contraindicated (see Contraindications).

P-glycoprotein Inducers: Potent P-gp inducers such as rifampicin and Saint John's Wort may reduce the systemic exposure of dabigatran. Less potent inducers such as tenofovir can potentially reduce systemic exposure. Caution is advised when co-administering these drug procucts.

P-glycoprotein Substrates: Dabigatran etexilate is not expected to have a clinically meaningful interaction with P-glycoprotein substrates that do not also act as inhibitors or inducers of P-gp.

Table 4: PRADAX

Summary of Drug-Drug Interactions

Proper Name	Ref[a]	Effect	Clinical Comment
Amiodarone	CT	When dabigatran etexilate was co-administered with a single oral dose of 600 mg amiodarone, the extent and rate of absorption of amiodarone and its active metabolite DEA were essentially unchanged. Dabigatran AUC and C_{max} were increased by about 60 % and 50 %, respectively.	Adjust dosing to 150 mg daily PRADAX with amiodarone. Caution should be exercised.
Antacids (aluminium compounds, sodium bicarbonate, calcium and/or magnesium compounds, or combinations of these)	CT	In population PK analyses, a reduction in dabigatran exposure by 35% was seen over the first 24 hours following surgery. Thereafter, (>24 hours after surgery), a reduction of about 11% was observed.	Diminished clinical effect may occur. Co-administration with PRADAX should be avoided within 24 hours after surgery.
Atorvastatin	CT	When dabigatran etexilate was co-administered with atorvastatin, exposure of atorvastatin, atorvastatin metabolites was not significantly changed. Dabigatran concentrations were decreased about 20%.	No dose adjustment is recommended.
Clarithromycin	CT	When clarithromycin 500 mg bid was administered together with dabigatran etexilate a modest PK-interaction was observed (increase of mean Cmax by about 19% and mean AUC of about 15%).	No dose adjustment is recommended. Caution should be exercised.
Diclofenac	CT	When dabigatran etexilate was co-administered with diclofenac, pharmacokinetics of both drugs appeared unchanged.	No dose adjustment is recommended.
Digoxin	CT	When dabigatran etexilate was co-administered with digoxin, no PK-interaction was observed.	No dose adjustment is recommended.
Pantoprazole	CT	When dabigatran etexilate was co-administered with pantoprazole, a decrease in dabigatran AUC of about 30 % was observed.	No dose adjustment is recommended. Diminished clinical effect may occur.
Verapamil	CT	When dabigatran etexilate was co-administered with oral verapamil, the Cmax and AUC of dabigatran were increased depending on timing of administration and formulation of verapamil. The greatest elevation of dabigatran exposure was observed with the first dose of an immediate release formulation of verapamil administered one hour prior to dabigatran etexilate intake (increase of Cmax by about 180% and AUC by about 150%). The effect was progressively decreased with administration of an extended release formulation (increase of Cmax by about 90% and AUC by about 70%) or administration of multiple doses of verapamil (increase of Cmax by about 60% and AUC by about 50%). This may be explained by the induction of P-gp in the gut by chronic verapamil treatment. There was no meaningful interaction observed when verapamil was given 2 hours after dabigatran etexilate (increase of Cmax by about 10% and AUC by about 20%). This is explained by essentially complete absorption of dabigatran etexilate after 2 hours. No data are available for the parenteral application of verapamil; based on the mechanism of the interaction, no meaningful interaction is expected.	Dosing should be reduced to 150 mg PRADAX daily in patients who concomitantly receive dabigatran etexilate and verapamil. Caution should be exercised.

(cont'd)

Table 4: PRADAX *(cont'd)*

Summary of Drug-Drug Interactions

Proper Name	Ref[a]	Effect	Clinical Comment
Quinidine	CT	When dabigatran etexilate was co-administered with 600 mg quinidine sulfate, the exposure to dabigatran was approximately twice expected, based on the limited data set (n=3 female subjects who received co-administration).	Co-administration with PRADAX is contraindicated.

[a] C=case study; CT=clinical trial; T=theoretical.

Drug-Food Interactions: Food does not affect the bioavailability of PRADAX but delays the time-to-peak plasma concentrations by 2 hours.

Drug-Herb Interactions: Drug-Herb Interactions have not been investigated. Potent P-gp inducers such as Saint John's Wort (Hypericum perforatum) may be expected to affect systemic exposure of dabigatran. Co-administration of these products is not recommended.

Drug-Laboratory Test Interactions: No single test (aPTT, INR, TT, ECT) is adequate to reliably assess the anticoagulant activity of dabigatran following PRADAX administration. However, in patients who are bleeding, an aPTT determination with values greater than 2.5 × control suggests excessive anticoagulation due to dabigatran. At therapeutic levels of dabigatran, thrombin time (TT) is the best measure of the pharmacodynamic effect of dabigatran because of its linear and sensitive relationship with dabigatran exposure (see Warnings and Precautions, Monitoring and Laboratory Tests; Action and Clinical Pharmacology, Pharmacodynamics). The ecarin clotting test (ECT) may also be useful in these circumstances.

Drug-Lifestyle Interactions: No direct interaction between dabigatran etexilate and alcohol was demonstrated pre-clinically or has been hypothesised. However, excessive use of alcohol may increase the likelihood of personal injury and should be avoided in patients taking any systemic anticoagulant, including PRADAX.

The effect of PRADAX on the ability to drive and use machines has not been investigated.

DOSAGE AND ADMINISTRATION: Recommended Dose and Dosage Adjustment: VTE Prevention Following Elective Knee Replacement Surgery: The recommended dose of PRADAX is 220 mg once daily taken orally as 2 capsules of 110 mg in patients with intact renal function. Treatment should normally be initiated within 1-4 hours of completed surgery once hemostasis is secured. Start with a single capsule of 110 mg, and continue with 2 capsules once daily thereafter for a total of 10 days. If hemostasis is not secured, initiation of treatment should be delayed. If treatment is not started on the day of surgery for whatever reason, then treatment should be initiated with 2 capsules at once.

VTE Prevention Following Elective Hip Replacement Surgery: The recommended dose of PRADAX is 220 mg once daily taken orally as 2 capsules of 110 mg in patients with intact renal function. Treatment should normally be initiated within 1-4 hours of completed surgery once hemostasis is secured. Start with a single capsule of 110 mg, and continue with 2 capsules once daily thereafter for a total of 28-35 days. If hemostasis is not secured, initiation of treatment should be delayed. If treatment is not started on the day of surgery for whatever reason, then treatment should be initiated with 2 capsules at once.

Renal Impairment: Following oral dosing with dabigatran etexilate, there is a direct correlation of systemic exposure to dabigatran with degree of renal impairment (see Warnings and Precautions, Renal). The kidneys account for 85% of dabigatran clearance.

Patients with moderate renal impairment (CrCL 30-50 mL/min) exposed to dabigatran etexilate appear to be at higher risk of bleeding. Accordingly, treatment with PRADAX should be initiated orally in these patients within 1-4 hours of completed surgery once hemostasis is secured. Start with 75 mg taken as a single capsule, and continued at 150 mg, taken as 2 capsules of 75 mg once daily thereafter.

There are no data to support use in patients with severe renal impairment (creatinine clearance <30 mL/min). Given the substantial increase in dabigatran exposure observed in this patient population, treatment with PRADAX is not recommended (see Contraindications, and Action and Clinical Pharmacology, Renal Insufficiency).

Creatinine clearance can be estimated using the Cockroft-Gault formula as follows:

Creatinine clearance (mL/min) =

$$\text{Males} = \frac{(140\text{-age (years)}) \times \text{weight (kg)}}{72 \times \text{serum creatinine (mg/100 mL)}}$$

$$\text{Females} = \frac{0.85 \times (140\text{-age (years)}) \times \text{weight (kg)}}{72 \times \text{serum creatinine (mg/100 mL)}}$$

Hepatic Impairment: Patients with moderate and severe hepatic impairment were excluded from clinical trials. Therefore, the use of PRADAX is not recommended in this population.

P-glycoprotein Inhibitors: Potent P-gp inhibitors like verapamil, clarithromycin and amiodarone may be expected to increase systemic exposure to dabigatran.

Dosing should be reduced to PRADAX 150 mg daily, taken as 2 capsules of 75 mg, in patients who concomitantly receive amiodarone or verapamil. Caution should be exercised (see Warnings and Precautions and Drug Interactions, P-glycoprotein Inhibitors).

Combination use with quinidine is contraindicated (see Contraindications).

Elderly: In patients >75 years of age, PRADAX should be used with caution, and a dose of 150 mg daily should be considered, taken as 2 capsules of 75 mg daily, since age-related compromise of renal function is frequently encountered (see Warnings and Precautions, Geriatrics (>65 years of age), and Renal).

Children: Since PRADAX has not been investigated in patients <18 years of age, treatment is not recommended.

Patient Body Weight: Population PK modelling shows that patients with a body weight of about 120 kg have about 20% lower drug exposure. Patients with a body weight of about 48 kg have about 25% higher drug exposure compared to patients with average weight.

Switching From PRADAX Treatment to Parenteral Anticoagulant: Wait 24 hours after the last dose of dabigatran etexilate before switching to a parenteral anticoagulant.

Switching From Parenteral Anticoagulants Treatment to PRADAX: No data are available, therefore it is not recommenced to start the administration of dabigatran etexilate before the next scheduled dose of the parenteral anticoagulant would have been due.

Missed Dose: Patients should be advised that if a dose is missed, they should not take a double dose.

Administration: PRADAX can be taken with food, or on an empty stomach with water.

OVERDOSAGE:

There is no antidote to dabigatran etexilate or dabigatran. Doses of PRADAX beyond those recommended expose the patient to increased risk of bleeding. In the event of hemorrhagic complications, treatment must be discontinued and the source of bleeding investigated. Since dabigatran is excreted predominantly by the renal route, adequate diuresis must be maintained. The initiation of appropriate treatment, e.g. surgical hemostasis or the transfusion of fresh frozen plasma, should be undertaken.

Dabigatran can be dialysed, although there is no clinical experience to demonstrate the utility of this approach.

For management of a suspected drug overdose, CPhA recommends that you contact your **regional Poison Control Centre**. See the *CPS* Directory section for a list of Poison Control Centres.

ACTION AND CLINICAL PHARMACOLOGY: Mechanism of Action: Dabigatran etexilate is a prodrug which does not exhibit anticoagulant activity itself. Following oral administration, dabigatran etexilate is rapidly absorbed and converted to dabigatran by esterase-catalysed hydrolysis in plasma and in the liver.

Dabigatran is a competitive, reversible direct thrombin inhibitor, and is the main active principle in plasma.

Since thrombin (serine protease) enables the conversion of fibrinogen into fibrin during the coagulation cascade, its inhibition prevents the development of thrombus. Dabigatran also inhibits free thrombin, fibrin-bound thrombin and thrombin-induced platelet aggregation.

In-vivo and ex-vivo animal studies have demonstrated antithrombotic efficacy and anticoagulant activity of dabigatran after intravenous administration and of dabigatran etexilate following oral administration in various animal models of thrombosis.

Pharmacodynamics: There is a clear correlation between plasma dabigatran concentration and degree of anticoagulant effect. The maximum effect (E_{max}) of dabigatran on pharmacodynamic (PD) parameters occurred at the same time as C_{max}, indicating that thrombin inhibition by dabigatran is a direct effect, linked to the central plasma compartment.

At recommended doses of dabigatran etexilate, dabigatran may prolong the activated partial thromboplastin time (aPTT) and prothrombin time (PT), as measured by INR, but these tests are relatively insensitive to the activity of dabigatran and are not suitable alone as measures of anticoagulant activity. However, in patients who are bleeding, aPTT may help determine an excess of anticoagulant activity.

PK/PD analyses suggested marked differences between the various assays in terms of sensitivity and precision with varying dabigatran plasma concentrations.

- A curvilinear relationship was shown between dabigatran plasma concentrations and aPTT. The flattening of the aPTT-plasma concentration response curve indicated that this assay was associated with low sensitivity at dabigatran plasma concentrations greater than 100 ng/mL, and well within the range observed following oral doses shown to be effective in the pivotal Phase III studies.
- The data suggest a linear relationship between plasma concentration and INR (<2.0); however, this assay lacked sensitivity within the clinically-relevant dabigatran plasma concentration range and showed high variability.
- The TT assay exhibited a linear relationship with plasma concentration with a high level of sensitivity. TT might be too sensitive to dabigatran plasma concentrations in the clinically relevant plasma concentration range. At dabigatran concentrations greater than 600 ng/mL, the thrombin clotting time frequently exceeded the maximum measurement time of the coagulometer. Hence, the TT assay may serve as a sensitive method for determining if any dabigatran is present. However, since the reagents used for determining TT at different laboratories are not standardised, the clinical utility of this test during dabigatran dosing remains to be established.
- The ECT assay displayed a linear relationship with drug plasma concentrations in the clinically-relevant drug concentration range and exhibited adequate sensitivity and precision. However, given lack of uniform standardisation of this assay, the clinical utility of this test remains to be established.

Pharmacokinetics: After oral administration of dabigatran etexilate in healthy volunteers, the pharmacokinetic profile of dabigatran in plasma is characterised by a rapid increase in plasma concentrations with C_{max} attained within 0.5 and 2.0 hours post-administration. After C_{max}, plasma concentrations of dabigatran showed a biexponential decline with a mean terminal half-life of approximately 11 hours in young healthy subjects and 14-17 hours in elderly subjects. The half-life was independent of dose. C_{max} and AUC were dose proportional. Food does not affect the bioavailability of dabigatran etexilate but delays the time to peak plasma concentrations by 2 hours.

The absolute bioavailability of dabigatran following oral administration of dabigatran etexilate was approximately 6.5 %. See Table 5.

Table 5: PRADAX

Summary of PK Parameters After Single and Repeated Oral Administration in Humans

	C_{max}	$t_{½}$ (h)	AUC	Clearance, Excretion	Volume of Distribution
Healthy volunteers	0.8–1.4 ng/mL/mg	11 hours	6–10 ng*h/mL/mg	Urine (85%) Fecal (6%) Total clearance (IV): about 120 mL/min	Vss=60–70 L
Patients	C_{max}:1.22 ng/mL/mg T_{max}: 7–9 hours following surgery	14–17 hours	9.7 ng*h/mL/mg	n/a (no IV data)	n/a (no IV data)

Absorption: A study evaluating post-operative absorption of PRADAX, 1-3 hours following surgery, demonstrated relatively slow absorption compared with that in healthy volunteers, showing a smooth plasma concentration-time profile without high peak plasma concentrations. Peak plasma concentrations are reached at 6 hours following administration, or at 7 to 9 hours following surgery. It is noted however that contributing factors such as anaesthesia, gastrointestinal paresis, and surgical effects will mean that a proportion of patients will experience absorption delay independent of the oral drug formulation. Although this study did not predict whether impaired absorption persists with subsequent doses, it was demonstrated in a further study that slow and delayed absorption is usually only present on the day of surgery. On subsequent days, absorption of dabigatran is rapid with peak plasma concentrations attained 2 hours after drug administration.

Distribution: Low (34-35%) concentration-independent binding of dabigatran to human plasma proteins was observed. The volume of distribution of dabigatran of 60-70 L exceeded the volume of total body water indicating moderate tissue distribution of dabigatran.

Metabolism: After oral administration, dabigatran etexilate is rapidly and completely converted to dabigatran, which is the active form in plasma. The cleavage of the prodrug dabigatran etexilate by esterase-catalysed hydrolysis to the active principle dabigatran is the predominant metabolic reaction. Dabigatran is subject to conjugation forming pharmacologically active acylglucuronides. Four positional isomers, 1-O, 2-O, 3-O, 4-O-acylglucuronide exist, each accounts for less than 10% of total dabigatran in plasma. Traces of other metabolites were only detectable with highly sensitive analytical methods.

Excretion: Metabolism and excretion of dabigatran were studied following a single intravenous dose of radiolabeled dabigatran in healthy male subjects. After an intravenous dose, the dabigatran-derived radioactivity was eliminated primarily in the urine (85%). Faecal excretion accounted for 6% of the administered dose. Recovery of the total radioactivity ranged from 88-94 % of the administered dose by 168 hours post dose.

Dabigatran is eliminated primarily in the unchanged form in the urine, at a rate of approximately 100 mL/min corresponding to the glomerular filtration rate.

Special Populations and Conditions: Pediatrics: Dabigatran has not been studied in the paediatric population.

Geriatrics: Specific pharmacokinetic studies with elderly subjects showed an increase of 40 to 60% in the AUC and of about 25 % in C_{max} compared to young subjects. Population-based pharmacokinetic studies have evaluated the pharmacokinetics of dabigatran after repeated doses in patients (up to 88 years of age). The observed increase of dabigatran exposure correlated with the age-related reduction in creatinine clearance.

Gender: There were no differences in the Phase 3 clinical studies for efficacy and safety data between men and women. Drug exposure in female patients is about 40 % to 50 % higher than in male patients.

Race: The pharmacokinetics of dabigatran were investigated in Caucasian and Japanese volunteers after single and multiple doses. Ethnic origin does not affect the pharmacokinetics of dabigatran in a clinically relevant manner. No pharmacokinetic data in black patients are available.

Hepatic Insufficiency: No change in dabigatran exposure was seen in 12 subjects with moderate hepatic insufficiency (Child Pugh B) compared to 12 controls.

Dabigatran is metabolised in the liver by conjugation with activated glucuronic acid. CYP 450 metabolic enzymes are not involved in dabigatran metabolism. Hepatic elimination via the bile represents a minor elimination pathway of dabigatran (approximately 20% of the dose is eliminated biliary).

Renal Insufficiency: The exposure (AUC) of dabigatran after the oral administration of dabigatran etexilate is approximately 2.7 fold higher in volunteers with moderate renal insufficiency (CrCL between 30-50 mL/min) than in those without renal insufficiency.

In a small number of volunteers with severe renal insufficiency (CrCL 10-30 mL/min), the exposure (AUC) to dabigatran was approximately 6 times higher and the half-life approximately 2 times longer than that observed in a population without renal insufficiency (see Contraindications; Warnings and Precautions, Renal; Dosage and Administration, Renal Impairment).

Body Weight: Population pharmacokinetic studies have evaluated the pharmacokinetics of dabigatran in patients of 48 to 120 kg body weight. Body weight had a minor effect on the plasma clearance of dabigatran resulting in slightly higher exposure in patients with low body weight.

STORAGE AND STABILITY: Blister: Store between 15-25°C. Store in the original package in order to protect from moisture. Bottle: Store between 15-30°C. Once opened, the product must be used within 30 days. Keep the bottle tightly closed. Store in the original package in order to protect from moisture.

SPECIAL HANDLING INSTRUCTIONS: Store in a safe place out of the reach of children!

INFORMATION FOR THE PATIENT: Published in e-CPS, available by subscription at www.e-cps.ca.

DOSAGE FORMS, COMPOSITION AND PACKAGING: 75 mg : Each imprinted hydroxypropylmethyl cellulose capsule with light blue, opaque cap and cream-colored, opaque body of size 2 filled with yellowish pellets contains: 86.48 mg of dabigatran etexilate mesilate corresponding to 75 mg of dabigatran etexilate base. The cap is imprinted with the Boehringer Ingelheim company symbol, the body with "R75". Nonmedicinal ingredients: acacia, dimeticone, hydroxypropyl cellulose, hypromellose, talc and tartaric acid; HPMC capsule shell: carragenan, hypromellose, Indigo Carmin (132), potassium chloride, purified water, Sunset Yellow (E110) and titanium dioxide; printing ink: iron oxide black, propylene glycol and shellac. Aluminium blister strips of 10×1 HPMC capsules, cartons containing 1, 3, or 6 blister strips (10×1, 30×1, or 60×1 HPMC capsules). Polypropylene bottles of 60 HMPC capsules.

110 mg : Each imprinted hydroxypropylmethyl cellulose capsule with light blue, opaque cap and cream-coloured, opaque body of size 1 filled with yellowish pellets contains: 126.83 mg of dabigatran etexilate mesilate corresponding to 110 mg of dabigatran etexilate base. The cap is imprinted with the Boehringer Ingelheim company symbol, the body with "R110". Nonmedicinal ingredients: acacia, dimeticone, hydroxypropyl cellulose, hypromellose, talc and tartaric acid; HPMC capsule shell: carragenan, hypromellose, Indigo Carmin (132), potassium chloride, purified water, Sunset Yellow (E110) and titanium dioxide; printing ink: iron oxide black, propylene glycol and shellac. Aluminium blister strips of 10×1 HPMC capsules, cartons containing 1, 3, or 6 blister strips (10×1, 30×1, or 60×1 HPMC capsules). Polypropylene bottles of 60 HMPC capsules.

(Shown in Product Identification Section)

The reader is invited to consult CPhA's monograph **HMG-CoA Reductase Inhibitors**.

Pravachol® Ⓟ

pravastatin sodium

Lipid Metabolism Regulator

Bristol-Myers Squibb

Date of Preparation: August 16, 1990
Date of Revision: December 9, 2008

SUMMARY PRODUCT INFORMATION:

Route of Administration	Dosage Form/ Strength	Clinically Relevant Nonmedicinal Ingredients
Oral	10, 20, 40 mg Tablets	Croscarmellose sodium, D&C yellow no. 10 (40 mg tablets), FD&C blue no. 1 (40 mg tablets), lactose, magnesium oxide, magnesium stearate, microcrystalline cellulose, povidone, red ferric oxide (10 mg tablets) and yellow ferric oxide (20 mg tablets) See Dosage Forms, Composition and Packaging.

INDICATIONS AND CLINICAL USE: Therapy with lipid-altering agents should be considered a component of multiple risk factor intervention in those individuals at increased risk for atherosclerotic vascular disease due to dyslipidemia. PRAVACHOL (pravastatin sodium) should be used in addition to a diet restricted in saturated fat and cholesterol when the response to diet and other non-pharmacological measures alone has been inadequate.

Hypercholesterolemia: PRAVACHOL is indicated as an adjunct to diet (at least an equivalent of the Adult Treatment Panel III [ATP III TLC diet]) for the reduction of elevated Total and Low Density Lipoprotein Cholesterol (LDL-C) levels in patients with primary hypercholesterolemia (Types IIa and IIb), when the response to diet and other non-pharmacologic measures alone has been inadequate.

Prior to initiating therapy with PRAVACHOL, secondary causes for hypercholesterolemia, such as obesity, poorly controlled diabetes mellitus, hypothyroidism, nephrotic syndrome, dysproteinemias, obstructive liver disease, other drug therapy or alcoholism, should be excluded and it should be determined that patients for whom treatment with PRAVACHOL is being considered have an elevated LDL-C level as the cause for an elevated total serum cholesterol. A lipid profile should be performed to measure Total Cholesterol, High Density Lipoprotein Cholesterol (HDL-C) and Triglycerides (TG).

For patients with total triglycerides less than 4.52 mmol/L (400 mg/dL), LDL-C can be estimated using the following equation:

LDL-C (mmol/L)=Total Cholesterol−[(0.37×triglycerides)+HDL-C]
LDL-C (mg/dL)=Total Cholesterol−[(0.16×triglycerides)+HDL-C]

When total triglyceride levels exceed 4.52 mmol/L (400 mg/dL), this equation is less accurate and LDL-C concentrations should be determined by ultracentrifugation.

As with other lipid-lowering therapy, PRAVACHOL is not indicated when hypercholesterolemia is due to hyperalphalipoproteinemia (elevated HDL-C). The efficacy of pravastatin has not been evaluated in conditions where the major abnormality is elevation of chylomicrons, VLDL or LDL (i.e. hyperlipoproteinemia or dyslipoproteinemia types I, III, IV or V).

Primary Prevention of Coronary Events: In hypercholesterolemic patients without clinically evident coronary heart disease, PRAVACHOL is indicated to:

- Reduce the risk of myocardial infarction;
- Reduce the risk for undergoing myocardial revascularization procedures;
- Reduce the risk of total mortality by reducing cardiovascular deaths.

Secondary Prevention of Cardiovascular Events: In patients with total cholesterol in the normal to moderately elevated range who have clinically evident coronary heart disease, PRAVACHOL is indicated to:

- Reduce the risk of total mortality
- Reduce the risk of death due to coronary heart disease
- Reduce the risk of myocardial infarction
- Reduce the risk of undergoing myocardial revascularization procedures
- Reduce the risk of stroke and transient ischemic attack (TIA)
- Reduce total hospitalization

PRAVACHOL was also found to reduce the rate of progression of atherosclerosis in patients with coronary heart disease as part of a treatment strategy to lower Total and LDL-cholesterol to desired levels. In two trials including this type of patients* (i.e. in a secondary prevention intervention), PRAVACHOL monotherapy was shown to reduce the rate of progression of atherosclerosis as evaluated by quantitative angiography and B-mode ultrasound. This effect may be associated with an improvement in the coronary endpoints (fatal or non fatal myocardial infarction). In these trials, however, no effect was observed in all cause mortality.

Pediatrics (<16 years of age): There is no experience to date with the use of PRAVACHOL in such patients. Treatment in these patients is not recommended at this time.

Geriatrics (≥65 years of age): Pharmacokinetic evaluation of pravastatin in patients over the age of 65 years indicates an increased AUC. As a precautionary measure, the lowest dose should be administered initially in these patients.

CONTRAINDICATIONS: Patients who are hypersensitive to this drug or to any ingredient in the formulation.

Active liver disease or unexplained persistent elevations of serum transaminases (see Warnings and Precautions).

In Pregnant and Nursing Women: Cholesterol and other products of cholesterol biosynthesis are essential components for fetal development (including synthesis of steroids and cell membranes). Since HMG-CoA reductase inhibitors such as PRAVACHOL (pravastatin sodium) decrease cholesterol synthesis and possibly the synthesis of other biologically active substances derived from cholesterol, they may cause fetal harm when administered to pregnant women. PRAVACHOL should be administered to women of childbearing age only when such patients are highly unlikely to conceive and have been informed of the possible harm. If the patient becomes pregnant while taking PRAVACHOL, the drug should be discontinued immediately and the patient apprised

* Pravastatin Limitation of Atherosclerosis in the Coronary/Carotid Arteries (PLAC I and II)

of the potential harm to the fetus. Atherosclerosis being a chronic process, discontinuation of lipid metabolism regulating drugs during pregnancy should have little impact on the outcome of longterm therapy of primary hypercholesterolemia (see Warnings and Precautions, Pregnant Women, Nursing Women).

WARNINGS AND PRECAUTIONS: Muscle Effects: Elevations of creatinine phosphokinase levels (CK [MM fraction]), have been reported with the use of HMG-CoA reductase inhibitors, including PRAVACHOL.

Effects on skeletal muscle such as myalgia, myopathy and, rarely, rhabdomyolysis have been reported in patients treated with PRAVACHOL.

Muscle weakness and rhabdomyolysis have been reported in patients receiving other HMG-CoA reductase inhibitors concomitantly with itraconozole and cyclosporine.

The benefits and risks of using HMG-CoA reductase inhibitors concomitantly with immunosuppressive drugs, fibrates, erythromycin, systemic azole derivative antifungal agents or lipid-lowering doses of niacin should be carefully considered.

Rare cases of rhabdomyolysis with acute renal failure secondary to myoglobinuria, have been reported with PRAVACHOL and with other HMG-CoA reductase inhibitors.

Myopathy, defined as muscle pain or muscle weakness in conjunction with increases in creatine phosphokinase (CK) values to greater than ten times the upper limit of normal, should be considered in any patient with diffuse myalgias, muscle tenderness or weakness, and/or marked elevation of CK. Patients should be advised to report promptly any unexplained muscle pain, tenderness or weakness, particularly if associated with malaise or fever. Patients who develop any signs or symptoms suggestive of myopathy should have their CK levels measured. PRAVACHOL therapy should be discontinued if markedly elevated CK levels are measured or myopathy is diagnosed or suspected.

As with other statins, the risk of myopathy including rhabdomyolysis may be substantially increased by concomitant immunosuppressive therapy including cyclosporines, and by concomitant therapy with gemfibrozil, erythromycin or niacin (see Warnings and Precautions).

Myopathy has not been observed in clinical trials involving small numbers of patients who were treated with PRAVACHOL together with immunosuppressants, fibric acid derivatives or niacin.

The use of fibrates alone is occasionally associated with myopathy. In a limited size clinical trial of combined therapy with pravastatin (40 mg/day) and gemfibrozil (1200 mg/day), myopathy was not reported, although a trend towards CK elevations and musculoskeletal symptoms was seen. **The combined use of pravastatin and fibrates should generally be avoided.**

No information is available on the combined therapy of pravastatin with erythromycin.

Pre-disposing Factors for Myopathy/Rhabdomyolysis: PRAVACHOL, as with other HMG-CoA reductase inhibitors, should be prescribed with caution in patients with pre-disposing factors for myopathy/rhabdomyolysis. Such factors include: personal or family history of hereditary muscular disorders; previous history of muscle toxicity with another HMG-CoA reductase inhibitor; concomitant use of a fibrate or niacin; hypothyroidism; alcohol abuse; excessive physical exercise; age >70 years; renal impairment; hepatic impairment; diabetes with hepatic fatty change; surgery and trauma; frailty; situation where an increase in plasma levels of active ingredient may occur.

PRAVACHOL therapy should be temporarily withheld or discontinued in any patient with an acute serious condition suggestive of myopathy or predisposing to the development of rhabdomyolysis (e.g. sepsis, hypotension, major surgery, trauma, severe metabolic endocrine and electrolyte disorders, or uncontrolled seizures).

Liver Dysfunction: HMG-CoA reductase inhibitors have been associated with biochemical abnormalities of liver function. As with other lipid-lowering agents, including non-absorbable bile acid-binding resins, increases in liver enzymes to **less than** three times the upper limit of normal have occurred during therapy with pravastatin. The significance of these changes, which usually appear during the first few months of treatment initiation, is not known. In the majority of patients treated with pravastatin, in clinical trials, these increased values declined to pretreatment levels despite continuation of therapy at the same dose.

Marked persistent increases (greater than three times the upper limit of normal) in serum transaminases were seen in 6 out of 1142 (0.5%) patients treated with pravastatin in clinical trials (see Adverse Reactions). The increases usually appeared 3 to 12 months after the start of therapy with PRAVACHOL (pravastatin sodium). These elevations were not associated with clinical signs and symptoms of liver disease and usually declined to pretreatment levels upon discontinuation of therapy. Patients rarely had persistent marked abnormalities possibly attributable to therapy. In the largest long-term placebo-controlled trial with pravastatin (Pravastatin Primary Prevention Study/WOSCOPS), no patient with normal liver function after 12 weeks of treatment (N=2875 pravastatin-treated patients) had subsequent ALT elevations greater than three times the upper limit of normal on two consecutive measurements. Two of these 2875 patients treated with pravastatin (0.07%) and one of 2919 placebo patients (0.03%) had elevations of AST greater than three times the upper limit of normal on two consecutive measurements during the 4.8 years (median treatment) of the study.

Liver function tests should be performed at baseline and at 12 weeks following initiation of therapy or the elevation of dose. Special attention should be given to patients who develop increased transaminase levels. Liver function tests should be repeated to confirm an elevation and subsequently monitored at more frequent intervals. **If increases in alanine aminotransferase (ALT) and aspartate aminotransferase (AST) equal or exceed three times the upper limit of normal and persist, therapy should be discontinued.**

PRAVACHOL, as well as other HMG-CoA reductase inhibitors should be used with caution in patients who consume substantial quantities of alcohol and/or have a past history of liver disease. Active liver disease or unexplained serum transaminase elevations are contraindications to the use of PRAVACHOL; if such condition develops during therapy, the drug should be discontinued.

General: Before instituting therapy with PRAVACHOL (pravastatin sodium), an attempt should be made to control hypercholesterolemia with appropriate diet, exercise, weight reduction in overweight and obese patients, and to treat other underlying medical problems (see Indications and Clinical Use). The patient should be advised to inform subsequent physicians of the prior use of PRAVACHOL.

Pravastatin may elevate creatine phosphokinase and transaminase levels. This should be considered in the differential diagnosis of chest pain in a patient on therapy with pravastatin.

Effect on the Lens: Current data from clinical trials do not indicate an adverse effect of pravastatin on the human lens.

Homozygous Familial Hypercholesterolemia: Pravastatin has not been evaluated in patients with rare homozygous familial hypercholesterolemia. Most HMG-CoA reductase inhibitors are less or not effective in this subgroup of hypercholesterolemic patients.

Effect on Lipoprotein (a): In some patients, the beneficial effect of lowered total cholesterol and LDL-C levels may be partly blunted by a concomitant increase in the Lipoprotein (a)[Lp(a)] level. Further research is ongoing to elucidate the significance of Lp(a) variations. Therefore, until further experience is obtained, where feasible, it is suggested that measurements of serum Lp(a) be followed up in patients placed on pravastatin therapy.

Effect on CoQ10 Levels (Ubiquinone): A significant short-term decrease in plasma CoQ10 levels in patients treated with PRAVACHOL has been observed. Longer clinical trials have also shown reduced serum ubiquinone levels during treatment with pravastatin and other HMG-CoA reductase inhibitors. The clinical significance of a potential long-term statin-induced deficiency of CoQ10 has not yet been established. It has been reported that a decrease in myocardial ubiquinone levels could lead to impaired cardiac function in patients with borderline congestive heart failure.

Carcinogenesis and Mutagenesis: A 21-month oral study in mice, with doses of 10 to 100 mg/kg daily of pravastatin did not demonstrate any carcinogenic potential. In a 2-year oral study in rats, a statistically significant increase in the incidence of hepatocellular carcinoma was observed in male rats given 100 mg/kg daily (60 times the maximum human dose) of pravastatin. This change was not seen in male rats given 40 mg/kg daily (25 times the recommended human dose) or less, or in female rats at any dose level.

Hypersensitivity: With lovastatin an apparent hypersensitivity syndrome has been reported rarely which has included one or more of the following features: anaphylaxis, angioedema, lupus-like syndrome, polymyalgia rheumatica, thrombocytopenia, leukopenia, hemolytic anemia, positive antinuclear antibody (ANA), erythrocytes sedimentation rate (ESR) increase, arthritis, arthralgia, urticaria, asthenia, photosensitivity, fever and malaise.

Although to date hypersensitivity syndrome has not been described as such, in few instances eosinophilia and skin eruptions appear to be associated with PRAVACHOL treatment. If hypersensitivity is suspected PRAVACHOL should be discontinued. Patients should be advised to report promptly any signs of hypersensitivity such as angioedema, urticaria, photosensitivity, polyarthralgia, fever, malaise.

Endocrine and Metabolism: HMG-CoA reductase inhibitors interfere with cholesterol synthesis and as such could theoretically blunt adrenal and/or gonadal steroid production.

In one long-term study investigating the endocrine function in hypercholesterolemic patients, PRAVACHOL exhibited no effect upon basal and stimulated cortisol levels, as well as on aldosterone secretion. Although no change was reported in the testicular function, conflicting results were observed in the analysis of sperm motility after administration of PRAVACHOL. A case of reversible impotence has been reported in a 57-year old man administered pravastatin 20 mg/day and metoprolol. A causal relationship to therapy with PRAVACHOL has not been established. Further studies are needed to clarify the effects of HMG-CoA reductase inhibitors on male fertility. Furthermore, the effects, if any, on the pituitary-gonadal axis in premenopausal women are unknown.

Patients treated with PRAVACHOL who develop clinical evidence of endocrine dysfunction should be evaluated appropriately. Caution should be exercised if an HMG-CoA reductase inhibitor or other agent used to lower cholesterol levels is administered to patients receiving other drugs (e.g. ketoconazole, spironolactone, or cimetidine) that may decrease the levels of endogenous steroid hormones.

Patients with Severe Hypercholesterolemia: Higher doses (≥40 mg/day) required for some patients with severe hypercholesterolemia are associated with increased plasma levels of pravastatin. **Caution should be exercised in such patients who are also significantly renally impaired or elderly** (see Warnings and Precautions, Muscle Effects).

Special Populations: Pregnant Women: PRAVACHOL is contraindicated during pregnancy (see Contraindications).

Safety in pregnant women has not been established. Although pravastatin was not teratogenic in rats at doses as high as 1000 mg/kg daily nor in rabbits at doses of up to 50 mg/kg daily, PRAVACHOL should be administered to women of childbearing age only when such patients are highly unlikely to conceive and have been informed of potential hazards. If a woman becomes pregnant while taking PRAVACHOL, PRAVACHOL should be discontinued and the patient advised again as to the potential hazards to the fetus.

Nursing Women: A negligible amount of pravastatin is excreted in human breast milk. Because of the potential for adverse reactions in nursing infants, if the mother is being treated with PRAVACHOL, nursing should be discontinued or treatment with PRAVACHOL stopped.

Pediatrics (<16 years of age): Only limited experience with the use of statins in children is available. There is no experience to date with the use of PRAVACHOL in such patients. Treatment in these patients is not recommended at this time.

Geriatrics (≥65 years of age): Pharmacokinetic evaluation of pravastatin in patients over the age of 65 years indicates an increased AUC. There were no reported increases in the incidence of adverse effects in these or other studies involving patients in that age group. As a precautionary measure, the lowest dose should be administered initially.

Elderly patients may be more susceptible to myopathy (see Warnings and Precautions, Muscle Effects, Pre-disposing Factors for Myopathy/Rhabdomyolysis).

Patients with Impaired Renal Function: There have been no studies on the use of pravastatin in patients with renal insufficiency. As a precautionary measure, the lowest dose should be used in these patients (see Warnings and Precautions, Muscle Effects).

ADVERSE REACTIONS: Adverse Drug Reaction Overview: Pravastatin is generally well tolerated. Adverse events have been usually mild to moderate and transient. Adverse events observed or reported in short- and long-term trials are as follows (see Table 1 and Table 2).

Clinical Trial Adverse Drug Reactions: Because clinical trials are conducted under very specific conditions the adverse reaction rates observed in the clinical trials may not reflect the rates observed in practice and should not be compared to the rates in the clinical trials of another drug. Adverse drug reaction information from clinical trials is useful for identifying drug-related adverse events and for approximating rates.

Short-term Controlled Trials: All adverse clinical events (regardless of attribution) reported in more than 2% of pravastatin treated patients in placebo-controlled trials of up to four months duration are identified in the following table; also shown are the percentages of patients in whom these medical events were believed to be related or possibly related to the drug (see Table 1).

Table 1: PRAVACHOL

Adverse Events in >2 Percent of Patients Treated with Pravastatin 10-40 mg in Short-term Placebo-controlled Trials

Body System/Event	All Events		Events Attributed to Study Drug	
	Pravastatin (N=900) % of patients	Placebo (N=411) % of patients	Pravastatin (N=900) % of patients	Placebo (N=411) % of patients
Cardiovascular				
Cardiac Chest Pain	4.0	3.4	0.1	0.0
Dermatologic				
Rash	4.0[a]	1.1	1.3	0.9
Gastrointestinal				
Nausea/Vomiting	7.3	7.1	2.9	3.4
Diarrhea	6.2	5.6	2.0	1.9
Abdominal Pain	5.4	6.9	2.0	3.9
Constipation	4.0	7.1	2.4	5.1
Flatulence	3.3	3.6	2.7	3.4
Heartburn	2.9	1.9	2.0	0.7
General				
Fatigue	3.8	3.4	1.9	1.0
Chest Pain	3.7	1.9	0.3	0.2
Influenza	2.4[a]	0.7	0.0	0.0
Musculoskeletal				
Localized Pain	10.0	9.0	1.4	1.5
Myalgia	2.7	1.0	0.6	0.0
Nervous System				
Headache	6.2	3.9	1.7[a]	0.2
Dizziness	3.3	3.2	1.0	0.5
Renal/Genitourinary				
Urinary Abnormality	2.4	2.9	0.7	1.2
Respiratory				
Common Cold	7.0	6.3	0.0	0.0
Rhinitis	4.0	4.1	0.1	0.0

(cont'd)

Table 1: PRAVACHOL *(cont'd)*

Adverse Events in >2 Percent of Patients Treated with Pravastatin 10-40 mg in Short-term Placebo-controlled Trials

	All Events		Events Attributed to Study Drug	
Body System/Event	**Pravastatin (N=900) % of patients**	**Placebo (N=411) % of patients**	**Pravastatin (N=900) % of patients**	**Placebo (N=411) % of patients**
Cough	2.6	1.7	0.1	0.0

[a] Statistically significantly different from placebo.

The safety and tolerability of PRAVACHOL at a dose of 80 mg in two controlled trials with a mean exposure of 8.6 months was similar to that of PRAVACHOL at lower doses except that 4 out of 464 patients taking 80 mg of pravastatin had a single elevation of CK >10×ULN compared to 0 out of 115 patients taking 40 mg of pravastatin.

Long-term Controlled Morbidity and Mortality Trials: In seven randomized double blind placebo-controlled trials involving over 21 500 patients treated with pravastatin (N=10 784) or placebo (N=10 719), the safety and tolerability in the pravastatin group was comparable to that of the placebo group. Over 19 000 patients were followed for a median of 4.8-5.9 years, while the remaining patients were followed for two years or more.

Clinical adverse events probably or possibly related, or of uncertain relationship to therapy, occurring in at least 0.5% of patients treated with pravastatin or placebo in these long-term morbidity/mortality trials are shown in Table 2.

Table 2: PRAVACHOL

Clinical Adverse Events Reported in Placebo-controlled Studies

	PRAVACHOL (N=10 784) %	**Placebo (N=10 719) %**
Cardiovascular		
Angina Pectoris	3.1	3.4
Disturbance Rhythm Subjective	0.8	0.7
Hypertension	0.7	0.9
Edema	0.6	0.6
Myocardial Infarction	0.5	0.7
Gastrointestinal		
Dyspepsia/Heartburn	3.5	3.7
Nausea/Vomiting	1.4	1.6
Flatulence	1.2	1.1
Constipation	1.2	1.3
Diarrhea	0.9	1.1
Abdominal Pain	0.9	1.0
Distention Abdomen	0.5	0.5
Musculoskeletal		
Musculoskeletal Pain (includes arthralgia)	5.9	5.7
Muscle Cramp	2.0	1.8
Myalgia	1.4	1.4
Musculoskeletal Trauma	0.5	0.3
Nervous System		
Dizziness	2.2	2.1
Headache	1.9	1.8
Sleep Disturbance	1.0	0.9
Depression	1.0	1.0
Anxiety/Nervousness	1.0	1.2
Paresthesia	0.9	0.9
Numbness	0.5	0.4
General		
Fatigue	3.4	3.3
Chest Pain	2.6	2.6
Weight Gain	0.6	0.7
Influenza	0.6	0.5
Special Senses		
Vision Disturbance (includes blurred vision)	1.5	1.3
Disturbance Eye (includes eye inflammation)	0.8	0.9
Hearing Abnormality (includes tinnitus and hearing loss)	0.6	0.5
Lens Opacity	0.5	0.4
Dermatologic		
Rash	2.1	2.2
Pruritus	0.9	1.0
Renal/Genitourinary		
Urinary Abnormality (includes dysuria and nocturia)	1.0	0.8
Respiratory		
Dyspnea	1.6	1.6
Upper Respiratory Infection	1.3	1.3
Cough	1.0	1.0
Sinus Abnormality (includes sinusitis)	0.8	0.8
Pharyngitis	0.5	0.6

Abnormal Hematologic and Clinical Chemistry Findings: Increases in serum transaminases and in creatine phosphokinase (CK) in patients treated with PRAVACHOL have been discussed (see Warnings and Precautions).

Post-Market Adverse Drug Reactions: The following adverse events have also been rarely reported during post-marketing experience with PRAVACHOL, regardless of causality assessment:

Cardiovascular: angioedema.

Dermatologic: a variety of skin changes (pruritus, scalp hair abnormalities, skin dryness and dermatitis).

Gastrointestinal: pancreatitis, hepatitis and fulminant hepatic necrosis, jaundice (including cholestatic), fatty change in liver, cirrhosis, thrombocytopenia, hepatoma, abnormal stool and appetite change. Liver Function Test (LFT) abnormalities have also been reported.

General: chest pain (non cardiovascular), weakness, excess sweating hot flashes and fever.

Hypersensitivity: anaphylaxis, lupus erythematosus-like syndrome, polymyalgia, rheumatica, dermatomyositis, vasculitis, purpura, hemolytic anemia, positive ANA, ESR increase, arthritis, arthralgia, asthenia, photosensitivity, chills, malaise, toxic epidermal necrolysis, erythema multiforme, including Stevens-Johnson syndrome.

Immunologic: allergy.

Musculoskeletal: myopathy, rhabdomyolysis.

Nervous System: dysfunction of certain cranial nerves (including alteration of taste, impairment of extra-ocular movement, facial paresis), peripheral nerve palsy, paresthesia equilibrium disturbance, vertigo, memory impairment, tremor, mood change.

Reproductive: gynecomastia, impotence (see Warnings and Precautions, Endocrine and Metabolism), urticaria, sexual dysfunction, libido change.

Special Senses: eye symptoms (including soreness, dryness or itching), tinnitus, taste disturbance.

The following have also been reported with other statins: hepatitis, cholestatic jaundice, anorexia, psychic disturbances including anxiety, hypospermia and hypersensitivity (see Warnings and Precautions).

Lens: Current data from clinical trials do not indicate an adverse effect of pravastatin on the human lens.

DRUG INTERACTIONS: Drug-Drug Interactions: Concomitant Therapy with Other Lipid Metabolism Regulators: Based on post-marketing surveillance, gemfibrozil, fenofibrate, other fibrates and lipid lowering doses of niacin (nicotinic acid) may increase the risk of myopathy when given concomitantly with HMG-CoA reductase inhibitors, probably because they can produce myopathy when given alone (see Warnings and Precautions, Muscle Effects). Therefore, combined drug therapy should be approached with caution.

Bile Acid Sequestrants: Preliminary evidence suggests that the cholesterol-lowering effects of PRAVACHOL and the bile acid sequestrants, cholestyramine/colestipol are additive.

When pravastatin was administered one hour before or four hours after cholestyramine or one hour before colestipol and a standard meal, there was no clinically significant decrease in bioavailability or therapeutic effect. Concomitant administration resulted in an approximately 40 to 50% decrease in the mean AUC of pravastatin (see Dosage and Administration, Concomitant Therapy).

Gemfibrozil and Nicotinic Acid: Gemfibrozil and nicotinic acid do not statistically significantly affect the bioavailability of pravastatin. However, in a limited size clinical trial, a trend toward CK elevations and musculoskeletal symptoms was seen in patients treated concurrently with pravastatin and gemfibrozil.

Myopathy, including rhabdomyolysis, has occurred in patients who were receiving coadministration of HMG-CoA reductase inhibitors with fibric acid derivatives and niacin, particularly in subjects with pre-existing renal insufficiency (see Warnings and Precautions, Muscle Effects).

Other Concomitant Therapy: The use of HMG-CoA reductase inhibitors has been associated with severe myopathy, including rhabdomyolysis, which may be more frequent when they are administered with drugs that inhibit the cytochrome P450 enzyme system. In vitro and in vivo data indicate that pravastatin is not metabolized by cytochrome P450 3A4 to a clinically significant extent. This has been shown in studies with known cytochrome P450 3A4 inhibitors.

Digoxin: Coadministration of digoxin and other HMG-CoA reductase inhibitors has been shown to increase the steady state digoxin concentrations. The potential effects of coadministration of digoxin and PRAVACHOL are not known. As a precautionary measure, patients taking digoxin should be closely monitored.

Antipyrine: Antipyrine was used as a model for drugs metabolized by the microsomal hepatic enzyme system (cytochrome P450 system). Pravastatin had no effect on the pharmacokinetics of antipyrine.

Coumarin Anticoagulants: Pravastatin had no clinically significant effect on prothrombin time when administered in a study to normal elderly subjects who were stabilized on warfarin.

Antacids and Cimetidine: On the average, antacids (one hour prior to PRAVACHOL) reduce and cimetidine increases the bioavailability of pravastatin. These changes were not statistically significant. The clinical significance of these interactions is not known but is probably minimal as judged from the interaction with food (see Action and Clinical Pharmacology, Human Pharmacology).

No information is available regarding interactions with erythromycin (see Warnings and Precautions, Muscle Effects).

Although specific interaction studies were not performed during clinical trials, no noticeable drug interactions were reported when PRAVACHOL was added to diuretics, antihypertensives, angiotensin converting-enzyme (ACE) inhibitors, calcium channel blockers, or nitroglycerin.

Propranolol: Co-administration of propranolol and pravastatin reduced the AUC values by 23% and 16% respectively.

Cyclosporine: In a multicentre study, the AUC values of pravastatin were shown to be five-fold higher in the presence of cyclosporine. There was no accumulation of pravastatin after multiple doses (see Dosage and Administration).

Drug-Laboratory Interactions: Pravastatin may elevate creatine phosphokinase and transaminase levels. This should be considered in the differential diagnosis of chest pain in a patient on therapy with pravastatin.

(cont'd)

DOSAGE AND ADMINISTRATION: **Dosing Considerations:** Patients should be placed on a standard cholesterol-lowering diet (at least equivalent to the Adult Treatment Panel III [ATP III TLC diet]) before receiving PRAVACHOL, and should continue on this diet during treatment with PRAVACHOL. If appropriate, a program of weight control and physical exercise should be implemented.

Prior to initiating therapy with PRAVACHOL, secondary causes for elevations in plasma lipid levels should be excluded. A lipid profile should also be performed.

Recommended Dose and Dosage Adjustment: Hypercholesterolemia and Coronary Heart Disease: The recommended starting dose is 20 mg once daily at bed time. Patients who require a large dose reduction in LDL-C may be started at 40 mg once daily. The dose of 80 mg once daily should be reserved for patients who do not achieve their treatment goal with lower doses. PRAVACHOL may be taken without regard to meals (see Action and Clinical Pharmacology).

In patients with a history of significant renal or hepatic dysfunction, a starting dose of 10 mg daily is recommended.

Concomitant Therapy: Some patients may require combination therapy with one or more lipid- lowering agents. Pharmacokinetic interaction with pravastatin administered concurrently with nicotinic acid, or gemfibrozil did not statistically significantly affect the bioavailability of pravastatin. The combined use of pravastatin and fibrates should however generally be avoided (see Warnings and Precautions, Muscle Effects).

The lipid-lowering effects of PRAVACHOL on Total and Low Density Lipoprotein Cholesterol are additive when combined with a bile acid- binding resin. However, when administering a bile acid-binding resin (e.g. cholestyramine, colestipol) and pravastatin, PRAVACHOL should not be administered concomitantly, but should be given either one hour or more before or at least four hours following the resin (see Drug Interactions, Concomitant Therapy with Other Lipid Metabolism Regulators).

In patients taking cyclosporine, with or without other immunosuppressive drugs, concomitantly with pravastatin, therapy should be initiated with 10 mg per day and titration to higher doses should be performed with caution. Most patients treated with this combination received a maximum pravastatin dose of 20 mg/day (see Warnings and Precautions and Drug Interactions, Other Concomitant Therapy, Cyclosporine).

The dosage of PRAVACHOL should be individualized according to baseline LDL-C, total- C/HDL-C ratio and/or TG levels to achieve the desired lipid values at the lowest possible dose.

OVERDOSAGE:

There have been two reports of overdosage with pravastatin, both of which were asymptomatic and not associated with clinical laboratory abnormalities.

In the event of overdosage, treatment should be symptomatic and supportive, and appropriate therapy instituted. Until further experience is obtained, no specific therapy of overdosage can be recommended. The dialyzability of pravastatin and its metabolites is not known.

> For management of a suspected drug overdose, CPhA recommends that you contact your **regional Poison Control Centre**. See the *CPS* Directory section for a list of Poison Control Centres.

ACTION AND CLINICAL PHARMACOLOGY: Mechanism of Action: PRAVACHOL (pravastatin sodium) is one of a new class of lipid-lowering compounds known as HMG-CoA reductase inhibitors (statins) that reduce cholesterol biosynthesis. These agents are competitive inhibitors of 3-hydroxy- 3-methylglutaryl-coenzyme A (HMG-CoA) reductase, the enzyme catalyzing the early rate-limiting step in cholesterol biosynthesis, conversion of HMG-CoA to mevalonate. Pravastatin is isolated from a strain of Penicillium citrinum. The active drug substance is the hydroxyacid form.

PRAVACHOL produces its lipid-lowering effect in two ways. First, as a consequence of its reversible inhibition of HMG-CoA reductase activity, it effects modest reductions in intracellular pools of cholesterol. This results in an increase in the number of Low Density Lipoproteins (LDL)-receptors on cell surfaces and enhanced receptor-mediated catabolism and clearance of circulating LDL. Second, pravastatin inhibits LDL production by inhibiting hepatic synthesis of Very Low Density Lipoproteins (VLDL), the LDL precursor.

Epidemiologic and clinical investigations have associated the risk of coronary artery disease (CAD) with elevated levels of Total-C, LDL-C and decreased levels of HDL-C. These abnormalities of lipoprotein metabolism are considered as major contributors to the development of the disease. Other factors, e.g. interactions between lipids/ lipoproteins and endothelium, platelets and macrophages, have also been incriminated in the development of human atherosclerosis and of its complications.

In long-term, prospective clinical trials effective treatment of hypercholesterolemia/ dyslipidemia has consistently been associated with a reduction in the risk of CAD.

Treatment with PRAVACHOL has been shown to reduce circulating Total-C, LDL-C, and apolipoprotein B, modestly reduce VLDL-C and triglycerides (TG) while producing increases of variable magnitude in HDL-C and apolipoprotein A. Clinical trials suggest that PRAVACHOL's effect on reducing clinical events appears to incorporate both cholesterol modification and some ancillary mechanism.

Pravastatin has complex pharmacokinetic characteristics.

Human Pharmacology: In both normal volunteers and patients with hypercholesterolemia, treatment with PRAVACHOL (pravastatin sodium) reduced total-C, LDL-C, apolipoprotein B, VLDL-C and TG while increasing HDL-C and apolipoprotein A. The mechanism of action of PRAVACHOL (pravastatin sodium) is complex. Inhibition of hepatic VLDL synthesis and/or secretion occurs, leading to a decrease in LDL precursor formation. The reduction in hepatic cellular pools of cholesterol, resulting from the specific and reversible inhibition of HMG-CoA reductase activity, leads to an increase in the fractional catabolic rate of IDL and LDL via increased expression of LDL receptors on the surface of hepatic cells. Through a combination of these and possibly other unknown metabolic effects, a decline in the serum level of cholesterol results.

Pharmacokinetics: Absorption: Pravastatin sodium is administered orally in the active form. Following oral ingestion, pravastatin is rapidly absorbed with peak plasma levels attained at about 1 to 1.5 hours. Average oral absorption of pravastatin, based on urinary recovery of radiolabelled drug after oral and intravenous dosing, is 34%; average absolute bioavailability of the parent drug is 17%. The therapeutic response to PRAVACHOL is similar, whether taken with meals or one hour prior to meals, even though the presence of food in the gastrointestinal tract causes a reduction in systemic bioavailability (see Table 3).

Table 3: PRAVACHOL

Percent Decrease in LDL-C

Pravastatin	10 mg bid	20 mg bid
With meals	−25%	−37%
Before meals[a]	−26%	−36%

[a] Administered one hour or more prior to eating.

Distribution: Pravastatin undergoes extensive first pass extraction in the liver (estimated hepatic extraction ratio, 66%), its primary site of action, and is excreted in the bile. Therefore, plasma levels of the drug are probably of limited value in predicting therapeutic effectiveness. Nevertheless, measurement of plasma pravastatin concentrations by gas chromatography and massspectrometry showed dose proportionality for area under the concentration-time curve (AUC) and maximum and steady-state plasma levels. Steady-state areas under the plasma concentrationtime- curves and maximum (C_{max}) or minimum (C_{min}) plasma concentrations showed no accumulation following once or twice-daily administration of PRAVACHOL tablets.

Metabolism: Pravastatin is extensively metabolized. The major metabolite is the 3 α-hydroxy isomer, which has one-tenth to one-fortieth of the inhibitory activity of the parent compound on HMG-CoA reductase.

Excretion: Protein binding of pravastatin is approximately 50%. The plasma elimination half-life of pravastatin is between 1.5 and 2 hours (2.5-3 hours in hypercholesterolemic subjects). Approximately 20% of a radiolabelled oral dose is excreted in the urine and 70% in the feces.

After intravenous administration to healthy subjects, approximately 47% of the total drug clearance occurs via renal excretion of intact pravastatin, and about 53% is cleared by non-renal routes, i.e. biliary excretion and biotransformation.

Special Populations and Conditions: Pediatrics: Only limited experience with the use of statins in children is available. There is no experience to date with the use of PRAVACHOL in such patients. Treatment in these patients is not recommended at this time.

Geriatrics: Studies of PRAVACHOL administered as a single dose to healthy elderly male and female subjects (age 65 to 78 years) indicated a 30-50% increase in plasma levels.

Renal Insufficiency: No studies have been carried out in patients with renal insufficiency.

STORAGE AND STABILITY: PRAVACHOL (pravastatin sodium) should be stored at room temperature (15-30°C). Protect from moisture and light.

INFORMATION FOR THE PATIENT: Published in e-CPS, available by subscription at www.e-cps.ca.

DOSAGE FORMS, COMPOSITION AND PACKAGING: 10 mg: Each pink to peach, rounded, rectangular-shaped, biconvex tablet, with a P embossed on one side and PRAVACHOL 10 engraved on the other, contains: pravastatin sodium 10 mg. Nonmedicinal ingredients: croscarmellose sodium, lactose, magnesium oxide, magnesium stearate, microcrystalline cellulose, povidone and red ferric oxide. Bottles of 90.

20 mg: Each yellow, rounded, rectangular-shaped, biconvex tablet, with a P embossed on one side and PRAVACHOL 20 engraved on the other, contains: pravastatin sodium 20 mg. Nonmedicinal ingredients: croscarmellose sodium, lactose, magnesium oxide, magnesium stearate, microcrystalline cellulose, povidone and yellow ferric oxide. Bottles of 90.

40 mg: Each green, rounded, rectangular-shaped, biconvex tablet, with a P embossed on one side and PRAVACHOL 40 engraved on the other, contains: pravastatin sodium 40 mg. Nonmedicinal ingredients: croscarmellose sodium, D&C yellow no. 10, FD&C blue no. 1, lactose, magnesium oxide, magnesium stearate, microcrystalline cellulose and povidone. Bottles of 90.

(Shown in Product Identification Section)

Pravastatin Ⓟ

CPhA Monograph

see *HMG-CoA Reductase Inhibitors*

Precedex™ Ⓟ

dexmedetomidine HCl

Alpha2-Adrenergic Agonist

Hospira

Date of Preparation: December 8, 2009

SUMMARY PRODUCT INFORMATION:

Route of Administration	Dosage Form/Strength	All Nonmedicinal Ingredients
IV infusion	Parenteral injection, 100 µg/mL in a 2 mL vial	Sodium Chloride 0.9%

INDICATIONS AND CLINICAL USE: Precedex (Dexmedetomidine Hydrochloride for Injection) is indicated for:

- **Intensive Care Unit Sedation:** Precedex is indicated for sedation of initially intubated and mechanically ventilated post-surgical patients during treatment in an intensive care setting by continuous intravenous infusion. The Precedex infusion must not exceed 24 hours.

  Precedex has been continuously infused in mechanically ventilated patients prior to extubation, during extubation, and post-extubation. It is not necessary to discontinue Precedex prior to extubation. After extubation, the dose of Precedex should be reduced by half. The mean time of continued infusion is approximately 6.6 hours.
- **Conscious Sedation:** Precedex is indicated for sedation of non-intubated patients prior to and/or during surgical and other procedures by continuous intravenous infusion for the following procedures:
  - Monitored Anesthesia Care (MAC) with an adequate nerve block and/or local infiltration; and
  - Awake Fiberoptic Intubation (AFI) with adequate topical preparation of the upper airway with local lidocaine formulations.

  Due to insufficient safety and efficacy data, Precedex is not recommended for use in procedures other than the two listed above.

Geriatrics (>65 years of age): Dosage adjustment in this population is recommended (see Dosage and Administration).

Pediatrics: There have been no clinical studies to establish the safety and efficacy of Precedex in pediatric patients younger than 18 years of age. Therefore, Precedex should not be used in this population.

CONTRAINDICATIONS:

- Patients who are hypersensitive to this drug or to any ingredient in the formulation or component of the container. For a complete listing, see Dosage Forms, Composition and Packaging.

WARNINGS AND PRECAUTIONS: General: Precedex should be administered only by persons skilled in the management of patients in the intensive care or operating room setting. Due to the known pharmacological effects of Precedex, patients should be continuously monitored while receiving Precedex.

Cardiovascular: Hypotension, Bradycardia and Sinus Arrest: Clinically significant episodes of bradycardia and sinus arrest have been reported with Precedex administration in young, healthy volunteers with high vagal tone or with different routes of administration including rapid intravenous or bolus administration.

Reports of hypotension and bradycardia have been associated with Precedex infusion. If medical intervention is required, treatment may include decreasing or stopping the infusion of Precedex, increasing the rate of intravenous fluid administration, elevation of the lower extremities, and use of pressor agents. Because Precedex has the potential to augment bradycardia induced by vagal stimuli; clinicians should be prepared to intervene. The intravenous administration of anticholinergic agents (e.g., glycopyrrolate, atropine) should be considered to modify vagal tone. In clinical trials, glycopyrrolate or atropine were effective in the treatment of most episodes of Precedex-induced bradycardia. However, in some patients with significant cardiovascular dysfunction, more advanced resuscitative measures were required.

Caution should be exercised when administering Precedex to patients with advanced heart block and/or severe ventricular dysfunction. Because Precedex decreases sympathetic nervous system activity, hypotension and/or bradycardia may be expected to be more pronounced in patients with hypovolemia, diabetes mellitus, or chronic hypertension and in elderly patients.

In situations where other vasodilators or negative chronotropic agents are administered, co-administration of Precedex could have an additive pharmacodynamic effect and should be administered with caution.

Transient Hypertension: Transient hypertension has been observed primarily during the loading dose in association with the initial peripheral vasoconstrictive effects of Precedex. Treatment of the transient hypertension has generally not been necessary, although reduction of the loading dose infusion rate may be desirable.

Dependence/Tolerance: Precedex is not a controlled substance. The dependence potential of Precedex has not been studied in humans.

Endocrine and Metabolism: The available evidence is inadequate to confirm if dexmedetomidine is associated with significant adrenocortical suppression. The adequacy of the adrenocortical function should be individually assessed and managed.

Hepatic/Biliary/Pancreatic: Since Precedex clearance decreases with severity of hepatic impairment, dose reduction should be considered in patients with impaired hepatic function.

Renal: Precedex is known to be substantially excreted by the kidney, and the risk of adverse reactions to this drug may be greater in patients with impaired renal function (see Dosage and Administration).

Peri-Operative Considerations: Arousability: Some patients receiving Precedex have been observed to be arousable and alert when stimulated. This alone should not be considered as evidence of lack of efficacy in the absence of other clinical signs and symptoms.

Withdrawal: Intensive Care Unit: Precedex is indicated only for sedation of initially intubated and mechanically ventilated post-operative patients recovering in a post-operative care unit or an intensive care unit. During the use of Precedex in an intensive care setting, the patients must be monitoring continuously, particularly for their cardiovascular safety indicators.

If Precedex were to be administered for more than 24 hours and stopped abruptly, withdrawal symptoms similar to those reported for other alpha[2]-adrenergic agents may result. These symptoms include nervousness, agitation, and headaches, accompanied or followed by a rapid rise in blood pressure and elevated catecholamine concentrations in the plasma. Precedex infusion must not exceed 24 hours.

Conscious Sedation: Withdrawal symptoms were not seen after discontinuation of short term infusion of Precedex (<6 hours).

Information to Be Provided to the Patient: Precedex is indicated for short-term intravenous sedation. Dosage must be individualized and titrated to the desired clinical effect. Blood pressure, heart rate and oxygen levels will be monitored both continuously during the infusion of Precedex and as clinically appropriate after discontinuation.

- When Precedex is infused for more than 6 hours, patients should be informed to report nervousness, agitation, and headaches that may occur for up to 48 hours.

- Additionally, patients should be informed to report symptoms that may occur within 48 hours after the administration of Precedex such as: weakness, confusion, excessive sweating, weight loss, abdominal pain, salt cravings, diarrhea, constipation, dizziness or light-headedness.

Special Populations: Pregnant Women: There are no adequate and well-controlled studies in pregnant women. Precedex should be used during pregnancy only if the potential benefits justify the potential risk to the fetus.

Labor and Delivery: The safety of Precedex during labor and delivery has not been studied. Therefore, Precedex is not recommended during labor and delivery including cesarean section deliveries.

Nursing Women: It is not known whether Precedex is excreted in human milk. Radio-labeled Precedex administered subcutaneously to lactating female rats was excreted in milk. Because many drugs are excreted in human milk, caution should be exercised when Precedex is administered to a nursing woman.

Pediatrics: There have been no clinical studies to establish the safety and efficacy of Precedex in pediatric patients below 18 years of age. Therefore, Precedex should not be used in this population.

Geriatrics: Precedex is known to be substantially excreted by the kidney, and the risk of adverse reactions to this drug may be greater in patients with impaired renal function. Because elderly patients are more likely to have decreased renal function, care should be taken in dose selection in elderly patients, and it may be useful to monitor renal function.

Intensive Care Unit Sedation: A total of 849 patients in the clinical studies were 65 years of age and over. A total of 242 patients were 75 years of age and over. In patients greater than 65 years of age, a higher incidence of bradycardia and hypotension was observed following administration of Precedex. Therefore a dose reduction should be considered in patients over 65 years of age (see Dosage and Administration).

Conscious Sedation: A total of 131 patients in the clinical studies were 65 years of age and over. A total of 47 patients were 75 years of age and over. Hypotension occurred in a higher incidence in Precedex-treated patients 65 years or older (72%) and 75 years or older (74%) as compared to patients <65 years (47%). Pre-specified criteria for the vital signs to be reported as adverse reactions are footnoted below Table 2 (see Adverse Reactions). A reduced loading dose of 0.5 µg/kg given over 10 minutes is recommended and a reduction in the maintenance infusion should be considered for patients greater than 65 years of age (see Dosage and Administration).

ADVERSE REACTIONS: Adverse Drug Reaction Overview: Use of Precedex has been associated with the following serious adverse reactions:

- Hypotension, bradycardia and sinus arrest (see Warnings and Precautions),
- Transient hypertension (see Warnings and Precautions).

Most common treatment-emergent adverse reactions, occurring in greater than 2% of patients in both Intensive Care Unit and conscious sedation studies include hypotension, bradycardia and dry mouth.

Clinical Trial Adverse Drug Reactions: Because clinical trials are conducted under very specific conditions the adverse reaction rates observed in the clinical trials may not reflect the rates observed in practice and should not be compared to the rates in the clinical trials of another drug. Adverse drug reaction information from clinical trials is useful for identifying drug-related adverse events and for approximating rates.

Intensive Care Unit Sedation: Adverse event information derived from the placebo-controlled, continuous infusion trials of Precedex for sedation in the surgical intensive care unit setting in which 387 patients received Precedex. In these studies, the mean total dose was 7.06 µg/kg (SD=2.86), mean dose per hour was 0.51 µg/kg/hr (SD=0.39) and the mean duration of infusion of 15.6 hours (range: 0.17 to 29.08). Midazolam or propofol was used as the rescue medication for patients on Precedex or placebo. The population was between 19 to 83 years of age, 43% ≥65 years of age, 73% male and 97% Caucasian. Overall, the most frequently observed treatment-emergent adverse events included hypotension, hypertension, nausea, bradycardia, fever, vomiting, hypoxia, tachycardia and anemia (see Table 1).

Table 1: Precedex

Treatment-Emergent Adverse Events Occurring in >1% of All Dexmedetomidine-Treated Patients in Placebo-controlled Continuous Infusion Short-Term Intensive Care Unit Sedation Studies

Adverse Event	Randomized Dexmedetomidine[a] (N=387)	Placebo with Midazolam Rescue (N=181)	Placebo with Propofol Rescue (N=198)
Hypotension	28%	15%	10%
Hypertension	16%	13%	23%
Nausea	11%	9%	10%
Bradycardia	7%	3%	2%
Fever	5%	6%	4%
Vomiting	4%	6%	6%
Atrial Fibrillation	4%	4%	3%
Hypoxia	4%	5%	3%
Tachycardia	3%	7%	3%
Hemorrhage	3%	6%	4%
Anemia	3%	4%	1%
Dry Mouth	3%	2%	<1%
Rigors	2%	3%	4%
Agitation	2%	3%	3%
Hyperpyrexia	2%	3%	2%
Pain	2%	3%	1%
Hyperglycemia	2%	3%	1%
Acidosis	2%	<1%	3%
Pleural Effusion	2%	<1%	2%
Oliguria	2%	1%	<1%
Thirst	2%	<1%	<1%

[a] Data combined from studies conducted in post-surgical patients recovering in an ICU setting.

Conscious Sedation: Adverse event information is derived from the two trials for conscious sedation in which 318 patients received Precedex. Midazolam was used as the rescue medication for patients on Precedex or placebo. The mean total dose was 1.6 µg/kg (range: 0.5 to 6.7), mean dose per hour was 1.3 µg/kg/hr (range: 0.3 to 6.1) and the mean duration of infusion of 1.5 hours (range: 0.1 to 6.2). The population was between 18 to 93 years of age, 30% ≥65 years of age, 52% male and 61% Caucasian.

Treatment-emergent adverse events occurring at an incidence of >2% are provided in Table 2. The most frequent adverse events were hypotension, bradycardia, and dry mouth. Pre-specified criteria for the vital signs to be reported as adverse reactions are footnoted below the table. The decrease in respiratory rate and hypoxia was similar between Precedex and comparator groups in both studies.

Table 2: Precedex

Adverse Events with an Incidence >2%—Conscious Sedation Population

Body System/Adverse Event	Precedex N=318 n (%)	Placebo N=113 n (%)
Vascular Disorders		
Hypotension[a]	173 (54%)	34 (30%)
Hypertension[b]	41 (13%)	27 (24%)
Respiratory, Thoracic and Mediastinal Disorders		
Respiratory depression[e]	117 (37%)	36 (32%)
Hypoxia[f]	7 (2%)	3 (3%)
Bradypnea	5 (2%)	5 (4%)
Cardiac Disorders		
Bradycardia[c]	45 (14%)	4 (4%)
Tachycardia[d]	17 (5%)	19 (17%)
Gastrointestinal Disorders		
Nausea	10 (3%)	2 (2%)
Dry mouth	8 (3%)	1 (1%)

[a] Hypotension was defined in absolute and relative terms as Systolic blood pressure of <80 mmHg or ≤30% lower than pre-study drug infusion value, or Diastolic blood pressure of <50 mmHg.
[b] Hypertension was defined in absolute and relative terms as Systolic blood pressure >180 mmHg or ≥30% higher than pre-study drug infusion value or Diastolic blood pressure of >100 mmHg.
[c] Bradycardia was defined in absolute and relative terms as <40 bpm or ≤30% lower than pre-study drug infusion value.
[d] Tachycardia was defined in absolute and relative terms as >120 bpm or ≥30% greater than pre-study drug infusion value.
[e] Respiratory Depression was defined in absolute and relative terms as respiratory rate (RR) <8 bpm or >25% decrease from baseline.
[f] Hypoxia was defined in absolute and relative terms as SpO_2 <90% or 10% decrease from baseline.

Post-Market Adverse Drug Reactions: The following adverse reactions have been identified during post approval use of Precedex. Because these reactions are reported voluntarily from a population of uncertain size, it is not always possible to reliably estimate their frequency or establish a causal relationship to drug exposure.

Hypotension and bradycardia were the most common adverse reactions associated with the use of Precedex during post approval use of the drug. See Table 3.

Table 3: Precedex

Adverse Events Experienced During Post Approval Use of Precedex

Body System	Preferred Term
Body as a Whole	Fever, hyperpyrexia, hypovolemia, light anesthesia, pain, rigors
Cardiovascular Disorders, General	Blood pressure fluctuation, heart disorder, hypertension, hypotension, myocardial infarction
Central and Peripheral Nervous System Disorders	Dizziness, headache, neuralgia, neuritis, speech disorder, convulsion
Gastrointestinal System Disorders	Abdominal pain, diarrhea, vomiting, nausea
Heart Rate and Rhythm Disorders	Arrhythmia, ventricular arrhythmia, bradycardia, hypoxia, atrioventricular block, cardiac arrest, extrasystoles, atrial fibrillation, heart block, T wave inversion, tachycardia, supraventricular tachycardia, ventricular tachycardia
Liver and Biliary System Disorders	Increased gamma-glutamyl transpeptidase, hepatic function abnormal, hyperbilirubinemia, increased alanine transaminase, increased aspartate aminotransferase
Metabolic and Nutritional Disorders	Acidosis, respiratory acidosis, hyperkalemia, increased alkaline phosphatase, thirst, hypoglycemia
Psychiatric Disorders	Agitation, confusion, delirium, hallucination, illusion
Red Blood Cell Disorders	Anemia
Renal Disorders	Blood urea nitrogen increased, oliguria
Respiratory System Disorders	Apnea, bronchospasm, dyspnea, hypercapnia, hypoventilation, hypoxia, pulmonary congestion
Skin and Appendages Disorders	Increased sweating
Vascular Disorders	Hemorrhage
Vision Disorders	Photopsia, abnormal vision

DRUG INTERACTIONS: Drug-Drug Interactions: Anesthetics, Sedatives, Hypnotics, Opioids: Co-administration of Precedex with anesthetics, sedatives, hypnotics, and opioids is likely to lead to an enhancement of effects. Specific studies have confirmed these effects with sevoflurane, isoflurane, propofol, alfentanil, and midazolam. No pharmacokinetic interactions between Precedex and isoflurane, propofol, alfentanil and midazolam have been demonstrated. However, due to possible pharmacodynamic interactions, when co-administered with Precedex, a reduction in dosage of Precedex or the concomitant anesthetic, sedative, hypnotic or opioid may be required.

Neuromuscular Blockers: In one study of 10 healthy volunteers, administration of Precedex for 45 minutes at a plasma concentration of 1 (one) ng/mL resulted in no clinically meaningful increases in the magnitude of neuromuscular blockade associated with rocuronium administration.

Cytochrome P-450: In vitro studies in human liver microsomes demonstrated no evidence of cytochrome P450 mediated drug interactions that are likely to be of clinical relevance.

DOSAGE AND ADMINISTRATION: Dosing Considerations:

- Precedex should be used in only facilities adequately staffed and equipped for anesthesia, resuscitation, and cardiovascular monitoring.
- Precedex dosing should be individualized and titrated to the desired clinical response.
- Precedex is not indicated for infusions lasting longer than 24 hours.
- Precedex should be administered using a controlled infusion device with adequate precision.

Recommended Dose and Dosage Adjustment: Intensive Care Unit Sedation:

- Precedex is indicated for post-surgical patients in an intensive care setting, e.g. in Post Anesthesia Care Unit or Intensive Care Unit.
- An assessment of the level of sedation and the need for Precedex should precede the initiation of Precedex.
- Another intravenous sedative (e.g. midazolam or propofol) may be added if Precedex provides inadequate sedation at the highest recommended dose level.
- The need for Precedex continuous infusion post-extubation must be assessed individually. If the continuous infusion is needed post-extubation, the infusion speed should be reduced by half. The mean time of continued infusion is approximately 6.6 hours.
- Precedex use should not exceed 24 hours in an ICU setting.

A dose reduction for both the loading and maintenance infusions should be considered in patients with impaired hepatic or renal function and in patients over 65 years of age.

Initiation: For adult patients, Precedex is generally initiated with a loading infusion of up to one µg/kg over 10 to 20 minutes, if needed.

For patients being converted from alternate sedative therapy a loading dose may not be required.

Maintenance: Adult patients will generally require a maintenance infusion of 0.2 to 0.7 µg/kg/hr. The rate of the maintenance infusion should be adjusted to achieve the desired level of sedation.

Conscious Sedation:

- Based on the Ramsay and Observer's Assessment of Alertness/Sedation Scales, the loading infusion provides clinically effective onset of sedation 10 to 15 minutes after start of infusion.
- For use in Monitored Anesthesia Care, an adequate nerve block and/or local infiltration should be used.
- For Awake Fiberoptic Intubation, the upper airway should be topicalized with proper lidocaine formulations.

Initiation: For adult patients, Precedex is generally initiated with a loading infusion of one µg/kg over 10 minutes.

For patients over 65 years of age or those undergoing less invasive procedures such as ophthalmic surgery, a loading infusion of 0.5 µg/kg over 10 minutes may be suitable.

Maintenance: The maintenance infusion of Precedex is generally initiated at 0.6 µg/kg/hr and titrated to achieve desired clinical effect with doses ranging from 0.2 to 1 µg/kg/hr. The rate of the maintenance infusion should be adjusted to achieve the targeted level of sedation.

Following the load in awake fiberoptic intubation, a fixed maintenance dose of 0.7 µg/kg/hr is recommended until the endotracheal tube is secured.

Dosage Adjustment: Due to possible pharmacodynamic interactions, a reduction in dosage of Precedex or other concomitant anesthetics, sedatives, hypnotics or opioids may be required when co-administered.

A dose reduction for both the loading and maintenance infusions should be considered in patients with impaired hepatic or renal function and in patients over 65 years of age.

Administration: Precedex must be diluted in 0.9% sodium chloride solution to achieve required concentration (4 µg/mL) prior to administration. Preparation of solutions is the same, whether for the loading dose or maintenance infusion.

Strict aseptic technique must always be maintained during handling of Precedex.

To prepare the infusion, withdraw 2 mL of Precedex and add to 48 mL of 0.9% sodium chloride injection to a total of 50 mL. Shake gently to mix well.

Parenteral drug products should be inspected visually for particulate matter and discoloration prior to administration, whenever solution and container permit.

Compatibility with Other Fluids: Precedex has been shown to be compatible when administered with the following intravenous fluids: Lactated Ringers, 5% Glucose in Water, 0.9% Sodium Chloride in Water, 20% Mannitol in Water.

Dexmedetomidine has been found to be compatible with water solutions of the following drugs when administered via Y-site injections: thiopental sodium, vecuronium bromide, pancuronium bromide, glycopyrrolate bromide, phenylephrine hydrochloride.

Compatibility with Natural Rubber: Compatibility studies have demonstrated the potential for absorption of Precedex to some types of natural rubber. Although Precedex is dosed to effect, it is advisable to use administration components made with synthetic or coated natural rubber gaskets.

Incompatibilities: Precedex infusion should not be co-administered through the same IV catheter with blood, serum, or plasma because physical compatibility has not been established.

Precedex has been shown to be incompatible when administered with the following drugs: amphotericin B, diazepam.

OVERDOSAGE:

The tolerability of Precedex was studied in one study in which healthy subjects were administered doses at and above the recommended dose of 0.2 to 0.7 µg/kg/hr. The maximum blood concentration achieved in this study was approximately 13 times the upper boundary of the therapeutic range. The most notable effects observed in two subjects who achieved the highest doses were first degree atrioventricular block and second degree heart block. No hemodynamic compromise was noted with the atrioventricular block and the heart block resolved spontaneously within one minute.

Five patients received an overdose of Precedex in the intensive care unit sedation studies. Two of these patients had no symptoms reported; one patient received a 2 µg/kg loading dose over 10 minutes (twice the recommended loading dose) and one patient received a maintenance infusion of 0.8 µg/kg/hr. Two other patients who received a 2 µg/kg loading dose over 10 minutes, experienced bradycardia and/or hypotension. One patient who received a loading bolus dose of undiluted Precedex (19.4 µg/kg), had cardiac arrest from which he was successfully resuscitated.

> For management of a suspected drug overdose, CPhA recommends that you contact your **regional Poison Control Centre**. See the *CPS* Directory section for a list of Poison Control Centres.

ACTION AND CLINICAL PHARMACOLOGY: Mechanism of Action: General: Precedex is a relatively selective $alpha_2$-adrenergic agonist with sedative properties. $Alpha_2$ selectivity is observed in animals following slow intravenous infusion of low and medium doses (10-300 µg/kg). Both $alpha_1$ and $alpha_2$ activity is observed following slow intravenous infusion of high doses (≥1000 µg/kg) or with rapid intravenous administration.

In a study in healthy volunteers (N=10), respiratory rate and oxygen saturation remained within normal limits and there was no evidence of respiratory depression when Precedex was administered by intravenous infusion at doses within the recommended dose range (0.2-0.7 µg/kg/hr).

Pharmacokinetics: Following intravenous administration, dexmedetomidine exhibits the following pharmacokinetic parameters: a rapid distribution phase with a distribution half-life ($t_{½}$) of approximately 6 minutes; a terminal elimination half-life ($t_{½}$) of approximately 2 hours; and steady-state volume of distribution (V_{ss}) of approximately 118 liters. Clearance is estimated to be approximately 39 L/h. The mean body weight associated with this clearance estimate was 72 kg.

Dexmedetomidine exhibits linear pharmacokinetics in the dosage range of 0.2 to 0.7 µg/kg/hr when administered by intravenous infusion for up to 24 hours. Table 4 shows the main pharmacokinetic parameters when Precedex was infused (after appropriate loading doses) at maintenance infusion rates of 0.17 µg/kg/hr (target plasma concentration of 0.3 ng/mL) for 12 and 24 hours, 0.33 µg/kg/hr (target plasma concentration of 0.6 ng/mL) for 24 hours, and 0.70 µg/kg/hr (target plasma concentration of 1.25 ng/mL) for 24 hours.

Distribution: The steady-state volume of distribution (V_{ss}) of dexmedetomidine is approximately 118 liters. Dexmedetomidine protein binding was assessed in the plasma of normal healthy male and female subjects. The average protein binding was 94% and was constant across the different plasma concentrations tested. Protein binding was similar in males and females. The fraction of dexmedetomidine that was bound to plasma proteins was significantly decreased in subjects with hepatic impairment compared to healthy subjects.

The potential for protein binding displacement of dexmedetomidine by fentanyl, ketorolac, theophylline, digoxin and lidocaine was explored in vitro, and negligible changes in the plasma protein binding of dexmedetomidine were observed. The potential for protein binding displacement of phenytoin, warfarin, ibuprofen, propranolol, theophylline and digoxin by dexmedetomidine was explored in vitro and none of these compounds appeared to be significantly displaced by dexmedetomidine.

Metabolism: Dexmedetomidine undergoes almost complete biotransformation with very little unchanged dexmedetomidine excreted in urine and feces. Biotransformation involves both direct glucuronidation as well as cytochrome P450 mediated metabolism. The major metabolic pathways of dexmedetomidine are: direct N-glucuronidation to inactive metabolites; aliphatic hydroxylation (mediated primarily by CYP2A6) of dexmedetomidine to generate 3-hydroxy-dexmedetomidine, the glucuronide of 3-hydroxy-dexmedetomidine, and 3-carboxy-dexmedetomidine; and N methylation of dexmedetomidine to generate 3-hydroxy N-methyl-dexmedetomidine, 3-carboxy N-methyl-dexmedetomidine, and dexmedetomidine-N-methyl O-glucuronide.

Table 4: Precedex

Mean±SD Pharmacokinetic Parameters

	Loading Infusion (min)/Total infusion Duration (hrs)			
	10 min/12 hrs	**10 min/24 hrs**	**10 min/24 hrs**	**35 min/24 hrs**
	Dexmedetomidine Target Concentration (ng/mL) and Dose (µg/kg/hr)			
Parameter	**0.3/0.17**	**0.3/0.17**	**0.6/0.33**	**1.25/0.70**
$t_{½}$[a], hour	1.78±0.30	2.22±0.59	2.23±0.21	2.50±0.61
CL, liter/hour	46.3±8.3	43.1±6.5	35.3±6.8	36.5±7.5
V_{ss}, liter	88.7±22.9	102.4±20.3	93.6±17.0	99.6±17.8
Avg Css [b], ng/mL	0.27±0.05	0.27±0.05	0.67±0.10	1.37±0.20

[a] Presented as harmonic mean and pseudo standard deviation.
[b] Avg Css=Average steady-state concentration of dexmedetomidine. (2.5-9 hour samples for 12 hour infusion and 2.5-18 hour samples for 24 hour infusions).

Excretion: The terminal elimination half-life ($t_{½}$) of dexmedetomidine is approximately 2 hours and clearance is estimated to be approximately 39 L/h. A mass balance study demonstrated that after nine days an average of 95% of the radioactivity, following intravenous administration of radiolabeled dexmedetomidine, was recovered in the urine and 4% in the feces. No unchanged dexmedetomidine was detected in the urine. Approximately 85% of the radioactivity recovered in the urine was excreted within 24 hours after the infusion. Fractionation of the radioactivity excreted in urine demonstrated that products of N-glucuronidation accounted for approximately 34% of the cumulative urinary excretion. In addition, aliphatic hydroxylation of parent drug to form 3-hydroxy-dexmedetomidine, the glucuronide of 3-hydroxy-dexmedetomidine, and 3-carboxylic acid-dexmedetomidine together represented approximately 14% of the dose in urine. N-methylation of dexmedetomidine to form 3-hydroxy N-methyl dexmedetomidine, 3-carboxy N-methyl dexmedetomidine, and N-methyl O-glucuronide dexmedetomidine accounted for approximately 18% of the dose in urine. The N-Methyl metabolite itself was a minor circulating component and was undetected in urine. Approximately 28% of the urinary metabolites have not been identified.

Special Populations and Conditions: Pediatrics: The pharmacokinetic profile of Precedex has not been studied in pediatric patients.

Geriatrics: The pharmacokinetic profile of Precedex was not altered by age. There were no differences in the pharmacokinetics of Precedex in young (18-40 years), middle age (41-65 years), and elderly (>65 years) subjects. However, in clinical trials an increased incidence of adverse events was observed in the elderly, and a dose reduction for both the loading and maintenance infusions should be considered in patients over 65 years of age. (See Dosage and Administration.)

Gender: There was no observed difference in Precedex pharmacokinetics due to gender.

Hepatic Insufficiency: In subjects with varying degrees of hepatic impairment (Child-Pugh Class A, B, or C), clearance values for Precedex were lower than in healthy subjects. The mean clearance values for patients with mild, moderate, and severe hepatic impairment were 74%, 64% and 53% of those observed in the normal healthy subjects, respectively. Mean clearances for free drug were 59%, 51% and 32% of those observed in the normal healthy subjects, respectively. In clinical trials an increased incidence of adverse events was observed in these patients, and a dose reduction for both the loading and maintenance infusions should be considered in patients with impaired hepatic function. (See Dosage and Administration.)

Renal Insufficiency: Precedex pharmacokinetics (C_{max}, T_{max}, AUC, $t_{½}$, CL, and V_{ss}) were not significantly different in patients with severe renal impairment (creatinine clearance: <30 mL/min) compared to healthy subjects. Precedex is known to be substantially excreted by the kidney, and the risk of adverse reactions to this drug may be greater in patients with impaired renal function. Because elderly patients are more likely to have decreased renal function, care should be taken in dose selection in elderly patients, and it may be useful to reduce the dose and monitor renal function. (See Dosage and Administration.)

Concomitant Opioid Use: In Intensive Care Unit, 41-44% of Precedex treated patients received no morphine sulfate for pain versus 15-19% in the placebo-treated patients.

In conscious sedation, 39.6-56.6% of Precedex treated patients received no fentanyl for pain versus 11.1% of placebo-treated patients.

STORAGE AND STABILITY: Store at controlled room temperature, 25°C with excursions allowed from 15 to 30°C. [See USP.]

INFORMATION FOR THE PATIENT: Published in e-CPS, available by subscription at www.e-cps.ca.

DOSAGE FORMS, COMPOSITION AND PACKAGING: Each mL of a sterile, nonpyrogenic solution suitable for intravenous infusion following dilution contains: dexmedetomidine hydrochloride 118 µg equivalent to dexmedetomidine 100 µg and sodium chloride in water 9 mg. The solution is preservative-free and contains no additives or chemical stabilizers. Clear glass vials of 2 mL (200 µg/2 mL). Vials are intended for single use only.

Pred Forte® Pr

prednisolone acetate

Ophthalmic Corticosteroid

Allergan

Pred Mild® Pr

prednisolone acetate

Ophthalmic Corticosteroid

Allergan

SUPPLIED: Each 5 mL (Pred Forte only) and 10 mL plastic dropper bottle contains: prednisolone acetate (microfine suspension) 1% (Pred Forte) or 0.12% (Pred Mild). Nonmedicinal ingredients: benzalkonium chloride, boric acid, disodium edetate, hydroxypropyl methylcellulose, polysorbate 80, purified water, sodium bisulfite, sodium chloride and sodium citrate.

Prednicarbate Pr

CPhA Monograph

see *Corticosteroids: Topical*

Prednisolone

CPhA Monograph

see *Corticosteroids: Eye Ear Nose*

see *Corticosteroids: Systemic*

Prednisone

CPhA Monograph

see *Corticosteroids: Systemic*

PregVit®

multiple vitamins and minerals

Prenatal/Postpartum Vitamin-Mineral Supplement

Duchesnay

PregVit folic 5®

multiple vitamins and minerals

Prenatal High Dose Folic Acid Vitamin-Mineral Supplement

Duchesnay

Date of Revision: January 7, 2009

SUMMARY PRODUCT INFORMATION:

Route of Administration	Dosage Form/Strength			Clinically Relevant Nonmedicinal Ingredients
Oral	**Each pink (a.m.) tablet contains (organized alphabetically)**	**PregVit**	**PregVit folic 5**	None For a complete listing, see Dosage Forms, Composition and Packaging.
	Beta-Carotene (source of vitamin A)	2700 IU	2700 IU	
	Vitamin B_1 (thiamine mononitrate)	3 mg	3 mg	
	Vitamin B_2 (riboflavin)	3.4 mg	3.4 mg	
	Niacinamide	20 mg	20 mg	
	Pantothenic Acid (calcium pantothenate)	5 mg	5 mg	
	Vitamin B_6 (pyridoxine HCl)	10 mg	10 mg	
	Vitamin C (ascorbic acid)	120 mg	120 mg	
	Vitamin E (dl-alpha tocopheryl acetate)	30 IU	30 IU	
	Copper (cupric oxide)	2 mg	2 mg	
	Iodine (potassium iodide)	0.15 mg	0.15 mg	
	Iron (ferrous fumarate)[a,b,c]	35 mg	35 mg	
	Magnesium (magnesium oxide)	50 mg	50 mg	
	Zinc (zinc oxide)	15 mg	15 mg	
	Each blue/dark blue (p.m.) tablet contains			None For a complete listing, see Dosage Forms, Composition and Packaging.
	Folic Acid[b]	1.1 mg	5 mg	
	Vitamin B_{12} (cyanocobalamin)	12 µg	12 µg	
	Vitamin D_3 (cholecalciferol)	250 IU	250 IU	
	Calcium (calcium carbonate)[a,c]	300 mg	300 mg	

[a] The purpose of taking the two tablets at different times is to prevent calcium inhibition on the absorption of iron.

[b] The purpose of taking the two tablets at different times is to prevent folic acid from interacting with iron resulting in their decreased intestinal absorption.

[c] Elemental amount as iron from ferrous fumarate; as calcium from calcium carbonate.

INDICATIONS AND CLINICAL USE: PregVit is a vitamin-mineral supplement specially formulated for use in women at least 2-3 months prior to conception, throughout pregnancy and during the postnatal period. PregVit folic 5 is a prenatal high dose folic acid vitamin-mineral supplement formulated for use in women who are planning pregnancy or pregnant and have had a previous pregnancy affected by a neural tube defect (NTD), women who have a family history of neural tube defects, have diabetes or malabsorption disorders (e.g., inflammatory bowel disease), who are taking folic acid antagonists (e.g., methotrexate) or anticonvulsant drugs (e.g., carbamazepine, phenobarbital, phenytoin, primidone, valproic acid), or require a high dose folic acid supplement in the opinion of their physician. Women are to take one pink (a.m.) and one dark blue (p.m.) PregVit folic 5 tablet daily at least 2-3 months prior to conception, continuing up to 10 to 12 weeks after the last menstrual period, or throughout pregnancy, if, in the judgment of the attending physician, the benefits of continued high dose folic acid supplementation outweigh potential risks.

Women who have poor folate status from multifactorial dietary and environmental conditions, including poor eating habits, stringent dieting for weight loss, drug and alcohol abuse, and cigarette smoking should discuss folate supplementation with their physician.

Oral contraceptive users may also have lower folate concentrations than non-users as estrogen and progesterone could lower plasma and erythrocyte folate levels. Supplementation with folic acid may theoretically reduce the occurrence of maternal folic acid deficiency.

The physiological changes of pregnancy call for extra nutrients and energy to meet demands of an expanding blood supply, the growth of maternal tissues, a developing fetus, loss of maternal tissues at birth and preparation for lactation. During pregnancy, special attention should be given to folate, calcium, vitamin D and iron intakes because there is a potential for inadequate intakes in some groups of women.

Taking vitamin and mineral supplements does not eliminate the need for a balanced nutrition.

PregVit and PregVit folic 5 are both formulated as two tablets in order to optimize the absorption of iron, calcium and folic acid; one pink (a.m.) tablet (with iron) is to be taken in the morning and a distinctly different blue/dark blue (p.m.) tablet (with calcium and folic acid) is to be taken in the evening. The rationale for this two tablet approach is to enhance bioavailability of iron; adjust the iron content so that it reduces adverse effects such as nausea, constipation, fatigue, diarrhea and headache associated with supplements containing higher levels of iron (60 mg) and; therefore increase compliance to the PregVit and PregVit folic 5. Calcium is provided separately from iron to avoid calcium inhibition of iron absorption from the gastrointestinal tract. A higher dose of vitamin C is also present in the morning tablet to facilitate iron absorption. Manganese was purposely excluded from these tablets so as not to affect iron absorption.

Concurrent ingestion of folic acid and iron may result in the formation of stable complexes. Folic acid is provided separately from iron to prevent their decreased intestinal absorption.

CONTRAINDICATIONS: These products are contraindicated in patients with known hypersensitivity to any of the ingredients in the formulation or component of the container. For a complete listing, see Dosage Forms, Composition and Packaging.

WARNINGS AND PRECAUTIONS: General: Although it has been suggested that high doses of folate may mask manifestations of vitamin B_{12} deficiency, a study by Metz et al. (2004) could not demonstrate that high serum folate levels masked the macrocytosis of cobalamin deficiency whether the serum folate was low, normal or high.

To address potential concerns regarding the masking of vitamin B_{12} deficiency and the potential precipitation or exacerbation of the progression of neurological complications associated with vitamin B_{12} deficiency, the use of folic acid in conjunction with vitamin B_{12} as a supplement should be recommended. Vitamin B_{12} levels may be monitored if, in the opinion of the healthcare professional, it is warranted.

Keep this product out of the reach of children. Accidental overdose of iron-containing products is a leading cause of fatal poisoning in children under 6. In case of accidental overdose, call a regional poison control centre immediately (see Overdosage).

Do not exceed the recommended dose.

Dependence/Tolerance: There is no information to indicate that abuse or dependency occurs at the concentration of vitamins and minerals found in PregVit and PregVit folic 5.

Hematologic: Folic acid should be used in conjunction with vitamin B_{12} in order to avoid potential neurologic complications. Any dose of folic acid over 1 mg per day may require monitoring for vitamin B_{12} deficiency by a healthcare provider.

Neurologic: Women with seizure disorders controlled on anticonvulsant medications (e.g., carbamazepine, phenobarbital, phenytoin, primidone, valproic acid) may have exacerbation of seizures when folic acid is taken.

Special Populations: Pregnant Women: Although the use of a folic acid supplement during the periconceptional period reduces the number of NTDs, they cannot be completely avoided through folate supplementation due to their multifactorial origin.

Taking vitamin and mineral supplements does not eliminate the need for a balanced nutrition.

Baseline Risk: The background baseline risk of major malformations for all pregnancies is approximately 1-3%. This is the risk of having a child with a birth defect when no teratogenic exposure occurs in pregnancy. This underlying risk may be increased due to maternal age, medical or family history, or exposures to certain drugs, chemicals or levels of radiation known to cause birth defects.

Each year, a quarter of a million pregnancies worldwide result in the birth of an infant with a neural tube defect (NTD) or an abortion performed because of such effect. In a recent study, a total of 2446 subjects with NTDs were recorded among 1.9 million births from 1993 to 2002 in seven Canadian provinces. The prevalence of NTDs was 0.86 per 1000 births.

Nursing Women: PregVit is specifically indicated in the postpartum period. The decision to continue use of PregVit folic 5 during lactation should be made by a healthcare professional.

The passage of vitamins and minerals into breast milk can be expected. Folic acid is actively excreted into breast milk. Accumulation of folate in milk takes precedence over maternal folate needs. Levels of folic acid are relatively low in colostrum but as lactation proceeds, concentrations of the vitamin rise. Folate levels in newborns and breast-fed infants are consistently higher than those in mothers and normal adults. In Japanese mothers, mean breast milk folate concentrations were 141.4 ng/mL, resulting in a total intake by the infant of 14-25 µg/kg/day. Much lower mean levels were measured in pooled human milk in an English study examining preterm (26 mothers, 29-34 weeks) and term (35 mothers, 39 weeks or longer) patients. Preterm milk folate concentrations rose from 10.6 ng/mL (colostrum) to 30.5 ng/mL post-natal (16-196 days), whereas term milk folate concentrations increased during the same period from 17.6 to 42.3 ng/mL.

In one study, maternal serum and red blood cell folate levels increased significantly after 1 mg of folic acid/day for 4 weeks, but milk folate levels remained unchanged. Investigators gave well-nourished lactating women a multivitamin preparation containing 0.8 mg of folic acid. At 6 months postpartum, milk concentrations of folate did not differ significantly from those of controls who were not receiving supplements. Other investigators measured more than adequate blood folate levels in American breast-fed infants during the 1st year of life. The mean milk concentration of folate consumed by these infants was 85 ng/mL.

In a study of lactating mothers with megaloblastic anemia treated with 5 mg/day of folic acid for 3 days, breast milk folate rose from 7-9 ng/mL to 15-40 ng/mL 1 day after treatment began. The elevated levels were maintained for 3 weeks without further treatment. Nine lower-socioeconomic status women were treated with multivitamins containing 0.8 mg of folic acid and were compared with seven untreated controls. Breast milk folate was significantly higher in the treated women. In another study of lactating women with low nutritional status, supplementation with folic acid, 0.2-10.0 mg/day, resulted in mean milk concentrations of 2.3-5.6 ng/mL. Milk concentrations were directly proportional to dietary intake.

Monitoring and Laboratory Tests: To address potential concerns that high doses of folate may mask manifestations of vitamin B_{12} deficiency, signs or symptoms of vitamin B_{12} deficiency should be considered before initiating folic acid supplementation if doses are greater than 1.0 mg. Vitamin B_{12} levels may be monitored before and during PregVit and PregVit folic 5 therapies if in the opinion of the healthcare professional it is warranted.

Monitor folate level when drugs known to interact with folic acid are taken concomitantly (see Drug Interactions, Table 3).

ADVERSE REACTIONS: Adverse Drug Reaction Overview: Allergic sensitization has been reported following both oral and parenteral administration of folic acid.

At high doses (e.g. 15 mg/day) folic acid has been associated on rare occasion with various gastrointestinal symptoms and CNS effects such as sleep disturbances, difficulty concentrating, irritability, hyperactivity, excitement, mental depression, confusion, and impaired judgment. In general, adverse reactions associated with iron supplements whether alone or in a multivitamin are: constipation, nausea, fatigue, diarrhea and headache.

Clinical Trial Adverse Drug Reactions: Because clinical trials are conducted under very specific conditions the adverse reaction rates observed in the clinical trials may not reflect the rates observed in practice and should not be compared to the rates in the clinical trials of another drug. Adverse drug reaction information from clinical trials is useful for identifying drug-related adverse events and for approximating rates.

A randomized, crossover open labelled study in 138 pregnant women attending outpatient clinics was conducted to compare tolerability and compliance with PregVit (a.m. and p.m. tablets) versus a supplement with high iron content in pregnant women. An equal number of pregnant women suffering from nausea and vomiting of pregnancy (NVP) and pregnant women without NVP were randomized to receive either PregVit or a supplement with high iron content for one month. The primary end point of interest was the mean rate of adverse events including decreased compliance. The mean rate of adverse event was collected for nausea, constipation and other adverse drug events and is illustrated in Table 1. Incidence of nausea was approximately 9% in PregVit group versus 10% in the supplement with high iron content group (p=0.71); incidence of constipation was 22.5% in PregVit group versus 34.8% in the supplement with high iron content group (p=0.03) and for other adverse events, the average number of events was 10.4 for the PregVit group versus 9.9 for the supplement with high iron content group (p=0.95).

In a single-dose crossover pharmacokinetic study conducted with the PregVit blue (p.m.) tablet in 6 healthy non-pregnant women (18-45 years), no adverse reactions were reported.

In another study of similar design, 12 healthy women were administered high iron and calcium and low iron without calcium [PregVit pink (a.m.) tablet] separately on two different occasions. No adverse reactions were reported.

Abnormal Hematologic and Clinical Chemistry Findings: None reported.

Post-Market Adverse Drug Reactions: PregVit and PregVit folic 5 have the same medicinal ingredients and strengths with the exception of the amount of folic acid (1.1 mg vs. 5 mg). Spontaneous adverse reactions reported for these products are summarized in Table 2. Reactions are presented by MedDRA System Organ Class (SOC) and Preferred Terms (signs, symptoms and diagnosis) from spontaneous notification.

DRUG INTERACTIONS: Overview: No formal vitamin/mineral-drug interaction studies have been performed with PregVit or PregVit folic 5.

Iron supplements may decrease absorption of thyroid hormone medications. Therefore, iron supplements whether alone or as part of a prenatal supplement, should not be taken at the same time as levothyroxine or other thyroid hormone medications (Synthroid, Eltroxin, Levo-T, Levothroid, Levoxyl, Euthroid, Thyrolar, etc.). Allow at least four (4) hours between taking iron and thyroid hormones. Calcium can also interfere with the absorption of thyroid drugs. Allow at least four (4) hours between taking calcium and thyroid hormones.

Table 1: PregVit/PregVit folic 5

Overall Study Results, Comparing PregVit (low iron) to a Supplement with a High Iron Content Over a Month Administration in a Cross-Over Design

Adverse Events (n=138)	PregVit (SD)	Supplement with High Iron Content (SD)	p value
Adverse events (%)	17.6±.24	20.3±24	0.14
Nausea (%)	9.3±19	10.1±18	0.71
Constipation time length (%)	3.1±8	4.7±11	**0.05**
Other adverse events	10.4±21	9.9±20	0.95
Nausea Rate (%)	41.3 (57/81)	45.7 (63/75)	0.54
Constipation Rate (%)	22.5% (31/107)	34.8% (48/90)	**0.03**

Table 2: PregVit/PregVit folic 5

Cumulative Summary of PregVit and PregVit folic 5 Adverse Reactions from Spontaneous Reports to Duchesnay Inc. and Regulatory Authority (Health Canada) from Launching Date to September 30th, 2008

MedDRA Preferred Term	PregVit Spontaneous Reports	PregVit folic 5 Spontaneous Reports
SOC: Eye Disorders (n=2)		
Eye pruritus	1	0
Visual impairment	0	1
SOC: Gastrointestinal Disorders (n=45)		
Nausea	10	4
Vomiting	8	1
Constipation	3	0
Diarrhea	3	0
Stomach discomfort	2	1
Abdominal pain upper	2	0
Dyspepsia	2	0
Abdominal distension	1	1
Infrequent bowel movement	1	1
Chelitis	1	0
Heartburn	1	0
Lip dry	1	0
Retching	1	0
Abdominal pain lower	0	1
SOC: General Disorders and Administration Site Conditions (n=7)		
Feeling abnormal	2	0
Asthenia	1	0
Fatigue	1	0
Hunger	1	0
Pyrexia	1	0
Thirst	1	0
SOC: Metabolism and Nutrition Disorders (n=4)		
Decreased appetite	2	0
Dehydration	1	0
Hyperglycemia	1	0
SOC: Musculoskeletal and Connective Tissue Disorders (n=1)		
Myalgia	1	0
SOC: Nervous System Disorders (n=5)		
Headache	1	1
Dizziness	1	0
Lethargy	1	0
Migraine	0	1
SOC: Pregnancy, Puerperium and Perinatal Conditions (n=2)		

(cont'd)

Table 2: PregVit/PregVit folic 5 *(cont'd)*

Cumulative Summary of PregVit and PregVit folic 5 Adverse Reactions from Spontaneous Reports to Duchesnay Inc. and Regulatory Authority (Health Canada) from Launching Date to September 30th, 2008

MedDRA Preferred Term	PregVit Spontaneous Reports	PregVit folic 5 Spontaneous Reports
Vomiting in pregnancy	2	0
SOC: Psychiatric Disorders (n=4)		
Insomnia	2	1
Nervousness	1	0
SOC: Renal and Urinary System Disorders (n=5)		
Chromaturia	3	2
SOC: Respiratory and Thoracic Disorders (n=2)		
Dyspnea	1	0
Throat tightness	1	0
SOC: Skin and Subcutaneous Tissue Disorders (n=2)		
Urticaria	1	0
Rash macular	0	1

Due to the inhibitory effect of calcium on iron absorption, women should be encouraged to take these supplements at different time. A high intake of iron can interfere with zinc absorption therefore; 15 mg of supplemental zinc should be taken when elemental iron supplementation exceeds 30 mg per day. When supplemental zinc is taken, concurrent supplementation with 2 mg copper is advised.

Concurrent ingestion of folic acid and iron may result in the formation of stable complexes with iron, resulting in their decreased intestinal absorption.

Several other drugs have reduced bioavailability when ingested with iron preparations. These include carbidopa, ciprofloxacin, levodopa, methyldopa, penicillamine, tetracyclines. A large number of drugs form stable complexes with iron, however, little is known about the clinical consequences of this binding. Further investigation is required to determine the clinical interactions between iron and drug molecules.

Drugs including, antibiotic therapies, bisphosphonates, carbidopa, fluoroquinolone antibiotics, levodopa, methyldopa and penicillamine should be taken at least two (2) hours apart from PregVit and PregVit folic 5.

Drugs including, cholestyramine, colestipol, levothyroxine and mycophenolate mofetil should be taken at least four (4) hours apart from PregVit and PregVit folic 5.

Vitamin/Mineral-Drug Interactions: See Table 3.

Table 3: PregVit/PregVit folic 5

Vitamin/Mineral—Drug Interactions for PregVit and PregVit folic 5

Vitamin/Mineral	Drugs	Effect	Clinical Comment
Folic Acid	Antacids	Can reduce folic acid absorption.	
	Antibiotic therapy	Can disrupt the normal gastrointestinal (GI) flora, interfering with absorption of folic acid.	
	Antiepileptic drugs (carbamazepine, phenobarbital, phenytoin, primidone, valproic acid)	Antiepileptic drugs can reduce serum folate levels, occasionally leading to megaloblastic anemia. Folic acid supplements have also decreased seizure control in some people with epilepsy.	Seizure activity should be monitored closely. Monitor folate levels, particularly in pregnant women, who are at risk of reduced folate.
	Chloramphenicol	May antagonize some effects of folic acid on the blood (hematopoietic system).	
	Cholestyramine	When administered together, there may be reduction or delay in folic acid absorption.	If concomitant therapy is required, folic acid should be administered at least one (1) hour before or four (4) to six (6) hours after cholestyramine.
	Colestipol	Can interfere with absorption of folic acid, and reduced serum folate levels may occur.	
	Dihydrofolate reductase inhibitors (sulphasalazine, triamterene, trimethoprim)	Inhibit absorption and metabolism of folic acid.	Monitor serum and red blood cell folate levels.
	H2 blockers (cimetidine, famotidine, nizatidine, ranitidine) and Proton Pump Inhibitors (esomeprazole, lansoprazole, omeprazole, pantoprazole, rabeprazole)	Folic acid absorption from the small intestine is optimal at pH 5.5 to 6. The increased pH associated with H2 blockers may therefore reduce folic acid absorption.	Monitor for folate deficiency.
	Malaria drugs (sulfadoxine-pyrimethamine)	Prevents conversion of folic acid to its active form.	Monitor for folate deficiency.
	Methotrexate	Methotrexate is a folate antagonist which prevents conversion of folic acid to its active form, and lowers plasma and red blood cell folate levels.	Monitor for folate deficiency.
	NSAIDs (ibuprofen, indomethacin, naproxen, sulindac)	Folate-dependent enzymes have been inhibited in laboratory experiments by certain NSAIDs.	Monitor for folate deficiency.

(cont'd)

Table 3: PregVit/PregVit folic 5 *(cont'd)*

Vitamin/Mineral—Drug Interactions for PregVit and PregVit folic 5

Vitamin/Mineral	Drugs	Effect	Clinical Comment
	Pancreatic extracts (Cotazym, Creon, Pancrease, Ultrase, Viokase)	May possibly reduce folic acid absorption.	Folate levels should be checked in patients taking pancreatic enzymes for prolonged periods.
	Pyrimethamine	Pyrimethamine is a folate antagonist that prevents conversion of folic acid to its active form.	Monitor for folate deficiency.
Iron	Acetohydroxamic acid	Iron supplements may cause medication to be less effective.	
	Allopurinol	May cause an increase in iron storage in the liver.	Do not use allopurinol with iron supplements.
	Aminosalicylic acid	May cause malabsorption syndrome (including iron depletion).	
	Antacids	May reduce iron absorption and reduce efficacy.	Separate the doses of antacids and iron.
	Antibiotic therapy (doxycycline, methacycline, oxytetracycline, tetracycline)	Forms iron-drug complexes reducing the extent of drug absorption.	It is recommended to take iron supplements and these drugs at least two (2) hours apart.
	Aspirin and NSAIDs	Can cause mucosal damage and bleeding throughout the gastrointestinal tract. Chronic blood loss may contribute to iron deficiency. Iron supplements may also irritate the gastrointestinal tract.	
	Bisphosphonates (alendronate, etidronate, risedronate, tiludronate)	Iron can decrease absorption of bisphosphonates by forming insoluble complexes.	Take bisphosphonates and iron at least two (2) hours apart.
	Carbidopa, levodopa	Forms iron-drug complexes reducing the extent of drug absorption.	It is recommended to take iron supplements and these drugs at least two (2) hours apart.
	Chloramphenicol	Can reduce the response to iron therapy in iron deficiency anemia.	
	Cholestyramine, colestipol	May bind iron in the gut, reducing its absorption.	Take cholestyramine or colestipol at least four (4) hours apart.
	Fluoroquinolone antibiotics (ciprofloxacin, levofloxacin, ofloxacin)	Iron decreases absorption of fluoroquinolone antibiotics.	Take fluoroquinolone antibiotics and iron at least two (2) hours apart.
	H2 blockers (cimetidine, ranitidine, famotidine, nizatidine) and Proton Pump Inhibitors (esomeprazole, iansoprazole, omeprazole, pantoprazole, rabeprazole)	Gastric acid is important for the absorption of iron.	
	Levothyroxine (e.g. Synthroid) (Please also see Calcium-Levothyroxine interaction)	Iron reduces the absorption of thyroid hormones.	It is recommended to take iron supplements and levothyroxine at least four (4) hours apart. Thyroid levels should be monitored regularly during pregnancy and in the first few months postpartum.
	Methyldopa	Forms iron-drug complex reducing the extent of drug absorption.	It is recommended to take iron supplements and methyldopa at least two (2) hours apart.
	Mycophenolate mofetil	Iron can markedly reduce absorption of mycophenolate mofetil.	Iron should be taken at least four (4) to six (6) hours before, or two (2) hours after mycophenolate mofetil.
	Pancreatic enzymes (Pancrease, Cotazym, Viokase, Creon, Ultrase)	Can reduce iron absorption, possibly by binding iron or altering pH.	
	Penicillamine	Forms iron-drug complex reducing the extent of drug absorption.	It is recommended to take iron supplements and penicillamine at least two (2) hours apart.
Calcium	Levothyroxine (e.g. Synthroid) (Please also see Iron-levothyroxine interaction)	Calcium supplements reduce the effectiveness of levothyroxine.	It is recommended to take calcium supplements and levothyroxine at least four (4) hours apart. Thyroid levels should be monitored regularly during pregnancy and in the first few months postpartum.

(cont'd)

Table 3: PregVit/PregVit folic 5 *(cont'd)*

Vitamin/Mineral—Drug Interactions for PregVit and PregVit folic 5

Vitamin/Mineral	Drugs	Effect	Clinical Comment
	Tetracycline	Calcium interferes with absorption of tetracycline.	It is recommended to take tetracycline one (1) hour before or two (2) hours after calcium supplements.

Vitamin/Mineral-Food Interactions: Interactions with food have been established with iron and calcium.

Iron: Factors that enhance non-heme iron absorption include: meat, poultry, fish and vitamin C. Factors that inhibit non-heme iron absorption include: polyphenols in tea, coffee; phytate in legumes, soybeans, whole grains; oxalate in spinach, chard, beet greens, rhubarb, sweet potato and calcium in both food and supplements.

Due to the inhibitory effect of calcium on iron absorption, women should be encouraged to take these supplements at different times.

Calcium: Compounds such as oxalate and phytate reduce calcium absorption. These compounds are found in foods such as legumes, grains, spinach, chard, beet greens, sweet potatoes and rhubarb.

Absorption of calcium carbonate can be improved when food has increased gastric acid levels.

Vitamin/Mineral-Vitamin/Mineral Interactions: Vitamin/mineral-vitamin/mineral interactions are important for the PregVit and PregVit folic 5 formulations, the dosing regimen itself [pink a.m. and blue/dark blue p.m. tablets at least four (4) hours apart] as well as the timing of administration of external sources of vitamins and minerals.

Concurrent ingestion of folic acid and iron may result in the formation of stable complexes with iron, decreasing their intestinal absorption. Vitamin C is known to increase the absorption of iron. Calcium has an inhibitory effect on iron absorption. Manganese also interferes with iron absorption. Vitamin D metabolites enhance calcium absorption.

These same interactions are seen with external sources of vitamins and minerals including supplements.

High intake of iron can interfere with zinc absorption. For this reason, 15 mg per day supplemental zinc should be taken when elemental iron supplementation exceeds 30 mg per day. When supplemental zinc is taken, concurrent supplementation with 2 mg copper is advised.

Table 4: PregVit/PregVit folic 5

Vitamin/Mineral—Vitamin/Mineral Interactions for PregVit and PregVit folic 5

Vitamin/Mineral	Vitamin/Mineral	Effect	Clinical Comment
Folic Acid	Iron	Forms stable complexes with iron and decreases intestinal absorption of iron.	Take at different times in the day.
Iron	Zinc	Iron inhibits absorption of zinc.	Take 15 mg per day supplemental zinc when elemental iron supplementation exceeds 30 mg per day. When supplemental zinc is taken, concurrent supplementation with 2 mg copper is advised.
	Manganese	Inhibits absorption of iron.	
	Vitamin C	Facilitates iron absorption.	
Calcium	Iron	Calcium inhibits absorption of iron.	Take at different times in the day.
	Vitamin D	Vitamin D metabolites enhance calcium absorption.	

Vitamin/Mineral-Herb Interactions: Interactions with herbal products have not been established.

Vitamin/Mineral-Laboratory Interactions: Interactions with laboratory tests have not been established.

DOSAGE AND ADMINISTRATION: Recommended Dose and Dosage Adjustment: For PregVit or PregVit folic 5 take one pink (a.m.) tablet in the morning and one blue/dark blue (p.m.) tablet in the evening at least four (4) hours apart. The purpose of taking the two tablets at different times is to prevent calcium inhibition on the absorption of iron and to prevent folic acid from interacting with iron resulting in their decreased intestinal absorption.

For PregVit, take at least 2-3 months prior to conception, throughout pregnancy and during the postnatal period.

For PregVit folic 5 take at least 2-3 months prior to conception, continuing up to 10-12 weeks after last menstrual period, or throughout pregnancy, if, in the judgment of the attending physician, the benefits of continued high dose folic acid supplementation outweigh potential risks.

It is preferable to take the PregVit/PregVit folic 5 pink (a.m.) tablet on an empty stomach with a glass of water and to wait at least one (1) hour before taking any food to optimize iron absorption, and to take the PregVit/PregVit folic 5 blue/dark blue (p.m.) tablet within one (1) hour of an evening meal to optimize calcium absorption.

The schedule may be individualized according to a woman's specific condition:

- For **women taking calcium rich food for breakfast**, the PregVit/PregVit folic 5 **pink (a.m.)** tablet may be taken two (2) hours or more after breakfast. Following administration of the **pink (a.m.)** tablet a wait of one (1) additional hour is recommended before eating in order to optimize the absorption of iron.
- For **women suffering from nausea and/or vomiting in the morning** where it is difficult to take vitamin-mineral supplements on an empty stomach, the PregVit/PregVit folic 5 **pink (a.m.)** tablet may be taken two (2) hours or more after breakfast. Following administration of the **pink (a.m.)** tablet a wait of one (1) additional hour is recommended before eating in order to optimize the absorption of iron.
- For **women taking levothyroxine hormone in the morning**, it is recommended to take the PregVit/PregVit folic 5 **pink (a.m.)** tablet at least four (4) hours apart to optimize the absorption of **levothyroxine hormone**. For **women taking levothyroxine hormone at bedtime**, it is recommended to take the PregVit **blue (p.m.)** or PregVit folic 5 **dark blue (p.m.)** tablet at least four (4) hours apart to optimize the absorption of **levothyroxine hormone**.

There is no specific recommendation to support a different dosage of vitamin-mineral supplement in **multiple pregnancies**.

Missed Dose: When a dose has been missed, it should be taken as soon as possible: one pink (a.m.) and one blue/dark blue (p.m.) tablets should be taken within a 24 hour period. It is recommended that PregVit/PregVit folic 5 pink (a.m.) and blue/dark blue (p.m.) tablets be taken at least four (4) hours apart in order to optimize the absorption of nutrients.

The prescribed dosing schedule should then continue as directed by physician or healthcare professional.

Administration: PregVit/PregVit folic 5 tablets are to be taken orally.

Tablets are not intended to be crushed or split. No stability and absorption data is available for crushed or split PregVit/PregVit folic 5 tablets.

OVERDOSAGE:

Accidental overdose of iron-containing products is a leading cause of fatal poisoning in children under 6.

PregVit and PregVit folic 5 are supplied in a 30-day blister pack containing 30 oval, pink (a.m.) tablets and 30 oval, blue/dark blue (p.m.) tablets. Each PregVit/PregVit folic 5 pink (a.m.) tablet contains 35 mg of elemental iron. No iron is contained in the PregVit blue (p.m.) tablet or PregVit folic 5 dark blue (p.m.) tablet. The amount of elemental iron in one box or a 30-day supply of PregVit/PregVit folic 5 is 1050 mg.

> For management of a suspected drug overdose, contact your **regional Poison Control Centre**. See the *CPS* Directory section for a list of Poison Control Centres.

ACTION AND CLINICAL PHARMACOLOGY: Mechanism of Action: PregVit/PregVit folic 5 provide a supplement of vitamins and minerals in an immediate release dosage form. Administration of the pink (a.m.) and the blue/dark blue (p.m.) tablets at two different times helps to maximize the absorption of iron, calcium and folic acid.

Clinical Pharmacology: Folic acid, also known as folate, pteroylglutamic acid or vitamin B_9, is a water-soluble B complex vitamin. After absorption from the gastrointestinal tract, folic acid is converted in the liver to tetrahydrofolic acid, which is a cofactor in the biosynthesis of purines and thymidylates of nucleic acids. An exogenous source of folic acid is necessary for the synthesis of nucleoproteins and maintenance of normal erythropoiesis. There is strong evidence that prophylactic therapy with folic acid, prior to and during pregnancy, can reduce the risk of fetal neural tube defects (NTDs). NTDs result from improper development and closure of the neural tube during the third and fourth weeks of gestation. Pregnancies affected by an NTD may result in a miscarriage or stillbirth, and children born with a NTD may have mild to severe disability or die in early childhood. NTDs include spina bifida, anencephaly and encephalocele.

Although the use of a folic acid supplement during the periconceptional period reduces the number of NTDs, they cannot be completely avoided through folate supplementation because of their multifactorial origin. For women who had prior history of NTDs, the recurrence rate is 2-3%. Consuming 5 mg of folic acid daily has the potential of reducing the incidence of another NTD pregnancy by up to 72%, i.e., down to 1%.

There is evidence that an increase of 0.4 mg/day of folic acid would reduce the risk of neural tube defects for all women planning a pregnancy by about 36%, 1 mg per day would reduce the risk by about 57%, 1.1 mg per day would reduce the risk by about 59% and the use of a 5 mg tablet daily would reduce the risk by about 85%.

Pharmacokinetics: PregVit and PregVit folic 5 are both multivitamin-mineral preparations containing the same active ingredients in a pink (a.m.) and blue/dark blue (p.m.) tablet presentation. The pink (a.m.) tablets are exactly the same for both preparations. In the blue and dark blue (p.m.) tablets, the amount of folic acid is different: PregVit blue (p.m.) tablets contain 1.1 mg of folic acid and PregVit folic 5 dark blue (p.m.) tablets contain 5 mg of folic acid.

The absorption of iron following the administration of PregVit/PregVit folic 5 pink (a.m.) tablets was measured in twelve healthy, non-pregnant women. The area under the concentration-time curve (AUC) for serum iron was 79.1±36.0 µM*h. Upon standardizing the AUC for dose, the relative absorption over the 8-hour time period was 2.3±1.0 µM*h/mg.

There is no evidence of circadian rhythm variation in folate pharmacokinetics. In a crossover design, six healthy, non-pregnant women were randomized to receive 1 PregVit blue (p.m.) tablet, containing 1.1 mg of folic acid, in the morning or evening. Serum folate levels were measured over 10 hours. The area under the concentration-time curve (AUC) was used to compare the extent of absorption between the two time periods. The mean AUC values for serum folate after administration of the PregVit blue (p.m.) tablets were 334.5±119.6 nM*h and 283.1±64.3 nM*h for morning and evening, respectively (p=0.17). The morning and evening peak serum folate concentrations (C_{max}) were also similar (135.3±41.7 nM and 130.3±14.2 nM, respectively) (p=0.75). There was no difference in the time to peak concentration (T_{max}) for the morning (1±0.5 hour) and the evening (1±0.4 hour) administration. Folic acid contained in the PregVit blue (p.m.) tablet was absorbed similarly whether administered in the morning or in the evening.

A study comparing folic acid pharmacokinetics was completed where serum folate levels of single dose PregVit and PregVit folic 5 were measured pre-dose and up to 10 hours post dose in healthy non-pregnant fertile women between the ages of 18 and 45 years. The mean area under the curve (AUC) of 1.1 mg and 5 mg folic acid were 147.6±52.8 (ng/mL)·hr and 997.5±271.9 (ng/mL)·hr, respectively (p<0.0002). An approximate 5-fold difference was detected in the peak concentrations (C_{max}) between the 2 groups (p<0.0005), alongside a slight difference in the times to peak (T_{max}) (p=0.02). The estimated steady-state serum folate concentrations produced by 1.1 mg and 5 mg folic acid were 6.2±2.2 ng/mL and 41.6±11.3 ng/mL, respectively (p<0.0002), prior to its summation with initial (baseline) steady-state levels. Single dose administration between 1.1 mg and 5 mg folic acid demonstrated linear pharmacokinetics, with approximately a 5-fold difference between the 2 doses in serum folate contribution to steady-state levels, under ideal adherence.

The study results are summarized in Table 5.

Table 5: PregVit/PregVit folic 5

Single Dose Pharmacokinetic Comparison of PregVit folic 5 (5 mg) Versus PregVit (1.1 mg) Folic Acid Ingestion, Among Non-Pregnant Women of Childbearing Age

	5 mg Folic Acid (n=6)	1.1 mg Folic Acid (n=6)	p-value (Student's t-test)
Baseline (fasting) serum folate concentration, at time=0 (ng/mL)	11.2±3.9	13.2±4.0	0.41
Area under the curve, AUC [(ng/mL)·hr]	997.5±271.9	147.6±52.8	<0.0002
C_{max}, peak serum folate concentration (ng/mL)	273.3±56.3	59.7±18.4	<0.0005
T_{max}, time to achieve peak concentration (hr)	1.8±0.4	1.2±0.4	0.02
Apparent clearance (mL/min)	91.7±37.2	143.6±66.6	0.13
Estimated steady-state serum folate concentration produced by supplemental folic acid (ng/mL)	41.6±11.3	6.2±2.2	<0.0002
Overall estimated steady-state serum folate concentration[a] (ng/mL)	52.8±12.6	19.3±4.2	<0.0001

[a] Overall estimated steady-state serum folate concentration = baseline concentration + estimated steady-state serum folate concentration produced by supplemental folic acid.
Note: Data presented as mean ± standard deviation.

Special Populations and Conditions: Race: No data is available on differences in the pharmacokinetics of either PregVit/PregVit folic 5 pink (a.m.) or blue/dark blue (p.m.) tablet in different races.

Hepatic Insufficiency: No data is available on differences in the pharmacokinetics of either PregVit/PregVit folic 5 pink (a.m.) or blue/dark blue (p.m.) tablet in patients with hepatic insufficiency.

Renal Insufficiency: No data is available on differences in the pharmacokinetics of either PregVit/PregVit folic 5 pink (a.m.) or blue/dark blue (p.m.) tablet in renal insufficiency.

Genetic Polymorphism: No data is available on differences in the pharmacokinetics of either PregVit/PregVit folic 5 pink (a.m.) or blue/dark blue (p.m.) tablet in patients with genetic polymorphism.

STORAGE AND STABILITY: Store at room temperature (15 to 30°C).

Protect from moisture. Contact with moisture may produce surface discoloration or erosion of the tablet.

Keep in a safe place out of reach of children.

SPECIAL HANDLING INSTRUCTIONS: No special handling instructions are required.

INFORMATION FOR THE PATIENT: Published in e-CPS, available by subscription at www.e-cps.ca.

DOSAGE FORMS, COMPOSITION AND PACKAGING: 30-day blister packs containing 30 oval, pink tablets (a.m.) and 30 oval, blue tablets (p.m.).

Tablets are imprinted with the pink image of a pregnant woman 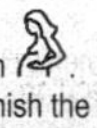.

The indicia of the pregnant woman serves as a method to diminish the incidence of erroneous ingestion by pregnant women or erroneous dispensing by pharmacists of therapeutic agents not prescribed or labeled for pregnant women. Noncompliance in the use of prescription medications is common among pregnant women owing to fear over fetal exposure and safety even in the case of drugs with appropriate safety data.

An observational, prospective cross-sectional study was conducted by the manufacturer to determine the teratogenic risk perception of pregnant women when viewing a plain tablet and a tablet imprinted with the image of a pregnant woman. The difference in teratogenic risk perception was highly significant (p<0.0001). In the survey group of 132 pregnant women the mean perception of teratogenic risk was decreased by 23.4% when viewing tablets imprinted with the image of a pregnant woman. By reducing the perception of teratogenic risk by pregnant women the pregnancy indicia may increase patient compliance and thus the effectiveness of the treatment.

Each oval shaped, pink (a.m.), film-coated, immediate release tablet contains:

	PregVit	PregVit folic 5
Beta-Carotene (source of vitamin A)	2700 IU	2700 IU
Vitamin B_1 (thiamine mononitrate)	3 mg	3 mg
Vitamin B_2 (riboflavin)	3.4 mg	3.4 mg
Niacinamide	20 mg	20 mg
Pantothenic Acid (calcium pantothenate)	5 mg	5 mg
Vitamin B_6 (pyridoxine HCl)	10 mg	10 mg
Vitamin C (ascorbic acid)	120 mg	120 mg
Vitamin E (dl-alpha tocopheryl acetate)	30 IU	30 IU
Copper (cupric oxide)	2 mg	2 mg
Iodine (potassium iodide)	0.15 mg	0.15 mg
Iron (ferrous fumarate)[a]	35 mg	35 mg
Magnesium (magnesium oxide)	50 mg	50 mg
Zinc (zinc oxide)	15 mg	15 mg

[a] Elemental amount.

Each oval shaped, blue/dark blue (p.m.), film-coated, immediate release tablet contains:

	PregVit	PregVit folic 5
Folic Acid	1.1 mg	5.0 mg
Vitamin B_{12} (cyanocobalamin)	12 µg	12 µg
Vitamin D_3 (cholecalciferol)	250 IU	250 IU
Calcium (calcium carbonate)[a]	300 mg	300 mg

[a] Elemental amount.

Nonmedicinal Ingredients: PregVit pink (a.m.) tablet: ammonium hydroxide, N-butyl alcohol, carnauba wax, D&C Red #27, FD&C Blue #1, FD&C Blue #2, FD&C Red #40, FD&C Yellow #6, isopropyl alcohol, macrogol/PEG 3350, magnesium stearate, microcrystalline cellulose, polyvinyl alcohol, propylene glycol, shellac glaze, simethicone, sodium croscarmellose, sodium lauryl sulfate, starch (corn starch), talc and titanium dioxide.

PregVit blue (p.m.) tablet: ammonium hydroxide, N-butyl alcohol, carnauba wax, D&C Red #27, FD&C Blue #2, FD&C Red #40, FD&C Yellow #6, isopropyl alcohol, macrogol/PEG 3350, magnesium stearate, polyvinyl alcohol, propylene glycol, shellac glaze, simethicone, sodium croscarmellose, sodium lauryl sulfate, talc and titanium dioxide.

PregVit folic 5 pink (a.m.) tablet: ammonium hydroxide, N-butyl alcohol, carnauba wax, D&C Red #27, FD&C Blue #1, FD&C Blue #2, FD&C Red #40, FD&C Yellow #6, isopropyl alcohol, macrogol/PEG 3350, magnesium stearate, microcrystalline cellulose, polyvinyl alcohol, propylene glycol, shellac glaze, simethicone, sodium croscarmellose, sodium lauryl sulfate, starch (corn starch), talc and titanium dioxide.

PregVit folic 5 dark blue (p.m.) tablet: ammonium hydroxide, N-butyl alcohol, carnauba wax, D&C Red #27, FD&C Blue #1, FD&C Blue #2, isopropyl alcohol, macrogol/PEG 3350, magnesium stearate, polyvinyl alcohol, propylene glycol, shellac glaze, simethicone, sodium croscarmellose, sodium lauryl sulfate, talc and titanium dioxide.

These products do not contain lactose, gliadin-gluten or tartrazine.

These products are certified Kosher and Halal.

Premarin® Intravenous Pr

conjugated estrogens

Estrogenic Hormones

Pfizer

Date of Revision: December 5, 2008

Warning: The Women's Health Initiative (WHI) study results indicated increased risk of myocardial infarction (MI), stroke, invasive breast cancer, pulmonary emboli and deep venous thrombosis in postmenopausal women receiving treatment with oral combined conjugated estrogens and medroxyprogesterone acetate compared to those receiving placebo tablets. Other combinations and dosage forms of estrogens and progestins were not studied. In the absence of comparable data, these risks should be assumed to be similar. Therefore, the following should be considered when estrogens and progestins are prescribed:

- Estrogens with or without progestins should not be prescribed for primary or secondary prevention of cardiovascular diseases.
- Estrogens with or without progestins should be prescribed at **the lowest effective dose** for the approved indication.
- Estrogens with or without progestins should be prescribed for **the shortest period** possible for the recognized indication.

PHARMACOLOGY: By a direct action, endogenous estrogens cause growth and development of the uterus, fallopian tubes, and vagina. With other hormones, such as pituitary hormones and progesterone, they cause enlargement of the breasts through promotion of ductal growth, stromal development, and the accretion of fat. Estrogens are intricately involved with other hormones, especially progesterone, in the processes of the ovulatory menstrual cycle and pregnancy, and affect the release of pituitary gonadotropins. Indirectly, they also contribute to the shaping of the skeleton, maintenance of tone and elasticity through the increase of collagen production in the supportive tissues of the heart, skin and urogenital structures, changes in the epiphyses of the long bones that allow for the pubertal growth spurt and its termination, growth of axillary and pubic hair and pigmentation of the nipples and genital tissues. Decline of ovarian estrogenic and progestogenic activity at the end of the menstrual cycle can result in menstruation, although the cessation of progesterone secretion is the most important factor in the mature ovulatory cycle. However, in the preovulatory or nonovulatory cycle, estrogen is the primary determinant in the onset of menstruation.

Although circulating estrogens exist in a dynamic equilibrium of metabolic interconversions, estradiol is the principal intracellular human estrogen and is substantially more potent than estrone or estriol at the receptor level. The primary source of estrogen in normally cycling adult women is the ovarian follicle, which secretes 70 to 500 µg of estradiol daily, depending on the phase of the menstrual cycle. After menopause, most endogenous estrogen is produced by conversion of androstenedione, secreted by the adrenal cortex, to estrone by peripheral tissues. Thus, estrone and the sulfate conjugated form, estrone sulfate, are the most abundant circulating estrogens in postmenopausal women.

Circulating estrogens modulate pituitary gonadotropins, luteinizing hormone (LH) and follicle stimulating hormone (FSH) through a negative feedback mechanism. Estrogen therapy acts to reduce elevated levels of these hormones seen in postmenopausal women.

Estrogen drug products act by regulating the transcription of a limited number of genes. They may act directly at the cell's surface via non "estrogen receptor" mechanism or directly with the estrogen receptor inside the cell. Estrogens diffuse through cell membranes, distribute themselves throughout the cell, and bind to and activate the nuclear estrogen receptor, a DNA-binding protein which is found in estrogen-responsive tissues. The activated estrogen receptor binds to specific DNA sequences, or hormone-response elements, which enhance the transcription of adjacent genes and in turn lead to the observed effects. Estrogen receptors have been identified in the wall of blood vessels, in tissues of the reproductive tract, breast, pituitary, hypothalamus, liver, and bone of women.

Conjugated estrogens are soluble in water and are well absorbed through the skin, mucous membranes, and gastrointestinal tract after release from the drug formulation. Some estrogens are excreted in bile; however, they are reabsorbed from the intestine and returned to the liver through the portal venous system. Water-soluble estrogen conjugates are strongly acidic and are ionized in body fluids, which favours excretion through the kidneys since tubular reabsorption is minimal.

When applied for a local action, absorption is usually sufficient to cause systemic effects. When conjugated with aryl and alkyl groups for parenteral administration, the rate of absorption of oily preparations is slowed with a prolonged duration of action, such that a single intramuscular injection of estradiol valerate or estradiol cypionate is absorbed over several weeks.

Administered estrogens and their esters are handled within the body essentially the same way as the endogenous hormones. Women's Health Initiative Study: The Women's Health Initiative (WHI) enrolled approximately 27 000 predominantly healthy postmenopausal women in two substudies to assess the risks and benefits of oral conjugated estrogens (CEE) [0.625 mg daily] alone or in combination with medroxyprogesterone acetate (MPA) [0.625 mg/2.5 mg daily] compared to placebo. The primary endpoint was the incidence of coronary heart disease (CHD), i.e. non-fatal myocardial infarction (MI), silent MI and coronary death. The primary safety endpoint was incidence of invasive breast cancer. The substudy did not evaluate the effects of hormone therapy on menopausal symptoms.

The oral estrogen-alone substudy was stopped early because an increased risk of stroke was observed, and it was deemed that no further information would be obtained regarding the risks and benefits of estrogen alone in predetermined primary endpoints. Results of the estrogen-alone substudy which included 10,739 women (average age of 63 years, range 50 to 79; 75.3% White, 15.1% Black, 6.1% Hispanic, 3.6% Other), after an average follow-up of 6.8 years are presented in Table 1.

In the oral estrogen-alone substudy of WHI, there was no significant overall effect on the relative risk (RR) of CHD (RR 0.95, 95% nominal confidence interval [nCI] 0.79-1.16); a slightly elevated RR of CHD was reported in the early follow-up period and diminished over time. There was no significant effect on the RR of invasive breast cancer (RR 0.80, 95% nCI 0.62-1.04) or colorectal cancer (RR 1.08, 95% nCI 0.75-1.55) reported. Estrogen use was associated with a statistically significant increased risk of stroke (RR 1.37, 95% nCI 1.09-1.73) and deep vein thrombosis (DVT) (RR 1.47, 95% nCI 1.06-2.06). The RR of PE (RR 1.37, 95% nCI 0.90-2.07) was not significantly increased. A statistically significant reduced risk of hip, vertebral and total fractures was reported with estrogen use (RR 0.65, 95% nCI 0.45-0.94), (RR 0.64, 95% nCI 0.44-0.93), and (RR 0.71, 95% nCI 0.64-0.80), respectively. The estrogen-alone substudy did not report a statistically significant effect on death due to other causes (RR 1.08, 95% nCI 0.88-1.32). There was no effect on overall mortality risk (RR 1.04, 95% nCI 0.88-1.22). These confidence intervals are unadjusted for multiple looks and multiple comparisons.

Table 1: Premarin Intravenous

Relative and Absolute Risk Seen in the Oral Estrogen-Alone Substudy of WHI

Event	Relative Risk Oral ERT vs Placebo (95% nCI[a])	Absolute Risk Per 10 000 Person-years	
		ERT (n=5310)	Placebo (n=5429)
CHD Events[b]	0.95 (0.79–1.16)	53	56
Non-fatal MI[b]	0.91 (0.73–1.14)	40	43
CHD Death[b]	1.01 (0.71–1.43)	16	16
Stroke[c]	1.37 (1.09[b]1.73)	45	33
Deep Vein Thrombosis[b]	1.47 (1.06–2.06)	23	15
Pulmonary Embolism[b]	1.37 (0.90–2.07)	14	10
Invasive Breast Cancer[b]	0.80 (0.62–1.04)	28	34
Colorectal Cancer[c]	1.08 (0.75–1.55)	17	16
Hip Fracture[c]	0.65 (0.45–0.94)	12	19
Vertebral Fractures[c]	0.64 (0.44–0.93)	11	18
Total Fractures[c]	0.71 (0.64–0.80)	144	197
Death Due to Other Causes[c,d]	1.08 (0.88–1.32)	53	50
Overall Mortality[c]	1.04 (0.88–1.22)	81	78

[a] Nominal confidence intervals unadjusted for multiple looks and multiple comparisons.
[b] Results are based on centrally adjudicated data for an average follow-up of 7.1 years.
[c] Results are based on an average follow-up of 7.1 years.
[d] All deaths, except from breast or colorectal cancer, definite/probable CHD, PE, or cerebrovascular disease.

Final adjudicated results for CHD events from the estrogen-alone substudy, after an average follow-up of 7.1 years, reported no overall difference for primary CHD events (nonfatal MI, silent MI and CHD death) in women receiving CEE alone compared with placebo.

The oral estrogen-plus-progestin substudy was also stopped early. According to the predefined stopping rule, after an average follow-up of 5.2 years of treatment, the increased risk of breast cancer and cardiovascular events, at that time, exceeded the specified benefits (such as the reduction of colorectal cancer and hip fracture). Results of the estrogen-plus-progestin substudy of WHI, which included 16 608 women (average age of 63 years, range 50 to 79) after an average follow-up of 5.6 years are presented in Table 2. These results reflect centrally adjudicated data after an average follow-up of 5.6 years.

In the WHI oral estrogen-plus-progestin substudy, an increase in CHD risk was associated with combined hormone therapy (RR 1.24, 95% nCI 1.00-1.54). This was most apparent in the first year of the study (RR 1.81, 95% nCI 1.09-3.01). The RR of invasive breast cancer (RR 1.24, 95% nCI 1.01-1.54) was increased in women on combined hormone therapy. The substudy also reported a statistically significant increased RR of overall stroke (RR 1.31, 95% nCI 1.02-1.68), ischemic stroke (RR 1.44, 95% nCI 1.09-1.90), DVT (RR 1.95, 95% nCI 1.43-2.67), and PE (RR 2.13, 95% nCI 1.45-3.11). Estrogen plus progestin was found to increase bone mineral density vs placebo (3.7% vs 0.14%, P<0.001) after three years. A statistically significant reduced RR of hip (RR 0.67, 95% nCI 0.47-0.96), vertebral (RR 0.65, 95% nCI 0.46-0.92), lower arm/wrist (RR 0.71, 95% nCI 0.59-0.85), and total fractures (RR 0.76, 95% nCI 0.69-0.83) was associated with estrogen plus progestin use.

Oral estrogen plus progestin use was associated with a statistically significant decreased risk of invasive colorectal cancer (RR 0.56, 95% nCI 0.38-0.81) although when colorectal cancers were diagnosed in combined hormone users, they were more advanced. Additional analyses showed no statistically significant differences in relative risk of endometrial (RR 0.81, 95% nCI 0.48-1.36) or cervical (RR 1.44, 95% nCI 0.47-4.42) cancers in patients on combined hormone replacement therapy vs placebo. After an average of 5.2 years of follow-up, the estrogen-plus-progestin substudy did not report a statistically significant effect on death due to other causes (RR 0.92, 95% nCI 0.74-1.14), and there was no effect on overall mortality risk (RR 0.98, 95% nCI 0.82-1.18). These confidence intervals are unadjusted for multiple looks and multiple comparisons.

Pharmacokinetics: Distribution: The distribution of exogenous estrogens is similar to that of endogenous estrogens. Estrogens are widely distributed in the body and are generally found in higher concentration in the sex hormone target organs. Estrogens circulate in the blood largely bound to sex hormone-binding globulin (SHBG) and albumin.

Metabolism: Metabolic conversion of estrogens occurs primarily in the liver (first pass effect), but also at local target tissue sites. Complex metabolic processes result in a dynamic equilibrium of circulating conjugated and unconjugated estrogenic forms which are continually interconverted, especially between estrone and estradiol and between esterified and non-esterified forms.

Table 2: Premarin Intravenous

Relative and Absolute Risk Seen in the Oral Estrogen Plus Progestin Subset of WHI at an Average of 5.6 Years[a]

Event	Relative Risk HRT[d] vs Placebo (95% nCI[b])	Absolute Risk Per 10 000 Person-years	
		HRT (n=8506)	Placebo (n=8102)
CHD Events	1.24 (1.00–1.54)	39	33
Non-fatal MI	1.28 (1.00–1.63)	31	25
CHD Death	1.10 (0.70–1.75)	8	8
All Strokes	1.31 (1.02–1.68)	31	24
Ischemic Stroke	1.44 (1.09–1.90)	26	18
Deep Vein Thrombosis	1.95 (1.43–2.67)	26	13
Pulmonary Embolism	2.13 (1.45–3.11)	18	8
Invasive Breast Cancer[c]	1.24 (1.01–1.54)	41	33
Invasive Colorectal Cancer	0.56 (0.38–0.81)	9	16
Endometrial Cancer	0.81 (0.48–1.36)	6	7
Cervical Cancer	1.44 (0.47–4.42)	2	1
Hip Fracture	0.67 (0.47–0.96)	11	16
Vertebral Fractures	0.65 (0.46–0.92)	11	17
Lower Arm/Wrist Fractures	0.71 (0.59–0.85)	44	62
Total Fractures	0.76 (0.69–0.83)	152	199

[a] Results are based on centrally adjudicated data. Mortality data was not part of the adjudicated data; however, data at 5.2 years of follow-up showed no difference between the groups in terms of all-cause mortality (RR 0.98, 95% nCI 0.82–1.18).
[b] Nominal confidence intervals unadjusted for multiple looks and multiple comparisons.
[c] Includes metastatic and non-metastatic breast cancer with the exception of in situ breast cancer.
[d] Conjugated equine estrogen tablets, 0.625 mg, and medroxyprogesterone acetate tablets, 2.5 mg.

Estrogen drug products administered by non-oral routes while not subject to true "first-pass" metabolism, do undergo significant hepatic uptake, metabolism, and enterohepatic recycling. Metabolism and inactivation occur primarily in the liver. Some estrogens are excreted into the bile; however, they are re-absorbed from the intestine and returned to the liver through the portal venous system. Water-soluble estrogen conjugates are strongly acidic and are ionized in body fluids, which favour excretion through the kidneys since tubular re-absorption is minimal.

Excretion: A certain proportion of the estrogen is excreted into the bile, then reabsorbed from the intestine and returned to the liver through the portal venous system. During this enterohepatic recirculation, estrogens are desulfated and resulfated and undergo degradation through conversion to less active estrogens (estriol and other estrogens), oxidation to nonestrogenic substances (catecholestrogens, which interact with catecholamine metabolism, especially in the central nervous system), and conjugation with glucuronic acids (which are then rapidly excreted in the urine).

INDICATIONS: For abnormal uterine bleeding due to hormonal imbalance in the absence of organic pathology.

CONTRAINDICATIONS: Estrogens should not be used in women with any of the following conditions:

- Liver dysfunction or disease as long as liver function tests have failed to return to normal.
- Known, suspected, or past history of breast cancer.
- Known or suspected estrogen-dependent neoplasia (e.g., endometrial cancer).
- Endometrial hyperplasia.
- Known or suspected pregnancy (see Warnings, Pregnancy).
- Undiagnosed abnormal genital bleeding.
- Active or past history of confirmed venous thromboembolism (such as deep venous thrombosis or pulmonary embolism) or active thrombophlebitis.
- Active or past history of arterial thromboembolic disease (e.g. stroke, myocardial infarction, coronary heart disease).
- Partial or complete loss of vision due to ophthalmic vascular disease.
- Premarin Intravenous should not be used in patients hypersensitive to any of the ingredients.

WARNINGS: See Boxed Warning.

Failure to control abnormal uterine bleeding or its unexpected recurrence is an indication for curettage.

Premarin Intravenous is indicated for short-term use. However, warnings, precautions and adverse reactions associated with oral CEE treatment should be taken into account.

Estrogen Replacement Therapy (ERT) and Hormone Replacement Therapy (HRT) have been associated with increased risks of certain cancers and cardiovascular diseases. The use of unopposed estrogens in women with an intact uterus is associated with an increased risk of endometrial cancer.

Cardiovascular Risk: **ERT has been associated with an increased risk of stroke and deep venous thrombosis (DVT).**

HRT has been associated with an increased risk of cardiovascular events such as myocardial infarction (MI), as well as stroke, venous thrombosis and pulmonary embolism (PE).

The physician should be aware of the possibility of thrombotic disorders (thrombophlebitis, retinal thrombosis, cerebral embolism, and pulmonary embolism) during estrogen replacement therapy and be alert to their earliest manifestations. Should any of these occur or be suspected, estrogen replacement therapy should be discontinued immediately.

Risk factors for cardiovascular disease (e.g. hypertension, diabetes mellitus, tobacco use, hypercholesterolemia, and obesity) should be managed appropriately.

Stroke: In the oral estrogen-alone substudy of the Women's Health Initiative (WHI) (see Pharmacology, Women's Health Initiative Study), a statistically significant increased risk of stroke was reported in women receiving estrogen alone compared to women receiving placebo (45 vs 33 per 10 000 person-years). The increase in risk was observed during year one and persisted.

In the oral estrogen-plus-progestin substudy of WHI, a statistically significant increased risk of stroke was reported in women receiving the estrogen/progestin combination compared to women receiving placebo (31 vs 24 per 10 000 person-years). The increase in risk was demonstrated after the first year and persisted.

Coronary Heart Disease: In the oral estrogen-alone substudy of WHI (see Pharmacology, Women's Health Initiative Study), no overall effect on coronary heart disease (CHD) events (defined as non-fatal myocardial infarction (MI), silent MI or death due to CHD) was reported in women receiving estrogen-alone compared to placebo.

In the oral estrogen-plus-progestin substudy of WHI, no statistically significant increase of coronary heart disease (CHD) events was reported in women receiving the oral estrogen/progestin combination (CE 0.625 mg plus MPA 2.5 mg daily) compared to women receiving placebo (39 vs 33 per 10 000 person-years—7 more cases). An increase in relative risk was demonstrated in year one and a trend toward decreasing relative risk was reported in years 2 through 5.

In post-menopausal women with documented heart disease (n=2763, average age 66.7 years) a controlled clinical trial of secondary prevention of cardiovascular disease (Heart and Estrogen/progestin Replacement Study; HERS) treatment with oral conjugated estrogens plus medroxyprogesterone acetate demonstrated no cardiovascular benefit. During an average follow-up of 4.1 years, treatment with oral conjugated estrogens plus medroxyprogesterone acetate did not reduce the overall rate of CHD events in postmenopausal women with established coronary heart disease. There were more CHD events in the hormone-treated group than in the placebo group in year one, but not during the subsequent years.

From the original HERS trial, 2321 women agreed to participate in an open label extension of HERS, HERS II. Average follow-up in HERS II was an additional 2.7 years, for a total of 6.8 years overall. Rates of CHD events were comparable among women in the hormone-treated group in the HERS, the HERS II, and overall.

Venous Thromboembolism: In the oral estrogen-alone substudy of WHI, the risk of VTE (deep venous thrombosis [DVT] and PE) was reported to be increased for women taking conjugated estrogens (30 vs 22 per 10 000 person-years), although only the increased risk of DVT reached statistical significance (23 vs 15 per 10 000 person-years). The increase in VTE risk was observed during the first two years.

In the oral estrogen-plus-progestin substudy of WHI (see Pharmacology, Women's Health Initiative Study), a statistically significant 2-fold greater rate of VTE, was reported in women receiving the oral estrogen/progestin combination, compared to women receiving placebo (35 vs 17 per 10 000 person-years). Statistically significant increases in risk for both DVT (26 vs 13 per 10 000 person-years) and PE (18 vs 8 per 10 000 person-years) were also demonstrated. The increase in VTE risk was observed during the first year and persisted.

Generally recognized risk factors for VTE include a personal history, a family history (the occurrence of VTE in a direct relative or at a relatively early age may indicate genetic predisposition), systemic lupus erythematosus, and severe obesity (body mass index >30 kg/m²). The risk of VTE also increases with age and smoking (see Precautions).

Malignant Neoplasms: Breast Cancer: In some studies, use of oral ERT and HRT is associated with an increased risk of breast cancer.

In the oral estrogen-alone substudy of WHI, after an average of 7.1 years of follow-up, CEE (0.625 mg per day) was not associated with an increased risk of invasive breast cancer (RR 0.80, 95% nCI 0.62-1.04).

In the oral estrogen-plus-progestin substudy of WHI, after a mean follow-up of 5.6 years, the WHI substudy reported an increased risk of invasive breast cancer (RR 1.24, 95% nCI 1.01-1.54); invasive breast cancers were larger and diagnosed at a more advanced stage in the active therapy group compared to those in the placebo group. The absolute risk was 41 vs 33 cases per 10 000 person-years, for estrogen plus progestin compared with placebo, respectively. Metastatic disease was rare with no apparent difference between groups. Other prognostic factors such as histologic subtype, grade and hormone receptor status did not differ between groups.

Epidemiologic studies have reported an increased risk of breast cancer in women taking estrogens or estrogen/progestin combinations for HRT for several years. The excess risk increases with duration of use and seems to return to baseline in the course of about five years after stopping treatment. These studies also suggest that the risk of breast cancer is greater and becomes apparent earlier with estrogen/progestin combination therapy as compared to the use of estrogens alone.

Studies evaluating various HRT formulations did not show significant variation in the relative risk of breast cancer among formulations regardless of the estrogen/progestin components, doses, regimens, or route of administration.

According to data from epidemiologic studies, about 32 women in every 1000 women who never used HRT are expected to have breast cancer diagnosed between the ages of 50 and 65 years. Among 1000 current or recent users of estrogen-only preparations, it is estimated that 5 and 10 years of use beginning at age 50 result in 1.5 (95% confidence interval (CI), 0-3) and 5 (95% CI, 3-7), respectively, additional breast cancers diagnosed by age 65 years. The corresponding numbers for those using estrogen/progestins combinations are 6 (95% CI, 5-7) and 19 (95% CI, 18-20), respectively.

Use of estrogen alone and estrogen plus progestin has been reported to result in an increase in abnormal mammograms requiring further evaluation.

All women should receive yearly breast examinations by a health care provider and perform monthly breast self-examinations. In addition, mammography examinations should be scheduled based on patient age, risk factors, and prior mammogram results.

Endometrial Cancer: The use of unopposed estrogens in women with an intact uterus has been associated with an increased risk of endometrial cancer.

The reported endometrial cancer risk among unopposed estrogen users is about 2- to 12-fold greater than in non-users, and appears dependent on duration of treatment and on estrogen dose. Most studies show no significant increased risk associated with use of estrogens for less than 1 year. The greatest risk appears associated with prolonged use, with increased risks of 15- to 24-fold for 5 to 10 years or more, and this risk has been shown to persist for at least 8 to 15 years after ERT is discontinued.

Ovarian Cancer: In some epidemiologic studies, use of estrogen-only products has been associated with an increased risk of ovarian cancer over multiple years of use. Other epidemiologic studies have not found these associations. The analysis of the WHI data suggested that oral estrogen plus progestin therapy may increase the risk of ovarian cancer.

Pregnancy: Estrogens/progestins should not be used during pregnancy (see Contraindications).

Gallbladder Disease: A 2- to 4-fold increase in the risk of surgically confirmed gallbladder disease requiring surgery has been reported in postmenopausal women receiving ERT/HRT.

Visual Abnormalities: Retinal vascular thrombosis has been reported in patients receiving estrogens. Discontinue medication pending examination if there is sudden partial or complete loss of vision, or a sudden onset of proptosis, diplopia, or migraine. If examination reveals papilledema or retinal vascular lesions, medication should be withdrawn.

PRECAUTIONS: General: Premarin Intravenous is indicated for short-term use only. However, warnings, precautions and adverse reactions associated with oral CEE treatment should be taken into account.

When bleeding has stopped in cases of suspected uterine bleeding due to hormonal imbalance, a complete physical examination should be performed with special reference to pelvic and breast examinations. If the diagnosis is confirmed, appropriate measures should be taken to prevent a recurrence.

Hypertriglyceridemia: Women with pre-existing hypertriglyceridemia need special surveillance during estrogen replacement or hormone replacement therapy. Caution should be exercised in patients with pre-existing hypertriglyceridemia since rare cases of large increases of plasma triglycerides leading to pancreatitis have been reported with estrogen replacement therapy in this population.

Porphyria: Women with porphyria may need special surveillance during estrogen replacement or hormone replacement therapy since estrogens may exacerbate this condition.

Impaired Liver Function: Liver function tests should be done periodically in subjects who are suspected of having hepatic disease (see Contraindications). Oral estrogens/progestins may be poorly metabolised in patients with impaired liver function. When liver or endocrine function tests are indicated, or surgical procedures are performed, the laboratory should be advised of the patient's therapy before specimens are forwarded. For information on endocrine and liver function tests, see section under Laboratory Test Interactions.

Past History of Cholestatic Jaundice: Caution is advised in patients with a history of estrogen- or pregnancy-related cholestatic jaundice. If cholestatic jaundice develops during treatment, medication should be discontinued, and appropriate investigations carried out.

Elevated Blood Pressure: In a small number of case reports, substantial increases in blood pressure during ERT have been attributed to idiosyncratic reactions to estrogens. In a large, randomized, placebo-controlled clinical trial, a generalized effect of ERT on blood pressure was not seen. Blood pressure should be monitored at regular intervals with HRT use. Elevation of blood pressure in previously normotensive or hypertensive patients should be investigated and HRT therapy may have to be discontinued.

Hypocalcemia: Estrogens should be used with caution in individuals with severe hypocalcemia.

Fluid Retention: Because estrogens/progestins may cause some degree of fluid retention, patients with conditions which might be influenced by this factor, such as cardiac or renal dysfunction, warrant careful observation when estrogens are prescribed.

Exacerbation of Other Conditions: Estrogen/hormone replacement therapy may cause an exacerbation of asthma, epilepsy, migraine, diabetes mellitus with or without vascular involvement, systemic lupus erythematosus, and hepatic hemangiomas, and should be used with caution in women with these conditions.

Symptoms and physical findings associated with a previous diagnosis of endometriosis may reappear or be exacerbated with administration of ERT/HRT. Addition of a progestin should be considered in women who have undergone a hysterectomy but are known to have residual endometriosis, since malignant transformation after estrogen-only therapy has been reported.

Hypothyroidism: Patients dependent on thyroid hormone therapy may require increased doses in order to maintain their free thyroid hormone levels in an acceptable range (see Laboratory Test Interactions).

Pregnancy: Estrogens should not be used during pregnancy.

Lactation: Estrogens should not be used during lactation.

Children: Premarin Intravenous is not indicated in children.

Drug Interactions: Estrogens may diminish the effectiveness of anticoagulants, antidiabetics and antihypertensive drugs.

Preparations affecting liver enzymes (e.g., barbiturates, hydantoins, carbamazepine, meprobamate, phenylbutazone or rifampicin) may interfere with the activity of estrogens.

Data from a drug-drug interaction study involving oral conjugated estrogens and medroxyprogesterone acetate indicate that the pharmacokinetic disposition of both drugs is not altered when the drugs are coadministered. Other clinical drug-drug interaction studies have not been conducted with conjugated estrogens.

In vitro and in vivo studies have shown that 17 β-estradiol, one of the components of conjugated estrogens, is metabolized partially by Cytochrome P450 3A4 (CYP3A4). Therefore, strong CYP3A4 inducers such as phenobarbital, phenytoin, carbamazepine, rifampicin and dexamethasone may reduce plasma concentrations of 17 β-estradiol. This may lead to a decreased effect and/or changes in the uterine bleeding profile. CYP3A4 inhibitors such as cimetadine, erythromycin, ketoconazole, clarithromycin, itraconazole, ritonavir, and grapefruit juice may increase plasma concentrations of 17 β-estradiol and may result in side effects.

It was found that some herbal products (e.g., St. John's wort) which are available as OTC products might affect metabolism, and, potentially, efficacy and safety of ERT/HRT products. Hot flashes and vaginal bleeding have been reported in patients taking estrogen/progestin and St. John's wort. St. John's wort may induce hepatic microsomal enzymes which theoretically may result in reduced efficacy of estrogen/progestin.

Physicians and other health care providers should be aware of other non-prescription products concomitantly used by the patient including herbal and natural products, obtained from the widely spread Health Stores.

Laboratory Test Interactions: The results of certain endocrine and liver function tests may be affected by estrogen-containing products:

- Accelerated prothrombin time, partial thromboplastin time, and increased norepinephrine-induced platelet aggregation time; increased platelet count; increased platelet factors II, VII antigen, VIII coagulant activity, IX, X, XII, VII-X complex, II, VII, X complex and beta-thromboglobulin; decreased levels of anti-factor Xa and antithrombin III, decreased antithrombin III activity; increased levels of fibrinogen and fibrinogen activity; increased plasminogen antigen and activity;
- Increased thyroid-binding globulin (TBG) levels leading to increased circulating total thyroid hormone (T_4) as measured by protein-bound iodine (PBI), T_4 levels determined either by column or radioimmunoassay or T_3 levels by radioimmunoassay; free T_3 resin uptake is decreased, reflecting the elevated TBG; free T_4 and free T_3 concentrations are unaltered;
- Other binding proteins may be elevated in serum, i.e., corticosteroid binding globulin (CBG), sex hormone-binding globulin (SHBG), leading to increased circulating corticosteroids and sex steroids respectively. Free or biologically active hormone concentrations are unchanged. Other plasma proteins may be increased (angiotensinogen/renin substrate, alpha-1-antitrypsin, ceruloplasmin);
- Impaired glucose tolerance. For this reason, diabetic patients should be carefully observed while receiving estrogen/progestin replacement therapy;
- Increased plasma HDL and HDL-2 subfraction concentrations, reduced LDL cholesterol concentration, increased triglyceride levels.

The results of the above laboratory tests may not be reliable unless therapy has been discontinued for two to four weeks. The pathologist should be informed that the patient is receiving ERT/HRT therapy when relevant specimens are submitted.

ADVERSE EFFECTS: The most serious adverse reactions associated with the use of estrogens are indicated under Warnings and Precautions.

The following adverse reactions have been reported with intravenous conjugated estrogens.

Reproductive System and Breast Disorders: Very rare: breast pain.

Gastrointestinal Disorders: Rare: ischemic colitis. Very rare: nausea, vomiting, bloating, abdominal pain.

Nervous System Disorders: Rare: possible growth potentiation of benign meningioma. Very rare: dizziness, headache, migraine, nervousness.

Vascular Disorders: Rare: pulmonary embolism, venous thrombosis. Very rare: superficial thrombophlebitis, hypotension, phlebitis (injection site).

General Disorders and Administration Site Conditions: Rare: injection site pain, injection site edema, edema.

Skin and Subcutaneous Tissue Disorders: Very rare: rash.

Immune System Disorders: Very rare: urticaria, angioedema, anaphylactic/anaphylactoid reactions.

OVERDOSE:

Symptoms: Symptoms of overdosage of estrogen-containing products in adults and children when the drug is taken orally may include nausea, vomiting, breast tenderness, dizziness, abdominal pain, drowsiness/fatigue; withdrawal bleeding may occur in females.

Treatment: There is no specific antidote and further treatment if necessary should be symptomatic.

For management of a suspected drug overdose, CPhA recommends that you contact your **regional Poison Control Centre**. See the *CPS* Directory section for a list of Poison Control Centres.

DOSAGE: Abnormal Uterine Bleeding Due to Hormonal Imbalance: One 25 mg injection, intravenously or intramuscularly. Intravenous use is preferred since a more rapid response can be expected from this mode of administration. Repeat in 6-12 hours if necessary. The use of Premarin Intravenous does not preclude the advisibility of other appropriate measures.

Immediately start an estrogen-progestogen cyclic regimen such as conjugated estrogens 3.75 mg to 7.5 mg daily in divided doses (as tablets), for 20 days. During the last 5 to 10 days of therapy, an oral progestogen should be given. Withdrawal bleeding may be expected in the next 2 to 5 days. It is important that therapy be continued and dosage not be reduced, otherwise breakthrough bleeding will occur. The above oral estrogen-progestogen regimen should be repeated, beginning on day 5 of the cycle, for up to three additional cycles after which medication should be withdrawn and the patient's requirement for therapy reassessed. Should breakthrough bleeding occur before the end of a 20-day regimen, therapy should be stopped and then resumed on the fifth day of flow.

The usual precautionary measures governing intravenous administration should be adhered to. Injection should be made **slowly** to obviate the occurrence of flushes.

Infusion of Premarin Intravenous with other agents is not generally recommended. In emergencies, however, when an infusion has already been started, it may be expedient to make the injection into the tubing just distal to the infusion needle. If so used, compatibility of solutions must be considered.

Compatibility of Solutions: Premarin Intravenous is compatible with normal saline and dextrose 10% infusions in a ratio of 1:1. **It is not compatible with protein hydrolysate, ascorbic acid, or any other infusion solutions with an acid pH.**

To reconstitute: Immediate use: Reconstitute Premarin Intravenous with 5 mL of Sterile Water for Injection U.S.P. to obtain approximately 5.0 mL of straw-coloured solution at 5 mg/mL. Diluent should be added slowly, letting it flow against the side of the vial. Agitate gently. Do not shake violently. **Use immediately after reconstitution.**

SUPPLIED: Each vial contains: conjugated estrogens CSD 25 mg, in a sterile lyophilized cake. Nonmedicinal ingredients: lactose, simethicone and sodium citrate. The pH is adjusted to 7.3 with sodium hydroxide or hydrochloric acid. The reconstituted solution is suitable for intravenous or intramuscular injection. Store in refrigerator, 2-8°C.

Premarin® Tablets Ⓟ

conjugated estrogens

Estrogenic Hormones

Pfizer

Date of Revision: March 19, 2009

SUMMARY PRODUCT INFORMATION:

Route of Administration	Dosage Form/ Strength	Clinically Relevant Nonmedicinal Ingredients
Oral	Conjugated estrogens tablets 0.3 mg, 0.625 mg and 1.25 mg	Lactose For a complete listing see Dosage Forms, Composition and Packaging.

INDICATIONS AND CLINICAL USE: Premarin (conjugated estrogens tablets, C.S.D.) is indicated for the following:

1. The relief of menopausal and postmenopausal symptoms occurring in naturally or surgically induced estrogen deficiency states including vulvar and vaginal atrophy.
2. The prevention of osteoporosis in naturally occurring or surgically induced estrogen-deficiency states. When prescribing solely for the prevention of postmenopausal osteoporosis, therapy with Premarin should be considered in light of other available therapies (see Boxed Serious Warnings and Precautions) and should only be considered for women at significant risk of osteoporosis. Non-estrogen medications should be carefully considered. For older women who are not experiencing any more acute symptoms of menopause, use in combination with a progestin should only be considered for women who failed on, or were intolerant of, non-estrogen medication. Adequate diet, calcium and vitamin D intake, cessation of smoking, as well as regular physical weight-bearing exercise are required in addition to the administration of Premarin. Postmenopausal women require an average of 1000 mg to 1500 mg/day of elemental calcium. Therefore, when not contraindicated, calcium supplementation may be helpful for women with suboptimal dietary intake. Vitamin D supplementation of 400-800 IU/day may also be required to ensure adequate daily intake in postmenopausal women.
3. Hypoestrogenism due to hypogonadism, castration, or primary ovarian failure.
4. Atrophic vaginitis.
5. Vulvar atrophy (with or without pruritus). **When prescribing solely for the treatment of symptoms of vulvar and vaginal atrophy, topical vaginal products should be considered.**

In patients with an intact uterus, Premarin should be prescribed with an appropriate dosage of a progestin for women with intact uteri, in order to prevent endometrial hyperplasia/carcinoma.

Geriatrics (>65 years of age): See above Indications.

Pediatrics (<16 years of age): Premarin is not indicated for use in children.

CONTRAINDICATIONS: Premarin (conjugated estrogens tablets, C.S.D.) should not be administered to patients with any of the following conditions:

- Patients who are hypersensitive to this drug or to any ingredient in the formulation or component of the container. For a complete listing, see Dosage Forms, Composition and Packaging.
- Liver dysfunction or disease as long as liver function tests have failed to return to normal.
- Known or suspected estrogen-dependent malignant neoplasia (e.g. endometrial cancer).
- Endometrial hyperplasia.
- Known, suspected, or past history of breast cancer.
- Undiagnosed abnormal genital bleeding.
- Known or suspected pregnancy (see Warnings and Precautions, Special Populations, Pregnant Women)
- Active or past history of confirmed venous thromboembolism (such as deep venous thrombosis or pulmonary embolism) or active thrombophlebitis.
- Active or past history of arterial thromboembolic disease (e.g. stroke, myocardial infarction, coronary heart disease).
- Partial or complete loss of vision due to ophthalmic vascular disease.

WARNINGS AND PRECAUTIONS:

Serious Warnings and Precautions

The Women's Health Initiative (WHI) trial examined the health benefits and risks of oral combined estrogen plus progestin therapy (n=16 608) and oral estrogen-alone therapy (n=10 739) in postmenopausal women aged 50 to 79 years.

The estrogen plus progestin arm of the WHI trial (mean age 63.3 years) indicated an increased risk of myocardial infarction (MI), stroke, invasive breast cancer, pulmonary emboli and deep vein thrombosis in postmenopausal women receiving treatment with combined conjugated equine estrogens (CEE, 0.625 mg/day) and medroxyprogesterone acetate (MPA, 2.5 mg/day) for 5.2 years compared to those receiving placebo.

The estrogen-alone arm of the WHI trial (mean age 63.6 years) indicated an increased risk of stroke and deep vein thrombosis in hysterectomized women treated with CEE-alone (0.625 mg/day) for 6.8 years compared to those receiving placebo.

Therefore, the following should be given serious consideration at the time of prescribing:

- Estrogens with or without progestins **should not** be prescribed for primary or secondary prevention of cardiovascular diseases.
- Estrogens with or without progestins should be prescribed at **the lowest effective dose** for the approved indication.
- Estrogens with or without progestins should be prescribed for the **shortest period possible** for the approved indication.
- The use of Premarin for the prevention of osteoporosis should be considered in light of other available therapies.

General: Combined Estrogen and Progestin Therapy: There are additional and/or increased risks that may be associated with the use of combination estrogen-plus-progestin therapy compared with using estrogen-alone regimens. These include an increased risk of myocardial infarction, pulmonary embolism, invasive breast cancer and ovarian cancer.

Carcinogenesis and Mutagenesis: Breast Cancer: Available epidemiological data indicate that the use of combined estrogen plus progestin by postmenopausal women is associated with an increased risk of invasive breast cancer.

In the estrogen plus progestin arm of the WHI trial, among 10 000 women over a one-year period, there were:

- 8 more cases of invasive breast cancer (38 on combined HRT versus 30 on placebo).

The WHI study also reported that the invasive breast cancers diagnosed in the estrogen plus progestin group were similar in histology but were larger (mean [SD], 1.7 cm [1.1] vs 1.5 cm [0.9], respectively; P=0.04) and were at a more advanced stage compared with those diagnosed in the placebo group. The percentage of women with abnormal mammograms (recommendations for short-interval follow-up, a suspicious abnormality, or highly suggestive of malignancy) was significantly higher in the estrogen plus progestin group versus the placebo group. This difference appeared at year one and persisted in each year thereafter.

In the estrogen-alone arm of the WHI trial, there was no statistically significant difference in the rate of invasive breast cancer in hysterectomized women treated with conjugated equine estrogens versus women treated with placebo.

It is recommended that estrogens not be given to women with existing breast cancer or those with a previous history of the disease (see Contraindications).

There is a need for caution in prescribing estrogens for women with known risk factors associated with the development of breast cancer, such as strong family history of breast cancer (first degree relative) or who present a breast condition with an increased risk (abnormal mammograms and/or atypical hyperplasia at breast biopsy).

Other known risk factors for the development of breast cancer such as nulliparity, obesity, early menarche, late age at first full term pregnancy and at menopause should also be evaluated.

It is recommended that women undergo mammography prior to the start of HRT treatment and at regular intervals during treatment, as deemed appropriate by the treating physician and according to the perceived risks for each patient.

The overall benefits and possible risks of hormone replacement therapy should be fully considered and discussed with patients. It is important that the modest increased risk of being diagnosed with breast cancer after 4 years of treatment with combined estrogen plus progestin HRT (as reported in the results of the WHI trial) be discussed with the patient and weighed against its known benefits.

Instructions for regular self-examination of the breasts should be included in this counselling.

Endometrial Hyperplasia and Endometrial Carcinoma: Estrogen-only HRT increases the risk of endometrial hyperplasia/carcinoma if taken by women with intact uteri. Estrogen should be prescribed with an appropriate dosage of a progestin for women with intact uteri in order to prevent endometrial hyperplasia/carcinoma.

The reported endometrial cancer risk among unopposed estrogen users is about 2- to 12-fold or greater than in non-users and appears to be dependent on duration of treatment and on estrogen dose. The greatest risk appears associated with prolonged use, with increased risks of 15- to 24-fold for five years or more, and this risk has been shown to persist for at least 8 to15 years after ERT is discontinued.

Clinical surveillance of all women taking combined estrogen plus progestin HRT is important. Adequate diagnostic measures, including endometrial sampling when indicated, should be undertaken to rule out malignancy in all cases of undiagnosed persistent or recurring abnormal vaginal bleeding.

Ovarian Cancer: In some epidemiologic studies, the use of estrogen-only products has been associated with an increased risk of ovarian cancer over multiple years of use. Other epidemiologic studies have not found these associations.

Cardiovascular: Cardiovascular Risk: ERT has been reported to increase the risk of stroke and deep venous thrombosis (DVT).

Risk factors for cardiovascular disease (e.g., hypertension, diabetes mellitus, tobacco use, hypercholesterolemia, and obesity) should be managed appropriately.

General: The results of the Heart and Estrogen/progestin Replacement Studies (HERS and HERS II) and the Women's Health Initiative (WHI) trial indicate that the use of estrogen plus progestin is associated with an increased risk of coronary heart disease (CHD) in postmenopausal women. The results of the WHI trial indicate that the use of estrogen-alone and estrogen plus progestin is associated with an increased risk of stroke in postmenopausal women.

WHI Trial Findings: In the combined estrogen plus progestin arm of the WHI trial, among 10 000 women over a one-year period, there were:

- 8 more cases of stroke (29 on combined HRT versus 21 on placebo)
- 7 more cases of CHD (37 on combined HRT versus 30 on placebo).

In the estrogen-alone arm of the WHI trial of women with prior hysterectomy, among 10 000 women over a one-year period, there were/was:

- 12 more cases of stroke (44 on estrogen-alone therapy versus 32 on placebo)
- no statistically significant difference in the rate of CHD.

HERS and HERS II Findings: In the Heart and Estrogen/progestin Replacement Study (HERS) of postmenopausal women with documented heart disease (n=2763, average age 66.7 years), a randomized placebo-controlled clinical trial of secondary prevention of coronary heart disease (CHD), treatment with 0.625 mg/day oral conjugated equine estrogen (CEE) plus 2.5 mg oral medroxyprogesterone acetate (MPA) demonstrated no cardiovascular benefit. Specifically, during an average follow-up of 4.1 years, treatment with CEE plus MPA did not reduce the overall rate of CHD events in postmenopausal women with established coronary heart disease. There were more CHD events in the hormone-treated group than in the placebo group in year 1, but not during the subsequent years.

From the original HERS trial, 2321 women consented to participate in an open label extension of HERS known as HERS II. Average follow-up in HERS II was an additional 2.7 years, for a total of 6.8 years overall. After 6.8 years, hormone therapy did not reduce the risk of cardiovascular events in women with CHD.

Blood Pressure: Women using hormone replacement therapy sometimes experience increased blood pressure. Blood pressure should be monitored with HRT use. Elevation of blood pressure in previously normotensive or hypertensive patients should be investigated and HRT may have to be discontinued.

Endocrine and Metabolism: Glucose and Lipid Metabolism: A worsening of glucose tolerance and lipid metabolism has been observed in a significant percentage of peri- and post-menopausal patients. Therefore, diabetic patients, or those with a predisposition to diabetes, should be observed closely to detect any alterations in carbohydrate or lipid metabolism, especially in triglyceride blood levels.

Women with familial hyperlipidemias need special surveillance. Lipid-lowering measures are recommended additionally, before treatment is started.

Caution should be exercised in patients with pre-existing hypertriglyceridemia since rare cases of large increases of plasma triglycerides leading to pancreatitis have been reported with estrogen therapy in this population.

Women with porphyria need special surveillance.

Estrogens should be used with caution in individuals with pre-existing severe hypocalcemia.

Calcium and Phosphorus Metabolism: Because the prolonged use of estrogens influences the metabolism of calcium and phosphorus, estrogens should be used with caution in patients with metabolic and malignant bone diseases associated with hypercalcemia and in patients with renal insufficiency.

Hypothyroidism: Patients who require thyroid hormone replacement therapy and who are also taking estrogen should have their thyroid function monitored regularly to assure that thyroid hormone levels remain in an acceptable range (see Drug Interactions, Drug-Laboratory Test Interactions).

Other Conditions: Premarin contains lactose. In patients with rare hereditary galactose intolerance, lactase deficiency or glucose-galactose malabsorption, the severity of the condition should be taken into careful consideration before prescribing Premarin. The patient should be closely monitored.

Genitourinary: Endometriosis: Symptoms and physical findings associated with a previous diagnosis of endometriosis may reappear or become aggravated with estrogen use.

Addition of a progestin should be considered in women who have undergone a hysterectomy but are known to have residual endometriosis, since a few cases of malignant transformation after estrogen-only therapy have been reported.

Uterine Leiomyomata: Pre-existing uterine leiomyomata may increase in size during estrogen use. Growth, pain or tenderness of uterine leiomyomata requires discontinuation of medication and appropriate investigation.

Vaginal Bleeding: Abnormal vaginal bleeding, due to its prolongation, irregularity or heaviness, occurring during therapy should prompt appropriate diagnostic measures to rule out the possibility of uterine malignancy and the treatment should be re-evaluated.

Hematologic: Venous Thromboembolism: Available epidemiological data indicate that use of estrogen with or without progestin by postmenopausal women is associated with an increased risk of developing venous thromboembolism (VTE).

In the estrogen plus progestin arm of the WHI trial, among 10 000 women on combined HRT over a one-year period, there were 18 more cases of venous thromboembolism, including 8 more cases of pulmonary embolism.

In the estrogen-alone arm of the WHI trial, among 10 000 women on estrogen therapy over a one-year period, there were 7 more cases of venous thromboembolism, although there was no statistically significant difference in the rate of pulmonary embolism.

Generally recognized risk factors for VTE include a personal history, a family history (the occurrence of VTE in a direct relative at a relatively early age may indicate genetic predisposition), severe obesity (body mass index >30 kg/m²) and systemic lupus erythematosus. The risk of VTE also increases with age and smoking.

The risk of VTE may be temporarily increased with prolonged immobilization, major surgery or trauma. In women on HRT, attention should be given to prophylactic measures to prevent VTE following surgery. Also, patients with varicose veins should be closely supervised. The physician should be alert to the earliest manifestations of thrombotic disorders (thrombophlebitis, retinal thrombosis, cerebral embolism and pulmonary embolism). If these occur or are suspected, hormone therapy should be discontinued immediately, given the risks of long-term disability or fatality.

If feasible, estrogens should be discontinued at least 4 weeks before major surgery which may be associated with an increased risk of thromboembolism, or during periods of prolonged immobilization.

Hepatic/Biliary/Pancreatic: Gallbladder Diseases: A 2 to 4-fold increase in the risk of gallbladder disease requiring surgery in women receiving postmenopausal estrogens has been reported.

Hepatic Hemangiomas: Particular caution is indicated in women with hepatic hemangiomas, as HRT may cause an exacerbation of this condition.

Jaundice: Caution is advised in patients with a history of liver and/or biliary disorders. If cholestatic jaundice develops during treatment, the treatment should be discontinued and appropriate investigations carried out.

Liver Function Tests: Liver function tests should be done periodically in subjects who are suspected of having hepatic disease. For information on endocrine and liver function tests, see Monitoring and Laboratory Tests.

Immune: Particular caution is indicated in women with systemic lupus erythematosus, as HRT may cause an exacerbation of this condition.

Neurologic: Cerebrovascular Insufficiency: Patients who develop visual disturbances, classical migraine, transient aphasia, paralysis or loss of consciousness should discontinue medication.

Patients with a previous history of classical migraine and who develop a recurrence or worsening of migraine symptoms should be reevaluated.

Dementia: Available epidemiological data indicate that the use of combined estrogen plus progestin in women age 65 and over may increase the risk of developing probable dementia.

The Women's Health Initiative Memory Study (WHIMS), a clinical substudy of the WHI, was designed to assess whether postmenopausal hormone replacement therapy (oral estrogen plus progestin or oral estrogen-alone) reduces the risk of dementia in women aged 65 and over (age range 65-79 years) and free of dementia at baseline.

In the estrogen plus progestin arm of the WHIMS (n=4532), women with intact uteri were treated with daily 0.625 mg conjugated equine estrogens (CEE) plus 2.5 mg medroxyprogesterone acetate (MPA) or placebo for an average of 4.05 years. The results, when extrapolated to 10 000 women treated over a one-year period showed:

- 23 more cases of probable dementia (45 on combined HRT versus 22 on placebo).

In the estrogen-alone arm of the WHIMS (n=2947), women with prior hysterectomy were treated with daily 0.625 mg CEE or placebo for an average of 5.21 years. The results, when extrapolated to 10 000 women treated over a one-year period showed:

- 12 more cases of probable dementia (37 on estrogen-alone versus 25 on placebo), although this difference did not reach statistical significance.

When data from the estrogen plus progestin arm of the WHIMS and the estrogen-alone arm of the WHIMS were combined, as per the original WHIMS protocol, in 10 000 women over a one-year period, there were:

- 18 more cases of probable dementia (41 on estrogen plus progestin or estrogen-alone versus 23 on placebo).

Epilepsy: Particular caution is indicated in women with epilepsy, as HRT may cause an exacerbation of this condition.

Ophthalmologic: Visual Abnormalities: Retinal vascular thrombosis has been reported in patients receiving estrogens. Discontinue medication pending examination if there is sudden partial or complete loss of vision, or a sudden onset of proptosis, diplopia, or migraine. If examination reveals papilledema or retinal vascular lesions, medication should be withdrawn.

Psychiatric: Depression: Patients who are taking progestogens and have a history of depression should be observed. If the depression occurs to a serious degree, the drug should be discontinued.

Renal: Fluid Retention: Estrogens may cause fluid retention.

Therefore, particular caution is indicated in cardiac, renal dysfunction, or asthma. If, in any of the above-mentioned conditions, a worsening of the underlying disease is diagnosed or suspected during treatment, the benefits and risks of treatment should be reassessed based on the individual case.

Special Populations: Pregnant Women: Estrogens/progestins should not be used during pregnancy (see Contraindications).

Nursing Women: Estrogen administration to nursing mothers has been shown to decrease the quantity and quality of breast milk. Detectable amounts of estrogens have been identified in the milk of mothers receiving the drug. Caution should be exercised when estrogens are administered to a nursing woman.

Pediatrics (<16 years of age): Premarin is not indicated for use in children.

Geriatrics (>65 years of age): The estrogen-alone substudy of the Women's Health Initiative (WHI) reported an increased risk of stroke compared with placebo in postmenopausal women 65 years of age or older.

Monitoring and Laboratory Tests: Before Premarin is administered, the patient should have a complete physical examination including blood pressure determination. Breasts and pelvic organs should be appropriately examined and a Papanicolaou smear should be performed. Endometrial biopsy should be done only when indicated. Baseline tests should include mammography, measurements of blood glucose, calcium, triglycerides and cholesterol, and liver function tests. Before starting treatment pregnancy should be excluded. Periodic check-ups and careful benefit/risk evaluations should be undertaken in women treated with ERT/HRT therapy. The first follow-up examination should be done within three to six months of initiation of treatment to assess response to treatment. Thereafter, examinations should be made at intervals of at least once a year. Appropriate investigations should be arranged at regular intervals as determined by the physician.

Mammography examinations should be scheduled based on patient age, risk factors and prior mammogram results.

The importance of regular self-examination of the breasts should be discussed with the patient.

ADVERSE REACTIONS: Adverse Drug Reaction Overview: See Warnings and Precautions regarding potential induction of malignant neoplasia and other adverse effects similar to those observed with oral contraceptives.

The following additional adverse reactions have been reported with estrogen replacement therapy or are undesirable effects associated with hormone replacement therapy:

Blood and Lymphatic System Disorders: Altered coagulation tests (see Drug Interactions, Drug-Laboratory Test Interactions).

Cardiac Disorders: palpitations; increase in blood pressure (see Warnings and Precautions); coronary thrombosis, myocardial infarction.

Endocrine Disorders: increased blood sugar levels; decreased glucose tolerance, carbohydrate tolerance.

Eye Disorders: neuro-ocular lesions (e.g. retinal vascular thrombosis, optic neuritis); visual disturbances; steepening of the corneal curvature; intolerance to contact lenses.

Gastrointestinal Disorders: nausea; vomiting; abdominal discomfort (cramps, pressure, pain), bloating, pancreatitis, gallbladder disorder; ischemic colitis.

General Disorders and Administration Site Conditions: fatigue; changes in appetite; changes in body weight; changes in libido. exacerbation of porphyria, hypocalcemia (in patients with disease that can predispose to severe hypocalcemia), exacerbation of asthma, angioedema, hypersensitivity; anaphylactic/anaphylactoid reactions, increased triglycerides.

Hepatobiliary Disorders: gallbladder disorder; cholestatic jaundice.

Musculoskeletal and Connective Tissue Disorders: Musculoskeletal pain including leg pain not related to thromboembolic disease (usually transient, lasting 3-6 weeks) may occur, arthralgias, leg cramps.

Neoplasms, benign: fibrocystic breast changes; enlargement of hepatic hemangiomas.

Nervous System Disorders: aggravation of migraine episodes; headaches; dizziness; cerebrovascular accident/stroke, exacerbation of epilepsy, stroke, exacerbation of chorea, somnolence, insomnia.

Psychiatric Disorders: mental depression; nervousness; irritability, anxiety, mood disturbances, dementia, fatigue.

Renal and Urinary Disorders: cystitis; dysuria; sodium retention; edema.

Reproductive System and Breast Disorders: breakthrough bleeding; spotting; change in menstrual flow and abnormal withdrawal bleeding or flow, dysmenorrhea/pelvic pain; vaginal itching/discharge; dyspareunia; endometrial hyperplasia; pre-menstrual-like syndrome; reactivation of endometriosis; changes in cervical erosion and amount of cervical secretion; vaginal candidiasis, amenorrhea, vaginitis, increase in size of uterine leiomyomata, breast swelling and tenderness, breast pain, enlargement, galactorrhea, breast discharge; growth potentiation of benign meningioma; leukorrhea.

Skin and Subcutaneous Tissue Disorders: Chloasma or melasma, which may persist when drug is discontinued; erythema multiforme; erythema nodosum; haemorrhagic eruption; loss of scalp hair; hirsutism and acne, urticaria, pruritus, generalized rash, rash (allergic) with without pruritus, alopecia.

Vascular Disorders: Isolated cases of: thrombophlebitis; thromboembolic disorders, venous thrombosis.

Clinical Trial Adverse Drug Reactions: Because clinical trials are conducted under very specific conditions the adverse drug reaction rates observed in the clinical trials may not reflect the rates observed in practice and should not be compared to the rates in the clinical trials of another drug. Adverse drug reaction information from clinical trials is useful for identifying drug-related adverse events and for approximating rates.

A phase III double-blind, randomized study was conducted to compare the efficacy and safety of various regimens of Premarin (conjugated estrogens) and medroxyprogesterone acetate (MPA). Efficacy was determined by the incidence of endometrial hyperplasia at the twelve month evaluation. A total of 1724 generally healthy postmenopausal women (mean age, 54.0 years±SD 4.6) participated in the study. The patients were considered as having completed the study if they participated in all 13 cycles (28 days/cycle). The five arms in the study were: 2 for Premplus, 2 for Premplus Cycle, and 1 for Premarin alone.

Prior to treatment, the following were performed: physical examinations, vital signs, papanicolaou smear, laboratory safety screen, mammography, follicle stimulating hormone (FSH), and endometrial biopsy. During the patient visit for Cycle 6, all but the mammography and FSH were performed. At the end of the study, Cycle 13, all but the FSH were performed.

No dose-dependent incidence of adverse experiences was seen in the multicenter efficacy and safety study. Significantly ($p < 0.05$) fewer (12%) Premarin treated patients reported breast pain than in the Premarin/MPA groups. Headache was the most common drug-related study event in the Premarin alone group, reported by 69 (20%) patients. Table 1 summarizes the treatment-emergent drug-related study events reported by 2% or more of the patients.

Table 1: Premarin Tablets

Treatment-emergent Drug-related Study Events with an Incidence of ≥2%

Study Event	Premarin 0.625 mg CE (n=347) No. (%) of Patients*
General Disorders and Administration Site Conditions	
Asthenia	18 (5)
Chest pain	2 (<1)
Generalized edema	9 (3)
Edema	5 (1)
Peripheral edema	11 (3)
Pain	11 (3)
Vascular Disorders	
Hypertension	7 (2)
Vasodilatation	9 (3)
Gastrointestinal Disorders	
Diarrhea	6 (2)
Dyspepsia	4 (1)
Flatulence	14 (4)[b]
Nausea	19 (5)
Abdominal pain	46 (13)
Musculoskeletal Connective Tissue, and Bone Disorders	
Leg cramps	8 (2)
Back pain	13 (4)
Nervous System Disorders	
Headache	69 (20)
Depression	22 (6)
Migraine	7 (2)
Dizziness	10 (3)
Emotional lability	4 (1)
Insomnia	2 (<1)
Nervousness	1 (<1)[b,d]
Skin and Subcutaneous Tissue Disorders	
Acne	6 (2)
Pruritus	6 (2)[a,b]
Rash	5 (1)
Reproductive System and Breast Disorders	
Breast enlargement	4 (1)[a,b]
Breast pain*	40 (12)[a,b,d]
Cervix disorder**	12 (3)
Dysmenorrhea	17 (5)[d]
Endometrial hyperplasia	57 (20)
Leukorrhea	24 (7)
Menstrual disorder	3 (<1)
Pelvic pain	16 (5)
Uterine spasm	0 (0)[a,d]
Vaginal bleeding***	28 (8)[b]
Vaginitis	4 (1)[a,b]
Investigations	
Pap smear abnormal†	0 (0)[a]
Weight increased	10 (3)
Psychiatric Disorders	
Depression	22 (6)
Emotional lability	4 (1)
Nervousness	1 (<1)[b,d]

(cont'd)

*Patients were counted only once for a particular study event.

*Breast pain also includes breast discomfort, breast soreness, breast tenderness, mastodynia, nipple soreness and nipple tenderness.

**Cervix disorder includes cervical dysplasia, cervical erosion, cervical hypersecretion.

†Pap smear abnormal refers to positive Pap smear class II through V.

***Vaginal bleeding includes menorrhagia, metrorrhagia, uterine hemorrhage, and vaginal hemorrhage.

[a,b,d]=Significant difference ($p < 0.05$) from treatment group Premplus (0.625/2.5 mg), Premplus (0.625/5.0 mg), Premplus Cycle (0.625/10.0 mg) and Premarin (0.625 mg) respectively.

Table 1 summarizes the treatment-emergent drug-related study events reported by greater than 2% of the patients. The number of patients with any study event is not necessarily the sum of the individual events since a patient might have reported two or more different study events. The addition of progestin to estrogen replacement therapy may contribute to breast pain. This s reflected by the greater percentage of patients with breast pain on combination therapy than on Premarin alone.

If adverse symptoms persist, the prescription of HRT should be re-considered.

DRUG INTERACTIONS: Overview: In vitro and in vivo studies have shown that 17 β-estradiol, one of the components of conjugated estrogens, is metabolized partially by cytochrome P450 3A4 (CYP3A4). Therefore, strong CYP3A4 inducers such as phenobarbitol, phenytoin, carbamazepine, rifampicin and dexamethasome may reduce plasma concentrations of 17 β-estradiol. This may lead to a decreased effect and/or changes in the uterine bleeding profile. CYP3A4 inhibitors such as cimetidine, erythromycin, ketoconazole, clarithromycin, itraconazole, ritonavir may increase plasma concentrations of 17 β-estradiol and may result in side effects.

Data from a drug-drug interaction study involving conjugated estrogens and medroxyprogesterone acetate indicate that the pharmacokinetic disposition of both drugs are not altered when the drugs are co-administered. Other clinical drug-drug interaction studies have not been conducted with conjugated estrogens.

Estrogens may diminish the effectiveness of anticoagulant, antidiabetic and antihypertensive agents.

Drug-Drug Interactions: The following section contains information on drug interactions with ethinyl estradiol-containing products (specifically, oral contraceptives) that have been reported in the public literature. **It is unknown whether such interactions occur with drug products containing other types of estrogens.**

Hepatic Metabolism: Interactions can occur with drugs that induce microsomal enzymes which can decrease ethinyl estradiol concentrations (eg., rifampin, barbiturates, phenytoin, carbamazepine, troglitazone).

Gastrointestinal Wall: Sulfation of ethinyl estradiol has been shown to occur in the gastrointestinal (GI) wall. Therefore, drugs which act as competitive inhibitors for sulfation in the GI wall may increase ethinyl estradiol bioavailability (eg., ascorbic acid, acetaminophen).

Interference in the Metabolism of Other Drugs: Ethinyl estradiol may interfere with the metabolism of other drugs by inhibiting hepatic microsomal enzymes or by inducing hepatic drug conjugation, particularly glucuronidation. Increased plasma concentrations of cyclosporin, prednisolone, and theophylline have been reported with concomitant administration of certain drugs containing ethinyl estradiol (eg., oral contraceptives containing ethinyl estradiol). In addition, products containing ethinyl estradiol may induce the conjugation of other compounds.

Decreased plasma concentrations of acetaminophen and increased clearance of temazepam, salicylic acid, morphine, and clofibric acid have been noted when these drugs were administered with certain ethinyl estradiol-containing drug products (eg., oral contraceptives containing ethinyl estradiol).

Other Interactions with Ethinyl Estradiol: Coadministration of atorvastatin and certain ethinyl estradiol-containing drug products (eg., oral contraceptives) increase AUC values for ethinyl estradiol by 20 percent.

Clinical pharmacokinetic studies have not demonstrated any consistent effect of antibiotics (other than rifampin) on plasma concentrations of synthetic steroids.

Drug-Food Interactions: CYP3A4 inhibitors such as grapefruit juice may increase plasma concentrations of 17 β-estradiol and may result in side effects.

A single dose study in healthy, postmenopausal women was conducted to investigate any potential drug interaction when 2×0.625 mg Premarin (conjugated estrogens) and 2.5 mg medroxyprogesterone acetate (MPA) tablets were administered immediately following a high-fat breakfast. Administration with food slowed the absorption of the conjugated estrogens, thereby reducing the C_{max} of the various estrogens by 25% to 30%, and increasing MPA C_{max} by 89% and $AUC_{0-\infty}$ by 28%. Thus, food slightly lowered the C_{max}, but did not affect the AUC, of the estrogens from a 0.625 mg Premarin tablet; food significantly increased the C_{max} and AUC of MPA from a 2.5-mg tablet.

Drug-Herb Interactions: It was found that some herbal products (e.g., St. John's wort), which are available as over-the-counter (OTC) products, might interfere with steroid metabolism, and therefore alter the efficacy and safety of estrogen/progestin products. Hot flashes and vaginal bleeding have been reported in patients taking estrogen replacement therapy (ERT) and combined estrogen plus progestin therapy (HRT) and St. John's wort. St. John's wort may induce hepatic microsomal enzymes, which theoretically may result in reduced efficacy of ERT and HRT.

Physicians and other health care providers should be made aware of other non-prescription products concomitantly used by the patient, including herbal and natural products, obtained from the widely spread Health Stores.

Drug-Laboratory Test Interactions: The results of certain endocrine and liver function tests may be affected by estrogen-containing products:

- increased prothrombin time and partial thromboplastin time; increased levels of fibrinogen and fibrinogen activity, increased coagulation factors VII, VIII, IX, X; increased norepinephrine-induced platelet aggregability; decreased antithrombin III;
- increased thyroid-binding globulin (TBG) levels leading to increased circulating total thyroid hormone (T4), as measured by column or radioimmunoassay; T3 resin uptake is decreased, reflecting the elevated TBG; free T4 concentration is unaltered;
- impaired glucose tolerance;
- increased serum triglycerides and phospholipids concentration;
- other binding proteins may be elevated in serum i.e., corticosteroid binding globulin (CBG), sex-hormone binding globulin (SHBG), leading to increased circulating corticosteroids and sex steroids respectively; free or biologically active hormone concentrations are unchanged.

The results of the above laboratory tests should not be considered reliable unless therapy has been discontinued for two to four weeks.

The pathologist should be informed that the patient is receiving hormone replacement therapy (HRT) when relevant specimens are submitted.

DOSAGE AND ADMINISTRATION:

Dosing Considerations: Use of estrogens alone or in combination with progestins therapy should be limited to the shortest duration consistent with treatment goals and risks for the individual woman. Patients should be re-evaluated periodically as clinically appropriate to determine if treatment is still necessary (see Boxed Serious Warnings and Precautions). For women who have intact uteri, adequate diagnostic measures, such as endometrial sampling, when indicated, should be undertaken to rule out malignancy in cases of undiagnosed persistent or recurring abnormal vaginal bleeding.

Recommended Dose and Dosage Adjustment: Premarin therapy may be given continuously with no interruption in therapy, or in cyclical regimens (regimens such as 25 days on drug followed by five days off drug) as is medically appropriate on an individualized basis.

Continuous, non-cyclic therapy may be indicated in hysterectomized women or in cases where the signs and symptoms of estrogen deficiency become problematic during the treatment-free interval. In women with an intact uterus, a progestin should be coadministered for a **minimum** of 10, but preferably at least 12 to 14 days per cycle to avoid overstimulation of the endometrium. In addition, progestin should be administered to minimize the occurrence of endometrial hyperplasia. Unexpected or abnormal vaginal bleeding in such patients requires institution of prompt diagnostic measures, such as endometrial biopsy or curettage to rule out the possibility of uterine malignancy. Since progestins are administered to reduce the risk of hyperplastic changes of the endometrium, patients without a uterus do not require a progestin for this purpose.

Usual Dosage Range: Menopausal Symptoms: 0.625-1.25 mg daily, cyclically or continuously as is medically required. Adjust dosage upward or downward according to severity of symptoms and response of the patient. For maintenance, adjust dosage to lowest level providing effective control.

Osteoporosis (loss of bone mass): 0.625 mg daily.

Hypoestrogenism due to:

1. **Female Hypogonadism:** 0.3 mg to 0.625 mg daily, administered cyclically (e.g., 3 weeks on and 1 week off) or continuously as required. Doses are adjusted depending on the severity of symptoms and responsiveness of the endometrium.
2. **Female Castration or Primary Ovarian Failure:** 1.25 mg daily, cyclically or continuously as required. Adjust dosage upward or downward according to severity of symptoms and response of the patient. For maintenance, adjust dosage to lowest level that will provide effective control.

Atrophic Vaginitis: 0.3 mg to 1.25 mg daily depending upon the tissue response of the individual patient. Administer cyclically or continuously as required.

Vulvar Atrophy: 0.3 mg to 1.25 mg daily depending upon the tissue response of the individual patient. Administer cyclically or continuously as required.

Missed Dose: If a patient misses a dose, it should be taken as soon as possible. If it is close to the patient's next scheduled dose, the missed dose should be skipped, and the patient should continue with her normal schedule. The patient should not take two doses at the same time.

Administration: Oral: Premarin should be prescribed with an appropriate dosage of a progestin for women with intact uteri in order to prevent endometrial hyperplasia/carcinoma. Progestin therapy is not required as part of hormone replacement therapy in women who have had a previous hysterectomy.

OVERDOSAGE:

Symptoms of Overdose: Numerous reports of ingestion of large doses of estrogen products and estrogen-containing oral contraceptives by young children have not revealed acute serious ill effects.

Overdosage with estrogen may cause nausea, breast discomfort, fluid retention, bloating or vaginal bleeding in women.

Treatment of Overdose: There is no specific antidote and further treatment if necessary should be symptomatic.

> For management of a suspected drug overdose, CPhA recommends that you contact your **regional Poison Control Centre**. See the *CPS* Directory section for a list of Poison Control Centres.

ACTION AND CLINICAL PHARMACOLOGY: Mechanism of Action: Estrogens generally act through binding to nuclear receptors in estrogen-responsive tissues. To date, two estrogen receptors have been identified. These vary in proportion from tissue to tissue. Circulating estrogens modulate the pituitary secretion of the gonadotropins, luteinizing hormone (LH) and follicle stimulating hormone (FSH), through a negative feedback mechanism. Estrogens act to reduce the elevated levels of these gonadotropins seen in postmenopausal women.

Pharmacodynamics: Conjugated estrogens used in therapy are soluble in water and are well absorbed through the skin, mucous membranes, and gastrointestinal tract after release from the drug formulation.

Effects on Vasomotor Symptoms Associated with Estrogen Deficiency: Hot flushes, feelings of intense heat over the upper trunk and face, with flushing of the skin and sweating occur in approximately 80% of women as a result of the decrease in ovarian hormones. These vasomotor symptoms are seen in women whether menopause is surgically induced or spontaneous. However, hot flushes may be more severe in women who undergo surgical menopause. Hot flushes can begin before the cessation of menses.

Effects on Osteoporosis Associated with Estrogen Deficiency: For several years following natural or induced menopause, the rate of bone mass decline is accelerated. Conjugated estrogens reduce bone resorption and retard postmenopausal bone loss. Case-control studies have shown a reduction of up to 60% in hip and wrist fractures in women whose estrogen replacement was begun within a few years of menopause. Studies also suggest that estrogen reduces the rate of vertebral fractures. One clinical study demonstrated that even when estrogen was started as late as fifteen years after menopause, further loss of bone mass was prevented, but was not restored to premenopausal levels. The effect on bone mass conservation is sustained only as long as conjugated estrogens therapy is continued.

Effects on Female Hypogonadism: In clinical studies of delayed puberty due to female hypogonadism, breast development was induced by doses as low as 0.15 mg. The dosage may be gradually titrated upward at 6 to 12-month intervals as needed to achieve appropriate bone age advancement and eventual epiphyseal closure. Available data suggest that chronic dosing with 0.625 mg is sufficient to induce artificial cyclic menses with sequential progestin treatment and to maintain bone mineral density after skeletal maturity is achieved.

Effects on the Endometrium: The use of unopposed estrogen therapy has been associated with an increased risk of endometrial hyperplasia, a possible precursor of endometrial adenocarcinoma. The results of clinical studies indicate that the addition of a progestin to an estrogen replacement regimen for more than 10 days per cycle reduces the incidence of endometrial hyperplasia and the attendant risk of adenocarcinoma in women with intact uteri. The addition of a progestin into an estrogen replacement regimen has not been shown to interfere with the efficacy of estrogen replacement therapy for its approved indications.

Effect on Bleeding Patterns: With a continuous therapy, several bleeding patterns may occur. These may range from absence of bleeding to irregular bleeding. If bleeding occurs, it is frequently light spotting or moderate bleeding.

Pharmacokinetics: Absorption: Conjugated estrogens are soluble in water and are well absorbed through the skin, mucous membranes, and the gastrointestinal tract after release from the drug formulation. However, Premarin contains a modified-release formulation of conjugated estrogens that slowly releases estrogens over several hours. Maximum plasma concentrations of the various conjugated and unconjugated estrogens are attained within 4 to 10 hours after dose administration.

Distribution: The distribution of exogenous estrogens is similar to that of endogenous estrogens. Estrogens are widely distributed in the body and are generally found in higher concentration in the sex hormone target organs. Estrogens circulate in the blood largely bound to sex hormone binding globulin (SHBG) and albumin.

Metabolism: Metabolic conversion of estrogens occurs primarily in the liver (first pass effect), but also at local target tissue sites. Complex metabolic processes result in a dynamic equilibrium of circulating conjugated and unconjugated estrogenic forms which are continually interconverted, especially between estrone and estradiol and between esterified and non-esterified forms.

Estrogen drug products administered by non-oral routes, while not subject to true "first-pass" metabolism, do undergo significant hepatic uptake, metabolism, and enterohepatic recycling. Metabolism and inactivation occur primarily in the liver. Some estrogens are excreted into the bile; however, they are re-absorbed from the intestine and returned to the liver through the portal venous system. Water-soluble estrogen conjugates are strongly acidic and are ionized in body fluids, which favour excretion through the kidneys since tubular re-absorption is minimal.

When given orally, naturally-occurring estrogens and their esters are extensively metabolized (first pass effect) and circulate primarily as estrone sulfate, with smaller amounts of other conjugated and unconjugated estrogenic species. This results in limited oral potency. By contrast, synthetic estrogens, such as ethinyl estradiol and the nonsteroidal estrogens, are degraded very slowly in the liver and other tissues, which results in their high intrinsic potency.

Excretion: During this enterohepatic recirculation, estrogens are desulfated and resulfated and undergo degradation through conversion to less active estrogens (estriol and other estrogens), oxidation to nonestrogenic substances (catecholestrogens, which interact with catecholamine metabolism, especially in the central nervous system), and conjugation with glucuronic acids (which are then rapidly excreted in the urine).

Estradiol, estrone, and estriol are excreted in the urine, along with glucuronide and sulfate conjugates.

Special Populations and Conditions: No pharmacokinetic studies were conducted in special populations, including patients with renal or hepatic impairment.

STORAGE AND STABILITY: Store at 15-30°C. Keep out of reach of children.

SPECIAL HANDLING INSTRUCTIONS: None required.

INFORMATION FOR THE PATIENT: Published in e-CPS, available by subscription at www.e-cps.ca.

DOSAGE FORMS, COMPOSITION AND PACKAGING: 0.3 mg: Each green, oval, sugar-coated tablet contains: conjugated estrogens CSD 0.3 mg. Nonmedicinal ingredients: calcium sulfate anhydrous, carnauba wax, edible ink, FD&C Blue No. 2, glyceryl monooleate, iron oxide yellow, lactose, magnesium stearate, methyl parahydroxybenzoate, methylcellulose, methylparaben, microcrystalline cellulose, pharmaceutical glaze, polyethylene glycol, polyvinylpyrrolidone, propyl parahydroxybenzoate, povidone, sodium benzoate, stearic acid, sucrose and titanium dioxide. Bottles of 100 and 500.

0.625 mg: Each maroon, oval, sugar-coated tablet contains: conjugated estrogens CSD 0.625 mg. Nonmedicinal ingredients: calcium sulfate anhydrous, carnauba wax, edible ink, erythrosine aluminum lake, FD&C Blue No. 2, FD&C Yellow No. 6, glyceryl monooleate, gum acacia, lactose, magnesium stearate, methylcellulose, microcrystalline cellulose, pharmaceutical glaze, polyethylene glycol, povidone, sodium benzoate, stearic acid, sucrose and titanium dioxide. Bottles of 100 and 1000.

1.25 mg: Each yellow, oval, sugar-coated tablet contains: conjugated estrogens CSD 1.25 mg. Nonmedicinal ingredients: calcium sulfate anhydrous, carnauba wax, edible ink, FD&C Yellow No. 6, glyceryl monooleate, lactose, magnesium stearate, methylcellulose, microcrystalline cellulose, pharmaceutical glaze, polyethylene glycol, quinoline yellow lake, stearic acid, sucrose and titanium dioxide. Bottles of 100.

(Shown in Product Identification Section)

Premarin® Vaginal Cream Ⓟ

conjugated estrogens

Estrogenic Hormones

Pfizer

Date of Revision: March 19, 2009

SUMMARY PRODUCT INFORMATION:

Route of Administration	Dosage Form/ Strength	Clinically Relevant Nonmedicinal Ingredients
Vaginal	Conjugated estrogens vaginal cream 0.625 mg/g	For a complete listing see Dosage Forms, Composition and Packaging.

INDICATIONS AND CLINICAL USE: Premarin Vaginal Cream is indicated in the treatment of atrophic vaginitis, dyspareunia, and kraurosis vulvae.

Premarin Vaginal Cream has not been shown to be effective for any purpose during pregnancy and its use may cause severe harm to the fetus.

Premarin Vaginal Cream should be prescribed with an appropriate dose of a progestin for women with intact uteri in order to prevent endometrial hyperplasia/carcinoma.

Geriatrics (>65 years of age): See above indications.

Pediatrics (<16 years of age): Premarin Vaginal Cream is not indicated for use in children.

CONTRAINDICATIONS: Premarin Vaginal Cream should not be administered to patients with any of the following conditions:

- Patients who are hypersensitive to this drug or to any ingredient in the formulation or component of the container. For a complete listing, see Dosage Forms, Composition and Packaging.
- Liver dysfunction or disease as long as liver function tests have failed to return to normal.
- Known or suspected estrogen-dependent malignant neoplasia (e.g. endometrial cancer).
- Endometrial hyperplasia.
- Known, suspected, or past history of breast cancer.
- Undiagnosed abnormal genital bleeding.
- Known or suspected pregnancy (see Warnings and Precautions, Special populations, Pregnant Women).
- Active or past history of confirmed venous thromboembolism (such as deep venous thrombosis or pulmonary embolism) or active thrombophlebitis.
- Partial or complete loss of vision due to ophthalmic vascular disease.

WARNINGS AND PRECAUTIONS:

Serious Warnings and Precautions
The Women's Health Initiative (WHI) trial examined the health benefits and risks of oral combined estrogen plus progestin therapy (n=16 608) and oral estrogen-alone therapy (n=10 739) in postmenopausal women aged 50 to 79 years.

The estrogen plus progestin arm of the WHI trial (mean age 63.3 years) indicated an increased risk of myocardial infarction (MI), stroke, invasive breast cancer, pulmonary emboli and deep vein thrombosis in postmenopausal women receiving treatment with combined conjugated equine estrogens (CEE, 0.625 mg/day) and medroxyprogesterone acetate (MPA, 2.5 mg/day) for 5.2 years compared to those receiving placebo.

The estrogen-alone arm of the WHI trial (mean age 63.6 years) indicated an increased risk of stroke and deep vein thrombosis in hysterectomized women treated with CEE-alone (0.625 mg/day) for 6.8 years compared to those receiving placebo.

Therefore, the following should be given serious consideration at the time of prescribing:
- Estrogens with or without progestins **should not** be prescribed for primary or secondary prevention of cardiovascular diseases.
- Estrogens with or without progestins should be prescribed at **the lowest effective dose** for the approved indication.
- Estrogens with or without progestins should be prescribed for the **shortest period possible** for the approved indication.

General: Systemic absorption may occur with the use of conjugated estrogens (CE) vaginal cream. Warnings and precautions associated with oral CE treatment should be taken into account.

Latex Condoms: Note: Preliminary studies conducted by the Health Products and Food Branch have demonstrated that PREMARIN Vaginal Cream may react with the latex rubber of certain mechanical barrier devices used for prevention of sexually transmitted diseases and pregnancy (diaphragms and condoms). In additional studies, Premarin Vaginal Cream has been shown to weaken latex condoms. The potential for Premarin Vaginal Cream to weaken and contribute to the failure of condoms, diaphragms, or cervical caps made of latex or rubber should be considered.

Carcinogenesis and Mutagenesis: Breast Cancer: Available epidemiological data indicate that the use of combined estrogen plus progestin by postmenopausal women is associated with an increased risk of invasive breast cancer.
In the estrogen plus progestin arm of the WHI trial, among 10 000 women over a one-year period, there were:
- 8 more cases of invasive breast cancer (38 on combined HRT versus 30 on placebo).

The WHI study also reported that the invasive breast cancers diagnosed in the estrogen plus progestin group were similar in histology but were larger (mean [SD], 1.7 cm [1.1] vs 1.5 cm [0.9], respectively; P=0.04) and were at a more advanced stage compared with those diagnosed in the placebo group. The percentage of women with abnormal mammograms (recommendations for short-interval follow-up, a suspicious abnormality, or highly suggestive of malignancy) was significantly higher in the estrogen plus progestin group versus the placebo group. This difference appeared at year one and persisted in each year thereafter.

In the estrogen-alone arm of the WHI trial, there was no statistically significant difference in the rate of invasive breast cancer in hysterectomized women treated with conjugated equine estrogens versus women treated with placebo.

It is recommended that estrogens not be given to women with existing breast cancer or those with a previous history of the disease (see Contraindications).

There is a need for caution in prescribing estrogens for women with known risk factors associated with the development of breast cancer, such as strong family history of breast cancer (first degree relative) or who present a breast condition with an increased risk (abnormal mammograms and/or atypical hyperplasia at breast biopsy).

Other known risk factors for the development of breast cancer such as nulliparity, obesity, early menarche, late age at first full term pregnancy and at menopause should also be evaluated.

It is recommended that women undergo mammography prior to the start of HRT treatment and at regular intervals during treatment, as deemed appropriate by the treating physician and according to the perceived risks for each patient.

The overall benefits and possible risks of hormone replacement therapy should be fully considered and discussed with patients. It is important that the modest increased risk of being diagnosed with breast cancer after 4 years of treatment with combined estrogen plus progestin HRT (as reported in the results of the WHI trial) be discussed with the patient and weighed against its known benefits.

Instructions for regular self-examination of the breasts should be included in this counselling.

Endometrial Hyperplasia and Endometrial Carcinoma: Estrogen-only HRT increases the risk of endometrial hyperplasia/carcinoma if taken by women with intact uteri. Estrogen should be prescribed with an appropriate dosage of a progestin for women with intact uteri in order to prevent endometrial hyperplasia/carcinoma.

The reported endometrial cancer risk among unopposed estrogen users is about 2- to 12-fold or greater than in non-users and appears to be dependent on duration of treatment and on estrogen dose. The greatest risk appears associated with prolonged use, with increased risks of 15- to 24-fold for five years or more, and this risk has been shown to persist for at least 8 to15 years after ERT is discontinued.

Clinical surveillance of all women taking combined estrogen plus progestin HRT is important. Adequate diagnostic measures, including endometrial sampling when indicated, should be undertaken to rule out malignancy in all cases of undiagnosed persistent or recurring abnormal vaginal bleeding.

Ovarian Cancer: In some epidemiologic studies, the use of estrogen-only products has been associated with an increased risk of ovarian cancer over multiple years use. Other epidemiologic studies have not found these associations.

Cardiovascular: Cardiovascular Risk: ERT has been reported to increase the risk of stroke and deep venous thrombosis (DVT).

Risk factors for cardiovascular disease (e.g., hypertension, diabetes mellitus, tobacco use, hypercholesterolemia, and obesity) should be managed appropriately.

General: The results of the Heart and Estrogen/progestin Replacement Studies (HERS and HERS II) and the Women's Health Initiative (WHI) trial indicate that the use of estrogen plus progestin is associated with an increased risk of coronary heart disease (CHD) in postmenopausal women. The results of the WHI trial indicate that the use of estrogen-alone and estrogen plus progestin is associated with an increased risk of stroke in postmenopausal women.

WHI Trial Findings: In the combined estrogen plus progestin arm of the WHI trial, among 10 000 women over a one-year period, there were:
- 8 more cases of stroke (29 on combined HRT versus 21 on placebo).
- 7 more cases of CHD (37 on combined HRT versus 30 on placebo).

In the estrogen-alone arm of the WHI trial of women with prior hysterectomy, among 10 000 women over a one-year period, there were/was:
- 12 more cases of stroke (44 on estrogen-alone therapy versus 32 on placebo)
- no statistically significant difference in the rate of CHD.

HERS and HERS II Findings: In the Heart and Estrogen/progestin Replacement Study (HERS) of postmenopausal women with documented heart disease (n=2763, average age 66.7 years), a randomized placebo-controlled clinical trial of secondary prevention of coronary heart disease (CHD), treatment with 0.625 mg/day oral conjugated equine estrogen (CEE) plus 2.5 mg oral medroxyprogesterone acetate (MPA) demonstrated no cardiovascular benefit. Specifically, during an average follow-up of 4.1 years, treatment with CEE plus MPA did not reduce the overall rate of CHD events in postmenopausal women with established coronary heart disease. There were more CHD events in the hormone-treated group than in the placebo group in year 1, but not during the subsequent years.

From the original HERS trial, 2321 women consented to participate in an open label extension of HERS known as HERS II. Average follow-up in HERS II was an additional 2.7 years, for a total of 6.8 years overall. After 6.8 years, hormone therapy did not reduce the risk of cardiovascular events in women with CHD.

Blood Pressure: Women using hormone replacement therapy sometimes experience increased blood pressure. Blood pressure should be monitored with HRT use. Elevation of blood pressure in previously normotensive or hypertensive patients should be investigated and HRT may have to be discontinued.

Endocrine and Metabolism: Glucose and Lipid Metabolism: A worsening of glucose tolerance and lipid metabolism has been observed in a significant percentage of peri- and post-menopausal patients. Therefore, diabetic patients, or those with a predisposition to diabetes, should be observed closely to detect any alterations in carbohydrate or lipid metabolism, especially in triglyceride blood levels.

Women with familial hyperlipidemias need special surveillance. Lipid-lowering measures are recommended additionally, before treatment is started.

Caution should be exercised in patients with pre-existing hypertriglyceridemia since rare cases of large increases of plasma triglycerides leading to pancreatitis have been reported with estrogen therapy in this population.

Women with porphyria need special surveillance.

Estrogens should be used with caution in individuals with pre-existing severe hypocalcemia.

Calcium and Phosphorus Metabolism: Because the prolonged use of estrogens influences the metabolism of calcium and phosphorus, estrogens should be used with caution in patients with metabolic and malignant bone diseases associated with hypercalcemia and in patients with renal insufficiency.

Hypothyroidism: Patients who require thyroid hormone replacement therapy and who are also taking estrogen should have their thyroid function monitored regularly to assure that thyroid hormone levels remain in an acceptable range (see Drug-Laboratory Test Interactions).

Genitourinary: Endometriosis: Symptoms and physical findings associated with a previous diagnosis of endometriosis may reappear or become aggravated with estrogen use.

Addition of a progestin should be considered in women who have undergone a hysterectomy but are known to have residual endometriosis, since malignant transformation after estrogen-only therapy has been reported.

Uterine Leiomyomata: Pre-existing uterine leiomyomata may increase in size during estrogen use. Growth, pain or tenderness of uterine leiomyomata requires discontinuation of medication and appropriate investigation.

Vaginal Bleeding: Abnormal vaginal bleeding, due to its prolongation, irregularity or heaviness, occurring during therapy should prompt appropriate diagnostic measures to rule out the possibility of uterine malignancy and the treatment should be re-evaluated.

Hematologic: Venous Thromboembolism: Available epidemiological data indicate that use of estrogen with or without progestin by postmenopausal women is associated with an increased risk of developing venous thromboembolism (VTE).

In the oral estrogen plus progestin arm of the WHI trial, among 10 000 women on combined HRT over a one-year period, there were 18 more cases of venous thromboembolism, including 8 more cases of pulmonary embolism.

In the oral estrogen-alone arm of the WHI trial, among 10 000 women on estrogen therapy over a one-year period, there were 7 more cases of venous thromboembolism, although there was no statistically significant difference in the rate of pulmonary embolism.

Generally recognized risk factors for VTE include a personal history, a family history (the occurrence of VTE in a direct relative at a relatively early age may indicate genetic predisposition), severe obesity (body mass index >30 kg/m^2) and systemic lupus erythematosus. The risk of VTE also increases with age and smoking.

The risk of VTE may be temporarily increased with prolonged immobilization, major surgery or trauma. In women on HRT, attention should be given to prophylactic measures to prevent VTE following surgery. Also, patients with varicose veins should be closely supervised. The physician should be alert to the earliest manifestations of thrombotic disorders (thrombophlebitis, retinal thrombosis, cerebral embolism and pulmonary embolism). If these occur or are suspected, hormone therapy should be discontinued immediately, given the risks of long-term disability or fatality.

If feasible, estrogens should be discontinued at least 4 weeks before major surgery which may be associated with an increased risk of thromboembolism, or during periods of prolonged immobilization.

Hepatic/Biliary/Pancreatic: Gallbladder Diseases: A 2- to 4-fold increase in the risk of gallbladder disease requiring surgery in women receiving postmenopausal estrogens has been reported.

Hepatic Hemangiomas: Particular caution is indicated in women with hepatic hemangiomas, as HRT may cause an exacerbation of this condition.

Jaundice: Caution is advised in patients with a history of liver and/or biliary disorders. If cholestatic jaundice develops during treatment, the treatment should be discontinued and appropriate investigations carried out.

Liver Function Tests: Liver function tests should be done periodically in subjects who are suspected of having hepatic disease. For information on endocrine and liver function tests, see Monitoring and Laboratory Tests.

Immune: Particular caution is indicated in women with systemic lupus erythematosus, as HRT may cause an exacerbation of this condition.

Neurologic: Cerebrovascular Insufficiency: Patients who develop visual disturbances, classical migraine, transient aphasia, paralysis or loss of consciousness should discontinue medication.

Patients with a previous history of classical migraine and who develop a recurrence or worsening of migraine symptoms should be reevaluated.

Dementia: Available epidemiological data indicate that the use of combined estrogen plus progestin in women age 65 and over may increase the risk of developing probable dementia.

The Women's Health Initiative Memory Study (WHIMS), a clinical substudy of the WHI, was designed to assess whether postmenopausal hormone replacement therapy (oral estrogen plus progestin or oral estrogen-alone) reduces the risk of dementia in women aged 65 and over (age range 65-79 years) and free of dementia at baseline.

In the estrogen plus progestin arm of the WHIMS (n=4532), women with intact uteri were treated with daily 0.625 mg conjugated equine estrogens (CEE) plus 2.5 mg medroxyprogesterone acetate (MPA) or placebo for an average of 4.05 years. The results, when extrapolated to 10 000 women treated over a one-year period showed:
- 23 more cases of probable dementia (45 on combined HRT versus 22 on placebo).

In the estrogen-alone arm of the WHIMS (n=2947), women with prior hysterectomy were treated with daily 0.625 mg CEE or placebo for an average of 5.21 years. The results, when extrapolated to 10 000 women treated over a one-year period showed:
- 12 more cases of probable dementia (37 on estrogen-alone versus 25 on placebo), although this difference did not reach statistical significance.

When data from the estrogen plus progestin arm of the WHIMS and the estrogen-alone arm of the WHIMS were combined, as per the original WHIMS protocol, in 10 000 women over a one-year period, there were:
- 18 more cases of probable dementia (41 on estrogen plus progestin or estrogen-alone versus 23 on placebo).

Epilepsy: Particular caution is indicated in women with epilepsy, as HRT may cause an exacerbation of this condition.

Ophthalmologic: Visual Abnormalities: Retinal vascular thrombosis has been reported in patients receiving estrogens. Discontinue medication pending examination if there is sudden partial or complete loss of vision, or a sudden onset of proptosis, diplopia, or migraine. If examination reveals papilledema or retinal vascular lesions, medication should be withdrawn.

Psychiatric: Depression: Patients who are taking progestogens and have a history of depression should be observed. If the depression occurs to a serious degree, the drug should be discontinued.

Renal: Fluid Retention: Estrogens may cause fluid retention.

Therefore, particular caution is indicated in cardiac, renal dysfunction, or asthma. If, in any of the above-mentioned conditions, a worsening of the underlying disease is diagnosed or suspected during treatment, the benefits and risks of treatment should be reassessed based on the individual case.

Special Populations: Pregnant Women: Estrogens/progestins should not be used during pregnancy (see Contraindications).

Nursing Women: Estrogen administration to nursing mothers has been shown to decrease the quantity and quality of breast milk. Detectable amounts of estrogens have been identified in the milk of mothers receiving the drug. Caution should be exercised when estrogens are administered to a nursing woman.

Pediatrics (<16 years of age): Premarin Vaginal Cream is not indicated for use in children.

Geriatrics (>65 years of age): The estrogen-alone substudy of the Women's Health Initiative (WHI) reported an increased risk of stroke compared with placebo in postmenopausal women 65 years of age or older (see Warnings and Precautions, Cardiovascular).

Monitoring and Laboratory Tests: Before Premarin Vaginal Cream is administered, the patient should have a complete physical examination including blood pressure determination. Breasts and pelvic organs should be appropriately examined and a Papanicolaou smear should be performed. Endometrial biopsy should be done only when indicated. Baseline tests should include mammography, measurements of blood glucose, calcium, triglycerides and cholesterol, and liver function tests. Before starting treatment pregnancy should be excluded. Periodic check-ups and careful benefit/risk evaluations should be undertaken in women treated with ERT/HRT therapy. The first follow-up examination should be done within three to six months of initiation of treatment to assess response to treatment. Thereafter, examinations should be made at intervals of at least once a year. Appropriate investigations should be arranged at regular intervals as determined by the physician.

Mammography examinations should be scheduled based on patient age, risk factors and prior mammogram results.

The importance of regular self-examination of the breasts should be discussed with the patient.

ADVERSE REACTIONS: Adverse Drug Reaction Overview: See Warnings and Precautions regarding potential induction of malignant neoplasia and other adverse effects similar to those observed with oral contraceptives.

The following additional adverse reactions have been reported with conjugated estrogens vaginal cream or are undesirable effects associated with ET/HT:

Blood and Lymphatic System Disorders: altered coagulation tests (see Drug Interactions, Drug-Laboratory Test Interactions).
Cardiac Disorders: palpitations; increase in blood pressure (see Warnings and Precautions); coronary thrombosis, pulmonary embolism, venous thrombosis, myocardial infarction.
Endocrine Disorders: increased blood sugar levels; decreased glucose tolerance, precocious puberty.
Eye Disorders: neuro-ocular lesions (e.g. retinal vascular thrombosis, optic neuritis); visual disturbances; steepening of the corneal curvature; intolerance to contact lenses.
Gastrointestinal Disorders: nausea; vomiting; abdominal discomfort (cramps, pressure, pain, bloating), pancreatitis, ischemic colitis.
General Disorders and Administration Site Conditions: fatigue; changes in appetite; changes in body weight; changes in libido, aggravation of porphyria, hypocalcemia (in patients with pre-existing conditions of hypocalcemia), angioedema, hypersensitivity, anaphylactic/anaphylactoid reactions, increased triglycerides.
Hepatobiliary Disorders: gallbladder disorder; cholestatic jaundice.
Musculoskeletal and Connective Tissue Disorders: musculoskeletal pain including leg pain not related to thromboembolic disease (usually transient, lasting 3-6 weeks) may occur, arthralgias, leg cramps.
Neoplasms, benign: fibrocystic breast changes; enlargement of hepatic hemangiomas; growth potentiation of benign meningioma.
Nervous System Disorders: aggravation of migraine episodes; headaches; migraines, dizziness; cerebrovascular accident/stroke; exacerbation of chorea.
Psychiatric Disorders: mental depression; nervousness; irritability, mood disturbances, dementia.
Renal and Urinary Disorders: cystitis-like syndrome; dysuria; sodium retention; edema.
Reproductive System and Breast Disorders: abnormal uterine bleeding; change in menstrual flow; dysmenorrhea/pelvic pain; vaginal itching/discharge; dyspareunia; endometrial hyperplasia; pre-menstrual-like syndrome; reactivation of endometriosis; changes in cervical erosion and amount of cervical secretion; breast swelling and tenderness, galactorrhea, breast discharge, amenorrhea, increase in size of uterine leiomyomata, vaginitis, application site reactions of vulvovaginal discomfort including burning, irritation and genital pruritus, vaginal candidiasis; leukorrhea.
Skin and Subcutaneous Tissue Disorders: chloasma or melasma, which may persist when drug is discontinued; erythema multiforme; erythema nodosum; haemorrhagic eruption; loss of scalp hair; hirsutism and acne, allergic reactions and rashes, generalized rash, urticaria, pigmentation of the skin, pruritus.
Vascular Disorders: isolated cases of: thrombophlebitis; thromboembolic disorders.

Clinical Trial Adverse Drug Reactions: Because clinical trials are conducted under very specific conditions the adverse drug reaction rates observed in the clinical trials may not reflect the rates observed in practice and should not be compared to the rates in the clinical trials of another drug. Adverse drug reaction information from clinical trials is useful for identifying drug-related adverse events and for approximating rates.

A phase III double-blind, randomized study was conducted to compare the efficacy and safety of various regimens of Premarin (conjugated estrogens) and medroxyprogesterone acetate (MPA). Efficacy was determined by the incidence of endometrial hyperplasia at the twelve month evaluation. A total of 1724 generally healthy postmenopausal women (mean age, 54.0 years±SD 4.6) participated in the study. The patients were considered as having completed the study if they participated in all 13 cycles (28 days/cycle). The five arms in the study were: 2 for Premplus, 2 for Premplus Cycle, and 1 for Premarin tablets alone.

Prior to treatment, the following were performed: physical examinations, vital signs, Papanicolaou smear, laboratory safety screen, mammography, follicle stimulating hormone (FSH), and endometrial biopsy. During the patient visit for Cycle 6, all but the mammography and FSH were performed. At the end of the study, Cycle 13, all but the FSH were performed.

No dose-dependent incidence of adverse experiences was seen in the multicenter efficacy and safety study. Significantly ($p<0.05$) fewer (12%) Premarin treated patients reported breast pain than in the Premarin/MPA groups. Headache was the most common drug-related study event in the Premarin alone group, reported by 69 (20%) patients. Table 1 summarizes the treatment-emergent drug-related study events reported by 2% or more of the patients.

Table 1: Premarin Vaginal Cream

Treatment-emergent Drug-related Study Events with an Incidence of ≥2% for Premarin Tablets

Study Event	Premarin 0.625 mg CE (n=347) No. (%) of Patients+
General Disorders and Administration Site Conditions	
Asthenia	18 (5)
Chest pain	2 (<1)
Generalized edema	9 (3)
Edema	5 (1)
Peripheral edema	11 (3)
Pain	11 (3)
Vascular Disorders	
Hypertension	7 (2)
Vasodilatation	9 (3)
Gastrointestinal Disorders	
Diarrhea	6 (2)
Dyspepsia	4 (1)
Flatulence	14 (4)[b]
Nausea	19 (5)
Abdominal pain	46 (13)
Musculoskeletal Connective Tissue, and Bone Disorders	
Leg cramps	8 (2)
Back pain	13 (4)
Nervous System Disorders	
Headache	69 (20)
Depression	22 (6)
Migraine	7 (2)
Dizziness	10 (3)
Emotional lability	4 (1)
Insomnia	2 (<1)
Nervousness	1 (<1)[b,d]
Skin and Subcutaneous Tissue Disorders	
Acne	6 (2)
Pruritus	6 (2)[a,b]
Rash	5 (1)
Reproductive System and Breast Disorders	
Breast enlargement	4 (1)[a,b]
Breast pain*	40 (12)[a,b,d]
Cervix disorder**	12 (3)
Dysmenorrhea	17 (5)[d]
Endometrial hyperplasia	57 (20)
Leukorrhea	24 (7)
Menstrual disorder	3 (<1)
Pelvic pain	16 (5)
Uterine spasm	0 (0)[a,d]
Vaginal bleeding***	28 (8)[b]
Vaginitis	4 (1)[a,b]
Investigations	
Pap smear abnormal†	0 (0)[a]
Weight increased	10 (3)
Psychiatric Disorders	
Depression	22 (6)
Emotional lability	4 (1)
Nervousness	1 (<1)[b,d]

(cont'd)

Table 1: Premarin Vaginal Cream *(cont'd)*

Treatment-emergent Drug-related Study Events with an Incidence of ≥2% for Premarin Tablets

+ Patients were counted only once for a particular study event.
* Breast pain also includes breast discomfort, breast soreness, breast tenderness, mastodynia, nipple soreness and nipple tenderness.
** Cervix disorder includes cervical dysplasia, cervical erosion, cervical hypersecretion.
† Pap smear abnormal refers to positive Pap smear class III through V.
*** Vaginal bleeding includes menorrhagia, metrorrhagia, uterine hemorrhage, and vaginal hemorrhage.
a,b,d= Significant difference ($p<0.05$) from treatment group Premplus (0.625/2.5 mg), Premplus (0.625/5.0 mg), Premplus Cycle (0.625/10.0 mg) and Premarin (0.625 mg) respectively.

Table 1 summarizes the treatment-emergent drug-related study events reported by greater than 2% of the patients. The number of patients with any study event is not necessarily the sum of the individual events since a patient might have reported two or more different study events. The addition of progestin to estrogen replacement therapy may contribute to breast pain. This is reflected by the greater percentage of patients with breast pain on combination therapy than on Premarin alone.

If adverse symptoms persist, the prescription of HRT should be re-considered.

DRUG INTERACTIONS: Overview: In vitro and in vivo studies have shown that 17 β-estradiol, one of the components of conjugated estrogens, is metabolized partially by cytochrome P450 3A4 (CYP3A4). Therefore, strong CYP3A4 inducers such as phenobarbitol, phenytoin, carbamazepine, rifampicin and dexamethasome may reduce plasma concentrations of 17 β-estradiol. This may lead to a decreased effect and/or changes in the uterine bleeding profile. CYP3A4 inhibitors such as cimetidine, erythromycin, ketoconazole, clarithromycin, itraconazole, and ritonavir may increase plasma concentrations of 17 β-estradiol and may result in side effects.

Data from a drug-drug interaction study involving conjugated estrogens and medroxyprogesterone acetate indicate that the pharmacokinetic disposition of both drugs are not altered when the drugs are coadministered. Other clinical drug-drug interaction studies have not been conducted with conjugated estrogens.

Estrogens may diminish the effectiveness of anticoagulant, antidiabetic and antihypertensive agents.

Drug-Drug Interactions: The following section contains information on drug interactions with ethinyl estradiol-containing products (specifically, oral contraceptives) that have been reported in the public literature. **It is unknown whether such interactions occur with drug products containing other types of estrogens.**

Hepatic Metabolism: Interactions can occur with drugs that induce microsomal enzymes which can decrease ethinyl estradiol concentrations (eg., rifampin, barbiturates, phenytoin, carbamazepine, troglitazone).

Gastrointestinal Wall: Sulfation of ethinyl estradiol has been shown to occur in the gastrointestinal (GI) wall. Therefore, drugs which act as competitive inhibitors for sulfation in the GI wall may increase ethinyl estradiol bioavailability (e.g., ascorbic acid, acetaminophen).

Interference in the Metabolism of Other Drugs: Ethinyl estradiol may interfere with the metabolism of other drugs by inhibiting hepatic microsomal enzymes or by inducing hepatic drug conjugation, particularly glucuronidation. Increased plasma concentrations of cyclosporin, prednisolone, and theophylline have been reported with concomitant administration of certain drugs containing ethinyl estradiol (e.g., oral contraceptives containing ethinyl estradiol). In addition, products containing ethinyl estradiol may induce the conjugation of other compounds.

Decreased plasma concentrations of acetaminophen and increased clearance of temazepam, salicylic acid, morphine, and clofibric acid have been noted when these drugs were administered with certain ethinyl estradiol-containing drug products (e.g., oral contraceptives containing ethinyl estradiol).

Other Interactions with Ethinyl Estradiol: Coadministration of atorvastatin and certain ethinyl estradiol-containing drug products (e.g., oral contraceptives) increase AUC values for ethinyl estradiol by 20 percent.

Clinical pharmacokinetic studies have not demonstrated any consistent effect of antibiotics (other than rifampin) on plasma concentrations of synthetic steroids.

Drug-Food Interactions: CYP3A4 inhibitors such as grapefruit juice may increase plasma concentrations of 17 β-estradiol and may result in side effects.

Drug-Herb Interactions: It was found that some herbal products (e.g., St. John's wort), which are available as over-the-counter (OTC) products, might interfere with steroid metabolism, and therefore alter the efficacy and safety of estrogen/progestin products. Hot flashes and vaginal bleeding have been reported in patients taking estrogen replacement therapy (ERT) and combined estrogen plus progestin therapy (HRT) and St. John's wort. St. John's wort may induce hepatic microsomal enzymes, which theoretically may result in reduced efficacy of ERT and HRT.

Physicians and other health care providers should be made aware of other non-prescription products concomitantly used by the patient, including herbal and natural products, obtained from the widely spread Health Stores.

Drug-Laboratory Test Interactions: The results of certain endocrine and liver function tests may be affected by estrogen-containing products:

- increased prothrombin time and partial thromboplastin time; increased levels of fibrinogen and fibrinogen activity, increased coagulation factors VII, VIII, IX, X; increased norepinephrine-induced platelet aggregability; decreased antithrombin III;
- impaired glucose tolerance;
- increased serum triglycerides and phospholipids concentration;
- increased thyroid-binding globulin (TBG) levels leading to increased circulating total thyroid hormone (T4), as measured by column or radioimmunoassay; T3 resin uptake is decreased, reflecting the elevated TBG; free T4 concentration is unaltered.
- other binding proteins may be elevated in serum i.e., corticosteroid binding globulin (CBG), sex-hormone binding globulin (SHBG), leading to increased circulating corticosteroids and sex steroids respectively, free or biologically active hormone concentrations are unchanged.

The results of the above laboratory tests should not be considered reliable unless therapy has been discontinued for two to four weeks.

The pathologist should be informed that the patient is receiving hormone replacement therapy (HRT) when relevant specimens are submitted.

DOSAGE AND ADMINISTRATION:

Dosing Considerations: Use of Premarin Vaginal Cream, alone, or in combination with a progestin, should be limited to the shortest duration consistent with treatment goals and risks for the individual woman. Patients should be re-evaluated periodically to determine if treatment for symptoms is still necessary.

Recommended Dose and Dosage Adjustment: Premarin Vaginal Cream should be administered cyclically for short-term use only for the treatment of atrophic vaginitis, dyspareunia or kraurosis vulvae.

In patients with severe cases of atrophic vaginitis, the mucosa should first be conditioned with a short course of oral therapy—1.25 mg daily for approximately 10 days. Vaginal treatment should be instituted at the lowest effective dosage, and the requirement for estrogen therapy reassessed regularly.

In patients already receiving oral therapy, the oral dosage may be reduced taking into account the potential absorption from the vaginal medication. The degree of atrophy is directly responsible for the level of absorption and should be the guiding factor in dose adjustment.

In women with an intact uterus, a progestin should be coadministered for a minimum of 10, but preferably at least 12 to 14 days per cycle to avoid overstimulation of the endometrium. In addition, progestin should be administered to minimize the occurrence of endometrial hyperplasia. Unexpected or abnormal vaginal bleeding in such patients requires institution of prompt diagnostic measures, such as endometrial biopsy or curettage to rule out the possibility of uterine malignancy. Since progestins are administered to reduce the risk of hyperplastic changes of the endometrium, patients without a uterus do not require a progestin for this purpose.

Usual Dosage Range: The lowest dose that will control symptoms should be chosen and medication should be discontinued as promptly as possible.

0.5 g to 2 g daily, intravaginally or topically depending on the severity of the condition. Administration should be cyclic (e.g., three weeks on and one week off).

Appropriate diagnostic measures should be taken to rule out malignancy in the event of persistent or recurring abnormal vaginal bleeding.

Instructions for Use of Applicator:

1. Remove cap.
2. Screw nozzle end of applicator onto the tube.
3. Gently squeeze tube to force sufficient cream into the barrel to provide the prescribed dose.
4. Unscrew applicator from tube.
5. Place the applicator into the vaginal opening.
6. To release medication, press plunger downward.

To Cleanse: Pull plunger out from barrel. Wash with mild soap and warm water. **Do not boil.**

Missed Dose: If a patient misses a dose, it should be taken as soon as possible. If it is close to the patient's next scheduled dose, the missed dose should be skipped, and the patient should continue with her normal schedule. The patient should not take two doses at the same time.

Administration: Vaginal: Premarin Vaginal Cream should be prescribed with an appropriate dosage of a progestin for women with intact uteri in order to prevent endometrial hyperplasia/carcinoma. Progestin therapy is not required as part of hormone replacement therapy in women who have had a previous hysterectomy.

OVERDOSAGE:

Symptoms: Numerous reports of ingestion of large doses of estrogen products and estrogen-containing oral contraceptives by young children have not revealed acute serious ill effects.

Overdosage with estrogen may cause nausea, breast discomfort, fluid retention, bloating or vaginal bleeding in women.

Treatment: There is no specific antidote and further treatment if necessary should be symptomatic.

> For management of a suspected drug overdose, CPhA recommends that you contact your **regional Poison Control Centre**. See the *CPS* Directory section for a list of Poison Control Centres.

ACTION AND CLINICAL PHARMACOLOGY: Mechanism of Action: Estrogens generally act through binding to nuclear receptors in estrogen-responsive tissues. To date, two estrogen receptors have been identified. These vary in proportion from tissue to tissue. Circulating estrogens modulate the pituitary secretion of the gonadotropins, luteinizing hormone (LH) and follicle stimulating hormone (FSH), through a negative feedback mechanism. Estrogens act to reduce the elevated levels of these gonadotropins seen in postmenopausal women.

Endogenous estrogens are largely responsible for the development and maintenance of the female reproductive system and secondary sex characteristics. By a direct action, they cause growth and development of the uterus, Fallopian tubes, and vagina. With other hormones, such as pituitary hormones and progesterone, they cause enlargement of the breasts through promotion of ductal growth, stromal development, and the accretion of fat. Estrogens are intricately involved with other hormones, especially progesterone, in the processes of the ovulatory menstrual cycle and pregnancy, and affect the release of pituitary gonadotropins. Indirectly, they also contribute to the shaping of the skeleton, maintenance of tone and elasticity through the increase of collagen production in the supportive tissues of the heart, skin and urogenital structures, changes in the epiphyses of the long bones that allow for the pubertal growth spurt and its termination, growth of axillary and pubic hair, and pigmentation of the nipples and genitals. Decline of ovarian estrogenic and progestogenic activity at the end of the menstrual cycle can result in menstruation, although the cessation of progesterone secretion is the most important factor in the mature ovulatory cycle. However, in the preovulatory or anovulatory cycle, estrogen is the primary determinant in the onset of menstruation.

Although circulating estrogens exist in a dynamic equilibrium of metabolic interconversions, estradiol is the principal intracellular human estrogen and is substantially more potent than its metabolites, estrone and estriol at the receptor level. The primary source of estrogen in normally cycling adult women is the ovarian follicle, which secretes 70 to 500 µg of estradiol daily, depending on the phase of the menstrual cycle. After menopause, most endogenous estrogen is produced by conversion of androstenedione, secreted by the adrenal cortex, to estrone by peripheral tissues. Thus, estrone and the sulfate conjugated form, estrone sulfate, are the most abundant circulating estrogens in postmenopausal women.

Circulating estrogens modulate pituitary gonadotropins, luteinizing hormone (LH) and follicle stimulating hormone (FSH) through a negative feedback mechanism. Estrogen therapy acts to reduce elevated levels of these hormones seen in postmenopausal women.

Estrogen drug products act by regulating the transcription of a limited number of genes. They may act directly at the cell's surface via non "estrogen receptor" mechanism or directly with the estrogen receptor inside the cell. Estrogens diffuse through cell membranes, distribute themselves throughout the cell, and bind to and activate the nuclear estrogen receptor, a DNA-binding protein which is found in estrogen-responsive tissues. The activated estrogen receptor binds to specific DNA sequences, or hormone-response elements, which enhance the transcription of adjacent genes and in turn lead to the observed effects. Estrogen receptors have been identified in the wall of blood vessels, in tissues of the reproductive tract, breast, pituitary, hypothalamus, liver, and bone of women.

Conjugated estrogens used in therapy are soluble in water and are well absorbed through the skin, mucous membranes, and the gastrointestinal tract after release from the drug formulation. Some estrogens are excreted in bile; however, they are reabsorbed from the intestine and returned to the liver through the portal venous system. Water-soluble estrogen conjugates are strongly acidic and are ionized in body fluids, which favours excretion through the kidneys since tubular reabsorption is minimal.

Estrogens used in therapy are also well absorbed through the skin and mucous membranes. When applied for a local action, absorption is usually sufficient to cause systemic effects. When conjugated with aryl and alkyl groups for parenteral administration, the rate of absorption of oily preparations is slowed with a prolonged duration of action, such that a single intramuscular injection of estradiol valerate or estradiol cypionate is absorbed over several weeks.

Administered estrogens and their esters are handled within the body essentially the same way as the endogenous hormones.

Pharmacodynamics: Conjugated estrogens used in therapy are soluble in water and are well absorbed through the skin, mucous membranes, and gastrointestinal tract after release from the drug formulation.

Effects on Vasomotor Symptoms Associated with Estrogen Deficiency: Hot flushes, feelings of intense heat over the upper trunk and face, with flushing of the skin and sweating occur in approximately 80% of women as a result of the decrease in ovarian hormones. These vasomotor symptoms are seen in women whether menopause is surgically induced or spontaneous. However, hot flushes may be more severe in women who undergo surgical menopause. Hot flushes can begin before the cessation of menses.

Effect on Bleeding Patterns: With a continuous therapy, several bleeding patterns may occur. These may range from absence of bleeding to irregular bleeding. If bleeding occurs, it is frequently light spotting or moderate bleeding.

Pharmacokinetics: Absorption: Conjugated estrogens are soluble in water and are well absorbed through the skin, mucous membranes, and the gastrointestinal tract after release from the drug formulation.

Distribution: The distribution of exogenous estrogens is similar to that of endogenous estrogens. Estrogens are widely distributed in the body and are generally found in higher concentration in the sex hormone target organs. Estrogens circulate in the blood largely bound to sex hormone binding globulin (SHBG) and albumin.

Metabolism: Metabolic conversion of estrogens occurs primarily in the liver (first pass effect), but also at local target tissue sites. Complex metabolic processes result in a dynamic equilibrium of circulating conjugated and unconjugated estrogenic forms which are continually interconverted, especially between estrone and estradiol and between esterified and non-esterified forms.

Estrogen drug products administered by non-oral routes, while not subject to true "first-pass" metabolism, do undergo significant hepatic uptake, metabolism, and enterohepatic recycling. Metabolism and inactivation occur primarily in the liver. Some estrogens are excreted into the bile; however, they are re-absorbed from the intestine and returned to the liver through the portal venous system. Water-soluble estrogen conjugates are strongly acidic and are ionized in body fluids, which favour excretion through the kidneys since tubular re-absorption is minimal.

When given orally, naturally-occurring estrogens and their esters are extensively metabolized (first-pass effect) and circulate primarily as estrone sulfate, with smaller amounts of other conjugated and unconjugated estrogenic species. This results in limited oral potency. By contrast, synthetic estrogens, such as ethinyl estradiol and the nonsteroidal estrogens, are degraded very slowly in the liver and other tissues, which results in their high intrinsic potency.

Excretion: A certain proportion of the estrogen is excreted into the bile, then reabsorbed from the intestine and returned to the liver through the portal venous system. During this enterohepatic recirculation, estrogens are desulfated and resulfated and undergo degradation through conversion to less active estrogens (estriol and other estrogens), oxidation to nonestrogenic substances (catecholestrogens, which interact with catecholamine metabolism, especially in the central nervous system), and conjugation with glucuronic acids (which are then rapidly excreted in the urine).

Estradiol, estrone, and estriol are excreted in the urine, along with glucuronide and sulfate conjugates.

Special Populations and Conditions: No pharmacokinetic studies were conducted in special populations, including patients with renal or hepatic impairment.

STORAGE AND STABILITY: Store at 15-30°C. Keep out of reach of children.

SPECIAL HANDLING INSTRUCTIONS: None required.

INFORMATION FOR THE PATIENT: Published in e-CPS, available by subscription at www.e-cps.ca.

DOSAGE FORMS, COMPOSITION AND PACKAGING: Each g of white, vaginal cream contains: 0.625 mg of conjugated estrogens CSD. Nonmedicinal ingredients: cetyl alcohol, cetyl esters wax, glycerin, glyceryl monostearate, methyl stearate, mineral oil, phenylethyl alcohol, propylene glycol monostearate, sodium lauryl sulfate, water purified and white wax. Gluten-, paraben-, sugar-, sulfite- and tartrazine-free. Tubes of 14 g with calibrated plastic applicator.

(Shown in Product Identification Section)

Premplus® Ⓟ

conjugated estrogens + medroxyprogesterone acetate

Estrogenic Hormones—Progestin

Pfizer

Date of Revision: July 23, 2010

SUMMARY PRODUCT INFORMATION:

Route of Administration	Dosage Form/ Strength	Clinically Relevant Nonmedicinal Ingredients
Premplus oral	Conjugated estrogens tablets 0.625 mg and medroxyprogesterone acetate tablets 2.5 mg, 5.0 mg	Lactose For a complete listing see Dosage Forms, Composition and Packaging.

INDICATIONS AND CLINICAL USE: Premplus therapy is indicated in women with intact uteri for the following:

- relief of moderate to severe vasomotor symptoms associated with menopause, occurring in naturally or surgically induced estrogen deficiency states;
- prevention of osteoporosis in naturally occurring or surgically induced estrogen-deficiency states. When prescribing solely for the prevention of postmenopausal osteoporosis, therapy with Premplus should be considered in light of other available therapies (please see the Serious Warnings and Precautions box), and should only be considered in women at significant risk of osteoporosis and for whom non-estrogen medications are not considered to be appropriate. Adequate diet, calcium and vitamin D intake, cessation of smoking, as well as regular physical weight-bearing exercise are required in addition to the administration of Premplus.
- treatment of vulvar and vaginal atrophy associated with menopause. **When prescribing solely for the treatment of symptoms of vulvar and vaginal atrophy, topical vaginal products should be considered.**

Premplus therapy is recommended for the above indications only in women with intact uteri since the regimen includes a progestin whose role is to prevent endometrial hyperplasia.

Geriatrics (>65 years of age): See above indications.

Pediatrics: Clinical studies have not been conducted in the pediatric population. Premplus is not indicated for use in children.

CONTRAINDICATIONS:

- Patients who are hypersensitive to this drug or to any ingredient in the formulation or component of the container. For a complete listing, see Dosage Forms, Composition and Packaging.
- Liver dysfunction or disease as long as liver function tests have failed to return to normal.
- Known or suspected estrogen-dependent or progestin-dependent malignant neoplasia (e.g. endometrial cancer).
- Endometrial hyperplasia.

- Known, suspected, or past history of breast cancer.
- Undiagnosed abnormal genital bleeding.
- Known or suspected pregnancy.
- Active or past history of confirmed venous thromboembolism (such as deep venous thrombosis or pulmonary embolism) or active thrombophlebitis.
- Active or past history of arterial thromboembolic disease (e.g. stroke, myocardial infarction, coronary heart disease).
- Partial or complete loss of vision due to ophthalmic vascular disease.

WARNINGS AND PRECAUTIONS:

Serious Warnings and Precautions

The Women's Health Initiative (WHI) trial examined the health benefits and risks of oral combined estrogen plus progestin therapy (n=16 608) and oral estrogen-alone therapy (n=10 739) in postmenopausal women aged 50 to 79 years.

The estrogen plus progestin arm of the WHI trial (mean age 63.3 years) indicated an increased risk of myocardial infarction (MI), stroke, invasive breast cancer, pulmonary emboli and deep vein thrombosis in postmenopausal women receiving treatment with combined conjugated equine estrogens (CEE, 0.625 mg/day) and medroxyprogesterone acetate (MPA, 2.5 mg/day) for 5.2 years compared to those receiving placebo.

The estrogen-alone arm of the WHI trial (mean age 63.6 years) indicated an increased risk of stroke and deep vein thrombosis in hysterectomized women treated with CEE-alone (0.625 mg/day) for 6.8 years compared to those receiving placebo.

Therefore, the following should be given serious consideration at the time of prescribing:

- Estrogens with or without progestins **should not** be prescribed for primary or secondary prevention of cardiovascular diseases.
- Estrogens with or without progestins should be prescribed at **the lowest effective dose** for the approved indication.
- Estrogens with or without progestins should be prescribed for the **shortest period possible** for the approved indication.
- The use of Premplus for the prevention of osteoporosis should be considered in light of other available therapies.

General: Combined Estrogen and Progestin Therapy: The benefits and risks of HRT must always be carefully weighed, including consideration of the emergence of risks as therapy continues.

There are additional and/or increased risks that may be associated with the use of combination estrogen-plus-progestin therapy compared with using estrogen-alone regimens. These include an increased risk of myocardial infarction, pulmonary embolism, invasive breast cancer and ovarian cancer.

Carcinogenesis and Mutagenesis: Breast Cancer: Available epidemiological data indicate that the use of combined estrogen plus progestin by postmenopausal women is associated with an increased risk of invasive breast cancer.

The use of estrogen and progestin has been reported to result in an increase in abnormal mammograms requiring further evaluation.

In the estrogen plus progestin arm of the WHI trial, among 10 000 women over a one-year period, there were:

- 8 more cases of invasive breast cancer (38 on combined HRT versus 30 on placebo).

The WHI study also reported that the invasive breast cancers diagnosed in the estrogen plus progestin group were similar in histology but were larger (mean [SD], 1.7 cm [1.1] vs 1.5 cm [0.9], respectively; p=0.04) and were at a more advanced stage compared with those diagnosed in the placebo group. The percentage of women with abnormal mammograms (recommendations for short-interval follow-up, a suspicious abnormality, or highly suggestive of malignancy) was significantly higher in the estrogen plus progestin group versus the placebo group. This difference appeared at year one and persisted in each year thereafter.

In the estrogen-alone arm of the WHI trial, there was no statistically significant difference in the rate of invasive breast cancer in hysterectomized women treated with conjugated equine estrogens versus women treated with placebo.

It is recommended that estrogens with or without progestins not be given to women with existing breast cancer or those with a previous history of the disease (see Contraindications).

There is a need for caution in prescribing estrogens with or without progestins for women with known risk factors associated with the development of breast cancer, such as strong family history of breast cancer (first degree relative) or who present a breast condition with an increased risk (abnormal mammograms and/or atypical hyperplasia at breast biopsy).

Other known risk factors for the development of breast cancer such as nulliparity, obesity, early menarche, late age at first full term pregnancy and at menopause should also be evaluated.

It is recommended that women undergo mammography prior to the start of HRT treatment and at regular intervals during treatment, as deemed appropriate by the treating physician and according to the perceived risks for each patient.

The overall benefits and possible risks of hormone replacement therapy should be fully considered and discussed with patients. It is important that the modest increased risk of being diagnosed with breast cancer after 4 years of treatment with combined estrogen plus progestin HRT (as reported in the results of the WHI trial) be discussed with the patient and weighed against its known benefits.

Instructions for regular self-examination of the breasts should be included in this counselling.

Endometrial Hyperplasia and Endometrial Carcinoma: The role of progestin, when combined with estrogen, is to help prevent endometrial hyperplasia/carcinoma in women with intact uteri.

The reported endometrial cancer risk among unopposed estrogen users is about 2- to 12-fold or greater than in non-users and appears to be dependent on duration of treatment and on estrogen dose. Most studies show no significant increased risk associated with the use of estrogens for less than one year. The greatest risk appears associated with prolonged use, with increased risks of 15- to 24-fold for five years or more, and this risk has been shown to persist for at least 8 to15 years after estrogen therapy is discontinued.

In a subset of WHI no increased risk of endometrial cancer after an average of 5.6 years of treatment with combined estrogen plus progestin HRT compared to placebo was observed.

Endometrial hyperplasia (a possible precursor of endometrial cancer) has been reported to occur at a rate of approximately 1% or less with CEE or CEE/MPA in two large clinical trials [Health and Osteoporosis, Progestin and Estrogen (n=2153) and Menopausal Study Group (n=1385)]. In these two clinical trials two cases of endometrial cancer were reported to occur among women taking combination CEE/MPA.

Clinical surveillance of all women taking combined estrogen plus progestin HRT is important. Adequate diagnostic measures, including endometrial sampling when indicated, should be undertaken to rule out malignancy in all cases of undiagnosed persistent or recurring abnormal vaginal bleeding.

Ovarian Cancer: Some recent epidemiologic studies have found that the use of hormone replacement therapy (estrogen-alone and estrogen plus progestin therapies), in particular for five or more years, has been associated with an increased risk of ovarian cancer.

The estrogen plus progestin substudy of WHI (CE/MPA versus placebo) reported a non-statistically significant increased risk of ovarian cancer. However, limitations of this study include only 5.6 years of follow-up, and the low number of ovarian cancer cases (20 of 8506 subjects in the estrogen plus progestin group and 12 of 8102 subjects in the placebo group were diagnosed with invasive ovarian cancer).

Cardiovascular: Cardiovascular Risk: HRT has been associated with an increased risk of cardiovascular events such as myocardial infarction and stroke, as well as venous thrombosis and pulmonary embolism (venous thromboembolism or VTE). Should any of these occur or be suspected, HRT should be discontinued immediately.

Estrogen Replacement Therapy (ERT) has been reported to increase the risk of stroke and deep venous thrombosis (DVT).

Risk factors for cardiovascular disease (e.g., hypertension, diabetes mellitus, tobacco use, hypercholesterolemia, and obesity) should be managed appropriately.

General: The results of the Heart and Estrogen/progestin Replacement Studies (HERS and HERS II) and the Women's Health Initiative (WHI) trial indicate that the use of estrogen plus progestin is associated with an increased risk of coronary heart disease (CHD) in postmenopausal women. The results of the WHI trial indicate that the use of estrogen-alone and estrogen plus progestin is associated with an increased risk of stroke in postmenopausal women.

WHI Trial Findings: In the combined estrogen plus progestin arm of the WHI trial, among 10 000 women over a one-year period, there were:

- 8 more cases of stroke (29 on combined HRT versus 21 on placebo)
- 7 more cases of CHD (37 on combined HRT versus 30 on placebo).

In the estrogen-alone arm of the WHI trial of women with prior hysterectomy, among 10 000 women over a one-year period, there were/was:

- 12 more cases of stroke (44 on estrogen-alone therapy versus 32 on placebo)
- no statistically significant difference in the rate of CHD.

In the WHI estrogen-alone substudy, a statistically significant increased risk of stroke was reported in women 50 to 79 years of age receiving daily CE (0.625 mg) compared to women in the same age group receiving placebo (45 versus 33 per 10 000 women-years). The increase in risk was demonstrated in year one and persisted.

Subgroup analyses of women 50 to 59 years of age suggest no increased risk of stroke for those women receiving CE (0.625 mg) versus those receiving placebo (18 versus 21 per 10 000 women-years).

Subgroup analyses of women 50 to 59 years of age suggest a statistically non-significant reduction in CHD events (CE 0.625 mg compared to placebo) in women with less than 10 years since menopause (8 versus 16 per 10 000 women-years).

HERS and HERS II Findings: In the Heart and Estrogen/progestin Replacement Study (HERS) of postmenopausal women with documented heart disease (n=2763, average age 66.7 years), a randomized placebo-controlled clinical trial of secondary prevention of coronary heart disease (CHD), treatment with 0.625 mg/day oral conjugated equine estrogen (CEE) plus 2.5 mg oral medroxyprogesterone acetate (MPA) demonstrated no cardiovascular benefit. Specifically, during an average follow-up of 4.1 years, treatment with CEE plus MPA did not reduce the overall rate of CHD events in postmenopausal women with established coronary heart disease. There were more CHD events in the hormone-treated group than in the placebo group in year 1, but not during the subsequent years.

From the original HERS trial, 2321 women consented to participate in an open label extension of HERS known as HERS II. Average follow-up in HERS II was an additional 2.7 years, for a total of 6.8 years overall. After 6.8 years, hormone therapy did not reduce the risk of cardiovascular events in women with CHD.

Blood Pressure: Women using hormone replacement therapy sometimes experience increased blood pressure. Blood pressure should be monitored with HRT use. Elevation of blood pressure in previously normotensive or hypertensive patients should be investigated and HRT may have to be discontinued.

Endocrine and Metabolism: Glucose and Lipid Metabolism: A worsening of glucose tolerance and lipid metabolism has been observed in a significant percentage of peri- and post-menopausal patients. Therefore, diabetic patients, or those with a predisposition to diabetes, should be observed closely to detect any alterations in carbohydrate or lipid metabolism, especially in triglyceride blood levels.

Women with familial hyperlipidemias need special surveillance. Lipid-lowering measures are recommended additionally, before treatment is started.

Women with porphyria need special surveillance.

Caution should be exercised in patients with pre-existing hypertriglyceridemia since rare cases of large increases of plasma triglycerides leading to pancreatitis have been reported with estrogen therapy in this population. Estrogen-containing products have been shown to increase plasma HDL and HDL-2 subfraction concentrations, reduce LDL cholesterol concentration, and increase triglyceride levels.

Calcium and Phosphorus Metabolism: Because the prolonged use of estrogens with or without progestins influences the metabolism of calcium and phosphorus, estrogens with or without progestins should be used with caution in patients with metabolic and malignant bone diseases associated with hypercalcemia and in patients with renal insufficiency. Estrogen therapy should be used with caution in women with hypoparathyroidism, as estrogen-induced hypocalcemia may occur.

Hypothyroidism: Estrogen administration leads to increased thyroid-binding globulin (TBG) levels. Women dependent on thyroid hormone replacement therapy, who are also receiving estrogens, may require increased doses of their thyroid replacement therapy. These women should have their thyroid function monitored in order to maintain their free thyroid hormone levels in an acceptable range (see Drug Interactions, Drug-Laboratory Test Interactions).

Other Conditions: Premplus contains lactose. In patients with rare hereditary galactose intolerance, lactase deficiency or glucose-galactose malabsorption, the severity of the condition should be taken into careful consideration before prescribing Premplus. The patients should be closely monitored.

Genitourinary: Endometriosis: Symptoms and physical findings associated with a previous diagnosis of endometriosis may reappear or become aggravated with estrogen use.

Uterine Leiomyomata: Pre-existing uterine leiomyomata may increase in size during estrogen use. Growth, pain or tenderness of uterine leiomyomata may require discontinuation of medication and appropriate investigation.

Vaginal Bleeding: Abnormal vaginal bleeding, due to its prolongation, irregularity or heaviness, occurring during therapy should prompt appropriate diagnostic measures to rule out the possibility of uterine malignancy and the treatment should be re-evaluated.

Hematologic: Venous Thromboembolism: Available epidemiological data indicate that use of estrogen with or without progestin by postmenopausal women is associated with an increased risk of developing venous thromboembolism (VTE).

In the estrogen plus progestin arm of the WHI trial, among 10 000 women on combined HRT over a one-year period, there were 18 more cases of venous thromboembolism, including 8 more cases of pulmonary embolism.

In the estrogen-alone arm of the WHI trial, among 10 000 women on estrogen therapy over a one-year period, there were 7 more cases of venous thromboembolism, although there was no statistically significant difference in the rate of pulmonary embolism.

Generally recognized risk factors for VTE include a personal history, a family history (the occurrence of VTE in a direct relative at a relatively early age may indicate genetic predisposition), severe obesity (body mass index >30 kg/m²) and systemic lupus erythematosus. The risk of VTE also increases with age and smoking.

The risk of VTE may be temporarily increased with prolonged immobilization, major surgery or trauma. In women on HRT, attention should be given to prophylactic measures to prevent VTE following surgery. Also, patients with varicose veins should be closely supervised. The physician should be alert to the earliest manifestations of thrombotic disorders (thrombophlebitis, retinal thrombosis, cerebral embolism and pulmonary embolism). If these occur or are suspected, hormone therapy should be discontinued immediately, given the risks of long-term disability or fatality.

If feasible, estrogens with or without progestins should be discontinued at least 4 weeks before major surgery which may be associated with an increased risk of thromboembolism, or during periods of prolonged immobilization.

Hepatic/Biliary/Pancreatic: Gallbladder Diseases: A 2 to 4-fold increase in the risk of gallbladder disease requiring surgery in women receiving postmenopausal estrogens has been reported.

Hepatic Hemangiomas: Particular caution is indicated in women with hepatic hemangiomas, as HRT may cause an exacerbation of this condition.

Jaundice: Caution is advised in patients with a history of liver and/or biliary disorders. If cholestatic jaundice develops during treatment, the treatment should be discontinued and appropriate investigations carried out.

Liver Function Tests: Liver function tests should be done periodically in subjects who are suspected of having hepatic disease. For information on endocrine and liver function tests, see Monitoring and Laboratory Tests.

Immune: Systemic lupus erythematosus: Particular caution is indicated in women with systemic lupus erythematosus, as HRT may cause an exacerbation of this condition.

Angioedema: Exogenous estrogens may induce or exacerbate symptoms of angioedema, particularly in women with hereditary angioedema.

Neurologic: Cerebrovascular Insufficiency: Patients who develop visual disturbances, classical migraine, transient aphasia, paralysis or loss of consciousness should discontinue medication.

Patients with a previous history of classical migraine and who develop a recurrence or worsening of migraine symptoms should be reevaluated.

Dementia: Available epidemiological data indicate that the use of combined estrogen plus progestin in women age 65 and over may increase the risk of developing probable dementia.

The Women's Health Initiative Memory Study (WHIMS), a clinical substudy of the WHI, was designed to assess whether postmenopausal hormone replacement therapy (oral estrogen plus progestin or oral estrogen-alone) reduces the risk of dementia in women aged 65 and over (age range 65-79 years) and free of dementia at baseline.

In the estrogen plus progestin arm of the WHIMS (n=4532), women with intact uteri were treated with daily 0.625 mg conjugated equine estrogens (CEE) plus 2.5 mg medroxyprogesterone acetate (MPA) or placebo for an average of 4.05 years. The results, when extrapolated to 10 000 women treated over a one-year period showed:

- 23 more cases of probable dementia (45 on combined HRT versus 22 on placebo).

In the estrogen-alone arm of the WHIMS (n=2947), women with prior hysterectomy were treated with daily 0.625 mg CEE or placebo for an average of 5.21 years. The results, when extrapolated to 10 000 women treated over a one-year period showed:

- 12 more cases of probable dementia (37 on estrogen-alone versus 25 on placebo), although this difference did not reach statistical significance.

When data from the estrogen plus progestin arm of the WHIMS and the estrogen-alone arm of the WHIMS were combined, as per the original WHIMS protocol, in 10 000 women over a one-year period, there were:

- 18 more cases of probable dementia (41 on estrogen plus progestin or estrogen-alone versus 23 on placebo).

Since this study was conducted in women aged 65-79 years, it is unknown whether these findings apply to younger postmenopausal women.

Epilepsy: Particular caution is indicated in women with epilepsy, as HRT may cause an exacerbation of this condition.

Ophthalmologic: Visual Abnormalities: Retinal vascular thrombosis has been reported in patients receiving estrogens. Discontinue medication pending examination if there is sudden partial or complete loss of vision, or a sudden onset of proptosis, diplopia, or migraine. If examination reveals papilledema or retinal vascular lesions, medication should be withdrawn.
Psychiatric: Depression: Patients who are taking progestogens and have a history of depression should be observed. If the depression occurs to a serious degree, the drug should be discontinued.
Renal: Fluid Retention: Estrogens with or without progestins may cause fluid retention.

Therefore, particular caution is indicated in cardiac, renal dysfunction, or asthma. If, in any of the above-mentioned conditions, a worsening of the underlying disease is diagnosed or suspected during treatment, the benefits and risks of treatment should be reassessed based on the individual case.
Special Populations: Pregnant Women: Estrogens/progestins should not be used during pregnancy.
Nursing Women: Estrogen should not be used during lactation.
Pediatrics: Clinical studies have not been conducted in the pediatric population. Premplus is not indicated for use in children.
Geriatrics (>65 years of age): There have not been sufficient numbers of geriatric women involved in clinical studies utilizing CE + MPA to determine whether those over 65 years of age differ from younger subjects in their response to CE + MPA.
The Women's Health Initiative Study: In the Women's Health Initiative (WHI) estrogen plus progestin substudy (daily conjugated estrogens 0.625 mg plus medroxyprogesterone acetate 2.5 mg), there was a higher relative risk of nonfatal stroke and invasive breast cancer in women greater than 65 years of age.

In the WHI estrogen-alone substudy (daily CE [0.625 mg] versus placebo), there was a higher relative risk of stroke in women greater than 65 years of age.
The Women's Health Initiative Memory Study: In the Women's Health Initiative Memory Study (WHIMS) of postmenopausal women 65 to 79 years of age, there was an increased risk of developing probable dementia in women receiving estrogen plus progestin or estrogen-alone when compared to placebo.

Since both ancillary studies were conducted in women 65 to 79 years of age, it is unknown whether these findings apply to younger postmenopausal women.
Monitoring and Laboratory Tests: Before Premplus is administered, the patient should have a complete physical examination including blood pressure determination. Breasts and pelvic organs should be appropriately examined and a Papanicolaou smear should be performed. Endometrial biopsy should be done only when indicated. Baseline tests should include mammography, measurements of blood glucose, calcium, triglycerides and cholesterol, and liver function tests. The first follow-up examination should be done within three to six months of initiation of treatment to assess response to treatment. Thereafter, examinations should be made at intervals of at least once a year. Appropriate investigations should be arranged at regular intervals as determined by the physician.

Mammography examinations should be scheduled based on patient age, risk factors and prior mammogram results.

The importance of regular self-examination of the breasts should be discussed with the patient.

ADVERSE REACTIONS: Adverse Drug Reaction Overview: See Warnings and Precautions regarding potential induction of malignant neoplasia and other adverse effects similar to those observed with oral contraceptives.

The following adverse reactions have been reported with estrogen/progestin combination in general:
Blood and Lymphatic System Disorders: altered coagulation tests (see Warnings and Precautions and Drug Interactions, Drug-Laboratory Test Interactions).
Cardiac Disorders: palpitations; increase in blood pressure (see Warnings and Precautions); coronary thrombosis.
Endocrine Disorders: increased blood sugar levels; decreased glucose tolerance.
Eye Disorders: neuro-ocular lesions (e.g. retinal thrombosis, optic neuritis); visual disturbances; steepening of the corneal curvature; intolerance to contact lenses.
Gastrointestinal Disorders: nausea; vomiting; abdominal discomfort (cramps, pressure, pain, bloating).
General Disorders and Administration Site Conditions: fatigue; changes in appetite; changes in body weight; changes in libido.
Hepatobiliary Disorders: gallbladder disorder; asymptomatic impaired liver function; cholestatic jaundice.
Musculoskeletal and Connective Tissue Disorders: musculoskeletal pain including leg pain not related to thromboembolic disease (usually transient, lasting 3-6 weeks) may occur.
Nervous System Disorders: aggravation of migraine episodes; headaches; dizziness; neuritis.
Psychiatric Disorders: mental depression; nervousness; irritability.
Renal and Urinary Disorders: cystitis; dysuria; sodium retention; edema.
Reproductive System and Breast Disorders: breakthrough bleeding; spotting; change in menstrual flow; dysmenorrhea; vaginal itching/discharge; dyspareunia; endometrial hyperplasia; pre-menstrual-like syndrome; reactivation of endometriosis; changes in cervical erosion and amount of cervical secretion; breast swelling and tenderness.
Skin and Subcutaneous Tissue Disorders: chloasma or melasma, which may persist when drug is discontinued; erythema multiforme; erythema nodosum; haemorrhagic eruption; loss of scalp hair; hirsutism and acne.
Vascular Disorders: isolated cases of: thrombophlebitis; thromboembolic disorders.
Clinical Trial Adverse Drug Reactions: Because clinical trials are conducted under very specific conditions the adverse reaction rates observed in the clinical trials may not reflect the rates observed in practice and should not be compared to the rates in the clinical trials of another drug. Adverse drug reaction information from clinical trials is useful for identifying drug-related adverse events and for approximating rates.

A phase III double-blind, randomized study was conducted to compare the efficacy and safety of various regimens of Premarin (conjugated estrogens) and medroxyprogesterone acetate (MPA). Efficacy was determined by the incidence of endometrial hyperplasia at the twelve month evaluation. A total of 1724 generally healthy postmenopausal women (mean age, 54.0 years ± SD 4.6) participated in the study. The patients were considered as having completed the study if they participated in all 13 cycles (28 days/cycle). The five arms in the study were: 2 for Premplus, 2 for Premplus Cycle, and 1 for Premarin alone.

Prior to treatment, the following were performed: physical examinations, vital signs, papanicolaou smear, laboratory safety screen, mammography, follicle stimulating hormone (FSH), and endometrial biopsy. During the patient visit for Cycle 6, all but the mammography and FSH were performed. At the end of the study, Cycle 13, all but the FSH were performed.

No dose-dependent incidence of adverse experiences was seen in the multicenter efficacy and safety study. In the Premarin/MPA groups, the most frequent treatment-emergent drug-related study event was breast pain (32 to 36%), reported by approximately one third of the patients in each of the three groups. By comparison, significantly ($p < 0.05$) fewer (12%) Premarin-treated patients reported breast pain. Headache was the most common drug-related study event in the Premarin alone group, reported by 69 (20%) patients, and the second most common event in the Premarin/MPA groups (16 to 26%). Table 1 summarizes the treatment-emergent drug-related study events reported by 2% or more of the patients.

Table 1 summarizes the treatment-emergent drug-related study events reported by greater than 2% of the patients. The number of patients with any study event is not necessarily the sum of the individual events since a patient might have reported two or more different study events. The addition of progestin to estrogen replacement therapy may contribute to breast pain. This is reflected by the greater percentage of patients with breast pain on combination therapy than on Premarin alone.

Table 1: PREMPLUS

Treatment-emergent Drug-related Study Events with an Incidence of ≥2%

Study Event	Premplus 0.625 mg CE /2.5 mg MPA (n=340)	Premplus 0.625 mg CE /5.0 mg MPA (n=338)	Premplus Cycle 0.625 mg CE /10.0 mg MPA (n=348)	Premarin 0.625 mg CE (no MPA) (n=347)
	No. (%) of Patients[+]			
General Disorders and Administration Site Conditions				
Asthenia	13 (4)	18 (5)	16 (5)	18 (5)
Chest pain	5 (1)	5 (1)	7 (2)	2 (<1)
Generalized edema	12 (4)	12 (4)	8 (2)	9 (3)
Edema	5 (1)	6 (2)	5 (1)	5 (1)
Peripheral edema	11 (3)	10 (3)	7 (2)	11 (3)
Pain	12 (4)	15 (4)	17 (5)	11 (3)
Vascular Disorders				
Hypertension	7 (2)	7 (2)	11 (3)	7 (2)
Vasodilatation	2 (<1)	8 (2)	4 (1)	9 (3)
Gastrointestinal Disorders				
Diarrhea	4 (1)	3 (<1)	11 (3)	6 (2)
Dyspepsia	5 (1)	5 (1)	7 (2)	4 (1)
Flatulence	26 (8)	27 (8)[e]	23 (7)	14 (4)[b]
Nausea	26 (8)	21 (6)	25 (7)	19 (5)
Abdominal pain	36 (11)	53 (16)	63 (18)	46 (13)
Musculoskeletal Connective Tissue, and Bone Disorders				
Leg cramps	8 (2)	11 (3)	7 (2)	8 (2)
Back pain	19 (6)	16 (5)	26 (7)	13 (4)
Nervous System Disorders				
Headache	69 (20)	54 (16)[d]	90 (26)[b]	69 (20)
Depression	14 (4)[b]	28 (8)[a]	22 (6)	22 (6)
Migraine	6 (2)	9 (3)	9 (3)	7 (2)
Dizziness	9 (3)	8 (2)	14 (4)	10 (3)
Emotional lability	5 (1)	6 (2)	7 (2)	4 (1)
Insomnia	7 (2)	6 (2)	9 (3)	2 (<1)
Nervousness	4 (1)	9 (3)[e]	10 (3)[e]	1 (<1)[b,d]
Skin and Subcutaneous Tissue Disorders				
Acne	1 (<1)	5 (1)	7 (2)	6 (2)
Pruritus	20 (6)[e]	19 (6)[e]	15 (4)	6 (2)[a,b]
Rash	8 (2)	6 (2)	6 (2)	5 (1)
Reproductive System and Breast Disorders				
Breast enlargement	14 (4)[e]	14 (4)[e]	10 (3)	4 (1)[a,b]
Breast pain*	110 (32)[e]	123 (36)[e]	115 (33)[e]	40 (12)[a,b,d]
Cervix disorder**	10 (3)	6 (2)	12 (3)	12 (3)
Dysmenorrhea	26 (8)[d]	18 (5)[d]	46 (13)[a,b,e]	17 (5)[d]
Endometrial hyperplasia	2 (<1)	0 (0)	0 (0)	57 (20)
Leukorrhea	19 (6)	13 (4)	21 (6)	24 (7)
Menstrual disorder	7 (2)	1 (<1)	2 (<1)	3 (<1)
Pelvic pain	11 (3)	13 (4)	22 (6)	16 (5)
Uterine spasm	7 (2)[e]	4 (1)	8 (2)[e]	0 (0)[a,d]
Vaginal bleeding***	19 (6)[b]	9 (3)[d,e]	22 (6)[b]	28 (8)[b]
Vaginitis	13 (4)[e]	13 (4)[e]	10 (3)	4 (1)[a,b]
Investigations				
Pap smear abnormal†	5 (1)[e]	0 (0)	2 (<1)	0 (0)[a]
Weight increased	9 (3)	10 (3)	10 (3)	10 (3)
Psychiatric Disorders				
Depression	14 (4)[b]	28 (8)[a]	22 (6)	22 (6)
Emotional lability	5 (1)	6 (2)	7 (2)	4 (1)

(cont'd)

Table 1: **PREMPLUS** *(cont'd)*

Treatment-emergent Drug-related Study Events with an Incidence of ≥2%

Study Event	Premplus 0.625 mg CE /2.5 mg MPA (n=340)	Premplus 0.625 mg CE /5.0 mg MPA (n=338)	Premplus Cycle 0.625 mg CE /10.0 mg MPA (n=348)	Premarin 0.625 mg CE (no MPA) (n=347)
	No. (%) of Patients+			
Nervousness	4 (1)	9 (3)	10 (3)[e]	1 (<1)[b,d]

+Patients were counted only once for a particular study event.
*Breast pain also includes breast discomfort, breast soreness, breast tenderness, mastodynia, nipple soreness and nipple tenderness.
**Cervix disorder includes cervical dysplasia, cervical erosion, cervical hypersecretion.
†Pap smear abnormal refers to positive Pap smear class III through V.
***Vaginal bleeding includes menorrhagia, metrorrhagia, uterine hemorrhage, and vaginal hemorrhage.
a, b, d, e = Significant difference (p<0.05) from treatment group Premplus (0.625/2.5 mg), Premplus (0.625/5.0 mg), Premplus Cycle (0.625/10.0 mg) and Premarin (0.625 mg) respectively.

Less Common (<2%) Clinical Trial Adverse Drug Reactions: General Disorders and Administration Site Conditions: fever, hypothermia, malaise, moniliasis, ulcer.

Cardiac Disorders: angina pectoris, extrasystoles, palpitation, phlebitis, postural hypotension, spider angioma, tachycardia, varicose vein.

Gastrointestinal Disorders: colitis, constipation, dry mouth, enterocolitis, eructation, gastritis, gingivitis, glossitis, increased appetite, mouth ulceration, periodontal abscess, rectal hemorrhage, salivary gland enlargement, stomach ulcer, taste perversion, tenesmus, thirst, tongue edema, vomiting.

Endocrine Disorders: goiter, hypothyroidism, pituitary activity increased.

Hepatobiliary Disorders: cholecystitis, cholelithiasis.

Immune System Disorders: allergic reaction, face edema.

Metabolism and Nutrition Disorders: anorexia, bilirubinemia, hypercholesteremia, hyperglycemia, hyperkalemia, hyperlipemia, hypocalcemia, obesity, increased appetite.

Musculoskeletal and Connective Tissue Disorders: arthralgia, arthritis, bursitis, myalgia, myasthenia, tenosynovitis, muscle twitching, neck pain.

Neoplasms Benign and Malignant: breast neoplasm, cervix neoplasm.

Nervous System Disorders: abnormal dreams, agitation, amnesia, anxiety, hyperesthesia, hypoesthesia, neurosis, paresthesia, reflexes decreased, somnolence, tinnitus, thinking abnormal, tremor, vertigo.

Renal and Urinary Tract Disorders: bladder pain, cystitis.

Respiratory, Thoracic and Mediastinal Disorders: asthma, bronchitis, dyspnea, epistaxis, pharyngitis, pneumonia, rhinitis, sinusitis.

Skin and Subcutaneous Tissue Disorders: contact dermatitis, dry skin, eczema, fungal dermatitis, hair discolouration, herpes simplex, herpes zoster, hirsutism, maculopapular rash, skin carcinoma, skin discoloration, skin benign neoplasm, skin hypertrophy, sweating, urticaria.

Eye Disorders: abnormal vision, abnormality of accommodation, amblyopia, conjunctivitis, diplopia, dry eyes, eye haemorrhage, eye pain, lacrimation, visual field defect.

Renal and Urinary Disorders: hematuria, nocturia, oliguria, polyuria, urinary incontinence, urinary tract infection, urinary urgency.

Reproductive System and Breast Disorders: anorgasmia, breast engorgement, cervix carcinoma, endometrial carcinoma, endometrial hyperplasia, fibrocystic breast, genital edema, labial edema, mastitis, salpingitis, uterine enlargement, uterine fibroids enlarged, uterine neoplasm, vulvovaginitis.

Blood and Lymphatic System Disorders: anaemia, hypochromic anaemia, leucopenia, lymphocytosis, lymphadenopathy.

Investigations: fibrinolysis increased, aspartate transferase (AST) increased.

Psychiatric Disorders: hostility, libido decreased, anorgasmia.

Vascular Disorders: hypertension, vasodilatation, thrombophlebitis.

Infections and Infestations: flu syndrome.

Post-Market Adverse Drug Reactions: enlargement of hepatic hemangiomas; angioedema, increased triglycerides; ischemic colitis, growth potentiation of benign meningioma.

If adverse symptoms persist, the prescription of HRT should be re-considered.

DRUG INTERACTIONS: Overview: In vitro and in vivo studies have shown that estrogens are metabolized partially by cytochrome P450 3A4 (CYP3A4). Therefore, inducers or inhibitors of CYP3A4 may affect estrogen drug metabolism. Inducers of CYP3A4, such as St. John's wort (Hypericum perforatum) preparations, phenobarbitol, phenytoin, carbamazepine, rifampicin and dexamethasome may reduce plasma concentrations estrogens, possibly resulting in a decrease in the therapeutic effects and/or changes in the uterine bleeding profile. Inhibitors of CYP3A4, such as cimetidine, erythromycin, ketoconazole, clarithromycin, itraconazole, ritonavir, and grapefruit juice, may increase plasma concentrations of estrogens and may result in side effects.

Data from a drug-drug interaction study involving conjugated estrogens and medroxyprogesterone acetate indicate that the pharmacokinetic disposition of both drugs are not altered when the drugs are co-administered. Other clinical drug-drug interaction studies have not been conducted with conjugated estrogens.

Estrogens may diminish the effectiveness of anticoagulant, antidiabetic and antihypertensive agents.

Preparations inducing liver enzymes (e.g. barbiturates, hydantoins, carbamazepine, meprobamates, phenylbutazone or rifampicin) may interfere with the activity of orally administered estrogens.

Drug-Drug Interactions: Aminoglutethimide administered concomitantly with MPA may significantly depress the bioavailability of MPA.

Drug-Food Interactions: CYP3A4 inhibitors such as grapefruit juice may increase plasma concentrations of 17β-estradiol and may result in side effects.

A single dose study in healthy, postmenopausal women was conducted to investigate any potential drug interaction when 2×0.625 mg Premarin (conjugated estrogens) and 2.5 mg medroxyprogesterone acetate (MPA) tablets were administered immediately following a high-fat breakfast. Administration with food slowed the absorption of the conjugated estrogens, thereby reducing the C_{max} of the various estrogens by 25 to 30%, and increasing MPA C_{max} by 89% and $AUC_{0-\infty}$ by 28%. Thus, food slightly lowered the C_{max}, but did not affect the AUC, of the estrogens from a 0.625 mg Premarin tablet; food significantly increased the C_{max} and AUC of MPA from a 2.5 mg tablet.

Drug-Herb Interactions: It was found that some herbal products (e.g., St. John's wort), which are available as over-the-counter (OTC) products, might interfere with steroid metabolism, and therefore alter the efficacy and safety of estrogen/progestin products. Hot flashes and vaginal bleeding have been reported in patients taking estrogen replacement therapy (ERT) and combined estrogen plus progestin therapy (HRT) and St. John's wort. St. John's wort may induce hepatic microsomal enzymes, which theoretically may result in reduced efficacy of ERT and HRT.

Physicians and other health care providers should be made aware of other non-prescription products concomitantly used by the patient, including herbal and natural products, obtained from the widely spread Health Stores.

Drug-Laboratory Test Interactions: The results of certain endocrine and liver function tests may be affected by estrogen-containing products:

- increased prothrombin time and partial thromboplastin time; increased levels of fibrinogen and fibrinogen activity, increased coagulation factors VII, VIII, IX, X; increased norepinephrine-induced platelet aggregability; decreased antithrombin III;
- impaired glucose tolerance;
- increased serum triglycerides and phospholipids concentration;
- increased thyroid-binding globulin (TBG) levels leading to increased circulating total thyroid hormone (T_4), as measured by column or radioimmunoassay; T_3 resin uptake is decreased, reflecting the elevated TBG; free T_4 concentration is unaltered;
- other binding proteins may be elevated in serum i.e., corticosteroid binding globulin (CBG), sex-hormone binding globulin (SHBG), leading to increased circulating corticosteroids and sex steroids respectively, free or biologically active hormone concentrations are unchanged;

The results of the above laboratory tests should not be considered reliable unless therapy has been discontinued for two to four weeks.

The pathologist should be informed that the patient is receiving hormone replacement therapy **(HRT) when relevant specimens are submitted**.

DOSAGE AND ADMINISTRATION: Dosing Considerations: Use of estrogens alone or in combination with progestins therapy should be limited to the shortest duration consistent with treatment goals and risks for the individual woman. Patients should be re-evaluated periodically as clinically appropriate to determine if treatment is still necessary (see boxed Serious Warnings and Precautions). For women who have intact uteri, adequate diagnostic measures, such as endometrial sampling, when indicated, should be undertaken to rule out malignancy in cases of undiagnosed persistent or recurring abnormal vaginal bleeding.

Recommended Dose and Dosage Adjustment: Premplus 0.625 mg conjugated estrogens tablet and 2.5 mg medroxyprogesterone acetate (MPA) tablet and Premplus 0.625 mg conjugated estrogens tablet and 5.0 mg MPA tablet, continuous therapy: The starting dose is one maroon 0.625 mg conjugated estrogens (Premarin) tablet plus one white 2.5 mg MPA tablet taken at the same time once daily for 28 days, or one maroon 0.625 mg conjugated estrogens tablet plus one purple 5.0 mg MPA tablet taken at the same time once daily every 28 days. There is no need for the patient to count days between cycles because there are no off-tablet days.

A starting dose of Premplus 0.625 mg/2.5 mg is appropriate for most women entering menopause. Consider increasing the dose to the Premplus 0.625 mg/5.0 mg therapy if amenorrhea is not achieved within a few months of initiating therapy. Once amenorrhea is achieved, consider dose reduction of MPA to 2.5 mg.

Additional factors, which should be taken into consideration when adjusting the dose, should include the patient's medical history, occurrence of adverse events, laboratory results and physical and gynecological examination. Patients should be re-evaluated at regular intervals.

Missed Dose: If a patient misses a dose, it should be taken as soon as possible. If it is close to the patient's next scheduled dose, the missed dose should be skipped, and the patient should continue with her normal schedule. The patient should not take two doses at the same time.

Administration: Oral.

OVERDOSAGE:

Symptoms of Overdose: Numerous reports of ingestion of large doses of estrogen products and estrogen-containing oral contraceptives by young children have not revealed acute serious ill effects.

Overdosage with estrogen may cause nausea, breast discomfort, fluid retention, bloating or vaginal bleeding in women. Overdosage with MPA, in female patients, may result in a period of amenorrhea of variable length and may be followed by irregular menses for several cycles. No cases of overdosage in male patients have been reported. However, such overdosage, if it were to occur, would not likely result in any particular symptomatology.

Treatment of Overdose: Symptomatic treatment should be given in the case of estrogen overdosage. There is no known therapy for overdosage of medroxyprogesterone. Doses as high as 1000 mg of medroxyprogesterone for the therapy of endometrial carcinoma have been used without adverse effect.

For management of a suspected drug overdose, contact your regional Poison Control Centre. See the *CPS* Directory section for a list of Poison Control Centres.

ACTION AND CLINICAL PHARMACOLOGY: Mechanism of Action: By a direct action, endogenous estrogens cause growth and development of the uterus, fallopian tubes, and vagina. With other hormones, such as pituitary hormones and progesterone, they cause enlargement of the breasts through promotion of ductal growth, stromal development, and the accretion of fat. Estrogens are intricately involved with other hormones, especially progesterone, in the processes of the ovulatory menstrual cycle and pregnancy and affect the release of pituitary gonadotropins. Indirectly, they also contribute to the shaping of the skeleton, maintenance of tone and elasticity through the increase of collagen production in the supportive tissues of the heart, skin and urogenital structures, changes in the epiphyses of the long bones that allow for the pubertal growth spurt and its termination, growth of axillary and pubic hair and pigmentation of the nipples and genital tissues. Decline of ovarian estrogenic and progestogenic activity at the end of the menstrual cycle can result in menstruation, although the cessation of progesterone secretion is the most important factor in the mature ovulatory cycle. However, in the preovulatory or anovulatory cycle, estrogen is the primary determinant in the onset of menstruation.

Estrogen products act by regulating the transcription of a limited number of genes. Estrogens diffuse through cell membranes, distribute themselves throughout the cell, and bind to and activate the nuclear estrogen receptor, a DNA-binding protein which is found in estrogen-responsive tissues. The activated estrogen receptor binds to specific DNA sequences, or hormone-response elements, which enhance the transcription of adjacent genes and in turn lead to the observed effects. Estrogen receptors have been identified in tissues of the reproductive tract, breast, pituitary, hypothalamus, liver and bone of women.

Progesterone is secreted by the ovary mainly from the corpus luteum during the second half of the menstrual cycle. Progesterone released during the luteal phase of the cycle leads to the development of a secretory endometrium. Estrogen precedes and accompanies progesterone in its action upon the endometrium and is essential to the development of the normal endometrial pattern.

Pharmacodynamics: Currently, there are no pharmacodynamic data known for CE/MPA or CE plus MPA.

Conjugated estrogens used in therapy are soluble in water and are well absorbed through the skin, mucous membranes, and gastrointestinal tract after release from the drug formulation. Like estrogens, progestogens diffuse freely into the cell nucleus where they bind to the progesterone receptor and influence the transcription of a limited set of genes. Progesterone receptors are primarily located in the female reproductive tract. Medroxyprogesterone acetate (MPA) differs considerably in its metabolic and pharmacologic effects from natural progesterone. Androgenic and anabolic effects of MPA have been noted with high doses, but the drug is apparently devoid of significant estrogenic activity.

Timing of the initiation of estrogen therapy relative to the start of menopause may affect the overall risk benefit profile. The WHI estrogen plus progestin substudy stratified by age showed in women 50-59 years of age, a non-significant trend toward reduced risk for overall mortality [HR 0.69 (95 percent CI 0.44-1.07)] when compared to the 60-69 year-old and 70-79 year-old groups with hazard ratios of 1.09 (95 percent CI 0.83-1.44) and 1.06 (95 percent CI 0.80-1.41) respectively.

Effects on Vasomotor Symptoms Associated with Estrogen Deficiency: Hot flushes, feelings of intense heat over the upper trunk and face, with flushing of the skin and sweating occur in approximately 80% of women as a result of the decrease in ovarian hormones. These vasomotor symptoms are seen in women whether menopause is surgically induced or spontaneous. However, hot flushes may be more severe in women who undergo surgical menopause. Hot flushes can begin before the cessation of menses. A double-blind, randomized, parallel study has confirmed a significant reduction in hot flushes experienced by menopausal women taking Premplus.

Effects on Osteoporosis Associated with Estrogen Deficiency: For several years following natural or induced menopause, the rate of bone mass decline is accelerated. Conjugated estrogens reduce bone resorption and retard postmenopausal bone loss. Case-control studies have shown a reduction of up to 60% in hip and wrist fractures in women whose estrogen replacement was begun within a few years of menopause. Studies also suggest that estrogen reduces the rate of vertebral fractures. One clinical study demonstrated that even when estrogen was started as late as fifteen years after menopause, further loss of bone mass was prevented, but was not restored to premenopausal levels. The effect on bone mass conservation is sustained only as long as conjugated estrogens therapy is continued.

Studies to date suggest that the addition of MPA to estrogen replacement therapy does not interfere with the beneficial effects of Premarin on bone.

Effects on the Endometrium: The use of unopposed estrogen therapy has been associated with an increased risk of endometrial hyperplasia, a possible precursor of endometrial adenocarcinoma. The results of clinical studies indicate that the addition of a progestin to an estrogen replacement regimen for more than 10 days per cycle reduces the incidence of endometrial hyperplasia and the attendant risk of adenocarcinoma in women with intact uteri. The addition of a progestin into an estrogen replacement regimen has not been shown to interfere with the efficacy of estrogen replacement therapy for its approved indications. Data from a large clinical trial indicate that MPA administered in the recommended dose to women receiving Premarin 0.625 mg reduces the incidence of hyperplastic changes and hence reduces the risk of developing adenocarcinoma. This is the clinical rationale for combining conjugated estrogens found in Premarin tablets with MPA in product presentations of Premplus.

Effect on Bleeding Patterns: With a continuous therapy, several bleeding patterns may occur. These may range from absence of bleeding to irregular bleeding. If bleeding occurs, it is frequently light spotting or moderate bleeding. These bleeding patterns may resolve with the continued use of Premplus. During a 1-year clinical trial the occurrence of bleeding or spotting was measured for the last 7 cycles of treatment with a continuous regimen of Premarin and MPA. Results demonstrated that a significantly greater percentage of women taking Premarin and MPA (0.625 mg/5.0 mg) continuous therapy had no bleeding or spotting compared to the Premarin and MPA (0.625 mg/2.5 mg) continuous therapy.

With a cyclic therapy of Premarin and MPA, it is customary to experience withdrawal bleeding or withdrawal spotting. This withdrawal bleeding or spotting may begin between day 20 of one 28-day cycle and day 5 of the next 28-day cycle. During a 1-year clinical trial, the overall incidence of withdrawal bleeding (with or without spotting) or withdrawal spotting was 62.6% of cycles.

In addition to withdrawal bleeding, irregular bleeding may occur with cyclic therapy. In a 1-year clinical trial, the reported mean number of days of irregular bleeding and irregular spotting for each cycle were 4.8 days and 2.5 days, respectively.

Pharmacokinetics: Coadministration of conjugated estrogens with MPA does not affect the pharmacokinetic profile of MPA; similarly, MPA does not affect the pharmacokinetic profile of the conjugated or unconjugated estrogens.

Absorption: Conjugated estrogens are soluble in water and are well absorbed through the skin, mucous membranes, and the gastrointestinal tract after release from the drug formulation. However, Premplus contains a modified-release formulation of conjugated estrogens that slowly releases estrogens over several hours. Maximum plasma concentrations of the various conjugated and unconjugated estrogens are attained within 4 to 10 hours after dose administration. MPA is rapidly absorbed from the gastrointestinal tract, and maximum MPA plasma concentrations are attained within 2 to 4 hours after dose administration.

An open-label, three period crossover study was conducted to investigate any potential pharmacokinetic interaction between Premarin (conjugated estrogens) and MPA. Fifty-four women received single oral doses each of two 0.625 mg Premarin tablets, two 5.0 mg MPA tablets in a capsule, and two 0.625 mg Premarin tablets and two 5.0 mg MPA tablets in a capsule concomitantly.

The pharmacokinetic data obtained from this study is presented in Table 2. The data are presented for individual components of Premarin and for MPA. The pharmacokinetic profiles of exogenous estrone and total estrone are based on plasma concentrations that are adjusted for baseline concentrations.

Table 2: PREMPLUS

Pharmacokinetic Parameters[b] for Unconjugated and Conjugated Estrogens[a] and Medroxyprogesterone Acetate (2×0.625 mg/5.0 mg)

		PK Parameter—result and standard deviation			
Drug	**Treatment**	C_{max} (pg/mL)	t_{max} (h)	AUC_T (pg·h/mL)	$AUC_{0-\infty}$ (pg·h/mL)
Unconjugated Estrogens					
estrone	Premarin	179±60	8.5±2.2	4009±1321	5700±2152
	Premarin + MPA	181±70	8.3±2.6	3978±1473	5621±2366
estrone BA[c]	Premarin	159±58	8.5±2.2	3065±1112	3757±1510
	Premarin + MPA	160±68	8.3±2.6	2961±1211	3618±1679
equilin	Premarin	76±29	7.8±2.8	1100±532	1327±578
	Premarin + MPA	77±35	7.2±2.3	1051±535	1289±609
Conjugated Estrogens					
total estrone	Premarin	7.01±4.16	7.0±2.0	107±59	124±72
	Premarin + MPA	7.11±4.11	7.5±2.1	108±60	126±77
total estrone BA[c]	Premarin	6.82±4.04	7.0±2.0	97±52	109±61
	Premarin + MPA	6.91±4.03	7.5±2.1	98±55	109±65
total equilin	Premarin	5.18±2.83	5.5±1.9	64.9±39.2	69.1±44.7
	Premarin + MPA	5.36±3.24	5.9±1.9	66.0±42.2	70.3±48.2
Medroxyprogesterone Acetate					
MPA	Premarin	33.3±1.30	2.7±1.7	49.7±16.2	58.0±16.7
	Premarin + MPA	2.84±1.02	2.6±1.7	42.2±11.7	49.4±13.0

a Estrogen (unconjugated and conjugated) source is Premarin 0.625 mg tablets
b Values are mean±SD.
c BA=Baseline adjusted.

This pharmacokinetic study was conducted to investigate potential interactions between single doses of Premarin and MPA given concomitantly. The results demonstrated that single-dose coadministration of 2×0.625 mg Premarin tablets with 2×5.0 mg MPA encapsulated tablets does not significantly affect the pharmacokinetics of estrone, equilin, total estrone, total equilin, or MPA.

Distribution: The distribution of exogenous estrogens is similar to that of endogenous estrogens. Estrogens are widely distributed in the body and are generally found in higher concentrations in the sex hormone target organs. Estrogens circulate in the blood largely bound to sex hormone binding globulin (SHBG) and albumin albumin (50-80% bound to plasma proteins). MPA is approximately 90% bound to plasma proteins but does not bind to SHBG.

Metabolism: Metabolism and inactivation of estrogens occur primarily in the liver. Metabolism and elimination of MPA occurs primarily in the liver via hydroxylation, with subsequent conjugation and elimination in the urine.

Excretion: Some estrogens are excreted in bile; however, they are reabsorbed from the intestine and returned to the liver through the portal venous system.

Estradiol, estrone, and estriol are excreted in the urine along with glucuronide and sulfate conjugates. Most metabolites of MPA are excreted as glucuronide conjugates with only minor amounts excreted as sulfates.

The apparent terminal-phase disposition half-life ($t_{½}$) of the various estrogens is prolonged by the slow absorption from Premarin/MPA and ranges from 10 to 24 hours. MPA has a mean $t_{½}$ of 38 hours.

Special Populations and Conditions: No pharmacokinetic studies were conducted in special populations, including patients with renal or hepatic impairment.

Estrogen Pharmacology: Endogenous estrogens are largely responsible for the development and maintenance of the female reproductive system and secondary sexual characteristics. Although circulating estrogens exist in a dynamic equilibrium of metabolic interconversions, estradiol is the principal intracellular human estrogen and is substantially more potent than its metabolites, estrone and estriol, at the receptor level.

The primary source of estrogen in normally cycling adult women is the ovarian follicle, which secretes 70 to 500 µg of estradiol daily, depending on the phase of the menstrual cycle. After menopause, most endogenous estrogen is produced by conversion of androstenedione, secreted by the adrenal cortex, to estrone by peripheral tissues. Thus, estrone and the sulfate-conjugated form, estrone sulfate, are the most abundant circulating estrogens in postmenopausal women.

Estrogens act through binding to nuclear receptors in estrogen-responsive tissues. To date, two estrogen receptors have been identified. These vary in proportion from tissue to tissue.

Circulating estrogens modulate the pituitary secretion of the gonadotropins, luteinizing hormone (LH) and follicle stimulating hormone (FSH) through a negative feedback mechanism. Estrogens act to reduce the elevated levels of these gonadotropins seen in postmenopausal women.

Progestin Pharmacology: Parenterally administered medroxyprogesterone acetate (MPA) inhibits gonadotropin production, which in turn prevents follicular maturation and ovulation, although available data indicate that this does not occur when the usually recommended oral dosage is given as single daily doses. MPA may achieve its beneficial effect on the endometrium in part by decreasing nuclear estrogen receptors and suppression of epithelial DNA synthesis in endometrial tissue. Androgenic and anabolic effects of MPA have been noted, but the drug is apparently devoid of significant estrogenic activity.

The purpose of adding a progestin medication to long-term estrogen therapy is to reduce the risk of endometrial hyperplasia in women with intact uteri.

STORAGE AND STABILITY: Store at 15-25°C.

Keep out of reach of children.

SPECIAL HANDLING INSTRUCTIONS: None required.

INFORMATION FOR THE PATIENT: Published in e-CPS, available by subscription at www.e-cps.ca.

DOSAGE FORMS, COMPOSITION AND PACKAGING: 0.625 mg/2.5 mg: Each oval, maroon tablet, branded "0.625" on one side in white ink, contains: conjugated estrogens C.S.D. 0.625 mg. Each oval, white MPA tablet, scored on one side, debossed with 2 opposing "C"s on the other side, contains: medroxyprogesterone acetate 2.5 mg. Nonmedicinal ingredients: maroon Premarin tablet: calcium sulfate, carnauba wax, edible ink, erythrosine aluminum lake, FD&C Blue No. 2, FD&C Yellow No. 6, glyceryl monooleate, lactose, magnesium stearate, methylcellulose, microcrystalline cellulose, pharmaceutical glaze, polyethylene glycol, povidone, sodium benzoate, stearic acid, sucrose and titanium dioxide; white MPA tablet: lactose, magnesium stearate, methylcellulose and microcrystalline cellulose. Blister cards (×2) of 14 Premarin and 14 MPA, cartons totalling 56 tablets.

0.625 mg/5 mg: Each oval, maroon tablet, branded "0.625" on one side in white ink, contains: conjugated estrogens C.S.D. 0.625 mg. Each oval, purple MPA tablet, scored on one side, debossed with 2 opposing "C"s on the other side, contains: medroxyprogesterone acetate 5 mg. Nonmedicinal ingredients: maroon Premarin tablet: calcium sulfate, carnauba wax, edible ink, erythrosine aluminum lake, FD&C Blue No. 2, FD&C Yellow No. 6, glyceryl monooleate, lactose, magnesium stearate, methylcellulose, microcrystalline cellulose, pharmaceutical glaze, polyethylene glycol, povidone, sodium benzoate, stearic acid, sucrose and titanium dioxide; purple MPA tablet: D&C Blue No. 1 aluminum lake, D&C Red No. 30 aluminum lake, lactose, magnesium stearate, methylcellulose and microcrystalline cellulose. Blister cards (×2) of 14 Premarin and 14 MPA, cartons totalling 56 tablets.

(Shown in Product Identification Section)

Preparation H® Cooling Gel
phenylephrine HCl—hamamelis water
Hemorrhoid Therapy

Pfizer Consumer Healthcare

Preparation H® Cream
live yeast derivative (bio-Dyne)—shark liver oil
Hemorrhoid Therapy

Pfizer Consumer Healthcare

Preparation H® Ointment
live yeast derivative (bio-Dyne)—shark liver oil
Hemorrhoid Therapy

Pfizer Consumer Healthcare

Preparation H® Suppositories
live yeast derivative (bio-Dyne)—shark liver oil
Hemorrhoid Therapy

Pfizer Consumer Healthcare

INDICATIONS: Ointment/Cream/Suppositories/Cooling Gel: To help shrink swelling of hemorrhoidal tissues caused by inflammation and to give prompt temporary relief from pain and itching. Preparation H is of considerable value as a lubricant in easing painful bowel movements by protecting and soothing the painful area.

PRECAUTIONS: In case of bleeding or if irritation/condition persists, patient should be instructed to discontinue use and contact physician.

Keep out of reach of children.
May stain clothing.

OVERDOSE:

If accidently ingested or misused, CPhA recommends that you contact your **regional Poison Control Centre**. See the *CPS* Directory section for a list of Poison Control Centres.

DOSAGE: Ointment/Cream/Cooling Gel: Apply freely morning, night, after each bowel movement and whenever symptoms occur. Lubricate applicator before each application and thoroughly cleanse after use.

Suppositories: Remove wrapper and insert one suppository morning, night, after each bowel movement and whenever symptoms occur.

SUPPLIED: Cooling Gel: Each tube contains: phenylephrine HCl 0.25% w/w and hamamelis water (witch hazel) 50% w/w in a nonstaining clear gel base. Nonmedicinal ingredients: edetate disodium, hydroxyethyl cellulose, parabens, propylene glycol, sodium citrate, sodium metabisulfite and water. Tubes of 25 g. Store at room temperature (15-25°C).

Cream: Each tube contains: yeast as a live cell derivative (Bio-Dyne: Skin Respiratory Factor) 1% and shark liver oil 3% in a nonstaining cream base. Nonmedicinal ingredients: butylated hydroxyanisole, cellulose, cetyl alcohol, citric acid, disodium edetate, glycerin, glyceryl monostearate, glycerol oleate, lanolin, parabens, petrolatum, propyl gallate, propylene glycol, simethicone emulsion, sodium benzoate, sodium lauryl sulfate, stearyl alcohol, water and xanthan gum. Tubes of 25 and 50 g. Store at room temperature (15-30°C).

Ointment: Each tube contains: yeast as a live cell derivative (Bio-Dyne: Skin Respiratory Factor) 1% and shark liver oil 3%. Nonmedicinal ingredients: beeswax, chlorhexidine gluconate, fragrance, lanolin, mineral oil, paraffin wax and petrolatum. Tubes of 25, 50 and 75 g. Store at room temperature (15-30°C).

Suppositories: Each 2.2 g suppository contains: yeast as a live cell derivative (Bio-Dyne: Skin Respiratory Factor) 22 mg (1%) and shark liver oil 66 mg (3%). Nonmedicinal ingredients: chlorhexidine gluconate, cocoa butter, glycerin, polyethylene glycol, wax and witepsol. Packages of 12, 24 and 48. Store at room temperature (15-30°C).

Prepidil® Ⓟ
dinoprostone
Prostaglandin

Paladin

SUPPLIED: Each prefilled syringe of translucent sterile gel with an accompanying catheter contains: dinoprostone (PGE_2) 0.5 mg. Nonmedicinal ingredients: colloidal silicon dioxide and triacetin. Syringes of 3 g (2.5 mL). Available to hospitals only. This product has a shelf life of 24 months when stored at 4°C, under continuous refrigeration.

Pressyn® Ⓟ
vasopressin
Antidiuretic

Ferring

PHARMACOLOGY: Pressyn is a synthetic water-soluble pressor principle identical in sequence to lysine vasopressin.

Vasopressin exerts its antidiuretic action by increasing the reabsorption of water by the renal tubules. The drug can also cause contraction of smooth muscle of the gastrointestinal tract and all parts of the vascular beds, especially the capillaries, small arterioles, and venules, with less effect on the smooth musculature of the large veins.

The direct effect on the contractile elements is neither antagonized by adrenergic blocking agents nor prevented by vascular denervation.

Vasopressin injection USP is intended for i.m. or s.c. injection.

INDICATIONS: For the prevention or treatment of postoperative abdominal distention, dispelling of gas shadows in abdominal roentgenography and symptomatic control of diabetes insipidus.

CONTRAINDICATIONS: Should not be used in patients having cardiorenal disease with hypertension, advanced arteriosclerosis, coronary thrombosis, angina pectoris, epilepsy or toxemia of pregnancy. Anaphylaxis or hypersensitivity to the drug or its components are also contraindications.

Chronic nephritis with nitrogen retention may be a contraindication (see Precautions).

WARNINGS: The drug should not be used except with extreme caution in patients with vascular disease, especially disease of the coronary arteries. In such patients even small doses of the drug may precipitate anginal pain and with larger doses, the possibility of myocardial infarction should be considered.

Vasopressin may produce water intoxication. The early signs of drowsiness, listlessness and headaches should be recognized to prevent convulsions and terminal coma.

PRECAUTIONS: Vasopressin should be used cautiously in the presence of epilepsy, migraine, asthma, heart failure, or any state in which a rapid addition to extracellular water may produce hazard for an already overburdened system.

Chronic nephritis with nitrogen retention contraindicates the use of vasopressin until reasonable nitrogen blood levels have been attained.

ADVERSE EFFECTS: Local or systemic allergic reactions may occur in hypersensitive individuals. The following side effects have been reported following the administration of vasopressin: tremor, sweating, vertigo, circumoral pallor, "pounding" in the head, abdominal cramps, passage of gas, nausea, vomiting, urticaria, bronchial constriction.

Anaphylaxis (cardiac arrest and/or shock) has been observed shortly after injection of vasopressin.

OVERDOSE:
No data supplied by the manufacturer.

> For management of a suspected drug overdose, CPhA recommends that you contact your **regional Poison Control Centre**. See the *CPS* Directory section for a list of Poison Control Centres.

DOSAGE: Dosage should be individualized: 0.25 to 0.5 mL i.m. or s.c. at intervals of 3 to 4 hours, as required. Children's dosages in proportion.
Abdominal Distension: Adults, 0.25 to 0.5 mL.
Abdominal Roentgenography: Adults, 0.5 mL given 2 hours and 0.5 hours before exposure of films.
Diabetes Insipidus: The dose by i.m. or s.c. injection is 0.25 to 0.5 mL repeated 2 or 3 times daily as required.

SUPPLIED: Each mL of aqueous solution contains: vasopressin 20 USP pressor units, chlorobutanol 0.5% as a preservative, and sodium chloride 9 mg/mL. The acidity of the solution is adjusted, if necessary to 2.5 to 4.5 with acetic acid. Ampuls of 5 mL, boxes of 1. Store at room temperature (15-30°C).

Pressyn® AR
vasopressin
Antidiuretic
Ferring

PHARMACOLOGY: Pressyn AR is a synthetic water-soluble pressor principle identical in sequence to arginine vasopressin.

Vasopressin is considered to exert its diuretic action by increasing the reabsorption of water by the renal tubules. The drug also can cause contraction of smooth muscle of the gastrointestinal tract and of all parts of the vascular beds, especially the capillaries, small arterioles, and venules, with less effect on the smooth musculature of the large veins.

The direct effect on the contractile elements is neither antagonized by adrenergic blocking agents nor prevented by vascular denervation.

Vasopressin Injection is intended for intramuscular (IM) or subcutaneous (SC) injection.

INDICATIONS: Vasopressin is intended for use in the prevention or treatment of post-operation abdominal distension, dispelling of gas shadows in abdominal roentgenography and symptomatic control of diabetes insipidus.

CONTRAINDICATIONS: Vasopressin should not be used in patients having cardiorenal disease with hypertension, advanced arteriosclerosis, coronary thrombosis, angina pectoris, epilepsy or toxemia of pregnancy. Anaphylaxis or hypersensitivity to the drug or its components are also contraindications.

Chronic nephritis with nitrogen retention may be a contraindication, see Precautions.

WARNINGS: Vasopressin should not be used except with extreme caution in patients with vascular disease, especially disease of the coronary arteries. In such patients even small doses of the drug may precipitate anginal pain and with larger doses, the possibility of myocardial infarction should be considered.

Vasopressin may produce water intoxication. The early signs of drowsiness, listlessness, and headaches should be recognized to prevent convulsions and terminal coma.

PRECAUTIONS: Vasopressin should be used cautiously in the presence of epilepsy, migraine, asthma, heart failure, or any state in which a rapid addition to extracellular water may produce hazard for an already overburdened system.

Chronic nephritis with nitrogen retention contraindicates the use of Vasopressin until reasonable nitrogen blood levels have been attained.

ADVERSE EFFECTS: Local or systemic allergic reactions may occur in hypersensitive individuals. The following side-effects have been reported following the administration of Vasopressin: tremor, sweating, vertigo, circumoral pallor, "pounding" in the head, abdominal cramps, passage of gas, nausea, vomiting, urticaria, bronchial constriction.

Anaphylaxis (cardiac arrest and/or shock) have been observed shortly after injection of Vasopressin.

OVERDOSE:
No data supplied by the manufacturer.

> For management of a suspected drug overdose, CPhA recommends that you contact your **regional Poison Control Centre**. See the *CPS* Directory section for a list of Poison Control Centres.

DOSAGE: The dosage of Vasopressin Injection should be individualized: 0.25 to 0.5 mL IM or SC at intervals of 3-4 hours, as required. Children's dosages in proportion.
Abdominal Distension: Adults: 0.25 to 0.5 mL.
Abdominal Roentgenography: Adults: 0.5 mL given 2 hours and 0.5 hours before exposure of films.
Diabetes Insipidus: The dose by IM or SC injection is 0.25 to 0.5 mL repeated 2 or 3 times daily as required.

SUPPLIED: Each mL of sterile aqueous solution contains: vasopressin (arginine), 20 USP pressor units, chlorobutanol 5 mg as a preservative and sodium chloride 9 mg. The acidity of the solution is adjusted, if necessary, to pH 2.5-4.5 with acetic acid. Cartons containing 1 x 5 mL ampul or 10 x 2 mL ampuls. Single dose use. Discard unused portion. Store at room temperature (15 to 30°C).

Prevacid®
lansoprazole
H+, K+-ATPase Inhibitor
Takeda

Prevacid® FasTab
lansoprazole
H+, K+-ATPase Inhibitor
Takeda

Date of Preparation: May 12, 1995
Date of Revision: September 25, 2008

SUMMARY PRODUCT INFORMATION:

Route of Administration	Dosage Form/ Strength	Clinically Relevant Nonmedicinal Ingredients
Oral	Capsules 15 mg, 30 mg	Cellulosic polymers, colloidal silicon dioxide, D&C Red No. 28, FD&C Blue No. 1, FD&C Green No. 3 (15 mg capsules only), FD&C Red No. 40, gelatin, magnesium carbonate, methacrylic acid copolymer, starch, talc, sugar spheres, sucrose, polyethylene glycol, polysorbate 80, and titanium dioxide
	Tablets 15 mg, 30 mg	Lactose monohydrate, microcrystalline cellulose, magnesium carbonate, hydroxypropyl cellulose, hydroxypropyl methylcellulose, titanium dioxide, talc, mannitol, methacrylic acid, polyacrylate, polyethylene glycol, glyceryl monostearate, polysorbate 80, triethyl citrate, ferric oxide, citric acid, crospovidone, aspartame[a], strawberry flavor and magnesium stearate

[a] Phenylketonurics: Contains Phenylalanine 2.5 mg per 15 mg tablet and 5.1 mg per 30 mg tablet.

INDICATIONS AND CLINICAL USE: Note: When used in combination with antimicrobials for the eradication of *H. pylori*, the product monograph for those agents should be consulted.

Oral Administration: Adults: PREVACID (lansoprazole delayed-release capsules), and PREVACID FasTab (lansoprazole delayed-release tablets) are indicated in the treatment of conditions where a reduction of gastric acid secretion is required, such as:

1. Duodenal ulcer.
2. Gastric ulcer.
3. Reflux esophagitis including patients with Barrett's esophagus, and patients poorly responsive to an adequate course of therapy with histamine H_2-receptor antagonists.
4. Healing of NSAID-Associated Gastric Ulcer; treatment of NSAID-associated gastric ulcer in patients who continue NSAID use. (Controlled studies did not extend beyond 8 weeks.)
5. Reduction of Risk of NSAID-Associated Gastric Ulcers in patients with a history of gastric ulcers who require to continue taking a NSAID. (A controlled study did not extend beyond 12 weeks.)
6. Symptomatic Gastroesophageal reflux disease (sGERD); treatment of heartburn and other symptoms associated with GERD.
7. Pathological hypersecretory conditions including Zollinger-Ellison Syndrome (see Dosage and Administration).
8. Eradication of *H. pylori*.

Triple Therapy: Lansoprazole, in combination with clarithromycin plus amoxicillin as triple therapy, is indicated for the treatment of patients with *H. pylori* infection and active duodenal ulcer disease. Eradication of *H. pylori* has been shown to reduce the risk of duodenal ulcer recurrence (see Dosage and Administration).

(For additional information on triple therapy for the treatment of *H. pylori* infection and active duodenal ulcer recurrence, refer to the Hp-PAC Product Monograph.)

In patients with a recent history of duodenal ulcers who are *H. pylori* positive, eradication therapy may reduce the rate of recurrence of duodenal ulcers. The optimal timing for eradication therapy for such patients remains to be determined.

In patients who fail a therapy combination containing clarithromycin, susceptibility testing should be done. If resistance to clarithromycin is demonstrated or susceptibility testing is not possible, an alternative therapy combination is recommended.

Resistance to amoxicillin has not been demonstrated in clinical studies with lansoprazole delayed-release capsules and amoxicillin.

Table 1 summarizes the eradication rates for the *H. pylori* Triple Therapy treatment regimens.

Table 1: PREVACID

Eradication Rates for the *H. pylori* Triple Therapy Treatment Regimens

Treatment Regimen	Days/Study No.	Evaluable (per protocol)[a] % (n/N)	ITT (all data)[b] % (n/N)	ITT (worst case)[c] % (n/N)
PREVACID 30 mg capsules/Clarithromycin 500 mg/Amoxicillin 1 g (all b.i.d.)	14/M93-131 14/M95-392	92 (44/48) 86 (57/66)	94 (47/50) 87 (58/67)	86 (47/55) 83 (58/70)
PREVACID 30 mg capsules/Clarithromycin 500 mg/Amoxicillin 1 g (all b.i.d.)	10/M95-399	84 (103/123)	86 (110/128)	81 (110/135)
PREVACID 30 mg capsules/Clarithromycin 250 mg/Amoxicillin 1 g (all b.i.d.)	7/GB 94/110	90 (103/114)	90 (104/116)	86 (104/121)

[a] Based on evaluable patients with confirmed duodenal ulcer and/or gastritis and *H. pylori* infection at baseline defined as at least 2 of 3 positive endoscopic tests from CLOtest, histology and/or culture. Patients were included in the analysis if they completed the study. Additionally, if patients dropped out of the study due to an adverse event related to the study drug, they were included in the analysis as failures of therapy.

[b] Patients were included in the analysis if they had documented *H. pylori* infection at baseline as defined above and had a confirmed duodenal ulcer.

[c] "Worst case" included patients with no available data as failures.

Patients were included in the analysis if they had documented duodenal ulcer (active) and *H. pylori* infection at baseline defined as at least 2 of 3 positive endoscopic tests from CLOtest, histology and/or culture.
Legend: ITT=intent-to-treat patients.

Pediatric GERD (erosive and non-erosive esophagitis) (1 to 17 years of age): PREVACID is indicated for treatment of erosive and non-erosive GERD in children, aged 1 to 17 years. The clinical trial treatment period did not extend beyond 12 weeks.

CONTRAINDICATIONS:

- Patients with known hypersensitivity to any component of the formulations. For a complete listing, see Dosage Forms, Composition and Packaging.
- Amoxicillin is contraindicated in patients with a known hypersensitivity to any penicillin. (Please refer to the Amoxicillin Product Monograph before prescribing.)

- Clarithromycin is contraindicated in patients with known hypersensitivity to clarithromycin, erythromycin or other macrolide antibacterial agents. Clarithromycin is also contraindicated in patients receiving concurrent therapy with astemizole, terfenadine, cisapride or pimozide. (Please refer to the Clarithromycin tablets Product Monograph before prescribing.)

WARNINGS AND PRECAUTIONS:

Serious Warnings and Precautions
Clarithromycin should not be used in pregnancy except where no alternative therapy is appropriate, particularly during the first 3 months of pregnancy. If pregnancy occurs while taking the drug, the patient should be apprised of the potential hazard to the fetus. Clarithromycin has demonstrated adverse effects on pregnancy outcome and/or embryo-fetal development in monkeys, mice, rats and rabbits at doses that produced plasma levels 2 to 17 times the serum levels obtained in humans treated at the maximum recommended doses (see Warnings and Precautions section in the Clarithromycin Product Monograph).

General: Symptomatic response to therapy with lansoprazole does not preclude the presence of gastric malignancy.

Pseudomembranous colitis has been reported with nearly all antibacterial agents, including clarithromycin and amoxicillin, and may range in severity from mild to life threatening. Therefore, it is important to consider this diagnosis in patients who present with diarrhea subsequent to the administration of antibacterial agents.

Treatment with antibacterial agents alters the normal flora of the colon and may permit overgrowth of clostridia. Studies indicate that a toxin produced by Clostridium difficile is a primary cause of "antibiotic-associated colitis".

After the diagnosis of pseudomembranous colitis has been established, therapeutic measures should be initiated. Mild cases of pseudomembranous colitis usually respond to discontinuation of the drug alone. In moderate to severe cases, consideration should be given to management with fluids and electrolytes, protein supplementation, and treatment with an antibacterial drug effective against *C. difficile*.

***H. pylori* Eradication and Compliance:** To avoid failure of the eradication treatment with a potential for developing antimicrobial resistance and a risk of failure with subsequent therapy, patients should be instructed to follow closely the prescribed regimen.

For the eradication of *H. pylori*, amoxicillin and clarithromycin should not be administered to patients with renal impairment since the appropriate dosage in this patient population has not yet been established.

Carcinogenesis and Mutagenesis: Safety concerns of long-term treatment relate to hypergastrinemia, possible enterochromaffin-like (ECL) effect and carcinoid formation. ECL cell hyperplasia and gastric carcinoid tumours were observed in four animal studies.

In two 24-month carcinogenicity studies, Sprague-Dawley rats were treated orally with doses of 5 to 150 mg/kg/day about 1 to 40 times the exposure on a body surface (mg/m^2) basis, of a 50 kg person of average height (1.46 m^2 body surface area) given the recommended human dose of 30 mg/day (22.2 mg/m^2). Lansoprazole produced dose-related gastric entero-chromaffin-like (ECL) cell hyperplasia and ECL cell carcinoids in both male and female rats. It also increased the incidence of intestinal metaplasia of the gastric epithelium in both sexes. In male rats, lansoprazole produced a dose related increase of testicular interstitial cell adenomas. The incidence of these adenomas in rats receiving doses of 15 to 150 mg/kg/day (4 to 40 times the recommended human dose based on body surface area) exceeded the low background incidence (range=1.4 to 10%) for this strain of rats. Testicular interstitial cell adenoma also occurred in 1 of 30 rats treated with 50 mg/kg/day (13 times the recommended human dose based on body surface area) in a one year toxicity study.

In a 24-month carcinogenicity study, CD-1 mice were treated orally with doses of 15 to 600 mg/kg/day, 2 to 80 times the recommended human dose based on body surface area. Lansoprazole produced a dose-related increased incidence of gastric ECL cell hyperplasia. Lansoprazole also induced a low, non-dose-related incidence of carcinoid tumours in the gastric mucosa in several dose groups (one female mouse in the 15 mg/kg/day group, one male mouse in the 150 mg/kg/day group, and 2 males and 1 female in the 300 mg/kg/day group). It also produced an increased incidence of liver tumours (hepatocellular adenoma plus carcinoma). The tumour incidences in male mice treated with 300 and 600 mg/kg/day (40 to 80 times the recommended human dose based on body surface area) and female mice treated with 150 to 600 mg/kg/day (20 to 80 times the recommended human dose based on body surface area) exceeded the ranges of background incidences in historical controls for this strain of mice. Lansoprazole treatment produced adenoma of rete testis in male mice receiving 75 to 600 mg/kg/day (10 to 80 times the recommended human dose based on body surface area).

Analysis of gastric biopsy specimens from patients after short-term treatment of proton pump inhibitors have not detected ECL cell effects similar to those seen in animal studies. Longer term studies in humans revealed a slight increase in the mean ECL-cell density, although there was no microscopic evidence of cell hyperplasia. Similar results were seen in the maintenance treatment studies, where patients received up to 15 months of lansoprazole therapy. Serum gastrin values increased significantly from their baseline values but reached a plateau after two months of therapy. By one month post-treatment, fasting serum gastrin values returned to lansoprazole therapy baseline. Moreover, results from gastric biopsies from short-term, long-term and maintenance treatment studies indicate that there are no clinically meaningful effects on gastric mucosa morphology among lansoprazole-treated patients.

Gastrointestinal: When gastric ulcer is suspected, the possibility of malignancy should be excluded before therapy with lansoprazole delayed-release capsules or lansoprazole delayed-release tablets are instituted as treatment with these drugs may alleviate symptoms and delay diagnosis.

Genitourinary: In the 24-month toxicology study in rats, after 18 months of treatment, Leydig cell hyperplasia increased above the concurrent and historical control level at dosages of 15 mg/kg/day or higher.

Testicular interstitial cell adenoma also occurred in 1 of 30 rats treated with 50 mg/kg/day (13 times the recommended human dose based on body surface area) in a one-year toxicity study.

These changes are associated with endocrine alterations which have not been, to date, observed in humans.

Hepatic/Biliary/Pancreatic: Use in Patients with Hepatic Impairment: It is recommended that the initial dosing regimen need not be altered for patients with mild or moderate liver disease, but for patients with moderate impairment, doses higher than 30 mg per day should not be administered unless there are compelling clinical indications. Dose reduction in patients with severe hepatic disease should be considered.

Immune: Allergic reactions (including anaphylaxis) have been reported in patients receiving clarithromycin orally.

Serious and occasionally fatal hypersensitivity (anaphylactic) reactions have been reported in patients on penicillin therapy. These reactions are more apt to occur in individuals with a history of penicillin hypersensitivity and/or a history of sensitivity to multiple allergens.

There have been well documented reports of individuals with a history of penicillin hypersensitivity reactions who have experienced severe hypersensitivity reactions when treated with a cephalosporin. Before initiating therapy with any penicillin, careful inquiry should be made concerning previous hypersensitivity reactions to penicillins, cephalosporins, and other allergens. If an allergic reaction occurs, amoxicillin should be discontinued and the appropriate therapy instituted.

Serious anaphylactic reactions require immediate emergency treatment with epinephrine, oxygen, corticosteroids, and airway management, including intubation, as indicated.

Ophthalmologic: Retinal Atrophy: In animal studies, retinal atrophy was observed in rats dosed orally for 2 years with lansoprazole at doses of 15 mg/kg/day and above. These changes in rats are believed to be associated with the effects of taurine imbalance and phototoxicity in a susceptible animal model.

Clinical data available from long-term PREVACID (lansoprazole delayed-release capsules) studies are not suggestive of any drug-induced eye toxicity in humans. In humans, there are presently no concerns for ocular safety with short-term lansoprazole treatment and the risks associated with long-term use for nearly five years appear to be negligible.

The finding of drug-induced retinal atrophy in the albino rat is considered to be species-specific with little relevance for humans.

Renal: No dosage modification of lansoprazole is required in patients with renal insufficiency.

For the eradication of *H. pylori*, amoxicillin and clarithromycin should not be administered to patients with renal impairment since the appropriate dosage in this patient population has not yet been established.

Sensitivity/Resistance: Antibiotic Resistance in Relation to *H. pylori* Eradication: Three patients 3/82 (3.7%) who had isolates susceptible to clarithromycin pretreatment and were treated with the triple therapy regimen remained *H. pylori* positive posttreatment. None of the isolates from these three patients had susceptibility results available after treatment with triple therapy; therefore, it is unknown whether or not these patients developed resistance to clarithromycin. Sixteen percent of the patients treated with the dual therapy regimen developed clarithromycin resistance post-treatment. Therefore, development of clarithromycin resistance should be considered as a possible risk.

Use in Women: Over 4000 women were treated with lansoprazole. Ulcer healing rates in females are similar to those in males. The incidence rates of adverse events are also similar to those seen in males.

Special Populations: Pregnant Women: Reproductive studies conducted in pregnant rats at oral doses up to 150 mg/kg/day (40 times the recommended human dose based on body surface area), and in rabbits at oral doses up to 30 mg/kg/day (16 times the recommended human dose based on body surface area), did not disclose any evidence of a teratogenic effect. Maternal toxicity and a significant increase in fetal mortality were observed in the rabbit study at doses above 10 mg/kg/day. In rats, maternal toxicity and a slight reduction in litter survival and weights were noted at doses above 100 mg/kg/day.

There are no adequate or well-controlled studies in pregnant women. Therefore, lansoprazole should be used during pregnancy only if the potential benefit justifies the potential risk to the fetus.

Nursing Women: Lansoprazole or its metabolites are excreted in the milk of rats. It is not known whether lansoprazole is excreted in human milk. Because drugs are excreted in human milk, lansoprazole should not be given to nursing mothers unless its use is considered essential.

Pediatrics (1 to 17 years of age): Safety and effectiveness have been established in pediatric patients 1 year to 17 years for short-term up to 12 weeks of symptomatic GERD and erosive esophagitis. Use of lansoprazole in this population is supported by evidence of adequate and well controlled studies of lansoprazole in adults with additional clinical, pharmacokinetic, pharmacodynamic, and safety studies performed in pediatric patients. The adverse events (AEs) profile in pediatric patients is similar to that of adults. There were no adverse events reported in U.S. clinical studies that were not previously observed in adults. Dose safety and effectiveness have not been established in patients <1 year.

Geriatrics: Ulcer healing rates in elderly patients are similar to those in younger age groups. The incidence rates of adverse events and laboratory test abnormalities are also similar to those seen in other age groups. The initial dosing regimen need not be altered for elderly patients, but subsequent doses higher than 30 mg per day should not be administered unless additional gastric acid suppression is necessary.

ADVERSE REACTIONS: Adverse Drug Reaction Overview: Since 1991, lansoprazole has been approved in over 100 countries around the world, and about 250 million patients have been treated. Worldwide, over 10 000 patients have been treated with lansoprazole during Phase II-III short-term and long-term clinical trials involving various dosages and duration of treatment. In general, lansoprazole treatment has been well tolerated.

Clinical Trial Adverse Drug Reactions: Because clinical trials are conducted under very specific conditions the adverse reaction rates observed in the clinical trials may not reflect the rates observed in practice and should not be compared to the rates in the clinical trials of another drug. Adverse drug reaction information from clinical trials is useful for identifying drug-related adverse events and for approximating rates.

PREVACID (lansoprazole delayed-release capsules): Short-term Studies: The following adverse events were reported to have a possible or probable relationship to drug as described by the treating physician in 1% or more of lansoprazole delayed-release capsules-treated patients who participated in placebo- and positive-controlled trials (Table 2 and Table 3, respectively). Numbers in parentheses indicate the percentage of the adverse events reported.

Table 2: PREVACID

Incidence of Possibly or Probably Treatment-related Adverse Events in Short-term, Placebo-controlled Studies in Takeda[a] Safety Database

Body System/Adverse Event[b]	PREVACID[c] (n=817), N (%)	Placebo (n=254), N (%)
Body as a Whole		
Headache	63 (7.7)	31 (12.2)
Abdominal Pain	19 (2.3)	3 (1.2)
Digestive System		
Diarrhea	29 (3.5)	6 (2.4)
Nausea	9 (1.1)	5 (2.0)
Vomiting	7 (0.9)	3 (1.2)
Liver Function Tests Abnormal	2 (0.2)	3 (1.2)
Nervous System		
Dizziness	8 (1.0)	2 (0.8)

[a] Takeda Pharmaceuticals America Inc.
[b] Events reported by at least 1% of patients on either treatment are included.
[c] Doses 15 mg, 30 mg and 60 mg q.d. for 4-8 weeks.

In the Takeda Safety Database, all short-term, Phase II/III studies, one or more treatment-emergent AEs were reported by 715/1359 (52.6%) PREVACID-treated patients; of those considered to be possibly or probably treatment-related AEs, one or more were reported by 276/1359 (20.3%) PREVACID-treated patients. In all short-term, Phase II/III studies, one or more treatment-emergent AEs were reported by 150/254 (59.1%) placebo-treated patients; of those considered to be possibly or probably treatment-related AEs, one or more were reported by 56/254 (22.0%).

The most frequent AEs reported in the European short-term studies were diarrhea (3.3%), laboratory test abnormal (2.3%), headache (1.5%), constipation (1.2%), asthenia (1.1%), dizziness (1.1%), and abdominal pain (1.0%). The most frequent AEs reported in the Asian short-term studies were unspecified laboratory test abnormalities (7.3%), eosinophilia (1.0%), and increased ALT (1.0%).

Table 3: PREVACID

Incidence of Possibly or Probably Treatment-related Adverse Events in Short-term, Positive-controlled Studies in Takeda Safety Database

Body System/Adverse Event[a]	PREVACID[b] (n=647), N (%)	Ranitidine (n=393), N (%)
Body as a Whole		
Headache	26 (4.0)	14 (3.6)
Abdominal Pain	8 (1.2)	3 (0.8)
Digestive System		
Diarrhea	27 (4.2)	8 (2.0)
Nausea	7 (1.1)	4 (1.0)
Nervous System		
Dizziness	8 (1.2)	3 (0.8)
Skin and Appendages		

(cont'd)

Table 3: PREVACID *(cont'd)*

Incidence of Possibly or Probably Treatment-related Adverse Events in Short-term, Positive-controlled Studies in Takeda Safety Database

Body System/Adverse Event[a]	PREVACID[b] (n=647), N (%)	Ranitidine (n=393), N (%)
Rash	7 (1.1)	1 (0.3)

[a] Events reported by at least 1% of patients on either treatment are included.
[b] Doses 15 mg, 30 mg and 60 mg q.d. for 4-8 weeks.

NSAID-associated Gastric Ulcer Studies: The following tables summarize the most frequently reported treatment-emergent AEs in the two (2) Healing studies and the Reduction of Risk study (Table 4 and Table 5, respectively).

Table 4: PREVACID

Most Frequently Reported[a] Treatment-emergent AEs by Treatment Group and Dose in the Principal Healing of NSAID-associated Gastric Ulcer Studies[b]

Body System/ COSTART Term	Treatment Group % (n)		
	Ranitidine 150 mg b.i.d. (N=235)	Lansoprazole 15 mg q.d. (N=235)	Lansoprazole 30 mg q.d. (N=231)
Any Event	47% (110)	43% (102)	52% (120)
Body as a Whole			
Abdominal Pain	7% (17)	3% (7)	5% (11)
Digestive System			
Diarrhea	8% (19)	11% (25)	9% (21)
Respiratory System			
Pharyngitis	7% (16)	6% (13)	7% (17)

[a] Reported by ≥5% of patients in any treatment group.
[b] Treatment duration: 8 weeks.

Table 5: PREVACID

Most Frequently Reported[a] Treatment-emergent Adverse Events by Treatment Group and Dose in the Principal Reduction of Risk of NSAID-associated Gastric Ulcer Study[e]

Body System/ COSTART Term	Treatment Group % (n)			
	Placebo (N=133)	Misoprostol 200 µg q.i.d. (N=134)	Lansoprazole 15 mg q.d. (N=136)	Lansoprazole 30 mg q.d. (N=132)
Body as a Whole				
Abdominal Pain	7% (9)	10% (14)	7% (9)	6% (8)
Digestive System				
Diarrhea	7% (9)	25% (33)[b,c,d]	10% (14)	13% (17)
Nausea	5% (6)	6% (8)	1% (2)	5% (6)
Respiratory System				
Pharyngitis	3% (4)	9% (12)	7% (10)	9% (12)[b]
Sinusitis	2% (3)	2% (3)	5% (7)	6% (8)
Urogenital System				
Urinary Tract Infection	2% (2)	7% (9)[d]	4% (6)	1% (1)

[a] Reported by ≥5% of patients in any treatment group.
[b] Statistically significant difference vs placebo (p≤0.05).
[c] Statistically significant difference vs lansoprazole 15 mg q.d. (p≤0.05).
[d] Statistically significant difference vs lansoprazole 30 mg q.d. (p≤0.05).
[e] Treatment duration: 12 weeks.

Gastroesophageal Reflux Disease (GERD) Studies: U.S. Placebo-controlled Studies: All adverse events considered possibly/probably treatment-related with an incidence of at least 5% in any treatment group are displayed by COSTART body system and term and by treatment group in Table 6.

Table 6: PREVACID

Adverse Events Possibly/Probably Related to Treatment, Reported by ≥5% of Patients in the US Placebo-controlled Non-erosive GERD Studies

Body System/ COSTART Term	Placebo N=71 % (n)	Lansoprazole[b] N=249 % (n)
Total Patients		
Any Event	16.9 (12)	28.5 (71)[a]
Body as a Whole		
Abdominal Pain	1.4 (1)	6.0 (15)
Headache	7.0 (5)	7.6 (19)
Digestive System		
Diarrhea	2.8 (2)	5.2 (13)

[a] Statistically significantly different vs placebo at p=0.05 level.
[b] Doses 15 mg and 30 mg q.d. for 8 weeks.

The most commonly reported (incidence ≥5% in any treatment group) treatment-emergent adverse events for lansoprazole patients were headache (14.9%), pharyngitis (9.6%), abdominal pain (8.8%), diarrhea (7.6%) and rhinitis (6.4%) and for placebo patients were headache (9.9%) and pharyngitis (9.9%). There were no clinically or statistically significant differences between lansoprazole and placebo when evaluated for treatment-emergent adverse events.

U.S. Positive-controlled Studies: All possibly/probably treatment-related adverse events with an incidence of at least 5% in either treatments are displayed by body system, COSTART term, and treatment in Table 7.

Table 7: PREVACID

Most Frequently[a] Reported Possibly/Probably Treatment-related Adverse Events by Treatment in the Positive-controlled Non-erosive GERD Studies

Body System/ COSTART Term	Treatment % (n)	
	RAN (N=283)	LAN[c] (N=572)
Any Event	17 (49)	16 (91)
Body as a Whole		
Abdominal Pain	2 (5)	5 (29)[b]
Digestive System		
Diarrhea	6 (18)	4 (23)

[a] Reported by ≥5% of patients in any treatment.
[b] Statistically significantly different vs ranitidine at p=0.05 level.
[c] Doses 15 mg and 30 mg q.d. for 8 weeks.
Legend: RAN=ranitidine 150 mg b.i.d.; LAN=lansoprazole 15 mg and 30 mg daily.

The most frequently reported (≥5% of patients in any treatment) treatment-emergent adverse events for lansoprazole-treated patients were abdominal pain (9%), diarrhea (7%), and headache (6%) and for ranitidine-treated patients were diarrhea (9%), abdominal pain (7%), and headache (7%). There were no clinically or statistically significant differences between lansoprazole- and ranitidine-treated patients in the percentage of patients reporting specific treatment-emergent adverse events.

Maintenance Studies: U.S. Studies: Treatment-emergent AEs with an incidence of at least 2% in any treatment group of the maintenance treatment studies occurring from the start of maintenance treatment to the first recurrence of disease are displayed by body system and COSTART term, and by treatment group in Table 8.

There were no frequently reported (≥2.0%, incidence) severe AEs in the treatment-emergent or the possibly/probably treatment-related event categories with onset at any point from the start of maintenance treatment to the time of first recurrence of disease.

Table 8: PREVACID

Treatment-emergent Adverse Effects Reported by ≥2% of the Placebo and Lansoprazole Patients to the Time of First Recurrence of Disease[a] in the Maintenance Treatment Studies

Treatment Group	Placebo	Lansoprazole
Mean Exposure (Days)	CUM[b] N=236 105.4	CUM[b] N=386 267.5
Body System/COSTART Term	**% (n)**	**% (n)**
Total Patients		
Any Event	39.4 (93)	70.5 (272)
Body as a Whole		
Abdominal Pain	3.0 (7)	5.2 (20)
Accidental Injury	2.1 (5)	5.4 (21)
Back Pain	4.2 (10)	3.1 (12)
Chest Pain	0.8 (2)	2.3 (9)
Flu Syndrome	3.8 (9)	7.3 (28)
Headache	6.4 (15)	11.4 (44)
Infection	1.3 (3)	2.1 (8)
Pain	0.8 (2)	2.6 (10)
Digestive System		
Diarrhea	5.5 (13)	9.8 (38)
Gastrointestinal Anomaly (polyp)	0.8 (2)	4.4 (17)
Nausea	1.3 (3)	2.8 (11)
Tooth Disorder	0.4 (1)	2.1 (8)
Vomiting	0.4 (1)	3.4 (13)
Musculoskeletal System		

(cont'd)

Table 8: PREVACID *(cont'd)*

Treatment-emergent Adverse Effects Reported by ≥2% of the Placebo and Lansoprazole Patients to the Time of First Recurrence of Disease[a] in the Maintenance Treatment Studies

Treatment Group	Placebo	Lansoprazole
	CUM[b] N=236	CUM[b] N=386
Mean Exposure (Days)	105.4	267.5
Body System/COSTART Term	% (n)	% (n)
Arthralgia	1.3 (3)	4.4 (17)
Myalgia	1.3 (3)	2.1 (8)
Nervous System		
Dizziness	0.4 (1)	2.8 (11)
Respiratory System		
Bronchitis	1.3 (3)	3.1 (12)
Cough Increased	0	2.3 (9)
Pharyngitis	9.3 (22)	17.1 (66)
Rhinitis	1.3 (3)	5.7 (22)
Sinusitis	2.5 (6)	6.5 (25)
Skin and Appendages		
Rash	3.0 (7)	4.7 (18)
Urogenital System		
Urinary Tract Infection	2.5 (6)	4.1 (16)

[a] Until time of first recurrence, withdrawal or end of maintenance treatment.
[b] CUM=cumulative.

European Studies: The AEs reported by at least 2% of patients in any treatment group are displayed by COSTART body system and term and by treatment group for controlled long-term European Studies in Table 9.

Table 9: PREVACID

Treatment-emergent Adverse Effects Reported by ≥2% of Patients Treated with H_2-Receptor Antagonists or Lansoprazole in Long-term, Phase II/III H_2-Receptor Antagonist Controlled European Studies

Treatment Group	Lansoprazole (N=263)	H_2-Receptor Antagonists (N=161)
Body System/COSTART Term	% (n)	% (n)
Total Patients		
Any Event	49.8 (131)	46.6 (75)
Body as a Whole		
Abdominal Pain	3.0 (8)	3.7 (6)
Back Pain	2.3 (6)	0.6 (1)
Accidental Injury	1.5 (4)	2.5 (4)
Infection	1.1 (3)	3.1 (5)
Cardiovascular System		
Hypertension	1.9 (5)	2.5 (4)
Digestive System		
Diarrhea	9.1 (24)	4.3 (7)
Gastritis	5.3 (14)	1.2 (2)
Constipation	2.7 (7)	2.5 (4)
Vomiting	1.9 (5)	3.1 (5)
Dyspepsia	1.1 (3)	3.1 (5)
Musculoskeletal System		
Arthralgia	1.9 (5)	2.5 (4)
Nervous System		
Dizziness	1.9 (5)	2.5 (4)
Respiratory System		
Respiratory Disorder	2.3 (6)	3.1 (5)
Cough Increased	1.1 (3)	2.5 (4)

The AEs reported by at least 1% of patients receiving lead-in open-label lansoprazole treatment in long-term European Studies are diarrhea (5.7%), esophagitis (2.5%), abdominal pain (2.1%), gastritis (2.1%), flatulence (1.3%), headache (1.1%), constipation (1.0%), and nausea (1.0%). The incidence of AEs reported in the lead-in open-label period of the European studies was similar to that seen in controlled studies, however, the overall incidence was lower for the lead-in open-label studies than for the H_2-RA controlled studies (27.5% versus 49.8%, respectively).

PREVACID FasTab (lansoprazole delayed-release tablets): Adverse events from two bioequivalency studies performed in healthy volunteers are listed in Table 10.

The incidence of adverse events between the test 15 mg lansoprazole delayed-release orally disintegrating tablets and the reference 15 mg lansoprazole delayed-release capsule (8% and 3%, respectively) was similar and are summarized in Table 10.

The incidence of adverse events between the test 30 mg lansoprazole delayed-release orally disintegrating tablets and the reference 30 mg lansoprazole delayed-release capsule (0% and 2%, respectively) was similar and are summarized in Table 10.

Table 10: PREVACID FasTab

Summary of Adverse Events by Regimen, COSTART Term, Number of Subjects, Percentage, and Incidence

Regimen/N	COSTART term	N [percentage]	Overall N [incidence]
15 mg lansoprazole delayed-release orally disintegrating tablets (test)/60	Headache	4 [7%]	5 [8%]
	Nausea	2 [3%]	
	Epistaxis	1 [2%]	
15 mg lansoprazole delayed-release capsules (reference)/60	Headache	2 [3%]	2 [3%]
	Nausea	1 [2%]	
30 mg lansoprazole delayed-release orally disintegrating tablets (test)/60	N/A	0 [0%]	0 [0%]
30 mg lansoprazole delayed-release capsules (reference)/60	Hyperlipemia	1 [2%]	1 [2%]

Pediatrics: The adverse event profile in pediatric patients resembled that of adults taking lansoprazole. The most frequently reported (2 or more patients) treatment-related adverse events in patients 1 to 11 years of age (N=66) were constipation (5%) and headache (3%). There were no adverse events reported in this U.S. clinical study that were not previously observed in adults.

The most frequently reported (at least 3%) treatment-related adverse events in patients 12-17 years of age (N=87) were headache (7%), abdominal pain (5%), nausea (3%) and dizziness (3%). Treatment-related dizziness, reported as occurring in <1% of adult patients, was reported in this study by 3 adolescent patients with nonerosive GERD, who had dizziness concurrently with other events (such as migraine, dyspnea, and vomiting).

In another study, an 8½-year-old female experienced moderate hot flashes and arterial hypertension after receiving lansoprazole 17.7 mg/m² for 5 days. However, blood pressure values were not recorded. The investigator considered the event possibly related to study drug. Study drug was discontinued and the symptoms resolved. This child experienced the same side effects at a later date when treated with ranitidine.

Less Common Clinical Trial Adverse Drug Reactions (<1%): PREVACID (lansoprazole delayed-release capsules) and PREVACID FasTab (lansoprazole delayed-release tablets): Additional adverse experiences occurring in <1% of patients or subjects in domestic and/or international trials, or occurring since the drug was marketed, are shown below within each body system. (Other adverse reactions have been observed during post-marketing surveillance. Please also refer to Post-market Adverse Drug Reactions.)

Body as a Whole: abdomen enlarged, allergic reaction, asthenia, candidiasis, carcinoma, chest pain (not otherwise specified), chills, edema, fever, flu syndrome, general pain, halitosis, infection (not otherwise specified), malaise, neck pain, neck rigidity, pelvic pain.

Cardiovascular System: angina, arrhythmia, bradycardia, cerebrovascular accident/cerebral infarction, hypertension/hypotension, migraine, myocardial infarction, palpitations, shock (circulatory failure), tachycardia, vasodilation.

Digestive System: abnormal stools, anorexia, bezoar, carcinoid, cardiospasm, cholelithiasis, colitis, constipation, dry mouth/thirst, dyspepsia, dysphagia, enteritis, eructation, esophageal stenosis, esophageal ulcer, esophagitis, fecal discoloration, flatulence, gastric nodules/fundic gland polyps, gastroenteritis, gastrointestinal disorder, gastrointestinal hemorrhage, glossitis, gum hemorrhage, hematemesis, increased appetite, increased salivation, melena, mouth ulceration, oral monoliasis, rectal disorder, rectal hemorrhage, stomatitis, tenesmus, tongue disorder, ulcerative colitis, ulcerative stomatitis.

Endocrine System: diabetes mellitus, goiter, hyperglycemia/hypoglycemia, hypothyroidism.

Hematologic and Lymphatic Systems: *anemia, hemolysis, lymphadenopathy.

Metabolic and Nutritional Disorders: gout, dehydration, peripheral edema, weight gain/loss.

Musculoskeletal System: arthritis/arthralgia, bone disorder, joint disorder, leg cramps, musculoskeletal pain, myalgia, myasthenia, synovitis.

Nervous System: abnormal dreams, agitation, amnesia, anxiety, apathy, confusion, convulsion, depersonalization, depression, diplopia, dizziness, emotional lability, hallucinations, hemiplegia, hostility aggravated, hyperkinesia, hypertonia, hypesthesia, insomnia, libido decreased, libido increased, nervousness, neurosis, paresthesia, sleep disorder, somnolence, syncope, thinking abnormality, tremor, vertigo.

Respiratory System: asthma, bronchitis, cough increased, dyspnea, epistaxis, hemoptysis, hiccup, laryngeal neoplasia, pleural disorder, pneumonia, stridor, upper respiratory inflammation/infection.

Skin and Appendages: acne, alopecia, contact dermatitis, dry skin, fixed eruption, hair disorder, maculopapular rash, nail disorder, pruritus, rash, skin carcinoma, skin disorder, sweating, urticaria.

Special Senses: abnormal vision, blurred vision, conjunctivitis, deafness, dry eyes, ear disorder, eye pain, ophthalmologic disorders, otitis media, parosmia, photophobia, retinal degeneration, taste loss, taste perversion, tinnitus, visual field defect.

Urogenital System: abnormal menses, breast enlargement/gynecomastia, breast tenderness, dysmenorrhea, dysuria, impotence, kidney calculus, kidney pain, leukorrhea, menorrhagia, menstrual disorder, penis disorder, polyuria, testis disorder, urethral pain, urinary frequency, urination impaired, urinary urgency, vaginitis.

Combination Therapy with Clarithromycin and Amoxicillin: In clinical trials using combination therapy with lansoprazole delayed-release capsules plus clarithromycin and amoxicillin, and lansoprazole delayed-release capsules plus amoxicillin, no adverse reactions related to these drug combinations were observed. Adverse reactions that have occurred have been limited to those that have been previously reported with lansoprazole delayed-release capsules, clarithromycin, or amoxicillin.

For more information on adverse reactions with clarithromycin or amoxicillin, refer to their respective Product Monographs, under the Adverse Reactions section.

Triple Therapy: PREVACID/clarithromycin/amoxicillin: The most frequently reported adverse events for patients who received triple therapy were diarrhea (7%), headache (6%), and taste perversion (5%). Patients in the 7-day triple therapy regimen reported fewer adverse events than those in the 10 and/or 14-day triple therapy regimens. There were no statistically significant differences in the frequency of reported adverse events between the 10 and 14-day triple therapy regimens.

Abnormal Hematologic and Clinical Chemistry Findings: In addition, the following changes in laboratory parameters were reported as adverse events. Abnormal liver function tests, increased AST, increased ALT, increased creatinine, increased alkaline phosphatase, increased gamma globulins, increased GGTP, increased/decreased/abnormal WBC, abnormal AG ratio, abnormal RBC, bilirubinemia, eosinophilia, hyperlipemia, increased/decreased electrolytes, increased/decreased cholesterol, increased glucocorticoids, increased LDH, increased/decreased/abnormal platelets, and increased gastrin levels. Urine abnormalities such as albuminuria, glycosuria, and hematuria were also reported. Additional isolated laboratory abnormalities were reported.

In the placebo controlled studies, when AST and ALT were evaluated, 0.4% (4/978) placebo patients and 0.3% (11/2677) lansoprazole patients had enzyme elevations greater than three times the upper limit of normal range at the final treatment visit. None of these lansoprazole patients reported jaundice at any time during the study.

For more information on laboratory value changes with clarithromycin or amoxicillin, refer to their respective Product Monographs, under the Adverse Reactions section.

* The majority of hematologic cases received were foreign-sourced and their relationship to lansoprazole was unclear.

The rate of increased liver function results in the U.S. clinical studies is low: 4.5% in EE patients and 3.6% in healthy subjects. Only 3 of the LFT abnormals were >3× of upper normal limit, and only one of them was considered possibly related to the study drug. However, a repeat of the laboratory tests for this subject revealed results within normal laboratory range.

Post-market Adverse Drug Reactions: These events were reported during postmarketing surveillance. Estimates of frequency cannot be made since such events are reported voluntarily from a population of unknown size. Due to the uncontrolled nature of spontaneous reports, a clear causal relationship to lansoprazole cannot be established.

Body as a Whole: hypersensitivity reactions, including anaphylaxis.

Digestive System: colitis, hepatotoxicity, pancreatitis, vomiting.

Hematologic and Lymphatic Systems: agranulocytosis, aplastic anemia, hemolytic anemia, leukopenia, neutropenia, pancytopenia, thrombocytopenia, and thrombotic thrombocytopenic purpura.

Musculoskeletal System: myositis.

Skin and Appendages: severe dermatologic reactions including erythema multiforme, Stevens-Johnson syndrome, toxic epidermal necrolysis (some fatal).

Special Senses: speech disorder.

Urogenital System: urinary retention, interstitial nephritis.

In an estimated exposure of 240 million patients worldwide (in both postmarketing surveillance and the clinical trials), the most commonly reported ophthalmic adverse events are amblyopia (13) and vision blurred (67) according to the MedDRA terminology. All the 13 cases of amblyopia had the reported term/verbatim "blurred or smeary vision". Only two of these 13 reports were considered serious, and both are foreign-sourced reports with very little information provided. Among the 67 reports with the "vision blurred", 10 were considered serious and might be related to optic neuritis/neuropathy, whether or not believed related to the drug. In two of these ten cases, one of the examining ophthalmologists proposed a diagnosis of AION. Eight out of the ten cases were foreign-sourced. Only two US-sourced serious cases involved the report of blurred vision. Both were consumer reports without any detailed information. No physician assessed any causality in either case.

DRUG INTERACTIONS: Overview: Lansoprazole is metabolized through the cytochrome P450 system, specifically through CYP3A and CYP2C19. Studies have shown that lansoprazole does not have clinically significant interactions with other drugs metabolized by the cytochrome P450 system such as warfarin, antipyrine, indomethacin, acetylsalicylic acid, ibuprofen, phenytoin, prednisone, antacids (Maalox and Riopan), diazepam, clarithromycin, propranolol, amoxicillin or terfenadine in healthy subjects. These compounds are metabolized through various cytochrome P450 isozymes including CYP1A2, CYP2C9, CYP2C19, CYP2D6, and CYP3A.

Lansoprazole causes a profound and long lasting inhibition of gastric acid secretion; therefore, it is theoretically possible that lansoprazole may interfere with the absorption of drugs where gastric pH is an important determinant of bioavailability (e.g., ketoconazole, ampicillin esters, iron salts, digoxin).

Drug-Drug Interactions: When lansoprazole was administered concomitantly with theophylline (CYP1A2, CYP3A), a minor increase (10%) in the clearance of theophylline was seen, which is unlikely to be of clinical concern. Nonetheless, individual patients may require adjustment of their theophylline dosage when lansoprazole is started or stopped to ensure clinically effective blood levels.

In a single-dose crossover study when 30 mg of lansoprazole was administered concomitantly with one gram of sucralfate in healthy volunteers, absorption of lansoprazole was delayed and its bioavailability was reduced. The value of lansoprazole AUC was reduced by 17% and that for C_{max} was reduced by 21%.

In a similar study when 30 mg of lansoprazole was administered concomitantly with 2 grams of sucralfate, lansoprazole AUC and C_{max} were reduced by 32% and 55%, respectively. When lansoprazole dosing occurred 30 minutes prior to sucralfate administration, C_{max} was reduced by only 28% and there was no statistically significant difference in lansoprazole AUC. Therefore, lansoprazole may be given concomitantly with antacids but should be administered at least 30 minutes prior to sucralfate.

Lansoprazole causes long-lasting inhibition of gastric acid secretion. Lansoprazole substantially decreases the systemic concentrations of the HIV protease inhibitor atazanavir, which is dependent upon the presence of gastric acid for absorption, and may result in a loss of therapeutic effect of atazanavir and the development of HIV resistance. Therefore, lansoprazole should not be co-administered with atazanavir. This appears to be a class effect. It is theoretically possible that lansoprazole may also interfere with the absorption of other drugs where gastric pH is an important determinant of bioavailability (e.g., ketoconazole, ampicillin esters, iron salts, digoxin).

In a study of healthy subjects neither the pharmacokinetics of warfarin enantiomers nor prothrombin time were affected following single or multiple 60 mg doses of lansoprazole. However, there have been reports of increased International Normalized Ratio (INR) and prothrombin time in patients receiving proton pump inhibitors, including lansoprazole, and warfarin concomitantly. Increases in INR and prothrombin time may lead to abnormal bleeding and even death. Patients treated with proton pump inhibitors and warfarin concomitantly may need to be monitored for increases in INR and prothrombin time.

Combination Therapy with Clarithromycin and/or Amoxicillin: For more information on drug interactions for clarithromycin and amoxicillin, refer to their respective Product Monographs, under Drug Interactions.

Drug-Food Interactions: Food reduces the peak concentration and the extent of absorption by about 50% to 70%. Therefore, it is recommended that lansoprazole delayed-release capsules be administered in the morning prior to breakfast.

DOSAGE AND ADMINISTRATION: Dosing Considerations: Duodenal Ulcer: *H. pylori* Eradication to Reduce the Risk of Duodenal Ulcer Recurrence: Triple Therapy: PREVACID/clarithromycin/amoxicillin: For the eradication of *H. pylori*, amoxicillin and clarithromycin should not be administered to patients with renal impairment since the appropriate dosage in this patient population has not yet been established.

Gastric Ulcer: Lansoprazole is not indicated for maintenance therapy in the treatment of patients with gastric ulcer.

Recommended Dose and Dosage Adjustment: Oral Administration: PREVACID (lansoprazole delayed-release capsules) and PREVACID FasTab (lansoprazole delayed-release tablets) should be taken daily before breakfast. Where the product may be used twice daily, it should be taken prior to breakfast and another meal. PREVACID capsules and PREVACID FasTab **should not be crushed or chewed**.

Duodenal Ulcer: The recommended adult oral dose is 15 mg daily before breakfast for two to four weeks (see Indications and Clinical Use).

A small percentage of patients that are *H. pylori* negative will experience a disease recurrence and will require maintenance treatment with an antisecretory agent. Lansoprazole 15 mg daily before breakfast may be used up to one year for the maintenance treatment of recurrent duodenal ulcers.

***H. pylori* Eradication to Reduce the Risk of Duodenal Ulcer Recurrence: Triple Therapy: PREVACID/clarithromycin/amoxicillin:** The recommended adult oral dose is 30 mg lansoprazole, 500 mg clarithromycin, and 1 g amoxicillin, all given twice daily for 7, 10 or 14 days (see Indications and Clinical Use). Daily doses should be taken before meals. **(For additional information on triple therapy for the treatment of *H. pylori* infection and active duodenal ulcer recurrence, refer to the Hp-PAC Product Monograph.)**

Gastric Ulcer: The recommended adult oral dose is 15 mg daily before breakfast for four to eight weeks.

No dosage adjustment is necessary in patients with renal insufficiency. No dosage adjustment is necessary in the initial lansoprazole dosing regimen for older patients and for patients with mild to moderate hepatic impairment. Dosing recommendations described in the labelling should be adhered to for older patients and patients with hepatic impairment.

NSAID-associated Gastric Ulcer: The issue of whether or not eradication of *H. pylori* in patients with NSAID-associated ulcers might have beneficial effects remains unresolved (Chan et al, 2001).

Healing of NSAID-associated Gastric Ulcer: The recommended adult oral dose is 15 mg to 30 mg once daily before breakfast for up to 8 weeks. A trend for higher healing rates (4% and 12%, two studies) was observed with the 30 mg dose, as compared to the 15 mg dose.

Reduction of Risk of NSAID-associated Gastric Ulcer: The recommended adult oral dose is 15 mg once daily before breakfast for up to 12 weeks.

Reflux Esophagitis or Poorly Responsive Reflux Esophagitis Including Patients with Barrett's Esophagus: The recommended adult oral dose is 30 mg daily before breakfast for four to eight weeks (see Indications and Clinical Use).

Maintenance Treatment of Healed Reflux Esophagitis: For the long-term management of patients with healed reflux esophagitis, 15 mg lansoprazole given once daily before breakfast has been found to be effective in controlled clinical trials of 12 months' duration.

The recommended adult oral dose of lansoprazole for maintenance treatment of patients with healed reflux esophagitis is 15 mg daily before breakfast (see Indications and Clinical Use).

Treatment and Maintenance of Pathological Hypersecretory Conditions Including Zollinger-Ellison Syndrome: The dosage of lansoprazole in patients with pathologic hypersecretory conditions varies with the individual patient. The recommended adult oral starting dose is 60 mg once a day. Doses should be adjusted to individual patient needs and should continue for as long as clinically indicated. Dosages up to 90 mg b.i.d. have been administered. Daily dosages of greater than 120 mg should be administered in divided doses. Some patients with Zollinger-Ellison syndrome have been treated continuously with lansoprazole for more than four years.

Gastroesophageal Reflux Disease (GERD): Short-term Treatment of Symptomatic GERD: The recommended adult oral dose for the treatment of heartburn and other symptoms associated with GERD is 15 mg daily before breakfast for up to 8 weeks. If significant symptom relief is not obtained within 4 to 8 weeks, further investigation is recommended.

Pediatric GERD (erosive and non-erosive esophagitis): Children 1 to 11 Years of Age: The recommended pediatric oral dose for children 1 to 11 years of age is 15 mg (≤30 kg) and 30 mg (>30 kg) once daily for up to 12 weeks. An increase in dose may be beneficial in some children.

Children 12 to 17 Years of Age: For adolescents of 12 to 17 years, the same approved regimen for adults can be used.

Patients with Hepatic Impairment: The daily dose of lansoprazole should not exceed 30 mg (see Warnings and Precautions).

Patients with Renal Impairment: No dosage modification of lansoprazole is necessary (see Warnings and Precautions).

Elderly Patients: The daily dose should not exceed 30 mg (see Warnings and Precautions).

Administration: Oral Formulation: PREVACID (lansoprazole delayed-release capsules) and PREVACID FasTab (lansoprazole delayed-release tablets) should be taken daily before breakfast. Where the product may be used twice daily, it should be taken prior to breakfast and another meal. PREVACID capsules and PREVACID FasTab **should not be crushed or chewed**.

Alternative Administration Options: For adults and children who have difficulty swallowing capsules, there are 2 options.

Option 1. PREVACID (lansoprazole delayed-release capsules): Lansoprazole delayed-release capsules can be opened, and the intact granules contained within can be sprinkled on one tablespoon of applesauce and swallowed immediately. The granules should not be chewed or crushed.

For patients who have a nasogastric tube in place, lansoprazole delayed-release capsules can be opened and the intact granules mixed in 40 mL of apple juice or water and injected through the nasogastric tube into the stomach. After administering the granules, the nasogastric tube should be flushed with additional apple juice or water to clear the tube.

The granules have also been shown in vitro to remain intact for up to 30 minutes when exposed to apple, cranberry, grape, orange, pineapple, prune, tomato, and V-8 vegetable juice.

Option 2. PREVACID FasTab (lansoprazole delayed-release tablets): Lansoprazole delayed-release tablets are available in 15 mg and 30 mg strengths. PREVACID FasTab should not be chewed. Place the tablet on the tongue and allow it to disintegrate with or without water until the particles can be swallowed. Lansoprazole delayed-release tablets are not designed to be swallowed intact or chewed. The tablet typically disintegrates in less than 1 minute.

Do not chew the granules.

Alternatively, for children or other patients who have difficulty swallowing tablets, PREVACID FasTab can also be delivered in two different ways.

PREVACID FasTab—Oral Syringe: For administration via oral syringe, PREVACID FasTab can be administered as follows:

- Place a 15 mg tablet in oral syringe and draw up approximately 4 mL of water, or place a 30 mg tablet in oral syringe and draw up approximately 10 mL of water.
- Shake gently to allow for a quick dispersal.
- After the tablet has dispersed, administer the contents within 15 minutes.
- Refill the syringe with approximately 2 mL (5 mL for the 30 mg tablet) of water, shake gently, and administer any remaining contents.

PREVACID FasTab—Nasogastric Tube Administration (≥8 French): For administration via a nasogastric tube, PREVACID FasTab can be administered as follows:

- Place a 15 mg tablet in a syringe and draw up 4 mL of water, or place a 30 mg tablet in a syring and draw up 10 mL of water.
- Shake gently to allow for a quick dispersal.
- After the tablet has dispersed, inject through the nasogastric tube into the stomach within 15 minutes.
- Refill the syringe with approximately 5 mL of water, shake gently, and flush the nasogastric tube.

Concomitant Antacid Use: Simultaneous administration of lansoprazole with Maalox (aluminum and magnesium hydroxide) or Riopan (magaldrate) results in lower peak plasma levels, but does not significantly reduce bioavailability. Antacids may be used concomitantly if required. If sucralfate is to be given concomitantly, lansoprazole should be administered at least 30 minutes prior to sucralfate (see Actions and Clinical Pharmacology, Absorption with Antacids). In clinical trials, antacids were administered concomitantly with lansoprazole delayed-release capsules; this did not interfere with its effect.

OVERDOSAGE:

As in all cases where overdosing is suspected, treatment should be supportive and symptomatic. Any unabsorbed material should be removed from the gastrointestinal tract, and the patient should be carefully monitored. Lansoprazole is not removed from the circulation by hemodialysis. In one reported case of overdose, the patient consumed 600 mg of lansoprazole with no adverse reaction

Oral Administration: Oral doses up to 5000 mg/kg in rats (approximately 1300 times the recommended human dose based on body surface area) and mice (about 675.7 times the recommended human dose based on body surface area) did not produce deaths or any clinical signs.

For management of a suspected drug overdose, CPhA recommends that you contact your **regional Poison Control Centre**. See the *CPS* Directory section for a list of Poison Control Centres.

ACTION AND CLINICAL PHARMACOLOGY: Mechanism of Action: PREVACID (lansoprazole delayed-release capsules) and PREVACID FasTab (lansoprazole delayed-release tablets inhibit the gastric H^+, K^+-ATPase (the proton pump) which catalyzes the exchange of H^+ and K^+. They are effective in the inhibition of both basal acid secretion and stimulated acid secretion.

Pharmacodynamics: In healthy subjects, single and multiple doses of lansoprazole delayed-release capsules (15 mg to 60 mg) have been shown to decrease significantly basal gastric acid output and to increase significantly mean gastric pH and percent of time at pH >3 and 4. These doses have also been shown to reduce significantly meal-stimulated gastric acid output and gastric secretion volume. Single or multiple doses of lansoprazole delayed-release capsules (10 mg to 60 mg) reduced pentagastrin-stimulated acid output. In addition, lansoprazole delayed-release capsules have been demonstrated to reduce significantly basal and pentagastrin-stimulated gastric acid secretion among Duodenal Ulcer (DU) and hypersecretory patients, and basal gastric acid secretion among patients with Gastric Ulcer (GU) disease.

A dose-response effect was analyzed by considering the results from clinical pharmacology studies that evaluated more than one dose of lansoprazole delayed-release capsules. The results indicated that, in general, as the dose was increased from 7.5 mg to 30 mg, there was a decrease in mean gastric acid secretion and an increase in the average time spent at higher pH values (pH >4).

The results of pharmacodynamic studies with lansoprazole delayed-release capsules in normal subjects suggest that doses of 7.5 to 10 mg are substantially less effective in inhibiting gastric acid secretion than doses of 15 mg or greater. In view of these results, the doses of lansoprazole delayed-release capsules evaluated in the principal clinical trials ranged from 15 mg to 60 mg daily.

Eradication of *H. pylori*: *H. pylori* is considered to be a major factor in the etiology of duodenal ulcer disease. The presence of *H. pylori* may damage the mucosal integrity due to the production of enzymes (catalase, lipases, phospholipases, proteases, and urease), adhesins and toxins; the inflammatory response generated in this manner contributes to mucosal damage.

The concomitant administration of an antimicrobial(s) and an antisecretory agent such as lansoprazole, improves the eradication of *H. pylori* as compared to individual drug administration. The higher pH resulting from antisecretory treatment, optimizes the environment for the pharmacologic action of the antimicrobial agent(s) against *H. pylori*.

Pharmacokinetics: Lansoprazole delayed-release capsules and lansoprazole delayed-release tablets contain an enteric-coated granule formulation of lansoprazole to ensure that absorption of lansoprazole begins only after the granules leave the stomach (lansoprazole is acid-labile). Peak plasma concentrations of lansoprazole (C_{max}) and the area under the plasma concentration curve (AUC) of lansoprazole are approximately proportional in doses from 15 mg to 60 mg after single-oral administration. Lansoprazole pharmacokinetics are unaltered by multiple dosing and the drug does not accumulate.

Lansoprazole delayed-release capsules are highly bioavailable when administered orally. In a definitive absolute bioavailability study, the absolute bioavailability was shown to be 86% for a 15 mg capsule and 80% for a 30-mg capsule. First pass effect is apparently minimal.

Lansoprazole Delayed-release Capsules: Table 11 summarizes the pharmacokinetic parameters (T_{max}, $T_{1/2}$, AUC and C_{max}) of lansoprazole delayed-release capsules in healthy subjects.

Lansoprazole Delayed-release Tablets: In two bioavailability studies, lansoprazole delayed-release orally disintegrating 15 mg and 30 mg tablets were found to be bioequivalent to the lansoprazole delayed-release 15 mg and 30 mg capsules, respectively with respect to C_{max}, AUC_t, and AUC_∞.

Absorption: The absorption of lansoprazole is rapid, with mean peak plasma levels of lansoprazole occurring at approximately 1.7 hours. Peak plasma concentrations of lansoprazole (C_{max}) and the area under the plasma concentration curve (AUC) are approximately proportional to dose throughout the range that has been studied (up to 60 mg).

Table 11: PREVACID

Pharmacokinetic Parameters of Lansoprazole Delayed-release Capsules Pooled Across Phase I Studies

Parameter	T_{max} (h)	$T_{½}$ (h)	AUC[a] (ng·h/mL)	C_{max}[a] (ng/mL)
Mean	1.68	1.53	2133	824
Median	1.50	1.24	1644	770
SD	0.80	1.01	1797	419
% CV	47.71	65.92	84.28	50.81
Min	0.50	0.39	213	27
Max	6.00	8.50	14 203	2440
N[b]	345	285	513	515

[a] Normalized to a 30 mg dose.
[b] Number of dosages associated with a parameter.

Absorption with Food: Food reduces the peak concentration and the extent of absorption by about 50% to 70%. Moreover, the results of a pharmacokinetic study that compared the bioavailability of lansoprazole following a.m. dosing (fasting) versus p.m. dosing (three hours after a meal) indicated that both C_{max} and AUC values were increased by approximately two-fold or more with a.m. dosing. Therefore, it is recommended that lansoprazole delayed-release capsules be administered in the morning prior to breakfast.

Absorption with Antacids: Simultaneous administration of lansoprazole delayed-release capsules with Maalox (aluminum and magnesium hydroxide) or Riopan (magaldrate) resulted in lower peak serum levels, but did not significantly reduce the bioavailability of lansoprazole.

In a single-dose crossover study when 30 mg of lansoprazole was administered concomitantly with one gram of sucralfate in healthy volunteers, absorption of lansoprazole was delayed and its bioavailability was reduced. The value of lansoprazole AUC was reduced by 17% and that for C_{max} was reduced by 21%.

In a similar study when 30 mg of lansoprazole was administered concomitantly with 2 grams of sucralfate, lansoprazole AUC and C_{max} were reduced by 32% and 55%, respectively. When lansoprazole dosing occurred 30 minutes prior to sucralfate administration, C_{max} was reduced by only 28% and there was no statistically significant difference in lansoprazole AUC. Therefore, lansoprazole may be given concomitantly with antacids but should be administered at least 30 minutes prior to sucralfate.

Distribution: The apparent volume of distribution of lansoprazole is approximately 15.7 (±1.9) L, distributing mainly in extracellular fluid. Lansoprazole is 97% bound to plasma proteins. The mean total body clearance (CL) of lansoprazole was calculated at 31±8 L/h, and the volume of distribution (V_{ss}) was calculated to be 29 (±4) L.

Metabolism: Lansoprazole is extensively metabolized in the liver. Two metabolites have been identified in measurable quantities in plasma; the hydroxylated sulfinyl and the sulfone derivatives of lansoprazole. These metabolites have very little or no antisecretory activity. Within the parietal cell canaliculus, lansoprazole is thought to be transformed into two active metabolites that inhibit acid secretion by H^+, K^+-ATPase, but these metabolites are not present in the systemic circulation. The plasma elimination half-life of lansoprazole does not reflect the duration of suppression of gastric acid secretion. Thus, the plasma elimination half-life is less than two hours while the acid inhibitory effect lasts over 24 hours.

Excretion: Following single dose oral administration of lansoprazole, virtually no unchanged lansoprazole was excreted in the urine. After a 30 mg single oral dose of ^{14}C-lansoprazole, approximately one-third of the dose was excreted in the urine and approximately two-thirds were recovered in the feces. This implies a significant biliary excretion of the metabolites of lansoprazole.

Following a 30 mg single intravenous dose of lansoprazole, the mean clearance was 11.1 (±3.8) L/h.

Special Populations and Conditions: Pediatrics: The pharmacokinetics of lansoprazole were studied in pediatric patients with Gastroesophageal Reflux Disease (GERD) aged 1 to 11 years, with lansoprazole doses of 15 mg q.d. for subjects weighing ≤30 kg and 30 mg q.d. for subjects weighing >30 kg. The pharmacokinetics were also studied in adolescents aged 12-17 years with GERD following 15 mg or 30 mg q.d.of lansoprazole.

Pharmacokinetic parameters for lansoprazole following 15 or 30 mg q.d. doses of lansoprazole to children aged 1 to 11 years and adolescents aged 12 to 17 years, as well as those observed from healthy adult subjects, are summarized in Table 12.

Table 12: PREVACID

Mean±SD Pharmacokinetic Parameters of Lansoprazole in Children, Adolescents and Adults

Pharmacokinetic Parameter	Children Aged 1 to 11 yrs (M97-808)		Adolescents Aged 12 to 17 yrs (M97-640)		Healthy Adults Aged ≥18 yrs
	15 mg[a]	30 mg[a]	15 mg	30 mg	30 mg[b]
T_{max} (h)	1.5±0.7	1.7±0.7	1.6± 0.7	1.7± 0.7	1.7± 0.8
C_{max} (ng/mL)	790.9± 435.4	898.5± 437.7	414.8± 215.5	1005± 604.9	824± 419
C_{max}/D (ng/mL/mg)	—	—	27.7± 14.4	33.5± 20.2	27.5± 14.0
AUC (ng·h/mL)	1707± 1689	1883± 1159	1017± 1737	2490± 2522	2133± 1797
AUC/D (ng·h/mL/mg)	—	—	67.8± 115.8	83.0± 84.1	71.1± 59.9
$t_{1/2}$ (h)[c]	0.68± 0.21	0.71± 0.22	0.84± 0.26	0.95± 0.31	1.19± 0.52

[a] Subjects with a body weight of ≤30 kg were administered a 15-mg dose; subjects with a body weight of >30 kg were administered a 30-mg dose.
[b] Data obtained from healthy adult subjects normalized to a 30-mg dose.
[c] Harmonic mean ± Pseudo Standard Deviation.

In general, the pharmacokinetics of lansoprazole in children and adolescents (aged 1 to 17 years) with GERD were similar to those observed in healthy adult subjects.

Children 1 to 11 years old weighing ≤30 kg received a 15 mg dose and children weighing >30 kg received a 30 mg dose. When normalized for body weight, the mean lansoprazole dose was similar for the two dosing groups (0.82 mg/kg for 15 mg dose group and 0.74 mg/kg for 30 mg dose group). The C_{max} and AUC values were therefore similar for both the 15 mg and 30 mg dose groups.

In adolescent subjects aged 12 to 17 years, a nearly proportional increase in plasma exposure was observed between 15 mg and 30 mg q.d. dosing groups. Plasma exposure of lansoprazole was not affected by body weight or age; and nearly dose-proportional increases in plasma exposure were observed between the two dose groups in the study. The results of the study in adolescents demonstrated that the pharmacokinetics of lansoprazole in this group is similar to that previously reported in healthy adult subjects.

Geriatrics: The results from the studies that evaluated the pharmacokinetics of lansoprazole following oral administration in an older population revealed that in comparison with younger subjects, older subjects exhibited significantly larger AUCs and longer $t_{½}$s. Lansoprazole did not accumulate in the older subjects upon multiple dosing since the longest mean $t_{½}$ in the studies was 2.9 hours, and lansoprazole is dosed once daily. C_{max} in the elderly was comparable to that found in adult subjects.

† Phenylketonurics: Contains Phenylalanine 2.5 mg per 15 mg Tablet.

Gender: In a study with oral lansoprazole comparing 12 male and 6 female subjects, no gender differences were found in pharmacokinetics or intragastric pH results (see Precautions; Use in Women).

Race: The pooled pharmacokinetic parameters of oral administered lansoprazole from twelve U.S. Phase I studies (N=513) were compared to the mean pharmacokinetic parameters from two Asian studies (N=20). The mean AUCs of lansoprazole in Asian subjects are approximately twice that seen in pooled U.S. data, however, the inter-individual variability is high. The C_{max} values are comparable.

Hepatic Insufficiency: As would be expected with a drug that is primarily metabolized by the liver, in patients with mild (Child-Pugh Class A) or moderate (Child-Pugh Class B) chronic hepatic disease, the plasma half-life of the drug after oral administration increased to 5.2 hours compared to the 1.5 hours half-life in healthy subjects. An increase in AUC of 3.4 fold was observed in patients with hepatic impairment versus healthy subjects (7096 versus 2645 ng·h/mL) which was due to slower elimination of lansoprazole; however, C_{max} was not significantly affected. Dose reduction in patients with severe hepatic disease should be considered.

Renal Insufficiency: In patients with mild (Cl_{cr} 40 to 80 mL/min), moderate (Cl_{cr} 20 to 40 mL/min) and severe (Cl_{cr} <20 mL/min) chronic renal impairment, the disposition of lansoprazole after oral administration was very similar to that of healthy volunteers.

The impact of dialysis on lansoprazole was evaluated from a pharmacokinetic standpoint, and there were no significant differences in AUC, C_{max} or $t_{½}$ between dialysis day and dialysis-free day. Dialysate contained no measurable lansoprazole or metabolite. Lansoprazole is not significantly dialysed.

STORAGE AND STABILITY: PREVACID (lansoprazole delayed-release capsules): Lansoprazole delayed-release capsules should be stored in a tight container protected from light and moisture. Store between 15-25°C.

PREVACID FasTab (lansoprazole delayed-release tablets): Lansoprazole delayed-release tablets should be stored in the original container. Store between 15-25°C.

INFORMATION FOR THE PATIENT: Published in e-CPS, available by subscription at www.e-cps.ca.

DOSAGE FORMS, COMPOSITION AND PACKAGING: PREVACID: 15 mg: Each pink and green-colored, opaque, hard gelatin, delayed-release capsule of enteric-coated granules contains: lansoprazole 15 mg. Nonmedicinal ingredients: cellulosic polymers, colloidal silicon dioxide, D&C Red No. 28, FD&C Blue No. 1, FD&C Green No. 3, FD&C Red No. 40, gelatin, magnesium carbonate, methacrylic acid copolymer, polyethylene glycol, polysorbate 80, starch, sucrose, sugar spheres, talc and titanium dioxide. Bottles of 30 and 100.

30 mg: Each pink and black-colored, opaque, hard gelatin, delayed-release capsule of enteric-coated granules contains: lansoprazole 30 mg. Nonmedicinal ingredients: cellulosic polymers, colloidal silicon dioxide, D&C Red No. 28, FD&C Blue No. 1, FD&C Red No. 40, gelatin, magnesium carbonate, methacrylic acid copolymer, polyethylene glycol, polysorbate 80, starch, sucrose, sugar spheres, talc and titanium dioxide. Bottles of 30 and 100.

PREVACID FasTab: 15 mg: Each white to yellowish white with orange to dark brown speckles, round, flat-faced, bevel-edged, uncoated, orally disintegrating tablet of enteric-coated microgranules, with "15" debossed on one side and measuring approximately 9 mm (side to side) with a strawberry flavor, contains: lansoprazole 15 mg. Nonmedicinal ingredients: aspartame†, citric acid, crospovidone, ferric oxide, glyceryl monostearate, hydroxypropyl cellulose, hydroxypropyl methylcellulose, lactose monohydrate, magnesium carbonate, magnesium stearate, mannitol, methacrylic acid, microcrystalline cellulose, polyacrylate, polyethylene glycol, polysorbate 80, strawberry flavor, talc, titanium dioxide and triethyl citrate. May also contain soya lecithin. Unit dose blister packages of 30.

30 mg: Each white to yellowish white, with orange to dark brown speckles, round, flat-faced, bevel-edged, uncoated, orally disintegrating tablet of enteric-coated microgranules, with "30" debossed on one side and measuring approximately 12 mm (side to side) with a strawberry flavor, contains: lansoprazole 30 mg. Nonmedicinal ingredients: aspartame‡, citric acid, crospovidone, ferric oxide, glyceryl monostearate, hydroxypropyl cellulose, hydroxypropyl methylcellulose, lactose monohydrate, magnesium carbonate, magnesium stearate, mannitol, methacrylic acid, microcrystalline cellulose, polyacrylate, polyethylene glycol, polysorbate 80, strawberry flavor, talc, titanium dioxide and triethyl citrate. May also contain soya lecithin. Unit dose blister packages of 30.

Prevex® B ℞

betamethasone valerate

Topical Corticosteroid

Stiefel, a GSK company

SUPPLIED: Each g of cream contains: betamethasone valerate USP 1.22 mg equivalent to 1 mg or 0.1% betamethasone in an anhydrous base containing highly refined petrolatum and dimethicone. Nonmedicinal ingredients: microcrystalline wax. Tubes of 30 g. Store below 25°C.

Prevex® Cream

petrolatum

Emollient—Skin Protectant

Stiefel, a GSK company

SUPPLIED: Each tube contains: petrolatum 67%, specially refined in an anhydrous base containing dimethicone. Nonmedicinal ingredients: microcrystalline wax. Perfume-free and preservative-free. Tubes of 15 and 60 g.

Prevex® HC ℞

hydrocortisone

Topical Corticosteroid

Stiefel, a GSK company

SUPPLIED: Each tube of cream contains: hydrocortisone USP 1% in an highly refined petrolatum and dimethicone base. Nonmedicinal ingredients: microcrystalline wax. Tubes of 30 g. Store below 25°C.

Prevnar®

pneumococcal 7-valent conjugate vaccine (diphtheria CRM197 protein)

Active Immunizing Agent

Pfizer

Date of Preparation: June 7, 2001
Date of Revision: September 26, 2008

PHARMACOLOGY: *S. pneumoniae* is an important cause of morbidity and mortality in persons of all ages worldwide. The organism causes invasive infections, such as bacteremia and meningitis, as well as pneumonia, and upper respiratory tract infections including otitis media and sinusitis. In children older than 1 month, *S. pneumoniae* is the most common cause of invasive disease. Data from community-based studies performed between 1986 and 1995 indicate that the overall annual incidence of invasive pneumococcal disease in the US is an estimated 10 to 30 cases per 100 000 population with the highest risk being in children aged less than or equal to 2 years of age (140 to 160 cases per 100 000 population).

In the Greater Toronto and Peel regions of Ontario, Canada, overall incidences of invasive pneumococcal disease were determined to be 14.4 per 100 000 population in 1995, 16.1 per 100 000 in 1996, and 11.8 per 100 000 in 1997. Rates of disease were markedly higher in the elderly, and most of the decrease in incidence from 1995 to 1997 was in this age group. In another Canadian study, 2040 consecutive cases of invasive pneumococcal infection seen at 11 pediatric centres across Canada during

‡ Phenylketonurics: Contains Phenylalanine 5.1 mg per 30 mg Tablet.

1991 to 1998 were analyzed. An overall annual incidence could not be established. Age distribution was determined to be as follows: 61.5% of cases occurred before age 2 years, 26.1% between 2 and 5 years, while 12.3% occurred between 6 and 16 years.

Children in day care have an increased risk for invasive pneumococcal disease. Immunocompromised individuals with neutropenia, asplenia, sickle cell disease, disorders of complement and humoral immunity, Human Immunodeficiency Virus (HIV) infections, or chronic underlying disease are also at increased risk for invasive pneumococcal disease. It was shown in the Canadian multicentre pediatric study that the proportion of children with an underlying condition increased with age, from 15.9% in those under 2 years of age, to 30.4% in those 2 to 5 years of age, and to 44.5% in those over 5 years of age (p<0.001). Conditions known to predispose to invasive pneumococcal infection were reported in 16.9% of cases, while other conditions were present in 6.4%.

S. pneumoniae is the most common cause of bacterial meningitis in the United States. The annual incidence of pneumococcal meningitis in children between 1 to 23 months of age is approximately 7 cases per 100 000 people. Pneumococcal meningitis in childhood has been associated with 8% mortality and may result in neurological sequelae (25%) and hearing loss (32%) in survivors.

S. pneumoniae is an important cause of acute otitis media, identified in 20 to 40% of middle ear fluid cultures. The 7 serotypes account for approximately 60% of acute otitis media due to *S. pneumoniae* (12 to 24% of all acute otitis media). The exact contribution of *S. pneumoniae* to childhood pneumonia is unknown, as it is often not possible to identify the causative organisms. In studies of children less than 5 years of age with community-acquired pneumonia, where diagnosis was attempted using serologic methods, antigen testing and culture data, 30% of cases were classified as bacterial pneumonia, and 70% of these (21% of total community-acquired pneumonia) were found to be due to *S. pneumoniae*.

In the past decade the portion of *S. pneumoniae* isolates resistant to antibiotics has been on the rise in the US and worldwide. In a multicentre US surveillance study, the prevalence of penicillin and cephalosporin-nonsusceptible (intermediate or high level resistance) invasive disease isolates from children was 21% (range <5% to 38% among centres), and 9.3% (range 0 to 18%), respectively. Over the 3-year surveillance period (1993 to 1996), there was a 50% increase in penicillin-nonsusceptible *S. pneumoniae* (PNSP) strains and a 3-fold rise in cephalosporin-nonsusceptible strains. Although generally less common than PNSP, pneumococci resistant to macrolides and trimethoprin-sulfazoxole have also been observed. Day care attendance, a history of ear infection, and a recent history of antibiotic exposure have also been associated with invasive infections with PNSP in children 2 months to 59 months of age. There has been no difference in mortality associated with PNSP strains. However, the American Academy of Pediatrics (AAP) revised the antibiotic treatment guidelines in 1997 in response to the increased prevalence of antibiotic-resistant pneumococci.

In 1992 the rate of reduced susceptibility to penicillin in Canada was thought to be less than 5%. Since 1994, reports from eastern Canada have identified rates of 7.3 to 8.1% and 1 recent national survey reported a rate of 11.7%. In Canada, from April 1993 through March 1994, 154 isolates from blood were evaluated for susceptibility to 9 antibiotics. Of these 40 (26%) were found to have reduced susceptibility to one or more of the drugs.

Approximately 90 serotypes of *S. pneumoniae* have been identified based on antigenic differences in their capsular polysaccharides. The serotypes responsible for disease differ with age and geographic location.

Serotypes 4, 6B, 9V, 14, 18C, 19F, and 23F are responsible for approximately 80% of invasive pneumococcal disease in children <6 years of age in the US. These 7 serotypes also accounted for 74% of PNSP and 100% of pneumococci isolated from children <6 years with invasive disease during a 1993 to 1994 surveillance by the Centers for Disease Control.

In the Canadian multicentre pediatric study, of the 2040 cases of invasive pneumococcal infection, serotype data were available for 1528 isolates, representing 74.9% of cases. Children 6 months to 5 years of age had the highest proportion of serotypes matched by the 7-valent vaccine, at 85.8%. The reduced match among children 0 to 5 months of age (65.7%) resulted mainly from fewer type 14 isolates, while that among children over 5 years of age (63.6%) resulted mainly from reduced prevalence of types 14 and 6B. Across all age groups, the match with 7-valent vaccine serotypes was better in previously healthy children than in those with underlying conditions. This rate difference was greatest among those 2 to 5 years of age (13.6%, P<0.001), and not significant in those 6 to 23 months of age. No differences were found over large geographic areas: in western and eastern Canada 80.6% and 81.7% of isolates matched vaccine types, respectively.

The match between 7-valent vaccine serotypes and those encountered with various infection syndromes differed as follows: isolated bacteremia cases, 83.4%; meningitis, 78.9%; pneumonia, 78.3%. Cases with shock matched least well (74.1%) but included 43 typed isolates. Among 27 typed isolates from fatal cases, 20 (74.1%) matched the 7-valent vaccine.

Results of Clinical Evaluations: Efficacy: Efficacy was assessed in a randomized, double-blinded clinical trial in a multiethnic population at Northern California Kaiser Permanente (NCKP), beginning in October 1995, in which 37 816 infants were randomized to receive either Prevnar or a control vaccine (an investigational meningococcal group C conjugate vaccine [MnCC]) at 2, 4, 6 and 12 to 15 months of age. Prevnar was administered to 18 906 children and the control vaccine to 18 910 children. Routinely recommended vaccines were also administered which changed during the trial to reflect changing AAP and Advisory Committee on Immunization Practices (ACIP) recommendations. A planned analysis was performed upon accrual of 17 cases of invasive disease due to vaccine-type *S. pneumoniae* (August 1998). Ancillary endpoints for evaluation of efficacy against pneumococcal disease were also assessed in this trial.

Efficacy Against Invasive Disease: Invasive disease was defined as isolation and identification of *S. pneumoniae* from normally sterile body sites in children presenting with an acute illness consistent with pneumococcal disease. Weekly surveillance of listings of cultures from the NCKP Regional Microbiology database was conducted to assure ascertainment of all cases. The primary endpoint was efficacy against invasive pneumococcal disease due to vaccine serotypes. The per-protocol analysis of the primary endpoint included cases which occurred ≥14 days after the third dose. The intent-to-treat (ITT) analysis included all cases of invasive pneumococcal disease due to vaccine serotypes in children who received at least 1 dose of vaccine. Secondary analysis of efficacy against all invasive pneumococcal disease, regardless of serotype were also performed according to these same per-protocol and ITT definitions. Results of these analyses are presented in Table 1.

Table 1: Prevnar

Efficacy of Prevnar Against Invasive Disease Due to *S. pneumoniae* in Cases Accrued From October 15, 1995 Through April 20, 1999

	Prevnar Number of Cases	Control[a] Number of Cases	Efficacy (%)	95% CI
Vaccine Serotypes				
Per-protocol	1	39	97.4	84.8, 99.9
Intent-to-treat	3	49	93.9	81, 98.8
All Pneumococcal Serotypes				
Per-protocol	3	42	92.9	77.6, 98.6
Intent-to-treat	6	55	89.1	74.7, 96.2

[a] Investigational meningococcal group C conjugate vaccine (MnCC).
Legend: CI=Confidence Interval.

Efficacy Against Otitis Media (OM): Physician visits for any OM were identified by physician coding of outpatient encounter forms. Because visits may have included both acute and follow-up care, a new visit or "episode" was defined as at least 21 days following a previous OM visit. Data on placement of ear tubes were collected from automated databases. No routine tympanocenesis was performed. Table 2 presents the results of these OM analyses for both the per-protocol and intent-to-treat analyses.

A significant risk reduction was seen in Prevnar recipients for clinically diagnosed acute otitis media (AOM) episodes, visits, frequent AOM, and the placement of tympanostomy tubes. The estimated reductions for all AOM episodes was 7% which corresponds to 12 episodes prevented per 100 child years. There is evidence of an increased vaccine effect in reducing the risk of more severe cases of recurrent otitis media with the estimated reduction of tympanostomy tube placement of 20.3%.

In a second efficacy study for otitis media performed in Finland, the vaccine was compared to a control vaccine (Hepatitis B vaccine, HBV) when administered at 2, 4, 6 and 12 months of age. In this study, an episode was defined as a visit to a study clinic at which time acute otitis media was diagnosed by defined symptom criteria and a period of 30 days had elapsed since the previous visit for AOM. Table 3 presents the results of the Finnish efficacy trial analyses.

A significant risk reduction was seen in the incidence of AOM in the Prevnar group vs the control vaccine group regardless of the endpoint assessed. The reduction in all episodes of AOM regardless of etiology in this trial (6%) was similar to that in the Kaiser efficacy study (7%).

Efficacy Against Pneumonia: Children with a clinical diagnosis of any pneumonia were identified by physician coding of outpatient encounter forms. Subjects for whom chest x-rays were obtained with −1 to +5 days of clinical diagnosis were identified. Films were defined as abnormal if consolidation, infiltrate, or effusion was present according to the radiology department report. Table 4 presents the results of the pneumonia analyses.

Table 2: Prevnar

Summary of Vaccine Effects on Acute Otitis Media (AOM)

	Per-protocol Analysis		Intent-to-treat Analysis	
Acute Otitis Media Outcome	**Estimated Risk Reduction (95% CI)**	**P-value**	**Estimated Risk Reduction (95% CI)**	**P-value**
All AOM Episodes-Primary Variable	7% (4.1%, 9.7%)	<0.0001	6.4% (3.9%, 8.7%)	<0.0001
First AOM Episodes	5.4% (2.3%, 8.4%)	0.0008	4.9% (2.3%, 7.5%)	0.0003
Frequent AOM	9.5% (3.2%, 15.3%)	0.0035	9.2% (4.3%, 13.9%)	0.0004
Tympanostomy Tube Placement	20.3% (1.8%, 35.4%)	0.0335	20.6% (4%, 34.3%)	0.0171
All AOM Visits	8.9% (5.8%, 11.8%)	<0.0001	7.8% (5.2%, 10.5%)	<0.0001
Ruptured Ear Drum with Vaccine Serotype Isolates	55.6% (−59.3%, 90%)	0.267	57.1% (−18.7%, 86.5%)	0.115

Legend: CI=Confidence Interval.

Table 3: Prevnar

Summary of Vaccine Efficacy in the Finnish Otitis Media Study

		Episodes		Rate/Person-year		Vaccine Efficacy	
Episode (follow-up)	**Analysis**	**HBV**	**Prevnar**	**HBV**	**Prevnar**	**Estimate**	**95% CI**
Vaccine Serotype AOM	(PP)	250	107	0.21	0.09	0.57	(0.44, 0.67)
Vaccine Serotype AOM	(ITT)	292	135	0.2	0.09	0.54	(0.41, 0.64)
Pneumococcal Culture-confirmed AOM	(PP)	414	271	0.36	0.23	0.34	(0.21, 0.45)
AOM with Middle Ear Fluid	(PP)	1267	1177	1.16	1.09	0.07	(−0.05, 0.17)
AOM Regardless of Etiology	(PP)	1345	1251	1.24	1.16	0.06	(−0.04, 0.16)

Legend: CI=Confidence Interval; AOM: Acute Otitis Media.

Table 4: Prevnar

Summary of Vaccine Effect on Pneumonia

	Per-protocol Analysis			Intent-to-treat Analysis		
Pneumonia Outcome	**Cases in 7VPnC/ MnCC**	**Estimated Risk Reduction (95% CI)**	**P-value[a]**	**Cases in 7VPnC/ MnCC**	**Estimated Risk Reduction (95% CI)**	**P-value[a]**
Clinical Pneumonia	500/566	11% (0.8, 21.1)	0.067	615/694	10% (0.1, 19.8)	0.019
Clinical Pneumonia with X-ray Taken	323/372	12% (2.2, 24.7)	0.091	393/456	13% (0.2, 24.1)	0.035
Clinical Pneumonia with Abnormal X-ray	45/70	35% (4.2, 56.4)	0.028	61/91	33% (6.2, 52.3)	0.033
Clinical Pneumonia with Consolidation	7/19	63% (8.87)	0.03	7/26	73% (36, 90)	0.001

[a] P-value calculated using the Exact binomial test (p=0.4975 for per-protocol and 0.4997 for intent-to-treat).
Legend: CI=Confidence Interval.

Immunogenicity: Routine Schedule: Subjects from a subset of selected study sites in the NCKP efficacy study were approached for participation in the immunogenicity portion of the study on a volunteer basis. Immune responses following 3 or 4 doses of Prevnar or the control vaccine were evaluated in children who received either concurrent diphtheria and tetanus toxoids and pertussis vaccine adsorbed and Haemophilus b conjugate vaccine (diphtheria CRM_{197} protein conjugate) (DTP-HbOC), or diphtheria and tetanus toxoids and acellular pertussis vaccine adsorbed (DTaP), and Haemophilus b conjugate vaccine (diphtheria CRM_{197} protein conjugate) (HbOC) vaccines at 2, 4, and 6 months of age. The use of hepatitis B (Hep B), oral polio vaccine (OPV), inactivated polio vaccine (IPV), measles-mumps-rubella (MMR) and varicella vaccines were permitted according to the AAP and ACIP recommendations.

Table 5 presents the geometric mean concentrations (GMC) of pneumococcal antibodies following the third and fourth doses of Prevnar or the control vaccine when administered concurrently with DTP-HbOC vaccine in the efficacy study.

In another randomized study (Manufacturing Bridging Study, 118-16), immune responses were evaluated following 3 doses of Prevnar administered concomitantly with DTaP and HbOC vaccines at 2, 4 and 6 months of age, IPV at 2 and 4 months of age, and Hep B at 2 and 6 months of age. The control group received concomitant vaccines only. Table 6 presents the immune responses to pneumococcal polysaccharides observed in both this study and in the subset of subjects from the efficacy study that received concomitant DTaP and HbOC vaccines.

Table 5: Prevnar

Geometric Mean Concentrations (µg/mL) of Pneumococcal Antibodies Following the Third and Fourth Doses of Prevnar or Control[a] When Administered Concurrently with DTP-HbOC in the Efficacy Study

	Post Dose 3 GMC[b] (95% CI for Prevnar)		Post Dose 4 GM[c] (95% CI for Prevnar)	
	Prevnar[d]	Control[a]	Prevnar[d]	Control[a]
Serotype	N=88	N=92	N=68	N=61
4	1.46 (1.19, 1.78)	0.03	2.38 (1.88, 3.03)	0.04
6B	4.7 (3.59, 6.14)	0.08	14.45 (11.17, 18.69)	0.17
9V	1.99 (1.64, 2.42)	0.05	3.51 (2.75, 4.48)	0.06
14	4.6 (3.70, 5.74)	0.05	6.52 (5.18, 8.21)	0.06
18C	2.16 (1.73, 2.69)	0.04	3.43 (2.7, 4.37)	0.07
19F	1.39 (1.16, 1.68)	0.09	2.07 (1.66, 2.57)	0.18
23F	1.85 (1.46, 2.34)	0.05	3.82 (2.85, 5.11)	0.09

[a] Control was investigational meningococcal group C conjugate vaccine (MnCC).
[b] Mean age of Prevnar group was 7.8 months and of control group was 7.7 months. N is slightly less for some serotypes in each group.
[c] Mean age of Prevnar group was 14.2 months and of control group was 14.4 months. N is slightly less for some serotypes in each group.
[d] $p<0.001$ when Prevnar compared to control for each serotype using a Wilcoxon's test.
Legend: CI=Confidence Interval; GMC=Geometric Mean Concentrations.

Table 6: Prevnar

Geometric Mean Concentrations (µg/mL) of Pneumococcal Antibodies Following the Third Dose of Prevnar or Control[a] When Administered Concurrently with DTaP and HbOC in the Efficacy Study[b] and Manufacturing Bridging Study

	Efficacy Study		Manufacturing Bridging Study	
	Post Dose 3 GMC[c] (95% CI for Prevnar)		Post Dose 3 GMC[d] (95% CI for Prevnar)	
	Prevnar[e]	Control[a]	Prevnar[e]	Control[a]
Serotype	N=32	N=32	N=159	N=83
4	1.47 (1.08, 2.02)	0.02	2.03 (1.75, 2.37)	0.02
6B	2.18 (1.2, 3.96)	0.06	2.97 (2.43, 3.65)	0.07
9V	1.52 (1.04, 2.22)	0.04	1.18 (1.01, 1.39)	0.04
14	5.05 (3.32, 7.7)	0.04	4.64 (3.8, 5.66)	0.04
18C	2.24 (1.65, 3.02)	0.04	1.96 (1.66, 2.3)	0.04
19F	1.54 (1.09, 2.17)	0.1	1.91 (1.63, 2.25)	0.08
23F	1.48 (0.97, 2.25)	0.05	1.71 (1.44, 2.05)	0.05

[a] Control in efficacy study was investigational meningococcal group C conjugate vaccine (MnCC) and in Manufacturing Bridging Study was concomitant vaccines only.
[b] Sufficient data are not available to reliably assess GMCs following 4 doses of Prevnar when administered with DTaP in the NCKP efficacy study.
[c] Mean age of Prevnar group was 7.4 months and of the control group was 7.6 months. N is slightly less for some serotypes.
[d] Mean age of Prevnar group and of the control group was 7.2 months.
[e] $p<0.001$ when Prevnar compared to control for each serotype using a Wilcoxon's test in the efficacy study and 2-sample t-test in the Manufacturing Bridging Study.
Legend: CI=Confidence Interval; GMC=Geometric Mean Concentration.

In all studies in which the immune responses to Prevnar were compared to a control, a significant antibody response was seen to all vaccine serotypes following 3 or 4 doses, although geometric mean concentrations varied among serotypes. The minimum serum antibody concentration necessary for protection against invasive pneumococcal disease has not been determined for any serotype. Prevnar induces functional antibodies to all vaccine serotypes, as measured by opsonophagocytosis following 3 doses.
Previously Unvaccinated Older Infants and Children: To determine an appropriate schedule for children 7 months of age or older at the time of the first immunization with Prevnar, 483 children in 4 ancillary studies received Prevnar at various schedules. GMCs attained using the various schedules among older infants and children were comparable to immune responses of children, who received concomitant DTaP, in the NCKP efficacy study (D118-P8) after 3 doses for most serotypes, as shown in Table 7. This data supports the schedule for previously unvaccinated older infants and children who are beyond the age of the infant schedule.
For usage in older infants and children, see Dosage, Previously Unvaccinated Older Infants and Children.

Table 7: Prevnar

Geometric Mean Concentrations (µg/mL) of Pneumococcal Antibodies Following Immunization of Children From 7 Months Through 9 Years of Age with Prevnar

Age Group, Vaccinations	Study	Sample Size(s)	4	6B	9V	14	18C	19F	23F
7–11 months, 3 doses	118-12	22	**2.34**	**3.66**	**2.11**	**9.33**	**2.31**	1.6	2.5
	118-16	39	**3.6**	**4.63**	**2.04**	**5.48**	**1.98**	**2.15**	**1.93**
12–17 months, 2 doses	118-15[a]	82–84[b]	**3.91**	**4.67**	**1.94**	**6.92**	**2.25**	**3.78**	**3.29**
	118-18	33	**7.02**	**4.25**	**3.26**	**6.31**	**3.6**	**3.29**	**2.92**
18–23 months, 2 doses	118-15[a]	52–54[b]	**3.36**	**4.92**	**1.8**	**6.69**	**2.65**	**3.17**	**2.71**
	118-18	45	**6.85**	**3.71**	**3.86**	**6.48**	**3.42**	**3.86**	**2.75**
24–35 months, 1 dose	118-18	53	**5.34**	**2.9**	**3.43**	**1.88**	**3.03**	**4.07**	**1.56**

(cont'd)

Table 7: Prevnar *(cont'd)*

Geometric Mean Concentrations (µg/mL) of Pneumococcal Antibodies Following Immunization of Children From 7 Months Through 9 Years of Age with Prevnar

Age Group, Vaccinations	Study	Sample Size(s)	4	6B	9V	14	18C	19F	23F
36–59 months, 1 dose	118-18	52	**6.27**	**6.4**	**4.62**	**5.95**	**4.08**	**6.37**	**2.95**
5–9 years, 1 dose	118-18	101	**6.92**	**20.84**	**7.49**	**19.32**	**6.72**	**12.51**	**11.57**
118-8, DTap	Post dose 3	31–32[b]	1.47	2.18	1.52	5.05	2.24	1.54	1.48

[a] Study in Navajo and Apache populations.
[b] Numbers vary with serotype.
Legend: Bold=GMC not inferior to 118-8, DTaP post dose 3 (one sided lower limit of the 95% CI of GMC ratio≥0.5).

The immunogenicity of Prevnar has been investigated in an open label, multicenter study in 49 infants with sickle cell disease. Children were vaccinated with Prevnar (3 doses one month apart from the age of 2 months) and 46 of these children also received a 23-valent pneumococcal polysaccharide vaccine at the age of 15-18 months. After primary immunization, 95.6% of the subjects had antibody levels of at least 0.35 µg/mL for all seven serotypes found in Prevnar. A significant increase was seen in the concentrations of antibodies against the seven serotypes after the polysaccharide vaccination, suggesting that immunological memory was well established.

INDICATIONS: Active immunization of infants and children from 6 weeks until 9 years of age against invasive disease, pneumonia and otitis media caused by *S. pneumoniae* due to the capsular serotypes included in the vaccine (4, 6B, 9V, 14, 18C, 19F and 23F). The routine schedule is 2, 4, 6, and 12 to 15 months of age. For additional information on usage, see Dosage.

CONTRAINDICATIONS: This vaccine should not be used in any patient demonstrating hypersensitivity to any component of the vaccine, including diphtheria toxoid.

This vaccine should not be given to infants or children with thrombocytopenia or any coagulation disorder that would contraindicate i.m. injection. (See Warnings.)

This vaccine is not intended to be used for treatment of active infection.

WARNINGS: Prevnar (pneumococcal 7-valent conjugate vaccine) will not help to protect against *S. pneumoniae* disease other than that caused by the 7 serotypes included in the vaccine, nor will it protect against other microorganisms that cause invasive infection such as bacteremia and meningitis, or otitis media and pneumonia.

This vaccine should not be given to infants or children with thrombocytopenia or any coagulation disorder that would contraindicate i.m. injection unless the potential benefit clearly outweighs the risk of administration. If the decision is made to administer this vaccine to children with coagulation disorders, it should be given with caution (see Precautions, Drug Interactions).

Immunization with Prevnar does not substitute for routine diphtheria immunization.

As with all injectable pediatric vaccines, the potential risk of apnea should be considered when administering the primary immunization series to premature infants. The need for monitoring for at least 48 hours after vaccination should be considered for very premature infants (born ≤30 weeks of gestation), who remain hospitalized at the time of the recommended administration. As the benefit of vaccination is high in this group of infants, vaccination should not be withheld or delayed.

PRECAUTIONS: General: Minor illnesses, such as mild respiratory infection with or without low-grade fever, are not generally contraindications to vaccination. The decision to administer or delay vaccination because of a current or recent febrile illness depends largely on the severity of the symptoms and their etiology. The administration of Prevnar should be postponed in subjects suffering from acute severe febrile illness. Prior to administration of any dose of Prevnar (pneumococcal 7-valent conjugate vaccine), the parent, guardian, or adult patient should be asked about the personal history, family history, recent health status, and immunization history of the patient to be immunized to determine the existence of any contraindication to immunization with pneumococcal vaccine (see Contraindications and Warnings).

The healthcare professional should also take all known precautions for the prevention of allergic or any other reactions. This includes: a review of the patient's history regarding possible sensitivity, the ready availability of epinephrine 1:1000 and other appropriate agents used for control of immediate allergic reactions; and a knowledge of the recent literature pertaining to use of the biological concerned, including the nature of side effects and adverse reactions that may follow its use (see Adverse Effects).

A separate sterile syringe and needle or a sterile disposable unit should be used for each individual patient to prevent transmission of infectious agents from one person to another. Needles should be disposed of properly and should not be recapped.

Special care should be taken to prevent injection into or near a blood vessel or nerve.

Children with impaired immune responsiveness, whether due to the use of immunosuppressive therapy (including irradiation, corticosteroids, antimetabolites, alkylating agents, and cytotoxic agents), a genetic defect, HIV infection, or other causes, may have a reduced antibody response to active immunization (see Drug Interactions).

As with any vaccine, Prevnar may not protect 100% of individuals receiving the vaccine.

Prophylactic antipyretic medication is recommended for all children receiving Prevnar simultaneously with vaccines containing whole cell pertussis. Prophylactic antipyretic medication should be considered in children at higher risk for seizures than the general population.

The use of pneumococcal conjugate vaccine does not replace the use of 23-valent pneumococcal polysaccharide vaccine in children ≥24 months of age with sickle cell disease, asplenia, HIV infection, chronic illness or who are immunocompromised, placing them at higher risk for invasive disease due to *S. pneumoniae*. Data on sequential vaccination with Prevnar followed by 23-valent pneumococcal polysaccharide vaccine are limited. In a randomized study, 23 subjects >2 years of age with sickle cell disease were administered either 2 doses of Prevnar followed by a dose of polysaccharide vaccine or a single dose of polysaccharide vaccine alone. In this small study, safety and immune responses with the combined schedule were similar to polysaccharide vaccine alone.

Children: Prevnar has been shown to be usually well-tolerated and immunogenic in infants. The safety and effectiveness of Prevnar in children below the age of 6 weeks or on or after the 10th birthday have not been established. Immune responses elicited by Prevnar among infants born prematurely have not been studied. See Dosage for the recommended pediatric dosage.

Geriatrics: Prevnar is not recommended for use in adult populations and it is not to be used as a substitute for the pneumococcal polysaccharide vaccine, 23-valent in geriatric populations.

Pregnancy: Safety during pregnancy has not been established.

Animal reproductive studies have not been conducted with Prevnar. It is also not known whether Prevnar can cause fetal harm when administered to a pregnant woman or whether it can affect reproductive capacity. Prevnar is not recommended for use in pregnant women.

Lactation: It is not known whether vaccine antigens or antibodies are excreted in human milk. Prevnar is not recommended for use in a nursing mother. Safety during lactation has not been established.

Carcinogenesis, Mutagenesis, Impairment of Fertility: Prevnar has not been evaluated for its carcinogenic or mutagenic potential, or impairment of fertility.

Drug Interactions: Children receiving therapy with immunosuppressive agents (large amounts of corticosteroids, antimetabolites, alkylating agents, cytotoxic agents) may not respond optimally to active immunization procedures (see Precautions).

As with other i.m. injections, Prevnar should be given with caution to children on anticoagulant therapy.

Simultaneous Administration with Other Vaccines: During clinical studies, Prevnar was administered simultaneously with DTP-HbOC or DTaP and HbOC, OPV or IPV, Hepatitis B Vaccine(s), meningococcal serogroup C conjugate vaccine, MMR and Varicella vaccine. Thus, the safety experience with Prevnar reflects the use of this product as part of the routine immunization schedule. In some studies, differences in antibody response to some of the antigens have been inconsistently found, however, it is not anticipated to be of any clinical relevance.

Data on concomitant administration of Prevnar with Meningitec (meningococcal C CRM197 protein conjugate vaccine) have shown no clinically relevant interference in the antibody response to each of the individual antigens when given as primary series vaccinations.

Table 8: Prevnar

Concurrent Administration of Prevnar with Other Vaccines to Infants in Non-efficacy Studies

Antigen[a]		GMC[a]		% Responders[b]		Study	Vaccine Schedule[c] (months)	N	
		Prevnar	Control[e]	Prevnar	Control[e]			Prevnar	Control[d]
Hib		6.2	4.4	99.5, 88.3	97, 88.1	118-12	2, 4, 6	214	67
Diphtheria		0.9	0.8	100	97.0				
Tetanus		3.5	4.1[e]	100	100				
PT		19.1	17.8	74	69.7				
FHA		43.8	46.7	66.4	69.7				
Pertactin		40.1	50.9	65.6	77.3				
Fimbriae 2		3.3	4.2	44.7	62.5[e]				
Hib		11.9	7.8[e]	100, 96.9	98.8, 92.8	118-16	2, 4, 6	159	83
Hep B		—	—	99.4	96.2	118-16	0, 2, 6	156	80
IPV	Type 1	—	—	89	93.6[f]	118-16	2, 4	156	80
	Type 2	—	—	94.2	93.6				
	Type 3	—	—	83.8	80.8				

a Hib vaccine was HibTiter, DTaP vaccine was Acel-Imune. Hib (μg/mL); Dip, Tet (IU/mL); pertussis antigens (PT, FHA, Ptn, Fim) (U/mL).
b Responders=Hib (≥0.15 μg/mL, ≥1 μg/mL); Dip, Tet (≥0.1 IU/mL); pertussis antigens (PT, FHA, Ptn, Fim) [4-fold rise]; IPV (≥1:10); Hep B(≥10 mIU/mL).
c Schedule for concurrently administered vaccines; Prevnar administered at 2, 4, 6 months; blood for antibody assessment attained 1 month after third dose, except for IPV (3 months post-immunization).
d Concurrent vaccines only.
e p<0.05 when Prevnar compared to control group using the following tests: ANCOVA for GMCs in 118-12; ANOVA for GMCs in 118-16; and Fisher's Exact test for % Responders in 118-12.
f Lower bound of 90% CI of difference >10%.
Legend: GMC=Geometric Mean Concentrations.

Table 9: Prevnar

Concurrent Administration of Prevnar with Other Vaccines to Toddlers in a Non-efficacy Study

Antigen[a]	GMC[a]		% Responders[b]		Study[c]	Vaccine Schedule[d] (months)	N	
	Prevnar	Control[e]	Prevnar	Control[e]			Prevnar	Control[e]
Hib	22.7	47.9[f]	100, 97.9	100, 100	118-7	12–15	47	26
Diphtheria	2	3.2[f]	100	100				
Tetanus	14.4	18.8	100	100				
PT	68.6	121.2[f]	68.1	73.1				
FHA	29	48.2[f]	68.1	84.6				
Pertactin	84.4	83	83	96.2				
Fimbriae2	5.2	3.8	63.8	50.0				

a Hib vaccine was HibTiter, DTaP vaccine was Acel-Imune. Hib (μg/mL); Dip, Tet (IU/mL); pertussis antigens (PT,FHA, Ptn, Fim) (U/mL).
b Responders=Hib (≥0.15 μg/mL, ≥1 μg/mL); Dip, Tet (≥0.1 IU/mL); pertussis antigens (PT, FHA, Ptn, Fim) [4-fold rise].
c Children received a primary series of DTP-HbOC (Tetramune).
d Blood for antibody assessment obtained 1 month after dose.
e Concurrent vaccines only.
f p<0.05 when Prevnar compared to control group using a 2-sample t-test.
Legend: GMC=Geometric Mean Concentrations.

Concurrent administration of Prevnar with DTaP-IPV/PRP-T vaccine (Pentacel, Sanofi-Aventis) and hepatitis B virus vaccine (Recombivax, Merck), at 2, 4 and 6 months of age, (concurrent administration in two groups of 126 subjects each) was compared to the sequential administration of DTaP-IPV/PRP-T vaccine and hepatitis B virus vaccine at 2, 4 and 6 months of age and Prevnar at 3, 5 and 7 months of age (sequential administration in 124 subjects). There were no significant differences in the antibody response to any Prevnar serotype in either the concurrent (N=123) or the sequential (N=121) group. A significantly lower percentage of responders to hepatitis B (seroprotective level equal to or greater than 10 mIU/mL, measured at 8 weeks post third dose) was noted in the concurrent group, 87.2% (95% CI: 79.7-92.6%), compared to that seen in the sequential group, 96.7% (95% CI: 91.8-99.1%) and statistically significant (p=0.006) higher antibody levels were reported in the sequential group for hepatitis B antibodies. The GMC response to the *H. influenza* type b (Hib) antigen was statistically higher in the concurrent group (1.11 mg/mL, CI: 0.82-1.50) compared to the sequential administration group (0.64 mg/mL, CI: 0.48-0.85). The clinical significance of these data is unknown.

The immune response to routine vaccines when administered with Prevnar (at separate sites) was assessed in 3 clinical studies in which there was a control group for comparison. Results for the concurrent immunizations in infants are shown in Table 8 and for toddlers in Table 9. Enhancement of antibody response to HbOC in the infant series was observed. Some suppression of *H. influenzae* type b (Hib) response was seen at the 4th dose, but over 97% of children achieved titres ≥1 μg/mL. Although some inconsistent differences in response to pertussis antigens were observed, the clinical relevance is unknown. The response to 2 doses of IPV given concomitantly with Prevnar, assessed 3 months after the second dose, was equivalent to controls for poliovirus Types 2 and 3, but slightly lower for types 1. MMR and varicella immunogenicity data from controlled clinical trials with concurrent administration of Prevnar are not available.

ADVERSE EFFECTS: Pre-licensure Clinical Trial Experience: Adverse reactions identified from clinical trial experience are listed below:

Administration Site Conditions: Very common: (≥10%): injection site erythema, induration/swelling, pain/tenderness. Common (≥1% and <10%): injection site induration/swelling or erythema greater than 2.4 cm, pain/tenderness interfering with movement.
Gastrointestinal Disorders: Very common: (≥10%): diarrhea, vomiting.
General Disorders: Very common: (≥10%): fever. Common (≥1% and <10%): fever greater than 39°C.
Metabolism and Nutrition Disorders: Very common: (≥10%): decreased appetite.
Nervous System Disorders: Very common: (≥10%): drowsiness, restless sleep. Rare: (≥0.01% and <0.1%): seizures (including febrile seizures): hypotonic-hyporesponsive episode.
Psychiatric Disorders: Very common: (≥10%): irritability.
Skin and Subcutaneous Tissue Disorders: Uncommon: (≥0.1% and <1%): rash, urticaria or urticaria type rash.

The majority of the safety experience with Prevnar comes from the NCKP efficacy trial in which 17 066 infants received 55 352 doses of Prevnar, along with other routine childhood vaccines through April 1998 (see Pharmacology). The number of Prevnar recipients in the safety analysis differs from the number included in the efficacy analysis due to the different lengths of follow-up for these study endpoints. Safety was monitored in this study using several modalities. Local reactions and systemic events occurring within 48 hours of each dose of vaccine were ascertained by scripted telephone interview on a randomly selected subset of approximately 3000 children in each vaccine group. The rate of relatively rare events requiring medical attention was evaluated across all doses in all study participants using automated databases. Specifically, rates of hospitalization within 3, 14, 30 and 60 days of immunization, and of emergency room visits within 3, 14, and 30 days of immunization were assessed and compared between vaccine groups for each diagnosis. Seizures within 3 and 30 days of immunization were ascertained across multiple settings (hospitalizations, emergency room or clinic visits, telephone interviews). Deaths and SIDS were ascertained through April 1999. Hospitalizations due to diabetes, autoimmune disorders, and blood disorders were ascertained through August 1999.

In Table 10 and Table 11, the rate of local reactions that were common during the first 2 days at the Prevnar injection site (erythema, induration/swelling and pain/tenderness) is compared at each dose to the DTP or DTaP injection site in the same children.

Table 12 presents the rates of local reactions in previously unvaccinated older infants and children.

Table 13 and Table 14 present the rates of systemic events observed in the efficacy study when Prevnar was administered concomitantly with DTP or DTaP.

Table 15 presents results from a second study (Manufacturing Bridging Study) conducted at Northern California and Denver Kaiser sites, in which children were randomized to receive 1 of 3 lots of Prevnar with concomitant vaccines including DTaP, or the same concomitant vaccines alone. Information was ascertained by scripted telephone interview, as described above.

Fever (≥38°C) within 48 hours of a vaccine dose was reported by a greater proportion of subjects who received Prevnar, compared to control (investigational meningococcal group C conjugate vaccine [MnCC]), after each dose when administered concurrently with DTP-HbOC or DTaP in the efficacy study. In the Manufacturing Bridging Study, fever within 48 to 72 hours was also reported more commonly after each dose compared to infants in the control group who received only recommended vaccines. When administered concurrently with DTaP in either study, fever rates among Prevnar recipients ranged from 15 to 34%, and were greatest after the 2nd dose. Table 16 presents the frequencies of systemic reactions in previously unvaccinated older infants and children.

Of the 17 066 subjects who received at least 1 dose of Prevnar in the efficacy trial, there were 24 hospitalizations (for 29 diagnoses) within 3 days of a dose from October 1995 through April 1998. Diagnoses were as follows: bronchiolitis (5); congenital anomaly (4); elective procedure, UTI (3 each); acute gastroenteritis, asthma, pneumonia (2 each); aspiration, breath holding, influenza, inguinal hernia repair, otitis media, febrile seizure, viral syndrome, well child/reassurance (1 each). There were 162 visits to the emergency room (for 182 diagnoses) within 3 days of a dose from October 1995 through April 1998. Diagnoses were as follows: febrile illness (20); acute gastroenteritis (19); trauma, URI (16 each); otitis media (15); well child (13); irritable child, viral syndrome (10 each); rash (8); croup, pneumonia (6 each); poisoning/ingestion (5); asthma, bronchiolitis (4 each); febrile seizure, UTI (3 each); thrush, wheezing, breath holding, choking, conjunctivitis, inguinal hernia repair, pharyngitis (2 each); colic, colitis, congestive heart failure, elective procedure, hives, influenza, ingrown toenail, local swelling, roseola, sepsis (1 each).

Table 10: Prevnar

Percentage of Subjects Experiencing Local Reactions Within 2 Days Following Immunization with Prevnar and DTP-HbOC[a] Vaccines at 2, 4, 6 and 12-15 Months of Age

	Dose 1		Dose 2		Dose 3		Dose 4	
	Prevnar Site	DTP-HbOC Site[b]	Prevnar Site	DTP-HbOC Site[b]	Prevnar Site	DTP-HbOC Site[b]	Prevnar Site	DTP-HbOC Site[b]
Reaction	N=2890	N=2890	N=2725	N=2725	N=2538	N=2538	N=599	N=599
Erythema								
Any	12.4	21.9	14.3	25.1	15.2	26.5	12.7	23.4
>2.4 cm	1.2	4.6	1	2.9	2	4.4	1.7	6.4
Induration								
Any	10.9	22.4	12.3	23	12.8	23.3	11.4	20.5
>2.4 cm	2.6	7.2	2.4	5.6	2.9	6.7	2.8	7.2
Tenderness								
Any	28	36.4	25.2	30.5	25.6	32.8	36.5	45.1
Interfered with Limb Movement	7.9	10.7	7.4	8.4	7.8	10.0	18.5	22.2

[a] If Hep B vaccine was administered simultaneously, it was administered into the same limb as the DTP-HbOC vaccine. If reactions occurred at either or both sites on that limb, the most severe reaction was recorded.
[b] p<0.05 when Prevnar site compared to the DTP-HbOC site using the sign test.

Table 11: Prevnar

Percentage of Subjects Reporting Local Reactions Within 2 Days Following Immunization with Prevnar[a] and DTaP Vaccines[b] at 2, 4, 6 and 12-15 Months of Age

	Dose 1		Dose 2		Dose 3		Dose 4	
	Prevnar Site	DTaP Site	Prevnar Site	DTaP Site	Prevnar Site	DTaP Site	Prevnar Site	DTaP Site[c]
Reaction	N=693	N=693	N=526	N=526	N=422	N=422	N=165	N=165
Erythema								
Any	10	6.7[d]	11.6	10.5	13.8	11.4	10.9	3.6[d]
>2.4 cm	1.3	0.4[d]	0.6	0.6	1.4	1	3.6	0.6
Induration								
Any	9.8	6.6[d]	12	10.5	10.4	10.4	12.1	5.5[d]
>2.4 cm	1.6	0.9	1.3	1.7	2.4	1.9	5.5	1.8
Tenderness								
Any	17.9	16.0	19.4	17.3	14.7	13.1	23.3	18.4
Interfered with Limb Movement	3.1	1.8[d]	4.1	3.3	2.9	1.9	9.2	8

[a] HbOC was administered in the same limb as Prevnar. If reactions occurred at either or both sites on that limb, the more severe reaction was recorded.
[b] If Hep B vaccine was administered simultaneously, it was administered into the same limb as DTaP. If reactions occurred at either or both sites on that limb, the more severe reaction was recorded.
[c] Subjects may have received DTP or a mixed DTP/DTaP regimen for the primary series. Thus, this is the 4th dose of a pertussis vaccine, but not a 4th dose of DTaP.
[d] p<0.05 when Prevnar site compared to DTaP site using the sign test.

Table 12: Prevnar

Percentage of Subjects Reporting Local Reactions Within 3 Days of Immunization with Prevnar in Infants and Children from 7 Months Through 9 Years of Age

Age at 1st Vaccination	7–11 Months						12–23 Months			24–35 Months	36–59 Months	5–9 Years
Study No.	118–12			118–16			118–9[a]	118–18		118–18	118–18	118–18
Dose Number	1	2	3[b]	1	2	3[b]	1	1	2	1	1	1
Number of Subjects	54	51	24	81	76	50	60	114	117	46	48	49
Reaction												
Erythema												
Any	16.7	11.8	20.8	7.4	7.9	14	48.3	10.5	9.4	6.5	29.2	24.2
>2.4 cm[c]	1.9	0	0	0	0	0	6.7	1.8	1.7	0	8.3	7.1
Induration												
Any	16.7	11.8	8.3	7.4	3.9	10	48.3	8.8	6	10.9	22.9	25.5
>2.4 cm[c]	3.7	0	0	0	0	0	3.3	0.9	0.9	2.2	6.3	9.3
Tenderness												
Any	13	11.8	12.5	8.6	10.5	12	46.7	25.7	26.5	41.3	58.3	82.8
Interfered with Limb Movements[d]	1.9	2	4.2	1.2	1.3	0	3.3	6.2	8.5	13	20.8	39.4

[a] For 118-9, 2 of 60 subjects were ≥24 months of age.
[b] For 118-12, dose 3 was administered at 15 to 18 mos. of age. For 118-16, dose 3 was administered at 12 to 15 mos. of age.
[c] For 118-16 and 118-18, ≥2 cm.
[d] Tenderness interfering with limb movement.

Table 13: Prevnar

Percentage of Subjects[a] Reporting Systemic Events Within 2 Days Following Immunization with Prevnar or Control[b] Vaccine Concurrently with DTP-HbOC Vaccine at 2, 4, 6, and 12-15 Months of Age

Reaction	Dose 1		Dose 2		Dose 3		Dose 4	
	Prevnar	Control[b]	Prevnar	Control[b]	Prevnar	Control[b]	Prevnar	Control[b]
	N=2998	N=2982	N=2788	N=2761	N=2596	N=2591	N=709	N=733
Fever								
≥38°C	33.4	28.7[c]	34.7	27.4[c]	40.6	32.4[c]	41.9	36.9
>39°C	1.3	1.3	3	1.6[c]	5.3	3.4[c]	4.5	4.5
Irritability	71.3	67.9[c]	69.4	63.8[c]	68.9	61.6[c]	72.8	65.8[c]
Drowsiness	49.2	50.6	32.5	33.6	25.9	23.4[c]	21.3	22.7
Restless Sleep	18.1	17.9	27.3	24.3[c]	33.3	30.1[c]	29.9	28
Decreased Appetite	24.7	23.6	22.8	20.3[c]	27.7	25.6	33	27.4[c]
Vomiting	17.9	14.9[c]	16.2	14.4	15.5	12.7[c]	9.6	6.8
Diarrhea	12	10.7	10.9	9.9	11.5	10.4	12.1	11.2
Rash or Hives	0.7	0.6	0.8	0.8	1.4	1.1	1.4	0.8

[a] Approximately 90% of subjects received prophylactic or therapeutic antipyretics within 48 hours of each dose.
[b] Investigational meningococcal group C conjugate vaccine (MnCC).
[c] p<0.05 when Prevnar compared to control group using a Chi-Square test.

Table 14: Prevnar

Percentage of Subjects[a] Reporting Systemic Reactions Within 2 Days Following Immunization with Prevnar or Control[b] Vaccine Concurrently with DTaP Vaccine at 2, 4, 6, and 12-15 Months of Age

Reaction	Dose 1		Dose 2		Dose 3		Dose 4[c]	
	Prevnar	Control[b]	Prevnar	Control[b]	Prevnar	Control[b]	Prevnar	Control[b]
	N=710	N=711	N=559	N=508	N=461	N=414	N=224	N=230
Fever								
≥38°C	15.1	9.4[d]	23.9	10.8[d]	19.1	11.8[d]	21	17
>39°C	0.9	0.3	2.5	0.8[d]	1.7	0.7	1.3	1.7
Irritability	48	48.2	58.7	45.3[d]	51.2	44.8	44.2	42.6
Drowsiness	40.7	42.0	25.6	22.8	19.5	21.9	17	16.5
Restless Sleep	15.3	15.1	20.2	19.3	25.2	19[d]	20.2	19.1
Decreased Appetite	17	13.5	17.4	13.4	20.7	13.8[d]	20.5	23.1
Vomiting	14.6	14.5	16.8	14.4	10.4	11.6	4.9	4.8
Diarrhea	11.9	8.4[d]	10.2	9.3	8.3	9.4	11.6	9.2
Rash or Hives	1.4	0.3[d]	1.3	1.4	0.4	0.5	0.5	1.7

[a] Approximately 75% of subjects received prophylactic or therapeutic antipyretics within 48 hours of each dose.
[b] Investigational meningococcal group C conjugate vaccine (MnCC).
[c] Most of these children had received DTP for the primary series. Thus, this is a 4th dose of a pertussis vaccine, but not a DTaP.
[d] p<0.05 when Prevnar compared to control group using a Chi-Square test.

One case of a hypotonic-hyporesponsive episode (HHE) was reported in the efficacy study following Prevnar and concurrent DTP vaccines in the study period from October 1995 through April 1998. Two additional cases of HHE were reported in 4 other studies and these also occurred in children who received Prevnar concurrent with DTP vaccine.

In the Kaiser efficacy study in which 17 066 children received a total of 55 352 doses of Prevnar and 17 080 children received a total of 55 387 doses of the control vaccine (investigational meningococcal group C conjugate vaccine [MnCC]), seizures (including febrile seizures) were reported in 8 Prevnar recipients and 4 control vaccine recipients within 3 days of immunization from October 1995 through April 1999. Of the 8 Prevnar recipients, 7 received concomitant DTP-containing vaccines and 1 received DTaP. Of the 4 control vaccine recipients, 3 received concomitant DTP-containing vaccines and 1 received DTaP. In the other 4 studies combined, in which 1102 children were immunized with 3347 doses of Prevnar and 408 children were immunized with 1310 doses of control vaccine (either investigational meningococcal group C conjugate vaccine [MnCC] or concurrent vaccines), there was 1 seizure event reported within 3 days of immunization. This subject received Prevnar concurrent with DTaP vaccine.

Twelve deaths (5 SIDS and 7 with clear alternative cause) occurred among subjects receiving Prevnar, of which 11 (4 SIDS and 7 clear alternative cause) occurred in the Kaiser efficacy study from October 1995 until April 20, 1999. In comparison, 21 deaths (8 SIDS, 12 with clear alternative cause and one SIDS-like death in an older child) occurred in the control vaccine group during the same time period in the efficacy study. The number of SIDS deaths in the efficacy study from October 1995 until April 20, 1999 was similar to or lower than the age and season-adjusted expected rate from the California State data from 1995 to 1997 and are presented in Table 17.

In a review of all hospitalizations that occurred between October 1995 and August 1999 in the efficacy study for the specific diagnoses of aplastic anemia, autoimmune disease, autoimmune hemolytic anemia, diabetes mellitus, neutropenia, and thrombocytopenia, the numbers of such cases were either equal to or less than the expected numbers based on the 1995 Kaiser Vaccine Safety Data Link (VSD) data set.

Overall, the safety of Prevnar has been evaluated in a total of five clinical studies in which 18 168 infants and children received a total of 58 699 doses of vaccine at 2, 4, 6 and 12-15 months of age. In addition, the safety of Prevnar was evaluated in 560 children from 4 ancillary studies who started immunization at 7 months to 9 years of age. Table 18 and Table 19 summarize systemic reactogenicity data within 2 or 3 days across 4748 subjects (13 039 infant doses and 1706 toddler doses) for whom these data were collected and according to the pertussis vaccine administered concurrently.

With vaccines in general, including Prevnar, it is not uncommon for patients to note within 48 to 72 hours at or around the injection site the following minor reactions: edema; pain or tenderness; redness, inflammation or skin discoloration; mass; or local hypersensitivity reaction. Such local reactions are usually self-limited and require no therapy.

As with other aluminum-containing vaccines, a nodule may occasionally be palpable at the injection site for several weeks.

Post-marketing Experience: Additional adverse reactions identified from post-marketing experiences are listed below:

Administration Site Conditions: Very rare: (<0.01%): injection site dermatitis, injection site urticaria, injection site pruritus.

Blood and Lymphatic System Disorders: Very rare: (<0.01%): lymphadenopathy localized to the region of the injection site.

Immune System Disorders: Very rare: (<0.01%): hypersensitivity reaction including face edema, dyspnea, bronchospasm; anaphylactic/anaphylactoid reaction including shock.

Skin and Subcutaneous Tissues Disorders: Very rare: (<0.01%): angioneurotic edema, erythema multiforme.

Psychiatric Disorders: Very common: (10%): crying.

Table 15: Prevnar

Percentage of Subjects[a] Reporting Systemic Reactions Within 3 Days Following Immunization with Prevnar, DTaP, HbOC, Hep B and IPV vs Control[b] in Manufacturing Bridging Study

Reaction	Dose 1		Dose 2		Dose 3	
	Prevnar	Control[b]	Prevnar	Control[b]	Prevnar	Control[b]
	N=498	N=108	N=452	N=99	N=445	N=89
Fever						
≥38°C	21.9	10.2[c]	33.6	17.2[c]	28.1	23.6
>39°C	0.8	0.9	3.8	0	2.2	0
Irritability	59.7	60.2	65.3	52.5[c]	54.2	50.6
Drowsiness	50.8	38.9[c]	30.3	31.3	21.2	20.2
Decreased Appetite	19.1	15.7	20.6	11.1[c]	20.4	9[c]

[a] Approximately 72% of subjects received prophylactic or therapeutic antipyretics within 48 hours of each dose.
[b] Control group received concomitant vaccines only in the same schedule as the Prevnar group (DTaP, HbOC at dose 1, 2, 3; IPV at doses 1 and 2; Hep B at doses 1 and 3).
[c] p<0.05 when Prevnar compared to control group using Fisher's Exact test.

Table 16: Prevnar

Percentage of Subjects Reporting Systemic Reactions Within 3 Days of Immunization in Infants and Children From 7 Months Through 9 Years of Age

Age at 1st Vaccination	7–11 Months					12–23 Months				24–35 Months	36–59 Months	5–9 Years
Study No.	118–12			118–16			118–9[a]	118–18		118–18	118–18	118–18
Dose Number	1	2	3[b]	1	2	3[b]	1	1	2	1	1	1
Number of Subjects	54	51	24	85	80	50	60	120	117	47	52	100
Reaction												
Fever												
≥38°C	20.8	21.6	25	17.6	18.8	22	36.7	11.7	6.8	14.9	11.5	7
>39°C	1.9	5.9	0	1.6	3.9	2.6	0	4.4	0	4.2	2.3	1.2
Fussiness	29.6	39.2	16.7	54.1	41.3	38	40	37.5	36.8	46.8	34.6	29.3
Drowsiness	11.1	17.6	16.7	24.7	16.3	14	13.3	18.3	11.1	12.8	17.3	11
Decreased Appetite	9.3	15.7	0	15.3	15	30	25	20.8	16.2	23.4	11.5	9

[a] For 118-9, 2 of 60 subjects were ≥24 months of age.
[b] For 118-12, dose 3 was administered at 15 to 18 months of age. For 118-16, dose 3 was administered at 12-15 months of age.

Table 17: Prevnar

Age and Season Adjusted Comparison with SIDS Rates in the NCKP Efficacy Trial with the Expected Rate From the California State Data for 1995-1997

	<1 Week After Immunization		≤2 Weeks After Immunization		≤1 Month After Immunization		≤1 Year After Immunization	
Vaccine	**Exp**	**Obs**	**Exp**	**Obs**	**Exp**	**Obs**	**Exp**	**Obs**
Prevnar	1.06	1	2.09	2	4.28	2	8.08	4
Control[a]	1.06	2	2.09	3[b]	4.28	3[b]	8.08	8[b]

[a] Investigational meningococcal group C conjugate vaccine (MnCC).
[b] Does not include 1 additional case of SIDS-like death in a child older than the usual SIDS age (448 days).

Table 18: Prevnar

Overall Percentage of Doses Associated with Systemic Events Within 2 or 3 Days for Efficacy Study and All Ancillary Studies When Prevnar Administered to Infants as a Primary Series at 2, 4 and 6 Months of Age

Systemic Event	Prevnar Concurrently with DTP-HbOC (9191 Doses)[a]	Prevnar Concurrently with DTaP-HbOC (3848 Doses)[b]	DTaP and HbOC Control (538 Doses)[c]
Fever			
≥38°C	35.6	21.1	**14.2**
>39°C	3.1	1.8	**0.4**
Irritability	69.1	52.5	**45.2**
Drowsiness	36.9	32.9	**27.7**
Restless Sleep	25.8	20.6	**22.3**
Decreased Appetite	24.7	18.1	**13.6**
Vomiting	16.2	13.4	**9.8**
Diarrhea	11.4	9.8	**4.4**
Rash or Hives	0.9	0.6	**0.3**

[a] Total from which reaction data are available varies between reactions from 8874-9191 doses. Data from studies 118-3, 118-7, 118-8.
[b] Total from which reaction data are available varies between reactions from 3121-3848 doses. Data from studies 118-8, 118-12, 118-16.
[c] Total from which reaction data are available varies between reactions from 295 to 538 doses. Data from studies 118-12 and 118-16.

Table 19: Prevnar

Overall Percentage of Doses Associated with Systemic Events Within 2 or 3 Days for Efficacy Study and All Ancillary Studies when Prevnar Administered to Toddlers as a Fourth Dose at 12 to 15 Months of Age

Systemic Event	Prevnar Concurrently with DTP-HbOC (709 Doses)[a]	Prevnar Concurrently with DTaP and HbOC (270 Doses)[b]	Prevnar Only No Concurrent Vaccines (727 Doses)[c]
Fever			
≥38°C	41.9	19.6	**13.4**
>39°C	4.5	1.5	**1.2**
Irritability	72.8	45.9	**45.8**
Drowsiness	21.3	17.5	**15.9**
Restless Sleep	29.9	21.2	**21.2**
Decreased Appetite	33	21.1	**18.3**

(cont'd)

Table 19: Prevnar *(cont'd)*

Overall Percentage of Doses Associated with Systemic Events Within 2 or 3 Days for Efficacy Study and All Ancillary Studies when Prevnar Administered to Toddlers as a Fourth Dose at 12 to 15 Months of Age

Systemic Event	Prevnar Concurrently with DTP-HbOC (709 Doses)[a]	Prevnar Concurrently with DTaP and HbOC (270 Doses)[b]	Prevnar Only No Concurrent Vaccines (727 Doses)[c]
Vomiting	9.6	5.6	**6.3**
Diarrhea	12.1	13.7	**12.8**
Rash or Hives	1.4	0.7	**1.2**

[a] Total from which reaction data are available varies between reactions from 706-709 doses. Data from study 118-8.
[b] Total from which reaction data are available varies between reactions from 269-270 doses. Data from studies 118-7 and 118-8.
[c] Total from which reaction data are available varies between reactions from 725-727 doses. Data from studies 118-7 and 118-8.

Respiratory: There have been spontaneous reports of apnoea in temporal association with the administration of Prevnar. In most cases Prevnar was administered concomitantly with other vaccines including diptheria tetanus pertussis vaccine (DTP), diptheria tetanus acellular pertussis vaccine (DTaP), hepatitis B vaccines, inactivated polio vaccine (IPV), *H. influenzae* type B vaccine (Hib), measles-mumps-rubella vaccine (MMR), and/or varicella vaccine. In addition, in most of the reports, existing medical conditions such as history of apnoea, infection, prematurity, and/or seizure were present.

A large-scale post-marketing surveillance study examined healthcare utilization for adverse reactions occurring in infants (N=65 927) after Prevnar was given concomitantly with other recommended vaccines (diphtheria, tetanus, acellular pertussis, inactivated polio, *H. influenzae* type b, and hepatitis B) in the course of routine care. The primary safety outcomes analyses included an evaluation of pre-defined adverse events occurring in temporal relationship to immunization. The secondary safety outcomes analyses included comparisons to a historical control population of infants (1995-1996, N=40 223) who received diphtheria, tetanus, whole-cell pertussis, oral polio, *H. influenzae* type b, and hepatitis B vaccines prior to the introduction of Prevnar, as well as long-term follow-up of subjects originally enrolled in the NCKP Efficacy Trial (N=37 866).

The primary safety outcomes analyses support the known safety profile of Prevnar. The primary analyses did not demonstrate an increased risk of healthcare utilization for "wheezing diagnoses" in the first thirty days post-vaccination. Analyses of secondary safety outcomes indicated that there was a modest increase in the relative risk of hospitalization for "wheezing diagnoses" including asthma, bronchiolitis and pneumonia, among infants receiving Prevnar in comparison to historical controls. The relative risk of occurrence of these events after Prevnar, compared to historical controls was 1.23 (95% CI: 1.11, 1.35: p<0.001) after adjusting for age at first dose, length of follow-up, gender, race and seasonality. Potential confounders, such as concomitantly administered vaccines, changes in vaccine recommendations, yearly variation in respiratory syncytial virus (RSV) or influenza infections, or secular trends in respiratory disease incidence, could not be controlled. The long-term follow-up of subjects originally enrolled in the NCKP Efficacy Trial did not confirm this observation.

OVERDOSE:

There have been reports of overdose with Prevnar, including cases of administration of a higher than recommended dose and cases of subsequent doses administered closer than recommended to the previous dose. Most individuals were asymptomatic. In general, adverse events reported with overdose have also been reported with recommended single doses of Prevnar.

For management of a suspected drug overdose, CPhA recommends that you contact your **regional Poison Control Centre**. See the *CPS* Directory section for a list of Poison Control Centres.

DOSAGE: Administration: Parenteral products should be inspected visually for particulate matter and discoloration prior to administration. This product should not be used if particulate matter or discoloration is found.

Prevnar is a suspension containing an adjuvant. Shake vigorously immediately prior to use to obtain a uniform suspension in the vaccine container. After shaking, the vaccine is a homogeneous, white suspension. The vaccine should not be used if it cannot be resuspended.

The vaccine is to be administered immediately after being drawn up into a syringe. The recommended dose is 0.5 mL given i.m. This vaccine should not be injected intradermally, s.c. or i.v. since the safety and immunogenicity of these routes have not been evaluated.

The preferred sites are the anterolateral aspect of the thigh in infants or in the deltoid muscle of the upper arm in toddlers and young children. The vaccine should not be injected in the gluteal area or areas where there may be a major nerve trunk and/or blood vessel. The needle should be long enough to reach the muscle mass and prevent the vaccine from seeping into subcutaneous tissue; but not so long as to involve underlying nerves and blood vessels or bone. Healthcare professionals should be familiar with the anatomy of the area into which they are injecting vaccine. An individual decision on needle size and site of injection must be made for each person on the basis of age, the volume of the material to be administered, the size of the muscle, and the depth below the muscle surface into which the material is to be injected.

Prevnar should not be mixed with other vaccines or products in the same syringe. Before injection, the skin at the injection site should be cleansed and prepared with a suitable germicide. After insertion of the needle, aspirate and wait to see if any blood appears in the syringe; this will help avoid inadvertent injection into a blood vessel. If blood appears, withdraw the needle, discard the syringe and prepare for a new injection at another site.

Vaccination Schedule: Infants: For infants, the immunization series of Prevnar consists of 3 doses of 0.5 mL each, at approximately 2 month intervals, followed by a fourth dose of 0.5 mL at 12 to 15 months of age. The customary age for the first dose is 2 months of age, but it can be given as young as 6 weeks of age. The recommended dosing interval is 4 to 8 weeks. The fourth dose should be administered at least 2 months after the third dose. In 1 study, a small subpopulation was administered the fourth dose from 15 to 18 months, and Prevnar was found to be both safe and immunogenic.

Previously Unvaccinated Older Infants and Children: For previously unvaccinated older infants and children, who are beyond the age of the routine infant schedule, the following applies: see Table 20.

Table 20: Prevnar

Vaccination Schedule for Previously Unvaccinated Older Infants and Children

Age at First Dose	Total Number of 0.5 mL Doses
7–11 months of age	3[a]
12–23 months of age	2[b]
≥24 months through 9 years of age	1

[a] 2 doses at least 4 weeks apart; third dose after the 1-year birthday, separated from the second dose by at least 2 months.
[b] 2 doses at least 2 months apart.

Limited safety data and limited immunogenicity data are available for patients treated with the previous vaccination schedule for older children (see Pharmacology and Adverse Effects).

Safety and immunogenicity data are either limited or not available for children in specific high risk groups for invasive pneumococcal disease (e.g., persons with sickle cell disease, asplenia, HIV-infected).

SUPPLIED: Prevnar is a sterile solution of saccharides of the capsular antigen of *S. pneumoniae* serotypes 4, 6B, 9V, 14, 18C, 19F and 23F and diphtheria CRM_{197} protein. Individual polysaccharides are prepared from purification of the culture broth of each serotype. The saccharides are directly conjugated to the protein carrier CRM_{197} protein by reductive amination. CRM_{197} is a nontoxic variant of diphtheria toxin isolated from cultures of *C. diphtheriae* strain C7 (β197) and/or *C. diphtheriae* strain C7 (β197) pPx 350 grown in a casamino acids and yeast extract-based medium. CRM_{197} is purified through ultrafiltration, ammonium sulfate precipitation, and iron-exchange chromatography to high purity. Each serotype is conjugated as a monovalent preparation prior to compounding as a multivalent vaccine. Individual glycoconjugates are analyzed for saccharide to protein ratios, for molecular size, free saccharide and free protein.

Each dose (0.5 mL) contains: 2 µg of each saccharide for serotypes 4, 9V, 14, 18C, 19F and 23F, and 4 µg of serotype 6B (16 µg total saccharides); and approximately 20 µg of CRM_{197} carrier protein. Nonmedicinal ingredients: aluminum phosphate adjuvant, sodium chloride and water for injection. Single dose vials of 0.5 mL, packages of 1 and 5.

Store between 2 to 8°C. Stability studies indicate that potency of unopened vaccine is not significantly affected by exposure to temperatures between 8 and 37°C for up to one week; however, this is not a storage or shipping recommendation. Do not freeze. Discard if the vaccine has been frozen. Prevnar is stable until the expiration date indicated on the container label.

Prevnar® 13

pneumococcal 13-valent conjugate vaccine (diphtheria CRM197 protein)

Active Immunizing Agent

Pfizer

Date of Preparation: December 21, 2009

SUMMARY PRODUCT INFORMATION:

Route of Administration	Dosage Form/ Strength	Clinically Relevant Nonmedicinal Ingredients
Intramuscular injection	Suspension for injection 1 dose (0.5 mL pre-filled syringe) contains: Pneumococcal polysaccharide serotype 1: 2.2 µg[a] Pneumococcal polysaccharide Serotype 3: 2.2 µg[a] Pneumococcal polysaccharide Serotype 4: 2.2 µg[a] Pneumococcal polysaccharide Serotype 5: 2.2 µg[a] Pneumococcal polysaccharide Serotype 6A: 2.2 µg[a] Pneumococcal polysaccharide Serotype 6B: 4.4 µg[a] Pneumococcal polysaccharide Serotype 7F: 2.2 µg[a] Pneumococcal polysaccharide Serotype 9V: 2.2 µg[a] Pneumococcal polysaccharide Serotype 14: 2.2 µg[a] Pneumococcal polysaccharide Serotype 18C: 2.2 µg[a] Pneumococcal polysaccharide Serotype 19A: 2.2 µg[a] Pneumococcal polysaccharide Serotype 19F: 2.2 µg[a] Pneumococcal polysaccharide Serotype 23F: 2.2 µg[a]	Sodium chloride, succinic acid, polysorbate 80, water for injection

[a] Conjugated to CRM197.

INDICATIONS AND CLINICAL USE: Prevnar 13, Pneumococcal 13-valent Conjugate Vaccine (Diphtheria CRM_{197} Protein), is indicated for the active immunization against *S. pneumoniae* serotypes 1, 3, 4, 5, 6A, 6B, 7F, 9V, 14, 18C, 19A, 19F and 23F, causing invasive pneumococcal disease (including sepsis, meningitis, bacteraemic pneumonia, pleural empyema and bacteraemia), in infants and children from 6 weeks through 5 years of age.

CONTRAINDICATIONS: Hypersensitivity to any component of the vaccine, including diphtheria toxoid.

(For a complete listing, see Dosage Forms, Composition and Packaging.)

WARNINGS AND PRECAUTIONS:

> **Serious Warnings and Precautions**
> Safety and immunogenicity data on Prevnar 13 are not available for children in specific groups at higher risk for invasive pneumococcal disease (e.g., children with congenital or acquired splenic dysfunction, HIV infection, malignancy, nephrotic syndrome). Children in these groups may have reduced antibody response to active immunization due to impaired immune responsiveness. Vaccination in high-risk groups should be considered on an individual basis.

General:

- As with all injectable vaccines, appropriate medical treatment and supervision must always be readily available in case of a rare anaphylactic event following the administration of the vaccine.
- Minor illnesses, such as mild respiratory infection, with or without low-grade fever, are not generally contraindications to vaccination. The decision to administer or delay vaccination because of a current or recent febrile illness depends largely on the severity of the symptoms and their etiology. The administration of Prevnar 13 should be postponed in subjects suffering from acute severe febrile illness.
- As with any intramuscular injection, Prevnar 13 should be given with caution to infants or children with thrombocytopenia or any coagulation disorder, or to those receiving anticoagulant therapy.
- Prevnar 13 will not protect against *S. pneumoniae* serotypes not included in the vaccine. Prevnar 13 will not protect against other microorganisms that cause invasive disease, pneumonia, or otitis media. This vaccine is not intended to be used for treatment of active infection.
- As with any vaccine, Prevnar 13 may not protect all individuals receiving the vaccine from pneumococcal disease.
- The use of pneumococcal conjugate vaccine does not replace the use of 23-valent pneumococcal polysaccharide vaccine (PPV23) in children ≥24 months of age with sickle cell disease, asplenia, HIV infection, chronic illness, or who are otherwise immunocompromised. Data on sequential vaccination with Prevnar 13 followed by 23-valent pneumococcal polysaccharide vaccine are not available; data on sequential vaccination with Prevnar (7-valent) vaccine followed by PPV23 are limited.
- As with all injectable pediatric vaccines, the potential risk of apnea should be considered when administering the primary immunization series to premature infants. The need for monitoring for at least 48 hours after vaccination should be considered for very premature infants (born ≤30 weeks of gestation) who remain hospitalized at the time of the recommended administration. As the benefit of vaccination is high in this group of infants, vaccination should not be withheld or delayed.
- Immunization with Prevnar 13 does not substitute for routine diphtheria immunization.

Special Populations: Pregnant Women: Safety during pregnancy has not been established.

Nursing Women: Safety during lactation has not been established.

It is not known whether vaccine antigens or antibodies are excreted in human milk.

Pediatrics: The safety and immunogenicity of Prevnar 13 in children below the age of 6 weeks or on or after the 6th birthday have not been established.

Geriatrics: The safety and immunogenicity of Prevnar 13 in geriatric populations have not been established.

ADVERSE REACTIONS: Adverse Drug Reaction Overview: Clinical Trial Adverse Drug Reactions: The safety of the vaccine was assessed in 13 controlled clinical trials where approximately 15 000 doses were given to 4729 healthy infants in ages ranging in age from 6 weeks to 16 months of age. In all trials, Prevnar 13 was co-administered with routine pediatric vaccines. In a catch-up study, 354 children (7 months to 5 years of age) receiving at least one dose of Prevnar 13 were also assessed for safety.

Expected frequency of adverse reactions is presented in CIOMS frequency categories: Very common ≥10%. Common: ≥1 % and <10 %. Uncommon: ≥0.1% and <1%. Rare: ≥0.01% and <0.1%. Very rare: <0.01%. See Table 1.

Table 1: Prevnar 13

Adverse Reactions

System Organ Class	Adverse Reaction
Metabolism and Nutrition Disorders	
Very common	Decreased appetite
Psychiatric Disorders	
Very common	Irritability
Uncommon	Crying
Nervous System Disorders	
Very common	Drowsiness/increased sleep; restless sleep/decreased sleep
Uncommon	Seizures (including febrile seizures)
Gastrointestinal Disorders	
Common	Diarrhea; vomiting
Immune System Disorders	
Rare	Hypersensitivity reaction including face edema, dyspnea, bronchospasm
Skin and Subcutaneous Tissue Disorders	
Common	Rash
Uncommon	Urticaria or urticaria-like rash
General Disorders and Administration Site Conditions	
Very common	Fever; any injection-site erythema, induration/swelling or pain/tenderness; Injection-site erythema or induration/swelling 2.5 cm-7.0 cm (after toddler dose and in older children [age 2 to 5 years]).
Common	Fever greater than 39°C; injection-site erythema or induration/swelling 2.5 cm-7.0 cm (after infant series); injection-site pain/tenderness interfering with movement
Uncommon	Injection-site induration/swelling or erythema greater than 7.0 cm

Additional Adverse Reactions from Prevnar (7-valent): Although the following adverse drug reactions were not observed in the clinical trials for Prevnar 13, they are considered adverse drug reactions for Prevnar (7-valent) and are considered adverse drug reactions for Prevnar 13 as well. These reactions are listed as follows with the frequency seen with Prevnar (7-valent).

Adverse Reactions from Prevnar (7-valent) Clinical Trials: See Table 2.

Table 2: Prevnar 13

Adverse Reactions

System Organ Class	Adverse Reaction
Nervous System Disorders	
Rare	Hypotonic-hyporesponsive episode

Post-Market Adverse Drug Reactions from Prevnar (7-valent): These frequencies are based on spontaneous reporting rates for Prevnar (7-valent) and have been calculated using number of reports and number of doses distributed. See Table 3.

Table 3: Prevnar 13

Adverse Reactions

System Organ Class	Adverse Reaction
Blood and Lymphatic System Disorders	
Very rare	Lymphadenopathy localized to the region of the injection-site
Immune System Disorders	
Very rare	Anaphylactic/anaphylactoid reaction including shock

(cont'd)

Table 3: Prevnar 13 *(cont'd)*

Adverse Reactions

System Organ Class	Adverse Reaction
Skin and Subcutaneous Tissue Disorders	
Very rare	Angioneurotic edema; erythema multiforme
General Disorders and Administration Site Conditions	
Very rare	Injection-site dermatitis; injection-site urticaria; injection-site pruritus

Serious Adverse Events (SAEs): During the 13 controlled clinical trials, SAEs that the investigator considered related to study vaccine were reported for 11 out of 7489 total subjects (0.1%); 6 out of 4729 subjects (0.1%) in the Prevnar 13 group and 5 out of 2760 (0.2%) in Prevnar (7-valent) group. Of these 11 cases, there were 3 cases of febrile convulsions and 4 cases of fever. Out of the 4 cases with fever, 1 subject had diffuse body rash, 1 subject had respiratory distress, and 1 subject had tense fontanelle. The remaining related SAE cases were crying (1), bronchitis (1), infantile spasms (1) and nephroblastoma (1).

Deaths: During the 13 controlled clinical trials, death occurred in 4 (out of 7489) infants. All 4 cases were attributable to Sudden Infant Death Syndrome (SIDS). Three (out of 4729 cases receiving 15 739 doses) cases were among Prevnar 13 recipients, and one (out of 2760 cases receiving 9030 doses) was in the Prevnar (7-valent) group. None of these cases were assessed by the investigator as causally related to vaccination.

DRUG INTERACTIONS: Overview: Prevnar 13 can be given, at a different injection site, with any of the following vaccine antigens, either as monovalent or combination vaccines: diphtheria, tetanus, acellular pertussis, *H. influenzae* type b, inactivated poliomyelitis, hepatitis B, meningococcal serogroup C, measles, mumps, rubella and varicella. Clinical studies demonstrated that the immune responses and the safety profiles of the administered vaccines were unaffected.

In the clinical trials, some infants and children were given rotavirus vaccine (oral administration) or hepatitis A vaccine (at a different site) with Prevnar 13. The safety profiles were comparable for these children but immunogenicity data were not available.

Different injectable vaccines should always be given at different injection-sites.

DOSAGE AND ADMINISTRATION: For intramuscular use only.

The dose is 0.5 mL given intramuscularly, with care to avoid injection into or near nerves and blood vessels. The preferred sites are the anterolateral aspect of the thigh in infants or the deltoid muscle of the upper arm in older children. The vaccine should not be injected in the gluteal area. **Do not administer Prevnar 13 intravascularly.**

The vaccine should not be injected intradermally, subcutaneously or intravenously, since the safety and immunogenicity of these routes have not been evaluated.

Parenteral products should be inspected visually for particulate matter or discoloration prior to use.

Data on the interchangeability of Prevnar 13 with other pneumococcal conjugate vaccines containing a protein carrier different from CRM_{197} are not available.

It is recommended that infants who receive a first dose of Prevnar 13 complete the vaccination course with Prevnar 13.

The vaccine is not to be mixed with other vaccines/products in the same syringe.

Vaccination Schedule: Primary Immunization: For infants, the recommended immunization series of Prevnar 13 consists of three doses of 0.5 mL each, at approximately 2-month intervals, followed by a fourth dose (booster) of 0.5 mL at 12-15 months of age (3+1 schedule). The customary age for the first dose is 2 months of age, but it can be given as young as 6 weeks of age. The recommended dosing interval is 4 to 8 weeks. The fourth dose should be administered at approximately 12-15 months of age, and at least 2 months after the third dose. See Table 4.

Table 4: Prevnar 13

Prevnar 13 Vaccine Schedule for Infants and Toddlers

Dose	Dose 1[a]	Dose 2[b]	Dose 3[b]	Dose 4[c]
Age at Dose	2 months	4 months	6 months	12–15 months

[a] Dose 1 may be given as early as 6 weeks of age.
[b] The recommended dosing interval is 4 to 8 weeks.
[c] The fourth dose should be administered at approximately 12-15 months of age, and at least 2 months after the third dose.

Previously Unvaccinated Older Infants and Children: For children who are beyond the age of routine infant schedule, the following Prevnar 13 schedule applies: see Table 5.

Table 5: Prevnar 13

Prevnar 13 Schedule for Previously Unvaccinated Children ≥7 Months through 5 Years of Age

Age at First Dose	Total Number of 0.5 mL Doses
7–11 months of age	3[a]
12–23 months of age	2[b]
≥24 months through 5 years of age (prior to the 6th birthday)	1

[a] 2 doses at least 4 weeks apart; third dose after the one-year birthday, separated from the second dose by at least 2 months.
[b] 2 doses at least 2 months apart.

If Prevnar 13 is given as part of a routine infant immunization program, a three dose (2+1) schedule may be considered. The first dose may be given from the age of 2 months, with a second dose 2 months later, and a third (booster) dose is recommended between 11-12 months of age. Lower immunogenicity responses for serotypes 6B and 23F were observed when Prevnar 13 is given as a 2-dose (e.g., at 2 and 4 months of age, or at 3 and 5 months of age) schedule in infants up to 6 months of age. After the booster dose, all vaccine serotypes had immune responses consistent with adequate priming with a two-dose primary series.

Infants and Children Previously Vaccinated with Prevnar (7-valent) (*S. pneumoniae* serotypes 4, 6B, 9V, 14, 18C, 19F, and 23F): Prevnar 13 contains the same 7 serotypes contained in Prevnar (7-valent) and is manufactured based on the same conjugate technology using the CRM_{197} carrier protein. A booster dose of Prevnar 13 in children (n=100) previously vaccinated with 3 doses of Prevnar (7-valent) elicited anti-capsular antibody levels (GMCs) to each of the seven common serotypes that were comparable to those elicited by 4 doses of Prevnar (7-valent).

Children who have completed the infant series with Prevnar (7-valent) can receive a single dose of Prevnar 13 in the second year of life. A single dose of Prevnar 13 in children >1 year of age elicits immune responses to the six additional serotypes that are comparable to those elicited by a 3-dose infant series of Prevnar 13, but are generally lower than those elicited by a 3 infant doses + 1 toddler dose schedule of Prevnar 13.

OVERDOSAGE:

Overdose with Prevnar 13 is unlikely due to its presentation as a pre-filled syringe. However, there have been reports of overdose with Prevnar 13 defined as subsequent doses administered closer than recommended to the previous dose. In general, adverse events reported with overdose are consistent with those that have been reported with doses given in the recommended schedules of Prevnar 13.

For management of a suspected drug overdose, CPhA recommends that you contact your **regional Poison Control Centre**. See the *CPS* Directory section for a list of Poison Control Centres.

ACTION AND CLINICAL PHARMACOLOGY: Mechanism of Action: Prevnar 13 contains the 7 pneumococcal capsular polysaccharides that are in Prevnar (7-valent) (4, 6B, 9V, 14, 18C, 19F, 23F) plus 6 additional polysaccharides (1, 3, 5, 6A, 7F, 19A) all conjugated to CRM_{197} carrier protein. B-cells produce antibodies in response to antigenic stimulation via T-dependent and T-independent mechanisms. The immune response to most antigens is T-dependent and involves the collaboration of CD4+ T-cells and B-cells, recognizing the antigen in a linked fashion. CD4+ T-cells (T-helper cells) provide signals to B-cells directly through cell surface protein interactions, and indirectly through the release of cytokines. These signals result in proliferation and differentiation of the B-cells, and production of high-affinity antibodies. CD4+ T-cell signaling is a requisite for the generation of long-lived B-cells called plasma cells, which continuously produce antibodies of several isotypes (with an IgG component) and memory B-cells that rapidly mobilize and secrete antibodies upon re-exposure to the same antigen.

Bacterial capsular polysaccharides (PSs), while varied in chemical structure, share the common immunological property of being largely T-independent antigens. In the absence of T-cell help, PS stimulated B-cells predominantly produce IgM antibodies; there is generally no affinity maturation of the antibodies, and no memory B-cells are generated. As vaccines, PSs are associated with poor or absent immunogenicity in infants less than 24 months of age and failure to induce immunological memory at any age. Conjugation of PSs to a protein carrier overcomes the T-cell–independent nature of PS antigens. Protein carrier-specific T-cells provide the signals needed for maturation of the B-cell response and generation of B-cell memory. Conversion of *S. pneumoniae* PSs to a T cell dependent antigen by covalent coupling to the immunogenic protein carrier CRM_{197} enhances the antibody response, induces immune memory, and elicits booster responses on re-exposure in infants and young children to pneumococcal polysaccharides.

Pharmacodynamics: Disease Burden: *S. pneumoniae* is an important cause of morbidity and mortality in persons of all ages worldwide. The organism causes invasive infections, such as bacteremia and meningitis, as well as pneumonia and upper respiratory tract infections, including otitis media and sinusitis. In 2002, the World Health Organization (WHO) estimated that pneumococcal disease was the most common vaccine-preventable cause of death among children <5 years of age worldwide, causing an estimated 716 000 deaths in this age group.

Prior to the licensure of 7-valent pneumococcal conjugate vaccine (Prevnar) in Canada in 2001, the observed incidence rates of invasive pneumococcal disease (IPD) among children <2 years of age and <5 years of age were 58.8-112.2 per 100 000 and 35.0 to 63.8 per 100 000 per year, respectively. 47 The overall fatality rate was 2.0%. The incidence rate of pneumococcal meningitis among children <2 years of age was 9.0 per 100 000 per year, with a case fatality rate of 5.9%.

Pneumonia may be accompanied by bacteremia or complicated by empyema, a local invasion into a normally sterile space; both of these invasive manifestations of pneumonia are more severe and are associated with higher morbidity and mortality than noninvasive pneumonia. Prior to the introduction of Prevnar (7-valent), the estimated incidence of children <2 years who were hospitalized with pneumococcal pneumonia in Canada was 2.25/1000 persons per year.

Since the introduction of Prevnar (7-valent) in Canada in 2001, it has been shown that the incidence of IPD caused by Prevnar (7-valent) serotypes decreased by 92% in Vancouver, 94% in Calgary and by 72% in Quebec.

A ten-year population-based surveillance of all cases of invasive pneumococcal infection occurring in the Calgary Health Region reported a decrease of 92% in 2007 vs. 1998-2001 in Prevnar (7-valent) serotypes among adults 65 years and older suggesting a herd immunity, a phenomenon that occurs via interruption of transmission of disease to otherwise susceptible populations.

Point-prevalence surveys conducted in Calgary have showed that routine Prevnar (7-valent) vaccination led to significant reductions in nasopharyngeal colonization of vaccine-serotype strains of *S. pneumoniae* in both vaccinated and unvaccinated children, indicating a direct and herd effect.

A laboratory-based surveillance study in Quebec showed that the resistance rates to penicillin G decreased from 17.6% in 2004, the year Prevnar (7-valent) was introduced, to 8.1% in 2007. Resistance rates to erythromycin decreased from 43.4% in 2004 to 21.6% in 2007. In Alberta, resistance rates to penicillin G dropped significantly from 14% in 2000 to 4.6% in 2006 (p<0.0001).

Data from the International Circumpolar Surveillance System for Invasive Pneumococcal Disease, 1999-2005, showed that in northern Canada, incidence of IPD among all indigenous persons decreased from 44.2 cases/100 000 persons in the pre- Prevnar (7-valent) period (1999-2002) to 25.0 cases/100 000 persons in the vaccine implementation period (2003-2005; p=0.0005). Among Canadian indigenous children <2 years of age, incidence decreased from 229.3/100 000 persons in the pre- Prevnar (7-valent) period to 92.6/100 000 persons in the vaccine implementation period (2003-2005; p=0.01). The incidence of serotypes in Prevnar (7-valent) in all age groups decreased from 12.6 cases/100 000 persons in the pre- Prevnar (7-valent) period (1999-2002) to 3.8 cases/100 000 persons in the vaccine implementation period (2003-2005; p<0.0001).

While the effect of routine use of the Prevnar (7-valent) in infants and young children has been dramatic, with a near-total elimination of the serotypes contained in this vaccine, an increase in other serotypes causing IPD has been observed (as an increasing percentage of residual disease). Data from Canadian surveillance systems (National Centre for Streptococcus [NCS]; Immunization Monitoring Program, Active [IMPACT]; and Institut National de Santé Publique du Québec [INSPQ]) showed that serotypes 19A, 6A and 3 have emerged as the predominant pneumococcal serotypes causing IPD in Canadian children, accounting for approximately one-third of the residual IPD in 2007 in children <5 years of age. The 6 additional serotypes included in Prevnar 13 caused up to 48% of residual IPD. Compounding the issue of the predominance of emerging serotype 19A is that it is increasingly likely to be nonsusceptible to commonly used first-line antimicrobial agents.

STORAGE AND STABILITY: Store refrigerated at +2 to +8°C.

Do not freeze. Discard if the vaccine has been frozen.

Store in original package.

Prevnar 13 has been shown to be stable at temperatures of up to 40°C for 4 days. These data are not recommendations for shipping or storage, but may guide decisions for use in case of temporary temperature excursions.

Do not use after the expiry date shown on the label.

SPECIAL HANDLING INSTRUCTIONS: Prevnar 13 is a suspension containing an adjuvant. The vaccine should be shaken well to obtain a homogeneous white suspension prior to expelling air from the syringe, and should be inspected visually for any particulate matter and/or variation of physical aspect prior to administration. Do not use if the content appears otherwise.

The vaccine is not to be mixed with other vaccines/products in the same syringe.

INFORMATION FOR THE PATIENT: Published in e-CPS, available by subscription at www.e-cps.ca.

DOSAGE FORMS, COMPOSITION AND PACKAGING: The vaccine is a white suspension for injection and provided in a single-dose, pre-filled syringe (0.5 mL). Pack size of 10, without needles.

Prezista® Ⓟ

darunavir

Human Immunodeficiency Virus (HIV) Protease Inhibitor

Janssen-Ortho

Date of Preparation: July 27, 2006
Date of Revision: July 6, 2010

SUMMARY PRODUCT INFORMATION:

Route of Administration	Dosage Form/ Strength	Clinically Relevant Nonmedicinal Ingredients
Oral	Tablet, 75 mg, 300 mg, 400 mg, 600 mg	None For a complete listing see Dosage Forms, Composition and Packaging.

INDICATIONS AND CLINICAL USE: PREZISTA (darunavir), co-administered with 100 mg ritonavir, and with other antiretroviral agents, is indicated for the treatment of HIV infection.

Pediatrics (from 6 to <18 years of age): PREZISTA, co-administered with low-dose ritonavir, and with other antiretroviral agents, is indicated for the treatment of HIV infection in treatment-experienced pediatric patients 6 years of age and above (see Warnings and Precautions and Dosage and Administration). This indication is based on 24-week analyses of plasma HIV RNA levels and CD4+ cell counts from an ongoing open-label Phase 2 trial in antiretroviral treatment-experienced pediatric patients 6 to <18 of age.

Geriatrics (>65 years of age): Clinical studies of PREZISTA did not include sufficient numbers of subjects aged 65 and over to determine whether they respond differently from younger subjects. In general, caution should be exercised in the administration and monitoring of PREZISTA in elderly patients, reflecting the greater frequency of decreased hepatic, renal or cardiac function and of concomitant disease or other drug therapy (see Warnings and Precautions, Dosage and Administration and Action and Clinical Pharmacology).

CONTRAINDICATIONS: PREZISTA is contraindicated in patients who are hypersensitive to this drug or to any ingredient in the formulation or component of the container. For a complete listing, see Dosage Forms, Composition and Packaging.

PREZISTA is contraindicated in patients with severe (Child-Pugh Class C) hepatic insufficiency.

Co-administration of PREZISTA/rtv is contraindicated with drugs that are highly dependent on CYP3A4 for clearance and for which elevated plasma concentrations are associated with serious and/or life-threatening events (narrow therapeutic index). These drugs are listed in Table 1 (also see Drug Interactions, Drug-Drug Interactions, Table 6).

Table 1: PREZISTA

Drugs That Are Contraindicated with PREZISTA/RTV

Drug Class	Drugs Within Class That Are Contraindicated with PREZISTA/RTV
Alpha1-Adrenoreceptor Antagonists	Alfuzosin
Antiarrhythmics	Amiodarone, bepridil[a], lidocaine (systemic), quinidine
Antihistamines	Astemizole[a], terfenadine[a]
Ergot Derivatives	Dihydroergotamine, ergonovine, ergotamine, methylergonovine
GI Motility Agents	Cisapride[a]
Neuroleptics	Pimozide
Sedatives/Hypnotics	Midazolam, triazolam
Herbal Products	St. John's Wort
HMG-CoA Reductase Inhibitors	Lovastatin, simvastatin
Antimycobacterial	Rifampin

[a] Bepridil, astemizole, terfenadine and cisapride are no longer marketed in Canada.

WARNINGS AND PRECAUTIONS: General: PREZISTA (darunavir) must be administered with low-dose ritonavir to ensure its therapeutic effect (see Drug Interactions, Drug-Drug Interactions, Table 8, Dosage and Administration and Action and Clinical Pharmacology, Pharmacokinetics). Failure to correctly co-administer PREZISTA with ritonavir will result in reduced plasma levels of PREZISTA that may be insufficient to achieve the desired antiviral effect. Patients should be instructed accordingly. Please refer to the ritonavir Product Monograph for additional information on precautionary measures.

PREZISTA is not a cure for HIV-1 infection or AIDS. Patients receiving darunavir or any other antiretroviral therapy may continue to develop opportunistic infections and other complications of HIV-1 infection.

PREZISTA therapy has not been shown to reduce the risk of transmission of HIV-1 to others.

Carcinogenesis and Mutagenesis: Darunavir was evaluated for carcinogenic potential by oral gavage administration to mice and rats up to 104 weeks. A dose-related increase in the incidence of hepatocellular adenomas and carcinomas were observed in males and females of both species as well as an increase in thyroid follicular cell adenomas in male rats. These findings are considered to be of limited relevance to humans. Based on AUC measurements, exposure to darunavir at the dose levels studied were below or approximately equivalent to exposure in humans at the recommended therapeutic dose.

Darunavir was not mutagenic or genotoxic in a battery of in vitro and in vivo assays including bacterial reverse mutation (Ames), chromosomal aberration in human lymphocytes and in vivo micronucleus test in mice.

Endocrine and Metabolism: Diabetes Mellitus/Hyperglycemia: New onset diabetes mellitus, exacerbation of pre-existing diabetes mellitus, and hyperglycemia have been reported during postmarketing surveillance in HIV-infected patients receiving PI therapy. Some patients required either initiation or dose adjustments of insulin or oral hypoglycemic agents for treatment of these events. In some cases, diabetic ketoacidosis has occurred. In those patients who discontinued PI therapy, hyperglycemia persisted in some cases. Because these events have been reported voluntarily during clinical practice, estimates of frequency cannot be made and causal relationships between PI therapy and these events have not been established.

Fat Distribution: Redistribution/accumulation of body fat, including central obesity, dorsocervical fat enlargement (buffalo hump), peripheral wasting, facial wasting, breast enlargement, and "cushingoid appearance" have been observed in patients receiving antiretroviral therapy. The mechanism and long-term consequences of these events are currently unknown. A causal relationship has not been established.

Hematologic: There have been reports of increased bleeding, including spontaneous skin hematomas and hemarthrosis, in patients with hemophilia type A and B treated with protease inhibitors. In some patients, additional factor VIII was given. In more than half of the reported cases, treatment with protease inhibitors was continued or reintroduced. A causal relationship between protease inhibitor therapy and these events has not been established; however, the frequency of bleeding episodes should be closely monitored in patients on PREZISTA/rtv.

Hepatic/Biliary/Pancreatic: Hepatic: PREZISTA is contraindicated in patients with severe hepatic insufficiency (Child-Pugh Class C) (see Contraindications). Patients with mild or moderate hepatic impairment (Child-Pugh Class A or B, respectively) should be closely monitored.

Patients with chronic hepatitis B or C and treated with combination antiretroviral therapy are at an increased risk for severe and potentially fatal hepatic adverse events. Limited data are currently available for the use of PREZISTA co-administered with low dose ritonavir, in patients co-infected with hepatitis B or C.

Patients with pre-existing liver dysfunction including chronic hepatitis B or C have an increased frequency of liver function abnormalities during combination antiretroviral therapy. Appropriate monitoring should be conducted prior to initiating therapy with PREZISTA/rtv and increased monitoring should be considered in patients with elevated baseline transaminase levels, active hepatitis B or C and in patients with underlying liver disease, especially during the first several months of PREZISTA/rtv treatment. Evidence of new or worsening liver dysfunction (including clinically significant elevation of liver enzymes and/or symptoms such as fatigue, anorexia, nausea, jaundice, dark urine, liver tenderness, hepatomegaly) in patients on PREZISTA/rtv, should prompt consideration to interrupt or discontinue treatment.

Drug-induced hepatitis (e.g., acute hepatitis, cytolytic hepatitis) has been reported with PREZISTA/rtv. During the clinical development program (N=3063), hepatitis has been reported in 0.5% of patients receiving combination therapy with PREZISTA/rtv.

Post-marketing cases of clinical hepatitis and hepatic decompensation, including some fatalities have been reported. These have generally occurred in patients with advanced HIV disease taking multiple concomitant medications, having co-morbidities including hepatitis B or C co-infection, and/or developing immune reconstitution syndrome. A causal relationship with PREZISTA/rtv therapy has not been established.

For information on the multi-dose pharmacokinetics of darunavir in hepatically impaired patients, see Action and Clinical Pharmacology.

Pancreatic: Pancreatitis has been observed in patients receiving PREZISTA/rtv therapy, including those who developed marked triglyceride elevations. Although a causal relationship to PREZISTA has not been established, marked triglyceride elevation is a risk factor for development of pancreatitis (see Warnings and Precautions, Lipid Elevations). Patients with advanced HIV disease may be at risk of elevated triglycerides and pancreatitis, and patients with a history of pancreatitis may be at increased risk for recurrence during PREZISTA/rtv therapy.

Immune: Immune Reconstitution Syndrome: During the initial phase of treatment, patients responding to antiretroviral therapy may develop an inflammatory response to indolent or residual opportunistic infections (such as MAC, CMV, PCP, and TB), which may necessitate further evaluation and treatment.

Lipid Elevations: Treatment with PREZISTA has resulted in increases in the concentration of total cholesterol and triglycerides. Triglyceride and cholesterol testing should be performed prior to initiating PREZISTA therapy and at periodic intervals during therapy. Lipid disorders should be managed as clinically appropriate. See Table 6 and Table 7 for additional information on potential drug interactions with PREZISTA and HMG-CoA reductase inhibitors.

Renal: Renal Impairment: Population pharmacokinetic analysis showed that the pharmacokinetics of darunavir were not significantly affected in HIV infected subjects with moderate renal impairment (CrCL between 30-60 mL/min, n=20). There are no pharmacokinetic data available in HIV-1 infected patients with severe renal impairment or end stage renal disease. However, since the renal clearance of darunavir is limited, a decrease in total body clearance is not expected in patients with renal impairment. As darunavir and ritonavir are highly bound to plasma proteins, it is unlikely that they will be significantly removed by hemodialysis or peritoneal dialysis (see Dosage and Administration and Action and Clinical Pharmacology, Special Populations and Conditions, Renal Insufficiency).

Sensitivity/Resistance: Darunavir contains a sulfonamide moiety. PREZISTA (darunavir) should be used with caution in patients with a known sulfonamide allergy. The potential for cross-sensitivity between drugs in the sulfonamide class and darunavir is unknown. In clinical studies with darunavir/ritonavir, the incidence and severity of rash was similar in subjects with or without a history of sulphonamide allergy.

Skin: During the clinical development program (n=3063), rash (all grades, regardless of causality) occurred in 10.3% of patients treated with PREZISTA/rtv (see Adverse Reactions). Rash was mostly mild-to-moderate, often occurring within the first four weeks of treatment and resolving with continued dosing. The discontinuation rate due to rash in patents using PREZISTA/rtv was 0.5%.

Severe skin reactions, which may be accompanied with fever and/or elevations of transaminases, have been reported in 0.4% of patients (Stevens-Johnson Syndrome has been rarely (<0.1%) reported). Both toxic epidermal necrolysis and Stevens-Johnson Syndrome have been reported from post-marketing experience. Discontinue PREZISTA/rtv immediately if signs or symptoms of severe skin reactions develop. These can include but are not limited to severe rash or rash accompanied with fever, general malaise, fatigue, muscle or joint aches, blisters, oral lesions, conjunctivitis, hepatitis and/or eosinophilia.

Special Populations: Pregnant Women: There are no adequate and well-controlled studies with darunavir in pregnant women. Studies in animals have not shown evidence of developmental toxicity or effect on reproductive function and fertility. However, due to limited bioavailability and/or dosing limitations, animal exposures (based on AUC) were only 50% (mice and rats) and 5% (rabbit) of those obtained in humans at the recommended clinical dose boosted with ritonavir.

PREZISTA should be used during pregnancy only if the potential benefit justifies the potential risk.

Antiretroviral Pregnancy Registry: To monitor maternal-fetal outcomes of pregnant women exposed to PREZISTA, an Antiretroviral Pregnancy Registry has been established. Physicians are encouraged to register patients by calling 1-800-258-4263.

Nursing Women: HIV-infected mothers should not breast-feed their infants to avoid risking postnatal transmission of HIV. It is not known whether darunavir is excreted in human milk. Studies in rats have demonstrated that darunavir is excreted into the milk of lactating rats and at high levels (1000 mg/kg/day) resulted in toxicity. Because of both the potential for HIV transmission and the potential for serious adverse events in nursing infants, mothers should be instructed not to breast-feed if they are receiving PREZISTA.

Pediatrics (<6 years of age): The pharmacokinetics, safety, tolerability and efficacy of PREZISTA in antiretroviral treatment-experienced pediatric patients 3 to <6 years of age have not been established.

PREZISTA should not be used in pediatric patients below 3 years of age in view of toxicity and mortality observed in juvenile rats dosed with darunavir (from 20 mg/kg to 1000 mg/kg) up to days 23 to 26 of age (see Action and Clinical Pharmacology, Special Populations and Conditions, Pediatrics).

Treatment-Naïve Pediatric Patients: The pharmacokinetics, safety, tolerability and efficacy of PREZISTA in antiretroviral treatment-naïve pediatric patients have not been established.

Geriatrics (>65 years of age): Clinical studies of PREZISTA did not include sufficient numbers of subjects aged 65 and over to determine whether they respond differently from younger subjects. In general, caution should be exercised in the administration and monitoring of PREZISTA in elderly patients, reflecting the greater frequency of decreased hepatic, renal or cardiac function and of concomitant disease or other drug therapy.

ADVERSE REACTIONS: Adverse Drug Reaction Overview: During the clinical development program (N=3063), 65.9% of subjects experienced at least 1 ADR. The total mean exposure for subjects was 57.5 weeks. The most common ADRs were diarrhea (23.7%), nausea (14.9%), headache (13.8%), and rash (10.3%). The majority of ADRs were mild or moderate in severity. The overall incidence of any grade 3 or 4 ADR was 15.1%. The most common grade 3 or 4 ADRs were diarrhea (1.3%) and those related to laboratory abnormalities, i.e., hepatic enzyme increased (3.4%), hypertriglyceridemia (2.9%), pancreatic enzyme increased (2.7%), and hypercholesterolemia (1.4%). Treatment discontinuation due to ADRs was infrequent (2.5%). The most common ADRs leading to treatment discontinuation were rash (0.5%), hepatic enzyme increased (0.6%), diarrhea (0.3%), and nausea (0.3%).

Clinical Trial Adverse Drug Reactions: Because clinical trials are conducted under very specific conditions the adverse reaction rates observed in the clinical trials may not reflect the rates observed in practice and should not be compared to the rates in the clinical trials of another drug. Adverse drug reaction information from clinical trials is useful for identifying drug-related adverse events and for approximating rates.

Antiretroviral Treatment-Naïve Adult Subjects: The safety assessment is based on all safety data from the randomized, controlled, open-label Phase 3 trial TMC114-C211 comparing PREZISTA/rtv 800/100 mg q.d. versus lopinavir/ritonavir 800/200 mg per day in antiretroviral treatment-naïve HIV-1-infected adult subjects. The total mean exposure in weeks for subjects in the PREZISTA/rtv 800/100 mg q.d. arm and the lopinavir/ritonavir 800/200 mg per day arm was 95.0 and 91.4, respectively.

Discontinuation due to adverse events/HIV-related events occurred in 3.8% of subjects in the PREZISTA/rtv group and in 9.2% of subjects in the LPV/rtv group.

The majority of the ADRs reported during treatment with PREZISTA/rtv 800/100 mg q.d. were mild in severity. The most common ADRs to PREZISTA/rtv 800/100 mg q.d. (≥5%) of at least moderate intensity (≥Grade 2) were diarrhea, headache, and abdominal pain.

ADRs to PREZISTA/rtv 800/100 mg q.d. of at least moderate intensity (≥Grade 2) in antiretroviral treatment naïve HIV-1-infected adult subjects are presented in Table 2.

Table 2: PREZISTA

Adverse Drug Reactions[a] of at Least Moderate Intensity (≥Grade 2) Reported in Antiretroviral Treatment-Naïve HIV-1-Infected Adult Subjects Who Received PREZISTA/rtv 800/100 mg q.d.

	Randomized Study TMC114-C211 (through 96 weeks)	
System Organ Class, Preferred Term, %	PREZISTA/rtv 800/100 mg q.d. + TDF/FTC N=343	Lopinavir/Ritonavir 800/200 mg per day + TDF/FTC N=346
Gastrointestinal Disorders		
Abdominal pain	5.2%	5.8%
Acute pancreatitis	0.3%	0.6%
Diarrhea	7.6%	14.7%
Dyspepsia	0.3%	0%
Flatulence	0.9%	0.9%
Nausea	2.6%	3.5%
Vomiting	1.5%	3.2%
General Disorders and Administration Site Conditions		
Asthenia	0.9%	0%

(cont'd)

Table 2: PREZISTA *(cont'd)*

Adverse Drug Reactions[a] of at Least Moderate Intensity (≥Grade 2) Reported in Antiretroviral Treatment-Naïve HIV-1-Infected Adult Subjects Who Received PREZISTA/rtv 800/100 mg q.d.

System Organ Class, Preferred Term, %	Randomized Study TMC114-C211 (through 96 weeks)	
	PREZISTA/rtv 800/100 mg q.d. + TDF/FTC N=343	Lopinavir/Ritonavir 800/200 mg per day + TDF/FTC N=346
Fatigue	0.3%	2.6%
Hepatobiliary Disorders		
Acute hepatitis	0.3%	0.6%
Immune System Disorders		
(Drug) hypersensitivity[b]	0.6%	1.4%
Immune reconstitution syndrome	0.3%	0.3%
Metabolism and Nutrition Disorders		
Anorexia	1.5%	0.9%
Diabetes mellitus	0.6%	0.6%
Musculoskeletal and Connective Tissue Disorders		
Myalgia	0.6%	1.2%
Nervous System Disorders		
Headache	5.8%	4.6%
Psychiatric Disorders		
Abnormal dreams	0.3%	0.3%
Skin and Subcutaneous Tissue Disorders		
Angioedema[b]	0.3%	0%
Lipodystrophy (lipohypertrophy, lipodystrophy, and lipoatrophy)	0.3%	0.3%
Pruritus	0.9%	0.6%
Rash	5.0%	6.0%
Stevens-Johnson Syndrome	0.3%	0%
Urticaria[b]	0.9%	0.3%

[a] Excluding laboratory abnormalities reported as ADRs.
[b] Adverse drug reaction also identified from post-marketing experience.
Legend: N=total number of subjects per treatment group; TDF=tenofovir disoproxil fumarate; FTC=emtricitabine.

Abnormal Hematologic and Clinical Chemistry Findings: Laboratory Abnormalities: The percentages of antiretroviral treatment-naïve HIV-1-infected adult subjects treated with PREZISTA/rtv 800/100 mg q.d. with Grade 2 to 4 laboratory abnormalities, considered ADRs, are presented in Table 3.

Table 3: PREZISTA

Grade 2 to 4 Laboratory Abnormalities Observed in Antiretroviral Treatment-Naïve HIV-1-Infected Adult Subjects

Laboratory Parameter Preferred Term, %	Limit	Randomized Study TMC114-C211 (through 96 weeks)	
		PREZISTA/rtv 800/100 mg q.d. + TDF/FTC N=343	Lopinavir/Ritonavir 800/200 mg per day + TDF/FTC N=346
Biochemistry			
Alanine Aminotransferase			
Grade 2	>2.5 to ≤5.0×ULN	7.3%	6.1%
Grade 3	>5.0 to ≤10.0×ULN	2.9%	2.6%
Grade 4	>10.0×ULN	0.9%	2.9%
Aspartate Aminotransferase			
Grade 2	>2.5 to ≤5.0×ULN	6.1%	6.1%
Grade 3	>5.0 to ≤10.0×ULN	4.1%	1.8%
Grade 4	>10.0×ULN	1.2%	2.3%
Alkaline Phosphatase			
Grade 2	>2.5 to ≤5.0×ULN	1.5%	1.2%
Grade 3	>5.0 to ≤10.0×ULN	0%	0.3%
Grade 4	>10.0×ULN	0%	0%

(cont'd)

Table 3: PREZISTA *(cont'd)*

Grade 2 to 4 Laboratory Abnormalities Observed in Antiretroviral Treatment-Naïve HIV-1-Infected Adult Subjects

Laboratory Parameter Preferred Term, %	Limit	Randomized Study TMC114-C211 (through 96 weeks)	
		PREZISTA/rtv 800/100 mg q.d. + TDF/FTC N=343	Lopinavir/Ritonavir 800/200 mg per day + TDF/FTC N=346
Hyperbilirubinemia			
Grade 2	>1.5 to ≤2.5×ULN	0.9%	4.4%
Grade 3	>2.5 to ≤5.0×ULN	0.3%	0.6%
Grade 4	>5.0×ULN	0%	0%
Triglycerides			
Grade 2	5.65–8.48 mmol/L 500–750 mg/dL	2.6%	7.9%
Grade 3	8.49–13.56 mmol/L 751–1200 mg/dL	1.2%	4.7%
Grade 4	>13.56 mmol/L >1200 mg/dL	0.6%	0.9%
Total Cholesterol[a]			
Grade 2	6.20–7.77 mmol/L 240–300 mg/dL	16.4%	23.0%
Grade 3	>7.77 mmol/L >300 mg/dL	1.2%	4.7%
Low-Density Lipoprotein[a] Cholesterol			
Grade 2	4.13–4.90 mmol/L 160–190 mg/dL	13.5%	9.6%
Grade 3	≥4.91 mmol/L ≥191 mg/dL	4.7%	5.0%
Elevated Glucose Levels			
Grade 2	6.95–13.88 mmol/L 126–250 mg/dL	7.3%	7.6%
Grade 3	13.89–27.75 mmol/L 251–500 mg/dL	0.9%	0%
Grade 4	>27.75 mmol/L >500 mg/dL	0%	0%
Pancreatic Lipase			
Grade 2	>1.5 to ≤3.0×ULN	1.8%	1.2%
Grade 3	>3.0 to ≤5.0×ULN	0.6%	0.6%
Grade 4	>5.0×ULN	0%	0.6%
Pancreatic Amylase			
Grade 2	>1.5 to ≤2.0×ULN	4.7%	1.7%
Grade 3	>2.0 to ≤5.0×ULN	2.6%	2.9%
Grade 4	>5.0×ULN	0%	0.6%

[a] Grade 4 data not applicable in Division of AIDS grading scale.
Legend: N=total number of subjects per treatment group; TDF=tenofovir disoproxil fumarate; FTC=emtricitabine.

Antiretroviral Treatment-Experienced Adult Subjects: The safety assessment is based on all safety data from the randomized, controlled, open-label Phase 3 trial TMC114-C214 comparing PREZISTA/rtv 600/100 mg b.i.d. versus lopinavir/ritonavir 400/100 mg b.i.d. in antiretroviral treatment-experienced HIV-1-infected adult subjects. The total mean exposure in weeks for subjects in the PREZISTA/rtv 600/100 mg b.i.d. arm and the lopinavir/ritonavir 400/100 mg b.i.d. arm was 80.7 and 76.4, respectively.

Discontinuation due to adverse events/HIV-related events occurred in 7.7% of subjects in the PREZISTA/rtv group and in 8.1% of subjects in the LPV/rtv group.

The majority of the ADRs reported during treatment with PREZISTA/rtv 600/100 mg b.i.d. were mild in severity. The most common ADRs to PREZISTA/rtv 600/100 mg b.i.d. (≥5%) of at least moderate intensity (≥Grade 2) were diarrhea, hypertriglyceridemia, hypercholesterolemia, nausea, abdominal pain, vomiting, lipodystrophy, hepatic enzymes increased and rash.

ADRs of at least moderate intensity (≥Grade 2) and reported in ≥1% of subjects treated with PREZISTA/rtv 600/100 mg b.i.d. in antiretroviral treatment-experienced HIV-1 infected adult subjects are presented in Table 4.

Less Common Clinical Trial Adverse Drug Reactions (<1%): Adverse drug reactions occurring in less than 1% of patients receiving PREZISTA/rtv, considered at least possibly related to treatment and of at least moderate intensity are listed below by body system:

Gastrointestinal Disorders: acute pancreatitis, flatulence.

Immune System Disorders: immune reconstitution syndrome.

Psychiatric Disorders: abnormal dreams.

Table 4: PREZISTA

Adverse Drug Reactions[a] of at Least Moderate Intensity (≥Grade 2) Reported in ≥1% of Antiretroviral Treatment-Experienced HIV-1-Infected Adult Subjects Who Received PREZISTA/rtv 600/100 mg b.i.d.

System Organ Class, Preferred Term, %	Randomized Study TMC114-C214 (through 96 weeks)	
	PREZISTA/rtv 600/100 mg b.i.d. + OBR N=298	Lopinavir/rtv 400/100 mg b.i.d. + OBR N=297
Gastrointestinal Disorders		
Abdominal distension	2.0%	0.3%
Abdominal pain	5.7%	2.7%
Diarrhea	14.4%	19.9%
Dyspepsia	2.0%	1.0%
Nausea	7.0%	6.4%
Vomiting	5.4%	2.7%
General Disorders and Administration Site Conditions		
Asthenia	3.0%	1.0%
Fatigue	1.3%	1.3%
Metabolism and Nutrition Disorders		
Anorexia	1.7%	2.0%
Diabetes mellitus	1.7%	0.3%
Musculoskeletal and Connective Tissue Disorders		
Myalgia	1.0%	0.7%
Nervous System Disorders		
Headache	2.7%	3.0%
Skin and Subcutaneous Tissue Disorders		
Lipodystrophy (lipohypertrophy, lipodystrophy, and lipoatrophy)	5.4%	4.4%
Pruritus	1.0%	1.0%
Rash	7.0%	3.0%

[a] Excluding laboratory abnormalities reported as ADRs.
Legend: N=total number of subjects per treatment group; OBR=optimized background regimen.

Reproductive and Breast Disorders: gynecomastia.
Skin and Subcutaneous Tissue Disorders: urticaria*.
Abnormal Hematologic and Clinical Chemistry Findings: Laboratory Abnormalities: The percentages of antiretroviral treatment-experienced HIV-1-infected adult subjects treated with PREZISTA/rtv 600/100 mg b.i.d. with Grade 2 to 4 laboratory abnormalities, considered ADRs, are presented in Table 5.

Table 5: PREZISTA

Grade 2 to 4 Laboratory Abnormalities Observed in Antiretroviral Treatment-Experienced HIV-1-Infected Adult Subjects

Laboratory Parameter Preferred Term, %	Limit	Randomized Study TMC114-C214 (through 96 weeks)	
		PREZISTA/rtv 600/100 mg b.i.d. + OBR N=298	Lopinavir/rtv 400/100 mg b.i.d. + OBR N=297
Biochemistry			
Alanine Aminotransferase			
Grade 2	>2.5 to ≤5.0×ULN	6.9%	4.8%
Grade 3	>5.0 to ≤10.0×ULN	2.4%	2.4%
Grade 4	>10.0×ULN	1.0%	1.7%
Aspartate Aminotransferase			
Grade 2	>2.5 to ≤5.0×ULN	5.5%	6.2%
Grade 3	>5.0 to ≤10.0×ULN	2.4%	1.7%
Grade 4	>10.0×ULN	0.7%	1.7%
Alkaline Phosphatase			
Grade 2	>2.5 to ≤5.0×ULN	0.3%	0%
Grade 3	>5.0 to ≤10.0×ULN	0.3%	0.3%
Grade 4	>10.0×ULN	0%	0%

* Adverse drug reaction also identified from post-marketing experience.

(cont'd)

Table 5: PREZISTA *(cont'd)*

Grade 2 to 4 Laboratory Abnormalities Observed in Antiretroviral Treatment-Experienced HIV-1-Infected Adult Subjects

Laboratory Parameter Preferred Term, %	Limit	Randomized Study TMC114-C214 (through 96 weeks)	
		PREZISTA/rtv 600/100 mg b.i.d. + OBR N=298	Lopinavir/rtv 400/100 mg b.i.d. + OBR N=297
Hyperbilirubinemia			
Grade 2	>1.5 to ≤2.5×ULN	0.3%	1.7%
Grade 3	>2.5 to ≤5.0×ULN	0.3%	0.3%
Grade 4	>5.0×ULN	0.3%	0%
Triglycerides			
Grade 2	5.65–8.48 mmol/L 500–750 mg/dL	10.4%	11.4%
Grade 3	8.49–13.56 mmol/L 751–1200 mg/dL	6.9%	9.7%
Grade 4	>13.56 mmol/L >1200 mg/dL	3.1%	6.2%
Total Cholesterol[a]			
Grade 2	6.20–7.77 mmol/L 240–300 mg/dL	24.9%	23.2%
Grade 3	>7.77 mmol/L >300 mg/dL	9.7%	13.5%
Low-Density Lipoprotein[a] Cholesterol			
Grade 2	4.13–4.90 mmol/L 160–190 mg/dL	14.4%	13.5%
Grade 3	≥4.91 mmol/L ≥191 mg/dL	7.7%	9.3%
Elevated Glucose Levels			
Grade 2	6.95–13.88 mmol/L 126–250 mg/dL	10.0%	11.4%
Grade 3	13.89–27.75 mmol/L 251–500 mg/dL	1.4%	0.3%
Grade 4	>27.75 mmol/L >500 mg/dL	0.3%	0%
Pancreatic Lipase			
Grade 2	>1.5 to ≤3.0×ULN	2.8%	3.5%
Grade 3	>3.0 to ≤5.0×ULN	2.1%	0.3%
Grade 4	>5.0×ULN	0.3%	0%
Pancreatic Amylase			
Grade 2	>1.5 to ≤2.0×ULN	6.2%	7.3%
Grade 3	>2.0 to ≤5.0×ULN	6.6%	2.8%
Grade 4	>5.0×ULN	0%	0%

[a] Grade 4 data not applicable in Division of AIDS grading scale.
Legend: N=total number of subjects per treatment group; OBR=optimized background regimen.

Except for a lower incidence of diarrhea and of grade 3 or 4 increases in triglycerides, and for a higher incidence of rash-related AEs with DRV/RTV than with LPV/RTV, there were no clinically relevant differences in the overall safety profile for DRV/RTV 600/100 mg b.i.d. and LPV/RTV 400/100 mg b.i.d in the TMC114-C214 study.

Additional ADRs to PREZISTA/rtv Identified in Other Clinical Trials: The additional ADRs of interest identified from other clinical trials were lipodystrophy and osteonecrosis (0.4%).

Patients Co-Infected with Hepatitis B and/or Hepatitis C Virus: The incidence of adverse events or clinical chemistry abnormalities, except for increased hepatic enzymes, was comparable in patients co-infected with hepatitis B or C virus and patients who were not co-infected. Patients co-infected with hepatitis B or C virus receiving PREZISTA/rtv were more likely to have baseline and treatment emergent hepatic transaminase elevations than those without chronic viral hepatitis. Patients with chronic hepatitis B and/or C co-infection should be monitored appropriately.

Clinical Trial Experience in Pediatric Patients: Study TMC114-C212: The safety assessment in children and adolescents is based on the safety data from the Phase 2 DELPHI trial (TMC114-C212) in which 80 antiretroviral treatment-experienced HIV-1-infected pediatric subjects 6 to <18 years of age and weighing at least 44 lbs (20 kg) received PREZISTA/RTV in combination with other antiretroviral agents (see Action and Clinical Pharmacology, Special Populations and Conditions, Pediatrics).

The mean duration of patient exposure to DRV/rtv at the time of the data cut-off for the Week 24 analysis was 39.5 (±11.02) weeks. Total patient years of exposure was 60.8 years. Frequency, type and severity of adverse drug reactions in pediatric subjects were comparable to those observed in adults. The overall incidence of ADRs was 40%. The most common ADRs in the TMC114-C212 trial were GI-related: vomiting (12.5%), diarrhea (11.3%), and abdominal pain (10.0%). The majority of ADRs were mild or moderate in severity. The overall incidence of any ADR of at least grade 2 was 13.8%. There were no ADRs leading to treatment discontinuation in the Week 24 analysis of the TMC114-C212 trial.

Post-Market Adverse Drug Reactions: In addition to adverse events identified in clinical trials, the following post-marketing events have been included due to their seriousness, frequency of reporting, potential causal association with PREZISTA/rtv, or a combination of these factors. Because they are reported spontaneously from a population of unknown size, estimates of incidence cannot be made.

Blood and Lymphatic System Disorders: anemia, pancytopenia.
Cardiac Disorders: bradycardia, myocarditis.
Eye Disorders: eye swelling.
Gastrointestinal Disorders: pancreatitis, pancreatitis relapsing, rectal hemorrhage.
Hepatobiliary Disorders: bile duct obstruction, hepatic cirrhosis, hepatic failure, hepatitis, hepatotoxicity, jaundice.
Infections and Infestations: clostridial infection, cryptosporidiosis infection, cytomegalovirus encephalitis, hepatitis B, esophageal candidiasis, progressive multifocal leukoencephalopathy, sepsis.
Investigations: blood alkaline phosphatase increased, blood bilirubin increased, abnormal liver function test.
Immune System Disorder: drug hypersensitivity, immune reconstitution syndrome.
Injury, Poisoning and Procedural Complications: drug toxicity.
Metabolism and Nutrition Disorders: dehydration, hyperkalemia, metabolic acidosis.
Musculoskeletal and Connective Tissue Disorders: myositis, osteonecrosis, rhabdomyolysis, sensation of heaviness.
Neoplasms Benign, Malignant and Unspecified: diffuse large B-cell neoplasm, malignant hepatic neoplasm, lymphoma.
Nervous System Disorders: altered state of consciousness, cerebrovascular accident, dizziness, facial palsy, grand mal convulsion, ischemic cerebral infarction, nervous system disorder, neuromyopathy, petit mal epilepsy.
Psychiatric Disorders: completed suicide.
Renal and Urinary Disorders: acute renal failure, hematuria, renal tubular necrosis.
Respiratory, Thoracic and Mediastinal Disorders: acute respiratory distress syndrome, pharyngeal lesion, pneumothorax, respiratory failure.
Skin and Subcutaneous Tissue Disorders: angioedema, rash, swelling face, Stevens-Johnson syndrome, toxic epidermal necrolysis, urticaria.

DRUG INTERACTIONS: Overview: Darunavir and ritonavir are both inhibitors of the cytochrome P450 isoform CYP3A4. Co-administration of darunavir and ritonavir with drugs primarily metabolized by CYP3A4 may result in increased plasma concentrations of such drugs, which could increase or prolong their therapeutic effect and adverse events (see Contraindications and Drug-Drug Interactions, Table 6 and Table 7).

Drug-Drug Interactions: Drugs that are contraindicated and not recommended for co-administration with PREZISTA/rtv are included in Table 6. These recommendations are based on either drug interaction studies or predicted interactions due to the expected magnitude of interaction and potential for serious events or loss of efficacy.

Table 6: PREZISTA

Drugs That Should Not Be Co-administered with PREZISTA/RTV

Drug Class: Drug Name	Clinical Comment
Alpha1-Adrenoreceptor Antagonists: alfuzosin	**Contraindicated** due to potential for serious reactions such as hypotension.
Antiarrhythmics: bepridil[a] lidocaine (systemic) quinidine amiodarone	**Contraindicated.** Concentrations of bepridil, lidocaine, quinidine and amiodarone may be increased when co-administered with PREZISTA/rtv.
Anticonvulsants: phenobarbital phenytoin	Phenobarbital and phenytoin are inducers of CYP450 enzymes. PREZISTA/rtv should not be used in combination with phenobarbital, or phenytoin as co-administration may cause significant decreases in darunavir plasma concentrations. This may result in loss of therapeutic effect of PREZISTA.
Antihistamines: astemizole[a] terfenadine[a]	**Contraindicated** due to potential for serious and/or life-threatening reactions such as cardiac arrhythmias.
Antimycobacterials: rifampin	**Contraindicated.** Rifampin is a potent inducer of CYP450 metabolism. PREZISTA/rtv should not be used in combination with rifampin, as this may cause significant decreases in darunavir plasma concentrations. This may result in loss of therapeutic effect of PREZISTA.
Ergot Derivatives: dihydroergotamine ergonovine ergotamine methylergonovine	**Contraindicated** due to potential for serious and/or life-threatening reactions such as acute ergot toxicity characterized by peripheral vasospasm and ischemia of the extremities and other tissues.
Gastrointestinal Motility Agents: cisapride[a]	**Contraindicated** due to potential for serious and/or life-threatening reactions such as cardiac arrhythmias.
Herbal Products: St. John's wort (Hypericum perforatum)	**Contraindicated.** PREZISTA/rtv should not be used concomitantly with products containing St. John's wort (Hypericum perforatum) because co-administration may cause significant decreases in darunavir plasma concentrations. This may result in loss of therapeutic effect of PREZISTA.
HIV-Protease Inhibitor: lopinavir/ritonavir	Results of interaction trials with PREZISTA with or without ritonavir and lopinavir/ritonavir (1200 mg darunavir b.i.d. with or without 100 mg ritonavir b.i.d. and lopinavir/ritonavir 400/100 mg b.i.d. or 533/133.3 mg b.i.d.) demonstrated a decrease in the exposure (AUC) of darunavir by 40%. The appropriate doses of the combination have not been established. Hence, it is not recommended to co-administer PREZISTA/rtv with lopinavir/ritonavir.
HIV-Protease Inhibitor: saquinavir	An interaction trial between darunavir (400 mg b.i.d.), saquinavir (1000 mg b.i.d.), and low-dose ritonavir (100 mg b.i.d.) demonstrated that darunavir exposure was decreased by 26% when co-administered with saquinavir and ritonavir; saquinavir exposure was not affected when administered concomitantly with darunavir/ritonavir. It is not recommended to co-administer saquinavir and PREZISTA, with or without low-dose ritonavir.
HMG-CoA Reductase Inhibitors: lovastatin simvastatin	**Contraindicated.** HMG-CoA reductase inhibitors, such as lovastatin and simvastatin, which are highly dependent on CYP3A4 metabolism, are expected to have markedly increased plasma concentrations when co-administered with darunavir/ritonavir. Increased concentrations of HMG-CoA reductase inhibitors may cause myopathy, including rhabdomyolysis. Concomitant use of PREZISTA/rtv with lovastatin or simvastatin is not recommended.

(cont'd)

Table 6: PREZISTA *(cont'd)*

Drugs That Should Not Be Co-administered with PREZISTA/RTV

Drug Class: Drug Name	Clinical Comment
pravastatin	An interaction trial between darunavir (600 mg b.i.d.), low dose ritonavir (100 mg b.i.d.) and pravastatin (40 mg single dose) demonstrated that DRV/rtv did not increase exposure to a single dose of pravastatin in most subjects but up to 5-fold in a limited subset of subjects. When administration of pravastatin and PREZISTA/rtv is required, it is recommended to start with the lowest possible dose of pravastatin and titrate up to the desired clinical effects while monitoring safety. For information regarding atorvastatin, see Table 7.
Neuroleptics: pimozide	**Contraindicated** due to the potential for serious and/or life-threatening reactions such as cardiac arrhythmias.
Sedatives/Hypnotics: midazolam triazolam	**Contraindicated** due to the potential for serious and/or life-threatening reactions such as prolonged or increased sedation or respiratory depression.

[a] Bepridil, astemizole, terfenadine and cisapride are no longer marketed in Canada.

Established and other potentially significant drug interactions with PREZISTA/RTV are included in Table 7. These recommendations are based on either drug interaction studies or predicted interactions due to the expected magnitude of interaction and potential for serious events or loss of efficacy.

Other NRTIs: Based on the different elimination pathways of the other NRTIs (zidovudine, zalcitabine, emtricitabine, stavudine, lamivudine and abacavir) that are primarily renally excreted, no drug interactions are expected for these drugs and PREZISTA/rtv.

Other Protease Inhibitors: The co-administration of PREZISTA/rtv and PIs other than lopinavir/ritonavir, saquinavir, atazanavir, and indinavir has not been studied. Therefore, such co-administration is not recommended.

CCR5 Antagonist: When used in combination with PREZISTA/rtv, the dose of maraviroc should be 150 mg twice daily.

An interaction trial between PREZISTA/rtv (600/100 mg b.i.d.) and maraviroc (150 mg b.i.d.) demonstrated that in the presence of PREZISTA/rtv the exposure of maraviroc was increased by 305%. There was no apparent effect of maraviroc on darunavir/ritonavir exposure.

Table 7: PREZISTA

Established and Other Potentially Significant Drug Interactions: Alterations in Dose or Regimen May be Recommended Based on Drug Interaction Studies or Predicted Interaction (see Table 8 and Table 9)

Concomitant Drug Class: Drug Name	Effect on Concentration of Darunavir or Concomitant Drug	Clinical Comment
HIV-Antiviral Agents: Non-Nucleoside Reverse Transcriptase Inhibitors (NNRTIs)		
efavirenz	↓ darunavir ↑ efavirenz	An interaction trial between darunavir (300 mg twice daily [b.i.d.]), low-dose ritonavir (100 mg b.i.d.), and efavirenz (600 mg once daily [q.d.]) has been performed. In the presence of efavirenz, a decrease of 13% for darunavir exposure was observed. Exposure to efavirenz increased by 21% when administered in combination with darunavir and ritonavir. Since this difference is not considered to be clinically relevant, the combination of PREZISTA/rtv and efavirenz can be used without dose adjustments.
etravirine	↔ darunavir ↓ etravirine	In an interaction trial between PREZISTA/rtv (600/100 mg b.i.d.) and etravirine (100 mg b.i.d.), there was a 37% decrease in etravirine exposure in the presence of PREZISTA/rtv and no relevant change in exposure to darunavir. Therefore, PREZISTA/rtv can be co-administered with etravirine at the recommended therapeutic dose of 200 mg b.i.d. without dose adjustments.
nevirapine	↔ darunavir ↑ nevirapine	The results of an interaction trial with darunavir (400 mg b.i.d.), low-dose ritonavir (100 mg b.i.d.), and nevirapine (200 mg b.i.d.) demonstrated that darunavir exposure was not affected when administered concomitantly with nevirapine. Exposure to nevirapine increased by 27% (compared to historical controls) when administered in combination with darunavir and ritonavir. No dose adjustment is currently recommended for the combination of PREZISTA/rtv and nevirapine. However, the literature indicates that changes in plasma exposure of nevirapine can lead to significant safety concerns, specifically hepatotoxicity. For further information, please refer to the nevirapine Product Monograph.
HIV-Antiviral Agents: Nucleoside Reverse Transcriptase Inhibitors (NRTIs)		
didanosine	↔ darunavir ↔ didanosine	PREZISTA/rtv (600/100 mg b.i.d.) did not significantly affect didanosine exposure. The combination of PREZISTA co-administered with 100 mg ritonavir and didanosine can be used without dose adjustments. Dosing of enteric-coated didanosine and darunavir, co-administered with low-dose ritonavir, should be separated by at least 2 hours to avoid formulation incompatibility (see Drug-Food Interactions and Dosage and Administration, Dosing Considerations).
tenofovir disoproxil fumarate	↔ darunavir ↑ tenofovir	The results of an interaction trial between darunavir (300 mg b.i.d.), low-dose ritonavir (100 mg b.i.d.), and tenofovir disoproxil fumarate (300 mg q.d.) demonstrated that darunavir exposure was not significantly affected when administered concomitantly with tenofovir disoproxil fumarate. Exposure to tenofovir disoproxil fumarate increased by 22% when administered in combination with darunavir and ritonavir. This finding is not considered to be clinically relevant. There was no change in the urinary excretion of tenofovir disoproxil fumarate or darunavir during co-administration. The combination of PREZISTA/rtv and tenofovir disoproxil fumarate can be used without dose adjustments.
HIV-Antiviral Agents: HIV-Protease Inhibitors (PIs)		

(cont'd)

Table 7: PREZISTA *(cont'd)*

Established and Other Potentially Significant Drug Interactions: Alterations in Dose or Regimen May be Recommended Based on Drug Interaction Studies or Predicted Interaction (see Table 8 and Table 9)

Concomitant Drug Class: Drug Name	Effect on Concentration of Darunavir or Concomitant Drug	Clinical Comment
ritonavir	↑ darunavir	The overall pharmacokinetic enhancement effect by ritonavir was an approximate 14-fold increase in the systemic exposure of darunavir when a single dose of 600 mg darunavir was given orally in combination with ritonavir at 100 mg b.i.d. Therefore, PREZISTA should only be used in combination with 100 mg of ritonavir as a pharmacokinetic enhancer (see Warnings and Precautions, General and Action and Clinical Pharmacology, Pharmacokinetics, Absorption).
atazanavir	↔ darunavir ↔ atazanavir	An interaction trial between darunavir (400 mg b.i.d.), low-dose ritonavir (100 mg b.i.d.), and atazanavir (300 mg q.d.) demonstrated that exposure to darunavir and atazanavir was not significantly affected when co-administered. Atazanavir can be co-administered with PREZISTA/rtv.
indinavir	↑ darunavir ↑ indinavir	An interaction trial between darunavir (400 mg b.i.d.), low-dose ritonavir (100 mg b.i.d.), and indinavir (800 mg b.i.d.) demonstrated that darunavir exposure was increased by 24% when co-administered with indinavir and ritonavir; indinavir exposure was increased by 23% when administered concomitantly with darunavir/ritonavir. When used in combination with PREZISTA/rtv, dose adjustment of indinavir may be warranted in case of intolerance.
HIV-Antiviral Agents: CCR5 Antagonist		
maraviroc	↔ darunavir ↑ maraviroc	An interaction trial between darunavir (600 mg b.i.d.), low dose ritonavir (100 mg b.i.d.), and maraviroc (150 mg b.i.d.) demonstrated that in the presence of PREZISTA/rtv the exposure of maraviroc was increased by 305%. There was no apparent effect of maraviroc on darunavir/ritonavir exposure. When used in combination with PREZISTA/rtv, the dose of maraviroc should be 150 mg twice daily.
Other Agents		
Antiarrythmics: digoxin	↑ digoxin	An interaction trial with PREZISTA/rtv (600/100 mg b.i.d.) and a single dose of digoxin (0.4 mg) showed an increase of digoxin AUC_{last} of 77% (ratio of Least Square Means was 1.77 with a 90% CI of 0.90 to 3.50). It is recommended that the lowest dose of digoxin should initially be prescribed and digoxin dose should be titrated to obtain the desired clinical effect when co-administered with PREZISTA/rtv. Serum digoxin concentrations should be monitored to assist in the titration.
Anticoagulants: warfarin	↓ warfarin ↔ darunavir	Warfarin concentrations may be affected when co-administered with PREZISTA/rtv. It is recommended that the international normalized ratio (INR) be monitored when warfarin is combined with PREZISTA/rtv.
Anticonvulsants: carbamazepine	↔ darunavir ↑ carbamazepine	An interaction trial between darunavir/rtv (600/100 mg b.i.d.) and carbamazepine (200 mg b.i.d.) showed that the exposure to darunavir, co-administered with ritonavir, was unaffected by carbamazepine. Ritonavir exposure (AUC_{12h}) was decreased by 49%. For carbamazepine, AUC_{12h} was increased by 45%. No dose adjustment for PREZISTA/rtv is recommended. If there is a need to combine PREZISTA/rtv and carbamazepine, patients should be monitored for potential carbamazepine-related adverse events. Carbamazepine concentrations should be monitored and its dose should be titrated for adequate response.
Anti-infectives: clarithromycin	↔ darunavir ↑ clarithromycin	An interaction trial between darunavir (400 mg b.i.d.), low-dose ritonavir (100 mg b.i.d.), and clarithromycin (500 mg b.i.d.) demonstrated an increase in exposure to clarithromycin by 57%, while exposure to darunavir was not affected. For patients with renal impairment, the following dose adjustments should be considered: • For subjects with CLcr of 30–60 mL/min, the dose of clarithromycin should be reduced by 50%. • For subjects with CLcr of <30 mL/min, the dose of clarithromycin should be reduced by 75%.
Antifungals: ketoconazole, itraconazole (not studied)	↑ ketoconazole ↑ darunavir itraconazole (not studied)	Ketoconazole and itraconazole are potent inhibitors as well as substrates of CYP3A4. Concomitant systemic use of ketoconazole or itraconazole, and darunavir and ritonavir may increase plasma concentrations of both darunavir and ketoconazole, or itraconazole. In an interaction trial, concomitant administration of ketoconazole (200 mg b.i.d.) with darunavir (400 mg b.i.d.) and ritonavir (100 mg b.i.d.) increased exposure of ketoconazole and darunavir by 212% and 42%, respectively. When co-administration is required, the daily dose of ketoconazole or itraconazole should not exceed 200 mg.
voriconazole (not studied)	voriconazole (not studied)	Co-administration of voriconazole with PREZISTA/rtv has not been studied. Administration of voriconazole with ritonavir (100 mg twice daily) decreased the AUC of voriconazole by an average of 39%. Voriconazole should not be administered to patients receiving darunavir/ritonavir unless an assessment of the benefit/risk ratio justifies the use of voriconazole.

(cont'd)

Table 7: PREZISTA *(cont'd)*

Established and Other Potentially Significant Drug Interactions: Alterations in Dose or Regimen May be Recommended Based on Drug Interaction Studies or Predicted Interaction (see Table 8 and Table 9)

Concomitant Drug Class: Drug Name	Effect on Concentration of Darunavir or Concomitant Drug	Clinical Comment
Antimycobacterials: rifabutin	↑ darunavir ↑ rifabutin ↑ 25-O-desacetyl-rifabutin	Rifabutin is a substrate of CYP450 enzymes. In an interaction trial, an increase of systemic exposure to darunavir by 57% was observed when PREZISTA/rtv (600/100 mg b.i.d.) was administered with rifabutin (150 mg once every other day [q.o.d.]). Based on the safety profile of PREZISTA/rtv, the increase in darunavir exposure in the presence of rifabutin does not warrant a dose adjustment for PREZISTA/rtv. The interaction trial showed a comparable systemic exposure for rifabutin between treatment at 300 mg q.d. alone and at 150 mg q.o.d. in combination with PREZISTA/rtv (600/100 mg b.i.d.) with an increase in exposure to the active metabolite 25-O-desacetyl-rifabutin. A dosage reduction of rifabutin by 75% of the usual dose of 300 mg/day (i.e., rifabutin 150 mg every other day) is warranted if rifabutin is co-administered with PREZISTA/rtv. Increased monitoring for rifabutin-related adverse events is warranted in patients receiving the combination.
Calcium Channel Blockers: felodipine nifedipine nicardipine	↑ calcium channel blockers	Plasma concentrations of calcium channel blockers (e.g. felodipine, nifedipine, nicardipine) may increase when PREZISTA/rtv are co-administered. Caution is warranted and clinical monitoring of patients is recommended.
Corticosteroids: dexamethasone fluticasone	↓ darunavir ↑ fluticasone	Use with caution. Systemic dexamethasone induces CYP3A4 and can thereby decrease darunavir plasma concentrations. This may result in loss of therapeutic effect to PREZISTA. Concomitant use of inhaled fluticasone and PREZISTA/rtv may increase plasma concentrations of fluticasone. Alternatives should be considered, particularly for long-term use.
Estrogen-Based Contraceptives: ethinyl estradiol norethindrone	↓ ethinyl estradiol ↓ norethindrone	The results of an interaction trial between PREZISTA/rtv (600/100 mg b.i.d.) and ethinyl estradiol and norethindrone demonstrated that at steady-state, systemic exposures to ethinyl estradiol and norethindrone are decreased by 44% and 14%, respectively. Therefore, alternative methods of non-hormonal contraception are recommended.
HMG-CoA Reductase Inhibitors: atorvastatin	↑ HMG-CoA reductase inhibitors	An interaction trial between darunavir (300 mg b.i.d.), low-dose ritonavir (100 mg b.i.d.), and atorvastatin (10 mg q.d.) demonstrated that exposure to atorvastatin was only 15% lower when co-administered with darunavir and ritonavir than when atorvastatin (40 mg q.d.) was administered alone. When administration of atorvastatin and PREZISTA/rtv is desired, it is recommended to start with an atorvastatin dose of 10 mg q.d. A gradual dose increase of atorvastatin may be tailored to the clinical response.
H2-Receptor Antagonists and Proton Pump Inhibitors: omeprazole ranitidine	↔ darunavir	Co-administration of omeprazole (20 mg q.d.) or ranitidine (150 mg b.i.d.) and darunavir (400 mg b.i.d.) in the presence of low-dose ritonavir (100 mg b.i.d.) did not affect the exposure to darunavir. Based on these results, PREZISTA/rtv can be co-administered with H2-receptor antagonists and proton pump inhibitors without dose adjustments. The effects of PREZISTA/rtv on omeprazole or ranitidine exposures were not evaluated.
Immunosuppressants: cyclosporine tacrolimus sirolimus	↑ immunosuppressants	Plasma concentrations of cyclosporine, tacrolimus or sirolimus may be increased when co-administered with PREZISTA/rtv. Therapeutic concentration monitoring of the immunosuppressive agent is recommended for immunosuppressant agents when co-administered with PREZISTA/rtv.
Narcotic Analgesics: methadone	↓ methadone	An interaction trial investigating the effect of PREZISTA/rtv (600/100 mg b.i.d.) on a stable methadone maintenance therapy showed an AUC decrease of 16% for R-methadone. Based on pharmacokinetic and clinical findings, no adjustment of methadone dosage is required when initiating co-administration of PREZISTA/rtv. However, clinical monitoring is recommended, as maintenance therapy may need to be adjusted in some patients.
meperidine	↓ meperidine	PREZISTA/rtv is expected to decrease meperidine concentrations and increase normeperidine metabolite concentrations. Dosage increase and long-term use of meperidine and PREZISTA/rtv are not recommended due to the increased concentrations of the metabolite normeperidine, which has both analgesic and CNS stimulant activity (e.g. seizures).
buprenorphine/naloxone	↑ norbuprenorphine	The results of an interaction trial with PREZISTA/rtv and buprenorphine/naloxone demonstrated that buprenorphine exposure was not affected when administered with PREZISTA/rtv. Exposure of the active metabolite, norbuprenorphine, increased by 46%. No dose adjustment for buprenorphine was required. Careful clinical monitoring is recommended if PREZISTA/rtv and buprenorphine are co-administered.

(cont'd)

Table 7: PREZISTA *(cont'd)*

Established and Other Potentially Significant Drug Interactions: Alterations in Dose or Regimen May be Recommended Based on Drug Interaction Studies or Predicted Interaction (see Table 8 and Table 9)

Concomitant Drug Class: Drug Name	Effect on Concentration of Darunavir or Concomitant Drug	Clinical Comment
PDE-5 Inhibitors: sildenafil tadalafil	↑ PDE-5 inhibitors	In an interaction trial, a comparable systemic exposure to sildenafil was observed for a single dose of 100 mg sildenafil alone and a single dose of 25 mg sildenafil co-administered with darunavir (400 mg b.i.d.) and low-dose ritonavir (100 mg b.i.d.). Concomitant use of PDE-5 inhibitors should be done with caution. Co-administration of darunavir and low-dose ritonavir with sildenafil or tadalafil is expected to substantially increase the PDE-5 concentration and may result in an increase in PDE-5 inhibitor-associated adverse events including hypotension, visual changes and priapism. If concomitant use of PREZISTA/rtv with sildenafil or tadalafil is required, sildenafil at a single dose not exceeding 25 mg in 48 hours or tadalafil at a single dose not exceeding 10 mg in 72 hours is recommended.
vardenafil		Vardenafil should not be used with PREZISTA/rtv.
Selective Serotonin Reuptake Inhibitors (SSRIs): sertraline paroxetine	↔ darunavir ↓ sertraline ↓ paroxetine	An interaction trial between paroxetine (20 mg q.d.) or sertraline (50 mg q.d.) and darunavir (400 mg b.i.d.) and low-dose ritonavir (100 mg b.i.d.) demonstrated that exposure to darunavir was not affected by the co-administration of sertraline or paroxetine. Exposure to sertraline or paroxetine decreased by 49% and 39%, respectively, when co-administered with darunavir and ritonavir. If sertraline or paroxetine is co-administered with PREZISTA/rtv, the recommended approach is a careful dose titration of the SSRI based on a clinical assessment of antidepressant response. In addition, patients on a stable dose of sertraline or paroxetine who start treatment with PREZISTA/ritonavir should be monitored for antidepressant response.

(cont'd)

Drug interaction studies were performed with darunavir and other drugs likely to be co-administered and some drugs commonly used as probes for pharmacokinetic interactions. The effects of co-administration of darunavir on the AUC, C_{max}, and C_{min} values are summarized in Table 8 and Table 9.

Table 8: PREZISTA

Drug Interactions: Pharmacokinetic Parameters for Darunavir in the Presence of Co-administered Drugs

Co-administered Drug	Dose/Schedule: Co-administered Drug	Dose/Schedule: Darunavir/rtv	N	PK	LS Mean Ratio % (90% CI) of Darunavir Pharmacokinetic Parameters With/Without Co-administered Drug No Effect=100%: C_{max}	AUC	C_{min}
Co-administration with Other Protease Inhibitors							
Atazanavir	300 mg q.d.	400/100 mg b.i.d.	13	↔	102 (96–109)	103 (94–112)	101 (88–116)
Indinavir	800 mg b.i.d.	400/100 mg b.i.d.	9	↑	111 (98.2–126)	124 (109–142)	144 (113–182)
Lopinavir/ Ritonavir	400/100 mg b.i.d.	1200/100 mg b.i.d.	14	↓	0.79 (0.67–0.92)	0.62 (0.53–0.73)	0.49 (0.39–0.63)
	533/133.3 mg b.i.d.	1200 mg b.i.d.	15	↓	0.79 (0.64–0.97)	0.59 (0.50–0.70)	0.45 (0.38–0.52)
Ritonavir	Titrated: 300 to 600 mg b.i.d. over 6 days	Darunavir 800 mg single dose	9	↑	197 (140–277)	923 (662–1288)	—
Saquinavir hard gel capsule	1000 mg b.i.d.	400/100 mg b.i.d.	14	↓	83 (75–92)	74 (63–86)	58 (47–72)
Co-administration with Other Antiretrovirals							
Didanosine	400 mg q.d.	600/100 mg b.i.d.	17	↔	0.93 (0.86–1.00)	1.01 (0.95–1.07)	1.07 (0.95–1.21)
Efavirenz	600 mg q.d.	300/100 mg b.i.d.	12	↓	85 (72–100)	87 (75–101)	69 (54–87)
Etravirine	100 mg b.i.d.	600/100 mg b.i.d.	14	↔	1.03 (0.98–1.09)	1.06 (1.00–1.13)	1.02 (0.89–1.17)
Nevirapine	200 mg b.i.d.	400/100 mg b.i.d.	8	↑	140[a] (114–173)	124[a] (97–157)	102[a] (79–132)
Tenofovir Disoproxil Fumarate	300 mg q.d.	300/100 mg b.i.d.	12	↑	116 (94–142)	121 (95–154)	124 (90–169)
Co-administration with Other Drugs							
Clarithromycin	500 mg b.i.d.	400/100 mg b.i.d.	17	↔	83 (72–96)	87 (75–101)	101 (81–126)
Carbamazepine	200 mg b.i.d.	600/100 mg b.i.d.	16	↔	1.04 (0.93–1.16)	0.99 (0.90–1.08)	0.85 (0.73–1.00)
Ketoconazole	200 mg b.i.d.	400/100 mg b.i.d.	14	↑	121 (104–140)	142 (123–165)	173 (139–214)
Omeprazole	20 mg q.d.	400/100 mg b.i.d.	16	↔	102 (95–109)	104 (96–113)	108 (93–125)
Paroxetine	20 mg q.d.	400/100 mg b.i.d.	16	↔	97 (92–102)	102 (95–110)	107 (96–119)
Ranitidine	150 mg b.i.d.	400/100 mg b.i.d.	16	↔	96 (89–105)	95 (90–101)	94 (90–99)
Rifabutin	150 mg q.o.d.	600/100 mg b.i.d.	11	↑	1.42 (1.21–1.67)	1.57 (1.28–1.93)	1.75 (1.28–2.37)
Sertraline	50 mg q.d.	400/100 mg b.i.d.	13	↔	101 (89–114)	98 (84–114)	94 (76–116)

[a] Ratio based on between-study comparison.
Legend: N=number of subjects with data; —=no information available.

Table 9: PREZISTA

Drug Interactions: Pharmacokinetic Parameters for Co-administered Drugs in the Presence of Darunavir/Ritonavir

Co-administered Drug	Dose/Schedule: Co-administered Drug	Dose/Schedule: Darunavir/rtv	N	PK	LS Mean Ratio % (90% CI) of Co-administered Drug Pharmacokinetic Parameters With/Without Darunavir No Effect=100%: C_{max}	AUC	C_{min}
Co-administration with Other Protease Inhibitors							
Atazanavir	300 mg q.d.	400/100 mg b.i.d.	13	↔	89 (78–101)	108 (94–124)	152 (99–234)
Indinavir	800 mg b.i.d.	400/100 mg b.i.d.	9	↑	108 (95–122)	123 (106–142)	225 (163–310)
Lopinavir/ Ritonavir	400/100 mg b.i.d.	1200/100 mg b.i.d.	14	↔	0.98 (0.78–1.22)	1.09 (0.86–1.37)	1.23 (0.90–1.69)

(cont'd)

Table 9: PREZISTA *(cont'd)*

Drug Interactions: Pharmacokinetic Parameters for Co-administered Drugs in the Presence of Darunavir/Ritonavir

	Dose/Schedule				LS Mean Ratio % (90% CI) of Co-administered Drug Pharmacokinetic Parameters With/Without Darunavir No Effect=100%		
Co-administered Drug	**Co-administered Drug**	**Darunavir/rtv**	**N**	**PK**	**C_{max}**	**AUC**	**C_{min}**
	533/133.3 mg b.i.d.	1200 mg b.i.d.	15	↔	1.11 (0.96–1.30)	1.09 (0.96–1.24)	1.13 (0.90–1.42)
Saquinavir hard gel capsule	1000 mg b.i.d.	400/100 mg b.i.d.	12	↔	94 (78–113)	94 (76–117)	82 (52–130)
Co-administration with Other Antiretrovirals							
Didanosine	400 mg q.d.	600/100 mg b.i.d.	17	↔	0.84	0.91	—
Efavirenz	600 mg q.d.	300/100 mg b.i.d.	12	↑	115 (97–135)	121 (108–136)	117 (101–136)
Etravirine	100 mg b.i.d.	600/100 mg b.i.d.	14	↓	0.68 (0.57–0.82)	0.63 (0.54–0.73)	0.51 (0.44–0.61)
Nevirapine	200 mg b.i.d.	400/100 mg b.i.d.	8	↑	118 (102–137)	127 (112–144)	147 (120–182)
Tenofovir Disoproxil Fumarate	300 mg q.d.	300/100 mg b.i.d.	12	↑	124 (108–142)	122 (110–135)	137 (119–157)
Maraviroc	150 mg b.i.d.	600/100 mg b.i.d.	15	↑	229 (146–359)	405 (294–559)	—
Co-administration with Other Drugs							
Atorvastatin[a]	10 mg q.d.[a]	300/100 mg b.i.d.	15	↑[a]	56 (48–67)	85 (76–97)	181 (137–240)
Buprenorphine[c]	24 mg q.d.[c]	600/100 mg b.i.d	17	↔	92 (79–108)	89 (78–102)	98 (82–116)
Norbuprenorphine				↑	136 (106–174)	146 (115–185)	171 (129–227)
Carbamazepine	200 mg b.i.d.	600/100 mg b.i.d.	16	↑	1.43 (1.34–1.53)	1.45 (1.35–1.57)	1.54 (1.41–1.68)
Carbamazepine epoxide			16	↓	0.46 (0.43–0.49)	0.46 (0.44–0.49)	0.48 (0.45–0.51)
Clarithromycin	500 mg b.i.d.	400/100 mg b.i.d.	17	↑	126 (103–154)	157 (135–184)	274 (230–326)
Digoxin	0.4 mg	600/100 mg b.i.d.	8	↑	1.15 (0.89–1.48)	1.36 (0.81–2.27)	—
Ethinyl Estradiol (EE)	Ortho-Novum 1/35	600/100 mg b.i.d.	11	↓	0.68 (0.61–0.74)	0.56 (0.50–0.63)	0.38 (0.27–0.54)
Norethindrone (NE)	(35 µg EE/1 mg NE)		11	↓	0/90 (0.83–0.97)	0.86 (0.75–0.98)	0.70 (0.51–0.97)
Ketoconazole	200 mg b.i.d.	400/100 mg b.i.d.	15	↑	211 (181–244)	312 (265–368)	968 (644–1455)
R-Methadone	55–150 mg q.d.	600/100 mg b.i.d.	16	↓	0.76 (0.71–0.81)	0.84 (0.78–0.91)	0.85 (0.77–0.94)
Paroxetine	20 mg q.d.	400/100 mg b.i.d.	16	↓	64 (59–71)	61 (56–66)	63 (55–73)
Pravastatin	40 mg single dose	600/100 mg b.i.d.	14	↑	163 (95–282)	181 (123–266)	—
Rifabutin	150 mg q.o.d.[d]	600/100 mg b.i.d.	11	↑	0.72 (0.55–0.93)	0.93 (0.80–1.09)	1.64 (1.48–1.81)
25-O-desacetyl-rifabutin			11	↑	4.77 (4.04–5.63)	9.81 (8.09–11.9)	27.1 (22.2–33.2)
Sertraline	50 mg q.d.	400/100 mg b.i.d.	13	↓	56 (49–63)	51 (46–58)	51 (45–57)
Sildenafil[b]	25 mg[b] single dose	400/100 mg b.i.d.	16	↑[b]	62 (55–70)	97 (86–109)	—

[a] Atorvastatin 10 mg q.d. with darunavir/ritonavir 300/100 mg b.i.d. was compared to atorvastatin 40 mg q.d. alone.
[b] Sildenafil 25 mg (single dose) with darunavir/ritonavir 400/100 mg b.i.d. was compared to sildenafil 100 mg alone (single dose).
[c] When co-administered with naloxone as buprenorphine/naloxone 24/6 mg q.d.
[d] In comparison to rifabutin 300 mg q.d.
Legend: N=number of subjects with data; —=no information available.

Drug-Food Interactions: Darunavir, when given as a tablet and co-administered with low-dose ritonavir as a pharmacokinetic enhancer, should be taken with food. The type of food does not affect the exposure to darunavir.

Drug-Herb Interactions: Concomitant use of PREZISTA/rtv and St. John's wort (Hypericum perforatum) or products containing St. John's wort is contraindicated. Co-administration of PIs, including PREZISTA/rtv, with St. John's wort is expected to substantially decrease PI concentrations and may result in suboptimal concentrations of darunavir and lead to loss of virologic response and possible resistance to PREZISTA/rtv or to the class of PIs (see Drug-Drug Interactions, Table 6).

Interactions with other herbal products have not been established.

Drug-Laboratory Test Interactions: Interactions with laboratory tests have not been established.

DOSAGE AND ADMINISTRATION:

Dosing Considerations: PREZISTA must always be given with 100 mg ritonavir as a pharmacokinetic enhancer, and in combination with other antiretroviral medicinal products. The prescribing information of ritonavir must, therefore, be consulted prior to initiation of therapy with PREZISTA/rtv.

Recommended Dose and Dosage Adjustment: Adults: Treatment Naïve Adult Patients: The recommended oral dose of PREZISTA tablets is 800 mg (two 400 mg tablets) once daily taken with ritonavir 100 mg once daily and with food. The type of food does not affect exposure to darunavir.

Treatment Experienced Adult Patients: The recommended oral dose of PREZISTA tablets is 600 mg (one 600 mg tablet or two 300 mg tablets) twice daily (b.i.d.) taken with ritonavir 100 mg b.i.d. and with food. The type of food does not affect exposure to darunavir. Ritonavir (100 mg b.i.d.) is used as a pharmacokinetic enhancer of PREZISTA (see Drug Interactions, Drug-Drug Interactions and Action and Clinical Pharmacology, Pharmacokinetics). A further increase in the dose of darunavir or ritonavir is not likely to result in any clinically relevant increase in antiviral activity.

Geriatric Patients: In general, caution should be exercised in the administration and monitoring of PREZISTA in elderly patients, reflecting the greater frequency of decreased hepatic, renal or cardiac function, and of concomitant disease or other drug therapy (see Indications and Clinical Use, Warnings and Precautions and Action and Clinical Pharmacology).

Pediatric Patients: Antiretroviral Treatment-Experienced Pediatric Patients 6 to <18 Years of Age: The recommended dose of PREZISTA for pediatric patients (6 to <18 years of age and weighing at least 44 lbs (20 kg)) is based on body weight (see Table 10) and should not exceed the recommended adult dose (PREZISTA/rtv 600/100 mg b.i.d.). PREZISTA tablets should be taken with ritonavir twice daily and with food. The type of food does not affect exposure to darunavir (see Action and Clinical Pharmacology, Pharmacokinetics).

Table 10: PREZISTA

Recommended Dose for Antiretroviral Treatment-Experienced Pediatric Patients (6 to <18 years of age) for PREZISTA Tablets with Ritonavir

Body Weight	Dose
≥20 kg–<30 kg	375 mg PREZISTA/50 mg ritonavir twice daily
≥30 kg–<40 kg	450 mg PREZISTA/60 mg ritonavir twice daily
≥40 kg	600 mg PREZISTA/100 mg ritonavir twice daily

Antiretroviral Treatment-Experienced Pediatric Patients <6 years of age and Antiretroviral Treatment-Naïve Pediatric Patients: The safety and efficacy of PREZISTA/rtv in antiretroviral treatment-experienced pediatric patients 3 to <6 years of age and in antiretroviral treatment-naïve pediatric patients have not been established.

PREZISTA/rtv should not be used in pediatric patients below 3 years of age (see Warnings and Precautions).

Hepatic Impairment: The safety and efficacy of PREZISTA have not been established in patients with severe hepatic insufficiency (see Contraindications). No dose adjustment is required in patients with mild or moderate hepatic impairment (see Action and Clinical Pharmacology, Pharmacokinetics).

Renal Impairment: No dose adjustment is required in patients with renal impairment (see Warnings and Precautions, Renal and Action and Clinical Pharmacology, Pharmacokinetics).

Dosing with Didanosine: Dosing of enteric-coated didanosine and darunavir, co-administered with low-dose ritonavir, should be separated by at least 2 hours to avoid formulation incompatibility.

Missed Dose: Patients Taking 600 mg of PREZISTA Twice Daily: The missed dose (one 600 mg tablet or two 300 mg tablets) should be taken as soon as possible, if the dose was missed by less than 6 hours. The next dose of PREZISTA (one 600 mg tablet or two 300 mg tablets) and ritonavir should be taken at the regularly scheduled time. If the dose of PREZISTA (one 600 mg tablet or two 300 mg tablets) or ritonavir was missed by more than 6 hours, the next dose of PREZISTA (one 600 mg tablet or two 300 mg tablets) and ritonavir should be taken at the regularly scheduled time. Doses should not be doubled.

Patients Taking 800 mg of PREZISTA Once Daily: The missed dose (two 400 mg tablets) should be taken as soon as possible, if the dose was missed by less than 12 hours. The next dose of PREZISTA (two 400 mg tablets) and ritonavir should be taken at the regularly scheduled time. If the dose of PREZISTA (two 400 mg tablets) or ritonavir was missed by more than 12 hours, the next dose of PREZISTA (two 400 mg tablets) and ritonavir should be taken at the regularly scheduled time. Doses should not be doubled.

OVERDOSAGE:
Human experience of acute overdose with PREZISTA/rtv is limited. Single doses up to 3200 mg of the oral solution of darunavir alone and up to 1600 mg of the tablet formulation of darunavir co-administered with ritonavir have been administered to healthy volunteers without untoward symptomatic effects.

There is no specific antidote for overdose with PREZISTA. Treatment of overdose with PREZISTA consists of general supportive measures including monitoring of vital signs and observation of the clinical status of the patient. Administration of activated charcoal may be used to aid in removal of unabsorbed active substance. Since PREZISTA is highly protein bound, dialysis is unlikely to be beneficial in significant removal of the active substance.

For management of a suspected drug overdose, contact your regional Poison Control Centre. See the *CPS Directory* section for a list of Poison Control Centres.

ACTION AND CLINICAL PHARMACOLOGY: Mechanism of Action: Darunavir is an inhibitor of the dimerization and of the catalytic activity of the HIV-1 protease. It selectively inhibits the cleavage of HIV encoded Gag-Pol polyproteins in virus-infected cells, thereby preventing the formation of mature infectious virus particles.

Darunavir tightly binds to the HIV-1 protease with a K_D of 4.5×10^{-12} M.

Darunavir is not an inhibitor of any of 13 tested human cellular proteases.

Pharmacodynamics: The pharmacokinetic properties of darunavir, co-administered with ritonavir, have been evaluated in healthy adult volunteers and in HIV-1 infected patients. Exposure to darunavir was higher in HIV-1 infected patients than in healthy subjects. Darunavir is primarily metabolized by CYP3A. Ritonavir inhibits CYP3A, thereby increasing the plasma concentrations of darunavir considerably.

Table 11 displays the mean plasma concentrations of darunavir at steady-state for the darunavir/ritonavir 800/100 mg q.d. dose.

Table 11: PREZISTA

Mean Steady-State Plasma Concentration-Time Profiles of Darunavir and Ritonavir at 800/100 mg q.d. at Week 4 (Study TMC114-C211)

	Darunavir		Ritonavir	
Scheduled Time	**Mean±SD (ng/mL)**	**CV (%)**	**Mean±SD (ng/mL)**	**CV (%)**
0 h	1826 ±1003	54.92	141.2±156.0	110.5
1 h	3964 ±1805	45.52	154.4±122.6	79.36
2 h	4692±1135	24.19	264.5±247.2	93.46
3 h	4949±1344	27.15	386.8±357.6	92.45
4 h	4426±1300	29.38	465.9±256.5	55.06
6 h	3532±1065	30.16	463.1± 205.3	44.33
9 h	2664±1002	37.59	282.7±137.5	48.64
12 h	2353±919.6	39.08	229.4±159.8	69.67
24 h	1440±513.9	35.68	97.10±99.08	102.0

Table 12 displays the mean plasma concentrations of darunavir and ritonavir at steady-state for the darunavir/ritonavir 600/100 mg b.i.d. dose.

Table 12: PREZISTA

Mean Steady-State Plasma Concentration-Time Profiles of Darunavir and Ritonavir at 600/100 mg b.i.d. at Week 4 (Integrated Data from POWER 1 and POWER 2, Primary 24-Week Analysis)

	Darunavir		Ritonavir	
Scheduled Time	**Mean±SD (ng/mL)**	**CV (%)**	**Mean±SD (ng/mL)**	**CV (%)**
0 h	4010±1635	40.78	495.6±258.6	52.18
1 h	5386±1538	28.55	634.0±462.2	72.9
2 h	6125±1750	28.57	658.1±439.7	66.81
3 h	6471±2066	31.92	713.8±371.5	52.04
4 h	5307±1796	33.84	719.5±274.7	38.18
6 h	4856±2007	41.33	701.9±318.3	45.36
9 h	3618±1893	52.33	516.9±224.4	43.42
12 h	2813±1612	57.3	321.9±180.1	55.97

Electrocardiogram: Effect on QT intervals: In an open-label, randomized, placebo- and active-controlled, four-way crossover trial, 40 healthy subjects were administered supratherapeutic doses of darunavir/ritonavir 1600/100 mg once daily and 800/100 mg twice daily for seven days.

At the mean maximum darunavir concentration of 6599 ng/mL observed in this study, the mean increase in QTcF was 2.2 ms with a 90% two-sided confidence interval (CI) of −2.0 to 6.3 ms. When evaluating the 2-sided 90% CI on the time-matched mean changes in QTcF versus placebo control, the upper bounds of both darunavir/ritonavir groups never exceeded the 10 ms boundary. In the setting of this trial, darunavir/ritonavir did not appear to prolong the QTc interval.

Pharmacokinetics: Absorption: Darunavir was rapidly absorbed following oral administration. Maximum plasma concentration of darunavir in the presence of low-dose ritonavir is generally achieved within 2.5-4.0 hours.

The absolute oral bioavailability of a single 600 mg dose of darunavir alone was approximately 37% and increased to approximately 82% in the presence of 100 mg b.i.d. ritonavir. The overall pharmacokinetic enhancement effect by ritonavir was an approximate 14-fold increase in the systemic exposure of darunavir when a single dose of 600 mg darunavir was given orally co-administered with ritonavir at 100 mg b.i.d. Therefore, PREZISTA should only be co-administered with 100 mg of ritonavir as a pharmacokinetic enhancer. See Table 13.

Table 13: PREZISTA

Pharmacokinetic Parameters of Darunavir 600 mg and Darunavir/rtv at 600/100 mg b.i.d.

Pharmacokinetics of darunavir (mean±SD, t_{max}: median [range])	Darunavir 600 mg Oral	Darunavir 600 mg Oral + RTV 100 mg b.i.d.
N	7	7
t_{max}, h	2.00 (1.00–4.00)	4.00 (2.00–5.00)
C_{max}, ng/Ml	2204±1071	5627±923.5
AUC_{last}, ng·h/mL	7748±4867	91 390±20 050
AUC_{∞}, ng·h/mL	10 990±4061	92 340±20 020
Bioavailability (F) (%)	36.93	81.93

Increasing the dose of ritonavir to above 100 mg b.i.d. did not significantly affect darunavir concentrations and is not recommended.

Effects of Food on Oral Absorption: When administered without food, the relative bioavailability of darunavir in the presence of low-dose ritonavir is 30% lower as compared to intake with food. Therefore, PREZISTA tablets should be taken with ritonavir and with food. The type of food does not affect exposure to darunavir.

Distribution: Darunavir is approximately 95% bound to plasma proteins. Darunavir binds primarily to plasma AAG (alpha-1-acid glycoprotein).

Metabolism: In vitro experiments with human liver microsomes (HLMs) indicate that darunavir primarily undergoes oxidative metabolism. Darunavir is extensively metabolized by the hepatic CYP system, and almost exclusively by isozyme CYP3A4. A ^{14}C-darunavir trial in healthy volunteers showed that a majority of the radioactivity in plasma after a single 400/100 mg darunavir/ritonavir dose was due to the parent drug. At least 3 oxidative metabolites of darunavir have been identified in humans; all showed activity that was at least 10-fold less than the activity of darunavir against wild-type HIV.

Excretion: After a 400/100 mg ^{14}C-darunavir/ritonavir dose, approximately 79.5% and 13.9% of the administered dose of ^{14}C-darunavir could be retrieved in feces and urine, respectively. Unchanged darunavir accounted for approximately 41.2% and 7.7% of the administered dose in feces and urine, respectively. The terminal elimination half-life of darunavir was approximately 15 hours when combined with ritonavir. The intravenous clearance of darunavir alone (150 mg) and in the presence of low-dose ritonavir was 32.8 L/h and 5.9 L/h, respectively.

Special Populations and Conditions: Pediatrics: The pharmacokinetics of darunavir in combination with ritonavir in 74 antiretroviral treatment-experienced HIV-1-infected pediatric subjects 6 to <18 years of age and weighing at least 44 lbs (20 kg) showed that the administered weight-based dosages resulted in darunavir exposure comparable to that in adults receiving PREZISTA/rtv 600/100 mg b.i.d. (see Dosage and Administration).

Table 14: PREZISTA

Population Pharmacokinetic Estimates of Darunavir (Study TMC114-C212, Primary 24-Week Analysis)

Parameter Median (Range)	Darunavir/Ritonavir N=74
AUC_{12h} (ng·h/mL)	63670 (33527–115360)
C_{0h} (ng/mL)	3888 (1836–7821)

Legend: N=number of subjects with data.

Geriatrics: Population pharmacokinetic analysis in HIV-infected patients showed that darunavir pharmacokinetics are not considerably different in the age range (18 to 75 years) evaluated in HIV-infected patients (n=12, age ≥65) (see Warnings and Precautions, Special Populations, Geriatrics (>65 years of age)).

Gender: Population pharmacokinetic analysis showed a slightly higher darunavir exposure (16.8%) in HIV-infected females (n=68) compared to males. This difference is not considered clinically relevant.

Race: Population pharmacokinetic analysis of darunavir in HIV-infected patients indicated that race had no apparent effect on the exposure to darunavir.

Hepatic Insufficiency: Hepatic Impairment: In a multiple dose study with PREZISTA co-administered with ritonavir (600/100 mg) twice daily, it was demonstrated that the steady-state pharmacokinetic parameters of darunavir in subjects with mild (Child-Pugh Class A, n=8) and moderate (Child-Pugh Class B, n=8) hepatic impairment were comparable with those in healthy subjects.

The effect of severe hepatic impairment on the pharmacokinetics of darunavir has not been studied (see Contraindications, Warnings and Precautions and Dosage and Administration).

Hepatitis B or Hepatitis C Virus Co-infection: The primary 48-week analysis of the data from Study TMC114-C211 and TMC114-C214 in HIV-1-infected patients indicated that hepatitis B and/or hepatitis C virus co-infection status had no apparent effect on the exposure to darunavir.

Renal Insufficiency: Results from a mass balance study with ^{14}C-darunavir/ritonavir showed that approximately 7.7% of the administered dose of darunavir is excreted in the urine as unchanged drug. As darunavir and ritonavir are highly bound to plasma proteins, it is unlikely that they will be significantly removed by hemodialysis or peritoneal dialysis. Although darunavir has not been studied in patients with renal impairment, population pharmacokinetic analysis showed that the pharmacokinetics of darunavir were not significantly affected in HIV-infected patients with moderate renal impairment (CrCL between 30-60 mL/min, n=20) (see Warnings and Precautions, Renal and Dosage and Administration, Recommended Dose and Dosage Adjustment, Renal Impairment).

STORAGE AND STABILITY: Store PREZISTA tablets between 15-30°C.

INFORMATION FOR THE PATIENT: Published in e-CPS, available by subscription at www.e-cps.ca.

DOSAGE FORMS, COMPOSITION AND PACKAGING: 75 mg : Each white, caplet-shaped, film-coated tablet, debossed with "75" on one side and "TMC" on the other side, contains: darunavir 75 mg (corresponding to darunavir ethanolate 81.31). Nonmedicinal ingredients: colloidal silicon dioxide, crospovidone, magnesium stearate and microcrystalline cellulose; film coating: polyethylene glycol, polyvinyl alcohol - partially hydrolyzed, talc and titanium dioxide. Bottles of 480.

300 mg: Each orange, oval-shaped, film-coated tablet, debossed with "300MG" on one side and "TMC114" on the other side, contains: darunavir 300 mg (corresponding to darunavir ethanolate 325.23 mg). Nonmedicinal ingredients: colloidal silicon dioxide, crospovidone, magnesium stearate and microcrystalline cellulose; film coating: polyethylene glycol, polyvinyl alcohol - partially hydrolyzed, sunset yellow FCF aluminum lake, talc and titanium dioxide. Bottles of 120.

400 mg: Each light orange, oval-shaped, film-coated tablet, debossed with "400MG" on one side and "TMC" on the other side, contains: darunavir ethanolate equivalent to darunavir 400 mg. Nonmedicinal ingredients: colloidal silicon dioxide, crospovidone, magnesium stearate and microcrystalline cellulose; film coating: polyethylene glycol, polyvinyl alcohol - partially hydrolyzed, sunset yellow FCF aluminum lake, talc and titanium dioxide. Bottles of 60.

600 mg: Each orange, oval-shaped, film-coated tablet, debossed with "600MG" on one side and "TMC" on the other side, contains: darunavir ethanolate equivalent to darunavir 600 mg. Nonmedicinal ingredients: colloidal silicon dioxide, crospovidone, magnesium stearate and microcrystalline cellulose; film coating: polyethylene glycol, polyvinyl alcohol - partially hydrolyzed, sunset yellow FCF aluminum lake, talc and titanium dioxide. Bottles of 60.

(Shown in Product Identification Section)

Primaquine ℞
primaquine phosphate
Antimalarial

sanofi-aventis

Date of Revision: May 23, 2006

PHARMACOLOGY: Primaquine is an 8-aminoquinoline anti-protozoal agent which is highly active against exo-erythrocytic stages of *P. vivax*, *P. ovale* and against the primary exo-erythrocytic stages of *P. falciparum*.

Primaquine is also highly active against gametocytes of Plasmodia, especially *P. falciparum*.

Primaquine is readily absorbed from the gastro-intestinal tract and extensively distributed into body tissues.

Peak plasma concentration occurs about 1 to 3 hours after a dose is taken and then rapidly diminishes with a reported elimination half-life of 3 to 6 hours.

Primaquine is rapidly metabolized in the liver, its principal metabolite being carboxyprimaquine. Little unchanged drug is excreted in the urine.

INDICATIONS: For the radical cure (prevention of relapse) of vivax and ovale malaria.

CONTRAINDICATIONS: In patients who are hypersensitive to primaquine.

In acutely ill patients suffering from systemic disease manifested by tendency to granulocytopenia, such as rheumatoid arthritis and lupus erythematosus.

In patients receiving concurrently other potentially hemolytic drugs or depressants of myeloid elements of the bone marrow.

Quinacrine appears to potentiate the toxicity of antimalarial compounds which are structurally related to primaquine; therefore, the use of quinacrine in patients receiving primaquine is contraindicated. Similarly, primaquine should not be administered to patients who have received quinacrine recently, as toxicity is increased.

WARNINGS: General: Discontinue the use of primaquine promptly if signs suggestive of hemolytic anemia occur (such as darkening of the urine or a sudden decrease in hemoglobin concentration or erythrocyte count), or if there is a sudden decrease in leukocyte count.

Use in Special Groups: Observe particular caution in individuals with a personal or family history of favism, hemolytic anemia, or glucose-6-phosphate dehydrogenase (G-6-PD) deficiency or nicotinamide adenine dinucleotide (NADH) methemoglobin reductase deficiency.

Pregnancy: The safety of primaquine in human pregnancy has not been established. It should therefore be avoided during pregnancy unless in the judgment of the physician the benefits outweigh the possible hazard.

Lactation: It is not known whether primaquine is excreted in breast milk.

Because of the potential of primaquine to produce serious adverse reactions in nursing infants, a decision should be made whether to discontinue breast-feeding or to discontinue the drug.

PRECAUTIONS: Anemia, methemoglobinemia and leukopenia have been observed following administration of large doses of primaquine; therefore, the adult dosage of 1 tablet daily for 14 days should not be exceeded. It is also advisable to make routine blood examinations, particularly blood cell counts and hemoglobin determinations, during therapy.

ADVERSE EFFECTS: Gastrointestinal: nausea, vomiting, epigastric distress, and abdominal pain.

Hematologic: leukopenia, hemolytic anemia especially in G-6-PD deficient individuals and methemoglobinemia especially in NADH methemoglobin reductase deficient individuals.

OVERDOSE:

Symptoms: Abdominal cramps, vomiting, jaundice, burning epigastric distress, CNS and cardiovascular disturbances, cyanosis, methemoglobinemia, moderate leukocytosis or leukopenia, and anemia. The most striking changes are granulocytopenia and acute hemolytic anemia in sensitive persons. Acute hemolysis often occurs, but complete recovery can be expected if primaquine is discontinued.

Treatment: Management should include appropriate attempts to recover primaquine from the stomach by emesis or gastric lavage and provision of respiratory and cardiovascular support.

Sodium lactate i.v. may be used to counter the depressant effects of primaquine on the heart. Electrical pacing of the heart may be needed.

Ammonium chloride in doses up to 12 g daily orally may be given to enhance urinary excretion.

Symptomatic methemoglobinemia should be treated with 1 to 2 mg per kg of methylene blue.

For management of a suspected drug overdose, CPhA recommends that you contact your **regional Poison Control Centre**. See the *CPS* Directory section for a list of Poison Control Centres.

DOSAGE: Primaquine is recommended only for the radical cure of vivax and ovale malaria, the prevention of relapse in vivax and ovale malaria, or following the termination of chloroquine phosphate suppressive therapy in an area where vivax or ovale malaria are endemic.

Patients suffering from an attack of vivax or ovale malaria or having parasitized red blood cells should initially receive a course of a blood schizontocide, which quickly destroys the erythrocytic parasites and terminates the paroxysm. Primaquine phosphate should then be administered in order to eradicate the exo-erythrocytic parasites.

When primaquine is indicated for the prevention of delayed primary attacks and relapse of *P. vivax* or *P. ovale* malaria in individuals who have returned home from areas where these plasmodial species are endemic, primaquine is generally initiated during the last 2 weeks of, or immediately following, therapy with chloroquine or another suitable antimalarial agent.

Adults: 1 tablet (15 mg primaquine base) daily for 14 days.

Children: 0.39 mg primaquine base per kg daily for 14 days.

Note: For radical cure of some strains of *P. vivax*, higher doses or longer courses may be required to overcome resistance.

Taking primaquine after a meal may reduce abdominal pain or cramps associated with ingestion of the drug.

SUPPLIED: Each pink, film-coated tablet, imprinted W on one side and P97 on the other, contains: primaquine phosphate USP 26.3 mg (equivalent to primaquine base 15 mg). Nonmedicinal ingredients: black ink SW-9031 and SW-9032, carnauba wax, ferric oxide, lactose, magnesium stearate, microcrystalline cellulose, polyethylene glycol, pregelatinized starch and talc. Gluten- and tartrazine-free. Bottles of 100.

(Shown in Product Identification Section)

Primaxin® ℞
imipenem—cilastatin sodium
Antibiotic

Merck Frosst

Date of Revision: February 19, 2010

PHARMACOLOGY: Imipenem exerts a bactericidal action by inhibiting cell wall synthesis in aerobic and anaerobic gram-positive and gram-negative bacteria.

Primaxin (imipenem and cilastatin sodium) consists of two components: (1) imipenem, a derivative of thienamycin, a carbapenem antibiotic; and (2) cilastatin sodium, a specific inhibitor of dehydropeptidase-I a renal enzyme which metabolizes and inactivates imipenem. Cilastatin blocks the metabolism of imipenem in the kidney, so that concomitant administration of imipenem and cilastatin allows antibacterial levels of imipenem to be attained in the urine.

Inhibition of cell-wall synthesis is achieved in gram-negative bacteria by the binding of imipenem to penicillin binding proteins (PBPs). In the case of *E. coli* and selected strains of *P. aeruginosa*, imipenem has been shown to have highest affinity for PBP-2, PBP-1a and PBP-1b, with lower activity against PBP-3. The preferential binding of imipenem on PBP-2 and PBP-1b leads to direct conversion of the individual cell to a spheroplast resulting in rapid lysis and cell death without filament formation. When imipenem is removed prior to complete killing of gram-negative species, the remaining viable cells show a measurable lag, termed a "post-antibiotic effect" (PAE), prior to resumption of new growth.

Pharmacokinetics: Primaxin (imipenem and cilastatin sodium) was administered via i.v. infusion over 20 minutes at a single dose of 250/250 mg to 4 male subjects (mean age: 31.5±0.6 years), at a single dose of 500/500 mg to 20 male subjects (mean age: 26.8±4.1 years), and at a single dose of 1000/1000 mg to 8 male subjects (mean age: 24.8±3.7 years). Peak plasma levels of imipenem and of cilastatin were measured at the end of a 20 minute infusion, and are presented in Table 1. Plasma levels of imipenem antimicrobial activity are proportional to the dose and decline to below 1 µg/mL or less in 4 to 6 hours.

Table 1: Primaxin

Range of Peak Plasma Levels of Imipenem and Cilastatin Following a 20 Minute I.V. Infusion of Primaxin

	250/250 mg	500/500 mg	1000/1000 mg
Imipenem (µg/mL)	12–20	21–58	41–83
Cilastatin (µg/mL)	21–26	21–55	56–88

Primaxin was administered via the i.v. route, over a 30 minute period, every 6 hours, for a period of 10 days, at a dose of 1000/1000 mg, to a group of 6 male volunteers (mean age 28.2±5).

The pharmacokinetic parameters for imipenem and cilastatin, when Primaxin was administered at a dose of 1000/1000 mg, are summarized in Table 2.

Table 2: Primaxin

Pharmacokinetic Parameters of Imipenem and Cilastatin when Primaxin Is Administered at a Dose of 1000/1000 mg by I.V. Infusion Over 30 min (N=6)

Time (days)	Volume of Distribution (L)	Area Under the Plasma Concentration Time Curve Between 0 and 6 h (µg·h/mL)	Plasma Half-Lives (min)[a]	Dose Recovered in Urine Through 6 h (mg)	Cumulative Renal Clearance (mL/min)	Plasma Clearance (mL/min)
			Imipenem			
Day 1	13.6 (±3.7)	73.3 (±10.4)	59.6	540.2 (±54.1)	126.5 (±29.9)	227.7 (±30.9)
Day 5	11.4 (±3.8)	74.5 (±10.9)	61.3	651.8 (±148.1)	139.9 (±27.4)	227.8 (±36.1)
Day 10	10.9 (±1.6)	79.7 (±7.1)	59.4	626.5 (±77.2)	131.3 (±21.0)	210.4 (±18.3)
			Cilastatin			
Day 1	10.3 (±3.9)	82.1 (±19.3)	57.5	698.6 (±33.9)	142.7 (±33.6)	208.9 (±43.0)
Day 5	9.5 (±1.4)	73.0 (±16.1)	50.7	ND	ND	236.5 (±44.9)
Day 10	9.7 (±2.1)	77.4 (±15.1)	50.8	ND	ND	221.6 (±38.6)

[a] Harmonic means.

Excretion and Metabolism: Imipenem, when administered alone, is metabolized in the kidneys by dehydropeptidase-I and therefore achieves relatively low levels in urine.

Cilastatin sodium is a specific inhibitor of this enzyme and it prevents renal metabolism of imipenem. When imipenem and cilastatin are given concomitantly, approximately 70% of the administered imipenem and cilastatin are recovered unchanged in the urine within 10 hours of administration, after which no further urinary excretion is detectable. Urine concentrations of imipenem in excess of 10 µg/mL can be maintained for up to 8 hours with Primaxin at the 500 mg dose.

The remainder of the administered dose of imipenem is recovered in the urine as antibacterially inactive metabolites, and fecal elimination of imipenem is essentially nil.

Approximately 10% of the cilastatin sodium administered is found as the N-acetyl metabolite, which has inhibitory activity against dehydropeptidase comparable to that of the parent drug. Activity of dehydropeptidase-I in the kidney returns to normal levels within approximately 8 to 12 hours after the elimination of cilastatin from the bloodstream.

No accumulation of imipenem and cilastatin in plasma is observed with regimens of Primaxin administered at therapeutic doses, in patients with normal renal function.

Serum Protein Binding: At serum concentration of 25 mg/L the human serum protein binding of imipenem is 20%. Cilastatin binding to protein was found to be approximately 35% in the human serum.

Impaired Renal Function: Primaxin was administered to 6 healthy male volunteers and 25 patients with different degrees of renal impairment at a dose of 250/250 mg, in single i.v. infusions over 5 minutes.

The pharmacokinetic parameters for imipenem and cilastatin are summarized in Table 3.

Table 3: Primaxin

Pharmacokinetic Parameters for Imipenem and Cilastatin in Patients with Renal Failure (Single Dose 250/250 mg by I.V. Infusion Over 5 Min)

Group No.	No. Pts	Mean Age (yrs)	Creatinine Clearance mL/min/1.73 m² (mL/s/1.73 m²)	% Dose Urinary Recovery	Renal Clear-ance (mL/min)	Plasma Clear-ance (mL/min)	[AUC][c] (µg·h/mL)	T½[d] (min)
				Imipenem				
I	6	22.8	>100 (>1.7)	46.2	101.9	219.5	19.8	56
II	6	41.8	31–99 (0.52–1.65)	51.0[e]	77.7[e]	157.2	30.3	92
III	9	50.8	10–30 (0.17–0.50)	26.1[g]	24.2[g]	86.2	51.6	139
IV	2	32 & 67	<10 (<0.17)	11.3	8.5	69.3	60.6	160
V[a]	4	42.3	Hemodialysis[a]			184.0	23.1	74
V[b]	4	61.5	Hemodialysis[b]	3.4	1.8	59.1	73.1	181
				Cilastatin				

(cont'd)

Table 3: Primaxin *(cont'd)*

Pharmacokinetic Parameters for Imipenem and Cilastatin in Patients with Renal Failure (Single Dose 250/250 mg by I.V. Infusion Over 5 Min)

Group No.	No. Pts	Mean Age (yrs)	Creatinine Clearance mL/min/1.73 m² (mL/s/1.73 m²)	% Dose Urinary Recovery	Renal Clearance (mL/min)	Plasma Clearance (mL/min)	[AUC][c] (µg·h/mL)	T½[d] (min)
I	6	22.8	>100 (>1.7)	59.4	100.7	168.5	25.4	54
II	6	41.8	31–99 (0.52–1.65)	71.2[e]	71.3[e]	99.9	45.7	84
III	9	50.8	10–30 (0.17–0.50)	61.9[f]	23.9[g]	38.4	135.3	198
IV	2	32 & 67	<10 (<0.17)	39.4	6.5	16.2	261.4	462
V[a]	4	42.3	Hemodialysis[a]			74.9	56.7	132
V[b]	4	61.5	Hemodialysis[b]	17.9	2.0	11.4	416.8	696

[a] Received dose during hemodialysis.
[b] Measurements done between dialysis sessions.
[c] AUC normalized to a 250 mg dose.
[d] Harmonic means.
[e] n=5.
[f] n=6.
[g] n=8.

INDICATIONS: Primaxin (imipenem and cilastatin sodium) may be indicated in the treatment of serious infections when caused by sensitive strains of bacteria. Where considered necessary, therapy may be initiated on the basis of clinical judgment before results of sensitivity testings are available. Continuation of therapy should be reevaluated on the basis of bacteriological findings and of the patient's clinical condition.

Imipenem is active in vitro against a wide range of gram-positive and gram-negative aerobic and anaerobic bacteria, including most strains which are beta-lactamase producing. Patients have responded while under treatment with Primaxin for single or mixed infections of the following body systems, when they were associated with a number of pathogenic species and strains of the genera listed: 1. lower respiratory tract infections; 2. urinary tract infections; 3. intra-abdominal infections; 4. gynecological infections; 5. septicemia; 6. endocarditis caused by *S. aureus*; 7. bone and joint infections; 8. skin structure infections.

Primaxin is not indicated for the treatment of meningitis.

Gram-positive Aerobes: *L. monocytogenes*, *N. asteroides*, Staphylococcus (excluding many strains which are methicillin resistant), Streptococcus [*E. faecium* (formerly *S. faecium*) is not susceptible to Primaxin.]

Gram-negative Aerobes: Acinetobacter, Citrobacter, Enterobacter, *E. coli*, *H. influenzae*, *H. parainfluenzae*, Klebsiella, *M. morganii*, Neisseria, Proteus (indole positive and indole negative strains), Providencia, *P. aeruginosa*, *S. marcescens*.

Gram-positive Anaerobes: Clostridium (excluding *C. difficile*), Peptococcus, Peptostreptococcus.

Gram-negative Anaerobes: *B. fragilis*, Bacteroides (non fragilis).

CONTRAINDICATIONS: Primaxin (imipenem and cilastatin sodium) is contraindicated in patients who have shown hypersensitivity to either component of this product.

WARNINGS: Primaxin (imipenem and cilastatin sodium) should be administered with caution to any patient who has demonstrated some form of allergy, particularly to structurally-related drugs. If an allergic reaction to Primaxin occurs, discontinue the drug. Serious hypersensitivity reactions may require epinephrine and other emergency measures.

C. difficile-associated disease: *C. difficile*-associated disease (CDAD) has been reported with the use of many antibacterial agents, including Primaxin. CDAD may range in severity from mild diarrhea to fatal colitis. It is important to consider this diagnosis in patients who present with diarrhea, or symptoms of colitis, pseudomembranous colitis, toxic megacolon, or perforation of colon subsequent to the administration of any antibacterial agent. CDAD has been reported to occur over 2 months after the administration of antibacterial agents.

Treatment with antibacterial agents may alter the normal flora of the colon and may permit overgrowth of *C. difficile*. *C. difficile* produces toxins A and B, which contribute to the development of CDAD. CDAD may cause significant morbidity and mortality. CDAD can be refractory to antimicrobial therapy.

If the diagnosis of CDAD is suspected or confirmed, appropriate therapeutic measures should be initiated. Mild cases of CDAD usually respond to discontinuation of antibacterial agents not directed against *C. difficile*. In moderate to severe cases, consideration should be given to management with fluids and electrolytes, protein supplementation, and treatment with an antibacterial agent clinically effective against *C. difficile*. Surgical evaluation should be instituted as clinically indicated, as surgical intervention may be required in certain severe cases (see Adverse Effects).

PRECAUTIONS: General: Prolonged use may result in overgrowth of resistant organisms. Repeated evaluation of the patient's condition is essential. If superinfection occurs during therapy, appropriate measures should be taken.

Case reports in the literature have shown that co-administration of carbapenems, including imipenem, to patients receiving valproic acid or divalproex sodium results in a reduction in serum valproic acid concentrations. The valproic acid concentrations may drop below the therapeutic range as a result of this interaction. In some cases of co-administration of imipenem with valproic acid, breakthrough seizures have occurred. Increasing the dose of valproic acid or divalproex sodium may not be sufficient to overcome this interaction. The concomitant use of imipenem and valproic acid/divalproex sodium is generally not recommended. Anti-bacterials other than carbapenems should be considered to treat infections in patients whose seizures are well controlled on valproic acid or divalproex sodium. If administration of Primaxin is necessary, supplemental anti-convulsant therapy should be considered (see Drug-Drug Interactions).

CNS adverse experiences such as myoclonic activity, confusional states, or seizures have been reported especially when recommended dosages based on renal function and body weight were exceeded. These experiences have occurred most commonly in patients with CNS disorders (e.g., brain lesions or history of seizures) and/or who have compromised renal function. However, there were rare reports in which there was no recognized or documented underlying CNS disorder. Close adherence to recommended dosage schedules is urged especially in patients with known factors that predispose to seizures (see Dosage).

Anticonvulsant therapy should be continued in patients with a known seizure disorder. If focal tremors, myoclonus, or seizures occur, patients should be evaluated neurologically and placed on anticonvulsant therapy if not already instituted. If CNS symptoms continue, the dosage should be decreased or discontinued (see Drug-Drug Interactions).

Impaired Renal Function: Dosage in patients with impaired renal function is based on the severity of infection but the maximum daily dose varies with the degree of renal functional impairment (see Dosage, Renal Insufficiency).

Pregnancy: Use in pregnant women has not been studied, therefore, Primaxin should be used during pregnancy only if clearly needed. Use of this drug in women of childbearing potential requires that the anticipated benefits be weighed against possible hazards.

Reproduction studies with bolus i.v. doses suggest an apparent intolerance to Primaxin (including emesis, inappetence, body weight loss, diarrhea and death) at doses equivalent to the average human dose in pregnant rabbits and cynomolgus monkeys that is not seen in non-pregnant animals in these or other species. In other studies, Primaxin was well tolerated in equivalent or higher doses (up to 11 times the average human dose) in pregnant rats and mice.

Lactation: Imipenem has been detected in human milk. If use of Primaxin is deemed essential, the patient should stop nursing.

Children: Efficacy and tolerability in infants under the age of 3 months have not yet been established; therefore, Primaxin is not recommended in the pediatric age group below the age of 3 months.

Drug Interactions: Drug-Drug Interactions: Generalized seizures have been reported in patients who received ganciclovir and Primaxin. These drugs should not be used concomitantly unless the potential benefits outweigh the risks.

Case reports in the literature have shown that co-administration of carbapenems, including imipenem, to patients receiving valproic acid or divalproex sodium results in a reduction of serum valproic acid concentrations. The valproic acid concentrations may drop below the therapeutic range as a result of this interaction. In some cases of co-administration of imipenem with valproic acid, breakthrough seizures have occurred. The mechanism of this interaction is unknown (see Precautions, General).

Concomitant administration of Primaxin and probenecid results in only minimal increases in plasma levels of imipenem and plasma half-life. It is not recommended that probenecid be given with Primaxin.

Primaxin should not be mixed with or physically added to other antibiotics. Primaxin has been administered concomitantly with some antibiotics, such as aminoglycosides.

There is no evidence to suggest that association of Primaxin with any other beta-lactam antibiotics has any therapeutic advantage.

ADVERSE EFFECTS: Primaxin is generally well tolerated. The following adverse reactions were reported on 1723 patients treated in clinical trials. Many of these patients were severely ill and had multiple background diseases and physiological impairments, making it difficult to determine causal relationship of adverse experiences to therapy with Primaxin.

Local Adverse Reactions: Adverse local clinical reactions that were reported as possibly, probably or definitely related to therapy with Primaxin were:

	Incidence (%)
Phlebitis/thrombophlebitis	1.7
Infused vein pain	0.6
Vein induration	0.2
Infused vein infection	0.1

Systemic Adverse Reactions: Adverse clinical reactions that were reported as possibly, probably or definitely related to Primaxin were: see Table 4.

Table 4: Primaxin

Systemic Adverse Reactions

	Incidence (%)
Gastrointestinal	
Nausea	2.0
Diarrhea	1.7
Vomiting	1.6
Tongue papillar hypertrophy	0.2
Pseudomembranous colitis (see Warnings)	0.1
Hemorrhagic colitis	<0.1
Gastroenteritis	<0.1
Abdominal pain	<0.1
Glossitis	<0.1
Heartburn	<0.1
Pharyngeal pain	<0.1
Increased salivation	<0.1
CNS	
Fever	0.4
Dizziness	0.3
Seizures (see Precautions)	0.2
Somnolence	0.2
Confusion	0.2
Myoclonus	0.1
Vertigo	0.1
Headache	0.1
Encephalopathy	<0.1
Paresthesia	<0.1
Special Senses	
Transient hearing loss in patients with impaired hearing	<0.1
Tinnitus	<0.1
Respiratory	
Dyspnea	0.1
Hyperventilation	<0.1
Thoracic spine pain	<0.1
Cardiovascular	
Hypotension	0.4
Palpitations	0.1
Tachycardia	<0.1

(cont'd)

Table 4: Primaxin *(cont'd)*

Systemic Adverse Reactions

	Incidence (%)
Renal	
Oliguria/anuria	<0.1
Polyuria	<0.1
Skin	
Rash	0.9
Pruritus	0.3
Urticaria	0.2
Skin texture changes	0.1
Candidiasis	0.1
Erythema multiforme	<0.1
Facial edema	<0.1
Flushing	<0.1
Cyanosis	<0.1
Hyperhidrosis	<0.1
Pruritus vulvae	<0.1
Body as a Whole	
Polyarthralgia	<0.1
Asthenia/weakness	<0.1

Adverse Laboratory Changes: Adverse laboratory changes, without regard to drug relationship, that were reported during clinical trials were:
Hepatic: increased ALT, AST, alkaline phosphatase, bilirubin and LDH.
Hemic: increased eosinophils, positive Coombs' test, decreased WBC and neutrophils, increased WBC, increased platelets, decreased platelets, decreased hemoglobin and hematocrit, increased monocytes, abnormal prothrombin time, increased lymphocytes, increased basophils.
Electrolytes: decreased serum sodium, increased potassium, increased chloride.
Renal: increased BUN, creatinine.
Urinalysis: presence of urine protein, urine red blood cells, urine white blood cells, urine casts, urine bilirubin, and urine urobilinogen.
Post-Market Adverse Drug Reactions: The following reactions have been reported since the drug was marketed, but occurred under circumstances where a causal relationship could not be established. However, in these rarely reported events, that possibility cannot be excluded. Therefore, these observations are listed to serve as alerting information to physicians and pharmacists: acute renal failure. The role of Primaxin in changes in renal function is difficult to assess, since factors predisposing to pre-renal azotemia or to impaired renal function usually have been present; anaphylactic reactions; bone marrow depression; exfoliative dermatitis; hallucinations, hearing loss, hemolytic anemia; hepatic failure; hepatitis; fulminant hepatitis; pancytopenia; psychic disturbances; staining of teeth; Stevens-Johnson syndrome; taste perversion; toxic epidermal necrolysis; urine discoloration.

OVERDOSE:

There are no data available on overdosage. Primaxin is cleared by hemodialysis.

For management of a suspected drug overdose, contact your **regional Poison Control Centre**. See the *CPS* Directory section for a list of Poison Control Centres.

DOSAGE: The dosage recommendations for Primaxin (imipenem and cilastatin sodium) represent the quantity of imipenem to be administered by i.v. infusion only. An equivalent amount of cilastatin is also present in the solution.

The dosage of Primaxin should be determined by the severity of the infection, renal function, body weight, the antibiotic susceptibility of the causative organism(s) and the condition of the patient. Doses cited are based on body weight of 70 kg.

The median duration of treatment with Primaxin in clinical trials for infections of the various body systems ranged from 6 to 10 days except for endocarditis and bone and joint infections for which the median duration of treatment was 4 weeks.

Adults: The recommended daily dose is 1 to 2 g administered in equally divided doses every 6 to 8 hours (see Table 5).

Table 5: Primaxin

Adult Dosage of Primaxin

	I.V. Administration		
Severity of Infection	**Dose (mg of Imipenem)**	**Dosage Interval**	**Daily Dose**
Mild	250 mg	6 h	1 g
Moderate	500 mg	8 h	1.5 g
Severe (fully susceptible)	500 mg	6 h	2 g
Severe[a] infections due to less susceptible organisms or life-threatening conditions	1000 mg	8 h	3 g
	1000 mg	6 h	4 g

[a] Primarily some strains of *P. aeruginosa*.

The maximum daily dose should not exceed 4 g or 50 mg/kg, whichever is less.

Geriatrics: The recommended dosage of Primaxin in elderly patients with normal renal function is the same as given for adults above. Renal status of elderly patients may not be accurately portrayed by measurement of BUN or creatinine alone. Determination of creatinine clearance is suggested to provide guidance for dosing in such patients.

Renal Insufficiency: Patients with creatinine clearances of ≤5 mL/min/1.73 m² (≤0.08 mL/s/1.73 m²) should not receive Primaxin unless hemodialysis is instituted within 48 hours. Both imipenem and cilastatin are cleared from the circulation during hemodialysis. The patient should receive Primaxin after hemodialysis and at 12 hour intervals timed from the end of that hemodialysis session (see Table 6). Dialysis patients, especially those with background CNS disease, should be carefully monitored; for patients on hemodialysis, Primaxin is recommended only when the benefit outweighs the potential risk of seizures (see Precautions). Currently, there are inadequate data to recommend the use of Primaxin in patients undergoing peritoneal dialysis.

Table 6: Primaxin

Maximum Dosage of Primaxin in Relation to Renal Function

Renal Function	**Creatinine Clearance mL/min/1.73 m² (mL/s/1.73 m²)**	**Maximum Total Daily Dosage for Infections Due to Fully Susceptible Organisms**	**Maximum Total Daily Dosage for Infections Due to Less Susceptible Organisms[b]**
Mild impairment	31–70 (0.52–1.17)	1.5 g (0.5 g q8h)	2.0 g (0.5 g q6h)
Moderate impairment	21–30 (0.35–0.50)	1.0 g (0.5 g q12h)	1.5 g (0.5 g q8h)
Severe impairment[a]	0–20 (0–0.33)	0.5 g (0.25 g q12h)	1.0 g (0.5 g q12h)

[a] Patients with creatinine clearance of 6 to 20 mL/min/1.73 m² (0.1 to 0.3 mL/s/1.73 m²) should be treated with 250 mg (or 3.5 mg/kg whichever is lower) every 12 hours for most pathogens. When the 500 mg dose is used in these patients, there may be an increased risk of seizures.
[b] Primarily some strains of *P. aeruginosa*.

A further proportionate reduction in dose administered must be made for patients with a body weight <70 kg.

When only the serum creatinine level is available, the following formula (based on sex, weight, and age of the patient) may be used to convert this value into creatinine clearance (mL/min). The serum creatinine should represent a steady state of renal function.

$$\text{Males} = \frac{\text{Weight (kg)} \times (140-\text{age})}{72 \times \text{serum creatinine (mg/100 mL)}}$$

$$\text{Females} = 0.85 \times \text{above value}$$

When using the International System of units (SI), the estimated creatinine clearance (mL/s) in males can be calculated as follows:

$$\text{Males} = \frac{\text{(lean body weight, kg)} \times (140-\text{age, years}) \times 1.4736}{(72) \times (\text{serum creatinine concentration, } \mu\text{mol/L})}$$

and in females the estimated creatinine clearance (mL/s) is:

$$\text{Females} = \frac{\text{(lean body weight, kg)} \times (140-\text{age, years}) \times 1.2526}{(72) \times (\text{serum creatinine concentration, } \mu\text{mol/L})}$$

Primaxin is cleared by hemodialysis. After each dialysis session the dosage schedule should be restarted.

Dosage in Infants and Children: The recommended total daily dosage of Primaxin in children and infants 3 months of age and older is 60 to 100 mg/kg of body weight divided into 4 equal doses given at six hour intervals. The higher dosages should be used for infants and young children. The total daily dosage should not exceed 2 grams. Clinical data are insufficient to recommend an optimum dose for infants and children with impaired renal function.

Primaxin is not recommended for the therapy of meningitis. If meningitis is suspected, an appropriate antibiotic should be used.

Primaxin may be used in children with sepsis as long as they are not suspected of having meningitis.

Administration: **Caution: Contents of vials not for direct infusion.**

Each reconstituted 250 mg or 500 mg dose should be given by i.v. infusion over 20 to 30 minutes. Each 1000 mg dose should be infused over 40 to 60 minutes. In patients who develop nausea during the infusion, the rate of infusion may be slowed (for reconstitution, see Reconstitution).

Reconstitution: Primaxin is supplied in vials of either 250 mg or 500 mg imipenem equivalent and cilastatin equivalent when reconstituted.

Vials—Primaxin: Contents of the vials must be suspended and transferred to 100 mL of an appropriate infusion solution.

A suggested procedure is to transfer approximately 10 mL from the 100 mL of the appropriate infusion solution to the vial (see list of diluents under Compatibility and Stability). Shake well. Return the resulting 10 mL of suspension to the remaining 90 mL of the infusion solution.

Repeat, using 10 mL of the diluted suspension, to ensure complete transfer of the contents of the vial to the infusion solution.

Caution: Contents of vials not for direct infusion.

Compatibility and Stability: List of Diluents: 0.9% Sodium Chloride Injection, 5% Or 10% Dextrose Injection, 5% Dextrose Injection with 0.02% sodium bicarbonate solution, 5% Dextrose with 0.9% Sodium Chloride Injection, 5% Dextrose with 0.225% or 0.45% saline solution, 5% Dextrose with 0.15% potassium chloride solution, Mannitol 5% and 10%.

Reconstituted Solutions: Solutions range from colorless to yellow. Variations of color within this range do not affect the potency of the product.

Primaxin, as supplied in vials and reconstituted as above maintains satisfactory potency for **4 hours at room temperature and for 24 hours under refrigeration (4°C)**.

SUPPLIED: 250 mg: Each vial of sterile powder mixture contains: imipenem anhydrous equivalent to imipenem 250 mg and cilastatin sodium equivalent to cilastatin 250 mg. Also contains sodium bicarbonate buffer. The dry powder should be stored at 15-30°C.

500 mg: Each vial of sterile powder mixture contains: imipenem anhydrous equivalent to imipenem 500 mg and cilastatin sodium equivalent to cilastatin 500 mg. Also contains sodium bicarbonate buffer. The dry powder should be stored at 15-30°C.

Primidone P

CPhA Monograph

see *Barbiturates*

Primovist®

gadoxetate disodium

Intravenous Contrast Enhancement Agent for Magnetic Resonance Imaging (MRI)

Bayer

Date of Preparation: January 13, 2010

SUMMARY PRODUCT INFORMATION:

Route of Administration	Dosage Form/ Strength	Clinically Relevant Nonmedicinal Ingredients
Intravenous	Solution/181.43 mg/mL gadoxetate disodium injection (0.25 mmol/mL)	None For a complete listing see Dosage Forms, Composition and Packaging.

INDICATIONS AND CLINICAL USE: PRIMOVIST (gadoxetate disodium injection) is a gadolinium-based contrast agent indicated for intravenous use in T1-weighted magnetic resonance imaging (MRI) of the liver to detect and characterize lesions in adults with known or suspected focal liver disease.

Geriatrics (>65 years of age): In clinical studies of PRIMOVIST, 37% of the patients were 65 years of age and over, while 7% were 75 years of age and over. No overall differences in safety or effectiveness were observed between these subjects and younger subjects, and other reported clinical experience has not identified differences in responses between the elderly and younger patients.

However, the elderly may be at particular risk of NSF due to impaired ability of their kidneys to clear gadolinium from the body (see Warnings and Precautions, Serious Warnings and Precautions and General).

Pediatrics (<18 years of age): The safety and effectiveness of PRIMOVIST have not been established in pediatric patients.

CONTRAINDICATIONS:

- Patients who are hypersensitive to this drug or to any ingredient in the formulation or component of the container. For a complete listing, see Dosage Forms, Composition and Packaging.

WARNINGS AND PRECAUTIONS:

Serious Warnings and Precautions

Nephrogenic Systemic Fibrosis: Gadolinium-based contrast agents (GBCAs) increase the risk for Nephrogenic Systemic Fibrosis (NSF) in patients with:

- acute or chronic severe renal insufficiency (glomerular filtration rate <30 mL/min/1.73 m^2), or
- acute renal insufficiency of any severity due to the hepato-renal syndrome or in the perioperative liver transplantation period.

In these patients, avoid use of GBCAs unless the diagnostic information is essential and not available with noncontrast-enhanced magnetic resonance imaging (MRI). NSF may result in fatal or debilitating systemic fibrosis affecting the skin, muscle, and internal organs. Screen all patients for renal dysfunction by obtaining a history and/or laboratory tests. When administering a GBCA, do not exceed the recommended dose (see Dosage and Administration) and allow a sufficient period of time for elimination of the agent from the body prior to any readministration. (See Warnings and Precautions, General, Skin, and Renal; and Adverse Reactions, Post-Market Adverse Drug Reactions.)

General: The usual safety rules for magnetic resonance imaging must be observed, eg, exclusion of cardiac pacemakers and ferromagnetic implants.

Intramuscular administration should be strictly avoided, because it may cause local intolerance reactions including focal necrosis.

Severe renal or hepatic failure may impair PRIMOVIST imaging performance. In patients with end-stage renal failure, hepatic contrast was reduced and was attributed to elevated serum ferritin levels. In patients with abnormally high (>3 mg/dL) serum bilirubin, reduced hepatic contrast was observed. If PRIMOVIST is used in these patients, complete Magnetic Resonance (MR) imaging no later than 60 minutes after PRIMOVIST administration period.

Nephrogenic Systemic Fibrosis (NSF): Gadolinium-based contrast agents (GBCAs) increase the risk for Nephrogenic Systemic Fibrosis (NSF) in patients with acute or chronic severe renal insufficiency (glomerular filtration rate <30 mL/min/1.73 m^2), and in patients with acute renal insufficiency of any severity due to the hepato-renal syndrome, or in the perioperative liver transplantation period. In these patients, avoid use of GBCAs unless the diagnostic information is essential and not available with noncontrast-enhanced magnetic resonance imaging (MRI). For patients receiving hemodialysis, healthcare professionals may consider prompt hemodialysis following GBCA administration in order to enhance the contrast agent's elimination. However, it is unknown if hemodialysis prevents NSF.

Among the factors that may increase the risk for NSF are repeated or higher than recommended doses of a GBCA and the degree of renal function impairment at the time of exposure.

NSF development is considered a potential class-related effect of all GBCAs.

Postmarketing reports have identified the development of NSF following single and multiple administrations of GBCAs. These reports have not always identified a specific agent. Where a specific agent was identified, the most commonly reported agent was gadodiamide (OMNISCAN), followed by gadopentetate dimeglumine (MAGNEVIST) and gadoversetamide (OPTIMARK). NSF has also developed following the sequential administration of gadodiamide with gadobenate dimeglumine (MULTIHANCE) or gadoteridol (PROHANCE). The number of postmarketing reports is subject to change over time and may not reflect the true proportion of cases associated with any specific GBCA.

The extent of risk for NSF following exposure to any specific GBCA is unknown and may vary among the agents. Published reports are limited and predominantly estimate NSF risks with gadodiamide. In one retrospective study of 370 patients with severe renal insufficiency who received gadodiamide, the estimated risk for development of NSF was 4%. The risk, if any, for the development of NSF among patients with mild to moderate renal insufficiency or normal renal function is unknown, and the cautious utilization of the lowest possible dose of GBCA is preferable.

Screen all patients for renal dysfunction by obtaining a history and/or laboratory tests. When administering a GBCA, do not exceed the recommended dose and allow a sufficient period of time for elimination of the agent from the body prior to any readministration. (See Action and Clinical Pharmacology and Dosage and Administration.)

A skin biopsy is necessary in order to exclude the diagnosis of similarly presenting skin disorders (eg, scleromyxedema). (See Warnings and Precautions, Serious Warnings and Precautions, Renal, and Skin; and Adverse Reactions, Post-Market Adverse Drug Reactions.)

Cardiovascular: Caution should be exercised when PRIMOVIST is administered to patients with severe cardiovascular problems because only limited data are available so far.

Hypersensitivity Reactions: As with other intravenous contrast agents, anaphylactoid and anaphylactic reactions with cardiovascular, respiratory, and cutaneous manifestations, ranging from mild to severe reactions, including shock have occurred very rarely following PRIMOVIST administration (see Adverse Reactions).

- Before PRIMOVIST administration, assess all patients for any history of a reaction to contrast media, a history of bronchial asthma, and/or a history of allergic disorders. These patients may have an increased risk for a hypersensitivity reaction to PRIMOVIST.
- Administer PRIMOVIST only in situations where trained personnel and therapies are promptly available for the treatment of hypersensitivity reactions, including personnel trained in resuscitation.

Most hypersensitivity reactions to PRIMOVIST have occurred within half an hour after administration. Delayed reactions (hours up to several days) may occur. Observe patients for signs and symptoms of hypersensitivity reactions during and following PRIMOVIST administration for at least 30 minutes and longer if clinically required.

Treat these reactions with standard medications for hypersensitivity reactions.

Patients taking beta blockers who experience such reactions may be resistant to treatment with beta agonists.

Renal: Exposure to GBCAs increase the risk for NSF in patients with:

- acute or chronic severe renal insufficiency (glomerular filtration rate <30 mL/min/1.73 m^2), or
- acute renal insufficiency of any severity due to the hepato-renal syndrome or in the perioperative liver transplantation period.

Screen all patients for renal dysfunction by obtaining a history and/or laboratory tests.

The risk, if any, for the development of NSF among patients with mild to moderate renal insufficiency or normal renal function is unknown, and the cautious utilization of the lowest possible dose of GBCA is preferable.

There is a possibility that NSF may occur with PRIMOVIST. Therefore, PRIMOVIST should only be used in these patients after careful risk/benefit assessment.

See Warnings and Precautions, Serious Warnings and Precautions, and Skin; and Adverse Reactions, Post-Market Adverse Drug Reactions.)

For patients receiving hemodialysis, healthcare professionals may consider prompt hemodialysis following GBCA administration in order to enhance the contrast agent's elimination. However, it is unknown if hemodialysis prevents NSF.

Skin: NSF was first identified in 1997 and has so far, been observed only in patients with renal disease. This is a systemic disorder with the most prominent and visible effects on the skin. Cutaneous lesions associated with this disorder are caused by excessive fibrosis and are usually symmetrically distributed on the limbs and trunk. Involved skin becomes thickened which may inhibit flexion and extension of joints and result in severe contractures. The fibrosis associated with NSF can extend beyond dermis and involve subcutaneous tissues, striated muscles, diaphragm, pleura, pericardium, and myocardium. NSF may be fatal. (See Warnings and Precautions, Serious Warnings and Precautions, General, and Renal; and Adverse Reactions, Post-Market Adverse Drug Reactions.)

Special Populations: Pregnant Women: For gadoxetate disodium, no clinical study data on exposed pregnancies are available. Animal studies showed no evidence for a risk of teratogenic action or influences on fertility, fetal as well as pre- and postnatal development. PRIMOVIST should only be used in pregnant women after a clear benefit-to-risk analysis.

Nursing Women: It is unknown whether gadoxetate disodium is excreted in human milk. There is evidence from non-clinical data in rats that minimal amounts of gadoxetate disodium transfer from maternal blood into milk (less than 0.5 % of the dose administered). PRIMOVIST should only be used in nursing women after a clear benefit-to-risk analysis.

Pediatrics (<18 years of age): The safety and effectiveness of PRIMOVIST have not been established in pediatric patients.

Geriatrics (>65 years of age): In clinical studies of PRIMOVIST, 37% of the patients were 65 years of age and over, while 7% were 75 years of age and over. No overall differences in safety or effectiveness were observed between these subjects and younger subjects, and other reported clinical experience has not identified differences in responses between the elderly and younger patients.

However, the elderly may be at particular risk of NSF due to impaired ability of their kidneys to clear gadolinium from the body (see Warnings and Precautions, Serious Warnings and Precautions and General).

Hepatic Insufficiency: Severe hepatic impairment may impair PRIMOVIST imaging performance. In patients with abnormally high (>3 mg/dL) serum bilirubin, reduced hepatic contrast was observed. If PRIMOVIST is used in these patients, complete MR imaging no later than 60 minutes after PRIMOVIST administration (see Warnings and Precautions, General and Action and Clinical Pharmacology). A dose adjustment is not necessary for patients with hepatic impairment.

Renal Insufficiency: Severe renal failure may impair PRIMOVIST imaging performance (see Warnings and Precautions, Serious Warnings and Precautions). In patients with end-stage renal failure, hepatic contrast was reduced and was attributed to elevated serum ferritin levels. If PRIMOVIST is used in these patients, complete MR imaging no later than 60 minutes after PRIMOVIST administration (see Warnings and Precautions, General and Action and Clinical Pharmacology). A dose adjustment is not necessary for patients with renal impairment.

ADVERSE REACTIONS: Adverse Drug Reaction Overview: Most adverse drug reactions reported with PRIMOVIST were of mild to moderate intensity, and did not require a discontinuation of the procedure. The most frequently reported adverse reactions in clinical trials were headache (0.6%; mild intensity), nausea (0.7%; usually occurring just after injection and resolving quickly), and feeling hot (0.7%: usually occurring during injection).

Clinical Trial Adverse Drug Reactions: Because clinical trials are conducted under very specific conditions, the adverse reaction rates observed in the clinical trials may not reflect the rates observed in practice and should not be compared to the rates in the clinical trials of another drug. Adverse drug reaction information from clinical trials is useful for identifying drug-related adverse events and for approximating rates.

PRIMOVIST was studied for use in MRI in phase II and phase III studies in 1755 patients. The average age was 58 years (range from 19 to 84 years). The dose of PRIMOVIST administered ranged from 0.003 to 0.1 mmol/kg body weight for most patients (1728 patients; 98.4%), with the majority (1347 patients; 76.8%) receiving the recommended dose of 0.025 mmol/kg body weight. Higher doses (0.2-0.5 mmol/kg body weight) were used in only a very few patients (27 patients; 1.5%). The ethnic distribution was 72% Caucasian, 12% Asian, 3% Hispanic, 2% Black, and 0.6% patients of other ethnic groups.

The clinical trials were predominantly of intrapatient-controlled design with nonactive comparators (precontrast MRI and contrast-enhanced CT).

A total of 76 patients (4.3%) had adverse drug reactions. The follow-up period for most subjects extended over 24 hours after PRIMOVIST administration. Most of the adverse drug reactions were of mild to moderate intensity.

No individual adverse drug reaction reached a frequency greater than "uncommon". No adverse drug reactions occurred at a rate greater than 1%.

Less Common Clinical Trial Adverse Drug Reactions: Table 1 lists all adverse drug reactions observed in <1% of patients.

Table 1 reports adverse reactions by MedDRA system organ classes (MedDRA SOCs).

Table 1: PRIMOVIST

All Adverse Drug Reactions Reported by <1% of Patients During Clinical Trials (N=1755)

System Organ Class	Uncommon (≥0.1% and <1%)	Rare (<0.1%)
General disorders and administration site conditions	chest pain, feeling hot, injection site reactions (various kinds)[a]	chills, discomfort, fatigue, feeling abnormal, malaise
Cardiac disorders		bundle branch block, palpitation
Gastrointestinal disorders	nausea, vomiting	dry mouth, oral discomfort, salivary hypersecretion
Musculoskeletal, connective tissue and bone disorders		back pain
Nervous system disorders	dizziness, dysgeusia, headache, paresthesia, parosmia	akathisia, vertigo, tremor
Respiratory, thoracic and mediastinal disorders	respiratory disorders (dyspnea, respiratory distress)	
Skin and subcutaneous tissue disorders	rash, pruritus[b]	hyperhidrosis , maculopapular rash
Vascular disorders	blood pressure increased, flushing	

[a] Injection site reactions (various kinds) comprise the following terms: injection site extravasation, injection site burning, injection site coldness, injection site irritation, injection site pain.

[b] Pruritus (eye pruritus, generalized pruritus).

The most appropriate MedDRA term is used to describe a certain reaction and its synonyms and related conditions. ADR term representation is based on MedDRA version 9.0.

As with other contrast agents, in very rare cases, anaphylactoid reactions ranging to shock may occur (see Warnings and Precautions, Hypersensitivity Reactions).

Abnormal Hematologic and Clinical Chemistry Findings: Elevation of serum iron values and serum bilirubin laboratory values were reported in less than 1% of patients after administration of PRIMOVIST. The values did not exceed more than 2 to 3 times the baseline values and returned to baseline within 1 to 4 days without other signs or symptoms of other abnormalities. All clinically significant changes in laboratory values observed during clinical trials with PRIMOVIST (0.025 mmol/kg bw) have been summarized in Table 2.

Post-Market Adverse Drug Reactions: In general, following single and multiple administrations of gadolinium-based contrast agents (GBCAs), postmarketing reports have identified the development of NSF. These reports have not always identified a specific agent. Where a specific agent was identified, the most commonly reported agent was gadodiamide (OMNISCAN), followed by gadopentetate dimeglumine (MAGNEVIST) and gadoversetamide (OPTIMARK). NSF has also developed following the sequential administration of gadodiamide with gadobenate dimeglumine (MULTIHANCE) or gadoteridol (PROHANCE). The number of postmarketing reports is subject to change over time and may not reflect the true proportion of cases associated with any specific GBCA. The extent of risk for NSF following exposure to any specific GBCA is unknown and may vary among the agents. Published reports are limited and predominantly estimate NSF risks with gadodiamide. In one retrospective study of 370 patients with severe renal insufficiency who received gadodiamide, the estimated risk for development of NSF was 4%. The risk, if any, for the development of NSF among patients with mild to moderate renal insufficiency or normal renal function is unknown, and the cautious utilization of the lowest possible dose of GBCA is preferable (see also Warnings and Precautions, Serious Warnings and Precautions, General, Skin and Renal).

The following additional adverse drug reactions have been reported during the postmarketing use of PRIMOVIST: anaphylactic reactions including shock, tachycardia, and restlessness.

Table 2: PRIMOVIST
Treatment-Emergent Laboratory Abnormalities in Clinical Trials With PRIMOVIST

Laboratory Parameter	Number of Patients with Changes	Magnitude of Change From Baseline Values
Alpha-amylase increased	2	1 time
Bilirubin increased	8	Up to 3 times
Gamma GT increased	1	1 time
Inorganic phosphate decreased	1	10% below the lower limit of the normal change
Potassium decreased	2	10% below the lower limit of the normal change
Serum iron increased	3	Up to 3 times
Sodium decreased	1	3% below the lower limit of the normal range
Total protein decreased	1	10% below the lower limit of the normal change

DRUG INTERACTIONS: Overview: Elevated levels of bilirubin or ferritin can reduce the hepatic contrast effect of PRIMOVIST.
Drug-Drug Interactions: Anionic drugs primarily excreted into the bile (such as rifampicin) may compete with the hepatic contrast enhancement and the biliary excretion of PRIMOVIST. Animal studies demonstrated that compounds belonging to the class of rifamycins block the hepatic uptake of gadoxetate disodium, thus reducing the hepatic contrast effect. In this case, the expected benefit of an injection of PRIMOVIST might be limited.

Interactions with other medications are not known.

Drug-Food Interactions: Interactions with food have not been studied.
Drug-Herb Interactions: Interactions with herbal medicines have not been studied.
Drug-Laboratory Test Interactions: Serum iron determination using complexometric methods (eg, Ferrocine complexation method) may result in falsely high and low values for up to 24 hours after the examination with PRIMOVIST because of the caloxetate trisodium excipients.

DOSAGE AND ADMINISTRATION: Dosing Considerations: Nausea and vomiting are known adverse reactions associated with the administration of contrast media. The patient should therefore refrain from eating for two hours prior to the MRI investigation in order to minimize the risk of vomiting and possible aspiration.

Whenever possible, the contrast agent should be administered with the patient lying down. After the injection, the patient should be kept under observation for at least 30 minutes. Delayed reactions may also occur (see also Warnings and Precautions, Hypersensitivity Reactions).

The safety and effectiveness of PRIMOVIST have not been established in pediatric patients.

Recommended Dose and Dosage Adjustment: The recommended dose of PRIMOVIST is 0.1 mL/kg body weight (equivalent to 0.025 mmol/kg body weight).
Imaging: Liver lesions are detected and characterized with precontrast MR images and PRIMOVIST MR images obtained during dynamic and hepatocyte imaging phases. During the dynamic imaging phases, use the temporal enhancement and washout pattern of intravascular PRIMOVIST to assess lesions.

Further assess lesions during a hepatocyte imaging phase based upon the pattern of PRIMOVIST accumulation within hepatocytes. The enhancement of liver parenchyma during this phase assists in the identification of the number, segmental distribution, visualisation, and delineation of liver lesions, thus improving lesion detection.

Perform a precontrast MRI, inject PRIMOVIST and begin dynamic imaging approximately 15 to 25 seconds after completion of the injection. Dynamic imaging consists of the arterial, the porto-venous (approximately 60 seconds post injection), and the blood equilibrium (approximately 120 seconds) phases. Begin the hepatocyte imaging phase at approximately 20 minutes post injection. Hepatocyte phase imaging may be performed up to 120 minutes post injection.

Elevated intrinsic levels of bilirubin (>3 mg/dL) or ferritin can reduce the hepatic contrast effect of PRIMOVIST. Perform MR imaging no later than 60 minutes following PRIMOVIST administration to patients with elevated bilirubin or ferritin levels (see Warnings and Precautions, Special Populations and Drug Interactions).

Lesions with no or minimal hepatocyte function (cysts, metastases, and the majority of hepatocellular carcinomas) generally will not accumulate PRIMOVIST. Well-differentiated hepatocellular carcinoma may contain functioning hepatocytes and can show some enhancement in the hepatocyte imaging phase. Additional clinical information is therefore needed to support a diagnosis of hepatocellular carcinoma.

Administration: PRIMOVIST is a ready-to-use solution. Visually inspect PRIMOVIST for particulate matter and discoloration prior to administration. Do not use the solution if it is discolored or if particulate matter is present. Do not use if the PRIMOVIST container is defective. PRIMOVIST should not be mixed with other drugs. PRIMOVIST is intended for single use and should be used immediately after opening.

Vials containing PRIMOVIST are not intended for the withdrawal of multiple doses. The rubber stopper should never be pierced more than once. Administer PRIMOVIST undiluted as an intravenous bolus injection at a flow rate of approximately 2 mL/second through a large-bore needle or indwelling catheter. Flush the intravenous cannula with physiological saline solution after the injection. Discard any unused portion of a PRIMOVIST vial.

OVERDOSAGE:
The maximum dose studied in MR imaging was 0.4 mL/kg (0.1 mmol/kg) body weight and was tolerated in a manner similar to lower doses. In a limited number of patients, a dose of 2.0 mL/kg (500 µmol/kg) body weight was tested in clinical trials; more frequent occurrences of adverse events but no new adverse events were found in these patients.

In view of the low volume (max. 10 mL) and the extremely low gastrointestinal absorption rate of PRIMOVIST, and based on acute toxicity data, intoxication due to inadvertent oral ingestion of the contrast medium is extremely improbable.

In the event of excessive inadvertent overdosage in patients with substantially impaired renal and hepatic function, PRIMOVIST can be removed by hemodialysis.

For management of a suspected drug overdose, contact your **regional Poison Control Centre**. See the *CPS Directory* section for a list of Poison Control Centres.

ACTION AND CLINICAL PHARMACOLOGY: Mechanism of Action: Gadoxetate disodium (Gd-EOB-DTPA) is a paramagnetic compound and develops a magnetic moment when placed in a magnetic field. The relatively large magnetic moment produced by gadoxetate disodium results in a local magnetic field, yielding enhanced relaxation rates (shortening of relaxation times) of water protons in the vicinity of the paramagnetic agent, which leads to an increase in signal intensity (brightening) of blood and tissue.

In MRI, visualization of normal and pathological tissue depends in part on variations in the radiofrequency signal intensity that occur with 1) differences in proton density; 2) differences of the spin-lattice or longitudinal relaxation times (T1); and 3) differences in the spin-spin or transverse relaxation time (T2). When placed in a magnetic field, gadoxetate disodium decreases the T1 and T2 relaxation time in target tissue. At the recommended dose, the effect is observed with greatest sensitivity in T1-weighted MR sequences.

Pharmacodynamics: EOB-DTPA forms a stable complex with the paramagnetic gadolinium ion with a high thermodynamic stability of log K_{GdL} = 23.46, and high stability in human serum, determined in vitro at pH 7.4 and 37°C (initial Gd^{3+} release rate: 0.07% per day and a total release of 1.1% Gd^{3+} after 15 days).

Gadoxetate disodium is a highly water-soluble, hydrophilic, linear ionic compound with a lipophilic moiety, the ethoxybenzyl group (EOB).

Gadoxetate disodium shows a weak (<10%), transient protein binding and the relaxivity in plasma is about 6.9 L/mmol/sec at pH 7, 37°C and 1.5 Tesla; 6.2 L/mmol/sec at pH 7, 37°C and 3.0 Tesla. The relaxivity in blood is about 7.3 L/mmol/sec at pH 7, 37°C and 1.5 T. The relaxivity displays only slight dependency on the strength of the magnetic field.

Gadoxetate disodium is selectively taken up by hepatocytes resulting in increased signal intensity in liver tissue. PRIMOVIST exhibits a biphasic mode of action: first, distribution in the extracellular space after bolus injection and subsequently, selective uptake by hepatocytes (and biliary excretion) due to the lipophilic (EOB) moiety.

Pharmacokinetics: Distribution: After intravenous administration, the plasma concentration time profile of gadoxetate disodium is characterized by a bi-exponential decline. The total distribution volume of gadoxetate disodium at steady state is about 0.21 L/kg (extracellular space); plasma protein binding is less than 10%. Gadoxetate disodium does not pass the intact blood-brain barrier and diffuses through the placental barrier.

Excretion: Gadoxetate disodium is equally eliminated via the renal (approximately 50%) and hepatobiliary (approximately 50%) routes. The mean terminal elimination half-life of gadoxetate disodium (0.01 to 0.1 mmol/kg) has been observed in healthy volunteers of 22 to 39 years of age to be 55 to 57 minutes. Clearance appeared to decrease slightly with increasing age. The pharmacokinetics are dose-linear up to a dose of 0.4 mL/kg (0.1 mmol/kg), which is 4 times the recommended dose.

The total serum clearance (Cl_{tot}) was 250 mL/min, whereas the renal clearance (Cl_r) corresponds to about 120 mL/min, a value similar to the glomerular filtration rate in healthy subjects.

Metabolism: Gadoxetate disodium is not metabolized.
Special Populations and Conditions: Hepatic Insufficiency: In patients with mild or moderate hepatic impairment, a slight to moderate increase in plasma AUC, half-life and urinary excretion, as well as decrease in hepatobiliary excretion was observed in comparison to healthy subjects with normal liver function. In patients with severe hepatic impairment, especially in patients with abnormally high (>3 mg/dL) serum bilirubin levels, the AUC was increased up to 60% and the elimination half-life was increased up to 49%. The hepatobiliary excretion substantially decreased to about 5% of the administered dose.

Renal Insufficiency: In patients with moderate renal impairment, a moderate increase in AUC and terminal half-life was observed in comparison to healthy volunteers with normal renal function. In patients with end-stage renal failure, the terminal half-life was prolonged about 12-fold and the AUC was increased about 6-fold.

STORAGE AND STABILITY: PRIMOVIST is chemically and physically stable. PRIMOVIST should be used immediately after opening.

PRIMOVIST should be stored at temperatures between 15 to 30°C.

INFORMATION FOR THE PATIENT: Published in e-CPS, available by subscription at www.e-cps.ca.

DOSAGE FORMS, COMPOSITION AND PACKAGING: Each mL of sterile, nonpyrogenic, clear, colorless to pale yellow aqueous solution contains: gadoxetate disodium 181.43 mg (0.25 mmol). Nonmedicinal ingredients: caloxetate trisodium, trometamol and water for injection. Sodium hydroxide and/or hydrochloric acid are added to adjust pH. No preservative is added. Single-use vials of 10 mL containing 7.5 mL and 10 mL of solution. Discard unused portion.

The reader is invited to consult CPhA's monograph **ACE Inhibitors**.

Prinivil® Pr

lisinopril

Angiotensin-Converting Enzyme Inhibitor

Merck Frosst

Date of Revision: April 22, 2010

PHARMACOLOGY: Lisinopril is an angiotensin-converting enzyme (ACE) inhibitor which is used in the treatment of hypertension, congestive heart failure and following myocardial infarction in hemodynamically stable patients.

Angiotensin-converting enzyme is a peptidyl dipeptidase which catalyzes the conversion of angiotensin I to the pressor substance, angiotensin II. Inhibition of ACE results in decreased plasma angiotensin II, which leads to increased plasma renin activity (due to removal of negative feedback of renin release) and decreased aldosterone secretion. Although the latter decrease is small, it results in a small increase in serum K+. In patients treated with lisinopril and a thiazide diuretic there was essentially no change in serum potassium (see Precautions).

ACE is identical to kininase II. Thus, lisinopril may also block the degradation of bradykinin, a potent vasodilator peptide. However, the role that this plays in the therapeutic effects of lisinopril is unknown.

While the mechanism through which lisinopril lowers blood pressure is believed to be primarily the suppression of the renin-angiotensin-aldosterone system, lisinopril also lowers blood pressure in patients with low-renin hypertension.

Pharmacodynamics: Administration of lisinopril to patients with hypertension results in a reduction of both supine and standing blood pressure. Abrupt withdrawal of lisinopril has not been associated with a rapid increase in blood pressure. In most patients studied, after oral administration of an individual dose of lisinopril, the onset of antihypertensive activity is seen at 1 hour with peak reduction of blood pressure achieved by 6 hours. Although an antihypertensive effect was observed 24 hours after dosing with recommended single daily doses, the effect was more consistent and the mean effect was considerably larger in some studies with doses of 20 mg or more than with lower doses. However, at all doses studied, the mean antihypertensive effect was substantially smaller 24 hours after dosing than it was 6 hours after dosing. On occasion, achievement of optimal blood pressure reduction may require 2 to 4 weeks of therapy.

In a clinical study involving 115 hypertensive pediatric patients 6 to 16 years of age, patients who weighed <50 kg received either 0.625, 2.5, or 20 mg of lisinopril daily and patients who weighed ≥50 kg received either 1.25, 5, or 40 mg of lisinopril daily. At the end of 2 weeks, lisinopril administered once daily lowered trough blood pressure in a dose-dependent manner with consistent antihypertensive efficacy demonstrated at doses >1.25 mg (0.02 mg/kg). This effect was confirmed in a withdrawal phase, where the diastolic pressure rose by about 9 mmHg more in patients randomized to placebo than it did in patients who were randomized to remain on the middle and high doses of lisinopril. The dose-dependent antihypertensive effect of lisinopril was consistent across several demographic subgroups: age, Tanner stage, gender, race. In this study, lisinopril was generally well-tolerated.

In hemodynamic studies in patients with essential hypertension, blood pressure reduction was accompanied by a reduction in peripheral arterial resistance with little or no change in cardiac output and in heart rate. In a study in 9 hypertensive patients, following administration of lisinopril, there was an increase in mean renal blood flow that was not significant. Data from several small studies are inconsistent with respect to the effect of lisinopril on glomerular filtration rate in hypertensive patients with normal renal function, but suggest that changes, if any, are not large.

When lisinopril is given together with thiazide-type diuretics, its blood pressure lowering effect is approximately additive.

The antihypertensive effect of angiotensin converting enzyme inhibitors is generally lower in Black than in non-Black patients.

Administration of lisinopril to patients with congestive heart failure reduces afterload and preload of the heart, resulting in an increase in cardiac output, without reflex tachycardia. Exercise tolerance is improved.

Pharmacokinetics: Following oral administration of lisinopril, peak serum concentrations of lisinopril occur within about 7 hours, although patients with recent myocardial infarction have demonstrated an increase in time to peak serum concentration to about 8 to 10 hours. Declining serum concentrations exhibit a prolonged terminal phase which does not contribute to drug accumulation. This terminal phase probably represents saturable binding to ACE and is not proportional to dose. Lisinopril does not bind serum proteins other than ACE.

Lisinopril does not undergo metabolism and is excreted unchanged entirely in the urine. Based on urinary recovery, the extent of absorption of lisinopril is approximately 25%, with large intersubject variability (6 to 60%) at all doses tested (5 to 80 mg). Lisinopril absorption is not influenced by the presence of food in the gastrointestinal tract.

Following multiple doses of lisinopril, the effective half-life of accumulation is 12 hours.

In a study in elderly healthy subjects (65 years and above), a single dose of lisinopril 20 mg produced higher serum concentrations than those seen in young healthy adults given a similar dose. In another study, single daily doses of lisinopril 5 mg were given for 7 consecutive days to young and elderly healthy volunteers and to elderly patients with congestive heart failure. Maximum serum concentrations of lisinopril on Day 7 were higher in the elderly volunteers than in the young, and still higher in the elderly patients with congestive heart failure. Renal clearance of lisinopril was decreased in the elderly, particularly in the presence of congestive heart failure.

The elimination of lisinopril in patients with renal insufficiency is similar to that in patients with normal renal function until the glomerular filtration rate is 30 mL/min or less. With renal function ≤30 mL/min, peak and trough lisinopril levels increase, time to peak concentration increases and time to steady-state is prolonged (see Dosage).

The pharmacokinetics of lisinopril were studied in 29 pediatric hypertensive patients between 6 years and 16 years with glomerular filtration rate >30 mL/min/1.73 m². After doses of 0.1 to 0.2 mg/kg, steady state peak plasma concentrations of lisinopril occured within 6 hours and the extent of absorption based on urinary recovery was about 28%. These values are similar to those obtained previously in adults. The typical value of lisinopril oral clearance (systemic clearance/absolute bioavailability) in a child weighing 30 kg is 10 L/h, which increases in proportion to renal function.

Studies in rats indicate that lisinopril crosses the blood-brain barrier poorly.

INDICATIONS: Hypertension: In the treatment of essential hypertension and in renovascular hypertension. It may be used alone or concomitantly with thiazide diuretics. A great majority of patients (>80%) with severe hypertension required combination therapy. Lisinopril has been used concomitantly with beta-blockers and calcium antagonists, but the data on such use are limited.

Heart Failure: Lisinopril is indicated in the management of symptomatic congestive heart failure as adjunctive treatment with diuretics and, where appropriate, digitalis. Treatment with lisinopril should be initiated under close medical supervision, usually in a hospital.

Treatment Following Acute Myocardial Infarction: Lisinopril is indicated in the treatment of hemodynamically stable patients as early as within 24 hours following acute myocardial infarction, to improve survival. Patients should receive, as appropriate, the standard recommended treatments such as thrombolytics, ASA and beta-blocker(s).

Therapy with lisinopril should be reassessed after 6 weeks. If there is no evidence of symptomatic or asymptomatic left ventricular dysfunction, treatment with lisinopril can be stopped.

Lisinopril should not be used if systolic blood pressure is less than 100 mmHg, if clinically relevant renal failure is present, if there is a history of bilateral stenosis of the renal arteries (see Precautions, Hypotension Following Acute Myocardial Infarction, Renal Impairment).

In using lisinopril, attention should be given to the risk of angioedema (see Warnings).

CONTRAINDICATIONS: In patients who are hypersensitive to any component of this product; have a history of angioneurotic edema relating to previous treatment with an angiotensin converting enzyme inhibitor; have hereditary or idiopathic angioedema.

WARNINGS:

Serious Warnings and Precautions

When used in pregnancy, angiotensin-converting enzyme (ACE) inhibitors can cause injury or even death of the developing fetus. When pregnancy is detected, Prinivil should be discontinued as soon as possible.

Angioedema: Angioedema has been reported in patients treated with lisinopril. This may occur at any time during treatment. Angioedema associated with shock may be fatal. If angioedema occurs, lisinopril should be promptly discontinued and the patient should be observed until the swelling subsides. Even in those instances where swelling of only the tongue is involved, without respiratory distress, patients may require prolonged observation since treatment with antihistamines and corticosteroids may not be sufficient. Very rarely, fatalities have been reported due to angioedema associated with laryngeal edema or tongue edema. Patients with involvement of the tongue, glottis or larynx are likely to experience airway obstruction, especially those with a history of airway surgery. When there is airway obstruction, emergency therapy should be administered promptly when indicated. This includes giving subcutaneous adrenaline (0.5 mL 1:1000), and/or maintaining a patent airway. The patient should be under close medical supervision until complete and sustained symptom resolution has occurred.

The incidence of angioedema during ACE inhibitor therapy has been reported to be higher in Black than in non-Black patients.

Patients with a history of angioedema unrelated to ACE inhibitor therapy may be at increased risk of angioedema while receiving an ACE inhibitor (see Contraindications).

Hypotension: Symptomatic hypotension has occurred after administration of lisinopril, usually after the first or second dose or when the dose was increased. It is more likely to occur in patients who are volume-depleted by diuretic therapy, dietary salt restriction, dialysis, diarrhea, vomiting, or possibly in patients with renin-dependent renovascular hypertension (see Dosage). In patients with severe congestive heart failure, with or without associated renal insufficiency, excessive hypotension has been observed and may be associated with oliguria and/or progressive azotemia, and rarely with acute renal failure and/or death. Because blood pressure could potentially fall, patients at risk for hypotension should start therapy under very close medical supervision, usually in a hospital. Such patients should be followed closely for the first 2 weeks of treatment and whenever the dose of lisinopril and/or diuretic is increased. Similar considerations apply to patients with ischemic heart or cerebrovascular disease in whom an excessive fall in blood pressure could result in a myocardial infarction or cerebrovascular accident (see Adverse Effects).

If hypotension occurs, the patient should be placed in supine position and, if necessary, receive an i.v. infusion of normal saline. A transient hypotensive response may not be a contraindication to further doses. These can usually be given to hypertensive patients without difficulty once the blood pressure has increased after volume expansion. However, lower doses of lisinopril and/or reduced concomitant diuretic therapy should be considered.

If hypotension occurs during treatment following acute myocardial infarction, consideration should be given to lisinopril discontinuation (see Adverse Effects and Dosage, Treatment Following Acute Myocardial Infarction).

In some patients with congestive heart failure who have normal or low blood pressure, additional lowering of systemic blood pressure may occur with lisinopril. If hypotension occurs, a reduction of dose or discontinuation of therapy should be considered.

Neutropenia/Agranulocytosis: Agranulocytosis and bone marrow depression have been caused by angiotensin converting enzyme inhibitors. Several cases of agranulocytosis and neutropenia have been reported in which a causal relationship to lisinopril cannot be excluded. Current experience with the drug shows the incidence to be rare. Periodic monitoring of white blood cell counts should be considered, especially in patients with collagen vascular disease and renal disease.

Pregnancy: ACE inhibitors can cause fetal and neonatal morbidity and mortality when administered to pregnant women. When pregnancy is detected, lisinopril should be discontinued as soon as possible.

The use of ACE inhibitors during the second and third trimesters of pregnancy has been associated with fetal and neonatal injury including hypotension, neonatal skull hypoplasia, anuria, reversible or irreversible renal failure, and death. Oligohydramnios has also been reported, presumably resulting from decreased fetal renal function, associated with fetal limb contractures, craniofacial deformation, and hypoplastic lung development.

Prematurity, and patent ductus arteriosus and other structural cardiac malformations, as well as neurologic malformations, have also been reported following exposure in the first trimester of pregnancy.

Infants with a history of in utero exposure to ACE inhibitors should be closely observed for hypotension, oliguria and hyperkalemia. If oliguria occurs, attention should be directed toward support of blood pressure and renal perfusion. Exchange transfusion or dialysis may be required as a means of reversing hypotension and/or substituting for impaired renal function; however, limited experience with those procedures has not been associated with significant clinical benefit.

Lisinopril has been removed from the neonatal circulation by peritoneal dialysis with some clinical benefit and may, theoretically, be removed by exchange transfusion, although there is no experience with the latter procedure.

Animal Data: Lisinopril was not teratogenic in mice treated on days 6 to 15 of gestation with up to 1000 mg/kg/day (625 times the maximum recommended human dose). There was an increase in fetal resorptions at doses down to 100 mg/kg; at doses of 1000 mg/kg this was prevented by saline supplementation. There was no fetotoxicity or teratogenicity in rats treated with up to 300 mg/kg/day (188 times the maximum recommended dose) of lisinopril at days 6 to 17 of gestation. In rats receiving lisinopril from day 15 of gestation through day 21 postpartum, there was an increased incidence in pup deaths on days 2 to 7 postpartum and a lower average body weight of pups on day 21 postpartum. The increase in pup deaths and decrease in pup weight did not occur with maternal saline supplementation.

Lisinopril, at doses up to 1 mg/kg/day, was not teratogenic when given throughout the organogenic period in saline supplemented rabbits. Saline supplementation (physiologic saline in place of tap water) was used to eliminate maternotoxic effects and enable evaluation of the teratogenic potential at the highest possible dosage level. The rabbit has been shown to be extremely sensitive to angiotensin converting enzyme inhibitors (captopril and enalapril) with maternal and fetotoxic effects apparent at or below the recommended therapeutic dosage levels in man.

Fetotoxicity was demonstrated in rabbits by an increased incidence of fetal resorptions at an oral dose of lisinopril of 1 mg/kg/day and by an increased incidence of incomplete ossification at the lowest dose tested (0.1 mg/kg/day). A single i.v. dose of 15 mg/kg of lisinopril administered to pregnant rabbits on gestation days 16, 21 or 26 resulted in 88 to 100% fetal death.

By whole body autoradiography, radioactivity was found in the placenta following administration of labelled lisinopril to pregnant rats, but none was found in the fetuses.

Lactation: The presence of concentrations of ACE inhibitor have been reported in human milk. Use of ACE inhibitors is not recommended during breast-feeding.

PRECAUTIONS: Renal Impairment: As a consequence of inhibiting the renin-angiotensin-aldosterone system, changes in renal function have been seen in susceptible individuals. In patients whose renal function may depend on the activity of the renin-angiotensin-aldosterone system, such as patients with bilateral renal artery stenosis, unilateral renal artery stenosis to a solitary kidney, or severe congestive heart failure, treatment with agents that inhibit this system has been associated with oliguria, progressive azotemia and, rarely, acute renal failure and/or death. In susceptible patients, concomitant diuretic use may further increase risk.

In acute myocardial infarction, treatment with lisinopril should not be initiated in patients with evidence of renal dysfunction, defined as serum creatinine concentration exceeding 177 µmol/L and/or proteinuria exceeding 500 mg/24 hours. If renal dysfunction develops during treatment with lisinopril (serum creatinine concentration exceeding 265 µmol/L or a doubling from the pretreatment value), then the physician should consider withdrawal of lisinopril.

Use of lisinopril should include appropriate assessment of renal function.

Hypotension Following Acute Myocardial Infarction: Lisinopril treatment following acute myocardial infarction must not be initiated in patients at risk of further serious hemodynamic deterioration after vasodilator treatment. These include patients with systolic blood pressure of 100 mmHg or lower or those in cardiogenic shock.

During the first 3 days following the infarction, dosage reduction should occur if systolic blood pressure is between 100 and 120 mmHg (see Dosage, Treatment Following Acute Myocardial Infarction).

Patients with myocardial infarction in the GISSI-3 study treated with lisinopril had a higher (9.0% vs 3.7%) incidence of persistent hypotension (systolic blood pressure less than 90 mmHg for more than 1 hour) than patients treated with placebo.

Hyperkalemia: In clinical trials hyperkalemia (serum potassium >5.7 mEq/L) occurred in approximately 2.2% of hypertensive patients and 4.0% of patients with congestive heart failure. In most cases these were isolated values which resolved despite continued therapy. Hyperkalemia was a cause of discontinuation of therapy in approximately 0.1% of hypertensive patients. Risk factors for the development of hyperkalemia include renal insufficiency, diabetes mellitus and concomitant use of potassium-sparing diuretics (e.g., spironolactone, triamterene, or amiloride), potassium supplements or potassium-containing salt substitutes (see also Drug Interactions, Agents Increasing Serum Potassium).

The use of potassium supplements, potassium-sparing diuretics, or potassium-containing salt substitutes particularly in patients with impaired renal function may lead to a significant increase in serum potassium. Hyperkalemia can cause serious, sometimes fatal, arrhythmias.

If concomitant use of Prinivil and any of the above-mentioned agents is deemed appropriate, they should be used with caution and with frequent monitoring of serum potassium.

Hypoglycemia: Diabetic patients treated with oral antidiabetic agents or insulin starting an ACE inhibitor should be told to closely monitor for hypoglycemia, especially during the first month of combined use. In addition, hypoglycemia appeared to be more likely to occur during the first weeks of combined treatment and in patients with renal impairment (see Drug Interactions).

Valvular Stenosis, Hypertrophic Cardiomyopathy: There is concern on theoretical grounds that patients with aortic stenosis or hypertrophic cardiomyopathy might be at particular risk of decreased coronary perfusion when treated with vasodilators.

Lisinopril should be given with caution to these patients.

Surgery/Anesthesia: In patients undergoing major surgery or during anesthesia with agents that produce hypotension, lisinopril blocks angiotensin II formation, secondary to compensatory renin release. If hypotension occurs and is considered to be due to this mechanism, it can be corrected by volume expansion.

Patients with Impaired Liver Function: Hepatitis, jaundice (hepatocellular and/or cholestatic), elevations of liver enzymes and/or serum bilirubin have occurred during therapy with lisinopril in patients with or without pre-existing liver abnormalities (see Adverse Effects). In most cases the changes were reversed on discontinuation of the drug.

Should the patient receiving lisinopril experience any unexplained symptoms (see Information to Be Provided to the Patient), particularly during the first weeks or months of treatment, it is recommended that a full set of liver function tests and any other necessary investigation be carried out. Discontinuation of lisinopril should be considered when appropriate.

There are no adequate studies in patients with cirrhosis and/or liver dysfunction. Lisinopril should be used with particular caution in patients with pre-existing liver abnormalities. In such patients baseline liver function tests should be obtained before administration of the drug and close monitoring of response and metabolic effects should apply.

Cough: A dry, persistent cough, which usually disappears only after withdrawal or lowering of the dose of lisinopril, has been reported.

Such possibility should be considered as part of the differential diagnosis of the cough.

Geriatrics: In general, blood pressure response and adverse experiences were similar in younger and older patients given similar doses of lisinopril. Pharmacokinetic studies, however, indicate that maximum blood levels and area under the plasma concentration time curve (AUC) are doubled in older patients so that dosage adjustments should be made with particular caution (see Dosage).

Children: Antihypertensive effects of lisinopril have been established in hypertensive pediatric patients aged 6 to 16 years. There are no data of the effects of lisinopril in hypertensive patients under the age of 6 or in patients with glomerular filtration rate <30 mL/min/1.73 m². (See Pharmacology, Pharmacodynamics, and Pharmacokinetics, and Dosage, Pediatric Patients.)

Anaphylactoid Reactions during Membrane Exposure: Anaphylactoid reactions have been reported in patients dialysed with high-flux membranes (e.g., polyacrylonitrile [PAN]) and treated concomitantly with an ACE inhibitor. Dialysis should be stopped immediately if symptoms such as nausea, abdominal cramps, burning, angioedema, shortness of breath and severe hypotension occur. Symptoms are not relieved by antihistamines. In these patients consideration should be given to using a different type of dialysis membrane or a different class of antihypertensive agent.

Anaphylactoid Reactions during LDL Apheresis: Rarely, patients receiving ACE inhibitors during low density lipoprotein (LDL) apheresis with dextran sulfate have experienced life-threatening anaphylactoid reactions. These reactions were avoided by temporarily withholding ACE inhibitor therapy prior to each apheresis.

Anaphylactoid Reactions during Hymenoptera Desensitization: There have been isolated reports of patients experiencing sustained life-threatening anaphylactoid reactions while receiving ACE inhibitors during desensitizing treatment with hymenoptera (bees, wasps) venom. In the same patients, these reactions have been avoided when ACE inhibitors were temporarily withheld for at least 24 hours, but they have reappeared upon inadvertent rechallenge.

Drug Interactions: Hypotension: Patients on Diuretic Therapy: Patients on diuretics and especially those in whom diuretic therapy was recently instituted may occasionally experience an excessive reduction of blood pressure after initiation of therapy with lisinopril. The possibility of symptomatic hypotension with lisinopril can be minimized by discontinuing the diuretic prior to initiation of treatment with lisinopril and/or lowering the initial dose of lisinopril (see Warnings, Hypotension and Dosage).

Agents Increasing Serum Potassium: Since lisinopril decreases aldosterone production, elevation of serum potassium may occur. Potassium-sparing diuretics, such as spironolactone, triamterene or amiloride, or potassium supplements should be given only for documented hypokalemia and with caution and with frequent monitoring of serum potassium since they may lead to a significant increase in serum potassium. Potassium-containing salt substitutes should also be used with caution (see also Precautions, Hyperkalemia).

Gold: Nitritoid reactions (symptoms include facial flushing, nausea, vomiting and hypotension) have been reported rarely in patients on therapy with injectable gold (sodium aurothiomalate) and concomitant ACE inhibitor therapy including lisinopril.

Agents Causing Renin Release: The antihypertensive effect of lisinopril is augmented by antihypertensive agents that cause renin release (e.g., diuretics).

Agents Affecting Sympathetic Activity: Agents affecting sympathetic activity (e.g., ganglionic blocking agents or adrenergic neuron blocking agents) may be used with caution. Beta-adrenergic blocking drugs add some further antihypertensive effect to lisinopril.

NSAIDs: Non-steroidal anti-inflammatory drugs (NSAIDs) including selective cyclooxygenase-2 inhibitors (COX-2 inhibitors) may reduce the effect of diuretics and other antihypertensive drugs. Therefore, the antihypertensive effect of ACE inhibitors or angiotensin II receptor antagonists may be attenuated by NSAIDs including selective COX-2 inhibitors.

In some patients with compromised renal function (e.g., elderly patients or patients who are volume-depleted including those on diuretic therapy) who are being treated with NSAIDs including selective COX-2 inhibitors, the co-administration of ACE inhibitors or angiotensin II receptor antagonists may result in further deterioration of renal function. Cases of acute renal failure, usually reversible, have been reported. This combination should therefore be administered with caution in this patient population.

Indomethacin may diminish the antihypertensive efficacy of concomitantly administered lisinopril.

Lithium Salts: As with other drugs which eliminate sodium, the lithium elimination may be reduced. Therefore, the serum lithium levels should be monitored carefully if lithium salts are to be administered.

Information to Be Provided to the Patient: Angioedema: Angioedema, including laryngeal edema, may occur especially following the first dose of lisinopril. Patients should be so advised and told to report immediately any signs or symptoms suggesting angioedema (swelling of face, extremities, eyes, lips, tongue, difficulty in breathing) and to take no more drug until they have consulted with the prescribing physician.

Hypotension: Patients should be cautioned to report lightheadedness especially during the first few days of therapy. If actual syncope occurs, the patients should be told to discontinue the drug until they have consulted with the prescribing physician.

All patients should be cautioned that excessive perspiration and dehydration may lead to an excessive fall in blood pressure because of reduction in fluid volume. Other causes of volume-depletion such as vomiting or diarrhea may also lead to a fall in blood pressure; patients should be advised to consult with their physician.

Neutropenia: Patients should be told to report promptly any indication of infection (e.g., sore throat, fever) which may be a sign of neutropenia.

Impaired Liver Function: Patients should be advised to return to the physician if he/she experiences any symptoms possibly related to liver dysfunction. This would include "viral-like symptoms" in the first weeks to months of therapy (such as fever, malaise, muscle pain, rash or adenopathy which are possible indicators of hypersensitivity reactions), or if abdominal pain, nausea or vomiting, loss of appetite, jaundice, itching or any other unexplained symptoms occur during therapy.
Hyperkalemia: Patients should be told not to use salt substitutes containing potassium without consulting their physician.
Pregnancy: Patients should be advised to stop taking the medication and to report promptly to their physician if they become pregnant, since the use of Prinivil during pregnancy can cause injury and even death of the developing fetus.
Lactation: Patients should be advised not to breast-feed while taking Prinivil, as it is possible that Prinivil passes into breast milk.
Note: As with many other drugs, certain advice to patients being treated with Prinivil is warranted. This information is intended to aid in the safe and effective use of this medication. It is not a disclosure of all possible adverse or intended effects.

ADVERSE EFFECTS: In controlled clinical trials involving 3269 patients (2633 patients with hypertension and 636 patients with congestive heart failure), the most frequent clinical adverse reactions were: dizziness (4.4%), headache (5.6%), asthenia/fatigue (2.7%), diarrhea (1.8%) and cough (3.0%), all of which were more frequent than in placebo-treated patients. Discontinuation of therapy was required in 5.9% of patients.

For adverse reactions which occurred in hypertensive patients and patients with congestive heart failure treated with lisinopril in controlled clinical trials, comparative incidence data are listed in Table 1.

Table 1: Prinivil
Incidence of Adverse Reactions Occurring in Patients Treated with Prinivil in Controlled Clinical Trials

	Hypertension (2633 Patients) %	Congestive Heart Failure (636 Patients) %
Cardiovascular		
Hypotension	0.8	5.2
Orthostatic Effects	0.9	1.3
Chest Pain	1.1	7.4
Angina	0.3	3.8
Edema	0.6	2.5
Palpitation	0.8	1.9
Rhythm Disturbances	0.5	0.6
Gastrointestinal		
Diarrhea	1.8	6.1
Nausea	1.9	4.9
Vomiting	1.1	2.4
Dyspepsia	0.5	1.9
Anorexia	0.4	1.4
Constipation	0.2	0.8
Flatulence	0.3	0.5
Nervous System		
Dizziness	4.4	14.2
Headache	5.6	4.6
Paresthesia	0.5	2.8
Depression	0.7	1.1
Somnolence	0.8	0.6
Insomnia	0.3	2.4
Vertigo	0.2	0.2
Respiratory		
Cough	3.0	6.4
Dyspnea	0.4	7.4
Orthopnea	0.1	0.9
Dermatologic		
Rash	1.0	5.0
Pruritus	0.5	1.4
Musculoskeletal		
Muscle Cramps	0.5	2.2
Back Pain	0.5	1.7
Leg Pain	0.1	1.3
Shoulder Pain	0.2	0.8
Other		
Asthenia/Fatigue	2.7	7.1
Blurred Vision	0.3	1.1
Fever	0.3	1.1
Flushing	0.3	0.3
Gout	0.2	1.7
Decreased Libido	0.2	0.2
Malaise	0.3	1.1

Angioedema: Angioedema has been reported in patients receiving lisinopril (0.1%). Angioedema associated with laryngeal edema may be fatal. If angioedema of the face, extremities, lips, tongue, glottis and/or larynx occurs, treatment with lisinopril should be discontinued and appropriate therapy instituted immediately (see Warnings, Angioedema).

In very rare cases intestinal angioedema has been reported with angiotensin converting enzyme inhibitors, including lisinopril.
Hypotension: In hypertensive patients, hypotension occurred in 0.8% and syncope occurred in 0.2% of patients. Hypotension or syncope was a cause for discontinuation of therapy in 0.3% of hypertensive patients (see Warnings).

In patients with congestive heart failure, hypotension occurred in 5.2% and syncope occurred in 1.7% of patients. Hypotension and dizziness were causes for discontinuation of therapy in 1.7% of these patients.
Treatment Following Acute Myocardial Infarction: In a controlled, open trial, involving 19 394 acute myocardial infarction patients (GISSI-3, see Indications, Treatment Following Acute Myocardial Infarction), comparing lisinopril alone, transdermal glycerol trinitrate, lisinopril and transdermal glycerol trinitrate, or control (no treatment), the most frequent in-hospital adverse events at 6 weeks were as follows: See Table 2.

Table 2: Prinivil
Adverse Events—Treatment Following Acute Myocardial Infarction

Event	Control n=4729 (%)	Lisinopril n=4713 (%)	Lisinopril +GTN n=4722 (%)	GTN Alone n=4731 (%)
Persistent Hypotension	3.6	8.8	9.3	3.9
Shock	2.5	2.8	2.2	1.9
Renal Dysfunction	1.1	2.4	2.4	1.1
Stroke	0.6	0.6	0.9	0.8
Re-infarction	2.2	2.2	2.2	1.9
Hemorrhagic Events	1.2	1.3	1.1	0.9
Post-infarction Angina	13.2	13.9	12.3	11.8
Ventricular Fibrillation	3.1	2.5	2.4	2.2
Sustained Ventricular Tachycardia	2.5	2.1	1.8	2.3
Atrial Flutter or Fibrillation	6.4	6.3	5.3	5.7
Complete Atrioventricular Block	2.4	2.9	2.5	2.1
Asystole	1.2	1.2	1.3	1.2
Intraventricular Septal Rupture	0.3	0.4	0.2	0.2
Papillary Muscle Rupture	0.3	0.4	0.5	0.4
Late CHF (>4 days)	4.5	4.5	4.2	4.2

Other Events in Controlled Clinical Trials or Postmarketing Experience: Additional adverse reactions which were reported rarely, either during controlled clinical trials or after the drug was marketed, include:
Cardiovascular: myocardial infarction or cerebrovascular accident possibly secondary to excessive hypotension in high-risk patients (see Warnings, Hypotension), tachycardia.
Dermatologic: alopecia, diaphoresis, pruritus, urticaria.
Severe Skin Disorders: erythema multiforme, pemphigus, Stevens-Johnson syndrome, toxic epidermal necrolysis, cutaneous pseudolymphoma.
Endocrine: syndrome of inappropriate antidiuretic hormone secretion (SIADH).
Gastrointestinal: abdominal pain and indigestion, dry mouth, pancreatitis, vomiting.
Hematologic: hemolytic anemia.
Hepatic: hepatitis, jaundice (hepatocellular and/or cholestatic), liver function abnormalities, hepatic failure.
Metabolic: Cases of hypoglycemia in diabetic patients on oral antidiabetic agents or insulin have been reported (see Drug Interactions).
Nervous System: mental confusion, mood alterations, paresthesia, vertigo.
Respiratory: bronchospasm, rhinitis, sinusitis.
Special Senses: taste disorders.
Urogenital: acute renal failure, impotence, oliguria/anuria, renal dysfunction, uremia.

A symptom complex has been reported which may include fever, vasculitis, myalgia, arthralgia/arthritis, a positive ANA, elevated ESR, eosinophilia and leukocytosis. Rash, photosensitivity or other dermatologic manifestations may also occur.
Pediatric Patients: The adverse experience profile for pediatric patients appears to be similar to that seen in adult patients.
Laboratory Test Findings: Serum Electrolytes: Hyperkalemia and hyponatremia have occurred (see Precautions).
Creatinine, Blood Urea Nitrogen: Increases in blood urea nitrogen and serum creatinine, usually reversible upon discontinuation of therapy, were observed in 1.1 and 1.6% of patients, respectively, with essential hypertension treated with lisinopril alone. Increases were more common in patients receiving concomitant diuretics and in patients with renal artery stenosis (see Precautions). Reversible increases in blood urea nitrogen (14.5%) and serum creatinine (11.2%) were observed in approximately 12.0% of patients with congestive heart failure on concomitant diuretic therapy. Frequently, these abnormalities resolved when the dosage of the diuretic was decreased.
Hematology: Decreases in hemoglobin and hematocrit (mean decreases of approximately 0.9 g % and 0.6 vol % respectively) occurred frequently in patients treated with lisinopril but were rarely of clinical importance in patients without some other cause of anemia.

Rarely, hemolytic anemia has been reported.

Agranulocytosis and bone marrow depression, manifested as anemia, thrombocytopenia or leukopenia, have been caused by angiotensin converting enzyme inhibitors, including lisinopril. Several cases of agranulocytosis and neutropenia have been reported in which a causal relationship to lisinopril cannot be excluded (see Warnings, Neutropenia/Agranulocytosis).
Hepatic: Elevations of liver enzymes and/or serum bilirubin have occurred (see Precautions).
Discontinuations: Overall, 1% of patients discontinued therapy due to laboratory adverse experiences, principally elevations in blood urea nitrogen (0.8%), serum creatinine (0.1%) and serum potassium (0.1%).

OVERDOSE:

Symptoms: The most likely manifestation of overdosage would be hypotension, for which the usual treatment would be i.v. infusion of normal saline solution. If available, angiotensin II may be beneficial.

Lisinopril may be removed from the general circulation by hemodialysis (see Precautions, Anaphylactoid Reactions during Membrane Exposure).

Treatment: See Symptoms.

> For management of a suspected drug overdose, contact your regional Poison Control Centre. See the *CPS* Directory section for a list of Poison Control Centres.

DOSAGE: Since absorption of lisinopril is not affected by food, the tablets may be administered before, during or after meals. Lisinopril should be administered in a single daily dose. Lisinopril should be taken at the same time each day. The splitting of Prinivil tablets is not advised.

Dosage must be individualized.

Essential Hypertension: In patients with essential hypertension, not on diuretic therapy, the usual recommended starting dose is 10 mg once a day. Dosage should be adjusted according to blood pressure response: the usual dosage range is 10 to 40 mg/day, administered in a single daily dose. In some patients, achievement of optimal blood pressure reduction may require 2 to 4 weeks of therapy. The antihypertensive effect may diminish toward the end of the dosing interval regardless of the administered dose, but most commonly with a dose of 10 mg daily. This can be evaluated by measuring blood pressure just prior to dosing to determine whether satisfactory control is being maintained for 24 hours. If it is not, an increase in dose should be considered. The maximum dose used in long-term controlled clinical trials was 80 mg/day. If blood pressure is not controlled with lisinopril alone, a low dose of a diuretic may be added. Hydrochlorothiazide 12.5 mg has been shown to provide an additive effect. After the addition of a diuretic, it may be possible to reduce the dose of lisinopril.

Diuretic Treated Patients: In hypertensive patients who are currently being treated with a diuretic, symptomatic hypotension may occur occasionally following the initial dose of lisinopril. The diuretic should be discontinued, if possible, for 2 to 3 days before beginning therapy with lisinopril to reduce the likelihood of hypotension (see Warnings). The dosage of lisinopril should be adjusted according to blood pressure response. If the patient's blood pressure is not controlled with lisinopril alone, diuretic therapy may be resumed as described above.

If the diuretic cannot be discontinued, an initial dose of 5 mg should be used under medical supervision for at least 2 hours and until blood pressure has stabilized for at least an additional hour (see Warnings, Hypotension and Precautions, Drug Interactions).

A lower starting dose is required in the presence of renal impairment, in patients in whom diuretic therapy cannot be discontinued, in patients who are volume and/or salt-depleted for any reason, and in patients with renovascular hypertension.

Dosage Adjustment in Renal Impairment: Dosage in patients with renal impairment should be based on creatinine clearance as outlined in Table 3.

Table 3: Prinivil

Dosage Adjustment in Renal Impairment

Creatinine Clearance	Starting Dose
≤70 ≥30 mL/min (≤1.17 ≥0.5 mL/s)	5.0–10.0 mg/day
≤30 ≥10 mL/min (≤0.5 ≥0.17 mL/s)	2.5–5.0 mg/day
<10 mL/min (<0.17 mL/s)	2.5 mg/day[a] (including patients on dialysis)

[a] Dosage and/or frequency of administration should be adjusted depending on the blood pressure response.

The dosage may be titrated upward until blood pressure is controlled or to a maximum of 40 mg daily.

Anaphylactoid reactions have been reported in patients dialysed with high-flux membranes (e.g., polyacrylonitrile [PAN]) and treated concomitantly with an ACE inhibitor (see Precautions, Anaphylactoid Reactions during Membrane Exposure).

Geriatrics: In general, blood pressure response and adverse experiences were similar in younger and older patients given similar doses of lisinopril. Pharmacokinetic studies, however, indicate that maximum blood levels and area under the plasma concentration time curve (AUC) are doubled in older patients so that dosage adjustments should be made with particular caution.

Renovascular Hypertension: Some patients with renovascular hypertension, especially those with bilateral renal artery stenosis or stenosis of the artery to a solitary kidney, may develop an exaggerated response to the first dose of lisinopril. Therefore, a lower starting dose of 2.5 or 5 mg is recommended. Thereafter, the dosage may be adjusted according to the blood pressure response.

Congestive Heart Failure: Lisinopril is to be used in conjunction with a diuretic and, where appropriate, digitalis. Therapy must be initiated under close medical supervision, usually in a hospital. Blood pressure and renal function should be monitored, both before and during treatment with lisinopril, because severe hypotension and, more rarely, consequent renal failure have been reported (see Warnings, Hypotension and Precautions, Renal Impairment).

Initiation of therapy requires consideration of recent diuretic therapy and the possibility of severe salt-/volume-depletion. If possible, the dose of diuretic should be reduced before beginning treatment.

The recommended initial dose is 2.5 mg/day. If required, the dose should be increased gradually, depending on the patient response. The usual effective dosage range is 5-20 mg/day administered in a single daily dose. Dose titration may be performed over a 2-4 week period, or more rapidly if indicated by the presence of residual signs and symptoms of heart failure.

Treatment Following Acute Myocardial Infarction: Treatment of hemodynamically stable patients may be started as early as within 24 hours following the onset of symptoms of myocardial infarction. Patients should receive, as appropriate, standard recommended treatments (see Indications, Treatment Following Acute Myocardial Infarction).

The first dose of lisinopril is 5 mg given orally, followed by 5 mg after 24 hours, 10 mg after 48 hours and then 10 mg once daily thereafter.

Patients with a low systolic blood pressure (between 100 and 120 mmHg) when treatment is started or during the first 3 days after the infarct should be given a lower dose, 2.5 mg orally. (Treatment with lisinopril must not be initiated in patients who are at risk of serious hemodynamic deterioration [see Precautions, Hypotension Following Acute Myocardial Infarction.]) After 3 days if hypotension occurs (systolic blood pressure less than or equal to 100 mmHg), a daily maintenance dose of 5 mg may be given with temporary reductions to 2.5 mg if needed. If prolonged hypotension occurs (systolic blood pressure less than 90 mmHg for more than 1 hour), lisinopril should be withdrawn.

Renal function should be assessed before and during therapy with lisinopril (see Precautions, Renal Impairment).

Dosing should normally continue for 6 weeks. At that time, patients with signs or symptoms of heart failure should continue with lisinopril (see Congestive Heart Failure).

Lisinopril is compatible with i.v. or transdermal glyceryl trinitrate.

Pediatric Patients: For patients who can swallow tablets, the dose should be individualized according to patient profile and blood pressure response. The recommended initial dose is 2.5 mg in patients 20 to <50 kg and 5 mg in patients ≥50 kg. Lisinopril is given once daily. The dosage should be adjusted according to the needs of the patient to a maximum of 20 mg daily in patients 20 to <50 kg and 40 mg in patients ≥50 kg (see Pharmacology, Pharmacodynamic, and Pharmacokinetics).

Lisinopril is not recommended in pediatric patients <6 years or with glomerular filtration rate <30 mL/min/1.73 m^2 (see Pharmacology, Pharmacodynamics, and Pharmacokinetics).

INFORMATION FOR THE PATIENT: Published in e-CPS, available by subscription at www.e-cps.ca.

SUPPLIED: 5 mg: Each white, oval-shaped, compressed tablet, with code MSD 19 on one side and scored on the other, contains: lisinopril 5 mg. Nonmedicinal ingredients: calcium phosphate, cornstarch, magnesium stearate and mannitol. Bottles of 100. Blister packages of 28. The splitting of Prinivil tablets is not advised. Store at room temperature (15 to 30°C).

10 mg: Each light yellow, oval-shaped, compressed tablet, engraved MSD 106 on one side and scored on the other, contains: lisinopril 10 mg. Nonmedicinal ingredients: calcium phosphate, cornstarch, iron oxide, magnesium stearate and mannitol. Blister packages of 28. The splitting of Prinivil tablets is not advised. Store at room temperature (15 to 30°C).

20 mg: Each peach, oval-shaped, compressed tablet, engraved MSD 207 on one side and scored on the other, contains: lisinopril 20 mg. Nonmedicinal ingredients: calcium phosphate, cornstarch, iron oxide, magnesium stearate and mannitol. Bottles of 100. Blister packages of 28. The splitting of Prinivil tablets is not advised. Store at room temperature (15 to 30°C).

(Shown in Product Identification Section)

> The reader is invited to consult CPhA's monograph **ACE Inhibitors** and **Thiazide Diuretics**.

Prinzide®

lisinopril—hydrochlorothiazide

Angiotensin Converting Enzyme Inhibitor—Diuretic

Merck Frosst

Date of Revision: December 24, 2009

PHARMACOLOGY: PRINZIDE combines the action of an angiotensin-converting enzyme (ACE) inhibitor, lisinopril, and a diuretic, hydrochlorothiazide.

Lisinopril: Angiotensin-converting enzyme is a peptidyl dipeptidase which catalyzes the conversion of angiotensin I to the pressor substance, angiotensin II. Inhibition of ACE results in decreased plasma angiotensin II, which leads to increased plasma renin activity (due to removal of negative feedback of renin release) and decreased aldosterone secretion. Although the latter decrease is small, it results in a small increase in serum potassium. In patients treated with lisinopril plus a thiazide diuretic, there was essentially no change in serum potassium (see Precautions).

ACE is identical to kininase II. Thus, lisinopril may also block the degradation of bradykinin, a potent vasodilator peptide. However, the role that this plays in the therapeutic effects of lisinopril is unknown.

While the mechanism through which lisinopril lowers blood pressure is believed to be primarily the suppression of the renin-angiotensin-aldosterone system, lisinopril also lowers blood pressure in patients with low-renin hypertension.

Pharmacodynamics: Lisinopril: Administration of lisinopril to patients with hypertension results in a reduction of both supine and standing blood pressure. Abrupt withdrawal of lisinopril has not been associated with a rapid increase in blood pressure. In most patients studied, after oral administration of an individual dose of lisinopril, the onset of antihypertensive activity is seen at 1 hour with peak reduction of blood pressure achieved by 6 hours. Although an antihypertensive effect was observed 24 hours after dosing with recommended single daily doses, the effect was more consistent and the mean effect was considerably larger in some studies with doses of 20 mg or more than with lower doses. However, at all doses studied, the mean antihypertensive effect was substantially smaller 24 hours after dosing than it was 6 hours after dosing. On occasion, achievement of optimal blood pressure reduction may require 2 to 4 weeks of therapy.

In hemodynamic studies in patients with essential hypertension, blood pressure reduction was accompanied by a reduction in peripheral arterial resistance with little or no change in cardiac output and in heart rate. In a study in 9 hypertensive patients, following administration of lisinopril, there was an increase in mean renal blood flow that was not significant. Data from several small studies are inconsistent with respect to the effect of lisinopril on glomerular filtration rate in hypertensive patients with normal renal function, but suggest that changes, if any, are not large.

When lisinopril is given together with thiazide-type diuretics, its blood pressure lowering effect is approximately additive.

The antihypertensive effect of angiotensin-converting enzyme inhibitors is generally lower in Black than in non-Black patients.

Hydrochlorothiazide: Hydrochlorothiazide is a diuretic and antihypertensive which interferes with the renal tubular mechanism of electrolyte reabsorption. It increases excretion of sodium and chloride in approximately equivalent amounts. Natriuresis may be accompanied by some loss of potassium and bicarbonate. While this compound is predominantly a saluretic agent, in vitro studies have shown that it has a carbonic anhydrase inhibitory action which seems to be relatively specific for the renal tubular mechanism. It does not appear to be concentrated in erythrocytes or the brain in sufficient amounts to influence the activity of carbonic anhydrase in those tissues.

Hydrochlorothiazide is useful in the treatment of hypertension. It may be used alone or as an adjunct to other antihypertensive drugs. Hydrochlorothiazide does not affect normal blood pressure. The mechanism of its antihypertensive action is not known. Lowering of the sodium content of arteriolar smooth muscle cells and diminished response to norepinephrine have been postulated.

Onset of the diuretic action following oral administration occurs in 2 hours and the peak action in about 4 hours. Diuretic activity lasts about 6 to 12 hours.

Pharmacokinetics: Lisinopril: Following oral administration of lisinopril, peak serum concentrations occur within about 7 hours. Declining serum concentrations exhibit a prolonged terminal phase which does not contribute to drug accumulation. This terminal phase probably represents saturable binding to ACE and is not proportional to dose. Lisinopril does not bind to plasma proteins other than ACE.

Lisinopril does not undergo metabolism and is excreted unchanged entirely in the urine. Based on urinary recovery, the extent of absorption of lisinopril is approximately 25%, with large inter-subject variability (6-60%) at all doses tested (5-80 mg).

Lisinopril absorption is not influenced by the presence of food in the gastrointestinal tract.

Upon multiple dosing, lisinopril exhibits an effective half-life of accumulation of 12 hours.

In a study in elderly healthy subjects (65 years and above), a single dose of lisinopril 20 mg produced higher serum concentrations than those seen in young healthy adults given a similar dose. In another study, single daily doses of lisinopril 5 mg were given for 7 consecutive days to young and elderly healthy volunteers. Maximum serum concentrations of lisinopril on Day 7 were higher in the elderly volunteers than in the young.

The elimination of lisinopril in patients with renal insufficiency is similar to that in patients with normal renal function until the glomerular filtration rate is 30 mL/min or less. With renal function ≤30 mL/min, peak and trough lisinopril levels increase, time to peak concentration increases and time to steady state may be prolonged (see Dosage).

Studies in rats indicate that lisinopril crosses the blood-brain barrier poorly.

Hydrochlorothiazide: Hydrochlorothiazide is not metabolized but is eliminated rapidly by the kidney. The plasma half-life is 5.6-14.8 hours when the plasma levels can be followed for at least 24 hours. At least 61% of the oral dose is eliminated unchanged within 24 hours. Hydrochlorothiazide crosses the placental but not the blood-brain barrier and is excreted in breast milk.

Lisinopril—Hydrochlorothiazide: Concomitant administration of lisinopril and hydrochlorothiazide has little or no effect on the bioavailability of either drug. The combination tablet is bioequivalent to concomitant administration of the separate entities.

INDICATIONS: For the treatment of essential hypertension in patients for whom combination therapy is appropriate.

In using PRINZIDE, consideration should be given to the risk of angioedema (see Warnings).

PRINZIDE is not indicated for initial therapy. Patients in whom lisinopril and diuretic are initiated simultaneously can develop symptomatic hypotension (see Precautions, Drug Interactions).

Patients should be titrated on the individual drugs. If the fixed combination represents the dosage determined by this titration, the use of PRINZIDE may be more convenient in the management of patients. If during maintenance therapy dosage adjustment is necessary, it is advisable to use individual drugs.

CONTRAINDICATIONS: In patients who are hypersensitive to any component of this product; have a history of angioneurotic edema relating to previous treatment with an angiotensin-converting enzyme inhibitor; and have hereditary or idiopathic angioedema.

Because of the hydrochlorothiazide component, this product is contraindicated in patients with anuria or hypersensitivity to other sulfonamide-derived drugs.

WARNINGS:

> **Serious Warnings and Precautions**
> When used in pregnancy, angiotensin-converting enzyme (ACE) inhibitors can cause injury or even death of the developing fetus. When pregnancy is detected, PRINZIDE should be discontinued as soon as possible.

Angioedema: Angioedema has been reported in patients treated with PRINZIDE (lisinopril and hydrochlorothiazide tablets). This may occur at any time during treatment. Angioedema associated with shock may be fatal. If angioedema occurs, PRINZIDE should be promptly discontinued and appropriate monitoring should be instituted to ensure complete resolution of symptoms prior to dismissing the patient. Even in those instances where swelling of only the tongue is involved, without respiratory distress, patients may require prolonged observation since treatment with antihistamines and corticosteroids may not be sufficient. Very rarely, fatalities have been reported due to angioedema associated with laryngeal edema or tongue edema. Patients with involvement of the tongue, glottis or larynx are likely to experience airway obstruction, especially those with a history of airway surgery. When there is airway obstruction, emergency therapy should be administered promptly when indicated. This includes giving subcutaneous adrenaline (0.5 mL 1:1000), and/or maintaining a patent airway. The patient should be under close medical supervision until complete and sustained symptom resolution has occurred.

The incidence of angioedema during ACE inhibitor therapy has been reported to be higher in Black than in non-Black patients.

Patients with a history of angioedema unrelated to ACE inhibitor therapy may be at increased risk of angioedema while receiving an ACE inhibitor (see Contraindications).

Hypotension: Symptomatic hypotension has occurred after administration of lisinopril, usually after the first or second dose or when the dose was increased. It is more likely to occur in patients who are volume-depleted by diuretic therapy, dietary salt restriction, dialysis, diarrhea or vomiting. Therefore, PRINZIDE should not be used to start therapy or when a dose change is needed. In patients with severe congestive heart failure, with or without associated renal insufficiency, excessive hypotension has been observed and may be associated with oliguria and/or progressive azotemia, and rarely with acute renal failure and/or death. Because blood pressure could potentially fall, patients at risk for hypotension should start therapy with lisinopril under very close medical supervision, usually in a hospital. Such patients should be followed closely for the first 2 weeks of treatment and whenever the dose of lisinopril and/or hydrochlorothiazide is increased. In patients with ischemic heart or cerebrovascular disease, an excessive fall in blood pressure could result in a myocardial infarction or cerebrovascular accident (see Adverse Effects).

If hypotension occurs, the patient should be placed in supine position and, if necessary, receive an i.v. infusion of normal saline. A transient hypotensive response may not be a contraindication to further doses. These can usually be given to hypertensive patients without difficulty once the blood pressure has increased after volume expansion. However, lower doses of lisinopril and/or concomitant diuretic therapy should be considered.

Neutropenia/Agranulocytosis: Agranulocytosis and bone marrow depression have been caused by angiotensin-converting enzyme inhibitors. Several cases of agranulocytosis and neutropenia have been reported in which a causal relationship to lisinopril cannot be excluded. Current experience with the drug shows the incidence to be rare. Periodic monitoring of white blood cell counts should be considered, especially in patients with collagen vascular disease and renal disease.

Azotemia: Azotemia may be precipitated or increased by hydrochlorothiazide. Cumulative effects of the drug may develop in patients with impaired renal function. If increasing azotemia and oliguria occur during treatment of severe progressive renal disease the diuretic should be discontinued.

Patients with Impaired Liver Function: Hepatitis, jaundice (hepatocellular and/or cholestatic), elevations of liver enzymes and/or serum bilirubin have occurred during therapy with lisinopril in patients with or without pre-existing liver abnormalities (see Adverse Effects). In most cases the changes were reversed on discontinuation of the drug.

Should the patient receiving PRINZIDE experience any unexplained symptoms (see Precautions, Information to Be Provided to the Patient), particularly during the first weeks or months of treatment, it is recommended that a full set of liver function tests and any other necessary investigation be carried out. Discontinuation of PRINZIDE should be considered when appropriate.

There are no adequate studies in patients with cirrhosis and/or liver dysfunction. PRINZIDE should be used with particular caution in patients with pre-existing liver abnormalities. In such patients baseline liver function tests should be obtained before administration of the drug and close monitoring of response and metabolic effects should apply.

Thiazides should be used with caution in patients with impaired hepatic function or progressive liver disease, since minor alterations of fluid and electrolyte balance may precipitate hepatic coma.

Hypersensitivity Reactions: Sensitivity reactions to hydrochlorothiazide may occur in patients with or without a history of allergy or bronchial asthma.

The possibility of exacerbation or activation of systemic lupus erythematosus has been reported in patients treated with hydrochlorothiazide.

Pregnancy: ACE inhibitors can cause fetal and neonatal morbidity and mortality when administered to pregnant women. When pregnancy is detected, PRINZIDE should be discontinued as soon as possible.

The use of ACE inhibitors during the second and third trimesters of pregnancy has been associated with fetal and neonatal injury including hypotension, neonatal skull hypoplasia, anuria, reversible or irreversible renal failure, and death. Oligohydramnios has also been reported, presumably resulting from decreased fetal renal function, associated with fetal limb contractures, craniofacial deformation, and hypoplastic lung development.

Prematurity, and patent ductus arteriosus and other structural cardiac malformations, as well as neurologic malformations, have also been reported following exposure in the first trimester of pregnancy.

Infants with a history of in utero exposure to ACE inhibitors should be closely observed for hypotension, oliguria, and hyperkalemia. If oliguria occurs, attention should be directed toward support of blood pressure and renal perfusion. Exchange transfusion or dialysis may be required as a means of reversing hypotension and/or substituting for impaired renal function; however, limited experience with those procedures has not been associated with significant clinical benefit.

Lisinopril has been removed from the neonatal circulation by peritoneal dialysis with some clinical benefit and may, theoretically, be removed by exchange transfusion, although there is no experience with the latter procedure.

Animal Data: Lisinopril was not teratogenic in mice treated on days 6-15 of gestation with up to 1000 mg/kg/day (625 times the maximum recommended human dose). There was an increase in fetal resorptions at doses down to 100 mg/kg; at doses of 1000 mg/kg, this was prevented by saline supplementation. There was no fetotoxicity or teratogenicity in rats treated with up to 300 mg/kg/day (188 times the maximum recommended dose) of lisinopril at days 6-17 of gestation. In rats receiving lisinopril from day 15 of gestation through day 21 postpartum, there was an increased incidence in pup deaths on days 2-7 postpartum and a lower average body weight of pups on day 21 postpartum. The increase in pup deaths and decrease in pup weight did not occur with maternal saline supplementation.

Lisinopril, at doses up to 1 mg/kg/day, was not teratogenic when given throughout the organogenic period in saline supplemented rabbits. Saline supplementation (physiologic saline in place of tap water) was used to eliminate maternotoxic effects and enable evaluation of the teratogenic potential at the highest possible dosage level. The rabbit has been shown to be extremely sensitive to angiotensin-converting enzyme inhibitors (captopril and enalapril) with maternal and fetotoxic effects apparent at or below the recommended therapeutic dosage levels in man.

Fetotoxicity was demonstrated in rabbits by an increased incidence of fetal resorptions at an oral dose of lisinopril of 1 mg/kg/day and by an increased incidence of incomplete ossification at the lowest dose tested (0.1 mg/kg/day). A single i.v. dose of 15 mg/kg of lisinopril administered to pregnant rabbits on gestation days 16, 21 or 26 resulted in 88% to 100% fetal death.

By whole body autoradiography, radioactivity was found in the placenta following administration of labeled lisinopril to pregnant rats, but none was found in the fetuses.

Lactation: The presence of concentrations of ACE inhibitor have been reported in human milk. Use of ACE inhibitors is not recommended during breast-feeding.

PRECAUTIONS: Renal Impairment: As a consequence of inhibiting the renin-angiotensin-aldosterone system, changes in renal function have been seen in susceptible individuals. In patients whose renal function may depend on the activity of the renin-angiotensin-aldosterone system, such as patients with bilateral renal artery stenosis, unilateral renal artery stenosis to a solitary kidney, or severe congestive heart failure, treatment with agents that inhibit this system has been associated with oliguria, progressive azotemia, and rarely, acute renal failure and/or death. In susceptible patients, concomitant diuretic use may further increase risk.

Use of PRINZIDE should include appropriate assessment of renal function.

Thiazides may not be appropriate diuretics for use in patients with renal impairment and are ineffective at creatinine clearance values of 30 mL/min or below (i.e., moderate to severe renal insufficiency).

Hyperkalemia: In clinical trials hyperkalemia (serum potassium >5.7 mEq/L) occurred in approximately 1.4% of hypertensive patients. In most cases these were isolated values which resolved despite continued therapy. Hyperkalemia was not a cause of discontinuation of therapy. Risk factors for the development of hyperkalemia include renal insufficiency, diabetes mellitus, and concomitant use of potassium-sparing diuretics (e.g., spironolactone, triamterene, or amiloride), potassium supplements, or potassium-containing salt substitutes (see also Drug Interactions, Agents Increasing Serum Potassium).

The use of potassium supplements, potassium-sparing diuretics, or potassium-containing salt substitutes particularly in patients with impaired renal function may lead to a significant increase in serum potassium. Hyperkalemia can cause serious, sometimes fatal, arrhythmias.

If concomitant use of PRINZIDE and any of the above-mentioned agents is deemed appropriate, they should be used with caution and with frequent monitoring of serum potassium.

Valvular Stenosis, Hypertrophic Cardiomyopathy: There is concern on theoretical grounds that patients with aortic stenosis or hypertrophic cardiomyopathy might be at particular risk of decreased coronary perfusion when treated with vasodilators.

PRINZIDE should be given with caution to these patients.

Metabolism: Hyperuricemia may occur, or acute gout may be precipitated in certain patients receiving thiazide therapy.

Thiazides may decrease serum protein-bound iodine (PBI) levels without signs of thyroid disturbance.

Thiazides have been shown to increase excretion of magnesium; this may result in hypomagnesemia.

Thiazides may decrease urinary calcium excretion. Thiazides may cause intermittent and slight elevation of serum calcium in the absence of known disorders of calcium metabolism. Marked hypercalcemia may be evidence of hidden hyperparathyroidism. Thiazides should be discontinued before carrying out tests for parathyroid function.

Increases in cholesterol, triglyceride and glucose levels may be associated with thiazide diuretic therapy.

Surgery/Anesthesia: In patients undergoing major surgery or during anesthesia with agents that produce hypotension, lisinopril blocks angiotensin II formation, secondary to compensatory renin release. If hypotension occurs and is considered to be due to this mechanism, it can be corrected by volume expansion.

Thiazides may increase the responsiveness to tubocurarine.

Cough: A dry, persistent cough, which usually disappears only after withdrawal or lowering of the dose of PRINZIDE, has been reported.

Such a possibility should be considered as part of the differential diagnosis of the cough.

Geriatrics: In general, blood pressure response and adverse experiences were similar in younger and older patients given similar doses of lisinopril. Pharmacokinetic studies, however, indicate that maximum blood levels and area under the plasma concentration time curve (AUC) are doubled in older patients so that dosage adjustments should be made with particular caution.

Children: PRINZIDE has not been studied in children and, therefore, use in this age group is not recommended.

Anaphylactoid Reactions during Membrane Exposure: Anaphylactoid reactions have been reported in patients dialyzed with high-flux membranes (e.g. polyacrylonitrile [PAN]) and treated concomitantly with an ACE inhibitor. Dialysis should be stopped immediately if symptoms such as nausea, abdominal cramps, burning, angioedema, shortness of breath and severe hypotension occur. Symptoms are not relieved by antihistamines. In these patients consideration should be given to using a different type of dialysis membrane or a different class of antihypertensive agent.

Anaphylactoid Reactions during LDL Apheresis: Rarely, patients receiving ACE inhibitors during low density lipoprotein (LDL)-apheresis with dextran sulfate have experienced life-threatening anaphylactoid reactions. These reactions were avoided by temporarily withholding ACE inhibitor therapy prior to each apheresis.

Anaphylactoid Reactions during Hymenoptera Desensitization: There have been isolated reports of patients experiencing sustained life-threatening anaphylactoid reactions while receiving ACE inhibitors during desensitizing treatment with hymenoptera (bees, wasp) venom. In the same patients, these reactions have been avoided when ACE inhibitors were temporarily withheld for at least 24 hours, but they have reappeared upon inadvertent rechallenge.

Drug Interactions: Hypotension—Patients on Diuretic Therapy: Patients on diuretics, and especially those in whom diuretic therapy was recently instituted, may occasionally experience an excessive reduction of blood pressure after initiation of therapy with lisinopril. The possibility of hypotensive effects with lisinopril can be minimized by either discontinuing the diuretic or increasing the salt intake prior to initiation of treatment with lisinopril (see Warnings and Dosage).

Agents Increasing Serum Potassium: Since lisinopril decreases aldosterone production, elevation of serum potassium may occur. Potassium sparing diuretics, such as spironolactone, triamterene or amiloride, or potassium supplements should be given only for documented hypokalemia and with caution and with frequent monitoring of serum potassium since they may lead to a significant increase in serum potassium. Salt substitutes which contain potassium should also be used with caution (see also Precautions, Hyperkalemia).

Agents Causing Renin Release: The antihypertensive effect of PRINZIDE is augmented by antihypertensive agents that cause renin release (e.g., diuretics).

Agents Affecting Sympathetic Activity: Agents affecting sympathetic activity (e.g., ganglionic blocking agents or adrenergic neuron blocking agents) may be used with caution. Beta-adrenergic blocking drugs add some further antihypertensive effect to lisinopril.

Lithium: Lithium generally should not be given with diuretics or ACE inhibitors. Diuretic agents and ACE inhibitors reduce the renal clearance of lithium and add a high risk of lithium toxicity.

d-tubocurarine: Thiazide drugs may increase the responsiveness to tubocurarine.

Insulin: Insulin requirements in diabetic patients treated with thiazide diuretics may be increased. Diabetes mellitus which has been latent may become manifest during thiazide administration.

Alcohol, Barbiturates or Narcotics: In the presence of thiazide diuretics, potentiation of orthostatic hypotension may occur.

Corticosteroids, ACTH: Intensified electrolyte depletion, particularly hypokalemia may occur when given concomitantly with thiazide diuretics.

Pressor Amines (e.g., norepinephrine): In the presence of thiazide diuretics, possible decreased response to pressor amines but not sufficient to preclude their use.

Nonsteroidal Anti-inflammatory Drugs: Non-steroidal anti-inflammatory drugs (NSAIDs) including selective cyclooxygenase-2 inhibitors (COX-2 inhibitors) may reduce the effect of diuretics and other antihypertensive drugs. Therefore, the antihypertensive effect of ACE inhibitors or angiotensin II receptor antagonists may be attenuated by NSAIDs including selective COX-2 inhibitors.

The antihypertensive effect of lisinopril may be diminished with concomitant non-steroidal anti-inflammatory drug use. In some patients with compromised renal function (e.g., elderly patients or patients who are volume-depleted including those on diuretic therapy) who are being treated with NSAIDS drugs including selective COX-2 inhibitors, the co-administration of ACE inhibitors or angiotensin II receptor antagonists may result in further deterioration of renal function. Cases of acute renal failure, usually reversible, have been reported. This combination should therefore be administered with caution in this patient population.

Therefore, when PRINZIDE and non-steroidal anti-inflammatory agents are used concomitantly, the patient should be observed closely to determine if the desired antihypertensive effect is obtained.

Gold: Nitritoid reactions (symptoms include facial flushing, nausea, vomiting and hypotension) have been reported rarely in patients on therapy with injectable gold (sodium aurothiomalate) and concomitant ACE inhibitor therapy including lisinopril.

Information to Be Provided to the Patient: Angioedema: Angioedema, including laryngeal edema, may occur during treatment with PRINZIDE. Patients should be so advised and told to report immediately any signs or symptoms suggesting angioedema (swelling of face, extremities, eyes, lips, tongue, difficulty in breathing) and to take no more drug until they have consulted with the prescribing physician.

Hypotension: Patients should be cautioned to report lightheadedness especially during the first few days of therapy. If actual syncope occurs, the patients should be told to discontinue the drug until they have consulted with the prescribing physician.

All patients should be cautioned that excessive perspiration and dehydration may lead to an excessive fall in blood pressure because of reduction in fluid volume. Other causes of volume-depletion such as vomiting or diarrhea may also lead to a fall in blood pressure; patients should be advised to consult with their physician.

Neutropenia: Patients should be told to report promptly any indication of infection (e.g., sore throat, fever) which may be a sign of neutropenia.

Impaired Liver Function: Patients should be advised to return to the physician if he/she experiences any symptoms possibly related to liver dysfunction. This would include "viral-like symptoms" in the first weeks to months of therapy (such as fever, malaise, muscle pain, rash or adenopathy which are possible indicators of hypersensitivity reactions), or if abdominal pain, nausea or vomiting, loss of appetite, jaundice, itching or any other unexplained symptoms occur during therapy.

Hyperkalemia: Patients should be told not to use salt substitutes containing potassium without consulting their physician.

Pregnancy: Patients should be advised to stop taking the medication and to report promptly to their physician if they become pregnant, since the use of PRINZIDE during pregnancy can cause injury and even death of the developing fetus.

Nursing Mothers: Patients should be advised not to breast-feed while taking PRINZIDE , as it is possible that PRINZIDE passes into breast milk.

Note: As with many other drugs, certain advice to patients being treated with PRINZIDE is warranted. This information is intended to aid in the safe and effective use of this medication. It is not a disclosure of all possible adverse or intended effects.

ADVERSE EFFECTS: In clinical trials involving 930 patients, including 100 patients treated for 50 weeks or more, the most severe clinical adverse reactions were syncope (0.8%) and hypotension (1.9%). The most frequent clinical adverse reactions were: dizziness (7.5%), headache (5.2%), cough (3.9%), fatigue (3.7%) and orthostatic effects (3.2%).

Discontinuation of treatment due to adverse reactions occurred in 4.4% of patients, mainly because of dizziness, cough, fatigue or muscle cramps.

Adverse reactions that have occurred in clinical trials or in marketing experience are those which have been previously reported with lisinopril and hydrochlorothiazide when used separately for the treatment of hypertension.

Adverse reactions occurring in hypertensive patients treated with lisinopril and hydrochlorothiazide in controlled trials are shown in Table 1.

Table 1: PRINZIDE

Incidence of Adverse Reactions Occurring in Hypertensive Patients Treated with Lisinopril and Hydrochlorothiazide in Controlled Trials

	Lisinopril 2633 Patients (%)	Lisinopril Plus Hydrochlorothiazide 930 Patients (%)
Cardiovascular		
Hypotension	1.4	1.9
Orthostatic effects	0.9	3.2
Chest pain	1.1	1.0
Syncope	0.2	0.8
Angina	0.3	0.1
Edema	0.6	0.1
Palpitation	0.8	0.9
Rhythm disturbances	0.5	0.1
Chest discomfort	—	0.6
Gastrointestinal		
Diarrhea	1.8	2.5
Nausea	1.9	2.2
Vomiting	1.1	1.4
Dyspepsia	0.5	1.3
Anorexia	0.4	0.2
Constipation	0.2	0.3
Flatulence	0.3	0.2
Abdominal pain	1.4	0.9
Dry mouth	0.5	0.2
Nervous System		
Dizziness	4.4	7.5
Headache	5.6	5.2
Paresthesia	0.5	1.5
Depression	0.7	0.5
Somnolence	0.8	0.4
Insomnia	0.3	0.2
Vertigo	0.2	0.9
Respiratory		
Cough	3.0	3.9
Dyspnea	0.4	0.4
Upper respiratory infection	2.1	2.2
Dermatologic		
Rash	1.0	1.2
Pruritus	0.5	0.4
Flushing	0.3	0.8
Angioedema	0.1	—[a]
Musculoskeletal		
Muscle cramps	0.5	2.0
Back pain	0.5	0.8
Shoulder pain	0.2	0.5
Other		
Fatigue	—	3.7
Asthenia	2.7	1.8
Decreased libido	0.2	1.0

(cont'd)

Table 1: PRINZIDE *(cont'd)*

Incidence of Adverse Reactions Occurring in Hypertensive Patients Treated with Lisinopril and Hydrochlorothiazide in Controlled Trials

	Lisinopril 2633 Patients (%)	Lisinopril Plus Hydrochlorothiazide 930 Patients (%)
Fever	0.3	0.5
Impotence	0.7	1.2
Gout	0.2	0.2

[a] See PRINZIDE (Marketing Experience Only).

Laboratory Test Findings: Hypokalemia, Hyperkalemia: See Precautions.
Creatinine, Blood Urea Nitrogen: Minor increases in blood urea nitrogen (3.8%) and serum creatinine (4.2%) were observed in patients with essential hypertension treated with PRINZIDE. More marked increases have also been reported and were more likely to occur in patients with bilateral renal artery stenosis (see Precautions).

Increases in blood urea nitrogen and serum creatinine, usually reversible upon discontinuation of therapy, were observed in 1.1 and 1.6% of patients, respectively, with essential hypertension treated with lisinopril alone.

Serum Uric Acid, Glucose, Magnesium, Cholesterol, Triglycerides and Calcium: See Precautions.
Hemoglobin and Hematocrit: Small decreases in hemoglobin and hematocrit (mean decreases of approximately 0.5 g % and 1.5 vol %, respectively) occurred frequently in hypertensive patients treated with PRINZIDE but were rarely of clinical importance unless another cause of anemia coexisted. In clinical trials, 0.4% of patients discontinued therapy due to anemia.

Rarely, hemolytic anemia has been reported.

Agranulocytosis and bone marrow depression, manifested as anemia, thrombocytopenia or leukopenia, have been caused by angiotensin-converting enzyme inhibitors, including lisinopril. Several cases of agranulocytosis and neutropenia have been reported in which a causal relationship to lisinopril cannot be excluded (see Warnings, Neutropenia/Agranulocytosis).

Other (Causal Relationship Unknown): Rarely, elevations of liver enzymes and/or serum bilirubin have occurred.
Adverse Reactions Reported in Uncontrolled Trials and/or Marketing Experience: PRINIVIL:
Cardiovascular: Myocardial infarction or cerebrovascular accident possibly secondary to excessive hypotension in high-risk patients (see Warnings), tachycardia.
Dermatologic: alopecia, urticaria, pruritus, diaphoresis.
Severe Skin Disorders: erythema multiforme, pemphigus, Stevens-Johnson syndrome, toxic epidermal necrolysis, cutaneous pseudolymphoma.
Gastrointestinal: abdominal pain and indigestion, dry mouth, pancreatitis, vomiting.
Hematologic: hemolytic anemia.
Hepatic: liver function abnormalities, hepatitis, jaundice (hepatocellular and/or cholestatic), hepatic failure.
Metabolic: Cases of hypoglycemia in diabetic patients on oral antidiabetic agents or insulin have been reported.
Nervous System: mood alterations, mental confusion, paresthesia, vertigo.
Respiratory: bronchospasm, rhinitis, sinusitis.
Special Senses: taste disorder.
Urogenital: uremia, oliguria/anuria, renal dysfunction, acute renal failure, impotence.

A symptom complex has been reported which may include fever, vasculitis, myalgia, arthralgia/arthritis, a positive ANA, elevated ESR, eosinophilia and leukocytosis. Rash, photosensitivity or other dermatologic manifestations may also occur.

PRINZIDE (Marketing Experience Only): Angioedema of the face, extremities, lips, tongue, glottis and/or larynx has been reported (see Warnings).

In very rare cases, intestinal angioedema has been reported with angiotensin converting enzyme inhibitors, including lisinopril.

Cases of pancreatitis have been reported.

Endocrine: Syndrome of inappropriate antidiuretic hormone secretion (SIADH).

No other adverse events have been reported with PRINZIDE which have not been reported with lisinopril or hydrochlorothiazide individually.

OVERDOSE:

Symptoms: No specific information is available on the treatment of overdosage with PRINZIDE. Treatment is symptomatic and supportive. Therapy with PRINZIDE should be discontinued and the patient observed closely. Suggested measures include induction of emesis and/or gastric lavage, if ingestion is recent, and correction of dehydration, electrolyte imbalance and hypotension by established procedures.
Lisinopril: The most likely feature of overdosage would be hypotension, for which the usual treatment would be i.v. infusion of normal saline solution. Lisinopril may be removed from general circulation by hemodialysis.
Hydrochlorothiazide: The most common signs and symptoms observed are those caused by electrolyte depletion (hypokalemia, hypochloremia, hyponatremia) and dehydration resulting from excessive diuresis. If digitalis has also been administered, hypokalemia may accentuate cardiac arrhythmias.
Treatment: See Symptoms.

> For management of a suspected drug overdose, contact your regional Poison Control Centre. See the *CPS* Directory section for a list of Poison Control Centres.

DOSAGE: Dosage must be individualized. The fixed combination is not for initial therapy. The dose of PRINZIDE should be determined by the titration of the individual components. The splitting of PRINZIDE tablets is not advised.

Once the patient has been successfully titrated with the individual components as described below, either one PRINZIDE 10 mg/12.5 mg or, one or two 20 mg/12.5 mg tablets once daily may be substituted if the titrated doses are the same as those in the fixed combination (see Indications and Warnings).

Patients usually do not require doses in excess of 50 mg of hydrochlorothiazide daily, particularly when combined with antihypertensive agents.

For lisinopril monotherapy the recommended initial dose in patients not on diuretics is 10 mg of lisinopril once a day. Dosage should be adjusted according to blood pressure response. The usual dosage range of lisinopril is 10 to 40 mg administered in a single daily dose. The antihypertensive effect may diminish toward the end of the dosing interval regardless of the administered dose, but most commonly with a dose of 10 mg daily. This can be evaluated by measuring blood pressure just prior to dosing to determine whether satisfactory control is being maintained for 24 hours. If it is not, an increase in dose should be considered. The maximum dose used in long-term controlled clinical trials was 80 mg/day. If blood pressure is not controlled with lisinopril alone, a low dose of a diuretic may be added. Hydrochlorothiazide 12.5 mg has been shown to provide an additive effect. After the addition of a diuretic, it may be possible to reduce the dose of lisinopril.

Diuretic Treated Patients: In patients who are currently being treated with a diuretic, symptomatic hypotension occasionally may occur following the initial dose of lisinopril. The diuretic should, if possible, be discontinued for 2 to 3 days before beginning therapy with lisinopril to reduce the likelihood of hypotension (see Warnings). The dosage of lisinopril should be adjusted according to blood pressure response. If the patient's blood pressure is not controlled with lisinopril alone, diuretic therapy may be resumed as described above.

If the diuretic cannot be discontinued, an initial dose of 5 mg of lisinopril alone should be administered and the patient remain under medical supervision for at least 2 hours, and until blood pressure has stabilized for at least an additional hour (see Warnings and Precautions, Drug Interactions).

Dosage Adjustment in Renal Impairment: In patients with creatinine clearance greater than 30 mL/min, the usual dose titration of the individual components is required.

For patients with creatinine clearance between 10 and 30 mL/min, the starting dose of lisinopril is 2.5 to 5 mg/day. The dosage may then be titrated upward until blood pressure is controlled or to a maximum of 40 mg daily.

When concomitant diuretic therapy is required in patients with moderate to severe renal impairment (creatinine clearance <30 mL/min), a loop diuretic, rather than a thiazide diuretic, is preferred for use with lisinopril. Therefore, for patients with moderate or severe renal dysfunction the lisinopril-hydrochlorothiazide combination tablet is not recommended (see Precautions, Renal Impairment—Anaphylactoid Reactions during Membrane Exposure).

INFORMATION FOR THE PATIENT: Published in e-CPS, available by subscription at www.e-cps.ca.

SUPPLIED: 10 mg/12.5 mg: Each blue, hexagon-shaped tablets, engraved 145 on one side and plain on the other, contains: lisinopril 10 mg and hydrochlorothiazide 12.5 mg. Nonmedicinal ingredients: calcium phosphate, cornstarch, indigotine on aluminum substrate, magnesium stearate and mannitol. Bottles of 100. The splitting of PRINZIDE tablets is not advised. Store at controlled room temperature (15 to 30°C). Protect from moisture.

20 mg/12.5 mg: Each yellow, hexagon-shaped tablets, engraved MSD 140 on one side and scored on the other, contains: lisinopril 20 mg and hydrochlorothiazide 12.5 mg. Nonmedicinal ingredients: calcium phosphate, cornstarch, iron oxide, magnesium stearate and mannitol. Bottles of 100. The splitting of PRINZIDE tablets is not advised. Store at controlled room temperature (15 to 30°C). Protect from moisture.

(Shown in Product Identification Section)

Priorix®

measles, mumps and rubella vaccine, combined, live, attenuated

Active Immunizing Agent

GlaxoSmithKline

Date of Revision: November 3, 2008

SUMMARY PRODUCT INFORMATION:

Route of Administration	Dosage Form/ Strength	Clinically Relevant Nonmedicinal Ingredients
Subcutaneous or Intramuscular injection	Lyophilized powder for injection/Not less than: $10^{3.0}$ $CCID_{50}$ of the Schwarz measles; $10^{3.7}$ $CCID_{50}$ of the RIT 4385 mumps; and $10^{3.0}$ $CCID_{50}$ of the Wistar RA 27/3 rubella virus strains/per 0.5 mL dose	Amino acids, lactose, mannitol, neomycin sulphate and sorbitol

DESCRIPTION: PRIORIX is a lyophilized mixed preparation of the attenuated Schwarz measles, RIT 4385 mumps (derived from Jeryl Lynn strain) and Wistar RA 27/3 rubella strains of viruses, separately obtained by propagation either in chick embryo tissue cultures (mumps and measles) or MRC_5 human diploid cells (rubella).

INDICATIONS AND CLINICAL USE: PRIORIX (combined measles, mumps and rubella vaccine, live, attenuated) is indicated for:

- active immunization against infection by measles, mumps and rubella.

Pediatrics: A single dose is recommended routinely for children on, or as soon as practicable after, their first birthday. Older children who have no documented evidence of having received the vaccine should also be vaccinated.

CONTRAINDICATIONS: PRIORIX (combined measles, mumps and rubella vaccine, live, attenuated):

- as with other vaccines, administration of PRIORIX should be postponed in subjects suffering from acute severe febrile illness. The presence of a minor infection, however, is not a contraindication for vaccination.
- is contraindicated in subjects with known systemic hypersensitivity to neomycin or to any other component of the vaccine (see also Warnings and Precautions). A history of contact dermatitis to neomycin is not a contraindication.
- is contraindicated for the re-immunization of subjects with a previous anaphylactic reaction to this vaccine.
- should not be given to subjects with impaired immune function. These include patients with primary or secondary immunodeficiencies. However, measles, mumps, and rubella combined vaccines can be given to asymptomatic HIV-infected persons without adverse consequences to their illness and may be considered for those who are symptomatic.
- is contraindicated in pregnant women. Women of child-bearing potential should be advised to avoid pregnancy for three months following vaccination (see also Warnings and Precautions).

When other susceptible persons with immune deficiencies are exposed to measles, passive immunization with immune globulin [human (IG)] should be given as soon as possible. It is desirable to immunize close contacts of immunocompromised individuals in order to minimize the risk of exposure of the latter to measles.

WARNINGS AND PRECAUTIONS: General: PRIORIX (combined measles, mumps and rubella vaccine, live, attenuated) **should under no circumstances be administered intravenously.**

A limited number of subjects received PRIORIX intramuscularly. An adequate immune response was obtained for all three components.

Alcohol and other disinfecting agents must be allowed to evaporate from the skin before injection of the vaccine since they may inactivate the attenuated viruses in the vaccine.

Limited protection against measles may be obtained by vaccination up to 72 hours after exposure to natural measles.

As with all injectable vaccines, appropriate medical treatment and supervision should be readily available in case of a rare anaphylactic event following the administration of the vaccine.

The measles and mumps components of the vaccine are produced in chick embryo cell culture and may therefore contain traces of egg protein. Persons with a history of anaphylactic, anaphylactoid, or other immediate reactions (e.g. generalized urticaria, swelling of the mouth and throat, difficulty breathing, hypotension or shock) subsequent to egg ingestion may be at an enhanced risk of immediate-type hypersensitivity reactions after vaccination, although these types of reactions have been shown to be very rare. Individuals who have experienced anaphylaxis after egg ingestion should be vaccinated with extreme caution, with adequate treatment for anaphylaxis on hand should such a reaction occur.

No special precautions are necessary for children with minor egg hypersensitivity who are able to ingest small quantities of egg uneventfully. No special measures are necessary in children who have never been fed eggs before MMR immunization. Prior egg ingestion should not be a prerequisite for MMR immunization.

PRIORIX should be given with caution to persons with a history or family history of allergic diseases or those with a history or family history of convulsions.

Transmission of measles and mumps virus from vaccinees to susceptible contacts has not been documented. Pharyngeal excretion of the rubella virus is known to occur approximately 7 to 28 days after vaccination, with peak excretion around the 11th day. However there is no evidence of transmission of this excreted vaccine virus to susceptible contacts.

Hematologic: Individuals with current thrombocytopenia may develop more severe thrombocytopenia following vaccination with measles-mumps-rubella vaccines. In addition, individuals who experienced thrombocytopenia with the first dose of vaccine may develop thrombocytopenia with repeat doses. Serologic status may be evaluated to determine whether or not additional doses of vaccine are needed. The potential risk to benefit ratio should be carefully evaluated before considering vaccination in such cases (see Adverse Reactions).

Special Populations: Pregnant Women: PRIORIX is contraindicated in pregnant women. Women of child-bearing potential should be advised to avoid pregnancy for three months following vaccination.

Nursing Women: There is no human data regarding use in breastfeeding women. Nursing mothers may be vaccinated where, in the judgement of the health professional, the benefit outweighs the risk.

Pediatrics: Infants below 12 months of age may not respond sufficiently to the measles component of the vaccine, due to the possible persistence of maternal measles antibodies. This should not preclude the use of the vaccine in younger infants (<12 months) since vaccination may be indicated in some situations such as high risk areas. In these circumstances revaccination at or after 12 months of age should be considered.

Febrile seizures occasionally follow vaccination, particularly in children who have previously had convulsions or whose sibling or parents have a history of convulsions. However, the risk is low and the benefit of immunizing children greatly outweighs any potential risk associated with febrile seizures.

Under certain conditions, the vaccine may be recommended for children <1 year of age. When an infant <12 months of age is at high risk of exposure for measles or is travelling abroad to an area where measles is common, measles vaccine alone or as MMR may be given as early as 6 months of age.

Under these circumstances, or if vaccine was inappropriately given before the child's first birthday, such children should receive two additional doses of MMR after the first birthday.

Susceptible persons >12 months of age who are exposed to measles may be protected from disease if measles vaccine is given within 72 hours after exposure. There are no known adverse effects of vaccine given to persons incubating measles. However, immune globulin (IG) given within 6 days after exposure can modify or prevent disease and may be used for this purpose in infants <12 months of age, persons for whom vaccine is contraindicated or those for whom more than 72 hours but less than 1 week have elapsed since exposure. Unless contraindicated, individuals who receive IG should receive measles vaccine later, at the intervals specified in the Canadian Immunization Guide.

PRIORIX is indicated for most infants infected with the human immunodeficiency virus (HIV) whose immune function at 12 to 15 months of age is compatible with safe MMR vaccination. Consultation with an expert is required in the case of HIV-infected children to determine the presence or absence of significant immunodeficiency in individual cases. Measles revaccination may still be appropriate for HIV-infected persons with moderate immunodeficiency if there is a high risk of measles in the local community or travel to an area where measles is endemic. Consultation with local public health authorities will help determine the local level of measles activity and risk to travellers abroad. Because the response to prior immunization may be impaired, HIV-infected children should receive IG after recognized exposure to measles.

Monitoring and Laboratory Tests: If tuberculin testing is required, it should be carried out before or simultaneously with vaccination since it has been reported that live measles (and possibly mumps) vaccine may cause a temporary depression of tuberculin skin sensitivity. This anergy may last for 4-6 weeks and tuberculin testing should not be performed within that period after vaccination in order to avoid false negative results.

ADVERSE REACTIONS: Adverse Drug Reaction Overview: Frequencies are reported as: Very common: ≥10%. Common: ≥1% and <10%. Uncommon: ≥0.1% and <1%. Rare: ≥0.01% and <0.1%. Very rare: <0.01%.

Clinical Trial Adverse Drug Reactions: Because clinical trials are conducted under very specific conditions the adverse reaction rates observed in the clinical trials may not reflect the rates observed in practice and should not be compared to the rates in the clinical trials of another drug. Adverse drug reaction information from clinical trials is useful for identifying drug-related adverse events and for approximating rates.

In controlled clinical studies, signs and symptoms were actively monitored during a 42-day follow-up period. The vaccinees were also requested to report any clinical events during the study period.

There were no major study-to-study differences with regards to the frequency of adverse events.

The safety profile presented below is based on a total of approximately 12 000 subjects administered PRIORIX in clinical trials.

Very common: ≥10%: General Disorders and Administration Site Conditions: redness at the injection site, fever ≥38°C (rectal) or ≥37.5°C (axillary/oral).

Common: ≥1% and <10%: Infections and Infestations: upper respiratory tract infection.

Skin and Subcutaneous Tissue Disorders: rash.

General Disorders and Administration Site Conditions: pain and swelling at the injection site, fever >39.5°C (rectal) or >39°C (axillary/oral).

Uncommon: ≥0.1% and <1%: Infections and Infestations: otitis media.

Blood and Lymphatic System Disorders: lymphadenopathy.

Metabolism and Nutrition Disorders: anorexia.

Psychiatric Disorders: nervousness, abnormal crying, insomnia.

Eye Disorders: conjunctivitis.

Respiratory, Thoracic and Mediastinal Disorders: bronchitis, cough.

Gastrointestinal Disorders: parotid gland enlargement, diarrhoea, vomiting.

Rare: ≥0.01% and <0.1%: Immune System Disorders: allergic reactions.

Nervous System Disorders: febrile convulsions.

There is no difference between the first and second vaccine doses with regard to the frequency category for the adverse reactions, except for pain which was "Common" after the first vaccine dose and "Very common" after the second vaccine dose.

Nevertheless, despite being classified in the same frequency category, higher incidences of temperature and rash were observed after the first vaccine dose as compared to the second vaccine dose. Likewise, the incidences of redness and swelling were higher after the second vaccine dose as compared to the first vaccine dose.

A total of 10 serious adverse events that were considered as at least possibly related to vaccination have been reported after the first vaccine dose (N=10 267). None have been reported following the administration of the second vaccine dose (N=1909).

In the comparative studies, a statistically significant lower incidence of local pain, redness and swelling was reported with PRIORIX compared with the comparator. The incidence of other adverse reactions listed above were similar in both vaccines.

Post-Market Adverse Drug Reactions: During post-marketing surveillance, the following reactions have been reported additionally in temporal association with PRIORIX vaccination:

Infections and Infestations: meningitis.

Blood and Lymphatic System Disorders: thrombocytopenia, thrombocytopenic purpura.

Immune System Disorders: anaphylactic reactions.

Nervous System Disorders: aseptic meningitis, transverse myelitis, Guillain Barré syndrome, peripheral neuritis, encephalitis*.

Skin and Subcutaneous Tissue Disorders: erythema multiforme.

Musculoskeletal and Connective Tissue Disorders: arthralgia, arthritis.

General Disorders and Administration Site Conditions: Kawasaki syndrome.

In rare cases a mumps-like condition with an abbreviated incubation period cannot be ruled out. In isolated cases, transient, painful swelling of the testicles has been reported after combined mumps, measles, rubella vaccination.

In rare cases a measles-like syndrome has been reported following vaccination with PRIORIX.

Accidental intravascular administration may give rise to severe reactions or even shock. Immediate measures depend on the severity of the reaction (see Warnings and Precautions).

DRUG INTERACTIONS: Overview: Although data on the concomitant administration of PRIORIX (combined measles, mumps and rubella vaccine, live, attenuated) and other vaccines are not yet available, it is generally accepted that measles, mumps and rubella combined vaccine may be given at the same time as the oral polio vaccine (OPV) or inactivated polio vaccine (IPV), the injectable trivalent diphtheria, tetanus and pertussis vaccines (DTPw/DTPa) and *H. influenzae* type b (Hib) if they are administered at separate injection sites.

If it is not possible to administer PRIORIX at the same time as other live attenuated vaccines, such as VARILRIX, it is recommended that an interval of at least one month should be left between vaccinations.

Administration of PRIORIX to subjects who have received human gammaglobulins or a blood transfusion should be delayed for a minimum of three months as there is a possibility of vaccine failure due to passively acquired mumps, measles and rubella antibodies.

According to the Canadian Immunization Guide, if administration of an IG preparation becomes necessary after MMR vaccine or its individual component vaccines have been given, interference can also occur. If the interval between administration of any of these vaccines and subsequent administration of an IG preparation is <14 days, immunization should be repeated at 3 months or longer, unless serologic test results indicate that antibodies were produced. If the IG product is given more than 14 days after the vaccine, immunization does not have to be repeated.

PRIORIX may be given as a booster dose in subjects who have previously been vaccinated with another measles, mumps and rubella combined vaccine.

PRIORIX should not be mixed with other vaccines in the same syringe.

DOSAGE AND ADMINISTRATION: Recommended Dose and Dosage Adjustment: The Canadian Immunization Guide recommends immunization at 12 months of age, or as soon as practicable thereafter. A second dose of MMR is recommended at least 1 month after the first dose for the purpose of better measles protection. For convenience, options include giving it with the next scheduled vaccination at 18 months of age or with school entry (4-6 years) vaccinations (depending on the provincial/territorial policy), or at any intervening age that is practicable. The need for a second dose of mumps and rubella vaccine is not established but may benefit (given for convenience as MMR).

A single 0.5 mL dose of the reconstituted vaccine is recommended.

Administration: It is recommended that PRIORIX (combined measles, mumps and rubella vaccine, live, attenuated) be given by subcutaneous injection, although it may also be given by intramuscular injection. PRIORIX should under no circumstances be administered intravenously.

Reconstitution: The diluent (sterile water for injection) and reconstituted vaccine should be inspected visually for any foreign particulate matter and/or variation of physical aspects prior to administration. In the event of either being observed, discard the diluent or reconstituted vaccine as appropriate.

Withdrawing the Sterile Diluent From the Ampoule: Disinfect the neck of the ampoule of sterile diluent and allow to dry. Using a sterile towel, break off the top of the ampoule at the scored line. Using a sterile syringe and needle, withdraw the diluent from the ampoule, ensuring that the point remains immersed throughout the withdrawal.

* Encephalitis has been reported with a frequency below 1 per 10 million doses. The risk of encephalitis following administration of the vaccine is far below the risk of encephalitis caused by natural diseases (measles: 1 in 1000 to 2000 cases; rubella: approximately 1 in 6000 cases).

Cartons Containing a Syringe of Diluent: Syringe is ready for use in reconstituting the lyophilized vaccine.
Reconstitution of the Lyophilized Vaccine: The vaccine should be reconstituted by adding the entire contents of the supplied container of diluent to the vial containing the pellet. Disinfect the rubber stopper of the vial of vaccine and allow to dry. Holding the plunger of the syringe containing the diluent, pierce the center of the rubber stopper of the vial and inject the sterile diluent into the vial containing the lyophilized vaccine. Shake the vial gently until the pellet is completely dissolved in the diluent.

Inject the entire contents of the vial, using a new needle for administration.

Reconstituted vaccine should be injected as soon as possible, within 8 hours of reconstitution.

OVERDOSAGE:
Cases of overdose (up to 2 times the recommended dose) have been reported during post-marketing surveillance. No adverse events have been associated to the overdose.

> For management of a suspected drug overdose, CPhA recommends that you contact your **regional Poison Control Centre**. See the *CPS* Directory section for a list of Poison Control Centres.

ACTION AND CLINICAL PHARMACOLOGY: Duration of Effect: All subjects followed up to 12 months after vaccination remained seropositive for anti-measles and anti-rubella antibodies. At month 12, 88.4% were still seropositive for anti-mumps antibody. This percentage is comparable to that observed for the commercially available measles, mumps and rubella combined vaccine (87%).
STORAGE AND STABILITY: The vaccine should not be used beyond the expiry date stamped on the vial label and outer packaging. The diluent should not be used beyond the expiry date stamped on the syringe or ampoule label and outer packaging.

PRIORIX (combined measles, mumps and rubella vaccine, live, attenuated) should be stored in a refrigerator at 2 to 8°C. Care should be taken to ensure appropriate storage conditions during transport.

The reconstituted vaccine should be administered as soon as possible. It may be kept up to 8 hours in the refrigerator. Store in the original packaging in order to protect from light.

To conserve refrigerator space, the diluent may be stored separately at room temperature.
INFORMATION FOR THE PATIENT: Published in e-CPS, available by subscription at www.e-cps.ca.
DOSAGE FORMS, COMPOSITION AND PACKAGING: After reconstitution, 1 dose (0.5 mL) contains: not less than $10^{3.0}$ $CCID_{50}$ of the live attenuated measles virus (Schwarz strain), not less than $10^{3.7}$ $CCID_{50}$ of the live attenuated mumps virus (RIT 4385 strain, derived from Jeryl Lynn strain), and not less than $10^{3.0}$ $CCID_{50}$ of the live attenuated rubella virus (Wistar RA 27/3 strain). Excipients: Vaccine: Amino acids, lactose, mannitol, neomycin sulphate and sorbitol. Diluent: Water for injection.

PRIORIX meets the World Health Organization requirements for manufacture of biological substances and for measles, mumps and rubella vaccines and combined vaccines (live).

Monodose vials of 0.5 mL. Boxes of monodose vials of vaccine with 10 ampuls of diluent.

Priorix-Tetra™

measles, mumps, rubella and varicella vaccine, combined, live, attenuated
Active Immunizing Agent

GlaxoSmithKline

Date of Revision: May 6, 2010

SUMMARY PRODUCT INFORMATION:

Route of Administration	Dosage Form/ Strength per 0.5 mL dose	Clinically Relevant Nonmedicinal Ingredients
Subcutaneous injection (SC) or Intramuscular injection (IM)	Powder and solution for injection/live, attenuated measles virus (Schwarz strain) not less than $10^{3.0}$ $CCID_{50}$; live, attenuated mumps virus (RIT 4385 strain, derived from Jeryl Lynn strain) not less than $10^{4.4}$ $CCID_{50}$; live, attenuated rubella virus (Wistar RA 27/3 strain) not less than $10^{3.0}$ $CCID_{50}$; live, attenuated varicella virus (OKA strain) not less than $10^{3.3}$ PFU	Amino acids for injection, lactose, mannitol, neomycin sulphate, sorbitol, water for injections

DESCRIPTION: PRIORIX-TETRA (combined measles, mumps, rubella and varicella vaccine, live, attenuated) is a lyophilized mixed preparation of the attenuated Schwarz measles, RIT 4385 mumps (derived from Jeryl Lynn strain), Wistar RA 27/3 rubella and OKA varicella strains of viruses.
INDICATIONS AND CLINICAL USE: PRIORIX-TETRA (combined measles, mumps, rubella and varicella vaccine, live, attenuated) is indicated for active immunization against measles, mumps, rubella and varicella in individuals from 9 months to 6 years of age. Efficacy has not been evaluated in subjects above 6 years of age.

PRIORIX-TETRA may be used in individuals up to 12 years of age based upon previous experience with the separate component vaccines, PRIORIX (combined measles, mumps and rubella vaccine, live attenuated) and VARILRIX [varicella virus vaccine, live, attenuated (OKA-strain)].
CONTRAINDICATIONS: PRIORIX-TETRA (combined measles, mumps, rubella and varicella vaccine, live, attenuated):
- Is contraindicated in subjects with known hypersensitivity to neomycin or to any other component of the vaccine (for egg allergy, see Warnings and Precautions). A history of contact dermatitis to neomycin is not a contraindication. For a complete listing of excipients, see Dosage Forms, Composition and Packaging.
- Is contraindicated in subjects having shown signs of hypersensitivity after previous administration of measles, mumps, rubella and/or varicella vaccines.
- Is contraindicated to be administered to pregnant females. Furthermore, pregnancy should be avoided for three months after vaccination (see Warnings and Precautions, Special Populations).
- Should not be given to subjects with impaired immune function. These include patients with primary or secondary immunodeficiencies.

WARNINGS AND PRECAUTIONS: General: PRIORIX-TETRA (combined measles, mumps, rubella and varicella vaccine, live, attenuated) **should under no circumstances be administered intravascularly or intradermally.**

As with other vaccines, the administration of PRIORIX-TETRA should be postponed in subjects suffering from acute severe febrile illness. However, the presence of a minor infection, such as a cold, should not result in the deferral of vaccination.

As with all injectable vaccines, appropriate medical treatment and supervision should always be readily available in case of a rare anaphylactic event following the administration of the vaccine.

Alcohol and other disinfecting agents must be allowed to evaporate from the skin before injection of the vaccine since they can inactivate the attenuated viruses in the vaccine.

A history of febrile convulsions or a family history of convulsions does not constitute a contraindication for the use of PRIORIX-TETRA. Vaccinees with a history of febrile convulsions should be closely followed up as vaccine related fever may occur during the period ranging from 4 to 12 days after vaccination.

Transmission of measles, mumps and rubella viruses from vaccinees to susceptible contacts has never been documented, although pharyngeal excretion of the rubella virus is known to occur about 7 to 28 days after vaccination with peak excretion around the 11th day. Post-marketing experience suggests that transmission of varicella vaccine virus may occur very rarely between healthy vaccinees who develop a varicella-like rash and susceptible contacts.

The measles and mumps components of the vaccine are produced in chick embryo cell culture and may therefore contain traces of egg protein. Persons with a history of anaphylactic, anaphylactoid, or other immediate reactions (e.g. generalized urticaria, swelling of the mouth and throat, difficulty breathing, hypotension, or shock) subsequent to egg ingestion may be at an enhanced risk of immediate-type hypersensitivity reactions after vaccination, although these types of reactions have been shown to be very rare. Individuals who have experienced anaphylaxis after egg ingestion should be vaccinated with extreme caution, with adequate treatment for anaphylaxis on hand should such a reaction occur.

* Following the administration of the first dose of PRIORIX-TETRA, higher incidences of fever (approximately 1.5 fold) were observed when compared to the concomitant administration of PRIORIX and VARILRIX vaccines at separate injection sites.

Immune: As with any vaccine, a protective immune response may not be elicited in all vaccinees.

Cases of worsening of thrombocytopenia and recurrence of thrombocytopenia in subjects who suffered thrombocytopenia after the first dose have been reported following vaccination with live measles, mumps and rubella vaccines. In such cases, the risk-benefit of immunising with PRIORIX-TETRA should be carefully evaluated.

The use of PRIORIX-TETRA in asymptomatic HIV subjects has not been studied. Administration of PRIORIX-TETRA may be considered with caution in this population when, in the opinion of the physician, withholding the vaccine entails a greater risk.
Special Populations: Pregnant Women: It is contraindicated to administer PRIORIX-TETRA to pregnant females. Furthermore, pregnancy should be avoided for three months after vaccination. Adequate human data on the use of PRIORIX-TETRA during pregnancy are not available and animal studies on reproductive toxicity have not been conducted.
Nursing Women: Adequate human data on the use of PRIORIX-TETRA during lactation are not available.

ADVERSE REACTIONS: Clinical Trial Adverse Drug Reactions: Because clinical trials are conducted under very specific conditions the adverse reaction rates observed in the clinical trials may not reflect the rates observed in practice and should not be compared to the rates in the clinical trials of another drug. Adverse drug reaction information from clinical trials is useful for identifying drug-related adverse events and for approximating rates.

The safety profile presented below is based on data from more than 6700 doses of PRIORIX-TETRA (combined measles, mumps, rubella and varicella vaccine, live, attenuated) administered subcutaneously to children from 9 to 27 months of age. Events were recorded for up to 42 days after vaccination.
Very Common Clinical Trial Adverse Drug Reactions ≥1/10: General Disorders and Administration Site Conditions: pain and redness at the injection site, fever (rectal ≥38°C and ≤39.5°C; axillary/oral: ≥37.5°C and ≤39°C).
Common Clinical Trial Adverse Drug Reactions ≥1/100 to <1/10: General Disorders and Administration Site Conditions: swelling at the injection site, fever (rectal >39.5°C; axillary/oral >39°C)*.
Psychiatric Disorders: irritability.
Skin and Subcutaneous Tissue Disorders: rash including measles-like, rubella-like and varicella-like rash.
Uncommon Clinical Trial Adverse Drug Reactions ≥1/1000 to <1/100: Blood and Lymphatic System Disorders: lymphadenopathy.
Endocrine Disorders: parotid swelling.
Gastrointestinal Disorders: diarrhea, vomiting.
General Disorders and Administration Site Conditions: lethargy, malaise, fatigue.
Infections and Infestations: upper respiratory tract infection.
Metabolism and Nutrition Disorders: anorexia.
Psychiatric Disorders: crying, insomnia, nervousness.
Respiratory, Thoracic and Mediastinal Disorders: rhinitis.
Rare Clinical Trial Adverse Drug Reactions ≥1/10 000 to <1/1000: General Disorders and Administration Site Conditions: injection site bruising.
Infections and Infestations: otitis media.
Nervous System Disorders: febrile convulsions.
Respiratory, Thoracic and Mediastinal Disorders: cough, bronchitis.
Post-Market Adverse Drug Reactions: The post-market information of PRIORIX-TETRA (combined measles, mumps, rubella and varicella vaccine, live, attenuated) is not yet available. The following post-market safety information is of the separate components of the vaccines, PRIORIX (combined measles, mumps and rubella vaccine, live attenuated) and VARILRIX [varicella virus vaccine, live, attenuated (OKA-strain)].

The safety of measles-mumps-rubella and varicella vaccines has been well characterised in clinical trials and post-marketing surveillance. PRIORIX and VARILRIX have been used in Canadian market since 2002 and 2003 respectively. Over 144 million doses of PRIORIX and 14 million doses of VARILRIX have been distributed worldwide since 1997 and 1994 respectively. No safety concerns outside the recognized and reported safety profile has been identified to date.

During post-marketing surveillance, the following additional reactions have been reported after measles-mumps-rubella and varicella vaccination:

Because these reactions were reported spontaneously, it is not possible to reliably estimate their frequency.
Blood and Lymphatic System Disorders: thrombocytopenia, thrombocytopenic purpura.
General Disorders and Administration Site Conditions: Kawasaki syndrome.
Immune System Disorders: allergic reactions (including anaphylactic and anaphylactoid reactions).
Infections and Infestations: meningitis.
Musculoskeletal and Connective Tissue Disorders: arthralgia, arthritis.
Nervous System Disorders: encephalitis, Guillain Barré syndrome, peripheral neuritis, Transverse myelitis.
Skin and Subcutaneous Tissue Disorders: erythema multiforme.

In rare cases a mumps-like condition with an abbreviated incubation period cannot be ruled out. In isolated cases transient, painful swelling of the testicles has been reported after combined mumps, measles, rubella vaccination.

DRUG INTERACTIONS: Administration with Other Vaccines: PRIORIX-TETRA (combined measles, mumps, rubella and varicella vaccine, live, attenuated) can be given simultaneously (but at separate injection sites) with any of the following monovalent or combination vaccines [including hexavalent vaccines (DTPa-HBV-IPV/Hib, Infanrix-hexa)]: diphtheria-tetanus-acellular pertussis vaccine (DTPa), *H. influenzae* type b vaccine (Hib), inactivated polio vaccine (IPV), Hepatitis B vaccine (HBV).
Drug-Drug Interactions: In subjects who have received human gammaglobulins or a blood transfusion, vaccination should be delayed for at least three months because of the likelihood of vaccine failure due to passively acquired antibodies.

Salicylates should be avoided for 6 weeks after each vaccination as Reye's Syndrome has been reported following the use of salicylates during natural varicella infection.
Drug-Food Interactions: Interactions with food have not been established.
Drug-Herb Interactions: Interactions with herbal products have not been established.
Drug-Laboratory Test Interactions: If tuberculin testing has to be done it should be carried out before or simultaneously with vaccination since it has been reported that combined measles, mumps and rubella vaccines may cause a temporary depression of tuberculin skin sensitivity. As this anergy may last up to a maximum of 6 weeks, tuberculin testing should not be performed within that period after vaccination to avoid false negative results.

DOSAGE AND ADMINISTRATION: Recommended Dose and Dosage Adjustment: Primary immunization consists of two doses of PRIORIX-TETRA (combined measles, mumps, rubella and varicella vaccine, live, attenuated) vaccine. An interval of at least 6 weeks between doses is preferable and in no circumstances should this interval be less than 4 weeks.

If official recommendations call for a second dose of varicella, PRIORIX-TETRA can be used in lieu of separate MMR and varicella vaccines. Refer to the Canadian Immunization Guide for current recommendations.
Administration: PRIORIX-TETRA is to be injected subcutaneously (SC), or intramuscularly (IM) in the deltoid region of the upper arm.

The vaccine should be administered subcutaneously in subjects with bleeding disorders (eg. thrombocytopenia or any coagulation disorder).

Alcohol and other disinfecting agents must be allowed to evaporate from the skin before injection of the vaccine since they can inactivate the attenuated viruses in the vaccine.
Directions for Reconstitution: The reconstituted vaccine should be inspected visually for any foreign particulate matter and/or abnormal physical appearance. In the event of either being observed, the vaccine should be discarded.

The vaccine is reconstituted by adding the entire contents of the supplied container of diluent to the vial containing the powder. After the addition of the diluent to the powder, the mixture should be well shaken until the powder is completely dissolved.

The colour of the reconstituted vaccine may vary from clear peach to fuchsia pink (bright pink) due to minor variations of its pH. This is normal and does not impair the performance of the vaccine. In the event of other variation being observed, discard the vaccine.

Reconstituted vaccine should be injected as soon as possible, within 8 hours of reconstitution if it is stored refrigerated (2 to 8°C).

Any unused product or waste material should be disposed of in accordance with local requirements.

OVERDOSAGE:
Insufficient data are available.

> For management of a suspected drug overdose, CPhA recommends that you contact your **regional Poison Control Centre**. See the *CPS* Directory section for a list of Poison Control Centres.

ACTION AND CLINICAL PHARMACOLOGY: Mechanism of Action: Measles: Measles is the most contagious vaccine-preventable infection in humans. The disease is spread by airborne or droplet exposure. There has been a marked reduction in incidence in countries where vaccine has been widely used. Complications such as otitis media and bronchopneumonia occur in about 10% of the reported cases. Measles encephalitis occurs in approximately 1 of every 1000 reported cases and may result in permanent brain damage. In Canada, death is estimated to occur once in 3000 cases.

Before the introduction of the vaccine, there were between 300 000 to 400 000 cases occurring annually. In Canada, since the introduction of the two doses of measles in the routine immunization schedule in every province and territory in 1997, endemic measles appears to have been eliminated

Mumps: Mumps is an acute infectious disease caused by the mumps virus. Before the widespread use of mumps vaccine, mumps was a major cause of viral meningitis. Since the licensure of vaccine in 1969, the number of reported mumps cases in Canada has decreased >99%. The number of cases ranged from 402 in 1995 to 90 in 1999 with average of 237 per year. Children <5 years accounted for 17% of cases and those aged 4 to 14 years accounted for 44%.

Rubella: Rubella is a viral disease that results in a transient exanthematous rash, post auricular or suboccipital lymphadenopathy, arthralgia and low grade fever. The main goal of immunization is the prevention of rubella infection in pregnancy which may give rise to congenital rubella syndrome (CRS). The risk of fetal damage following maternal infection is particularly high in the earliest months after conception (85%) in the first trimester. Since the introduction of an immunization program for rubella in Canada, reported cases of CRS have dropped throughout the country.

Varicella: Varicella zoster virus (VZV) causes a primary illness chickenpox, established latency in the sensory nerve ganglia and may be reactivated later as herpes zoster (shingles). VZV is spread by direct contact with the virus shed from skin lesions or in oral secretions as well as by the airborne route. The lifetime risk of developing varicella is 95% and having at least one reactivation to herpes zoster is 15 to 20%. The case fatality rates for varicella are highest among young adults. In Canada, 71% of the 59 reported chickenpox deaths from 1987 to 1997 occurred in those >15 years of age.

Duration of Effect: Long term persistence of anti-measles, anti-mumps, anti-rubella and anti-varicella antibodies are currently under evaluation in the follow up phase of studies. At the one year follow-up after a second dose of PRIORIX-TETRA (combined measles, mumps, rubella, varicella vaccine, live, attenuated), more than 98.8% of all children were seropositive for anti-measles, anti-rubella and anti-varicella antibodies, and 90.6% were seropositive for the anti-mumps antibodies.

STORAGE AND STABILITY: Store PRIORIX-TETRA (combined measles, mumps, rubella and varicella vaccine, live, attenuated) at 2 to 8°C (in a refrigerator). Do not freeze. Store in the original packaging in order to protect from light.

The reconstituted vaccine should be administered as soon as possible. It may be kept up to 8 hours in the refrigerator (2 to 8°C).

The expiry date of the vaccine is indicated on the label and packaging.

INFORMATION FOR THE PATIENT: Published in e-CPS, available by subscription at www.e-cps.ca.

DOSAGE FORMS, COMPOSITION AND PACKAGING: Each 0.5 mL dose of the reconstituted vaccine contains not less than $10^{3.0}$ $CCID_{50}$ of the live, attenuated measles virus (Schwarz strain), not less than $10^{4.4}$ $CCID_{50}$ of the live, attenuated mumps virus (RIT 4385 strain, derived from Jeryl Lynn strain), not less than $10^{3.0}$ $CCID_{50}$ live, attenuated rubella virus (Wistar RA 27/3 strain) and not less than $10^{3.3}$ PFU Live, attenuated varicella virus (OKA strain). The virus also contains amino acids, lactose, mannitol, neomycin sulphate, sorbitol, water for injections.

Monodose vials of 0.5 mL, pack sizes of 1, 10, 20, 50 and 100. The diluent is available as 0.5 mL of solution in: ampoules in pack sizes of 1, 10 or 100; prefilled syringes with rubber stopper, pack sizes of 1 or 10 with 2 separate needles and pack sizes of 1, 10, 20 or 50 without needles; vials with stopper in pack sizes of 1 or 100.

Pristiq™ ℞

desvenlafaxine succinate

Antidepressant

Pfizer

Date of Revision: August 26, 2009

SUMMARY PRODUCT INFORMATION:

Route of Administration	Dosage Form/ Strength	Nonmedicinal Ingredients
Oral	Extended-release tablet (50 and 100 mg desvenlafaxine as desvenlafaxine succinate)	Inactive ingredients consist of hypromellose, magnesium stearate, microcrystalline cellulose, talc, and film coating which consists of dextrose, maltodextrin, sodium carboxymethylcellulose, stearic acid, iron oxides and titanium dioxide.

INDICATIONS AND CLINICAL USE: Adults: PRISTIQ desvenlafaxine Extended-release Tablets is indicated for the symptomatic relief of major depressive disorder.

The short-term efficacy of PRISTIQ desvenlafaxine succinate Extended-release Tablets has been demonstrated in placebo-controlled trials of up to 8 weeks.

Pediatrics (<18 years of age): PRISTIQ is not indicated for use in children under the age of 18. Safety and effectiveness in the pediatric population have not been established (see Warnings and Precautions, Potential Association with Behavioral and Emotional Changes, Including Self-harm).

CONTRAINDICATIONS:

- Desvenlafaxine must not be used concomitantly in patients taking monoamine oxidase inhibitors (MAOIs, including linezolid, an antibiotic) or in patients who have taken MAOIs within the preceding 14 days due to the risk of serious, sometimes fatal, drug interactions with selective serotonin reuptake inhibitor (SSRI) or serotonin norepinephrine reuptake inhibitor (SNRI) treatment or with other serotonergic drugs. These interactions have been associated with symptoms that include tremor, myoclonus, diaphoresis, nausea, vomiting, flushing, dizziness, hyperthermia with features resembling neuroleptic malignant syndrome, seizures, rigidity, autonomic instability with possible rapid fluctuations of vital signs, and mental status changes that include extreme agitation progressing to delirium and coma. Based on the half-life of desvenlafaxine succinate, at least 7 days should be allowed after stopping desvenlafaxine succinate and before starting an MAOI.
- Hypersensitivity to desvenlafaxine succinate extended-release, venlafaxine hydrochloride or to any excipients in the desvenlafaxine formulation (see Dosage Forms, Composition and Packaging).

WARNINGS AND PRECAUTIONS: Potential Association with Behavioral and Emotional Changes, Including Self-harm: Pediatrics: Placebo-controlled Clinical Trial Data: Recent analyses of placebo-controlled clinical trial safety databases from Selective Serotonin Reuptake Inhibitors (SSRIs) and other newer anti-depressants suggest that use of these drugs in patients under the age of 18 may be associated with behavioural and emotional changes, including an increased risk of suicidal ideation and behaviour over that of placebo.

The small denominators in the clinical trial database, as well as the variability in placebo rates, preclude reliable conclusions on the relative safety profiles among the drugs in the class.

Adults and Pediatrics: Additional Data: There are clinical trial and post-marketing reports with SSRIs and other newer antidepressants, in both pediatrics and adults, of severe agitation-type adverse events coupled with self-harm or harm to others. The agitation-type events include: akathisia, agitation, disinhibition, emotional lability, hostility, aggression, depersonalization. In some cases, the events occurred within several weeks of starting treatment.

Rigorous clinical monitoring for suicidal ideation or other indicators of potential for suicidal behaviour is advised in patients of all ages especially when initiating therapy or during any change in dose or dosage regimen. This includes monitoring for agitation-type emotional and behavioural changes.

Patients currently taking PRISTIQ should NOT be discontinued abruptly, due to risk of discontinuation symptoms (see Warnings and Precautions, Discontinuation Symptoms). At the time that a medical decision is made to discontinue an SSRI or other newer antidepressant drug, a gradual reduction in the dose, rather than an abrupt cessation, is recommended (see Dosage and Administration).

Concomitant Use of PRISTIQ with Venlafaxine: Since desvenlafaxine is the major active metabolite of venlafaxine, concomitant use of PRISTIQ with products containing **venlafaxine** is not recommended since the combination of the two will lead to additive desvenlafaxine exposure.

Psychiatric: Mania/Hypomania: Mania/hypomania may occur in a small proportion of patients with mood disorders who have received medication to treat depression, including desvenlafaxine succinate. During phase 2 and phase 3 studies, mania was reported for approximately 0.1% of patients treated with PRISTIQ. Activation of mania/hypomania has also been reported in a small proportion of patients with major affective disorder who were treated with other marketed antidepressants. As with all antidepressants, PRISTIQ should be used cautiously in patients with a history or family history of mania or hypomania.

Neurologic: Seizures: Cases of seizures have been reported in pre-marketing trials with PRISTIQ. Desvenlafaxine succinate should be prescribed with caution in patients with a seizure disorder. Desvenlafaxine has not been systematically evaluated in patients with a seizure disorder.

Serotonin Syndrome: As with other serotonergic agents, serotonin syndrome, a potentially life-threatening condition, may occur with desvenlafaxine treatment, particularly with concomitant use of other agents that may affect the serotonergic neurotransmitter systems (such as triptans, serotonin reuptake inhibitors, sibutramine, MAOIs (including linezolid, an antibiotic), St. John's Wort (Hypericum perforatum) and/or lithium) and with drugs that impair metabolism of serotonin. Serotonin syndrome symptoms may include mental status changes (e.g., agitation, hallucinations, and coma), autonomic instability (e.g., tachycardia, labile blood pressure, and hyperthermia), neuromuscular aberrations (e.g., hyperreflexia, incoordination) and/or gastrointestinal symptoms (e.g., nausea, vomiting, and diarrhea).

If concomitant treatment with desvenlafaxine and other agents that may affect the serotonergic neurotransmitter system (such as an other SSRI, a Selective Serotonin and Norepinephrine Reuptake Inhibitor (SNRI) or a 5-hydroxytryptamine receptor agonist (triptan) is clinically warranted, careful observation of the patient is advised, particularly during treatment initiation and dose increases. The concomitant use of desvenlafaxine with serotonin precursors (such as tryptophan supplements) is not recommended (see Drug Interactions, Serotonin Syndrome).

Ophthalmologic: Narrow Angle Glaucoma: Mydriasis has been reported in association with desvenlafaxine; therefore, patients with raised intraocular pressure or those at risk of acute narrow-angle glaucoma (angle-closure glaucoma) should be monitored (see Adverse Reactions).

Gastrointestinal: Potential for Gastrointestinal Obstruction: Because the PRISTIQ tablet does not appreciably change in shape in the gastrointestinal tract, PRISTIQ should not be administered to patients with pre-existing gastrointestinal narrowing (pathologic or iatrogenic, such as small bowel inflammatory disease, "short gut" syndrome due to adhesions or decreased transit time, past history of peritonitis, cystic fibrosis, chronic intestinal pseudo-obstruction, or Meckel's diverticulum). There have been rare reports of obstructive symptoms in patients with known strictures in association with the ingestion of other drugs in nondeformable controlled-release formulations, and very rare reports of obstructive symptoms associated with the use of nondeformable controlled-release formulations in patients without known gastrointestinal stricture. Due to the controlled-release design, PRISTIQ tablets should only be used in patients who are able to swallow the tablets whole. (See Dosage and Administration, Recommended Dose and Dosage Adjustment.)

Cardiovascular/Cerebrovascular: Caution is advised in administering PRISTIQ to patients with cardiovascular, cerebrovascular, or lipid metabolism disorders (see Clinical Trial Adverse Drug Reactions). Increases in blood pressure and heart rate were observed in clinical trials with PRISTIQ. PRISTIQ has not been evaluated systematically in patients with a recent history of myocardial infarction, unstable heart disease, uncontrolled hypertension, or cerebrovascular disease. Patients with these diagnoses, except for cerebrovascular disease, were excluded from clinical trials.

Effects on Blood Pressure: Increases in blood pressure were observed in some patients in clinical trials, particularly with higher doses. Caution should be exercised in treating patients with underlying conditions that might be compromised by increases in blood pressure (see Adverse Reactions, Vital Sign Changes). Pre-existing hypertension should be controlled before treatment with PRISTIQ. Patients receiving PRISTIQ should have regular monitoring of blood pressure. Cases of elevated blood pressure requiring immediate treatment have been reported with desvenlafaxine. Sustained blood pressure increases could have adverse consequences. For patients who experience a sustained increase in blood pressure while receiving PRISTIQ, either dose reduction or discontinuation should be considered.

Treatment with PRISTIQ at all doses from 50 mg/day to 400 mg/day in controlled studies was associated with sustained hypertension (defined as treatment-emergent supine diastolic blood pressure ≥90 mm Hg and ≥10 mm Hg above baseline for 3 consecutive visits). Table 1 provides the incidence of patients meeting criteria for sustained hypertension.

Table 1: PRISTIQ

Incidence (%) of Patients with Sustained Hypertension for All Short-term Fixed-Dose Clinical Trials

		PRISTIQ			
	Placebo	**50 mg**	**100 mg**	**200 mg**	**400 mg**
Sustained hypertension	0.5	1.3	0.7	1.1	2.3

Endocrine and Metabolism: Serum Cholesterol Elevation: Increases in cholesterol (total and LDL) and triglycerides were observed in some patients treated with desvenlafaxine succinate in placebo-controlled pre-marketing clinical trials, particularly with higher doses. Measurement of serum lipid levels should be considered during treatment.

Hyponatremia: Cases of hyponatremia and/or the Syndrome of Inappropriate Antidiuretic Hormone (SIADH) secretion have been described with SNRIs and SSRIs, usually in volume-depleted or dehydrated patients, including elderly patients and patients taking diuretics.

Discontinuation Symptoms: At the time that a medical decision is made to discontinue PRISTIQ, a gradual reduction in the dose, rather than an abrupt cessation, is recommended.

During marketing of SNRIs, and SSRIs, there have been spontaneous reports of adverse events occurring upon discontinuation of these drugs, particularly when abrupt, including the following: dysphoric mood, irritability, agitation, dizziness, sensory disturbances (e.g., paraesthesias, such as electric shock sensations), anxiety, confusion, headache, lethargy, emotional lability, insomnia, hypomania, tinnitus, and seizures. While these events are generally self-limiting, there have been reports of serious discontinuation symptoms.

Patients should be monitored for these symptoms when discontinuing treatment with PRISTIQ. A gradual reduction in the dose rather than abrupt cessation is recommended whenever possible. If intolerable symptoms occur following a decrease in the dose or upon discontinuation of treatment, then resuming the previously prescribed dose may be considered. Subsequently, the physician may continue decreasing the dose but at a more gradual rate (see Adverse Reactions, Discontinuation Symptoms and Dosage and Administration, Discontinuing PRISTIQ).

Hematologic: Abnormal Bleeding: Drugs that inhibit serotonin uptake in platelets may lead to abnormalities of platelet aggregation. As with other agents that inhibit serotonin-reuptake, desvenlafaxine succinate should be used cautiously in patients predisposed to bleeding, including patients on anticoagulants and platelet inhibitors.

Special Populations: Pregnant Women: The safety of desvenlafaxine in human pregnancy has not been established. The extent of exposure to PRISTIQ in pregnancy during clinical trials was very limited. There are no adequate and well-controlled studies in pregnant women. Therefore, desvenlafaxine should be used during pregnancy only if the potential benefits justify the potential risks. If desvenlafaxine succinate is used until or shortly before birth, discontinuation effects in the newborn should be considered.

Post-marketing reports indicate that some neonates exposed to SNRIs, SSRIs, or other newer antidepressants late in the third trimester have developed complications requiring prolonged hospitalization, respiratory support, and tube feeding. Such complications can arise immediately upon delivery. Reported clinical findings have included respiratory distress, cyanosis, apnea, seizures, temperature instability, feeding difficulty, vomiting, hypoglycemia, hypotonia, hypertonia, hyper-reflexia, tremor, jitteriness, irritability, and constant crying. These features are consistent with either a direct toxic effect of SNRIs, SSRIs and other newer antidepressants, or, possibly a drug discontinuation syndrome. It should be noted that, in some cases, the clinical picture is consistent with serotonin syndrome (see Drug Interactions). When treating a pregnant woman with PRISTIQ during the third trimester, the physician should carefully consider the potential risks and benefits of treatment.

Patients should be advised to notify their physician if they become pregnant or intend to become pregnant during therapy.

Labour and Delivery: The effect of desvenlafaxine on labour and delivery in humans is unknown. PRISTIQ should be used during labour and delivery only if the potential benefits justify the potential risks.

Nursing Women: Desvenlafaxine (O-desmethylvenlafaxine) is excreted in human milk. Because of the potential for serious adverse reactions in nursing infants from PRISTIQ, a decision should be made whether or not to discontinue nursing or to discontinue the drug, taking into account the importance of the drug to the mother. Only administer PRISTIQ to breastfeeding women if the expected benefits outweigh any possible risk.

Pediatrics: Safety and effectiveness in patients less than 18 years of age have not been established.

Geriatrics (≥65 years of age): Of the 3292 patients in clinical trials with PRISTIQ, 5% were 65 years of age or older. No overall differences in safety or efficacy were detected between these subjects and younger subjects; however in the short-term placebo-controlled trials, there was a higher incidence of systolic orthostatic hypotension in patients ≥65 years of age compared to all adults treated with desvenlafaxine. For elderly patients, possible reduced renal clearance of desvenlafaxine should be considered when determining dose (see Dosing Considerations, Geriatrics (≥65 years of age) and Action and Clinical Pharmacology, Special Populations and Conditions, Geriatrics). Greater sensitivity of some older individuals cannot be ruled out.

Dependence/Tolerance: Although desvenlafaxine succinate has not been systematically studied in preclinical or clinical trials for its potential for abuse, no indication of drug-seeking behavior was seen in the clinical trials.

Allergic Reactions: Patients should be advised to notify their physician if they develop a rash, hives or a related allergic phenomenon.

Interstitial Lung Disease and Eosinophilic Pneumonia: Interstitial lung disease and eosinophilic pneumonia associated with venlafaxine (the parent drug of PRISTIQ) therapy have been rarely reported. The possibility of these adverse events should be considered in patients treated with PRISTIQ who present with progressive dyspnea, cough, or chest discomfort. Such patients should undergo a prompt medical evaluation, and discontinuation of PRISTIQ should be considered.

Monitoring and Laboratory Tests: Serum Lipids: Increases in cholesterol (total and LDL) and triglycerides were observed in some patients treated with desvenlafaxine succinate in placebo-controlled pre-marketing clinical trials, particularly with higher doses. Measurement of serum lipid levels should be considered during treatment.

Heart Rate and Blood Pressure: Increases in heart rate and blood pressure were observed in some patients in clinical trials, particularly with higher doses. Measurement of blood pressure is recommended prior to initiating treatment and regularly during treatment with desvenlafaxine succinate (see Adverse Reactions, Vital Sign Changes).

Self-harm: Rigorous clinical monitoring for suicidal ideation or other indicators of potential for suicidal behaviour is advised in patients of all ages. Patients, their families, and their caregivers should be encouraged to be alert to the emergence of anxiety, agitation, panic attacks, insomnia, irritability, hostility, aggressiveness, impulsivity, akathisia (psychomotor restlessness), hypomania, mania, other unusual changes in behavior, worsening of depression, and suicidal ideation, especially when initiating therapy or during any change in dose or dosage regimen. (See Warnings and Precautions, Potential Association with Behavioral and Emotional Changes, Including Self-harm.)

ADVERSE REACTIONS: Adverse Drug Reaction Overview: The safety of PRISTIQ in major depressive disorder was evaluated in 3292 patients exposed to at least one dose of PRISTIQ.

The most commonly observed adverse reactions (incidence of 5% or greater for the DVS SR pooled 50- to 400-mg doses, and incidence higher than placebo) in DVS SR-treated MDD patients in short-term placebo controlled trials were: nausea, headache, dry mouth, hyperhydrosis, dizziness, insomnia, constipation, decreased appetite, somnolence, fatigue, tremor, and vomiting, and, in men, erectile dysfunction and ejaculation delayed.

Adverse Events Reported as Reasons for Discontinuation of Treatment in MDD Clinical Trials: In the 8-week placebo-controlled, pre-marketing trials for MDD, 12% of the 1834 patients who received PRISTIQ (50-400 mg/day) discontinued treatment due to an adverse experience, compared with 3% of the 1116 placebo-treated patients in those trials.

At the recommended dose of 50 mg, the discontinuation rate due to an adverse experience for PRISTIQ (4.1%) was similar to the rate for placebo (3.8%) and only 1% of patients discontinued due to nausea.

The most common adverse reactions leading to discontinuation (i.e., leading to discontinuation in at least 2% and incidence higher than placebo) of the PRISTIQ-treated patients in short-term trials of up to 8 weeks were: nausea (4%); dizziness, headache and vomiting (2% each).

Clinical Trial Adverse Drug Reactions: Because clinical trials are conducted under very specific conditions the adverse reaction rates observed in the clinical trials may not reflect the rates observed in practice and should not be compared to the rates in the clinical trials of another drug. Adverse drug reaction information from clinical trials is useful for identifying drug-related adverse events and for approximating rates.

Adverse Reactions in MDD Clinical Trials: PRISTIQ was evaluated for safety in 3292 patients diagnosed with major depressive disorder who participated in multiple-dose pre-marketing trials, representing 1289 patient-years of exposure. Among these 3292 PRISTIQ-treated patients, 1834 patients participated in 8-week, placebo-controlled trials at doses ranging from 50 to 400 mg/day. Of the total 3292 subjects exposed to at least 1 dose of PRISTIQ, 1070 were exposed to PRISTIQ for greater than 6 months and 274 were exposed for 1 year.

Adverse Reactions Occurring at an Incidence of ≥1% among PRISTIQ-treated Patients in Short-term Placebo-controlled Trials: The following adverse reactions (Table 2) occurred at ≥1% and are listed alphabetically by body system.

Reported adverse events were classified using a standard MedDRA-based Dictionary terminology.

Table 2: PRISTIQ

Adverse Reactions (≥1% in Any PRISTIQ Group): Percentage of Subjects in Short-term, Placebo-controlled MDD Studies

System Organ Class Preferred Term	Placebo[a] n=1116	DVS SR 50 mg[b] n=317	DVS SR 100 mg[b] n=424	DVS SR 200 mg[b] n=307	DVS SR 400 mg[b] n=317	DVS SR 50–400 mg[a] n=1834
Cardiac Disorders						
Palpitations	2	1	3	2	3	2
Tachycardia	1	1	<1	1	2	1
Ear and Labyrinth Disorders						
Tinnitus	1	2	1	1	2	1
Eye Disorders						
Mydriasis	<1	2	2	6	6	4
Vision blurred	1	3	4	4	4	4
Gastrointestinal Disorders						
Nausea	11	22	26	36	41	32
Dry mouth	8	11	17	21	25	20
Constipation	4	9	9	10	14	11
Diarrhoea	9	11	9	7	5	8
Vomiting	2	3	4	6	9	6
General Disorders and Administration Site Conditions						
Fatigue	4	7	7	10	11	8
Chills	1	1	<1	3	4	2
Feeling jittery	1	1	2	3	3	2
Asthenia	1	1	2	1	1	1
Investigations						
Blood pressure increased	1	1	1	2	2	2
Weight decreased	1	2	1	1	2	1
Metabolism and Nutrition Disorders						
Decreased appetite	2	5	8	10	10	9
Musculoskeletal and Connective Tissue Disorders						
Musculoskeletal stiffness	1	1	<1	1	1	1
Nervous System Disorders						
Headache	25	20	22	29	25	25
Dizziness	6	13	10	15	16	13
Somnolence	4	4	9	12	12	9
Tremor	2	2	3	9	9	6
Paraesthesia	1	2	2	1	3	2
Dysgeusia	1	1	1	1	2	2
Disturbance in attention	<1	<1	1	2	1	1
Psychiatric Disorders						
Insomnia	6	9	12	14	15	12
Anxiety	3	3	5	4	4	4
Abnormal dreams	2	2	3	2	4	3
Anorgasmia	0	<1	2	2	6	2
Libido decreased	1	2	3	3	2	2
Orgasm abnormal	<1	1	1	1	2	1
Nervousness	1	<1	1	2	2	1
Renal and Urinary Disorders						
Urinary hesitation	<1	<1	1	2	2	1
Respiratory, Thoracic and Mediastinal Disorders						
Yawning	<1	1	1	4	3	3
Skin and Subcutaneous Tissue Disorders						
Hyperhidrosis	4	10	11	18	21	15
Rash	1	1	1	2	<1	1
Vascular Disorders						
Hot flush	<1	1	1	2	2	2

[a] Includes data from all short-term, placebo-controlled studies including fixed-dose and flexible-dose studies.
[b] Only includes data from short-term, placebo-controlled, fixed-dose studies.
Classifications of adverse events are based on the Medical Dictionary for Regulatory Activities (MedDRA).
Note: <1% indicates an incidence less than 0.5%, but greater than zero.
Legend: MDD=major depressive disorder.

Sexual Function Adverse Reactions: Table 3 shows the incidence of sexual function adverse reactions that occurred in 1% or more of PRISTIQ-treated MDD patients in the 50 mg dose group (8-week, placebo-controlled, fixed and flexible-dose, pre-marketing clinical trials).

Table 3: PRISTIQ

Sexual Dysfunction Adverse Reactions (≥1% in Men or Women in Any PRISTIQ Group) During the On-Therapy Period: Percentage) of Subjects in Short-term, Placebo-controlled MDD Studies

Preferred Term[a]	Placebo[b]	DVS SR 50 mg[c]	DVS SR 100 mg[c]	DVS SR 200 mg[c]	DVS SR 400 mg[c]	DVS SR 50–400 mg[b]
Men only[d]						
Erectile dysfunction	1	3	6	8	11	7
Ejaculation delayed	<1	1	5	7	6	5
Anorgasmia	0	0	3	5	8	4
Libido decreased	1	4	5	6	3	4

(cont'd)

Table 3: PRISTIQ *(cont'd)*

Sexual Dysfunction Adverse Reactions (≥1% in Men or Women in Any PRISTIQ Group) During the On-Therapy Period: Percentage) of Subjects in Short-term, Placebo-controlled MDD Studies

Preferred Term[a]	Placebo[b]	DVS SR 50 mg[c]	DVS SR 100 mg[c]	DVS SR 200 mg[c]	DVS SR 400 mg[c]	DVS SR 50–400 mg[b]
Ejaculation disorder	<1	0	1	2	5	2
Ejaculation failure	0	1	0	2	2	1
Orgasm abnormal	0	0	1	2	3	1
Women only[e]						
Anorgasmia	0	1	1	0	3	1
Libido decreased	<1	1	2	1	1	1
Orgasm abnormal	<1	1	1	1	1	1

[a] Medical Dictionary for Regulatory Activities (MedDRA) terms.
[b] Includes data from all short-term, placebo-controlled studies including fixed-dose and flexible-dose studies.
[c] Only includes data from short-term, placebo-controlled, fixed-dose studies.
[d] Percentage based on the number of men (placebo, n=403; DVS SR 50 mg, n=108; DVS SR 100 mg, n=157; DVS SR 200 mg, n=131; DVS SR 400 mg= 154; DVS SR 50-400 mg, n=723).
[e] Percentage based on the number of women (placebo, n=713; DVS SR 50 mg, n=209; DVS SR 100 mg, n=267; DVS SR 200 mg, n=176; DVS SR 400 mg= 163; DVS SR 50-400 mg, n=1111).

Adverse Drug Reactions—All MDD Clinical Trials: A total of 3292 subjects were exposed to at least 1 dose of PRISTIQ ranging from 50 to 400 mg/day in MDD clinical trials. Long-term safety was evaluated in 1070 subjects in MDD who were exposed to desvenlafaxine succinate for at least 6 months (180 days) and 274 subjects in MDD who were exposed for 1 year (356 days).

The following list is a list of MedDRA preferred terms that reflect adverse events that have been determined to be adverse drug reactions throughout the dose range studied (50 to 400 mg) during any premarketing MDD trials.

Adverse reactions are categorized by system organ class and listed in order of decreasing frequency using the following definitions: very common: ≥10% of patients; common: ≥1% and <10% of patients; uncommon: ≥0.1% and <1% of patients; rare: ≥0.01% and <0.1% of patients; very rare: <0.01% of patients.

Cardiac Disorders: Common: palpitations, tachycardia.
Ear and Labyrinth Disorders: Common: tinnitus.
Eye Disorders: Common: mydriasis, vision blurred.
Gastrointestinal Disorders: Very common: nausea, dry mouth, constipation; Common: vomiting, diarrhea.
General Disorders and Administration Site Conditions: Very common: fatigue; Common: asthenia, chills, feeling jittery, irritability; Uncommon: drug withdrawal syndrome.
Immune System Disorders: Uncommon: hypersensitivity.
Investigations: Common: weight decreased, weight increased, blood pressure increased; Uncommon: blood cholesterol increased, blood prolactin increased, blood triglycerides increased, liver function test abnormal.
Metabolism and Nutrition Disorders: Very common: decreased appetite.
Musculoskeletal, Connective Tissue, and Bone Disorders: Common: musculoskeletal stiffness.
Nervous System Disorders: Very common: headache, dizziness; Common: somnolence, tremor, disturbance in attention, paraesthesia, dysgeusia; Uncommon: syncope; Rare: convulsion, dystonia.
Psychiatric Disorders: Very common: insomnia; Common: orgasm abnormal, anorgasmia, anxiety, nervousness, libido decreased, abnormal dreams; Uncommon: depersonalization, hypomania.
Renal and Urinary Disorders: Common: urinary hesitation; Rare: proteinuria.
Reproductive System and Breast Disorders: Common: erectile dysfunction*, ejaculation delayed*, ejaculation disorder*, ejaculation failure*; Uncommon: sexual dysfunction.
Respiratory, Thoracic, and Mediastinal Disorders: Common: yawning; Uncommon: epistaxis.
Skin and Subcutaneous Tissue Disorders: Very common: hyperhidrosis; Common: rash.
Vascular Disorders: Common: hot flush; Uncommon: orthostatic hypotension.
Ischemic Cardiac Adverse Events: In clinical trials, there were uncommon reports of ischemic cardiac adverse events, including myocardial ischemia, myocardial infarction, and coronary occlusion requiring revascularization; these patients had multiple underlying cardiac risk factors. More patients experienced these events during desvenlafaxine treatment as compared to placebo (see Warnings and Precautions, Cardiovascular/Cerebrovascular).
Discontinuation Symptoms: Adverse drug reactions reported in association with abrupt discontinuation, dose reduction or tapering of treatment in MDD clinical trials at a rate of ≥5% include: dizziness, nausea, headache, irritability, diarrhea, anxiety, abnormal dreams, fatigue, and hyperhidrosis. In general, discontinuation events occurred more frequently with longer duration of therapy (see Dosage and Administration and Warnings and Precautions).
Orthostatic Hypotension: Of the 3292 patients in clinical trials with PRISTIQ, 5% were 65 years of age or older. No overall differences in safety or efficacy were detected between these subjects and younger subjects; however, in the short term placebo-controlled trials, there was a higher incidence of orthostatic hypotension in patients ≥65 years of age compared to patients <65 years of age treated with desvenlafaxine. Greater sensitivity of some older individuals cannot be ruled out. For elderly patients, possible reduced renal clearance of desvenlafaxine should be considered when determining dose (see Dosage and Administration, Dosing Considerations, Geriatrics (≥65 years of age) and Action and Clinical Pharmacology, Geriatrics).
ECG Changes: Electrocardiograms were obtained from 1492 PRISTIQ-treated patients with major depressive disorder and 984 placebo-treated patients in clinical trials lasting up to 8 weeks. No clinically relevant differences were observed between PRISTIQ-treated and placebo-treated patients for QT, QTc, PR, and QRS intervals. In a thorough QTc study with prospectively determined criteria, desvenlafaxine did not cause QT prolongation. No difference was observed between placebo and desvenlafaxine treatments for the QRS interval (see Action and Clinical Pharmacology).

A thorough QTc study was designed to assess the potential effect of 200 and 600 mg of PRISTIQ on QT interval prolongation.

Table 4: PRISTIQ

Estimated and 90% Confidence Interval for QTc Changes from Time-matched Baseline Relative to Placebo at Hour 8 after Dose with Different Heart Rate Corrections[a]

Treatment	Fridericia's QT Correction (ms)	Population QT Correction (ms)
PRISTIQ 200 mg[b]	1.5 (−0.88, 3.88)	3.18 (0.87, 5.50)
PRISTIQ 600 mg[b]	−2.43 (−4.90, 0.04)	0.98 (−1.42, 3.38)
Moxifloxacin 400 mg (Active control)	10.80 (8.44, 13.16)	10.92 (8.62, 13.22)

[a] Mean (90% confidence intervals).
[b] The PRISTIQ doses of 200 and 600 mg were 2 and 6 times the maximum recommended dose, respectively.

Abnormal Hematologic and Clinical Chemistry Findings: Serum Lipids: Elevations in fasting serum total cholesterol, LDL cholesterol, and triglycerides occurred in the controlled trials. Some of these abnormalities were considered potentially clinically significant (see Warnings and Precautions, Serum Cholesterol Elevation and Monitoring and Laboratory Tests, Serum Lipids).

The percentage of subjects who exceeded a predetermined threshold for values of outliers is represented in Table 5.

* Frequency is calculated based on men only.

Table 5: PRISTIQ

Proportion (%) of Subjects With Lipid Abnormalities of Potential Clinical Significance for All Short-term, Placebo-controlled Clinical Trials

		PRISTIQ				
	Placebo[a]	50 mg	100 mg	200 mg	400 mg	50–400 mg[a]
Total Cholesterol Increase ≥1.29 mmol/L and absolute value ≥6.75 mmol/L	2	3	4	4	10	5
LDL Cholesterol Increase ≥1.29 mmol/L and absolute value ≥4.91 mmol/L	<1	1	0	1	2	1
Triglycerides ≥3.7 mmol/L	3	2	1	4	6	3

[a] Includes data from all short-term, placebo-controlled studies including fixed-dose and flexible-dose studies.

Proteinuria: In placebo-controlled studies 6.4% of subjects treated with PRISTIQ, had treatment-emergent proteinuria. Proteinuria was usually of trace amounts, and was not associated with increases in BUN or creatinine or adverse events. The mechanism of the enhanced protein excretion is not clear but may be related to noradrenergic stimulation.
Vital Sign Changes: Table 6 and Table 7 summarize the changes that were observed in placebo-controlled, short-term, premarketing trials with PRISTIQ in patients with MDD.

Table 6: PRISTIQ

Mean Changes, Vital Signs, at Final On-Therapy for All Short-term, Fixed-dose Controlled Trials

		PRISTIQ			
	Placebo	50 mg	100 mg	200 mg	400 mg
Blood Pressure					
Supine systolic bp (mm Hg)	−1.4	1.2	2.0	2.5	2.1
Supine diastolic bp (mm Hg)	−0.6	0.7	0.8	1.8	2.3
Pulse Rate Supine pulse (bpm)	−0.3	1.3	1.3	0.9	4.1
Weight (kg)	0.0	−0.4	−0.6	−0.9	−1.1

At the final on-therapy assessment in the 6-month, double-blind, placebo-controlled phase of a long-term trial in patients who had responded to PRISTIQ during the initial 12-week, open-label phase, there was no statistical difference in mean weight change between PRISTIQ- and placebo-treated patients.

Table 7 provides the incidence of patients meeting criteria for sustained hypertension (defined as treatment-emergent supine diastolic blood pressure ≥90 mm Hg and ≥10 mm Hg above baseline for 3 consecutive visits).

Table 7: PRISTIQ

Incidence (%) of Patients with Sustained Hypertension for All Short-term Fixed-Dose Clinical Trials

		PRISTIQ			
	Placebo	50 mg	100 mg	200 mg	400 mg
Sustained hypertension	0.5	1.3	0.7	1.1	2.3

DRUG INTERACTIONS:

Serious Drug Interactions
Monoamine Oxidase Inhibitors: See Contraindications and Drug-Drug Interactions.

Overview: Selected drug interaction studies were performed. The combination of linear pharmacokinetics, a simple metabolic profile without the potential for CYP polymorphism factors, weak interactions with selected probe substrates, and low protein binding results in a low potential for the interaction of desvenlafaxine with other prescribed medications.
Drug-Drug Interactions: Monoamine Oxidase Inhibitors: Desvenlafaxine succinate is contraindicated in patients taking MAOIs. Desvenlafaxine succinate must not be used in combination with a monoamine oxidase inhibitor (MAOI), or within at least 14 days of discontinuing treatment with an MAOI. Based on the half-life of desvenlafaxine succinate, at least 7 days should be allowed after stopping desvenlafaxine succinate before starting an MAOI (see Contraindications).
Serotonin Syndrome: As with other serotonergic agents, serotonin syndrome, a potentially life-threatening condition, may occur with desvenlafaxine treatment, particularly with concomitant use of other agents that may affect the serotonergic neurotransmitter system (including triptans, SSRIs, other SNRIs, linezolid [an antibiotic which is a reversible non-selective MAOI], lithium, sibutramine, tramadol, or St. John's Wort [Hypericum perforatum], with drugs which impair metabolism of serotonin (including MAOIs; see Contraindications), or with serotonin precursors (such as tryptophan supplements). Serotonin syndrome symptoms may include mental status changes, autonomic instability, neuromuscular aberrations and/or gastrointestinal symptoms (see Warnings and Precautions).

If concomitant treatment of desvenlafaxine with an SSRI, an SNRI or a 5-hydroxytryptamine receptor agonist (triptan) is clinically warranted, careful observation of the patient is advised, particularly during treatment initiation and dose increases. The concomitant use of desvenlafaxine with serotonin precursors is not recommended.
Central Nervous System (CNS) Active Agents: The risk of using desvenlafaxine succinate in combination with other CNS-active drugs has not been systematically evaluated. Consequently, caution is advised when desvenlafaxine succinate is taken in combination with other CNS-active drugs.
Drugs that Interfere with Hemostasis (e.g., NSAIDs, Aspirin, and Warfarin): Serotonin release by platelets plays an important role in hemostasis. Epidemiological studies of case-control and cohort design that have demonstrated an association between use of psychotropic drugs that interfere with serotonin reuptake and the occurrence of upper gastrointestinal bleeding. These studies have also shown that concurrent use of an NSAID or aspirin may potentiate this risk of bleeding. Altered anticoagulant effects, including increased bleeding, have been reported when SSRIs and SNRIs are coadministered with warfarin. Patients receiving warfarin therapy should be carefully monitored when PRISTIQ is initiated or discontinued.
Potential for Other Drugs to Affect Desvenlafaxine Succinate (see also Action and Clinical Pharmacology): Inhibitors of CYP3A4: CYP3A4 is a minor pathway for the metabolism of PRISTIQ. In a clinical study, ketoconazole (200 mg BID) increased the area under the concentration vs. time curve AUC of PRISTIQ (400 mg single dose) by about 43% and C_{max} by about 8%. Concomitant use of PRISTIQ with potent inhibitors of CYP3A4 may result in higher concentrations of PRISTIQ.
Inhibitors of Other CYP Enzymes: Based on in vitro data, drugs that inhibit CYP isozymes 1A1, 1A2, 2A6, 2D6, 2C8, 2C9, 2C19, and 2E1 are not expected to have significant impact on the pharmacokinetic profile of desvenlafaxine.
Potential for Desvenlafaxine to Affect Other Drugs (see also Action and Clinical Pharmacology): Drugs Metabolized by CYP2D6: Clinical studies have shown that desvenlafaxine does not have a clinically relevant effect on CYP2D6 metabolism at the dose of 100 mg daily. When desvenlafaxine succinate was administered at a dose of 100 mg daily in conjunction with a

single 50 mg dose of desipramine, a CYP2D6 substrate, the AUC of desipramine increased approximately 17%. When 400 mg of desvenlafaxine was administered (8 times the recommended 50 mg dose), the AUC of desipramine increased approximately 90%. Concomitant use of desvenlafaxine with a drug metabolized by CYP2D6 may result in higher concentrations of that drug.

Drugs Metabolized by CYP3A4: In vitro, desvenlafaxine does not inhibit or induce the CYP3A4 isozyme.

In a clinical study, PRISTIQ (400 mg daily) was coadministered with a single 4 mg dose of midazolam (a CYP3A4 substrate). The AUC and C_{max} of midazolam decreased by approximately 31% and 16%, respectively. Concomitant use of PRISTIQ with a drug metabolized by CYP3A4 may result in lower exposure to that drug.

Drugs Metabolized by CYP1A2, 2A6, 2C8, 2C9 and 2C19: In vitro, desvenlafaxine does not inhibit CYP1A2, 2A6, 2C8, 2C9, and 2C19 isozymes and would not be expected to affect the pharmacokinetics of drugs that are metabolized by these CYP isozymes.

P-glycoprotein Transporter: In vitro, desvenlafaxine is not a substrate or an inhibitor for the P-glycoprotein transporter.

The pharmacokinetics of desvenlafaxine are unlikely to be affected by drugs that inhibit the P-glycoprotein transporter and desvenlafaxine is not likely to affect the pharmacokinetics of drugs that are substrates of the P-glycoprotein transporter.

Drug-Food Interactions: Food does not alter the bioavailability of desvenlafaxine.

Drug-Herb Interactions: St. John's Wort: In common with SSRIs, pharmacodynamic interactions between PRISTIQ and the herbal remedy St. John's Wort may occur and may result in an increase in undesirable effects (see Drug Interactions, Serotonin Syndrome).

Drug-Lifestyle Interactions: Ethanol: As with all CNS-active drugs, patients should be advised to avoid alcohol consumption while taking desvenlafaxine succinate.

Interference with Cognitive and Motor Performance: A clinical study that assessed the effects of desvenlafaxine on behavioral performance of healthy individuals did not reveal clinically significant impairment of psychomotor, cognitive, or complex behavior performance. However, since any CNS-active drug may impair judgment, thinking, or motor skills, patients should be cautioned about operating hazardous machinery, including automobiles, until they are reasonably certain that PRISTIQ therapy does not adversely affect their ability to engage in such activities.

DOSAGE AND ADMINISTRATION:

General: PRISTIQ is not indicated for use in children under 18 years of age (see Warnings and Precautions, Potential Association with Behavioral and Emotional Changes, Including Self-harm).

Recommended Dose and Dosage Adjustment: Initial Treatment: The recommended dose of PRISTIQ desvenlafaxine succinate extended-release tablets is 50 mg once daily, with or without food. In clinical studies, no additional benefit was demonstrated at doses greater than 50 mg/day. In clinical studies, doses of 50-400 mg/day were shown to be effective, although no additional benefit was demonstrated at doses greater than 50 mg/day, and adverse events and discontinuations were more frequent at higher doses. If the physician, based on clinical judgment, decides a dose increase above 50 mg/day is warranted for an individual patient the maximum dose should not exceed 100 mg/day. Patients should be periodically reassessed to determine the need for continued treatment.

It is recommended that PRISTIQ be taken at approximately the same time each day.

PRISTIQ tablets must be swallowed whole with liquids, and must not be chewed, divided or crushed. The medication is contained within a non-absorbable shell designed to release the drug at a controlled rate. The tablet shell, along with insoluble core components, is eliminated from the body; patients should not be concerned if they occasionally notice something that looks like a tablet in their stool. Due to the controlled-release design, PRISTIQ tablets should only be used in patients who are able to swallow the tablets whole.

Missed Dose: A patient missing a dose should take it as soon as they remember to. If it is almost time for the next dose, the missed dose should be skipped. The patient should be cautioned against taking two doses concomitantly to "make up" for the missed dose.

Discontinuing PRISTIQ: Symptoms associated with discontinuation of PRISTIQ, other SNRIs and SSRIs have been reported (see Warnings and Precautions, Discontinuation Symptoms and Adverse Reactions, Discontinuation Symptoms). Patients should be monitored for these symptoms when discontinuing treatment. A gradual reduction in the dose rather than abrupt cessation is recommended whenever possible. If intolerable symptoms occur following a decrease in the dose or upon discontinuation of treatment, then resuming the previously prescribed dose may be considered. Subsequently, the physician may continue decreasing the dose, but at a more gradual rate. As the lowest dosage strength of PRISTIQ is 50 mg, it is recommended that dose reduction from 50 mg/day should proceed to 50 mg every other day before discontinuation.

Dosing Considerations: Patients with Severe Renal Impairment and End-stage Renal Disease: The recommended dose in patients with severe renal impairment (24-hr CrCl <30 mL/min) or end-stage renal disease (ESRD) is 50 mg every other day. Because of individual variability in clearance in these patients, individualization of dosage may be desirable. Supplemental doses should not be given to patients after dialysis (see Action and Clinical Pharmacology, Renal Insufficiency).

Use in Patients with Hepatic Impairment: No dosage adjustment is necessary for patients with hepatic impairment (see Action and Clinical Pharmacology, Hepatic Insufficiency).

Geriatrics (≥65 years of age): No dosage adjustment is required solely on the basis of age; however, possible reduced clearance of PRISTIQ should be considered when determining dose (see Action and Clinical Pharmacology, Geriatrics).

Switching Patients To or From a Monoamine Oxidase Inhibitor: At least 14 days should elapse between discontinuation of an MAOI and initiation of therapy with desvenlafaxine succinate. In addition, based on the half-life of desvenlafaxine succinate, at least 7 days should be allowed after stopping desvenlafaxine succinate before starting an MAOI.

Discontinuation of Therapy: A gradual reduction in the dose rather than abrupt cessation is recommended whenever possible. Discontinuation regimens should take into account the individual circumstances of the patient, such as duration of treatment and dose at discontinuation (see Warnings and Precautions and Adverse Reactions).

OVERDOSAGE:

Human Experience: There is limited clinical experience with desvenlafaxine succinate overdosage in humans. In pre-marketing clinical trials, no cases of fatal acute overdose of desvenlafaxine succinate were reported.

Among the patients included in the pre-marketing major depressive disorder trials of desvenlafaxine succinate, there were four adults who ingested doses over 800 mg of desvenlafaxine (4000 mg [desvenlafaxine alone], 900, 1800 and 5200 mg [in combination with other drugs]); all patients recovered. In addition, a patient's 11 month-old child accidentally ingested 600 mg of desvenlafaxine, was treated and recovered.

The adverse reactions reported within 5 days of an overdose >600 mg that were possibly related to desvenlafaxine included: headache, vomiting, agitation, dizziness, nausea, constipation, diarrhea, dry mouth, paresthesia, and tachycardia.

Desvenlafaxine is the major active metabolite of venlafaxine. Overdose experience reported with venlafaxine (the parent drug of desvenlafaxine) is presented below; the identical information can be found in the Overdosage section of the venlafaxine package insert Product Monograph.

Post-marketing Experience with EFFEXOR: In post-marketing experience, overdose with venlafaxine was reported predominantly in combination with alcohol and/or other drugs. The most commonly reported events in overdose include tachycardia, changes in level of consciousness (ranging from somnolence to coma), mydriasis, convulsion, and vomiting. Electrocardiographic changes (e.g., prolongation of QT interval, bundle branch block, QRS prolongation), ventricular tachycardia, bradycardia, hypotension, delayed rise in plasma creatine kinase levels, rhabdomyolysis, liver necrosis, serotonin syndrome, vertigo, and death have been reported. Muscle enzymes should be monitored in patients with venlafaxine overdose to detect development of rhabdomyolysis at an early stage and to initiate appropriate treatment. According to post-marketing overdose reports with venlafaxine (where overdose amounts were provided) fatal acute overdoses have been reported with venlafaxine alone at doses as low as approximately 1 gram.

Published retrospective studies report that venlafaxine overdosage may be associated with an increased risk of fatal outcomes compared to that observed with SSRI antidepressant products, but lower than that for tricyclic antidepressants. Epidemiological studies have shown that venlafaxine-treated patients have a higher burden of suicide risk factors than SSRI patients. The extent to which the finding of an increased risk of fatal outcomes can be attributed to the toxicity of venlafaxine in overdosage as opposed to some characteristics of venlafaxine-treated patients is not clear.

Prescriptions for PRISTIQ should be written for the smallest quantity of drug consistent with good patient management, in order to reduce the risk of overdose.

Management of Overdosage: Treatment should consist of those general measures employed in the management of overdosage with any SSRI/SNRI.

Induction of emesis is not recommended. Because of the moderate volume of distribution of this drug, forced diuresis, dialysis, hemoperfusion, and exchange transfusion are unlikely to be of benefit. No specific antidotes for desvenlafaxine are known.

Ensure an adequate airway, oxygenation, and ventilation. Monitor cardiac rhythm and vital signs. General supportive and symptomatic measures are also recommended. Gastric lavage with a large-bore orogastric tube with appropriate airway protection, if needed, may be indicated if performed soon after ingestion or in symptomatic patients. Activated charcoal should be administered.

In managing an overdose, consider the possibility of multiple drug involvement. The physician should consider contacting a poison control center for additional information on the treatment of any overdose.

> For management of a suspected drug overdose, CPhA recommends that you contact your **regional Poison Control Centre**. See the *CPS* Directory section for a list of Poison Control Centres.

ACTION AND CLINICAL PHARMACOLOGY: Mechanism of Action: Desvenlafaxine is the major active metabolite of venlafaxine which is also approved for treatment of depression. Preclinical studies have shown that desvenlafaxine succinate is a selective serotonin and norepinephrine reuptake inhibitor. The clinical efficacy of desvenlafaxine succinate is thought to be related to the potentiation of these neurotransmitters in the central nervous system.

Pharmacodynamics: Desvenlafaxine lacked significant affinity for numerous receptors, including muscarinic-cholinergic, H_1-histaminergic, or α_1-adrenergic receptors in vitro. Desvenlafaxine also lacked significant affinity for various ion channels, including calcium, chloride, potassium and sodium ion channels and also lacked monoamine oxidase (MAO) inhibitory activity. Desvenlafaxine lacked significant activity in the in vitro cardiac potassium channel (hERG) assay.

Pharmacokinetics: The single dose pharmacokinetics of desvenlafaxine are linear and dose-proportional in a dose range of 100 to 600 mg/day. The mean terminal half-life, $t_{1/2}$, is approximately 11 hours. With once-daily dosing, steady-state plasma concentrations are achieved within approximately 4-5 days. At steady state, multiple-dose accumulation of desvenlafaxine is linear and predictable from the single-dose pharmacokinetic profile.

The pharmacokinetics of desvenlafaxine have been thoroughly evaluated in women and men. There are minimal differences based on gender; data from all subjects are presented below.

Absorption and Distribution: The absolute oral bioavailability of PRISTIQ after oral administration is about 80%. Mean time to peak plasma concentrations (t_{max}) is about 7.5 hours after oral administration.

A food-effect study involving administration of PRISTIQ to healthy volunteers under fasting and fed conditions (high-fat meal) indicated that the C_{max} was increased about 16% in the fed state, while the AUCs were similar. This difference is not clinically significant; therefore, PRISTIQ can be taken without regard to meals.

The plasma protein binding of desvenlafaxine is low (30%) and is independent of drug concentration. Desvenlafaxine's volume of distribution at steady-state following intravenous administration is 3.4 L/kg, indicating distribution into nonvascular compartments.

Metabolism and Excretion: Desvenlafaxine is primarily metabolized by conjugation (mediated by UGT isoforms) and, to a minor extent, through oxidative metabolism. CYP3A4 is the cytochrome P450 isozyme mediating the oxidative metabolism (N-demethylation) of desvenlafaxine. Approximately 45% of desvenlafaxine is excreted unchanged in urine at 72 hours after oral administration. Approximately 19% of the administered dose is excreted as the glucuronide metabolite and <5% as the oxidative metabolite (N,O-didesmethylvenlafaxine) in urine.

Residual Inert Matrix Tablet: Patients receiving PRISTIQ may notice an inert matrix tablet passing in the stool or via colostomy. Patients should be informed that the active medication has already been absorbed by the time the patient sees the inert matrix tablet.

Special Populations and Conditions: Gender: In a trial of healthy subjects administered doses up to of 300 mg, women had an approximately 25% higher C_{max} and an approximately 10% higher AUC than age-matched men. No adjustment of dosage on the basis of gender is needed.

Pediatrics: PRISTIQ is not indicated for use in children and adolescents.

Geriatrics: In a trial of healthy subjects administered doses of up to 300 mg, there was an approximate 32% increase in C_{max} and a 55% increase in AUC in subjects older than 75 years of age (n=17), compared with subjects 18 to 45 years of age (n=16). Subjects 65 to 75 years of age (n=15) had no change in C_{max} but an approximately 32% increase in AUC, compared to subjects 18 to 45 years of age. No dosage adjustment is required solely on the basis of age; however, possible reduced renal clearance of desvenlafaxine should be considered when determining dose.

Race: Pharmacokinetic analysis on the basis of race (White, N=466; Black, N=97; Hispanic, N=39; Other, N=33) did not demonstrate an effect on the pharmacokinetics of PRISTIQ. No adjustment of dosage on the basis of race is needed.

Hepatic Insufficiency: The disposition of desvenlafaxine succinate after administration of 100 mg was studied in subjects with mild (Child-Pugh A, n=8), moderate (Child-Pugh B, n=8), and severe (Child-Pugh C, n=8) hepatic impairment and to healthy subjects (n=12). Average AUC was increased by approximately 31% and 35% in patients with moderate and severe hepatic impairment, respectively, as compared to healthy subjects. Average AUC values were similar in subjects with mild hepatic impairment and healthy subjects (<5% difference).

Systemic clearance (CL/F) was decreased by approximately 20% and 36% in patients with moderate and severe hepatic impairment, respectively, as compared to healthy subjects. CL/F values were comparable in mild hepatic impairment and healthy subjects (<5% difference).

The mean $t_{1/2}$ changed from approximately 10 hours in healthy subjects and subjects with mild hepatic impairment to 13 and 14 hours in moderate and severe hepatic impairment, respectively. No dosage adjustment is necessary for patients with hepatic impairment.

Renal Insufficiency: The disposition of desvenlafaxine after administration of 100 mg was studied in subjects with mild (n=9), moderate (n=8), severe (n=7) and end-stage renal disease (ESRD) requiring dialysis (n=9) and in healthy, age-matched control subjects (n=8). Elimination was significantly correlated with creatinine clearance. Increases in AUCs of about 42% in mild renal impairment, about 56% in moderate renal impairment, about 108% in severe renal impairment, and about 116% in ESRD subjects were observed, compared with healthy, age-matched, control subjects.

The mean terminal half-life ($t_{1/2}$) was prolonged from 11.1 hours in the control subjects to approximately 13.5, 15.5, 17.6, and 22.8 hours in mild, moderate, severe renal impairment and ESRD subjects, respectively. Less than 5% of the drug in the body was cleared during a standard 4-hour hemodialysis procedure. Therefore, supplemental doses should not be given to patients after dialysis.

Dosage adjustment is recommended in patients with significant impairment of renal function (see Dosage and Administration, Patients with Severe Renal Impairment and End-stage Renal Disease).

STORAGE AND STABILITY: Store at 15 to 30°C; excursions permitted to 40°C.

SPECIAL HANDLING INSTRUCTIONS: None.

INFORMATION FOR THE PATIENT: Published in e-CPS, available by subscription at www.e-cps.ca.

DOSAGE FORMS, COMPOSITION AND PACKAGING: 50 mg: Each extended-release, light pink, square pyramid tablet debossed with "W" over "50" on the flat side, contains: desvenlafaxine succinate 50 mg. Nonmedicinal ingredients: hypromellose, magnesium stearate, microcrystalline cellulose and talc; film coating: dextrose, iron oxides, maltodextrin, sodium carboxymethylcellulose, stearic acid and titanium dioxide. HDPE bottles of 14, 30 and 90. Unit dose blisters of 7, 14 and 28.

100 mg: Each extended-release, reddish-orange, square pyramid tablet debossed with "W" over "100" on the flat side, contains: desvenlafaxine succinate 100 mg. Nonmedicinal ingredients: hypromellose, magnesium stearate, microcrystalline cellulose and talc; film coating: dextrose, iron oxides, maltodextrin, sodium carboxymethylcellulose, stearic acid and titanium dioxide. HDPE bottles of 14, 30 and 90. Unit dose blisters of 7, 14 and 28.

Privigen®

immune globulin intravenous (human)

Passive Immunizing Agent

CSL Behring

Date of Revision: February 9, 2010

SUMMARY PRODUCT INFORMATION:

Route of Administration	Dosage Form/ Strength	Clinically Relevant Nonmedicinal Ingredients
Intravenous	10% Solution for infusion	L-Proline For a complete listing see Dosage Forms, Composition and Packaging.

DESCRIPTION: Privigen, Immune Globulin Intravenous (Human), is a ready-to-use, sterile, 10% protein liquid preparation of polyvalent human immunoglobulin G (IgG) for intravenous administration. Privigen is prepared from large pools of human plasma by a combination of cold ethanol fractionation, octanoic acid fractionation, combined with a filter aid-assisted depth filtration, and anion exchange chromatography.

INDICATIONS AND CLINICAL USE: Privigen (Immune Globulin Intravenous (Human)) is indicated for:

- The treatment of patients with primary immune deficiency (PID) and secondary immune deficiency (SID). This includes, but is not limited to, common variable immunodeficiency (CVID), X-linked agammaglobulinemia, congenital agammaglobulinemia, secondary hypogammaglobulinemia, Wiskott-Aldrich syndrome, and severe combined immunodeficiencies.
- The treatment of patients with immune thrombocytopenic purpura (ITP) to rapidly raise platelet counts to prevent bleeding.

Geriatrics: See Warnings and Precautions, Special Populations.
Pediatrics: See Warnings and Precautions, Special Populations.

CONTRAINDICATIONS: Privigen is contraindicated in individuals with selective IgA deficiency with known anti-IgA antibodies. Privigen contains trace amounts of IgA (average 2.7 μg/mL).

Privigen is contraindicated in patients who have had an anaphylactic or severe systemic reaction to the administration of human immune globulin.

Because it contains the stabilizer L-proline, Privigen is contraindicated in patients with hyperprolinemia.

WARNINGS AND PRECAUTIONS:

Serious Warnings and Precautions
Immune Globulin Intravenous (Human) (IGIV) products have been reported to be associated with renal dysfunction, acute renal failure, osmotic nephrosis, and death. Patients predisposed to acute renal failure include patients with any degree of pre-existing renal insufficiency, diabetes mellitus, age greater than 65, volume depletion, sepsis, paraproteinemia, or patients receiving known nephrotoxic drugs. In such patients, IGIV products should be administered at the minimum rate of infusion practicable. While these reports of renal dysfunction and acute renal failure have been associated with the use of many of the licensed IGIV products, those containing sucrose as a stabilizer accounted for a disproportionate share of the total number. Privigen does not contain carbohydrates as stabilizers (e.g., sucrose, maltose). (See Dosage and Administration and Warnings and Precautions for important information intended to reduce the risk of acute renal failure.)

General: Privigen is made from human plasma. Products made from human plasma may contain infectious agents, e.g., viruses, and theoretically the Creutzfeldt-Jakob disease (CJD) agent, that can cause disease. The risk that such products will transmit an infectious agent has been reduced by screening plasma donors for prior exposure to certain viruses, by testing for the presence of certain current virus infections, and by removing certain viruses during manufacturing through a four step process: octanoic acid fractionation combined with a filter aid-assisted depth filtration, virus filtration and inactivation by pH 4 incubation as well as additional depth filtration.

Despite these measures, such products can still potentially transmit disease. There is also the possibility that unknown infectious agents may be present in such products. All infections thought by a physician possibly to have been transmitted by this product should be reported by the physician or other healthcare provider to CSL Behring at 1-613-783-1892. The physician should discuss the risks and benefits of this product with the patient.

Cardiovascular: Thrombotic events have been reported in association with IGIV. Patients at risk may include those with a history of atherosclerosis, hypercoagulable disorders, prolonged periods of immobilization, multiple cardiovascular risk factors, advanced age, impaired cardiac output, and/or known or suspected hyperviscosity. The potential risks and benefits of IGIV should be weighed against those of alternative therapies in all patients for whom IGIV administration is being considered.

Because of the potentially increased risk of thrombosis, baseline assessment of blood viscosity should be considered in patients at risk of hyperviscosity, including those with cryoglobulins, fasting chylomicronemia/markedly high triglycerides, or monoclonal gammopathies.

Hematologic: IGIV products can contain blood group antibodies that may act as hemolysins and induce in vivo coating of red blood cells (RBCs) with immunoglobulin, causing a positive direct antiglobulin reaction. Hemolysis, possibly intravascular, occurred in two subjects treated with Privigen in the ITP study. These cases resolved uneventfully. Six other subjects experienced hemolysis in the ITP study as documented from clinical laboratory data.

IGIV recipients should be monitored for clinical signs and symptoms of hemolysis. If signs and/or symptoms of hemolysis are present after IGIV infusion, appropriate confirmatory laboratory testing should be performed.

Neurologic: Aseptic Meningitis Syndrome (AMS) has been reported to occur infrequently in association with IGIV treatment. The syndrome usually begins within several hours to 2 days following IGIV treatment. AMS is characterized by signs and symptoms including severe headache, nuchal rigidity, drowsiness, fever, photophobia, painful eye movements, nausea, and vomiting. Cerebrospinal fluid (CSF) studies are frequently positive with pleocytosis up to several thousand cells per cubic millimeter, predominantly from the granulocyte series, and with elevated protein levels up to several hundred mg/dL. Patients exhibiting such signs and symptoms should receive a thorough neurological examination, including CSF studies, to rule out other causes of meningitis. AMS may occur more frequently in association with high doses (2 g/kg bw) and/or rapid infusion of IGIV. Discontinuation of IGIV treatment has resulted in remission of AMS within several days without sequelae.

Renal: Patients should not be volume depleted prior to the initiation of the infusion of Privigen. Periodic monitoring of renal function and urine output is particularly important in patients judged to have a potential increased risk of developing acute renal failure. Renal function, including measurement of blood urea nitrogen (BUN) and serum creatinine, should be assessed before the initial infusion of Privigen and at appropriate intervals thereafter. For patients judged to be at risk of developing renal dysfunction, Privigen should be administered at the minimum rate of infusion practicable (see Dosage and Administration). If renal function deteriorates, consider discontinuing Privigen.

Respiratory: There have been reports of noncardiogenic pulmonary edema in patients administered IGIV. Transfusion-related Acute Lung Injury (TRALI) is characterized by severe respiratory distress, pulmonary edema, hypoxemia, normal left ventricular function, and fever and typically occurs within 1 to 6 hours following transfusion. IGIV recipients should be monitored for pulmonary adverse reactions. Patients with TRALI may be managed using oxygen therapy with adequate ventilatory support.

If TRALI is suspected, appropriate tests should be performed for the presence of antineutrophil antibodies in both product and the patient's serum.

Special Populations: Pregnant Women: The safety of Privigen for use in human pregnancy has not been established in controlled clinical trials; consequently, it should only be used in pregnant women when the benefits outweigh the risks associated with its use.

Nursing Women: Immunoglobulins are excreted into the milk. Privigen should only be used in nursing woman when the benefits outweigh the risk associated with its use.

Pediatrics (3-16 years of age): Treatment of Primary and Secondary Immune Deficiency: In the pivotal study, Privigen was evaluated in 31 pediatric subjects (19 children and 12 adolescents) with PID. In the extension study, there were 21 pediatric subjects evaluated (13 children and 8 adolescents) of which 19 were carried forward from the pivotal study. There were no apparent differences in the safety and efficacy profiles as compared to adult subjects. No pediatric-specific dose requirements were necessary to achieve the desired serum IgG levels. The safety and efficacy of Privigen has not been established in pediatric subjects with PID who are under the age of 3.

Treatment of Immune Thrombocytopenic Purpura: The safety and effectiveness of Privigen has not been established in pediatric subjects with ITP who are under the age of 15.

Geriatrics: Privigen should be used with caution in patients over 65 years of age who are judged to be at increased risk of developing renal insufficiency (see Box Serious Warnings and Warnings and Precautions). For those patients with the risk of renal insufficiencies, Privigen must be infused at the minimum practicable rate.

Clinical studies of Privigen did not include sufficient numbers of subjects aged 65 and over to determine whether they respond differently from younger subjects.

Monitoring and Laboratory Tests: The patient's vital signs should be observed and monitored carefully throughout the infusion. If side effects occur, the infusion should be slowed or stopped until the symptoms subside. The infusion may then be resumed at a lower rate that is comfortable for the patient. After infusion of IgG, the transitory rise of the various passively transferred antibodies in the patient's blood may yield positive serological testing results, with the potential for misleading interpretation. Passive transmission of antibodies to erythrocyte antigens (e.g., A, B, and D) may cause a positive direct or indirect antiglobulin (Coombs') test.

ADVERSE REACTIONS: Adverse Drug Reaction Overview: In clinical trials undertaken with Privigen, the most serious adverse reactions observed in patients receiving Privigen for the PID were hypersensitivity in one subject. The most serious adverse reactions observed in patients receiving Privigen for ITP were aseptic meningitis syndrome in one subject and anemia in two other ITP subjects (see Warnings and Precautions). The most common adverse reaction observed for both PID and ITP was headache. In general, reported adverse reactions to Privigen in subjects with either PID or ITP were similar in kind and frequency to those observed with other IGIV products.

Clinical Trial Adverse Drug Reactions: Because clinical studies are conducted under widely varying conditions, adverse reaction rates observed cannot be directly compared to rates in other clinical trials and may not reflect the rates observed in practice.

Treatment of Primary and Secondary Immune Deficiency: Pivotal Study: In a prospective, open-label, single-arm, multicenter clinical study, 80 subjects with PID received median doses of Privigen ranging from 200 to 888 mg/kg bw every 3 weeks (median dose 428.3 mg/kg bw) or 4 weeks (median dose 440.6 mg/kg bw) for up to 12 months.

Routine premedication was not allowed. However, subjects who experienced two consecutive infusion-related adverse events (AEs) that were likely to be prevented by premedication were permitted to receive antipyretics, antihistamines, NSAIDs, or antiemetic agents. During the study, 8 (10%) subjects received premedication prior to 51 (4.9%) of the 1038 infusions administered.

The safety endpoint of the study was the proportion of infusions with one or more temporally associated AEs. Temporally associated AEs are those occurring during or within 72 hours after the end of an infusion, irrespective of causality.

A target for this safety endpoint is an upper 1-sided confidence limit of less than 40%. In this study, the upper bound of the 1-sided 97.5% confidence interval for the proportion of Privigen infusions with temporally associated AEs was 23.8%, thus well below the target for this safety endpoint.

Table 1 summarizes the proportion of Privigen infusions resulting in temporally associated AEs and the number and rate of temporally associated AEs, **irrespective of causality**.

Table 1: Privigen

Privigen Infusions with Temporally Associated Adverse Events[a] (TAAEs) in Subjects with PID, Irrespective of Causality

	TAAEs[a] Occurring During or Within the Specified Number of Hours After the End of an Infusion		
Total Number of Infusions: 1038	**24 Hours**	**48 Hours**	**72 Hours**
Proportion of infusions with TAAEs	16%	19%	21%
Upper bound of 1-sided 97.5% confidence interval for the proportion of infusions with TAAEs	18.7%	21.5%	23.8%
Total number of TAAEs	282	353	396
Rate of TAAEs (per total number of infusions)	0.27	0.34	0.38

[a] Including infections.

Table 2 lists the temporally associated AEs that occurred in more than 5% of subjects during or within 72 hours after the end of a Privigen infusion, **irrespective of causality**.

Table 2: Privigen

Temporally Associated Adverse Events[a] (TAAEs) in >5% of Subjects with PID During or Within 72 Hours After the End of an Privigen Infusion, Irrespective of Causality

TAAE[a]	Subjects (%) (n=80)	Infusions (%) (n=1038)
Headache	35 (43.8)	90 (8.7)
Fatigue	13 (16.3)	29 (2.8)
Nausea	10 (12.5)	22 (2.1)
Chills	9 (11.3)	15 (1.4)
Back pain	8 (10.0)	14 (1.3)
Pain	7 (8.8)	14 (1.3)
Vomiting	7 (8.8)	13 (1.3)
Pyrexia	6 (7.5)	11 (1.1)
Cough	5 (6.3)	5 (0.5)
Diarrhea	5 (6.3)	5 (0.5)
Stomach discomfort	5 (6.3)	5 (0.5)

[a] Excluding infections.

Table 3 lists the **related** temporally associated AEs that occurred in more than 5% of subjects with PID during or within 72 hours after the end of a Privigen infusion. Related AEs were defined as those judged by the investigators to be "at least possibly" causally related to the infusion of Privigen.

Table 3: Privigen

Related Temporally Associated Adverse Events (TAAEs) in >5% of Subjects with PID During or Within 72 Hours After the End of a Privigen Infusion

Related TAAE	Subjects (%) (n=80)	Infusions (%) (n=1038)
Headache	23 (28.8)	64 (6.2)
Nausea	9 (11.3)	20 (1.9)
Fatigue	9 (11.3)	18 (1.7)
Chills	9 (11.3)	15 (1.4)
Pain	5 (6.3)	9 (0.9)

Sixteen subjects (20%) experienced 38 serious AEs. Five of these were severe AEs (hypersensitivity, chills, fatigue, dizziness, and increased body temperature) that occurred in one subject. All five were related to Privigen and resulted in the subject's withdrawal from the study. Two other subjects withdrew from the study due to AEs related to Privigen (chills and headache in one subject; vomiting in the other). One subject died due to multiple organ system failure, which was not related to Privigen.

Of the 1330 AEs reported, the investigators judged 215 to be related to the infusion of Privigen (including the five serious, severe AEs described above). Of the 210 non-serious AEs, 104 were mild, 89 were moderate, 16 were severe, and 1 was not ranked ("unknown").

During this study, no subjects tested positive for infection due to human immunodeficiency virus (HIV), hepatitis B virus (HBV), hepatitis C virus (HCV), or B19 virus (B19V).

Extension Study: During an extension of the pivotal study, higher infusion rates were permitted and additional efficacy, safety and tolerability data were collected. This study included original subjects from the pivotal study (n=45) and new subjects who were previously receiving another IGIV product (n=10). Only subjects who continued from the pivotal study were permitted to receive a Higher Infusion Rate (HIR) at the discretion of the investigator. Twenty-three of 45 subjects (51.1%) received 265 (38.4%) infusions at a maximum rate greater than 8 mg/kg/min (median: 12 mg/kg/min; maximum: 16 mg/kg/min) with 97% of infusions in the HIR group reaching a maximum infusion rate of 12 mg/kg/min.

When analyzed by infusion rate class (i.e., LIR vs. HIR), the proportion of infusions with TAAEs (72 hours) was considerably lower with HIR infusions than with LIR infusions (0.072 vs. 0.192), as was also seen in the rate of TAAEs per infusion. Overall, this reflects both the study design and the clinical practice to increase the infusion rate according to patient tolerance.

Twenty-two subjects remained on the high infusion rate; one subject withdrew from the study due to urticaria, which was mild, but was considered drug-related. Due to the small population size in the clinical trial, the safety and tolerability of Privigen administered at a higher infusion rate of 12 mg/kg/min should be monitored by users.

Treatment of Immune Thrombocytopenic Purpura: In a prospective, open-label, single-arm, multicenter clinical study, 57 subjects with ITP received a 2 g/kg bw dose of Privigen administered as two 1 g/kg bw intravenous infusions on two consecutive days.

Two of the 57 ITP subjects experienced hemolysis. These cases resolved uneventfully. Six other subjects experienced laboratory signs for hemolysis without clinical relevance. All 8 subjects developed a transient positive direct Coombs´ test.

Concomitant medications affecting platelets or other treatments for ITP were not allowed. Thirty-two (56.1%) subjects received premedication with acetaminophen and/or an antihistamine.

Table 4 lists the temporally associated AEs that occurred in more than 5% of subjects with ITP during or within 72 hours after the end of a treatment cycle (two consecutive infusions) with Privigen, **irrespective of causality**.

Table 4: Privigen

Temporally Associated Adverse Events (TAAEs) in >5% Subjects with ITP During or Within 72 hours After the End of a Treatment Cycle[a] with Privigen, Irrespective of Causality

TAAE	Subjects (%) (n=57)
Headache	37 (64.9)
Pyrexia	14 (24.6)
Nausea	6 (10.5)
Vomiting	6 (10.5)
Epistaxis	6 (10.5)
Hyperthermia	5 (8.8)
Bilirubin conjugated increased	5 (8.8)
Blood bilirubin unconjugated increased	5 (8.8)
Hyperbilirubinemia	3 (5.3)
Hematocrit decreased	3 (5.3)

[a] Two consecutive infusions.

Table 5 lists all **related** AEs that occurred in more than 5% of subjects with ITP during and/or following a treatment cycle with Privigen. Related AEs were defined as those judged by the investigators to be "at least possibly" causally related to the infusion of Privigen.

Table 5: Privigen

Related Adverse Events[a] in >5% of Subjects with ITP During and/or Following a Treatment Cycle[b] with Privigen

Related AE[a]	Subjects (%) (n=57)
Headache	37 (64.9)
Pyrexia	14 (24.6)
Anemia	6 (10.5)
Hyperthermia	5 (8.8)
Nausea	5 (8.8)
Vomiting	5 (8.8)
Bilirubin conjugated increased	5 (8.8)
Blood bilirubin unconjugated increased	5 (8.8)
Blood lactate dehydrogenase increased	3 (5.3)
Coombs' direct test positive	3 (5.3)
Coombs' test positive	3 (5.3)
Hematocrit decreased	3 (5.3)
Hyperbilirubinemia	3 (5.3)

[a] Includes all related AEs, including those beyond 72 hours after end of last infusion.
[b] Two consecutive infusions.

Three subjects experienced three serious AEs, one of which (aseptic meningitis) was related to the infusion of Privigen. One subject withdrew from the study due to gingival bleeding, which was not related to Privigen. Two subjects experienced transient drug-related non-serious hemolytic reactions manifested as anemia and a positive direct Coombs' test.

Of the 270 AEs reported, 256 (94.8%) were mild to moderate in severity and transient in nature. The investigators judged 174 of the 270 AEs reported to be related to the infusion of Privigen.

Post-Market Adverse Drug Reactions: Adverse reactions reported during worldwide post-marketing use of Privigen do not differ from what is known for IGIV products or from what has been observed in clinical studies with Privigen.

The following mild to moderate reactions may occur with the administration of IGIV products: headache, diarrhea, tachycardia, fever, fatigue, dizziness, malaise, chills, flushing, skin reactions, wheezing or chest tightness, nausea, vomiting, rigors, back pain, chest pain, myalgia, arthralgia, and changes in blood pressure. Immediate hypersensitivity and anaphylactic reactions are also a possibility.

The following adverse reactions have been identified and reported during the postapproval use of IGIV products.

Respiratory: apnea, Acute Respiratory Distress Syndrome (ARDS), TRALI, cyanosis, hypoxemia, pulmonary edema, dyspnea, bronchospasm.
Cardiovascular: cardiac arrest, thromboembolism, vascular collapse, hypotension.
Neurological: coma, loss of consciousness, seizures, tremor, aseptic meningitis.
Integumentary: Stevens-Johnson syndrome, epidermolysis, erythema multiforme, bullous dermatitis.
Hematologic: pancytopenia, leukopenia, hemolysis, positive direct antiglobulin (Coombs') test, hemolytic anemia.
General/Body as a Whole: pyrexia, rigors.
Musculoskeletal: back pain.
Gastrointestinal: hepatic dysfunction, abdominal pain.

Because postmarketing reporting of adverse reactions is voluntary and from a population of uncertain size, it is not always possible to reliably estimate the frequency of these reactions or establish a causal relationship to drug exposure. Evaluation and interpretation of these postmarketing reactions is confounded by underlying diagnosis, concomitant medications, pre-existing conditions, and inherent limitations of passive surveillance.

DRUG INTERACTIONS: Overview: Immunoglobulin administration may transiently impair the efficacy of live attenuated virus vaccines such as measles, mumps, and rubella. The immunizing physician should be informed of recent therapy with Privigen so that appropriate measures may be taken.
Drug-Drug Interactions: See Overview.
Drug-Food Interactions: Interactions with food have not been established.
Drug-Herb Interactions: Interactions with herbal products have not been established.
Drug-Laboratory Test Interactions: See Monitoring and Laboratory Tests.

DOSAGE AND ADMINISTRATION: Ensure that patients with pre-existing renal insufficiency and those predisposed to acute renal failure are not volume depleted before administering Privigen (see Box Serious Warnings and Precautions and Warnings and Precautions).

The patient's vital signs should be observed and monitored carefully throughout the infusion. If side effects occur, the infusion should be slowed or stopped until the symptoms subside. The infusion may then be resumed at a lower rate that is comfortable for the patient.

Recommended Dose and Dosage Adjustment: Treatment of Primary and Secondary Immune Deficiency: The usual dose of Privigen for patients with PID and SID is 200 to 800 mg/kg body weight (bw), administered every 3 to 4 weeks. A target serum immunoglobulin G (IgG) trough level of at least 5 g/L has been proposed. However, an optimum level has not been established in randomized, controlled clinical studies. Doses should be adjusted to achieve the desired serum trough levels and clinical responses.

Treatment of Immune Thrombocytopenic Purpura: The usual dose of Privigen for patients with ITP is 1 g/kg bw administered for 2 consecutive days, resulting in a total dosage of 2 g/kg bw.

Missed Dose: A missed dose should be administered as soon as possible to ensure an adequate IgG serum level.

Administration: Infusion Rate: The recommended initial infusion rate of Privigen is 0.5 mg/kg/min (0.3 mL/kg/hr). If well tolerated, the rate of administration may gradually be increased up to an infusion rate of 12 mg/kg/min (7.2 mL/kg/hr).

As with other IgG products, patients who are receiving IgG for the first time, who have received another IgG, or who have not received IgG in more than 8 weeks may be at risk of developing inflammatory reactions on rapid infusion of Privigen (greater than 4 mg/kg/min [2.4 mL/kg/hr]). These patients should be started at a slow rate of infusion (e.g., 0.5 mg/kg/min [0.3 mL/kg/hr] or less) for at least 30 min. and gradually advanced to the maximum rate as tolerated. When high doses (≥1 g/kg bw) are administered it is recommended not to exceed the rate of 4 mg/kg/min. The initial infusion rate for patients who have previously received Privigen for three or more consecutive infusions can be individualized based on the rate the patient previously tolerated.

For patients judged to be at risk of renal dysfunction or thrombotic events, Privigen should be administered at the minimum infusion rate practicable (see Warnings and Precautions).

Infusion Parameters: Privigen is for intravenous administration and should be given by a separate infusion line. An infusion pump may be used to control the rate of administration.

Do not mix Privigen with other IGIV products or other intravenous medications. If necessary, Privigen can be diluted with Dextrose Injection, USP (D5W). As well Privigen can be flushed with Dextrose Injection, USP (D5W) or 0.9% Sodium Chloride for injection, USP.

If large doses of Privigen are to be administered, several vials may be pooled using aseptic technique. Because the solution contains no preservative, discard partially used product after 24 hours.

Reconstitution: Not applicable. Privigen is a ready to use solution of human immunoglobulin for intravenous infusion.

OVERDOSAGE:
Consequences of an overdose are not known.

For management of a suspected drug overdose, CPhA recommends that you contact your **regional Poison Control Centre**. See the *CPS* Directory section for a list of Poison Control Centres.

ACTION AND CLINICAL PHARMACOLOGY: Mechanism of Action: Treatment of Primary and Secondary Immune Deficiency: Privigen contains a broad spectrum of antibody specificities against bacterial, viral, parasitic, and mycoplasma agents that are capable of both opsonization and neutralization of pathogens and toxins. Appropriate doses of Privigen should restore abnormally low IgG levels to the normal range.

Treatment of Immune Thrombocytopenic Purpura: The mechanism of action of immunoglobulins in the treatment of ITP is not fully understood. One possible mechanism may be the inhibition of the elimination of autoantibody-reacted platelets from the blood circulation by IgG-induced Fc-receptor blockade of phagocytes. Another proposed mechanism is the down-regulation of platelet autoantibody-producing B cells by anti-idiotypic antibodies in IGIV.

Pharmacokinetics: Treatment of Primary and Secondary Immune Deficiency: In the clinical study assessing the efficacy and safety of Privigen in 80 subjects with PID, serum concentrations of total IgG and IgG subclasses were measured in 25 subjects (ages 12 to 65) following the 7th infusion for the 3 subjects on the 3-week dosing interval and following the 5th infusion for the 22 subjects on the 4-week dosing interval. Blood samples were taken 10 to 30 minutes before the infusion and 3 to 20 minutes, 24±2 hours, 3 days, 7 days, 10 days, 14±1 days, and 21±1 days after the infusion. For subjects on the 4-week dosing interval, an additional sample was taken 28±1 days after the infusion.

Table 6 presents the pharmacokinetic parameters of Privigen, measured as serum concentrations of total IgG.

Table 6: Privigen

Pharmacokinetic Parameters of Privigen

Parameter	No. of Subjects	Median (Range)
C_{max} (peak, mg/dL)	25	2340 (1040–3460)
C_{min} (trough, mg/dL)	25	1023 (579–1469)
$t_{½}$ (days)	25	36.6 (20.6–96.6)
AUC_{0-t} (day × mg/dL)[a]		
3-week dosing interval	3	29 860 (28 580–40 010)
4-week dosing interval	22	36 670 (19 680–44 340)

[a] Calculated by log-linear trapezoidal rule.
Legend: C_{max}, maximum serum concentration; C_{min}, trough (minimum level) serum concentration; $t_{½}$, elimination half-life; AUC_{0-t}, area under the curve from 0 hour to last sampling time.

The median half-life of Privigen of 36.6 days is representative of half-lives in the PID patient population receiving immunoglobulins.

The IgG subclass levels observed in the pharmacokinetic population were consistent with a physiologic distribution pattern (mean trough values): IgG_1, 564.91 mg/dL; IgG_2, 394.15 mg/dL; IgG_3, 30.16 mg/dL; IgG_4, 10.88 mg/dL.

In the extension study, mean trough levels of total IgG serum concentrations achieved in subjects with PID were 1115±297 mg/dL for the 3-week dosing interval and 931±181 mg/dL for the 4-week dosing interval, comparable to the results from the pivotal study.

Treatment of Immune Thrombocytopenic Purpura: Pharmacokinetic studies with Privigen were not performed in patients with chronic ITP.

STORAGE AND STABILITY: Privigen can be stored at room temperature (up to 25°C) until the expiration date printed on the outer carton and vial label. Do not freeze. Keep Privigen in its original carton to protect it from light.

SPECIAL HANDLING INSTRUCTIONS: Privigen is a clear or slightly opalescent, colorless to pale yellow solution. As with all parenteral solutions, Privigen should be inspected visually for particulate matter and discoloration prior to administration. Do not use if the solution is cloudy or contains particulates. Any solution that has been frozen must not be used. **Do not shake.**

Do not mix Privigen with other IGIV products or other intravenous medications. If necessary, Privigen can be diluted with Dextrose Injection, USP (D5W). If large doses of Privigen are to be administered, several vials may be pooled using aseptic technique.

The Privigen vial is for single use only. Once the vial has been entered under aseptic conditions, its contents should be used promptly. Because the solution contains no preservative, discard partially used product after 24 hours. Any unused product or waste material should be disposed of in accordance with local requirements.

INFORMATION FOR THE PATIENT: Published in e-CPS, available by subscription at www.e-cps.ca.

DOSAGE FORMS, COMPOSITION AND PACKAGING: Each single-use, tamper-evident vial contains: human immunoglobulin 100 g/L, L-proline 28.8 g/L (250 mmol/L), HCl and/or NaOH for pH adjustment to 4.8 and Water for Injection, USP q.s. Vials of 25, 50, 100 and 200 mL. The components used in the packaging for Privigen are latex-free. Each vial has an integral suspension band and a label with two peel-off strips showing the product name, lot number, and expiration date.

Probenecid

Uricosuric

CPhA Monograph

Date of Preparation: August 2006
Date of Revision: June 2009

This monograph has been compiled by CPhA and reviewed by experts. It may contain information different from that found in Health Canada-approved Product Monographs. The reader is referred to the *CPS* Editorial Policy for more information.

SUMMARY PRODUCT INFORMATION:

Route of Administration	Dosage Form	Strength
Oral	Tablet	500 mg

INDICATIONS AND CLINICAL USE: Probenecid is indicated for:

- Chronic treatment of gouty arthritis or treatment of hyperuricemia

Probenecid is recommended in patients who are hyperuricemic as a result of underexcretion (24-hour renal urate excretion ≤800 mg) with the objective of reducing the number of acute gout attacks by lowering urate levels. Probenecid is not effective in the presence of renal insufficiency or in patients who are hyperuricemic due to overproduction [*Ann Rheum Dis* 2006;65(10):1312-24].

Probenecid is not effective in treating acute gout attacks; nonsteroidal anti-inflammatory agents (NSAIDs) and/or colchicine are effective treatments.

- Treatment of hyperuricemia secondary to the administration of thiazides, loop diuretics, pyrazinamide, ethambutol.

In clinical practice, asymptomatic hyperuricemia secondary to the aforementioned drugs may not require treatment with a uricosuric agent unless there is a personal or family history of gouty arthritis.

Probenecid is not indicated for the treatment of hyperuricemia secondary to cancer chemotherapy, radiation or myeloproliferative neoplastic diseases due to increased risk of uric acid nephropathy.

Cyclosporine-induced hyperuricemia may be more common in transplant patients, placing them at a higher risk of symptomatic gout [*Am J Med* 1992;92(2):141-6]. Probenecid is not indicated in this setting.

Other Clinical Uses:

Probenecid has a long history of use in combination with β-lactam antibacterial agents for the treatment of particular infectious diseases. Probenecid has no intrinsic clinically antibacterial properties; however, the drug retards renal excretion of many β-lactam antibacterial agents. When administered together the serum concentrations of the antibacterial agent are sustained and allow for decreased clearance. Currently, the combinations of probenecid plus β-lactam antibacterials are used as an inexpensive antibacterial regimen for outpatient treatment of certain infections:

- According to the 2008 update of the Canadian guidelines on sexually transmitted infections, the combination of oral probenecid and cefoxitin, as a single dose in combination with doxycycline for 14 days, is used as an alternative to ceftriaxone for outpatient treatment regimen for pelvic inflammatory disease [www.phac-aspc.gc.ca/std-mts/sti_2006/pdf/404_Pelvic_Inflammatory_Disease.pdf].
- According to the 2005 Anti-infective guidelines for community-acquired infections, the combination of cefazolin with oral probenecid (given 30 minutes prior to cefazolin) is used as an alternative treatment regimen for severe non-facial uncomplicated cellulitis [*Clin Infect Dis* 2002;34(11):1440-8].
- According to the 2009 Guidelines for prevention and treatment of opportunistic infections in HIV-infected adults and adolescents, oral probenecid is administered in combination with cidofovir (administered iv) for the prevention of cidofovir-related nephrotoxicity. Cidofovir is used for the treatment of cytomegalovirus (CMV) retinitis in patients with AIDS in whom other drugs are inappropriate [www.cdc.gov/mmwr/pdf/rr/rr5804.pdf].

CONTRAINDICATIONS:

- Patients who are hypersensitive to probenecid or to any ingredient in the formulation.
- Patients who are at increased risk of uric acid renal calculus formation or urate nephropathy such as those undergoing cancer chemotherapy with rapidly cytolytic antineoplastic agents, radiation therapy for malignancy, history of renal calculi (especially uric acid calculi), urate excretion >800 mg/24 hour, history of urate nephropathy, moderate to severe renal impairment.
- Patients with blood dyscrasias as these may be exacerbated.
- Patients with a history of peptic ulcers which may result in gastrointestinal side effects with concomitant use.

WARNINGS AND PRECAUTIONS:

Serious Warnings and Precautions

- Probenecid increases the concentration of uric acid in urine and can promote formation of kidney stones, particularly in the early phases of treatment.
- Antineoplastic drugs increase serum urate concentrations and uricosuric agents increase the risk of uric acid precipitation and renal stone formation. For this reason probenecid should not be used in patients receiving cancer chemotherapy.
- Peptic ulcer disease.

Special Populations: Pregnant Women: Pregnancy Category C. Probenecid crosses the placenta and is detectable in umbilical cord blood. There are no data to suggest that probenecid is associated with an increased incidence of congenital abnormalities. Human data are limited.

Nursing Women: Because of its low molecular weight, probenecid is excreted into breast milk. There are no reports of the effects of probenecid on the infant during breastfeeding; human data are limited. Caution is advised when using it during lactation because of potential toxicity to the infant.

ADVERSE REACTIONS: Adverse Drug Reactions Overview: The most common adverse reactions associated with probenecid include headache, anorexia, nausea and vomiting. Initiating treatment with low doses and increasing the dose as tolerance develops is recommended.

Cardiovascular: hypotension, flushing.
Dermatologic: rash, dermatitis, pruritus, alopecia.
Ear/Nose/Throat: sore gums.
Gastrointestinal: anorexia, nausea, vomiting.
Genitourinary: formation of uric acid stones.
Hematologic: anemia, aplastic anemia, hemolytic anemia, leukopenia.
Hepatic/Biliary/Pancreatic: hepatic necrosis.
Immune: anaphylaxis, hypersensitivity reactions.
Musculoskeletal: acute gouty arthritis.
Neurologic: headache, dizziness.

DRUG INTERACTIONS: Overview: Probenecid inhibits excretion of weak organic acids in the proximal and distal convoluted tubules, altering the pharmacokinetics of many drugs. It also inhibits glucuronidation of some drugs. Probenecid inhibits renal tubular excretion of many β-lactam antibacterial agents (e.g., cephalosporins and penicillins), an interaction that has been exploited clinically to maintain serum levels of the antibacterial agent, thereby reducing the frequency of administration. Probenecid does not alter serum levels of ceftriaxone or ceftazidime. Probenecid does not alter the pharmacokinetics of digoxin or theophylline.

Drug-Drug Interactions: See Table 1.

Table 1: Probenecid

Drug-Drug Interactions

Interacting Drug	Effect	Clinical Comment
Acetaminophen	Decreased clearance of acetaminophen.	Clinical significance not known. Avoid use of high doses of acetaminophen during treatment with probenecid.
Acyclovir	Increased serum levels of acyclovir probably due to decreased renal excretion. Valacyclovir is a prodrug of acyclovir.	Not of clinical significance because of the wide therapeutic index of acyclovir.
Allopurinol	Probenecid increases renal excretion of oxypurinol, the active metabolite of allopurinol. Allopurinol decreases metabolism of probenecid.	Not clinically significant. Has not been reported to increase precipitation of uric acid.
Aminosalicylates	Serum levels of aminosalicylic acid are increased two- to four-fold by probenecid.	Avoid use of probenecid if possible. If the combination is used, consider adjusting the dose of the aminosalicylate and monitor the patient for signs of toxicity.
Benzodiazepines (i.e., lorazepam, midazolam)	Probenecid decreases clearance and prolongs the elimination half-life of lorazepam. The onset of midazolam-induced "sleep" is faster in the presence of probenecid.	Consider reducing the dose of the benzodiazepine. Warn patients about, and/or monitor for the signs of benzodiazepine excess including rapid onset, pronounced sedation. Patients receiving probenecid may require lower doses of midazolam to induce anesthesia.
Captopril	Probenecid decreases renal clearance of captopril.	Unknown if interaction occurs with other angiotensin converting enzyme inhibitors. Monitor patients for signs of increased hypotensive effects.
Cephalosporin antibiotics	Probenecid increases the serum levels of many cephalosporin antibiotics by inhibiting urinary excretion.	Generally not of clinical significance. The interaction between probenecid and cefazolin, and probenecid and cefoxitin are exploited in order to reduce the frequency of administration of cefazolin (see CPhA monographs, Cefazolin and Cefoxitin).
Chlorpropamide	Probenecid increases the elimination half-life of chlorpropamide.	Monitor blood sugar levels in patients receiving probenecid and chlorpropamide and adjust the dose of chlorpropamide if necessary.
Dapsone	Probenecid reduces urinary excretion of dapsone and its metabolites resulting in a marked increase in the serum levels of dapsone.	Clinical significance unknown. Monitor patients for signs and symptoms of hematologic toxicity associated with dapsone.
Famotidine	Serum levels of famotidine are increased when administered with probenecid.	Unlikely to be of clinical significance
Fexofenadine	Probenecid significantly decreases renal clearance of fexofenadine.	Clinical significance unknown
Furosemide	Probenecid decreases renal clearance of furosemide but does not impair the diuretic effects of the drug.	Clinical significance unknown
Ganciclovir	Increased serum levels of ganciclovir probably due to decreased renal excretion.	Clinical significance uncertain. Monitor patients for adverse events of ganciclovir.
Heparin	Limited evidence suggests that probenecid may potentiate the anticoagulant effects of heparin.	Monitor aPTT and adjust the dose of heparin accordingly. Monitor patients for bleeding.
Morphine	Probenecid significantly decreased clearance of morphine-6-glucuronide, a pharmacologically active metabolite of morphine.	Patients receiving probenecid may require lower or less frequent doses of morphine. Monitor patients receiving the combination closely.
Mycophenolate mofetil	Probenecid inhibits renal tubular secretion of mycophenolic acid, a pharmacologically active metabolite of mycophenolate mofetil thereby increasing its plasma concentrations.	Monitor mycophenolate levels and monitor for signs and symptoms of mycophenolate toxicity, e.g., gastrointestinal intolerance, hematologic abnormalities such as neutropenia. Adjust the dose of mycophenolate, if necessary.
NSAIDs	Probenecid inhibits conjugation of ketoprofen and diflunisal and excretion of naproxen. The serum half life is prolonged and serum levels of ketorolac and tenoxicam increase when co-administered with probenecid.	Avoid concurrent use of ketorolac and probenecid. The clinical significance of other interactions is not established.

(cont'd)

Table 1: Probenecid *(cont'd)*

Drug-Drug Interactions

Interacting Drug	Effect	Clinical Comment
Nucleoside reverse transcriptase inhibitors (zalcitabine, zidovudine)	Retards elimination of zalcitabine and zidovudine. Probenecid is assumed to retard renal excretion of zalcitabine and to inhibit glucuronidation of zidovudine.	The combination of zalcitabine and probenecid is reported to be well tolerated. The incidence of zidovudine-related adverse events (rash, malaise, fever and myalgia) increases when the drug is co-administered with probenecid. Avoid use of probenecid in patients receiving zidovudine. If concurrent use cannot be avoided, monitor patients for adverse events of zidovudine.
Olanzapine	Probenecid significantly increases C_{max} and AUC_{0-24h}, without affecting clearance of olanzapine, presumably because of inhibition of UDP glucuronosyltransferase and a resulting decrease in the rate of glucuronidation.	Monitor patients for signs of olanzapine excess.
Oseltamivir	Probenecid completely blocks renal excretion of oseltamivir. Systemic exposure to oseltamivir increases by 2.5-fold.	Clinical significance unknown
Penicillins (e.g., amoxicillin, ampicillin, piperacillin, ticarcillin)	Probenecid inhibits renal tubular excretion of penicillins.	This interaction has been exploited to increase serum levels of penicillins.
Pramipexole	Probenecid reduces clearance of pramipexole by approximately one-third.	Clinical significance uncertain. Monitor patients receiving the combination for adverse events of pramipexole.
Pyrazinamide	Pyrazinamide inhibits renal excretion of uric acid. Pyrazinamide also reduces metabolism of probenecid and probenecid retards elimination of pyrazinamide. The net effect of these changes is a reduced uricosuric effect of probenecid.	Consider alternative antitubercular agents in patients with gout. If probenecid is used to treat pyrazinamide-induced hyperuricemia, higher dosages of probenecid may be required.
Quinolone antibacterial agents (ciprofloxacin, levofloxacin, moxifloxacin, norfloxacin, ofloxacin)	Probenecid reduces renal clearance of ciprofloxacin, levofloxacin, norfloxacin and ofloxacin, but not moxifloxacin.	Unlikely to be clinically significant
Salicylates including acetylsalicylic acid (ASA)	The uricosuric effects of salicylates, (with the exception of low dose ASA ≤325 mg/day) including high dose ASA, antagonize those of probenecid.	Avoid concurrent use of salicylates including high dose ASA in patients receiving probenecid (use an alternative if possible). Concurrent use of ASA 325 mg/day or less is compatible with probenecid.
Sulfinpyrazone	Probenecid inhibits renal tubular excretion of sulfinpyrazone with no changes in the uricosuric effect compared with administering either drug alone.	Clinical significance is unknown. Concomitant use for the treatment of gout is not recommended.
Thiopental	Probenecid prolongs the duration of thiopental-induced anesthesia, possibly because of competitive binding to albumin.	Reduced dosages of anesthetic may be required in patients receiving probenecid.
Valacyclovir	See Acyclovir.	See Acyclovir.

DOSAGE AND ADMINISTRATION: Recommended Dose and Dosage Adjustment: Adults: See Table 2.

Table 2: Probenecid

Dose in Adult Patients

Indication	Dose	Duration of Therapy	Clinical Comment
Gouty arthritis, chronic	Initial dose: 250 mg po BID for 1 week. Increase to 500 mg/day after 1 week. If symptoms persist, increase dose every 4 weeks in 500 mg increments. Maintenance dose: 500 to 1000 mg po BID to TID. Maximum dose: 3 g/day.	If no acute attacks of gout have occurred for 6 months or longer and serum uric acid concentrations are controlled, it may be possible to decrease the dosage by 500 mg/day at 6-month intervals.	Start with a low dose to avoid marked uricosuria and possible stone formation. Maintain hydration (about 2 L/day). Avoid use in patients with ClCr <50 mL/min.
Cellulitis, moderate to severe (nonfacial) (combination with cefazolin)	1 g po once daily	Given 30 minutes prior to cefazolin administration.	Switch cefazolin to an oral antibiotic as soon as feasible.
Pelvic inflammatory disease, outpatient treatment (combination with cefoxitin)	1 g as a single dose	Single dose in combination with cefoxitin 2 g IM **plus** doxycycline 100 mg po BID for 14 days	An alternate regimen is ceftriaxone given as a single dose plus doxycycline.

(cont'd)

Table 2: Probenecid *(cont'd)*

Dose in Adult Patients

Indication	Dose	Duration of Therapy	Clinical Comment
Prevention of cidofovir-related nephrotoxicity in CMV retinitis	2 g 3 hours before cidofovir infusion, then 1 g at 2 hours and 1 g at 8 hours after the end of the cidofovir infusion		Along with saline hydration before cidofovir infusion.

Adult Patients with Renal Impairment: Avoid use of probenecid in patients with creatinine clearance <50 mL/min. As a uricosuric agent, the drug is ineffective in these individuals.

Administration: Gastrointestinal adverse events may be minimized by taking probenecid with food or antacids. Maintain fluid intake to ensure urinary output of 2 to 3 L/day. Alkalinization of the urine, for example with sodium bicarbonate, during the first few days of therapy is desirable as it may prevent stone formation.

OVERDOSAGE:

For management of a suspected drug overdose, CPhA recommends that you contact your **regional Poison Control Centre**. See the *CPS* Directory section for a list of Poison Control Centres.

ACTION AND CLINICAL PHARMACOLOGY: Mechanism of Action: Probenecid, a sulfonamide derivative, competitively inhibits active reabsorption of uric acid at the level of the proximal convoluted tubule. This promotes excretion of uric acid, thereby reducing serum urate concentrations.

Pharmacokinetics: Adults: Absorption: Probenecid is rapidly and completely absorbed from the gastrointestinal tract. Plasma concentrations in the range of 100 to 200 mg/L produce a uricosuric effect while lower concentrations (40 to 60 mg/L) inhibit penicillin excretion.

After a single 2 g oral dose, peak plasma concentrations of 150 to 200 mg/L are achieved within 4 hours and concentrations remain above 50 mg/L for up to 8 hours.

Distribution: Approximately 75% of probenecid is bound to plasma proteins.

Metabolism and Excretion: Probenecid is secreted into the proximal convoluted tubule and then nearly completely reabsorbed from acidic urine. Alkalinization of urine decreases renal tubular reabsorption and results in an increase in the excreted fraction of unchanged drug. This does not alter the uricosuric efficacy of the drug.

Probenecid undergoes hepatic metabolism and, in addition to formation of a glucuronide conjugate, there are 4 oxidative metabolites formed by phase II reactions.

Prochlorperazine

Phenothiazine

CPhA Monograph

Date of Preparation: November 2007

This monograph has been compiled by CPhA and reviewed by experts. It may contain information different from that found in Health Canada-approved Product Monographs. The reader is referred to the *CPS* Editorial Policy for more information.

SUMMARY PRODUCT INFORMATION:

Route of Administration	Dosage Form	Strength
Parenteral	Injectable solution	5 mg/mL (2 mL)
Oral	Tablet	5 mg, 10 mg
Rectal	Suppository	10 mg

INDICATIONS AND CLINICAL USE: Prochlorperazine is indicated for:

- treatment of nausea and vomiting due to stimulation of the chemoreceptor trigger zone (CTZ). The CTZ is located proximal to the area postrema on the floor of the fourth ventricle outside of the blood-brain barrier. It detects drugs or toxins in blood and sends impulses to vomiting centre.

  Postoperative nausea and vomiting as well as that caused by toxins, radiation, drugs or uremia are amenable to treatment with prochlorperazine. In contrast, the drug is generally not effective for prevention of nausea associated with motion sickness, vertigo, or local irritation of the gastrointestinal tract.

Prochlorperazine is also classified as a phenothiazine antipsychotic agent and is approved for the treatment of schizophrenia. However, it is generally not used for this indication because of the availability of other more effective and better tolerated agents.

CONTRAINDICATIONS:

- Hypersensitivity to prochlorperazine or to any ingredient in the formulation or component of the container. Cross-sensitivity may occur among phenothiazines.
- Circulatory collapse.
- Coma and/or severe CNS depression, particularly when due to intoxication with CNS depressants (e.g., alcohol, hypnotics, narcotics). Patients receiving large doses of hypnotics should not receive prochlorperazine because of the possibility of potentiation of sedation.
- Children undergoing surgery
- Children under two years of age or weight <10 kg.

WARNINGS AND PRECAUTIONS: General: The signs and symptoms of some medical conditions (e.g., brain tumour, intestinal obstruction) or of overdose with other drugs may be masked by the antiemetic effect of prochlorperazine. The etiology of nausea and vomiting should be established before administering the drug.

Use with caution in patients with conditions associated with CNS depression.

The parenteral formulation may contain bisulfites, which may cause hypersensitivity reactions in susceptible patients.

Phenothiazines impair adaptive thermoregulatory responses. Use prochlorperazine with caution in patients who might be exposed for prolonged periods to extremes of heat or cold.

Cardiovascular: Phenothiazines, including prochlorperazine, can cause orthostatic hypotension; thus, they should not be used in patients with hemodynamic instability or severe cardiac disease. Phenothiazines, including prochlorperazine, have been associated with QT interval prolongation.

Gastrointestinal: The anticholinergic effects of phenothiazines decrease gastrointestinal motility and can lead to constipation and paralytic ileus, especially in the elderly.

Genitourinary: Urinary retention associated with benign prostatic hyperplasia may be worsened by phenothiazines through their anticholinergic effects.

Neurologic: Phenothiazines including prochlorperazine may lower the seizure threshold and should be used with caution in patients with a history of seizures. Patients using opioids, local anesthetics or other drugs that also decrease seizure threshold may be at increased risk. This caution also applies to patients with head trauma or alcoholism.

Prolonged use of prochlorperazine may be associated with emergence of tardive dyskinesia. The lowest effective dose should be used for the shortest period of time.

Prochlorperazine may be associated with neuroleptic malignant syndrome. Patients should be monitored for fever, muscle rigidity, autonomic instability and/or changes in mental status, particularly during prolonged use. The drug should be discontinued and supportive measures should be instituted if the syndrome is suspected.

Phenothiazines may cause extrapyramidal symptoms such as drug-induced parkinsonism, akathisia, tardive dyskinesia and acute dystonic reactions.

The drug should be used with caution in patients with subcortical brain damage. The cause of nausea and vomiting should be diagnosed before using high doses of prochlorperazine as the antiemetic properties can mask the symptoms of increased intracranial pressure.

Ophthalmic: Phenothiazines have anticholinergic effects and should be used with caution in patients with glaucoma.

Special Populations: Pregnant Women: Prochlorperazine crosses the placenta when it is used as an antiemetic in pregnant women. There are isolated reports of congenital abnormalities in infants born to women who received the drug during pregnancy, although large surveillance studies have not shown an increase in the incidence of birth defects.

Nursing Women: The extent to which prochlorperazine is excreted in breast milk is unknown. However, occasional short-term use of prochlorperazine for the treatment of nausea and vomiting appears to pose little risk to the breastfed infant. With repeated doses the infant should be monitored for excess sedation.

Pediatrics: Use of prochlorperazine should be avoided in children less than two years of age as there is a potential for respiratory depression. It has been hypothesized that phenothiazines depress arousal and respiratory mechanisms in sleeping infants. Because of the potential for extrapyramidal symptoms, prochlorperazine should not be given to children with signs and symptoms of Reye's syndrome since it may obscure the diagnosis of this condition.

Geriatrics: Phenothiazines, including prochlorperazine, can cause orthostatic hypotension and have anticholinergic effects (especially sedative effects and confusion) which are of particular concern in the elderly.

Occupational Hazards: Patients should be cautioned about performing tasks which require mental alertness, such as driving or operating heavy machinery, as prochlorperazine can cause drowsiness or dizziness.

ADVERSE REACTIONS: Cardiovascular: hypotension, orthostatic hypotension and tachycardia. Bradycardia, nonspecific QT changes, hypertension. Cardiac arrest.

Central Nervous System: drowsiness, dizziness, and headache are common. Neuroleptic malignant syndrome, seizures, confusion, insomnia. Extrapyramidal symptoms (akathisia, dystonia, pseudoparkinsonism, tardive dyskinesia). Temperature dysregulation.

Allergic/Dermatologic: rash, photosensitivity, slate gray skin pigmentation.

Endocrine and Metabolism: hypoglycemia, hyperglycemia, galactorrhea, lactation, amenorrhea, gynecomastia, breast engorgement, syndrome of inappropriate anti-diuretic hormone secretion.

Gastrointestinal: Dry mouth is a common anticholinergic side effect. Constipation, weight gain, nausea and vomiting.

Genitourinary: urinary retention.

Hematologic: agranulocytosis, leucopenia, eosinophilia, hemolytic anemia, thrombocytopenia, pancytopenia (rare).

Hepatic/Biliary/Pancreatic: cholestatic jaundice.

Neurologic: incoordination, tremor.

Ophthalmologic: corneal and lenticular changes, diplopia, pigmentary retinopathy, blurred vision (rare).

Respiratory: nasal congestion.

Sexual Function/Reproduction: impotence, ejaculatory disorder.

DRUG INTERACTIONS: Overview: If used with other CNS depressant drugs (e.g., ethanol, narcotics) prochlorperazine may cause additive CNS depressant effects. Concurrent use of prochlorperazine and metoclopramide may result in additive anti-dopaminergic adverse events and an increased risk of extrapyramidal symptoms. Through antagonistic effects at CNS dopamine receptors, prochlorperazine may interfere with the antiparkinsonian effect of levodopa and the ability of bromocriptine to lower serum prolactin levels.

Drug-Drug Interactions: See Table 1.

Table 1: Prochlorperazine

Drug-Drug Interactions

Interacting Drug	Effect	Clinical Comment
Anticholinergic agents	Additive anticholinergic effects	Of particular concern in certain individuals, e.g., patients with benign prostatic hyperplasia or angle-closure glaucoma or older individuals.
CNS depressants	Additive sedative and respiratory effects with other CNS depressants including alcohol	Monitor the patient for excessive sedation. Adjust the dose of the interacting agent accordingly.
Fluoroquinolone antibiotics (e.g.,levofloxacin, moxifloxacin)	Possible ↑ risk of cardiac arrhythmias including torsades de pointes.	Avoid coadministration of drugs that may prolong the QT interval such as levofloxacin. Use gatifloxacin and moxifloxacin with caution.

DOSAGE AND ADMINISTRATION: Recommended Dose and Dosage Adjustment: Adults: See Table 2.

Table 2: Prochlorperazine

Dose in Adult Patients

Indication	Route	Usual Dose	Maximum Daily Dose
Antiemetic	Oral	5–10 mg 3–4 times daily PRN	40 mg
	IM, IV	5-10 mg 2–3 times daily PRN	40 mg
	Rectal	5-10 mg 3–4 times daily PRN	40 mg
Sedative-hypnotic	Oral, IM, IV	25–50 mg per dose; repeat every 4–6 hours as needed. Not to exceed 100 mg daily.	

Pediatrics: See Table 3.

Table 3: Prochlorperazine

Dose in Pediatric Patients

Indication	Weight	Route	Dose	Maximum Daily Dose
Antiemetic	9–14 kg	Oral or rectal	2.5 mg once or twice daily PRN	7.5 mg
		IM	0.13 mg/kg	
	> 14–18 kg	Oral or rectal	2.5 mg 2–3 times daily PRN	10 mg
		IM	0.13 mg/kg	
	> 18–39 kg	Oral or rectal	2.5 mg 3 times daily PRN, or 5 mg twice daily PRN	15 mg
		IM	0.13 mg/kg	

Renal Impairment: No specific dosage adjustment is recommended in renal insufficiency. Prochlorperazine is not removed by hemodialysis.

Missed Dose: If a dose is missed, patients should be instructed to take the missed dose as soon as they remember. If it is close to time for the next dose patients should be instructed to wait until then and return to their regular schedule. Doses should **not** be doubled.

Administration: Prochlorperazine may be given orally, rectally, or by im or iv injection. When given orally, the drug may be given with food or water.

For iv administration the infusion rate should not exceed 5 mg/minute.

OVERDOSAGE:

For management of a suspected drug overdose, CPhA recommends that you contact your **regional Poison Control Centre**. See the *CPS* Directory section for a list of Poison Control Centres.

ACTION AND CLINICAL PHARMACOLOGY: Mechanism of Action: Like all phenothiazines, prochlorperazine is an antagonist at dopamine receptors in the central nervous system, and has antipsychotic properties. Prochlorperazine also has anticholinergic effects and is an antagonist at peripheral alpha-adrenergic receptors.

Pharmacokinetics: Adults: The onset of action after oral administration of prochlorperazine is 30 to 40 minutes; 60 minutes after rectal administration and 10 to 20 minutes after im injection.

Oral bioavailability of prochlorperazine is low. After administration of a single 5 mg oral dose, the absolute bioavailability of prochlorperazine was 5.7% relative to a single 5 mg iv dose in healthy male and female volunteers. No gender-based differences in pharmacokinetics have been reported for prochlorperazine. [*J Clin Pharmacol* 2005;45(12):1383-90]

Distribution: Prochlorperazine is widely distributed into body tissues and crosses the blood brain barrier. The volume of distribution was 12.9 L/kg after a single iv dose in healthy young male volunteers. Prochlorperazine is > 90% bound to plasma proteins, primarily alpha-1 acid glycoprotein.

Metabolism: Prochlorperazine undergoes extensive hepatic metabolism to inactive metabolites including N-desmethyl-prochlorperazine, prochlorperazine-sulfoxide, prochlorperazine-7-hydroxide and prochlorperazine-sulfoxide-4-N-oxide [*J Clin Pharmacol* 2005;45(12):1383-90]. Plasma clearance of prochlorperazine was 1.62±0.3 L/hr/kg in healthy volunteers.

Excretion: Prochlorperazine undergoes enterohepatic recirculation and is excreted in bile and feces. Urinary recovery of unchanged drug and metabolites is low. The terminal elimination half-life ($t_{1/2}$) of prochlorperazine has been reported to be 6.8±0.7 to 9.0±0.1 hours after single iv doses of 6.25 to 12.5 mg in healthy volunteers [*Br J Clin Pharmacol* 1987;23(2):137-42; *Br J Clin Pharmacol* 1991;32(6):677-84]; 7.5±1.8 hours after a single 3.125 mg iv dose in elderly female volunteers [*Age Ageing* 1992;21(1):27-31]; and 7.6±0.4 hours after a single iv dose of 0.2 to 1.2 mg/kg in patients receiving cytotoxic chemotherapy [*Eur J Clin Oncol* 1989;25(10):1457-61]. More recently, the $t_{1/2}$ of prochlorperazine in healthy volunteers was reported to be 15.8±2.1 hours after a single 5 mg iv dose and 17.0±6.1 hours after a single 5 mg oral dose [*J Clin Pharmacol* 2005;45(12):1383-90]. The large discrepancy between the older and more recent estimates may be attributable to increased sensitivity of the assay used in the more recent study.

Prochlorperazine Mesylate Injection

prochlorperazine mesylate

Antiemetic—Antipsychotic

Sandoz

Sandoz® Prochlorperazine Suppository

prochlorperazine

Antiemetic—Antipsychotic

Sandoz

SUPPLIED: Injection: Each mL contains prochlorperazine mesylate 7.6 mg equivalent to prochlorperazine base 5 mg. Nonmedicinal ingredients: sodium metabisulfite 0.2% in a sodium phosphate buffer and water for injection. Ampoules of 2 mL, boxes of 10. Store between 15 and 30°C. Protect from light.

Suppository: Each suppository contains: prochlorperazine base 10 mg. Boxes of 10. Store in a cool place. Protect unwrapped suppository from exposure to light.

Proctodan™-HC

pramoxine HCl—hydrocortisone acetate—zinc sulfate monohydrate

Anorectal Therapy

Odan

SUPPLIED: Ointment: Each g of ointment contains: pramoxine HCl 1%, hydrocortisone acetate 0.5% and zinc sulfate monohydrate 0.5%. Nonmedicinal ingredients: methylparaben, propylparaben and petrolatum. Tubes of 15 and 30 g with rectal applicator.

Suppositories: Each suppository contains: pramoxine HCl 20 mg, zinc sulfate monohydrate 10 mg, hydrocortisone acetate 10 mg in a triglyceride base. Nonmedicinal ingredients: dibasic calcium phosphate, magnesium stearate, methylparaben, propylparaben and triglyceride. Boxes of 12. Store between 15 and 30°C. Avoid freezing.

Proctofoam®-HC

hydrocortisone acetate—pramoxine HCl

Anorectal Therapy

Duchesnay

PHARMACOLOGY: Proctofoam-HC combines the anti-inflammatory action of hydrocortisone with the surface anesthetic effect of pramoxine HCl.

INDICATIONS: The temporary relief of anorectal inflammation, pruritus, pain and swelling associated with hemorrhoids, proctitis, cryptitis, fissures, postoperative pain and pruritus ani.

CONTRAINDICATIONS: The presence of active infection, abscess, extensive fistulas or sinus tracts, tuberculosis, varicella, vaccinia, acute herpes simplex, fungal infections, patients with a known sensitivity to any of the product's components.

WARNINGS: Contents are flammable and the aerosol container may explode if heated.

Do not insert any part of the aerosol container into the anus. Do not use in presence of open flame or spark. Contents under pressure. Do not refrigerate. Do not place in hot water or near radiators, stoves or other sources of heat. Do not puncture or incinerate container or store at temperatures over 50°C.

PRECAUTIONS: General: A complete rectal examination to rule out serious pathology should be completed before instituting therapy. Do no use on infected lesions unless accompanied by anti-infective agents. Discontinue use if sensitivity develops. Prolonged use of Proctofoam-HC could produce systemic corticosteroid effects.

Pregnancy: The safety of topical corticosteroids during pregnancy and lactation has not been established. The potential benefit to the mother should be weighed against possible hazards to the fetus or the nursing infant. A study to evaluate the safety of Proctofoam-HC in the third trimester of pregnancy is on-going.

Lactation: See Pregnancy.

ADVERSE EFFECTS: Occasionally, patients may experience itching, burning and/or pain upon application of Proctofoam-HC. The following local adverse reactions have been reported with the use of topical corticosteroids: dryness, itching, burning, local irritation, striae, skin atrophy, hypertrichosis, hypopigmentation and secondary infection. When occlusive dressings are used, pustules, miliaria, folliculitis and pyoderma may occur.

Investigations of Proctofoam-HC have demonstrated very few side effects with this drug. All effects were very minor and it cannot be shown conclusively whether they were caused by the drug or were symptoms of the underlying problem.

In one study of 174 patients 2 complained of irritation. In another investigation of 109 cases of anorectal disorders, there were 18 reports of minor side effects such as itching, burning, urge to defecate and pain on insertion, and 3 reports of allergic responses. These responses were not unexpected due to the sensitization characteristics of the anorectal area; many therapeutic agents applied to this area result in allergic response. In another report of 100 patients, 3 reported burning, 1 had slight itching and 1 had irritation. Three of 92 proctologic patients in another study reported a burning sensation from the medication. A study of 50 postpartum patients who had undergone episiotomies showed that application of Proctofoam-HC led to rapid healing, with no reports of sensitivity reactions and no complications that could be attributed to the drug. Extensive clinical investigations of a 1% pramoxine HCl solution have shown an absence of primary sensitivity or cross-sensitivity in patients using this drug.

OVERDOSE:

Symptoms: No specific symptoms or therapy known. However, overdosage is improbable at the concentrations of pramoxine and hydrocortisone per 18 g unit of Proctofoam-HC.

Treatment: In case of accidental ingestion, institute symptomatic treatment.

For management of a suspected drug overdose, CPhA recommends that you contact your **regional Poison Control Centre**. See the *CPS* Directory section for a list of Poison Control Centres.

DOSAGE: Shake the aerosol container before using. Insert 1 applicatorful into anus 2 or 3 times daily and after bowel evacuation. The foam may also be placed on a perianal pad and applied externally as needed to relieve pain or itching.

SUPPLIED: Each aerosol container with anal and topical applicator contains: 18 g of a mixture of hydrocortisone acetate USP 1%, pramoxine HCl USP 1% in a water-miscible mucoadhesive foam base formulated with cetyl alcohol, emulsifying wax, methylparaben, propylene glycol, propylparaben, steareth-10, triethanolamine, water and inert propellants, isobutane and propane. Each application provides 375 mg of mucoadhesive base containing 1% hydrocortisone acetate USP (3.75 mg/dose) and 1% pramoxine HCl USP (3.75 mg/dose). The aerosol container contains approximately 36 applications.

Proctol™ Ⓟ

hydrocortisone—cinchocaine HCl—framycetin sulfate—esculin

Anorectal Therapy

Odan

SUPPLIED: Ointment: Each g of translucent ointment contains: hydrocortisone 5 mg, cinchocaine HCl 5 mg, framycetin sulfate 10 mg and esculin 10 mg in a petrolatum ointment base. Nonmedicinal ingredients: anhydrous lanolin and white petrolatum. Tubes of 15 and 30 g with rectal applicator. Store between 15 and 22°C.

Suppositories: Each white to off-white torpedo-shaped suppository contains: hydrocortisone 5 mg, cinchocaine HCl 5 mg, framycetin sulfate 10 mg and esculin 10 mg in a triglyceride base. Nonmedicinal ingredients: methylparaben, propylparaben and triglyceride. Boxes of 12 and 24. Store between 15 and 30°C. Avoid freezing.

Proctosedyl® Ⓟ

hydrocortisone—framycetin sulfate—cinchocaine HCl—esculin

Anorectal Therapy

Axcan Pharma

Date of Revision: June 2010

INDICATIONS: The reduction of swelling, pain and inflammation of hemorrhoids and other rectal lesions. The management of acute and chronic nonspecific proctitis, acute internal hemorrhoids, cryptitis, fissures and incomplete fistulas, internal and external pruritus ani. May be used in pre- and postoperative hemorrhoidectomy and repair of fissures.

CONTRAINDICATIONS: Hydrocortisone must not be used in the presence of tuberculosis, fungal and viral infections. Sensitivity to any of the components.

PRECAUTIONS: Discontinue use if sensitization occurs. Hydrocortisone should not be used until an adequate proctologic examination is completed and a diagnosis made. Other specific measures against infections, allergy, and other causal factors must not be neglected. The possibility, however rare, that prolonged use of this preparation might produce systemic corticosteroid effects, should be borne in mind. Patients should be advised to inform subsequent physicians of the previous use of hydrocortisone.

Pregnancy: The safe use of topical corticosteroids during pregnancy has not been fully established. Therefore, during pregnancy, they should not be used unnecessarily on extended areas, in large amounts or for prolonged periods of time.

ADVERSE EFFECTS: Certain patients may experience burning upon application, especially if the mucous membrane is not intact.

OVERDOSE:

For management of a suspected drug overdose, contact your **regional Poison Control Centre**. See the *CPS* Directory section for a list of Poison Control Centres.

DOSAGE: Ointment: For external treatment: Apply a small quantity morning and evening and after each bowel movement, to the affected area. For internal application: attach rectal cannula to tube, insert to full extent and squeeze tube gently from lower end while withdrawing.

Suppositories: 1 suppository morning and evening and after each bowel movement.

SUPPLIED: Ointment: Each g contains: hydrocortisone BP 5 mg (0.5%), framycetin sulfate BP 10 mg (equivalent to 7 mg of framycetin base-1%), cinchocaine HCl BP 5 mg (0.5%), esculin 10 mg (1%). Also contains 10% w/w anhydrous lanolin. Tubes of 15 and 30 g with rectal cannula. Store between 15 and 30ºC.

Suppositories: Each rectal suppository contains: hydrocortisone BP 5 mg (0.5 %), framycetin sulfate BP 10 mg (equivalent to 7 mg of framycetin base-1%), cinchocaine HCl BP 5 mg (0.5%), esculin 10 mg (1%). Boxes of 12 and 24. Store between 15 and 30°C.

Procyclidine Ⓟ

Antiparkinsonian Agent

CPhA Monograph

Date of Revision: November 2005

This monograph has been compiled by CPhA and reviewed by experts. It may contain information different from that found in Health Canada-approved Product Monographs. The reader is referred to the *CPS* Editorial Policy for more information.

SUMMARY PRODUCT INFORMATION:

Route of Administration	Dosage Form	Strength
Oral	Tablet	2.5 mg, 5 mg
Oral	Elixir	2.5 mg/5 mL

INDICATIONS AND CLINICAL USE: Procyclidine is indicated for the treatment of Parkinson's disease and the prevention and treatment of drug-induced extrapyramidal symptoms.

Procyclidine and other anticholinergics (e.g., benztropine, trihexyphenidyl, orphenadrine) are generally used in younger patients with Parkinson's disease (i.e., less than 60 years of age) whose dominant symptom is tremor and who have good cognitive function. They are less effective against other symptoms of Parkinson's disease (e.g., rigidity, akinesia) than they are against tremor. They may be used as monotherapy in mild to moderate disease or as an adjunct to levodopa. There is no evidence that either of the drugs listed above is any better than the other. Use of anticholinergics may be limited by their adverse effects (see Adverse Effects).

Procyclidine may also be used to treat drug-induced parkinsonian symptoms.

CONTRAINDICATIONS: Procyclidine is contraindicated in myasthenia gravis, angle-closure glaucoma, severe ulcerative colitis or toxic megacolon complicating ulcerative colitis, or obstructive uropathy.

WARNINGS AND PRECAUTIONS: Cardiovascular: Use with caution in patients with tachyarrhythmias, congestive heart failure, ischemic heart disease, hypertension or hypotension.

Dependence/Tolerance/Withdrawal: Procyclidine has been abused for its euphoric effects. Clinicians should remain aware of this possibility.

Endocrine and Metabolism: Procyclidine, alone or in combination with antipsychotics or other anticholinergics, may cause anhidrosis and/or hyperthermia, which may be fatal. Patients should avoid becoming overheated from prolonged exposure to high environmental temperatures and/or sustained heavy exercise. The elderly, the chronically ill, alcoholics and those with CNS disease may be particularly vulnerable. If there is evidence of anhidrosis, dosage should be reduced so that the ability to maintain body temperature equilibrium by perspiration is not impaired. Procyclidine should also be used with caution in patients experiencing fever.

Gastrointestinal: Use procyclidine with extreme caution in patients with mild to moderate ulcerative colitis since antimuscarinic agents may suppress intestinal motility and produce paralytic ileus with resultant precipitation or aggravation of toxic megacolon. Use procyclidine cautiously in patients with known or suspected gastrointestinal infections since it may decrease gastrointestinal motility and prolong symptomatology by causing retention of the causative organism or toxin. In patients with gastric ulcer antimuscarinics in general may delay gastric emptying with possible antral stasis; therefore, procyclidine should be used cautiously in these patients. Antimuscarinics may also relax the lower esophageal sphincter. This, combined with their effect on gastric emptying, may result in increased gastroesophageal reflux in patients with GERD or hiatus hernia associated with reflux esophagitis.

Genitourinary: Use with caution in patients with prostatic hypertrophy or partial obstruction of the genitourinary tract.

Hepatic/Biliary/Pancreatic: Use with caution in patients with hepatic disease.

Neurologic: Procyclidine should be used with extreme caution in patients with autonomic neuropathy or other dementias.

Ophthalmologic: Procyclidine is contraindicated in patients with angle-closure glaucoma. Patients with primary open-angle glaucoma controlled with medications are at minimal risk of induction of an increase in intraocular pressure and many clinicians do not consider this condition a contraindication to therapy with procyclidine.

Psychiatric: When procyclidine is used to treat parkinsonian symptoms caused by antipsychotic therapy in patients with a psychiatric illness, there may be an intensification of psychiatric illness. When using procyclidine in these patients, they should be carefully observed, especially at the beginning of treatment or if dosage is increased. Tardive dyskinesia may appear in some patients on long-term treatment with antipsychotics or related agents, or may occur after these drugs are discontinued. Anticholinergic agents such as procyclidine usually do not alleviate these symptoms and in some instances may aggravate or unmask them. Procyclidine is not recommended in tardive dyskinesia.

Renal: Use with caution in patients with renal disease.

Respiratory: Due to its drying effects on bronchial secretions, procyclidine should be used with caution in patients with COPD.

Special Populations: Pregnant Women: It is not known if procyclidine crosses the placenta. The safe use of procyclidine in pregnancy has not been established. The use of procyclidine during pregnancy requires that potential benefits be weighed against the possible hazards to the mother and fetus.

Nursing Women: It is not known if procyclidine is excreted into breast milk.

Pediatrics: Safety and efficacy in the pediatric population have not been established. Children are especially sensitive to anticholinergic drug effects. The use of procyclidine in this age group requires that potential benefits be weighed against the possible hazards to the child.

Geriatrics: Geriatric patients are particularly susceptible to the adverse effect of anticholinergic agents, including procyclidine. These patients may require lower doses, especially at the onset of therapy, and slower dose titration than younger adults. In many instances, other therapeutic classes may be preferred. Some clinicians recommend that baseline cognitive evaluations, psychiatric history, and supine and standing blood pressure be obtained in older patients before initiation of anticholinergic therapy.

Occupational Hazards: Since antimuscarinics may produce drowsiness, dizziness or blurred vision, patients should be warned not to engage in activities that require mental alertness or visual acuity while taking procyclidine.

DRUG INTERACTIONS: See Table 1.

Table 1: Procyclidine

Drug-Drug Interactions

Interacting Drug	Effect	Clinical Comment
Alcohol	Increased CNS depressant effect.	
Amantadine	Procyclidine and other anticholinergics may increase the CNS side effects of amantadine. (Also see Anticholinergic agents below.)	Monitor patients for this effect and reduce the dose of one or both drugs as necessary.
Anticholinergic Agents	Additive anticholinergic effects may occur when procyclidine is administered concurrently with other drugs having anticholinergic effects (e.g., amantadine, some antihistamines, phenothiazines, tricyclic antidepressants)	
Cholinesterase Inhibitors	Theoretically, procyclidine and other anticholinergics that readily penetrate the blood-brain barrier may interfere with the action of cholinesterase inhibitors (e.g., donepezil, galantamine, rivastigmine). In addition, cholinesterase inhibitors have the potential to interfere with the activity of anticholinergic medications.	
CNS Depressants	Procyclidine may enhance the CNS depressant effects of drugs including alcohol, antiepileptic drugs, barbiturates, benzodiazepines, MAO inhibitors, opioids, phenothiazines and tricyclic antidepressants.	
Levodopa	The effect of levodopa may be reduced. This is probably due to decreased gastric motility resulting in increased gastric deactivation of levodopa and decreased absorption.	Monitor patients for this effect if an anticholinergic is added to levodopa therapy. The dose of levodopa may need to be increased or the dose of anticholinergic decreased.

Table 2: Procyclidine

Dose in Adult Patients

Indication	Route	Initial Dose	Titrate	Usual Dose	Maximum Dose	Duration of Treatment	Detailed Information
Drug-induced parkinsonian symptoms	Oral	2.5 mg TID after meals	Increase by 2.5 mg increments until symptoms are relieved	10–20 mg/day		Attempt to taper and discontinue procyclidine 6–12 weeks after symptoms have resolved. If symptoms reappear, some clinicians recommend switching to an atypical antipsychotic if possible.	
Parkinson's disease	Oral	2.5 mg TID after meals	If well-tolerated, dose can be gradually increased to 5 mg three times daily. A bedtime dose can also be added if necessary		60 mg/day		If transferring from prior therapy for Parkinson's disease, initially substitute 2.5 mg TID for all or part of the original agent. Increase as necessary while tapering the dose of the original drug.

ADVERSE REACTIONS: Adverse Drug Reaction Overview: The adverse effects of procyclidine are usually an extension of its pharmacologic action. They are usually dose related and may be reduced by lowering the dosage and administering the drug after meals. Children and the elderly may be particularly susceptible (see Warnings and Precautions, Geriatrics and Warnings and Precautions, Pediatrics).

Cardiovascular: Tachycardia, palpitations or orthostatic hypotension may occur.

CNS: Disorientation, confusion, memory loss, hallucinations, agitation, nervousness, depression, drowsiness, giddiness and lightheadedness may occur.

Dermatologic: Rash, urticaria and decreased sweating have been reported.

Endocrine and Metabolism: Hyperthermia has occurred secondary to decreased sweating.

Gastrointestinal: Dry mouth is common. Saliva substitutes may be helpful if this occurs. Nausea, vomiting, epigastric distress, constipation and paralytic ileus have also occurred.

Ophthalmologic: Mydriasis and blurred vision may occur.

Genitourinary: Urinary retention and urinary hesitancy may occur.

DOSAGE AND ADMINISTRATION: Dosing Considerations: See Table 2.

OVERDOSAGE:

Signs and Symptoms: Symptoms of overdose are primarily extensions of procyclidine's anticholinergic actions. Tachycardia; Flushed, hot, dry skin, tachycardia, dry mucous membranes, mydriasis and blurred vision are common. Drowsiness, lightheadedness and nervousness may progress to or alternate with agitation, confusion, delirium and hallucinations, especially in children or the elderly. Urinary retention, hypertension, hyperthermia, photophobia, thirst and decreased gastrointestinal motility are also seen. Pupils may be fixed. In severely poisoned patients coma or seizures may occur. Psychosis, rash, dystonic reactions, ataxia, weakness, respiratory depression, cardiac arrhythmias and rhabdomyolysis have been reported.

Recommended Management: Treatment is symptomatic and supportive. Consider the use of activated charcoal in significant ingestions. Do not induce vomiting due to the possible rapid onset of CNS and cardiovascular symptoms. Monitor the patient's urine output, vital signs and bowel sounds. If poisoning is severe, monitor the ECG. Maintain the patient's fluid and electrolyte balance. Mydriasis and cycloplegia may be treated with a local miotic such as pilocarpine. Manage hyperthermia with physical measures and control of agitation. Treat agitation and seizures with i.v. benzodiazepines. Avoid the use of physical restraints in agitated patients due to the risk of hyperthermia and rhabdomyolysis. Also avoid the use of antipsychotics and other drugs with anticholinergic effects. If patients have severe CNS symptoms without evidence of AV widening or block and it is certain they have not ingested other medications, especially tricyclic antidepressants, a small dose of physostigmine can be slowly infused. (Physostigmine is not currently marketed in Canada but is available through the Special Access Program—Appendix 2.)

> For management of a suspected drug overdose, CPhA recommends that you contact your **regional Poison Control Centre**. See the *CPS* Directory section for a list of Poison Control Centres.

ACTION AND CLINICAL PHARMACOLOGY: Procyclidine is a synthetic tertiary amine antimuscarinic agent, structurally and pharmacologically related to trihexyphenidyl. It has an atropine-like action on parasympathetic-innervated peripheral structures including smooth muscle, is a potent mydriatic and inhibits salivation. It has no ganglionic blocking activity in doses as high as 4 mg/kg.

Pharmacokinetics: Procyclidine hydrochloride is well-absorbed from the GI tract. Its bioavailability ranges from 52% to 97% and its T_{max} from 1.1 to 2 hours. Its elimination half-life has been reported to range from 11.5 to 12.6 hours and its duration of action is approximately 4 hours.

Procytox® Ⓟ

cyclophosphamide

Antineoplastic

Baxter

Cyclophosphamide is a potent drug that should only be used by physicians experienced with cancer chemotherapeutic drugs or immunosuppressive therapy.

Extreme caution is recommended in the use of cyclophosphamide for non-neoplastic conditions, because of potential carcinogenicity with long-term use of this agent.

PHARMACOLOGY: Cyclophosphamide, a nitrogen mustard derivative, is a polyfunctional alkylating agent. The parent drug is inactive in vitro, when tested on cultures of human leukocytes or carcinomatous cells of human origin. The active metabolite of cyclophosphamide, phosphoramide mustard, exhibits the alkylating action. Phosphoramide mustard is formed, following the biological transformation through oxidation by hepatic microsomal enzymes under spontaneous ß-elimination of acrolein from aldophosphamide. The cytotoxic action of the active metabolite is primarily due to crosslinking of DNA and RNA strands, as well as inhibition of DNA synthesis. Cyclophosphamide is a potent immunosuppressive agent that also causes marked and persistent inhibition of cholinesterase activity. Alkylating metabolites of cyclophosphamide have been measured in cerebrospinal fluid, but, only a small fraction crosses the brain barrier.

Pharmacokinetics: See Table 1. Absorption: Cyclophosphamide is well absorbed from the gastrointestinal tract and from parenteral sites. Topical cyclophosphamide, applied to external (body surface) neoplastic tissues, appears to be absorbed. The following demonstrates that **cyclophosphamide can be absorbed through intact human skin**; therefore, requiring the protective use of unpowdered latex gloves (see Dosage, Special Instructions).

Table 1: Procytox

Urinary Excretion of CP[a] (µg) after Topical Application (20 mg/mL)

Chemotherapy: volunteers in remission	Time after drug application (hours)				
	0–6	6–12	12–18	18–24	Total
A ♂	0	0	0	0	0
B ♀	0.83	2.16	2.16	6.30	11.90
C ♀	0	0	0.50	0.94	1.44
D ♀	0	2.41	5.50	—	7.9
E ♀	0	0.97	11.19	4.31	16.47

[a] CP: cyclophosphamide.

Bioavailability: The systemic availability, estimated from the ratio of areas under serum-concentration-time curves following oral and intravenous cyclophosphamide (CP), was reported as 97% for a 100 mg, and 74% for a 300 mg dose.

Oral CP is approximately 75% absorbed from the gastrointestinal tract. Oral administration demonstrated 3.5 times more alkylating activity than following an intravenous dose.

In all the pharmacokinetic measurements in man, large inter-individual variations must be considered.

Distribution: A mean apparent volume of distribution of cyclophosphamide was 0.56 L/kg in adults and 0.67 L/kg in children.

Tissue Distribution of CP after i.v. administration to cancer patients indicated that both unchanged parent drug and metabolites in small quantities penetrate the blood brain barrier; brain tissue concentrations being similar to those in blood. Biopsies, performed 2 hours after CP infusion, indicated approximately 30% more radioactivity in lymph nodes compared to muscle, adipose tissue or skin, but relative proportions of unchanged drug metabolites were not established.

Protein Binding: 12 to 14% of unchanged cyclophosphamide is protein-bound; the alkylating metabolites, however, are more extensively bound, namely 67% of the total plasma alkylating activity, and in another study, 39% of phosphamide mustard was protein-bound.

Metabolism: While chemically not reactive, the primary metabolites 4-hydroxycyclophosphamide and aldophosphamide are cytotoxic in vitro, and may represent transport forms of the alkylating moiety, phosphoramide mustard. The two primary metabolites can be further oxidized into the major urinary metabolites 5-ketocyclophosphamide and carboxyphosphamide. Nor-nitrogen mustard, a decomposition product of carboxyphosphamide, is an active alkylating agent with cytotoxicity in vivo and in vitro, however, little antitumor activity could be demonstrated; yet, it may play a role in the hematopoietic and other toxicities of cyclophosphamide. Another metabolite formed from aldophosphamide is acrolein, which has been identified as the most urotoxic species.

Disposition Kinetics: The decline in CP plasma levels following an i.v. dose is biexponential with terminal half-life averaging 7 hours (1.8 to 12.4) for adults, and 4 hours (2.4 to 6.5) for children; daily administration of approximately 50 mg/kg bid or qid (i.v. infusion) to children significantly decreased both plasma half life and urinary excretion of CP. With daily exposure or repeated high-dose administration (i.v.) of cyclophosphamide to adult patients, the half-life of CP decreased without an increase in urinary excretion, suggesting that the drug induces its own metabolism. After an i.v. dose, the NBP [4-(nitrobenzyl)-pyridine] plasma alkylating activity peaks 2 hours after administration, and declines with a half-life of 7.7 hours. Phosphoramide mustard in 3 patients, receiving 60-75 mg/kg cyclophosphamide, peaked 2 to 3 hours after the administration of CP at levels 10 to 20% of the unchanged drug, and declined slowly with levels still detectable at 24 hours.

Even with doses as high as 80 mg/kg, the plasma half-life of CP does not increase.

The $t_{½}$ and AUC of cyclophosphamide after a 5-day continuous infusion schedule of 300-400 mg/m²/day, were similar to the $t_{½}$ and AUC of a 1500 mg/m² i.v. bolus. The AUC of the alkylating activity after 5-day i.v. infusion, however, was three times higher than the AUC of alkylating activity after 1500 mg/m² i.v. bolus administration of cyclophosphamide. After CP administration to man and laboratory animals, significant differences in the pharmacokinetic parameters of the active metabolite 4-hydroxycyclophosphamide in both man and animals were found. In man, the active metabolite in blood was found at only low but longer lasting concentrations compared to the high and relatively short time concentration in blood of mice and rats, after a comparable dose.

Elimination: In man, a generally higher proportion of the administered CP is excreted as metabolites in urine. Urinary recovery of radioactivity after intravenously administered ^{14}C-cyclophosphamide to patients ranged from 59 to 82% after 4 days, while not more than 20% of i.v. cyclophosphamide was excreted unchanged in urine at any dose level.

Renal clearance estimates of between 5.3 and 11 mL/min indicate substantial renal tubular reabsorption.

Pharmacokinetics in Renal Function Impairment: Patients with severe renal function impairment have a normal biotransformation of cyclophosphamide, but impaired excretion of metabolites with significantly higher plasma alkylating activity. Dose modification of cyclophosphamide, related to the degree of renal dysfunction, may be advised. Patients with moderate to severe renal impairment receiving high doses of cyclophosphamide or those with severe renal impairment receiving conventional doses may require dose reduction, e.g., a dose reduction of 50% for a glomerular filtration rate below 10 mL/minute is recommended.

Cyclophosphamide is dialysable with a high extraction efficiency.

Pharmacokinetics in Hepatic Function Impairment: A patient with Hodgkin's disease showing jaundice, markedly elevated alkaline phosphatase and filling defects on liver scan had the longest cyclophosphamide half life (8.4 hrs) and lowest peak plasma alkylating metabolite level (4.2 µmoles/mL) of 12 patients having received 40 mg/kg CP. Prior hepatic dysfunction and/or hepatotoxic medication might predispose the patient to oral cyclophosphamide toxicity by altering the balance between the enzymatic production of non-toxic metabolites (carboxyphosphamide) and the decomposition of aldophosphamide to the effective alkylating agent phosphoramide mustard.

INDICATIONS: A. Frequently responsive myeloproliferative and lymphoproliferative disorders:

1. Malignant lymphomas (see also Dosage):
   a. Hodgkin's disease [Cotswold stages II & III (massive mediastinal disease) and $IIIA_{1,2}$ - IV E]
      Non-Hodgkin's lymphomas (Working Formulation. Low Grade A,B,C; Intermediate Grade D,E,F,G; High Grade H,I,J)
   b. Follicular lymphoma (B,C,D)
   c. Lymphocytic lymphoma (A,B,E; mixed histiocytic, C,F)
      Note: Type A, small diffuse and well differentiated malignant lymphocytic lymphoma is consistent with chronic lymphocytic leukemia, to be considered a heterogenous group of chronic B-cell disorders.
   d. Diffuse histiocytic lymphoma (G,H)
   e. Lymphoblastic lymphoma (I)
   f. Burkitt's lymphoma (J)
2. Multiple myeloma (Myeloma stages II, IIIA, IIIB) (see also Dosage).
3. Leukemias (see also Dosage):
   a. Chronic lymphocytic leukemia (CLL) (Rai Stages II, III, IV) (Binet Stages B, C)
      Note: Chronic lymphocytic leukemias are considered to be a heterogenous group of chronic B-cell disorders.
   b. Chronic Myelogenous Leukemia (CML) (Ineffective in acute blastic crises)

c. Acute Myelogenous Leukemia (AML) (M0-M7) (Also called acute nonlymphocytic leukemia) Acute Myelomonocytic Leukemia (AMML) (Type M4)
d. Acute Lymphoblastic (Stem Cell) Leukemia (ALL) in children (Cyclophosphamide given during remission is effective in prolonging remission duration)
4. Mycosis Fungoides (Advanced disease) (Stages III, IVA, IVB) (see also Dosage).
B. Frequently responsive solid malignancies (see also Dosage):
1. Neuroblastoma (in patients with disseminated disease, Stage IV)
2. Carcinoma of the Breast (Stages II-IV)
3. Retinoblastoma (St. Jude Stages II-IV)
C. Malignant neoplasms of the lung (T N M Staging) (see also Dosage):
Frequently responsive.

CONTRAINDICATIONS: Cyclophosphamide is contraindicated in patients with severely depressed bone marrow function; particularly after previous or during concurrent chemo- and/or radiation therapy without appropriate reduction in dosage.

Caution is indicated, when administering cyclophosphamide to patients with severe leukopenia, thrombocytopenia, and tumor cell infiltration of bone marrow.

Cyclophosphamide is contraindicated in patients who have demonstrated hypersensitivity to this drug or its metabolites, alone or as part of combination chemotherapy.

Because of the mutagenic and teratogenic potential of cyclophosphamide adequate methods of contraception should be used by patients (both female and male) during treatment with cyclophosphamide. The duration of contraception in men and women after the end of chemotherapy depends on the prognosis of the primary disease and on the intensity of the parents' desire for a child. Men should be informed about sperm preservation prior to initiation of treatment with cyclophosphamide. Cyclophosphamide-induced malignancy, mutagenicity, or impairment of fertility must be considered in any risk/benefit assessment.

Use during pregnancy; primarily during the first trimester. If pregnancy occurs during cyclophosphamide treatment, the patient must be informed about the possible risks to the fetus.

Use during breast feeding. Since cyclophosphamide is distributed into breast milk, breast-feeding is not recommended during chemotherapy, due to the potential risks to the infant (adverse effects, carcinogenicity, mutagenicity).

Since varicella-zoster infections appear to be particularly dangerous, concomitant use of cyclophosphamide must be avoided. With all acute infections, caution is indicated when administering cyclophosphamide.

Use in patients with inflammation of the bladder (cystitis).

Use in patients with urinary outflow obstructions.

In combined chemotherapy regimen, the contraindications for each individual drug must be identified.

WARNINGS: Extreme caution is recommended in the use of cyclophosphamide for non-neoplastic conditions, because of potential carcinogenicity with long-term use of this agent.

Since cyclophosphamide is an inhibitor of serum cholinesterase, patients receiving this drug may exhibit increased sensitivity to neuromuscular blocking agents, such as succinylcholine. If a patient who is to undergo surgery is receiving cyclophosphamide or has been treated with cyclophosphamide within 10 days of general anesthesia, the anesthetist should be so advised prior to surgery.

The rate of metabolism and the leucopenic activity of cyclophosphamide are increased by chronic administration of phenobarbital.

Cyclophosphamide has been shown to be more toxic in adrenalectomized dogs. Dose adjustments of cyclophosphamide may be necessary for adrenalectomized patients.

Treatment with cyclophosphamide may cause significant suppression of immune responses. **Dose modification should be considered for patients who develop bacterial, fungal or viral infections.**

Prior to initiating treatment with cyclophosphamide, it is necessary to exclude or correct any obstructions of the efferent urinary tract, cystitis, infections and electrolyte imbalances.

Bladder injury such as hemorrhagic cystitis, or fibrosis of the bladder may develop in patients on long-term cyclophosphamide therapy. Should a cystitis in connection with micro- or macrohematuria appear during treatment with cyclophosphamide, therapy must be interrupted until normalization.

PRECAUTIONS: Cyclophosphamide is a potent drug that should only be used by physicians experienced with cancer chemotherapeutic drugs or immunosuppressive therapy.

The patient's hematologic, hepatic and urinary profile must regularly be monitored.

Leukocyte counts must be conducted regularly during treatment: at intervals of 5-7 days when starting treatment and every 2 days if the counts drop below 3000/mm³. Daily counts may be necessary under certain circumstances. In patients receiving long-term treatment, counts every two weeks are usually sufficient. If signs of myelosuppression become evident, it is recommended to check the red blood count and the platelet count. Urinary sediment should also be checked regularly for the presence of erythrocytes.

General: Each individual component of a cyclophosphamide-containing poly-chemotherapy regimen must have its precaution profile reviewed.

Since cyclophosphamide is highly toxic with a relatively low therapeutic index, and a therapeutic response is not likely to occur without some evidence of toxicity, the drug must only be used under constant supervision of the attending physician.

Due to potential adverse effects of cyclophosphamide such as nausea and vomiting which may result in vasomotor ataxia, caution should be advised when driving or operating machinery.

Geriatrics: While age-related renal and/or hepatic impairment may require cautious dose adjustment, no geriatrics-specific problems are expected to limit the usefulness of cyclophosphamide in the elderly.

Children: No pediatrics-specific problems are documented that would limit the usefulness of cyclophosphamide in children. With or without renal and/or hepatic impairment, dosage adjustment in this patient group is necessary.

Patients with Special Diseases and Conditions: Previous therapy with other cytotoxic agents, previous X-ray therapy, hyperuricemia (gout and/or urate renal stones or history thereof).

Drug Interactions: Cyclophosphamide (<10 mg/kg i.v.) and indomethacin (50 mg p.o. qid). Four (4) cases of severe pulmonary edema and acute life-threatening water intoxication. Appropriate supportive measures should be employed if water intoxication occurs.

Cyclophosphamide (100-150 mg p.o.) and prednisone (20-80 mg p.o.). Four (4) cases of acute respiratory failure; three patients died.

Cyclophosphamide (10 mg/kg infusion) and succinylcholine anesthesia. Post-operative apnea, which is not reduced with smaller doses of cyclophosphamide.

Prior or concurrent treatment with hepatic enzyme inducers such as phenobarbital, phenytoin, benzodiazepines and/or chloral hydrate may induce microsomal metabolism to increase formation of alkylating metabolites of cyclophosphamide, thereby reducing the half-life and increasing the activity of cyclophosphamide.

Cyclophosphamide (15-20 mg/kg ^{14}C) and phenobarbitone (60 mg p.o. tid). Cyclophosphamide half-life decreased from 4.3 hours to 1.6 hours; however, in another study, cyclophosphamide biotransformation was increased 2 to 3 fold after phenobarbitone. In these studies, urinary excretion of metabolites over 48 hours was unchanged.

Alcohol consumption is not recommended in patients treated with cyclophosphamide.

Concurrent cyclophosphamide with allopurinol or hydrochlorothiazide may enhance the bone marrow toxicity of cyclophosphamide. If concurrent use is unavoidable, frequent monitoring for toxic effects is strongly recommended.

Concurrent cyclophosphamide with anthracyclines, (e.g., doxorubicin, daunorubicin, epirubicin, idarubicin) may result in increased cardiotoxicity. It is recommended that the total dose of doxo- or daunorubicin does not exceed 400 mg/m² of body surface. Specific dosing instructions for idarubicin and epirubicin are not available, and their concurrent use with cyclophosphamide should be undertaken with caution after consulting the relevant product information for each product. Pentostatin or radiation towards the cardiac region may result in increased cardiotoxicity in the presence of cyclophosphamide. Concurrent administration of methotrexate and cyclophosphamide may result in the inhibition of the metabolism of cyclophosphamide.

The blood glucose-lowering effect of sulfonyl ureas may be intensified when administered concomitantly with cyclophosphamide.

Since cyclophosphamide has immunosuppressive effects, the patient can be expected to exhibit a diminished response to any vaccination; injection with activated vaccines may be accompanied by vaccine-induced infection.

Concomitant administration of chloramphenicol leads to a prolonged half-life of cyclophosphamide and to a delayed metabolism.

Concomitant administration of grapefruit or grapefruit juice is not recommended since grapefruit contains a compound that may impair the activation of cyclophosphamide, and thereby its efficacy.

It is prudent to monitor, among others, the following drugs if administered concurrent with cyclophosphamide: Colchicine, Probenecid, Sulfinpyrazone, Cytarabine, Azathioprine, Chlorambucil, Corticosteroids, Glucocorticoid, Cyclosporine, Mercaptopurine, ACE-inhibitors (Pancytopenia is a known ADR of this latter combination), Indomethacin, (see also above EDI-Evaluation of drug interactions-reference).

Concurrent use in cardiac transplant patients of cyclophosphamide with the antihyperlipidemic HMG-CoA reductase inhibitor lovastatin may be associated with an increased risk of rhabdomyolysis and acute renal failure.

Laboratory Tests: During treatment, the patient's hematologic profile (particularly neutrophils and platelets) should be monitored regularly, to determine the degree of hematopoietic suppression.

Urine should also be examined regularly for red cells, a possible indicator for hemorrhagic cystitis.

Frequent liver function tests (LFT's) are advised.

The following laboratory alterations have been reported in the literature and are potentially clinically significant:

- Positive reactions may be suppressed: Candida skin test, mumps skin test, trichophyton skin test, tuberculin PPD skin test
- False-positive results may be produced: Papanicolaou (PAP) test
- Serum concentrations may be decreased: Pseudocholinesterase
- Blood and urine concentrations may be increased: Uric acid

Information to Be Provided to the Patient: Patients should be fully informed as to treatment options, risks, and safety of cyclophosphamide, both alone, or as component of a polychemotherapy regimen (see Dosage).

Present information listed in this monograph under Contraindications, Warnings, Precautions, and Adverse Effects.

Patients must strictly respect dosage instructions and treatment schedules, to ensure efficacy and tolerability of cyclophosphamide.

Prevention of drug interactions and reporting of moderate to severe side effects must carefully be advised.

Importance of ample fluid intake - some patients may require up to 3000 mL (3 quarts) - and subsequent increase in urine output, as well as frequent voiding to prevent accumulation in the bladder of the toxic metabolite acrolein, suspected of causing hemorrhagic cystitis, and to aid in excretion of uric acid.

Importance of continuing medication despite stomach upset; patients should be advised about the administration of antiemetics.

To avoid bruising or injury (accidental cuts). Caution in the use of instruments of dental hygiene, or when dental work is done. Physician may suggest alternatives.

Wearing a facial mask (nose and mouth), to prevent exposure to persons with bacterial infections, as well as avoiding persons (including family members) who were immunized with oral polio-virus vaccine.

Not to touch the eyes or inside of nose, unless hands were washed immediately before.

To notify the attending physician or nurse of any upcoming surgery including dental surgery, to prevent cyclophosphamide (use within 10 days of general anesthesia) interactions with general anesthetic medications.

To notify the attending physician or nurse of any upcoming immunizations.

Patients should be informed about the importance of meticulous oral hygiene.

The recommended storage temperature for the cyclophosphamide dosage forms should not exceed 25°C.

ADVERSE EFFECTS: Note: Many side effects of cancer chemotherapy are unavoidable, since they represent the drug's pharmacologic action. Leukopenia and thrombocytopenia are used as guidelines, among others, to aid in individual dosage titration.

The following is a summary of adverse reactions reported with cyclophosphamide either alone or in combination with other chemotherapeutic agents. In the case of a polychemotherapy regimen, the adverse reaction profile of each drug component should be reviewed.

Anaphylactic and Hypersensitivity Reactions: **Note: Anaphylaxis has resulted in death.** Case of cyclophosphamide-induced fulminating anaphylaxis. Hypersensitivity reactions accompanied by fever, extending to shock in isolated cases. Generalized urticaria and pruritus. Possibility of cross-sensitivity with other alkylating agents must also be considered.

Patients receiving cyclophosphamide may experience the following dose-dependent side effects which are reversible in most cases:

Hematopoietic System: Depending on the dose of cyclophosphamide administered, different degrees of myelosuppression may occur, involving leukocytopenia, thrombocytopenia, hypothrombinemia, and anaemia. It can commonly be expected that leukocytopenia with and without fever and the risk of secondary (sometimes life-threatening) infections will occur, as will thrombocytopenia associated with the higher risk of a bleeding event. The leukocyte and platelet nadirs are usually reached in week 1 and 2 of treatment. They usually recover within 3 to 4 weeks after the initiation of treatment. Anaemia will usually not develop until after several treatment cycles. Pancytopenia is a known ADR of cyclophosphamide in combination with, for instance, etoposide and cisplatin, where individual drug cause is difficult to identify. More severe myelosuppression is to be expected in patients who have been pre-treated with chemo- and/or radiotherapy and in patients with renal impairment. A combination treatment with other myelopsuppressive agents may require dose adjustments.

Leukopenia of less than 2000 cells/mm³ develops commonly in patients treated with an initial loading dose of the drug.

Thrombocytopenia nadirs occur within 10-15 days after administration.

The degree of neutropenia is particularly important because it correlates with a reduction in resistance to infection.

Thrombocytopenia, hypothrombinemia, and anemia occasionally develops in patients treated with cyclophosphamide. These toxic effects can usually be reversed by reducing the drug dose or through interruption of treatment.

Cardiopulmonary: Cardiotoxicity, which is uncommon at usual cyclophosphamide dosages, has been reported at high doses of between 120 and 180 mg/kg to as high as 270 mg/kg within a period of 4 to 6 days. This dosage range is usually part of an intensive polychemotherapy regimen, or is given in conjunction with transplantation procedures. This secondary cardiomyopathy may manifest as arrhythmias, ECG changes and/or LVEF (e.g., myocardial infarction). Cases of severe and sometimes fatal congestive heart failure have occurred within a few days after the first dose of a high-dose course of cyclophosphamide. Histopathologic examination revealed primarily hemorrhagic myocarditis. A fatal high-dose cyclophosphamide-induced cardiomyopathy, characterized by hemorrhagic myocardial necrosis has been reported.

There is evidence that the cardiotoxic effect of cyclophosphamide may be enhanced in patients who have received previous radiation treatment of the heart region and/or adjuvant treatment with anthracyclines or pentostatin. In this context, regular electrolyte monitoring is necessary and special caution is advised in patients with pre-existing heart disease.

Sudden weight gain, ECG abnormalities, dyspnea and/or other signs of congestive heart failure should be monitored. The antidiuretic effect, occasionally seen with cyclophosphamide alone, and as drug interaction with indomethacin (the latter manifesting itself as severe water intoxication-SIADH), may contribute to the cardiopulmonary pathology.

Pulmonary toxicity due to cyclophosphamide is a recognized entity. Interstitial pulmonary fibrosis, which can be fatal, has been reported with long-term high-dose cyclophosphamide. Careful monitoring is advised, since in some cases the discontinuance of the drug and administration of corticosteroids have failed to reverse this syndrome. In isolated cases, pneumonitis may develop.

Urogenital: There have been isolated reports of hemorrhagic cystitis resulting in death.

Sterile hemorrhagic cystitis, which can become a severe to fatal condition, mainly due to long-term daily low-dose, or short-term high-dose cyclophosphamide, is thought to be secondary to the formation/concentration of the toxic metabolite acrolein during prolonged contact with the bladder epithelium. Changes in the efferent urinary tract may also occur. Hemorrhagic cystitis, microhematuria and macrohematuria are the most common dose-dependent complications of treatment with cyclophosphamide. Cystitis is initially abacterial; secondary bacterial colonization may follow. Reduction or interruption of cyclophosphamide, forced diuresis, hydration may limit the time of contact between the metabolite acrolein and the bladder epithelium. Prophylactic Mesna treatment is effective in many patients. Hematuria usually resolves spontaneously within a few days after interruption of cyclophosphamide therapy, but may persist for several months.

Cyclophosphamide-related non-hemorrhagic cystitis, edema of the bladder wall, suburethral bleeding, interstitial inflammation, and at times extensive fibrosis of the bladder with atypical cells in the urinary sediment have also been reported. A potential for sclerosis of the bladder wall also exists. Cryosurgery and other methods have been used in protracted cases.

Renal lesions (particularly in patients with a history of impaired renal function) are a rare side effect after high doses of cyclophosphamide. Interruption of therapy may, in most cases, resolve the lesion.

Second malignancy of the urinary bladder may develop, generally in patients who previously developed hemorrhagic cystitis, and may in some cases not be detected until several years after discontinuance of cyclophosphamide. Studies in animals have demonstrated that the risk of bladder cancer can be markedly reduced by an adequate administration of Mesna treatment.

Sterility in both sexes may result from cyclophosphamide treatment, depending on dose, duration of therapy, and state of gonadal function at time of treatment. By virtue of its alkylating mode of action, cyclophosphamide can be assumed to cause partially irreversible disturbances of spermatogenesis and the resulting azoospermia or persistent oligospermia. Ovulation disorders, that sometimes take an irreversible course, with the resulting amenorrhoea and lower levels of female sex hormones occur with a rarer frequency. Ovarian atrophy, fibrosis and complete absence of follicular structures are reported histologic features in some cyclophosphamide-treated women, where regaining reproductive function is unpredictable.

Gastrointestinal: Nausea and vomiting are common with cyclophosphamide treatment and are dose-dependent. Moderate to severe forms occur in approximately 50% of patients. Anorexia and, less frequently, abdominal discomfort or pain, diarrhea or obstipation, constipation and inflammatory conditions of the mucosa (mucositis), ranging from stomatitis to ulcerations may occur. There have been isolated reports of hemorrhagic colitis, oral mucosal ulceration (stomatitis), and jaundice occurring during therapy. These adverse events generally remit when cyclophosphamide is stopped.

Metabolic Effects: As a result of rapid cellular destruction (tumor lysis), especially in non-Hodgkin's lymphomas or leukemias, hyperuricemia may occur in some patients being treated with cyclophosphamide. Hyperuricemia may be minimized by adequate hydration, alkalinization of the urine, and/or administration of allopurinol. If allopurinol is decided upon, the patient must carefully be monitored to prevent severe cyclophosphamide toxicity (see Precautions, Drug Interactions). Cyclophosphamide-related hyperkalemia may also be due to tumorlysis.

A syndrome of inappropriate antidiuretic hormone secretion (SIADH) with hyponatremia and water retention has occurred in patients on high-dose cyclophosphamide therapy. Careful monitoring of this condition is advised.

Rare cases of disturbances of hepatic function have been reported that are reflected by an increase in the corresponding laboratory test values (AST, ALT, gamma-GT, alkaline phosphatase and/or bilirubin).

Veno-occlusive disease (VOD) is observed in approximately 15-50 % of the patients receiving high-dose cyclophosphamide in combination with busulfan or whole-body irradiation during allogenic bone marrow transplantation. By contrast, VOD is only rarely observed in patients with aplastic anaemia who are receiving high dose cyclophosphamide alone. The syndrome typically develops 1-3 weeks after the transplantation and is characterized by sudden weight gain, hepatomegaly, ascites and hyperbilirubinaemia. Hepatic encephalopathy may also develop. Known risk factors predisposing a patient to the development of VOD are pre-existing disturbances of hepatic function, hepatotoxic drug therapy concurrently with high-dose (chemo)therapy and especially when the alkylating agent busulfan is an element of the conditioning therapy.

Dermatologic Effects: Alopecia occurs commonly in patients treated with even low doses of cyclophosphamide. With large parenteral doses, considerable hair loss (5-30%, with possible total alopecia) is to be expected. The hair can be expected to grow back after or even during continued treatment; it may, however be different in texture and/or colour.

Skin rash occurs occasionally. Pigmentation of skin and changes in nails may occur.

A case of a variant of CHOP-associated erythrodysesthesia syndrome (identified as a variant of palmar-plantar erythema) related to high-dose cyclophosphamide has been reported.

Other Adverse Effects: Nadir fever, headache, dizziness, diabetes mellitus, blurring of vision and myopia. Rare cases of rhabdomyolysis have been reported. Acute pancreatitis may occur in isolated cases. In rare cases, severe skin reactions like Stevens Johnson Syndrome and toxic epidermal necrolysis have been reported under cyclophosphamide therapy. Cyclophosphamide may impair wound healing, which can be alleviated by supplemental vitamin "A"; **monitoring the patient is necessary, to prevent a possible drug interaction.**

There are certain complications, such as thromboembolism, DIC (disseminated intravascular coagulation), or hemolytic uremic syndrome (HUS), that may also be induced by the underlying disease, but that might occur with an increased frequency under chemotherapy that includes cyclophosphamide.

Carcinogenesis: As with cytotoxic therapy in general, treatment with cyclophosphamide involves the risk of secondary tumours and their precursors as late sequelae. The risk of developing urinary tract cancer as well as myelodysplastic alterations partly progressing to acute leukemias, or non-malignant disease in which immune processes are believed to be involved pathologically is increased. Urinary bladder malignancies have usually occurred in patients who previously had hemorrhagic cystitis. Animal studies demonstrate that the risk of bladder cancer can be markedly reduced by an adequate administration of mesna.

OVERDOSE:

Symptoms: Limited information on acute overdosage of cyclophosphamide is available.

Since no specific antidote for cyclophosphamide is known, great caution is advised each time it is used. If overdose of cyclophosphamide is known or suspected, the patient should be hospitalized for general supportive therapy. Cyclophosphamide can be dialysed. Therefore, rapid hemodialysis is indicated when treating any suicidal or accidental overdose or intoxication. A dialysis clearance of 78 mL/min was calculated from the concentration of non-metabolized cyclophosphamide in the dialysate (normal renal clearance is around 5 - 11 mL/min). A second working group reported a value of 194 mL/min. After 6 hours of dialysis, 72% of the dose of cyclophosphamide administered was found in the dialysate. In the case of overdose, myelosuppression, mostly leukocytopenia, is to be expected, among other reactions. The severity and duration of the myelosuppression depends on the extent of the overdose. Frequent checks of the blood count and monitoring of the patient are necessary. If neutropenia develops, infection prophylaxis must be given and infections must be treated adequately with antibiotics. If thrombocytopenia develops, thrombocyte replacement should be ensured according to need. It is essential that cystitis prophylaxis with mesna be undertaken to avoid any urotoxic effects.

Cardiotoxicity may also occur with overdosage. In patients who received 4 to 10-day courses of cyclophosphamide with total dosage per course exceeding 140 mg/kg or 5.2 g/m^2, cardiac damage manifested by heart failure occurred within 15 days of the initial dose. Impairment of water excretion with hyponatremia, weight gain, and inappropriately concentrated urine has been reported after cyclophosphamide doses exceeding 50 mg/kg (2 g/m^2).

At least one fatal case of cyclophosphamide overdosage had been reported; potentially fatal cardiotoxicity was the most serious consequence of overdosage. The risk of overdose with high-dose cyclophosphamide concomitantly with radiation therapy or other potentially cardiotoxic drugs (e.g: anthracyclines) must carefully be taken into consideration.

If a cyclophosphamide solution is inadvertently administered by paravenous injection, there is usually no danger of cytostatic tissue damage since such damage is not expected before cyclophosphamide has been bioactivated in the liver. Nevertheless, if paravasation should occur, stop the infusion immediately and aspirate the paravasate with the cannula in place, irrigate the area with saline solution and immobilize the extremity.

Treatment: See Symptoms.

For management of a suspected drug overdose, CPhA recommends that you contact your **regional Poison Control Centre**. See the *CPS* Directory section for a list of Poison Control Centres.

DOSAGE: Cyclophosphamide is a drug with the potential for fatal complications, and should, therefore, be only used by a physician experienced with cancer chemotherapeutic drugs and/or immunosuppressive therapy.

Parenteral products prior to administration need to be visually inspected for discolouration and particulate matter. After reconstitution, this parenteral dosage form represents a colourless and clear solution.

During or immediately after the administration of cyclophosphamide, adequate amounts of fluid should be ingested and the patient should empty his/her bladder at regular intervals. Prophylactic treatment with Mesna is recommended for protection of the bladder (see Warnings; Precautions, Information to Be Provided to the Patient; and Adverse Effects).

Initial Loading Dose: Cyclophosphamide: Patients with normal hematologic and bone marrow function: Adults: i.v. 40-50 mg/kg (1.5-1.8 g/m^2) as 10 to 20 mg/kg/day for 2-5 days. Children: i.v. 2 - 8 mg/kg (60-250 mg/m^2) in divided doses for six or more days.

Patients with compromised bone marrow function due to prior radiation therapy, poly-chemotherapy, or tumour cell infiltration, must have their initial loading dose reduced by 30-50%. Dosage adjustment must also be considered for children and adults with concurrent disease or special conditions. Adults: p.o. 1-5 mg/kg/day depending upon the tolerance of the patient. Children: p.o. 2-8 mg/kg (60-250 mg/m^2) in divided doses for six or more days. Morning administration of cyclophosphamide is recommended.

The leukocyte count generally serves as a guide to dosage adjustments, and maintaining a range of 2500-4000 cells/mm^3 is recommended to possibly avoid infection.

The above initial loading doses may lead to transient or more persistent reduction to 200 cells/mm^3. The patient's hematologic profile must carefully be monitored.

Maintenance Dose: Cyclophosphamide: It is generally advisable to administer the largest maintenance dose that can reasonably be tolerated by the patient, unless the disease is unusually sensitive to cyclophosphamide. Adults: i.v. 10-15 mg/kg (350-550 mg/m^2) every 7-10 days; i.v. 3- 5 mg/kg (110-185 mg/m^2) twice weekly; p.o. 1- 5 mg/kg/day. Children: i.v. 10-15 mg/kg every 7-10 days, or 30 mg/kg at three- to four-week intervals or when bone marrow recovery occurs. p.o. 2- 5 mg/kg (50-150 mg/m^2) twice weekly. Concurrent disease, special conditions including performance index must lead to dosage adjustment.

Polychemotherapy Regimen: As with monotherapy, it is advisable that treatment-related emergency measures and equipment, including pathology-specific antibiotics be physically present during polychemotherapy.

It should be noted that regular and high-dose cyclophosphamide as monotherapy or as component of polychemotherapy are being effectively used in patients resistant to first line treatment such as melphalan or busulfan. Objective responses in a variety of different forms of cancer, plus its relative platelet-sparing effect make cyclophosphamide an alternate drug of choice. Cyclophosphamide as 60 mg/kg i.v. for 2 days may be administered for bone marrow transplant conditioning. In patients with multiple transfusions, cyclophosphamide is not adequately immunosuppressive, requiring the addition of AT to the retransplant cytoreduction conditioning.

Note: Due to constant new developments in cancer chemotherapy, any presentation can only be viewed as an example of effective treatments. For additional details, the physician is referred to the Product Monograph and the literature cited therein.

Stability and Storage Recommendations: The recommended storage temperature for the cyclophosphamide dosage forms is 15-25°C (do not exceed 25°C). The dosage forms should be protected from direct light

During transport or storage of Procytox injection vials, temperature fluctuations can lead to melting of the active ingredient, cyclophosphamide. Vials containing melted substance are easily noticeable, since the powder becomes a clear or viscous yellow liquid (seen as droplets or a connected phase in the affected vials). Do not use vials with melted content.

Reconstituted Solutions: The following solutions have been recommended as diluents for intravenous infusion: 5% dextrose USP in 0.9% sodium chloride USP, 5% dextrose USP in sterile water for injection USP, 0.9% sodium chloride USP.

Such solutions are chemically stable for 24 hours at 15-25°C, or 72 hours under refrigeration (4°C). Unless prepared under aseptic conditions, such solutions should be used within 8 hours after dilution.

An oral elixir may be prepared by dissolving the Procytox dry powder contents of the vials in "Aromatic Elixir USP" shortly before administration. This liquid oral formulation, if refrigerated at 4°C, should be used within 14 days.

Solutions of Procytox for parenteral use should be prepared by adding isotonic, sterile, Sodium Chloride Injection USP to the vial, and shaking the contents until dissolution and a clear solution is obtained.

Procytox should not be reconstituted with benzyl alcohol-preserved diluent solution such as bacteriostatic sodium chloride when used in children or infants, due to toxicity concerns in this age group (i.e., gasping syndrome in infants). Further, Procytox should not be reconstituted or diluted with benzyl alcohol-containing diluents, as benzyl alcohol may catalyse the decomposition of cyclophosphamide. Therefore, it is recommended to reconstitute Procytox with isotonic, sterile, Sodium Chloride Injection USP.

Heating should not be used to facilitate dissolution.

Solutions prepared with isotonic, sterile, Sodium Chloride Injection USP should only be used for a single dose administration, and any unused portion should be discarded (see Special Instructions).

Parenteral Products: Reconstitution Table: See Table 2.

Table 2: Procytox
Reconstitution Table

Vial Size Cyclophosphamide (mg)	Volume of Diluent to be Added to Vial (mL)	Nominal Concentration (mg/mL)
200	10	20
500	25	20
1000	50	20
2000	100	20

As with all parenteral drug products, intravenous admixtures should be inspected visually for clarity, particulate matter, precipitate, discolouration and leakage prior to administration, whenever solution and container permit. Solutions showing haziness, particulate matter, precipitate, discolouration or leakage should not be used. Discard unused portion.

Since it has been reported that immersion of a needle with an aluminum component into cyclophosphamide resulted in a slight darkening of the aluminum and gas production after a few days at 24°C with protection from light, it is recommended to avoid the use of utensils, needles or parts of infusion pumps made of aluminum in the presence of Procytox.

Special Instructions: Cyclophosphamide is cytotoxic, carcinogenic, mutagenic and teratogenic. Avoid ingestion, inhalation, or skin and eye contact. Mandatory washing of hands before and after using gloves must be advised. If necessary, consult the Company's Material Safety Data Sheet.

Personnel, regularly handling these agents should have frequent hematologic examinations (CBC), and frequently be screened for urine mutagenesis.

Work-practice guidelines for personnel dealing with and handling cytotoxic and hazardous preparations must be respected, to minimize unnecessary exposure to cyclophosphamide in physicians, nurses, pharmacists, and technicians.

Appropriate Personal Protective Equipment (PPE) must be available in all areas where cyclophosphamide is handled. See Table 3.

Table 3: Procytox
Personal Protective Equipment (PPE)

Activity (when to wear)	Personal Protective Equipment (PPE) Gloves: Surgical Latex (7–9 mil thickness) or material which provides equal or better protection. Gloves must be changed at least hourly or immediately if contaminated, torn or punctured. Wash hands with soap and water after removal of gloves.	Gown: Moisture-resistant, long-sleeved gown with cuffs. Gowns must be changed daily, immediately if contaminated and immediately after spill clean-up.	Eye Protection: Eye/face protection (e.g., chemical splash goggles) must be worn when there is hazard of eye contact.	Mask: (As approved by Workers Compensation Board)
Preparation	Always	Always	If preparing outside a biological safety cabinet	No
Administration	Always	Always	If hazard of eye contact	No
Spill Clean-up	Always	Always	Always	Yes
Waste Disposal	Always	If waste uncontained	If waste uncontained	No

Preparation of Procytox must take place in a Pharmacy or, in facilities where there is not a Pharmacy, in a Class II Type B or better, externally-vented biological safety cabinet. The biological safety cabinet should have airflow monitoring devices and should be certified at least annually. Only luer-lock connections should be used in the preparation of Procytox.

Disposal of cyclophosphamide-contaminated clothing, gloves, utensils, broken glass etc. must be considered as hazardous waste. It must be deposited into a 4 mil thick polypropylene hospital trash bag (properly labelled), or be otherwise segregated and incinerated at above 1000°C. Chemical inactivation should, if possible, be avoided, since it is often ineffective and may produce byproducts that are more mutagenic than the parent drug.

Spills: Cleaning up immediately, and decontaminating areas of spills and breakage by experienced and well-protected personnel is of utmost importance. Contaminated areas including hood interiors must have clearly worded warning labels posted. It is suggested that spill kits be easily accessible, and include replacement hood filters, a respirator ("P3" filter, Manufacturer's current recommendation for cyclophosphamide powder spills), chemical splash goggles, at least 2 pairs of protective gloves, at least 2 sheets (31 cm x 33 cm/12" x 13") of absorbent material, 250 mL and 1 Liter spill-control pillows, a small scoop, spatula, forceps or tweezers to collect glass fragments, and at least two large polypropylene hospital trash bags 4 mil or thicker, or other cytotoxic drug waste-disposal bags, puncture- and leak-resistant waste container for sharp or breakable objects or spilled liquid, and warning sign (e.g., " Danger - Cytotoxic Agent Spill"). Absorbents should be incinerable.

SUPPLIED: Injection: Each vial contains: cyclophosphamide 200, 500, 1000 and 2000 mg. No excipients. Single vials. Protect from direct light.

Tablets: 25 mg: Each round, deeply biconvex, white to off-white, sugar-coated tablet contains: 26.7 mg cyclophosphamide monohydrate equivalent to 25 mg anhydrous cyclophosphamide. Nonmedicinal ingredients: calcium carbonate, cellulose, dibasic calcium phosphate, gelatin, glycerin, lactose, magnesium stearate, polyethylene glycol, polysorbate, povidone, silicon dioxide, starch (corn), sucrose, talc, titanium dioxide and wax. Bottles of 200.

50 mg: Each round, deeply biconvex, off-white, sugar-coated tablet contains: 53.5 mg cyclophosphamide monohydrate equivalent to 50 mg anhydrous cyclophosphamide. Nonmedicinal ingredients: calcium carbonate, cellulose, dibasic calcium phosphate, gelatin, glycerin, lactose, magnesium stearate, polyethylene glycol, polysorbate, povidone, silicon dioxide, starch (corn), sucrose, talc, titanium dioxide and wax. Blister packs of 10, boxes 100.

Proferrin®

heme iron polypeptide

Natural Health Product

Medical Futures

PHARMACOLOGY: Proferrin is a heme iron polypeptide, a naturally sourced form of iron derived from bovine hemoglobin. Heme iron is essentially the iron in hemoglobin with part of its protein removed during normal digestion or during the processing of Proferrin. Heme iron is readily absorbed throughout the small intestine and is absorbed more efficiently than other forms of oral iron. Heme iron absorption is not affected by foods such as: phytates (bran or wheat), polyphenols (compounds in tea or coffee), calcium, or by achlorhydria (low stomach acid) that reduce the absorption of other oral irons.

INDICATIONS: For adults 18 and over: To prevent or treat those at risk of iron deficiency.

CONTRAINDICATIONS: Before using heme iron polypeptide individuals should tell their pharmacist or doctor if using methyldopa, or other iron-containing products, iron supplements can decrease the absorption of drugs such as tetracycline antibiotics, penicillamine, cefdinir, chloramphenicol, levothyroxine, levodopa and quinolone antibiotics. Therefore, doses of these medications should be spaced as far as possible.

This product may interfere with certain laboratory tests (including testing for blood in stool) possibly causing false test results. Make sure laboratory personnel and all doctors know a patient is using this drug.

This product should not be used if you have certain medical conditions.

WARNINGS: Keep away from children. Accidental overdose of iron-containing products is a leading cause of fatal poisoning in children younger than 6 years. If accidental overdose does occur, call a doctor or poison centre immediately.

PRECAUTIONS: *Pregnancy:* Individuals who are pregnant, breastfeeding or have hemochromatosis, other types of anemia, repeated blood transfusions, or stomach/intestinal problems should tell their pharmacist or doctor before using Proferrin.
Lactation: See Pregnancy.

ADVERSE EFFECTS: Constipation, diarrhea, nausea, upset stomach and stomach/abdominal cramping may occur. The incidence of these adverse events is less than that of ionic iron. Iron may cause your stools to turn black, an effect that is not harmful. A very serious allergic reaction to this product is rare. Do not use if you have any allergy to cow products.

OVERDOSE:

> For management of a suspected drug overdose, CPhA recommends that you contact your **regional Poison Control Centre**. See the *CPS* Directory section for a list of Poison Control Centres.

DOSAGE: Take 1-3 tablets daily in divided doses with a glass of water, with or without food. Do not lie down for 30 minutes after taking Proferrin.

SUPPLIED: Each tablet contains: 11 mg elemental iron from heme iron polypeptide (bovine). Nonmedicinal ingredients: calcium stearate, cellulose, chlorophyllin, croscarmellose sodium, hydrogenated vegetable oils, pharmaceutical glaze, polyethylene glycol, polyvinyl alcohol, povidone, protease, silicon dioxide, sucrose, talc and titanium dioxide. Store at room temperature between 15-30°C, away from light and moisture.

Proflavanol 90

vitamin C—grape seed extract

Vitamin Supplement

USANA Health Sciences

SUPPLIED: Each tablet contains: vitamin C (ascorbates of calcium, magnesium, potassium, and zinc) 300 mg and grape seed extract (Vitis vinifera, 120:1, 80% procyanidins) 90 mg. Nonmedicinal ingredients: ascorbyl palmitate, croscarmellose sodium, dextrin, dextrose, microcrystalline cellulose, silicon dioxide, soy lecithin and starch. Bottles of 56. Safety seal under cap. Store below 25°C.

(Shown in Product Identification Section)

Progesterone Injection USP Ⓟ

progesterone

Progestogen

Cytex

SUPPLIED: Each mL contains: progesterone 50 mg, benzyl alcohol 10% as preservative in sesame oil q.s. Multiple dose vials of 10 mL.

Proglycem® Ⓟ

diazoxide

Hyperglycemic Agent

Schering-Plough

PHARMACOLOGY: Diazoxide administered orally produces a prompt dose-related increase in blood glucose level, due primarily to an inhibition of insulin release from the pancreas and also to an extrapancreatic effect.

The hyperglycemic effect begins within an hour and generally lasts no more than 8 hours in the presence of normal renal function.

Diazoxide decreases the excretion of sodium and water, resulting in fluid retention which may be clinically significant.

The effects on blood pressure are usually not marked with the oral preparation. This contrasts with the i.v. preparation (see Adverse Effects). Other pharmacologic actions include increased pulse rate; increased serum uric acid levels due to decreased excretion; increased serum levels of free fatty acids; decreased chloride excretion; decreased para-aminohippuric acid (PAH) clearance with no appreciable effect on glomerular filtration rate. The concomitant administration of a benzothiazide diuretic may intensify the hyperglycemic and hyperuricemic effects of diazoxide. In the presence of hypokalemia, hyperglycemic effects are also potentiated. Diazoxide-induced hyperglycemia is reversed by the administration of insulin or tolbutamide.

The inhibition of insulin release by diazoxide is antagonized by alpha-adrenergic blocking agents. Diazoxide is extensively bound (more than 90%) to serum proteins and is excreted by the kidneys. The plasma half-life following i.v. administration is about 28+/−8.3 hours. Limited data on oral administration revealed a half-life of 24 and 36 hours in 2 adults. In 4 children aged 4 months to 6 years, the plasma half-life varied from 9.5 to 24 hours on long-term oral administration. The half-life may be prolonged following overdosage and in patients with impaired renal function.

INDICATIONS: Oral diazoxide is useful in the management of hypoglycemia due to hyperinsulinism associated with the following conditions:
Adults: inoperable islet cell adenoma or carcinoma or extrapancreatic malignancy.
Children: leucine sensitivity, islet cell hyperplasia, nesidioblastosis, extrapancreatic malignancy, islet cell adenoma, or adenomatosis. It may be used preoperatively as a temporary measure and post-operatively if hypoglycemia persists.

Diazoxide should be used only after a diagnosis of hypoglycemia due to one of the above conditions has been definitely established. When other specific medical therapy or surgical management either has been unsuccessful or is not feasible, treatment with diazoxide should be considered.

CONTRAINDICATIONS: The use of diazoxide for functional hypoglycemia is contraindicated. The drug should not be used in patients hypersensitive to diazoxide or to other thiazides unless the potential benefits outweigh the possible risks.

WARNINGS: *Pregnancy:* Diazoxide should not be used in women of child-bearing age except in life-threatening situations. Reproduction studies using the oral preparation in rats have revealed increased fetal resorptions and delayed parturition, as well as fetal skeletal anomalies. Evidence of skeletal and cardiac teratogenic effects in rabbits has been noted with the i.v. administration. The drug has also been demonstrated to cross the placental barrier in animals and cause degeneration of the fetal pancreatic beta cells. Since there are no **adequate** data on fetal effects of this drug when given to pregnant women, safety in pregnancy has not been established.

When its use in pregnant women is considered, the indications should be limited to those specified above for adults (see Indications) and the potential benefits to the mother must be weighed against possible harmful effects to the fetus.
Lactation: Diazoxide may pass into the breast milk of nursing mothers.

The antidiuretic property of diazoxide may lead to significant fluid retention, which in patients with compromised cardiac reserve may precipitate congestive heart failure. The fluid retention will respond to conventional therapy with diuretics.

It should be noted that concomitantly administered thiazides may potentiate the hyperglycemic and hyperuricemic actions of diazoxide (see Precautions, Drug Interactions).

Ketoacidosis and non-ketotic hyperosmolar coma have been reported in patients treated with recommended doses, usually during intercurrent illness. Prompt recognition and treatment are essential (see Overdose) and prolonged surveillance following the acute episode is necessary because of the long drug half-life of approximately 30 hours. The occurrence of these serious events may be reduced by careful education of patients regarding the need for monitoring the urine for sugar and ketones and for prompt reporting of abnormal findings and unusual symptoms to the physician.

In the presence of hypokalemia, the hyperglycemia effects of diazoxide are potentiated.

Transient cataracts occurred in association with hyperosmolar coma in an infant and subsided on correction of the hyperosmolarity. Cataracts have been observed in several animals receiving daily doses of i.v. or oral diazoxide.

PRECAUTIONS: Treatment should be initiated under close clinical supervision, with careful monitoring of blood glucose and clinical response until the patient's condition has stabilized. This usually requires several days. If not effective in 2 or 3 weeks, the drug should be discontinued.

Prolonged treatment requires regular monitoring of the urine for sugar and ketones, especially under stress conditions, with prompt reporting of any abnormalities to the physician. Additionally, blood sugar levels should be monitored periodically by the physician to determine the need for dose adjustment.

The effects of diazoxide on the hematopoietic system and the level of serum uric acid should be kept in mind; the latter should be considered particularly in patients with hyperuricemia or a history of gout.

In some patients, higher blood levels have been observed with the liquid than with the capsule formulation. Dosage should be adjusted as necessary in individual patients if changed from 1 formulation to the other.

Since the plasma half-life of diazoxide is prolonged in patients with impaired renal function, a reduced dosage should be considered. Serum electrolyte levels should also be evaluated for such patients.

The antihypertensive effect of other drugs may be enhanced by diazoxide and this should be kept in mind when administering it concomitantly with antihypertensive agents.

Because of protein binding, administration of diazoxide with coumarin or its derivatives may require reduction in the dosage of the anticoagulant, although there has been no reported evidence of excessive anticoagulant effect. In addition, it may possibly displace bilirubin from albumin; this should be kept in mind particularly when treating newborns with increased bilirubinemia.

Drug Interactions: Diuretics: The hyperglycemic and hyperuricemic actions of diazoxide may be potentiated by the concomitant administration of thiazides or other commonly used diuretics.
Coumarin Anticoagulants: The administration of diazoxide to patients treated with coumarin and its derivatives may result in potentiation of hypoprothrombic action and may necessitate a decrease of anticoagulant dosage.
Diphenyldydantoin: The concomitant administration of diazoxide to diphenyldydantoin treated patients can cause loss of seizure control.
Chlorpromazine: The hyperglycemic action of diazoxide may be enhanced by concomitant administration of chlorpromazine.

ADVERSE EFFECTS: Frequent and serious: Sodium and fluid retention is most common in young infants and in adults and may precipitate congestive heart failure in patients with compromised cardiac reserve. It usually responds to diuretic therapy (see Precautions, Drug Interactions).
Infrequent but serious: Diabetic ketoacidosis and hyperosmolar non-ketotic coma may develop very rapidly. Conventional therapy with insulin and restoration of fluid and electrolyte balance are usually effective if instituted promptly. Prolonged surveillance is essential in view of the long half-life of diazoxide (see Overdose).

Other frequent adverse reactions: Hirsutism of the lanugo type mainly on the forehead, back and limbs which occurs most commonly in children and women may be cosmetically unacceptable. It subsides on discontinuation of the drug.

Hyperglycemia or glycosuria may require reduction in dosage in order to avoid progression to ketoacidosis or hyperosmolar coma.

Gastrointestinal intolerance may include anorexia, nausea, vomiting, abdominal pain, ileus, diarrhea, transient loss of taste. Tachycardia, palpitations, increased levels of serum uric acid are common.

Thrombocytopenia with or without purpura may require discontinuation of the drug. Neutropenia is transient, is not associated with increased susceptibility to infection and ordinarily does not require discontinuation of the drug. Skin rash, headache, weakness and malaise may also occur.

Other adverse reactions which have been observed:
Cardiovascular: hypotension occurs occasionally which may be augmented by thiazide diuretics given concurrently. A few cases of transient hypertension, for which no explanation is apparent have been noted. Chest pain has been reported rarely.
Hematologic: eosinophilia; decreased hemoglobin/hematocrit; excessive bleeding; decreased IgG.
Hepato-Renal: increased AST, alkaline phosphatase, azotemia, decreased creatinine clearance, reversible nephrotic syndrome, decreased urinary output, hematuria, albuminuria.
Neurologic: anxiety, dizziness, insomnia, polyneuritis, paresthesia, pruritus, extrapyramidal signs.
Ophthalmologic: transient cataracts, subconjunctival hemorrhage, ring scotoma, blurred vision, diplopia, lacrimation.
Skeletal/Integumentary: monilial dermatitis, herpes, advance in bone age; loss of scalp hair.
Systemic: fever, lymphadenopathy.
Other: gout, acute pancreatitis/pancreatic necrosis, galactorrhea, enlargement of lump in breast.

OVERDOSE:

Symptoms: An overdose of diazoxide causes marked hyperglycemia which may be associated with ketoacidosis.

Treatment: It will respond to prompt insulin administration and restoration of fluid and electrolyte balance. Because of the drug's long half-life (approximately 30 hours), the symptoms of overdosage require prolonged surveillance for periods up to 7 days, until the blood sugar level stabilizes within the normal range. One investigator reported successful lowering of diazoxide blood levels by peritoneal dialysis in 1 patient and by hemodialysis in another.

> For management of a suspected drug overdose, CPhA recommends that you contact your **regional Poison Control Centre**. See the *CPS* Directory section for a list of Poison Control Centres.

DOSAGE: Patients should be under close clinical observation when treatment is initiated. The clinical response and blood glucose level should be carefully monitored until the patient's condition has stabilized satisfactorily; in most instances, this may be accomplished in several days. If administration of diazoxide is not effective after 2 or 3 weeks, the drug should be discontinued.

The dosage must be individualized based on the severity of the hypoglycemic condition and the blood glucose level and the clinical response of the patient. The dosage should be adjusted until the desired clinical and laboratory effects are produced with the least amount of the drug. Special care should be taken to assure accuracy of dosage in infants and young children.
Adults and Children: The usual daily dosage is 3 to 8 mg/kg, divided into 2 or 3 equal doses every 8 or 12 hours. In certain instances, patients with refractory hypoglycemia may require higher dosages. Ordinarily, an appropriate starting dosage is 3 mg/kg/day, divided into 3 equal doses every 8 hours. Thus, an average adult would receive a starting dosage of approximately 200 mg daily.

SUPPLIED: Each opaque orange capsule, contains: diazoxide USP 100 mg. Nonmedicinal ingredients: lactose and magnesium stearate. Tartrazine-free. Bottles of 100. Store between 15 and 30°C.

(Shown in Product Identification Section)

Prograf® Ⓟ

tacrolimus

Immunosuppressant

Astellas

Date of Revision: August 27, 2009

SUMMARY PRODUCT INFORMATION:

Route of Administration	Dosage Form/ Strength	Clinically Relevant Nonmedicinal Ingredients
Oral	Capsules/0.5 mg, 1 mg and 5 mg	Lactose monohydrate, NF For a complete listing see Dosage Forms, Composition and Packaging.
Intravenous	Injection/5 mg/mL	Polyoxyl 60 hydrogenated castor oil (HCO-60) For a complete listing see Dosage Forms, Composition and Packaging.

INDICATIONS AND CLINICAL USE: Transplantation: Prograf (tacrolimus) is indicated for:

- prophylaxis of organ rejection in patients receiving allogeneic liver, kidney or heart transplants.
- treatment of refractory rejection in patients receiving allogeneic liver or kidney transplants.

Prograf is to be used concomitantly with adrenal corticosteroids and other immunosuppressive agents. The safety and efficacy of the use of Prograf with sirolimus has not been established.

Only physicians experienced in immunosuppressive therapy and management of organ transplant should prescribe Prograf (tacrolimus). Patients receiving the drug should be managed in facilities equipped and staffed with adequate laboratory and supportive medical resources. The physician responsible for maintenance therapy should have complete information requisite for the follow-up of the patient.

Rheumatoid Arthritis: Prograf (tacrolimus immediate release capsules) is indicated for:

- treatment of active rheumatoid arthritis in adult patients for whom disease modifying anti-rheumatic drug (DMARD) therapy is ineffective or inappropriate.

Prograf may be used as monotherapy or in combination with non-steroidal anti-inflammatory drugs (NSAIDs) and/or steroids, although the possibility of increased toxicity has not been fully explored (see Warnings and Precautions and Drug Interactions).

Combined use of Prograf with gold, penicillamine, hydroxychloroquine, sulfasalazine or azathioprine has not been studied.

There is currently insufficient data to support the concomitant use of Prograf and methotrexate.

Careful monitoring of Prograf treated patients is mandatory. Prograf should only be prescribed for rheumatoid arthritis by physicians experienced with the use of immunosuppressants.

Geriatrics (>65 years of age): The safety and efficacy of Prograf in patients older than 65 years of age has not been established.

Pediatrics (<18 years of age): Experience with Prograf in pediatric kidney and heart transplant patients is limited. Successful liver transplants have been performed in pediatric patients (ages 4 months up to 16 years) using Prograf, with the majority of these patients under 5 years of age (see Warnings and Precautions).

Prograf is not indicated for the use of rheumatoid arthritis in children younger than 18 years of age.

CONTRAINDICATIONS:

- Prograf (tacrolimus) is contraindicated in patients with a hypersensitivity to tacrolimus or to any ingredient in the formulation or component of the capsules. For a complete listing, see Dosage Forms, Composition and Packaging.
- Prograf (tacrolimus for injection) is contraindicated in patients with a hypersensitivity to HCO-60 (polyoxyl 60 hydrogenated castor oil).

WARNINGS AND PRECAUTIONS:

> **Serious Warnings and Precautions**
> **Increased susceptibility to infection and the possible development of lymphoma may result from immunosuppression.**
> **Transplant Patients: Only physicians experienced in immunosuppressive therapy and management of organ transplant patients should prescribe Prograf (tacrolimus). Patients receiving the drug should be managed in facilities equipped and staffed with adequate laboratory and supportive medical resources. The physician responsible for maintenance therapy should have complete information requisite for the follow-up of the patient.**
> **Rheumatoid Arthritis: Careful monitoring of Prograf treated patients is mandatory. Prograf should only be prescribed for rheumatoid arthritis by physicians experienced with the use of immunosuppressants. Prograf is indicated for the treatment of active rheumatoid arthritis in adult patients for whom disease modifying anti-rheumatic drug (DMARD) therapy is ineffective or inappropriate.**

General: Tacrolimus is extensively metabolized by the mixed-function oxidase system, primarily the cytochrome P450 system (CYP3A). Prograf does not induce or inhibit CYP3A4 or any other major CYP isoenzymes.

Since tacrolimus is metabolized mainly by the cytochrome P450 3A enzyme systems, substances known to inhibit these enzymes may decrease the metabolism or increase bioavailability of tacrolimus with resultant increases in whole blood or plasma levels. Drugs known to induce these enzyme systems may result in an increased metabolism of tacrolimus or decreased bioavailability as indicated by decreased whole blood or plasma levels. Monitoring of blood levels and appropriate dosage adjustments in transplant patients are essential when such drugs are used concomitantly (see Drug Interactions).

Prograf contains lactose and is not recommended for patients with rare hereditary disease of galactose intolerance, the Lapp lactase deficiency or glucose-galactose malabsorption.

For Transplant Patients: Patients receiving Prograf for injection should be under continuous observation for at least the first 30 minutes following the start of the infusion and at frequent intervals thereafter. If signs or symptoms of anaphylaxis occur, the infusion should be stopped. An aqueous solution of epinephrine 1:1000 should be available at the bedside as well as a source of oxygen.

Prograf, when given orally, is a twice-a-day formulation of tacrolimus. Prograf therapy requires careful monitoring by adequately qualified and equipped personnel. The medicinal product should only be prescribed, and changes in immunosuppressive therapy initiated, by physicians experienced in immunosuppressive therapy and the management of transplant patients.

Inadvertent, unintentional or unsupervised switching of Prograf (immediate release formulation) to Advagraf (extended-release formulation) of tacrolimus is unsafe. This can lead to graft rejection or increased incidence of side effects, including under- or overimmunosuppression, due to clinically relevant differences in systemic exposure to tacrolimus. Patients should be maintained on a single formulation of tacrolimus with the corresponding daily dosing regimen; alterations in formulation or regimen should only take place under the close supervision of a transplant specialist (see Dosage and Administration). **Following conversion to any alternative formulation, therapeutic drug monitoring must be performed and dose adjustments made to ensure that systemic exposure to tacrolimus is maintained.**

Carcinogenesis and Mutagenesis: An increased incidence of malignancy is a recognized complication of immunosuppression in recipients of organ transplants. The most common forms of neoplasms are non-Hodgkin's lymphomas and carcinomas of the skin. As with other immunosuppressive therapies, the risk of developing lymphomas and other malignancies, particularly of the skin, may be higher in Prograf recipients than in the normal, healthy population. The risk appears to be related to the intensity and duration of immunosuppression rather than to the use of any specific agent.

Lymphoproliferative disorders associated with Epstein-Barr virus infection have been seen. It has been reported that reduction or discontinuation of immunosuppression may cause the lesions to regress.

Cardiovascular: Hypertension is a common side effect of Prograf (tacrolimus) therapy (see Adverse Reactions). Mild or moderate hypertension is more frequently reported than severe hypertension. The incidence of hypertension decreases over time. Antihypertensive therapy may be required; the control of blood pressure can be accomplished with any of the common antihypertensive agents. Since tacrolimus may cause hyperkalemia, potassium-sparing diuretics should be avoided.

While calcium channel blocking agents can be effective in treating Prograf-associated hypertension, care should be taken since interference with tacrolimus metabolism may require a dosage reduction in the transplant patient (see Drug Interactions). Hypertension and hyperkalemia has also been noted in patients with rheumatoid arthritis. Tacrolimus should be discontinued in patients in whom hypertension and hyperkalemia cannot be controlled.

Heart failure, myocardial hypertrophy and arrhythmia have been reported in association with the administration of Prograf. Myocardial hypertrophy is generally manifested by echocardiographically demonstrated concentric increases in left ventricular posterior wall and interventricular septum thickness. Hypertrophy has been observed in infants, children and adults. This condition appears reversible in most cases following dose reduction or discontinuance of therapy. In a group of 20 transplant patients with pre- and post-treatment echocardiograms who showed evidence of myocardial hypertrophy, mean tacrolimus whole blood concentrations during the period prior to diagnosis of myocardial hypertrophy ranged from 11 to 53 ng/mL in infants (N=10) age 0.4 to 2 years, 4-46 ng/mL in children (n=7) age 2-15 years and 11-24 ng/mL in adults (N=3) age 37-53 years.

Hepatic/Biliary: The use of Prograf in liver transplant recipients experiencing post-transplant hepatic impairment may be associated with increased risk of developing renal insufficiency related to high whole blood levels of tacrolimus. These patients should be monitored closely and dosage adjustments should be considered. Some evidence suggests that the use of lower doses may be warranted in these patients. (See Dosage and Administration.)

Immune/Infection: A lymphoproliferative disorder (LPD) related to Epstein-Barr Virus (EBV) infection has been reported in immunosuppressed organ transplant recipients. The risk of LPD appears greatest in young children who are at risk for primary EBV infection while immunosuppressed, or who are switched to Prograf following long-term immunosuppression therapy. Experience on combining Prograf with immunosuppressive drugs other than adrenal corticosteroids, azathioprine and mycophenolate mofetil is limited because of the potency of Prograf and the risk of over immunosuppression and such combinations are not recommended.

Immunosuppressed patients are at increased risk for opportunistic infections, including activation of latent viral infections. These include BK virus associated nephropathy and JC virus associated progressive multifocal leukoencephalopathy (PML) which have been observed in patients receiving tacrolimus. These infections are often related to a high immunosuppressive burden and may lead to serious or fatal conditions that physicians should consider in the differential diagnosis in immunosuppressed patients with deteriorating renal function or neurological symptoms.

A few patients receiving Prograf injection have experienced anaphylactic reactions. Although the exact cause of these reactions is not known, other drugs with castor oil derivatives in the formulation have been associated with anaphylaxis in a small percentage of patients. Because of this potential risk of anaphylaxis, Prograf injection should be reserved for patients who are unable to take Prograf capsules.

Neurologic: Prograf may cause neurotoxicity, particularly when used at high doses.

Neurotoxicity, including tremor, headache, and other changes in motor function, mental status and sensory function were reported in approximately 55% of liver transplant recipients in the two randomized studies. Tremor occurred more often in Prograf-treated kidney transplant patients in the U.S. and European studies (54 and 35%, respectively), and heart transplant patients (15%) compared with cyclosporine-treated patients. The incidence of other neurological events in the two treatment groups in both kidney studies and heart transplant patients was similar. Tremor and headache have been associated with high whole blood concentrations of tacrolimus and may respond to dosage adjustment. Seizures have occurred in adult and pediatric patients receiving Prograf. Coma and delirium also have been associated with high plasma concentrations of tacrolimus.

Patients treated with tacrolimus have been reported to develop posterior reversible encephalopathy syndrome (PRES). Symptoms indicating PRES include headache, altered mental status, seizures and visual disturbances. Diagnosis should be confirmed by radiological procedure (e.g., MRI). If PRES is suspected or diagnosed, blood pressure and seizure control and immediate discontinuation of immunosuppression is advised. Most patients completely recover after appropriate measures are taken.

Pancreatic: Insulin-dependent post-transplant diabetes mellitus (PTDM) was reported in 20% and 6% of Prograf-treated kidney transplant patients in the U.S. and European studies respectively. Since the development of PTDM is related to increased whole blood trough concentrations of tacrolimus and higher doses of corticosteroids, trough concentrations of tacrolimus and/or steroid doses may be decreased if the risk/benefit assessment permits. In the U.S. multicenter trial, Black and Hispanic kidney transplant patients were at an increased risk of development of PTDM, regardless of randomized treatment. Insulin-dependence was reversible in some patients without discontinuation of Prograf or steroids, and therefore, the need for insulin therapy should be reassessed periodically. In the Phase IV kidney transplant study, PTDM was reported in 11.9% of patients. Insulin dependence was reversible in 40% of these PTDM patients at one year post transplant. See Table 1.

Table 1: Prograf

The Incidence of Post Transplant Diabetes Mellitus and Insulin Use at One Year in the Kidney Transplant Phase IV Study

Status of PTDM[a]	Prograf + AZA[b]	Prograf + MMF 1 g[c]	Prograf + MMF 2 g[c]
Patients without pretransplant history of diabetes mellitus	42	41	43
New onset insulin-dependent PTDM[a]	8 (19%)	5 (12%)	2 (5%)
Patients with PTDM[a] at 1 year	6 (14%)	2 (5%)	1 (2%)

[a] PTDM=Post-Transplant Diabetes Mellitus. Use of insulin for 30 or more consecutive days, with <5 day gap, without a prior history of insulin dependent diabetes mellitus or non insulin dependent diabetes mellitus.
[b] AZA=azathioprine.
[c] MMF=mycophenolate mofetil.

Hyperglycemia was associated with the use of Prograf in 47% and 33% of liver transplant recipients in the U.S. and European randomized studies, respectively, and may require treatment (see Adverse Reactions). **Insulin dependent diabetes was associated with the use of Prograf. This may reverse with dose decrease, however, it may be irreversible after prolonged tacrolimus administration.**

In de novo heart transplant recipients, new onset glucose intolerance (no history/no diabetes at baseline; fasting plasma glucose ≥126 mg/dL; oral hypoglycemic agent use; and/or insulin use ≥30 days) was observed in 63% (83/132) of transplant recipients in the tacrolimus group and 54% (74/138) in the cyclosporine group in the European trial (p=0.139, Fisher's exact test). In the US trial in de novo heart transplant recipients, new onset glucose intolerance was observed in 68% (58/85) of transplant recipients in the tacrolimus/sirolimus group, 61% (46/75) in the tacrolimus/MMF group and 58% (48/83) in the cyclosporine/MMF group.

Hyperglycemia, elevations in HbA_{1c}, and overt diabetes have also been noted in rheumatoid arthritis patients treated with tacrolimus. Tacrolimus should be discontinued in patients in whom blood sugars cannot be controlled.

Renal: Prograf may cause nephrotoxicity, and the likelihood increases with higher blood levels.

Nephrotoxicity has been noted in approximately 52% and 57% of kidney transplantation patients and in 40% and 36% of liver transplantation patients receiving Prograf in the U.S. and European randomized trials, respectively, and in 59% of heart transplantation patients in a European randomized trial (see Adverse Reactions). More overt nephrotoxicity is seen early after transplantation, characterized by increasing serum creatinine and a decrease in urine output. Impaired renal function requires close monitoring and may necessitate Prograf dosage reduction. In patients with persistent elevations of serum creatinine who are unresponsive to dosage adjustments, consideration should be given to changing to other immunosuppressive therapy. Care should be taken in using tacrolimus with other nephrotoxic drugs. **In particular, to avoid excess nephrotoxicity, when switching patients from a cyclosporine-based regimen to a Prograf-based regimen, cyclosporine should be discontinued at least 24 hours prior to initiating Prograf. Prograf dosing may be further delayed in the presence of elevated cyclosporine levels (see Drug Interactions). When switching from tacrolimus to cyclosporine, tacrolimus should be discontinued for at least 24 hours before initiating the other medication.**

For patients with renal insufficiency some evidence suggests that the use of lower doses may be warranted. (See Action and Clinical Pharmacology and Dosage and Administration.)

Mild to severe hyperkalemia was reported in 31% and 21% of kidney transplant patients and in 45% and 13% of liver transplant recipients treated with Prograf in the U.S. and European randomized trials, respectively, and in 8% of heart transplant recipients in a European randomized trial and may require treatment (see Adverse Reactions). **Serum potassium levels should be monitored and potassium sparing diuretics should not be used during Prograf therapy. (See Warnings and Precautions, Monitoring and Laboratory Tests.)**

Hyperkalemia has also been noted in patients with rheumatoid arthritis. Tacrolimus should be discontinued in patients in whom hypertension and hyperkalemia cannot be controlled. The adverse events associated with Prograf treatment in rheumatoid arthritis patients occurred at a lower rate of incidence than seen in transplant patients receiving Prograf. The majority of adverse events were mild or moderate in intensity, of limited duration and did not result in discontinuation of the study drug.

Sexual Function/Reproduction: No impairment of fertility was demonstrated in studies of male and female rats. In reproduction studies in rats and rabbits, adverse effects on the fetus were observed mainly at dose levels that were toxic to dams. However, in female rats dosed during organogenesis, embryo toxicity (expressed as reduced pup weights) was seen at a dose which was one-third of the maternally toxic dose. At this same dose, when administered prior to mating and during gestation, tacrolimus was associated with adverse effects on female reproductive parameters and embryolethality. This dose was equivalent to 0.5× the clinical dose. (See Warnings and Precautions.)

Special Populations: Pregnant Women: Tacrolimus at oral doses of 0.32 and 1.0 mg/kg during organogenesis in rabbits, was associated with maternal toxicity as well as an increase in incidence of abortions; these doses are equivalent to 0.33× and 1.0× (based on body surface area corrections) the recommended clinical dose (0.3 mg/kg). At the higher dose only, an increased incidence of malformations and developmental variations was also seen. Tacrolimus, at oral doses of 3.2 mg/kg during organogenesis in rats, was associated with maternal toxicity and caused an increase in late resorptions, decreased numbers of live births, and decreased pup weight and viability.

Tacrolimus, given orally at 1.0 and 3.2 mg/kg (equivalent to 0.5× and 1.5×), the recommended clinical dose based on body surface area corrections to pregnant rats after organogenesis and during lactation, was associated with reduced pup weights.

Tacrolimus, given orally at 1.0 mg/kg (0.5× the recommended clinical dose based on body surface area corrections) to male and female rats, prior to and during mating, as well as to dams during gestation and lactation, was associated with adverse effects on female reproduction and embryo lethality. Effects on female reproductive function (parturition) and embryo lethal effects were indicated by a higher rate of pre-implantation loss and increased numbers of undelivered and nonviable pups. When given at 3.2 mg/kg (1.5× the recommended clinical dose based on body surface area correction), tacrolimus was associated with maternal and paternal toxicity as well as reproductive toxicity including marked adverse effects on estrous cycles, parturition, pup viability and pup malformations. Toxicities to parental rats were indicated by tremors and circling, as well as reduced weight gains and food consumption in males; and reduced food consumption during gestation and lactation in females. Adverse effects on reproductive parameters included: 1) increased copulatory intervals, 2) increased pre- and post-implantation loss of fetuses (resulting in smaller litter sizes), and 3) decreased numbers of dams delivering. No reduction in male or female fertility was evident. Adverse effects seen in pups were markedly reduced viability and a slight increase in the incidence of malformation (3 pups from 3 dams).

There are no adequate and well-controlled studies in pregnant women. Tacrolimus is transferred across the placenta. The use of tacrolimus during pregnancy has been associated with neonatal hyperkalemia and renal dysfunction. Prograf should be used during pregnancy only if the potential benefit to the mother justifies potential risk to the fetus.

In experience reported by the University of Pittsburgh, eleven female transplant patients maintained on tacrolimus therapy throughout pregnancy delivered twelve babies, with one patient conceiving twice. These patients received tacrolimus from week one to 20 months prior to conception. Ten of the pregnancies were successful, four with C-sections. The neonates showed no growth retardation or congenital anomalies. Hyperkalemia was observed in the majority of babies, but resolved within 24-48 hours without adverse effects. Two babies (both premature 22 and 24 weeks) died shortly after birth. One pregnancy was complicated by diabetes, hypertension and proteinuria, the other by CMV infection requiring ganciclovir therapy. Additional information includes a report of one newborn who had temporary anuria associated with high cord blood tacrolimus concentration, however, renal function was normal within one week. Another reference reports on the successful pregnancy (normal healthy male) in a 28 year old female with bolus steroids and increased doses of tacrolimus for liver graft rejection. In this case, the cord blood plasma concentration was approximately one half that noted in maternal plasma.

Nursing Women: Since tacrolimus is excreted in human milk, nursing should be avoided.

Pediatrics (<18 years of age): Heart failure, cardiomegaly and increased thickness of the myocardium have been reported in patients taking Prograf. Patients at risk for these effects are primarily children younger than 5 years undergoing liver "rescue", small bowel or multivisceral transplantation with trough whole blood tacrolimus levels exceeding 25 ng/mL. Also, these patients at risk often have experienced fluid overload, renal and/or hepatic dysfunction, hypertension and are receiving large doses of corticosteroids and other concomitant medications. Cardiovascular function for such patients should be carefully monitored. In addition, tacrolimus trough whole blood levels should be maintained below 25 ng/mL. If cardiac abnormalities develop, dose reduction or discontinuation of Prograf should be considered in cases where the perceived risk to the patient outweighs the benefit.

The two randomized active-controlled trials of Prograf in primary liver transplantation included 56 pediatric patients. Thirty-one patients were randomized to Prograf and 25 to cyclosporine-based therapies. Additionally, a minimum of 120 pediatric patients (median age 22.5 months) who underwent 122 liver transplants were studied in an uncontrolled published trial of tacrolimus in living related donor liver transplantation. Pediatric patients generally required higher doses of Prograf to maintain blood trough concentrations of tacrolimus similar to adult patients (see Dosage and Administration). This is thought to be a result of age related differences in the oxidative capacity of the cytochrome P450 enzyme system (CYP3A) used to metabolize tacrolimus.

Geriatrics (>65 years of age): No formal studies have been performed to evaluate the effect of Prograf specifically in the geriatric patient population.

Monitoring and Laboratory Tests: Serum creatinine, potassium and fasting glucose should be assessed regularly. Routine monitoring of metabolic and hematologic systems should be performed as clinically warranted.

Blood Level Monitoring in Transplant Patients: Monitoring of tacrolimus blood levels in conjunction with other laboratory and clinical parameters is considered an essential aid to transplant patient management. During the immediate post-operative period trough blood concentrations should be measured every 1-3 days. In patients with hepatic or renal dysfunction or in those receiving or discontinuing concomitant interacting medications, more intensive monitoring may be required, since tacrolimus clearance may be affected under each of these circumstances. More frequent monitoring may also be required in patients early after transplantation since it is at this time patients experience the highest risk of rejection. Blood concentration monitoring is not a replacement for renal and liver function monitoring and tissue biopsies. Following discharge from the hospital, the frequency of patient monitoring will decrease with time post-transplant.

Although there is a lack of direct correlation between tacrolimus levels and drug efficacy, data from Phase II and III studies of kidney and liver transplant patients has shown an increasing incidence of adverse events with increasing trough blood concentrations. Most stable patients are maintained with 12 hour trough whole blood levels of 5 to 20 ng/mL. Long term post-transplant patients often are maintained at the low end of this target range.

Two methods are available for the assay of tacrolimus: 1) microparticle enzyme immuno assay (MEIA) and 2) enzyme linked immuno sorbent assay (ELISA). Both methods use the same monoclonal anti-body for the tacrolimus parent compound. Whole blood is the matrix of choice and specimens should be collected into tubes containing ethylene diamine tetraacetic acid (EDTA) anti-coagulant. Heparin anti-coagulation is not recommended because of the tendency to form clots on storage. Samples which are not analyzed immediately should be stored in a refrigerator and assayed within 3 days; if samples are to be kept longer they should be deep frozen −20°C for up to 12 months.

Kidney Transplantation: Data from the U.S. and European Phase III studies indicate that trough concentrations of tacrolimus in whole blood, as measured by IMx, were most variable during the first week of dosing. During the first three months, 80% of the patients maintained trough concentrations between 7-20 ng/mL, and then between 5-15 ng/mL, through one year.

The relative risk of toxicity is increased with higher trough concentrations. Therefore, monitoring of whole blood trough concentrations is recommended to assist in the clinical evaluation of toxicity.

Liver Transplantation: Data from the U.S. clinical trial show that tacrolimus whole blood concentrations, as measured by ELISA, were most variable during the first week post-transplantation. After this early period, the median trough blood concentrations, measured at intervals from the second week to one year post-transplantation, ranged from 9.8 ng/mL to 19.4 ng/mL.

Heart Transplantation: Data from a European Phase III study indicates that trough concentrations of tacrolimus in whole blood, as measured by IMx were most variable during the first week of dosing. From 1 week to 3 months, 80% of patients maintained trough concentrations between 8-20 ng/mL and, from 3 months through 18 months, 80% of patients maintained trough concentrations between 6-18 ng/mL.

The relative risk of toxicity is increased with higher trough concentrations. Therefore, monitoring of whole blood trough concentrations is recommended to assist in the clinical evaluation of toxicity.

Blood Level Monitoring in Rheumatoid Arthritis Patients: Prograf used in the treatment of rheumatoid arthritis patients has resulted in a lower incidence rate of adverse events than previously seen in transplant patients. Trough blood levels of tacrolimus in this patient population have been demonstrated to be very close to the lower limit of quantitation in assays used to evaluate tacrolimus levels. The lower incidence rates of adverse events as well as the lower levels of tacrolimus detected in rheumatoid arthritis patients may be due to the lower daily dose of Prograf administered to this patient population. Consequently, monitoring tacrolimus trough levels in rheumatoid arthritis patients has not proven to be the most effective approach of managing this patient population. Management of these patients has proven to be effective based on the incidence of adverse events and monitoring serum creatinine levels. Current data further supports the fact that nephrotoxicity associated with Prograf is predictable and can be managed through the careful monitoring of serum creatinine, adjustments of concomitant medications and if necessary, withdrawal of due to the treatment. Since Prograf can impair renal function, a reliable baseline level of serum creatinine should be established by at least two measurements prior to treatment. Serum creatinine should be monitored every 2 weeks during the first month of therapy and every four weeks for the next three months, then quarterly thereafter.

If serum creatinine is increased by more than 40% above baseline, the serum creatinine should be repeated in one week. If the repeated serum creatinine remains increased by more than 40% from baseline, dosing of Prograf should be interrupted for 14 days and the serum creatinine measurement should again be repeated. If the serum creatinine returns to a value less than a 40% increase from baseline, dosing with Prograf may be resumed. If the serum creatinine remains elevated by more than 40% from baseline, Prograf should be discontinued. These recommendations apply even if the patient's values still lie within the laboratory normal range.

ADVERSE REACTIONS: Kidney Transplantation: The most common adverse reactions reported were infection, tremor, hypertension, decreased renal function, constipation, diarrhea, headache, abdominal pain and insomnia. Many of these adverse reactions were mild and responded to a reduction in dosage. Insulin-dependent post-transplant diabetes mellitus (PTDM) was related to increased whole blood trough concentrations of tacrolimus and higher doses of corticosteroids. The median time to onset of PTDM was 68 days.

Liver Transplantation: The principal adverse reactions of Prograf (tacrolimus) are tremor, headache, diarrhea, hypertension, nausea, and renal dysfunction. These occur with oral and intravenous administration of Prograf and may respond to a reduction in dosing. Diarrhea was sometimes associated with other gastrointestinal complaints such as nausea and vomiting. Hyperkalemia and hypomagnesemia have occurred in patients receiving Prograf therapy. Hyperglycemia has been noted in many patients; some may require insulin therapy.

Heart Transplantation: The more common adverse reactions in Prograf-treated heart transplant recipients were kidney function abnormal, hypertension, diabetes mellitus, CMV infection, tremor, hyperglycemia, leukopenia, infection, and hyperlipemia.

Rheumatoid Arthritis : The adverse events associated with Prograf treatment in rheumatoid arthritis patients, occurred at a lower rate of incidence than seen in transplant patients receiving Prograf. The majority of adverse events were mild or moderate in intensity, of limited duration and did not result in discontinuation of the study drug.

Clinical Trial Adverse Drug Reactions: Because clinical trials are conducted under very specific conditions the adverse reaction rates observed in the clinical trials may not reflect the rates observed in practice and should not be compared to the rates in the clinical trials of another drug. Adverse drug reaction information from clinical trials is useful for identifying drug-related adverse events and for approximating rates.

Kidney Transplantation: The incidence of adverse events was determined in two randomized Phase III comparative kidney transplant studies involving 508 patients receiving Prograf and 352 patients receiving cyclosporine. Adverse events that occurred in ≥15% of Prograf-treated patients (combined study results) are presented in Table 2 for the two controlled trials in kidney transplantation:

Table 2: Prograf

Kidney Transplantation: Treatment-Emergent Adverse Events Occurring in ≥15% of Prograf-treated Patients

	U.S. Study		European Study	
Body System	**Prograf N=205 %**	**CBIR[a] N=207 %**	**Prograf N=303 %**	**CBIR[a] N=145 %**
Nervous System				
Tremor[b]	54	34	35	12
Headache[b]	44	38	21	14
Insomnia	32	30	24	26
Gastrointestinal				
Diarrhea	44	41	22	10
Nausea	38	36	17	16
Constipation	35	43	31	35
Vomiting	29	23	13	8
Dyspepsia	28	20	16	13
Cardiovascular				
Hypertension[b]	50	52	37	39
Urogenital				
Creatinine Increased[b]	45	42	35	21
Metabolic and Nutritional				
Hypophosphatemia	49	53	3	5
Hypomagnesemia	34	17	4	1
Hyperkalemia[b]	31	32	21	16
Diabetes Mellitus[b]	24	9	12	2
Hyperglycemia[b]	22	16	16	7
Hemic and Lymphatic				
Anemia	30	24	18	17
Leukopenia	15	17	17	15
Body as a Whole				
Infection	45	49	76	75
Peripheral Edema	36	48	16	16
Asthenia	34	30	7	4
Abdominal Pain	33	31	27	23
Pain	32	30	21	23

(cont'd)

Table 2: Prograf *(cont'd)*

Kidney Transplantation: Treatment-Emergent Adverse Events Occurring in ≥15% of Prograf-treated Patients

	U.S. Study		European Study	
Body System	**Prograf N=205 %**	**CBIR[a] N=207 %**	**Prograf N=303 %**	**CBIR[a] N=145 %**
Fever	29	29	8	9
Respiratory System				
Dyspnea	22	18	12	11
Musculoskeletal				
Arthralgia	25	24	9	10

[a] Cyclosporine-based immunosuppressive regimen.
[b] See Warnings and Precautions.

Tacrolimus has been studied in combination with azathioprine and steroids (triple therapy) in recipients of kidney transplants. In a Phase II European trial, tacrolimus triple therapy was administered to 31 adults receiving deceased donor kidney transplants. Within six weeks post-transplant there were no deaths or graft losses. Six patients (19.4%) experienced acute rejection, with one patient experiencing corticosteroid resistant rejection. Three patients (9.7%) developed transient hyperglycemia, but no patient required long-term therapy for diabetes. Other adverse events reported frequently included infections (51.6%), minor neurological disorders (54.8%), and hypertension (48.8%) (Transpl Int 1995;8:86-90). The University of Pittsburgh has studied double therapy (tacrolimus and steroids) compared to triple therapy in 204 adult recipients of kidney transplants between August 1991 and October 1992 (Clin Transplantation 1994;8:508-515). The one year actuarial patient and graft survival of double therapy were 95 and 90% versus 91 and 82% for triple therapy (p=NS). The incidence of rejection was significantly lower with triple therapy in deceased donor recipients (39% versus 58%) but not significantly different in recipients from living related donors. New onset diabetes was seen in 20.2% of double therapy patients versus 7.7% of triple therapy patients. A U.S. Phase II trial studied 92 adult recipients of deceased donor kidney transplants randomized to three target whole blood concentration ranges of tacrolimus. All patients received antilymphoblast globulin induction with azathioprine and steroids followed by tacrolimus triple therapy initiated within 2 weeks post-transplant. With follow-up to six weeks post-transplant there were no patient deaths, and one graft loss. The incidence of rejection was 14% combining all tacrolimus treatment groups. Adverse events requiring dose reduction were significantly associated with target tacrolimus blood concentrations (36%-62%).

Data on the safety and efficacy of tacrolimus in combination with immunosuppressants other than steroids in liver transplant patients is more limited. In the European multicentre liver transplant study, many patients received azathioprine or ATG/ALG when tacrolimus therapy was withheld. Seven patients received azathioprine in combination with tacrolimus and steroids. Of these 7 patients, one died and one lost their graft in the first year post-transplant.

Liver Transplantation: The incidence of adverse events reported in two randomized comparative liver transplant trials was determined in 514 patients receiving tacrolimus and steroids and 515 patients receiving a cyclosporine-based regimen (CBIR). The proportion of patients reporting more than one adverse event was 99.8% in the tacrolimus group and 99.6% in the CBIR group. Precautions must be taken when comparing the incidence of adverse events in the U.S. Study to that in the European Study. The 12 month posttransplant information from the U.S. study and from the European study is presented below. The two studies included different patient populations and patients were treated with immunosuppressive regimens of differing intensities. Adverse events reported in ≥15% in tacrolimus patients (combined study results) are presented in Table 3 for the two controlled trials in liver transplantation.

Table 3: Prograf

Liver Transplantation: Treatment-Emergent Adverse Events Occurring in ≥15% of Prograf-treated Patients

	U.S. Study		European Study	
	Prograf N=250 (%)	**CBIR[a] N=250 (%)**	**Prograf N=264 (%)**	**CBIR[a] N=265 (%)**
Nervous System				
Headache	64	60	37	26
Tremor	56	46	48	32
Insomnia	64	68	32	23
Paresthesia	40	30	17	17
Gastrointestinal				
Diarrhea	72	47	37	27
Nausea	46	37	32	27
Constipation	24	27	23	21
Liver Function Test Abnormal	36	30	6	5
Anorexia	34	24	7	5
Vomiting	27	15	14	11
Cardiovascular				
Hypertension	47	56	38	43
Urogenital				
Kidney Function Abnormal	40	27	36	23
Creatinine Increased	39	25	24	19
Hyperkalemia	45	26	13	9
Hypokalemia	29	34	13	16
BUN Increased	30	22	12	9
Urinary Tract Infection	16	18	21	19

(cont'd)

Table 3: Prograf *(cont'd)*

Liver Transplantation: Treatment-Emergent Adverse Events Occurring in ≥15% of Prograf-treated Patients

	U.S. Study		European Study	
	Prograf N=250 (%)	**CBIR[a] N=250 (%)**	**Prograf N=264 (%)**	**CBIR[a] N=265 (%)**
Oliguria	18	15	19	12
Metabolic and Nutritional				
Hyperglycemia	47	38	33	22
Hypomagnesemia	48	45	16	9
Peripheral Edema	26	26	12	14
Hemic and Lymphatic				
Anemia	47	38	5	1
Leukocytosis	32	26	8	8
Thrombocytopenia	24	20	14	19
Body as a Whole				
Abdominal Pain	59	54	29	22
Pain	63	57	24	22
Fever	48	56	19	22
Asthenia	52	48	11	7
Back Pain	30	29	17	17
Ascites	27	22	7	8
Respiratory System				
Pleural Effusion	30	32	36	35
Atelectasis	28	30	5	4
Dyspnea	29	23	5	4
Skin and Appendages				
Pruritus	36	20	15	7
Rash	24	19	10	4

[a] Cyclosporine-based immunosuppressive regimen.

Heart Transplantation: The more common adverse reactions in Prograf-treated heart transplant recipients were kidney function abnormal, hypertension, diabetes mellitus, CMV infection, tremor, hyperglycemia, leukopenia, infection, and hyperlipemia.

Adverse events in heart transplant patients in the European trial are presented in Table 4.

Table 4: Prograf

Heart Transplantation: Treatment-Emergent Adverse Events Occurring ≥15% of Prograf-treated Patients

COSTART Body System **COSTART Term**	**Prograf N=157 %**	**CBIR N=157 (%)**
Cardiovascular System		
Hypertension[a]	62	69
Pericardial Effusion	15	14
Body as a Whole		
CMV Infection	32	30
Infection	24	21
Metabolic and Nutritional Disorders		
Hyperlipemia	18	27
Diabetes Mellitus[a]	26	16
Hyperglycemia[a]	23	17
Hemic and Lymphatic System		
Leukopenia	48	39
Anemia	50	36
Urogenital System		
Kidney Function Abnormal[a]	56	57
Urinary Tract Infection	16	12
Respiratory System		

(cont'd)

Table 4: Prograf *(cont'd)*

Heart Transplantation: Treatment-Emergent Adverse Events Occurring ≥15% of Prograf-treated Patients

COSTART Body System COSTART Term	Prograf N=157 %	CBIR N=157 (%)
Bronchitis	17	18
Nervous System		
Tremor[a]	15	6

[a] See Warnings and Precautions.

The incidence of hyperlipidemia or hypercholesteremia as an adverse event at any time during the 18 month study was significantly lower in the tacrolimus group (45/157, 28.7%) than in the cyclosporine group (63/157, 40.1%) (p=0.043, Fisher's exact test).

In the US study, mean serum creatinine levels at 1 year posttransplant were significantly lower in the tacrolimus/MMF group compared with those in either the cyclosporine/MMF group (p=0.002, one-way ANOVA) or the tacrolimus/sirolimus group (p=0.020, one-way ANOVA).

Rheumatoid Arthritis : In a long-term study of rheumatoid arthritis patients receiving Prograf treatment, the adverse events seen in this patient population were similar in nature to those previously reported for patients receiving liver or kidney transplants. In this study, as well as two other studies, the incidence of treatment emergent adverse events seen in the rheumatoid arthritis patient, has a lower incidence of occurrence than seen in the transplant patient.

A summary of treatment-emergent adverse events experienced by at least 5% of patients in any treatment group is presented in Table 5 and Table 6.

Table 5: Prograf

Summary of Common Treatment-emergent Adverse Events (≥5%) in Rheumatoid Arthritis Patients

	Phase II Study FK506RA-001			
Body System	**Placebo N=71 %**	**Prograf 1 mg N=69 %**	**Prograf 3 mg N=64 %**	**Prograf 5 mg N=64 %**
Body as a Whole				
Flu Syndrome	19.7	26.1	20.3	15.6
Accidental Injury	1.4	10.1	3.1	7.8
Abdominal Pain	4.2	7.2	9.4	9.4
Asthenia	4.2	2.9	4.7	6.3
Allergic Reaction	2.8	5.8	6.3	1.6
Infection	2.8	1.4	6.3	1.6
Digestive System				
Diarrhea	11.3	11.6	15.6	28.1
Nausea	5.6	15.9	18.8	14.1
Dyspepsia	7.0	17.4	20.3	9.4
Vomiting	1.4	7.2	6.3	6.3
Gastroenteritis	1.4	4.3	7.8	7.8
Nervous System				
Headache	11.3	10.1	20.3	15.6
Tremor	0	4.3	3.1	21.9
Paresthesia	1.4	2.9	3.1	9.4
Anxiety	1.4	1.4	1.6	10.9
Cardiovascular System				
Hypertension	4.2	5.8	3.1	4.7
Migraine	2.8	1.4	6.3	3.1
Vasodilatation	0	2.9	1.6	6.3
Respiratory System				
Pharyngitis	2.8	10.1	3.1	3.1
Sinusitis	0	4.3	7.8	3.1
Dyspnea	0	5.8	0	1.6
Metabolic and Nutritional Disorders				
Creatinine Increased	0	2.9	3.1	6.3
Musculoskeletal System				
Arthralgia	5.6	5.8	4.7	4.7
Urogenital System				
Urinary Tract Infection	1.4	0	12.5	9.4

Table 6: Prograf

Phase III Studies: Summary of Common Treatment-emergent Adverse Events (≥5%) in Rheumatoid Arthritis Patients

	Study 98-0-049			Study 98-0-51
Body System	**Placebo N=157 %**	**Prograf 2 mg N=154 %**	**Prograf 3 mg N=153 %**	**Prograf 3 mg N=896 %**
Body as a Whole				
Flu Syndrome	16.6	16.2	16.3	26.2
Accidental Injury	5.1	7.8	6.5	8.7
Abdominal Pain	4.5	6.5	7.8	13.5
Asthenia	3.2	4.5	8.5	8.5
Back Pain	2.5	3.2	4.6	6.4
Insomnia	5.1	3.9	2.6	4.2
Digestive System				
Diarrhea	5.1	13.0	13.7	19.9
Nausea	6.4	11.7	10.5	14.6
Dyspepsia	3.2	11.0	6.5	13.1
Vomiting	1.3	2.6	5.2	6.6
Nervous System				
Headache	8.9	8.4	9.2	15.1
Dizziness	3.8	4.5	7.2	7.1
Tremor	1.9	4.5	8.5	10.5
Cardiovascular				
Hypertension	4.5	5.8	7.8	8.5
Respiratory System				
Pharyngitis	2.5	6.5	2.0	5.5
Sinusitis	3.2	4.5	3.9	6.0
Skin and Appendages				
Rash	6.4	7.1	3.3	6.8
Metabolic and Nutritional Disorders				
Creatinine Increased	1.9	1.9	6.5	6.7
Musculoskeletal System				
Cramps	0	2.6	5.2	5.6
Urogenital System				
Urinary Tract Infection	2.5	3.2	4.6	5.9

The overall incidence of treatment-emergent adverse events for any treatment group for the three studies (RA-001, 049, and 051) ranged from 72.0% to 90.6%. In the placebo-controlled studies (RA-001 and 049), the overall incidence of treatment-emergent adverse events for the tacrolimus-treated groups was significantly different from placebo. In the tacrolimus-treated groups, the most common adverse events seen across the three studies were flu syndrome, diarrhea, nausea, abdominal pain, dyspepsia, and tremor.

In the case of gastrointestinal events, the incidence of diarrhea in the tacrolimus-treated groups in the three studies varied from 13.0% to 28.1%, with incidence increasing with dose. Tacrolimus 5 mg/day in the RA-001 study elicited the highest incidence of diarrhea (28.1%); the next highest incidence of diarrhea was 19.9% in the 3 mg/day group in the 051 study. The incidences of diarrhea in the tacrolimus 5 mg/day group in the RA-001 study, and in the 2 mg and 3 mg groups in the 049 study were significantly different from placebo. Nausea was seen in the tacrolimus-treated groups with incidences of 10.5% to 18.8%. Only the incidence of nausea in the tacrolimus 3 mg/day group in the RA-001 study was significantly different from placebo, and the incidence did not increase with an increasing dose. Dyspepsia was observed in the tacrolimus-treated groups with incidences of 6.5% to 20.3%. In the three studies, the incidence of dyspepsia in patients taking 3 mg tacrolimus/day were 6.5% (049), 13.1% (051), and 20.3% (RA-001). The incidences of dyspepsia in the 2 mg tacrolimus/day group in the 049 study and in the tacrolimus 3 mg/day group in the RA-001 study were significantly different from placebo. No increase in incidence was seen with increasing dose in any study. Abdominal pain was reported in the tacrolimus-treated groups with incidences of 6.5% to 13.5%. There was no increase in incidence with increasing doses, and there was no significant difference from placebo in either placebo-controlled study.

The incidence of vasodilatation in the tacrolimus-treated groups varied from 1.6% to 6.3%. There was an increased incidence of vasodilatation with higher doses of tacrolimus. The incidences of vasodilatation in the tacrolimus 3 mg/day group in the 049 study and in the tacrolimus 5 mg/day group in the RA-001 study were significantly different from placebo.

Tremor occurred in the tacrolimus-treated groups with incidences of 3.1% to 21.9%. The incidence of tremor increased with an increasing dose, and in the tacrolimus 5 mg/day group in the RA-001 study, the incidence of tremor (21.9%) was more than twice the incidence of tremor seen with tacrolimus 3 mg/day in any of the three studies. The incidences of tremor in the tacrolimus 3 mg/day group in the 049 study and in the tacrolimus 5 mg/day group in the RA-001 study were significantly different from placebo. Paresthesia was seen in the tacrolimus-treated groups with incidences of 2.6% to 9.4%. The incidence of paresthesia increased with increasing dose, and in the tacrolimus 5 mg/day group in the RA-001 study, the incidence of paresthesia (9.4%) was more than twice the incidence of tremor seen with tacrolimus 3 mg/day in any of the three studies. The incidence of paresthesia in the tacrolimus 5 mg/day group in the RA-001 study was significantly different from placebo.

The incidence of urinary tract infections in the tacrolimus-treated groups varied from 3.2% to 12.5%. The incidence of urinary tract infection in the tacrolimus 3 mg/day group in the RA-001 study was significantly different from placebo; however, the incidence did not increase with increasing doses. The incidence of flu-like syndrome in the tacrolimus-treated groups ranged from

15.6% to 26.2%. There was no increase in incidence with larger doses, and no difference from placebo in any tacrolimus-treated group. The incidence of other infections was between 1.6% and 3.3% in the tacrolimus-treated groups. Increasing dose did not influence the incidence of infection, and there was no difference seen from placebo.

Comparisons of patient subpopulations were performed on data from patients in the 051 study, all of whom received tacrolimus 3 mg/day. In general, the incidence of adverse events was similar in patients <65 years of age and ≥65 years of age, in patients with and without hypertension, in patients with and without hyperlipidemia, and in patients with and without diabetes.

A total of 213 patients (23.8%) were at least 65 years of age at study entry. The overall incidence of adverse events for patients ≥65 years of age (86.9%) was similar to that for patients <65 years of age (88.7%). There were no notable differences between patients ≥65 years of age and those <65 years of age for the incidence of any specific adverse events. The more common adverse events occurring in at least 10% of patients ≥65 years of age were flu syndrome (18.3%), diarrhea (16.9%), tremor (15.0%), nausea (13.6%), headache (12.7%), accidental injury (12.2%), hypertension (12.2%), dyspepsia (11.7%), and abdominal pain (11.3%). For patients <65 years of age, the more common adverse events were occurring in at least 10% of patients were flu syndrome (28.7%), diarrhea (20.8%), headache (15.8%), nausea (14.9%), abdominal pain (14.2%), and dyspepsia (13.5%). The incidences of tremor, accidental injury, and hypertension among these patients were 9.1%, 7.6%, and 7.3%, respectively.

Three hundred fifty patients (39.1%) had a history of hypertension at the time they entered the study. The overall incidence of adverse events for patients with a history of hypertension (91.1%) was similar to that for patients without a history of hypertension (86.4%). Among adverse events reported for at least 5% of patients with a history of hypertension, the incidences of bronchitis (6.9%) and peripheral edema (6.0%) were more than twice the incidences (3.1% and 2.4%, respectively) reported for patients without a history of hypertension. The more common adverse events occurring in at least 10% of patients with a history of hypertension were flu syndrome (26.9%), diarrhea (18.3%), nausea (15.7%), headache (13.4%), dyspepsia (13.1%), tremor (13.1%), abdominal pain (13.1%), and hypertension (11.7%). For patients without a history of hypertension, the more common adverse events occurring in at least 10% of patients were flu syndrome (25.8%), diarrhea (20.9%), headache (16.1%), nausea (13.9%), abdominal pain (13.7%), and dyspepsia (13.0%). The incidences of tremor and hypertension among these patients were 8.8% and 6.4%, respectively.

A total of 271 patients (30.2%) had a history of hyperlipidemia at the time they entered the study. The overall incidence of adverse events for patients with a history of hyperlipidemia (92.6%) was similar to that for patients without a history of hyperlipidemia (86.4%). There were no notable differences between patients with a history of hyperlipidemia and those without a history of hyperlipidemia for the incidence of any specific adverse events. The more common adverse events occurring in at least 10% of patients with a history of hyperlipidemia were flu syndrome (26.2%), diarrhea (18.1%), nausea (15.9%), dyspepsia (14.0%), headache (12.9%), tremor (12.2%), abdominal pain (11.8%), and asthenia (10.3%). For patients without a history of hyperlipidemia, the more common adverse events occurring in at least 10% of patients were flu syndrome (26.2%), diarrhea (20.6%), headache (16.0%), abdominal pain (14.2%), nausea (14.1%), and dyspepsia (12.6%). The incidences of tremor and asthenia among these patients were 9.8% and 7.7%, respectively. Hypercholesterolemia and hyperlipemia were reported as adverse events in 3.0% and 2.2%, respectively, of patients with a history of hyperlipidemia, and in 1.4% and 1.0%, respectively, of patients without a history of hyperlipidemia.

Seventy-five patients (8.4%) had a history of diabetes at the time of study entry. The overall incidence of adverse events for patients with a history of diabetes (89.3%) was similar to that for patients without a history of diabetes (88.2%). Among adverse events reported for at least 5% of patients with a history of diabetes, the incidences of urinary tract infection (13.3%), hyperglycemia (9.3%), and infection (8.0%) were more than twice the incidences (5.2%, 1.8%, and 2.9%, respectively) reported for patients without a history of diabetes, and the incidence of headache (6.7%) in patients with a history of diabetes was less than half the incidence (15.8%) reported for patients without a history of diabetes. The more common adverse events occurring in at least 10% of patients with a history of diabetes were flu syndrome (26.7%), diarrhea (18.7%), tremor (17.3%), dyspepsia (16.0%), urinary tract infection (13.3%), nausea (13.3%), and hypertension (12.0%). The incidences of headache and abdominal pain among these patients were 6.7% and 8.0% respectively. For patients without a history of diabetes, the more common adverse events occurring in at least 10% of patients were flu syndrome (26.2%), diarrhea (20.0%), headache (15.8%), nausea (14.7%), abdominal pain (14.0%), and dyspepsia (12.8%). The incidences of tremor and urinary tract infection among these patients were 9.9% and 5.2%, respectively.

In some Rheumatoid Arthritis patients, an increase in serum creatinine levels has been detected. In the long-term safety study (98-0-051), in which patients were treated with Prograf for up to 18 months, 65.5% of all patients who had increases in serum creatinine ≥30% to <40% above baseline had levels return to baseline during the study. For the remaining patients, creatinine levels either did not return to baseline or no documentation of follow-up levels was available. Patients with increases in serum creatinine levels, ≥40% above baseline, had their levels return to baseline in 56.3% of all patients. These included patients who continued study drug therapy and patients who discontinued study drug therapy during the recovery period. For those patients whose creatinine levels returned to baseline, the median time to return to baseline creatinine levels was 40.5 days for patients with ≥30% to <40% increase from baseline and 32.0 days for patient with ≥40% increases from baseline.

In Study FK506RA-001, patients who experienced an increase from baseline in serum creatinine levels of ≥30% and <40%, 50% of the patients in the placebo group, 80% of patients in the 1 mg Prograf treatment group, 89% in the 3 mg Prograf treatment group and 78% patients in the 5 mg Prograf treatment group experienced a return to baseline serum creatinine levels within 56 days for placebo treated patients, 33 days for patients treated with 1 mg Prograf, 29 days for those treated with 3 mg and 57 days for those treated with 5 mg.

In those patients experiencing a serum creatinine increase of ≥40%, above baseline, 50% of placebo treated patients, 20% of the 1 mg treated patents, 75% of the patients treated with 3 mg Prograf and 31% of patients treated with 5 mg Prograf experienced a subsequent return to baseline creatinine levels. The duration of time for serum creatinine levels to return to baseline for this patient population occurred sooner than those patients experiencing a serum creatinine increase of ≥30% and <40%. Patients treated with placebo demonstrated a return to baseline of serum creatinine levels within 28 days, an average of 6 days for patients treated with 1 mg, 20 days for those treated with 3 mg and 38 days for those treated with 5 mg. There were however, eight of nine patients with elevated creatinine levels (>40%) who discontinued the study. These patients had creatinine values return to below a 40% increase from baseline and within normal limits (0.7-1.4 mg/dL) post discontinuation, with one patient lost to follow-up.

In study 98-0-049, of those patients who experienced an increase from baseline in creatinine of ≥30% to <40%, 63.6% of these patients in the placebo treatment group, 50.0% of patients in the 2 mg Prograf treatment group, and 77. 8% of patients in the 3 mg Prograf treatment group, experienced a documented subsequent return to baseline creatinine values, within 36 days for placebo treated patients, 43 days for 2 mg treated patients and 41 days for 3 mg patients treated with Prograf. For those patients with a ≥40% increase from baseline, 33.3% of patients in the placebo treatment group, 53.3% of patients in the 2 mg Prograf treatment group, and 45.5% of patients in the 3 mg Prograf treatment group experienced a documented subsequent return to baseline creatinine values. Serum creatinine levels in this patient population returned to baseline levels sooner, than patients who experienced an increase from baseline of ≥30% to <40%. Patients with a serum creatinine increase >40% demonstrated a return to baseline at 20 days for placebo treated patients, 33 days for patients treated with 2 mg and 38 days for those patients treated with 3 mg Prograf per day. The remaining patients either had creatinine levels that did not return to baseline during the follow-up period or were not monitored for return to baseline values.

For 88.5% (139/157) of placebo-treated patients, 87.0% (134/154) of patients treated with 2 mg/day Prograf and 86.3% (132/153) of patients treated with 3 mg/day Prograf, creatinine levels were within the normal range at baseline, and remained within the normal range throughout the study. In total, four patients all treated with 3 mg Prograf, discontinued treatment as a result of a reported adverse event of increased serum creatinine. See Table 7.

Table 7: Prograf

Number of Patients with at Least a 30% Baseline Increase in Serum Creatinine That Returned to Baseline

Evaluated Study Groups	Increase in Serum Creatinine Levels Above Baseline ≥30% to <40%[a]	≥40%[a]
Study 98-0-051		
Combined De Novo[b] (n=685)	46/78 (59.0%)	90/177 (50.8%)
2 mg[c] (n=103)	8/11 (72.7%)	20/37 (54.1%)
3 mg[d] (n=108)	20/24 (83.3%)	37/47 (78.7%)
Total (n=896)	74/113 (65.5%)	147/261 (56.3%)

(cont'd)

Table 7: Prograf *(cont'd)*

Number of Patients with at Least a 30% Baseline Increase in Serum Creatinine That Returned to Baseline

Evaluated Study Groups	Increase in Serum Creatinine Levels Above Baseline ≥30% to <40%[a]	≥40%[a]
Study FK506RA-001		
Placebo (n=71)	1/2 (50%)	2/4 (50%)
1 mg (n=69)	4/5 (80%)	1/5 (20%)
3 mg (n=64)	8/9 (88.9%)	9/12 (75%)
5 mg (n=64)	7/9 (77.8%)	4/13 (30.8%)
Study 98-0-049		
Placebo (n=157)	7/11 (63.6%)	5/15 (33.3%)
2 mg (n=154)	4/8 (50%)	16/30 (53.3%)
3 mg (n=153)	7/9 (77.8%)	20/44 (45.5%)

[a] Percent increase from baseline during treatment. A patient could have been represented in both percentage increase groups if their creatinine increased, returned to baseline levels, and subsequently increased into the other percentage increase group.

[b] All de novo patients for study 98-0-051, all patients from study FK506RA-001, and all placebo rollover patients from study 98-0-049.

[c] All 2 mg tacrolimus rollover patient from study 98-0-049.

[d] All 3 mg tacrolimus rollover patients from study 98-0-049.

Patient base: Full analysis set; all patients who received at least one dose of the study drug in study 98-0-051.

Less Common Clinical Trial Adverse Drug Reactions: The following adverse events were reported in either liver, kidney, and/or heart transplant recipients who were treated with tacrolimus in clinical trials.

Nervous System: (See Warnings and Precautions) abnormal dreams, agitation, amnesia, anxiety, confusion, crying, convulsion, depression, dizziness, elevated mood, emotional lability, encephalopathy, hemorrhagic stroke, hallucinations, hypertonia, incoordination, monoparesis, myoclonus, nerve compression, nervousness, neuralgia, neuropathy, paralysis flaccid, paresthesia, psychomotor skills impaired, psychosis, quadriparesis somnolence, thinking abnormal, vertigo, writing impaired.

Special Senses: abnormal vision, amblyopia, ear pain, otitis media, tinnitus.

Gastrointestinal: anorexia, cholangitis, cholestatic jaundice, dyspepsia, duodenitis, dysphagia, esophagitis, flatulence, gastritis, gastrointestinal hemorrhage, gastroesophagitis, GGT increase, GI disorder, GI perforation, hepatitis, hepatitis granulomatous, ileus, increased appetite, jaundice, liver damage, liver function test abnormal, esophagitis ulcerative, oral moniliasis, pancreatic pseudocyst, rectal disorder, stomatitis.

Cardiovascular: abnormal ECG, angina pectoris, arrhythmia, atrial fibrillation, atrial flutter, bradycardia, cardiac fibrillation, cardiopulmonary failure, cardiovascular disorder, chest pain, congestive heart failure, deep thrombophlebitis, echocardiogram abnormal, electrocardiogram QRS complex abnormal, electrocardiogram ST segment abnormal, heart rate decreased, heart failure, hemorrhage, hypotension, postural hypotension, peripheral vascular disorder, phlebitis, syncope, tachycardia, thrombosis, vasodilatation.

Urogenital: (See Warnings and Precautions) acute kidney failure, albuminuria, BK nephropathy, bladder spasms cystitis, dysuria, hematuria, hydronephrosis, kidney failure, kidney tubular necrosis, nocturia, oliguria, pyuria, toxic nephropathy, urge incontinence, urinary frequency, urinary tract infection, urinary incontinence, urinary retention, vaginitis.

Metabolic/Nutritional: acidosis, alkaline phosphatase increased, alkalosis, AST increased, ALT increased, bicarbonate decreased, bilirubinemia, BUN increased, dehydration, edema, GGT increased, gout, healing abnormal, hypercalcemia, hypercholesterolemia, hyperlipemia, hypertriglyceridemia, hyperphosphatemia, hyperuricemia, hypocalcemia, hypervolemia, hypoglycemia, hypokalemia, hypophosphatemia, hyponatremia, hypoproteinemia, lactic dehydrogenase increase, weight gain.

Endocrine System: (See Warnings and Precautions) diabetes mellitus, Cushing's Syndrome.

Hemic/Lymphatic: coagulation disorder, ecchymosis, hematocrit increased, hemoglobin abnormal, hypochromic anemia, leukopenia, prothrombin decreased, leukocytosis, polycythemia, serum iron decreased, thrombocytopenia.

Body as a Whole: abdomen enlarged, abscess, accidental injury, allergic reaction, back pain, cellulitis, chills, fall, feeling abnormal, flu syndrome, generalized edema, hernia, mobility decreased, peritonitis, photosensitivity reaction, sepsis, temperature intolerance, ulcer, pain.

Musculoskeletal: arthralgia, cramps, generalized spasm, joint disorder, leg cramps, myalgia, myasthenia, osteoporosis.

Respiratory System: asthma, bronchitis, cough increased, emphysema, hiccups, lung disorder, lung function decreased, pharyngitis, pneumothorax, pneumonia, pulmonary edema, respiratory disorder, rhinitis, sinusitis, voice alteration.

Skin and Appendages: acne, alopecia, exfoliative dermatitis, fungal dermatitis, herpes simplex, herpes zoster, hirsutism, pruritus, rash, neoplasm skin benign, skin discolouration, skin disorder, skin ulcer, sweating.

The following nervous system adverse events were also reported at a frequency (<3%): acute brain syndrome (0.2%), coma (2.1%), delirium (1.2%), dysarthria (0.4%), dystonia (0.4%), encephalopathy (2.5%), flaccid paralysis (0.4%), hemiplegia (0.8%), nystagmus (0.8%), paralysis (0.4%) and stupor (0.2%).

Abnormal Hematologic and Clinical Chemistry Findings: Refer to Warnings and Precautions (Hepatic/Biliary, Renal, and Monitoring and Laboratory Tests).

Post-Market Adverse Drug Reactions: The following adverse events have been reported from worldwide marketing experience with Prograf. Because these events are reported voluntarily from a population of uncertain size, are associated with concomitant diseases and multiple drug therapies and surgical procedures, it is not always possible to reliably estimate their frequency or establish a causal relationship to drug exposure. Decisions to include these events in labeling are typically based on one or more of the following factors: (1) seriousness of the event, (2) frequency of the reporting, or (3) strength of causal connection to the drug:

Cardiovascular: atrial fibrillation, atrial flutter, cardiac arrhythmia, cardiac arrest, electrocardiogram T wave abnormal, flushing, myocardial infarction, myocardial ischemia, pericardial effusion, QT prolongation with or without Torsade de Pointes, venous thrombosis deep limb, ventricular extrasystoles, ventricular fibrillation.

Gastrointestinal: bile duct stenosis, colitis, enterocolitis, gastroenteritis, gastrooesophageal reflux disease, hepatic cytolysis, hepatic necrosis, hepatotoxicity, impaired gastric emptying, liver fatty, mouth ulceration, pancreatitis hemorrhagic, pancreatitis necrotizing, stomach ulcer, venoocclusive liver disease.

Hemic/Lymphatic: disseminated intravascular coagulation, neutropenia, pancytopenia, thrombocytopenic purpura, thrombotic thrombocytopenic purpura.

Metabolic/Nutritional: glycosuria, increased amylase including pancreatitis, weight decreased.

Miscellaneous: feeling hot and cold, feeling jittery, hot flushes, multi-organ failure, primary graft dysfunction.

Nervous System: carpal tunnel syndrome, cerebral infarction, hemiparesis, leukoencephalopathy, mental disorder, mutism, posterior reversible encephalopathy syndrome (PRES), progressive multifocal leukoencephalopathy (PML), quadriplegia, speech disorder, syncope, polyneuropathy, neuropathy peripheral, peripheral sensory neuropathy, mononeuropathy multiplex.

Respiratory: acute respiratory distress syndrome, interstitial lung disease (predominantly in rheumatoid arthritis), lung infiltration, respiratory distress, respiratory failure.

Skin: Stevens-Johnson syndrome, toxic epidermal necrolysis.

Special Senses: blindness, blindness cortical, hearing loss including deafness, photophobia.

Urogenital: acute renal failure, cystitis hemorrhagic, hemolytic-uremic syndrome, micturition disorder.

There have been rare spontaneous reports of myocardial hypertrophy associated with clinically manifested ventricular dysfunction in patients receiving Prograf therapy (see Warnings and Precautions).

There have been reports of pure red cell aplasia in patients receiving tacrolimus.

DRUG INTERACTIONS: Overview: Tacrolimus is extensively metabolized by the mixed-function oxidase system, primarily the cytochrome P450 system (CYP3A). Prograf does not induce or inhibit CYP3A4 or any other major CYP isoenzymes.

Drug-Drug Interactions: Drug Interactions Potentially Affecting Renal Function: Due to the potential for additive or synergistic impairment of renal function, care should be taken when administering Prograf with drugs that may be associated with renal dysfunction. These include, and are not limited to, aminoglycosides, amphotericin B, ganciclovir, acyclovir and cisplatin.

NSAIDs may interact with Prograf causing deteriorations in blood pressure (BP) control and serum creatinine levels. Initial clinical experience with Prograf and cyclosporine resulted in additive/synergistic nephrotoxicity when both agents were co-administered. Patients switched from cyclosporine to Prograf should receive the first Prograf dose no sooner than 24 hours after the last cyclosporine dose. Dosing may be further delayed in the presence of elevated cyclosporine levels.

Drug Interactions Potentially Affecting Tacrolimus Blood Concentrations: Since tacrolimus is metabolized mainly by the cytochrome P450 3A enzyme systems, substances known to inhibit these enzymes may decrease the metabolism or increase bioavailability of tacrolimus with resultant increases in whole blood or plasma levels. Drugs known to induce these enzyme systems may result in an increased metabolism of tacrolimus or decreased bioavailability as indicated by decreased whole blood or plasma levels.

Monitoring of blood levels and appropriate dosage adjustments in transplant patients are essential when such drugs (Table 8) are used concomitantly with Prograf.

Lack of Drug Interaction With Prograf : At a given mycophenolate mofetil (MMF) dose, mycophenolic acid (MPA) exposure is higher with Prograf co-administration than with cyclosporine co-administration due to the inhibitory action of cyclosporine on biliary excretion of MPA-glucuronide by MRP-2 and the resulting reduction in enterohepatic recirculation of MPA. As a result, exposure to MPA when mycophenolate mofetil is given in combination with cyclosporine is approximately 30-40% lower than that observed when given alone or with tacrolimus. No effect on enterohepatic MPA-glucuronide recirculation is exerted by tacrolimus; thus, clinicians should be aware that there is a potential for increased MPA exposure after crossover from cyclosporine to tacrolimus in patients concomitantly receiving MMF or mycophenolate sodium (MPS). Conversely, there is a potential for decreased MPA exposure after crossover from tacrolimus to cyclosporine in patients concomitantly receiving MMF or MPS.

Prograf and Vaccinations: Immunosuppressants may affect vaccination. Therefore, during treatment with Prograf, vaccination may be less effective. The use of live vaccines should be avoided; live vaccines may include, but are not limited to: measles, mumps, rubella, oral polio, BCG, yellow fever and TY 21a typhoid.

Drug-Food Interactions: Grapefruit juice affects P450 3A-mediated metabolism and should be avoided.

Drug-Herb Interactions: St. John's Wort (Hypericum perforatum) induces CYP3A4 and P-glycoprotein. Since tacrolimus is a substrate for CYP3A4, there is the potential that the use of St. John's Wort in patients receiving Prograf could result in reduced tacrolimus levels.

Drug-Laboratory Test Interactions: Interactions with laboratory tests have not been established.

Drug-Lifestyle Interactions: As with other immunosuppressive agents, owing to the potential risk of malignant skin changes, exposure to sunlight and ultraviolet (UV) light should be limited by wearing protective clothing and using sunscreen with a high protection factor.

Table 8: Prograf

Established or Potential Drug-Drug Interactions

Concomitant Drug Class: Drug Name	Reference	Effect on Concentration of Prograf	Comment
Antacid: magnesium-aluminium-hydroxide	CT	↑ Prograf	In a single-dose crossover study in healthy volunteers, co-administration of tacrolimus and magnesium-aluminium-hydroxide resulted in a 21% increase in the mean tacrolimus AUC and a 10% decrease in the mean tacrolimus C_{max} relative to tacrolimus administration alone.
Azole antifungals: ketoconazole†	CT	↑ Prograf	In a study of 6 normal volunteers, a significant increase in tacrolimus oral bioavailability (14±5% vs 30±8%) was observed with concomitant administration of ketoconazole (200 mg), a strong CYP3A4 and P-glycoprotein inhibitor. The apparent clearance of oral tacrolimus during ketoconazole administration was significantly decreased compared to tacrolimus alone (0.430+0.129 L/hr/kg vs. 0.148+0.043 L/hr/kg). Overall, clearance of IV tacrolimus was not significantly changed by ketoconazole co-administration, although it was highly variable between patients. †When co-administered with ketoconazole, a dose adjustment of tacrolimus is required in most patients.
clotrimazole fluconazole† itraconazole† voriconazole†	T	↑ Prograf	The concomitant use of Prograf with azole antifungals that are strong or moderate CYP3A4 and P-glycoprotein inhibitors (e.g. itraconazole, fluconazole, voriconazole) might lead to an increased Prograf concentration. †When co-administered with fluconazole, itraconazole and voriconazole, a dose adjustment of tacrolimus is required in most patients.
Calcium channel blockers: diltiazem nicardipine nifedipine verapamil	T	↑ Prograf	Co-administration of substrates and/or inhibitors of CYP3A4 and P-glycoprotein with Prograf might increase blood concentrations of tacrolimus.
GI Prokinetic Agents: cisapride[a] metoclopramide	T	↑ Prograf	Co-administration of Prograf with substrates of CYP3A4 might increase blood concentrations of tacrolimus.
Macrolide antibiotics: erythromycin† clarithromycin troleandomycin	T	↑ Prograf	Co-administration of Prograf with substrates and/or inhibitors of CYP3A4 and P-glycoprotein might increase blood concentrations of tacrolimus. †When co-administered with erythromycin, a dose adjustment of tacrolimus is required in most patients.
Proton pump inhibitor: lansoprazole omeprazole	T	↑ Prograf	Lansoprazole and omeprazole (CYP2C19 and CYP3A4 substrate, inhibitor) may potentially inhibit CYP3A4-mediated metabolism of tacrolimus and thereby substantially increase tacrolimus whole blood concentrations, especially in transplant patients who are intermediate or poor CYP2C19 metabolizers, as compared to those patients who are efficient CYP2C19 metabolizers.
Other drugs: bromocriptine cimetidine chloramphenicol cyclosporine danazol ethinyl estradiol methylprednisolone nefazodone	T	↑ Prograf	Co-administration of Prograf with substrates and/or inhibitors of CYP3A4 and P-glycoprotein might increase blood concentrations of tacrolimus.

(cont'd)

Table 8: Prograf *(cont'd)*

Established or Potential Drug-Drug Interactions

Concomitant Drug Class: Drug Name	Reference	Effect on Concentration of Prograf	Comment
Protease inhibitors nelfinavir ritonavir saquinavir	T	↑ Prograf	Interaction studies with drugs used in HIV therapy have not been conducted. However, care should be exercised when drugs that are metabolized by CYP3A4 (e.g., nelfinavir, ritonavir, saquinavir) are administered concomitantly with tacrolimus. Based on a clinical study of 5 liver transplant recipients, co-administration of tacrolimus with nelfinavir increased blood concentrations of tacrolimus significantly and, as a result, a reduction in the tacrolimus dose by an average of 16-fold was needed to maintain mean trough tacrolimus blood concentrations of 9.7 ng/mL. Thus, frequent monitoring of tacrolimus blood concentrations and appropriate dosage adjustments are essential when nelfinavir is used concomitantly.
Anticonvulsants: carbamazepine phenobarbital phenytoin†	T	↓ Prograf	Co-administration of Prograf with inducers of CYP3A4 and P-glycoprotein might decrease blood concentrations of tacrolimus. †When co-administered with phenytoin, a dose adjustment of tacrolimus is required in most patients.
Anti-Infectives: rifampicin†	CT	↓ Prograf	In a study of 6 normal volunteers, a significant decrease in tacrolimus oral bioavailability (14±6% vs 7±3%) was observed with concomitant administration of rifampicin (600 mg), a strong CYP3A4 and P-glycoprotein inducer. In addition, there was a significant increase in tacrolimus clearance (0.036±0.008 L/hr/kg vs. 0.053±0.010 L/hr/kg) with concomitant rifampicin administration. In a study of 9 normal volunteers, concomitantly administered 10 mL doses of aluminum hydroxide or milk of magnesia antacids did not affect the rate and extent of absorption of orally administered tacrolimus, as indicated by C_{max}, T_{max} and AUC_{0-t}. †When co-administered with rifampicin, a dose adjustment of tacrolimus is required in most patients.
caspofungin rifabutin	T	↓ Prograf	Co-administration of Prograf with inducers of CYP3A4 and P-glycoprotein might decrease blood concentrations of tacrolimus.
Calcineurin inhibitor: sirolimus	CT	↓ Prograf	Following 14 days co-administration of tacrolimus and sirolimus (2 mg/day or 5 mg/day; a substrate for both CYP3A4 and P-glycoprotein) in stable renal transplant patients, tacrolimus AUC and C_{min} decreased approximately 30% relative to tacrolimus alone. Mean tacrolimus AUC_{0-12} and C_{min} following co-administration of 1 mg/day of sirolimus decreased approximately 3% and 11%, respectively. The safety and efficacy of the use of tacrolimus with sirolimus has not been established.
Herbal preparation: St. John's Wort	T	↓ Prograf	St. John's Wort (Hypericum perforatum) induces CYP3A4 and P-glycoprotein. Since tacrolimus is a substrate for CYP3A4, there is the potential that the use of St. John's Wort in patients receiving Prograf could result in reduced tacrolimus levels.

[a] No longer marketed in Canada.
Legend: CT=Clinical Trial. T=Theoretical.

DOSAGE AND ADMINISTRATION: Dosing Considerations: Due to intersubject variability following dosing with tacrolimus, individualization of the dosing regimen is necessary for optimal therapy.

Additional factors that may impact dosing include, pre-existing conditions, such as renal or hepatic impairment, race, pediatric use and the concomitant use of other medications.

Prograf has been used in combination with azathioprine. Prograf has been used in combination with mycophenolate mofetil (MMF) in patients receiving deceased donor kidney transplants and heart transplants. Because of the risk of anaphylaxis, intravenous Prograf should be reserved for patients unable to take Prograf capsules orally.

Medication errors, including inadvertent, unintentional or unsupervised substitution of Prograf (immediate release)—or Advagraf (extended-release) tacrolimus formulations, have been observed. This has led to serious adverse events, including graft rejection, or other side effects which could be a consequence of either under- or over-exposure to tacrolimus. Patients should be maintained on a single formulation of tacrolimus with the corresponding daily dosing regimen; alterations in formulation or regimen should only take place under the close supervision of a transplant specialist.

Recommended Dose and Dosage Adjustment: Prograf (tacrolimus for injection) is for intravenous (IV) use in transplant patients only. **Anaphylactic reactions have occurred with injectables containing castor oil derivatives (see Warnings and Precautions).**

In patients unable to take oral Prograf (tacrolimus immediate release capsules), therapy may be initiated with IV Prograf (tacrolimus for injection). The initial dose of Prograf should be administered no sooner than 6 hours after transplantation. The recommended starting dose of Prograf given intravenously is 0.01 mg/kg/day (heart) or 0.03-0.05 mg/kg/day (liver, kidney) as a continuous intravenous infusion (see Table 10). Adult patients should receive doses at the lower end of the dosing range. Concomitant adrenal corticosteroid therapy is recommended early post transplantation.

Continuous intravenous infusion of Prograf (tacrolimus for injection) should be continued until the patient can tolerate oral administration of Prograf (immediate release capsules).

Kidney Transplantation: The recommended starting oral dose of Prograf is 0.2-0.3 mg/kg/day administered every 12 hours in two divided doses. The initial dose of Prograf may be administered within 24 hours of transplantation but should be delayed until renal function has recovered (as indicated for example by a serum creatinine ≤4 mg/dL). Black patients may require higher doses to achieve comparable blood levels. Dosage and typical tacrolimus whole blood trough concentrations are shown in Table 9; blood concentration details are described under Warnings and Precautions.

Table 9: Prograf

Recommended Tacrolimus Oral Dosing in Kidney Transplant Patients

Dosage	
Initial Oral Dose	0.2–0.3 mg/kg/day

(cont'd)

Table 9: Prograf *(cont'd)*

Recommended Tacrolimus Oral Dosing in Kidney Transplant Patients

Dosing Regimen	2 divided doses, q12h
Tacrolimus whole blood trough concentration	
Month 1–3	7–20 ng/mL
Month 4–12	5–15 ng/mL

Liver Transplantation: It is recommended that patients be converted from IV to oral Prograf as soon as oral therapy can be tolerated. This usually occurs within 2-3 days. The first dose of oral therapy should be given 8-12 hours after discontinuing the IV infusion. The recommended starting oral dose of Prograf capsules is 0.1-0.15 mg/kg/day administered in two divided daily doses every 12 hours. The initial dose of Prograf should be administered no sooner than 6 hours after transplantation. Adult patients should receive doses at the lower end of the dosing range.

Some centres use lower Prograf doses during maintenance therapy post transplantation. Dosing should be titrated based on clinical assessment of rejection and tolerability. Adjunct therapy with adrenal corticosteroids is recommended early post transplant.

Heart Transplantation: The recommended starting oral dose of Prograf is 0.075 mg/kg/day administered every 12 hours in two divided doses. It is recommended that patients initiate oral therapy with Prograf capsules if possible. If IV therapy is necessary, conversion from IV to oral Prograf is recommended as soon as oral therapy can be tolerated. This usually occurs within 2-3 days. The initial dose of Prograf should be administered no sooner than 6 hours after transplantation. In a patient receiving an IV infusion, the first dose of oral therapy should be given 8-12 hours after discontinuing the IV infusion.

Dosing should be titrated based on clinical assessments of rejection and tolerability. Lower Prograf dosages may be sufficient as maintenance therapy. Adjunct therapy with adrenal corticosteroids is recommended early post transplant.

Rheumatoid Arthritis: The recommended adult oral dose of Prograf is 3 mg, administered once a day. Regular monitoring of Prograf treated patients for occurrence of adverse events is mandatory.

Patients with Hepatic or Renal Dysfunction: Due to the potential for nephrotoxicity, patients with renal or hepatic impairment should receive doses at the lowest value of the recommended intravenous and oral dosing ranges. Further reductions in dose below these ranges may be required.

Conversion to Prograf from Cyclosporine: Patients converted from cyclosporine to Prograf should receive the first Prograf dose no sooner than 24 hours after the last cyclosporine dose. Dosing may be further delayed in the presence of elevated cyclosporine levels. Patients converted from Prograf to cyclosporine should receive the first cyclosporine dose no sooner than 24 hours after the last Prograf dose. Dosing may be further delayed in the presence of elevated tacrolimus levels.

Pediatric Patients: Pediatric liver transplantation patients without pre-existing renal or hepatic dysfunction have required and tolerated higher doses than adults to achieve similar blood concentrations. Therefore, it is recommended that therapy be initiated in pediatric patients at a starting IV dose of 0.03-0.05 mg/kg/day and a starting oral dose of 0.15-0.20 mg/kg/day. Dose adjustments may be required. Experience in pediatric kidney and heart transplantation patients is limited.

Race: Although a formal study to evaluate the pharmacokinetics of tacrolimus in Black transplant patients has not been conducted, a retrospective comparison of Black and Caucasian kidney transplant patients indicated that Black patients required higher tacrolimus doses to attain similar trough concentrations.

Missed Dose: Transplant and Rheumatoid Arthritis: If a dose is missed, contact your physician or pharmacist immediately.

Administration: Prograf (tacrolimus for injection)—Intravenous Administration: Patients receiving Prograf intravenously (tacrolimus for injection) should be under continuous observation for at least the first 30 minutes following the start of the infusion and at frequent intervals thereafter. If signs or symptoms of anaphylaxis occur, the intravenous infusion should be stopped. An aqueous solution of epinephrine 1:1000 should be available at the bedside as well as a source of oxygen.

Reconstitution:

Table 10: Prograf

Reconstitution of Prograf Injection 5 mg/mL

Vial Size	Diluent to Be Added to Vial	Approximate Available Volume in Ampoule	Nominal Concentration per mL
1 mL (2 mL capacity)	0.9% Sodium Chloride or 5% Dextrose Injection	1 mL	Dilute to between 0.004 mg/mL and 0.02 mg/mL

Prograf (tacrolimus for injection) must be diluted with 0.9% Sodium Chloride Injection or 5% Dextrose Injection to a concentration between 0.004 mg/mL and 0.02 mg/mL prior to use. Diluted infusion solution should be stored in glass or polyethylene containers and should be discarded after 24 hours. The diluted infusion solution should not be stored in a PVC container due to poor stability and the potential for extraction of phthalates. In situations where more dilute solutions are utilized (e.g., pediatric dosing, etc.), PVC-free tubing should likewise be used to minimize the potential for significant drug adsorption onto the tubing. Parenteral drug products should be inspected visually for particulate matter and discoloration prior to administration, whenever solution and container permit. Due to the chemical instability of tacrolimus in alkaline media, Prograf injection should not be mixed or coinfused with solutions of pH 9 or greater (e.g., ganciclovir or acyclovir). Prograf injection is administered as a continuous intravenous infusion.

Prograf (tacrolimus immediate release capsules)—Oral Administration: Prograf (tacrolimus immediate release capsules) should be administered whole and should not be cut, crushed or chewed. Prograf can be administered with or without food however doses should be administered in a consistent manner, with doses spaced evenly throughout the day.

OVERDOSAGE:

Limited overdosage experience is available. Acute overdosages of up to 30 times the intended dose have been reported. All patients recovered with no sequelae. Acute overdosage has been followed by adverse reactions consistent with those listed in the Adverse Reactions section, including mild elevations of renal function markers (creatinine), nausea, headache, hyperreflexia, oliguria, hypotension, tremor and elevations in liver enzymes. In one case transient urticaria and lethargy were observed and in another case acute anuric renal insufficiency developed. Based on the poor aqueous solubility and extensive erythrocyte and plasma protein binding, it is anticipated that tacrolimus is not dialyzable to any significant extent; there is no experience with charcoal hemoperfusion. The oral use of activated charcoal has been reported in treating acute overdoses, but experience has not been sufficient to warrant recommending its use. General supportive measures and treatment of specific symptoms should be followed in all cases of overdosage.

In acute oral and intravenous toxicity studies, mortalities were seen at or above the following doses: in adult rats, 52× the recommended human oral dose: in immature rats, 16× the recommended oral dose and in adult rats, 16× the recommended human intravenous dose (all based on body surface area corrections).

For management of a suspected drug overdose, contact your **regional Poison Control Centre**. See the *CPS* Directory section for a list of Poison Control Centres.

ACTION AND CLINICAL PHARMACOLOGY: Mechanism of Action/Pharmacodynamics: Tacrolimus, the active ingredient in Prograf, is a macrolide immunosuppressant produced by *S. tsukubaensis*.

Tacrolimus prolongs the survival of the host and transplanted graft in animal transplant models of liver, kidney, heart, bone marrow, small bowel and pancreas, lung and trachea, skin, cornea and limb.

Tacrolimus has been demonstrated to suppress some humoral immunity and, to a greater extent, cell-mediated reactions such as allograft rejection, delayed type hypersensitivity, Freund's adjuvant arthritis, experimental allergic encephalomyelitis and graft versus host disease in several animal species.

Tacrolimus inhibits T-lymphocyte activation, although the exact mechanism of action is not known. The minimum inhibitory tissue culture level of tacrolimus that prevents antigen stimulation of T-lymphocytes is 0.1 nM-0.3 nM. Experimental evidence suggests that tacrolimus binds to an intracellular protein, FKBP-12. A complex of tacrolimus-FKBP-12, calcium, calmodulin and calcineurin is then formed and the phosphatase activity of calcineurin inhibited. This effect may prevent the generation of nuclear factor of activated T-cells (NF-AT), a nuclear component thought to initiate the gene transcription for the formation of lymphokines (interleukin-2, gamma interferon). The net result is the inhibition of T-lymphocyte activation (i.e., immunosuppression).

Pharmacokinetics: Tacrolimus activity is primarily due to the parent drug. After oral administration, absorption of tacrolimus into the systemic circulation from the gastrointestinal tract is incomplete and can be variable. Elimination of tacrolimus is via hepatic metabolism with a mean terminal elimination half-life of 18.8 hours in kidney transplant patients, 11.7 hours in liver transplant patients, 23.6 hours in heart transplant patients receiving a single intravenous dose of Prograf and 34.2 hours in healthy volunteers following intravenous administration. In rheumatoid arthritis patients the administration of a single intravenous and oral dose of Prograf, produced a mean terminal elimination half-life of 34.9 and 35.2 hrs respectively.

In transplant patients the intersubject variability in tacrolimus pharmacokinetics, has resulted in the need for the dosing regimen to be individualized. Dosing individualization can be achieved by therapeutic drug monitoring of tacrolimus blood concentrations and evaluation of clinical status (see Dosage and Administration). Pharmacokinetic data indicate that whole blood concentrations rather than plasma concentrations serve as the more appropriate sampling compartment to describe tacrolimus pharmacokinetics.

Absorption: Absorption of tacrolimus from the gastrointestinal tract after oral administration is incomplete and can be variable. Mean (±S.D.) pharmacokinetic parameters of tacrolimus in whole blood after oral administration to volunteers in two studies are presented in Table 11.

Table 11: Prograf

Mean (±S.D.) Pharmacokinetic Parameters of Tacrolimus in Whole Blood after Oral Administration

Parameter	Bioequivalence Study		Pharmacokinetic Study
Age	19–53 yrs		19–50 yrs
Number	62	59	16
Dose	5×1 mg single dose	1×5 mg single dose	5×1 mg single dose
Absolute Bioavailability (%)	—	—	17.8±5.0
C_{max} (ng/mL)	25.2±9.7	26.5±10.8	29.7±7.2
T_{max} (h)	1.2±0.4	1.4±0.6	1.6±0.7
AUC_{0-t} (ng·h/mL)	196±93[a]	209±97[a]	243±73[b]

[a] $AUC_{(0-72)}$.
[b] $AUC_{(0-120)}$.

The 1 mg and 5 mg dose strengths of tacrolimus capsules are bioequivalent as indicated in Table 11.

Bioequivalence Study 0.5 mg Capsule: An open label, four period, four sequence, randomized crossover study was done to determine the bioequivalence of the 0.5 mg Prograf capsule to the 1 mg Prograf capsule. In two periods of the study, a single dose of 6×0.5 mg capsules were consumed by healthy volunteers. In the two other periods of the study, 3×1 mg capsules were consumed in a single dose. The pharmaceutical parameters derived from this bioequivalence study are outlined in Table 12 and Table 13.

Table 12: Prograf

Bioequivalence of the 0.5 mg Prograf (tacrolimus) Capsule to the 1 mg Prograf (tacrolimus) Capsule in Healthy Volunteers: From Measured and Log Transformed Data, Uncorrected for Potency, Geometric Mean, Arithmetic Mean (CV %)

	Test (6×0.5 mg capsules)		Reference (3×1 mg capsules)		% Ratio of Geometric Means
Parameter	A1	A2	B1	B2	
AUC_T (ng·h/mL)	140±52.4	122±40.1	133±53.9	125±46.5	102.6
AUC_I (ng·h/mL)	168±66.3	148±50.4	160±70.9	152±62.1	102.9
C_{max} (ng/mL)	20.3±6.94	18.7±6.55	19.0±6.91	18.7±6.43	103.4
T_{max}[a] (h)	1.4±0.61	1.3±0.44	1.4±0.51	1.5±0.50	92.5
$T_{1/2}$[a] (h)	34.4±9.12	35.4±11.1	32.6±7.86	35.8±9.10	102.2

[a] Expressed as arithmetic mean (CV%) only.

Legend: A1 and A2 refer to data from 2 different study periods for test drug; B1 and B2 refer to data from 2 different study periods for reference drug.

Table 13: Prograf

Bioequivalence of the 0.5 mg Prograf (Tacrolimus) Capsule to the 1 mg Prograf (Tacrolimus) Capsule in Healthy Volunteers: Corrected for Potency, Geometric Mean

Parameter	Test	Reference	% Ratio of Geometric Means
AUC_T (ng·h/mL)	121.1[a]	116.3[a]	104.2
AUC_I (ng·h/mL)	145.5[a]	139.2[a]	104.5
C_{max} (ng/mL)	18.1[a]	17.3[a]	105.0

[a] Values calculated using LS Means of log-transformed data.

Potency corrections made using potencies of 100.8% for the 0.5 mg capsule and 102.3% for the 1 mg capsule.

In 26 kidney transplant patients, peak concentrations (C_{max}) were achieved at approximately 1-3 hours. The absorption half-life of tacrolimus in 17 liver transplant patients averaged 0.6 hour (S.D. 1.0 hour) with peak concentrations (C_{max}) in blood and plasma being achieved at approximately 1.5-3.5 hours. In rheumatoid arthritis patients peak concentrations (C_{max}) were achieved within 1.3 hours. Mean (±S.D.) pharmacokinetic parameters of tacrolimus in whole blood after initial dose in adult kidney and liver transplant patients and in rheumatoid arthritis patients are presented in Table 14.

The absolute bioavailability of tacrolimus is approximately 17% in kidney transplant patients, 22% in adult liver transplant patients, 34% in pediatric liver transplant patients, and approximately 25% in rheumatoid arthritis patients. In healthy volunteers the absolute bioavailability of tacrolimus was found to be approximately 18% (Table 14).

Food Effects: The rate and extent of tacrolimus absorption is greatest under fasted conditions. The presence and composition of food decreased both the rate and extent of tacrolimus absorption when administered to healthy volunteers, see Table 15.

The effect was most pronounced with the high-fat meal: mean area under the curve (AUC_{0-96}) and C_{max} were decreased 37% and 77%, respectively; T_{max} was lengthened 5-fold. The high-carbohydrate meal decreased AUC_{0-96} and C_{max} by 28% and 65%, respectively.

The effect of food was also studied in 11 liver transplant patients. Prograf was administered in the fasted state or 15 minutes after a breakfast of known fat content (34% of 400 total calories). The results indicate that the presence of food reduces the absorption of tacrolimus in these patients (decrease in AUC and C_{max} and increase in T_{max}). The relative oral bioavailability (whole blood) was reduced by 27.0 (±18.2)% compared to administration in the fasting state.

In healthy volunteers, the time of the meal also affected tacrolimus bioavailability. Relative to the fasted state, there was little effect on tacrolimus bioavailability when administered one hour prior to a high-fat breakfast, whereas bioavailability (both extent and rate of absorption) was greatly reduced when the drug was administered immediately or 1.5 hours after the meal. When given immediately following the meal, C_{max} was reduced 71%, $AUC_{0\text{-}96}$ was reduced by 39%, and T_{max} was delayed 1.6 hours relative to the fasting condition. When administered 1.5 hours following the meal, C_{max} was reduced 63%, $AUC_{0\text{-}96}$ was reduced 39%, and T_{max} was delayed 1.4 hours relative to the fasted condition.

Table 14: Prograf

Mean (±S.D.) Pharmacokinetic Parameters of Tacrolimus in Whole Blood after Initial Dose in Adult Transplant and Rheumatoid Arthritis Patients

Population	N	Route (Dose)	Pharmacokinetic Parameters C_{max} (ng/mL)	T_{max} (h)	AUC (ng·h/mL)
Kidney Transplant Patients	26	IV (0.02 mg/kg/12 h)	—	—	294[c]±262
		PO (0.2 mg/kg/day)	19.2±10.3	3	203[c]±42
		PO (0.3 mg/kg/day)	24.2±15.8	1.5	288[c]±93
Liver Transplant Patients	17	IV (0.05 mg/kg/12 h)	—	—	3300[c]±2130
		PO (0.3 mg/kg/day)	68.5±30.0	2.3±1.5	519[c]±179
Heart Transplant Patients	11	IV (0.01 mg/kg/day as a continuous infusion)	—	—	954[d]±334
		PO (0.075 mg/kg/day)	24.9±7.72	1.0	175[e]±49.8
Rheumatoid Arthritis Patients	12	PO (3×1 mg single dose)	19.64±6.32	1.3±0.58	192.88±86.42

a $AUC_{0\text{-}120}$.
b $AUC_{0\text{-}72}$.
c $AUC_{0\text{-}inf}$.
d $AUC_{0\text{-}t}$.
e $AUC_{0\text{-}12}$.
Legend: PO: oral; IV: intravenous; —: not applicable; NA: not available.

Table 15: Prograf

Food Effects on the Rate and Extent of Tacrolimus Absorption in Healthy Volunteers

Parameter	Fasted (n=15)	High Carbohydrate[a] (n=15)	High Fat[b] (n=15)
C_{max} (ng/mL)	25.6±11.4	9.0±3.8	5.9±2.3
T_{max} (h)	1.4±0.6	3.2±1.1	6.5±3.0
$AUC_{0\text{-}t}$ (ng·h/mL)	233±121[c]	168±59[c]	147±56[c]

a 668 kcal (4% fat; 85% carbohydrate).
b 848 kcal (46% fat, 39% carbohydrate).
c $AUC_{(0\text{-}96)}$.

In fasted healthy volunteers given a single dose, the absorption of tacrolimus was proportional to dose; see Table 16.

Table 16: Prograf

Absorption of Tacrolimus in Fasted Healthy Volunteers

Parameter	Dose 3 mg n=18	7 mg n=18	10 mg n=18
C_{max} (ng/mL)	14.5±5.8	31.2±10.1	45.1±15.0
	14.5±5.8[a]	13.4±4.3[a]	13.5±4.5[a]
T_{max} (h)	1.4±0.4	1.4±0.5	1.3±0.4
$AUC_{0\text{-}96}$ (ng·h/mL)	131±77	303±138	420±166
	131±77[a]	130±59[a]	126±50[a]

a Adjusted to 3 mg dose.

Distribution: The apparent volume of distribution (based on whole blood concentrations) of tacrolimus is approximately 1.41, 1.91 , 0.85 and 2.37 L/kg in kidney transplant patients, healthy volunteers, adult liver transplant patients and adult rheumatoid arthritis patients, respectively (see Table 17).

The plasma protein binding of tacrolimus is approximately 99% and is independent of concentration over a range of 5-50 ng/mL. Tacrolimus is bound to proteins, mainly albumin and alpha-1-acid glycoprotein, and has a high level of association with erythrocytes. The distribution of tacrolimus between whole blood and plasma depends on several factors, such as hematocrit, temperature at the time of plasma separation, drug concentration, and plasma protein concentration. In a U.S. study, the ratio of whole blood concentration to plasma concentration ranged from 12 to 67 (mean 35).

In 18 kidney transplant patients, tacrolimus trough concentrations from 3 to 30 ng/mL measured at 10-12 hours post dose (C_{min}) correlated well with the $AUC_{0\text{-}12}$ (correlation coefficient 0.93). In 24 liver transplant patients over a concentration range of 10 to 60 ng/mL, the correlation coefficient was 0.94. In 25 heart transplant patients, the correlation coefficient was 0.89 after an oral dose of 0.075 or 0.15 mg/kg/day at steady-state.

Metabolism: Tacrolimus is extensively metabolized by the mixed-function oxidase system, primarily the cytochrome P450 enzyme system (CYP3A). A metabolic pathway leading to the formation of 8 possible metabolites has been proposed. Demethylation and hydroxylation were identified as the primary mechanisms of biotransformation in vitro. The major metabolite identified in incubations with human liver microsomes is 13-demethyl tacrolimus. In in vitro studies, a 31-demethyl metabolite has been reported to have the same activity as tacrolimus; the 13-demethyl, 15-demethyl and 15- and 31- double-demethylated metabolites were shown to retain an activity of less than 10%.

Excretion: The clearance of tacrolimus is 0.040, 0.083, 0.042 and 0.049 L/h/kg in healthy volunteers, adult kidney transplant patients, adult liver transplant patients, and adult rheumatoid arthritis patients, respectively. In man, less than 1% of the dose administered is excreted unchanged in urine.

Table 17: Prograf

Volume of Distribution and Clearance in Transplant and Rheumatoid Arthritis Patients

Parameter	Volunteers (n=8)	Kidney Transplant Patients (n=26)	Liver Transplant Patients (Adults, n=17)	Heart Transplant Patient (n=11)	Rheumatoid Arthritis Patients (Adults, n=12)
Mean IV Dose	0.025 mg/kg/4 h	0.02 mg/kg/4 h	0.05 mg/kg/12 h	0.01 mg/kg/day as a continuous infusion	0.015 mg/kg/4 h
V (L/kg)	1.91±0.31	1.41±0.66	0.85±0.3	NA	2.37±0.45
Cl (L/h/kg)	0.040±0.009	0.083±0.050	0.053±0.017	0.051±0.015	0.049±0.014

Special Populations and Conditions: Pediatrics: A study in liver transplantation has been conducted in sixteen pediatric patients (age range: 0.7-13.2 years). A mean terminal elimination half-life of 11.5 hours was determined following an intravenous dose of 0.037 mg/kg/day in twelve patients; the volume of distribution was 2.6 L/kg, whereas clearance was 0.135 L/h/kg. In nine patients receiving capsule formulation, a mean C_{max} of 48.4 ng/mL was attained at a mean T_{max} of 2.7 hours following an oral dose of 0.152 mg/kg as Prograf capsules. The $AUC_{(0\text{-}72\ h)}$ was 337 ng·h/mL. The absolute bioavailability was 31%.

Whole blood trough concentrations from 31 pediatric patients (less than 12 years old) showed that pediatric patients need higher doses than adults to achieve similar tacrolimus trough concentrations, suggesting that the pharmacokinetic characteristics of tacrolimus are different in pediatric patients compared to adults (see Dosage and Administration).

Geriatrics: The pharmacokinetics of tacrolimus has not been established in the geriatric population.

Gender: A formal study to evaluate the effect of gender on tacrolimus pharmacokinetics has not been conducted however, there was no differences noted in dosing by gender in the kidney transplant trial. A retrospective comparison of pharmacokinetics in healthy volunteers, and in kidney and liver transplant patients indicated no gender-based differences.

Race: A formal study to evaluate the pharmacokinetic disposition of tacrolimus in Black transplant patients has not been conducted. However, a retrospective comparison of Black and Caucasian kidney transplant patients indicated that Black patients required higher tacrolimus doses to attain similar trough concentrations. (See Dosage and Administration.)

Hepatic Insufficiency: Tacrolimus pharmacokinetics have been determined in six patients with mild hepatic dysfunction (mean Pugh score: 6.2) following single intravenous and oral administrations. The pharmacokinetic parameters obtained were as follows (see Table 18).

Table 18: Prograf

Tacrolimus Pharmacokinetics in Patients with Mild Hepatic Impairment

Parameter (N=6)	Dose and Route 7.7 mg PO	1.3 mg IV
Age Range (yrs)	52–63	
Absolute Bioavailability (%)	22.3± 11.4	—
C_{max} (ng/mL)	48.2±17.9	
T_{max} (h)	1.5±0.6	
$AUC_{0\text{-}72}$ (ng·h/mL)	488±320	367±107
V (L/kg)	3.7±4.7[a]	3.1±1.6
Cl (L/h/kg)	0.034±0.019[a]	0.042±0.020
$t_{1/2}$ (h)	66.1±44.8	60.6±43.8

a Corrected for bioavailability.

The disposition of tacrolimus in patients with mild hepatic dysfunction was not substantially different from that in normal volunteers (see previous tables). In general, tacrolimus elimination half-life was longer and volume of distribution larger in patients with mild hepatic dysfunction compared to normal volunteers. The clearance in both populations was similar and since tacrolimus is extensively metabolized at multiple sites, patients with mild hepatic dysfunction may not require lower maintenance doses of tacrolimus than patients with normal hepatic function.

Tacrolimus pharmacokinetics were studied in 6 patients with severe hepatic dysfunction (mean Pugh score: >10). The mean clearance was substantially lower in patients with severe hepatic dysfunction, irrespective of the route of administration. See Table 19.

Table 19: Prograf

Tacrolimus Pharmacokinetics in Patients with Severe Hepatic Impairment

Route, N	Dose	AUC ng· h/mL (0-t)	$T_{1/2}$ (h)	V L/kg	Cl (L/h/kg)
IV, n=6	0.02 mg/kg/4 h IV (n=2)	762 (t=120 h)	198±158 Range: 81–436	—	—
	0.01 mg/kg/8 h IV (n=4)	289±117 (t=144 h)		3.9±1.0	0.017±0.013
PO, n=5[a]	8 mg PO (n=1)	658 (t=120 h)	119±35 Range: 85–178	3.1±3.4	0.016±0.011
	5 mg PO (n=4)	533±156 (t=144 h)			
	4 mg PO (n=1)	—			

a 1 patient did not receive the PO dose.

Renal Insufficiency: Tacrolimus pharmacokinetics following a single intravenous administration have been determined in 12 patients (7 not on dialysis and 5 on dialysis) prior to their kidney transplant. The pharmacokinetic parameters obtained are presented in Table 20.

The disposition of tacrolimus in patients with renal dysfunction was not different from that in normal volunteers (see previous tables). The clearance was similar whereas volume of distribution was smaller and the mean terminal elimination half-life shorter than that of normal volunteers.

Table 20: Prograf
Tacrolimus Pharmacokinetics in Patients with Renal Insufficiency

Serum Creatinine (mg/dL)	3.9±1.6 (not on dialysis)
	12.0±2.4 (on dialysis)
Age range (yrs)	25–65
Route	IV
Dose (mg)	1.17±0.28
AUC_{0-60} (ng·h/mL)	393±123
AUC_{0-inf} (ng·h/mL)	499±155
V (L/kg)	1.07±0.20
Cl (L/h/kg)	0.038±0.014
$t_{1/2}$ (h)	26.3±9.2

STORAGE AND STABILITY: Prograf (immediate release capsules): Store and dispense at controlled room temperature, 15-30°C.

Prograf (tacrolimus for injection): Store in the carton and protect from light. Dispense Prograf ampoules between 15 and 25°C.

Prograf (tacrolimus for injection) must be diluted to a concentration between 0.004 mg/mL and 0.02 mg/mL with 0.9% Sodium Chloride Injection or 5% Dextrose Injection before use. The diluted infusion solution should be stored at 15-25°C in glass or polyethylene containers and should be discarded after 24 hours. The diluted infusion solution should not be stored in a PVC container due to poor stability and the potential for extraction of phthalates. Parenteral drug products should be inspected visually for particulate matter and discoloration prior to administration, whenever solution and container permit.

SPECIAL HANDLING INSTRUCTIONS: None required.

INFORMATION FOR THE PATIENT: Published in e-CPS, available by subscription at www.e-cps.ca.

DOSAGE FORMS, COMPOSITION AND PACKAGING: Capsules: 0.5 mg: Each oblong, light yellow, immediate release capsule, branded with red "0.5 mg" on cap and "▣ 607" on capsule body contains: anhydrous tacrolimus 0.5 mg. Nonmedicinal ingredients: croscarmellose sodium, hydroxypropylmethylcellulose, lactose and magnesium stearate; capsule shell: ferric oxide, gelatin and titanium dioxide. Bottles of 100 or 10 blister packs of 10.

1 mg: Each oblong, white, immediate release capsule, branded with red "1 mg" on cap and "▣ 617" on capsule body contains: anhydrous tacrolimus 1 mg. Nonmedicinal ingredients: croscarmellose sodium, hydroxypropylmethylcellulose, lactose and magnesium stearate; capsule shell: gelatin and titanium dioxide. Bottles of 100 or 10 blister packs of 10.

5 mg: Each oblong, greyish/red, immediate release capsule, branded with white "5 mg" on cap and "▣ 657" on capsule body, contains: anhydrous tacrolimus 5 mg. Nonmedicinal ingredients: croscarmellose sodium, hydroxypropylmethylcellulose, lactose and magnesium stearate; capsule shell: gelatin, ferric oxide and titanium dioxide. Bottles of 100 or 10 blister packs of 10.

Injection: Each mL of sterile solution contains: the equivalent of anhydrous tacrolimus 5 mg. Nonmedicinal ingredients: dehydrated alcohol, USP, 83% v/v and polyoxyl 60 hydrogenated castor oil (HCO-60). Ampuls of 1 mL, boxes of 10.

(Shown in Product Identification Section)

Prolastin®-C

alpha1-proteinase inhibitor (human), highly purified

Alpha1-antitrypsin Replenisher

Talecris

Date of Revision: February 15, 2010

SUMMARY PRODUCT INFORMATION:

Route of Administration	Dosage Form/ Strength	Clinically Relevant Nonmedicinal Ingredients
Intravenous injection	Lyophilized powder for injection 1000 mg/vial	For a complete listing see Dosage Forms, Composition and Packaging.

DESCRIPTION: PROLASTIN-C ($Alpha_1$-Proteinase Inhibitor [Human]) is a sterile, stable, lyophilized preparation of highly purified human $Alpha_1$-Proteinase Inhibitor ($alpha_1$-PI), also known as $alpha_1$-antitrypsin. $Alpha_1$-Proteinase Inhibitor (Human) is intended for use in therapy of congenital $alpha_1$-antitrypsin deficiency.

PROLASTIN-C is prepared from pooled human plasma of normal donors by modification and refinements of the cold ethanol method of Cohn. PROLASTIN-C is produced through a modification of the Prolastin manufacturing process that results in improved product purity and a higher concentration of the same active substance, $alpha_1$-PI, in the reconstituted product.

INDICATIONS AND CLINICAL USE: Congenital $Alpha_1$-Antitrypsin Deficiency: PROLASTIN-C is indicated for chronic replacement therapy of individuals having congenital deficiency of $alpha_1$-PI ($alpha_1$-antitrypsin deficiency) with clinically demonstrable panacinar emphysema. Clinical and biochemical studies have demonstrated that with such therapy, it is possible to increase plasma levels of $alpha_1$-PI, and that levels of functionally active $alpha_1$-PI in the lung epithelial lining fluid are increased proportionately. As some individuals with $alpha_1$-antitrypsin deficiency will not go on to develop panacinar emphysema, only those with evidence of such disease should be considered for chronic replacement therapy with $Alpha_1$-Proteinase Inhibitor (Human). Subjects with the PiMZ or PiMS phenotypes of $alpha_1$-antitrypsin deficiency should not be considered for such treatment as they appear to be at small risk for panacinar emphysema. Clinical data are not available as to the long-term effects derived from chronic replacement therapy of individuals with $alpha_1$-antitrypsin deficiency with $Alpha_1$-Proteinase Inhibitor (Human). Only adult subjects have received $Alpha_1$-Proteinase Inhibitor (Human) to date.

$Alpha_1$-Proteinase Inhibitor (Human) is not indicated for use in patients other than those with PiZZ, PiZ (null) or Pi (null) (null) phenotypes.

CONTRAINDICATIONS:

- PROLASTIN-C should not be given to patients who are hypersensitive to $Alpha_1$-Proteinase Inhibitor (Human) or to any ingredient in the formulation or component of the container. For a complete listing, see Dosage Forms, Composition and Packaging.
- PROLASTIN-C should not be given to individuals with selective immunoglobulin A (IgA) deficiencies, since these patients may experience severe reactions, including anaphylaxis, to IgA which may be present.

WARNINGS AND PRECAUTIONS: General: Because this product is made from human blood, it may carry the risk of transmitting infectious agents, e.g. viruses, and theoretically, the Creutzfeldt-Jakob Disease (CJD) or Creutzfeldt-Jakob Disease variant (vCJD) agents. The risk that such products will transmit an infectious agent has been reduced by screening plasma donors for prior exposure to certain viruses, by testing for the presence of certain current virus infections, and by inactivating and/or removing certain viruses. Despite these measures, such products can still potentially transmit disease. There is also the possibility that unknown infectious agents may be present in such products. Individuals who receive infusions of blood or plasma products may develop signs and/or symptoms of some viral infections, particularly hepatitis C. All infections thought by a physician possibly to have been transmitted by this product should be reported by the physician or other healthcare provider to Talecris Biotherapeutics Ltd. (1-866-482-5226).

The physician should discuss the risks and benefits of this product with the patient, before prescribing or administering to the patient.

Administer only by the intravenous route.

As with any colloid solution, there will be an increase in plasma volume following intravenous administration of $Alpha_1$-Proteinase Inhibitor (Human). Caution should therefore be used in patients at risk for circulatory overload.

Product administration and handling of the needles must be done with caution. Percutaneous puncture with a needle contaminated with blood can transmit infectious virus including HIV (AIDS) and hepatitis. Obtain immediate medical attention if injury occurs.

Place needles in sharps container after single use. Discard all equipment including any reconstituted PROLASTIN-C product in accordance with biohazard procedures.

Carcinogenesis and Mutagenesis: Long-term studies in animals to evaluate carcinogenesis and mutagenesis have not been conducted.

Sexual Function/Reproduction: Long-term studies in animals to evaluate impairment of fertility have not been conducted.

Special Populations: Pregnant Women: Animal reproduction studies have not been conducted with PROLASTIN-C. It is also not known whether PROLASTIN-C can cause fetal harm when administered to a pregnant woman or can affect reproduction capacity. PROLASTIN-C should be given to a pregnant woman only if clearly needed.

Nursing Women: It is not known whether $Alpha_1$-Proteinase Inhibitor (Human) is excreted in human milk. Because many drugs are excreted in human milk, caution should be exercised when PROLASTIN-C is administered to a nursing woman.

Pediatrics: Safety and effectiveness in the pediatric population have not been established.

ADVERSE REACTIONS: Adverse Drug Reaction Overview: Therapeutic administration of PROLASTIN-C 60 mg/kg weekly, has been demonstrated to be well-tolerated.

Clinical Trial Adverse Drug Reactions: Because clinical trials are conducted under very specific conditions the adverse reaction rates observed in the clinical trials may not reflect the rates observed in practice and should not be compared to the rates in the clinical trials of another drug. Adverse drug reaction information from clinical trials is useful for identifying drug-related adverse events and for approximating rates.

Two separate clinical studies were conducted with PROLASTIN-C: Study 11815, a 20 week, open-label, safety study in 38 subjects, and Study 11816, a 16 week, randomized, double-blind, cross-over pharmacokinetic comparability study vs. Prolastin (original product) in 24 subjects, followed by an 8 week open label treatment with PROLASTIN-C. Thus, 62 subjects were exposed to PROLASTIN-C in clinical trials, receiving a total of 1132 infusions.

Table 1: PROLASTIN-C
Adverse Event Frequency as a % of All Infusions (>0.5%) Irrespective of Causality

	PROLASTIN-C No. of infusions: 1132	Prolastin No. of infusions: 192
Adverse Event	**No. of AE (percentage of all infusions)**	**No. of AE (percentage of all infusions)**
Upper respiratory tract infection	9 (0.8%)	1 (0.5%)
Urinary tract infection	8 (0.7%)	0
Nausea	7 (0.6%)	0
Headache	4 (0.4%)	3 (1.6%)
Arthralgia	2 (0.2%)	2 (1.0%)

The most common drug related adverse event was chills, which occurred in 3.2% of PROLASTIN-C patients (n=2). The following drug related adverse events were reported in 1.6% of patients (one subject each) treated with PROLASTIN-C: malaise, headache, rash (severe), hot flush and pruritus.

In clinical studies with Prolastin, six reactions were observed with 517 infusions of $Alpha_1$-Proteinase Inhibitor (Human), or 1.16%. None of the reactions was severe. The adverse reactions reported included delayed fever (maximum temperature rise was 38.9°C, resolving spontaneously over 24 hours) occurring up to 12 hours following treatment (0.77%), light-headedness (0.19%), and dizziness (0.19%). Mild transient leukocytosis and dilutional anemia several hours after infusion have also been noted.

Post-Market Adverse Drug Reactions: Additionally, since market entry of $Alpha_1$-Proteinase Inhibitor (Human), occasional reports of the following events have been received: flu-like symptoms, allergic-like reactions, dyspnea, tachycardia, shortness of breath, bronchospasm, wheezing, urticaria, back pain, clamminess, sweating, diarrhea, and fatigue.

Less frequently, the following have also been reported: hypotension, anxiety, cyanosis, swelling of hands and feet, angio-, facial and lip edema, nasal congestion, sinusitis, abdominal pains or cramps, pallor, and weakness.

Rare cases of transient increase in blood pressure or hypertension and chest pain have also been reported.

DRUG INTERACTIONS: Drug-Drug Interactions: No drug-drug interactions are known.

DOSAGE AND ADMINISTRATION: Recommended Dose and Dosage Adjustment: Each vial of PROLASTIN-C ($Alpha_1$-Proteinase Inhibitor [Human]), has the functional activity, as determined by inhibition of porcine pancreatic elastase, stated on the label of the vial.

The "threshold" level of $alpha_1$-PI in the serum believed to provide adequate anti-elastase activity in the lung of individuals with $alpha_1$-antitrypsin deficiency is 80 mg/dL (based on commercial standards for $alpha_1$-PI immunologic assay). However, assays of $alpha_1$-PI based on commercial standards measure antigenic activity of $alpha_1$-PI, whereas the labeled potency value of $alpha_1$-PI is expressed as actual functional activity, i.e., actual capacity to neutralize porcine pancreatic elastase. As functional activity may be less than antigenic activity, serum levels of $alpha_1$-PI determined using commercial immunologic assays may not accurately reflect actual functional $alpha_1$-PI levels.

Therefore, although it may be helpful to monitor serum levels of $alpha_1$-PI in individuals receiving PROLASTIN-C, using currently available commercial assays of antigenic activity, results of these assays should not be used to determine the required therapeutic dosage.

The recommended dosage of PROLASTIN-C is 60 mg/kg body weight administered once weekly. This dose is intended to increase and maintain a level of functional $alpha_1$-PI in the epithelial lining of the lower respiratory tract, providing adequate anti-elastase activity in the lung of individuals with $alpha_1$-antitrypsin deficiency.

PROLASTIN-C may be given at a rate of 0.08 mL/kg/min or greater and must be administered intravenously. The recommended dosage of 60 mg/kg takes approximately 15 minutes to infuse.

Administration: For intravenous use only.

Parenteral drug products should be inspected visually for particulate matter and discoloration prior to administration, whenever solution and container permit.

Reconstituted PROLASTIN-C should be given alone, without mixing with other agents or diluting solutions.

Reconstitution: PROLASTIN-C should be reconstituted with Sterile Water for Injection, USP (see Table 2). PROLASTIN-C and diluent should be brought to room temperature prior to reconstitution. PROLASTIN-C should be filtered through a sterile filter needle as supplied in the package prior to use.

Table 2: PROLASTIN-C
Reconstitution of PROLASTIN-C

Approximate $Alpha_1$-PI Functional Activity	Volume of Diluent Provided (To be Added to Vial)
1000 mg	20 mL

Administer within 3 hours after reconstitution. Do not refrigerate after reconstitution.

Vacuum Transfer: Aseptic technique should be followed.

1. Warm the PROLASTIN-C (Product) and sterile water (diluent) to room temperature (25°C) before reconstitution.
2. Remove the plastic flip-top caps from each vial. Swab the exposed stopper surfaces with alcohol and allow surface to dry.
3. Carefully remove the plastic sheath from the short end of the transfer needle. Insert the exposed needle into the center of the stopper in the diluent vial.

4. Carefully grip the sheath of the other end of the transfer needle and twist to remove it.
5. Invert the diluent vial and insert the attached needle into the PROLASTIN-C vial at a 45° angle. This will direct the stream of diluent against the wall of the Product vial and minimize foaming. The vacuum will draw the diluent into the Product vial. Because the vial of PROLASTIN-C is under vacuum, the stopper must only be pierced one time by the needle, to ensure complete transfer of diluent.
6. Remove the diluent vial and transfer needle.
7. Immediately after adding the diluent, swirl vigorously for 10-15 seconds to thoroughly break-up cake then swirl continuously until the powder is completely dissolved. Some foaming will occur, but this does not affect the quality of the product. The vial should then be visually inspected for particulate matter and discoloration prior to administration.
8. Attach the filter needle (from the package) to sterile syringe. Withdraw the PROLASTIN-C solution into the syringe through the filter needle.
9. Remove the filter needle from the syringe and replace with an appropriate injection needle for administration. Discard filter needle into a puncture-proof container.
10. The contents of more than one vial of PROLASTIN-C may be drawn into the same syringe before administration. If more than one vial of PROLASTIN-C is used, withdraw contents from vial using aseptic technique. Place contents into a sterile I.V. administration container (plastic or glass) using a syringe. Avoid pushing a large I.V. spike into the product container stopper as this has been known to force the stopper into the vial, with a resulting loss of sterility.

Described above is one acceptable method of reconstitution. The product may also be reconstituted with other appropriate transfer devices according to the manufacturer's accepted procedure.

OVERDOSAGE:
To date, there have been no reported cases of overdose for PROLASTIN-C or other Alpha$_1$-Proteinase Inhibitor (Human) manufactured by Talecris. No data are available in regard to overdosage in humans.

For management of a suspected drug overdose, CPhA recommends that you contact your **regional Poison Control Centre**. See the *CPS* Directory section for a list of Poison Control Centres.

ACTION AND CLINICAL PHARMACOLOGY: Mechanism of Action: Alpha$_1$-antitrypsin deficiency is a chronic, hereditary, usually fatal, autosomal co-dominant disorder in which a low concentration of alpha$_1$-PI (alpha$_1$-antitrypsin)* is associated with slowly progressive severe panacinar emphysema that most often manifests itself in the third to fourth decades of life. The emphysema is typically worse in the lower lung zones. The pathogenesis of development of emphysema in alpha$_1$-antitrypsin deficiency is not well understood at this time. It is believed, however, to be due to a chronic biochemical imbalance between elastase (an enzyme capable of degrading elastin tissues, released by inflammatory cells, primarily neutrophils, in the lower respiratory tract) and alpha$_1$-PI (the principal inhibitor of neutrophil elastase), which is deficient in alpha$_1$-antitrypsin disease. As a result, it is believed that alveolar structures are unprotected from chronic exposure to elastase released from a chronic, low-level burden of neutrophils in the lower respiratory tract, resulting in progressive degradation of elastin tissues. The eventual outcome is the development of emphysema. Neonatal hepatitis with cholestatic jaundice appears in approximately 10% of newborns with alpha$_1$-antitrypsin deficiency. In some adults, alpha$_1$-antitrypsin deficiency is complicated by cirrhosis. Since severe alpha$_1$-PI deficiency is one of the most common serious genetic conditions, it is recommended that families of index cases also be screened for alpha1-PI deficiency.

A large number of phenotypic variants of alpha$_1$-antitrypsin deficiency exists. The most severely affected individuals are those with the PiZZ variant, typically characterized by alpha$_1$-PI serum levels <35% normal. Epidemiologic studies of individuals with various phenotypes of alpha$_1$-antitrypsin deficiency have demonstrated that individuals with endogenous serum levels of alpha$_1$-PI ≤50 mg/dL (based on commercial standards) have a risk of >80% of developing emphysema over a lifetime. However, individuals with endogenous alpha$_1$-PI levels >80 mg/dL, in general, do not manifest an increased risk for development of emphysema above the general population background risk. From these observations, it is believed that the "threshold" level of alpha$_1$-PI in the serum required to provide adequate anti-elastase activity in the lung of individuals with alpha$_1$-antitrypsin deficiency is about 80 mg/dL (11 μM), based on commercial standards for immunologic assay of alpha$_1$-PI. The maintenance of blood serum levels of alpha$_1$-PI above 80 mg/dL (11 μM) is historically thought to provide therapeutically relevant anti-neutrophil elastase protection.

Pharmacodynamics: In clinical studies, patients received Alpha$_1$-Proteinase Inhibitor (Human) replacement therapy, 60 mg/kg body weight, once weekly for up to 26 weeks (average 24 weeks of therapy). With this schedule of replacement therapy, blood levels of alpha$_1$-PI were maintained above 80 mg/dL (based on the commercial standards for alpha$_1$-PI immunologic assay).

Pharmacokinetics: In clinical studies, the mean in vivo recovery of alpha$_1$-PI was 4.2 mg (immunologic)/dL per mg (functional)/kg body weight administered. The half-life of alpha$_1$-PI in vivo was approximately 6 days.

Duration of Effect: See Action and Clinical Pharmacology, Pharmacokinetics.

STORAGE AND STABILITY: PROLASTIN-C should be stored at temperatures not to exceed 25°C. Freezing should be avoided as breakage of the diluent vial might occur. Administer within 3 hours after reconstitution.

INFORMATION FOR THE PATIENT: Published in e-CPS, available by subscription at www.e-cps.ca.

DOSAGE FORMS, COMPOSITION AND PACKAGING: A sterile, white to beige, lyophilized powder in single use vials with the total alpha$_1$-PI functional activity, in milligrams, stated on the label of each vial (approximate functional activity of 1000 mg per vial; see Table 2). A suitable volume of Sterile Water for Injection USP (20 mL), a sterile double-ended transfer needle and a sterile filter needle are provided.

Proleukin® Ⓟ
aldesleukin
Biological Response Modifier

Novartis Pharmaceuticals

Date of Revision: May 19, 2010

PHARMACOLOGY: Aldesleukin an analogue of human interleukin-2 produced by recombinant DNA technology, has been shown to possess the biological activities of human native interleukin-2. Aldesleukin exhibits antitumor activity; the exact mechanism by which aldesleukin mediates its antitumor activity in animals and humans is unknown. In vitro studies performed on human cell lines demonstrate the immunoregulatory properties of aldesleukin, including: a) enhance-ment of lymphocyte mitogenesis and stimulation of long-term growth of human interleukin-2 dependent cell lines; b) enhancement of lymphocyte cytotoxicity; c) induction of killer cell (lymphokine-activated (LAK) and natural (NK)) activity; and d) induction of interferon-gamma production.

The in vivo administration of aldesleukin in animals and humans produces multiple immunological effects in a dose dependent manner. These effects include activation of cellular immunity with profound lymphocytosis, eosinophilia, and thrombocytopenia, and the production of cytokines including tumor necrosis factor, IL-1 and gamma interferon. In vivo experiments in murine tumor models have shown inhibition of tumor growth.

Pharmacokinetics: Aldesleukin exists as biologically active, non-covalently bound microaggregates with an average size of 27 recombinant interleukin-2 molecules. The solubilizing agent, sodium dodecyl sulfate, may have an effect on the kinetic properties of this product. The pharmacokinetic profile of aldesleukin is characterized by high plasma concentrations following a short i.v. infusion, rapid distribution into the extravascular space and elimination from the body by metabolism in the kidneys with little or no bioactive protein excreted in the urine.

Studies of i.v. aldesleukin in sheep and humans indicated that upon completion of infusion, approximately 30% of the administered dose is detectable in plasma. This finding is consistent with studies in rats using radiolabeled aldesleukin, which demonstrate a rapid (<1 minute) uptake of the majority of the label into the lungs, liver, kidney, and spleen.

The serum half-life ($t_{½}$) curves of aldesleukin remaining in the plasma are derived from studies done in 52 cancer patients following a 5-minute i.v. infusion. These patients were shown to have a distribution and elimination $t_{½}$ of 13 and 85 minutes, respectively.

The relatively rapid clearance rate of aldesleukin has led to dosage schedules characterized by frequent, short infusions. Observed serum levels are proportional to the dose of aldesleukin.

* Although the terms "Alpha$_1$-Proteinase Inhibitor" and "alpha$_1$-antitrypsin" are used interchangeably in the scientific literature, the hereditary disorder associated with a reduction in the serum level of alpha$_1$-PI is conventionally referred to as "alpha$_1$-antitrypsin deficiency" while the deficient protein is referred to as "Alpha$_1$-Proteinase Inhibitor".

Following the initial rapid organ distribution, the primary route of clearance of circulating aldesleukin is the kidney. In humans and animals, aldesleukin is cleared from the circulation by both glomerular filtration and peritubular extraction in the kidney. This dual mechanism for delivery of aldesleukin to the proximal tubule may account for the preservation of clearance in patients with rising serum creatinine values. Greater than 80% of the amount of aldesleukin distributed to plasma, cleared from the circulation and presented to the kidney is metabolized to amino acids in the cells lining the proximal convoluted tubules. In humans, the mean clearance rate in cancer patients is 268 mL/min.

Immunogenicity: Fifty-seven of 77 (74%) metastatic renal cell carcinoma patients treated with an every 8-hour aldesleukin regimen and 33 of 50 (66%) metastatic malignant melanoma patients treated with a variety of i.v. regimens developed low titers of nonneutralizing anti-aldesleukin antibodies. Neutralizing antibodies were not detected in this group of patients, but have been detected in 1/106 (<1%) patients treated with i.v. aldesleukin using a wide variety of schedules and doses. The clinical significance of anti-aldesleukin antibodies is unknown.

Clinical Experience: Two hundred fifty-five patients with metastatic renal cell cancer (metastatic RCC) were treated with single agent aldesleukin in 7 clinical studies conducted at 21 institutions. Two hundred seventy patients with metastatic malignant melanoma were treated with single agent aldesleukin in 8 clinical studies conducted at 22 institutions. Patients enrolled in trials of single agent aldesleukin were required to have an Eastern Cooperative Oncology Group (ECOG) Performance Status (PS) of 0 or 1 and normal organ function as determined by cardiac stress test, pulmonary function tests, and creatinine ≤1.5 mg/dL. Patients with brain metastases, active infections, organ allografts and diseases requiring steroid treatment were excluded.

Aldesleukin was given by 15 min i.v. infusion every 8 hours for up to 5 days (maximum of 14 doses). No treatment was given on days 6 to 14 and then dosing was repeated for up to 5 days on days 15 to 19 (maximum of 14 doses). These 2 cycles constituted 1 course of therapy. Patients could receive a maximum of 28 doses during a course of therapy. In practice >90% of patients had doses withheld. Metastatic RCC patients received a median of 20 of 28 scheduled doses of aldesleukin. Metastatic malignant melanoma patients received a median of 18 of 28 scheduled doses of aldesleukin during the first course of therapy. Doses were withheld for specific toxicities (see Dosage, Dose Modifications and Adverse Effects).

In the renal cell cancer studies (n=255), objective response was seen in 37 (15%) patients, with 17 (7%) complete and 20 (8%) partial responders. The 95% confidence interval for objective response was 11 to 20%. Onset of tumor regression was observed as early as 4 weeks after completion of the first course of treatment, and in some cases, tumor regression continued for up to 12 months after the start of treatment. The median duration of response for all responding patients is 54 months (3 to 131+ months). The median duration for patients with complete responses has not been observed and for patients with partial response was 20 months. Twelve patients who achieved a complete response and 6 patients who achieved a partial response had responses ongoing at the time of last contact. The median progression-free survival for all responding patients was 55 months. Responses were observed in both lung and non-lung sites (e.g., liver, lymph node, renal bed occurrences, and soft tissue). Of the 37 responding patients, 12 patients with individual bulky lesions (largest lesion ≥25 cm²) and 22 patients with large cumulative tumor burden (total ≥25 cm²) achieved responses.

In the metastatic malignant melanoma studies (n=270), objective response was seen in 43 (16%) patients, with 17 (6%) complete and 26 (10%) partial responders. The 95% confidence interval for objective response was 12% to 21%. The median duration of response for all responding patients was 9 months (1 to 122+ months); the median duration of objective complete responses has not been observed and the median duration for partial response was 6 months. Ten patients who achieved a complete response and 3 patients who achieved a partial response had responses ongoing at the time of last contact. The median progression-free survival for the 43 responding patients was 13 months. Responses in metastatic malignant melanoma patients were observed in both visceral and nonvisceral sites (e.g., lung, liver, lymph node, soft tissue, adrenal, subcutaneous). Of the 43 responding patients, 14 patients with individual bulky lesions (largest lesion ≥25 cm²) and 21 patients with large cumulative tumor burden (total ≥25 cm²) achieved responses. See Table 1.

Table 1: Proleukin
Proleukin Clinical Response Data

	Metastatic RCC		Metastatic Malignant Melanoma	
	Number of Responding Patients (response rate)	**Median Response Duration in Months (range)**	**Number of Responding Patients (response rate)**	**Median Response Duration in Months (range)**
CR	17 (7%)	80+[a] (7 to 131+)	17 (6%)	59+[a] (3 to 122+)
PR	20 (8%)	20 (3 to 126+)	26 (10%)	6 (1 to 111+)
PR+CR	37 (15%)	54 (3 to 131+)	43 (16%)	9 (1 to 122+)

[a] Median duration not yet observed; a conservative value is presented which represents the minimum median duration of response.
Legend: (+) sign means ongoing; CR=complete response; PR=partial response.

INDICATIONS: For the treatment of adults (≥18 years of age) with metastatic renal cell carcinoma (metastatic RCC). Aldesleukin is indicated for the treatment of adults (≥18 years of age) with metastatic malignant melanoma.

In the renal cell cancer studies (n=255), objective response was seen in 37 (15%) patients, with 17 (7%) complete and 20 (8%) partial responders. In the metastatic malignant melanoma studies (n=270), objective response was seen in 43 (16%) patients, with 17 (6%) complete and 26 (10%) partial responders. Prior to enrollment into the studies, patients had progression of disease after prior therapies. A majority (96%) of patients had previous surgical resection of their primary lesions, lymph node dissections, or area of relapse.

Careful patient selection is mandatory prior to the administration of aldesleukin. See Contraindications, Warnings and Precautions sections regarding patient screening, including recommended cardiac and pulmonary function tests and laboratory tests.

Evaluation of clinical studies to date reveals that patients with more favorable ECOG performance status (ECOG PS 0) at treatment initiation respond better to aldesleukin, with a higher response rate and lower toxicity (see Adverse Effects). Therefore, selection of patients for treatment should include assessment of performance status. Experience in patients with ECOG PS >1 is limited. See Table 2.

Table 2: Proleukin
Proleukin Clinical Response by ECOG Performance Status (PS)

	Metastatic RCC		Metastatic Malignant Melanoma	
Pretreatment ECOG PS	**CR**	**PR**	**CR**	**PR**
0	14/166 (8%)	16/166 (10%)	14/191 (7%)	22/191 (12%)
≥1	3/89 (3%)	4/89 (4%)	3/79 (4%)	4/79 (5%)

CONTRAINDICATIONS: In patients with a known history of hypersensitivity to interleukin-2 or any component of the aldesleukin formulation.

Aldesleukin is contraindicated in patients with an abnormal thallium stress test or abnormal pulmonary function tests and those with organ allografts. Retreatment with aldesleukin is contraindicated in patients who experienced the following drug related toxicities while receiving an earlier course of therapy: sustained ventricular tachycardia (≥5 beats); cardiac arrhythmias not controlled or unresponsive to management; chest pain with ECG changes, consistent with angina or myocardial infarction; cardiac tamponade; intubation required >72 hours; renal failure requiring dialysis >72 hours; coma or toxic psychosis lasting >48 hours; repetitive or difficult to control seizures; bowel ischemia/perforation; GI bleeding requiring surgery.

WARNINGS: Aldesleukin should be administered only to well informed patients in a hospital setting under the supervision of a qualified physician experienced in the use of anticancer agents. An intensive care facility and specialists skilled in cardiopulmonary or intensive care medicine must be available.

Aldesleukin administration has been associated with capillary leak syndrome (CLS) which is characterized by a loss of vascular tone and extravasation of plasma proteins and fluid into the extravascular space. CLS results in hypotension and reduced organ perfusion, which may be severe and can result in death. CLS may be associated with cardiac arrhythmias (supraventricular and ventricular), angina, myocardial infarction, respiratory insufficiency requiring intubation, gastrointestinal bleeding or infarction, renal insufficiency, edema and mental status changes.

Because of the severe adverse events which generally accompany aldesleukin therapy at the recommended dosages, thorough clinical evaluation should be performed to identify patients with significant cardiac, pulmonary, renal, hepatic, or CNS impairment; aldesleukin is contraindicated in these patients.

Therapy with aldesleukin should be restricted to patients with normal cardiac and pulmonary functions as defined by thallium stress testing and formal pulmonary function testing. Extreme caution should be used in patients with normal thallium stress tests and pulmonary function tests who have a history of prior cardiac or pulmonary disease.

Patients with normal cardiovascular, pulmonary, hepatic and CNS function may experience serious, life threatening or fatal adverse events. Adverse events are frequent, often serious, and sometimes fatal.

Should adverse events, which require dose modification occur, dosage should be withheld rather than reduced (see Dosage, Dose Modifications).

Aldesleukin has been associated with exacerbation of pre-existing or initial presentation of autoimmune disease and inflammatory disorders. Exacerbation of Crohn's disease, scleroderma, thyroiditis, inflammatory arthritis, diabetes mellitus, oculo-bulbar myasthenia gravis, crescentic IgA glomerulonephritis, cholecystitis, cerebral vasculitis, Stevens-Johnson syndrome and bullous pemphigoid, has been reported following treatment with IL-2.

All patients should have thorough evaluation and treatment of CNS metastases and have a negative scan prior to receiving aldesleukin therapy. New neurologic signs, symptoms, and anatomic lesions following aldesleukin therapy have been reported in patients without evidence of CNS metastases. Clinical manifestations included changes in mental status, speech difficulties, cortical blindness, limb or gait ataxia, hallucinations, agitation, obtundation, and coma. Radiological findings included multiple and, less commonly, single cortical lesions on MRI and evidence of demyelination. Neurologic signs and symptoms associated with aldesleukin therapy usually improve after discontinuation of aldesleukin therapy; however, there are reports of permanent neurologic defects. One case of possible cerebral vasculitis, responsive to dexamethasone, has been reported. In patients with known seizure disorders, extreme caution should be exercised as aldesleukin may cause seizures.

Aldesleukin administration should be held in patients developing moderate to severe lethargy or somnolence; continued administration may result in coma.

Aldesleukin treatment is associated with impaired neutrophil function (reduced chemotaxis) and with an increased risk of disseminated infection, including sepsis and bacterial endocarditis. Consequently, pre-existing bacterial infections should be adequately treated prior to initiation of aldesleukin therapy. Patients with indwelling central lines are particularly at risk for infection with gram-positive microorganisms. Antibiotic prophylaxis with oxacillin, nafcillin, ciprofloxacin, or vancomycin has been associated with a reduced incidence of staphylococcal infections. Disseminated infections acquired in the course of aldesleukin treatment are a major contributor to treatment morbidity, and use of antibiotic prophylaxis and aggressive treatment of suspected and documented infections may reduce the morbidity of aldesleukin treatment. Note: Prior to the use of any product mentioned in this paragraph, the physician should refer to the Product Monograph for the respective product.

PRECAUTIONS: General: Patients should have normal cardiac, pulmonary, hepatic, and CNS function at the start of therapy. Metastatic renal cell carcinoma patients who have had a nephrectomy are eligible for treatment if they have serum creatinine levels ≤1.5 mg/dL.

Patients with normal cardiovascular, pulmonary, hepatic, and CNS function may experience serious life threatening or fatal adverse events. Adverse events are frequent, often serious, and sometimes fatal.

Capillary leak syndrome (CLS) begins immediately after aldesleukin treatment starts and is marked by increased capillary permeability to protein and fluids and reduced vascular tone. In most patients, this results in a concomitant drop in mean arterial blood pressure within 2 to 12 hours after the start of treatment. With continued therapy, clinically significant hypotension (defined as systolic blood pressure below 90 mmHg or a 20 mmHg drop from baseline systolic pressure) and hypoperfusion will occur. In addition, extravasation of protein and fluids into the extravascular space will lead to the formation of edema and creation of new effusions.

Medical management of CLS begins with careful monitoring of the patient's fluid and organ perfusion status. This is achieved by frequent determination of blood pressure and pulse, and by monitoring organ function, which includes assessment of mental status and urine output. Hypovolemia is assessed by catheterization and central pressure monitoring.

Flexibility in fluid and pressor management is essential for maintaining organ perfusion and blood pressure. Consequently, extreme caution should be used in treating patients with fixed requirements for large volumes of fluid (e.g., patients with hypercalcemia).

Administration of i.v. fluids, either colloids or crystalloids is recommended for treatment of hypovolemia. I.V. fluids are usually given when the central venous pressure (CVP) is below 3 to 4 mmH_2O. Correction of hypovolemia may require large volumes of i.v. fluids but caution is required because unrestrained fluid administration may exacerbate problems associated with edema formation or effusions.

With extravascular fluid accumulation, edema is common and ascites, pleural or pericardial effusions may develop. Management of these events depends on a careful balancing of the effects of fluid shifts so that neither the consequences of hypovolemia (e.g., impaired organ perfusion) nor the consequences of fluid accumulations (e.g., pulmonary edema) exceeds the patient's tolerance.

Clinical experience has shown that early administration of dopamine (1 to 5 μg/kg/min) to patients manifesting capillary leak syndrome, before the onset of hypotension, can help to maintain organ perfusion particularly to the kidney and thus preserve urine output. Weight and urine output should be carefully monitored. If organ perfusion and blood pressure are not sustained by dopamine therapy, clinical investigators have increased the dose of dopamine to 6 to 10 μg/kg/min or have added phenylephrine HCl (1 to 5 μg/kg/min) to low dose dopamine. Prolonged use of pressors, either in combination or as individual agents, at relatively high doses, may be associated with cardiac rhythm disturbances. If there has been excessive weight gain or edema formation, particularly if associated with shortness of breath from pulmonary congestion, use of diuretics, once blood pressure has normalized, has been shown to hasten recovery. Note: Prior to the use of any product mentioned, the physician should refer to the Product Monograph for the respective product.

Aldesleukin treatment should be withheld for failure to maintain organ perfusion, as demonstrated by altered mental status, reduced urine output, a fall in the systolic blood pressure below 90 mmHg or onset of cardiac arrhythmias (see Dosage, Dose Modifications). Recovery from CLS begins soon after cessation of aldesleukin therapy. Usually, within a few hours, the blood pressure rises, organ perfusion is restored and reabsorption of extravasated fluid and protein begins.

Oxygen is given to the patient if pulmonary function monitoring confirms that PaO_2 is decreased.

Aldesleukin administration may cause anemia and/or thrombocytopenia. Packed red blood cell transfusions have been given both for relief of anemia and to insure maximal oxygen carrying capacity. Platelet transfusions have been given to resolve absolute thrombocytopenia and to reduce the risk of gastrointestinal bleeding. In addition, leukopenia and neutropenia are observed.

Aldesleukin administration results in fever, chills, rigors, pruritus, and gastrointestinal side effects in most patients treated at recommended doses. These side effects have been aggressively managed as described in Adverse Effects.

Kidney and liver function are impaired during aldesleukin treatment. Use of concomitant nephrotoxic or hepatotoxic medications may further increase toxicity to the kidney or liver.

Mental status changes including irritability, confusion, or depression which occur while receiving aldesleukin may be indicators of bacteremia or early bacterial sepsis, hypoperfusion, occult CNS malignancy, or direct aldesleukin-induced CNS toxicity. Alterations in mental status due solely to aldesleukin may progress for several days before recovery begins. Rarely, patients have sustained permanent neurologic deficits (see Adverse Effects).

Exacerbation of preexisting autoimmune disease or initial presentation of autoimmune and inflammatory disorders has been reported following aldesleukin alone or in combination with interferon (see Adverse Effects). Impairment of thyroid function, sometimes preceded by hyperthyroidism, has been reported following aldesleukin treatment. Some of these patients required thyroid replacement therapy. Changes in thyroid function may be a manifestation of autoimmunity. Onset of symptomatic hyperglycemia and/or diabetes mellitus has been reported during aldesleukin therapy.

Aldesleukin enhancement of cellular immune function may increase the risk of allograft rejection in transplant patients.

Laboratory Tests: The following clinical evaluations are recommended for all patients, prior to beginning treatment and then daily during drug administration: standard hematologic tests—including complete blood count (CBC), differential and platelet counts; blood chemistries—including electrolytes, renal and hepatic function tests; and chest x-rays.

Serum creatinine should be ≤1.5 mg/dL prior to initiation of aldesleukin treatment. All patients should have baseline pulmonary function tests with arterial blood gases. Adequate pulmonary function should be documented (FEV_1 >2 L or ≥75% of predicted for height and age) prior to initiating therapy. All patients should be screened with a stress thallium study. Normal ejection fraction and unimpaired wall motion should be documented. If a thallium stress test suggests minor wall motion abnormalities, further testing is suggested to exclude significant coronary artery disease.

Daily monitoring during therapy with aldesleukin should include vital signs (temperature, pulse, blood pressure, and respiration rate), weight, and fluid intake and output. In a patient with a decreased systolic blood pressure, especially less than 90 mmHg, constant cardiac rhythm monitoring should be conducted. If an abnormal complex or rhythm is seen, an ECG should be performed. Vital signs in these hypotensive patients should be taken hourly.

During treatment, pulmonary function should be monitored on a regular basis by clinical examination, assessment of vital signs and pulse oximetry. Patients with dyspnea or clinical signs of respiratory impairment (tachypnea or rales) should be further assessed with arterial blood gas determination. These tests are to be repeated as often as clinically indicated.

Cardiac function should be assessed daily by clinical examination and assessment of vital signs. Patients with signs or symptoms of chest pain, murmurs, gallops, irregular rhythm or palpitations should be further assessed with an ECG examination and cardiac enzyme evaluation. Evidence of myocardial injury, including findings compatible with myocardial infarction or myocarditis, has been reported. Ventricular hypokinesia due to myocarditis may be persistent for several months. If there is evidence of cardiac ischemia or congestive heart failure, aldesleukin therapy should be held, and a repeat thallium study should be done.

Drug Interactions: Aldesleukin may affect central nervous function. Therefore, interactions could occur following concomitant administration of psychotropic drugs (e.g., narcotics, analgesics, antiemetics, sedatives, and tranquilizers).

Concurrent administration of drugs possessing nephrotoxic (e.g., aminoglycosides, indomethacin), myelotoxic (e.g., cytotoxic chemotherapy), cardiotoxic (e.g., doxorubicin) or hepatotoxic (e.g., methotrexate, asparaginase) effects with aldesleukin may increase toxicity in these organ systems. The safety and efficacy of aldesleukin in combination with any antineoplastics have not been established.

In addition, reduced kidney and liver function secondary to aldesleukin treatment may delay elimination of concomitant medications and increase the risk of adverse events from those drugs.

Hypersensitivity reactions have been reported in patients receiving combination regimens containing sequential high dose aldesleukin and antineoplastic agents, specifically, dacarbazine, cis-platinum, tamoxifen and interferon-alfa. These reactions consisted of erythema, pruritus, and hypotension and occurred within hours of administration of chemotherapy. These events required medical intervention in some patients. Myocardial injury, including myocardial infarction, myocarditis, ventricular hypokinesia, and severe rhabdomyolysis appear to be increased in patients receiving aldesleukin and interferon-alfa concurrently.

Exacerbation or the initial presentation of a number of autoimmune and inflammatory disorders has been observed following concur-rent use of interferon-alfa and aldesleukin, including crescentic IgA glomerulonephritis, oculo-bulbar myasthenia gravis, inflammatory arthritis, thyroiditis, bullous pemphigoid, and Stevens-Johnson syndrome.

Although glucocorticoids have been shown to reduce aldesleukin-induced side effects including fever, renal insufficiency, hyperbilirubinemia, confusion, and dyspnea, concomitant administration of these agents with aldesleukin may reduce the antitumor effectiveness of aldesleukin and thus should be avoided.

Beta-blockers and other antihypertensives may potentiate the hypotension seen with aldesleukin.

Delayed adverse reactions to iodinated contrast media: A review of the literature revealed that 12.6% (range 11 to 28%) of 501 patients treated with various interleukin-2 containing regimens who were then subsequently administered radiographic iodinated contrast media experienced acute, atypical adverse reactions. The onset of symptoms usually occurred within hours (most commonly 1 to 4 hours) following the administration of contrast media. These reactions include fever, chills, nausea, vomiting, pruritus, rash, diarrhea, hypotension, edema and oliguria. Some clinicians have noted that these reactions resemble the immediate side effects caused by interleukin-2 administration, however the cause of contrast reactions after interleukin-2 therapy is unknown. Most events were reported to occur when contrast media was given within 4 weeks after the last dose of interleukin-2. These events were also reported to occur when contrast media was given several months after interleukin-2 treatment.

Carcinogenesis, Mutagenesis, Impairment of Fertility: There have been no studies conducted assessing the carcinogenic or mutagenic potential of aldesleukin.

There have been no studies conducted assessing the effect of aldesleukin on fertility. It is recommended that this drug not be administered to fertile persons of either gender not practicing effective contraception.

Pregnancy: Aldesleukin has been shown to have embryolethal effects in rats when given in doses at 27 to 36 times the human dose (scaled by body weight). Significant maternal toxicities were observed in pregnant rats administered aldesleukin by i.v. injection at doses 2.1 to 36 times higher than the human dose during critical period of organogenesis. No evidence of teratogenicity was observed other than that attributed to maternal toxicity. There are no adequate well-controlled studies of aldesleukin in pregnant women. Aldesleukin should be used during pregnancy only if the potential benefit justifies the potential risk to the fetus.

Lactation: It is not known whether this drug is excreted in human milk. Because many drugs are excreted in human milk and because of the potential for serious adverse reactions in nursing infants from aldesleukin, a decision should be made whether to discontinue nursing or to discontinue the drug, taking into account the importance of the drug to the mother.

Children: Safety and effectiveness in children under 18 years of age have not been established.

ADVERSE EFFECTS: The rate of drug-related deaths in the 255 metastatic RCC patients who received single-agent aldesleukin was 4% (11/255); the rate of drug-related deaths in the 270 metastatic malignant melanoma patients who received single-agent aldesleukin was 2% (6/270).

The following data on common adverse events (reported in greater than 10% of patients, any grade), presented by body system, decreasing frequency and by preferred term (COSTART) are based on 525 patients (255 with renal cell cancer and 270 with metastatic malignant melanoma) treated with the recommended infusion dosing regimen. See Table 3.

Table 3: Proleukin

Adverse Events Occurring in ≥10% of Patients (n=525)

Body System	% of Patients
Body as a Whole	
Chills	52
Fever	29
Malaise	27
Asthenia	23
Infection	13
Pain	12
Abdominal pain	11
Abdomen enlarged	10
Cardiovascular	
Hypotension	71
Tachycardia	23
Vasodilation	13
Supraventricular tachycardia	12
Cardiovascular disorder[a]	11
Arrhythmia	10
Digestive	
Diarrhea	67
Vomiting	50

(cont'd)

Table 3: Proleukin *(cont'd)*

Adverse Events Occurring in ≥10% of Patients (n=525)

Body System	**% of Patients**
Nausea	35
Stomatitis	22
Anorexia	20
Nausea and vomiting	19
Hemic and Lymphatic	
Thrombocytopenia	37
Anemia	29
Leukopenia	16
Metabolic and Nutritional Disorders	
Bilirubinemia	40
Creatinine increased	33
Peripheral edema	28
AST increased	23
Weight gain	16
Edema	15
Acidosis	12
Hypomagnesemia	12
Hypocalcemia	11
Alkaline phosphatase increased	10
Nervous	
Confusion	34
Somnolence	22
Anxiety	12
Dizziness	11
Respiratory	
Dyspnea	43
Lung disorder[b]	24
Respiratory disorder[c]	11
Cough increase	11
Rhinitis	10
Skin and Appendages	
Rash	42
Pruritus	24
Exfoliative dermatitis	18
Urogenital	
Oliguria	63

[a] Cardiovascular disorder: fluctuations in blood pressure, asymptomatic ECG changes, CHF.
[b] Lung disorder: physical findings associated with pulmonary congestion, rales, and rhonchi.
[c] Respiratory disorder: ARDS, CXR infiltrates, unspecified pulmonary changes.

The following data on life-threatening adverse events (reported in greater than 1% of patients, grade 4), presented by body system, and by preferred term (COSTART) are based on 525 patients (255 with renal cell cancer and 270 with metastatic malignant melanoma) treated with the recommended infusion dosing regimen. See Table 4.

Table 4: Proleukin

Life-threatening (Grade 4) Adverse Events (n=525)

Body System	**# (%) of Patients**
Body as a Whole	
Fever	5 (1%)
Infection	7 (1%)
Sepsis	6 (1%)
Cardiovascular	

(cont'd)

Table 4: Proleukin *(cont'd)*

Life-threatening (Grade 4) Adverse Events (n=525)

Body System	**# (%) of Patients**
Hypotension	15 (3%)
Supraventricular tachycardia	3 (1%)
Cardiovascular disorder[a]	7 (1%)
Myocardial infarct	7 (1%)
Ventricular tachycardia	5 (1%)
Heart arrest	4 (1%)
Digestive	
Diarrhea	10 (2%)
Vomiting	7 (1%)
Hemic and Lymphatic	
Thrombocytopenia	5 (1%)
Coagulation disorder[b]	4 (1%)
Metabolic and Nutritional Disorders	
Bilirubinemia	13 (2%)
Creatinine increased	5 (1%)
AST increased	3 (1%)
Acidosis	4 (1%)
Nervous	
Confusion	5 (1%)
Stupor	3 (1%)
Coma	8 (2%)
Psychosis	7 (1%)
Respiratory	
Dyspnea	5 (1%)
Respiratory disorder[c]	14 (3%)
Apnea	5 (1%)
Urogenital	
Oliguria	33 (6%)
Anuria	25 (5%)
Acute kidney failure	3 (1%)

[a] Cardiovascular disorder: fluctuations in blood pressure.
[b] Coagulation disorder: intravascular coagulopathy.
[c] Respiratory disorder: ARDS, respiratory failure, intubation.

The following life-threatening (grade 4) adverse events were reported by <1% of the 525 patients: reaction unevaluable, hypothermia, shock, bradycardia, ventricular extrasystoles, myocardial ischemia, syncope, hemorrhage, atrial arrhythmia, phlebitis, AV block 2nd degree, endocarditis, pericardial effusion, peripheral gangrene, thrombosis, coronary artery disorder, stomatitis, nausea and vomiting, liver function tests abnormal, gastrointestinal hemorrhage, hematemesis, bloody diarrhea, gastrointestinal disorder, intestinal perforation, pancreatitis, anemia, leukopenia, leukocytosis, hypocalcemia, alkaline phosphatase increased, BUN increased, hyperuricemia, NPN increase, respiratory acidosis, somnolence, agitation, neuropathy, paranoid reaction, convulsion, grand mal convulsion, delirium, lung edema, hyperventilation, hypoxia, hemoptysis, hypoventilation, pneumothorax, mydriasis, pupillary disorder, kidney function abnormal, kidney failure, acute tubular necrosis.

In an additional population of greater than 1800 patients treated with aldesleukin-based regimens using a variety of doses and schedules (e.g., s.c., continuous infusion, administration with LAK cells), the following serious adverse events were reported: duodenal ulceration, bowel necrosis, myocarditis, supraventricular tachycardia, permanent or transient blindness secondary to optic neuritis, transient ischemic attacks, meningitis, cerebral edema, pericarditis, allergic interstitial nephritis, tracheo-esophageal fistula.

In the same clinical population, the following events which were fatal or resulted in death each occurred with a frequency of <1%: liver or renal failure; intestinal perforation, cardiac arrest, myocardial infarction, malignant hyperthermia, pulmonary edema, respiratory arrest, respiratory failure, stroke, pulmonary emboli, severe depression leading to suicide.

Postmarketing Experience: The reactions reported in the post market setting are reported voluntarily from a population of uncertain size, therefore it is not always possible to reliably estimate their frequency or establish a causal relationship to drug exposure.

In world-wide post approval experience, the following serious adverse events have been reported in a variety of treatment regimens that include interleukin-2: hypertension, pneumonia (bacterial, fungal, viral), neutropenia, cholecystitis, colitis, gastritis, hepatitis, hepatosplenomegaly, intestinal obstruction, retroperitoneal hemorrhage, cerebral lesions, intracranial/cerebral hemorrhage, encephalopathy, extrapyramidal syndrome, neuralgia, neuritis, neuropathy (demyelination), rhabdomyolysis, myopathy, myositis, hyperthyroidism, anaphylaxis, cellulitis, injection site necrosis, insomnia, neutropenic fever, leukoencephalopathy, cardiac arrest, pericardial effusion, cardiac tamponade, gastrointestinal perforation including necrosis/gangrene, cardiomyopathy, fatal endocarditis, hypothyroidism and urticaria.

There have been rare reports of leukoencephalopathy associated with interleukin-2 in the literature, mostly in patients treated for HIV infection. The role of interleukin-2 in elucidating this event remains uncertain. However opportunistic infections, co-administration of interferons as well as multiple courses of chemotherapy are other factors that may pre-dispose the treated population to such event. Proleukin should not be used in the HIV indication.

Exacerbation or initial presentations of a number of autoimmune and inflammatory disorders have been reported (see Warnings). Persistent but non-progressive vitiligo has been observed in metastatic malignant melanoma patients treated with interleukin-2. Synergistic, additive and novel toxicities have been reported with aldesleukin used in combination with other drugs. Novel toxicities include delayed adverse reactions to iodinated contrast media and hypersensitivity reactions to antineoplastic agents (see Precautions).

Experience has shown the following concomitant medications to be useful in the management of patients on aldesleukin therapy: a) standard antipyretic therapy, including NSAIDs, started immediately prior to aldesleukin to reduce fever. Renal function should be monitored as some NSAIDs may cause synergistic nephrotoxicity; b) meperidine used to control the rigors associated with fever; c) H_2 antagonists given for prophylaxis of gastrointestinal irritation and bleeding; d) antiemetics and antidiarrheals used as needed to treat other gastrointestinal side effects. Generally these medications were discontinued 12 hours after the last dose of aldesleukin.

Patients with in-dwelling central lines have a higher risk of infection with gram-positive organisms. A reduced incidence of staphylococcal infections in aldesleukin studies has been associated with the use of antibiotic prophylaxis which includes the use of oxacillin, nafcillin, ciprofloxacin, or vancomycin. Hydroxyzine or diphenhydramine have been used to control symptoms from pruritic rashes and continued until resolution of pruritus. Topical creams and ointments should be applied as needed for skin manifestations. Preparations containing a steroid (e.g., hydrocortisone) should be avoided. Note: Prior to the use of any product mentioned, the physician should refer to the Product Monograph for the respective product.

OVERDOSE:

Symptoms: Side effects following the use of aldesleukin appear to be dose-related. Exceeding the recommended dose has been associated with a more rapid onset of expected dose-limiting toxicities.

Treatment: Symptoms which persist after cessation of aldesleukin should be monitored and treated supportively. Life-threatening toxicities may be ameliorated by the i.v. administration of dexamethasone, which may result in loss of the therapeutic effects of aldesleukin. Note: Prior to the use of dexamethasone, the physician should refer to the Product Monograph for this product.

For management of a suspected drug overdose, CPhA recommends that you contact your **regional Poison Control Centre**. See the *CPS* Directory section for a list of Poison Control Centres.

DOSAGE: The recommended aldesleukin treatment regimen is administered by a 15-minute i.v. infusion every 8 hours. Before initiating treatment, carefully review the Indications, Contraindications, Warnings, Precautions and Adverse Effects, particularly regarding patient selection, possible serious adverse events, patient monitoring and withholding dosage.

The following schedule has been used to treat adult patients with metastatic renal cell carcinoma (metastatic RCC) or metastatic malignant melanoma. Each course of treatment consists of two 5-day treatment cycles separated by a rest period.

600 000 IU/kg (0.037 mg/kg) dose administered every 8 hours by a 15-minute i.v. infusion for a maximum of 14 doses. Following 9 days of rest, the schedule is repeated for another 14 doses, for a maximum of 28 doses per course, as tolerated. During clinical trials, doses were frequently withheld for toxicity (see Pharmacology, Clinical Experience Dosage, Dose Modifications). Metastatic RCC patients treated with this schedule received a median of 20 of the 28 doses during the first course of therapy. Metastatic malignant melanoma patients received a median of 18 doses during the first course of therapy.

Retreatment: Patients should be evaluated for response approximately 4 weeks after completion of a course of therapy and again immediately prior to the scheduled start of the next treatment course. Additional courses of treatment should be given to patients only if there is some tumor shrinkage following the last course and retreatment is not contraindicated (see Contraindications). Each treatment course should be separated by a rest period of at least 7 weeks from the date of hospital discharge.

Dose Modifications: Dose modification for toxicity should be accomplished by withholding or interrupting a dose rather than reducing the dose to be given. Decisions to stop, hold, or restart aldesleukin therapy must be made after a global assessment of the patient. With this in mind, the following guidelines should be used:

Retreatment with aldesleukin is contraindicated in patients who experience the following toxicities: See Table 5.

Table 5: Proleukin

Toxicities for Which Retreatment is Contraindicated

Body System	Toxicity
Cardiovascular	Sustained ventricular tachycardia (≥5 beats) Cardiac rhythm disturbances not controlled or unresponsive to management Chest pain with ECG changes, consistent with angina or myocardial infarction Cardiac tamponade
Respiratory	Intubation for >72 hours
Urogenital	Renal failure requiring dialysis >72 hours
Nervous	Coma or toxic psychosis lasting >48 hours Repetitive or difficult to control seizures
Digestive	Bowel ischemia/perforation Gastrointestinal bleeding requiring surgery

Doses should be held and restarted according to the following: See Table 6.

Stability and Storage Recommendations: Store vials of lyophilized aldesleukin in a refrigerator at 2 to 8°C. Avoid exposure to heat and light.

Reconstituted or diluted aldesleukin is stable for up to 48 hours at refrigerated and room temperatures, 2 to 25°C. However, since this product contains no preservatives, the reconstituted and diluted solutions should be stored in the refrigerator.

Table 6: Proleukin

Toxicities for Which Doses Should Be Held and Restarted

Body System	Hold Dose For	Subsequent Doses May Be Given If
Cardiovascular	Atrial fibrillation, supraventricular tachycardia, or bradycardia that requires treatment or is recurrent or persistent Systolic bp ≥90 mmHg and stable or improving requirements for pressors Any ECG change consistent with MI, ischemia or myocarditis with or without chest pain; suspicion of cardiac ischemia	Patient is asymptomatic with full recovery to normal sinus rhythm Systolic bp <90 mmHg with increasing requirements for pressors Patient is asymptomatic, MI and myocarditis have been ruled out, clinical suspicion of angina is low; there is no evidence of ventricular hypokinesia
Respiratory	O_2 saturation <94% on room air or <90% with 2 L O_2 by nasal prongs	O_2 saturation >94% on room air or >90% with 2 L O_2 by nasal prongs
Nervous	Mental status changes, including moderate confusion or agitation	Mental status changes completely resolved
Body as a Whole	Sepsis syndrome, patient is clinically unstable	Sepsis syndrome has resolved, patient is clinically stable, infection is under treatment
Urogenital	Serum creatinine >4.5 mg/dL or a serum creatinine of ≥4 mg/dL in the presence of severe volume overload, acidosis, or hyperkalemia Persistent oliguria, urine output of <10 mL/h for 16 to 24 hours with rising serum creatinine	Serum creatinine <4 mg/dL and fluid and electrolyte status is stable Urine output >10 mL/h with a decrease of serum creatinine >1.5 mg/dL or normalization of serum creatinine

(cont'd)

Table 6: Proleukin *(cont'd)*

Toxicities for Which Doses Should Be Held and Restarted

Body System	Hold Dose For	Subsequent Doses May Be Given If
Digestive	Signs of hepatic failure including encephalopathy, increasing ascites, liver pain, hypoglycemia	All signs of hepatic failure have resolved[a]
	Stool guaiac repeatedly >3-4+	Stool guaiac negative
Skin	Bullous dermatitis or marked worsening of pre-existing skin condition, avoid topical steroid therapy	Resolution of all signs of bullous dermatitis

[a] Discontinue all further treatment for that course. A new course of treatment, if warranted, should be initiated no sooner than 7 weeks after cessation of adverse event and hospital discharge.

Do not use beyond the expiration date printed on the vial. Note: This product contains no preservative.

Reconstitution: Reconstitution and dilution procedures other than those recommended may alter the delivery and/or pharmacology of aldesleukin and thus should be avoided.

1. Proleukin is a sterile, white to off-white preservative-free, lyophilized powder suitable for i.v. infusion upon reconstitution and dilution. **Each vial contains 22 million IU (1.3 mg) of aldesleukin and should be reconstituted aseptically with 1.2 mL of Sterile Water for Injection, USP. When reconstituted as directed, each mL contains 18 million IU (1.1 mg) of aldesleukin.** The resulting solution should be a clear, colorless to slightly yellow liquid. The vial is for single-use only and any unused portion should be discarded.
2. During reconstitution the Sterile Water for Injection, USP should be directed at the side of the vial and the contents gently swirled to avoid excess foaming. **Do not shake.**
3. The dose of aldesleukin, reconstituted in Sterile Water for Injection, USP (without preservative) should be diluted aseptically in 50 mL of 5% Dextrose Injection, USP and infused over a 15-minute period.

In cases where the total dose of Proleukin is 1.5 mg or less (e.g., a patient with a body weight of less than 40 kg), the dose of Proleukin should be diluted in a smaller volume of D5W.

Concentrations of Proleukin below 30 µg/mL and above 70 µg/mL have shown increased variability in drug delivery. Dilution and delivery of Proleukin outside of this concentration range should be avoided.

4. Glass bottles and plastic (polyvinyl chloride) bags have been used in clinical trials with comparable results; it is recommended that plastic bags be used as the dilution container since experimental studies suggest that use of plastic containers results in more consistent drug delivery. **In-line filters should not be used when administering aldesleukin.**
5. Before and after reconstitution and dilution, store in a refrigerator at 2 to 8°C. Do not freeze. Administer Proleukin within 48 hours of reconstitution. The solution should be brought to room temperature prior to infusion in the patient.
6. Reconstitution or dilution with Bacteriostatic Water for Injection, USP, or 0.9% Sodium Chloride Injection, USP should be avoided because of increased aggregation. Proleukin should not be coadministered with other drugs in the same container.
7. Parenteral drug products should be inspected visually for particulate matter and discoloration prior to administration, whenever solution and container permit.

SUPPLIED: When reconstituted with 1.2 mL Sterile Water for Injection, USP, each mL contains: aldesleukin 18 million IU (1.1 mg), mannitol 50 mg and sodium dodecyl sulfate 0.18 mg, buffered with approximately 0.17 mg monobasic sodium phosphate and 0.89 mg dibasic sodium phosphate to a pH of 7.5 (range 7.2 to 7.8). Preservative-free. Single-use vials of 22 million IU (1.3 mg). Discard unused portion. Before and after reconstitution and dilution, store in a refrigerator at 2 to 8°C.

Prolia™ Ⓟ

denosumab

RANK Ligand Inhibitor—Bone Metabolism Regulator

Amgen

Date of Preparation: August 6, 2010

SUMMARY PRODUCT INFORMATION:

Route of Administration	Dosage Form/ Strength	Clinically Relevant Nonmedicinal Ingredients
Subcutaneous	Solution for injection/ 60 mg denosumab in 1 mL solution in a single use prefilled syringe	Single use prefilled syringe: sorbitol, acetate, polysorbate 20, water for injection (USP) and sodium hydroxide For a complete listing see Dosage Forms, Composition and Packaging.

DESCRIPTION: PROLIA (denosumab) is a human IgG2 monoclonal antibody with affinity and specificity for human RANK ligand (RANKL) that inhibits RANKL from activating its receptor, RANK, on the surface of osteoclasts and their precursors. Prevention of RANKL-RANK interaction inhibits osteoclast formation, function and survival, thereby decreasing bone resorption. Denosumab has an approximate molecular weight of 147 kDa and is produced in genetically engineered mammalian (Chinese Hamster Ovary) cells.

PROLIA is supplied as a single use, sterile, preservative-free, clear, colourless to slightly yellow solution formulated at pH 5.2. PROLIA is supplied in a 60 mg/mL prefilled syringe (PFS) with a 1.0 mL volume intended for delivery by subcutaneous injection.

INDICATIONS AND CLINICAL USE: Postmenopausal Osteoporosis: PROLIA (denosumab) is indicated for the treatment of postmenopausal women with osteoporosis at high risk for fracture, defined as a history of osteoporotic fracture, or multiple risk factors for fracture; or patients who have failed or are intolerant to other available osteoporosis therapy. In postmenopausal women with osteoporosis, PROLIA reduces the incidence of vertebral, nonvertebral and hip fractures.

Geriatrics (≥65 years of age): The majority of patients treated with PROLIA in the PMO clinical trial were 65 years and over (see Warnings and Precautions, Special Populations, Geriatrics (≥65 years of age)).

Pediatrics: The safety and efficacy of PROLIA have not been studied in pediatric populations. PROLIA is not indicated for use in pediatric patients (see Warnings and Precautions, Special Populations, Pediatrics).

CONTRAINDICATIONS:

- Patients who are hypersensitive to the drug or any component of the product. For a complete listing, see Dosage Forms, Composition and Packaging.
- Hypocalcemia

WARNINGS AND PRECAUTIONS: General: Adequate intake of calcium and vitamin D is important in all patients.

Endocrine and Metabolism: Hypocalcemia: Hypocalcemia must be corrected by adequate intake of calcium and vitamin D prior to initiating therapy with PROLIA. Other disorders affecting mineral metabolism (such as vitamin D deficiency) should be treated. In patients predisposed to hypocalcemia (eg, history of hypoparathyroidism, thyroid surgery, parathyroid surgery, malabsorption syndromes, excision of small intestine, severe renal impairment [creatinine clearance <30 mL/min] or receiving dialysis), clinical monitoring of calcium levels is recommended (see Monitoring and Laboratory Tests). Patients should be advised to report to their physicians any symptoms of hypocalcemia, such as paresthesias or muscle spasms (see Adverse Reactions, Hypocalcemia).

Infections: In a 3-year clinical trial in women with postmenopausal osteoporosis, serious infections leading to hospitalization were reported more frequently in the PROLIA group (4.1%) than in the placebo group (3.4%). Skin infections leading to hospitalization were reported more frequently in the PROLIA (0.4%) versus the placebo (<0.1%) groups. These cases were predominantly cellulitis. As well, infections of the abdomen, urinary tract, and ear, were more frequent in patients treated with PROLIA. Endocarditis was also reported more frequently in PROLIA-treated patients (<0.1% PROLIA group; 0% placebo group). The incidence of opportunistic infections was balanced between PROLIA and placebo groups and the overall incidence of skin infections was similar between the PROLIA (1.5%) and placebo (1.2%) groups. Patients should be advised to seek prompt medical attention if they develop signs or symptoms of severe infection, including cellulitis and erysipelas (see Adverse Reactions, Infections).

Patients on concomitant immunosuppressant agents or with impaired immune systems may be at increased risk for serious infections. Consider the benefit-risk profile in such patients before treating with PROLIA. In patients who develop serious infections while on PROLIA, prescribers should assess the need for continued PROLIA therapy.

Dermatologic: In a large, 3-year clinical trial of over 7800 women with postmenopausal osteoporosis, epidermal and dermal adverse events such as dermatitis, eczema, and rashes occurred at a significantly higher rate in the PROLIA (10.8%) group compared to the placebo (8.2%) group. Most of these events were not specific to the injection site. Consider discontinuing PROLIA if severe symptoms develop (see Adverse Reactions, Dermatologic).

Osteonecrosis of the Jaw (ONJ): Osteonecrosis of the jaw (ONJ) has been reported in patients treated with denosumab or bisphosphonates, another class of anti-resorptive agents. Most cases have been in cancer patients; however some have occurred in patients with osteoporosis. ONJ has been reported in clinical studies in patients receiving denosumab at a dose of 60 mg every 6 months for osteoporosis. There have been reports of ONJ in clinical studies in patients with advanced cancer treated with denosumab at the studied dose of 120 mg administered every 4 weeks.

Known risk factors for ONJ include a diagnosis of cancer with bone lesions, concomitant therapies (eg, chemotherapy, antiangiogenic biologics, corticosteroids, radiotherapy to head and neck), poor oral hygiene, dental extractions, and co-morbid disorders (eg, pre-existing dental disease, anemia, coagulopathy, infection).

A dental examination with appropriate preventative dentistry should be considered prior to treatment with PROLIA in patients with risk factors for ONJ such as invasive dental procedures (eg, tooth extraction, dental implants, oral surgery), diagnosis of cancer, concomitant therapies (eg, chemotherapy, corticosteroids) poor oral hygiene, and co-morbid disorders (eg, periodontal and/or other pre-existing dental disease, anemia, coagulopathy, infection, ill-fitting dentures).

Good oral hygiene practices should be maintained during treatment with PROLIA. If ONJ occurs during treatment with PROLIA, use clinical judgment and guide the management plan of each patient based on individual benefit/risk evaluation (see Adverse Reactions, Osteonecrosis of the Jaw (ONJ).

Suppression of Bone Turnover: In clinical trials in women with postmenopausal osteoporosis, treatment with PROLIA resulted in significant suppression of bone remodeling as evidenced by markers of bone turnover and bone histomorphometry. The significance of these findings and the effect of long-term treatment with PROLIA are unknown. Monitor patients for osteonecrosis of the jaw, atypical fractures, and delayed fracture healing (see Adverse Reactions, Fracture Healing, Osteonecrosis of the Jaw (ONJ); Action and Clinical Pharmacology, Pharmacodynamics).

Malignancies: See Adverse Reactions, Clinical Trial Adverse Drug Reactions.

Special Populations: Pregnant Women: There have been no studies in pregnant women.

PROLIA is indicated only for women who are postmenopausal (see also Pediatrics) and is not recommended for women who could become pregnant. Women who become pregnant during PROLIA treatment are encouraged to enrol in Amgen's Pregnancy Surveillance Program. Patients or their physicians should call 1-866-51-AMGEN (1-866-512-6436) to enrol.

Developmental toxicity studies have been performed in cynomolgus monkeys at AUC exposures of up to 100-fold higher than the human exposure. No evidence of impaired fertility or harm to the fetus was observed. Studies in mice suggest that absence of RANKL could interfere with the development of lymph nodes in the fetus and may impair postnatal dentition and bone growth.

Studies in mice suggest absence of RANKL during pregnancy may interfere with maturation of the mammary gland leading to impaired lactation postpartum.

Nursing Women: PROLIA is not recommended for use in nursing women (see also Pediatrics). It is not known whether PROLIA is excreted into human milk. Because PROLIA has the potential to cause adverse reactions in nursing infants, a decision should be made whether to discontinue nursing or discontinue the drug.

Pediatrics: The safety and effectiveness of PROLIA in pediatric patients have not been studied.

PROLIA is not recommended in pediatric patients. Adolescent primates (cynomolgus monkeys) dosed with denosumab at 27 and 150 times (10 and 50 mg/kg dose) the clinical exposure based on AUC had abnormal growth plates. In neonatal rats, inhibition of RANKL (target of denosumab therapy) with a construct of osteoprotegerin bound to Fc (OPG-Fc) at high doses was associated with inhibition of bone growth and tooth eruption. Therefore, treatment with PROLIA may inhibit bone growth in children with open growth plates and may inhibit eruption of dentition.

Geriatrics (≥65 years of age): In the PMO clinical trial, 94.7% of the patients who received PROLIA were 65 years and over and 31.6% were 75 years and over. No overall differences in safety or efficacy were observed between patients 65 years and older and patients 75 years and older. Other reported clinical experience has not identified differences in responses between the elderly and younger patients, but greater sensitivity of some older individuals cannot be ruled out.

Renal Impairment: In a study of 55 patients with varying degrees of renal function, including patients on dialysis, the degree of renal impairment had no effect on the pharmacokinetics of denosumab; thus, dose adjustment for renal impairment is not necessary.

In clinical studies, patients with severe renal impairment (creatinine clearance <30 mL/min) or receiving dialysis were at greater risk of developing hypocalcemia. Adequate intake of calcium and vitamin D is important in patients with severe renal impairment or receiving dialysis (see Warnings and Precautions, Endocrine and Metabolism, Hypocalcemia).

Hepatic Impairment: The safety and efficacy of PROLIA have not been studied in patients with hepatic impairment.

Monitoring and Laboratory Tests: In patients with a history of hypocalcemia, or signs and symptoms of hypocalcemia or predisposed to hypocalcemia (eg, history of hypoparathyroidism, thyroid surgery, parathyroid surgery, malabsorption syndromes, excision of small intestine, severe renal impairment [creatinine clearance <30 mL/min] or receiving dialysis), clinical monitoring of calcium levels is recommended (see Warnings and Precautions, Renal Impairment).

Information to Be Provided to the Patient: Patients must be adequately supplemented with calcium and vitamin D. All patients should be instructed on the importance of calcium and vitamin D supplementation in maintaining serum calcium levels. Patients should be advised to seek prompt medical attention if they develop signs or symptoms of hypocalcemia (eg, paresthesias or muscle spasms) (see Information for the Patient).

Patients should be advised to seek prompt medical attention if they develop signs or symptoms of cellulitis.

Patients should be aware of the most commonly associated side effects of PROLIA therapy.

If a dose of PROLIA is missed, the injection should be administered as soon as convenient. Thereafter, injections should be scheduled every 6 months from the date of the last injection.

Latex Sensitivity Allergies: The patient or caregiver should be informed that the needle cap on the single use prefilled syringe contains dry natural rubber (a derivative of latex), which should not be handled by persons with a known sensitivity to latex.

ADVERSE REACTIONS: Adverse Drug Reaction Overview: A total of 8091 women (4050 PROLIA vs. 4041 placebo) were enrolled in placebo-controlled studies of women with postmenopausal osteoporosis or low bone mass (Study 1 and Study 2).

Clinical Trial Adverse Drug Reactions: Because clinical trials are conducted under very specific conditions, the adverse reaction rates observed in the clinical trials may not reflect the rates observed in practice and should not be compared to the rates in the clinical trials of another drug. Adverse drug reaction information from clinical trials is useful for identifying drug-related adverse events and for approximating rates.

Treatment of Postmenopausal Osteoporosis: The safety of PROLIA was assessed in clinical studies of up to 5 years in duration.

The safety of PROLIA in the treatment of postmenopausal osteoporosis was assessed in a large, 3-year, randomized, double-blind, placebo-controlled, multinational study of 7808 postmenopausal women aged 60 to 91 years with osteoporosis (Study 1). A total of 3886 women received placebo and 3876 women received PROLIA administered once every 6 months as a single 60 mg subcutaneous (SC) dose. All women received calcium (at least 1000 mg) and vitamin D (at least 400 IU) supplementation per day. The incidence of adverse events was 93% in both treatment groups (n=3605 in the PROLIA group and 3607 in the placebo group). The 3 most common adverse events overall were back pain (1347 [34.7%] PROLIA, 1340 [34.6%] placebo), arthralgia (784 [20.2%] PROLIA, 782 [20.2%] placebo), and hypertension (614 [15.8%] PROLIA, 636 [16.4%] placebo). The most common adverse events (>5% and more common than placebo) were back pain (1347 [34.7%] PROLIA, 1340 [34.6%] placebo), pain in extremity (453 [11.7%] PROLIA, 430 [11.1%] placebo), hypercholesterolemia (280 [7.2%] PROLIA, 236 [6.1%] placebo), musculoskeletal pain (297 [7.6%] PROLIA, 291 [7.5%] placebo) and cystitis (228 [5.9%] PROLIA, 225 [5.8%] placebo). The incidence of serious adverse events was 25.8% (n=1004) in the PROLIA group and 25.1% (n=972) in the placebo group. The 3 most common serious adverse events were osteoarthritis (63 [1.6%] PROLIA, 79 [2.0%] placebo), atrial fibrillation (36 [0.9%] PROLIA, 33 [0.9%] placebo), and pneumonia (34 [0.9%] PROLIA, 36 [0.9%] placebo). Deaths occurred in 70 subjects (1.8%) in the denosumab group and 90 subjects (2.3%) in the placebo group. Adverse events leading to treatment discontinuation occurred in 192 (4.9%) women in the PROLIA group and 202 (5.2%) women in the placebo group. The 3 most common adverse events leading to treatment discontinuation were breast cancer (including patients with a history of breast cancer) (20 [0.5%] PROLIA, 10 [0.3%] placebo), back pain (6 [0.2%] PROLIA, 10 [0.3%] placebo), and constipation (6 [0.2%] PROLIA, 6 [0.2%] placebo). Cardiac disorders leading to discontinuation were reported in 14 patients (0.4%) in the PROLIA group and 3 patients (<0.1%) in the placebo group.

Adverse events reported in ≥1% of postmenopausal women with osteoporosis are shown in Table 1.

Table 1: PROLIA

Adverse Events Occurring in ≥1% of Patients with Postmenopausal Osteoporosis

System Organ Class Preferred Term	PROLIA (N=3886) n (%)	Placebo (N=3876) n (%)
Blood and Lymphatic System Disorders		
Anemia	129 (3.3)	107 (2.8)
Cardiac Disorders		
Angina pectoris	101 (2.6)	87 (2.2)
Atrial fibrillation	79 (2.0)	77 (2.0)
Palpitations	59 (1.5)	59 (1.5)
Cardiac failure	53 (1.4)	38 (1.0)
Arrhythmia	41 (1.1)	41 (1.1)
Ear and Labyrinth Disorders		
Vertigo	195 (5.0)	187 (4.8)
Tinnitus	35 (0.9)	55 (1.4)
Endocrine Disorders		
Hypothyroidism	62 (1.6)	59 (1.5)
Eye Disorders		
Cataract	229 (5.9)	253 (6.5)
Glaucoma	59 (1.5)	64 (1.7)
Conjunctivitis	48 (1.2)	59 (1.5)
Gastrointestinal Disorders		
Constipation	355 (9.1)	361 (9.3)
Diarrhea	228 (5.9)	236 (6.1)
Dyspepsia	178 (4.6)	212 (5.5)
Nausea	178 (4.6)	193 (5.0)
Abdominal pain	146 (3.8)	149 (3.8)
Abdominal pain upper	129 (3.3)	111 (2.9)
Gastritis	99 (2.5)	109 (2.8)
Vomiting	91 (2.3)	93 (2.4)
Flatulence	84 (2.2)	53 (1.4)
Gastroesophageal reflux disease	80 (2.1)	66 (1.7)
Hemorrhoids	55 (1.4)	50 (1.3)
Hiatus hernia	49 (1.3)	56 (1.4)
General Disorders and Administration Site Conditions		
Edema peripheral	189 (4.9)	155 (4.0)
Fatigue	115 (3.0)	127 (3.3)
Asthenia	90 (2.3)	73 (1.9)
Noncardiac chest pain	84 (2.2)	90 (2.3)
Pain	47 (1.2)	55 (1.4)
Pyrexia	45 (1.2)	40 (1.0)
Hepatobiliary Disorders		
Cholelithiasis	52 (1.3)	69 (1.8)
Infections and Infestations		
Nasopharyngitis	563 (14.5)	600 (15.5)
Influenza	331 (8.5)	335 (8.6)
Bronchitis	301 (7.7)	301 (7.8)
Urinary tract infection	245 (6.3)	253 (6.5)
Cystitis	228 (5.9)	225 (5.8)
Upper respiratory tract infection	190 (4.9)	167 (4.3)
Pneumonia	152 (3.9)	150 (3.9)

(cont'd)

Table 1: PROLIA *(cont'd)*

Adverse Events Occurring in ≥1% of Patients with Postmenopausal Osteoporosis

System Organ Class Preferred Term	PROLIA (N=3886) n (%)	Placebo (N=3876) n (%)
Sinusitis	101 (2.6)	121 (3.1)
Pharyngitis	91 (2.3)	78 (2.0)
Gastroenteritis	81 (2.1)	94 (2.4)
Herpes zoster	79 (2.0)	72 (1.9)
Lower respiratory tract infection	69 (1.8)	86 (2.2)
Viral infection	66 (1.7)	72 (1.9)
Rhinitis	63 (1.6)	84 (2.2)
Respiratory tract infection	55 (1.4)	69 (1.8)
Ear infection	43 (1.1)	21 (0.5)
Tooth infection	26 (0.7)	41 (1.1)
Injury, Poisoning and Procedural Complications		
Fall	205 (5.3)	250 (6.4)
Contusion	162 (4.2)	192 (5.0)
Radius fracture	104 (2.7)	116 (3.0)
Joint sprain	60 (1.5)	65 (1.7)
Procedural pain	57 (1.5)	54 (1.4)
Humerus fracture	42 (1.1)	49 (1.3)
Rib fracture	40 (1.0)	33 (0.9)
Ulna fracture	37 (1.0)	39 (1.0)
Foot fracture	34 (0.9)	39 (1.0)
Lumbar vertebral fracture	25 (0.6)	72 (1.9)
Thoracic vertebral fracture	22 (0.6)	53 (1.4)
Investigations		
Weight decreased	41 (1.1)	49 (1.3)
Metabolism and Nutrition Disorders		
Hypercholesterolemia	280 (7.2)	236 (6.1)
Diabetes mellitus	62 (1.6)	58 (1.5)
Hyperlipidemia	45 (1.2)	35 (0.9)
Musculoskeletal and Connective Tissue Disorders		
Back pain	1347 (34.7)	1340 (34.6)
Arthralgia	784 (20.2)	782 (20.2)
Pain in extremity	453 (11.7)	430 (11.1)
Osteoarthritis	436 (11.2)	442 (11.4)
Musculoskeletal pain	297 (7.6)	291 (7.5)
Muscle spasms	167 (4.3)	182 (4.7)
Bone pain	142 (3.7)	117 (3.0)
Neck pain	129 (3.3)	136 (3.5)
Myalgia	114 (2.9)	94 (2.4)
Spinal osteoarthritis	82 (2.1)	64 (1.7)
Musculoskeletal chest pain	61 (1.6)	63 (1.6)
Tendonitis	56 (1.4)	47 (1.2)
Joint swelling	55 (1.4)	66 (1.7)
Arthritis	48 (1.2)	53 (1.4)
Nervous System Disorders		
Headache	237 (6.1)	258 (6.7)
Dizziness	217 (5.6)	218 (5.6)

* **Terms designated by investigators as related to study drugs.**

(cont'd)

Table 1: PROLIA *(cont'd)*

Adverse Events Occurring in ≥1% of Patients with Postmenopausal Osteoporosis

System Organ Class Preferred Term	PROLIA (N=3886) n (%)	Placebo (N=3876) n (%)
Sciatica	178 (4.6)	149 (3.8)
Syncope	67 (1.7)	71 (1.8)
Paraesthesia	63 (1.6)	56 (1.4)
Memory impairment	52 (1.3)	37 (1.0)
Psychiatric Disorders		
Depression	213 (5.5)	221 (5.7)
Insomnia	126 (3.2)	122 (3.1)
Anxiety	123 (3.2)	123 (3.2)
Renal and Urinary Disorders		
Urinary incontinence	39 (1.0)	40 (1.0)
Renal cyst	23 (0.6)	39 (1.0)
Respiratory, Thoracic and Mediastinal Disorders		
Cough	224 (5.8)	238 (6.1)
Dyspnea	93 (2.4)	105 (2.7)
Asthma	66 (1.7)	65 (1.7)
Pharyngolaryngeal pain	52 (1.3)	67 (1.7)
Chronic obstructive pulmonary disease	38 (1.0)	39 (1.0)
Skin and Subcutaneous Tissue Disorders		
Rash	96 (2.5)	79 (2.0)
Pruritus	87 (2.2)	82 (2.1)
Eczema	50 (1.3)	25 (0.6)
Alopecia	31 (0.8)	41 (1.1)
Vascular Disorders		
Hypertension	614 (15.8)	636 (16.4)
Varicose vein	58 (1.5)	60 (1.5)
Hematoma	38 (1.0)	51 (1.3)

Legend: N=Number of subjects who received ≥1 dose of investigational product; n=Number of subjects reporting ≥1 event.
Includes only treatment-emergent adverse events.

Less Common Clinical Trial Adverse Drug Reactions* (<1%): Musculoskeletal and Connective Tissue Disorders: arthralgia, muscle spasms, pain in extremity, bone pain, myalgia, musculoskeletal stiffness, musculoskeletal pain, osteoarthritis, neck pain, exostosis, joint swelling, muscle fatigue, limb discomfort, tendonitis, joint stiffness, muscular weakness, nodule on extremity, fistula, groin pain, joint ankylosis, limb deformity, muscle hemorrhage, rheumatoid arthritis, spinal deformity, spondylitis, polymyalgia rheumatica, sensation of heaviness, arthritis, bone callus excessive, foot deformity, muscle atrophy, osteitis, renal rickets, resorption bone increased, synovitis, tendon pain, tenosynovitis.

Gastrointestinal Disorders: nausea, constipation, diarrhea, vomiting, abdominal pain, flatulence, abdominal pain upper, dry mouth, gastritis, dyspepsia, stomach discomfort, abdominal distension, abdominal discomfort, abdominal pain lower, coeliac disease, faecalith, frequent bowel movements, gastric ulcer, gastritis erosive, gastrooesophageal reflux disease, gingivitis, glossodynia, hemorrhoids, irritable bowel syndrome, oral cavity fistula, pancreatitis, pancreatitis acute, rectal hemorrhage, aphthous stomatitis, change of bowel habit, enterocolitis, gastroduodenitis, gastrointestinal hemorrhage, lip swelling, melaena, oesophageal spasm, rectal prolapse, reflux oesophagitis, tongue ulceration.

Infections and Infestations: nasopharyngitis, respiratory tract infection, upper respiratory tract infection, influenza, urinary tract infection, rhinitis, lower respiratory tract infection, pneumonia, bronchitis, cystitis, sinusitis, herpes zoster, oral herpes, pharyngitis, herpes virus infection, tinea pedis, viral infection, chlamydial infection, eczema infected, gastroenteritis viral, herpes ophthalmic, laryngitis, liver abscess, lung infection, viremia, borrelia infection, chronic sinusitis, diverticulitis, furuncle, genital infection fungal, gingival infection, hematoma infection, helicobacter infection, herpes simplex, sialoadenitis, tracheitis.

Nervous System Disorders: headache, dizziness, paraesthesia, lethargy, somnolence, hypoaesthesia, ischemic stroke, dysgeusia, sciatica, tremor, parosmia, syncope, transient ischemic attack, disturbance in attention, epilepsy, freezing phenomenon, global amnesia, Guillain-Barré syndrome, head discomfort, hemicephalalgia, hypotonia, poor quality sleep, trigeminal neuralgia, hypersomnia, loss of consciousness, memory impairment, ageusia, amnesia, anosmia, dyskinesia, formication, intercostal neuralgia, migraine, muscle contractions involuntary, neuritis cranial, Parkinson's disease, Parkinsonism, restless legs syndrome.

General Disorders and Administration Site Conditions: asthenia, fatigue, injection site pain, edema peripheral, injection site erythema, pain, influenza like illness, injection site irritation, feeling hot, malaise, injection site bruising, injection site reaction, injection site hematoma, injection site rash, pyrexia, noncardiac chest pain, peripheral coldness, chills, injection site warmth, chest discomfort, feeling cold, gait disturbance, hernia, impaired healing, injection site discomfort, injection site mass, injection site swelling, irritability, injection site pruritus, fat tissue increased, injection site scab, thirst.

Skin and Subcutaneous Tissue Disorders: pruritus, rash, alopecia, hyperhidrosis, eczema, dermatitis allergic, erythema, dry skin, rash macular, rash pruritic, onychomadesis, ecchymosis, pruritus generalised, dermatitis, rosacea, subcutaneous nodule, blister, dermatitis atopic, hair growth abnormal, heat rash, hyperkeratosis, lichen planus, nail disorder, psoriasis, rash generalised, skin exfoliation, skin warm, urticaria, acne, night sweats, pigmentation disorder, purpura, rash maculo-papular, skin lesion, skin nodule, skin wrinkling, swelling face, vasculitic rash.

Vascular Disorders: hypertension, hot flush, aortic calcification, deep vein thrombosis, flushing, hematoma, varicose vein, arteriosclerosis, aortic stenosis, orthostatic hypotension, peripheral ischemia, vasculitis, hypotension, thrombophlebitis, hypertensive crisis, venous thrombosis.

Respiratory, Thoracic and Mediastinal Disorders: cough, pharyngolaryngeal pain, dyspnea, dysphonia, nasal congestion, epistaxis, rhinorrhea, pulmonary embolism, asthma, dyspnea exertional, nocturnal dyspnea, sinus congestion, sneezing, vasomotor rhinitis, acute pulmonary edema, nasal dryness, pleurisy, productive cough, rhinitis allergic.

Cardiac Disorders: palpitations, angina pectoris, cardiac failure, arrhythmia, acute myocardial infarction, extrasystoles, ventricular extrasystoles, atrial fibrillation, myocardial infarction, cardiac failure chronic, coronary artery disease, hypertensive cardiomyopathy, ischemic cardiomyopathy, supraventricular extrasystoles, tachycardia, mitral valve incompetence, tachyarrhythmia.

Eye Disorders: cataract, glaucoma, conjunctivitis allergic, dry eye, ocular discomfort, eyelid pain, lacrimation increased, visual disturbance, vitreous disorder, conjunctivitis, eye pain, arteriosclerotic retinopathy, blepharitis, blepharospasm, eyelids pruritus, lacrimal gland enlargement, photophobia, vision blurred, vitreous hemorrhage.
Ear and Labyrinth Disorders: vertigo, ear pain, ear discomfort, tinnitus, cerumen impaction, ear congestion, ear disorder, otosalpingitis, tympanic membrane perforation.
Neoplasms Benign, Malignant and Unspecified (Incl Cysts and Polyps): breast cancer, ovarian cancer, basal cell carcinoma, benign neoplasm of thyroid gland, benign soft tissue neoplasm, cerebellar tumour, cervix carcinoma, lipoma, multiple myeloma, uterine leiomyoma, benign breast neoplasm, acral lentiginous melanoma stage unspecified, adenocarcinoma, benign bone neoplasm, benign neoplasm, bladder neoplasm, colon cancer, diffuse large B-cell lymphoma recurrent, hemangioma, hemangioma of liver, lipoma of breast, melanocytic naevus.
Blood and Lymphatic System Disorders: eosinophilia, leukopenia, thrombocytopenia, anemia, leukocytosis, lymphadenopathy, lymphocytosis, neutrophilia, pancytopenia, neutropenia, bone marrow failure, lymphopenia.
Investigations: weight decreased, blood pressure increased, alanine aminotransferase increased, coagulation time shortened, red blood cell sedimentation rate increased, blood chloride decreased, blood sodium decreased, weight increased, cardiac murmur, aspartate aminotransferase increased, hemoglobin decreased, international normalised ratio increased, platelet count decreased, red blood cell count decreased, rheumatoid factor positive.
Metabolism and Nutrition Disorders: hypercalcemia, anorexia, hypercholesterolemia, decreased appetite, diabetes mellitus, glucose tolerance impaired, hypomagnesemia.
Psychiatric Disorders: depression, depressed mood, insomnia, apathy, dysthymic disorder, sleep disorder, restlessness.
Renal and Urinary Disorders: dysuria, hematuria, nephrolithiasis, acute prerenal failure, polyuria, urge incontinence, urine abnormality, pollakiuria, nephrosclerosis, nocturia, proteinuria, renal impairment, urine odour abnormal.
Reproductive System and Breast Disorders: breast pain, vulvovaginal pruritus, breast disorder, vaginal hemorrhage, breast discomfort, vulvovaginal dryness, breast mass, fibrocystic breast disease, breast necrosis, breast tenderness, vulvovaginal burning sensation.
Endocrine Disorders: goitre, hyperthyroidism, hypothyroidism, hyperparathyroidism.
Injury, Poisoning and Procedural Complications: thoracic vertebral fracture, clavicle fracture, femoral neck fracture, post procedural hemorrhage, lumbar vertebral fracture, fall, anastomotic ulcer hemorrhage, contusion, humerus fracture, ilium fracture, joint dislocation, joint sprain, post concussion syndrome, radius fracture, scratch.
Hepatobiliary Disorders: liver disorder, hepatic cyst, cholecystitis, cholelithiasis.
Immune System Disorders: hypersensitivity, drug hypersensitivity.
Congenital, Familial and Genetic Disorders: familial tremor.
Surgical and Medical Procedures: fistula repair.
Hypocalcemia: In postmenopausal women with osteoporosis in Study 1, declines of serum calcium concentrations to less than the normal range were reported in 15 (0.4%) women in the placebo group and 63 (1.6%) women in the PROLIA group. Declines of serum calcium concentrations to <7.5 mg/dL (<1.88 mmol/L) were reported in 2 (<0.1%) women in the placebo group and 1 (<0.1%) in the PROLIA group. In clinical studies, subjects with impaired renal function were more likely to have greater reductions in serum calcium levels compared to subjects with normal renal function. In a study of 55 patients with varying degrees of renal function who did not receive calcium and vitamin D supplementation, symptomatic hypocalcemia or serum calcium levels <7.5 mg/dL was observed in 5 subjects, including no subjects in the normal renal function group, 10% (1 out of 10) of subjects in the CrCL 50 to 80 mL/min group, 29% (2 out of 7) of subjects in the CrCL <30 mL/min group, and 29% (2 out of 7) of subjects in the hemodialysis group (see Warnings and Precautions).
Infections: Receptor activator of nuclear factor kappa-B ligand (RANKL) is expressed on activated T and B lymphocytes and in lymph nodes. Therefore, a RANKL inhibitor such as PROLIA may increase the risk of infection. In the clinical study of 7808 postmenopausal women with osteoporosis, the incidence of infections resulting in death was 6 (0.2%) in both placebo and PROLIA treatment groups. The incidence of nonfatal serious infections was 3.3% (n=128) in the placebo group and 4.0% (n=154) in the PROLIA group. Hospitalizations due to serious infections in the abdomen 28 (0.7%) placebo vs. 36 (0.9%) PROLIA, urinary tract 20 (0.5%) placebo vs. 29 (0.7%) PROLIA, and ear 0 (0.0%) placebo vs. 5 (0.1%) PROLIA were reported. Endocarditis was reported in 0 (0.0%) placebo patients and 3 (0.1%) patients receiving PROLIA.

Overall skin infections leading to hospitalization were reported more frequently in patients treated with PROLIA (2 [<0.1%] placebo vs. 15 [0.4%] PROLIA) among women with postmenopausal osteoporosis in Study 1. These events were predominantly comprised of erysipelas (0 [0%] placebo and 7 [0.2%] PROLIA) and cellulitis (1 [<0.1%] placebo and 6 [0.2%] PROLIA) (see Warnings and Precautions).

The overall incidence of infections was similar between the PROLIA and placebo groups (2055 [52.9%] PROLIA, 2108 [54.4%] placebo). The incidence of specific infection types was as follows: urinary tract infections (245 [6.3%] PROLIA, 253 [6.5%] placebo), upper respiratory infections (190 [4.9%] PROLIA, 167 [4.3%] placebo), ear infections (43 [1.1%] PROLIA, 21 [0.5%] placebo), and diverticulitis (28 [0.7%] PROLIA, 22 [0.6%] placebo).

There was no imbalance in the reporting of opportunistic infections (4 [0.1%] PROLIA, 3 [0.1%] placebo).
Dermatologic: A significantly higher number of patients treated with PROLIA developed epidermal and dermal adverse events (such as dermatitis, eczema, and rashes), with these events reported in 8.2% (n=316) of placebo and 10.8% (n=421) of PROLIA group (p <0.0001). Most of these events were not specific to the injection site (see Warnings and Precautions, Dermatologic).
Osteonecrosis of the Jaw (ONJ): ONJ has been reported rarely in the open-label osteoporosis clinical trial program in patients treated with PROLIA (see Warnings and Precautions).
Cardiovascular Disorders: The incidence of positively adjudicated cardiovascular serious adverse events was 186 (4.8%) PROLIA and 178 (4.6%) placebo, with a hazard ratio (95% confidence interval) of 1.02 (0.83, 1.25). Adjudicated cardiovascular events were further sub-categorized as follows: cardiovascular death, acute coronary syndrome, stroke/transient ischemic attack, congestive heart failure, other vascular event, and arrhythmia. The incidence of these subcategories was 23 (0.6%) PROLIA and 31 (0.8%) placebo for cardiovascular death, 47 (1.2%) PROLIA and 39 (1.0%) placebo for acute coronary syndrome, 56 (1.4%) PROLIA and 54 (1.4%) placebo for stroke/transient ischemic attack, 27 (0.7%) PROLIA and 22 (0.6%) placebo for congestive heart failure, 31 (0.8%) PROLIA and 30 (0.8%) placebo for other vascular event, and 52 (1.3%) PROLIA and 45 (1.2%) placebo for arrhythmia.
Fracture Healing: Delayed fracture healing of nonvertebral fractures was reported in 2 out of 303 (0.7%) subjects in the PROLIA group (3 out of 386 [0.8%] nonvertebral fractures) and 2 out of 364 (0.5%) subjects in the placebo group (2 out of 465 [0.4%] nonvertebral fractures). In addition, nonunion of nonvertebral fractures was reported in 0 out of 303 (0%) subjects in the PROLIA group (0 out of 386 [0%] nonvertebral fractures) and 1 out of 364 (0.3%) subjects in the placebo group (1 out of 465 [0.2%] nonvertebral fractures). For fractures that occurred near the final study closure, additional follow-up after study closure identified 2 additional subjects in the placebo group and 0 in the PROLIA group with delayed fracture healing. Of the subjects with a distal radius fracture, 1 out of 104 (1.0%) subjects in the PROLIA group (1 out of 106 [0.9%] distal radius fractures) and 0 out of 116 (0%) subjects in the placebo group (0 out of 118 [0%] distal radius fractures) had delayed fracture healing.
Malignancies: The overall incidence of new malignancies was 188 (4.8%) in the PROLIA and 166 (4.3%) in the placebo groups. The most common malignancies (≥0.2%) included: breast cancer (28 [0.7%] PROLIA, 26 [0.7%] placebo), colon cancer (11 [0.3%] PROLIA, 8 [0.2%] placebo), lung neoplasm malignant (9 [0.2%] PROLIA, 9 [0.2%] placebo), gastric cancer (7 [0.2%] PROLIA, 3 [0.1%] placebo), pancreatic carcinoma (7 [0.2%] PROLIA, 3 [0.1%] placebo), squamous cell carcinoma of skin (6 [0.2%] PROLIA, 8 [0.2%] placebo), and recurrent breast cancer (6 [0.2%] PROLIA, 2 [0.1%] placebo). Other malignancies reported include: thyroid cancer (2 [0.1%] PROLIA, 0 [0%] placebo), carcinoid of the stomach (1 [<0.1%] PROLIA, 0 [0%] placebo), uterine cancer (3 [0.1%] PROLIA, 1 [<0.1%] placebo), ovarian cancer metastatic (2 [0.1%] PROLIA, 0 [0%] placebo), ovarian epithelial cancer (2 [0.1%] PROLIA, 0 [0%] placebo), vulval cancer (2 [0.1%] PROLIA, 0 [0%] placebo), and lentigo maligna stage unspecified (3 [0.1%] PROLIA, 0 [0%] placebo). A causal relationship to drug exposure has not been established.
Hypersensitivity Reactions: The incidence of adverse drug reactions potentially associated with hypersensitivity was 50 (1.3%) in the PROLIA group and 50 (1.3%) in the placebo group. The most common adverse event potentially associated with hypersensitivity was urticaria (27 [0.7%] PROLIA, 27 [0.7%] placebo).
Pancreatitis: Pancreatitis was reported in 4 patients (0.1%) in the placebo and 8 patients (0.2%) in the PROLIA groups. Of these reports, one patient in the placebo group and all 8 patients in the PROLIA group had serious events including 2 deaths in the PROLIA group. Several patients had a prior history of pancreatitis or a confounding event (eg, gallstones). The time from product administration to event occurrence was variable.
Abnormal Hematologic and Clinical Chemistry Findings: The most frequent laboratory abnormalities were changes in serum calcium with compensatory physiological changes in serum phosphorus. The median percent change from baseline (interquartile range) at month 1 for serum calcium was −2.1% (−5.2% to 1.0%) for PROLIA and 1.0% (−2.0% to 3.2%) for placebo. The median percent change from baseline (interquartile range) at month 1 for serum phosphorus was −8.3% (−15.8% to 0%) for PROLIA and 0% (−5.6% to 8.3%) for placebo. Alkaline phosphatase was also reduced, by month 6, which reflects reduced osteoclast activity in bone, with a decrease from baseline of 25% in PROLIA subjects compared to 3% to 8% in placebo subjects.

Serum phosphorous levels were between 2.0 and 2.5 mg/dL in 2.0% (n=82) of patients in the placebo group and 7.0% (n=263) of patients in the denosumab group. Decrease in platelet levels to between 50 000/mm³ and 75 000/mm³ was reported at 0.2% (n=7) in the placebo group and 0.4% (n=14) in the denosumab group, and decrease in platelet levels to <25 000/mm³ was reported at <0.1% (n=2) in the placebo group and at 0.1% (n=4) in the denosumab group. Increase in asparate aminotransferase (AST) levels to between 1.0 and 2.5 × the upper limit of normal (ULN) was reported at 5.0% (n=206) in the placebo group and 7.0% (n=264) in the denosumab group, and increase in alanine aminotransferase levels (ALT) to between 2.5 and 5.0 × ULN were reported at 0.5% (n=21) in the placebo group and 1.0% (n=37) in the denosumab group. Increase in total bilirubin value to between 3.0 and 10.0 × ULN was reported at 0.0% (n=0) in the placebo group and 0.1% (n=5) in the denosumab group.
Other Studies in Postmenopausal Women: The safety of PROLIA was assessed in a 2 year, randomized, double-blind, placebo-controlled, multinational study of 332 postmenopausal women aged 43 to 83 years with low bone mass (Study 2). A total of 165 women received placebo and 164 women received PROLIA administered once every 6 months as a single 60 mg SC dose. All women received calcium (at least 1000 mg) and vitamin D (at least 400 IU) supplementation per day. The incidence of adverse events was 156 (95%) in the PROLIA group and 157 (95%) in the placebo group. The incidence of serious adverse events was 11% (n=18) in the PROLIA group and 6% (n=9) in the placebo group. No subject died during the study. The 3 most common adverse events were arthralgia (26% (n=43) PROLIA vs. 26% (n=42) placebo), nasopharyngitis (22% (n=36) PROLIA vs. 19% (n=32) placebo), and back pain (20% (n=33) PROLIA vs. 21% (n=34) placebo).

Two randomized, double-blind, active-controlled studies (Study 3 and Study 4) assessed the safety of PROLIA compared with alendronate. In Study 3, a total of 1179 postmenopausal women with low bone mass who were treatment naive (593 randomized to PROLIA 60 mg SC once every 6 months, 586 randomized to alendronate tablets 70 mg once weekly) received investigational product and were evaluated for safety. All women received daily supplemental calcium (at least 1000 mg) and vitamin D (at least 400 IU). The incidence of adverse events was 81% (n=480) in the PROLIA group and 82% (n=482) in the alendronate group. The incidence of serious adverse events was 6% (n=34) in the PROLIA group and 6% (n=37) in the alendronate group. One subject in each treatment group died during the study. The 3 most frequent adverse events were arthralgia (13% (n=75) PROLIA vs. 10% (n=56) alendronate), nasopharyngitis (8% (n=45) PROLIA vs. 7% (n=43) alendronate), and back pain (7% (n=42) PROLIA vs. 10% (n=56) alendronate).

In Study 4, a total of 502 postmenopausal women with low bone mass who were being treated with alendronate for a median duration of 3 years (253 PROLIA 60 mg SC every 6 months, 249 alendronate tablets 70 mg once weekly) received investigational product and were evaluated for safety. All women received daily supplemental calcium (at least 1000 mg) and vitamin D (at least 400 IU). The incidence of adverse events was 78% (n=197) in the PROLIA group and 79% (n=196) in the alendronate group. The incidence of serious adverse events was 6% (n=15) in the PROLIA group and 6% (n=16) in the alendronate group. One subject in the PROLIA treatment group died during the study. The 3 most frequent adverse events were nasopharyngitis (13% (n=34) PROLIA vs. 11% (n=27) alendronate), back pain (11% (n=27) PROLIA vs. 12% (n=29) alendronate), and arthralgia (6% (n=15) PROLIA vs. 10% (n=26) alendronate).

The safety profile of denosumab in women with postmenopausal osteoporosis was consistent with results in these 3 studies among women with postmenopausal bone loss. No notable differences were observed between those women who had received prior osteoporosis therapy versus those who had not received prior osteoporosis therapy (ie, alendronate).
Immunogenicity: Denosumab is a human monoclonal antibody. As with all therapeutic proteins, there is potential for immunogenicity with PROLIA. More than 13 000 patients were screened for binding antibodies using a sensitive electrochemiluminescent bridging immunoassay. Less than 1% (55 out of 8113) of patients treated with PROLIA for up to 5 years tested positive for antibodies (including pre existing, transient, and developing antibodies). The patients that tested positive for binding antibodies were further evaluated for neutralizing antibodies using a chemiluminescent cell-based in vitro biological assay and none of them tested positive. No evidence of altered pharmacokinetic profile, toxicity profile, or clinical response was associated with binding antibody development.

The detection of antibody formation is dependent on the sensitivity and specificity of the assay. The observed incidence of antibody positivity in an assay may be influenced by factors such as sample handling, concomitant medications, and underlying disease. For these reasons, comparison of antibodies to denosumab with the incidence of antibodies to other products may be misleading.
DRUG INTERACTIONS: Overview: No formal drug interaction studies have been conducted with PROLIA.
Drug-Drug Interactions: Interactions with other drugs have not been established.

The pharmacokinetics and pharmacodynamics of PROLIA were similar in postmenopausal women with osteoporosis transitioning from alendronate therapy compared to those who had not received prior alendronate therapy.
Drug-Food Interactions: Interactions with food have not been established.
Drug-Herb Interactions: Interactions with herbal products have not been established.
Drug-Laboratory Test Interactions: Interactions with laboratory tests have not been established.

DOSAGE AND ADMINISTRATION: Dosing Considerations: PROLIA is intended for use under the guidance and supervision of physicians who have fully familiarized themselves with the efficacy/safety profile of PROLIA. After an initial training in proper subcutaneous injection technique, patients with PMO may self-inject PROLIA if a physician determines that is appropriate and with medical follow-up as necessary.

Patients must be adequately supplemented with calcium and vitamin D at the recommended doses†.

PROLIA is indicated for the treatment of osteoporosis in postmenopausal women at high risk for fracture, defined as a history of osteoporotic fracture, or multiple risk factors for fracture; or patients who have failed or are intolerant to other available osteoporosis therapy. In postmenopausal women with osteoporosis, PROLIA reduces the incidence of vertebral, nonvertebral and hip fractures.
Recommended Dose and Dosage Adjustment: The recommended dose of PROLIA (denosumab) is a single SC injection of 60 mg, once every 6 months.
Administration: Administration of PROLIA should be performed by an individual who has been adequately trained in injection techniques.

Parenteral drug products should be inspected visually for particulate matter and discolouration prior to administration, whenever solution and container permit. PROLIA is a clear, colourless to slightly yellow solution that may contain trace amounts of translucent to white proteinaceous particles. Do not use if the solution is cloudy.

Prior to administration, PROLIA may be allowed to reach room temperature (up to 25°C) in the original container.

Administer PROLIA via SC injection in the upper arm, the upper thigh, or the abdomen.

OVERDOSAGE:
There is no experience with overdosage with PROLIA.

> For management of a suspected drug overdose, contact your regional Poison Control Centre. See the *CPS* Directory section for a list of Poison Control Centres.

ACTION AND CLINICAL PHARMACOLOGY: Mechanism of Action: PROLIA is a RANK ligand (RANKL) inhibitor. RANKL exists as a transmembrane or soluble protein. RANKL ligand is essential for the formation, function and survival of osteoclasts, the sole cell type responsible for bone resorption. Osteoclasts play an important role in bone loss associated with postmenopausal osteoporosis. Denosumab targets and binds with high affinity and specificity to RANKL, preventing RANKL from activating its only receptor, RANK, on the surface of osteoclasts and their precursors, independent of bone surface. Prevention of RANKL-RANK interaction inhibits osteoclast formation, function and survival, thereby decreasing bone resorption and increasing bone mass and strength in both cortical and trabecular bone throughout the skeleton.
Pharmacodynamics: In clinical studies, treatment with 60 mg of PROLIA resulted in rapid reduction in the bone resorption marker serum type 1 C-telopeptide (CTX) within 6 hours of SC administration by approximately 70%, with reductions of approximately 85% occurring by 3 days. CTX levels were below the limit of assay quantitation (0.049 ng/mL) in 39 to 68% of subjects 1 to 3 months after dosing of PROLIA. CTX reductions were maintained over the 6-month dosing interval. At the end of each dosing interval, CTX reductions were partially attenuated from maximal reduction of ≥87% to ≥45% (range 45% to 80%), as serum denosumab levels diminished, reflecting the reversibility of the effects of PROLIA on bone remodelling. These effects were maintained with continued treatment. Consistent with the physiological coupling of bone formation and resorption in skeletal remodeling, subsequent reductions in bone formation markers were observed beginning 1 month after the first dose of PROLIA.

Bone turnover markers (bone resorption and formation markers) generally reached pre-treatment levels within 9 months after the last 60 mg SC dose. Upon re-initiation, the degree of inhibition of CTX by PROLIA was similar to that observed in patients initiating PROLIA treatment.

† Canadian Consensus Conference on Osteoporosis 2006 Update, Society of Obstetrician and Gynecologists of Canada, SOGC.

In a clinical study of postmenopausal women with low bone mass (N=504) who were previously treated with alendronate for a median duration of 3 years, those transitioning to receive PROLIA experienced additional reductions in serum CTX, compared with women who remained on alendronate. In this study, the changes in serum calcium were similar between the 2 groups.

Pharmacokinetics: In dose ranging studies, denosumab exhibited nonlinear, dose-dependent pharmacokinetics for doses between 0.01 mg/kg to 3.0 mg/kg inclusive. Clearance or apparent clearance (mL/hr/kg) was higher at lower doses and had a linear inverse relationship with dose on a log-log plot. Exposures (SC dosing) based on area under the serum denosumab concentration-time curve (AUC) increased greater than dose-proportionally from 0.01 to 1 mg/kg (700-fold for the 100 fold increase in dose), but approximately dose-proportionally from 1 to 3 mg/kg (3.9 fold for the 3-fold increase in dose).

Figure 1: PROLIA

Individual Serum Denosumab Concentration-Time Profiles Following Single Dose SC Administration at 1.0 mg/kg to Healthy Postmenopausal Women

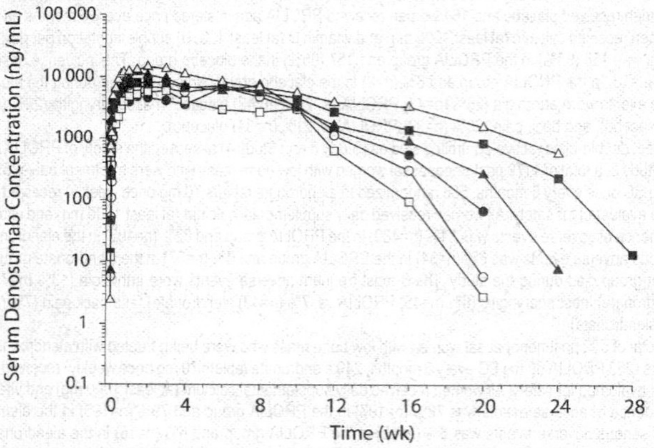

Table 2: PROLIA

Mean (SD) Denosumab Pharmacokinetic Parameters Following Single Dose SC Administration of 1.0 mg/kg Denosumab to Healthy Postmenopausal Women (N=6)

T_{max} (days)	C_{max} (µg/mL)	$AUC_{0\text{-}inf}$ (µg×day/mL)	CL/F (mL/hr)	MRT (days)	$t_{½}$ (days)	$t_{½,z}$ (days)
17.5 (7–42)	8.99 (3.34)	538 (224)	6.61 (2.93)	44.2 (6.96)	30.2 (7.04)	8 (0.975)

Legend: SD=standard deviation; C_{max}=maximum observed concentration; T_{max}=time of C_{max} (range reported instead of SD); $AUC_{0\text{-}inf}$=area under the serum concentration-time curve from pre-dose to infinity; CL/F=apparent clearance; MRT=mean residence time; $t_{½}$=half-life following C_{max}; $t_{½,z}$=terminal-phase half-life.

Table 3: PROLIA

Mean (SD) Denosumab Pharmacokinetic Parameters Following SC Administration of 60 mg Denosumab Every 6 Months to Postmenopausal Women with Low BMD (n=32-46)[a]

Dose	T_{max} (days)	C_{max} (µg/mL)	$AUC_{0\text{-}tau}$ (µg×day/mL)	CL/F (mL/hr)	MRT (days)	$t_{½}$ (days)	C_{min} (µg/mL)
1st	26 (2.9–32)	7.93 (2.95)	503 (239)	6.71 (5.00)	44.2 (9.48)	25.4 (8.47)	0.137 (0.334)
2nd	29 (1.9–42)	6.94 (3.18)	448 (239)	7.50 (5.04)	45.0 (9.99)	27.1 (8.99)	0.132 (0.334)

[a] 1st dose: n=46 for T_{max}, C_{max}, $AUC_{0\text{-}tau}$, CL/F, & MRT; n=32 for $t_{½}$; n=38 for C_{min}.
2nd dose: n=44 for T_{max}, C_{max}, $AUC_{0\text{-}tau}$, CL/F, & MRT; n=33 for $t_{½}$; n=39 for C_{min}.

Legend: SD=standard deviation; C_{max}=maximum observed concentration; T_{max}=time of C_{max} (range reported instead of SD); $AUC_{0\text{-}tau}$=area under the serum denosumab concentration-time curve over the dosing interval; CL/F=apparent clearance; MRT=mean residence time; $t_{½}$=half-life following C_{max}; C_{min}=trough serum denosumab concentration.

Denosumab pharmacokinetic parameters were not affected by the formation of binding antibodies to denosumab.

At the level of the administered dose, the pharmacokinetics of denosumab do not appear to be affected by gender, age (28 to 87 years), race, or disease state.

Special Populations and Conditions: Geriatrics: The pharmacokinetics of denosumab were not affected by age.

Pediatrics: The pharmacokinetics of denosumab in pediatric patients has not been assessed.

Race: The pharmacokinetics of denosumab were not affected by race in postmenopausal women.

Hepatic Insufficiency: No clinical studies have been conducted to evaluate the effect of hepatic impairment on the pharmacokinetics of denosumab.

Renal Insufficiency: In a study of 55 patients with varying degrees of renal function, including patients on dialysis, the degree of renal impairment had no effect on the pharmacokinetics of denosumab; thus, dose adjustment for renal impairment is not necessary.

STORAGE AND STABILITY: Store PROLIA in a refrigerator at 2°C to 8°C in the original carton. Do not freeze.

If removed from the refrigerator, PROLIA should be kept at controlled room temperature (up to 25°C) in the original carton and must be used within 30 days.

Protect PROLIA from light and do not expose to temperatures above 25°C.

Avoid vigorous shaking of PROLIA.

Do not use PROLIA beyond the expiry date stamped on the label.

INFORMATION FOR THE PATIENT: Published in e-CPS, available by subscription at www.e-cps.ca.

DOSAGE FORMS, COMPOSITION AND PACKAGING: Each 1 mL single use prefilled syringe of sterile, preservative-free, clear, colourless to slightly yellow solution contains: 60 mg denosumab, 4.7% sorbitol, 17 mM acetate, 0.01% polysorbate 20, water for injection (USP), and sodium hydroxide to a pH of 5.2. Dispensing packs containing one prefilled syringe with a safety guard.

Prolopa® Ⓟ

levodopa—benserazide HCl

Antiparkinsonian Agent

Roche

Date of Preparation: April 5, 1977
Date of Revision: May 14, 2008

SUMMARY PRODUCT INFORMATION:

Route of Administration	Dosage Form/ Strength	Clinically Relevant Nonmedicinal Ingredients
Oral	Capsule 50-12.5, 100-25, 200-50	Mannitol For a complete listing see Dosage Forms, Composition and Packaging.

INDICATIONS AND CLINICAL USE: Adults >25 years of age: PROLOPA (levodopa and benserazide combination) is indicated for the treatment of Parkinson's disease with the exception of drug-induced parkinsonism.

The administration of PROLOPA is associated with amelioration of the symptoms of Parkinson's disease with the advantage that combined therapy significantly diminishes the incidence of the levodopa-induced peripheral side-effects of nausea, vomiting and possibly cardiac arrhythmias.

This results in an advantage for those patients who previously were unable to tolerate an optimal daily dosage of levodopa. Improved gastrointestinal tolerance also provides for a more rapid induction of therapy, e.g., optimum dosage can in most cases be achieved within two to three weeks.

However, combined therapy with levodopa and benserazide increases the incidence of centrally mediated abnormal movements earlier in therapy and can lead to an earlier appearance of oscillations in performance. Thus, when combined therapy with levodopa and benserazide is instituted it is important to strive at using and maintaining a dosage regimen which balances efficacy with freedom from dyskinesias.

Despite the dramatic symptomatic improvement it produces in many patients with Parkinson's disease, levodopa does not arrest the progression of the disease and there is evidence to indicate that drug adverse effects increase with continuing use. Combined therapy, because of the advantages already described, is therefore indicated only when its use is capable of improving the quality of life of the patient. However, there is little to be gained by substituting combined therapy for levodopa in patients already on stable, effective and well-tolerated levodopa therapy.

Pediatrics and Young Adults (<25 years of age): The safety and effectiveness of PROLOPA have not been established in these populations. Animal studies have suggested the possibility of skeletal abnormalities when beserazide is administered before ossification is complete. Therefore PROLOPA must not be given to patients less than 25 years of age (see Contraindications and Warnings and Precautions).

CONTRAINDICATIONS: As with levodopa, PROLOPA should not be given when administration of a sympathomimetic amine is contraindicated (e.g., epinephrine, norepinephrine or isoproterenol).

Monoamine oxidase inhibitors cannot be given concomitantly and should be withdrawn at least two weeks prior to initiating therapy with PROLOPA, otherwise, unwanted effects such as hypertensive crises are likely to occur.

PROLOPA is contraindicated in patients with clinical or laboratory evidence of uncompensated cardiovascular, endocrine, renal, hepatic, hematologic, or pulmonary disease. PROLOPA is also contraindicated in patients with narrow angle glaucoma.

PROLOPA is contraindicated in patients with a known hypersensitivity to levodopa, benserazide or to any ingredient in the formulation or component of the container. For a complete listing, see Dosage Forms, Composition and Packaging.

PROLOPA is contraindicated in patients with decompensated endocrine, renal or hepatic function, cardiac disorders, psychiatric diseases with a psychiatric component or closed angle glaucoma.

PROLOPA is contraindicated in patients less than 25 years old (skeletal development must be complete). See Warnings and Precautions.

PROLOPA is contraindicated in pregnant women or to women of childbearing potential in the absence of adequate contraception. If pregnancy occurs in a woman taking PROLOPA, the drug must be discontinued via tapering, as advised by the prescribing physician. PROLOPA must not be withdrawn abruptly (see Warnings and Precautions, Neurologic, Neuroleptic Malignant Syndrome).

WARNINGS AND PRECAUTIONS:

Serious Warnings and Precautions

Patients receiving treatment with PROLOPA (levodopa and berserazide combination) and other dopaminergic agents have reported suddenly falling asleep while engaged in activities of daily living, including the driving of a car, which has sometimes resulted in accidents. Although some of the patients reported somnolence while on PROLOPA, others perceived that they had no warning signs, such as excessive drowsiness, and believed that they were alert immediately prior to the event.

Physicians should alert patients of the reported cases of sudden onset of sleep, bearing in mind that these events are **not** limited to initiation of therapy. Patients should also be advised that sudden onset of sleep has occurred without warning signs and should be specifically asked about factors that may increase the risk with PROLOPA such as concomitant medications or the presence of sleep disorders. Given the reported cases of somnolence and sudden onset of sleep (not necessarily preceded by somnolence), physicians should caution patients about the risk of operating hazardous machinery, including driving motor vehicles, while taking PROLOPA. If drowsiness or sudden onset of sleep should occur, patients should be informed to immediately contact their physician.

Episodes of falling asleep while engaged in activities of daily living have also been reported in patients taking other dopaminergic agents, therefore, symptoms may not be alleviated by substituting these products.

Currently, the precise cause of this event is unknown. It is known that many Parkinson's disease patients experience alterations in sleep architecture, which results in excessive daytime sleepiness or spontaneous dozing, and that dopaminergic agents can also induce sleepiness. There is insufficient information to determine whether this event is associated specifically with PROLOPA, all dopaminergic agents, or Parkinson's disease itself.

General: Before initiating therapy in patients already receiving levodopa, this drug should be discontinued at least 12 hours before PROLOPA (levodopa and benserazide combination) is started. Therapy with PROLOPA should be instituted at a level that will provide approximately 15% of the previous dosage of levodopa (see Dosage and Administration).

Regular assessment of cardiovascular, hepatic, hematopoietic and renal function should be performed in all patients during the dosage stabilization period.

Hypersensitivity reactions may occur in susceptible individuals.

Patients with severe parkinsonism who improve on therapy with PROLOPA should be advised to resume normal activities gradually and with caution as rapid mobilization may increase the risk of injury, especially in those patients with osteoporosis or phlebothrombosis. Physiotherapy and appropriate safeguards may be useful during this phase.

Cardiovascular: Care should be exercised in administering PROLOPA to patients with a history of myocardial infarction or who have atrial, nodal or ventricular arrhythmias. Patients with cardiac abnormalities should have their treatment with PROLOPA initiated in a facility with adequate monitoring equipment and provision for intensive care.

Dependence/Tolerance: A small sub-group of Parkinson's disease patients suffer from cognitive and behavioural disturbance that can be directly attributed to taking increasing quantities of dopaminergic medication against medical advice and well beyond the dose required to treat their motor disabilities.

Endocrine and Metabolism: Patients with diabetes should undergo frequent blood sugar tests, and the dosage of antidiabetic agents should be adjusted to blood sugar levels.

Gastrointestinal: The possibility of upper gastrointestinal hemorrhage occurring in patients with a history of peptic ulcer must be borne in mind when treating them with PROLOPA.

Neurologic: PROLOPA is not indicated in the management of intention tremor, Huntington's chorea, or drug-induced extrapyramidal effects.

Since PROLOPA may induce central nervous system side effects shortly after beginning its use, and at lower doses than levodopa, it is important to administer the dosage in careful increments and to observe patients carefully for the development of abnormal involuntary movements. These movements and oscillations in performance may appear earlier with combination therapy. Should they occur, a reduction of dosage is indicated.

Patients with a history of convulsive disorders should be treated cautiously if PROLOPA is incorporated into their treatment regimen.

Neuroleptic Malignant Syndrome: PROLOPA must not be withdrawn abruptly. A symptom complex resembling the neuroleptic malignant syndrome, characterized by elevated temperature, muscular rigidity, altered consciousness, autonomic instability, possible psychological changes and elevated serum creatinine phosphokinase has been reported in association with rapid dose reduction, withdrawal of, or changes in antiparkinsonian therapy. Should a combination of such symptoms occur, the patient should be kept under medical surveillance, hospitalized if necessary, and appropriate symptomatic treatment given. This may include resumption of therapy with PROLOPA after appropriate evaluation.

Ophthalmologic: Patients with chronic wide-angle glaucoma can be treated cautiously with PROLOPA, provided the intraocular pressure is well controlled. The intraocular pressure should be monitored carefully during therapy as levodopa theoretically has the potential to raise intraocular pressure. Rarely pupillary dilatation and activation of latent Horner's syndrome have been reported during levodopa treatment.

Peri-Operative Considerations: If a patient on levodopa requires general anesthetics, the normal PROLOPA regimen should be continued as close to surgery as possible, except in the case of halothane (see Drug Interactions).

In general anesthesia with halothane, PROLOPA should be discontinued 12-48 hours before surgical interventions as fluctuations in blood pressure and/or arrhythmias may occur in patients being treated with PROLOPA. Therapy with PROLOPA may be resumed following surgery; the dosage should be increased gradually to the preoperative level (see Drug Interactions).

Psychiatric: Depression may occur in patients treated with PROLOPA, but may also be an effect of the underlying disease. All patients should be carefully observed for signs of depression with suicidal tendencies or other serious behavioural changes. Extreme caution should be used in treating patients with a history of psychotic disorders or who are receiving psychotherapeutic agents such as reserpine, phenothiazines or tricyclic antidepressants.

Psychomotor Performance: Patients being treated with levodopa and presenting with somnolence and/or sudden onset sleep episodes should be advised to refrain from driving or engaging in activities where impaired alertness may put themselves or others at risk of serious injury or death (e.g., operating machines) until such recurrent episodes and somnolence have resolved (see Warnings and Precautions, Serious Warnings and Precautions).

Behavioural Changes: Patients and prescribers should be aware that impulse control symptoms such as pathological (compulsive) gambling and hypersexuality have been sporadically reported in patients treated with dopaminergic agents, including levodopa. Dose reduction/taper discontinuation should be considered in management of this behaviour (see Adverse Reactions).

Hallucinations: Hallucinations and confusion are known side effects of treatment with dopaminergic agents, including levodopa. Patients should be aware of the fact that hallucinations (mostly visual) can occur.

Skin: Care should be exercised in administering this drug to patients with a history of melanoma or with suspicious undiagnosed skin lesions.

Some epidemiological studies have shown that patients with Parkinson's disease have a higher risk (perhaps 2- to 4-fold higher) of developing melanoma than the general population. Whether the observed increased risk was due to Parkinson's disease or other factors, such as drugs used to treat Parkinson's disease, was unclear. PROLOPA is one of the drugs used to treat Parkinson's disease. Although PROLOPA has not been associated with an increased risk of melanoma specifically, its potential role as a risk factor has not been systematically studied. Patients treated with PROLOPA should be made aware of these results and should undergo periodic dermatologic screening.

Special Populations: Pregnant Women: Although the effects of PROLOPA on human pregnancy are unknown, levodopa has caused visceral and skeletal malformations in rabbits. Therefore, PROLOPA is completely contraindicated during pregnancy and in women of childbearing potential in the absence of adequate contraception (see Contraindications).

Nursing Women: Since it is not known whether benserazide passes into breast milk, mothers requiring treatment with PROLOPA should not nurse their infants, since the occurrence of skeletal malformations in infants cannot be excluded.

Pediatrics and Young Adults (<25 years of age): The safety and effectiveness of PROLOPA have not been established in these populations. Animal studies have suggested the possibility of skeletal abnormalities when benserazide is administered before ossification is complete. Therefore PROLOPA must not be given to patients less than 25 years of age (see Contraindications).

It should also be borne in mind that PROLOPA stimulates human growth hormone secretion.

Monitoring and Laboratory Tests: Liver and kidney function tests and monitoring of blood cell counts should be performed during the dosage stabilization period and periodically during extended treatment.

Patients with diabetes should undergo frequent blood sugar tests, and the dosage of antidiabetic agents should be adjusted to blood sugar levels.

ADVERSE REACTIONS: Adverse Drug Reaction Overview: The most common serious adverse reactions occurring with PROLOPA (levodopa and benserazide combination) are abnormal involuntary movements and dyskinesias. Dosage reduction can diminish those reactions though often at the expense of increasing parkinsonism. Other serious adverse reactions are oscillations in performance, psychiatric disorders and, less frequently, cardiovascular effects.

Involuntary Movements: choreiform, dystonic, athetotic and other involuntary movements. Muscle twitching and blepharospasm occur less often and may be taken as early signs of overdosage. The appearance of these reactions can usually be eliminated or made tolerable by adjusting the dosage and by giving smaller single doses more frequently. The incidence of involuntary movements reported by several investigators was 30 to 40% in the first month and 50 to 60% or more by six to nine months.

Oscillations in Performance: Periodic oscillations in performance constitute the most serious problem encountered after prolonged levodopa therapy and appear earlier with combined therapy than when levodopa is used alone. Three types have been described:

End-of-dose Akinesia: episodic re-emergence of Parkinsonian symptoms three or more hours after each dose of levodopa, often following a period of dyskinesia. This type of akinesia tends to occur progressively earlier after each dose during prolonged therapy and is regarded as resulting from a temporary insufficiency of dopamine at the appropriate receptor sites.

On-off Phenomenon: a rapid alternation between a state of satisfactory motility, usually with oral-facial dyskinesias and a rigid akinetic state without dyskinesias. This oscillation of performance is also regarded as being associated with a temporary insufficiency of dopamine.

Akinesia Paradoxica (Hypotonic Freezing): irregular episodes of sudden freezing, usually short duration, with the patient unable to move, accompanied by hypotonia and postural instability. These episodes are at times accompanied by autonomic symptoms. Hypotonic freezing is regarded as possibly associated with a severe temporary deficiency in noradrenaline in progressively depleted and damaged noradrenaline pathways.

Psychiatric Disorders: paranoid ideation, psychotic episodes, depression (with or without development of suicidal tendencies) and dementia. In depressed patients, levodopa may give rise to an improvement in mood in a small number of individuals. However, when administered to patients with bipolar depression, it tends regularly to produce hypomania. Various psychiatric disturbances have been reported in about 20% of patients.

Gastrointestinal Effects: Undesirable gastrointestinal effects, which may occur mainly in the early stages of the treatment, can largely be controlled by taking PROLOPA with a small snack (e.g., biscuits) or liquid, or by increasing the dose slowly.

Other adverse reactions that have been reported less frequently are:

Cardiovascular: arrhythmias and orthostatic hypotensive episodes, hypertension, non-specific ECG changes, flushing, phlebitis and angina pectoris.

Dermatologic: dark sweat, sweating, edema, hair loss, pallor, rash, pruritus.

Gastrointestinal: nausea and vomiting, constipation, diarrhea, epigastric and abdominal distress or pain, flatulence, eructation, hiccups, sialorrhea, difficulty in swallowing, bitter taste, dry mouth, duodenal ulcer, gastrointestinal bleeding, burning sensation of the tongue.

General: fever, weight variation, anorexia, isolated cases of loss of taste.

Genitourinary: dark urine, hematuria, nocturia and urinary frequency, retention or incontinence and changes in libido.

Hematologic: hemolytic anemia, transient leukopenia, agranulocytosis, thrombocytopenia.

Intellectual Function: Progressive impairment of intellectual and autonomic functions has been described, particularly in akinetic patients, after prolonged levodopa therapy.

Musculoskeletal: low back pain, muscle spasm and twitching, musculoskeletal pain.

Neurologic: ataxia, faintness, impairment of gait, headache, increased hand tremor, akinetic episodes, torticollis, trismus, tightness of the mouth, lips or tongue, oculogyric crisis, weakness, numbness, bruxism and convulsions.

Ophthalmologic: blurred vision, diplopia, dilated pupils, activation of latent Horner's syndrome.

Psychiatric: increased libido with serious antisocial behaviour, euphoria, lethargy, sedation, stimulation, fatigue and malaise, confusion, insomnia, nightmares, hallucinations and delusions, agitation, temporal disorientation and anxiety, somnolence and very rarely excessive daytime somnolence and sudden sleep onset episodes. Agitation, anxiety, insomnia, hallucinations, delusions and temporal disorientation may occur particularly in elderly patients and in patients with a history of such disorders.

Respiratory: cough, hoarseness, bizarre breathing pattern, post nasal drip.

Pathological (compulsive) gambling has been reported in post-marketing data, including those in the literature, for antiparkinsonian drugs. Sporadic cases of pathological (compulsive) gambling have been reported in patients treated with dopaminergic agents including levodopa. Dosage adjustments should be considered in the management of this behaviour.

Abnormal Hematologic and Clinical Chemistry Findings: Elevations of BUN, serum uric acid, AST, ALT, LDH, bilirubin, alkaline phosphatase or PBI have been observed. Positive Coombs' tests have been observed during extended therapy, both with PROLOPA and with levodopa alone but hemolytic anemia is extremely rare.

DRUG INTERACTIONS: Drug-Drug Interactions: Cardiovascular Drugs: Postural hypotensive episodes have been reported; therefore, PROLOPA (levodopa and benserazide combination) should be administered cautiously and blood pressure monitored in patients on antihypertensive medication. It may be necessary to adjust the dosage of the latter particularly during the initial stages of therapy with PROLOPA. Antihypertensive medications containing reserpine inhibit the action of PROLOPA.

MAO Inhibitors: See Contraindications.

Psychoactive Drugs: If concomitant administration of psychoactive drugs is necessary, they should be administered with great caution. Patients should be carefully observed for unusual untoward drug effects (see Contraindications and Warnings and Precautions, Psychiatric). Neuroleptics and opioids inhibit the action of PROLOPA.

Anesthetics: If a patient on levodopa requires general anesthetics, the normal PROLOPA regimen should be continued as close to surgery as possible, except in the case of halothane (see Warnings and Precautions). PROLOPA should be discontinued 12-48 hours before surgical intervention requiring general anesthesia with halothane as fluctuations in blood pressure and/or arrhythmias may occur in patients being treated with PROLOPA. Therapy with PROLOPA may be resumed following surgery; the dosage should be increased gradually to the preoperative level (see Warnings and Precautions).

Sympathomimetics: PROLOPA should not be administered concomitantly with sympathomimetics (agents such as epinephrine, norepinephrine, isoproterenol or amphetamine which stimulate the sympathetic nervous system) as levodopa may potentiate their effects (see Contraindications). Should concomitant administration prove necessary, close surveillance of the cardiovascular system is essential, and the dose of the sympathomimetic agents may need to be reduced.

Trihexyphenidyl: Coadministration of the anticholinergic drug trihexyphenidyl with PROLOPA reduces the rate, but not the extent, of levodopa absorption.

Ferrous Sulphate: Ferrous sulphate decreases the maximum plasma concentration and the AUC of levodopa by 30% to 50%. The pharmacokinetic changes observed during co-treatment with ferrous sulphate appear to be clinically significant in some but not all patients.

Metoclopramide: Metoclopramide increases the rate of absorption.

Other Compounds: There are no pharmacokinetic interactions between levodopa and the following: bromocriptine, amantidine, selegiline, and domperidone.

Other Anti-Parkinsonian Agents: Combination with other anti-parkinsonian agents (anticholinergics, amantadine, dopamine agonists) is permissible, though both the desired and undesired effects of treatment may be intensified. It may be necessary to reduce the dosage of PROLOPA or the other substance. When initiating an adjuvant treatment with a COMT inhibitor, a reduction of the dosage of PROLOPA may be necessary. Anticholinergics should not be withdrawn abruptly when therapy with PROLOPA is instituted, as levodopa does not begin to take effect for some time.

Drug-Food Interactions: Since certain amino acids can compete with the absorption of levodopa, the absorption of levodopa may be impaired and its effects may be diminished when administered with a protein-rich meal in some patients.

Taking PROLOPA with a small snack (e.g., biscuits) or liquid does not impair absorption and may help to control gastrointestinal side effects.

Drug-Herb Interactions: No drug-herb interactions have been established.

Drug-Laboratory Test Interactions: Levodopa may affect the results of laboratory tests for catecholamines, creatinine, uric acid and glucose.

DOSAGE AND ADMINISTRATION: Dosing Considerations: General: In order to achieve maximal benefit and reduce the incidence of adverse reactions, therapy with PROLOPA (levodopa and benserazide combination) should be introduced gradually and must be individualized. Drug administration must be continuously matched to the needs and tolerance of the patient. The following dosing instructions should therefore be regarded as guidelines. Because of the increased availability of levodopa to the central nervous system when administered in combined therapy, titration and adjustments of dosage should be made in small steps and the dosage ranges recommended should usually not be exceeded. The appearance of involuntary movements should be regarded as a sign of levodopa toxicity and as an indication of overdosage, usually requiring a reduction in dosage. Treatment should aim at maximal benefit without dyskinesias. Patients should be carefully observed for possible undesirable psychiatric symptoms (see Warnings and Precautions, Psychiatric).

Levodopa should be discontinued for at least twelve (12) hours before initiating therapy with PROLOPA (see Warnings and Precautions, General).

PROLOPA must not be withdrawn abruptly, due to risk of neuroleptic malignant syndrome (see Warnings and Precautions, Neurologic, Neuroleptic Malignant Syndrome).

Geriatrics: Dosage must be carefully titrated in the elderly.

Pediatrics and Young Adults (<25 years of age): The safety and effectiveness of PROLOPA have not been established in these populations (see Contraindications and Warnings and Precautions).

Recommended Dose and Dosage Adjustment: Initiation of Treatment in Patients Not on Levodopa Therapy: The initial recommended dose is one capsule of PROLOPA 100-25 once or twice a day. This dose may be carefully increased by one capsule every third or fourth day until an optimal therapeutic effect is obtained without dyskinesias. Near the upper limits of dosage, the increments should be made slowly, at two to four week intervals for example. The dosage should be divided, aiming at a frequency of dosing of at least four times daily taken with or immediately after meals.

The optimal dosage for most patients is usually four to eight capsules of PROLOPA 100-25 daily (400 mg to 800 mg of levodopa) divided into four to six doses. Most patients require no more than six capsules of PROLOPA 100-25 (600 mg of levodopa) per day.

Individual patient response varies. Some patients, e.g., post-encephalitic Parkinson patients, may only tolerate a slower rate of increase in dosage, e.g., one capsule of PROLOPA 100-25 at weekly intervals, since these patients are more sensitive to levodopa and usually only tolerate lower dosages.

PROLOPA 200-50 capsules are intended only for maintenance therapy once the optimal dosage has been determined using PROLOPA 100-25 capsules. No patient should receive more than five to six capsules of PROLOPA 200-50 daily (1000 mg to 1200 mg of levodopa in combined therapy) during the first year of therapy.

Treatment should be continued for at least three to six weeks before it is concluded that therapy with PROLOPA has not benefited the patient.

Initiation of Treatment in Patients on Levodopa Therapy: Allow at least twelve (12) hours or more to elapse between the last dose of levodopa and the first dose of PROLOPA. A dosage of PROLOPA should be used that will provide approximately 15% of the previous levodopa daily dosage. For example, if a patient is receiving 4000 mg of levodopa per day, the dosage of PROLOPA 100-25 should not exceed six capsules (600 mg of levodopa) divided into four to six doses.

Adjustment and Maintenance of Therapy in All Patients: PROLOPA 200-50 capsules may be used for maintenance therapy once the optimal dosage has been determined using PROLOPA 100-25 capsules. PROLOPA 50-12.5 capsules should be used when frequent dosing is required to minimize adverse effects. During the first year of treatment, the total daily dosage should not exceed 1000 mg to 1200 mg of levodopa in combined therapy.

The variability in dosage response of patients is considerable. Some individuals may experience oscillations in performance with a diurnal rhythm of periods of symptomatic control alternating with periods of akinesia (end-of-dose), with return of Parkinson's symptoms, which can frequently be corrected by re-scheduling individual doses. A low protein diet tends to potentiate and stabilize the effects of levodopa, whereas a high protein diet may decrease the effect of levodopa, although with combined therapy this effect may be less prominent. The predominant limiting factor in treatment with PROLOPA is the occurrence of involuntary movements. These frequently can be controlled by reducing the dosage of levodopa and varying the frequency of individual doses. A progressive decrease in the threshold for dyskinetic manifestations and an increase in the incidence of oscillations in performance have been reported after a certain time on levodopa therapy. These appear earlier in the course of combined treatment with PROLOPA than with levodopa alone.

In an attempt to avoid the emergence, or decrease the incidence of these manifestations, it is recommended that, after the initial period, the daily maintenance dosage of levodopa as combined therapy should be reduced slowly (at a rate of about 50 mg a month) over a period of a few months, to a maintenance level without dyskinesias. After one year of therapy, the patient should usually receive not more than six capsules of PROLOPA 100-25 daily (600 mg of levodopa) divided into at least four to six doses.

Other antiparkinson agents, e.g., anticholinergics, amantadine, and dopamine agonists may be continued during therapy with PROLOPA (although both the desired and undesired effects of treatment may be intensified) and should not be abruptly withdrawn. However, as treatment proceeds, their dosage may need to be altered (see Drug Interactions).

Interruption of Therapy: If therapy with PROLOPA is interrupted for a brief period, the previous dosage may be administered as soon as the patient is again able to take oral medication. If, however, therapy is interrupted for a longer period, a lower dosage should be given and the dosage should be adjusted gradually. In many cases, patients can be returned rapidly to their previous therapeutic dosage.

Administration: PROLOPA should be taken orally in divided doses.

It is recommended that the capsules be swallowed whole and not be opened or dissolved in liquid.

OVERDOSAGE:

Symptoms and Signs: Symptoms and signs of overdose are qualitatively similar to the side effects of PROLOPA (levodopa and benserazide) in therapeutic doses but may be of greater severity. Overdose may lead to: cardiovascular side effects (e.g. cardiac arrhythmias), psychiatric disturbances (e.g. confusion and insomnia), gastro-intestinal effects (e.g. nausea and vomiting) and abnormal involuntary movements (see Warnings and Precautions, Neurologic).

Treatment: Monitor the patient's vital signs and institute supportive measures as indicated by the patient's clinical state. Intravenous fluids should be administered judiciously and an adequate airway maintained. Monitoring of respiratory function is recommended. It may be necessary to administer respiratory stimulants, or where appropriate, neuroleptics. ECG monitoring should be instituted and the patient carefully observed for the development of arrhythmias and if required appropriate anti-arrhythmic therapy should be provided. To date, the value of dialysis in the treatment of PROLOPA (levodopa and benserazide combination) overdosage is not known. Consideration should be given to the possibility of multiple drug ingestion by the patient. Pyridoxine is ineffective in reversing the effects of PROLOPA overdosage.

> For management of a suspected drug overdose, CPhA recommends that you contact your **regional Poison Control Centre**. See the *CPS* Directory section for a list of Poison Control Centres.

ACTION AND CLINICAL PHARMACOLOGY: Mechanism of Action: The symptoms of Parkinson's disease are to a high degree associated with striatal dopamine deficiency and degeneration of the dopamine containing neurons in the nigro-striatal bundle. Levodopa (INN) or L-DOPA (3,4-dihydroxy L-henylalanine) is an intermediate in dopamine biosynthesis. Levodopa (dopamine precursor) is used as a prodrug to increase dopamine levels since it is able to cross the blood-brain barrier whereas dopamine itself cannot. Once levodopa has entered the central nervous system (CNS), it is metabolized to dopamine by aromatic L-amino acid decarboxylase.

Levodopa, which does permeate the blood-brain barrier, appears to correct the akinesia of Parkinson's disease by the formation of dopamine at nigro-striatal dopaminergic sites that remain functional. While rigidity and tremor also improve with levodopa therapy, these symptoms seem to be related to a disturbed balance of neurotransmitters.

When levodopa is given alone, a large proportion of it does not reach the brain, because it is rapidly converted to dopamine by aromatic acid decarboxylase at extracerebral sites. Large doses must therefore be given in order to allow for sufficient levodopa to reach the brain and provide the dopamine needed to correct the deficiency observed in patients with Parkinson's disease. These large doses of levodopa result in a sharp increase in the levels of circulating dopamine and other dopa metabolites, and the excessive quantities of these substances in extracerebral tissues may explain in part some of the side effects of levodopa, such as nausea, vomiting and cardiac arrhythmias. The high incidence of these adverse effects requires a very slow titration of levodopa and may interfere with the administration of an effective drug dosage.

The decarboxylase inhibitor, benserazide, at the recommended therapeutic doses, does not cross the blood-brain barrier. Thus, administration of this agent makes it possible to inhibit the peripheral decarboxylation of levodopa without significantly affecting its metabolism in the brain.

In this way, the formation of circulating dopamine is minimized and the incidence of extracerebral side effects may thereby be reduced while at the same time permitting more levodopa to reach the brain. Combined therapy with levodopa and benserazide reduces the amount of levodopa required for optimum therapeutic benefit and permits an earlier response to therapy.

Nevertheless, combined therapy does not decrease the adverse reactions due to central effects of levodopa. In fact, dyskinesias and oscillations in performance occur at lower dosages of levodopa and earlier in treatment during combined therapy.

Plasma levels of levodopa are markedly increased when the drug is given in combination with benserazide compared to those obtained after levodopa alone. There is also a reduction in the level of dopa metabolites when levodopa is combined with benserazide. Clinical trials have suggested that the combination of levodopa and benserazide in a 4 to 1 ratio is effective in reducing peripheral side effects and the amount of levodopa required for therapeutic improvement.

Pharmacokinetics: The pharmacokinetics of ^{14}C-benserazide administered alone and in combination with levodopa has been studied in six patients with Parkinson's disease. Three of these patients were administered 50 mg of the inhibitor by both intravenous and oral routes. Three additional patients received oral doses of 50 mg ^{14}C-benserazide alone and also in combination with 200 mg of levodopa.

Comparison of the time-plasma concentration curves of total radioactivity in the patients receiving oral and intravenous ^{14}C-benserazide indicated that between 66 and 74% of the administered dose was absorbed from the gastrointestinal tract. Peak plasma concentrations of radioactivity were detected one hour after oral administration in five of the six patients.

Elimination of the ^{14}C-label was primarily by urinary excretion with 86% to 90% of an intravenous dose recovered in the urine while 53 to 64% of the oral dose was detected in the urine. The majority of the ^{14}C radioisotope was accounted for in the urine within 48 hours after administration. Fecal recovery studies conducted over five to eight days accounted for the majority (approximately 30%) of the remainder of administered ^{14}C-benserazide.

In still another experiment in man, where ^{14}C-dopa had been administered either intravenously (0.1 mg/kg) or orally (3 mg/kg), the administration of benserazide (16 to 24 mg orally) enhanced the ^{14}C dopa and ^{14}C-methyldopa plasma concentrations 6 to 10 fold over those observed with the administration of ^{14}C-dopa alone. Also, the ^{14}C-phenolcarboxylic acid concentration was 1/5 to 1/10th that which was observed when ^{14}C-dopa was administered alone.

Absorption: Levodopa is mainly absorbed from the upper regions of the small intestine. Maximum plasma concentrations of levodopa are reached approximately one hour after ingestion of PROLOPA (levodopa and benserazide combination). The bioavailability of levodopa from PROLOPA is 98% (range 74-112%).

Food intake impairs or reduces the rate and extent of levodopa absorption. The peak levodopa plasma concentration is 30% lower and occurs later when PROLOPA is administered after a standard meal. The extent of levodopa absorption is reduced by 15% due to an increase in gastric emptying time.

Distribution: Levodopa crosses the blood-brain barrier by a saturable transport system. It is not bound to plasma proteins, and its volume of distribution is 57 litres. In contrast to levodopa, benserazide does not penetrate the blood-brain barrier at therapeutic doses. It is concentrated mainly in the kidneys, lungs, small intestine and liver.

Metabolism: Levodopa is metabolized by two major pathways (decarboxylation and O-methylation) and two minor ones (transamination and oxidation).

Aromatic amino acid decarboxylase converts levodopa to dopamine. The major end-products of this pathway are homovanillic acid and dihydroxyphenylacetic acid.

Catechol-O-methyltransferase methylates levodopa to 3-O-methyldopa. This major plasma metabolite has an elimination half-life of 15 hours and accumulates in patients who are treated with therapeutic doses of PROLOPA.

Decreased peripheral decarboxylation of levodopa when it is administered with benserazide is reflected in higher plasma levels of levodopa and 3-O-methyldopa and lower plasma levels of catecholamines (dopamine, noradrenaline) and phenolcarboxylic acids (homovanillic acid and dihydroxyphenylacetic acid).

Benserazide is hydroxylated to trihydroxybenzylhydrazine in the intestinal mucosa and the liver. This metabolite is a potent inhibitor of the aromatic amino acid decarboxylase.

Pyridoxine hydrochloride (Vitamin B_6) accelerates the decarboxylation of levodopa and is therefore contraindicated in patients on levodopa alone.

Excretion: In the presence of peripherally inhibited levodopa decarboxylase, the elimination half-life of levodopa is approximately 1.5 hours. The elimination half-life is slightly longer in elderly patients with Parkinson's disease. The clearance of levodopa in plasma is about 430 mL/min.

Benserazide is almost entirely eliminated by metabolism. The metabolites are mainly excreted in the urine (64%) and to a smaller extent in feces (24%).

STORAGE AND STABILITY: Keep in a tightly closed, light-resistant container. Store at 15-30°C.

INFORMATION FOR THE PATIENT: Published in e-CPS, available by subscription at www.e-cps.ca.

DOSAGE FORMS, COMPOSITION AND PACKAGING: Prolopa 50-12.5: Each light grey and blue capsule, size #4, imprinted ROCHE (black ink) on both body and cap, contains: levodopa 50 mg and benserazide base 12.5 mg in the form of benserazide HCl. Nonmedicinal ingredients: gelatin, indigotine, iron oxide, magnesium stearate, mannitol, microcrystalline cellulose, povidone, talc and titanium dioxide. Energy: 0.7 kJ (0.2 kcal). Gluten-, lactose-, paraben-, sodium-, sulfite- and tartrazine-free. Bottles of 100.

Prolopa 100-25: Each blue and pale pink colored capsule, size #2, imprinted ROCHE (black ink) on both body and cap, contains: levodopa 100 mg and benserazide base 25 mg in the form of benserazide HCl. Nonmedicinal ingredients: gelatin, indigotine, iron oxide, magnesium stearate, microcrystalline cellulose, povidone, talc and titanium dioxide. Energy-, gluten-, lactose-, paraben-, sodium-, sulfite- and tartrazine-free. Bottles of 100.

Prolopa 200-50: Each blue and caramel colored capsule, size #1, imprinted ROCHE (black ink) on both body and cap, contains: levodopa 200 mg and benserazide base 50 mg in the form of benserazide HCl. Nonmedicinal ingredients: gelatin, indigotine, iron oxide, magnesium stearate, microcrystalline cellulose, povidone, talc and titanium dioxide. Energy-, gluten-, lactose-, paraben-, sodium-, sulfite- and tartrazine-free. Bottles of 100.

(Shown in Product Identification Section)

Promethazine

promethazine HCl

Phenothiazine Antihistamine

CPhA Monograph

Date of Preparation: September 2007

> This monograph has been compiled by CPhA and reviewed by experts. It may contain information different from that found in Health Canada-approved Product Monographs. The reader is referred to the *CPS* Editorial Policy for more information.

SUMMARY PRODUCT INFORMATION:

Route of Administration[a]	Dosage Form[a]	Strength[a]
Parenteral	Injectable solution	25 mg/mL (1 mL, 2 mL)
Oral	Syrup	2 mg/mL
Oral	Tablet	25 mg, 50 mg

[a] For specific product information consult Health Canada's Drug Product Database http://www.hc-sc.gc.ca/dhp-mps/prodpharma/databasdon/index_e.html.

INDICATIONS AND CLINICAL USE: Promethazine is indicated for:

- Treatment of allergic reactions including hay fever, urticaria, pruritus, poison ivy, insect bites, skin allergies and vasomotor rhinitis. However, use as an antihistamine in ambulatory patients is limited by pronounced sedative effects. Promethazine is also used for the treatment of allergic reactions to blood or plasma and as adjunctive therapy in anaphylactic reactions.
- Treatment of nausea and vomiting associated with surgery, anesthesia, centrally-acting emetics, gastroenteritis, radiation sickness, metabolic or endocrine disorders. It is also effective in the management of motion sickness, unlike most other phenothiazines.
- Promethazine is used as a sedative in insomnia or anxiety and as an anesthetic potentiator.

CONTRAINDICATIONS:

- Patients who are hypersensitive to promethazine or to any ingredient in the formulation or component of the container. Cross-reactivity may occur among phenothiazines.
- Children under two years of age because of the risk of potentially fatal respiratory depression.
- Patients who are comatose and/or have received large doses of other CNS depressants.
- Lower respiratory tract symptoms including asthma.

WARNINGS AND PRECAUTIONS: General: Use with caution in patients with conditions associated with CNS depression. The parenteral formulation may contain sodium metabisulfite that may cause allergic-type reactions in susceptible patients.

It should **not** be administered by subcutaneous or intra-arterial injection. Severe tissue damage is possible with the intravenous route of administration. Discontinue immediately if pain or burning occur.

Because of the potential for extrapyramidal symptoms, promethazine should not be given to children with signs and symptoms of Reye's syndrome since diagnosis of this condition may be obscured.

Phenothiazines affect thermoregulation. Use promethazine with caution in patients who might be exposed to extreme heat or cold.

Cardiovascular: Promethazine should not be used in patients with hemodynamic instability or severe cardiac disease. Because life-threatening arrhythmias have occurred in patients taking therapeutic doses of phenothiazines the drug should not be used in patients with cardiac conduction abnormalities. Promethazine should also be used cautiously in patients with hypotension or those unable to tolerate hypotensive episodes (e.g., cerebrovascular disease) as it can cause orthostatic hypotension.

Gastrointestinal: Because of possible anticholinergic effects monitor patients with decreased gastrointestinal motility. The antiemetic properties of promethazine can mask the symptoms of intestinal obstruction.

Genitourinary: Urinary retention associated with benign prostatic hyperplasia may be worsened by phenothiazines through their anticholinergic effects.

Hematologic: Use promethazine with caution in patients with bone marrow suppression as it has been reported to cause blood dyscrasias.

Hepatic/Biliary/Pancreatic: Use with caution in patients with severe hepatic disease.

Neurologic: Use with caution in patients with Parkinson's disease as the drug may cause anticholinergic effects. It may cause extrapyramidal symptoms such as akathisia, tardive dyskinesia or acute dystonic reactions.

Promethazine may also be associated with neuroleptic malignant syndrome. Monitor the patient for fever, muscle rigidity, autonomic instability and/or changes in mental status. Cholinergic blockade may also worsen myasthenia gravis.

Promethazine should be used cautiously in patients with seizure disorder as it may lower seizure threshold. Patients using opioids, local anesthetics or other drugs that also decrease seizure threshold may be at increased risk. These cautions also apply to patients with head trauma or alcoholism.

The drug should be used with caution in subcortical brain damage. The cause of nausea and vomiting should be diagnosed before using high doses of promethazine as the antiemetic properties can mask the symptoms of increased intracranial pressure.

Ophthalmic: Because it is a phenothiazine with possible anticholinergic effects, promethazine should be used with caution in patients with angle-closure glaucoma. Screening is often recommended.

Renal: The drug should be used with caution in patients with severe renal disease.

Special Populations: Pregnant Women: Promethazine crosses the placenta. In a few cases, administration during delivery has been associated with respiratory depression in the newborn. However, in larger series no evidence of respiratory depression was found. Use during labour has also been associated with impaired platelet aggregation in the newborn. Clinical significance is unknown but the degree of impairment is similar to the amount seen in diseases associated with a definite bleeding risk.

Promethazine has been used as an antiemetic in pregnant women. It has also been used as an adjunct to opioid analgesics during labour. Transient EEG and behavioural changes were seen in a small series of newborns whose mothers received meperidine in combination with either promethazine or phenobarbital at term.

Animal studies did not reveal teratogenic effects.

Nursing Women: Excretion in breast milk is unknown. Because of its low molecular weight, passage into breast milk should be expected. The American Academy of Pediatrics classifies promethazine as a drug whose effect on nursing infants is unknown but may be of concern. Based on the minimal excretion of other phenothiazine derivatives, occasional short-term use of promethazine for the treatment of nausea and vomiting poses little risk. However, with repeated doses the infant should be monitored for excess sedation. Promethazine can lower basal prolactin secretion. As such, if it is given in the early postpartum period the drug may interfere with the establishment of breastfeeding.

Pediatrics: Because respiratory fatalities have been reported in children less than two years of age the drug should not be used in this age group.

Promethazine should be used with caution in children with a history of sleep apnea or family history of SIDS. It has been hypothesized that phenothiazines depress arousal and respiratory mechanisms in normal sleeping infants.

Children over two years of age should be given the lowest effective dose. Avoid concomitant use of other drugs with respiratory depressant effects.

Children performing hazardous activities such as bicycle riding while receiving promethazine should be supervised.

Geriatrics: Clinical studies of promethazine did not include significant numbers of subjects over 65 years of age. Because of the risk of sedative effects and confusion, older individuals should probably have therapy initiated with doses in the lower end of the dosage range. Promethazine is included as a drug of concern on the Beers list of potentially harmful drugs in the elderly because of its propensity to cause sedation and adverse anticholinergic effects.

Occupational Hazards: Caution patients about performing tasks which require mental alertness such as driving or operating heavy machinery as the drug can cause drowsiness or dizziness.

ADVERSE REACTIONS: Cardiovascular: bradycardia, nonspecific QT changes, hypertension. Hypotension and tachycardia are seen rarely but may occur at the beginning of parenteral therapy. Rapid intravenous administration may result in transient hypotension. This can usually be avoided by giving the drug slowly.

Central Nervous System: Drowsiness, sedation and confusion are the most common adverse effects of promethazine; paradoxical reactions such as hyperexcitability and/or nightmares are seen especially in children (rare). Akathisia, catatonic states, hallucinations, dizziness, neuroleptic malignant syndrome, seizure, tardive dyskinesia, confusion, euphoria, lassitude, insomnia, oculogyric crises and dystonias including extremity tremor and torticollis have all been reported. The risk for dystonias appears to be increased in dehydrated children.

Extrapyramidal symptoms may occur with higher doses of promethazine and generally remit with dosage reduction.

With parenteral administration of promethazine patients with untreated pain have displayed athetoid-like movements of the upper extremities. These usually subside with adequate pain control.

Allergic/Dermatologic: allergic reactions including contact dermatitis, urticaria (common) and slate gray skin pigmentation. Photosensitivity may be a contraindication to continued therapy.

Local reactions including severe chemical irritation and tissue damage can occur with parenteral therapy. These reactions range from burning, pain, swelling and erythema to phlebitis, abscesses and tissue necrosis. Inadvertent intra-arterial injection must be avoided as it has resulted in gangrene requiring amputation. Nerve damage from parenteral administration has been reported as temporary sensory loss to paralysis.

Ear/Nose/Throat: tinnitus.

Endocrine and Metabolism: amenorrhea, gynecomastia, breast engorgement, fever, heat stroke.

Gastrointestinal: Nausea and vomiting may accompany hypotension usually with parenteral therapy. Dry mouth is a common anticholinergic side effect. Constipation has been reported.

Genitourinary: urinary retention.

Hematologic: agranulocytosis, eosinophilia, hemolytic anemia, thrombocytopenia, thrombocytopenia purpura, aplastic anemia, leukopenia (rare).

Hepatic/Biliary/Pancreatic: Jaundice has been reported with high doses of promethazine.

Immune: angioedema.

Neurologic: incoordination, tremor.

Ophthalmologic: corneal and lenticular changes, diplopia, pigmentary retinopathy, blurred vision (rare).

Respiratory: respiratory depression, apnea, nasal congestion, asthma.

Sexual Function/Reproduction: impotence, ejaculatory disorder.

DRUG INTERACTIONS: Overview: Promethazine is a substrate of CYP2B6 and CYP2D6. CYP2B6 inhibitors such as desipramine and sertraline may increase the expected and adverse effects of promethazine. The same might be expected for CYP2D6 inhibitors such as paroxetine and fluoxetine. Promethazine is also a weak inhibitor of CYP2D6. CYP2B6 inducers such as carbamazepine and phenytoin may decrease the effects of promethazine.

Drug-Drug Interactions: See Table 1.

Table 1: Promethazine

Drug-Drug Interactions

Interacting Drug	Effect	Clinical Comment
Anticholinergic agents	Additive anticholinergic effects. It is also possible that the therapeutic effects of promethazine may be decreased by centrally acting anticholinergics.	Of particular concern in certain individuals, e.g., patients with benign prostatic hyperplasia or angle-closure glaucoma or older individuals
CNS depressants	Additive sedative and respiratory effects with other CNS depressants including alcohol	If promethazine is used concomitantly with barbiturates dosage of the latter should be reduced by at least 50%. Opioid doses should be reduced by 25-50% when used with promethazine.
Epinephrine	Possible reversal of vasopressor effect of epinephrine	Patients receiving promethazine and requiring a vasopressor agent should be given norepinephrine or phenylephrine.
Fluoroquinolone antibiotics (gatifloxacin, levofloxacin, moxifloxacin)	Possible ↑ risk of cardiac arrhythmias including torsades de pointes.	Avoid coadministration of drugs that may prolong the QT interval such as levofloxacin. Use gatifloxacin and moxifloxacin with caution.
Monoamine oxidase (MAO) inhibitors	↑ extrapyramidal effects	

Drug-Herb Interactions: Valerian, St John's wort and gotu kola may increase the CNS depressant effects of promethazine.

Drug-Laboratory Interactions: Promethazine may interfere with ABO blood grouping. It inhibits the wheal and flare response during allergy skin testing.

Promethazine use may result in false positives on urine salicylate assays that are based upon the Trinder method.

It may also interfere with several immunologic urinary pregnancy tests based on human chorionic gonadotropin, yielding either false positive or false negative results.

Glucose tolerance tests may yield falsely elevated serum glucose concentrations.

DOSAGE AND ADMINISTRATION: Recommended Dose and Dosage Adjustment: Adults: See Table 2.

Table 2: Promethazine

Dose in Adult Patients

Indication	Route	Usual Dose
Anesthesia, adjunct	IM, IV[a]	25–50 mg prior to surgery
Antiemetic	Oral, IM, IV[a]	Oral: 12.5–25 mg Q4–6H prn IM, IV: 25 mg; may repeat within 2 hours if needed
Allergic conditions	Oral, IM, IV[a]	Oral: 6.25–12.5 mg before meals and at bedtime OR 25 mg QHS IM, IV: 25 mg; may repeat in 2 hours when necessary. Switch to oral therapy as soon as possible Prevention or control of minor transfusion reactions: 25 mg prior to or during blood transfusion
Motion sickness	Oral	25 mg twice daily with the first dose 30 minutes to 1 hour before departure, then repeat 8–12 hours later as needed
Postoperative pain, adjunct	IM, IV[a]	25–50 mg combined with appropriately reduced dose of analgesic
Sedative-hypnotic	Oral, IM, IV[a]	25–50 mg per dose; repeat every 4–6 hours as needed. Not to exceed 100 mg daily.

[a] IV administration is not the preferred route as tissue damage may occur.

Geriatrics: See Table 3.

Table 3: Promethazine

Dose in Geriatric Patients

Indication	Initial Dose	Usual Dose
All indications	IV[a]: To limit the risk of perivascular extravasation in elderly patients, the Institute for Safe Medication Practices recommends a starting dose of 6.25–12.5 mg.	Dosage should be lower in elderly patients.

[a] IV administration is not the preferred route as tissue damage may occur.

Pediatrics: See Table 4.

Table 4: Promethazine

Dose in Pediatric Patients Over Two Years of Age

Indication	Route	Age/Weight	Initial Dose	Usual Dose	Maximum Dose
Allergic conditions	Oral	Only for children over 2 years of age	Use with extreme caution, administering the lowest effective dose	0.1 mg/kg/dose Q6H prn during the day; and 0.5 mg/kg/dose prn at bedtime	Not to exceed 12.5 mg per dose during the day Not to exceed 25 mg per dose at bedtime
Antiemetic	Oral, IM, IV[a]	See Allergic conditions	See Allergic conditions	0.25–1 mg/kg Q4–6H prn	Not to exceed 25 mg per dose
Motion sickness	Oral	See Allergic conditions	See Allergic conditions	0.5 mg/kg 30 minutes to 1 hour before departure then every 12 hours as needed	Not to exceed 25 mg per dose
Postoperative pain, adjunct	Oral	See Allergic conditions	See Allergic conditions	12.5–25 mg combined with appropriately reduced doses of analgesics	
Sedative-hypnotic	Oral, IM, IV[a]	See Allergic conditions	See Allergic conditions	0.5–1 mg/kg/dose every 6 hours as needed	Not to exceed 50 mg per dose

[a] IV administration is not the preferred route as tissue damage may occur.

Renal Impairement: No specific dosage adjustment is recommended in renal insufficiency.

Missed Dose: If a dose is missed patients should be instructed to take the missed as soon as they remember. If it is close to time for the next dose patients should be instructed to wait until then and return to their regular schedule. Doses should **not** be doubled.

Administration: Promethazine is a chemical irritant capable of causing necrosis.3 Deep im injection is the preferred parenteral route of administration.

Avoid iv use if possible. For iv administration the infusion rate should not exceed 25 mg/minute. Consider administration over 10 to 15 minutes. Dilute to a maximum concentration of 25 mg/mL; more dilute solutions are recommended. Injection should be into the tubing of a running infusion when possible at the point furthest from the patient's vein or through a large bore vein. Avoid perivascular extravasation. Do not administer intra-arterially or subcutaneously. Ensure patency of the site before the drug is administered. Blood can become discoloured on contact with promethazine so aspiration of dark blood does not rule out inadvertent intra-arterial placement. Patients should be instructed to report any burning or pain during injection.

To decrease gastrointestinal discomfort administer oral doses with food, milk or water.

OVERDOSAGE:

Signs and Symptoms: Clinical manifestations of overdose are generally extensions of adverse effects seen with therapeutic use. Symptoms of promethazine toxicity include respiratory and CNS depression, and the anticholinergic toxidrome which includes tachycardia, hyperthermia, mydriasis, dry mouth, dry flushed skin and urinary retention. In addition to CNS depression, other CNS toxicity includes hallucinations, seizures, delirium and myoclonic or choreoathetoid movements. CNS stimulation is seen more often in young children and the elderly.

Recommended Management: Monitor patient's vital signs and mental status. Initiate supportive treatment. Isotonic iv fluids (e.g., 0.9% sodium chloride or lactated Ringer solution) or Trendelenburg positioning should correct hypotension. For hypotension that does not respond to these measures, use norepinephrine or phenylephrine. Patients should have cardiac monitoring to observe for signs of sodium channel blockade (i.e., increased QRS duration) and potassium channel blockade (i.e., prolonged QTc interval). Sodium channel blockade is treated with sodium bicarbonate 1 to 2 mEq/kg iv. QTc prolongation and torsades may respond to magnesium sulfate 2 g iv or overdrive pacing if necessary. When treatment is required benzodiazepines can be administered for seizures. Barbiturates (e.g., phenobarbital, pentobarbital) or propofol are other options for seizure control.

Hyperthermic patients should be treated with benzodiazepines to control psychomotor agitation and external cooling measures (e.g., mist, fan, ice packs). Hyperthermia can cause multisystem organ failure and disseminated intravascular coagulation.

Extrapyramidal symptoms such as dystonic reactions can be treated with diphenhydramine 0.5 to 1 mg/kg in adults up to a maximum of 50 mg im or slow iv push or benztropine mesylate 1 to 2 mg iv (adults). These agents usually show effects within 2 to 5 minutes.

Activated charcoal 1 g/kg po may be considered in patients who present within one hour of overdose and who have no contraindications to its administration.

Promethazine is not dialyzable. Measurement of promethazine concentrations in body fluids is not widely available and unnecessary for assessment and management.

For management of a suspected drug overdose, CPhA recommends that you contact your **regional Poison Control Centre**. See the *CPS* Directory section for a list of Poison Control Centres.

ACTION AND CLINICAL PHARMACOLOGY: Mechanism of Action: Although promethazine is a phenothiazine derivative, it is structurally unlike the antipsychotic phenothiazines. Antihistamine, antiemetic and sedative effects come from its histamine H_1 receptor-blocking properties. It does not block the secretion of histamine. It also depresses the release of hypothalamic and hypophyseal hormones.

Pharmacokinetics: Adults: Absorption: Oral: Promethazine exhibits rapid and complete oral absorption with a large first pass effect.

Metabolism: Promethazine undergoes hepatic metabolism mainly through oxidation. Inactive metabolites include sulfoxides of promethazine and N-desmethylpromethazine.

Excretion: The half-life is 9 to 16 hours. Excretion is primarily by urine and feces as inactive metabolites.

Prometrium® Ⓟ
progesterone
Progestin

Schering-Plough

Date of Preparation: May 5, 1995
Date of Revision: May 24, 2005

SUMMARY PRODUCT INFORMATION:

Route of Administration	Dosage Form/ Strength	Clinically Relevant Nonmedicinal Ingredients
Oral	Capsule 100 mg	For a complete listing see Dosage Forms, Composition and Packaging.

INDICATIONS AND CLINICAL USE: PROMETRIUM (micronized progesterone) is indicated for:
- women with an intact uterus as an adjunct to postmenopausal estrogen replacement therapy to significantly reduce the risk of endometrial hyperplasia and carcinoma.

CONTRAINDICATIONS: Prometrium (micronized progesterone) is contraindicated in patients with any of the following disorders:
- hypersensitivity to this drug or to any ingredient in the formulation of the capsule. **PROMETRIUM (micronized progesterone) contains peanut oil and should never be used by patients allergic to peanuts.** For a complete listing, see Dosage Forms, Composition and Packaging;
- active hepatic dysfunction or disease, especially of the obstructive type;
- personal history of known or suspected estrogen-dependent or progestin-dependent malignant neoplasia (e.g. breast cancer or endometrial cancer);
- endometrial hyperplasia;
- undiagnosed abnormal genital bleeding;
- known or suspected pregnancy;
- active or past history of arterial thromboembolic disease (e.g. stroke, myocardial infarction, coronary heart disease);
- classical migraine;
- active or past history of confirmed venous thromboembolism (such as deep venous thrombosis or pulmonary embolism) or active thrombophlebitis;
- partial or complete loss of vision due to ophthalmic vascular disease.

WARNINGS AND PRECAUTIONS:

> **Serious Warnings and Precautions**
> The Women's Health Initiative (WHI) trial examined the health benefits and risks of combined estrogen plus progestin therapy (n=16 608) and estrogen-alone therapy (n=10 739) in postmenopausal women aged 50 to 79 years.
> The estrogen plus progestin arm of the WHI trial indicated an increased risk of myocardial infarction (MI), stroke, invasive breast cancer, pulmonary emboli and deep vein thrombosis in postmenopausal women receiving treatment with combined conjugated equine estrogens (CEE, 0.625 mg/day) and medroxyprogesterone acetate (MPA, 2.5 mg/day) for 5.2 years compared to those receiving placebo.
> The estrogen-alone arm of the WHI trial indicated an increased risk of stroke and deep vein thrombosis in hysterectomized women treated with CEE-alone (0.625 mg/day) for 6.8 years compared to those receiving placebo.
> Therefore, the following should be given serious consideration at the time of prescribing:
> - Estrogens with or without progestins **should not** be prescribed for primary or secondary prevention of cardiovascular diseases.
> - Estrogens with or without progestins should be prescribed at **the lowest effective dose** for the approved indication.
> - Estrogens with or without progestins should be prescribed for **the shortest period** possible for the approved indication.

Some of the information presented in the Warnings and Precautions section is provided in light of the fact that progestin medication is often prescribed concomitantly with an estrogen medication. Information in this section pertaining to combined estrogen-progestin therapy may therefore not apply to progestin-only therapy. Physician discretion is advised.

General: Occupational Hazards: Effects on ability to drive and use machines: Transient and occasional somnolence or dizziness may occur in some patients 1-4 hours after ingestion of PROMETRIUM, particularly if administered with food. Activities requiring concentration, good attention, good coordination or reflex action should be avoided when the above-mentioned neurological symptoms occur. In most cases, these problems can be avoided by taking the capsules at the recommended times. The 200 mg dosage should be taken at bedtime. The 300 mg dosage should be divided into two doses, 100 mg 2 hours after breakfast and 200 mg at bedtime.

Carcinogenesis and Mutagenesis: Breast Cancer: Available epidemiological data indicate that the use of combined estrogen plus progestin by postmenopausal women is associated with an increased risk of invasive breast cancer.

In the estrogen plus progestin arm of the WHI trial (conjugated equine estrogens (CEE), 0.625 mg/day plus medroxyprogesterone acetate (MPA) 2.5 mg/day), among 10 000 women over a one-year period, there were:
- 8 more cases of invasive breast cancer (38 on combined HRT versus 30 on placebo).

The WHI study also reported that the invasive breast cancers diagnosed in the estrogen plus progestin group were similar in histology but were larger (mean [SD], 1.7 cm [1.1] vs. 1.5 cm [0.9], respectively; p=0.04) and were at a more advanced stage compared with those diagnosed in the placebo group. The percentage of women with abnormal mammograms (recommendations for short-interval follow-up, a suspicious abnormality, or highly suggestive of malignancy) was significantly higher in the estrogen plus progestin group versus the placebo group. This difference appeared at year one and persisted in each year thereafter.

In the estrogen-alone arm of the WHI trial (CEE at 0.625 mg/day), there was no statistically significant difference in the rate of invasive breast cancer in hysterectomized women treated with conjugated equine estrogens versus women treated with placebo.

It is recommended that estrogens with or without progestins not be given to women with existing breast cancer or those with a previous history of the disease. There is a need for caution in prescribing estrogens with or without progestins for women with known risk factors associated with the development of breast cancer, such as strong family history of breast cancer (first degree relative) or who present a breast condition with an increased risk (abnormal mammograms and/or atypical hyperplasia at breast biopsy). Other known risk factors for the development of breast cancer such as nulliparity, obesity, early menarche, late age at first full term pregnancy and at menopause should also be evaluated.

It is recommended that women undergo mammography prior to the start of HRT treatment and at regular intervals during treatment, as deemed appropriate by the treating physician and according to the perceived risks for each patient.

The overall benefits and possible risks of hormone replacement therapy should be fully considered and discussed with patients. It is important that the modest increased risk of being diagnosed with breast cancer after 4 years of treatment with combined estrogen plus progestin HRT (as reported in the results of the WHI trial) be discussed with the patient and weighed against its known benefits.

Instructions for regular self-examination of the breasts should be included in this counselling.

Cardiovascular: The results of the Heart and Estrogen/progestin Replacement Studies (HERS and HERS II) and the Women's Health Initiative (WHI) trial indicate that the use of estrogen plus progestin is associated with an increased risk of coronary heart disease (CHD) in postmenopausal women. The results of the WHI trial indicate that the use of estrogen-alone and estrogen plus progestin is associated with an increased risk of stroke in postmenopausal women.

WHI trial findings: In the combined estrogen plus progestin arm of the WHI trial, among 10 000 women over a one-year period, there were:
- 8 more cases of stroke (29 on combined HRT versus 21 on placebo)
- 7 more cases of CHD (37 on combined HRT versus 30 on placebo).

In the estrogen-alone arm of the WHI trial of women with prior hysterectomy, among 10 000 women over a one-year period, there were/was:
- 12 more cases of stroke (44 on estrogen-alone therapy versus 32 on placebo)
- no statistically significant difference in the rate of CHD.

HERS and HERS II findings: In the Heart and Estrogen/progestin Replacement Study (HERS) of postmenopausal women with documented heart disease (n=2763, average age 66.7 years), a randomized placebo-controlled clinical trial of secondary prevention of coronary heart disease (CHD), treatment with 0.625 mg/day oral conjugated equine estrogen (CEE) plus 2.5 mg medroxyprogesterone acetate (MPA) demonstrated no cardiovascular benefit. Specifically, during an average follow-up of 4.1 years, treatment with CEE plus MPA did not reduce the overall rate of CHD events in postmenopausal women with established coronary heart disease. There were more CHD events in the hormone-treated group than in the placebo group in year 1, but not during the subsequent years.

From the original HERS trial, 2321 women consented to participate in an open label extension of HERS known as HERS II. Average follow-up in HERS II was an additional 2.7 years, for a total of 6.8 years overall. After 6.8 years, hormone therapy did not reduce the risk of cardiovascular events in women with CHD.

High Blood Pressure: Women using hormonal replacement therapy (HRT) sometimes experience increased blood pressure. Blood pressure should be monitored with HRT use. Elevation of blood pressure in previously normotensive or hypertensive patients should be investigated and HRT may have to be discontinued.

Endocrine and Metabolism: Glucose and Lipid Metabolism: A worsening of glucose tolerance and lipid metabolism has been observed in a significant percentage of peri- and post-menopausal patients. Therefore, diabetic patients or those with a predisposition to diabetes should be observed closely to detect any alterations in carbohydrate or lipid metabolism, especially in triglyceride blood levels.

Calcium and Phosphorus Metabolism: Because the prolonged use of estrogens, with or without progestins, influences the metabolism of calcium and phosphorus, estrogens should be used with caution in patients with metabolic and malignant bone diseases associated with hypercalcemia and in patients with renal insufficiency.

Familial Hyperlipidemias or Porphyria: Women with familial hyperlipidemias or porphyria need special surveillance. Lipid-lowering measures are recommended additionally as appropriate.

Genitourinary: Vaginal Bleeding: Abnormal vaginal bleeding, due to its prolongation, irregularity or heaviness, occurring during therapy should prompt diagnostic measures like hysteroscopy, endometrial biopsy or curettage to rule out the possibility of uterine malignancy and the treatment should be re-evaluated.

Hematologic: Venous Thromboembolism: Available epidemiological data indicate that use of estrogen with or without progestin by postmenopausal women is associated with an increased risk of developing venous thromboembolism (VTE).

In the estrogen plus progestin arm of the WHI trial, among 10 000 women on combined HRT over a one-year period, there were 18 (34 on combined HRT versus 16 on placebo) more cases of venous thromboembolism, including 8 (16 on combined HRT versus 8 on placebo) more cases of pulmonary embolism.

In the estrogen-alone arm of the WHI trial, among 10 000 women on estrogen therapy over a one-year period, there were 7 (28 on estrogen therapy versus 21 on placebo) more cases of venous thromboembolism, although there was no statistically significant difference in the rate of pulmonary embolism.

Generally recognized risk factors for VTE include a personal history, a family history (the occurrence of VTE in a direct relative at a relatively early age may indicate genetic predisposition) and severe obesity (body mass index >30 kg/m²). The risk of VTE also increases with age and smoking.

The risk of VTE may be temporarily increased with prolonged immobilization, major surgery or trauma. In women on HRT, attention should be given to prophylactic measures to prevent VTE following surgery. Also, patients with varicose veins should be closely supervised. The physician should be alert to the earliest manifestations of thrombotic disorders (thrombophlebitis, retinal thrombosis, cerebral embolism and pulmonary embolism). If these occur or are suspected, hormone therapy should be discontinued immediately, given the risks of long-term disability or fatality.

If feasible, estrogens with or without progestins should be discontinued at least 4 weeks before major surgery which may be associated with an increased risk of thromboembolism, or during periods of prolonged immobilization.

Hepatic/Biliary/Pancreatic: Liver Function Test: Liver function tests should be done periodically in subjects who are suspected of having hepatic disease. For information on endocrine and liver function tests, see Drug Interactions, Drug-Laboratory Interactions, Laboratory Tests.

Neurologic: Cerebrovascular Insufficiency: Patients who develop visual disturbances, classical migraine, transient aphasia, paralysis, or loss of consciousness should discontinue medication.

Dementia: Available epidemiological data indicate that the use of combined estrogen plus progestin in women age 65 and over may increase the risk of developing probable dementia.

The Women's Health Initiative Memory Study (WHIMS), a clinical substudy of the WHI, was designed to assess whether postmenopausal hormone replacement therapy (estrogen plus progestin or estrogen-alone) reduces the risk of dementia in women aged 65 and over and free of dementia at baseline.

In the estrogen plus progestin arm of the WHIMS (n=4532), women with an intact uterus were treated with daily 0.625 mg conjugated equine estrogens (CEE) plus 2.5 mg medroxyprogesterone acetate (MPA) or placebo for an average of 4.05 years. The results, when extrapolated to 10 000 women treated over a one-year period showed:
- 23 more cases of probable dementia (45 on combined HRT versus 22 on placebo).

In the estrogen-alone arm of the WHIMS (n=2947), women with prior hysterectomy were treated with daily 0.625 mg CEE or placebo for an average of 5.21 years. The results, when extrapolated to 10 000 women treated over a one-year period showed:
- 12 more cases of probable dementia (37 on estrogen-alone versus 25 on placebo), although this difference did not reach statistical significance.

When data from the estrogen plus progestin arm of the WHIMS and the estrogen-alone arm of the WHIMS were combined, as per the original WHIMS protocol, in 10 000 women over a one-year period, there were:
- 18 more cases of probable dementia (41 on estrogen plus progestin or estrogen-alone versus 23 on placebo).

Renal: Fluid Retention: Estrogens, with or without progestins, may cause fluid retention. Therefore, particular caution is indicated in cardiac or renal dysfunction, epilepsy or asthma. Treatment should be stopped if there is an increase in epileptic seizures. If, in any of the above-mentioned conditions, a worsening of the underlying disease is diagnosed or suspected during treatment, the benefits and risks of treatment should be reassessed based on the individual case.

Special Populations: Pregnant Women: If the patient is exposed to PROMETRIUM (micronized progesterone) capsules during the first 4 months of pregnancy or if she becomes pregnant while taking this drug she should be informed of the potential risks to the fetus.

A case of cleft palate was reported. Additionally rare cases of fetal death (causality not established) have been reported when PROMETRIUM was used for unapproved indications.

Cases of hepatocellular disease have been reported rarely in women treated with PROMETRIUM during the second and third trimester (see Adverse Reactions).

Nursing Women: Detectable amounts of progesterone have been identified in the milk of mothers receiving progesterone. The possible effects of progesterone on the nursing infant have not been determined.

Monitoring and Laboratory Tests: Physical Examination: Before PROMETRIUM (micronized progesterone) is administered, the patient should have a complete physical examination including a blood pressure determination. Breasts and pelvic organs should be appropriately examined and a Papanicolaou smear should be performed. Endometrial biopsy should be done when indicated. Baseline tests should include mammography, measurements of blood glucose, calcium, triglycerides, cholesterol, and liver function tests.

The first follow-up examination should be done within 3-6 months after initiation of treatment to assess response to treatment. Thereafter, examinations should be made at intervals at least once a year. Appropriate investigations should be arranged at regular intervals as determined by the physician.

It is important that patients are encouraged to practice frequent self-examination of the breasts.

ADVERSE REACTIONS: Adverse Drug Reaction Overview: See Warnings and Precautions regarding potential induction of malignant neoplasms and adverse effects similar to those of oral contraceptives.

Adverse events that could be considered to be possibly associated with PROMETRIUM (micronized progesterone) therapy are: breakthrough bleeding, spotting, and menstrual irregularity.

Under the recommended conditions of use (200 mg HS), dizziness, somnolence, cramps or nausea have been reported occasionally.

Fatigue, headache, vertigo, lightheadedness or migraine have been reported rarely.

Breast: Breast tenderness may occur with the use of PROMETRIUM.

Other adverse events which are generally attributed to synthetic progestins and which may possibly occur during PROMETRIUM treatment include: chloasma, pruritus, jaundice, rash, fluid retention, mental depression and thrombotic disorders.

The following adverse reactions have been reported with estrogen/progestin combinations in general:

Blood and Lymphatic System Disorders: altered coagulation tests (see Drug Interactions, Drug-Laboratory Interactions, Laboratory Tests).

Cardiac Disorders: palpitations; increase in blood pressure (see Warnings and Precautions); coronary thrombosis.

Endocrine Disorders: increased blood sugar levels; decreased glucose tolerance.

Eye Disorders: neuro-ocular lesions (e.g. retinal thrombosis, optic neuritis); visual disturbances; steepening of the corneal curvature; intolerance to contact lenses.
Gastrointestinal Disorders: nausea; vomiting; abdominal discomfort (cramps, pressure, pain, bloating).
General Disorders and Administration Site Conditions: fatigue; changes in appetite; changes in body weight; change in libido.
Hepatobiliary Disorders: gallbladder disorder; asymptomatic impaired liver function; cholestatic jaundice.
Musculoskeletal and Connective Tissue Disorders: musculoskeletal pain including leg pain not related to thromboembolic disease (usually transient, lasting 3-6 weeks) may occur.
Nervous System Disorders: aggravation of migraine episodes; headaches; dizziness; neuritis.
Psychiatric Disorders: mental depression; nervousness; irritability.
Renal and Urinary Disorders: cystitis; dysuria; sodium retention; edema.
Reproductive System and Breast Disorders: breakthrough bleeding; spotting; change in menstrual flow; dysmenorrhea; vaginal itching/discharge; dyspareunia; endometrial hyperplasia; pre-menstrual-like syndrome; reactivation of endometriosis; changes in cervical erosion and amount of cervical secretion; breast swelling and tenderness.
Skin and Subcutaneous Tissue Disorders: chloasma or melasma, which may persist when drug is discontinued; erythema multiforme; erythema nodosum; haemorrhagic eruption; loss of scalp hair; hirsutism and acne.
Vascular Disorders: isolated cases of: thrombophlebitis; thromboembolic disorders.

If adverse symptoms persist, the prescription of HRT should be re-considered.

Clinical Trial Adverse Drug Reactions: Because clinical trials are conducted under very specific conditions the adverse reaction rates observed in the clinical trials may not reflect the rates observed in practice and should not be compared to the rates in the clinical trials of another drug. Adverse drug reaction information from clinical trials is useful for identifying drug-related adverse events and for approximating rates.

Table 1 lists adverse reactions experienced in a double-blind, randomized, parallel-group study compared the efficacy and safety of PROMETRIUM 200 mg and 300 mg with placebo. Two patients withdrew from the study prior to receiving study drug. The majority of adverse reactions experienced are those resulting from the pharmacological action of progesterone as well as from the onset of withdrawal bleeding. These events include cramping, nausea, abdominal pain and/or bloating and tender or swollen breasts.

Table 1: PROMETRIUM

Adverse Reactions Reported in a 60 Patient Double-blind, Randomized, Parallel-group Study [Percentage (%) of Patients Reporting]

	PROMETRIUM 200 mg N=19 %	PROMETRIUM 300 mg N=20 %	Placebo N=21 %
Cramps	58	35	29
Nausea	5	15	10
Breast Tenderness	5	10	19
Abdominal Discomfort	5	10	14
Dizziness	11	15	14
Tired/Lethargy	21	20	14

Dupont et al conducted a single-blind, randomized, controlled study that compared percutaneous estradiol and oral conjugated estrogens as replacement therapy (with or without PROMETRIUM) in sixty-three healthy postmenopausal women. In this study, serum aldosterone concentrations were slightly elevated in subjects receiving PROMETRIUM independent of the form of estrogen therapy administered. The increase in aldosterone was not associated with any clinical symptoms or side effects. There was no significant change in diastolic and systolic blood pressure.

Table 2 lists adverse experiences which were reported in ≥2% of patients (regardless of relationship to treatment) who received cyclic PROMETRIUM Capsules, 200 mg daily (12 days per calendar month cycle) with daily 0.625 mg conjugated estrogen, in a multicenter, randomized, double-blind, placebo-controlled clinical trial (Postmenopausal Estrogen and Progestin Interventions (PEPI) Trial) in 875 postmenopausal women. Table 2 also lists adverse experiences reported in the conjugated estrogen-alone group and placebo group of the PEPI trial.

Table 2: PROMETRIUM

Adverse Experiences (≥2%) Reported in an 875 Patient Placebo-controlled Trial in Postmenopausal Women Over a 3-Year Period [Percentage (%) of Patients Reporting]

	PROMETRIUM Capsules 200 mg with Conjugated Estrogens 0.625 mg (N=178) %	Conjugated Estrogens 0.625 mg (only) (N=175) %	Placebo (N=174) %
Headache	31	30	27
Breast Tenderness	27	16	6
Joint Pain	20	22	29
Depression	19	18	12
Dizziness	15	5	9
Abdominal Bloating	12	10	5
Hot Flashes	11	14	35
Urinary Problems	11	10	9
Abdominal Pain	10	13	10
Vaginal Discharge	10	10	3
Nausea/Vomiting	8	6	7
Worry	8	5	4
Chest Pain	7	4	5
Diarrhea	7	7	4
Night Sweats	7	5	17

(cont'd)

Table 2: PROMETRIUM *(cont'd)*

Adverse Experiences (≥2%) Reported in an 875 Patient Placebo-controlled Trial in Postmenopausal Women Over a 3-Year Period [Percentage (%) of Patients Reporting]

	PROMETRIUM Capsules 200 mg with Conjugated Estrogens 0.625 mg (N=178) %	Conjugated Estrogens 0.625 mg (only) (N=175) %	Placebo (N=174) %
Breast Pain	6	6	2
Swelling of Hands and Feet	6	9	9
Vaginal Dryness	6	8	10
Constipation	3	3	2

Post-market Adverse Drug Reactions: During the marketing of PROMETRIUM internationally, cases of hepatocellular liver disease have been reported rarely. Most of these occurred in women treated outside of the approved indications, i. e., during the second and third trimester of pregnancy when premature labour was threatened.

Additional adverse experiences have been observed in women taking progestins in general: anaphylaxis and anaphylactoid reaction, rash with and without pruritus, confusion, speech disorder, impaired concentration, and hot flashes. Additionally, rare instances of syncope have been reported.

DRUG INTERACTIONS: Overview: Drugs Inducing Liver Enzymes: Preparations inducing liver enzymes (e.g., barbiturates, hydantoins, carbamazepine, meprobamates, phenylbutazone or rifampin) may interfere with the activity of orally administered progestins.
Drugs Inhibiting Liver Enzymes: Metabolism of progesterone capsules by human liver microsomes was inhibited by ketoconazole (IC50 <0.1 microM; ketoconazole is a known inhibitor of cytochrome P450 3A4). These data therefore suggest that ketoconazole may increase the bioavailability of progesterone. The clinical relevance of the in vitro findings is unknown.

Clinical pharmacokinetic studies have not demonstrated any consistent effect of antibiotics (other than rifampin) on plasma concentrations of synthetic steroids.

Concomitant administration of aminoglutethimide with MPA may significantly reduce the bioavailability of MPA. It is unknown whether this interaction occurs with micronized progesterone.
Drug-Food Interactions: Concomitant food ingestion increased the AUC and Cmax values of PROMETRIUM Capsules, with no effect on Tmax relative to a fasting state when administered to postmenopausal women at a dose of 200 mg, for information see Action and Clinical Pharmacology, Pharmacokinetics.
Drug-Herb Interactions: It was found that some herbal products (e.g. St-John's wort), which are available as OTC products, might affect metabolism, and therefore, efficacy and safety of estrogen/progestin products.

Physicians and other health care providers should be aware of other non-prescription products concomitantly used by the patient, including herbal and natural products, obtained from the widely spread Health Stores.
Drug-Laboratory Interactions: Laboratory Tests: The following laboratory results may be altered by the use of progesterone: levels of gonadotropin, plasma progesterone, and urinary pregnanediol.
The results of certain endocrine and liver function tests may be affected by progestin-containing products:

- impaired glucose tolerance;
- reduced serum folate concentration;
- change in plasma lipoprotein levels.

The results of the above laboratory tests should not be considered reliable unless therapy has been discontinued for two to four weeks. The pathologist should be informed that the patient is receiving HRT therapy when relevant specimens are submitted.

DOSAGE AND ADMINISTRATION: Recommended Dose and Dosage Adjustment: Hormone Replacement Therapy: In general, the dosage of PROMETRIUM (micronized progesterone) is 200 mg daily for the last 14 days of estrogen treatment per cycle (i.e. from day 8 to day 21 for a 28-day cycle, and from day 12 to day 25 for a 30-day cycle). Estrogens should be administered daily at the lowest effective dose. Patients being treated with high dosages of estrogen (equivalent to 1.25 mg conjugated estrogens or higher) should be administered 300 mg daily for the last 12-14 days of estrogen treatment.

The dosage of PROMETRIUM should be proportional to the dosage of estrogen. With adequate adjustment of the dosage of PROMETRIUM, patients should experience either regular withdrawal uterine bleeding or cessation of bleeding (amenorrhea).
Missed Dose: If a patient is treated with 200 mg daily (total dose at bedtime) and she forgets to take this dose, she should take an extra dose of one capsule (100 mg) the following morning and continue taking the rest of the capsules as prescribed. If a patient is treated with 300 mg daily, and she forgets to take a morning or evening dose, she should not take the missed dose.
Administration: The 200 mg daily dosage of PROMETRIUM should be taken at bedtime. Patients receiving 300 mg PROMETRIUM daily should take one capsule (100 mg) in the morning and two capsules (200 mg) at bedtime. The morning dose should be taken 2 hours after breakfast.

OVERDOSAGE:
Symptoms: The toxicity of progesterone is very low. Symptoms that may occur are: nausea, vomiting, somnolence and dizziness.

Progestin (norethindrone acetate) overdosage has been characterized by depressed mood, tiredness, acne and hirsutism.
Treatment: Symptomatic treatment should be given.

> For management of a suspected drug overdose, CPhA recommends that you contact your **regional Poison Control Centre**. See the *CPS* Directory section for a list of Poison Control Centres.

ACTION AND CLINICAL PHARMACOLOGY: Mechanism of Action: PROMETRIUM (micronized progesterone) is an oral dosage form of the naturally occurring steroid; it is chemically identical to progesterone of ovarian origin.

Progestins are used in combination with estrogens to prevent estrogen-induced endometrial hyperplasia and reduce the risk of endometrial carcinoma to that of untreated women.
Clinical Pharmacology: PROMETRIUM is intended for use in women with an intact uterus as an adjunct to estrogen replacement therapy. Progesterone exerts significant anti-proliferative effects on the estrogenized endometrium and maintains sufficient control of endometrial mitotic activity through suppression of nuclear estradiol receptors, significant reduction in epithelial and stromal DNA synthesis and induction of 17ß-estradiol dehydrogenase and isocitric dehydrogenase activity.

PROMETRIUM administered per os is a physiologic inhibitor of aldosterone and thus increases the sodium excretion rate. A 200 mg dose of micronized progesterone is equivalent to a dose of 25 to 50 mg of spironolactone as an aldosterone inhibitor.

PROMETRIUM has no significant effect on carbohydrate metabolism, even when administered to non-insulin dependent diabetics. PROMETRIUM does not negate the beneficial oral or transdermal estrogen-induced effect on lipoprotein profiles. In general, administration of PROMETRIUM (with or without estrogen) does not lead to significant changes in systolic and diastolic blood pressure or heart rate in normotensive women. Administration of PROMETRIUM does not lead to any significant change in renin substrate, even when administered to diabetic patients. Administration of PROMETRIUM in combination with percutaneous estradiol produces a decrease in blood platelet aggregation in perimenopausal women. In combination with oral conjugated estrogens, PROMETRIUM does not negatively affect the balance between the vasoactive prostanoids PGI_2 and TxA_2.
Pharmacokinetics: Absorption and Distribution: Pharmacokinetic studies indicate that plasma progesterone levels within the luteal range are achieved with peak levels (mean 77.3 nmol/L) at 2-4 hours following oral administration to postmenopausal women of PROMETRIUM 200 mg (see Table 3).

The plasma concentration of progesterone then declines slowly but remains within the range found in the mid-luteal phase for approximately 9 to 12 hours after administration. Plasma progesterone levels remain above baseline 84 hours after administration of the final dosage. Ingestion of food following administration of PROMETRIUM significantly increases AUC and Cmax values, with no effect on Tmax. Bioavailability (defined as area under the curve, AUC) is linearly related to the dose.

Table 3: PROMETRIUM

Mean Pharmacokinetic Parameters in Postmenopausal Women After Five Daily Doses of PROMETRIUM Capsules

Mean (n=15) Day 5 Progesterone C_{max} and AUC Values after Administration of Prometrium 200 and 300 mg once Daily		
	Prometrium Dose (mg/day)	
	200	300
Cmax (nmol/L)	121.2	192.7
AUC_{0-10} (nmol·h/L)	321.8	558.7

Progesterone concentrations measured in the endometrium after 8 days of treatment with PROMETRIUM either 200 mg/day or 300 mg/day are comparable to physiologic levels during the luteal phase even 12 hours after administration. This fact demonstrates the strong retention of this hormone in target tissue, which is responsible for its biological action during 24 hours. Similarly, significant increases in progesterone concentrations occur in breast tissue.

Intestinal absorption is rapid. Micronization of progesterone improves its absorption by the digestive tract by increasing the surface area in contact between the steroid and the mucous membrane.

Metabolism and Excretion: Following administration of PROMETRIUM 300 mg, the major inactive metabolite (pregnanediol-3 α glucuronide) and the 2 major active metabolites (17-hydroxyprogesterone, 20 α dihydroprogesterone) show similar plasma profiles to progesterone. Twenty-four hours following oral administration of 200 mg of PROMETRIUM to postmenopausal women, 22.8 mg of pregnanediol glucuronide are eliminated in urine. The second major excretion pathway is via the bile and the feces.

Since PROMETRIUM is metabolized primarily by the liver and is excreted mainly in the urine, patients with illness related to the liver and/or kidneys should be monitored closely.

STORAGE AND STABILITY: Store at controlled room temperature 15-30°C. Protect from light.

Keep in a safe place out of the reach of children and pets.

INFORMATION FOR THE PATIENT: Published in e-CPS, available by subscription at www.e-cps.ca.

DOSAGE FORMS, COMPOSITION AND PACKAGING: Each capsule contains: micronized progesterone 100 mg. Nonmedicinal ingredients: arachis (peanut) oil, gelatin, glycerin, lecithin and titanium dioxide. Unit dose blister packages of 28. Bottles of 100.

(Shown in Product Identification Section)

The reader is invited to consult CPhA's monograph **Corticosteroids: Eye, Ear and Nose.**

Propaderm® 🅿

beclomethasone dipropionate

Topical Corticosteroid

Paladin

SUPPLIED: Each g of cream contains: beclomethasone dipropionate 0.025%. Cartoned tubes of 15 and 45 g.

Propafenone 🅿

Antiarrhythmic

CPhA Monograph

Date of Preparation: September 2010

This monograph has been compiled by CPhA and reviewed by experts. It may contain information different from that found in Health Canada-approved Product Monographs. The reader is referred to the *CPS* Editorial Policy for more information.

SUMMARY PRODUCT INFORMATION:

Route of Administration	Dosage Form	Strength
Oral	Tablet	150 mg, 300 mg

INDICATIONS AND CLINICAL USE: Health Canada-approved Indications Include:

- treatment of documented life-threatening ventricular arrhythmias, such as sustained ventricular tachycardia. Propafenone therapy should be initiated in the hospital.
- treatment of patients with documented symptomatic ventricular arrhythmias when the symptoms are severe enough to require treatment.

Uses Without Health Canada Approval:

- treatment and prevention of supraventricular arrhythmias including atrial flutter, atrial fibrillation, Wolff-Parkinson-White syndrome and supraventricular tachycardia in patients without structural heart disease.
- management of supraventricular arrhythmias (e.g., paroxysmal supraventricular tachycardia, junctional ectopic tachycardia and atrial fibrillation/flutter) in infants and children.

CONTRAINDICATIONS: Propafenone is contraindicated in:

- Patients who are hypersensitive to propafenone or to any ingredient in the formulation or component of the container.
- Severe or uncontrolled heart failure (see Warnings and Precautions)
- Cardiogenic shock
- Sinoatrial, atrioventricular and intraventricular disorders of impulse conduction and sinus node dysfunction (e.g., sick sinus syndrome) in the absence of an artificial pacemaker
- Severe bradycardia
- Marked hypotension
- Bronchospastic disorders
- Severe disorders of electrolyte balance
- Severe hepatic failure (see Warnings and Precautions)

WARNINGS AND PRECAUTIONS:

Serious Warnings and Precautions
No antiarrhythmic drug has been shown to reduce the incidence of sudden death in patients with asymptomatic ventricular arrhythmias. Most antiarrhythmic drugs have the potential to cause dangerous arrhythmias; some have been associated with an increased incidence of sudden death. In light of the above, physicians should carefully consider the risks and benefits of antiarrhythmic therapy for all patients with ventricular arrhythmias.

General: It is important to look for and treat electrolyte imbalances, especially hypokalemia or hypomagnesemia, before initiating and during propafenone therapy.

Cardiovascular: Mortality: Use of antiarrhythmic agents in recent myocardial infarction patients with asymptomatic ventricular arrhythmias is associated with increased risk of mortality or nonfatal cardiac arrest as evidenced in the Cardiac Arrhythmia Suppression Trial (CAST) [*N Engl J Med* 1991;324(12):781-8].

Proarrhythmic effects, or worsening of arrhythmias, can occur and are more likely in patients with sustained ventricular arrhythmias and left ventricular dysfunction. In general, proarrhythmic effects occur in the first week of therapy, although increased risk of proarrhythmic effects applies throughout propafenone therapy. Clinical and ECG monitoring should be performed to detect arrhythmias and to assess the need for propafenone therapy.

Heart Failure: Propafenone is associated with new or worsened heart failure. Propafenone shows weak beta-blockade and a dose-related direct negative inotropic effect on myocardium. Propafenone should not be used in patients with uncontrolled heart failure where left ventricular ejection fraction is below 35%. Use propafenone with caution in patients taking drugs that have negative inotropic effect, or in patients with minimal cardiac reserve.

Effects on Cardiac Conduction: Propafenone slows cardiac conduction which can lead to a dose-related prolongation of PR interval and QRS complex, development of first or higher degree AV block, bundle branch block and intraventricular conduction delay. If depression of cardiac conductivity is observed, decrease the dose or discontinue propafenone.

Effects on Pacemaker Threshold: Propafenone may increase endocardial stimulation threshold. Pacemaker adjustment may be necessary.

Hematologic: Propafenone infrequently induces reversible agranulocytosis (<0.1%), generally within 4-6 weeks of initiating therapy. Instruct patients to immediately report any symptoms of agranulocytosis such as fever, fatigue, malaise or any other manifestations of infection especially in the first 3 months of therapy. Discontinue propafenone if other signs and symptoms of agranulocytosis (e.g., decreased white blood cell count) are confirmed.

Hepatic/Biliary/Pancreatic: In patients with impaired hepatic function, reduce the dose of propafenone to compensate for accumulation of the parent drug (see Dosage and Administration). Hepatocellular injury, cholestasis or both have been reported in patients taking propafenone (see Adverse Reactions).

Respiratory: Propafenone should in general not be used in patients with bronchospastic disease since its beta-blockade effects may precipitate or worsen bronchospasm (see Contraindications).

Special Populations: Pregnant Women: Use only if the potential benefit outweighs the risk. When administered to a pregnant woman near term, detectable serum concentrations were produced in the newborn without harm to the newborn.

Nursing Women: Propafenone is excreted in breast milk with a milk:plasma ratio of 0.25. If propafenone therapy is considered necessary in a breastfeeding mother, consider advising the mother to stop breastfeeding.

Occupational Hazards: Due to adverse reactions such as blurred vision, dizziness, fatigue and postural hypotension, propafenone may impair mental or physical abilities required to operate machinery or drive a motor vehicle.

ADVERSE REACTIONS: Adverse Drug Reactions Overview: The most common adverse reactions occurring in approximately 10% of patients are dizziness, nausea and/or vomiting, unusual taste and constipation. The most serious adverse reactions are new or worsened arrhythmia, heart failure and ventricular tachycardia. These serious reactions are more common in patients with a history of myocardial infarction. Adverse reactions occur mostly within the first month of therapy and are dose-related.

More Common Adverse Drug Reactions (≥1%): Table 1 lists the more common adverse effects of propafenone.

Table 1: Propafenone

More Common Adverse Drug Reactions (≥1%)

Body System	Effect
Cardiovascular	Conduction abnormalities: bundle branch block, first degree AV block, intraventricular conduction delay, prolonged QRS duration Proarrhythmic effects: premature ventricular contractions, ventricular tachycardia Angina, atrial fibrillation, bradycardia, chest pain, edema, heart failure, hypotension, palpitations, syncope
CNS	Anxiety, ataxia, dizziness, drowsiness, fatigue, headache, insomnia
Dermatologic	Diaphoresis, rash
GI	Abdominal pain, anorexia, constipation, diarrhea, dry mouth, dyspepsia, flatulence, nausea/vomiting, unusual taste
Musculoskeletal	Joint pain, tremor, weakness
Ophthalmologic	Blurred vision
Respiratory	Dyspnea

Less Common Adverse Drug Reactions (<1%): Cardiovascular: AV dissociation, AV block (second or third degree), cardiac arrest, sick sinus syndrome, torsades de pointes, ventricular fibrillation, supraventricular tachycardia.

Central Nervous System: confusion, depression, memory loss, psychosis/mania, seizure, tinnitus, vertigo, coma.

Allergic/Dermatologic: alopecia, pruritus.

Endocrine and Metabolism: hyperglycemia, syndrome of inappropriate antidiuretic hormone (SIADH) secretion.

Hematologic: agranulocytosis (see Warnings and Precautions), anemia, granulocytopenia, leukopenia, purpura, thrombocytopenia, increased bleeding time.

Hepatic/Biliary/Pancreatic: cholestasis, hepatitis.

Immune: systemic lupus erythematosis, positive ANA.

Neurologic: numbness, paresthesias.

Renal: nephrotic syndrome, renal failure.

Respiratory: apnea.

Sexual Function/Reproduction: impotence.

DRUG INTERACTIONS: Overview: Inhibitors of CYP2D6, 1A2 and 3A4 may increase plasma concentrations of propafenone.

Drug-Drug Interactions: Drug-drug interactions involving propafenone are listed in Table 2.

Table 2: Propafenone

Drug-Drug Interactions

Interacting Drug	Effect	Clinical Comment
Amiodarone	Enhanced proarrhythmic effect.	Adjust dose of both amiodarone and propafenone as necessary.
Beta-adrenergic blockers	Propafenone may increase plasma concentrations of propranolol and metoprolol.	Dose of metoprolol/propranolol may need to be reduced.
Cimetidine	Cimetidine may increase plasma concentrations of propafenone.	Monitor for signs of propafenone toxicity. Adjust dose of propafenone as necessary.

(cont'd)

Table 2: Propafenone *(cont'd)*
Drug-Drug Interactions

Interacting Drug	Effect	Clinical Comment
Desipramine	Propafenone may increase serum concentrations of desipramine; additive QTc prolongation.	Avoid combination.
Digoxin	Propafenone may increase serum concentrations of digoxin.	Monitor plasma concentrations of digoxin. Adjust dose of digoxin as necessary.
Lidocaine	Propafenone increases the frequency and severity of CNS side effects of lidocaine (e.g., lightheadedness, dizziness, paresthesia, lethargy and somnolence) [*Clin Pharmacol Ther* 1993;53(1):38-48].	Monitor for CNS side effects of lidocaine.
Phenobarbital	Phenobarbital may reduce plasma concentrations of propafenone by inducing metabolism of propafenone.	Monitor efficacy of propafenone.
Quinidine	Quinidine, an inhibitor of CYP2D6, increases plasma concentrations of propafenone; additive QTc prolongation.	Reduce dose of propafenone as necessary.
Quinine	Additive QTc prolongation.	Avoid combination.
Rifampin	Rifampin decreases plasma concentrations of propafenone by inducing metabolism of propafenone.	Higher doses of propafenone may be required in patients receiving rifampin.
Ritonavir	Ritonavir may increase plasma concentrations of propafenone by reducing metabolism of propafenone.	Avoid combination.
SSRIs (e.g., fluoxetine, paroxetine)	SSRIs may increase plasma concentrations of propafenone by inhibiting CYP2D6.	Reduce dose of propafenone as necessary.
Theophylline	Propafenone may increase concentrations of theophylline.	Monitor for theophylline toxicity.
Venlafaxine	Propafenone may increase concentrations of venlafaxine by inhibiting CYP2D6 or P-glycoprotein.	Monitor for hallucinations and psychomotor agitation.
Warfarin	Propafenone may increase plasma concentrations of warfarin and prothrombin time.	Monitor prothrombin time. Adjust dose of warfarin as necessary.

Table 3: Propafenone
Dose in Adult Patients

Indication	Route	Initial Dose	Dose Titration	Usual Dose	Maximum Dose	Clinical Comment
Ventricular arrhythmia	Oral	150 mg q8h	Increase to 300 mg q12h, then to 300 mg q8h at 3–4 day intervals	600–900 mg/day	300 mg q8h	Reduce dose if QRS interval is prolonged >20% from baseline.
Supraventricular arrhythmia (Not an approved use in Canada)	Oral	150 mg q8h	Increase to 300 mg q12h, then to 300 mg q8h at 3–4 day intervals		300 mg q8h	Reduce dose if QRS interval is prolonged >20% from baseline.
Recent-onset atrial fibrillation[a] (Not an approved use in Canada)	Oral	450 mg (weight <70 kg), or 600 mg (≥70 kg)				May not repeat in 24 hours. "Pill-in-the-pocket" dose.

[a] Guidelines on the management of atrial fibrillation are published [*J Am Coll Cardiol* 2006;48(4):854-906] or available from www.heart.org/HEARTORG/.

Table 4: Propafenone
Dose in Pediatric Patients

Indication	Route	Initial Dose	Dose Titration	Maximum Dose	Clinical Comment
Supraventricular arrhythmia (Not an approved use in Canada)	Oral	8–10 mg/kg/day divided in 3–4 doses	Increase daily dose by 2 mg/kg	20 mg/kg/day	Limited experience in pediatric patients. Consider other agents (e.g., adenosine, digoxin) first.

Drug-Food Interactions: Grapefruit juice may increase concentrations of propafenone by inhibiting CYP3A4, especially in individuals who are poor metabolizers of CYP2D6 [*Am J Cardiovasc Drugs* 2004;4(5):281-97].

DOSAGE AND ADMINISTRATION: Recommended Dose and Dosage Adjustment: Adults: See Table 3.
Pediatrics: See Table 4.
Hepatic Impairment: The dose should be decreased by 70-80% in patients with hepatic impairment. See Table 5.

Table 5: Propafenone
Dose in Adult Patients with Hepatic Impairment

Indication	Route	Initial Dose	Dosage Titration	Clinical Comment
Ventricular arrhythmia	Oral	150 mg once daily	Increase to 150 mg BID, then to 150 mg q8h, then to 300 mg q12h at a minimum of 4 day intervals	Monitor for signs of toxicity (e.g., hypotension, bradycardia, somnolence, conduction disturbances, seizures and/or ventricular arrhythmias).

Renal Impairment: Dosage adjustment is not necessary in renal impairment.
Genetic Polymorphism: Dosage adjustment is not necessary in patients with varying capacity for CYP2D6 metabolism.

OVERDOSAGE:

For management of a suspected drug overdose, CPhA recommends that you contact your **regional Poison Control Centre**. See the *CPS* Directory section for a list of Poison Control Centres.

ACTION AND CLINICAL PHARMACOLOGY: Mechanism of Action: Propafenone is a class Ic antiarrhythmic agent with local anesthetic and membrane stabilizing properties. The drug markedly slows the rate of increase of phase 0 of the action potential by blocking the fast inward sodium current. Propafenone prolongs PR and QRS intervals in a dose-dependent manner, prolongs effective refractory period and reduces spontaneous automaticity. Propafenone is a weak inhibitor of beta-adrenergic receptors and weakly inhibits calcium influx.

Propafenone prolongs atrioventricular conduction. Occasionally propafenone significantly lengthens sinus nodal recovery times with a non-significant effect on sinus cycle length. Both atrioventricular (AV) nodal conduction time (AH interval) and His-Purkinje conduction time (HV interval) are prolonged. Propafenone increases atrial, AV nodal and ventricular effective refractory periods. Non-significant increases in the QTc interval and occasional slowing of the heart rate have also been observed.

Pharmacokinetics: Adults: Absorption: Propafenone is almost completely absorbed. The drug undergoes extensive first-pass effect with a bioavailability of <40%. Peak plasma concentrations occur within 3 hours. Fast metabolizers exhibit nonlinear kinetics where a 300 mg dose gives plasma concentrations 6 times that of a 150 mg dose. Slow metabolizers exhibit linear kinetics. Steady-state is achieved in 3-4 days.

Distribution: Propafenone is 97% protein bound; this decreases to 88% if the liver is severely impaired. The drug is highly lipophilic with a volume of distribution of about 3 L/kg.

Metabolism: Propafenone undergoes extensive hepatic metabolism. The major active metabolites are 5-hydroxypropafenone formed by CYP2D6 and N-depropylpropafenone formed by CYP1A2 and 3A4. 5-hydroxypropafenone is equipotent to propafenone, while N-depropylpropafenone is much less potent. These two metabolites account for about 20% of the parent compound.

A well-described polymorphism in the gene that produces CYP2D6 affects the metabolism of propafenone. In individuals who lack the gene for CYP2D6 ("poor metabolizers"), propafenone does not undergo hydroxylation so there will be a relatively higher proportion of circulating propafenone. Beta blocking and adverse effects will therefore present more often. The frequency of the poor metabolizer phenotype is variable within any given population, but is generally reported to be <10%. Elimination half-life is 2-10 hours and 10-32 hours for extensive and poor metabolizers of CYP2D6, respectively.

Excretion: <1% renally excreted unchanged. 20-40% of the administered dose is renally excreted as active metabolites.

Propecia® ℞
finasteride
Type II 5 Alpha-reductase Inhibitor

Merck Frosst

Date of Preparation: May 30, 2005
Date of Revision: July 24, 2006

SUMMARY PRODUCT INFORMATION:

Route of Administration	Dosage Form/ Strength	Clinically Relevant Nonmedicinal Ingredients
Oral	Tablet 1 mg	Lactose monohydrate For a complete listing see Dosage Forms, Composition and Packaging.

INDICATIONS AND CLINICAL USE: PROPECIA (finasteride, USP) is indicated for the treatment of male pattern hair loss (androgenetic alopecia) in **men** who have mild to moderate scalp hair loss of the vertex and anterior mid-scalp. Clinical studies were conducted in men between 18 to 41 years of age.

PROPECIA is **not** indicated for use in women (see Warnings and Precautions) or children.

CONTRAINDICATIONS: PROPECIA (finasteride, USP) is contraindicated in the following:

- Pregnancy: Use in women when they are or may potentially be pregnant (see Warnings and Precautions, Exposure to Finasteride—Risk to Male Fetus);
- Hypersensitivity to any component of this product.

PROPECIA is not indicated for use in women or children.

WARNINGS AND PRECAUTIONS: General: Caution should be used in the administration of PROPECIA (finasteride, USP) in patients with liver function abnormalities, as finasteride is metabolized in the liver.

Other causes of alopecia should be ruled out prior to prescribing PROPECIA. Efficacy and duration of treatment should be assessed periodically by the treating physician.

Special Populations: Pregnant Women: PROPECIA (finasteride, USP) is not indicated for use in women. Women should not handle crushed or broken PROPECIA tablets when they are or may potentially be pregnant (see Contraindications). Because of the ability of Type II 5 alpha-reductase inhibitors such as finasteride to inhibit conversion of testosterone to dihydrotestosterone, PROPECIA may cause abnormalities of the external genitalia of a male fetus when administered to a pregnant woman.

Nursing Women: It is not known whether PROPECIA is excreted in human milk.

Exposure to Finasteride—Risk to Male Fetus: Women should not handle crushed or broken tablets of PROPECIA when they are or may potentially be pregnant because of the possibility of absorption of finasteride and the subsequent potential risk to a male fetus (see Pregnant Women). PROPECIA tablets are coated and will prevent contact with the active ingredient during normal handling, provided that the tablets have not been broken or crushed.
Pediatrics: PROPECIA is not indicated for use in children.
Geriatrics (>65 years of age): Clinical studies with PROPECIA have not been conducted in elderly men with male pattern hair loss.
Use in Postmenopausal Women: Results of a one year placebo-controlled study, enrolling 137 healthy postmenopausal women with androgenetic alopecia (age range: 41-60 years), showed no benefit of treatment with PROPECIA 1 mg daily on scalp hair growth.

ADVERSE REACTIONS: Adverse Drug Reaction Overview: Finasteride for male pattern hair loss has been evaluated for safety in clinical studies involving more than 3200 men and is generally well tolerated. In three 12-month, placebo-controlled, double-blind, multicenter studies of comparable design, the overall safety profiles of PROPECIA (finasteride, USP) and placebo were similar. Discontinuation of therapy due to any clinical adverse experience occurred in 1.7% of 945 men treated with PROPECIA and 2.1% of 934 men treated with placebo.

In these studies, the following drug-related adverse experiences were reported in ≥1% of men treated with PROPECIA or placebo, respectively: decreased libido (1.8%, 1.3%), erectile dysfunction (1.3%, 0.7%) and ejaculation disorder (1.2%, 0.7%; primarily decreased volume of ejaculate: [0.8%, 0.4%]). Integrated analysis of clinical adverse experiences showed that during treatment with PROPECIA, 36 (3.8%) of 945 men had reported one or more of these adverse experiences as compared to 20 (2.1%) of 934 men treated with placebo (p=0.04). Resolution of these adverse reactions occurred in men who discontinued therapy with PROPECIA and in most who continued therapy. In a separate study, the effect of PROPECIA on ejaculate volume was measured and was not different from that seen with placebo.

The incidence of each of the above side effects decreased to ≤0.3% by the fifth year of treatment with PROPECIA.

A sexual function questionnaire was self-administered by patients participating in the two vertex baldness trials to detect more subtle changes in sexual function. At Month 12, statistically significant differences were found in 3 of 4 domains (sexual interest, erections, and perception of sexual problems) when compared to placebo. However, no significant difference was seen in the question on overall satisfaction with sex life.

The following adverse experiences have been reported in postmarketing use: ejaculation disorder; breast tenderness and enlargement; hypersensitivity reactions including rash, pruritus, urticaria, and swelling of the lips and face; and testicular pain.
Laboratory Tests: No difference in standard laboratory parameters was observed between patients treated with placebo or PROPECIA.

DRUG INTERACTIONS: Overview: No drug interactions of clinical importance have been identified. Finasteride does not appear to affect significantly the cytochrome P450-linked drug metabolizing enzyme system. Compounds which have been tested in man have included antipyrine, digoxin, glyburide, propranolol, theophylline, and warfarin and no interactions were found. However, patients on medication with narrow therapeutic indices, such as phenytoin, should be carefully monitored when treatment with PROPECIA is initiated.
Other Concomitant Therapy : Although specific interaction studies were not performed, in clinical studies finasteride doses of 1 mg or more were used concomitantly with ACE inhibitors, acetaminophen, alpha blockers, benzodiazepines, beta blockers, calcium-channel blockers, cardiac nitrates, diuretics, H_2 antagonists, HMG-CoA reductase inhibitors, prostaglandin synthetase inhibitors (NSAIDs), and quinolones, without evidence of clinically significant adverse interactions.
Drug-Laboratory Test Interactions: In clinical studies with PROPECIA in men 18-41 years of age, the mean value of serum prostate-specific antigen (PSA) decreased from 0.7 ng/mL at baseline to 0.5 ng/mL at month 12. When finasteride is used in older men who have benign prostatic hyperplasia (BPH), PSA levels are decreased by approximately 50%. Until further information is gathered in men >41 years of age without BPH, consideration should be given to doubling the PSA level in men undergoing this test while taking PROPECIA.

DOSAGE AND ADMINISTRATION: Recommended Dose and Dosage Adjustment: The recommended dosage is one 1 mg tablet daily. PROPECIA (finasteride, USP) may be taken with or without food.

In general, daily use for three months or more is necessary before hair growth is increased and/or further hair loss is prevented. Continued use is recommended to obtain maximum benefit. Withdrawal of treatment leads to reversibility of effect within 12 months.
Dosage in Renal Insufficiency: Adjustments in dosage are not necessary in patients with varying degrees of renal insufficiency (creatinine clearances as low as 0.15 mL/s [9 mL/min]) as pharmacokinetic studies did not indicate any change in the disposition of finasteride.
Missed Dose: If a tablet is missed at its usual time, an extra dose should not be taken. The next dose should be taken as usual.

OVERDOSAGE:
Patients have received single doses of finasteride up to 400 mg and multiple doses of finasteride up to 80 mg/day for three months without adverse reactions.

No specific treatment for overdosage with PROPECIA (finasteride, USP) is recommended.

For management of a suspected drug overdose, CPhA recommends that you contact your **regional Poison Control Centre**. See the *CPS* Directory section for a list of Poison Control Centres.

ACTION AND CLINICAL PHARMACOLOGY: Mechanism of Action: PROPECIA (finasteride, USP) is a competitive and specific inhibitor of Type II 5 alpha-reductase, an intracellular enzyme that converts the androgen testosterone into dihydrotestosterone (DHT). Two distinct isozymes of 5 alpha-reductase are found in mice, rats, monkeys, and humans: Type I and II. Each of these isozymes is differentially expressed in tissues and developmental stages. In humans, Type I 5 alpha-reductase is predominant in the sebaceous glands of most regions of skin, including scalp, and liver. Type I 5 alpha-reductase is responsible for approximately one-third of circulating DHT. The Type II 5a-reductase isozyme is primarily found in prostate, seminal vesicles, epididymides, and hair follicles as well as liver, and is responsible for two-thirds of circulating DHT.

In humans, the mechanism of action of finasteride is based on its preferential inhibition of the Type II isozyme. Using native tissues (scalp and prostate), in vitro binding studies examining the potential of finasteride to inhibit either isozyme revealed a 100-fold selectivity for the human Type II 5 alpha-reductase over Type I isozyme (IC_{50}=500 and 4.2 nM for Type I and II, respectively). For both isozymes, the inhibition by finasteride is accompanied by reduction of the inhibitor to dihydrofinasteride and adduct formation with NADP+. The turnover for the enzyme complex is slow ($t_{1/2}$ approximately 30 days for the Type II enzyme complex and 14 days for the Type I complex).

Finasteride has no affinity for the androgen receptor and has no androgenic, antiandrogenic, estrogenic, antiestrogenic, or progestational effects. Inhibition of Type II 5 alpha-reductase blocks the peripheral conversion of testosterone to DHT, resulting in significant decreases in serum and tissue DHT concentrations. Finasteride produces a rapid reduction in serum DHT concentration, reaching 65% suppression within 24 hours of oral dosing with a 1 mg tablet.

In men with male pattern hair loss (androgenetic alopecia), the balding scalp contains miniaturized hair follicles and increased amounts of DHT compared with hairy scalp. Administration of finasteride decreases scalp and serum DHT concentrations in these men. By this mechanism, finasteride interrupts a key factor in the development of androgenetic alopecia in those patients genetically predisposed.
Pharmacokinetics: In a study in 15 healthy male subjects, the mean bioavailability of finasteride 1 mg tablets was 65% (range, 26-170%), based on the ratio of AUC relative to a 5 mg intravenous dose infused over 60 minutes. Following the intravenous infusion, mean plasma clearance was 165 mL/min (range, 70-279 mL/min) and mean steady-state volume of distribution was 76 L (range, 44-96 L). In a separate study, the bioavailability of finasteride was not affected by food.

Approximately 90% of circulating finasteride is bound to plasma proteins. Finasteride has been found to cross the blood-brain barrier.

STORAGE AND STABILITY: Store at room temperature 15-30°C and protect from moisture.

SPECIAL HANDLING INSTRUCTIONS: Crushed or broken Tablets PROPECIA should not be handled by women when they are or may potentially be pregnant (see Warnings and Precautions, Special Populations, Exposure to Finasteride—Risk to Male Fetus).

INFORMATION FOR THE PATIENT: Published in e-CPS, available by subscription at www.e-cps.ca.

DOSAGE FORMS, COMPOSITION AND PACKAGING: Each tan-colored, 8-sided, film-coated convex tablet, with the code "P" logo on one side and PROPECIA on the other, contains: finasteride 1 mg. Nonmedicinal ingredients: docusate sodium, hydroxypropylcellulose, lactose monohydrate, magnesium stearate, methylhydroxypropylcellulose, microcrystalline cellulose, pregelatinized starch, red ferric oxide, sodium starch glycolate, talc, titanium dioxide and yellow ferric oxide. Blister packages of 28.

(Shown in Product Identification Section)

Propofol Injection ℞
propofol
I.V. Emulsion—Anesthetic—Sedative

Hospira

PHARMACOLOGY: Propofol is an i.v. hypnotic agent for use in the induction and maintenance of general anesthesia or sedation. The drug, an alkylphenol formulated in an oil-in-water emulsion, is chemically distinct from currently available i.v. anesthetic agents. I.V. injection of a therapeutic dose of propofol produces hypnosis rapidly and smoothly, usually within 40 seconds from the start of an injection (one arm-brain circulation time), although induction times >60 seconds have been observed.
Pharmacokinetics: Adults: The pharmacokinetic profile of propofol can be described by a 3-compartment open model. After a single bolus dose, there is fast distribution from blood into tissues ($t_{1/2}\alpha$: 1.8 to 8.3 min), high metabolic clearance ($t_{1/2}\beta$: 34 to 66 min) and a terminal slow elimination from poorly perfused tissues ($t_{1/2}\gamma$: 184 to 480 min). With 12- and 24-hour samplings, $t_{1/2}\gamma$ values of 502 and 674 minutes, respectively, were observed.

Propofol has large volumes of distribution as would be expected with a highly lipophilic anesthetic agent. The volume of central compartment (V_c) is between 21 and 56 L (0.35 to 0.93 L/kg based on a 60 kg patient), and the volume of distribution at steady state (V_{ss}) is between 171 and 364 L (2.85 to 6.07 L/kg). Values for volume of distribution during the terminal phase (V_d) are 2 to 3 times the corresponding V_{ss} values.

The termination of the anesthetic or sedative effects of propofol after a single i.v. bolus or a maintenance infusion is due to extensive redistribution from the CNS to other tissues and high metabolic clearance, both of which will decrease blood concentrations. The mean propofol concentration at time of awakening is 1 µg/mL (range: 0.74 to 2.2 µg/mL). Recovery from anesthesia or sedation is rapid. When propofol is used for both induction (2 to 2.5 mg/kg) and maintenance (0.1 to 0.2 mg/kg/min) of anesthesia, the majority of patients are generally awake, responsive to verbal command and oriented in approximately 7 to 8 min. Recovery from the effects of propofol occurs due to rapid metabolism and is not dependent on the terminal elimination half-life since the blood levels achieved in this phase are not clinically significant.

A study in 6 subjects showed that 72% and 88% of the administered radio-labeled dose was recovered in the urine within 24 hours and 5 days, respectively. Less than 2% was excreted in the feces. Unchanged drug was less than 0.3%. Propofol is chiefly metabolized by conjugation in the liver to inactive metabolites which are excreted by the kidney. Propofol glucuronide accounts for about 50% of the administered dose. The remainder consists of the 1- and 4-glucuronide and 4-sulfate conjugates of 2,6 diisopropyl-1,4-quinol.

The total body clearance (Cl) of propofol ranges from 1.6 L/min to 2.3 L/min (0.026 to 0.038 L/min/kg based on a 60 kg patient). This clearance exceeds estimates of hepatic blood flow, suggesting possible extrahepatic metabolism.

The pharmacokinetics of propofol do not appear to be altered by gender or chronic hepatic cirrhosis. The effects of acute hepatic failure on the pharmacokinetics of propofol have not been studied. In renal failure, the data are based on very limited findings. There was a trend towards longer half-lives, although the differences versus control patients did not reach statistical significance. With increasing age, the dose of propofol needed to achieve a defined anesthetic endpoint (dose-requirement) decreases. Elderly patients had higher propofol blood concentrations at 2 minutes than young ones (6.07 vs 4.15 µg/mL), probably due to a significantly lower initial distribution volume (20 vs 26 L). The relatively high blood concentrations during the first few minutes can predispose elderly patients to cardiorespiratory effects including hypotension, apnea, airway obstruction and/or oxygen desaturation. The clearance of propofol also decreased from a mean±S.D. of 1.8±0.4 L/min in young patients (18 to 35 years) to 1.4±0.4 L/min in elderly patients (65 to 80 years). The reduced clearance could decrease maintenance propofol requirements and prolong recovery if inappropriate infusions are used. Obesity is associated with significantly larger volumes of distribution (399 vs 153 L) and clearance rates (2.8 vs 1.8 L/min) but there is no change in the elimination half-life.

When given by an infusion for up to 2 hours, the pharmacokinetics of propofol appear to be independent of dose (0.05 to 0.15 mg/kg/minute: 3 to 9 mg/kg/h) and similar to i.v. bolus pharmacokinetics. Pharmacokinetics are linear over recommended infusion rates. The steady-state propofol blood concentrations are proportional to the rate of administration.

Propofol is highly protein-bound (97 to 99%): the degree of binding seems to be unrelated to either sex or age.

In the presence of propofol, alfentanil concentrations are generally higher than expected based upon the rate of infusion. However, alfentanil is not known to affect the pharmacokinetics of propofol.
Pharmacokinetics in Adult Patients in Intensive Care Unit (ICU): Regarding most parameters, the pharmacokinetics of propofol in these patients are similar to those of patients undergoing anesthesia/sedation for short surgical procedures. However, the terminal half-life ($t_{1/2}\gamma$) is substantially prolonged after long-term infusion, reflecting extensive tissue distribution.
Pharmacokinetics in Children: The results were obtained in ASA I children, ranging in age from 3 to 10 years, who received a single bolus dose of propofol, 2.5 mg/kg. Propofol was rapidly distributed from blood into tissue ($t_{1/2}\alpha$: 1.5 to 4.1 min), metabolic clearance was high ($t_{1/2}\beta$: 9.3 to 56.1 min) and terminal elimination slow ($t_{1/2}\gamma$: 209 to 735 min). The volume of central compartment (V_c) ranged between 0.53 to 0.72 L/kg, the volume of distribution at steady state (V_{ss}) was between 2.1 to 10.9 L/kg and clearance (Cl) ranged between 0.032 to 0.040 L/min/kg. The mean plasma concentration of propofol at awakening was 2.3 µg/mL.
Clinical Pharmacology: Propofol induces anesthesia in a dose-dependent manner. In unpremedicated, ASA I or II patients, propofol induced anesthesia in 87% and 95% of patients at doses of 2 and 2.5 mg/kg, respectively. Elderly patients require lower doses; for unpremedicated patients older than 55 years of age, the mean dose requirement was 1.66 mg/kg. Premedication profoundly alters dose requirements: at 1.75 mg/kg, propofol induced anesthesia in 65% of patients who had no premedication and in 85% and 100% of patients who received diazepam or papaveretum-hyoscine premedication, respectively.

During induction of anesthesia, the hemodynamic effects of propofol vary. If spontaneous ventilation is maintained, the major cardiovascular effects are arterial hypotension (sometimes greater than a 30% decrease) with little or no change in heart rate and no appreciable decrease in cardiac output. If ventilation is assisted or controlled (positive pressure ventilation), the degree and incidence of decrease in cardiac output are accentuated. Maximal fall in blood pressure occurs within the first few minutes of the administration of a bolus dose. The fall in arterial pressure is greater under propofol anesthesia than under anesthesia induced by thiopental or methohexital. Increases in heart rate with propofol are generally less pronounced or absent after an induction dose, than after equivalent doses of these other 2 agents.

During maintenance of anesthesia with propofol, systolic and diastolic blood pressures generally remain below pre-anesthetic levels, although the depth of anesthesia, the rate of maintenance infusion as well as stimulation from tracheal intubation and/or surgery may increase or decrease blood pressure. Heart rate may also vary as a function of these factors but will generally remain below pre-anesthetic levels.

In the presence of potent opioid (e.g., fentanyl), the blood pressure lowering effect of propofol is substantially increased. Fentanyl also decreases heart rate and this might lead to a significant decrease in cardiac output.

Age is highly correlated with the fall in blood pressure. In elderly subjects, both the incidence and degree of hypotension are greater than in younger subjects. Thus, a lower induction dose and a slower maintenance rate of administration should be used in the elderly (see Dosage). Particular caution should be exercised in elderly patients with severe coronary and/or cerebral arteriosclerosis: reduction in perfusion pressure may impair adequate blood supply to these organs.

Insufficient data are available regarding the cardiovascular effects of propofol when used for induction and/or maintenance of anesthesia or sedation in elderly, hypotensive, debilitated or other ASA III and IV patients. However, limited information suggests that these patients may have more profound cardiovascular responses. It is recommended that if propofol is used in these patients, a lower induction dose and a slower maintenance rate of administration of the drug be used (see Warnings and Dosage).

The first respiratory disturbance after a bolus dose of propofol is a profound fall in tidal volume leading to apnea in many patients. There has been no accompanying cough or hiccough and otherwise anesthesia is smooth. However, there might be some difficulty in uptake of volatile agents if respiration is not assisted.

In unpremedicated, healthy patients, there is a steep dose-response relationship regarding apnea: 0% and 44% of patients had apnea after receiving 2 and 2.5 mg/kg of propofol, respectively. Fentanyl enhanced both the incidence and the onset of apnea and the episode lasted for >60 seconds in the majority of patients.

Opioid premedication-in the presence of hyoscine-affected respiratory function (rate of respiration and minute volume) substantially more than atropine premedication. Respiratory function was more depressed when these premedicants were combined with propofol than when they were combined with thiopental. Enhanced respiratory depression with propofol and an opioid has been observed in the postoperative period.

During maintenance, propofol (0.1 to 0.2 mg/kg/min: 6 to 12 mg/kg/h) caused a decrease in ventilation usually associated with an increase in carbon dioxide tension which may be marked depending upon the rate of administration and other concurrent medication (e.g., narcotics, sedatives, etc.). Propofol was not evaluated in patients with any respiratory dysfunction.

During sedation, attention must be given to the cardiorespiratory effects of propofol. Hypotension, apnea, airway obstruction, and/or oxygen desaturation can occur, especially with a rapid bolus injection. During initiation of sedation, slow infusion or slow injection techniques are preferable over rapid bolus administration, and during maintenance of sedation, a variable rate infusion is preferable over intermittent bolus administration in order to minimize undesirable cardiorespiratory effects. In the elderly, debilitated, ASA III or IV patients, rapid (single or repeated) bolus dose administration should not be used for sedation (see Warnings).

Clinical and preclinical studies suggest that propofol is rarely associated with elevation of plasma histamine levels and does not cause signs of histamine release.

Clinical and preclinical studies show that propofol does not suppress the adrenal response to ACTH.

Preliminary findings in patients with normal intraocular pressure indicate that propofol anesthesia produces a decrease in intraocular pressure which may be associated with a concomitant decrease in systemic vascular resistance.

Propofol is devoid of analgesic or antalgesic activity.

INDICATIONS: Induction and Maintenance of General Anaesthesia: Propofol is a short-acting i.v. general anesthetic agent that can be used for both induction and maintenance of anesthesia as part of a balanced anesthesia technique, including total i.v. anesthesia (TIVA), for inpatient and outpatient surgery.

Propofol is also indicated for pediatric anesthesia in children 3 years of age and older.

Conscious Sedation for Surgical and Diagnostic Procedures: Adults: Propofol, when administered i.v. as directed, can be used to initiate and maintain sedation in conjunction with local/regional anesthesia in patients undergoing surgical procedures. Propofol may also be used for sedation during diagnostic procedures (see Warnings and Precautions).

Children: Propofol is not recommended for sedation in children under the age of 18 during surgical/diagnostic procedures as safety and efficacy have not been established.

Sedation During Intensive Care: Adults: Propofol should only be administered to intubated, mechanically ventilated patients in the Intensive Care Unit (ICU) to provide continuous sedation and control of stress responses. In this setting, propofol should be administered only by or under the supervision of persons trained in general anesthesia or critical care medicine.

Children: See Contraindications.

CONTRAINDICATIONS: When general anesthesia or sedation are contraindicated. In patients with a known allergy and/or hypersensitivity to propofol or to lipid emulsions. For the sedation of children 18 years or younger receiving intensive care.

WARNINGS: For general anesthesia or sedation for surgical/diagnostic procedures, propofol should be administered only by persons trained in the administration of general anesthesia and not involved in the conduct of surgical/diagnostic procedures. Patients should be continuously monitored and facilities for maintenance of a patent airway, artificial ventilation, and oxygen enrichment and circulatory resuscitation must be immediately available.

For sedation of intubated, mechanically ventilated, adult patients in the Intensive Care Unit (ICU), propofol should be administered only by persons trained in general anesthesia or critical care medicine.

In the elderly, debilitated and ASA III or IV patients, rapid (single or repeated) bolus administration should not be used during general anesthesia or sedation in order to minimize undesirable cardiorespiratory depression including hypotension, apnea, airway obstruction and/or oxygen desaturation.

Propofol should not be coadministered through the same i.v. catheter with blood or plasma because compatibility has not been established. In vitro tests have shown that aggregates of the globular component of the emulsion vehicle have occurred with blood/plasma/serum from humans and animals. The clinical significance is not known.

The neuromuscular blocking agents, atracurium and mivacurium should not be given through the same i.v. line as propofol without prior flushing.

Propofol should not be used in obstetrics including Cesarean section deliveries, because propofol crosses the placenta and may be associated with neonatal depression.

Propofol should not be used for Intensive Care Unit (ICU) sedation in patients who have severely disordered fat metabolism because the vehicle of propofol is similar to that of Intralipid 10%. The restrictions that apply to Intralipid 10% should also be considered when using propofol in the ICU.

Extreme care should be used in administering propofol in patients with impaired left ventricular function because propofol may produce a negative inotropic effect.

Extreme care should be used in administering propofol in patients who are hypotensive, hypovolemic or in shock because propofol may cause excessive arterial hypotension.

Extreme care should be used in administering propofol in elderly, debilitated or other ASA III or IV patients.

Strict aseptic techniques must always be maintained during handling as propofol is a single-use parenteral product, for use in an individual patient, and contains no antimicrobial preservatives. The vehicle is capable of supporting rapid growth of microorganisms (see Precautions and Dosage). Failure to follow aseptic handling procedures may result in microbial contamination causing fever/infection/sepsis which could lead to life-threatening illness.

Propofol lacks vagolytic activity and has been associated with reports of bradycardia, (occasionally profound) and also asystole. The i.v. administration of an anticholinergic agent before induction, or during maintenance of anesthesia should be considered, especially in situations where vagal tone is likely to predominate or when propofol is used in conjunction with other agents likely to cause a bradycardia.

Since various manifestations of seizures have been reported during propofol anesthesia, special care should be taken when giving the drug to epileptic patients.

Occupational Hazards: Patients receiving propofol on an outpatient basis should not engage in hazardous activities requiring complete mental alertness such as driving a motor vehicle or operating machinery until the effects of propofol have completely subsided. Alcohol must be avoided.

PRECAUTIONS: General: In adults and children, attention should be paid to minimize pain on administration of propofol. Transient local pain during intravenous injection may be reduced by prior injection of i.v. lidocaine (1.0 mL of a 1% solution).

Patients should be continuously monitored for early signs of significant hypotension and/or bradycardia. Treatment may include increasing the rate of i.v. fluid, elevation of lower extremities, use of pressor agents or administration of anticholinergic agents (e.g., atropine) or use of plasma volume expanders. Apnea often occurs during induction and may persist for more than 60 seconds. Ventilatory support may be required. Because propofol is a lipid emulsion, caution should be exercised in patients with disorders of lipid metabolism such as primary hyperlipoproteinemia, diabetic hyperlipemia and pancreatitis.

When propofol is administered as a sedative for surgical or diagnostic procedures, patients should be continuously monitored by persons not involved in the conduct of the surgical/diagnostic procedure. Oxygen supplementation should be immediately available and provided where clinically indicated; and oxygen saturation should be monitored in all patients. Patients should be continuously monitored for early signs of hypotension, apnea, airway obstruction and/or oxygen desaturation. These cardiorespiratory effects are more likely to occur following rapid initiation (loading) boluses or during supplemental maintenance boluses, especially in the elderly, debilitated and ASA III or IV patients.

Since propofol is rarely used alone, an adequate period of evaluation of the awakened patient is indicated to ensure satisfactory recovery from general anesthesia or sedation prior to discharge of the patient from the recovery room or to home. Very rarely the use of propofol may be associated with the development of a period of post-operative unconsciousness, which may be accompanied by an increase in muscle tone. This may or may not be preceded by a period of wakefulness. Although recovery is spontaneous, appropriate care of an unconscious patient should be administered.

Intensive Care Unit (ICU) Sedation: Adults: Strict aseptic techniques must be followed when handling propofol as the vehicle is capable of supporting rapid growth of microorganisms (see Warnings and Dosage).

The administration of propofol should be initiated as a continuous infusion and changes in the rate of administration made slowly (>5 min) in order to minimize hypotension and avoid acute overdosage.

Patients should be monitored for early signs of significant hypotension and/or cardiovascular depression, which may be profound. These effects are responsive to discontinuation of propofol, i.v. fluid administration, and/or vasopressor therapy.

As with other sedative medications, there is wide interpatient variability in propofol dosage requirements, and these requirements may change with time.

Patients who receive large doses of narcotics during surgery may require very small doses of propofol for appropriate sedation.

Abrupt discontinuation of propofol infusion prior to weaning should be avoided since, due to the rapid clearance of propofol, it may result in rapid awakening with associated anxiety, agitation and resistance to mechanical ventilation. Infusions of propofol should be adjusted to maintain a light level of sedation throughout the weaning process.

Since propofol is formulated in an oil-water emulsion, elevations in serum triglycerides may occur when propofol injection is administered for extended periods of time. Patients at risk of hyperlipidemia should be monitored for increases in serum triglycerides or serum turbidity. Administration of propofol should be adjusted if fat is being inadequately cleared from the body. A reduction in the quantity of concurrently administered lipids is indicated to compensate for the amount of lipid infused as part of the propofol formulation: 1 mL of propofol contains approximately 0.1 g of fat (1.1 kcal).

The long-term administration of propofol to patients with renal failure and/or hepatic insufficiency has not been evaluated.

Children Under 18 years of Age: Intensive Care Unit (ICU) Sedation: See Contraindications.

Sedation During Surgical/Diagnostic Procedures in Children Under 18 Years of Age: Propofol is not recommended for sedation during surgical/diagnostic procedures, in children under the age of 18, as safety and efficacy have not been established. See Adverse Effects.

Pediatric Use for General Anaesthesia: In the absence of sufficient clinical experience, propofol is not recommended for anaesthesia in children less than 3 years of age (see Indications and Dosage).

Pregnancy: Propofol should not be used during pregnancy. Propofol has been used during termination of pregnancy in the first trimester. Teratology studies in rats and rabbits show some evidence of delayed ossification or abnormal cranial ossification, however such developmental delays are not considered indicative of a teratogenic effect. Reproductive studies in rats suggest that administration of propofol to the dam adversely affects perinatal survival of the offspring.

Lactation: Propofol is not recommended for use in nursing mothers because preliminary findings indicate that it is excreted in human milk and the effects of oral absorption of small amounts of propofol are not known.

Geriatrics: Elderly patients may be more sensitive to the effects of propofol; therefore, the dosage of propofol should be reduced in these patients according to their condition and clinical response (see Pharmacology, Pharmacokinetics and Dosage).

Cardiac Anesthesia: Propofol was evaluated in 328 patients undergoing coronary artery bypass graft (CABG). Of these patients 85% were males (mean age 61, range 32 to 83) and 15% were females (mean age 65, range 42 to 86).

The majority of patients undergoing CABG had good left ventricular function. Experience in patients with poor left ventricular function, as well as, in patients with hemodynamically significant valvular or congenital heart disease is limited.

Slower rates of administration should be utilized in premedicated patients, geriatric patients, patients with recent fluid shift, or patients who are hemodynamically unstable. Any fluid deficits should be corrected prior to administration of propofol. In those patients where additional fluid therapy may be contraindicated, other measures, e.g., elevation of lower extremities, or use of pressor agents, may be useful to offset the hypotension which is associated with the induction of anesthesia with propofol.

Neurosurgical Anesthesia: When using propofol in patients with increased intracranial pressure (ICP) or impaired cerebral circulation, significant decreases in mean arterial pressure should be avoided because of the resultant decreases in cerebral perfusion pressure. When increased ICP is suspected, hyperventilation and hypocarbia should accompany the administration of propofol (see Dosage).

Drug Interactions: Propofol has been used in association with spinal and epidural anaesthesia and with a range of premedicants, muscle relaxants, inhalational agents, analgesic agents and with local anaesthetic agents; no significant adverse interactions have been observed.

The induction dose requirements of propofol injection may be reduced in patients with i.m. or i.v. premedication, particularly with narcotics and combinations of opioids and sedatives. These agents may increase the anesthetic or sedative effects of propofol and may result in more pronounced decreases in systolic, diastolic, and mean arterial pressures and cardiac output.

Other drugs that cause CNS depression (hypnotics/sedatives, inhalational anesthetics and opioids) can increase CNS depression induced by propofol. Morphine premedication with nitrous oxide in oxygen has been shown to decrease the necessary propofol injection maintenance infusion rate and therapeutic blood concentrations when compared to non-narcotic (lorazepam) premedication.

After suxamethonium and neostigmine, bradycardia and cardiac arrest may occur.

Leukoencephalopathy has been reported with administration of lipid emulsions such as propofol in patients on cyclosporine.

ADVERSE EFFECTS: Anesthesia and Sedation for Surgical/Diagnostic Procedures: During induction of anesthesia in clinical trials, hypotension and apnea occurred in the majority of patients. The incidence of apnea varied considerably, occurring in between 30 and 100% of patients depending upon premedication, speed of administration and dose (see Pharmacology). Decreases in systolic and diastolic pressures ranged between 10 and 28%, but were more profound in the elderly and in ASA III and IV patients. Excitatory phenomena occurred in up to 14% of adult patients and in 33 to 90% of pediatric patients: they consisted most frequently of spontaneous musculoskeletal movements and twitching and jerking of the hands, arms, feet or legs. Epileptiform movements including convulsions, myoclonus and opisthotonus have occurred rarely, but a causal relationship with propofol has not been established. Flushing and rash have occurred in 10 to 25% of pediatric patients. Local pain occurred during i.v. injection of propofol at an incidence of 28% when veins of the dorsum of the hand were used and 5% when the larger veins of the forearm and the antecubital fossa were used. Propofol increased plasma glucose concentrations significantly, but no other significant changes in hematological or biochemical values were observed.

In the sedation clinical trials, the adverse reaction profile of propofol was similar to that seen during anesthesia. The most common adverse reactions included hypotension, nausea, pain and/or hotness at injection site and headache. Respiratory events included upper airway obstruction, apnea, hypoventilation, dyspnea and cough.

Rarely, clinical features of anaphylaxis, which may include angioedema, bronchospasm, erythema and hypotension, occur following propofol administration.

There have been reports of post-operative fever.

Pulmonary edema may be a potential side effect associated with the use of propofol.

As with other anesthetics, sexual disinhibition may occur during recovery.

Intensive Care Unit (ICU) Sedation: Adults: The most frequent adverse reactions during Intensive Care Unit (ICU) sedation were hypotension (31.5%), hypoxia (6.3%), and hyperlipemia (5.5%). In some patients, hypotension was severe. Other reactions considered severe were observed in single patients and included ventricular tachycardia, decreased cardiac output, decrease in vital capacity and negative inspiratory force, increase in triglycerides and agitation. Two patients with head injury suffered renal failure with severe increases in BUN accompanied in 1 patient by an increase in creatinine.

There have been rare reports of rhabdomyolysis when propofol has been administered at doses greater than 4 mg/kg/hr for ICU sedation.

Very rarely pancreatitis has been observed following the use of propofol for induction and maintenance of anaesthesia, and for intensive care sedation. A causal relationship has not been clearly established.

Table 1 compares the overall occurrence rates of adverse reactions in propofol patients from non-ICU and ICU clinical trials where the rate of occurrence was greater than 1%. Major differences include lack of metabolic/nutritional (hyperlipemia) and respiratory events in the non-ICU group and lack of nausea, vomiting, headache, movement and injection site events in the ICU group.

Adverse Reactions Reported at an Incidence of 1% or Less During Anesthesia and Sedation for Surgical/Diagnostic Procedures: Body as a Whole: asthenia, awareness, chest pain, extremity pain, increased drug effect, neck rigidity/stiffness, trunk pain, perinatal disorder.

Cardiovascular System: significant hypotension, premature atrial contractions, premature ventricular contractions, tachycardia, syncope, abnormal ECG, bigeminy, edema, AV heart block, bleeding, bundle branch block, myocardial infarction, myocardial ischemia, ST segment depression, ventricular fibrillation.

Table 1: Propofol Injection

Non-ICU vs ICU Adverse Events Occurring in Greater than 1% of Propofol Injection Patients

Body System	Event	Non-ICU (%)	ICU (%)
Number of Patients		**2588**	**127**
Cardiovascular	Hypotension	7.38	31.50
	Bradycardia	2.82	3.94
	Hypertension	2.82	1.57
	Arrhythmia	1.24	0.79
	Tachycardia	0.81	3.15
	Cardiovascular Disorder	0.23	2.36
	Hemorrhage	0.23	1.57
	Atrial Fibrillation	0.15	1.57

(cont'd)

Table 1: Propofol Injection *(cont'd)*
Non-ICU vs ICU Adverse Events Occurring in Greater than 1% of Propofol Injection Patients

Body System	Event	Non-ICU (%)	ICU (%)
Number of Patients		**2588**	**127**
	Cardiac Arrest	0.12	3.15
	Ventricular Tachycardia	0.08	1.57
Digestive	Nausea	14.57	0.0
	Vomiting	8.31	0.0
	Abdominal Cramping	1.24	0.0
Nervous	Movement	4.44	0.0
	Headache	1.78	0.0
	Dizziness	1.70	0.0
	Twitching	1.47	0.0
	Agitation	0.19	2.36
	Intracranial Hypertension	0.0	3.94
Metabolic/Nutritional	Hyperlipemia	0.08	5.51
	Acidosis	0.04	1.57
	Creatinine Increased	0.0	2.36
	BUN Increased	0.0	1.57
	Hyperglycemia	0.0	1.57
	Hypernatremia	0.0	1.57
	Hypokalemia	0.0	1.57
Respiratory	Dyspnea	0.43	1.57
	Hypoxia	0.08	6.30
	Acidosis	0.0	1.57
	Pneumothorax	0.0	1.57
Other	Injection Site:		
	Pain	8.11	0.0
	Burning/Stinging	7.77	0.0
	Fever	1.89	2.36
	Hiccough	1.78	0.0
	Cough	1.55	0.0
	Rash	1.20	1.57
	Anemia	0.35	1.57
	Kidney Failure	0.0	1.57

Respiratory System: burning in throat, tachypnea, dyspnea, upper airway obstruction, wheezing, bronchospasm, laryngospasm, hypoventilation, hyperventilation, sneezing, pharyngitis.
Excitatory: hypertonia, dystonia, rigidity, tremor.
Central Nervous System: confusion, dizziness, paresthesia, somnolence, shivering, abnormal dreams, agitation, delirium, euphoria, fatigue, amorous behavior, anxiety, bucking/jerking/thrashing, combativeness, depression, emotional lability, hallucinations, hypotonia, hysteria, insomnia, moaning, neuropathy, tremor.
Injection Site: phlebitis, thrombosis, hives/itching, redness/discoloration.
Digestive System: hypersalivation, dry mouth, diarrhea, enlarged parotid, swallowing.
Hematologic/Lymphatic: coagulation disorder, leukocytosis.
Metabolic/Nutritional: hyperkalemia.
Skin and Appendages: flushing/rash (for incidence in children, see above), urticaria, pruritus, conjunctival hyperemia, diaphoresis.
Special Senses: diplopia, amblyopia, tinnitus, ear pain, eye pain, nystagmus, taste perversion.
Musculoskeletal: myalgia.
Urogenital: urine retention, discoloration of urine.
Adverse Reactions Reported at an Incidence of 1% or Less During ICU Sedation:
Cardiovascular: arrhythmia, extrasystole, heart block, right heart failure, bigeminy, ventricular fibrillation, heart failure, myocardial infarction.
Respiratory: lung function decreased, respiratory arrest.
Central Nervous System: seizure, thinking abnormal, akathisia, chills, anxiety, confusion, hallucinations.
Digestive: ileus, hepatomegaly.
Metabolic/Nutritional: osmolality increased, dehydration.
Urogenital: green urine, urination disorder, oliguria.
Body as a Whole: sepsis, trunk pain, whole body weakness.
Post-marketing Experience: Clinical trial: A randomized, controlled, clinical trial that evaluated the safety and effectiveness of propofol versus standard sedative agents (SSA) in pediatric ICU patients has been conducted. In that study a total of 327 pediatric patients were randomized to receive either propofol 2% (113 patients), propofol 1% (109 patients),or an SSA (e.g, lorazepam, chloral hydrate, fentanyl, ketamine, morphine, or phenobarbital).

Propofol therapy was initiated at an infusion rate of 5.5 mg/kg/hr and titrated as needed to maintain sedation at a standardized level. The results of the study showed an increase in the number of deaths in patients treated with propofol as compared to SSAs. A total of 25 patients died during the trial or within the 28-day follow-up period: 12 (11%) in the propofol 2% treatment group, 9 (8%) in the propofol 1% treatment group, and 4 (4%) in the SSA treatment group.

Spontaneous reports and publications: There are several publications identifying an association in adults between high infusion rates (greater than 5 mg/kg/h) of propofol for more than 48 hours in ICUs and a potentially fatal constellation of adverse events characterized by metabolic acidosis, rhabdomyolysis and cardiovascular collapse.

The majority of the above-reported cases occurred in adults with head injury. These patients were treated with propofol at infusion rates greater than 5 mg/kg/h in an attempt to control intracranial hypertension. It is unclear at this time whether propofol at these high infusion rates can provide enhanced intracranial pressure reduction. A causal relationship between these adverse events and propofol and/or the lipid carrier cannot yet be established.

Similar findings were first reported in the literature in 1992 in children who received high doses of propofol in the ICU. Since the 1992 publication, several similar reports have been published, including an article that summarized 18 cases of children who received propofol infusions and suffered serious adverse events, including death.

Drug Abuse and Dependence: Rare cases of self administration of propofol by health care professionals have been reported, including some fatalities.

OVERDOSE:

Symptoms: To date, there is no known case of acute overdosage, and no specific information on emergency treatment of overdosage is available. If accidental overdosage occurs, propofol administration should be discontinued immediately. Overdosage is likely to cause cardiorespiratory depression. Respiratory depression should be treated by artificial ventilation with oxygen. Cardiovascular depression may require repositioning of the patient by raising the patient's legs, increasing the flow rate of i.v. fluids and if severe may require the administration of plasma volume expanders and/or pressor agents.

Treatment: See Symptoms.

> For management of a suspected drug overdose, CPhA recommends that you contact your **regional Poison Control Centre**. See the *CPS* Directory section for a list of Poison Control Centres.

DOSAGE: Strict aseptic techniques must always be maintained during handling as propofol is a single-use parenteral product, for use in an individual patient, and contains no antimicrobial preservatives. The vehicle is capable of supporting rapid growth of microorganisms. Failure to follow aseptic handling procedures may result in microbial contamination causing fever/infection/sepsis which could lead to life-threatening illness.

Propofol should be shaken well before use.

General: Dosage and rate of administration should be individualized and titrated to the desired effect according to clinically relevant factors including preinduction and concomitant medications, age, ASA status and level of debilitation of the patient. In heavily premedicated patients, both the induction and maintenance doses should be reduced.

Induction of General Anesthesia: Most **adult patients** under 55 years of age and classified ASA I and II are likely to require 2 to 2.5 mg/kg of propofol for induction when unpremedicated or when premedicated with oral benzodiazepines or i.m. narcotics. For induction, it is recommended that propofol should be titrated (approximately 40 mg every 10 seconds by bolus injection or infusion) against the response of the patient until the clinical signs show the onset of general anesthesia.

It is important to be familiar and experienced with the appropriate i.v. use of propofol before treating **elderly, debilitated and/or adult patients in ASA Physical Status Classes III and IV.** These patients may be more sensitive to the effects of propofol; therefore, the dosage of propofol should be reduced in these patients by approximately 50% (20 mg every 10 seconds) according to their condition and clinical response. A rapid bolus should not be used as this will increase the likelihood of undesirable cardiorespiratory depression including hypotension, apnea, airway obstruction and/or oxygen desaturation (see Warnings, Precautions and Table 2, Dosage Guide).

During **cardiac anesthesia**, a rapid bolus induction should be avoided. A slow rate of approximately 20 mg every 10 seconds until induction onset (0.5 to 1.5 mg/kg) should be used.

Most **children** over 8 years of age require approximately 2.5 mg/kg of propofol for induction of anesthesia. Children 3 to 8 years of age may require somewhat higher doses, however the dose should be titrated by administering propofol slowly until the clinical signs show the onset of anesthesia. Propofol is not recommended for induction of anesthesia in children less than 3 years of age. Reduced dosage is recommended for children in ASA Classes III and IV.

Additionally, as with most anesthetic agents, the effects of propofol may be potentiated in patients who have received i.v. sedative or narcotic premedications shortly prior to induction.

Maintenance of General Anesthesia: Anesthesia can be maintained by administering propofol by infusion or intermittent i.v. bolus injection. The patient's clinical response will determine the infusion rate or the amount and frequency of incremental injections.

When administering propofol by infusion, drop counters, syringe pumps or volumetric pumps must be used to provide controlled infusion rates.

Continuous Infusion: Propofol 0.1 to 0.2 mg/kg/min (6 to 12 mg/kg/h) administered in a variable rate infusion with 60 to 70% nitrous oxide and oxygen provides anesthesia for patients undergoing general surgery. Maintenance by infusion of propofol should immediately follow the induction dose in order to provide satisfactory or continuous anesthesia during the induction phase. During this initial period following the induction injection higher rates of infusion are generally required (0.15 to 0.2 mg/kg/min; 9 to 12 mg/kg/h) for the first 10 to 15 minutes. Infusion rates should subsequently be decreased by 30 to 50% during the first half-hour of maintenance. Changes in vital signs (increases in pulse rate, blood pressure, sweating and/or tearing) that indicate a response to surgical stimulation or lightening of anesthesia may be controlled by the administration of propofol 25 mg (2.5 mL) to 50 mg (5 mL) incremental boluses and/or by increasing the infusion rate. If vital sign changes are not controlled after a 5-minute period, other means such as a narcotic, barbiturate, vasodilator or inhalation agent therapy should be initiated to control these responses.

For minor surgical procedures (i.e., body surface) 60 to 70% nitrous oxide can be combined with a variable rate propofol infusion to provide satisfactory anesthesia. With more stimulating surgical procedures (i.e., intra-abdominal) supplementation with i.v. analgesic agents should be considered to provide a satisfactory anesthetic and recovery profile. When supplementation with nitrous oxide is not provided, administration rate(s) of propofol and/or opioids should be increased in order to provide adequate anesthesia.

Infusion rates should always be titrated downward in the absence of clinical signs of light anesthesia until a mild response to surgical stimulation is obtained in order to avoid administration of propofol at rates higher than are clinically necessary. Generally, rates of 0.05 to 0.1 mg/kg/minute should be achieved during maintenance in order to optimize recovery times.

During **cardiac anesthesia**, when propofol is used as the primary agent, maintenance infusion rates should not be less than 0.1 mg/kg/min and should be supplemented with analgesic levels of continuous opioid administration. When an opioid is used as the primary agent, propofol maintenance rates should not be less than 0.05 mg/kg/min. Higher doses of propofol will reduce the opioid requirements.

For **children**, the average rate of administration varies considerably but rates between 0.1 to 0.25 mg/kg/min (6 to 15 mg/kg/h) should achieve satisfactory anesthesia. These infusion rates may be subsequently reduced depending on patient response and concurrent medication.

Intermittent Bolus: Increments of propofol 25 mg (2.5 mL) to 50 mg (5 mL) may be administered with nitrous oxide in patients undergoing general surgery. The incremental boluses should be administered when changes in vital signs indicate a response to surgical stimulation or light anesthesia.

Propofol has been used in conjunction with a wide variety of agents commonly used in anesthesia such as atropine, scopolamine, glycopyrrolate, diazepam, depolarizing and nondepolarizing muscle relaxants, and narcotic analgesics, as well as with inhalational and regional anesthetic agents. No pharmacological incompatibilities have been encountered.

Lower doses of propofol may be required when used as an adjunct to regional anaesthesia.

Sedation During Surgical or Diagnostic Procedures: Adults: When propofol is administered for sedation, rates of administration should be individualized and titrated to clinical response. In most patients, the rates of propofol administration will be approximately 25 to 30% of those used for maintenance of general anesthesia.

During initiation of sedation, slow injection or slow infusion techniques are preferable over rapid bolus administration. During maintenance of sedation, a variable rate infusion is preferable over intermittent bolus dose administration.

Initiation of Sedation: **Slow Injection:** Most adult patients will generally require 0.5 to 1 mg/kg administered over 3 to 5 minutes and titrated to clinical response.

In the elderly, debilitated, hypovolemic and ASA III or IV patients, the dosage of propofol should be reduced to approximately 70 to 80% of the adult dosage and administered over 3 to 5 minutes.

Infusion: Sedation may be initiated by infusing propofol at 0.066 to 0.1 mg/kg/min (4 to 6 mg/kg/h) and titrating to the desired level of sedation while closely monitoring respiratory function.

Maintenance of Sedation: Patients will generally require maintenance rates of 0.025 to 0.075 mg/kg/min (1.5 to 4.5 mg/kg/h) during the first 10 to 15 minutes of sedation maintenance.

Infusion rates should always be titrated downward in the absence of clinical signs of light sedation until mild responses to stimulation are obtained in order to avoid sedative administration of propofol at rates higher than are clinically necessary.

In addition to the infusion, bolus administration of 10 to 15 mg may be necessary if a rapid increase in sedation depth is required.

In the elderly, debilitated, hypovolemic and ASA III or IV patients, the rate of administration and the dosage of propofol should be reduced to approximately 70 to 80% of the adult dosage according to their condition, responses, and changes in vital signs. Rapid (single or repeated) bolus dose administration should not be used for sedation in these patients (see Warnings).

Intensive Care Unit (ICU) Sedation: Propofol should be individualized according to the patient's condition and response, blood lipid profile, and vital signs.

Adults: For intubated, mechanically ventilated, adult patients, Intensive Care Unit (ICU) sedation should be initiated slowly with a continuous infusion in order to titrate to desired clinical effect and minimize hypotension. When indicated, initiation of sedation should begin at 0.005 mg/kg/min (0.3 mg/kg/h). The infusion rate should be increased by increments of 0.005 to 0.01 mg/kg/min (0.3 to 0.6 mg/kg/h) until the desired level of sedation is achieved. A minimum period of 5 minutes between adjustments should be allowed for onset of peak drug effect.

Most adult patients require maintenance rates of 0.005 to 0.05 mg/kg/min (0.3 to 3 mg/kg/h). Dosages of propofol should be reduced in patients who have received large dosages of narcotics. As with other sedative medications, there is interpatient variability in dosage requirements and these requirements may change with time (see Table 2, Dosage Guide).

Bolus administration of 10 to 20 mg should only be used to rapidly increase sedation depth in patients where hypotension is not likely to occur. A rapid bolus should not be used as this will increase the likelihood of hypotension. Patients with compromised myocardial function, intravascular volume depletion or abnormally low vascular tone (e.g., sepsis) may be more susceptible to hypotension.

Children under 18 years of age: Propofol is contraindicated for the sedation of children 18 years or younger receiving intensive care.

Compatibility and Stability: Propofol should not be mixed with other therapeutic agents prior to administration.

The neuromuscular blocking agents, atracurium and mivacurium should not be given through the same i.v. line as propofol without prior flushing.

Dilution Prior to Administration: When propofol is diluted prior to administration, it should only be diluted with 5% Dextrose Injection, USP, and it should not be diluted to a concentration less than 2 mg/mL because it is an emulsion. Dilutions should be prepared aseptically immediately before administration and should not be used beyond 6 hours of preparation. In diluted form it has been shown to be more stable when in contact with glass than with plastic (95% potency after 2 hours of running infusion in plastic).

Administration Into a Running I.V. Catheter: Compatibility of propofol with the coadministration of blood/serum/plasma has not been established (see Warnings). Propofol has been shown to be compatible with the following i.v. fluids when administered into a running i.v. catheter: 5% Dextrose Injection, USP; Lactated Ringers Injection, USP; Lactated Ringers and 5% Dextrose Injection; 5% Dextrose and 0.45% Sodium Chloride Injection, USP; 5% Dextrose and 0.2% Sodium Chloride Injection, USP.

Table 2: Propofol Injection

Dosage Guide

Indication	Dosage and Administration
Induction of General Anesthesia	
	Dosage should be individualized.
	Adult Patients Less than 55 Years of Age: Are likely to require 2 to 2.5 mg/kg (approximately 40 mg every 10 seconds until induction onset).
	Elderly, Debilitated and/or Adult ASA III or IV Patients: Are likely to require 1 to 1.5 mg/kg (approximately 20 mg every 10 seconds until induction onset) but dose should be carefully titrated to effect.
	Cardiac Anesthesia: Patients are likely to require 0.5 to 1.5 mg/kg (approximately 20 mg every 10 seconds until induction onset).
	Neurosurgical Patients: Are likely to require 1 to 2 mg/kg (approximately 20 mg every 10 seconds until induction onset).
	Pediatric Patients: Children over 8 years of age require approximately 2.5 mg/kg. Children 3 to 8 years of age may require somewhat higher doses but doses should be titrated slowly to the desired effect. In the absence of sufficient clinical experience, propofol is not recommended for anesthesia in children less than 3 years of age (see Indications and Precautions). Reduced dosage is recommended for children of ASA Classes III and IV.
Maintenance of General Anesthesia	
Infusion:	**Variable rate infusion titrated to the desired clinical effect.**
	Adult Patients Less than 55 Years of Age: Generally, 0.1 to 0.2 mg/kg/min (6 to 12 mg/kg/h).
	Elderly, Debilitated and/or Adult ASA III or IV Patients: Generally, 0.05 to 0.1 mg/kg/min (3 to 6 mg/kg/h).
	Cardiac Anesthesia: Most patients require: primary propofol with secondary opioid: 0.1 to 0.15 mg/kg/min (6 to 9 mg/kg/h); low dose propofol with primary opioid: 0.05 to 0.1 mg/kg/min (3 to 6 mg/kg/h).
	Neurosurgical Patients: Generally, 0.1 to 0.2 mg/kg/min (6 to 12 mg/kg/h).
	Pediatric Patients: Generally, 0.1 to 0.25 mg/kg/min (6 to 15 mg/kg/h).
Intermittent Bolus:	Increments of 25 mg to 50 mg, as needed.
Surgical/Diagnostic Sedation:	
	Dosage and rate should be individualized and titrated to the desired clinical effect.
	Adult Patients Less than 55 Years of Age: Are likely to require 0.5 to 1 mg/kg over 3 to 5 minutes to initiate sedation, followed by 0.025 to 0.075 mg/kg/min (1.5 to 4.5 mg/kg/h) for continued sedation.
	Elderly, Debilitated, Hypovolemic and/or ASA III or IV Patients: The dosage and rate of administration may need to be reduced in these patients by approximately 20 to 30% (see previous section for details).
	Pediatric Patients: Propofol is not recommended for sedation during surgical/diagnostic procedures in children under the age of 18, as safety and efficacy have not been established (see Indications).
Initiation and Maintenance of ICU Sedation in Intubated, Mechanically Ventilated, Adult Patients	
	Dosage and rate of infusion should be individualized.
	Adult Patients: For initiation, most patients require an infusion of 0.005 mg/kg/min (0.3 mg/kg/h) for at least 5 minutes. Subsequent increments of 0.005 to 0.010 mg/kg/min (0.3 - 0.6 mg/kg/h) over 5 to 10 minutes may be used until desired level of sedation is achieved.
	For maintenance, most patients require 0.005 to 0.05 mg/kg/min (0.3 to 3 mg/kg/h).
	The long-term administration of propofol to patients with renal failure and/or hepatic insufficiency has not been evaluated.
	Pediatric Patients: (see Contraindications).

When administering propofol injection by infusion, drop counters, syringe pumps or volumeric pumps must be used to provide controlled infusion rates.

Handling Procedures: Parenteral drug products should be inspected visually for particulate matter and discoloration prior to administration whenever solution and container permit.

Do not freeze. Do not use if there is evidence of separation of the phases of the emulsion.

Aseptic techniques must be applied to the handling of the drug. Propofol contains no antimicrobial preservatives and the vehicle supports growth of microorganisms. When propofol is to be aspirated it should be drawn aseptically into a sterile syringe or i.v. administration set immediately after breaking the ampul or breaking the vial seal. Administration should commence without delay. Asepsis must be maintained for both propofol and the infusion equipment throughout the infusion period. Any drugs or fluids added to the infusion line must be administered close to the cannula site. Propofol must not be administered via a microbiological filter.

Propofol and any syringe containing propofol are for single-use in an individual patient only. The contents of a propofol ampul must be used within 6 hours of opening or discarded thereafter. If a vial is utilized for infusion, both the reservoir of propofol and the infusion line must be discarded and replaced as appropriate at the end of the procedure or at 12 hours, whichever is sooner. (When using **diluted** propofol, see Dilution Prior to Administration.)

Since Propofol contains no preservative or bacteriostatic agents, any unused portions of propofol or solutions containing propofol should be discarded at the end of the surgical procedure.

SUPPLIED: Each mL of white, oil in water emulsion contains: propofol 10 mg for i.v. administration. Nonmedicinal ingredients: egg phosphatide, glycerin, sodium hydroxide to adjust pH, soybean oil and water for injection. It is isotonic with a pH of 6.5 to 8.5. Ready-to-use 20 mL ampuls, trays of 5. Glass infusion vials of 20, 50 and 100 mL, cartons of 5, 1, and 1 respectively. Store between 15 and 25°C; do not freeze. The emulsion should be visually inspected for particulate matter, emulsion separation and discoloration prior to use. Any unused portions or solutions containing propofol should be discarded at the end of the surgical procedure.

Propoxyphene Ⓝ

CPhA Monograph

see *Opioids*

Propranolol 🄿

Beta-adrenergic Receptor Blocking Agent, Nonselective

CPhA Monograph

Date of Preparation: November 2005
Date of Revision: December 2009

This monograph has been compiled by CPhA and reviewed by experts. It may contain information different from that found in Health Canada-approved Product Monographs. The reader is referred to the *CPS* Editorial Policy for more information.

SUMMARY PRODUCT INFORMATION:

Route of Administration	Dosage Form	Strength
Oral, immediate release	Tablet	10 mg, 20 mg, 40 mg, 80 mg, 120 mg
Oral, extended-release[a]	Capsule	60 mg, 80 mg, 120 mg, 160 mg
Intravenous	Vial	1 mg/mL

[a] Bioavailability significantly reduced with extended release formulations. Dose re-titration may be required if switching between immediate and extended release preparations.

INDICATIONS AND CLINICAL USE: Health Canada-approved indications include:

- treatment of hypertension and cardiac arrhythmias (including supraventricular and ventricular tachycardias)
- prevention of stable angina pectoris, migraine headache and essential tremor
- reduction of cardiovascular mortality post-myocardial infarction
- management of hypertrophic subaortic stenosis
- as an adjunct in the treatment of pheochromocytoma and thyrotoxicosis

Uses Without Health Canada Approval: Propranolol can be used in the management of aggression in patients with a brain injury, situational anxiety and tetralogy of Fallot hypercynanotic spells. In patients with portal hypertension, propranolol has been used for the primary or secondary prevention of bleeding esophageal varices.

CONTRAINDICATIONS:

- Patients who are hypersensitive to propranolol or to any ingredient in the formulation
- Bronchospasm, including asthma and COPD; patients with allergic rhinitis during pollen season
- Sinus bradycardia, second or third degree AV block, cardiogenic shock, right ventricular failure secondary to pulmonary hypertension and heart failure, unless the failure is secondary to a tachyarrhythmia treatable with propranolol (see Warnings and Precautions)
- Pregnancy (second and third trimesters)
- Raynaud's disease

WARNINGS AND PRECAUTIONS:

Serious Warnings and Precautions
Abrupt discontinuation of propranolol therapy in patients with angina pectoris can lead to exacerbation of angina and in some cases, myocardial infarction. If propranolol is to be discontinued, gradually reduce the dose over a period of 2 weeks and observe the patient closely.

General: Propranolol may be associated with a wider variety of adverse reactions than other beta-adrenergic receptor blocking drugs due to its ability to distribute into the CNS. Significant problems can develop as a result of its mechanism of action. Adverse reactions are more frequent and severe with iv propranolol than oral propranolol.

Cardiovascular: In patients with heart failure, beta blockade may precipitate more severe failure. In patients with no history of heart failure, continued use of beta-blockers can lead to cardiac failure in rare instances. If heart failure develops discontinue propranolol, treat if required and monitor the patient for resolution of symptoms.

Severe bradycardia can occur and may lead to vertigo, syncope or orthostatic hypotension. A reduction in the dose of propranolol may be necessary.

Endocrine and Metabolism: Use beta-blockers with caution in diabetic patients, especially those with labile diabetes or those prone to hypoglycemia. Propranolol can mask some of the symptoms of hypoglycemia such as tachycardia and blood pressure changes, but not dizziness and sweating. Propranolol may mask the signs of hyperthyroidism in patients with thyrotoxicosis. Abrupt withdrawal of propranolol may exacerbate the symptoms of hyperthyroidism, including thyroid storm. Propranolol may alter thyroid function tests, increasing T_4 and rT_3, and decreasing T_3.

Hepatic: Use propranolol with caution in patients with impaired hepatic function.

Perioperative Considerations: The need to discontinue propranolol prior to major surgery is controversial. There have been cases of protracted severe hypotension and difficulty in restarting and maintaining the heartbeat in patients receiving beta-adrenergic blocking agents. If necessary, the effects of propranolol can be reversed with beta-agonists such as dobutamine or isoproterenol.

Renal: Use propranolol with caution in patients with impaired renal function.

Respiratory: Beta-blocking agents may inhibit bronchodilation and increase airway resistance and bronchospasm. Patients with bronchospastic disease should in general not use propranolol. Use with caution in patients with nonallergic bronchospasm (e.g., chronic bronchitis, emphysema).

Special Populations: Pregnant Women: The safety of propranolol in pregnancy has not been established. Low birth weight, respiratory distress and hypoglycemia have been reported in neonates born to women using propranolol during pregnancy. Propranolol should be used during pregnancy only when the possible benefits outweigh the potential risks.

Nursing Women: Propranolol is excreted in breast milk. Although there are no reports, potential adverse effects to the nursing infant include respiratory depression, bradycardia and hypoglycemia. The American Academy of Pediatrics considers propranolol to be compatible with breast feeding.

Pediatrics: The safety and efficacy of propranolol has not been studied as extensively in children as in adults. The recommended doses are estimates from medical literature and have been reasonably studied. Propranolol should be used with caution in children with Down syndrome since the oral bioavailability may be increased in this group of patients.

Geriatrics: Lower doses of propranolol should be used in the elderly.

ADVERSE REACTIONS: Cardiovascular: bradycardia, cardiogenic shock, chest pain, exacerbation of symptoms of peripheral vascular disease including intermittent claudication and cold extremities, hypotension, impaired myocardial contractility, mesenteric thrombosis (rare), pulmonary edema, syncope, worsening of AV conduction disturbance.

Central Nervous System: amnesia, cognitive dysfunction, confusion, depression, dizziness, emotional lability, fatigue, hallucinations, insomnia, lethargy, lightheadedness, paresthesia, psychosis, vivid dreams, vertigo.

Dermatologic: alopecia, contact dermatitis, exfoliative dermatitis, eczematous eruptions, hyperkeratosis, nail changes, pruritus, psoriasiform eruptions, rash, urticaria.

Endocrine and Metabolism: hyperglycemia, hyperkalemia, hyperlipidemia, hypoglycemia.

Gastrointestinal: anorexia, constipation, diarrhea, ischemic colitis (rare), nausea, vomiting.

Genitourinary: impotence, interstitial nephritis (rare), oliguria (rare), Peyronie's disease, proteinuria (rare).

Hematologic: agranulocytosis, eosinophilia, thrombocytopenia, thrombocytopenic purpura.

Musculoskeletal: arthropathy, carpal tunnel syndrome (rare), myotonus, polyarthritis.

Ophthalmologic: decreased visual acuity, dry eyes, hyperemia of the conjunctiva, mydriasis.

Respiratory: bronchospasm, pharyngitis, wheezing.

DRUG INTERACTIONS: Overview: Propranolol is a substrate of CYP1A2, CYP2D6 and CYP2C19, and an inhibitor of CYP1A2, CYP2D6 and CYP3A4. Some of the drug interactions in Table 1 involve these isoenzymes.

Drug-Drug Interactions: See Table 1.

Table 1: Propranolol HCl

Drug-Drug Interactions

Interacting Drug	Effect	Clinical Comment
Amiodarone	Increased bradycardic effect of propranolol; can be significant	Mechanism may involve hepatic metabolism; consider therapy modification or monitor for signs of bradycardia.
Barbiturates	Decreased serum levels of propranolol	Monitor for decrease in propranolol efficacy. Consider using beta-blockers that are primarily excreted unchanged by the kidneys (e.g., atenolol).
$Beta_2$-agonists (e.g., albuterol, fenoterol, formoterol, salmeterol, terbutaline)	Diminished bronchodilatory effect of $beta_2$-agonist	Combination of a nonselective beta-blocker and a $beta_2$-agonist should be avoided when possible.
Cimetidine	Inhibits hepatic metabolism of propranolol	Use alternative H_2-antagonist such as ranitidine.
Cholinesterase Inhibitors	Increased bradycardic effect of propranolol	Monitor for bradycardia.
Clonidine	Increased blood pressure possibly due to unopposed alpha activity	Closely monitor blood pressure after initiation or discontinuation of either drug. Discontinue propranolol several days before stopping clonidine.
Digoxin	Bradycardia, heart block, heart failure	Monitor for bradycardia and arrhythmias.
Diltiazem	Increased effect of propranolol	Monitor efficacy of propranolol. If an interaction is suspected, consider decreasing the dose of propranolol, or use alternative therapy.
Epinephrine	Hypertension and bradycardia	Caution when larger doses used as a local anesthetic.
Ergotamine	Increased vasoconstrictive action of ergotamine	Monitor for signs of peripheral ischemia.
Fluoxetine	Increased bradycardic effect of propranolol	Monitor for changes in heart rate if fluoxetine therapy started or stopped.
Insulin	Propranolol prolongs and masks the signs of hypoglycemia	Avoid combination or use with caution. Monitor for signs of hypoglycemia not masked by beta-blockers (e.g., sweating).
Lidocaine	Increased effects of lidocaine	Monitor lidocaine levels and adjust if necessary.
Methacholine	Increased effects of methacholine	Avoid combination or use with caution.
NSAIDs	Decreased antihypertensive effect of propranolol	Monitor blood pressure and adjust propranolol dose as necessary when either starting or stopping an NSAID.
Phenothiazines	Increased effects of both drugs	The dosage of both drugs may need to be decreased. Consider using a beta-blocker with greater renal elimination, e.g. atenolol or nadolol.
Prazosin	Increased hypotension with first prazosin dose	Minimize first prazosin dose.
Propafenone	Decreased first pass metabolism of propranolol	Monitor patient and adjust dose of propranolol if necessary.
Rifampin	Decreased propranolol levels	Monitor clinical response to propranolol and adjust dose if necessary.
Rizatriptan	Decreased clearance of rizatriptan; magnitude of effect unpredictable	Rizatriptan product monograph recommends no more than 5 mg per dose, at least 2 hours between doses, and a maximum of 10 mg/day, in patients taking propranolol.
Theophylline	Increased serum theophylline levels	Monitor serum theophylline levels and observe carefully for reduced bronchodilator response; consider using a cardioselective beta-blocker such as metoprolol.
Verapamil	Increased effects of both drugs	Monitor cardiac function and decrease the doses if necessary.

DOSAGE AND ADMINISTRATION: Recommended Dose and Dosage Adjustment: Adults: See Table 2.

Dose in Geriatric Patients: Initiate therapy at reduced doses and titrate slowly.

Pediatrics: See Table 3.

Hepatic Impairment: Bradycardia may occur in patients with hepatic dysfunction. Initiate propranolol at lower doses and monitor heart rate regularly.

OVERDOSAGE:

For management of a suspected drug overdose, CPhA recommends that you contact your **regional Poison Control Centre**. See the *CPS* Directory section for a list of Poison Control Centres.

ACTION AND CLINICAL PHARMACOLOGY: Mechanism of Action: As a nonselective beta-adrenergic blocking agent, propranolol competitively blocks the response to adrenergic stimuli of beta receptors in the myocardium, and in bronchial and vascular smooth muscle. Effects on the myocardium include decreased heart rate, contractility, cardiac output and conduction velocity. Propranolol's clinical usefulness in the management of angina is likely related to effects such as decreased myocardial oxygen consumption and enhanced oxygen delivery to tissues; propranolol may also affect platelet aggregation through a mechanism unrelated to beta blockade.

The proposed mechanism of propranolol's antihypertensive action involves an overlap among various effects such as decreased cardiac output, decreased sympathetic outflow from the CNS and decreased renin release.

Table 2: Propranolol HCl

Dose in Adult Patients

Indication	Route	Initial Dose	Titrate	Usual Dose	Clinical Comment
Aggression following acquired brain injury (Not an approved use in Canada)	Oral	20–40 mg daily	20 mg per day	40–640 mg daily in divided doses	Monitor heart rate and blood pressure.
Angina pectoris	Oral	20–40 mg BID	Increase to 80 mg BID in 1 week if necessary	80–320 mg daily in 2–4 divided doses	If propranolol is to be discontinued, taper slowly over 2 weeks (see Warnings and Precautions).
Arrhythmias	Oral	10–30 mg 3–4 times daily			In older individuals, start with 10 mg twice daily and titrate up at 3- to 7-day intervals.
	IV	1–3 mg	Repeat after 2 min	Additional doses after 4 hours if required	Close cardiovascular monitoring.
Essential tremor	Oral	40 mg BID		120–320 mg daily in 3 divided doses	Individualize dosage.
Hypertension[a]	Oral	Extended release: 80 mg once daily	Extended release: increase to 160 mg daily in 1 week if necessary	Extended release: 160–320 mg once daily	Individualize dosage. Immediate-release formulations not recommended for hypertension. Doses of greater than 320 mg may be needed, but it may be preferable to add another antihypertensive.
Hypertrophic subaortic stenosis	Oral	20–40 mg TID or QID			
Migraine prophylaxis	Oral	40 mg BID	Gradually increase dose	80–240 mg daily in 1–4 divided doses	Individualize dosage.
Pheochromocytoma	Oral	60 mg daily in divided doses, for 3 days prior to surgery			Give with an alpha-receptor blocker.
Post-myocardial infarction	Oral	40 mg TID	Increase to 60 mg TID in 1–2 weeks	180–240 mg daily in 2–4 divided doses	Continue therapy for at least 3 years. Some experts recommend treating indefinitely in patients with no contraindications.
Prevention of bleeding esophageal varices (Not an approved use in Canada)	Oral	10 mg TID	Titrate to resting heart rate of 55–60, a reduction in resting heart rate of 20–25%, or occurrence of adverse effects		Assess portal pressures to identify patients who do not adequately respond to beta-blocker alone.

(cont'd)

Table 2: Propranolol HCl *(cont'd)*

Dose in Adult Patients

Indication	Route	Initial Dose	Titrate	Usual Dose	Clinical Comment
Situational anxiety (Not an approved use in Canada)	Oral	10 mg 30 minutes prior to event (e.g., public speaking, performance)			
Thyrotoxicosis	Oral	10–40 mg Q6H			
	IV	1–3 mg single dose			

[a] Canadian guidelines on the management of hypertension are published [*Can J Cardiol* 2008;24(6):465-75] or available at www.hypertension.ca.

Table 3: Propranolol HCl

Oral Dose in Pediatric Patients

Indication	Initial Dose	Titrate	Usual Dose	Maximum Dose
Arrhythmia	0.5–1 mg/kg/day in 3–4 divided doses	Titrate at 3- to 7-day intervals as necessary to control arrhythmia	2–6 mg/kg/day in divided doses	16 mg/kg/day not to exceed 60 mg, in 4 divided doses
Hypertension	0.5–1 mg/kg/day in 2 divided doses	Titrate according to blood pressure and tolerance	2–4 mg/kg/day in 2 divided doses	16 mg/kg daily
Migraine prophylaxis	2–4 mg/kg/day OR 10–20 mg TID if ≤35 kg, 20–40 mg TID if >35 kg			
Tetralogy spells (Not an approved use in Canada)	1 mg/kg/day in 4 divided doses	Increase dose after 1 week in 1 mg/kg/day increments if not effective	1–6 mg/kg/day in 3 or 4 divided doses	10–15 mg/kg/day in 3 or 4 divided doses
Thyrotoxicosis	2 mg/kg/day in 3–4 divided doses			In adolescents use adult doses

Pharmacokinetics: Adults: Absorption: Propranolol is well absorbed following oral administration. Large interindividual differences in hepatic extraction result in widely varying plasma concentrations. The presence of food increases its bioavailability.
Distribution: Propranolol is widely distributed throughout the body including the CNS, and is >90% bound to plasma proteins.
Metabolism: Both protein-bound and free propranolol are hepatically metabolized, partly by cytochrome P450 enzymes. The elimination half-life is 3–6 hours with chronic oral administration of immediate-release formulations, 12 hours for controlled-release capsules and 2–3 hours following intravenous doses.
Excretion: Propranolol and its metabolites are excreted mainly in the urine. About 1–4% appears in the feces. In patients with significant renal impairment, fecal excretion increases. Propranolol is not substantially removed by hemodialysis.
Special Populations: Geriatrics: Plasma levels and half-life may be increased in older individuals.

Propylthiouracil Ⓟ
Antithyroid Therapy

CPhA Monograph

Date of Preparation: October 2007
Date of Revision: June 2009

This monograph has been compiled by CPhA and reviewed by experts. It may contain information different from that found in Health Canada-approved Product Monographs. The reader is referred to the *CPS* Editorial Policy for more information.

SUMMARY PRODUCT INFORMATION:

Route of Administration	Dosage Form	Strength
Oral	Tablet	50 mg, 100 mg

INDICATIONS AND CLINICAL USE: Propylthiouracil is indicated for:
- medical treatment of hyperthyroidism in patients with Graves' disease
- preparative therapy to render patients euthyroid prior to receiving radioactive iodine (RAI) treatment or while awaiting ablative effects of radioactive iodine
- preparative therapy for stabilizing thyroid function prior to a thyroidectomy
- treatment of thyroid storm in addition to other therapeutic measures (e.g., beta-adrenergic blockers)

Propylthiouracil is used to control the symptoms in Graves' disease until spontaneous remission occurs. The recommended treatment duration with antithyroid drugs in adults with Graves' disease is 12-18 months. A longer duration of therapy may be required in patients whose disease is well controlled with a low dose of antithyroid drug.

Factors that may reduce the likelihood of remission include severe hyperthyroidism, large goiters, higher triiodothyronine (T_3):thyroxine (T_4) ratio, low antithyroid receptor levels and higher baseline levels of antithyrotropin-receptor antibodies. Patients may relapse at the end of treatment, even if they have normal antibody titers.

Propylthiouracil is not recommended in patients with hyperthyroidism caused by toxic multinodular goiters or solitary autonomous nodules as spontaneous remission rarely occurs in these conditions. A more definitive treatment such as RAI or surgery may be required.

Propylthiouracil is given prior to RAI administration to deplete thyroid hormones. RAI treatment damages the thyroid gland allowing leakage of thyroid hormones into the circulation; pretreatment with propylthiouracil prevents thyroid storm after RAI treatment.

Propylthiouracil is the preferred antithyroid agent in pregnant and nursing women with hyperthyroidism. (See Warnings and Precautions, Special Populations, Pregnant Women.)

Pediatrics: Long-term propylthiouracil treatment can be used in children and adolescents with hyperthyroidism to achieve and maintain a euthyroid state in an attempt to delay the need for ablative therapy with RAI. Neonatal hyperthyroidism can also be treated with propylthiouracil; once a euthyroid state is achieved, the dose should be gradually tapered to the lowest effective maintenance dose. It has been recommended that propylthiouracil use in children be avoided if possible because of concerns that propylthiouracil may induce liver failure in some children [*N Engl J Med* 2009;360(15):1574-5]. Methimazole should be the preferred alternative in children.

CONTRAINDICATIONS:
- Patients who are hypersensitive to propylthiouracil or to any ingredient in the formulation.

WARNINGS AND PRECAUTIONS:

Serious Warnings and Precautions
- Agranulocytosis (<0.5×10⁹ WBC/mm³) is a serious adverse reaction with an estimated frequency 0.1-0.5%. Though agranulocytosis can occur at any time, this adverse reaction typically develops within the first 3 months of therapy with propylthiouracil. The reaction is dose-related and reversible upon discontinuation. Patients >40 years and receiving other drugs known to cause agranulocytosis may be more susceptible. Instruct patients to immediately report any symptoms such as sore throat, fever or flu-like symptoms, and to discontinue propylthiouracil. Sepsis is suspected if there is rapid onset of fever, chills and prostration. Discontinue propylthiouracil treatment. Monitor CBC with differential at baseline and during the first 3 months of therapy. Agranulocytosis is a contraindication to further thionamide treatment because cross-reactivity between propylthiouracil and methimazole has been reported.
- Hepatotoxicity, a rare adverse reaction, has an estimated frequency of 0.1-0.2% in patients treated with propylthiouracil. Propylthiouracil-induced hepatotoxicity is not dose-related and is thought to be idiosyncratic with an autoimmune component. Hepatocellular necrosis and fulminant hepatic failure have been reported in patients treated with propylthiouracil. Typically these reactions occur within the first two months of propylthiouracil treatment. Injury is reversible upon discontinuation of propylthiouracil although encephalopathy and/or substantial hepatic necrosis have been reported. Routine monitoring of serum transaminases is not required but may be recommended for patients with a history of liver disease or for those who have other risk factors for hepatitis, e.g., alcohol use. Discontinue propylthiouracil when signs and symptoms of hepatic injury are present. Further thionamide therapy is contraindicated as death has resulted upon rechallenge.

General: Signs of hypothyroidism such as increased vascularity and size of the thyroid gland may manifest with antithyroid therapy. This is indicative of overtreatment and the dose of propylthiouracil should be reduced or temporarily discontinued.
Special Populations: Pregnant Women: Propylthiouracil readily crosses the placenta. Maternal therapy can cause fetal goiter and hypothyroidism. The effects on fetal thyroid, however, are often mild. Follow-up studies of children exposed in utero have shown normal intellectual and physiological development. Pregnant women should receive the lowest dose of propylthiouracil needed to control symptoms and to achieve and maintain serum free thyroxine (FT_4) in the upper half of the normal range. As pregnancy progresses, especially in the 3rd trimester, it is common for those with Graves' disease to experience a significant improvement in their condition, and the dose may need to be significantly reduced or the drug discontinued. Frequent monitoring of thyroid function (FT_4 levels) is important for detecting any changes in the mother's condition so dosing can be adjusted accordingly. Do not administer thyroxine concurrently with propylthiouracil. Thyroxine does not cross the placenta in sufficient amounts to reverse the effects of fetal hypothyroidism and can necessitate the need for higher maternal doses of propylthiouracil, further increasing the risk to the fetus.
Nursing Women: Propylthiouracil is classified as compatible with breastfeeding by the American Academy of Pediatrics and is considered to be the preferred antithyroid therapy during breastfeeding. Ionized at physiologic pH and highly protein bound, propylthiouracil transfer into breast milk is minimal. Infant exposure through breastfeeding has not shown any adverse effects on thyroid function. Follow-up studies have demonstrated no subsequent impairment in intellectual development. Monitor the infant's serum T_4 and thyroid stimulating hormone (TSH) levels every 2-4 weeks.
Monitoring and Laboratory Tests: Obtain baseline FT_4 and TSH levels prior to initiating propylthiouracil treatment. Monitor thyroid function every 4-6 weeks until a euthyroid state is achieved, then monitor thyroid function every 2-3 months for 6 months and then every 4-6 months for the duration of therapy. For all patients who enter remission, the risk of spontaneously redeveloping hyperthyroidism years after discontinuing therapy requires that lifelong thyroid assessment be routinely performed.

A baseline CBC count with differential is recommended at the start of propylthiouracil treatment. Hyperthyroid-induced leukopenia can be differentiated from leukopenia and/or agranulocytosis that may develop as a result of propylthiouracil therapy. Baseline serum transaminases may be useful in identifying the development of drug-induced hepatotoxicity.

ADVERSE REACTIONS: Adverse Drug Reactions Overview: Most common adverse reactions include gastrointestinal upset and skin rash, which frequently resolve with continued propylthiouracil therapy. Urticaria or arthralgia may be the harbinger of a serious hypersensitivity reaction and warrants prompt discontinuation of treatment. The more serious adverse reactions associated with propylthiouracil are agranulocytosis, hepatotoxicity and rarely, systemic vasculitis. Recovery is often possible following immediate cessation of the drug. (See Warnings and Precautions.)
More Common Adverse Drug Reactions: See Table 1.

Table 1: Propylthiouracil

More Common Adverse Drug Reactions (≥1%)

Body System	Effect	Clinical Comment
Central Nervous System	Headache	
Dermatologic	Skin rash	Commonly manifests as pruritic and maculopapular (occurs early in treatment) but may also be urticarial. Often maculopapular rash will resolve spontaneously but may be treated with antihistamines and/or topical corticosteroids. Discontinuing propylthiouracil treatment is not required unless the rash manifests as urticaria or is associated with other systemic symptoms, e.g., fever. Cross sensitivity for this adverse reaction is not common; consider continuing treatment with an alternative thionamide.
Gastrointestinal	Nausea and dyspepsia	
Musculoskeletal	Arthralgia and polyarthritis	Manifestation of arthralgia warrants immediate drug cessation as this symptom may herald the development of a severe transient migratory polyarthritis known as the "antithyroid arthritis syndrome."

Less Common Adverse Drug Reactions (<1%): Cardiovascular: edema.
Central Nervous System: dizziness, drowsiness, depression.
Allergic/Dermatologic: hair loss, depigmentation, erythema nodosum, vesicular eruption in newborns.
Ear/Nose/Throat: unilateral sensorineural hearing impairment.
Endocrine and Metabolism: sialadenopathy (enlargement of salivary glands). Hypothyroidism may develop with excessive dosage. Dose should be reduced or therapy temporarily discontinued. (See Warnings and Precautions, General.)
Gastrointestinal: vomiting, loss of taste.
Hematologic: agranulocytosis (see Warnings and Precautions), aplastic anemia, granulocytopenia, hemolytic anemia, hyperglobulinemia, hypoprothrombinemia, leukopenia, myeloblastic leukemia and thrombocytopenia.
Hepatic/Biliary/Pancreatic: hepatotoxicity.
Immune: drug fever, lupus-like syndrome (e.g., splenomegaly, skin ulcers, pericarditis), lymphadenopathy and polyarteritis.

The mechanism of propylthiouracil-induced, anti-neutrophil cytoplasmic autoantibody (ANCA)-positive vasculitis is unknown. The renal, musculoskeletal and dermatologic systems are affected. Characterized by inflammation and destruction of the blood vessels, clinical presentation is variable and may include fever, fatigue, skin ulcerations, pulmonary edema, nephritis and/or complications involving other organs. Time to develop vasculitis varies from months to years. Patients are at an increased risk if they are Asian or if they are receiving therapy for an extended duration. Discontinue propylthiouracil if this occurs.
Neurologic: neuritis, paresthesia.
Ophthalmologic: recurrent keratitis, conjunctival disorders.
Renal: nephritis.
Abnormal Hematologic and Clinical Chemistry Findings: See Table 2.

Table 2: Propylthiouracil
Abnormal Hematologic and Clinical Chemistry Findings

Test	Effect	Clinical Comment
CBC count with differential	leukopenia, agranulocytosis	Drug-induced leukopenia is often transient and is not associated with the development of agranulocytosis. Presentation does not warrant discontinuation of therapy. A granulocyte count of less than 1000/mm³ indicates impending agranulocytosis (<500/mm³). Discontinue propylthiouracil treatment immediately. Monitor closely if count is greater than 1000/mm³ but less than 1500/mm³.
TSH, FT_4	↑ TSH plasma concentration and/or ↓ FT_4 plasma concentration	Indicates development of hypothyroidism and is likely due to overtreatment. Reduce dose of propylthiouracil or temporarily discontinue. (See Warnings and Precautions, General.)
ALT, AST, bilirubin, LDH	↑ concentration	May indicate an adverse reaction, in particular hepatotoxicity.
INR	↑/↓ prothrombin time	May indicate an adverse reaction/drug interaction.

Abbreviations: ALT=alanine aminotransferase; AST=aspartate aminotransferase; CBC=complete blood cell; FT_4=free thyroxine; INR=international normalized ratio; LDH=lactate dehydrogenase; TSH=thyroid stimulating hormone.

DRUG INTERACTIONS: Drug-Drug Interactions: See Table 3.

Table 3: Propylthiouracil
Drug-Drug Interactions

Interacting Drug	Effect	Clinical Comment
Beta-blockers, e.g., metoprolol, propranolol	↑ clearance of beta-blocker in hyperthyroidism	Hyperthyroidism is associated with the ↑ clearance of beta-blockers with high extraction ratios. Liver blood flow, first pass metabolism and volume of distribution are increased in hyperthyroid states. These changes selectively affect beta-blockers that have a significant first pass effect. ↓ in beta-blocker dose may be necessary once a euthyroid state is achieved with propylthiouracil.
Digoxin	↑ serum digoxin levels when a euthyroid state is reached	Patients with hyperthyroidism may eliminate digoxin faster than euthyroid patients. Higher doses of digoxin may be required due to the ↑ clearance. May require a ↓ in digoxin dose once a euthyroid state is achieved. Monitor digoxin levels and adjust dose as necessary.

(cont'd)

Table 3: Propylthiouracil *(cont'd)*
Drug-Drug Interactions

Interacting Drug	Effect	Clinical Comment
Radioactive iodine (RAI, ¹³¹I)	↓ uptake of radioactive iodine by the thyroid gland pretreated with propylthiouracil	Propylthiouracil given a week before or after radioactive iodine reduced RAI effectiveness. Increased failure rates and reduced hypothyroidism rates have resulted. Discontinue propylthiouracil treatment at least 7 days before receiving RAI treatment. ↑ in RAI dose may be required if given concomitantly with propylthiouracil.
Theophylline	↑ clearance of theophylline in hyperthyroidism	Monitor theophylline serum levels when initiating, discontinuing or changing dose of propylthiouracil. Adjust theophylline dose as required.
Warfarin	↑ INR, enhanced anticoagulant response	Hyperthyroidism induces metabolism of vitamin K-dependent clotting factors (II, VII, IX, X) (↑ clearance, shorter plasma half-lives). Warfarin inhibits clotting factor synthesis by interfering with regeneration of reduced vitamin K. This may result in an enhanced anticoagulant response to warfarin. Patients with hyperthyroidism may require a ↓ in warfarin dose. Monitor INR and observe for signs of ↑ or ↓ response to warfarin therapy when initiating, discontinuing or changing doses of propylthiouracil. Adjust warfarin dose as needed.

Drug-Laboratory Interactions: Propylthiouracil may decrease the optimal uptake and retention of ¹³¹I by the thyroid gland. Thus, when performing a thyroid scan or assessing gland function through RAI uptake, propylthiouracil treatment should be temporarily discontinued at least 7 days before scheduled examination. Propylthiouracil may be reinitiated after RAI administration.

DOSAGE AND ADMINISTRATION:

Recommended Dose and Dosage Adjustment: Adults: See Table 4.
Pediatrics: See Table 5.
Renal Impairment: No dose adjustment needed in renal impairment.
Hepatic Impairment: No dose adjustment needed in hepatic impairment.
Administration: Tablets are for oral administration. If oral administration is not possible, the tablets may be crushed and administered rectally as a mineral oil or sodium phosphate enema or as a suppository. Patients should be instructed to retain the solution in the rectum for several hours following administration.

OVERDOSAGE:

For management of a suspected drug overdose, CPhA recommends that you contact your **regional Poison Control Centre**. See the *CPS* Directory section for a list of Poison Control Centres.

ACTION AND CLINICAL PHARMACOLOGY: Mechanism of Action: Propylthiouracil reduces plasma concentrations of thyroid hormones (T_3, T_4). The drug is actively transported into the thyroid gland. Propylthiouracil depletes preformed thyroid hormone stores and inhibits synthesis of thyroid hormones. It inhibits thyroid hormone synthesis by interfering with the coupling of iodotyrosine and the incorporation of iodine onto tyrosine residues in thyroglobulin. Propylthiouracil is suspected of inhibiting thyroid peroxidase thereby preventing the oxidation of iodide ions and iodotyrosyl groups required for the production of active thyroid hormone. Before a euthyroid state is achieved, a lag time of 3-4 weeks may occur, as it takes time for T_4 to be depleted.

Propylthiouracil inhibits the peripheral conversion of T_4 (produced solely by the thyroid gland) to T_3 (which is metabolically more active than T_4) by inhibiting 5′-monodeiodinase in a rapid dose-related manner.

Propylthiouracil does not inhibit the pharmacologic effect on thyroid hormone already formed and present in the thyroid gland or circulation nor will it interfere with the effect of exogenously administered thyroid hormone.
Pharmacokinetics: Adults: See Table 6.
Absorption: Following oral administration, approximately 75% of the dose is rapidly absorbed from the gastrointestinal tract. Absorption is unaffected by concomitant food intake.
Distribution: Propylthiouracil is widely distributed throughout the body. It crosses the placenta and is minimally distributed into milk. In serum, propylthiouracil is 75% to 80% protein-bound.

Table 4: Propylthiouracil
Dose in Adult Patients

Indication	Initial Dose (maximum dose)	Maintenance Dose	Duration of Therapy	Clinical Comment
Hyperthyroidism secondary to Graves' disease	300 mg po daily divided every 8 hours (max. 900–1200 mg po daily)	100–150 mg po daily divided every 8–12 hours	Recommended treatment duration is 12–18 months. Therapy extending beyond recommended treatment duration has shown no additional benefit.	For doses >300 mg po daily, administer in divided doses every 4–6 hours. Monitor thyroid function (FT_4 levels, TSH levels) every 4–6 weeks. If no improvement occurs after 4–6 weeks of treatment, consider ↑ the propylthiouracil dose. Symptom improvement should occur within 1–3 weeks of therapy and achieve euthyroidism after 6–8 weeks of therapy. Once thyroid function normalizes, dose may be gradually reduced by 33% every 4–6 weeks to the lowest effective maintenance dose. Response to treatment may be delayed in patients with abnormally large thyroid glands or if iodine therapy has been previously administered.
Thyroid Storm or Thyrotoxicosis	600–1200 mg po daily divided every 4–6 hours	N/A	As symptoms resolve, gradually ↓ dose to maintenance dose	Preferred agent in thyroid storm as it inhibits peripheral FT_4 conversion to T_3. Propylthiouracil can be given rectally as an enema or suppository.

Abbreviations: N/A=not applicable; FT_4=free thyroxine.

Table 5: Propylthiouracil
Dose in Pediatric Patients

Indication	Age	Initial Dose	Duration of Therapy	Clinical Comment
Hyperthyroidism, congenital	Neonate	5–10 mg/kg daily divided every 8 hours	Hyperthyroidism in neonates may remit within 3–4 months; however, remission can vary depending on the levels of thyroid receptor stimulating antibodies transferred from the mother. Occasionally hyperthyroidism will persist into childhood.	Not preferred agent: see Indications and Clinical Use, Pediatrics May add oral administration of Lugol solution (aqueous solution of iodine 5% and potassium iodide 10%) 1 drop every 8 hours, in addition to propylthiouracil therapy. Once thyroid function normalizes, dose may be gradually reduced to the lowest effective maintenance dose (e.g., ⅓ to ½ of the initial dose). Once a euthyroid state is achieved, gradually taper the dose to determine the lowest effective maintenance dose.
	6–10 years	50–150 mg daily divided every 8 hours or 5–10 mg/kg daily divided every 8 hours	There appears to be a remission rate of 25% every 2 years associated with childhood and adolescence and long-term treatment up to 6 years may be recommended.	Not preferred agent: see Indications and Clinical Use, Pediatrics Prolonged therapy may be required for the purpose of allowing the child to reach a more appropriate age to receive ablation therapy. Once thyroid function normalizes, the dose may be gradually reduced to the lowest effective maintenance dose (e.g., ⅓ to ½ of the initial dose). Once a euthyroid state is achieved, gradually taper the dose to achieve a lowest effective maintenance dose.
	>10 years	150–300 mg daily divided every 8 hours or 5–10 mg/kg daily divided every 8 hours		

Table 6: Propylthiouracil

Summary of Pharmacokinetic Parameters

T_{max}	Duration of Action	Elimination $t_{1/2}$	Clearance	Volume of Distribution
1–1.5 h	2–3 h	1–2 h	10 L/h	0.3–0.4 L/kg

Metabolism: The liver rapidly metabolizes propylthiouracil to a glucuronide conjugate and other minor metabolites.
Excretion: Approximately 35% of the drug and its metabolites are excreted in the urine within 24 hours.
STORAGE AND STABILITY: Store at a temperature less than 40°C, preferably between 15 and 30°C, in a closed container.

Propyl-Thyracil® Ⓟ
propylthiouracil
Hyperthyroidism Therapy

Paladin

SUPPLIED: Each white, phi-marked, scored tablet contains: propylthiouracil 50 or 100 mg. Gluten-, lactose- and tartrazine-free. Bottles of 100.

Proscar® Ⓟ
finasteride
Type II 5 Alpha-reductase Inhibitor

Merck Frosst

Date of Revision: April 27, 2007

SUMMARY PRODUCT INFORMATION:

Route of Administration	Dosage Form/ Strength	Clinically Relevant Nonmedicinal Ingredients
Oral	Film-coated tablet 5 mg	Lactose, starch glycolate For a complete listing see Dosage Forms, Composition and Packaging.

INDICATIONS AND CLINICAL USE:
- PROSCAR (finasteride, USP) as monotherapy is indicated for the treatment and control of benign prostatic hyperplasia (BPH) and for the prevention of urologic events to:
  - Reduce the risk of acute urinary retention;
  - Reduce the risk of surgery including transurethral resection of the prostate (TURP) and prostatectomy.
- PROSCAR causes regression of the enlarged prostate, improves urinary flow and improves the symptoms associated with BPH.
- PROSCAR administered in combination with the alpha-blocker doxazosin is indicated to reduce the risk of symptomatic progression of BPH (a confirmed ≥4 point increase in AUA symptom score).

Patients with an enlarged prostate are the appropriate candidates for therapy with PROSCAR. PROSCAR is not indicated to reduce the risk of developing prostate cancer in healthy men.

CONTRAINDICATIONS: PROSCAR is not indicated for use in women or children.
PROSCAR is contraindicated in the following:
- Pregnant Women—Use in women when they are or may potentially be pregnant (see Warnings and Precautions, Exposure to Finasteride—Risk to Male Fetus);
- Hypersensitivity to any component of this product.

WARNINGS AND PRECAUTIONS: General: Patients with large residual urine volume and/or severely diminished urinary flow should be carefully monitored for obstructive uropathy.

PROSCAR is not indicated for those patients who are candidates for immediate surgery.

No studies have been conducted to determine if PROSCAR can be used for the control of prostatic hyperplasia in asymptomatic patients.

The long term (>10 years) beneficial and adverse effects of PROSCAR have not yet been established.

Prior to treatment with PROSCAR, the patient should undergo a thorough urological evaluation to determine the severity of the condition, and to exclude the need for immediate surgery or the possibility of carcinoma of the prostate. Periodic follow-up evaluations should be performed to determine whether a clinical response has occurred.

Effects on PSA and Prostate Cancer Detection: No clinical benefit has yet been demonstrated in patients with prostate cancer treated with PROSCAR. Patients with BPH and elevated prostate-specific antigen (PSA) were monitored in controlled clinical studies with serial PSAs and prostate biopsies. In these studies, PROSCAR did not appear to alter the rate of prostate cancer detection. The overall incidence of prostate cancer was not significantly different in patients treated with PROSCAR or placebo.

Digital rectal examinations, as well as other evaluations for prostate cancer are recommended prior to initiating therapy with PROSCAR and periodically thereafter. Serum PSA is also used as one of the components of the screening process to detect prostate cancer. Generally, a baseline PSA >10 ng/mL (Hybritech) prompts further evaluation and consideration of biopsy; for PSA levels between 4 and 10 ng/mL, further evaluation is generally considered advisable. There is considerable overlap in PSA levels among men with and without prostate cancer. Therefore, in men with BPH, PSA values within the normal reference range do not rule out prostate cancer, regardless of treatment with PROSCAR. A baseline PSA <4 ng/mL does not exclude prostate cancer.

PROSCAR causes a decrease in serum PSA concentrations by approximately 50% in patients with BPH, even in the presence of prostate cancer (see Adverse Reactions, Laboratory Tests). This decrease in serum PSA levels in patients with BPH treated with PROSCAR should be considered when evaluating PSA data and does not rule out concomitant prostate cancer. This decrease is predictable over the entire range of PSA values, although it may vary in individual patients. Analysis of PSA data from over 3000 patients in the 4-year, double-blind, placebo-controlled PROSCAR Long-Term Efficacy and Safety Study (PLESS) confirmed that in typical patients treated with PROSCAR for six months or more, PSA values should be doubled for comparison with normal ranges in untreated men. This adjustment preserves the sensitivity and specificity of the PSA assay and maintains its ability to detect prostate cancer.

Any sustained increases in PSA levels of patients treated with finasteride should be carefully evaluated, including consideration of non-compliance to therapy with PROSCAR.

Clinical experience with finasteride in men with prostate cancer (n=72) suggests that the reduction in PSA from malignant prostate disease appears to be no greater than the percentage reduction of PSA from benign prostate disease.

Special Populations: Pregnant Women: Pregnant Women and Nursing Women: PROSCAR is contraindicated for use in women when they are or may potentially be pregnant (see Contraindications). Because of the ability of Type II 5 alpha-reductase inhibitors such as finasteride to inhibit conversion of testosterone to dihydrotestosterone, PROSCAR may cause abnormalities of the external genitalia of a male fetus when administered to a pregnant woman. It is not known whether finasteride is excreted in human milk. In female rats, low doses of finasteride administered during pregnancy have produced abnormalities of the external genitalia in male offspring. Therefore, if this drug is used during pregnancy or if pregnancy occurs while taking or exposed to this drug, the pregnant woman should be apprised of the potential hazard to the male fetus.

Nursing Women: See Pregnant Women.

Exposure to Finasteride—Risk to Male Fetus: Women should not handle crushed or broken tablets of PROSCAR when they are or may potentially be pregnant because of the possibility of absorption of finasteride and the subsequent potential risk to a male fetus (see Warnings and Precautions, Pregnant Women). PROSCAR tablets are coated and will prevent contact with the active ingredient during normal handling, provided that the tablets have not been broken or crushed.

Pediatrics: PROSCAR is not indicated for use in children. Safety and effectiveness in children have not been established.

Monitoring and Laboratory Tests: Effect on Levels of PSA: Serum PSA concentration is correlated with patient age and prostatic volume, and prostatic volume is correlated with patient age. When PSA laboratory determinations are evaluated, consideration should be given to the fact that PSA levels decrease in patients treated with PROSCAR.

ADVERSE REACTIONS: Adverse Drug Reaction Overview: PROSCAR is well tolerated.

Clinical Trial Adverse Drug Reactions: In PLESS, 1524 patients treated with PROSCAR 5 mg daily and 1516 patients treated with placebo were evaluated for safety over a period of 4 years. 4.9% (74 patients) were discontinued from treatment due to side effects associated with PROSCAR compared with 3.3% (50 patients) treated with placebo. 3.7% (57 patients) treated with PROSCAR and 2.1% (32 patients) treated with placebo discontinued therapy as a result of side effects related to sexual function, which were the most frequently reported side effects.

Table 1 presents the only clinical adverse reactions considered possibly, probably or definitely drug related by the investigator, for which the incidence on PROSCAR was ≥1% and greater than placebo over the 4 years of the study. In years 2-4 of the study, there was no significant difference between treatment groups in the incidences of impotence, decreased libido and ejaculation disorder.

Table 1: PROSCAR

Drug-related Adverse Experiences

	Treatment	Year 1 (%)	Years 2, 3 and 4[a] (%)
Impotence	Placebo Finasteride	3.7 8.1	5.1 5.1
Decreased Libido	Placebo Finasteride	3.4 6.4	2.6 2.6
Decreased Volume of Ejaculate	Placebo Finasteride	0.8 3.7	0.5 1.5
Ejaculation Disorder	Placebo Finasteride	0.1 0.8	0.1 0.2
Breast Enlargement	Placebo Finasteride	0.1 0.5	1.1 1.8
Breast Tenderness	Placebo Finasteride	0.1 0.4	0.3 0.7
Rash	Placebo Finasteride	0.2 0.5	0.1 0.5

[a] Combined years 2–4.

Table 2: PROSCAR

Incidence ≥2% in One or More Treatment Groups. Drug-Related Clinical Adverse Experiences in MTOPS

Adverse Experience	Placebo (N=737) (%)	Doxazosin 4 mg or 8 mg[a] (N=756) (%)	Finasteride (N=768) (%)	Combination (N=786) (%)
Body as a Whole				
Asthenia	7.1	15.7	5.3	16.8
Headache	2.3	4.1	2.0	2.3
Cardiovascular				
Hypotension	0.7	3.4	1.2	1.5
Postural Hypotension	8.0	16.7	9.1	17.8
Metabolic and Nutritional				
Peripheral Edema	0.9	2.6	1.3	3.3
Nervous				
Dizziness	8.1	17.7	7.4	23.2
Libido Decreased	5.7	7.0	10.0	11.6
Somnolence	1.5	3.7	1.7	3.1
Respiratory				
Dyspnea	0.7	2.1	0.7	1.9
Rhinitis	0.5	1.3	1.0	2.4
Urogenital				
Abnormal Ejaculation	2.3	4.5	7.2	14.1
Gynecomastia	0.7	1.1	2.2	1.5
Impotence	12.2	14.4	18.5	22.6
Sexual Function Abnormal	0.9	2.0	2.5	3.1

[a] Doxazosin dose was achieved by weekly titration (1 to 2 to 4 to 8 mg). The final tolerated dose (4 mg or 8 mg) was administered at end-Week 4. Only those patients tolerating at least 4 mg were kept on doxazosin. The majority of patients received the 8-mg dose over the duration of the study.

The adverse experience profile in the one-year, placebo-controlled, Phase III studies and the five-year extensions, including 853 patients treated for 5 to 6 years, was similar to that reported in years 2-4 in PLESS. There is no evidence of increased adverse experiences with increased duration of treatment with PROSCAR. The incidence of new drug related sexual adverse experiences decreased with duration of treatment.

The following additional adverse reactions have been reported in post-marketing experience:
- hypersensitivity reactions, including pruritus, urticaria and swelling of the lips and face;
- and testicular pain

Medical Therapy of Prostatic Symptoms (MTOPS): The MTOPS study compared finasteride 5 mg/day (n=768), doxazosin 4 or 8 mg/day (n=756), combination therapy of finasteride 5 mg/day and doxazosin 4 or 8 mg/day (n=786), and placebo (n=737). In this study, the safety and tolerability profile of the combination therapy was generally consistent with the profiles of the individual components. The incidence of ejaculation disorder in patients receiving combination therapy was comparable to the sum of incidences of this adverse experience for the two monotherapies. The individual adverse effects that occurred more frequently in the combination group compared to either drug alone were: asthenia, postural hypotension, peripheral edema, dizziness, decreased libido, rhinitis, abnormal ejaculation, impotence and abnormal sexual function (see Table 2).

Four patients in MTOPS reported the adverse experience breast cancer. Three of these patients were on finasteride only and one was on the combination therapy. During the four year, placebo-controlled PLESS study, which enrolled 3040 men, there were 2 cases of breast cancer in the placebo treated men, but no cases were reported in men treated with finasteride. The relationship between the long-term use of finasteride and male breast cancer is currently unknown.

Other Long-Term Data: In a 7-year placebo-controlled trial that enrolled 18 882 healthy men, of whom 9060 had prostate needle biopsy data available for analysis, prostate cancer was detected in 803 (18.4%) men receiving PROSCAR and 1147 (24.4%) men receiving placebo. The clinical significance of this observation on the occurrence of prostate cancer in men treated with PROSCAR is unknown. In the PROSCAR group, 280 (6.4%) men had prostate cancer with Gleason scores of 7-10 detected on needle biopsy vs. 237 (5.1%) men in the placebo group. The mechanism of an increased occurrence of high-grade prostate cancers in men treated with PROSCAR in this study is unknown. Additional analyses have indicated that the observation of an increase in high-grade prostate tumors in men treated with PROSCAR may be due to a detection bias that could be mediated through an effect on the volume of the prostate induced by long term PROSCAR treatment. Of the total cases of prostate cancer diagnosed in this study, approximately 98% were classified as intracapsular (clinical stage T1 or T2) at diagnosis. The clinical significance of the Gleason 7-10 data is unknown. **PROSCAR is not indicated to reduce the risk of developing prostate cancer in healthy men.**

Laboratory Tests: When PSA laboratory determinations are evaluated, consideration should be given to the fact that PSA levels are decreased in patients treated with PROSCAR (see Warnings and Precautions, Effects on PSA and Prostate Cancer Detection).

In most patients, a rapid decrease in PSA is seen within the first months of therapy, after which time PSA levels stabilize to a new baseline. The post-treatment baseline approximates half of the pre-treatment value. Therefore, in typical patients treated with PROSCAR for six months or more, PSA values should be doubled for comparison to normal ranges in untreated men. For clinical interpretation, see Warnings and Precautions, Effects on PSA and Prostate Cancer Detection.

No other difference in standard laboratory parameters was observed between patients treated with placebo or PROSCAR.

DRUG INTERACTIONS: Overview: No drug interactions of clinical importance have been identified. PROSCAR, at prescribed doses, does not appear to affect significantly the cytochrome P450-linked drug metabolizing enzyme system. Compounds which have been tested in man have included propranolol, digoxin, glyburide, warfarin, theophylline and antipyrine and no clinically meaningful interactions were found. However, patients on medications with narrow therapeutic indices, such as phenytoin, should be carefully monitored when treatment with PROSCAR is initiated.

Drug-Drug Interactions: Although specific interaction studies were not performed, in clinical studies PROSCAR was used concomitantly with ACE-inhibitors, acetaminophen, acetylsalicylic acid, alpha-blockers, beta-blockers, calcium channel blockers, cardiac nitrates, diuretics, H_2 antagonists, HMG-CoA reductase inhibitors, nonsteroidal anti-inflammatory drugs (NSAIDs), quinolones and benzodiazepines without evidence of clinically significant adverse interactions.

DOSAGE AND ADMINISTRATION: Dosing Considerations:

- PROSCAR as monotherapy is indicated for the treatment and control of benign prostatic hyperplasia (BPH) and for the prevention of urologic events to:
  - Reduce the risk of acute urinary retention;
  - Reduce the risk of surgery including transurethral resection of the prostate (TURP) and prostatectomy.
- PROSCAR causes regression of the enlarged prostate, improves urinary flow and improves the symptoms associated with BPH.
- PROSCAR administered in combination with the alpha-blocker doxazosin is indicated to reduce the risk of symptomatic progression of BPH (a confirmed ≥4 point increase in AUA symptom score).

Recommended Dose and Dosage Adjustment: The recommended dosage of PROSCAR is one 5 mg tablet daily with or without food (for information on doxazosin, see a doxazosin Product Monograph).

Dosage in Renal Insufficiency: No adjustment in dosage is required in patients with varying degrees of renal insufficiency (creatinine clearances as low as 0.15 mL/s [9 mL/min]) as pharmacokinetic studies did not indicate any change in the disposition of finasteride.

Dosage in Geriatrics: No adjustment in dosage is required although pharmacokinetic studies indicated the elimination of finasteride is decreased in patients more than 70 years of age.

Missed Dose: If a tablet is missed at its usual time, an extra dose should not be taken. The next dose should be taken as usual.

OVERDOSAGE:

Patients have received single doses of PROSCAR up to 400 mg and multiple doses of PROSCAR up to 80 mg/day for three months without adverse effects.

No specific treatment of overdosage with PROSCAR is recommended.

> For management of a suspected drug overdose, CPhA recommends that you contact your **regional Poison Control Centre**. See the *CPS* Directory section for a list of Poison Control Centres.

ACTION AND CLINICAL PHARMACOLOGY: Mechanism of Action: PROSCAR a synthetic 4-azasteroid compound, is an inhibitor of Type II 5 alpha-reductase, an intracellular enzyme which metabolizes testosterone into the more potent androgen dihydrotestosterone (DHT). In benign prostatic hyperplasia (BPH), enlargement of the prostate gland is dependent upon the conversion of testosterone to DHT within the prostate. PROSCAR is highly effective in reducing circulating and intraprostatic DHT. Finasteride has very low affinity for the androgen receptor.

In the PROSCAR Long-Term Efficacy and Safety Study (PLESS), the effect of therapy with PROSCAR on BPH-related urologic events (surgical intervention [e.g., transurethral resection of the prostate and prostatectomy] or acute urinary retention requiring catheterization) was assessed over a 4-year period in 3016 patients with moderate to severe symptoms of BPH. In this double-blind, randomized, placebo-controlled multicenter study, treatment with PROSCAR reduced the risk of total urologic events by 51% and was also associated with a marked and sustained regression in prostate volume, and a sustained increase in maximum urinary flow rate and improvement in symptoms.

Pharmacokinetics: In a study in 15 healthy male subjects, the mean bioavailability of a 5 mg PROSCAR tablet was 63% (range, 34-108%), based on the ratio of the area under the curve (AUC) relative to a 5 mg intravenous dose infused over 60 minutes. Maximum finasteride plasma concentration averaged 37 ng/mL (range, 27-49 ng/mL) and was reached 1 to 2 hours postdose. The mean plasma half-life of elimination was 6 hours (range, 3-16 hours). Following the intravenous infusion, mean plasma clearance was 2.75 mL/s (range, 1.17-4.65 mL/s) (165 mL/min, range, 70-279 mL/min) and mean steady-state volume of distribution was 76 L (range, 44-96 L). In a separate study, the bioavailability of finasteride was not affected by food.

Approximately 90% of circulating finasteride is bound to plasma proteins. Finasteride has been found to cross the blood-brain barrier.

Special Populations and Conditions: Geriatrics: No dosage adjustment is necessary for the elderly or patients with renal insufficiency.

STORAGE AND STABILITY: Store at room temperature (15-30°C) and protect from light to prevent discoloration.

SPECIAL HANDLING INSTRUCTIONS: Women should not handle crushed or broken tablets of PROSCAR when they are or may potentially be pregnant (see Warnings and Precautions, Special Populations, Exposure to Finasteride—Risk to Male Fetus).

INFORMATION FOR THE PATIENT: Published in e-CPS, available by subscription at www.e-cps.ca.

DOSAGE FORMS, COMPOSITION AND PACKAGING: Each blue, apple-shaped, film-coated tablet, with the code MSD 72 on one side and PROSCAR on the other, contains: finasteride 5 mg. Nonmedicinal ingredients: cellulose and cellulose derivatives, cornstarch, docusate sodium, FD&C Blue 2 Aluminum Lake, lactose, magnesium stearate, sodium starch glycolate, talc, titanium dioxide and yellow ferric oxide. Blister packages of 28.

(Shown in Product Identification Section)

Prostigmin® Ⓟ

neostigmine bromide

Parasympathomimetic Agent

Valeant

PHARMACOLOGY: Neostigmine inhibits the destruction of acetylcholine by cholinesterase, thus permitting freer transmission of nerve impulses across the neuromuscular junction. It also has a direct effect on voluntary muscle fibres and possibly on autonomic ganglion cells and neurons of the CNS.

After absorption or i.v. administration, 80% of a dose is excreted by the kidney in the unchanged (50%) and metabolized (30%) forms in 24 hours. The elimination half-life is approximately 51 to 91 minutes.

INDICATIONS: Myasthenia gravis.

CONTRAINDICATIONS: Bronchial asthma or mechanical obstruction of intestinal or urinary tract. Known hypersensitivity to neostigmine.

WARNINGS: No data supplied by the manufacturer.

PRECAUTIONS: When large doses are given, simultaneous administration of atropine sulfate may be advisable. Because of the possibility of hypersensitivity in an occasional patient, atropine should always be at hand, together with antishock medications. Hypotension and bradycardia may occur if the effect of gallamine or curare is antagonized by neostigmine.

ADVERSE EFFECTS: The untoward effects of neostigmine are most commonly related to overdosage and generally are of 2 varieties: muscarinic and nicotinic. Among the former group are nausea, vomiting, diarrhea, abdominal cramps, increased salivation, increased bronchial secretions, miosis, and diaphoresis. Muscarinic untoward effects can usually be counteracted by atropine. Nicotinic untoward effects are chiefly muscle cramps, fasciculation and weakness, which can be difficult to distinguish from exacerbation of underlying myasthenia gravis.

OVERDOSE:

Symptoms: Muscarinic and nicotinic effects (see Adverse Effects). Distinguish from myasthenic crisis with edrophonium chloride, if necessary.

Treatment: Control muscarinic effects with i.v. atropine, followed by i.m. atropine every 2 to 4 hours. Assist ventilation and treat convulsions or shock if necessary.

> For management of a suspected drug overdose, CPhA recommends that you contact your **regional Poison Control Centre**. See the *CPS* Directory section for a list of Poison Control Centres.

DOSAGE: Myasthenia Gravis: 75 to 300 mg, spaced over 24 hours as required.

SUPPLIED: Each white, round, flat-faced tablet with bevelled edges, "Prostigmin" engraved on the perimeter and "15" in the centre of one face, partially scored and engraved "V" on the other, contains: neostigmine bromide 15 mg. Also contains lactose, gelatin, sugar and starch. Gluten-, paraben-, sodium-, sulfite- and tartrazine-free. Bottles of 100. Protect from excessive heat (40°C), and keep in a tightly closed container.

Prostin® E2 Tablets Ⓟ

dinoprostone

Prostaglandin

Paladin

SUPPLIED: Available to hospitals only. Each white rectangular compressed tablet imprinted "U" on one side and "76" on the other side contains: dinoprostone 0.5 mg. Nonmedicinal ingredients: cornstarch, lactose, magnesium stearate, microcrystalline cellulose and silicon dioxide. Gluten-free. Glass bottles of 10. Tablets are stable for at least 2 years if stored under normal refrigeration (2 to 8°C). Once bottle is opened, use tablets within 90 days.

Prostin® E2 Vaginal Gel Ⓟ

dinoprostone

Prostaglandin

Paladin

SUPPLIED: Each syringe of semi-translucent viscous vaginal gel contains: dinoprostone 1 mg or 2 mg/3 g (2.5 mL). Nonmedicinal ingredients: colloidal silicon dioxide and triacetin gel. The contents of one syringe (a single dose container/closure system) to be used for one patient. Discard after use. The gel has a shelf-life of 24 months when stored at 2 to 8°C, under continuous refrigeration.

Prostin® VR Ⓟ

alprostadil

Prostaglandin

Pfizer

PHARMACOLOGY: Alprostadil (also known as prostaglandin E_1) relaxes the ductus arteriosus in early postnatal life and supports its patency when continuously infused i.v. or intra-arterially in neonates with congenital heart defects who depend on a patent ductus for survival. The desired pharmacological effects are obtained with an initial dosage of 0.1 µg/kg/minute. Higher doses do not offer added benefit. Postnatally the ductus arteriosus rapidly loses its responsiveness to alprostadil and consequently alprostadil appears to be most effective within 96 hours after birth, particularly when the pre-infusion arterial pO_2 is less than 40 mm Hg.

The estimated half-life of alprostadil is 5 to 10 minutes. I.V. administered alprostadil is rapidly distributed and metabolized and the pulmonary vascular bed removes about 68% of the drug in a single pass. Alprostadil is weakly bound to serum albumin. The major route of elimination of alprostadil and its metabolites is via the kidneys. In laboratory animals and humans, alprostadil can lower blood pressure, probably by relaxing the smooth muscle of the cardiovascular system. Alprostadil can elevate body temperature and this effect has been observed in some neonates receiving the drug.

INDICATIONS: To temporarily maintain the patency of the ductus arteriosus until corrective or palliative surgery can be performed in neonates who have congenital heart defects and who depend upon a patent ductus arteriosus for survival.

Alprostadil should be administered only by medically trained personnel in facilities in which pediatric patients can receive or have access to pediatric intensive care.

CONTRAINDICATIONS: In the following patients: Cyanotic neonates with persistent fetal circulation. Neonates with total anomalous pulmonary venous return below the diaphragm, neonates with polysplenia or asplenia in whom pulmonary atresia is combined with anomalous pulmonary venous return which may be obstructed.

In such patients alprostadil may precipitate pulmonary edema because of increased pulmonary blood flow.

WARNINGS: Approximately 10 to 12% of neonates treated with alprostadil experienced apnea. Apnea is seen most often in neonates weighing less than 2 kg at birth and usually appears during the first hour of drug infusion. Therefore alprostadil should be used in facilities with immediately available intensive care for intubation and assisted ventilation.

Pathologic studies of the ductus arteriosus and pulmonary arteries of infants treated with prostaglandin E_1 have disclosed histologic changes compatible with a weakening effect upon these structures. The specificity or clinical relevance of these findings is not known.

Cortical proliferation of the long bones has followed long-term infusions of alprostadil in infants. The proliferation appeared to regress after withdrawal of the drug.

The administration of alprostadil to neonates may result in gastric outlet obstruction secondary to antral hyperplasia. This effect appears to be related to duration of therapy and cumulative dose of the drug. Neonates receiving alprostadil at recommended doses for more than 120 hours should be closely monitored for evidence of antral hyperplasia and gastric outlet obstruction.

Alprostadil should be infused for the shortest period of time at the lowest dose which will produce the desired effects. Risk of long-term treatment infusion of alprostadil should be weighed against the possible benefits that critically ill infants may derive from its administration.

PRECAUTIONS: Alprostadil should be used with caution in infants with suspected bleeding tendencies.

Care should be taken to avoid the use of alprostadil in neonates with respiratory distress syndrome (hyaline membrane disease), which sometimes can be confused with cyanotic heart disease. If full diagnostic facilities are not immediately available, cyanosis (pO_2 less than 40 mmHg) and restricted pulmonary blood flow apparent on an x-ray are good indicators of congenital heart defects.

In all neonates, blood pressure should be monitored by appropriate methods such as an umbilical artery catheter, or by a Doppler transducer. **Should arterial pressure fall significantly, reduce the rate of infusion immediately.**

Since alprostadil appears most effective within 96 hours after birth due to a decreasing responsiveness of the ductus arteriosus with time after birth, every effort should be made to start infusion of the drug during this period.

Long-term carcinogenicity and fertility studies have not been done.

The Ames and Alkaline Elution assays reveal no potential for mutagenesis.

In infants with restricted pulmonary blood flow, the increase in blood oxygenation is inversely proportional to pre-treatment pO_2 values; that is, patients with low pO_2 values (less than 40 torr) respond best, and patients with high pO_2 values (greater than 40 torr) usually have little response.

In infants with restricted pulmonary blood flow, measure efficacy of alprostadil by monitoring an improvement in blood oxygenation. In infants with restricted systemic blood flow, measure efficacy by monitoring improvement of systemic blood pressure and blood pH.

Drug Interactions: No drug interactions have been reported to occur between alprostadil and the standard therapy employed in neonates with congenital heart defects. Standard therapy includes antibiotics, such as penicillin or gentamicin; vasopressors, such as dopamine or isoproterenol; cardiac glycosides; and diuretics, such as furosemide.

ADVERSE EFFECTS: In infants whose ductus arterious must be kept patent, the most frequent adverse reactions observed with alprostadil infusion are related to its known pharmacological effects. The following incidences are based on experience in 436 patients.

Cardiovascular System: The most common adverse reactions reported in these patients were flushing 10.1%, bradycardia 6.7%, hypotension 3.9%, tachycardia 2.8%, cardiac arrest 1.1% and edema 1.1%. The following reactions were reported in less than 1% of patients: congestive heart failure, hyperemia, pneumopericardium, second degree heart block, shock, spasm of the right infundibulum (conus arteriosus), supraventricular tachycardia, ventricular fibrillation, ventricular hypertrophy, tachyphylaxis.

CNS: The most common adverse reactions reported were fever in 13.8% and seizures in 4.1% of patients. The following reactions were reported in less than 1% of patients: intracranial bleeding, hyperextension of neck, hyperirritability, hypothermia, jitteriness, lethargy, stiffness.

Respiratory System: The most common adverse reaction reported was apnea in 11.5% of patients. The following reactions were reported in less than 1% of patients: bradypnea, bronchial wheezing, hypercapnia, pneumothorax, respiratory depression, respiratory distress, tachypnea.

Gastrointestinal System: The most common adverse reaction reported was diarrhea in 2.6% of patients. The following reactions were reported in less than 1% of patients: gastric regurgitation, hyperbilirubinemia, peritonitis.

Hematologic: The most common adverse reaction reported was disseminated intravascular coagulation in 1.1% of patients. The following reactions were reported in less than 1% of patients: anemia, bleeding, thrombocytopenia, hypochromic anemia.

Urinary tract: The following reactions were reported in less than 1% of patients: anuria, hematuria, renal failure.

Metabolic: The most common adverse reaction reported was hypokalemia in 1.1% of patients. The following reactions were reported in less than 1% of patients: hypoglycemia, hyperkalemia.

Infection: Sepsis was reported in 1.6% and peritonsillitis in less than 1% of patients.

Ductus arteriosus histological changes: One group of investigators reported edema of the media, separation of the medial components by clear spaces, pathological interruption of the internal elastic lamina, and intimal lacerations some of which extended into the media in the ductus arteriosus of 4 patients.

Cortical proliferation of long bones: Following long-term infusion of alprostadil, cortical proliferation of long bones has been reported.

This hypertrophic osteoarthropathy appeared to be reversible on discontinuation of the drug.

OVERDOSE:

Symptoms: Apnea, bradycardia, pyrexia, hypotension and flushing may be signs of drug overdose.

Treatment: If apnea or bradycardia occur, the infusion should be discontinued and the appropriate medical treatment initiated. Caution should be used if the infusion is restarted. If pyrexia or hypotension occur, the infusion rate should be reduced until these symptoms subside. Flushing is usually attributed to incorrect intra-arterial catheter placement and is usually alleviated by repositioning the tip of the catheter.

For management of a suspected drug overdose, CPhA recommends that you contact your **regional Poison Control Centre**. See the *CPS* Directory section for a list of Poison Control Centres.

DOSAGE: The initial infusion rate of alprostadil should be 0.1 µg/kg of body weight/minute. When the desired effect on the ductus arteriosus is achieved, decrease infusion to the lowest possible dose while maintaining the desired effect. This may be accomplished by reducing the dosage from 0.1 to 0.05 to 0.025 to 0.01 µg/kg of body weight/minute. Although doses up to 0.4 µg/kg of body weight/minute have been used, doses above 0.1 µg/kg of body weight/minute generally do not offer additional benefits.

The preferred route of administration of alprostadil is by continuous i.v. infusion into a large vein. Alternatively, alprostadil may be administered through an umbilical artery catheter placed at the ductal opening. Adverse effects have occurred with both routes of administration, but higher incidence of flushing has been associated with intra-arterial than with i.v. administration.

If undiluted alprostadil comes in direct contact with a plastic container, plasticizers are leached from the sidewalls. The solution may turn hazy and the appearance of the container may change. Should this occur, the solution should be discarded and the plastic container replaced. This appears to be a concentration-dependent phenomenon. To minimize the possibility of haze formation, alprostadil should be added directly to the i.v. infusion solution avoiding contact with the walls of plastic containers (refer to Dilution Instructions).

Dilution Instructions: To prepare infusion solutions, dilute 1 mL of Prostin VR with sterile Sodium Chloride Injection or sterile Dextrose Injection. Dilute to volumes appropriate for the pump delivery system available. Prepare fresh infusion solution every 24 hours. **Discard any solution more than 24 hours old.**

For administration using a **pump capable of delivering small volume constant infusions** (i.e., not limited to discrete infusion rates) dissolve 1 mL Prostin VR (500 µg alprostadil) in 25 to 100 mL sterile 0.9% Sodium Chloride injection USP or sterile 5% Dextrose Injection USP to provide a solution containing 500 µg alprostadil. The infusion rate to deliver 0.1 µg/kg of body weight/minute can be calculated as follows:

$$\text{Infusion rate (mL/hr)} = \frac{\text{Volume containing 500 µg alprostadil} \times \text{body weight (kg)}}{83.3}$$

For administration using an infusion pump limited to discrete infusion rates, infuse 2 to 4 mL/hour. The volume of saline or glucose to be added to the 1 mL Prostin VR is to be calculated as follows:

$$\text{Volume of saline or glucose needed (mL)} = \frac{\text{Pump rate (mL/hr)} \times 83.3}{\text{body weight (kg)}} - 1$$

The infusion solution may be mixed conveniently in a graduated mixing chamber inserted between the i.v. bottle and the pump.

Change the dosage from 0.1 µg/kg of body weight/minute to 0.05 µg/kg of body weight/minute by reducing the pump rate to one-half the original rate.

SUPPLIED: Each 1 mL ampul contains: alprostadil 500 µg in anhydrous ethanol. Ampuls of 1 mL. Cartons of 5. Store in a refrigerator at 2 to 8°C. Prepare fresh dilutions every 24 hours. Discard any dilution more than 24 hours old.

Protamine Sulfate Injection USP

protamine sulfate

Heparin Antagonist

Sandoz

SUPPLIED: Each mL of preservative-free, sterile, isotonic solution contains: protamine sulfate 10 mg. Nonmedicinal ingredients: sodium chloride, sulfuric acid and/or dibasic sodium phosphate to adjust pH and water for injection. Single use vials of 5 and 25 mL, boxes of 10 and 1, respectively. Discard unused portion. Store between 15 and 30°C. Do not freeze.

Protopic® Ⓟ

tacrolimus

Topical Calcineurin Inhibitor

Astellas

Date of Revision: April 13, 2006

SUMMARY PRODUCT INFORMATION:

Route of Administration	Dosage Form/ Strength	Clinically Relevant Nonmedicinal Ingredients
Topical	Ointment/0.03% and 0.1%	For a complete listing of nonmedicinal ingredients see Dosage Forms, Composition and Packaging.

INDICATIONS AND CLINICAL USE: Protopic (tacrolimus ointment), both 0.03% and 0.1% for adults and only 0.03% for children aged 2 to 15 years, is indicated as a second-line therapy for short and long-term intermittent treatment of moderate to severe atopic dermatitis in non-immunocompromised patients, in whom the use of conventional therapies are deemed inadvisable because of potential risks, or who are not adequately responsive to or intolerant of conventional therapies. For additional safety information, please refer to Warnings and Precautions.

Geriatrics (>65 years of age): Four hundred and four (404) patients ≥65 years old received Protopic Ointment in phase 3 studies. The adverse event profile for these patients was consistent with that for other adult patients.

Pediatrics (2 to 15 years): Protopic, 0.03% strength only, is indicated for use in children aged 2 to 15 years. The safety and efficacy of Protopic have not been established in pediatric patients below 2 years of age, and its use in this age group is not recommended.

CONTRAINDICATIONS:

- Protopic (tacrolimus ointment) is contraindicated in patients with a history of hypersensitivity to tacrolimus or to any other component of the preparation. For a complete listing, see Dosage Forms, Composition and Packaging.

WARNINGS AND PRECAUTIONS:

Long-term safety of topical calcineurin inhibitors has not been established. Although a causal relationship has not been established, rare cases of skin malignancy and lymphoma have been reported in patients treated with topical calcineurin inhibitors, including Protopic ointment 0.1% and 0.03%.

Therefore:

- Continuous long-term use of topical calcineurin inhibitors including Protopic ointment 0.1% and 0.03% should be avoided, and application limited to areas of involvement with atopic dermatitis.
- Protopic ointment is not indicated in children less than 2 years of age. Only 0.03% Protopic ointment is indicated for use in children 2-15 years of age.

General: Patients using Protopic should receive the following information and instructions:

- Patients should use Protopic as directed by the physician. Protopic is for external use only. As with any topical medication, patients should wash hands after application if hands are not an area for treatment.
- Patients should minimize or avoid exposure to natural or artificial sunlight (tanning beds or UVA/B treatment) while using Protopic.
- Patients should not use this medication for any disorder other than that for which it was prescribed.
- Patients should report any signs of adverse reactions to their physician.
- Before applying Protopic after a bath or shower, be sure your skin is completely dry.

Immune: In clinical studies, cases of lymphadenopathy were reported and were usually related to infections and noted to resolve upon appropriate antibiotic therapy. The majority of these cases had either a clear etiology or were known to resolve. Transplant patients receiving immunosuppressive regimens (e.g. systemic tacrolimus) are at increased risk for developing lymphoma; therefore, patients who receive Protopic and who develop lymphadenopathy should have the etiology of their lymphadenopathy investigated. In the absence of a clear etiology for the lymphadenopathy or in the presence of acute infectious mononucleosis, discontinuation of Protopic should be considered. Patients who develop lymphadenopathy should be monitored to ensure that the lymphadenopathy resolves.

Sexual Function/Reproduction: Reproductive toxicology studies were not performed with tacrolimus ointment. In studies of oral tacrolimus no impairment of fertility was seen in male and female rats. Tacrolimus, given orally at 1.0 mg/kg to male and female rats, prior to and during mating, as well as to dams during gestation and lactation, was associated with embryolethality and with adverse effects on female reproduction. Effects on female reproductive function (parturition) and embryolethal effects were indicated by a higher rate of pre-implantation loss and increased numbers of undelivered and nonviable pups. When given at 3.2 mg/kg, tacrolimus was associated with maternal and paternal toxicity as well as reproductive toxicity including marked adverse effects on estrus cycles, parturition, pup viability, and pup malformations.

Skin: The use of Protopic may cause local symptoms of short duration, such as skin burning (burning sensation, stinging, soreness) or pruritus. Localized symptoms are most common during the first few days of Protopic application and typically resolve as the lesions of atopic dermatitis heal.

Protopic (tacrolimus ointment) has not been studied for its efficacy and safety in the treatment of clinically infected atopic dermatitis. Patients with atopic dermatitis are predisposed to superficial skin infections. Treatment with Protopic may be associated with an increased risk of varicella zoster virus infection (chickenpox or shingles), herpes simplex virus infection, or eczema herpeticum. In the presence of infections, the balance of risks and benefits associated with Protopic use should be evaluated.

The enhancement of ultraviolet carcinogenicity is not necessarily dependent on phototoxic mechanisms. Despite the absence of observed phototoxicity in humans, Protopic shortened the time to skin tumour formation in an animal photocarcinogenicity study. Therefore, it is prudent for patients to minimize or avoid natural or artificial sunlight exposure.

The use of Protopic in patients with Netherton's syndrome is not recommended due to the potential for increased systemic absorption of tacrolimus. The safety of Protopic has not been established in patients with generalized erythroderma.

Special Populations: Pregnant Women: There are no studies on the use of Protopic in pregnant women. Reproduction studies were carried out with systemically administered tacrolimus in rats and rabbits. Adverse effects on the fetus were observed mainly at oral dose levels that were toxic to dams. Tacrolimus at oral doses of 0.32 and 1.0 mg/kg during organogenesis in rabbits was associated with maternal toxicity as well as an increase in incidence of abortions. At the higher dose only, an increased incidence of malformations and developmental variations was also seen. Tacrolimus, at oral doses of 3.2 mg/kg during organogenesis in rats, was associated with maternal toxicity and caused an increase in late resorptions, decreased numbers of live births, and decreased pup weight and viability. Tacrolimus, given orally at 1.0 and 3.2 mg/kg to pregnant rats after organogenesis and during lactation, was associated with reduced pup weights. No reduction in male or female fertility was evident.

There are no adequate and well-controlled studies of systemically administered tacrolimus in pregnant women. Tacrolimus is transferred across the placenta. The use of systemically administered tacrolimus during pregnancy has been associated with neonatal hyperkalemia and renal dysfunction. Protopic should be used during pregnancy only if the potential benefit to the mother justifies a potential risk to the fetus.

Nursing Women: Although systemic absorption of tacrolimus following topical applications of Protopic is minimal relative to systemic administration, it is known that tacrolimus is excreted in milk. Therefore, breast feeding should be avoided during use of Protopic.

Pediatrics: Protopic 0.03% may be used in pediatric patients 2 years of age and older.

The safety and efficacy of Protopic have not been established in pediatric patients below 2 years of age, and its use in this age group is not recommended.

Geriatrics (>65 years of age): Four hundred and four (404) patients ≥65 years old received Protopic Ointment in phase 3 studies. The adverse event profile for these patients was consistent with that for other adult patients.

ADVERSE REACTIONS: Adverse Drug Reaction Overview: In normal volunteer dermal safety studies, Protopic (tacrolimus ointment) was neither phototoxic, nor photoallergenic, nor a contact sensitizer.

Overall, 2716 patients treated with Protopic were evaluated in phase 3 studies: 655 in three randomized vehicle-controlled studies, 759 in two randomized active-controlled studies and 571 in two long-term safety studies.

Clinical Trial Adverse Drug Reactions: Because clinical trials are conducted under very specific conditions the adverse reaction rates observed in the clinical trials may not reflect the rates observed in practice and should not be compared to the rates in the clinical trials of another drug. Adverse drug reaction information from clinical trials is useful for identifying drug-related adverse events and for approximating rates.

Clinical Trials with Protopic Compared to Active Comparators: In the active comparator studies using topical corticosteroids with Protopic, the duration of treatment was 3 weeks. In the adult study, the most common adverse events experienced were skin burning and pruritus, which were primarily application-site events caused by the medication. In total, 35.5% of patients in the 0.1% hydrocortisone butyrate group, 63.7% of patients in the 0.03% Protopic group and 68.6% of patients in the 0.1% Protopic group experienced an application-site adverse event. Both skin burning and pruritus tended to be brief; the occurrence of which decreased with time, lasting approximately 4-7 days.

The occurrence of other adverse events were reported in this clinical trial included flu-like symptoms, folliculitis, headache, allergic reaction, skin erythema, maculopapular rash, nausea, diarrhea and paresthesia. None of these adverse events showed a significant difference in incidence among the treatment groups. Herpes simplex, a less common adverse reaction (<5%), was more frequent in patients treated with Protopic compared to 0.1% hydrocortisone butyrate group.

As in the adult study, skin burning and pruritus comprised the most common application site adverse events and tended to occur only during the first few days of treatment in this pediatric comparator study. In this study population, 21.1% of patients in the 1% hydrocortisone acetate group, 38.1% of patients in the 0.03% Protopic group, and 36.6% of patients in the 0.1% Protopic group experienced an application site adverse event. There was a marked decrease in the prevalence of skin burning over time, particularly in the Protopic treatment groups. Pruritus also decreased over time in the Protopic treatment groups but not in the hydrocortisone acetate group.

The incidence of other adverse events that may be associated with treatment was similar among all study groups and included flu-like symptoms, fever, abdominal pain, increased cough, rhinitis, diarrhea and headache.

Clinical Trials with Protopic Compared to Vehicle Ointment: See Table 1.

Table 1: Protopic

12-Week Incidence Rate of Common Adverse Events in Three Phase III Studies

Body System	Protopic 0.03% N=328	Protopic 0.1% N=327	Vehicle (placebo) N=328
Skin			
Skin Burning	45%	49%	27%
Pruritus	44%	41%	33%
Respiratory System			
Flu-like Symptoms (eg. common cold, congestion, upper respiratory track infection)	25%	31%	22%
Nervous System			
Headache	14%	17%	10%

In the three controlled clinical trials, the most frequent adverse experiences associated with Protopic were limited to local irritation of the skin. For the most common events, the incidence rate within 12 weeks, by treatment group (vehicle, Protopic 0.03%, and Protopic 0.1%, respectively) were 27%, 45%, 49% for skin burning and 33%, 44%, 41% for pruritus. These events were typically observed during the first few days of treatment, tended to be mild or moderate in severity, and diminished in prevalence after the first few days of treatment.

The 12-week incidence rate for other common events that may be associated with Protopic, by treatment group (vehicle, Protopic 0.03%, and Protopic 0.1%, respectively) were 22%, 25%, 31% for flu-like symptoms (e.g. common cold, congestion, upper respiratory infection) and 10%, 14%, 17% for headache.

In the two long-term safety studies, 255 pediatric patients and 316 adult patients applied Protopic 0.1% for up to 1 year. The incidence of adverse events did not increase with increased duration of study drug exposure or amount of ointment used.

Less Common Clinical Trial Adverse Drug Reactions: Less common events occurring in 1%-5% of patients in order of decreasing frequency include skin tingling, acne, folliculitis, hyperesthesia (sensitive skin, increased sensitivity to hot/cold temperature), alcohol intolerance (skin/facial flushing, redness, heat sensation), dyspepsia, myalgia, and cyst.

The incidence of herpes zoster (chickenpox) occurred less frequently in patients treated with vehicle (0 cases) and Protopic 0.1% (1 case) than in patients treated with Protopic 0.03% (4 cases).

Post-Market Adverse Drug Reactions: The following adverse reactions have been reported from post-marketing surveillance for patients also having used Protopic ointment 0.1% and 0.03%. Since these events are reported voluntarily from a population of uncertain size it is not always possible to reliably estimate their frequency or establish a causal relationship to drug exposure.

Hematology/Oncology: Isolated cases of malignant neoplasms were reported from post-marketing surveillance for patients also having used Protopic ointment 0.1% and 0.03%. The malignancies included lymphomas, skin neoplasms (basal cell carcinoma, squamous cell carcinoma and melanoma).

Urology: Rare occurrences of acute renal failure in patients with or without Netherton's syndrome and renal impairment, have been reported during post marketing use of Protopic ointment.

DRUG INTERACTIONS: Overview: Formal topical drug interaction studies with Protopic have not been conducted. Based on its minimal extent of absorption, interactions of Protopic with systemically administered drugs cannot be ruled out, but are unlikely to occur.

Drug-Drug Interactions: Interactions with other drug products have not been established.

Drug-Food Interactions: There are no known interactions with food.

Drug-Herb Interactions: Interactions with herbal products have not been established.

Drug-Laboratory Test Interactions: Interactions with laboratory tests have not been established.

Drug-Lifestyle Interactions: Patients should minimize or avoid exposure to natural or artificial sunlight (tanning beds or UVA/B treatment) while using Protopic.

DOSAGE AND ADMINISTRATION: Dosing Considerations: Not applicable.

Recommended Dose and Dosage Adjustment: Adults (age 16 and over): Protopic (tacrolimus ointment) 0.03% and 0.1%.

Pediatrics (2-15 years of age): Protopic (tacrolimus ointment) 0.03% only.

Missed Dose: If you forget to use Protopic as directed, apply it as soon as possible, then go back to your regular schedule.

Administration: Protopic 0.03% and 0.1% should be applied topically morning and evening twice daily as a thin layer to affected areas of skin, including the face, neck and eyelids.

Therapy should be stopped upon clearance of the signs and symptoms of atopic dermatitis (e.g. pruritus, inflammation and erythema). Treatment should be discontinued if resolution of disease occurs. If no improvement occurs after 6 weeks of therapy or in case of disease exacerbation, Protopic therapy should be discontinued and patients should consult their physicians.

The use of Protopic under occlusion has not been studied, therefore occlusive dressings are not recommended.

OVERDOSAGE:
Protopic (tacrolimus ointment) is not for oral use. Oral ingestion of Protopic may lead to adverse effects associated with systemic administration of tacrolimus. If oral ingestion occurs, medical advice should be sought.

> For management of a suspected drug overdose, CPhA recommends that you contact your **regional Poison Control Centre**. See the *CPS* Directory section for a list of Poison Control Centres.

ACTION AND CLINICAL PHARMACOLOGY: Mechanism of Action/Pharmacodynamics: The exact mechanism of action of tacrolimus in atopic dermatitis is not known. However, It has been demonstrated that tacrolimus inhibits T-lymphocyte activation by first binding, an intracellular protein, FKBP-12. A complex of tacrolimus-FKBP-12, calcium, calmodulin, and calcineurin is then formed and the phosphatase activity of calcineurin is inhibited. This effect has been shown to prevent the dephosphorylation and translocation of nuclear factor of activated T-cells (NF-AT), a nuclear component thought to initiate gene transcription for the formation of lymphokines (such as interleukin-2, gamma interferon). Tacrolimus also inhibits the transcription for genes which encode for IL-3, IL-4, IL-5, GM-CSF, and TNF-α, all of which are involved in the early stages of T-cell activation and have been postulated to play significant roles in the pathogenesis of atopic dermatitis. Additionally, tacrolimus has been shown to inhibit the release of pre-formed mediators from skin mast cells and basophils, and to downregulate the expression of FcεRI on Langerhans cells.

Application of tacrolimus ointment (0.03%-0.3%) did not affect cutaneous pigmentation in micropigs. Tacrolimus ointment does not affect collagen synthesis, reduce skin thickness or cause skin atrophy in humans.

Pharmacokinetics: A pharmacokinetic study in 21 adult patients with atopic dermatitis demonstrated that tacrolimus is absorbed into the systemic circulation following single or repeated application of tacrolimus ointment in 0.1% concentration. Peak tacrolimus blood concentrations ranged from undetectable to 20 ng/mL. A blood concentration of 20 ng/mL was detected in two patients in both the single dosing group and the multiple dosing group, both of whom had severe disease and were applying ointment to almost the entire body. These concentrations were transient and decreased to 2.9 ng/mL (72 hour) and 3.9 ng/mL (day 7), respectively. Eight pediatric patients (5 to 12 years of age), with moderate atopic dermatitis, received 0.3% tacrolimus ointment. Peak tacrolimus blood concentrations ranged from 0.14 to 3.28 ng/mL. Similarly to the adult results, these peak concentrations were transient. There was no systemic accumulation of tacrolimus in both adult and pediatric patients.

Although a direct determination of bioavailability was not performed, a comparison of area under the curve (AUC) data following topical administration to historical AUC data after oral and intravenous administration indicates that the bioavailability of tacrolimus ointment applied to damaged skin (atopic dermatitis) relative to oral administration is <3%; the absolute bioavailability is <0.5%. Despite prolonged and repeated topical application for periods of up to 1 year, there is no evidence based on blood concentrations that tacrolimus accumulates systemically.

Special Populations and Conditions: Not applicable.

STORAGE AND STABILITY: Store between 15 and 30°C.

SPECIAL HANDLING INSTRUCTIONS: None required.

INFORMATION FOR THE PATIENT: Published in e-CPS, available by subscription at www.e-cps.ca.

DOSAGE FORMS, COMPOSITION AND PACKAGING: 0.03%: Each g of white to slightly yellowish ointment contains: tacrolimus 0.03% in a base of white petrolatum, mineral oil, propylene carbonate, white wax and paraffin. Laminate tubes of 10, 30, 60 and 100 g.

0.1%: Each g of white to slightly yellowish ointment contains: tacrolimus 0.1% in a base of white petrolatum, mineral oil, propylene carbonate, white wax and paraffin. Laminate tubes of 10, 30, 60 and 100 g.

Provera® Ⓟ
medroxyprogesterone acetate
Progestin

Pfizer

Date of Preparation: September 24, 2003
Date of Revision: December 9, 2009

SUMMARY PRODUCT INFORMATION:

Route of Administration	Dosage Form/ Strength	Clinically Relevant Nonmedicinal Ingredients
Oral	Tablets 2.5, 5, 10 and 100 mg	Lactose, sucrose, cornstarch, FD&C colour For a complete listing see Dosage Forms, Composition and Packaging.

INDICATIONS AND CLINICAL USE: PROVERA (medroxyprogesterone acetate) is indicated for:

- Hormonal replacement therapy, to oppose the effects of estrogen on the endometrium and significantly reduce the risk of hyperplasia and carcinoma;
- Functional menstrual disorders due to hormonal imbalance in non-pregnant women, in the absence of organic pathology;
- Adjunctive and/or palliative treatment of recurrent and/or metastatic endometrial carcinoma;
- Adjunctive and/or palliative treatment of hormonally-dependent, recurrent metastatic breast cancer in postmenopausal women.

For indications not including breast cancer, PROVERA should be prescribed only to women with intact uteri.

Pediatrics (<16 years of age): PROVERA is not intended for pediatric use and no clinical data has been collected in children.

CONTRAINDICATIONS: Estrogens & estrogen/progestin combinations are contraindicated in patients with any of the following disorders:

- Patients who are hypersensitive to this drug or to any ingredient in the formulation or component of the container. For a complete listing, see Dosage Forms, Composition and Packaging.
- Liver dysfunction or disease as long as liver function tests have failed to return to normal;
- Known or suspected estrogen-dependent or progestin-dependent malignant neoplasia (e.g. endometrial cancer), unless PROVERA is being used as a treatment for endometrial or breast cancer, as outlined in Indications and Clinical Use;
- Known, suspected, or past history of breast cancer, unless PROVERA is being used as a treatment for breast cancer in postmenopausal women, as outlined in Indications and Clinical Use;
- Undiagnosed abnormal genital bleeding;
- Known or suspected pregnancy;
- Active or past history of arterial thromboembolic disease (e.g. stroke, myocardial infarction, coronary heart disease);
- Active or past history of confirmed venous thromboembolism (such as deep vein thrombosis or pulmonary embolism) or active thrombophlebitis;
- Partial or complete loss of vision due to ophthalmic vascular disease.

WARNINGS AND PRECAUTIONS:

> **Serious Warnings and Precautions**
> The Women's Health Initiative (WHI) trial examined the health benefits and risks of oral combined estrogen plus progestin therapy (n=16 608) and oral estrogen-alone therapy (n=10 739) in postmenopausal women aged 50 to 79 years.
>
> The estrogen plus progestin arm of the WHI trial (mean age 63.3 years) indicated an increased risk of myocardial infarction (MI), stroke, invasive breast cancer, pulmonary emboli and deep vein thrombosis in postmenopausal women receiving treatment with combined conjugated equine estrogens (CEE, 0.625 mg/day) and medroxyprogesterone acetate (MPA, 2.5 mg/day) for 5.2 years compared to those receiving placebo.
>
> The estrogen-alone arm of the WHI trial (mean age 63.6 years) indicated an increased risk of stroke and deep vein thrombosis in hysterectomized women treated with CEE-alone (0.625 mg/day) for 6.8 years compared to those receiving placebo.

Therefore, the following should be given serious consideration at the time of prescribing:

- Estrogens with or without progestins **should not** be prescribed for primary or secondary prevention of cardiovascular diseases.
- Estrogens with or without progestins should be prescribed at **the lowest effective dose** for the approved indication.
- Estrogens with or without progestins should be prescribed for **the shortest period** possible for the approved indication.

General: Some information presented in Warnings and Precautions is provided in light of the fact that a progestin medication is often prescribed concomitantly with an estrogen medication. Information in this section pertaining to combined estrogen-progestin therapy may therefore not apply to progestin-only therapy. Physician discretion is advised.

When PROVERA is used for adjunctive and/or palliative treatment of recurrent and/or metastatic endometrial or hormonally-dependent, recurrent metastatic carcinoma of the breast in post-menopausal women, the risks outlined in Warnings and Precautions (including cardiovascular disorders and breast and ovarian cancer), should be weighed against the potential benefits of this treatment to the patient.

Carcinogenesis and Mutagenesis: Breast Cancer: Available epidemiological data indicate that the use of combined estrogen plus progestin by postmenopausal women is associated with an increased risk of invasive breast cancer. In the estrogen plus progestin arm of the WHI trial, among 10 000 women over a one-year period, there were:

- 8 more cases of invasive breast cancer (38 on combined HRT versus 30 on placebo).

The WHI study also reported that the invasive breast cancers diagnosed in the estrogen plus progestin group were similar in histology but were larger (mean [SD], 1.7 cm [1.1] vs 1.5 cm [0.9], respectively; P=0.04) and were at a more advanced stage compared with those diagnosed in the placebo group. The percentage of women with abnormal mammograms (recommendations for short-interval follow-up, a suspicious abnormality, or highly suggestive of malignancy) was significantly higher in the estrogen plus progestin group versus the placebo group. This difference appeared at year one and persisted in each year thereafter.

In the estrogen-alone arm of the WHI trial, there was no statistically significant difference in the rate of invasive breast cancer in hysterectomized women treated with conjugated equine estrogens versus women treated with placebo.

It is recommended that estrogens with or without progestins not be given to women with existing breast cancer or those with a previous history of the disease (see Contraindications). There is a need for caution in prescribing estrogens with or without progestins for women with known risk factors associated with the development of breast cancer, such as strong family history of breast cancer (first degree relative) or who present a breast condition with an increased risk (abnormal mammograms and/or atypical hyperplasia at breast biopsy). Other known risk factors for the development of breast cancer such as nulliparity, obesity, early menarche, late age at first full term pregnancy and at menopause should also be evaluated.

It is recommended that women undergo a mammography prior to the start of HRT treatment and at regular intervals during treatment, as deemed appropriate by the treating physician and according to the perceived risks for each patient.

The overall benefits and possible risks of hormone replacement therapy should be fully considered and discussed with patients. It is important that the modest increased risk of being diagnosed with breast cancer after 4 years of treatment with combined estrogen plus progestin HRT (as reported in the results of the WHI trial) be discussed with the patient and weighed against its known benefits.

Instructions for regular self-examination of the breasts should be included in this counselling.

Endometrial Hyperplasia & Endometrial Carcinoma: The incidence of estrogen-associated endometrial hyperplasia was assessed in 2 large, long-term, randomized clinical trials. The first study demonstrated that combining conjugated estrogens with medroxyprogesterone acetate or micronized progesterone protected the endometrium from hyperplastic changes associated with estrogen-only therapy. In the second study, the endometrial hyperplasia incidence was significantly lower in women treated with conjugated estrogen and medroxyprogesterone acetate (P<0.001) than in women treated with conjugated estrogen alone.

Ovarian Cancer: Some recent epidemiologic studies have found that the use of postmenopausal hormone replacement therapy (estrogen alone and estrogen plus progestin therapies) in particular for five or more years has been associated with an increased risk of ovarian cancer.

Cardiovascular: The results of the Heart and Estrogen/progestin Replacement Studies (HERS and HERS II) and the Women's Health Initiative (WHI) trial indicate that the use of estrogen plus progestin is associated with an increased risk of coronary heart disease (CHD) in postmenopausal women. The results of the WHI trial indicate that the use of estrogen-alone and estrogen plus progestin is associated with an increased risk of stroke in postmenopausal women.

WHI Trial Findings: In the combined estrogen plus progestin arm of the WHI trial, among 10 000 women over a one-year period, there were:

- 8 more cases of stroke (29 on combined HRT versus 21 on placebo)
- 7 more cases of CHD (37 on combined HRT versus 30 on placebo).

In the estrogen-alone arm of the WHI trial of women with prior hysterectomy, among 10 000 women over a one-year period, there were/was:

- 12 more cases of stroke (44 on estrogen-alone therapy versus 32 on placebo)
- no statistically significant difference in the rate of CHD.

HERS and HERS II Findings: In the Heart and Estrogen/progestin Replacement Study (HERS) of postmenopausal women with documented heart disease (n=2763, average age 66.7 years), a randomized placebo-controlled clinical trial of secondary prevention of coronary heart disease (CHD), treatment with 0.625 mg/day oral conjugated equine estrogen (CEE) plus 2.5 mg oral medroxyprogesterone acetate (MPA) demonstrated no cardiovascular benefit. Specifically, during an average follow-up of 4.1 years, treatment with CEE plus MPA did not reduce the overall rate of CHD events in postmenopausal women with established coronary heart disease. There were more CHD events in the hormone treated group than in the placebo group in year 1, but not during the subsequent years.

From the original HERS trial, 2321 women consented to participate in an open label extension of HERS known as HERS II. Average follow-up in HERS II was an additional 2.7 years, for a total of 6.8 years overall. After 6.8 years, hormone therapy did not reduce the risk of cardiovascular events in women with CHD.

Blood Pressure: Women using hormone replacement therapy sometimes experience increased blood pressure. Blood pressure should be monitored with HRT use. Elevation of blood pressure in previously normotensive or hypertensive patients should be investigated and HRT may have to be discontinued.

Endocrine and Metabolism: Adrenocortical Function: Clinical suppression of adrenocortical function has not been observed at low dose levels. However, the high doses of PROVERA used in the treatment of certain cancers may, in some cases, produce Cushingoid symptoms (e.g., "moon" facies, fluid retention, glucose intolerance, and blood pressure elevation).

Glucose and Lipid Metabolism: A worsening of glucose tolerance and lipid metabolism have been observed in a significant percentage of peri- and post-menopausal patients. Therefore, diabetic patients or those with a predisposition to diabetes should be observed closely to detect any alterations in carbohydrate or lipid metabolism, especially in triglyceride blood levels.

Women with familial hypertriglyceridemia need special surveillance. Lipid-lowering measures are recommended additionally, before treatment is started.

Heme Metabolism: Women with porphyria need special surveillance.

Other Conditions: PROVERA contains lactose. In patients with rare hereditary galactose intolerance, lactase deficiency or glucose-galactose malabsorption, the severity of the condition should be taken into careful consideration before prescribing PROVERA. The patients should be closely monitored.

Calcium and Phosphorus Metabolism: Because the prolonged use of estrogens with or without progestins influences the metabolism of calcium and phosphorus, estrogens with or without progestins should be used with caution in patients with metabolic and malignant bone diseases associated with hypercalcemia and in patients with renal insufficiency.

Decrease in Bone Mineral Density: There are no available studies on the effects of orally administered medroxyprogesterone acetate (MPA) as a single agent, on bone mineral density (BMD).

However, it may be suspected that for specific medical conditions, when MPA is administered over a prolonged period of time at a dose that is high enough to suppress endogenous estrogen production e.g., pre-menopausal women), it could result in a decrease in bone mineral density (BMD). In these circumstances, adequate calcium and vitamin D intake should be considered.

Hypothyroidism: Patients who require thyroid hormone replacement therapy and who are also taking estrogen should have their thyroid function monitored regularly to assure that thyroid hormone levels remain in an acceptable range (see Drug Interactions, Drug-Laboratory Test Interactions).

Genitourinary: Vaginal Bleeding: Abnormal vaginal bleeding, due to its prolongation, irregularity or heaviness, occurring during therapy should prompt appropriate diagnostic measures to rule out the possibility of uterine malignancy and the treatment should be reevaluated.

Uterine Leiomyomata: Pre-existing uterine leiomyomata may increase in size during estrogen use. Growth, pain or tenderness of uterine leiomyomata requires discontinuation of medication and appropriate investigation.

Endometriosis: Symptoms and physical findings associated with a previous diagnosis of endometriosis may reappear or become aggravated with estrogen use.

Menstrual Bleeding Patterns: Patients should be advised of the menstrual bleeding patterns expected with the sequential regimen (see Dosage and Administration).

Upon sequential administration of PROVERA to women with adequate levels of estrogen (endogenous or exogenous), withdrawal bleeding usually occurs within 7 days after stopping PROVERA. Bleeding that occurs during PROVERA administration period indicates a need for a longer duration, or a higher dose of PROVERA.

Hematologic: Venous Thromboembolism: Available epidemiological data indicate that use of estrogen with or without progestin by postmenopausal women is associated with an increased risk of developing venous thromboembolism (VTE).

In the estrogen plus progestin arm of the WHI trial, among 10 000 women on combined HRT over a one-year period, there were 18 more cases of venous thromboembolism, including 8 more cases of pulmonary embolism.

In the estrogen-alone arm of the WHI trial, among 10 000 women on estrogen therapy over a one-year period, there were 7 more cases of venous thromboembolism, although there was no statistically significant difference in the rate of pulmonary embolism.

Generally recognized risk factors for VTE include a personal history, a family history (the occurrence of VTE in a direct relative at a relatively early age may indicate genetic predisposition) and severe obesity (body mass index >30 kg/m^2) and systemic lupus erythematosus. The risk of VTE also increases with age and smoking.

The risk of VTE may be temporarily increased with prolonged immobilization, major surgery or trauma. In women on HRT, attention should be given to prophylactic measures to prevent VTE following surgery. Also, patients with varicose veins should be closely supervised. The physician should be alert to the earliest manifestations of thrombotic disorders (thrombophlebitis, retinal thrombosis, cerebral embolism and pulmonary embolism). If these occur or are suspected, hormone therapy should be discontinued immediately, given the risks of long-term disability or fatality.

If feasible, estrogens with or without progestins should be discontinued at least 4 weeks before major surgery which may be associated with an increased risk of thromboembolism, or during periods of prolonged immobilization.

Hepatic/Biliary/Pancreatic: Gallbladder Diseases: A 2- to 4-fold increase in the risk of gallbladder disease requiring surgery in women receiving postmenopausal estrogens has been reported.

Jaundice: Caution is advised in patients with a history of liver and/or biliary disorders. If cholestatic jaundice develops during treatment, the treatment should be discontinued and appropriate investigations carried out.

Liver Function Tests: Liver function tests should be done periodically in subjects who are suspected of having hepatic disease. For information on endocrine and liver function tests, see Monitoring and Laboratory Tests.

Immune: Anaphylactic/Anaphylactoid Reactions: Anaphylactic and anaphylactoid reactions have occasionally been reported in patients treated with PROVERA.

Neurologic: Cerebrovascular Insufficiency: Patients who develop visual disturbances (including sudden partial or complete loss of vision or sudden onset of proptosis, diplopia), classical migraine, transient aphasia, paralysis, or loss of consciousness should discontinue medication.

Patients with a previous history of classical migraine and who develop a recurrence or worsening of migraine symptoms should be reevaluated.

Dementia: Available epidemiological data indicate that the use of combined estrogen plus progestin in women age 65 and over may increase the risk of developing probable dementia.

The Women's Health Initiative Memory Study (WHIMS), a clinical substudy of the WHI, was designed to assess whether postmenopausal hormone replacement therapy (oral estrogen plus progestin or oral estrogen-alone) reduces the risk of dementia in women aged 65 and over (age range 65-79 years) and free of dementia at baseline.

In the estrogen plus progestin arm of the WHIMS (n=4532), women with intact uteri were treated with daily 0.625 mg conjugated equine estrogens (CEE) plus 2.5 mg medroxyprogesterone acetate (MPA) or placebo for an average of 4.05 years. The results, when extrapolated to 10 000 women treated over a one-year period showed:

- 23 more cases of probable dementia (45 on combined HRT versus 22 on placebo).

In the estrogen-alone arm of the WHIMS (n=2947), women with prior hysterectomy were treated with daily 0.625 mg CEE or placebo for an average of 5.21 years. The results, when extrapolated to 10 000 women treated over a one-year period showed:

- 12 more cases of probable dementia (37 on estrogen-alone versus 25 on placebo), although this difference did not reach statistical significance.

When data from the estrogen plus progestin arm of the WHIMS and the estrogen alone arm of the WHIMS were combined, as per the original WHIMS protocol, in 10 000 women over a one-year period, there were:

- 18 more cases of probable dementia (41 on estrogen plus progestin or estrogen-alone versus 23 on placebo).

In addition, conjugated equine estrogens and medroxyprogesterone acetate (CEE/MPA) therapy did not prevent mild cognitive impairment (MCI) in post-menopausal women 65 years of age or older. Use of hormone therapy to prevent dementia or MCI in women 65 years or older is not recommended.

Epilepsy: Particular caution is indicated in women with epilepsy, as estrogens with or without progestins may cause an exacerbation of this condition.

Psychiatric: Depression: Patients who have a history of mental depression should be carefully monitored while receiving therapy with PROVERA. Some patients may complain of premenstrual like depression while on PROVERA.

Renal: Fluid Retention: Estrogens with or without progestins may cause fluid retention. Therefore, particular caution is indicated in cardiac or renal dysfunction or asthma. If, in any of the above-mentioned conditions, a worsening of the underlying disease is diagnosed or suspected during treatment, the benefits and risks of treatment should be reassessed based on the individual case.

Sexual Function/Reproduction: Menopause: The age of the patient constitutes no absolute limiting factor although treatment with progestins may mask the onset of the climacteric.

Special Populations: Pregnant Women: Usage in pregnancy is not recommended. Progestational agents are also not recommended as a diagnostic test for pregnancy. If the patient is exposed to PROVERA (medroxyprogesterone acetate) during pregnancy or if she becomes pregnant while taking the drug, she should be apprised of the potential risk to the fetus.

Nursing Women: Detectable amounts of progestin have been identified in the milk of mothers receiving the drug. Infants exposed to medroxyprogesterone via breast milk have been studied for developmental and behavioral effects through puberty. No adverse effects have been noted.

Pediatrics (<16 years of age): PROVERA is not intended for pediatric use and no clinical data has been collected in children.

Geriatrics (>65 years of age): Of the total number of subjects in the estrogen plus progestin substudy of the Women's Health Initiative (WHI), 21.5 percent (n=3576) were 70 to 79 years old at baseline.

No significant differences in relative risks of stroke and invasive breast cancer were observed between subjects 70 years and over compared to younger subjects. However, there was a higher relative risk of stroke and invasive breast cancer in women 75 and over compared to younger subjects.

Monitoring and Laboratory Tests: Before PROVERA is administered, the patient should have a complete physical examination including a blood pressure determination. Breasts and pelvic organs should be appropriately examined and a Papanicolaou smear should be performed. Endometrial biopsy should be done only when indicated. Baseline tests should include mammography, measurements of blood glucose, calcium, triglycerides and cholesterol, and liver function tests.

The first follow-up examination should be done within 3-6 months after initiation of treatment to assess response to treatment. Thereafter, examinations should be made at intervals at least once a year. Appropriate investigations should be arranged at regular intervals as determined by the physician.

The importance of regular self-examination of the breasts should be discussed with the patient.

ADVERSE REACTIONS: Adverse Drug Reaction Overview: See Warnings and Precautions regarding potential induction of malignant neoplasms and adverse effects similar to those of oral contraceptives.

Overview of Adverse Drug Reactions with PROVERA Use: The following adverse reactions have been reported with the use of PROVERA (medroxyprogesterone acetate):

Breast: tenderness, galactorrhea.

Reproductive System: breakthrough bleeding, spotting, change in menstrual flow, amenorrhea, changes in cervical erosion and cervical secretions.

Central Nervous System: headache, nervousness, dizziness, depression, insomnia, somnolence, fatigue, premenstrual syndrome-like symptoms.

Thromboembolic Phenomena: including thrombophlebitis and pulmonary embolism.

Skin and Mucous Membranes: sensitivity reactions ranging from pruritus, urticaria, angioneurotic edema to generalized rash and anaphylaxis; acne, alopecia, hirsutism.

Gastrointestinal: abdominal discomfort, nausea, bloating.

Miscellaneous: pyrexia, increase in weight, peripheral edema, "moon" facies.

Overview of Adverse Drug Reactions with Estrogen/Progestin Combination Use: The following adverse reactions have been reported with estrogen/progestin combination in general:

Blood and Lymphatic Systems Disorders: altered coagulation tests (see Warnings and Precautions and Drug Interactions, Drug-Laboratory Test Interactions).

Cardiac Disorders: palpitations; increase in blood pressure (see Warnings and Precautions); coronary thrombosis.
Endocrine Disorders: increased blood sugar levels; decreased glucose tolerance.
Eye Disorders: neuro-ocular lesions (e.g., retinal thrombosis, optic neuritis); visual disturbances; steepening of the corneal curvature; intolerance to contact lenses.
Gastrointestinal Disorders: nausea; vomiting; abdominal discomfort (cramps, pressure, pain); bloating.
General Disorders and Administration Site Conditions: fatigue; changes in appetite; changes in body weight; change in libido.
Hepatobiliary Disorders: gallbladder disorder; asymptomatic impaired liver function; cholestatic jaundice.
Musculoskeletal and Connective Tissue Disorders: musculoskeletal pain including leg pain not related to thromboembolic disease (usually transient, lasting 3-6 weeks) may occur.
Nervous System Disorders: aggravation of migraine episodes; headaches; dizziness; neuritis.
Psychiatric Disorders: mental depression; nervousness; irritability.
Renal and Urinary Disorders: cystitis; dysuria; sodium retention; edema.
Reproductive System and Breast Disorders: breakthrough bleeding; spotting; change in menstrual flow; dysmenorrhea; vaginal itching/discharge; dyspareunia; endometrial hyperplasia; pre-menstrual-like syndrome; reactivation of endometriosis; changes in cervical erosion and amount of cervical secretion; breast swelling and tenderness.
Skin and Subcutaneous Tissue Disorders: chloasma or melasma; which may persist when drug is discontinued; erythema multiform; erythema nodosum; haemorrhagic eruption; loss of scalp hair; hirsutism and acne.
Vascular Disorders: isolated cases of: thrombophlebitis; thromboembolic disorders.
Post-Market Adverse Drug Reactions: Adverse events reported during worldwide post-marketing experience, regardless of causality and frequency, are listed below. It should be noted that the nature of post-marketing surveillance makes it difficult to determine if a reported event was actually caused by PROVERA.
Musculoskeletal and Connective Tissue Disorders: muscle spasms.
Nervous System Disorders: cerebral infarction.
Pregnancy, Puerperium and Perinatal Conditions: abortion spontaneous.
Respiratory, Thoracic and Mediastinal Disorders: dyspnea.
Vascular Disorders: hemorrhage.

The following post-market ADRs have been observed with PROVERA indicated for oncology:
Cardiac Disorders: myocardial infarction, congestive heart failure.
Eye Disorders: diabetic cataract.
Gastrointestinal Disorders: constipation, diarrhea, dry mouth.
Investigations: elevation of white blood cells and platelet counts.
Nervous System Disorders: loss of concentration, adrenergic-like effects (e.g. fine-hand tremors, sweating, cramps in calves in night).
Psychiatric Disorders: euphoria.
Renal and Urinary System Disorders: glycosuria.

If adverse symptoms persist, the prescription of the HRT should be re-considered.

DRUG INTERACTIONS: Overview: Preparations inducing liver enzymes (e.g., barbiturates, hydantoins, carbamazepine, meprobamates, phenylbutazone or rifampicin) may interfere with the activity of orally administered progestins.
Drug-Drug Interactions: Concomitant administration of aminoglutethimide with medroxyprogesterone acetate (MPA) may significantly reduce the bioavailability of MPA.
Drug-Food Interactions: Administration with food increases the bioavailability of MPA. A 10 mg dose of oral MPA, taken immediately before or after a meal, increased average MPA C_{max} (51 and 77%, respectively) and average AUC (18 and 33%, respectively). The half-life of MPA was not changed with food. MPA can be taken with or without food.
Drug-Herb Interactions: It was found that some herbal products (e.g., St. John's wort) which are available as over-the-counter (OTC) products might interfere with steroid metabolism, and therefore, alter the efficacy and safety of estrogen/progestin products.

Physicians and other health care providers should made be aware of other non-prescription products concomitantly used by the patient, including herbal and natural products, obtained from the widely spread Health Stores.
Drug-Laboratory Test Interactions: The results of certain endocrine and liver function tests may be affected by estrogen/progestin-containing products:

- increased sulfobromophthalein retention;
- increased prothrombin time and partial thromboplastin time; increased levels of fibrinogen and fibrinogen activity; increased coagulation factors VII, VIII, IX, X; increased norepinephrine-induced platelet aggregability; decreased antithrombin III;
- increased thyroxine-binding globulin (TBG), leading to increased circulating total thyroid hormone (T_4) as measured by column or radioimmunoassay; T_3 resin uptake is decreased, reflecting the elevated TBG; free T_4 concentration is unaltered;
- other binding proteins may be elevated in serum i.e., corticosteroid binding globulin (CBG), sex-hormone binding globulin (SHBG), leading to increased circulating corticosteroids and sex steroids, respectively; free or biologically active hormone concentrations are unchanged;
- impaired glucose tolerance;
- reduced serum folate concentration;
- increased serum triglycerides and phospholipids concentration.

The following laboratory tests may be affected by the use of PROVERA: gonadotropin levels; plasma progesterone levels; urinary pregnanediol levels; plasma testosterone levels (in the male); plasma estrogen levels (in the female); plasma cortisol levels; glucose tolerance test.

The results of the above laboratory tests should not be considered reliable unless therapy has been discontinued for 2 to 4 weeks. The pathologist should be informed that the patient is receiving HRT therapy when relevant specimens are submitted.

DOSAGE AND ADMINISTRATION:

Dosing Considerations: When estrogen is prescribed for a postmenopausal woman with a uterus, a progestin should also be initiated to reduce the risk of endometrial cancer. A woman without a uterus does not need progestin. Use of estrogen, alone or in combination with a progestin, should be with the lowest effective dose and for the shortest duration consistent with treatment goals and risks for the individual woman. Patients should be reevaluated periodically as clinically appropriate (for example, 3-month to 6-month intervals) to determine if treatment is still necessary (see Warnings and Precautions). For women with intact uteri, adequate diagnostic measures, such as endometrial sampling, when indicated, should be undertaken to rule out malignancy in cases of undiagnosed persistent or recurring abnormal vaginal bleeding. Patients should be started at the lowest dose. The lowest effective dose of PROVERA has not been determined.
Recommended Dose and Dosage Adjustment: Hormone Replacement Therapy: (a) Progestin Challenge Test: The progestin challenge test may be considered for amenorrheic women with intact uteri. PROVERA 10 mg daily should be administered for 10 days.

A negative test is identified by the absence of withdrawal bleeding, and implies the absence of endometrial stimulation due to insufficient estrogen secretion.

A positive test is indicated by the presence of withdrawal bleeding which occurs within 7 days after stopping PROVERA treatment. Withdrawal bleeding implies the presence of sufficient endogenous estrogen to stimulate the endometrium.
(b) Sequential Therapy: See Figure 1.

Figure 1: PROVERA
Sequential Therapy

Days of the Month 1 2 3 4 5 6 7 8 9 10 11	12 13 14	15 16 17 18 19 20 21 22 23 24 25	26 27 28 29 30 31
Sequential Estrogen — 25 days			
	Start	PROVERA 5–10 mg/day	
Continuous Estrogen — everyday			
PROVERA 5–10 mg/day	Stop		

In women with intact uteri receiving estrogen replacement therapy, PROVERA tablets may be given in a dosage of 5-10 mg daily for 12-14 days. The recommended starting dose for PROVERA should be 10 mg/day, administered for 12-14 days. A dose of 5 mg/day PROVERA for 12-14 days may be appropriate for some women.
Note: The lowest dose of PROVERA required to protect the endometrium from estrogenic-hyperstimulation should be used. A good indicator is the lowest dose of PROVERA that will consistently result in withdrawal bleeding within 7 days after stopping PROVERA treatment. Bleeding that occurs during the PROVERA treatment indicates a need for a longer duration, or higher dose of PROVERA.
Functional Menstrual Disorders: (a) Secondary Amenorrhea: After ruling out pregnancy, PROVERA (medroxyprogesterone acetate) may be administered in doses ranging from 5-10 mg daily depending upon the degree of progestational effect desired. The dose should be given daily for 12-14 days every month.
Note: In patients with poorly developed endometria, conventional estrogen therapy should be given in conjunction with PROVERA.
(b) Dysfunctional Uterine Bleeding: In dysfunctional uterine bleeding, PROVERA may be given in doses ranging from 5-10 mg/day, for 10-14 days, beginning on the assumed or calculated 12-16th day of the cycle. This regimen should be repeated for 2 subsequent cycles or longer if necessary.

When bleeding is due to a deficiency of both ovarian hormones, as indicated by a poorly developed proliferative endometrium, conventional estrogen therapy should be given in conjunction with PROVERA. If bleeding is controlled satisfactorily, at least 2 subsequent cycles of treatment should be given.

If dysfunctional uterine bleeding is not controlled by hormone therapy, appropriate diagnostic measures should be undertaken to rule out uterine pathology.
Endometrial Cancer: 200-400 mg/day is the usual dose. It is suggested that if neither subjective nor objective improvement is noted within 2 to 3 months, therapy should be discontinued. Where improvement is noted and the disease process appears to be stabilized, it may be possible to maintain this improvement with a 200 mg/day dose.
Breast Cancer: The recommended dose is 400 mg daily, given in divided doses. The patient should be continued on therapy as long as she is responding to treatment. Although doses of up to 2400 mg daily have been reported, controlled studies using 800 mg daily did not demonstrate any appreciable increase in response rates compared to the 400 mg daily dose.

PROVERA is not recommended as primary therapy, but as adjunctive and palliative treatment in advanced, inoperable cases including those with recurrent metastatic disease.
Note: Response to hormonal therapy for endometrial or breast cancer may not be evident until 8 to 10 weeks of therapy. Rapid progression of disease at any time during therapy should result in termination of treatment with PROVERA.
Missed Dose: If a dose of this medication has been missed, it should be taken as soon as possible. However, if it is almost time for the next dose, skip the missed dose and go back to the regular dosing schedule. Do not double doses.
Administration: PROVERA (medroxyprogesterone acetate) is administered orally.

OVERDOSAGE:
Symptoms of Overdose: Progestin (e.g., norethindrone acetate) overdosage has been characterized by depressed mood, tiredness, acne and hirsutism.

In female patients, overdosage may result in a period of amenorrhea of a variable length and may be followed by irregular menses for several cycles.

No cases of overdosage in male patients have been reported. However, such overdosage, if it were to occur, would not likely result in any particular symptomatology.
Treatment of Overdose: There is no known therapy for overdosage of medroxyprogesterone. Doses as high as 1000 mg for the therapy of endometrial carcinoma have been used without adverse effect.

> For management of a suspected drug overdose, contact your regional Poison Control Centre. See the *CPS Directory* section for a list of Poison Control Centres.

ACTION AND CLINICAL PHARMACOLOGY: Mechanism of Action: PROVERA (medroxyprogesterone acetate) is an orally-active progestational steroid (progestin) derived from a natural source (soybeans) and devoid of androgenic and estrogenic activity.
Pharmacodynamics: Osteoporosis/Osteopenia: Presently there are no conclusive data concerning the mechanism of action of progestins on bone.

Clinically, research to date has shown women treated with medroxyprogesterone acetate to prevent estrogenic hyperstimulation of the endometrium do not lose protection against osteoporosis.
Urogenital Symptoms: Medroxyprogesterone acetate, when administered to women with adequate levels of estrogen (endogenous or exogenous), transforms a proliferative endometrium into a secretory endometrium. Withdrawal bleeding is anticipated within 7 days after stopping medroxyprogesterone acetate.

Microscopically, the secretory change is associated with glycoprotein-rich stromal cells which surround the glands and vessels and assist them in maintaining their integrity during hormonal withdrawal. The result is an orderly regression and remodelling, and preservation of the functional layer of the endometrium.

Medroxyprogesterone acetate decreases both cytoplasmic and nuclear estrogen receptors in endometrial cells. In addition, medroxyprogesterone acetate induces estradiol dehydrogenase (E_2DH) activity, the enzyme mechanism by which endometrial cells metabolize and excrete estrogens.

Oral medroxyprogesterone acetate also produces typical progestational changes in the cervical mucous (inhibits ferning) and increases the intermediate cell count in the maturation index of the vaginal epithelium.
Metabolism: In studies which examined metabolic changes, a decrease in glucose tolerance has been associated with progestins, including medroxyprogesterone acetate.

Medroxyprogesterone acetate shows small or undetectable effects on lipoproteins when used at therapeutic dosages. Furthermore, research demonstrates that the use of medroxyprogesterone acetate with estrogen in hormone replacement therapy maintains the estrogenic effects on lipid profile.
Hemostatic Factors: There is no conclusive evidence that medroxyprogesterone acetate produces adverse coagulation changes in women receiving the progestin alone, or as part of a sequential regimen with estrogen.
Endocrine: Medroxyprogesterone acetate in appropriate doses, suppresses the secretion of pituitary gonadotropins which in turn, prevents follicular maturation, producing anovulation in the pre-menopausal woman.

The anti-cancer activity of medroxyprogesterone acetate at pharmacologic doses may be dependent upon its effect on the hypothalamic/pituitary/gonadal axis, estrogen receptors and the metabolism of steroids at the tissue level.

Like progesterone, medroxyprogesterone acetate is thermogenic. At the very high dosage levels used in the treatment of certain cancers (500 mg/day or more), corticoid-like activity may be manifest.

Medroxyprogesterone acetate in appropriate doses suppresses the Leydig cell function in the male (ie, suppresses endogenous testosterone production).
Pharmacokinetics: In a randomized, cross-over study using 22 healthy male volunteers, the pharmacokinetics of PROVERA 2.5 mg and PROVERA 10 mg tablets was studied following 10 mg single oral doses in the following regimens:

a. four PROVERA 2.5 mg tablets or
b. one PROVERA 10 mg tablet as a single dose during a fasting period which began 9 hours before and lasted until 4 hours after the dose. Treatment phases were separated by a 14-day washout period. Blood samples were collected prior to and at the following times after drug administration: 0.5, 1.0, 2.0, 3.0, 4.0, 6.0, 8.0, 10.0, 12.0, 16.0, 24.0, 36.0, 72.0, 96.0, and 120.0 hours. The resulting serum samples were analyzed for medroxyprogesterone using a radioimmunoassay procedure.

Relevant bioavailability parameters are included in Table 1.

Table 1: PROVERA
Pharmacokinetic Parameters of Medroxyprogesterone Acetate Following Oral Administration

PROVERA Dose (mg)	T_{max} (hr)	C_{max} (ng/mL)	AUC (ng/hr/mL)
2.5 mg (4 tablets)	1.68	22.10	390.66–466.62
10 mg (1 tablet)	1.91	19.26	399.95–471.96

Legend: Dose=single oral dose; T_{max}=time to reach peak serum concentration; C_{max}=peak serum concentration; AUC=area under the curve.

The pharmacokinetics of PROVERA 100 mg tablets was assessed in a clinical study using 16 healthy, male volunteers. A single dose of medroxyprogesterone acetate 100 mg was administered orally to subjects who fasted overnight and for 2 hours after the dose was administered. Blood samples were collected prior to, and at the following times, after drug administration: 0.5, 1.0, 2.0, 3.0, 4.0, 6.0, 8.0, 10.0, 12.0, 26.0, 32.0, 50.0, 74.0, 98.0, and 170.0 hours. Serum samples were analyzed for medroxyprogesterone using a radioimmunoassay procedure.

Relevant bioavailability parameters are included in Table 2.

Table 2: PROVERA

Pharmacokinetic Parameters of Medroxyprogesterone Acetate Following Oral Administration

PROVERA Dose (mg)	T_{max} (hr)	C_{max} (ng/mL)	AUC (ng/hr/mL)
100 mg (1 tablet)	4.1	35.2	974.2

Legend: Dose=single oral dose; T_{max}=time to reach peak serum concentration; C_{max}=peak serum concentration; AUC=area under the curve.

Absorption: Medroxyprogesterone acetate is rapidly absorbed from the gastrointestinal tract, and maximum concentrations are obtained between 2 to 4 hours after oral administration.

Distribution: MPA is approximately 90% protein bound, primarily to albumin; no MPA binding occurs with sex hormone binding globulin.

Metabolism: Medroxyprogesterone acetate is metabolized in the liver to several progestin metabolites. The major drug-related material found in circulation following oral administration has been characterized as both free and glucuronide-conjugated metabolites of medroxyprogesterone acetate.

Excretion: Medroxyprogesterone acetate has an apparent half-life of about 30 hours and is primarily eliminated via fecal excretion, to which biliary secretion may contribute. Approximately 44% of an oral dose is eliminated through urinary excretion in the form of metabolites.

The only metabolite of medroxyprogesterone acetate that has been isolated and unequivocally identified is 6α-methyl-6β,17α,21-trihydroxy-4-pregnene-3,20-dione-17-acetate, and appears to be the primary urinary metabolite. This metabolite accounts for approximately 8% of an oral dose, and is found to be excreted as a glucuronide conjugate.

Special Populations and Conditions: Hepatic Insufficiency: No clinical studies have evaluated the effect of hepatic disease on the pharmacokinetics of PROVERA. However, MPA is almost exclusively eliminated by hepatic metabolism and steroid hormones may be poorly metabolized in patients with severe liver insufficiency (see Contraindications).

Progestin Pharmacology: Medroxyprogesterone acetate significantly reduces the risk of endometrial hyperplasia in women with intact uteri. See Pharmacodynamics for specific information on the pharmacology of medroxyprogesterone acetate.

STORAGE AND STABILITY: Store at controlled room temperature (15-30°C). Keep in a safe place out of the reach of children.

INFORMATION FOR THE PATIENT: Published in e-CPS, available by subscription at www.e-cps.ca.

DOSAGE FORMS, COMPOSITION AND PACKAGING: 2.5 mg: Each circular, orange tablet, embossed with "U 64" on one side and scored on the other, contains: medroxyprogesterone acetate 2.5 mg. Nonmedicinal ingredients: calcium stearate, corn starch, FD&C Yellow No. 6, lactose monohydrate, mineral oil, sucrose and talc. Bottles of 100 and 500. Blisters of 30, cartons of 3.

5 mg: Each circular, blue tablet, embossed "U 286" on one side and scored on the other, contains: medroxyprogesterone acetate 5 mg. Nonmedicinal ingredients: calcium stearate, corn starch, lactose monohydrate, mineral oil, sucrose and talc. Bottles of 100 and 500.

10 mg: Each circular, white tablet, embossed "Upjohn 50" on one side and scored on the other, contains: medroxyprogesterone acetate 10 mg. Nonmedicinal ingredients: calcium stearate, corn starch, lactose monohydrate, mineral oil, sucrose and talc. Bottles of 100 and 500.

100 mg: Each circular, white tablet, embossed "U 467" on one side and scored on the other, contains: medroxyprogesterone acetate 100 mg. Nonmedicinal ingredients: calcium stearate, corn starch, lactose monohydrate, sodium lauryl sulphate, sucrose and talc. Bottles of 100.

(Shown in Product Identification Section)

Proviodine

povidone-iodine

Antiseptic—Anti-infective

Rougier Pharma

SUPPLIED: Detergent: Each mL of red-brown liquid having an abundant foam after stirring and the iodine odor, contains: povidone-iodine USP 7.5% (0.75% free iodine). Nonmedicinal ingredients: polyethylene glycol, purified water, sodium lauryl ether sulphate, sorbitol solution and tribasic sodium phosphate. Bottles of 115 mL, 500 mL and 5 L. Use only in a well-ventilated area.

Solution: Each mL of red-brown liquid, with iodine odor, contains: povidone-iodine USP 10% (1% free iodine). Nonmedicinal ingredients: octoxynol-8, purified water and tribasic sodium phosphate. Bottles of 115 mL, 500 mL and 5 L. Use only in a well-ventilated area.

The reader is invited to consult CPhA's monograph **Selective Serotonin Reuptake Inhibitors**.

Prozac®

fluoxetine HCl

Antidepressant—Antiobsessional—Antibulimic

Lilly

Date of Revision: September 30, 2009

SUMMARY PRODUCT INFORMATION:

Route of Administration	Dosage Form/Strength	Nonmedicinal Ingredients
Oral	Capsules/ 10 mg and 20 mg	Benzyl alcohol, butyl paraben, carboxymethylcellulose sodium, edetate calcium disodium, FD&C Blue No. 1, gelatin, iron oxide yellow, methylparaben, propylparaben, silicone, sodium propionate, sodium lauryl sulfate, starch and titanium dioxide There is no gluten, lactose, sulfite, or tartrazine in PROZAC.

INDICATIONS AND CLINICAL USE: Adults: Depression: PROZAC (fluoxetine) is indicated for the symptomatic relief of Major Depressive Disorder (MDD).

Bulimia Nervosa: PROZAC has been shown to significantly decrease binge-eating and purging activity when compared with placebo treatment.

Obsessive-Compulsive Disorder: PROZAC is indicated for the symptomatic treatment of obsessive-compulsive disorder (OCD).

The obsessions or compulsions must be experienced as intrusive, markedly distressing, time consuming, or interfering significantly with the person's social or occupational functioning.

The efficacy of PROZAC in hospitalized patients has not been adequately studied.

Long-Term Use of PROZAC: The effectiveness of PROZAC in long-term use in bulimia nervosa (i.e. for more than 16 weeks) and in obsessive-compulsive disorder (i.e. for more than 13 weeks) has not been systematically evaluated in controlled trials. Therefore, the physician who elects to use PROZAC in these indications for extended periods should periodically re-evaluate the long-term usefulness of the drug for the individual patient.

Geriatrics (≥60 years of age): Evidence from clinical studies and experience suggests that use in the geriatric population may be associated with differences in safety or effectiveness, and a brief discussion can be found in the appropriate sections (Warnings and Precautions, Special Populations, Geriatrics (≥60 years of age); Dosage and Administration).

Pediatrics (<18 years of age): PROZAC is not indicated for use in patients below the age of 18 years. See Warnings and Precautions, General, Potential Association with Behavioural and Emotional Changes, Including Self-Harm; see also Adverse Reactions, Potential for Effects on Growth in Pediatric Patients.

CONTRAINDICATIONS: Hypersensitivity: PROZAC (fluoxetine) is contraindicated in patients with known hypersensitivity to the drug or the excipients of the product. For a complete listing, see Dosage Forms, Composition and Packaging.

Monoamine Oxidase Inhibitors: There have been reports of serious, sometimes fatal, reactions (including hyperthermia, rigidity, myoclonus, autonomic instability with possible rapid fluctuations of vital signs, and mental status changes that include extreme agitation progressing to delirium and coma) in patients receiving PROZAC, or other serotonin reuptake inhibitors (SSRIs), in combination with a monoamine oxidase inhibitor (MAOI), and in patients who have recently discontinued PROZAC and then started on an MAOI. Some cases presented with features resembling neuroleptic malignant syndrome (e.g., serotonin syndrome). Therefore, **PROZAC should not be used in combination with an MAOI, including either within a minimum of 14 days of discontinuing therapy with an MAOI, or a minimum of 5 weeks of discontinuing therapy with PROZAC.** Since fluoxetine and its major metabolite have very long elimination half-lives, at least 5 weeks should be allowed after stopping PROZAC before starting an MAOI. Limited reports suggest that intravenously administered dantrolene (Dantrium) or orally administered cyproheptadine (Periactin) may benefit patients experiencing such reactions. See Drug Interactions.

Thioridazine: Thioridazine should not be administered concomitantly with PROZAC or within a minimum of 5 weeks after PROZAC has been discontinued, nor should PROZAC be administered within 2 weeks after thioridazine has been discontinued.

Thioridazine administration alone produces prolongation of the QTc interval, which is associated with serious ventricular arrhythmias, such as torsades de pointes-type arrhythmias, and sudden death. This effect appears to be dose-related.

An in vivo study suggests that drugs which inhibit $P4502D_6$, including certain SSRIs such as paroxetine, fluoxetine and fluvoxamine, will elevate plasma levels of thioridazine. Therefore, PROZAC should not be used in combination with thioridazine. See Drug Interactions.

WARNINGS AND PRECAUTIONS: General: Potential Association with Behavioural and Emotional Changes, Including Self-Harm: Pediatrics: Placebo-Controlled Clinical Trial Data: Recent analyses of placebo-controlled clinical trial safety databases from selective serotonin reuptake inhibitors (SSRIs) and other newer anti-depressants suggests that use of these drugs in patients under the age of 18 may be associated with behavioural and emotional changes, including an increased risk of suicidal ideation and behaviour over that of placebo.

The small denominators in the clinical trial database, as well as the variability in placebo rates, preclude reliable conclusions on the relative safety profiles among these drugs.

Adults and Pediatrics: Additional Data: There are clinical trial and post-marketing reports with SSRIs and other newer anti-depressants, in both pediatrics and adults, of severe agitation-type adverse events coupled with self-harm or harm to others. The agitation-type events include: akathisia, agitation, disinhibition, emotional lability, hostility, aggression, depersonalization. In some cases, the events occurred within several weeks of starting treatment.

Rigorous clinical monitoring for suicidal ideation or other indicators of potential for suicidal behaviour is advised in patients of all ages. This includes monitoring for agitation-type emotional and behavioural changes.

Discontinuation Symptoms: Patients currently taking SSRIs or newer anti-depressants should not be discontinued abruptly, due to risk of discontinuation symptoms. PROZAC has only rarely been associated with such symptoms. At the time that a medical decision is made to discontinue an SSRI or other newer anti-depressant drug, a gradual reduction in the dose rather than an abrupt cessation, except for fluoxetine, is recommended. Plasma fluoxetine and norfluoxetine concentrations decrease gradually at the conclusion of therapy which makes dose tapering unnecessary in most patients taking this drug (see Warnings and Precautions, Dependence and Adverse Reactions, Adverse Events Subsequent to Discontinuation and Dosage and Administration, Discontinuation of Treatment).

Implications of the Long Elimination Half-Life of Fluoxetine: Because of the long elimination half-lives of fluoxetine and its major active metabolite norfluoxetine, changes in dose will not be fully reflected in plasma for several weeks, affecting both strategies for titration to final dose and withdrawal from treatment (see Action and Clinical Pharmacology and Dosage and Administration). Even when dosing is stopped, active drug substance will persist in the body for weeks due to the long elimination half-lives of fluoxetine and norfluoxetine. This is of potential consequence when drug discontinuation is required or when drugs are prescribed that might interact with fluoxetine and norfluoxetine following discontinuation of PROZAC.

Safety of PROZAC in Pregnant Women: Effects on Newborns: Post-marketing reports indicate that some neonates exposed to PROZAC, other SSRIs (selective serotonin reuptake inhibitors), or newer anti-depressants late in the third trimester have developed complications requiring prolonged hospitalization, respiratory support, and tube feeding. Such complications can arise immediately upon delivery. When treating a pregnant woman with PROZAC during the third trimester, the physician should carefully consider the potential risks and benefits of treatment (see Warnings and Precautions, Special Populations, Pregnant Women and Dosage and Administration).

Weight Change: Significant weight loss, especially in underweight depressed patients and the elderly, may be an undesirable result of treatment with PROZAC. PROZAC should be given with caution to patients suffering from anorexia nervosa and only if the expected benefits (e.g. co-morbid depression) markedly outweigh the potential weight reducing effect of the drug.

Psychomotor Impairment: Patients should be cautioned against driving an automobile or performing hazardous tasks until they are reasonably certain that treatment with PROZAC does not affect them adversely.

Allergic Reactions (Rash and Accompanying Events): During premarketing testing, 7% of 10,782 patients developed various types of rashes and/or urticaria. Among these cases, almost a third were withdrawn from treatment because of the rash and/or systemic signs or symptoms associated with the rash. Clinical findings reported in association with these allergic reactions include rash, fever, leukocytosis, arthralgias, edema, carpal tunnel syndrome, respiratory distress, lymphadenopathy, proteinuria, and mild transaminase elevation. Most patients improved promptly with discontinuation of fluoxetine and/or adjunctive treatment with antihistamines or steroids, and all patients experiencing these events were reported to recover completely.

In premarketing clinical trials two patients are known to have developed a serious cutaneous systemic illness. In neither patient was there an unequivocal diagnosis, but one was considered to have a leukocytoclastic vasculitis, and the other severe desquamation that was considered variously to be a vasculitis or erythema multiforme. Other patients have had systemic manifestations suggestive of serum sickness.

Since the introduction of fluoxetine, systemic events, possibly related to vasculitis, and including lupus-like syndrome, have developed in patients with rash. Although these events are rare, they may be serious, involving the lung, kidney, or liver. Death has been reported to occur in association with these systemic events.

Anaphylactoid events, including bronchospasm, angioedema, laryngospasm and urticaria alone and in combination, have been reported.

Pulmonary events, including inflammatory processes of varying histopathology and/or fibrosis, have been reported rarely. These events have occurred with dyspnea as the only preceding symptom.

Whether these systemic events and rash have a common underlying cause or are due to different etiologies or pathogenic processes is not known. Furthermore, a specific underlying immunologic basis for these events has not been identified. Upon the appearance of rash or of other possibly allergic phenomena for which an alternative etiology cannot be identified, PROZAC should be discontinued. Particular caution should be exercised in patients with a history of allergic reactions.

The following additional Precautions are listed alphabetically.

Cardiovascular: PROZAC has not been evaluated or used to any appreciable extent in patients with a recent history of myocardial infarction or unstable heart disease. Patients with these diagnoses were systematically excluded from premarketing clinical studies. Retrospective evaluation of EKGs in some of these studies showed no conduction abnormalities that resulted in heart block. The mean heart rate was reduced by approximately 3 beats/minute.

Hypokalemia: Self-induced vomiting often leads to hypokalemia which may lower seizure threshold and/or may lead to cardiac conduction abnormalities. Electrolyte levels of bulimic patients should be assessed prior to initiation of treatment.

Concomitant Illness: Clinical experience with PROZAC in patients with concomitant systemic illness is limited and it should be used cautiously in such patients, especially those with diseases or conditions that could affect metabolism or hemodynamic responses.

Dependence: Discontinuation of Treatment with PROZAC (Post-Marketing and Clinical Trials): When discontinuing treatment, patients should be monitored for symptoms which may be associated with discontinuation (e.g. headache, insomnia, paresthesias, nervousness, anxiety, nausea, sweating, numbness, dizziness, jitteriness, asthenia or other symptoms which may be of clinical significance).

PROZAC (fluoxetine) has been only rarely associated with such symptoms. Plasma fluoxetine and norfluoxetine concentrations decrease gradually at the conclusion of therapy, which makes dose tapering unnecessary in most patients (see Warnings and Precautions, General; Adverse Reactions and Dosage and Administration).

Dependence Liability: PROZAC has not been systematically studied, in animals or humans, for its potential for abuse, tolerance, or physical dependence. Physicians should carefully evaluate patients for history of drug abuse and follow such patients closely, observing them for signs of misuse or abuse of PROZAC.

Endocrine and Metabolism: Diabetes: In patients with diabetes, fluoxetine may alter glycemic control. Hypoglycemia has occurred during therapy with fluoxetine, and hyperglycemia has developed following discontinuation of the drug. As is true with many other types of medication when taken concurrently by patients with diabetes, insulin and/or oral hypoglycemic dosage may need to be adjusted when therapy with fluoxetine is instituted or discontinued.

Hematologic: Abnormal Bleeding: There have been rare reports of altered platelet function and/or abnormal results from laboratory studies in patients taking fluoxetine. While there have been reports of abnormal bleeding in several patients taking fluoxetine, it is unclear whether fluoxetine had a causative role.

Hepatic/Biliary/Pancreatic: Hepatic Impairment: Since clearances of fluoxetine and norfluoxetine may be decreased in patients with impaired liver function including cirrhosis, a lower or less frequent dose should be used in such patients. See Action and Clinical Pharmacology.

Neurologic: Seizures: PROZAC should be used with caution in patients with a history of convulsive disorders. The incidence of seizures associated with fluoxetine during clinical trials did not appear to differ from that reported with other marketed antidepressants; however, patients with a history of convulsive disorders were excluded from these trials.

Concurrent administration with electroshock therapy should be avoided because of the absence of experience in this area. There have been rare reports of prolonged seizures in patients on fluoxetine receiving ECT treatment.

Serotonin Syndrome/Neuroleptic Malignant Syndrome: On rare occasions serotonin syndrome or neuroleptic malignant syndrome-like events have occurred in association with treatment with SSRIs, including PROZAC, particularly when given in combination with other serotonergic and/or neuroleptic drugs. As these syndromes may result in potentially life-threatening conditions, treatment with PROZAC should be discontinued if such events (characterized by clusters of symptoms such as hyperthermia, rigidity, myoclonus, autonomic instability with possible rapid fluctuations of vital signs, mental status changes including confusion, irritability, extreme agitation progressing to delirium and coma) occur and supportive symptomatic treatment should be initiated. PROZAC should not be used in combination with MAO inhibitors or serotonin-precursors (such as L-tryptophan, oxitriptan) and should be used with caution in combination with other serotonergic drugs (triptans, certain tricyclic antidepressants, lithium, tramadol, St. John's Wort) due to the risk of serotonergic syndrome (see Contraindications and Drug Interactions).

Psychiatric: Suicide Risk: The possibility of a suicide attempt is inherent in depression and other psychiatric disorders and may persist until significant remission occurs. As with other drugs with similar pharmacological action (antidepressants), isolated cases of suicidal ideation and suicidal behaviors have been reported during fluoxetine therapy or early after treatment discontinuation.

Although a causal role for fluoxetine in inducing such events has not been established, an FDA analysis from pooled studies of antidepressants in psychiatric disorders found an increased risk for suicidal ideation and/or suicidal behaviors in pediatric and young adult (<25 years of age) patients compared to placebo.

Close supervision of high-risk patients should accompany drug therapy and consideration should be given to the possible need for hospitalization. Physicians should encourage patients of all ages to report any new or worsened distressing thoughts or feelings occurring at any time. In order to minimize the opportunity for overdosage, prescriptions for fluoxetine should be written for the smallest quantity of drug consistent with good patient management.

Because of the well established comorbidity between depression and other psychiatric disorders, the same precautions observed when treating patients with depression should be observed when treating patients with other psychiatric disorders (see Warnings and Precautions, General, Potential Association with Behavioural and Emotional Changes, Including Self-Harm).

Activation of Mania/Hypomania: During premarketing clinical trials in a patient population comprised primarily of unipolar depressed patients, hypomania or mania occurred in approximately 1% of fluoxetine treated patients. The incidence in a general patient population which might also include bipolar depressives is unknown. The likelihood of hypomanic or manic episodes may be increased at the higher dosage levels. Such reactions require a reduction in dosage or discontinuation of the drug.

A major depressive episode may be the initial presentation of bipolar disorder. Patients with bipolar disorder may be at an increased risk of experiencing manic episodes when treated with antidepressants alone. Therefore, the decision to initiate symptomatic treatment of depression should only be made after patients have been adequately assessed to determine if they are at risk for bipolar disorder.

Electroconvulsive Therapy (ECT): There are no clinical studies to support the safety and efficacy of combined use of ECT and fluoxetine. There have been rare reports of prolonged seizures in patients on fluoxetine receiving ECT treatment.

Renal: Severe Renal Impairment: Since fluoxetine is extensively metabolized, excretion of unchanged drug in urine is a minor route of elimination. However, until an adequate number of patients with severe renal impairment have been evaluated in the course of chronic treatment, fluoxetine should be used with caution in such patients.

Hyponatremia: Several cases of hyponatremia (some with serum sodium lower than 110 mmol/L) have been reported. The hyponatremia appeared to be reversible when PROZAC was discontinued. Although these cases were complex with varying possible etiologies, some were possibly due to the syndrome of inappropriate antidiuretic hormone secretion (SIADH). The majority of these occurrences have been in older patients and in patients taking diuretics or who were otherwise volume depleted.

In two 6-week controlled studies in patients ≥60 years of age, 10 of 323 fluoxetine patients and 6 of 327 placebo recipients had a lowering of serum sodium below the reference range; this difference was not statistically significant. The lowest observed concentration of sodium in a fluoxetine treated patient was 129 mmol/L. The observed decreases were not clinically significant.

Special Populations: Pregnant Women: Safe use of fluoxetine during pregnancy has not been established. Therefore PROZAC should not be administered to women of childbearing potential unless, in the opinion of the treating physician, the expected benefits to the patient markedly outweigh the possible hazards to the fetus or the child.

Post-marketing reports indicate that some neonates exposed to PROZAC, other SSRIs (selective serotonin reuptake inhibitors), or newer anti-depressants late in the third trimester have developed complications requiring prolonged hospitalization, respiratory support, and tube feeding. Such complications can arise immediately upon delivery. Reported clinical findings have included respiratory distress, cyanosis, apnea, seizures, temperature instability, feeding difficulty, vomiting, hypoglycemia, hypotonia, hypertonia, hyperreflexia, tremor, jitteriness, irritability, and constant crying. These features are consistent with either a direct toxic effect of SSRIs and other newer anti-depressants or, possibly, a drug discontinuation syndrome. It should be noted that, in some cases, the clinical picture is consistent with serotonin syndrome (see Contraindications, Monoamine Oxidase Inhibitors). When treating a pregnant woman with PROZAC during the third trimester, the physician should carefully consider the potential risks and benefits of treatment (see Dosage and Administration).

Nursing Women: PROZAC and its metabolites are excreted in breast milk, and have been observed to reach high levels in the plasma of nursing infants. Women who are taking PROZAC should not breast feed unless, in the opinion of the treating physician, breast feeding is necessary, in which case the infant should be closely monitored.

In one breast milk sample, the concentration of fluoxetine plus norfluoxetine was 70.4 ng/mL. The concentration in the mother's plasma was 295.0 ng/mL. No adverse effects on the infant were reported. In another case, a 6-week infant, nursed by a mother on PROZAC, developed crying, decreased sleep, vomiting and watery stools. The breast milk showed concentrations of 69 ng/mL for fluoxetine and 90 ng/mL for norfluoxetine. In the infant's plasma, the concentrations of fluoxetine and norfluoxetine on the second day of feeding were 340 and 208 ng/mL, respectively.

Pediatrics (<18 years of age): PROZAC is not indicated for use in patients below the age of 18 years. See Warnings and Precautions, General, Potential Association with Behavioural and Emotional Changes, Including Self-Harm. See also Adverse Reactions, Potential for Effects on Growth in Pediatric Patients.

Geriatrics (≥60 years of age): Evaluation of patients over the age of 60 who received PROZAC 20 mg daily revealed no unusual pattern of adverse events relative to the clinical experience in younger patients. These data are however insufficient to rule out possible age-related differences during chronic use, particularly in elderly patients who have concomitant systemic illnesses or who are receiving concomitant drugs. See Indications and Clinical Use and Dosage and Administration.

ADVERSE REACTIONS: Overview: Commonly Observed: In clinical trials, the most commonly observed adverse events associated with the use of PROZAC (fluoxetine) and not seen at an equivalent incidence among placebo treated patients were: central nervous system complaints, including headache, nervousness, insomnia, drowsiness, fatigue or asthenia, anxiety, tremor, and dizziness or lightheadedness; gastrointestinal complaints, including nausea, diarrhea, dry mouth and anorexia; and excessive sweating.

Adverse Events Leading to Discontinuation of Treatment: Fifteen percent of approximately 4000 patients who received PROZAC in North American clinical trials discontinued treatment due to an adverse event. The more common events causing discontinuation from depression trials in adults and elderly, included: psychiatric, primarily nervousness, anxiety, and insomnia; digestive, primarily nausea; nervous system, primarily dizziness, asthenia, and headaches; skin, primarily rash and pruritus.

In obsessive compulsive disorder studies, 12.1% of fluoxetine treated patients discontinued treatment early because of adverse events. Anxiety and rash, at incidences of less than 2%, were the most frequently reported events. In bulimia nervosa studies, 10.2% of fluoxetine treated patients discontinued treatment early because of adverse events. Insomnia, anxiety and rash, at incidences of less than 2%, were the most frequently reported events.

Adverse Events Subsequent to Discontinuation: Symptoms associated with discontinuation of PROZAC have been reported in clinical trials and post-marketing (e.g. headache, insomnia, paresthesias, nervousness, anxiety, nausea, sweating, numbness, dizziness, jitteriness, asthenia, or other symptoms which may be of clinical significance). The majority of these are mild and self-limiting. PROZAC (fluoxetine) has been only rarely associated with such symptoms. Plasma fluoxetine and norfluoxetine concentrations decrease gradually at the conclusion of therapy, which makes dose tapering unnecessary in most patients. See Warnings and Precautions, General and Dosage and Administration.

Serious Adverse Reactions: Suicidal thoughts and acts are far more common among depressed patients than in the general population. It is estimated that suicide is 22 to 36 times more prevalent in depressed persons than in the general population. A comprehensive meta-analysis of pooled data from 17 double blind clinical trials in patients with major depressive disorder compared fluoxetine (n=1765) with a tricyclic antidepressant (n=731) or placebo (n=569), or both. The pooled incidence of emergence of substantial suicidal ideation was 1.2% for fluoxetine, 2.6% for placebo, and 3.6% for tricyclic antidepressants.

In countries where the drug has already been marketed, the following potentially serious adverse reactions have been reported; interactions with MAO inhibitors and possibly other drugs, allergic reactions, cardiovascular reactions, syndrome of inappropriate ADH secretion, and grand mal seizure. Death and life-threatening events have been associated with some of these reactions, although causal relationship to PROZAC has not necessarily been established.

Post-marketing experience also confirms the profile of adverse reactions commonly reported during clinical trials with PROZAC including allergic skin reactions.

Clinical Trial Adverse Drug Reactions: Because clinical trials are conducted under very specific conditions the adverse drug reaction rates observed in the clinical trials may not reflect the rates observed in practice and should not be compared to the rates in the clinical trials of another drug. Adverse drug reaction information from clinical trials is useful for identifying drug-related adverse events and for approximating rates.

Multiple doses of PROZAC had been administered to 10 782 patients with various diagnoses in US clinical trials as of May 8, 1995. Adverse events were recorded by clinical investigators using descriptive terminology of their own choosing. Consequently, it is not possible to provide a meaningful estimate of the proportion of individuals experiencing adverse events without first grouping similar types of events into a limited (i.e., reduced) number of standardized event categories.

Adults: In Table 1, Table 2 and Table 3 and tabulations that follow, COSTART Dictionary terminology has been used to classify reported adverse events. The stated frequencies represent the proportion of individuals who experienced, at least once, a treatment-emergent adverse event of the type listed. An event was considered treatment-emergent if it occurred for the first time or worsened while receiving therapy following baseline evaluation. It is important to emphasize that events reported during therapy were not necessarily caused by it.

The prescriber should be aware that the figures in the tables and tabulations cannot be used to predict the incidence of side effects in the course of usual medical practice where patient characteristics and other factors differ from those that prevailed in the clinical trials. Similarly, the cited frequencies cannot be compared with figures obtained from other clinical investigations involving different treatments, uses, and investigators. The cited figures, however, do provide the prescribing physician with some basis for estimating the relative contribution of drug and nondrug factors to the side effect incidence rate in the population studied. See Table 1.

Table 1: PROZAC

Treatment-Emergent Adverse Events Incidence in Fluoxetine versus Placebo Trials Listed by Indication

	Percentage of Patients Reporting Event							
	Depression[a] (Adults)		Depression (Elderly)		OCD[a]		Bulimia[a]	
Body System/ Adverse Event	**Fluoxetine (N=1728)**	**Placebo (N=975)**	**Fluoxetine (N=335)**	**Placebo (N=336)**	**Fluoxetine (N=266)**	**Placebo (N=89)**	**Fluoxetine (N=450)**	**Placebo (N=267)**
Nervous System								
Headache	—	—	28	24	—	—	—	—
Nervousness	14	9	12	7	14	15	11	5
Insomnia	16	9	18	12	28	22	33	13
Somnolence	13	6	9	6	17	7	13	5
Anxiety	12	7	13	8	14	7	15	19
Tremor	10	3	8	4	9	1	13	1
Dizziness	—	—	11	10	—	—	—	—
Libido, decreased	3	0	—	—	11	2	5	1
Abnormal dreams	1	1	—	—	5	2	5	3

(cont'd)

Table 1: PROZAC *(cont'd)*

Treatment-Emergent Adverse Events Incidence in Fluoxetine versus Placebo Trials Listed by Indication

Body System/ Adverse Event	Percentage of Patients Reporting Event							
	Depression[a] (Adults)		Depression (Elderly)		OCD[a]		Bulimia[a]	
	Fluoxetine (N=1728)	Placebo (N=975)	Fluoxetine (N=335)	Placebo (N=336)	Fluoxetine (N=266)	Placebo (N=89)	Fluoxetine (N=450)	Placebo (N=267)
Digestive System								
Nausea	21	9	17	7	26	13	29	11
Diarrhea	—	—	14	9	—	—	—	—
Dry Mouth	10	7	7	5	12	3	9	6
Anorexia	11	2	11	2	17	10	8	4
Dyspepsia	7	5	11	5	10	4	10	6
Constipation	—	—	7	6	—	—	—	—
Flatulence	—	—	7	2	—	—	—	—
Skin and Appendages								
Sweating	8	3	7	3	7	0	8	3
Rash	4	3	—	—	6	3	4	4
Body as a Whole								
Asthenia	9	5	13	10	15	11	21	9
Flu Syndrome	3	4	—	—	10	7	8	3
Back Pain	—	—	7	9	—	—	—	—
Abdominal Pain	—	—	6	6	—	—	—	—
Myalgia	—	—	3	5	—	—	—	—
Respiratory System								
Rhinitis	—	—	9	14	—	—	—	—
Pharyngitis	3	3	—	—	11	9	10	5
Sinusitis	1	4	3	7	5	2	6	4
Yawn	—	—	—	—	7	—	11	—
Cardiovascular System								
Vasodilatation	3	2	—	—	5	0	2	1
Urogenital System								
Abnormal Ejaculation[b]	—	—	—	—	7	—	7	—
Impotence[b]	2	—	—	—	—	—	7	—

[a] The most common treatment-emergent adverse events associated with the use of PROZAC (incidence of at least 5% for PROZAC and at least twice that for placebo within at least one of the indications) for the treatment of depression, OCD, and bulimia in US controlled clinical trials.
[b] Denominator used was for males only (N=690 PROZAC depression; N=410 placebo depression; N=116 PROZAC OCD; N=43 placebo OCD; N=14 PROZAC bulimia; N=1 placebo bulimia).
Legend: — =incidence less than 1%.

Table 2 enumerates treatment-emergent adverse events that occurred in 2% or more patients treated with PROZAC and with incidence greater than placebo who participated in US controlled clinical trials comparing PROZAC with placebo in the treatment of depression, OCD, or bulimia. Table 2 provides combined data for the pool of studies that are provided separately by indication in Table 1.

Table 3 lists the adverse events associated with discontinuation of PROZAC treatment (incidence at least twice that for placebo and at least 1% for PROZAC in clinical trials collecting only a primary event associated with discontinuation) in depression, OCD, and bulimia. For symptoms associated with discontinuation of PROZAC in clinical trials and post-marketing, see Adverse Reaction, Post-Market Adverse Drug Reactions.

Male and Female Sexual Dysfunction with SSRIs: Although changes in sexual desire, sexual performance, and sexual satisfaction often occur as manifestations of a psychiatric disorder, they may also be a consequence of pharmacologic treatment. In particular, some evidence suggests that SSRIs can cause such untoward sexual experiences.

Reliable estimates of the incidence and severity of untoward experiences involving sexual desire, performance, and satisfaction are difficult to obtain, however, in part because patients and physicians may be reluctant to discuss them. Accordingly, estimates of the incidence of untoward sexual experience and performance, cited in product labeling, are likely to underestimate their actual incidence. In patients enrolled in depression, OCD, and bulimia placebo-controlled clinical trials, decreased libido was the only sexual side effect reported by at least 2% of patients taking fluoxetine (4% fluoxetine, <1% placebo). There have been spontaneous reports in women taking fluoxetine of orgasmic dysfunction, including anorgasmia.

There are no adequate and well-controlled studies examining sexual dysfunction with fluoxetine treatment. Priapism has been reported with all SSRIs. While it is difficult to know the precise risk of sexual dysfunction associated with the use of SSRIs, physicians should routinely inquire about such possible side effects.

Treatment-Emergent Adverse Events: Following is a list of all treatment-emergent adverse events reported at anytime by individuals taking fluoxetine in US clinical trials (10 782 patients) except: (1) those listed in the body or footnotes of Table 1 or Table 2 above or elsewhere in labelling; (2) those for which the COSTART terms were uninformative or misleading; (3) those events for which a causal relationship to PROZAC use was considered remote; and (4) events occurring in only 1 patient treated with PROZAC and which did not have a substantial probability of being acutely life-threatening.

Events are further classified within body system categories and enumerated in order of decreasing frequency using the following definitions: frequent adverse events are defined as those occurring on 1 or more occasions in at least 1/100 patients; infrequent adverse events are those occurring in less than 1/100 but at least 1/1000 patients; rare events are those occurring in less than 1/1000 patients.

Body as a Whole: Frequent: chills. Infrequent: chills and fever, face edema, feeling abnormal, intentional overdose, malaise, pelvic pain, suicide attempt. Rare: abdominal syndrome acute, hypothermia, intentional injury, neuroleptic malignant syndrome* (characterized by the clustering of clinical features of changes in mental state and neuromuscular activity, in combination with autonomic nervous system dysfunction), photosensitivity reaction.

* Neuroleptic malignant syndrome is the COSTART term which best captures serotonin syndrome.

Table 2: PROZAC

Combined Treatment-Emergent Adverse Events Incidence for Patients Treated with PROZAC versus Placebo

Body System/ Adverse Event[a]	Percentage of Patients Reporting Event	
	Depression, OCD, and Bulimia Combined	
	PROZAC (N=2444)	Placebo (N=1331)
Body as a Whole		
Headache	21	20
Asthenia	12	6
Flu Syndrome	5	4
Fever	2	1
Cardiovascular System		
Vasodilatation	3	1
Palpitation	2	1
Digestive System		
Nausea	23	10
Diarrhea	12	8
Anorexia	11	3

(cont'd)

Table 2: PROZAC *(cont'd)*

Combined Treatment-Emergent Adverse Events Incidence for Patients Treated with PROZAC versus Placebo

Body System/ Adverse Event[a]	Percentage of Patients Reporting Event — Depression, OCD, and Bulimia Combined	
	PROZAC (N=2444)	**Placebo (N=1331)**
Dry Mouth	10	7
Dyspepsia	8	5
Flatulence	3	2
Vomiting	3	2
Metabolic and Nutritional Disorders		
Weight Loss	2	1
Nervous System		
Insomnia	20	11
Anxiety	13	8
Nervousness	13	9
Somnolence	13	6
Dizziness	10	7
Tremor	10	3
Libido, decreased	4	—
Respiratory System		
Pharyngitis	5	4
Yawn	3	—
Skin and Appendages		
Sweating	8	3
Rash	4	3
Pruritus	3	2
Special Senses		
Abnormal Vision	3	1

[a] Included are events reported by at least 2% of patients taking PROZAC, except the following events, which had an incidence on placebo >PROZAC (depression, OCD, and bulimia combined): abdominal pain, abnormal dreams, accidental injury, back pain, chest pain, constipation, cough increased, depression (includes suicidal thoughts), dysmenorrhea, gastrointestinal disorder, infection, myalgia, pain, paresthesia, rhinitis, sinusitis, thinking abnormal.

Legend: — =incidence less than 1%.

Table 3: PROZAC

Adverse Events Associated with Discontinuation of PROZAC Treatment

Depression, OCD, and Bulimia Combined (N=1108)	Depression (N=392)	OCD (N=266)	Bulimia (N=450)
—	—	Anxiety (2%)	—
Insomnia (1%)	—	—	Insomnia (2%)
—	Nervousness (1%)	—	—
—	—	Rash (1%)	—

Cardiovascular System: Frequent: hemorrhage, hypertension. Infrequent: angina pectoris, arrhythmia, congestive heart failure, hypotension, migraine, myocardial infarct, postural hypotension, syncope, tachycardia, vascular headache. Rare: atrial fibrillation, bradycardia, cerebral embolism, cerebral ischemia, cerebrovascular accident, extrasystoles, heart arrest, heart block, pallor, peripheral vascular disorder, phlebitis, shock, thrombophlebitis, thrombosis, vasospasm, ventricular arrhythmia, ventricular extrasystoles, ventricular fibrillation.

Digestive System: Frequent: increased appetite, nausea and vomiting. Infrequent: aphthous stomatitis, cholelithiasis, colitis, dysphagia, eructation, esophagitis, gastritis, gastroenteritis, glossitis, gum hemorrhage, hyperchlorhydria, increased salivation, liver function tests abnormal, melena, mouth ulceration, nausea/vomiting/diarrhea, stomach ulcer, stomatitis, thirst. Rare: biliary pain, bloody diarrhea, cholecystitis, duodenal ulcer, enteritis, esophageal ulcer, fecal incontinence, gastrointestinal hemorrhage, hematemesis, hemorrhage of colon, hepatitis, intestinal obstruction, liver fatty deposit, oesophageal pain, pancreatitis, peptic ulcer, rectal hemorrhage, salivary gland enlargement, stomach ulcer hemorrhage, tongue edema.

Endocrine System: Infrequent: hypothyroidism. Rare: diabetic acidosis, diabetes mellitus.

Hemic and Lymphatic Systems: Infrequent: anemia, ecchymosis. Rare: blood dyscrasia, hypochromic anemia, leukopenia, lymphedema, lymphocytosis, petechia, purpura, thrombocythemia, thrombocytopenia.

Metabolic and Nutritional: Frequent: weight gain. Infrequent: dehydration, generalized edema, gout, hypercholesteremia, hyperlipemia, hypokalemia, peripheral edema. Rare: alcohol intolerance, alkaline phosphatase increased, BUN increased, creatine phosphokinase increased, hyperkalemia, hyperuricemia, hypocalcemia, iron deficiency anemia, ALT increased.

Musculoskeletal System: Infrequent: arthritis, bone pain, bursitis, leg cramps, tenosynovitis. Rare: arthrosis, chondrodystrophy, myasthenia, myopathy, myositis, osteomyelitis, osteoporosis, rheumatoid arthritis.

Nervous System: Frequent: abnormal movement/tremor†, agitation, amnesia, confusion, emotional lability, fatigue‡, headache, sleep abnormalities§. Infrequent: abnormal gait, acute brain syndrome, akathisia, apathy, balance disorder, bruxism, CNS depression, CNS stimulation, depersonalization, euphoria, hallucinations, hostility, hyperkinesia, hypertonia, hypesthesia, incoordination, libido increased, neuralgia, neuropathy, neurosis, paranoid reaction, personality disorder¶, psychosis, vertigo. Rare: abnormal electroencephalogram, antisocial reaction, circumoral paresthesia, coma, delusions, dysarthria, dystonia, extrapyramidal syndrome, foot drop, hyperesthesia, neuritis, paralysis, reflexes decreased, reflexes increased, stupor.

Respiratory System: Infrequent: asthma, epistaxis, hiccup, hyperventilation. Rare: apnea, atelectasis, cough decreased, emphysema, hemoptysis, hypoventilation, hypoxia, larynx edema, lung edema, pneumothorax, stridor.

Skin and Appendages: Infrequent: acne, alopecia, contact dermatitis, eczema, maculopapular rash, skin discoloration, skin ulcer, vesiculobullous rash. Rare: furunculosis, herpes zoster, hirsutism, petechial rash, psoriasis, purpuric rash, pustular rash, seborrhea.

Special Senses: Frequent: ear pain, taste perversion, tinnitus. Infrequent: conjunctivitis, dry eyes, mydriasis, photophobia. Rare: blepharitis, deafness, diplopia, exophthalmos, eye hemorrhage, glaucoma, hyperacusis, iritis, parosmia, scleritis, strabismus, taste loss, visual field defect.

Urogenital System: Frequent: gynaecological bleeding**, sexual dysfunction**,††, urinary frequency. Infrequent: abortion**, albuminuria, amenorrhea, breast enlargement, breast pain, cystitis, dysuria, female lactation**, fibrocystic breast**, hematuria, leukorrhea**, menorrhagia**, metrorrhagia**, nocturia, polyuria, urinary incontinence, urinary retention, urinary urgency. Rare: breast engorgement, glycosuria, hypomenorrhea**, kidney pain, oliguria, priapism**, uterine fibroids enlarged**.

Special Populations: (Only adverse events that are different from the above events are listed under special populations.)

Pediatrics (<18 years of age): Frequent: epistaxis.

Potential for Effects on Growth in Pediatric Patients: PROZAC is not indicated for use in patients below the age of 18 years (see Warnings and Precautions, General, Potential Association with Behavioural and Emotional Changes, Including Self-Harm).

Decreased weight gain and a lesser gain in height have been observed in association with the use of fluoxetine in children and adolescent patients. After 19 weeks of treatment in a clinical trial, pediatric subjects treated with fluoxetine (n=88) were recorded as gaining an average of 1.1 cm less in height than subjects treated with placebo (n=75). However, the study was not designed for a rigorous assessment of growth (e.g., heights were recorded to the nearest rounded inch), and thus a definite interpretation of this finding was compromised. This is exemplified by the reported outcome of a loss in height for 17 of the patients. Notwithstanding these limitations, an attenuation of height gain with acute fluoxetine treatment cannot be excluded. Fluoxetine treatment was also associated with a decrease in serum alkaline phosphatase levels in this study. Limited evidence is available concerning the longer-term effects of fluoxetine on the development and maturation of children and adolescent patients. Height and weight should be monitored periodically in pediatric patients receiving fluoxetine.

Post-Market Adverse Drug Reactions: Voluntary reports of adverse events temporally associated with PROZAC that have been received since market introduction and that may have no causal relationship with the drug include the following: aplastic anemia, atrial fibrillation, cataract, cerebral vascular accident, cholestatic jaundice, confusion, dyskinesia (including, for example, a case of buccal-lingual- masticatory syndrome with involuntary tongue protrusion reported to develop in a 77-year-old female after 5 weeks of fluoxetine therapy and which completely resolved over the next few months following drug discontinuation), eosinophilic pneumonia, epidermal necrolysis, erythema multiforme, erythema nodosum, exfoliative dermatitis, gynecomastia, heart arrest, hepatic failure/necrosis, hyperprolactinemia, hypoglycemia, immune-related hemolytic anemia, kidney failure, misuse/abuse, movement disorders developing in patients with risk factors including drugs associated with such events and worsening of preexisting movement disorders, neuroleptic malignant syndrome-like events, optic neuritis, pancreatitis, pancytopenia, priapism, pulmonary embolism, pulmonary hypertension, QT prolongation, serotonin syndrome (a range of signs and symptoms that can rarely, in most severe cases, resemble neuroleptic malignant syndrome), Stevens-Johnson syndrome, sudden unexpected death, suicidal ideation, thrombocytopenia, thrombocytopenic purpura, vaginal bleeding after drug withdrawal, ventricular tachycardia (including torsades de pointes-type arrhythmias) and violent behaviours.

DRUG INTERACTIONS:

Serious Drug Interactions
Monoamine Oxidase Inhibitors: See Contraindications.
Thioridazine: See Contraindications.

Overview: PROZAC, like other agents that are metabolized by the P4502D6 system, inhibits the activity of this isoenzyme. Therefore, co-therapy with medications that are predominantly metabolized by the P4502D6 system and that have a relatively narrow therapeutic index (e.g. flecainide, encainide, vinblastine, carbamazepine and tricyclic antidepressants) should be initiated at the low end of the dose range if a patient is receiving fluoxetine concurrently, or has taken it in the previous 5 weeks. If fluoxetine is added to the treatment regimen of a patient already receiving a drug metabolized by P4502D6, the need for decreased dose of the original medication should be considered. The aforementioned drugs with a narrow therapeutic index represent the greatest concern.

Other drugs that have demonstrated increased plasma values or magnified effects when co-administered with fluoxetine include: phenytoin, antipsychotics, benzodiazepines, thioridazine (see Contraindications), St. John's Wort and warfarin.

As fluoxetine is highly bound to plasma proteins, co-administration with another drug which is also highly bound (e.g. warfarin, digitoxin) may result in adverse effects due to an increase in plasma levels of either unbound drug.

There are little data available on the concomitant use of fluoxetine and alcohol.

Drug-Drug Interactions: Monoamine Oxidase Inhibitors: Combined use of PROZAC and MAO inhibitors is contraindicated due to the potential for serious reactions with features resembling serotonin syndrome or neuroleptic malignant syndrome (see Contraindications; Warnings and Precautions, Serotonin Syndrome/Neuroleptic Malignant Syndrome).

Thioridazine: Potential Interactions with thioridazine (see also Contraindications): In a study of 19 healthy male subjects, which included 6 slow and 13 rapid hydroxylators of debrisoquin, a single 25 mg oral dose of thioridazine produced a 2.4-fold higher C_{max} and a 4.5-fold higher AUC for thioridazine in the slow hydroxylators compared to the rapid hydroxylators. The rate of debrisoquin hydroxylation is felt to depend on the level of cytochrome P4502D6 isozyme activity. Thus, this study suggests that drugs which inhibit P4502D6, such as certain SSRIs, including fluoxetine, will produce elevated plasma levels of thioridazine.

Thioridazine administration produces a dose-related prolongation of the QTc interval which is associated with serious ventricular arrhythmias, such as torsades de pointes-type arrhythmias, and sudden death. This risk is expected to increase with fluoxetine-induced inhibition of thioridazine metabolism. Due to the risk of serious ventricular arrhythmias and sudden death potentially associated with elevated plasma levels of thioridazine, thioridazine should not be concomitantly administered, nor within a minimum of 5 weeks after fluoxetine has been discontinued, nor should PROZAC be administered within 2 weeks after thioridazine has been discontinued (see Contraindications).

Drugs Tightly Bound to Plasma Protein: Because fluoxetine is highly bound to plasma protein, the administration of fluoxetine to a patient taking another drug which is tightly bound to protein (e.g. warfarin, digitoxin) may cause a shift in plasma concentrations potentially resulting in an adverse effect. Conversely, adverse effects may result from displacement of protein bound fluoxetine by other tightly bound drugs.

Drugs Metabolized by P4502D6 Isoenzyme: Approximately 3 to 10% of the normal population has a genetic defect that leads to reduced levels of activity of the cytochrome P450 isoenzyme P4502D6. Such individuals have been referred to as "poor metabolizers" of drugs such as debrisoquine, dextromethorphan, sparteine, tricyclic antidepressants (e.g. nortryptiline, amitriptyline, imipramine, and desipramine), phenothiazine neuroleptics (e.g. perphenazine and thioridazine) and Type 1C antiarrhythmics (e.g. propafenone and flecainide).

Conversely, approximately 90 to 97% of the normal population do not have this genetic defect, and are known as "extensive metabolizers". PROZAC, like other agents that are metabolized by the P4502D6 system, inhibits the activity of this isoenzyme, and thus may make normal "extensive" metabolizers resemble "poor metabolizers". Therapy with medications that are predominantly metabolized by the P4502D6 system and that have a relatively narrow therapeutic index (e.g. flecainide, encainida, vinblastine, carbamazepine and tricyclic antidepressants) should be initiated at the low end of the dose range if a patient is receiving fluoxetine concurrently, or has taken it in the previous 5 weeks.

If fluoxetine is added to the treatment regimen of a patient already receiving a drug metabolized by P4502D6 the need for decreased dose of the original medication should be considered. The aforementioned drugs with a narrow therapeutic index represent the greatest concern.

Drugs Metabolized by Cytochrome P4503A4: In an in vivo interaction study involving co-administration of fluoxetine with single doses of terfenadine (a cytochrome P4503A4 substrate), no increase in plasma terfenadine concentrations occurred with concomitant fluoxetine. In addition, in vitro studies have shown ketoconazole, a potent inhibitor of P4503A4 activity, to be at least

† COSTART group term **abnormal movement/tremor** includes the independent terms: frequent: tremor; infrequent: ataxia, buccoglossal, myoclonus; rare: twitching.
‡ COSTART group term **fatigue** includes the independent terms: frequent: asthenia, somnolence.
§ COSTART group term **sleep abnormalities** includes the independent terms: frequent: insomnia; rare: abnormal dreams.
¶ Personality disorder is the COSTART term for designating non-aggressive objectionable behavior.
** Adjusted for gender.

†† COSTART group term **sexual dysfunction** includes the independent terms: frequent: impotence, libido decreased; infrequent: anorgasmia, delayed or absent ejaculation.

100 times more potent than fluoxetine or norfluoxetine as an inhibitor of the metabolism of several substrates for this enzyme, including astemizole, cisapride, and midazolam. These data indicate that fluoxetine's extent of inhibition of cytochrome P4503A4 activity is not likely to be of clinical significance.
Tricyclic Antidepressants: In two studies, previously stable plasma levels of imipramine and desipramine have increased greater than 2 to 10-fold when fluoxetine has been administered in combination. This influence may persist for three weeks or longer after fluoxetine is discontinued. Thus, the dose of tricyclic antidepressant (TCA) may need to be reduced and plasma TCA concentrations may need to be monitored temporarily when fluoxetine is coadministered or has been recently discontinued. See Warnings and Precautions and Action and Clinical Pharmacology, Accumulation and Slow Elimination.
Lithium: There have been reports of both increased and decreased lithium levels when lithium was used concomitantly with fluoxetine. Cases of lithium toxicity have been reported. Lithium levels should be monitored when these drugs are administered concomitantly.
Tryptophan: Five patients receiving PROZAC in combination with tryptophan experienced adverse reactions, including agitation, restlessness and gastrointestinal distress.
Benzodiazepines: The half-life of concurrently administered diazepam may be prolonged in some patients.
Coadministration of alprazolam and fluoxetine has resulted in increased alprazolam plasma concentrations and in further psychomotor performance decrement due to increased alprazolam levels. Consideration should be given to monitoring of clinical status. Experience with the use of PROZAC in combination with other CNS-active drugs is limited and caution is advised if such concomitant medication is required.
Alcohol: The concomitant use of fluoxetine and alcohol on cognitive and psychomotor effects in depressed, panic disorder or OCD patients is not known and is not recommended.
St. John's Wort: In common with other SSRIs, pharmacodynamic interactions between fluoxetine and the herbal remedy St. John's Wort may occur and may result in an increase in undesirable effects.
Antipsychotics: Elevation of blood levels of haloperidol and clozapine and in some cases, clinical manifestations of toxicity have been observed with coadministration of fluoxetine. Consideration should be given to monitoring of clinical status.
Serotonergic Drugs: Based on the mechanism of action of fluoxetine and the potential for serotonin syndrome, caution is advised when PROZAC is coadministered with other drugs or agents that may affect the serotonergic neurotransmitter systems, such as tryptophan, triptans, serotonin reuptake inhibitors, linezolid (an antibiotic which is a reversible non-selective MAOI), lithium, tramadol, or St. John's Wort (see Warnings and Precautions, Serotonin Syndrome/Neuroleptic Malignant Syndrome).
Triptans (5HT$_1$ agonists): There have been rare postmarketing reports describing patients with weakness, hyperreflexia, and incoordination following the use of a selective serotonin reuptake inhibitor (SSRI) and the 5HT$_1$ agonist, sumatriptan. If concomitant treatment with triptan and an SSRI (e.g. fluoxetine, fluvoxamine, paroxetine, sertraline, or citalopram) is clinically warranted, appropriate observation of the patient is advised. The possibility of such interactions should also be considered if other 5HT$_1$ agonists are to be used in combination with SSRIs (see Warnings and Precautions, Serotonin Syndrome/Neuroleptic Malignant Syndrome).
Phenytoin: In patients on stable, maintenance doses of phenytoin, plasma phenytoin concentrations increased substantially and symptoms of phenytoin toxicity appeared (nystagmus, diplopia, ataxia and CNS depression) following initiation of concomitant fluoxetine treatment.
Carbamazepine: Patients on stable doses of phenytoin and carbamazepine have developed elevated plasma anticonvulsant concentrations and clinical anticonvulsant toxicity following initiation of concomitant fluoxetine treatment. Consideration should be given to monitoring of clinical status when fluoxetine treatment is initiated in these patients.
Warfarin: Altered anti-coagulant effects, including increased bleeding, have been reported when fluoxetine is co-administered with warfarin. Serious bleeding events have been reported including five with outcome of death. However, a causal relationship to the bleeding events cannot be established. Therefore, patients receiving warfarin therapy should receive careful coagulation monitoring when fluoxetine is initiated or stopped.
Drug-Food Interactions: Absorption of fluoxetine is not affected by food.
Drug-Herb Interactions: Interactions with PROZAC and herbal remedy St. John's Wort may occur (see Drug-Drug Interactions).
Drug-Laboratory Interactions: Interactions with laboratory tests have not been established.
Drug-Lifestyle Interactions: Interaction with lifestyle interactions have not been established.

DOSAGE AND ADMINISTRATION:

Dosing Considerations: PROZAC (fluoxetine) is not indicated for use in children under 18 year of age (see Warnings and Precautions, General, Potential Association with Behavioural and Emotional Changes, Including Self-Harm).
General: For any indication, the total fluoxetine dosage should not exceed a maximum of 80 mg per day since clinical experience with doses above 80 mg per day is very limited.
During maintenance therapy, the dosage should be kept at the lowest effective level.
Dose Adjustment: Since it may take up to four or five weeks to reach steady-state plasma levels of PROZAC (fluoxetine), sufficient time should be allowed to elapse before dosage is gradually increased. Higher dosages are usually associated with an increased incidence of adverse reactions.
Switching Patients to a Tricyclic Antidepressant (TCA): Dosage of a TCA may need to be reduced and plasma TCA concentrations may need to be monitored temporarily when fluoxetine is coadministered or has been recently discontinued (see Drug Interactions, Tricyclic Antidepressants).
Switching Patients to or from a Monoamine Oxidase Inhibitor (MAOI): At least 14 days should elapse between discontinuation of an MAOI and initiation of therapy with PROZAC. In addition, at least 5 weeks, perhaps longer, should be allowed after stopping PROZAC before starting MAOI (see Contraindications).
Discontinuation of Treatment: When dosing is stopped, active drug substances will persist in the body for weeks. This should be borne in mind when starting or stopping treatment. Dosage tapering is unnecessary in most patients.
Despite its long-half life, symptoms associated with the discontinuation of PROZAC have been reported in clinical trials and post-marketing. Patients should be monitored for these and other symptoms when discontinuing treatment, regardless of the indication for which PROZAC is being prescribed. PROZAC (fluoxetine) has been only rarely associated with such symptoms. Plasma fluoxetine and norfluoxetine concentrations decrease gradually at the conclusion of therapy, which makes dose tapering unnecessary in most patients (see Warnings and Precautions and Adverse Reactions).
Adults: Depression: Initial Adult Dosage: The usual initial dosage is 20 mg administered once daily in the morning. A gradual dose increase should be considered only after a trial period of several weeks if the expected clinical improvement does not occur. Dosage should not exceed a maximum of 80 mg per day since clinical experience with doses above 80 mg per day is very limited.
Long-Term: The efficacy of PROZAC in maintaining an antidepressant response for up to 38 weeks following 12 weeks of open-label acute treatment (50 weeks total) was demonstrated in a placebo-controlled trial. The usefulness of the drug in patients receiving PROZAC for extended periods should be reevaluated periodically.
Bulimia Nervosa: Adult Dosage: The recommended dosage is 60 mg per day, although studies show that lower doses may also be efficacious. Electrolyte levels should be assessed prior to initiation of treatment.
Obsessive-Compulsive Disorder: A dose range of 20 mg/day to 60 mg/day is recommended for the treatment of obsessive-compulsive disorder.
Special Patient Populations: For Any Indication: Treatment of Pregnant Women During the Third Trimester: Post-marketing reports indicate that some neonates exposed to PROZAC, SSRIs or other newer anti-depressants, late in the third trimester have developed complications requiring prolonged hospitalization, respiratory support, and tube feeding (see Warnings and Precautions). When treating pregnant women with PROZAC during the third trimester, the physician should carefully consider the potential risks and benefits of treatment. The physician may consider tapering PROZAC in the third trimester.
Geriatrics: Fluoxetine was evaluated in depressed elderly patients only at a dosage of 20 mg/day. A lower or less frequent dosage may be effective and should be considered in elderly patients with concurrent disease or on multiple medications.
Pediatrics: PROZAC (fluoxetine) is not indicated for use in children under 18 year of age (see Warnings and Precautions, General, Potential Association with Behavioural and Emotional Changes, Including Self-Harm).
Debilitated Patients: A lower or less frequent dosage should be used in patients with renal and/or hepatic impairment and in those on multiple medications.

OVERDOSAGE:

Signs and Symptoms: Cases of overdose of fluoxetine alone usually have a mild course. Symptoms of overdose included nausea, vomiting, seizures, cardiovascular dysfunction ranging from asymptomatic arrhythmias to cardiac arrest, pulmonary dysfunction, and signs of altered CNS status ranging from excitation to coma. Fatalities attributed to overdose of fluoxetine alone have been reported. (Please refer to Human Experience and Animal Experience).
Management of Overdosage: There are no specific antidotes for PROZAC.
Treatment should consist of those general measures employed in the management of overdosage with any antidepressant.
Establish and maintain an airway; ensure adequate oxygenation and ventilation.
Cardiac and vital signs monitoring is recommended, along with general symptomatic and supportive measures.
Induction of emesis is not recommended.
Gastric lavage with a large-bore orogastric tube with appropriate airway protection, if needed, may be indicated if performed soon after ingestion, or in symptomatic patients.
Activated charcoal should be considered in treating overdose.
Due to the large volume of distribution of PROZAC, forced diuresis, dialysis, hemoperfusion, and exchange transfusion are unlikely to be of benefit.
A specific caution involves patients who are taking or have recently taken fluoxetine and might ingest excessive quantities of a TCA. In such a case, accumulation of the parent tricyclic and/or an active metabolite may increase the possibility of clinically significant sequelae and extend the time needed for close medical observation.
Fluoxetine-induced seizures which fail to remit spontaneously may respond to diazepam. (See Product Monograph for diazepam.)
In managing overdosage, consider the possibility of multiple drug involvement. The physician should consider contacting a poison control centre on the treatment of any overdosage.
Human Experience: Worldwide exposure to fluoxetine hydrochloride is estimated to be over 38 million patients (circa 1999). Of the 1578 cases of overdose involving fluoxetine hydrochloride, alone or with other drugs, reported from this population, there were 195 deaths.
Among 633 adult patients who overdosed on fluoxetine hydrochloride alone, 34 resulted in a fatal outcome, 378 completely recovered, and 15 patients experienced sequelae after overdosage, including abnormal accommodation, abnormal gait, confusion, unresponsiveness, nervousness, pulmonary dysfunction, vertigo, tremor, elevated blood pressure, impotence, movement disorder, and hypomania. The remaining 206 patients had an unknown outcome. The most common signs and symptoms associated with non-fatal overdosage were seizures, somnolence, nausea, tachycardia, and vomiting. The largest known ingestion of fluoxetine hydrochloride in adult patients was 8 grams in a patient who took fluoxetine alone and who subsequently recovered. However, in an adult patient who took fluoxetine alone, an ingestion as low as 520 mg has been associated with lethal outcome, but causality has not been established.
Among pediatric patients (ages 3 months to 17 years), there were 156 cases of overdose involving fluoxetine alone or in combination with other drugs. Six patients died, 127 patients completely recovered, 1 patient experienced renal failure, and 22 patients had an unknown outcome. One of the six fatalities was a 9-year-old boy who had a history of OCD, Tourette's syndrome with tics, attention deficit disorder, and fetal alcohol syndrome. He had been receiving 100 mg of fluoxetine daily for 6 months in addition to clonidine, methylphenidate, and promethazine. Mixed-drug ingestion or other methods of suicide complicated all six overdoses in children that resulted in fatalities. The largest ingestion in pediatric patients was 3 grams which was non-lethal.
Other important adverse events reported with fluoxetine overdose (single and multiple drugs) include coma, delirium, ECG abnormalities (such as QT interval prolongation and ventricular tachycardia, including torsades de pointes-type arrhythmias), hypotension, mania, neuroleptic malignant syndrome-like events, pyrexia stupor, and syncope.
Animal Experience: Studies in animals do not provide precise or necessarily valid information about the treatment of human overdose.
However, animal experiments can provide useful insights into possible treatment strategies.
The oral median lethal dose in rats and mice was found to be 452 and 248 mg/kg, respectively. Acute high oral doses produced hyper-irritability and convulsions in several animal species.
Among six dogs purposely overdosed with oral fluoxetine, five experienced grand mal seizures. Seizures stopped immediately upon the bolus intravenous administration of a standard veterinary dose of diazepam. In this short-term study, the lowest plasma concentration at which a seizure occurred was only twice the maximum plasma concentration seen in humans taking 80 mg/day, chronically.
In a separate single-dose study, the ECG of dogs given high doses did not reveal prolongation of the PR, QRS, or QT intervals. Tachycardia and an increase in blood pressure were observed. Consequently, the value of the ECG in predicting cardiac toxicity is unknown. Nonetheless, the ECG should ordinarily be monitored in cases of human overdose.

> For management of a suspected drug overdose, CPhA recommends that you contact your **regional Poison Control Centre**. See the *CPS* Directory section for a list of Poison Control Centres.

ACTION AND CLINICAL PHARMACOLOGY: Pharmacodynamics: The antidepressant, antiobsessional, and antibulimic actions of PROZAC (fluoxetine) are presumed to be linked to its ability to selectively inhibit the neuronal reuptake of serotonin. At clinically relevant doses fluoxetine blocks the uptake of serotonin into human platelets. Antagonism of muscarinic, histaminergic and α_1-adrenergic receptors has been hypothesized to be associated with various anticholinergic, sedative and cardiovascular effects of classical tricyclic antidepressant drugs. In vitro receptor binding studies have demonstrated that fluoxetine binds to these and other membrane receptors [opiate, serotonergic (5-HT$_1$, 5-HT$_2$), adrenergic (α_1,α_2,β) and dopaminergic] much less potently than do the tricyclic drugs.
Pharmacokinetics: Absorption, Distribution, Metabolism, and Excretion: Fluoxetine is well absorbed after oral administration. In man, following a single oral 40 mg dose, peak plasma concentrations of fluoxetine from 15 to 55 ng/mL are observed after 6 to 8 hours. The capsule and oral solution dosage forms of PROZAC are bioequivalent. Food does not appear to affect the systemic bioavailability of fluoxetine, although it may delay its absorption inconsequentially. Thus, PROZAC may be administered with or without food.
Fluoxetine is extensively metabolized in the liver to norfluoxetine, and other unidentified metabolites. The pharmacological activity of norfluoxetine, which is formed by demethylation of fluoxetine appears to be similar to that of the parent drug. Norfluoxetine contributes to the long duration of action of PROZAC. The primary route of elimination appears to be hepatic metabolism to inactive metabolites excreted by the kidney. The elimination half-life of fluoxetine is 4 to 6 days and that of its active metabolite is 4 to 16 days.
Clinical Issues Related to Metabolism/Elimination: Variability in Metabolism: The metabolism of fluoxetine, like that of a number of other compounds, including tricyclic antidepressants and some selective serotonin reuptake inhibitors (SSRIs), involves the P4502D6 system. Concomitant therapy with fluoxetine and the aforementioned drugs may lead to clinically significant drug interactions (see Drug Interactions).
Accumulation and Slow Elimination: The relatively slow elimination of fluoxetine and its active metabolite, norfluoxetine, results in significant accumulation of these active moieties in chronic use. Therefore, it may take up to 1 to 2 months for the active drug substance(s) to disappear from the body. This persistence of active moieties is important to keep in mind when PROZAC is discontinued, or when drugs that are predicted to interact with PROZAC are to be administered soon after its discontinuation (see Warnings and Precautions, General, Implications of the Long Elimination Half-Life of Fluoxetine and Drug Interactions).
Kinetic Data: After 30 days of dosing at 20 mg/day, mean plasma concentrations of fluoxetine 79.1±33.4 ng/mL and of norfluoxetine 129±42.0 ng/mL have been observed. Plasma concentrations of fluoxetine (elimination half-life of 1 to 3 days after acute administration and 4 to 6 days after chronic administration) were higher than those predicted by single-dose studies. Norfluoxetine appears to have linear pharmacokinetics. Its mean terminal half-lives after a single dose and multiple doses were 8.6 days and 9.3 days, respectively.
Steady state plasma levels are attained after 4 to 5 weeks of continuous drug administration. Patients receiving fluoxetine at doses of 40 to 80 mg/day over periods as long as 3 years exhibited, on average, plasma concentrations similar to those seen among patients treated for 4 to 5 weeks at the same dose.
Protein Binding: Approximately 94% of fluoxetine is protein bound. The interaction between fluoxetine and other highly protein bound drugs has not been fully evaluated, but may be important (see Drug Interactions).
Special Populations and Conditions: Age: The effects of age upon the metabolism of fluoxetine have been investigated in a subset of 260 elderly, but otherwise healthy, depressed patients (mean age: 67.4 yr, range 60 to 85 yr) who received 20 mg PROZAC for 6 weeks. Mean plasma concentrations were found to be 89.5±53.6 ng/mL for fluoxetine and 119±51.3 ng/mL for norfluoxetine. However, the effects of concomitant illness and/or concomitant drugs have not been evaluated.
Hepatic Insufficiency: In patients with cirrhosis, the elimination half-life of fluoxetine was prolonged, with a mean of 7.6 days compared to a range of 2 to 3 days seen in healthy subjects; norfluoxetine half-life was also prolonged, with a mean of 12 days compared to a range of 7 to 9 days in healthy subjects. Fluoxetine should therefore be used with caution in patients with liver disease (see Warnings and Precautions, Hepatic Impairment and Dosage and Administration).
Renal Insufficiency: In single dose studies, the pharmacokinetics of fluoxetine and norfluoxetine were similar among subjects with all levels of impaired renal function including anephric patients on chronic hemodialysis. However, with chronic administration, additional accumulation of fluoxetine or its metabolites (possibly including some not yet identified) may occur in patients with severely impaired renal function, and the use of a lower or less frequent dose is advised (see Warnings and Precautions, Renal and Dosage and Administration).

STORAGE AND STABILITY: Store PROZAC capsules at 15-30°C.

INFORMATION FOR THE PATIENT: Published in e-CPS, available by subscription at www.e-cps.ca.

DOSAGE FORMS, COMPOSITION AND PACKAGING: 10 mg: Each green capsule, printed with Dista 3104 and PROZAC 10 mg, contains: fluoxetine HCl equivalent to fluoxetine 10 mg (32.3 μmoles). Nonmedicinal ingredients: silicone and starch; capsule shell: benzyl alcohol, butylparaben, carboxymethylcellulose sodium, edetate calcium disodium, FD&C Blue No. 1, gelatin, iron oxide yellow, methylparaben, propylparaben, sodium lauryl sulfate, sodium propionate and titanium dioxide. Amber HDPE bottles of 100.

20 mg: Each green and yellow capsule, printed with Dista 3105 and PROZAC 20 mg, contains: fluoxetine HCl equivalent to fluoxetine 20 mg (64.7 μmoles). Nonmedicinal ingredients: silicone and starch; capsule shell: benzyl alcohol, butylparaben, carboxymethylcellulose sodium, edetate calcium disodium, FD&C Blue No. 1, gelatin, iron oxide yellow, methylparaben, propylparaben, sodium lauryl sulfate, sodium propionate and titanium dioxide. Amber HDPE bottles of 100.

Pseudofrin
pseudoephedrine HCl
Decongestant

Trianon

SUPPLIED: Each white round flat-faced tablet, scored on one side and engraved TRIANON on the other, contains: pseudoephedrine HCl 60 mg. Nonmedicinal ingredients: lactose, magnesium stearate, povidone, starch and stearic acid. Alcohol-, gluten-, sulfite- and tartrazine-free. Blister packs of 12 and 24, in boxes.

Pulmicort® Nebuamp® Ⓟ
budesonide
Glucocorticosteroid for the Treatment of Bronchial Asthma

AstraZeneca

Date of Preparation: January 19, 2000
Date of Revision: January 14, 2009

PHARMACOLOGY: The active ingredient of PULMICORT NEBUAMP, budesonide, is a potent non-halogenated synthetic glucocorticosteroid with strong topical and weak systemic effects.

PULMICORT NEBUAMP has a high topical anti-inflammatory potency and it is rapidly biotransformed in the liver. This favorable separation between topical anti-inflammatory activity and systemic effect is due to strong glucocorticosteroid receptor affinity and an effective first pass metabolism with a short half-life.

The late reaction can be significantly inhibited if PULMICORT NEBUAMP is given at least 2 hours before a bronchial challenge. Pretreatment for 1 to 4 weeks with inhaled budesonide may inhibit the immediate bronchial reaction.

After therapeutic use of orally inhaled budesonide, several weeks may pass before the full effect is obtained.

INDICATIONS: Patients with bronchial asthma, who require maintenance treatment with inhaled glucocorticosteroids for control of the underlying airways inflammation and who are unable to efficiently use other inhaled formulations.

CONTRAINDICATIONS:

1. Status asthmaticus; not to be used in primary treatment of acute episodes of asthma or in patients with moderate to severe bronchiectasis;
2. Known hypersensitivity to any components;
3. Active or quiescent pulmonary tuberculosis;
4. Untreated fungal, bacterial or viral infections of the respiratory system.

WARNINGS: Deaths due to adrenal insufficiency have occurred in asthmatic patients during and after transfer from systemic corticosteroids to inhaled corticosteroids. Particular care is needed in patients who are transferred from systemically active corticosteroids to PULMICORT NEBUAMP and in patients who required high dose emergency corticosteroid therapy. This is important as deaths due to adrenal insufficiency have occurred in asthmatic patients during and after transfer from systemic corticosteroids to inhaled corticosteroids. Patients receiving prolonged treatment at the highest recommended dose of inhaled corticosteroids may also be at risk for adrenal insufficiency. After withdrawal from systemic corticosteroids, a number of months are required for recovery of hypothalamic-pituitary-adrenal (HPA) function. During this period of HPA suppression, patients may exhibit signs and symptoms of adrenal insufficiency when exposed to severe stress including worsening of asthma attacks, trauma, surgery or infections, particularly gastroenteritis, or other conditions associated with severe electrolyte loss. Although PULMICORT NEBUAMP may provide control of asthmatic symptoms during these episodes, it does **not** provide the systemic steroid which is necessary for coping with these emergencies. Additional systemic corticosteroid should be considered during periods of stress or elective surgery.

During periods of stress or a severe asthmatic attack, patients who have been withdrawn from systemic corticosteroids should be instructed to resume systemic steroids (in large dosages) immediately and to contact their physicians for further instruction. These patients should also be instructed to carry a warning card indicating that they may need supplementary systemic steroids during periods of stress or a severe asthma attack. To assess the risk of adrenal insufficiency in emergency situations, routine tests of adrenal cortical function, including measurement of early morning and evening cortisol levels, should be performed periodically in all patients. An early morning resting cortisol level may be accepted as normal only if it falls at or near the normal mean level.

Patients previously on high doses of systemic steroids may regain earlier symptoms not related to asthma such as rhinitis and eczema when transferred from oral therapy to PULMICORT NEBUAMP. These allergies should be symptomatically treated with antihistamine and/or topical preparations, including topical steroids. These symptoms are a result of the generally lower systemic steroid action which will be experienced. Patients may also suffer from tiredness, headache, pain in muscles and joints and, occasionally, nausea and vomiting. Temporary resumption of systemic steroids may be necessary to treat these conditions.

The development of pharyngeal and laryngeal candidiasis is cause for concern because the extent of its penetration of the respiratory tract is unknown. If oral pharyngeal candidiasis develops, appropriate antifungal therapy should be implemented to eradicate the infection. The incidence of candidiasis can generally be held to a minimum by having patients rinse their mouths out with water after each nebulization treatment (see Dosage).

Glucocorticosteroids may mask some signs of infection and new infections may appear during its use.

PULMICORT NEBUAMP is not to be regarded as a bronchodilator and is not indicated for rapid relief of bronchospasm.

The nebulizer chamber should be cleaned after every administration. Wash the nebulizer chamber and mouthpiece or face mask in hot tap water using a mild detergent. Rinse well and dry by connecting the nebulizer chamber to the compressor or air inlet.

Due to a low output of budesonide, ultrasonic nebulizers should not be used for administration of PULMICORT NEBUAMP.

PRECAUTIONS: Two cases of mortality due to cerebral edema and encephalopathy were reported during clinical trials. There was no apparent cause and effect relationship.

There is still insufficient data for the long-term systemic effect of PULMICORT NEBUAMP. The long-term effects of budesonide in developmental or immunologic processes in the mouth, pharynx, trachea, eyes and lungs are unknown. With the recommended therapeutic doses, the risk/benefit ratio seems to be very low. However, as with any other glucocorticosteroid, patients should be carefully followed up for systemic adverse effects, particularly during long-term therapy.

In transferring patients from a systemic steroid to PULMICORT NEBUAMP, the reduction of the systemic steroid must be very gradual and carefully supervised by the physician since systemic withdrawal symptoms (e.g. joint and/or muscular pain, lassitude, depression) may occur in spite of maintenance or improvement of respiratory functions (see Dosage).

It is essential that the patient be instructed that PULMICORT NEBUAMP is a preventative agent which must be taken at regular intervals and is not to be used to relieve an acute asthmatic attack.

Treatment with PULMICORT NEBUAMP should not be stopped abruptly, but tapered off gradually (see Dosage, Clinical Management).

Pulmonary infiltrates with eosinophilia may occur in patients on PULMICORT NEBUAMP therapy. The causative role of inhalational steroids cannot be ruled out.

Pregnancy: In experimental animal studies, budesonide was found to cross the placental barrier. Like other glucocorticosteroids, budesonide is teratogenic to rodent species. High doses of budesonide administered subcutaneously produced fetal malformations, primarily skeletal defects, in rabbits, rats, and in mice. Results from world-wide post marketing experience indicate inhaled budesonide during pregnancy has no adverse effects on the health of the fetus/new born child. Review of published literature of orally inhaled budesonide, including results from a large case control study performed with cases identified from 3 Swedish health registers showed that there was no association between exposure to inhaled budesonide and overall congenital malformations. Results from a similar study performed with intranasal budesonide, using the same 3 Swedish health registers showed that the use of intranasal budesonide was associated with a subgroup "less severe cardiovascular defects"; however there was no statistically significant association between the use of intranasal budesonide during pregnancy and overall congenital malformations, or overall frequency of cardiovascular defects in the offspring. Budesonide should be used during pregnancy only if the potential benefits clearly outweigh the risk to the fetus. Infants born of mothers who have received substantial doses of corticosteroids, especially oral steroids, during pregnancy should be carefully observed for hypoadrenalism.

Lactation: Budesonide is excreted in breast milk. The administration of PULMICORT NEBUAMP to women who are breast feeding should only be considered if the expected benefit to the mother is greater than any possible risk to the child.

Corticosteroids may mask some signs of infections and new infections may appear. A decreased resistance to localized infection has been observed during corticosteroid therapy. During long-term therapy, pituitary-adrenal function and height (in children) should be periodically assessed.

Patients should be advised to inform subsequent physicians of the prior use of corticosteroids.

There may be enhanced systemic effects of budesonide in patients with an advanced liver cirrhosis, and in those with hypothyroidism.

ASA should be used cautiously in conjunction with corticosteroids in hypoprothrombinemia.

Special care is needed in patients with lung tuberculosis and fungal and viral infections. Children who are on immunosuppressant drugs are more susceptible to infections than healthy children. Chickenpox and measles, for example, can have a more serious or fatal course in children on immunosuppressant corticosteroids. In such children, or in adults who have not had these diseases, particular care should be taken to avoid exposure. If exposed, therapy with varicella zoster immune globulin (VZIG) or pooled i.v. immunoglobulin (IVIG), as appropriate, may be indicated. If chickenpox develops, treatment with antiviral agents may be considered.

If, however, a viral upper respiratory infection is present, the patient should adhere to the regular asthma medication. In patients who are known to deteriorate rapidly when they have a viral respiratory infection, a short course of oral corticosteroid therapy should be considered.

Clinical studies have shown that viral upper respiratory infections cause significantly fewer problems in patients who are on regular treatment with topical glucocorticosteroids.

To ensure the proper dosage and administration of the drug, the patient should be instructed by a physician or other health professional in the use of PULMICORT NEBUAMP and the nebulizing equipment.

Adequate oral hygiene is of primary importance in minimizing overgrowth of microorganisms such as *C. albicans* (see Dosage).

Drug Interactions: Cimetidine: The kinetics of budesonide were investigated in a study of healthy subjects without and with cimetidine, 1000 mg daily. After a 4 mg oral dose the values for C_{max} (nmol/L) and systemic availability (%) of budesonide without and with cimetidine (3.3 vs 5.1 nmol/L and 10 vs 12%, respectively) indicated a slight inhibitory effect on hepatic metabolism of budesonide, caused by cimetidine. This should be of little clinical importance.

CYP3A4 Inhibitors: The metabolism of budesonide is primarily mediated by CYP3A4, a subfamily of cytochrome P450. CYP3A4 inhibitors like ritonavir and azole antifungals (e.g. ketoconazole and itraconazole) increase the systemic exposure to budesonide. Therefore, concomitant use of budesonide and ritonavir or azole antifungals should be avoided, unless the potential benefit outweighs the risk of systemic corticosteroid side-effects.

ADVERSE EFFECTS: During clinical trials, the most common side effects were cough, throat irritation, and hoarseness (2 to 4%). Bad taste, headache, nausea and dryness of the throat were reported less frequently. Other side effects reported on occasion during budesonide treatment were tiredness, thirst, and diarrhea. In rare cases, anaphylactic reactions have been reported following the use of PULMICORT NEBUAMP. Facial skin irritation has occurred in a few cases when a nebulizer with a face mask has been used. To prevent irritation, the facial skin should be washed after use of the face mask. Skin reactions (urticaria, rash, dermatitis, etc.) may, in rare cases, occur in association with local corticosteroid therapy.

Psychiatric symptoms such as nervousness, restlessness and depression as well as behavioral disturbances in children have been observed.

As with other inhalation therapy, the potential for paradoxical bronchospasm should be kept in mind. If it occurs, the preparation should be discontinued immediately and alternative therapy instituted.

Systemic effects and oropharyngeal complications caused by budesonide were found to be dose-dependent. Candidiasis has been reported by some patients and may occur at therapeutic doses. In rare cases, PULMICORT NEBUAMP may provoke bronchoconstriction in hyperreactive patients.

In patients in whom systemic steroids are reduced or stopped, withdrawal symptoms due to decreased systemic activity occur frequently (see Dosage, Clinical Management).

OVERDOSE:

Symptoms: Occasional overdosing will not give any obvious symptoms in most cases but it will decrease the plasma cortisol level. Other pharmacological effects are an increase in the number and percentage of circulating neutrophils, while the number and percentage of eosinophils will decrease concurrently. Stopping the treatment or decreasing the dose will abolish the induced effects.

Habitual overdosing may cause hypercorticism and hypothalamic-pituitary-adrenal (HPA) suppression. Decreasing the dose or stopping the therapy will abolish these effects, although the restitution of the HPA-axis may be a slow process, and during periods with pronounced physical stress (severe infections, trauma, surgical operations, etc.) it may be advisable to supplement with systemic steroids.

Treatment: See Symptoms.

> For management of a suspected drug overdose, CPhA recommends that you contact your **regional Poison Control Centre**. See the *CPS* Directory section for a list of Poison Control Centres.

DOSAGE: PULMICORT NEBUAMP should be administered from suitable nebulizers. Due to a low output of budesonide, ultrasonic nebulizers should not be used.

The amount of budesonide suspension delivered to the patient in a nebulizer is variable and dependent upon several factors, including the following: nebulization time, volume fill, the characteristics of the nebulizing equipment, the inspiratory/expiratory ratio and tidal volume of the patient, the use of either a face-mask or a mouth piece.

Data from ex vivo studies have estimated that the dose of nebulized budesonide delivered to the patient varies between 9 to 19% of the nominal dose.

The nebulization time and the dose delivered are dependent on flow rate, volume of nebulizer chamber and volume fill.

Nebulization should take place using a gas flow (oxygen or compressed air) of 6 to 10 L/minute and the suspension nebulized over a 10 to 15 minute period. A suitable volume fill for most nebulizers is 2 to 4 mL. The manufacturer's instructions concerning cleaning and maintenance of the nebulizer should be strictly followed.

Initial Dose: The dosage of PULMICORT NEBUAMP is individual. The initial dose should be: Children (3 months to 12 years): 0.25 to 0.5 mg twice daily. In some cases, the dosage may be further increased up to 1 mg twice daily.

Adults: usually 1 to 2 mg twice daily. In some cases, the dosage may be further increased.

Maintenance Dose: The maintenance dose is individual. After the desired clinical effect has been obtained, the maintenance dose should be gradually reduced to the smallest amount necessary for control of symptoms.

See Table 1.

In patients where an increased therapeutic effect is desired, an increased dose of PULMICORT NEBUAMP is recommended because of the lower risk of systemic effects as compared with a combined treatment with oral glucocorticosteroids.

If only half the contents of an ampul are used, add sterile normal saline to make up the required volume fill.

Clinical Management: Patients—Nonsteroid Dependent: Treatment with the recommended doses of PULMICORT NEBUAMP usually gives a therapeutic effect within 10 days. However, certain patients might have an excessive collection of mucous secretion in the bronchi which reduces the penetration of the active substance in PULMICORT NEBUAMP into the bronchial mucosa. In these cases, it is desirable to initially give a short (about 2 weeks) oral corticosteroid regimen in addition to PULMICORT NEBUAMP. The oral treatment is started on a rather large dose which is then gradually reduced. Thereafter, treatment with PULMICORT NEBUAMP only is sufficient. Exacerbations of the asthma caused by bacterial infections are controlled by adequate antibiotic regimens and also by increasing the PULMICORT NEBUAMP dosage.

Table 1: PULMICORT NEBUAMP

Dosage

Dose (mg)	Volume of PULMICORT NEBUAMP 0.125 mg/mL	0.25 mg/mL	0.5 mg/mL
0.125	1 mL[a]	—	—
0.25	2 mL	1 mL[a]	—
0.5	4 mL	2 mL	—
0.75	—	3 mL	—
1	—	—	2 mL
1.5	—	—	3 mL
2	—	—	4 mL

[a] This should be mixed with 0.9% saline to a volume of 2 mL.

Patients—Steroid Dependent: Transferal of patients dependent upon oral steroids to treatment with PULMICORT NEBUAMP demands special care mainly because of the slow restitution of the disturbed hypothalamic-pituitary-adrenal function caused by extended treatment with oral corticosteroids. When PULMICORT NEBUAMP treatment is initiated, the patient should be in a relatively stable phase. PULMICORT NEBUAMP is then given in combination with the previously used oral steroid dose for about 10 days. After this period of time, reduction of the oral corticoid dose may be started gradually. The oral dose is thus reduced to the lowest level which, in combination with PULMICORT NEBUAMP, gives a stable respiratory capacity. In adults, the usual rate of withdrawal of the systemic corticosteroid is the equivalent of 2.5 mg of prednisone every 4 days if the patient is under close observation. **If continuous supervision is not feasible, the withdrawal of the systemic steroid should be slower**, approximately 2.5 mg of prednisone (or equivalent) every 10 days. A slow rate of withdrawal cannot be overemphasized. If withdrawal symptoms appear, the previous dosage of the systemic drug should be resumed for a week before further decrease is attempted. During withdrawal, some patients may experience symptoms of systemically active steroid withdrawal, e.g., joint and/or muscular pain, lassitude and depression, despite maintenance or even improvement of respiratory function. Such patients should be encouraged to continue with PULMICORT NEBUAMP, but should be watched carefully for objective signs of adrenal insufficiency such as hypotension and weight loss. If evidence of adrenal insufficiency occurs, the systemic steroid dosage should be boosted temporarily and thereafter further withdrawal should continue more slowly. In many cases it may be possible to completely replace the oral steroid with PULMICORT NEBUAMP treatment. In other patients, a low oral steroid maintenance dosage may be required. The length of time needed for the body to regain its natural production of corticosteroid in sufficient quantity is often extended. **Thus, during severe asthma attacks or physically stressing situations such as severe infections, trauma and surgical operations, it is necessary to resume systemic steroids (in large dosages) in order to avoid adrenocorticoid insufficiency.** Acute exacerbations, especially in connection with increased viscosity and mucous plugging, may require complementary treatment with a short course of oral corticosteroids which are gradually tapered as symptoms subside.

During transfer from oral therapy to PULMICORT NEBUAMP, a lower general steroid action is experienced. The patients might regain earlier symptoms (rhinitis, eczema) or suffer from tiredness, headache, pain in muscles and joints and, occasionally, nausea and vomiting. In these cases, further medical support may be required.

Note: Patients should be instructed to rinse their mouths out with water after each nebulization treatment. This will help prevent the occurrence of candidiasis and potential systemic effects. Cleansing dentures has the same effect.

INFORMATION FOR THE PATIENT: Published in e-CPS, available by subscription at www.e-cps.ca.

SUPPLIED: Each ampul contains: budesonide 0.125 mg/mL, 0.25 mg/mL and 0.5 mg/mL. Nonmedicinal ingredients: citric acid, disodium edetate, polysorbate 80, sodium chloride, sodium citrate and water, purified. LD-polyethylene ampuls of 2 mL. Sheets of 5 ampuls packed in foil-laminate envelopes. Cartons of 4 envelopes. Store at 5 to 30°C in an upright position. Keep protected from light. Once envelope is opened, use ampuls within 3 months. Opened ampuls must be used within 12 hours.

(Shown in Product Identification Section)

Pulmicort® Turbuhaler® ℞

budesonide

Glucocorticosteroid for the Treatment of Bronchial Asthma

AstraZeneca

Date of Preparation: January 19, 2000
Date of Revision: January 14, 2009

PHARMACOLOGY: Budesonide is a potent synthetic glucocorticosteroid with strong topical and weak systemic effects.

Budesonide has a high topical anti-inflammatory potency and it is rapidly biotransformed in the liver. This favorable separation between topical anti-inflammatory activity and systemic effect is due to strong glucocorticosteroid receptor affinity and an effective first pass metabolism with a short half-life.

The late reaction can be significantly inhibited if budesonide is given at least 2 hours before a bronchial challenge. Pretreatment for 1 to 4 weeks with inhaled budesonide may inhibit the immediate bronchial reaction. After initiation of therapeutic use of orally inhaled budesonide, 1 to 2 weeks may pass before the full effect is obtained.

INDICATIONS: Patients with bronchial asthma: in patients who require inhaled steroids and in patients for whom a reduction of systemic glucocorticoids is desirable.

CONTRAINDICATIONS: Status asthmaticus; not to be used in primary treatment of acute episodes of asthma or in patients with moderate to severe bronchiectasis. Hypersensitivity to budesonide. Active or quiescent pulmonary tuberculosis. Untreated fungal, bacterial or viral infections of the respiratory system.

WARNINGS: Budesonide is not intended for rapid relief of acute episodes of asthma where an inhaled short-acting bronchodilator is required. If patients find short-acting bronchodilator treatment ineffective, or they need more inhalations than usual, medical attention must be sought. In this situation consideration should be given to the need for increased anti-inflammatory therapy, e.g., higher doses of inhaled budesonide or a course of oral corticosteroid.

Particular care is needed in patients who are transferred from systemically active corticosteroids to budesonide and in patients who have required high dose emergency corticosteroid therapy. This is important as deaths due to adrenal insufficiency have occurred in asthmatic patients during and after transfer from systemic corticosteroids to inhaled corticosteroids. Patients receiving proloned treatment at the highest recommended dose of inhaled corticosteroids, may also be at risk for adrenal insufficiency. After withdrawal from systemic corticosteroids, a number of months are required for recovery of hypothalamic-pituitary-adrenal (HPA) function. During this period of HPA suppression, patients may exhibit signs and symptoms of adrenal insufficiency when exposed to severe stress including worsening of asthma attacks, trauma, surgery or infections, particularly gastroenteritis, or other conditions associated with severe electrolyte loss. Additional systemic corticosteroid should be considered during periods of stress or elective surgery.

Although budesonide may provide control of asthmatic symptoms during these episodes, it does **not** provide the systemic steroid which is necessary for coping with these emergencies.

During periods of stress or a severe asthmatic attack, patients who have been withdrawn from systemic corticosteroids should be instructed to resume systemic steroids (in large dosages) immediately and to contact their physicians for further instruction. These patients should also be instructed to carry a warning card indicating that they may need supplementary systemic steroids during periods of stress or a severe asthma attack. To assess the risk of adrenal insufficiency in emergency situations, routine tests of adrenal cortical function, including measurement of early morning and evening cortisol levels, should be performed periodically in all patients. An early morning resting cortisol level may be accepted as normal only if it falls at or near the normal mean level.

Patients previously on high doses of systemic steroids may regain earlier symptoms not related to asthma such as rhinitis and eczema when transferred from oral therapy to inhaled budesonide. These allergies should be symptomatically treated with anti-histamine and/or topical preparations, including topical steroids. These symptoms are a result of the generally lower systemic steroid action which will be experienced. Patients may also suffer from tiredness, headache, pain in muscles and joints and, occasionally, nausea and vomiting.

Temporary resumption of systemic steroids may be necessary to treat these conditions.

The development of pharyngeal and laryngeal candidiasis is cause for concern because the extent of its penetration of the respiratory tract is unknown. If oral pharyngeal candidiasis develops, appropriate antifungal therapy should be implemented to eradicate the infection. The incidence of candidiasis can generally be held to a minimum by having patients rinse their mouths out with water after each inhalation (see Dosage).

Glucocorticosteroids may mask some signs of infection and new infections may appear during their use.

There is no evidence that control of asthma can be achieved by administration of budesonide in doses higher than those recommended. During such periods, patients may require therapy with systemic corticosteroids.

PRECAUTIONS: In transferring patients from a systemic steroid to budesonide, the reduction of the systemic steroid must be very gradual and carefully supervised by the physician since systemic withdrawal symptoms (e.g., joint and/or muscular pain, lassitude, depression), may occur in spite of maintenance or improvement of respiratory functions (see Dosage).

It is essential that the patient be instructed that budesonide is a preventative agent which must be taken at regular intervals and is not to be used to relieve an acute asthmatic attack.

The long-term effects of budesonide on developmental or immunologic processes in the mouth, pharynx, trachea, eyes and lungs are unknown. With the recommended therapeutic doses of budesonide, there is little risk of adverse systemic effects.

In children aged 3 to 13 years (mean 8.7 years), treated for 3 to 13 years (mean 9.2 years), with budesonide via Turbuhaler at a mean daily dose of 412 µg, no effect was demonstrated on long-term statural growth compared to nonsteroidal therapy. During the course of the corticosteroid therapy, a reduction in growth velocities was observed only during the initial 2 years of treatment which may be a result of the severity of asthma or from use of the corticosteroid. Nonetheless, in the long-term, children receiving treatment with inhaled budesonide attained normal adult height. However, it is recommended that height is monitored in children taking corticosteroids by any route.

Treatment with budesonide should not be stopped abruptly, but tapered off gradually.

Pulmonary infiltrates with eosinophilia may occur in patients on budesonide therapy. Although this is possible in some patients who are administered inhalational steroids, their causative role cannot be ruled out.

Pregnancy: In experimental animal studies, budesonide was found to cross the placental barrier. Like other glucocorticosteroids, budesonide is teratogenic to rodent species. High doses of budesonide administered s.c. produced fetal malformations, primarily skeletal defects, in rabbits, rats, and in mice. Results from world-wide post-marketing experience indicate inhaled budesonide during pregnancy has no adverse effects on the health of the fetus/new born child. Review of published literature of orally inhaled budesonide, including results from a large case control study performed with cases identified from 3 Swedish health registers showed that there was no association between exposure to inhaled budesonide and overall congenital malformations. Results from a similar study performed with intranasal budesonide, using the same 3 Swedish health registers showed that the use of intranasal budesonide was associated with a subgroup "less severe cardiovascular defects"; however there was no statistically significant association between the use of intranasal budesonide during pregnancy and overall frequency of cardiovascular defects in the offspring. Budesonide should be used during pregnancy only if the potential benefits clearly outweigh the risk to the fetus. Infants born of mothers who have received substantial doses of corticosteroids, especially oral steroids, during pregnancy should be carefully observed for hypoadrenalism.

Lactation: Budesonide is excreted in breast milk. The administration of Pulmicort Turbuhaler to women who are breast feeding should only be considered if the expected benefit to the mother is greater than any possible risk to the child.

Children Under 6 Years of Age: Budesonide Turbuhaler is not presently recommended for children younger than 6 years of age due to limited clinical data in this age group.

Corticosteroids may mask some signs of infections and new infections may appear. A decreased resistance to localized infection has been observed during corticosteroid therapy. During long-term therapy, pituitary-adrenal function and height (in children) should be periodically assessed.

Patients should be advised to inform subsequent physicians of the prior use of corticosteroids.

There may be enhanced systemic effects of budesonide in patients with an advanced liver cirrhosis, and in those with hypothyroidism. Reduced liver function may affect the elimination of corticosteroids. The i.v. pharmacokinetics of budesonide however, are similar in cirrhotic patients and in healthy subjects. The pharmacokinetics after oral ingestion of budesonide were affected by compromised liver function as evidenced by increased systemic availability. This is however, of limited importance for budesonide, as after inhalation the oral contribution to the systemic availability is very small.

ASA should be used cautiously in conjunction with corticosteroids in hypoprothrombinemia.

Special care is needed in patients with lung tuberculosis and fungal and viral infections. Children who are on immunosuppressant drugs are more susceptible to infections than healthy children. Chickenpox and measles, for example, can have a more serious or fatal course in children on immunosuppressant corticosteroids. In such children, or in adults who have not had these diseases, particular care should be taken to avoid exposure. If exposed, therapy with varicella zoster immune globulin (VZIG) or pooled i.v. immunoglobulin (IVIG), as appropriate, may be indicated. If chickenpox develops treatment with antiviral agents may be considered.

If, however, a viral upper respiratory infection is present, the patient should adhere to the regular asthma medication. In patients who are known to deteriorate rapidly when they have a viral respiratory infection, a short course of oral corticosteroid therapy should be considered.

Clinical studies have shown that viral upper respiratory infections cause significantly fewer problems in patients who are on regular treatment with topical glucocorticosteroids.

To ensure the proper dosage and administration of the drug, the patient should be instructed by a physician or other health professional in the use of Pulmicort Turbuhaler.

Adequate oral hygiene is of primary importance in minimizing overgrowth of microorganisms such as *C. albicans* (see Dosage).

Drug Interactions: Budesonide has not been observed to interact with any drug used for the treatment of asthma.

Cimetidine: The kinetics of budesonide were investigated in a study of healthy subjects without and with cimetidine, 1000 mg daily. After a 4 mg oral dose the values for C_{max} (nmol/L) and systemic availability (%) of budesonide without and with cimetidine (3.3 vs 5.1 nmol/L and 10 vs 12%, respectively) indicated a slight inhibitory effect on hepatic metabolism of budesonide, caused by cimetidine. This should be of little clinical importance.

CYP3A4 Inhibitors: The metabolism of budesonide is primarily mediated by CYP3A4, a subfamily of cytochrome P450. CYP3A4 inhibitors like ritonavir and azole antifungals (e.g. ketoconazole and itraconazole) increase the systemic exposure to budesonide. Therefore, concomitant use of budesonide and ritonavir or azole antifungals should be avoided, unless the potential benefit outweighs the risk of systemic corticosteroid side-effects.

Omeprazole: At recommended doses, omeprazole has no effect on the pharmacokinetics of oral budesonide.

ADVERSE EFFECTS: No major side effects attributable to the use of budesonide, in all dosage forms, have been reported. During clinical trials, the frequency of subjectively reported side effects was low.

Clinical trials, literature reports and postmarketing experience suggest that the following adverse drug reactions may occur:

The most common side effects were cough, throat irritation, and hoarseness (2 to 4%).

Bad taste, headache, nausea and dryness of the throat were reported less frequently. Other side effects reported on occasion during budesonide treatment were tiredness, thirst, and diarrhea. Rare cases of anaphylactic reaction have been reported following the use of PULMICORT TURBUHALER. Skin reactions (urticaria, rash, dermatitis, angioedema, etc.) may, in rare cases, occur in association with local corticosteroid therapy. In rare cases, skin bruising has been reported following treatment with inhaled glucocorticosteroids.

Psychiatric symptoms such as nervousness, restlessness and depression, as well as behavioral disturbances in children, have been observed.

As with other inhalation therapy, the potential for paradoxical bronchospasm should be kept in mind. If it occurs, the preparation should be discontinued immediately and alternative therapy instituted.

In rare cases, signs or symptoms of systemic glucocorticosteroid effect including hypofunction of the adrenal gland and oropharyngeal complications may occur, depending on dose, exposure time, concomitant and previous steroid exposure, and individual sensitivity. Candidiasis has been reported by some patients and may occur at therapeutic doses.

In patients in whom systemic steroids are reduced or stopped, withdrawal symptoms due to decreased systemic activity occur frequently (see Dosage, Clinical Management).

OVERDOSE:

Symptoms: Occasional overdosing will not give any obvious symptoms in most cases but it will decrease the plasma cortisol level. Other pharmacological effects are an increase in the number and percentage of circulating neutrophils, while the number and percentage of eosinophils will decrease concurrently. Stopping the treatment or decreasing the dose will abolish the induced effects.

Habitual overdosing may cause hypercorticism and hypothalamic-pituitary-adrenal suppression. Decreasing the dose or stopping the therapy will abolish these effects, although the restitution of the HPA-axis may be a slow process and during periods with pronounced physical stress (severe infections, trauma, surgical operations, etc.) it may be advisable to supplement with systemic steroids.

Treatment: See Symptoms.

For management of a suspected drug overdose, CPhA recommends that you contact your **regional Poison Control Centre**. See the *CPS* Directory section for a list of Poison Control Centres.

DOSAGE: Adults and Children Over 12 Years of Age: When treatment with inhaled glucocorticosteroids is started, during periods of severe asthma, and while reducing or discontinuing oral glucocorticosteroids the dosage should be 400 to 2400 µg daily divided into 2 to 4 administrations.

The maintenance dose is usually 200 to 400 µg of budesonide twice daily but higher doses may be necessary for longer or shorter periods of time in some patients. The dose of budesonide should be individualized to the patient's need and should be the lowest possible dose that fills the therapeutic objective.

Once daily dosing may be considered in patients who require a dosage of 400 µg budesonide per day. The dose may then be given in the morning or in the evening. If deterioration of asthma occurs, the frequency of dosing and the daily dose should be increased.

Treatment with budesonide should not be stopped abruptly, but tapered off gradually.

Children 6 to 12 years: When starting therapy with budesonide in children, during periods of severe asthma and while reducing or discontinuing oral corticosteroids, the dosage should be 200 to 400 µg daily, given in divided doses twice daily at 100 to 200 µg per inhalation.

The maintenance dose is individual and should be the lowest dose which keeps the patient symptom-free. Administration twice daily is usually adequate in stable asthmatics.

Children Under 6 Years of Age: Budesonide via Turbuhaler is not recommended for children in this age group.

Clinical studies in man have shown an improved efficacy for the same amount of budesonide delivered via Turbuhaler inhaler as compared with the pressurized aerosol with Nebuhaler spacer device. It may be possible to reduce the dose of Pulmicort Turbuhaler when the patient is in a stable phase.

In patients where an increased therapeutic effect is desired, an increased dose of budesonide Turbuhaler is recommended because of the lower risk of systemic effects as compared with a combined treatment with oral glucocorticosteroids.

Since the effect of budesonide depends on its regular use and on the proper technique of inhalation, patients must be instructed to use their Pulmicort Turbuhaler daily, as prescribed by their physician and not as they feel necessary. They must also be instructed in the correct method which is described in Information for the Patient.

Turbuhaler: Turbuhaler is a breath-activated dry powder inhaler which does not require a coordinated inhalation technique. It contains only the active ingredient budesonide—no propellants or preservatives, and as such, offers those patients sensitive to excipients, an alternate dosage form. Note: The patient may not taste or feel any medication when inhaling from budesonide Turbuhaler. This lack of feeling does not mean that the patient is not receiving benefit from Pulmicort Turbuhaler.

Clinical Management: Patients—Nonsteroid Dependent: Treatment with the recommended doses of budesonide usually gives a therapeutic effect within 10 days. However, certain patients might have an excessive collection of mucous secretion in the bronchi which reduces the penetration of budesonide into the bronchial mucosa. In these cases, it is desirable to initially give a short (about 2 weeks) oral corticosteroid regimen in addition to budesonide. The oral treatment is started on a rather large dose which is then gradually reduced. Thereafter, treatment with budesonide only is sufficient. Exacerbations of the asthma caused by bacterial infections are controlled by adequate antibiotic regimens and also by increasing the budesonide dosage.

Patients—Steroid Dependent: Transferal of patients dependent upon oral steroids to treatment with budesonide demands special care mainly because of the slow restitution of the disturbed hypothalamic-pituitary-adrenal function caused by extended treatment with oral corticosteroids. When treatment is initiated, the patient should be in a relatively stable phase. Budesonide is then given in combination with the previously used oral steroid dose for about 10 days. After this period of time, reduction of the oral corticoid dose may be started gradually. The oral dose is thus reduced to the lowest level which, in combination with budesonide, gives a stable respiratory capacity.

In adults, the usual rate of withdrawal of the systemic corticosteroid is the equivalent of 2.5 mg of prednisone every 4 days if the patient is under close observation. **If continuous supervision is not feasible, the withdrawal of the systemic steroid should be slower**, approximately 2.5 mg of prednisone (or equivalent) every 10 days. A slow rate of withdrawal cannot be overemphasized. If withdrawal symptoms appear, the previous dosage of the systemic drug should be resumed for a week before further decrease is attempted. During withdrawal, some patients may experience symptoms of systemically active steroid withdrawal, e.g., joint and/or muscular pain, lassitude, and depression, despite maintenance or even improvement of respiratory function. Such patients should be encouraged to continue with budesonide, but should be watched carefully for objective signs of adrenal insufficiency such as hypotension and weight loss. If evidence of adrenal insufficiency occurs, the systemic steroid dosage should be boosted temporarily and thereafter further withdrawal should continue more slowly.

In many cases it may be possible to completely replace the oral steroid with budesonide treatment. In other patients, a low oral steroid maintenance dosage may be required. The length of time needed for the body to regain its natural production of corticosteroid in sufficient quantity is often extended. **Thus, during severe asthma attacks or physically stressing situations such as severe infections, trauma, and surgical operations, it is necessary to resume systemic steroids (in large dosages) in order to avoid adrenocorticoid insufficiency.** Acute exacerbations, especially in connection with increased viscosity and mucous plugging, may require complementary treatment with a short course of oral corticosteroids which are gradually tapered as symptoms subside.

During transfer from oral therapy to budesonide, a lower general steroid action is experienced. The patients might regain earlier symptoms (rhinitis, eczema) or suffer from tiredness, headache, pain in muscles and joints and, occasionally, nausea and vomiting. In these cases, further medical support may be required.

Note: The medication from budesonide Turbuhaler is delivered to the lungs as the patient inhales and, therefore, it is important to instruct the patient to breathe in forcefully and deeply through the mouthpiece. When prescribing Turbuhaler to young children it is necessary to ascertain that they can follow the instructions for use. The patient may not taste or feel any medication when using budesonide Turbuhaler due to the small amount of drug dispensed.

Patients should be instructed to rinse their mouths out with water after each inhalation. This will help prevent the occurrence of candidiasis. Cleansing dentures has the same effect.

INFORMATION FOR THE PATIENT: Published in e-CPS, available by subscription at www.e-cps.ca.

SUPPLIED: Each dry powder inhaler contains: 200 doses of 100, 200 and 400 µg of micronized budesonide. Each inhalation from Pulmicort Turbuhaler will provide either 100, 200 or 400 µg of budesonide active substance; no additives or carrier substances are included. Pulmicort Turbuhaler cannot be refilled and should be discarded when empty. Store with the cover tightened, at room temperature (15 to 30°C), in a dry place, away from moisture.

(Shown in Product Identification Section)

Pulmozyme®

dornase alfa recombinant

Enzyme that Cleaves DNA

Roche

Date of Preparation: December 24, 1993
Date of Revision: August 15, 2006

SUMMARY PRODUCT INFORMATION:

Route of Administration	Dosage Form/Strength	Clinically Relevant Nonmedicinal Ingredients
Inhalation (using a nebulizer)	Solution/1 mg/mL	None For a complete listing see Dosage Forms, Composition and Packaging.

INDICATIONS AND CLINICAL USE: Daily administration of PULMOZYME (dornase alfa) for inhalation in conjunction with standard therapies is indicated in the management of cystic fibrosis patients to reduce the frequency of respiratory infections requiring parenteral antibiotics and to improve pulmonary function. Safety and efficacy of daily administration have not been demonstrated in patients with FVC<40% of predicted, or for longer than twelve months.

CONTRAINDICATIONS: PULMOZYME (dornase alfa) is contraindicated in patients with known hypersensitivity to dornase alfa, Chinese Hamster Ovary cell products or any component of the product. For a complete listing, see Dosage Forms, Composition and Packaging.

WARNINGS AND PRECAUTIONS: General: PULMOZYME (dornase alfa) should be used in conjunction with standard therapies for CF.

Patients should be instructed in the proper use and maintenance of the nebulizer and compressor system used in its delivery.

Carcinogenesis and Mutagenesis: There is no evidence of oncogenic or mutagenic potential.

Sexual Function/Reproduction: Fertility and reproductive performance were not affected in animal studies.

Special Populations: Pregnant Women: The safety of PULMOZYME has not been established in pregnant women. Animal studies do not indicate direct or indirect harmful effects with respect to pregnancy, or embryofoetal development. Caution should be exercised when prescribing PULMOZYME to pregnant women.

Nursing Women: As it is not known whether dornase alfa is excreted in human milk, caution should be exercised when PULMOZYME is administered to a nursing woman.

Pediatrics (< 5 years of age): There is limited experience in the use of PULMOZYME in patients under the age of 5 years. The clinical efficacy in patients under the age of 5 years is not established.

ADVERSE REACTIONS: Adverse Drug Reaction Overview: The adverse event data reflect the clinical trial and post-marketing experience of using PULMOZYME (dornase alfa) at the recommended dose regimen.

Adverse reactions attributed to PULMOZYME are rare (<1/1000). In most cases, the adverse reactions are mild and transient in nature and do not require alterations in the dosing of PULMOZYME.

Body as a Whole: chest pain (pleuritic/non-cardiac), fever.

Gastrointestinal System: dyspepsia.

Respiratory System: voice alteration (hoarseness), pharyngitis (inflammation of the throat), dyspnea, laryngitis, rhinitis, decreased lung function.

Skin and Appendages: rash, urticaria.

Special Senses: conjunctivitis.

Patients who experience adverse events common to cystic fibrosis can, in general, safely continue administration of PULMOZYME as evidenced by the high percentage of patients completing clinical trials with PULMOZYME.

Upon initiation of therapy with PULMOZYME, as with any aerosol, pulmonary function may decline and expectoration of sputum may increase.

Clinical Trial Adverse Drug Reactions: Because clinical trials are conducted under very specific conditions the adverse reaction rates observed in the clinical trials may not reflect the rates observed in practice and should not be compared to the rates in the clinical trials of another drug. Adverse drug reaction information from clinical trials is useful for identifying drug-related adverse events and for approximating rates.

In clinical trials, few patients experienced adverse events resulting in permanent discontinuation from PULMOZYME, and the discontinuation rate was observed to be similar between placebo (2%) and PULMOZYME (3%).

Mortality rates observed in a controlled trial were similar for the placebo (1%) and PULMOZYME (1%). Causes of death were consistent with progression of cystic fibrosis and included apnea, cardiac arrest, cardiopulmonary arrest, cor pulmonale, heart failure, massive hemoptysis, pneumonia, pneumothorax, and respiratory failure.

The safety of PULMOZYME, 2.5 mg by inhalation, was studied with 2 weeks of daily administration in 98 patients with cystic fibrosis (65 aged 3 months to <5 years, 33 aged 5 to ≤10 years) all of whom received bronchoalveolar lavage on the first day of therapy (Z0644g). The number of patients reporting cough was higher in the younger age group as compared to the older age group (29/65, 45% compared to 10/33, 30%) as was the number reporting moderate to severe cough (24/65, 37% as compared to 6/33, 18%). Other events tended to be of mild to moderate severity. The number of patients reporting rhinitis was higher in the younger age group as compared to the older age group (23/65, 35% compared to 9/33, 27%) as was the number reporting rash (4/65, 6% as compared to 0/33). Adverse events were common in this study and some were considered to be due to bronchoalveolar lavage. The nature of adverse drug reactions was similar to that seen in the larger trials of PULMOZYME.

In this phase II uncontrolled study (Z0644g), 98 patients aged 3 months to 9 years were treated with PULMOZYME by inhalation daily at a dose of 2.5 mg (the recommended dose). Data presented in Table 1 are based on adverse drug reactions reported in Study Z0644g.

Table 1: PULMOZYME

Adverse Drug Reactions Occurring in ≥1% of Patients and Occurring in >1 Patient in Study Z0644g

Adverse Event System Organ Class (MedDRA)	Number	Percentage (n=98)
Infections And Infestations		
Rhinitis	12	12.2
Pharyngitis	7	7.1
Psychiatric Disorders		
Nervousness	4	4.1
Nervous System Disorders		
Headache	4	4.1
Hyperkinesias	2	2.0
Eye Disorders		
Conjunctivitis	2	2.0
Respiratory, Thoracic And Mediastinal Disorders		
Cough increased	35	35.7
Lung disorder	3	3.1
Hyperventilation	2	2.0
Voice alteration	14	14.3
Gastrointestinal Disorders		

(cont'd)

Table 1: PULMOZYME *(cont'd)*

Adverse Drug Reactions Occurring in ≥1% of Patients and Occurring in >1 Patient in Study Z0644g

Adverse Event System Organ Class (MedDRA)	Number	Percentage (n=98)
Abdominal pain	2	2.0
Nausea	2	2.0
Vomiting	7	7.1
Skin And Subcutaneous Tissue Disorders		
Rash	2	2.0
General Disorders And Administration Site Conditions		
Pyrexia	7	7.1
Unevaluable reaction	5	5.1
Investigations		
Sputum increased	6	6.1

Allergic Reactions: There have been no reports of anaphylaxis attributed to the administration of PULMOZYME to date. Skin rash and urticaria have been observed, and were mild and transient in nature. Less than 5% of patients treated with PULMOZYME have developed antibodies to the drug and none of these patients have developed IgE antibodies to PULMOZYME. Improvement in pulmonary function tests has still occurred even after the development of antibodies to PULMOZYME.

DRUG INTERACTIONS: Clinical trials have indicated that PULMOZYME can be effectively and safely used in conjunction with standard cystic fibrosis therapies including oral, inhaled and parenteral antibiotics, bronchodilators, enzyme supplements, vitamins, oral and inhaled corticosteroids, and analgesics. No formal drug interaction studies have been performed.

DOSAGE AND ADMINISTRATION: Recommended Dose and Dosage Adjustment: The recommended dose for use in most cystic fibrosis patients is one 2.5 mg single use ampoule inhaled once daily using a recommended nebulizer. Some patients may benefit from twice daily administration.

Missed Dose: The missed dose should be taken as soon as remembered, then the regular dosing schedule should be continued. Two doses of PULMOZYME should not be taken at the same time.

Administration: PULMOZYME should not be diluted or mixed with other drugs in the nebulizer. Mixing of PULMOZYME with other drugs could lead to adverse physicochemical and/or functional changes in PULMOZYME or the admixed compound.

Patients should be advised to squeeze each ampoule prior to use in order to check for leaks.

Clinical trials have been performed with the following nebulizers and compressors: the disposable jet nebulizer Hudson T Up draft II and disposable jet nebulizer Marquest Acorn II in conjunction with a Pulmo Aide compressor, and with the reusable PARI LC Jet + nebulizer, in conjunction with the PARI PRONEB compressor. Patients who are unable to inhale or exhale orally throughout the entire nebulization period may use the reusable PARI BABY nebulizer with a tight fitting face mask. It is recommended that patients <5 years of age use the PARI BABY nebulizer. Safety and efficacy have been demonstrated only with these recommended nebulizer systems.

No clinical data are currently available that support the safety and efficacy of administration of PULMOZYME (dornase alfa) with other nebulizer systems. The patient should follow the manufacturer's instructions on the use and maintenance of the equipment.

OVERDOSAGE:

Single dose inhalation studies in rats and monkeys at doses up to 180 times higher than doses routinely used in clinical studies are well tolerated. Single dose oral administration of PULMOZYME (dornase alfa) in doses up to 200 mg/kg are also well tolerated by rats.

Cystic fibrosis patients have received up to 20 mg BID for up to 6 days and 10 mg BID intermittently (2 weeks on/2 weeks off drug) for 168 days. These doses were well tolerated.

No data are available specifically for patients <5 years of age.

> For management of a suspected drug overdose, CPhA recommends that you contact your **regional Poison Control Centre**. See the *CPS* Directory section for a list of Poison Control Centres.

ACTION AND CLINICAL PHARMACOLOGY: Mechanism of Action: PULMOZYME (dornase alfa) for inhalation is a sterile, clear, colourless, highly purified solution of recombinant human deoxyribonuclease I (rhDNase), an enzyme which selectively cleaves DNA. The protein is produced by genetically engineered Chinese Hamster Ovary (CHO) cells containing DNA encoding for the native human protein, deoxyribonuclease I (DNase). The product is purified by tangential flow filtration and column chromatography.

PULMOZYME is administered by inhalation of an aerosol mist produced by a compressed air driven nebulizer system (see Dosage and Administration). Each single use ampoule will deliver 2.5 mL of the solution to the nebulizer bowl.

In cystic fibrosis (CF) patients, retention of viscous purulent secretions in the airways contributes both to reduced pulmonary function and to exacerbations of infection.

Purulent pulmonary secretions contain very high concentrations of extracellular DNA released by degenerating leukocytes that accumulate in response to infection. In vitro, PULMOZYME hydrolyzes the DNA in sputum of CF patients and reduces sputum viscoelasticity.

Pharmacokinetics: When 2.5 mg dornase alfa was administered by inhalation to eighteen CF patients, mean sputum concentrations of 3 µg/mL DNase were measurable within 15 minutes. Mean sputum concentrations declined to an average of 0.6 µg/mL two hours following inhalation. Inhalation of up to 10 mg TID of PULMOZYME by 4 CF patients for six consecutive days, did not result in a significant elevation of serum concentrations of DNase above normal endogenous levels. After administration of up to 2.5 mg of PULMOZYME twice daily for six months to 321 CF patients, no accumulation of serum DNase was noted.

STORAGE AND STABILITY: PULMOZYME must be stored in the refrigerator at 2-8°C and protected from light. It should be kept refrigerated during transport and should not be exposed to room temperatures for a total time of 24 hours. The solution should be discarded if it is cloudy or discoloured. PULMOZYME contains no preservative and, once opened, the entire ampoule must be used or discarded.

INFORMATION FOR THE PATIENT: Published in e-CPS, available by subscription at www.e-cps.ca.

DOSAGE FORMS, COMPOSITION AND PACKAGING: Each ampoule of sterile, clear, colorless, aqueous solution contains: dornase alfa 1 mg/mL (2.5 mg), formulated in calcium chloride dihydrate, sodium chloride, and Sterile Water for Injection. Nominal pH is 6.3. Preservative-free. Sterile, single-use ampoules of 2.5 mL. Cartons of 30 (5 foil pouches of 6 ampoules).

Puregon® Ⓟ

follitropin beta

Human Gonadotropin

Schering-Plough

Date of Preparation: February 13, 2006
Date of Revision: February 4, 2009

SUMMARY PRODUCT INFORMATION:

Route of Administration	Dosage Form/ Strength	Clinically Relevant Nonmedicinal Ingredients
Subcutaneous injection	Solution in cartridges: 300 IU/0.36 mL, 600 IU/0.72 mL and 900 IU/1.08 mL at a concentration of 833 IU recFSH /mL	Not applicable For a complete listing see Dosage Forms, Composition and Packaging.
Subcutaneous or Intramuscular injection	Solution in vials: 50 and 100 IU FSH activity/vial.	Not applicable For a complete listing see Dosage Forms, Composition and Packaging.

INDICATIONS AND CLINICAL USE: In the Female: PUREGON (follitropin beta) is indicated for:

- development of multiple follicles in ovulatory patients participating in an Assisted Reproduction Technology (ART) program
- induction of ovulation and pregnancy in anovulatory infertile females in whom the cause of infertility is functional and not due to primary ovarian failure

In the Male: PUREGON (follitropin beta) is indicated for:

- deficient spermatogenesis due to hypogonadotrophic hypogonadism

CONTRAINDICATIONS: Patients who are hypersensitive to this drug or to any ingredient in the formulation or component of the container. For a complete listing, see Dosage Forms, Composition and Packaging.

PUREGON (follitropin beta) is contraindicated in women who exhibit:

- a high circulating FSH level indicating primary ovarian failure.
- uncontrolled thyroid or adrenal dysfunction.
- tumour of the ovary, breast, uterus, hypothalamus or pituitary gland.
- pregnancy and lactation.
- heavy or irregular vaginal bleeding of undetermined origin.
- ovarian cysts or enlargement not due to polycystic ovary syndrome (PCOD).
- conditions incompatible with pregnancy (e.g. malformation of sexual organs or fibroid tumours of the uterus).

PUREGON (follitropin beta) is contraindicated in men who exhibit:

- primary testicular failure.

PUREGON (follitropin beta) is contraindicated in children.

WARNINGS AND PRECAUTIONS: General: PUREGON (follitropin beta) is a potent gonadotropic agent that is capable of causing severe adverse effects in women. It should be used only by physicians who are experienced in the management of fertility disorders and only when facilities for appropriate clinical and endocrinologic evaluations are available.

A thorough gynecologic and endocrinologic evaluation must be performed prior to treatment with PUREGON (follitropin beta). The evaluation may include hysterosalpinography to detect uterine and tubal pathology. Anovulation should be confirmed by menstrual history, observation of the basal body temperature pattern, determination of serum progesterone concentration in the luteal phase, or an endometrial biopsy. Tumours of the thyroid, adrenals, pituitary, and ovary may cause anovulation and patients with such tumours should be excluded from follitropin beta therapy.

Determination of serum gonadotropin concentrations should be obtained to rule out primary ovarian failure.

The presence of early pregnancy should be ruled out by a biochemical pregnancy test. Evaluation of the fertility potential of the male sexual partner should also be performed (a semen analysis) before starting PUREGON therapy.

Overstimulation of the Ovary During Therapy: To minimize the risk associated with abnormal ovarian enlargement in women receiving PUREGON and hCG for the induction of ovulation and pregnancy, the drugs should be administered at the lowest possible effective dosage. Since PUREGON may cause ovarian enlargement and/or hyperstimulation, patients should be assessed for signs of excessive ovarian stimulation during therapy and for a 2-week post-treatment period. Careful monitoring of ovarian response (i.e. ultrasonography and/or estradiol level determination) can minimize the risk of overstimulation.

Mild to moderate uncomplicated ovarian enlargement, which may be accompanied by abdominal distension and/or abdominal pain, occurs in approximately 20% of patients treated with gonadotropins and hCG, and generally regresses without treatment within 2 to 3 weeks. If unwanted hyperstimulation occurs, the administration of PUREGON should be discontinued immediately. In this case, hCG must not be given, because the administration of an LH active gonadotropin at this stage may induce ovarian hyperstimulation syndrome, in addition to multiple ovulations. This warning is particularly important with respect to patients with anovulation or oligoovulation (polycystic ovarian disease and hypothalamic hypogonadism).

Clinical symptoms of mild ovarian hyperstimulation syndrome are gastrointestinal problems (abdominal distention, nausea, diarrhea), painful breasts, and mild to moderate enlargement of ovaries because of ovarian cysts.

Severe ovarian hyperstimulation syndrome (OHSS) is characterized by ovarian enlargement (large cysts prone to rupture) accompanied by hemoconcentration, decreased urinary output, ascites with or without pain and/or pleural effusion.

If severe OHSS occurs, treatment should be stopped and the patient hospitalized. Ovarian hyperstimulation syndrome develops rapidly within 3 to 4 days and generally during the 2-week period following the hCG injection.

Hemoconcentration associated with fluid loss into the abdominal cavity has been observed to occur and should be thoroughly assessed as follows: 1) fluid intake and output; 2) weight and abdominal girth; 3) hematocrit; 4) serum and urinary electrolytes; and 5) urine specific gravity. Other monitoring should include serum albumin and total proteins. These determinations should be performed daily or more often if needed. Treatment consists of primarily bed rest, fluid, electrolyte and albumin replacement, and analgesics as needed. Generally, removal of ascitic fluid (paracentesis) should be reserved for the more severe cases of third space fluid shift or abdominal discomfort.

Hemoperitoneum may occur from ruptured ovarian cysts. This is usually the result of sexual intercourse or a vigorous pelvic examination. Should this occur and be accompanied by bleeding to the extent that surgery is necessary, partial resection of the enlarged ovary or ovaries may be required. Intercourse should be prohibited in those patients in whom significant ovarian enlargement occurs after ovulation due to the risk of hemoperitoneum resulting from ruptured ovarian cysts.

Liver Function Test Abnormalities: Transient liver function test abnormalities suggestive of hepatic dysfunction, which may be accompanied by morphologic changes on liver biopsy, have been reported in association with ovarian hyperstimulation syndrome.

PUREGON may contain traces of streptomycin and/or neomycin. These antibiotics may cause hypersensitivity reactions in susceptible persons.

No effects on ability to drive and use machines have been observed.

Carcinogenesis and Mutagenesis: PUREGON displays no mutagenic potential. Carcinogenicity studies have not been performed.

Cardiovascular: Thromboembolism: Thromboembolism has been reported in patients who have received gonadotropin and hCG, both in association with and separate from ovarian hyperstimulation syndrome. Complications resulting from thromboembolism have included venous thrombophlebitis, pulmonary embolism, pulmonary infarction, stroke, arterial occlusion necessitating limb amputation, and (rarely) death.

Women with generally recognized risk factors for thrombosis, such as a personal or family history, severe obesity (Body Mass Index >30 kg/m^2) or thrombophilia, may have an increased risk of venous or arterial thromboembolic processes upon treatment with gonadotropins. In these women the benefits of IVF treatment need to be weighed against the risks. It should be noted, however, that pregnancy itself also carries an increased risk of thrombosis.

Sexual Function/Reproduction: Other Reproductive Complications: Multiple ovulations with resulting multiple births occur (mostly twins) frequently (~20% of pregnancies) following treatment with gonadotropins and hCG. Prior to gonadotropin and hCG therapy, the patient and her male sexual partner should be informed of the possibility and potential risks associated with multiple births.

Spontaneous abortion rates have been reported from 10 to 25% of all patients following gonadotropin treatment. Increased abortion rates are more common in women over 35 years of age, in women with polycystic ovarian disease, and are more common in the infertile couple. The increased frequency of multiple pregnancy is also associated with an increased rate of abortion.

Since infertile women undergoing assisted reproduction, and particularly IVF, often have tubal abnormalities the incidence of ectopic pregnancies might be increased. Early ultrasound confirmation that a pregnancy is intrauterine is therefore important.

In the Male: Semen analysis is recommended 4 to 6 months after the beginning of treatment to assess the response.

Special Populations: Pregnant Women: PUREGON is not intended for use during pregnancy.

Nursing Women: PUREGON is not intended for use during lactation.

Pediatrics: There is no relevant indication for use of PUREGON in children.

ADVERSE REACTIONS: Adverse Drug Reaction Overview: Clinical Trial Adverse Drug Reactions: The following adverse events, listed by body system, have been reported in clinical studies evaluating the efficacy and safety of PUREGON (follitropin beta) in women: See Table 1 and Table 2.

Table 1: PUREGON

% Incidence of Most Frequently (≥1%) Reported Adverse Events (AEs) in Clinical Trials

	PUREGON (n=1074)	Urinary Gonadotropin (n=498)
Body System	%	
Patients with at least one AE	17.3	19.7
Patients with known severe AE	5.0	6.2
Patients with drug-related AEs[a]	8.7	8.2
Reproductive System	**8.8**	**9.4**
Ovarian hyperstimulation syndrome	5.0	4.0
Ectopic pregnancy	2.1	3.4
Vaginal hemorrhage	1.0	1.0
Gastrointestinal System	**3.6**	**4.2**
Abdominal pain	2.0	2.4
Fetal Disorders	**3.1**	**4.2**
Miscarriage	3.1	4.2
Body as a Whole	**1.2**	**1.0**
Application Site Disorders	**1**	**0.6**
Injection site pain	1	0.6
Hearing/Vestibular Disorders	**0**	**0.2**

[a] **Related:** Definitely, probably, or possibly related to the study drug.

Table 2: PUREGON

% Incidence of Most Frequently (<1%) Reported Adverse Events (AEs) in Clinical Trials

	PUREGON (n=1074)	Urinary Gonadotropin (n=498)
Body System	%	
Reproductive System		
Vaginitis	0.4	0.2
Gastrointestinal System		
Abdominal pain-upper/lower	0.7	0.6
Nausea	0.5	0.8
Abdominal discomfort	0.4	0.2
Urinary System	**0.8**	**0.4**
Urinary tract infection	0.5	0.2
Neoplasms	**0.8**	**0.8**
Ovarian cyst	0.7	0.8
Central and Peripheral Nervous Systems	**0.7**	**0.6**
Headache	0.7	0.4
Resistance Mechanism Disorders	**0.5**	**0.2**
Skin and Appendages	**0.4**	**0.6**
Autonomous Nervous System (hyperemesis, loose stools, vasovagal syncope)	**0.4**	**0**
Respiratory System (dyspnea, rhinitis, sore throat, upper respiratory tract infection)	**0.4**	**0.6**
Platelet/Bleeding, Clotting Disorders	**0.2**	**0**
Psychiatric Disorders (Nervousness)	**0.1**	**0**
Vision/Eye Abnormalities	**0.1**	**0.2**
Hearing/Vestibular Disorders	**0**	**0.2**

Less Common Clinical Trial Adverse Drug Reactions (<1%): Reproductive Disorder Women: premature labour, menorrhagia, ovarian disorder, vaginal discharge, vulvovaginitis, genital infection, genital herpes.
Skin and Appendages: eczema, itching, rash, hematoma, abscess, Herpes zoster.
Respiratory System: dyspnea, otitis media.
Gastrointestinal: bloating, constipation, gastroesophageal reflux, vomiting, increased bilirubin, swollen abdomen.
Urinary System: dysuria, cystitis, frequent micturition.
Body as a Whole, General Disorders: back pain, feeling unwell, influenza-like symptoms, face edema, lumbar pain, pain, sepsis, tooth disorder, hydatidiform mole.
Autonomous Nervous System: hypermesis, hot flashes, syncope.
Abnormal Hematologic and Clinical Chemistry Findings: Post-treatment sera were analysed following three treatment cycles and no evidence of induction of anti-FSH or anti-CHO cell-derived protein antibodies were found.
In Males: The safety of PUREGON was examined in a clinical trial that enrolled 49 male patients for the indication of spermatogenesis, of whom 30 received PUREGON. Two subjects in the treatment period each reported one serious event, which were judged not related to study drug by the investigator. The events involved a pilonidal cyst and hemorrhoids. Both subjects recovered from these adverse events. In the PUREGON treatment phase, no patients discontinued due to an adverse event.

In total, 21 patients in the treatment phase experienced at least one adverse event. Nine were reported by the investigator to be possibly related to study drug. These include: two cases of acne, two cases of injection site reaction, two cases of injection site pain, and single case of varicose veins, gynecomastia, and a dermoid cyst.

Post-Market Adverse Drug Reactions: Clinical use of PUREGON by the intramuscular or subcutaneous routes may lead to local reactions at the site of injection: bruising, pain, redness, swelling and itching, are commonly reported (3% of all patients treated). The majority of these local reactions are mild and transient in nature. Generalised hypersensitivity reactions including erythema, urticaria, rash and pruritus have been observed uncommonly (approximately 0.1% of all patients treated with PUREGON).

Treatment of Women: In approximately 4% of the women treated with PUREGON in clinical trials, signs and symptoms related to ovarian hyperstimulation syndrome (OHSS) have been reported. Other undesirable effects related to this syndrome were observed in clinical studies. These include pelvic pain and/or congestion, abdominal pain and/or distension, breast complaints (breast tenderness, pain and/or engorgement), ovarian enlargement, and spontaneous abortion. They were all reported at an incidence of approximately 1% (pelvic pain and abdominal distension) or less.

A slightly increased risk of ectopic pregnancy and multiple gestations has been seen.

Other more general symptoms that have been reported include headache and nausea (in up to 1.0% of the women treated with PUREGON).

In rare instances, thromboembolism has been associated with PUREGON/hCG treatment as with other gonadotrophins.

Number (%) of Female Subjects with at Least One AE per MedDRA Body System and Preferred Term. Trials: All female studies (Europe, US and Japan): See Table 3.

Table 3: PUREGON

Reported Adverse Drug Reactions in Clinical Trials with Incidence of >1%

MedDRA System Organ Class MedDRA Preferred Term	Treatment Group PUREGON N=3535 All n (%)	Drug Related n (%)
Gastrointestinal Disorders		
Abdominal distension	42 (1.2)	38 (1.1)
Abdominal pain	43 (1.2)	19 (0.5)
Nausea	44 (1.2)	19 (0.5)
General Disorders and Administration Site Conditions		
Injection site pain	71 (2.0)	68 (1.9)
Nervous System Disorders		
Headache	96 (2.7)	37 (1.0)
Pregnancy, Puerperium and Perinatal Conditions		
Abortion spontaneous	113 (3.2)	24 (0.7)
Ectopic pregnancy	44 (1.2)	7 (0.2)
Reproductive System and Breast Disorders		
Ovarian hyperstimulation syndrome	138 (3.9)	129 (3.6)
Pelvic pain	67 (1.9)	44 (1.2)

Note: Coded with MedDRA version 8.1.

Treatment of Men: Gynaecomastia and acne may occur occasionally during PUREGON/hCG therapy. These are known effects of hCG treatment.

In one subject an epididymal cyst was observed.

Number (%) of Male Subjects with at Least One AE per MedDRA Body System and Preferred Term. Trials: P37618 (male trial): See Table 4.

DRUG INTERACTIONS: Overview: Concurrent use of PUREGON and clomifene may enhance the follicular response. After pituitary desensitization effected by a GnRH agonist, a higher dose of PUREGON may be necessary to elicit an adequate follicular response.

DOSAGE AND ADMINISTRATION: Dosing Considerations: PUREGON may be given alone, or in combination with clomifene citrate to stimulate the endogenous production of gonadotropins or in combination with a GnRH agonist to prevent premature luteinization (see Drug Interactions).
Recommended Dose and Dosage Adjustment: Dosage: In the Female: There are great inter- and intra-individual variations in the response of the ovaries to exogenous gonadotrophins. This makes it impossible to set a uniform dosage scheme. The dosage should, therefore, be adjusted individually depending on the ovarian response. This requires ultrasonography and monitoring of estradiol levels.

In comparative clinical studies with PUREGON and urinary FSH it was shown that PUREGON is more effective than urinary FSH in terms of a lower total dose and a shorter treatment period needed to achieve pre-ovulatory conditions. Therefore, it is considered appropriate to give a lower dosage of PUREGON than generally used for urinary FSH, not only in order to optimise follicular development but also to minimise the risk of unwanted ovarian hyperstimulation.

After pituitary desensitisation induced by GnRH agonist a higher dose of PUREGON may be necessary to achieve an adequate follicular response. Clinical experience with PUREGON is based on up to three treatment cycles in both indications. Overall experience with IVF indicates that in general the treatment success rate remains stable during the first four attempts and gradually declines thereafter.

Ovulation Induction: A sequential treatment scheme is recommended starting with daily administration of 50 IU PUREGON. The starting dose is maintained for at least 7 days. If there is no ovarian response, the daily dose is then gradually increased until follicle growth and/or plasma estradiol levels indicate an adequate pharmacodynamic response. A daily increase of estradiol levels of 40-100% is considered to be optimal. The daily dose is then maintained until pre-ovulatory conditions are reached. Pre-ovulatory conditions are reached when there is ultrasonographic evidence of a dominant follicle of at least 18 mm in diameter and/or when plasma estradiol levels of 300-900 picograms/mL (1000-3000 pmol/L) are attained. Usually, 7 to 14 days of treatment is sufficient to reach this state. The administration of PUREGON is then discontinued and ovulation can be induced by administering human chorionic gonadotrophin (hCG).

Table 4: PUREGON

Reported Adverse Drug Reactions in Clinical Trials with Incidence of >1%

MedDRA System Organ Class MedDRA Preferred Term	Treatment Group PUREGON N=30 All n (%)	 Drug Related n (%)
Blood and Lymphatic System Disorders		
Leukopenia	1 (3.3)	0 (0.0)
Lymphadenopathy	1 (3.3)	0 (0.0)
Neutropenia	1 (3.3)	0 (0.0)
Gastrointestinal Disorders		
Haemorrhoids	1 (3.3)	0 (0.0)
General Disorders and Administration Site Conditions		
Injection site bruising	2 (6.7)	2 (6.7)
Injection site haemorrhage	1 (3.3)	0 (0.0)
Injection site induration	1 (3.3)	1 (3.3)
Injection site pain	2 (6.7)	2 (6.7)
Pyrexia	2 (6.7)	0 (0.0)
Infections and Infestations		
Bronchitis	1 (3.3)	0 (0.0)
Influenza	5 (16.7)	0 (0.0)
Nasopharyngitis	1 (3.3)	0 (0.0)
Pilonidal cyst	1 (3.3)	0 (0.0)
Viral infection	2 (6.7)	0 (0.0)
Injury, Poisoning and Procedural Complications		
Upper limb fracture	1 (3.3)	0 (0.0)
Investigations		
Aspartate aminotransferase increased	1 (3.3)	0 (0.0)
Blood lactate dehydrogenase increased	1 (3.3)	0 (0.0)
Blood urea increased	1 (3.3)	0 (0.0)
Red blood cells semen positive	1 (3.3)	0 (0.0)
Musculoskeletal and Connective Tissue Disorders		
Back pain	2 (6.7)	0 (0.0)
Nervous System Disorders		
Headache	2 (6.7)	0 (0.0)
Reproductive System and Breast Disorders		
Epididymal cyst	1 (3.3)	1 (3.3)
Gynaecomastia	1 (3.3)	1 (3.3)
Varicocele	1 (3.3)	1 (3.3)
Respiratory, Thoracic and Mediastinal Disorders		
Cough	1 (3.3)	0 (0.0)
Pharyngolaryngeal pain	1 (3.3)	0 (0.0)
Skin and Subcutaneous Tissue Disorders		
Acne	2 (6.7)	2 (6.7)
Rash	1 (3.3)	0 (0.0)

Note: Coded with MedDRA version 8.1.

If the number of responding follicles is too high or estradiol levels increase too rapidly, i.e. more than a daily doubling for estradiol for 2 or 3 consecutive days, the daily dose should be decreased. Since follicles of over 14 mm may lead to pregnancies, multiple pre-ovulatory follicles exceeding 14 mm carry the risk of multiple gestations. In that case hCG should be withheld and pregnancy should be avoided in order to prevent multiple gestations.

Controlled Ovarian Hyperstimulation in Medically Assisted Reproduction Programs: The dosage regimen may vary according to the physician's preference or the patient's response. In general, stimulation of follicular growth is achieved by starting with daily s.c. or i.m. (see Administration) administration of 150-225 IU PUREGON for a period of 4 days. Thereafter, the dose may be adjusted according to the individual's ovarian response.

Maturation of follicles is monitored by pelvic ultrasonography and measurement of plasma estrogen levels. In responding patients, daily maintenance doses of 75 to 300 IU for 6 to 12 days are usually sufficient, although longer treatment may be necessary. The maximum individualized daily dose safely used in clinical studies was 450 IU. There is limited experience with higher doses. When ultrasonic evaluation indicates the presence of at least three follicles of sufficient size and there is evidence of a good estradiol response, the final phase of maturation of the follicles is induced by administration of hCG. HCG is given 30-40 hours after the last administration of PUREGON in a dose of 5000-10 000 IU.

After embryo transfer, up to three repeat injections of 1000 to 3000 IU hCG each, may be given within the following 9 days to provide luteal phase support.

Dosage in the Male: PUREGON should be given at a dosage of 450 IU/week, preferably divided in 3 dosages of 150 IU (two doses of 225 IU per week is considered to be equivalent) concomitantly with hCG. Please note that the intramuscular route of administration of PUREGON in males has not been evaluated. The treatment should be continued for at least 3 to 4 months before any improvement in spermatogenesis can be expected. If a patient has not responded after this period, the combination therapy may be continued. **The efficacy and safety of PUREGON have not been established beyond a treatment period of 48 weeks. Clinical experience with other gonadotropins suggests that a treatment for up to 18 months or longer may be necessary to achieve spermatogenesis.**

Administration: PUREGON (follitropin beta) Solution for Injection in Cartridges: PUREGON (follitropin beta) solution for injection in cartridges has been developed for use with the PUREGON Pen (a pen-injector) and should be administered subcutaneously. The injection site should be alternated to prevent lipoatrophy.

When using the pen-injector, it should be realized that the pen is a precision device which accurately delivers the dose to which it is set. It was shown that on average an 18% higher amount of FSH is given with the pen compared with a conventional syringe. Since the daily dose of PUREGON is determined by the patient's individual ovarian response, the slightly higher dose delivered by the PUREGON Pen is unlikely to affect clinical outcome. It may however be of relevance when switching between the pen-injector and a conventional syringe within one treatment cycle. Especially when switching from a syringe to the PUREGON Pen, small dose adjustments may be needed to prevent too high of a dose being given.

In view of loss of the active ingredient because of priming and dead volume, the 300 IU/0.36 mL cartridge contains a minimum of 400 IU/0.48 mL which is sufficient for a net deliverable dose of 300 IU. The 600 IU/0.72 mL cartridge contains a minimum of 700 IU/0.84 mL which is sufficient for a net deliverable dose of 600 IU and the 900 IU/1.08 mL cartridge contains a minimum of 1025 IU/1.23 mL which is sufficient for a net deliverable dose of 900 IU.

The net deliverable dose of 300 IU, 600 IU and 900 IU are based upon a maximum of six 50 IU injections, six 100 IU injections and nine 100 IU injections respectively.

When more injections are given, the net total dose of active ingredient may be lowered, because each injection has to be preceded by an air shot.

The instructions for using the pen must be followed carefully.

PUREGON (follitropin beta) Solution for Injection in Vials: Administer the PUREGON solution either subcutaneously or intramuscularly. Any unused solution should be discarded.

Subcutaneous Administration: The best site for subcutaneous injection is in the abdomen around the navel (an alternate site is the upper thigh). Pinch up a large area of skin between the finger and thumb. Vary the injection site with each injection. The needle should be inserted at a 90° angle to the skin surface. The first injection of PUREGON should be performed under direct medical supervision. Subcutaneous administration of PUREGON can be carried out by the patients or by their partners, provided that proper instructions are given by the physician. Self-administration of PUREGON should only be performed by patients who are well motivated, adequately trained and with access to expert advice.

Intramuscular Administration: The best site for intramuscular administration is the upper outer quadrant of the buttock muscle. Stretching the skin helps the needle to go in more easily and pushes the tissue beneath the skin out of the way. This helps the solution to disperse correctly. The needle should be inserted right up to the hilt at an angle of 90° to the skin surface. Pushing in with a quick thrust causes the least discomfort.

OVERDOSAGE:

The acute toxicity of gonadotropin preparations has been shown to be very low. However, too high a dosage for more than one day may lead to hyperstimulation of the ovaries (see Warnings and Precautions).

> For management of a suspected drug overdose, CPhA recommends that you contact your **regional Poison Control Centre**. See the *CPS* Directory section for a list of Poison Control Centres.

ACTION AND CLINICAL PHARMACOLOGY: Pharmacodynamics: PUREGON (follitropin beta) is a sterile solution containing highly purified human follicle- stimulating hormone (hFSH) prepared by recombinant DNA technology. The active substance, follitropin beta, is a heterodimeric glycoprotein with a molecular mass of approximately 35-45 kD. It is produced by a Chinese hamster ovary (CHO) cell line transfected with a plasmid containing two subunit genes encoding human FSH. Structural analysis has shown that the amino acid sequence of follitropin beta is identical to that of natural hFSH. The oligosaccharide side chains are very similar to those reported for natural hFSH but not completely identical. These small differences do not affect the degree of charge heterogeneity, receptor binding affinity and bioactivity of follitropin relative to natural hFSH. Follitropin beta, as purified from the CHO cell culture supernatant, is of high biochemical purity (≥99%), high specific biological activity (approximately 10 000 IU/mg protein), and devoid of luteinizing hormone (LH) activity.

Follicle-stimulating Hormone (FSH) is essential for normal female and male gamete growth and maturation, and gonadal steroid production. Deficiencies in the endogenous production of FSH may lead to infertility.

FSH is critical for the onset and duration of follicular development, and consequently for the timing and number of follicles reaching maturity in females. The primary action of follitropin beta in women with gonadal dysfunction, is the stimulation of follicular development and steroid production. Follitropin may also be used to promote multiple follicular development in medically assisted reproduction programs (i.e. IVF/ET/ISCI) and gamete or zygote intra-fallopian transfer (GIFT/ZIFT). In order to induce ovulation, in the absence of an endogenous LH surge, human chorionic gonadotropin (hCG) must be given after follitropin beta administration once follicular maturation has occurred.

Pharmacokinetics: See Table 5.

Absorption: After i.m. or s.c. administration of follitropin beta, high concentrations of FSH are reached within about 12 hours. After intramuscular administration of PUREGON, the maximum FSH concentrations are higher and reached earlier in men as compared to women. FSH levels remain high for 24-48 hours due to follitropin beta's relatively long elimination half-life of about 40 hours (ranging from 12 to 70 hours). Plasma FSH concentrations, after repeated administration of PUREGON, are approximately 1.5-2.5 times higher than after single dose administration.

The bioavailability of PUREGON following subcutaneous and intramuscular administration was investigated in healthy, pituitary-suppressed, female subjects given a single 300 IU dose. After subcutaneous or intramuscular injection the apparent dose absorbed was 77.8% and 76.4%, respectively.

The subcutaneous (455.6±141.4 IU·h/L) and intramuscular (455.7±135.7 IU·h/L) routes of administration were equivalent with respect area under the curve (AUC) in healthy, pituitary-suppressed, female subjects given a single 300 IU dose. However, equivalence could not be established for C_{max} between the subcutaneous (5.41±0.72 IU/L) and intramuscular (6.86±2.90 IU/L) routes of administration.

The pharmacokinetics and pharmacodynamics of a single, intramuscular dose (300 IU) of PUREGON were also investigated in a group of gonadotropin-deficient, but otherwise healthy women. Peak (C_{max}) serum FSH levels in these women were 4.3±1.7 IU/L (mean±SD) and they occurred approximately 27 hours after intramuscular administration.

Table 5: PUREGON

Pharmacokinetics

	C_{max} (IU/L)[a]	$t_{1/2}$ (h)[b]	$AUC_{0-\infty}$ (IU· h/L)[a]	Clearance (L/h)[a] (intravenous)	Volume of Distribution (L)[c]
Single dose mean	SC: 5.4 IM: 6.9	34	SC: 456 IM: 446	0.51	25

a Taken from trial 37614 (n=13).
b Taken from trial 37626 (n=22).
c Volume of distribution during terminal phase calculated as CL.

A multiple, dose proportionality, pharmacokinetic study of PUREGON was completed in healthy, pituitary-suppressed, female subjects given intramuscular doses of 75 IU, 150 IU or 225 IU for 7 days. Steady-state blood concentrations of FSH were reached with all the doses after 4 days of treatment based on the minimum concentrations of FSH just prior to dosing (C_{min}). Peak blood concentrations with the 75 IU, 150 IU, and 225 IU dose were 4.65±1.49 IU/L, 9.46±2.57 IU/L and 11.30±1.77 IU/L, respectively.

A multiple, dose proportionality, pharmacokinetic study of PUREGON was completed in healthy, pituitary-suppressed, female subjects given subcutaneous doses of 75 IU, 150 IU, or 225 IU for 7 days. Steady-state blood concentrations of FSH were reached with all the doses after 5 days of treatment based on the minimum concentrations of FSH just prior to dosing (C_{min}). Peak blood concentrations with the 75 IU, 150 IU, and 225 IU dose were 4.30±0.60 IU/L, 8.51±1.16 IU/L and 13.92±1.81 IU/L, respectively.

Distribution: The volume of distribution of PUREGON in healthy, pituitary-suppressed, female subjects following intravenous administration of 300 IU dose was approximately 8 L.

Metabolism: The recombinant FSH in PUREGON is biochemically very similar to urinary FSH and it is therefore anticipated that it is metabolized in the same manner.

Excretion: The elimination half-life following a single intramuscular dose (300 IU) of PUREGON in female subjects was 43.9±14.1 hours (mean±SD). The elimination half-life following a 7-day intramuscular treatment with 75 IU, 150 IU or 225 IU was 26.9±7.8 hours (mean±SD), 30.1±6.2 hours (mean±SD) and 28.9±6.5, respectively.

There are no significant pharmacokinetic differences between intramuscular and subcutaneous administration of PUREGON. Both have an absolute bioavailability of approximately 77%. Recombinant FSH is biochemically very similar to urinary human FSH and is distributed, metabolised, and excreted in the same way.

Special Populations and Conditions: No studies have been conducted with special populations and conditions.

STORAGE AND STABILITY: Pharmacist: Store in a refrigerator at 2-8°C. Keep the vial(s)/cartridge(s) in the outer carton. Do not freeze. Protect from light.

Patient: Store in a refrigerator (2-8°C) **or** store at or below 25°C for a maximum of 3 months. Keep the vial(s)/cartridge(s) in the outer carton. Do not use past expiry date. Protect from light.

PUREGON Solution for Injection in Cartridges: Once the rubber inlay of a cartridge is pierced by a needle, the product may be stored for a maximum of 28 days.

PUREGON Solution for Injection in Vials: The contents of a vial should be used immediately after piercing of the rubber stopper.

Route of Administration: PUREGON Solution for Injection in Cartridges: For subcutaneous injection only.

PUREGON Solution for Injection in Vials: For intramuscular or subcutaneous injection. For single use only. Once solution has been taken from a vial, any unused drug (solution) should be discarded.

SPECIAL HANDLING INSTRUCTIONS: The instructions for the pen must be followed carefully (see PUREGON Pen booklet).

Do not use the cartridge if the solution contains particles or if the solution is not clear. Air bubbles must be removed from the cartridge before injection (see instructions for using the pen).

Empty cartridges must not be refilled.

PUREGON cartridges are not designed to allow any other drug to be mixed in the cartridges. Discard used needles immediately after injection.

Discard used cartridges (including the remaining volume) after the last injection of the treatment cycle.

INFORMATION FOR THE PATIENT: Published in e-CPS, available by subscription at www.e-cps.ca.

DOSAGE FORMS, COMPOSITION AND PACKAGING: Solution for Injection in Cartridges: Solution for injection in cartridges - 833 IU/mL. Cartridges contain a minimum of 400 IU FSH activity in 0.48 mL aqueous solution which is sufficient for a net deliverable dose of 300 IU, a minimum of 700 IU FSH activity in 0.84 mL aqueous solution which is sufficient for a net deliverable dose of 600 IU or a minimum of 1025 IU FSH activity in 1.23 mL which is sufficient for a net dose of 900 IU. Nonmedicinal ingredients: benzyl alcohol, L-methionine, polysorbate 20, sodium citrate and sucrose. Hydrochloric acid 0.1 N and sodium hydroxide 0.1 N (trace amounts for pH adjustment to pH 7.0). Boxes of Puregon solution for injection contain 1 cartridge of Puregon and 6 (300 IU and 600 IU cartridges) or 9 (900 IU cartridges) needles to be used with the Puregon Pen. The cartridges are of colourless hydrolytic (class 1) glass, with a rubber piston and an aluminium crimp-cap with a rubber inlay.

The net deliverable dose of 300 IU, 600 IU and 900 IU are based upon a maximum of six 50 IU injections, six 100 IU injections and nine 100 IU injections respectively.

When more injections are given the net total dose may be lowered, because each injection has to be preceded by an air shot.

Cartridges contain 833 IU of FSH activity per mL aqueous solution. Cartridges with a net dose of 300 IU contain a minimum of 400 IU in 0.48 mL; those of 600 IU contain a minimum of 700 IU in 0.84 mL; those of 900 IU contain a minimum of 1025 IU in 1.23 mL.

Solution for Injection in Vials: Each vial of sterile solution for injection contains: follitropin beta (recombinant FSH) 50 or 100 IU. 50 or 100 FSH activity/0.5 mL. Nonmedicinal ingredients: L-methionine, polysorbate 20, sodium citrate, sucrose. Hydrochloric acid 0.1 N and sodium hydroxide 0.1 N (trace amounts for pH adjustment). Boxes of 1, 5 or 10 vial(s) of PUREGON in 0.5 mL aqueous solution. PUREGON solution for injection is filled in colourless, 3 mL vials of hydrolytic resistant glass, Type 1, and closed with chlorobutyl rubber closures.

PureTrim® Mediterranean Wellness Shake

multiple vitamins and minerals

High Protein Meal Replacement Shake

Awareness Corporation/dba AwarenessLife

SUPPLIED: Chocolate: One pack of Mediterranean Wellness Shake contains: vitamin A (as retinyl palmitate with lemongrass) 2000 IU, vitamin C (as sodium ascorbate and ascorbic acid with camu fruit and wolf berrie) 19 mg, vitamin D (as cholecalciferol with brewer's yeast) 90 IU, vitamin E (as d-alpha-tocopheryl acetate) 4.5 IU, thiamin (as thiamin mononitrate with brown rice) 700 µg, riboflavin (with brown rice) 750 µg, niacin (as niacinamide with brown rice) 11 mg, vitamin B_6 (as pyridoxine HCl with brown rice) 700 µg, folate (as folic acid with brown rice) 110 µg, vitamin B_{12} (as cyanocobalamin with brown rice) 0.70 µg, biotin (with brown rice) 70 µg, pantothenic acid (as calcium pantothenate with brown rice) 2 mg, calcium (from green plants, sesame seeds, kale leaf, and spinach leaf) 400 mg, phosphorus (as potassium phosphate, magnesium phosphate and ocean plant) 250 mg, iodine (as potassium iodide) 100 µg, magnesium (as magnesium phosphate and ocean plant) 110 mg, zinc (as zinc oxide)5.5 mg, selenium (as sodium selenite) 19 µg, copper (as copper oxide) 1 mg, manganese (as manganese sulfate) 1 mg, chromium (as chromium dinicotinate glycinate) 19 µg, molybdenum (as sodium molybdate) 37.5 µg, sodium 250 mg, potassium 375 mg.

Nonmedicinal ingredients: protein complex: non-GMO vegetable pea protein concentrate and non-GMO brown rice protein; mediterranean essential fatty acid blend: (containing omega 3,6 fatty acids) safflower oil complex, almond oil, flaxseed oil, grape seed oil, olive oil, and sesame seed oil; prebiotic and enzyme blend: fibersol-2t (soluble fibre glucose polymer complex), bromelain, guar gum, gum acacia, inulin, lipase, and protease; ionic plant trace mineral blend (from ocean plant); anti-stress & energy blend: green tea leaf extract, passionflower (whole plant and flower), cinnamon twig extract, greater galangal root extract, american ginseng root extract, apple pectin, cayenne fruit, chamomile flower, citrus pectin, jujube fruit, lemon balm leaf, licorice root extract, asian ginseng root extract, peppermint leaf, rhodiola root extract, and maté leaf extract; mediterranean skin & digestion blend: olive leaf 4:1 extract, artichoke leaf 4:1 extract, grape leaf extract, pomegranate fruit extract; super greens blend: alfalfa leaf, asparagus spear extract, barley grass, bitter melon fruit extract, broccoli floret, brussels sprout leaf, cabbage leaf, cauliflower floret, chlorella, mustard seed, nettle leaf, spirulina, cocoa (bean), natural & artificial flavors, gum blend (cellulose gum, xanthan gum, and carrageenan), salt, silica, acesulfame potassium, sucralose, stevia leaf extract.

Aspartame-, dairy-, soy-, sucrose- and whey-free. Serving size 1 pack (56 g).

Vanilla: One pack of Mediterranean Wellness Shake contains: vitamin A (as retinyl palmitate with lemongrass) 2000 IU, vitamin C (as sodium ascorbate and ascorbic acid with camu fruit and wolf berrie) 19 mg, vitamin D (as cholecalciferol with brewer's yeast) 90 IU, vitamin E (as d-alpha-tocopheryl acetate) 4.5 IU, thiamin (as thiamin mononitrate with brown rice) 700 µg, riboflavin (with brown rice) 750 µg, niacin (as niacinamide with brown rice) 11 mg, vitamin B_6 (as pyridoxine HCl with brown rice) 700 µg, folate (as folic acid with brown rice) 110 µg, vitamin B_{12} (as cyanocobalamin with brown rice) 0.70 µg, biotin (with brown rice) 70 µg, pantothenic acid (as calcium pantothenate with brown rice) 2 mg, calcium (from green plants, sesame seeds, kale leaf, and spinach leaf) 400 mg, phosphorus (as potassium phosphate, magnesium phosphate and ocean plant) 260 mg, iodine (as potassium iodide) 100 µg, magnesium (as magnesium phosphate and ocean plant) 110 mg, zinc (as zinc oxide) 5.5 mg, selenium (as sodium selenite) 19 µg, copper (as copper oxide) 1 mg, manganese (as manganese sulfate) 1 mg, chromium (as chromium dinicotinate glycinate) 19 µg, molybdenum (as sodium molybdate) 37.5 µg, sodium 250 mg, potassium 375 mg.

Nonmedicinal ingredients: protein complex: non-GMO vegetable pea protein concentrate and non-GMO brown rice protein; mediterranean essential fatty acid blend: (containing omega 3,6 fatty acids) safflower oil complex, almond oil, flaxseed oil, grape seed oil, olive oil, and sesame seed oil; prebiotic and enzyme blend: fibersol-2t (soluble fibre glucose polymer complex), bromelain, guar gum, gum acacia, inulin, lipase, and protease; ionic plant trace mineral blend (from ocean plant); anti-stress & energy blend: green tea leaf extract, passionflower (whole plant and flower), cinnamon twig extract, greater galangal root extract, american ginseng root extract, apple pectin, cayenne fruit, chamomile flower, citrus pectin, jujube fruit, lemon balm leaf, licorice root extract, asian ginseng root extract, peppermint leaf, rhodiola root extract, and maté leaf extract; mediterranean skin & digestion blend: olive leaf 4:1 extract, artichoke leaf 4:1 extract, grape leaf extract, pomegranate fruit extract; super greens blend: alfalfa leaf, asparagus spear extract, barley grass, bitter melon fruit extract, broccoli floret, brussels sprout leaf, cabbage leaf, cauliflower floret, chlorella, mustard seed, nettle leaf, spirulina, natural & artificial flavors, gum blend (cellulose gum, xanthan gum, and carrageenan), salt, silica, acesulfame potassium, sucralose, stevia leaf extract, sodium phosphate.

Aspartame-, dairy-, soy-, sucrose- and whey-free. Serving size 1 pack (56 g).

(Shown in Product Identification Section)

Purg-Odan™

picosulfate sodium—magnesium oxide—citric acid

Purgative

Odan

SUPPLIED: Purg-Odan: Each sachet contains: sodium picosulfate 10 mg, magnesium oxide 3.5 g and citric acid 12 g. Nonmedicinal ingredients: orange flavor, potassium bicarbonate and sodium saccharin. Cartons of 2. Store between 15 and 30°C. Keep out of reach of children.

Purg-Odan Solo: Each sachet contains: sodium picosulfate 10 mg, magnesium oxide 3.5 g and citric acid 12 g. Nonmedicinal ingredients: orange flavor, potassium bicarbonate and sodium saccharin. Cartons of 1. Store between 15 and 30°C. Keep out of reach of children.

Purinethol® Ⓟ

mercaptopurine

Antileukemic

Teva Canada

SUPPLIED: Each pale yellow to buff, scored tablet, imprinted with "PURINETHOL" and "O4A", contains: mercaptopurine 50 mg. Nonmedicinal ingredients: corn starch, lactose, magnesium stearate, potato starch and stearic acid. Bottles of 25. Store in a dry place between 15 and 25°C, protected from light.

Pyridoxine

CPhA Monograph

see *Vitamin B6*

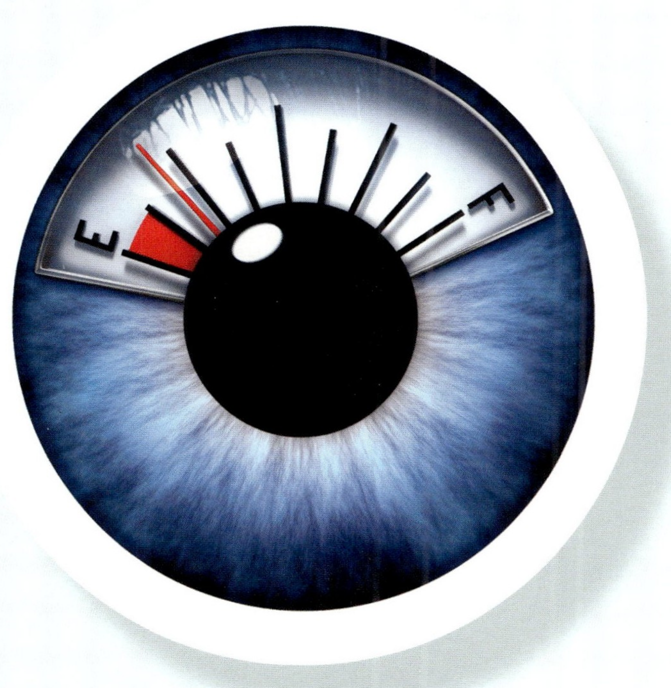

Restasis®
(Cyclosporine Ophthalmic Emulsion) 0.05% w/v

A New Treatment Option for Aqueous Deficient Dry Eye Disease is Available in Canada*[1]

Restasis® (cyclosporine) is thought to act as a partial immunomodulator in patients whose tear production is presumed to be suppressed due to ocular inflammation associated with *keratoconjunctivitis sicca* (KCS).[§1]

- The exact mechanism of action is not known.[1]

Restasis® may help improve tear production in patients with Level 2–3 aqueous deficient Dry Eye disease:*[†1]

- A statistically significant greater proportion of Restasis® patients were Schirmer's with anesthesia score responders vs. the vehicle group at Month 6 (17.1% [22/129] vs. 6.2% [9/146]; p=0.005).[1]
  - Complete Schirmer's with anesthesia score responder: a patient with an increase from baseline ≥10 mm/5 min at Month 6 (Month 6 minus baseline)[1]

*Restasis® (cyclosporine) ophthalmic emulsion, 0.05% w/v is indicated for the treatment of moderate to moderately severe (Level 2–3 severity by DEWS Guidelines) aqueous deficient Dry Eye disease, characterized by moderate to moderately severe: ocular staining, reduction in tear production and fluctuating visual symptoms, such as blurred vision. The efficacy of Restasis® alone has not been demonstrated in patients with more severe disease (Level 4 DEWS classification).[‡1]

Restasis® is contraindicated in patients with active ocular infections and in patients who are hypersensitive to this drug or to any ingredient in the formulation or component of the container.[1]

Warnings: Restasis® is for ophthalmic use only. Restasis® has not been studied in patients with a history of *herpes keratitis*, end stage lacrimal gland disease, *keratoconjunctivitis sicca* (KCS) secondary to the destruction of conjunctival goblet cells such as occurs with Vitamin A deficiency, or scarring, such as occurs with cicatricial pemphigoid, alkali burns, Stevens Johnson syndrome, trachoma, or irradiation.[1]

Precautions: Patients should be advised to avoid touching the tip of the vial to the eye or any surface, as this may contaminate the emulsion. To avoid the potential for injury to the eye, patients should be advised to be careful not to touch the vial container to the eye. Restasis® should not be administered while the patient is wearing contact lenses. If contact lenses are worn, they should be removed prior to the administration of the emulsion. Lenses may be reinserted 15 minutes after the administration of Restasis®. Restasis® may cause transient blurred vision due to its emulsion formulation. If patients experience blurred vision, they should be advised not to drive or operate machinery until vision has cleared.[1]

There are no adequate data from the use of Restasis® in pregnant women. Studies in animals have shown reproductive toxicity at high maternotoxic doses. Restasis® should not be used during pregnancy unless the benefits outweigh the risks and caution should be exercised when Restasis® is administered to a nursing woman. The safety and efficacy of Restasis® has only been studied in adults.[1]

The most commonly reported adverse events following the use of Restasis® were ocular burning (17%), eye irritation (3%), foreign body sensation (2.8%), conjunctival hyperaemia (2.5%), eye pain (2.3%), and eye stinging (2.3%). The majority were ocular, mild or moderate in severity, and none was serious.[1]

[†] In three six-month, phase-3, multicentre, double-masked, randomized, vehicle-controlled studies, 1,315 patients with moderate to severe *keratoconjunctivitis sicca* were administered cyclosporine emulsion via the ophthalmic route on a twice-daily schedule. Refresh® use could continue during this treatment phase, however, patients were asked to discontinue Refresh® use one week before the Month 4 visit and try to restrict Refresh® usage for the remainder of the trial to less than 8 times daily. Although many findings in each of the individual clinical trials showed numerical superiority for cyclosporine over vehicle, the relatively large standard deviations encountered meant that statistical significance was not usually demonstrated. A post-hoc meta-analysis of these studies evaluated efficacy in a subpopulation characterized as having Level 2–Level 3 dry eye disease (n=316); this classification was based on the Dry Eye Workshop (DEWS) guidelines (2007). Schirmer test with anesthesia score was >2 mm/5 min at baseline. The Schirmer's with anesthesia score at baseline in the pooled studies was similar in the cyclosporine 0.05% and vehicle groups (p=0.494): 6.2 and 6.5, respectively.[1]

[‡] This indication is based on a pooled analysis of a subpopulation of patients from three pivotal studies.[1]

[§] Clinical significance unknown.

1. Restasis® Product Monograph. August 16, 2010.

ALLERGAN

PAAB

Q
R

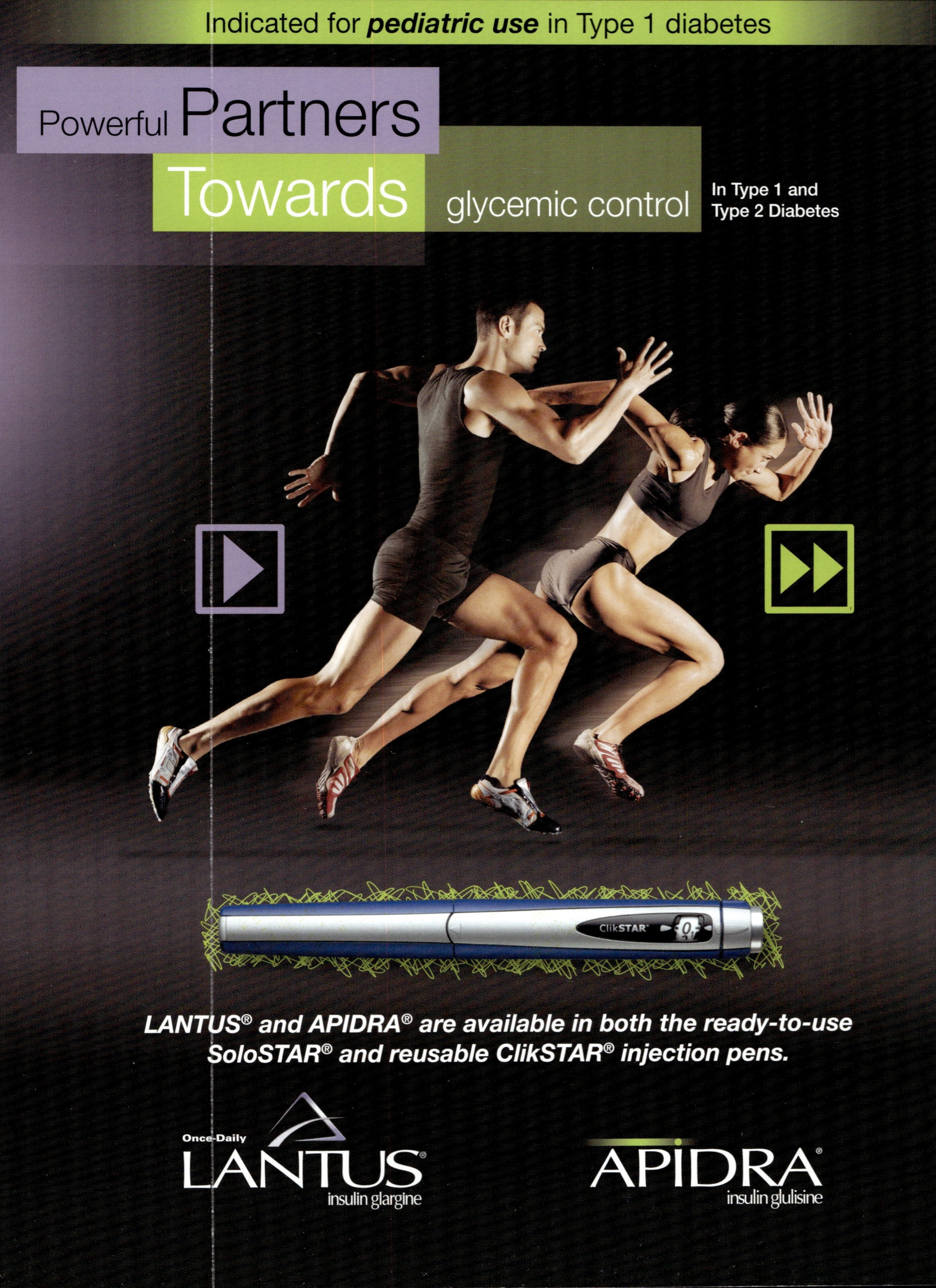

Indicated for *pediatric use* in Type 1 diabetes
Powerful Partners
Towards glycemic control
In Type 1 and Type 2 Diabetes
ClikSTAR
LANTUS® and APIDRA® are available in both the ready-to-use SoloSTAR® and reusable ClikSTAR® injection pens.
Once-Daily
LANTUS®
insulin glargine
APIDRA®
insulin glulisine

LANTUS® (insulin glargine [rDNA origin]) is a novel recombinant human insulin analogue indicated for once-daily subcutaneous administration in the treatment of Type 1 or Type 2 diabetes in patients over 17 years of age who require basal (long-acting) insulin. LANTUS® is also indicated in the treatment of pediatric patients with Type 1 diabetes mellitus who require basal (long-acting) insulin for the control of hyperglycemia. Safety and efficacy have been established in children over 6 years of age.

LANTUS® is contraindicated in patients hypersensitive to insulin glargine or the excipients.

As with all insulin preparations, hypoglycemic reactions may be associated with the administration of LANTUS®. Hypoglycemia is the most common adverse effect of insulins; other adverse effects may include allergic reactions, injection site reactions, lipodystrophy, pruritus, rash and antibody formation. With LANTUS®, the most common adverse reactions in a pediatric clinical trial were infection (13.8%), upper respiratory infection (13.8%), pharyngitis (7.5%), rhinitis (5.2%), gastroenteritis (4.6%) and injection site mass (4.6%). Incidence of serious hypoglycemic reaction was reported at 1.7%.

APIDRA® (insulin glulisine [rDNA origin]) is a recombinant human insulin analogue indicated for the treatment of adult patients with diabetes mellitus where treatment with insulin is required; and pediatric patients with Type 1 diabetes mellitus who require a short-acting insulin. There is insufficient clinical data on the use of APIDRA® in children below the age of 6 years.

The safety and effectiveness of APIDRA® have been investigated in pediatric patients age 4 to 17 years with Type 1 diabetes. APIDRA® has not been studied in pediatric patients younger than 4 years of age.

APIDRA® has a more rapid onset of action and a shorter duration of action than regular human insulin. APIDRA® should normally be used in regimens that include a longer-acting insulin or basal insulin analogue to maintain adequate glucose control. APIDRA® can be used with oral hypoglycemic agents.

APIDRA® is contraindicated in patients who are hypersensitive to insulin glulisine or any ingredient in the formulation or component of the container.

Hypoglycemia is the most common adverse effect of insulin therapy. As with all insulin preparations, hypoglycemic reactions may be associated with the administration of APIDRA®. Overall, clinical studies comparing APIDRA® with short-acting insulins did not demonstrate a difference in frequency of adverse events. Other adverse reactions may include local or systemic allergy; localized reactions and generalized myalgias have been reported with the use of cresol as an injectable excipient.

Adverse events reported from a trial in children and adolescents with Type 1 diabetes were: injection site hypertrophy (1.1%); hypoglycemia (not otherwise specified) (2.2%); hypoglycemic seizure (6.1%); hypoglycemic coma (0.4%).

In pooled studies in Type 1 and Type 2 diabetes, adverse events with APIDRA® were: injection site hypertrophy (0.5%), hypoglycemia (4.5%), hypoglycemic seizure (0.9%), hypoglycemic unawareness (0.1%) and hypoglycemic coma (2.7%).

Glucose monitoring is recommended for all patients with diabetes. Insulin dosage should be individualized for each patient. As in adults, the dosage of APIDRA® must be individualized in pediatric patients based on metabolic needs and frequent monitoring of blood glucose.

LANTUS® and APIDRA® Product Monographs available upon request or at **www.sanofi-aventis.ca**.

REFERENCES:
1. LANTUS® Product Monograph, July 2007. 2. APIDRA® Product Monograph, April 2010.

sanofi aventis

Because health matters

Member R&D PAAB

CDN.GLU.10.05.02E

ClikSTAR®

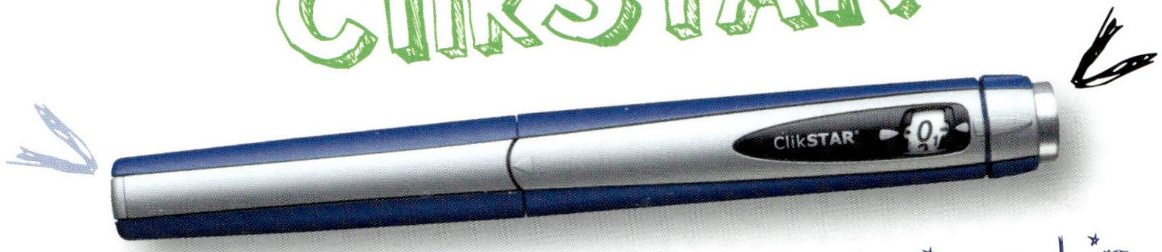

the reusable injection pen designed in partnership with nearly 2,000 patients*

The result is a convenient pen that's easy to learn and easy to use[1]

- Dosing increments of 1 U, to a maximum of 80 U
- Audible click when selecting dose
- Dial-back safety feature to correct dose selection errors
- One-step push-back plunger reset for cartridge exchange
- Available in grey and blue

ClikSTAR®

For simple insulin delivery

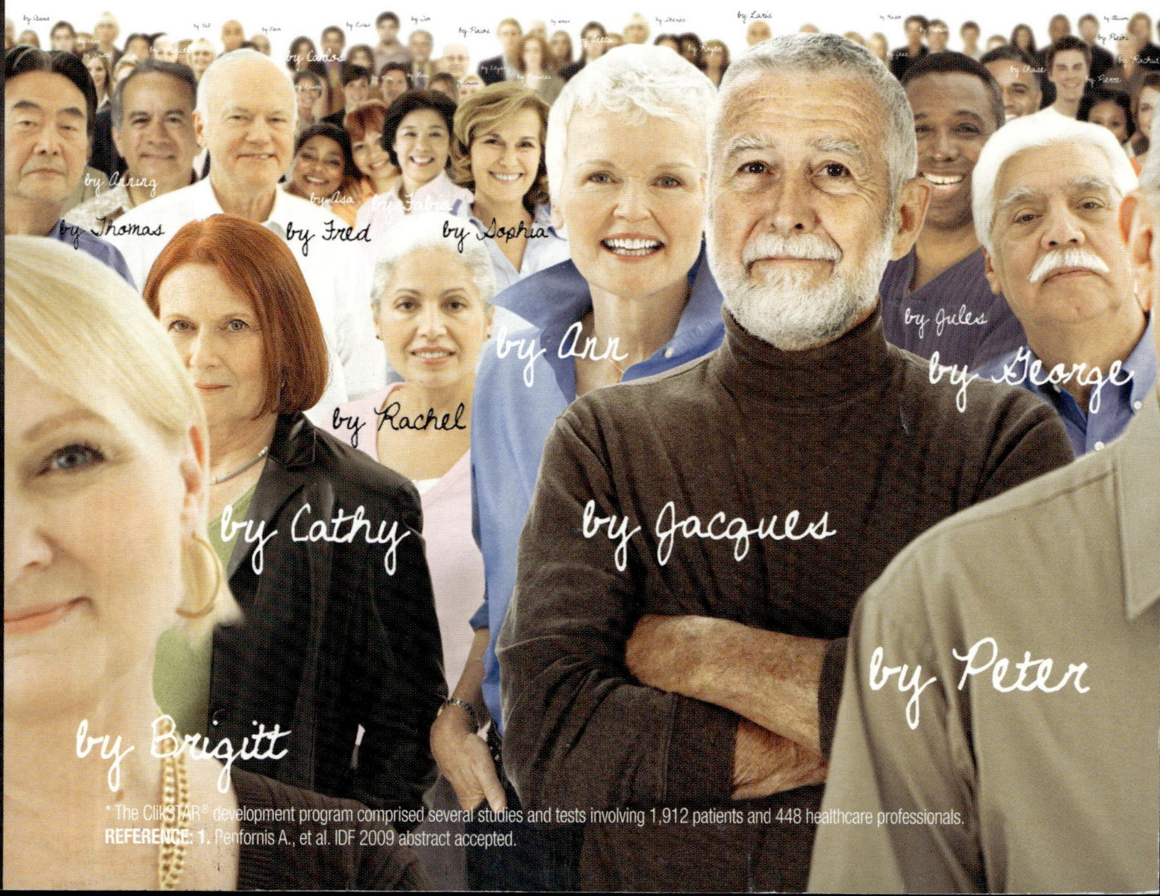

* The ClikSTAR® development program comprised several studies and tests involving 1,912 patients and 448 healthcare professionals.

REFERENCE: 1. Penfornis A., et al. IDF 2009 abstract accepted.

Q

Quadracel®

diphtheria and tetanus toxoids and acellular pertussis vaccine adsorbed combined with inactivated poliomyelitis vaccine

Active Immunizing Agent

sanofi pasteur

Date of Revision: July 2, 2008

SUMMARY PRODUCT INFORMATION:

Route of Administration	Dosage Form/ Strength	Clinically Relevant Nonmedicinal Ingredients
Intramuscular injection	Suspension for injection Each dose is formulated to contain: **Active Ingredients:** Diphtheria toxoid, tetanus toxoid, acellular pertussis [pertussis toxoid (PT), filamentous haemagglutinin (FHA), pertactin (PRN), fimbriae types 2 and 3 (FIM)], inactivated poliomyelitis vaccine (IPV) type 1 (Mahoney), type 2 (MEF-1) and type 3 (Saukett)].	Excipients: Aluminum phosphate (adjuvant), 2-phenoxyethanol, polysorbate 80 Manufacturing process residuals: Bovine serum albumin (BSA), formaldehyde, glutaraldehyde, neomycin and polymyxin B may be present in trace amounts. For a complete listing see Dosage Forms, Composition and Packaging.

DESCRIPTION: QUADRACEL [Diphtheria and Tetanus Toxoids and Acellular Pertussis Vaccine Adsorbed Combined with Inactivated Poliomyelitis Vaccine] is a sterile, uniform, cloudy, white to off-white suspension of diphtheria and tetanus toxoids and acellular pertussis vaccine adsorbed separately on aluminum phosphate combined with inactivated poliomyelitis virus types 1, 2 and 3 and suspended in water for injection. The acellular pertussis vaccine is composed of 5 purified pertussis antigens (PT, FHA, PRN and FIM).

INDICATIONS AND CLINICAL USE: QUADRACEL is indicated for primary immunization of infants, from the age of 2 months and in children up to 6 years of age (prior to their 7th birthday), against diphtheria, tetanus, pertussis and poliomyelitis. (See Dosage and Administration.)

When both vaccines are indicated, QUADRACEL may be used to reconstitute Act-HIB [Haemophilus b Conjugate Vaccine (Tetanus Protein-Conjugate)] for simultaneous administration of all 5 antigens in a single injection.

According to the National Advisory Committee on Immunization (NACI) children who have had diphtheria, tetanus, or pertussis, should still be immunized since these clinical infections do not always confer immunity.

NACI recommends that Human Immunodeficiency Virus (HIV)-infected persons, both asymptomatic and symptomatic, should be immunized against diphtheria, pertussis, tetanus and poliomyelitis according to standard schedules.

QUADRACEL is not to be used for the treatment of diseases caused by *C. diphtheriae*, *C. tetani*, *B. pertussis* or poliovirus infections.

Pediatrics: QUADRACEL is not indicated for persons less than 2 months of age or persons 7 years of age or older.

Geriatrics: QUADRACEL is not indicated for use in adult and elderly populations.

CONTRAINDICATIONS: Hypersensitivity: NACI recommends that known systemic hypersensitivity reaction to any component of QUADRACEL or a life-threatening reaction after previous administration of the vaccine or a vaccine containing one or more of the same components are contraindications to vaccination. (See Summary Product Information.) Because of uncertainty as to which component of the vaccine may be responsible, none of the components should be administered. Alternatively, such persons may be referred to an allergist for evaluation if further immunizations are considered.

Neurological Disorders: According to the US Advisory Committee on Immunization Practices (ACIP), the following events are contraindications to administration of any pertussis-containing vaccine, including QUADRACEL:

Encephalopathy (e.g., coma, decreased level of consciousness, prolonged seizures) within 7 days of a previous dose of a pertussis-containing vaccine that is not attributable to another identifiable cause.

Progressive neurologic disorder, including infantile spasms, uncontrolled epilepsy, progressive encephalopathy. Pertussis vaccine should not be administered to persons with such conditions until a treatment regimen has been established and the condition has stabilized.

WARNINGS AND PRECAUTIONS: General: Before administration of QUADRACEL, health-care providers should inform the parent or guardian of the recipient of the benefits and risks of immunization, inquire about the recent health status of the recipient, review the recipient's history concerning possible hypersensitivity to the vaccine or similar vaccine, previous immunization history, the presence of any contraindications to immunization and comply with any local requirements with respect to information to be provided to the parent or guardian before immunization and the importance of completing the immunization series.

It is extremely important that the parent or guardian be questioned concerning any symptoms and/or signs of an adverse reaction after a previous dose of vaccine. (See Contraindications and Adverse Reactions.)

The rates and severity of adverse events in recipients of tetanus toxoid are influenced by the number of prior doses and level of pre-existing antitoxins.

As with any vaccine, QUADRACEL may not protect 100% of susceptible individuals.

Administration Route-Related Precautions: Do not administer QUADRACEL by intravascular injection: ensure that the needle does not penetrate a blood vessel.

Intradermal or subcutaneous routes of administration are not to be utilized.

QUADRACEL should not be administered into the buttocks.

Febrile or Acute Disease: ACIP recommends that vaccination should be postponed in cases of acute or febrile disease. However, a disease with low-grade fever should not usually be a reason to postpone vaccination.

ACIP recommends that if any of the following events occur within the specified period after administration of a whole-cell pertussis vaccine or a vaccine containing an acellular pertussis component, the decision to administer QUADRACEL should be based on careful consideration of potential benefits and possible risks.

- Temperature of ≥40.5°C within 48 hours, not attributable to another identifiable cause;
- Collapse or shock-like state (hypotonic-hyporesponsive episode) within 48 hours;
- Persistent crying lasting ≥3 hours within 48 hours;
- Convulsions with or without fever within 3 days.

Hematologic: Because any intramuscular injection can cause an injection site hematoma in persons with any bleeding disorders, such as hemophilia or thrombocytopenia, or in persons on anticoagulant therapy, intramuscular injections with QUADRACEL should not be administered to such persons unless the potential benefits outweigh the risk of administration. If the decision is made to administer any product by intramuscular injection to such persons, it should be given with caution, with steps taken to avoid the risk of hematoma formation following injection.

Immune: The possibility of allergic reactions in persons sensitive to components of the vaccine should be evaluated. Hypersensitivity reactions may occur following the use of QUADRACEL even in persons with no prior history of hypersensitivity to the product components. Cases of allergic or anaphylactic reaction have been reported after receiving some preparations containing diphtheria and tetanus toxoids and/or pertussis antigens.

As recommended by NACI epinephrine hydrochloride solution (1:1000) and other appropriate agents should be available for immediate use in case an anaphylactic or acute hypersensitivity reaction occurs. Health-care providers should be familiar with current recommendations for the initial management of anaphylaxis in non-hospital settings including proper airway management. For instructions on recognition and treatment of anaphylactic reactions, see the current edition of the Canadian Immunization Guide or visit the Health Canada website.

According to NACI immunocompromised persons (whether from disease or treatment) may not obtain the expected immune response. If possible, consideration should be given to delaying vaccination until after the completion of any immunosuppressive treatment. Nevertheless, ACIP advises that vaccination of persons with chronic immunodeficiency such as HIV infection is recommended even if the antibody response might be limited.

Neurologic: A review by the US Institute of Medicine (IOM) found evidence for a causal relationship between tetanus toxoid and both brachial neuritis and Guillain-Barré syndrome (GBS). ACIP recommends that if GBS occurred within 6 weeks of receipt of prior vaccine containing tetanus toxoid, the decision to give QUADRACEL or any vaccine containing tetanus toxoid should be based on careful consideration of potential benefits and possible risks.

ACIP recommends that for infants or children at higher risk for seizures than the general population that an appropriate antipyretic may be administered (in the dosage recommended in its prescribing information) at the time of vaccination with a vaccine containing an acellular pertussis component (including QUADRACEL) and for the following 24 hours, to reduce the possibility of post-vaccination fever.

Hypotonic-hyporesponsive episodes (HHEs) rarely follow vaccination with whole-cell pertussis containing DTP vaccines and occur even less commonly after acellular pertussis-containing DTP vaccines and DT vaccines. NACI states that a history of HHEs is not a contraindication to the use of acellular pertussis vaccines but recommends caution in these cases.

Special Populations: Pregnant Women: The vaccine should not be administered to pregnant women.

Nursing Women: The vaccine should not be administered to nursing women.

ADVERSE REACTIONS: Clinical Trial Adverse Drug Reactions: Because clinical trials are conducted under widely varying conditions, adverse reaction rates observed in the clinical trials of a vaccine cannot be directly compared to rates in the clinical trials of another vaccine and may not reflect rates observed in practice. The adverse reaction information from clinical trials does, however, provide a basis for identifying the adverse events that appear to be related to vaccine use and for approximating rates of those events.

In clinical trials conducted in Canada, more than 3000 children have received QUADRACEL alone or used to reconstitute Act-HIB. Adverse reactions are generally mild and self-limiting. Serious adverse events are rare.

In a randomized, controlled clinical trial conducted in Canada, 113 infants were immunized with QUADRACEL at 2, 4 and 6 months of age. In addition, 104 of these children were immunized as toddlers at 18 months. In another randomized, controlled Canadian trial, 130 children 4 to 6 years of age, previously immunized with a whole-cell DTP vaccine, were immunized with QUADRACEL. Table 1 provides a summary of the frequency of solicited reactions observed within 24 hours following each dose of QUADRACEL. Injection site reactions were generally mild and occurred in approximately a quarter of infants receiving QUADRACEL. The size and frequency of the injection site reactions was higher after the 4th and 5th doses, however severe tenderness did not increase. Similar observations have been made with other acellular pertussis combination (DTaP) vaccines.

In a recent study involving 800 children 4 to 6 years old immunized at public health units in British Columbia, the extent of local reactions 48 to 96 hours after immunization was evaluated by means of a cross-sectional telephone survey. Among the 398 children who had previously received PENTACEL [Haemophilus b Conjugate Vaccine (Tetanus Protein-Conjugate) Reconstituted with Diphtheria and Tetanus Toxoids and Acellular Pertussis Vaccine Adsorbed Combined with Inactivated Poliomyelitis Vaccine] at 2, 4, 6 and 18 months of age, 24% experienced moderate to severe redness (≥46 mm), 16% reported moderate to severe swelling (≥46 mm), and only 7% had severe tenderness or marked limitation of movement.

Table 1: QUADRACEL

Frequency (%) of Solicited Reactions Following a Single Dose of QUADRACEL Administered at 2, 4, 6, 18 Months and 4-6 Years of Age

Solicited Reactions	2 Months[a] (N=113)	4 Months[a] (N=111)	6 Months[a] (N=111)	18 Months[a] (N=104)	4–6 Years[b] (N=130)
Injection Site Reactions					
Redness/Erythema	0.9	8.1	12.6	18.3	18.5
Swelling	5.3	3.6	7.2	13.5	18.5
Tenderness	18.6	18.0	9.0	28.8	74.6
Systemic Reactions					
Fever >38.0°C	22.1	21.1	18.0	24.0	17.3
Less Active	51.3	27.9	21.6	16.3	23.1
Eating Less	34.5	20.7	16.2	20.2	23.1
Fussiness	46.0	45.0	35.1	33.7	20.0
Crying	31.0	28.8	23.4	19.2	N.S.[c]
Diarrhea	6.2	7.2	9.9	2.9	2.3
Vomiting	8.0	2.7	6.3	6.7	4.6

[a] Act-HIB was administered concurrently at a separate site.
[b] Previously immunized with a whole-cell DTP vaccine.
[c] N.S.: not solicited.

Post-Market Adverse Drug Reactions: The following additional adverse events have been spontaneously reported during the post-marketing use of QUADRACEL worldwide. Because these events are reported voluntarily from a population of uncertain size, it is not always possible to reliably estimate their frequency or establish a causal relationship to vaccine exposure. Decisions to include these events in labelling were based on one or more of the following factors: 1) severity of the event, 2) frequency of reporting, or 3) strength of causal connection to QUADRACEL.

Immune System Disorders: anaphylactic reaction, hypersensitivity and allergic reactions (such as rash, urticaria, dyspnoea).

Psychiatric Disorders: screaming.

Nervous System Disorders: somnolence, convulsion, febrile convulsion, HHE, hypotonia.

Cardiac Disorders: cyanosis.

Vascular Disorders: pallor.

General Disorders and Administration Site Conditions: Injection site reactions (including inflammation, mass, abscess and sterile abscess), edema.

Very rarely, large injection site reactions (>50 mm), including limb swelling which may extend from the injection site beyond one or both joints have been reported in children following QUADRACEL administration. These reactions usually start within 24-72 hours after vaccination, may be associated with erythema, warmth, tenderness or pain at the injection site, and resolve spontaneously within 3-5 days. The risk appears to be dependent on the number of prior doses of d/DTaP vaccine, with a greater risk following the 4th and 5th doses.

Listlessness.

Physicians, nurses and pharmacists should report any adverse occurrences temporally related to the administration of the product in accordance with local requirements and report to the Global Pharmacovigilance Department, Sanofi Pasteur Limited, 1755 Steeles Avenue West, Toronto, ON, M2R 3T4, Canada. 1-888-621-1146 (phone) or 416-667-2435 (fax).

DRUG INTERACTIONS: Vaccine-Drug Interactions: Immunosuppressive treatments may interfere with the development of the expected immune response. (See Warnings and Precautions.)

Topical use of lidocaine-prilocaine patches to reduce injection site pain has no adverse effect on antibody response to QUADRACEL.

Concomitant Vaccine Administration: NACI states that administering the most widely used live and inactivated vaccines during the same patient visit has produced seroconversion rates and rates of adverse reactions similar to those observed when the vaccines are administered separately. Simultaneous administration is suggested, particularly when there is concern that a person may not return for subsequent vaccination. Simultaneous administration of childhood vaccines such as QUADRACEL, Hib, MMR, varicella, pneumococcal conjugate and hepatitis B vaccines, is encouraged for children who are at the recommended age to receive these vaccines and for whom no contraindications exist.

Clinical trials have shown that QUADRACEL is safe and immunogenic if administered at the same time as other vaccines (including meningococcal C conjugate vaccine and hepatitis B vaccine). When both vaccines are indicated, QUADRACEL may be used to reconstitute Act HIB for administration of both vaccines in a single injection.

NACI recommends that unless otherwise indicated, vaccines administered simultaneously should be given using separate syringes at separate sites.

QUADRACEL should not be mixed in the same syringe with other parenterals, with the exception of Act-HIB when both vaccines are indicated.

DOSAGE AND ADMINISTRATION: Recommended Dose and Dosage Adjustment: For routine immunization, QUADRACEL is recommended as a 4-dose series, with a single dose of 0.5 mL of QUADRACEL at 2, 4, 6 and 18 months of age.

If for any reason this schedule is delayed, it is recommended that 3 doses be administered with an interval of 2 months between each dose, followed by a fourth dose administered approximately 6 to 12 months after the third dose.

Whenever feasible, QUADRACEL should be used for all 4 doses in the vaccination series as there are no clinical data to support the use of QUADRACEL with any other licensed acellular pertussis combination vaccine in a mixed sequence. For situations where a different brand of DTaP, DTaP-IPV or DTaP-IPV/Hib vaccine was originally used, or where the brand is unknown, please refer to the latest edition of the Canadian Immunization Guide.

NACI recommends that premature infants whose clinical condition is satisfactory should be immunized with full doses of vaccine at the same chronological age and according to the same schedule as full-term infants, regardless of birth weight.

Fractional doses (doses <0.5 mL) should not be given. The effect of fractional doses on the safety and efficacy has not been determined.

In compliance with NACI's recommended immunization schedule, the childhood immunization series should be completed with a single booster dose of 0.5 mL of QUADRACEL administered between 4 and 6 years of age (i.e., at the time of school entry). Alternatively, ADACEL [Tetanus Toxoid, Reduced Diphtheria Toxoid and Acellular Pertussis Vaccine Adsorbed] and IPV may be administered at separate sites for this booster at 4 to 6 years of age. This booster dose is unnecessary if the fourth dose of QUADRACEL was administered after the child's fourth birthday.

QUADRACEL should not be administered to persons less than 2 months or to persons 7 years of age or older. (See Indications and Clinical Use.)

Administration: Inspect for extraneous particulate matter and/or discolouration before use. If these conditions exist, the product should not be administered.

Shake the vial well until a uniform, cloudy, suspension results. Cleanse the vial stopper with a suitable germicide prior to withdrawing the dose. Do not remove either the stopper or the metal seal holding it in place.

Aseptic technique must be used. Use a separate, sterile syringe and needle, or a sterile disposable unit, for each individual patient to prevent disease transmission. Needles should not be recapped but should be disposed of according to biohazard waste guidelines.

Before injection, the skin over the site to be injected should be cleansed with a suitable germicide. Administer the total volume of 0.5 mL **intramuscularly** (I.M.). In infants younger than 1 year, the anterolateral aspect of the thigh provides the largest muscle and is the preferred site of injection. In older children, the deltoid muscle is usually large enough for injection.

Give the patient a permanent personal immunization record. In addition, it is essential that the physician or nurse record the immunization history in the permanent medical record of each patient. This permanent office record should contain the name of the vaccine, date given, dose, manufacturer and lot number.

ACTION AND CLINICAL PHARMACOLOGY: Diphtheria and Tetanus: Strains of *C. diphtheriae* that produce diphtheria toxin can cause severe or fatal illness characterized by membranous inflammation of the upper respiratory tract and toxin-induced damage to the myocardium and nervous system. Protection against disease attributable to *C. diphtheriae* is due to the development of neutralizing antibodies to diphtheria toxin. A serum diphtheria antitoxin level of 0.01 IU/mL is the lowest level giving some degree of protection. Antitoxin levels of at least 0.1 IU/mL are generally regarded as protective. Levels of 1.0 IU/mL have been associated with long-term protection.

Tetanus is an acute and often-fatal disease caused by an extremely potent neurotoxin produced by *C. tetani*. The toxin causes neuromuscular dysfunction, with rigidity and spasms of skeletal muscles. Protection against disease attributable to *C. tetani* is due to the development of neutralizing antibodies to tetanus toxin. A serum tetanus antitoxin level of at least 0.01 IU/mL, measured by neutralization assay, is considered the minimum protective level. A tetanus antitoxin level of at least 0.1 IU/mL as measured by the ELISA used in clinical studies of QUADRACEL is considered protective for tetanus. Levels of 1.0 IU/mL have been associated with long-term protection.

In a clinical trial in Canada, after 4 doses of QUADRACEL, 100% (N=104) of immunized children achieved serum diphtheria and tetanus antitoxin levels of at least 0.01 IU/mL. 99.0% and 100% of these children achieved serum antitoxin levels of at least 0.1 IU/mL for diphtheria and tetanus, respectively. After a booster dose of QUADRACEL at 4 to 6 years of age, in a clinical trial in Canada, 100% (N=125) of children achieved serum diphtheria and tetanus antitoxin levels of at least 0.1 IU/mL.

After completion of the childhood immunization series, circulating antibodies to diphtheria and tetanus toxoids gradually decline but are thought to persist at protective levels for up to 10 years. NACI recommends diphtheria and tetanus toxoids boosters every 10 years.

Pertussis: Pertussis (whooping cough) is a respiratory disease caused by *B. pertussis*. This Gram-negative coccobacillus produces a variety of biologically active components, though their role in either the pathogenesis of, or immunity to, pertussis has not been clearly defined. The mechanism of protection from *B. pertussis* disease is not well understood. However, in a clinical trial in Sweden (Sweden I Efficacy Trial), pertussis components in QUADRACEL (i.e., PT, FHA, PRN and FIM) have been shown to prevent pertussis in infants with a protective efficacy of 85.2% using the World Health Organization (WHO) case definition (≥21 consecutive days of paroxysmal cough with culture or serologic confirmation or epidemiological link to a confirmed case). In the same study, the protective efficacy against mild disease was 77.9%.

Minimum serum antibody levels to specific pertussis vaccine components that confer protection against the development of clinical pertussis have not been identified. Nevertheless, a number of studies have demonstrated a correlation between the presence of serum antibody responses to pertussis vaccine components and protection against clinical disease. In a controlled clinical trial in Sweden (Sweden II Trial), the efficacy of a DTaP vaccine with the same formulation of five pertussis antigens as QUADRACEL was demonstrated to provide a two-fold to three-fold higher protection against pertussis with any cough compared to the vaccine containing three pertussis antigens. The observed difference supports the role of FIM in the protection against colonization of *B. pertussis* and mild disease.

In a recent publication, Bettinger et al reviewed pertussis cases during 1991-2004 using surveillance data from the Canadian Immunization Monitoring Program, Active (IMPACT), an active surveillance network based in 12 pediatric tertiary-care hospitals across Canada. Overall, the data show declining rates of pertussis during the years in which PENTACEL (QUADRACEL in combination with Act-HIB) has been used (1999-2004) compared to the period when whole-cell pertussis vaccine was used (1991-1996). Among children 1-4 years of age, incidence of pertussis declined 85%. Data from the Northwest Territories, Newfoundland and Labrador and British Columbia support national and IMPACT data demonstrating a progressive decline of pertussis cases among infants and children through 9 years of age.

Poliomyelitis: Inactivated poliomyelitis vaccine induces the production of detectable levels of neutralizing antibodies against each type of poliovirus. The detection of type-specific neutralizing antibodies has been correlated with protection. A clinical study of QUADRACEL in 104 Canadian infants showed that, after 4 doses, 100% of vaccinated children achieved protective antibody levels (titres ≥1:8) to poliovirus types 1, 2, and 3 following the primary series. In a clinical study in Canada, 100% (N=125) of children immunized with QUADRACEL at 4 to 6 years of age achieved protective antibody levels (titres ≥1:8) to poliovirus types 1, 2, and 3.

Duration of Effect: To ensure optimal protection during childhood, 4 consecutive doses should be given at 2, 4, 6 and 18 months of age. A booster with a vaccine containing diphtheria, tetanus, acellular pertussis with or without IPV is required at 4 to 6 years.

STORAGE AND STABILITY: Store at 2 to 8°C. **Do not freeze.** Discard product if exposed to freezing.

Do not use vaccine after expiration date.

INFORMATION FOR THE PATIENT: Published in e-CPS, available by subscription at www.e-cps.ca.

DOSAGE FORMS, COMPOSITION AND PACKAGING: Each dose (0.5 mL) of sterile, uniform, cloudy, white to off-white suspension contains: diphtheria toxoid 15 Lf, tetanus toxoid 5 Lf, pertussis toxoid (PT) 20 µg, filamentous haemagglutinin (FHA) 20 µg, pertactin (PRN) 3 µg, fimbriae types 2 and 3 (FIM) 5 µg, inactivated poliomyelitis vaccine type 1 (Mahoney) 40 D-antigen units, type 2 (MEF-1) 8 D-antigen units, type 3 (Saukett) 32 D-antigen units, aluminum phosphate (adjuvant) (aluminum 0.33 mg) 1.5 mg, 2-phenoxyethanol 0.6% v/v, polysorbate 80 10 ppm (by calculation). Manufacturing Process Residuals: BSA, formaldehyde, glutaraldehyde, neomycin and polymyxin B may be present in trace amounts.

Single dose vials of 0.5 mL; packages of 1 and 5. Packages of 5 doses containing QUADRACEL (5×0.5 mL vials) for reconstitution of Act-HIB (5×1 dose vials) sold under the tradename PENTACEL. The stoppers of the vials for QUADRACEL do not contain latex (natural rubber).

Quelicin® Injection ℞

succinylcholine chloride

Neuromuscular Blocking Agent

Hospira

SUPPLIED: 20 mg/mL: Each mL contains: succinylcholine chloride 20 mg with methylparaben and propylparaben as preservatives contains also sodium chloride for tonicity and water for injection. May contain sodium hydroxide and/or hydrochloric acid to adjust pH at approximately 4. Multidose vials of 10 and 20 mL, boxes of 25.

100 mg/mL: Each mL contains: succinylcholine chloride 100 mg, water for injection and sodium hydroxide and/or hydrochloric acid to adjust pH to about 4. This solution **must be diluted** for i.v. use. Any unused reconstituted portion should be discarded. Vials of 10 mL containing 5 mL solution, boxes of 25.

All units must be kept refrigerated (2 to 8°C) to prevent loss of potency. These products are stable for up to 14 days at room temperature without significant loss of potency.

Quinapril ℞

CPhA Monograph

see *ACE Inhibitors*

Quinidine

quinidine gluconate

quinidine sulfate

Antiarrhythmic—Antimalarial

CPhA Monograph

Date of Revision: July 2010

This monograph has been compiled by CPhA and reviewed by experts. It may contain information different from that found in Health Canada-approved Product Monographs. The reader is referred to the *CPS* Editorial Policy for more information.

SUMMARY PRODUCT INFORMATION:

Drug[a]	Route of Administration	Dosage Form	Strength
Quinidine gluconate	Intravenous	Solution	80 mg/mL
Quinidine sulphate	Oral	Tablet	200 mg, 300 mg

[a] Quinidine is available in Canada through the Special Access Programme (see Appendix 2).

PHARMACOLOGY: Quinidine is a class IA antiarrhythmic agent according to the Vaughan-Williams classification. It depresses most cardiac tissues by a direct action on cardiac cells.

Quinidine depresses the rapid inward depolarizing sodium current, thereby reducing the amplitude of the action potential without affecting the resting potential. The slope of the slow depolarization phase of Purkinje fibres is reduced, and the threshold voltage for reactivation is increased by an effect on the sodium current. The result is a reduction in excitability, conduction velocity and contractility in most parts of the heart, with an increase in the refractory periods and duration of action potential in the atria, ventricles and Purkinje tissues.

In addition, quinidine inhibits many potassium channels, suppressing the repolarizing delayed rectifier current; this action may contribute to quinidine's beneficial effects in atrial fibrillation. Quinidine also raises the ventricular defibrillation threshold.

Quinidine has anticholinergic activity, and acts peripherally as an α-adrenergic antagonist (i.e., a vasodilator).

By slowing conduction and prolonging the effective refractory period, quinidine can interrupt or prevent re-entrant arrhythmias, including atrial flutter, atrial fibrillation and paroxysmal supraventricular tachycardia.

In patients with sick sinus syndrome, quinidine may cause marked sinus node depression and bradycardia. In most patients, however, quinidine is associated with an increase in sinus rate and AV conduction, presumably through the combination of its anticholinergic effects and reflex increases in sympathetic activity.

Quinidine prolongs the QT interval in a dose-related fashion. Even at therapeutic serum concentrations, and especially in the presence of hypokalemia, this may lead to increased ventricular automaticity and polymorphic ventricular tachycardias, including torsades de pointes.

In patients with normal conduction time, a 50% increase in QRS duration indicates cardiotoxicity, and therefore, the increase in the QRS interval should not exceed 25% of the control value.

Quinidine has antimalarial activity and is used iv to treat severe and complicated *P. falciparum* malaria. It has been associated with clearing of parasitemia and high rates of survival.

Quinidine is available in Canada as the gluconate and sulfate salts (see Table 1).

Table 1: Quinidine

Comparison of Available Salts

Quinidine Salt	Equivalent Dose (mg)	% Quinidine Base
Quinidine gluconate	267	62
Quinidine sulfate	200	83

Pharmacokinetics: Each salt dissociates in the gastrointestinal tract to release quinidine base, which is rapidly and almost completely absorbed from the small intestine. The different salts of the drug are absorbed at different rates. Quinidine concentrations are generally higher and appear earlier when the drug is administered on an empty stomach, but the amount of drug absorbed is not diminished by the presence of food in the digestive tract.

Quinidine tablets have a bioavailability of approximately 70%. Peak plasma concentrations will vary among individuals primarily as a result of individual variations in first pass metabolism. Quinidine is widely distributed to all tissues except the brain. Quinidine crosses the placenta and is distributed into breast milk. At therapeutic plasma concentrations, the plasma protein binding of quinidine is 70% to 90% in adults and older children, but in infants and neonates it may be as low as 50% to 70%.

The onset of action of quinidine is 1 to 3 hours, with therapeutic cardiovascular effects lasting for 6 to 8 hours following an oral dose.

The elimination half-life is approximately 6 to 8 hours in adults and 3 to 4 hours in children but varies considerably among individuals. Quinidine is metabolized in the liver by the cytochrome P450 isoenzyme, CYP3A4. Some of its metabolites may be therapeutically active. Decreased liver function does not seem to significantly affect the plasma clearance of the drug. Approximately 10% to 50% is excreted unchanged in the urine within 24 hours. Renal excretion is by glomerular filtration and secretion by proximal renal tubules. Renal clearance diminishes as urinary pH increases. Fecal excretion accounts for less than 5% of the oral dose.

Traditionally, the average therapeutic range for quinidine has been 6 to 15 µmol/L (2 to 5 µg/mL). Toxicity was generally associated with a serum quinidine concentration above 15 µmol/L (5 µg/mL). However, values differ based on the assay method used. Currently available methods which are more specific than older methods report lower serum quinidine concentrations.

The concentration necessary to produce a therapeutic effect will depend on the individual as well as the type, severity and duration of the arrhythmia. When efficacy is established a serum drug concentration should be determined, against which future concentrations should be compared if arrhythmia recurs or the dose is altered. Sampling is usually done just prior to the next dose.

Small amounts of quinidine are removed by hemodialysis; the drug is not removed by peritoneal dialysis.

INDICATIONS:

> No antiarrhythmic drug has been shown to reduce the incidence of sudden death in patients with asymptomatic ventricular arrhythmias. Most antiarrhythmic drugs have the potential to cause dangerous arrhythmias; some have been shown to be associated with an increased incidence of sudden death. In light of the above, physicians should carefully consider the risks and benefits of antiarrhythmic therapy for all patients with ventricular arrhythmias.

Health Canada-approved indications include:

- treatment and prevention of recurrence of atrial fibrillation or flutter. Current guidelines do not recommend quinidine as a first line agent for this indication [*Circulation* 2006;114;700-52].
- treatment of other supraventricular arrythmias, e.g., paroxysmal atrial or AV junctional tachycardia. Other treatment options are preferred over quinidine [*Circulation* 2003;108(15):1871-909].
- treatment of documented life-threatening ventricular arrhythmias, such as sustained ventricular tachycardia. Quinidine may also be used for the treatment of patients with documented symptomatic ventricular arrhythmias when the symptoms are of sufficient severity to require treatment. Other treatments should be considered before using quinidine [*J Am Coll Cardiol* 2006;48(5):1064-108].
- parenteral administration for the treatment of life-threatening *P. falciparum* malaria. For more information, consult the *Canadian Recommendations for the Prevention and Treatment of Malaria Among International Travellers,* available from: www.phac-aspc.gc.ca/publicat/ccdr-rmtc/04vol30/30s1/index-eng.php.

CONTRAINDICATIONS: Second-degree or complete atrioventricular block, junctional or idioventricular conduction disturbance that might be aggravated by quinidine, uncompensated heart failure, digitalis intoxication, prolonged QT interval (see also Warnings); patients manifesting clinical signs or having a past history of idiosyncrasy or hypersensitivity to quinidine or other cinchona derivatives (e.g., febrile reactions, skin eruptions, thrombocytopenic purpura, systemic lupus erythematosus-like syndrome); history of drug-induced torsades de pointes; myasthenia gravis.

WARNINGS: Mortality: The results of the Cardiac Arrhythmia Suppression Trial (CAST) in postmyocardial infarction patients with asymptomatic ventricular arrhythmias showed a significant increase in mortality and in nonfatal cardiac arrest rate in patients treated with certain antiarrhythmic agents compared with a matched placebo group. Whether these results apply to other patient populations, or to other antiarrhythmic agents such as quinidine, is uncertain, but it is prudent to consider these results when using any antiarrhythmic agent [*N Engl J Med* 1991;324(12):781-8].

Quinidine should be used with extreme caution in the presence of: incomplete AV block (since a complete block and asystole may result); digitalized patients (quinidine may cause unpredictable abnormalities of rhythm); partial bundle branch block; severe heart failure, cardiogenic shock, severe bradycardia and hypotensive states (quinidine may have a depressant effect on myocardial contractility and arterial pressure); hepatic and renal insufficiency (especially renal tubular acidosis, because of the potential for quinidine accumulation).

In the treatment of atrial fibrillation or flutter, conversion to sinus rhythm may be preceded by an extremely rapid ventricular rate as AV conduction is enhanced. Agents that inhibit AV node conduction such as digoxin, beta-blockers or verapamil should be used prior to the initiation of quinidine therapy for atrial fibrillation or flutter.

Conversion of atrial fibrillation may be associated with embolism; therefore, anticoagulant treatment may be necessary before administration of quinidine.

Cardiotoxicity: Quinidine cardiotoxicity may be manifested by increased PR and QT intervals, 50% widening of QRS, ventricular ectopic beats or tachycardia. Appearance of these toxic signs during quinidine administration mandates immediate discontinuation of the drug and close clinical and ECG monitoring.

Digitalis Intoxication: Quinidine slows the elimination of digoxin and simultaneously reduces digoxin's apparent volume of distribution. As a result, serum digoxin concentration may double or even triple. When used concurrently, digoxin dosage should be reduced by approximately 50%, plasma concentrations should be monitored and patients observed closely for digoxin toxicity.

Hepatotoxicity: A few cases of hepatotoxicity, including granulomatous hepatitis, due to quinidine hypersensitivity have been reported. Unexplained fever and/or elevation of hepatic enzymes, particularly in the early stages of therapy, warrant consideration of possible hepatotoxicity. Cessation of quinidine in these cases usually results in the disappearance of toxicity.

Syncopal Episodes: Quinidine syncope may occur as a complication of long-term therapy. It is manifested by sudden loss of consciousness and ventricular arrhythmias with bizarre QRS complexes of the torsades de pointes type. This syndrome does not appear to be related to dose or plasma concentration, but occurs more often with prolonged QT intervals. Syncopal episodes frequently terminate spontaneously, but sometimes are fatal. If quinidine-induced syncope occurs, the drug should be discontinued immediately.

Vagal Stimulation: Because quinidine antagonizes the effect of vagal excitation upon the atrium and the AV node, the administration of parasympathomimetic drugs or the use of any other procedure to enhance vagal activity may fail to terminate paroxysmal supraventricular tachycardia in patients receiving quinidine.

PRECAUTIONS: Proarrhythmic effects, or worsening of arrhythmias, can occur and are more likely in patients with sustained ventricular arrhythmias and left ventricular dysfunction.

Quinidine can have proarrhythmic effects in patients who have survived cardiac arrest or had previous MI and is not recommended in these patients.

An oral test dose of quinidine should be given initially in order to identify possible hypersensitivity to quinidine. Although rare, the possibility of hypersensitivity should be constantly considered, especially during the first week of therapy.

When initiating therapy, hospitalization for close clinical observation and ECG monitoring is indicated when large doses (>2 g/day) are used, or in patients at increased risk such as those with a history of syncope or presyncope due to ventricular arrhythmias.

Patients should be instructed to notify their physician immediately if they experience fever, unusual bleeding or bruising, rash, ringing in the ears or visual disturbances.

Complete blood counts, liver and renal function tests should be performed periodically during chronic quinidine therapy, especially during the first 4 to 8 weeks of therapy.

Serum Potassium: Quinidine's activity is enhanced by potassium and reduced if hypokalemia is present.

Established Atrial Fibrillation: The use of quinidine in established atrial fibrillation is controversial. Weigh the benefits of such use in each patient against possible hazards.

Parenteral Administration: Overly rapid infusion of quinidine may cause peripheral vascular collapse and severe hypotension. Blood pressure and ECG should be monitored continuously during iv administration; quinidine administration should be discontinued if there is a significant fall in blood pressure. Because the kinetics of absorption may vary with the patient's peripheral perfusion, im injection of quinidine is not recommended. IM injections are typically followed by moderate to severe local pain. Some patients will develop tender nodules at the site of injection that persist for several weeks.

P. falciparum Malaria: Complicated *P. falciparum* infection represents a medical emergency, and prompt administration of a schizonticidal drug is essential. All patients with severe *P. falciparum* malaria requiring iv administration of quinidine should be treated in an intensive care facility where hemodynamic and ECG monitoring is available. Even in patients without pre-existing cardiac disease, antimalarial use of quinidine has occasionally been associated with hypotension, QT prolongation and cinchonism.

Pregnancy: Quinidine has been used during pregnancy, dating back at least to the 1920s, to treat a variety of maternal and fetal arrhythmias and malaria. There have been no reports linking quinidine to congenital defects. Neonatal thrombocytopenia has been reported after maternal use of quinidine; however, among class IA antiarrhythmic agents, quinidine is considered to be relatively well tolerated during pregnancy.

Lactation: Whether quinidine is safe during lactation is controversial. Quinidine is present in breast milk at concentrations slightly lower than those in maternal serum. Because of the potential accumulation of the drug in neonates due to the immature liver, some expert groups recommend avoiding breast-feeding during quinidine therapy. Others consider quinidine compatible with breast-feeding.

Children: Safety and efficacy of antiarrhythmic use of quinidine in children has not been established. In antimalarial trials, quinidine was as safe and effective in pediatric patients as in adults. Children in these trials received the same doses (on a mg/kg basis) as adults.

Drug Interactions: In addition to being a substrate of CYP3A4, quinidine is an inhibitor of CYP3A4 and CYP2D6 and can decrease the clearance of other substrates of these isoenzymes, potentially increasing their toxicity. Table 2 presents many of the possible drug interactions involving quinidine.

Table 2: Quinidine

Drug Interactions

Interacting Drug	Potential Effect
Amiloride	Increased prolongation of QRS interval
Amiodarone	Increased quinidine plasma concentration and prolonged cardiac conduction
Antiarrhythmics (e.g., disopyramide, flecainide, mexiletine)	Increased serum concentrations of several antiarrhythmics; enhanced cardiac depressant effects and potential toxicity
β-blockers	Decreased metabolism of some β-blockers; additive cardiac depressant effects
Cholinergic drugs (e.g., neostigmine, edrophonium, pyridostigmine)	Quinidine may antagonize cholinergic effects. May result in failure of quinidine to terminate PSVT
Codeine, hydrocodone[a]	Blocked analgesic effect of codeine or hydrocodone
Colchicine	Increased colchicine serum concentrations
Digoxin	Markedly increased digoxin plasma concentration (see Warnings)
Grapefruit juice	Increased plasma concentrations of quinidine
Hepatic enzyme inducers (e.g., barbiturates, phenytoin, rifampin)	Enhanced hepatic metabolism and decreased plasma concentration of quinidine
Hepatic enzyme inhibitors (e.g., cimetidine, erythromycin, fluconazole)	Reduced hepatic metabolism and increased plasma concentration of quinidine
Neuromuscular blockers (e.g., pancuronium, succinylcholine, tubocurarine)	Potentiation of neuromuscular blockade
Nifedipine	Decreased quinidine plasma concentration
Potassium	Quinidine effects enhanced by potassium and reduced by hypokalemia
QT prolonging agents (e.g., erythromycin, haloperidol)	Additive QT prolongation. Potential for serious arrythmias
Quinine	Additive effects of both drugs
Tamoxifen	Decreased hepatic production of active tamoxifen metabolites
Tricyclic antidepressants	Decreased clearance of some tricyclic antidepressants; additive QT prolongation
Urinary alkalinizers (e.g., acetazolamide, sodium bicarbonate, some antacids)	Decreased renal excretion of quinidine and increased blood concentration
Verapamil	Increased quinidine plasma concentration, hypotension
Warfarin	Enhanced hypoprothrombinemic effect and bleeding

[a] Codeine's analgesic effect is mainly due to its metabolism by the hepatic isoenzyme CYP2D6 to morphine. Quinidine inhibits this enzyme. Hydrocodone may depend on the same isoenzyme for conversion to active metabolites.

Drug-Food Interactions: see Table 2, Grapefruit juice.

ADVERSE EFFECTS: Cardiac: ventricular tachycardia (most frequently torsades de pointes or ventricular fibrillation), bradycardia, decreased contractility, reduction in blood pressure, syncope (see Warnings, Syncopal Episodes) and ECG abnormalities (marked increase in PR, QRS and QT intervals) can occur.

Central Nervous System: headache, vertigo, apprehension, excitement, confusion, delirium, ataxia, mental depression.

Gastrointestinal: The most frequent adverse reactions occurring in approximately 30% of patients are gastrointestinal disorders (diarrhea, nausea, vomiting, esophagitis, abdominal cramps and anorexia). These can occur as isolated reactions to therapeutic plasma concentrations of quinidine, but they may also be the first signs of cinchonism. Gastrointestinal side effects may be less severe with extended-release formulations.

Hearing: tinnitus, decreased auditory capacity, transitory deafness.

Hematologic: hemolytic anemia, aplastic anemia, thrombocytopenia, neutropenia, leukocytosis, leukopenia, agranulocytosis, hemolysis in patients with G-6-PD deficiency.

Hepatic: increased hepatic enzyme serum concentrations, hepatitis (see Warnings).

Hypersensitivity: fever, urticaria, flushing, exfoliative rash, bronchospasm, psoriasiform rash, photosensitivity, pruritus, lymphadenopathy, vasculitis, hepatotoxicity, thrombocytopenic purpura, uveitis, angioedema, Sjögren's syndrome and SLE-like syndrome. Serious reactions are manifested by respiratory arrest or cardiovascular collapse.

Musculoskeletal: arthralgia, myalgia, increased serum skeletal muscle creatine phosphokinase.

Ophthalmic: mydriasis, blurred vision, disturbed color perception, photophobia, diplopia, night blindness, scotomata, reduced visual fields, optic neuritis.

Miscellaneous: Cinchonism is most often a sign of chronic toxicity but may appear in sensitive patients after a single dose. Symptoms include tinnitus and other hearing disturbances, nausea, diarrhea, vertigo, blurred vision, headache, dizziness, confusion and tremor.

OVERDOSE:

For management of a suspected drug overdose, CPhA recommends that you contact your **regional Poison Control Centre**. See the *CPS* Directory section for a list of Poison Control Centres.

DOSAGE: Equivalent doses for each of the available quinidine salts can be found in Table 1.
Oral: Dosage based on quinidine sulfate equivalent. Administer a preliminary test dose of a single tablet of quinidine sulfate to determine whether the patient has a quinidine idiosyncrasy. Continuous or frequent ECG monitoring is desirable when quinidine therapy is initiated, especially if using large doses (>2 g quinidine sulfate daily). Gastrointestinal symptoms such as nausea, vomiting, diarrhea and colic may be minimized by giving the drug with food.
Premature Atrial and Ventricular Contractions: 200 to 300 mg of quinidine sulfate 3 or 4 times daily. Alternatively, a loading dose of 12 mg/kg, followed by a maintenance dose of 6 mg/kg every 4 to 6 hours has been recommended.
Paroxysmal Supraventricular Tachycardia: 400 to 600 mg of quinidine sulfate every 2 or 3 hours until the paroxysm is terminated.
Atrial Fibrillation or Flutter: Various schedules of quinidine administration have been utilized. One widely used technique is to give 200 mg of quinidine sulfate orally every 2 or 3 hours for up to 8 doses, with subsequent daily increase of the individual dose until sinus rhythm is restored or toxic effects occur. Most clinicians recommend, however, that 300 to 400 mg of quinidine sulfate be given every 6 hours for conversion of atrial fibrillation. The total daily dose should not exceed 3 to 4 g of quinidine sulfate in any regimen.
The patient should be anticoagulated before conversion of atrial fibrillation. Ventricular rate should be brought under control with digoxin, verapamil or β blockers. Heart failure should be controlled if present. Patients should be digitalized before quinidine administration for atrial flutter.
Maintenance Therapy: 200 to 300 mg of quinidine sulfate 3 or 4 times daily.
Parenteral: Specialized references should be consulted for information on the use of parenteral quinidine in the treatment of arrhythmias or malaria.

Quinine-Odan™
quinine sulfate
Antimalarial

Odan

SUPPLIED: Capsules: 200 mg: Each clear capsule imprinted ODAN 200 contains: quinine sulfate USP 200 mg. Nonmedicinal ingredients: croscarmellose sodium, gelatin, microcrystalline cellulose, sodium lauryl sulfate, starch, stearic acid and talc. Gluten-, lactose-, paraben-, sodium-, sulfite- and tartrazine-free. Bottles of 100 and 500.
300 mg: Each clear capsule imprinted ODAN 300 contains: quinine sulfate USP 300 mg. Nonmedicinal ingredients: croscarmellose sodium, gelatin, microcrystalline cellulose, sodium lauryl sulfate, starch, stearic acid and talc. Gluten-, lactose-, paraben-, sodium-, sulfite- and tartrazine-free. Bottles of 100 and 500.
Tablets: Each white, round, scored tablet, monogrammed ODAN/300, contains: quinine sulfate USP 300 mg. Nonmedicinal ingredients: colloidal silicon dioxide, croscarmellose sodium, gelatin, hydroxypropyl methylcellulose, microcrystalline cellulose, PEG 400, sodium lauryl sulfate, starch, stearic acid and talc. Bottles of 100.

Quinine Sulfate
Antimalarial

CPhA Monograph

Date of Revision: October 2006

This monograph has been compiled by CPhA and reviewed by experts. It may contain information different from that found in Health Canada-approved Product Monographs. The reader is referred to the *CPS* Editorial Policy for more information.

PHARMACOLOGY: Quinine, an alkaloid derived from the bark of the cinchona tree, decreases the response of skeletal muscle to tetanic stimulation by increasing the refractory period of the muscle and affecting calcium distribution in individual muscle fibres. The excitability of the motor end-plate is also decreased causing a reduction in the response of the muscle to acetylcholine and repetitive nerve stimulation.
Quinine has antimalarial activity and is used orally in combination with a second drug to treat nonsevere *P. falciparum* infections acquired in zones where chloroquine resistance has been reported. Patients with nonsevere infections unable to tolerate oral therapy or those patients with severe and complicated *P. falciparum* infections should receive iv drug therapy. Quinine and its optical isomer, quinidine, are both effective in the treatment of *P. falciparum* malaria. Neither is available parenterally through the usual procurement channels. For information on obtaining parenteral quinine or quinidine, contact the Special Access Programme, Health Canada (see Appendix 2).
Quinine is also contained in some commercial nonalcoholic beverages, such as tonic water, as a flavoring agent.
Pharmacokinetics: Following oral administration, quinine is rapidly and almost completely absorbed from the gastrointestinal tract. It is widely distributed to body tissues and approximately 70% protein bound. Quinine readily crosses the placenta and is excreted into breast milk. Concentrations in CSF are 2 to 7% of plasma levels. Quinine is metabolized in the liver by the cytochrome P450 isoenzyme CYP3A4, and excreted mainly in the urine. Less than 5% is excreted unchanged in the urine. Renal excretion of the drug is enhanced at low urinary pH. The elimination half-life of quinine in healthy individuals ranges from 7 to 12 hours. Plasma concentrations of the drug may be higher and the half-life longer in patients with malaria due to impaired hepatic metabolism of the drug.
INDICATIONS: Health Canada-approved indications include:
- orally, in combination with a second drug, in the treatment of uncomplicated chloroquine-resistant *P. falciparum* malaria.
- iv quinine or iv quinidine, in combination with a second drug, for those patients unable to tolerate oral therapy or those with severe *P. falciparum* infections.
- treatment of chloroquine-resistant *P. vivax* malaria (higher doses may be required). Expert advice from an infectious or tropical disease specialist should be sought for the management of these cases.

Uses Not Approved in Canada: Quinine has also been used to prevent nocturnal recumbency leg muscle cramps, although its efficacy and safety for this indication have not been well established [*Cochrane Database Syst Rev* 2009;(1):CD005044].
CONTRAINDICATIONS: Quinine is contraindicated in patients who have a known hypersensitivity to the drug. Cross-sensitivity between quinine and quinidine may occur.
Quinine should not be used in patients with G-6-PD deficiency; tinnitus; optic neuritis; myasthenia gravis; hypoglycemia; history of blackwater fever and thrombocytopenic purpura (associated with previous quinine ingestion).
WARNINGS: See Precautions.
PRECAUTIONS: Quinine has quinidine-like activity; the same precautions should be taken with quinine as with quinidine in patients with atrial fibrillation. Advise patients to notify physician if cutaneous, angioedematous, visual or auditory symptoms occur. If evidence of hemolysis appears, stop the drug immediately.
Patients with hypersensitivity to quinine should be advised to avoid beverages such as tonic water that contain quinine as a flavoring agent.
Drug Interactions: Antacids: Concomitant administration of antacids and quinine may decrease or delay the absorption of oral quinine.
Anticoagulants, warfarin: Quinine may enhance the anticoagulant effects of warfarin.
Cimetidine: Cimetidine may inhibit the metabolism of quinine and increase the risk of quinine toxicity.
Digitalis Glycosides: Quinine increases plasma concentrations of digoxin. Monitor digoxin and digitoxin serum concentrations in patients receiving quinine.
Mefloquine: Concomitant use of quinine and mefloquine may cause ECG abnormalities or cardiac arrest. The risk of seizures may also be increased. Quinine therapy for malaria should be initiated with caution in patients who have received mefloquine for prophylaxis.
Neuromuscular blockers: Quinine may potentiate the effects of neuromuscular blockers such as pancuronium, succinylcholine and tubocurarine resulting in respiratory difficulties.
Urinary alkalinizers: Agents such as sodium bicarbonate and acetazolamide which increase urinary pH may inhibit the renal excretion of quinine and increase the risk of quinine toxicity.
Pregnancy: Quinine use during pregnancy should be avoided when possible, but may be considered necessary to treat chloroquin-resistant malaria in certain patients.
Lactation: Quinine is distributed into breast milk. No adverse effects have been reported in healthy infants exposed to quinine through breast milk. Infants with G-6-PD deficiency should not be exposed quinine through breast-feeding.
Children: Quinine is considered safe for use in children at recommended doses for the treatment of malaria.
ADVERSE EFFECTS: Cardiovascular: Conduction disturbances, ventricular tachycardia and anginal symptoms have occurred with prolonged quinine therapy in highly sensitive patients.
Endocrine: Hypoglycemia, which may be severe and recurrent, has been reported in some patients with severe malaria caused by *P. falciparum* who received quinine therapy, and there was some evidence that quinine-induced insulin secretion may have been one of several possible precipitating factors.
Eyes: Quinine can affect the retina and optic nerve, causing symptoms such as photophobia, night blindness, disturbed color perception, blurred or double vision. Quinine's effect on the eye can occur in overdose or at therapeutic doses, and may or may not be reversible.
Hematologic: Thrombocytopenic purpura, leukopenia, pancytopenia, coagulopathy, hypoprothrombinemia and agranulocytosis have been reported. Massive hemolysis is a rare complication of quinine therapy.
Hypersensitivity Reactions: Cutaneous flushing, pruritus, scarlatiniform, maculopapular or urticarial skin eruptions, fever, facial edema, gastrointestinal distress, dyspnea, tinnitus and impairment of vision have been reported. Extreme flushing of the skin with intense, generalized pruritus is most common. Hemoglobinuria and asthma have been reported rarely.
Miscellaneous: Cinchonism: A syndrome known as cinchonism, named for the tree from which quinine is derived, can occur during prolonged therapy or following excessive doses of quinine. Symptoms can include tinnitus, headache, impaired hearing, nausea and blurred vision; in severe cases, vomiting, abdominal pain, diarrhea, dysrhythmias and hypotension can occur.

OVERDOSE:

Symptoms: In overdose, symptoms of "cinchonism" may be more pronounced. This includes auditory symptoms (e.g., tinnitus, vertigo), visual disturbances (e.g., blurring, diplopia, acute blindness — transitory, rarely permanent, may occur 24 h after overdose) and CNS symptoms (e.g., headache and confusion). Because of its antidysrhythmic effects on the heart, cardiovascular toxicity may include conduction disturbances and arrhythmias. Hypotension may lead to cardiac arrest and circulatory collapse. Gastrointestinal effects may occur in severe cases and include nausea, vomiting, abdominal pain and diarrhea. Other symptoms include coma, convulsions, respiratory depression and hypokalemia.
Treatment: It is recommended that a Poison Control Centre be contacted to obtain expert advice on the management of quinine overdose.
General management of quinine overdose includes supportive care with focus on maintaining ventilation, monitoring vital signs, fluid and electrolyte balance and ECG and correcting hypoglycemia, if it occurs. If ingestion of quinine is recent, consider administration of multiple dose therapy of activated charcoal every 2–4 hours to reduce quinine absorption. Hypotension unreponsive to iv fluids and patient positioning may be treated with vasopressor therapy such as dopamine or norepinephrine. Sodium bicarbonate iv can be used to treat QRS widening; monitor potassium level. Ventricular dysrhythmias unresponsive to alkalinization may respond to lidocaine, phenytoin or overdrive pacing. Seizures can be treated with iv benzodiazepines. Avoid class 1A and 1C antiarrhythmics, beta-blockers and calcium channel blockers because they may aggravate conduction abnormalities. Quinine is not removed by hemodialysis, peritoneal dialysis or charcoal hemoperfusion.

For management of a suspected drug overdose, CPhA recommends that you contact your **regional Poison Control Centre**. See the *CPS* Directory section for a list of Poison Control Centres.

DOSAGE: Quinine sulfate 300 mg is approximately equivalent to quinine base 250 mg. Quinine dihydrochloride 300 mg is approximately equivalent to quinine base 250 mg.
Malaria: Oral: Uncomplicated chloroquine-resistant P. falciparum malaria: quinine sulfate should be administered in conjunction with doxycycline, clindamycin or the combination product pyrimethamine/sulfadoxine.
Adults: Quinine sulfate 600 mg 3 times daily, after meals, for 3 to 7 days.
Children: Quinine sulfate 9 mg/kg to a maximum of 600 mg, 3 times daily, after meals, for 3 to 7 days.
Parenteral: Information on obtaining parenteral quinine can be found by contacting the Special Access Programme, Health Canada (see Appendix 2). Parenteral quinidine gluconate may also be used to treat severe, life-threatening *P. falciparum* malaria (see Quinidine, General Monograph).
Severe *P. falciparum* malaria: The 2 dosage regimens listed below are equally effective. Either regimen should be administered in conjunction with doxycycline, clindamycin or the combination product pyrimethamine/sulfadoxine. Therapy should be switched to oral quinine sulfate when the patient can swallow, to complete a 7-day treatment course. If parenteral therapy is required for more than 48 hours, the maintenance dose of quinine should be reduced by one-third to one-half.
a) If an infusion pump is available: Quinine dihydrochloride 7 mg/kg iv. over 30 minutes, followed immediately by quinine dihydrochloride 10 mg/kg diluted in 10 mL/kg isotonic fluid, iv over 4 hours; repeat every 8 hours until oral therapy can be instituted.
b) Without an infusion pump: Quinine dihydrochloride 20 mg/kg iv over 4 hours, then quinine dihydrochloride 10 mg/kg diluted in 10 mL/kg isotonic fluid, iv over 4 hours; repeat every 8 hours until oral therapy can be instituted.
Nocturnal Recumbency Leg Cramps (not an approved use in Canada): Oral: Quinine sulfate 200 to 300 mg at bedtime. If leg cramps do not occur for several consecutive nights during therapy, quinine may be discontinued to assess the need for continued therapy.

Quinolones ℞

CPhA Monograph

see *Fluoroquinolones*

The reader is invited to consult CPhA's monograph **Corticosteroids: Inhaled.**

Qvar™ ℞
beclomethasone dipropionate
Corticosteroid for Oral Inhalation

Graceway

Date of Preparation: April 13, 2000
Date of Revision: March 30, 2007

PHARMACOLOGY: Beclomethasone dipropionate is a diester of beclomethasone, a synthetic corticosteroid chemically related to dexamethasone. Beclomethasone differs from dexamethasone in having a chlorine at the 9-alpha carbon in place of a fluorine, and in having a 16 beta-methyl group instead of a 16 alpha-methyl group.

Bronchial inflammation is known to be an important component in the pathogenesis of asthma, occurring in both large and small airways. Glucocorticoids have multiple anti-inflammatory effects, inhibiting both inflammatory cells and release of inflammatory mediators. It is presumed that these anti-inflammatory actions play an important role in the efficacy of beclomethasone dipropionate (BDP) in controlling symptoms and improving lung function in asthma. Inhaled BDP probably acts as a topical anti-inflammatory agent at the site of deposition in the bronchial tree.

In two studies evaluating the deposition pattern of technetium-99m labeled QVAR (beclomethasone dipropionate), approximately 50-60% of the dose from the actuator (40% of the dose from the valve) of QVAR was deposited in the lungs. The imaging data suggest that QVAR, beclomethasone dipropionate formulated in hydrofluoroalkane-134a (HFA-BDP), deposited widely throughout the central, intermediate, and peripheral airways. In contrast, approximately 4-7% dose from the actuator (5% of the dose from the valve) of beclomethasone dipropionate formulated in chlorofluorocarbons (CFC-BDP) was deposited in the lungs, and deposition was limited to the central airways. Over 90% of the CFC-BDP dose was deposited in the oropharynx. The smaller particle size of QVAR explains the different deposition patterns compared with CFC-BDP. This accounts for the dosage adjustment recommended when switching patients from CFC-BDP to QVAR (see Dosage).

INDICATIONS: QVAR (beclomethasone dipropionate) is indicated for the prophylactic management of steroid-responsive bronchial asthma in patients 5 years and older.

QVAR may be effective in the management of asthmatics dependent or maintained on systemic corticosteroids and may permit replacement or significant reduction in the dosage of systemic corticosteroids.

Beclomethasone dipropionate is **not** indicated for the relief of acute bronchospasm.

CONTRAINDICATIONS: QVAR (beclomethasone dipropionate) is contraindicated in the primary treatment of status asthmaticus or other acute episodes of asthma or in patients with moderate to severe bronchiectasis where intensive measures are required.

QVAR is contraindicated in patients with untreated fungal, bacterial or tuberculous infections of the respiratory tract.

Hypersensitivity to any of the ingredients of this preparation contraindicates its use.

WARNINGS: For the transfer of patients being treated with oral corticosteroids, QVAR (beclomethasone dipropionate) should first be added to the existing oral steroid therapy, which is then gradually withdrawn.

After withdrawal from systemic corticosteroids, a number of months are required for recovery of hypothalamic-pituitary-adrenal (HPA) function. Particular care is needed in patients who are transferred from systemically active corticosteroids to inhaled corticosteroids. Deaths due to adrenal insufficiency have occurred in asthmatic patients during and after transfer from systemic corticosteroids to less systemically available inhaled corticosteroids.

Patients who have been previously maintained on 20 mg or more per day of prednisone (or its equivalent) may be most susceptible to problems associated with adrenal insufficiency, particularly when their systemic corticosteroids have been almost completely withdrawn. During this period of HPA suppression, patients may exhibit signs and symptoms of adrenal insufficiency when exposed to trauma, surgery, or infections, particularly gastroenteritis or other conditions with severe electrolyte loss. Although inhaled corticosteroids may provide control of asthmatic symptoms during these episodes, they do **not** provide systemically available steroid which is necessary for coping with these emergencies.

Transfer of patients from systemic steroid therapy to inhaled corticosteroids may unmask allergic conditions previously suppressed by the systemic steroid therapy, e.g., rhinitis, conjunctivitis, and eczema.

During periods of stress or severe asthmatic attack, patients who have been withdrawn from systemic corticosteroids should be instructed to resume systemic steroids (in large doses) immediately and to contact their physician for further instruction. These patients should also be instructed to carry a warning card indicating that they may need supplementary systemic steroids during periods of stress or severe asthma attack.

As with other inhalation therapy, paradoxical bronchospasm may occur characterized by an immediate increase in wheezing after dosing. This should be treated immediately with a fast-acting inhaled bronchodilator to relieve acute asthmatic symptoms. QVAR should be discontinued immediately, the patient assessed, and if necessary, alternative therapy instituted.

Increasing use of short-acting inhaled bronchodilators to control symptoms indicates deterioration of asthma control. Sudden and progressive deterioration in asthma control is potentially life-threatening and consideration should be given to increasing corticosteroid dosage. Patients should be instructed to contact their physicians if they find that relief with short-acting bronchodilator treatment becomes less effective or they need more inhalations than usual. During such episodes, patients may require therapy with systemic corticosteroids.

QVAR is not indicated for rapid relief of bronchospasm but for regular daily treatment of the underlying inflammation. Patients will require a fast and short acting inhaled bronchodilator to relieve acute asthmatic symptoms. There is no evidence that control of bronchial asthma can be achieved by the administration of QVAR in amounts greater than the recommended dosages.

Lack of response or severe exacerbations of asthma should be treated by increasing the dose of QVAR and, if necessary, by giving a systemic steroid and/or an antibiotic if there is an infection.

Persons who are on drugs that suppress the immune system are more susceptible to infections than healthy individuals. Chickenpox and measles, for example, can have a more serious or even fatal course in non-immune children or adults on corticosteroids. In children or adults who have not had these diseases, particular care should be taken to avoid exposure. It is not known how the dose, route and duration of corticosteroid administration affects the risk of developing a disseminated infection. Nor is the contribution of the underlying disease and/or prior corticosteroid treatment known. If exposed to chickenpox, prophylaxis with varicella-zoster immune globulin (VZIG) may be indicated. If exposed to measles, prophylaxis with pooled intramuscular immunoglobulin (IG) may be indicated. (See the respective package inserts for complete VZIG and IG prescribing information.) If chickenpox develops, treatment with antiviral agents may be considered.

Therapeutic dosages frequently cause the appearance of *C. albicans* (thrush) in the mouth and throat. The development of pharyngeal and laryngeal candidiasis is a cause for concern because the extent of its penetration into the respiratory tract is unknown. Patients may find it helpful to rinse out their mouths with water after using beclomethasone dipropionate. Symptomatic candidiasis can be treated with topical antifungal therapy while still continuing to use QVAR (see Precautions).

PRECAUTIONS: General: It is essential that the patients be instructed that QVAR (beclomethasone dipropionate) is a preventative agent which must be taken daily at the intervals recommended by their doctors and is not to be used as acute treatment for an asthmatic attack.

Patients should be advised to inform subsequent physicians of the prior use of corticosteroids.

Treatment with QVAR should not be stopped abruptly, but tapered off gradually.

The replacement of a systemic steroid with inhaled steroid must be gradual and carefully supervised by the physician since upon withdrawal systemic symptoms (e.g. joint and/or muscular pain, lassitude, depression) may occur despite maintenance or improvement of respiratory function. (See Dosage for details.)

Doses of QVAR up to 800 µg/day may permit control of asthmatic symptoms without clinically meaningful suppression of HPA function. Doses of QVAR exceeding 800 µg/day may cause clinically meaningful HPA suppression.

Systemic effects may occur with any inhaled corticosteroid, particularly at high doses prescribed for long periods; these effects are much less likely to occur than with oral corticosteroids. Possible systemic effects include adrenal suppression, growth retardation in children and adolescents, decrease in bone mineral density, cataract and glaucoma. It is important, therefore, that the dose of QVAR is titrated to the lowest dose at which effective control is maintained (see Adverse Effects).

Certain individuals can show greater susceptibility to the effects of inhaled corticosteroid than do most patients.

The long-term and systemic effects of BDP in human subjects are still not fully known. In particular, the effects resulting from chronic use of the agent on developmental or immunologic processes in the mouth, pharynx, trachea, and lung are unknown. During long-term therapy, HPA-axis function and hematological status should be assessed periodically.

Rare instances of glaucoma, increased intraocular pressure, and cataracts have been reported following the administration of very high doses of inhaled corticosteroids.

Eosinophilic Conditions: In rare cases, patients on inhaled beclomethasone dipropionate may present with systemic eosinophilic conditions, with some patients presenting with clinical features of vasculitis consistent with Churg-Strauss syndrome, a condition that is often treated with systemic corticosteroid therapy. These events usually, but not always, have been associated with the reduction and/or withdrawal of oral corticosteroid therapy following the introduction of beclomethasone dipropionate. Cases of serious eosinophilic conditions have also been reported with other inhaled corticosteroids in this clinical setting. Physicians should be alert to eosinophilia, vasculitic rash, worsening pulmonary symptoms, cardiac complications, and/or neuropathy presenting in their patients. A causal relationship between beclomethasone dipropionate and these underlying conditions has not been established.

Children: Eight-hundred and forty-three (843) children between the ages of 5 and 12 were treated with HFA beclomethasone diproprionate (HFA-BDP) in clinical trials.

Pregnancy: There are no adequate and well controlled studies of BDP in pregnant women. The use of BDP in pregnancy, nursing mothers, or women of childbearing potential requires that the possible benefits of the drug be weighed against the potential hazards to the mother, embryo, or fetus. Infants born of mothers who have received substantial doses of corticosteroids during pregnancy should be carefully observed for hypoadrenalism.

Labor and Delivery: Use of QVAR during labor and delivery has not been studied.

Lactation: Glucocorticoids are secreted in human milk. Because of the potential for serious adverse reactions in nursing infants from BDP, a decision should be made whether to discontinue nursing or to discontinue the drug, taking into account the importance of the drug to the mother.

Carcinogenesis, Mutagenesis, Impairment of Fertility: Glucocorticoids are known teratogens in rodent species and BDP is no exception. Teratology studies were done in rats, mice, and rabbits treated with subcutaneous BDP. Beclomethasone dipropionate was found to produce fetal resorptions, cleft palate, agnathia, microstomia, absence of tongue, delayed ossification, and partial agenesis of the thymus in these species. Well-controlled trials relating to fetal risk in humans are not available.

Effect on Infection: Corticosteroids may mask some signs of infections and new infections may appear. A decreased resistance to localised infection has been observed during corticosteroid therapy. This may require treatment with appropriate therapy or stopping the administration of beclomethasone dipropionate until the infection is eradicated.

Hypothyroidism and Cirrhosis: There is an enhanced effect of corticosteroids on patients with hypothyroidism and in those with cirrhosis.

Use of Corticosteroids and Acetylsalicylic Acid: Acetylsalicylic acid should be used cautiously in conjunction with corticosteroids in hypoprothrombinemia.

Proper Use of the Inhalation Device: To ensure the proper dosage and administration of the drug, the patient must be instructed by a physician or other health professional in the use of the inhalation aerosol (see Information for the Patient). Inhaler actuation should be synchronised with inspiration to ensure optimum delivery of the drug to the lungs.

Oral Hygiene: In some patients, corticosteroids may cause hoarseness or candidiasis of the mouth and throat (thrush). Adequate oral hygiene is of primary importance in minimizing overgrowth of micro-organisms such as *C. albicans*. Patients may find it helpful to rinse out their mouth with water after using the inhaler (see Dosage). Symptomatic candidiasis can be treated with topical anti-fungal therapy while still continuing treatment with QVAR.

Information to Be Provided to the Patient: See the illustrated Information for the Patient insert that is dispensed with the product. For patients switching from a CFC-BDP inhaler, the following should be mentioned:

You may notice a different taste or spray force with QVAR compared to beclomethasone dipropionate aerosol inhalers that contain CFC propellants. Laboratory tests using instruments (not on people) show that QVAR delivers a softer spray force (less than 1/3 the maximum impact force) and warmer spray temperature (more than 30°C warmer) than beclomethasone dipropionate aerosol inhalers containing CFC propellants.

There is no tail-off phenomenon observed for QVAR since the propellant and drug exhaust simultaneously, providing consistent dosing from priming through to a few sprays beyond the planned maximum number of doses. Tail-off means that as most inhalers approach empty, the delivered dose becomes unpredictable and subject to wide variation.

ADVERSE EFFECTS: In general, inhaled corticosteroid therapy may be associated with dose dependent increases in the incidence of ocular complications, reduced bone density, suppression of HPA-axis responsiveness to stress, and inhibition of growth velocity in children.

Glaucoma may be exacerbated by inhaled corticosteroid treatment for asthma or rhinitis. In patients with established glaucoma who require long-term inhaled corticosteroid treatment, it is prudent to measure intraocular pressure before commencing the inhaled corticosteroid and to monitor it subsequently. In patients without established glaucoma, but with a potential for developing intraocular hypertension (e.g. the elderly), intraocular pressure should be monitored at appropriate intervals.

In elderly patients treated with inhaled corticosteroids, the prevalence of posterior subcapsular and nuclear cataracts is probably low but increases in relation to the daily and cumulative lifetime dose. Cofactors such as smoking, ultraviolet B exposure, or diabetes may increase the risk. Children may be less susceptible.

A reduction of growth velocity in children or teenagers may occur as a result of inadequate control of chronic diseases such as asthma or from use of corticosteroids for treatment. Physicians should closely follow the growth of adolescents taking corticosteroids by any route and weigh the benefits of corticosteroid therapy and asthma control against the possibility of growth suppression if any adolescent's growth appears slowed.

Osteoporosis and fracture are the major complications of long-term asthma treatment with parenteral or oral steroids. Inhaled corticosteroid therapy is also associated with dose-dependent bone loss although the degree of risk is very much less than with oral steroid. This risk may be offset by estrogen replacement in post-menopausal women, and by titrating the daily dose of inhaled steroid to the minimum required to maintain optimal asthma control. It is not yet known whether the peak bone density achieved during youth is adversely affected if substantial amounts of inhaled corticosteroid are administered prior to 30 years of age. Failure to achieve maximal bone density during youth could increase the risk of osteoporotic fracture when those individuals reach 60 years of age and older.

Eosinophilic conditions: See Precautions, Eosinophilic Conditions.

The following reporting rates of common adverse experiences are based upon three clinical trials in which 940 patients (544 female and 396 male adults previously treated with as-needed bronchodilators and/or inhaled corticosteroids) were treated with QVAR (beclomethasone dipropionate) (doses of 50, 100, 200, or 400 µg twice daily) or CFC-BDP (doses of 50, 200, or 400 µg twice daily) or placebo. Table 1 includes all events reported by patients taking QVAR (whether considered drug related or not) that occurred at a rate over 3% and more frequently than placebo, or at a rate that significantly differed across treatment groups.

Table 1: QVAR

Adverse Events Reported in ≥3% of the Patients in the QVAR Group (%)

Adverse Events	QVAR N=453	CFC-BDP N=283	HFA-placebo N=204	Overall N=940	Overall P-value[a]
Inhalation Route Effects	7	11[d]	4	7	**0.028**
Oral Symptoms	3	6	2	4	0.085
General	8	11	8	9	0.290
Pain	3	3	<1	2	0.143
Central and Peripheral Nervous Systems	20	20	16	19	0.442
Headache	17	15	11	15	0.213
Gastrointestinal	6	9	4	6	0.771
Nausea	2	3[d]	0	2	**0.032**
Vomiting	<1[b]	2	<1	<1	**0.022**
Musculoskeletal	4	5	2	4	0.275
Reproductive	4	2	2	3	0.545
Dysmenorrhea	3	<1	2	2	0.131
Respiratory	30[b,c]	37	45	36	**0.001**
Increased Asthma Symptoms	4[b,c]	8[d]	22[e]	9	**<0.001**
Pharyngitis	10	10	5	9	0.054
Respiratory Disorder	0	1	0	<1	**0.037**
Sinusitis	4	4	2	4	0.599
Skin and Appendage	5	5	2	5	0.254

(cont'd)

Table 1: QVAR *(cont'd)*

Adverse Events Reported in ≥3% of the Patients in the QVAR Group (%)

Adverse Events	QVAR N=453	CFC-BDP N=283	HFA-placebo N=204	Overall N=940	Overall P-value[a]
Vision					
Eye Abnormality	0	1	0	<1	0.037

[a] The p-value for the overall comparison is a 2-sided Fisher's Exact Test.
[b] The pairwise comparison between HFA-BDP and CFC-BDP was statistically significant (p≤0.05) based on the two-sided Fisher's Exact Test.
[c] The pairwise comparison between HFA-BDP and HFA-placebo was statistically significant (p≤0.05) based on the two-sided Fisher's Exact Test.
[d] The pairwise comparison between CFC-BDP and HFA-placebo was statistically significant (p≤0.05) based on the two-sided Fisher's Exact Test.
[e] The higher incidence of increased asthma symptoms for the placebo-treated patients is not unexpected in a population requiring inhaled corticosteroids.

No patients treated with QVAR in the clinical program developed symptomatic oropharyngeal candidiasis. If such an infection develops, treatment with appropriate antifungal therapy or discontinuance of treatment with QVAR may be required.

Rare cases of immediate and delayed hypersensitivity reactions, including urticaria, angioedema, rash, and bronchospasm, have been reported following the oral and intranasal inhalation of BDP.

Pediatric Studies: In two 12-week placebo controlled studies in pediatric patients 5 to 12 years of age, no clinically relevant differences were found in the pattern, severity, or frequency of adverse events compared with those reported in adults, with the exception of conditions which are more prevalent in a pediatric population generally.

OVERDOSE:

Symptoms: Chronic overdosage of inhaled steroids, as a class, may cause manifestation of Cushing's syndrome, including truncal obesity, hypertension, fatigability and weakness, menstrual irregularities, hirsutism, purplish abdominal striae, edema, glucosuria, osteoporosis, etc.

Treatment: Managing chronic overdosage requires gradual reduction of the dose of inhaled steroid. Gradual reduction is emphasized, because chronic overdosage with inhaled steroids must be recognized as possibly causing suppression of endogenous adrenal production of corticosteroids. Careful titration downward of inhaled steroids, with monitoring of asthma control, is required. Periodic evaluation of the function of the hypothalamic-pituitary-adrenal axis is prudent during this down titration process to ensure that endogenous production of adrenal corticosteroids has resumed. It is expected that HFA-BDP will have the same potential for causing chronic overdosage as other inhaled steroids.

For management of a suspected drug overdose, CPhA recommends that you contact your **regional Poison Control Centre**. See the *CPS* Directory section for a list of Poison Control Centres.

DOSAGE: It is important that children be adequately instructed in the correct use of the pressurized metered-dose inhaler.

General: The lowest dose of beclomethasone dipropionate required to maintain good asthma control should be used. When the patient's asthma is well controlled, a reduction in the dose of beclomethasone dipropionate should be attempted in order to identify the lowest possible dose required to maintain control. Such an attempt at dose reduction should be carried out on a regular basis.

QVAR (beclomethasone dipropionate) Inhalation Aerosol is to be administered by oral inhalation only.

Since the effect of QVAR depends on its regular use and on the proper technique of inhalation, the patient should be made aware of the prophylactic nature of therapy with inhaled beclomethasone dipropionate, and that for optimum benefit QVAR should be taken regularly, even when the patient is asymptomatic. Improvement in asthma symptoms should be expected within the first or second week of starting treatment.

If patients find that relief with short-acting bronchodilator treatment becomes less effective or they need more inhalations than usual, medical attention should be sought.

Patients using inhaled bronchodilators should be advised to use the bronchodilator before the QVAR in order to enhance the penetration of QVAR into the bronchial tree. Several minutes should lapse between the use of the two inhalers to allow for some bronchodilation to occur.

In the presence of excessive mucous secretion, the drug may fail to reach the bronchioles. Therefore, if an obvious response is not obtained after ten days, attempts should be made to remove the mucous with expectorants and/or with a short course of systemic corticosteroid treatment.

As a general rule, rinsing the mouth and gargling after each inhalation with water can help in preventing the occurrence of candidiasis. Cleansing dentures has the same effect.

Treatment with QVAR should not be stopped abruptly, but tapered off gradually.

QVAR (beclomethasone dipropionate) is indicated for the prophylactic management of steroid-responsive bronchial asthma in patients 5 years and older. More clinical safety and efficacy studies are required to support an indication for use in younger children.

The recommended dosing range for QVAR is 100 to 800 µg/day. Each actuation of QVAR 50 µg delivers 50 µg of BDP from the valve, equivalent to 40 µg of BDP from the actuator. Each actuation of QVAR 100 µg delivers 100 µg of BDP from the valve, equivalent to 80 µg of BDP from the actuator.

Pediatric Patients (5–11 Years Old):		
Previous Therapy	**Recommended Starting Dose**	**Highest Recommended Dose**
Bronchodilators Alone	50 µg of QVAR twice daily	100 µg of QVAR twice daily
Inhaled Corticosteroids	50 µg of QVAR twice daily	100 µg of QVAR twice daily
Oral Corticosteroids	The highest recommended dose in children is 100 µg of QVAR twice daily.	
Patients 12 Years and Older:		
Mild Asthma Patients:		
50 to 100 µg of QVAR twice daily (total daily dose of 100 to 200 µg).		
Moderate Asthma Patients:		
100 to 250 µg of QVAR twice daily (total daily dose of 200 to 500 µg).		
In More Severe Cases:		
300 to 400 µg twice daily of QVAR (total daily dose of 600 to 800 µg).		

The recommended total daily dose of QVAR is lower than that recommended for current CFC-BDP products because of increased lung deposition. Dosage should be adjusted to the individual patient (see Table 2).

Table 2: QVAR

Suggested Conversion of Doses for Patients Switching from CFC-BDP to QVAR

CFC-BDP Dose (µg/day)	200	400–500	600–750	800–1000
	↓	↓	↓	↓
QVAR Dose (µg/day)	100	200	300	400

[a] Note: The conversion to the QVAR dose should be based on the dose of CFC-BDP that would be appropriate for the patient at the time of the switch. Symptomatic patients may require an increased dose of CFC-BDP and this increased dose should be considered in transferring patients to QVAR.

Patients Switched From Systemic to Inhaled Corticosteroids: Patients who require maintenance therapy of their asthma may benefit from treatment with QVAR at the doses recommended in Table 2. In patients who respond to QVAR, improvement in pulmonary function is usually apparent within 1 to 4 weeks after the start of therapy. Once the desired effect is achieved, consideration should be given to tapering to the lowest effective dose.

Particular care is needed in patients who are transferred from systemic corticosteroids to inhaled corticosteroids mainly because recovery from impaired adrenocortical function caused by prolonged systemic steroid therapy is slow.

The patient's asthma should be stable before treatment with QVAR is started. Initially, QVAR should be used concurrently with the patient's usual maintenance dose of systemic corticosteroids. After approximately one week, gradual withdrawal of the systemic corticosteroids is started by reducing the daily or alternate daily dose. Reductions may be made after an interval of one or two weeks, depending on the response of the patient. A slow rate of withdrawal is strongly recommended. Gradual withdrawal of the systemic steroid is started by reducing the daily dose by 1.0 mg of prednisone, or its equivalent of other corticosteroid, at not less than weekly intervals, if the patient is under close observation. During withdrawal, some patients may experience symptoms of systemic corticosteroid withdrawal, e.g. joint and/or muscular pain, lassitude and depression, despite maintenance or even improvement in pulmonary function. Such patients should be encouraged to continue with the inhaler but should be monitored for objective signs of adrenal insufficiency. If evidence of adrenal insufficiency occurs, the systemic corticosteroid doses should be increased temporarily and thereafter withdrawal should continue more slowly.

During periods of stress or a severe asthma attack, patients who have been withdrawn from systemic corticosteroids should be instructed to resume systemic steroids immediately and to contact their physician for further instruction. These patients should also be instructed to carry a warning card indicating that they may need supplementary systemic steroid during periods of stress or a severe asthma attack.

Patients who have been treated with systemic steroids for long periods of time or at high dose may have adrenocortical suppression. In these patients, adrenocortical function should be monitored regularly and their dose of systemic steroid reduced cautiously.

There are some patients who cannot completely discontinue the oral steroid. In these cases, a minimum maintenance dosage should be given in addition to QVAR.

Administration: QVAR should be administered by the oral inhaled route in patients 5 years of age and older. The onset and degree of symptom relief will vary in individual patients. Improvement in asthma symptoms should be expected within the first or second week of starting treatment, but maximum benefit should not be expected until 3-4 weeks of therapy. After asthma stability has been achieved at the starting dose, it is always desirable to titrate to the lowest effective dose to reduce the possibility of side effects. For patients who do not respond adequately to the starting dose after 3-4 weeks of therapy, higher doses may provide additional asthma control. The safety and efficacy of QVAR when administered in excess of recommended doses has not been established.

As with all inhalation aerosol medications, it is recommended that patients "test spray" QVAR before using for the very first time after purchase. If QVAR has not been used for over 14 days, four "test sprays" are again recommended prior to use (see Information for the Patient).

QVAR is a solution aerosol that does not require shaking. Consistent dose delivery is assured, whether using 50 or 100 µg strengths, due to good proportionality of the solution aerosol. Dose proportionality means that the 100 µg/actuation strength provides twice as much medication as the 50 µg/actuation strength. Consistent dosing can be assured as doses are adjusted and different product strengths are used. QVAR provides consistent medication delivery actuation to actuation regardless of storage position. This allows reliable dosing with a single actuation. Consistent medication delivery is also ensured throughout the labeled product life. When the canister is nearly empty, the spray from the mouthpiece will decrease sharply and will be obvious to the patient.

No clinical trials have been conducted using a spacer with QVAR; however, in vitro studies indicate that AeroChamber is compatible with QVAR

Use of a Spacer: QVAR has been developed to be used without a spacer device being necessary. Where a spacer is considered necessary the AeroChamber is a suitable device for use with QVAR MDI as the extrafine particle fraction is maintained.

INFORMATION FOR THE PATIENT: Published in e-CPS, available by subscription at www.e-cps.ca.

SUPPLIED: 50 µg: Each pressurized, metered-dose inhaler actuation, intended for oral inhalation only, delivers: beclomethasone dipropionate 50 µg from the valve, equivalent to beclomethasone dipropionate 40 µg from the actuator. Nonmedicinal ingredients: HFA-134a propellant (hydrofluoroalkane-134a or 1,1,1,2 tetrafluoroethane) and ethanol. Chlorofluorocarbons (CFCs)-free. Particle size of the emitted aerosol spray is 1 to 1.2 microns. Canisters of 6.5 and 12.4 g containing 100 and 200 actuations respectively, with a beige plastic oral actuator, Patient's Instruction; boxes of 1.

100 µg: Each pressurized, metered-dose inhaler actuation, intended for oral inhalation only, delivers: beclomethasone dipropionate 100 µg from the valve, equivalent to beclomethasone dipropionate 80 µg from the actuator. Nonmedicinal ingredients: HFA-134a propellant (hydrofluoroalkane-134a or 1,1,1,2 tetrafluoroethane) and ethanol. Chlorofluorocarbons (CFCs)-free. Particle size of the emitted aerosol spray is 1 to 1.2 microns. Canisters of 6.5 and 12.4 g containing 100 and 200 actuations respectively, with a dark mauve plastic oral actuator and Patient's Instruction; boxes of 1.

Contents under pressure. Do not puncture. Do not use or store near heat or open flame. Exposure to temperatures above 50°C may cause bursting. Never throw container into fire or incinerator. Keep out of reach of children. Store between 15 and 30°C. If the canister is subjected to cold temperatures (as low as −10°C), it will not adversely affect delivery of medication.

(Shown in Product Identification Section)

R

R & C® Shampoo/Conditioner

pyrethrins—piperonyl butoxide

Pediculicide—Ovicide

GlaxoSmithKline Consumer Healthcare

INDICATIONS: For the treatment of infestations with head lice (*P. capitis*), crab lice (*P. pubis*) and their nits.

CONTRAINDICATIONS: Should not be used by persons allergic to chrysanthemum, pyrethrins or synthetic pyrethroids. Do not use on eyelashes or eyebrows. Do not exceed 2 applications within 24 hours.

WARNINGS: Do not use on eyelashes or eyebrows. Do not exceed 2 applications within 24 hours.

PRECAUTIONS: For external use only. Harmful if swallowed. It should not be inhaled. During shampooing, contact should be avoided with eyelashes, eyes, nose and mouth and other mucous areas. If contact does take place, flush with water.

If accidental ingestion should occur, call a physician or Poison Control Centre immediately. Drink a large amount of milk or water. Do not induce vomiting.

In case of infection or skin irritation, discontinue use and consult a physician. Consult a physician if an infestation of lice to eyebrows or eyelashes occurs.

ADVERSE EFFECTS: In case of infection or skin irritation, discontinue use and consult a physician. Consult a physician if an infestation of lice to eyebrows or eyelashes occurs.

OVERDOSE:

Treatment: If accidental ingestion should occur, call a physician or Poison Control Centre immediately. Drink a large amount of milk or water. Do not induce vomiting.

> For management of a suspected drug overdose, CPhA recommends that you contact your **regional Poison Control Centre**. See the *CPS* Directory section for a list of Poison Control Centres.

DOSAGE: Apply R & C Shampoo/Conditioner to dry hair. (Do not use any product before applying R & C Shampoo/Conditioner.) Thoroughly soak the hair and skin of the infested areas with R & C Shampoo/Conditioner (min 25 mL). For thicker and longer hair, it is recommended to use more than 25 mL. Allow the shampoo/conditioner to remain on the area for 10 minutes. Add small quantities of water, working the shampoo/conditioner into the hair and skin until a lather forms. Rinse thoroughly. The dead lice and their nits should be removed with the in-pack nit comb. A second application of R & C is recommended 7-10 days after the first application to kill any newly hatched nymphs (young lice). Do not exceed 2 applications within 24 hours.

Lice infestations are spread by contact. Each family member and sexual partner should be examined carefully. If infested, they should be treated immediately to prevent the spread of the infestation or cause a reinfestation with previously treated family members. All contaminated clothing and other articles such as combs, brushes, hats, etc. should be dry cleaned or washed in hot water (above 54°C). Upholstery, carpets and other areas where lice may linger and cause a reinfestation should be sprayed with R & C II Spray Insecticide.

SUPPLIED: Each plastic bottle contains: pyrethrins 0.33%; piperonyl butoxide technical 3.0%. Nonmedicinal ingredients: fragrance, isocetyl alcohol, isopropyl alcohol, lauryl dimethyl amine oxide, mineral oil white, polyoxyethylene 4 lauryl ether, polyoxyethylene 23 lauryl ether, polyquaternium-11, purified water and triethanolamine lauryl sulphate. Plastic bottles of 50 and 200 mL, each with a nit comb and applicator cap.

RabAvert®

rabies vaccine

Active Immunizing Agent

Novartis Pharmaceuticals

Date of Preparation: April 29, 2005
Date of Revision: November 2009

SUMMARY PRODUCT INFORMATION:

Route of Administration	Dosage Form/Strength	Clinically Relevant Nonmedicinal Ingredients (per 1 mL)
Intramuscular (IM) Injection	Freeze-dried vaccine for reconstitution with a diluent/ ≥2.5 IUs of rabies antigen per 1 mL	Polygeline <12 mg; human serum albumin <0.3 mg; neomycin <1 µg; chlortetracycline <20 ng; amphotericin B <2 ng; ovalbumin <3 ng

DESCRIPTION: RabAvert (Rabies Vaccine) produced by Novartis Vaccines and Diagnostics GmbH & Co KG is a sterile freeze-dried vaccine obtained by growing the fixed-virus strain Flury LEP in primary cultures of chicken fibroblasts. The strain Flury LEP was obtained from American Type Culture Collection as the 59th egg passage. The growth medium for propagation of the virus is a synthetic cell culture medium with the addition of human albumin, polygeline (processed bovine gelatin) and antibiotics.

The virus is inactivated with β-propiolactone, and further processed by zonal centrifugation in a sucrose density-gradient. The vaccine is lyophilized after addition of a stabilizer solution which consists of buffered polygeline and potassium glutamate.

One dose of reconstituted vaccine contains less than 12 mg polygeline (processed bovine gelatin), less than 0.3 mg human serum albumin, 1 mg potassium glutamate and 0.3 mg sodium EDTA. Small quantities of bovine serum are used in the cell culture process. Bovine components originate only from source countries known to be free of bovine spongiform encephalopathy. Minimal amounts of chicken protein may be present in the final product; ovalbumin content is less than 3 ng/dose (1 mL), based on ELISA. In the final vaccine, neomycin is present at <1 µg, chlortetracycline at <20 ng, and amphotericin B at <2 ng per dose.

RabAvert is intended for intramuscular (IM) injection. The vaccine contains no preservative and should be used immediately after reconstitution with the supplied Sterile Diluent for RabAvert (Water for Injection).

The potency of the final product is determined by the US National Institute of Health (NIH) mouse potency test using the US reference standard. The potency of one dose (1.0 mL) RabAvert is at least 2.5 IU of rabies antigen.

RabAvert is a white, freeze-dried vaccine for reconstitution with the water for injection diluent prior to use; the reconstituted vaccine is a clear to slightly opaque, colorless solution.

INDICATIONS AND CLINICAL USE: RabAvert is indicated for:

- Pre-exposure vaccination, in both primary series and booster doses against rabies in all age groups.
- Post-exposure prophylaxis against rabies in all age groups.

Pre-Exposure Vaccination: Primary immunization: Pre-exposure rabies immunization is an elective procedure and should be offered to people at potential risk of contact with rabid animals, e.g., certain laboratory workers, veterinarians, animal control and wildlife workers, spelunkers, and hunters and trappers in high-risk areas such as the far north. Travellers to endemic areas where there is not likely to be access to adequate and safe post-exposure measures should consider pre-travel immunization. As well, children who are too young to understand either the need to avoid animals or to report a traumatic contact are considered at greater risk of rabid animal exposure and should be offered pre-exposure immunization when travelling to endemic areas.

Booster doses: People with continuing high risk of exposure, such as certain veterinarians, should have their serum tested for rabies antibodies every 2 years (RFFIT); others working with live rabies virus in laboratories or vaccine production facilities who are at risk of unapparent exposure should be tested every 6 months.

Those with inadequate titres should be given a booster dose of RabAvert.

Alternatively, booster doses may be given every 2-5 years, if situation does not warrant continual serological control and depending on the level of exposure risk.

Post-Exposure Prophylaxis: Table 1 outlines the recommendations for the management of people after possible exposure to rabies. These recommendations are intended as a guide and may need to be modified in accordance with the specific circumstances of the exposure.

Immediate washing and flushing with soap and water and a virucidal agent is imperative. Suturing the wound should be avoided if possible. Tetanus prophylaxis and antibacterial drugs should be given as required.

Table 1: RabAvert

Post-exposure Prophylaxis for People Not Previously Immunized Against Rabies

Animal Species	Condition of Animal at Time of Exposure	Management of Exposed Person
Dog or cat	Healthy, and available for 10 days observation	1. Local wound treatment 2. At first sign of rabies in animal, give RIG and start RabAvert
	Rabid or suspected to be rabid[a] Unknown or escaped	1. Local wound treatment 2. RIG and RabAvert
Skunk, bat, fox, coyote, raccoon and other carnivores. Included bat found in room when a person was sleeping unattended.	Regard as rabid unless geographic area is known to be rabies free[a]	1. Local wound treatment 2. RIG and RabAvert
Livestock, rodents or lagomorphs (hares and rabbits)	Consider individually. Consult appropriate public health and Food Inspection Agency officials. Bites of squirrels, chipmunks, rats, mice, hamsters, gerbils, other rodents, rabbits and hares may warrant post-exposure rabies prophylaxis if the behavior of the biting animal was highly unusual.	

[a] If possible, the animal should be humanely killed and the brain tested for rabies as soon as possible; holding for observation is not recommended. Discontinue vaccination if fluorescent antibody test of animal brain is negative.
Legend: RIG=(human) rabies immune globulin.

The following factors should be considered before antirabies treatment is initiated.

Species of Biting Animal: The animals in Canada most often proven rabid are wild terrestrial carnivores (raccoons, foxes, and skunks), wild dogs and cats, bats, and cattle. The distribution of animal rabies and the species involved vary considerably across Canada by region and over time, so in cases of possible exposure it is important to consult the local medical officer or government veterinarian. Human exposures to livestock are usually confined to salivary contamination with the exception of horses and swine, for which bites have been reported. Risk of infection after exposure to rabid cattle is low. Squirrels, hamsters, guinea-pigs, gerbils, chipmunks, rats, mice, other rodents, rabbits and hares are only rarely found to be infected with rabies and are not known to have caused human rabies in North America; post-exposure prophylaxis should be considered only if the animal's behavior was highly unusual.

The manifestations of rabies and the incubation periods vary in different species. The length of time virus may be excreted in saliva before the development of symptoms has not been determined for the purpose of defining rabies exposure except in domestic dogs, cats and ferrets. In these animals, rabies virus excretion does not generally preceed symptom development beyond 10 days. It remains unclear as to whether asymptomatic carriage of rabies virus in animals in the wild is possible.

Circumstances of Biting Incident: An **unprovoked** attack is more likely than a provoked attack to indicate the animal is rabid. Nevertheless, rabid cats and dogs may become uncharacteristically quiet. Bites inflicted on a person attempting to feed or handle an apparently healthy animal should generally be regarded as **provoked**. A currently vaccinated dog, cat or ferret is unlikely to become infected with rabies.

Type of Exposure: Rabies is transmitted when the virus is inoculated into tissue. This occurs most commonly when rabies virus in saliva is introduced into tissues by bites. Transmission can also occur when cuts or wounds of skin or mucous membranes are contaminated with virus in saliva or infected tissues. Rarely, transmission has been recorded when virus was inhaled, or infected corneal grafts or solid organs were transplanted into patients. Thus, two broad categories of exposure are recognized as warranting post-exposure prophylaxis:

Bite: This is defined as any penetration of skin by teeth. Bites inflicted by most animals are readily apparent. However, bites inflicted by bats to a sleeping person may not be felt, and may leave no visible bite marks. Hence, when people are sleeping unattended in a room where a bat is or was present or where the possibility of a bite cannot be reasonably excluded (e.g., if a bat is discovered in proximity to an individual who is cognitively impaired) post-exposure prophylaxis should be initiated.

Non-bite: This category includes contamination of scratches, abrasions or cuts of skin or mucous membranes by saliva or other potentially infectious material, such as the brain tissue of a rabid animal. Petting a rabid animal or handling its blood, urine or feces is not considered to be an exposure nor is being sprayed by a skunk. These incidents do not warrant post-exposure prophylaxis.

Post-exposure prophylaxis is warranted and recommended in rare instances of non-bite exposure, such as inhalation of aerosolized virus by spelunkers exploring caves inhabited by infected bats or by laboratory technicians homogenizing tissues infected with rabies virus; however, the efficacy of prophylaxis after such exposures is unknown. Stringent guidelines concerning the suitability of tissue donors have almost eliminated the possibility that rabies virus may be transmitted iatrogenically.

Exposures incurred in the course of caring for humans with rabies could theoretically transmit the infection. No case of rabies acquired in this way has been documented, but post-exposure prophylaxis should be considered for exposed individuals.

Because some bat bites may be less severe, and therefore more difficult to recognize, than bites by larger mammalian carnivores, rabies post-exposure prophylaxis should be considered for any physical contact with bats when bites or mucous membrane contacts cannot be excluded.

Vaccination Status of Biting Animal: A small number of vaccinated animals have developed rabies. Therefore, symptoms suggesting rabies, even in a vaccinated animal, must be carefully evaluated. The vaccination history in itself should not influence the need for post-exposure prophylaxis nor the need to sacrifice the animal for assessment.

Geriatrics (65 years and over): Clinical studies of RabAvert did not include sufficient numbers of subjects aged 65 and over to determine whether they respond differently from younger subjects. Other reported clinical experience has not identified differences in responses between the elderly and younger patients.

Pediatrics (under 18 years): The indication for children and infants is the same as for adults (see Action and Clinical Pharmacology).

CONTRAINDICATIONS: In view of the almost invariably fatal outcome of rabies, there is no contraindication to post-exposure prophylaxis, including pregnancy.

Hypersensitivity: History of anaphylaxis to the vaccine or any of the vaccine components, including the container, constitutes a contraindication to pre-exposure vaccination with this vaccine.

In the case of post-exposure prophylaxis, if an alternative product is not available, the patient should be vaccinated with caution with the necessary medical equipment and emergency supplies available and observed carefully after vaccination. A patient's risk of acquiring rabies must be carefully considered before deciding to discontinue vaccination. Advice and assistance on the management of serious adverse reactions for persons receiving rabies vaccines may be sought from the appropriate health department.

WARNINGS AND PRECAUTIONS:

> **Serious Warnings and Precautions**
> Anaphylaxis and neuroparalytic events such as transient paralysis or Guillain-Barré-Syndrome have been reported to be temporally associated with the use of RabAvert. See Precautions and Adverse Reactions.
> A patient's risk of developing rabies must be carefully considered, however, before deciding to discontinue immunization.

General: Care is to be taken by the health-care provider for the safe and effective use of the product. The health-care provider should also question the patient, parent or guardian about:

1. the current health status of the vaccinee; and
2. reactions to a previous dose of RabAvert, or a similar product.

Pre-exposure vaccination should be postponed in the case of sick and convalescent persons, and those considered to be in the incubation stage of an infectious disease.

A separate, sterile syringe and needle or a sterile disposable unit should be used for each patient to prevent transmission of hepatitis and other infectious agents from person to person. Needles should not be recapped and should be properly disposed of.

As with any rabies vaccine, vaccination with RabAvert may not protect 100% of susceptible individuals.

RabAvert must not be used subcutaneously and should not be used intradermally.

Intradermal administration requires highly experienced personnel, in order to use the correct technique and to ensure that the exact dose is given. Furthermore, the sterility of the administered dose cannot be guaranteed, if another dose has already been withdrawn from the vial.

RabAvert must be injected intramuscularly. For adults, the **deltoid area** is the preferred site of immunization; for small children and infants, administration into the anterolateral zone of the thigh is preferred. The use of the gluteal region should be avoided, since administration in this area may result in lower neutralizing antibody titres.

Do not inject intravascularly.

Unintentional intravascular injection may result in systemic reactions, including shock. Immediate measures include catecholamines, volume replacement, high doses of corticosteroids, and oxygen.

Development of active immunity after vaccination may be impaired in immuno-compromised individuals. Please refer to Drug Interactions.

This product contains albumin, a derivative of human blood. It is present in RabAvert at concentrations of less than 0.3 mg/dose. Based on effective donor screening and product manufacturing processes, it carries an extremely remote risk for transmission of viral diseases. A theoretical risk for transmission of variant Creutzfeld-Jakob disease (vCJD) also is considered extremely remote. No cases of transmission of viral diseases or vCJD have ever been identified for albumin.

A history of allergy to eggs or a positive skin test to ovalbumin does not necessarily indicate that a subject will be allergic to RabAvert. However, subjects who have a history of a severe hypersensitivity reaction to eggs or egg products should not receive the vaccine for pre-exposure vaccination. Such subjects should also not receive the vaccine for post-exposure prophylaxis unless a suitable alternative vaccine is not available, in which case all injections should be administered with close monitoring and with facilities for emergency treatment.

Similarly, subjects with a history of a severe hypersensitivity reaction to any of the other ingredients in RabAvert such as polygeline (stabilizer), or to amphotericin B, chlortetracycline or neomycin (which may be present as trace residues) should not receive the vaccine for pre-exposure vaccination. The vaccine should also not be given to such persons for post-exposure prophylaxis unless a suitable alternative vaccine is not available, in which case precautions should be taken as above.

Carcinogenesis and Mutagenesis: Long-term studies with RabAvert have not been conducted to assess the potential for carcinogenesis, mutagenesis, or impairment of fertility.

Special Populations: Pregnant Women: Animal reproductive studies have not been conducted with RabAvert. It is also not known whether RabAvert can cause fetal harm when administered to a pregnant woman or can affect reproduction capacity. No reports on adverse effects associated with the use of RabAvert in pregnancy have been received.

Because of the potential consequences of inadequately treated rabies exposure, pregnancy is not considered a contraindication to post-exposure prophylaxis. If there is a substantial risk of exposure to rabies, pre-exposure vaccination may also be indicated during pregnancy.

Nursing Women: It is not known whether RabAvert is excreted in animal or human milk.

Because of the potential consequences of inadequately treated rabies exposure, nursing is not considered a contraindication to post-exposure prophylaxis. If there is a substantial risk of exposure to rabies, pre-exposure vaccination may also be indicated during nursing.

Monitoring and Laboratory Tests: When rabies post-exposure prophylaxis is administered to persons receiving corticosteroids or other immunosuppressive therapy, or who are immunosuppressed, it is important that a serum sample on Day 14 (the day of the fourth vaccination) be tested for rabies antibody to ensure that an acceptable antibody response has been induced (RFFIT).

ADVERSE REACTIONS: As with all vaccines and as outlined below, RabAvert administration may cause unintended reactions. However, not all events occurring after vaccination are causally related to the vaccine. For any unexpected effects while taking RabAvert, contact your physician or pharmacist.

Adverse Drug Reaction Overview: In very rare cases, neurological and neuroparalytical events and cases of hypersensitivity have been reported in temporal association with administration of RabAvert.

The most commonly occurring adverse reactions are injection-site reactions, such as injection-site erythema, induration and pain; flu-like symptoms, such as asthenia, fatigue, fever, headache, myalgia and malaise; arthralgia, dizziness, lymphadenopathy, nausea, and rash.

A patient's risk of acquiring rabies must be carefully considered before deciding to discontinue vaccination. Advice and assistance on the management of serious adverse reactions for persons receiving rabies vaccines may be sought from the health department.

Clinical Trial Adverse Drug Reactions: As clinical trials are conducted under widely varying conditions, adverse reaction rates observed in the clinical trials of a vaccine cannot be directly compared to rates in the clinical trials of another vaccine and may not reflect the rates observed in practice. The adverse reaction information from clinical trials does, however, provide a basis for identifying the adverse events that appear to be related to vaccine use and for approximating rates.

The data from clinical trials described below (Table 2) reflect exposure to RabAvert in 1307 subjects, including 355 subjects in pre-exposure vaccination settings and 952 patients, who received RabAvert for post-exposure prophylaxis. RabAvert was studied primarily in single-blind, randomized controlled trials. The population studied was mainly Caucasian and Asian, ranging from healthy infants to healthy adults with an equal gender distribution. Patients only received IM administration of RabAvert.

Table 2: RabAvert
Adverse Reactions Information (clinical trials)

Body System	Frequency	Adverse Reactions (Clinical Trials, n=1307)
General disorders and administration-site condition	Very common >10%	Injection-site pain, injection-site reaction, injection-site induration
	Common >1%, <10%	Asthenia, malaise, fever, fatigue, influenza-like illness, injection-site erythema
Blood and lymphatic system disorders	Common >1%, <10%	Lymphadenopathy
Nervous system disorders	Common >1%, <10%	Dizziness, headache
Skin disorders	Common >1%, <10%	Rash
Musculosceletal and connective tissue disorders	Common >1%, <10%	Myalgia, arthralgia
Gastrointestinal disorders	Common >1%, <10%	Gastrointestinal disorders (such as nausea or abdominal pain)

Post-Market Adverse Drug Reactions: Those adverse reactions identified during post-approval use of RabAvert can be found in the following (Table 3). As these reactions are reported voluntarily from a population of uncertain size, it is not always possible to reliably estimate their frequency or establish a causal relationship to vaccine exposure. Decisions to include these reactions in labelling are typically based on one or more of the following factors: 1) seriousness of the reaction, 2) frequency of reporting, or 3) strength of causal connection to vaccine exposure, or a combination of these factors.

Table 3: RabAvert
Adverse Reactions Information (post-marketing)

Body System	Adverse Reactions (only observed in postapproval use, n≥10 000 000); frequency <1:1 000 for all events
General disorders and administration-site condition	Chills, sweating
Cardiac disorders	Circulatory reactions (such as palpitations or hot flush)
Ear and labyrinth disorders	Vertigo
Eye disorders	Visual disturbance
Nervous system disorders	Paraesthesia
	Nervous system disorders (such as encephalitis, transient paralysis or Guillain-Barré-Syndrome)
Immune system disorders	Allergic reactions (such as anaphylaxis, bronchospasm, oedema, urticaria or pruritus)
	Type III hypersensitivity-like symptoms
Musculosceletal and connective tissue disorders	Pain in limbs, limb swelling

Once initiated, rabies prophylaxis should not be interrupted or discontinued because of local or mild systemic adverse reactions to rabies vaccine. Usually such reactions can be successfully managed with anti-inflammatory and antipyretic agents.

In addition to the reactions outlined above, the following adverse events have been reported very rarely following widespread use of the vaccine. A causal relationship to the vaccine has not been established for any of these events: aphasia, cardiovascular disorder, conversion disorder, convulsion, diabetes mellitus, encephalitis, eye disorder, hearing impaired, meningitis, multiple sclerosis, nephritis, pneumonia, polymyalgia rheumatica, respiratory disorder, somnolence, spontaneous abortion, thrombocytopenia.

Adherence to treatment guidelines, as outlined below, are of utmost importance in order to minimize risk of rabies disease. However, in very few cases development of rabies disease despite correct treatment has been reported. Direct inoculation of the rabies virus into nerve endings has been discussed as an explanation for these rare cases.

In very rare cases immediate-type allergic reactions may occur even after the first application of RabAvert, e.g. when pre-sensitisation occurred with a different product with similar excipients.

DRUG INTERACTIONS:

> **Serious Drug Interactions**
> Radiation therapy, antimalarials, corticosteroids, other immunosuppressive agents and immunosuppressive illnesses can interfere with the development of active immunity after vaccination, and may diminish the protective efficacy of the vaccine.

Overview: Pre-exposure vaccination may be administered to persons under radiation therapy, antimalarials, corticosteroids, other immunosuppressive agents, and persons with immunosuppressive illnesses with the awareness that the immune response may be inadequate.

Immunosuppressive agents should not be administered during post-exposure prophylaxis unless essential for the treatment of other conditions. When rabies post-exposure prophylaxis is administered to persons receiving corticosteroids or other immunosuppressive therapy, or who are immunosuppressed, it is important that a serum sample on Day 14 (the day of the fourth vaccination) be tested for rabies antibody to ensure that an acceptable antibody response has been induced (RFFIT).

RIG must not be administered at more than the recommended dose, and not later than eight days after administration of first RabAvert dose since active immunization to the vaccine may be impaired.

No clinical trial data are available regarding the concurrent administration of RabAvert with other vaccines. Other essential inactivated vaccines may be given at the same time as RabAvert. Different injectable inactivated vaccines should be administered into separate injection sites.

Drug-Food Interactions: Interactions with food have not been established.
Drug-Herb Interactions: Interactions with herbal products have not been established.
Drug-Laboratory Test Interactions: Interactions with laboratory tests have not been established.

DOSAGE AND ADMINISTRATION: Dosing Considerations:

- Pre-exposure vaccination—primary series and booster doses.
- Post-exposure prophylaxis.

Recommended Dose and Dosage Adjustment: The individual dose for adults, children, and infants is 1 mL, given intramuscularly. In adults, administer vaccine by IM injection into the **deltoid muscle**. In small children and infants, administer vaccine into the anterolateral zone of the thigh. The gluteal area should be avoided for vaccine injections, since administration in this area may result in lower neutralizing antibody titres.

Care should be taken to avoid injection into or near blood vessels and nerves. After aspiration, if blood or any suspicious discoloration appears in the syringe, do not inject but discard contents and repeat procedure using a new dose of vaccine, at a different site.

Pre-exposure Dosage: Primary Immunization: Three intramuscular injections of 1.0 mL each: One injection on each of **Days 0, 7, and 21 (or 28)**.

Healthy people immunized with an appropriate regimen will develop rabies antibodies, and therefore routine post-immunization antibody determinations are not recommended. Neutralizing antibodies develop 7 days after the second dose of primary immunization and persist for at least 2 years after the third dose.

The Canadian national rabies reference laboratory considers an acceptable antibody response to be a titre of ≥0.5 IU/mL by the Rapid Fluorescent-Focus Inhibition Test (RFFIT). Post-immunization antibody titre determination may be advisable for those anticipating frequent exposure or whose immune response may be reduced by illness, medication or advanced age.

Booster Immunization: The individual booster dose is 1 mL, given intramuscularly.

People with continuing high risk of exposure, such as certain veterinarians, should have their serum tested for rabies antibodies every 2 years (RFFIT); others working with live rabies virus in laboratories or vaccine production facilities who are at risk of unapparent exposure should be tested every 6 months.

Those with inadequate titres should be given a booster dose of RabAvert.

Alternatively, booster doses may be given every 2-5 years, if situation does not warrant continual serological control and depending on the level of exposure risk.

Post-exposure Dosage for Previously Unvaccinated Persons: Immunization should begin as soon as possible after exposure. A complete course of immunization consists of a total of 5 injections of 1 mL each: One injection on each of **Days 0, 3, 7, 14 and 28**.

In conjunction with the administration of human rabies-specific immuno globulin (RIG) on Day 0. Other immunization schedules have also been validated by the World Health Organization (WHO).

Post-exposure prophylaxis should be started as soon as possible after exposure and should be offered to exposed individuals regardless of the elapsed interval. If the suspect animal is domestic and is available for quarantine, then immunization may be withheld pending the animal's status after the 10-day observation period. However, if the bite wound is to the head and neck region, prophylaxis should begin immediately and not be delayed until after the 10-day period. When notification of an exposure is delayed, prophylaxis may be started as late as 6 or more months after exposure.

Begin with the administration of (human) RIG. Give 20 IU/kg body weight. This formula is applicable to all age groups, including infants and children. The recommended dosage of human RIG should not exceed 20 IU/kg body weight as it may otherwise interfere with active antibody production. For both human and non-human RIG administration and dosage, please refer to package information leaflet of respective product.

Since vaccine-induced antibody appears within 1 week, RIG is not indicated more than 8 days after initiating post-exposure prophylaxis with RabAvert. If anatomically feasible, the full dose of RIG should be thoroughly infiltrated in the area around and into the wounds. Any remaining volume of RIG should be injected IM at a site distant from rabies vaccine administration. RIG should never be administered in the same syringe or in the same anatomical site as the rabies vaccine.

Because the antibody response following the recommended immunization regimen with RabAvert has been satisfactory, routine post-immunization serologic testing is not recommended. Serologic testing is indicated in unusual circumstances, as when the patient is known to be immunosuppressed (RFFIT).

Post-exposure Dosage for Previously Immunized Persons: When rabies exposure occurs in a **previously vaccinated** person, that person should receive two IM (deltoid) doses (1.0 mL each) of RabAvert: One injection on **Day 0 (immediately after exposure) and Day 3**.

RIG should not be given in these cases. Persons considered to have been immunized previously are those a) who received a complete pre-exposure vaccination or post-exposure prophylaxis with RabAvert or other tissue culture vaccines; or b) who have been documented to have had a protective antibody response to another rabies vaccine or to unapproved schedules or routes of administration. If the immune status of a previously vaccinated person is not known, full post-exposure antirabies prophylaxis (RIG plus 5 doses of vaccine) is recommended. In such cases, if protective levels of neutralizing antibodies can be demonstrated in a serum sample collected before vaccine is given (RFFIT), treatment can be discontinued after at least two doses of vaccine.

Administration: Using the longer of the 2 needles supplied, withdraw the entire contents of the Sterile Diluent for RabAvert into the syringe. Insert the needle at a 45° angle and slowly inject the entire contents of the diluent vial into the vaccine vial. Mix gently to avoid foaming. The white, freeze-dried vaccine dissolves to give a clear or slightly opaque solution. Withdraw the total amount of dissolved vaccine into the syringe and replace the long needle with the smaller needle for IM injection. The reconstituted vaccine should be used immediately.

Parenteral drug products should be inspected visually for particulate matter and discoloration prior to administration. If either of these conditions exists, the vaccine should not be administered. A separate, sterile syringe and needle or a sterile disposable unit should be used for each patient to prevent transmission of hepatitis and other infectious agents from person to person. Needles should not be recapped and should be properly disposed of.

The lyophilization of the vaccine is performed under reduced pressure and the subsequent closure of the vials needs to be done under vacuum. Additionally, if there is no negative pressure in the vial, injection of Sterile Diluent for RabAvert would lead to an excess positive pressure in the vial. After reconstitution of the vaccine, it is recommended to unscrew the syringe from the needle to eliminate the negative pressure. After that, the vaccine can be easily withdrawn from the vial. It is not recommended to induce excess pressure, since over-pressurization will create problems in withdrawing the proper amount of the vaccine.

Table 4: RabAvert

Administration Volume

Vial	Volume of Diluent to be Added to Vial	Approximate Available Volume	Nominal Concentration per mL
Freeze-dried vaccine containing 1 dose	1 mL	1 mL	≥2.5 IU/mL of rabies antigen

OVERDOSAGE:
No symptoms of overdose are known.

For management of a suspected drug overdose, CPhA recommends that you contact your **regional Poison Control Centre**. See the *CPS* Directory section for a list of Poison Control Centres.

ACTION AND CLINICAL PHARMACOLOGY: Mechanism of Action: Intramuscular injection of RabAvert induces lymphocytes to produce virus neutralizing antibodies that provide adequate protection against rabies virus.

Pharmacodynamics: Pre-exposure Vaccination: The immunogenicity of RabAvert has been demonstrated in clinical trials conducted in Europe, North America and Asia. When administered according to the recommended immunisation schedule (days 0, 7, 21 or 28), 100% of subjects attained an adequate titre of 0.5 IU/mL by day 28 or earlier. Persistence of antibody titres ≥0.5 IU/mL for up to 2 years after immunisation of RabAvert has been measured in clinical trials.

Pre-exposure Vaccination in Children: Pre-exposure administration of RabAvert in 11 Thai children from the age of 2 years and older resulted in antibody levels higher than 0.5 IU/mL on Day 14 in all children.

Post-exposure Prophylaxis: Clinical studies in patients exposed to rabies virus have demonstrated that RabAvert, when used in the recommended post-exposure WHO schedule of 5 to 6 IM injections of 1 ML (on days 0, 3, 7, 14, 28), provided protective titres of neutralising antibodies (>0.5 IU/mL) in 98% of patients within 14 days and in 100% of patients by Day 30. Similar results were obtained in several studies with healthy volunteers who had been given the WHO recommended post-exposure regimen ("simulated" post-exposure immunisation).

Failures have occurred, almost always after deviation from the recommended post-exposure prophylaxis protocol. However, in very few cases development of rabies disease despite correct treatment has been reported. Direct inoculation of the rabies virus into nerve endings has been discussed as an explanation for these rare cases.

Post-exposure Prophylaxis in Children: In a 10-year serosurveillance study, RabAvert has been administered to 91 children aged 1 to 5 years and 436 children and adolescents aged 6 to 20 years. The vaccine was effective in both age groups. None of these patients developed rabies.

Pharmacokinetics: Not applicable.

STORAGE AND STABILITY: RabAvert should be stored protected from light at 2 to 8°C. After reconstitution the vaccine is to be used immediately. The vaccine may not be used after the expiration date given on package and container.

SPECIAL HANDLING INSTRUCTIONS: The vaccine should be visually inspected both before and after reconstitution for any foreign particulate matter and or change in physical appearance. The vaccine must not be used if any change in the appearance of the vaccine has taken place. For appearance see Description.

The powder for solution should be reconstituted using the diluent supplied and carefully agitated prior to injection. The reconstituted vaccine should be used immediately.

Any unused vaccine or waste material should be disposed of in accordance with local requirements.

INFORMATION FOR THE PATIENT: Published in e-CPS, available by subscription at www.e-cps.ca.

DOSAGE FORMS, COMPOSITION AND PACKAGING: RabAvert, Rabies Vaccine, produced by Chiron Behring GmbH & Co KG is a sterile freeze-dried vaccine obtained by growing the fixed-virus strain Flury LEP in primary cultures of chicken fibroblasts. The strain Flury LEP was obtained from American Type Culture Collection as the 59th egg passage. The growth medium for propagation of the virus is a synthetic cell culture medium with the addition of human albumin, polygeline (processed bovine gelatin) and antibiotics.

The virus is inactivated with beta-propiolactone, and further processed by zonal centrifugation in a sucrose density-gradient. The vaccine is lyophilized after addition of a stabilizer solution which consists of buffered polygeline and potassium glutamate. One dose of reconstituted vaccine contains less than 12 mg polygeline (processed bovine gelatin), less than 0.3 mg human serum albumin, 1 mg potassium glutamate and 0.3 mg sodium EDTA. Small quantities of bovine serum are used in the cell culture process. Bovine components originate only from source countries known to be free of bovine spongiform encephalopathy. Minimal amounts of chicken protein may be present in the final product; ovalbumin content is less than 3 ng/dose (1 mL), based on ELISA. Antibiotics (neomycin, chlortetracycline, amphotericin B) added during cell and virus propagation are largely removed during subsequent steps in the manufacturing process. In the final vaccine, neomycin is present at <1 µg, chlortetracycline at <20 ng, and amphotericin B at <2 ng per dose.

RabAvert is a white, freeze-dried vaccine for reconstitution with the diluent prior to use; the reconstituted vaccine is a clear to slightly opaque, colorless solution. RabAvert is intended for intramuscular (IM) injection. The vaccine contains no preservative and should be used immediately after reconstitution with the supplied Sterile Diluent for RabAvert (Water for Injection). Single dose vial of freeze-dried vaccine, 1 mL vial of Sterile Diluent, 1 disposable syringe, 1 smaller needle for injection, 25 gauge×1", 1 longer needle for reconstitution, 21 gauge×1.5".

The potency of the final product is determined by the NIH mouse potency test using the US reference standard. The potency of one dose (1.0 mL) RabAvert is at least 2.5 IU of rabies antigen.

Viral Inactivation: Only human serum albumin (HSA) approved for sale in Canada is used for the production of RabAvert. Therefore, the HSA complies with the requirements of the USP regarding viral inactivation.

Ralivia™ Ⓟ
tramadol HCl
Opioid Analgesic

Biovail Pharmaceuticals

Date of Preparation: August 30, 2007
Date of Revision: July 26, 2010

SUMMARY PRODUCT INFORMATION:

Route of Administration	Dosage Form/ Strength	Clinically Relevant Nonmedicinal Ingredients
Oral	Extended-release tablets: 100 mg, 200 mg and 300 mg	Tablet components: colloidal silicon dioxide, ethylcellulose, dibutyl sebacate, polyvinyl alcohol, polyvinyl pyrrolidone, sodium stearyl fumarate, black ink (containing: shellac glaze, isopropyl alcohol, iron oxide black, n-butyl alcohol, propylene glycol and ammonium hydroxide) For Complete Information see Dosage Forms, Composition and Packaging.

INDICATIONS AND CLINICAL USE: Adults: Ralivia (tramadol hydrochloride) extended-release tablets are indicated for the management of moderate to moderately severe pain in adults who require continuous treatment for several days or more.

Geriatrics (>65 years of age): Healthy elderly subjects aged 65 to 75 years administered tramadol have plasma concentrations and elimination half-lives comparable to those observed in healthy subjects less than 65 years of age. Ralivia should be administered with greater caution in patients older than 75 years, due to the greater potential for adverse events in this population (see Warnings and Precautions and Dosage and Administration).

Pediatrics (<18 years of age): The safety and efficacy of Ralivia in patients under 18 years of age have not been established. The use of Ralivia in the pediatric population is not recommended.

CONTRAINDICATIONS:

- Patients who have previously demonstrated hypersensitivity to tramadol, opioids or any other component of this product. For a complete listing of nonmedicinal ingredients, see Dosage Forms, Composition and Packaging.
- In any situation where opioids are contraindicated, including acute intoxication with any of the following: alcohol, hypnotics, centrally acting analgesics, opioids or psychotropic drugs. Ralivia may worsen central nervous system and respiratory depression in these patients.
- With concomitant MAO inhibitors (or within 14 days of such therapy).
- In severe renal or hepatic impairment (creatinine clearance of less than 30 mL/min and/or Child-Pugh Class C).

WARNINGS AND PRECAUTIONS: General: Ralivia (tramadol hydrochloride) extended-release tablets must be swallowed whole and should not be broken, chewed or crushed, since this can lead to the rapid release of tramadol and absorption of a potentially fatal dose of tramadol.

Seizure Risk: Seizures have been reported in patients receiving tramadol within the recommended dosage range. Spontaneous post-marketing reports indicate that seizure risk is increased with doses of tramadol above the recommended range. Concomitant use of tramadol increases the seizure risk in patients taking:

- Selective serotonin re-uptake inhibitors (SSRI antidepressants or anorectics), or
- Tricyclic antidepressants (TCAs), and other tricyclic compounds (e.g., cyclobenzaprine, promethazine, etc.), or
- opioids.

Administration of tramadol may enhance the seizure risk in patients taking:

- MAO inhibitors (see Contraindications),
- Neuroleptics,
- Other drugs that reduce the seizure threshold.

Risk of convulsions may also increase in patients with epilepsy, those with a history of seizures, or in patients with a recognized risk for seizure (such as head trauma, metabolic disorders, alcohol and drug withdrawal, CNS infections). In tramadol overdose, naloxone administration may increase the risk of seizure.

Anaphylactoid Reactions: Serious and rarely fatal anaphylactoid reactions have been reported in patients receiving therapy with tramadol. When these events do occur it is often following the first dose. Other reported allergic reactions include pruritus, hives, bronchospasm, angioedema, toxic epidermal necrolysis and Stevens-Johnson syndrome. Patients with a history of anaphylactoid reactions to codeine and other opioids may be at increased risk and therefore should not receive Ralivia (see Contraindications).

Drug Abuse, Addiction and Dependence: Tramadol has a potential to cause psychic and physical dependence of the morphine-type (µ-opioid). The drug has been associated with craving, drug-seeking behaviour and tolerance development. Cases of abuse and dependence on tramadol have been reported. Ralivia tablets should not be used in opioid-dependent patients. Tramadol can re-initiate physical dependence in patients who have been previously dependent or chronically using other opioids. In patients with a tendency to abuse drugs or a history of drug dependence, and in patients who are chronically abusing opioids, treatment with Ralivia is not recommended.

Proper assessment of the patient, proper prescribing practices, periodic re-evaluation of therapy, and proper dispensing and storage are appropriate measures that help to limit abuse of opioid drugs.

A Risk Management program to support the safe and effective use of Ralivia has been established. The following are considered to be the essential components of the Risk Management program: a) Commitment to not emphasize or highlight the scheduling status of Ralivia (i.e., not listed under a schedule to the CDSA) in its advertising or promotional activities; b) Inclusion of a PAAB-approved fair balance statement in all Ralivia advertising and promotional materials; c) Provision of progress reports to TPD, MHPD and HECSB from a drug abuse surveillance program for Ralivia; d) Assurance that health-care education activities on pain management with Ralivia include balanced, evidence-based and current information. Commitment to take reasonable actions to inform health-care professionals that there is Health Canada-approved patient information on benefits and risks, and to ensure that this information can be readily accessed through electronic and/or hard copy sources; e) Reassessment of the risk management program 2 years post product launch.

Ralivia is intended for oral use only. Ralivia could be abused by breaking, crushing, chewing, snorting, or injecting the dissolved product. These practices will result in the uncontrolled delivery of tramadol, and pose a significant risk to the abuser that could result in seizures, overdose, and death. These risks are increased with concurrent abuse of alcohol and other substances. With parenteral abuse, the tablet excipients can be expected to result in local tissue necrosis, infection, pulmonary granulomas, and increased risk of endocarditis and valvular heart injury.

Ralivia should not be used in opioid-dependent patients since it cannot suppress morphine withdrawal symptoms, even though it is an opioid agonist.

Abuse and addiction are separate and distinct from physical dependence and tolerance. In addition, abuse of opioids can occur in the absence of true addiction and is characterized by misuse for non-medical purposes, often in combination with other psychoactive substances. Tolerance as well as both physical and psychological dependence may develop upon repeated administration of opioids, and are not by themselves evidence of an addictive disorder or abuse.

Concerns about abuse, addiction, and diversion should not prevent the proper management of pain. The development of addiction to opioid analgesics in properly managed patients with pain has been reported to be rare. However, data are not available to establish the true incidence of addiction in chronic pain patients.

Careful record-keeping of prescribing information, including quantity, frequency, and renewal requests is strongly advised.

Withdrawal Symptoms: Withdrawal symptoms may occur following abrupt discontinuation of therapy. These symptoms may include anxiety, sweating, insomnia, rigors, pain, nausea, tremors, diarrhea, upper respiratory symptoms, piloerection and rarely hallucinations. Other symptoms that have been seen less frequently with tramadol discontinuation include: panic attacks, severe anxiety and paresthesias.

Patients on prolonged therapy should be withdrawn gradually from the drug if it is no longer required for pain control. Clinical experience suggests that withdrawal symptoms may be relieved by reinstitution of tramadol therapy followed by a gradual, tapered dose reduction of the medication combined with symptomatic support.

Risk of Overdosage: Serious potential consequences of overdosage with Ralivia are seizures, central nervous system depression, respiratory depression, and death. In treating an overdose, primary attention should be given to maintaining adequate ventilation along with general supportive treatment (see Overdosage).

Do not prescribe Ralivia for patients who are suicidal or addiction prone.

Ralivia should not be taken in doses higher than those recommended by the physician. The judicious prescribing of tramadol is essential to the safe use of this drug. With patients who are depressed or suicidal, consideration should be given to the use of non-narcotic analgesics. Patients should be cautioned about the concomitant use of tramadol products and alcohol because of potentially serious CNS-additive effects of these agents. Because of its added depressant effects, tramadol should be prescribed with caution for those patients whose medical condition requires the concomitant administration of sedatives, tranquilizers, muscle relaxants, antidepressants, or other CNS-depressant drugs. Patients should be advised of the additive depressant effects of these combinations.

Increased Intracranial Pressure or Head Trauma: Ralivia should be used with caution in patients with increased intracranial pressure or head injury, since the respiratory depressant effects of opioid receptor agonism include carbon dioxide retention and secondary elevation of cerebrospinal fluid pressure, and such effects may be markedly exaggerated in these patients. Also, pupillary changes (miosis) from tramadol may obscure the existence, extent or course of intracranial pathology. Clinicians should also maintain a high index of suspicion for adverse drug reaction when evaluating altered mental status in these patients if they are receiving tramadol (see Warnings and Precautions, Respiratory Depression).

Respiratory Depression: Administer Ralivia cautiously in patients at risk for respiratory depression. In these patients alternative non-opioid analgesics should be considered. When large doses of tramadol are administered with anesthetic medications or alcohol, respiratory depression may result. Respiratory depression should be treated as an overdose. If naloxone is to be administered, use cautiously because it may precipitate seizures (see Warnings and Precautions, Seizure Risk and Overdosage).

Interaction with Central Nervous System (CNS) Depressants: Ralivia should be used with caution and in reduced dosages when administered to patients receiving CNS depressants such as alcohol, opioids, anesthetic agents, narcotics, phenothiazines, tranquilizers or sedative hypnotics. Ralivia increases the risk of CNS and respiratory depression in these patients.

Ralivia may be expected to have additive effects when used in conjunction with alcohol, other opioids, or illicit drugs that cause central nervous system depression.

"In Vitro" Dissolution Studies of Interaction with Alcohol: As drugs may be abused in conjunction with alcohol, the effect of alcohol on the rate of drug release from Ralivia tablets was evaluated in dissolution studies using the product dissolution medium compared to 60% 0.1N HCl: 40% ethanol. Dissolution profiles for all tablet strengths in the alcohol medium were found to be within proposed dissolution specifications. The 60% 0.1N HCl: 40% ethanol medium resulted in a slight decrease in the rate of release of tramadol from Ralivia tablets. The clinical significance of the slight decrease in dissolution rate is unknown.

Use with Alcohol: Ralivia should not be used concomitantly with alcohol consumption. The use of Ralivia in patients with severe hepatic impairment is contraindicated. (See Contraindications.)

Use in Ambulatory Patients: Ralivia may impair the mental or physical abilities required for the performance of potentially hazardous tasks such as driving a car or operating machinery. Patients using Ralivia should be cautioned accordingly.

Use with Serotonin Re-uptake Inhibitors: Use Ralivia with great caution in patients taking SSRIs. Concomitant use of Ralivia with SSRIs increases the risk of adverse events, including seizure and serotonin syndrome. (See Warnings and Precautions, Seizure Risk and Drug Interactions.)

Acute Abdominal Conditions: The administration of Ralivia may complicate the clinical assessment of patients with acute abdominal conditions (e.g., cholecystitis, appendicitis, acute pancreatitis, etc.).

Use in Drug and Alcohol Addiction: Ralivia is an opioid with no approved use in the management of addictive disorders.

Special Populations: Renal Impairment: Impaired renal function results in a decreased rate and extent of excretion of tramadol and its active metabolite, M1. Ralivia has not been studied in patients with severe renal impairment (CLcr <30 mL/min). Ralivia is contraindicated in patients with severe renal impairment (see Contraindications; Action and Clinical Pharmacology and Dosage and Administration).

Hepatic/Biliary/Pancreatic Impairment: Use in Hepatic Disease: Metabolism of tramadol and it's M1 metabolite is reduced in patients with advanced cirrhosis of the liver. The pharmacokinetics of Ralivia has not been studied in patients with severe hepatic impairment (Child-Pugh Class C). Ralivia is contraindicated in patients with severe hepatic impairment (see Contraindications; Action and Clinical Pharmacology and Dosage and Administration).

Pregnant Women: There are no adequate and well-controlled studies in pregnant women. Safe use in pregnancy has not been established. Ralivia should not be used during pregnancy, prior to or during labor, unless in the opinion of the physician, the expected benefit to the patient outweighs the possible risk to the fetus. Chronic use during pregnancy may lead to physical dependence and post-partum withdrawal symptoms in the newborn (see Drug Abuse, Addiction and Dependence). Tramadol has been shown to cross the placenta. The mean ratio of serum tramadol in the umbilical veins compared to maternal veins was 0.83 for 40 women given tramadol during labour. Neonatal seizures, neonatal withdrawal syndrome, fetal death and stillbirth have been reported during post-marketing reports with tramadol HCl immediate-release products. The effect of Ralivia, if any, on the later growth, development, and functional maturation of the child is unknown.

Nursing Women: Tramadol and its metabolites are found in small amounts in human breast milk. Ralivia is not recommended for obstetrical preoperative medication, for post-delivery analgesia or at any time in nursing mothers because its safety in infants and newborns has not been studied.

Pediatrics (<18 years of age): The safety and efficacy of Ralivia has not been studied in the pediatric population. Therefore, use of Ralivia is not recommended in patients under 18 years of age.

Geriatrics (>65 years of age): In general, caution should be used when selecting the dose for an elderly patient. The elimination half-life of tramadol may be prolonged in patients over 75 years, thereby increasing the potential for adverse events. Usually, dose administration should start at the low end of the dosing range, reflecting the greater frequency of decreased hepatic, renal or cardiac function and of concomitant disease or other drug therapy (see Dosage and Administration).

Nine hundred-one elderly (≥65 years of age) subjects were exposed to Ralivia in clinical trials. Of those subjects, 156 were ≥75 years of age. Based on all dosage groups combined, the incidence of adverse events was similar for patients ≥65 years, compared with patients <65 years, except for constipation which was higher, and headache which was lower, in patients ≥65 years of age.

ADVERSE REACTIONS: Adverse Drug Reaction Overview: Ralivia was administered to a total of 3108 patients in four double-blind studies in patients with chronic pain of osteoarthritis or low back pain, and one 1-year open-label study in patients with chronic non-malignant pain. A total of 901 patients were ≥65 years.

Incidence of Commonly Observed Adverse Events in Controlled Clinical Trials: The most common adverse events with Ralivia were dizziness, nausea, constipation, and headache.

Clinical Trial Adverse Drug Reactions: Because clinical trials are conducted under very specific conditions, the adverse reaction rates observed in the clinical trials may not reflect the rates observed in practice and should not be compared to the rates in the clinical trials of another drug. Adverse drug reaction information from clinical trials is useful for identifying drug-related adverse events and for approximating rates.

Table 1 shows incidence of all adverse events ≥1% in the four randomized, placebo- controlled studies, whether considered by the clinical investigator to be related to the study drug or not. The adverse events observed in the open label study were similar to those seen in the 4 randomized, placebo-controlled, clinical trials.

Table 1: Ralivia

Adverse Events: Placebo-Controlled Studies

Treatment-emergent Adverse Experiences Occurring in ≥1% of Patients Taking Ralivia (with an incidence greater than placebo)							
		Ralivia					
	MedDRA Preferred Term	Flexible[a] (N=133) n (%)	100 mg QD (N=403) n (%)	200 mg QD (N=529) n (%)	300 mg QD (N=528) n (%)	Total (N=1795) n (%)	Placebo (N=664) n (%)
Eye Disorders	Vision blurred	0 (0.0)	4 (1.0)	2 (0.4)	5 (0.9)	14 (0.8)	3 (0.5)
Gastrointestinal Disorders	Nausea	33 (24.8)	61 (15.1)	102 (19.3)	128 (24.2)	377 (21.0)	51 (7.7)
	Constipation	32 (24.1)	49 (12.2)	76 (14.4)	104 (19.7)	321 (17.9)	25 (3.8)
	Diarrhea NOS	12 (9.0)	15 (3.7)	38 (7.2)	43 (8.1)	118 (6.6)	29 (4.4)
	Vomiting NOS	10 (7.5)	20 (5.0)	36 (6.8)	44 (8.3)	129 (7.2)	13 (2.0)
	Dry mouth	4 (3.0)	20 (5.0)	29 (5.5)	39 (7.4)	110 (6.1)	8 (1.2)
	Abdominal pain upper	3 (2.3)	5 (1.2)	12 (2.3)	16 (3.0)	41 (2.3)	5 (0.8)
	Abdominal pain NOS	3 (2.3)	5 (1.2)	6 (1.1)	6 (1.1)	24 (1.3)	3 (0.5)
	Dyspepsia	2 (1.5)	7 (1.7)	10 (1.9)	14 (2.7)	38 (2.1)	8 (1.2)
	Sore throat NOS	3 (2.3)	6 (1.5)	5 (0.9)	5 (0.9)	22 (1.2)	9 (1.4)
General Disorders and Administration Site Conditions	Asthenia	10 (7.5)	14 (3.5)	29 (5.5)	32 (6.1)	98 (5.5)	10 (1.5)
	Feeling hot	4 (3.0)	7 (1.7)	7 (1.3)	7 (1.3)	28 (1.6)	3 (0.5)
	Rigors	3 (2.3)	3 (0.7)	3 (0.6)	11 (2.1)	27 (1.5)	2 (0.3)
	Influenza-like illness	3 (2.3)	1 (0.2)	7 (1.3)	8 (1.5)	23 (1.3)	4 (0.6)
	Chest pain NEC	3 (2.3)	3 (0.7)	4 (0.8)	4 (0.8)	17 (0.9)	4 (0.6)
	Lethargy	3 (2.3)	4 (1.0)	4 (0.8)	1 (0.2)	14 (0.8)	3 (0.5)
	Pain NOS	2 (1.5)	10 (2.5)	16 (3.0)	16 (3.0)	49 (2.7)	14 (2.1)
	Fall	2 (1.5)	5 (1.2)	5 (0.9)	5 (0.9)	19 (1.1)	3 (0.5)
	Malaise	2 (1.5)	0 (0.0)	1 (0.2)	5 (0.9)	10 (0.6)	0 (0.0)
	Drug withdrawal syndrome	2 (1.5)	1 (0.2)	2 (0.4)	0 (0.0)	7 (0.4)	0 (0.0)
	Weakness	1 (0.8)	3 (0.7)	11 (2.1)	15 (2.8)	39 (2.2)	5 (0.8)

(cont'd)

Table 1: Ralivia *(cont'd)*

Adverse Events: Placebo-Controlled Studies

Treatment-emergent Adverse Experiences Occurring in ≥1% of Patients Taking Ralivia (with an incidence greater than placebo)							
		Ralivia					
	MedDRA Preferred Term	Flexible[a] (N=133) n (%)	100 mg QD (N=403) n (%)	200 mg QD (N=529) n (%)	300 mg QD (N=528) n (%)	Total (N=1795) n (%)	Placebo (N=664) n (%)
Infections and Infestations	Influenza	9 (6.8)	4 (1.0)	4 (0.8)	3 (0.6)	23 (1.3)	3 (0.5)
	Upper respiratory tract infection NOS	5 (3.8)	15 (3.7)	12 (2.3)	13 (2.5)	49 (2.7)	20 (3.0)
	Sinusitis NOS	3 (2.3)	7 (1.7)	13 (2.5)	12 (2.3)	40 (2.2)	12 (1.8)
Investigations	Weight decreased	3 (2.3)	0 (0.0)	4 (0.8)	10 (1.9)	23 (1.3)	1 (0.2)
	Blood creatine phosphokinase increased	0 (0.0)	7 (1.7)	8 (1.5)	10 (1.9)	28 (1.6)	6 (0.9)
Metabolism and Nutrition Disorcers	Anorexia	3 (2.3)	3 (0.7)	7 (1.3)	23 (4.4)	48 (2.7)	1 (0.2)
	Appetite decreased NOS	2 (1.5)	5 (1.2)	9 (1.7)	8 (1.5)	31 (1.7)	3 (0.5)
	Gout	2 (1.5)	1 (0.2)	0 (0.0)	1 (0.2)	5 (0.3)	2 (0.3)
Musculoskeletal, Connective Tissue and Bone Disorders	Back pain	3 (2.3)	11 (2.7)	9 (1.7)	8 (1.5)	36 (2.0)	10 (1.5)
	Muscle spasms	3 (2.3)	4 (1.0)	2 (0.4)	3 (0.6)	12 (0.7)	4 (0.6)
Nervous System Disorders	Dizziness (exc vertigo)	46 (34.6)	64 (15.9)	95 (18.0)	108 (20.5)	370 (22.6)	54 (8.1)
	Headache NOS	18 (13.5)	49 (12.2)	78 (14.7)	65 (12.3)	242 (13.5)	77 (11.6)
	Somnolence	10 (7.5)	33 (8.2)	46 (8.7)	32 (6.1)	162 (9.0)	11 (1.7)
	Insomnia NEC	8 (6.0)	26 (6.5)	42 (7.9)	54 (10.2)	152 (8.5)	22 (3.3)
	Paresthesia NEC	3 (2.3)	1 (0.2)	3 (0.6)	3 (0.6)	15 (0.8)	7 (1.1)
	Irritability	3 (2.3)	2 (0.5)	3 (0.6)	3 (0.6)	12 (0.7)	3 (0.5)
	Tremor NEC	1 (0.8)	3 (0.7)	4 (0.8)	14 (2.7)	24 (1.3)	1 (0.2)
	Dizziness aggravated	0 (0.0)	2 (0.5)	7 (1.3)	3 (0.6)	16 (0.9)	2 (0.3)
Psychiatric Disorders	Restlessness	2 (1.5)	3 (0.7)	2 (0.4)	10 (1.9)	18 (1.0)	2 (0.3)
	Nervousness	0 (0.0)	7 (1.7)	13 (2.5)	20 (3.8)	48 (2.7)	5 (0.8)
	Anxiety NEC	0 (0.0)	2 (0.5)	9 (1.7)	15 (2.8)	28 (1.6)	4 (0.6)
	Depression NEC	0 (0.0)	2 (0.5)	4 (0.8)	8 (1.5)	17 (0.9)	2 (0.3)
Renal and Urinary Disorders	Hematuria	3 (2.3)	1 (0.2)	2 (0.4)	6 (1.1)	13 (0.7)	1 (0.2)
	Difficulty in micturition	2 (1.5)	2 (0.5)	0 (0.0)	5 (0.9)	11 (0.6)	2 (0.3)
Respiratory, Thoracic and Mediastinal Disorders	Sneezing	0 (0.0)	10 (2.5)	10 (1.9)	12 (2.3)	36 (2.0)	2 (0.3)
	Rhinorrhea	1 (0.8)	8 (2.0)	11 (2.1)	7 (1.3)	28 (1.6)	5 (0.8)
Skin and Subcutaneous Tissue Disorders	Pruritus NOS	9 (6.8)	25 (6.2)	36 (6.8)	31 (5.9)	125 (7.0)	6 (0.9)
	Sweating increased	5 (3.8)	6 (1.5)	9 (1.7)	18 (3.4)	51 (2.8)	1 (0.2)
	Dermatitis NOS	5 (3.8)	5 (1.2)	9 (1.7)	13 (2.5)	35 (1.9)	10 (1.5)
	Urticaria NOS	2 (1.5)	1 (0.2)	2 (0.4)	1 (0.2)	8 (0.4)	3 (0.5)
	Contusion	1 (0.8)	5 (1.2)	6 (1.1)	4 (0.8)	17 (0.9)	1 (0.2)
Vascular Disorders	Flushing	13 (9.8)	31 (7.7)	47 (8.9)	42 (8.0)	165 (9.2)	26 (3.9)
	Postural hypotension	3 (2.3)	7 (1.7)	21 (4.0)	18 (3.4)	60 (3.3)	15 (2.3)
	Vasodilatation	2 (1.5)	1 (0.2)	4 (0.8)	2 (0.4)	14 (0.8)	3 (0.5)
	Hot flushes NOS	0 (0.0)	4 (1.0)	11 (2.1)	13 (2.5)	32 (1.8)	5 (0.8)

[a] Patients in the flexible dose study received Ralivia 200 to 400 mg per day.

The following listings include adverse events for the four placebo-controlled studies and the open-label study (N=3108):

Adverse Events with Incidence Rates ≥1.0% and Not Noted in the Placebo-controlled Studies: General Disorders: pyrexia.

Infections and Infestations: bronchitis, viral gastroenteritis, nasopharyngitis.

Musculoskeletal, Connective Tissue and Bone Disorders: neck pain, arthralgia.

Nervous System Disorders: hypoaesthesia.

Respiratory, Thoracic and Mediastinal Disorders: dyspnoea, nasal congestion, sinus congestion.

Adverse Events with Incidence Rates <1.0%: Cardiac Disorders: palpitations, myocardial infarction.

Ear and Labyrinth Disorders: tinnitus.

Gastrointestinal Disorders: flatulence, constipation aggravated, toothache, pancreatitis.

General Disorders: feeling jittery, edema lower limb, shivering, joint swelling, malaise, drug withdrawal syndrome, peripheral swelling.

Hepato-biliary Disorders: cholelithiasis, cholecystitis.

Infections and Infestations: appendicitis, cellulitis, ear infection, gastroenteritis, pneumonia, urinary tract infection, viral infection.

Injury and Poisoning: joint sprain, muscle injury.

Investigations: heart rate increased, liver function tests abnormal, blood pressure increased, alanine aminotransferase increased, aspartate aminotransferase increased, blood glucose increased.

Musculoskeletal, Connective Tissue and Bone Disorders: joint stiffness, myalgia, muscle cramps, muscle spasms, muscle twitching, osteoarthritis aggravated.

Nervous System Disorders: migraine, syncope, disturbance in attention, dizziness aggravated, vertigo, sedation.

Psychiatric Disorders: irritability, libido decreased, euphoric mood, sleep disorder, agitation, disorientation, abnormal dreams.

Renal and Urinary Disorders: difficulty in micturition, urinary frequency, urinary retention, dysuria, haematuria.

Respiratory, Thoracic and Mediastinal Disorders: yawning.

Skin and Subcutaneous Tissue Disorders: contusion, clamminess, night sweats, urticaria, piloerection.

Vascular Disorders: hypertension aggravated, hypertension, peripheral ischaemia.

Abnormal Hematologic and Clinical Chemistry Findings: In clinical trials where clinical abnormalities were recorded (n=230), the following clinical laboratory abnormalities were reported: alanine aminotransferase increased (0.8%), aspartate aminotransferase increased (0.7%), liver function tests NOS abnormal (0.4%), blood lactate dehydrogenase increased (0.3%), white blood cell count increased (0.3%), blood alkaline phosphatase NOS increased (0.3%), hematocrit decreased (0.3%), rectal hemorrhage (0.3%), and hypokalemia (0.3%).

The following abnormalities occurred in 0.2% of patients: red blood cell count decreased, hemoglobin decreased, blood calcium increased, blood creatinine increased, anemia NOS, blood potassium decreased, and neutrophil count increased.

The following abnormalities occurred in 0.1% of patients: thrombocythemia, blood potassium increased, blood bilirubin increased, blood in stool, hemoglobin increased, hypercalcemia, hematocrit increased, eosinophil count increased, blood sodium increased, and hyponatremia.

The following abnormalities were single occurrences in patients: blood sodium decreased, hyperkalemia, blood calcium decreased, hypophosphatemia, hemoptysis, hematemesis, red blood cell count increased, band neutrophil count increased, monocyte count increased, and lymphocyte count increased.

Other Adverse Experiences Previously Reported in Clinical Trials or Post-Marketing Reports with Tramadol Hydrochloride: Adverse events which have been reported with the use of tramadol products include: allergic reactions (including anaphylaxis, angioneurotic edema and urticaria, Stevens-Johnson syndrome), bradycardia, convulsions, drug dependence, hyperactivity, hypoactivity, and respiratory depression. Other adverse events which have been reported with the use of tramadol products and for which a causal association has not been determined include: difficulty concentrating, hepatitis, liver failure, pulmonary edema, and suicidal tendency.

Serotonin syndrome (whose symptoms may include mental status change, hyperreflexia, fever, shivering, tremor, agitation, diaphoresis, seizures and coma) has been reported with tramadol when used concomitantly with other serotonergic agents such as SSRIs and MAOIs.

Drug Abuse, Addiction and Dependence: Tramadol may induce psychic and physical dependence of the morphine-type (μ-opioid) (see Warnings and Precautions, Drug Abuse, Addiction and Dependence). Dependence and abuse, including drug-seeking behaviour and taking illicit actions to obtain the drug, are not limited to those patients with a prior history of opioid dependence. The risk in patients with substance abuse has been observed to be higher. Tramadol is associated with craving and tolerance development.

A Risk Management program to support the safe and effective use of Ralivia has been established. The following are considered to be the essential components of the Risk Management program: a) commitment to not emphasize or highlight the scheduling status of Ralivia (i.e., not listed under a schedule to the CDSA) in its advertising or promotional activities; b) inclusion of a PAAB-approved fair balance statement in all Ralivia advertising and promotional materials; c) provision of progress reports to TPD, MHPD and HECSB from a drug abuse surveillance program for Ralivia; d) assurance that health-care education activities on pain management with Ralivia include balanced, evidence-based and current information. Commitment to take reasonable actions to inform health-care professionals that there is Health Canada approved patient information on benefits and risks, and to ensure that this information can be readily accessed through electronic and/or hard copy sources; e) reassessment of the risk management program 2 years post product launch.

Withdrawal Symptoms: Withdrawal symptoms may occur if tramadol is discontinued abruptly. These symptoms may include: anxiety, sweating, insomnia, rigors, pain, nausea, tremors, diarrhea, upper respiratory symptoms, piloerection, and rarely, hallucinations. Other symptoms that have been seen less frequently with Ralivia discontinuation include: panic attacks, severe anxiety, and paresthesias. Clinical experience suggests that withdrawal symptoms may be relieved by reinstitution of opioid therapy followed by a gradual, tapered dose reduction of the medication combined with symptomatic support.

DRUG INTERACTIONS: Overview: In vitro studies indicated that tramadol is unlikely to inhibit the CYP3A4-mediated metabolism of other drugs when tramadol is administered concomitantly at therapeutic doses.

Tramadol does not appear to induce its own metabolism in humans, since observed maximal plasma concentrations after multiple oral doses are higher than expected based on single dose data.

Tramadol is a mild inducer of selected drug metabolism pathways measured in animals.

Drug-Drug Interactions: MAO Inhibitors: Tramadol is contraindicated in patients receiving MAO inhibitors or who have used them within the previous 14 days (see Contraindications and Warnings and Precautions).

Drugs that Lower Seizure Threshold: Tramadol can increase the potential for selective serotonin re-uptake inhibitors (SSRIs), tricyclic anti-depressants (TCAs), anti-psychotics and other seizure threshold lowering drugs to cause convulsions (see Warnings and Precautions).

CNS Depressants: Concurrent administration of tramadol with other centrally acting drugs, including alcohol, centrally acting analgesics, opioids and psychotropic drugs may potentiate CNS depressant effects.

Carbamazepine: Carbamazepine, a CYP3A4 inducer, increases tramadol metabolism. Patients taking carbamazepine may have a significantly reduced analgesic effect of tramadol. Because of the seizure risk associated with tramadol, concomitant administration of Ralivia and carbamazepine is not recommended (see Warnings and Precautions).

Quinidine: Tramadol is metabolized to M1 by CYP2D6. A study was conducted to examine the effect of quinidine, a selective inhibitor of CYP2D6, on the pharmacokinetics of tramadol by administering 200 mg of quinidine two hours before the administration of Ralivia 100 mg. The results demonstrated that the exposure of tramadol increased 50-60% and the exposure of M1 decreased 60-65%. In vitro drug interaction studies in human liver microsomes indicate that tramadol has no effect on quinidine metabolism.

Inhibitors of CYP2D6: Inhibitors of CYP2D6 (e.g., quinidine, fluoxetine, paroxetine, amitriptyline) may inhibit the metabolism of tramadol, resulting in increased serum concentrations of tramadol and decreased concentrations of its O-demethylated metabolite (M1). Co-administration of quinidine did not diminish the analgesic effect of tramadol in human experimental pain models.

Inhibitors or Inducers of CYP3A4: Administration of CYP3A4 inhibitors, such as ketoconazole and erythromycin, or inducers, such as rifampin and St. John's Wort may affect the metabolism of tramadol, leading to altered tramadol exposure.

Cimetidine: Concomitant administration of tramadol immediate-release tablets with cimetidine does not result in clinically significant changes in tramadol pharmacokinetics. No alteration of the Ralivia dosage regimen with cimetidine is recommended.

Digoxin: Digoxin toxicity has occurred rarely during co-administration of digoxin and tramadol.

Protease Inhibitors, e.g., ritonavir: Co-administered ritonavir may increase the serum concentration of tramadol, resulting in tramadol toxicity.

Warfarin and Other Coumarin Anticoagulants: Alteration of the effect of warfarin, including elevation of prothrombin times, has been reported rarely during co-administration of warfarin and tramadol. While such changes have been generally of limited clinical significance for the individual products, periodic evaluation of prothrombin time should be performed when Ralivia tablets and warfarin-like compounds are administered concurrently.

Drug-Food Interactions: After a single dose administration of 200 mg Ralivia tablet with a high fat meal, the C_{max} and $AUC_{0-\infty}$ of tramadol decreased 28% and 14%, respectively, compared to fasting conditions. Mean T_{max} was increased by 3 h (from 14 h under fasting conditions to 17 h under fed conditions). While Ralivia may be taken without regard to food, it is recommended that it be taken in a consistent manner.

DOSAGE AND ADMINISTRATION: Dosing Considerations: Ralivia (tramadol hydrochloride extended-release tablets) is not recommended for minor pain, or acute short-term pain that may be treated adequately through lesser means where benefit does not outweigh the possible opioid-related side effects.

Due to possible differences in pharmacokinetic properties, Ralivia tablets are not interchangeable with other tramadol extended-release formulations.

The maximum recommended daily dose of Ralivia should not be exceeded.

Ralivia can be administered without regard to food.

Administration: Ralivia tablets are a once-daily extended-release formulation that must be swallowed whole and should not be broken, chewed or crushed, since this can lead to the rapid release of tramadol and absorption of a potentially fatal dose of tramadol.

Recommended Dose and Dosage Adjustment: General: Ralivia is designed for once-daily dosing, i.e., dosing at 24-hourly intervals. Treatment with Ralivia should be initiated at the lowest available dose (100 mg). Clinical studies of Ralivia have not demonstrated a clinical benefit at a total daily dose exceeding 300 mg. The maximum dose is 300 mg daily.

The correct dosage for any individual patient is that which controls the pain for a full 24 hours, with no or tolerable side effects.

As with all analgesic drugs, the dose of tramadol should be adjusted according to the severity of the pain and the clinical response of the individual patient. It is recommended that doses be slowly titrated (dosage adjustments generally separated by five days), to higher doses to minimize side effects.

Patients Not Receiving Opioids at the Time of Initiation of Tramadol Treatment: The usual initial dose of Ralivia for patients who have not previously received opioid analgesics is 100 mg q24h.

Patients Currently Receiving Other Tramadol Formulations: Patients currently receiving oral immediate-release tramadol preparations may be transferred to Ralivia tablets at the same or lowest nearest total daily tramadol dosage.

Adults (18 years of age and older): Ralivia should be initiated at a dose of 100 mg once daily and may be titrated up by 100 mg increments every five days, as necessary and depending on tolerability, to relief of pain. Ralivia should not be administered at doses exceeding 300 mg per day.

Geriatric Patients (>65 years old): In general, dose selection for patients over 65 years of age, who may have decreased hepatic or renal function, or other concomitant diseases, should be initiated cautiously, usually starting at the low end of the dosing range. Ralivia should be administered with greater caution at the lowest effective dose in patients over 75 years, due to the potential for greater frequency of adverse events in this population.

Pediatrics (<18 years old): The safety and efficacy of Ralivia has not been studied in the pediatric population. Therefore, Ralivia is not indicated for use in children under 18 years of age.

Patients with Renal or Hepatic Insufficiency: The elimination half-life of tramadol and its active metabolite may be prolonged in these patient populations. A starting dose of 100 mg daily is recommended. Upward dosage titration should be done with careful monitoring. Tramadol is contraindicated in patients with severe renal impairment and/or severe hepatic impairment (creatinine clearance less than 30 mL/min and/or Child-Pugh Class C, see Contraindications).

Management of Patients Requiring Rescue Medication: If rescue medications are warranted for episodes of pain in the course of appropriate adjustments of Ralivia dose, acetaminophen or ibuprofen may be given. If immediate release tramadol is used as rescue medication, the total daily dose of tramadol should not exceed 300 mg. Selection of rescue medication should be based on individual patient conditions. Fentanyl products should not be used as rescue medication in patients taking Ralivia.

Missed Dose: If a patient forgets to take one or more doses, they should take their next dose at the normal time and in the normal amount.

Discontinuation: Withdrawal symptoms may occur if Ralivia is discontinued abruptly. These symptoms may include: anxiety, sweating, insomnia, rigors, pain, nausea, tremors, diarrhea, upper respiratory symptoms, piloerection, and rarely hallucinations. Clinical experience suggests that withdrawal symptoms may be reduced by tapering Ralivia.

OVERDOSAGE:
Deaths due to overdose have been reported with abuse and misuse of tramadol, by ingesting, inhaling, or injecting the crushed tablets. Review of case reports has indicated that the risk of fatal overdose is further increased when tramadol is abused concurrently with alcohol or other CNS depressants, including other opioids.

Symptoms: Acute overdosage with tramadol can be manifested by respiratory depression, somnolence progressing to stupor or coma, skeletal muscle flaccidity, cold and clammy skin, constricted pupils, bradycardia, hypotension, and death.

Deaths due to overdose have been reported with abuse and misuse of tramadol, by ingesting, inhaling, or injecting the crushed tablets. Review of case reports has indicated that the risk of fatal overdose is further increased when tramadol is abused concurrently with alcohol or other CNS depressants, including other opioids.

Treatment: In the treatment of tramadol overdosage, primary attention should be given to the re-establishment of a patent airway and institution of assisted or controlled ventilation. Supportive measures (including oxygen and vasopressors) should be employed in the management of circulatory shock and pulmonary edema accompanying overdose as indicated. Cardiac arrest or arrhythmias may require cardiac massage or defibrillation.

While naloxone will reverse some, but not all, symptoms caused by overdosage with tramadol, the risk of seizures is also increased with naloxone administration. Seizures may be controlled with diazepam.

In animals, convulsions following the administration of toxic doses of Ralivia could be suppressed with barbiturates or benzodiazepines but were increased with naloxone. Naloxone administration did not change the lethality of an overdose in mice.

Hemodialysis is not expected to be helpful in an overdose because it removes less than 7% of the administered dose in a 4-hour dialysis period.

Emptying of the gastric contents is useful to remove any unabsorbed drug.

> For management of a suspected drug overdose, CPhA recommends that you contact your **regional Poison Control Centre**. See the *CPS* Directory section for a list of Poison Control Centres.

ACTION AND CLINICAL PHARMACOLOGY: Mechanism of Action: Tramadol is a centrally acting synthetic opioid analgesic. Although its mode of action is not completely understood, animal tests suggest that at least two complementary mechanisms appear applicable: binding of parent and M1 metabolite to μ-opioid receptors and weak inhibition of reuptake of norepinephrine and serotonin.

Opioid activity is due to both low affinity binding of the parent compound and higher affinity binding of the O-demethylated metabolite M1 to μ-opioid receptors. In animal models, M1 is up to 6-times more potent than tramadol in producing analgesia and 200-times more potent in μ-opioid binding. Tramadol-induced analgesia is only partially antagonized by the opiate antagonist naloxone in several animal tests. The relative contribution of both tramadol and M1 to human analgesia is dependent upon the plasma concentrations of each compound.

Tramadol has been shown to inhibit reuptake of norepinephrine and serotonin in vitro, as have some other opioid analgesics. These mechanisms may contribute independently to the overall analgesic profile of tramadol. The relationship between exposure of tramadol and M1 and efficacy has not been evaluated in the Ralivia clinical studies.

Apart from analgesia, tramadol administration may produce a constellation of symptoms (including dizziness, somnolence, nausea, constipation, sweating and pruritus) similar to that of other opioids. In contrast to morphine, tramadol has not been shown to cause histamine release. Tramadol produces less respiratory depression than other opioids and has no significant cardiac effects. At therapeutic doses, tramadol has no effect on heart rate, left-ventricular function or cardiac index. Orthostatic hypotension has been observed.

Pharmacodynamics: The administration of naloxone only partially antagonizes tramadol's antinociceptive and analgesic effects in animals and man, indicating a contribution from non-opioid analgesic mechanisms. In animals and man the effect of tramadol is attenuated by the α_2-adrenoceptor antagonist, yohimbine, and in animals, the serotonin antagonist rianserin reduces the antinociceptive effect of tramadol. This indicates the potential for a contribution to the analgesic effect of tramadol through modulation of monaminergic inhibitory pain pathways in the dorsal horn of the spinal cord, in addition to an opioidergic effect.

Pharmacokinetics: The analgesic activity of tramadol is due to both parent drug and the M1 metabolite. Ralivia is administered as a racemate and both the [−] and [+] forms of both tramadol and M1 are detected in the circulation.

The pharmacokinetics of Ralivia is approximately dose-proportional over a 100-400 mg dose range in healthy subjects. However, the observed tramadol AUC values for the 400-mg dose were 26% higher than predicted based on the AUC values for the 200-mg dose. The clinical significance of this finding has not been studied and is not known.

Absorption: Consistent with the extended-release nature of the formulation, there is a lag time in drug absorption following Ralivia administration. The mean peak plasma concentrations of tramadol and M1 after administration of Ralivia tablets to healthy volunteers are attained at about 12 h and 15 h, respectively, after dosing. Following administration of the Ralivia, steady-state plasma concentrations of both tramadol and M1 are achieved within four days with once daily dosing.

Food Effects: After a single dose administration of 200 mg Ralivia tablet with a high fat meal, the C_{max} and $AUC_{0-\infty}$ of tramadol decreased 28% and 14%, respectively, compared to fasting conditions. Mean T_{max} was increased by 3 h (from 14 h under fasting conditions to 17 h under fed conditions). While Ralivia may be taken without regard to food, it is recommended that it be taken in a consistent manner.

Distribution: The volume of distribution of tramadol was 2.6 and 2.9 L/kg in male and female subjects, respectively, following a 100 mg intravenous dose. The binding of tramadol to human plasma proteins is approximately 20% and binding also appears to be independent of concentration up to 10 μg/mL. Saturation of plasma protein binding occurs only at concentrations outside the clinically relevant range.

Metabolism: Tramadol is extensively metabolized after oral administration. The major metabolic pathways appear to be N- (mediated by CYP3A4 and CYP2B6) and O- (mediated by CYP2D6) demethylation and glucuronidation or sulfation in the liver. One metabolite (O-desmethyl tramadol, denoted M1) is pharmacologically active in animal models. Formation of M1 is dependent on CYP2D6 and as such is subject to inhibition, which may affect the therapeutic response (see Drug Interactions).

Excretion: Tramadol is eliminated primarily through metabolism by the liver and the metabolites are eliminated primarily by the kidneys. Approximately 30% of the dose is excreted in the urine as unchanged drug, whereas 60% of the dose is excreted as metabolites. The remainder is excreted either as unidentified or as unextractable metabolites. The mean terminal plasma elimination half-lives of racemic tramadol and racemic M1 after administration of Ralivia are approximately 7.9 and 8.8 h, respectively.

Special Populations and Conditions: Pediatrics: The pharmacokinetics of Ralivia in individuals under 18 years old has not been evaluated. Therefore, its use is not recommended in patients under 18 years of age.

Geriatrics (>65 years of age): Healthy elderly subjects aged 65 to 75 years administered tramadol have plasma concentrations and elimination half lives comparable to those observed in healthy subjects less than 65 years of age. Ralivia should be administered with greater caution in patients older than 75 years due to the greater potential for adverse events in this population (see Warnings and Precautions and Dosage and Administration).

Gender: Based on pooled multiple-dose pharmacokinetics studies for Ralivia in 166 healthy subjects (111 males and 55 females), the dose-normalized AUC values for tramadol were somewhat higher in females than in males. There was a considerable degree of overlap in dose-normalized AUC values for males and females, thus, dosage adjustment based on gender is not recommended.

Race: Due to the small sample size for Asian, Hispanic, and other populations, conclusions cannot be drawn about the pharmacokinetics of tramadol in these populations.

Hepatic Insufficiency: Pharmacokinetics of tramadol was studied in patients with mild or moderate hepatic impairment after receiving multiple doses of Ralivia 100 mg. The exposure of (+)- and (−)-tramadol was similar in mild and moderate hepatic impairment patients in comparison to patients with normal hepatic function. However, exposure of (+)- and (−)-M1 decreased ~50% with increased severity of the hepatic impairment (from normal to mild and moderate). The pharmacokinetics of tramadol after the administration of Ralivia has not been studied in patients with severe hepatic impairment (Child-Pugh Class C). After the administration of tramadol immediate-release tablets to patients with advanced cirrhosis of the liver, tramadol AUC was larger and the tramadol and M1 half-lives were longer than subjects with normal hepatic function. Ralivia is contraindicated in patients with severe hepatic impairment (see Contraindications; Warnings and Precautions, Hepatic/Biliary/Pancreatic Impairment and Dosage and Administration).

Renal Insufficiency: Impaired renal function results in a decreased rate and extent of excretion of tramadol and its active metabolite, M1. The pharmacokinetics of tramadol were studied in patients with mild or moderate renal impairment after receiving multiple doses of Ralivia 100 mg. There is no consistent trend observed for tramadol exposure related to renal function in patients with mild (CLcr: 50-80 mL/min) or moderate (CLcr: 30-50 mL/min) renal impairment in comparison to patients with normal renal function. However, exposure of M1 increased 20-40% with increased severity of the renal impairment (from normal to mild and moderate). Ralivia has not been studied in patients with severe renal impairment (CLcr <30 mL/min). Ralivia is contraindicated in patients with severe renal impairment (see Contraindications; Warnings and Precautions, Renal Impairment and Dosage and Administration). The total amount of tramadol and M1 removed during a 4-hour dialysis period is less than 7% of the administered dose.

STORAGE AND STABILITY: Store at room temperature (15-30°C).

INFORMATION FOR THE PATIENT: Published in e-CPS, available by subscription at www.e-cps.ca.

DOSAGE FORMS, COMPOSITION AND PACKAGING: 100 mg: Each round, white, extended-release tablet, imprinted with "100" over "ER" in black ink, contains: tramadol hydrochloride 100 mg. Nonmedicinal ingredients: colloidal silicon dioxide, dibutyl sebacate, ethylcellulose, polyvinyl alcohol, polyvinyl pyrrolidone, sodium stearyl fumarate and black ink (containing: shellac glaze, isopropyl alcohol, iron oxide black, n-butyl alcohol, propylene glycol and ammonium hydroxide). Bottles of 30, 90 and 500.
200 mg: Each round, white, extended-release tablet, imprinted with "200" over "ER" in black ink, contains: tramadol hydrochloride 200 mg. Nonmedicinal ingredients: colloidal silicon dioxide, dibutyl sebacate, ethylcellulose, polyvinyl alcohol, polyvinyl pyrrolidone, sodium stearyl fumarate and black ink (containing: shellac glaze, isopropyl alcohol, iron oxide black, n-butyl alcohol, propylene glycol and ammonium hydroxide). Bottles of 30, 90 and 500.
300 mg: Each round, white, extended-release tablet, imprinted with "300" over "ER" in black ink, contains: tramadol hydrochloride 300 mg. Nonmedicinal ingredients: colloidal silicon dioxide, dibutyl sebacate, ethylcellulose, polyvinyl alcohol, polyvinyl pyrrolidone, sodium stearyl fumarate and black ink (containing: shellac glaze, isopropyl alcohol, iron oxide black, n-butyl alcohol, propylene glycol and ammonium hydroxide). Bottles of 30, 90 and 500.

(Shown in product Identification Section)

Ramipril P

CPhA Monograph

see ACE Inhibitors

The reader is invited to consult CPhA's monograph **Calcium Channel Blockers**.

RAN™-Amlodipine P

amlodipine besylate

Antihypertensive—Antianginal

Ranbaxy

SUPPLIED: 5 mg: Each white to off-white, octagonal, flat, uncoated tablet, debossed with "RI63" on one side and break line on the other side, contains: amlodipine 5 mg (as amlodipine besylate). Nonmedicinal ingredients: colloidal silicon dioxide, magnesium stearate, mannitol, microcrystalline cellulose and sodium starch glycolate. Bottles of 100 and 500. Store at 15-30°C. Protect from light.
10 mg: Each white to off-white, octagonal, flat, uncoated tablet, debossed with "RI64" on one side and plain on the other side, contains: amlodipine 10 mg (as amlodipine besylate). Nonmedicinal ingredients: colloidal silicon dioxide, magnesium stearate, mannitol, microcrystalline cellulose and sodium starch glycolate. Bottles of 100 and 500. Store at 15-30°C. Protect from light.

RAN™-Atenolol P

atenolol

Beta-adrenergic Receptor Blocking Agent

Ranbaxy

SUPPLIED: 50 mg: Each round, white, biconvex, film-coated tablet, engraved "rbx R14" on one side and bisected on the other, contains: atenolol 50 mg. Blisters of 30. Bottles of 100 and 500. Store at room temperature (15-30°C). Protect from light and moisture. Keep away from children.
100 mg: Each round, white, biconvex, film-coated tablet, engraved "rbx R15" on one side and bisected on the other, contains: atenolol 100 mg. Blisters of 30. Bottles of 100 and 500. Store at room temperature (15-30°C). Protect from light and moisture. Keep away from children.

The reader is invited to consult CPhA's monograph **HMG-CoA Reductase Inhibitors**.

RAN™-Atorvastatin P

atorvastatin calcium

Lipid Metabolism Regulator

Ranbaxy

SUPPLIED: 10 mg: Each white, elliptical, film-coated tablet, debossed "AT 10" on one side and "RBX" on the other, contains: atorvastatin 10 mg. Nonmedicinal ingredients: calcium carbonate, candelilla wax, croscarmellose sodium, hydroxypropyl cellulose, hydroxypropyl methylcellulose, lactose monohydrate, magnesium stearate, microcrystalline cellulose, polyethylene glycol, polysorbate 80, simethicone emulsion, talc and titanium dioxide. Bottles of 90 and 500. Store at room temperature (15 to 25°C).
20 mg: Each white, elliptical, film-coated tablet, debossed "AT 20" on one side and "RBX" on the other, contains: atorvastatin 20 mg. Nonmedicinal ingredients: calcium carbonate, candelilla wax, croscarmellose sodium, hydroxypropyl cellulose, hydroxypropyl methylcellulose, lactose monohydrate, magnesium stearate, microcrystalline cellulose, polyethylene glycol, polysorbate 80, simethicone emulsion, talc and titanium dioxide. Bottles of 90 and 500. Store at room temperature (15 to 25°C).
40 mg: Each white, elliptical, film-coated tablet, debossed "AT 40" on one side and "RBX" on the other, contains: atorvastatin 40 mg. Nonmedicinal ingredients: calcium carbonate, candelilla wax, croscarmellose sodium, hydroxypropyl cellulose, hydroxypropyl methylcellulose, lactose monohydrate, magnesium stearate, microcrystalline cellulose, polyethylene glycol, polysorbate 80, simethicone emulsion, talc and titanium dioxide. Bottles of 90 and 500. Store at room temperature (15 to 25°C).
80 mg: Each white, elliptical, film-coated tablet, debossed "AT 80" on one side and "RBX" on the other, contains: atorvastatin 80 mg. Nonmedicinal ingredients: calcium carbonate, croscarmellose sodium, hydroxypropyl cellulose, hydroxypropyl methylcellulose, lactose monohydrate, magnesium stearate, microcrystalline cellulose, polyethylene glycol, polysorbate 80, simethicone emulsion, talc, and titanium dioxide. Bottles of 90 and 500. Store at room temperature (15 to 25°C).

RAN™-Carvedilol P

carvedilol

Congestive Heart Failure Agent

Ranbaxy

SUPPLIED: 3.125 mg: Each white, oval, biconvex, film-coated tablet, embossed 482A on one side and rbx on the other, contains: carvedilol 3.125 mg. Bottles of 100. Store between 15-30°C in tightly closed, light-resistant container. Protect from humidity.
6.25 mg: Each white, oval, biconvex, film-coated tablet, embossed 482B on one side and rbx on the other, contains: carvedilol 6.25 mg. Bottles of 100. Store between 15-30°C in tightly closed, light-resistant container. Protect from humidity.
12.5 mg: Each white, oval, biconvex, film-coated tablet, embossed 482C on one side and rbx on the other, contains: carvedilol 12.5 mg. Bottles of 100. Store between 15-30°C in tightly closed, light-resistant container. Protect from humidity.
25 mg: Each white, oval, biconvex, film-coated tablet, embossed 482D on one side and rbx on the other, contains: carvedilol 25 mg. Bottles of 100. Store between 15-30°C in tightly closed, light-resistant container. Protect from humidity.

RAN™-Cefprozil P

cefprozil

Antibiotic

Ranbaxy

SUPPLIED: Powder For Solution: 250 mg/5 mL: Yellowish pink colored granular powder forming yellowish pink colored suspension on constitution with water. The resulting suspension has a characteristic fruity flavor. Bottles of 75 and 100 mL. Store the dry powder at room temperature (15 to 30°C). Protect from light. Protect from excessive humidity. The constituted oral suspension must be stored in the refrigerator (2-8°C) for up to 14 days. Keep container tightly closed. Discard unused portion after 14 days.
Tablets: 250 mg: Each oval, white to off-white, film-coated tablet, debossed with "RB 41" on one side and plain on the other side, contains: cefprozil 250 mg. Bottles of 100. Store at room temperature (15 to 30°C). Protect from light. Protect from excessive humidity.
500 mg: Each oval, white to off-white, film-coated tablet, debossed with "RB 42" on one side and plain on the other side, contains: cefprozil 500 mg. Bottles of 100. Store at room temperature (15 to 30°C). Protect from light. Protect from excessive humidity.

The reader is invited to consult CPhA's monograph **Fluoroquinolones**.

RAN™-Ciproflox P

ciprofloxacin HCl

Antibacterial

Ranbaxy

SUPPLIED: 250 mg: Each white to off-white, round, film-coated tablet, debossed with "RX709" on one side and plain on the other side, contains: ciprofloxacin 250 mg (as ciprofloxacin HCl). Nonmedicinal ingredients: colloidal silicon dioxide, hypromellose, magnesium stearate, microcrystalline cellulose, polyethylene glycol, sodium starch glycolate, starch (corn), talc and titanium dioxide. Bottles of 100. Store at room temperature (15-30°C).
500 mg: Each white to off-white, caplet shaped, film-coated tablet, debossed with "RX710" on one side and plain on the other side, contains: ciprofloxacin 500 mg (as ciprofloxacin HCl). Nonmedicinal ingredients: colloidal silicon dioxide, hypromellose, magnesium stearate, microcrystalline cellulose, polyethylene glycol, sodium starch glycolate, starch (corn), talc and titanium dioxide. Bottles of 100. Store at room temperature (15-30°C).
750 mg: Each white to off-white, caplet shaped, film-coated tablet, debossed with "RX711" on one side and plain on the other side, contains: ciprofloxacin 750 mg (as ciprofloxacin HCl). Nonmedicinal ingredients: colloidal silicon dioxide, hypromellose, magnesium stearate, microcrystalline cellulose, polyethylene glycol, sodium starch glycolate, starch (corn), talc and titanium dioxide. Bottles of 100. Store at room temperature (15-30°C).

The reader is invited to consult CPhA's monograph **Selective Serotonin Reuptake Inhibitors**.

RAN™-Citalo P

citalopram HBr

Antidepressant

Ranbaxy

SUPPLIED: 20 mg: Each white to off-white, oval shaped, biconvex, film-coated tablet, debossed with "RB31" on one side and score line on the other side, contains: citalopram 20 mg (as citalopram HBr). Nonmedicinal ingredients: copovidone, corn starch, croscarmellose sodium, hydroxypropyl cellulose, hypromellose, lactose monohydrate, magnesium stearate, microcrystalline cellulose (Avicel PH 101 and 102), propylene glycol, talc and titanium dioxide. Bottles of 30, 100, 500 and 1000. Store in a dry place at room temperature between 15 and 30°C.
40 mg: Each white to off-white, oval shaped, biconvex, film-coated tablet, debossed with "RB32" on one side and score line on the other side, contains: citalopram 40 mg (as citalopram HBr). Nonmedicinal ingredients: copovidone, corn starch, croscarmellose sodium, hydroxypropyl cellulose, hypromellose, lactose monohydrate, magnesium stearate, microcrystalline cellulose (Avicel PH 101 and 102), propylene glycol, talc and titanium dioxide. Bottles of 30, 100 and 1000. Store in a dry place at room temperature between 15 and 30°C.

RAN™-Domperidone P

domperidone maleate

Upper Gastrointestinal Motility Modifier

Ranbaxy

SUPPLIED: Each round, plain-coated, biconvex, white tablet, engraved "R113" on one side and plain on the other side, contains: domperidone maleate 12.72 mg (equivalent to domperidone 10 mg). Bottles of 500. Store at room temperature (15-30°C). Protect from light and moisture.

RAN™-Fentanyl Transdermal System Ⓝ

fentanyl

Opioid Analgesic

Ranbaxy

SUPPLIED: 2.5 mg: Each rectangular, multilayer, transparent, 10 cm² transdermal system contains: fentanyl 2.5 mg for nominal in-vivo delivery of 25 µg/h fentanyl for 72 hours. Nonmedicinal ingredients: alcohol (less than 0.2 mL is released from the system during a 72-hour use). Cartons containing 5 individually packaged systems.

5 mg: Each rectangular, multilayer, transparent, 20 cm² transdermal system contains: fentanyl 5 mg for nominal in-vivo delivery of 50 µg/h fentanyl for 72 hours. Nonmedicinal ingredients: alcohol (less than 0.2 mL is released from the system during a 72-hour use). Cartons containing 5 individually packaged systems.

7.5 mg: Each rectangular, multilayer, transparent, 30 cm² transdermal system contains: fentanyl 7.5 mg for nominal in-vivo delivery of 75 µg/h fentanyl for 72 hours. Nonmedicinal ingredients: alcohol (less than 0.2 mL is released from the system during a 72-hour use). Cartons containing 5 individually packaged systems.

10 mg: Each rectangular, multilayer, transparent, 40 cm² transdermal system contains: fentanyl 10 mg for nominal in-vivo delivery of 100 µg/h fentanyl for 72 hours. Nonmedicinal ingredients: alcohol (less than 0.2 mL is released from the system during a 72-hour use). Cartons containing 5 individually packaged systems.

RAN™-Fentanyl Matrix Patch Ⓝ

fentanyl

Opioid Analgesic

Ranbaxy

SUPPLIED: RAN-Fentanyl Matrix Patch is a transdermal patch providing continuous systemic delivery of fentanyl, a potent opioid analgesic, for 72 hours.

The construction of the fentanyl transdermal system is a typical matrix-based system where the matrix acts simultaneously as drug reservoir and as adhesive layer. The resorption of the active ingredient to the systemic circulation is controlled by the contact area with the skin. There is no release-controlling element in this type of system. The matrix is covered by a flexible transparent foil (backing foil) which enables a comfortable wearing of the system and protects the matrix from outer influences during application.

RAN-Fentanyl Matrix Patch is available in five different strengths. Each system is labelled with a nominal flux which represents the average amount of drug delivered to the systemic circulation per hour across average skin. The active component of the system is fentanyl. The amount of fentanyl released from each system per hour is proportional to the surface area. The release rate of fentanyl in [µg/h] correlates directly to the fentanyl content (2.1 mg, 4.2 mg, 8.4 mg, 12.6 mg and 16.8 mg) and to the effective release area of the patches (5.25 cm², 10.5 cm², 21 cm², 31.5 cm² and 42 cm²).

Total fentanyl contents and system sizes for the five strengths are summarized in Table 1.

Table 1: RAN-Fentanyl Matrix Patch

Total Fentanyl Contents and System Sizes for the Five Strengths

System	Nominal Fentanyl Delivery Rate (µg/h)	Total Fentanyl Content (mg)	System Size (cm²)
RAN-Fentanyl Matrix Patch	12[a]	2.1	5.25
RAN-Fentanyl Matrix Patch	25	4.2	10.5
RAN-Fentanyl Matrix Patch	50	8.4	21
RAN-Fentanyl Matrix Patch	75	12.6	31.5
RAN-Fentanyl Matrix Patch	100	16.8	42

[a] Nominal delivery rate 12.5 µg/hr.

Nonmedicinal ingredients: acrylic-vinylacetate copolymer adhesive, polyethyleneterephthalate backing foil and siliconized polyethyleneterephthalate release liner.

RAN-Fentanyl Matrix Patch is supplied in cartons containing 5 individually packaged systems. Each patch system is packaged in foil paper/PE/AL/PE sachets.

RAN-Fentanyl Matrix Patch should be kept out of the reach of children before and after use. Do not cut RAN-Fentanyl Matrix Patch.

The opposite side of the matrix is covered by a siliconized, easy removable protective foil (release liner), which has to be removed prior to application.

Used systems should be folded so that the adhesive side of the system adheres to itself, then flushed down the toilet immediately upon removal. If the drug adhesive layer accidentally contacts the skin, the area should be washed with clear water. Do not use soap, alcohol or other solvents because they may enhance the drug's ability to penetrate the skin. Patients should dispose of any systems remaining from a prescription as soon as they are no longer needed. Unused systems should be removed from their protective pouch, folded so that the adhesive side of the patch adheres to itself and flushed down the toilet.

Wash hands, with water only, after applying or removing the patch.

Store in original sealed sachet pouch between 15 and 25°C. Do not refrigerate. Protect from freezing.

Ranitidine Injection USP Ⓟ

ranitidine HCl

Histamine H2-Receptor Antagonist

Sandoz

SUPPLIED: Each mL contains: ranitidine (as hydrochloride) 25 mg. Nonmedicinal ingredients: dibasic sodium phosphate, monobasic potassium phosphate, phenol (as preservative), hydrochloric acid and/or sodium hydroxide to adjust pH and water for injection. Single dose vials of 2 mL, boxes of 10. Pharmacy Bulk Vials **(discard unused portion)** of 50 and 100 mL, boxes of 1. Store between 15 and 25°C. Do not autoclave. Protect from light and excessive heat.

The reader is invited to consult CPhA's monograph **ACE Inhibitors**.

RAN™-Lisinopril Ⓟ

lisinopril

Angiotensin Converting Enzyme Inhibitor

Ranbaxy

SUPPLIED: 5 mg: Each light pink colored, round flat face, beveled edge bisect tablet, debossed with "RX" above the bisect and "532" below the bisect on one side and plain on the other side, contains: lisinopril 5 mg (as lisinopril dihydrate). Nonmedicinal ingredients: corn starch, dibasic calcium phosphate (anhydrous), magnesium stearate, mannitol, pregelatinized starch and red iron oxide. Bottles of 30 and 1000. Store at room temperature (15-30°C). Protect from light.

10 mg: Each light pink colored, round flat face, beveled edge tablet debossed with "RX533" on one side and plain on the other side, contains: lisinopril 10 mg (as lisinopril dihydrate). Nonmedicinal ingredients: corn starch, dibasic calcium phosphate (anhydrous), magnesium stearate, mannitol, pregelatinized starch and red iron oxide. Bottles of 30 and 1000. Store at room temperature (15-30°C). Protect from light.

20 mg: Each light rust colored, round flat face, beveled edge tablet debossed with "RX534" on one side and plain on the other side, contains: lisinopril 20 mg (as lisinopril dihydrate). Nonmedicinal ingredients: corn starch, dibasic calcium phosphate (anhydrous), magnesium stearate, mannitol, pregelatinized starch and red iron oxide. Bottles of 30 and 1000. Store at room temperature (15-30°C). Protect from light.

The reader is invited to consult CPhA's monograph **HMG-CoA Reductase Inhibitors**.

RAN™-Lovastatin Ⓟ

lovastatin

Lipid Metabolism Regulator

Ranbaxy

SUPPLIED: 20 mg: Each light blue colored, octagon-shaped, biconvex, film-coated tablet, scored on one side and "RBX" on the other side, contains: lovastatin 20 mg. Bottles of 100 and 500. Container must be tightly closed. Store at room temperature (15-30°C). Protect from light.

40 mg: Each mint green colored, octagon-shaped, biconvex, film-coated tablet, plain on one side and "RBX" on the other side, contains: lovastatin 40 mg. Bottles of 100. Container must be tightly closed. Store at room temperature (15-30°C). Protect from light.

RAN™-Metformin Ⓟ

metformin HCl

Antihyperglycemic

Ranbaxy

SUPPLIED: 500 mg: Each white, round, biconvex, film-coated tablet, embossed R12 on one side and RBX and score-line on the other, contains: metformin HCl 500 mg. Bottles of 100 and 500. Store at room temperature (15-30°C) in well closed containers. Protect from light.

850 mg: Each white, oblong, biconvex, film-coated tablet, embossed R22 on one side and RBX on the other, contains: metformin HCl 850 mg. Bottles of 100. Store at room temperature (15-30°C) in well closed containers. Protect from light.

RAN™-Ondansetron Ⓟ

ondansetron HCl

Antiemetic

Ranbaxy

SUPPLIED: 4 mg: Each oval shaped, yellow, film-coated tablet, engraved "ROn 4" on one face, contains: ondansetron 4 mg (as ondansetron hydrochloride). Nonmedicinal ingredients: croscarmellose sodium, iron oxide yellow, lactose, magnesium stearate, methyl hydroxypropyl cellulose, microcrystalline cellulose, pregelatinised starch, titanium dioxide and triacetin. Bottles of 100. Blister packs of 10. Store at room temperature (15-30°C) in a dry place.

8 mg: Each oval shaped, yellow, film-coated tablet, engraved "ROn 8" on one face, contains: ondansetron 8 mg (as ondansetron hydrochloride). Nonmedicinal ingredients: croscarmellose sodium, iron oxide yellow, lactose, magnesium stearate, methyl hydroxypropyl cellulose, microcrystalline cellulose, pregelatinised starch, titanium dioxide and triacetin. Bottles of 100. Blister packs of 10. Store at room temperature (15-30°C) in a dry place.

RAN™-Pantoprazole Ⓟ

pantoprazole sodium

H+, K+-ATPase Inhibitor

Ranbaxy

SUPPLIED: 20 mg: Each enteric-coated, yellow, oval, biconvex tablet, marked P20 on one side, contains: pantoprazole 20 mg (22.6 mg pantoprazole sodium sesquihydrate). Bottles of 100. Store at 15 to 30°C in the recommended packaging.

40 mg: Each enteric-coated, yellow, oval, biconvex tablet, marked P40 on one side, contains: pantoprazole 40 mg (45.1 mg pantoprazole sodium sesquihydrate). Bottles of 100. Store at 15 to 30°C in the recommended packaging.

The reader is invited to consult CPhA's monograph **HMG-CoA Reductase Inhibitors**.

RAN™-Pravastatin Ⓟ

pravastatin sodium

Lipid Metabolism Regulator

Ranbaxy

SUPPLIED: 10 mg: Each pink to peach coloured mottled, rounded, rectangular shaped biconvex, uncoated tablet, debossed with 'RE25' on one side and plain on the other side, contains: pravastatin sodium 10 mg. Nonmedicinal ingredients: D&C yellow no. 10 aluminum lake, FD&C blue no. 1 aluminum lake, ferric oxide (red), ferric oxide (yellow), lactose anhydrous and sodium stearyl fumarate. Blister cartons of 30. Bottles of 30 and 2500. Store at room temperature (15-30°C). Protect from moisture and light.

20 mg: Each yellow coloured mottled, rounded, rectangular shaped biconvex, uncoated tablet debossed with 'RE26' on one side and plain on the other side, contains: pravastatin sodium 20 mg. Nonmedicinal ingredients: D&C yellow no. 10 aluminum lake, FD&C blue no. 1 aluminum lake, ferric oxide (red), ferric oxide (yellow), lactose anhydrous and sodium stearyl fumarate. Blister cartons of 30. Bottles of 30 and 2500. Store at room temperature (15-30°C). Protect from moisture and light.

40 mg: Each green coloured mottled, rounded, rectangular shaped biconvex, uncoated tablet debossed with 'RE27' on one side and plain on the other side, contains: pravastatin sodium 40 mg. Nonmedicinal ingredients: D&C yellow no. 10 aluminum lake, FD&C blue no. 1 aluminum lake, ferric oxide (red), ferric oxide (yellow), lactose anhydrous and sodium stearyl fumarate. Blister cartons of 30. Bottles of 30 and 2500. Store at room temperature (15-30°C). Protect from moisture and light.

RAN™-Rabeprazole ℞

rabeprazole sodium

H+, K+-ATPase Inhibitor

Ranbaxy

SUPPLIED: 10 mg: Each pink enteric-coated tablet, printed "€ 241" on one side, contains: rabeprazole sodium 10 mg. Bottles of 100. Store at room temperature (15 to 25°C) protected from moisture.
20 mg: Each light yellow film-coated bi-convex tablet, imprinted with "RAB 20" on one side, contains: rabeprazole sodium 20 mg. Bottles of 100. Store at room temperature (15 to 25°C) protected from moisture.

The reader is invited to consult CPhA's monograph **ACE Inhibitors**.

RAN™-Ramipril ℞

ramipril

Angiotensin Converting Enzyme Inhibitor

Ranbaxy

SUPPLIED: 1.25 mg: Each yellow opaque cap and white opaque body, self lock hard gelatin capsule of size '4' imprinted with "RANBAXY" on cap and "R-1.25" on body containing white to off-white powder, contains: ramipril 1.25 mg. Nonmedicinal ingredients: black iron oxide, gelatin, iron oxide yellow, potassium hydroxide, pre-gelatinized starch, propylene glycol, shellac, sodium lauryl sulfate and titanium dioxide. Bottles of 100. Store in original container at room temperature 15-30°C. Protect from light and moisture.
2.5 mg: Each orange opaque cap and white opaque body, self lock hard gelatin capsule of size '4' imprinted with "RANBAXY" on cap and "R-2.5" on body containing white to off-white powder, contains: ramipril 2.5 mg. Nonmedicinal ingredients: black iron oxide, D&C Yellow 10, FD&C Red 40, gelatin, potassium hydroxide, pre-gelatinized starch, propylene glycol, shellac, sodium lauryl sulfate and titanium dioxide. Bottles of 100 and 500. Store in original container at room temperature 15-30°C. Protect from light and moisture.
5 mg: Each red opaque cap and white opaque body, self lock hard gelatin capsule of size '4' imprinted with "RANBAXY" on cap and "R-5" on body containing white to off-white powder, contains: ramipril 5 mg. Nonmedicinal ingredients: black iron oxide, FD&C Blue 1, FD&C Red 40, gelatin, potassium hydroxide, pre-gelatinized starch, propylene glycol, shellac, sodium lauryl sulfate and titanium dioxide. Bottles of 100 and 500. Store in original container at room temperature 15-30°C. Protect from light and moisture.
10 mg: Each blue opaque cap and white opaque body, self lock hard gelatin capsule of size '4' imprinted with "RANBAXY" on cap and "R-10" on body containing white to off-white powder, contains: ramipril 10 mg. Nonmedicinal ingredients: black iron oxide, D&C Yellow 10, FD&C Blue 2, FD&C Red 3, gelatin, potassium hydroxide, pre-gelatinized starch, propylene glycol, shellac, sodium lauryl sulfate and titanium dioxide. Bottles of 30, 100 and 500. Store in original container at room temperature 15-30°C. Protect from light and moisture.

RAN™-Risperidone ℞

risperidone

Antipsychotic

Ranbaxy

SUPPLIED: 0.25 mg: Each yellowish ochre, film-coated, oblong, biconvex tablet, engraved with "RAN 0.25" on one side and blank on the other side, contains: risperidone 0.25 mg. Bottles of 100. Store at room temperature (15-30°C). Protect from light and moisture. Keep out of the reach of children.
0.5 mg: Each brownish-red, film-coated, oblong, biconvex tablet, engraved with "RAN" and "0.5", separated by a score on one side and blank on the other side, contains: risperidone 0.5 mg. Bottles of 100. Store at room temperature (15-30°C). Protect from light and moisture. Keep out of the reach of children.
1 mg: Each white, oblong, biconvex, film-coated tablet, engraved with "RAN 1" on one side and blank on the other side, contains: risperidone 1 mg. Blister cartons of 60. Bottles of 500. Store at room temperature (15-30°C). Protect from light and moisture. Keep out of the reach of children.
2 mg: Each orange, oblong, biconvex, film-coated tablet, engraved with "RAN" and "2" separated by a score on one side and blank on the other side, contains: risperidone 2 mg. Blister cartons of 60. Bottles of 500. Store at room temperature (15-30°C). Protect from light and moisture. Keep out of the reach of children.
3 mg: Each yellow, oblong, biconvex, film-coated tablet, engraved with "RAN" and "3" separated by a score on one side and blank on the other side, contains: risperidone 3 mg. Blister cartons of 60. Bottles of 250. Store at room temperature (15-30°C). Protect from light and moisture. Keep out of the reach of children.
4 mg: Each green, oblong, biconvex, film-coated tablet, engraved with "RAN" and "4" separated by a score on one side and blank on the other side, contains: risperidone 4 mg. Bottles of 60. Store at room temperature (15-30°C). Protect from light and moisture. Keep out of the reach of children.

RAN™-Ropinirole ℞

ropinirole HCl

Antiparkinsonian Agent—Dopamine Agonist

Ranbaxy

SUPPLIED: 0.25 mg: Each white to off-white, film coated, pentagonal, centrally tipped tablet, debossed with "R" on one side and "6" on the other side, contains: ropinirole hydrochloride 0.25 mg. Nonmedicinal ingredients: cellulose microcrystalline, croscarmellose sodium, hypromellose, lactose anhydrous, lactose monohydrate, magnesium stearate, macrogol/polyethylene glycol 400, titanium dioxide and talc. Bottles of 100. Keep at room temperature (between 15-30°C), protect from light and moisture. Close container tightly after each use.
1 mg: Each light green to green coloured, film coated, pentagonal, centrally tipped tablet, debossed with 'R' on one side '8' on the other side, contains: ropinirole hydrochloride 1 mg. Nonmedicinal ingredients: cellulose microcrystalline, croscarmellose sodium, FD&C Blue No. 2/lake colour of indigo carmine, hypromellose, iron oxide black lactose anhydrous, iron oxide yellow, lactose monohydrate, magnesium stearate, macrogol/polyethylene glycol 400 and titanium dioxide. Bottles of 100. Keep at room temperature (between 15-30°C), protect from light and moisture. Close container tightly after each use.
2 mg: Each pink coloured, film coated, pentagonal, centrally tipped tablet debossed with 'R' on one side and '9' on the other side, contains: ropinirole hydrochloride 2 mg. Nonmedicinal ingredients: cellulose microcrystalline, croscarmellose sodium, hypromellose, iron oxide red, lactose anhydrous, lactose monohydrate, magnesium stearate, macrogol/polyethylene glycol 400 and titanium dioxide. Bottles of 100. Keep at room temperature (between 15-30°C), protect from light and moisture. Close container tightly after each use.
5 mg: Each blue coloured, film coated, pentagonal, centrally tipped tablet debossed with 'R' on one side and '11' on the other side, contains: ropinirole hydrochloride 5 mg. Nonmedicinal ingredients: cellulose microcrystalline, croscarmellose sodium, FD&C Blue No. 2/lake colour of indigo carmine, hypromellose, lactose anhydrous, lactose monohydrate, macrogol/polyethylene glycol 400, macrogol/polyethylene glycol 4000, magnesium stearate, talc and titanium dioxide. Bottles of 100. Keep at room temperature (between 15-30°C), protect from light and moisture. Close container tightly after each use.

The reader is invited to consult CPhA's monograph **HMG-CoA Reductase Inhibitors**.

RAN™-Simvastatin ℞

simvastatin

Lipid Metabolism Regulator

Ranbaxy

SUPPLIED: 5 mg: Each buff colored, film coated, oval-shaped tablet, debossed with "SST" on one side and "5" on other side with intact coating, contains: simvastatin 5 mg. Nonmedicinal ingredients: ascorbic acid, butylated hydroxyanisole, citric acid, hydroxypropyl cellulose, hydroxypropyl methylcellulose, lactose monohydrate, magnesium stearate, microcrystalline cellulose, pregelatinized starch, talc, titanium dioxide and yellow ferric oxide. Bottles of 100. Store at room temperature (15-30°C), in the original package, away from heat and direct light, and out of damp places, such as the bathroom or kitchen.
10 mg: Each peach colored, film coated, oval-shaped tablet, debossed with 'SST' on one side and '10' on other side with intact coating, contains: simvastatin 10 mg. Nonmedicinal ingredients: ascorbic acid, butylated hydroxyanisole, citric acid, hydroxypropyl cellulose, hydroxypropyl methylcellulose, lactose monohydrate, magnesium stearate, microcrystalline cellulose, pregelatinized starch, talc, titanium dioxide, yellow ferric oxide and red ferric oxide. Bottles of 100 and 500. Store at room temperature (15-30°C), in the original package, away from heat and direct light, and out of damp places, such as the bathroom or kitchen.
20 mg: Each tan colored, film coated, oval-shaped tablet, debossed with 'SST' on one side and '20' on other side with intact coating, contains: simvastatin 20 mg. Nonmedicinal ingredients: ascorbic acid, butylated hydroxyanisole, citric acid, hydroxypropyl cellulose, hydroxypropyl methylcellulose, lactose monohydrate, magnesium stearate, microcrystalline cellulose, pregelatinized starch, talc, titanium dioxide, yellow ferric oxide and red ferric oxide. Bottles of 100 and 500. Store at room temperature (15-30°C), in the original package, away from heat and direct light, and out of damp places, such as the bathroom or kitchen.
40 mg: Each brick red colored, film coated, oval-shaped tablet, debossed with 'SST' on one side and '40' on other side with intact coating, contains: simvastatin 40 mg. Nonmedicinal ingredients: ascorbic acid, butylated hydroxyanisole, citric acid, hydroxypropyl cellulose, hydroxypropyl methylcellulose, lactose monohydrate, magnesium stearate, microcrystalline cellulose, pregelatinized starch, talc, titanium dioxide, yellow ferric oxide and red ferric oxide. Bottles of 100. Store at room temperature (15-30°C), in the original package, away from heat and direct light, and out of damp places, such as the bathroom or kitchen.
80 mg: Each brick red colored, film coated, capsule-shaped tablet, debossed with 'SST' on one side and '80' on other side with intact coating, contains: simvastatin 80 mg. Nonmedicinal ingredients: ascorbic acid, butylated hydroxyanisole, citric acid, hydroxypropyl cellulose, hydroxypropyl methylcellulose, lactose monohydrate, magnesium stearate, microcrystalline cellulose, pregelatinized starch, talc, titanium dioxide, yellow ferric oxide and red ferric oxide. Bottles 100. Store at room temperature (15-30°C), in the original package, away from heat and direct light, and out of damp places, such as the bathroom or kitchen.

RAN™-Tamsulosin ℞

tamsulosin HCl

Selective Antagonist of Alpha1A Adrenoreceptor Subtype in the Prostate

Ranbaxy

SUPPLIED: Each sustained-release capsule for oral administration contains: tamsulosin HCl 0.4 mg. Nonmedicinal ingredients: Eudragit L30 D55, Eudragit L100-55, magnesium stearate, microcrystalline cellulose, sodium hydroxide, talc, titanium dioxide and triacetin. Blister cartons of 100 (10×10's). Bottles of 100. Store at room temperature (15-30°C).

RAN™-Zopiclone ℞

zopiclone

Hypnotic

Ranbaxy

SUPPLIED: 5 mg: Each white, round, biconvex, film-coated tablet, embossed "312R" on one side and "RBX" on the other, contains: zopiclone 5 mg. Bottles of 100. Keep in a dry place. Store at room temperature (15-30°C). Protect from light.
7.5 mg: Each blue, oval, film-coated tablet, marked with "RBX 312" on one side and a score line on the other, contains: zopiclone 7.5 mg. Bottles of 100 and 500. Keep in a dry place. Store at room temperature (15-30°C). Protect from light.

Rapamune® ℞

sirolimus

Immunosuppressive Agent

Pfizer

Date of Preparation: December 27, 2000
Date of Revision: June 2, 2010

SUMMARY PRODUCT INFORMATION:

Route of Administration	Dosage Form/ Strength	Clinically Relevant Nonmedicinal Ingredients
Oral	Solution: 1 mg/mL	Ethanol For a complete listing see Dosage Forms, Composition and Packaging.
	Tablets: 1 mg	Lactose monohydrate For a complete listing see Dosage Forms, Composition and Packaging.

INDICATIONS AND CLINICAL USE: Rapamune (sirolimus oral solution and tablets) is indicated for the prophylaxis of organ rejection in patients receiving allogeneic renal transplants:

- **In patients at low to moderate immunological risk**, it is recommended that Rapamune be used initially in a regimen with cyclosporine and corticosteroids. Cyclosporine should be withdrawn 2 to 4 months after transplantation and the Rapamune dose should be increased to reach recommended blood concentrations (see Dosage and Administration).
- **In patients at high immunologic risk** (defined as Black transplant recipients and/or repeat renal transplant recipients who lost a previous allograft for immunologic reason and/or patients with high-panel reactive antibodies (PRA; peak PRA level >80%), it is recommended that Rapamune be used in combination with cyclosporine and corticosteroids for the first year following transplantation (see Dosage and Administration). Thereafter, any adjustments to the immunosuppressive regimen should be considered on the basis of the clinical status of the patient.

Geriatrics (>65 years of age): Clinical studies of Rapamune did not include sufficient numbers of patients aged 65 and over to determine whether safety and efficacy differ in this population from younger patients. Based on the finding that blood clearance decreases linearly with age, consideration should be given to reducing the Rapamune dose in patients 65 years of age and over.
Pediatrics (<13 years of age): The safety and efficacy of Rapamune in pediatric patients below the age of 13 years have not been established.

CONTRAINDICATIONS:

- Rapamune is contraindicated in patients with a hypersensitivity to sirolimus or its derivatives or any component of the drug product. For a complete listing, see Dosage Forms, Composition and Packaging.
- For information on use during pregnancy and contraceptive requirements see Warnings and Precautions, Special Populations.

WARNINGS AND PRECAUTIONS:

Serious Warnings and Precautions

- Increased susceptibility to infection and the possible development of lymphoma may result from immunosuppression.
- Only physicians experienced in immunosuppressive therapy and management of organ transplant patients should use Rapamune. Patients receiving the drug should be managed in facilities equipped and staffed with adequate laboratory and supportive medical resources. The physician responsible for maintenance therapy should have complete information requisite for the follow-up of the patient.
- Hypersensitivity reactions, including anaphylactic/anaphylactoid reactions, angioedema, exfoliative dermatitis, and hypersensitivity vasculitis, have been associated with the administration of sirolimus.
- The safety and efficacy of sirolimus as immunosuppressive therapy have not been established in liver or lung transplant patients, and therefore, such use is not recommended.

General: Rapamune is intended for oral administration only.

Rapamune has been approved to be administered concurrently with cyclosporine (liquid and microemulsion) and corticosteroids. The efficacy and safety of the use of Rapamune in combination with other immunosuppressive agents has not been established.

Use in High Risk Patients: The safety and efficacy of cyclosporine withdrawal in high-risk patients have not been adequately studied and it is therefore not recommended. This includes patients with Banff grade III acute rejection or vascular rejection prior to cyclosporine withdrawal, those who are dialysis-dependent, or with serum creatinine >400 μmol/L (4.5 mg/dL), black patients, re-transplants, multi-organ transplants, and patients with high panel of reactive antibodies. It is recommended that Rapamune be used in combination with cyclosporine and corticosteroids for the first year following transplantation.

The safety and efficacy of this combination in high-risk renal transplant patients have not been studied beyond one year. Therefore, after the first year following transplantation any adjustments to the immunosuppressive regimen should be considered on the basis of the clinical status of the patient (see Indications and Clinical Use and Dosage and Administration).

Antimicrobial Prophylaxis: Cytomegalovirus (CMV) prophylaxis is recommended for 3 months after transplantation, particularly for patients at increased risk for CMV infection.

Cases of *P. carinii* pneumonia have been reported in patients not receiving antimicrobial prophylaxis. Therefore, antimicrobial prophylaxis for *P. carinii* pneumonia should be administered for 1 year following transplantation.

Carcinogenesis and Mutagenesis: Patients receiving immunosuppression regimens involving combinations of drugs, including Rapamune, as part of an immunosuppression regimen are at increased risk of developing lymphomas and other malignancies, particularly of the skin. The risk appears to be related to the intensity and duration of immunosuppression rather than to the use of any specific agent. As with all patients at an increased risk for skin cancer, exposure to sunlight and UV light should be limited by wearing protective clothing and using a sunscreen with a high protection factor.

Endocrine and Metabolism: Co-administration of Rapamune with strong inhibitors of CYP3A4 and/or P-glycoprotein (P-gp) (such as ketoconazole, voriconazole, itraconazole, telithromycin, or clarithromycin) or strong inducers of CYP3A4 and/or P-gp (such as rifampicin or rifabutin) is not recommended. Sirolimus is extensively metabolized by the CYP3A4 isozyme in the intestinal wall and liver. Inhibitors of CYP3A4 decrease the metabolism of sirolimus and increase sirolimus whole blood concentrations. Inducers of CYP3A4 increase the metabolism of sirolimus and decrease sirolimus whole blood concentrations (see Drug Interactions).

Hematologic: Patients receiving immunosuppressive agents such as Rapamune may develop leukopenia. The development of leukopenia may be related to Rapamune itself, concomitant medications, viral infection, or some combination of these causes. If leukopenia develops, dose reduction of Rapamune and/or other immunosuppressive agents should be considered.

Hepatic/Biliary/Pancreatic: Liver Transplantation—Excess Mortality, Graft Loss, and Hepatic Artery Thrombosis (HAT): The use of Rapamune in combination with tacrolimus was associated with excess mortality and graft loss in a study in de novo liver transplant recipients. Many of these patients had evidence of infection at or near the time of death. In this and another study in de novo liver transplant recipients, the use of Rapamune in combination with cyclosporine or tacrolimus was associated with an increase in HAT; most cases of HAT occurred within 30 days post-transplantation and most led to graft loss or death.

Hepatic impairment: When compared to normal subjects, the clearance of sirolimus is significantly decreased in patients with impaired hepatic function. Accordingly, the blood concentration of Rapamune should be closely monitored and the dose of Rapamune should be adjusted based on the blood concentration. It is not necessary to modify the loading dose (see Action and Clinical Pharmacology and Dosage and Administration).

Immune: Oversuppression of the immune system can increase susceptibility to opportunistic infections, sepsis, and fatal infections. Mucosal herpes simplex infections were significantly more frequent in the 5 mg/day Rapamune-treated patients compared to other treatment groups (see Adverse Reactions). Activation of latent viral infections was reported, including BK virus associated nephropathy and JC virus associated progressive multifocalleukoencephalopathy (PML). These infections are often related to a high immunosuppressive burden and may lead to serious or fatal conditions.

Vaccinations: Immunosuppressants may affect response to vaccination (see Drug Interactions, Overview, Vaccination).

Concomitant Use of Angiotensin-Converting Enzyme (ACE) Inhibitors: In rare cases, the concomitant administration of Rapamune and ACE inhibitors has resulted in angioneurotic edema-type reactions.

Musculoskeletal: Rhabdomyolysis: In clinical trials, the concomitant administration of Rapamune and HMG-CoA reductase inhibitors and/or fibrates was well tolerated. During Rapamune therapy with cyclosporine, patients administered an HMG-CoA reductase inhibitor and/or fibrate should be monitored for the possible development of rhabdomyolysis and other adverse effects as described in the respective labelling for these agents.

Post-Operative Complications: mTOR inhibitors such as sirolimus have been shown in vitro to inhibit production of certain growth factors that may affect angiogenesis, fibroblast proliferation, and vascular permeability, which may be associated with impaired or delayed wound healing and/or fluid accumulation.

Impaired Wound Healing: Studies showed that in comparison with other immunosuppressive regimens the use of sirolimus-based immunosuppressive regimens was associated with a significantly higher incidence of wound-healing complications, including wound dehiscence, incisional herniae, anastomotic disruption, and lymphocele (see Adverse Reactions, Post-Market Adverse Drug Reactions, Skin and Appendages). Greater post-operative measures should be taken to minimize this complication.

Fluid Accumulation: Use of sirolimus is associated with an increased incidence of fluid accumulation, including peripheral edema, lymphedema, pleural effusion and pericardial effusions (including hemodynamically significant effusions in children and adults).

Renal: Renal Function: Patients treated with cyclosporine and Rapamune were noted to have higher serum creatinine levels, lower glomerular filtration rates, and a more rapid rate of decline in renal function compared with patients treated with cyclosporine and placebo or azathioprine controls (Studies 1 and 2) or patients continuing treatment with Rapamune following withdrawal of cyclosporine (Rapamune Maintenance Regimen: Study 4). In the Rapamune Maintenance Regimen Study that compared a regimen of Rapamune, cyclosporine and steroids to one in which cyclosporine was withdrawn 2-4 months post-transplantation, those in whom cyclosporine was not withdrawn had significantly higher serum creatinine levels and significantly lower glomerular filtration rates at 12 months through 60 months, and significantly lower graft survival at 48 months, the point at which it was decided by the sponsor to discontinue subjects from assigned therapy in the Rapamune and cyclosporine arm. When the protocol was amended all subjects had reached 48 months and some completed the 60 months of the study. In patients at low to moderate immunologic risk continuation of combination therapy with cyclosporine beyond 4 months following transplantation should only be considered when the benefits outweigh the risks of this combination for the individual patients.

In patients with delayed graft function, Rapamune may delay recovery of renal function.

Proteinuria: In a study evaluating conversion from calcineurin inhibitors to sirolimus in maintenance renal transplant patients 6-120 months post-transplant, conversion was associated with significantly increased urinary protein excretion. Periodic quantitative monitoring of urinary protein excretion is recommended. The safety and efficacy of conversion from calcineurin inhibitors to sirolimus in maintenance renal transplant population has not been established.

Renal function should be closely monitored during the administration of Rapamune in combination with cyclosporine. Appropriate adjustment of the immunosuppression regimen, including discontinuation of cyclosporine and/or Rapamune, should be considered in patients with elevated or increasing serum creatinine levels. Caution should be exercised when using agents (e.g., aminoglycosides and amphotericin B) that are known to have a deleterious effect on renal function.

De novo Use Without Calcineurin Inhibitor (CNI): The safety and efficacy of de novo use of Rapamune, mycophenolate mofetil (MMF), and corticosteroids, in combination with interleukin-2 receptor antibody induction is not established and is not recommended in de novo renal transplant patients.

Hemolytic Uremic Syndrome/Thrombotic Thrombocytopenic Purpura/Thrombotic Microangiopathy (HUS/TTP/TMA): The concomitant use of sirolimus with a calcineurin inhibitor may increase the risk of calcineurin inhibitor-induced HUS/TTP/TMA.

Respiratory: Lung Transplantation—Bronchial Anastomotic Dehiscence: Cases of bronchial anastomotic dehiscence, most fatal, have been reported in de novo lung transplant patients when Rapamune has been used as part of an immunosuppressive regimen.

Interstitial Lung Disease: Cases of interstitial lung disease [including pneumonitis, and infrequently bronchiolitis obliterans organizing pneumonia (BOOP) and pulmonary fibrosis], some fatal, with no identified infectious etiology have occurred in patients receiving immunosuppressive regimens including sirolimus. In some cases, the interstitial lung disease has resolved upon discontinuation or dose reduction of sirolimus. The risk may be increased as the sirolimus trough concentration increases.

Special Populations: Pregnant Women: Because sirolimus is embryo/fetal toxic in rats at dosages of 0.1 mg/kg and above (approximately 1.4 times the maximum recommended human dose [MRHD]), it may cause fetal harm when administered to pregnant women. In animal studies, embryo/fetal toxicity was manifested as mortality and reduced fetal weights (with associated delays in skeletal ossification). However, no teratogenesis was evident. There were no effects on rabbit development at the maternally toxic dosage of 0.05 mg/kg (approximately 0.7 times the MRHD).

There are no adequate and well-controlled studies of Rapamune use in pregnant women. Consequently, use of Rapamune during pregnancy should be considered only if the potential benefit outweighs the potential risk to the embryo/fetus.

Effective contraception must be used before beginning Rapamune therapy, during Rapamune therapy and for 12 weeks after Rapamune has been stopped.

Nursing Women: Studies in rats have shown that sirolimus is excreted in milk. It is not known whether sirolimus is excreted in human milk. A decision should be made whether to discontinue nursing or to discontinue the drug, taking into account the importance of the drug to the mother.

Pediatrics (<13 years of age): The safety and efficacy of Rapamune in pediatric patients have not been established. Therefore, Rapamune is not recommended for use in pediatric renal transplant patients.

Safety and efficacy information from a controlled clinical trial in pediatric and adolescent (<18 years of age) renal transplant recipients judged to be at **high immunologic risk**, defined as a history of one or more acute rejection episodes and/or the presence of chronic allograft nephropathy, do not support the chronic use of the combination of Rapamune oral solution or tablets in combination with calcineurin inhibitors and corticosteroids, due to the increased risk of lipid abnormalities and deterioration of renal function associated with these immunosuppressive regimens, without increased benefit with respect to acute rejection, graft survival, or patient survival.

Geriatrics (>65 years of age): Clinical studies of Rapamune did not include sufficient numbers of patients aged 65 and over to determine whether safety and efficacy differ in this population from younger patients. Based on the finding that blood clearance decreases linearly with age, consideration should be given to reducing the Rapamune dose in patients 65 years of age and over.

Monitoring and Laboratory Tests: Blood Concentration Monitoring: Whole blood trough concentrations of sirolimus should be monitored in patients receiving concentration-controlled Rapamune. Monitoring is also necessary in patients likely to have altered drug metabolism; in patients with hepatic impairment; in pediatric patients; during concurrent administration of inhibitors and inducers of CYP3A4 and P-glycoprotein; and if the cyclosporine dosage is markedly changed or discontinued. It is recommended that a whole blood trough concentration be measured 1 to 2 weeks after altering the total daily dose of Rapamune, after switching between the solution and the tablet formulation, or switching from one tablet strength (1 mg, 2 mg or 5 mg) to another, to confirm that the trough concentration is within the desired target range.

In controlled clinical trials, with concomitant cyclosporine (Studies 1 and 2), mean sirolimus whole blood trough concentrations through month 6 following transplantation, expressed as chromatographic assay value, were approximately 7.2 ng/mL (range 3.6-11 ng/mL [10th to 90th percentile]) for the 2 mg/day treatment group (n=226), and 14 ng/mL (range 8.0-22 ng/mL [10th to 90th percentile]) for the 5 mg/day dose (n=219; values were obtained using a research immunoassay, but are expressed as chromatographic equivalent values, using a +20% bias for the immunoassay).

In a controlled clinical trial with cyclosporine withdrawal (Study 4), the mean sirolimus whole blood trough concentrations during months 4 through 12 following transplantation, expressed as chromatographic assay values, were approximately 8.6 ng/mL (range 5.2-12 ng/mL [10th to 90th percentile]) in the concomitant Rapamune, cyclosporine and corticosteroid treatment group (n=205) and were 19 ng/mL (range 14-24 ng/mL [10th to 90th percentile]) in the Rapamune maintenance group after withdrawal of cyclosporine (n=201). By month 60, the mean sirolimus whole blood trough concentrations remained stable in the concomitant Rapamune, cyclosporine and corticosteroid group (n=71) at 8.6 ng/mL (range 5.0 to 12 ng/mL [10th to 90th percentile]). For the cyclosporine withdrawal group (n=104) by month 60, the mean sirolimus whole blood concentration had fallen to 15 ng/mL (range 9.4 to 19 ng/mL [10th to 90th percentile]).

In a concentration-controlled clinical trial in high-risk adult patients (Study 5), the mean whole blood sirolimus trough concentrations, during months 9 through 12 months following transplantation, as measured by chromatography, were 11.2 ng/mL (range 6.8-15.9 ng/mL [10th to 90th percentile]) (n=127), and the mean whole blood trough concentrations of cyclosporine were 133 ng/mL (range 54-215 ng/mL [10th to 90th percentile]).

Results from other assays may differ from those with an immunoassay. On average, chromatographic methods [high-performance liquid chromatography with ultraviolet detection (HPLC UV) or liquid chromatography with tandem mass spectrometric detection (LC/MS/MS)] yield results that are approximately 20% (range 10%-29%) lower than the immunoassay whole blood concentration determinations. The recommended 24-hour trough concentration ranges for sirolimus are based on chromatographic methods. Several assay methodologies have been used to measure the whole blood concentrations of sirolimus. Currently in clinical practice, sirolimus whole blood concentrations are being measured by both chromatographic and immunoassay methodologies. The concentration values obtained by these different methodologies are not interchangeable. Adjustments to the targeted range should be made according to the assay being utilized to determine the sirolimus trough concentration. A discussion of different assay methods is contained in Clinical Therapeutics 2000; 22 Suppl B:B1-B132. Since assay results are also laboratory dependent, adjustment to the targeted therapeutic range must be made with a detailed knowledge of the site-specific assay used.

Lipids: The use of Rapamune may lead to increased serum cholesterol and triglycerides that may require treatment. Patients must be monitored for hyperlipidemia. In studies 1 and 2, high fasting triglyceride levels (>11.3 mmol/L [1000 mg/dL]) were observed in 0.8% of patients receiving Rapamune 2 mg/day and 3% of patients receiving Rapamune 5 mg/day. Monitoring of triglycerides should be included as part of routine post-transplant patient management, particularly in patients with antecedent dyslipidemia. Elevated triglycerides can be managed by appropriate medical therapy, dose reduction or, for severe elevations, discontinuation of Rapamune.

In Study 4 during the pre-randomization period, mean fasting serum cholesterol and triglyceride values rapidly increased, and peaked at 2 months with mean cholesterol values >6.2 mmol/L (240 mg/dL) and triglycerides >2.8 mmol/L (250 mg/dL). After 3 years, mean fasting cholesterol (5.9 versus 6.3 mmol/L; p=0.059) trended higher in the cyclosporine withdrawal arm, whereas HDL cholesterol, LDL cholesterol, and triglycerides were similar in the two groups.

ADVERSE REACTIONS: Adverse Drug Reaction Overview:

- Increased susceptibility to infection and the possible development of lymphoma may result from immunosuppression.
- Hypersensitivity reactions, including anaphylactic/anaphylactoid reactions, angioedema, exfoliative dermatitis, and hypersensitivity vasculitis, have been associated with the administration of sirolimus.

Clinical Trial Adverse Drug Reactions: Because clinical trials are conducted under very specific conditions the adverse reaction rates observed in the clinical trials may not reflect the rates observed in practice and should not be compared to the rates in the clinical trials of another drug. Adverse drug reaction information from clinical trials is useful for identifying drug-related adverse events and for approximating rates.

Rapamune and Cyclosporine Combination Therapy: Rapamune Oral Solution: The incidence of adverse reactions was determined in two randomized, double-blind, multicentre controlled trials (Studies 1 and 2) in which 499 renal transplant patients received Rapamune (sirolimus oral solution) 2 mg/day, 477 received Rapamune oral solution 5 mg/day, 160 received azathioprine 2-3 mg/kg/day, and 124 received placebo. All patients were treated with cyclosporine and corticosteroids.

Adverse reactions associated with the administration of Rapamune which occurred at a significantly higher frequency than placebo or azathioprine control group include arthralgia, hirsutism, diarrhea, hypertension, hypokalemia, lymphocele, peripheral edema, rash, tachycardia, and some infections. In general, adverse events related to administration of Rapamune were dependent on dose/concentration. Dose related elevations of triglycerides and cholesterol and decreases in platelets and hemoglobin have occurred in patients receiving Rapamune.

The data presented by study group in Table 1 show the adverse reactions that occurred in any treatment group with an incidence of ≥10%.

Table 1: Rapamune

Adverse Events Occurring at a Frequency Of ≥10% in Any Treatment Group in Prevention of Acute Renal Rejection Trials (%) at 12 Months Post-Transplantation for Studies 1 and 2[a]

Body System Adverse Event	Rapamune Oral Solution 2 mg/day		Rapamune Oral Solution 5 mg/day		Azathioprine 2–3 mg/kg/day	Placebo
	Study 1	Study 2	Study 1	Study 2	Study 1	Study 2
	(n=281)	(n=218)	(n=269)	(n=208)	(n=160)	(n=124)
Body as a Whole						
Abdomen Enlarged	15	8	9	13	9	10
Abdominal Pain	20	26	24	31	22	23
Accidental Injury	8	11	9	8	9	10
Asthenia	27	17	32	23	23	19
Back Pain	13	20	21	15	19	17
Chest Pain	10	16	15	18	12	16
Chills	7	5	8	12	2	8
Face Edema	5	5	11	10	4	4
Fever	19	18	22	27	19	23
Headache	18	30	23	30	10	20
Lymphocele	12	11	15	13	3	6
Overdose	10	17	11	17	6	10
Pain	19	29	25	23	20	21
Transplant Rejection	2	3	3	7	3	15
Cardiovascular System						
Hypertension	38	39	34	43	23	41
Tachycardia	10	10	12	12	4	4
Hypotension	3	4	8	4	10	6
Digestive System						
Constipation	25	34	30	34	34	28
Diarrhea	20	18	32	28	14	14
Dyspepsia	12	21	20	22	21	25
Liver Function Tests Abnormal	9	7	11	11	9	7
Nausea	25	21	28	25	31	22
Vomiting	16	17	17	18	25	16
Endocrine System	15	15	20	20	12	15
Hemic and Lymphatic Systems						
Anemia	21	18	31	28	22	14
Leukopenia	6	7	12	9	12	2
Ecchymosis	5	6	6	12	7	3
Thrombocytopenia	10	12	18	24	7	3
Metabolic and Nutritional						
Creatinine Increased	28	32	28	38	22	33
Edema	20	17	14	14	15	7
Healing Abnormal	8	7	10	12	4	6
Hypercholesterolemia	33	41	37	46	24	20
Hyperglycemia	13	11	16	14	13	10
Hyperkalemia	13	14	10	12	19	23
Hyperlipemia	34	42	42	55	24	20
Hypokalemia	12	7	17	15	9	6
Hypophosphatemia	16	14	21	17	18	18

(cont'd)

Table 1: Rapamune *(cont'd)*

Adverse Events Occurring at a Frequency Of ≥10% in Any Treatment Group in Prevention of Acute Renal Rejection Trials (%) at 12 Months Post-Transplantation for Studies 1 and 2[a]

Body System Adverse Event	Rapamune Oral Solution 2 mg/day		Rapamune Oral Solution 5 mg/day		Azathioprine 2–3 mg/kg/day	Placebo
	Study 1	Study 2	Study 1	Study 2	Study 1	Study 2
	(n=281)	(n=218)	(n=269)	(n=208)	(n=160)	(n=124)
Lactic Dehydrogenase Increased	10	11	13	18	6	5
Peripheral Edema	53	48	56	51	48	42
Weight Gain	17	8	11	6	13	13
Musculoskeletal System						
Arthralgia	18	21	23	25	13	15
Nervous System						
Dizziness	10	9	13	13	11	8
Hypesthesia	5	7	7	10	6	5
Insomnia	10	10	20	11	13	8
Tremor	23	17	26	17	18	11
Paresthesia	7	10	8	9	4	6
Respiratory System						
Cough Increased	14	8	16	15	13	17
Dyspnea	17	20	22	24	14	23
Epistaxis	4	4	6	11	<1	0
Pulmonary Physical Finding	9	13	11	11	5	12
Rhinitis	12	11	14	13	8	8
Skin and Appendages						
Acne	25	19	19	19	11	14
Rash	10	5	9	15	2	5
Hirsutism	5	8	12	8	3	8
Special Senses						
Abnormal Vision	9	8	11	12	8	6
Urogenital System						
Dysuria	9	10	13	17	10	6
Hematuria	11	14	15	17	13	9
Oliguria	5	4	4	7	6	10
Kidney Tubular Necrosis	9	9	10	10	7	4
Study Event Associated with Miscellaneous Factors	41	37	42	40	34	35
Local Reaction to Procedure	40	37	42	40	34	34

[a] All patients in Study 1 and 2 received cyclosporine and corticosteroids.

Table 2 summarizes the incidence rates at 6 months for clinically important opportunistic or common transplant-related infections across treatment groups Studies 1 and 2. There were no significant differences in incidence rates between treatment groups, with the exception of mucosal infections with Herpes simplex, which occurred at a significantly greater rate in patients treated with Rapamune 5 mg/day.

Table 2: Rapamune

Incidence (%) of Selected Clinically Important Infections in Prevention of Acute Renal Rejection for Studies 1 and 2[a,b]

Infection	Sirolimus 2 mg/day (n=511)	Sirolimus 5 mg/day (n=493)	Azathioprine 2–3 mg/kg/day (n=161)	Placebo (n=130)
Sepsis	6.3	6.7	3.7	6.9
CMV Infection (generalized)	2.9	4.1	3.7	5.4
CMV Infection (tissue-invasive)	0.4	1.0	1.2	0.8

(cont'd)

Table 2: Rapamune *(cont'd)*

Incidence (%) of Selected Clinically Important Infections in Prevention of Acute Renal Rejection for Studies 1 and 2[a,b]

Infection	Sirolimus 2 mg/day (n=511)	Sirolimus 5 mg/day (n=493)	Azathioprine 2–3 mg/kg/day (n=161)	Placebo (n=130)
Pneumonia	2.5	4.3	1.2	3.9
P. carinii Pneumonia	0.4	0	0	0
Herpes Simplex	5.3	12.2	3.7	6.2
Herpes Zoster	1.8	2.2	1.9	3.1
Urinary Tract Infection/ Pyelonephritis	19.8	23.1	23	21.5
Wound Infection	6.5	8.3	5.0	6.9
Epstein-Barr Virus	0.6	0.6	0	0

a Analysis performed on the intent-to-treat patient populations.
b All patients in Study 1 and 2 received cyclosporine and corticosteroids.

Table 3 summarizes the incidence of malignancies in Studies 1 and 2. At 12 months following transplantation there was a very low incidence of malignancies and there were no significant differences between treatment groups.

Table 3: Rapamune

Incidence (%) of Malignancy (Studies 1 and 2 Combined, 12 Months)

Malignancy	Rapamune 2 mg/day (n=511)	Rapamune 5 mg/day (n=493)	Placebo (n=130)	Azathioprine (n=161)
Lymphoma/PTLD[a,b]	0.4	1.4	0	0.6
Skin (excluding melanoma)[c]	0.4	1.4	3.1	1.2
Other	0.6	0.6	0	0

a Lymphoma/Post-transplant lymphoproliferative disorder.
b p>0.05 across treatment groups.
c p<0.05, placebo vs Rapamune 2 mg/day.

The following reactions (listed alphabetically by body system) were reported with a ≥1% incidence in patients treated with Rapamune in combination with cyclosporine and corticosteroids: see Table 4.

In general, adverse events related to administration of Rapamune were dependent on dose/concentration.

Table 4: Rapamune

Adverse Reactions

Body as a Whole	Lymphocele, peripheral edema, generalized edema, hernia, hormone level altered, lab test abnormal, malaise, pelvic pain, abnormal healing, fever, fungal, viral and bacterial infections (such as Mycobacterial infections, Epstein-Barr virus, CMV, and Herpes zoster), herpes simplex, sepsis
Cardiovascular System	Arterial anomaly, cardiomegaly, cardiovascular physical finding, congestive heart failure, hemorrhage, hypervolemia, palpitation, peripheral vascular disorder, postural hypotension, thrombophlebitis, thrombosis, vascular disorder, vasodilatation, venous thromboembolism (including pulmonary embolism, deep vein thrombosis), tachycardia
Digestive System	Anorexia, eructation, esophagitis, flatulence, gingivitis, gum hyperplasia, ileus, increased appetite, mouth ulceration, rectal disorder, stomatitis, abdominal pain, diarrhea
Endocrine System	Cushing's syndrome, diabetes mellitus, glycosuria, parathyroid disorder
Hemic and Lymphatic System	Leukocytosis, neutropenia, polycythemia, thrombotic thrombocytopenic purpura/hemolytic uremic syndrome, anemia, leukopenia, thrombocytopenia
Metabolic and Nutritional	Acidosis, alkaline phosphatase increased, bilirubinemia, urea/BUN increased, creatine phosphokinase increased, dehydration, hypercalcemia, hypophosphatemia, hypocalcemia, hyperglycemia, hypomagnesemia, hyponatremia, hypoproteinemia, AST increased, ALT increased, weight loss, hypercholesterolemia, hypertriglyceridemia (hyperlipemia), hypokalemia, increased lactic dehydrogenase (LDH)
Musculoskeletal System	Bone necrosis, bone pain, joint disorder, leg cramps, myalgia, osteoporosis, tetany, arthralgia
Nervous System	Agitation, anxiety, circumoral paresthesia, confusion, depression, hallucinations, hypertonia, hypesthesia, hypotonia, nervousness, neuropathy, somnolence
Respiratory System	Asthma, atelectasis, hemoptysis, hiccup, hypoxia, lung edema, pharyngitis, pleural effusion, pneumonitis, sinusitis, epistaxis, pneumonia
Skin and Appendages	Nail disorder, pruritus, skin benign neoplasm, skin disorder, skin hypertrophy, skin ulcer, sweating, acne, rash, squamous cell carcinoma, basal cell carcinoma
Special Senses	Cataract specified, conjunctivitis, ear pain, tinnitus
Urogenital System	Albuminuria, bladder pain, hydronephrosis, impotence, kidney function abnormal, kidney pain, nocturia, scrotal edema, testis disorder, toxic nephropathy, urinary frequency, urinary incontinence, urinary retention, urinary tract disorder, urine abnormality, urinary tract infection, pyelonephritis, proteinuria

Less frequently occurring adverse events included: pancreatitis, lymphoma/post-transplant lymphoproliferative disorder, pancytopenia, melanoma, exfoliative dermatitis (see Warnings and Precautions), nephrotic syndrome, pulmonary hemorrhage, and pericardial effusion (including hemodynamically significant effusions in children and adults).

Rapamune Tablets: The incidence of adverse reactions through 12 months was determined in a randomized, multicentre, controlled trial (Study 3) in which 229 renal transplant patients received Rapamune Oral Solution 2 mg once daily and 228 patients received Rapamune Tablets 2 mg once daily. All patients were treated with cyclosporine and corticosteroids.

The adverse reactions that occurred in either treatment group with an incidence of ≥10% in Study 3 were similar to those reported for Studies 1 and 2. There was no notable difference in the incidence of these adverse events between treatment groups (oral solution versus tablets) in Study 3, with the exception of acne and pharyngitis, which occurred more frequently in the oral solution group, and liver function abnormal and tremor which occurred more frequently in the tablet group.

The adverse events that occurred in patients with an incidence of ≥3% and <10% in either treatment group in Study 3 were similar to those reported in Studies 1 and 2. There was no notable difference in the incidence of these adverse events between treatment groups (oral solution versus tablets) in Study 3, with the exception of hypertonia and urinary incontinence, which occurred more frequently in the oral solution group and cataract, acidosis, ascites, and dysphagia which occurred more frequently in the tablet group. In Study 3 alone, menorrhagia, metrorrhagia, and polyuria occurred with an incidence of ≥3% and <10%.

The clinically important opportunistic or common transplant-related infections were identical in all three studies and the incidences of these infections were similar in Study 3 compared with Studies 1 and 2. The incidence rates of these infections were not significantly different between the oral solution and tablet treatment groups in Study 3.

In Study 3 (at 12 months), there were two cases of lymphoma or lymphoproliferative disorder in the oral solution treatment group (0.8%) and two reported cases of lymphoma or lymphoproliferative disorder in the tablet treatment group (0.8%). These differences were not statistically significant and were similar to the incidences observed in Studies 1 and 2.

Rapamune Maintenance Regimen (RMR): The incidence of adverse reactions was determined through 60 months in a randomized, multicentre controlled trial (Study 4). This study compared 430 renal transplant patients who were administered Rapamune, cyclosporine and corticosteroids for the first 3 months after transplantation (pre-randomization period) followed by a 1:1 randomization at 3 months ±2 weeks to the withdrawal of cyclosporine (Rapamune maintenance regimen) or the continuation of the Rapamune, cyclosporine and steroid regimen. The safety profile prior to randomization (start of cyclosporine withdrawal) was similar to that of the 2 mg Rapamune groups in Studies 1, 2, and 3.

Patients who had cyclosporine eliminated from their immunosuppressive therapy at 3 months ±2 weeks experienced significantly higher incidences of increased AST and increased ALT, liver damage, hypokalemia, thrombocytopenia, abnormal healing, acne, ileus, and joint disorder. Conversely, the incidence of acidosis, hypertension, cyclosporine toxicity, increased creatinine, abnormal kidney function, toxic nephropathy, edema, hyperkalemia, hyperuricemia, gout, benign skin neoplasm and gum hyperplasia was significantly higher in patients who remained on a Rapamune plus cyclosporine regimen. Mean systolic and diastolic blood pressure improved significantly following cyclosporine withdrawal.

The incidence of Herpes zoster infection (at 60 months) was significantly lower in patients receiving Rapamune following cyclosporine withdrawal compared with patients who continued to receive Rapamune and cyclosporine.

The incidence of malignancies at 60 months post-transplant following cyclosporine withdrawal, is presented in Table 5. The incidence of lymphoma or lymphoproliferative disease was similar in all treatment groups. The overall incidence of malignancy, based upon the number of patients who had one or more malignancy, was lower in patients receiving Rapamune as part of the Rapamune maintenance regimen as compared with patients receiving Rapamune and cyclosporine (10.7% versus 15.8%, respectively; p=0.155).

Table 5: Rapamune

Incidence (%) of Malignancies in Study 4 at 60 Months Post-transplant[a]

Malignancy[d]	Nonrandomized[b] (n=95)	Rapamune with Cyclosporine Therapy[c] (n=215)	Rapamune Following Cyclosporine Withdrawal[c] (n=215)
Lymphoma/ lymphoproliferative Disease	1.1	1.4	0.5
Skin Carcinoma			
Non-melanoma Skin Carcinoma	5.3	8.8	7.0
Melanoma	0.0	0.5	0.5
Other Malignancy	1.1	3.3	1.4

a Includes patients who prematurely discontinued treatment.
b Patients received Rapamune, cyclosporine and corticosteroids.
c Patients received Rapamune and corticosteroids.
d Patients may be counted in more than one category.

High-Risk Patients Study: Safety was assessed in a controlled trial (Study 5) in 224 patients who received at least one dose of sirolimus with cyclosporine. Overall, the incidence and nature of adverse events was similar to those seen in previous combination studies with Rapamune. The incidence of malignancy was 1.3% at 12 months.

Table 6 shows the adverse reactions that occurred with an incidence of ≥10%.

Table 6: Rapamune

Number (%) of Subjects Reporting Treatment-Emergent Adverse Events with an Incidence ≥10% for Study 5

Body System[a] Adverse Event, Preferred Term	SRL+CsA (n=224)
Body as a Whole	
Abdominal Pain	73 (32.6)
Asthenia	67 (29.9)
Back Pain	34 (15.2)
Chest Pain	36 (16.1)
Chills	28 (12.5)
Fever	93 (41.5)
Headache	57 (25.4)
Infection	48 (21.4)
Lymphocele	61 (27.2)
Overdose	32 (14.3)
Pain	88 (39.3)
Cardiovascular System	
Cardiovascular Physical Finding	24 (10.7)

(cont'd)

Table 6: Rapamune (cont'd)

Number (%) of Subjects Reporting Treatment-Emergent Adverse Events with an Incidence ≥10% for Study 5

Body System[a] Adverse Event, Preferred Term	SRL+CsA (n=224)
Hypertension	130 (58.0)
Hypervolemia	38 (17.0)
Hypotension	43 (19.2)
Tachycardia	48 (21.4)
Digestive System	
Abdominal Distension	45 (20.1)
Anorexia	24 (10.7)
Constipation	75 (33.5)
Diarrhea	80 (35.7)
Dyspepsia	25 (11.2)
Liver Function Tests Abnormal	31 (13.8)
Nausea	99 (44.2)
Vomiting	73 (32.6)
Endocrine System	
Diabetes Mellitus	28 (12.5)
Hemic and Lymphatic System	
Anemia	137 (61.2)
Leukopenia	78 (34.8)
Thrombocytopenia	55 (24.6)
Metabolic and Nutritional System	
Acidosis	54 (24.1)
Creatinine Increased	89 (39.7)
Edema	59 (26.3)
Healing Abnormal	49 (21.9)
Hypercholesterolemia	58 (25.9)
Hyperglycemia	65 (29.0)
Hyperkalemia	71 (31.7)
Hyperlipemia	97 (43.3)
Hyperphosphatemia	23 (10.3)
Hypocalcemia	39 (17.4)
Hypokalemia	53 (23.7)
Hypomagnesemia	50 (22.3)
Hypophosphatemia	78 (34.8)
Peripheral Edema	156 (69.6)
Weight Gain	45 (20.1)
Weight Loss	24 (10.7)
Musculoskeletal System	
Arthralgia	47 (21.0)
Nervous System	
Dizziness	38 (17.0)
Insomnia	45 (20.1)
Tremor	35 (15.6)

(cont'd)

Table 6: Rapamune (cont'd)

Number (%) of Subjects Reporting Treatment-Emergent Adverse Events with an Incidence ≥10% for Study 5

Body System[a] Adverse Event, Preferred Term	SRL+CsA (n=224)
Respiratory System	
Cough Increased	46 (20.5)
Dyspnea	75 (33.5)
Lung Edema	24 (10.7)
Pharyngitis	35 (15.6)
Pneumonia	17 (7.6)
Pulmonary Physical Finding	42 (18.8)
Rhinitis	49 (21.9)
Upper Respiratory Infection	33 (14.7)
Skin and Appendages	
Acne	42 (18.8)
Pruritus	22 (9.8)
Urogenital System	
Dysuria	40 (17.9)
Hematuria	49 (21.9)
Impotence[b]	16 (12.7)
Kidney Tubular Necrosis	103 (46.0)
Urinary Frequency	25 (11.2)
Urinary Tract Disorder	26 (11.6)
Urinary Tract Infection	67 (29.9)
Treatment-emergent Adverse Event Associated With Miscellaneous Factors	
Local Reaction to Procedure	133 (59.4)

[a] A subject may have reported 2 or more different adverse events in the same body system.
[b] Sex-related event; the percentage is calculated using as the denominator the number of men in group I (120) or group II (126).
Legend: CsA=cyclosporine; SRL=sirolimus.

Other Clinical Trial Adverse Drug Reactions: Safety was assessed in a controlled clinical trial in pediatric (<18 years of age) renal transplant patients considered high immunologic risk, defined as a history of one or more acute allograft rejection episodes and/or the presence of chronic allograft nephropathy on a renal biopsy. The use of Rapamune in combination with calcineurin inhibitors and corticosteroids was associated with an increased risk of deterioration of renal function, serum lipid abnormalities (including but not limited to increased serum triglycerides and cholesterol), and urinary tract infections.

The safety and efficacy of conversion from calcineurin inhibitors to Rapamune in maintenance renal transplant patients have not been established. In an ongoing study evaluating the safety and efficacy of conversion from calcineurin inhibitors to Rapamune (sirolimus target levels of 12-20 ng/mL by chromatographic assay) in maintenance renal transplant patients 6 months-10 years post-transplant, enrollment was stopped in the subset of patients (n=90) with a baseline glomerular filtration rate of less than 40 mL/min. There was a higher rate of serious adverse events including pneumonia, acute rejection, graft loss and death in this Rapamune treatment arm (n=60, median time post-transplant 36 months).

The concomitant use of Rapamune with a calcineurin inhibitor may increase the risk of calcineurin inhibitor-induced hemolytic uremic syndrome/thrombotic thrombocytopenic purpura/thrombotic microangiopathy.

In patients with delayed graft function, Rapamune may delay recovery of renal function (see Warnings and Precautions, Renal).

Abnormal Hematologic and Clinical Chemistry Findings: Abnormal hematologic and clinical chemistry findings are included in Clinical Trial Adverse Drug Reactions.

Post-Market Adverse Drug Reactions: Reporting rates determined on the basis of spontaneously reported post-marketing adverse events are generally presumed to underestimate the risks associated with drug treatments.

The following adverse events have been reported spontaneously during post-marketing experience with Rapamune. A causal relationship to Rapamune cannot be excluded for spontaneously reported events.

Body as a Whole: lymphedema, tuberculosis.

Cardiovascular System: pericardial effusion (including hemodynamically significant effusions in children and adults).

Digestive: Ascites reports have been common.

Hemic and Lymphatic System: pancytopenia.

Hepatobiliary Disorders: Hepatotoxicity has been reported, including fatal hepatic necrosis with elevated trough sirolimus concentrations (i.e., exceeding therapeutic levels).

Immune System: Hypersensitivity reactions, including anaphylactic/anaphylactoid reactions, angioedema, exfoliative dermatitis, and hypersensitivity vasculitis, have been associated with the administration of sirolimus (see Warnings and Precautions).

Metabolic and Nutritional: Fluid accumulation reports have been common.

Musculoskeletal: Rhabdomyolysis has been reported in patients administered Rapamune with HMG-CoA reductase inhibitors, with or without cyclosporine (See Warnings and Precautions, Special Populations; Musculoskeletal).

Respiratory System: Cases of interstitial lung disease [including pneumonitis, and infrequently bronchiolitis obliterans organizing pneumonia (BOOP) and pulmonary fibrosis], some fatal, with no identified infectious etiology have occurred in patients receiving immunosuppressive regimens including Rapamune. In some cases, the interstitial lung disease has resolved upon discontinuation or dose reduction of Rapamune. The risk may be increased as the sirolimus trough concentration increases. Occurrence of pulmonary hemorrhage coincident with sirolimus administration has been reported in selected patients. Symptomatic improvement or resolution were seen after withdrawal of sirolimus. Pleural effusion reports have been common. Rare reports of alveolar proteinosis have been received.

Skin and Appendages: Abnormal healing following transplant surgery has been reported, including fascial dehiscence, incisional hernia and anastomotic disruption (e.g., wound, vascular, airway, ureteral, biliary).

Urogenital System: Azoospermia reports have been uncommon. Azoospermia reported with the use of Rapamune has been reversible upon discontinuation of Rapamune in most cases. Focal segmental glomerulosclerosis (frequency unknown) has been reported.

DRUG INTERACTIONS:

Serious Drug Interactions

- Co-administration of Rapamune with strong inhibitors of CYP3A4 (such as ketoconazole, voriconazole, itraconazole, telithromycin, or clarithromycin) or inducers of CYP3A4 (such as rifampin or rifabutin) is not recommended.

Overview: Sirolimus is extensively metabolized by the CYP3A4 isozyme in the gut wall and liver and undergoes counter-transport from enterocytes of the small intestine by the P-glycoprotein drug-efflux pump. Therefore, absorption and the subsequent elimination of systemically absorbed sirolimus may be influenced by drugs that affect these proteins. A summary of the potential effects of these concomitantly administered drugs on the pharmacokinetics of sirolimus is given in Table 7.

Table 7: Rapamune

Ratios of Sirolimus Pharmacokinetic Parameters After Co-administration with Potentially Interacting Drugs

		Ratio of Sirolimus Pharmacokinetic Parameters[a,b]				
Population	**Interacting Drug**	t_{max}	C_{max}	$t_{1/2}$	**AUC**	**CL/F/W**
Healthy Subjects	Acyclovir	0.95	↔	↔	↔	↔
	Cyclosporine microemulsion (simultaneous dosing)[d]	1.92	2.16	↔	3.3	0.3
	Cyclosporine microemulsion (4 h dosing separation)[d]	1.58	1.37	1.1	1.8	0.56
	Cyclosporine microemulsion (simultaneous dosing)[e]	0.70	6.12	0.93	2.48	0.40
	Cyclosporine microemulsion (4 h dosing separation)[e]	0.67	1.33	0.90	1.33	0.75
	Cyclosporine microemulsion (simultaneous dosing)[f]	1.47	2.17	0.87	2.8	0.35
	Cyclosporine microemulsion (2 h after sirolimus dose)[f]	0.95	0.98	0.97	0.99	1.01
	Cyclosporine microemulsion (2 h before sirolimus dose)[f]	1.47	2.26	0.87	2.4	0.42
	Digoxin	1.03	↔	↔	↔	↔
	Diltiazem	1.29	1.43	0.85	1.6	0.38
	Glyburide	↔	↔	↔	↔	↔
	Ketoconazole	1.38	4.42	↔	10.9	0.085
	Nifedipine	↔	↔	↔	↔	↔
	Norgestrel/ethinyl estradiol	—	—	0.86	1.08	↔
	Rifampin	↔	0.29	↔	0.18	5.53
Renal Post-transplant	Sulfamethoxazole/trimethoprim	↔	↔	—	↔	—
Psoriasis	Cyclosporine liquid (simultaneous dosing)	—	—	—	1.75[c]	—

a Ratio=(sirolimus + drug): (sirolimus alone).
b ↔=no statistically significant change.
c Ratio of average sirolimus trough concentrations.
d 10 mg dose of sirolimus oral solution; 300 mg dose of cyclosporine microemulsion.
e 10 mg dose of sirolimus tablet; 300 mg dose of cyclosporine microemulsion.
f 5 mg dose of sirolimus oral solution given simultaneously, 2 hours before or 2 hours after 300 mg dose of cyclosporine microemulsion.

Inhibitors of CYP3A4 and P-glycoprotein may increase sirolimus levels. Inducers of CYP3A4 and P-glycoprotein may decrease sirolimus levels. In patients in whom strong inhibitors or inducers of CYP3A4 and P-glycoprotein are indicated, alternative therapeutic agents with less potential for inhibition or induction of CYP3A4 and P-glycoprotein should be considered.

Care should be exercised when drugs or other substances that are nephrotoxic (eg, ganciclovir) or that are metabolized by CYP3A4 are administered concomitantly with Rapamune.

Rhabdomyolysis HMG-CoA reductase inhibitors and/or fibrates: In clinical trials, the concomitant administration of Rapamune and HMG-CoA reductase inhibitors and/or fibrates was well tolerated. During Rapamune therapy with or without cyclosporine, patients should be monitored for elevated lipids and patients administered an HMG-CoA reductase inhibitor and/or fibrate should be monitored for the possible development of rhabdomyolysis and other adverse effects as described in the respective labeling for these agents. (See Warnings and Precautions, Special Populations; Musculoskeletal.)

Calcineurin Inhibitors: Calcineurin inhibitor-induced hemolytic uremic syndrome/thrombotic thrombocytopenic purpura/thrombotic microangiopathy (HUS/TTP/TMA) has been reported in patients receiving sirolimus with a calcineurin inhibitor.

Vaccination: Immunosuppressants may affect response to vaccination. Therefore, during treatment with Rapamune, vaccination may be less effective. The use of live vaccines should be avoided; live vaccines may include, but are not limited to measles, mumps, rubella, oral polio, BCG, yellow fever, varicella, and TY21a typhoid.

Drug-Drug Interactions: The drugs listed in Table 8 are based on either drug interaction case reports or studies, or potential interactions due to the expected magnitude and seriousness of the interaction (i.e., those identified as contraindicated).

Table 8: Rapamune

Established or Potential Drug-Drug Interactions

Drug Name	Ref	Effect	Clinical Comment
Cyclosporine (microemulsion)	CT	Multiple dose, staggered administration of Rapamune and cyclosporine ↓cyclosporine oral dose clearance	Based on dosing design of Phase III trials, it is recommended that Rapamune be administered 4 hours after cyclosporine microemulsion (Neoral); slightly lower doses of cyclosporine needed to meet target cyclosporine concentrations.
Diltiazem	CT	Co-administration of 10 mg Rapamune oral solution and diltiazem (120 mg) ↑ sirolimus C_{max}, T_{max}, AUC 1.4-, 1.3-, and 1.6-fold, respectively. Sirolimus did not affect the pharmacokinetics of either diltiazem or its metabolites desacetyldiltiazem and desmethyldiltiazem.	Sirolimus levels should be monitored and a dose adjustment of Rapamune may be necessary.
Erythromycin	CT	Multiple dose co-administration ↑ whole blood sirolimus C_{max}, T_{max}, and AUC 4.4-, 1.4-, and 4.2-fold, respectively, and ↑ C_{max}, T_{max}, and AUC of plasma erythromycin base 1.6-, 1.3-, and 1.7-fold, respectively	Sirolimus levels should be monitored and appropriate dose reductions of both medications should be considered.
Ketoconazole	CT	Multiple-dose co-administration of sirolimus ↑ sirolimus C_{max}, T_{max}, and AUC 4.4-, 1.4-, and 10.9-fold, respectively	Co-administration of Rapamune and ketoconazole is not recommended. Ketoconazole significantly affected the rate and extent of absorption and sirolimus exposure.
Rifampicin	CT	Pretreatment with multiple doses of rifampicin, 600 mg daily for 14 days, greatly ↓ sirolimus exposure following a single 10 mg dose of Rapamune oral solution	Co-administration of Rapamune and rifampicin is not recommended.
Verapamil	CT	Multiple-dose co-administration of verapamil and Rapamune oral solution ↑ sirolimus C_{max}, T_{max}, and AUC 2.3-, 1.1-, and 2.2-fold, respectively, and plasma S-(-) verapamil C_{max} and AUC were both increased 1.5-fold, and tmax ↓ 24%.	Sirolimus levels should be monitored and appropriate dose reductions of both medications should be considered.

Legend: C=Case Study; CT=Clinical Trial; T=Theoretical.

Other Inhibitors and Inducers of CYP3A4: Other substances, aside from those mentioned above, that inhibit CYP3A4 include but are not limited to: calcium channel blockers: nicardipine; antifungal agents: clotrimazole, fluconazole; antibiotics: troleandomycin; gastrointestinal prokinetic agents: cisapride, metoclopramide; other drugs: bromocriptine, cimetidine, cyclosporine, danazol, HIV-protease inhibitors (eg, ritonavir, indinavir); grapefruit juice.

Other substances, aside from those mentioned above, that induce CYP3A4 include but are not limited to: anticonvulsants: carbamazepine, phenobarbital, phenytoin; antibiotics: rifapentine.

This list is not all-inclusive.

There were no clinically significant drug-drug interactions between sirolimus and acyclovir, atorvastatin, digoxin, glyburide, nifedipine, norgestrel 0.3 mg/ethinyl estradiol 0.03 mg, methylprednisolone, sulfamethoxazole/trimethoprim or tacrolimus. Therefore, they may be co-administered without dose adjustments.

Drug interaction studies have not been conducted with other drugs that may be commonly administered to renal transplant patients.

Drug-Food Interactions: The bioavailability of sirolimus is affected by concomitant food intake after administration of Rapamune oral solution or tablet. Rapamune should be taken consistently, either with or without food to minimize blood level variability. Grapefruit juice reduces CYP3A4-mediated drug metabolism and potentially enhances P-glycoprotein-mediated drug counter-transport from enterocytes of the small intestine. Grapefruit juice must not be taken with Rapamune tablets or oral solution or be used for oral solution dilution.

Drug-Herb Interactions: St. John's Wort (Hypericum perforatum) induces CYP3A4 and P-glycoprotein. Since sirolimus is a substrate for both cytochrome CYP3A4 and P-glycoprotein, there is the potential that the use of St. John's Wort in patients receiving Rapamune could result in reduced whole blood sirolimus concentrations.

Drug-Laboratory Test Interactions: No studies have been conducted on the interactions of sirolimus in commonly employed clinical laboratory tests.

Drug-Lifestyle Interactions: No studies have been conducted on the interactions of sirolimus with lifestyle.

DOSAGE AND ADMINISTRATION: Dosing Considerations:

- **In patients at low to moderate immunological risk,** it is recommended that Rapamune should be used initially in a regimen with cyclosporine and corticosteroids. Cyclosporine withdrawal is recommended 2 to 4 months after transplantation in patients at low to moderate immunologic risk.
- **In patients at high immunologic risk,** it is recommended that Rapamune be used in combination with cyclosporine and corticosteroids for the first year following transplantation (see Dosage and Administration).
- To minimize the variability of exposure to Rapamune, this drug should be taken once daily, preferably at the same time of day, and consistently with or without food.
- Cyclosporine microemulsion enhances absorption of Rapamune (see Drug Interactions). It is recommended that sirolimus be taken 4 hours after cyclosporine microemulsion administration.
- A daily dose of 2 mg Rapamune Tablets has been demonstrated to be clinically equivalent to 2 mg Rapamune Oral Solution. However, it is not known if higher doses of Rapamune tablets and oral solution are clinically equivalent on a mg-to-mg basis. (See Action and Clinical Pharmacology.)
- It is recommended that a sirolimus trough concentration be taken 1 or 2 weeks after switching Rapamune formulations or tablet strengths or altering the total daily dose to confirm that the trough concentration is within the recommended target range (see Warnings and Precautions, Monitoring and Laboratory Tests, Blood Concentration Monitoring).
- Blood sirolimus trough levels should be monitored:
  - In patients receiving concentration-controlled Rapamune.
  - In pediatric patients
  - In patients with hepatic impairment.
  - During concurrent administration of inhibitors and inducers of CYP3A4 and P-glycoprotein.
  - If the cyclosporine dose is markedly reduced, or if cyclosporine is discontinued.
- The Rapamune dosage need not be adjusted because of **impaired renal function** (see Action and Clinical Pharmacology, Special Populations and Conditions, Renal Insufficiency).
- It is recommended that the maintenance dose of Rapamune be reduced by approximately one third to one-half in patients with **hepatic impairment**. It is not necessary to modify the Rapamune loading dose (see Action and Clinical Pharmacology, Special Populations and Conditions, Hepatic Insufficiency). In patients with hepatic impairment, it is recommended that sirolimus whole blood trough levels be monitored.
- Based on the finding that blood clearance decreases linearly with age, consideration should be given to reducing the Rapamune dose in patients 65 years of age and over. (See Pharmacokinetics, Special Populations and Conditions, Geriatrics (>65 years of age).)

- The safety and efficacy of Rapamune in pediatric patients below the age of 13 years have not been established. The initial loading dose should be 3 mg/m² in patients ≥13 years who weigh less than 40 kg. The maintenance dose should be adjusted, based on body surface area, to 1 mg/m²/day. It is recommended that sirolimus whole blood trough levels be monitored.
- The bioavailability of sirolimus (oral solution or tablet) is altered by concomitant food intake after administration. Rapamune should be taken consistently, either with or without food to minimize blood level variability.
- Bioavailability has not been determined for tablets after they have been crushed, chewed, or split and therefore this cannot be recommended. Patients unable to take the tablets should be prescribed the oral solution and instructed in its use.

Recommended Dose and Dosage Adjustment: Patients at Low to Moderate Immunological Risk: Rapamune and Cyclosporine Combination Therapy: The initial dose of Rapamune should be administered as soon as possible after transplantation. For de novo transplant recipients, a loading dose of Rapamune corresponding to 3 times the maintenance dose should be given. For most patients, the maintenance dose is 2 mg/day, with a loading dose of 6 mg.

Although a maintenance dose of 5 mg/day, with a loading dose of 15 mg, was used in clinical trials of the oral solution and was shown to be safe and effective, no efficacy advantage over the 2 mg dose could be established for renal transplant patients. Patients receiving 2 mg of Rapamune oral solution per day demonstrated an overall better safety profile than did patients receiving 5 mg of Rapamune oral solution per day.

It is recommended that Rapamune oral solution and tablets be used initially in a regimen with cyclosporine and corticosteroids. Cyclosporine should be withdrawn 2 to 4 months after renal transplantation in patients at low to moderate immunologic risk, and the Rapamune dose should be increased to reach recommended blood concentrations (see Rapamune Maintenance Regimen (RMR, Rapamune following cyclosporine withdrawal)). Cyclosporine withdrawal has not been studied in patients with Banff 93 grade III acute rejection or vascular rejection prior to cyclosporine withdrawal, those who are dialysis dependent, or with serum creatinine >4.5 mg/dL, Black patients, re-transplants, multi-organ transplants, or patients with high-panel reactive antibodies.

It is recommended that Rapamune be taken 4 hours after cyclosporine microemulsion [(cyclosporine, USP) MODIFIED] administration.

Rapamune Maintenance Regimen (RMR, Rapamune following cyclosporine withdrawal): Initially, patients considered for cyclosporine withdrawal should be receiving Rapamune and cyclosporine combination therapy. At 2 to 4 months following transplantation, cyclosporine should be progressively discontinued over 4 to 8 weeks and the Rapamune dose should be adjusted to obtain whole blood trough concentrations within the range of 16 to 24 ng/mL (chromatographic method) for the first year following transplantation. Thereafter, the target sirolimus concentrations should be 12 to 20 ng/mL (chromatographic method). The actual observations at year 1 and 5 were close to these ranges (see Warnings and Precautions, Monitoring and Laboratory Tests, Blood Concentration Monitoring).

Patients at High Immunological Risk: Rapamune Combination Therapy: It is recommended that Rapamune be used in combination with cyclosporine and corticosteroids for the first year following transplantation in patients at high immunologic risk (defined as Black transplant recipients and/or repeat renal transplant recipients who lost a previous allograft for immunologic reason and/or patients with high-panel reactive antibodies [PRA; peak PRA level >80%]).

The safety and efficacy of these combinations in high-risk patients have not been studied beyond one year. Therefore, after the first year following transplantation, any adjustments to the immunosuppressive regimen should be considered on the basis of the clinical status of the patient.

For patients receiving Rapamune with cyclosporine, Rapamune therapy should be initiated with a loading dose of up to 15 mg on day 1 post-transplantation. Beginning on day 2, an initial maintenance dose of 5 mg/day should be given. A trough level should be obtained between days 5 and 7, and the daily dose of Rapamune should thereafter be adjusted to achieve whole blood trough sirolimus concentrations of 10-15 ng/mL.

The starting dose of cyclosporine should be up to 7 mg/kg/day in divided doses, and the dose should subsequently be adjusted to achieve whole blood trough concentrations of 200-300 ng/mL through week 2, 150-200 ng/mL from week 2 to week 26, and 100-150 ng/mL from week 26 to week 52. Prednisone should be administered at a minimum of 5 mg/day.

Antibody induction therapy may be used.

Rapamune Dosage Adjustment: Therapeutic drug monitoring should not be the sole basis for adjusting Rapamune therapy. Careful attention should be made to clinical signs/symptoms, tissue biopsies, and laboratory parameters (see Drug Interactions).

Cyclosporine inhibits the metabolism and transport of sirolimus, and consequently, whole blood sirolimus concentrations will decrease when cyclosporine is discontinued unless the Rapamune dose is increased. The Rapamune dose will need to be approximately 4-fold higher to account for both the absence of the pharmacokinetic interaction with cyclosporine (approximately 2-fold increase) and the augmented immunosuppressive requirement in the absence of cyclosporine (approximately 2-fold increase).

Sirolimus has a long half-life; therefore frequent Rapamune dose adjustments based on non-steady-state sirolimus concentrations can lead to overdosing or underdosing. Once the Rapamune maintenance dose is adjusted, patients should be retained on the new maintenance dose for at least 7 to 14 days before further dosage adjustment with trough concentration monitoring.

In most patients dose adjustments can be based on simple proportion: New Rapamune dose = Current Dose × (Target Concentration ÷ Current Concentration).

A loading dose should be considered in addition to a new maintenance dose when it is necessary to considerably increase sirolimus trough concentrations: Rapamune Loading Dose = 3 × (New Maintenance Dose − Current Maintenance Dose).

The maximum Rapamune dose administered on any day **should not exceed 40 mg**. If an estimated daily dose would exceed 40 mg due to the addition of a loading dose, the loading dose should be administered over 2 days. Sirolimus trough concentrations should be monitored at least 3 to 4 days after a loading dose(s).

Missed Dose: A missed dose should be taken as soon as remembered, but not within 4 hours of the next dose of cyclosporine. Medicines can then be taken as usual. If a dose is missed completely, a double dose should not be taken to make up for a forgotten dose.

Administration: Instructions for Dilution and Administration of Rapamune Oral Solution: The amber oral dose syringe should be used to withdraw the prescribed amount of Rapamune from the bottle. Empty the correct amount of Rapamune from the syringe into a glass or plastic container holding at least two (2) ounces (¼ cup; 60 mL) of water or orange juice. No other liquids, including grapefruit juice, should be used for dilution. Stir vigorously and drink at once. Rinse the container with an additional volume (minimum of four [4] ounces; ½ cup; 120 mL) of water or orange juice, stir vigorously, and drink at once.

Rapamune oral solution contains polysorbate-80, which is known to increase the rate of di-(2- ethylhexyl)phthalate (DEHP) extraction from polyvinyl chloride (PVC). This should be considered during the preparation and administration of Rapamune oral solution. It is important that the recommendations in this section be followed closely.

Instructions for Rapamune Tablets: Rapamune tablets should be taken with orange juice or water only. Rapamune tablets should not be taken with grapefruit juice.

OVERDOSAGE:

There is limited experience with overdose. In general, the adverse effects of overdose are consistent with those listed in Adverse Reactions. During clinical trials, there were two accidental Rapamune (sirolimus oral solution) ingestions, of 120 mg and 150 mg. One patient, receiving 150 mg, experienced an episode of transient atrial fibrillation. The other patient experienced no adverse effects. General supportive measures should be followed in all cases of overdose. Based on the poor aqueous solubility and high erythrocyte and plasma protein binding of Rapamune, it is anticipated that Rapamune is not dialyzable to any significant extent.

In mice and rats, the acute oral LD_{50} was greater than 800 mg/kg.

> For management of a suspected drug overdose, contact your regional Poison Control Centre. See the *CPS* Directory section for a list of Poison Control Centres.

ACTION AND CLINICAL PHARMACOLOGY: Mechanism of Action: Rapamune is a potent immunosuppressive agent. Sirolimus is a macrocyclic lactone produced by *S. hygroscopicus*. Sirolimus inhibits T lymphocyte activation and proliferation that occurs in response to antigenic and cytokine (Interleukin [IL]-2, IL-4, IL-7, and IL-15) stimulation by a mechanism that is distinct from that of other immunosuppressants. Sirolimus also inhibits antibody production. In cells, sirolimus binds to the immunophilin, FK Binding Protein-12 (FKBP-12), to generate an immunosuppressive complex. Unlike cyclosporine and tacrolimus, the sirolimus:FKBP-12 complex has no effect on calcineurin activity. Rather, this complex binds to and inhibits the activation of a specific cell cycle regulatory protein called the mammalian Target Of Rapamycin (mTOR). mTOR is a key regulatory kinase and its inhibition by sirolimus suppresses cytokine-driven T-cell proliferation, inhibiting the progression from the G1 to the S phase of the cell cycle.

Pharmacodynamics: In in vitro studies, sirolimus inhibits proliferation of T lymphocytes, B lymphocytes, and vascular and bronchial smooth muscle cells induced by cytokines and growth factors. Because sirolimus affects lymphocyte activation by a different mechanism, activation stimuli that resist inhibition by cyclosporine and tacrolimus have been shown to be sensitive to sirolimus. Sirolimus also affects B cell activation and antibody production. These effects contribute to the immunosuppressive properties of sirolimus.

Sirolimus prolongs allograft survival in animal models of transplantation, ranging from rodents to primates, both for solid organ and for cellular allografts. In mice, sirolimus prolongs the survival of heart, skin and islet allografts. Sirolimus prevents acute rejection of heart, kidney, small bowel, and pancreatico-duodenal grafts in rats and induces long-term tolerance. In rats, sirolimus reverses ongoing acute rejection of heart, kidney, and pancreas allografts, and suppresses accelerated heart allograft rejection in presensitized hosts. Sirolimus also prevents acute rejection of kidney allografts in dogs, pigs and baboons, as well as pancreatic islet cell rejection in dogs. Although in animals, sirolimus improves allograft survival as a single agent, it is synergistic with cyclosporine and is effective in combination with tacrolimus.

In animal models of autoimmune disease, sirolimus suppresses immune-mediated events associated with systemic lupus erythematosus, collagen-induced arthritis, autoimmune type I diabetes, autoimmune myocarditis, experimental allergic encephalomyelitis, graft versus host disease, and autoimmune uveoretinitis.

In rodents and primates, sirolimus mitigates the progression of chronic rejection by reducing the vascular intimal proliferation that is characteristic of chronic vascular rejection. In a pig model of coronary restenosis after angioplasty, sirolimus reduces the vascular proliferative response to mechanical vascular injury.

Animal studies have shown that sirolimus-mediated immunosuppression is reversible.

Pharmacokinetics: Sirolimus pharmacokinetic activity has been determined following oral administration in healthy subjects, pediatric dialysis patients, hepatically impaired patients and renal transplant patients. Sirolimus is rapidly absorbed and undergoes extensive metabolism to seven major metabolites that do not contribute significantly to the pharmacological effect.

Absorption: Following administration of Rapamune oral solution, sirolimus is rapidly absorbed, with a time to peak concentration (t_{max}) of 1 hour in healthy subjects and 2-3 hours in renal transplant recipients. Following administration of Rapamune tablet, sirolimus t_{max} was approximately 3 hours after single doses in healthy volunteers and multiple doses in renal transplant patients. The systemic availability of sirolimus is approximately 14% after the administration of Rapamune Oral Solution. The mean bioavailability of sirolimus after administration of the Rapamune tablet is about 22% higher relative to the oral solution. Sirolimus tablets are not bioequivalent to the oral solution; however, clinical equivalence has been demonstrated at the 2 mg dose level over a 12-month period in renal allograft recipients, where clinical equivalence was measured as the rate of occurrence of the composite endpoint of first biopsy-proven acute rejection, graft loss, or death in the first 3 months after transplantation. (See Dosage and Administration.) Sirolimus concentrations are dose proportional between 3 and 12 mg/m² following the administration of Rapamune oral solution to stable renal transplant patients, and between 5 and 40 mg after administration of Rapamune tablets in healthy volunteers. Upon repeated administration to stable renal transplant patients, the average blood concentration of sirolimus was increased approximately 3-fold.

Bioequivalence testing of the various sirolimus tablet strengths in healthy volunteers (n=22) showed that 10 mg doses of the 1 mg, 2 mg, and 5 mg tablets were equivalent with respect to C_{max}, $AUC_{0\text{-}72h}$ and $AUC_{0\text{-}inf}$.

Food Effects: In 22 healthy volunteers receiving Rapamune oral solution, a high fat breakfast (861.8 kcal, 54.9% kcal from fat) altered the bioavailability characteristics of sirolimus. Compared with fasting, a 34% decrease in the peak blood sirolimus concentration (C_{max}), a 3.5-fold increase in the time to peak concentration (t_{max}), and a 35% increase in total exposure (AUC) was observed. The change in bioavailability is not clinically important. After administration of Rapamune tablets and a high-fat meal in 24 healthy volunteers, C_{max}, t_{max}, and AUC showed increases of 65%, 32%, and 23%, respectively. Thus, a high-fat meal produced differences in the two formulations with respect to rate of absorption but not in extent of absorption. Evidence from a large randomized multicentre controlled trial comparing Rapamune oral solution to tablets, supports that the differences in absorption rate do not affect the efficacy of the drug.

To minimize variability, both Rapamune oral solution and tablets should be taken consistently with or without food (see Dosage and Administration). Bioequivalence testing based on AUC and C_{max} showed that Rapamune administered with orange juice is equivalent to administration with water. Therefore, orange juice and water may be used interchangeably as administration liquids for Rapamune (see Dosage and Administration). Grapefruit juice reduces CYP3A4-mediated drug metabolism and potentially enhances P-glycoprotein-mediated drug counter-transport from enterocytes of the small intestine. Grapefruit juice must not be taken with Rapamune tablets or oral solution or be used for oral solution dilution.

Distribution: The mean (±SD) blood-to-plasma ratio of sirolimus was 36±17.9 in stable renal allograft recipients after administration of Rapamune oral solution, indicating that sirolimus is extensively partitioned into formed blood elements. The mean volume of distribution (V_{ss}/F) of sirolimus by Rapamune oral solution is 12±7.52 L/kg. Sirolimus is extensively bound (approximately 92%) to human plasma proteins. In man, the binding of sirolimus was shown mainly to be associated with serum albumin (97%), α_1-acid glycoprotein, and lipoproteins.

Metabolism: Sirolimus is a substrate for both cytochrome P450 IIIA4 (CYP3A4) and P-glycoprotein. Sirolimus is extensively metabolized by O-demethylation and/or hydroxylation. Seven major metabolites, including hydroxy, demethyl, and hydroxy-demethyl, are identifiable in whole blood. Some of these metabolites are also detectable in plasma, fecal, and urine samples. The glucuronide and sulfate conjugates are not present in any of the biologic matrices. The combined demethyl and hydroxy metabolites show ≤30% of the in vitro immunosuppressive activity of sirolimus.

Excretion: After a single dose of [^{14}C] sirolimus by oral solution in healthy volunteers, the majority (91%) of radioactivity was recovered from the feces, and only a minor amount (2.2%) was excreted in urine.

The mean ±SD terminal elimination half-life ($t_{½}$) of sirolimus after multiple dosing by Rapamune oral solution in stable renal transplant patients was estimated to be 62±16 hours.

Pharmacokinetics in Renal Transplant Patients: Rapamune Oral Solution: Mean (±SD) pharmacokinetic parameters for Rapamune oral solution given daily in combination with cyclosporine and corticosteroids in renal transplant patients were determined at months 1, 3, and 6 after transplantation (Study 1). There were no significant differences in any of these parameters with respect to treatment group or month. Whole blood sirolimus trough concentrations (mean±SD) for the 2 mg/day and 5 mg/day dose groups were 8.6±4.0 ng/mL (n=226) and 17.3±7.4 ng/mL (n=219), respectively. Whole blood trough sirolimus concentrations were significantly correlated (r^2=0.95) with $AUC_{\tau,ss}$. Table 9 provides a summary of these sirolimus pharmacokinetic parameters.

Table 9: Rapamune

Sirolimus Pharmacokinetic Parameters (Mean±SD) in Renal Transplant Patients (Multiple Dose Oral Solution)[a,b]

n	Dose	$C_{max,ss}$[c] (ng/mL)	$t_{max,ss}$ (h)	$AUC_{\tau,ss}$[c] (ng·h/mL)	CL/F[d] (mL/h/kg)
19	2 mg	12.2±6.2	3.01±2.40	158±70	182±72
23	5 mg	37.4±21	1.84±1.30	396±193	221±143

[a] Sirolimus administered four hours after cyclosporine microemulsion.
[b] As measured by the Liquid Chromatographic/Tandem Mass Spectrometric Method (LC/MS/MS).
[c] These parameters are dose normalized for the statistical comparison.
[d] CL/F=oral dose clearance.

Rapamune Tablets: Pharmacokinetic parameters for Rapamune tablets administered daily in combination with cyclosporine and corticosteroids in renal transplant patients are summarized in Table 10 based on data collected at months 1 and 3 after transplantation.

Table 10: Rapamune

Sirolimus Pharmacokinetic Parameters (Mean±SD) in Renal Transplant Patients (Multiple Dose Tablets)[a,b]

n	Dose (2 mg/day)	$C_{max,ss}$[c] (ng/mL)	$t_{max,ss}$ (h)	$AUC_{\tau,ss}$[c] (ng·h/mL)	CL/F[d] (mL/h/kg)
17	Oral solution	14.4±5.3	2.12±0.84	194±78	173±50
13	Tablets	15.0±4.9	3.46±2.40	230±67	139±63

[a] Sirolimus administered four hours after cyclosporine microemulsion.
[b] As measured by the Liquid Chromatographic/Tandem Mass Spectrometric Method (LC/MS/MS).
[c] These parameters are dose normalized for the statistical comparison.
[d] CL/F=oral dose clearance.

Whole blood sirolimus trough concentrations, (mean±SD), as measured by immunoassay, for 2 mg of oral solution and 2 mg of tablets over 6 months, were 8.9±4.4 ng/mL (n=172) and 9.5±3.9 ng/mL (n=179), respectively. Whole blood trough sirolimus concentrations, as measured by LC/MS/MS, were significantly correlated (r^2=0.85) with $AUC_{τ,ss}$. Mean whole blood sirolimus trough concentrations in patients receiving either Rapamune Oral Solution or Rapamune Tablets with a loading dose of three times the maintenance dose achieved steady-state concentrations within 24 hours after the start of dose administration.

Use of Rapamune Without Concomitant Cyclosporine Administration: Average Rapamune doses and sirolimus whole blood trough concentrations for Rapamune tablets administered daily in combination with cyclosporine and following cyclosporine withdrawal, in combination with corticosteroids in renal transplant patients are summarized in Table 11.

Table 11: Rapamune

Average Rapamune Doses and Sirolimus Trough Concentrations (Mean±SD) in Renal Transplant Patients After Multiple Dose Tablet Administration

	Rapamune with Cyclosporine Therapy[a]	Rapamune Following Cyclosporine Withdrawal[a]
Rapamune Dose (mg/day)		
Months 4 to 12	2.1±0.7	8.2±4.2
Months 12 to 24	2.0±0.8	6.4±3.0
Months 24 to 36	2.0±0.8	5.0±2.5
Months 36 to 48	2.0±0.8	4.8±2.2
Months 48 to 60	2.1±1.0	4.4±2.0
Sirolimus C_{min}, (ng/mL)[b]		
Months 4 to 12	10.7±3.8	23.3±5.0
Months 12 to 24	11.2±4.1	22.5±4.8
Months 24 to 36	11.4±4.2	20.4±5.4
Months 36 to 48	10.8±3.7	19.4±5.6
Months 48 to 60	10.7±4.1	18.2±5.3

a 215 patients were randomized to each group.
b Expressed by immunoassay and equivalence.

The time required for withdrawal of cyclosporine and concurrent increases in sirolimus trough concentrations to steady state was approximately 6 weeks. Larger Rapamune doses were required due to the absence of the inhibition of sirolimus metabolism and transport by cyclosporine and the need for higher target sirolimus concentrations during concentration-controlled administration of Rapamune following cyclosporine withdrawal.

Pharmacokinetics in high-risk patients: Average Rapamune doses and sirolimus whole blood trough concentrations for tablets administered daily in combination with cyclosporine and corticosteroids in high-risk renal transplant patients (Clinical Trials) are summarized in Table 12.

Table 12: Rapamune

Average Rapamune Doses and Sirolimus Trough Concentrations (Mean ± SD) in High-risk Renal Transplant Patients After Multiple-dose Tablet Administration

	Rapamune with Cyclosporine Therapy
Rapamune Dose (mg/day)	
Months 3 to 6[a]	5.1±2.4
Months 9 to 12[b]	5.0±2.3
Sirolimus C_{min} (ng/mL)[c]	
Months 3 to 6	11.8±4.2
Months 9 to 12	11.2±3.8

a n=109.
b n=127.
c Expressed by chromatography.

Special Populations and Conditions: Pediatrics (<13 years of age): Sirolimus pharmacokinetic data were collected in concentration-controlled trials of pediatric renal transplant patients who were also receiving cyclosporine and corticosteroids. The target ranges for trough concentrations were either 10-20 ng/mL for the 21 children receiving tablets, or 5-15 ng/mL for the one child receiving oral solution. The children aged 6-11 years (n=8) received mean±SD doses of 1.75±0.71 mg/day (0.064±0.018 mg/kg, 1.65±0.43 mg/m²). The children aged 12-18 years (n=14) received mean±SD doses of 2.79±1.25 mg/day (0.053±0.0150 mg/kg, 1.86±0.61 mg/m²). At the time of sirolimus blood sampling for pharmacokinetic evaluation, the majority (80%) of these pediatric patients received the sirolimus dose at 16 hours after the once daily cyclosporine dose. See Table 13.

Table 13: Rapamune

Sirolimus Pharmacokinetic Parameters (Mean±SD) in Pediatric Renal Transplant Patients (Multiple Dose Concentration Control)[a,b]

Age (y)	n	Body Weight (kg)	$C_{max,ss}$ (ng/mL)	$t_{max,ss}$ (h)	$C_{min,ss}$ (ng/mL)	$AUC_{τ,ss}$ (ng·h/mL)	CL/F[c] (mL/h/kg)	CL/F[c] (L/h/m²)
6–11	8	27±10	22.1±8.9	5.88±4.05	10.6±4.3	356± 127	214±129	5.4±2.8
12–18	14	52±15	34.5±12.2	2.7±1.5	14.7±8.6	466±236	136±57	4.7±1.9

a Sirolimus co-administered with cyclosporine oral solution (MODIFIED) (e.g., Neoral Oral Solution) and/or cyclosporine capsules (MODIFIED) (e.g., Neoral Soft Gelatin Capsules).
b As measured by Liquid Chromatographic/Tandem Mass Spectrometric Method (LC/MS/MS).
c Oral-dose clearance adjusted by either body weight (kg) or body surface area (m²).

Table 14 summarizes pharmacokinetic data obtained in pediatric dialysis patients with chronically impaired renal function receiving Rapamune by oral solution.

Geriatrics (>65 years of age): A decrease in CL/F of approximately 13% per decade was observed in population analyses. Clinical studies of Rapamune did not include a sufficient number of patients >65 years of age to determine whether they will respond differently than younger patients. After the administration of Rapamune oral solution, sirolimus trough concentration data in 35 renal transplant patients >65 years of age were similar to those in the adult population (n=822) 18 to 65 years of age. Similar results were obtained after the administration of Rapamune tablets to 12 renal transplant patients >65 years of age compared with adults (n=167) 18 to 65 years of age.

Table 14: Rapamune

Sirolimus Pharmacokinetic Parameters (Mean±SD) in Pediatric Patients with Stable Chronic Renal Failure Maintained on Hemodialysis or Peritoneal Dialysis (1, 3, 9, 15 mg/m² Single Dose)

Age Group (years)	n	t_{max} (h)	$t_{1/2}$ (h)	CL/F/WT (mL/h/kg)
5–11	9	1.1±0.5	71±40	580±450
12–18	11	0.79±0.17	55±18	450±232

Gender: The pharmacokinetic differences between males and females are relatively small. Rapamune oral dose clearance after Rapamune oral solution in males was 12% lower than that in females; male subjects had a significantly longer $t_{½}$ than did female subjects (72.3 hours versus 61.3 hours). A similar trend in the effect of gender on sirolimus oral dose clearance and $t_{½}$ was observed after the administration of Rapamune tablets. Dose adjustments based on gender are not recommended.

Race: In large phase 3 trials (Studies 1 and 2) using Rapamune and cyclosporine (microemulsion, Neoral), there were no significant differences in mean trough sirolimus concentrations or AUC over time between black (n=139) and non-black (n=724) patients during the first 6 months after transplantation at sirolimus doses of 2 mg/day and 5 mg/day by oral solution. Similarly, after administration of Rapamune Tablets (2 mg/day) in a phase 3 trial, mean sirolimus trough concentrations over 6 months were not significantly different among black (n=51) and non-black (n=128) patients. There is limited information on black patients from a Phase 3 trial (Study 4) using Rapamune with cyclosporine elimination. In a Phase 2 study of similar design to Study 4, mean dose-normalized sirolimus trough concentrations in the control group (sirolimus 2 mg/day+cyclosporine) over 12 months were significantly decreased by approximately 31% among black (n=17) patients compared with non-black (n=72) patients. The mean dose-normalized sirolimus trough concentrations over 12 months in the Rapamune (concentration-controlled 10-20 ng/mL) with cyclosporine elimination group were significantly decreased by approximately 15% among black (n=15) patients compared with non-black (n=76) patients.

Hepatic Insufficiency: Table 15 shows the mean (±SD) pharmacokinetic parameters for sirolimus following the administration of sirolimus to subjects with hepatic impairment and healthy subjects. Rapamune (15 mg) was administered as a single dose by oral solution to subjects with normal hepatic function and to patients with Child-Pugh classification A (mild), B (moderate) or C (severe) hepatic impairment, in which hepatic impairment was primary and not related to an underlying systemic disease.

Table 15: Rapamune

Sirolimus Pharmacokinetic Parameters (Mean±SD) in 18 Healthy Subjects and 18 Patients with Mild to Moderate Hepatic Impairment (15 mg Single Dose)

Population	$C_{max,ss}$[a] (ng/mL)	t_{max} (h)	$AUC_{0-∞}$ (ng·h/mL)	CL/F (mL/h/kg)
Healthy Subjects	78.2±18.3	0.83±0.17	970±272	215±76
Hepatic Impairment	77.9±23.1	0.84±0.17	1567±616	144±62

a As measured by LC/MS/MS.

Table 16: Rapamune

Whole Blood Sirolimus Pharmacokinetic Parameters (Mean±SD) in 9 Healthy Subjects and 9 Patients with Severe Hepatic Impairment (15 mg Single Dose)

Group[a]	C_{max} (ng/mL)	t_{max} (h)	$t_{½}$ (h)	AUC (ng·h/mL)	CL/F (mL/h/kg)	Vss/F (L/kg)	MRT (h)
Healthy subjects	72.3±16.6	0.78±0.16	80.0±5.4	838±277	300±66	34.5±7.2	77.5±6.4
Severe hepatic impairment	56.2±23.1	0.82±0.17	214.5±68.9	2597±1092	98.1±43.8	29.1±12.9	280±99
	p-Values from ANOVA						
	0.108	0.652	0.0001	0.0002	0.0001	0.286	0.0001

a Sirolimus was administered by oral solution.
Legend: ANOVA=analysis of variance; AUC=area under the concentration-time curve; CL/F=apparent oral dose clearance; C_{max}=peak concentration; MRT=mean residence time; SD=standard deviation; t_{max}=time peak concentration occurs; $t_{½}$=terminal-phase elimination half-life; V_{ss}/F=apparent oral-dose steady-state volume of distribution.

Compared with the values in the normal hepatic group, the hepatic impairment group had higher mean values for sirolimus AUC and $t_{½}$ and had lower mean values for sirolimus CL/F. Sirolimus absorption was not altered by hepatic disease, as evidenced by no changes in C_{max} and t_{max} values. The initial maintenance dose of Rapamune should be reduced by approximately one third in patients with mild to moderate hepatic impairment and by approximately one half in patients with severe hepatic impairment. In patients with hepatic impairment, it is recommended that sirolimus whole blood trough levels be monitored. However, hepatic diseases with varying etiologies may show different effects.

Renal Insufficiency: There is minimal (2.2%) renal excretion of the drug or its metabolites. The pharmacokinetics of sirolimus are very similar in various populations with renal function ranging from normal to absent (dialysis patients).

STORAGE AND STABILITY: Keep in a safe place out of the reach of children.

Rapamune Oral Solution: Rapamune Oral Solution bottles should be stored protected from exposure to light and refrigerated at 2 to 8°C. Do not freeze. Rapamune is stable until the expiration date indicated on the container label. Once the bottle is opened, it should be kept in a refrigerator and the contents used within one month. If not refrigerated, the opened bottles may be stored at room temperature (15 to 30°C) for up to 5 days.

An amber syringe and cap are provided for dosing and the product may be kept in the syringe for a maximum of 24 hours at room temperatures up to 30°C or refrigerated at 2to 8°C. The syringe should be discarded after one use. After dilution, the preparation should be used immediately.

Rapamune provided in bottles may develop a slight haze when refrigerated. If such a haze occurs allow the product to stand at room temperature and shake gently until the haze disappears. The presence of this haze does not affect the quality of the product.

Rapamune Tablets: Rapamune Tablets should be stored at 15 to 30°C. Dispense in a light-resistant container. Protect from exposure to light. Rapamune is stable until the expiration date indicated on the container label.

SPECIAL HANDLING INSTRUCTIONS: Since Rapamune is not absorbed through the skin, there are no special precautions. However, if direct contact with the skin or mucous membranes occurs, wash thoroughly with soap and water; rinse eyes with plain water.

INFORMATION FOR THE PATIENT: Published in e-CPS, available by subscription at www.e-cps.ca.

DOSAGE FORMS, COMPOSITION AND PACKAGING: Oral Solution: Each mL of oral solution contains: sirolimus 1 mg. Nonmedicinal ingredients: Phosal 50 PG (ascorbyl palmitate, ethanol, phosphatidylcholine, propylene glycol, soybean oil fatty acids and sunflower mono and diglycerides) and polysorbate 80. Amber glass bottles of 60 mL, with an oral syringe adapter for fitting into the neck of the bottle, 30 disposable amber oral syringes and 30 caps for daily dosing.

Tablets: Each white, triangular-shaped tablet, marked "RAPAMUNE 1 mg" on one side contains: sirolimus 1 mg. Nonmedicinal ingredients: calcium sulfate anhydrous, carnauba wax, glyceryl monooleate, ink, lactose monohydrate, magnesium stearate, microcrystalline cellulose, pharmaceutical glaze, polaxamer 188, polyethylene glycol 8000 powdered, polyethylene glycol type 20 000, povidone, sucrose, talc, titanium dioxide and vitamin E (dl-alpha tocopherol). Bottles of 100. Unit dose cartons of 100 (10 blister cards of 10 tablets).

(Shown in Product Identification Section)

Rasilez® Ⓟ

aliskiren fumarate

Renin Inhibitor

Novartis Pharmaceuticals

Date of Preparation: November 8, 2007
Date of Revision: August 10, 2010

SUMMARY PRODUCT INFORMATION:

Route of Administration	Dosage Form/ Strength	Clinically Relevant Nonmedicinal Ingredients
Oral	Tablet 150 mg, 300 mg	Colloidal silicon dioxide, crospovidone, hypromellose, iron oxide colorants, magnesium stearate, microcrystalline cellulose, polyethylene glycol, povidone, talc and titanium dioxide See Dosage Forms, Composition and Packaging.

INDICATIONS AND CLINICAL USE: RASILEZ (aliskiren) is indicated for the treatment of mild to moderate essential hypertension. It may be used alone or concomitantly with thiazide diuretics, angiotensin converting enzyme inhibitors, angiotensin II AT_1 receptor blockers or dihydropyridine calcium channel blockers.

Geriatrics (>65 years of age): Of the total number of patients receiving RASILEZ in clinical studies, 1275 (19 %) were 65 years or older and 231 (3.4%) were 75 years or older. No differences were observed in safety and efficacy of RASILEZ in older patients compared to those under age 65.

Pediatrics (<18 years of age): Safety and efficacy in children and adolescents have not been established. RASILEZ should not be given to this patient population.

CONTRAINDICATIONS:

- Patients who are hypersensitive to any component of this product (see Dosage Forms, Composition and Packaging).

WARNINGS AND PRECAUTIONS:

> **Serious Warnings and Precautions**
> Drugs that act directly on the renin-angiotensin system can cause fetal and neonatal morbidity and death when administered to pregnant women. When pregnancy is detected, RASILEZ should be discontinued as soon as possible (see Warnings and Precautions, Special Populations, Pregnant Women).

Information to Be Provided to the Patient: Pregnancy: Female patients of childbearing age should be told about the consequences of second- and third-trimester exposure to drugs that act on the renin-angiotensin system, and they should also be told that these consequences do not appear to have resulted from intrauterine drug exposure that has been limited to the first trimester. These patients should be asked to report pregnancies to their physicians as soon as possible.

Cardiovascular: Hypotension: Symptomatic hypotension was rarely seen (0.1%) in patients with uncomplicated hypertension treated with RASILEZ alone. Hypotension was also infrequent during combination therapy with other antihypertensive agents (<1%). Aliskiren-induced hypotension is more likely to occur in patients with an activated renin-angiotensin system, such as volume- or salt-depleted patients (possibly as a result of treatment with a diuretic), patients on dialysis or with fluid loss through diarrhea or vomiting. This condition should be corrected prior to administration of RASILEZ, or the treatment should start under close medical supervision.

If symptomatic hypotension occurs, the patient should be placed in the supine position and, if necessary, given an intravenous infusion of normal saline (see Dosage and Administration). A transient hypotensive response is not a contraindication to further treatment, which usually can be continued without difficulty once the blood pressure has stabilized. However, lower doses of RASILEZ and/or reduced concomitant diuretic therapy should be considered when symptoms re-occur.

Renal: Impaired Renal Function: Patients with greater than moderate renal dysfunction (creatinine ≥150 µmol/L for women and ≥176.8 µmol/L for men and/or eGFR <30 mL/min), a history of dialysis, nephrotic syndrome, or renovascular hypertension were excluded from clinical trials of RASILEZ. Caution should be exercised, due to the limited availability of safety information with RASILEZ in these patients, and the potential for other drugs acting on the renin-angiotensin system to increase serum creatinine and blood urea nitrogen.

Serum Electrolyte Changes: Based on experience with other substances that affect the RAAS, increases in serum potassium levels may be observed when aliskiren is taken concomitantly with another RAAS blocker (an angiotensin II AT_1 receptor blocker or an angiotensin converting enzyme inhibitor). Consistent with standard medical practice, periodic determination of serum electrolytes to detect possible electrolyte imbalances is advised, particularly in patients at risk for hyperkalemia such as those with renal impairment.

Renal Artery Stenosis: No data are available on the effects of RASILEZ on renal function in patients with uni-or bilateral renal artery stenosis.

Concomitant Use with Cyclosporine A: The concomitant use of aliskiren with cyclosporine, a highly potent P glycoprotein inhibitor, is not recommended (see Drug Interactions, Drug-Drug Interactions).

Gastrointestinal: In the event of severe and persistent diarrhea, RASILEZ therapy should be stopped (see Adverse Reactions, Clinical Trial Adverse Drug Reactions).

Special Populations: Pregnant Women: Drugs that act directly on the renin-angiotensin system can cause fetal and neonatal morbidity and death when administered to pregnant women. When pregnancy is detected, RASILEZ should be discontinued as soon as possible.

The use of drugs that act directly on the renin-angiotensin system during the second and third trimesters of pregnancy has been associated with fetal and neonatal injury, including hypotension, neonatal skull hypoplasia, anuria, reversible or irreversible renal failure, and death. Oligohydramnios has also been reported, presumably resulting from decreased fetal renal function; oligohydramnios in this setting has been associated with fetal limb contractures, craniofacial deformation, and hypoplastic lung development. Prematurity, intrauterine growth retardation, and patent ductus arteriosus have also been reported, although it is not clear whether these occurrences were due to exposure to the drug. These adverse effects do not appear to have resulted from intrauterine drug exposure that has been limited to the first trimester. Mothers whose embryos and fetuses are exposed to a renin inhibitor during the first trimester should be so informed. Nonetheless, when patients become pregnant, physicians should have the patient discontinue the use of RASILEZ as soon as possible.

Rarely (probably less often than once in every thousand pregnancies), no alternative to a drug acting on the renin-angiotensin system will be found. In these rare cases, the mothers should be apprised of the potential hazards to their fetuses, and serial ultrasound examinations should be performed to assess the intra-amniotic environment.

If oligohydramnios is observed, RASILEZ should be discontinued unless it is considered lifesaving for the mother. Contraction stress testing (CST), a nonstress test (NST), or biophysical profiling (BPP) may be appropriate, depending upon the week of pregnancy. Patients and physicians should be aware, however, that oligohydramnios may not appear until after the fetus has sustained irreversible injury.

There is no clinical experience with the use of RASILEZ in pregnant women. Infants with histories of in-utero exposure to a renin inhibitor should be closely observed for hypotension, oliguria, and hyperkalemia. If oliguria occurs, attention should be directed toward support of blood pressure and renal perfusion. Exchange transfusion or dialysis may be required as means of reversing hypotension and/or substituting for disordered renal function. Aliskiren is not removed by hemodialysis.

Reproductive toxicity studies did not reveal any evidence of embryofetal toxicity or teratogenicity at oral doses up to 600 mg/kg/day in rats or 100 mg/kg/day in rabbits. Aliskiren was present in the placenta, amniotic fluid and fetuses of pregnant rabbits. In rats, there were no adverse effects on fertility or early embryonic development or reproductive performance of the F1 generation.

Nursing Women: It is not known whether RASILEZ is excreted in human milk. RASILEZ was excreted in the milk of lactating rats. Because of the potential for adverse effects on the nursing infant, a decision should be made whether to discontinue nursing or discontinue the drug, taking into account the importance of the drug to the mother.

Pediatrics (<18 years of age): The safety and effectiveness of RASILEZ in children and adolescents have not been established.

Geriatrics (>65 years of age): Of the total number of patients receiving RASILEZ in clinical studies, 1275 (19 %) were 65 years or older and 231 (3.4%) were 75 years or older. No clinically significant differences were observed in safety and efficacy of RASILEZ in older patients compared to those under age 65.

ADVERSE REACTIONS: Adverse Drug Reaction Overview: RASILEZ has been evaluated for safety in more than 7440 patients, including at least 2580 treated for over 6 months, and at least 1730 for over 1 year. The incidence of adverse events showed no association with gender, age, body mass index, race, or ethnicity. Treatment with RASILEZ was well tolerated with an overall incidence of adverse events similar to placebo up to 300 mg. Adverse events have generally been mild and transient in nature and have only infrequently required discontinuation of therapy. In placebo-controlled clinical trials, discontinuation of therapy due to a clinical adverse event occurred in 2.2% of patients treated with RASILEZ versus 3.5% of patients given placebo. In long-term active controlled clinical trials discontinuation of therapy due to an adverse event occurred in 5.4% of RASILEZ treated patients versus 4.7% of ramipril treated patients and 7.3% of hydrochlorothiazide treated patients.

Clinical Trial Adverse Drug Reactions: Because clinical trials are conducted under very specific conditions the adverse reaction rates observed in the clinical trials may not reflect the rates observed in practice and should not be compared to the rates in the clinical trials of another drug. Adverse drug reaction information from clinical trials is useful for identifying drug-related adverse events and for approximating rates.

The following adverse events occurred in the short-term, placebo controlled clinical trials in patients treated with RASILEZ at a rate of ≥1% over that of placebo-treated patients (see Table 1).

Note that 600 mg is double the highest recommended dose. At 600 mg o.d., diarrhea has consistently been seen across trials.

The following adverse events of special interest occurred in two long-term double-blind studies (Table 2).

RASILEZ use in clinical trials was associated with a slightly increased incidence of dry cough, but less so than with angiotensin converting enzyme inhibitor use. In controlled, short-term clinical trials the incidence of cough was similar in placebo (0.6%) and RASILEZ (1.1%) patients.

In a short-term active controlled trial, peripheral edema occurred in 3.4% of patients treated with amlodipine 5 mg, 11.2% of patients treated with amlodipine 10 mg, and 2.1% of patients treated with the combination of amlodipine 5 mg and aliskiren 150 mg. In other controlled short-term clinical trials, the incidence of edema was similar in placebo (0.6%) and RASILEZ-treated patients (0.8% to 1.0%) except at a dose of 600 mg (2.0%).

Other adverse events that occurred in short-term, controlled clinical trials of patients treated with RASILEZ (>0.5% RASILEZ patients) are listed below. It cannot be determined whether these events were causally related to RASILEZ.

Digestive: nausea, dyspepsia, abdominal pain.
Musculoskeletal: muscle spasms, arthralgia, pain in extremity, neck pain, shoulder pain.
Neurologic and Psychiatric: vertigo, insomnia.
Respiratory: bronchitis, pharyngolaryngeal pain, epistaxis.
Urinary: urinary tract infection.

Table 1: RASILEZ

Number (%) of Patients with Frequent AEs (at least 1% over placebo in any group) by Preferred Term—Placebo Controlled, Short-Term Studies (pooled safety population)

	Placebo N= 781 n (%)	Ali 75 mg N=478 n (%)	Ali 150 mg N=774 n (%)	Ali 300 mg N=768 n (%)	Ali 600 mg N=296 n (%)	Ali /HCTZ N=1464 n (%)	HCTZ N=555 n (%)
Any Adverse Event	314 (40.2)	193 (40.4)	290 (37.5)	309 (40.2)	130 (43.9)	591 (40.4)	226 (40.7)
Preferred Term							
Nasopharyngitis	45 (5.8)	34 (7.1)	33 (4.3)	29 (3.8)	5 (1.7)	56 (3.8)	21 (3.8)
Diarrhea	9 (1.2)	6 (1.3)	9 (1.2)	18 (2.3)	28 (9.5)	24 (1.6)	11 (2.0)
Edema Peripheral	5 (0.6)	5 (1.0)	6 (0.8)	7 (0.9)	6 (2.0)	13 (0.9)	6 (1.1)
Constipation	5 (0.6)	5 (1.0)	1 (0.1)	5 (0.7)	6 (2.0)	12 (0.8)	3 (0.5)
Influenza	5 (0.6)	1 (0.2)	9 (1.2)	5 (0.7)	2 (0.7)	33 (2.3)	6 (1.1)
Asthenia	1 (0.1)	6 (1.3)	4 (0.5)	4 (0.5)	0 (0.0)	19 (1.3)	6 (1.1)
Rash	0 (0.0)	0 (0.0)	2 (0.3)	3 (0.4)	3 (1.0)	7 (0.5)	1 (0.2)
Rhinitis	1 (0.1)	1 (0.2)	3 (0.4)	2 (0.3)	0 (0.0)	7 (0.5)	5 (1.1)

Legend: Ali=aliskiren; HCTZ=hydrochlorothiazide.

Table 2: RASILEZ

Number (%) of Patients with Adverse Events of Special Interest During the Double-Blind Active Controlled Periods of Two Long-Term Studies

Preferred Term	Aliskiren Regimen[a] N=566 n (%)	HCTZ Regimen[a] N=558 n (%)	Aliskiren Regimen[b] N=419 n (%)	Ramipril Regimen[b] N=422 n (%)
Any Adverse Event	369 (65.2)	343 (61.5)	257 (61.3)	255 (60.4)
Headache	38 (6.7)	53 (9.5)	47 (11.2)	35 (8.3)
Nasopharyngitis	25 (4.4)	30 (5.4)	25 (6.0)	26 (6.2)
Bronchitis	16 (2.8)	16 (2.9)	13 (3.1)	4 (0.9)
Cough	16 (2.8)	22 (3.9)	17 (4.1)	40 (9.5)
Back Pain	27 (4.8)	25 (4.5)	15 (3.6)	13 (3.1)
Diarrhea	16 (2.8)	16 (2.9)	16 (3.8)	7 (1.7)
Edema Peripheral	30 (5.3)	31 (5.6)	16 (3.8)	13 (3.1)

[a] In this 12-month study, the treatment regimen was aliskiren or HCTZ with forced titration and optional add-on of amlodipine.
[b] In this 6-month study, the treatment regimen was aliskiren or ramipril with optional titration and optional add-on of HCTZ.

Diarrhea was reported by 2.3% of patients at 300 mg, compared to 1.2% in placebo patients. In women and the elderly (age ≥65) increases in diarrhea rates were evident starting at a dose of 150 mg daily, with rates for these subgroups at 150 mg comparable to those seen at 300 mg for men or younger patients (all rates about 2.0%-2.3%). Other GI symptoms included abdominal pain, dyspepsia, and gastroesophageal reflux, although increased rates for abdominal pain and dyspepsia were distinguished from placebo only at 600 mg daily. Diarrhea and other GI symptoms were typically mild and rarely led to discontinuation.

Rare cases of colonic cancer (0.05%) were reported in the clinical trials with RASILEZ. The incidence is consistent with the expected prevalence rates of 0.1-0.3% in this patient population.

Angioedema: Angioedema, including edema of the larynx, has occurred during treatment with RASILEZ. In controlled clinical trials, angioedema occurred rarely during treatment with RASILEZ with rates comparable to treatment with placebo or hydrochlorothiazide. Patients should discontinue the treatment and should report immediately to the physician any signs suggesting allergic reactions, in particular, difficulties in breathing or swallowing, swelling of face, extremities, eyes, lips, tongue.

Abnormal Hematologic and Clinical Chemistry Findings: In short-term, controlled clinical trials, clinically relevant changes in standard laboratory parameters were rarely associated with the administration of RASILEZ. In multiple dose studies in hypertensive patients RASILEZ had no clinically important effects on total cholesterol, HDL, fasting triglycerides, fasting glucose, or uric acid.

In a 1-year open label safety study of the aliskiren/valsartan combination, elevations of serum triglycerides above 3.4 mmol/L were observed in 7% of patients who had triglyceride values of 3.4 mmol/L or below prior to treatment. It could not be determined whether this would have been different from placebo, as the study had no control arm.

No special monitoring is necessary in patients receiving RASILEZ.

Blood Urea Nitrogen, Creatinine: Minor increases in blood urea nitrogen (BUN) were observed in less than 7% of patients with essential hypertension treated with RASILEZ alone vs. 6% on placebo. RASILEZ alone increased creatinine slightly (by ~1 μmol/L), but this effect increased (to 2.4 μmol/L) with co-administration of HCTZ.

In an active controlled, double-blind 1-year clinical trial, 13.4% of RASILEZ-treated patients compared to 15.8% of hydrochlorothiazide-treated patients experienced >50% increases in blood urea nitrogen (BUN). In another active controlled, double-blind trial, >50% increases in BUN occurred in 15.5% of RASILEZ-treated patients and 16.0% of ramipril-treated patients. Increases in serum creatinine (>50%) were less frequent, occurring in 2.7% of RASILEZ-treated patients in the one-year study compared to 1.1% of patients treated with hydrochlorothiazide, and 1.7% of RASILEZ-treated patients and 1.4% of ramipril-treated patients in the other trial.

Hemoglobin and Hematocrit: Small decreases in hemoglobin and hematocrit (mean decreases of approximately 0.8 g/L and 0.16 volume percent, respectively) were observed with RASILEZ monotherapy. These decreases led to slight increases in the rate of anemia with aliskiren: 0.1% for any aliskiren use, 0.3% for aliskiren 600 mg o.d., vs. 0% for placebo). No patients discontinued therapy due to anemia. This effect is also seen with other agents acting on the renin-angiotensin system, such as angiotensin converting enzyme inhibitors and angiotensin receptor blockers, and may be mediated by reduction of angiotensin II which stimulates erythropoietin production via the AT_1 receptor.

Serum Potassium: In short-term placebo controlled clinical trials, increases in serum potassium were minor and infrequent in patients with essential hypertension treated with RASILEZ alone (0.9% patients had serum potassium levels >5.5 mmol/L compared to 0.6% with placebo). In combination with the angiotensin receptor blocker valsartan, transient increases in potassium (>5.5 mmol/L) not reported as adverse events occurred in 3.4% of patients compared to 2.1% for placebo. Significant potassium elevations (>6.0 mmol/L) occurred in 0.3% and 1.0% of patients in the aliskiren/valsartan and placebo groups, respectively.

However, when used in combination with an angiotensin converting enzyme inhibitor in a diabetic population, increases in serum potassium were more frequent (5.5%). Routine monitoring of electrolytes and renal function is indicated in this population.

In an active controlled, double-blind, 1-year clinical trial in patients with essential hypertension, increases in serum potassium (>5.5 mmol/L) occurred in 36/550 (6.5%) of patients on RASILEZ compared to 20/535 (3.7%) on hydrochlorothiazide and decreases in serum potassium (<3.5 mmol/L) occurred in 5/550 (0.9%) patients on RASILEZ compared to 96/535 (17.9%) on hydrochlorothiazide. In a 1-year trial of aliskiren and valsartan alone and in combination with HCTZ, elevated serum potassium (>5.5 mmol/L) occurred in 4.1% and 2.0% of patients respectively. In another active controlled, double-blind trial, increases in serum potassium (>5.5 mmol/L) occurred in 8/412 (1.9%) of RASILEZ-treated patients compared to 4/417 (1.0%) on ramipril and decreases in potassium (<3.5 mmol/L) occurred in 22/412 (5.3%) on RASILEZ compared to 19/417 (4.6%) on ramipril.

Creatine Kinase: In the short-term, placebo-controlled clinical trials, increases in creatine kinase of >300% were found in 22 of the 2233 (~1%) patients on aliskiren monotherapy vs. in 4/746 (0.5%) of patients on placebo. The effect, suggesting to be dose-related, seemed more common in men, and at ages <65 years. No cases were associated with renal dysfunction.

In an active controlled, double-blind, 1-year clinical trial, 21 of 543 patients (3.9%) on an aliskiren regimen and 9/535 patients (1.7%) on an HCTZ regimen had >300% increases in creatine kinase. This increase was seen more often in men than in women. In another long term study almost no elevations in CKs were seen in patients (0.5%) on an aliskiren regimen vs. in 1.3% of the patients on a ramipril regimen.

Post-Market Adverse Drug Reactions: Cases of peripheral edema have been reported at a frequency of 0.31 per 1000 patient treatment years.

DRUG INTERACTIONS: Overview: Aliskiren has low potential for drug interactions. Aliskiren is mainly excreted as unchanged drug within the feces and is minimally metabolized in man. Only 1.4% of the total dose is metabolized by the enzyme CYP3A4 of the cytochrome P450 system. RASILEZ is poorly absorbed (bioavailability ~2.6% of an oral dose). Metabolism accounted for up to 20% of the absorbed dose in the systemic circulation. A quarter of the absorbed fraction in the systemic circulation is excreted unchanged in the urine. In vitro studies have shown that aliskiren does not inhibit the CYP450 isoenzymes (CYP1A2, 2C8, 2C9, 2C19, 2D6, 2E1, and CYP3A) or induce CYP3A4. As CYP3A4 is the major enzyme responsible for metabolism of aliskiren, complete inhibition may be expected to result in increased plasma levels of aliskiren (see Action and Clinical Pharmacology, Pharmacokinetics).

Drug-Drug Interactions: Effects of Other Drugs on Aliskiren: Co-administration of aliskiren with amlodipine, digoxin, furosemide, hydrochlorothiazide, metformin, ramipril and valsartan did not result in clinically significant changes in aliskiren exposure.

Co-administration with irbesartan reduced aliskiren C_{max} up to 50% after multiple dosing with little effect on AUC (up to a 20% decrease).

Effects of Aliskiren on Other Drugs: Co-administration of aliskiren did not affect the steady-state pharmacokinetics of amlodipine, digoxin, hydrochlorothiazide, metformin, ramipril, ramiprilat or valsartan.

Co-administration of aliskiren with furosemide resulted in reductions of furosemide C_{max} and AUC of 49% and 28%, respectively. It is therefore recommended that the effects be monitored when initiating and adjusting furosemide therapy to avoid possible under-dosing.

Potential Mechanisms of Drug-Drug Interaction: Based on in vitro studies, aliskiren is metabolised by the CYP3A4 enzyme system. However, pharmacokinetic studies in human volunteers seem to indicate that metabolism does not play a clinically significant role in the elimination of aliskiren.

P glycoprotein Interactions: In vitro studies indicate that MDR1 (Pgp) is the major efflux transporter involved in absorption and disposition of aliskiren in preclinical studies. The potential for drug interactions at the Pgp site will likely depend on the degree of inhibition of this transporter.

Pgp Substrates or Weak-Moderate Inhibitors: No relevant interactions with atenolol, digoxin, amlodipine, and cimetidine have been observed. When administered with atorvastatin (80 mg), steady-state aliskiren (300 mg) AUC and C_{max} increased by 50%.

Moderate Pgp Inhibitors: Co-administration of ketoconazole (200 mg b.i.d.) with aliskiren (300 mg) resulted in a 80% increase in plasma levels of aliskiren (AUC and C_{max}). Preclinical studies indicate that aliskiren and ketoconazole co-administration enhances aliskiren gastrointestinal absorption and decreases biliary excretion. In healthy volunteers, co-administration of a single oral dose of 300 mg aliskiren with 240 mg verapamil increased AUC and C_{max} of aliskiren by ~2-fold. The change in plasma levels of aliskiren in the presence of ketoconazole or verapamil is expected to be within the range that would be achieved if the dose of aliskiren were doubled; aliskiren doses of up to 600 mg, or twice the highest recommended therapeutic dose, have been found to be well tolerated in controlled clinical trials. As a result no dose adjustment for aliskiren is necessary.

Potent Pgp Inhibitors: A single dose drug interaction study in healthy subjects has shown that cyclosporine (200 and 600 mg) increases C_{max} of aliskiren 75 mg by approximately 2.5 fold and the AUC by approximately 5 fold. Therefore, the concomitant use of both drugs is not recommended (see Warnings and Precautions, Renal, Concomitant Use with Cyclosporine A).

Potassium and Potassium-Sparing Diuretics: Based on experience with the use of other drugs that affect the renin-angiotensin system, concomitant use of aliskiren with the following medicines may lead to increases in serum potassium: Potassium-sparing diuretics, potassium supplements, or salt substitutes containing potassium. If comedication is considered necessary, caution is advisable.

Drug-Food Interactions: When taken with food, mean AUC and C_{max} of aliskiren were decreased by 71% and 85%, respectively (see Dosage and Administration). There was a delay in median t_{max} by 1 h.

Drug-Herb Interactions: The interaction of aliskiren with herbal medications or supplements has not been studied.

Drug-Lifestyle Interactions: There are no physical restrictions for patients who receive aliskiren.

DOSAGE AND ADMINISTRATION: Recommended Dose and Dosage Adjustment: The usual recommended starting dose of RASILEZ is 150 mg once daily. In patients whose blood pressure is not adequately controlled, the daily dose may be increased to 300 mg. RASILEZ may be used over a dosage range of 150 mg to 300 mg administered once daily.

The antihypertensive effect is substantially present (85%-90%) within 2 weeks after initiating therapy with 150 mg per day with the maximum effect reached after 4 weeks.

RASILEZ may be administered alone or concomitantly with thiazide diuretics or angiotensin converting enzyme inhibitors. Co-administration of 150 mg aliskiren and 5 mg amlodipine has been shown to be safe and effective; higher doses and other calcium channel blockers have not been tested.

RASILEZ may be administered with or without food, although a high fat meal decreases drug absorption significantly. Patients should establish a convenient daily schedule of drug-intake and maintain a steady temporal relationship with food intake.

No initial dosage adjustment is required for elderly patients, for patients with mild-to-severe renal impairment, or for patients with mild to severe hepatic impairment. Care should be exercised when dosing RASILEZ in patients with severe renal impairment as clinical experience is limited.

Missed Dose: If one or several doses of RASILEZ are missed, patients should be advised to take the dose as soon as they remember. If it is almost time for the next dose, patients should skip the missed dose and go back to their regular schedule. Patients should not increase the dose of RASILEZ to compensate for the missed dose(s).

OVERDOSAGE:

Limited data are available related to overdosage in humans. The most likely manifestation of overdosage would be hypotension. If symptomatic hypotension should occur, supportive treatment should be initiated.

For management of a suspected drug overdose, contact your regional Poison Control Centre. See the *CPS Directory* section for a list of Poison Control Centres.

ACTION AND CLINICAL PHARMACOLOGY: Mechanism of Action: Aliskiren has a novel mechanism of action which differs in pharmacologic action from the angiotensin converting enzyme inhibitors, angiotensin receptor blockers, aldosterone blockers, beta blockers, alpha blockers, diuretics and calcium channel blockers.

Aliskiren is an orally active, nonpeptide, highly specific and potent direct renin inhibitor. Aliskiren targets the renin angiotensin system (RAS) at its point of activation by binding to the renin enzyme, thereby blocking the conversion of angiotensinogen to angiotensin I (Ang I). Renin is secreted by the kidney in response to decreases in blood volume and renal perfusion. This response initiates a cycle that includes the renin angiotensin system (RAS) and a homeostatic feedback loop. Renin cleaves angiotensinogen to form the inactive decapeptide angiotensin I (Ang I). Ang I is converted to the active octapeptide angiotensin II (Ang II) by angiotensin converting enzyme (ACE) and non-ACE pathways. Ang II is a powerful vasoconstrictor and leads to the release of catecholamines from the adrenal medulla and prejunctional nerve endings. It also promotes aldosterone secretion and sodium reabsorption. Together, these effects increase blood pressure. Chronic increases in Ang II result in the expression of markers and mediators of inflammation and fibrosis that are associated with end organ damage.

Aliskiren is a direct renin inhibitor that inhibits the production of Ang I, Ang II by acting at the point of activation of the renin cycle, inhibiting the conversion of angiotensinogen to Ang I and Ang II. This action suppresses the entire system, resulting in a reduction in plasma renin activity (PRA), Ang I, Ang II and aldosterone.

All agents that inhibit the RAS system suppress the negative feedback loop and lead to a compensatory rise in plasma renin concentration. When this rise occurs, it is accompanied by increased levels of PRA. However, treatment with aliskiren neutralizes the feedback loop effects. As a result, despite an elevation of the plasma renin concentration, PRA, Ang I and Ang II are all reduced, whether aliskiren is used as monotherapy or in combination with other antihypertensive agents.

Pharmacodynamics: Treatment with aliskiren decreases plasma renin activity (PRA) and increases plasma renin concentration (PRC) in hypertensive patients. In clinical trials, PRA reductions ranged from approximately 50%-80%. PRA reductions occurred with aliskiren monotherapy or when aliskiren was combined with other antihypertensive drugs. There was no rebound increase in PRA or blood pressure either acutely or over a 4-week period after aliskiren discontinuation. There was a weak correlation between the magnitudes of PRC elevation and blood pressure reduction.

Antihypertensive Effect: In hypertensive patients, once-daily administration of RASILEZ at doses of 150 mg and 300 mg provided dose-dependent reductions in both systolic and diastolic blood pressure that were maintained over the entire 24-hour dose interval (maintaining benefit in the early morning) with a mean trough to peak ratio for diastolic response of up to 98% for the 300 mg dose.

Type 2 Diabetes Mellitus: There are presently no clinical outcome studies indicating beneficial effects of aliskiren in diabetic patients with nephropathy. Clinical data have shown that aliskiren reduces the urinary albumin to creatinine ratio (UACR) in these patients, but whether a reduction in this surrogate marker for nephropathy leads to improved cardio-renal outcomes has not been validated.

Cardiac Electrophysiology: The potential of aliskiren to affect cardiac conduction and repolarisation was studied in a randomized, double-blind, placebo and active-controlled (moxifloxacin), repeat dosing, parallel group study, conducted for 7 days in 283 subjects. Twelve lead Holter ECGs were monitored over the entire dosing interval. No effect of aliskiren on the QT interval was seen.

Pharmacokinetics: Absorption: Following oral administration, peak plasma concentrations of aliskiren are reached within 1-3 hours. The approximate bioavailability of aliskiren is 2.6%. Peak plasma concentrations (C_{max}) and exposure (AUC) are expected to increase 2.6-fold and 2.4-fold when doubling the dose of aliskiren. When taken with food with a high fat content, mean AUC and C_{max} of aliskiren are decreased by 71% and 85%, respectively, and t_{max} is delayed by 1 h. Steady state plasma concentrations are reached within 5 to 7 days after starting once daily administration, and steady state levels are approximately 2-fold greater than following a single dose.

Distribution: Aliskiren is evenly distributed systemically after oral administration. Following intravenous administration, mean volume of distribution at steady state is approximately 135 L indicating that aliskiren distributes extensively into extravascular space. Aliskiren plasma protein binding is moderate (47%-51%) and concentration independent.

Metabolism: Aliskiren is mainly eliminated as unchanged drug within feces (91% of an oral dose), mainly as unchanged drug (86% of an oral dose as adjusted for extraction efficiency). How much of the absorbed dose is metabolized is unknown. The enzyme responsible for this metabolism is CYP3A4.

Excretion: Approximately 0.6% of the dose is recovered in urine following oral administration. Following intravenous administration, the mean plasma clearance is approximately 9 L/h. The mean elimination half-life is about 40 hours (range 34-41 hours).

Special Populations and Conditions: Pediatrics: The pharmacokinetics of aliskiren have not been investigated in patients <18 years of age.

Geriatrics: The pharmacokinetics of aliskiren were studied in the elderly (≥65 years). The exposure (measured by AUC) and C_{max} of aliskiren is increased in elderly by 57% and 28%, respectively. Adjustment of the starting dose is not required in these patients (see Dosage and Administration).

Gender: Males have slightly lower AUC (24%) than females. This difference is not clinically significant.

Race: The pharmacokinetics of aliskiren do not differ significantly among different races and ethnicities (Blacks, Caucasians, Hispanics, and Japanese).

Diabetes: The pharmacokinetics of aliskiren were similar between type 2 diabetics and healthy volunteers.

Hepatic Insufficiency: The pharmacokinetics of aliskiren were not significantly affected in patients with mild-to-severe liver disease. Consequently, adjustment of the starting dose is not required in these patients (see Dosage and Administration).

Renal Insufficiency: The pharmacokinetics of aliskiren were evaluated in patients with varying degrees of renal insufficiency. Relative AUC and C_{max} of aliskiren in subjects with renal impairment ranged between 0.8- to 2-fold those observed in healthy subjects following single dose administration and at steady state. These observed changes, however, did not correlate with the severity of renal impairment. Consequently, adjustment of the starting dose is not required in patients with mild-to-severe renal impairment (see Dosage and Administration).

STORAGE AND STABILITY: Do not store above 30°C. Protect from moisture.

INFORMATION FOR THE PATIENT: Published in e-CPS, available by subscription at www.e-cps.ca.

DOSAGE FORMS, COMPOSITION AND PACKAGING: 150 mg: Each light-pink, biconvex, round, film-coated tablet, imprinted NVR on one side and IL on the other side, contains: aliskiren 150 mg (as aliskiren fumarate). Nonmedicinal ingredients: colloidal silicon dioxide, crospovidone, hypromellose, iron oxide colorants, magnesium stearate, microcrystalline cellulose, polyethylene glycol, povidone, talc and titanium dioxide. Blister packages (4 strips of 7 tablets).

300 mg: Each light-red, biconvex, ovaloid, film-coated tablet, imprinted NVR on one side and IU on the other side, contains: aliskiren 300 mg (as aliskiren fumarate). Nonmedicinal ingredients: colloidal silicon dioxide, crospovidone, hypromellose, iron oxide colorants, magnesium stearate, microcrystalline cellulose, polyethylene glycol, povidone, talc and titanium dioxide. Blister packages (4 strips of 7 tablets).

(Shown in Product Identification Section)

Rasilez HCT® Ⓟ

aliskiren fumarate—hydrochlorothiazide

Renin Inhibitor—Diuretic

Novartis Pharmaceuticals

Date of Preparation: September 2, 2009
Date of Revision: August 10, 2010

SUMMARY PRODUCT INFORMATION:

Route of Administration	Dosage Form/Strength	Nonmedicinal Ingredients
Oral	Tablet 150 mg/12.5 mg, 150 mg/25 mg, 300 mg/12.5 mg and 300 mg/25 mg	Cellulose, microcrystalline, crospovidone, hypromellose, iron oxide black (E 172), iron oxide red (E 172), iron oxide yellow (E 172) lactose monohydrate, macrogol, magnesium stearate, povidone, silica colloidal anhydrous, talc, titanium dioxide (E 171) and wheat starch

INDICATIONS AND CLINICAL USE: RASILEZ HCT is indicated for the treatment of mild to moderate essential hypertension in patients for whom combination therapy is appropriate.

RASILEZ HCT is indicated as replacement therapy in patients already receiving aliskiren and hydrochlorothiazide from separate tablets at the same dose levels. RASILEZ HCT is not indicated for initial therapy.

Geriatrics (>65 years of age): Of the total number of patients receiving RASILEZ HCT in short-term controlled clinical studies, 529 (18.3 %) were 65 years or older and 71 (2.5%) were 75 years or older. No additional safety findings were observed with RASILEZ HCT in older patients compared to those under age 65. However, as with other antihypertensive agents, a greater sensitivity in some older patients cannot be ruled out. Appropriate caution in dosing these patients is recommended.

Pediatrics (<18 years of age): Safety and efficacy in children and adolescents have not been established. RASILEZ HCT should not be given to this patient population.

CONTRAINDICATIONS:

- Patients who are hypersensitive to aliskiren or hydrochlorothiazide (see Dosage Forms, Composition and Packaging).
- Because of the hydrochlorothiazide component, it is also contraindicated in patients with anuria, and in patients who are hypersensitive to other sulfonamide-derived drugs.
- RASILEZ HCT is also contraindicated in pregnant women.

WARNINGS AND PRECAUTIONS:

> **Serious Warnings and Precautions**
> Drugs that act directly on the renin-angiotensin system can cause fetal and neonatal morbidity and death when administered to pregnant women. When pregnancy is detected, RASILEZ HCT should be discontinued as soon as possible (see Warnings and Precautions, Special Populations, Pregnant Women).

Information to Be Provided to the Patient: Pregnancy: Female patients of childbearing age should be told about the consequences of second- and third-trimester exposure to drugs that act on the renin-angiotensin system, and they should also be told that these consequences do not appear to have resulted from intrauterine drug exposure that has been limited to the first trimester. These patients should be asked to report pregnancies to their physicians as soon as possible.

Cardiovascular: Hypotension: In placebo-controlled clinical trials, dizziness and vertigo occurred in 1.5% of the patients on placebo or aliskiren monotherapy, in 2.5 to 4.0% of the patients on hydrochlorothiazide monotherapy, and in 1.1 to 6.7% of the patients on aliskiren/hydrochlorothiazide therapy.

Hypotension is more likely to occur in patients with an activated renin-angiotensin system, such as volume- or salt-depleted patients (possibly as a result of treatment with a diuretic), patients on dialysis or with fluid loss through diarrhea or vomiting. This condition should be corrected prior to administration of RASILEZ HCT, or the treatment should start under close medical supervision.

If symptomatic hypotension occurs, the patient should be placed in the supine position and, if necessary, given an intravenous infusion of normal saline (see Dosage and Administration). A transient hypotensive response is not a contraindication to further treatment, which usually can be continued without difficulty once the blood pressure has stabilized. However, lower doses of RASILEZ HCT should be considered when symptoms re-occur.

Renal: Impaired Renal Function: Aliskiren: Patients with greater than moderate renal dysfunction (creatinine ≥150 µmol/L for women and ≥176.8 µmol/L for men and/or eGFR <30 mL/min), a history of dialysis, nephrotic syndrome, or renovascular hypertension were excluded from clinical trials of RASILEZ. Caution should be exercised, due to the limited availability of safety information with RASILEZ in these patients, and the potential for other drugs acting on the renin-angiotensin system to increase serum creatinine and blood urea nitrogen.

In patients with mild to moderate renal impairment (30 mL/min≤GFR<60 mL/min) RASILEZ HCT should be administered with caution. Periodic monitoring of blood urea nitrogen, creatinine and uric acid is recommended.

Hydrochlorothiazide: Thiazide should be used with caution. Because of the hydrochlorothiazide component, RASILEZ HCT is not recommended in patients with severe renal impairment (creatinine clearance ≤30 mL/min).

Renal Artery Stenosis: No data are available on the use of RASILEZ HCT in patients with unilateral or bilateral renal artery stenosis or stenosis of the artery to a solitary kidney.

Gastrointestinal: Aliskiren: In the event of severe and persistent diarrhea, RASILEZ therapy should be stopped (see Adverse Reactions, Clinical Trial Adverse Drug Reactions).

Immune: Hypersensitivity Reaction: Sensitivity reactions to hydrochlorothiazide may occur in patients with or without a history of allergy or bronchial asthma.

Systemic Lupus Erythematosus: Thiazide diuretics have been reported to cause exacerbation or activation of systemic lupus erythematosus.

Serum Electrolyte Changes: Based on experience with the use of other substances that affect the renin-angiotensin system (RAS), concomitant use with potassium supplements, potassium sparing diuretics, salt substitutes containing potassium, or other drugs that may increase potassium levels should be used with caution. Hypokalaemia has been reported under treatment with thiazide diuretics including hydrochlorothiazide. The renin-aldosterone link is mediated by angiotensin II, so with co-administration of aliskiren the reduction in serum potassium is less pronounced than observed under monotherapy with hydrochlorothiazide (see Adverse Reactions).

Treatment with thiazide diuretics, including hydrochlorothiazide, has been associated with hyponatremia and hypochloremic alkalosis. Patients receiving thiazides should be carefully observed for clinical signs of fluid and electrolyte imbalance (hyponatremia, hypochloremic alkalosis and hypokalemia). Periodic determinations of serum electrolytes to detect possible electrolyte disturbance should be performed at appropriate intervals, particularly when the patient is vomiting excessively or receiving parenteral fluids. Warning signs or symptoms of fluid and electrolyte imbalance include dryness of the mouth, thirst, weakness, lethargy, drowsiness, restlessness, muscle pains or cramps, muscular fatigue, hypotension, oliguria, tachycardia, and gastrointestinal disturbances such as nausea and vomiting.

Hyperuricemia may occur or acute gout may be precipitated in certain patients receiving thiazide therapy.

Thiazides may decrease serum protein-bound iodine (PBI) levels without signs of thyroid disturbance. Thiazides have been shown to increase excretion of magnesium; this may result in hypomagnesia.

Thiazides may decrease urinary calcium excretion. Thiazides may cause intermittent and slight elevation of serum calcium in the absence of known disorders of calcium metabolism. Marked hypercalcemia may be evidence of hidden hyperparathyroidism. Thiazides should be discontinued before carrying out tests for parathyroid function.

Increases in cholesterol, triglyceride and glucose levels may be associated with thiazide diuretic therapy, including hydrochlorothiazide.

Cyclosporine: The concomitant use of aliskiren with cyclosporine, a highly potent P glycoprotein inhibitor, is not recommended (see Drug Interactions, Drug-Drug Interactions).

Special Populations: Pregnant Women: Drugs that act directly on the renin-angiotensin system can cause fetal and neonatal morbidity and death when administered to pregnant women. When pregnancy is detected, RASILEZ HCT should be discontinued as soon as possible.

The use of drugs that act directly on the renin-angiotensin system during the second and third trimesters of pregnancy has been associated with fetal and neonatal injury, including hypotension, neonatal skull hypoplasia, anuria, reversible or irreversible renal failure, and death. Oligohydramnios has also been reported, presumably resulting from decreased fetal renal function; oligohydramnios in this setting has been associated with fetal limb contractures, craniofacial deformation, and hypoplastic lung development. Prematurity, intrauterine growth retardation, and patent ductus arteriosus have also been reported, although it is not clear whether these occurrences were due to exposure to the drug. These adverse effects do not appear to have resulted from intrauterine drug exposure that has been limited to the first trimester. Mothers whose embryos and fetuses are exposed to a renin inhibitor during the first trimester should be so informed. Nonetheless, when patients become pregnant, physicians should have the patient discontinue the use of RASILEZ HCT as soon as possible.

Rarely (probably less often than once in every thousand pregnancies), no alternative to a drug acting on the renin-angiotensin system will be found. In these rare cases, the mothers should be apprised of the potential hazards to their fetuses, and serial ultrasound examinations should be performed to assess the intra-amniotic environment.

If oligohydramnios is observed, RASILEZ HCT should be discontinued unless it is considered life-saving for the mother. Contraction stress testing (CST), a nonstress test (NST), or biophysical profiling (BPP) may be appropriate, depending upon the week of pregnancy. Patients and physicians should be aware, however, that oligohydramnios may not appear until after the fetus has sustained irreversible injury.

Thiazides cross the placental barrier and appear in cord blood. The routine use of diuretics, including hydrochlorothiazide, in otherwise healthy pregnant women is not recommended and exposes mother and fetus to unnecessary hazard including fetal or neonatal jaundice, thrombocytopenia and possibly other adverse experiences which have occurred in the adult. Diuretics do not prevent development of toxemia of pregnancy and there is no satisfactory evidence that they are useful in the treatment of toxemia.

There is no clinical experience with the use of RASILEZ HCT in pregnant women. Infants with histories of in-utero exposure to a renin inhibitor should be closely observed for hypotension, oliguria, and hyperkalemia. If oliguria occurs, attention should be directed toward support of blood pressure and renal perfusion. Exchange transfusion or dialysis may be required as means of reversing hypotension and/or substituting for disordered renal function. Aliskiren is not removed by hemodialysis.

Reproductive toxicity studies did not reveal any evidence of embryofetal toxicity or teratogenicity at oral doses up to 600 mg/kg/day in rats or 100 mg/kg/day in rabbits. Aliskiren was present in the placenta, amniotic fluid and fetuses of pregnant rabbits. In rats, there were no adverse effects on fertility or early embryonic development or reproductive performance of the F1 generation.

Nursing Women: RASILEZ HCT is not recommended during lactation. Hydrochlorothiazide is excreted into breast milk. It is not known whether aliskiren is excreted in human milk. Aliskiren was secreted in the milk of lactating rats. Because of the potential for adverse effects on the nursing infant, a decision should be made whether to discontinue nursing or discontinue the drug, taking into account the importance of the drug to the mother.

Pediatrics (<18 years of age): The safety and effectiveness of RASILEZ HCT in children and adolescents have not been established.

Geriatrics (>65 years of age): Of the total number of patients receiving RASILEZ HCT in short-term controlled clinical studies, 529 (18.3 %) were 65 years or older and 71 (2.5%) were 75 years or older. No differences were observed in the safety of RASILEZ HCT in older patients compared to those under age 65. However, as with other antihypertensive agents, a greater sensitivity of elderly patients cannot be ruled out.

ADVERSE REACTIONS: Adverse Drug Reaction Overview: The safety of RASILEZ HCT has been evaluated in 9 clinical trials with more than 3900 patients, including over 700 treated for over 6 months, and 190 for over 1 year. The incidence of adverse events showed no association with gender, age, body mass index, race or ethnicity. Treatment with RASILEZ HCT had an overall incidence of adverse experiences at doses up to 300 mg/25 mg similar to placebo. Adverse events have generally been mild and transient in nature and have only infrequently required discontinuation of therapy (in short term controlled studies 2.9% of patients on RASILEZ HCT discontinued therapy due to an adverse event versus 4.1% for placebo). The most frequent adverse drug reaction with aliskiren/hydrochlorothiazide is diarrhea.

Clinical Trial Adverse Drug Reactions: Because clinical trials are conducted under very specific conditions the adverse reaction rates observed in the clinical trials may not reflect the rates observed in practice and should not be compared to the rates in the clinical trials of another drug. Adverse drug reaction information from clinical trials is useful for identifying drug-related adverse events and for approximating rates.

The following adverse events occurred in the short-term, placebo-controlled clinical trials in patients treated with RASILEZ HCT at a rate of ≥1% over that of placebo-treated patients (see Table 1).

Table 1: RASILEZ HCT

Number (%) of Patients with Frequent AEs (at least 1% over placebo in any group) by Preferred Term—Placebo-Controlled, Short-Term Studies (pooled safety population)

Preferred Term	Placebo (N=193) n (%)	Ali/HCTZ 150/12.5 mg (N=184) n (%)	Ali/HCTZ 150/25 mg (N=188) n (%)	Ali/HCTZ 300/12.5 mg (N=181) n (%)	Ali/HCTZ 300/25 mg (N=173) n (%)
Influenza	3 (1.6)	1 (0.5)	6 (3.2)	2 (1.1)	7 (4.0)
Vertigo	1 (0.5)	1 (0.5)	3 (1.6)	3 (1.7)	5 (2.9)
Diarrhoea	1 (0.5)	1 (0.5)	6 (3.2)	6 (3.3)	3 (1.7)

(cont'd)

Table 1: RASILEZ HCT *(cont'd)*

Number (%) of Patients with Frequent AEs (at least 1% over placebo in any group) by Preferred Term—Placebo-Controlled, Short-Term Studies (pooled safety population)

Preferred Term	Placebo (N=193) n (%)	Ali/HCTZ 150/12.5 mg (N=184) n (%)	Ali/HCTZ 150/25 mg (N=188) n (%)	Ali/HCTZ 300/12.5 mg (N=181) n (%)	Ali/HCTZ 300/25 mg (N=173) n (%)
Dizziness	2 (1.0)	6 (3.3)	3 (1.6)	9 (5.0)	3 (1.7)
Edema peripheral	1 (0.5)	2 (1.1)	1 (0.5)	3 (1.7)	3 (1.7)
Abdominal pain upper	1 (0.5)	3 (1.6)	4 (2.1)	1 (0.6)	2 (1.2)
Asthenia	0 (0.0)	1 (0.5)	3 (1.6)	2 (1.1)	2 (1.2)
Cerumen impaction	0 (0.0)	0 (0.0)	0 (0.0)	0 (0.0)	2 (1.2)
Dry mouth	0 (0.0)	1 (0.5)	0 (0.0)	2 (1.1)	2 (1.2)
Rash	0 (0.0)	2 (1.1)	0 (0.0)	1 (0.6)	2 (1.2)
Somnolence	0 (0.0)	0 (0.0)	0 (0.0)	1 (0.6)	2 (1.2)
Tendonitis	0 (0.0)	0 (0.0)	0 (0.0)	0 (0.0)	2 (1.2)
Cough	1 (0.5)	2 (1.1)	4 (2.1)	2 (1.1)	1 (0.6)
Influenza like illness	0 (0.0)	0 (0.0)	2 (1.1)	2 (1.1)	1 (0.6)
Myalgia	0 (0.0)	2 (1.1)	0 (0.0)	0 (0.0)	1 (0.6)
Non-cardiac chest pain	0 (0.0)	2 (1.1)	2 (1.1)	2 (1.1)	1 (0.6)
Palpitations	3 (1.6)	2 (1.1)	5 (2.7)	2 (1.1)	1 (0.6)
Pyrexia	0 (0.0)	1 (0.5)	0 (0.0)	2 (1.1)	1 (0.6)
Rhinitis	0 (0.0)	0 (0.0)	2 (1.1)	2 (1.1)	1 (0.6)
Sinusitis	1 (0.5)	1 (0.5)	0 (0.0)	3 (1.7)	1 (0.6)
Dyspnoea	0 (0.0)	1 (0.5)	2 (1.1)	0 (0.0)	0 (0.0)
Eczema	0 (0.0)	2 (1.1)	0 (0.0)	0 (0.0)	0 (0.0)
Flushing	0 (0.0)	2 (1.1)	0 (0.0)	0 (0.0)	0 (0.0)
Hypokalaemia	0 (0.0)	0 (0.0)	1 (0.5)	2 (1.1)	0 (0.0)
Migraine	0 (0.0)	1 (0.5)	2 (1.1)	1 (0.6)	0 (0.0)
Pain in extremity	0 (0.0)	0 (0.0)	3 (1.6)	2 (1.1)	0 (0.0)
Pharyngolaryngeal pain	0 (0.0)	1 (0.5)	2 (1.1)	3 (1.7)	0 (0.0)
Urinary tract infection	3 (1.6)	3 (1.6)	0 (0.0)	5 (2.8)	0 (0.0)

The following adverse events of special interest occurred in two long-term open-label studies (Table 2).

Table 2: RASILEZ HCT

Number (%) of Patients with AEs of Interest (≥2% for any group) by Preferred Term in Long-Term Open-Label Studies (safety population)

Preferred Term	Mono Ali N=1955 n (%)	Ali/HCTZ 300/12.5 mg N=843 n (%)	Ali/HCTZ 300/25 mg N=454 n (%)	All Ali/HCTZ N=871 n (%)
Dizziness	75 (3.8)	21 (2.5)	11 (2.4)	31 (3.6)
Back pain	68 (3.5)	22 (2.6)	5 (1.1)	28 (3.2)
Headache	153 (7.8)	12 (1.4)	10 (2.2)	22 (2.5)
Arthralgia	36 (1.8)	8 (0.9)	11 (2.4)	19 (2.2)
Cough	30 (1.5)	15 (1.8)	4 (0.9)	19 (2.2)
Diarrhea	69 (3.5)	12 (1.4)	6 (1.3)	18 (2.1)
Fatigue	41 (2.1)	10 (1.2)	2 (0.4)	12 (1.4)
Nausea	42 (2.1)	0 (0.0)	5 (1.1)	5 (0.6)

Additional Information on the Combination: Diarrhea: Diarrhea is a dose-related adverse drug reaction for aliskiren. In controlled clinical trials, the incidence of diarrhea in RASILEZ HCT treated patients was low and not more than that in aliskiren or hydrochlorothiazide treated patients.

Serum Potassium: In a placebo controlled, 8-week study of various doses of aliskiren/HCTZ, hyperkalemia (K^+ >5.5 mmol/L) occurred in 0.6% of the patients on placebo, and in 0% to 1.4% of the patients receiving aliskiren/HCTZ at doses varying between 75/6.25 and 300/25 mg. Hypokalemia (K^+ <3.5 mmol/L) occurred in 1.3% of patients on placebo and between 0.7% and 3.4% in patients on aliskiren/HCTZ. No patients discontinued based on extreme potassium values.

Periodic determinations of serum potassium to detect possible electrolyte imbalance should be performed at appropriate intervals.

Additional Information on Individual Components: RASILEZ use was associated with a slightly increased incidence of dry cough, but less so than with angiotensin converting enzyme inhibitor use. In controlled, short-term clinical trials the incidence of cough was similar in placebo (0.6%) and RASILEZ (1.1%) patients.

In a short-term active controlled trial, peripheral edema occurred in 3.4% of patients treated with amlodipine 5 mg, 11.2% of patients treated with amlodipine 10 mg, and 2.1% of patients treated with the combination of amlodipine 5 mg and aliskiren 150 mg. In other controlled short-term clinical trials, the incidence of edema was similar in placebo (0.6%) and RASILEZ treated patients (0.8% to 1.0%) except at a dose of 600 mg (2.0%).

Other adverse events that occurred in short-term, controlled clinical trials of patients treated with RASILEZ (>0.5% RASILEZ patients) are listed below. It cannot be determined whether these events were causally related to RASILEZ.

Digestive: nausea, dyspepsia, abdominal pain.

Musculoskeletal: muscle spasms, arthralgia, pain in extremity, neck pain, shoulder pain.

Neurologic and Psychiatric: vertigo, insomnia.

Respiratory: bronchitis, pharyngolaryngeal pain, epistaxis.

Urinary: urinary tract infection.

Diarrhea was reported by 2.3% of patients at 300 mg, compared to 1.2% in placebo patients. In women and the elderly (age ≥65) increases in diarrhea rates were evident starting at a dose of 150 mg daily, with rates for these subgroups at 150 mg comparable to those seen at 300 mg for men or younger patients (all rates about 2.0%-2.3%). Other GI symptoms included abdominal pain, dyspepsia, and gastroesophageal reflux, although increased rates for abdominal pain and dyspepsia were distinguished from placebo only at 600 mg daily. Diarrhea and other GI symptoms were typically mild and rarely led to discontinuation.

Rare cases of colonic cancer (0.05%) were reported in the clinical trials with RASILEZ. The incidence is consistent with the expected prevalence rates of 0.1-0.3% in this patient population.

Angioedema: Angioedema, including edema of the larynx, has occurred during treatment with RASILEZ. In controlled clinical trials, angioedema occurred rarely during treatment with RASILEZ with rates comparable to treatment with placebo or hydrochlorothiazide. Patients should discontinue the treatment and should report immediately to the physician any signs suggesting allergic reactions, in particular, difficulties in breathing or swallowing, swelling of face, extremities, eyes, lips, tongue.

Abnormal Hematologic and Clinical Chemistry Findings: In short-term, controlled clinical trials, clinically relevant changes in standard laboratory parameters were rarely associated with the administration of RASILEZ. In multiple dose studies in hypertensive patients RASILEZ had no clinically important effects on total cholesterol, HDL, fasting triglycerides, fasting glucose, or uric acid.

Blood Urea Nitrogen, Creatinine: Minor increases in blood urea nitrogen (BUN) were observed in less than 7% of patients with essential hypertension treated with RASILEZ alone vs 6% on placebo. RASILEZ alone increased creatinine slightly (by ~1 µmol/L), but this effect increased (to 2.4 µmol/L) with co-administration of HCTZ.

In an active controlled, double-blind 1-year clinical trial, 13.4% of RASILEZ-treated patients compared to 15.8% of hydrochlorothiazide-treated patients experienced >50% increases in blood urea nitrogen (BUN). In another active controlled, double-blind trial, >50% increases in BUN occurred in 15.5% of RASILEZ-treated patients and 16.0% of ramipril-treated patients. Increases in serum creatinine (>50%) were less frequent, occurring in 2.7% of RASILEZ-treated patients in the one-year study compared to 1.1% of patients treated with hydrochlorothiazide, and 1.7% of RASILEZ-treated patients and 1.4% of ramipril-treated patients in the other trial.

Hemoglobin and Hematocrit: Small decreases in hemoglobin and hematocrit (mean decreases of approximately 0.8 g/L and 0.16 volume percent, respectively) were observed with RASILEZ monotherapy. These decreases led to slight increases in the rate of anemia with aliskiren: 0.1% for any aliskiren use, 0.3% for aliskiren 600 mg o.d., vs 0% for placebo). No patients discontinued therapy due to anemia. This effect is also seen with other agents acting on the renin-angiotensin system, such as angiotensin converting enzyme inhibitors and angiotensin receptor blockers, and may be mediated by reduction of angiotensin II which stimulates erythropoietin production via the AT_1 receptor.

Serum Potassium: In short-term placebo controlled clinical trials, increases in serum potassium were minor and infrequent in patients with essential hypertension treated with RASILEZ alone (0.9% patients had serum potassium levels >5.5 mmol/L compared to 0.6% with placebo). However, when used in combination with an angiotensin converting enzyme inhibitor in a diabetic population, increases in serum potassium were more frequent (5.5%). Routine monitoring of electrolytes and renal function is indicated in this population.

In an active controlled, double-blind, 1-year clinical trial in patients with essential hypertension, increases in serum potassium (>5.5 mmol/L) occurred in 36/550 (6.5%) of patients on RASILEZ compared to 20/535 (3.7%) on hydrochlorothiazide and decreases in serum potassium (<3.5 mmol/L) occurred in 5/550 (0.9%) patients on RASILEZ compared to 96/535 (17.9%) on hydrochlorothiazide. In another active controlled, double-blind trial, increases in serum potassium (>5.5 mmol/L) occurred in 8/412 (1.9%) of RASILEZ-treated patients compared to 4/417 (1.0%) on ramipril and decreases in potassium (<3.5 mmol/L) occurred in 22/412 (5.3%) on RASILEZ compared to 19/417 (4.6%) on ramipril.

Creatine Kinase: In the short-term, placebo-controlled clinical trials, increases in creatine kinase of >300% were found in 22 of the 2233 (~1%) patients on aliskiren monotherapy vs in 4/746 (0.5%) of patients on placebo. The effect, suggesting to be dose-related, seemed more common in men, and at ages <65 years. No cases were associated with renal dysfunction.

In an active controlled, double-blind, 1-year clinical trial, 21 of 543 patients (3.9%) on an aliskiren regimen and 9/535 patients (1.7%) on an HCTZ regimen had >300% increases in creatine kinase. This increase was seen more often in men than in women. In another long term study almost no elevations in CKs were seen in patients (0.5%) on an aliskiren regimen vs in 1.3% of the patients on a ramipril regimen.

Hydrochlorothiazide: Hydrochlorothiazide has been extensively prescribed for many years, frequently in higher doses than those contained in RASILEZ HCT. The following adverse experiences have been reported in patients treated with thiazide diuretics alone, including hydrochlorothiazide, irrespective of their causal association with the study drug:

Electrolytes and Metabolic Disorders (see Warnings and Precautions).

Common: urticaria and other forms of rash, decreased appetite, mild nausea and vomiting, orthostatic hypotension, which may be aggravated by alcohol, anaesthetics or sedatives, and erectile dysfunction.

Rare: photosensitivity reaction, abdominal discomfort, constipation, diarrhoea, cholestasis or jaundice, arrhythmia, headache, dizziness, sleep disorder, depression, paresthesia, visual disturbance, thrombocytopenia, sometimes with purpura.

Very Rare: vasculitis necrotising and toxic epidermal necrolysis, cutaneous lupus erythematous-like reactions, reactivation of cutaneous lupus erythematous, pancreatitis, leukopenia, agranulocytosis, bone marrow depression, haemolytic anaemia, hypersensitivity reactions, respiratory distress including pneumonitis and pulmonary edema.

Post-Market Adverse Drug Reactions: Cases of peripheral edema have been reported with aliskiren at a frequency of 0.31 per 1000 patient treatment years.

DRUG INTERACTIONS: Overview: Aliskiren has low potential for drug interactions. Aliskiren is mainly excreted as unchanged drug within the feces and is minimally metabolized in man. Only 1.4% of the total dose is metabolized by the enzyme CYP3A4 of the cytochrome P450 system. RASILEZ is poorly absorbed (bioavailability ~2.6% of an oral dose). Metabolism accounted for up to 20% of the absorbed dose in the systemic circulation. A quarter of the absorbed fraction in the systemic circulation is excreted unchanged in the urine. In vitro studies have shown that Aliskiren does not inhibit the CYP450 isoenzymes (CYP1A2, 2C8, 2C9, 2C19, 2D6, 2E1, and CYP3A) or induce CYP3A4. As CYP3A4 is the major enzyme responsible for metabolism of aliksiren, complete inhibition may be expected to result in increased plasma levels of aliskiren (see Action and Clinical Pharmacology, Pharmacokinetics). No relevant pharmacokinetic interactions have been reported between hydrochlorothiazide and other drugs and, particularly, no drug interactions of hydrochlorothiazide via CYP450 enzymes have been observed. Since hydrochlorothiazide is excreted largely unchanged into urine, no significant effect on hydrochlorothiazide pharmacokinetics is expected by inhibitors of metabolism or biliary excretion.

Drug-Drug Interactions: RASILEZ HCT: Co-administration of aliskiren and hydrochlorothiazide does not cause meaningful changes in the steady-state pharmacokinetic exposure (AUC) and the maximum concentration (C_{max}) of both components in healthy volunteers.

Aliskiren: Effects of Other Drugs on Aliskiren: P Glycoprotein (Pgp) Interactions: In vitro studies indicate that MDR1 (Pgp) is the major efflux transporter involved in absorption and disposition of aliskiren. The potential for drug interactions at the Pgp site will likely depend on the degree of inhibition of this transporter.

Pgp Substrates or Weak Inhibitors: No relevant interactions with atenolol, digoxin amlodipine, and cimetidine have been observed. When administered with atorvastatin (80 mg), steady-state aliskiren (300 mg) AUC and C_{max} increased by 50%.

Moderate Pgp Inhibitors: Co-administration of ketoconazole (200 mg) with aliskiren (300 mg) resulted in a 80% increase in plasma levels of aliskiren (AUC and C_{max}). Preclinical studies indicate that aliskiren and ketoconazole co-administration enhances aliskiren gastrointestinal absorption and decreases biliary excretion. In healthy volunteers, co-administration of a single oral dose of 300 mg aliskiren with 240 mg verapamil increased AUC and C_{max} of aliskiren by ~2-fold. The change in plasma levels of aliskiren in the presence of ketoconazole or verapamil is expected to be within the range that would be achieved if the dose of aliskiren were doubled; aliskiren doses of up to 600 mg, or twice the highest recommended therapeutic dose, have been found to be well tolerated in controlled clinical trials. As a result no dose adjustment for aliskiren is necessary.

Potent Pgp Inhibitors: A single dose drug interaction study in healthy subjects has shown that cyclosporine A (200 and 600 mg) increases C_{max} of aliskiren 75 mg by approximately 2.5 fold and the AUC by approximately 5-fold. Therefore, the concomitant use of both drugs is not recommended (see Warnings and Precautions).

Co-administration of aliskiren with amlodipine, digoxin, furosemide, metformin, ramipril and valsartan did not result in clinically significant changes in aliskiren exposure.

Co-administration with irbesartan reduced aliskiren C_{max} up to 50% after multiple dosing with little effect on AUC (up to a 20% decrease).

Potassium and Potassium Sparing Diuretics: Based on experience with the use of other drugs that affect the renin-angiotensin system, concomitant use of aliskiren with the following medicines may lead to increases in serum potassium: Potassium-sparing diuretics, potassium supplements, or salt substitutes containing potassium. If comedication is considered necessary, caution is advisable.

Effects of Aliskiren on Other Drugs: Co-administration of aliskiren did not affect the steady-state pharmacokinetics of amlodipine, digoxin, metformin, ramipril, ramiprilat or valsartan.

Co-administration of aliskiren with furosemide resulted in reductions of furosemide C_{max} and AUC of 49% and 28%, respectively. It is therefore recommended that the effects be monitored when initiating and adjusting furosemide therapy to avoid possible under-dosing.

Hydrochlorothiazide: Lithium: Reversible increases in serum lithium concentrations and toxicity have been reported during concurrent use of ACE inhibitors and thiazides. There is no experience with concomitant use of aliskiren and lithium. Therefore, monitoring of serum lithium concentrations is recommended during concurrent use.

Curare Derivatives: Thiazide drugs, including hydrochlorothiazide, may increase the responsiveness to curare derivatives such as d-tubocurarine.

Non Steroidal Anti-Inflammatory Drugs: In some patients, the administration of a non-steroidal anti-inflammatory agent can reduce the diuretic, natriuretic, and antihypertensive effects of loop, potassium-sparing and thiazide diuretics. Therefore, when RASILEZ HCT and non-steroidal anti-inflammatory agents are used concomitantly, the patient should be observed closely to determine if the desired effect of the diuretic is obtained.

Digitalis Glycosides: Thiazide-induced hypokalemia or hypomagnesemia may occur as unwanted effects, favouring the onset of digitalis-induced cardiac arrhythmias.

Insulin: Insulin requirements in diabetic patients treated with diuretics may be increased, decreased or unchanged. Diabetes mellitus which has been latent may become manifest during thiazide administration.

Alcohol, Barbiturates, or Narcotics: Diuretic potentiation of orthostatic hypotension may occur.

Corticosteroids, ACTH: Intensified electrolyte depletion, particularly hypokalemia, may occur when steroids are given concomitantly with diuretics.

Pressor Amines (e.g. norepinephrine): In the presence of diuretics possible decreased response to pressor amines may be seen but not sufficient to preclude use.

Anticholinergic Agents: The bioavailability of thiazide-type diuretics may be increased by anticholinergic agents (e.g. atropine, biperiden), apparently due to a decrease in gastrointestinal motility and the stomach emptying rate.

Methyldopa: There have been reports in the literature of haemolytic anaemia occurring with concomitant use of hydrochlorothiazide and methyldopa.

Cholestyramine: Absorption of thiazide diuretics, including hydrochlorothiazide, is decreased by cholestyramine.

Vitamin D and Calcium Salts: Administration of thiazide diuretics, including hydrochlorothiazide, with vitamin D or with calcium salts may potentiate the rise in serum calcium.

Cyclosporine: Concomitant treatment with cyclosporine may increase the risk of hyperuricemia and gout-type complications.

Carbamazepine: Patients receiving hydrochlorothiazide concomitantly with carbamazepine may develop hyponatremia. Such patients should therefore be advised about the possibility of hyponatremic reactions, and should be monitored accordingly.

Other Interactions: Co-administration of thiazide diuretics, including hydrochlorothiazide, may increase the incidence of hypersensitivity reactions to allopurinol, may increase the risk of adverse effects caused by amantadine, may enhance the hyperglycemic effect of diazoxide, and may reduce the renal excretion of cytotoxic drugs (e.g. cyclophosphamide, methotrexate) and potentiate their myelosuppressive effects.

Drug-Food Interactions: Following oral administration of RASILEZ HCT with food , mean AUC and C_{max} of aliskiren are decreased by 60% and 82%, respectively; mean AUC and C_{max} of hydrochlorothiazide increased by 13% and 10%, respectively.

Drug-Herb Interactions: The interaction of aliskiren-hydrochlorothiazide with herbal medications or supplements has not been studied.

Drug-Lifestyle Interactions: There are no physical restrictions for patients who receive aliskiren-hydrochlorothiazide.

DOSAGE AND ADMINISTRATION: Dosage must be individualized. RASILEZ HCT is not for initial therapy. The appropriate dose of RASILEZ HCT should be determined by titration of the individual components aliskiren and hydrochlorothiazide.

The recommended dose is one tablet per day. RASILEZ HCT may be used over a dosage range of 150 mg/12.5 mg to 300 mg/25 mg administered once daily.

The antihypertensive effect is substantially present within 1 week and the maximum effect is generally seen within 4 weeks.

RASILEZ HTC may be administered with or without food, although a high fat meal decreases the absorption of aliskiren significantly. Patients should establish a convenient daily schedule of drug-intake and maintain a steady temporal relationship with food intake.

Patients not Adequately Treated on Monotherapy: A patient whose blood pressure is not adequately controlled on either aliskiren or hydrochlorothiazide monotherapy may be switched to the combination therapy with RASILEZ HCT using the lowest dose of the added component. When clinically appropriate direct change from monotherapy to RASILEZ HCT fixed combination may be considered.

Patients Receiving Aliskiren Monotherapy: The recommended starting dose of RASILEZ is 150 mg once daily. The antihypertensive effect is present within 2 weeks and maximal reduction is usually attained within 4 weeks after initiation of therapy. In patients whose blood pressure is not adequately controlled, the daily dose may be increased to 300 mg, or a low-dose thiazide diuretic may be added.

Patients Receiving Diuretics: In patients receiving diuretics, aliskiren therapy should be initiated with caution, since these patients may be volume-depleted and thus more likely to experience hypotension after adding another anti-hypertensive agent. Whenever possible, diuretics should be discontinued 2-3 days prior to the initiation of RASILEZ HCT to reduce the likelihood of hypotension. If this is not possible because of the patient's condition, RASILEZ HCT should be initiated with caution and the blood pressure monitored closely.

Patients Adequately Treated with Separate Tablets of Aliskiren and Hydrochlorothiazide: For convenience and optimal compliance, patients already receiving aliskiren and hydrochlorothiazide from separate tablets may be switched to a single tablet of RASILEZ HCT containing the same component doses.

Renal Impairment: No adjustment of the initial dose is required for patients with mild to moderate renal impairment. Due to the hydrochlorothiazide component, RASILEZ HCT is contraindicated in patients with severe renal impairment (creatinine clearance <30 mL/min).

Hepatic Impairment: No adjustment of the initial dose is required for patients with mild to moderate hepatic impairment. Due to the hydrochlorothiazide component, RASILEZ HCT is contraindicated in patients with severe hepatic impairment.

Elderly Patients (over 65 years): No adjustment of the initial dose is required for elderly patients.

Paediatric Patients (below 18 years): RASILEZ HCT is not recommended for use in children and adolescents below age 18 due to insufficient data on safety and efficacy.

Missed Dose: If one or several doses of RASILEZ HCT are missed, patients should be advised to take the dose as soon as they remember. If it is almost time for the next dose, patients should skip the missed dose and go back to their regular schedule. Patients should not increase the dose of RASILEZ HCT to compensate for the missed dose(s).

OVERDOSAGE:

No data is available related to overdose in humans. The most likely manifestation of overdosage would be hypotension. If symptomatic hypotension should occur, supportive treatment should be initiated.

> For management of a suspected drug overdose, contact your regional Poison Control Centre. See the *CPS* Directory section for a list of Poison Control Centres.

ACTION AND CLINICAL PHARMACOLOGY: Mechanism of Action: Aliskiren: Aliskiren has a novel mechanism of action which differs in pharmacologic action from the angiotensin converting enzyme inhibitors, angiotensin receptor blockers, aldosterone blockers, beta blockers, alpha blockers, diuretics and calcium channel blockers.

Aliskiren is an orally active, nonpeptide, highly specific and potent direct renin inhibitor. Aliskiren targets the renin angiotensin system (RAS) at its point of activation by binding to the renin enzyme, thereby blocking the conversion of angiotensinogen to angiotensin I (Ang I). Renin is secreted by the kidney in response to decreases in blood volume and renal perfusion. This response initiates a cycle that includes the renin angiotensin system (RAS) and a homeostatic feedback loop. Renin cleaves angiotensinogen to form the inactive decapeptide angiotensin I (Ang I). Ang I is converted to the active octapeptide angiotensin II (Ang II) by angiotensin converting enzyme (ACE) and non-ACE pathways. Ang II is a powerful vasoconstrictor and leads to the release of catecholamines from the adrenal medulla and prejunctional nerve endings. It also promotes aldosterone secretion and sodium reabsorption. Together, these effects increase blood pressure. Chronic increases in Ang II result in the expression of markers and mediators of inflammation and fibrosis that are associated with end organ damage.

Aliskiren is a direct renin inhibitor that inhibits the production of Ang I, Ang II by acting at the point of activation of the renin cycle, inhibiting the conversion of angiotensinogen to Ang I and Ang II. This action suppresses the entire system, resulting in a reduction in plasma renin activity (PRA), Ang I, Ang II and aldosterone.

All agents that inhibit the RAS system suppress the negative feedback loop and lead to a compensatory rise in plasma renin concentration. When this rise occurs, it is accompanied by increased levels of PRA. However, treatment with aliskiren neutralizes the feedback loop effects. As a result, despite an elevation of the plasma renin concentration, PRA, Ang I and Ang II are all reduced, whether aliskiren is used as monotherapy or in combination with other antihypertensive agents.

Hydrochlorothiazide: Hydrochlorothiazide is a thiazide diuretic. Thiazides affect the renal tubular mechanism of electrolyte reabsorption, directly increasing excretion of sodium and chloride in approximately equivalent amounts. Indirectly, the diuretic action of hydrochlorothiazide reduces plasma volume with consequent increases in plasma renin activity, increases in aldosterone secretion, increases in urinary potassium loss, and decreases in serum potassium. The renin-aldosterone link is mediated by angiotensin II, therefore co-administration of the renin-inhibitor, aliskiren, tends to reverse the potassium loss associated with thiazide diuretics.

Hydrochlorothiazide is useful in the treatment of hypertension. It may be used alone or as an adjunct to other antihypertensive drugs. Hydrochlorothiazide does not affect normal blood pressure.

Pharmacodynamics: RASILEZ HCT: In placebo-controlled clinical trials, plasma renin activity (PRA) was decreased with aliskiren monotherapy (ranging from 54% to 65%) and increased with hydrochlorothiazide monotherapy (ranging from 4% to 72%). Treatment with RASILEZ HCT resulted in PRA reductions ranging from approximately 46% to 63% in various doses, despite the increase in PRA with hydrochlorothiazide treatment.

In a placebo-controlled, 8-week study, plasma renin concentration (PRC) was found increased on average 1.3-fold in patients on placebo. Average 1.1- to 2.1-fold increases were found in 3 dose groups of patients on hydrochlorothiazide, 2.6- to 4.5-fold in 3 dose groups on aliskiren, and 3.0- to 13.1-fold in 8 dose groups on aliskiren/HCTZ. Individual changes in PRC in a group of 38 patients on aliskiren/HCTZ 300/25 mg in this 8-week study varied between 0.7-fold and 86.3-fold. 34.2% of these patients had a >20-fold increase in their PRC levels.

While rises in PRC have been observed with angiotensin converting enzyme inhibitors and angiotensin receptor blockers without recognised detrimental effects, the potential consequence of long-term exposure to high levels of plasma renin is presently unknown, but under investigation. There is no evidence that the increase in PRC leads to loss of efficacy over time. In a one year open label study, RASILEZ HCT use was associated with sustained blood pressure reduction.

Aliskiren: Treatment with aliskiren decreases plasma renin activity (PRA) and increases plasma renin concentration (PRC) in hypertensive patients. In clinical trials, PRA reductions ranged from approximately 50%-80%. PRA reductions occurred with aliskiren monotherapy or when aliskiren was combined with other antihypertensive drugs. There was no rebound increase in PRA or blood pressure either acutely or over a 4-week period after aliskiren discontinuation. There was a weak correlation between the magnitudes of PRC elevation and blood pressure reduction.

Antihypertensive Effect: RASILEZ HCT: RASILEZ HCT combines two antihypertensive compounds to control blood pressure in patients with essential hypertension: The combination of these substances with complementary mechanisms of action provides an additive antihypertensive effect, reducing blood pressure to a greater degree than either component alone. In hypertensive patients, once-daily administration of RASILEZ HCT provided dose-dependent reductions in both systolic and diastolic blood pressure that were maintained over the entire 24-hour dose interval. The antihypertensive effect is largely manifested within 1 week and the maximum effect is generally seen within 4 weeks. The blood-pressure-lowering effect was sustained during long-term treatment, and was largely independent of age, gender, body mass index and ethnicity. The antihypertensive effect of a single dose of the combination persisted for 24 hours.

Aliskiren: In hypertensive patients, once-daily administration of RASILEZ at doses of 150 mg and 300 mg provided dose-dependent reductions in both systolic and diastolic blood pressure that were maintained over the entire 24-hour dose interval (maintaining benefit in the early morning) with a mean trough to peak ratio for diastolic response of up to 98% for the 300 mg dose.

Cardiac Electrophysiology: The potential of aliskiren to affect cardiac conduction and repolarisation was studied in a randomized, double-blind, placebo and active-controlled (moxifloxacin), repeat dosing, parallel group study, conducted for 7 days in 283 subjects. Twelve lead Holter ECGs were monitored over the entire dosing interval. No effect of aliskiren on the QT interval was seen.

Hydrochlorothiazide: Onset of the diuretic action following oral administration occurs in 2 hours and the peak action in about 4 hours. Diuretic activity lasts about 6-12 hours.

Pharmacokinetics: RASILEZ HCT: Following oral administration of RASILEZ HCT combination tablets, the median peak plasma concentration time are within 1 hour for aliskiren and 2.5 hours for hydrochlorothiazide. The rate and extent of absorption of RASILEZ HCT are equivalent to the bioavailability of aliskiren and hydrochlorothiazide when administered as individual monotherapies. Similar food effect was observed for RASILEZ HCT as for the individual monotherapies.

Aliskiren: Absorption: Following oral administration, peak plasma concentrations of aliskiren are reached within 1-3 hours. The approximate bioavailability of aliskiren is 2.6%. Peak plasma concentrations (C_{max}) and exposure (AUC) are expected to increase 2.6-fold and 2.4-fold when doubling the dose of aliskiren. When taken with food with a high fat content, mean AUC and C_{max} of aliskiren are decreased by 71% and 85%, respectively, and t_{max} is delayed by 1 h. Steady state plasma concentrations are reached within 5 to 7 days after starting once daily administration, and steady state levels are approximately 2-fold greater than following a single dose.

Distribution: Aliskiren is evenly distributed systemically after oral administration. Following intravenous administration, mean volume of distribution at steady state is approximately 135 L indicating that aliskiren distributes extensively into extravascular space. Aliskiren plasma protein binding is moderate (47%-51%) and concentration independent.

Metabolism: Aliskiren is predominantly eliminated as unchanged drug within feces (91% of an oral dose), mainly as unchanged drug (86% of an oral dose as adjusted for extraction efficiency). How much of the absorbed dose is metabolized is unknown. The enzyme responsible for this metabolism is CYP3A4 (see Drug Interactions, Drug-Drug Interactions, P glycoprotein inhibitors).

Excretion: Approximately 0.6% of the dose is recovered in urine following oral administration. Following intravenous administration, the mean plasma clearance is approximately 9 L/h. The mean elimination half-life is about 40 hours (range 34-41 hours).

Hydrochlorothiazide: The absorption of hydrochlorothiazide following an oral dose is rapid with a t_{max} of approximately 2 hours. The distribution and elimination kinetics have generally been described by a bi-exponential decay function, with a terminal half-life of 6-15 hours.

Absolute bioavailability of hydrochlorothiazide is 60-80% after oral administration, with >95% of the absorbed dose being excreted unchanged in the urine.

Hydrochlorothiazide crosses the placental but not the blood-brain barrier and is excreted in breast milk.

Special Populations and Conditions: Pediatrics: The pharmacokinetics of aliskiren or aliskiren-hydrochlorothiazide have not been investigated in patients <18 years of age.

Geriatrics: No adjustment of the initial dose of RASILEZ HCT is required for elderly patients, although some may be more sensitive to the drug combination (see Dosage and Administration).

Gender: Males have slightly lower AUC (24%) for aliskiren than females. This difference is not clinically significant.

Race: The pharmacokinetics of aliskiren do not differ significantly among different races and ethnicities (Blacks, Caucasians, Hispanics, and Japanese).

Diabetes: The pharmacokinetics of aliskiren were similar between type 2 diabetics and healthy volunteers.

Hepatic Insufficiency: The pharmacokinetics of aliskiren and hydrochlorothiazide are not significantly affected in patients with mild to moderate liver disease. Consequently, adjustment of the starting dose is not required in patients with mild to moderate hepatic impairment (see Dosage and Administration). However, because of hydrochlorothiazide, RASILEZ HCT is contraindicated in patients with severe hepatic impairment.

Renal Insufficiency: No dose adjustment is required for patients with mild to moderate renal impairment (see Dosage and Administration). No data are available for RASILEZ HCT in patients with severe renal impairment (creatinine clearance <30 mL/min). However, as expected for a compound which is cleared almost exclusively via the kidneys, renal function has a marked effect on the kinetics of hydrochlorothiazide. Therefore, RASILEZ HCT is not recommended for use in patients with severe renal impairment (creatinine clearance <30 mL/min).

STORAGE AND STABILITY: Do not store above 30°C. Protect from moisture.

INFORMATION FOR THE PATIENT: Published in e-CPS, available by subscription at www.e-cps.ca.

DOSAGE FORMS, COMPOSITION AND PACKAGING: 150 mg/12.5 mg: Each white, biconvex, ovaloid, film-coated tablet, imprinted with LCI on one side and NVR on the other side, contains: aliskiren 150 mg (as aliskiren fumarate) and hydrochlorothiazide 12.5 mg. Nonmedicinal ingredients: cellulose, crospovidone, hypromellose, lactose monohydrate, macrogol, magnesium stearate, microcrystalline, povidone, silica colloidal anhydrous, talc, titanium dioxide (E 171) and wheat starch. Blister cards of 28.
150 mg/25 mg: Each pale yellow, biconvex, ovaloid, film-coated tablet, imprinted with CLL on one side and NVR on the other side, contains: aliskiren 150 mg (as aliskiren fumarate) and hydrochlorothiazide 25 mg. Nonmedicinal ingredients: cellulose, crospovidone, hypromellose, iron oxide red (E 172), iron oxide yellow (E172), lactose monohydrate, macrogol, magnesium stearate, microcrystalline, povidone, silica colloidal anhydrous, talc, titanium dioxide (E 171) and wheat starch. Blister cards of 28.
300 mg/12.5 mg: Each violet white, biconvex, ovaloid, film-coated tablet, imprinted with CVI on one side and NVR on the other side, contains: aliskiren 300 mg (as aliskiren fumarate) and hydrochlorothiazide 12.5 mg. Nonmedicinal ingredients: cellulose, crospovidone, hypromellose, iron oxide black (E 172), iron oxide red (E 172), lactose monohydrate, macrogol, magnesium stearate, microcrystalline, povidone, silica colloidal anhydrous, talc, titanium dioxide (E 171) and wheat starch. Blister cards of 28.
300 mg/25 mg: Each light yellow, biconvex, ovaloid, film-coated tablet, imprinted with CVV on one side and NVR on the other side, contains: aliskiren 300 mg (as aliskiren fumarate) and hydrochlorothiazide 25 mg. Nonmedicinal ingredients: cellulose, crospovidone, hypromellose, iron oxide red (E 172), iron oxide yellow (E172), lactose monohydrate, macrogol, magnesium stearate, microcrystalline, povidone, silica colloidal anhydrous, talc, titanium dioxide (E 171) and wheat starch. Blister cards of 28.

(Shown in Product Identification Section)

ratio-Aclavulanate Ⓟ
amoxicillin trihydrate—clavulanate potassium
Antibiotic—Beta-lactamase Inhibitor

ratiopharm

SUPPLIED: Tablets: 500 mg/125 mg: Each white to off-white, oval, film-coated tablet contains: amoxicillin 500 mg as the trihydrate and clavulanic acid 125 mg as the potassium salt (in a ratio of 4:1). Nonmedicinal ingredients: colloidal silica, dimethicone 500, hydroxypropyl methylcellulose, magnesium stearate, microcrystalline cellulose, polyethylene glycol, sodium starch glycolate and titanium dioxide. Bottles of 100. Store in a dry place at room temperature (15-25°C).
875 mg/125 mg: Each white to off-white capsule-shaped, film-coated tablet, breakline on one side and monogrammed "AC", contains: amoxicillin 875 mg as the trihydrate and clavulanic acid 125 mg as the potassium salt (in a ratio of 7:1). Nonmedicinal ingredients: colloidal silica, dimethicone 500, hydroxypropyl methylcellulose, magnesium stearate, microcrystalline cellulose, polyethylene glycol, sodium starch glycolate and titanium dioxide. Bottles of 60. Store in a dry place at room temperature (15-25°C).
Oral Suspensions: 125F: Each 5 mL of reconstituted suspension contains: amoxicillin 125 mg as the trihydrate and clavulanic acid 31.25 mg as the potassium salt (in a ratio of 4:1). Nonmedicinal ingredients: aspartame, colloidal silica, golden syrup dry flavor, hydroxypropyl methylcellulose, orange dry flavor 1, orange dry flavor 2, raspberry dry flavor, silicon dioxyde, succinic acid and xanthan gum. Bottles of 100 and 150 mL. The reconstituted oral suspension should be stored under refrigeration and should be used within 10 days. Keep bottle closed at all times.
250F: Each 5 mL of reconstituted suspension contains: amoxicillin 250 mg as the trihydrate and clavulanic acid 62.5 mg as the potassium salt (in a ratio of 4:1). Nonmedicinal ingredients: aspartame, colloidal silica, golden syrup dry flavor, hydroxypropyl methylcellulose, orange dry flavor 1, orange dry flavor 2, raspberry dry flavor, silicon dioxyde, succinic acid and xanthan gum. Bottles of 100 and 150 mL. The reconstituted oral suspension should be stored under refrigeration and should be used within 10 days. Keep bottle closed at all times.

ratio-Acyclovir Ⓟ
acyclovir
Antiviral Agent

ratiopharm

SUPPLIED: 200 mg : Each blue, round, biconvex, scored tablet, imprinted with "ACV" above "200" on one side and plain on the other side contains: acyclovir 200 mg. Nonmedicinal ingredients: cellulose, indigotine, lactose, magnesium stearate, povidone and sodium starch glycolate. Bottles of 100. The tablets may be mottled. Tablets should be stored at controlled room temperature (15 to 25°C) in a dry place and protected from light.
400 mg: Each pink, round, biconvex, scored tablet, imprinted with "ACV" above "400" on one side and plain on the other side contains: acyclovir 400 mg. Nonmedicinal ingredients: cellulose, iron oxide, magnesium stearate, povidone and sodium starch glycolate. Bottles of 100. The tablets may be mottled. Tablets should be stored at controlled room temperature (15 to 25°C) in a dry place and protected from light.
800 mg: Each blue, oval, scored tablet, imprinted with "ACV" above "800" on one side and plain on the other contains: acyclovir 800 mg. Nonmedicinal ingredients: cellulose, indigotine, magnesium stearate, povidone and sodium starch glycolate. Bottles of 100. The tablets may be mottled. Tablets should be stored at controlled room temperature (15 to 25°C) in a dry place and protected from light.

The reader is invited to consult CPhA's monograph **Bisphosphonates: Oral.**

ratio-Alendronate Ⓟ
alendronate sodium
Bone Metabolism Regulator

ratiopharm

SUPPLIED: Each white, oval-shaped, biconvex tablet debossed with "rph" logo on one side and "A101" on the other side, contains: alendronate sodium 91.37 mg equivalent to alendronate USP 70 mg. Nonmedicinal ingredients: magnesium stearate, mannitol, microcrystalline cellulose, sodium starch glycolate and starch. High-density polyethylene (HDPE) bottles of 100. Blisters of 4 (1×4). Store at room temperature (15-30°C).

The reader is invited to consult CPhA's monograph **Corticosteroids: Topical.**

ratio-Amcinonide Ⓟ
amcinonide
Topical Corticosteroid

ratiopharm

SUPPLIED: Cream: Each g contains: amcinonide 1 mg (0.1%). Nonmedicinal ingredients: benzyl alcohol 2.2 % as the preservative, ethoxylated stearyl alcohol, glycerin, isopropyl palmitate, lactic acid, purified water and sorbitol solution. Lanolin-, propylene glycol-, tartrazine- and urea-free. Tubes of 15, 30, 60 g. Store between 15-30°C. Avoid freezing.
Lotion: Each bottle contains: amcinonide 0.1%. Nonmedicinal ingredients: benzyl alcohol as a preservative, emulsifying wax, glycerin, isopropyl palmitate, lactic acid, purified water and sorbitol solution. Lanolin-, propylene glycol-, tartrazine- and urea-free. Plastic squeezes bottles of 20 and 60 mL. Store between 15-30°C. Avoid freezing. Shake well.
Ointment: Each g contains: amcinonide 1 mg (0.1%) in a formulated base. Nonmedicinal ingredients: benzyl alcohol, emulsifying wax, Tenox II and white petrolatum. Tartrazine-free. Tubes of 15, 30, 60 g. Store between 15-30°C. Avoid freezing.

ratio-Amiodarone Ⓟ
amiodarone HCl
Antiarrhythmic

ratiopharm

SUPPLIED: Each round, flat, pink tablet, engraved with "200" in depressed center on one side and engraved with "ALTI" and "200" above and below the score line on the other side contains: amiodarone HCl 200 mg. Nonmedicinal ingredients: colloidal silicon dioxide, cornstarch, FD&C Red #40 Lake, lactose, magnesium stearate and povidone. Bottles of 100. Keep bottle tightly closed. Store at room temperature, 15 to 30°C. Protect from light.

The reader is invited to consult CPhA's monograph **Calcium Channel Blockers.**

ratio-Amlodipine Ⓟ
amlodipine besylate
Antihypertensive—Antianginal

ratiopharm

SUPPLIED: 5 mg: Each white, octagonal tablet, scored and engraved "rph" on one side and "A72" on the other, contains: amlodipine besylate equivalent to amlodipine 5 mg. Nonmedicinal ingredients: calcium phosphate dibasic anhydride, magnesium stearate, microcrystalline cellulose and sodium starch glycolate. HDPE bottles of 100. Store between 15 and 30°C in a tightly closed light-resistant container. Protect from humidity.
10 mg: Each white, octagonal tablet, engraved "rph" on one side and "A71" on the other, contains: amlodipine besylate equivalent to amlodipine 10 mg. Nonmedicinal ingredients: calcium phosphate dibasic anhydride, magnesium stearate, microcrystalline cellulose and sodium starch glycolate. HDPE bottles of 100. Store between 15 and 30°C in a tightly closed light-resistant container. Protect from humidity.

ratio-Atenolol Ⓟ
atenolol
Beta-adrenergic Receptor Blocking Agent

ratiopharm

SUPPLIED: 50 mg: Each white, round, biconvex tablet, engraved with rphA52 on one side and bisected on the other side, contains: atenolol 50 mg. Nonmedicinal ingredients: hydroxypropyl methylcellulose, macrogol/PEG, magnesium stearate, magnesium trisilicate, microcrystalline cellulose, polydextrose, polyethylene glycol, polyvinyl alcohol, sodium croscarmellose, talc, titanium dioxide and triacetin. Compliance packs of 30. Bottles of 100 and 500.
100 mg: Each white, round, biconvex tablet, engraved with rphA51 on one side and bisected on the other side, contains: atenolol 100 mg. Nonmedicinal ingredients: hydroxypropyl methylcellulose, macrogol/PEG, magnesium stearate, magnesium trisilicate, microcrystalline cellulose, polydextrose, polyethylene glycol, polyvinyl alcohol, sodium croscarmellose, talc, titanium dioxide and triacetin. Compliance packs of 30. Bottles of 100 and 500.
Store at room temperature (15 to 30°C). Protect from light and moisture.

The reader is invited to consult CPhA's monograph **HMG-CoA Reductase Inhibitors.**

ratio-Atorvastatin Ⓟ
atorvastatin calcium
Lipid Metabolism Regulator

ratiopharm

SUPPLIED: 10 mg: Each white, film-coated, elliptic tablet, with "10" engraved on one side and "rph" on the other contains: atorvastatin calcium equivalent to atorvastatin 10 mg. Nonmedicinal ingredients: croscarmellose sodium, crospovidone, hydroxypropyl methylcellulose, magnesium stearate, microcrystalline cellulose, lactose monohydrate, polyethylene glycol, polysorbate 80, polyvinyl alcohol, purified water, talc and titanium dioxide. Blister packs of 30. Bottles of 100 and 500. Store at controlled room temperature (15-30°C). Protect from moisture, heat and light. Keep container tightly closed.
20 mg: Each white, film-coated, elliptic tablet, with "20" engraved on one side and "rph" on the other contains: atorvastatin calcium equivalent to atorvastatin 20 mg. Nonmedicinal ingredients: croscarmellose sodium, crospovidone, hydroxypropyl methylcellulose, magnesium stearate, microcrystalline cellulose, lactose monohydrate, polyethylene glycol, polysorbate 80, polyvinyl alcohol, purified water, talc, and titanium dioxide. Blister packs of 30. Bottles of 100 and 500. Store at controlled room temperature (15-30°C). Protect from moisture, heat and light. Keep container tightly closed.
40 mg: Each white, film-coated, elliptic tablet, with "40" engraved on one side and "rph" on the other contains: atorvastatin calcium equivalent to atorvastatin 40 mg. Nonmedicinal ingredients: croscarmellose sodium, crospovidone, hydroxypropyl methylcellulose, magnesium stearate, microcrystalline cellulose, lactose monohydrate, polyethylene glycol, polysorbate 80, polyvinyl alcohol, purified water, talc, and titanium dioxide. Blister packs of 30. Bottles of 100 and 500. Store at controlled room temperature (15-30°C). Protect from moisture, heat and light. Keep container tightly closed.
80 mg: Each white, film-coated, elliptic tablet, with "80" engraved on one side and "rph" on the other contains: atorvastatin calcium equivalent to atorvastatin 80 mg. Nonmedicinal ingredients: croscarmellose sodium, crospovidone, hydroxypropyl methylcellulose, magnesium stearate, microcrystalline cellulose, lactose monohydrate, polyethylene glycol, polysorbate 80, polyvinyl alcohol, purified water, talc, and titanium dioxide. Blister packs of 30. Bottles of 100. Store at controlled room temperature (15-30°C). Protect from moisture, heat and light. Keep container tightly closed.

ratio-Azithromycin Ⓟ
azithromycin monohydrate hemiethanolate
Antibiotic

ratiopharm

SUPPLIED: Each dark pink, modified capsule-shaped, film-coated tablet, engraved with "rph" logo on one side and "A91" on the other, contains: azithromycin $*1H_2O*0.5EtOH$ equivalent to azithromycin 250 mg (as azithromycin monohydrate hemiethanolate). Nonmedicinal ingredients: croscarmellose sodium, D&C red #27, FD&C blue #2, FD&C red #40, FD&C yellow #6, hydroxypropylmethyl cellulose, lactose, magnesium stearate, poloxamer 188, polydextrose, polyethylene glycol, povidone, silicified microcrystalline cellulose, talc, titanium dioxide and triacetin. HPDE bottles of 30 and 100. Blister packs of 6. Store at controlled room temperature (15 to 30°C).

ratio-Baclofen ℞
baclofen
Muscle Relaxant—Antispastic

ratiopharm

SUPPLIED: 10 mg: Each flat, white, oval shaped tablet scored on one side and debossed "TEC 102A" on the other, contains: baclofen USP 10 mg. Nonmedicinal ingredients: colloidal silicon dioxide, dibasic calcium phosphate, lactose, magnesium stearate, microcrystalline cellulose and sodium starch glycolate. Bottles of 100 and 500.
20 mg: Each white, capsule shaped tablet scored on one side and debossed "TEC 102B" on the other, contains: baclofen USP 20 mg. Nonmedicinal ingredients: colloidal silicon dioxide, dibasic calcium phosphate, lactose, magnesium stearate, microcrystalline cellulose and sodium starch glycolate. Bottles of 100.
Store between 15 and 30°C. Protect from heat and humidity.

ratio-Bicalutamide ℞
bicalutamide
Nonsteroidal Antiandrogen

ratiopharm

SUPPLIED: Each white, film coated tablet, imprinted with "rph" on one side and "B31" on the other side, contains: bicalutamide 50 mg. Nonmedicinal ingredients: colloidal silicon dioxide, hydroxypropyl methylcellulose, lactose monohydrate, magnesium stearate, polydextrose, polyethylene glycol, povidone, sodium lauryl sulfate, sodium starch glycolate, titanium dioxide and triethyl citrate. White high density polyethylene bottles of 100 and 500. Blister strips of 15 and 30 per package. Store at room temperature (15-30°C). Protect from light.

ratio-Bisacodyl
bisacodyl
Laxative

ratiopharm

SUPPLIED: Each white to creamy white rectal suppository contains: bisacodyl 10 mg. Nonmedicinal ingredients: semisynthetic glycerides. Boxes of 100. Preserve in well-closed container at a temperature not exceeding 30°C.

ratio-Brimonidine ℞
brimonidine tartrate
Elevated Intraocular Pressure Therapy

ratiopharm

SUPPLIED: Each mL of sterile ophthalmic solution contains: brimonidine tartrate 2 mg (0.2%). Nonmedicinal ingredients: 0.005% benzalkonium chloride as preservative, citric acid, polyvinyl alcohol, purified water, sodium chloride and sodium citrate. Hydrochloric acid and/or sodium hydroxide may be added to adjust pH. White, opaque plastic dropper bottles with Cap Compliance Cap b.i.d. (twice daily) of 5 and 10 mL. Store at 15 to 25°C. Keep the container tightly closed.

ratio-Bupropion SR ℞
bupropion HCl
Antidepressant

ratiopharm

SUPPLIED: 100 mg: Each aquamarine, film-coated, round, biconvex, sustained release tablet, engraved "B42" over the tablet score on one side and "rph" on the other side, contains: bupropion HCl 100 mg. Nonmedicinal ingredients: carnauba wax, FD&C blue #1, hydrochloric acid, hydroxypropyl cellulose, hydroxypropyl methylcellulose, magnesium stearate, microcrystalline cellulose, polyethylene glycol, polysorbate, titanium dioxide and water. Bottles of 30 and 60. Store between 15 and 25°C in a dry place. Keep tightly close. Protect from light.
150 mg: Each plum, film-coated, round, biconvex, sustained release tablet, engraved "B41" over the tablet score on one side and "rph" on the other side, contains: bupropion HCl 150 mg. Nonmedicinal ingredients: carnauba wax, FD&C blue #2, FD&C red #40, hydrochloric acid, hydroxypropyl cellulose, hydroxypropyl methylcellulose, magnesium stearate, microcrystalline cellulose, polyethylene glycol, polysorbate, titanium dioxide and water. Bottles of 30 and 60. Store between 15 and 25°C in a dry place. Keep tightly close. Protect from light.

ratio-Calmydone Ⓝ
hydrocodone bitartrate—etafedrine HCl—doxylamine succinate
Antihistaminic—Antitussive—Decongestant

ratiopharm

SUPPLIED: Each mL of red, limpic, cherry flavor syrup, contains: hydrocodone bitartrate 0.33 mg, etafedrine HCl 3.33 mg and doxylamine succinate 1.2 mg. Nonmedicinal ingredients: alcohol, artificial coloring and flavoring, caramel, FD&C Yellow #6, glycerin, menthol, methylparaben, natural flavoring, propylparaben, purified water, sodium citrate and sucrose. Alcohol: 4.1% w/v. Sucrose: 0.6 g/mL. Bottles of 500 mL and 2 L. Store between 15 and 30°C.

ratio-Carvedilol ℞
carvedilol
Congestive Heart Failure Agent

ratiopharm

SUPPLIED: 3.125 mg: Each white, oval, biconvex, film-coated tablet, embossed with "284W" on one side and "rph" on the other side, contains: carvedilol 3.125 mg. Nonmedicinal ingredients: colloidal silicon dioxide, copolyvidone, crospovidone, lactose monohydrate, magnesium stearate, microcrystalline cellulose, polyethylene glycol, polyvinyl alcohol, talc and titanium dioxide. Bottles of 100. Store between 15-30°C in tightly closed containers or dispensed in a tight, light-resistant container. Protect from high humidity.
6.25 mg: Each white, oval, biconvex, film-coated tablet, embossed with "284X" on one side and "rph" on the other side, contains: carvedilol 6.25 mg. Nonmedicinal ingredients: colloidal silicon dioxide, copolyvidone, crospovidone, lactose monohydrate, magnesium stearate, microcrystalline cellulose, polyethylene glycol, polyvinyl alcohol, talc and titanium dioxide. Bottles of 100. Store between 15-30°C in tightly closed containers or dispensed in a tight, light-resistant container. Protect from high humidity.
12.5 mg: Each white, oval, biconvex, film-coated tablet, embossed with "284Y" on one side and "rph" on the other side, contains: carvedilol 12.5 mg. Nonmedicinal ingredients: colloidal silicon dioxide, copolyvidone, crospovidone, lactose monohydrate, magnesium stearate, microcrystalline cellulose, polyethylene glycol, polyvinyl alcohol, talc and titanium dioxide. Bottles of 100. Store between 15-30°C in tightly closed containers or dispensed in a tight, light-resistant container. Protect from high humidity.
25 mg: Each white, oval, biconvex, film-coated tablet, embossed with "284Z" on one side and "rph" on the other side, contains: carvedilol 25 mg. Nonmedicinal ingredients: colloidal silicon dioxide, copolyvidone, crospovidone, lactose monohydrate, magnesium stearate, microcrystalline cellulose, polyethylene glycol, polyvinyl alcohol, talc and titanium dioxide. Bottles of 100. Store between 15-30°C in tightly closed containers or dispensed in a tight, light-resistant container. Protect from high humidity.

ratio-Cefuroxime ℞
cefuroxime axetil
Antibiotic

ratiopharm

SUPPLIED: 250 mg: Each white to off-white, film-coated, capsule-shaped, biconvex tablet, plain on one side and engraved GXES7 on the other side, contains: 250 mg of cefuroxime (as cefuroxime axetil). Nonmedicinal ingredients: colloidal silicon dioxide, croscarmellose sodium, hydrogenated vegetable oil, hydroxypropyl methylcellulose, methylparaben, microcrystalline cellulose, propylene glycol, propylparaben, sodium benzoate, sodium lauryl sulfate and titanium dioxide. Bottles of 60. Store between 15 and 30°C.
500 mg: Each white to off-white, film-coated, capsule-shaped, biconvex tablet, plain on one side and engraved GXEG2 on the other side, contains: 500 mg of cefuroxime (as cefuroxime axetil). Nonmedicinal ingredients: colloidal silicon dioxide, croscarmellose sodium, hydrogenated vegetable oil, hydroxypropyl methylcellulose, methylparaben, microcrystalline cellulose, propylene glycol, propylparaben, sodium benzoate, sodium lauryl sulfate and titanium dioxide. Bottles of 60. Store between 15 and 30°C.

The reader is invited to consult CPhA's monograph **Fluoroquinolones.**

ratio-Ciprofloxacin ℞
ciprofloxacin HCl
Antibacterial

ratiopharm

SUPPLIED: 250 mg: Each white, round, coated tablet, engraved with "C93" on one side and "rph" on the other side, contains: ciprofloxacin HCl equivalent to ciprofloxacin 250 mg. Nonmedicinal ingredients: hydroxypropyl methylcellulose, magnesium stearate, microcrystalline cellulose, polydextrose, polyethylene glycol, pregelatinized corn starch, silicon dioxide, sodium starch glycolate, titanium dioxide and triacetin. Bottles of 100. Store between 15-30°C.
500 mg: Each white, oblong, coated tablet, engraved with "C92" on one side and "rph" on the other side, contains: ciprofloxacin HCl equivalent to ciprofloxacin 500 mg. Nonmedicinal ingredients: hydroxypropyl methylcellulose, magnesium stearate, microcrystalline cellulose, polydextrose, polyethylene glycol, pregelatinized corn starch, silicon dioxide, sodium starch glycolate, titanium dioxide and triacetin. Unit dose packages of 100. Bottles of 100. Store between 15-30°C and protect from light for blisters. Store between 15-30°C for bottles.
750 mg: Each white, oblong, coated tablet, engraved with "C91" on one side and "rph" on the other side, contains: ciprofloxacin HCl equivalent to ciprofloxacin 750 mg. Nonmedicinal ingredients: hydroxypropyl methylcellulose, magnesium stearate, microcrystalline cellulose, polydextrose, polyethylene glycol, pregelatinized corn starch, silicon dioxide, sodium starch glycolate, titanium dioxide and triacetin. Bottles of 50. Store between 15-30°C.

The reader is invited to consult CPhA's monograph **Selective Serotonin Reuptake Inhibitors.**

ratio-Citalopram ℞
citalopram HBr
Antidepressant

ratiopharm

SUPPLIED: 20 mg: Each white color, oval, biconvex, film-coated tablet, with bisect on one side and rph 285X on the other side, contains: citalopram HBr corresponding to citalopram 20 mg. Nonmedicinal ingredients: colloidal silicon dioxide, croscarmellose sodium, hydroxypropyl methylcellulose, lactose monohydrate, magnesium stearate, microcrystalline cellulose, polydextrose, polyethylene glycol, titanium dioxide and triacetin. Bottles of 100 and 500. Blister packages of 30. Store in a dry place at room temperature between 15 and 30°C.
40 mg: Each white color, oval, biconvex, film-coated tablet, with bisect on one side and rph 285Y on the other side, contains: citalopram HBr corresponding to citalopram 40 mg. Nonmedicinal ingredients: colloidal silicon dioxide, croscarmellose sodium, hydroxypropyl methylcellulose, lactose monohydrate, magnesium stearate, microcrystalline cellulose, polydextrose, polyethylene glycol, titanium dioxide and triacetin. Bottles of 100. Blister packages of 30. Store in a dry place at room temperature between 15 and 30°C.

ratio-Clarithromycin ℞
clarithromycin
Antibiotic

ratiopharm

SUPPLIED: 250 mg: Each oval, biconvex, yellow, film-coated tablet, marked "rph" on one side and "C112" on the other side, contains: clarithromycin 250 mg. Nonmedicinal ingredients: D&C yellow #10 lake, hydroxypropyl methylcellulose, hydroxypropyl methylcellulose/hypromellose, magnesium stearate, maltodextrin, microcrystalline cellulose, polydextrose, polyethylene glycol, povidone, pregelatinized corn starch, silicon dioxide, sodium croscarmellose, titanium dioxide, triacetin and vanillin. HDPE bottles of 100 and 500. Store between 15-30°C in a tightly closed light-resistant container. Protect from humidity.
500 mg: Each oval, biconvex, yellow, film-coated tablet, marked "rph" on one side and "C111" on the other side, contains: clarithromycin 500 mg. Nonmedicinal ingredients: D&C yellow #10 lake, hydroxypropyl methylcellulose, hydroxypropyl methylcellulose/hypromellose, magnesium stearate, maltodextrin, microcrystalline cellulose, polydextrose, polyethylene glycol, povidone, pregelatinized corn starch, silicon dioxide, sodium croscarmellose, titanium dioxide, triacetin and vanillin. HDPE bottles of 100 and 500. Store between 15-30°C in a tightly closed light-resistant container. Protect from humidity.

The reader is invited to consult CPhA's monograph **Corticosteroids: Topical**.

ratio-Clobetasol

clobetasol 17-propionate

Topical Anti-inflammatory Corticosteroid

ratiopharm

SUPPLIED: Cream: Each g of homogenous, odorless white cream, contains: clobetasol 17-propionate 0.05% w/w in a cream base. Nonmedicinal ingredients: ceteareth-20, chlorocresol, citric acid, glyceryl stearate, polyethylene glycol, propylene glycol, purified water, sodium citrate and stearyl alcohol. Aluminum tubes of 15 and 50 g. Polypropylene jars of 450 g. Store between 15 and 30°C.
Ointment: Each g of homogeneous, smooth yellow, translucent ointment, odorless, contains: clobetasol 17-propionate 0.05% w/w in an ointment base. Nonmedicinal ingredients: light mineral oil and petrolatum. Aluminum tubes of 15 and 50 g. Polypropylene jars of 450 g. Store between 15 to 30°C.
Scalp Lotion: Each mL of homogeneous, translucent lotion, with a characteristic odor of alcohol, contains: clobetasol 17-propionate 0.05% w/w in a hydroalcoholic solution. Nonmedicinal ingredients: carbomer, isopropyl alcohol, purified water and triethanolamine. Bottles of 20 and 60 mL.

ratio-Clonazepam

clonazepam

Anticonvulsant

ratiopharm

SUPPLIED: 0.5 mg: Each orange, round, biplane, beveled-edge tablet, engraved "rph" scored and "180" on one side and "0.5" on the other side, contains: clonazepam 0.5 mg. Nonmedicinal ingredients: cornstarch, FD&C Yellow #6 Lake, lactose, magnesium stearate and microcrystalline cellulose. Sodium-, and tartrazine-free. Bottles of 100 and 500.
2 mg: Each white, round, biplane, beveled-edge tablet, engraved "rph" scored and "180" on one side and "2" on the other side, contains: clonazepam 2 mg. Nonmedicinal ingredients: cornstarch, lactose, magnesium stearate and microcrystalline cellulose. Sodium-, and tartrazine-free. Bottles of 100 and 500.
Keep in a tightly closed, light-resistant container. Store at 15 to 30°C.

ratio-Codeine

codeine phosphate

Opioid Analgesic—Antitussive

ratiopharm

SUPPLIED: Tablets: 15 mg: Each round, biconvex, white tablet, imprinted with "TEC 15" on one side and plain on the other side, contains: codeine phosphate 15 mg. Nonmedicinal ingredients: colloidal silicon dioxide, lactose, magnesium stearate, microcrystalline cellulose and stearic acid. Gluten-, paraben-, sodium- and sulfite-free. Bottles of 100. Store between 15-30°C.
30 mg: Each round, biconvex, white tablet, imprinted with "TEC 30" on one side and bisected on the other side, contains: codeine phosphate 30 mg. Nonmedicinal ingredients: colloidal silicon dioxide, lactose, magnesium stearate, microcrystalline cellulose and stearic acid. Gluten-, paraben-, sodium- and sulfite-free. Bottles of 100 and 500. Store between 15-30°C.
Syrup: Each mL of clear, colorless, syrupy liquid contains: codeine phosphate 5 mg. Nonmedicinal ingredients: 0.61% w/v alcohol, purified water, sodium benzoate, sodium bisulfite and sucrose. Bottles of 500 mL and 2 L. Store between 15-30°C.

ratio-Coristex-DH

phenylephrine HCl—hydrocodone bitartrate

Antitussive—Decongestant

ratiopharm

SUPPLIED: Each 5 mL of red liquid with a raspberry flavor contains: hydrocodone bitartrate 5 mg and phenylephrine HCl 20 mg. Nonmedicinal ingredients: alcohol, artificial coloring and flavorings, eucalyptol, menthol, methylparaben, propylparaben, purified water, simethicone and sucrose. Bottles of 500 mL. Store between 15 and 30°C. Protect from light and freezing.

ratio-Cotridin

triprolidine HCl—pseudoephedrine HCl—codeine phosphate

Antitussive—Decongestant

ratiopharm

ratio-Cotridin Expectorant

triprolidine HCl—pseudoephedrine HCl—codeine phosphate—guaifenesin

Antitussive—Expectorant—Decongestant

ratiopharm

SUPPLIED: ratio-Cotridin: Each 5 mL of red syrupy liquid with a cherry odor contains: triprolidine HCl 2 mg, pseudoephedrine HCl 30 mg and codeine phosphate 10 mg. Nonmedicinal ingredients: artificial coloring and flavorings, glycerin, methylparaben, propylparaben, purified water, sorbitol and sucrose. Bottles of 100 mL and 2 L.
ratio-Cotridin Expectorant: Each 5 mL of clear, orange syrupy liquid with a fruit odor contains: triprolidine HCl 2 mg, pseudoephedrine HCl 30 mg, guaifenesin 100 mg and codeine phosphate 10 mg. Nonmedicinal ingredients: artificial flavorings, citric acid, FD&C Yellow #6, maltitol, menthol, methylparaben, polyethylene glycol, propylene glycol, propylparaben, purified water, sodium citrate and sodium cyclamate. Bottles of 500 mL and 2 L.
Protect from light. Store between 15 and 30°C. Do not refrigerate.

ratio-Cyclobenzaprine

cyclobenzaprine HCl

Skeletal Muscle Relaxant

ratiopharm

SUPPLIED: Each butterscotch yellow, D-shaped, film-coated tablet, with a debossed "TEC" on one side and "10" on the other side, contains: cyclobenzaprine HCl USP 10 mg. Nonmedicinal ingredients: colloidal silicon dioxide, hydroxypropylcellulose, lactose, magnesium stearate, pregelatinized starch, purified water and synthetic yellow iron oxide. Bottles of 100 and 500. Store between 15 and 30°C in tightly sealed containers. Protect from heat.

ratio-Dexamethasone

dexamethasone

Corticosteroid

ratiopharm

SUPPLIED: 0.5 mg: Each white pentagonal, flat, beveled, bisected tablet, with TEC 0.50 on one side, contains: dexamethasone 0.5 mg. Nonmedicinal ingredients: dicalcium phosphate dihydrate, lactose, magnesium stearate and pregelatinized cornstarch. Bottles of 100. Store between 15 and 30°C.
4 mg: Each white pentagonal, flat, beveled, bisected tablet, with TEC 4 on one side, contains: dexamethasone 4 mg. Nonmedicinal ingredients: dicalcium phosphate dihydrate, lactose, magnesium stearate and pregelatinized cornstarch. Bottles of 50 and 100. Store between 15 and 30°C.

The reader is invited to consult CPhA's monograph **Calcium Channel Blockers**.

ratio-Diltiazem CD

diltiazem HCl

Antianginal—Antihypertensive

ratiopharm

SUPPLIED: 120 mg: Each hard gelatin controlled delivery capsule, with a light turquoise blue opaque body and a light turquoise blue opaque cap, imprinted "Dilt CD 120 mg" and "rph" with white spherical bead fill, contains: diltiazem HCl 120 mg. Nonmedicinal ingredients: acetyl tributyl citrate, ethylcellulose, magnesium stearate, methylacrylic acid copolymer Type B, polysorbate, sugar spheres and talc; capsule shell: FD&C Blue #1, gelatin and titanium dioxide. Bisulfites-, gluten- and tartrazine-free. Bottles of 100 and 500. Store in tight containers between 15 and 30°C. Protect from light.
180 mg: Each hard gelatin controlled delivery capsule, with a light turquoise blue opaque body and a light blue opaque cap, imprinted "Dilt CD 180 mg" and "rph" with white spherical bead fill, contains: diltiazem HCl 180 mg. Nonmedicinal ingredients: acetyl tributyl citrate, ethylcellulose, magnesium stearate, methylacrylic acid copolymer Type B, polysorbate, sugar spheres and talc; capsule shell: FD&C Blue #1, gelatin and titanium dioxide. Bisulfites-, gluten- and tartrazine-free. Bottles of 100 and 500. Store in tight containers between 15 and 30°C. Protect from light.
240 mg: Each hard gelatin controlled delivery capsule, with a light blue opaque body and a light blue opaque cap, imprinted "Dilt CD 240 mg" and "rph" with white spherical bead fill, contains: diltiazem HCl 240 mg. Nonmedicinal ingredients: acetyl tributyl citrate, ethylcellulose, magnesium stearate, methylacrylic acid copolymer Type B, polysorbate, sugar spheres and talc; capsule shell: FD&C Blue #1, gelatin and titanium dioxide. Bisulfites-, gluten- and tartrazine-free. Bottles of 100 and 500. Store in tight containers between 15 and 30°C. Protect from light.
300 mg: Each hard gelatin controlled delivery capsule, with a light grey opaque body and a light blue opaque cap, imprinted "Dilt CD 300 mg" and "rph" with white spherical bead fill, contains: diltiazem HCl 300 mg. Nonmedicinal ingredients: acetyl tributyl citrate, ethylcellulose, magnesium stearate, methylacrylic acid copolymer Type B, polysorbate, sugar spheres and talc; capsule shell: black iron oxide, FD&C Blue #1, gelatin and titanium dioxide. Bisulfites-, gluten- and tartrazine-free. Bottles of 100 and 500. Store in tight containers between 15 and 30°C. Protect from light.

ratio-Docusate Calcium

docusate calcium

Stool Softener—Laxative

ratiopharm

SUPPLIED: Each red, odorless, oblong soft gel capsule, imprinted "TEC" in white ink, contains: docusate calcium USP 240 mg. Nonmedicinal ingredients: corn oil, D&C Red #33, FD&C Red #40, gelatin, glycerin, purified water, and sorbitol. Lactose-, sodium- and tartrazine-free. Bottles of 1000. Store the capsules in the container in which they were purchased. Do not expose container or contents to humidity, sources of heat or direct light. Store at controlled room temperature, below 25°C.

ratio-Docusate Sodium

docusate sodium

Stool Softener

ratiopharm

SUPPLIED: Capsules: Each red, oblong, soft gel capsule, imprinted with "TEC" with white ink, filled with red oily liquid and with the potential presence of gelatinous substance in the capsule, contains: docusate sodium USP 100 mg. Nonmedicinal ingredients: FD&C blue #1, FD&C red #40, gelatin, glycerin, paraben, polyethylene glycol, propylene glycol, purified water, sorbitol and white ink. Bottles of 1000. Safety sealed cap for protection.
Syrup: 5 mL of clear, dark pink to red syrup, contains: docusate sodium USP 20 mg. Nonmedicinal ingredients: alcohol, artificial flavoring, citric acid, D&C red #33, FD&C red #40, menthol, methylparaben, peppermint oil, poloxamer, polyethylene glycol, propylparaben, purified water, sodium citrate and sucrose. Bottles of 500 mL. Safety sealed bottle for protection.
Unit dose: Each unit dose (25 mL) container filled with a clear, dark pink to red syrup, contains: docusate sodium USP 100 mg. Nonmedicinal ingredients: alcohol, artificial flavoring, citric acid, D&C red #33, FD&C red #40, menthol, methylparaben, peppermint oil, poloxamer, polyethylene glycol, propylparaben, purified water, sodium citrate and sucrose.
Store at approximately 25°C. Avoid freezing or excessive heat. Keep out of the reach of children.

ratio-Domperidone

domperidone maleate

Upper Gastrointestinal Motility Modifier

ratiopharm

SUPPLIED: Each white, film-coated, round, biconvex tablet, engraved with "rph D51" on one side and plain on the other side, contains: domperidone maleate 12.72 mg (equivalent to domperidone 10 mg). Nonmedicinal ingredients: cornstarch, hydroxypropyl methylcellulose, lactose, magnesium stearate, microcrystalline cellulose, polydextrose, polyethylene glycol, povidone, sodium benzoate and docusate sodium, sodium croscarmellose, titanium dioxide and triacetin. Bisulfite-, gluten- and tartrazine-free. HDPE bottles of 100 and 500. Store at room temperature between 15 and 30°C. Protect from light and moisture.

ratio-Ectosone ℞

betamethasone valerate

Topical Corticosteroid

ratiopharm

SUPPLIED: Regular Cream: Each g of white, homogeneous smooth, odorless cream, contains: betamethasone 0.1% (as betamethasone valerate USP) in a water-miscible base. Nonmedicinal ingredients: caprylic/capric triglyceride, ceteareth-12, ceteareth-20, cetearyl alcohol, glycerin, methylparaben, propylparaben and purified water. Jars of 450 g.
Mild Cream: Each g of white, homogeneous smooth, odorless cream, contains: betamethasone 0.05% (as betamethasone valerate USP) in a water-miscible base. Nonmedicinal ingredients: caprylic/capric triglyceride, ceteareth-12, ceteareth-20, cetearyl alcohol, glycerin, methylparaben, propylparaben and purified water. Jars of 450 g.
Regular Lotion: Each g of white, homogeneous, odorless lotion, contains: betamethasone valerate USP 1.22 mg (equivalent to betamethasone 1 mg [0.1%]). Nonmedicinal ingredients: ceteareth-20, cetearyl alcohol, glycerin, glycol distearate, guar gum, isopropyl alcohol, isopropyl myristate, methylparaben, propylparaben and purified water. Bottles of 60 mL.
Mild Lotion: Each g of white, homogeneous, odorless lotion, contains: betamethasone valerate USP 0.61 mg (equivalent to betamethasone 0.5 mg [0.05%]). Nonmedicinal ingredients: ceteareth-20, cetearyl alcohol, glycerin, glycol distearate, guar gum, isopropyl alcohol, isopropyl myristate, methylparaben, propylparaben and purified water. Bottles of 60 mL.
Scalp Lotion: Each g of translucid, homogeneous lotion with a strong odor of alcohol, contains: betamethasone valerate USP 1.22 mg (equivalent to betamethasone 1 mg [0.1%]). Nonmedicinal ingredients: butylated hydroxytoluene, carbomer, EDTA disodium, isopropyl alcohol, purified water and triethanolamine. Plastic squeeze bottles of 30 and 75 mL.

Store at room temperature between 15 to 30°C. Protect from freezing.

ratio-Emtec-30 Ⓝ

acetaminophen—codeine phosphate

Analgesic—Antipyretic—Antitussive

ratiopharm

SUPPLIED: Each round, biplane tablet, beveled-edged, peach-colored tablet, imprinted with «Emtec-30» on one side and bisected on the other side, contains: acetaminophen 300 mg and codeine phosphate 30 mg. Nonmedicinal ingredients: crospovidone, FD&C Ysellow #6 aluminum lake, magnesium stearate, microcrystalline cellulose, povidone, pregelatinized cornstarch, sodium starch glycolate and stearic acid. Sodium: <1 mmol. Bottles of 500. Store between 15 and 30°C.

The reader is invited to consult CPhA's monograph **ACE Inhibitors**.

ratio-Enalapril ℞

enalapril maleate

Angiotensin Converting Enzyme Inhibitor

ratiopharm

SUPPLIED: 2.5 mg: Each white, oval-shaped tablet with "rph" on one side and "E24" on the other side and breaking line, contains: enalapril maleate 2.5 mg that appears as enalapril sodium 2 mg. Nonmedicinal ingredients: corn starch, lactose monohydrate, magnesium stearate, pregelatinized starch and sodium bicarbonate. Bottles of 100 and 500. Store at controlled room temperature (15-25°C). Keep container tightly closed. Protect from moisture. Discard remaining tablets six months after opening the bottle.
5 mg: Each white, arc triangle tablet, with "rph" on one side and "E23" on the other side and breaking line, contains: enalapril maleate 5 mg that appears as enalapril sodium 4 mg. Nonmedicinal ingredients: corn starch, lactose monohydrate, magnesium stearate, pregelatinized starch and sodium bicarbonate. Bottles of 100 and 500. Store at controlled room temperature (15-25°C). Keep container tightly closed. Protect from moisture. Discard remaining tablets six months after opening the bottle.
10 mg: Each red, arc triangle tablet, with "rph" on one side and "E22" on the other side and breaking line, contains: enalapril maleate 10 mg that appears as enalapril sodium 8 mg. Nonmedicinal ingredients: corn starch, lactose monohydrate, magnesium stearate, pregelatinized starch, red iron oxide and sodium bicarbonate. Bottles of 100 and 500. Store at controlled room temperature (15-25°C). Keep container tightly closed. Protect from moisture. Discard remaining tablets six months after opening the bottle.
20 mg: Each peach, arc triangle tablet, with "rph" on one side and "E21" on the other side and breaking line, contains: enalapril maleate 20 mg that appears as enalapril sodium 16 mg. Nonmedicinal ingredients: corn starch, lactose monohydrate, magnesium stearate, pregelatinized starch, red iron oxide, sodium bicarbonate and yellow iron oxide. Bottles of 100 and 500. Store at controlled room temperature (15-25°C). Keep container tightly closed. Protect from moisture. Discard remaining tablets six months after opening the bottle.

ratio-Fenofibrate MC ℞

fenofibrate nanocrystals

Lipid Metabolism Regulator

ratiopharm

SUPPLIED: Each hard gelatin capsule, with an orange opaque body and cap imprinted "rph 183" on the body and "200" on the cap, filled with white beige homogeneous mass, wax-like, no apparent crystals, contains: fenofibrate 200 mg. Nonmedicinal ingredients: hydroxypropyl cellulose, lauroyl macrogolglyceride and polyethylene glycol; capsule shell: FD&C Red no. 3, gelatin, titanium dioxide and yellow iron oxide. Bottles of 100. Packages of 30. Store between 15-30°C in tightly closed containers. Avoid excessive humidity. Protect from freezing.

ratio-Fentanyl Ⓝ

fentanyl

Opioid Analgesic

ratiopharm

Date of Revision: May 27, 2010

SUMMARY PRODUCT INFORMATION:

Route of Administration	Dosage Form/ Strength	Clinically Relevant Nonmedicinal Ingredients
Transdermal	Patch Five strengths with 2.063, 4.125, 8.25, 12.375 and 16.5 mg fentanyl per patch, delivering 12, 25, 50, 75, 100 µg/h fentanyl respectively for 72 hours	For a complete listing see Dosage Forms, Composition and Packaging.

INDICATIONS AND CLINICAL USE: Adults: ratio-FENTANYL (fentanyl transdermal system) is indicated in the management of **persistent**, moderate to severe chronic pain that cannot be managed by other means such as opioid combination products or immediate-release opioids, and only in patients:

- who require continuous around-the-clock opioid analgesia for an extended period of time and
- who are already receiving opioid therapy at a total daily dose of at least 60 mg/day Morphine Equivalents.

The initial dose of ratio-FENTANYL should be obtained or calculated from the conversion tables (see Dosage and Administration), and must **not** be higher than that dose which is equivalent to the total dose of opioids the patient is receiving at the time of the switch to the patch.

Because serious or life-threatening hypoventilation could occur, ratio-FENTANYL should not be used in:

- non-opioid-tolerant patients
- the management of postoperative pain

Special Populations: Pediatrics: The use of ratio-FENTANYL in children under 18 years of age is not recommended, as dosage requirements for the safe and efficacious use of fentanyl transdermal system have not been established for this patient population. Life-threatening hypoventilation has been reported in some pediatric patients receiving fentanyl transdermal systems.
Elderly and Debilitated Patients: In elderly, cachectic, or debilitated patients, ratio-FENTANYL may have altered pharmacokinetics due to poor fat stores, muscle wasting or altered clearance (see Dosage and Administration). Therefore, it may be appropriate, according to clinical judgment, to initiate these patients on a lower ratio-FENTANYL dose than that which the conversion tables recommend, including the use of the 12 µg/h dose by itself or in combination with another dose, provided the patient is not opioid-naïve (see Contraindications). The 12 µg/h strength may also be used for dose titration up or down, as using small increments for dose adjustment is recommended to enhance tolerability of opioid therapy (see Dosage and Administration).

CONTRAINDICATIONS: Because serious or life-threatening hypoventilation could occur, ratio-FENTANYL is contraindicated in:

1. patients with acute or perioperative pain, especially use in out-patient or day surgeries (see Warnings and Precautions, Peri-Operative Considerations);
2. patients with mild, intermittent or short duration pain that can otherwise be managed;
3. opioid-naïve patients at any dose;
4. situations of significant respiratory depression, especially in unmonitored settings where there is a lack of resuscitative equipment; and
5. patients who have acute or severe bronchial asthma.

Because serious or life-threatening hypoventilation could occur, the **maximum initiation dose** of ratio-FENTANYL should not be higher than that equivalent to the total dose of opioids the patient is receiving at the time of the switch (see conversion tables in Dosage and Administration).

ratio-FENTANYL is contraindicated in patients who have or are suspected of having paralytic ileus.

ratio-FENTANYL is contraindicated in patients with known hypersensitivity to fentanyl, or to the adhesives present in the system.

WARNINGS AND PRECAUTIONS: General: Use in non-opioid-tolerant patients, or use of an initiating dose which is higher than the opioid equivalent to which the patient is tolerant at the time of the switch, may lead to fatal respiratory depression.

The following contraindications reduce the potential risk of serious or life-threatening hypoventilation: ratio-FENTANYL should not be used in the management of acute or postoperative pain since there is no opportunity for dose titration during short-term use and serious or life-threatening hypoventilation could result. Similarly, ratio-FENTANYL should not be administered to patients who do not have some degree of tolerance to opioid-induced side effects. ratio-FENTANYL should only be prescribed to patients who require continuous opioids for pain management, and who are tolerant to at least the morphine equivalent of the lowest initiating ratio-FENTANYL dose.

The initial dose of ratio-FENTANYL should be obtained from the conversion tables in Dosage and Administration, and must not be higher than that dose which is equivalent to the total dose of opioids the patient is receiving at the time of the switch to the patch. It may be appropriate, according to clinical judgment, to initiate some patients on a lower ratio-FENTANYL dose than that which the conversion tables recommend, which may include use of the 12 µg/h dose. Opioid-naïve patients should not be given ratio-FENTANYL at any dose, inclusive of 12 µg/h (see Contraindications). In general, the 12 µg/h dose, which allows for smaller dose increases than does the 25 µg/h patch, is to be used for titration/adjustments of dosage (see Dosage and Administration).

The use of ratio-FENTANYL in children under 18 years of age is not recommended as dosage requirements for the safe and efficacious use of ratio-FENTANYL have not been established for this patient population. Life-threatening hypoventilation has been reported in some pediatric patients receiving fentanyl transdermal systems.

ratio-FENTANYL should only be prescribed by persons knowledgeable in the continuous administration of potent opioids, in the management of patients receiving potent opioids for treatment of pain and in the detection and management of respiratory depression including the use of opioid antagonists.

Since serum fentanyl concentrations decline gradually after system removal, patients who have experienced serious adverse events should be monitored for at least 24 hours after ratio-FENTANYL removal or until the adverse reaction has subsided.

As with other CNS depressants, patients who have received ratio-FENTANYL should be closely monitored especially for signs of respiratory depression until a stable maintenance dose is reached.

Due to the formation of a subcutaneous depot of fentanyl, not only does continued exposure occur after system removal but, in the case of removal prior to attainment of peak fentanyl exposure, fentanyl plasma levels may, in fact, continue to increase after removal of ratio-FENTANYL patches.

ratio-FENTANYL patches are intended for transdermal use on intact skin only; use on compromised skin can lead to increased exposure to fentanyl.

Placing ratio-FENTANYL transdermal systems in the mouth, chewing it, swallowing it, or using it in any ways other than indicated may cause choking or overdose that could result in death.

Risk of Unintentional Increase in Drug Exposure: Patients with Fever: Serum fentanyl concentrations could theoretically increase by approximately one-third for patients with a body temperature of 40°C due to temperature-dependent increases in fentanyl release from the system and increased skin permeability. Patients who develop fever should be monitored for opioid side effects and have their ratio-FENTANYL dose adjusted if necessary.
External Heat Sources: All patients should be advised to avoid exposing the ratio-FENTANYL application site to direct external heat sources, such as heating pads, electric blankets, heated water beds, heat lamps, hot water bottles, saunas and hot whirlpool spa baths, intensive sunbathing, etc.
Accidental Exposure to ratio-FENTANYL: Serious medical consequences, including death, have occurred when people were accidentally exposed to fentanyl transdermal system. Examples of accidental exposure include transfer of a fentanyl transdermal system while hugging, sharing a bed, or moving a patient.
Disposal of ratio-FENTANYL: ratio-FENTANYL should be kept out of the reach of children before and after use.

Used systems should be folded so that the adhesive side of the system adheres to itself, then flushed down the toilet immediately upon removal. If the drug adhesive layer accidentally contacts the skin, the area should be washed with clear water. Patients should dispose of any systems remaining from a prescription as soon as they are no longer needed. Unused systems should be removed from their pouch, folded so that the adhesive side of the system adheres to itself, and flushed down the toilet (see Dosage and Administration and Special Handling Instructions).

Cardiovascular: Intravenous fentanyl may produce bradycardia. Fentanyl should be administered with caution to patients with bradyarrhythmias.
Concomitant Use of Central Nervous System Depressants: When patients are receiving ratio-FENTANYL, the dose of additional opioids or other CNS-depressant drugs (including alcohol beverages, benzodiazepines, general anesthetics, muscle relaxants and sedating over-the-counter antihistamines) should be reduced by at least 50%. The concomitant use of CNS depressants may result in hypotension, respiratory depression and profound sedation, coma or death (see Drug Interactions).
Concomitant Use of CYP3A4 Inhibitors: The concomitant use of ratio-FENTANYL with potent cytochrome P450 3A4 inhibitors (ritonavir, ketoconazole, itraconazole, troleandomycin, clarithromycin, nelfinavir, nefazodone, verapamil, diltiazem, amiodarone, amprenavir, fosamprenavir, aprepitant, fluconazole, erythromycin and grapefruit juice) may result in an increase in fentanyl plasma concentrations, which could increase or prolong adverse drug effects and may cause potentially fatal respiratory depression. In this situation special patient care and observation are appropriate. Therefore, the concomitant use of transdermal fentanyl and CYP3A4 inhibitors is not recommended unless the patient is closely monitored, for an extended period of time, for signs of respiratory depression, with dosage adjustments made as warranted (see Drug Interactions).
Potential for Abuse and Diversion: ratio-FENTANYL contains a high concentration of a potent opioid, fentanyl, which along with other opioids of the morphine type has high potential for abuse and associated risk of fatal overdose due to respiratory depression. The high fentanyl content in ratio-FENTANYL may be a particular target for abuse and diversion, with alternative routes of administration potentially resulting in overdose from uncontrolled delivery of the opioid.

This risk should be considered when administering, prescribing, or dispensing ratio-FENTANYL in situations where the health-care professional is concerned about increased risk of misuse, abuse or diversion.

Concerns about abuse, addiction and diversion should not prevent the proper management of pain. Patients should be assessed for their clinical risks for opioid abuse or addiction prior to being prescribed opioids. All patients receiving opioids should be routinely monitored for signs of misuse and abuse.

Since ratio-FENTANYL may be diverted for non-medical use, careful record keeping of prescribing information, including quantity, frequency, and renewal requests is strongly advised. Proper assessment of the patient, proper prescribing practices, periodic re-evaluation of therapy, and proper dispensing and storage are appropriate measures that help to limit abuse of opioid drugs (see Dependence/Tolerance).

Dependence/Tolerance: Drug Dependence vs Abuse: Fentanyl is an opioid substance and can produce drug dependence similar to that produced by morphine. ratio-FENTANYL, therefore, has the potential for abuse. However, tolerance as well as both physical and psychological dependence may develop upon repeated administration of opioids, and are not by themselves evidence of an addictive disorder or abuse. Iatrogenic addiction following appropriate opioid administration for relief of severe pain is relatively rare. Physicians should not let concerns of physical dependence deter them from using adequate amounts of opioids in the management of severe pain when such use is indicated. Patients at increased risk of opioid abuse may still be appropriately treated with modified-release opioid formulations; however, these patients will require monitoring for signs of misuse, abuse, or addiction.

Drug or Alcohol Dependence: Use of ratio-FENTANYL in combination with CNS depressants, including alcohol, can result in increased risk to the patient (see Drug Interactions).

ratio-FENTANYL should be used with caution in individuals who have a history of drug or alcohol abuse, especially those outside a medically controlled environment. While the management of severe pain in patients with a history of addiction requires special consideration, the use of opioids is not necessarily contraindicated in these patients. There may also be an increased risk of diversion in this population; this risk may be decreased by attention to patterns of prescription requests, and by prescribing opioids only as part of an ongoing relationship between a patient and a healthcare provider.

"Drug seeking" behaviour includes emergency calls or visits near the end of office hours; refusal to undergo appropriate examination, testing or referral; repeated "loss" of prescriptions; tampering with prescriptions; "doctor shopping" to obtain additional prescriptions; and reluctance to provide prior medical records or contact information for other treating physician(s).

Head Injuries and Increased Intracranial Pressure: ratio-FENTANYL should not be used in patients who may be particularly susceptible to the intracranial effects of CO_2 retention such as those with evidence of increased intracranial pressure, impaired consciousness, or coma. Opioids may obscure the clinical course of patients with head injury. ratio-FENTANYL should be used with caution in patients with brain tumours.

Peri-Operative Considerations: ratio-FENTANYL is contraindicated for peri-operative pain relief, especially in the elective surgical setting. In the case of planned chordotomy, or other pain-relieving operations, patients should not be treated with ratio-FENTANYL within 72 hours before the operation and should not be used in the immediate post-operative period. Thereafter, if ratio-FENTANYL is to be continued after the patient recovers from the post-operative period, a new dosage should be administered in accordance with the changed need for pain relief, if needed, and to reduce the risk of withdrawal in highly opioid-tolerant patients. The administration of analgesics in the perioperative period should be managed by health care providers with adequate training and experience (e.g., an anaesthesiologist) (see Contraindications).

Hepatic/Biliary/Pancreatic: Because of the hepatic metabolism of fentanyl, ratio-FENTANYL should be used with caution in patients with liver dysfunction.

ratio-FENTANYL may cause spasm of the sphincter of Oddi and should be used with caution in patients with biliary tract disease, including acute pancreatitis. Opioids like ratio-FENTANYL may cause increases in the serum amylase concentration.

Psychomotor Impairment: ratio-FENTANYL may impair mental and/or physical ability required for the performance of potentially hazardous tasks such as driving a car or operating machinery. Patients using ratio-FENTANYL should not drive or operate dangerous machinery unless they are tolerant to the effects of the drug.

Renal: Because of the renal excretion of fentanyl, ratio-FENTANYL should be used with caution in patients with kidney dysfunction.

Respiratory: Respiratory Depression: As with all potent opioids, some patients may experience significant respiratory depression (including respiratory distress, apnea, bradypnea, hypoventilation, dyspnea) with ratio-FENTANYL; caution must be exercised and patients carefully observed for untoward reactions. While most patients using fentanyl transdermal systems chronically develop tolerance to fentanyl-induced hypoventilation, episodes of slowed respiration may occur at any time during therapy. A small number of patients have experienced clinically significant hypoventilation with fentanyl transdermal system; medical intervention generally was not required in these instances. The incidence of respiratory depression increases as the fentanyl transdermal system dose is increased.

Hypoventilation can occur throughout the therapeutic range of fentanyl serum concentrations. However, the risk of hypoventilation increases at serum fentanyl concentrations greater than 2 ng/mL in non-opioid-tolerant patients, especially for patients who have an underlying pulmonary condition or who receive usual doses of opioids or other CNS drugs associated with hypoventilation in addition to ratio-FENTANYL (see Drug Interactions regarding the use of concomitant CNS active drugs). The use of ratio-FENTANYL should be monitored by clinical evaluation. As with other drug-level measurements, serum fentanyl concentrations may be useful clinically, although they do not reflect patients' sensitivity to fentanyl and should not be used by physicians as a sole indicator of effectiveness or toxicity.

The duration of the respiratory depressant effect of ratio-FENTANYL may extend beyond the removal of the system (see also Overdosage concerning respiratory depression).

Use in Patients with Chronic Pulmonary Disease: Fentanyl should be used with caution in patients with chronic pulmonary disease, patients with decreased respiratory reserve and others with potentially compromised respiration. Normal analgesic doses of opioids may further decrease respiratory drive in these patients to the point of respiratory failure.

Information to Be Provided to the Patient: A patient information sheet is included in the package of ratio-FENTANYL patches dispensed to the patient.

Patients receiving ratio-FENTANYL patches should be given the following instructions by the physician:

1. Patients should be informed that accidental ingestion or use by individual (including children) other than the patient for whom it was originally prescribed, may lead to severe, even fatal, consequences.
2. Patients should be advised that ratio-FENTANYL patches contain fentanyl, an opioid pain medicine similar to morphine, hydromorphone, methadone, oxycodone, and oxymorphone.
3. Patients should be advised that each ratio-FENTANYL patch may be worn continuously for 72 hours, and that each patch should be applied to a different skin site after removal of the previous transdermal patch.
4. Patients should be advised that ratio-FENTANYL patches should be applied to intact, non-irritated, and non-irradiated skin on a flat surface such as the chest, back, flank, or upper arm. Additionally, patients should be advised of the following:
   - In young children or persons with cognitive impairment, the patch should be put on the upper back to lower the chances that the patch will be removed and placed in the mouth.
   - Hair at the application site should be clipped (not shaved) prior to patch application.
   - If the site of ratio-FENTANYL application must be cleansed prior to application of the patch, do so with clear water.
   - Do not use soaps, oils, lotions, alcohol, or any other agents that might irritate the skin or alter its characteristics.
   - Allow the skin to dry completely prior to patch application.
5. Patients should be advised that ratio-FENTANYL should be applied immediately upon removal from the sealed package and after removal of the protective liner. Additionally the patient should be advised of the following:
   - The ratio-FENTANYL patch should not be used if the seal is broken, or if it is altered, cut, or damaged in any way prior to application. The transdermal patch should be pressed firmly in place with the palm of the hand for 30 seconds, making sure the contact is complete, especially around the edges.
   - The patch should not be folded so that only part of the patch is exposed.
6. Patients should be advised that, while wearing the patch, they should avoid exposing the ratio-FENTANYL application site to direct external heat sources, such as:
   - heating pads,
   - electric blankets,
   - heat lamps,
   - saunas,
   - hot tubs, and
   - heated water beds, etc.
7. Patients should be advised that there is a potential for temperature-dependent increase in fentanyl release from the patch that could result in an overdose of fentanyl; therefore, if patients develop a high fever while wearing the patch they should contact their physician.
8. Patients should be advised that if they experience problems with the adhesion of the ratio-FENTANYL patch, they may tape the edges of the patch with first aid tape. If problems with adhesion persist, patients may overlay the patch with a transparent adhesive film dressing.
9. Patients should be advised that if the patch falls off before 72 hours a new patch may be applied to a different skin site.
10. Patients should be advised to fold (so that the adhesive side adheres to itself) and immediately flush down the toilet used ratio-FENTANYL patches after removal from the skin.
11. Patients should be instructed that, if the drug adhesive layer accidentally contacts the skin, the area should be washed clean with clear water and not soap, alcohol, or other chemicals, because these products may increase the ability of fentanyl to go through the skin.
12. Patients should be advised that the dose of ratio-FENTANYL should **never** be adjusted without the prescribing health care professional's instruction.
13. Patients should be advised that ratio-FENTANYL may impair mental and/or physical ability required for the performance of potentially hazardous tasks (e.g., driving, operating machinery).
14. Patients should be advised to refrain from any potentially dangerous activity when starting on ratio-FENTANYL or when their dose is being adjusted, until it is established that they have not been adversely affected.
15. Patients should be advised that ratio-FENTANYL should not be combined with alcohol or other CNS depressants (e.g. sleep medications, tranquilizers) because dangerous additive effects may occur, resulting in serious injury or death.
16. Patients should be advised to consult their physician or pharmacist if other medications are being or will be used with ratio-FENTANYL.
17. Patients should be advised of the potential for severe constipation.
18. Patients should be advised that if they have been receiving treatment with ratio-FENTANYL and cessation of therapy is indicated, it may be appropriate to taper the ratio-FENTANYL dose, rather than abruptly discontinue it, due to the risk of precipitating withdrawal symptoms.
19. Patients should be advised that ratio-FENTANYL contains fentanyl, is a drug with high potential for abuse.
20. Patients, family members and caregivers should be advised to protect ratio-FENTANYL from theft or misuse in the work or home environment.
21. Patients should be advised that ratio-FENTANYL should never be given to anyone other than the individual for whom it was prescribed because of the risk of death or other serious medical problems to that person for whom it was not intended.
22. Patients should be instructed to keep ratio-FENTANYL in a secure place out of the reach of children due to the high risk of **fatal respiratory depression**.
23. When ratio-FENTANYL is no longer needed, the unused patches should be removed from their pouches, folded so that the adhesive side of the patch adheres to itself, and flushed down the toilet.
24. Women of childbearing potential who become or are planning to become pregnant should be advised to consult a physician prior to initiating or continuing therapy with ratio-FENTANYL.
25. Patients should be informed that accidental exposure or misuse may lead to death or other serious medical problems.
26. Patients should be informed that, if the patch dislodges and accidentally sticks to the skin of another person, they should immediately take the patch off, wash the exposed area with water and seek medical attention for the accidentally exposed individual.

Special Populations: Pregnant Women: Fentanyl has been shown to impair fertility and to have an embryocidal effect in rats when given in intravenous doses 0.3 times the human dose for a period of 12 days. No evidence of teratogenic effects has been observed after the administration of fentanyl to rats. The safe use of fentanyl has not been established with respect to possible adverse effects upon human fetal development. Neonatal withdrawal syndrome has been reported in newborn infants with chronic maternal use of fentanyl transdermal systems during pregnancy. Therefore, ratio-FENTANYL should not be used in women of childbearing potential unless, in the judgement of the physician, the potential benefits outweigh the possible hazards.

Use of ratio-FENTANYL during childbirth is not recommended because fentanyl passes through the placenta and may cause respiratory depression in the newborn child.

Nursing Women: Fentanyl is excreted in human milk, therefore ratio-FENTANYL is not recommended for use in nursing women because of the possibility of effects in their infants.

Pediatrics (<18 years of age): The use of ratio-FENTANYL in children under 18 years of age is not recommended as dosage requirements for the safe and efficacious use of ratio-FENTANYL have not been established for this patient population. Life-threatening hypoventilation has been reported in some pediatric patients receiving fentanyl transdermal systems.

Elderly and Debilitated Patients: In elderly, cachectic, or debilitated patients, ratio-FENTANYL may have altered pharmacokinetics due to poor fat stores, muscle wasting or altered clearance (see Dosage and Administration). Therefore, it may be appropriate, according to clinical judgment, to initiate these patients on a lower ratio-FENTANYL dose than that which the conversion tables recommend, including the use of the 12 µg/h dose by itself or in combination with another dose, provided the patient is not opioid-naïve (see Contraindications). The 12 µg/h strength may also be used for dose titration up or down, as using small increments for dose adjustment is recommended to enhance tolerability of opioid therapy (see Dosage and Administration). As with all ratio-FENTANYL patients, they should be carefully monitored for pain levels and adverse events, particularly hypoventilation.

ADVERSE REACTIONS: Clinical Trial Adverse Drug Reactions: Cancer Trials—Adults: Open-Label and Active-Control Double-Blind Studies: The safety of fentanyl transdermal systems have been evaluated in 153 cancer patients and 357 post-operative patients. The duration of fentanyl transdermal system use varied in cancer patients; 56% of patients used fentanyl transdermal systems for over 30 days, 28% continued treatment for more than 4 months, and 10% used fentanyl transdermal systems for more than 1 year. In cancer patients, fentanyl transdermal systems were administered in doses of 25 µg/h to 600 µg/h. Patients with acute pain used fentanyl transdermal systems for 1 to 3 days.

Respiratory depression, the most serious adverse reaction, was observed in 3 (2%) of the cancer patients and 13 (4%) of postoperative patients. Hypotension and hypertension were observed in 11 (3%) and 4 (1%) of the opioid-naïve patients.

Placebo-Controlled Study: Adverse events occurring at a greater frequency than placebo were identified in a placebo-controlled clinical trial of fentanyl transdermal systems (25 µg/h to100 µg/h) in cancer patients. Patients were stabilized on morphine for 7 days, and those who achieved adequate pain relief (n=131) were then switched to fentanyl transdermal systems. During the initial open-label dose-titration and stabilization period of 15 days, a total of 43 patients dropped out; four experienced dyspnea, three nausea and one severe hallucinations.

Following this stabilization period, the nine-day double-blind period began, with patients randomized to either continue the dose of fentanyl transdermal systems achieved during stabilization (n=47) or to switch to placebo (n=48). Rescue morphine was available. The median dose of fentanyl transdermal systems was 50 µg/h. Adverse events during this period, as reported by at least 1 fentanyl transdermal system patient (2.1%), and with a higher frequency of occurrence versus placebo include: vomiting (4.3% vs 0%), and the following events at 2.1% vs 0%: abscess, vertigo, hemorrhage, abdominal pain and jaundice.

Chronic Non-Cancer Pain Trials—Adults: The safety findings from the two primary trials (FEN-INT-12, n=248 patients, and FEN-INT-13, n=532 patients) are described below.

Safety Findings: Adverse events related to respiratory depression (reported as either bradypnea or hypoventilation) have been reported in 3/780 (0.4%) of the CNCP patients, leading to discontinuation in all three cases.

There were nine deaths (all in the one-year trial): four were due to cardiac events, three to pneumonia, one to a cerebrovascular event, and one to cancer.

The discontinuation rates were 16% for the one-month crossover trial (FEN-INT-12) and 43% for the one-year trial (FEN-INT-13).

Of the 780 patients, 149 (19%) received less than one month fentanyl transdermal system treatment, 272 (35%) used fentanyl transdermal systems for one to six months, 137 (18%) for six months to one year and 222 patients (28%) continued treatment for more than one year.

Among patients who completed the one-year trial (n=301 of 530 ITT patients), the mean dose at the 12-month endpoint was 90.4 µg/h, with the most common dose being 75 µg/h.

Most Common Adverse Events: A causal relationship of adverse events to fentanyl transdermal systems was not always determined. The most commonly observed adverse events in the non-cancer chronic pain clinical trials, regardless of causal relationship, are: nausea or vomiting, somnolence, constipation, sweating, headache, dizziness, pruritus and depression.

Other reported adverse reactions occurring in >1% of patients that are probably or likely related to fentanyl transdermal systems treatment are:

Application Site: application site reaction.

Body as a Whole: fatigue, pain, malaise, asthenia, hot flushes, withdrawal syndrome, back pain, rigors, temperature changed sensation.

Central and Peripheral Nervous Systems: tremor, vertigo, hypertonia.

Gastrointestinal System: dry mouth, diarrhea, abdominal pain, dyspepsia.

Heart Rate and Rhythm: palpitation.

Liver and Biliary System: hepatic enzymes increased, gamma-GT increased.

Metabolic and Nutritional: weight decreased, LDH increased.
Psychiatric: anorexia, anxiety, confusion, insomnia, nervousness, agitation, hallucination, concentration impaired, emotional lability, amnesia.
Respiratory System: dyspnea.
Skin and Appendages: rash erythematous, skin disorder.
Chronic Pain Trials—Pediatrics: The safety of fentanyl transdermal systems has been evaluated in 293 opioid-tolerant pediatric patients (age 18 years or less) with chronic pain, with n=63 receiving fentanyl transdermal system for at least 2 months. Approximately 60% of the patients had underlying pain due to malignancy. The number of patients in the lower age ranges were as follows: n=2 patients <2 years old; n=65 patients 2 to <6 years old; n=100 patients 6 to <12 years old. The most commonly reported adverse events regardless of causality include: vomiting (14.3%), nausea (11.6%), constipation (9.2%), pruritus (8.2%), and somnolence (5.8%). Three patients experienced respiratory depression within 96 hours of beginning the fentanyl transdermal system treatment; two of these patients died. The underlying condition of the patients contributed to the deaths. The third patient's decreased respiratory rate was resolved after temporary discontinuation of fentanyl transdermal system.

Dosing recommendations for the safe and effective use of ratio-FENTANYL in this patient population have not been established, in view of the combination of:

i. the variety of factors which could lead to overexposure from ratio-FENTANYL in children as compared to adults (including smaller body weight and significantly different body surface area; differential skin characteristics; potential for magnification, compared to adults, of the impact of amount of body fat stores, muscle wasting, fever, external heat), and
ii. the limitations in both formal PK data (see Action and Clinical Pharmacology, Pharmacokinetics, Special Populations and Conditions) and exposure data (as above).

Post-Market Adverse Drug Reactions: In post-marketing experience, deaths from hypoventilation have been reported in cases of inappropriate use of fentanyl transdermal systems.

Other opioid-related adverse reactions include: nausea, vomiting, constipation, hypotension, bradycardia, somnolence, headache, confusion, hallucination, euphoria, pruritus, sweating, tachycardia, paresthesia, sexual dysfunction, and urinary retention.

Skin reactions such as rash, erythema and itching have occasionally been reported. These reactions usually resolve within 24 hours or upon removal of the patch.

There have been very rare reports of anaphylactic and anaphylactoid reaction, including Stevens-Johnson syndrome, airway constriction, swelling, anaphylactic shock, and two deaths that occurred within 24 hours of the anaphylactic reaction. In one case, it was the care-giver of the patient who experienced dyspnea, urticaria and swelling, within ten minutes of applying the patch to the patient.

There have also been rare reports of convulsions, including clonic convulsions and grand mal convulsions. In two cases, vegetative state or coma was reported to immediately follow the convulsions.

Opioid withdrawal symptoms, such as nausea, vomiting, diarrhea, anxiety and shivering are possible in some patients after conversion from their previous opioid analgesic to ratio-FENTANYL or if therapy is stopped suddenly. There have been very rare reports of newborn infants experiencing neonatal withdrawal syndrome when mothers chronically used fentanyl transdermal systems during pregnancy (see Warnings and Precautions, Special Populations, Pregnant Women).

DRUG INTERACTIONS: Overview: Additive Effects of Other CNS Depressants: Hypoventilation, hypotension and profound sedation or coma may occur with the concomitant use of other central nervous system depressants (including other opioids, sedatives or hypnotics, general anesthetics, phenothiazines, tranquilizers); skeletal muscle relaxants, sedating antihistamines, and alcoholic beverages may produce additive depressant effects. When combined therapy is contemplated, the dose of each agent should be reduced by at least 50%.
Drug-Drug Interactions: CYP 3A4 Inhibitors: Fentanyl, a high clearance drug, is rapidly and extensively metabolized mainly by the human cytochrome P450 3A4 isoenzyme system (CYP3A4); therefore, potential interactions may occur when ratio-FENTANYL is given concurrently with agents that affect CYP3A4 activity. Coadministration with agents that **induce** 3A4 activity may reduce the efficacy of ratio-FENTANYL. The concomitant use of transdermal fentanyl with ritonavir or other potent **3A4 inhibitors** such as ketoconazole, itraconazole, troleandomycin, clarithromycin, nelfinavir, nefazodone, verapamil, diltiazem, amiodarone, amprenavir, fosamprenavir, aprepitant, fluconazole, erythromycin and grapefruit juice may result in an increase in fentanyl plasma concentrations which could increase or prolong adverse drug effects and may cause serious respiratory depression (see also Warnings and Precautions, Concomitant Use of CYP3A4 Inhibitors). In this situation, special patient care and observation are appropriate. The concomitant use of CYP3A4 inhibitors and ratio-FENTANYL is not recommended, unless the patient is closely monitored.
MAO Inhibitors: Severe and unpredictable potentiation by MAO inhibitors has been reported with opioid analgesics. Since the safety of fentanyl in this regard has not been established, the use of fentanyl in patients who have received MAO inhibitors during the previous 14-day period is not recommended. Conversely, the use of MAO inhibitors in patients who have received fentanyl in the previous 14-day period is not recommended.

DOSAGE AND ADMINISTRATION: **General: ratio-FENTANYL should only be prescribed by persons knowledgeable in the continuous administration of potent opioids, in the management of patients receiving potent opioids for treatment of pain and in the detection and management of respiratory depression including the use of opioid antagonists.**

At the time of the switch to ratio-FENTANYL from other opioids, patients must be tolerant to opioid therapy of comparable potency to that of the intended initiating dose. Use of ratio-FENTANYL in patients who are non-opioid-tolerant, or insufficiently tolerant, may lead to fatal respiratory depression.
Dosing Considerations: ratio-FENTANYL doses must be individualized based upon the status of each patient and should be assessed at regular intervals after application. Proper optimization of doses scaled to the relief of the individual's pain should aim at the regular administration of the lowest dose of ratio-FENTANYL which will achieve the overall treatment goal of satisfactory pain relief with acceptable side effects. Dosage of the drug must be individualized according to the response and tolerance of the patient. The most important factor to be considered in determining the appropriate dose is the extent of pre-existing opioid tolerance. Reduced doses of ratio-FENTANYL are suggested for the elderly and other groups discussed in Warnings and Precautions.

There has been no systematic evaluation of ratio-FENTANYL as an initial opioid analgesic in the management of chronic pain. Most patients in the clinical trials were converted to the fentanyl transdermal systems from other opioid therapies on which inadequate to moderate pain control had been experienced prior to conversion.

Initiation of ratio-FENTANYL in patients who are opioid-naïve is contraindicated at any dose (see Contraindications). The initial dose of ratio-FENTANYL should be obtained from the conversion tables in Dosage and Administration, and must not be higher than that dose which is equivalent to the total dose of opioids the patient is receiving at the time of the switch to the patch. It may be appropriate, according to clinical judgement, to initiate some patients on a lower ratio-FENTANYL dose than that which the conversion tables recommend, including the use of 12 µg/h dose by itself or in combination with another dose, provided the patient is not opioid-naïve (see Contraindications).

In general the 12 µg/h dose, which allows for smaller dose increases than does the 25 µg/h patch, is to be used for titration/adjustments of dosage (For oral morphine equivalency in dose adjustment, see Recommended Dose and Dosage Adjustment, Titration Dose Increment). The 12 µg/h dose is not included in the conversion table (Table 1 and Table 2) because it is generally not to be used as the initiating dose.

Opioid analgesics may be only partially effective in relieving dysesthetic pain, postherpetic neuralgia, stabbing pains, activity-related pain and some forms of headache. That is not to say that patients with these types of pain should not be given an adequate trial of opioid analgesics, but it may be necessary to refer such patients at an early time to other forms of pain therapy.

ratio-FENTANYL has a high potential for abuse and diversion (see Warnings and Precautions).
Concomitant Use of CYP3A4 Inhibitors: The concomitant use of ratio-FENTANYL with potent cytochrome P450 3A4 inhibitors (ritonavir, ketoconazole, itraconazole, troleandomycin, clarithromycin, nelfinavir, nefazodone, verapamil, diltiazem, amiodarone, amprenavir, fosamprenavir, aprepitant, fluconazole, erythromycin and grapefruit juice) may result in an increase in fentanyl plasma concentrations, which could increase or prolong adverse drug effects and may cause potentially fatal respiratory depression. Patients concomitantly exposed to ratio-FENTANYL and potent CYP3A4 inhibitors should be carefully monitored for an extended period of time and dosage adjustments should be made if warranted (see Drug Interactions).
Recommended Dose and Dosage Adjustment: Pediatrics: The use of ratio-FENTANYL in children under 18 years of age is not recommended as dosage requirements for the safe and efficacious use of fentanyl transdermal system have not been established for this patient population. Life-threatening hypoventilation has been reported in some pediatric patients receiving fentanyl transdermal system.

Adults: Initial Dose Selection: In selecting an initial ratio-FENTANYL dose, attention should be given to 1) the daily dose, potency, and characteristics of the opioid the patient has been taking previously (e.g. whether it is a pure agonist or mixed agonist-antagonist), 2) the reliability of the relative potency estimates used to calculate the ratio-FENTANYL dose needed (potency estimates may vary with the route of administration), 3) the degree of opioid tolerance, and 4) the general condition and medical status of the patient.

At the time of the switch to ratio-FENTANYL, patients must be tolerant to opioid therapy of comparable potency to that of the intended initiating dose. It may be appropriate, according to clinical judgment, to initiate some patients on a lower ratio-FENTANYL dose than that which the conversion tables recommend, which may include use of the 12 µg/h dose. The 12 µg/h dose is not included in the conversion tables (Table 1 and Table 2), because it is generally to be used for dose adjustment rather than as the initiation dose, except in the case of patients who, because of their clinical status, are to be initiated on a lower dose than that which the conversion tables recommend. Overestimating the ratio-FENTANYL dose when converting patients from another opioid medication can result in fatal overdose with the first dose. Due to the mean elimination half-life of 17 hours of ratio-FENTANYL, patients who are thought to have had a serious adverse event, including overdose, will require monitoring and treatment for at least 24 hours or until the adverse event has subsided.

To convert patients from oral or parenteral opioids to ratio-FENTANYL, refer to Table 1 (entitled: Dose Conversion Guidelines, to be used to convert from current opioid analgesic to the Fentanyl Transdermal Systems (FTS)). Alternatively, for patients taking opioids or doses not listed in Table 1, use Table 2 (entitled: Recommended Initial ratio-FENTANYL Dose Based Upon Daily Oral Morphine Dose).
Parenteral/Oral/Rectal Equianalgesic Potency Conversion: To convert adult patients from oral or parenteral opioids to ratio-FENTANYL, use Table 1.

Alternatively, for adult patients taking opioids or doses not listed in Table 1, use the following methodology:

1. Calculate the previous 24-hour analgesic requirement expressed in morphine equivalents.
2. Use Table 2 to convert this equianalgesic morphine dose to the recommended initial ratio-FENTANYL dose. **This conversion recommendation is intentionally conservative to minimize the potential for ratio-FENTANYL overdosage.**

For delivery rates in excess of 100 µg/h, multiple systems may be applied.

Because of the gradual increase in serum fentanyl concentration over the first 24 hours following initial system application, the initial evaluation of the maximum analgesic effect of ratio-FENTANYL cannot be made before 24 hours of wearing. Patients should use short-acting analgesics after the initial dose application as needed until analgesic efficacy with ratio-FENTANYL is attained.
Initial Dose Selection in Elderly, Cachectic, or Debilitated Patients: In patients from these populations, ratio-FENTANYL may have altered pharmacokinetics due to poor fat stores, muscle wasting or altered clearance. Therefore, it may be appropriate, according to clinical judgment, to initiate these patients on ratio-FENTANYL at a dose level lower than that which the conversion tables recommend, including the use of the 12 µg/h dose by itself or in combination with another dose, provided the patient is not opioid-naïve (see Contraindications). As with all ratio-FENTANYL patients, they should be carefully monitored for pain levels and adverse events, particularly hypoventilation.
Dosage Adjustment: Dose titration is the key to success with opioid analgesic therapy. The recommended initial ratio-FENTANYL dose based upon the daily morphine dose is conservative, and 50% of patients are likely to require a dose increase after initial application of ratio-FENTANYL. If analgesia is insufficient after the initial application, the first dosage increase should occur three days after application, while all subsequent dosage increases should occur six days following the previous application.
Initial Dosage Increase: The initial ratio-FENTANYL dosage may be increased after 3 days based on the daily dose of supplemental analgesics required by the patients in the second or third day of the initial application.
All Other Dosage Increases: Physicians are advised that it may take up to 6 days after increasing the dose of ratio-FENTANYL for the patient to reach equilibrium on the new dose. Therefore, patients should wear a higher dose through two applications before any further increase in dosage is made on the basis of the average daily use of a supplemental analgesic.
Titration Dose Increment: Dosage of ratio-FENTANYL must be individualized according to the pain relief and tolerance of the patient. Appropriate dosage increase increments should be based on the daily dose of supplementary opioids, using the ratio of 45-59 mg/24 hours of oral morphine to a 12 µg/h increase in ratio-FENTANYL dose. For example, if at the end of the required 6-day duration with a new patch strength, a patient is consuming an average daily dose of 150 mg of oral morphine, then the recommended ratio-FENTANYL dose increase would be 3×12 µg/h, which can be achieved by three 12 µg/h patches, or one of 25 µg/h and one of 12 µg/h. The use of 12 µg/h in the ratio for calculation of ratio-FENTANYL dose increases allows for achieving smaller increments when needed, i.e. increments that are as close as possible to the actual average amount of supplementary oral morphine. Some patients may continue to require periodic supplemental doses of short-acting analgesic for "breakthrough" pain.
Maintenance: The majority of patients are adequately maintained with ratio-FENTANYL administered every 72 hours. A small number of patients may not achieve adequate analgesia using this dosing interval and may require systems to be applied every 48 hours rather than every 72 hours. If breakthrough pain repeatedly occurs at the end of the dosing interval, it is generally an indication for a dosage increase rather than more frequent administration. An increase in the ratio-FENTANYL dose should be considered before changing dosing intervals in order to maintain patients on a 72-hour regimen.

Some patients may require additional or alternative methods of opioid administration when the ratio-FENTANYL dose exceeds 300 µg/h.
Decreased Dosing or Discontinuation of ratio-FENTANYL: Following the successful relief of severe pain, periodic attempts should be made to reduce the opioid dose. Lower doses or complete discontinuation of the opioid analgesic may become feasible due to physiological change or improved mental state of the patient.

Opioid withdrawal symptoms, such as nausea, vomiting, diarrhea, anxiety and shivering, are possible in some patients after conversion or dose decrease. For patients requiring discontinuation of opioids, a gradual downward titration is recommended since it is not known at what dose level the opioid may be discontinued without producing the signs and symptoms of abrupt withdrawal (see Dosage Adjustment, Titration Dose Increment).

For all downward titration, it is important to note that it takes 17 hours or more for the fentanyl serum concentration to fall by 50% after system removal.
Safe Use of Table 1 and Table 2: To convert patients to another opioid, remove ratio-FENTANYL and titrate the dose of the new analgesic, based upon the patient's report of pain, until adequate analgesia has been attained.

Table 1 and Table 2 should not be used to convert from ratio-FENTANYL to other opioid therapies. Because the conversion to ratio-FENTANYL is conservative, use of Table 1 and Table 2 for conversion to other analgesic therapies can overestimate the dose of the new agent. Overdosage of the new analgesic agent is possible.

Table 1: [a]ratio-FENTANYL

Dose Conversion Guidelines, To be Used to Convert From Current Opioid Analgesic to the Fentanyl Transdermal Systems (FTS)

Current Analgesic	Daily Dosage (mg/d)						
Oral morphine	60–134	135–179	180–224	225–269	270–314	315–359	360–404
IM/IV morphine (based on a 1:3 IM:PO ratio)	20–44	45–60	61–75	76–90	NA[b]	NA[b]	NA[b]
Oral oxycodone	30–66	67–90	91–112	113–134	135–157	158–179	180–202
Oral codeine	150–447	448–597	598–747	748–897	898–1047	1048–1197	1198–1347
Oral hydromorphone	8–16	17–22	23–28	29–33	34–39	40–45	46–51

(cont'd)

Table 1: [a]ratio-FENTANYL (cont'd)

Dose Conversion Guidelines, To be Used to Convert From Current Opioid Analgesic to the Fentanyl Transdermal Systems (FTS)

Current Analgesic	Daily Dosage (mg/d)						
IV hydro-morphone[c]	4.0–8.4	8.5–11.4	11.5–14.4	14.5–16.5	16.6–19.5	19.6–22.5	22.6–25.5
	↓	↓	↓	↓	↓	↓	↓
Recom-mended Fentanyl Transder-mal Sys-tem (FTS) Dose	**25 µg/h**	**37 µg/h**	**50 µg/h**	**62 µg/h**	**75 µg/h**	**87 µg/h**	**100 µg/h**

[a] **Table 1 should not be used to convert from ratio-FENTANYL and other FTS to other therapies because this conversion to ratio-FENTANYL and other FTS is conservative. Use of Table 1 for conversion to other analgesic therapies can overestimate the dose of the new agent. Overdosage of the new analgesic agent is possible (see Dosage and Administration, Safe Use of Table 1 and Table 2).**

[b] NA (not applicable) reflects insufficient data available for guidance. If needed, prescribers should make these conversions very carefully and conservatively.

[c] The conversion ratio of parenteral hydromorphone to oral hydromorphone of 1:2 is based on clinical experience in patients with chronic pain. Reference: Parenteral Drug Therapy Manual, Vancouver General Hospital, Pharmaceutical Sciences Clinical Services. 2006: Available from: http://www.vhpharmsci.com/PDTM/APDX11.htm.

Table 2: [b]ratio-FENTANYL

Recommended Initial ratio-FENTANYL Dose Based Upon Daily Oral Morphine Dose[a]

	Oral 24-hour morphine (mg/day)	ratio-FENTANYL Dose (µg/h)
Dose Adjustment	45–59	12
Initiation Dose	60–134	25
	135–179	25+12
	180–224	50
	225–269	50+12
	270–314	75
	315–359	75+12
	360–404	100
	405–494	125
	495–584	150
	585–674	175
	675–764	200
	765–854	225
	855–944	250
	945–1034	275
	1035–1124	300

[a] In clinical trials these ranges of chronic daily oral morphine doses were used as a basis for conversion to fentanyl transdermal system (see Recommended Dose and Dosage Adjustment, Dosage Adjustment).

[b] 12 µg/h dose is included in this table for dose adjustment. 12 µg/h dose generally should not be used as the initiating dose, except in the case of patients for whom clinical judgment deems it appropriate to start ratio-FENTANYL at less than 25 µg/h; ratio-FENTANYL at any dose is contraindicated in opioid-naïve patients (see Contraindications).

Administration: Application of ratio-FENTANYL Patch: ratio-FENTANYL should be applied to non-irritated and non-irradiated skin on a flat surface such as the chest, back, flank, or upper arm. Hair at the application site should be clipped (not shaved) prior to application. If the site of ratio-FENTANYL application must be cleansed prior to application of the system, do so with clear water. Do not use soaps, oils, lotions, alcohol, or any other agents that might irritate the skin or alter its characteristics. Allow the skin to dry completely prior to system application.

ratio-FENTANYL should be applied immediately upon removal from the sealed package. The system should not be altered, e.g. cut, in any way prior to its application. The transdermal system should be pressed firmly in place with the palm of the hand for 30 seconds, making sure the contact is complete, especially around the edges.

Each ratio-FENTANYL system may be worn continuously for 72 hours. A new system should be applied on a different skin site after removal of the previous transdermal system.

Disposal of ratio-FENTANYL Patch: Used systems should be folded so that the adhesive side of the system adheres to itself, then flushed down the toilet immediately upon removal (see Special Handling Instructions).

OVERDOSAGE:

Symptoms: The manifestations of fentanyl overdosage are an extension of its pharmacologic actions with the most serious effect being respiratory depression.

Treatment: For management of respiratory depression, immediate countermeasures include removing ratio-FENTANYL and physically or verbally stimulating the patient. These actions can be followed by administration of a specific opioid antagonist such as naloxone. The duration of respiratory depression following an overdose may be longer than the effects of the opioid antagonist's action (the half-life of naloxone ranges from 30 to 81 minutes). The interval between IV antagonist doses should be carefully chosen because of the possibility of re-narcotization after system removal; repeated administration of naloxone may be necessary. Reversal of the opioid effect may result in acute onset of pain and release of catecholamines.

If the clinical situation warrants, establish and maintain a patent airway, administer oxygen and assist or control respiration as indicated, and use an oropharyngeal airway or endotracheal tube if necessary. If depressed respiration is associated with muscular rigidity, an intravenous neuromuscular blocking agent may be required to facilitate assisted or controlled respiration. Adequate body temperature and fluid intake should be maintained.

If severe or persistent hypotension occurs, the possibility of hypovolemia should be considered, and managed with appropriate parenteral fluid therapy.

For management of a suspected drug overdose, contact your regional Poison Control Centre immediately. See the *CPS* Directory section for a list of Poison Control Centres.

ACTION AND CLINICAL PHARMACOLOGY: Pharmacodynamics: Fentanyl is an opioid analgesic which interacts predominantly with the µ-opioid receptor. Fentanyl produces analgesia, sedation, respiratory depression, constipation, and physical dependence but appears to have less emetic activity than other opioid analgesics. Fentanyl may produce muscle rigidity, miosis, cough reflex suppression, alterations in mood, bradycardia and bronchoconstriction.

Analgesic blood levels of fentanyl may cause nausea and vomiting directly by stimulating the chemoreceptor trigger zone, but nausea and vomiting are significantly more common in ambulatory than in recumbent patients, as is postural syncope.

Opioids increase the tone and decrease the propulsive contractions of the smooth muscle of the gastrointestinal tract. The resultant prolongation in gastrointestinal transit time may be responsible for the constipating effect of fentanyl. Because opioids may increase biliary tract pressure, some patients with biliary colic may experience worsening rather than relief of pain.

While opioids generally increase the tone of urinary tract smooth muscle, the net effect tends to be variable, in some cases producing urinary urgency, in others, difficulty in urination.

At therapeutic dosages, fentanyl usually does not exert major effects on the cardiovascular system. However, some patients may exhibit orthostatic hypotension and fainting.

Histamine assays and skin wheal testing in man indicate that histamine release rarely occurs with fentanyl. Assays in man show no clinically significant histamine release in dosages up to 50 µg/kg.

Both the minimum effective concentration and the concentration at which toxicity occurs rise with increasing tolerance. The rate of development of tolerance varies widely among individuals.

Pharmacokinetics: ratio-FENTANYL provides continuous systemic delivery of fentanyl for up to 72 hours. Fentanyl is released along the concentration gradient existing between the drug adhesive layer of the system and the lower concentration in the skin.

Adults: Fentanyl Transdermal System: Absorption: Following initial ratio-FENTANYL administration, serum fentanyl concentrations increase gradually, generally levelling off between 12 and 24 hours and remaining relatively constant for the remainder of the 72-hour application period. Peak serum levels of fentanyl generally occur between 24 and 72 hours after the first application.

Serum fentanyl concentrations achieved are proportional to the ratio-FENTANYL delivery rate (see Table 3). With continuous use, serum fentanyl concentrations continue to rise for the first few system applications. After several sequential 72-hour applications, patients reach and maintain a steady-state serum concentration that is determined by individual variation in skin permeability and body clearance of fentanyl.

Table 3: ratio-FENTANYL

Pharmacokinetic Parameters of a Fentanyl Transdermal System in Adults

	Mean (SD) Maximal Concentration C_{max} (ng/mL)	Mean (SD) Time to Maximal Concentration T_{max} (h)
Fentanyl transdermal system 12 µg/h	0.3 (0.2)	27.5 (9.6)
Fentanyl transdermal system 25 µg/h	0.6 (0.3)	38.1 (18.0)
Fentanyl transdermal system 50 µg/h	1.4 (0.5)	34.8 (15.4)
Fentanyl transdermal system 75 µg/h	1.7 (0.7)	33.5 (14.5)
Fentanyl transdermal system 100 µg/h	2.5 (1.2)	36.8 (15.7)

After fentanyl transdermal system removal, serum fentanyl concentrations decline gradually, falling about 50% in approximately 17 (range 13-22) hours. Continued absorption of fentanyl from the skin accounts for a slower disappearance of the drug from the serum than is seen after an IV infusion, where the apparent half-life ranges from 3-12 hours.

Distribution: The average volume of distribution for fentanyl is 6 L/kg (range 3-8, n=8). The average clearance in patients undergoing various surgical procedures is 46 L/h (range 27-75, n=8). Mean values for unbound fractions of fentanyl in plasma are estimated to be between 13% and 21%.

Metabolism: Skin does not appear to metabolize fentanyl delivered transdermally. Fentanyl is metabolized primarily in the liver. In humans, the drug is metabolized primarily by N-dealkylation to norfentanyl and other inactive metabolites.

Excretion: Approximately 75% of an IV fentanyl dose is excreted in urine, mostly as metabolites, with less than 10% representing unchanged drug. Approximately 9% of the dose is recovered in the feces, primarily as metabolites.

Special Populations and Conditions: Pediatrics Under 18 Years of Age: In a pharmacokinetic study with non-opioid-tolerant patients, 8 children aged 1.5 to 5 years old on **25 µg/h** patches were compared to 8 adults on **50 µg/h** patches. The comparative "dose per mean body weight" i.e. µg/h/kg was 1.67 for children vs 0.67 for adults. Mean C_{max} was 50% higher in the children and mean AUC ~25% higher, with both mean T_{max} and mean half-life shorter (approx. 50% and 75% of the adult values, respectively). For 6 of the 8 children, there was no apparent plateau in plasma concentrations. Adjusting for either body weight or body surface area, clearance in pediatric subjects was found to be about 20%-40% higher than in adults.

Analyses of population pharmacokinetics data in pediatrics indicate that the variability in fentanyl AUC and C_{max} values at steady state (C_{ss}) correlated with changes in body surface area (BSA) values observed in subjects. An increase in BSA of 0.1 m^2 is predicted to result in a 4.8% increase in clearance and 4.6% decrease in C_{ss}.

Dosing recommendations for the safe and effective use of ratio-FENTANYL in this patient population have not been established, in view of the combination of:

i. the variety of factors which could lead to overexposure from ratio-FENTANYL in children as compared to adults (including smaller body weight and significantly different body surface area; differential skin characteristics; potential for magnification, compared to adults, of the impact of amount of body fat stores, muscle wasting, fever, external heat), and
ii. the limitations in both formal PK data (as above) and exposure data (see Adverse Reactions, Clinical Trial Adverse Drug Reactions, Chronic Pain Trials—Pediatrics).

Elderly or Debilitated patients: In elderly, cachectic, or debilitated patients, ratio-FENTANYL may have altered pharmacokinetics due to poor fat stores, muscle wasting or altered clearance. The clearance of fentanyl may be reduced, and the terminal half-life prolonged (see Dosage and Administration).

Hepatic Insufficiency: No data available.

Renal Insufficiency: No data available.

STORAGE AND STABILITY: ratio-FENTANYL is stable for 2 years from date of manufacturing when stored in sealed pouch between 15 and 25°C.

SPECIAL HANDLING INSTRUCTIONS: ratio-FENTANYL should be kept out of the reach of children before and after use.

Do not cut ratio-FENTANYL patches.

Used systems should be folded so that the adhesive side of the system adheres to itself, then flushed down the toilet immediately upon removal. If the drug adhesive layer accidentally contacts the skin, the area should be washed with clear water. Do not use soap, alcohol or other solvents as they may enhance the drug's ability to penetrate the skin. Patients should dispose of any systems remaining from a prescription as soon as they are no longer needed. Unused systems should be removed from their protective pouch, folded so that the adhesive side of the patch adheres to itself, and flushed down the toilet.

Wash hands, with water only, after applying or removing the patch.

INFORMATION FOR THE PATIENT: Published in e-CPS, available by subscription at www.e-cps.ca.

DOSAGE FORMS, COMPOSITION AND PACKAGING: ratio-FENTANYL is a transdermal patch providing continuous systemic delivery of fentanyl, a potent opioid analgesic, for 72 hours.

ratio-FENTANYL is a rectangular unit comprising a release liner, adhesive drug containing matrix, a backing and a cover sheet. Proceeding from the outer surface toward the surface adhering to the skin, ratio-FENTANYL is made up of: 1) the cover sheet which comprises Polyethyleneterepthalate (PET or PETP) foil, with one side siliconized, 2) a backing made of Trespaphane which is in contact with the self adhesive drug containing matrix, 3) a self adhesive drug containing the matrix of Fentanyl, Polybutyltitanate, and Duro-Tak. 4) A peelable release liner covering the adhesive layer must be removed before the system can be applied. The protective liner comprises Polyethyleneterepthalate (siliconized on the one side in contact with the matrix) and is printed with blue ink.

ratio-FENTANYL is available in five different strengths. Each system is labelled with a nominal flux which represents the average amount of drug delivered to the systemic circulation per hour across average skin. The active component of the system is fentanyl. The amount of fentanyl released from each system per hour is proportional to the surface area (25 µg/h per 7.5 cm^2). The 3.75, 7.5, 15, 22.5 and 30 cm^2 systems are designed to deliver 12, 25, 50, 75 or 100 µg/h fentanyl to the systemic circulation, representing approximately 0.3, 0.6, 1.2, 1.8 or 2.4 mg per day, respectively. The remaining components are pharmacologically inactive. The composition per unit area of all system sizes is identical.

Total fentanyl contents and system sizes for the five strengths are summarized in Table 4.

Table 4: ratio-FENTANYL

Total Fentanyl Contents and System Sizes for the Five Strengths

System	Nominal Fentanyl Delivery Rate (µg/h)	Total Fentanyl Content (mg)	System Size (cm^2)	System Dimensions (without release liner)	Print in blue ink on backing film (outside layer of system)
ratio-FENTANYL 12	12.5	2.063	3.75	20×20 mm	"fentanyl 12 µg/h"
ratio-FENTANYL 25	25	4.125	7.5	30×26 mm	"ratio-fentanyl 25 µg/h"
ratio-FENTANYL 50	50	8.25	15	30×51 mm	"ratio-fentanyl 50 µg/h"
ratio-FENTANYL 75	75	12.375	22.5	47.5×48 mm	"ratio-fentanyl 75 µg/h"
ratio-FENTANYL 100	100	16.5	30	47.5×64 mm	"ratio-fentanyl 100 µg/h"

ratio-FENTANYL is supplied in cartons containing 5 individually packaged systems.

ratio-Finasteride ℞
finasteride
Type II Alpha-reductase Inhibitor

ratiopharm

SUPPLIED: Each blue, rounded triangle shaped, film-coated tablet, with "RG" on one side, contains: finasteride 5 mg. Nonmedicinal ingredients: FD&C blue No. 2, hydroxypropyl cellulose, hypromellose, lactose monohydrate, macrogol, magnesium stearate, microcrystalline cellulose, pregelatinised starch, sodium starch glycolate, talc and titanium dioxide. Blisters of 30. HDPE bottles of 100. Store between 15 and 30°C and protect from light to prevent discoloration.

ratio-Fluoxetine ℞
fluoxetine HCl
Antidepressant—Antiobsessional—Antibulimic

ratiopharm

SUPPLIED: 10 mg: Each grey and green capsule, filled with white powder, imprinted in black ink with "TEC 137A", contains: fluoxetine HCl 11.18 mg equivalent to fluoxetine base 10 mg. Nonmedicinal ingredients: black ink, black iron oxide, D&C Yellow #10, FD&C Blue #1, FD&C Yellow #6, gelatin, pregelatinized cornstarch, silicon dioxide, sodium lauryl sulfate and titanium dioxide. HDPE bottles of 100.
20 mg: Each ivory and green capsule, filled with white powder, imprinted in black ink with "TEC 137B", contains: fluoxetine HCl 22.36 mg equivalent to fluoxetine base 20 mg. Nonmedicinal ingredients: black ink, D&C Yellow #10, FD&C Blue #1, FD&C Yellow #6, gelatin, pregelatinized cornstarch, silicon dioxide, sodium lauryl sulfate and titanium dioxide. HDPE bottles of 100 and 500.

Store between 15 and 30°C. Keep tightly closed. Protect from light.

> The reader is invited to consult CPhA's monograph **Corticosteroids: Eye, Ear, Nose.**

ratio-Fluticasone ℞
fluticasone propionate
Corticosteroid for Nasal Use

ratiopharm

SUPPLIED: Each 100 mg of spray delivered by the nasal adaptor (1 actuation), contains: micronised fluticasone propionate 50 µg. Nonmedicinal ingredients: benzalkonium chloride, dextrose, microcrystalline cellulose and carboxymethylcellulose sodium, phenylethyl alcohol, polysorbate 80 and purified water. Amber glass bottles containing sufficient formulation for 120 metered sprays (16 g net weight). Store between 4 and 30°C. Shake gently before use.

> The reader is invited to consult CPhA's monograph **Selective Serotonin Reuptake Inhibitors.**

ratio-Fluvoxamine ℞
fluvoxamine maleate
Antidepressant—Antiobsessional

ratiopharm

SUPPLIED: 50 mg: Each biconvex, round, scored, film-coated, white to off-white tablet, symbol "s" on one side and on the other side "291" on both sides of the score, contains: fluvoxamine maleate 50 mg. Nonmedicinal ingredients: colloidal anhydrous silica, hydroxypropyl methylcellulose, maize starch, mannitol, polyethylene glycol, pregelatinized starch, sodium stearyl fumarate, talc and titanium dioxide. Gluten-, lactose-, sodium metabisulfite- and tartrazine-free. Bottles of 100.
100 mg: Each biconvex, oval, scored, film-coated, white to off-white tablet, symbol "s" on one side and on the other side "313" on both sides of the score, contains: fluvoxamine maleate 100 mg. Nonmedicinal ingredients: colloidal anhydrous silica, hydroxypropyl methylcellulose, maize starch, mannitol, polyethylene glycol, pregelatinized starch, sodium stearyl fumarate, talc and titanium dioxide. Gluten-, lactose-, sodium metabisulfite- and tartrazine-free. Bottles of 100.

Preserve in well closed containers. Store in a dry place between 0 and 30°C.

ratio-Gabapentin ℞
gabapentin
Antiepileptic

ratiopharm

SUPPLIED: Capsules: 100 mg: Each hard gelatin Coni-Snap capsule with white opaque body and cap, printed "rph" on one side and "G43" on the other in blue ink, contains: gabapentin 100 mg. Nonmedicinal ingredients: cornstarch, lactose and talc; capsule shell: gelatin, silicon dioxide, sodium lauryl sulfate and titanium dioxide, may contain red iron oxide and yellow iron oxide. Bottles of 100 and 500. Keep out of the reach of children. Store at controlled room temperature 15-30°C.
300 mg: Each hard gelatin Coni-Snap capsule with yellow opaque body and cap, printed "rph" on one side and "G42" on the other in blue ink, contains: gabapentin 300 mg. Nonmedicinal ingredients: cornstarch, lactose and talc; capsule shell: gelatin, silicon dioxide, sodium lauryl sulfate and titanium dioxide, may contain red iron oxide and yellow iron oxide. Bottles of 100 and 500. Keep out of the reach of children. Store at controlled room temperature 15-30°C.
400 mg: Each hard gelatin Coni-Snap capsule with orange opaque body and cap, printed "rph" on one side and "G41" on the other in blue ink, contains: gabapentin 400 mg. Nonmedicinal ingredients: cornstarch, lactose and talc, capsule shell: gelatin, silicon dioxide, sodium lauryl sulfate and titanium dioxide, may contain red iron oxide and yellow iron oxide. Bottles of 100 and 500. Keep out of the reach of children. Store at controlled room temperature 15-30°C.
Tablets: 600 mg: Each white to off-white, elliptical in shape, film-coated tablet, embossed "rph" on one side and "G32" on the other side, contains: gabapentin 600 mg. Nonmedicinal ingredients: carnauba wax, copovidone, dehydrated alcohol, hydroxypropyl cellulose, hydroxypropyl methylcellulose, magnesium stearate, microcrystalline cellulose, polyethylene glycol, sodium starch glycolate and talc. Bottles of 100 and 500. Keep out of the reach of children. Store at controlled room temperature 15-30°C.
800 mg: Each white to off-white, elliptical in shape, film-coated tablet, embossed "rph" on one side and "G31" on the other side, contains: gabapentin 800 mg. Nonmedicinal ingredients: carnauba wax, copovidone, dehydrated alcohol, hydroxypropyl cellulose, hydroxypropyl methylcellulose, magnesium stearate, microcrystalline cellulose, polyethylene glycol, sodium starch glycolate and talc. Bottles of 100. Keep out of the reach of children. Store at controlled room temperature 15-30°C.

ratio-Gentamicin ℞
gentamicin sulfate
Topical Antibiotic

ratiopharm

SUPPLIED: Cream: Each g of homogeneous white cream, odorless, contains: gentamicin (as sulfate USP) 1 mg (0.1%). Nonmedicinal ingredients: cetyl alcohol, chlorocresol, glyceryl stearate, heavy mineral oil, polysorbate 60, polysorbate 80, propylene glycol and purified water. Tubes of 15 g. Store between 15 and 30°C.
Ointment: Each g of homogeneous yellowish ointment with a characteristic odor, contains: gentamicin (as sulfate USP) 1 mg (0.1%). Nonmedicinal ingredients: light mineral oil, methylparaben, petrolatum and propylparaben. Tubes of 15 g. Store between 15 and 30°C.

> The reader is invited to consult CPhA's monograph **Sulfonylureas.**

ratio-Glimepiride ℞
glimepiride
Oral Hypoglycemic Agent (Sulfonylurea)

ratiopharm

SUPPLIED: 1 mg: Each pink, flat-faced, oblong tablet with notched sides at the bisect imprinted with "W" on one side of the bisect and "03" on the other side of the bisect and plain on both sides of the bisect on the other side, contains: glimepiride 1 mg. Nonmedicinal ingredients: ferric oxide. Bottles of 30. Store between 15 and 30°C. Dispense in well-closed container.
2 mg: Each green, flat-faced, oblong tablet with notched sides at the bisect imprinted with "W" on one side of the bisect and "03" on the other side of the bisect and plain on both sides of the bisect on the other side, contains: glimepiride 2 mg. Nonmedicinal ingredients: FD&C Blue #2 Aluminum Lake and ferric oxide. Bottles of 30. Store between 15 and 30°C. Dispense in well-closed container.
4 mg: Each blue, flat-faced, oblong tablet with notched sides at the bisect imprinted with "W" on one side of the bisect and "03" on the other side of the bisect and plain on both sides of the bisect on the other side, contains: glimepiride 4 mg. Nonmedicinal ingredient: FD&C Blue #2 Aluminum Lake. Bottles of 30. Store between 15 and 30°C. Dispense in well-closed container.

> The reader is invited to consult CPhA's monograph **Sulfonylureas.**

ratio-Glyburide ℞
glyburide
Oral Hypoglycemic Agent

ratiopharm

SUPPLIED: 2.5 mg: Each white, cylindrical, biplane tablet, with a face with a scored-line and an embossed "GLY" on each side of the scored-line and the other face, an embossed "A" in a debossed circle in an embossed square, contains: glyburide 2.5 mg. Nonmedicinal ingredients: colloidal silicon dioxide, cornstarch, lactose hydrous, magnesium stearate, purified water and talc. Plastic bottles of 300.
5 mg: Each almost white, oblong, biplane tablet, with a face with a scored-line and an embossed "5" on one side of the score and on the other side, an embossed "A" in a debossed circle in an embossed square, contains: glyburide 5 mg. Nonmedicinal ingredients: colloidal silicon dioxide, cornstarch, lactose hydrous, magnesium stearate, purified water and talc. Cartons of 30 (3×10 blister packed) or plastic bottles of 300.

Store at room temperature, below 25°C.

ratio-Hemcort-HC ℞
hydrocortisone acetate—zinc sulfate monohydrate
Anorectal Therapy

ratiopharm

SUPPLIED: Ointment: Each g of transparent, homogeneous, smooth white odorless ointment, contains: hydrocortisone acetate 0.5% and zinc sulfate monohydrate 0.5%. Nonmedicinal ingredients: light mineral oil and petrolatum. Tubes of 15 and 30 g with applicator.
Suppositories: Each homogeneous, smooth white odorless suppository, contains: hydrocortisone acetate 10 mg and zinc sulfate monohydrate 10 mg. Nonmedicinal ingredients: semisynthetic glycerides. Boxes of 12.

Store between 15 and 30°C.

ratio-Indomethacin ℙ
indomethacin
Anti-inflammatory—Analgesic

ratiopharm

SUPPLIED: Each yellowish to beige torpedo-shaped suppository with a homogeneous texture, smooth surfaced without crumbling, contains: indomethacin USP 100 mg. Nonmedicinal ingredients: butylated hydroxyanisole, butylated hydroxytoluene, EDTA, glycerin, polyethylene glycol and sodium chloride. Boxes of 30. Store below 30°C. Protect from light and elevated humidity. Keep away from excessive heat. Preserve in well-closed containers, at controlled room temperature.

ratio-Ipra Sal UDV ℙ
ipratropium bromide—salbutamol sulfate
Bronchodilator

ratiopharm

SUPPLIED: Each single dose unit of clear, colourless or almost colourless liquid, free from suspended particles, filled into a polyethylene unit-dose vial (UDV), contains: ipratropium bromide anhydrous 0.5 mg (as monohydrate) and salbutamol sulfate 3 mg (equivalent to 2.5 mg salbutamol base) in a 2.5 mL isotonic preservative-free solution for inhalation. Nonmedicinal ingredients: hydrochloric acid, purified water and sodium chloride. Plastic single dose units, strips of 10. Unopened unit dose vials should be stored at controlled room temperature (between 15 and 25°C) and protected from light and heat. Do not use if solution is discoloured. Keep out of reach of children.

ratio-Ipratropium ℙ
ipratropium bromide
Bronchodilator

ratiopharm

ratio-Ipratropium UDV ℙ
ipratropium bromide
Bronchodilator

ratiopharm

SUPPLIED: ratio-Ipratropium: Each mL of clear, colorless or almost colorless solution contains: ipratropium bromide 250 µg (0.025%). Nonmedicinal ingredients: benzalkonium chloride, edetate disodium, purified water and sodium chloride. Amber glass bottles of 20 mL with screwcap.
ratio-Ipratropium UDV: 125 µg/mL: Each mL of clear, colorless or almost colorless solution contains: ipratropium bromide 125 µg (0.0125%). Nonmedicinal ingredients: hydrochloric acid, purified water and sodium chloride. Plastic single use vials of 2 mL.
250 µg/mL: Each mL of clear, colorless or almost colorless solution contains: ipratropium bromide 250 µg (0.025%). Nonmedicinal ingredients: hydrochloric acid, purified water and sodium chloride. Plastic single use vials of 1 and 2 mL.

ratio-Ketorolac ℙ
ketorolac tromethamine
Anti-inflammatory

ratiopharm

SUPPLIED: Each bottle of ophthalmic solution contains: ketorolac tromethamine 0.5%. Nonmedicinal ingredients: benzalkonium chloride solution (50% aqueous solution), edetate disodium, octoxynol 40 (70% aqueous solution), purified water, sodium chloride and sodium hydroxide and/or hydrochloric acid solution to adjust to pH 7.4. White opaque plastic bottles of 5 and 10 mL with a controlled dropper tip. Store between 15 to 30 °C. Protect from light.

ratio-Lactulose
lactulose
Portal-systemic Encephalopathy Therapy—Laxative

ratiopharm

SUPPLIED: Each mL of orange, clear sirupy liquid contains: lactulose 667 mg. Nonmedicinal ingredients: FD&C Yellow #6 and purified water. Bottles of 500 mL and 1 L. Store between 15 and 30°C.

ratio-Lamotrigine ℙ
lamotrigine
Antiepileptic

ratiopharm

SUPPLIED: 25 mg: Each white, flat-faced, bevelled edges, shield-shaped tablet, engraved "ALTI" over "25" on one side and scored on the other side, contains: lamotrigine 25 mg. Nonmedicinal ingredients: cellulose, lactose, magnesium stearate, povidone and sodium starch glycolate. Bottles of 100. Store between 15-30°C, in a dry place and protected from light.
100 mg: Each peach, flat-faced, bevelled edges, shield-shaped tablet, engraved "ALTI" over "100" on one side and scored on the other side, contains: lamotrigine 100 mg. Nonmedicinal ingredients: cellulose, lactose, magnesium stearate, povidone, sodium starch glycolate and sunset Yellow FCF Lake. Bottles of 100. Store between 15-30°C, in a dry place and protected from light.
150 mg: Each cream, flat-faced, bevelled edges, scored, shield-shaped tablet, engraved "ALTI" over "150" on one side and scored on the other side, contains: lamotrigine 150 mg. Nonmedicinal ingredients: cellulose, ferric oxide yellow, lactose, magnesium stearate, povidone and sodium starch glycolate. Bottles of 60. Store between 15-30°C, in a dry place and protected from light.

ratio-Lenoltec No. 1, 2 & 3 Ⓝ
acetaminophen—caffeine—codeine phosphate
Analgesic—Antipyretic

ratiopharm

ratio-Lenoltec No. 4 Ⓝ
acetaminophen—codeine phosphate
Analgesic—Antipyretic

ratiopharm

SUPPLIED: ratio-Lenoltec No. 1: Caplets: Each white, oblong, biconvex caplet, engraved TEC and 1 on one side, reverse side plain, contains: acetaminophen 300 mg, caffeine 15 mg and codeine phosphate 8 mg. Nonmedicinal ingredients: colloidal silicon dioxide, crospovidone, magnesium stearate, microcrystalline cellulose, povidone, pregelatinized cornstarch, sodium croscarmellose and stearic acid. Bottles of 30, 100 and 200.
Tablets: Each round, white, biplane tablet with beveled edges, engraved TEC and 1 on one side, reverse side plain, contains: acetaminophen 300 mg, caffeine 15 mg and codeine phosphate 8 mg. Nonmedicinal ingredients: colloidal silicon dioxide, crospovidone, magnesium stearate, microcrystalline cellulose, povidone, pregelatinized cornstarch, sodium croscarmellose and stearic acid. Bottles of 100.
ratio-Lenoltec No. 2: Each round, white, biplane tablet with beveled edges, engraved TEC and 2 on one side, reverse side plain, contains: acetaminophen 300 mg, caffeine 15 mg and codeine phosphate 15 mg. Nonmedicinal ingredients: colloidal silicon dioxide, crospovidone, magnesium stearate, microcrystalline cellulose, povidone, pregelatinized cornstarch, sodium croscarmellose and stearic acid. Bottles of 500.
ratio-Lenoltec No. 3: Each round, white, biplane tablet with beveled edges, engraved TEC and 3 on one side, reverse side plain, contains: acetaminophen 300 mg, caffeine 15 mg and codeine phosphate 30 mg. Nonmedicinal ingredients: colloidal silicon dioxide, crospovidone, magnesium stearate, microcrystalline cellulose, povidone, pregelatinized cornstarch, sodium croscarmellose and stearic acid. Bottles of 500.
ratio-Lenoltec No. 4: Each round, white, biplane tablet with beveled edges, engraved TEC and 4 on one side, reverse side plain, contains: acetaminophen 300 mg and codeine phosphate 60 mg. Nonmedicinal ingredients: colloidal silicon dioxide, crospovidone, magnesium stearate, microcrystalline cellulose, povidone, pregelatinized cornstarch, sodium croscarmellose and stearic acid. Bottles of 100.

Alcohol-, gluten-, paraben-, sucrose-, sulfite- and tartrazine-free. Keep bottle tightly closed. Store at room temperature. Do not use if neckband is damaged.

ratio-Levobunolol ℙ
levobunolol HCl
Glaucoma Therapy

ratiopharm

SUPPLIED: 0.25%: Each mL of sterile, ophthalmic solution contains: levobunolol HCl 2.5 mg. Nonmedicinal ingredients: benzalkonium chloride 0.004% (as preservative), edetate disodium, polyvinyl alcohol (Liquifilm), potassium phosphate monobasic, sodium chloride, sodium metabisulfite, sodium phosphate dibasic and sodium hydroxide or hydrochloric acid to adjust pH. Plastic dropper bottles of 10 mL.
0.5%: Each mL of sterile, ophthalmic solution contains: levobunolol HCl 5 mg. Nonmedicinal ingredients: benzalkonium chloride 0.004% (as preservative), edetate disodium, polyvinyl alcohol (Liquifilm), potassium phosphate monobasic, sodium chloride, sodium metabisulfite, sodium phosphate dibasic and sodium hydroxide or hydrochloric acid to adjust pH. Plastic dropper bottles of 5, 10 and 15 mL.

Protect from light and excessive heat.

The reader is invited to consult CPhA's monograph **ACE Inhibitors**.

ratio-Lisinopril P ℙ
lisinopril
Angiotensin Converting Enzyme Inhibitor

ratiopharm

SUPPLIED: 5 mg: Each white, shield-shaped, compressed tablet, with "rph" on one side and "L63" on the other, contains: lisinopril 5 mg. Nonmedicinal ingredients: dibasic calcium phosphate dihydrate, lactose monohydrate, magnesium stearate, povidone and pregelatinized starch. Bottles of 100 and 500. Blister packages of 30. Store at room temperature between 15 and 25°C. Protect from moisture and humidity.
10 mg: Each yellow, shield-shaped, compressed tablet, with "rph" on one side and "L62" on the other, contains: lisinopril 10 mg. Nonmedicinal ingredients: dibasic calcium phosphate dihydrate, lactose monohydrate, magnesium stearate, povidone, pregelatinized starch and yellow iron oxide. Bottles of 100 and 500. Blister packages of 30. Store at room temperature between 15 and 25°C. Protect from moisture and humidity.
20 mg: Each peach, shield-shaped, compressed tablet, with "rph" on one side and "L61" on the other, contains: lisinopril 20 mg. Nonmedicinal ingredients: dibasic calcium phosphate dihydrate, lactose monohydrate, magnesium stearate, povidone, pregelatinized starch, red iron oxide and yellow iron oxide. Bottles of 100 and 500. Blister packages of 30. Store at room temperature between 15 and 25°C. Protect from moisture and humidity.

The reader is invited to consult CPhA's monograph **ACE Inhibitors**.

ratio-Lisinopril Z ℙ
lisinopril
Angiotensin Converting Enzyme Inhibitor

ratiopharm

SUPPLIED: 5 mg: Each pink, round tablet, scored on one side and marked "rph L53" on the other side, contains: lisinopril 5 mg. Nonmedicinal ingredients: dibasic calcium phosphate dihydrate, lactose monohydrate, magnesium stearate, povidone, pregelatinized starch and red iron oxide. Bottles of 100 and 500. Blister packages of 30. Store at room temperature (15 to 25°C). Protect from moisture and humidity.
10 mg: Each pink, round tablet, marked "rph" on one side and "L52" on the other side, contains: lisinopril 10 mg. Nonmedicinal ingredients: dibasic calcium phosphate dihydrate, lactose monohydrate, magnesium stearate, povidone, pregelatinized starch and red iron oxide. Bottles of 100 and 500. Blister packages of 30. Store at room temperature (15 to 25°C). Protect from moisture and humidity.
20 mg: Each pink, round tablet, marked "rph" on one side and "L51" on the other side, contains: lisinopril 20 mg. Nonmedicinal ingredients: dibasic calcium phosphate dihydrate, lactose monohydrate, magnesium stearate, povidone, pregelatinized starch and red iron oxide. Bottles of 100 and 500. Blister packages of 30. Store at room temperature (15 to 25°C). Protect from moisture and humidity.

The reader is invited to consult CPhA's monograph **HMG-CoA Reductase Inhibitors**.

ratio-Lovastatin Ⓟ
lovastatin
Lipid Metabolism Regulator

ratiopharm

SUPPLIED: 20 mg: Each light blue colored, octagon-shaped, biconvex, film-coated tablet, scored on one side, and "TEC" on the other side, contains: lovastatin 20 mg. Nonmedicinal ingredients: butylhydroxyanisole, FD&C Blue No. 2 lake, hydroxypropylcellulose, hydroxypropyl methylcellulose, lactose anhydrous, magnesium stearate, microcrystalline cellulose, pregelatinized cornstarch, talc and titanium dioxide. Bottles of 100 and 500.
40 mg: Each mint green colored, octagon-shaped, biconvex, film-coated tablet, plain on one side, and "TEC" on the other side, contains: lovastatin 40 mg. Nonmedicinal ingredients: butylhydroxyanisole, D&C Yellow No. 10 lake, FD&C Blue No. 1 lake, hydroxypropylcellulose, hydroxypropyl methylcellulose, lactose anhydrous, magnesium stearate, microcrystalline cellulose, pregelatinized cornstarch, talc and titanium dioxide. Bottles of 100.
Keep container tightly closed and store between 15 to 30°C. Protect from light.

ratio-Meloxicam Ⓟ
meloxicam
Anti-inflammatory—Analgesic

ratiopharm

SUPPLIED: 7.5 mg: Each round, biconvex, pastel yellow tablet, identified with "rph" on one side and "306X" on the other side, contains: meloxicam 7.5 mg. Nonmedicinal ingredients: anhydrous colloidal silica, crospolyvidone, lactose, magnesium stearate, microcrystalline cellulose, polyvidone and sodium citrate. Bottles of 100 and 500. Keep out of the reach of children. Store at 15-30°C. Store in a dry place.
15 mg: Each round, pastel yellow snap-tab tablet, impressed with "306Y" on both sides of a broad score line on its concave side and "rph" on the convex side, contains: meloxicam 15 mg. Nonmedicinal ingredients: anhydrous colloidal silica, crospolyvidone, lactose, magnesium stearate, microcrystalline cellulose, polyvidone and sodium citrate. Bottles of 100 and 500. Keep out of the reach of children. Store at 15-30°C. Store in a dry place.

ratio-Memantine Ⓟ
memantine HCl
N-methyl-D-aspartate (NMDA) Receptor Antagonist

ratiopharm

SUPPLIED: Each white to off-white, capsule shaped film-coated tablet, embossed with "rph" and a break line on one side and "M111" on the other side, contains: memantine hydrochloride 10 mg. Nonmedicinal ingredients: colloidal silicon dioxide, lactose anhydrous, lecithin (soya), magnesium stearate, microcrystalline cellulose, polysorbate, polyvinyl alcohol, pregelatinised starch, talc, titanium dioxide and xanthan gum. Bottles of 30 and 500. Store in a dry place at room temperature between 15 and 30°C. Protect from moisture.

ratio-Metformin Ⓟ
metformin HCl
Antihyperglycemic

ratiopharm

SUPPLIED: 500 mg: Each white, round, biconvex, film-coated tablet with a partial scored-line on one side and with "rph M12" on the other side, contains: metformin HCl 500 mg. Nonmedicinal ingredients: hydroxypropyl methylcellulose, magnesium stearate, maltodextrin, polyethylene glycol and povidone. Bottles of 100, 360 and 500. Store between 15 and 30°C in well-closed containers. Protect from light.
850 mg: Each white, oval, biconvex, film-coated tablet with "rph M11" on one side and plain on the other side, contains: metformin HCl 850 mg. Nonmedicinal ingredients: hydroxypropyl methylcellulose, magnesium stearate, maltodextrin, polyethylene glycol and povidone. Bottles of 100 and 500. Store between 15 and 30°C in well-closed containers. Protect from light.

ratio-Methotrexate Sodium Ⓟ
methotrexate sodium
Antimetabolite

ratiopharm

SUPPLIED: Each yellow, round, convex tablet, imprinted "M" and "l" on the scored side and 2.5 on the other side, contains: methotrexate sodium equivalent to methotrexate 2.5 mg. Nonmedicinal ingredients: cornstarch, lactose and magnesium stearate. Dye-free. Bottles of 100. Store between 15 to 30°C. Protect from light. Keep the container tightly closed. Keep out of reach of children.

The reader is invited to consult CPhA's monograph **Tetracyclines**.

ratio-Minocycline Ⓟ
minocycline HCl
Antibiotic

ratiopharm

SUPPLIED: 50 mg: Each opaque orange, hard-shell capsule, printed "AltiMed M2" and "MIN 50 mg", contains: minocycline HCl equivalent to minocycline 50 mg. Nonmedicinal ingredients: FD&C Blue #1, FD&C Yellow 6, gelatin, microcrystalline cellulose, silicon dioxide, sodium lauryl sulfate and titanium dioxide. Energy: <4.2 kJ (1 kcal). Tartrazine-free. Bottles of 100.
100 mg: Each opaque orange-purple, hard-shell capsule, printed "AltiMed M4" and "MIN 100 mg", contains: minocycline HCl equivalent to minocycline 100 mg. Nonmedicinal ingredients: FD&C Blue #1, FD&C Red #3, FD&C Yellow #6, gelatin, microcrystalline cellulose, silicon dioxide, sodium lauryl sulfate and titanium dioxide. Energy: <4.2 kJ (1 kcal). Tartrazine-free. Bottles of 100.

Store between 15-30°C. Protect from light.

ratio-Mirtazapine Ⓟ
mirtazapine
Antidepressant

ratiopharm

SUPPLIED: Each red brown, oval shaped, film-coated tablet, debossed "M101" on one side and bisected on the other side contains: mirtazapine 30 mg. Nonmedicinal ingredients: colloidal silicon dioxide, FD&C yellow No. 6, hydroxypropyl methylcellulose, iron oxide red, lactose monohydrate, magnesium stearate, polyethylene glycol 400, polysorbate 80, pregelatinized starch and titanium dioxide. HDPE bottles of 100. Store between 15 to 30°C. Dispense in a tight, light resistant container.

The reader is invited to consult CPhA's monograph **Corticosteroids: Topical**.

ratio-Mometasone Ⓟ
mometasone furoate
Topical Corticosteroid

ratiopharm

SUPPLIED: Each g of homogeneous, smooth, translucent and odourless white ointment contains: 1 mg of mometasone furoate. Nonmedicinal ingredients: hexylene glycol, propylene glycol monostearate, white petrolatum and white wax. Tubes of 15 and 50 g. Store between 15 and 30°C.

ratio-Morphine Ⓝ
morphine HCl
Opioid Analgesic

ratiopharm

SUPPLIED: 1 mg/mL: Each mL of orange-flavored, light yellow limpid syrup, contains: morphine HCl 1 mg. Nonmedicinal ingredients: artificial and natural orange flavoring, calcium cyclamate, FD&C Yellow #5, glycerin, methylparaben, propylparaben, purified water and sorbitol. Energy: 1.844 kcal/mL. Alcohol- and sucrose-free. Plastic bottles of 200 and 450 mL.
5 mg/mL: Each mL of orange-flavored, light yellow limpid syrup, contains: morphine HCl 5 mg. Nonmedicinal ingredients: artificial and natural orange flavoring, calcium cyclamate, FD&C Yellow #5, glycerin, methylparaben, propylparaben, purified water and sorbitol. Energy: 1.844 kcal/mL. Alcohol- and sucrose-free. Plastic bottles of 200 and 450 mL.
10 mg/mL: Each mL of orange-flavored, light yellow limpid syrup, contains: morphine HCl 10 mg. Nonmedicinal ingredients: artificial and natural orange flavoring, calcium cyclamate, FD&C Yellow #5, glycerin, methylparaben, propylparaben, purified water and sorbitol. Energy: 1.848 kcal/mL. Alcohol- and sucrose-free. Plastic bottles of 200 mL.
20 mg/mL: Each mL of unflavored, light yellow limpid syrup, contains: morphine HCl 20 mg. Nonmedicinal ingredients: calcium cyclamate, FD&C Yellow #5, glycerin, methylparaben, propylparaben, purified water and sorbitol. Energy: 1.848 kcal/mL. Alcohol- and sucrose-free. Plastic bottles of 50 mL with calibrated glass dropper.
Store at room temperature. Protect from freezing and light. Keep container well closed.

ratio-Morphine SR Ⓝ
morphine sulfate
Opioid Analgesic

ratiopharm

SUPPLIED: 15 mg: Each green, oval, sustained-release, biconvex tablet, imprinted "15" on one side and "TC" on the other side, contains: morphine sulfate 15 mg. Nonmedicinal ingredients: carnauba wax, FD&C Blue No.1 Brilliant Blue FCF lake, FD&C Blue No. 2 indigo carmine lake, FD&C Yellow No. 5 tartrazine lake, hydroxypropyl methylcellulose, lactose, magnesium stearate, polyethylene glycol, purified water, stearic acid and titanium dioxide. Bottles of 100.
30 mg: Each purple, oval, sustained-release biconvex tablet, imprinted "30" on one side and "TC" on the other side, contains: morphine sulfate 30 mg. Nonmedicinal ingredients: carnauba wax, D&C Red No. 7 lithol rubin B CA lake, FD&C Blue No.1 Brilliant Blue FCF lake, hydroxypropyl methylcellulose, lactose, magnesium stearate, polyethylene glycol, purified water, stearic acid and titanium dioxide. Bottles of 100.
60 mg: Each orange, oval, sustained-release, biconvex tablet, imprinted "60" on one side and "TC" on the other side, contains: morphine sulfate 60 mg. Nonmedicinal ingredients: carnauba wax, FD&C Yellow No.6 sunset Yellow FCF lake, hydroxypropyl methylcellulose, lactose, magnesium stearate, polyethylene glycol, polysorbate 80, purified water, stearic acid and titanium dioxide. Bottles of 100.
Store at room temperature (15 to 30°C) in a dry place. Protect from light and moisture. Keep the container tightly closed. Keep out of reach of children.

ratio-Nystatin
nystatin
Antifungal Antibiotic

ratiopharm

INDICATIONS: Oral Suspension: Monilial infections of the mouth (thrush) and intestinal moniliasis in infants and children.
Oral Tablets: Prevention and treatment of intestinal moniliasis. Prevention or treatment of lower intestinal and anal infections caused by *C. albicans* (monilia).
Powder: For the treatment of infections of the oral cavity caused by *C. albicans* (monilia).
Topical Cream and Ointment: Treatment of cutaneous or mucocutaneous mycotic infections caused by Candida (monilia) species. For dermatological use only.
Vaginal Cream: Local treatment of vaginal mycotic infections caused by *C. albicans*.
PRECAUTIONS: Little activity against bacteria, protozoa and viruses. Discontinue medication if irritation should occur from topical or intravaginal use.
Pregnancy: During pregnancy, the vaginal applicators should be used only on the advice of a physician.
Appropriate measures should be taken to avoid reinfection during sexual intercourse.
ADVERSE EFFECTS: High oral dosage may produce nausea, vomiting and diarrhea.
Tachycardia, bronchospasm, facial swelling, urticaria and nonspecific myalgia have been reported rarely.
OVERDOSE:

For management of a suspected drug overdose, CPhA recommends that you contact your **regional Poison Control Centre**. See the *CPS* Directory section for a list of Poison Control Centres.

DOSAGE: Therapy should generally be continued for at least 48 hours after clinical cure to prevent relapse. When oral nystatin is given concomitantly with an oral antibacterial agent, oral nystatin should be continued at least as long as the antibacterial agent. Local treatment of chronic or resistant vaginal, oral or cutaneous moniliasis with nystatin may be supplemented with oral nystatin administration.

Oral Suspension: Infants and children: 100 000 units 3 to 4 times daily for oral (thrush) and intestinal moniliasis. For treatment of infections of the oral cavity, the medication should be dropped directly on the tongue by means of the calibrated dropper and retained in the mouth for as long as possible before swallowing. For treatment of intestinal infections, may be dropped directly on the tongue by means of the calibrated dropper, or may be mixed with milk, lukewarm formula, or other nonacid vehicles, or incorporated in honey, jelly or peanut butter.

Oral Tablets: 500 000 units 3 times daily. Double dosage, if necessary, for adults.

Powder: Children and adults: Oral suspension: 400 000 to 600 000 units 4 times daily.

Topical Cream and Ointment: Apply cream or ointment liberally to affected areas twice daily or as prescribed by the physician.

Vaginal Cream (100 000 units/g): 1 applicatorful (5 g of cream) daily. In cases of severe infection, repeat application every 12 hours. Generally 2 weeks therapy will be sufficient; however, more prolonged therapy may be necessary. Therapy should be continued during menstruation.

SUPPLIED: Oral Suspension Ⓟ: Each mL of light yellow suspension with cherry-like odor contains: nystatin 100 000 units. Nonmedicinal ingredients: artificial flavoring, calcium disodium EDTA, D&C Yellow #10, magnesium aluminum silicate, methylparaben, polysorbate 80, propylparaben, purified water and sucrose. Energy: <12.6 kJ (3 kcal)/mL. Bottles of 24, 48, 100 and 1000 mL with calibrated dropper. Store between 15 and 30°C.

Oral Tablets Ⓟ: Each round, film-coated, biconvex, pink tablet, imprinted with "TEC" on one side, contains: nystatin 500 000 units. Nonmedicinal ingredients: cornstarch, D&C red #30 aluminum lake, ethylcellulose, hydroxypropyl methylcellulose, magnesium stearate, mineral oil, sodium lauryl sulfate, stearic acid and titanium dioxide. Bottles of 100. Store between 15 and 30°C.

Powder: For use only in extemporaneous prescription compounding of oral and topical preparations. Nonmedicinal ingredients: none. Bottles of 1 billion units. Nonsterile. The resultant suspension contains no preservatives and should be used immediately. Protect from light. Store under refrigeration between 2 and 8°C.

Topical Cream: Each g of light yellow cream with a characteristic odor contains: nystatin 100 000 units. Nonmedicinal ingredients: emulsifying wax, glycerin, isopropyl myristate, lactic acid, purified water and sorbic acid. Tubes of 15 and 30 g. Jars of 450 g. Store between 15 and 30°C.

Topical Ointment: Each g of yellow, smooth, homogenous ointment contains: nystatin 100 000 units. Nonmedicinal ingredients: mineral oil and polyethylene. Tubes of 30 g. Store between 15 and 30°C.

Vaginal Cream (100 000 units/g) Ⓟ: Each g of light yellow cream with a characteristic odor contains: nystatin 100 000 units. Nonmedicinal ingredients: emulsifying wax, glycerin, isopropyl myristate, purified water and sorbic acid. Tubes of 75 g with reusable applicator. Store between 15 and 30°C.

ratio-Omeprazole Ⓟ
omeprazole magnesium
H+, K+-ATPase Inhibitor

ratiopharm

SUPPLIED: Each red-brown, circular, biconvex, film-coated tablet contains: omeprazole magnesium anhydrous 20.6 mg equivalent to omeprazole 20 mg. Nonmedicinal ingredients: hydroxypropyl methylcellulose, iron oxide, mannitol, methacrylic acid copolymer, microcrystalline cellulose, paraffin, polyethylene glycol, sodium starch glycolate, sodium stearyl fumarate, talc and titanium dioxide. Press-through blister compliance strips in cartons of 28. High-density polyethylene (HDPE) bottles of 100 and 500. Store in a dry place at controlled room temperature (15-30°C).

ratio-Ondansetron Ⓟ
ondansetron HCl dihydrate
Antiemetic

ratiopharm

SUPPLIED: 4 mg: Each oval shaped, yellow film-coated tablet, imprinted "rph" on one side and "O72" on the other, contains: ondansetron 4 mg (as hydrochloride dihydrate). Nonmedicinal ingredients: cornstarch, croscarmellose sodium, lactose, magnesium stearate and microcrystalline cellulose; film-coating: iron oxide yellow, PEG 3350, polyvinyl alcohol-part hydrolyzed, talc and titanium dioxide. HDPE containers of 30 and 100. Blister packages of 10 (2×5). Store protected from light, between 2 and 30°C.

8 mg: Each oval shaped, yellow, film-coated tablet, imprinted "rph" on one side and "O71" on the other, contains: ondansetron 8 mg (as hydrochloride dihydrate). Nonmedicinal ingredients: cornstarch, croscarmellose sodium, lactose, magnesium stearate and microcrystalline cellulose; film-coating: iron oxide yellow, PEG 3350, polyvinyl alcohol-part hydrolyzed, talc and titanium dioxide. HDPE containers of 10, 30 and 100. Blister packages of 10 (2×5). Store protected from light, between 2 and 30°C.

ratio-Oxycocet Ⓝ
oxycodone HCl—acetaminophen
Opioid Analgesic

ratiopharm

SUPPLIED: Each white, round, biconvex tablet, imprinted with "TEC" on one side and single score on the other side, contains: oxycodone HCl 5 mg and acetaminophen 325 mg. Nonmedicinal ingredients: colloidal silicon dioxide, crospovidone, magnesium stearate, microcrystalline cellulose, povidone, pregelatinized cornstarch, sodium starch glycolate and stearic acid. Bottles of 100 and 500. Unit push-thru doses of 100. Store at controlled room temperature (15 to 30°C).

ratio-Oxycodan Ⓝ
oxycodone HCl—ASA
Opioid Analgesic

ratiopharm

SUPPLIED: Each yellow, biconvex tablet, imprinted with "TEC" on one side and with a single score on the other side, contains: oxycodone HCl 5 mg and ASA 325 mg. Nonmedicinal ingredients: colloidal silicon dioxide, FD&C Yellow #5 aluminum lake, lactose, microcrystalline cellulose, sodium starch glycolate and stearic acid. Bottles of 100 and 500. Store at controlled room temperature (15 to 30°C).

ratio-Pantoprazole Ⓟ
pantoprazole sodium
H+, K+-ATPase Inhibitor

ratiopharm

SUPPLIED: 20 mg: Each yellow, oval, biconvex, coated tablet with ink-printed "P22" on one side and "rph" on the other contains: pantoprazole sodium sesquihydrate 20 mg. Nonmedicinal ingredients: colloidal anhydrous silica, crospovidone, glyceryl behenate, hydroxypropyl methylcellulose, iron oxide black, iron oxide yellow, lactose monohydrate, methacrylic acid copolymer, polyethylene glycol, polyvinyl alcohol, propylene glycol, sodium bicarbonate, sodium lauryl sulphate, talc, titanium dioxide and triacetin. Bottles of 100. Store at room temperature, between 15 and 30°C. Protect from moisture.

40 mg: Each yellow, oval, biconvex, coated tablet with ink-printed "P21" on one side and "rph" on the other contains: pantoprazole sodium sesquihydrate 40 mg. Nonmedicinal ingredients: colloidal anhydrous silica, crospovidone, glyceryl behenate, hydroxypropyl methylcellulose, iron oxide black, iron oxide yellow, lactose monohydrate, methacrylic acid copolymer, polyethylene glycol, polyvinyl alcohol, propylene glycol, sodium bicarbonate, sodium lauryl sulphate, talc, titanium dioxide and triacetin. Bottles of 100 and 500. Store at room temperature, between 15 and 30°C. Protect from moisture.

The reader is invited to consult CPhA's monograph **Selective Serotonin Reuptake Inhibitors**.

ratio-Paroxetine Ⓟ
paroxetine HCl
Antidepressant —Antiobsessional—Antipanic—Anxiolytic—Social Phobia (Social Anxiety Disorder)—Post-traumatic Stress Disorder Therapy

ratiopharm

SUPPLIED: 10 mg: Each yellow, scored, film-coated, oval tablet, engraved with "10" on one side and scored, contains: paroxetine HCl equivalent to paroxetine free base 10 mg. Nonmedicinal ingredients: dibasic calcium phosphate dihydrate, hydroxypropyl methylcellulose, hypromellose, magnesium stearate, polyethylene glycol, polysorbate 80, sodium starch glycolate and titanium dioxide. May also contain one or more of the following: FD&C Yellow no. 6 aluminum lake, D&C Red no. 30 aluminum lake, D&C Yellow no. 10 aluminum lake, FD&C Blue no. 2 aluminum lake. Bottles 30.

20 mg: Each pink, scored, film-coated, oval tablet, engraved with "20" on one side and scored, contains: paroxetine HCl equivalent to paroxetine free base 20 mg. Nonmedicinal ingredients: dibasic calcium phosphate dihydrate, hydroxypropyl methylcellulose, hypromellose, magnesium stearate, polyethylene glycol, polysorbate 80, sodium starch glycolate and titanium dioxide. May also contain one or more of the following: FD&C Yellow no. 6 aluminum lake, D&C Red no. 30 aluminum lake, D&C Yellow no. 10 aluminum lake, FD&C Blue no. 2 aluminum lake. Bottles 100 and 500. Cartons of 6 cp blister cards (30 tablets each).

30 mg: Each blue, film-coated, oval tablet, engraved with "30" on one side, contains: paroxetine HCl equivalent to paroxetine free base 30 mg. Nonmedicinal ingredients: dibasic calcium phosphate dihydrate, hydroxypropyl methylcellulose, hypromellose, magnesium stearate, polyethylene glycol, polysorbate 80, sodium starch glycolate and titanium dioxide. May also contain one or more of the following: FD&C Yellow no. 6 aluminum lake, D&C Red no. 30 aluminum lake, D&C Yellow no. 10 aluminum lake, FD&C Blue no. 2 aluminum lake. Bottles 30.

Store between 15-30°C.

ratio-Pentoxifylline Ⓟ
pentoxifylline
Vasoactive Agent

ratiopharm

SUPPLIED: Each pink, oblong, film-coated tablet, one face is embossed with "Pentox", the other face is embossed with "Alti", contains: pentoxifylline 400 mg. Nonmedicinal ingredients: FD&C red no. 3, hydroxyethyl cellulose, hydroxypropyl methyl cellulose, magnesium stearate, polyethylene glycol, povidone, talc, titanium dioxide. Packed in unit pack boxes of 60 [6×10 blister-packed] tablets, or plastic bottles of 500 and 100 tablets. Store between 15 and 30°C.

ratio-Pioglitazone Ⓟ
pioglitazone HCl
Antidiabetic Agent—Insulin Resistance Reducing Agent

ratiopharm

SUPPLIED: 15 mg: Each white to off-white, round, convex, non-scored tablet, engraved "P33" on one side and "rph" on the other, contains: pioglitazone HCl equivalent to pioglitazone 15 mg. Nonmedicinal ingredients: carboxymethylcellulose calcium, hydroxypropylcellulose, lactose monohydrate and magnesium stearate. Bottles of 100 and 500. Store at controlled room temperature (15-30°C). Keep container tightly closed and protect from moisture and humidity.

30 mg: Each white to off-white, round, flat, non-scored tablet, engraved "P32" on one side and "rph" on the other, contains: pioglitazone HCl equivalent to pioglitazone 30 mg. Nonmedicinal ingredients: carboxymethylcellulose calcium, hydroxypropylcellulose, lactose monohydrate and magnesium stearate. Bottles of 100 and 500. Store at controlled room temperature (15-30°C). Keep container tightly closed and protect from moisture and humidity.

45 mg: Each white to off-white, round, flat, non-scored tablet, engraved "P31" on one side and "rph" on the other, contains: pioglitazone HCl equivalent to pioglitazone 45 mg. Nonmedicinal ingredients: carboxymethylcellulose calcium, hydroxypropylcellulose, lactose monohydrate and magnesium stearate. Bottles of 100 and 500. Store at controlled room temperature (15-30°C). Keep container tightly closed and protect from moisture and humidity.

The reader is invited to consult CPhA's monograph **HMG-CoA Reductase Inhibitors**.

ratio-Pravastatin Ⓟ
pravastatin sodium
Lipid Metabolism Regulator

ratiopharm

SUPPLIED: 10 mg: Each rounded, rectangular, pink to peach, biconvex tablet, engraved "rph" over "10" on one side and plain on the other side, contains: pravastatin sodium 10 mg. Nonmedicinal ingredients: croscarmellose sodium, lactose monohydrate, magnesium stearate, microcrystalline cellulose and red ferric oxide. Bottles of 100. Unit dose packages of 30. Store between 15-30°C. Protect from moisture and light.

20 mg: Each rounded, rectangular-shaped, yellow, biconvex tablet, engraved "rph" over "20" on one side and plain on the other side, contains: pravastatin sodium 20 mg. Nonmedicinal ingredients: croscarmellose sodium, lactose monohydrate, magnesium stearate, microcrystalline cellulose and yellow ferric oxide. Bottles of 100 and 500. Unit dose packages of 30. Store between 15-30°C. Protect from moisture and light.

40 mg: Each rounded, rectangular-shaped, green, biconvex tablet, engraved "rph" over "40" on one side and plain on the other side, contains: pravastatin sodium 40 mg. Nonmedicinal ingredients: croscarmellose sodium, D&C Yellow #10, FD&C Blue #1, lactose monohydrate, magnesium stearate and microcrystalline cellulose. Bottles of 100. Unit dose packages of 30. Store between 15-30°C. Protect from moisture and light.

ratio-Prednisolone P
prednisolone acetate
Ophthalmic Corticosteroid

ratiopharm

SUPPLIED: Each mL of suspension contains: prednisolone acetate 1%. Nonmedicinal ingredients: benzalkonium chloride 0.004% (as preservative), boric acid, disodium edetate, hydroxypropyl methylcellulose, polysorbate 80, purified water, sodium bisulfite, sodium chloride and sodium citrate. Plastic dropper bottles of 5 and 10 mL.

ratio-Proctosone P
hydrocortisone acetate—framycetin sulfate—cinchocaine HCl—esculin
Antibacterial—Corticosteroid—Anorectal Therapy

ratiopharm

SUPPLIED: Ointment: Each g of ointment contains: hydrocortisone (as acetate) 5 mg, framycetin sulfate 10 mg (equivalent to 7 mg of framycetin base), cinchocaine HCl 5 mg and esculin 10 mg. Nonmedicinal ingredients: lanolin, light mineral oil and petrolatum. Tubes of 15 and 30 g with rectal canula.
Suppositories: Each rectal suppository contains: hydrocortisone (as acetate) 5 mg, framycetin sulfate 10 mg (equivalent to 7 mg of framycetin base), cinchocaine HCl 5 mg and esculin 10 mg. Nonmedicinal ingredients: semisynthetic glycerides. Boxes of 12.
Store between 15 to 30°C.

ratio-Quetiapine P
quetiapine fumarate
Antipsychotic

ratiopharm

SUPPLIED: 25 mg: Each peach, round, biconvex, film-coated tablet, identified with "Q" and "25" on one side and plain on the other, contains: quetiapine fumarate 25 mg. Nonmedicinal ingredients: calcium hydrogen phosphate dihydrate, hydryoxypropyl methylcellulose, lactose monohydrate, magnesium stearate, microcrystalline cellulose, polyethylene glycol, povidone, red ferric oxide, sodium starch glycolate, titanium dioxide and yellow ferric oxide. Bottles of 100 and 500. Store at room temperature, between 15 and 30°C.
100 mg: Each yellow, round, biconvex, film-coated tablet, identified with "Q" and "100" on one side and plain on the other, contains: quetiapine fumarate 100 mg. Nonmedicinal ingredients: calcium hydrogen phosphate dihydrate, hydryoxypropyl methylcellulose, lactose monohydrate, magnesium stearate, microcrystalline cellulose, polyethylene glycol, povidone, sodium starch glycolate, titanium dioxide and yellow ferric oxide. Bottles of 100 and 500. Store at room temperature, between 15 and 30°C.
200 mg: Each white, round, biconvex, film-coated tablet, identified with "Q" and "200" on one side and plain on the other, contains: quetiapine fumarate 200 mg. Nonmedicinal ingredients: calcium hydrogen phosphate dihydrate, hydryoxypropyl methylcellulose, lactose monohydrate, magnesium stearate, microcrystalline cellulose, polyethylene glycol, povidone, sodium starch glycolate and titanium dioxide. Bottles of 100 and 500. Store at room temperature, between 15 and 30°C.
300 mg: Each white, capsule-shaped, biconvex, film-coated tablet, identified with "Q" and "300" on one side and plain on the other, contains: quetiapine fumarate 300 mg. Nonmedicinal ingredients: calcium hydrogen phosphate dihydrate, hydryoxypropyl methylcellulose, lactose monohydrate, magnesium stearate, microcrystalline cellulose, polyethylene glycol, povidone, sodium starch glycolate and titanium dioxide. Bottles of 100 and 500. Store at room temperature, between 15 and 30°C.

> The reader is invited to consult CPhA's monograph **ACE Inhibitors.**

ratio-Ramipril P
ramipril
Angiotensin Converting Enzyme Inhibitor

ratiopharm

SUPPLIED: 1.25 mg: Each hard gelatin capsule size no. 4, with opaque white body imprinted with "Ramipril" and yellow opaque cap imprinted with "1.25" containing a white powder mixture (the printing on the head and body can be reversed), contains: ramipril 1.25 mg. Nonmedicinal ingredients: pre-gelatinized starch; hard capsule: gelatin, titanium dioxide and yellow iron oxide. Cartons of 30 (2×15 blister-packed). White high-density polyethylene (HDPE) bottles of 100. Store in original container at room temperature (15-30°C).
2.5 mg: Each hard gelatin capsule size no. 4, with white body imprinted with "Ramipril" and medium orange opaque cap imprinted with "2.5" containing a white powder mixture (the printing on the head and body can be reversed), contains: ramipril 2.5 mg. Nonmedicinal ingredients: pre-gelatinized starch; hard capsule: FD&C red no. 3, gelatin, titanium dioxide and yellow iron oxide. Cartons of 30 (2×15 blister-packed). White high-density polyethylene (HDPE) bottles of 100 and 500. Store in original container at room temperature (15-30°C).
5 mg: Each hard gelatin capsule size no. 4, with white body imprinted with "Ramipril" and Swedish orange opaque cap imprinted with "5" containing a white powder mixture (the printing on the head and body can be reversed), contains: ramipril 5 mg. Nonmedicinal ingredients: pre-gelatinized starch; hard capsule: FD&C blue no. 2, FD&C red no. 3, gelatin and titanium dioxide. Cartons of 30 (2×15 blister-packed). White high-density polyethylene (HDPE) bottles of 100 and 500. Store in original container at room temperature (15-30°C).
10 mg: Each hard gelatin capsule size no. 4, with white body imprinted with "Ramipril" and blue opaque cap imprinted with "10" containing a white powder mixture (the printing on the head and body can be reversed), contains: ramipril 10 mg. Nonmedicinal ingredients: pre-gelatinized starch; hard capsule: black iron oxide, FD&C blue no. 2, FD&C red no. 3, gelatin and titanium dioxide. Cartons of 30 (2×15 blister-packed). White high-density polyethylene (HDPE) bottles of 100 and 500. Store in original container at room temperature (15-30°C).
15 mg: Each hard gelatin capsule size no. 3, with grey opaque body imprinted with "Ramipril" and powder blue opaque cap imprinted with "15" containing a white powder mixture (the printing on the head and body can be reversed), contains ramipril 15 mg. Nonmedicinal ingredients: pre-gelatinized starch; hard capsule: black iron oxide, D&C red no. 28, FD&C blue no. 1, gelatin and titanium dioxide. Cartons of 30 (2×15 blister-packed). White high-density polyethylene (HDPE) bottles of 100 and 500. Store in original container at room temperature (15-30°C).

ratio-Ranitidine P
ranitidine HCl
Histamine H2-Receptor Antagonist

ratiopharm

SUPPLIED: 150 mg: Each white to off-white, round, biconvex, film-coated tablet, embossed "rph" on one side and "r12" on the other side, contains: ranitidine HCl 168 mg (equivalent to ranitidine anhydrous free base 150 mg). Nonmedicinal ingredients: calcium hydrogen phosphate, colloidal anhydrous silica, magnesium stearate, maize starch, microcrystalline cellulose and sodium starch glycolate; film-coating suspension: hydroxypropyl methylcellulose, lactose, macrogol 4000 and titanium dioxide. Gluten- and tartrazine-free. Packs of 60. Bottles of 60 and 500.
300 mg: Each white to off-white, oblong, film-coated tablet, embossed "rph" on one side and "r11" on the other side, contains: ranitidine HCl 335 mg (equivalent to ranitidine anhydrous free base 300 mg). Nonmedicinal ingredients: calcium hydrogen phosphate, colloidal anhydrous silica, magnesium stearate, maize starch, microcrystalline cellulose and sodium starch glycolate; film-coating suspension: hydroxypropyl methylcellulose, lactose, macrogol 4000 and titanium dioxide. Gluten- and tartrazine-free. Packs of 30.
Store between 15-30°C. Protect from light and moisture.

> The reader is invited to consult CPhA's monograph **Bisphosphonates: Oral.**

ratio-Risedronate P
risedronate sodium hemi-pentahydrate
Bone Metabolism Regulator

ratiopharm

SUPPLIED: Each light orange, caplet shaped, film-coated tablet, with "rph" engraved on one side and "R51" on the other side contains: the equivalent of 35 mg of anhydrous risedronate sodium in the form of the hemi-pentahydrate with small amounts of monohydrate. Nonmedicinal ingredients: colloidal silicon dioxide, crospovidone, FD&C yellow No. 6 aluminum lake, ferric oxide red, ferric oxide yellow, hydroxypropyl methylcellulose, lactose monohydrate, magnesium stearate, microcrystalline cellulose, polyethylene glycol and titanium dioxide. Blister package of 4. Store at controlled room temperature (15-30°C). Protect from moisture.

ratio-Rivastigmine P
rivastigmine hydrogen tartrate
Cholinesterase Inhibitor

ratiopharm

SUPPLIED: 1.5 mg: Each yellow opaque/yellow opaque, hard gelatin capsule, radially imprinted with "1.5" on body and "rph R64" on cap in red ink, filled with white to off-white free flowing powder contains: rivastigmine 1.5 mg (as rivastigmine hydrogen tartrate). Nonmedicinal ingredients: colloidal silicon dioxide, hypromellose, magnesium stearate and microcrystalline cellulose; capsule: gelatin, titanium dioxide and yellow iron oxide. Red ink: ammonium hydroxide, iron oxide red, isopropyl alcohol, N-Butyl alcohol, propylene glycol and Shellac glaze. Bottles of 100 and 500. Store at room temperature (15-30°C).
3 mg: Each orange opaque/orange opaque, hard gelatin capsule, radially imprinted with "3" on body and "rph R63" on cap in red ink, filled with white to off-white free flowing powder, contains: rivastigmine 3 mg (as rivastigmine hydrogen tartrate). Nonmedicinal ingredients: colloidal silicon dioxide, hypromellose, magnesium stearate and microcrystalline cellulose; capsule: gelatin, red iron oxide, titanium dioxide and yellow iron oxide. Red ink: ammonium hydroxide, iron oxide red, isopropyl alcohol, N-Butyl alcohol, propylene glycol and Shellac glaze. Bottles of 100 and 500. Store at room temperature (15-30°C).
4.5 mg: Each red opaque/red opaque, hard gelatin capsule, radially imprinted with "4.5" on body and "rph R62" on cap in white ink, filled with white to off-white free flowing powder, contains: rivastigmine 4.5 mg (as rivastigmine hydrogen tartrate). Nonmedicinal ingredients: colloidal silicon dioxide, hypromellose, magnesium stearate and microcrystalline cellulose; capsule: gelatin, red iron oxide and titanium dioxide. White ink: butyl alcohol, dehydrated alcohol, isopropyl alcohol, povidone, propylene glycol, Shellac, sodium hydroxide and titanium dioxide. Bottles of 100 and 500. Store at room temperature (15-30°C).
6 mg: Each orange opaque/red opaque, hard gelatin capsule, radially imprinted with "6" on body and "rph R61" on cap in white ink, filled with white to off-white free flowing powder, contains: rivastigmine 6 mg (as rivastigmine hydrogen tartrate). Nonmedicinal ingredients: colloidal silicon dioxide, hypromellose, magnesium stearate and microcrystalline cellulose; capsule: gelatin, red iron oxide, titanium dioxide and yellow iron oxide. White ink: butyl alcohol, dehydrated alcohol, isopropyl alcohol, povidone, propylene glycol, Shellac, sodium hydroxide and titanium dioxide. Bottles of 100 and 500. Store at room temperature (15-30°C).

ratio-Salbutamol P
salbutamol sulfate
Bronchodilator—Beta2-adrenergic Stimulant

ratiopharm

SUPPLIED: Bottles: Each mL of isotonic solution contains: salbutamol sulfate, equivalent to salbutamol base 5 mg. Adjusted to pH 3.4 to 4.4. Preserved with benzalkonium chloride 0.01% w/v, sulfuric acid and purified water. Amber colored glass bottles of 10 mL. Store between 15-30°C. Protect from light.
Unit Dose Ampuls: 1 mg/mL: Each ampul of sterile, isotonic solution contains: salbutamol sulfate equivalent to salbutamol base 2.5 mg in 2.5 mL and sodium chloride, sulfuric acid and purified water. Adjusted to pH 3.5 to 4.5. Boxes of 20. Overwrapped nebule: store below 25°C. Nebule removed from overwrap: store below 25°C. Protect from light. Use within 3 months.
0.5 mg/mL: Each unit dose of sterile, isotonic solution contains: salbutamol sulfate equivalent to 0.5 mg/mL salbutamol base. Nonmedicinal ingredients: purified water, sodium chloride and sulfuric acid (0.IN) for pH adjustment. Boxes of 20 unit doses. Store between 15 and 25°C. Protect from light.
2 mg/mL: Each unit dose of sterile, isotonic solution contains: salbutamol sulfate equivalent to 2 mg/mL salbutamol base. Nonmedicinal ingredients: purified water, sodium chloride and sulfuric acid (0.IN) for pH adjustment. Boxes of 20 unit doses. Store between 15 and 25°C. Protect from light.

> The reader is invited to consult CPhA's monograph **Selective Serotonin Reuptake Inhibitors.**

ratio-Sertraline P
sertraline HCl
Antidepressant—Antipanic—Antiobsessional

ratiopharm

SUPPLIED: 25 mg: Each yellow capsule, imprinted in black ink with "ratio-Sertraline 25" and "rph 297A", contains: sertraline HCl equivalent to sertraline 25 mg. Nonmedicinal ingredients: cornstarch, lactose, magnesium stearate and sodium lauryl sulfate; capsule shell: D&C Yellow No. 10, FD&C Red No. 40, FD&C Yellow No. 6, gelatin and titanium dioxide. White HDPE bottles of 100.
50 mg: Each white and yellow capsule, imprinted in black ink with "ratio-Sertraline 50" and "rph 297B", contains: sertraline HCl equivalent to sertraline 50 mg. Nonmedicinal ingredients: cornstarch, lactose, magnesium stearate and sodium lauryl sulfate; capsule shell: D&C Yellow No. 10, FD&C Red No. 40, FD&C Yellow No. 6, gelatin and titanium dioxide. White HDPE bottles of 100 and 250.

100 mg: Each orange capsule, imprinted in black ink with "ratio-Sertraline 100" and "rph 297C", contains: sertraline HCl equivalent to sertraline 100 mg. Nonmedicinal ingredients: cornstarch, lactose, magnesium stearate and sodium lauryl sulfate; capsule shell: D&C Yellow No. 10, FD&C Red No. 40, FD&C Yellow No. 6, gelatin and titanium dioxide. White HDPE bottles of 100 and 250.

Store at room temperature (15 to 30°C) in a dry place. Keep the container tightly closed. Keep out of reach of children.

ratio-Sildenafil R

sildenafil citrate

cGMP-Specific Phosphodiesterase Type 5 Inhibitor—Treatment of Pulmonary Arterial Hypertension

ratiopharm

SUPPLIED: Each white, circular, biconvex, film-coated tablet, embossed with "rph" on one side and "20" on the other side contains: sildenafil citrate equivalent to sildenafil 20 mg. Nonmedicinal ingredients: calcium hydrogen phosphate, croscarmellose sodium, hydroxypropyl methylcellulose, magnesium stearate, microcrystalline cellulose, polyethylene glycol, talcum and titanium dioxide. Blister packs of 30 and 90. Bottles of 30 and 100. Store at 25°C (excursions are permitted to 15-30°C).

> The reader is invited to consult CPhA's monograph **HMG-CoA Reductase Inhibitors**.

ratio-Simvastatin

simvastatin

Lipid Metabolism Regulator

ratiopharm

SUPPLIED: 10 mg: Each light pink, shield-shaped, biconvex, film-coated tablet, engraved with "rph" on one side and "10" on the other side, contains: simvastatin 10 mg. Nonmedicinal ingredients: colloidal silicon dioxide, crospovidone, hydroxyethyl cellulose, microcrystalline cellulose, polyethylene glycol, red ferric oxide, titanium dioxide, yellow ferric oxide and zinc stearate. Unit dose packages of 30. Bottles of 100 and 250.

20 mg: Each peach, shield-shaped, biconvex, film-coated tablet, engraved with "rph" on one side and "20" on the other side, contains: simvastatin 20 mg. Nonmedicinal ingredients: colloidal silicon dioxide, crospovidone, hydroxyethyl cellulose, microcrystalline cellulose, polyethylene glycol, red ferric oxide, titanium dioxide and zinc stearate Unit dose packages of 30. Bottles of 100 and 250.

40 mg: Each dusty-rose, shield-shaped, biconvex, film-coated tablet, engraved with "rph" on one side and "40" on the other side, contains: simvastatin 40 mg. Nonmedicinal ingredients: colloidal silicon dioxide, crospovidone, hydroxyethyl cellulose, microcrystalline cellulose, polyethylene glycol, red ferric oxide, titanium dioxide and zinc stearate. Unit dose packages of 30. Bottles of 100.

80 mg: Each dusty-rose, capsule-shaped, biconvex, film-coated tablet, engraved with "rph" on one side and "80" on the other side, contains: simvastatin 80 mg. Nonmedicinal ingredients: colloidal silicon dioxide, crospovidone, hydroxyethyl cellulose, microcrystalline cellulose, polyethylene glycol, red ferric oxide, titanium dioxide and zinc stearate. Unit dose packages of 30.

ratio-Sotalol

sotalol HCl

Antiarrhythmic

ratiopharm

SUPPLIED: 80 mg: Each blue caplet, plain on one side and debossed "rph" on the left and "S22" on the right side of a score line on the other side, contains: sotalol HCl 80 mg. Nonmedicinal ingredients: colloidal silicon dioxide, FD&C Blue No. 2 aluminum lake, lactose, magnesium stearate, microcrystalline cellulose, starch and stearic acid. Bottles of 100.

160 mg: Each blue caplet, plain on one side and debossed "rph" on the left and "S21" on the right side of a score line on the other side, contains: sotalol HCl 160 mg. Nonmedicinal ingredients: colloidal silicon dioxide, FD&C Blue No. 2 aluminum lake, lactose, magnesium stearate, microcrystalline cellulose, starch and stearic acid. Bottles of 100.

Store at room temperature (15 to 30°C).

ratio-Tamsulosin

tamsulosin HCl

Selective Antagonist of Alpha1A Adrenoreceptor Subtype in the Prostate

ratiopharm

SUPPLIED: Each hard gelatin sustained-release capsule with an orange coloured body and olive coloured cap, with a black line at the top of the cap and of the body, imprinted with the code "TSL 0.4" with black ink on the cap and filled with white to off-white pellets, contains: tamsulosin HCl 0.4 mg. Nonmedicinal ingredients: methacrylic acid-ethyl acrylate copolymer (polysorbate 80, sodium lauryl sulphate), microcrystalline cellulose, talc and triethylcitrate; shell: black iron oxide, FD&C Blue No. 2, gelatin, red iron oxide, titanium dioxide and yellow iron oxide; imprinting ink: antifoam, black iron oxide, shellac glaze and soya lecithin. Bottles of 100 and 500. Blister packages of 30. Store between 15 and 30°C.

ratio-Tecnal

ASA—caffeine—butalbital

Analgesic—Sedative

ratiopharm

ratio-Tecnal C¼, C½

ASA—caffeine—codeine phosphate—butalbital

Analgesic—Sedative

ratiopharm

SUPPLIED: ratio-Tecnal: Capsules: Each white powder in hard gelatine capsule with a blue opaque cap and purple body, imprinted in white ink "Tecnal: Technilab", contains: butalbital USP 50 mg, caffeine USP 40 mg and ASA USP 330 mg. Nonmedicinal ingredients: ammonium hydroxide, FD&C Blue #1, FD&C Red #3, gelatin, microcrystalline cellulose, pregelatinized cornstarch, propylene glycol, shellac, simethicone and titanium dioxide. Bottles of 100 and 500.

Tablets: Each white, round, biplane tablet with bevelled edges engraved "TEC" on one side contains: butalbital USP 50 mg, caffeine USP 40 mg and ASA USP 330 mg. Nonmedicinal ingredients: microcrystalline cellulose, povidone, simethicone, sodium croscarmellose and stearic acid. Bottles of 100 and 500.

ratio-Tecnal C¼: Each white powder in hard gelatine capsule with a blue opaque cap and white opaque body, imprinted in black ink "Tecnal C ¼ Technilab", contains: butalbital USP 50 mg, caffeine USP 40 mg, ASA USP 330 mg and codeine phosphate USP 15 mg. Nonmedicinal ingredients: black iron oxide, D&C Yellow #10 lake, FD&C Blue #1 lake, FD&C Blue #2 lake, FD&C Red #3, FD&C Red #40 lake, gelatin, microcrystalline cellulose, pregelatinized cornstarch, propylene glycol, shellac and titanium dioxide. Bottles of 100 and 500.

ratio-Tecnal C½: Each white powder in hard gelatine capsule with a blue opaque cap and powder blue opaque body, imprinted in black ink "Tecnal C ½: Technilab", contains: butalbital USP 50 mg, caffeine USP 40 mg, ASA USP 330 mg and codeine phosphate USP 30 mg. Nonmedicinal ingredients: black iron oxide, D&C Yellow #10 lake, FD&C Blue #1 lake, FD&C Blue #2 lake, FD&C Red #3, FD&C Red #40 lake, gelatin, microcrystalline cellulose, pregelatinized cornstarch, propylene glycol, shellac and titanium dioxide. Bottles of 100 and 500.

ratio-Temazepam

temazepam

Hypnotic

ratiopharm

SUPPLIED: 15 mg: Each maroon and peach, hard shell gelatin capsule, printed in white ink with "TEC 185A", contains: temazepam 15 mg. Nonmedicinal ingredients: ammonium hydroxide, D&C Red #28, D&C Red #33, D&C Yellow #10, FD&C Blue #1, FD&C Yellow #6, gelatin, isopropyl alcohol, lactose, magnesium stearate, n-butyl alcohol, propylene glycol, shellac, silicon dioxide, simethicone, sodium lauryl sulfate and titanium dioxide. Bottles of 100 and 500. Store in a dry place, between 15-30°C. Protect from light.

30 mg: Each maroon and blue, hard shell gelatin capsule, printed in white ink with "TEC 185B", contains: temazepam 30 mg. Nonmedicinal ingredients: ammonium hydroxide, D&C Red #28, D&C Red #33, D&C Yellow #10, FD&C Blue #1, gelatin, isopropyl alcohol, lactose, magnesium stearate, n-butyl alcohol, propylene glycol, shellac, silicon dioxide, simethicone, sodium lauryl sulfate and titanium dioxide. Bottles of 100 and 500. Store in a dry place, between 15-30°C. Protect from light.

ratio-Terazosin

terazosin HCl

Antihypertensive—Symptomatic Treatment of Benign Prostatic Hyperplasia (BPH)

ratiopharm

SUPPLIED: 1 mg: Each white, round, flat, beveled-edged tablet embossed with "74" on one side and "ZA" on the other, contains: terazosin 1 mg (as terazosin HCl). Nonmedicinal ingredients: cornstarch, lactose, magnesium stearate, povidone and talc. Alcohol-, gluten-, paraben-, sodium-, sucrose-, sulfite- and tartrazine-free. Bottles of 100.

2 mg: Each orange, round, flat, beveled-edged tablet embossed with "74" on one side and "ZB" on the other, contains: terazosin 2 mg (as terazosin HCl). Nonmedicinal ingredients: cornstarch, FD&C yellow No. 6, lactose, magnesium stearate, povidone and talc. Alcohol-, gluten-, paraben-, sodium-, sucrose-, sulfite- and tartrazine-free. Bottles of 100.

5 mg: Each tan, round, flat, beveled-edged tablet embossed with "74" on one side and "ZC" on the other, contains: terazosin 5 mg (as terazosin HCl). Nonmedicinal ingredients: cornstarch, iron oxide, lactose, magnesium stearate, povidone and talc. Alcohol-, gluten-, paraben-, sodium-, sucrose-, sulfite- and tartrazine-free. Bottles of 100.

10 mg: Each blue, round, flat, beveled-edged tablet, with "74" on one side and "ZD" on the other, contains: terazosin 10 mg (as terazosin HCl). Nonmedicinal ingredients: cornstarch, FD&C Blue No. 2, lactose, magnesium stearate and talc. Alcohol-, gluten-, paraben-, sodium-, sucrose-, sulfite- and tartrazine-free. Bottles of 100.

Store at controlled room temperature (15 to 30°C).

ratio-Theo-Bronc

theophylline—potassium iodide—guaifenesin—mepyramine maleate

Bronchodilator—Expectorant

ratiopharm

SUPPLIED: Each 5 mL of clear, colorless to slightly yellow, bitter tasting syrup, cherry and menthol odor, contains: guaifenesin 50 mg, potassium iodide 80 mg, theophylline (base) 35 mg and mepyramine maleate 6 mg. Nonmedicinal ingredients: alcohol, inverted sugar/honey, menthol, purified water, sucrose, wild cherry and citrus flavoring. Energy: 56.6 kJ (13.33 kcal)/5 mL. Bottles of 250 mL and 2 L.

ratio-Topilene

betamethasone dipropionate

Topical Corticosteroid

ratiopharm

SUPPLIED: Cream: Each g contains: betamethasone (as dipropionate USP) 0.5 mg (0.05%). Nonmedicinal ingredients: ceteareth-20, cetyl alcohol, glyceryl stearate, light mineral oil, methylparaben, petrolatum, polysorbate 60, propylene glycol, propylene glycol monostearate, propylparaben and purified water. Tubes of 15 and 50 g.

Lotion: Each g contains: betamethasone (as dipropionate USP) 0.5 mg (0.05%). Nonmedicinal ingredients: carbomer, isopropyl alcohol, propylene glycol, purified water, sodium phosphate monobasic and triethanolamine. Plastic squeeze bottles of 30 and 60 mL.

Ointment: Each g contains: betamethasone (as dipropionate USP) 0.5 mg (0.05%). Nonmedicinal ingredients: petrolatum, propylene glycol and propylene glycol monostearate. Tubes of 15 and 50 g.

Store between 15 and 30°C.

ratio-Topiramate

topiramate

Antiepileptic

ratiopharm

SUPPLIED: 25 mg: Each white, round, biconvex, beveled-edge coated tablet, engraved "T63" on one side and "rph" on the other side, contains: topiramate 25 mg. Nonmedicinal ingredients: colloidal silicon dioxide, hydroxypropyl methylcellulose, lactose monohydrate, magnesium stearate, microcrystalline cellulose, polydextrose, polyethyleneglycol, pregelatinized starch, sodium starch glycolate, titanium dioxide and triacetin. Bottles of 100. Keep out of the reach of children. Store at 15-30°C in tightly closed, light resistant container. Protect from humidity.

100 mg: Each yellow, round, biconvex, beveled-edge coated tablet, engraved "T62" on one side and "rph" on the other side, contains: topiramate 100 mg. Nonmedicinal ingredients: colloidal silicon dioxide, hydroxypropyl methylcellulose, lactose monohydrate, magnesium stearate, microcrystalline cellulose, polydextrose, polyethyleneglycol, pregelatinized starch, sodium starch glycolate, titanium dioxide, triacetin and yellow iron oxide. Bottles of 100. Keep out of the reach of children. Store at 15-30°C in tightly closed, light resistant container. Protect from humidity.

200 mg: Each salmon colored, round, biconvex, coated tablet, engraved "T61" on one side and "rph" on the other side, contains: topiramate 200 mg. Nonmedicinal ingredients: colloidal silicon dioxide, hydroxypropyl methylcellulose, lactose monohydrate, magnesium stearate, microcrystalline cellulose, polydextrose, polyethyleneglycol, pregelatinized starch, red iron oxide, sodium starch glycolate, titanium dioxide and triacetin. Bottles of 100. Keep out of the reach of children. Store at 15-30°C in tightly closed, light resistant container. Protect from humidity.

ratio-Topisalic

betamethasone dipropionate—salicylic acid

Topical Corticosteroid—Keratolytic

ratiopharm

SUPPLIED: Each g of translucent, homogeneous lotion with a strong alcoholic odor, contains: betamethasone dipropionate 0.64 mg, equivalent to 0.5 mg of betamethasone and salicylic acid 20 mg. Nonmedicinal ingredients: hydroxyethyl cellulose, isopropanol, purified water and triethanolamine. Plastic squeeze bottles of 30 and 60 mL. Store between 15-30°C.

ratio-Topisone

betamethasone dipropionate

Topical Corticosteroid

ratiopharm

SUPPLIED: Cream: Each g contains: betamethasone 0.5 mg (0.05%) (as dipropionate USP) in a miscible base. Nonmedicinal ingredients: ceteareth-20, cetyl alcohol, glyceryl stearate, light mineral oil, methylparaben, polysorbate 60, propylene glycol, propylparaben and purified water. Tubes of 15 and 50 g. Plastic jars of 450 g.
Lotion: Each g contains: betamethasone 0.5 mg (0.05%) (as dipropionate USP). Nonmedicinal ingredients: carbomer, isopropyl alcohol, purified water and triethanolamine. Plastic bottles of 30 and 75 mL.
Ointment: Each g contains: betamethasone 0.5 mg (0.05%) (as dipropionate USP). Nonmedicinal ingredients: light mineral oil and petrolatum. Tubes of 15 and 50 g. Plastic jars of 450 g.
Store between 15 and 30°C.

ratio-Trazodone

trazodone HCl

Antidepressant

ratiopharm

SUPPLIED: 50 mg: Each light orange, round, standard convex, film-coated, single-scored tablet, with one side imprinted with "rph" and "T43" on the other side contains: trazodone hydrochloride 50 mg. Nonmedicinal ingredients: colloidal silicon dioxide, FD&C yellow No. 6 aluminum lake, hydroxypropyl methylcellulose, lactose monohydrate, magnesium stearate, microcrystalline cellulose, polyethylene glycol, pregelatinized starch and sodium starch glycolate. Bottles of 100 and 500. Store between 15 and 30°C. Protect from light.
100 mg: Each white, round, standard convex, film-coated, single-scored tablet, with one side imprinted with "rph" and "T42" on the other side contains: trazodone hydrochloride 100 mg. Nonmedicinal ingredients: colloidal silicon dioxide, hydroxypropyl methylcellulose, lactose monohydrate, magnesium stearate, microcrystalline cellulose, polyethylene glycol, pregelatinized starch and sodium starch glycolate. Bottles of 100. Store between 15 and 30°C. Protect from light.
150 mg (DIVIDOSE): Each light orange, rectangular-shaped, trisected and bisected tablet, with one side imprinted with "rph" and "T41" on the other side contains: trazodone hydrochloride 150 mg. Nonmedicinal ingredients: croscarmellose sodium, FD&C yellow No. 6 aluminum lake, lactose monohydrate, magnesium stearate, microcrystalline cellulose and pregelatinized starch. Bottles of 100. The DIVIDOSE 150 mg tablet design makes dosage adjustments easy. Each tablet can be broken accurately to provide any of the following dosage: 50 mg (one-third of a tablet); 75 mg (one-half of a tablet); 100 mg (two-thirds of a tablet); 150 mg (the entire tablet). Store between 15 and 30°C. Protect from light.

ratio-Triacomb

triamcinolone acetonide—nystatin—neomycin sulfate—gramicidin

Corticosteroid—Antifungal—Antibacterial

ratiopharm

SUPPLIED: Each g of cream contains: triamcinolone acetonide USP 1 mg, nystatin USP 100 000 units, neomycin base (in sulfate) USP 2.5 mg and gramicidin USP 0.25 mg in a vanishing cream base. Nonmedicinal ingredients: aluminum hydroxide, ceteareth-20, cetearyl alcohol, glyceryl monostearate, glyceryl stearate, methylparaben, petrolatum, polysorbate 60, propylene glycol, propylene glycol monostearate, propylparaben, purified water, sorbitol and titanium dioxide. Jars of 450 g. Tubes of 15, 30 and 60 g. Keep tube and jar tightly closed. Store between 15-30°C. Keep from freezing and store away from heat and direct light.

ratio-Tryptophan

L-tryptophan

Adjunct in the Management of Affective Disorders

ratiopharm

SUPPLIED: Capsules: Each white, hard gelatin capsule, opaque, size No. 00, imprinted "ALTI500" on capsule cap and body, contains: L-tryptophan, USP 500 mg. Nonmedicinal ingredients: magnesium stearate and talc. Bottles of 100. Store between 15 and 30°C. Protect from heat and light.
Tablets: 500 mg: Each white, oval-shaped, smooth, film-coated tablet, embossed with "ALTIMED" on one side and with "500 mg" on the other side, contains: L-tryptophan, USP 500 mg. Nonmedicinal ingredients: acetylated monoglyceride, calcium phosphate, carnauba wax, hydroxypropyl methylcellulose, magnesium stearate, methylcellulose, opaspray white, povidone, sodium croscarmellose, titanium dioxide and white wax solution. Bottles of 100. Store between 15 and 30°C. Protect from heat and light.
1 g: Each white, oval-shaped, smooth film-coated tablet, embossed "ALTI-TRYP" 1 g on one side, contains: L-tryptophan, USP 1 g. Nonmedicinal ingredients: acetylated monoglyceride, calcium phosphate, carnauba wax, hydroxypropyl methylcellulose, magnesium stearate, methylcellulose, opaspray white, povidone, sodium croscarmellose, titanium dioxide and white wax solution. Bottles of 100. Store between 15 and 30°C. Protect from heat and light.

ratio-Valproic

valproic acid

Anticonvulsant

ratiopharm

SUPPLIED: Capsules: 250 mg: Each orange, opaque soft gelatin capsule, imprinted with "K", contains: valproic acid 250 mg. Nonmedicinal ingredients: corn oil, ethyl vanillin, FD&C yellow no. 6, gelatin, glycerin, methylparaben, propylparaben and titanium dioxide. Alcohol-, gluten-, lactose-, sucrose-, sulfite- and tartrazine-free. Bottles of 100 and 500. Store between 15-25°C.
500 mg: Each pale-yellow, oval, soft, smooth gelatin, enteric-coated capsule contains: valproic acid 500 mg. Nonmedicinal ingredients: cellulose acetate phthalate, dextrose, diethyl phthalate, ethyl acetate, gelatin, glycerin, methylparaben, propylparaben, tartrazine and titanium dioxide. Alcohol-, gluten-, lactose-, sucrose- and sulfite-free. Bottles of 100 and 500. Store between 15-25°C.
Syrup: Each 5 mL of red syrup contains: the equivalent of 250 mg valproic acid, as the sodium salt. Nonmedicinal ingredients: artificial cherry flavor, FD&C No. 40 red dye, glycerin, methylparaben, propylparaben, purified water, sorbitol, sucrose, vanillin, and hydrochloric acid and sodium hydroxide for pH adjustment. Alcohol-, gluten-, lactose-, sulfite- and tartrazine-free. Bottles of 480 mL. Store between 15-25°C.

ratio-Venlafaxine XR

venlafaxine HCl

Antidepressant

ratiopharm

SUPPLIED: 37.5 mg: Each extended-release hard gelatin capsule with light grey cap and peach body filled with white to off-white pellets, with "rph" and "v23" written in red ink on the cap and "37.5" written in red ink on the body, contains: venlafaxine HCl equivalent to venlafaxine base 37.5 mg. Nonmedicinal ingredients: dibutyl sebecate, ethyl cellulose, povidone and sugar spheres; capsule: black iron oxide, gelatin, red iron oxide, titanium dioxide and yellow iron oxide; red ink: ammonium hydroxide, isopropyl alcohol, N-butyl alcohol, propylene glycol, red iron oxide, shellac glaze and simethicone. Bottles of 100 and 500. Store at room temperature (15-30°C), in a dry place.
75 mg: Each extended-release hard gelatin capsule with peach cap and body filled with white to off-white pellets, with "rph" and "v22" written in red ink on the cap and "75" written in red ink on the body, contains: venlafaxine HCl equivalent to venlafaxine base 75 mg. Nonmedicinal ingredients: dibutyl sebecate, ethyl cellulose, povidone and sugar spheres; capsule: gelatin, global red iron oxide, global yellow iron oxide and titanium dioxide; red ink: ammonium hydroxide, isopropyl alcohol, N-butyl alcohol, propylene glycol, red iron oxide, shellac glaze and simethicone. Bottles of 100 and 500. Store at room temperature (15-30°C), in a dry place.
150 mg: Each extended release hard gelatin capsule with dark orange cap and body filled with white to off-white pellets, with "rph" and "v21" written in white ink on the cap and "150" written in white ink on the body, contains: venlafaxine HCl equivalent to venlafaxine base 150 mg. Nonmedicinal ingredients: dibutyl sebecate, ethyl cellulose, povidone and sugar spheres; capsule: gelatin, global red iron oxide, global yellow iron oxide and titanium dioxide; white ink: butyl alcohol, dehydrated alcohol, isopropyl alcohol, povidone, propylene glycol, shellac, sodium hydroxide and titanium dioxide. Bottles of 100 and 500. Store at room temperature (15-30°C), in a dry place.

ratio-Zopiclone

zopiclone

Hypnotic

ratiopharm

SUPPLIED: 5 mg: Each white, round, biconvex, film-coated tablet, imprinted "TEC" on one side and "213C" on the other, contains: zopiclone 5 mg. Nonmedicinal ingredients: calcium phosphate dihydrate, cornstarch, hydroxypropyl methylcellulose, lactose, magnesium stearate, maltodextrin, polydextrose, polyethylene glycol, sodium croscarmellose, titanium dioxide and triacetin. Bottles of 100. Store in a dry place, at room temperature (15 to 30°C). Protect from light.
7.5 mg: Each oval, film-coated blue tablet, marked "TEC 213" on one side and with a scored line on the other, contains: zopiclone 7.5 mg. Nonmedicinal ingredients: calcium phosphate dihydrate, cornstarch, D&C Yellow No. 10 aluminum lake, FD&C Blue No. 1 aluminum lake, FD&C Blue No. 2 aluminum lake, hydroxypropyl methylcellulose, lactose, magnesium stearate, maltodextrin, polydextrose, polyethylene glycol, sodium croscarmellose, titanium dioxide and triacetin. Bottles of 100 and 500. Store in a dry place, at room temperature (15 to 30°C). Protect from light.

Reactine®

cetirizine HCl

Histamine H1-Receptor Antagonist

McNeil Consumer Healthcare

Date of Revision: April 26, 2007

SUMMARY PRODUCT INFORMATION:

Route of Administration	Dosage Form/ Strength	Clinically Relevant Nonmedicinal Ingredients
Oral	Nonprescription tablet 5 mg, 10 mg Prescription tablet 20 mg Syrup 5 mg/5 mL	Tablets: lactose Syrup: parabens, sucrose For a complete listing see Dosage Forms, Composition and Packaging.

INDICATIONS AND CLINICAL USE: Patient Subsets: Adults and Children 12 Years of Age and Over: REACTINE (cetirizine hydrochloride) is indicated for the fast relief of nasal and non-nasal symptoms associated with seasonal and perennial allergic rhinitis (i.e. sneezing, rhinorrhea, post-nasal discharge, nasal congestion/stuffiness, tearing and redness of the eyes, itchy nose/throat) and chronic idiopathic urticaria (e.g. pruritus and hives).
Pediatrics—Children 2-12 Years of Age: REACTINE Syrup is indicated for the relief of the symptoms associated with seasonal allergic rhinitis. REACTINE Syrup is also indicated for the fast and long-lasting relief of itching due to allergic skin reactions such as hives.

The nasal congestion/stuffiness and itchy nose/throat symptoms have not been adequately studied in the pediatric 2-12 years of age patient subset. The effectiveness of REACTINE Syrup in treating symptoms associated with perennial allergic rhinitis and chronic idiopathic urticaria has not been established in this age group.

CONTRAINDICATIONS: REACTINE (cetirizine hydrochloride) is contraindicated in those patients with a known hypersensitivity to it or to its parent compound, hydroxyzine, in patients who are hypersensitive to any other ingredient in the formulation, or in patients with severe renal impairment (less than 10 mL/min creatinine clearance).

WARNINGS AND PRECAUTIONS: General: Activities Requiring Mental Alertness: Studies using objective measurements have shown no effect of REACTINE (cetirizine hydrochloride) on cognitive function, motor performance or sleep latency in healthy volunteers. However, in clinical trials the appearance of some CNS effects, particularly somnolence, have been observed. If drowsiness occurs, do not drive or operate machinery and avoid concurrent use of REACTINE with sedating substances because additional reductions in alertness and additional impairment of CNS performance may occur. (See Drug Interactions.)
Special Populations: Pregnant Women: No teratogenic effects were caused by oral doses as high as 60, 188 and 133 times the maximum clinically studied human dose in mice, rats and rabbits, respectively. No effects on reproduction and fertility were observed at doses as high as 40 and 10 times the maximum recommended human dose in male and female mice, respectively. An oral dose 60 times the maximum clinically studied human dose in female mice did not affect parturition or lactation. Although the animal studies are not indicative of any adverse effects during pregnancy at clinically relevant doses, such studies are not always predictive of a human response. There are no adequate and well-controlled studies in pregnant women. Until such data become available, REACTINE (cetirizine hydrochloride) should not be used during pregnancy, unless advised otherwise by a physician.

Nursing Women: Studies in beagle dogs indicate that approximately 3% of the dose is excreted in milk. The extent of excretion in human milk is unknown. Use of REACTINE in nursing mothers is not recommended, unless directed otherwise by a physician.
Pediatrics: Unless directed otherwise by a physician, REACTINE should not be administered to children below 2 years of age. (See Dosage and Administration.)
Geriatrics: REACTINE (cetirizine hydrochloride) was well tolerated by patients aged 65 and over. Clearance of REACTINE is reduced in proportion to creatinine clearance. In patients whose creatinine clearance is reduced (i.e., those with moderate renal impairment), a starting dose of 5 mg/day is recommended.

Occasional instances of liver function test (transaminase) elevations have occurred during REACTINE (cetirizine hydrochloride) therapy. This incidence was 1.6% in the short-term trials and 4.4% in the 6 month trials. These liver enzyme elevations, mainly ALT, were generally reversible. There was no evidence of jaundice or hepatitis, and the clinical significance is presently unknown. Consequently, REACTINE should be used with caution in patients with pre-existing liver disease. In patients with moderate hepatic impairment, a starting dose of 5 mg is recommended.
Use in Asthmatics: REACTINE has been safely administered to patients with mild to moderate asthma. REACTINE did not cause exacerbation of asthma symptoms.

ADVERSE REACTIONS: Clinical Trial Adverse Drug Reactions: Because clinical trials are conducted under very specific conditions the adverse reaction rates observed in the clinical trials may not reflect the rates observed in practice and should not be compared to the rates in the clinical trials of another drug. Adverse drug reaction information from clinical trials is useful for identifying drug-related adverse events and for approximating rates.

In clinical development programs (domestic and international), REACTINE (cetirizine hydrochloride) has been evaluated in more than 6000 treated patients at daily doses ranging from 5 to 20 mg. The most common adverse reactions were headache and somnolence (see paragraph below). The incidence of headache associated with REACTINE (cetirizine hydrochloride) was not different from placebo. The incidence of somnolence associated with REACTINE was dose related and predominantly mild to moderate. The adverse reaction profile in children shows a lower incidence of somnolence.

Incidence of somnolence reported in placebo controlled efficacy trials with cetirizine should not be misinterpreted as these studies were not designed or powered to assess somnolence or lack of somnolence. Several placebo controlled studies involving objective and subjective tests in healthy volunteers have demonstrated that REACTINE at doses up to 10 mg did not significantly differ from placebo with respect to CNS impairment or task performance.

Most adverse reactions reported during REACTINE (cetirizine hydrochloride) therapy in clinical trials were mild to moderate. The incidence of discontinuation due to adverse reactions in patients receiving REACTINE was not significantly different from placebo (1.0% vs 0.6%, respectively, in placebo-controlled trials). There was no difference by gender or by body weight with regard to the incidence of adverse reactions.

Occasional instances of transient, reversible hepatic transaminase elevations have occurred during REACTINE therapy, without evidence of jaundice, hepatitis or other clinical findings.

Adverse events which were reported at an incidence of greater than 1/50 (2%) in clinical trials are listed in Table 1 and Table 2.

Table 1: REACTINE

Adverse Reactions Reported in Placebo-Controlled REACTINE Trials (Maximum Dose of 10 mg) at Rates of 2% or Greater (Percent Incidence)

Adverse Experience	REACTINE (N=3260)	Placebo (N=3061)	Difference of Percentage
Headache	7.42	8.07	(0.65)[a]
Dry Mouth	2.09	0.82	1.27
Somnolence	9.63	5.00	4.63

[a] ( )=Higher frequency in placebo group.

Table 2: REACTINE

Adverse Reactions Reported in Placebo-Controlled U.S. REACTINE Trials (Total Daily of 20 mg) at Rates of 2% or Greater (Percent Incidence)

Adverse Experience	REACTINE 20 mg (N=272)	Placebo (N=671)	Difference of Percentage
Somnolence	23.9%	7.7%	16.2
Headache	16.5	18.8	(2.3)[a]
Dry Mouth	7.7	1.5	6.2
Fatigue	7.0	2.4	4.6
Nausea	2.9	4.2	(1.3)[a]

[a] ( )=Higher frequency in placebo group.

The following events were observed infrequently (equal to or less than 2%), in 3982 patients who received REACTINE in worldwide trials, including an open study of 6 months duration; a causal relationship with REACTINE administration has not been established.
Application Site: application site reaction, injection site inflammation.
Autonomic Nervous System: anorexia, urinary retention, flushing, saliva increased.
Cardiovascular: palpitation, tachycardia, hypertension, arrhythmia, cardiac failure.
Central and Peripheral Nervous Systems: fatigue, dizziness, insomnia, nervousness paresthesia, confusion, hyperkinesia, hypertonia, migraine, tremor, vertigo, leg cramps, ataxia, dysphonia, coordination abnormal, hyperesthesia, hypoesthesia, myelitis, paralysis, ptosis, speech disorder, twitching, visual field defect.
Endocrine: thyroid disorder.
Gastrointestinal: nausea, pharyngitis, appetite increased, dyspepsia, abdominal pain, diarrhea, flatulence, constipation, vomiting, stomatitis ulcerative, tongue disorder, tooth caries aggravated, stomatitis, tongue discoloration, tongue edema, gastritis, hemorrhage rectum, hemorrhoids, melena, hepatic function abnormal.
Genitourinary: polyuria, urinary tract infection, cystitis, dysuria, hematuria, urine abnormal.
Hearing and Vestibular: earache, tinnitus, deafness, ototoxicity.
Metabolic/Nutritional: thirst, edema, dehydration, diabetes mellitus.
Musculoskeletal: myalgia, arthralgia, bone disorder, arthrosis, tendon disorder, arthritis, muscle weakness.
Psychiatric: depression, emotional lability, concentration impaired, anxiety, depersonalization, paroniria, thinking abnormal, agitation, amnesia, libido decreased, euphoria.
Resistance Mechanism: healing impaired, herpes simplex, infection, infection fungal, infection viral.
Respiratory System: epistaxis, rhinitis, coughing, respiratory disorder, bronchospasm, dyspnea, upper respiratory tract infection, hyperventilation, sinusitis, sputum increased, bronchitis, pneumonia.
Reproductive: dysmenorrhea, menstrual disorder, breast pain female, intermenstrual bleeding, leukorrhea, menorrhagia, pregnancy unintended, vaginitis, testes disorder.
Reticuloendothelial: lymphadenopathy.
Skin: pruritus, rash, skin disorder, skin dry, urticaria, acne, dermatitis, rash erythematous, sweating increased, alopecia, angioedema, furunculosis, bullous eruption, eczema, hyperkeratosis, hypertrichosis, photosensitivity reaction, photosensitivity toxic reaction, rash maculopapular, seborrhea, purpura.
Special Senses: taste perversion, taste loss, parosmia.
Vision: eye abnormality, vision abnormal, eye pain, conjunctivitis, xerophthalmia, glaucoma, ocular hemorrhage.
Body as a Whole: weight increase, back pain, malaise, pain, chest pain, fever, asthenia, edema generalized, edema periorbital, edema peripheral, rigors, edema legs, face edema, hot flushes, abdomen enlarged, allergic reaction, nasal polyp.

The adverse reaction profile in children is similar to the one in adults with, however, a lower incidence of somnolence (3.7% overall vs 0.84% for children receiving placebo) and higher incidences of abdominal pain, pharyngitis, coughing and epistaxis, as indicated in Table 3. Adverse drug reactions at rates of 1 % or greater in children aged from 6 months to 12 years, included in placebo-controlled clinical or pharmacoclinical trials are: see Table 3.

Table 3: REACTINE

Most Common Adverse Reactions Reported in Placebo-Controlled Pediatric Trials

Adverse Experience	Placebo (N=239)	Cetirizine 5 mg (N=161)	Cetirizine 10 mg (N=144)
Headache	10.9	11.2	12.5
Abdominal Pain	2.1	4.4	6.3
Pharyngitis	3.8	6.2	4.2
Coughing	3.4	4.4	3.5
Epistaxis	2.5	3.7	2.8
Somnolence	0.8	1.9	4.2
Nausea	2.1	1.9	4.2

Less Common Clinical Trial Adverse Drug Reactions (<1%): Weight gain was reported as an adverse event in 0.4% of cetirizine patients in placebo controlled trials. In an open study of 6 months duration, the mean weight gain was 2.8% after 20 weeks, with no further increase at 26 weeks.

In a 6-week, placebo-controlled study of 186 patients with allergic rhinitis and mild to moderate asthma, REACTINE 10 mg o.d. improved rhinitis symptoms and did not alter pulmonary function. This study supports the safety of administering REACTINE to allergic rhinitis patients with mild to moderate asthma.
Abnormal Hematologic and Clinical Chemistry Findings: Occasional instances of transient, reversible hepatic transaminase elevations have occurred during cetirizine therapy.
Post-Market Adverse Drug Reactions: In post-marketing experience the following additional rare, but potential severe adverse events have been reported: hemolytic anemia, thrombocytopenia, orofacial dyskinesia, severe hypotension, anaphylaxis, hepatitis, glomerulonephritis, stillbirth, and cholestasis. In addition, isolated cases of the following adverse drug reactions have been reported: convulsions, syncope, aggression, and hypersensitivity.
DRUG INTERACTIONS: Overview: Interaction studies with REACTINE and alcohol or diazepam indicate that at therapeutic doses, REACTINE does not increase alcohol-induced or diazepam-induced impairment of motor and mental performance.
Drug-Drug Interactions: No clinically significant drug interactions have been found with theophylline, pseudoephedrine, cimetidine, erythromycin and ketoconazole. Epidemiologic data suggests that there also would not be interaction with other macrolide antibiotics or imidazole antifungals. In clinical trials, REACTINE (cetirizine hydrochloride) has been safely administered with beta-agonists, nonsteroidal anti-inflammatory drugs, oral contraceptives, narcotic analgesics, corticosteroids, H_2-antagonists, cephalosporins, penicillins, thyroid hormones and thiazide diuretics. If drowsiness occurs, concurrent use of REACTINE with sedating substances should be avoided because additional reductions in alertness and additional impairment of CNS performance may occur. (See Warnings and Precautions, Activities Requiring Mental Alertness.)

Based on (1) its relatively low level of metabolic elimination, (2) no effect on corrected QT intervals at plasma concentrations three times the maximal therapeutic levels, and (3) no apparent interactions with ketoconazole or erythromycin, cetirizine is unlikely to have clinically significant interactions with other macrolides such as clarithromycin or other imidazole antifungals such as itraconazole in patients with normal renal and hepatic function. Although no data with these other drugs are available at the present time, there is no epidemiological evidence (the safety database comprised 6490 patients evaluated in U.S. and Canadian studies) of interactions between macrolide antibiotics and/or imidazole antifungals taken orally, and cetirizine/hydroxyzine. The epidemiologic data do not suggest an increase of adverse events, cardiac or non-cardiac, in patients treated with cetirizine and concomitant macrolide or imidazole antifungal medication.

DOSAGE AND ADMINISTRATION: Recommended Dose and Dosage Adjustment: Adults and Children 12 Years of Age and Over: The recommended initial dose of REACTINE (cetirizine hydrochloride) is 5 to 10 mg, depending on symptom severity, given as a single daily dose, with or without food. If sufficient response is not obtained with the nonprescription strengths of 5 or 10 mg, the dose may be increased and prescribed as necessary to the maximum recommended daily dose of 20 mg. The time of administration, with or without food, may be varied to suit individual patient needs.

Clinical studies to date support treatment for up to 6 months thus medical recommendation is advised for long-term use.
Children Aged 6-12 Years of Age: 10 mg (one 10 mg tablet or 2 teaspoons of syrup) once daily, or one 5 mg tablet or 5 mL syrup in the morning and one 5 mg tablet or 5 mL syrup in the evening, with or without food.
Children Aged 2-6 Years of Age: 5 mg or 5 mL (1 teaspoon) given once daily, or 2.5 mg or 2.5 mL (one-half teaspoon) syrup in the morning and 2.5 mg or 2.5 mL (one-half teaspoon) syrup in the evening, with or without food.

Do not give to children under 2 years of age, unless advised by physician.
Adults 65 Years of Age and Over: In patients with moderate hepatic and/or renal impairment, a starting dose of 5 mg/day is recommended.

OVERDOSAGE:
Overdose has been reported with REACTINE (cetirizine hydrochloride). Symptoms observed after an overdose of cetirizine are mainly associated with CNS effects or with symptoms that could suggest an anticholinergic effect. Adverse events reported after an intake of at least 5 times the recommended daily dose are: confusion, diarrhea, dizziness, fatigue, headache, malaise, mydriasis, pruritus, restlessness, sedation, somnolence, stupor, tachycardia, tremor, and urinary retention. If an acute overdose occurs, evacuation of the stomach should be considered during the first few hours after this overdose. Treatment should be symptomatic and supportive taking into account any concomitantly ingested medications. There is no known specific antidote to REACTINE (cetirizine hydrochloride). REACTINE (cetirizine hydrochloride) is not effectively removed by dialysis, and dialysis will be ineffective unless a dialyzable agent has been concomitantly ingested. The minimal lethal oral dose in rodents is at least 590 times the maximum clinically studied dose.

For management of a suspected drug overdose, CPhA recommends that you contact your **regional Poison Control Centre**. See the *CPS* Directory section for a list of Poison Control Centres.

ACTION AND CLINICAL PHARMACOLOGY: Mechanism of Action: REACTINE (cetirizine hydrochloride), an active human metabolite of hydroxyzine, is a histamine H_1 receptor antagonist anti-allergic compound; its principal effects are mediated via selective inhibition of peripheral H_1 receptors. REACTINE (cetirizine hydrochloride) is distinguished from other histamine H_1 receptor antagonists by the presence of a carboxylic acid function. This difference may be partly responsible for the selectivity of REACTINE (cetirizine hydrochloride) seen in pharmacologic models and its distinctive pharmacokinetic properties in humans.
Pharmacodynamics: The antihistaminic activity of REACTINE has been well documented in a variety of animal and human models. In vivo animal models have shown negligible anticholinergic or antiserotonergic activity. In vitro receptor binding studies have detected no measurable affinity for other than H_1 receptors. Autoradiographic studies have shown negligible penetration into the brain. Systemically administered cetirizine does not significantly occupy cerebral H_1 receptors. Several studies involving objective and subjective tests in healthy volunteers have demonstrated that REACTINE at doses up to 10 mg did not significantly differ from placebo with respect to CNS impairment, daytime drowsiness, reaction times, mental alertness, task performance, objective CNS depression and various other tests of cognitive function.

REACTINE (cetirizine hydrochloride) does not exacerbate asthma and is effective in a variety of histamine mediated disorders. In adults, oral doses of 5-20 mg in humans strongly inhibit the skin wheal and flare response caused by the intradermal injection of histamine. The onset of activity occurs within 20 (50% of subjects) to 60 (95% of subjects) minutes and persists for at least 24 hours following a single dose. The effects of intradermal injection of various other mediators or histamine releasers as well as components of the allergy cascade, including allergic inflammatory response to cutaneous antigen challenge are also inhibited.

In children aged 2-12 years, with a documented history of pollen-induced allergic rhinitis, once daily treatment with 5 mg or 10 mg cetirizine significantly suppressed the wheal and flare response to histamine, with onset of action occurring within 1 hour and persisting for 24 hours following the initial dose; significant suppression of the wheal and flare response persisted on repeated once daily treatment for 35 days and was accompanied by significant improvements in nasal and ocular symptoms.

Pharmacokinetics: Absorption: In adults, REACTINE is rapidly absorbed after oral administration. Peak plasma levels after a 10 mg dose are approximately 300 ng/mL and occur at about 1 hour. Co-administration of REACTINE with food does not affect bioavailability as measured by AUC but absorption is delayed by about 1 hour, with 23% lower C_{max}.

Distribution: Plasma protein binding is 93% in the concentration range observed in clinical studies.

Metabolism: In adults, REACTINE is less extensively metabolized than other antihistamines and approximately 60% of an administered dose is excreted unchanged in 24 hours. High bioavailability is associated with generally low inter-subject variation in blood levels. It is attributable primarily to low first-pass metabolism. Only one metabolite has been identified in humans—the product of oxidative dealkylation of the terminal carboxymethyl group. The antihistaminic activity of this metabolite is negligible.

Excretion: The plasma elimination half-life is approximately 8 to 9 hours and does not change with multiple dosing. Pharmacokinetics are dose independent and plasma levels are proportional to the dose administered over the clinically studied range of 5 to 20 mg.

In children, when compared to adults, the observed C_{max} and AUC increases with decreasing age, in inverse relationship to body weight. Based on cross-study comparison, the elimination half-life was 33-41% shorter in children than in adults, with weight-normalized total body clearance 33% greater in 7-12 year olds and 88-111% greater in younger children than in adults. The nature of the metabolites formed in children is unknown at present. Table 4 compares typical pharmacokinetic parameters in children vs adults.

Table 4: REACTINE

Typical Pharmacokinetic Parameters of Cetirizine in Children and in Adults

Parameter	Adults 10 mg Single Dose	Children 6–12 years 5 mg Single Dose
C_{max} (ng/mL)	300	275
T_{max} (hr)	1.1	1.1
t½ (hr)	8.0	5.6
AUC (ng·hr/mL)	2871	2201
Urinary Recovery (%)	60	40–50

Special Populations and Conditions: Hepatic Insufficiency/Renal Insufficiency: In patients with mild to moderate hepatic and renal impairment, total body clearance of REACTINE is reduced and AUC and half-life increased by about 2 to 3 fold. Clearance is reduced in proportion to the decline in creatinine clearance. Plasma levels are unaffected by hemodialysis. The plasma elimination half-life in dialysis patients is approximately 20 hours and the plasma AUC is increased by about threefold.

STORAGE AND STABILITY: Recommended storage: Store between 15-30°C.

INFORMATION FOR THE PATIENT: Published in e-CPS, available by subscription at www.e-cps.ca.

DOSAGE FORMS, COMPOSITION AND PACKAGING: Syrup: Each 5 mL of colorless, banana-grape flavored preparation contains: cetirizine HCl 5 mg. Nonmedicinal ingredients: acetic acid, artificial grape flavour, artificial banana flavour, glycerin, methyl paraben, propyl paraben, propylene glycol, purified water, sodium acetate and sugar syrup (sucrose). Amber glass bottles of 100 mL.

Tablets: 5 mg: Each white (dye-free), film-coated, scored, ovoid tablet contains: cetirizine HCl 5 mg. Nonmedicinal ingredients: cornstarch, hypromellose, lactose, magnesium stearate, polyethylene glycol, povidone and titanium dioxide. Blister packages (for OTC use) of 24 and 36.

10 mg: Each white (dye-free), film-coated, scored, ovoid tablet contains: cetirizine HCl 10 mg. Nonmedicinal ingredients: cornstarch, hypromellose, lactose, magnesium stearate, polyethylene glycol, povidone and titanium dioxide. Bottles of 100 and 500. Blister packages (for OTC use) of 10, 20, 30 and 48.

20 mg Pr: Each white (dye-free), film-coated, scored, ovoid tablet contains: cetirizine HCl 20 mg. Nonmedicinal ingredients: cornstarch, hypromellose, lactose, magnesium stearate, polyethylene glycol, povidone and titanium dioxide. Plastic bottles of 100.

Reactine™ Allergy & Sinus

cetirizine HCl—pseudoephedrine HCl

Histamine H1-Receptor Antagonist—Sympathomimetic Amine

McNeil Consumer Healthcare

Date of Revision: July 19, 2005

SUMMARY PRODUCT INFORMATION:

Route of Administration	Dosage Form/Strength	Clinically Relevant Nonmedicinal Ingredients
Oral	Nonprescription tablet containing 5 mg cetirizine hydrochloride in an immediate release layer and 120 mg pseudoephedrine hydrochloride in an extended release layer	Lactose For a complete listing see Dosage Forms, Composition and Packaging.

INDICATIONS AND CLINICAL USE: Patient Subsets: Adults: REACTINE ALLERGY & SINUS Extended Release Tablets (cetirizine hydrochloride 5 mg/pseudoephedrine hydrochloride 120 mg) are indicated for the relief of symptoms associated with seasonal allergic rhinitis and perennial allergic rhinitis. Symptoms treated effectively include: sneezing, rhinorrhea, post nasal discharge, tearing and redness of the eyes and nasal congestion.

Pediatrics (Children 12 years of age and over): REACTINE ALLERGY & SINUS Extended Release Tablets are indicated for the relief of symptoms associated with seasonal allergic rhinitis and perennial allergic rhinitis. Symptoms treated effectively include: sneezing, rhinorrhea, post nasal discharge, tearing and redness of the eyes and nasal congestion. Refer to Warnings and Precautions for additional information regarding pediatric patients.

CONTRAINDICATIONS: REACTINE ALLERGY & SINUS Extended Release Tablets (cetirizine hydrochloride/pseudoephedrine hydrochloride) are contraindicated in those patients with a known hypersensitivity to cetirizine or to its parent compound, hydroxyzine, those with a known hypersensitivity or idiosyncrasy to pseudoephedrine hydrochloride, to adrenergic agents, to other drugs of similar chemical structures, or to any of the ingredients in the formulation or components of the container. Manifestations of patient idiosyncrasy to adrenergic agents include: insomnia, dizziness, weakness, tremor, or arrhythmias. For a complete listing, see Dosage Forms, Composition and Packaging.

Due to its pseudoephedrine hydrochloride component, REACTINE ALLERGY & SINUS is contraindicated in patients with narrow-angle glaucoma or urinary retention, and in patients receiving monoamine oxidase (MAO) inhibitor therapy or within 14 days of stopping such treatment. It is also contraindicated in patients with severe hypertension, or severe coronary artery disease, and in patients with hyperthyroidism.

The use of cetirizine/pseudoephedrine should be avoided in children under 12 years of age.

WARNINGS AND PRECAUTIONS: General: Sympathomimetics should be used with caution in patients with stenosing peptic ulcer, pyloroduodenal obstruction, prostatic hypertrophy, or bladder neck obstruction, cardiovascular disease, arrhythmia, tachycardia, hypertension, hyperthyroidism, increased intraocular pressure, renal or hepatic insufficiency or diabetes mellitus. Sympathomimetics should be used with caution in patients receiving decongestants, appetite suppressants, psychostimulants (such as amphetamines), tricyclic antidepressants, and digitalis. Sympathomimetics may cause central nervous system (CNS) stimulation and convulsions or cardiovascular collapse with accompanying hypotension.

Activities Requiring Mental Alertness: Studies using objective measurements have shown no effect of cetirizine hydrochloride on cognitive function, motor performance or sleep latency in healthy volunteers. However, in clinical trials the appearance of some CNS effects, particularly somnolence, have been observed. If drowsiness occurs, do not drive or operate machinery.

Special Populations: Pregnant Women: There are no adequate and well-controlled studies in pregnant women. Until such data become available, REACTINE ALLERGY & SINUS (cetirizine hydrochloride/pseudoephedrine hydrochloride) should not be used during pregnancy, unless advised otherwise by a physician.

Nursing Women: Cetirizine has been reported to be excreted in human breast milk. For pseudoephedrine hydrochloride administered alone, about 0.5% of the dose has been reported to be excreted in human breast milk. Because cetirizine and pseudoephedrine are excreted in milk, use of REACTINE ALLERGY & SINUS in nursing mothers is not recommended.

Pediatrics: REACTINE ALLERGY & SINUS contains a fixed dose of pseudoephedrine hydrochloride 120 mg in an extended release formulation. This dose of pseudoephedrine hydrochloride is not recommended for pediatric patients under 12 years of age. The safety and effectiveness of REACTINE ALLERGY & SINUS in pediatric patients under the age of 12 years has not been established.

Geriatrics: In elderly patients, sympathomimetics are more likely to cause adverse reactions such as confusion, hallucination, convulsions, and/or CNS depression.

Cetirizine hydrochloride was well tolerated by patients aged 65 and over. Clearance of cetirizine hydrochloride is reduced in proportion to creatinine clearance. In patients whose creatinine clearance is reduced (i.e., those with moderate renal impairment), a starting dose of 5 mg/day (one REACTINE ALLERGY & SINUS tablet) is recommended.

Pseudoephedrine is incompletely metabolized (less than 1%) in the liver by N-demethylation to an inactive metabolite. The drug and its metabolite are excreted in urine; 55-96% of a dose is excreted unchanged. Therefore, pseudoephedrine may accumulate in patients with renal insufficiency.

Occasional instances of liver function test (transaminase) elevations have occurred during cetirizine hydrochloride therapy. This incidence was 1.6% in the short-term trials and 4.4% in the 6 month trials. These liver enzyme elevations, mainly ALT, were generally reversible. There was no evidence of jaundice or hepatitis, and the clinical significance is presently unknown. Consequently, cetirizine hydrochloride should be used with caution in patients with pre-existing liver disease. In patients with moderate hepatic impairment, a starting dose of 5 mg is recommended.

The effect of hepatic impairment on pseudoephedrine hydrochloride pharmacokinetics is unknown.

ADVERSE REACTIONS: Clinical Trial Adverse Drug Reactions: Because clinical trials are conducted under very specific conditions the adverse reaction rates observed in the clinical trials may not reflect the rates observed in practice and should not be compared to the rates in the clinical trials of another drug. Adverse drug reaction information from clinical trials is useful for identifying drug-related adverse events and for approximating rates.

In controlled clinical trials, adverse reactions reported in more than 1% of the patients receiving the combination cetirizine/pseudoephedrine, were not different from those reported for cetirizine or pseudoephedrine alone. They included: dry mouth, headache, insomnia, somnolence, asthenia, tachycardia, nervousness, dizziness, vertigo, and nausea. Sympathomimetic drugs have also been associated with certain untoward reactions, including fear, anxiety, tenseness, restlessness, tremor, weakness, pallor, respiratory difficulty, dysuria, hallucinations, convulsions, CNS depression, arrhythmias and cardiovascular collapse with hypotension.

Hypersensitivity reactions, including skin reactions and angioedema, may occur.

Cetirizine HCl: In clinical development programs (domestic and international), cetirizine hydrochloride has been evaluated in more than 6000 treated patients at daily doses ranging from 5 to 20 mg. The most common adverse reactions were headache and somnolence (see paragraph below). The incidence of headache associated with cetirizine hydrochloride was not different from placebo. The incidence of somnolence associated with cetirizine hydrochloride was dose related and predominantly mild to moderate. The adverse reaction profile in children shows a lower incidence of somnolence.

Incidence of somnolence reported in placebo controlled efficacy trials with cetirizine should not be misinterpreted as these studies were not designed or powered to assess somnolence or lack of somnolence. Several placebo controlled studies involving objective and subjective tests in healthy volunteers have demonstrated that cetirizine hydrochloride at doses up to 10 mg did not significantly differ from placebo with respect to CNS impairment or task performance.

Most adverse reactions reported during cetirizine hydrochloride therapy in clinical trials were mild to moderate. The incidence of discontinuation due to adverse reactions in patients receiving cetirizine hydrochloride was not significantly different from placebo (1.0% vs 0.6%, respectively, in placebo-controlled trials). There was no difference by gender or by body weight with regard to the incidence of adverse reactions.

Adverse events which were reported at an incidence of greater than 1/50 (2%) in clinical trials are listed in Table 1.

Table 1: REACTINE ALLERGY & SINUS

Adverse Effects Reported in Placebo-Controlled REACTINE Trials (Maximum Dose of 10 mg) at Rates of 1% or Greater (Percent Incidence)

Adverse Experience	Cetirizine HCl (n=3260)	Placebo (n=3061)	Difference of Percentage
Headache	7.42	8.07	(0.65)[a]
Dry Mouth	2.09	0.82	1.27
Somnolence	9.63	5.00	4.63

[a] Higher frequency in placebo group.

The following events were observed infrequently (equal to or less than 2%), in 3982 patients who received cetirizine hydrochloride in worldwide trials, including an open study of 6 months duration; a causal relationship with cetirizine hydrochloride administration has not been established.

Autonomic Nervous System: anorexia, urinary retention, flushing, saliva increased.

Cardiovascular: palpitation, tachycardia, hypertension, arrhythmia, cardiac failure.

Central and Peripheral Nervous Systems: fatigue, dizziness, insomnia, nervousness, paresthesia, confusion, hyperkinesia, hypertonia, migraine, tremor, vertigo, cramps legs, ataxia, dysphonia, coordination abnormal, hyperesthesia, hypoesthesia, myelitis, paralysis, ptosis, speech disorder, twitching, visual field defect.

Endocrine: thyroid disorder.

Gastrointestinal: nausea, pharnyngitis, appetite increased, dyspepsia, abdominal pain, diarrhea, flatulence, constipation, vomiting, stomatitis ulcerative, tongue disorder, tooth caries aggravated, stomatitis, tongue discoloration, tongue edema, gastritis, hemorrhage rectum, hemorrhoids, melena, hepatic function abnormal.

Genitourinary: polyuria, urinary tract infection, cystitis, dysuria, hematuria, urine abnormal.

Hearing and Vestibular: earache, tinnitus, deafness, ototoxicity.

Metabolic/Nutritional: thirst, edema, dehydration, diabetes mellitus.

Musculoskeletal: myalgia, arthralgia, bone disorder, arthrosis, tendon disorder, arthritis, muscle weakness.

Psychiatric: depression, emotional lability, concentration impaired, anxiety, depersonalization, paroniria, thinking abnormal, agitation, amnesia, libido decreased, euphoria.

Resistance Mechanism: healing impaired, herpes simplex infection, infection fungal, infection viral.

Respiratory System: epistaxis, rhinitis, coughing, respiratory disorder bronchospasm, dyspnea, upper respiratory tract infection, hyperventilation, sinusitis, sputum increased, bronchitis, pneumonia.

Reproductive: dysmenorrhea, menstrual disorder, breast pain female, intermenstrual bleeding, leukorrhea, menorrhagia, pregnancy unintended, vaginitis, testes disorder.

Reticuloendothelial: lymphadenopathy.

Skin: pruritus, rash, skin disorder, skin dry, urticaria, acne, dermatitis, rash erythematous, sweating increased, alopecia, angioedema, furunculosis, bullous eruption, eczema, hyperkeratosis, hypertrichosis, photosensitivity reaction, photosensitivity toxic reaction, rash maculopapular, seborrhea, purpura.

Special Senses: taste perversion, taste loss, parosmia.

Vision: eye abnormality, vision abnormal, eye pain, conjunctivitis, xerophthalmia, glaucoma, ocular hemorrhage.

Body as a Whole: weight increase, back pain, malaise, pain, chest pain, fever, asthenia, edema generalized, edema periorbital, edema peripheral, rigors, edema legs, face edema, hot flushes, abdomen enlarged, allergic reaction, nasal polyps.

Less Common Clinical Trial Adverse Drug Reactions (<1%): Cetirizine HCl: Weight gain was reported as an adverse event in 0.4% of cetirizine patients in placebo controlled trials. In an open study of 6 months duration, the mean weight gain was 2.8% after 20 weeks, with no further increase at 26 weeks.

Occasional instances of transient, reversible hepatic transaminase elevations have occurred during cetirizine therapy.

In a 6-week, placebo-controlled study of 186 patients with allergic rhinitis and mild to moderate asthma, cetirizine hydrochloride 10 mg o.d. improved rhinitis symptoms and did not alter pulmonary function. This study supports the safety of administering cetirizine hydrochloride to allergic rhinitis patients with mild to moderate asthma.

Abnormal Hematologic and Clinical Chemistry Findings: Occasional instances of transient, reversible hepatic transaminase elevations have occurred during cetirizine hydrochloride therapy, without evidence of jaundice, hepatitis or other clinical findings.

Post-Market Adverse Drug Reactions: Cetirizine HCl: In post-marketing experience the following additional rare, but potential severe adverse events have been reported: hemolytic anemia, thrombocytopenia, orofacial dyskinesia, severe hypotension, anaphylaxis, hepatitis, glomerulonephritis, stillbirth, and cholestasis. In addition, isolated cases of the following adverse drug reactions have been reported: convulsions, syncope, aggression, and hypersensitivity.

Pseudoephedrine HCl: Pseudoephedrine hydrochloride may cause mild CNS stimulation in hypertensive patients. As with other sympathomimetic amines, CNS stimulation, muscular weakness, tightness in the chest and syncope may also be encountered. Nervousness, excitability, restlessness, dizziness, weakness, or insomnia may occur. Headache, nausea, drowsiness, tachycardia, palpitation, pressor activity, and cardiac arrhythmias have been reported. Sympathomimetic drugs have also been associated with other untoward effects such as fear, anxiety, confusion, tenseness, tremor, hallucinations, seizures, dry mouth, difficulty in micturition, vomiting, pallor, respiratory difficulty, dysuria, fixed drug eruption, and cardiovascular collapse.

DRUG INTERACTIONS: Overview: Interaction studies with cetirizine hydrochloride and alcohol or diazepam indicate that cetirizine hydrochloride does not increase alcohol-induced or diazepam-induced impairment of motor and mental performance.

Drug-Drug Interactions: Cetirizine HCl: No clinically significant drug interactions have been found with cetirizine hydrochloride and theophylline, pseudoephedrine hydrochloride, cimetidine, erythromycin and ketoconazole. Epidemiologic data suggests that there also would not be interaction with other macrolide antibiotics or imidazole antifungals. In clinical trials, cetirizine hydrochloride has been safely administered with beta-agonists, non-steroidal anti-inflammatory drugs, oral contraceptives, narcotic analgesics, corticosteroids, H_2-antagonists, cephalosporins, penicillins, thyroid hormones and thiazide diuretics.

Based on: (a) its relatively low level of metabolic elimination, (b) no effect on corrected QT intervals at plasma concentrations three times the maximal therapeutic levels, and (c) no apparent interactions with ketoconazole or erythromycin, cetirizine hydrochloride is unlikely to have clinically significant interactions with other macrolides such as clarithromycin or other imidazole antifungals such as itraconazole in patients with normal renal and hepatic function. Although no data with these other drugs are available at the present time, there is no epidemiological evidence (the safety database comprised 6490 patients evaluated in U.S. and Canadian studies) of interactions between macrolide antibiotics and/or imidazole antifungals taken orally, and cetirizine hydrochloride/hydroxyzine. The epidemiologic data do not suggest an increase of adverse events, cardiac or non-cardiac, in patients treated with cetirizine hydrochloride and concomitant macrolide or imidazole antifungal medication.

Pseudoephedrine HCl: Monoamine oxidase (MAO) inhibitors potentiate effects of sympathomimetic drugs such as pseudoephedrine hydrochloride. When sympathomimetic drugs are given to patients receiving MAO inhibitors, hypertensive crises may result. Pseudoephedrine hydrochloride should therefore be avoided in patients receiving drugs with MAO inhibiting activity. Pseudoephedrine hydrochloride may reduce the antihypertensive effects of methyldopa, mecamylamine, guanethidine, reserpine, and veratrum alkaloids. Beta adrenergic blocking agents may also interact with sympathomimetics. Increased ectopic pacemaker activity can occur when pseudoephedrine hydrochloride is used concomitantly with digitalis. Therefore, use of REACTINE ALLERGY & SINUS should be avoided in patients on digitalis. The antibacterial agent, furazolidone, is known to cause a dose-related inhibition of MAO. Although there are no reports of a hypertensive crisis caused by the concurrent administration of pseudoephedrine hydrochloride and furazolidone, they should not be taken together. Care should be taken in the administration of REACTINE ALLERGY & SINUS concomitantly with other sympathomimetic amines because combined effects on the cardiovascular system may be harmful to the patient (see Contraindications). Antacids increase the rate of pseudoephedrine absorption; kaolin decreases it.

DOSAGE AND ADMINISTRATION: Recommended Dose and Dosage Adjustment: Adults and children 12 years of age and over: The recommended dose of REACTINE ALLERGY & SINUS (cetirizine hydrochloride/pseudoephedrine hydrochloride) is one tablet every 12 hours. REACTINE ALLERGY & SINUS may be given with or without food.

Adults 65 years of age and over: In patients with moderate hepatic and/or renal impairment, a dose of one tablet once daily is recommended.

OVERDOSAGE:

Acute overdosage with cetirizine/pseudoephedrine may produce tachycardia, arrhythmia, hypertension, signs of CNS depression (sedation, apnea, unconsciousness, cyanosis and cardiovascular collapse) or stimulation (insomnia, hallucinations, tremor, seizures), which could be fatal. Treatment, preferably in a hospital setting, should be symptomatic and supportive, taking into account any concomitantly ingested medications. Should vomiting not occur spontaneously, it should be induced. Gastric lavage is recommended.

There are no known antidotes. Sympathomimetic amines should not be used. Hypertension can be controlled with alpha blockers and tachycardia with beta blockers. Seizures can be treated with intravenous diazepam (or diazepam given rectally in the case of children).

Cetirizine and pseudoephedrine are poorly eliminated by hemodialysis.

> For management of a suspected drug overdose, CPhA recommends that you contact your **regional Poison Control Centre**. See the *CPS* Directory section for a list of Poison Control Centres.

ACTION AND CLINICAL PHARMACOLOGY: Mechanism of Action: Cetirizine hydrochloride, an active human metabolite of hydroxyzine, is a histamine H_1 receptor antagonist anti-allergic compound; its principal effects are mediated via selective inhibition of peripheral H_1 receptors. Cetirizine hydrochloride is distinguished from other histamine H_1 receptor antagonists by the presence of a carboxylic acid function. This difference may be partly responsible for the selectivity of cetirizine hydrochloride seen in pharmacologic models and its distinctive pharmacokinetic properties in humans.

Pharmacodynamics: The antihistaminic activity of cetirizine hydrochloride has been well documented in a variety of animal and human models. In vivo animal models have shown negligible anticholinergic or antiserotonergic activity. In vitro receptor binding studies have detected no measurable affinity for other than H_1 receptors. Autoradiographic studies have shown negligible penetration into the brain. Systemically administered cetirizine does not significantly occupy cerebral H_1 receptors. Several studies involving objective and subjective tests in healthy volunteers have demonstrated that cetirizine hydrochloride at doses up to 10 mg did not significantly differ from placebo with respect to CNS impairment, daytime drowsiness, reaction times, mental alertness, task performance, objective CNS depression and various other tests of cognitive function.

Cetirizine hydrochloride does not exacerbate asthma and is effective in a variety of histamine mediated disorders. In adults, oral doses of 5-20 mg in humans strongly inhibit the skin wheal and flare response caused by the intradermal injection of histamine. The onset of activity occurs within 20 (50% of subjects) to 60 (95% of subjects) minutes and persists for at least 24 hours following a single dose. The effects of intradermal injection of various other mediators or histamine releasers as well as components of the allergic inflammatory response to cutaneous antigen challenge are also inhibited.

Pseudoephedrine hydrochloride is an orally active sympathomimetic amine and is recognized as an effective agent for the relief of nasal congestion due to allergic rhinitis. Pseudoephedrine acts directly on α-adrenergic receptors in the mucosa of the respiratory tract producing vasoconstriction which results in shrinkage of swollen nasal mucous membranes, reduction of tissue hyperemia, edema, and nasal congestion, and an increase in nasal airway patency. Drainage of sinus secretions is increased and obstructed eustachian ostia may be opened. Pseudoephedrine produces peripheral effects similar to those of ephedrine and has the potential for excitatory side effects.

Pharmacokinetics: Absorption: The bioavailability of cetirizine hydrochloride and pseudoephedrine hydrochloride from REACTINE ALLERGY & SINUS Extended Release Tablets is not significantly different from that achieved with separate administration of cetirizine hydrochloride 5 mg tablets and pseudoephedrine hydrochloride 120 mg extended release caplets. Co-administration of cetirizine hydrochloride and pseudoephedrine hydrochloride does not significantly affect the bioavailability of either component.

Following a single dose of the REACTINE ALLERGY & SINUS Tablet, cetirizine hydrochloride was rapidly absorbed and produced a mean peak plasma concentration (Cmax) of 114 ng/mL at a time (Tmax) 2.2 hours postdose. Pseudoephedrine hydrochloride produced a mean peak plasma concentration of 309 ng/mL at 4.4 hours postdose.

When healthy volunteers were administered multiple doses of the REACTINE ALLERGY & SINUS Tablet to reach steady state concentrations (cetirizine hydrochloride 5 mg/pseudoephedrine hydrochloride 120 mg twice daily for seven days), a mean peak plasma concentration (Cmax) of 178 ng/mL was observed for cetirizine and 526 ng/mL for pseudoephedrine.

Food had no significant effect on the extent of cetirizine hydrochloride absorption (AUC), but Tmax was delayed by 1.8 hours and Cmax was decreased by 30%. Food had no significant effect on the pharmacokinetics of pseudoephedrine hydrochloride. REACTINE ALLERGY & SINUS Tablets may be given with or without food.

Distribution: Plasma protein binding of cetirizine hydrochloride is 93% in the concentration range observed in clinical studies.

Metabolism: In adults, cetirizine hydrochloride is less extensively metabolized than other antihistamines and approximately 60% of an administered dose is excreted unchanged in 24 hours. The high bioavailability associated with generally low inter-subject variation in blood levels is attributable primarily to low first-pass metabolism. Only one metabolite has been identified in humans—the product of oxidative dealkylation of the terminal carboxymethyl group. The antihistaminic activity of this metabolite is negligible.

Excretion: After administration of the REACTINE ALLERGY & SINUS Tablet, the mean elimination half-life of cetirizine was 7.9 hours and the mean elimination half-life of pseudoephedrine was 6.0 hours.

Special Populations and Conditions: Hepatic Insufficiency: Hepatic Insufficiency/Renal Insufficiency: In patients with mild to moderate hepatic and renal impairment, total body clearance of cetirizine hydrochloride is reduced and AUC and half-life increased by about 2 to 3 fold. Clearance is reduced in proportion to the decline in creatinine clearance. Plasma levels are unaffected by hemodialysis. The plasma elimination half-life in dialysis patients is approximately 20 hours and the plasma AUC is increased by about threefold.

Renal Insufficiency: See Hepatic Insufficiency.

STORAGE AND STABILITY: Recommended Storage: Store between 15-30°C.

INFORMATION FOR THE PATIENT: Published in e-CPS, available by subscription at www.e-cps.ca.

DOSAGE FORMS, COMPOSITION AND PACKAGING: Each white, round, biconvex, extended release tablet, debossed with " REACTINE + " on one side, contains: cetirizine HCl 5 mg in an immediate release layer and pseudoephedrine HCl 120 mg in an extended release layer. Nonmedicinal ingredients: colloidal silicon dioxide, croscarmellose sodium, hydroxypropyl methylcellulose, lactose, magnesium stearate, microcrystalline cellulose, polyethylene glycol and titanium dioxide. PVC film and aluminum foil blister packages of 10, 20 and 30.

Rebif® Ⓟ

interferon beta-1a

Immunomodulator

EMD Canada

Date of Revision: March 5, 2010

SUMMARY PRODUCT INFORMATION:

Route of Administration	Dosage Form/ Strength	Clinically Relevant Nonmedicinal Ingredients
Subcutaneous	Interferon beta-1a Solution for Injection in Pre-filled Syringe/8.8 µg/0.2 mL, 22 µg/0.5 mL, 44 µg/0.5 mL	Mannitol, benzyl alcohol, poloxamer-188, methionine, 0.01 M sodium acetate pH 4.2 buffer For a complete listing see Dosage Forms, Composition and Packaging.
	Interferon beta-1a Solution for Injection in a Pre-filled Cartridge/22 µg×3 (66 µg/1.5 mL), 44 µg×3 (132 µg/1.5 mL)	Mannitol, benzyl alcohol, poloxamer-188, methionine, 0.01 M sodium acetate pH 3.9 buffer For a complete listing see Dosage Forms, Composition and Packaging.

DESCRIPTION: REBIF (Interferon beta-1a) is a purified, sterile glycoprotein product produced by recombinant DNA techniques and formulated for use by injection. The active ingredient of REBIF is produced by genetically engineered Chinese Hamster Ovary (CHO) cells. Interferon beta-1a is a highly purified glycoprotein that has 166 amino acids and an approximate molecular weight of 22 500 daltons. It contains a single N-linked carbohydrate moiety attached to Asn-80 similar to that of natural human Interferon beta.

INDICATIONS AND CLINICAL USE: REBIF is indicated for the treatment of relapsing forms of multiple sclerosis (MS), to:

- reduce the number and severity of clinical exacerbations,
- slow the progression of physical disability,
- reduce the requirement for steroids,
- reduce the number of hospitalizations for treatment of multiple sclerosis, and
- reduce T1-Gd enhanced and T2 (burden of disease) lesions as seen on MRI.

Relapsing forms of multiple sclerosis include the subgroups of MS in which patients still experience recurrent attacks of neurological dysfunction including traditional RRMS but also SPMS patients still experiencing relapses.

Although REBIF did not affect progression of disability in SPMS, the clinical trial has shown that secondary progressive MS patients who still experience relapses, had a statistically significant improvement on relapse rate and on MRI measures of disease activity as compared to patients on placebo.

REBIF has not yet been investigated in patients with primary progressive multiple sclerosis and should not be administered to such patients.

CONTRAINDICATIONS: REBIF (Interferon beta-1a) is contraindicated in patients with a known hypersensitivity to natural or recombinant interferon beta, or any other component of the formulation.

REBIF is contraindicated in pregnant patients (see Warnings and Precautions).

WARNINGS AND PRECAUTIONS: REBIF (Interferon beta-1a) should be used under the supervision of a physician. The first injection should be performed under the supervision of an appropriately qualified health care professional.

Fertile women receiving REBIF should be advised to take adequate contraceptive measures. It is not known if interferon alters the efficacy of oral contraceptives. Patients planning for pregnancy and those becoming pregnant should be informed of the potential hazards of interferons to the fetus including an increased risk of early miscarriage. In theses patients discontinuation of therapy should be considered (see Contraindications and also Warnings and Precautions, Information to Be Provided to the Patient).

General: Patients should be informed of the most common adverse reactions associated with interferon beta administration, including symptoms of the flu-like syndrome (see Adverse Reactions). These symptoms tend to be most prominent at the initiation of therapy and may decrease in frequency and severity with continued treatment.

Endocrine and Metabolism: Patients treated with REBIF may develop new or worsening thyroid laboratory abnormalities. Caution should be exercised when administering REBIF to patients with pre-existing thyroid disorders. Patients treated with REBIF should be carefully monitored for evidence of thyroid dysfunction (most often presenting as hypothyroidism or hyperthyroidism), and development of thyroid auto-antibodies. Thyroid testing is recommended at baseline and if abnormal, every 6-12 months following initiation of therapy. If normal, routine testing is not needed but should be performed if clinical findings of thyroid dysfunction appear.

Neurologic (including seizures): Caution should be exercised when administering REBIF (interferon-beta-1a) to patients with pre-existing seizures disorder. For patients without a pre-existing seizure disorder who develop seizures during therapy, an etiologic basis should be established and appropriate anti-convulsant therapy instituted prior to continuing treatment with REBIF. The effect of REBIF administration on the medical management of patients with seizure disorder is unknown.

Depression: REBIF should be used with caution in patients with depression, a condition that is common in people with multiple sclerosis. Depression, suicidal ideation, and suicide attempts have been reported to occur with increased frequency in patients receiving interferon products, including REBIF. Depressive symptoms associated with interferon beta may often be an atypical syndrome, occurring more frequently early in the course of treatment and not associated with all of the usual clinical symptoms of depression. Patients treated with REBIF should be advised to immediately report any symptoms of depression and/or suicidal ideation to their prescribing physician. Patients developing depression during REBIF therapy should be monitored closely and cessation of therapy should be considered.

Hepatic/Biliary/Pancreatic: Isolated, life-threatening cases of acute hepatic failure have been reported with REBIF therapy. Symptomatic hepatic dysfunction, primarily presenting as jaundice, has been reported as a rare complication of REBIF therapy. Several possible mechanisms may explain the effect of REBIF on the liver (including direct toxicity, indirect toxicity via release of cytokines and/or autoimmunity). Asymptomatic elevations of transaminases (particularly ALT) is common with interferon therapy. (see Adverse Reactions). In clinical trials with REBIF, the majority of these elevations were below 2.5 times the upper limit of normal [ULN] with 1-3% of patients developing elevations above 5 times ULN. In the absence of clinical symptoms, serum ALT levels should be monitored at baseline, every month for the first 6 months and every 6 months thereafter. REBIF should be initiated with caution in patients with a history of significant liver disease, clinical evidence of active liver disease, alcohol abuse or increased serum ALT (>2.5 times ULN). Dose reduction or discontinuation should be considered if ALT rises 5 times above the ULN and gradually re-escalated when enzyme levels have normalized. Treatment with REBIF should be stopped if icterus or other clinical symptoms of hepatic dysfunction appear.

Immune (including hypersensitivity, autoimmunity, immunogenicity): Anaphylaxis has been reported as a rare complication of REBIF use. Other allergic reactions have included skin rash, angioedema, and urticaria, and have ranged from mild to severe without a clear relationship to dose or duration of exposure. Several allergic reactions, some severe, have occurred after prolonged use.

Neutralising antibodies (NAbs) to REBIF may develop during the first 24 months of therapy in a small proportion of patients, the precise incidence of which is uncertain. Neutralising antibodies have been associated with a reduced clinical benefit, as evaluated by MRI parameters and multiple sclerosis relapse rate; however, the clinical significance of NAbs development in individual patients remains uncertain. Treatment decisions should be based on the assessment of clinical efficacy by the clinician in view of available NAbs data. A poor clinical course associated with persistent NAbs should prompt reconsideration of REBIF therapy. Neutralising antibodies to REBIF are cross-reactive to different forms of interferon beta.

Cardiac Disease: Patients with cardiac disease, such as angina, congestive heart failure or arrhythmia, should be closely monitored for worsening of their clinical condition during initiation and continued therapy with REBIF. Symptoms of the flu-like syndrome associated with REBIF may prove stressful to patients with cardiac conditions.

Special Populations: Pregnant Women: REBIF should not be administered in case of pregnancy and lactation. There are no adequate and well-controlled clinical studies of REBIF in pregnant women. In cynomolgous monkeys administered doses approximately 2 times the cumulative weekly human dose (based on either body weight or surface area), REBIF treatment was associated with significant increases in embryolethal or abortifacient effects either during the period of organogenesis (gestation day 21-89) or later in pregnancy. There were no fetal malformations or other evidence of teratogenesis noted in these studies; however, it is not known if teratogenic effects can occur in humans. These effects are consistent with the abortifacient effects of other type I interferons. Patients should be advised about the abortifacient potential of REBIF.

Nursing Women: It is not known whether REBIF is excreted in human milk and is not known if interferon beta-1a can cross the gastrointestinal mucosa. Because of the potential for serious adverse reactions in nursing infants, a decision should be made either to discontinue nursing or to discontinue REBIF therapy.

Pediatrics: There is limited experience with REBIF in children under 18 years of age with MS.

Geriatrics: There is no controlled clinical experience with REBIF in patients with multiple sclerosis over 65 years of age.

Patients with Special Diseases and Conditions: Caution should be exercised and close monitoring conducted when administering REBIF to patients with severe renal failure, or severe myelosuppression, or cardiac disease.

Monitoring and Laboratory Tests: Laboratory abnormalities are associated with the use of interferons. Therefore, in addition to those laboratory tests normally required for monitoring patients with multiple sclerosis, when initiating REBIF therapy, liver enzymes should be monitored at baseline, every month for the first 6 months and every 6 months thereafter (see Warnings and Precautions, Hepatic/Biliary/Pancreatic). Complete blood cell counts with white blood cell differential, and platelet counts are also recommended at baseline 1, 3 and 6 months, and every 6 months thereafter in the absence of clinical symptoms. As patients being treated with REBIF may develop new or worsening thyroid abnormalities (see Warnings and Precautions, Endocrine and Metabolism), testing of thyroid function should be performed at baseline and every 6 months. In case of abnormal results or in patients with a past history of thyroid dysfunction, any necessary treatment should be administered and more frequent testing should be performed as clinically indicated (see Adverse Reactions).

Information to Be Provided to the Patient: Patients should be advised not to stop or modify their treatment unless instructed by their physician.

Patients should be informed of the potential risk of liver injury during REBIF therapy, and be informed about the signs and symptoms of such injury, such as loss of appetite with malaise, fatigue, nausea, vomiting, abdominal pain, dark urine, jaundice or pruritus, and be informed of the requirement for frequent laboratory testing (see Warnings and Precautions, Hepatic/Biliary/Pancreatic). They should be advised to consult their physician immediately if such symptoms arise.

Flu-like symptoms (fever, headache, chills, muscle and joint aches, and fatigue) are the most common adverse reactions following initiation of therapy with REBIF. Acetaminophen or ibuprofen may be used for relief of flu-like symptoms. Patients should contact their physician or pharmacist if they experience any undesirable effects.

Depression may occur in patients with multiple sclerosis and may occur while patients are taking REBIF. Patients receiving REBIF should be instructed to inform their doctor immediately if they have feelings of sadness, unusual tiredness, trouble concentrating, or if they think about committing suicide.

Female patients should be advised about the abortifacient potential of REBIF and instructed to take adequate contraceptive measures (see Contraindications and Warnings and Precautions).

Injection site reactions are commonly experienced by patients during therapy (see Adverse Reactions). In general, they do not require discontinuation of therapy, but the nature and severity of all reported reactions should be carefully assessed. Patient understanding and use of aseptic self-injection technique and procedures should be periodically re-evaluated.

Instruction on Self-injection Technique and Procedures: Patients should be instructed in the use of aseptic technique when administering REBIF. Appropriate instruction for self-injection should be given including careful review of the REBIF patient leaflet. The first injection should be performed under the supervision of an appropriately qualified health care professional. Patients should be advised of the importance of rotating sites of injection with each dose, to minimize the likelihood of severe injection site reactions or necrosis and not to inject into an area that appears abnormal. Patients should be advised to consult with their physician should they develop multiple lesions and/or experience any break in the skin, which may be associated with swelling or drainage of fluid from the injection site, as a decision may be required to discontinue REBIF until healing has occurred. Patients with single lesions may be advised to continue provided that necrosis is not too extensive. Patients should be cautioned against the re-use of needles or syringes and instructed in safe disposal procedures. A puncture resistant container for disposal of used needles and syringes should be supplied to the patient along with instructions for safe disposal of full containers.

Certain laboratory tests may change. The number of white blood cells or platelets may decrease, but no increased risk of infections or bleeding has been observed.

As REBIF may cause changes in thyroid function, patients should be informed of the symptoms of thyroid dysfunction such as difficulty concentrating, feeling abnormally cold or hot, gaining or losing weight unexpectedly, feeling unusually tired or nervous and unusual very dry skin.

REBIF may cause skin reactions such as rash, hives or urticaria, and itching or pruritus associated with redness, which may be a local allergic reaction. Rarely (in less than 1% of patients) these skin and/or allergic reactions can become generalized and very severe, associated with difficulty breathing, cough, swelling of the mouth or throat, fainting, dizziness, low blood pressure, heart palpitations, hives, itching, abdominal pain, vomiting and diarrhea. Patients should be informed that if this occurs, REBIF should be discontinued and prompt medical care is needed, since severe allergic reactions may be potentially life threatening.

ADVERSE REACTIONS: Adverse Drug Reaction Overview: The most common adverse reactions which can occur during REBIF therapy are mild to moderate flu-like symptoms, injection site reactions, reduction in white blood cell count and elevation of liver enzymes. Depending on the severity and persistence of the reactions, the dose may be lowered or temporarily interrupted, at the discretion of the physician.

Less common reactions include erythematous skin rash with pruritus, anemia, depression and thyroid dysfunction. Uncommonly, cases of infection and skin ulceration/necrosis at the site of injection have been reported with long term treatment (see Warnings and Precautions, Information to Be Provided to the Patient).

Serious adverse hepatic reactions such as hepatitis, with or without jaundice, have been rarely (≤1/1000 to ≥1/10 000) reported and isolated cases of acute hepatic failure have been reported (see Warnings and Precautions).

Thyroid dysfunction, may present as hypothyroidism or hyperthyroidism, is generally transient and mild, and may occur during the first year of treatment, particularly in patients with pre-existing thyroiditis (see Warnings and Precautions, Monitoring and Laboratory Tests).

Anaphylaxis has very rarely (≤1/10 000) been observed with the use of REBIF (see Warnings and Precautions).

Clinical Trial Adverse Drug Reactions: Because clinical trials are conducted under very specific conditions the adverse reaction rates observed in the clinical trials may not reflect the rates observed in practice and should not be compared to the rates in the clinical trials of another drug. Adverse drug reaction information from clinical trials is useful for identifying drug-related adverse events and for approximating rates.

Study 25632 (REBIF New HSA-free Formulation): Adverse Drug Reactions: Study 25632 was performed to assess the immunogenicity and safety of the New FBS-free/HSA-free Formulation of interferon beta-1a (REBIF New HSA-free Formulation), administered subcutaneously three times per week in accordance with the current product label.

The adverse events experienced during ninety-six weeks of Study 25632 are listed in below, by MedDRA (Version 8.0) System Organ Class. See Table 1.

Table 1: REBIF

Adverse Events[a] Experienced by at Least 1% of the Patients Enrolled in Study 25632 for Ninety-six Weeks

System Organ Class/Preferred Term	RNF 44 µg TIW Subjects (n=260)
General Disorders and Administration Site Conditions	
Influenza like illness	176 (67.7)
Injection site erythema	63 (24.2)
Injection site haemorrhage	25 (9.6)
Fatigue	24 (9.2)
Chills	18 (6.9)
Pyrexia	18 (6.9)
Injection site pain	17 (6.5)
Asthenia	16 (6.2)
Injection site pruritus	5 (1.9)
Pain	5 (1.9)
Hyperthermia	4 (1.5)
Injection site rash	3 (1.2)
Injection site swelling	3 (1.2)
Nervous System Disorders	
Headache	98 (37.7)
Dizziness	19 (7.3)
Hypoaesthesia	8 (3.1)
Migraine	8 (3.1)
Burning sensation	4 (1.5)
Paraesthesia	4 (1.5)
Hypertonia	3 (1.2)
Tremor	3 (1.2)
Infections and Infestations	
Upper respiratory tract infection	23 (8.8)
Nasopharyngitis	17 (6.5)
Viral upper respiratory tract infection	15 (5.8)
Urinary tract infection	14 (5.4)
Rhinitis	12 (4.6)
Influenza	10 (3.8)
Sinusitis	8 (3.1)
Tonsillitis	8 (3.1)
Herpes simplex	6 (2.3)
Dental caries	4 (1.5)
Ear infection	4 (1.5)
Cystitis	3 (1.2)
Pharyngitis	3 (1.2)
Gastrointestinal Disorders	
Nausea	26 (10.0)
Diarrhoea	17 (6.5)
Vomiting	13 (5.0)
Dyspepsia	12 (4.6)
Abdominal pain	10 (3.8)
Abdominal pain upper	10 (3.8)
Toothache	7 (2.7)
Constipation	6 (2.3)
Flatulence	5 (1.9)

(cont'd)

Table 1: REBIF *(cont'd)*

Adverse Events[a] Experienced by at Least 1% of the Patients Enrolled in Study 25632 for Ninety-six Weeks

System Organ Class/Preferred Term	RNF 44 µg TIW Subjects (n=260)
Gastritis	3 (1.2)
Musculoskeletal and Connective Tissue Disorders	
Back pain	26 (10.0)
Arthralgia	21 (8.1)
Pain in extremity	20 (7.7)
Myalgia	12 (4.6)
Muscle spasms	9 (3.5)
Osteochondrosis	4 (1.5)
Neck pain	3 (1.2)
Investigations	
Alanine aminotransferase increased	19 (7.3)
Aspartate aminotransferase increased	15 (5.8)
Blood creatine phosphokinase increased	8 (3.1)
White blood cell count decreased	8 (3.1)
Hepatic enzyme increased	7 (2.7)
Body temperature increased	5 (1.9)
Neutrophil count decreased	5 (1.9)
Transaminases increased	4 (1.5)
Weight decreased	4 (1.5)
Anti-thyroid antibody positive	3 (1.2)
Blood thyroid stimulating hormone increased	3 (1.2)
Psychiatric Disorders	
Insomnia	13 (5.0)
Anxiety	12 (4.6)
Depression	9 (3.5)
Depressed mood	5 (1.9)
Blood and Lymphatic System Disorders	
Neutropenia	18 (6.9)
Lymphopenia	9 (3.5)
Leukopenia	7 (2.7)
Anaemia	4 (1.5)
Iron deficiency anaemia	4 (1.5)
Skin and Subcutaneous Tissue Disorders	
Urticaria	5 (1.9)
Dermatitis contact	4 (1.5)
Erythema	4 (1.5)
Night sweats	3 (1.2)
Pruritus	3 (1.2)
Injury, Poisoning and Procedural Complications	
Contusion	7 (2.7)
Limb injury	4 (1.5)
Joint sprain	3 (1.2)
Reproductive System and Breast Disorders	
Breast pain	3 (1.2)
Menstruation irregular	3 (1.2)
Respiratory, Thoracic and Mediastinal Disorders	
Pharyngolaryngeal pain	6 (2.3)
Epistaxis	5 (1.9)
Dyspnoea	4 (1.5)
Eye Disorders	
Eye pain	6 (2.3)
Vision blurred	5 (1.9)
Vascular Disorders	
Hypertension	6 (2.3)
Hypotension	6 (2.3)
Cardiac Disorders	
Palpitations	5 (1.9)
Ear and Labyrinth Disorders	
Ear pain	4 (1.5)
Vertigo	3 (1.2)
Endocrine Disorders	
Hyperthyroidism	4 (1.5)

[a] Treatment Emergent Adverse Events.

No new or unexpected treatment emergent adverse events (TEAEs) were observed in the REBIF New HSA-free Formulation Cohort compared to the Historical HSA-containing Formulation Cohort (Historical Cohort). The Historical Cohort consisted of patients from three phase III clinical trials (Study GF6789, Study GF6954 and Study 21125) who were administered identical dosing of the previous HSA- and FBS-containing formulation of interferon beta 1a (44 µg tiw) during the 24-month/96-week period. For the purposes of these comparisons, the Historical Cohort TEAE data for 24-months/96-weeks of treatment was recoded in MedDRA version 8.0 (Clinical Trial Report Study 25632: 96-week Analysis). Overall, the proportion of subjects experiencing TEAEs was similar between the REBIF New HSA-free Formulation Cohort (95.0%) and the Historical Cohort (99.7%). With regard to severity, the majority (97%) of AEs in the REBIF New HSA-free Formulation Cohort were mild (70%) or moderate (27%). To facilitate comparison of the REBIF New HSA-free Formulation Cohort safety profile with that of the Historical Cohort the common AEs of interferon beta-1a were pre-specified into groups of MedDRA preferred terms. The pre-specified AE groups were "cytopenia", "flu like syndrome", "hepatic disorders", "hypersensitivity reactions", "injection site reactions", "depression and suicidal ideation," "skin rashes" and "thyroid disorders". Specific differences were observed in some of these eight pre-specified AE groups known to be associated with interferon beta-1a. The adverse event profile of REBIF New HSA-free Formulation was generally comparable with that observed in the historical trials with the original formulation of interferon-beta-1a. Events related to the flu-like syndrome were reported in 71.5% of REBIF New HSA-free Formulation subjects and in 69.0%, 55.4% and 49.0% of subjects in protocols 6789, 6954 and 21125 respectively. Local injection site reactions were 30.8% in REBIF New HSA-free Formulation Cohort and in 85.8% to 92.4% in the historical trials. Events related to depression and suicidal ideation were reported in 6.5% of REBIF New HSA-free Formulation subjects compared with 22.7% to 36.3% in the historical trials.

In addition to the above listed adverse events, the following events have been experienced less frequently (i.e. in less than 1% of the study population) during the 96 weeks of treatment. See Table 2.

Table 2: REBIF

Adverse Events[a] Experienced by Less Than 1% of Patients Enrolled in Study 25632 During Ninety-six Weeks of Follow-up

System Organ Class/Preferred Term	RNF 44 µg TIW Subjects (n=260)
General Disorders and Administration Site Conditions	
Feeling cold	2 (0.8)
Injection site inflammation	2 (0.8)
Injection site irritation	2 (0.8)
Oedema peripheral	2 (0.8)
Chest pain	1 (0.4)
Cyst	1 (0.4)
Feeling hot	1 (0.4)
Infusion site pain	1 (0.4)
Injection site desquamation	1 (0.4)
Injection site induration	1 (0.4)
Injection site necrosis	1 (0.4)
Injection site oedema	1 (0.4)
Injection site reaction	1 (0.4)
Malaise	1 (0.4)
Non-cardiac chest pain	1 (0.4)
Thirst	1 (0.4)

(cont'd)

Table 2: REBIF *(cont'd)*

Adverse Events[a] Experienced by Less Than 1% of Patients Enrolled in Study 25632 During Ninety-six Weeks of Follow-up

System Organ Class/Preferred Term	RNF 44 μg TIW Subjects (n=260)
General Disorders and Administration Site Conditions	
Nervous System Disorders	
Coordination abnormal	2 (0.8)
Hemiparesis	2 (0.8)
Muscle spasticity	2 (0.8)
Sinus headache	2 (0.8)
Somnolence	2 (0.8)
Syncope	2 (0.8)
Amnesia	1 (0.4)
Autonomic nervous system imbalance	1 (0.4)
Cognitive disorder	1 (0.4)
Dysgeusia	1 (0.4)
Dysgraphia	1 (0.4)
Lethargy	1 (0.4)
Loss of consciousness	1 (0.4)
Motor dysfunction	1 (0.4)
Neuralgia	1 (0.4)
Optic neuritis	1 (0.4)
Restless legs syndrome	1 (0.4)
Syncope vasovagal	1 (0.4)
Tension headache	1 (0.4)
Infections and Infestations	
Bronchitis acute	2 (0.8)
Gastroenteritis	2 (0.8)
Otitis externa	2 (0.8)
Pharyngitis streptococcal	2 (0.8)
Pneumonia	2 (0.8)
Pulpitis dental	2 (0.8)
Salpingitis	2 (0.8)
Acute sinusitis	1 (0.4)
Acute tonsillitis	1 (0.4)
Bacterial food poisoning	1 (0.4)
Blister infected	1 (0.4)
Bronchitis	1 (0.4)
Campylobacter infection	1 (0.4)
Cervicitis	1 (0.4)
Dry socket	1 (0.4)
Furuncle	1 (0.4)
Gastroenteritis *E. coli*	1 (0.4)
Genital candidiasis	1 (0.4)
Gingival abscess	1 (0.4)
Hordeolum	1 (0.4)
Injection site infection	1 (0.4)
Kidney infection	1 (0.4)
Laryngitis	1 (0.4)
Localised infection	1 (0.4)
Lower respiratory tract infection	1 (0.4)

(cont'd)

Table 2: REBIF *(cont'd)*

Adverse Events[a] Experienced by Less Than 1% of Patients Enrolled in Study 25632 During Ninety-six Weeks of Follow-up

System Organ Class/Preferred Term	RNF 44 μg TIW Subjects (n=260)
General Disorders and Administration Site Conditions	
Nail candida	1 (0.4)
Onychomycosis	1 (0.4)
Oral fungal infection	1 (0.4)
Osteomyelitis acute	1 (0.4)
Paronychia	1 (0.4)
Parotitis	1 (0.4)
Penile infection	1 (0.4)
Periodontal infection	1 (0.4)
Peritonsillar abscess	1 (0.4)
Pilonidal cyst	1 (0.4)
Pyelonephritis	1 (0.4)
Pyelonephritis acute	1 (0.4)
Pyelonephritis chronic	1 (0.4)
Tinea versicolour	1 (0.4)
Tooth infection	1 (0.4)
Tracheitis	1 (0.4)
Vaginal candidiasis	1 (0.4)
Vaginal mycosis	1 (0.4)
Gastrointestinal Disorders	
Coeliac disease	2 (0.8)
Abdominal discomfort	1 (0.4)
Abdominal distension	1 (0.4)
Aerophagia	1 (0.4)
Anal haemorrhage	1 (0.4)
Colitis	1 (0.4)
Faecal incontinence	1 (0.4)
Food poisoning	1 (0.4)
Gastritis erosive	1 (0.4)
Gastroduodenitis	1 (0.4)
Gingival bleeding	1 (0.4)
Gingival oedema	1 (0.4)
Gingivitis	1 (0.4)
Mouth ulceration	1 (0.4)
Odynophagia	1 (0.4)
Pancreatitis	1 (0.4)
Periodontitis	1 (0.4)
Periproctitis	1 (0.4)
Peritonitis	1 (0.4)
Stomach discomfort	1 (0.4)
Tongue discolouration	1 (0.4)
Tooth impacted	1 (0.4)
Musculoskeletal and Connective Tissue Disorders	
Chest wall pain	2 (0.8)
Musculoskeletal stiffness	2 (0.8)
Sensation of heaviness	2 (0.8)
Arthropathy	1 (0.4)

(cont'd)

Table 2: REBIF *(cont'd)*

Adverse Events[a] Experienced by Less Than 1% of Patients Enrolled in Study 25632 During Ninety-six Weeks of Follow-up

System Organ Class/Preferred Term	RNF 44 µg TIW Subjects (n=260)
General Disorders and Administration Site Conditions	
Bone pain	1 (0.4)
Bursitis	1 (0.4)
Fibromyalgia	1 (0.4)
Groin pain	1 (0.4)
Joint stiffness	1 (0.4)
Muscle fatigue	1 (0.4)
Muscle tightness	1 (0.4)
Muscle twitching	1 (0.4)
Musculoskeletal pain	1 (0.4)
Myositis	1 (0.4)
Night cramps	1 (0.4)
Osteoarthritis	1 (0.4)
Osteopenia	1 (0.4)
Osteoporosis	1 (0.4)
Shoulder pain	1 (0.4)
Investigations	
Lymphocyte count decreased	2 (0.8)
Thyroid function test abnormal	2 (0.8)
Weight increased	2 (0.8)
Blood cholesterol increased	1 (0.4)
Blood creatinine increased	1 (0.4)
Blood thyroid stimulating hormone decreased	1 (0.4)
Haemoglobin decreased	1 (0.4)
Heart rate increased	1 (0.4)
Hepatic enzyme abnormal	1 (0.4)
Red blood cell count decreased	1 (0.4)
Serum ferritin increased	1 (0.4)
Thyroxine free decreased	1 (0.4)
Tri-iodothyronine free decreased	1 (0.4)
Psychiatric Disorders	
Dyssomnia	2 (0.8)
Panic attack	2 (0.8)
Sleep disorder	2 (0.8)
Hypomania	1 (0.4)
Irritability	1 (0.4)
Tension	1 (0.4)
Blood and Lymphatic System Disorders	
Lymphadenopathy	2 (0.8)
Skin and Subcutaneous Tissue Disorders	
Acne	2 (0.8)
Alopecia	2 (0.8)
Dermatitis allergic	2 (0.8)
Rash	2 (0.8)
Anhidrosis	1 (0.4)
Dermal cyst	1 (0.4)
Dermatitis atopic	1 (0.4)

(cont'd)

Table 2: REBIF *(cont'd)*

Adverse Events[a] Experienced by Less Than 1% of Patients Enrolled in Study 25632 During Ninety-six Weeks of Follow-up

System Organ Class/Preferred Term	RNF 44 µg TIW Subjects (n=260)
General Disorders and Administration Site Conditions	
Eczema	1 (0.4)
Exanthem	1 (0.4)
Haemorrhage subcutaneous	1 (0.4)
Heat rash	1 (0.4)
Hypotrichosis	1 (0.4)
Livedo reticularis	1 (0.4)
Pigmentation disorder	1 (0.4)
Pityriasis	1 (0.4)
Pruritus generalised	1 (0.4)
Skin irritation	1 (0.4)
Skin ulcer	1 (0.4)
Injury, Poisoning and Procedural Complications	
Fall	2 (0.8)
Post procedural pain	2 (0.8)
Arthropod bite	1 (0.4)
Back injury	1 (0.4)
Caustic injury	1 (0.4)
Concussion	1 (0.4)
Drug toxicity	1 (0.4)
Excoriation	1 (0.4)
Face injury	1 (0.4)
Humerus fracture	1 (0.4)
Injury	1 (0.4)
Joint dislocation	1 (0.4)
Ligament sprain	1 (0.4)
Muscle strain	1 (0.4)
Near drowning	1 (0.4)
Radius fracture	1 (0.4)
Reproductive System and Breast Disorders	
Amenorrhoea	2 (0.8)
Dysmenorrhoea	2 (0.8)
Erectile dysfunction	2 (0.8)
Menorrhagia	2 (0.8)
Ovarian cyst	2 (0.8)
Premenstrual syndrome	2 (0.8)
Breast discharge	1 (0.4)
Cervical polyp	1 (0.4)
Endometriosis	1 (0.4)
Fibrocystic breast disease	1 (0.4)
Menometrorrhagia	1 (0.4)
Menstrual disorder	1 (0.4)
Ovarian cyst ruptured	1 (0.4)
Uterine cervical erosion	1 (0.4)
Respiratory, Thoracic and Mediastinal Disorders	
Cough	2 (0.8)
Haemoptysis	1 (0.4)

(cont'd)

Table 2: REBIF *(cont'd)*

Adverse Events[a] Experienced by Less Than 1% of Patients Enrolled in Study 25632 During Ninety-six Weeks of Follow-up

System Organ Class/Preferred Term	RNF 44 µg TIW Subjects (n=260)
General Disorders and Administration Site Conditions	
Increased upper airway secretion	1 (0.4)
Pulmonary congestion	1 (0.4)
Rhinitis allergic	1 (0.4)
Rhinitis seasonal	1 (0.4)
Rhinorrhoea	1 (0.4)
Sleep apnoea syndrome	1 (0.4)
Upper respiratory tract congestion	1 (0.4)
Eye Disorders	
Blepharitis	2 (0.8)
Eye irritation	2 (0.8)
Conjunctivitis	1 (0.4)
Diplopia	1 (0.4)
Dry eye	1 (0.4)
Myopia	1 (0.4)
Retinal degeneration	1 (0.4)
Visual brightness	1 (0.4)
Vitreous disorder	1 (0.4)
Vitreous floaters	1 (0.4)
Vascular Disorders	
Essential hypertension	1 (0.4)
Flushing	1 (0.4)
Haematoma	1 (0.4)
Hot flush	1 (0.4)
Peripheral coldness	1 (0.4)
Raynaud's phenomenon	1 (0.4)
Cardiac Disorders	
Angina pectoris	2 (0.8)
Tachycardia	2 (0.8)
Angina unstable	1 (0.4)
Renal and Urinary Disorders	
Nocturia	2 (0.8)
Renal colic	2 (0.8)
Dysuria	1 (0.4)
Micturition urgency	1 (0.4)
Neurogenic bladder	1 (0.4)
Pollakiuria	1 (0.4)
Proteinuria	1 (0.4)
Urinary hesitation	1 (0.4)
Urine odour abnormal	1 (0.4)
Ear and Labyrinth Disorders	
Ear discomfort	1 (0.4)
Middle ear effusion	1 (0.4)
Endocrine Disorders	
Goitre	2 (0.8)
Cushing's syndrome	1 (0.4)
Hypothyroidism	1 (0.4)

(cont'd)

Table 2: REBIF *(cont'd)*

Adverse Events[a] Experienced by Less Than 1% of Patients Enrolled in Study 25632 During Ninety-six Weeks of Follow-up

System Organ Class/Preferred Term	RNF 44 µg TIW Subjects (n=260)
General Disorders and Administration Site Conditions	
Thyroiditis chronic	1 (0.4)
Hepatobiliary Disorders	
Cholecystitis	2 (0.8)
Cholecystitis chronic	1 (0.4)
Hepatic function abnormal	1 (0.4)
Hepatic pain	1 (0.4)
Hepatic steatosis	1 (0.4)
Hepatitis toxic	1 (0.4)
Hepatotoxicity	1 (0.4)
Metabolism and Nutrition Disorders	
Anorexia	2 (0.8)
Dehydration	1 (0.4)
Diabetes mellitus non-insulin-dependent	1 (0.4)
Hyperglycaemia	1 (0.4)
Hypokalaemia	1 (0.4)
Lactose intolerance	1 (0.4)
Neoplasms Benign, Malignant and Unspecified (incl cysts and polyps)	
Uterine leiomyoma	2 (0.8)
Fallopian tube neoplasm	1 (0.4)
Tracheal neoplasm	1 (0.4)
Immune System Disorders	
Seasonal allergy	2 (0.8)
Congenital, Familial and Genetic Disorders	
Factor VIII deficiency	1 (0.4)

[a] Treatment Emergent Adverse Events.

Study 25827 (REBIF New HSA-free Formulation): Adverse Drug Reactions: The safety and tolerability of the New HSA-free Formulation of interferon beta-1a was compared to the previously marketed HSA- and FBS-containing formulation of REBIF as a secondary objective of the study. Both formulations were well tolerated when administered in subcutaneous doses of 44 µg in this study. There were no deaths or SAEs. All subjects who were administered with either study drug experienced mild Treatment Emergent Adverse Events (TEAEs). Of those TEAEs reported, 59.3% and 65.7% were probably related to the administration of the previously marketed REBIF formulation and the New HSA-free Formulation of interferon beta-1a, respectively. The nature and severities of AEs were similar for both study drugs, and were consistent with the known safety profile of previously marketed REBIF formulation. There appeared to be a higher frequency of pain associated TEAEs after administration of previously marketed REBIF formulation, and more episodes of pyrexia, and associated symptoms, after administration of the HSA-free interferon beta-1a. Injection site reactions, particularly redness, were observed after administration of both of the study drugs. Pain at the administration site and the incidence of injection site reactions however lower after injection of the HSA-free interferon beta-1a compared to previously marketed REBIF formulation.

Study GF6789 (PRISMS): Adverse Reactions: The adverse events experienced during the first two years of Study GF6789 are listed below, by WHOART System Organ Class. The most common amongst the injection site reactions was in the form of injection site inflammation. The majority of the other injection site reactions were also mild in the 2 REBIF groups. Necrosis was reported in 8 patients treated with REBIF. Two of these patients were in the 66 µg weekly and six in the 132 µg weekly groups. All patients completed the planned treatment period, with only 1 requiring temporary dose reductions and another patient stopping treatment for 2 weeks. Those that required treatments, received antibiotics.

Long-term Follow-up (LTFU) data up to 8 years for the PRISMS study has been collected in the retrospective study 22930. LTFU was attended by 68.2% of the original PRISMS study cohort (382/560 patients). 72.0% (275/382) were still receiving IFN-beta-1a s.c., with 74.3% (101/136) of those originally randomized to receive the 44 microg dose and 70.7% (87/123) the 22 microg dose. Overall, 19.7% of patients progressed to secondary progressive MS between baseline and LTFU (75/381). No new safety concerns were identified and treatment was generally well tolerated. See Table 3.

Table 3: REBIF

Adverse Events Experienced by at Least 1% of the Patients Enrolled in Study GF6789 (PRISMS—Year 1 and 2)

Body System/Preferred Term	Placebo (n=187)	REBIF 66 µg Weekly (n=189)	REBIF 132 µg Weekly (n=184)
Application Site Disorders			
Injection Site Inflammation	15.0%	65.6%	65.8%
Injection Site Reaction	13.4%	31.2%	34.8%
Injection Site Pain	14.4%	20.1%	22.8%
Injection Site Bruising	11.2%	3.7%	5.4%

(cont'd)

Table 3: REBIF *(cont'd)*

Adverse Events Experienced by at Least 1% of the Patients Enrolled in Study GF6789 (PRISMS—Year 1 and 2)

Body System/Preferred Term	Placebo (n=187)	REBIF 66 µg Weekly (n=189)	REBIF 132 µg Weekly (n=184)
Injection Site Mass	0.5%	3.2%	3.8%
Injection Site Bleeding	0.5%	2.1%	2.2%
Injection Site Necrosis		1.1%	3.3%
Injection Site Abscess		1.1%	2.2%
Body as a Whole—General Disorders			
Influenza-Like Symptoms	51.3%	56.1%	58.7%
Fatigue	35.8%	32.8%	41.3%
Fever	15.5%	24.9%	27.7%
Leg Pain	14.4%	10.1%	13.0%
Rigors	5.3%	6.3%	13.0%
Sweating Increased	6.4%	6.9%	8.2%
Chest Pain	5.3%	5.8%	7.6%
Allergic Reaction	5.3%	4.8%	6.0%
Pain	6.4%	2.6%	2.7%
Malaise	1.1%	4.2%	5.4%
Asthenia	2.1%	3.2%	2.2%
Hot Flushes	2.1%	1.6%	2.7%
Back Pain	2.7%	2.1%	1.1%
Temperature Changed Sensation	1.1%	0.5%	0.5%
Oedema Peripheral	1.1%		0.5%
Necrosis Ischaemic			1.1%
Cardiovascular Disorders, General			
Hypotension	3.2%	1.6%	1.6%
Hypertension	2.7%	1.1%	1.6%
Heart Murmur	0.5%	1.1%	0.5%
Oedema Dependent		2.1%	
Centr & Periph Nervous System Disorders			
Headache	62.6%	64.6%	70.1%
Paraesthesia	18.7%	19.6%	16.3%
Dizziness	17.6%	14.3%	16.3%
Hypoaesthesia	12.8%	12.2%	7.6%
Migraine	9.1%	6.3%	7.6%
Hypertonia	5.3%	7.4%	6.0%
Vertigo	7.0%	5.8%	5.4%
Ataxia	7.5%	4.2%	4.9%
Muscle Contractions Involuntary	7.5%	4.2%	3.3%
Dysaesthesia	4.8%	3.2%	4.9%
Coordination Abnormal	2.1%	5.3%	3.8%
Convulsions	2.1%	4.8%	3.8%
Gait Abnormal	2.7%	4.2%	3.8%
Sensory Disturbance	4.8%	3.2%	1.6%
Cramps Legs	3.2%	2.1%	2.7%
Tremor	0.5%	3.2%	1.6%
Speech Disorder	2.7%	1.1%	1.1%
Dysphonia	1.1%	0.5%	2.2%
Trigeminal Neuralgia	0.5%	0.5%	1.6%
Dyskinesia		0.5%	1.6%

(cont'd)

Table 3: REBIF *(cont'd)*

Adverse Events Experienced by at Least 1% of the Patients Enrolled in Study GF6789 (PRISMS—Year 1 and 2)

Body System/Preferred Term	Placebo (n=187)	REBIF 66 µg Weekly (n=189)	REBIF 132 µg Weekly (n=184)
Faecal Incontinence		2.1%	
Convulsions Grand Mal		1.1%	
Collagen Disorders			
Auto-Antibody Response	1.1%	0.5%	1.1%
Endocrine Disorders			
Thyroid Disorder	3.2%	4.2%	6.0%
T4 Increased	2.1%	2.6%	2.2%
Thyroid Stim. Hormone Decreased	1.1%	1.1%	2.2%
T3 Increased	0.5%	2.1%	1.1%
T4 Decreased	1.1%	2.1%	0.5%
Gastro-Intestinal System Disorders			
Nausea	23.0%	24.9%	24.5%
Abdominal Pain	17.1%	22.2%	19.6%
Diarrhoea	18.7%	17.5%	19.0%
Vomiting	12.3%	12.7%	12.0%
Constipation	10.2%	10.1%	7.1%
Dyspepsia	9.6%	5.8%	8.2%
Tooth Disorder	5.9%	5.8%	7.6%
Tooth Ache	6.4%	5.8%	6.0%
Gastroenteritis	7.5%	5.8%	4.3%
Mouth Dry	1.1%	0.5%	4.9%
Gastritis	2.7%	1.1%	2.2%
Flatulence	2.7%	2.1%	0.5%
Gastro-Intestinal Disorder Nos	2.7%	2.1%	0.5%
Gingivitis	2.1%	0.5%	2.2%
Stomatitis Ulcerative	1.1%	3.2%	0.5%
Dysphagia	1.6%	1.1%	1.1%
Haemorrhoids		2.1%	0.5%
Change in Bowel Habits		1.1%	1.1%
Haemorrhage Rectum	1.6%	0.5%	
Appendicitis	1.1%	0.5%	
Enteritis	0.5%		1.1%
Glossitis		1.6%	
Melaena			1.6%
Tongue Ulceration		1.6%	
Eructation		1.1%	
Hearing and Vestibular Disorders			
Ear Ache	7.5%	3.2%	4.9%
Tinnitus	3.2%	2.6%	1.6%
Ear Disorder Nos	1.1%	2.1%	1.1%
Vestibular Disorder	1.1%		1.1%
Heart Rate and Rhythm Disorders			
Palpitation	4.3%	2.1%	2.7%
Tachycardia	2.1%	1.1%	1.6%
Liver and Biliary System Disorders			
ALT Increased	4.3%	19.6%	27.2%
AST Increased	3.7%	10.1%	17.4%

(cont'd)

Table 3: REBIF *(cont'd)*

Adverse Events Experienced by at Least 1% of the Patients Enrolled in Study GF6789 (PRISMS—Year 1 and 2)

Body System/Preferred Term	Placebo (n=187)	REBIF 66 µg Weekly (n=189)	REBIF 132 µg Weekly (n=184)
Hepatic Function Abnormal	1.6%	3.7%	9.2%
Bilirubinaemia	0.5%	2.6%	2.2%
Hepatomegaly			1.1%
Metabolic and Nutritional Disorders			
Phosphatase Alkaline Increased	3.7%	4.8%	3.3%
Weight Decrease	3.2%	4.8%	3.8%
Hypocalcaemia	4.8%	4.2%	2.2%
Weight Increase	3.2%	2.6%	1.6%
Hypoglycaemia	1.6%	1.1%	1.6%
Hypokalaemia	3.2%		
Oedema Legs	2.1%	0.5%	0.5%
Serum Iron Decreased	2.1%	1.1%	
Blood Urea Decreased	0.5%	1.6%	0.5%
Bun Increased	0.5%	1.1%	1.1%
Glycosuria	1.1%	0.5%	1.1%
Hypoproteinaemia		1.6%	
Hypercalcaemia			1.1%
Npn Increased	1.1%		
Musculo-Skeletal System Disorders			
Myalgia	19.8%	24.9%	25.0%
Back Pain	19.8%	23.3%	24.5%
Arthralgia	17.1%	15.3%	19.0%
Skeletal Pain	10.2%	14.8%	9.8%
Muscle Weakness	13.4%	8.5%	8.7%
Arthrosis	2.1%	2.1%	2.7%
Tendinitis	0.5%	2.6%	1.1%
Arthritis	0.5%	2.6%	
Bursitis	0.5%	2.1%	0.5%
Arthropathy		1.1%	0.5%
Torticollis		0.5%	1.1%
Platelet, Bleeding & Clotting Disorders			
Thrombocytopenia	1.6%	1.6%	8.2%
Epistaxis	3.2%	2.6%	2.2%
Purpura	2.7%	0.5%	1.1%
Haematoma	1.1%	1.6%	
Thrombocythaemia		1.1%	
Psychiatric Disorders			
Depression	27.8%	20.6%	23.9%
Insomnia	21.4%	19.6%	23.4%
Anxiety	5.9%	4.8%	7.6%
Nervousness	6.4%	5.3%	6.0%
Anorexia	3.7%	4.8%	3.3%
Somnolence	0.5%	3.7%	4.9%
Sleep Disorder	2.1%	3.7%	2.2%
Emotional Lability	3.2%	2.1%	1.1%
Amnesia	1.6%	2.1%	1.1%
Suicide Attempt	1.6%	1.6%	1.6%

(cont'd)

Table 3: REBIF *(cont'd)*

Adverse Events Experienced by at Least 1% of the Patients Enrolled in Study GF6789 (PRISMS—Year 1 and 2)

Body System/Preferred Term	Placebo (n=187)	REBIF 66 µg Weekly (n=189)	REBIF 132 µg Weekly (n=184)
Agitation	0.5%	0.5%	2.2%
Libido Decreased	1.1%	1.1%	1.1%
Concentration Impaired	0.5%	1.6%	0.5%
Confusion	1.6%		1.1%
Paroniria		0.5%	1.1%
Red Blood Cell Disorders			
Anaemia	2.7%	2.6%	4.9%
Polycythaemia	0.5%	1.6%	
Reproductive Disorders, Female			
Menstrual Disorder	3.7%	4.8%	4.3%
Vaginitis	5.9%	2.6%	3.3%
Dysmenorrhoea	4.8%	2.6%	1.1%
Menorrhagia	1.1%	0.5%	2.7%
Intermenstrual Bleeding	1.6%	1.6%	0.5%
Amenorrhoea	1.6%	1.1%	0.5%
Breast Neoplasm Female	1.6%	0.5%	1.1%
Leukorrhoea		1.6%	
Ovarian Cyst	0.5%		1.1%
Pregnancy Unintended	1.1%		0.5%
Uterine Fibroid	0.5%	1.1%	
Breast Neoplasm Malignant Female	1.1%		
Mastitis	1.1%		
Reproductive Disorders, Male			
Impotence	2.1%	2.1%	2.7%
Resistance Mechanism Disorders			
Herpes Simplex	8.0%	4.8%	5.4%
Infection Fungal	7.5%	3.7%	5.4%
Infection	6.4%	5.8%	3.3%
Otitis Media	5.3%	3.2%	1.6%
Moniliasis	1.6%	2.6%	3.3%
Infection Viral	2.1%	2.1%	2.2%
Herpes Zoster	1.1%	1.1%	2.2%
Abscess	1.1%	1.1%	
Infection Parasitic			1.1%
Respiratory System Disorders			
Rhinitis	59.9%	52.4%	50.5%
Pharyngitis	38.5%	34.9%	28.3%
Upper Resp Tract Infection	32.6%	36.0%	29.3%
Coughing	21.4%	14.8%	19.0%
Sinusitis	15.5%	7.9%	9.8%
Bronchitis	9.6%	10.6%	9.2%
Tracheitis	5.9%	2.6%	6.5%
Laryngitis	3.2%	2.6%	3.8%
Dyspnoea	2.1%	1.6%	2.2%
Throat Tightness		3.2%	1.1%
Asthma	1.6%		2.2%
Bronchospasm	0.5%	1.1%	1.6%

(cont'd)

Table 3: REBIF *(cont'd)*

Adverse Events Experienced by at Least 1% of the Patients Enrolled in Study GF6789 (PRISMS—Year 1 and 2)

Body System/Preferred Term	Placebo (n=187)	REBIF 66 µg Weekly (n=189)	REBIF 132 µg Weekly (n=184)
Hyperventilation	2.1%		1.1%
Pneumonia	2.7%	0.5%	
Secondary Terms			
Fall	16.0%	16.9%	15.8%
Bite	3.2%	3.2%	
Food Poisoning		1.6%	
Varicella			1.1%
Skin and Appendages Disorders			
Pruritus	11.8%	9.0%	12.5%
Rash	6.4%	6.9%	8.2%
Rash Erythematous	3.2%	6.9%	4.9%
Alopecia	5.3%	4.2%	3.3%
Eczema	3.7%	5.3%	3.3%
Skin Dry	3.7%	3.2%	5.4%
Rash Maculo-Papular	1.6%	4.8%	4.3%
Acne	3.7%	2.1%	3.3%
Skin Disorder	2.1%	3.7%	3.3%
Skin Hypertrophy	3.2%	1.1%	4.3%
Skin Discolouration	4.3%	1.1%	2.7%
Dermatitis Fungal	2.1%	2.1%	0.5%
Urticaria	2.7%	1.1%	0.5%
Nail Disorder	1.1%	1.1%	0.5%
Onychomycosis	1.1%	0.5%	1.1%
Folliculitis	0.5%	1.6%	
Psoriasis	0.5%	1.6%	
Dermatitis		0.5%	1.1%
Furunculosis	0.5%		1.1%
Hair Disorder Nos		1.6%	
Photosensitivity Reaction	0.5%	1.1%	
Pityriasis Rosea	0.5%		1.1%
Verruca	1.1%		0.5%
Dermatitis Lichenoid	1.1%		
Rash Pustular	1.1%		
Vitiligo	1.1%		
Urinary System Disorders			
Urinary Tract Infection	18.7%	18.0%	16.8%
Cystitis	12.3%	5.8%	6.5%
Micturition Frequency	3.7%	1.6%	6.5%
Haematuria	3.7%	2.6%	2.7%
Urinary Incontinence	1.6%	3.7%	1.6%
Albuminuria	1.6%	3.2%	1.6%
Micturition Disorder	1.6%	2.1%	2.2%
Dysuria	1.1%	1.6%	2.2%
Renal Pain	2.1%		2.2%
Urinary Retention	2.1%	2.1%	
Urine Abnormal	1.1%	1.1%	1.6%
Face Oedema	1.6%		1.6%

(cont'd)

Table 3: REBIF *(cont'd)*

Adverse Events Experienced by at Least 1% of the Patients Enrolled in Study GF6789 (PRISMS—Year 1 and 2)

Body System/Preferred Term	Placebo (n=187)	REBIF 66 µg Weekly (n=189)	REBIF 132 µg Weekly (n=184)
Micturition Urgency	1.1%	1.1%	1.1%
Nocturia		0.5%	1.1%
Vascular (extracardiac) Disorders			
Flushing	3.2%	1.6%	2.2%
Vascular Disorder		0.5%	1.1%
Peripheral Ischaemia	1.1%		
Vision Disorders			
Vision Abnormal	7.0%	7.4%	13.0%
Eye Pain	8.0%	6.3%	4.9%
Conjunctivitis	6.4%	5.8%	4.9%
Diplopia	3.2%	1.6%	2.2%
Xerophthalmia		2.6%	0.5%
Eye Infection	1.1%	0.5%	1.1%
Photophobia	0.5%	1.1%	1.1%
Conjunctival Discolouration	1.1%		
Photopsia	1.1%		
White Cell and Res Disorders			
Lymphopenia	11.2%	20.1%	28.8%
Leucopenia	3.7%	12.7%	22.3%
Lymphadenopathy	8.0%	11.1%	12.0%
Granulocytopenia	3.7%	11.6%	15.2%
Leukocytosis	4.3%	5.3%	4.3%
Monocytosis	2.7%	4.8%	4.3%
Eosinophilia	2.1%	3.7%	1.1%
Wbc Abnormal Nos	0.5%	3.2%	2.7%
Lymphadenopathy Cervical	1.6%	1.6%	1.6%
Lymphocytosis	1.1%	1.6%	0.5%

In addition to the above listed adverse events, the following events have been experienced less frequently (i.e. in less than 1% of the study population) during years 1 and 2 of treatment. See Table 4.

After 2 years, the placebo patients were switched to REBIF, and along with the patients for the REBIF treatment groups, they were treated for an additional two years. Listed below by WHOART System Organ Class, are the proportion of patients reporting the most common adverse events ongoing from years 1 and 2 or started during years 3 and 4 of treatment. The results are similar to those obtained in the original phase of the study. The findings indicate that the incidence of interferon-related adverse events diminishes somewhat with continued exposure to the medication.

Cases of necrosis were rare and not a cause of drop-out. For REBIF 66 µg weekly, there was one episode of skin necrosis per 92 years of exposure or per 14 100 injections. The comparable figures for REBIF 132 µg weekly are 1 episode of necrosis per 61 years of exposure or per 9 300 injections. See Table 5.

In addition to the above listed adverse events, the following events have been experienced less frequently (i.e. in less than 1% of the study population) ongoing from years 1 and 2 or started during years 3 and 4 of treatment. See Table 6.

Table 4: REBIF

Adverse Events Experienced by Less Than 1% of the Patients Enrolled in Study GF6789 (PRISMS—Year 1 and 2)

Body System	Preferred Term
Application Site Disorders	Injection Site Atrophy
Body as a Whole—General Disorders	Scar
	Oedema
	Syncope
	Abdomen Enlarged
	Anaphylactoid Reaction
	Carpal Tunnel Syndrome
	Nasal Polyp
	Oedema Genital
Cardiovascular Disorders, General	Hypotension Postural

(cont'd)

Table 4: REBIF *(cont'd)*

Adverse Events Experienced by Less Than 1% of the Patients Enrolled in Study GF6789 (PRISMS—Year 1 and 2)

Body System	Preferred Term
Centr & Periph Nervous System Disorders	Convulsions Local
	Extrapyramidal Disorder
	Hypotonia
	Nerve Root Lesion
	Neuralgia
	Optic Neuritis
	Paralysis
	Paresis
	Scotoma
	Visual Field Defect
Endocrine Disorders	Hypothyroidism
	Sialoadenitis
Foetal Disorders	Hernia Congenital
	Death Foetal
Gastro-Intestinal System Disorders	Appetite Increased
	Saliva Increased
	Tooth Caries
	Colitis
	Crohn's Disease
	Gastroesophageal Reflux
	Gi Neoplasm Benign
	Gum Hyperplasia
	Hiccup
	Intestinal Obstruction
	Irritable Bowel Syndrome
	Rectal Prolapse
	Stomatitis
	Stomatitis Aphthous
Hearing and Vestibular Disorders	Hearing Decreased
	Hyperacusis
	Motion Sickness
	Deafness
Heart Rate and Rhythm Disorders	Arrhythmia
	Bradycardia
	Cardiac Arrest
	Extrasystoles
	Sick Sinus Syndrome
Liver and Biliary System Disorders	Cholecystitis
	Cholelithiasis
	Gamma-Gt Increased
Metabolic and Nutritional Disorders	Hypercholesterolaemia
	Thirst
	Hyperlipaemia
	Hypernatraemia
	Oedema Generalised
Musculo-Skeletal System Disorders	Malformation Foot
	Osteoporosis
Myo Endo Pericardial & Valve Disorders	Angina Pectoris

(cont'd)

Table 4: REBIF *(cont'd)*

Adverse Events Experienced by Less Than 1% of the Patients Enrolled in Study GF6789 (PRISMS—Year 1 and 2)

Body System	Preferred Term
Neoplasm	Basal Cell Carcinoma
	Colon Carcinoma
	Lipoma
Platelet, Bleeding & Clotting Disorders	Dissem. Intravasc. Coagulation
	Embolism Arterial
	Embolism Pulmonary
	Thrombosis Arterial Arm
Psychiatric Disorders	Apathy
	Dreaming Abnormal
	Hallucination
	Psychosis Manic-Depressive
	Thinking Abnormal
Red Blood Cell Disorders	Hyperhaemoglobinaemia
	Splenomegaly
Reproductive Disorders, Female	Cervicitis
	Endometriosis
	Lactation Nonpuerperal
	Vaginal Haemorrhage
	Bacterial Growth Genital Asymptom
	Breast Neoplasm Benign Female
	Cervical Dysplasia
	Endometrial Disorder
	Menopausal Symptoms
	Ovarian Disorder
	Premenstrual Tension
	Uterovaginal Prolapse
Reproductive Disorders, Male	Breast Discharge
	Epididymitis
	Sexual Function Abnormal
	Testicular Pain
	Testis Disorder
Resistance Mechanism Disorders	Infection Bacterial
	Moniliasis Genital
	Sepsis
Respiratory System Disorders	Sputum Increased
	Atelectasis
	Pneumonitis
	Stridor
Secondary Terms	Cyst Nos
	Heat Intolerance
	Spinal Cord Compression
	Abrasion Nos
	Asthma Extrinsic
	Cytomegalus Virus Infection
	Heat Stroke
	Lumbar Disc Lesion
	Malaria

(cont'd)

Table 4: REBIF *(cont'd)*

Adverse Events Experienced by Less Than 1% of the Patients Enrolled in Study GF6789 (PRISMS—Year 1 and 2)

Body System	Preferred Term
Skin and Appendages Disorders	Pigmentation Abnormal
	Rosacea
	Bullous Eruption
	Hair Texture Abnormal
	Hyperkeratosis
	Hypertrichosis
	Paronychia
	Rhagades
	Seborrhoea
	Skin Reaction Localised
	Skin Ulceration
	Sweat Gland Disorder
	Vesicular Rash
Special Senses Other, Disorders	Taste Perversion
Urinary System Disorders	Pyelonephritis
	Polyuria
Vascular (extracardiac) Disorders	Thrombophlebitis Arm Superficial
	Vein Distended
	Claudication Intermittent
	Thrombophlebitis
	Vascular Malformation Cerebral
Vision Disorders	Accommodation Abnormal
	Conjunctival Haemorrhage
	Blindness
	Blindness Temporary
	Cataract
	Iritis
	Keratitis
	Meibomianitis
	Retinal Disorder
	Uveitis
White Cell and Res Disorders	Immunoglobulins Increased

Table 5: REBIF

Adverse Events Experienced by at Least 1% of the Patients Enrolled in Study GF6789 (PRISMS—Ongoing from Year 1 and 2 or Started During Year 3 and 4)

Body System/Preferred Term	Placebo/66 (n=85)	Placebo/132 (n=87)	REBIF 66 µg Weekly (n=167)	REBIF 132 µg Weekly (n=167)
Application Site Disorders				
Injection Site Inflammation	65.9%	65.5%	56.9%	66.5%
Injection Site Reaction	28.2%	37.9%	29.9%	31.7%
Injection Site Pain	18.8%	21.8%	15.0%	13.8%
Injection Site Bruising	5.9%	6.9%	2.4%	6.0%
Injection Site Mass	3.5%	4.6%	4.8%	3.6%
Injection Site Necrosis	2.4%	1.1%	1.8%	3.0%
Injection Site Abscess	1.2%	2.3%	1.8%	1.2%
Injection Site Bleeding	2.4%		0.6%	1.8%
Skin Nodule				1.2%
Body as a Whole—General Disorders				

(cont'd)

Table 5: REBIF *(cont'd)*

Adverse Events Experienced by at Least 1% of the Patients Enrolled in Study GF6789 (PRISMS—Ongoing from Year 1 and 2 or Started During Year 3 and 4)

Body System/Preferred Term	Placebo/66 (n=85)	Placebo/132 (n=87)	REBIF 66 µg Weekly (n=167)	REBIF 132 µg Weekly (n=167)
Influenza-Like Symptoms	42.4%	60.9%	50.3%	42.5%
Fatigue	34.1%	36.8%	24.6%	27.5%
Fever	14.1%	14.9%	15.6%	12.0%
Leg Pain	8.2%	12.6%	6.6%	7.8%
Pain	4.7%	14.9%	4.2%	4.2%
Rigors	5.9%	6.9%	4.2%	7.8%
Sweating Increased	5.9%	3.4%	5.4%	3.6%
Malaise	3.5%	3.4%	3.0%	5.4%
Asthenia	1.2%	2.3%	4.8%	3.6%
Chest Pain	2.4%	5.7%	3.6%	2.4%
Allergic Reaction	2.4%	4.6%	3.0%	2.4%
Hot Flushes	3.5%	1.1%	1.8%	2.4%
Oedema Peripheral	3.5%	2.3%	0.6%	0.6%
Temperature Changed Sensation	1.2%		1.2%	2.4%
Scar		2.3%	1.2%	1.2%
Carpal Tunnel Syndrome		1.1%	0.6%	
Anaphylactic Shock		1.1%		
Choking		1.1%		
Necrosis Ischaemic	1.2%			
Pallor	1.2%			
Cardiovascular Disorders, General				
Hypertension	3.5%	5.7%	4.2%	4.2%
Hypotension	1.2%	1.1%	1.8%	2.4%
Oedema Dependent	3.5%	1.1%	1.2%	0.6%
Cardiac Failure Left	1.2%			
Hypotension Postural		1.1%		
Centr & Periph Nervous System Disorders				
Headache	44.7%	55.2%	46.7%	46.7%
Dizziness	4.7%	11.5%	13.2%	12.6%
Hypertonia	14.1%	11.5%	10.8%	9.6%
Paraesthesia	15.3%	13.8%	10.2%	7.8%
Hypoaesthesia	7.1%	13.8%	7.2%	9.0%
Migraine	8.2%	9.2%	6.6%	5.4%
Ataxia	2.4%	8.0%	5.4%	7.2%
Vertigo	7.1%	8.0%	3.6%	3.0%
Muscle Contractions Involuntary	4.7%	3.4%	5.4%	2.4%
Gait Abnormal	2.4%	2.3%	4.8%	2.4%
Dysaesthesia	2.4%	3.4%	2.4%	2.4%
Tremor	2.4%	2.3%	3.6%	1.8%
Convulsions	2.4%	1.1%	3.0%	2.4%
Coordination Abnormal	4.7%		3.6%	0.6%
Cramps Legs	1.2%	2.3%	1.2%	3.0%
Sensory Disturbance	4.7%	1.1%	1.2%	1.2%
Speech Disorder		4.6%	1.8%	1.2%
Faecal Incontinence			3.0%	0.6%
Paresis		1.1%	1.2%	1.2%

(cont'd)

Table 5: REBIF *(cont'd)*

Adverse Events Experienced by at Least 1% of the Patients Enrolled in Study GF6789 (PRISMS—Ongoing from Year 1 and 2 or Started During Year 3 and 4)

Body System/Preferred Term	Placebo/66 (n=85)	Placebo/132 (n=87)	REBIF 66 µg Weekly (n=167)	REBIF 132 µg Weekly (n=167)
Extrapyramidal Disorder	1.2%			0.6%
Hyperkinesia		1.1%		0.6%
Ms Aggravated	1.2%			0.6%
Paralysis	1.2%			0.6%
Ptosis				1.2%
Aphasia	1.2%			
Hemiplegia		1.1%		
Visual Field Defect		1.1%		
Collagen Disorders				
Auto-Antibody Response		1.1%	1.2%	1.8%
Arthritis Rheumatoid Aggravated		1.1%		
Endocrine Disorders				
Thyroid Disorder	4.7%	8.0%	4.2%	6.6%
T4 Increased	4.7%	1.1%	3.0%	2.4%
Thyroid Stim. Hormone Decreased	3.5%	1.1%	0.6%	3.0%
Hypothyroidism	2.4%		0.6%	1.8%
T3 Increased		1.1%	1.2%	1.2%
T4 Decreased	2.4%		1.2%	0.6%
Goitre	1.2%		1.2%	0.6%
Hyperthyroidism			1.2%	1.2%
Foetal Disorders				
Hernia Congenital		1.1%	1.2%	
Gastro-Intestinal System Disorders				
Nausea	12.9%	19.5%	10.8%	11.4%
Abdominal Pain	8.2%	16.1%	13.2%	10.8%
Diarrhoea	5.9%	8.0%	12.0%	9.0%
Constipation	14.1%	9.2%	6.0%	7.2%
Vomiting	3.5%	9.2%	3.0%	6.0%
Dyspepsia	7.1%	5.7%	3.0%	3.6%
Gastroenteritis	2.4%	4.6%	4.2%	4.2%
Tooth Ache	2.4%	4.6%	3.0%	4.8%
Tooth Disorder	1.2%	3.4%	3.0%	6.0%
Haemorrhoids	1.2%	1.1%	2.4%	1.8%
Dysphagia	1.2%	2.3%	0.6%	1.2%
Gastritis	1.2%		1.2%	1.2%
Gastro-Intestinal Disorder Nos		4.6%	0.6%	
Stomatitis Ulcerative	1.2%	1.1%	1.2%	0.6%
Flatulence	2.4%	1.1%		0.6%
Gastroesophageal Reflux		2.3%	0.6%	0.6%
Appendicitis	1.2%		0.6%	0.6%
Melaena		2.3%	0.6%	
Mouth Dry				1.8%
Colitis				1.2%
Enterocolitis				1.2%
Eructation	1.2%		0.6%	
Gingivitis		1.1%		0.6%

(cont'd)

Table 5: REBIF *(cont'd)*

Adverse Events Experienced by at Least 1% of the Patients Enrolled in Study GF6789 (PRISMS—Ongoing from Year 1 and 2 or Started During Year 3 and 4)

Body System/Preferred Term	Placebo/66 (n=85)	Placebo/132 (n=87)	REBIF 66 µg Weekly (n=167)	REBIF 132 µg Weekly (n=167)
Glossitis				1.2%
Irritable Bowel Syndrome		1.1%	0.6%	
Oesophagitis		1.1%		0.6%
Stomatitis		1.1%		0.6%
Abdominal Adhesions	1.2%			
Achalasia Cardiae		1.1%		
Crohn's Disease	1.2%			
Gi Haemorrhage		1.1%		
Peptic Ulcer		1.1%		
Saliva Increased		1.1%		
Hearing and Vestibular Disorders				
Tinnitus	2.4%	3.4%	3.6%	1.8%
Ear Ache	4.7%	3.4%	1.2%	1.2%
Ear Disorder Nos	2.4%	1.1%		1.8%
Hearing Decreased	1.2%		0.6%	1.2%
Deafness		2.3%		0.6%
Hyperacusis	1.2%	1.1%		
Deafness Nerve	1.2%			
Otosclerosis	1.2%			
Heart Rate and Rhythm Disorders				
Palpitation	2.4%	2.3%	3.0%	2.4%
Tachycardia	1.2%	2.3%	1.2%	
Liver and Biliary System Disorders				
ALT Increased	11.8%	14.9%	13.8%	12.6%
AST Increased	4.7%	9.2%	6.6%	6.0%
Hepatic Function Abnormal	7.1%	4.6%	2.4%	3.0%
Bilirubinaemia	1.2%		1.2%	0.6%
Hepatic Enzymes Increased	1.2%	1.1%		
Gamma-Gt Increased	1.2%			
Hepatitis	1.2%			
Jaundice		1.1%		
Metabolic and Nutritional Disorders				
Weight Increase	4.7%	9.2%	3.6%	1.8%
Phosphatase Alkaline Increased	8.2%	1.1%	2.4%	4.8%
Weight Decrease	3.5%	4.6%	3.6%	3.6%
Blood Urea Decreased	3.5%		2.4%	1.2%
Hypoglycaemia	2.4%	1.1%	2.4%	0.6%
Oedema Legs	2.4%	1.1%	2.4%	0.6%
Glycosuria			1.8%	1.2%
Hypercholesterolaemia		1.1%	1.2%	1.2%
Hyperproteinaemia			0.6%	1.8%
Npn Increased	2.4%		0.6%	0.6%
Hyperglycaemia			1.8%	
Hypocalcaemia	1.2%		0.6%	0.6%
Hypoproteinaemia	2.4%		0.6%	
Serum Iron Decreased	2.4%	1.1%		

(cont'd)

Table 5: REBIF *(cont'd)*

Adverse Events Experienced by at Least 1% of the Patients Enrolled in Study GF6789 (PRISMS—Ongoing from Year 1 and 2 or Started During Year 3 and 4)

Body System/Preferred Term	Placebo/66 (n=85)	Placebo/132 (n=87)	REBIF 66 µg Weekly (n=167)	REBIF 132 µg Weekly (n=167)
Hypokalaemia		2.3%		
Hyperkalaemia		1.1%		
Hyperlipaemia	1.2%			
Musculo-Skeletal System Disorders				
Back Pain	14.1%	20.7%	20.4%	22.2%
Myalgia	21.2%	23.0%	15.6%	14.4%
Arthralgia	16.5%	18.4%	12.6%	18.0%
Muscle Weakness	12.9%	17.2%	7.2%	9.6%
Skeletal Pain	8.2%	11.5%	7.2%	6.6%
Arthritis		5.7%	2.4%	2.4%
Arthrosis	1.2%	2.3%	1.8%	2.4%
Tendinitis	2.4%		1.2%	1.2%
Bursitis			1.8%	0.6%
Arthropathy			1.2%	0.6%
Bone Disorder		1.1%		
Ischial Neuralgia		1.1%		
Malformation Foot	1.2%			
Neoplasm				
Breast Fibroadenosis	1.2%		0.6%	
Platelet, Bleeding & Clotting Disorder				
Thrombocytopenia	3.5%	1.1%	1.8%	3.6%
Haematoma	3.5%	1.1%	1.8%	1.8%
Epistaxis		2.3%	1.8%	0.6%
Thrombocythaemia	1.2%		1.2%	
Thrombosis	1.2%			
Psychiatric Disorders				
Depression	29.4%	27.6%	23.4%	25.1%
Insomnia	22.4%	21.8%	16.2%	21.6%
Nervousness	7.1%	8.0%	6.6%	4.8%
Anxiety	3.5%	6.9%	4.8%	3.0%
Emotional Lability	4.7%	3.4%	3.0%	2.4%
Sleep Disorder	1.2%	5.7%	3.6%	1.8%
Anorexia	4.7%	1.1%	3.0%	2.4%
Somnolence	2.4%		2.4%	4.2%
Amnesia	1.2%	2.3%	3.0%	0.6%
Depression Aggravated			2.4%	0.6%
Concentration Impaired			1.2%	1.2%
Suicide Attempt	1.2%			1.8%
Agitation			1.8%	
Confusion		2.3%		0.6%
Libido Decreased	1.2%	1.1%	0.6%	
Apathy	1.2%			
Paroniria	1.2%			
Personality Disorder		1.1%		
Psychosis Manic-Depressive	1.2%			
Teeth-Grinding	1.2%			

(cont'd)

Table 5: REBIF *(cont'd)*

Adverse Events Experienced by at Least 1% of the Patients Enrolled in Study GF6789 (PRISMS—Ongoing from Year 1 and 2 or Started During Year 3 and 4)

Body System/Preferred Term	Placebo/66 (n=85)	Placebo/132 (n=87)	REBIF 66 µg Weekly (n=167)	REBIF 132 µg Weekly (n=167)
Red Blood Cell Disorders				
Anaemia	7.1%	9.2%	3.6%	6.6%
Polycythaemia	1.2%		1.8%	
Anaemia Hypochromic	1.2%			
Marrow Hyperplasia		1.1%		
Reproductive Disorders, Female				
Menstrual Disorder	5.9%	6.9%	6.6%	2.4%
Amenorrhoea	3.5%		0.6%	1.8%
Breast Neoplasm Female	2.4%	2.3%	1.2%	0.6%
Menorrhagia	1.2%	1.1%	1.8%	0.6%
Vaginitis		3.4%	1.2%	0.6%
Dysmenorrhoea	1.2%	2.3%	1.2%	
Intermenstrual Bleeding		2.3%	1.8%	
Uterine Fibroid	1.2%		1.2%	1.2%
Menopausal Symptoms	1.2%		1.8%	
Vaginal Haemorrhage	1.2%	1.1%	0.6%	0.6%
Ovarian Cyst	1.2%		0.6%	0.6%
Breast Neoplasm Malignant Female		2.3%		
Endometriosis	1.2%		0.6%	
Pregnancy Unintended	1.2%			0.6%
Breast Neoplasm Benign Female	1.2%			
Cervicitis		1.1%		
Uterine Inflammation		1.1%		
Reproductive Disorders, Male				
Impotence	7.1%		3.0%	2.4%
Epididymitis		1.1%	0.6%	
Testicular Pain		1.1%		
Resistance Mechanism Disorders				
Infection Fungal	4.7%	1.1%	6.6%	5.4%
Herpes Simplex	2.4%	6.9%	5.4%	1.2%
Infection	3.5%	1.1%	4.8%	2.4%
Infection Viral	4.7%		3.0%	3.0%
Otitis Media	4.7%		1.2%	2.4%
Herpes Zoster			1.2%	1.8%
Moniliasis		1.1%	0.6%	1.8%
Abscess		1.1%		0.6%
Infection Parasitic	1.2%			0.6%
Moniliasis Genital		1.1%		
Sepsis	1.2%			
Respiratory System Disorders				
Rhinitis	38.8%	29.9%	39.5%	33.5%
Upper Resp Tract Infection	18.8%	14.9%	22.8%	20.4%
Pharyngitis	23.5%	12.6%	19.8%	15.0%
Coughing	5.9%	11.5%	8.4%	13.8%
Sinusitis	8.2%	11.5%	5.4%	10.2%
Bronchitis	1.2%	9.2%	4.2%	8.4%

(cont'd)

Table 5: REBIF *(cont'd)*

Adverse Events Experienced by at Least 1% of the Patients Enrolled in Study GF6789 (PRISMS—Ongoing from Year 1 and 2 or Started During Year 3 and 4)

Body System/Preferred Term	Placebo/66 (n=85)	Placebo/132 (n=87)	REBIF 66 µg Weekly (n=167)	REBIF 132 µg Weekly (n=167)
Tracheitis	1.2%		2.4%	3.0%
Laryngitis		3.4%	3.6%	
Dyspnoea	2.4%	2.3%	1.2%	1.2%
Asthma	1.2%	1.1%		0.6%
Hyperventilation	2.4%			0.6%
Pneumonia			1.2%	0.6%
Bronchospasm			1.2%	
Pneumonitis	1.2%			
Secondary Terms				
Trauma Nos	15.3%	5.7%	14.4%	11.4%
Fall	3.5%	5.7%	2.4%	4.8%
Cyst Nos	2.4%	1.1%	1.2%	2.4%
Bite	2.4%	2.3%	0.6%	1.8%
Post-Operative Wound Infection	1.2%	2.3%	1.2%	
Post-Operative Pain	1.2%	1.1%	0.6%	0.6%
Food Poisoning		1.1%	0.6%	
Post-Operative Haemorrhage	2.4%			
Surgical Procedure			1.2%	
Metastases Nos		1.1%		
Skin and Appendages Disorders				
Pruritus	3.5%	5.7%	7.8%	9.6%
Rash	3.5%	8.0%	6.5%	6.0%
Skin Disorder	2.4%	4.6%	7.2%	3.0%
Eczema	2.4%	3.4%	7.2%	3.0%
Skin Dry	2.4%	3.4%	3.0%	5.4%
Acne	4.7%	1.1%	3.6%	3.0%
Alopecia	4.7%	2.3%	3.6%	1.8%
Rash Erythematous	3.5%	2.3%	4.8%	1.2%
Dermatitis Fungal	1.2%	2.3%	2.4%	0.6%
Rash Maculo-Papular	2.4%	1.1%	1.2%	1.8%
Skin Hypertrophy	1.2%	2.3%	0.6%	1.8%
Psoriasis	1.2%	2.3%	1.8%	
Verruca	1.2%	1.1%		2.4%
Onychomycosis		1.1%	1.2%	1.2%
Folliculitis		1.1%	1.8%	
Furunculosis		1.1%		1.8%
Nail Disorder		1.1%		1.8%
Photosensitivity Reaction	1.2%		0.6%	1.2%
Urticaria	1.2%	1.1%		1.2%
Dermatitis	1.2%			1.2%
Rosacea		1.1%	0.6%	0.6%
Skin Discolouration			0.6%	1.2%
Hair Disorder Nos		1.1%	0.6%	
Papilloma	1.2%	1.1%		
Pilonidal Cyst	1.2%		0.6%	
Bullous Eruption	1.2%			

(cont'd)

Table 5: REBIF *(cont'd)*

Adverse Events Experienced by at Least 1% of the Patients Enrolled in Study GF6789 (PRISMS—Ongoing from Year 1 and 2 or Started During Year 3 and 4)

Body System/Preferred Term	Placebo/66 (n=85)	Placebo/132 (n=87)	REBIF 66 µg Weekly (n=167)	REBIF 132 µg Weekly (n=167)
Dermographia		1.1%		
Hyperkeratosis		1.1%		
Special Senses Other, Disorders				
Taste Perversion	1.2%			1.8%
Urinary System Disorders				
Urinary Tract Infection	8.2%	14.9%	16.2%	13.8%
Cystitis	5.9%	6.9%	9.6%	6.6%
Haematuria	1.2%	4.6%	3.0%	4.8%
Micturition Frequency	1.2%	3.4%	1.8%	4.8%
Urinary Incontinence		5.7%	3.0%	1.8%
Urinary Retention	2.4%	2.3%	2.4%	0.6%
Urine Abnormal	4.7%		1.8%	1.2%
Dysuria	1.2%		1.8%	1.8%
Micturition Disorder	1.2%	1.1%	1.2%	1.8%
Albuminuria	1.2%	1.1%	1.2%	1.2%
Micturition Urgency	1.2%	1.1%	1.2%	1.2%
Renal Calculus			1.2%	2.4%
Pyelonephritis			1.2%	1.2%
Renal Pain	1.2%	1.1%		1.2%
Creatinine Decrease	1.2%			1.2%
Face Oedema		1.1%		
Pyuria	1.2%			
Vascular (extracardiac) Disorders				
Peripheral Ischaemia	1.2%	2.3%	1.8%	1.8%
Flushing	1.2%	2.3%	1.8%	
Telangiectasis			1.8%	
Vascular Disorder			0.6%	1.2%
Vein Varicose	1.2%	1.1%	0.6%	
Thrombophlebitis			1.2%	
Thrombophlebitis Deep		1.1%		
Vision Disorders				
Vision Abnormal	5.9%	4.6%	4.2%	9.0%
Eye Pain	1.2%	4.6%	5.4%	5.4%
Conjunctivitis	1.2%	3.4%	3.6%	3.6%
Xerophthalmia		1.1%	3.0%	0.6%
Diplopia			1.8%	1.2%
Eye Infection			0.6%	1.2%
Lacrimal Duct Obstruction	1.2%		0.6%	
Meibomianitis	1.2%	1.1%		
Accommodation Abnormal		1.1%		
Conjunctival Discolouration	1.2%			
Keratitis	1.2%			
Lacrimation Abnormal	1.2%			
White Cell and Res Disorders				
Lymphopenia	22.4%	23.0%	19.8%	25.7%
Leucopenia	16.5%	14.9%	12.0%	13.8%

(cont'd)

Table 5: REBIF *(cont'd)*

Adverse Events Experienced by at Least 1% of the Patients Enrolled in Study GF6789 (PRISMS—Ongoing from Year 1 and 2 or Started During Year 3 and 4)

Body System/Preferred Term	Placebo/66 (n=85)	Placebo/132 (n=87)	REBIF 66 µg Weekly (n=167)	REBIF 132 µg Weekly (n=167)
Granulocytopenia	9.4%	10.3%	7.8%	12.0%
Lymphadenopathy	2.4%	14.9%	8.4%	10.2%
Leukocytosis	3.5%	3.4%	6.0%	3.6%
Monocytosis	4.7%	1.1%	1.8%	2.4%
Eosinophilia	3.5%	1.1%	1.2%	2.4%
Wbc Abnormal Nos	1.2%	1.1%	2.4%	1.2%
Lymphadenopathy Cervical		1.1%	0.6%	2.4%
Lymphocytosis	1.2%		1.8%	0.6%

Table 6: REBIF

Adverse Events Experienced by Less Than 1% of the Patients Enrolled in Study GF6789 (PRISMS—Ongoing from Year 1 and 2 or Started During Year 3 and 4)

Body System	Preferred Term
Application Site Disorders	Injection Site Atrophy
	Cellulitis
	Injection Site Fibrosis
	Skin Necrosis
Body as a Whole—General Disorders	Chest Pain Substernal
	Sarcoidosis
Cardiovascular Disorders, General	Aneurysm
	Circulatory Failure
	Heart Murmur
Centr & Periph Nervous System Disorders	Trigeminal Neuralgia
	Dyskinesia
	Dysphonia
	Nerve Root Lesion
	Neuralgia
	Neuropathy
	Scotoma
Collagen Disorders	Antinuclear Factor Test Positive
Endocrine Disorders	Glucocorticoids Increased
Gastro-Intestinal System Disorders	Change in Bowel Habits
	Enanthema
	Haemorrhage Rectum
	Hiccup
	Oesophageal Ulceration
	Periodontal Destruction
	Tongue Ulceration
	Tooth Caries
Heart Rate and Rhythm Disorders	Arrhythmia
	Extrasystoles
Liver and Biliary System Disorders	Cholelithiasis
	Hepatomegaly
Metabolic and Nutritional Disorders	Bun Increased
	Diabetes Mellitus
	Hypercalcaemia
	Oedema Generalised
	Vitamin B12 Deficiency

(cont'd)

Table 6: REBIF *(cont'd)*

Adverse Events Experienced by Less Than 1% of the Patients Enrolled in Study GF6789 (PRISMS—Ongoing from Year 1 and 2 or Started During Year 3 and 4)

Body System	Preferred Term
Musculo-Skeletal System Disorders	Myopathy
	Osteoporosis
Myo Endo Pericardial & Valve Disorders	Myocardial Infarction
Neoplasm	Bladder Carcinoma
	Ovarian Carcinoma
	Renal Carcinoma
Platelet, Bleeding & Clotting Disorders	Purpura
Psychiatric Disorders	Depression Psychotic
	Drug Dependence
Red Blood Cell Disorders	Hyperhaemoglobinaemia
	Packed Cell Volume Increased
Reproductive Disorders, Female	Cervical Uterine Polyp
	Cervix Lesion
	Fertility Decreased Female
	Premenstrual Tension
	Vulva Discomfort
Reproductive Disorders, Male	Hernia Inguinal
	Semen Abnormal
	Sexual Function Abnormal
	Testis Disorder
Resistance Mechanism Disorders	Toxoplasmosis
Respiratory System Disorders	Pleural Pain
	Pleurisy
	Pulmonary Congestion
Secondary Terms	Abrasion Nos
	Heat Intolerance
	Lumbar Disc Lesion
	Medication Reaction Nos
	Nasal Septum Deviation
Skin and Appendages Disorders	Dermatitis Contact
	Pigmentation Abnormal
	Pityriasis Rosea
	Hair Texture Abnormal
	Hypertrichosis
	Livedo Reticularis
	Photosensitivity Allergic React
	Rash Pustular
	Rhagades
	Skin Malformation
	Skin Reaction Localised
	Vesicular Rash
	Vitiligo
Urinary System Disorders	Nocturia
	Cystitis Haemorrhagic
	Polyuria
	Renal Cyst
	Urethral Disorder

(cont'd)

Table 6: REBIF *(cont'd)*

Adverse Events Experienced by Less Than 1% of the Patients Enrolled in Study GF6789 (PRISMS—Ongoing from Year 1 and 2 or Started During Year 3 and 4)

Body System	Preferred Term
Vascular (extracardiac) Disorders	Claudication Intermittent
	Ocular Haemorrhage
	Vascular Malformation Cerebral
	Vascular Malformation Peripheral
	Vein Distended
Vision Disorders	Blepharitis
	Corneal Ulceration
	Herpes Ocular
	Lacrimal Gland Disorder
	Mydriasis
	Retinal Disorder
	Uveitis

Asymptomatic laboratory abnormalities were reported frequently with interferon dosing over the 4 years. Of the abnormalities noted, the cytopenias and abnormalities of liver function showed dose-related differences. Lymphopenia occurred in 35% of high dose patients and 27% of low dose patients. Thrombocytopenia was seen in 2.6% of patients on low dose, and 8.2% of patients on high dose. Differences in the frequency of abnormal liver enzymes were seen which included elevated ALT (24% for low dose vs. 30% for high dose, p=0.07) and elevated AST (11% vs. 20%, p=0.03). Severe elevations are uncommon and not different between dose groups. These data suggest that there is only minimal evidence of significant dose-dependent lab abnormalities with interferon therapy in MS patients.

After 4 years of therapy, 23.7% of the low dose and 14.3% of the high-dose patients had developed persistent neutralising antibodies (p=0.024, 44 µg vs. 22 µg), the vast majority of which (91%) developed within 24 months. The lower incidence in the high dose group may be due to the phenomenon of high-zone tolerance. While continuing interferon treatment, 20.0% of low-dose NAb+ patients reverted, while 25.7% of high-dose NAb+ patients reverted. The neutralising antibodies were associated with reduced clinical efficacy during years 3 and 4 and reduced MRI efficacy over 4 years.

Study GF6954 (SPECTRIMS): Adverse Reactions: Table 7 presents adverse events that were reported in at least 1% of the patients in any treatment group of Study GF6954; the AEs are listed by WHOART system organ class and preferred term (sorted by preferred term in order of frequency). The most frequently reported adverse event was injection site inflammation, which occurred in 67% of both treated groups compared to 16% for placebo. Lower frequencies of the closely associated but more symptomatic injection site reactions were reported in 3 to 4 times as many treated patients as placebo patients. Injection site necrosis was seen in 3.3% and 6.9% of patients in the 22 µg and 44 µg groups respectively, but almost always as a single event per patient. The rate of necrosis was 1/3 800 injections for high-dose and 1/9 600 for low-dose therapy. Liver function abnormalities were also reported 3 to 4 times more commonly with active therapy. The haematopoietic system was also affected, with increased reports of leucopenia, granulocytopenia and lymphopenia associated with active therapy and most prominently with the higher dose. These haematopoietic abnormalities are expected side-effects of interferon therapy. Increased reports of anaemia and thrombocytopenia were noted with treatment, but these events occurred in less than 10% of patients.

Table 7: REBIF

Adverse Events Experienced by at Least 1% of the Patients Enrolled in Study GF6954 (SPECTRIMS—Year 3)

Body System/Preferred Term	Placebo (n=205)	REBIF 66 µg Weekly (n=209)	REBIF 132 µg Weekly (n=204)
Application Site Disorders			
Injection Site Inflammation	15.6%	66.5%	67.2%
Injection Site Reaction	7.8%	21.1%	31.9%
Injection Site Pain	18.0%	17.2%	22.5%
Injection Site Bruising	16.1%	8.1%	9.8%
Injection Site Necrosis		3.3%	6.9%
Injection Site Mass	1.0%	1.9%	2.5%
Injection Site Abscess		2.4%	2.5%
Injection Site Bleeding		2.4%	1.5%
Autonomic Nervous System Disorders			
Flushing	1.5%	1.9%	2.9%
Body as a Whole—General Disorders			
Headache	56.6%	52.2%	63.2%
Influenza-Like Symptoms	52.2%	50.7%	49.5%
Fatigue	32.2%	33.0%	43.1%
Fever	11.7%	14.4%	19.1%
Leg Pain	9.3%	11.5%	12.3%
Asthenia	9.8%	5.7%	12.3%
Rigors	5.4%	7.7%	7.8%

(cont'd)

Table 7: REBIF *(cont'd)*

Adverse Events Experienced by at Least 1% of the Patients Enrolled in Study GF6954 (SPECTRIMS—Year 3)

Body System/Preferred Term	Placebo (n=205)	REBIF 66 µg Weekly (n=209)	REBIF 132 µg Weekly (n=204)
Chest Pain	5.9%	7.2%	6.4%
Sweating Increased	4.4%	9.1%	5.4%
Malaise	5.9%	4.3%	7.8%
Pain	4.9%	5.3%	5.4%
Allergic Reaction	5.9%	2.4%	3.9%
Hot Flushes	3.4%	4.3%	2.5%
Temperature Changed Sensation	3.4%	2.4%	3.9%
Syncope	1.0%	2.4%	1.5%
Scar	1.5%	0.5%	1.5%
Cardiovascular Disorders, General			
Hypertension	2.9%	7.7%	7.8%
Oedema Dependent	4.9%	5.7%	5.4%
Oedema Peripheral	4.9%	5.7%	3.4%
Oedema Legs	4.9%	1.9%	2.0%
Hypotension	1.0%	1.9%	1.0%
Centr & Periph Nervous System Disorders			
Hypertonia	26.8%	24.4%	30.4%
Dizziness	18.0%	16.3%	17.2%
Paraesthesia	13.2%	8.1%	9.3%
Hypoaesthesia	9.3%	10.0%	8.3%
Dysaesthesia	9.8%	6.2%	5.9%
Ataxia	7.3%	6.7%	5.9%
Gait Abnormal	6.8%	6.7%	5.9%
Vertigo	5.9%	3.3%	4.9%
Tremor	5.4%	3.8%	4.4%
Migraine	3.4%	4.3%	4.9%
Paresis	3.4%	3.3%	3.9%
Muscle Contractions Involuntary	2.4%	3.8%	3.4%
Ms Aggravated	1.5%	3.3%	3.4%
Speech Disorder	2.4%	1.4%	1.0%
Confusion	2.9%	1.5%	
Coordination Abnormal	1.0%	1.4%	2.0%
Convulsions	1.0%	2.4%	0.5%
Dysphonia	1.0%	1.0%	1.5%
Sensory Disturbance	0.5%	0.5%	2.5%
Trigeminal Neuralgia	2.4%	0.5%	0.5%
Hyperkinesia	1.0%	1.4%	0.5%
Endocrine Disorders			
Thyroid Disorder	3.4%	3.3%	5.4%
T4 Increased	0.5%	3.8%	2.0%
Gastro-Intestinal System Disorders			
Nausea	26.3%	23.9%	17.6%
Abdominal Pain	18.0%	14.8%	15.2%
Diarrhoea	15.6%	18.7%	13.7%
Constipation	19.0%	14.8%	13.2%
Vomiting	8.3%	7.2%	6.9%
Dyspepsia	7.3%	7.2%	5.9%

(cont'd)

Table 7: REBIF *(cont'd)*

Adverse Events Experienced by at Least 1% of the Patients Enrolled in Study GF6954 (SPECTRIMS—Year 3)

Body System/Preferred Term	Placebo (n=205)	REBIF 66 µg Weekly (n=209)	REBIF 132 µg Weekly (n=204)
Tooth Disorder	4.4%	5.3%	6.9%
Anorexia	5.4%	5.3%	4.9%
Gastroenteritis	7.3%	2.9%	5.4%
Tooth Ache	3.4%	3.3%	2.5%
Gastro-Intestinal Disorder Nos	3.9%	1.4%	2.9%
Faecal Incontinence	3.9%	0.5%	3.4%
Dysphagia	2.4%	2.4%	2.5%
Mouth Dry	3.4%	1.9%	0.5%
Gastritis	1.5%	1.4%	1.0%
Flatulence	1.5%		1.5%
Appetite Increased	1.0%	1.4%	
Hiccup	1.0%		1.5%
Oesophagitis	1.5%	0.5%	0.5%
Gingival Bleeding		1.4%	
Gingivitis	1.5%		
Hearing and Vestibular Disorders			
Ear Ache	1.0%	2.4%	4.9%
Tinnitus	2.0%	1.4%	2.0%
Ear Disorder Nos	2.9%	1.4%	
Heart Rate and Rhythm Disorders			
Palpitation	1.5%	3.3%	3.4%
Tachycardia	0.5%	1.4%	0.5%
Liver and Biliary System Disorders			
ALT Increased	7.3%	21.1%	23.0%
AST Increased	3.4%	11.5%	13.2%
Hepatic Enzymes Increased	1.0%	5.3%	6.4%
Phosphatase Alkaline Increased	1.5%	3.8%	2.9%
Hepatic Function Abnormal	1.5%	2.4%	3.4%
Cholelithiasis		0.5%	1.5%
Metabolic and Nutritional Disorders			
Weight Decrease	6.3%	4.8%	8.3%
Weight Increase	3.4%	3.3%	2.0%
Glycosuria	1.0%	1.4%	1.5%
Hypercholesterolaemia	1.0%	1.0%	2.0%
Hyperproteinaemia	1.0%	1.9%	0.5%
Musculo-Skeletal System Disorders			
Myalgia	23.9%	24.9%	27.9%
Arthralgia	25.4%	24.4%	23.0%
Back Pain	22.4%	21.5%	22.1%
Muscle Weakness	18.0%	17.2%	16.7%
Skeletal Pain	8.8%	9.1%	7.4%
Arthropathy	3.4%	3.8%	2.9%
Tendinitis	2.0%	2.9%	3.9%
Arthritis	2.0%	1.4%	2.9%
Bursitis	2.0%	2.9%	1.0%
Arthrosis	0.5%	3.3%	1.0%
Neoplasm			
Cervical Smear Test Positive			1.5%
Platelet, Bleeding & Clotting Disorders			
Thrombocytopenia	0.5%	3.3%	6.4%
Thrombocythaemia	1.5%	1.0%	1.5%
Psychiatric Disorders			
Depression	28.8%	32.1%	34.8%
Insomnia	22.0%	20.6%	23.5%
Anxiety	7.3%	4.3%	5.4%
Depression Aggravated	1.5%	7.2%	5.4%
Somnolence	4.4%	4.3%	4.4%
Nervousness	2.4%	1.9%	2.0%
Emotional Lability	1.5%	2.4%	2.0%
Amnesia	2.4%	1.0%	0.5%
Suicide Attempt	1.5%	1.4%	1.0%
Agitation	1.0%	0.5%	2.0%
Libido Decreased		2.4%	
Cyclothymic Reaction			1.5%
Red Blood Cell Disorders			
Anaemia	3.9%	2.4%	9.3%
Reproductive Disorders, Female			
Menstrual Disorder	5.4%	2.9%	3.4%
Menorrhagia	2.9%	2.4%	2.5%
Vaginitis	2.4%	1.4%	2.0%
Amenorrhoea	0.5%	2.9%	0.5%
Dysmenorrhoea	2.4%	1.0%	0.5%
Menopausal Symptoms	0.5%	1.9%	1.5%
Vaginal Haemorrhage	2.0%	0.5%	1.0%
Breast Neoplasm Benign Female	1.5%	0.5%	0.5%
Leukorrhoea		1.4%	
Reproductive Disorders, Male			
Impotence	1.5%	1.0%	2.9%
Resistance Mechanism Disorders			
Infection	3.9%	5.3%	6.4%
Herpes Simplex	4.4%	6.2%	3.4%
Infection Fungal	2.9%	2.9%	2.9%
Moniliasis	2.0%	1.4%	3.4%
Abscess	1.0%	2.4%	2.0%
Infection Viral	1.5%	1.4%	2.0%
Otitis Media	1.0%	0.5%	2.9%
Herpes Zoster	0.5%	1.9%	0.5%
Moniliasis Genital	1.0%	1.4%	0.5%
Respiratory System Disorders			
Rhinitis	41.5%	38.3%	33.3%
Upper Resp Tract Infection	33.2%	31.1%	26.0%
Pharyngitis	20.0%	19.6%	17.2%
Sinusitis	6.8%	7.2%	8.8%
Coughing	6.3%	6.7%	5.4%

(cont'd)

Table 7: REBIF *(cont'd)*

Adverse Events Experienced by at Least 1% of the Patients Enrolled in Study GF6954 (SPECTRIMS—Year 3)

Body System/Preferred Term	Placebo (n=205)	REBIF 66 µg Weekly (n=209)	REBIF 132 µg Weekly (n=204)
Bronchitis	5.9%	3.8%	7.8%
Tracheitis	6.3%	7.2%	3.9%
Dyspnoea	3.9%	4.3%	0.5%
Pneumonia	1.0%	2.9%	2.9%
Epistaxis	2.0%	1.0%	3.4%
Laryngitis	2.9%	1.4%	1.0%
Secondary Terms			
Trauma Nos	28.3%	24.3%	23.0%
Fall	7.3%	5.7%	6.9%
Post-Operative Pain	3.4%	1.9%	2.5%
Bite	1.0%	2.4%	2.0%
Food Poisoning	0.5%	2.4%	2.0%
Abrasion Nos	0.5%	1.4%	1.5%
Cyst Nos	0.5%	1.4%	0.5%
Eye Burns	0.5%	1.4%	
Skin and Appendages Disorders			
Rash	6.3%	5.7%	8.8%
Pruritus	5.9%	5.7%	8.8%
Alopecia	4.9%	8.1%	4.4%
Rash Erythematous	2.4%	8.6%	6.4%
Eczema	5.9%	4.3%	2.9%
Skin Dry	1.0%	5.7%	4.9%
Skin Disorder	2.0%	4.3%	3.9%
Dermatitis	2.9%	1.0%	1.5%
Rash Maculo-Papular	2.0%	1.9%	1.5%
Acne	1.0%	2.4%	1.5%
Pruritic Rash	1.0%	1.9%	1.0%
Skin Ulceration		1.4%	2.5%
Seborrhoea	0.5%	1.4%	1.5%
Skin Discolouration	1.5%	0.5%	1.5%
Dermatitis Fungal	1.0%		2.0%
Furunculosis	1.0%	1.4%	0.5%
Nail Disorder		1.4%	1.5%
Urticaria	2.4%	0.5%	
Rosacea	0.5%	0.5%	1.5%
Verruca	0.5%		1.5%
Special Senses Other, Disorders			
Taste Perversion	0.5%	1.9%	0.5%
Urinary System Disorders			
Urinary Tract Infection	26.3%	34.4%	27.0%
Cystitis	12.7%	17.2%	10.8%
Haematuria	4.4%	6.2%	5.4%
Micturition Frequency	2.9%	5.3%	3.9%
Urinary Incontinence	6.3%	3.3%	2.0%
Albuminuria	3.4%	3.3%	3.4%
Urinary Retention	4.4%	3.8%	1.0%
Micturition Disorder	2.9%	3.3%	1.5%

(cont'd)

Table 7: REBIF *(cont'd)*

Adverse Events Experienced by at Least 1% of the Patients Enrolled in Study GF6954 (SPECTRIMS—Year 3)

Body System/Preferred Term	Placebo (n=205)	REBIF 66 µg Weekly (n=209)	REBIF 132 µg Weekly (n=204)
Creatinine Decrease	2.4%	1.4%	2.5%
Dysuria	3.4%	1.9%	0.5%
Micturition Urgency	2.0%	0.5%	0.5%
Pyelonephritis	2.0%		1.0%
Bun Increased		0.5%	1.5%
Vascular (extracardiac) Disorders			
Haematoma	6.3%	1.4%	3.4%
Thrombophlebitis Deep		1.4%	0.5%
Vision Disorders			
Vision Abnormal	11.7%	10.5%	4.9%
Eye Pain	5.9%	6.7%	7.4%
Conjunctivitis	3.4%	4.8%	2.5%
Diplopia	2.9%	1.9%	2.0%
Xerophthalmia	1.0%	1.9%	1.0%
Eye Infection	2.0%	0.5%	1.0%
Meibomianitis		1.4%	2.0%
White Cell and Res Disorders			
Lymphopenia	15.1%	21.5%	26.0%
Leucopenia	4.9%	11.0%	21.1%
Granulocytopenia	2.0%	9.1%	13.2%
Lymphadenopathy	3.9%	5.3%	7.8%
Leukocytosis	4.4%	0.5%	2.9%
Monocytosis	1.5%	1.4%	2.0%
Eosinophilia	1.0%	1.4%	2.0%

In addition to the above listed adverse events, the following events have been experienced less frequently (i.e. in less than 1% of the study population) during the 3 years of treatment. See Table 8.

Table 8: REBIF

Adverse Events Experienced by Less Than 1% of the Patients Enrolled in Study GF6954 (SPECTRIMS—Year 3)

Body System	Preferred Term
Application Site Disorders	Cellulitis
	Otitis Externa
	Skin Nodule
Body as a Whole—General Disorders	Allergy
	Choking
	Face Oedema
	Carpal Tunnel Syndrome
	Condition Aggravated
	Granulomatous Lesion
	Halitosis
	Necrosis Ischaemic
	Oedema
	Pallor
Cardiovascular Disorders, General	Heart Murmur
	Cyanosis
	Oedema Periorbital

(cont'd)

Table 8: REBIF *(cont'd)*

Adverse Events Experienced by Less Than 1% of the Patients Enrolled in Study GF6954 (SPECTRIMS—Year 3)

Body System	Preferred Term
Centr & Periph Nervous System Disorders	Anaesthesia Mouth
	Cramps Legs
	Neuralgia
	Coma
	Dyskinesia
	Lower Motor Neurone Lesion
	Neuropathy
	Paralysis
	Paraplegia
	Convulsions Grand Mal
	Hemianopia
	Hyperaesthesia
	Nystagmus
	Optic Atrophy
	Scotoma
	Stupor
	Visual Field Defect
Collagen Disorders	Auto-Antibody Response
Endocrine Disorders	Thyroid Stim. Hormone Decreased
	Hypothyroidism
	T3 Increased
	Goitre
	Hyperthyroidism
	T4 Decreased
	Thyroiditis
Foetal Disorders	Hernia Congenital
Gastro-Intestinal System Disorders	Stomatitis Ulcerative
	Appendicitis
	Gastroesophageal Reflux
	Haemorrhoids
	Change in Bowel Habits
	Enteritis
	Abdomen Enlarged
	Colitis
	Gastric Ulcer
	Haemorrhage Rectum
	Melaena
	Tenesmus
	Tongue Discolouration
	Abdominal Adhesions
	Anus Disorder
	Duodenal Ulcer
	Faeces Discoloured
	Gi Haemorrhage
	Leukoplakia Oral
	Mucositis Nos
	Oesophagospasm
	Saliva Altered

(cont'd)

Table 8: REBIF *(cont'd)*

Adverse Events Experienced by Less Than 1% of the Patients Enrolled in Study GF6954 (SPECTRIMS—Year 3)

Body System	Preferred Term
	Saliva Increased
	Salivary Duct Obstruction
	Salivary Gland Enlargement
	Stomatitis
	Teeth-Grinding
	Tongue Ulceration
Hearing and Vestibular Disorders	Hearing Decreased
	Deafness
	Motion Sickness
	Vestibular Disorder
Heart Rate and Rhythm Disorders	Fibrillation Atrial
	Arrhythmia
	Bradycardia
Liver and Biliary System Disorders	Bilirubinaemia
	Hepatomegaly
	Cholangitis
	Gall Bladder Disorder
	Gamma-Gt Increased
Metabolic and Nutritional Disorders	Blood Urea Decreased
	Hypercalcaemia
	Hyperkalaemia
	Thirst
	Vitamin B12 Deficiency
	Hypokalaemia
	Oedema Generalised
	Dehydration
	Gout
	Hyperglycaemia
	Hyperuricaemia
	Hypocalcaemia
	Hypoglycaemia
	Hypoglycaemic Reaction
	Lipodystrophy
	Npn Increased
Musculo-Skeletal System Disorders	Osteoporosis
	Torticollis
	Avascular Necrosis Femoral Head
	Myositis
	Synovitis
Myo Endo Pericardial & Valve Disorders	Angina Pectoris
Neoplasm	Basal Cell Carcinoma
	Brain Neoplasm Benign
	Breast Neoplasm Malignant Female
	Cervical Uterine Polyp
	Gi Neoplasm Benign
	Lipoma
	Thyroid Neoplasm Malignant

(cont'd)

Table 8: REBIF *(cont'd)*

Adverse Events Experienced by Less Than 1% of the Patients Enrolled in Study GF6954 (SPECTRIMS—Year 3)

Body System	Preferred Term
Psychiatric Disorders	Concentration Impaired
	Aggressive Reaction
	Paroniria
	Depersonalization
	Drug Abuse
	Euphoria
	Paranoid Reaction
	Sleep Disorder
	Snoring
Red Blood Cell Disorders	Anaemia Hypochromic
	Polycythaemia
	Packed Cell Volume Increased
	Splenomegaly
Reproductive Disorders, Female	Cervical Dysplasia
	Intermenstrual Bleeding
	Mastitis
	Uterine Fibroid
	Breast Discharge
	Endometrial Hyperplasia
	Ovarian Cyst
	Uterine Haemorrhage
	Uterovaginal Prolapse
	Vaginal Discomfort
	Vaginal Neoplasm Benign
Reproductive Disorders, Male	Prostatic Disorder
	Semen Abnormal
	Ejaculation Failure
	Epididymitis
	Hernia Inguinal
	Testicular Pain
Resistance Mechanism Disorders	Infection Bacterial
	Sepsis
Respiratory System Disorders	Asthma
	Bronchospasm
	Pneumonitis
	Chronic Obstruct Airways Disease
	Pleurisy
	Pulmonary Congestion
	Respiratory Insufficiency
	Sleep Apnoea
	Pleural Effusion
	Pulmonary Eosinophilia
	Pulmonary Oedema
	Sputum Increased
	Throat Tightness
Secondary Terms	Post-Operative Haemorrhage
	Post-Operative Wound Infection

(cont'd)

Table 8: REBIF *(cont'd)*

Adverse Events Experienced by Less Than 1% of the Patients Enrolled in Study GF6954 (SPECTRIMS—Year 3)

Body System	Preferred Term
	Surgical Procedure
	Asthma Extrinsic
	Bone Metastases
	Lumbar Disc Lesion
	Nasal Septum Deviation
	Varicella
Skin and Appendages Disorders	Photosensitivity Reaction
	Psoriasis
	Rash Psoriaform
	Bullous Eruption
	Rash Pustular
	Hyperkeratosis
	Onychomycosis
	Dermatitis Contact
	Hypertrichosis
	Skin Odor Abnormal
	Vesicular Rash
	Chloasma
	Erythema Induratum
	Erythema Multiforme
	Erythema Nodosum
	Folliculitis
	Hair Disorder Nos
	Heat Rash
	Livedo Reticularis
	Melanosis
	Nail Discolouration
	Photosensitivity Allergic React
	Piloerection
	Pilonidal Cyst
	Pruritus Genital
	Skin Atrophy
	Skin Hypertrophy
	Sweating Decreased
Special Senses Other, Disorders	Parosmia
Urinary System Disorders	Polyuria
	Renal Pain
	Nocturia
	Urethral Disorder
	Urine Abnormal
	Bladder Discomfort
	Cystitis Haemorrhagic
	Hydronephrosis
	Renal Calculus
	Renal Cyst
	Renal Function Abnormal

(cont'd)

Table 8: REBIF *(cont'd)*

Adverse Events Experienced by Less Than 1% of the Patients Enrolled in Study GF6954 (SPECTRIMS—Year 3)

Body System	Preferred Term
Vascular (extracardiac) Disorders	Peripheral Ischaemia
	Embolism Pulmonary
	Vascular Disorder
	Vasculitis
	Vein Distended
	Cerebral Haemorrhage
	Cerebrovascular Disorder
	Phlebitis
	Subarachnoid Haemorrhage
	Thrombophlebitis
	Vascular Malformation Peripheral
	Vein Varicose
Vision Disorders	Blepharitis
	Photophobia
	Accommodation Abnormal
	Cataract
	Retinal Disorder
	Blindness
	Glaucoma
	Blepharospasm
	Blindness Temporary
	Conjunctival Discolouration
	Conjunctival Haemorrhage
	Corneal Deposits
	Corneal Opacity
	Exophthalmos
	Eyelid Retraction
	Herpes Ocular
	Uveitis
White Cell and Res Disorders	Lymphadenopathy Cervical
	Wbc Abnormal Nos
	Basophilia

Study GF7480 (ETOMS): Adverse Reactions: In Study GF7480, adverse events were reported more frequently in patients assigned REBIF than in those assigned placebo. These events included injection-site inflammation (60% vs 12%), fever (28% vs 12%), myalgia (17% vs 9%) and chills (11% vs 5%). Serious adverse events were reported in five patients in the placebo group and six in the interferon beta-1a group.

Study 21125 (EVIDENCE): Adverse Reactions: Study 21125 was a direct comparative trial of IFN beta-1a 44 µg tiw (REBIF) vs. IFN beta-1a 30 µg im qw (Avonex) in RRMS patients. Of the 677 patients randomized, 339 patients received REBIF 44 µg sc tiw and 338 patients were randomized to AVONEX 30 µg im qw. The following tables present AE frequencies for only the REBIF-treated group coded in MedDRA version 8.0.

There were a total of 2682 AEs reported by the subjects who received REBIF, the majority of which were mild in severity. The most commonly reported AEs were injection site disorders, flu-like symptoms (headache, fever, chills, fatigue, malaise, arthralgia and myalgia), white blood cell abnormalities and elevated hepatic transaminases (AST and ALT), all of which are well-known reactions to interferon and are included in the product label for REBIF. See Table 9.

Table 9: REBIF

Adverse Events[a] Experienced by at Least 1% of the REBIF-Treated Patients Enrolled in Study 21125 (EVIDENCE) During Forty-Eight Weeks

System Organ Class/Preferred Term	REBIF 44 µg TIW Subjects (n=339)
General Disorders and Administration Site Conditions	
Injection site erythema	45.1%
Influenza like illness	44.2%
Injection site reaction	27.1%
Fatigue	17.1%
Injection site pain	14.2%
Injection site haemorrhage	10.0%
Injection site irritation	8.3%
Pain	5.0%
Pyrexia	5.0%
Asthenia	3.5%
Chest pain	3.2%
Chills	3.2%
Injection site inflammation	2.4%
Gait disturbance	1.2%
Injection site mass	1.2%
Injection site pruritus	1.2%
Malaise	1.2%
Infections and Infestations	
Rhinitis	17.7%
Upper respiratory tract infection	15.9%
Sinusitis	11.2%
Viral infection	8.0%
Urinary tract infection	7.4%
Bronchitis	5.0%
Gastroenteritis viral	4.1%
Ear infection	2.9%
Herpes simplex	2.1%
Localised infection	1.8%
Lower respiratory tract infection	1.8%
Pharyngitis	1.8%
Tooth abscess	1.8%
Vaginal candidiasis	1.5%
Acute tonsillitis	1.2%
Eye infection	1.2%
Gastroenteritis	1.2%
Otitis media	1.2%
Vaginal infection	1.2%
Nervous System Disorders	
Headache	37.5%
Dizziness	9.1%
Hypoaesthesia	5.6%
Migraine	4.7%
Paraesthesia	4.7%
Hemiparesis	2.7%
Muscle spasticity	2.7%
Balance disorder	2.1%
Sinus headache	1.8%
Paresis	1.5%
Tremor	1.5%
Musculoskeletal and Connective Tissue Disorders	
Arthralgia	10.6%

(cont'd)

Table 9: REBIF *(cont'd)*

Adverse Events[a] Experienced by at Least 1% of the REBIF-Treated Patients Enrolled in Study 21125 (EVIDENCE) During Forty-Eight Weeks

System Organ Class/Preferred Term	REBIF 44 μg TIW Subjects (n=339)
Back pain	8.8%
Myalgia	8.8%
Pain in extremity	3.8%
Musculoskeletal stiffness	3.5%
Muscle spasms	2.9%
Musculoskeletal pain	2.4%
Neck pain	1.8%
Tendonitis	1.5%
Arthritis	1.2%
Psychiatric Disorders	
Depression	15.9%
Insomnia	14.2%
Anxiety	3.5%
Mood swings	1.5%
Affect lability	1.2%
Depressed mood	1.2%
Irritability	1.2%
Nervousness	1.2%
Sleep disorder	1.2%
Investigations	
Alanine aminotransferase increased	12.1%
Aspartate aminotransferase increased	7.7%
Hepatic enzyme increased	3.8%
White blood cell count decreased	3.8%
Blood creatine phosphokinase increased	3.2%
Lymphocyte count decreased	2.4%
Neutrophil count decreased	2.4%
Weight decreased	2.4%
Blood pressure increased	1.5%
Thyroxine increased	1.5%
Weight increased	1.5%
Blood alkaline phosphatase increased	1.2%
Blood calcium decreased	1.2%
Red blood cell count decreased	1.2%
Gastrointestinal Disorders	
Nausea	10.3%
Diarrhoea	5.9%
Constipation	5.0%
Abdominal pain upper	4.4%
Abdominal pain	2.7%
Vomiting	2.7%
Toothache	1.8%
Dyspepsia	1.5%
Faecal incontinence	1.2%
Gastroesophageal reflux disease	1.2%
Stomach discomfort	1.2%
Skin and Subcutaneous Tissue Disorders	

(cont'd)

Table 9: REBIF *(cont'd)*

Adverse Events[a] Experienced by at Least 1% of the REBIF-Treated Patients Enrolled in Study 21125 (EVIDENCE) During Forty-Eight Weeks

System Organ Class/Preferred Term	REBIF 44 μg TIW Subjects (n=339)
Rash	4.1%
Pruritus	3.2%
Alopecia	2.4%
Dry skin	1.8%
Hyperhidrosis	1.2%
Night sweats	1.2%
Rash pruritic	1.2%
Respiratory, Thoracic and Mediastinal Disorders	
Pharyngolaryngeal pain	5.0%
Cough	4.4%
Nasal congestion	2.7%
Sinus congestion	2.7%
Dyspnoea	2.1%
Epistaxis	1.8%
Injury, Poisoning and Procedural Complications	
Traumatic haematoma	4.4%
Joint sprain	1.8%
Laceration	1.2%
Reproductive System and Breast Disorders	
Dysmenorrhoea	2.7%
Menstruation irregular	2.7%
Menorrhagia	1.5%
Amenorrhoea	1.2%
Metrorrhagia	1.2%
Eye Disorders	
Eye pain	2.4%
Vision blurred	2.1%
Conjunctivitis	1.5%
Blood and Lymphatic System Disorders	
Lymphadenopathy	2.7%
Leukopenia	2.4%
Anaemia	2.1%
Lymphopenia	1.5%
Renal and Urinary Disorders	
Micturition urgency	1.5%
Urinary incontinence	1.5%
Pollakiuria	1.2%
Ear and Labyrinth Disorders	
Vertigo	1.8%
Tinnitus	1.2%
Vascular Disorders	
Hypertension	2.7%
Hot flush	1.5%
Cardiac Disorders	
Palpitations	1.8%
Metabolism and Nutrition Disorders	

(cont'd)

Table 9: REBIF *(cont'd)*

Adverse Events[a] Experienced by at Least 1% of the REBIF-Treated Patients Enrolled in Study 21125 (EVIDENCE) During Forty-Eight Weeks

System Organ Class/Preferred Term	REBIF 44 µg TIW Subjects (n=339)
Anorexia	1.2%

[a] Treatment Emergent Adverse Events.

In addition to the above listed adverse events, the following events have been experienced less frequently (i.e. in less than 1% of the study population) during the 48 weeks of treatment. See Table 10.

Table 10: REBIF

Adverse Events[a] Experienced by Less than 1% of the REBIF-Treated Patients Enrolled in Study 21125 (EVIDENCE) During Forty-Eight Weeks

System Organ Class	Preferred Term
General Disorders and Administration Site Conditions	Chest discomfort
	Injection site discolouration
	Injection site rash
	Injection site swelling
	Nodule
	Feeling hot
	Injection site vesicles
	Temperature intolerance
	Thirst
	Circadian rhythm sleep disorder
	Cyst
	Difficulty in walking
	Drug withdrawal syndrome
	Facial pain
	Feeling jittery
	Hernia
	Injection site induration
	Injection site necrosis
	Injection site photosensitivity reaction
	Injection site ulcer
	Oedema peripheral
Infections and Infestations	Fungal infection
	Onychomycosis
	Vaginal mycosis
	Abscess limb
	Cystitis
	Dental caries
	Nasopharyngitis
	Paronychia
	Pharyngitis streptococcal
	Pneumonia
	Abscess
	Bacterial infection
	Bacteriuria
	Fungal skin infection
	Gastrointestinal fungal infection
	Herpes zoster
	Infection parasitic
	Injection site cellulitis
	Laryngitis

(cont'd)

Table 10: REBIF *(cont'd)*

Adverse Events[a] Experienced by Less than 1% of the REBIF-Treated Patients Enrolled in Study 21125 (EVIDENCE) During Forty-Eight Weeks

System Organ Class	Preferred Term
	Malaria
	Postoperative infection
	Skin candida
	Skin infection
	Tinea infection
	Tonsillitis
	Tooth infection
	Wound infection
Nervous System Disorders	Coordination abnormal
	Dysgeusia
	Neuralgia
	Restless legs syndrome
	Amnesia
	Carpal tunnel syndrome
	Cognitive disorder
	Disturbance in attention
	Hyperaesthesia
	Multiple sclerosis
	Sciatica
	Somnolence
	Syncope
	Aphasia
	Burning sensation
	Dizziness postural
	Dyskinesia
	Dystonia
	Head discomfort
	Lethargy
	Muscle contractions involuntary
	Myoclonus
	Sensory disturbance
	Syncope vasovagal
Musculoskeletal and Connective Tissue Disorders	Muscle twitching
	Sensation of heaviness
	Arthropathy
	Bone pain
	Bursitis
	Intervertebral disc disorder
	Joint stiffness
	Bone disorder
	Costochondritis
	Flank pain
	Ganglion
	Joint effusion
	Osteoporosis
	Pain in jaw

(cont'd)

Table 10: REBIF *(cont'd)*

Adverse Events[a] Experienced by Less than 1% of the REBIF-Treated Patients Enrolled in Study 21125 (EVIDENCE) During Forty-Eight Weeks

System Organ Class	Preferred Term
	Periarthritis
	Spinal osteoarthritis
	Torticollis
Psychiatric Disorders	Apathy
	Confusional state
	Suicidal ideation
	Anxiety disorder
	Libido decreased
	Nightmare
	Suicide attempt
	Tension
Investigations	Anti-thyroid antibody
	Blood glucose increased
	Blood thyroid stimulating hormone decreased
	Blood urine present
	Blood albumin increased
	Blood thyroid stimulating hormone increased
	Glucose urine
	Haematocrit decreased
	Haemoglobin decreased
	Neutrophil count
	Thyroid function test abnormal
	Tri-iodothyronine increased
	Blood iron decreased
	Blood phosphorus decreased
	Blood potassium increased
	Lymphocyte count abnormal
	Monocyte count increased
	Neutrophil count increased
	Platelet count decreased
	Platelet count increased
	Protein total increased
	Thyroxine decreased
	White blood cell count
	White blood cell count increased
Gastrointestinal Disorders	Dry mouth
	Mouth ulceration
	Abdominal distension
	Abdominal pain lower
	Dysphagia
	Gastritis
	Abdominal tenderness
	Anorectal disorder
	Aphthous stomatitis
	Change of bowel habit
	Colitis
	Colonic polyp

(cont'd)

Table 10: REBIF *(cont'd)*

Adverse Events[a] Experienced by Less than 1% of the REBIF-Treated Patients Enrolled in Study 21125 (EVIDENCE) During Forty-Eight Weeks

System Organ Class	Preferred Term
	Diverticulum
	Enteritis
	Flatulence
	Gingivitis
	Halitosis
	Irritable bowel syndrome
	Oesophagitis
	Oral pain
	Salivary hypersecretion
	Stomatitis
	Tongue discolouration
	Tooth disorder
Skin and Subcutaneous Tissue Disorders	Acne
	Rash erythematous
	Dermatitis allergic
	Livedo reticularis
	Rash maculo-papular
	Skin disorder
	Urticaria
	Alopecia areata
	Blister
	Cold sweat
	Dermatitis
	Dermatitis bullous
	Dermatitis contact
	Eczema
	Ephelides
	Erythema
	Exanthem
	Hypotrichosis
	Nail disorder
	Onychorrhexis
	Palmar erythema
	Photosensitivity allergic reaction
	Pruritus allergic
	Rash scaly
	Rash vesicular
	Rosacea
	Skin discolouration
	Skin nodule
Respiratory, Thoracic and Mediastinal Disorders	Rhinitis allergic
	Rhinorrhoea
	Asthma
	Dysphonia
	Postnasal drip
	Rales
	Wheezing

(cont'd)

Table 10: REBIF *(cont'd)*

Adverse Events[a] Experienced by Less than 1% of the REBIF-Treated Patients Enrolled in Study 21125 (EVIDENCE) During Forty-Eight Weeks

System Organ Class	Preferred Term
	Breath sounds decreased
	Nasal discomfort
	Nasopharyngeal disorder
	Pleurisy
	Productive cough
	Rhinitis seasonal
	Rhonchi
Injury, Poisoning and Procedural Complications	Arthropod bite
	Excoriation
	Fall
	Pain trauma activated
	Animal bite
	Joint dislocation
	Joint injury
	Post procedural pain
	Tooth injury
	Accident
	Anaemia postoperative
	Ankle fracture
	Arthropod sting
	Foot fracture
	Hand fracture
	Injury
	Limb injury
	Muscle injury
	Muscle strain
	Nerve injury
	Post procedural complication
	Sunburn
	Thermal burn
Reproductive System and Breast Disorders	Breast mass
	Sexual dysfunction
	Breast pain
	Endometriosis
	Genital disorder female
	Oligomenorrhoea
	Ovarian cyst
	Pelvic pain
	Pruritus genital
	Scrotal pain
	Vaginal discharge
	Vaginal prolapse
	Vulvovaginal discomfort
Eye Disorders	Photopsia
	Visual disturbance
	Diplopia
	Dry eye

(cont'd)

Table 10: REBIF *(cont'd)*

Adverse Events[a] Experienced by Less than 1% of the REBIF-Treated Patients Enrolled in Study 21125 (EVIDENCE) During Forty-Eight Weeks

System Organ Class	Preferred Term
	Eye disorder
	Vitreous floaters
	Accommodation disorder
	Conjunctivitis allergic
	Eye irritation
	Ocular hyperaemia
	Optic atrophy
	Visual acuity reduced
Blood and Lymphatic System Disorders	Neutropenia
	Bone marrow depression
	Lymphadenitis
	Microcytic anaemia
	Monocytosis
Renal and Urinary Disorders	Glycosuria
	Dysuria
	Nocturia
	Urine odour abnormal
	Bladder disorder
	Ketonuria
	Proteinuria
	Renal colic
	Stress incontinence
	Urinary retention
	Urinary tract disorder
Ear and Labyrinth Disorders	Ear disorder
	Ear pain
	Meniere's disease
	Motion sickness
	Vertigo positional
Vascular Disorders	Flushing
	Haematoma
	Phlebitis
	Varicose vein
Cardiac Disorders	Tachycardia
	Arrhythmia
	Bundle branch block right
	Supraventricular tachycardia
Metabolism and Nutrition Disorders	Hypokalaemia
	Diabetes mellitus
	Hypercholesterolaemia
	Hypertriglyceridaemia
	Hypocalcaemia
	Hypoglycaemia
	Increased appetite
	Ketoacidosis

(cont'd)

Table 10: REBIF *(cont'd)*

Adverse Events[a] Experienced by Less than 1% of the REBIF-Treated Patients Enrolled in Study 21125 (EVIDENCE) During Forty-Eight Weeks

System Organ Class	Preferred Term
Neoplasms Benign, Malignant and Unspecified (incl cysts and polyps)	Thyroid neoplasm
	Basal cell carcinoma
	Breast cancer
	Breast neoplasm
	Fibroadenoma of breast
	Uterine leiomyoma
Immune System Disorders	Hypersensitivity
	Seasonal allergy
Hepatobiliary Disorders	Hepatitis
	Cholecystitis
	Hepatocellular damage
Endocrine Disorders	Hypothyroidism
	Goitre
Congenital, Familial and Genetic Disorders	Colour blindness
Pregnancy, Puerperium and Perinatal Conditions	Abortion spontaneous

[a] Treatment Emergent Adverse Events.

Clinical Trials: Summary of Adverse Reactions: Studies with REBIF have included patients with Relapsing Remitting Multiple Sclerosis and secondary progressive forms of MS, disability ranging from none to severe, and age ranging from 18 to 60 at study start.

Post-Market Adverse Drug Reactions: The vast majority of the adverse reactions of REBIF in multiple sclerosis have been identified from the clinical trials and are summarized in the above placebo-controlled study tables. The adverse reactions reported with marketed use of REBIF that are not already mentioned in the clinical study tables are shown below. These reactions have been identified during post-marketing surveillance and their exact frequency is unknown.

General Disorders and Administration Site Conditions: injection site necrosis.
Infections and Infestations: injection site infections, including cellulitis which could be severe and injection site abscesses.
Immune System Disorders: anaphylactic reaction.
Psychiatric Disorders: suicide attempt.
Nervous System Disorders: seizures, transient neurological symptoms (i.e. hypoesthesia, muscle spasm, paresthesia, difficulty in walking, musculoskeletal stiffness) that may mimic multiple sclerosis exacerbations.
Vascular Disorders: thromboembolic events.
Blood and Lymphatic System Disorders: thrombotic thrombocytopenic purpura, haemolytic uraemic syndrome.
Eye Disorders: retinal vascular disorders (i.e. retinopathy, cotton wool spots, obstruction of retinal artery or vein).
Hepatobiliary Disorders: hepatitis with or without icterus.
Skin and Subcutaneous Tissue Disorders: angioedema (Quincke's edema), urticaria, erythema multiforme, erythema multiforme-like skin reactions, hair loss, Stevens-Johnson Syndrome.

DRUG INTERACTIONS: No formal drug interaction studies have been conducted with REBIF in humans. Interferons have been reported to reduce the activity of hepatic cytochrome P450-dependent enzymes in humans and animals. Caution should be exercised when administering REBIF in combination with medicinal products that have a narrow therapeutic index and are largely dependent on the hepatic cytochrome P450 system for clearance, e.g. antiepileptics and some classes of antidepressants. The interaction of REBIF with corticosteroids or ACTH has not been studied systematically. Clinical studies indicate that multiple sclerosis patients can receive REBIF and corticosteroids or ACTH during relapses. REBIF should not be mixed with other drugs in the same syringe.

DOSAGE AND ADMINISTRATION: Relapsing Forms of Multiple Sclerosis: Before initiating a patient on REBIF therapy, please review completely the Contraindications.

Recommended Dose and Dosage Adjustment: The recommended dose is 44 µg given 3 times per week by subcutaneous injection. The dose can be reduced to 22 µg tiw if the patient is not able to tolerate the higher dose.

Treatment should be initiated under supervision of a physician experienced in the treatment of the disease. When first starting treatment with REBIF, in order to allow tachyphylaxis to develop thus reducing adverse events, it is recommended that 20% of the total dose be administered during the initial 2 weeks of therapy, 50% of total dose be administered in week 3 and 4, and the full dose from the fifth week onwards.

Please also review the Warnings and Precautions section and ensure appropriate monitoring of patients with depression, hepatic dysfunction, a history of seizures, cardiac disease, renal dysfunction, thyroid dysfunction, myelosuppression, and female patients of child-bearing potential.

At the present time, it is not known for how long patients should be treated. Safety and efficacy with REBIF have been demonstrated following 4 years of treatment. Therefore, it is recommended that patients should be evaluated after 4 years of treatment with REBIF and a decision for longer-term treatment be made on an individual basis by the treating physician.

Missed Dose: Should a dose be missed, the patient should be advised to continue to inject from the day of the next scheduled dose. The patient should not take a double dose to make up for the missed dose.

Administration: Patients should be advised of REBIF side-effects and instructed on the use of aseptic technique when administering REBIF. The REBIF Patient Leaflet should be carefully reviewed with all patients, and patients should be educated on self-care and advised to keep the Leaflet for continued reference during REBIF therapy.

Preparation of Solution: Liquid formulation in a Pre-filled Syringe: The liquid formulation in a pre-filled syringe is ready for use. These syringes are graduated to facilitate therapy initiation. The pre-filled syringes contain 8.8 µg, 22 µg and 44 µg of REBIF New HSA-free Formulation respectively. The pre-filled syringes are ready for subcutaneous use only.

Preparation of Solution: Liquid formulation in a Pre-filled Cartridge: The liquid formulation in a pre-filled cartridge is ready for use with the RebiSmart autoinjection device. For administration, follow the instructions given in the package leaflet and in the instructions manual which is provided with each RebiSmart autoinjection device. The pre-filled cartridge that contains 66 µg/1.5 mL is designed to deliver three doses of 22 µg/0.5 mL and the pre-filled cartridge that contains 132 µg/1.5 mL is designed to deliver three doses of 44 µg/0.5 mL of REBIF. The pre-filled cartridges are for subcutaneous use only.

OVERDOSAGE:

One medically-confirmed case of REBIF overdose has been reported in over 450 000 patient-years of exposure to REBIF, and concerned a subject who injected himself with seven syringes of REBIF 44 µg (total dose of 308 µg) in a suicide attempt. Symptoms included a modest rise in body temperature (to 37.5°C), diffuse erythema of the limbs and abdomen with rigors. The subject was treated with 500 mg of acetyl-salicylic acid dl-lysine intravenously, and haematologic screening revealed no abnormalities of hepatic function, thyroid function, or indices of inflammation. The event was not considered serious. There is no known antidote for an overdose of REBIF. The subject should be hospitalised for observation and appropriate supportive treatment administered.

For management of a suspected drug overdose, CPhA recommends that you contact your **regional Poison Control Centre**. See the *CPS* Directory section for a list of Poison Control Centres.

ACTION AND CLINICAL PHARMACOLOGY: REBIF (Interferon beta-1a) is a purified, sterile glycoprotein product produced by recombinant DNA techniques and formulated for use by injection. The active ingredient of REBIF is produced by genetically engineered Chinese Hamster Ovary (CHO) cells. Interferon beta-1a is a highly purified glycoprotein that has 166 amino acids and an approximate molecular weight of 22 500 daltons. It contains a single N-linked carbohydrate moiety attached to Asn-80 similar to that of natural human Interferon beta.

The specific activity of REBIF is approximately 0.27 million international units (MIU)/µg Interferon beta-1a. The unit measurement is derived by comparing the antiviral activity of the product to an in-house natural hIFN-β NIH standard that is obtained from human fibroblasts (BILS 11), which has been calibrated against the NIH natural hIFN-β standard (GB 23-902-531).

General: Interferons are a family of naturally occurring proteins, which have molecular weights ranging from 15 000 to 21 000 daltons. Three major classes of interferons have been identified: alpha, beta, gamma. Interferon beta, Interferon alpha and Interferon gamma have overlapping yet distinct biologic activities.

Mechanism of Action: Interferon beta-1a acts through various mechanisms:

- Immunomodulation through an induction of cell membrane components of the major histocompatibility complex i.e., MHC Class I antigens, an increase in natural killer (NK) cell activity, and an inhibition of IFN-γ induced MHC Class II antigen expression, as well as a sustained reduction in TNF level.
- Antiviral effect through the induction of proteins like 2'-5' oligoadenylate synthetase and p78.
- Antiproliferative effect through direct cytostatic activity and indirect through antitumoral immune response enhancement.

The mechanism of action of REBIF in relapsing forms of multiple sclerosis is still under investigation.

STORAGE AND STABILITY: Refer to the date indicated on the labels for the expiry date. REBIF New HSA-free Formulation liquid in a pre-filled syringe or pre-filled cartridge should be stored at 2-8°C. REBIF New HSA-free Formulation in pre-filled syringes or in pre-filled cartridges may be stored for a limited period at room temperature (up to 25°C), but not more than 1 month. Do not freeze.

SPECIAL HANDLING INSTRUCTIONS: The liquid in the pre-filled syringe is ready for use.

The liquid in the pre-filled cartridge is ready for use with the RebiSmart autoinjection device. The RebiSmart autoinjection device should be stored in the device storage box when stored with a REBIF pre-filled cartridge.

INFORMATION FOR THE PATIENT: Published in e-CPS, available by subscription at www.e-cps.ca.

DOSAGE FORMS, COMPOSITION AND PACKAGING: Pre-filled Syringes: Each pre-filled syringe with 0.5 mL of solution contains: interferon beta-1a 22 µg or 44 µg. Nonmedicinal ingredients: benzyl alcohol, mannitol, methionine, poloxamer-188 and sodium acetate buffer. Packs of 3. The pre-filled syringes are for subcutaneous use only.

Initiation packs are available for the initial 4 weeks of treatment (see Dosage and Administration). The initiation pack contains six syringes of 8.8 µg/0.2 mL and six syringes of 22 µg/0.5 mL.

Pre-filled Cartridges: Each pre-filled cartridge of 1.5 mL of solution contains: interferon beta-1a 66 µg or 132 µg. Nonmedicinal ingredients: benzyl alcohol, mannitol, methionine, poloxamer-188 and sodium acetate buffer. The pre-filled cartridge that contains 66 µg/1.5 mL is designed to deliver three doses of 22 µg/0.5 mL and the pre-filled cartridge that contains 132 µg/1.5 mL is designed to deliver three doses of 44 µg/0.5 mL of REBIF. Boxes of 4. The pre-filled cartridge is ready for use with the RebiSmart autoinjection device for subcutaneous administration only.

Initiation packs are available for the initial 4 weeks of treatment (see Dosage and Administration). The initiation pack for the recommended therapeutic dose of 44 µg contains two cartridges of 132 µg/1.5 mL. The cartridges provided in the initiation pack will be injected with the RebiSmart autoinjection device. The RebiSmart autoinjection device is programmed to deliver 20% of the total dose during the initial 2 weeks of therapy (6 injections in total) and 50% of the total dose in the week 3 and 4 (6 injections in total).

The route of administration for Relapsing forms of Multiple Sclerosis is subcutaneous.

(Shown in Product Identification Section)

Recombivax HB®

hepatitis B vaccine (recombinant)

Vaccine

Merck Frosst

Date of Revision: March 23, 2009

SUMMARY PRODUCT INFORMATION:

Route of Administration	Dosage Form/ Strength	Clinically Relevant Nonmedicinal Ingredients
Intramuscular injection	Suspension for injection Pediatric: single-dose vial containing 5 µg hepatitis B surface antigen (HBsAg)/0.5 mL dose Adult: single-dose and multi-dose vials containing 10 µg HBsAg/1 mL dose Adult dialysis: single-dose vial containing 40 µg HBsAg/1 mL dose	Aluminum hydroxyphosphate, thimerosal (adult multi-dose vial only) For a complete listing see Dosage Forms, Composition and Packaging.

DESCRIPTION: RECOMBIVAX HB (hepatitis B vaccine [recombinant]) is a non-infectious subunit viral vaccine consisting of surface antigen (HBsAg or Australia antigen) of hepatitis B virus produced in yeast cells. A portion of the hepatitis B virus gene, coding for HBsAg, is cloned into yeast and the vaccine for hepatitis B is produced from cultures of this recombinant yeast strain according to methods developed in the Merck Research Laboratories.

INDICATIONS AND CLINICAL USE: RECOMBIVAX HB (hepatitis B vaccine [recombinant]) is indicated for immunization against infection caused by all known subtypes of hepatitis B virus.

RECOMBIVAX HB will not prevent hepatitis caused by other agents, such as hepatitis A virus, non-A, non-B hepatitis viruses, or other viruses known to infect the liver.

Vaccination with RECOMBIVAX HB is recommended in persons of all ages, especially those who are or will be at increased risk of infection with hepatitis B virus. In areas with low prevalence like Canada, universal immunization before adolescence is recommended. Special efforts should also target the high-risk populations.

A. **Infants Born to HBsAg-Positive Mothers**
B. **Children <7 years of age whose families have immigrated** to Canada from areas where there is a high prevalence of hepatitis B, and who are exposed to hepatitis B virus carriers through their extended families.
C. **Adolescents**
D. **Health-Care Personnel:** Dentists and oral surgeons. Physicians and surgeons. Nurses. Paramedical personnel and custodial staff who may be exposed to the virus via blood or other patient specimens (i.e., body fluids and tissues). Dental hygienists and dental nurses. Laboratory personnel handling blood, blood products and other patient specimens (i.e., body fluids and tissues). Dental, medical and nursing students, preferably soon after acceptance in the university.
E. **Selected Patients and Patient Contacts:** Patients and staff in hemodialysis units and hematology/oncology units. Patients requiring frequent and/or large-volume blood transfusions or clotting factor concentrates (e.g., persons with hemophilia, thalassemia). Patients (residents) and staff of institutions for the mentally handicapped. Classroom contacts of deinstitutionalized mentally handicapped persons who have persistent hepatitis B antigenemia and who show aggressive behavior. Household and other intimate contacts of persons with persistent hepatitis B antigenemia. Children in child-care settings in which there is a hepatitis B virus-infected child. These children should receive serious consideration for immunization against hepatitis B virus.
F. **Travellers to Hepatitis B Endemic Areas**
G. **Military Personnel Identified as Being at Increased Risk**
H. **Emergency Service Workers (police, firefighters)**
I. **Morticians and Embalmers**

J. **Blood Bank and Plasma Fractionation Workers**
K. **Persons at Increased Risk of the Disease Due to Their Sexual Practices** such as: persons who have heterosexual activity with multiple partners; persons who repeatedly contract sexually transmitted diseases; homosexually active males; female prostitutes.
L. **Prisoners**
M. **Users of Illicit Injectable Drugs**

CONTRAINDICATIONS: Patients who are hypersensitive to this drug or to any ingredient in the formulation or component of the container. For a complete listing, see Dosage Forms, Composition and Packaging.

WARNINGS AND PRECAUTIONS: Because of the long incubation period for hepatitis B, it is possible for unrecognized infection to be present at the time RECOMBIVAX HB (hepatitis B vaccine [recombinant]) is given. RECOMBIVAX HB may not prevent hepatitis B in such patients.

Patients who develop symptoms suggestive of hypersensitivity after an injection should not receive further injections of RECOMBIVAX HB (see Contraindications).

General: Persons with immunodeficiency or those receiving immunosuppressive therapy require larger vaccine doses and respond less well than healthy individuals.

As with any parenteral vaccine, epinephrine should be available for immediate use should an anaphylactoid reaction occur.

Any serious active infection is reason for delaying use of RECOMBIVAX HB, except when, in the opinion of the physician, withholding the vaccine entails a greater risk.

Caution and appropriate care should be exercised in administering RECOMBIVAX HB to individuals with severely compromised cardiopulmonary status or to others in whom a febrile or systemic reaction could pose a significant risk.

Special Populations: Pregnant Women: Animal reproduction studies have not been conducted with RECOMBIVAX HB. It is also not known whether RECOMBIVAX HB can cause fetal harm when administered to a pregnant woman or can affect reproductive capacity. RECOMBIVAX HB should be given to a pregnant woman only if clearly needed.

Nursing Women: It is not known whether RECOMBIVAX HB is excreted in human milk. However, studies with RECOMBIVAX HB in 12 lactating women have failed to reveal evidence of this vaccine being secreted.

Pediatrics: RECOMBIVAX HB has been shown to be generally well-tolerated and highly immunogenic in infants and children of all ages. Newborns have responded well; maternally transferred antibodies did not interfere with the active immune response to the vaccine. See Dosage and Administration for recommended pediatric dosage and recommended dosage for infants born to HBsAg-positive mothers. The safety profile and effectiveness of the dialysis formulation in children have not been established.

ADVERSE REACTIONS: Adverse Drug Reaction Overview: RECOMBIVAX HB (hepatitis B vaccine [recombinant]) is generally well-tolerated. No adverse reactions were reported during clinical trials which could be related to changes in the titers of antibodies to yeast. As with any vaccine, there is the possibility that broad use of the vaccine could reveal rare adverse reactions not observed in clinical trials.

Clinical Trial Adverse Drug Reactions: Because clinical trials are conducted under very specific conditions the adverse reaction rates observed in the clinical trials may not reflect the rates observed in practice and should not be compared to the rates in the clinical trials of another vaccine. Adverse drug reaction information from clinical trials is useful for identifying vaccine-related adverse events and for approximating rates.

In a group of studies, 3258 doses of RECOMBIVAX HB, 10 µg, were administered to 1252 healthy adults. Vaccine recipients were monitored for 5 days after each dose, and the following adverse reactions were reported:

Incidence Equal to or Greater Than 10% of Injections: Local Reactions at Injection Site: Injection site reactions (consisting principally of local pain, soreness and tenderness and including pruritus, erythema, ecchymoses, swelling, warmth and nodule formation).

Incidence Equal to or Greater Than 1% and Less Than 10% of Injections: Body as a Whole: fatigue/asthenia, malaise, fever ≥38°C.

Digestive System: nausea, diarrhea.
Nervous System: headache.
Respiratory System: pharyngitis, upper respiratory infection (NOS).
Incidence Less Than 1% of Injections: Body as a Whole: sweating, chills, flushing, aching, sensation of warmth.
Integumentary System: pruritus, rash, urticaria, angioedema.
Digestive System: vomiting, abdominal pains/cramps, dyspepsia, diminished appetite.
Musculoskeletal System: myalgia, arthralgia, back pain, neck pain, shoulder pain, neck stiffness.
Nervous System: lightheadedness, vertigo/dizziness, paresthesia.
Respiratory System: rhinitis, cough, influenza.
Special Senses: earache.
Hemic/Lymphatic System: lymphadenopathy.
Psychiatric/Behavioral: insomnia/disturbed sleep.
Urogenital System: dysuria.
Cardiovascular System: hypotension.

In a study that compared the three-dose regimen (5 µg) with the two-dose regimen (10 µg) of RECOMBIVAX HB in adolescents, the overall frequency of adverse reactions was generally similar.

Post-Market Adverse Drug Reactions: The following additional adverse reactions have been reported with use of the marketed vaccine; however, in many instances a causal relationship to the vaccine has not been established.

Hematologic: increased erythrocyte sedimentation rate.
Hypersensitivity: Anaphylaxis and symptoms of immediate hypersensitivity reactions including edema, dyspnea, chest discomfort, bronchial spasm, or palpitation have been reported within the first few hours after vaccination. An apparent hypersensitivity syndrome (serum-sickness-like) of delayed onset has been reported days to weeks after vaccination, including: arthritis (usually transient), and dermatologic reactions such as erythema multiforme, ecchymoses and erythema nodosum (see Warnings and Precautions).
Immune System: vasculitis, polyarteritis nodosa.
Integumentary System: alopecia, eczema.
Musculoskeletal System: arthritis, pain in extremity.
Nervous System: peripheral neuropathy including Bell's Palsy, Guillain-Barré syndrome, exacerbation of multiple sclerosis, multiple sclerosis, optic neuritis, seizure, febrile seizure, encephalitis, vasovagal syncope.
Special Senses: tinnitus.

DRUG INTERACTIONS: Use With Other Vaccines: According to the National Advisory Committee on Immunization (NACI), RECOMBIVAX HB (hepatitis B vaccine [recombinant]) may be administered simultaneously with other vaccines at different sites. A separate needle and syringe should be used for each vaccine.

The safety and immunogenicity of co-administration of RECOMBIVAX HB with GARDASIL (quadrivalent human papillomavirus [types 6, 11, 16, 18] recombinant vaccine) (same visit, injections at separate sites) were evaluated in a randomized study of 1871 women aged 16 to 24 years at enrolment. Immune response and safety profile to both RECOMBIVAX HB and GARDASIL were similar whether they were administered at the same visit or at a different visit.

Results from published clinical studies indicate that RECOMBIVAX HB can be administered concomitantly with DTaP-IPV-Hib (diphtheria, tetanus, acellular pertussis, inactivated poliomyelitis, and *H. influenzae* type b conjugate vaccine), or M-M-R II (measles, mumps and rubella virus vaccine, live, attenuated, Merck Frosst Std.), using separate syringes and injection sites for each vaccine. No impairment of immune response to individually tested vaccine antigens was seen in these studies.

In addition, an HBsAg-containing product, COMVAX (Haemophilus b conjugate vaccine [meningococcal protein conjugate] and hepatitis B [recombinant] vaccine) was given concomitantly with M-M-R II and VARIVAX III (varicella virus vaccine, live, attenuated [Oka/Merck]), using separate syringes and injection sites for each vaccine. No impairment of immune response to these individually tested vaccine antigens was demonstrated.

Another randomized study conducted in 1993 with COMVAX, administered concurrently with routine pediatric vaccines (DTP, OPV/IPV, M-M-R II, booster dose of DTaP) in 94 infants who completed the study, showed an acceptable response rate for most antigens but a lower response than pre-specified to polio antigens type 1 and type 3, pertussis antigens and rubella. However, the assays, endpoints and time points used differ from currently used criteria. The response to polio was assessed on sera at week-12 (instead of week-4) post-dose 2 and not after the third dose.

DOSAGE AND ADMINISTRATION: Recommended Dose and Dosage Adjustment: Three-Dose Regimen: The vaccination regimen consists of three doses of vaccine given according to the following schedule:
First injection: at elected date.
Second injection: ≥1 month after first injection.
Third injection: ≥1 month after second injection.

Within limits, the timing of successive injections may be adjusted to accommodate a variety of needs, such as coadministration with other vaccines.

For infants born of mothers who are HbsAg positive or mothers of unknown HBsAg status, treatment recommendations are described in Dosage for Infants Born to HBsAg-positive Mothers.

A minimum of one month should separate successive injections of vaccine. Accelerated three-dose regimens (e.g., 0, 1, 2 months; 0, 2, 4 months) may induce protective antibody earlier in a slightly larger proportion of vaccinees. However, regimens that extend the time interval between the second and third injections (e.g., 0, 1, 6 months; 0, 1, 12 months) will ultimately seroconvert a similar proportion of vaccinees while inducing substantially higher antibody titers than accelerated regimens.

The dose of vaccine to be given on each occasion is as follows: see Table 1.

Table 1: RECOMBIVAX HB

Three-dose Regimen

Group	Regimen
Infants[a]/children (birth to 10 years of age)	3×2.5 µg
Adolescents (11–19 years of age)	3×5 µg
Adults (≥20 years)	3×10 µg

[a] Infants born of HBsAg-negative mothers.

Two-Dose Regimen: Adolescents (11 to 15 years of age).

An alternate two-dose regimen is available for routine vaccination of adolescents (11 to 15 years of age). The regimen consists of two doses of vaccine (10 µg) given according to the following schedule:
1st dose: at elected date.
2nd dose: 4 to 6 months after the first dose.
See Table 2.

Table 2: RECOMBIVAX HB

Two-dose Regimen

Group	Initial	4–6 Months
Adolescents[a] (11–15 years of age)	10 µg	10 µg

[a] Adolescents (11 to 15 years of age) may receive either regimen, the 3×5 µg or the 2×10 µg (see Dosage and Administration, Three-Dose Regimen and Two-Dose Regimen).

RECOMBIVAX HB Dialysis 40 µg/mL Formulation: RECOMBIVAX HB dialysis formulation (40 µg/mL) is intended only for adult predialysis/dialysis patients.

The recommended vaccination regimen for predialysis/dialysis patients is as follows: see Table 3.

Table 3: RECOMBIVAX HB

Recommended Vaccination Regimen for Predialysis/Dialysis Patients

Group	Initial	1 Month	6 Months
Predialysis/dialysis Adult dialysis presentation 40 µg/1 mL	40 µg	40 µg	40 µg

RECOMBIVAX HB Preservative-free (thimerosal-free) Formulations: RECOMBIVAX HB Preservative-free formulations are available for use in individuals for whom a thimerosal-free vaccine may be desired. These formulations are intended for single-use only.

Revaccination of Nonresponders: When persons who do not respond (anti-HBs <10 IU/L) to the primary vaccine series are revaccinated, 15-25% produce an adequate antibody response after one additional dose and 30-50% after three additional doses. However, because data are insufficient concerning the safety of hepatitis B vaccine when additional doses in excess of the recommended two- or three-dose series are administered, revaccination following completion of the primary series is not routinely recommended. Revaccination should only be considered for high-risk individuals, after weighing the benefits of vaccination against the potential risk of experiencing increased local or systemic adverse reactions.

Dosage for Infants Born to HBsAg-positive Mothers: Infants born to HBsAg-positive mothers are at high risk of becoming chronic carriers of hepatitis B virus and of developing the chronic sequelae of hepatitis B virus infection. Well-controlled studies have shown that administration of three 0.5 mL doses of hepatitis B immune globulin starting at birth is 75% effective in preventing establishment of the chronic carrier state in these infants during the first year of life. Protection is transient under these circumstances and the effectiveness of the passively administered hepatitis B immune globulin declines thereafter. Results from clinical studies indicate that administration of one 0.5 mL dose of hepatitis B immune globulin at birth and three 5 µg (0.5 mL) doses of RECOMBIVAX HB, the first dose given within one week after birth, was 96% effective in preventing establishment of the chronic carrier state in infants born to HBsAg- and HBeAg-positive mothers. Testing for HBsAg and anti-HBs is recommended at 12-15 months to monitor the final success or failure of therapy. If HBsAg is not detectable, and anti-HBs is present, the child has been protected.

The recommended dosage for infants born to HBsAg-positive mothers is as follows: see Table 4.

Table 4: RECOMBIVAX HB

Recommended Dosage for Infants Born to HBsAg-positive Mothers

Treatment	Birth	1 Month	6 Months
RECOMBIVAX HB	5 µg[a]	5 µg	5 µg
Hepatitis B immune globulin	0.5 mL		

[a] The first dose of RECOMBIVAX HB (5 µg) may be given at birth at the same time as hepatitis B immune globulin, but should be administered in the opposite anterolateral thigh. This procedure may be preferable to ensure absorption of the vaccine.

Acute Exposure to Blood Containing HBsAg: There are no prospective studies directly testing the efficacy of a combination of hepatitis B immune globulin and RECOMBIVAX HB in preventing clinical hepatitis B following percutaneous, ocular or mucous membrane exposure to hepatitis B virus. However, recent studies have established the relative efficacies of immune globulins and/or hepatitis B vaccine in various exposure situations. Since most persons with such exposures (e.g., health-care workers) are candidates for the hepatitis B vaccine and since combined hepatitis B immune globulin plus vaccine is more efficacious than hepatitis B immune globulin alone in perinatal exposures, the following guidelines are recommended for persons who have been exposed to hepatitis B virus such as through (1) percutaneous (needlestick), ocular, mucous membrane exposure to blood known or presumed to contain HBsAg, (2) human bites by known or presumed HBsAg carriers, that penetrate the skin, or (3) following intimate sexual contact with known or presumed HBsAg carriers.

Hepatitis B immune globulin (0.06 mL/kg) should be given as soon as possible after exposure and within 24 hours if possible. Hepatitis B vaccine should be given intramuscularly within 7 days of exposure and second and third doses given one and six months, respectively, after the first dose.

Administration: The deltoid muscle is the preferred site for intramuscular injection in adults. The anterolateral thigh is the recommended site for intramuscular injection in infants and children. Data suggest that injections given in the buttocks are given frequently into fatty tissue instead of into muscle. Such injections may result in a lower seroconversion rate than is expected.

The vaccine should be used as supplied. No dilution or reconstitution is necessary. The full recommended dose of the vaccine should be used.

It is recommended to record lot numbers when the vaccine is administered to a recipient.

For Intramuscular Use: Do not inject intravenously or intradermally. RECOMBIVAX HB (hepatitis B vaccine [recombinant]) is for intramuscular injection. It may, however, be administered subcutaneously to persons at risk of hemorrhage following intramuscular injections. However, when other aluminum-adsorbed vaccines have been administered subcutaneously, an increased incidence of local reactions including subcutaneous nodules has been observed. Therefore, subcutaneous administration should be used only in persons (e.g., hemophiliacs) at risk of hemorrhage following intramuscular injections.

Shake well before withdrawal and use.

Thorough agitation at the time of administration is necessary to maintain suspension of the vaccine. Parenteral drug products should be inspected visually for particulate matter and discolouration prior to administration. After thorough agitation, RECOMBIVAX HB is a slightly opaque, white suspension.

It is important to use a separate sterile syringe and needle for each individual patient to prevent transmission of hepatitis and other infectious agents from one person to another.

For the preservative-free (thimerosal-free) formulations: Once the single-dose vial has been penetrated, the withdrawn vaccine should be used promptly, and the vial must be discarded.

For Syringe Use Only: Withdraw the recommended dose from the vial using a sterile needle and syringe free of preservatives, antiseptics, and detergents.

OVERDOSAGE:
There are no data with regard to overdose.

For management of a suspected drug overdose, CPhA recommends that you contact your **regional Poison Control Centre**. See the *CPS* Directory section for a list of Poison Control Centres.

ACTION AND CLINICAL PHARMACOLOGY: Hepatitis B virus is one of at least five hepatitis viruses that cause a systemic infection, with major pathology in the liver. The others are hepatitis A, hepatitis C, hepatitis D, and hepatitis E viruses.

Hepatitis B virus is an important cause of viral hepatitis. There is no specific treatment for this disease. The incubation period for type B hepatitis is relatively long; six weeks to six months may elapse between exposure and the onset of clinical symptoms. The prognosis following infection with hepatitis B virus is variable and dependent on at least three factors: (1) Age—Infants and younger children usually experience milder initial disease than older persons; (2) Dose of Virus—The higher the dose, the more likely acute icteric hepatitis B will result; and, (3) Severity of associated underlying disease—Underlying malignancy or pre-existing hepatic disease predisposes to increased morbidity and mortality.

Persistence of viral infection (the chronic hepatitis B virus carrier state) occurs in 5-10% of persons following acute hepatitis B, and occurs more frequently after initial anicteric hepatitis B than after initial icteric disease. Consequently, carriers of hepatitis B surface antigen (HBsAg) frequently give no history of recognized acute hepatitis. The World Health Organization estimated that more than 2 billion people worldwide have evidence of post or current hepatitis B virus infection, and 350 million are chronic carriers of the virus. The Centers for Disease Control (CDC) estimate that there are approximately 0.5 to 1 million chronic carriers of hepatitis B virus in the USA and that this pool of carriers grows by 2-3% (8000 to 16 000 individuals) annually. Chronic carriers represent the largest human reservoir of hepatitis B virus.

The serious complications and sequelae of hepatitis B virus infection include massive hepatic necrosis, cirrhosis of the liver, chronic active hepatitis, and hepatocellular carcinoma. Chronic carriers of HBsAg appear to be at increased risk of developing hepatocellular carcinoma, which accounts for 80 to 90% of primary liver carcinomas. Although a number of etiologic factors are associated with development of hepatocellular carcinoma, the single most important etiologic factor appears to be active infection with the hepatitis B virus. Globally, approximately one million individuals die each year as a direct result of HBV-induced cirrhosis or liver cancer. Based on death certificates, about 100 Canadians died in 1995 due to hepatitis B associated acute or chronic liver disease.

There is also evidence that several diseases other than hepatitis have been associated with hepatitis B virus infection through an immunologic mechanism involving antigen-antibody complexes. Such diseases include a syndrome with rash, urticaria and arthralgia resembling serum sickness; polyarteritis nodosa; membranous glomerulonephritis; and infantile papular acrodermatitis.

Although the vehicles for transmission of the virus are predominantly blood and blood products, viral antigen has also been found in tears, saliva, breast milk, urine, semen and vaginal secretions. Hepatitis B virus is capable of surviving for days on environmental surfaces. Infection may occur when hepatitis B virus, transmitted by infected body fluids, is implanted via mucous surfaces or percutaneously introduced through accidental or deliberate breaks in the skin.

Transmission of hepatitis B virus infection is often associated with close interpersonal contact with an infected individual and with crowded living conditions. In such circumstances, transmission by inoculation via routes other than overt parenteral ones may be quite common. Perinatal transmission of hepatitis B infection from infected mother to child, at, or shortly after birth, can occur if the mother is an HBsAg carrier or if the mother has an acute hepatitis B infection in the third trimester. Infection in infancy by the hepatitis B virus usually leads to the chronic carrier state. Among infants born to women whose sera are positive for both the hepatitis B surface antigen and the e antigen, 85-90% are infected and become chronic carriers.

Hepatitis B is endemic throughout the world, and is a serious medical problem in population groups at increased risk (see Indications and Clinical Use). The prevalence of HBsAg in the general population varies between less than 0.5% in the U.S., Canada and Western Europe, 1 to 2% in South America and Southern Europe, 3 to 5% in North Africa and in many parts of the Federation of Russia (formally known as USSR) and 9 to 10% and higher in sub Saharan Africa, Southeast Asia and Alaska. The overall prevalence of serologic markers of infection varies between 7 and 10% in the U.S. and 60 and 80% in Southeast Asia or Africa. Even in countries like those in Northern and Western Europe and other highly developed countries with a relatively low prevalence of hepatitis B, certain populations are at high risk of acquiring the disease and have cumulative infection rates of up to 70% (see Indications and Clinical Use). In countries or areas with a high prevalence rate, the entire population is at risk and infection tends to occur during childhood.

Numerous epidemiological studies have shown that persons who develop anti-HBs following active infection with the hepatitis B virus are protected against the disease on re-exposure to the virus.

Reports in the literature describe a more virulent form of hepatitis B associated with superinfections or coinfections by delta virus, an incomplete RNA virus. Delta virus can only infect and cause illness in persons infected with hepatitis B virus since the delta agent requires a coat of HBsAg in order to become infectious. Therefore, persons immune to hepatitis B virus infection should also be immune to delta virus infection.

STORAGE AND STABILITY: Store unopened and opened vials at 2-8°C. Storage above or below the recommended temperature may reduce potency.

Do not freeze because freezing destroys potency. Do not use vaccine after the expiration date.

INFORMATION FOR THE PATIENT: Published in e-CPS, available by subscription at www.e-cps.ca.

DOSAGE FORMS, COMPOSITION AND PACKAGING: Pediatric Presentation: Single-dose Type I glass vials of 3 mL containing one 0.5 mL dose (5 µg HBsAg), packages of 1. Nonmedicinal ingredients: aluminum (as amorphous aluminum hydroxyphosphate), sodium borate, sodium chloride and water for injection. The vial stopper contains latex.
Adult Presentation: Single-dose Type I glass vials of 3 mL containing one 1 mL dose (10 µg HBsAg), packages of 1 and 10. Nonmedicinal ingredients: aluminum (as amorphous aluminum hydroxyphosphate), sodium borate, sodium chloride and water for injection. Multi-dose Type I glass vials of 4 mL containing three 1 mL doses (10 µg HBsAg/dose), packages of 1 and 10. Nonmedicinal ingredients: aluminum (as amorphous aluminum hydroxyphosphate), sodium borate, sodium chloride, thimerosal and water for injection. The vial stoppers contain latex.
Adult Dialysis Presentation: Single-dose Type I glass vials of 3 mL containing one 1 mL dose (40 µg HBsAg), packages of 1. Nonmedicinal ingredients: aluminum (as amorphous aluminum hydroxyphosphate), sodium borate, sodium chloride and water for injection. The vial stopper contains latex.
Manufacturing Process Residuals: The vaccine contains no detectable yeast DNA but may contain <1% yeast protein. The vaccine also contain <15 µg/mL formaldehyde as all preparations have been treated with formaldehyde prior to adsorption onto amorphous aluminum hydroxyphosphate.

Recothrom®
thrombin alfa (recombinant)
Coagulation Factor

Bayer

Date of Preparation: December 15, 2009

SUMMARY PRODUCT INFORMATION:

Route of Administration	Dosage Form/ Strength	Clinically Relevant Nonmedicinal Ingredients
Topical	Lyophilized powder and sterile diluent for solution; 6000 IU/vial	For a complete listing of nonmedicinal ingredients see Dosage Forms, Composition and Packaging.

DESCRIPTION: RECOTHROM (Thrombin alfa [Recombinant]) is a coagulation factor produced via recombinant DNA technology from a modified Chinese hamster ovary (CHO) cell line that is extensively characterized and free of known infectious agents. RECOTHROM is identical in amino acid sequence to naturally occurring human thrombin and is purified by a chromatographic process that yields a high-purity active RECOTHROM.

RECOTHROM is not sourced from human or animal blood or plasma. RECOTHROM contains no added human or animal components, and is inherently free from the risk of transmission of human blood-borne pathogens, such as HIV, hepatitis, parvovirus, and the infectious agents associated with Creutzfeldt-Jakob Disease (CJD) and variant CJD.

INDICATIONS AND CLINICAL USE: RECOTHROM (Thrombin alfa [Recombinant]) is indicated as an aid to hemostasis whenever oozing blood and minor bleeding from capillaries and small venules is accessible and control of bleeding by standard surgical techniques is ineffective or impractical.

The effectiveness of RECOTHROM was evaluated in surgical settings where adjuncts to hemostasis are frequently required: hepatic resection, peripheral arterial bypass surgery, arteriovenous graft formation for hemodialysis access, and spinal surgery. The evidence to support the effectiveness of RECOTHROM was not established in spinal surgery.

RECOTHROM may be applied directly to the bleeding site or used in conjunction with a compatible absorbable gelatin sponge.

CONTRAINDICATIONS:

- Patients who are hypersensitive to this drug or to any ingredient in the formulation or component of the container. For a complete listing, see Dosage Forms, Composition and Packaging.
- Do not use in patients with known hypersensitivity to hamster protein.
- RECOTHROM (Thrombin alfa [Recombinant]) must not be injected directly into the circulatory system.
- RECOTHROM should not be used for the treatment of massive or brisk arterial bleeding.

WARNINGS AND PRECAUTIONS:

Serious Warnings and Precautions
Do not inject RECOTHROM directly into the bloodstream. Intravascular injection of thrombin-containing hemostats may result in life-threatening intravascular coagulation or death.

General: There is a potential risk of thrombosis if RECOTHROM (Thrombin alfa [Recombinant]) is absorbed systemically.
Sensitivity/Resistance: In patients with known hypersensitivity to snake proteins, there may be a potential for allergic reaction.
Special Populations: Pregnant Women: No human data are available for use of RECOTHROM in pregnant women.

It is not known whether RECOTHROM causes fetal harm when administered to a pregnant woman or can affect reproduction capacity. RECOTHROM should be given to a pregnant woman only after careful risk/benefit evaluation.
Nursing Women: Safe use during lactation has not been established.
Pediatrics (<18 years of age): Safety and effectiveness of RECOTHROM in pediatric patients have not been established.
Geriatrics (>65 years of age): No substantial differences in safety were observed between elderly and younger patients. No modification to dosing or administration is required (see Dosage and Administration).

ADVERSE REACTIONS: Adverse Drug Reaction Overview: The safety database for the RECOTHROM (Thrombin alfa [Recombinant]) clinical program reflects treatment with a solution at a nominal concentration of 1000 IU/mL in the 368 subjects: 163 from the phase I and phase II studies and 205 from the phase III study.

RECOTHROM was also administered as a spray in an open-label, noncomparative phase II study in 72 burn patients requiring wound excision and grafting.
Clinical Trial Adverse Drug Reactions: Because clinical trials are conducted under very specific conditions, the adverse reaction rates observed in the clinical trials may not reflect the rates observed in practice and should not be compared to the rates in the clinical trials of another drug. Adverse drug reaction information from clinical trials is useful for identifying drug-related adverse events and for approximating rates.

Among the 411 subjects treated with RECOTHROM or comparator in the pivotal phase III study, all but 2 subjects (1 subject/treatment group) reported adverse events. Most events were moderate in severity and had a similar incidence in the RECOTHROM and bovine thrombin treatment groups. The most common adverse events were incision site complication (63% for both treatment groups), procedural pain (RECOTHROM 29%; bovine thrombin 34%), and nausea (RECOTHROM 28%; bovine thrombin 35%). Serious adverse events were reported by 18% of subjects treated with RECOTHROM and 22% with bovine thrombin.

Based on analysis of the above database, no specific adverse events have been established as adverse reactions causally related to RECOTHROM administration.

Adverse events of special interest were prespecified, based on the thrombin mechanism of action, use of absorbable gelatin sponge, historical reporting in association with cross-reacting antibodies to bovine thrombin product, and results from RECOTHROM phase II clinical trials. The incidences of these prespecified events were similar between treatment groups (see Table 1).

Table 1: RECOTHROM

Events of Special Interest in the RECOTHROM Phase III Study

	RECOTHROM (N=205) n (%)	Bovine Thrombin (N=206) n (%)
Subjects with any event category[a]	124 (60)	136 (66)
Bleeding	27 (13)	24 (12)
Cardiac	41 (20)	38 (18)
Hypersensitivity	30 (15)	37 (18)
Nausea + vomiting	68 (33)	83 (40)
Other infection	26 (13)	31 (15)
Postoperative wound infection	19 (9)	22 (11)
Thromboembolic	12 (6)	10 (5)

[a] Adverse events were included in event categories based on a blinded review of the investigator verbatim and coded terms.

Immunogenicity: The development of anti-Thrombin alfa (Recombinant) product antibodies was monitored in the controlled phase III clinical study. Treatment with RECOTHROM resulted in a statistically significantly lower incidence of anti-Thrombin alfa (Recombinant) product antibody development than treatment with bovine thrombin, P <0.0001 (see Table 2). None of the anti-Thrombin alfa (Recombinant) product antibodies seen in the clinical program neutralized native human thrombin activity.

At baseline in the phase III study, 1.5% of patients (n=3/198) in the Thrombin alfa (Recombinant) group had positive anti-Thrombin alfa (Recombinant) product antibody titers compared with 5% of patients in the bovine thrombin group (n=10/200). Of the patients who had detectable anti-Thrombin alfa (Recombinant) product antibodies at baseline, 0 of 3 in the thrombin group and 8 of 10 in the bovine thrombin group exhibited ≥1.0 titer unit (≥10 fold) increases in antibody levels after study treatment.

In controlled phase II studies of RECOTHROM applied with a gelatin sponge, incidence of antibody development following treatment with Thrombin alfa (Recombinant) was 1.2% (95% CI, 0% to 6.5%) compared to 2.4% (95% CI, 0.1% to 12.9%) for placebo.

Table 2: RECOTHROM

Anti-rThrombin Product Antibody Development[a] Following Exposure to Thrombin alfa (Recombinant) or Bovine Thrombin

	RECOTHROM (N=205)	Bovine Thrombin (N=206)
Evaluable patients, n	198	200
Antibody development, n (%)	3 (1.5%)	43 (22%)
95% Confidence Interval (CI)	0%–4%	16%–28%

[a] As evidenced by seroconversion or ≥1.0 titer unit (≥10-fold) increase in antibody levels after study treatment.

DRUG INTERACTIONS: Interactions with other drugs, food, herbal preparations, or laboratory tests have not been established.

DOSAGE AND ADMINISTRATION: Dosing Considerations: Do not inject RECOTHROM directly into the bloodstream. Intravascular injection of thrombin-containing hemostats may result in life-threatening intravascular coagulation or death.

RECOTHROM (Thrombin alfa [Recombinant]) is for topical use only.

Apply on the surface of bleeding tissue only.

Recommended Dose and Dosage Adjustment: The volume of reconstituted RECOTHROM required will vary, depending on the size and number of bleeding sites to be treated and the method of application. The health care professional should determine the number of vials required to produce a sufficient volume of reconstituted product. The mean volume of RECOTHROM used in the pivotal phase III trial was 11.6 mL.

Administration: Inspect the integrity of the RECOTHROM package and contents. Do not use if the packaging or contents have been damaged or opened.

Reconstitution: NOTE: Use aseptic technique when handling vials and syringes.

1. Remove flip-off plastic cap from the top of the RECOTHROM vial.
2. Insert the sharp end of the needle-free transfer device into the center of the vial stopper until it snaps onto the vial.
3. Open the diluent container by twisting the closure.
4. Attach the sterile empty syringe (provided) to the luer lock of the diluent container and remove the diluent.
5. Detach the diluent-filled syringe from the luer lock container.
6. Attach the diluent-filled syringe to the needle-free transfer device valve port.
7. Inject diluent into the vial.
8. Gently swirl the vial until the powder is completely dissolved (avoid excessive agitation of the vial during reconstitution).
9. Invert the vial and withdraw the RECOTHROM solution for transfer.
10. Attach the adhesive label "Do not inject" provided onto the transfer syringe.

Application: Topically apply RECOTHROM solution directly to bleeding site or in conjunction with a compatible absorbable gelatin sponge.

For Use with Absorbable Gelatin Sponge:

1. Refer to the absorbable gelatin sponge labeling for instructions on appropriate use.
2. Transfer reconstituted solution from syringe to a sterile bowl or basin.
3. Place the desired size pieces of the absorbable gelatin sponge into the bowl containing reconstituted RECOTHROM to completely saturate the sponge(s).
4. Remove the saturated sponge(s) and squeeze gently to remove excess RECOTHROM solution.
5. Apply the saturated sponge to the bleeding site in a single layer.

The amount of RECOTHROM required depends upon the area of tissue to be treated and the method of application.

Vials are for single use only. Discard unused contents.

OVERDOSAGE:

A maximum dose of topically applied RECOTHROM (Thrombin alfa [Recombinant]) has not been established. In clinical studies, the maximum volume administered was 48 mL.

For management of a suspected drug overdose, CPhA recommends that you contact your **regional Poison Control Centre**. See the *CPS* Directory section for a list of Poison Control Centres.

ACTION AND CLINICAL PHARMACOLOGY: Mechanism of Action: RECOTHROM (Thrombin alfa [Recombinant]) efficiently activates platelets and catalyzes the conversion of fibrinogen to fibrin, which are steps that are essential for blood clot formation.

Pharmacodynamics: RECOTHROM is a highly specific serine protease that promotes hemostasis and acts locally when applied topically to a site of bleeding.

RECOTHROM was evaluated in a phase III study conducted in 411 subjects undergoing surgery in 1 of 4 surgical settings: spinal surgery, hepatic segment surgery, peripheral arterial bypass surgery, and arteriovenous graft formation for hemodialysis access. The study was a multiple-site, randomized, double-blind, controlled evaluation of RECOTHROM compared to bovine thrombin, each at a nominal concentration of 1000 IU/mL topically applied to bleeding sites with an absorbable gelatin sponge.

Pharmacokinetics: Not applicable.

RECOTHROM is intended for topical use only. Intravascular administration is contraindicated (see Contraindications). As a consequence, intravascular pharmacokinetic studies were not performed in humans.

STORAGE AND STABILITY: RECOTHROM (Thrombin alfa [Recombinant]) powder vials should be stored at 2 to 25°C. Do not store above 25°C. Do not freeze.

Reconstituted solutions of RECOTHROM prepared with sterile sodium chloride solution may be stored for up to 24 hours at 2 to 25°C.

SPECIAL HANDLING INSTRUCTIONS: Not applicable.

INFORMATION FOR THE PATIENT: Published in e-CPS, available by subscription at www.e-cps.ca.

DOSAGE FORMS, COMPOSITION AND PACKAGING: Each 8 mL clear colorless glass vial (type 1 glass) with a stopper, aluminium seal and plastic flip-off cap contains: thrombin alfa (recombinant) 6000 IU, one 5 mL sterile polyethylene luer-lock bottle containing 5 mL sterile sodium chloride 9 mg/mL (0.9%) solution, one sterile, needle-free transfer device, one 5 mL sterile empty syringe and adhesive label "Do not inject". The formulated product is a clear, colorless solution upon reconstitution and contains the following nonmedicinal ingredients: calcium chloride dihydrate, USP, histidine, mannitol, polyethylene glycol 3350, sodium chloride and sucrose. The sterile diluent for reconstitution contains sodium chloride and water for injection. Single-use, preservative-free vials of 8 mL.

Reconstituted RECOTHROM solution may be applied directly to the bleeding site or used with absorbable gelatin sponges.

Incompatibilities: RECOTHROM has been shown to be compatible with GELFOAM, SURGIFOAM, and SPONGOSTAN, and should only be used with these sponges. The use of RECOTHROM with other absorbable gelatin sponges is not recommended because potency may be affected.

Rectogel

zinc sulfate monohydrate—benzocaine

Anorectal Therapy

Riva

Rectogel HC 🅿

zinc sulfate monohydrate—benzocaine—hydrocortisone acetate

Anorectal Therapy

Riva

SUPPLIED: Rectogel: Each tube contains: zinc sulfate monohydrate 0.5% and benzocaine 10% in a petroleum base. Nonmedicinal ingredients: methyl- and propylparaben. Tubes of 15 and 30 g with applicator.

Store in a cool place under 22°C.

Rectogel HC: Each tube contains: zinc sulfate monohydrate 0.5%, benzocaine 10% and hydrocortisone acetate 1% in a petroleum base. Nonmedicinal ingredients: methyl- and propylparaben. Tubes of 15 and 30 g with applicator.

Store in a cool place under 22°C.

Redoxon®

multiple vitamins and minerals

Vitamin-Mineral Supplement

Bayer Consumer Care

SUPPLIED: Redoxon: Each cylindrical, biplane, rough-surfaced, effervescent tablet contains: vitamin C (ascorbic acid) 1000 mg. Orange Tablet (orange color, orange odor and taste): Nonmedicinal ingredients: acacia, acesulfame potassium, aspartame, beta-carotene, citric acid, dl-α-tocopherol, flavours (orange and tangerine), isomalt, maltodextrin, modified starch, partially hydrogenated soybean oil, sodium ascorbate, sodium bicarbonate, sodium carbonate, sodium chloride and sucrose. Lemon Tablet (lemon color, lemon odor and taste): Nonmedicinal ingredients: acacia, acesulfame potassium, aspartame, citric acid, isomalt, lemon flavour, malic acid, maltodextrin, modified starch, riboflavin, sodium bicarbonate, sodium carbonate, sodium chloride, sucrose and vegetable oil. Tubes of 10.

Redoxon-B: Each pale to light orange, mottled, orange-like odor, cylindrical, biplane, edges bevelled, rough-surfaced, orange-flavored, effervescent tablet contains: vitamin C (ascorbic acid) 1000 mg, thiamine (vitamin B_1) (thiamine monophosphate ester chloride) 11.8 mg, riboflavin (vitamin B_2) (riboflavin 5-phosphate sodium) 15 mg, niacinamide (niacinamide) 50 mg, vitamin B_6 (pyridoxine hydrochloride) 8.23 mg, pantothenic acid (calcium d-pantothenate) 23 mg, biotin (biotin) 150 µg, vitamin B_{12} (cyanocobalamin) 10 µg and magnesium (carbonate and sulfate) 100 mg. Nonmedicinal ingredients: acacia, alpha-tocopherol, aspartame, beta-carotene, calcium carbonate, citric acid, dl-α-tocopherol, maltodextrin, mannitol, orange flavour, partially hydrogenated soybean oil, red beet juice, sodium ascorbate, sodium bicarbonate, sodium chloride, sodium lauryl sulfate, sucrose and trisodium citrate. Tubes of 10.

Refludan® 🅿

lepirudin (rDNA)

Antithrombotic

Bayer

Date of Preparation: October 1, 1999
Date of Revision: May 29, 2007

PHARMACOLOGY: Lepirudin is a highly specific direct inhibitor of thrombin. Lepirudin (chemical designation [Leu^1, Thr^2]-63-desulfohirudin) is a recombinant hirudin produced in yeast cells. Natural hirudin is produced in trace amounts as a family of highly homologous isopolypeptides by the leech Hirudo medicinalis.

The activity of lepirudin is measured with a chromogenic assay. One anti-thrombin unit (ATU) is the amount of lepirudin that neutralizes 1 unit of World Health Organization preparation 89/588 of thrombin. The specific activity of lepirudin is approximately 16 000 ATU/mg. Its mode of action is independent of antithrombin III. Platelet factor 4 does not inhibit lepirudin. One molecule of lepirudin binds to one molecule of thrombin and thereby blocks the thrombogenic activity of thrombin. As a result, all thrombin dependent coagulation assays are affected, e.g., activated partial thromboplastin time (aPTT) and PT (INR) values increase in a dose-dependent fashion.

Pharmacodynamics: In clinical studies, the pharmacodynamic effect of lepirudin on the proteolytic activity of thrombin was routinely assessed as an increase in aPTT. This was observed with increasing plasma concentrations of lepirudin, with no saturable effect up to the highest tested dose (0.5 mg/kg body weight i.v. bolus). Thrombin time frequently exceeded 200 seconds, even at low plasma concentrations of lepirudin, which renders this test unsuitable for routine monitoring of lepirudin therapy.

The pharmacodynamic response defined by the aPTT increase depends on plasma drug levels, which in turn depend on the individual patient's renal function (see Pharmacokinetics). For patients undergoing additional thrombolysis, elevated aPTT ratios (aPTT at a time after lepirudin administration over an aPTT reference value, usually median of the laboratory normal range for aPTT) were already observed at low lepirudin plasma concentrations, and further response to increasing plasma concentrations was relatively flat. In other populations, the response was steeper. At plasma concentrations of 1500 ng/mL, aPTT ratios were nearly 3.0 for healthy volunteers, 2.3 for patients with heparin induced thrombocytopenia (HIT), and 2.1 for patients with deep venous thrombosis. In patients treated for acute coronary syndromes (ACS), a prolongation of the aPTT to 73 to 75 seconds (mean values during infusion period) was found at lepirudin plasma concentrations of 1400 ng/mL.

Pharmacokinetics: The pharmacokinetic properties of lepirudin following i.v. administration are well described by a 2-compartment model. Distribution is essentially confined to extracellular fluids and is characterized by an initial half-life of approximately 10 minutes. Elimination follows a first-order process and is characterized by a terminal half-life of about 1.3 hours in young healthy volunteers. As the i.v. dose is increased over the range of 0.1 to 0.4 mg/kg, the plasma concentration increases proportionally.

Lepirudin is probably partially hydrolyzed into amino acids in the kidney. Half of the dose administered is detectable in the urine. About 35% of the dose is excreted as unchanged compound. The systemic clearance of lepirudin is proportional to the glomerular filtration rate or creatinine clearance. Dose adjustment based on creatinine clearance is recommended (see Dosage, Monitoring and Adjustment of Therapy, Renal Impairment). In patients with marked renal insufficiency (creatinine clearance below 15 mL/min), elimination half-lives are prolonged up to 2 days.

The systemic clearance of lepirudin in women is about 25% lower than in men. In elderly patients, the systemic clearance of lepirudin is 20% lower than in younger patients. This may be explained by the lower creatinine clearance in elderly patients compared to younger patients. Table 1 summarizes the systemic clearance (Cl) and volume of distribution at steady state (Vss) of lepirudin for various study populations.

Table 1: Refludan

Systemic Clearance (Cl) and Volume of Distribution at Steady State (Vss) of Lepirudin

Population	Cl (mL/min) Mean (% CV)	Vss (L) Mean (% CV)
Healthy Young Subjects (n=18; 18–60 years)	164 (19.3%)	12.2 (16.4%)
Healthy Elderly Subjects (n=10; 65–80 years)	139 (22.5%)	18.7 (20.6%)
Renally Impaired Subjects (n=16; creatinine clearance <80 mL/min)	61 (89.4%)	18.0 (41.1%)
Heparin-induced Thrombocytopenia Patients (n=73)	114 (46.8%)	32.1 (98.9%)

Legend: CV=Coefficient of variation.

INDICATIONS: Acute Coronary Syndromes: Lepirudin for injection is indicated for anticoagulation in adult patients with acute coronary syndromes (ACS); i.e. unstable angina/acute myocardial infarction without ST elevation. In patients with ACS, lepirudin is intended for use with ASA.

Heparin Induced Thrombocytopenia: Lepirudin for injection is indicated for anticoagulation in patients with heparin induced thrombocytopenia (HIT) and associated thromboembolic disease in order to prevent further thromboembolic complications.

CONTRAINDICATIONS: Acute Coronary Syndromes: Lepirudin for injection is contraindicated in patients with a generalized hemostatic abnormality such as hemophilia, Christmas disease, idiopathic thrombocytopenic purpura and in patients with active bleeding from a local lesion such as acute ulcer or ulcerating carcinoma; in patients who have had recent cranial, spinal, eye or ear surgery or trauma; hypersensitivity to hirudins; shock.

Heparin Induced Thrombocytopenia: Lepirudin for injection is contraindicated in patients with known hypersensitivity to hirudins.

WARNINGS: Hemorrhagic Events: Due to the increased risk of bleeding, which may be life-threatening, concomitant use of lepirudin for injection with thrombolytic therapy is not recommended. There has been limited experience with concomitant thrombolytic therapy in patients with HIT; in the OASIS-1 and OASIS-2 clinical trials (in patients with ACS), concomitant treatment with thrombolytics was not studied (see Dosage, Monitoring and Adjustment of Therapy, Concomitant Use with Thrombolytic Therapy). In postmarketing experience, there have been rare reports of intracranial bleeding with lepirudin in the absence of concomitant thrombolytic therapy (see Adverse Effects).

In the setting of patients at risk for bleeding or bleeding risk, a careful assessment weighing the risk with lepirudin administration versus its anticipated benefit should be made by the treating physician. It may be necessary to exclude such patients from treatment with lepirudin. Situations with increased bleeding risk include: recent puncture of large vessels or organ biopsy; anomaly of vessels or organs; recent cerebrovascular accident, stroke or intracerebral surgery; severe uncontrolled hypertension; bacterial endocarditis; advanced renal impairment (see Warnings, Renal Impairment); hemorrhagic diathesis; recent major surgery; overt signs of bleeding; recent major bleeding (e.g., intracranial, gastrointestinal, intraocular or pulmonary bleeding); recent active peptic ulcer; age >65 (see Precautions, Geriatrics).

Patients who weigh less than 50 kg are at an especially high risk of bleeding unless appropriate dosage reductions are made. In the OASIS-2 clinical trial, the observed rate of bleeding events was higher in the subgroup of lepirudin patients who weighed less than 50 kg, compared to those who weighed greater than 50 kg. This is most likely attributable to the fact that there was no dosage adjustment for body weight made for patients weighing less than 55 kg. The initial dosage of lepirudin should be adjusted for all body weights less than 100 kg (see Dosage, Initial Dosage, Acute Coronary Syndromes).

Renal Impairment: With renal impairment, relative overdose might occur even with the standard dosage regimen. Therefore, the bolus dose and the rate of infusion must be reduced in patients with known or suspected renal insufficiency. In clinical trials, lepirudin was not evaluated in patients with ACS and a serum creatinine above 2.0 mg/dL (175 µmol/L) prior to initiation of treatment and dosage regimen was adjusted during treatment based on serum creatinine. With this regimen in the OASIS-2 clinical trial, an increased risk of hemorrhagic adverse events was observed in patients with serum creatinine above 1.5 mg/dL. Therefore, a careful assessment weighing the risk of lepirudin administration versus its anticipated benefit should be made by the treating physician. It may be necessary to exclude such patients from treatment with lepirudin (see Pharmacology, Pharmacokinetics, and Dosage, Monitoring and Adjustment of Therapy, Use in Renal Impairment).

PRECAUTIONS: General: Antibodies: Formation of anti-hirudin antibodies was observed in about 15% of ACS patients and 40% of HIT patients treated with lepirudin for injection during clinical development. Very few patients in the clinical trials received the drug on more than one occasion. Therefore, the true frequency of antibody formation in patients who may be exposed to repeat courses of therapy may be higher. These antibodies may **increase** the anticoagulant effect of lepirudin, possibly due to delayed renal elimination of active lepirudin-antihirudin complexes. Therefore, strict ongoing monitoring of aPTT is necessary during prolonged therapy (see Dosage, Monitoring and Adjustment of Therapy, Standard Recommendations). No evidence of neutralization of lepirudin was found with positive antibody test results.

Allergic Reactions: Allergic reactions occurred in some patients (see Adverse Effects) but were not found to be correlated with the presence of antibodies to lepirudin. However, because a causal relationship of the allergic reactions to lepirudin therapy cannot be excluded with certainty, it is recommended to monitor patients receiving lepirudin with regard to signs and symptoms of allergic reactions. Anaphylactic reactions have been reported in post-marketing experience, including rare reports of serious anaphylactic reactions that have resulted in shock or death. These reactions have been reported during initial administration or upon second or subsequent re-exposure(s).

Re-exposure: During the HAT-1 and HAT-2 clinical studies, a total of 13 patients were re-exposed to lepirudin. One of these patients experienced a mild allergic skin reaction during the second treatment cycle. In post marketing experience, anaphylaxis after re-exposure has been reported (see Adverse Effects, Allergic Reactions).

Liver Injury: Serious liver injury (e.g., liver cirrhosis) may enhance the anticoagulant effect of lepirudin due to coagulation defects secondary to reduced generation of vitamin K-dependent coagulation factors.

Laboratory Test Interactions: Heparin Induced Thrombocytopenia: In general, the dosage (infusion rate) should be adjusted to the aPTT ratio (patient aPTT at a given time over an aPTT reference value, usually median of the laboratory normal range for aPTT (see Dosage, Monitoring and Adjustment of Therapy, Standard Recommendations). Other thrombin-dependent coagulation assays are changed by lepirudin.

Drug Interactions: Concomitant use of lepirudin with the following agents has not been assessed and may increase the risk of bleeding complications:

- antiplatelet agents other than ASA such as ticlopidine or clopidogrel;
- GpIIb/IIIa-receptor antagonists such as eptifibatide, tirofiban, or abciximab;
- other thrombin inhibitors such as low-molecular-weight heparins.

Concomitant treatment with thrombolytics (e.g. recombinant tissue plasminogen activator [rt-PA] or streptokinase) may increase the risk of bleeding complications, and considerably enhance the effect of lepirudin on aPTT prolongation (see Warnings, Hemorrhagic Events; Adverse Effects, Adverse Events Reported in Other Populations, Intracranial Severe Bleeding and Dosage, Monitoring and Adjustment of Therapy, Concomitant Use with Thrombolytic Therapy).

Concomitant treatment with coumarin derivatives (warfarin or other vitamin K antagonists) or drugs that affect platelet function may also increase the risk of bleeding (see Dosage, Monitoring and Adjustment of Therapy, Use in Patients Scheduled for a Switch to Oral Anticoagulation).

Patients with a history of diabetes mellitus appeared to not respond to lepirudin as well as heparin in one clinical trial. The reason for this observation is unknown and may have been a chance finding.

Pregnancy: There are no adequate and well-controlled studies to evaluate the efficacy or safety of lepirudin in pregnancy. If the use of lepirudin is being considered, the treating physician must weigh the potential benefit of treatment versus any potential risks (including bleeding complications) that may occur during pregnancy.

Teratogenic effects have been studied in rats. Because animal reproductive studies are not always predictive of human response, this drug should be used during pregnancy only if clearly needed and potential benefits outweigh the risk. It is not known whether the drug crosses the placental barrier in humans.

Lactation: It is not known whether lepirudin is excreted in human milk. Because many drugs are excreted in human milk and because of the potential for serious adverse reactions in nursing infants from lepirudin, a decision should be made whether to discontinue nursing or to discontinue the drug, taking into account the importance of the drug to the mother.

Children: Safety and effectiveness in children have not been established. Two children, an 11 year old girl and a 12 year old boy, were treated with lepirudin in the HAT-2 study. Both children presented with thromboembolic complications at baseline. Lepirudin doses given ranged from 0.15 to 0.22 mg/kg/h for the girl and from 0.1 mg/kg/h (in conjunction with urokinase) to 0.7 mg/kg/h for the boy. Treatment with lepirudin was completed after 8 and 58 days, respectively, without serious adverse events.

Geriatrics: Lepirudin is known to be substantially excreted by the kidney, and the risk of adverse reactions to this drug may be greater in patients with impaired renal function. In clinical trials, the percentage of hemorrhagic events increased in patients over 65 years of age (from 6.7% to 11%). Decreased renal function is more frequent in elderly patients, so care should be taken in dose selection, and in monitoring renal function.

The frequency of nonhemorrhagic events also increased in elderly patients. Dosage adjustments, in both elderly and younger patients, should be made based on renal functions, weight and aPTT (see Dosage, Monitoring and Adjustment of Therapy).

ADVERSE EFFECTS: Severe Bleeding: In clinical trials, major bleeding events occurred in 1.2% of patients with acute coronary syndromes treated with lepirudin for injection, and in 0.7% of patients treated with unfractionated heparin. This difference was statistically significant (p=0.0243). In these trials, patients with aPTT values ≥100 seconds were at higher risk of major bleeding.

Severe bleeding may lead to hypovolemia, hypotension and shock and their clinical sequelae. Severe bleeding and, in particular, intracranial bleeding may be life threatening. Intracranial bleeding was the most serious adverse reaction found in populations other than HIT patients. Intracranial bleeding occurred in patients with acute myocardial infarction who received both lepirudin and thrombolytic therapy (rt-PA or streptokinase). The overall frequency of this potentially life-threatening complication among patients receiving both lepirudin and thrombolytic therapy was 0.6% (7 out of 1134 patients). Although no intracranial bleeding was observed in 1168 subjects or patients who did not receive concomitant thrombolysis, in postmarketing experience there have been rare reports of intracranial bleeding with lepirudin in the absence of concomitant thrombolytic therapy (see Warnings). The most frequently reported major bleeding in acute coronary syndrome patients were GI bleeds, the majority of which required blood transfusion. The frequency of life-threatening bleeding events was substantially reduced in clinical studies in patients with acute coronary syndrome in which concomitant thrombolysis was not administered.

Hypersensitivity and Injection Site Reactions: Based on clinical study data and postmarketing experience, hypersensitivity reactions may be assumed to occur in <1% of patients. These include: airway reactions (cough, bronchospasm, stridor, dyspnea), skin reactions (pruritus, urticaria, rash, flushes, chills), general allergic reactions (including anaphylactoid or anaphylactic reactions), edema (facial edema, tongue edema, larynx edema, angioedema), injection site reactions and injection site pain. Cases of shock and death from anaphylactic reactions have rarely been reported (see Precautions).

Adverse Events Reported in ACS Patients: The most frequently reported adverse events in the OASIS-1 and OASIS-2 clinical trials were bleeding events.

OASIS-2 Clinical Trial: The incidence rates in Table 2 and Table 3 reflect the scheduled 72-hour treatment period for lepirudin or heparin and a subsequent follow-up period until study Day 7. All patients were to receive concomitant ASA treatment.

Table 2: Refludan

Hemorrhagic Adverse Events: Minor, Major, Life-threatening and Fatal Bleeding Events in the OASIS-2 Clinical Trial, From Randomization to Day 7; Irrespective of causal Relationship to Treatment[a]

	OASIS-2 Clinical Trial	
	Refludan (n=5047) %	**Heparin (n=5033) %**
Minor Bleeding	7.7	4.5
Major Bleeding[b]	1.2	0.7
Life-threatening[c]	0.4	0.4
Fatal	0.1	0.1

[a] Patients may have experienced more than one event

[b] Major bleeding was defined as fatal, life-threatening, permanently or significantly disabling bleeding events, or events that required surgical intervention or transfusion of 2 or more units of packed red cells or equivalent.

[c] Life-threatening bleeding was defined as major bleeding events that were fatal, intracranial, required surgical intervention or transfusion of 4 or more units of blood products or plasma expanders.

Table 3: Refludan

Hemorrhagic Adverse Events with Incidences ≥1% in the OASIS-2 Clinical Trial From Randomization to Day 7; Irrespective of Causal Relationship to Treatment[a]

	OASIS-2 Clinical Trial	
	Refludan (n=5047) %	**Heparin (n=5033) %**
Hematuria	2.1	0.7
Injection site hemorrhage	2.1	1.9
Epistaxis	1.4	0.6
GI hemorrhage	1.3	0.7

[a] Patients may have experienced more than one event

Table 4: Refludan

Hemorrhagic Adverse Events in Patients According to Body Weight in the OASIS-2 Clinical Trial[a]

	OASIS-2 Clinical Trial			
Weight	**Refludan (n=5047)**	**Heparin (n=5033)**	**Total**	**p-value**
<50 kg	16/98 (16.33%)	4/77 (5.19%)	20/175 (11.43%)	0.0297
50–100 kg	408/4720 (8.64%)	244/4677 (5.22%)	652/9397 (6.94%)	0.0001
>100 kg	22/228 (9.65%)	15/279 (5.38%)	37/507 (7.30%)	0.0853

[a] The lepirudin dosage was not adjusted in patients with body weight <55 kg in the OASIS-2 clinical trial, which probably resulted in overdosage in this sub-group.

Other hemorrhagic adverse events reported in >0.2% of lepirudin patients in the OASIS-2 clinical trial included hemoptysis, gum hemorrhage, subcutaneous hematoma, and surgical bleeding.

Nonhemorrhagic Adverse Events: In the OASIS-2 clinical trial, nonhemorrhagic adverse events from randomization to Day 7 (irrespective of causal relationship to treatment) were reported with lepirudin and heparin at a similar frequency. Adverse events reported with lepirudin at an incidence from >0.2% to ≤0.5% included heart arrest, shock, MI, rash, confusion, and hypotension. There were no nonhemorrhagic adverse events at a frequency >0.5%.

OASIS-1 Clinical Trial: The incidence rates in Table 5 and subsequent text reflect the scheduled 72-hour treatment period for lepirudin or heparin and a subsequent follow-up period until study Day 7.

The types of hemorrhagic adverse events observed in lepirudin-treated patients in the OASIS-1 clinical trial were similar to those reported in the OASIS-2 clinical trial. From randomization to Day 7, the most frequent hemorrhagic adverse event (irrespective of causal relationship to treatment) was skin hemorrhage. Other hemorrhagic events that occurred in >1% of lepirudin-treated patients (either dose group; nor specifically listed in the OASIS-2 clinical trial data above) included hemoptysis, rectal bleeding, subcutaneous hematoma and hematemesis. More hemorrhagic adverse events occurred with lepirudin compared to heparin; this difference was primarily due to a higher incidence of epistaxis and hematuria in lepirudin-treated patients.

Nonhemorrhagic Adverse Events: In the OASIS-1 clinical trial, the nonhemorrhagic adverse events (possibly treatment related) that occurred in 1% to 3% of lepirudin patients (either dose group) included headache, nausea, diarrhea, bradycardia, hypotension, insomnia, dyspepsia, fever, pain, vasodilation, rash, increased serum creatinine, and ventricular tachycardia.

Adverse Reactions Reported in HIT Patients: The following safety information is based on 403 HIT patients treated in the two open, historically-controlled clinical studies (n=198) and in an additional uncontrolled study that was performed to increase the knowledge about the safety profile of patients with HIT (n=205).

Table 5: Refludan

Hemorrhagic Adverse Events: Minor, Major, Life-threatening and Fatal Bleeding Events in the OASIS-1 Clinical Trial From Randomization to Day 7; Irrespective of Causal Relationship to Treatment[a]

	OASIS-1 Clinical Trial		
	Refludan 0.2 mg/kg Bolus, 0.10 mg/kg/hour Infusion (n=270) %	**Refludan 0.4 mg/kg Bolus, 0.15 mg/kg/hour Infusion (n=265) %**	**Heparin (n=369) %**
Minor Bleeding	16.3	21.5	10.6
Major Bleeding[b]	0.7	1.1	1.1

(cont'd)

Table 5: Refludan *(cont'd)*

Hemorrhagic Adverse Events: Minor, Major, Life-threatening and Fatal Bleeding Events in the OASIS-1 Clinical Trial From Randomization to Day 7; Irrespective of Causal Relationship to Treatment[a]

	OASIS-1 Clinical Trial		
	Refludan 0.2 mg/kg Bolus, 0.10 mg/kg/hour Infusion (n=270) %	Refludan 0.4 mg/kg Bolus, 0.15 mg/kg/hour Infusion (n=265) %	Heparin (n=369) %
Life-threatening[c]	0.7	0.8	0.8
Fatal	0	0.4	0

[a] Patients may have experienced more than one event

[b] Major bleeding was defined as fatal, life-threatening, permanently or significantly disabling bleeding events, or events that required surgical intervention or transfusion of 2 or more units of packed red cells or equivalent.

[c] Life-threatening bleeding was defined as major bleeding events that were fatal, intracranial, required surgical intervention or transfusion of 4 or more units of blood products or plasma expanders.

Hemorrhagic Events: Bleeding was the most frequent adverse reaction observed in patients treated with lepirudin. Table 6 gives an overview of all hemorrhagic events which occurred in at least two patients receiving lepirudin in clinical studies HAT-1 and HAT-2.

Table 6: Refludan

Hemorrhagic Events Which Occurred in at Least Two Patients in Clinical Studies HAT-1 and HAT-2

		Patients with TECs	
Hemorrhagic Event	Clinical Studies HAT-1, HAT-2 (n=198) %	Refludan (n=113) %	Historical Control (n=91) %
Bleeding from puncture sites and wounds	14.1	10.6	4.4
Anemia or isolated drop in hemoglobin	13.1	12.4	1.1
Other hematoma and bleeding	11.1	10.6	4.4
Hematuria	6.6	4.4	0
Gastrointestinal and rectal bleeding	5.1	5.3	6.6
Epistaxis	3.0	4.4	1.1
Hemothorax	3.0	0	1.1
Vaginal bleeding	1.5	1.8	0
Intracranial bleeding	0	0	2.2

Other possibly related hemorrhagic events, which were reported in one patient each, were gastrointestinal hemorrhage, hematemesis, hemoperitoneum, hemoptysis, hemorrhagic gastritis, intracerebral bleeding, lung hemorrhage, mouth hemorrhage, retroperitoneal bleeding, and subcutaneous hematoma.

Nonhemorrhagic Events: Table 7 gives an overview of the most frequently observed nonhemorrhagic events in clinical studies HAT-1 and HAT-2.

Table 7: Refludan

Incidence of Most Frequent (≥1%) Nonhemorrhagic Events[a] Considered at Least Possibly Related to Refludan in Clinical Studies HAT-1 and HAT-2

Event	All Refludan Patients (n=198) %
AST increased	3.0
Fever	2.5
Prothrombin increased	1.5
Allergic reaction	1.0
Eczema	1.0
Rash	1.0

[a] Patients may have experienced more than one event.

The following other nonhemorrhagic events were assessed as at least possibly related, and occurred in 1 patient each among all 198 patients treated with lepirudin.

Body as a Whole: abscess, infection superimposed.

Cardiovascular: coronary thrombosis, pericardial effusion, vasodilatation, ventricular fibrillation.

Digestive: diarrhea, gastritis, liver function test abnormal, and vomiting.

Hemic and Lymphatic Systems: antinuclear antibody present and thrombocytopenia.

Nervous System: agitation, convulsion, and sweating increased.

Skin and Appendages: skin necrosis.

Thromboembolism: arterial thrombosis, pulmonary embolus, and thrombophlebitis of arm.

In the open multicenter trial HAT-3, a total of 54% (111/205) experienced adverse events. The following type of major bleedings were observed: Bleeding at invasive/instrumented sites gastrointestinal, urogenital, pericardial and intracerebral bleedings. One intracerebral bleeding occurred during the study. Four of the observed major bleeding events were fatal. The most frequent minor bleeding events were isolated drop in hemoglobin (6/205) hematuria, and hematomas (7/205). Of these, 53 patients (26%) had possibly related adverse events. The most frequently observed adverse events other than bleeding events previously described were the following: pneumonia (5%), new TEC-arterial peripheral (4%), multi organ failure (4%), fever (3%), sepsis (3%), and shock (2%). Eight patients (4%) experienced a total of 11 allergic reactions.

OVERDOSE:

Symptoms: In case of overdose, as suggested by excessively high aPTT values, the risk of bleeding is increased.

Treatment: No specific antidote for lepirudin is available. If life-threatening bleeding occurs and excessive plasma levels of lepirudin are suspected, the following steps should be followed: Immediately stop lepirudin administration. Determine aPTT and other coagulation parameters as appropriate. Determine hemoglobin and prepare for blood transfusion. Follow the current guidelines for treating patients with shock.

Individual clinical case reports and animal data suggest that either hemofiltration or hemodialysis (using high-flux dialysis membranes with a molecular weight cut-off point of 50 000 Daltons) may be useful in this situation.

In studies in pigs the application of von Willebrand Factor (vWF, 66 IU/kg) markedly reduced the bleeding time prolongation by lepirudin. The clinical significance of this data is unknown.

Coagulant complex anti-inhibitor was effective in completely inhibiting lepirudin induced prolongation of whole blood coagulation time (WBCT) in rabbits at a dose of 50 U/kg. The clinical significance of these data is unknown. Due to its procoagulant effects, the use of coagulant complex anti-inhibitor should only be considered in cases of life-threatening bleeding. As there is no experience in humans in the presence of lepirudin, no dosing recommendations can be given. Careful dose titration is necessary in order to avoid the risk of further thromboembolic complications or disseminated intravascular coagulation (DIC) caused by overdosage. The clinical usefulness of coagulation tests such as activated partial thromboplastin time, whole blood clotting time, activated clotting time, or bleeding time in this particular setting is not known.

For management of a suspected drug overdose, CPhA recommends that you contact your **regional Poison Control Centre**. See the *CPS* Directory section for a list of Poison Control Centres.

DOSAGE: Initial Dosage: Acute Coronary Syndromes: Anticoagulation in adult patients with acute coronary syndromes: 0.4 mg/kg body weight **(up to 100 kg)** slowly intravenously (eg. over 15 to 20 seconds) as a bolus dose, followed by 0.15 mg/kg body weight **(up to 100 kg)**/hour as a continuous intravenous infusion. Lepirudin should be infused for 72 hours. A bolus must not be given if, for any reason (eg, previous heparin treatment) the baseline aPTT is higher than 60 seconds, and infusion is not to be started if the aPTT is higher than 100 seconds. Heparin treatment must be discontinued before lepirudin treatment is started.

Normally the initial dosage depends on the patient's body weight. This is valid up to a body weight of 100 kg in patients with ACS. In ACS patients with a body weight exceeding 100 kg, the initial dosage should not be increased beyond the 100 kg body weight dose (maximal initial bolus dose of 40 mg, maximal initial infusion dose of 15 mg/hour). (See also Administration, Initial Intravenous Bolus, Table 10 and Administration, Intravenous Infusion, Table 11).

Heparin Induced Thrombocytopenia: Anticoagulation in Adult Patients with HIT and Associated Thromboembolic Disease: The initial dose of lepirudin is 0.4 mg/kg body weight (up to 110 kg) given as a slow (e.g., over 15 to 20 seconds) i.v. bolus injection. This is followed by a continuous i.v. infusion of 0.15 mg/kg/hour (up to 110 kg) for 2-10 days, or longer if clinically needed (see Administration for directions on preparation and dilution).

Normally, the initial dosage depends on the patient's body weight. This is valid up to a body weight of 110 kg in patients with HIT. In HIT patients with a body weight exceeding 110 kg, the initial dosage should not be increased beyond the 110 kg body weight dose (maximum initial bolus dose of 44 mg; maximum initial infusion dose of 16.5 mg/h; see Table 10 and Table 11 under Administration, Initial Intravenous Bolus and Intravenous Infusion).

Monitoring and Adjustment of Therapy: Standard Recommendations: Monitoring: Acute Coronary Syndromes: Any aPTT value out of the target range is to be confirmed at once before drawing conclusions with respect to dose modifications, unless there is a clinical need to react immediately. Target range (therapeutic window) for the aPTT is between 60 and 100 seconds. It is recommended that aPTT measurements be done before lepirudin treatment, 6 to 8 hours after the start of treatment, and daily thereafter for the duration of treatment in all patients. Heparin treatment must be discontinued before lepirudin treatment is started. The bolus must not be given if the aPTT is higher than 60 seconds and the infusion must not be started if the aPTT is higher than 100 seconds. The same applies to patients with elevated aPTT for other reasons. More frequent measurements may be required in the course of the treatment if the aPTT is too high or too low. These measurements will be used to adjust the infusion of lepirudin according to Table 8.

Dose Modifications—Acute Coronary Syndromes: Adjustments of the dose will be made according to Table 8.

Table 8: Refludan

Adjustment of Infusion Rate Based on Confirmed aPTT

Category	aPTT	Action
1[a]	<60 seconds	Increase hourly infusion rate by 20%. (If after 2 consecutive 20% increases in rate with aPTT still <60 seconds, maintain current rate)[b]
2	60 to 100 seconds	Maintain same infusion rate
3[a]	>100 seconds	Reduce hourly infusion rate by 20%
4	Still >100 seconds 6 to 8 hours after reducing infusion rate second time by 20% or if infusion rate is 0.09 mg/kg/hour or slower	**Stop** infusion

[a] It is recommended that for categories 1 and 3, aPTT is remeasured 6 to 8 hours later and appropriate readjustments made.

[b] An infusion rate of 0.21 mg/kg/hour should not be exceeded.

In case of minor bleeding, the infusion should be interrupted for about 2 hours and then restarted at a 20% lower infusion speed. In case of severe or major bleeding, the infusion must be terminated, and appropriate measures (eg, transfusion, surgery) must be taken.

Monitoring—Heparin Induced Thrombocytopenia: In general, the dosage (infusion rate) should be adjusted according to the aPTT ratio (patient aPTT at a given time over an aPTT reference value, usually median of the laboratory normal range for aPTT). Lepirudin should not be started in patients presenting with a baseline aPTT ratio of 2.5 or more, in order to avoid initial overdosing. The target range for the aPTT ratio during treatment (therapeutic window) should be 1.5 to 2.5. Data from clinical trials in HIT patients suggest that with aPTT ratios higher than this target range, the risk of bleeding increases, while there is no incremental increase in clinical efficacy.

A repeat aPTT determination should be performed one hour after stopping heparin, if the last available and elevated aPTT ratio is suspected to be caused by the recent heparin treatment which resulted in heparin induced thrombocytopenia.

The first aPTT determination for monitoring treatment should be done 4 hours after start of the infusion. Follow-up aPTT determinations are recommended at least once daily, as long as treatment is ongoing. More frequent aPTT monitoring is highly recommended in patients with renal impairment (see Monitoring and Adjustment of Therapy, Renal Impairment), serious liver injury or with an increased risk of bleeding.

Dose Modifications—Heparin Induced Thrombocytopenia: Any aPTT ratio out of the target range is to be confirmed at once before drawing conclusions with respect to dose modifications, unless there is a clinical need to react immediately. If the confirmed aPTT ratio is above the target range, the infusion should be stopped for two hours. At restart, the infusion rate should be decreased by 50% (no additional intravenous bolus should be administered). The aPTT ratio should be determined again 4 hours later.

If the confirmed aPTT ratio is below the target range, the infusion rate should be increased in steps of 20%. The aPTT ratio should be determined again 4 hours later. In general, an infusion rate of 0.21 mg/kg/h should not be exceeded without checking for coagulation abnormalities which might be preventative of an appropriate aPTT response.

Renal Impairment: As approximately 50% of lepirudin is excreted by the kidneys (see Pharmacology, Pharmacokinetics), renal function should be considered prior to administration. In case of renal impairment, relative overdose might occur even with the standard dosage regimen. Therefore, the bolus dose and the infusion rate must be reduced in case of known or suspected renal insufficiency (creatinine clearance below 60 mL/min or serum creatinine above 1.5 mg/dL). In all patients with renal insufficiency, the bolus dose is to be reduced to 0.2 mg/kg body weight (note: this reduced dose has not been evaluated in ACS patients) (see Warnings, Renal Impairment). The infusion rate is to be adjusted as follows in patients with ACS and in patients with HIT and thromboembolic disease.

Acute Coronary Syndromes: Starting treatment with lepirudin is not recommended in ACS patients with a baseline serum creatinine value >2.0 mg/dL. In ACS patients with a baseline serum creatinine value of >1.5 to 2.0 mg/dL, the recommended infusion rate is 0.075 mg/kg/hour (note: this reduced dose has not been evaluated in ACS patients). If during lepirudin treatment serum creatinine values in the range of >1.5 to 2.5 mg/dL are obtained in patients without an initial dose reduction, the infusion rate is to be reduced by 50% and the serum creatinine remeasured 6 to 8 hours later. In this group of patients, the infusion may be continued only if aPTTs are checked at least every 6 to 8 hours, serum creatinine is measured daily, and adjustments to treatment are made accordingly. Otherwise, discontinuation of the infusion is recommended. If at any time during treatment the serum creatinine is found to be >2.5 mg/dL, treatment with lepirudin is to be discontinued.

Heparin Induced Thrombocytopenia: There is only limited information on the therapeutic use of lepirudin in HIT patients with significant renal impairment. The following dosage recommendations are mainly based on single-dose studies in a small number of patients with renal impairment. These recommendations are only tentative.

Dose adjustments should be based on creatinine clearance values, whenever available, as obtained from a reliable method (e.g., 24-hour urine sampling). If creatinine clearance is not available, the dose adjustments should be based on the serum creatinine.

The standard initial infusion rate given in Table 11 must be reduced according to the recommendations given in Table 9. Additional aPTT monitoring is highly recommended.

Table 9: Refludan

Reduction of Infusion Rate in Patients with Renal Impairment

Creatinine Clearance (mL/min)	Serum Creatinine (mg/dL)	Adjusted Infusion Rate: % of Standard Initial Infusion Rate	Adjusted Infusion Rate: mg/kg/h
45–60	1.6–2.0	50	0.075
30–44	2.1–3.0	30	0.045
15–29	3.1–6.0	15	0.0225
below 15[a]	above 6.0[a]	Avoid or **stop** infusion![a]	

[a] In hemodialysis patients or in case of acute renal failure (creatinine clearance below 15 mL/min or serum creatinine above 6.0 mg/dL), infusion of Refludan is to be avoided or stopped. Additional i.v. bolus doses of 0.1 mg/kg body weight should be considered every other day only if the aPTT ratio falls below the lower therapeutic limit of 1.5 (see also Monitoring and Adjustment of Therapy, Standard Recommendations).

Concomitant Use with Thrombolytic Therapy: Acute Coronary Syndromes: In patients with acute coronary syndrome, concomitant treatment with thrombolytics was not studied. Concomitant use of lepirudin and thrombolytics is not recommended in patients with ACS.

Heparin Induced Thrombocytopenia: Clinical trials in HIT patients have provided only limited information on the combined use of lepirudin and thrombolytic agents. The following dosage regimen of lepirudin was used in a total of nine HIT patients in clinical studies who presented with thromboembolic complications at baseline and received both lepirudin and thrombolytic therapy (rt-PA, urokinase or streptokinase): initial intravenous bolus of 0.2 mg/kg body weight, followed by continuous intravenous infusion of 0.1 mg/kg/hour.

The number of patients receiving combined therapy was too small to identify differences in clinical outcome of patients who received both lepirudin and thrombolytic therapy as compared to those who received lepirudin alone. The combined incidences of death, limb amputation, or new thromboembolic complication were 22.2% and 20.7%, respectively. While there was a 47% relative increase in the overall bleeding rate in patients who were started on both lepirudin and thrombolytic therapy versus lepirudin alone (55.6% vs. 37.9%), there were no differences in the rates of major bleeding events (fatal or life-threatening bleeds, bleeds that were permanently or significantly disabling, overt bleeds requiring transfusion of two or more units of packed red blood cells, bleeds necessitating surgical intervention, intracranial bleeds) between the groups (11.1% vs. 11.2%). Although no intracranial bleeding has been observed in any of these patients, the risk of this potentially life-threatening complication may be increased in conjunction with thrombolytic agents (see Adverse Effects, Intracranial Bleeding).

Special attention should be paid to the fact that thrombolytic agents per se may increase the aPTT ratio. Therefore, aPTT ratios with a given plasma level of lepirudin are usually higher in patients who receive concomitant thrombolysis than in those who do not (see also Pharmacology, Pharmacodynamics).

Use in Patients Scheduled for a Switch to Oral anticoagulation: Lepirudin monotherapy influences the INR/prothrombin time in a dose dependent, gradual and linear fashion (mean INR increase +0.14 with aPTT in the recommended therapeutic range in the absence of other anticoagulants).

In lepirudin-treated patients with aPTT values within the recommended target range receiving overlapping therapy with oral anticoagulants and who had stable therapeutic INR values, a cumulative analysis of two prospective trials did not find evidence of a relevant decrease in INR values upon cessation of lepirudin treatment.

If a patient is scheduled to receive coumarin derivatives (vitamin K antagonists) for oral anticoagulation after lepirudin therapy, the following should apply: Coumarin derivatives should be initiated only when platelet counts are normalizing. The intended maintenance dose should be started with no loading dose. To avoid prothrombotic effects when initiating coumarin, continue parenteral anticoagulation for 4 to 5 days. The parenteral agent can be discontinued when INR stabilizes within the desired target range.

Acute Coronary Syndromes: In patients with acute coronary syndromes in the OASIS-2 clinical trial, warfarin treatment was initiated in a sub-group of patients 12 to 30 hours after starting lepirudin therapy. Warfarin was administered with a loading dose of 10 mg, followed by 3 mg/day for 3 days. Subsequent warfarin doses were adjusted by the treating physician to achieve an international normalized ratio (INR) of 2.5 (range 2 to 3).

Heparin Induced Thrombocytopenia: If a patient is scheduled to receive coumarin derivatives (vitamin K antagonists) for oral anticoagulation after lepirudin therapy, the dose of lepirudin should first be gradually reduced in order to reach an aPTT ratio just above 1.5 before initiating oral anticoagulation. As soon as an international normalized ratio (INR) of 2.0 is reached, lepirudin therapy should be stopped.

Administration: Directions on Preparation and Dilution: Lepirudin should not be mixed with other drugs or diluents except for Water for Injection USP, 0.9% Sodium Chloride Injection USP or 5% Dextrose Injection.

Reconstitution and further dilution are to be carried out under sterile conditions. For reconstitution, Water for Injection USP or 0.9% Sodium Chloride Injection USP are to be used. For further dilution, 0.9% Sodium Chloride Injection USP or 5% Dextrose Injection are suitable.

For rapid, complete reconstitution, inject 1 mL of diluent into the vial and shake it gently. After reconstitution, a clear, colorless solution is usually obtained in a few seconds, but definitely in less than 3 minutes.

Parenteral drug products should be inspected visually for particulate matter and discoloration prior to administration whenever solution and container permit. Do not use solutions that are cloudy or contain particles.

It is recommended that the reconstituted solution be used immediately. The diluted solution for i.v. administration remains stable for up to 24 hours at 2 to 25°C. The preparation should be allowed to reach room temperature before administration. Discard any unused solution appropriately.

Initial I.V. Bolus: For i.v. bolus injection, use a solution with a concentration of 5 mg/mL.

Preparation of a Lepirudin Solution with a Concentration of 5 mg/mL: Reconstitute 1 vial (50 mg of lepirudin) with 1 mL of Water for Injection USP or 0.9% Sodium Chloride Injection USP. The final concentration of 5 mg/mL is obtained by transferring the entire contents of the vial into a sterile, single-use syringe (of at least 10 mL capacity) and diluting the solution to a total volume of 10 mL, using Water for Injection USP, 0.9% Sodium Chloride Injection USP, or 5% Dextrose Injection.

The final solution is to be administered according to body weight (see Table 10 and Dosage, Initial Dosage). I.V. injection of the bolus is to be carried out slowly (over 15 to 20 seconds).

I.V. Infusion: For continuous i.v. infusion, solutions with concentrations of 0.2 or 0.4 mg/mL may be used.

Preparation of a Lepirudin Solution with a Concentration of 0.2 or 0.4 mg/mL: Reconstitute 2 vials (each containing 50 mg of lepirudin) with 1 mL each using either Water for Injection USP or 0.9% Sodium Chloride Injection USP. The final concentrations of 0.2 or 0.4 mg/mL are obtained by transferring the entire contents of both vials into an infusion bag containing 500 mL or 250 mL, respectively, of 0.9% Sodium Chloride Injection USP or 5% Dextrose Injection.

Table 10: Refludan

Standard Bolus Injection Volumes According to Body Weight for a 5 mg/mL Concentration

Body Weight (kg)	Injection Volume: Dosage 0.4 mg/kg (mL)	Injection Volume: Dosage 0.2 mg/kg[a] (mL)
<50	Adjust injection volume for body weight: (0.4×BW)/5=injection volume (mL)	Adjust injection volume for body weight: (0.2×BW)/5=injection volume (mL)
50	4.0	2.0
60	4.8	2.4
70	5.6	2.8
80	6.4	3.2
90	7.2	3.6
100[b]	8.0[b]	4.0[b]
≥110[c]	8.8[c]	4.4[c]

[a] Dosage recommended for all patients with renal insufficiency (see Monitoring and Adjustment of Therapy, Renal Impairment).
[b] Highest recommended initial dose in ACS patients.
[c] Highest recommended initial dose in HIT patients.

The infusion rate (mL/h) is to be set according to body weight (see Table 11 and Initial Dosage).

Table 11: Refludan

Standard Infusion Rates According to Body Weight[a]

Body Weight (kg)	Infusion Rate at 0.15 mg/kg/h: 500 mL Infusion Bag 0.2 mg/mL (mL/h)	Infusion Rate at 0.15 mg/kg/h: 250 mL Infusion Bag 0.4 mg/mL (mL/h)
<50	Adjust infusion rate for body weight: (0.15×BW)/0.2=infusion rate (mL/h)	Adjust infusion rate for body weight: (0.15×BW)/0.4=infusion rate (mL/h)
50	38	19
60	45	23
70	53	26
80	60	30
90	68	34
100[b]	75[b]	38[b]
≥110[c]	83[c]	41[c]

[a] For dosage adjustment in patients with renal impairment, please refer to Table 9.
[b] Highest recommended initial dose in ACS patients.
[c] Highest recommended initial dose in HIT patients.

The i.v. infusion solution remains stable for up to 24 hours at room temperature.

SUPPLIED: Each vial of sterile, white freeze-dried powder contains: lepirudin 50 mg. Nonmedicinal ingredients: mannitol and sodium hydroxide (for pH adjustment). pH of approximately 7. Preservative-free. Single use vials of 2 mL. Packages of 10. Do not use past expiry date on labels. Unopened vials should be stored between 2 to 25°C.

Refresh™
polyvinyl alcohol
Ocular Lubricant

Allergan

SUPPLIED: Each unit dose container of 0.4 mL contains: polyvinyl alcohol 1.4%. Also contains povidone, purified water and sodium chloride. May also contain hydrochloric acid or sodium hydroxide to adjust pH. Preservative-free. Use immediately after opening. Do not store opened container.

Refresh® Celluvisc®
carboxymethylcellulose sodium
Ocular Lubricant

Allergan

SUPPLIED: Each unit-dose container of 0.4 mL contains: carboxymethylcellulose sodium 1%. Nonmedicinal ingredients: calcium chloride, potassium chloride, sodium chloride and sodium lactate. Preservative-free.

Refresh® Eye Allergy Relief
antazoline phosphate—naphazoline HCl
Antihistamine—Ophthalmic Decongestant

Allergan

SUPPLIED: Sterile ophthalmic solution containing: antazoline phosphate 0.51% (w/v) and naphazoline hydrochloride 0.051% (w/v). Nonmedicinal ingredients: benzalkonium chloride 0.004% (as preservative), edetate disodium, Liquifilm (polyvinyl alcohol), povidone, sodium acetate and sodium chloride. Plastic dropper bottles of 15 mL. Protect from light. Keep bottle tightly closed. Keep out of reach of children.

Refresh® Lacri-Lube® S.O.P.®
white petrolatum—mineral oil—lanolin alcohols
Ocular Lubricant

Allergan

SUPPLIED: Each g of sterile, bland, nonmedicated, preservative-free ophthalmic ointment contains: white petrolatum USP, mineral oil USP and lanolin alcohols NF. Tubes of 3.5 and 7 g.

Refresh Liquigel™
carboxymethylcellulose sodium
Lubricant Eye Drops

Allergan

SUPPLIED: Each mL of sterile solution contains: carboxymethylcellulose sodium 1.0%. Nonmedicinal ingredients: boric acid, calcium chloride, magnesium chloride, potassium chloride, purified water, Purite (stabilized oxychloro complex), sodium borate and sodium chloride. May also contain sodium hydroxide to adjust pH. Plastic bottles of 15 and 30 mL. Boxes of 12×3 mL.

Refresh Plus™
carboxymethylcellulose sodium
Ocular Lubricant

Allergan

Refresh Tears™
carboxymethylcellulose sodium
Ocular Lubricant with Purite

Allergan

Refresh Contacts™
carboxymethylcellulose sodium
Ocular Lubricant with Purite

Allergan

SUPPLIED: Unit Dose: Each unit-dose container of 0.4 mL contains: carboxymethylcellulose sodium 0.5%. Nonmedicinal ingredients: calcium chloride, magnesium chloride, potassium chloride, sodium chloride and sodium lactate. Preservative-free. Boxes of 30.

Multi-dose: Each mL of sterile solution contains: carboxymethylcellulose sodium 0.5%. Nonmedicinal ingredients: boric acid, calcium chloride, magnesium chloride, potassium chloride, purified water, Purite (stabilized oxychloro complex) and sodium chloride. Plastic bottles of 3 and 15 mL and boxes of 4×15 mL.

Multi-dose: Each mL of sterile solution contains: carboxymethylcellulose sodium 0.5%. Nonmedicinal ingredients: boric acid, calcium chloride, magnesium chloride, potassium chloride, purified water, Purite (stabilized oxychloro complex) and sodium chloride. Plastic bottles of 15 mL.

Refresh Redness Relief
naphazoline HCl
Ophthalmic Decongestant

Allergan

SUPPLIED: Sterile ophthalmic solution containing: naphazoline hydrochloride 0.1% (w/v). Nonmedicinal ingredients: benzalkonium chloride 0.004% (as preservative), citric acid, edetate disodium, Liquifilm (polyvinyl alcohol), sodium chloride and sodium citrate. Plastic dropper bottles of 15 mL. Store between 15 and 25°C. Keep out of reach of children.

Refresh Ultra™
boric acid—castor oil—glycerin
Lubricant Eye Drops

Allergan

SUPPLIED: Each bottle of white, opaque emulsion contains the following nonmedicinal ingredients: boric acid, Carbomer, castor oil, glycerin, polysorbate 80, purified water, PURITE (stabilized oxychloro complex) and sodium hydroxide. Green opaque LDPE bottles of 15 and 30 mL.

Regranex® 🅿
becaplermin
Wound Healing Growth Factor

Janssen-Ortho

Date of Preparation: December 30, 1998
Date of Revision: July 15, 2009

PHARMACOLOGY: Becaplermin is a recombinant human platelet-derived growth factor (rhPDGF). It is a homodimer produced by insertion of the gene for the B chain of platelet-derived growth factor into the yeast, *S. cerevisiae*. Becaplermin has a molecular weight of approximately 25 kD and is composed of 2 identical polypeptide chains (each composed of 109 amino acids) that are bound together by disulfide bonds. It has biological activity similar to that of naturally occurring platelet-derived growth factor, which includes promoting the chemotactic recruitment and proliferation of cells involved in wound repair. In animal wound models, the predominant effect of becaplermin is to enhance the formation of granulation tissue.

REGRANEX is a preserved gel, containing 100 µg of becaplermin per g of gel. Becaplermin contains the following inactive ingredients: sodium carboxymethylcellulose, methylparaben, propylparaben, m-cresol and L-lysine HCl.

Becaplermin has been shown to be effective in increasing the incidence of complete wound healing and in decreasing the time to complete wound healing of full-thickness, lower extremity diabetic ulcers.

Pharmacokinetics: Ten patients with Stage III or IV [as defined in the International Association of Enterostomal Therapy (IAET) guide to chronic wound staging] lower extremity diabetic ulcers received topical applications of becaplermin at a dose of 0.32 to 2.95 µg/kg (7 µg/cm^2) daily for 14 days. Six patients had non-quantifiable PDGF levels at baseline and throughout the study, 2 patients had PDGF levels at baseline which did not increase substantially, and 2 patients had PDGF levels that increased sporadically above their baseline values during the 14-day study period.

INDICATIONS: REGRANEX becaplermin is indicated to promote healing of full-thickness, lower extremity diabetic ulcers. Becaplermin increases the incidence of complete wound healing and decreases the time to complete wound healing. 100% wound closure was more frequently observed in patients with ulcer size (length × width) <7 cm^2 (see Clinical Experience).

Becaplermin therapy should be used in conjunction with good wound care practices. A good wound care program consists of: initial debridement (to remove all callus and necrotic tissue), pressure relief, moist dressings changed at a frequency to sufficiently maintain a moist wound-healing environment, systemic treatment of wound-related infection if present, and additional debridement as necessary.

Clinical Experience: The effects of becaplermin therapy on the incidence of and time to complete healing in lower extremity diabetic ulcers were assessed in 4 randomized controlled studies. A total of 922 patients with diabetes, without severe peripheral arterial insufficiency, who had full-thickness, lower extremity diabetic ulcers were enrolled. Comparators were placebo gel and/or good wound care alone. In each trial, all patients received a standard regimen of good wound care. Becaplermin was applied once daily. Patients were treated until complete healing, or for a maximum period of 20 weeks. Data from the primary and integrated analyses are presented below.

Three hundred and eighty-two patients with Stage III or IV (IAET guide to chronic wound staging) lower extremity diabetic ulcers, over 90% of whom had Stage III ulcers, were enrolled in the pivotal double-blind study. The results from the study demonstrated that becaplermin treatment significantly increased the incidence of complete healing by 43% when compared to placebo gel (p=0.007, 50% in the becaplermin group vs 35% in the placebo group). Becaplermin treatment also significantly decreased the time to achieve complete healing by 32% (p=0.013; 86 days for becaplermin group vs 127 days for placebo gel, estimated 35th percentile). The best results were seen with ulcers sized <5 cm^2 measured by planimetry, which is equivalent to approximately 7 cm^2 when measured length × width.

An integrated analysis of the 4 controlled trials was conducted in patients with baseline ulcer areas (length x width) of up to approximately 7 cm^2. Seven hundred and seventy-four patients (84% of the study population) in the 4 trials had baseline ulcer areas within this range. In these patients, becaplermin treatment significantly increased the incidence of complete healing compared to placebo gel (p=0.009, logistic regression) and significantly reduced the time to complete healing by 30% (p=0.008; 92 days for becaplermin group vs 131 days for placebo gel, estimated 35th percentile).

CONTRAINDICATIONS: REGRANEX becaplermin is contraindicated in patients with known hypersensitivity to any component of this product (e.g., parabens); known neoplasm(s) at the site(s) of application.

WARNINGS AND PRECAUTIONS:

Serious Warnings and Precautions
Malignancies distant from the site of application have occurred in becaplermin users in both a clinical study and in postmarketing use.

An increased rate of mortality secondary to malignancy was observed in patients treated with 3 or more tubes of REGRANEX Gel in a post-marketing retrospective cohort study. REGRANEX Gel should only be used when the benefits can be expected to outweigh the risks. (See Contraindications and Warnings and Precautions.)

REGRANEX Gel contains becaplermin, a recombinant human platelet-derived growth factor, which promotes cellular proliferation and angiogenesis (see Pharmacology). Malignancies distant from the site of application have occurred in becaplermin users in both a clinical study and in postmarketing use, and an increased rate of death from systemic malignancies was seen in patients who have received 3 or more tubes of REGRANEX Gel. The benefits and risks of becaplermin treatment should be carefully evaluated before prescribing.

Application Site Reactions: If application site reactions occur, the possibility of sensitization or irritation caused by parabens or m-cresol should be considered.

Immunogenicity: Becaplermin may have a very small potential to elicit an antibody response when applied topically once daily for up to 20 weeks; however, none of the patients that received REGRANEX therapy developed neutralizing antibodies against becaplermin

Drug Interactions: It is not known whether becaplermin interacts with other topical medications applied to the ulcer site. Consequently, it is recommended that REGRANEX not be applied to the ulcer site in conjunction with other topical medications.

Carcinogenesis, Mutagenesis, Impairment of Fertility: Becaplermin was not genotoxic in a battery of in vitro assay testing including endpoints of bacterial and mammalian cell point mutation, chromosomal aberration, and DNA damage/repair. Becaplermin was also not mutagenic in an in vivo assay for the induction of micronuclei in mouse bone marrow cells.

Carcinogenesis and reproductive toxicity studies have not been conducted with becaplermin.

Pregnancy: Animal reproductive toxicity studies have not been conducted with becaplermin. There are no adequate and well-controlled studies in pregnant women. Therefore, REGRANEX therapy should not be used in pregnant women.

Lactation: It is not known whether becaplermin is excreted in human milk. Therefore, becaplermin therapy should be used with caution in nursing women.

Children: Safety and effectiveness in children and adolescents under the age of 18 years have not been established.

Potential Effect on Bones and Connective Tissues: The effects of becaplermin on exposed joints, tendons, ligaments and bone have not been established in humans. Data in rats suggest that, when injected near bones, becaplermin may cause a temporal and potentially reversible accelerated bone modeling.

ADVERSE EFFECTS: Clinical Trial Data: The safety of REGRANEX Gel was evaluated in 1883 adult patients who participated in 17 clinical trials (diabetic ulcer trials with 1292 patients and non-diabetic ulcer trials with 591 patients) of REGRANEX and placebo and/or standard therapy (saline dressing). These 1883 patients had at least one topical administration of REGRANEX and provided safety data.

Adverse drug reactions reported by ≥1% of patients treated with REGRANEX in these trials are shown in Table 1.

Table 1: REGRANEX

Adverse Drug Reactions Reported by ≥1% REGRANEX-treated Patients in 17 Clinical Trials of REGRANEX

System/Organ Class Adverse Reaction	REGRANEX (n=1883) %	Placebo (n=1069) %	Standard Therapy (n=190) %	p-value[a]
Infections and Infestations				
Infected skin ulcer	12.3	11.9	18.9	0.725
Cellulitis	10.3	7.5	18.9	0.011
Osteomyelitis	7.2	5.4	14.2	0.058

[a] Comparison between REGRANEX and placebo.

Postmarketing Data: Adverse drug reactions first identified during postmarketing experience with REGRANEX are included in Table 2. The frequencies are provided according to the following convention: Very common: ≥1/10. Common: ≥1/100 and <1/10. Uncommon: ≥1/1000 and <1/100. Rare: ≥1/10 000 and <1/1000. Very rare: <1/10 000, including isolated reports.

In Table 2, ADRs are presented by frequency category based on spontaneous reporting rates.

In a follow-up study, 491 (75%) of 651 subjects from two randomized, controlled trials of becaplermin gel 0.01% were followed for a median of approximately 20 months to identify malignancies diagnosed after the end of the trials. Eight of 291 subjects (3%) from the becaplermin group and two of 200 subjects (1%) from the vehicle/standard of care group were diagnosed with cancers during the follow-up period, a relative risk of 2.7, (95% confidence interval 0.6-12.8). The types of cancers varied and all were remote from the treatment site.

In a retrospective study of a medical claims database, patients who received REGRANEX between January 1, 1998 and June 30, 2003 were followed through December 31, 2003. Cancer rates and overall cancer mortality were compared between 1622 patients who used REGRANEX Gel and 2809 matched comparators. Estimates of the incidence rates reported below may be under-reported due to limited follow-up for each individual.

- The incidence rate for all cancers was 10.2 per 1000 person years for patients treated with REGRANEX Gel and 9.1 per 1000 person years for the comparators. Adjusted for several possible confounders, the rate ratio was 1.2, (95% confidence interval 0.7-1.9). Types of cancers varied and were remote from the site of treatment.
- The incidence rate for mortality from all cancers was 1.6 per 1000 person years for those who received REGRANEX Gel and 0.9 per 1000 person years for the comparators. The adjusted rate ratio was 1.8 (95% confidence interval 0.7-4.9). Additional follow-up (not part of the original study plan) to include deaths through 2006 changed these mortality estimates to a rate of 0.9 per 1000 person years for those who received REGRANEX gel, and 1.0 per 1000 person years for the comparators, an adjusted rate ratio of 1.0 (95% confidence interval 0.5-2.3).
- The incidence rate for mortality from all cancers among patients who received 3 or more tubes of REGRANEX gel was 3.9 per 1000 person years and 0.9 per 1000 person years in the comparators. The adjusted rate ratio for cancer mortality among those who received 3 or more tubes relative to those who received none was 5.2, (95% confidence interval 1.6-17.6). Additional follow-up (not part of the original study plan) to include deaths through 2006 changed these mortality estimates to a rate of 2.0 per 1000 person years for those who received three or more tubes, and 1.0 per 1000 person years for the comparators, an adjusted rate ratio of 2.4 (95% confidence interval 0.8-7.4).

Table 2: REGRANEX

Adverse Drug Reactions Identified During Postmarketing Experience with REGRANEX by Frequency Category Estimated from Spontaneous Reporting Rates

Nervous System Disorders	
Rare	Burning sensation[a]
Skin and Subcutaneous Tissue Disorders	
Very rare	Rash Erythema[b]

[a] The bundled term burning sensation consists of the preferred terms burning sensation, skin burning sensation, and application site irritation, all of which referred specifically to burning at the application site.
[b] Refers to erythema at the application site.

OVERDOSE:
There are limited data on the effects of becaplermin overdose.

For management of a suspected drug overdose, CPhA recommends that you contact your **regional Poison Control Centre**. See the *CPS* Directory section for a list of Poison Control Centres.

DOSAGE: Becaplermin should be applied topically as a continuous thin layer to the entire ulcerated area(s) once daily using a clean application aid (e.g., tongue depressor or cotton swab). The site(s) of application should then be covered with a saline dressing that maintains a moist wound-healing environment and left in place for approximately 12 hours. The dressing should then be removed and the ulcer rinsed with saline or water to remove residual gel and covered again with a second moist dressing (without REGRANEX Gel) for the remainder of the day.

Becaplermin treatment should continue once daily until complete healing is achieved. Becaplermin should be discontinued if complete healing has not occurred after 20 weeks of therapy or if a 30% reduction in ulcer size is not observed after 10 weeks of treatment (see Warnings and Precautions).

INFORMATION FOR THE PATIENT: Published in e-CPS, available by subscription at www.e-cps.ca.

SUPPLIED: Each g of clear, colorless to straw-colored preserved gel contains: becaplermin 100 µg (0.01%), rhPDGF-BB. Nonmedicinal ingredients: glacial acetic acid, L-lysine HCl, m-cresol, methylparaben, propylparaben, sodium acetate trihydrate, sodium carboxymethylcellulose, sodium chloride and water for injection. Tubes of 15 g. Store refrigerated at 2 to 8°C. **Do not freeze.**

(Shown in Product Identification Section)

Rejuva-A® Ⓟ

tretinoin

Agent for the Treatment of Photodamaged Skin

Stiefel, a GSK company

Date of Preparation: October 2, 1990
Date of Revision: January 22, 2002

PHARMACOLOGY: Tretinoin, a member of the retinoid class of compounds, is both pharmacologically and structurally related to vitamin A which regulates epithelial cell growth and differentiation. Retinoic acid may exert its effects at the molecular level by binding to specific steroid-like nuclear receptors known as retinoic acid receptors. Binding of retinoic acid to a retinoic acid receptor will promote events at the cellular level by regulating gene transcription and affecting activities such as cellular differentiation and proliferation but the exact mechanism underlying these processes remain to be elucidated.

Topical tretinoin has been reported to correct many of the structural abnormalities of photoaged skin. Tretinoin has been shown to produce epidermal and dermal changes. At the epidermal level, tretinoin increased the epidermal thickness (acanthosis) and the mean granular layer, decreased tonofilament and desmosome strength and increased secretion of a glycosaminoglycan-like substance into the intercellular space. In addition, the cohesion of the epidermal cells and activity of the melanocytes are reduced.

Functional changes in the epidermis include an increase in trans-epidermal water loss and permeability. At the level of the dermis, vasodilatation and angiogenesis of the superficial vasculature, along with increased papillary dermal collagen, have been reported.

The long-term (1 year) safety and efficacy of tretinoin cream in the treatment of photoaging was evaluated during a double-blind, randomized, parallel group, multicentre, placebo controlled study. A total of 147 patients (110 active, 37 placebo) were entered; all were caucasian with chronic, moderate to severe actinically damaged facial skin. The patients applied the medication over their entire face once a day before retiring and were evaluated by the investigators after 1, 3, 6, 9 and 12 months of therapy.

Among the various expressions of the entity of the disease, significant clinical benefits were demonstrated for tretinoin cream versus placebo for the following: reduction in fine wrinkles from Month 3; reduction in moderate, moderately severe and severe coarse wrinkles from Month 6; reduction in the severity of dermatosis at Month 9.

In addition, histological findings demonstrated that skin treated with tretinoin cream showed significant decrease in the thickness of the stratum corneum and increases in the thickness of the stratum granulosum and spinulosum. Skin receiving the placebo cream showed no significant difference in the thickness of the different epidermal strata.

INDICATIONS: For the treatment of photodamaged skin (heliodermatitis).

The safety and efficacy of tretinoin cream (0.025%) for the prevention and treatment of actinic keratosis has not been established.

CONTRAINDICATIONS: Patients with known hypersensitivity to retinoids or to any ingredient contained in the preparation.

WARNINGS: Tretinoin cream should be used as part of a comprehensive skin protection program, including use of sunscreen products and protective clothing.

Tretinoin cream is intended for external use only and should be kept away from the nostrils and other mucous membranes because of its irritant effect. Avoid the angles of the nose and nasolabial fold (if treatment in these areas is necessary, apply very sparingly). Topical use may induce severe local erythema and peeling at the site of application. If the degree of local irritation warrants, patients should be directed to use the medication less frequently, discontinue use temporarily or discontinue use altogether. Tretinoin has been reported to cause severe irritation of eczematous skin, and tretinoin cream should only be used with utmost caution in patients with this condition.

Pregnancy: **Topical tretinoin should be used by women of childbearing years only after contraceptive counseling. It is recommended that topical tretinoin should not be used by pregnant women.**

There have been rare reports of birth defects among babies born to women exposed to **topical** tretinoin during pregnancy. However, there are no well-controlled prospective studies of the use of topical tretinoin in pregnant women. A retrospective study of mothers exposed to topical tretinoin during the first trimester of pregnancy found no increase in the incidence of birth defects.

Topical retinoid teratology studies in rats and rabbits have been inconclusive. As with all retinoids, tretinoin administered **orally** at high doses is teratogenic.

Lactation: **It is not known whether tretinoin is excreted in human milk. Nevertheless, a decision should be made whether to discontinue nursing or to discontinue the drug, taking into account the importance of the drug to the mother.**

Children: **Safety and effectiveness in children have not been established.**

PRECAUTIONS: General: Care should be used when tretinoin cream is applied to treat wrinkles around the eyes (Crow's feet) and mouth.

Exposure to sunlight and sun lamps should be avoided or minimized during the use of REJUVA-A, because of heightened susceptibility to UV radiation as a result of the use of tretinoin.

If sunburn occurs, it is advisable to interrupt therapy until the severe erythema and peeling subside. **Patients whose occupations require considerable exposure to the sun and those inherently sensitive to the sun should exercise particular caution and are advised to use sunburn protectant products of at least SPF 15. Protective clothing over treated areas is recommended when sun exposure cannot be avoided.**

Carcinogenesis: Carcinogenic studies have not been conducted with tretinoin cream. Studies in hairless albino mice suggest that tretinoin may accelerate the tumorigenic potential of ultraviolet radiation. Although the significance of these studies to man is not clear, patients should avoid or minimize exposure to sun.

Information to Be Provided to the Patient: A patient information leaflet has been prepared and is included with each package of Rejuva-A (see Information for the Patient).

Drug Interactions: Concomitant topical medication should be used with caution during therapy with tretinoin cream because of possible intensified reactions. Particular caution should be exercised when using cosmetics with a strong drying effect and products with high concentration of alcohol, as well as those containing a peeling agent concomitantly (such as sulfur, resorcinol, benzoyl peroxide or salicylic acid) with tretinoin cream. It may be advisable to "rest" a patient's skin until the effects of previously used peeling agents subside before initiating tretinoin cream therapy.

Tretinoin is compatible with almost all oral drugs except for photosensitizers. In treating thin-skinned, sensitive regions such as the neck area with tretinoin, it is recommended to apply tretinoin cream thinly every third night, in the beginning, and then every other night as tolerance develops.

Avoid or minimize exposure to sunlight and sun lamps because REJUVA-A heightens the susceptibility of the skin to the adverse effects of the sun.

If sunburn occurs, it is advisable to interrupt therapy until the severe erythema and peeling subside. Patients whose occupations require considerable exposure to the sun should exercise particular caution and advised to use a sunscreen of at least SPF 15. Protective clothing over treated areas is recommended when exposure cannot be avoided.

ADVERSE EFFECTS: In the long-term clinical trial with tretinoin cream, erythema and peeling/dryness were the most reported side effects in the tretinoin cream group with only 5 of 110 patients from this group withdrawing because of adverse events (erythema and peeling).

The skin of certain sensitive individuals, particularly those with fair complexions, may become excessively red, edematous, blistered or crusted when exposed to tretinoin cream. Pain, burning sensation, tenderness, irritation or pruritus have also been occasionally reported. If any of these effects occur, the medication should be discontinued until the integrity of the skin has been restored or the treatment schedule adjusted to the level the patient can tolerate. Temporary hyper- or hypopigmentation has been reported with repeated application of tretinoin. To date, all adverse clinical effects of tretinoin encountered have been reversible upon discontinuance of therapy. In many instances, reinstitution of therapy with tretinoin failed to produce the adverse effect previously experienced.

OVERDOSE:

Symptoms: Topical: If medication is applied excessively, marked redness, peeling or discomfort may occur.

Inadvertent oral ingestion of tretinoin cream may lead to the same adverse effects as those associated with excessive oral intake of vitamin A including teratogenesis in women of childbearing years. Therefore, in such cases, pregnancy testing should be carried out in women of childbearing years.

For management of a suspected drug overdose, CPhA recommends that you contact your **regional Poison Control Centre**. See the *CPS* Directory section for a list of Poison Control Centres.

DOSAGE: Tretinoin cream is especially suitable for the treatment of sun sensitive Type I and II skin types e.g., fair skinned people with red or blond hair and blue or hazel eyes, who always burn easily, severely with no or minimal tanning.

Tretinoin cream should be applied to the affected area once a day just before retiring. The area under treatment should be thoroughly cleansed with a mild soap and water and patted dry with a soft towel followed by application of tretinoin cream with a gentle rubbing motion using the fingertips.

It is recommended to start the therapy by applying one pea-size amount to the forehead and spread it evenly over the entire face. After tolerance to the medication is established, the dose may be doubled by applying a pea-size amount to each temple. For those patients who experience excessive irritation or discomfort, the frequency of application should be decreased to every other night or even every third night.

Treatment should be discontinued if a severe local inflammatory response is experienced. In cases where it has been necessary to discontinue therapy or to reduce the frequency of application, therapy may be reinstituted when the adverse effects have ceased.

Therapeutic results will occur gradually. Nine to twelve months of therapy may be required before beneficial effects are seen. At that time, frequency of application may be reduced to 2 or 3 times/week.

INFORMATION FOR THE PATIENT: Published in e-CPS, available by subscription at www.e-cps.ca.

SUPPLIED: Rejuva-A Cream is available in Rejuva-A Skin Revitalizing System which also contains Rejuva Moisturizing Day Cream SPF 30.

Rejuva-A: Each g of cream contains: tretinoin 0.025% in a moisturizing cream base. Nonmedicinal ingredients: butylated hydroxytoluene, carbomer 934, cyclomethicone, diisopropyl adipate, germaben II, glycerin, light mineral oil, phenyl trimethicone, polysorbate 60, purified water, sodium hydroxide, sorbitan monostearate and stearyl alcohol. Tubes of 20 g. Store between 15 and 30°C.

Rejuva Moisturizing Day Cream SPF 30: Each g of cream contains: Parsol 1789, Parsol MCX and Parsol 5000. Nonmedicinal ingredients: butylated hydroxytoluene, carbomer 934, cyclomethicone, diisopropyl adipate, germaben II, glycerin, isoarachidyl neopentanoate, light mineral oil, phenyl trimethicone, polysorbate 60, purified water, sodium hydroxide and stearyl alcohol. Tubes of 40 g. Store between 15 and 30°C.

Relenza® ℞
zanamivir
Antiviral Agent

GlaxoSmithKline

Date of Revision: November 12, 2009

SUMMARY PRODUCT INFORMATION:

Route of Administration	Dosage Form/ Strength	Clinically Relevant Nonmedicinal Ingredients
Oral inhalation	Dry powder 5 mg/blister	Lactose

INDICATIONS AND CLINICAL USE: Treatment of Influenza: RELENZA (zanamivir) is indicated for treatment of uncomplicated acute illness due to influenza A and B virus in adults and pediatric patients 7 years of age and older, who have been symptomatic for no more than 2 days. No data are available to support zanamivir safety and efficacy in patients who receive treatment after 48 hours of symptoms.

This indication is based on placebo-controlled studies conducted in North America, the Southern Hemisphere, and Europe during their respective influenza seasons. The magnitude of treatment effect varied between studies, with possible relationships to population-related factors including amount of symptomatic relief medication used.

RELENZA, when taken as recommended for treatment of influenza, alleviates the symptoms and reduces their duration.

Prophylaxis of Influenza: RELENZA is indicated in adults and pediatric patients 7 years of age and older for prophylaxis of influenza.

Important Information on Use of RELENZA: RELENZA is not recommended for treatment or prophylaxis of influenza in individuals with underlying airways disease (such as asthma or chronic obstructive pulmonary disease [see Warnings and Precautions]) due to risk of serious bronchospasm.

RELENZA has not been proven effective for prophylaxis of influenza in the nursing home setting.

RELENZA is not a substitute for influenza vaccination on an annual basis as recommended by the National Advisory Committee on Immunization (NACI).

Geriatrics (≥65 years of age): In clinical trials, the safety profile of RELENZA did not appear to vary with increasing age and no overall differences in the safety and efficacy were observed between the elderly and younger patients. A brief discussion can be found in Warnings and Precautions, Special Populations, Geriatrics (≥65 years of age).

Pediatrics: Safety and effectiveness of RELENZA for treatment of influenza have not been established in pediatric patients under 7 years of age. Safety and effectiveness of RELENZA for prophylaxis of influenza have not been assessed in pediatric patients under 5 years of age. Efficacy data from the age of 5 to 7 years are limited.

CONTRAINDICATIONS: RELENZA (zanamivir) is contraindicated in patients with a known or suspected hypersensitivity to zanamivir or any component of the zanamivir inhalation powder (including lactose, which contains milk protein).

WARNINGS AND PRECAUTIONS:

Serious Warnings and Precautions
There have been reports of patients being treated for influenza who have experienced bronchospasm and decline in respiratory function. Many but not all of these patients had underlying airways disease such as asthma or chronic obstructive pulmonary disease. There have been cases of respiratory arrest, including deaths, in which a contribution from RELENZA (zanamivir) cannot be excluded. RELENZA should be discontinued in any patient who develops bronchospasm or a decline in respiratory function; immediate treatment and hospitalization may be required. All patients should be advised of the risk of bronchospasm with RELENZA.

RELENZA is not generally recommended for treatment of patients with severe underlying airways disease because of the risk of serious adverse events and because efficacy has not been demonstrated in this population (see Warnings and Precautions, Respiratory).

General: Due to the limited number of patients with severe asthma or other severe chronic respiratory diseases, patients with chronic illnesses or immunocompromised patients who have been treated, it has not been possible to demonstrate the efficacy and safety of RELENZA in these groups.

Vaccination of persons at high risk each year before the influenza season is currently recognized as the most effective measure for reducing the impact of influenza. The use of zanamivir should not affect the evaluation of individuals for annual influenza vaccination, in accordance to "Health Canada, An Advisory Committee Statement, National Advisory Committee on Immunization (NACI), Statement on Influenza Vaccination for the current Year/Season".

Patients should be instructed in the use of the DISKHALER inhalation device and instructions should include a demonstration wherever possible. Patients should be advised to read and follow carefully the patient instructions to ensure safe and effective use. Patients should be advised to finish the full course of treatment or prophylaxis therapy as prescribed.

Hepatic/Biliary/Pancreatic: The pharmacokinetics of zanamivir have not been investigated in patients with impaired hepatic function; doses of up to 1200 mg IV in healthy adults did not show evidence of hepatic metabolism.

Immune/Infection: Serious bacterial infections may begin with influenza-like symptoms or may co-exist with or occur as complications during the course of influenza. RELENZA has not been shown to prevent such complications.

Allergic-like reactions, including facial and oropharyngeal edema, bronchospasm, laryngospasm, dyspnea, urticaria, serious skin rashes and anaphylaxis have been reported in post-marketing experience. RELENZA should be discontinued and immediate medical attention sought by any patient who develops an allergic reaction or if one is suspected.

Neurologic: There have been post-marketing reports (mostly from Japan) of delirium and abnormal behaviour leading to injury in patients with influenza who were receiving neuraminidase inhibitors, including RELENZA. Because these events were reported voluntarily during clinical practice, estimates of frequency cannot be made, but they appear to be uncommon based on usage data for RELENZA. These events were reported primarily among pediatric patients and often had an abrupt onset. The contribution of RELENZA to these events has not been established. Patients with influenza receiving RELENZA should be closely monitored for signs of abnormal behaviour. If neuropsychiatric symptoms occur, the risks and benefits of continuing treatment should be evaluated for each patient.

It should be noted that influenza infection itself can be complicated with a variety of neurologic and behavioural symptoms which can include events such as seizures, hallucinations, delirium, and abnormal behaviour, in some cases resulting in fatal outcomes. These events may occur in the setting of encephalitis or encephalopathy but can occur without obvious severe disease.

Renal: At the therapeutic daily dose of 20 mg, bioavailability is low (10-20%), and as a result, systemic exposure of patients to RELENZA is limited. However, after a single IV dose of 4 mg or 2 mg of zanamivir in volunteers with mild or moderate, or severe renal impairment, respectively, significant decreases in renal clearance (and hence total clearance: normals 5.3 L/h, mild/moderate 2.7 L/h, and severe 0.8 L/h; median values) and significant increases in half-life (normals 3.1 h, mild/moderate 4.7 h, and severe 18.5 h; median values) and systemic exposure were observed. Safety and efficacy have not been documented in the presence of severe renal insufficiency after repeated dosing.

Respiratory: Safety and efficacy of RELENZA have not been demonstrated in patients with severe underlying chronic pulmonary disease or severe asthma due to limited number of patients treated. Therefore, RELENZA is not generally recommended for treatment in such patients. Serious adverse events have been reported in patients with underlying chronic pulmonary disease and in patients with severe or decompensated chronic obstructive pulmonary disease or asthma (see Serious Warnings and Precautions).

If treatment with RELENZA is considered for a patient with an underlying airway disease, the potential risks and benefits should be carefully weighed. The patients should be advised of the risk of bronchospasm. If a decision is made to prescribe RELENZA for such a patient, this should be done only under conditions of careful monitoring of respiratory function, close observation and appropriate supportive care including availability of fast-acting bronchodilators. Patients should be instructed to contact their physician if they experience increased respiratory symptoms during treatment such as worsening wheezing, shortness of breath, or other signs or symptoms of bronchospasm (see Serious Warnings and Precautions) and to discontinue RELENZA. Patients scheduled to take inhaled bronchodilators at the same time as RELENZA should be advised to use their bronchodilators before taking RELENZA.

In a placebo controlled study in patients with predominantly mild/moderate asthma and/or Chronic Obstructive Pulmonary Disease (COPD), RELENZA was shown to be effective and well tolerated for the treatment of influenza. There was no evidence of a difference between RELENZA and placebo in forced expiratory volume in one second (FEV_1) or peak expiratory flow rate (PEFR) measured after the end of treatment.

Skin: Severe skin reactions including erythema multiforme, Stevens-Johnson syndrome and toxic epidermal necrolysis have been reported in post-marketing experience.

Special Populations: Pregnant Women: The safe use of zanamivir during pregnancy has not been established. There are no adequate and well controlled studies of zanamivir in pregnant women. There is no information on placental transfer in humans. Reproductive studies performed in rats and rabbits indicated that placental transfer of zanamivir occurs. In these animals, fetal blood concentrations of zanamivir were significantly lower than zanamivir concentrations in the maternal blood. Studies in rats did not show any evidence of teratogenicity, impairment of fertility or malformations. One embryo/fetal study, was conducted using subcutaneous administration of zanamivir, 3 times daily at doses of 1, 9 or 80 mg/kg during days 7 to 17 of pregnancy. Based on AUC measurements, the high dose in the study produced an exposure greater than 1000 times the human exposure at the proposed clinical dose. There was an increase in the incidence rates of a variety of minor skeleton alterations and variants in the exposed offspring in this study. The individual incidence rates of each skeletal alteration or variant, in many but not in all cases, remained within the range of background rates of the historical occurrence in the rat strain studied.

RELENZA should not be used in pregnancy, especially during the first trimester, unless the possible benefit to the patient is thought to outweigh any possible risk to the fetus.

Nursing Women: Studies in rats have demonstrated that zanamivir is excreted in milk. Nursing mothers, however, should be instructed that it is not known whether zanamivir is excreted in human milk. Because many drugs are excreted in human milk, caution should be exercised when RELENZA is administered to a nursing mother.

Pediatrics: Safety and effectiveness of RELENZA for treatment of influenza have not been established in pediatric patients under 7 years of age. Safety and effectiveness of RELENZA for prophylaxis of influenza have not been assessed in pediatric patients under 5 years of age. Efficacy data from the age of 5 to 7 years are limited. Prescribers should carefully evaluate the ability of young children to use the delivery system if prescription of RELENZA is considered. When RELENZA is prescribed for children, it should be used only under adult supervision and with attention to proper use of the delivery system.

Geriatrics (≥65 years of age): At the therapeutic daily dose of 20 mg, bioavailability of zanamivir in young healthy adults is low (10-20%), and as a result systemic exposure of patients to zanamivir is limited. The bioavailability of zanamivir in elderly individuals has not been determined. However, a total of 83 elderly patients (aged ≥65 years old) received inhaled zanamivir at a dose of 10 mg twice daily, or greater, for the treatment of symptomatic influenza in completed clinical trials. Of the total number of patients who received zanamivir 10 mg once daily for prophylaxis of influenza in households and community settings in 4 clinical studies of RELENZA, 954 were aged 65 and over. The safety profile did not appear to vary with increasing age and no overall differences in the safety and efficacy were observed between the elderly and younger patients. However, greater sensitivity of some older patients to medications in general, cannot be ruled out. In 2 additional studies of RELENZA for prophylaxis of influenza in the nursing home setting, efficacy was not demonstrated. Elderly subjects may need assistance with use of the device.

ADVERSE REACTIONS: Adverse Drug Reaction Overview: See Warnings and Precautions for information about risk of serious adverse events such as bronchospasm and allergic-like reactions, and for safety information in patients with underlying respiratory disease.

Clinical Trial Adverse Drug Reactions: Because clinical trials are conducted under very specific conditions the adverse reaction rates observed in the clinical trials may not reflect the rates observed in practice and should not be compared to the rates in the clinical trials of another drug. Adverse drug reaction information from clinical trials is useful for identifying drug-related adverse events and for approximating rates.

Because the placebo consisted of inhaled lactose powder which is also the vehicle for the active drug, some adverse events occurring at similar frequencies in different treatment groups could be related to lactose vehicle inhalation.

Treatment of Influenza: Clinical studies were conducted predominately in young adults, in pediatric patients 5 to 12 years old, and in high risk patients (mostly patients with underlying respiratory disease and/or elderly ≥65 years old). The incidence of adverse events in these trials appeared similar in the RELENZA (zanamivir) and placebo groups. No differences in adverse reactions were observed between these patient groups.

Adverse events that occurred with an incidence ≥1.5% in treatment studies in adults and adolescents are listed in Table 1.

Table 1: RELENZA

Summary of Adverse Events ≥1.5% Incidence During Treatment in Adults and Adolescents

	RELENZA		
Adverse Event	**10 mg b.i.d. Inhaled (n=1132) %**	**All Dosing Regimens[a] (n=2289) %**	**Placebo (Lactose Vehicle) (n=1520) %**
Body as a Whole			
Headaches	2	2	3
Digestive			
Diarrhea	3	3	4
Nausea	3	3	3
Vomiting	1	1	2
Respiratory			
Nasal signs and symptoms	2	3	3
Bronchitis	2	3	3
Cough	2	2	3
Sinusitis	3	2	2
Ear, nose and throat infections	2	1	2
Nervous System			
Dizziness	2	1	<1

[a] Includes studies where RELENZA was administered intranasally (6.4 mg 2 to 4 times per day in addition to inhaled preparation) and/or inhaled more frequently (q.i.d.) than the currently recommended dose.

Additional adverse reactions occurring in less than 1.5% of patients receiving RELENZA and placebo included malaise, fatigue, fever, abdominal pain, myalgia, arthralgia, and urticaria. Other side effects that have been reported, but are not as common include allergic reactions and rashes.

Adverse events that occurred with an incidence ≥1.5% in children receiving treatment doses of RELENZA in two Phase 3 studies are listed in Table 2.

Prophylaxis of Influenza: Family/Household Prophylaxis Studies: Adverse events that occurred with an incidence of ≥1% in the 2 prophylaxis studies are listed in Table 3. This table shows adverse events occurring in patients ≥5 years of age receiving RELENZA 10 mg or placebo inhaled once daily for 10 days.

Community Prophylaxis Studies: Adverse events that occurred with an incidence of ≥1% in 2 prophylaxis studies are listed in Table 4. This table shows adverse events occurring in patients ≥12 years of age receiving RELENZA 10 mg or placebo inhaled once daily for 28 days.

Table 2: RELENZA

Summary of Adverse Events ≥1.5% Incidence During Treatment in Pediatric Patients[a]

Adverse Event	RELENZA 10 mg b.i.d. Inhaled (n=291) %	Placebo (Lactose Vehicle) (n=318) %
Respiratory		
Ear, nose, and throat infections	5	5
Ear, nose, and throat hemorrhage	<1	2
Asthma	<1	2
Cough	<1	2
Digestive		
Vomiting	2	3
Diarrhea	2	2
Nausea	<1	2

[a] Includes a subset of patients receiving RELENZA for treatment of influenza in a prophylaxis study.

Table 3: RELENZA

Summary of Adverse Events ≥1% Incidence During 10 Day Prophylaxis Studies in Adults and Pediatric Patients[a]

Adverse Event	Contact Cases: RELENZA (n=1068) %	Contact Cases: Placebo (n=1059) %
Lower Respiratory		
Viral respiratory infections	13	19
Cough	7	9
Neurologic		
Headaches	13	14
Ear, Nose, and Throat		
Nasal signs and symptoms	12	12
Throat and tonsil discomfort and pain	8	9
Nasal inflammation	1	2
Musculoskeletal		
Muscle pain	3	3
Musculoskeletal pain	1	1
Endocrine and Metabolic		
Feeding problems (decreased or increased appetite and anorexia)	2	2
Gastrointestinal		
Nausea and vomiting	1	2
Diarrhea	1	<1
Non-site Specific		
Malaise and fatigue	5	5
Temperature regulation disturbances (fever and/or chills)	5	4

[a] In prophylaxis studies, symptoms associated with influenza-like illness were captured as adverse events; subjects were enrolled during a winter respiratory season during which time any symptoms that occurred were captured as adverse events.

Table 4: RELENZA *(cont'd)*

Summary of Adverse Events ≥1% Incidence During 28 Day Prophylaxis Studies in Adults and Adolescents[a]

Adverse Event	RELENZA (n=2231) %	Placebo (n=2239) %
Neurologic		
Headaches	24	26
Ear, Nose, and Throat		
Throat and tonsil discomfort and pain	19	20
Nasal signs and symptoms	12	13
Ear, nose, and throat infections	2	2
Viral ear, nose, and throat infections	1	1
Sinusitis	1	1
Lower Respiratory		
Cough	17	18
Viral respiratory infections	3	4
Bronchitis	1	1
Asthma	<1	1
Musculoskeletal		
Muscle pain	8	8
Musculoskeletal pain	6	6
Arthralgia and articular rheumatism	2	<1
Endocrine and Metabolic		
Feeding problems (decreased or increased appetite and anorexia)	4	4
Gastrointestinal		
Nausea and vomiting	2	3
Diarrhea	2	2
Reproduction		
Menstruation symptoms	1	1
Non-site Specific		
Temperature regulation disturbances (fever and/or chills)	9	10
Malaise and fatigue	8	8

[a] In prophylaxis studies, symptoms associated with influenza like illness were captured as adverse events; subjects were enrolled during a winter respiratory season during which time any symptoms that occurred were captured as adverse events.

Abnormal Hematologic and Clinical Chemistry Findings: The most frequent laboratory abnormalities in Phase 3 treatment studies included elevations of liver enzymes and CPK, lymphopenia, and neutropenia. These were reported in similar proportions of zanamivir and lactose vehicle placebo recipients with acute influenza-like illness.

Post-Market Adverse Drug Reactions: Reporting rates determined on the basis of spontaneously reported post-marketing adverse events are generally presumed to underestimate the risks associated with drug treatments.

The following adverse events have been reported spontaneously during post-marketing experience with RELENZA. However, a causal relationship to RELENZA cannot be clearly established for spontaneously reported events.

Cardiac: arrhythmias, syncope, tachycardia.

Gastrointestina: diarrhea, nausea, vomiting.

General: allergic or allergic-like reactions, including facial and oropharyngeal oedema, laryngospasm (see Warnings and Precautions).

Neurologic: dizziness, headaches, insomnia, seizures.

Psychiatric: delirium, including symptoms such as altered level of consciousness, confusion, abnormal behaviour, delusions, hallucinations, agitation, anxiety, nightmares (see Warnings and Precautions).

Respiratory: bronchospasm, dyspnea (see Warnings and Precautions).

Skin: rash, urticaria, and severe skin reactions including erythema multiforme, Stevens-Johnson syndrome, toxic epidermal necrolysis (see Warnings and Precautions).

DRUG INTERACTIONS: Drug-Drug Interactions: Zanamivir is less than 15% protein bound. There is no evidence of hepatic metabolism, and zanamivir is not a substrate nor does it affect cytochrome P450 (CYP) isoenzymes (CYP1A1/2, 2A6, 2C9, 2C18, 2D6, 2E1, and 3A4) in human liver microsomes. Therefore, based on data from in-vitro studies, clinically significant drug interactions are unlikely. RELENZA (zanamivir), when given for 28 days (10 mg once daily), did not impair the immune response to the influenza vaccine.

Drug-Food Interactions: Interactions with food have not been established.

Drug-Herb Interactions: Interactions with herbal products have not been established.

Drug-Laboratory Test Interactions: Interactions with laboratory tests have not been established.

DOSAGE AND ADMINISTRATION: Recommended Dose and Dosage Adjustment: Treatment of Influenza: The recommended dose of RELENZA (zanamivir) for treatment of influenza in adults and pediatric patients ≥7 years of age is 2 inhalations (one 5 mg blister per inhalation for a total dose of 10 mg) twice daily (approximately 12 hours apart) for 5 days. A second dose should be taken on the first day of treatment whenever possible, provided there is at least 2 hours between doses. On subsequent days, doses should be about 12 hours apart (e.g., morning and evening) at approximately the same time each day. There are no data on the effectiveness of treatment with RELENZA when initiated more than 2 days after the onset of signs or symptoms. For maximum benefit, treatment must begin within two days, after the onset of symptoms.

Prophylaxis of Influenza: Household Setting: The recommended dose of RELENZA for prophylaxis of influenza in adults and pediatric patients 7 years of age and older in a household setting is 10 mg once daily for 10 days. The 10 mg dose is provided by 2 inhalations (one 5 mg blister per inhalation). The dose should be administered at approximately the same time each day. There are no data on the effectiveness of prophylaxis with RELENZA in a household setting when initiated more than 1.5 days after the onset of signs or symptoms in the index case.

Community Outbreaks: The recommended dose of RELENZA for prophylaxis of influenza in adults and adolescents in a community setting is 10 mg once daily for 28 days. The 10 mg dose is provided by 2 inhalations (one 5 mg blister per inhalation). The dose should be administered at approximately the same time each day. There are no data on the effectiveness of prophylaxis with RELENZA in a community outbreak when initiated more than 5 days after the outbreak was identified in the community. The safety and effectiveness of prophylaxis with RELENZA have not been evaluated for longer than 28 days duration.

Missed Dose: In case of a missed dose, RELENZA should be taken immediately, except if it is near the next dose (within 2 hours). Then, RELENZA should be continued at the usual times.

Administration: RELENZA is for administration to the respiratory tract by oral inhalation only. The contents of each blister are inhaled using a specially designed breath-activated plastic device for inhaling powder called the DISKHALER inhalation device.

(cont'd)

Patients scheduled to use an inhaled bronchodilator at the same time as RELENZA should use their bronchodilator before taking RELENZA (see Warnings and Precautions, Respiratory).

OVERDOSAGE:
There have been no reports of overdosage from the administration of RELENZA (zanamivir). Accidental overdose is unlikely due to the physical limitations of the presentation, the route of administration, and the poor oral bioavailability (2% to 3%) of RELENZA. Doses of RELENZA up to 64 mg/day (approximately 3 times the maximum daily recommended dose) have been administered by oral inhalation (by nebuliser). Additionally, systemic administration by intravenous route of up to 1200 mg/day for five days in 12 healthy adults caused no adverse effect.

For management of a suspected drug overdose, CPhA recommends that you contact your **regional Poison Control Centre**. See the *CPS* Directory section for a list of Poison Control Centres.

ACTION AND CLINICAL PHARMACOLOGY: Mechanism of Action: RELENZA (zanamivir) is a selective inhibitor of neuraminidase, the influenza virus surface enzyme. It is believed that viral neuraminidase aids the release of newly formed virus particles from infected cells and may facilitate access of virus through mucus to epithelial cell surfaces, to allow viral infection of other cells. It is believed that the inhibition of this enzyme is reflected in both in vitro and in vivo (in animals) activity against influenza A and B virus replication, and encompasses all of the known neuraminidase subtypes of influenza A viruses.

It is believed that the activity of zanamivir is extracellular. It reduces the propagation of both influenza A and B viruses by inhibiting the release of infectious influenza virions from the epithelial cells of the respiratory tract. Influenza viral replication is primarily confined to the superficial epithelium of the respiratory tract. The efficacy of topical administration of zanamivir to this site has been confirmed in clinical studies.

Pharmacokinetics: Absorption: Pharmacokinetic studies in humans have shown that the absolute oral absorption of zanamivir, as compared to IV administration of the drug, was low (mean 2%). Similar studies of orally inhaled RELENZA (zanamivir) indicate that approximately 10-20% of the dose is systemically absorbed, with serum concentrations generally peaking within 1-2 hours. The peak serum concentrations ranged from 17 to 142 ng/mL following a 10 mg dose. The area under the serum concentration versus time curve (AUC to infinity) ranged from 111 to 1364 ng·hr/mL.

Distribution: In healthy adults, after oral inhalation, RELENZA is widely deposited at high concentrations throughout the respiratory tract, thus delivering the drug to the site of influenza infection. The high concentrations of RELENZA in the respiratory tract will result in the rapid onset of inhibition of the viral neuraminidase. The two major sites of deposition are the oropharynx and the lungs (mean 77.6% and 13.2 %, respectively), from where zanamivir is eliminated via the gastrointestinal tract.

Metabolism: Zanamivir has been shown to be renally excreted as unchanged drug. There is no evidence of metabolism of orally inhaled drug.

Excretion: The serum half-life of zanamivir following administration by oral inhalation ranges from 2.6 to 5.05 hours. It is entirely excreted unchanged in the urine. Total clearance ranges from 2.5 to 10.9 L/h as approximated by urinary clearance. Renal elimination is completed within 24 hours. The unabsorbed drug is excreted in the feces.

Special Populations and Conditions: Pediatrics: The pharmacokinetics of zanamivir were evaluated in pediatric patients with signs and symptoms of respiratory illness. Sixteen patients, 6 to 12 years of age, received a single dose of 10 mg zanamivir dry powder via the DISKHALER inhalation device. Five patients had either undetectable zanamivir serum concentrations or had low drug concentrations (8.32 to 10.38 ng/mL) that were not detectable after 1.5 hours. Eleven patients had C_{max} median values of 43 ng/mL (range 15 to 74) and AUC_{∞} median values of 167 ng·hr/mL (range 58 to 279). Low or undetectable serum concentrations were related to lack of measurable peak inspiratory flow rates (PIFR) in individual patients (see Warnings and Precautions, Special Populations, Pediatrics).

Geriatrics: The bioavailability of zanamivir in elderly individuals has not been determined (see Warnings and Precautions).

Hepatic Insufficiency: The pharmacokinetics of zanamivir have not been investigated in patients with impaired hepatic function; doses of up to 1200 mg IV in healthy adults did not show evidence of hepatic metabolism.

Renal Insufficiency: At the therapeutic daily dose of 20 mg, bioavailability is low (10-20%), and as a result systemic exposure of patients to RELENZA is limited. However, after a single IV dose of 4 mg or 2 mg of zanamivir in volunteers with mild or moderate, or severe renal impairment, respectively, significant decreases in renal clearance (and hence total clearance: normal 5.3 L/h, mild/moderate 2.7 L/h, and severe 0.8 L/h; median values) and significant increases in half-life (normal 3.1 h, mild/moderate 4.7 h, and severe 18.5 h; median values) and systemic exposure were observed. Safety and efficacy have not been documented in the presence of severe renal insufficiency after repeated dosing.

STORAGE AND STABILITY: Store at room temperature (15 to 30°C) in a dry place.

SPECIAL HANDLING INSTRUCTIONS: Use the ROTADISK disks before the expiration date. Do not puncture any ROTADISK disk blister until taking a dose using the DISKHALER inhalation device.

INFORMATION FOR THE PATIENT: Published in e-CPS, available by subscription at www.e-cps.ca.

DOSAGE FORMS, COMPOSITION AND PACKAGING: RELENZA ROTADISKS consist of a circular foil disk with 4 regularly distributed blisters each containing 5 mg of zanamivir. A DISKHALER inhalation device is provided to administer the medication. Nonmedicinal ingredients: lactose (which contains milk protein). Boxes of 5 ROTADISK disks.

(Shown in Product Identification Section)

Relistor® Ⓟ

methylnaltrexone bromide

µ-opioid Receptor Antagonist

Pfizer

Date of Preparation: March 27, 2008
Date of Revision: February 3, 2010

SUMMARY PRODUCT INFORMATION:

Route of Administration	Dosage Form/ Strength	Clinically Relevant Nonmedicinal Ingredients
Subcutaneous	Methylnaltrexone bromide injection, 20 mg/mL	None For a complete listing see Dosage Forms, Composition and Packaging.

INDICATIONS AND CLINICAL USE: RELISTOR is indicated for the treatment of opioid-induced constipation in patients with advanced illness, receiving palliative care. When response to laxatives has been insufficient, RELISTOR should be used as an adjunct therapy to induce a prompt bowel movement.

- The majority of patients in the clinical studies had WHO performance status of 3 or greater.
- All patients maintained a stable regimen of laxatives and opiates during the studies.
- Most patients who responded to RELISTOR had a bowel movement within 4 hours (median 24 minutes).

Geriatrics (≥65 years of age): There was no difference in the efficacy or safety profile of these elderly patients when compared to younger patients. Therefore, no dose adjustment is recommended based on age.

Pediatrics: RELISTOR is not indicated for use in children and adolescents. Safety and efficacy of RELISTOR have not been established in pediatric patients.

CONTRAINDICATIONS:

- RELISTOR is contraindicated in patients who are hypersensitive to any of its components. For a complete listing of the components, see Dosage Forms, Composition and Packaging.
- Use of RELISTOR is contraindicated in patients with known or suspected mechanical gastrointestinal obstruction or acute surgical abdomen.

WARNINGS AND PRECAUTIONS: General: Patients should be seated or recumbent during dosing. Care should be taken when the patient stands following dosing.

RELISTOR should not be used for treatment of patients with constipation not related to opioid use.

Gastrointestinal: Severe Diarrhea: If severe or persistent diarrhea occurs during treatment, patients should be advised not to continue therapy with RELISTOR and consult their physician.

Special Populations: Pregnant Women: Pregnancy Category B Reproduction studies have been performed in pregnant rats and rabbits. There were no effects on fetal development at intravenous dosages of up to 25 mg/kg/day in the rat or up to 16 mg/kg/day in the rabbit. There are, however, no adequate and well-controlled studies in pregnant women. Because animal reproduction studies are not always predictive of human response, this drug should be used during pregnancy only if clearly needed. The potential for teratogenic effects of RELISTOR on a human fetus is unknown.

Labour and Delivery: Effects of RELISTOR on mother, fetus, duration of labor, and delivery are unknown. In a perinatal/postnatal reproduction study there were no effects on the mother, labor, delivery, or on offspring survival and growth in rats following subcutaneous injection of methylnaltrexone at dosages up to 25 mg/kg/day.

Nursing Women: Results from an animal study using ^{3}H-labeled methylnaltrexone indicate that methylnaltrexone is excreted via the milk of lactating rats. It is not known whether this drug is excreted in human milk. Because many drugs are excreted in human milk, caution should be exercised when RELISTOR is administered to a nursing woman.

Pediatrics: Safety and efficacy of RELISTOR have not been established in pediatric patients. Studies have been conducted in juvenile rats and dogs. Following intravenous injection of methylnaltrexone bromide, juvenile rats were found to be more sensitive than adult rats to methylnaltrexone-related toxicity.

Geriatrics (≥65 years of age): In the phase II and III double-blind studies, a total of 77 patients aged 65-74 years (54 RELISTOR, 23 placebo) and a total of 100 patients aged 75 years or older (61 RELISTOR, 39 placebo) were enrolled. There was no difference in the efficacy or safety profile of these elderly patients when compared to younger patients. Therefore, no dose adjustment is recommended based on age.

Renal Impairment: In patients with severe renal impairment (creatinine clearance less than 30 mL/min), dose reductions are recommended. (See Dosage and Administration.)

Monitoring and Laboratory Tests: None.

ADVERSE REACTIONS: Adverse Drug Reaction Overview: Two placebo-controlled Phase III studies (301 and 302) contributed 288 patients to the population evaluable for safety.

The adverse drug reactions (defined as undesirable effects, reasonably associated with the use of a drug, based on belief that there is a causal relationship between the drug and the occurrence of the adverse event) reported with RELISTOR are abdominal pain, flatulence, nausea, dizziness and diarrhea (see Table 1). All reports of diarrhea, flatulence, and dizziness in the placebo controlled studies were rated mild or moderate by the Investigators, as were most reports of abdominal pain and nausea. Abdominal pain was rated severe in 1.8% of the RELISTOR treated patients and 2.4% of the placebo-treated patients. Nausea was rated severe in 1.2% and 2.4%, respectively. None of the events was rated life-threatening.

All adverse events reported in at least 1 patient treated with RELISTOR in this population are summarized in Table 2.

Clinical Trial Adverse Drug Reactions: Because clinical trials are conducted under very specific conditions the adverse reaction rates observed in the clinical trials may not reflect the rates observed in practice and should not be compared to the rates in the clinical trials for another drug. Adverse drug reaction information from clinical trials is useful for identifying drug-related adverse events and for approximating rates.

The safety of RELISTOR was evaluated in two double blind, placebo controlled trials in patients receiving palliative care: Study 301 included a single dose double-blind, placebo controlled period, whereas study 302 included a 14 day multiple dose, double-blind, placebo controlled period. Both the RELISTOR and placebo patients were on a stable laxative regimen for at least 3 days prior to study entry, and continued on their regimen throughout the study.

Table 1: RELISTOR

Adverse Reactions From All Doses in Double-Blind, Placebo Controlled Clinical Studies of RELISTOR[a]

Adverse Reaction	RELISTOR N=165	Placebo N=123
Abdominal Pain	47 (28.5%)	12 (9.8%)
Flatulence	22 (13.3%)	7 (5.7%)
Nausea	19 (11.5%)	6 (4.9%)
Dizziness	12 (7.3%)	3 (2.4%)
Diarrhea	9 (5.5%)	3 (2.4%)

[a] Doses 0.075, 0.15, and 0.30 mg/kg. The data source is Study 301 (single dose) and Study 302 (7 doses over 14 days).
Note: A phase II study (251) not included in Table 1 was randomized double-blind, non-placebo controlled in which patients (N=33) were administered either 1, 5, 12.5, or 20 mg as a total SC dose three times in one week. The adverse drug reactions reported during study 251 for all doses pooled were abdominal pain (45%), flatulence (33%), nausea (24%), dizziness (9%), and diarrhea (30%).

Adverse Events: Table 2 presents treatment emergent adverse events in phase III placebo controlled double-blind studies. Adverse events included are those found in at least one patient in the RELISTOR group. The discontinuation rate due to adverse events was 1.2% for RELISTOR and 2.4% for placebo.

Table 2: RELISTOR

Treatment-Emergent Adverse Events that Occurred in ≥1% of Patients

	MNTX-301[a]			MNTX-302[b]	
Body System Preferred Term	**Placebo N=52**	**0.15 mg/kg N=47**	**0.3 mg/kg N=55**	**Placebo N=71**	**0.15 mg/kg N=63**
Blood and Lymphatic System Disorders					
Anaemia	1 (1.9%)	1 (2.1%)	1 (1.8%)	0	0
Cardiac Disorders					
Acute Coronary Syndrome	0	0	0	0	1 (1.6%)
Bradycardia	0	0	1 (1.8%)	0	0
Cardiac Failure Congestive	0	0	0	1 (1.4%)	1 (1.6%)
Cyanosis	0	0	0	1 (1.4%)	1 (1.6%)
Myocardial Ischaemia	0	0	0	0	1 (1.6%)
Tachycardia	1 (1.9%)	0	0	4 (5.6%)	2 (3.2%)
Ear and Labyrinth Disorders					
Cerumen Impaction	0	0	0	0	1 (1.6%)
Tinnitus	0	0	1 (1.8%)	0	0
Eye Disorders					
Lacrimation Increased	0	1 (2.1%)	1 (1.8%)	0	1 (1.6%)

(cont'd)

Table 2: RELISTOR *(cont'd)*

Treatment-Emergent Adverse Events that Occurred in ≥1% of Patients

Body System Preferred Term	MNTX-301[a]			MNTX-302[b]	
	Placebo N=52	0.15 mg/kg N=47	0.3 mg/kg N=55	Placebo N=71	0.15 mg/kg N=63
Visual Disturbance	0	0	0	0	1 (1.6%)
Gastrointestinal Disorders					
Abdominal Pain	3 (5.8%)	14 (29.8%)	21 (38.2%)	9 (12.7%)	12 (19.0%)
Flatulence	2 (3.8%)	6 (12.8%)	8 (14.5%)	5 (7.0%)	8 (12.7%)
Nausea	1 (1.9%)	3 (6.4%)	8 (14.5%)	5 (7.0%)	8 (12.7%)
Vomiting	1 (1.9%)	3 (6.4%)	3 (5.5%)	9 (12.7%)	8 (12.7%)
Diarrhea	0	3 (6.4%)	1 (1.8%)	3 (4.2%)	5 (7.9%)
Abdominal Pain Upper	1 (1.9%)	2 (4.3%)	3 (5.5%)	1 (1.4%)	1 (1.6%)
Abdominal Distension	1 (1.9%)	1 (2.1%)	1 (1.8%)	5 (7.0%)	1 (1.6%)
Abdominal Discomfort	0	0	1 (1.8%)	2 (2.8%)	1 (1.6%)
Abdominal Tenderness	0	0	0	4 (5.6%)	1 (1.6%)
Anal Haemorrhage	0	0	0	0	1 (1.6%)
Aphthous Stomatitis	0	0	0	0	1 (1.6%)
Ascites	0	0	1 (1.8%)	1 (1.4%)	0
Bowel Sounds Abnormal	0	0	0	4 (5.6%)	1 (1.6%)
Constipation	0	1 (2.1%)	0	3 (4.2%)	0
Dry Mouth	1 (1.9%)	0	0	2 (2.8%)	0
Dysphagia	0	1 (2.1%)	1 (1.8%)	0	0
Gastrooesophageal Reflux Disease	0	0	0	0	1 (1.6%)
Haemorrhoids	0	0	1 (1.8%)	0	0
Oral Mucosal Disorder	0	0	0	1 (1.4%)	1 (1.6%)
Proctalgia	0	0	1 (1.8%)	1 (1.4%)	1 (1.6%)
Rectal Haemorrhage	0	1 (2.1%)	0	1 (1.4%)	0
Retching	0	0	1 (1.8%)	0	1 (1.6%)
Salivary Hypersecretion	0	0	0	0	1 (1.6%)
Stomach Discomfort	0	0	0	0	2 (3.2%)
Stomatitis	0	0	1 (1.8%)	0	0
Tongue Coated	0	0	0	1 (1.4%)	1 (1.6%)
General Disorders and Administration Site Conditions					
Pain	5 (9.6%)	3 (6.4%)	7 (12.7%)	8 (11.3%)	3 (4.8%)
Injection Site Pain	0	1 (2.1%)	1 (1.8%)	0	1 (1.6%)
Asthenia	0	0	5 (9.1%)	5 (7.0%)	4 (6.3%)
Chest Pain	0	0	0	3 (4.2%)	4 (6.3%)
Chills	0	0	2 (3.6%)	1 (1.4%)	0
Concomitant Disease Progression	0	0	1 (1.8%)	0	2 (3.2%)
Drug Withdrawal Syndrome	1 (1.9%)	1 (2.1%)	0	0	0
Fatigue	1 (1.9%)	5 (10.6%)	1 (1.8%)	3 (4.2%)	0
Feeling Cold	0	1 (2.1%)	0	0	0
Generalised Oedema	0	0	0	0	1 (1.6%)
Infusion Related Reaction	0	0	0	0	1 (1.6%)
Injection Site Irritation	0	0	1 (1.8%)	1 (1.4%)	1 (1.6%)
Injection Site Vesicles	0	0	0	0	1 (1.6%)
Mucosal Inflammation	1 (1.9%)	0	0	0	1 (1.6%)
Oedema	0	0	0	0	1 (1.6%)
Oedema Peripheral	1 (1.9%)	2 (4.3%)	0	9 (12.7%)	5 (7.9%)
Pyrexia	0	0	0	2 (2.8%)	3 (4.8%)
Secretion Discharge	0	1 (2.1%)	0	0	0
Infections and Infestations					
Bacteraemia	0	0	0	0	1 (1.6%)
Bronchitis	0	0	0	1 (1.4%)	2 (3.2%)
Candidiasis	0	0	1 (1.8%)	1 (1.4%)	1 (1.6%)
Furuncle	0	0	0	0	1 (1.6%)
Infection	0	0	1 (1.8%)	0	0
Nasopharyngitis	0	0	0	0	1 (1.6%)
Oral Candidiasis	0	0	0	0	2 (3.2%)
Pneumonia	0	1 (2.1%)	0	1 (1.4%)	1 (1.6%)
Skin Infection	0	1 (2.1%)	0	0	0
Upper Respiratory Tract Infection	0	0	0	0	1 (1.6%)
Urinary Tract Infection	2 (3.8%)	0	0	3 (4.2%)	2 (3.2%)
Injury, Poisoning and Procedural Complications					
Contusion	1 (1.9%)	1 (2.1%)	2 (3.6%)	1 (1.4%)	0
Excoriation	0	0	1 (1.8%)	2 (2.8%)	0
Fall	0	0	1 (1.8%)	8 (11.3%)	1 (1.6%)
Post Procedural Nausea	0	0	1 (1.8%)	0	0
Skin Laceration	0	0	1 (1.8%)	3 (4.2%)	1 (1.6%)
Tooth Injury	0	1 (2.1%)	0	0	0
Wound	0	0	1 (1.8%)	0	0
Investigations					
Clinical Laboratory					
Alanine Aminotransferase Increased	0	0	0	0	1 (1.6%)
Aspartate Aminotransferase Increased	0	0	0	1 (1.4%)	1 (1.6%)
Bleeding Time Prolonged	0	0	1 (1.8%)	0	0
Blood Albumin Decreased	0	0	0	0	1 (1.6%)
Blood Calcium Decreased	0	0	1 (1.8%)	0	0
Blood Calcium Increased	0	0	0	0	1 (1.6%)
Blood Creatinine Increased	0	0	1 (1.8%)	0	0
Blood Potassium Decreased	0	0	0	0	1 (1.6%)
Blood Pressure Increased	0	1 (2.1%)	1 (1.8%)	0	0
Haemoglobin Decreased	0	0	0	0	1 (1.6%)
Monocyte Count Increased	0	0	1 (1.8%)	0	0
Platelet Count Decreased	0	0	1 (1.8%)	0	0
Protein Total Decreased	0	0	0	0	1 (1.6%)
White Blood Cell Count Increased	0	0	0	1 (1.4%)	1 (1.6%)
Physical Findings					
Breath Sounds Abnormal	0	0	1 (1.8%)	3 (4.2%)	1 (1.6%)
Cardiac Murmur	1 (1.9%)	0	0	0	1 (1.6%)
Gallop Rhythm Present	0	1 (2.1%)	0	0	0
Heart Sounds Abnormal	0	0	0	0	1 (1.6%)
Skin Turgor Decreased	0	0	0	1 (1.4%)	2 (3.2%)
Vital Signs					
Body Temperature Increased	0	0	1 (1.8%)	3 (4.2%)	5 (7.9%)
Heart Rate Irregular	1 (1.9%)	1 (2.1%)	0	2 (2.8%)	0

(cont'd)

Table 2: RELISTOR *(cont'd)*

Treatment-Emergent Adverse Events that Occurred in ≥1% of Patients

Body System Preferred Term	MNTX-301[a]			MNTX-302[b]	
	Placebo N=52	0.15 mg/kg N=47	0.3 mg/kg N=55	Placebo N=71	0.15 mg/kg N=63
Respiratory Rate Decreased	0	1 (2.1%)	0	0	0
Metabolism and Nutrition Disorders					
Dehydration	1 (1.9%)	0	2 (3.6%)	5 (7.0%)	2 (3.2%)
Hyperglycaemia	0	0	0	0	2 (3.2%)
Hypokalaemia	0	1 (2.1%)	0	0	0
Hyponatraemia	0	0	1 (1.8%)	0	0
Musculoskeletal and Connective Tissue Disorders					
Muscle Spasms	0	2 (4.3%)	1 (1.8%)	1 (1.4%)	2 (3.2%)
Arthalgia	1 (1.9%)	1 (2.1%)	0	0	1 (1.6%)
Back Pain	2 (3.8%)	2 (4.3%)	0	0	3 (4.8%)
Bunion	0	0	0	0	1 (1.6%)
Kyphosis	0	0	0	0	1 (1.6%)
Musculoskeletal Discomfort	0	0	0	0	1 (1.6%)
Neck Pain	0	1 (2.1%)	0	0	0
Sensation Of Heaviness	0	0	0	0	1 (1.6%)
Shoulder Pain	0	1 (2.1%)	0	1 (1.4%)	1 (1.6%)
Neoplasms Benign, Malignant and Unspecified (incl. cysts and polyps)					
Malignant Neoplasm Progression	2 (3.8%)	1 (2.1%)	4 (7.3%)	12 (16.9%)	7 (11.1%)
Cancer Pain	0	0	1 (1.8%)	2 (2.8%)	1 (1.6%)
Nervous System Disorders					
Dizziness	0	2 (4.3%)	5 (9.1%)	3 (4.2%)	5 (7.9%)
Lethargy	0	1 (2.1%)	2 (3.6%)	4 (5.6%)	4 (6.3%)
Somnolence	1 (1.9%)	3 (6.4%)	1 (1.8%)	4 (5.6%)	1 (1.6%)
Tremor	1 (1.9%)	1 (2.1%)	2 (3.6%)	1 (1.4%)	2 (3.2%)
Balance Disorder	0	0	0	0	1 (1.6%)
Convulsion	0	0	0	1 (1.4%)	1 (1.6%)
Coordination Abnormal	0	1 (2.1%)	0	0	0
Depressed Level of Consciousness	0	1 (2.1%)	0	2 (2.8%)	1 (1.6%)
Drooling	0	1 (2.1%)	0	0	0
Dysarthria	0	1 (2.1%)	0	0	0
Headache	1 (1.9%)	0	2 (3.6%)	1 (1.4%)	2 (3.2%)
Hypoaesthesia	0	1 (2.1%)	1 (1.8%)	0	0
Myoclonus	0	0	1 (1.8%)	0	1 (1.6%)
Poor Quality Sleep	0	0	1 (1.8%)	0	0
Sedation	1 (1.9%)	0	0	0	1 (1.6%)
Speech Disorder	0	0	1 (1.8%)	0	1 (1.6%)
Psychiatric Disorders					
Restlessness	4 (7.7%)	5 (10.6%)	4 (7.3%)	4 (5.6%)	2 (3.2%)
Anxiety	2 (3.8%)	1 (2.1%)	5 (9.1%)	3 (4.2%)	2 (3.2%)
Confusional State	2 (3.8%)	1 (2.1%)	4 (7.3%)	2 (2.8%)	2 (3.2%)
Agitation	2 (3.8%)	2 (4.3%)	1 (1.8%)	3 (4.2%)	2 (3.2%)
Delirium	0	1 (2.1%)	1 (1.8%)	0	0
Delusion	1 (1.9%)	1 (2.1%)	0	0	0
Depression	0	0	0	1 (1.4%)	2 (3.2%)
Disorientation	0	1 (2.1%)	0	2 (2.8%)	1 (1.6%)
Hallucination	1 (1.9%)	2 (4.3%)	0	1 (1.4%)	1 (1.6%)

(cont'd)

Table 2: RELISTOR *(cont'd)*

Treatment-Emergent Adverse Events that Occurred in ≥1% of Patients

Body System Preferred Term	MNTX-301[a]			MNTX-302[b]	
	Placebo N=52	0.15 mg/kg N=47	0.3 mg/kg N=55	Placebo N=71	0.15 mg/kg N=63
Insomnia	1 (1.9%)	0	1 (1.8%)	2 (2.8%)	2 (3.2%)
Nervousness	0	2 (4.3%)	1 (1.8%)	0	0
Suicidal Ideation	0	0	0	0	1 (1.6%)
Renal and Urinary Disorders					
Bladder Spasm	0	0	0	1 (1.4%)	1 (1.6%)
Renal Impairment	0	0	1 (1.8%)	0	0
Reproductive System and Breast Disorders					
Oedema Genital	0	0	1 (1.8%)	0	0
Respiratory, Thoracic and Mediastinal Disorders					
Rhinorrhoea	1 (1.9%)	4 (8.5%)	2 (3.6%)	2 (2.8%)	1 (1.6%)
Apnoea	0	1 (2.1%)	1 (1.8%)	0	0
Chronic Obstructive Pulmonary Disease	0	0	1 (1.8%)	1 (1.4%)	0
Cough	0	0	0	2 (2.8%)	1 (1.6%)
Dyspnoea	1 (1.9%)	0	2(3.6%)	5 (7.0%)	2 (3.2%)
Dyspnoea Exacerbated	0	0	0	2 (2.8%)	1 (1.6%)
Epistaxis	0	0	1 (1.8%)	0	0
Hypoventilation	0	0	0	0	1 (1.6%)
Hypoxia	0	0	1 (1.8%)	0	0
Increased Bronchial Secretion	0	1 (2.1%)	0	0	0
Increased Upper Airway Secretion	0	0	0	0	1 (1.6%)
Nasal Congestion	0	0	0	1 (1.4%)	1 (1.6%)
Nasal Mucosal Disorder	0	0	0	0	1 (1.6%)
Pharyngolaryngeal Pain	0	0	1 (1.8%)	1 (1.4%)	1 (1.6%)
Productive Cough	0	0	0	1 (1.4%)	2 (3.2%)
Pulmonary Congestion	1 (1.9%)	0	0	4 (5.6%)	1 (1.6%)
Pulmonary Embolism	0	0	0	1 (1.4%)	0
Pulmonary Fibrosis	0	0	0	0	1 (1.6%)
Pulmonary Oedema	0	1 (2.1%)	0	0	0
Rales	0	0	0	1 (1.4%)	1 (1.6%)
Respiratory Arrest	0	0	0	0	1 (1.6%)
Respiratory Tract Congestion	0	0	0	0	1 (1.6%)
Rhonchi	0	1 (2.1%)	0	2 (2.8%)	1 (1.6%)
Wheezing	0	0	0	1 (1.4%)	2 (3.2%)
Yawning	1 (1.9%)	0	1 (1.8%)	0	2 (3.2%)
Skin and Subcutaneous Tissue Disorders					
Hyperhidrosis	4 (7.7%)	4 (8.5%)	4 (7.3%)	4 (5.6%)	3 (4.8%)
Cold Sweat	0	0	1 (1.8%)	0	0
Decubitus Ulcer	0	0	1 (1.8%)	2 (2.8%)	2 (3.2%)
Ecchymosis	0	0	0	1 (1.4%)	1 (1.6%)
Erythema	0	0	1 (1.8%)	1 (1.4%)	0
Night Sweats	0	0	0	1 (1.4%)	0
Onychomadesis	0	0	0	0	1 (1.6%)
Piloerection	0	1 (2.1%)	0	1 (1.4%)	0
Pruritus	0	0	0	1 (1.4%)	2 (3.2%)
Psoriasis	0	0	0	0	1 (1.6%)
Skin Ulcer	0	0	0	1 (1.4%)	1 (1.6%)

(cont'd)

Table 2: RELISTOR *(cont'd)*

Treatment-Emergent Adverse Events that Occurred in ≥1% of Patients

Body System Preferred Term	MNTX-301[a]			MNTX-302[b]	
	Placebo N=52	0.15 mg/kg N=47	0.3 mg/kg N=55	Placebo N=71	0.15 mg/kg N=63
Yellow Skin	0	0	0	0	1 (1.6%)
Social Circumstances					
Bedridden	0	0	0	0	1 (1.6%)
Physical Abuse	0	0	0	0	1 (1.6%)
Verbal Abuse	0	0	0	0	1 (1.6%)
Vascular Disorders					
Aneurysm Ruptured	0	0	0	0	1 (1.6%)
Flushing	0	0	1 (1.8%)	0	0
Haematoma	0	0	0	1 (1.4%)	1 (1.6%)
Hot Flush	1 (1.9%)	0	0	0	1 (1.6%)
Hypotension	0	0	1 (1.8%)	4 (5.6%)	0
Orthostatic Hypotension	0	0	1 (1.8%)	0	0

[a] Study MNTX 301—Duration: 1 day; single dose only.
[b] Study MNTX 302—Duration 2 weeks; one dose every other day (7 doses).
Note: Adverse Events occurring during follow up from double-blind treatment or during the time prior to the first dose in an extension study have been attributed to the double-blind treatment.

Serious Adverse Events: Table 3 shows the incidence of Treatment-Emergent Serious Adverse Events reported in the double blind placebo controlled phase III clinical trials.

Table 3: RELISTOR

Incidence of Treatment-Emergent Serious Adverse Events in Phase III[a] Clinical Trials

Primary System Organ Class Preferred Term	Double-Blind Treatment	
	Placebo (N=123) n (%)	MNTX (N=165) n (%)
Cardiac Disorders		
Cardiac Failure Congestive	1 (0.8)	1 (0.6)
Myocardial Ischemia	0	1 (0.6)
General Disorders and Administration Site Conditions		
Concomitant Disease Progression	0	3 (1.8)
Drug Withdrawal Syndrome	0	1 (0.6)
Neoplasms benign, Malignant and Unspecified (incl. cysts and polyps)		
Malignant Neoplasm Progression	13 (10.6)	12 (7.3)
Psychiatric Disorders		
Suicidal Ideation	0	1 (0.6)
Respiratory, Thoracic and Mediastinal Disorders		
Dyspnoea Exacerbated	0	1 (0.6)
Pulmonary Fibrosis	0	1 (0.6)
Respiratory Arrest	0	1 (0.6)
Social Circumstances		
Physical abuse	0	1 (0.6)
Verbal abuse	0	1 (0.6)
Vascular Disorders		
Aneurysm Ruptured	0	1 (0.6)

[a] Study 301 and Study 302—Phase III Placebo controlled double-blind studies.
Note: The Serious Adverse Events reported during the double-blind period of the non-placebo-controlled Phase II study 251 (N=33) were: Neutropenia 1 (3.0%), Concomitant Disease Progression 6 (18.2%), Disease Progression 2 (6.1%), Intentional Overdose 1(3.0%), Depressed Level of Consciousness 1 (3.0%), Delirium 1(3.0%), and Lymphadenectomy 1 (3.0%).

Less Common Clinical Trial Adverse Drug Reactions (<1%): Please refer to Table 2 (based on the number of subjects studied, Table 2 includes any adverse event that occurred in at least 1 subject receiving RELISTOR).

Abnormal Hematologic and Clinical Chemistry Findings: Please refer to Table 2, section Metabolism and Nutritional Disorders and Investigations for information on Abnormal Hematologic and Clinical Chemistry findings.

Adverse Events that Led to Discontinuation: Among the 286 patients treated with RELISTOR in the phase II and III clinical studies, adverse events led to discontinuation in 23 (8.0%) patients. The only events that led to discontinuation of more than 1 patient were malignant neoplasm progression (6 patients), abdominal pain (3 patients), and vomiting (2 patients).

Deaths: Of the 286 advanced illness patients treated with RELISTOR in the phase II and III clinical studies, 138 died while on study, or during follow-up. The causes of death as assessed by investigators were the underlying primary disease or complications related to concurrent illnesses in all but 1 case. One patient with terminal breast cancer developed severe diarrhea and dehydration subsequent to treatment with study drug. In the investigator's opinion, this exacerbated her underlying cardiovascular status, which ultimately led to cardiovascular collapse. This death was deemed by the investigator to be related to treatment with RELISTOR.

Serious Adverse Events during Open-Label Treatment: The serious adverse events reported during uncontrolled open-label treatment in study extensions are reported below (n, %):

Very Common Serious Adverse Events (≥10%): Neoplasms Benign, Malignant and Unspecified: malignant neoplasm progression (82, 37.6%).

Common Serious Adverse Events (≥1% and ≤10%): Cardiac Disorders: congestive cardiac failure aggravated (4, 1.8%).
Gastrointestinal Disorders: abdominal pain NOS (3, 1.4%); nausea (4, 1.8%); vomiting NOS (4, 1.8%).
General Disorders and Administration Site Conditions: chest pain (4, 1.8%); concomitant disease progression (6, 2.8%); multi-organ failure (3, 1.4%); pain exacerbated (4, 1.8%).
Infections and Infestations: pneumonia NOS (4, 1.8%).
Injury, Poisoning and Procedural Complications: fall (4, 1.8%).
Metabolism and Nutritional Disorders: dehydration (3, 1.4%).
Nervous System Disorders: coma (6, 2.8%).
Psychiatric Disorders: delirium (4, 1.8%).
Respiratory, Thoracic and Mediastinal Disorders: chronic obstructive airways disease exacerbated (5, 2.3%); pneumonia aspiration (4, 1.8%); respiratory failure (3, 1.4%).

Uncommon Serious Adverse Events (≥0.1% and <1%): Blood and Lymphatic Disorders: disseminated intravascular coagulation (1, 0.5%); neutropenia (1, 0.5%).
Cardiac Disorders: cardiac arrest (1, 0.5%); cardiac failure congestive (2, 0.9%); myocardial infarction (2, 0.9%).
Gastrointestinal Disorders: constipation (2, 0.9%); diarrhea NOS (1, 0.5%); dysphagia (1, 0.5%); gastric ulcer haemorrhage (1, 0.5%); ileus (2, 0.9%); oesophageal obstruction (1, 0.5%); pancreatitis NOS (1, 0.5%).
General Disorders and Administration Site Conditions: asthenia (2, 0.9%); chest pain aggravated (1, 0.5%); drug withdrawal syndrome (1, 0.5%); intractable pain (1, 0.5%); oedema peripheral (2, 0.9%).
Infections and Infestations: abscess neck (1, 0.5%); bronchitis viral (1, 0.5%); cellulitis (2, 0.9%); clostridial infection NOS (1, 0.5%); infection NOS (1, 0.5%); Klebsiella bacteraemia (1, 0.5%); osteomyelitis NOS (1, 0.5%); pseudomonal sepsis (1, 0.5%); respiratory tract infection NOS (1, 0.5%); sepsis NOS (1, 0.5%); septic shock (1, 0.5%); urinary tract infection NOS (1, 0.5%).
Injury, Poisoning and Procedural Complications: femoral neck fracture (1, 0.5%); femur fracture (1, 0.5%); fractured pelvis NOS (1, 0.5%); hip fracture (1, 0.5%); laceration (1, 0.5%); wound dehiscence (1, 0.5%).
Investigations: weight increased (1, 0.5%).
Metabolism and Nutritional Disorders: failure to thrive (1, 0.5%); hyperkalaemia (1, 0.5%); hypoglycaemia NOS (1, 0.5%); hypoglycaemic seizure (1, 0.5%).
Musculoskeletal and Connective Tissue Disorders: arthralgia (1, 0.5%); back pain (1, 0.5%); fistula NOS (1, 0.5%); muscle spasms (1, 0.5%); myalgia (1, 0.5%); pathological fracture (1, 0.5%).
Neoplasms Benign, Malignant and Unspecified: cancer pain (2, 0.9%).
Nervous System Disorders: aphasia (1, 0.5%); cerebrovascular accident (2, 0.9%); paraparesis (1, 0.5%); simple partial seizures (1, 0.5%).
Psychiatric Disorders: agitation (2, 0.9%); confusional state (2, 0.9%); depression (1, 0.5%).
Renal and Urinary Disorders: haematuria (1, 0.5%); renal failure acute (2, 0.9%).
Respiratory, Thoracic and Mediastinal Disorders: breath sounds decreased (1, 0.5%); dyspnoea (1, 0.5%); dyspnoea exacerbated (1, 0.5%); hypoxia (1, 0.5%); lung infiltration NOS (1, 0.5%); pleural effusion (1, 0.5%); pulmonary embolism (1, 0.5%); pulmonary oedema NOS (1, 0.5%); respiratory arrest (1, 0.5%); respiratory distress (1, 0.5%).
Vascular Disorders: circulatory collapse (1, 0.5%); flushing (1, 0.5%); haemorrhage NOS (2, 0.9%); hypotension NOS (1, 0.5%).

DRUG INTERACTIONS: Overview: Methylnaltrexone is minimally metabolized by CYP isozymes. Methylnaltrexone does not affect the pharmacokinetics of drugs metabolized by cytochrome P450 (CYP) isozymes.

Drug-Drug Interactions: Drugs Metabolized by Cytochrome P450 Isozymes: Methylnaltrexone does not affect the pharmacokinetics of drugs metabolized by cytochrome P450 (CYP) isozymes. Methylnaltrexone is minimally metabolized by CYP isozymes. In vitro drug metabolism studies suggest that methylnaltrexone does not inhibit the activity of CYP1A2, CYP2A6, CYP2C9, CYP2C19 or CYP3A4 while it is a weak inhibitor of metabolism of a model CYP2D6 substrate. In a clinical drug interaction study in healthy adult male subjects, a subcutaneous dose of 0.3 mg/kg of methylnaltrexone did not significantly affect the metabolism of dextromethorphan, a CYP2D6 substrate.

The inhibitory effects of methylnaltrexone, at concentrations up to 100 μM, on the catalytic activities cytochrome P-450 (CYP) enzymes were determined in human liver microsomes. Data suggest that clinical metabolic drug drug interactions involving methylnaltrexone and CYP2D6 substrates are possible following intravenous administration, but not likely to occur for oral or subcutaneous administration of methylnaltrexone at therapeutic doses.

Drugs Renally Excreted: The potential for drug interactions between methylnaltrexone and drugs that are actively secreted by the kidney, such as cimetidine and metformin has not been investigated in humans.
Drug-Food Interactions: Interactions with food have not been established.
Drug-Herb Interactions: Interactions with herbal products have not been established.
Drug-Laboratory Test Interactions: Interactions with laboratory tests have not been established.

DOSAGE AND ADMINISTRATION: Dosing Considerations: For subcutaneous injection only.

RELISTOR should be injected in the upper arm, abdomen or thigh. Patients should be seated or recumbent during dosing. Care should be taken when the patient stands following dosing.

Dosing: RELISTOR is administered as a subcutaneous injection every other day, as needed. Physicians should consider discontinuing treatment in patients who fail to show an adequate response to RELISTOR after 4 doses (1 week).

Recommended Dose and Dosage Adjustment: The recommended dose of RELISTOR is 8 mg for patients weighing 38 to less than 62 kg or 12 mg for patients weighing 62 to 114 kg given as subcutaneous injection every other day as needed. See the table below to determine the correct injection volume.

Patient Weight (kilograms)	Injection Volume	Total Dose
38 to less than 62	**0.4 mL**	8 mg
62 to 114	**0.6 mL**	12 mg

Patients whose weight falls outside of the ranges in the table should be dosed at 0.15 mg/kg. The injection volume for these patients should be calculated using the following:

Multiply the patient's weight in kilograms by 0.0075 and round the volume to the nearest 0.1 mL.

For patients who cannot be weighed, an estimation of the patient's weight should be made by the clinician or the caregiver.

Use in Patients with Renal Impairment: For patients with severe renal impairment (creatinine clearance less than 30 mL/min), the dose of RELISTOR should be reduced by one-half. For those patients weighing 38 to less than 62 kg the injection volume should be 0.2 mL (4 mg) and for those weighing 62 to 114 kg the injection volume should be 0.3 mL (6 mg). For those patients outside of the weight bands, dosing should be 0.075 mg/kg. (See Special Populations and Conditions, Renal Insufficiency.)

Missed Dose: Not applicable.

Administration: Preparation for Injection: RELISTOR is a sterile clear, and colorless to pale yellow aqueous solution. Parenteral drug products should be inspected visually for particulate matter and discoloration prior to administration, whenever solution and container permit. If any of these are present the vial should not be used.

OVERDOSAGE:

Human Experience: During clinical trials of RELISTOR administered subcutaneously, no cases of overdose were reported. In a study of healthy volunteers (n=41), a single dose of 0.50 mg/kg administered as a subcutaneous injection was well-tolerated. A study of healthy volunteers noted orthostatic hypotension associated with a dose of 0.64 mg/kg administered as an IV bolus.

Management of Overdosage: No specific information is available on the treatment of overdose with RELISTOR. In the event of overdose, employ the usual supportive measures such as clinical monitoring and supportive therapy as dictated by the patient's clinical status and contact your local poison centre. Signs or symptoms of orthostatic hypotension should be monitored, and treatment should be initiated, as appropriate.

For management of a suspected drug overdose, CPhA recommends that you contact your **regional Poison Control Centre**. See the *CPS* Directory section for a list of Poison Control Centres.

ACTION AND CLINICAL PHARMACOLOGY: Mechanism of Action: Methylnaltrexone is a selective antagonist of opioid binding at the μ-opioid receptor. As a quaternary amine, the ability of methylnaltrexone to cross the blood brain barrier is restricted. This allows methylnaltrexone to function as a peripherally acting μ-opioid antagonist in tissues such as the gastrointestinal tract, without impacting opioid mediated analgesic effects on the central nervous system. Data from clinical studies 301 and 302, are consistent with a lack of central opioid antagonism by methylnaltrexone, and therefore with this mechanism of action.

Pharmacodynamics: Use of opioids induce slowing of gastrointestinal motility and transit. Antagonism of gastrointestinal μ-opioid receptors by methylnaltrexone inhibits opioid-induced delay of gastrointestinal transit time in a dose-dependent manner. In a clinical study of reversal of constipation due to chronic methadone use with intravenous methylnaltrexone at a dose of mean (±SD) 0.09±0.10 mg/kg, oral-cecal transit time for subjects in the methylnaltrexone group (n=11) decreased from 132.3±36 minutes at baseline to 54.5±19.3 minutes following methylnaltrexone administration, while that for the placebo group (n=11) remained essentially unchanged, with a mean value of 126.8±48.3 minutes at baseline and 125.3±45.0 minutes following placebo administration. These changes in transit time were accompanied by an immediate laxation response in 10 of 11 subjects in the methylnaltrexone group and none in the placebo group.

Dependence/Tolerance: RELISTOR is a peripherally acting μ-opioid receptor antagonist with no known risk of dependency.

Effect on Cardiac Electrophysiology: In a double-blind, randomized, parallel-group ECG study of single subcutaneous doses of methylnaltrexone (0.15, 0.30 and 0.50 mg/kg) in 207 healthy volunteers, no signal of prolongation of the QT/QTc interval, PR interval, or QRS duration was seen at any of the doses studied. Statistically significant increases in heart rate were observed at 0.25 to 0.75 h post-dosing in the 0.30 and 0.50 mg/kg treatment groups. The maximum mean increase was 6.05 (90% CI 2.62, 9.48) bpm (beats per minute) in the 0.30 mg/kg treatment group and 6.08 (90 % CI 2.67, 9.49) bpm in the 0.50 mg/kg arm. No significant effect on heart rate was observed in the 0.15 mg/kg group.

Pharmacokinetics: The pharmacokinetics of methylnaltrexone was characterized in healthy male and female adults and subjects with various degrees of renal or hepatic impairment. Peak plasma concentration and area under the plasma concentration-time curve (AUC) increase in a dose-proportional manner between 0.15 mg/kg and 0.5 mg/kg.

Absorption: Methylnaltrexone is absorbed rapidly, with (C_{max}) achieved at approximately 0.5 hours following subcutaneous administration. The mean (±SD) C_{max} and AUC values at doses of 0.15 mg/kg to 0.5 mg/kg are provided in the table below :

Dose (mg/kg)	N (female/male)	C_{max} (ng/mL)	AUC (ng·h/mL)
0.15	39 (20/19)	117±33	180±37
0.3	60 (25/35)	234±65	376±73
0.5	41 (20/21)	392±148	593±111

Absolute bioavailability of a 0.30 mg/kg subcutaneous dose versus a 0.30 mg/kg intravenous dose is 82% (n=5, males).

Distribution: Methylnaltrexone undergoes moderate tissue distribution. The steady-state volume of distribution (Vss) following 0.45 mg/kg IV q 6 hours for 5 doses was approximately 1.1 (±0.2) L/kg (n=8, males). In another study, after a single 0.3 mg/kg IV dose, Vss was found to be approximately 2.0±0.6 L/kg.

Methylnaltrexone is minimally bound to human plasma proteins (11.0% to 15.3%) as determined by equilibrium dialysis. Methylnaltrexone and metabolites in plasma are about twice those in whole blood, suggesting low penetration into blood cells.

Metabolism: Methylnaltrexone is metabolized in humans to a modest extent (n=6, males). Conversion to methyl-6-naltrexol isomers and methylnaltrexone sulfate appears to be the primary pathways of metabolism (<6.0%). N-demethylation of methylnaltrexone to produce naltrexone is not significant (0.06% of the administered dose).

Excretion: Methylnaltrexone is eliminated primarily as the unchanged drug. Approximately one-half of the dose is excreted in the urine and somewhat less in feces (n=11, males). The terminal disposition half-life ($t_{½}$) is approximately 8 hours (n=19, males). Renal clearance of methylnaltrexone exceeds creatinine clearance, indicating a significant extent of active renal secretion. Renal clearance of methylnaltrexone accounts for roughly half of the total clearance, suggesting appreciable non-renal elimination.

Special Populations and Conditions: Pediatrics: Safety and Efficacy of RELISTOR have not been established in pediatric patients. (See Warnings and Precautions.)

Geriatrics: In the phase II and III double-blind studies, a total of 77 patients aged 65-74 years (54 RELISTOR, 23 placebo) and a total of 100 patients aged 75 years or older (61 RELISTOR, 39 placebo) were enrolled. There was no difference in the efficacy or safety profile of these elderly patients when compared to younger patients. Therefore, no dose adjustment is recommended based on age.

Gender: No recommendations based on gender.

Race: No recommendations based on race.

Hepatic Insufficiency: No dose adjustment is required for patients with mild or moderate hepatic impairment. The effect of mild and moderate hepatic impairment on the systemic exposure to a single subcutaneous methylnaltrexone dose (0.3 mg/kg) has been studied in 8 subjects each, with Child-Pugh Class A (mild impairment: males/females=4/4) and B (moderate impairment: males/females=5/3), compared to healthy subjects (Normal status: males/females=5/3). Results showed no meaningful effect of hepatic impairment on the AUC or C_{max} of methylnaltrexone. The effect of severe hepatic impairment on the pharmacokinetics of methylnaltrexone has not been studied.

Renal Insufficiency: No dose adjustment is required in patients with mild or moderate renal impairment. In patients with severe renal impairment (creatinine clearance less than 30 mL/min), dose reductions are recommended. (See Dosage and Administration, Use in Patients with Renal Impairment.) In a study of volunteers with normal renal function and mild, moderate or severe renal impairment (8 male subjects each) receiving a single dose of 0.30 mg/kg methylnaltrexone, renal impairment had a marked effect on the renal excretion of methylnaltrexone. Severe renal impairment decreased the renal clearance of methylnaltrexone by 8-to 9-fold, however, this resulted in only a 2-fold increase in total methylnaltrexone exposure (AUC). C_{max} was not significantly changed. No studies were performed in patients with end-stage renal impairment requiring dialysis.

Effect of Body Weight on Exposure to Methylnaltrexone: An integrated analysis of pharmacokinetic data from 137 healthy subjects who received methylnaltrexone subcutaneously indicated that methylnaltrexone exposure per unit dose (mg/kg) increased as body weight increased. In addition, the analysis showed that equivalent methylnaltrexone exposure to that at 0.15 mg/kg can be achieved with a weight-band-based dosing regimen of an 8 mg dose for body weight 38 to less than 62 kg or a 12 mg dose for body weight 62 to 114 kg. (See Dosage and Administration.)

Safety in Patients with Potential for Impairment of Blood Brain Barrier Function: An evaluation of the type and incidence of adverse events reported for the 38 patients with documented baseline central nervous system metastases, that represents 13.3% of advanced illness patients studied in clinical trials, were similar to those reported for the aggregate trial population. This suggests that the safety and tolerability of methylnaltrexone in patients with potential impairment of blood brain barrier function secondary to CNS metastasis is not demonstrably different than that seen for the overall advanced illness population.

STORAGE AND STABILITY: RELISTOR should be stored at 20-25°C; excursions permitted to 15-30°C. Do not freeze. **Protect from light.**

SPECIAL HANDLING INSTRUCTIONS: RELISTOR should be inspected visually for particulate matter and discoloration prior to administration, whenever solution and container permit. If any of these are present, the vial should not be used.

INFORMATION FOR THE PATIENT: Published in e-CPS, available by subscription at www.e-cps.ca.

DOSAGE FORMS, COMPOSITION AND PACKAGING: Each mL of sterile, clear and colorless to pale yellow aqueous solution for injection contains: methylnaltrexone bromide 20 mg . Each vial contains 12 mg of methylnaltrexone bromide in 0.6 mL of sterile water for injection. Nonmedicinal ingredients: edetate calcium disodium, glycine hydrochloride, sodium chloride and sterile water for injection. The solution of RELISTOR is isotonic and the pH is adjusted during manufacture with hydrochloric acid and/or sodium hydroxide to approximately 3.4. Single-use vials, cartons of 1. Cartons of seven trays. Each tray (kit) contains: one sterile single use vial (20 mg/mL), one 1 cc (mL) syringe with retractable 27-gauge×½-inch needle, two alcohol swabs.

Relpax™ Ⓟ

eletriptan HBr

5-HT1 Receptor Agonist—Migraine Therapy

Pfizer

Date of Preparation: August 4, 2004

Date of Revision: April 20, 2009

SUMMARY PRODUCT INFORMATION:

Route of Administration	Dosage Form/Strength	All Nonmedicinal Ingredients
Oral	Tablets 20 mg, 40 mg	Croscarmellose sodium, FD&C Yellow No 6 aluminum lake, hypromellose, lactose monohydrate, microcrystalline cellulose, magnesium stearate, titanium dioxide and triacetin

INDICATIONS AND CLINICAL USE: Adults: RELPAX (eletriptan hydrobromide) is indicated for the acute treatment of migraine with or without aura in adults.

RELPAX tablets are not intended for the prophylactic therapy of migraine or for use in the management of hemiplegic, ophthalmoplegic or basilar migraine (see Contraindications). Safety and effectiveness of RELPAX tablets have not been established for cluster headache, which is present in an older, predominantly male population.

Pediatrics (<18 years of age): The safety and efficacy of RELPAX in children has not been established and its use in this age group is not recommended (see Warnings and Precautions).

Geriatrics (>65 years of age): Experience of the use of RELPAX in patients aged over 65 years is limited. Therefore the use of RELPAX in patients over 65 years is not recommended (see Warnings and Precautions).

CONTRAINDICATIONS: RELPAX (eletriptan hydrobromide) tablets are contraindicated in patients with history, symptoms, or signs of ischemic cardiac, cerebrovascular or peripheral vascular syndromes, valvular heart disease or cardiac arrhythmias (especially tachycardias). In addition, patients with other significant underlying cardiovascular diseases (e.g., atherosclerotic disease, congenital heart disease) should not receive eletriptan. Ischemic cardiac syndromes include, but are not restricted to, angina pectoris of any type (e.g., stable angina of effort and vasospastic forms of angina such as the Prinzmetal's variant), all forms of myocardial infarction, and silent myocardial ischemia. Cerebrovascular syndromes include, but are not limited to, strokes of any type as well as transient ischemic attacks (TIAs). Peripheral vascular disease includes, but is not limited to, ischemic bowel disease, or Raynaud's syndrome (see Warnings and Precautions).

Because RELPAX may increase blood pressure it is contraindicated in patients with uncontrolled or severe hypertension (see Warnings and Precautions).

CYP3A4 Inhibitors: RELPAX is contraindicated within 72 hours of treatment with the following potent CYP3A4 inhibitors: ketoconazole, itraconazole, nefazodone, troleandomycin, clarithromycin, ritonavir, and nelfinavir. RELPAX is contraindicated within 72 hours with drugs that have demonstrated potent CYP3A4 inhibition and have this potent effect described in the Contraindications, or Warnings and Precautions sections of their labeling (see Warnings and Precautions, Drug Interactions and Dosage and Administration).

RELPAX is contraindicated within 24 hours of treatment with another 5-HT$_1$ agonist, an ergotamine containing or ergot type medication such as dihydroergotamine (DHE) or methysergide.

RELPAX is contraindicated in patients with hemiplegic ophthalmoplegic or basilar migraine.

RELPAX tablets are contraindicated in patients with severe hepatic impairment.

RELPAX tablets are contraindicated in patients with known hypersensitivity to eletriptan or to any of its inactive ingredients.

WARNINGS AND PRECAUTIONS: General: RELPAX (eletriptan hydrobromide) tablets should only be used where a clear diagnosis of migraine has been established.

CYP3A4 Inhibitors: Eletriptan is metabolized by the CYP3A4 enzyme. RELPAX is contraindicated within 72 hours of treatment with the following potent CYP3A4 inhibitors: ketoconazole, itraconazole, nefazodone, troleandomycin, clarithromycin, ritonavir, and nelfinavir. RELPAX is contraindicated within 72 hours with drugs that have demonstrated potent CYP3A4 inhibition and have this potent effect described in the Contraindications or Warnings and Precautions sections of their labeling (see Drug Interactions and Dosage and Administration).

Cardiovascular: Risk of Myocardial Ischemia and/or Infarction and Other Cardiac Events: As with other triptans, eletriptan has been associated with transient pain or pressure sensation in the chest or throat. Because of the potential of 5-HT$_1$ agonists to cause coronary vasospasm, eletriptan should not be given to patients with documented ischemic or vasospastic coronary artery disease (CAD) (see Contraindications). It is strongly recommended that eletriptan not be given to patients in whom unrecognized CAD is predicted by the presence of risk factors (e.g., hypertension, hypercholesterolemia, smoker, obesity, diabetes, strong family history of CAD, female with surgical or physiological menopause, or male over 40 years of age) unless a cardiovascular evaluation provides satisfactory clinical evidence that the patient is reasonably free of coronary artery and ischemic myocardial disease, or other significant underlying cardiovascular disease. The sensitivity of cardiac diagnostic procedures to detect cardiovascular disease or predisposition to coronary artery vasospasm is modest, at best. If, during the cardiovascular evaluation, the patient's medical history, electrocardiographic, or other investigations reveal findings indicative of, or consistent with coronary artery vasospasm or myocardial ischemia, eletriptan should not be administered (see Contraindications).

These evaluations, however, may not identify every patient who has cardiac disease, and in very rare cases, serious cardiac events, such as myocardial infarction or coronary ischemia have occurred in patients without evidence of underlying cardiovascular disease.

For patients with risk factors predictive of CAD who are determined to have a satisfactory cardiovascular evaluation, it is strongly recommended that administration of the first dose of eletriptan take place in the setting of a physician's office or similar medically staffed and equipped facility unless the patient has previously received eletriptan. Because cardiac ischemia can occur in the absence of clinical symptoms, consideration should be given to obtaining, on the first occasion of use, an electrocardiogram (ECG) during the interval immediately following administration of eletriptan, in patients with risk factors. However, an absence of drug-induced cardiovascular effects on the occasion of the initial dose does not preclude the possibility of such effects occurring with subsequent administrations.

It is recommended that patients who are intermittent long-term users of 5-HT$_1$ agonists including eletriptan, and who have or acquire risk factors predictive of CAD, as described above, undergo periodic cardiovascular evaluation as they continue to use eletriptan.

If symptoms consistent with angina occur after the use of eletriptan, ECG evaluation should be carried out to look for ischemic changes.

The systematic approach described above is intended to reduce the likelihood that patients with unrecognized cardiovascular disease will be inadvertently exposed to therapy with eletriptan.

Discomfort in the chest, neck, throat and jaw (including pain, pressure, heaviness, and tightness) has been reported after administration of eletriptan. Because 5-HT$_1$ agonists may cause coronary vasospasm, patients who experience signs or symptoms suggestive of angina following eletriptan should be evaluated for the presence of CAD or a predisposition to variant angina before receiving additional doses, and should be monitored electrocardiographically if dosing is resumed and similar symptoms recur. Similarly, patients who experience other symptoms or signs suggestive of decreased arterial flow, such as ischemic bowel syndrome or Raynaud's syndrome following eletriptan should be evaluated for atherosclerosis or predisposition to vasospasm (see Contraindications and Warnings and Precautions and Adverse Reactions, Clinical Trial Adverse Drug Reactions).

Cardiac Events and Fatalities Associated with 5-HT$_1$ Agonists: As with other triptans, eletriptan may cause coronary artery vasospasm. Serious adverse cardiac events, including acute myocardial infarction, life-threatening disturbances of cardiac rhythm, and death have been reported within a few hours following the administration of other 5-HT$_1$ agonists. Considering the extent of use of 5-HT$_1$ agonists in patients with migraine, the incidence of these events is extremely low.

Patients with symptomatic Wolff-Parkinson-White syndrome or arrhythmias associated with other cardiac accessory conduction pathway disorders should not receive RELPAX.

As with other 5-HT$_1$ agonists, sensations of tightness, pain, pressure, and heaviness have been reported after treatment with RELPAX (eletriptan hydrobromide) tablets in the precordium, throat and jaw. Events that are localized to the chest, throat, neck and jaw have not been associated with arrhythmias or ischemic ECG changes in clinical trials.

Premarketing Experience with Eletriptan: In a clinical pharmacology study, in subjects undergoing diagnostic coronary angiography, a subject with a history of angina, hypertension and hypercholesterolemia, receiving intravenous eletriptan (C_{max} of 127 ng/mL equivalent to 60 mg oral eletriptan), reported chest tightness and experienced angiographically documented coronary vasospasm with no ECG changes indicative of ischemia. There was also 1 report of atrial fibrillation in a patient with a past history of atrial fibrillation.

Because 5-HT$_1$ agonists may cause coronary artery vasospasm, patients who experience signs or symptoms suggestive of angina following dosing should be evaluated for the presence of CAD or a predisposition to Prinzmetal's variant angina before receiving additional doses of medication, and should be monitored electrocardiographically if dosing is resumed and similar symptoms recur. Similarly, patients who experience other symptoms or signs suggestive of decreased arterial flow, such as ischemic bowel syndrome or Raynaud's syndrome, following the use of any 5-HT_1 agonist are candidates for further evaluation (see Contraindications).

In another coronary angiography study, supratherapeutic doses of eletriptan (comparable to 2×80 mg in the presence of a potent CYP3A4 inhibitor), administered as a rapid intravenous infusion, were compared with a standard formulation and dose of sumatriptan (6 mg sc) and placebo. There were 8 subjective reports of vasoconstriction in the eletriptan group (compared with no cases in the sumatriptan or placebo groups); however, mean change in coronary artery diameter, as determined by quantitative coronary angiography, did not differ in the 3 treatment groups.

Postmarketing Experience with Eletriptan: Cases of myocardial infarction and cardiac death have been reported in patients with cardiovascular risk factors (e.g. hypertension, hyperlipidemia, strong family history of CAD) or with inappropriate concomitant use of therapeutic doses of eletriptan and other triptans.

The uncontrolled nature of postmarketing surveillance, however, makes it impossible to determine definitively if the cases were actually caused by eletriptan or to reliably assess causation in individual cases.

Cerebrovascular Events and Fatalities Associated with 5-HT_1 Agonists: Cerebral hemorrhage, subarachnoid hemorrhage, stroke, and other cerebrovascular events have been reported in patients treated with 5-HT_1 agonists, and some have resulted in fatalities. In a number of cases, it appears possible that the cerebrovascular events were primary, the agonist having been administered in the incorrect belief that the symptoms experienced were a consequence of migraine, when they were not. It should be noted that patients with migraine may be at increased risk of certain cerebrovascular events (e.g., stroke, hemorrhage, transient ischemic attack).

Special Cardiovascular Pharmacology Studies with Another 5-HT_1 Agonist: In subjects (n=10) with suspected coronary artery disease undergoing angiography, a 5-HT_1 agonist at a subcutaneous dose of 1.5 mg produced an 8% increase in aortic blood pressure, an 18% increase in pulmonary artery blood pressure, and an 8% increase in systemic vascular resistance. In addition, mild chest pain or tightness was reported by 4 subjects. Clinically significant increases in blood pressure were experienced by 3 of the subjects (2 of whom also had chest pain/discomfort). Diagnostic angiogram results revealed that 9 subjects had normal coronary arteries and 1 had insignificant coronary artery disease.

In an additional study with this same drug, migraine patients (n=35) free of cardiovascular disease were subjected to assessments of myocardial perfusion by positron emission tomography while receiving a subcutaneous 1.5 mg dose in the absence of a migraine attack. Reduced coronary vasodilatory reserve (~10%), increased coronary resistance (~20%), and decreased hyperaemic myocardial blood flow (~10%) were noted. The relevance of these findings to the use of the recommended oral dose of this 5-HT_1 agonist is not known.

Other Vasospasm-Related Events: 5-HT_1 agonists may cause vasospastic reactions other than coronary artery spasm. Both peripheral vascular ischemia and colonic ischemia with abdominal pain, and bloody diarrhea have been reported with 5-HT_1 agonists.

Increase in Blood Pressure: Significant elevation in blood pressure, including hypertensive crisis, has been reported on rare occasions in patients receiving other 5-HT_1 agonists with and without a history of hypertension. In clinical pharmacology studies, oral eletriptan (at doses of 60 mg or more) was shown to cause small transient dose-related increases in blood pressure, predominantly diastolic, consistent with its mechanism of action and with other 5-$HT_{1B/1D}$ agonists. The effect was more pronounced in renally impaired and elderly subjects. A single patient with hepatic cirrhosis received eletriptan 80 mg and experienced a blood pressure of 220/96 mmHg 5 hours after dosing. The treatment-related event persisted for 7 hours.

RELPAX tablets are contraindicated in patients with uncontrolled or severe hypertension (see Contraindications).

Selective Serotonin Reuptake Inhibitors/Serotonin Norepinephrine Reuptake Inhibitors and Serotonin Syndrome: Cases of life-threatening serotonin syndrome have been reported during combined use of selective serotonin reuptake inhibitors (SSRIs)/serotonin norepinephrine reuptake inhibitors (SNRIs) and triptans. If concomitant treatment with RELPAX and SSRIs (e.g., fluoxetine, paroxetine, sertraline) or SNRIs (e.g., venlafaxine) is clinically warranted, careful observation of the patient is advised, particularly during treatment initiation and dose increases. Serotonin syndrome symptoms may include mental status changes (e.g., agitation, hallucinations, coma), autonomic instability (e.g., tachycardia, labile blood pressure, hyperthermia), neuromuscular aberrations (e.g., hyperreflexia, incoordination) and/or gastrointestinal symptoms (e.g., nausea, vomiting, diarrhea) (see Drug Interactions).

Dependence/Tolerance: Although the abuse potential of RELPAX tablets has not been assessed, no abuse of, tolerance to, or withdrawal from, or drug-seeking behavior was observed in patients who received RELPAX in clinical trials or their extensions. The 5-$HT_{1B/1D}$ agonists, as a class, have not been associated with drug abuse.

Hepatic/Biliary/Pancreatic: The effects of severe hepatic impairment on eletriptan metabolism were not evaluated. RELPAX tablets should not be given to patients with severe hepatic impairment.

Subjects with mild or moderate hepatic impairments demonstrated an increase in AUC (34%), C_{max} (18%) and in half-life. No dose adjustment is necessary in mild to moderate impairment (see Action and Clinical Pharmacology, Pharmacokinetics, and Dosage and Administration).

Neurologic: Care should be taken to exclude other potentially serious neurologic conditions before treating headache in patients not previously diagnosed with migraine headache or who experience a headache that is atypical for them. There have been rare reports where patients received 5-HT_1 agonists for severe headaches that were subsequently shown to have been secondary to an evolving neurologic lesion. For newly diagnosed patients or patients presenting with atypical symptoms, the diagnosis of migraine should be reconsidered if no response is seen after the first dose of eletriptan.

Seizures: Caution should be observed if eletriptan is to be used in patients with a history of seizures or other risk factors, such as structural brain lesions, which lower the convulsion threshold.

Ophthalmologic: Corneal Opacities: Transient corneal opacities were seen in dogs receiving oral eletriptan at 5 mg/kg and above. They were observed during the first week of treatment, but were not present thereafter despite continued treatment. Exposure at the no-effect dose level of 2.5 mg/kg exceeded that achieved in humans at the maximum recommended daily dose.

Preclinical Toxicology: Binding to Melanin-Containing Tissues: In rats treated with a single intravenous (3 mg/kg) dose of radiolabelled eletriptan, elimination of radioactivity from the retina was prolonged, suggesting that eletriptan and/or its metabolites may bind to the melanin of the eye. Because there could be accumulation in melanin-rich tissues over time, this raises the possibility that eletriptan could cause toxicity in these tissues after extended use. There were, however, no adverse ophthalmologic changes related to treatment with eletriptan in the 1-year dog toxicity study. Although no systematic monitoring of ophthalmologic function was undertaken in clinical trials, and no specific recommendations for ophthalmologic monitoring are offered, prescribers should be aware of the possibility of long-term ophthalmologic effects.

Carcinogenicity: Lifetime carcinogenicity studies, 104 weeks in duration, were carried out in mice and rats by administering eletriptan in the diet at doses of up to 400 mg/kg/day. In rats, the incidence of testicular interstitial cell adenomas was increased at the high dose of 75 mg/kg/day. The estimated exposure (AUC) to parent drug at that dose was approximately 6 times that achieved in humans receiving the maximum recommended daily dose (MRDD) of 80 mg, and at the no-effect dose of 15 mg/kg/day it was approximately 2 times the human exposure at the MRDD. In mice, the incidence of hepatocellular adenomas was increased at the high dose of 400 mg/kg/day. The exposure to parent drug (AUC) at that dose was approximately 18 times that achieved in humans receiving the MRDD, and the AUC at the no-effect dose of 90 mg/kg/day was approximately 7 times the human exposure at the MRDD.

Mutagenicity: Eletriptan was not mutagenic in bacterial or mammalian cell assays in vitro, testing negative in the Ames reverse mutation test and the hypoxanthineguanine phosphoribosyl transferase (HGPRT) mutation test in Chinese hamster ovary cells. It was not clastogenic in 2 in vivo mouse micronucleus assays. Results were equivocal in in vitro human lymphocyte clastogenicity tests, in which the incidence of polyploidy was increased in the absence of metabolic activation (-S9 conditions), but not in the presence of metabolic activation.

Psychomotor Effect: Patients should be advised to avoid driving a car or operating hazardous machinery until they are reasonably certain that RELPAX does not affect them adversely.

Renal: There was no significant change in clearance observed in subjects with mild, moderate or severe renal impairment. In some of these patients, an elevation in blood pressure was observed (see Action and Clinical Pharmacology, Pharmacokinetics and Dosage and Administration).

Sensitivity/Resistance: Hypersensitivity: Rare hypersensitivity (anaphylaxis/anaphylactoid) reactions have occurred in patients receiving other 5-HT_1 agonists. Such reactions can be life-threatening or fatal. In general, hypersensitivity reactions to drugs are more likely to occur in individuals with a history of sensitivity to multiple allergens. Owing to the possibility of cross-reactive hypersensitivity reactions, RELPAX should not be used in patients having a history of hypersensitivity to chemically-related 5-HT_1 receptor agonists (see Adverse Reactions).

Sexual Function/Reproduction: Impairment of Fertility: In a rat fertility and early embryonic development study, doses tested were 50, 100 and 200 mg/kg/day, resulting in systemic exposures to parent drug in rats, based on AUC, that were 4, 8, and 16 times MRDD, respectively, in males and 7, 14, and 28 times MRDD, respectively, in females. There was a prolongation of the estrous cycle at the 200 mg/kg/day dose due to an increase in duration of estrus, based on vaginal smears. There were also dose-related, statistically significant decreases in mean numbers of corpora lutea per dam at all 3 doses, resulting in decreases in mean numbers of implants and viable fetuses per dam. This suggests a partial inhibition of ovulation by eletriptan. There was no-effect on fertility of males and no other effect on fertility of females.

Special Populations: Pregnant Women: The safety of eletriptan in pregnant women has not been established. Administration of RELPAX tablets should only be considered if the expected benefit to the mother is greater than any possible risk to the fetus.

In reproductive toxicity studies in rats and rabbits, oral administration of eletriptan was associated with developmental toxicity (decreased fetal and pup weights) and an increased incidence of fetal structural abnormalities). Effects on fetal and pup weights were observed at doses that were, on a mg/m² basis, 6 to 12 times greater than the clinical MRDD of 80 mg. The increase in structural alterations occurred in the rat and rabbit at doses that, on a mg/m² basis, were 12 times greater than (rat) and approximately equal to (rabbit) the MRDD.

When pregnant rats were administered eletriptan during the period of organogenesis at doses of 10, 30 or 100 mg/kg/day, fetal weights were decreased and the incidences of vertebral and sternebral variations were increased at 100 mg/kg/day (approximately 12 times the MRDD on a mg/m² basis). The 100 mg/kg dose was also maternally toxic, as evidenced by decreased maternal body weight gain during gestation. The no-effect dose for developmental toxicity in rats exposed during organogenesis was 30 mg/kg, which is approximately 4 times the MRDD on a mg/m² basis.

When doses of 5, 10 or 50 mg/kg/day were given to New Zealand White rabbits throughout organogenesis, fetal weights were decreased at 50 mg/kg, which is approximately 12 times the MRDD on a mg/m² basis. The incidences of fused sternebrae and vena cava deviations were increased in all treated groups. Maternal toxicity was not produced at any dose. A no-effect dose for developmental toxicity in rabbits exposed during organogenesis was not established, and the 5 mg/kg dose is approximately equal to the MRDD on a mg/m² basis.

When female rats were treated with 5, 15 or 50 mg/kg/day during late gestation and lactation, in utero deaths were increased and pup weights were decreased postnatally at 50 mg/kg/day. The effect on pup weights persisted to adulthood. Exposure to parent drug (AUC) at that dose was approximately 4 times that achieved in humans receiving the MRDD. The 50 mg/kg/day dose was mildly maternally toxic, as evidenced by minimally decreased maternal body weight gain during gestation. The no-effect dose for developmental effects was 15 mg/kg, a dose that produced an AUC for parent drug approximately equal to that achieved in humans receiving the MRDD.

Nursing Women: Caution should be exercised when RELPAX tablets are administered to nursing women.

Eletriptan is excreted in human breast milk. In 1 study of 8 women given a single dose of 80 mg, the mean total amount of eletriptan in breast milk over 24 hours in this group was approximately 0.02% of the administered dose. The ratio of eletriptan mean concentration in breast milk to plasma was 1:4, but there was great variability. The resulting eletriptan concentration-time profile was similar to that seen in the plasma over 24 hours, with very low concentrations of drug (mean 1.7 ng/mL) still present in the milk 18-24 hours post-dose. The N-desmethyl active metabolite was not measured in the breast milk.

Pediatrics (<18 years of age): Safety and effectiveness of RELPAX tablets in pediatric patients have not been established; therefore, RELPAX is not recommended for use in patients under 18 years of age.

The efficacy of RELPAX tablets (40 mg) in patients 11-17 was not established in a randomized, placebo-controlled trial of 274 adolescent migraineurs, there were no statistically significant differences between treatment groups. The headache response rate at 2 hours was 57% for both RELPAX 40 mg tablets and placebo. Adverse events observed were similar in nature to those reported in clinical trials in adults. RELPAX is not recommended for use in patients under 18 years of age.

Geriatrics (>65 years of age): RELPAX has been given to only 50 patients over the age of 65. Blood pressure was increased to a greater extent in elderly subjects than in young subjects. The pharmacokinetic disposition of eletriptan in the elderly is similar to that seen in younger adults. There is a statistically significant increase in half-life (from about 4.4 hours to 5.7 hours) between elderly (65 to 93 years of age) and younger adult subjects (18 to 45 years of age) (see Action and Clinical Pharmacology, Special Populations and Conditions). Experience of the use of RELPAX in patients aged over 65 years is limited. Therefore the use of RELPAX in patients over 65 years is not recommended.

ADVERSE REACTIONS: Adverse Drug Reaction Overview: Serious cardiac events, including some that have been fatal, have occurred following the use of other 5-HT_1 agonists. These events are extremely rare and most have been reported in patients with risk factors of CAD. Events reported have included coronary artery vasospasm, transient myocardial ischemia, myocardial infarction, ventricular tachycardia, and ventricular fibrillation (see Contraindications and Warnings and Precautions).

Typical 5-HT_1 Agonist Adverse Reactions: As with other 5-HT_1 agonists, RELPAX has been associated with sensations of heaviness, pressure, tightness or pain which may be intense. These may occur in any part of the body including the chest, throat, neck, jaw and upper limbs.

Increases in Blood Pressure: Significant elevations in systemic blood pressure, including hypertensive crisis, have been reported on rare occasions in patients with and without a history of hypertension treated with other 5-HT_1 agonists. RELPAX is contraindicated in patients with uncontrolled hypertension (see Contraindications).

Clinical Trial Adverse Drug Reactions: In the clinical program, 7483 subjects have received RELPAX (eletriptan hydrobromide) tablets and 1595 have received placebo.

In Phase 2/3 clinical trials for the treatment of migraine, safety data were obtained for 6954 subjects treated with eletriptan and 1376 subjects treated with placebo. In the clinical pharmacology program, 529 subjects received eletriptan and 219 received placebo.

Among 5984 patients who treated a single migraine headache with RELPAX 20, 40 or 80 mg tablets in short-term, placebo-controlled trials, the most common and dose-related adverse events reported with treatment with RELPAX were asthenia (7.2%), nausea (7.8%), dizziness (5.7%) and somnolence (5.2%).

Table 1 lists the most common adverse events that occurred in the subset of 7131 patients with migraine who received eletriptan doses of 20 mg, 40 mg, 80 mg or placebo in worldwide, placebo-controlled clinical trials. Adverse events that were more frequent in a RELPAX treatment group compared to the placebo group with an incidence greater than 1% are included in Table 1. The events cited reflect experience gained under closely monitored conditions of clinical trials in a highly selected patient population. In actual clinical practice or in other clinical trials, those frequency estimates may not apply, as the conditions of use, reporting behavior, and the kinds of patients treated may differ.

RELPAX tablets are generally well tolerated. Across all doses, most adverse reactions were mild and transient. The frequency of adverse events in clinical trials did not increase when up to 2 doses of RELPAX tablets were taken within 24 hours. The incidence of adverse events in controlled clinical trials was not affected by gender, age, or race of patients. Adverse event frequencies were also unchanged by concomitant use of drugs commonly taken for migraine prophylaxis, (e.g., beta-blockers, calcium channel blockers, tricyclic antidepressants), estrogen replacement therapy and oral contraceptives.

Table 1: RELPAX

Treatment-Emergent Adverse Events by Initial Oral Dose of RELPAX and Placebo Reported by at Least 1% Patients with Migraine from Controlled Clinical Trials

	Placebo	20 mg	40 mg	80 mg
Number of Patients	1559	536	2951	2085
Symptoms of Potentially Cardiac Origin				
Chest Sensations[a]	1.1	0.4	2.2	4.4
Neck/Throat/Jaw Sensations[a]	0.2	0.2	1.4	2.2
Palpitations	0.9	0.7	1.3	1.8
Upper Limb Sensations[a]	0.1	0.2	0.6	1.1
Neurological				
Dizziness	2.8	2.4	5.1	7.2
Drowsiness	2.8	1.9	4.9	5.9
Head/Face Sensations[a]	0.7	1.5	1.2	1.8

(cont'd)

Table 1: RELPAX *(cont'd)*

Treatment-Emergent Adverse Events by Initial Oral Dose of RELPAX and Placebo Reported by at Least 1% Patients with Migraine from Controlled Clinical Trials

	Placebo	20 mg	40 mg	80 mg
Number of Patients	1559	536	2951	2085
Headache	2.4	2.8	2.8	3.5
Hypertonia	0.2	0.9	0.6	1.8
Vertigo	0.5	0.2	0.4	1.8
Digestive				
Abdominal Discomfort & Pain	0.7	0.9	1.7	2.2
Diarrhea	0.9	1.1	1.1	1.4
Gastrointestinal Discomfort & Pain	0.8	1.9	1.6	2.3
Hyposalivation	1.5	2.1	3.0	3.7
Nausea	7.8	3.9	6.9	10.4
Vomiting	5.7	0.6	3.0	4.0
Musculoskeletal				
Muscle Atrophy, Weakness & Tiredness	0.5	0.2	0.8	3.0
Muscle Pain	0.4	1.1	1.5	2.9
Ear, Nose & Throat				
Nasal Signs & Symptoms	0.6	0.9	1.0	1.5
Throat & Tonsil Symptoms	0.4	1.3	1.4	2.4
Respiratory				
Viral Infection	0.8	0.6	1.1	1.3
Non-Site Specific				
Chills	1.3	0.2	0.8	1.2
Malaise/Fatigue	1.9	2.6	4.5	9.4
Sensations[a]	2.1	2.6	3.6	5.6
Sweating	0.6	0.4	1.1	1.6

[a] The term "sensations" encompasses adverse events described as pain & discomfort, pressure, heaviness, constriction, tightness, heat/burning sensation, paresthesia, numbness, tingling and strange sensations.

Other Events Observed in Association with the Administration of RELPAX Tablets: The frequencies of less commonly reported adverse clinical events are listed below by body system in order of decreasing frequency. Because the reports include events observed in open studies, the role of RELPAX tablets in their causation cannot be reliably determined. Furthermore, variability associated with adverse event reporting, the terminology used to describe adverse events, etc., limit the value of the quantitative frequency estimates provided. Event frequencies are calculated as the number of patients reporting an event divided by the total number of patients (N=4719) exposed to RELPAX. All reported events are included except those already listed in Table 1, those too general to be informative, and those not reasonably associated with the use of the drug. Frequent adverse events are those occurring in at least 1/100 patients, infrequent adverse events are those occurring in 1/100 to 1/1000 patients, and rare adverse events are those occurring in fewer than 1/1000 patients.

General: Frequent: back pain, chills and pain. Infrequent: face edema and malaise. Rare: abdomen enlarged, abscess, accidental injury, allergic reaction, fever, flu syndrome, halitosis, hernia, hypothermia, lab test abnormal, moniliasis, rheumatoid arthritis and shock.

Cardiovascular: Frequent: palpitation. Infrequent: hypertension, migraine, peripheral vascular disorder and tachycardia. Rare: angina pectoris, arrhythmia, atrial fibrillation, AV block, bradycardia, hypotension, syncope, thrombophlebitis, cerebrovascular disorder, vasospasm and ventricular arrhythmia.

Digestive: Infrequent: anorexia, constipation, diarrhea, eructation, esophagitis, flatulence, gastritis, gastrointestinal disorder, glossitis, increased salivation and liver function tests abnormal. Rare: gingivitis, hematemesis, increased appetite, rectal disorder, stomatitis, tongue disorder, tongue edema and tooth disorder.

Endocrine: Rare: goiter, thyroid adenoma and thyroiditis.

Hemic and Lymphatic: Rare: anemia, cyanosis, leukopenia, lymphadenopathy, monocytosis and purpura.

Metabolic: Infrequent: creatine phosphokinase increased, edema, peripheral edema and thirst. Rare: alkaline phosphatase increased, bilirubinemia, hyperglycemia, weight gain and weight loss.

Musculoskeletal: Infrequent: arthralgia, arthritis, arthrosis, bone pain, myalgia and myasthenia. Rare: bone neoplasm, joint disorder, myopathy and tenosynovitis.

Neurological: Frequent: hypertonia, hypesthesia and vertigo. Infrequent: abnormal dreams, agitation, anxiety, apathy, ataxia, confusion, depersonalization, depression, emotional lability, euphoria, hyperesthesia, hyperkinesia, incoordination, insomnia, nervousness, speech disorder, stupor, thinking abnormal and tremor. Rare: abnormal gait, amnesia, aphasia, catatonic reaction, dementia, diplopia, dystonia, hallucinations, hemiplegia, hyperalgesia, hypokinesia, hysteria, manic reaction, neuropathy, neurosis, oculogyric crisis, paralysis, psychotic depression, sleep disorder and twitching.

Respiratory: Frequent: pharyngitis. Infrequent: asthma, dyspnea, respiratory disorder, respiratory tract infection, rhinitis, voice alteration and yawn. Rare: bronchitis, choking sensation, cough increased, epistaxis, hiccup, hyperventilation, laryngitis, sinusitis and sputum increased.

Skin and Appendages: Frequent: sweating. Infrequent: pruritus, rash and skin disorder. Rare: alopecia, dry skin, eczema, exfoliative dermatitis, maculopapular rash, psoriasis, skin discolouration, skin hypertrophy and urticaria.

Special Senses: Infrequent: abnormal vision, conjunctivitis, ear pain, eye pain, lacrimation disorder, photophobia, taste perversion and tinnitus. Rare: abnormality of accommodation, dry eyes, ear disorder, eye hemorrhage, otitis media, parosmia and ptosis.

Urogenital: Infrequent: impotence, polyuria, urinary frequency and urinary tract disorder. Rare: breast pain, kidney pain, leukorrhea, menorrhagia, menstrual disorder and vaginitis.

In postmarketing experience, the following additional undesirable effects have been reported:

Gastrointestinal Disorders: ischaemic colitis.

Nervous System Disorders: syncope.

Immune System Disorders: allergic reaction, some of which may be serious.

Skin and Subcutaneous Tissue Disorders: pruritus, rash, urticaria.

DRUG INTERACTIONS: Effects of Other Drugs on Eletriptan: CYP3A4 Inhibitors: In vitro studies have shown that eletriptan is metabolized by the CYP3A4 enzyme. A clinical study demonstrated about a 3-fold increase in C_{max} and about a 6-fold increase in the AUC of eletriptan when combined with ketoconazole. The half-life increased from 5 hours to 8 hours and the T_{max} increased from 2.8 hours to 5.4 hours. Another clinical study demonstrated about a 2-fold increase in C_{max} and about a 4-fold increase in AUC when erythromycin was co-administered with eletriptan. It has also been shown that co-administration of verapamil and eletriptan yields about a 2-fold increase in C_{max} and about a 3-fold increase in AUC of eletriptan, and that co-administration of fluconazole and eletriptan yields about a 1.4-fold increase in C_{max} and about a 2-fold increase in AUC of eletriptan.

RELPAX is contraindicated within 72 hours of treatment with the following potent CYP3A4 inhibitors: ketoconazole, itraconazole, nefazodone, troleandomycin, clarithromycin, ritonavir and nelfinavir. RELPAX is contraindicated within 72 hours with drugs that have demonstrated potent CYP3A4 inhibition and have this potent effect described in the Contraindications or Warnings and Precautions sections of their Product Monograph (see Contraindications, Warnings and Precautions and Dosage and Administration).

Ketoconazole: A clinical study demonstrated about a 3-fold increase in C_{max} and about a 6-fold increase in the AUC of eletriptan when co-administered with ketoconazole. The half-life of eletriptan increased from 5 hours to 8 hours and the T_{max} increased from 2.8 hours to 5.4 hours (see Action and Clinical Pharmacology, Pharmacokinetics).

Erythromycin: A clinical study demonstrated about a 2-fold increase in eletriptan C_{max} and about a 4-fold increase in AUC when erythromycin was co-administered with eletriptan. This increased exposure was associated with an increase in eletriptan $t_{½}$ from 4.6 hours to 7.1 hours (see Action and Clinical Pharmacology, Pharmacokinetics).

Fluconazole: Co-administration of fluconazole and eletriptan yields about a 1.4-fold increase in C_{max} and about a 2-fold increase in AUC of eletriptan.

Verapamil: It has also been shown that co-administration of verapamil and eletriptan yields about a 2-fold increase in C_{max} and about a 3-fold increase in AUC of eletriptan.

Ergot-Containing Drugs: Ergot-containing drugs have been reported to cause prolonged vasospastic reactions. Because these effects may be additive, use of ergotamine-containing or ergot-type medications (like dihydroergotamine [DHE] or methysergide) and RELPAX tablets within 24 hours is not recommended (see Action and Clinical Pharmacology, Pharmacokinetics and Contraindications).

Other 5-HT_1 Agonists: Concomitant use of other 5-HT_1 agonists within 24 hours of RELPAX treatment is not recommended (see Contraindications).

Selective Serotonin Reuptake Inhibitors (SSRIs)/Serotonin Norepinephrine Reuptake Inhibitors (SNRIs): Cases of life-threatening serotonin syndrome have been reported during combined use of selective serotonin reuptake inhibitors (SSRIs) or serotonin norepinephrine reuptake inhibitors (SNRIs) and triptans (see Warnings and Precautions).

Propranolol: The C_{max} and AUC of eletriptan were increased by 10% and 33%, respectively, following an 80 mg BID dose of propranolol administered for 7 days. No interactive increases in blood pressure were observed. No dose adjustment is necessary for patients also taking propranolol.

MAO Inhibitors: Eletriptan is not a substrate for monoamine oxidase (MAO) enzymes. Therefore there is no expectation of an interaction between RELPAX and MAO inhibitors.

The Effect of Eletriptan on Other Drugs: The effect of eletriptan on enzymes other than cytochrome P-450 has not been investigated. In vitro human liver microsome studies suggest that eletriptan has little potential to inhibit CYP1A2, 2C9, 2E1 and 3A4 at concentrations up to 100 μM. While eletriptan has an effect on CYP2D6 at high concentration (IC_{50} of about 41 μM), this effect should not interfere with metabolism of other drugs when eletriptan is used at recommended doses. There is no in vitro or in vivo evidence that clinical doses of eletriptan will induce drug metabolizing enzymes. Therefore, eletriptan is unlikely to cause clinically important drug interactions mediated by these enzymes.

Drug-Food Interactions: The AUC and C_{max} of eletriptan are increased by approximately 20 to 30% following oral administration with a high fat meal.

Drug-Herb Interactions: Interactions with herbal products have not been established.

Drug-Laboratory Test Interactions: Interactions with laboratory tests have not been established.

DOSAGE AND ADMINISTRATION:

Dosing Considerations: RELPAX (eletriptan hydrobromide) tablets should be taken as early as possible after the onset of a migraine attack, but are also effective if taken at a later stage. RELPAX tablets should not be used prophylactically.

Recommended Dose and Dosage Adjustment: Adult (18-65 years of age): In controlled clinical trials, single doses of 20 mg and 40 mg were effective for the acute treatment of migraine in adults. A greater proportion of patients had a response following a 40 mg dose than following a 20 mg dose. Individuals may vary in response to doses of RELPAX tablets.

When initiating treatment with RELPAX, a starting dose of 20 mg or 40 mg may be considered. Patients who do not obtain satisfactory efficacy after an initial trial of 20 mg may be effectively treated with 40 mg in subsequent migraine attacks. The choice of dose should therefore be made on an individual basis, according to the clinical status of the patient and weighing the possible risk/benefit of the 40 mg dose. A minimal effective dose should be used.

If after an initial dose of 20 mg, headache improves but then returns a repeat dose of 20 mg may be beneficial and should be taken at least 2 hours after the initial dose. If an initial dose of 40 mg is taken, a second dose is not recommended.

If the initial dose is ineffective, controlled clinical trials have not shown a benefit of a second dose to treat the same attack.

The maximum daily dose should not exceed 40 mg.

The safety of treating an average of more than 3 headaches in a 30-day period has not been established.

Patients Receiving Potent CYP3A4 Inhibitors: Eletriptan is metabolized by the CYP3A4 enzyme. Concomitant use of RELPAX and potent CYP3A4 inhibitors may lead to significant increases in AUC and C_{max}, therefore RELPAX tablets are contraindicated within 72 hours of treatment with the following potent CYP3A4 inhibitors: ketoconazole, itraconazole, clarithromycin, troleandomycin, ritonavir, nelfinavir and nefazodone. RELPAX is contraindicated within 72 hours with drugs that have demonstrated potent CYP3A4 inhibition and have this potent effect described in the Contraindications or Warnings and Precautions sections of their labeling (see Warnings and Precautions, Drug Interactions and Contraindications).

Patients with Hepatic Impairment: No dose adjustment is required in patients with mild or moderate hepatic impairment. As RELPAX has not been studied in patients with severe hepatic impairment, it is contraindicated in these patients (see Action and Clinical Pharmacology and Contraindications).

Patients with Renal Impairment: In some patients with renal impairment, an elevation in blood pressure was observed. A total daily dose of greater than 20 mg should be administered with caution (see Action and Clinical Pharmacology and Warnings and Precautions).

Administration: RELPAX tablets should be swallowed whole with water.

OVERDOSAGE:

Symptoms: No significant overdoses in clinical trials have been reported. Twenty-one (21) subjects have received single doses of 120 mg in Phase 1 trials and 427 in Phase 2/3 trials without significant adverse effects. Based on the pharmacology of 5-HT_1 agonists, hypertension or other more serious cardiovascular symptoms could occur on overdose.

Treatment: In case of overdose, standard supportive measures should be adopted. The elimination half-life of eletriptan is about 4 hours (see Action and Clinical Pharmacology), and therefore monitoring of patients after overdose with eletriptan should continue for at least 20 hours, or longer should symptoms or signs persist.

There is no specific antidote to eletriptan. In cases of severe intoxication, intensive care procedures are recommended, including establishing and maintaining a patent airway, ensuring adequate oxygenation and ventilation, and monitoring and support of the cardiovascular system.

It is unknown what effect hemodialysis or peritoneal dialysis has on the serum concentration of eletriptan.

> For management of a suspected drug overdose, CPhA recommends that you contact your **regional Poison Control Centre**. See the *CPS* Directory section for a list of Poison Control Centres.

ACTION AND CLINICAL PHARMACOLOGY: Mechanism of Action: Eletriptan binds with high affinity to 5-HT_{1B}, 5-HT_{1D} and 5-HT_{1F} receptors, has modest affinity for 5-HT_{1A}, 5-HT_{1E}, 5-HT_{2B} and 5-HT_7 receptors, and little or no affinity for 5-HT_{2A}, 5-HT_{2C}, 5-HT_3, 5-HT_4, 5-HT_{5A} and 5-HT_6 receptors.

Eletriptan has no significant affinity or pharmacological activity at adrenergic alpha$_1$, alpha$_2$, or beta; dopaminergic D_1 or D_2; muscarinic; or opioid receptors.

Two theories have been proposed to explain the efficacy of 5-HT receptor agonists in migraine. One theory suggests that activation of 5-HT_1 receptors located on intracranial blood vessels, including those on the arteriovenous anastomoses, leads to vasoconstriction, which is correlated with the relief of migraine headache. The other hypothesis suggests that activation of 5-HT_1 receptors on sensory nerve endings in the trigeminal system results in the inhibition of pro-inflammatory neuropeptide release.

In the anesthetized dog, eletriptan has been shown to reduce carotid arterial blood flow, with only a small increase in arterial blood pressure at high doses. While the effect on blood flow was selective for the carotid arterial bed, decreases in coronary artery diameter were observed. Eletriptan has also been shown to inhibit trigeminal nerve activity in the rat.

Pharmacokinetics: Absorption: Eletriptan is rapidly and well absorbed after oral administration with peak plasma levels occurring approximately 1.5 hours after dosing to healthy subjects. In patients with moderate to severe migraine, the median T_{max} is 2.0 hours. The mean absolute bioavailability of eletriptan is approximately 50%. The oral pharmacokinetics are slightly more than dose proportional over the clinical dose range. The AUC and C_{max} of eletriptan are increased by approximately 20 to 30% following oral administration with a high fat meal.

Distribution: The volume of distribution following IV administration is 138L. Plasma protein binding is moderate and approximately 85%.

Metabolism: The N-demethylated metabolite of eletriptan is the only known active metabolite. This metabolite causes vasoconstriction similar to eletriptan in animal models. Though the half-life of the metabolite is estimated to be about 13 hours, the plasma concentration of the N-demethylated metabolite is 10-20% of that of parent drug and is unlikely to contribute significantly to the overall effect of the parent compound. In vitro studies indicate that eletriptan is primarily metabolized by cytochrome P-450 enzyme CYP3A4 (see Contraindications, Warnings and Precautions and Drug Interactions).

Excretion: The elimination half-life of eletriptan is approximately 4 hours. Mean-renal clearance (CL_R) following oral administration is approximately 3.9 L/h. Non-renal clearance accounts for about 90% of the total clearance. The pharmacokinetic parameters while fasting are summarized in Table 2.

Table 2: RELPAX

Single Dose Pharmacokinetics of Eletriptan (N=18 patients, 9 males and 9 females)

Pharmacokinetic Parameter	Means[a]		
	20 mg	40 mg	80 mg
C_{max} (ng/mL)	37	82	188
AUC (ng·h/mL)	240	573	1218
AUC_t (ng·h/mL)	235	563	1198
T_{max} (h)	1.5	1.8	2.1
K_{el} (/h)	0.194	0.181	0.183
$t_{½}$ (h)	3.6	3.8	3.8

[a] Means are geometric for AUC, AUC_t and C_{max}, arithmetic for T_{max} and k_{el}, and harmonic for $t_{½}$.

Special Populations and Conditions: Pediatrics: The volume of distribution following oral administration is lower in children <12 years of age resulting in higher plasma concentrations than would be predicted following the same dose in adults. RELPAX is not recommended for use in patients under 18 years of age (see Warnings and Precautions, Special Populations).

Geriatrics: RELPAX (eletriptan hydrobromide) has been given to only 50 patients over the age of 65. There is a statistically significant increase in half-life (from about 4.4 hours to 5.7 hours) in the elderly compared to younger adult subjects based on population pharmacokinetic analysis (see Warnings and Precautions, Special Populations).

Blood pressure was increased to a greater extent in elderly subjects than in young subjects.

Gender: The pharmacokinetics of eletriptan are unaffected by gender.

Race: A comparison of the pharmacokinetic studies conducted in western countries and those conducted in Japan have indicated an approximate 35% reduction in the exposure of eletriptan in Japanese male volunteers compared to western males.

Population pharmacokinetic analysis of 2 clinical studies indicates no evidence of pharmacokinetic differences between Caucasians and non-Caucasian patients.

Menstrual Cycle: In a study of 16 healthy females, the pharmacokinetic profile of eletriptan remained consistent throughout the phases of the menstrual cycle.

Hepatic Insufficiency: The effects of severe hepatic impairment on eletriptan metabolism have not been evaluated. Subjects with mild or moderate hepatic impairment demonstrated an increase of eletriptan in AUC (34%), C_{max} (18%) and half-life (see Contraindications, Warnings and Precautions and Dosage and Administration for severe hepatic impairment).

Renal Insufficiency: There was no significant change in clearance observed in subjects with mild, moderate or severe renal impairment, though blood pressure elevations were observed in this population (see Warnings and Precautions and Dosage and Administration).

STORAGE AND STABILITY: Store at room temperature between 15-30°C. Protect from moisture.

INFORMATION FOR THE PATIENT: Published in e-CPS, available by subscription at www.e-cps.ca.

DOSAGE FORMS, COMPOSITION AND PACKAGING: 20 mg: Each orange, round, film-coated tablet, printed "REP20" on one side and PFIZER on the reverse, contains: eletriptan HBr 24.2 mg equivalent to eletriptan (base) 20 mg. Nonmedicinal ingredients: croscarmellose sodium, FD&C Yellow No. 6 aluminum lake, hypromellose, lactose monohydrate, microcrystalline cellulose, magnesium stearate, titanium dioxide and triacetin. Blister packs of 3.

40 mg: Each orange, round, film-coated tablet, printed "REP40" on one side and PFIZER on the reverse, contains: eletriptan HBr 48.5 mg equivalent to eletriptan (base) 40 mg. Nonmedicinal ingredients: croscarmellose sodium, FD&C Yellow No. 6 aluminum lake, hypromellose, lactose monohydrate, microcrystalline cellulose, magnesium stearate, titanium dioxide and triacetin. Blister packs of 3.

(Shown in Product Identification Section)

Remeron® Pr
mirtazapine
Antidepressant

Schering-Plough

Date of Preparation: May 7, 2001
Date of Revision: March 5, 2009

SUMMARY PRODUCT INFORMATION:

Route of Administration	Dosage Form/ Strength	Clinically Relevant Nonmedicinal Ingredients
Oral	Tablets, 30 mg	Lactose For a complete listing, see Dosage Forms, Composition and Packaging.

INDICATIONS AND CLINICAL USE: Adults: REMERON (mirtazapine) is indicated for the symptomatic relief of depressive illness.

Long-term Use of REMERON: The efficacy of REMERON in maintaining a response in patients with major depressive disorder for up to 40 weeks following 8-12 weeks of initial open-label treatment was demonstrated in a placebo-controlled trial. Nevertheless, the physician who elects to use REMERON for extended periods should periodically evaluate the long-term response of the individual patient to the drug.

Geriatrics (>65 years of age): Evidence from clinical trials and experience suggests that use in geriatric populations may be associated with differences in safety or effectiveness. A brief discussion can be found in the appropriate sections [see Warnings and Precautions, Neurologic, Somnolence; Special Populations, Geriatrics (>65 years of age); Dosage and Administration; Action and Clinical Pharmacology, Special Populations and Conditions, Geriatrics].

Pediatrics (<18 years of age): REMERON is not indicated for use in patients below the age of 18 years (see Warnings and Precautions, General, Potential Association with Behavioural and Emotional Changes, Including Self-Harm; and Dosage and Administration).

CONTRAINDICATIONS: Hypersensitivity: REMERON is contraindicated in patients who are known to be hypersensitive to the drug or any of its components. For a complete listing, see Dosage Forms, Composition and Packaging.

Monoamine Oxidase Inhibitors: In patients receiving agents that may affect the serotonergic neurotransmitter systems in combination with a monoamine oxidase (MAO) inhibitor, there have been reports of serious, sometimes fatal, reactions including hyperthermia, rigidity, myoclonus, autonomic instability with possible rapid fluctuations of vital signs, and mental status changes that include extreme agitation progressing to delirium and coma. These reactions have also been reported in patients who have recently discontinued SSRI treatment and have begun treatment on a MAO inhibitor. Some cases presented with features resembling serotonin syndrome or neuroleptic malignant syndrome (see Warnings and Precautions, Neurologic, Serotonin Syndrome/Neuroleptic Malignant Syndrome). Therefore, REMERON should not be used in combination with MAO inhibitors (including linezolid, an antibiotic which is a reversible non-selective MAO inhibitor) or within a minimum of 2 weeks of terminating treatment with MAO inhibitors. Treatment with REMERON should then be initiated cautiously and dosage increased gradually until optimal response is reached. MAO inhibitors should not be introduced within 2 weeks of cessation of therapy with REMERON.

WARNINGS AND PRECAUTIONS: General: Potential Association with Behavioural and Emotional Changes, Including Self-Harm: Pediatrics: Placebo-Controlled Clinical Trial Data:

- **Recent analyses of placebo-controlled clinical trial safety databases from SSRIs (Selective Serotonin Reuptake Inhibitors) and other newer antidepressants suggest that use of these drugs in patients under the age of 18 may be associated with behavioural and emotional changes, including an increased risk of suicidal ideation and behaviour over that of placebo.**
- **The small denominators in the clinical trial database, as well as the variability in placebo rates, preclude reliable conclusions on the relative safety profiles among these drugs.**

Adults and Pediatrics: Additional Data:

- **There are clinical trial and post-marketing reports with SSRIs and other newer antidepressants, in both pediatrics and adults, of severe agitation-type adverse events coupled with self-harm or harm to others. The agitation-type events include akathisia, agitation, disinhibition, emotional lability, hostility, aggression and depersonalization. In some cases, the events occurred within several weeks of starting treatment.**

Rigorous clinical monitoring for suicidal ideation or other indicators of potential for suicidal behaviour is advised in patients of all ages. This includes monitoring for agitation-type emotional and behavioural changes.

Discontinuation Symptoms: Patients currently taking REMERON should not discontinue treatment abruptly, due to risk of discontinuation symptoms. At the time that a medical decision is made to discontinue an SSRI or other newer antidepressant drug, a gradual reduction in the dose, rather than an abrupt cessation, is recommended.

Lactose: Lactose is a nonmedicinal ingredient in REMERON tablets. Therefore, patients with rare hereditary problems of galactose intolerance **or** glucose-galactose malabsorption should not take REMERON tablets.

Agranulocytosis: In pre-marketing clinical trials, two (one with Sjögren's Syndrome) out of 2796 patients treated with REMERON (mirtazapine) Tablets and one patient treated with imipramine developed agranulocytosis. In all three cases, the patients recovered after the drug with which they were being treated was stopped. In the post-marketing period with REMERON, very rare cases of agranulocytosis have been reported, mostly reversible, but in some cases fatal. All fatal cases concerned patients with an age above 65. If a patient develops a sore throat, fever, stomatitis or other signs of infection, along with a low WBC count, treatment with REMERON should be discontinued and the patient should be closely monitored.

Discontinuation of Treatment with REMERON: When discontinuing treatment, patients should be monitored for symptoms which may be associated with discontinuation, e.g., dizziness, abnormal dreams, sensory disturbances (including paraesthesia and electric shock sensations), agitation, anxiety, fatigue, confusion, headache, tremor, nausea, vomiting and sweating or other symptoms which may be of clinical significance (see Adverse Reactions). A gradual reduction in the dose over several weeks, rather than abrupt cessation, is recommended whenever possible. If intolerable symptoms occur following a decrease in the dose or upon discontinuation of treatment, dose titration should be managed on the basis of the patient's clinical response (see Adverse Reactions and Dosage and Administration).

The following additional precautions are listed alphabetically.

Cardiovascular: Cholesterol/Triglycerides: In U.S. short-term controlled studies, non-fasting cholesterol increases of >20% above the upper limits of normal were observed in 15% of patients taking REMERON compared to 7% for placebo. In these same studies, non-fasting triglycerides increased to >500 mg/dL in 6% of patients taking REMERON compared to 3% for placebo.

Concomitant Illness: Use in Patients with Concomitant Illness: Clinical experience with REMERON in patients with concomitant systemic illness is limited. Accordingly, care is advisable in prescribing REMERON for patients with diseases or conditions that affect metabolism or hemodynamic responses. REMERON has not been systematically evaluated or used to any appreciable extent in patients with a recent history of myocardial infarction or other significant heart disease. REMERON was associated with significant orthostatic hypotension in early clinical pharmacology trials with normal human volunteers. Orthostatic hypotension was infrequently observed in clinical trials with depressed patients. REMERON should be used with caution in patients with known cardiovascular or cerebrovascular disease that could be exacerbated by hypotension (history of myocardial infarction, angina or ischemic stroke) and conditions that would predispose patients to hypotension (dehydration, hypovolemia, and treatment with antihypertensive medication).

Dependence/Tolerance: Physical and Psychological Dependence: REMERON (mirtazapine) has not been systematically studied in animals or humans for its potential for abuse, tolerance or physical dependence. While the clinical trials did not reveal any tendency for any drug-seeking behaviour, these observations were not systematic and it is not possible to predict on the basis of this limited experience the extent to which a CNS-active drug will be misused, diverted and/or abused once marketed. Consequently, patients should be evaluated carefully for history of drug abuse, and such patients should be observed closely for signs of REMERON misuse or abuse (e.g., development of tolerance, incrementation of dose, drug-seeking behaviour).

Endocrine and Metabolism: Increased Appetite/Weight Gain: In U.S. short-term controlled studies, the use of REMERON was associated with increased appetite in 17% and the complaint of weight gain in 12 % of patients, compared to 2% for placebo in both cases. In these same trials, weight gain of ≥7% occurred in 7.5% of the patients taking REMERON compared to 0% in patients taking placebo. The average weight gain in the U.S. long-term controlled trials was 8 lb over 28 weeks.

Diabetes: Care should be taken in patients with diabetes mellitus.

Genitourinary: Care should be taken in patients with micturition disturbances like prostate hypertrophy.

Hematologic: Please refer to Warnings and Precautions, General, Agranulocytosis.

Hepatic/Biliary/Pancreatic: Hepatic Impairment: Increased plasma concentrations of mirtazapine occur in patients with moderate and severe hepatic impairment (see Action and Clinical Pharmacology, Special Populations and Conditions). In such patients, upward dose titration should be carefully monitored (see Dosage and Administration).

Transaminase Elevations: In U.S. short-term controlled studies, clinically significant ALT elevations (3 times the normal range) were noted in 2%, respectively, of patients treated with REMERON and in 0% of patients treated with placebo. Most patients did not develop signs or symptoms associated with compromised liver function. While some patients were discontinued due to ALT increases, other patients with elevations continued with enzyme levels returning to normal during ongoing treatment. Mirtazapine should be used with caution in patients with impaired hepatic function (see Dosage and Administration).

Jaundice: Treatment should be discontinued if jaundice occurs.

Neurologic: Somnolence: The use of REMERON (mirtazapine) Tablets was associated with somnolence in 54% of patients in U.S. short-term controlled studies, compared to 18% with placebo. In these studies, somnolence resulted in discontinuation of 10% of mirtazapine-treated patients compared to 2% of placebo-treated patients. REMERON may cause mental or motor impairment because of this prominent sedative effect. Thus, patients should be cautioned about engaging in hazardous activities, such as driving a car or operating dangerous machines, until they are reasonably certain that REMERON therapy does not adversely affect their ability to engage in such activities.

Dizziness: In U.S. short-term controlled studies, the use of REMERON was associated with dizziness in 7% of patients, compared to 3% for placebo.

Activation of Mania/Hypomania: Mania/hypomania occurred in approximately 0.2% (3/1299 patients) of REMERON-treated patients in all U.S. studies (controlled and non-controlled). Although the incidence of mania/hypomania was very low during treatment with REMERON, it should be used carefully in patients with a history of mania/hypomania.

Seizures: In pre-marketing clinical trials, only one seizure was reported in the 2796 U.S. and non-U.S. patients treated with REMERON. However, no controlled studies have been carried out in patients with a history of seizures. Therefore, care should be exercised when REMERON is used in these patients.

Serotonin Syndrome/Neuroleptic Malignant Syndrome: On rare occasions serotonin syndrome or neuroleptic malignant syndrome-like events have occurred in association with treatment of REMERON, particularly when given in combination with other serotonergic and/or neuroleptic/antipsychotic drugs. As these syndromes may result in potentially life-threatening conditions, treatment with REMERON should be discontinued if patients develop a combination of symptoms possibly including hyperthermia, rigidity, myoclonus, autonomic instability with possible rapid fluctuations of vital signs, mental status changes including confusion, irritability, extreme agitation progressing to delirium and coma and supportive symptomatic treatment should be initiated. Due to the risk of serotonergic syndrome or neuroleptic malignant syndrome REMERON should not be used in combination with MAO inhibitors or serotonin-precursors (such as L-tryptophan, oxitriptan) and should be used with caution in patients receiving other serotonergic drugs (triptans, lithium, tramadol, St. John's wort, most tricyclic antidepressants) or neuroleptics/antipsychotics (see Contraindications and Drug Interactions).

Ophthalmologic: Care should be taken in patients with acute narrow-angle glaucoma and increased intra-ocular pressure.

Psychiatric: Suicide: Suicidal ideation is inherent in depression and may persist until significant remission occurs. As with any patient receiving antidepressants, high-risk patients should be closely supervised during initial drug therapy. Prescriptions of REMERON should be written for the smallest quantity consistent with good patient management, in order to reduce the risk of overdose (see Warnings and Precautions, General, Potential Association with Behavioural and Emotional Changes, Including Self-Harm).

Renal: Renal and Hepatic Impairment: Increased plasma concentrations of mirtazapine occur in patients with moderate and severe renal impairment and, to a lesser extent, in patients with hepatic impairment (see Action and Clinical Pharmacology, Special Populations and Conditions). In such patients, upward dose titration should be carefully monitored (see Dosage and Administration).

Special Populations: Pregnant Women: Safe use of REMERON during pregnancy has not been established. Therefore, it should not be administered to women of childbearing potential or nursing mothers unless, in the opinion of the treating physician, the expected benefits to the patient outweigh the possible hazards to the child or fetus.

Post-marketing reports indicate that some neonates exposed to SSRIs or other newer antidepressants, such as REMERON, late in the third trimester have developed complications requiring prolonged hospitalization, respiratory support, and tube feeding. Such complications can arise immediately upon delivery. Reported clinical findings have included respiratory distress, cyanosis, apnea, seizures, temperature instability, feeding difficulty, vomiting, hypoglycemia, hypotonia, hypertonia, hyperreflexia, tremor, jitteriness, irritability and constant crying. The frequency of symptoms may vary with each drug. These features are consistent with either a direct toxic effect of SSRIs and other newer antidepressants, or, possibly, a drug discontinuation syndrome. It should be noted that, in some cases, the clinical picture is consistent with serotonin syndrome (see Warnings and Precautions, Neurologic, Serotonin Syndrome/Neuroleptic Malignant Syndrome). When treating a pregnant woman with REMERON during the third trimester, the physician should carefully consider the potential risks and benefits of treatment (see Dosage and Administration).

The extent of exposure in pregnancy during clinical trials: None.

Nursing Women: Safe use of REMERON during lactation has not been established.

Pediatrics (<18 years of age): Safety and effectiveness in children under 18 years of age have not been established.

Geriatrics (>65 years of age): Pharmacokinetic studies revealed a decreased clearance in the elderly, especially in elderly females. Elderly patients may be more susceptible to adverse events such as sedation, dizziness or confusion. Care should be exercised in dosage and titration to higher doses (see Action and Clinical Pharmacology; Dosage and Administration; Warnings and Precautions, Neurologic, Somnolence).

ADVERSE REACTIONS: Adverse Drug Reaction Overview: Adverse Events Leading to Discontinuation of Treatment: Sixteen percent of patients treated with REMERON (mirtazapine) Tablets in U.S. short-term controlled studies discontinued treatment due to an adverse event, compared to 7% of patients treated with placebo. The adverse event that accounted for more than 5% of discontinuations with REMERON was somnolence (10%).

Commonly Observed Adverse Events in U.S. Short-Term Controlled Clinical Trials: The most commonly observed adverse events related to the use of REMERON Tablets (5% or greater drug-related incidence for REMERON Tablets and at least twice that of placebo) were somnolence (54% vs. 18%), increased appetite (17% vs. 2%), weight gain (12% vs. 2%) and dizziness (7% vs. 3%).

Clinical Trial Adverse Drug Reactions: Adverse Events Occurring at an Incidence of 1% or More Among REMERON-Treated Patients: Table 1 enumerates adverse events that occurred at an incidence of 1% or more among REMERON-treated patients (and greater than the incidence in placebo-treated patients) who participated in U.S. short-term placebo-controlled trials, in which patients were dosed in a range of 5 to 60 mg/day. The investigators reported adverse clinical experiences using terms of their own choice. Reported adverse events were then classified using the standard COSTART-based dictionary terminology.

The prescriber should be aware that these figures cannot be used to predict the incidence of side effects in the course of usual medical practice where patient characteristics and other factors differ from those which prevailed in the clinical trials. Similarly, the cited frequencies cannot be compared with figures obtained from other investigations involving different treatments, uses and investigators. The cited figures, however, do provide the prescribing physician with some basis for estimating the relative contribution of drug and non-drug factors to the side effect incidence rate in the population studied.

Table 1: REMERON

Incidence of Adverse Clinical Experiences (≥1% for REMERON) in U.S. Short-Term Placebo-Controlled Studies[a,b,c]

Body System/Adverse Event N=Number of Patients	U.S. Studies REMERON N=453	 Placebo N=361
Body as a Whole		
Asthenia	34 (8%)	17 (5%)
Flu Syndrome	22 (5%)	9 (3%)
Back Pain	9 (2%)	3 (1%)
Digestive System		
Dry Mouth	112 (25%)	54 (15%)
Increased Appetite	76 (17%)	7 (2%)
Constipation	57 (13%)	24 (7%)
Metabolic and Nutritional Disorders		
Weight Gain	54 (12%)	6 (2%)
Peripheral Edema	11 (2%)	4 (1%)
Edema	6 (1%)	1 (0%)
Musculoskeletal System		
Myalgia	9 (2%)	3 (1%)
Nervous System		
Somnolence	243 (54%)	65 (18%)
Dizziness	33 (7%)	12 (3%)
Abnormal Dreams	19 (4%)	5 (1%)
Thinking Abnormal	15 (3%)	4 (1%)
Tremor	7 (2%)	2 (1%)
Confusion	9 (2%)	1 (0%)
Respiratory System		
Dyspnea	5 (1%)	1 (0%)
Urogenital System		
Urinary Frequency	8 (2%)	5 (1%)

[a] % rounded off to the nearest whole integer.
[b] Events which had an incidence on placebo >REMERON: infection, pain, headache, nausea, diarrhea and insomnia.
[c] Events which had an incidence of REMERON comparable to placebo: chest pain, palpitation, tachycardia, postural hypotension, dyspepsia, flatulence, libido decreased, hypertonia, nervousness, rhinitis, pharyngitis, sweating, amblyopia, tinnitus and taste perversion.

There was evidence of adaptation to some adverse events with continued therapy (e.g., increased appetite, dizziness and somnolence).

ECG Changes: The electrocardiograms for 338 patients who received REMERON and 261 patients who received placebo in the U.S. short-term controlled trials were analyzed, in which the QTc calculations using the method of Fridericia was employed . Prolongation in QTc ≥500 msec was not observed among mirtazapine-treated patients. Mean change in QTc was +1.6 msec for mirtazapine and −3.1 msec for placebo. Mirtazapine was associated with a mean increase in heart rate of 3.4 bpm, compared to 0.8 bpm for placebo. The clinical significance of these changes is unknown.

Less Common Clinical Trial Adverse Drug Reactions (<1%): During worldwide controlled and uncontrolled clinical trials, REMERON was administered to 2796 patients. The listing of events which follows includes those events which were judged by the investigator to be adverse clinical experiences. The investigators used terminology of their own choice to describe the adverse experiences. Consequently, it is not possible to provide a meaningful estimate of the proportion of individuals experiencing adverse events without first grouping similar types of untoward events into a smaller number of standardized categories. It is important to emphasize that although the events occurred during treatment with REMERON, they were not necessarily drug-related. Following the adverse experiences tabulations, the incidence of clinically significant laboratory values which occurred at a rate of ≥1% of patients is presented.

In the tabulations that follow, adverse events as reported by the investigator were classified using a standard COSTART-based dictionary terminology. Events are further categorized by body system and listed in order of decreasing frequency according to the following definitions: **frequent** adverse events are those occurring on one or more occasions in at least 1/100 patients, **infrequent** adverse events are those occurring in 1/100 to 1/1000 patients, and **rare** events are those occurring in fewer than 1/1000 patients. Only those events not already listed in Table 1 appear in this listing. Events of major clinical importance are also described in Warnings and Precautions.

Body as a Whole: Frequent: malaise, abdominal pain, abdominal syndrome acute. Infrequent: chills, fever, face edema, ulcer, photosensitivity reaction, neck rigidity, neck pain, abdomen enlarged. Rare: cellulitis, substernal chest pain.

Cardiovascular System: Frequent: hypertension, vasodilatation. Infrequent: angina pectoris, myocardial infarction, bradycardia, ventricular extrasystoles, syncope, migraine, hypotension. Rare: atrial arrhythmia, bigeminy, vascular headache, pulmonary embolus, cerebral ischemia, cardiomegaly, phlebitis, left heart failure.

Digestive System: Frequent: vomiting, anorexia. Infrequent: eructation, glossitis, cholecystitis, nausea and vomiting, gum hemorrhage, stomatitis, colitis, liver function tests abnormal. Rare: tongue discolouration, ulcerative stomatitis, salivary gland enlargement, increased salivation, intestinal obstruction, pancreatitis, aphthous stomatitis, cirrhosis of liver, gastritis, gastroenteritis, oral moniliasis, tongue edema.

Endocrine System: Rare: goiter, hypothyroidism.

Hemic and Lymphatic Systems: Rare: lymphadenopathy, leukopenia, petechia, anemia, thrombocytopenia, lymphocytosis, pancytopenia.

Metabolic and Nutritional Disorders: Frequent: thirst. Infrequent: dehydration, weight loss. Rare: gout, AST increased, healing abnormal, acid phosphatase increased, ALT increased, diabetes mellitus.

Musculoskeletal System: Frequent: myasthenia, arthralgia. Infrequent: arthritis, tenosynovitis. Rare: pathologic fracture, osteoporosis fracture, bone pain, myositis, tendon rupture, arthosis, bursitis.

Nervous System: Frequent: hypoesthesia, apathy, depression, hypokinesia, vertigo, twitching, agitation, anxiety, amnesia, hyperkinesia, paraesthesia. Infrequent: ataxia, delirium, delusions, depersonalization, dyskinesia, extrapyramidial syndrome, libido increased, coordination abnormal, dysarthria, hallucinations, manic reaction, neurosis, dystonia, hostility, reflexes increased, emotional lability, euphoria, paranoid reaction. Rare: aphasia, nystagmus, akathisia, stupor, dementia, diplopia, drug dependence, paralysis, grand mal convulsion, hypotonia, myoclonus, psychotic depression, withdrawal syndrome.

Respiratory System: Frequent: cough increased, sinusitis. Infrequent: epistaxis, bronchitis, asthma, pneumonia. Rare: asphyxia, laryngitis, pneumothorax, hiccup.

Skin and Appendages: Frequent: pruritus, rash. Infrequent: acne, exfoliative dermatitis, dry skin, herpes simplex, alopecia. Rare: urticaria, herpes zoster, skin hypertrophy, seborrhea, skin ulcer.

Special Senses: Infrequent: eye pain, abnormality of accommodation, conjunctivitis, deafness, keratoconjunctivitis, lacrimation disorder, glaucoma, hyperacusis, ear pain. Rare: blepharitis, partial transitory deafness, otitis media, taste loss, parosmia.

Urogenital System: Frequent: urinary tract infection. Infrequent: kidney calculus, cystitis, dysuria, urinary incontinence, urinary retention, vaginitis, hematuria, breast pain, amenorrhea, dysmenorrhea, leukorrhea, impotence. Rare: polyuria, urethritis, metrorrhagia, menorrhagia, abnormal ejaculation, breast engorgement, breast enlargement, urinary urgency.

Abnormal Hematologic and Clinical Chemistry Findings: Abnormal Laboratory Values: Elevated cholesterol, serum glucose and triglycerides were the most common blood chemistry parameters observed in U.S. studies.

The plasma samples were drawn from non-fasting patients, and these parameters are affected by diet. Patients taking REMERON had increased appetite and weight gain, and are likely to have had increased food intake. Increased food intake may account for the increased triglyceride and cholesterol values. Moreover, LDL:HDL ratio data from a limited number of patients suggest that fat metabolism does not change with REMERON treatment, further suggesting that the increase in triglyceride and cholesterol values reflected increased dietary intake.

Mild changes in liver function are shown by increases in liver enzymes. However, changes are temporary, mild, and are not expected to negatively influence liver function. Premature terminations due to liver enzyme abnormalities were, respectively, REMERON, 1.7% and placebo, 1.1%.

The incidence of neutropenias in all clinical studies for REMERON was 1.5%. Most of the observed cases of neutropenia were mild isolated and nonprogressive (see Warnings and Precautions).

Post-Market Adverse Drug Reactions: Adverse Events Observed During Post-Marketing Evaluation of REMERON: Adverse events reported since market introduction, which were temporally (but not necessary causally) related to mirtazapine therapy, include four cases of the ventricular arrhythmia torsades de pointes. In three of the four cases, however, concomitant drugs were implicated. All patients recovered.

Other adverse events observed post-marketing listed by System Organ Class and by frequency are found in Table 2.

Table 2: REMERON
Post-Marketing Adverse Events with REMERON

System Organ Class	Very Common (≥1/10)	Common (>1/100 to <1/10)	Uncommon (>1/1000 to ≤1/100)	Rare (>1/10 000 to ≤1/1000)	Very rare (≤1/10 000)
Blood and the Lymphatic System Disorders				- Bone marrow depression (granulocytopenia, agranulocytosis, aplastic anemia and thrombocytopenia) (see also Warnings and Precautions, Agranulocytosis) - Eosinophilia	
Metabolism and Nutrition Disorders		- Increase in appetite			
Psychiatric Disorders				- Nightmares/vivid dreams - Mania - Agitation - Confusion - Hallucinations - Anxiety[a] - Insomnia[a] - Psychomotor restlessness[b]	
Nervous System Disorders		- Somnolence (which can lead to impaired concentration), generally occurring during the first few weeks of treatment. (N.B.: Dose reduction generally does not lead to less sedation but can jeopardize antidepressant efficacy). - Dizziness - Headache		- Convulsions (insults), tremor, myoclonus - Paraesthesia - Restless legs - Syncope	- Oral paraesthesia - Serotonin syndrome
Vascular Disorders				- (Orthostatic) hypotension	
Gastrointestinal Disorders			- Nausea	- Dry mouth - Diarrhea	- Oral hypoesthesia - Mouth edema
Hepato-biliary Disorders				- Elevations in serum transaminase activities	
Skin and Subcutaneous Tissue Disorders				- Exanthema	
Musculoskeletal, Connective Tissue and Bone Disorders				- Arthralgia/myalgia	
General Disorders and Administration Site Conditions		- Generalised or local edema		- Fatigue	
Investigations		- Weight gain			

[a] Upon treatment with antidepressants in general, anxiety and insomnia (which may be symptoms of depression) can develop or become aggravated. Under REMERON treatment, development or aggravation of anxiety and insomnia has been reported very rarely.
[b] Incl. akathisia, hyperkinesia.

Adverse Reactions following Discontinuation of Treatment (or Dose Reduction): There have been reports of adverse reactions upon the discontinuation of REMERON (particularly when abrupt), including but not limited to the following: dizziness, abnormal dreams, sensory disturbances (including paraesthesia and electric shock sensations), agitation, anxiety, fatigue, confusion, headache, tremor, nausea, vomiting and sweating or other symptoms which may be of clinical significance (see Warnings and Precautions and Dosage and Administration).

Patients should be monitored for these or any other symptoms. A gradual reduction in the dosage over several weeks, rather than abrupt cessation, is recommended whenever possible. If intolerable symptoms occur following a decrease in dose or upon discontinuation of treatment, dose titration should be managed on the basis of the patient's clinical response. These events are generally self-limiting. Symptoms associated with discontinuation have been reported for other antidepressants with serotonergic effects (see Warnings and Precautions and Dosage and Administration).

DRUG INTERACTIONS:

Serious Drug Interactions
• **Monoamine Oxidase Inhibitors: See Contraindications.**

Overview: As with other drugs, the potential for interaction by a variety of mechanisms (e.g., pharmacodynamic, pharmacokinetic inhibition or enhancement, etc.) is a possibility (see Action and Clinical Pharmacology).

The metabolism and pharmacokinetics of mirtazapine may be affected by the induction or inhibition of drug-metabolizing enzymes.

Mirtazapine is extensively metabolized by CYP2D6, CYP3A4, and to a lesser extent by CYP1A2.

Drug-Drug Interactions: Monoamine Oxidase Inhibitors: Combined use of REMERON and monoamine oxidase inhibitors (including linezolid, an antibiotic which is a reversible non-selective MAO inhibitor) is contraindicated due to the potential for serious reactions with features resembling serotonin syndrome or neuroleptic malignant syndrome (see Contraindications and Warnings and Precautions, Neurologic, Serotonin Syndrome/Neuroleptic Malignant Syndrome).

Diazepam: The impairment of motor skills produced by REMERON has been shown to be additive with those caused by diazepam. Accordingly, patients should be advised to avoid diazepam and other similar drugs while taking REMERON.

CYP Enzyme Inducers: CYP3A4 Inducers (these studies used both drugs at steady state):

- **Phenytoin:** In healthy male patients (n=18), phenytoin (200 mg daily) increased mirtazapine (30 mg daily) clearance, resulting in about a twofold decrease in plasma mirtazapine concentrations. Mirtazapine did not significantly affect the pharmacokinetics of phenytoin. During combined use of mirtazapine and phenytoin, 3 out of 19 patients experienced fatigue and 1 out of 19 patients developed rash (and none had experienced either fatigue or rash with mirtazapine alone or phenytoin alone). The rash was severe enough to necessitate withdrawal from the study.
- **Carbamazepine:** In healthy male patients (n=24), carbamazepine (400 mg b.i.d.) increased mirtazapine (15 mg b.i.d.) clearance, resulting in about a twofold decrease in plasma mirtazapine concentrations.

When phenytoin, carbamazepine or another inducer of hepatic metabolism (such as rifampicin) is added to mirtazapine therapy, the mirtazapine dose may have to be increased. If treatment with such a medicinal product is discontinued, it may be necessary to reduce the mirtazapine dose.

CYP Enzyme Inhibitors: Cimetidine: In healthy male patients (n=12), when cimetidine (800 mg b.i.d.) at steady state was co-administered with mirtazapine (30 mg daily) at steady state, the Area Under the Curve (AUC) of mirtazapine increased by about 60%. Mirtazapine did not significantly change the pharmacokinetics of cimetidine. During combined use, side effects included somnolence [10 of 12 patients (including 1 of moderate severity) vs. 7 of 12 with mirtazapine alone and none with cimetidine alone], arrhythmia (2 of 12 patients vs. none with mirtazapine or cimetidine alone). The mirtazapine dose may have to be decreased when concomitant treatment with cimetidine is started, or increased when cimetidine treatment is discontinued.

Ketoconazole: In healthy, male, Caucasian patients (n=24), co-administration of the potent CYP3A4 inhibitor ketoconazole (200 mg b.i.d. for 6.5 days) increased the peak plasma levels and the AUC of a single 30 mg dose mirtazapine by approximately 40% and 50% respectively. During combined use, 2 severe adverse events have been reported: One patient experienced circulatory collapse and another patient experienced syncope. Both patients have lost consciousness for a brief period. Caution should be exercised when co-administering mirtazapine with potent CYP3A4 inhibitors, HIV protease inhibitors, azole antifungals, erythromycin or nefazodone.

Paroxetine: In an in vivo interaction study in healthy, CYP2D6 extensive metabolizer patients (n=24), mirtazapine (30 mg/day), at steady state, did not significantly change the pharmacokinetics of steady state paroxetine (40 mg/day), a CYP2D6 inhibitor. However, plasma concentrations of mirtazapine and its demethyl metabolite were slightly higher (about 18 and 25%, respectively) during combined administration with paroxetine. This difference is considered to be without clinical relevance. During combined use, side effects included exanthema (1 of 24 patients) that required withdrawal of the patient. Increases in AST and ALT were also reported, with a greater increase in men due to several outliers (including a patient that was withdrawn due to high AST (about 4 fold higher than the upper normal limit) and ALT (about 2 fold higher than the upper normal limit) levels; this patient also showed elevated WBC, neutrophils, decreased lymphocytes and basophils). AST/ALT levels returned to normal following the end of the treatment. Caution is advised for the co-administration of paroxetine with mirtazapine.

Other Drug-Drug Interactions: Amitriptyline: In healthy, CYP2D6 extensive metabolizer patients (n=32), amitriptyline (75 mg daily), at steady state, did not change the pharmacokinetics of steady state mirtazapine (30 mg daily) considerably and mirtazapine also did not change the pharmacokinetics of amitriptyline considerably. During combined use the following adverse reactions have been reported at considerably higher frequencies than with either drug alone: postural hypotension, impaired concentration (about 5 fold higher incidence), nausea (over 4 fold higher incidence) and dizziness (about 2 fold higher incidence). A CYP2D6 slow metabolizer patient experienced a serious adverse event following combined use of amitriptyline and mirtazapine. The subject complained of abdominal discomfort accompanied by dizziness and nausea and then leading to loss of consciousness for about 30 s. Apart from slight tremor (resembling myoclonic contractions) there were no other abnormalities. Caution is advised for the co-administration of amitriptyline with mirtazapine.

Warfarin: In healthy male subjects (n=16) mirtazapine (30 mg daily), at steady state, caused a small (0.2) but statistically significant increase in the International Normalised Ratio (INR) in subjects treated with warfarin to achieve subtherapeutic levels of prothrombin activity (1.5-2.0 INR) at steady state. As at a higher dose of mirtazapine, a more pronounced effect can not be excluded. It is advisable to monitor the INR in case of concomitant treatment of warfarin with mirtazapine.

Lithium: No relevant clinical effects or significant changes in pharmacokinetics have been observed in healthy male subjects on concurrent treatment with subtherapeutic levels of lithium (600 mg/day for 10 days) at steady state and a single 30 mg dose of mirtazapine. The serum levels of lithium were approximately 0.3 mmol/L 10 hrs after dosing. The effects of higher doses of lithium on the pharmacokinetics of mirtazapine are unknown.

Risperidone: In an in vivo non-randomized, interaction study subjects (n=6) in need of treatment with an antipsychiatric and antidepressant drug, the results of the effect of mirtazapine (30 mg daily) at steady state on the pharmacokinetics of risperidone (up to 3 mg b.i.d.) at steady state is inconclusive, due to high inter-patient variability and low number of patients. The study design does not permit conclusions to be made on the safety on the combined use of mirtazapine and risperidone. However, a case report of a male patient receiving combined treatment with mirtazapine (60 mg daily) and risperidone (3 mg daily) documents that, 6 weeks after initiation of this combination therapy, the patient developed pulmonary embolism and rhabdomyolysis. Caution is advised for the co-administration of risperidone with mirtazapine.

Serotonergic Drugs: Based on the mechanism of action of mirtazapine and the potential for serotonin syndrome, caution is advised when REMERON is coadministered with other drugs or agents that may affect the serotonergic neurotransmitter systems, such as tryptophan, triptans, serotonin reuptake inhibitors, lithium, tramadol or St. John's Wort (see Contraindications and Warnings and Precautions, Neurologic, Serotonin Syndrome/Neuroleptic Malignant Syndrome).

Drugs Bound to Plasma Protein: Because mirtazapine is bound to plasma proteins (85%), care should be exercised when REMERON is co-administered to a patient who may be receiving another drug which is highly protein-bound.

Drug-Herb Interactions: St. John's Wort: Pharmacodynamic interactions between REMERON and the herbal remedy St. John's Wort may occur and may result in an increase in undesirable effects. Dose adjustment of REMERON should be considered if clinically indicated.

Drug-Lifestyle Interactions: Alcohol: The impairment of mental and motor skills produced by REMERON have been shown to be additive with those produced by alcohol. Accordingly, patients should be advised to avoid alcohol while taking REMERON.

DOSAGE AND ADMINISTRATION: REMERON (mirtazapine) is not indicated for use in children under 18 years of age (see Warnings and Precautions, Potential Association with Behavioural and Emotional Changes, Including Self-Harm).

Dosing Considerations: Treatment of Pregnant Women During the Third Trimester: Post-marketing reports indicate that some neonates exposed to SSRIs or other newer antidepressants, such as REMERON, late in the third trimester have developed complications requiring prolonged hospitalization, respiratory support and tube feeding (see Warnings and Precautions). When treating pregnant women with REMERON during the third trimester, the physician should carefully consider the potential risks and benefits of treatment. The physician may consider tapering REMERON in the third trimester.

Children: See Warnings and Precautions, Potential Association with Behavioural and Emotional Changes, Including Self-Harm.

Elderly and Patients with Moderate to Severe Renal or Hepatic Impairment: In elderly patients, and patients with moderate to severe renal or hepatic impairment, limited pharmacokinetic data (see Action and Clinical Pharmacology) demonstrates increased serum concentration and/or reduced clearance of REMERON. REMERON should thus be dosed with care in these populations (see Action and Clinical Pharmacology, Pharmacokinetics).

Recommended Dose and Dosage Adjustment: Initial Treatment: Adults: REMERON (mirtazapine) Tablets should be administered as a single dose, preferably in the evening prior to sleep. The recommended initial dose is 15 mg daily. In clinical trials, patients generally received doses of REMERON in the range of 15-45 mg/day. While a relationship between dose and antidepressant response for REMERON has not been established, patients not responding to the initial 15 mg dose may benefit from dose increases up to a maximum of 45 mg/day. REMERON has an elimination half-life of approximately 20-40 hours, therefore, dose changes should occur in intervals of not less than one week. Dosage adjustments may be made according to the tolerance and based on the patient's response.

Longer-Term Treatment: It is generally agreed that acute episodes of depression require several months or longer of sustained therapy beyond response to the acute episode. Systematic evaluation of REMERON has demonstrated that its efficacy in major depressive disorder is maintained for periods of up to 40 weeks following 8-12 weeks of initial treatment at a dose 15-45 mg/day (see Action and Clinical Pharmacology). Based on these limited data, it is unknown whether or not the dose of REMERON needed for continuation treatment is identical to the dose needed to achieve an initial response. Patients should be periodically reassessed to determine the need for continuation treatment and the appropriate dose for such treatment.

Discontinuation of REMERON Treatment: Symptoms associated with the discontinuation or dose reduction of REMERON have been reported. Patients should be monitored for these and other symptoms when discontinuing treatment or during dosage reduction (see Warnings and Precautions and Adverse Reactions).

A gradual reduction in the dose over several weeks, rather than abrupt cessation, is recommended whenever is possible. If intolerable symptoms occur following a decrease in the dose or upon discontinuation of treatment, dose titration should be managed on the basis of the patient's clinical response (see Warnings and Precautions and Adverse Reactions).

Missed Dose: Do not take a double dose to make up for forgotten doses.

If a patient forgets to take the evening dose, advise the patient not to take the missed dose the next morning. Continue treatment in the evening (prior to sleep) with the normal dose.

Administration: Administration of REMERON (Mirtazapine) Tablets: Patients should be instructed to take the tablets at the same time each day, preferably as a single evening dose (prior to sleep). The tablets should be swallowed whole with water. The patient should be instructed not to chew the tablet (see Information for the Patient).

OVERDOSAGE:

Human Experience: In clinical trials, the only drug overdose death reported while taking REMERON (mirtazapine) Tablets was in combination with amitriptyline and chlorprohixene in a non-U.S. clinical study. Based on plasma levels, the REMERON dose taken was 30-45 mg, while plasma levels of amitriptyline and chlorprohixene were found to be at toxic levels. In other pre-marketing overdose cases with REMERON Tablets, the following signs and symptoms were reported: disorientation, drowsiness, impaired memory and tachycardia. There were no reports of ECG abnormalities, coma or convulsions following overdose with REMERON Tablets alone.

In post-marketing experience with more than 35 million patients exposed to REMERON (based on average treatment courses of 30 mg/day during 3 months), fatal cases of overdose with REMERON alone have been reported. In many cases details regarding the precise dose are lacking. Fatal acute overdoses with REMERON alone are documented at doses as low as approximately 440 mg, which is estimated from the post-mortem plasma levels, assuming linear pharmacokinetics. However, survival has also been reported with a single REMERON overdose as high as 1350 mg.

Present experience concerning overdose with REMERON alone indicates that symptoms are usually mild. Depression of the central nervous system with disorientation and prolonged sedation has been reported, together with tachycardia and mild hyper- or hypotension. However, there is a possibility of more serious outcomes (including fatalities) at dosages much higher than the therapeutic dose, especially with mixed overdosages.

Overdose Management: Treatment should consist of those general measures employed in the management of overdose with any antidepressant.

Ensure an adequate airway, oxygenation and ventilation. Monitor cardiac rhythm and vital signs. General supportive and symptomatic measures are also recommended. Induction of emesis is not recommended. Gastric lavage with a large-bore orogastric tube with appropriate airway protection, if needed, may be indicated if performed soon after ingestion, or in symptomatic patients.

Activated charcoal should be administered. There is no experience with the use of forced diuresis, dialysis, hemoperfusion or exchange transfusion in the treatment of mirtazapine overdosage. No specific antidotes for mirtazapine are known.

In managing overdosage, consider the possibility of multiple drug involvement. The physician should consider contacting a poison control centre for additional information on the treatment of any overdose.

> For management of a suspected drug overdose, CPhA recommends that you contact your **regional Poison Control Centre**. See the *CPS* Directory section for a list of Poison Control Centres.

ACTION AND CLINICAL PHARMACOLOGY: Mechanism of Action: The mechanism of action of REMERON (mirtazapine) Tablets, as with other drugs effective in the treatment of major depressive disorder, is unknown.

Evidence gathered in preclinical studies suggests that mirtazapine enhances central noradrenergic and serotonergic activity. These studies have shown that mirtazapine acts as an antagonist at central presynaptic α_2 adrenergic inhibitory autoreceptors and heteroreceptors, an action that is postulated to result in an increase in central noradrenergic and serotonergic activity. The clinical relevance of this finding is unknown.

Pharmacodynamics: REMERON acts as an antagonist at central presynaptic α_2 adrenergic inhibitory autoreceptors and heteroreceptors, which results in an increase in central noradrenergic and serotonergic activity. The clinical relevance of this finding is unknown, however, this action may explain its antidepressant activity.

REMERON is a potent antagonist of 5-HT_2 and 5-HT_3 receptors. The clinical relevance of this finding is unclear, however, the 5-HT_2 and 5-HT_3 antagonism by REMERON may account for its low rate of nausea, insomnia and anxiety as observed in clinical trials. REMERON has no significant direct effect on 5-HT_{1A} and 5-HT_{1B} receptors.

Both enantiomers of REMERON appear to contribute to its pharmacological activity. The (+)enantiomer blocks 5-HT_2 receptors as well as α_2 receptors, and the (−)enantiomer blocks 5-HT_3 receptors. The clinical relevance of this finding is unclear, but this may explain its antidepressant activity and side-effects profile.

REMERON is a potent histamine (H_1) receptor antagonist, which may contribute to its sedative effect and possibly to weight gain due to increased appetite.

REMERON is a moderate peripheral α_1 adrenergic antagonist, a property which may explain the occasional orthostatic hypotension reported in association with its use.

REMERON is a moderate antagonist at muscarinic receptors, a property that may explain the occasional occurrence of anticholinergic side effects associated with its use as shown in clinical trials.

Pharmacokinetics: REMERON is well absorbed following oral administration and its absolute bioavailability is approximately 50% after either single or multiple doses. Peak plasma concentrations are reached within about 2 hours following an oral dose. The time to peak plasma concentration is independent of dose. The presence of food in the stomach somewhat slows the rate but not the extent of absorption, and thus does not require a dosage adjustment.

Plasma levels are linear over a dose range of 30 to 80 mg. Steady-state plasma levels are attained within about 5 days. The half-life of elimination of REMERON after oral administration is approximately 20-40 hours.

Metabolism: REMERON is extensively metabolized and quantitatively eliminated via urine (75%) and feces (15%); approximately 90% of this elimination occurs within the first 72-96 hours. Major pathways of biotransformation are demethylation and oxidation followed by conjugation. In vitro data from human liver microsomes indicate that cytochrome 2D6 and 1A2 are involved in the formation of the 8-hydroxy metabolite of mirtazapine, whereas cytochrome 3A is considered to be responsible for the formation of the N-demethyl and N-oxide metabolite. The demethyl metabolite is pharmacologically active and appears to have a similar pharmacokinetic profile as that of the parent compound.

The (−)enantiomer has an elimination half-life that is approximately twice as long, and achieves plasma levels that are three times as high as that of the (+)enantiomer.

Protein Binding: REMERON is approximately 85% bound to plasma proteins over a concentration range of 10 to 1000 ng/mL. Binding appears to be both non-specific and reversible. The binding affinity of mirtazapine to human liver proteins is 2.8 times greater than to human plasma proteins. As with all drugs that are protein-bound, care should be exercised when co-administering medications that may interact with REMERON at protein-binding sites (see Warnings and Precautions).

Table 3: REMERON

Effect of Age and Gender on Plasma Half-Life of Mirtazapine

Group	$t_{1/2}$ (mean±SD)[a] Single Dose	Multiple Dose
Adult Male N=9	21.7±4.2	22.1±3.7
Adult Female N=9	37.7±13.3	35.4±13.7
Elderly[b] Male N=8	32.2±15.4	31.1±15.1
Elderly[b] Female N=8	40.6±12.8	39.0±10.8

[a] Expressed in hours.
[b] The "elderly" group consisted of subjects 55 and older (55-75; mean age 65).

Special Populations and Conditions: Pediatrics: REMERON is not indicated for use in patients below the age of 18 years (see Warnings and Precautions, General, Potential Association with Behavioural and Emotional Changes, Including Self-Harm; and Dosage and Administration).

Geriatrics: Following administration of REMERON 20 mg/day for 7 days, oral clearance was reduced in older subjects (mean age 65; range 55-75) compared to younger subjects (see Table 3). The difference was greatest in males, with a 40% lower clearance for REMERON in the older vs. younger group. Caution is indicated in administering REMERON (mirtazapine) Tablets in the elderly (see Warnings and Precautions and Dosage and Administration).

Gender: Age and Sex: In the same study above (see Action and Clinical Pharmacology, Special Populations and Conditions, Geriatrics) females of all ages (range 25-74) exhibited significantly longer elimination half-lives than males (mean half-life 37 hours for females vs. 26 hours for males) (see Table 3). Although these differences result on average in higher area-under-the-curve (AUC) for females compared to males, there is considerable overlap in individual AUCs between groups. Because of substantial individual variation of AUC and half-life, no specific dosage recommendations based on sex are indicated (see Dosage and Administration).

Hepatic Insufficiency: Liver Disease: In a single-dose study conducted with REMERON 15 mg, the elimination half-life of REMERON was increased 40% in mild to moderately hepatically impaired subjects as compared to subjects with normal hepatic function; this effect on elimination resulted in a 57% increase in AUC and a 33% decrease in clearance.

Renal Insufficiency: Renal Disease: In a single-dose study conducted with REMERON 15 mg, subjects with moderate and severe renal impairment showed a significant decrease in the clearance of ORG 3770 and a consequent increase in the AUC (54% and 215% for moderate and severe renal impairment, respectively). Subjects with severe renal impairment had significantly higher peak plasma levels of ORG 3770 (about double that of subjects without renal impairment). These results suggest that caution must be exercised in administering REMERON to patients who may have compromised renal function.

STORAGE AND STABILITY: Store at controlled room temperature, 15-30°C. Dispense in a tight, light-resistant container.

SPECIAL HANDLING INSTRUCTIONS: The tablets should be swallowed whole with water. The patient should be instructed not to chew the tablet.

INFORMATION FOR THE PATIENT: Published in e-CPS, available by subscription at www.e-cps.ca.

DOSAGE FORMS, COMPOSITION AND PACKAGING: Each oval, scored, red-brown, film-coated tablet, with "Organon" embossed on one side and "TZ5" on the other side, contains: mirtazapine 30 mg. Nonmedicinal ingredients: colloidal silicon dioxide, cornstarch, hydroxypropylcellulose, hydroxypropyl methylcellulose, lactose monohydrate, magnesium stearate, polyethylene glycol 8000, red iron oxide, titanium dioxide and yellow iron oxide. Blister packs of 10 tablets, cartons of 3 blister packs.

(Shown in Product Identification Section)

Remeron RD® Pr

mirtazapine

Antidepressant

Schering-Plough

Date of Preparation: December 16, 2003
Date of Revision: February 19, 2009

SUMMARY PRODUCT INFORMATION:

Route of Administration	Dosage Form/ Strength	Clinically Relevant Nonmedicinal Ingredients
Oral	Orally Disintegrating Tablets, 15, 30 and 45 mg	Aspartame and sucrose For a complete listing, see Dosage Forms, Composition and Packaging.

INDICATIONS AND CLINICAL USE: Adults: REMERON RD (mirtazapine) is indicated for the symptomatic relief of depressive illness.

Long-term Use of REMERON RD: The efficacy of REMERON RD (mirtazapine) Orally Disintegrating Tablets in maintaining a response in patients with major depressive disorder for up to 40 weeks following 8-12 weeks of initial open-label treatment was demonstrated in a placebo-controlled trial. Nevertheless, the physician who elects to use REMERON RD for extended periods should periodically evaluate the long-term response of the individual patient to the drug.

Geriatrics (>65 years of age): Evidence from clinical trials and experience suggests that use in geriatric populations may be associated with differences in safety or effectiveness. A brief discussion can be found in the appropriate sections [see Warnings and Precautions, Neurologic, Somnolence; Special Populations, Geriatrics (>65 years of age); Dosage and Administration; Action and Clinical Pharmacology, Special Populations and Conditions, Geriatrics].

Pediatrics (<18 years of age): REMERON RD is not indicated for use in patients below the age of 18 years (see Warnings and Precautions, General, Potential Association with Behavioural and Emotional Changes, Including Self-Harm; and Dosage and Administration).

CONTRAINDICATIONS: Hypersensitivity: REMERON RD is contraindicated in patients who are known to be hypersensitive to the drug or any of its components. For a complete listing, see Dosage Forms, Composition and Packaging.

Monoamine Oxidase Inhibitors: In patients receiving agents that may affect the serotonergic neurotransmitter systems in combination with a monoamine oxidase (MAO) inhibitor, there have been reports of serious, sometimes fatal, reactions including hyperthermia, rigidity, myoclonus, autonomic instability with possible rapid fluctuations of vital signs, and mental status changes that include extreme agitation progressing to delirium and coma. These reactions have also been reported in patients who have recently discontinued SSRI treatment and have begun treatment on a MAO inhibitor. Some cases presented with features resembling serotonin syndrome or neuroleptic malignant syndrome (see Warnings and Precautions, Neurologic, Serotonin Syndrome/Neuroleptic Malignant Syndrome). Therefore, REMERON RD should not be used in combination with MAO inhibitors (including linezolid, an antibiotic which is a reversible non-selective MAO inhibitor) or within a minimum of 2 weeks of terminating treatment with MAO inhibitors. Treatment with REMERON RD should then be initiated cautiously and dosage increased gradually until optimal response is reached. MAO inhibitors should not be introduced within 2 weeks of cessation of therapy with REMERON RD.

WARNINGS AND PRECAUTIONS: General: Potential Association with Behavioural and Emotional Changes, Including Self-Harm: Pediatrics: Placebo-Controlled Clinical Trial Data:

- **Recent analyses of placebo-controlled clinical trial safety databases from SSRIs (Selective Serotonin Reuptake Inhibitors) and other newer antidepressants suggest that use of these drugs in patients under the age of 18 may be associated with behavioural and emotional changes, including an increased risk of suicidal ideation and behaviour over that of placebo.**
- **The small denominators in the clinical trial database, as well as the variability in placebo rates, preclude reliable conclusions on the relative safety profiles among these drugs.**

Adults and Pediatrics: Additional Data:

- **There are clinical trial and post-marketing reports with SSRIs and other newer antidepressants, in both pediatrics and adults, of severe agitation-type adverse events coupled with self-harm or harm to others. The agitation-type events include: akathisia, agitation, disinhibition, emotional lability, hostility, aggression, and depersonalization. In some cases, the events occurred within several weeks of starting treatment.**

Rigorous clinical monitoring for suicidal ideation or other indicators of potential for suicidal behaviour is advised in patients of all ages. This includes monitoring for agitation-type emotional and behavioural changes.

Discontinuation Symptoms: Patients currently taking REMERON RD should not discontinue treatment abruptly, due to risk of discontinuation symptoms. At the time that a medical decision is made to discontinue an SSRI or other newer antidepressant drug, a gradual reduction in the dose, rather than an abrupt cessation, is recommended.

Sucrose: REMERON RD contains sucrose, therefore, patients with rare hereditary problems of fructose intolerance, glucose-galactose malabsorption or sucrase-isomaltase insufficiency should not take this medicine.

Aspartame: REMERON RD contains aspartame, a source of phenylalanine, therefore, may be harmful for people with phenylketonuria.

Agranulocytosis: In pre-marketing clinical trials, two (one with Sjögren's Syndrome) out of 2796 patients treated with REMERON (mirtazapine) Tablets and one patient treated with imipramine developed agranulocytosis. In all three cases, the patients recovered after the drug with which they were being treated was stopped. In the post-marketing period with REMERON, very rare cases of agranulocytosis have been reported, mostly reversible, but in some cases fatal. All fatal cases concerned patients with an age above 65. If a patient develops a sore throat, fever, stomatitis or other signs of infection, along with a low WBC count, treatment with REMERON RD (mirtazapine) Orally Disintegrating Tablets should be discontinued and the patient should be closely monitored.

Discontinuation of Treatment with REMERON RD: When discontinuing treatment, patients should be monitored for symptoms which may be associated with discontinuation, e.g., dizziness, abnormal dreams, sensory disturbances (including paraesthesia and electric shock sensations), agitation, anxiety, fatigue, confusion, headache, tremor, nausea, vomiting and sweating or other symptoms which may be of clinical significance (see Adverse Reactions). A gradual reduction in the dosage over several weeks, rather than abrupt cessation, is recommended whenever possible. If intolerable symptoms occur following a decrease in the dose or upon discontinuation of treatment, dose titration should be managed on the basis of the patient's clinical response (see Adverse Reactions and Dosage and Administration).

The following additional precautions are listed alphabetically.

Cardiovascular: Cholesterol/Triglycerides: In U.S. short-term controlled studies, non-fasting cholesterol increases of >20% above the upper limits of normal were observed in 15% of patients taking REMERON Tablets compared to 7% for placebo. In these same studies, non-fasting triglycerides increased to >500 mg/dl in 6% of patients taking REMERON Tablets compared to 3% for placebo.

Concomitant Illness: Use in Patients with Concomitant Illness: Clinical experience with mirtazapine in patients with concomitant systemic illness is limited. Accordingly, care is advisable in prescribing REMERON RD for patients with diseases or conditions that affect metabolism or hemodynamic responses. Mirtazapine has not been systematically evaluated or used to any appreciable extent in patients with a recent history of myocardial infarction or other significant heart disease. Mirtazapine was associated with significant orthostatic hypotension in early clinical pharmacology trials with normal human volunteers. Orthostatic hypotension was infrequently observed in clinical trials with depressed patients. REMERON RD should be used with caution in patients with known cardiovascular or cerebrovascular disease that could be exacerbated by hypotension (history of myocardial infarction, angina or ischemic stroke) and conditions that would predispose patients to hypotension (dehydration, hypovolemia and treatment with antihypertensive medication).

Dependence/Tolerance: Physical and Psychological Dependence: Mirtazapine has not been systematically studied in animals or humans for its potential for abuse, tolerance or physical dependence. While the clinical trials did not reveal any tendency for any drug-seeking behaviour, these observations were not systematic and it is not possible to predict on the basis of this limited experience the extent to which a CNS-active drug will be misused, diverted and/or abused once marketed. Consequently, patients should be evaluated carefully for history of drug abuse, and such patients should be observed closely for signs of REMERON RD misuse or abuse (e.g., development of tolerance, incrementation of dose, drug-seeking behaviour).

Endocrine and Metabolism: Increased Appetite/Weight Gain: In U.S. short-term controlled studies the use of REMERON Tablets was associated with increased appetite in 17% and the complaint of weight gain in 12% of patients, compared to 2% for placebo in both cases. In these same trials, weight gain of ≥7% occurred in 7.5% of the patients taking REMERON Tablets compared to 0% in patients taking placebo. The average weight gain in the U.S. long-term controlled trials was 8 lbs. over 28 weeks.

Diabetes: Care should be taken in patients with diabetes mellitus.

Genitourinary: Care should be taken in patients with micturition disturbances like prostate hypertrophy.

Hematologic: Please refer to Warnings and Precautions, General, Agranulocytosis.

Hepatic/Biliary/Pancreatic: Hepatic Impairment: Increased plasma concentrations of mirtazapine occur in patients with moderate and severe hepatic impairment (see Action and Clinical Pharmacology, Special Populations and Conditions). In such patients, upward dose titration should be carefully monitored (see Dosage and Administration).

Transaminase Elevations: In U.S. short-term controlled studies, clinically significant ALT elevations (3 times the normal range) were noted in 2%, respectively, of patients treated with REMERON Tablets and in 0% of patients treated with placebo. Most patients did not develop signs or symptoms associated with compromised liver function. While some patients discontinued treatment due to ALT increases, other patients with elevations continued with enzyme levels returning to normal during ongoing treatment. Mirtazapine should be used with caution in patients with impaired hepatic function (see Dosage and Administration).

Jaundice: Treatment should be discontinued if jaundice occurs.

Neurologic: Somnolence: The use of REMERON (mirtazapine) Tablets was associated with somnolence in 54% of patients in U.S. short-term controlled studies, compared to 18% with placebo. In these studies, somnolence resulted in of 10% of mirtazapine-treated patients discontinuing treatment compared to 2% of placebo-treated patients. REMERON RD (mirtazapine) Orally Disintegrating Tablets may cause mental or motor impairment because of this prominent sedative effect. Thus, patients should be cautioned about engaging in hazardous activities, such as driving a car or operating dangerous machines, until they are reasonably certain that REMERON RD therapy does not adversely affect their ability to engage in such activities.

Dizziness: In U.S. short-term controlled studies, the use of REMERON Tablets was associated with dizziness in 7% of patients, compared to 3% for placebo.

Activation of Mania/Hypomania: Mania/hypomania occurred in approximately 0.2% (3/1299 patients) of REMERON-treated patients in all U.S. studies (controlled and non-controlled). Although the incidence of mania/hypomania was very low during treatment with REMERON Tablets, it should be used carefully in patients with a history of mania/hypomania.

Seizures: In pre-marketing clinical trials, only one seizure was reported in the 2796 U.S. and non-U.S. patients treated with REMERON Tablets. However, no controlled studies have been carried out in patients with a history of seizures. Therefore, care should be exercised when REMERON RD is used in these patients.

Serotonin Syndrome/Neuroleptic Malignant Syndrome: On rare occasions serotonin syndrome or neuroleptic malignant syndrome-like events have occurred in association with treatment of REMERON RD, particularly when given in combination with other serotonergic and/or neuroleptic/antipsychotic drugs. As these syndromes may result in potentially life-threatening conditions, treatment with REMERON RD should be discontinued if patients develop a combination of symptoms possibly including hyperthermia, rigidity, myoclonus, autonomic instability with possible rapid fluctuations of vital signs, mental status changes including confusion, irritability, extreme agitation progressing to delirium and coma and supportive symptomatic treatment should be initiated. Due to the risk of serotonergic syndrome or neuroleptic malignant syndrome REMERON RD should not be used in combination with MAO inhibitors or serotonin-precursors (such as L-tryptophan, oxitriptan) and should be used with caution in patients receiving other serotonergic drugs (triptans, lithium, tramadol, St. John's wort, most tricyclic antidepressants) or neuroleptics/antipsychotics (see Contraindications and Drug Interactions).

Ophthalmologic: Care should be taken in patients with acute narrow-angle glaucoma and increased intra-ocular pressure.

Psychiatric: Suicide: Suicidal ideation is inherent in depression and may persist until significant remission occurs. As with any patient receiving antidepressants, high-risk patients should be closely supervised during initial drug therapy. Prescriptions of REMERON RD should be written for the smallest quantity consistent with good patient management, in order to reduce the risk of overdose (see Warnings and Precautions, General, Potential Association with Behavioural and Emotional Changes, Including Self-Harm).

Renal: Renal and Hepatic Impairment: Increased plasma concentrations of mirtazapine occur in patients with moderate and severe renal impairment and, to a lesser extent, in patients with hepatic impairment (see Action and Clinical Pharmacology, Special Populations and Conditions). In such patients, upward dose titration should be carefully monitored (see Dosage and Administration).

Special Populations: Pregnant Women: Safe use of REMERON RD during pregnancy has not been established. Therefore, it should not be administered to women of childbearing potential or nursing mothers unless, in the opinion of the treating physician, the expected benefits to the patient outweigh the possible hazards to the child or fetus.

Post-marketing reports indicate that some neonates exposed to SSRIs (Selective Serotonin Reuptake Inhibitors) or other newer antidepressants, such as REMERON RD, late in the third trimester have developed complications requiring prolonged hospitalization, respiratory support and tube feeding. Such complications can arise immediately upon delivery. Reported clinical findings have included respiratory distress, cyanosis, apnea, seizures, temperature instability, feeding difficulty, vomiting, hypoglycemia, hypotonia, hypertonia, hyperreflexia, tremor, jitteriness, irritability and constant crying. The frequency of symptoms may vary with each drug. These features are consistent with either a direct toxic effect of SSRIs and other newer antidepressants, or, possibly, a drug discontinuation syndrome. It should be noted that, in some cases, the clinical picture is consistent with serotonin syndrome (see Warnings and Precautions, Neurologic, Serotonin Syndrome/Neuroleptic Malignant Syndrome). When treating a pregnant woman with REMERON RD during the third trimester, the physician should carefully consider the potential risks and benefits of treatment (see Dosage and Administration).

The Extent of Exposure in Pregnancy During Clinical Trials: None.

Nursing Women: Safe use of REMERON RD during lactation has not been established.

Pediatrics (<18 years of age): Safety and effectiveness in children under 18 years of age have not been established.

Geriatrics (>65 years of age): Pharmacokinetic studies revealed a decreased clearance in the elderly, especially in elderly females. Elderly patients may be more susceptible to adverse events such as sedation, dizziness or confusion. Care should be exercised in dosage and titration to higher doses (see Action and Clinical Pharmacology; Dosage and Administration and Warnings and Precautions, Neurologic, Somnolence).

ADVERSE REACTIONS: Adverse Drug Reaction Overview: Adverse Events Leading to Discontinuation of Treatment: Sixteen percent of patients treated with REMERON (mirtazapine) Tablets in U.S. short-term controlled studies discontinued treatment due to an adverse event, compared to 7% of patients treated with placebo. The adverse event that accounted for more than 5% of discontinuations with REMERON Tablets was somnolence (10%).

Commonly Observed Adverse Events in U.S. Short-Term Controlled Clinical Trials: The most commonly observed adverse events related to the use of REMERON Tablets (5% or greater drug-related incidence for REMERON Tablets and at least twice that of placebo) were: somnolence (54% vs. 18%), increased appetite (17% vs. 2%), weight gain (12% vs. 2%), dizziness (7% vs. 3%).

Clinical Trial Adverse Drug Reactions: Adverse Events Occurring at an Incidence of 1% or More Among REMERON-Treated Patients: Table 1 enumerates adverse events that occurred at an incidence of 1% or more among REMERON-treated patients (and greater than the incidence in placebo-treated patients) who participated in U.S. short-term placebo-controlled trials, in which patients were dosed in a range of 5 to 60 mg/day. The investigators reported adverse clinical experiences using terms of their own choice. Reported adverse events were then classified using the standard COSTART-based dictionary terminology.

The prescriber should be aware that these figures cannot be used to predict the incidence of side effects in the course of usual medical practice, where patient characteristics and other factors differ from those which prevailed in the clinical trials. Similarly, the cited frequencies cannot be compared with figures obtained from other investigations involving different treatments, uses and investigators. The cited figures, however, do provide the prescribing physician with some basis for estimating the relative contribution of drug and non-drug factors to the side effect incidence rate in the population studied.

Table 1: REMERON RD

Incidence of Adverse Clinical Experiences (≥1% for REMERON Tablets) In U.S. Short-Term Placebo-Controlled Studies[a,b,c]

Body System Adverse Clinical Experience N=Number of Patients	U.S. Studies	
	REMERON Tablets N=453	Placebo N=361
Body as a Whole		
Asthenia	34 (8%)	17 (5%)
Flu Syndrome	22 (5%)	9 (3%)
Back Pain	9 (2%)	3 (1%)
Digestive System		
Dry Mouth	112 (25%)	54 (15%)
Increased Appetite	76 (17%)	7 (2%)
Constipation	57 (13%)	24 (7%)
Metabolic and Nutritional Disorders		
Weight Gain	54 (12%)	6 (2%)
Peripheral Edema	11 (2%)	4 (1%)
Edema	6 (1%)	1 (0%)
Musculoskeletal System		
Myalgia	9 (2%)	3 (1%)
Nervous System		
Somnolence	243 (54%)	65 (18%)
Dizziness	33 (7%)	12 (3%)
Abnormal Dreams	19 (4%)	5 (1%)
Thinking Abnormal	15 (3%)	4 (1%)
Tremor	7 (2%)	2 (1%)
Confusion	9 (2%)	1 (0%)
Respiratory System		
Dyspnea	5 (1%)	1 (0%)
Urogenital System		
Urinary Frequency	8 (2%)	5 (1%)

a % rounded off to the nearest whole integer.
b Events which had an incidence on placebo >REMERON Tablets: infection, pain, headache, nausea, diarrhea and insomnia.
c Events which had an incidence of REMERON Tablets comparable to placebo: chest pain, palpitation, tachycardia, postural hypotension, dyspepsia, flatulence, libido decreased, hypertonia, nervousness, rhinitis, pharyngitis, sweating, amblyopia, tinnitus and taste perversion.

There was evidence of adaptation to some adverse events with continued therapy (e.g., increased appetite, dizziness and somnolence).

ECG Changes: The electrocardiograms for 338 patients who received REMERON Tablets and 261 patients who received placebo in the U.S. short-term controlled trials were analyzed, in which the QTc calculations using the method of Fridericia was employed. Prolongation in QTc ≥500 msec was not observed among mirtazapine-treated patients. Mean change in QTc was +1.6 msec for mirtazapine and −3.1 msec for placebo. Mirtazapine was associated with a mean increase in heart rate of 3.4 bpm, compared to 0.8 bpm for placebo. The clinical significance of these changes is unknown.

Less Common Clinical Trial Adverse Drug Reactions (<1%): During worldwide controlled and uncontrolled clinical trials, REMERON Tablets were administered to 2796 patients. The listing of events which follows includes those events which were judged by the investigator to be adverse clinical experiences. The investigators used terminology of their own choice to describe the adverse experiences. Consequently, it is not possible to provide a meaningful estimate of the proportion of individuals experiencing adverse events without first grouping similar types of untoward events into a smaller number of standardized categories. It is important to emphasize that although the events occurred during treatment with REMERON Tablets, they were not necessarily drug-related. Following the adverse experience tabulations, the incidence of clinically significant laboratory values which occurred at a rate of ≥1% of patients is presented.

In the tabulations that follow, adverse events as reported by the investigator were classified using a standard COSTART-based Dictionary terminology. Events are further categorized by body system and listed in order of decreasing frequency according to the following definitions: **frequent** adverse events are those occurring on one or more occasions in at least 1/100 patients; **infrequent** adverse events are those occurring in 1/100 to 1/1000 patients; **rare** events are those occurring in fewer than 1/1000 patients. Only those events not already listed in Table 1 appear in this listing. Events of major clinical importance are also described in Warnings and Precautions.

Body as a Whole: Frequent: malaise, abdominal pain, abdominal syndrome acute. Infrequent: chills, fever, face edema, ulcer, photosensitivity reaction, neck rigidity, neck pain, abdomen enlarged. Rare: cellulitis, substernal chest pain.

Cardiovascular System: Frequent: hypertension, vasodilatation. Infrequent: angina pectoris, myocardial infarction, bradycardia, ventricular extrasystoles, syncope, migraine, hypotension. Rare: atrial arrhythmia, bigeminy, vascular headache, pulmonary embolus, cerebral ischemia, cardiomegaly, phlebitis, left heart failure.

Digestive System: Frequent: vomiting, anorexia. Infrequent: eructation, glossitis, cholecystitis, nausea and vomiting, gum hemorrhage, stomatitis, colitis, liver function tests abnormal. Rare: tongue discolouration, ulcerative stomatitis, salivary gland enlargement, increased salivation, intestinal obstruction, pancreatitis, aphthous stomatitis, cirrhosis of liver, gastritis, gastroenteritis, oral moniliasis, tongue edema.

Endocrine System: Rare: goiter, hypothyroidism.

Hemic and Lymphatic Systems: Rare: lymphadenopathy, leukopenia, petechia, anemia, thrombocytopenia, lymphocytosis, pancytopenia.

Metabolic and Nutritional Disorders: Frequent: thirst. Infrequent: dehydration, weight loss. Rare: gout, AST increased, healing abnormal, acid phosphatase increased, ALT increased, diabetes mellitus.

Musculoskeletal System: Frequent: myasthenia, arthralgia. Infrequent: arthritis, tenosynovitis. Rare: pathologic fracture, osteoporosis fracture, bone pain, myositis, tendon rupture, arthosis, bursitis.

Nervous System: Frequent: hypoesthesia, apathy, depression, hypokinesia, vertigo, twitching, agitation, anxiety, amnesia, hyperkinesia, paraesthesia. Infrequent: ataxia, delirium, delusions, depersonalization, dyskinesia, extrapyramidial syndrome, libido increased, coordination abnormal, dysarthria, hallucinations, manic reaction, neurosis, dystonia, hostility, reflexes increased, emotional lability, euphoria, paranoid reaction. Rare: aphasia, nystagmus, akathisia, stupor, dementia, diplopia, drug dependence, paralysis, grand mal convulsion, hypotonia, myoclonus, psychotic depression, withdrawal syndrome.

Respiratory Systems: Frequent: cough increased, sinusitis. Infrequent: epistaxis, bronchitis, asthma, pneumonia. Rare: asphyxia, laryngitis, pneumothorax, hiccup.

Skin and Appendages: Frequent: pruritus, rash. Infrequent: acne, exfoliative dermatitis, dry skin, herpes simplex, alopecia. Rare: urticaria, herpes zoster, skin hypertrophy, seborrhea, skin ulcer.

Special Senses: Infrequent: eye pain, abnormality of accommodation, conjunctivitis, deafness, keratoconjunctivitis, lacrimation disorder, glaucoma, hyperacusis, ear pain. Rare: blepharitis, partial transitory deafness, otitis media, taste loss, parosmia.

Urogenital System: Frequent: urinary tract infection. Infrequent: kidney calculus, cystitis, dysuria, urinary incontinence, urinary retention, vaginitis, hematuria, breast pain, amenorrhea, dysmenorrhea, leukorrhea, impotence. Rare: polyuria, urethritis, metrorrhagia, menorrhagia, abnormal ejaculation, breast engorgement, breast enlargement, urinary urgency.

Abnormal Hematologic and Clinical Chemistry Findings: Abnormal Laboratory Values: Elevated cholesterol, serum glucose and triglycerides were the most common blood chemistry parameters observed in U.S. studies.

The plasma samples were drawn from non-fasting patients, and these parameters are affected by diet. Patients taking REMERON Tablets had increased appetite and weight gain, and are likely to have had increased food intake. Increased food intake may account for the increased triglyceride and cholesterol values. Moreover, LDL:HDL ratio data from a limited number of patients suggest that fat metabolism does not change with REMERON treatment, further suggesting that the increase in triglyceride and cholesterol values reflected increased dietary intake.

Mild changes in liver function are shown by increases in liver enzymes. However, changes are temporary, mild, and are not expected to negatively influence liver function. Premature terminations due to liver enzyme abnormalities were, respectively, REMERON Tablets, 1.7% and placebo, 1.1%.

The incidence of neutropenias in all clinical studies for REMERON Tablets was 1.5%. Most of the observed cases of neutropenia were mild, isolated and nonprogressive (see Warnings and Precautions).

Post-Market Adverse Drug Reactions: Adverse Events Observed During Post-Marketing Evaluation of REMERON Tablets: Adverse events reported since market introduction, which were temporally (but not necessary causally) related to mirtazapine therapy, include four cases of the ventricular arrhythmia torsades de pointes. In three of the four cases, however, concomitant drugs were implicated. All patients recovered.

Other adverse events observed post-marketing, listed by system organ class and by frequency, are found in Table 2.

Adverse Reactions Following Discontinuation of Treatment (or Dose Reduction): There have been reports of adverse reactions upon the discontinuation of REMERON Tablets (particularly when abrupt), including but not limited to the following: dizziness, abnormal dreams, sensory disturbances (including paraesthesias and electric shock sensations), agitation, anxiety, fatigue, confusion, headache, tremor, nausea, vomiting and sweating or other symptoms which may be of clinical significance (see Warnings and Precautions and Dosage and Administration).

Patients should be monitored for these or any other symptoms. A gradual reduction in the dosage over several weeks, rather than abrupt cessation, is recommended whenever possible. If intolerable symptoms occur following a decrease in dose or upon discontinuation of treatment, dose titration should be managed on the basis of the patient's clinical response. These events are generally self-limiting. Symptoms associated with discontinuation have been reported for other antidepressants with serotonergic effects (see Warnings and Precautions and Dosage and Administration).

Table 2: REMERON RD

Post-Marketing Adverse Events with REMERON

System Organ Class	Very Common (≥1/10)	Common (>1/100 to <1/10)	Uncommon (>1/1000 to ≤1/100)	Rare (>1/10 000 to ≤1/1000)	Very Rare (≤1/10 000)
Blood and the Lymphatic System Disorders				- Bone marrow depression (granulocytopenia, agranulocytosis, aplastic anemia and thrombocytopenia) (see also Warnings and Precautions, Agranulocytosis) - Eosinophilia	
Metabolism and Nutrition Disorders		- Increase in appetite			
Psychiatric Disorders				- Nightmares/vivid dreams - Mania - Agitation - Confusion - Hallucinations - Anxiety[a] - Insomnia[a] - Psychomotor restlessness[b]	
Nervous System Disorders		- Somnolence (which can lead to impaired concentration), generally occurring during the first few weeks of treatment. (N.B.: Dose reduction generally does not lead to less sedation but can jeopardize antidepressant efficacy) - Dizziness - Headache		- Convulsions (insults), tremor, myoclonus - Paraesthesia - Restless legs - Syncope	- Oral paraesthesia - Serotonin syndrome
Vascular Disorders				- (Orthostatic) hypotension	
Gastrointestinal Disorders			- Nausea	- Dry mouth - Diarrhea	- Oral hypoaesthesia - Mouth oedema
Hepato-Biliary Disorders				- Elevations in serum transaminase activities	
Skin and Subcutaneous Tissue Disorders				- Exanthema	
Musculoskeletal, Connective Tissue and Bone Disorders				- Arthralgia/myalgia	
General Disorders and Administration Site Conditions		- Generalised or local edema		- Fatigue	
Investigations		- Weight gain			

[a] Upon treatment with antidepressants in general, anxiety and insomnia (which may be symptoms of depression) can develop or become aggravated. Under REMERON treatment, development or aggravation of anxiety and insomnia has been reported very rarely.
[b] Incl. akathisia, hyperkinesia.

DRUG INTERACTIONS:

Serious Drug Interactions
- **Monoamine Oxidase Inhibitors: See Contraindications.**

Overview: As with other drugs, the potential for interaction by a variety of mechanisms (e.g., pharmacodynamic, pharmacokinetic inhibition or enhancement, etc.) is a possibility (see Action and Clinical Pharmacology).

The metabolism and pharmacokinetics of mirtazapine may be affected by the induction or inhibition of drug-metabolizing enzymes.

Mirtazapine is extensively metabolized by CYP2D6, CYP3A4, and to a lesser extent by CYP1A2.

Drug-Drug Interactions: Monoamine Oxidase Inhibitors: Combined use of REMERON RD and monoamine oxidase inhibitors (including linezolid, an antibiotic which is a reversible non-selective MAO inhibitor) is contraindicated due to the potential for serious reactions with features resembling serotonin syndrome or neuroleptic malignant syndrome (see Contraindications and Warnings and Precautions, Neurologic, Serotonin Syndrome/Neuroleptic Malignant Syndrome).

Diazepam: The impairment of motor skills produced by mirtazapine has been shown to be additive with those caused by diazepam. Accordingly, patients should be advised to avoid diazepam and other similar drugs while taking REMERON RD.

CYP Enzyme Inducers: CYP3A4 Inducers (these studies used both drugs at steady state):
- **Phenytoin:** In healthy male patients (n=18), phenytoin (200 mg daily) increased mirtazapine (30 mg daily) clearance, resulting in about a twofold decrease in plasma mirtazapine concentrations. Mirtazapine did not significantly affect the pharmacokinetics of phenytoin. During combined use of mirtazapine and phenytoin, 3 out of 19 patients experienced fatigue and 1 out of 19 patients developed rash (and none had experienced either fatigue or rash with mirtazapine alone or phenytoin alone). The rash was severe enough to necessitate withdrawal from the study.
- **Carbamazepine:** In healthy male patients (n=24), carbamazepine (400 mg b.i.d.) increased mirtazapine (15 mg b.i.d.) clearance, resulting in about a twofold decrease in plasma mirtazapine concentrations.

When phenytoin, carbamazepine or another inducer of hepatic metabolism (such as rifampicin) is added to mirtazapine therapy, the mirtazapine dose may have to be increased. If treatment with such a medicinal product is discontinued, it may be necessary to reduce the mirtazapine dose.

CYP Enzyme Inhibitors: Cimetidine: In healthy male patients (n=12), when cimetidine (800 mg b.i.d.) at steady state was co-administered with mirtazapine (30 mg daily) at steady state, the Area Under the Curve (AUC) of mirtazapine increased by about 60%. Mirtazapine did not significantly change the pharmacokinetics of cimetidine. During combined use, side effects included somnolence [10 of 12 patients (including 1 of moderate severity) vs. 7 of 12 with mirtazapine alone and none with cimetidine alone], arrhythmia (2 of 12 patients vs. none with mirtazapine or cimetidine alone). The mirtazapine dose may have to be decreased when concomitant treatment with cimetidine is started, or increased when cimetidine treatment is discontinued.

Ketoconazole: In healthy, male, Caucasian patients (n=24), co-administration of the potent CYP3A4 inhibitor ketoconazole (200 mg b.i.d. for 6.5 days) increased the peak plasma levels and the AUC of a single 30 mg dose mirtazapine by approximately 40% and 50% respectively. During combined use, 2 severe adverse events have been reported: One patient experienced circulatory collapse and another patient experienced syncope. Both patients have lost consciousness for a brief period. Caution should be exercised when co-administering mirtazapine with potent CYP3A4 inhibitors, HIV protease inhibitors, azole antifungals, erythromycin or nefazodone.

Paroxetine: In an in vivo interaction study in healthy, CYP2D6 extensive metabolizer patients (n=24), mirtazapine (30 mg/day), at steady state, did not significantly change the pharmacokinetics of steady state paroxetine (40 mg/day), a CYP2D6 inhibitor. However, plasma concentrations of mirtazapine and its demethyl metabolite were slightly higher (about 18 and 25%, respectively) during combined administration with paroxetine. This difference is considered to be without clinical relevance. During combined use, side effects included exanthema (1 of 24 patients) that required withdrawal of the patient. Increases in AST and ALT were also reported, with a greater increase in men due to several outliers (including a patient that was withdrawn due to high AST (about 4 fold higher than the upper normal limit) and ALT (about 2 fold higher than the upper normal limit) levels; this patient also showed elevated WBC, neutrophils, decreased lymphocytes and basophils). AST/ALT levels returned to normal following the end of the treatment. Caution is advised for the co-administration of paroxetine with mirtazapine.

Other Drug-Drug Interactions: Amitriptyline: In healthy, CYP2D6 extensive metabolizer patients (n=32), amitriptyline (75 mg daily), at steady state, did not change the pharmacokinetics of steady state mirtazapine (30 mg daily) considerably and mirtazapine also did not change the pharmacokinetics of amitriptyline considerably. During combined use the following adverse reactions have been reported at considerably higher frequencies than with either drug alone: postural hypotension, impaired concentration (about 5 fold higher incidence), nausea (over 4 fold higher incidence) and dizziness (about 2 fold higher incidence). A CYP2D6 slow metabolizer patient experienced a serious adverse event following combined use of amitriptyline and mirtazapine. The subject complained of abdominal discomfort accompanied by dizziness and nausea and then leading to loss of consciousness for about 30 s. Apart from slight tremor (resembling myoclonic contractions) there were no other abnormalities. Caution is advised for the co-administration of amitriptyline with mirtazapine.

Warfarin: In healthy male subjects (n=16) mirtazapine (30 mg daily), at steady state, caused a small (0.2) but statistically significant increase in the International Normalised Ratio (INR) in subjects treated with warfarin to achieve subtherapeutic levels of prothrombin activity (1.5-2.0 INR) at steady state. As at a higher dose of mirtazapine, a more pronounced effect can not be excluded. It is advisable to monitor the INR in case of concomitant treatment of warfarin with mirtazapine.

Lithium: No relevant clinical effects or significant changes in pharmacokinetics have been observed in healthy male subjects on concurrent treatment with subtherapeutic levels of lithium (600 mg/day for 10 days) at steady state and a single 30 mg dose of mirtazapine. The serum levels of lithium were approximately 0.3 mmol/L 10 hrs after dosing. The effects of higher doses of lithium on the pharmacokinetics of mirtazapine are unknown.

Risperidone: In an in vivo non-randomized, interaction study subjects (n=6) in need of treatment with an antipsychiatric and antidepressant drug, the results of the effect of mirtazapine (30 mg daily) at steady state on the pharmacokinetics of risperidone (up to 3 mg b.i.d.) at steady state is inconclusive, due to high inter-patient variability and low number of patients. The study design does not permit conclusions to be made on the safety on the combined use of mirtazapine and risperidone. However, a case report of a male patient receiving combined treatment with mirtazapine (60 mg daily) and risperidone (3 mg daily) documents that, 6 weeks after initiation of this combination therapy, the patient developed pulmonary embolism and rhabdomyolysis. Caution is advised for the co-administration of risperidone with mirtazapine.

Serotonergic Drugs: Based on the mechanism of action of mirtazapine and the potential for serotonin syndrome, caution is advised when REMERON RD is co-administered with other drugs or agents that may affect the serotonergic neurotransmitter systems, such as tryptophan, triptans, serotonin reuptake inhibitors, lithium, tramadol or St. John's wort (see Contraindications and Warnings and Precautions, Neurologic, Serotonin Syndrome/Neuroleptic Malignant Syndrome).

Drugs Bound to Plasma Protein: Because mirtazapine is bound to plasma proteins (85%), care should be exercised when REMERON RD is co-administered to a patient who may be receiving another drug which is highly protein-bound.

Drug-Herb Interactions: St. John's Wort: Pharmacodynamic interactions between REMERON RD and the herbal remedy St. John's wort may occur and may result in an increase in undesirable effects. Dose adjustment of REMERON RD should be considered if clinically indicated.

Drug-Lifestyle Interactions: Alcohol: The impairment of mental and motor skills produced by mirtazapine has been shown to be additive with those produced by alcohol. Accordingly, patients should be advised to avoid alcohol while taking REMERON RD.

DOSAGE AND ADMINISTRATION: REMERON RD (mirtazapine) is not indicated for use in children under 18 years of age (see Warnings and Precautions, Potential Association with Behavioural and Emotional Changes, Including Self-Harm).

REMERON RD (mirtazapine) Orally Disintegrating Tablets are unique tablets that are designed to rapidly disintegrate on the tongue. No water is needed to take the tablets.

Dosing Considerations: Treatment of Pregnant Women During the Third Trimester: Post-marketing reports indicate that some neonates exposed to SSRI's or other newer antidepressants, such as REMERON RD, late in the third trimester have developed complications requiring prolonged hospitalization, respiratory support and tube feeding (see Warnings and Precautions). When treating pregnant women with REMERON RD during the third trimester, the physician should carefully consider the potential risks and benefits of treatment. The physician may consider tapering REMERON RD in the third trimester.

Children: (See Warnings and Precautions, Potential Association with Behavioural and Emotional Changes, Including Self-Harm.)

Elderly and Patients with Moderate to Severe Renal or Hepatic Impairment: In elderly patients, and patients with moderate to severe renal or hepatic impairment, limited pharmacokinetic data (see Action and Clinical Pharmacology) demonstrates increased serum concentration and/or reduced clearance of REMERON Tablets. REMERON RD should thus be dosed with care in these populations (see Action and Clinical Pharmacology, Pharmacokinetics).

Recommended Dose and Dosage Adjustment: Initial Treatment: Adults: REMERON RD (mirtazapine) Orally Disintegrating Tablets should be administered as a single dose, preferably in the evening prior to sleep. The recommended initial dose is 15 mg daily. In clinical trials, patients generally received doses of REMERON Tablets in the range of 15-45 mg/day. While a relationship between dose and antidepressant response for mirtazapine has not been established, patients not responding to the initial 15 mg dose may benefit from dose increases up to a maximum of 45 mg/day. Mirtazapine has an elimination half-life of approximately 20-40 hours, therefore, dose changes should occur in intervals of not less than one week. Dosage adjustments may be made according to the tolerance and based on the patient's response.

Longer-Term Treatment: It is generally agreed that acute episodes of depression require several months or longer of sustained therapy beyond response to the acute episode. Systematic evaluation of REMERON has demonstrated that its efficacy in major depressive disorder is maintained for periods of up to 40 weeks following 8-12 weeks of initial treatment at a dose of 15-45 mg/day (see Action and Clinical Pharmacology). Based on these limited data, it is unknown whether or not the dose of REMERON RD needed for continuation treatment is identical to the dose needed to achieve an initial response. Patients should be periodically reassessed to determine the need for continuation treatment and the appropriate dose for such treatment.

Discontinuation of REMERON RD Treatment: Symptoms associated with the discontinuation or dose reduction of REMERON RD Tablets have been reported. Patients should be monitored for these and other symptoms when discontinuing treatment or during dosage reduction of REMERON RD (see Warnings and Precautions and Adverse Reactions).

A gradual reduction in the dose over several weeks, rather than abrupt cessation, is recommended whenever is possible. If intolerable symptoms occur following a decrease in the dose or upon discontinuation of treatment, dose titration should be managed on the basis of the patient's clinical response (see Warnings and Precautions and Adverse Reactions).

Missed Dose: Do not take a double dose to make up for forgotten doses.

If a patient forgets to take the evening dose, advise the patient not to take the missed dose the next morning. Continue treatment in the evening (prior to sleep) with the normal dose.

Administration: Administration of REMERON RD (Mirtazapine) Orally Disintegrating Tablets: Patients should be instructed to open the tablet blister pack with dry hands and place the tablet on the tongue. The tablet should be used immediately after removal from the blister; once removed, it cannot be stored. REMERON RD will disintegrate rapidly on the tongue and can be swallowed with saliva. No water is needed for taking the tablet. Patients should not attempt to split the tablets (see Information for the Patient).

OVERDOSAGE:

Human Experience: In clinical trials, the only drug overdose death reported while taking REMERON (mirtazapine) Tablets was in combination with amitriptyline and chlorprohixene in a non-U.S. clinical study. Based on plasma levels, the REMERON dose taken was 30-45 mg, while plasma levels of amitriptyline and chlorprohixene were found to be at toxic levels. In other pre-marketing overdose cases with REMERON Tablets, the following signs and symptoms were reported: disorientation, drowsiness, impaired memory and tachycardia. There were no reports of ECG abnormalities, coma or convulsions following overdose with REMERON Tablets alone.

In post-marketing experience with more than 35 million patients exposed to REMERON (based on average treatment courses of 30 mg/day during 3 months), fatal cases of overdose with REMERON alone have been reported. In many cases details regarding the precise dose are lacking. Fatal acute overdoses with REMERON alone are documented at doses as low as approximately 440 mg, which is estimated from the post-mortem plasma levels, assuming linear pharmacokinetics. However, survival has also been reported with a single REMERON overdose as high as 1350 mg.

Present experience concerning overdose with REMERON alone indicates that symptoms are usually mild. Depression of the central nervous system with disorientation and prolonged sedation have been reported, together with tachycardia and mild hyper- or hypotension. However, there is a possibility of more serious outcomes (including fatalities) at dosages much higher than the therapeutic dose, especially with mixed overdosages.

Overdose Management: Treatment should consist of those general measures employed in the management of overdose with any antidepressant.

Ensure an adequate airway, oxygenation and ventilation. Monitor cardiac rhythm and vital signs. General supportive and symptomatic measures are also recommended. Induction of emesis is not recommended. Gastric lavage with a large-bore orogastric tube with appropriate airway protection, if needed, may be indicated if performed soon after ingestion, or in symptomatic patients.

Activated charcoal should be administered. There is no experience with the use of forced diuresis, dialysis, hemoperfusion or exchange transfusion in the treatment of mirtazapine overdosage. No specific antidotes for mirtazapine are known.

In managing overdosage, consider the possibility of multiple drug involvement. The physician should consider contacting a poison control centre for additional information on the treatment of any overdose.

For management of a suspected drug overdose, CPhA recommends that you contact your **regional Poison Control Centre**. See the *CPS* Directory section for a list of Poison Control Centres.

ACTION AND CLINICAL PHARMACOLOGY: Mechanism of Action: The mechanism of action of REMERON RD (mirtazapine) Tablets, as with other drugs effective in the treatment of major depressive disorder, is unknown.

Evidence gathered in preclinical studies suggests that mirtazapine enhances central noradrenergic and serotonergic activity. These studies have shown that mirtazapine acts as an antagonist at central presynaptic α_2 adrenergic inhibitory autoreceptors and heteroreceptors, an action that is postulated to result in an increase in central noradrenergic and serotonergic activity. The clinical relevance of this finding is unknown.

Pharmacodynamics: Mirtazapine acts as an antagonist at central presynaptic α_2 adrenergic inhibitory autoreceptors and heteroreceptors, which results in an increase in central noradrenergic and serotonergic activity. The clinical relevance of this finding is unknown, however, this action may explain its antidepressant activity.

Mirtazapine is a potent antagonist of 5-HT_2 and 5-HT_3 receptors. The clinical relevance of this finding is unclear, however, the 5-HT_2 and 5-HT_3 antagonism by mirtazapine may account for its low rate of nausea, insomnia and anxiety as observed in clinical trials. Mirtazapine has no significant effect on 5-HT_{1A} and 5-HT_{1B} receptors.

Both enantiomers of mirtazapine appear to contribute to its pharmacological activity. The (+)enantiomer blocks 5-HT_2 receptors as well as α_2 receptors, and the (−)enantiomer blocks 5-HT_3 receptors. The clinical relevance of this finding is unclear, but this may explain its antidepressant activity and side-effect profile.

Mirtazapine is a potent histamine (H_1) receptor antagonist, which may contribute to its sedative effect and possibly to weight gain due to increased appetite.

Mirtazapine is a moderate peripheral α_1 adrenergic antagonist, a property which may explain the occasional orthostatic hypotension reported in association with its use.

Mirtazapine is a moderate antagonist at muscarinic receptors, a property that may explain the occasional occurrence of anticholinergic side effects associated with its use as shown in clinical trials.

Pharmacokinetics: Mirtazapine is well absorbed following oral administration and its absolute bioavailability is approximately 50% after either single or multiple doses. Peak plasma concentrations are reached within about 2 hours following an oral dose. The time to peak plasma concentration is independent of dose. The presence of food in the stomach somewhat slows the rate but not the extent of absorption, and thus does not require a dosage adjustment.

Plasma levels are linear over a dose range of 30 to 80 mg. Steady-state plasma levels are attained within about 5 days. The half-life of elimination of mirtazapine after oral administration is approximately 20-40 hours.

REMERON RD (mirtazapine) Orally Disintegrating Tablets have been found to be bioequivalent to REMERON (mirtazapine) Tablets.

Metabolism: Mirtazapine is extensively metabolized and quantitatively eliminated via urine (75%) and feces (15%); approximately 90% of this elimination occurs within the first 72-96 hours. Major pathways of biotransformation are demethylation and oxidation followed by conjugation. In vitro data from human liver microsomes indicate that cytochrome 2D6 and 1A2 are involved in the formation of the 8-hydroxy metabolite of mirtazapine, whereas cytochrome 3A is considered to be responsible for the formation of the N-demethyl and N-oxide metabolite. The demethyl metabolite is pharmacologically active and appears to have a similar pharmacokinetic profile as that of the parent compound.

The (−)enantiomer has an elimination half-life that is approximately twice as long, and achieves plasma levels that are three times as high as that of the (+)enantiomer.

Protein Binding: Mirtazapine is approximately 85% bound to plasma proteins over a concentration range of 10 to 1000 ng/mL. Binding appears to be both non-specific and reversible. The binding affinity of mirtazapine to human liver proteins is 2.8 times greater than to human plasma proteins. As with all drugs that are protein-bound, care should be exercised when co-administering medications that may interact with mirtazapine at protein-binding sites (see Warnings and Precautions).

Table 3: REMERON RD

Effect of Age and Gender on Plasma Half-Life of Mirtazapine

Group	$t_{½}$ (mean±SD)[a]	
	Single Dose	Multiple Dose
Adult male N=9	21.7±4.2	22.1±3.7
Adult female N=9	37.7±13.3	35.4±13.7
Elderly[b] male N=8	32.2±15.4	31.1±15.1
Elderly[b] female N=8	40.6±12.8	39.0±10.8

[a] Expressed in hours.
[b] The "elderly" group consisted of subjects 55 and older (55-75; mean age 65).

Special Populations and Conditions: Pediatrics: REMERON RD is not indicated for use in patients below the age of 18 years (see Warnings and Precautions, General, Potential Association with Behavioural and Emotional Changes, Including Self-Harm; and Dosage and Administration).

Geriatrics: Following administration of mirtazapine 20 mg/day for 7 days, oral clearance was reduced in older subjects (mean age 65; range 55-75) compared to younger subjects (see Table 3). The difference was greatest in males, with a 40% lower clearance for mirtazapine in the older vs. younger group. Caution is indicated in administering REMERON RD (mirtazapine) Orally Disintegrating Tablets in the elderly (see Warnings and Precautions and Dosage and Administration).

Gender: Age and Sex: In the same study above (see Action and Clinical Pharmacology, Special Populations and Conditions, Geriatrics) females of all ages (range 25-74) exhibited significantly longer elimination half-lives than males (mean half-life of 37 hours for females vs. 26 hours for males) (see Table 3). Although these differences result on average in higher area-under-the-curve (AUC) for females compared to males, there is considerable overlap in individual AUCs between groups. Because of substantial individual variation of AUC and half-life, no specific dosage recommendations based on sex are indicated (see Dosage and Administration).

Hepatic Insufficiency: Liver Disease: In a single-dose study conducted with mirtazapine 15 mg, the elimination half-life of mirtazapine was increased 40% in mild to moderately hepatically impaired subjects as compared to patients with normal hepatic function; this effect on elimination resulted in a 57% increase in AUC and a 33% decrease in clearance.

Renal Insufficiency: Renal Disease: In a single-dose study conducted with mirtazapine 15 mg, subjects with moderate and severe renal impairment showed a significant decrease in the clearance of ORG 3770 and a consequent increase in AUC (54% and 215% for moderate and severe renal impairment, respectively). Subjects with severe renal impairment had significantly higher peak plasma levels of ORG 3770 (about double that of subjects without renal impairment). These results suggest that caution must be exercised in administering REMERON RD to patients who may have compromised renal function.

STORAGE AND STABILITY: Store at controlled room temperature, 15-30°C. Protect from light and moisture. Use immediately upon opening individual tablet blister.

SPECIAL HANDLING INSTRUCTIONS: Patients should be instructed to open the tablet blister pack with dry hands and place the tablet on the tongue. The tablet should be used immediately after removal from the blister; once removed, it cannot be stored. REMERON RD will disintegrate rapidly on the tongue and can be swallowed with saliva. No water is needed for taking the tablet. Patients should not attempt to split the tablets.

INFORMATION FOR THE PATIENT: Published in e-CPS, available by subscription at www.e-cps.ca.

DOSAGE FORMS, COMPOSITION AND PACKAGING: 15 mg: Each white, flat-faced, round, beveled edge, orally disintegrating tablet, coded with TZ1, with a characteristic orange odor, contains: mirtazapine 15 mg. Nonmedicinal ingredients: aspartame (contains phenylalanine), citric acid, crospovidone, hydroxypropyl methylcellulose, magnesium stearate, mannitol, microcrystalline cellulose, natural and artificial orange flavour, polymethyl acrylate, povidone, sodium bicarbonate, starch and sucrose. Boxes of 30 (5×6 unit Dose Blisters).

30 mg: Each white, flat-faced, round, beveled edge, orally disintegrating tablet, coded with TZ2, with a characteristic orange odor, contains: mirtazapine 30 mg. Nonmedicinal ingredients: aspartame (contains phenylalanine), citric acid, crospovidone, hydroxypropyl methylcellulose, magnesium stearate, mannitol, microcrystalline cellulose, natural and artificial orange flavour, polymethyl acrylate, povidone, sodium bicarbonate, starch and sucrose. Boxes of 30 (5×6 unit Dose Blisters).

45 mg: Each white, flat-faced, round, beveled edge, orally disintegrating tablet, coded with TZ4, with a characteristic orange odor, contains: mirtazapine 45 mg. Nonmedicinal ingredients: aspartame (contains phenylalanine), citric acid, crospovidone, hydroxypropyl methylcellulose, magnesium stearate, mannitol, microcrystalline cellulose, natural and artificial orange flavour, polymethyl acrylate, povidone, sodium bicarbonate, starch and sucrose. Boxes of 30 (5×6 unit Dose Blisters).

(Shown in Product Identification Section)

Remicade® Ⓟ

infliximab

Biological Response Modifier

Schering-Plough

Date of Revision: March 29, 2010

SUMMARY PRODUCT INFORMATION:

Route of Administration	Dosage Form/ Strength	Clinically Relevant Nonmedicinal Ingredients
Intravenous Injection	Injection/100 mg/vial	For a complete listing see Dosage Forms, Composition and Packaging.

INDICATIONS AND CLINICAL USE: REMICADE (infliximab) is indicated for:

- use in combination with methotrexate for the reduction in signs and symptoms, inhibition of the progression of structural damage and improvement in physical function in adult patients with moderately to severely active rheumatoid arthritis.
- the reduction of signs and symptoms and improvement in physical function in patients with active ankylosing spondylitis who have responded inadequately, or are intolerant to, conventional therapies.
- reduction of signs and symptoms and induction and maintenance of clinical remission in adult and pediatric patients with moderately to severely active Crohn's disease who have had an inadequate response to conventional therapy (i.e., aminosalicylate and/or corticosteroid and/or an immunosuppressant). The safety and efficacy of REMICADE is not established in patients less than 9 years of age.
- treatment of fistulising Crohn's disease, in adult patients who have not responded despite a full and adequate course of therapy with conventional treatment.
- reducing signs and symptoms, inducing and maintaining clinical remission, inducing and maintaining mucosal healing, and reducing or eliminating corticosteroid use in patients with moderately to severely active ulcerative colitis who have had an inadequate response to conventional therapy.
- reduction of signs and symptoms, induction of major clinical response, and inhibition of the progression of structural damage of active arthritis, and improvement in physical function in patients with psoriatic arthritis.
- treatment of adult patients with chronic moderate to severe plaque psoriasis who are candidates for systemic therapy. For patients with chronic moderate plaque psoriasis, REMICADE should be used after phototherapy has been shown to be ineffective or inappropriate. When assessing the severity of psoriasis, the physician should consider the extent of involvement, location of lesions, response to previous treatments, and impact of disease on the patient's quality of life.

REMICADE should be used by physicians who have sufficient knowledge of rheumatoid arthritis and/or ankylosing spondylitis and/or Crohn's disease and/or ulcerative colitis and/or psoriatic arthritis and/or plaque psoriasis and who have fully familiarized themselves with the efficacy/safety profile of REMICADE.

Geriatrics (≥65 years of age): Evidence from clinical studies suggests that the use in geriatric population is associated with no overall differences in safety and efficacy.

In rheumatoid arthritis clinical trials, (ATTRACT) and plaque psoriasis trials, no overall differences were observed in the effectiveness or safety in 181 patients with rheumatoid arthritis and 75 patients with plaque psoriasis, aged 65 or older compared to younger patients although the incidence of serious adverse events in patients aged 65 or older was higher in both REMICADE and control groups compared to younger patients. In Crohn's disease, ulcerative colitis, ankylosing spondylitis and psoriatic arthritis studies, there were insufficient numbers of patients aged 65 and over to determine whether they respond differently from patients aged 18 to 64. Because there is a higher incidence of infections in the elderly population in general, caution should be used in treating the elderly (see Adverse Reactions, Infections).

Pediatrics: REMICADE is indicated for reducing signs and symptoms and for inducing and maintaining clinical remission in pediatric patients with moderately to severely active Crohn's disease who have had an inadequate response to conventional therapy. In general, the adverse events in pediatric patients with Crohn's disease who received REMICADE were similar to those seen in adult patients with Crohn's disease. It should be noted that in the Phase 3 trial (REACH) of pediatric patients with Crohn's disease, all patients were required to be on a stable dose of either 6-mercaptopurine (6-MP), azathioprine (AZA), or methotrexate (MTX). (See Indications and Clinical Use; Warnings and Precautions, Special Populations, Pediatrics (9-17 years of age); Adverse Reactions, Adverse Reactions in Pediatric Patients, Crohn's Disease and Dosage and Administration.)

The safety and efficacy of REMICADE has not been established in children with Crohn's disease <9 years of age. The safety and efficacy of REMICADE in pediatric patients with ulcerative colitis, plaque psoriasis, psoriatic arthritis, ankylosing spondylitis, and in juvenile rheumatoid arthritis have not been established.

CONTRAINDICATIONS:

- Patients with severe infections such as sepsis, abscesses, tuberculosis and opportunistic infections (see Warnings and Precautions, Risk of Infections).
- Patients with moderate or severe (NYHA Class III/IV) congestive heart failure (see Warnings and Precautions, Cardiovascular and Adverse Reactions, Congestive Heart Failure).
- Patients with a history of hypersensitivity to infliximab, to other murine proteins, or to any of the excipients. For a complete listing, see Dosage Forms, Composition and Packaging.

WARNINGS AND PRECAUTIONS:

Serious Warnings and Precautions

Risk of infections: Tuberculosis (frequently disseminated or extrapulmonary at clinical presentation), invasive fungal infections, and other opportunistic infections, have been observed in patients receiving REMICADE (infliximab). Some of these infections have been fatal.

Patients must be evaluated for the risk of tuberculosis, including latent tuberculosis, prior to initiation of REMICADE. This evaluation should include a detailed medical history of tuberculosis or possible previous contact with tuberculosis and previous and/or current immunosuppressive therapy. Appropriate screening tests, i.e, tuberculin skin test and chest x-ray (if indicated), should be performed in all patients. Prescribers are reminded of the risk of false negative tuberculin skin test results especially in patients who are severely ill or immunocompromised. Treatment of latent tuberculosis infection should be initiated prior to therapy with REMICADE (see Warning and Precautions, Risk of Infections).

Hepatosplenic T-Cell Lymphoma: Postmarketing cases of hepatosplenic T-cell lymphoma have been reported in patients treated with TNF blockers including REMICADE. This rare type of T-cell lymphoma has a very aggressive disease course and is usually fatal. All REMICADE cases have occurred in patients with Crohn's disease or ulcerative colitis and the majority were reported in adolescent or young adult males. All of these patients had received treatment with azathioprine or 6-mercaptopurine concomitantly with or immediately prior to REMICADE (see Warning and Precautions, Carcinogenesis and Mutagenesis).

Pediatric Malignancy: Lymphoma and other malignancies, some fatal, have been reported in children and adolescent patients treated with TNF blockers, including REMICADE (see Warning and Precautions, Carcinogenesis and Mutagenesis).

Risk of Infections: Serious infections due to bacterial (including sepsis and pneumonia), invasive fungal, viral, and other opportunistic pathogens, have been reported in patients receiving TNF-blocking agents. Some of these infections have been fatal. Many of the serious infections in patients treated with REMICADE (infliximab) have occurred in patients on concomitant immunosuppressive therapy that, in addition to their underlying disease, could predispose them to infections.

REMICADE should not be given to patients with a clinically important, active infection. Caution should be exercised when considering the use of REMICADE in patients with a chronic infection or a history of recurrent infection. Patients should be monitored for signs and symptoms of infection while on or after treatment with REMICADE. New infections should be closely monitored. If a patient develops a serious infection, REMICADE therapy should be discontinued (see Adverse Reactions, Infections).

Cases of histoplasmosis, coccidioidomycosis, blastomycosis, listeriosis, pneumocystosis, and tuberculosis have been observed in patients receiving REMICADE. For patients who have resided in or travelled to regions where histoplasmosis, coccidioidomycosis, or blastomycosis are endemic, the benefits and risks of REMICADE treatment should be carefully considered before initiation or continuation of REMICADE therapy.

In at risk patients treated with REMICADE, an invasive fungal infection should be suspected if they develop a serious systemic illness. Invasive fungal infections may present as disseminated rather than localized disease, and antigen and antibody testing may be negative in some patients with active infection. Appropriate empiric antifungal therapy should be considered while a diagnostic workup is being performed. The decision to administer empiric antifungal therapy should be made in consultation with a physician with expertise in the diagnosis and treatment of invasive fungal infections and should take into account both the risk for severe fungal infection and the risks of antifungal therapy.

Patients receiving REMICADE should be monitored closely for signs and symptoms of active tuberculosis during and after treatment, including patients who tested negative for latent tuberculosis infection. The possibility of undetected latent tuberculosis should be considered, especially in patients who have immigrated from or traveled to countries with a high prevalence of tuberculosis or had close contact with a person with active tuberculosis. All patients treated with REMICADE should have a thorough history taken prior to initiating therapy. Some patients who have previously received treatment for latent or active tuberculosis have developed active tuberculosis while being treated with REMICADE. Anti-tuberculosis therapy should be considered prior to initiation of REMICADE in patients with a past history of latent or active tuberculosis in whom an adequate course of treatment cannot be confirmed. Anti-tuberculosis therapy prior to initiating REMICADE should also be considered in patients who have several or highly significant risk factors for tuberculosis infection and have a negative test for latent tuberculosis. The decision to initiate anti-tuberculosis therapy in these patients should only be made following consultation with a physician with expertise in the treatment of tuberculosis and taking into account both the risk for latent tuberculosis infection and the risks of anti-tuberculosis therapy.

Concurrent Administration of TNF-alpha Inhibitor and Anakinra: Serious infections and neutropenia were seen in clinical studies with concurrent use of anakinra and another TNFα-blocking agent, etanercept, with no added clinical benefit compared to etanercept alone. Because of the nature of the adverse events seen with combination of etanercept and anakinra therapy, similar toxicities may also result from the combination of anakinra and other TNFα-blocking agents. Therefore, the combination of REMICADE and anakinra is not recommended.

Concurrent Administration of REMICADE with Abatacept: In clinical studies, concurrent administration of TNF-blocking agents and abatacept have been associated with an increased risk of infections including serious infections compared with TNF-blocking agents alone, without increased clinical benefit. Because of the nature of the adverse events seen with the combination of TNF-blocking agents and abatacept therapy, the combination of REMICADE and abatacept is not recommended.

Switching between Biological DMARDS: When switching from one biologic to another, patients should continue to be monitored for signs of infection.

Carcinogenesis and Mutagenesis: Pediatric malignancy: Malignancies, some fatal, have been reported among children, adolescents and young adults who received treatment with TNF-blocking agents (initiation of therapy ≤18 years of age), including REMICADE. Approximately half of these cases were lymphomas, including Hodgkin's and non-Hodgkin's lymphoma. The other cases represented a variety of malignancies, including rare malignancies that are usually associated with immunosuppression and malignancies that are not usually observed in children and adolescents. The malignancies occurred after a median of 30 months (range 1 to 84 months) after the first dose of TNF blocker therapy. Most of the patients were receiving concomitant immunosuppressants. These cases were reported post-marketing and are derived from a variety of sources, including registries and spontaneous postmarketing reports.

Lymphoma: Lymphomas have been observed in patients treated with TNF blocking agents, including REMICADE. In clinical trials, patients treated with infliximab had a higher incidence of lymphoma than the expected rate in the general population. Patients with rheumatoid arthritis and Crohn's disease, particularly those with highly active disease and/or chronic exposure to immunosuppressant therapies, may be at a higher risk (up to several fold) for the development of lymphoma than the general population, even in the absence of TNF-blocking therapy. The role of TNF blockers in the development of malignancy is not known.

Hepatosplenic T-Cell Lymphoma: Rare postmarketing cases of hepatosplenic T-cell lymphoma have been reported in patients treated with TNF blockers including REMICADE. This rare type of T-cell lymphoma has a very aggressive disease course and is usually fatal. All REMICADE cases have occurred in patients with Crohn's disease or ulcerative colitis and the majority were reported in adolescent or young adult males. All of these patients had received treatment with azathioprine or 6-mercaptopurine concomitantly with or immediately prior to REMICADE. Cases of hepatosplenic T-cell lymphoma have also occurred in Crohn's disease and ulcerative colitis patients receiving azathioprine or 6-mercaptopurine who were not treated with REMICADE. Before initiating or continuing REMICADE therapy in a patient who has chronic inflammatory bowel disease and who is receiving an immunosuppressant such as azathioprine or 6-mercaptopurine, carefully assess the need for continuing the immunosuppressant therapy in light of the potential risks of concomitant treatment. The causal relationship of hepatosplenic T-cell lymphoma to REMICADE therapy remains unclear.

Leukemia: Cases of acute and chronic leukemia have been reported with postmarketing TNF-blocker use in rheumatoid arthritis and other indications. Even in the absence of TNF blocker therapy, patients with rheumatoid arthritis may be at a higher risk (approximately 2-fold) than the general population for the development of leukemia.

Non-Lymphoma Malignancy: In the controlled portions of clinical trials of some TNF-blocking agents, including REMICADE, more malignancies (excluding lymphoma and non-melanoma skin cancer [NMSC]) have been observed in patients receiving those TNF blockers compared with control patients (see Adverse Reactions, Malignancies/Lymphoproliferative Disease). The rate of non-lymphoma malignancies among REMICADE-treated patients was similar to that expected in the general population whereas the rate among control patients was lower than expected.

In an exploratory clinical trial evaluating the use of REMICADE in patients with moderate to severe chronic obstructive pulmonary disease (COPD), more malignancies were reported in REMICADE-treated patients compared with control patients. All patients had a history of heavy smoking.

Psoriasis patients should be monitored for nonmelanoma skin cancers (NMSCs), particularly those patients who have had prior prolonged phototherapy treatment. In the maintenance portion of clinical trials for REMICADE, NMSCs were more common in patients with previous phototherapy (see Adverse Reactions, Malignancies/Lymphoproliferative Disease).

The potential role of TNF-blocking therapy in the development of malignancies is not known. Caution should be exercised when considering TNF-blocking therapy for patients with a history of malignancy or when considering continuing treatment in patients who develop a malignancy. (See Adverse Reactions, Malignancies/Lymphoproliferative Disease.)

Long-term studies in animals have not been performed to evaluate the carcinogenic potential. No clastogenic or mutagenic effects of infliximab were observed in the in vivo mouse micronucleus test or the Salmonella–*E. coli* (Ames) assay, respectively. Chromosomal aberrations were not observed in an assay performed using human lymphocytes. Tumourigenicity studies in mice deficient in TNFα demonstrated no increase in tumours when challenged with known tumour initiators and/or promoters.

Cardiovascular: Doses greater than 5 mg/kg should not be administered to patients with congestive heart failure (CHF). REMICADE should be used with caution in patients with mild heart failure (NYHA Class I/II). Patients should be closely monitored, and REMICADE must not be continued in patients who develop new or worsening symptoms of heart failure (see Contraindications and Adverse Reactions, Congestive Heart Failure). The results of a randomized study evaluating the use of REMICADE in patients with heart failure (NYHA Functional Class III/IV) suggested higher mortality in patients who received 10 mg/kg REMICADE, and higher rates of cardiovascular adverse events at doses of 5 mg/kg and 10 mg/kg.

Hematologic: There have been reports of pancytopenia, leukopenia, neutropenia, and thrombocytopenia in patients receiving TNF-blockers, including REMICADE. Caution should be exercised in patients treated with REMICADE who have a current or past history of significant cytopenias.

Hepatic/Biliary/Pancreatic: Very rare cases of jaundice and non-infectious hepatitis, some with features of autoimmune hepatitis, have been observed in the postmarketing experience of REMICADE. Isolated cases of liver failure resulting in liver transplantation or death have occurred. A causal relationship between REMICADE and these events has not been established. Patients with symptoms or signs of liver dysfunction should be evaluated for evidence of liver injury. If jaundice and/or ALT elevations ≥5 times the upper limit of normal develop, REMICADE should be discontinued immediately, and a thorough investigation of the abnormality should be undertaken. As also observed with the use of other immunosuppressive drugs, reactivation of hepatitis B has occurred very rarely in patients receiving REMICADE who are chronic carriers of this virus (i.e., surface antigen positive). Patients at risk for HBV infection should be evaluated for prior evidence of HBV infection before initiating REMICADE. Chronic carriers of hepatitis B should be appropriately evaluated prior to the initiation of REMICADE therapy and monitored closely during treatment and for several months following discontinuation of therapy.

Immune: To minimize the incidence of hypersensitivity reactions, including infusion reactions and serum sickness-like reactions, REMICADE should be administered as regular maintenance therapy after an induction regimen at weeks 0, 2 and 6 (see Dosage and Administration).

Hypersensitivity Reactions: REMICADE has been associated with hypersensitivity reactions that vary in their time of onset. Most hypersensitivity reactions, which include urticaria, dyspnea, and/or hypotension, have occurred during or within 2 hours of infliximab infusion. However, in some cases, serum sickness-like reactions have been observed in Crohn's disease and rheumatoid arthritis patients 3 to 12 days after REMICADE therapy was reinstituted following an extended period without REMICADE treatment. Symptoms associated with these reactions include fever, rash, headache, sore throat, myalgias, polyarthralgias, hand and facial edema and/or dysphagia. These reactions were associated with marked increase in antibodies to infliximab, loss of detectable serum concentrations of REMICADE, and possible loss of drug efficacy. REMICADE should be discontinued for severe reactions. Medications for the treatment of hypersensitivity reactions (e.g., acetaminophen, antihistamines, corticosteroids and/or epinephrine) should be available for immediate use in the event of a reaction (see Adverse Reactions, Infusion-Related Reactions).

During clinical trials, REMICADE was sometimes readministered within 14 weeks following the last infusion. After a drug free interval of 15 weeks to 2 years, the risk of delayed hypersensitivity following readministration has not been accurately determined (see Adverse Reactions, Infusion-related Reactions, Delayed Hypersentivity/Reactions Following Readministration of REMICADE).

Infusion Reactions Following Readministration of REMICADE: In a rheumatoid arthritis clinical trial where subjects were receiving low dose methotrexate and in a psoriasis clinical trial, a 3-dose induction of REMICADE after a period of no treatment resulted in a higher incidence of serious and severe infusion reactions during the reinduction regimen than had been observed in rheumatoid arthritis, psoriasis and Crohn's disease trials in which a period of no drug treatment was followed by regular maintenance therapy without reinduction. Most of these reactions occurred during the second reinduction infusion at Week 2. The serious infusion reactions included anaphylaxis, urticaria, facial edema; chills and itching. Retreatment with a reinduction regimen after a period of no treatment is not recommended (see Adverse Reactions, Infusion-related Reactions, Infusion Reactions Following Readministration of REMICADE).

The BioAdvance Network has been established to facilitate the administration of REMICADE. BioAdvance Network clinics are staffed by qualified healthcare professionals specially trained in the administration of REMICADE infusions and are available across Canada. Information about the BioAdvance Network and location of the nearest BioAdvance Network clinic can be obtained by calling Schering-Plough Canada Inc. Medical Information at: 1-866-736-4223.

Autoimmunity: Treatment with REMICADE (infliximab) may result in the formation of autoantibodies and, rarely, in the development of a lupus-like syndrome. If a patient develops symptoms suggestive of a lupus-like syndrome following treatment with REMICADE, treatment should be discontinued (see Adverse Reactions, Autoantibodies/Lupus-like Syndrome).

Immunogenicity: Treatment with REMICADE can be associated with the development of antibodies to infliximab (see Warnings and Precautions, Hypersensitivity Reactions). Approximately 10% of patients were antibody positive. The majority of antibody positive patients had low titers. Patients who were antibody-positive were more likely to have higher rates of clearance, reduced efficacy and to experience an infusion reaction (see Adverse Reactions, Infusion-Related Reactions) than were patients who were antibody negative. Antibody development was lower among adult rheumatoid arthritis, Crohn's disease, and psoriatic arthritis patients receiving immunosuppressant therapies such as 6-mercaptopurine (6-MP), azathioprine (AZA), or methotrexate (MTX), although among patients with juvenile rheumatoid arthritis antibody development occurred in a high percentage of patients receiving 3 mg/kg REMICADE with concomitant MTX (see Adverse Reactions in Pediatric Patients, Juvenile Rheumatoid Arthritis).

With repeated dosing of REMICADE, serum concentrations of infliximab were higher in rheumatoid arthritis patients who received concomitant MTX. In the 2 Phase 3 studies of psoriasis (EXPRESS and EXPRESS II), REMICADE was administered as induction followed by maintenance and without concomitant immunosuppressive therapy. In these studies, antibodies occurred in approximately 26.5%-35.8% of patients who received 5 mg/kg every 8 week maintenance for 1 year and at higher rates (up to 1.4-fold) with other dose regimens (3 mg/kg q 8 week, 3 mg/kg dosed as needed, and 5 mg/kg dosed as needed). Despite the increase in the rate of antibody formation, the infusion reaction rates in the 2 psoriasis Phase 3 studies (EXPRESS and EXPRESS II) in patients treated with 5 mg/kg induction followed by every 8 week maintenance for 1 year (14.1% and 23.0%, respectively) and serious infusion reaction rates (<1%) were similar to those observed in other study populations. In the Phase 3 study of psoriatic arthritis (IMPACT 2), where patients received 5 mg/kg with and without MTX, antibodies to infliximab occurred in 15.4% of patients. Because immunogenicity analyses are product-specific, comparison of antibody rates to those from other products is not appropriate.

Vaccinations: No data are available on the response to vaccination or on the secondary transmission of infection by live vaccines in patients receiving anti-TNF therapy. It is recommended that live vaccines not be given concurrently. In a subset of 56 patients from the ASPIRE study, a similar proportion of patients in each treatment group mounted an effective two-fold increase in titers to a therapeutic 23-valent pneumococcal vaccine (which is not a live vaccine), indicating that REMICADE did not interfere with T-cell-dependent humoral immune response.

It is recommended that the vaccinations of pediatric patients with Crohn's disease, be brought up to date with all vaccination guidelines prior to initiating REMICADE therapy.

Neurological Events: Infliximab and other agents that inhibit TNF have been associated in rare cases with new onset or exacerbation of clinical symptoms and/or radiographic evidence of central nervous system demyelinating disorders, including multiple sclerosis, and peripheral demyelinating disorders, including Guillain-Barré syndrome. Rare cases of optic neuritis and seizure have been associated with REMICADE treatment. In patients with pre-existing or recent onset of demyelinating disorders, the benefits and risks of REMICADE treatment should be carefully considered before initiation of REMICADE therapy. Discontinuation of REMICADE should be considered in patients who develop significant central or peripheral nervous system reactions.

Physicians should alert patients to the presence of the Patient Package Insert, provide this information to them, and ensure full understanding of the content.

Peri-Operative Considerations: If a patient requires surgery while on infliximab therapy, appropriate precautions must be taken as necessary.

Sexual Function/Reproduction: It is not known whether infliximab can impair fertility in humans. No impairment of fertility was observed in a fertility and general reproduction toxicity study conducted in mice using an analogous antibody that selectively inhibits the functional activity of mouse TNFα.

Special Populations: Pregnant Women: Since infliximab does not cross-react with TNFα in species other than humans and chimpanzees, animal reproduction studies have not been conducted with REMICADE. No evidence of maternal toxicity, embryotoxicity or teratogenicity was observed in a developmental toxicity study conducted in mice using an analogous antibody that selectively inhibits the functional activity of mouse TNFα. Doses of 10 to 15 mg/kg in pharmacodynamic animal models with the anti-TNF analogous antibody produced maximal pharmacologic effectiveness. Doses up to 40 mg/kg were shown to produce no adverse effects in animal reproduction studies. It is not known whether REMICADE can cause fetal harm when administered to a pregnant woman or can affect reproduction capacity. Administration of REMICADE is not recommended during pregnancy. **Women of childbearing potential must use adequate contraception to prevent pregnancy and continue its use for at least 6 months after the last REMICADE treatment.**

Nursing Women: It is not known whether infliximab is excreted in human milk or absorbed systemically after ingestion. Because human immunoglobulins are excreted in milk, **women must not breast feed for at least 6 months after REMICADE treatment.**

Pediatrics (9-17 years of age): REMICADE is indicated for reducing signs and symptoms and for inducing and maintaining clinical remission in pediatric patients with moderately to severely active Crohn's disease who have had an inadequate response to conventional therapy. In general, the adverse events in pediatric patients with Crohn's disease who received REMICADE were similar to those seen in adult patients with Crohn's disease. It should be noted that in REACH, all patients were required to be on a stable dose of either 6-MP, AZA, or MTX. (See Indications and Clinical Use, Pediatrics, Adverse Reactions, Adverse Reactions in Pediatric Patients, Crohn's Disease, Dosage and Administration.) For additional pediatric information also see Warnings and Precautions, Immune, Vaccinations, and Action and Clinical Pharmacology, Pharmacokinetics, Special Populations).

The safety and efficacy of REMICADE has not been established in children with Crohn's disease <9 years of age. The safety and efficacy of REMICADE in pediatric patients with ulcerative colitis, plaque psoriasis, psoriatic arthritis, ankylosing spondylitis, and juvenile rheumatoid arthritis have not been established.

Geriatrics (65 years of age or older): In rheumatoid arthritis clinical trials, (ATTRACT) and in plaque psoriasis studies no overall differences were observed in the effectiveness or safety in 181 patients with rheumatoid arthritis and 75 patients with plaque psoriasis, aged 65 or older compared to younger patients although the incidence of serious adverse events in patients aged 65 or older was higher in both REMICADE and control groups compared to younger patients. Mean duration of REMICADE treatment in this population (154) was approximately 50 weeks. In Crohn's disease, ulcerative colitis, ankylosing spondylitis, and psoriatic arthritis studies, there were insufficient numbers of patients aged 65 and over to determine whether they responded differently from patients aged 18 to 64. Because there is a higher incidence of infections in the elderly population in general, caution should be used in treating the elderly (see Adverse Reactions, Infections).

ADVERSE REACTIONS: Adverse Drug Reaction Overview: The most common adverse drug reactions reported from both clinical trials and post-marketing reports are infections, allergic reactions and infusion-related reactions. Less common adverse drug reactions from these sources which may be serious and clinically relevant include hepatobiliary events (see Warnings and Precautions, Hepatic/Biliary/Pancreatic), demyelinating disorders (see Warnings and Precautions, Neurological Events), and lymphoma (see Warnings and Precautions, Carcinogenesis and Mutagenesis). One of the most common reasons for discontinuation of treatment in clinical trials was infusion-related reactions (dyspnea, flushing, headache and rash). (See Warnings and Precautions, Hypersensitivity Reactions.) Adverse events have been reported in a higher proportion of rheumatoid arthritis patients receiving the 10 mg/kg dose than the 3 mg/kg dose, however, no differences were observed in the frequency of adverse events between the 5 mg/kg dose and the 10 mg/kg dose in patients with Crohn's disease or ulcerative colitis and between the 3 mg/kg and 5 mg/kg dose in patients with plaque psoriasis.

Clinical Trial Adverse Drug Reactions: Because clinical trials are conducted under very specific conditions the adverse reaction rates observed in the clinical trials may not reflect the rates observed in practice and should not be compared to the rates in the clinical trials of another drug. Adverse drug reaction information from clinical trials is useful for identifying drug-related adverse events and for approximating rates.

Description of Data Sources: The data described herein reflect the exposure to REMICADE in 5157 patients in adequate and well-controlled studies. Infliximab was studied in patients with rheumatoid arthritis (1304 patients exposed), juvenile rheumatoid arthritis (117 patients exposed), Crohn's disease (1224 patients exposed, including 1085 adult and 139 pediatric patients), ulcerative colitis (484 patients exposed), plaque psoriasis (1373 patients exposed), psoriatic arthritis (293 patients exposed), ankylosing spondylitis (345 patients exposed) and other conditions (17 patients exposed), primarily in double-blind, placebo-controlled trials. In general, integration of data in the following sections is based on clinical trials in rheumatoid arthritis and adult Crohn's disease.

Relative Frequency of Adverse Drug Reactions: Adverse events occurring at a frequency of at least 5% in REMICADE-treated adult patients with rheumatoid arthritis, Crohn's disease, ankylosing spondylitis, plaque psoriasis, psoriatic arthritis, and ulcerative colitis are shown in Table 1. Adverse events occurring at a frequency of at least 5% in REMICADE-treated pediatric patients with Crohn's disease are shown in Table 2. Adverse events occurring at a frequency of ≥1% to <5% in REMICADE-treated adult patients are shown in Table 3. Adverse events occurring at a frequency of ≥1% to <5% in REMICADE-treated pediatric patients with Crohn's disease are shown in Table 4. Adverse events in a juvenile rheumatoid arthritis (JRA) trial are set forth in the section entitled Adverse Reactions in Pediatric Patients, Juvenile Rheumatoid Arthritis. In general, the adverse events in pediatric patients with Crohn's disease who received REMICADE were similar in frequency and type to those seen in adult patients with Crohn's disease. Differences from adults and other special considerations are discussed in the section, Adverse Reactions in Pediatric Patients, Crohn's Disease.

Table 1: REMICADE

Number of Subjects with 1 or More Adverse Events (with frequency of ≥5%) by WHOART System-Organ Class and Preferred Term; Treated Subjects ≥18 Years of Age[a,b]

	RA Studies		CD Studies		AS Studies		UC Studies		Psoriasis Studies		PsA Studies	
	Placebo	Infliximab	Placebo	Infliximab	Placebo	Infliximab	Placebo	Infliximab	Placebo	Infliximab	Placebo	Infliximab
Treated subjects ≥18 years of age	427	1304	56	1085	76	275	248	493	334	1373	98	191
Average Weeks of Follow-up	52.0	59.9	14.7	46.0	25.3	87.8	31.9	40.5	18.1	41.9	20.2	42.8
System-organ Class/Preferred Term												
Respiratory System Disorders												
Upper Respiratory Tract Infection	22%	29%	9%	26%	14%	49%	17%	18%	16%	25%	13%	24%
Pharyngitis	7%	12%	5%	14%	5%	20%	6%	10%	4%	9%	4%	10%
Sinusitis	7%	13%	2%	10%	1%	11%	5%	9%	3%	8%	4%	11%
Coughing	7%	12%	0%	7%	3%	13%	4%	6%	1%	5%	1%	7%
Rhinitis	4%	8%	4%	6%	5%	21%	2%	4%	1%	6%	2%	4%

(cont'd)

Table 1: REMICADE *(cont'd)*

Number of Subjects with 1 or More Adverse Events (with frequency of ≥5%) by WHOART System-Organ Class and Preferred Term; Treated Subjects ≥18 Years of Age[a,b]

	RA Studies		CD Studies		AS Studies		UC Studies		Psoriasis Studies		PsA Studies	
	Placebo	Infliximab	Placebo	Infliximab	Placebo	Infliximab	Placebo	Infliximab	Placebo	Infliximab	Placebo	Infliximab
Bronchitis	8%	9%	2%	6%	1%	8%	3%	4%	2%	4%	3%	6%
Gastrointestinal System Disorders												
Nausea	19%	19%	4%	20%	9%	11%	9%	11%	4%	8%	6%	5%
Abdominal Pain	7%	12%	4%	24%	4%	16%	13%	12%	1%	4%	2%	5%
Diarrhea	11%	11%	2%	8%	5%	20%	5%	5%	2%	5%	3%	2%
Vomiting	6%	7%	0%	12%	4%	6%	7%	6%	1%	3%	2%	1%
Dyspepsia	6%	9%	0%	6%	4%	4%	2%	3%	1%	2%	2%	2%
Skin and Appendages Disorders												
Pruritus	2%	6%	2%	7%	7%	12%	4%	6%	4%	9%	3%	6%
Rash	5%	9%	5%	12%	7%	10%	8%	8%	1%	2%	0%	2%
Body as a Whole—General Disorders												
Pain	7%	7%	5%	15%	5%	29%	12%	11%	5%	10%	1%	4%
Fatigue	6%	8%	5%	13%	4%	15%	8%	10%	2%	7%	3%	4%
Musculoskeletal System Disorders												
Arthralgia	6%	7%	2%	14%	1%	8%	10%	15%	2%	10%	2%	4%
Back Pain	4%	7%	4%	8%	3%	12%	8%	4%	3%	5%	6%	9%
Myalgia	3%	3%	5%	7%	3%	4%	5%	6%	1%	6%	0%	2%
Central and Peripheral Nervous Systems Disorders												
Headache	12%	17%	21%	26%	11%	20%	18%	19%	8%	17%	5%	10%
Dizziness	6%	7%	9%	11%	4%	10%	5%	6%	2%	4%	4%	4%
Resistance Mechanism Disorders												
Fever	4%	7%	7%	12%	0%	8%	9%	10%	1%	4%	1%	2%

a RA Studies include C0168T07, C0168T09, C0168T14, C0168T15, C0168T18, C0168T22, and C0168T29. CD Studies include C0168T08, C0168T11, C0168T16, C0168T20, C0168T21, and C0168T26. AS Studies include C0168T51. UC Studies include C0168T12, C0168T37, and C0168T46. Psoriasis Studies include C0168T31, C0168T38, and C0168T44. PsA Studies include C0168T50.

b The adverse events included in this table are determined by the frequency of events in the combined infliximab group over all indications in this table. Percentages are rounded to an integer value after the adverse event frequency is determined.

Table 2: REMICADE

Number of Subjects with 1 or More Adverse Events (with frequency of ≥5%) by WHOART System-Organ Class and Preferred Term; Treated Subjects <18 Years of Age[a,b] with Crohn's Disease

	CD Studies	
	Placebo	Infliximab
Treated subjects <18 years of age	0	139
Avg weeks of follow-up	NA	44.1
System-organ Class/Preferred Term		
Gastrointestinal System Disorders		
Crohn's Disease	NA	27%
Abdominal Pain	NA	22%
Vomiting	NA	22%
Nausea	NA	19%
Diarrhea	NA	13%
Blood in Stool	NA	7%
Constipation	NA	6%
Dyspepsia	NA	6%
Gastroenteritis	NA	5%
Respiratory System Disorders		
Upper Respiratory Tract Infection	NA	29%
Pharyngitis	NA	19%
Coughing	NA	11%
Rhinitis	NA	8%
Sinusitis	NA	8%

(cont'd)

Table 2: REMICADE *(cont'd)*

Number of Subjects with 1 or More Adverse Events (with frequency of ≥5%) by WHOART System-Organ Class and Preferred Term; Treated Subjects <18 Years of Age[a,b] with Crohn's Disease

	CD Studies	
	Placebo	Infliximab
Bronchitis	NA	5%
Resistance Mechanism Disorders		
Fever	NA	17%
Infection Viral	NA	6%
Flu Syndrome	NA	5%
Infection Bacterial	NA	5%
Skin and Appendages Disorders		
Rash	NA	10%
Pruritus	NA	9%
Central and Peripheral Nervous Systems Disorders		
Headache	NA	31%
Dizziness	NA	6%
Body as a Whole—General Disorders		
Pain	NA	9%
Fatigue	NA	5%
Musculoskeletal System Disorders		
Arthralgia	NA	9%
Bone fracture	NA	6%

(cont'd)

Table 2: REMICADE *(cont'd)*

Number of Subjects with 1 or More Adverse Events (with frequency of ≥5%) by WHOART System-Organ Class and Preferred Term; Treated Subjects <18 Years of Age[a,b] with Crohn's Disease

	CD Studies	
	Placebo	Infliximab
White Cell and RES Disorders		
Leukopenia	NA	8%
Neutropenia	NA	6%
Vascular (Extracardiac) Disorders		
Flushing	NA	8%
Red Blood Cell Disorders		
Anemia	NA	9%

[a] CD Studies include T23, T47, and T55.

[b] The adverse events included in this table are determined by the frequency of events in the combined infliximab group. Percentages are rounded to an integer value after the adverse event frequency is determined.

Table 3: REMICADE

Number of Subjects with 1 or More Adverse Events (with frequency of ≥1% to <5%) by WHOART System-Organ Class and Preferred Term; Treated Subjects ≥18 Years of Age[a,b]

	RA Studies		CD Studies		AS Studies		UC Studies		Psoriasis Studies		PsA Studies	
	Placebo	Infliximab	Placebo	Infliximab	Placebo	Infliximab	Placebo	Infliximab	Placebo	Infliximab	Placebo	Infliximab
Treated subjects ≥18 years of age	427	1304	56	1085	76	275	248	493	334	1373	98	191
Avg Weeks of Follow-up	52.0	59.9	14.7	46.0	25.3	87.8	31.9	40.5	18.1	41.9	20.2	42.8
System-organ Class/Preferred Term												
Respiratory System Disorders												
Dyspnea	2%	5%	0%	5%	3%	5%	2%	3%	1%	3%	1%	3%
Pneumonia	1%	4%	0%	1%	0%	1%	0%	2%	0%	1%	0%	3%
Respiratory Tract Allergic Reaction	1%	2%	0%	1%	0%	1%	0%	1%	0%	2%	1%	2%
Epitaxis	1%	1%	0%	1%	0%	2%	0%	1%	0%	1%	0%	1%
Gastrointestinal System Disorders												
Gastroenteritis	3%	4%	2%	4%	4%	7%	2%	3%	1%	3%	3%	1%
Stomatitis Ulcerative	5%	6%	4%	3%	1%	1%	1%	1%	0%	1%	1%	1%
Crohn's Disease	0%	0%	0%	13%	0%	0%	0%	0%	0%	0%	0%	0%
Flatulence	1%	2%	0%	6%	0%	1%	2%	4%	0%	0%	0%	1%
Constipation	3%	2%	0%	4%	1%	3%	1%	2%	0%	1%	2%	0%
Gastroesophageal Reflux	1%	2%	0%	2%	0%	3%	2%	1%	0%	1%	1%	2%
Colitis Ulcerative	0%	0%	0%	0%	0%	0%	25%	16%	0%	0%	0%	0%
Tooth Ache	0%	1%	2%	2%	0%	1%	0%	1%	1%	2%	0%	1%
Blood in Stool	1%	1%	0%	3%	0%	1%	1%	1%	0%	0%	0%	0%
Anorexia	1%	1%	0%	2%	0%	0%	1%	1%	0%	0%	0%	1%
Skin and Appendages Disorders												
Urticaria	1%	4%	0%	3%	0%	2%	0%	1%	1%	4%	0%	4%
Sweating Increased	0%	2%	0%	4%	5%	4%	3%	3%	0%	2%	0%	2%
Dermatitis	1%	2%	0%	2%	1%	7%	2%	1%	0%	2%	0%	1%
Alopecia	2%	3%	0%	2%	0%	1%	1%	3%	1%	1%	2%	3%
Dermatitis Fungal	1%	3%	0%	2%	0%	5%	3%	1%	0%	2%	1%	2%
Psoriasis	0%	0%	0%	1%	1%	5%	1%	0%	7%	5%	2%	4%
Eczema	1%	2%	0%	3%	0%	3%	3%	1%	1%	1%	0%	1%
Skin Dry	0%	1%	2%	2%	0%	7%	1%	3%	1%	1%	0%	0%
Acne	0%	1%	0%	3%	0%	3%	1%	2%	1%	1%	0%	0%
Skin Wound	2%	2%	0%	1%	0%	2%	0%	1%	0%	2%	0%	1%
Erythema	0%	2%	0%	2%	0%	3%	1%	1%	0%	1%	1%	0%
Rash Erythematous	1%	1%	2%	1%	1%	5%	0%	1%	0%	0%	0%	1%
Body as a Whole—General Disorders												
Chest Pain	3%	4%	5%	5%	1%	6%	2%	3%	0%	4%	2%	4%
Edema Peripheral	4%	4%	2%	6%	1%	4%	4%	4%	2%	3%	0%	3%
Chills	2%	3%	2%	3%	3%	3%	2%	4%	1%	3%	0%	1%
Infusion Syndrome	0%	2%	0%	1%	1%	3%	0%	2%	0%	3%	0%	2%

(cont'd)

Table 3: REMICADE *(cont'd)*

Number of Subjects with 1 or More Adverse Events (with frequency of ≥1% to <5%) by WHOART System-Organ Class and Preferred Term; Treated Subjects ≥18 Years of Age[a,b]

	RA Studies		CD Studies		AS Studies		UC Studies		Psoriasis Studies		PsA Studies	
	Placebo	Infliximab	Placebo	Infliximab	Placebo	Infliximab	Placebo	Infliximab	Placebo	Infliximab	Placebo	Infliximab
Wound	1%	1%	0%	1%	1%	3%	0%	1%	0%	3%	1%	3%
Hot Flushes	0%	2%	2%	2%	1%	3%	2%	1%	0%	1%	0%	2%
Allergic Reaction	0%	1%	0%	2%	0%	5%	0%	2%	1%	1%	1%	1%
Asthenia	1%	1%	0%	2%	0%	2%	0%	1%	0%	1%	1%	1%
Reaction Unvaluable	0%	1%	0%	2%	0%	2%	1%	1%	1%	1%	0%	0%
Musculoskeletal System Disorders												
Arthritis	1%	1%	2%	4%	5%	14%	1%	1%	3%	7%	5%	5%
Bone Fracture	3%	4%	0%	2%	0%	4%	0%	1%	1%	1%	0%	4%
Skeletal Muscle Strain	2%	2%	0%	1%	0%	1%	1%	0%	1%	3%	1%	2%
Tendinitis	2%	0%	0%	1%	1%	5%	1%	1%	0%	1%	2%	1%
Central and Peripheral Nervous Systems Disorders												
Paresthesia	2%	3%	0%	3%	0%	7%	3%	3%	1%	3%	0%	0%
Muscle Contractions Involuntary	2%	4%	0%	3%	1%	3%	3%	2%	0%	2%	1%	1%
Hypesthesia	1%	2%	0%	2%	4%	3%	1%	1%	0%	2%	1%	1%
Vertigo	2%	2%	0%	1%	3%	1%	1%	1%	0%	1%	1%	2%
Migraine	1%	1%	0%	2%	0%	1%	0%	1%	0%	1%	0%	1%
Resistance Mechanism Disorders												
Abscess	3%	4%	4%	10%	3%	6%	3%	3%	1%	3%	2%	2%
Flu Syndrome	3%	4%	4%	7%	1%	8%	2%	4%	1%	3%	0%	3%
Moniliasis	3%	5%	0%	6%	0%	5%	2%	3%	0%	1%	0%	1%
Influenza-like Symptoms	0%	2%	2%	3%	1%	2%	2%	3%	1%	2%	0%	2%
Herpes simplex	1%	2%	0%	1%	0%	9%	2%	1%	1%	2%	1%	4%
Infection	2%	3%	0%	1%	3%	4%	1%	1%	1%	2%	0%	1%
Influenza	1%	2%	2%	3%	1%	1%	2%	2%	1%	2%	0%	1%
Cellulitis	1%	2%	0%	1%	0%	2%	0%	1%	1%	1%	1%	3%
Infection Bacterial	1%	1%	0%	1%	0%	1%	0%	0%	0%	1%	0%	2%
Herpes Zoster	1%	1%	0%	1%	0%	0%	0%	1%	1%	1%	0%	2%
Psychiatric Disorders												
Insomnia	4%	4%	4%	7%	1%	4%	2%	4%	1%	2%	1%	0%
Depression	5%	5%	0%	4%	0%	4%	2%	3%	1%	3%	2%	3%
Anxiety	1%	3%	0%	2%	1%	2%	3%	2%	0%	2%	1%	0%
Liver and Biliary System Disorders												
ALT Increased	4%	5%	0%	3%	5%	12%	1%	1%	1%	4%	1%	8%
AST Increased	2%	3%	0%	2%	3%	9%	0%	1%	1%	3%	2%	5%
Hepatic Enzymes Increased	3%	4%	0%	1%	0%	2%	0%	1%	0%	4%	0%	2%
Hepatic Function Abnormal	1%	2%	0%	1%	0%	2%	0%	0%	0%	1%	1%	2%
Vascular (extracardiac) Disorders												
Flushing	0%	3%	2%	3%	3%	4%	1%	2%	0%	5%	0%	3%
Ecchymosis	2%	4%	0%	2%	0%	2%	1%	1%	0%	2%	0%	1%
Hemorrhoids	1%	1%	0%	2%	1%	3%	3%	1%	0%	0%	0%	1%
Urinary System Disorders												
Urinary Tract Infection	5%	7%	4%	4%	0%	2%	2%	2%	1%	2%	4%	3%
Metabolic and Nutritional Disorders												
Hypokalemia	0%	2%	0%	4%	0%	0%	0%	1%	0%	0%	0%	1%
Weight Increase	2%	2%	0%	0%	1%	3%	0%	0%	0%	1%	0%	0%
Phosphatase Alkaline Increased	0%	1%	0%	2%	1%	2%	0%	0%	0%	0%	2%	2%

(cont'd)

Table 3: REMICADE *(cont'd)*

Number of Subjects with 1 or More Adverse Events (with frequency of ≥1% to <5%) by WHOART System-Organ Class and Preferred Term; Treated Subjects ≥18 Years of Age[a,b]

	RA Studies		CD Studies		AS Studies		UC Studies		Psoriasis Studies		PsA Studies	
	Placebo	Infliximab	Placebo	Infliximab	Placebo	Infliximab	Placebo	Infliximab	Placebo	Infliximab	Placebo	Infliximab
Cardiovascular Disorders, General												
Hypertension	5%	6%	2%	3%	5%	8%	2%	2%	3%	4%	2%	3%
Hypotension	1%	2%	0%	2%	1%	3%	0%	2%	0%	1%	0%	2%
Eye and Vision Disorders												
Conjunctivitis	2%	4%	2%	4%	1%	4%	3%	1%	0%	1%	1%	1%
Vision Abnormal	1%	2%	0%	2%	0%	4%	2%	1%	0%	1%	0%	2%
Ear and Hearing Disorders												
Otitis	0%	2%	0%	1%	0%	2%	1%	1%	0%	1%	0%	0%
White Cell and RES Disorders												
Leukopenia	1%	2%	0%	1%	0%	2%	0%	2%	0%	1%	0%	1%
Lymphadenopathy	0%	1%	0%	2%	0%	2%	1%	1%	0%	1%	0%	1%
Neutropenia	0%	1%	0%	1%	0%	3%	0%	0%	0%	1%	0%	3%
Red Blood Cell Disorders												
Anemia	4%	4%	0%	4%	1%	4%	10%	5%	0%	1%	0%	0%
Heart Rate and Rhythm Disorders												
Tachycardia	2%	2%	2%	1%	1%	1%	2%	1%	1%	1%	1%	1%
Palpitation	1%	2%	0%	1%	0%	3%	1%	1%	0%	1%	0%	1%
Administration/Application Site Disorders												
Injection Site Infiltration	3%	2%	0%	2%	0%	0%	1%	0%	0%	2%	0%	0%
Collagen Disorders												
Arthritis Rheumatoid	6%	7%	0%	0%	0%	0%	0%	0%	0%	0%	0%	0%

[a] RA Studies include C0168T07, C0168T09, C0168T14, C0168T15, C0168T18, C0168T22, and C0168T29. CD Studies include C0168T08, C0168T11, C0168T16, C0168T20, C0168T21, and C0168T26. AS Studies include C0168T51. UC Studies include C0168T12, C0168T37, and C0168T46. Psoriasis Studies include C0168T31, C0168T38, and C0168T44. PsA Studies include C0168T50.

[b] The adverse events included in this table are determined by the frequency of events in the combined infliximab group over all indications in this table. Percentages are rounded to an integer value after the adverse event frequency is determined.

Table 4: REMICADE

Number of Subjects with 1 or More Adverse Events (with frequency of ≥1% to <5%) by WHOART System-Organ Class and Preferred Term; Treated Subjects <18 Years of Age[a,b] with Crohn's Disease

	CD Studies	
	Placebo	Infliximab
Treated Subjects <18 Years of Age	0	139
Avg Weeks of Follow-up	NA	44.1
System-organ class/Preferred Term		
Gastrointestinal System Disorders		
Flatulence	NA	4%
Anal Fistula	NA	3%
Anorexia	NA	3%
Enterocolitis	NA	3%
Intestinal Stenosis	NA	2%
Pancreatitis	NA	2%
Proctalgia	NA	2%
Stomatitis Ulcerative	NA	2%
Tooth Ache	NA	2%
Dysphagia	NA	1%
Hemorrhage Rectum	NA	1%
Intestinal Obstruction	NA	1%
Oral Pain	NA	1%
Respiratory System Disorders		
Dyspnea	NA	4%
Respiratory Tract Allergic Reaction	NA	4%

(cont'd)

Table 4: REMICADE *(cont'd)*

Number of Subjects with 1 or More Adverse Events (with frequency of ≥1% to <5%) by WHOART System-Organ Class and Preferred Term; Treated Subjects <18 Years of Age[a,b] with Crohn's Disease

	CD Studies	
	Placebo	Infliximab
Epistaxis	NA	3%
Pneumonia	NA	2%
Asthma	NA	1%
Bronchospasm	NA	1%
Resistance Mechanism Disorders		
Abscess	NA	4%
Moniliasis	NA	4%
Infection	NA	3%
Influenza	NA	3%
Cellulitis	NA	1%
Herpes zoster	NA	1%
Infectious Mononucleosis	NA	1%
Skin and Appendages Disorders		
Cracking of Skin	NA	4%
Eczema	NA	4%
Skin Lesion	NA	3%
Acne	NA	2%
Dermatitis Contact	NA	2%
Dermatitis Fungal	NA	2%

(cont'd)

Table 4: REMICADE *(cont'd)*

Number of Subjects with 1 or More Adverse Events (with frequency of ≥1% to <5%) by WHOART System-Organ Class and Preferred Term; Treated Subjects <18 Years of Age[a,b] with Crohn's Disease

	CD Studies	
	Placebo	**Infliximab**
Rash Erythematous	NA	2%
Skin Dry	NA	2%
Verruca	NA	2%
Alopecia	NA	1%
Skin Hypertrophy	NA	1%
Sweating Increased	NA	1%
Urticaria	NA	1%
Central and Peripheral Nervous Systems Disorders		
Paresthesia	NA	2%
Migraine	NA	1%
Body as a Whole—General Disorders		
Allergic Reaction	NA	4%
Chest Pain	NA	3%
Asthenia	NA	1%
Edema Peripheral	NA	1%
Musculoskeletal System Disorders		
Myalgia	NA	4%
Back Pain	NA	2%
Sprain	NA	1%
White Cell and RES disorders		
Eosinophilia	NA	3%
Lymphadenopathy	NA	1%
Monocytosis	NA	1%
Vascular (extracardiac) Disorders		
Ecchymosis	NA	4%
Psychiatric Disorders		
Insomnia	NA	4%
Somnolence	NA	3%
Anxiety	NA	2%
Depression	NA	2%
Irritability	NA	1%
Suicide Attempt	NA	1%
Eye and Vision Disorders		
Conjunctivitis	NA	4%
Eye Pain	NA	3%
Metabolic and Nutritional Disorders		
Weight Decrease	NA	3%
Dehydration	NA	2%
Liver and Biliary System Disorders		
Hepatic Enzymes Increased	NA	2%
Hepatic Function Abnormal	NA	2%
AST Increased	NA	1%
ALT Increased	NA	1%
Cardiovascular Disorders, General		
Syncope	NA	2%
Hypotension	NA	1%

(cont'd)

Table 4: REMICADE *(cont'd)*

Number of Subjects with 1 or More Adverse Events (with frequency of ≥1% to <5%) by WHOART System-Organ Class and Preferred Term; Treated Subjects <18 Years of Age[a,b] with Crohn's Disease

	CD Studies	
	Placebo	**Infliximab**
Administration/application Site Disorders		
Injection Site Infiltration	NA	4%
Ear and Hearing Disorders		
Earache	NA	2%
Otitis media	NA	2%
Reproductive Disorders		
Dysmenorrhea	NA	2%
Ovarian Cyst	NA	1%
Urinary System Disorders		
Dysuria	NA	1%
Collagen Disorders		
Antinuclear Factor Test Positive	NA	3%
Platelet, Bleeding and Clotting Disorders		
Thrombocytopenia	NA	1%

[a] CD Studies include T23, T47, and T55.
[b] The adverse events included in this table are determined by the frequency of events in the combined infliximab group. Percentages are rounded to an integer value after the adverse event frequency is determined.

Infusion-Related Reactions: Acute Infusion Reactions: An infusion reaction was defined in clinical trials as any adverse event occurring during an infusion or within 1 to 2 hours after an infusion. Approximately 20% of REMICADE-treated patients in clinical studies, primarily adult rheumatoid arthritis and Crohn's disease, experienced an infusion reaction compared with 7% of placebo-treated patients. In these clinical trials, approximately 3% of REMICADE infusions were accompanied by nonspecific symptoms such as fever or chills, 1% were accompanied by cardiopulmonary reactions (primarily chest pain, hypotension, hypertension or dyspnea), <1% were accompanied by pruritus, urticaria, or the combined symptoms of pruritus/urticaria and cardiopulmonary reactions. Serious infusion reactions occurred in less than 1% of patients and included anaphylaxis, convulsions, erythematous rash and hypotension. Approximately 3% of patients discontinued REMICADE because of infusion reactions, and all patients recovered with treatment and/or discontinuation of infusion. REMICADE infusions beyond the initial infusion were not associated with a higher incidence of reactions. In psoriatic arthritis (IMPACT 2), infusion reactions were reported in 12% of REMICADE-treated patients compared with 7% of placebo-treated patients. Among the 1376 REMICADE infusions, 2% of these led to an infusion reaction. In plaque psoriasis, infusion reactions were reported in 22% of REMICADE-treated patients compared with 5% of placebo-treated patients. Among the 8366 REMICADE infusions, 5% of these led to an infusion reaction. In the ankylosing spondylitis study ASSERT, infusion reactions were reported in 19% of REMICADE-treated patients compared with 9% of placebo-treated patients. Among the 4257 REMICADE infusions, 2% of these led to an infusion reaction.

In a clinical study of patients with early rheumatoid arthritis (ASPIRE), 66% percent of all treated patients (686 out of 1040) received at least one shortened infusion of 90 minutes or less and 44% of the patients (454 out of 1040) received at least one shortened infusion of 60 minutes or less. Of the REMICADE-treated patients who received at least one shortened infusion **of 90 minutes or less** at the dose of 3 mg/kg, infusion-related reactions occurred in 19% (48/248) of patients and serious infusion reactions occurred in 0.4% (1/248) of patients. Of the REMICADE-treated patients who received at least one shortened infusion **of 90 minutes or less** at the dose of 6 mg/kg, infusion-related reactions occurred in 11% (26/246) of patients and serious infusion reactions occurred in 0.4% (1/246) of patients. Shortened infusions at doses >6 mg/kg have not been studied.

In the UC studies ACT 1 and ACT 2 through Week 30, the proportion of subjects with infusion reactions was comparable in the placebo and combined infliximab treatment groups. Through Week 54, the proportion of subjects with infusion reactions rose and was greater in the combined infliximab treatment group than in the placebo treatment group (13.4% versus 9.4%, respectively). A greater proportion of subjects in the 10 mg/kg than in the 5 mg/kg infliximab treatment group (16.1% versus 10.7%) experienced an infusion reaction.

Patients who became positive for antibodies to infliximab were more likely to develop infusion reactions than were those who were negative (approximately 3-fold). Use of concomitant immunosuppressant agents appeared to reduce the frequency of antibodies to infliximab and infusion reactions (see Warnings and Precautions, Immunogenicity and Drug Interactions).

In post-marketing experience, cases of anaphylactic-like reactions, including laryngeal/pharyngeal edema and severe bronchospasm, and seizure have been associated with REMICADE administration (see Warnings and Precautions, Neurological Events). Very rare cases of transient visual loss and myocardial ischemia/infarction occurring during or within 2 hours of REMICADE infusion have also been reported.

Infusion Reactions Following Readministration of REMICADE: In rheumatoid arthritis, Crohn's disease and psoriasis clinical trials, readministration of REMICADE after a period of no treatment resulted in a higher incidence of infusion reactions relative to regular maintenance treatment.

In a clinical trial of patients with moderate to severe psoriasis designed to assess the efficacy of long-term maintenance therapy versus re-treatment with an induction cycle of REMICADE, 4% (8/219) of patients in the intermittent therapy arm experienced serious infusion reactions versus <1% (1/222) in the maintenance therapy arm. Patients enrolled in this trial did not receive any concomitant immunosuppressant therapy. Intermittent therapy in this trial was defined as the readministration of an induction cycle (maximum of four infusions at 0, 2, 6, and 14 weeks) of REMICADE upon disease flare after a period of no treatment. In this study, the majority of serious infusion reactions occurred during the second infusion at Week 2. Symptoms included, but were not limited to, dyspnea, urticaria, facial edema, and hypotension. In all cases, REMICADE treatment was discontinued and/or other treatment instituted with complete resolution of signs and symptoms (see Warnings and Precautions, Immune, Infusion Reactions Following Readministration of REMICADE).

Delayed Hypersentivity/Reactions Following Readministration of REMICADE: In a clinical study where 37 of 41 patients with Crohn's disease were retreated with infliximab following a 2 to 4 year period without infliximab treatment, 10 patients experienced adverse events manifesting 3 to 12 days following infusion of which 6 were considered serious. Signs and symptoms included myalgia and/or arthralgia with fever and/or rash, with some patients also experiencing pruritus, facial, hand or lip edema, dysphagia, urticaria, sore throat, and headache. Patients experiencing these adverse events had not experienced infusion-related adverse events associated with their initial infliximab therapy. Of these patients, adverse events occurred in 9 of 23 (39%) who had received liquid formulation which is no longer in use and 1 of 14 (7%) who received lyophilized formulation. The clinical data are not adequate to determine if occurrence of these reactions is due to differences in formulation. Patients' signs and symptoms improved substantially or resolved with treatment in all cases. There are insufficient data on the incidence of these events after drug-free intervals of 1 to 2 years. These events have been observed only infrequently in clinical studies and post-marketing surveillance with retreatment intervals up to 1 year.

In 3 other psoriasis studies, 1% (15/1373) of patients experienced a possible delayed hypersensitivity reaction with symptoms of arthralgia, myalgia, fever, and rash, often early in the treatment course following infliximab infusions. There were no possible delayed hypersensitivity reactions identified in the psoriatic arthritis study (IMPACT 2) (see Warnings and Precautions, Immune, Hypersensitivity Reactions).

Infections: In REMICADE clinical studies, primarily of RA and CD, treated infections were reported in 36% of REMICADE-treated patients (average of 53 weeks of follow-up) and in 28% of placebo-treated patients (average of 47 weeks of follow-up). In the ATTRACT* study, 60% of REMICADE-treated RA patients (average of 97 weeks of follow-up) had treated infections reported vs 43% of placebo-treated patients (average of 75 weeks of follow-up); treated infections were more common with higher doses of REMICADE. In the ASPIRE† study, 37% of REMICADE-treated RA patients (average of 54 weeks of follow-up) had treated infections reported vs 30% of placebo-treated patients (average of 52 weeks of follow-up). The infections most frequently reported in the RA studies were respiratory tract infections (including URI, sinusitis, pharyngitis, and bronchitis) and urinary tract infections. No increased risk of serious infections or sepsis was observed with REMICADE compared with placebo in the ATTRACT or ACCENT I ‡ and II § studies. However, in the ATTRACT study, the incidence of serious events of pneumonia and lobar pneumonia combined was higher in patients receiving infliximab plus MTX vs. MTX alone (2.6% vs. 1.2%, respectively). In the ASPIRE study, the incidence of serious pneumonia was also higher in patients receiving infliximab plus MTX vs. MTX alone (2.5% vs. 0%, respectively). In other RA trials, the incidence of serious infections including pneumonia was higher in infliximab plus MTX treated patients compared with methotrexate alone, especially at higher than recommended induction regimen of REMICADE 6 mg/kg or greater. Among REMICADE-treated patients, serious infections included pneumonia, cellulitis, abscess and sepsis. In ATTRACT, one patient died with miliary tuberculosis, one died with disseminated coccidioidomycosis and one died due to sepsis. In the ASPIRE study, four patients were diagnosed with tuberculosis. In the ACCENT I study, one patient was diagnosed with tuberculosis. In EXPRESS II¶, two patients with psoriasis were diagnosed with tuberculosis. Other cases of tuberculosis, including disseminated tuberculosis, also have been reported post-marketing. Most of the cases of tuberculosis occurred within the first two months after initiation of therapy with infliximab and may reflect recrudescence of latent disease (see Warnings and Precautions, Risk of Infections). In the ACCENT II study, serious infections of nocardiosis (one patient) and cytomegalovirus (one patient) were reported. Twelve percent of patients with fistulising Crohn's disease developed a new abscess 8 to 16 weeks after the last infusion of REMICADE in the T20 study. In the ACCENT II study, there was no difference between the REMICADE and placebo maintenance arms for proportions of patients with newly diagnosed fistula-related abscesses. In the psoriasis studies, 1.5% of patients (average of 41.9 weeks of follow up) receiving REMICADE and 0.6% of patients (average of 18.1 weeks of follow up) receiving placebo developed serious infections. In EXPRESS**, one patient died due to sepsis. In the IMPACT 2†† study of psoriatic arthritis, 1.6% of patients (average 42.8 weeks of follow-up) receiving REMICADE and 2.0% of patients (average 20.2 weeks of follow-up) receiving placebo developed serious infections.

In the REMICADE clinical studies in patients with ulcerative colitis (ACT 1 and ACT 2‡‡), the most frequently reported infections were upper respiratory infection (URI), sinusitis, pharyngitis, bronchitis and moniliasis. In the UC studies, infections were reported in 30.6% and 40.1% of REMICADE-treated patients at Week 30 (average 26.9 weeks of follow-up) and at Week 54 (average 41.1 weeks of follow-up) and in 29.5% and 32.8% of placebo-treated patients at Week 30 (average 22.2 weeks of follow up) and at Week 54 (average 32.2 weeks of follow-up). The types of infections, including serious infections, reported in patients with ulcerative colitis were similar to those reported in other clinical studies, and included one case of tuberculosis and a fatal case of histoplasmosis.

In post-marketing experience, infections have been observed with various pathogens including viral, bacterial, fungal, and protozoal organisms. Infections have been noted in all organ systems and have been reported in patients receiving REMICADE alone or in combination with immunosuppressive agents.

Autoantibodies/Lupus-like Syndrome: Approximately 55% of 1598 infliximab-treated patients in clinical trials (primarily RA and CD) who were antinuclear antibody (ANA) negative at baseline developed a positive ANA during the trial compared with approximately 20% of 265 placebo-treated patients. Anti-dsDNA antibodies were newly detected in approximately 19% of 2116 infliximab-treated patients compared with 0% of 422 placebo-treated patients. Reports of lupus and lupus-like syndromes, however, remain uncommon.

In the ATTRACT rheumatoid arthritis study through Week 102, 62% of REMICADE-treated patients developed antinuclear antibodies (ANA) between screening and last evaluation, compared with 27% of placebo-treated patients. In the ASPIRE study through Week 58, 66% of REMICADE-treated patients developed antinuclear antibodies (ANA) between screening and last evaluation, compared with 21% of placebo-treated patients. In both RA studies, anti-dsDNA antibodies developed in approximately 15% of REMICADE-treated patients, compared to none of the placebo-treated patients. No association was seen between REMICADE dose/schedule and development of ANA or anti-dsDNA antibodies.

Of Crohn's disease patients treated with REMICADE who were evaluated for antinuclear antibodies (ANA), 40% developed ANA between screening and last evaluation. Anti-dsDNA antibodies developed in approximately 20% of Crohn's disease patients treated with REMICADE. The development of anti-dsDNA antibodies was not related to either the dose or duration of REMICADE treatment. However, baseline therapy with an immunosuppressant in Crohn's disease patients was associated with reduced development of anti-dsDNA antibodies (3% compared to 21% in patients not receiving any immunosuppressant). Crohn's disease patients were approximately 2 times more likely to develop anti-dsDNA antibodies if they were ANA-positive at study entry.

In the EXPRESS plaque psoriasis study through Week 50, 59% of REMICADE-treated patients developed antinuclear antibodies following REMICADE treatment compared to 2% of placebo-treated patients. Anti-dsDNA antibodies developed in 16% of REMICADE-treated patients, compared to none of the placebo-treated patients. In the EXPRESS II plaque psoriasis study through Week 50, 65% of REMICADE-treated patients developed antinuclear antibodies following REMICADE treatment compared to 8% of placebo-treated patients. Anti-dsDNA antibodies developed in 27% of REMICADE-treated patients, compared to none of the placebo-treated patients. No association was seen between REMICADE dose/schedule and development of ANA or anti-dsDNA antibodies.

In the IMPACT 2 psoriatic arthritis study through Week 66, 59% of REMICADE-treated patients developed antinuclear antibodies following REMICADE treatment compared to 11% of placebo-treated patients. Anti-dsDNA antibodies developed in 12% of REMICADE-treated patients, compared to none of the placebo-treated patients.

In the ASSERT ankylosing spondylitis study through week 102, 35% of REMICADE-treated patients developed antinuclear antibodies following REMICADE treatment compared to 1% of placebo-treated patients. Anti-dsDNA antibodies developed in 30% of REMICADE-treated patients, compared to none of the placebo-treated patients.

In clinical studies, 22 patients were diagnosed with a possible lupus-like syndrome, four with Crohn's disease, eight patients with plaque psoriasis [seven (0.5%) patients treated with infliximab and one (0.3%) patient treated with placebo], 8 patients with ankylosing spondylitis, and two with rheumatoid arthritis. Twenty-one patients improved following discontinuation of therapy and/or appropriate medical treatment. One psoriasis patient on concomitant hydralazine had central nervous system involvement. No patients had renal involvement. No cases of lupus-like syndromes were reported in the psoriatic arthritis studies. The lupus-like syndrome in one patient with rheumatoid arthritis and one patient with ankylosing spondylitis remained ongoing at the end of the study. One case of a lupus-like reaction has been observed in a Crohn's disease patient in up to three years of long-term follow-up (see Warnings and Precautions, Autoimmunity).

Hepatobiliary Events: In post-marketing surveillance, very rare cases of jaundice and hepatitis, some with features of autoimmune hepatitis, have been reported in patients receiving REMICADE (see Warnings and Precautions, Hepatic/Biliary/Pancreatic).

In clinical trials, mild or moderate elevations of ALT and AST have been observed in patients receiving REMICADE without progression to severe hepatic injury. Elevations of aminotransferases were observed (ALT more common than AST) in a greater proportion of patients receiving REMICADE than in controls, both when REMICADE was given as monotherapy and when it was used in combination with other immunosuppressive agents. Most aminotransferase abnormalities were transient; however, a small number of patients experienced more prolonged elevations. In general, patients who developed ALT and AST elevations were asymptomatic, and the abnormalities decreased or resolved with either continuation or discontinuation of REMICADE, or modification of concomitant medications.

Malignancies/Lymphoproliferative Disease: In the controlled portions of clinical trials of all the TNF-blocking agents, more cases of lymphoma have been observed among patients receiving a TNF blocker compared with control patients. In the controlled and open-label portions of REMICADE clinical trials, 5 patients developed lymphomas among 5780 patients treated with REMICADE (median duration of follow-up 1.0 years) vs. 0 lymphomas in 1600 control patients (median duration of follow-up 0.4 years). In rheumatoid arthritis patients, 2 lymphomas were observed for a rate of 0.08 cases per 100 patient-years of follow-up, which is approximately 3-fold higher than expected in the general population. In the combined clinical trial population for rheumatoid arthritis, Crohn's disease, psoriatic arthritis, psoriasis, ankylosing spondylitis, and ulcerative colitis, 5 lymphomas were observed for a rate of 0.09 cases per 100 patient-years of follow-up, which is approximately 4-fold higher than expected in the general population. Patients with Crohn's disease or rheumatoid arthritis, particularly patients with highly active disease and/or chronic exposure to immunosuppressant therapies, may be at a higher risk (up to several fold) than the general population for the development of lymphoma, even in the absence of TNF-blocking therapy.

In the controlled portions of clinical trials of some TNF-blocking agents including REMICADE, more cases of non-lymphoma malignancies have been observed in patients receiving those TNF-blockers compared with control patients. During the controlled portions of REMICADE trials in patients with moderately to severely active rheumatoid arthritis, Crohn's disease, psoriatic arthritis, psoriasis, ankylosing spondylitis, and ulcerative colitis, 14 patients were diagnosed with non-lymphoma malignancies among 4019 REMICADE-treated patients vs 1 among 1597 control patients (at a rate of 0.52/100 patient-years among REMICADE-treated patients vs a rate of 0.11/100 patient-years among control patients), with median duration of follow-up 0.5 years for REMICADE-treated patients and 0.4 years for control patients. Of these, the most common malignancies were breast, colorectal, and melanoma. The rate of non-lymphoma malignancies among REMICADE-treated patients was similar to that expected in the general population whereas the rate in control patients was lower than expected.

The potential role of TNF-blocking therapy in the development of malignancies is not known. Rates in clinical trials for REMICADE cannot be compared to rates in clinical trials of other TNF-blockers and may not predict rates observed in a broader patient population. Caution should be exercised in considering REMICADE treatment in patients with a history of malignancy or in continuing treatment in patients who develop malignancy while receiving REMICADE.

Among the 345 patients who received REMICADE in ankylosing spondylitis trials, 3 patients developed malignancies (1 patient had a squamous cell and a basal cell carcinoma, 1 patient had a pulmonary carcinoma, and 1 patient had breast cancer). Additionally, 1 patient in ASSERT developed a nonseminoma testicular carcinoma after leaving the trial, approximately 1 year after his last dose of REMICADE.

In the IMPACT 2 study of psoriatic arthritis, 2 malignancies were reported through Week 54 (Stage I Hodgkin's lymphoma in a REMICADE-treated patient and basal cell carcinoma in a placebo-treated patient). No malignancies were reported through Week 50 of IMPACT. An adenocarcinoma of the pancreas was reported 2 months after completing the year 2 extension of IMPACT.

During the REMICADE plaque psoriasis trials, no patients developed lymphoma. In the placebo-controlled portions of the psoriasis studies, 7 of 1123 patients who received REMICADE at any dose (443 patient-years) were diagnosed with a non-melanoma skin cancer (NMSC) compared to 0 of 334 patients who received placebo (113 patient-years). Among the 1373 patients with psoriasis who received REMICADE at any dose in the controlled and uncontrolled portions of the psoriasis studies (1101 patient-years), a total of 17 were diagnosed with NMSC (12 basal cell cancers, 5 squamous cell cancers). The size of the placebo group and limited duration of the controlled portions of studies precludes the ability to draw firm conclusions. Patients on REMICADE should be monitored for the development of NMSC. Two noncutaneous malignancies (breast cancer and adenocarcinoma) were reported during the psoriasis clinical trials.

Congestive Heart Failure: In a phase II study evaluating REMICADE in NYHA Class III/IV CHF patients (left ventricular ejection fraction ≤35%), higher incidences of mortality and hospitalization due to worsening heart failure were seen in REMICADE-treated patients, especially those treated with 10 mg/kg. One hundred and fifty patients were treated with 3 infusions of REMICADE 5 mg/kg, 10 mg/kg, or placebo over 6 weeks. At 28 weeks, 4 of 101 patients treated with REMICADE (1 at 5 mg/kg and 3 at 10 mg/kg) died compared with no deaths among the 49 placebo-treated patients. In follow-up, at 38 weeks, 9 patients treated with REMICADE (2 at 5 mg/kg and 7 at 10 mg/kg) died compared with one death among the placebo-treated patients. At 28 weeks, 14 of 101 patients treated with REMICADE (3 at 5 mg/kg and 11 at 10 mg/kg) were hospitalized for worsening CHF compared with 5 of the 49 placebo-treated patients (see Contraindications and Warnings and Precautions, Cardiovascular).

Less Common Clinical Trial Adverse Drug Reactions: Other medically relevant adverse events occurring at a frequency <1% were as follows, presented by body system:

Administration/Application Site: injection site inflammation, injection site ecchymosis, injection site swelling, injection site infection.

Autonomic Nervous System: fecal incontinence.

Body as a Whole: anaphylactoid reaction, diaphragmatic hernia, generalized edema, surgical/procedural sequela, substernal chest pain, rigors.

Blood: pancytopenia, splenomegaly.

Cardiovascular: circulatory failure, hypotension postural, pallor.

Collagen: LE syndrome, anti-DNA antibodies, positive antinuclear factor test.

Ear and Hearing: otitis externa.

Endocrine: adrenal insufficiency, hypothyroidism.

Eye and Vision: lacrimation abnormal, iritis, scleritis, eye pain, glaucoma.

Gastrointestinal: ileus, intestinal stenosis, pancreatitis, peritonitis, rectal hemorrhage, appetite increased, anal fistula, diarrhea bloody, gastritis, intestinal obstruction, intestinal perforation.

Central and Peripheral Nervous: meningitis, neuritis, optic neuritis, peripheral neuropathy, neuralgia, ataxia, dysesthesia, tremor, hyperkinesia.

Heart Rate and Rhythm: arrhythmia, bradycardia, cardiac arrest, palpitations.

Liver and Biliary: cholelithiasis, hepatitis, bilirubinemia, cholecystitis, hepatocellular damage, elevated GGT, fatty liver, hepatomegaly.

Metabolic and Nutritional: hypercholesterolemia.

Musculoskeletal: intervertebral disk herniation, tendon disorder, joint stiffness.

Myo-, Endo-, Pericardial and Coronary Valve: myocardial infarction, mitral insufficiency, heart murmur, cardiac failure.

Platelet, Bleeding and Clotting: thrombocytopenia.

Neoplasms: adenocarcinoma, basal cell carcinoma, breast cancer, lymphoma, malignant melanoma, squamous cell carcinoma, bladder carcinoma, rectal carcinoma, uterine cancer, pulmonary carcinoma.

Psychiatric: confusion, suicide attempt, irritability, nervousness, amnesia.

Red Blood Cell: iron deficiency anemia, hemolytic anemia.

Reproductive: menstrual irregularity, dysmenorrhea, menorrhagia, breast fibroadenosis, amenorrhea, female breast pain.

Resistance Mechanism: sepsis, serum sickness, tuberculosis, fungal infection, viral infection.

Respiratory: Adult respiratory distress syndrome, respiratory tract infection, pleural effusion, lobar pneumonia, pulmonary edema, respiratory insufficiency, bronchospasm, asthma, hemoptysis, epistaxis, laryngitis.

Skin and Appendages: erythema nodosum, rash maculopapular, rash pustular, photosensitivity reaction, edema periorbital, fascitis.

Special Senses, Other: taste perversion, taste loss.

Urinary: renal failure, dysuria, renal calculus, pyelonephritis.

Vascular (Extracardiac): brain infarction, thrombophlebitis, vasculitis, brain ischemia, pulmonary embolism.

White Cell and Reticuloendothelial: neutropenia, neutrophilia, lymphocytosis.

Abnormal Hematologic and Clinical Chemistry Findings: Serious, medically relevant hematologic adverse events ≥0.2%, or clinically relevant hematologic adverse reactions observed in clinical trials include: pancytopenia, thrombocytopenia, anemia, hemolytic anemia, neutropenia and leukopenia.

Table 5: REMICADE

Proportion of Patients with Elevated ALT in Clinical Trials

	Proportion of Patients with Elevated ALT					
	>1 to <3×ULN		≥3×ULN		≥5×ULN	
	placebo	infliximab	placebo	infliximab	placebo	infliximab
Rheumatoid Arthritis[a]	24.0%	34.4%	3.2%	3.9%	0.8%	0.9%
Crohn's Disease[b]	34.1%	38.8%	3.5%	5.1%	0.0%	1.7%
Ulcerative Colitis[c]	12.4%	17.4%	1.2%	2.5%	0.4%	0.6%
Psoriatic Arthritis[d]	16.3%	49.5%	0.0%	6.8%	0.0%	2.1%
Plaque Psoriasis[e]	23.8%	49.4%	0.4%	7.7%	0.0%	3.4%

(cont'd)

* ATTRACT (the Anti-TNF Trial in Rheumatoid Arthritis with Concomitant Therapy).
† ASPIRE (the Active-controlled Study of Patients Receiving Infliximab for the Treatment of Rheumatoid Arthritis of Early Onset).
‡ ACCENT I (the Anti-TNF Trial in Long-term Treatment of Moderately to Severely Active Crohn's Disease).
§ ACCENT II (the Anti-TNF Trial in Long-term Treatment of Fistulising Crohn's Disease).
¶ EXPRESS II Evaluation of Infliximab for Psoriasis in a REMICADE Efficacy and Safety Study.
** EXPRESS European infliximab for Psoriasis (REMICADE) Efficacy and Safety Study.
†† IMPACT 2 Induction and Maintenance Psoriatic Arthritis Clinical Trial.
‡‡ ACT 1 and ACT 2 (the Anti-TNF Trials in moderately to severely active ulcerative colitis).

Table 5: REMICADE *(cont'd)*

Proportion of Patients with Elevated ALT in Clinical Trials

	Proportion of Patients with Elevated ALT					
	>1 to <3×ULN		≥3×ULN		≥5×ULN	
	placebo	infliximab	placebo	infliximab	placebo	infliximab
Pediatric Crohn's Disease[f]	n/a	18.2%	n/a	4.4%	n/a	1.5%
Ankylosing Spondylitis[g]	14.5%	51.1%	0.0%	9.5%	0.0%	3.6%

[a] Note that placebo patients received methotrexate while infliximab patients received both infliximab and methotrexate. Median follow-up was 58 weeks for placebo patients and infliximab-treated patients. RA trials include ATTRACT (T22) and ASPIRE (T29).
[b] Note that placebo patients in the 2 Phase III trials in Crohn's disease, ACCENT I and ACCENT II, received an initial dose of 5 mg/kg infliximab at study start and were on placebo in the maintenance phase. Patients who were randomized to the placebo maintenance group and then later crossed over to infliximab are included in the infliximab group in this table. Median follow-up time was 54 weeks.
[c] Ulcerative colitis trials include ACT I (C0168T37) through Week 54 and ACT II (C0168T46) through Week 30; median duration of follow up was 30.8 weeks for the infliximab group and 30.1 weeks for placebo group.
[d] IMPACT 2 median duration of follow up was 39.1 weeks for the infliximab group and 18.1 weeks for placebo group.
[e] EXPRESS and EXPRESS II median duration of follow up was 16.1 weeks for placebo and 50.1 weeks for infliximab groups.
[f] Patients from pediatric Crohn's disease trials T23, T55 and T47 (REACH). Median follow-up was 53.0 weeks.
[g] Patients from the ASSERT trial (T51); median duration of follow-up was 24.1 weeks for placebo and 101.9 weeks for the infliximab group.

The difference in rates of ALT elevations ≥3×ULN between infliximab and placebo treatment groups tended to be greater in ankylosing spondylitis, psoriasis and psoriatic arthritis clinical trials than in rheumatoid arthritis, Crohn's disease and ulcerative colitis clinical trials.

See Hepatobiliary Events.

Adverse Reactions in Pediatric Patients: Crohn's Disease: Adverse events occurring at a frequency of ≥5% or from ≥1% to <5% in REMICADE-treated pediatric patients with Crohn's disease are shown in Table 2 and Table 4, respectively. In general, the adverse events in pediatric patients who received REMICADE were similar in frequency and type to those seen in adult patients with Crohn's disease. Differences from adults and other special considerations are discussed in the following paragraphs.

The following adverse events were reported more commonly in the 103 randomised pediatric patients with Crohn's disease (Phase 3 Trial, REACH) who received 5 mg/kg REMICADE through 54 weeks than in the 385 adult patients with Crohn's disease (ACCENT I) where 193/385 patients received 5 mg/kg and 192/385 received 10 mg/kg REMICADE through 54 weeks: anemia (10.7%), blood in stool (9.7%), leukopenia (8.7%), flushing (8.7%), viral infection (7.8%), neutropenia (6.8%), bone fracture (6.8%), bacterial infection (6.8%), and respiratory tract allergic reaction (5.8%). The Phase 3 study (REACH) enrolled 112 pediatric patients 6 to 17 years old (median age 13.0 years) with moderately to severely active Crohn's disease and an inadequate response to conventional therapies.

Infections were reported in 56.3% of randomised pediatric patients in the REACH trial, and in 50.3% of patients in the ACCENT I Study. In the pediatric Phase 3 trial, infections were reported more frequently for subjects who received q8 week as opposed to q12 week infusions (73.6% and 38.0%, respectively), while serious infections were reported for 3 patients in the q8 week and 4 patients in the q12 week maintenance treatment group. The most commonly reported infections were upper respiratory tract infection and pharyngitis, and the most commonly reported serious infection was abscess. Pneumonia was reported for 3 patients, 2 in the q8 week and 1 in the q12 week maintenance treatment groups. Herpes zoster was reported for 2 patients in the q8 week maintenance treatment group.

In REACH, 17.5% of randomised patients experienced 1 or more infusion reactions, with no notable difference between treatment groups (17.0% and 18.0% of patients in the q8 week and q12 week maintenance treatment groups, respectively). There were no serious infusion reactions, and 2 patients had non-serious anaphylactic reactions.

Antibodies to REMICADE developed in 3 (2.9%) pediatric patients in the REACH trial and in none of the patients in the Phase 2 trial (T23).

Juvenile Rheumatoid Arthritis: The efficacy of REMICADE in the treatment of children with juvenile rheumatoid arthritis, JRA, has not been established. In a clinical trial where children were treated with either 3 mg/kg or 6 mg/kg of REMICADE, the proportion of children with infusion reactions, most commonly vomiting, fever, headache and hypotension, was 35% at a dosage of 3 mg/kg. Four of these reactions were serious, and three were considered to be possible anaphylactic reactions. Two of the 4 patients who experienced serious infusion reactions at a dose of 3 mg/kg received infliximab by rapid infusion (duration time less than 2 hours). Antibodies to infliximab developed in 37.7% of children receiving that dosage, but only in 12.2% receiving a higher dosage (6 mg/kg).

Post-Market Adverse Drug Reactions: Additional adverse events, some with fatal outcome, reported from worldwide post-marketing experience with REMICADE are included in Table 6 (see Adverse Reactions, Infections and Infusion-Related Reactions). Because these events are reported voluntarily from a population of uncertain size, it is not always possible to reliably estimate their frequency or establish a causal relationship to REMICADE exposure.

The most common serious adverse events reported in the post-marketing experience in children were infections (some fatal) including opportunistic infections and tuberculosis, infusion reactions, and hypersensitivity reactions. Spontaneous serious adverse events in the post-marketing experience with REMICADE in the pediatric population have also included malignancies, transient hepatic enzyme abnormalities, lupus-like syndromes, and the development of autoantibodies.

Rare post-marketing cases of hepatosplenic T-cell lymphoma have been reported in patients with Crohn's disease and ulcerative colitis treated with REMICADE, the majority of whom were adolescent or young adult males (see Warnings and Precautions, Carcinogenesis and Mutagenesis, Hepatosplenic T-Cell Lymphoma).

Table 6: REMICADE

Post-Marketing Reports

Blood and Lymphatic System Disorders	Agranulocytosis, idiopathic thrombocytopenic purpura, hemolytic anemia, pancytopenia, thrombotic thrombocytopenic purpura
General Disorders and Administration Site Conditions	Anaphylactic reactions, anaphylactic shock, infusion-related reactions, serum sickness
Cardiac Disorders	Pericardial effusion, very rare cases of myocardial ischemia/myocardial infarction occurring during or within 2 hours of infusion
Eye Disorders	Very rare transient visual loss occurring during or within 2 hours of infusion
Immune System Disorders	Vasculitis
Neoplasm Benign and Malignant	Hepatosplenic T-cell lymphoma (Crohn's disease and ulcerative colitis: primarily adolescents and young adults), pediatric malignancy, leukemia
Hepatobiliary System Disorders	Hepatocellular damage, hepatitis, jaundice, autoimmune hepatitis, liver failure
Nervous System Disorders	Central nervous system demyelinating disorders (such as multiple sclerosis and optic neuritis), peripheral demyelinating disorders (such as Guillain-Barré syndrome, chronic inflammatory demyelinating polyneuropathy, and multifocal motor neuropathy), neuropathies, numbness, seizure, tingling, transverse myelitis

(cont'd)

Table 6: REMICADE *(cont'd)*

Post-Marketing Reports

Infections and Infestations	Opportunistic infections (such as aspergillosis, atypical mycobacteria, coccidioidomycosis, cryptococcosis, candidiasis, histoplasmosis, listeriosis, pneumocystosis), salmonellosis, sepsis, tuberculosis, protozoal infections, and hepatitis B reactivation
Respiratory, Thoracic and Mediastinal Disorders	Interstitial lung disease, including pulmonary fibrosis/interstitial pneumonitis, and very rare rapidly progressive disease
Skin and Subcutaneous Tissue Disorders	Vasculitis (primarily cutaneous), psoriasis including new onset and pustular (primarily palmar/plantar), erythema multiforme, Stevens-Johnson Syndrome, toxic epidermal necrolysis

DRUG INTERACTIONS: Overview: Specific drug interaction studies have not been conducted. The majority of patients in rheumatoid arthritis, Crohn's disease or ulcerative colitis clinical trials received one or more concomitant medications. In rheumatoid arthritis, concomitant medications besides MTX were nonsteroidal anti-inflammatory agents, folic acid, corticosteroids and/or narcotics. Concomitant Crohn's disease medications were antibiotics, antivirals, corticosteroids, 6-MP/AZA, MTX, and aminosalicylates. Patients with Crohn's disease who received immunosuppressants tended to experience fewer infusion reactions compared to patients using no immunosuppressants (see Warnings and Precautions, Immunogenicity and Adverse Reactions, Infusion-Related Reactions).

Drug-Drug Interactions: Concurrent Use of REMICADE with Anakinra or Abatacept: The combination of REMICADE and anakinra or abatacept is not recommended (see Warnings and Precautions, Risk of Infections).

Interactions with other drugs have not been established.

Drug-Food Interactions: Interactions with food have not been established.

Drug-Herb Interactions: Interactions with herbal products have not been established.

Drug-Laboratory Test Interactions: Interactions with laboratory tests have not been established.

DOSAGE AND ADMINISTRATION: Recommended Dose and Dose Adjustment: For recommended infusion duration for patients with each of the indications described below, see Dosage and Administration, Preparation and Administration Instructions.

Rheumatoid Arthritis: The recommended dose of REMICADE (infliximab) is 3 mg/kg given as an intravenous infusion followed by additional 3 mg/kg doses at 2 and 6 weeks after the first infusion then every 8 weeks thereafter. REMICADE should be given in combination with methotrexate. For patients who have an incomplete response, consideration may be given to adjusting the dose up to 10 mg/kg and/or treating as often as every 4 weeks. Duration of treatment needed to achieve a response after dose escalation is not known. However, higher doses of REMICADE were associated with a slightly higher proportion of patients experiencing adverse events (97% for the 3 mg/kg dose given every 8 weeks vs. 100% for the 10 mg/kg dose given every 4 weeks), including infections (84% for the 3 mg/kg dose given every 8 weeks vs. 91% for the 10 mg/kg dose given every 4 weeks).

Ankylosing Spondylitis: The recommended dose of REMICADE is 5 mg/kg given as an intravenous infusion followed by additional 5 mg/kg doses at 2 and 6 weeks after the first infusion, then every 6 to 8 weeks thereafter.

Ulcerative Colitis: The recommended dose of REMICADE is 5 mg/kg given as an induction regimen at 0, 2 and 6 weeks followed by 5 mg/kg every 8 weeks thereafter, for the treatment of moderately to severely active ulcerative colitis. In some patients, consideration may be given to adjusting the dose up to 10 mg/kg to sustain clinical response and remission.

Crohn's Disease: Adults: The recommended dose of REMICADE is 5 mg/kg given as an induction regimen at 0, 2 and 6 weeks followed by a maintenance regimen of 5 mg/kg every 8 weeks thereafter for the treatment of moderate to severe, active Crohn's disease. For patients who have an incomplete response, consideration may be given to adjusting the dose up to 10 mg/kg.

The recommended dose of REMICADE is 5 mg/kg given as an induction regimen at 0, 2 and 6 weeks followed by a maintenance regimen of 5 mg/kg every 8 weeks thereafter for the treatment of fistulising Crohn's disease. Patients who do not respond by Week 14 are unlikely to respond with continued dosing and consideration should be given to discontinue REMICADE in these patients. For patients who respond and then lose their response, consideration may be given to treatment with 10 mg/kg. In the ACCENT II clinical study, among patients who lost response at 5 mg/kg REMICADE and re-established response following dose escalation to 10 mg/kg REMICADE, most had done so after 1 dose and all had done so after 2 doses of 10 mg/kg.

Pediatric: The recommended dose of REMICADE for children with moderately to severely active Crohn's disease is 5 mg/kg given as an induction regimen at 0, 2 and 6 weeks followed by a maintenance regimen of 5 mg/kg every 8 weeks. Patients who do not respond by week 14 are unlikely to respond with continued dosing and consideration should be given to discontinue REMICADE in these patients.

Psoriatic Arthritis: The recommended dose of REMICADE is 5 mg/kg given as an intravenous infusion followed with additional similar doses at 2 and 6 weeks after the first infusion then every 8 weeks thereafter. REMICADE can be used with or without methotrexate. If a patient shows no response at 24 weeks, no additional treatment with REMICADE should be given.

Plaque Psoriasis: The recommended dose of REMICADE is 5 mg/kg given as an intravenous infusion followed by additional 5 mg/kg doses at 2 and 6 weeks after the first infusion, then every 8 weeks thereafter. If a patient does not show an adequate response at Week 14, after infusions at weeks 0, 2, and 6, no additional treatment with REMICADE should be given.

The infusion solution must be administered over a period of not less than 2 hours. All patients administered REMICADE should be observed for at least 1-2 hours post-infusion for side effects. Emergency equipment, such as adrenaline, antihistamines, corticosteroids and an artificial airway must be available (see Adverse Reactions, Infusion-Related Reactions).

The BioAdvance Network has been established to facilitate the administration of REMICADE. BioAdvance Network clinics are staffed by qualified healthcare professionals specially trained in the administration of REMICADE infusions and are available across Canada. Information about the BioAdvance Network and location of the nearest BioAdvance Network clinic can be obtained by calling Schering-Plough Canada Inc. Medical Information at: 1-866-736-4223.

Reconstitution:

Table 7: REMICADE

Reconstitution

Vial Size	Volume of Diluent to be Added to Vial	Approximate Available Volume	Nominal Concentration per mL
100 mg as lyophilized powder	10 mL Sterile water for injection, USP The total dose of the reconstituted product must be further diluted to 250 mL with 0.9% Sodium Chloride Injection, USP	250 mL	Between 0.4 mg/mL and 4 mg/mL

Since no preservative is present, it is recommended that the REMICADE infusion be started within 3 hours of reconstitution and dilution.

Preparation and Administration Instructions: Use aseptic technique.

REMICADE vials do not contain antibacterial preservatives. Therefore, after reconstitution, the vials should be used immediately, not re-entered or stored. The diluent to be used for reconstitution is 10 mL of Sterile Water for Injection, USP. The total dose of the reconstituted product must be further diluted to 250 mL with 0.9% Sodium Chloride Injection, USP. The infusion concentration should range between 0.4 mg/mL and 4 mg/mL. Since no preservative is present, it is recommended that the REMICADE infusion be started within 3 hours of reconstitution and dilution.

1. Calculate the dose and the number of REMICADE vials needed. Each REMICADE vial contains 100 mg of infliximab. Calculate the total volume of reconstituted REMICADE solution required.
2. Reconstitute each REMICADE vial with 10 mL of Sterile Water for Injection, USP, using a syringe equipped with a 21-gauge or smaller needle. Remove the flip-top from the vial and wipe the top with an alcohol swab. Insert the syringe needle into the vial through the centre of the rubber stopper and direct the stream of Sterile Water for Injection, USP, to the glass wall of the vial. Gently swirl the solution by rotating the vial to dissolve the lyophilized powder. Avoid prolonged or vigorous agitation. **Do not shake.** Foaming of the solution on reconstitution is not unusual. Allow the reconstituted solution to stand for 5 minutes. The solution should be colourless to light yellow and opalescent, and the solution may develop a few translucent particles as infliximab is a protein. Do not use if opaque particles, discolouration, or other foreign particles are present.

3. Dilute the total volume of the reconstituted REMICADE solution dose to 250 mL with 0.9% Sodium Chloride Injection, USP, by withdrawing a volume of 0.9% Sodium Chloride Injection, USP, equal to the volume of reconstituted REMICADE from the 0.9% Sodium Chloride Injection, USP, 250 mL bottle or bag. Slowly add the total volume of reconstituted REMICADE solution to the 250 mL infusion bottle or bag. Gently mix.
4. For patients with Crohn's disease, ulcerative colitis, ankylosing spondylitis, psoriatic arthritis, and plaque psoriasis, the infusion solution must be administered over a period of not less than 2 hours.

   For patients with rheumatoid arthritis, the recommended infusion duration is over a period of not less than 2 hours in patients not previously treated with REMICADE. At the discretion of the treating physician, some patients with rheumatoid arthritis who have tolerated 3 initial 2-hour infusions of REMICADE may be considered for receiving subsequent infusions at the same dose over a period of not less than 1 hour (see Adverse Reactions, Infusion-Related Reactions). The safety of shortened infusions at doses >6 mg/kg has not been studied.

   Use only an infusion set with an in-line, sterile, non-pyrogenic, low-protein-binding filter (pore size of 1.2 µm or less). Any unused portion of the infusion solution should not be stored for reuse
5. Parenteral drug products should be inspected visually for particulate matter and discolouration prior to administration, whenever solution and container permit. If visibly opaque particles, discolouration or other foreign particulates are observed, the solution should not be used.
6. No physical biochemical compatibility studies have been conducted to evaluate the co-administration of REMICADE with other agents. REMICADE should not be infused concomitantly in the same intravenous line with other agents.

OVERDOSAGE:
Single doses up to 20 mg/kg have been administered without any direct toxic effect. In case of overdosage, it is recommended that the patient be monitored for any signs or symptoms of adverse reactions or effects and appropriate symptomatic treatment instituted immediately.

For management of a suspected drug overdose, CPhA recommends that you contact your **regional Poison Control Centre**. See the *CPS* Directory section for a list of Poison Control Centres.

ACTION AND CLINICAL PHARMACOLOGY: Mechanism of Action: Infliximab is a chimeric IgG1κ monoclonal antibody with an approximate molecular weight of 149 100 daltons. It is composed of human constant and murine variable regions. Infliximab binds specifically to human tumour necrosis factor alpha (TNFα) with an association constant of 10^{10} M^{-1}. Infliximab is produced by a recombinant cell line cultured by continuous perfusion and is purified by a series of steps that includes measures to inactivate and remove viruses.

Infliximab neutralises the biological activity of TNFα by binding with high affinity to the soluble and transmembrane forms of TNFα and inhibits binding of TNFα with its receptors. Infliximab does not neutralise TNFβ (lymphotoxin α), a related cytokine that utilises the same receptors as TNFα. Biological activities attributed to TNFα include: induction of pro-inflammatory cytokines such as interleukins (IL) 1 and 6, enhancement of leukocyte migration by increasing endothelial layer permeability and expression of adhesion molecules by endothelial cells and leukocytes, activation of neutrophil and eosinophil functional activity, and induction of acute phase reactants and other liver proteins. Cells expressing transmembrane TNFα bound by infliximab can be lysed in vitro by complement or effector cells. Infliximab inhibits the functional activity of TNFα in a wide variety of in vitro bioassays utilising human fibroblasts, endothelial cells, neutrophils, B and T lymphocytes and epithelial cells. Anti-TNFα antibodies reduce disease activity in a cotton-top tamarin colitis model, and decrease synovitis and joint erosions in a murine model of collagen-induced arthritis. Infliximab prevents disease in transgenic mice that develop polyarthritis as a result of constitutive expression of human TNFα, and, when administered after disease onset, facilitates eroded joints to heal.

Pharmacodynamics: Preclinical: Infliximab binds to the soluble and transmembrane forms of TNFα with high affinity and blocks the interaction of TNFα with its receptors, thereby neutralising the biological activity of TNFα. Cells expressing transmembrane TNFα can be lysed in vitro by complement or effector cell-mediated mechanisms after infliximab binds. Infliximab inhibits the functional activity of TNFα in a wide variety of in vitro bioassays utilising human fibroblasts, endothelial cells, neutrophils, B and T lymphocytes, and epithelial cells.

Infliximab specifically neutralises TNFα-induced cell cytotoxicity but not lymphotoxin α. Lymphotoxin α is a cytokine that shares 30% homology with TNFα and utilises the same receptors as TNFα. Species cross-reactivity of infliximab is limited to human and chimpanzee TNFα. In vivo, infliximab rapidly forms stable complexes with human TNFα, a process that parallels the loss of TNFα bioactivity.

In a transgenic mouse (Tg197) that constitutively expresses human TNFα, infliximab administered twice weekly at 5 mg/kg or once weekly at 10 mg/kg prevents the development of polyarthritis by Week 10, demonstrating that infliximab neutralises TNFα in vivo.

Clinical: Elevated concentrations of TNFα have been found in the joints of rheumatoid arthritis patients, in the joints of psoriatic arthritis patients, in the skin lesions of plaque psoriasis patients, and in the stools of Crohn's disease and ulcerative colitis patients. This correlates with elevated disease activity. In rheumatoid arthritis, treatment with REMICADE reduced infiltration of inflammatory cells into inflamed areas of the joint as well as expression of molecules mediating cellular adhesion [E-selectin, intercellular adhesion molecule-1 (ICAM-1) and vascular cell adhesion molecule-1 (VCAM-1)], chemoattraction [IL-8 and monocyte chemotactic protein (MCP-1)] and tissue degradation [matrix metalloproteinase (MMP) 1 and 3]. In Crohn's disease, treatment reduces infiltration of inflammatory cells and TNFα production in inflamed areas of the intestine, and reduces the proportion of mononuclear cells in the lamina propria able to express TNFα and interferon γ ex vivo. After treatment with REMICADE, patients with rheumatoid arthritis or Crohn's disease exhibited decreased levels of serum IL-6 and C-reactive protein compared to baseline. Peripheral blood lymphocytes from REMICADE-treated patients showed no decrease in proliferative responses to in vitro mitogenic stimulation when compared to cells from untreated patients. In psoriatic arthritis, treatment with REMICADE resulted in a reduction in the number of T cells and blood vessels in the synovium and psoriatic skin lesions as well as a reduction of macrophages in the synovium. Infliximab treatment alters the histopathological features of plaque psoriasis as demonstrated in lesional skin biopsies collected at baseline, day 3 and Week 10 following initiation of treatment. Infliximab treatment reduced epidermal thickness and infiltration of inflammatory cells, downregulated the percentage of activated and cutaneous lymphocyte antigen (CLA)-positive inflammatory cells, including CD3 , CD4-, and CD8-positive lymphocytes, and upregulated the percentage of CD1a-positive epidermal Langerhans cells. In ulcerative colitis, treatment with REMICADE showed changes consistent with histological healing and decreased expression of pharmacodynamic markers of tissue injury and inflammation in colonic biopsies. Treatment with REMICADE also decreased serum levels of the proinflammatory molecules with statistically significant and consistent decreases observed for IL-2R, and ICAM-1. In patients with ankylosing spondylitis, infliximab was more effective at decreasing levels of serum markers of inflammation (IL-6 and VEGF) at both weeks 2 and 24 than placebo. In addition, serum levels of markers of bone formation (bone alkaline phosphatase and osteocalcin) were increased at both weeks 2 and 24 in patients with ankylosing spondylitis treated with infliximab compared with patients receiving placebo.

Pharmacokinetics: Single intravenous infusions of 1 to 20 mg/kg showed a linear relationship between the dose administered and the maximum serum concentration. The volume of distribution at steady state was independent of dose and indicated that infliximab was distributed primarily within the vascular compartment. Median pharmacokinetic results for the doses of 3 mg/kg to 10 mg/kg in rheumatoid arthritis, 5 mg/kg in Crohn's disease and 3 mg/kg to 5 mg/kg in plaque psoriasis indicate that the terminal half life of infliximab is approximately 7.7 to 10 days. The terminal half-life in ulcerative colitis trials was 12.3 to 14.7 days. See Table 8.

Table 8: REMICADE
Pharmacokinetics

	Rheumatoid Arthritis		Crohn's Disease	
Study	**T09 (n=14)**	**T09 (n=29)**	**T11 (n=5)**	**T11 (n=5)**
Dose	3 mg/kg	10 mg/kg	5 mg/kg	10 mg/kg
C_{max} (µg/mL)	77.3	277	74.9	181.0
AUC (µg· day/mL)	461	2282	788	2038
CL (mL/day/kg)	6.4	4.4	6.3	4.9
V_{ss} (mL/kg)	67.5	57.2	80	65
$t_{½}$ (day)	8	9.1	7.8	10

(cont'd)

Table 8: REMICADE *(cont'd)*

Absorption: REMICADE is administered intravascularly and thus has no absorption profile.

Distribution: REMICADE is primarily distributed into the blood, its apparent median steady state volume of distribution of 57.2 to 80 mL/kg estimated to 4.0 to 5.60 litres in a 70 kg individual corresponds to the total blood volume.

Metabolism: It is believed that REMICADE is metabolized in a similar manner to other proteins in the body. It is probably hydrolysed into its component amino acids and recycled or catabolized.

Excretion: REMICADE as a whole molecule was not detected in the urine after its intravenous infusion.

Following an initial dose of REMICADE, repeated infusions at 2 and 6 weeks resulted in predictable concentration time profiles following each treatment. No systemic accumulation of infliximab occurred upon continued repeated treatment with 3 mg/kg or 10 mg/kg at 4- or 8- week intervals in rheumatoid arthritis patients or patients with moderate or severe Crohn's disease retreated with 4 infusions of 10 mg/kg REMICADE at 8 week intervals. No systemic accumulation of infliximab occurred upon continued repeated treatment with 3 mg/kg or 5 mg/kg at 8-week intervals in patients with psoriatic arthritis or plaque psoriasis. The proportion of patients with rheumatoid arthritis who had undetectable infliximab concentrations at 8 weeks following an infusion was approximately 25% for those receiving 3 mg/kg every 8 weeks, 15% for patients administered 3 mg/kg every 4 weeks, and 0% for patients receiving 10 mg/kg every 4 or 8 weeks. At steady state, the proportion of patients with plaque psoriasis who had undetectable infliximab concentrations at 8 weeks following an infusion ranged from 71.4% to 73.1% for patients receiving 3 mg/kg every 8 weeks (EXPRESS II), and from 25.9% to 46.4% for those administered 5 mg/kg every 8 weeks (EXPRESS and EXPRESS II). The proportion of patients with psoriatic arthritis who had undetectable infliximab concentrations was 15.8% at Week 38 when administered 5 mg/kg every 8 weeks (IMPACT 2). In IMPACT 2, approximately half of the patients received concomitant MTX.

Special Populations: No major differences in clearance or volume of distribution were observed in patient subgroups defined by age. It is not known if gender differences, genetic polymorphism, renal insufficiency or hepatic insufficiency have effects on clearance or volume of distribution of REMICADE.

The pharmacokinetics in pediatric patients with Crohn's disease (ages 6 to 17 years old) were similar to those of adult patients with Crohn's disease; the median terminal half-life for 5 mg/kg dose is 10.9 days (see Indications and Clinical Use, Pediatrics, and Warnings and Precautions, Special Populations, Pediatrics (9-17 years of age).

STORAGE AND STABILITY: Store the lyophilized product under refrigeration at 2 to 8 °C. Do not use beyond the expiration date. This product contains no preservative. Since no preservative is present, it is recommended that the administration of the infusion solution should begin within 3 hours of reconstitution and dilution.

SPECIAL HANDLING INSTRUCTIONS: Chemical and physical in-use stability of the reconstituted solution has been demonstrated for 24 hours at room temperature (25 °C). Diluted REMICADE infusion solution is stable for 24 hours when stored between 2 and 30 °C. If the infusion solution is not used immediately (i.e., within 3 hours of preparation), the in-use storage times and conditions prior to its use are the responsibility of the user and would not normally be longer than 24 hours at 2 to 8 °C, unless reconstitution and dilution have taken place in controlled and validated aseptic conditions.

INFORMATION FOR THE PATIENT: Published in e-CPS, available by subscription at www.e-cps.ca.

DOSAGE FORMS, COMPOSITION AND PACKAGING: Each vial of sterile white lyophilized powder for i.v. infusion contains: infliximab 100 mg. Nonmedicinal ingredients: dibasic sodium phosphate dihydrate, monobasic sodium phosphate monohydrate, polysorbate 80 and sucrose. Preservative-free. Single use vials, boxes of 1.

Reminyl® ER Pr
galantamine HBr
Cholinesterase Inhibitor

Janssen-Ortho

Date of Preparation: July 19, 2001
Date of Revision: April 26, 2010

SUMMARY PRODUCT INFORMATION:

Route of Administration	Dosage Form/ Strength	Clinically Relevant Nonmedicinal Ingredients
Oral	Extended release capsule 8 mg, 16 mg, 24 mg	None For a complete listing see Dosage Forms, Composition and Packaging.

INDICATIONS AND CLINICAL USE: REMINYL ER is indicated for the symptomatic treatment of patients with mild to moderate dementia of the Alzheimer's type. REMINYL ER has not been studied in controlled clinical trials for longer than 6 months.

REMINYL ER should only be prescribed by (or following consultation with) clinicians who are experienced in the diagnosis and management of Alzheimer's disease.

Geriatrics (≥85 years of age): There is limited safety information for REMINYL ER in this patient population (see Warnings and Precautions, Special Populations).

Pediatrics (<18 years of age): No data are available in children. Therefore, the use of REMINYL ER is not recommended in children under 18 years of age.

CONTRAINDICATIONS: REMINYL ER is contraindicated in patients with known hypersensitivity to galantamine hydrobromide, other tertiary alkaloid derivatives or to any excipients used in the formulation. For a complete listing, see Dosage Forms, Composition and Packaging.

WARNINGS AND PRECAUTIONS: Cardiovascular: Because of their pharmacological action, cholinesterase inhibitors have vagotonic effects on the sinoatrial and atrioventricular nodes, leading to bradycardia and heart block. These actions may be particularly important to patients with "sick sinus syndrome" or other supraventricular cardiac conduction disorders, or to patients taking other drugs concomitantly which significantly slow heart rate. In clinical trials, patients with serious cardiovascular disease were excluded. Caution should be exercised in treating patients with active coronary artery disease or congestive heart failure. It is recommended that REMINYL ER not be used in patients with cardiac conduction abnormalities (except for right bundle branch block) including "sick sinus syndrome" and those with unexplained syncopal episodes.

In randomized controlled trials, bradycardia was reported at 2-3% for galantamine doses up to 24 mg/day compared with <1% for placebo, but was rarely severe and rarely led to treatment discontinuation. No increased incidence of heart block was observed at the recommended doses. Patients treated with galantamine up to 24 mg/day at the recommended dosing schedule showed a dose-related increase in risk of syncope (placebo, 0.7% [2/286]; 4 mg b.i.d., 0.4% [3/692]; 8 mg b.i.d., 1.3% [7/552]; 12 mg b.i.d., 2.2% [6/273]).

A 6-week cardiovascular safety clinical trial (GAL-USA-16; n=139) was performed to investigate the effect of galantamine at doses up to 32 mg/day. This dosing regimen was: 8 mg/day in Week 1, 16 mg/day in Week 2, 24 mg/day in Weeks 3 and 4, and 32 mg/day in Weeks 5 and 6. Heart block/pauses greater than two seconds were more common in galantamine-treated patients than in placebo-treated patients. It should be noted that a forced 1-week dose escalation was used in this study, which is not recommended. Whether these cardiac effects are attenuated by slower titration rates is not known. Particular caution is warranted during titration where the majority of pauses occurred in the above study.

Metabolism: Cholinesterase inhibitors as well as Alzheimer's disease can be associated with significant weight loss. In controlled clinical trials, the use of REMINYL was associated with weight loss. Weight decrease occurred early during treatment and was related to dose. Weight loss of ≥7% occurred more frequently in patients treated with REMINYL and in female patients than in patients receiving placebo. Where weight loss may be of clinical concern, body weight should be monitored.

Gastrointestinal: Through their primary action, cholinesterase inhibitors may be expected to increase gastric acid secretion due to increased cholinergic activity. Therefore, patients should be monitored closely for symptoms of active or occult gastrointestinal bleeding, especially those with an increased risk for developing ulcers, e.g. those with a history of ulcer disease or patients using concurrent nonsteroidal anti-inflammatory drugs (NSAIDs). In controlled clinical studies with galantamine, patients with symptomatic peptic ulceration were excluded. Clinical studies of galantamine have shown no increase, relative to placebo, in the incidence of either peptic ulcer disease or gastrointestinal bleeding (see Adverse Reactions).

Galantamine, as a predictable consequence of its pharmacological properties, has been shown to produce nausea, vomiting and diarrhea, anorexia and weight loss. These effects appeared more frequently at higher doses (see Adverse Reactions), with nausea and vomiting being more prevalent in women and patients with lower body weight and correspondingly higher plasma drug concentrations. Females are more sensitive to the cholinergic adverse effects associated with cholinesterase inhibitors and in general are more likely to experience nausea and vomiting than are males. In most cases, these effects were of mild to moderate intensity and transient and have resolved during continued treatment or upon treatment discontinuation.

Genitourinary: Although not observed in clinical trials of galantamine, cholinomimetics may cause bladder outflow obstruction.

Neurologic: Seizures: In placebo-controlled trials with galantamine, cases of seizure were reported; there was no increase in incidence compared with placebo. Although cholinomimetics are believed to have some potential to cause seizures, seizure activity may also be a manifestation of Alzheimer's disease. The risk/benefit of REMINYL ER treatment for patients with a history of seizure disorder must therefore be carefully evaluated.

REMINYL ER has not been studied in patients with moderately severe or severe Alzheimer's disease, non-Alzheimer dementias or individuals with Parkinsonian features. The efficacy and safety of REMINYL ER in these patient populations is unknown.

Peri-Operative Considerations: Anesthesia: Galantamine, as a cholinesterase inhibitor, is likely to exaggerate succinylcholine-type muscle relaxation during anesthesia.

Respiratory: Like other cholinomimetic drugs, REMINYL ER should be prescribed with care for patients with a history of asthma or obstructive pulmonary disease.

Special Populations: Hepatic Impairment: There is limited information on the pharmacokinetics of galantamine in hepatically impaired patients (see Action and Clinical Pharmacology). It is therefore recommended that dose escalation with REMINYL ER in Alzheimer's disease patients with hepatic impairment be undertaken with caution and under conditions of close monitoring for adverse effects (see Dosage and Administration, Special Populations). Since no data are available on the use of REMINYL ER in patients with severe hepatic impairment (Child-Pugh score of 10-15), REMINYL ER is not recommended for this population.

Renal Impairment: There is limited information on the pharmacokinetics of galantamine in renally impaired patients (see Action and Clinical Pharmacology). It is therefore recommended that dose escalation with REMINYL ER in Alzheimer's disease patients with renal impairment (creatinine clearance of 9 to 60 mL/min) be undertaken with caution and under conditions of close monitoring for adverse effects (see Dosage and Administration, Special Populations). Since no data are available on the use of REMINYL ER in patients with a creatinine clearance of less than 9 mL/min, REMINYL ER is not recommended for this population.

Geriatrics (≥85 years of age): In controlled clinical studies, the number of patients aged 85 years or over who received REMINYL at therapeutic doses of 16 or 24 mg/day was 123. Of these patients, 70 received the maximum recommended dose of 24 mg/day. There is limited safety information for REMINYL ER in this patient population.

Since cholinomimetics as well as Alzheimer's disease can be associated with significant weight loss, caution is advised regarding the use of REMINYL ER in elderly patients with low body weight, especially in those ≥85 years old.

Use in Elderly Patients with Serious Comorbid Disease: There is limited information on the safety of galantamine treatment in patients with mild to moderate Alzheimer's disease and serious/significant comorbidity. The use of REMINYL ER in Alzheimer's disease patients with chronic illnesses common among the geriatric population, should be considered only after careful risk/benefit assessment and include close monitoring for adverse events. Dose escalation in this patient population should proceed with caution.

Patients with Mild Cognitive Impairment (MCI): Mortality in Investigational Trials in MCI: Two randomized, double-blind, placebo-controlled efficacy and safety studies of 2 years' duration were completed in non-demented subjects with MCI. Individuals with MCI demonstrate isolated memory impairment greater than expected for their age and education, but do not meet current diagnostic criteria for Alzheimer's Disease. In these trials, REMINYL was not shown to be effective in patients with MCI. In the double-blind portion of these two trials, a total of 13 deaths in subjects on REMINYL (n=1026) were recorded and 1 death in subjects on placebo (n=1022); the reason for this difference is currently unknown. This difference in mortality has not been observed in REMINYL studies in Alzheimer's Disease. Approximately half of the REMINYL deaths appeared to have resulted from various vascular causes (myocardial infarction, stroke, and sudden death); other deaths appeared to have resulted from infection, suicide and cancer. There is no evidence of an increased risk of mortality when REMINYL ER is used in patients with mild to moderate Alzheimer's Disease.

Pregnant Women: In a teratology study in which rats were dosed from Day 14 (females) or Day 60 (males) prior to mating through the period of organogenesis, a slightly increased incidence of skeletal variations was observed at doses of 8 mg/kg/day (3 times the MRHD on a mg/m[2] basis) and 16 mg/kg/day. In a study in which pregnant rats were dosed from the beginning of organogenesis through day 21 post-partum, pup weights were decreased at 8 and 16 mg/kg/day, but no adverse effects on other postnatal developmental parameters were seen. The doses causing the above effects in rats produced slight maternal toxicity. No major malformations were caused in rats given up to 16 mg/kg/day. No drug related teratogenic effects were observed in rabbits given up to 40 mg/kg/day (32 times the MRHD on a mg/m[2] basis) during the period of organogenesis.

The safety of REMINYL ER in pregnant women has not been established. REMINYL ER should not be used in women of childbearing potential unless, in the opinion of the physician, the potential benefit to the patient justifies the potential risk to the fetus.

Nursing Women: It is not known whether galantamine is excreted in human breast milk and therefore REMINYL ER should not be used in nursing mothers.

Pediatrics: The safety and effectiveness of REMINYL ER in any illness occurring in pediatric patients have not been established.

ADVERSE REACTIONS: Clinical Trial Adverse Drug Reactions: Because clinical trials are conducted under very specific conditions, the adverse drug reaction rates observed in the clinical trials may not reflect the rates observed in practice and should not be compared to the rates in the clinical trials of another drug. Adverse drug reaction information from clinical trials is useful for identifying drug-related adverse events and for approximating rates.

A total of 2287 patients with mild to moderate Alzheimer's disease were treated with REMINYL in Phase III controlled clinical studies using either a 1-week or 4-week dose-escalation period, and 761 patients received REMINYL 24 mg/day, the maximum recommended maintenance dose. The number of patients who completed the studies was 1686 (72%). The mean duration of treatment for all REMINYL groups was 130 days (range 1-214 days).

Adverse Events Leading to Discontinuation: Overall, 19% (441/2287) of patients treated with REMINYL discontinued from Phase III controlled clinical trials due to adverse events compared to 8% (98/1159) in the placebo group. For patients treated with REMINYL, the rate of discontinuation due to adverse events was 14% for males and 22% for females.

In the 4-week dose-escalation fixed-dose study (GAL-USA-10), 8% (55/692) of patients treated with REMINYL withdrew due to adverse events compared to 7% (20/286) in the placebo group. During the dose-escalation phase of this study the incidence of discontinuations due to adverse events was 4% for placebo, 5% for REMINYL 16 mg/day and 6% for REMINYL 24 mg/day. During the maintenance phase, 4% of patients who received placebo, 3% of patients who received REMINYL 16 mg/day and 4% of patients who received REMINYL 24 mg/day withdrew from this study due to adverse events.

Table 1 shows the most frequent adverse events leading to discontinuation for study GAL-USA-10, in which the recommended 4-week dose-escalation schedule was used.

Most Frequent Adverse Clinical Events Seen in Association with the Use of REMINYL: The most frequent adverse events, defined as those occurring at a frequency of at least 5% and at least twice the rate of placebo in study GAL-USA-10, in which the recommended 4-week dose-escalation schedule was used are shown in Table 2.

These events were primarily gastrointestinal and tended to occur at a lower rate with 16 mg/day, the initial recommended maintenance dose. Administration of REMINYL with food, the use of anti-emetic medication and ensuring adequate fluid intake may reduce the impact of these events.

The majority of these adverse events occurred during the dose-escalation period. Nausea and vomiting, the most frequent adverse events, occurred more frequently at higher doses, lasted 5-7 days in most cases, and the majority of patients had one episode. The incidence of weight loss in this study was, during dose escalation (Weeks 1-12): placebo, 1%; 16 mg/day, 3%; 24 mg/day, 2%; and during the maintenance phase (Weeks 13-21): placebo, <1%; 16 mg/day, 3%; 24 mg/day, 3%.

Dose-escalation should be cautious and maintenance dosing should remain flexible and be adjusted according to individual needs.

Table 1: REMINYL

Most Frequent Adverse Events Leading to Discontinuation in a Placebo-controlled, Double-blind Trial With a 4-week Dose-escalation Schedule (GAL-USA-10)

	Recommended 4-week Dose Escalation		
Adverse Events	**Placebo n=286 %**	**16 mg/day n=279 %**	**24 mg/day n=273 %**
Nausea	<1	2	4
Vomiting	0	1	3
Anorexia	<1	1	<1
Dizziness	<1	2	1
Syncope	0	0	1

Table 2: REMINYL

Most Frequent Adverse Events in a Randomized Placebo-controlled Clinical Trial with a 4-week Dose Increment During Dose-escalation and Maintenance Phases (GAL-USA-10)

	Week 1–12[a]			Week 13–21		
Adverse Events	**Placebo n=286 %**	**16 mg/day n=279 %**	**24 mg/day n=273 %**	**Placebo n=259 %**	**16 mg/day n=243 %**	**24 mg/day n=241 %**
Nausea	5	11	13	<1	4	6
Vomiting	<1	5	6	<1	2	6
Diarrhea	5	9	4	2	5	2
Anorexia	2	5	5	1	2	5

[a] Dose escalation occurred with 4 weeks per dose increment.

Adverse Events Reported in Controlled Trials: The reported adverse events in REMINYL trials reflect experience gained under closely monitored conditions in a highly selected patient population. In actual practice or in other clinical trials, these frequency estimates may not apply, as the conditions of use, reporting behaviour and the types of patients treated may differ.

Table 3 lists the most common adverse events (adverse events occurring with an incidence of 2% with REMINYL treatment and in which the incidence was greater than with placebo treatment) for four placebo-controlled trials for patients treated with 16 or 24 mg/day of REMINYL. The combined values presented in Table 3 were derived from trials using a 1-week or the recommended 4-week dose-escalation period.

Table 3: REMINYL

Adverse Events Reported in at Least 2% of Patients with Alzheimer's Disease Administered REMINYL and at a Frequency Greater Than with Placebo (Combined 1- and 4-week Dose-escalation Data)

Body System/Adverse Events	**Placebo (n=801) %**	**REMINYL[a] (n=1040) %**
Body as a Whole—General Disorders		
Fatigue	3	5
Syncope	1	2
Central and Peripheral Nervous System Disorders		
Dizziness	6	9
Headache	5	8
Tremor	2	3
Gastrointestinal System Disorders		
Nausea	9	24
Vomiting	4	13
Diarrhea	7	9
Abdominal Pain	4	5
Dyspepsia	2	5
Heart Rate and Rhythm Disorders		
Bradycardia	1	2
Metabolic and Nutritional Disorders		
Weight Decrease	2	7
Psychiatric Disorders		
Anorexia	3	9
Depression	5	7
Insomnia	4	5
Somnolence	3	4

(cont'd)

Table 3: REMINYL *(cont'd)*

Adverse Events Reported in at Least 2% of Patients with Alzheimer's Disease Administered REMINYL and at a Frequency Greater Than with Placebo (Combined 1- and 4-week Dose-escalation Data)

Body System/Adverse Events	Placebo (n=801) %	REMINYL[a] (n=1040) %
Red Blood Cell Disorders		
Anemia	2	3
Respiratory System Disorders		
Rhinitis	3	4
Urinary System Disorders		
Urinary Tract Infection	7	8
Hematuria	2	3

[a] Adverse events in patients treated with 16 or 24 mg/day of REMINYL in three placebo-controlled trials with a 1-week dose-escalation period and a 26-week fixed-dose REMINYL treatment, and one placebo-controlled trial with the recommended 4-week dose-escalation period and a 21-week fixed-dose REMINYL treatment are included.

No clinically relevant abnormalities in laboratory values were observed. In a cardiovascular safety clinical trial (GAL-USA-16), pauses greater than two seconds were more common in galantamine-treated patients than in placebo-treated patients during the dose-escalation period (see Warnings and Precautions).

Most Frequent Adverse Clinical Events Seen in Association with the Use of REMINYL ER: Adverse reactions in clinical trials of once-daily treatment with REMINYL ER extended release capsules were similar to those seen with REMINYL immediate release tablets (see Table 4).

Table 4: REMINYL ER

Adverse Events Reported in at Least 2% of Patients with Alzheimer's Disease Administered REMINYL or REMINYL ER and at a Frequency Greater Than Placebo

System Organ Class Preferred Term	Placebo (n=320) %	REMINYL (n=326) %	REMINYL ER (n=319) %
Body as a Whole—General Disorders			
Injury	6	4	8
Edema Peripheral	3	2	4
Fatigue	1	4	4
Syncope	1	1	2
Fever	1	2	1
Leg Pain	1	2	<1
Central and Peripheral Nervous System Disorders			
Dizziness	4	7	10
Headache	6	6	8
Tremor	0	1	2
Gastrointestinal System Disorders			
Nausea	5	14	17
Vomiting	2	9	7
Abdominal Pain	2	3	2
Dyspepsia	2	3	2
Heart Rate and Rhythm Disorders			
Bradycardia	2	2	3
Metabolic and Nutritional Disorders			
Weight Decrease	1	5	4
Hyperglycemia	1	2	2
Musculoskeletal System Disorders			
Arthralgia	2	2	3
Skeletal Pain	1	3	2
Arthritis	1	1	2
Myalgia	1	1	2
Psychiatric Disorders			
Anorexia	3	7	6
Depression	3	5	6
Anxiety	3	1	4

(cont'd)

Table 4: REMINYL ER *(cont'd)*

Adverse Events Reported in at Least 2% of Patients with Alzheimer's Disease Administered REMINYL or REMINYL ER and at a Frequency Greater Than Placebo

System Organ Class Preferred Term	Placebo (n=320) %	REMINYL (n=326) %	REMINYL ER (n=319) %
Somnolence	2	2	3
Depression Aggravated	1	2	2
Aggressive Reaction	1	2	2
Nervousness	1	2	1
Respiratory System Disorders			
Rhinitis	3	4	4
Pneumonia	1	2	2
Secondary Terms			
Abrasion nos[a]	1	1	2
Skin and Appendages Disorders			
Rash	1	<1	3
Urinary System Disorders			
Hematuria	1	1	2
Micturition Frequency	1	2	1
Vision Disorders			
Cataract	1	1	2

[a] Not otherwise specified.

Adverse Events Observed During the GAL-INT-6 Study: The frequencies of certain cardiovascular-related adverse events, including syncope, hypertension, arrhythmia and bundle branch block were increased in patients treated with galantamine compared to placebo. The increase was due primarily to events that occurred in the subgroup of Alzheimer's patients with concomitant cerebrovascular disease. Patients with Alzheimer's disease and concomitant cerebrovascular disease who were treated with galantamine experienced syncope (3%), hypertension (4%), arrhythmia (3%) and bundle branch block (2%), but these events were not reported in the placebo group.

In the vascular dementia subgroup syncope was reported for 2% of patients treated with galantamine and 2% of patients treated with placebo; hypertension was reported for 5% of patients treated with galantamine and 2% of patients treated with placebo. Arrhythmia and bundle branch block adverse events were not reported in the vascular dementia subgroup.

In the entire study population the most common treatment-emergent adverse events (nausea, dizziness, vomiting, abdominal pain, diarrhea, fatigue and upper respiratory tract infection) were consistent with what has been observed in previous REMINYL studies involving Alzheimer's disease patients (see Action and Clinical Pharmacology, Special Populations and Conditions).

Other Adverse Events Observed During Clinical Trials: REMINYL has been administered to 3055 patients with Alzheimer's disease during clinical trials worldwide.

A total of 2357 patients received galantamine in placebo-controlled trials and 761 patients with Alzheimer's disease received galantamine 24 mg/day, the maximum recommended maintenance dose. About 1000 patients received galantamine for at least one year and approximately 200 patients received galantamine for two years. To establish the rate of adverse events, data from all patients for any dose of REMINYL in 8 placebo-controlled trials and 6 open-label extension trials were pooled. The methodology to gather and codify these adverse events was standardized across trials, using WHO terminology. All events occurring in approximately 0.1% of patients are included, except for those already listed elsewhere in labelling, WHO terms too general to be informative, or relatively minor events. Events are classified by body system and listed using the following definitions: frequent adverse events—those occurring in at least 1/100 patients; infrequent adverse events—those occurring in 1/100 to 1/1000 patients; rare—those occurring in 1/1000 to 1/10 000 patients; very rare—those occurring in fewer than 1/10 000 patients. These adverse events are not necessarily related to REMINYL treatment and in most cases were observed at a similar frequency in placebo-treated patients in the controlled studies.

Body as a Whole—General Disorders: Frequent: chest pain, asthenia, fever, malaise.

Cardiovascular System Disorders: Frequent: hypertension; Infrequent: postural hypotension, hypotension, dependent edema, cardiac failure, myocardial ischemia or infarction.

Central and Peripheral Nervous System Disorders: Infrequent: vertigo, hypertonia, convulsions, involuntary muscle contractions, paresthesia, ataxia, hypokinesia, hyperkinesia, apraxia, aphasia, leg cramps, tinnitus, transient ischemic attack or cerebrovascular accident.

Gastrointestinal System Disorders: Frequent: flatulence; Infrequent: gastritis, melena, dysphagia, rectal hemorrhage, dry mouth, saliva increased, diverticulitis, gastroenteritis, hiccup; Rare: esophageal perforation.

Heart Rate and Rhythm Disorders: Infrequent: AV block, palpitation, atrial arrhythmias including atrial fibrillation and supraventricular tachycardia, QTc prolonged, bundle branch block, T-wave inversion, ventricular tachycardia; Rare: severe bradycardia.

Metabolic and Nutritional Disorders: Infrequent: hyperglycemia, alkaline phosphatase increased, NPN increased.

Platelet, Bleeding and Clotting Disorders: Infrequent: purpura, epistaxis, thrombocytopenia.

Psychiatric Disorders: Infrequent: apathy, paroniria, paranoid reaction, libido increased, delirium; Rare: suicidal ideation, suicide attempt.

Urinary System Disorders: Frequent: incontinence; Infrequent: hematuria, micturition frequency, cystitis, urinary retention, nocturia, renal calculi.

Hepatobiliary: There have been reports of hepatic-related adverse reactions including elevated liver enzymes and hepatitis, from both open-label studies of galantamine (duration up to 4 years) and post-marketing experience (see Post-Market Adverse Drug Reactions).

Post-Market Adverse Drug Reactions: Other adverse events from post-approval controlled and uncontrolled clinical trials and post-marketing experience observed in patients treated with REMINYL include:

Body as a Whole—General Disorders: dehydration (including rare, severe cases leading to renal insufficiency and renal failure).

Central and Peripheral Nervous System Disorders: behavioural disturbances including agitation, aggression and hallucinations.

Gastrointestinal: upper and lower GI bleeding.

Hepatobiliary: elevated liver enzymes, hepatitis.

Metabolic and Nutritional Disorders: hypokalemia.

Some of these adverse events may be attributable to cholinomimetic properties of REMINYL or in some cases may represent manifestations or exacerbations of the underlying disease processes common in the elderly population.

DRUG INTERACTIONS: Overview: Multiple metabolic pathways and renal excretion are involved in the elimination of galantamine so no single pathway appears predominant. Based on in vitro studies, CYP2D6 and CYP3A4 were the major enzymes involved in the metabolism of galantamine. CYP2D6 was involved in the formation of O-desmethyl-galantamine, whereas CYP3A4 mediated the formation of galantamine-N-oxide.

Use with Anticholinergics: Because of their mechanism of action, cholinesterase inhibitors have the potential to interfere with the activity of anticholinergic medications.
Use with Cholinomimetics and Other Cholinesterase Inhibitors: A synergistic effect may be expected when cholinesterase inhibitors are given concurrently with succinylcholine, similar neuromuscular blocking agents or cholinergic agonists such as bethanechol.
Use with Other Psychoactive Drugs: Few patients in the clinical trials received neuroleptics, antidepressants or anticonvulsants, there is thus limited information concerning the interaction of REMINYL ER with these drugs.
Drug-Drug Interactions: Effect of Other Drugs on the Metabolism of Galantamine: Pharmacokinetic studies to assess the potential of galantamine for interaction with cimetidine, ranitidine, ketoconazole, erythromycin, paroxetine, warfarin and digoxin were limited to short-term, mostly single-dose studies in young healthy volunteers. Similar studies in elderly patients were not done.
In vitro: CYP3A4 and CYP2D6 are the major enzymes involved in the metabolism of galantamine. CYP3A4 mediates the formation of galantamine-N-oxide, whereas CYP2D6 is involved in the formation of O-desmethyl-galantamine. Because galantamine is also glucuronidated and excreted unchanged in urine, no single pathway appears predominant.
In vivo: Cimetidine and Ranitidine: Galantamine was administered as a single dose of 4 mg on Day 2 of a 3-day treatment with either cimetidine (800 mg daily; n=6 males and 6 females) or ranitidine (300 mg daily; n=6 males and 6 females). Cimetidine increased the bioavailability of galantamine by approximately 16%. Ranitidine had no effect on the pharmacokinetics of galantamine.
Ketoconazole: Ketoconazole, a strong inhibitor of CYP3A4 and an inhibitor of CYP2D6, at a dose of 200 mg b.i.d. for 4 days, increased the AUC of galantamine by 30% when subjects were treated with galantamine 4 mg b.i.d. for 8 days (n=8 males and 8 females).
Erythromycin: Erythromycin, a moderate inhibitor of CYP3A4 at a dose of 500 mg q.i.d. for 4 days increased the AUC of galantamine by 10% when subjects received galantamine 4 mg b.i.d. for 6 days (n=8 males and 8 females).
Paroxetine: Paroxetine, a strong inhibitor of CYP2D6, increased the AUC of 4 mg b.i.d., 8 mg b.i.d. and 12 mg b.i.d. galantamine by 40%, 45% and 48 %, respectively, in 16 healthy volunteers (8 males and 8 females) who received galantamine together with 20 mg/day paroxetine.
Memantine: In a multiple dose pharmacokinetic study in healthy volunteers (n=15, age range 21-55 years), concurrent administration of memantine at a dose of 10 mg b.i.d. did not affect the pharmacokinetic profile of galantamine (16 mg daily) at steady state.

The safety of co-administering memantine and galantamine in patients with Alzheimer's disease has not been studied in clinical trials.
Effect of Galantamine on the Metabolism of Other Drugs: In vitro: Galantamine did not inhibit the metabolic pathways catalyzed by CYP1A2, CYP2A6, CYP3A4, CYP4A, CYP2C, CYP2D6 or CYP2E1. This indicates that the inhibitory potential of galantamine towards the major forms of cytochrome P450 is very low.
In vivo: Warfarin: Galantamine at 12 mg b.i.d. had no effect on the pharmacokinetics of R- and S- warfarin (25 mg single dose) or on the prothrombin time (n=16 males). The protein binding of warfarin was unaffected by galantamine.
Digoxin: Galantamine at 12 mg b.i.d. had no effect on the steady-state pharmacokinetics of digoxin (0.375 mg once daily) when they were co-administered. In this study, however, one healthy subject was hospitalized for 2nd and 3rd degree heart block and bradycardia (n=8 males and 8 females).
Nicotinic Receptor Modulation: Single in vitro applications of galantamine dose-dependently modulate the effect on nicotinic receptors, having a positive allosteric (sensitizing) effect at concentrations below 0.28 μg/mL (1 μM) and an inhibitory effect at higher concentrations. Chronic in vitro or in vivo studies on nicotinic receptor modulation have not been conducted.

It is unknown whether galantamine has an effect on the pharmacodynamic action of other drugs that act on cholinergic nicotinic receptors (see Action and Clinical Pharmacology).
Drug-Food Interactions: Interactions with food have not been established.
Drug-Herb Interactions: Interactions with herbal products have not been established.
Drug-Laboratory Test Interactions: Interactions with laboratory tests have not been established.

DOSAGE AND ADMINISTRATION: **REMINYL ER (galantamine hydrobromide) is not indicated for use in patients with mild cognitive impairment (see Warnings and Precautions, Special Populations, Patients with Mild Cognitive Impairment (MCI), Mortality in Investigational Trials in MCI).**

REMINYL ER should only be prescribed by (or following consultation with) clinicians who are experienced in the diagnosis and management of Alzheimer's disease.

REMINYL ER extended release capsules should be administered once daily in the morning, preferably with food. Patients and caregivers should be advised to ensure adequate fluid intake during treatment.
Dosing Considerations:
- **Concomitant Treatment:** In patients treated with potent CYP2D6 or CYP3A4 inhibitors, dose reductions can be considered.
- **Special Populations:** Dosage adjustments may be required for elderly patients (>85 years old) with low body weight (especially females), and patients with hepatic and/or renal impairment.
- **Missed Dose:** The missed dose should be taken at the next scheduled dose. Doses should not be doubled. If therapy has been interrupted for several days or longer, the patient should be restarted at the lowest dose and the dose escalated to the current dose.

Recommended Dose and Dosage Adjustment: The dosage of REMINYL shown to be effective in controlled clinical trials is 16-32 mg/day given as twice daily dosing. As the dose of 32 mg/day is less well tolerated than lower doses and does not provide increased effectiveness, the recommended dose range is 16-24 mg/day. The dose of 24 mg/day did not provide a statistically significant greater clinical benefit than 16 mg/day. It is possible, however, that a daily dose of 24 mg of REMINYL ER might provide additional benefit for some patients.

The recommended starting dose is 8 mg/day. The dose should be increased to the initial maintenance dose of 16 mg/day after 4 weeks. If this initial maintenance dose is well tolerated, a further increase to 24 mg/day may be considered only after a minimum of 4 weeks at 16 mg/day.

The abrupt withdrawal of REMINYL ER in those patients who had been receiving doses in the effective range was not associated with an increased frequency of adverse events in comparison with those continuing to receive the same doses of that drug. The beneficial effects of REMINYL ER are lost, however, when the drug is discontinued.
Special Populations: Dose escalation for elderly patients (>85 years old) with low body weight (especially females) or serious comorbid diseases should be undertaken with particular caution.
Hepatic Impairment: Galantamine plasma levels may be increased in patients with moderate to severe hepatic impairment. For REMINYL ER extended release capsules, based on pharmacokinetic modelling, dosing should begin with 8 mg every other day in the morning, preferably with food, for at least 1 week. Then the dosage should be increased to 8 mg once daily for at least 4 weeks. In these patients, daily doses should not exceed a total of 16 mg/day. Since no data are available on the use of REMINYL ER in patients with severe hepatic impairment (Child-Pugh score of 10-15), REMINYL ER is not recommended for this population (see Warnings and Precautions).
Renal Impairment: For patients with renal impairment (creatinine clearance of 9 to 60 mL/min), dose escalation should proceed cautiously and the maintenance dose should generally not exceed 16 mg/day. Since no data are available on the use of REMINYL ER in patients with a creatinine clearance less than 9 mL/min, REMINYL ER are not recommended for this population (see Warnings and Precautions).

In a population of cognitively-impaired individuals, safe use of this and all other medications may require supervision.

OVERDOSAGE:
Symptoms: Overdosage with cholinesterase inhibitors can result in cholinergic crisis characterized by severe nausea, vomiting, salivation, sweating, bradycardia, hypotension, respiratory depression, collapse and convulsions. Increasing muscle weakness is a possibility and may result in death if respiratory muscles are involved.

There have been post-marketing reports of Torsade de Pointes, QT prolongation, bradycardia, ventricular tachycardia and brief loss of consciousness in association with inadvertent overdoses of galantamine. In one case where the dose was known, eight 4 mg tablets (32 mg total) were ingested on a single day. Two additional cases of accidental ingestion of 32 mg (nausea, vomiting, and dry mouth; nausea, vomiting, and substernal chest pain) and one of 40 mg (vomiting), resulted in brief hospitalizations for observation with full recovery. One patient, who was prescribed 24 mg/day and had a history of hallucinations over the previous two years, mistakenly received 24 mg twice daily for 34 days and developed hallucinations requiring hospitalization. Another patient, who was prescribed 16 mg/day, inadvertently ingested 160 mg and experienced sweating, vomiting, bradycardia, and near-syncope one hour later, which necessitated hospital treatment. His symptoms resolved within 24 hours.
Treatment: Galantamine has a plasma half-life of approximately 7-8 hours. It is recommended that, in case of asymptomatic overdose, no further dose of REMINYL ER should be administered and the patient should be monitored.

As in any case of overdose, general supportive measures should be utilized. Signs and symptoms of significant overdosing of galantamine are predicted to be similar to those of overdosing of other cholinomimetics. These effects generally involve the central nervous system, the parasympathetic nervous system, and the neuromuscular junction. In addition to muscle weakness or fasciculations, some or all of the following signs of cholinergic crisis may develop: severe nausea, vomiting, gastrointestinal cramping, salivation, lacrimation, urination, defecation, sweating, bradycardia, hypotension, respiratory depression, collapse and convulsions. Increasing muscle weakness is a possibility and may result in death if respiratory muscles are involved.

Tertiary anticholinergics such as atropine may be used as an antidote for galantamine overdosage. Intravenous atropine sulphate titrated to effect is recommended at an initial dose of 0.5 to 1 mg i.v. with subsequent doses based upon clinical response. Atypical responses in blood pressure and heart rate have been reported with other cholinomimetics when co-administered with quaternary anticholinergics. It is not known whether galantamine and/or its metabolites can be removed by dialysis (hemodialysis, peritoneal dialysis, or hemofiltration). Dose-related signs of toxicity in animals included hypoactivity, tremors, clonic convulsions, salivation, lacrimation, chromodacryorrhea, mucoid feces, and dyspnea.

For management of a suspected drug overdose, contact your regional Poison Control Centre. See the *CPS* Directory section for a list of Poison Control Centres.

ACTION AND CLINICAL PHARMACOLOGY: Mechanism of Action: Although the etiology of cognitive impairment in Alzheimer's disease is not fully understood, it has been reported that acetylcholine-producing neurons degenerate in the brains of patients with Alzheimer's disease. The degree of this cholinergic loss has been correlated with degree of cognitive impairment and density of amyloid plaques (a neuropathological hallmark of Alzheimer's disease).

Galantamine, a tertiary alkaloid, is a competitive and reversible cholinesterase inhibitor. While the precise mechanism of galantamine's action is unknown, it is postulated to exert its therapeutic effect by enhancing cholinergic function. This is accomplished by increasing the concentration of acetylcholine through reversible cholinesterase inhibition. It has also been postulated, based on in vitro data, that galantamine enhances the action of acetylcholine through binding to an allosteric site on the nicotinic receptors (see Warnings and Precautions). The clinical relevance to humans of these in vitro findings is unknown.

If these mechanisms are correct, galantamine's effect may lessen as the disease process advances and fewer cholinergic neurons remain functionally intact. There is no evidence that galantamine alters the course of the underlying dementing process.
Pharmacokinetics: The summary of related pharmacokinetic parameters in healthy subjects is presented in Table 5.

Table 5: REMINYL
Pharmacokinetic Parameters of Galantamine After Single or Multiple Dose Administration

	C_{max} (ng/mL)	T_{max} (h)	$C_{ss,av}$ (ng/mL)	C_{min} (ng/mL)	AUC[a] (ng· h/mL)	$T_{1/2}$ (h)
Single dose, 12 healthy males						
8 mg, solution p.o.	42.6±13.1	1.2±0.6	—	—	427±102	7.3±1.7
8 mg, 1 h i.v. infusion	—	—	—	—	482±112	7.4±1.7
Food effect, single dose, 24 healthy elderly						
Fasted, 8 mg p.o.	57.5±15.8	1.1±0.5	—	—	562±180	9.7±3.1
Non-fasted, 8 mg p.o.	42.5±7.5	2.6±1.4	—	—	543±176	9.7±3.3
Multiple oral dose, 27 healthy males						
12 mg b.i.d. tablet	89.4±18.3	1.0±0.6	51.9±12.2	30.7±10.3	623±147	—
12 mg b.i.d. solution	87.6±20.5	1.1±0.5	50.5±13.0	29.8±10.2	606±156	—
Dose-proportionality, multiple oral dose, 18 healthy subjects						
4 mg b.i.d. tablet	30.7±6.2	1.9±0.8	17.7±4.6	10.6±4.0	212±56	—
8 mg b.i.d. tablet	63.8±14.2	1.7±0.8	36.6±9.8	20.6±6.8	439±117	—
12 mg b.i.d. tablet	97.4±31.4	1.9±1.1	53.1±12.7	29.1±9.3	637±152	—
16 mg b.i.d. tablet	137±36	1.7±0.9	76.5±20.3	41.5±14.2	918±244	7.9±0.8

[a] AUC=AUC_∞ after single dose and AUC=AUC_τ after multiple dose.

Absorption: After oral intake of a single 8 mg galantamine solution in 12 healthy males, absorption is rapid, with a peak plasma concentration (C_{max}) of 43±13 ng/mL, which is reached after 1.2 hours (T_{max}), and a mean AUC_∞ of 427±102 ng·h/mL.

The absolute oral bioavailability of galantamine is 88.5%. Bioavailability of the tablet was the same as the bioavailability of an oral solution in 27 healthy males. Food did not affect the AUC of galantamine but C_{max} decreased by 25% and T_{max} was delayed by 1.5 hours after repeated oral dosing of 12 mg galantamine b.i.d. in 24 healthy elderly subjects.

The maximum inhibition of cholinesterase activity of about 40% was achieved about one hour after a single oral dose of 8 mg galantamine in healthy male subjects.

In a steady-state bioavailability study, galantamine hydrobromide extended release capsules, 24 mg once daily, were shown to be bioequivalent to the 12 mg twice-daily galantamine tablets with respect to AUC_{24h} and C_{min}. The C_{max} value of the 24 mg once-daily extended release capsule, which is reached after 4.4 hours, was about 24% lower than that of the 12 mg twice-daily tablet. Food had no effect on the steady-state bioavailability of the 24 mg extended release capsules. In a dose-proportionality study of galantamine extended release capsules in healthy elderly and young subjects, steady-state plasma concentrations were achieved within 6 days at all doses (8 mg, 16 mg, and 24 mg) in both age groups. Steady-state pharmacokinetics were dose-proportional within the studied dose range of 8 mg to 24 mg in both age groups.
Distribution: Galantamine is a low-clearance drug (plasma clearance of approximately 300 mL/min) with a moderate volume of distribution (average Vdss of 175 L) after a one-hour i.v. infusion of 8 mg galantamine in 12 healthy males.

The plasma protein binding of galantamine is 18% at therapeutically relevant concentrations. In whole blood, galantamine is mainly distributed to blood cells (52.7%) and plasma water (39.0%), whereas the fraction of galantamine bound to plasma proteins is only 8.4%. The blood-to-plasma concentration ratio of galantamine is 1.2.
Metabolism: Galantamine is metabolized by hepatic cytochrome P450 enzymes, glucuronidated and excreted unchanged in the urine. In vitro studies indicate that cytochrome CYP2D6 and CYP3A4 are the major cytochrome P450 isoenzymes involved in the metabolism of galantamine, and inhibitors of both pathways increase oral bioavailability of galantamine modestly (see Drug Interactions, Drug-Drug Interactions). O-demethylation, mediated by CYP2D6 is greater in extensive metabolizers of CYP2D6 than in poor metabolizers. In plasma from both poor and extensive metabolizers, however, unchanged galantamine and its glucuronide accounted for most of the sample radioactivity.
Excretion: The elimination of galantamine is bi-phasic, with a terminal half-life in the order of 7-8 hours in young healthy subjects (n=4 males). Two studies in healthy elderly subjects indicated that the terminal half-life of galantamine is 8.5 hours (n=13 males and 16 females) and 9.7 hours (n=10 males and 14 females) after administering a single oral dose of 10 mg galantamine. Up

to 8 hours post-dose, unchanged galantamine accounted for 39-77% of the total radioactivity in the plasma, and galantamine glucuronide accounted for 14-24%. Seven days after a single oral dose of 4 mg 3H-galantamine, 93-99% of the radioactivity had been recovered, with about 95% in urine and about 5% in feces. Total urinary recovery of unchanged galantamine accounted for, on average, 32% of the dose, and that of galantamine glucuronide for another 12% on average.

After i.v. and oral administration, about 20% of the dose was excreted as unchanged galantamine in the urine in 24 hours, with a renal clearance of about 65 mL/min, which represents 20-25% of the total plasma clearance of about 300 mL/min.

Special Populations and Conditions: Patients with Alzheimer's Disease: Data from clinical trials in patients indicate that there is a difference in total clearance after oral administration between patients with Alzheimer's disease and healthy subjects (13.2 L/h versus 19.4 L/h) based on pooled population analysis. Therefore, the plasma concentrations of galantamine in elderly patients (median age 75) with Alzheimer's disease are 30-40% higher than in healthy young subjects (median age 28).

Patients with Alzheimer's Disease and Concomitant Cerebrovascular Disease and Patients with Vascular Dementia: A randomized, double-blind, placebo-controlled clinical trial (GAL-INT-6) was conducted in a study population consisting of two different types of dementia patients: patients with vascular dementia (VaD) and patients with Alzheimer's disease and concomitant cerebrovascular disease (AD+CVD).

Trial Design: VaD patients (n=282) were diagnosed according to NINDS-AIREN criteria for probable vascular dementia. Patients with AD+CVD (n=255) were required to meet NINCDS-ADRDA criteria for possible Alzheimer's disease and have radiological evidence (CAT or MRI) of relevant cerebrovascular disease for inclusion in the study. Patients were treated for 26 weeks with galantamine 12 mg b.i.d. (VaD n=173; AD+CVD n=186) or placebo (VaD n=82; AD+CVD n=86).

Safety Results: The frequencies of certain cardiovascular-related adverse events, including syncope, hypertension, arrhythmia and bundle branch block, were increased in patients treated with galantamine compared to placebo. Analyses of treatment-emergent adverse events by diagnostic subgroup indicated that the increase was due primarily to events that occurred in the subgroup of patients with AD+CVD (see Adverse Reactions).

Efficacy Results: Efficacy results for the entire study population showed that there were statistically significant treatment effects on both primary endpoints (ADAS-cog and CIBIC-Plus) for galantamine-treated patients compared to placebo. Because the study population consisted of two different types of dementia patients, these results cannot be extrapolated to either patient population. Pre-specified analyses, conducted on the two subgroups for exploratory purposes, indicated that for both primary endpoints treatment differences for galantamine compared to placebo were not statistically significant for patients with VaD (galantamine n=171, placebo n=81), but were statistically significant for patients with AD+CVD (galantamine n=188, placebo n=97).

Confounding factors that preclude regulatory endorsement of an Indication for either of the two dementia patient populations include:

1. Trial Design:
   a. The study population consisted of two clinically different dementia patient populations, included in a ratio of approximately 1:1. Separate exploratory analyses of efficacy data from the diagnostic subgroups were pre-specified in the study statistical analysis plan but exploratory analyses are not regarded as confirmatory and therefore are not supportive of an indication.
   b. The validity of the assessment scales used in this study (ADAS-cog and CIBIC-Plus) has not been established for evaluating treatment effects in VaD, but has been established for Alzheimer's disease.
   c. There are no established diagnostic criteria in clinical practice for the identification of patients with AD+CVD. In the primary care setting, without the use of radiological imaging (CAT or MRI), these patients may be difficult to distinguish from Alzheimer's disease patients.
2. Data Analyses:
   a. The overall positive efficacy results for the entire study population cannot be extrapolated to either of the two patient subgroups.
   b. The significance of the negative outcome from the exploratory analysis of the VaD patient subgroup is not known, in view of the unconfirmed validity of these assessment scales for evaluating efficacy in VaD.
   c. Positive results from the exploratory analysis of the subgroup of patients with AD+CVD, in a single study, are not sufficient to support a claim of efficacy for these patients.

Conclusion: The results of this single study do not support regulatory endorsement of an indication for either VaD or AD+CVD patient populations.

There are no criteria established for making a differential diagnosis between patients with Alzheimer's disease and patients with concomitant cerebrovascular disease in clinical practice. Under the currently approved Canadian indication, REMINYL ER is available for the treatment of patients with mild to moderate Alzheimer's disease, which in clinical practice is likely to also include the treatment of patients with Alzheimer's disease and concomitant cerebrovascular disease.

Gender: No specific pharmacokinetic study was performed to investigate the gender differences. A population pharmacokinetic analysis (n=539 males and 550 females) suggests that galantamine clearance is about 20% lower in females than in males, which is explained by lower body weight in females.

Race: Pharmacokinetic differences due to race have not been identified in a population pharmacokinetic analysis (n=1029 White, 24 Black, 13 Asian and 23 other).

Hepatic Impairment: Following a single 4 mg dose of galantamine, the pharmacokinetics of galantamine in subjects with mild hepatic impairment (n=8; Child-Pugh score of 5-6) were similar to those in healthy subjects. In patients with moderate hepatic impairment (n=8; Child-Pugh score of 7-9), AUC and half-life of galantamine were increased by about 30% compared to normal subjects (see Warnings and Precautions and Dosage and Administration).

Renal Impairment: In patients with renal insufficiency, elimination of galantamine decreases with decreasing creatinine clearance. Following a single 8 mg dose of galantamine, AUC increased by 37% and 67% in moderately (n=8; creatinine clearance of 30 to 60 mL/min/1.73 m^2) and severely (n=9; creatinine clearance of 5 to 29 mL/min/1.73 m^2) renal-impaired patients compared to normal volunteers (n=8) (see Warnings and Precautions and Dosage and Administration).

CYP2D6 Poor Metabolizers: Approximately 7% of the normal population has a genetic variation that leads to reduced levels of activity of the CYP2D6 isozyme. Such individuals have been referred to as poor metabolizers. After a single oral dose of 4 mg or 8 mg galantamine, CYP2D6 poor metabolizers demonstrated a similar C_{max} and about 35% AUC_{∞} increase of unchanged galantamine compared to extensive metabolizers.

A total of 356 patients with Alzheimer's disease enrolled in two Phase III studies were genotyped with respect to CYP2D6 (n=210 hetero-extensive metabolizers, 126 homo-extensive metabolizers, and 20 poor metabolizers). Population pharmacokinetic analysis indicated that there was a 25% decrease in median clearance in poor metabolizers compared to extensive metabolizers. Dosage adjustment is not necessary in patients identified as poor metabolizers as the dose of drug is individually titrated to tolerability due to observed inter-patient variability.

STORAGE AND STABILITY: REMINYL ER extended release capsules should be stored between 15-30°C.

INFORMATION FOR THE PATIENT: Published in e-CPS, available by subscription at www.e-cps.ca.

DOSAGE FORMS, COMPOSITION AND PACKAGING: 8 mg: Each white opaque, extended release capsule, containing white to off-white pellets, imprinted with "G 8", contains: galantamine 8 mg as galantamine HBr. Nonmedicinal ingredients: diethyl phthalate, ethylcellulose, gelatin, hypromellose, polyethylene glycol, sugar spheres (sucrose and starch) and titanium dioxide. Bottles of 30.

16 mg: Each pink opaque, extended release capsule, containing white to off-white pellets, imprinted with "G 16", contains: galantamine 16 mg as galantamine HBr. Nonmedicinal ingredients: diethyl phthalate, ethylcellulose, gelatin, hypromellose, polyethylene glycol, red ferric oxide, sugar spheres (sucrose and starch) and titanium dioxide. Bottles of 30.

24 mg: Each caramel opaque, extended release capsule, containing white to off-white pellets, imprinted with "G 24", contains: galantamine 24 mg as galantamine HBr. Nonmedicinal ingredients: diethyl phthalate, ethylcellulose, gelatin, hypromellose, polyethylene glycol, red ferric oxide, sugar spheres (sucrose and starch), titanium dioxide and yellow ferric oxide. Bottles of 30.

(Shown in Product Identification Section)

Renagel® Ⓟ

sevelamer HCl

Phosphate Binder

Genzyme

Date of Preparation: February 24, 2000
Date of Revision: May 26, 2009

SUMMARY PRODUCT INFORMATION:

Route of Administration	Dosage Form/ Strength	Clinically Relevant Nonmedicinal Ingredients
Oral	Tablet/800 mg	There are no clinically relevant nonmedicinal ingredients. Nonmedicinal ingredients include: hypromellose; diacetylated monoglyceride; colloidal silicon dioxide; and stearic acid. The tablet imprint contains iron oxide black ink. For a complete listing see Dosage Forms, Composition and Packaging.

INDICATIONS AND CLINICAL USE: RENAGEL (sevelamer hydrochloride) is indicated for:

- the control of hyperphosphatemia in patients with ESRD (End Stage Renal Disease) undergoing dialysis.

CONTRAINDICATIONS: RENAGEL (sevelamer hydrochloride) is contraindicated in the following situations:

- patients with hypophosphatemia
- patients with bowel obstruction
- patients hypersensitive to sevelamer hydrochloride or one of the other ingredients in the product (colloidal silicon dioxide, stearic acid).

WARNINGS AND PRECAUTIONS: General: RENAGEL (sevelamer hydrochloride) tablets should be swallowed intact and should not be crushed, chewed, or broken into pieces.

Patients with renal insufficiency may develop hypocalcemia. As RENAGEL does not contain calcium, serum calcium levels should be monitored and elemental calcium should be supplemented whenever considered necessary. In cases of hypocalcemia, patients should be given an evening calcium supplement. Approximately 1000 mg elemental calcium is recommended.

Caution should be exercised to avoid hypophosphatemia, a serum phosphorus of <0.8 mmol/L (see Dosage and Administration).

The safety and efficacy of RENAGEL in patients with renal disease who are not undergoing dialysis has not been studied.

Gastrointestinal: The safety and efficacy of RENAGEL in patients with dysphagia, swallowing disorders, severe gastrointestinal (GI) motility disorders including severe constipation, or major GI tract surgery have not been established. Caution should be exercised when RENAGEL is used in patients with these GI disorders.

Special Populations: Pregnant Women: The safety of RENAGEL has not been established in pregnant women. In preclinical studies, there was no evidence that RENAGEL induced embryolethality, fetotoxicity or teratogenicity at the doses tested (up to 1 g/kg/day in rabbits; up to 4.5 g/kg/day in rats). RENAGEL should only be given to pregnant women if the benefits outweigh the risks.

Nursing Women: There have been no adequate, well-controlled studies in lactating, or nursing women.

Pediatrics: The safety and efficacy of RENAGEL has not been established in pediatric patients. The minimum age of patients treated with RENAGEL in clinical trials was 18 years old.

Geriatrics: No special considerations are needed for elderly patients.

Monitoring and Laboratory Tests: Serum phosphorus and serum calcium should be monitored every 1 to 3 weeks until the target phosphorus level is reached. The dose of RENAGEL should be adjusted based on serum phosphorus concentration and titrated to a target serum phosphorus of ≤1.8 mmol/L.

RENAGEL does not contain calcium or alkali supplementation; serum calcium, bicarbonate, and chloride levels should be monitored.

ADVERSE REACTIONS: Clinical Trial Adverse Drug Reactions: Because clinical trials are conducted under very specific conditions the adverse reaction rates observed in the clinical trials may not reflect the rates observed in practice and should not be compared to the rates in the clinical trials of another drug. Adverse drug reaction information from clinical trials is useful for identifying drug-related adverse events and for approximating rates.

In a combined safety database comprised of 483 patients with end-stage renal disease undergoing hemodialysis, adverse events reported at an incidence ≥10% are provided in Table 1. From this database, adverse events are also presented separately from a single long-term randomized clinical study for RENAGEL and calcium. The adverse events presented in the table are not necessarily attributed to RENAGEL treatment. The incidence of these events was not dose related.

Table 1: RENAGEL

Adverse Events in Patients with End-Stage Renal Disease Undergoing Hemodialysis

	Total AEs Reported	52 Weeks Study of RENAGEL vs. Calcium (calcium acetate and calcium carbonate)	
System Organ Class Event	RENAGEL N=483 %	RENAGEL N=99 %	Calcium N=101 %
Gastrointestinal Disorders			
Vomiting	24.4	22.2	21.8
Nausea	25.3	20.2	19.8
Diarrhea	21.1	19.2	22.8
Dyspepsia	15.7	16.2	6.9
Constipation	13.3	8.1	11.9
Infections and Infestations			
Nasopharyngitis	13.9	14.1	7.9
Bronchitis	5.4	11.1	12.9
Upper Respiratory Tract Infection	7.0	5.1	10.9
Musculoskeletal, Connective Tissue and Bone Disorders			
Pain in Limb	13.7	13.1	14.9
Arthralgia	11.4	12.1	17.8
Back Pain	6.0	4.0	17.8
Skin Disorders			
Pruritus	10.4	13.1	9.9
Respiratory, Thoracic and Mediastinal Disorders			
Dyspnea	15.7	10.1	16.8
Cough	11.6	7.1	12.9
Vascular Disorders			

(cont'd)

Table 1: RENAGEL *(cont'd)*

Adverse Events in Patients with End-Stage Renal Disease Undergoing Hemodialysis

System Organ Class Event	Total AEs Reported RENAGEL N=483 %	52 Weeks Study of RENAGEL vs. Calcium (calcium acetate and calcium carbonate) RENAGEL N=99 %	 Calcium N=101 %
Hypertension	9.3	10.1	5.9
Nervous System Disorders			
Headache	18.4	9.1	15.8
General Disorders and Site Administration Disorders			
Dialysis Access Complication	4.3	6.1	10.9
Pyrexia	8.7	5.1	10.9

In one hundred and forty three patients with end-stage renal disease undergoing peritoneal dialysis with treatment duration of 12 weeks, adverse events reported at an incidence ≥10% are provided in Table 2. The adverse events presented in the table are not necessarily attributed to RENAGEL treatment. The incidence of these events was not dose related.

Table 2: RENAGEL

Adverse Events in Patients with End-Stage Renal Disease Undergoing Peritoneal Dialysis

System Organ Class Event	RENAGEL (N=97) %	Calcium (N=46) %
Gastrointestinal Disorders		
Dyspepsia	17.5	8.7
Vomiting	11.3	4.3
Peritonitis	11.3	4.3

The most frequently occurring serious adverse event with RENAGEL use was peritonitis at 8.2%, compared to 4.3 % with calcium. Patients receiving dialysis are subject to certain risks for infection specific to the dialysis modality. Peritonitis is a known complication in patients receiving peritoneal dialysis (PD). Therefore, patients on PD should be closely monitored to ensure the reliable use of appropriate aseptic technique with the prompt recognition and management of any signs and symptoms associated with peritonitis.

Less Common Clinical Trial Adverse Events: The following adverse events have been observed with RENAGEL use with an incidence of <10%, but greater than calcium and without attribution to causality, including: abdominal distension, constipation, diarrhea, nausea, chest pain, fatigue, pyrexia, catheter site infection, anorexia, headache, cough and pruritus.

Some patients experienced adverse events related to hypercalcemia in the calcium group but not in the RENAGEL group.

Post-Market Adverse Drug Reactions: During post-marketing experience with RENAGEL, the following have been reported without attribution to causality: pruritus, rash, abdominal pain and in very rare cases, intestinal obstruction, ileus and intestinal perforation.

DRUG INTERACTIONS: Drug-Drug Interactions: RENAGEL (sevelamer hydrochloride) was studied in human drug-drug interaction studies with digoxin, warfarin, enalapril, metoprolol and iron. RENAGEL had no effect on the bioavailability of these medications. However, in a study of 15 healthy subjects, a co-administered single dose of 7 RENAGEL Capsules (approximately 2.8 g) decreased the bioavailability of ciprofloxacin by approximately 50%. Consequently, RENAGEL should not be taken simultaneously with ciprofloxacin.

During post-marketing experience, very rare cases of increased TSH levels have been reported in patients co-administered RENAGEL and levothyroxine. Closer monitoring of TSH levels is therefore recommended for patients receiving both medications.

When administering any other medication where a reduction in the bioavailability of that medication would have a clinically significant effect on safety or efficacy, the physician should consider monitoring blood levels or dosing that medicine apart from RENAGEL (at least one hour before or three hours after RENAGEL). Patients taking anti-arrhythmic and anti-seizure medications were excluded from the clinical trials. Special precautions should be taken when prescribing RENAGEL to patients also taking these medications.

Drug-Food Interactions: There have been no adequate, well-controlled studies regarding the effect of a variety of foods on the intestinal phosphorus binding of RENAGEL.

Drug-Herb Interactions: There have been no adequate, well-controlled studies regarding drug-herb interactions.

Drug-Laboratory Test Interactions: There have been no adequate, well-controlled studies regarding drug-laboratory interactions.

Drug-Lifestyle Interactions: There have been no adequate, well-controlled studies regarding drug-lifestyle interactions.

DOSAGE AND ADMINISTRATION: Dosing Considerations:

- The tablets should not be bitten, chewed or broken apart prior to dosing.
- RENAGEL (sevelamer hydrochloride) should be taken immediately prior to or with meals, since its action is to bind ingested phosphate (see Action and Clinical Pharmacology, Mechanism of Action).
- When administering any other medication where a reduction in the bioavailability of that medication would have a clinically significant effect on safety or efficacy, the physician should consider monitoring blood levels or dosing that medicine apart from RENAGEL (at least one hour before or three hours after RENAGEL).

Recommended Dose and Dosage Adjustment: The recommended dosing to be used when initiating RENAGEL in patients not using another phosphate binder are outlined in Table 3.

Table 3: RENAGEL

Recommended Dosing to Be Used When Initiating RENAGEL in Patients Not Using Another Phosphate Binder

Initial Serum Phosphorus	Starting Dose RENAGEL Tablets 800 mg
>1.8 and <2.4 mmol/L	3 tablets/day (2.4 g)
≥2.4 mmol/L	6 tablets/day (4.8 g)

When switching from calcium-based phosphate binders to RENAGEL, an equivalent starting dose on a mg/weight basis of RENAGEL should be prescribed.

Dosage adjustments, when necessary should be recommended every 1 to 3 weeks by increasing one tablet per meal (3 per day) until the target serum phosphorus levels are met.

The total daily dose should be divided according to meal portions during the day.

Average Maintenance Dose: Dosage should be adjusted based upon the target serum phosphorus levels. The dose may be increased or decreased by one tablet per meal at two week intervals as necessary. The average final dose in the chronic phase of a 52 week Phase 3 clinical trial designed to lower serum phosphorous to 1.6 mmol/L or less was approximately 7.1 grams, (approximately nine 800 mg tablets per day equivalent to three 800 mg tablets per meal). The maximum average daily RENAGEL dose studied was 13 g.

Missed Dose: If a dose is forgotten, it should be skipped. Double dosing is not advisable.

OVERDOSAGE:

Since RENAGEL (sevelamer hydrochloride) is not absorbed, the risk of systemic toxicity is minimal. RENAGEL has been given to healthy volunteers at doses up to 14 grams per day for 8 days with no adverse effects. The maximum average daily dose of RENAGEL that has been given to hemodialysis patients is 13 grams.

> For management of a suspected drug overdose, CPhA recommends that you contact your **regional Poison Control Centre**. See the *CPS* Directory section for a list of Poison Control Centres.

ACTION AND CLINICAL PHARMACOLOGY: Patients with end-stage renal disease (ESRD) retain phosphorus and can develop hyperphosphatemia. High serum phosphorus can precipitate serum calcium resulting in ectopic calcification. When the product serum calcium and phosphorus concentrations (Ca×P) exceeds 4.4 mmol/L, there is an increased risk that ectopic calcification will occur. Hyperphosphatemia plays a role in the development of secondary hyperparathyroidism in renal insufficiency. An increase in parathyroid hormone (PTH) levels is characteristic of patients with chronic renal failure. Increased levels of PTH can lead to osteitis fibrosa, a bone disease. A decrease in serum phosphorus may decrease serum PTH levels.

Mechanism of Action: RENAGEL (sevelamer hydrochloride) is a nonabsorbed polymer phosphate binder. When taken with meals RENAGEL inhibits intestinal absorption of ingested phosphate.

RENAGEL binds bile acids and therefore lowers LDL serum cholesterol. Since RENAGEL does not contain aluminum or other metals, it does not cause aluminum or other metal intoxication.

Pharmacodynamics: A mass balance study using ^{14}C-sevelamer hydrochloride in 16 healthy male and female volunteers showed that sevelamer hydrochloride is not systemically absorbed. No absorption studies have been performed in patients with renal disease.

STORAGE AND STABILITY: Store at controlled room temperature 15 to 30°C. Protect from moisture.

SPECIAL HANDLING INSTRUCTIONS: None.

INFORMATION FOR THE PATIENT: Published in e-CPS, available by subscription at www.e-cps.ca.

DOSAGE FORMS, COMPOSITION AND PACKAGING: Each oval, film-coated tablet, imprinted with "RENAGEL 800", on the crown, single side, contains: sevelamer HCl 800 mg. Nonmedicinal ingredients: colloidal silicon dioxide and stearic acid; coating: diacetylated monoglyceride and hypromellose; printing ink: hypromellose (hydroxypropyl methylcellulose), iron oxide black (E172), isopropyl alcohol and propylene glycol. Bottles of 180.

(Shown in Product Identification Section)

> The reader is invited to consult CPhA's monograph **Calcium Channel Blockers**.

Renedil® Pr
felodipine
Antihypertensive

sanofi-aventis

SUPPLIED: 2.5 mg: Each yellow, circular, biconvex, film-coated, extended release tablet, engraved "H/FF" on one side and 2.5 on the other; contains: felodipine 2.5 mg. Nonmedicinal ingredients: aluminum silicate, carnauba wax, hydroxypropyl cellulose, hydroxypropyl methylcellulose, iron oxide, lactose, microcrystalline cellulose, polyethylene glycol, polyoxy 40 hydrogenated castor oil, propyl gallate, sodium stearyl fumarate and titanium dioxide. Gluten- and tartrazine-free. Compliance packages of 2×15. Note: These extended release tablets must not be divided, crushed or chewed. Store at 15 to 30°C.

5 mg: Each pink, circular, biconvex, film-coated, extended release tablet, engraved "H/FC" on one side and 5 on the other, contains: felodipine 5 mg. Nonmedicinal ingredients: aluminum silicate, carnauba wax, hydroxypropyl cellulose, hydroxypropyl methylcellulose, iron oxide, lactose, microcrystalline cellulose, polyethylene glycol, polyoxy 40 hydrogenated castor oil, propyl gallate, sodium stearyl fumarate and titanium dioxide. Gluten- and tartrazine-free. Compliance packages of 2×15. Note: These extended release tablets must not be divided, crushed or chewed. Store at 15 to 30°C.

10 mg: Each red-brown, circular, biconvex, film-coated, extended release tablet, engraved "H/FD" on one side and 10 on the other, contains: felodipine 10 mg. Nonmedicinal ingredients: aluminum silicate, carnauba wax, hydroxypropyl cellulose, hydroxypropyl methylcellulose, iron oxide, lactose, microcrystalline cellulose, polyethylene glycol, polyoxy 40 hydrogenated castor oil, propyl gallate, sodium stearyl fumarate and titanium dioxide. Gluten- and tartrazine-free. Compliance packages of 2×15. Note: These extended release tablets must not be divided, crushed or chewed. Store at 15 to 30°C.

(Shown in Product Identification Section)

ReoPro® Pr
abciximab
Chimeric Monoclonal Antiplatelet Antibody

Lilly

Date of Preparation: August 26, 2004

PHARMACOLOGY: General: ReoPro (abciximab) is the Fab fragment of the chimeric monoclonal antibody 7E3. It selectively binds to the glycoprotein IIb/IIIa (GPIIb/IIIa) receptor located on the surface of human platelets. ReoPro inhibits platelet aggregation by preventing the binding of fibrinogen, von Willebrand factor and other adhesive molecules to GPIIb/IIIa receptor sites on activated platelets. ReoPro also binds with similar affinity to the vitronectin ($\alpha_v\beta_3$) receptor found on platelets and vessel wall endothelial and smooth muscle cells. The vitronectin receptor mediates pro-coagulant properties of platelets and proliferative properties of vascular endothelial cells and smooth muscle cells.

Pharmacokinetics: Following i.v. administration of ReoPro, free plasma concentrations decreased very rapidly with an initial half-life of several minutes and a second phase half-life of about 30 minutes. This disappearance from the plasma is probably related to rapid binding to the platelet GPIIb/IIIa receptors (approximately 80 000 to 100 000 GPIIb/IIIa receptors on the surface of each platelet).

After a single bolus injection of ReoPro, the inhibitory effects on platelet function, as measured by inhibition of platelet aggregation, were evident within 10 minutes. The antibody remains in the circulation for 15 days or more in a platelet-bound state. Its disappearance follows a monoexponential time course.

I.V. administration of a 0.25 mg/kg bolus dose of ReoPro followed by continuous infusion of 5 or 10 µg/min for periods of 12 to 96 hours produced relatively constant total plasma concentrations from the first time point measured (usually 2 hours) for all infusion rates and durations. However, although the total plasma concentrations resulting from the 5 µg/min infusion were only slightly lower than those from the 10 µg/min infusion, the 5 µg/min infusion was ineffective in inhibiting platelet function over the whole infusion period. At the termination of the infusion period, plasma concentrations fell rapidly for approximately 6 hours, then declined at a much slower rate.

Pharmacodynamics: I.V. administration in humans of single bolus doses of ReoPro from 0.15 to 0.30 mg/kg resulted in a dose-dependent blockade of platelet GPIIb/IIIa receptors and produced dose-dependent inhibition of platelet function as measured by ex vivo platelet aggregation in response to ADP or by prolongation of bleeding time. At the 2 highest doses (0.25 and 0.30 mg/kg) at 2 hours post-injection, over 80% of the GPIIb/IIIa receptors were blocked and platelet aggregation in response to 20 µM ADP was almost abolished. The median bleeding time increased to over 30 minutes at both doses compared with a baseline value of approximately 5 minutes.

I.V. administration in humans of a single bolus dose of 0.25 mg/kg followed by a continuous infusion of 10 µg/min for periods of 12 to 96 hours produced sustained high-grade platelet inhibition (ex vivo platelet aggregation in response to 5 or 20 µM ADP less than 20% of baseline and bleeding time greater than 30 minutes) for the duration of the infusion in most patients. Equivalent results were obtained when a weight adjusted infusion dose (0.125 µg/kg/min to a maximum of 10 µg/min) was used in patients up to 80 kg. Results in patients who received the 0.25 mg/kg bolus followed by a 5 µg/min infusion for 24 hours showed a similar initial inhibition of platelet aggregation, but the response was not maintained throughout the infusion period. Following cessation of the infusion, platelet function typically returned to baseline values over a period of 24 to 48 hours.

INDICATIONS: ReoPro (abciximab) is indicated as an adjunct to percutaneous coronary intervention for the prevention of cardiac ischemic complications:

- in patients undergoing percutaneous coronary intervention
- in patients with unstable angina not responding to conventional medical therapy when percutaneous coronary intervention is planned within 24 hours.

ReoPro use in patients not undergoing percutaneous coronary intervention has not been studied.

ReoPro is intended for use with acetylsalicylic acid and heparin and has been studied only in that setting.

ReoPro has been studied in three pivotal clinical trials, all of which evaluated the effect of ReoPro in patients undergoing percutaneous coronary intervention: in patients at high risk for abrupt closure of the treated coronary vessel (EPIC), in a broader group of patients (EPILOG), and in unstable angina patients not responding to conventional medical therapy (CAPTURE). Percutaneous intervention included balloon angioplasty, atherectomy, or stent placement. All trials involved the use of various, concomitant heparin dose regimens and, unless contraindicated, acetylsalicylic acid (325 mg) was administered orally 2 hours prior to the planned procedure and then once daily. In each of the three pivotal trials, a statistically significant reduction in thrombotic complications of coronary intervention (the composite of death and MI or death, MI and urgent intervention) was observed within hours of the intervention and sustained for 30 days.

CONTRAINDICATIONS: ReoPro (abciximab) should not be administered to patients with known sensitivity to ReoPro, to any component of the product or to murine monoclonal antibodies.

ReoPro is contraindicated in the following clinical situations: active internal bleeding; recent (within 6 weeks) gastrointestinal or genitourinary bleeding of clinical significance; history of cerebrovascular accident (CVA) within 2 years or a CVA with a significant residual neurological deficit; recent (within 6 weeks) major surgery or trauma; intracranial neoplasm, arteriovenous malformation or aneurysm; known bleeding diathesis or severe uncontrolled hypertension; pre-existing thrombocytopenia; vasculitis; use of i.v. dextran before PTCA, or intent to use it during PTCA; administration of oral anticoagulants within 7 days unless prothrombin time is ≤1.2 times control.

WARNINGS: Requirement for Specialist Facilities: ReoPro (abciximab) should only be administered in conjunction with extensive specialist medical and nursing care. In addition, there must be availability of laboratory tests of hematology function and facilities for administration of blood products.

ReoPro has the potential to increase the risk of bleeding, particularly in the presence of excessive anticoagulation, e.g., from heparin or thrombolytics (see Adverse Effects, Bleeding).

The risks of major bleeds due to ReoPro therapy is increased in patients receiving thrombolytics and should be weighed against the anticipated benefits (see Thrombolytics, Anticoagulants and Other Antiplatelet Agents).

Should serious bleeding occur that is not controllable with pressure, the infusion of ReoPro and any concomitant heparin should be stopped (see also Restoration of Platelet Function).

Pulmonary hemorrhage associated with ReoPro use, although a very rare occurrence, can be a serious life-threatening complication that can be misdiagnosed and result in the patient not receiving timely treatment. Respiratory symptoms should be monitored closely for early detection of serious pulmonary hemorrhage in patients receiving ReoPro (see Precautions, Pulmonary (mostly alveolar) Hemorrhage).

Anaphylactic reactions have occurred very rarely in patients treated with ReoPro. Epinephrine, antihistamines and corticosteroids should be available for immediate use, in addition to equipment for resuscitation, in the event of a hypersensitivity reaction. Immediately, upon occurrence of anaphylaxis, administration of ReoPro should be stopped and appropriate resuscitative measures should be initiated.

PRECAUTIONS: Bleeding Precautions: Results of the EPILOG clinical trial show that bleeding can be reduced to the level of placebo by the use of low-dose, weight-adjusted heparin regimens, early sheath removal, careful patient and access site management and weight-adjustment of the ReoPro infusion dose.

Before infusion of ReoPro, platelet count, prothrombin time, ACT and APTT should be measured to identify pre-existing hemostatic abnormalities.

Low-dose, Weight-adjusted Heparin: Percutaneous Coronary Intervention: Heparin Bolus Pre-PTCA: If a patient's activated clotting time (ACT) is less than 200 seconds prior to the start of the PTCA procedure, an initial bolus of heparin should be given upon gaining arterial access according to the following algorithm: ACT <150 seconds: administer 70 U/kg; ACT 150-199 seconds: administer 50 U/kg.

The initial heparin bolus dose should not exceed 7000 U.

ACT should be checked a minimum of 2 minutes after the heparin bolus. If the ACT is <200 seconds, additional heparin boluses of 20 U/kg may be administered. Should the ACT remain <200 seconds, additional 20 U/kg boluses are to be given until an ACT ≥200 seconds is achieved.

Should a situation arise where higher doses of heparin are considered clinically necessary in spite of the possibility of a greater bleeding risk, it is recommended that heparin be carefully titrated using weight-adjusted boluses and that the target ACT not exceed 300 seconds.

Heparin Bolus during PTCA: During the PTCA procedure, ACT should be checked every 30 minutes. If ACT is <200 seconds, additional heparin boluses of 20 U/kg may be administered. Should the ACT remain <200 seconds, additional 20 U/kg boluses may be given until an ACT ≥200 seconds is achieved. ACT should be checked prior to and a minimum of 2 minutes after each heparin bolus.

Heparin Infusion after PTCA: Discontinuation of heparin immediately following completion of the procedure, with removal of the arterial sheath within 6 hours, is **strongly recommended**. In individual patients, if prolonged heparin therapy after PTCA or later sheath removal is used, then an initial infusion rate of 7 U/kg/h is recommended (see Bleeding Precautions, Femoral Artery Sheath Removal). In all circumstances, heparin should be discontinued at least 2 hours prior to arterial sheath removal.

Stabilization of Unstable Angina: Anticoagulation should be initiated with heparin to a target APTT of 60 to 85 seconds. The heparin infusion should be maintained during the ReoPro infusion. Following angioplasty, heparin management is outlined above under Percutaneous Coronary Intervention.

Femoral Artery Access Site: ReoPro is associated with an increase in bleeding rate particularly at the site of arterial access for femoral artery sheath placement. The following are specific recommendations for access site care: Femoral Artery Sheath Insertion: when appropriate, place only an arterial sheath for vascular access (avoid venous sheath placement); puncture only the anterior wall of the artery or vein when establishing vascular access; the use of a through and through technique to identify the vascular structure is **strongly discouraged**.

While Femoral Artery Sheath Is in Place: Check sheath insertion site and distal pulses of affected leg(s) every 15 minutes for 1 hour, then hourly for 6 hours; maintain complete bed rest with head of bed ≤30°; maintain affected leg(s) straight via sheet tuck method or soft restraint; medicate for back/groin pain as necessary; educate patient on post-PTCA care via verbal instructions.

Femoral Artery Sheath Removal: Heparin should be discontinued at least 2 hours prior to arterial sheath removal; check APTT or ACT prior to arterial sheath removal: do not remove sheath unless APTT ≤50 seconds or ACT ≤175 seconds; apply pressure to access site for at least 30 min following sheath removal, using either manual compression or a mechanical device; apply pressure dressing after hemostasis has been achieved.

After Femoral Artery Sheath Removal: Check groin for bleeding/hematoma and distal pulses every 15 minutes for the first hour or until stable, then hourly; continue complete bed rest with head of bed ≤30° and affected leg(s) straight for 6 to 8 hours following femoral artery sheath removal, 6 to 8 hours following discontinuation of abciximab or 4 hours following discontinuation of heparin, whichever is later; remove pressure dressing prior to ambulation; continue to medicate for discomfort.

Management of Femoral Access Site Bleeding/Hematoma Formation: In the event of groin bleeding with or without hematoma formation, the following procedures are recommended: Lower head of bed to 0°; apply manual pressure/compression device until hemostasis has been achieved; any hematoma should be measured and monitored for enlargement; change pressure dressing as needed; if heparin is being given, obtain APTT and adjust heparin as needed; maintain i.v. access if sheath has been removed.

If groin bleed continues or the hematoma expands during ReoPro infusion despite the above measures, the ReoPro infusion should be immediately discontinued and the arterial sheath removed according to the guidelines listed above. After sheath removal i.v. access should be maintained until bleeding is controlled.

Potential Bleeding Sites: Careful attention should be paid to all potential bleeding sites, including arterial and venous puncture sites, catheter insertion sites, cutdown sites, and needle puncture sites.

Retroperitoneal Bleeding: ReoPro is associated with an increased risk of retroperitoneal bleeding in association with femoral vascular puncture. The use of venous sheaths should be minimized and only the anterior wall of the artery or vein should be punctured when establishing vascular access.

Pulmonary (mostly alveolar) Hemorrhage: ReoPro has rarely been associated with pulmonary (mostly alveolar) hemorrhage. This can present with any or all of the following in close association with ReoPro administration: hypoxemia, alveolar infiltrates on chest x ray, hemoptysis, or an unexplained drop in hemoglobin. If confirmed, ReoPro and all anticoagulant and other antiplatelet drugs should immediately be discontinued.

Gastrointestinal Bleeding Prophylaxis: In order to prevent spontaneous gastrointestinal bleeding it is recommended that patients are pretreated with H_2-histamine receptor antagonists or liquid antacids. Antiemetics should be given as needed to prevent vomiting.

General Nursing Care: Unnecessary arterial and venous punctures, i.m. injections, routine use of urinary catheters, nasotracheal intubation, nasogastric tubes and automatic blood pressure cuffs should be avoided. When obtaining i.v. access, noncompressible sites (e.g., subclavian or jugular veins) should be avoided. Saline or heparin locks should be considered for blood drawing. Vascular puncture sites should be documented and monitored. Gentle care should be provided when removing dressings.

Patient Monitoring: Before administration of ReoPro, platelet count, ACT, prothrombin time (PT) and APTT should be measured to identify pre-existing coagulation abnormalities. Hemoglobin and hematocrit measurements should be obtained prior to the ReoPro administration, at 12 hours following the ReoPro bolus injection, and again at 24 hours following the bolus injection. Twelve lead electrocardiograms (ECG) should be obtained prior to the bolus injection of ReoPro, and repeated once the patient has returned to the hospital ward from the catheterization laboratory, and at 24 hours after the bolus injection of ReoPro. Vital signs (including blood pressure and pulse) should be obtained hourly for the first 4 hours following the ReoPro bolus injection, and then at 6, 12, 18 and 24 hours following the ReoPro bolus injection.

Thrombolytics, Anticoagulants and Other Antiplatelet Agents: Because ReoPro inhibits platelet aggregation, caution should be employed when used with other drugs affecting hemostasis such as heparin, oral anticoagulants such as warfarin, thrombolytics and antiplatelet agents other than ASA, such as dipyridamole, ticlopidine or low molecular weight dextrans.

Because of concern about observed synergistic effects on bleeding, ReoPro therapy should be used judiciously in patients who have received systemic thrombolytic therapy. The GUSTO V trial randomized patients with acute myocardial infarction to treatment with combined ReoPro and half-dose Reteplase, or full-dose Reteplase alone. In this trial, the incidence of moderate or severe non-intracranial bleeding was increased in those patients receiving ReoPro and half-dose Reteplase versus those receiving Reteplase alone (4.6% versus 2.3%, respectively). This increase was more pronounced in patients above age 75. Also noted in this age group, but not in other age groups, was a trend towards increased incidence of intracranial hemorrhage in those patients receiving ReoPro and half-dose Reteplase versus those receiving Reteplase alone.

If urgent intervention is required for refractory symptoms, it is recommended that PTCA using ReoPro be attempted first to salvage the situation. Should PTCA and any other appropriate procedures fail, and should the angiographic appearance suggest that the etiology is due to thrombosis, consideration may be given to the administration of adjunctive thrombolytic therapy via the intracoronary route. Prior to surgical interventions, the bleeding time should be determined by the Ivy method and should be 12 minutes or less (see Precautions, Restoration of Platelet Function).

Thrombocytopenia: To reduce the possibility of thrombocytopenia, platelet counts should be monitored prior to treatment, 2 to 4 hours following the bolus dose of ReoPro and at 24 hours or prior to discharge, whichever is first. If a patient experiences an acute platelet decrease, (e.g. a platelet decrease to less than 100,000 cells/µL and a decrease of at least 25% from pre-treatment value), additional platelet counts should be determined. These platelet counts should be drawn in 3 separate tubes containing ethylenediaminetetraacetic acid (EDTA), citrate and heparin, respectively, to exclude pseudothrombocytopenia due to in vitro anticoagulant interaction. If true thrombocytopenia is verified, ReoPro should be immediately discontinued and the condition appropriately monitored and treated. A daily platelet count should be obtained until it returns to normal. If a patient's platelet count drops to 60 000 cells/µL, heparin and ASA should be discontinued. If a patient's platelet count drops below 50 000 cells/µL, platelets should be transfused.

In a registry study of ReoPro readministration, a history of thrombocytopenia associated with prior use of ReoPro was predictive of an increased risk of recurrent thrombocytopenia. Readministration within 30 days was associated with an increased incidence and severity of thrombocytopenia, as was a positive human anti-chimeric antibody (HACA) test at baseline, compared to the rates seen in studies with first administration.

Restoration of Platelet Function: Transfusion of donor platelets has been shown to restore platelet function following ReoPro administration in animal studies and transfusions of fresh random donor platelets have been given empirically to restore platelet function in humans. In the event of serious uncontrolled bleeding or the need for surgery, a bleeding time should be determined. If the bleeding time is greater than 12 minutes, 10 units of platelets may be given. ReoPro may be displaced from endogenous platelet receptors and subsequently bind to platelets which have been transfused. Nevertheless, a single transfusion may be sufficient to reduce receptor blockade to 60 to 70% at which level platelet function is restored. Repeat platelet transfusions may be required to maintain the bleeding time at or below 12 minutes.

Readministration: Administration of ReoPro may result in human anti-chimeric antibody (HACA) formation (see Adverse Effects) that could potentially cause allergic or hypersensitivity reactions (including anaphylaxis), thrombocytopenia or diminished benefit upon readministration of ReoPro. Readministration of ReoPro to 29 patients known to be HACA-negative has not led to any change in ReoPro pharmacokinetics or to any reduction in antiplatelet potency.

Readministration of ReoPro to patients undergoing PCI was assessed in a registry that included 1342 treatments in 1286 patients. Most patients were receiving their second ReoPro exposure; 15% were receiving the third or subsequent exposure. The overall rate of HACA positivity prior to the readministration was 6% and increased to 27% post-readministration. There were no reports of serious allergic reactions or anaphylaxis. Thrombocytopenia was observed at higher rates in the readministration study than in the phase 3 studies of first-time administration (See Precautions, Thrombocytopenia), suggesting that readministration may be associated with an increased incidence and severity of thrombocytopenia.

Allergic Reactions (including anaphylaxis): Although anaphylaxis was not reported for ReoPro-treated patients in any of the pivotal clinical trials (EPIC, EPILOG, CAPTURE), suspected cases of anaphylaxis have been very rarely observed and reported following marketing of ReoPro.

Drug Interactions: Although drug interactions with ReoPro have not been studied systematically, ReoPro has been administered to patients with ischemic heart disease treated concomitantly with a broad range of medications used in the treatment of angina, myocardial infarction and hypertension. These medications have included heparin, warfarin, beta-adrenergic receptor blockers, calcium channel antagonists, angiotensin converting enzyme inhibitors, i.v. and oral nitrates, and ASA. Heparin, other anticoagulants, thrombolytics, and antiplatelet agents are associated with an increase in bleeding. Patients with HACA titres may have allergic or hypersensitivity reactions when treated with other diagnostic or therapeutic monoclonal antibodies.

Carcinogenesis and Mutagenesis: In vitro and in vivo mutagenicity studies have not demonstrated any mutagenic effect. Long-term studies in animals have not been performed to evaluate carcinogenic potential.

Children: Safety and effectiveness of ReoPro in children below the age of 18 have not been established.

Pregnancy: Animal reproduction studies have not been conducted with ReoPro and the effects on fertility in male or female animals are unknown. It is also not known whether ReoPro can cause fetal harm when administered to a pregnant woman or can affect reproduction capacity. ReoPro should be given to a pregnant woman only if clearly needed.

Lactation: It is not known if this drug is excreted in human milk. Because many drugs are excreted in human milk, caution should be exercised when ReoPro is administered to a nursing woman.

ADVERSE EFFECTS: Bleeding: Bleeding was classified as major or minor by the criteria of the Thrombolysis in Myocardial Infarction (TIMI) study group. Major bleeding events were defined as either an intracranial hemorrhage or decrease in hemoglobin greater than 5 g/dL. Minor bleeding events included spontaneous gross hematuria or hematemesis or observed blood loss with a hemoglobin decreasing more than 3 g/dL or with a decrease in hemoglobin of at least 4 g/dL with no observed blood loss.

In the EPIC trial, in which a non-weight-adjusted, standard heparin dose regimen was used, the most common complication during ReoPro (abciximab) therapy was bleeding during the first 36 hours. The incidences of major bleeding, minor bleeding and transfusion of blood products were approximately doubled. Approximately 70% of ReoPro-treated patients with major bleeding had bleeding at the arterial access site in the groin. ReoPro-treated patients also had a higher incidence of major bleeding events from gastrointestinal, genitourinary, retroperitoneal, and other sites.

In a subsequent clinical trial, EPILOG, using the heparin and ReoPro dosing, sheath removal and arterial access site guidelines described under Precautions, the incidence of major bleeding in patients treated with abciximab and low-dose, weight-adjusted heparin (1.8%) was not significantly different from patients receiving placebo (3.1%) and there was no significant increase in the incidence of intracranial hemorrhage. The reduction in bleeding observed in the EPILOG trial was achieved without loss of efficacy.

The rates of major bleeding, minor bleeding and bleeding events requiring transfusions in the EPIC, CAPTURE and EPILOG trials are shown in Table 1.

Table 1: ReoPro

Non-CABG Bleeding in the EPIC, EPILOG and CAPTURE Trials

	Number of Patients with Bleeds (%)		
	EPIC:		
	Placebo (n=696)	**ReoPro (Bolus + Infusion) (n=708)**	
Major[a]	23 (3.3)	75 (10.6)	
Minor	64 (9.2)	119 (16.8)	
Requiring Transfusion[b]	14 (2.0)	55 (7.8)	
	CAPTURE:		
	Placebo (n=635)	**ReoPro (n=630)**	
Major[a]	12 (1.9)	24 (3.8)	
Minor	13 (2.0)	30 (4.8)	
Requiring Transfusion[b]	9 (1.4)	15 (2.4)	
	EPILOG:		
	Placebo + Std-dose Heparin (n=939)	**ReoPro + Std-dose Heparin (n=918)**	**ReoPro + Low-dose Heparin (n=935)**
Major[a]	10 (1.1)	17 (1.9)	10 (1.1)
Minor	32 (3.4)	70 (7.6)	37 (4.0)
Requiring Transfusion[b]	10 (1.1)	7 (0.8)	6 (0.6)

[a] Patients who had bleeding in more than one classification are counted only once according to the most severe classification. Patients with multiple bleeding events of the same classification are also counted once within that classification.
[b] Packed red blood cells or whole blood.

Although data are limited, ReoPro treatment was not associated with excess major bleeding in patients who underwent CABG surgery. Some patients with prolonged bleeding times received platelet transfusions to correct the bleeding time prior to surgery (See Precautions, Restoration of Platelet Function).

The total incidence of intracranial hemorrhage and nonhemorrhagic stroke across all 3 trials was similar, 7/2225 (0.31%) for placebo patients and 10/3112 (0.32%) for ReoPro-treated patients. The incidence of intracranial hemorrhage was 0.13% in placebo patients and 0.19% in ReoPro patients.

Pulmonary hemorrhage with fatal outcomes following administration of ReoPro have been reported. In many cases, patients received at least two co-suspect or concomitant medications such as heparin or aspirin. Although the outcomes of most cases were not provided, approximately 2/3 had fatal outcomes. Based on exposure data, the reporting rate for pulmonary hemorrhage is less than 1 case report per 10 000 patients (see Warnings and Precautions, Pulmonary (mostly alveolar) Hemorrhage).

Thrombocytopenia: In the clinical trials, patients treated with ReoPro were more likely than patients treated with placebo to experience decreases in platelet counts. The overall rates of thrombocytopenia (platelet counts <100 000 cells/µL) in the EPIC, EPILOG and CAPTURE trials were 0.5% for placebo-treated patients and 2.9% for patients receiving ReoPro bolus plus infusion. The incidence of thrombocytopenia was lowest in the EPILOG trial (placebo: 1.5%; ReoPro and standard-dose, weight-adjusted heparin: 2.6%; ReoPro and low-dose, weight-adjusted heparin: 2.5%). The lowest rates of platelet transfusions in ReoPro-treated patients were also observed in the EPILOG trial, (placebo: 1.1%; ReoPro and standard-dose, weight-adjusted heparin: 1.6%; ReoPro and low-dose, weight-adjusted heparin: 0.9%).

In a readministration registry study of patients receiving a second or subsequent exposure to ReoPro (see Precautions, Readministration) the incidence of any degree of thrombocytopenia was 5%, with an incidence of profound thrombocytopenia of 2% (<20 000 cell/µL). Factors associated with an increased risk of thrombocytopenia were a history of thrombocytopenia on previous ReoPro exposure, readministration within 30 days, and a positive HACA assay prior to the readministration.

Among 14 patients who had thrombocytopenia associated with a prior exposure to ReoPro, 7 (50%) had recurrent thrombocytopenia. In 130 patients with a readministration interval of 30 days or less, 25 (19%) developed thrombocytopenia. Severe thrombocytopenia occurred in 19 of these patients. Among the 71 patients who had a positive HACA assay at baseline, 11 (15%) developed thrombocytopenia, 7 of which were severe.

Human Antichimeric Antibody (HACA): Human antichimeric antibody (HACA) may appear in response to the administration of ReoPro. In the EPIC, EPILOG, and CAPTURE trials, positive responses occurred in approximately 5.8% of the ReoPro-treated patients. There was no excess of hypersensitivity or allergic reactions related to ReoPro treatment compared with placebo treatment. See also Precautions, Allergic Reactions (including anaphylaxis).

In a study of readministration of ReoPro to patients (see Precautions, Readministration) the overall rate of HACA positivity prior to the readministration was 6% and increased post-readministration to 27%. Among the 36 subjects receiving a fourth or greater ReoPro exposure, HACA positive assays were observed post-readministration in 16 subjects (44%). There were no reports of serious allergic reactions or anaphylaxis. HACA positive status was associated with an increased risk of thrombocytopenia (see Precautions, Thrombocytopenia).

The data reflect the percentage of patients whose test results were considered positive for antibodies to ReoPro using an ELISA assay, and are highly dependent on the sensitivity and specificity of the assay. Additionally, the observed incidence of antibody positivity in an assay may be influenced by several factors including sample handling, timing of sample collection, concomitant medications, and underlying disease. For these reasons, comparison of the incidence of antibodies to ReoPro with the incidence of antibodies to other products may be misleading.

Other Adverse Events: Clinical toxicity has been infrequent with the administration of ReoPro. Adverse events reasonably related to study agent that were reported by investigators with at least a 0.2% greater incidence for ReoPro bolus plus infusion compared with placebo for the 5337 treated patients in the 3 pivotal clinical trials (EPIC, EPILOG and CAPTURE) are shown in Table 2.

Table 2: ReoPro

Patients Who Experienced Adverse Events Reasonably Related to Study Agent

	Placebo (n=2226)	ReoPro (n=3111)
Hypotension	35 (1.6%)	103 (3.3%)
Nausea	47 (2.1%)	95 (3.1%)
Vomiting	34 (1.5%)	59 (1.9%)
Bradycardia	9 (0.4%)	24 (0.8%)
Pseudoaneurysm	7 (0.3%)	16 (0.5%)
Rash	5 (0.2%)	11 (0.4%)

(cont'd)

Table 2: ReoPro *(cont'd)*

Patients Who Experienced Adverse Events Reasonably Related to Study Agent

	Placebo (n=2226)	ReoPro (n=3111)
Hematoma	4 (0.2%)	11 (0.4%)
Pain	3 (0.1%)	9 (0.3%)
Dizziness	1 (0.0%)	6 (0.2%)
Ventricular tachycardia	1 (0.0%)	5 (0.2%)
Circulatory failure	1 (0.0%)	5 (0.2%)
Epistaxis	1 (0.0%)	5 (0.2%)

The following adverse events from the EPIC, EPILOG and CAPTURE trials were reported for patients treated with ReoPro bolus plus infusion at incidences higher than for patients in the placebo arm, regardless of whether the investigator considered the event related to study agent: back pain (17.6%), hypotension (14.4%), nausea (13.6%), chest pain (11.4%), vomiting (7.3%), headache (6.4%), pain (5.4%), bradycardia (4.5%), puncture site pain (3.6%), thrombocytopenia (3.5%), abdominal pain (3.1%), dizziness (2.9%), dyspepsia (2.1%), anxiety (1.7%), peripheral edema (1.6%), ventricular tachycardia (1.4%), anemia (1.3%), abnormal thinking (1.3%), diarrhea (1.1%), sweating increased (1.0%), pseudoaneurysm (0.8%), urinary retention (0.7%), agitation (0.7%), asthenia (0.7%), hematoma (0.7%), hypesthesia (0.6%), incisional pain (0.6%), leukocytosis (0.5%), confusion (0.5%), palpitation (0.5%), pruritus (0.5%), arteriovenous fistula (0.4%), pneumonia (0.4%), rales (0.4%), muscle contractions (0.4%), dysuria (0.4%), abnormal renal function (0.4%), abnormal vision (0.3%), edema (0.3%), incomplete AV block (0.3%), pleural effusion (0.3%), bronchitis (0.3%), bronchospasm (0.3%), pleurisy (0.2%), pulmonary embolism (0.2%), myalgia (0.2%), coma (0.2%), hypertonia (0.2%), nodal arrhythmia (0.2%), petechiae (0.2%), wound (0.2%), abscess (0.2%), cellulitis (0.2%), peripheral coldness (0.2%), injection site pain (0.1%), dry mouth (0.1%), pallor (0.1%), diabetes mellitus (0.1%), hyperkalemia (0.1%), enlarged abdomen (0.1%), bullous eruption (0.1%), inflammation (0.1%), drug toxicity (0.1%), complete AV block (0.1%), ileus (0.1%), embolism (limb) (0.1%); thrombophlebitis (0.1%), gastroesophageal reflux (0.1%), diplopia (0.1%), rhonchi (0.1%), frequent micturition (0.1%), cystalgia (0.1%), urinary incontinence (0.1%), prostatitis (0.1%).

Although extremely unlikely, anaphylaxis may potentially occur at any time during administration. If it does, immediate cessation of infusion, s.c. administration of 0.3 to 0.5 mL of aqueous epinephrine (1:1000 dilution), corticosteroids, respiratory assistance and other resuscitative measures are essential.

OVERDOSE:
There has been no experience of overdosage with abciximab in human clinical trials. However, refer to Precautions, Restoration of Platelet Function.

For management of a suspected drug overdose, CPhA recommends that you contact your **regional Poison Control Centre**. See the *CPS* Directory section for a list of Poison Control Centres.

DOSAGE: The safety and efficacy of ReoPro (abciximab) have only been investigated with concomitant administration of heparin and acetylsalicylic acid.

Acetylsalicylic acid should be administered orally at a daily dose of 300 to 325 mg.

For heparin anticoagulation guidelines see Precautions, Bleeding Precautions, Heparin.

In patients with failed PTCAs, the continuous infusion of ReoPro should be stopped because there is no evidence for ReoPro efficacy in that setting.

In the event of serious bleeding that cannot be controlled by compression, ReoPro and heparin should be discontinued immediately (see Precautions, Restoration of Platelet Function).

Adults: The recommended dose of ReoPro is a 0.25 mg/kg i.v. bolus followed by a 0.125 µg/kg/min (to a maximum of 10 µg/min) continuous i.v. infusion.

For the stabilization of unstable angina patients, the bolus dose followed by the infusion should be started up to 24 hours prior to the possible intervention.

For the prevention of ischemic cardiac complications in patients undergoing percutaneous coronary intervention, and who are not currently receiving a ReoPro infusion, the bolus should be administered 10 to 60 minutes prior to the intervention, followed by the infusion for 12 hours.

Children: There is no experience on the use of ReoPro in children.

Administration Instructions: Parenteral drug products should be inspected visually for particulate matter prior to administration. Preparations of ReoPro containing visibly opaque particles should **not** be used.

Hypersensitivity reactions should be anticipated whenever protein solutions such as ReoPro are administered. Epinephrine, dopamine, theophylline, antihistamines and corticosteroids should be available for immediate use. If symptoms of an allergic reaction or anaphylaxis appear, the infusion should be stopped and appropriate treatment given.

As with all parenteral drug products, aseptic procedures should be used during the administration of ReoPro.

Withdraw the necessary amount of ReoPro for bolus injection into a syringe. Filter the bolus injection using a sterile, nonpyrogenic, low protein-binding 0.2 or 0.22 µm filter (Millipore SLGV025LS or equivalent).

Withdraw the necessary amount of ReoPro for the continuous infusion into a syringe. Inject into an appropriate container of sterile 0.9% saline or 5% dextrose and infuse at the calculated rate via a continuous infusion pump. The continuous infusion should be filtered either upon admixture using a sterile, nonpyrogenic, low protein-binding 0.2 or 0.22 µm syringe filter (Millipore SLGV025LS or equivalent) or upon administration using an in-line, sterile, nonpyrogenic, low protein-binding 0.2 or 0.22 µm filter (Abbott #4524 or equivalent).

Discard the unused portion at the end of the infusion.

Although incompatibilities have not been observed with i.v. infusion fluids or commonly used cardiovascular drugs, it is recommended that ReoPro be administered in a separate i.v. line whenever possible and not mixed with other medications.

No incompatibilities have been observed with glass bottles or polyvinyl chloride bags and administration sets.

SUPPLIED: Each mL of clear, colorless, sterile, nonpyrogenic solution for i.v. use contains: abciximab 2 mg. Nonmedicinal ingredients: polysorbate 80, sodium chloride and sodium phosphate. Preservative-free. Vials of 5 mL, packages of 1. Store at 2 to 8°C. Do not freeze. Do not shake. Do not use beyond the expiration date. Discard any unused portion left in the vial.

Replagal™

agalsidase alfa

Gene-Activated alpha-Galactosidase A for Enzyme Replacement Therapy of Fabry Disease

Paladin

Date of Revision: May 21, 2008

Replagal shows promising preliminary evidence of efficacy for the treatment of patients with Fabry Disease; however, the optimal individual dose requires further investigation. Studies are underway to evaluate more frequent and/or higher doses of Replagal therapy than used in clinical trials to date.

This product has been approved under the Notice of Compliance with Conditions (NOC/c) policy for one or all of its indicated uses.

What is a Notice of Compliance with Conditions (NOC/c)? An NOC/c is a form of market approval granted to a product on the basis of **promising** evidence of clinical effectiveness following review of the submission by Health Canada.

Products approved under Health Canada's NOC/c policy are intended for the treatment, prevention or diagnosis of a serious, life-threatening or severely debilitating illness. They have demonstrated promising benefit, are of high quality and possess an acceptable safety profile based on a benefit/risk assessment. In addition, they either respond to a serious unmet medical need in Canada or have demonstrated a significant improvement in the benefit/risk profile over existing therapies. Health Canada has provided access to this product on the condition that sponsors carry out additional clinical trials to verify the anticipated benefit within an agreed upon time frame.

SUMMARY PRODUCT INFORMATION:

Route of Administration	Pharmaceutical Form/Strength	Clinically Relevant Nonmedicinal Ingredients
Intravenous (IV)	1 mg/mL concentrate for solution for infusion	None

INDICATIONS AND CLINICAL USE: Replagal (agalsidase alfa) is indicated for:

- long-term enzyme replacement therapy in patients with a confirmed diagnosis of Fabry Disease (α-galactosidase A deficiency).

Replagal treatment should initially be supervised by a physician experienced in the management of patients with Fabry Disease or other inherited metabolic diseases.

CONTRAINDICATIONS:

- Life-threatening hypersensitivity (anaphylactic reaction) to the active substance or any of the excipients.
- Replagal should not be co-administered with chloroquine, amiodarone, benoquin or gentamicin since these substances have the potential to inhibit intra-cellular α-galactosidase activity.

WARNINGS AND PRECAUTIONS:

Serious Warnings and Precautions
• None

General: Occupational Hazards: Replagal has no or negligible influence on the ability to drive and use machines.
Hepatic: No studies have been performed in patients with hepatic impairment.
Immune: In approximately 10% of patients, Replagal has been associated with mild, acute idiosyncratic infusion reactions, during or within one hour following infusion. The most common symptoms have been chills and facial flushing. Severe infusion reactions have been reported uncommonly. Symptoms reported include nausea, pyrexia, rigors, tachycardia, urticaria and vomiting. Such reactions have generally occurred within the first 2-4 months after initiation of treatment with Replagal. If mild or moderate acute infusion reactions occur, medical attention must be sought immediately and appropriate actions instituted. The infusion can be temporarily interrupted (5 to 10 minutes) until symptoms subside and the infusion may then be restarted. Mild and transient effects may not require medical treatment or discontinuation of the infusion. In addition pre-treatment, generally with oral antihistamines and corticosteroids, from 1 to 3 hours prior to infusion has prevented subsequent reactions in those cases where symptomatic treatment was required.

As with any intravenous protein product, allergic-type hypersensitivity reactions are possible. If severe allergic or anaphylactic-type reactions occur, the administration of Replagal should be discontinued immediately and appropriate treatment initiated. The current medical standards for emergency treatment are to be observed.

As with all protein pharmaceutical products, patients may develop antibodies to the protein. A low titre IgG antibody response has been observed in approximately 55% of the patients treated with Replagal. The antibodies appear to develop following approximately 3 months of treatment. After 12 to 18 months of therapy, 60% of patients are antibody free and >80% of patients who were antibody positive showed evidence for the development of immunologic tolerance, based on the reduction of antibody titres over time. (See Adverse Reactions.)
Renal: No dose adjustment is necessary in patients with renal impairment.

The presence of extensive renal damage (eGFR <60 mL/min) may limit the renal response to enzyme replacement therapy. Limited data are available in patients on dialysis or post-kidney transplantation, no dose adjustment is required.
Special Populations: Pregnant Women: For Replagal, no clinical data on exposed pregnancies are available. Animal studies do not indicate direct or indirect harmful effects with respect to pregnancy or embryonal/foetal development when exposed during organogenesis.
Nursing Women: It is not known whether Replagal is excreted in human milk.
Pediatrics (0-17 years of age) and Geriatrics (>65 years of age): Replagal has been found to be safe and well tolerated following 12 months of therapy in children with Fabry disease and there is no evidence of any difference in the safety profile compared to the larger experience in treating adult patients. In the first six children studied there have been no reports of significant infusion related symptoms and no patients have developed IgG anti-agalsidase alfa antibodies following 12 months of therapy. Studies in patients over the age of 65 have not been performed.

The benefit versus risk balance should be considered carefully before prescribing Replagal to pregnant or nursing women, children or the elderly.
Monitoring and Laboratory Tests: No special laboratory tests are required for patients receiving Replagal, other than the usual tests that are required for monitoring patients with Fabry Disease.

ADVERSE REACTIONS: Adverse Drug Reaction Overview: The most commonly reported undesirable effects were associated with infusion reactions which occurred in approximately 10% of patients treated in clinical trials. Most undesirable effects were mild to moderate in severity and the majority were consistent with the natural course of Fabry Disease.
Adverse Drug Reactions: Table 1 lists those adverse drug reactions (ADRs) reported for the 55 patients treated with agalsidase alfa in clinical trials where causality is at least suspected in one or more cases. Information is presented by system organ class and frequency (very common >1/10; common >1/100 and <1/10). The occurrence of an event in a single patient is defined as common in view of the number of patients treated. A single patient could be affected by several ADRs.

Table 1: Replagal
Adverse Drug Reactions in Clinical Trials

		Replagal (n=55)	
		Patients (n)	%
Metabolism and Nutrition Disorders			
Common	edema	1	1.8
	peripheral edema	1	1.8
Psychiatric Disorders			
Common	panic attack	1	1.8
Nervous System Disorders			
Very Common	headache	6	10.9

(cont'd)

Table 1: Replagal *(cont'd)*
Adverse Drug Reactions in Clinical Trials

		Replagal (n=55)	
		Patients (n)	%
Common	dizziness	5	9.1
	dysgeusia	3	5.5
	neuropathic pain	3	5.5
	tremor	2	3.6
	hypersomnia	1	1.8
	hypoesthesia	1	1.8
	paraesthesia	1	1.8
	parosmia	1	1.8
	somnolence	1	1.8
Eye Disorders			
Common	lacrimation increased	1	1.8
	periorbital edema	1	1.8
Ear and Labyrinth Disorders			
Common	vertigo	1	1.8
Cardiac Disorders			
Common	tachycardia	2	3.6
	chest pain	1	1.8
Vascular Disorders			
Very Common	flushing	13	23.6
Common	hypertension	2	3.6
	peripheral coldness	1	1.8
Respiratory, Thoracic and Mediastinal Disorders			
Common	hoarseness	3	5.5
	throat tightness	3	5.5
	cough	2	3.6
	dyspnea	2	3.6
	nasopharyngitis	2	3.6
	pharyngitis	2	3.6
	nasal congestion	1	1.8
	snoring	1	1.8
	throat irritation	1	1.8
Gastrointestinal Disorders			
Common	nausea	5	9.1
	diarrhea	2	3.6
	vomiting	2	3.6
	abdominal pain	1	1.8
	dyspepsia	1	1.8
	gastrointestinal upset	1	1.8
	stomach cramps	1	1.8
	stomach discomfort	1	1.8
Skin and Subcutaneous Tissue Disorders			

(cont'd)

Table 1: Replagal *(cont'd)*

Adverse Drug Reactions in Clinical Trials

		Replagal (n=55)	
		Patients (n)	%
Common	acne	5	9.1
	erythema	4	7.3
	mottled skin	2	3.6
	pruritus	2	3.6
	dry skin	1	1.8
	eczema	1	1.8
	itchy rash	1	1.8
	rash	1	1.8
Musculoskeletal, Connective Tissue and Bone Disorders			
Common	myalgia	3	5.5
	musculoskeletal discomfort	1	1.8
	back pain	1	1.8
	limb pain	1	1.8
General Disorders and Administrative Site Conditions			
Very Common	rigors	11	20
	pyrexia	11	20
	infusion related reactions (see below)	7	12.7
Common	fatigue	5	9.1
	chest tightness	4	7.3
	pain and discomfort	4	7.3
	fatigue aggravated	4	7.3
	feeling hot	2	3.6
	asthenia	1	1.8
	chest pain	1	1.8
	influenza like illness	1	1.8
	edema	1	1.8

In pre-approval clinical trials approximately 10% of agalsidase alfa treated patients have experienced idiosyncratic infusion-reactions (see Warnings and Precautions). These effects have decreased with time. Symptoms have included predominantly rigors (chills) and facial flushing with a few patients experiencing headache, dyspnea, abdominal pain, nausea or chest pain. All symptoms resolved with appropriate intervention, such as, stopping the infusion prior to restarting or medical therapy with antihistamines and corticosteroids. Severe infusion reactions have been reported uncommonly. Symptoms reported include nausea, pyrexia, rigors, tachycardia, urticaria and vomiting.

Considering the rarity of Fabry Disease and the relatively limited number of patients exposed to agalsidase alfa to date, health-care professionals should be aware of the occurrence of the following very common adverse events observed in this patient population that were considered unrelated to agalsidase alfa: anorexia, insomnia, anxiety, depression, headache, dizziness, neuropathic pain, hypoesthesia, paraesthesia, syncope, vision blurred, vertigo, hypoacusis, ear pain, tinnitus, palpitations, nausea, diarrhoea, vomiting, abdominal pain, gastrointestinal upset, flatulence, abdominal distension, flu like illness, dyspnea, erythema, rash, contusion, musculoskeletal pain, pain exacerbated, chest pain, rigors, pyrexia, asthenia, malaise, peripheral edema, generalized infections, dysuria. An increase in the frequency of some events considered unrelated to treatment was reported following 6 to 12 months of therapy, none were considered serious. Most events were associated with Fabry Disease such as gastrointestinal disorders, changed temperature sensation/heat intolerance and dyspnea. Events that were not reported in placebo controlled trials but were observed after longer term treatment include asthenia.

Post-market Adverse Drug Reactions: The safety experience with the use of commercial Replagal is similar to that which has been reported in clinical trials. The most commonly reported adverse drug reactions have been infusion related reactions or infusion associated symptoms and were mild to moderate in severity. Symptoms have predominantly included chills (rigors) and facial flushing with a small number of patients experiencing headache, dyspnea, fever, urticaria and diarrhea. All symptoms resolved either with or without intervention. Reported intervention has included temporarily stopping the infusion for a few minutes prior to restarting, restarting the infusion at a slower rate, medical treatment with analgesics, antipyretics, antihistamines and or corticosteroids. In some cases subsequent infusions were premedicated, which after a limited period was successfully withdrawn.

DRUG INTERACTIONS:

> **Serious Drug Interactions**
> - **None**

Overview: Replagal should not be co-administered with chloroquine, amiodarone, benoquin or gentamicin since these substances have the potential to inhibit intra-cellular α-galactosidase activity.

As α-galactosidase A is itself an enzyme, it would be an unlikely candidate for cytochrome P450 mediated drug-drug interactions. In clinical studies, neuropathic pain medicinal products (such as carbamazepine, phenytoin and gabapentin) were administered concurrently to most patients without any evidence of interaction.

Drug-Drug Interactions: Replagal should not be co-administered with chloroquine, amiodarone, benoquin or gentamicin since these substances have the potential to inhibit intra-cellular α-galactosidase activity.
Drug-Herb Interactions: Interactions with herbal products have not been established.
Drug-Laboratory Interactions: Interactions with laboratory tests have not been established.

DOSAGE AND ADMINISTRATION: Dosing Considerations:
- Replagal (agalsidase alfa) is intended for long term, chronic use under the guidance and supervision of a physician; however, home infusion is permitted.
- Replagal is administered at a dose of 0.2 mg/kg body weight every other week by intravenous infusion over 40 minutes.
- For preparation and administration instructions, see Special Handling Instructions.

Recommended Dose and Dosage Adjustment: Replagal is administered at a dose of 0.2 mg/kg body weight every other week by intravenous infusion over 40 minutes. Replagal shows promising preliminary evidence of efficacy for the treatment of patients with Fabry Disease; however, the optimal individual dose requires further investigation. Studies are underway to evaluate more frequent and/or higher doses of Replagal therapy than used in clinical trials to date.
Administration: See Special Handling Instructions for method of dilution.

OVERDOSAGE:
No case of overdose has been reported.

> For management of a suspected drug overdose, CPhA recommends that you contact your **regional Poison Control Centre**. See the *CPS* Directory section for a list of Poison Control Centres.

ACTION AND CLINICAL PHARMACOLOGY: Mechanism of Action: Fabry Disease is a glycosphingolipid storage disorder that is caused by deficient activity of the lysosomal enzyme α-galactosidase A, resulting in accumulation of globotriaosylceramide (also referred to as Gb_3 or CTH), the glycosphingolipid substrate for this enzyme. Agalsidase alfa catalyzes the hydrolysis of Gb_3, cleaving a terminal galactose residue from the molecule. Treatment with the enzyme has been shown to reduce accumulation of Gb_3 in many cell types including endothelial and parenchymal cells. Agalsidase alfa has been produced in a human cell line to provide for a human glycosylation profile that can influence uptake by mannose-6-phosphate receptors on the surface of target cells.

Pharmacodynamics: Agalsidase alfa is a human α-galactosidase A produced by Gene Activation technology. Agalsidase alfa is a homodimer comprising 2 approximately 50,000 Dalton subunits, with each subunit containing 398 amino acid residues. The product is synthesized by a human cell line and has the identical amino acid sequence as that of α-galactosidase A produced in human tissues.

Agalsidase alfa is targeted to its lysosomal site of action by mannose-6-phosphate (M6P) residues on the agalsidase alfa molecule. The M6P moiety binds to a specific M6P receptor on the cell surface and is thus directed to the lysosomes. Many cells in the body contain M6P receptors, and agalsidase alfa has been shown to be taken up by the liver, kidney, heart, and blood vessels.

Agalsidase alfa is a highly purified preparation. Biological activity of agalsidase alfa is measured using the water soluble substrate 4-methylumbelliferyl-α-D-galactopyranoside (4-MUF-gal), and biological potency is measured based on its ability to be taken up by normal human cells.

Agalsidase alfa catalyzes the hydrolysis of Gb_3, cleaving a terminal galactose residue from the molecule. The hydrolysis of Gb_3 in affected individuals causes a reduction in the amount of Gb_3 in many cell types in the body, including cells in the liver, heart, kidney, and blood vessels, and in the plasma.

Pharmacokinetics: Single doses ranging from 0.007-0.2 mg enzyme per kg body weight were administered to adult male patients as 20-40 minute intravenous infusions while female patients received 0.2 mg enzyme per kg body weight as 40 minute infusions. The pharmacokinetic properties were essentially unaffected by the dose of the enzyme. Following a single intravenous dose of 0.2 mg/kg, agalsidase alfa had a biphasic distribution and elimination profile from the circulation. Pharmacokinetic parameters were not significantly different between male and female patients. Elimination half-lives were 108±17 minutes (1.8 hours) in males compared to 89±28 minutes (1.5 hours) in females and volume of distribution was approximately 17% body weight in both sexes. Clearance normalized for body weight was 2.66 and 2.10 mL/min/kg for males and females, respectively. Based on the similarity of pharmacokinetic properties of agalsidase alfa in both males and females, tissue distribution in major tissues and organs is also expected to be comparable in male and female patients.

Following six months of Replagal treatment 12 of 28 male patients showed altered pharmacokinetics including an apparent increase in clearance. These changes were associated with the development of low titre antibodies to agalsidase alfa.

Based on the analysis of pre- and post-dose liver biopsies in males with Fabry Disease, the tissue half-life has been estimated to be in excess of 24 hours and hepatic uptake of the enzyme estimated to be 10% of administered dose.

Agalsidase alfa is a protein and is therefore: 1) not expected to bind to proteins, 2) expected that metabolic degradation will follow the pathways of other proteins, i.e. peptide hydrolysis, and 3) unlikely to be a candidate for drug-drug interactions.

Renal elimination of agalsidase alfa is considered to be a minor clearance pathway since pharmacokinetic parameters are not altered by impaired renal function. As metabolism is expected to occur by peptide hydrolysis, impaired liver function is not expected to affect the pharmacokinetics of agalsidase alfa in a clinically significant manner.

A short-term study is being initiated to assess the pharmacodynamic and pharmacokinetic effects as well as the safety of alternative dosing regimens of Replagal in comparison to the current dosing regimen of 0.2 mg/kg every 2 weeks. Replagal doses between 0.1 and 0.4 mg/kg will be studied with weekly and biweekly infusions.

STORAGE AND STABILITY: Store at 2 to 8°C (in a refrigerator).

Replagal has a shelf life of 3 years.

After dilution, the product should be administered immediately (within 3 hours). The product does not contain any bacteriostatic preservative therefore storage of the diluted solution is not recommended; however, when prepared under aseptic conditions, the chemical and physical stability of the diluted solution has been demonstrated for 24 hours at 25°C.

SPECIAL HANDLING INSTRUCTIONS:
1. Calculate the dose and number of Replagal vials needed. Each Replagal vial contains 3.5 mg agalsidase alfa.
2. Dilute the total volume of Replagal concentrate required in 100 mL of 9 mg/mL (0.9%) sodium chloride solution for infusion. Care must be taken to ensure the sterility of the prepared solutions since Replagal does not contain any preservative or bacteriostatic agent; aseptic technique must be observed. Once diluted, the solution should be mixed gently but not shaken.
3. The solution should be inspected visually for particulate matter and discoloration prior to administration.
4. Administer the infusion solution over a period of 40 minutes using an intravenous line with an integral filter. After dilution, the product should be administered immediately (within 3 hours). The product does not contain any bacteriostatic preservative therefore storage of the diluted solution is not recommended; however, when prepared under aseptic conditions, the chemical and physical stability of the diluted solution has been demonstrated for 24 hours at 25°C.
5. Do not infuse Replagal concomitantly in the same intravenous line with other agents.
6. For single use only. Any unused product or waste material should be disposed of in accordance with local requirements.

INFORMATION FOR THE PATIENT: Published in e-CPS, available by subscription at www.e-cps.ca.

DOSAGE FORMS, COMPOSITION AND PACKAGING: Each vial contains 3.5 mg of agalsidase alfa.

Agalsidase alfa is the human protein α-galactosidase A produced by Gene Activation technology in a human cell line.

The concentrate must be diluted further, see Special Handling Instructions Procedures section.

Nonmedicinal ingredients: polysorbate 20, sodium chloride, sodium hydroxide, sodium phosphate monobasic, monohydrate and water for Injection. 3.5 mL of concentrate for solution for infusion in 5 mL vial (Type 1 glass) with a fluoro-resin coated butyl rubber stopper, a one piece aluminum seal and flip-off cap. Pack sizes of 1, 4 or 10 vials per carton. Not all pack sizes may be marketed.

Repronex™ Ⓟ

menotropins

Gonadotropins for Infertility

Ferring

PHARMACOLOGY: Repronex (menotropins for injection) administered for seven to twelve days, produces ovarian follicular growth in women who do not have primary ovarian failure. Treatment with menotropins in most instances results only in follicular growth and maturation. In order to effect ovulation, human chorionic gonadotropin (hCG) must be given following the administration of menotropins when clinical assessment of the patient indicates that sufficient follicular maturation has occurred.

Pharmacokinetics: In an early pharmacokinetic study including 16 healthy female volunteers, 300 IU menotropins were administered subcutaneously (SC) and intramuscularly (IM) in a crossover study, after patients' endogenous FSH and LH were suppressed. Measurements of serum FSH concentrations indicated that SC administration leads to higher values for both C_{max} and $AUC_{(0-\infty)}$ when compared to IM injections.

The subcutaneous and intramuscular routes were not bioequivalent. Compared to IM administration, the SC administration of menotropins results in an increase of FSH C_{max} and $AUC_{(0-\infty)}$ by 35 and 20% respectively.

Clinical studies for ovulation induction (in women with anovulatory or oligo-ovulatory infertility) and in vitro fertilization showed enhanced follicular development, induction of ovulation, and clinical pregnancies.

INDICATIONS: Repronex (menotropins for injection) and hCG given in a sequential manner are indicated for multiple follicular development (controlled ovarian stimulation) and induction of ovulation in infertile patients who have previously received pituitary suppression.

CONTRAINDICATIONS: Repronex (menotropins for injection) is contraindicated in women who have: a high FSH level indicating primary ovarian failure, uncontrolled thyroid and adrenal dysfunction, an organic intra cranial lesion such as a pituitary tumor, the presence of any cause of infertility other than anovulation unless they are candidates for in vitro-fertilization, abnormal bleeding of undetermined origin. ovarian cysts or enlargement not due to polycystic ovary syndrome, prior hypersensitivity to menotropins.

Repronex is contraindicated in women who are pregnant. There are limited human data on the effects of menotropins when administered during pregnancy.

WARNINGS: Repronex (menotropins for injection) is a drug that should only be used by physicians who are thoroughly familiar with infertility problems. It is a potent gonadotropic substance capable of causing mild to severe adverse reactions in women. Gonadotropin therapy requires a certain time commitment by physicians and supportive health professionals, and its use requires the availability of appropriate monitoring facilities (see Precautions, Laboratory Tests).

Overstimulation of the Ovary During Repronex Therapy: Ovarian Enlargement: Mild to moderate uncomplicated ovarian enlargement which may be accompanied by abdominal distension and/or abdominal pain, occurs in approximately 5 to 10% of those treated with Repronex and hCG, and generally regresses without treatment within two or three weeks.

In order to minimize the hazard associated with the occasional abnormal ovarian enlargement which may occur with Repronex -hCG therapy, the lowest dose consistent with expectation of good results should be used. Careful monitoring of ovarian response can further minimize the risk of overstimulation.

If the ovaries are abnormally enlarged on the last day of Repronex therapy, hCG should not be administered in this course of therapy; this will reduce the chances of development of the Ovarian Hyperstimulation Syndrome.

The Ovarian Hyperstimulation Syndrome (OHSS): OHSS is a medical event distinct from uncomplicated ovarian enlargement. OHSS may progress rapidly to become a serious medical event. It is characterized by an apparent dramatic increase in vascular permeability which can result in a rapid accumulation of fluid in the peritoneal cavity, thorax, and potentially, the pericardium. The early warning signs of development of OHSS are severe pelvic pain, nausea, vomiting, and weight gain. The following symptomatology has been seen with cases of OHSS: abdominal pain, abdominal distension, gastrointestinal symptoms including nausea, vomiting and diarrhea, severe ovarian enlargement, weight gain, dyspnea, and oliguria. Clinical evaluation may reveal hypovolemia, hemoconcentration, electrolyte imbalances, ascites, hemoperitoneum, pleural effusions, hydrothorax, acute pulmonary distress, and thromboembolic events (see Pulmonary and Vascular Complications). Transient liver function test abnormalities suggestive of hepatic dysfunction, which may be accompanied by morphologic changes on liver biopsy, have been reported in association with the Ovarian Hyperstimulation Syndrome (OHSS).

OHSS occurs in approximately 0.4% of patients when the recommended dose is administered and in 1.3% of patients when higher than recommended doses are administered. OHSS occurred in 3 of 125 (2.4%) Repronex treated women during the In Vitro Fertilization (IVF) clinical study. None of these cases was classified as severe. In the Ovulation Induction (OI) clinical study, 4 of 72 (5.5%) Repronex treated women developed OHSS and of this number, one case was classified as severe (1.4%). Cases of OHSS are more common, more severe and more protracted if pregnancy occurs. OHSS develops rapidly; therefore patients should be followed for at least two weeks after hCG administration. Most often, OHSS occurs after treatment has been discontinued and reaches its maximum at about seven to ten days following treatment. Usually, OHSS resolves spontaneously with the onset of menses. If there is evidence that OHSS may be developing prior to hCG administration (see Precautions, Laboratory Tests), the hCG should be withheld.

If OHSS occurs, treatment should be stopped and the patient hospitalized. Treatment is primarily symptomatic, consisting of bed rest, fluid and electrolyte management, and analgesics if needed. The phenomenon of hemoconcentration associated with fluid loss into the peritoneal cavity, pleural cavity, and the pericardial cavity has been seen to occur and should be thoroughly assessed in the following manner: 1) fluid intake and output, 2) weight, 3) hematocrit, 4) serum and urinary electrolytes, 5) urine specific gravity, 6) BUN and creatinine, and 7) abdominal girth. These determinations are to be performed daily or more often if the need arises.

With OHSS there is an increased risk of injury to the ovary. The ascitic, pleural, and pericardial fluid should not be removed unless absolutely necessary to relieve symptoms such as pulmonary distress or cardiac tamponade. Pelvic examination may cause rupture of an ovarian cyst, which may result in hemoperitoneum, and should therefore be avoided. If this does occur, and if bleeding becomes such that surgery is required, the surgical treatment should be designed to control bleeding and to retain as much ovarian tissue as possible. Intercourse should be prohibited in those patients in whom significant ovarian enlargement occurs after ovulation because of the danger of hemoperitoneum resulting from ruptured ovarian cysts.

The management of OHSS may be divided into three phases: the acute, the chronic, and the resolution phases. Because the use of diuretics can accentuate the diminished intravascular volume, diuretics should be avoided except in the late phase of resolution as described below.

Acute Phase: Management during the acute phase should be designed to prevent hemoconcentration due to loss of intravascular volume to the third space and to minimize the risk of thromboembolic phenomena and kidney damage. Treatment is designed to normalize electrolytes while maintaining an acceptable but somewhat reduced intravascular volume. Full correction of the intravascular volume deficit may lead to an unacceptable increase in the amount of third space fluid accumulation. Management includes administration of limited intravenous fluids, electrolytes, and human serum albumin. Monitoring for the development of hyperkalemia is recommended.

Chronic Phase: After stabilizing the patient during the acute phase, excessive fluid accumulation in the third space should be limited by instituting severe potassium, sodium, and fluid restriction.

Resolution Phase: A fall in hematocrit and an increasing urinary output without an increased intake are observed due to the return of third space fluid to the intravascular compartment. Peripheral and/or pulmonary edema may result if the kidneys are unable to excrete third space fluid as rapidly as it is mobilized. Diuretics may be indicated during the resolution phase if necessary to combat pulmonary edema.

Pulmonary and Vascular Complications: Serious pulmonary conditions (e.g. atelectasis, acute respiratory distress syndrome) have been reported. In addition, thromboembolic events both in association with, and separate from, the Ovarian Hyperstimulation Syndrome have been reported following menotropins therapy. Intravascular thrombosis and embolism, which may originate in venous or arterial vessels, can result in reduced blood flow to critical organs or the extremities. Sequelae of such events have included venous thrombophlebitis, pulmonary embolism, pulmonary infarction, cerebral vascular occlusion (stroke), and arterial occlusion resulting in loss of limb. In rare cases, pulmonary complications and/or thromboembolic events have resulted in death.

Multiple Births: Multiple pregnancies have occurred following treatment with Repronex IM and SC. In a clinical trial for ovulation induction in which Repronex IM and Repronex SC were directly compared, the rates of multiple pregnancies were as follows. Of the four clinical pregnancies with Repronex IM, two were single and two were multiple pregnancies. Both multiple pregnancies were triplet pregnancies. Of the six clinical pregnancies with Repronex SC, three were single and three were multiple pregnancies. The three multiple pregnancies included one twin pregnancy and two quadruplet pregnancies.

In a clinical trial of IVF patients in which Repronex IM and Repronex SC were directly compared, the rates of multiple pregnancies were as follows: Of the twenty four continuing pregnancies on Repronex IM, fourteen were single and ten were multiple pregnancies. The ten multiple pregnancies included three triplet and seven twin pregnancies. Of the twenty nine continuing pregnancies on Repronex SC, fourteen were single and fifteen were multiple pregnancies. The fifteen multiple pregnancies included three quadruplet, three triplet and nine twin pregnancies. The patient and her partner should be advised of the frequency and potential hazards of multiple gestation before starting treatment.

Hypersensitivity/Anaphylactic Reactions: Hypersensitivity/anaphylactic reactions associated with menotropins administration have been reported in some patients. These reactions presented as generalized urticaria, facial edema, angioneurotic edema, and/or dyspnea suggestive of laryngeal edema. The relationship of these symptoms to uncharacterized urinary proteins is uncertain.

PRECAUTIONS: General: Careful attention should be given to diagnosis in the selection of candidates for menotropins therapy (see Indications; Precautions).

Information to Be Provided to the Patient: Prior to therapy with Repronex(menotropins for injection), patients should be informed of the duration of treatment and the monitoring of their condition that will be required. Possible adverse reactions (see Adverse Effects) and the risk of multiple births should be discussed.

Selection of Patients: Before treatment with Repronex is instituted, a thorough gynecologic and endocrinologic evaluation must be performed. Except for those patients enrolled in an in vitro fertilization program, this should include a hysterosalpingogram (to rule out uterine and tubal pathology) and documentation of anovulation by means of basal body temperature, serial vaginal smears, examination of cervical mucus, determination of serum (or urine) progesterone, urinary pregnanediol and endometrial biopsy. Patients with tubal pathology should receive menotropins only if enrolled in an in vitro fertilization program.

Primary ovarian failure should be excluded by the determination of gonadotropin levels. Careful examination should be made to rule out the presence of an early pregnancy.

Patients in late reproductive life have a greater predilection to endometrial carcinoma as well as a higher incidence of anovulatory disorders. Cervical dilation and curettage should always be done for diagnosis before starting Repronex therapy in such patients who demonstrate abnormal uterine bleeding or other signs of endometrial abnormalities.

Evaluation of the partner's fertility potential should be included in the workup.

Pregnancy: See Contraindications.

Lactation: It is not known whether this drug is excreted in human milk. Because many drugs are excreted in human milk, caution should be exercised if menotropins are administered to a nursing woman.

Drug Interactions: No clinically significant drug/drug or drug/food adverse interactions have been reported during menotropins therapy.

Laboratory Tests: Treatment for Induction of Ovulation: In most instances, treatment with menotropins results only in follicular growth and maturation. In order to effect ovulation, hCG must be given following the administration of Repronex when clinical assessment of the patient indicates that sufficient follicular maturation has occurred. This may be directly estimated by measuring serum (or urinary) estrogen levels and sonographic visualization of the ovaries. The combination of both estradiol levels and ultrasonography are useful for monitoring the growth and development of follicles, timing hCG administration, as well as minimizing the risk of the Ovarian Hyperstimulation Syndrome and multiple gestation.

Other clinical parameters which may have potential use for monitoring menotropins therapy include: changes in the vaginal cytology; appearance and volume of the cervical mucus; spinnbarkeit; and ferning of the cervical mucus.

The above clinical indices provide an indirect estimate of the estrogenic effect upon the target organs, and therefore should only be used adjunctively with more direct estimates of follicular development, i.e. serum estradiol and ultrasonography.

The clinical confirmation of ovulation, with the exception of pregnancy, is obtained by direct and indirect indices of progesterone production. The indices most generally used are as follows: a rise in basal body temperature; increase in serum progesterone; and menstruation following the shift in basal body temperature.

When used in conjunction with indices of progesterone production, sonographic visualization of the ovaries will assist in determining if ovulation has occurred. Sonographic evidence of ovulation may include the following: fluid in the cul-de-sac, ovarian stigmata and collapsed follicle.

Because of the subjectivity of the various tests for the determination of follicular maturation and ovulation, it cannot be overemphasized that the physician should choose tests with which he/she is thoroughly familiar.

Carcinogenesis/Mutagenesis: Long-term toxicity studies in animals have not been performed to evaluate the carcinogenic potential of menotropins.

ADVERSE EFFECTS: The following adverse reactions, reported during menotropins therapy, are listed in decreasing order of potential severity: pulmonary and vascular complications (see Warnings), ovarian hyperstimulation syndrome (see Warnings), hemoperitoneum, adnexal torsion (as a complication of ovarian enlargement), mild to moderate ovarian enlargement; ovarian cysts, abdominal pain, sensitivity to menotropins (febrile reactions suggestive of allergic response have been reported following the administration of menotropins. Reports of flu-like symptoms including fever, chills, musculoskeletal aches, joint pains, nausea, headaches, and malaise have also been reported), gastrointestinal symptoms (nausea, vomiting, diarrhea, abdominal cramps, bloating), pain, rash, swelling and/or irritation at the site of injection, body rashes, dizziness, tachycardia, dyspnea, and tachypnea.

The following medical events have been reported subsequent to pregnancies resulting from menotropins therapy: ectopic pregnancy, congenital abnormalities.

From a study of 287 completed pregnancies following menotropins-hCG therapy, five incidents of birth defects were reported (1.7%). One infant had multiple congenital anomalies consisting of imperforate anus, aplasia of the sigmoid colon, third degree hypospadias, cecovesicle fistula, bifid scrotum, meningocele, bilateral internal tibial torsion, and right metatarsus adductus. Another infant was born with an imperforate anus and possible congenital heart lesions; another had a supernumerary digit; another was born with hypospadias and exstrophy of the bladder; and the fifth child had Down's syndrome. None of the investigators felt that these defects were drug-related. Subsequently one report of an infant death due to hydrocephalus and cardiac anomalies has been received.

There have been infrequent reports of ovarian neoplasms, both benign and malignant, in women who have undergone multiple drug regimens for ovulation induction; however, a causal relationship has not been established.

In the two randomized, controlled clinical studies, comparing Repronex (menotropins for injection) IM, Repronex SC and Pergonal IM in patients undergoing IVF and in patients with polycystic ovary disease and other diagnoses causing anovulation for ovulation induction, the adverse events occurring in ≥1% of patients exposed to Repronex IM or Repronex SC are described in Table 1.

Table 1: Repronex

Patients with Adverse Events ≥1%

Adverse Event	Repronex IM N=101	Repronex SC N=96
Injection Site AEs	n (%)	n (%)
Injection Site Edema	1 (1.0)	8 (8.3)[a]
Injection Site Reaction	2 (2.0)	8 (8.3)[a]
Genitourinary/Reproductive AEs		
OHSS	2 (2.0)	5 (5.2)
Vaginal Hemorrhage	8 (7.9)	3 (3.1)
Ovarian Disease	3 (3.0)	8 (8.3)
Ectopic Pregnancy	1 (1.0)	1 (1.0)
Pelvic Pain	3 (3.0)	1 (1.0)
Breast Tenderness	2 (2.0)	2 (2.1)
Gastrointestinal AEs		
Nausea	4 (4.0)	7 (7.3)
Vomiting	0 (0.0)	3 (3.1)
Diarrhea	0 (0.0)	2 (2.1)

(cont'd)

Table 1: Repronex *(cont'd)*

Patients with Adverse Events ≥1%

Adverse Event Injection Site AEs	Repronex IM N=101 n (%)	Repronex SC N=96 n (%)
Abdominal Cramping	7 (6.9)	5 (5.2)
Abdominal Pain	5 (5.0)	7 (7.3)
Enlarged Abdomen	6 (6.0)	2 (2.1)
Other Body System AEs		
Headache	6 (6.0)	5 (5.2)
Infection	1 (1.0)	0 (0.0)
Dyspnea	1 (1.0)	2 (2.1)

[a] Fisher's Exact/Chi-Squared Tests - significant for Repronex SC vs. Repronex IM.

Post-market Experience: Repronex has been marketed in the United States since 1997. All adverse events reported have been non-serious and expected reactions, and were predominantly injection site reactions, as well as fever, malaise and nausea. These reactions abated and resolved without sequelae.

OVERDOSE:

Symptoms: Aside from ovarian hyperstimulation (see Warnings), little is known concerning the consequences of acute overdosage with menotropins.

For management of a suspected drug overdose, CPhA recommends that you contact your **regional Poison Control Centre**. See the *CPS* Directory section for a list of Poison Control Centres.

DOSAGE: Infertile Patients with Oligo-Anovulation: The dose of Repronex (menotropins for injection) to produce maturation of the follicle must be individualized for each patient. It is recommended that the initial dose of Repronex to any patient should be 150 IU (for any patient receiving leuprolide or other GnRH therapy) of FSH/LH per day, for five days. Based on clinical monitoring (ultrasound results and serum estradiol concentrations) subsequent dosing should be adjusted according to individual patient response. Adjustments in dose should not be made more frequently than once every two days and should not exceed more than 75 to 150 IU per adjustment. The maximum daily dose of Repronex should not exceed 450 IU and dosing beyond 12 days is not recommended.

If patient response to Repronex is appropriate, hCG (5000 to 10 000 USP units) should be given one day following the last dose of Repronex. The hCG should be withheld if the serum estradiol is greater than 2000 pg/mL, if the ovaries are abnormally enlarged or if abdominal pain occurs, and the patient should be advised to refrain from intercourse. These precautions may reduce the risk of development of the Ovarian Hyperstimulation Syndrome and multiple gestation.

During treatment with both Repronex and hCG and during a two-week post-treatment period, patients should be examined at least every other day for signs of excessive ovarian stimulation. Most of the Ovarian Hyperstimulation Syndrome occurs after treatment has been discontinued and reaches its maximum at about seven to ten days post-ovulation. If there is inadequate follicle development, or follicle development or ovulation without subsequent pregnancy, the course of treatment with gonadotropins may be repeated.

The couple should be encouraged to have intercourse daily, beginning on the day prior to the administration of hCG until ovulation becomes apparent from the indices employed for the determination of progestational activity. Care should be taken to ensure insemination. In the light of the foregoing indices and parameters mentioned, it should become obvious that, unless a physician is willing to devote considerable time to these patients and be familiar with and conduct the necessary laboratory studies, he/she should not use Repronex.

Assisted Reproductive Technologies: The recommended initial dose of Repronex for patients who have received GnRH agonist or antagonist pituitary suppression is 225 IU. Based on clinical monitoring (including serum estradiol levels and vaginal ultrasound results) subsequent dosing should be adjusted according to individual patient response. Adjustments in dose should not be made more frequently than once every two days and should not exceed more than 75 to 150 IU per adjustment. The maximum daily dose of Repronex given should not exceed 450 IU and dosing beyond 12 days is not recommended.

Once adequate follicular development is evident, hCG (5000-10 000 USP units) should be administered to induce final follicular maturation in preparation for oocyte retrieval. The administration of hCG must be withheld in cases where the ovaries are abnormally enlarged on the last day of therapy. This should reduce the chance of developing OHSS.

Administration: Dissolve the contents of one to six vials of Repronex in one to two mL of 0.9% Sodium Chloride Injection and **administer subcutaneously or intramuscularly** immediately. Any unused reconstituted material should be discarded.

The lower abdomen (alternating sides) should be used for subcutaneous administration.

INFORMATION FOR THE PATIENT: Published in e-CPS, available by subscription at www.e-cps.ca.

SUPPLIED: Repronex (menotropins for injection) is a purified preparation of gonadotropins extracted from the urine of postmenopausal women. Each vial of a sterile, lyophilized, white to off-white powder, contains: follicle-stimulating hormone (FSH) 75 IU activity and luteinizing hormone (LH) 75 IU activity, plus 20 mg lactose monohydrate in a sterile, lyophilized form. By biological assay, one IU of LH for the Second International Reference Preparation for hMG is biologically equivalent to approximately 0.5 U of hCG. Boxes of 5 vials and 5 vials diluent (0.9% Sodium Chloride Injection, USP). Lyophilized powder may be stored at 3 to 25°C. Protect from light. Use immediately after reconstitution. Discard unused material.

ReQuip® Ⓟ

ropinirole HCl

Antiparkinsonian Agent—Dopamine Agonist

GlaxoSmithKline

Date of Revision: June 17, 2010

SUMMARY PRODUCT INFORMATION:

Route of Administration	Dosage Form/ Strength	Clinically Relevant Nonmedicinal Ingredients
Oral	Tablets 0.25 mg, 1 mg, 2 mg, 5 mg	Hydrous lactose For a complete listing see Dosage Forms, Composition and Packaging.

INDICATIONS AND CLINICAL USE: Adults: REQUIP (ropinirole hydrochloride) is indicated in the treatment of the signs and symptoms of idiopathic Parkinson's disease.

REQUIP can be used both as early therapy without concomitant levodopa and as an adjunct to levodopa.

Geriatrics (>65 years of age): Oral clearance of REQUIP is reduced in patients older than 65 years of age, however the dosing of ropinirole for elderly patients can be titrated in the normal manner. (See Action and Clinical Pharmacology, Special Populations and Conditions, Geriatrics.)

Pediatrics (≤18 years of age): The safety and efficacy of REQUIP have not been established in children under 18 years of age, therefore REQUIP is not recommended in this patient population.

CONTRAINDICATIONS: REQUIP is contraindicated in patients with a known hypersensitivity to ropinirole hydrochloride or the excipients of the drug product. For a complete listing of excipients, see Dosage Forms, Composition and Packaging.

WARNINGS AND PRECAUTIONS:

Serious Warnings and Precautions

Sudden Onset of Sleep: Patients receiving treatment with REQUIP and other dopaminergic agents have reported suddenly falling asleep while engaged in activities of daily living, including operating a motor vehicle, which has sometimes resulted in accidents. Although some of the patients reported somnolence while on REQUIP, others perceived that they had no warning signs, such as excessive drowsiness, and believed that they were alert immediately prior to the event.

Physicians should alert patients of the reported cases of sudden onset of sleep, bearing in mind that these events are **not** limited to initiation of therapy. Patients should also be advised that sudden onset of sleep has occurred without warning signs. If drowsiness or sudden onset of sleep should occur, patients should immediately contact their physician.

Until further information is available on the management of this unpredictable and serious adverse event, patients should be warned not to drive or engage in other activities where impaired alertness could put themselves and others at risk of serious injury or death (e.g., operating machines). Episodes of falling asleep while engaged in activities of daily living have also been reported in patients taking other dopaminergic agents, therefore, symptoms may not be alleviated by substituting these products.

Presently, the precise cause of this event is unknown. It is known that many Parkinson's disease patients experience alterations in sleep architecture, which results in excessive daytime sleepiness or spontaneous dozing, and that dopaminergic agents can also induce sleepiness. There is insufficient information to determine whether this event is associated with REQUIP, all dopaminergic agents or Parkinson's disease itself.

The following Warnings and Precautions are listed in alphabetical order.

Cardiovascular: Patients with Pre-existing Cardiovascular Conditions: Since REQUIP has not been studied in patients with a history or evidence of significant cardiovascular disease including myocardial infarction, unstable angina, cardiac decompensation, cardiac arrhythmias, vaso-occlusive disease (including cerebral) or cardiomyopathy, it should be used with caution in such patients.

There is limited experience with REQUIP in patients treated with antihypertensive and antiarrhythmic agents. Consequently, in such patients, the dose of REQUIP should be titrated with caution.

Orthostatic Hypotension: Dopamine agonists appear to impair the systemic regulation of blood pressure with resulting orthostatic symptoms of dizziness or lightheadedness, with or without documented hypotension. These symptoms appear to occur especially during dose initiation and escalation. Therefore, patients treated with REQUIP and other dopamine agonists should be carefully monitored for signs and symptoms of orthostatic hypotension, especially during dose initiation and escalation (see Dosage and Administration) and should be informed of this risk.

Connective Tissue: Fibrotic Complications: Cases of retroperitoneal fibrosis, pulmonary infiltrates, pleural effusion, pleural thickening, pericarditis, and cardiac valvulopathy have been reported in some patients treated with ergot-derived dopaminergic agents. While these complications may resolve when the drug is discontinued, complete resolution does not always occur.

Although these adverse events are believed to be related to the ergoline structure of these compounds, whether other, non-ergot-derived dopamine agonists can cause them is unknown.

A small number of reports have been received of possible fibrotic complications, including pleural effusion, pleural fibrosis, interstitial lung diseases, and cardiac valvulopathy, in the development program and postmarketing experience for REQUIP. While the evidence is not sufficient to establish a causal relationship between REQUIP and these fibrotic complications, a contribution of REQUIP cannot be completely ruled out in rare cases.

Neurologic: Neuroleptic Malignant Syndrome: A symptom complex resembling the neuroleptic malignant syndrome (characterized by elevated temperature, muscular rigidity, altered consciousness, and autonomic instability), with no other obvious aetiology, has been reported in association with rapid dose reduction, withdrawal of, or changes in antiparkinsonian therapy.

A single spontaneous report of a symptom complex resembling the neuroleptic malignant syndrome has been observed in a 66 year old diabetic male patient with Parkinson's disease, who developed fever, muscle stiffness, and drowsiness 8 days after beginning REQUIP treatment. The patient also experienced acute bronchitis, which did not respond to antibiotic treatment. REQUIP was discontinued three days before the patient died. The reporting physician considered these events to be possibly related to REQUIP treatment (see Dosage and Administration).

A single spontaneous report of severe muscle pain has been reported in a 66 year old male patient around his thigh. The reporting physician considered the event to be probably related to REQUIP treatment.

Dyskinesia with Adjunctive Levodopa: REQUIP may potentiate the dopaminergic side effects of levodopa and may cause or exacerbate pre-existing dyskinesia. Decreasing the dose of levodopa may ameliorate this side effect.

Ophthalmologic: Retinal Pathology in Rats: In a two year carcinogenicity study in albino Sprague-Dawley rats, retinal atrophy was observed at incidences of 0%, 1.4%, 1.4% and 10% of male rats and 0%, 4.4%, 2.9% and 12.9% of female rats dosed at 0, 1.5, 15 and 50 mg/kg/day respectively. The incidence was statistically significant at 50 mg/kg/day. This dose represents a 2.8 fold (AUC) and 13.1 fold (C_{max}) greater exposure to ropinirole in rats than the exposure in humans at the maximum recommended dose of REQUIP of 24 mg/day.

While the potential significance of this effect on humans has not been established, it cannot be excluded that human albinos (or people who suffer from albinismus oculi) might have an increased susceptibility to ropinirole compared to normally pigmented people. Therefore, such patients should take ropinirole only under ophthalmological control.

Psychiatric: Compulsive Behaviours: Impulse control symptoms including compulsive behaviours such as pathological gambling and hypersexuality have been reported in patients treated with dopaminergic agents, including ropinirole. As described in the literature, such behaviours have been reported principally in Parkinson's disease patients treated with dopaminergic agents, especially at higher doses, and were generally reversible upon dose reduction or treatment discontinuation. In some ropinirole cases, other factors were present such as a history of compulsive behaviours or concurrent dopaminergic treatment.

Hallucinations: Early Therapy: In placebo-controlled trials, REQUIP caused hallucinations in 5.1% of patients during early therapy (1.4% in the placebo group). Hallucinations were of sufficient severity to result in that it led to discontinuation in 1.3% of patients. The incidence of hallucinations was dose-dependent.

In a 5-year study comparing REQUIP with levodopa in early Parkinson's patients, the overall incidence of hallucinations was 17.3% (31/179) for patients treated with REQUIP and 5.6% (5/89) for levodopa patients. Hallucinations led to discontinuation of the study treatment in 5.0% of REQUIP and 2.2% of levodopa patients. In a 3-year study comparing REQUIP with another dopamine agonist, the overall incidence of hallucinations was 9.5% (16/168) for patients treated with REQUIP and 9.0% (15/167) for patients receiving active comparator. Hallucinations led to discontinuation of the study treatment in 2.4% of REQUIP patients and 3.0% of comparator patients.

Concomitant Selegiline: In a 5-year study, REQUIP patients receiving concomitant selegiline reported a higher incidence of hallucinations (23.5%) than did those without (12.2%); this subpopulation effect was not seen in the L-dopa arm (hallucinations with concomitant selegiline=2.0% vs. hallucinations without selegiline=8.0%).

Adjunct Therapy: Hallucinations were experienced by 10.1% of patients receiving REQUIP and levodopa, compared to 4.2% receiving placebo and levodopa. Hallucinations were of sufficient severity that it led to discontinuation in 1.9% of patients. The incidence of hallucinations was dose dependent.

Skin: Melanoma: Epidemiological studies have shown that patients with Parkinson's disease have a higher risk (2- to approximately 6-fold higher) of developing melanoma than the general population. Whether the increased risk observed was due to Parkinson's disease or other factors, such as drugs used to treat Parkinson's disease, is unclear. For the reasons stated above, patients and healthcare providers are advised to monitor for melanomas frequently and on a regular basis when using REQUIP for **any** indication. Ideally, periodic skin examinations should be performed by appropriately qualified individuals (e.g., dermatologists).

Special Populations: Pregnant Women: The use of REQUIP during pregnancy is not recommended. REQUIP given to pregnant rats during organogenesis (gestation days 8 through 15) resulted in decreased fetal body weight at 60 mg/kg/day (approximately 3-4 times the AUC at the maximal human dose of 8 mg t.i.d), increased fetal death at 90 mg/kg/day (approximately 5 times the AUC at the maximal human dose of 8 mg t.i.d) and digital malformations at 150 mg/kg/day (approximately 8-9 times the AUC at the maximal human dose of 8 mg t.i.d). These effects occurred at maternally toxic doses. There was no indication of an effect on development of the conceptus at a maternally toxic dose of 20 mg/kg/day in the rabbit. In a perinatal-postnatal study in rats, 10 mg/kg/day of REQUIP (approximately 0.5-0.6 times the AUC at the maximal human dose of 8 mg t.i.d) impaired growth and development of nursing offspring and altered neurological development of female offspring.

Nursing Women: Since REQUIP suppresses lactation, it should not be administered to mothers who wish to breast-feed infants.

Studies in rats have shown that REQUIP and/or its metabolites cross the placenta and are excreted in breast milk. Consequently, the human foetus and/or neonate may be exposed to dopamine agonist activity.

Use in Women Receiving Oestrogen Replacement Therapy: In female patients on long-term treatment with conjugated oestrogens, oral clearance was reduced and elimination half-life prolonged compared to patients not receiving oestrogens (see Action and Clinical Pharmacology, Special Populations and Conditions). In patients, already receiving oestrogen replacement therapy, REQUIP may be titrated in the recommended manner according to clinical response. However, if oestrogen replacement therapy is stopped or introduced during treatment with REQUIP, adjustment of the REQUIP dosage may be required.

Pediatrics: Safety and effectiveness in the paediatric population have not been established.

Renal Impairment: No dosage adjustment is needed in patients with mild to moderate renal impairment (creatinine clearance between 30 to 50 mL/min; see Action and Clinical Pharmacology).

Because the use of REQUIP in patients with severe renal impairment (creatinine clearance less than 30 mL/min without regular dialysis) has not been studied, administration of REQUIP to such patients is not recommended.

In patients with end stage renal disease (ESRD), a lower maximum dose is recommended which, compared to the maximum exposure evaluated in clinical trials, results in similar exposure to ropinirole, and to a 4.5-fold increased exposure to the N-despropyl inactive metabolite (see Dosage and Administration and Action and Clinical Pharmacology, Special Populations and Conditions). Caution should be taken with the use of concomitant CYP1A2 inhibitors in these patients.

Hepatic Impairment: The use of ropinirole in patients with hepatic impairment has not been studied. Administration of ropinirole to such patients is not recommended.

ADVERSE REACTIONS: Adverse Drug Reaction Overview: Most Frequent Adverse Events: Adverse events occurring with an incidence of greater than, or equal to, 10% were as follows: **Early therapy:** nausea, dizziness, somnolence, headache, peripheral oedema, vomiting, syncope, fatigue and viral infection. **Adjunct therapy:** dyskinesia, nausea, dizziness, somnolence and headache.

Adverse Reactions Associated with Discontinuation of Treatment: Of 1599 patients who received REQUIP during the premarketing clinical trials, 17.1% in early-therapy studies and 17.3% in adjunct-therapy studies discontinued treatment due to adverse reactions. The events resulting in discontinuation of REQUIP in 1% or more of patients were as follows: **Early therapy:** nausea (6.4%), dizziness (3.8%), aggravated Parkinson's disease (1.3%), hallucination (1.3%), headache (1.3%), somnolence (1.3%) and vomiting (1.3%). **Adjunct therapy:** dizziness (2.9%), dyskinesia (2.4%), confusion (2.4%), vomiting (2.4%), hallucination (1.9%), nausea (1.9%), anxiety (1.9%), and increased sweating (1.4%). Patients over 75 years of age (n=130) showed slightly higher incidences of withdrawal due to hallucination, confusion and dizziness than patients less than 75 years of age.

Clinical Trial Adverse Drug Reactions: Because clinical trials are conducted under very specific conditions the adverse reaction rates observed in the clinical trials may not reflect the rates observed in practice and should not be compared to the rates in the clinical trials of another drug. Adverse drug reaction information from clinical trials is useful for identifying drug-related adverse events and for approximating rates.

Incidence of Adverse Drug Reactions in Placebo Controlled Trials: The incidence of postural hypotension, an event commonly associated with initiation of dopamine agonist therapy, was not notably different from placebo in clinical trials. However, decreases in systolic blood pressure to <90 mmHg have been observed in 13% (<65 years), 16% (65-75 years) and 7.6% (>75 years) of patients treated with REQUIP.

Table 1 lists adverse events that occurred at an incidence of 1% or more among REQUIP-treated patients who participated in placebo-controlled trials for up to one year. Patients were dosed in a range of 0.75 mg to 24 mg/day. Reported adverse events were classified using a standard World Health Organization Reaction Term Thesaurus (WHO-ART).

Table 1: REQUIP

Adverse Events with Incidence >1% From All Placebo-controlled Early and Adjunct Therapy Studies

	Early Therapy		Adjunct Therapy	
	REQUIP N=157 % occurrence	**Placebo N=147 % occurrence**	**REQUIP N=208 % occurrence**	**Placebo N=120 % occurrence**
Autonomic Nervous System				
Sweating Increased	6.4	4.1	7.2	1.7
Mouth Dry	5.1	3.4	5.3	0.8
Flushing	3.2	0.7	1.4	0.8
Body as a Whole General				
Peripheral Edema	13.4	4.1	3.9	2.5
Fatigue	10.8	4.1	—	—
Injury	—	—	10.6	9.2
Pain	7.6	4.1	5.3	3.3
Asthenia	6.4	1.4	—	—
Drug Level Increased	4.5	2.7	6.7	3.3
Chest Pain	3.8	2.0	—	—
Malaise	3.2	0.7	1.4	0.8
Therapeutic Response Decreased	1.9	0.7	—	—
Cellulitis	1.3	0.0	—	—
Influenza-like Symptoms	—	—	1.0	0.0
Fever	—	—	1.4	0.0
Cardiovascular General				
Syncope	11.5	1.4	2.9	1.7
Hypotension Postural	6.4	4.8	—	—
Hypertension	4.5	3.4	3.4	3.3
Hypotension	1.9	0.0	2.4	0.8

(cont'd)

Table 1: REQUIP *(cont'd)*

Adverse Events with Incidence >1% From All Placebo-controlled Early and Adjunct Therapy Studies

	Early Therapy		Adjunct Therapy	
	REQUIP N=157 % occurrence	**Placebo N=147 % occurrence**	**REQUIP N=208 % occurrence**	**Placebo N=120 % occurrence**
Cardiac Failure	—	—	1.0	0.0
Central and Peripheral Nervous Systems				
Dizziness	40.1	21.8	26.0	15.8
Dyskinesia	—	—	33.7	12.5
Headache	17.2	17.0	16.8	11.7
Ataxia (Falls)	—	—	9.6	6.7
Tremor	—	—	6.3	2.5
Paresthesia	—	—	5.3	2.5
Hyperesthesia	3.8	2.0	—	—
Dystonia	—	—	4.3	4.2
Hypokinesia	—	—	5.3	4.2
Paresis	—	—	2.9	0.0
Speech Disorder	—	—	1.0	0.0
Vertigo	1.9	0.0	—	—
Carpal Tunnel Syndrome	1.3	0.7	—	—
Gastrointestinal				
Nausea	59.9	21.8	29.8	18.3
Vomiting	12.1	6.8	7.2	4.2
Dyspepsia	9.6	4.8	—	—
Constipation	8.3	7.5	5.8	3.3
Abdominal Pain	6.4	2.7	8.7	7.5
Diarrhea	—	—	4.8	2.5
Anorexia	3.8	1.4	—	—
Flatulence	2.5	1.4	1.9	0.8
Tooth Disorder	1.9	0.7	1.0	0.8
Saliva Increased	—	—	2.4	0.8
Colitis	1.3	0.0	—	—
Dysphagia	1.3	0.0	2.4	0.8
Periodontitis	1.3	0.0	1.4	0.8
Eructation	—	—	1.4	0.0
Fecal Incontinence	—	—	1.0	0.0
Hemorrhoids	—	—	1.0	0.0
Gastroesophageal Reflux	—	—	1.0	0.0
Gastrointestinal Disorder (NOS)	—	—	1.0	0.0
Tooth Ache	—	—	1.0	0.0
Hearing and Vestibular				
Tinnitus	1.3	0.0	—	—
Heart Rate and Rhythm				
Palpitation	3.2	2.0	2.9	2.5
Extrasystoles	1.9	0.7	—	—

(cont'd)

Table 1: REQUIP *(cont'd)*

Adverse Events with Incidence >1% From All Placebo-controlled Early and Adjunct Therapy Studies

	Early Therapy		Adjunct Therapy	
	REQUIP N=157 % occurrence	Placebo N=147 % occurrence	REQUIP N=208 % occurrence	Placebo N=120 % occurrence
Tachycardia	1.9	0.0	1.0	0.0
Fibrillation Atrial	1.9	0.0	—	—
Tachycardia Supraventricular	1.3	0.0	—	—
Bradycardia	—	—	1.0	0.0
Liver and Biliary				
Gamma-GT Increased	1.3	0.7	1.0	0.0
Hepatic Enzymes Increased	1.3	0.0	—	—
Metabolic and Nutritional				
Alkaline Phosphate Increased	2.5	1.4	1.0	0.0
Weight Decrease	—	—	2.4	0.8
Hypoglycemia	1.3	0.0	—	—
Musculoskeletal				
Arthralgia	—	—	6.7	5.0
Arthritis	—	—	2.9	0.8
Arthritis Aggravated	1.3	0.0	1.4	0.0
Myocardial, Endocardial, Pericardial Valve				
Myocardial Ischemia	1.3	0.7	—	—
Psychiatric				
Somnolence	40.1	6.1	20.2	8.3
Anxiety	—	—	6.3	3.3
Confusion	5.1	1.4	8.7	1.7
Hallucination	5.1	1.4	10.1	4.2
Nervousness	—	—	4.8	2.5
Yawning	3.2	0.0	—	—
Amnesia	2.5	1.4	4.8	0.8
Dreaming Abnormal	—	—	2.9	1.7
Depersonalization	—	—	1.4	0.0
Paranoid Reaction	—	—	1.4	0.0
Agitation	1.3	0.7	1.0	0.0
Concentration Impaired	1.9	0.0	1.0	0.0
Illusion	1.3	0.0	—	—
Thinking Abnormal	—	—	1.4	0.8
Apathy	—	—	1.0	0.0
Personality Disorder	—	—	1.0	0.0
Red Blood Cell				
Anemia	—	—	2.4	0.0
Reproductive Male				
Impotence	2.5	1.4	—	—
Prostatic Disorder	—	—	1.0	0.0
Penis Disorder	—	—	1.3	0.0

(cont'd)

Table 1: REQUIP *(cont'd)*

Adverse Events with Incidence >1% From All Placebo-controlled Early and Adjunct Therapy Studies

	Early Therapy		Adjunct Therapy	
	REQUIP N=157 % occurrence	Placebo N=147 % occurrence	REQUIP N=208 % occurrence	Placebo N=120 % occurrence
Resistance Mechanism				
Upper Respiratory Tract Infection	—	—	8.7	8.3
Infection Viral	10.8	3.4	7.2	6.7
Respiratory				
Pharyngitis	6.4	4.1		
Rhinitis	3.8	2.7		
Sinusitis	3.8	2.7		
Dyspnea	3.2	0.0	2.9	1.7
Bronchitis	2.5	1.4	—	—
Respiratory Disorder	1.9	1.4	1.9	0.0
Pneumonia	1.3	0.7	1.0	0.8
Coughing	—	—	1.4	0.8
Skin/Appendages				
Pruritus	—	—	1.0	0.0
Urinary				
Urinary Tract Infection	5.1	4.1	6.3	2.5
Cystitis	1.3	0.7	—	—
Micturition Frequency	—	—	1.4	0.0
Pyuria	—	—	1.9	0.8
Urinary Incontinence	—	—	1.9	0.8
Urinary Retention	1.3	0.7	—	—
Dysuria	—	—	1.0	0.0
Vascular Extracardiac				
Peripheral Ischemia	2.5	0.0	—	—
Vision				
Vision Abnormal	5.7	3.4	—	—
Eye Abnormality	3.2	1.4	—	—
Diplopia	—	—	1.9	0.8
Xerophthalmia	1.9	0.0	1.4	0.8
Cataract	—	—	1.4	0.8
Lacrimation Abnormal	—	—	1.4	0.0
White Cell and Reticuloendothelial System				
Eosinophilia	—	—	1.4	0.0

— Incidence of adverse event <1%.

In addition to the events listed in Table 1, the following adverse events were recorded with rates equal to, or more common in, placebo-treated patients:

Early Therapy: fever, hot flushes, injury, rigors, ataxia, dyskinesia, dystonia, hyperkinesia, involuntary muscle contractions, paresthesia, aggravated Parkinsonism, tremor, diarrhea, gingivitis, increased saliva, bradycardia, gout, hyperglycemia, decreased weight, arthralgia, arthritis, back pain, myalgia, basal cell carcinoma, anxiety, depression, abnormal dreaming, insomnia, nervousness, prostatic disorder, upper respiratory tract infection, coughing, rash, hematuria and leg cramps.

Adjunct Therapy: asthenia, chest pain, fatigue, hot flushes, postural hypotension, abnormal gait, hyperkinesia, aggravated Parkinsonism, vertigo, abdominal pain, constipation, back pain, myalgia, depression, insomnia, paroniria (WHO dictionary term for nightmares), viral infection, upper respiratory tract infection, pharyngitis, rhinitis, rash, rash erythematous, taste perversion, hematuria, leg cramps and diplopia, myocardial infarction, extrasystoles supraventricular.

Events Observed During the Pre-marketing Evaluation of REQUIP: Of the 1599 patients who received REQUIP in therapeutic studies, the following adverse events, which are not included in Table 1 or in the listing above, have been noted up to May 1996. In the absence of appropriate controls in some of the studies, a causal relationship between these events and treatment with REQUIP cannot be determined.

Events are categorized by body system and listed in order of decreasing frequency according to the following definitions: **"frequent"** adverse events are those occurring on one or more occasions in at least 1/100 patients; **"infrequent"** adverse events are those occurring in 1/100 to 1/1000 patients; **"rare"** events are those occurring in fewer than 1/1000 patients.

Table 2: REQUIP

Adverse Events Observed During the Pre-marketing Evaluation of REQUIP

Frequency	Frequent <10% and ≥1%	Infrequent <1% and ≥0.1%	Rare <0.1% and ≥0.01%
Body System			
Autonomic Nervous System			cold, clammy hands
Body as a Whole		pallor, allergy, enlarged abdomen, substernal chest pain, oedema allergic reaction, ascites, precordial chest pain, therapeutic response increased, ischemic necrosis, oedema generalized	periorbital oedema, face oedema, halitosis
Cardiovascular System		cardiac failure, heart disorder, specific abnormal ECG, aneurysm, cardiomegaly, abnormal ECG, aggravated hypertension	cyanosis, fluid overload, heart valve disorder
Central and Peripheral Nervous System	neuralgia	hypertonia, speech disorder, choreoathetosis, abnormal coordination, dysphonia, extrapyramidal disorder, migraine, aphasia, coma, convulsions, hypotonia, nerve root lesion, peripheral neuropathy, paralysis, stupor	cerebral atrophy, grand mal convulsions, hemiparesis, hemiplegia, hyperreflexia, neuropathy, ptosis, sensory disturbance, hydrocephaly
Collagen			rheumatoid arthritis
Endocrine System		gynaecomastia, hypothyroidism	SIADH (syndrome of inappropriate anti-diuretic hormone secretion), increased thyroxine, goiter, hyperthyroid
Gastrointestinal System	gastrointestinal disorder (NOS)	gastritis, gastroenteritis, gastroesophageal reflux, increased appetite, oesophagitis, peptic ulcer, diverticulitis, hemorrhoids, hiccup, tooth caries, increased amylase, duodenal ulcer, duodenitis, fecal incontinence, GI hemorrhage, glossitis, rectal hemorrhage, melena, pancreatitis, rectal disorder, altered saliva, stomatitis, ulcerative stomatitis, tongue oedema, gastric ulcer, tooth disorder	oesophageal stricture, oesophageal ulceration, hemorrhagic gastritis, gingival bleeding, haematemesis, lactose intolerance, salivary duct obstruction, tenesmus, tongue disorder, hemorrhagic duodenal ulcer, aggravated tooth caries
Hearing		earache, decreased hearing, vestibular disorder, ear disorder (NOS)	hyperacusis, deafness
Heart Rate and Rhythm		arrhythmia, bundle branch block, cardiac arrest, supraventricular extrasystoles, ventricular tachycardia	atrioventricular block
Liver and Biliary System		abnormal hepatic function, increased ALT, bilirubinemia, cholecystitis, cholelithiasis, hepatocellular damage, increased AST	biliary pain, aggravated bilirubinemia, gall bladder disorder
Metabolic and Nutritional System	increased blood urea nitrogen	increased LDH, increased NPN, hyperuricemia, increased weight, hyperphosphatemia, diabetes mellitus, glycosuria, hypercholesterolemia, acidosis, hypokalemia, hyponatremia, thirst, increased creatine phosphokinase, dehydration, aggravated diabetes mellitus, hyperkalemia	electrolyte abnormality, enzyme abnormality, hypochloremia, obesity, increased phosphatase acid, decreased serum iron
Musculoskeletal System	arthrosis	arthropathy, osteoporosis, tendonitis, bone disorder, bursitis, muscle weakness, polymyalgia rheumatica, skeletal pain, torticollis	muscle atrophy, myositis, Dupuytren's contracture, spine malformation
Myocardial, Endocardial, Pericardial Valve	angina pectoris	myocardial infarction, aggravated angina pectoris	mitral insufficiency

(cont'd)

Table 2: REQUIP *(cont'd)*

Adverse Events Observed During the Pre-marketing Evaluation of REQUIP

Frequency	Frequent <10% and ≥1%	Infrequent <1% and ≥0.1%	Rare <0.1% and ≥0.01%
Body System			
Neoplasm		carcinoma, malignant female breast neoplasm, dermoid cyst, malignant skin neoplasm, prostate adenocarcinoma, adenocarcinoma, neoplasm (NOS)	bladder carcinoma, benign brain neoplasm, breast fibroadenosis, malignant endometrial neoplasm, oesophageal carcinoma, malignant larynx neoplasm, malignant lymphoma, malignant neoplasm, neuroma , lipoma, rectal carcinoma, uterine neoplasm
Platelet Bleeding and Clotting		purpura, thrombocytopenia, haematoma	
Psychiatric	aggravated depression, agitation	sleep disorder, apathy, dementia, delirium, emotional lability, psychosis, aggressive reaction, delusion, psychotic depression, euphoria, decreased libido, manic reaction, neurosis, personality disorder, somnambulism	suicide attempt
Red Blood Cell		hypochromic anaemia, anaemia B_{12} deficiency	polycythemia
Female Reproductive		amenorrhea, menstrual disorder, vaginal hemorrhage, uterine disorders (NOS)	female breast enlargement, inter-menstrual bleeding, mastitis, uterine hemorrhage, dysmenorrhoea
Male Reproductive		epididymitis, balanoposthitis, ejaculation failure, penis disorder, perineal pain	Peyronie's disease, ejaculation disorder, testicular disorder
Resistance Mechanism	infection	herpes zoster, moniliasis, otitis media, sepsis, herpes simplex, fungal infection, abscess, bacterial infection, genital moniliasis	poliomyelitis
Respiratory System	pneumonia	asthma, epistaxis, laryngitis, pleurisy, increased sputum, pulmonary oedema	hypoxia, respiratory insufficiency, vocal cord paralysis
Skin and Appendages		dermatitis, alopecia, skin discoloration, dry skin, skin hypertrophy, skin ulceration, fungal dermatitis, eczema, hyperkeratosis, photosensitivity reaction, psoriasis, maculopapular rash, psoriaform rash, seborrhoea, skin disorder, urticaria, furunculosis	bullous eruption, nail disorder, nevus, photosensitivity allergic reaction, aggravated psoriasis, skin exfoliation, abnormal skin odour
Other Special Senses			parosmia
Urinary		albuminuria, dysuria, nocturia, polyuria, renal calculus, abnormal urine, micturition disorder	oliguria, pyelonephritis, renal cyst, acute renal failure, renal pain, uremia, urethral disorder, urinary casts, bladder calculus, nephritis
Vascular Extracariac		cerebrovascular disorder, vein disorder, varicose vein, peripheral gangrene, phlebitis, vascular disorder	atherosclerosis, limb embolism, pulmonary embolism, gangrene, superficial phlebitis, subarachnoid hemorrhage, deep thrombophlebitis, leg thrombophlebitis, thrombosis, arteritis
Vision		conjunctivitis, blepharitis, abnormal accommodation, blepharospasm, eye pain, glaucoma, photophobia, scotoma	blindness, blindness temporary, hemianopia, keratitis, photopsia, macula lutea degeneration, vitreous detachment, retinal disorder
White Cell and Reticuloendothelial System		leukocytosis, leukopenia, lymphopenia, lymphedema, lymphocytosis	lymphadenopathy, granulocytopenia

Events Observed During Long-term Therapy with REQUIP: In two long-term, comparator-controlled studies of early therapy (durations of three and five years), patients with mild to moderate Parkinson's Disease initiated treatment on REQUIP alone, with open L-dopa available as supplementary medication.

The overall rates of withdrawal due to adverse events were 27% for the five year study and 20% for the three year one. Table 3 lists the adverse events that occurred at an incidence of 5% or more in these two studies.

Concomitant Selegiline and Associated Hallucination Rates: In the five year study, REQUIP patients receiving concomitant selegiline reported a higher incidence of hallucination (23.5%) than did those without (12.2%); this subpopulation effect was not seen in the L-dopa arm (hallucination with concomitant selegiline=2.0% vs hallucination without selegiline=8.0%).

Adverse Drug Reactions from Post-Market Experience and Post-Launch Clinical Trials: The following section enumerates potentially important adverse drug reactions that have been reported spontaneously to various surveillance systems and have also occurred in post-launch clinical trials. The events enumerated represent reports arising from both domestic and nondomestic use of ropinirole. These events do not include those already listed in Adverse Reactions above.

Patients treated with REQUIP have rarely reported suddenly falling asleep while engaged in activities of daily living, including operation of motor vehicles which has sometimes resulted in accidents (see Warnings and Precautions).

Pathological (compulsive) gambling has been reported in post-market data, including those in the literature, for antiparkinson drugs. Sporatic cases of pathological (compulsive) gambling have been reported in patients treated with REQUIP. Dosage adjustment should be considered in the management of this behaviour.

Table 3: REQUIP

Adverse Events with Incidence of >5% from 2 Long-term Comparator-controlled Early Therapy Studies (regardless of the presence or absence of concomitant L-dopa)

	Three-year Study		Five-year Study	
	REQUIP (N=168) % occurrence	**Dopamine Agonist (N=167) % occurrence**	**REQUIP (N=179) % occurrence**	**L-dopa (N=89) % occurrence**
Autonomic Nervous System				
Mouth Dry	5.4	4.8	6.1	5.6
Sweating Increased	—	—	6.1	10.1
Body as a Whole General				
Asthenia	8.9	3.0	7.8	5.6
Chest Pain	—	—	8.4	9.0
Edema, Dependent	6.0	6.6	—	—
Edema, Legs	6.5	5.4	14.0	5.6
Fatigue	8.9	4.8	7.3	5.6
Injury	7.1	11.4	19.0	19.1
Pain	11.3	3.6	11.7	15.7
Cardiovascular General				
Hypertension	5.4	6.0	7.8	4.5
Hypotension Postural	9.5	13.2	11.2	12.4
Syncope	6.5	4.2	7.8	6.7
Central and Peripheral Nervous System				
Ataxia	5.4	4.2	14.0	9.0
Dizziness	22.6	19.8	20.1	19.1
Dyskinesia[a]	—	—	8.9	25.8
Dystonia	—	—	6.7	12.4
Headache	10.7	15.6	14.0	18.0
Hyperkinesia	—	—	0.0	5.6
Hypokinesia	—	—	8.4	9.0
Paresthesia	—	—	3.4	6.7
Parkinsonism Aggravated	8.9	12.0	22.3	20.2
Tremor	—	—	16.2	12.4
Vertigo	7.1	7.8	—	—
Gastrointestinal System				
Abdominal Pain	10.7	15.6	15.1	14.6
Anorexia	—	—	8.9	9.0
Constipation	7.7	12.0	9.5	12.4
Diarrhea	5.4	4.8	4.5	10.1
Dyspepsia	5.4	7.8	20.7	16.9
Nausea	40.5	25.1	48.6	49.4
Vomiting	14.9	7.2	16.2	11.2
Heart Rate and Rhythm				
Palpitation	—	—	5.0	3.4
Liver and Biliary System				
Hepatic Enzymes Increased	—	—	6.1	5.6
Musculoskeletal System				
Arthralgia	7.1	8.4	15.1	13.5
Arthritis	—	—	7.8	7.9

(cont'd)

Table 3: REQUIP *(cont'd)*

Adverse Events with Incidence of >5% from 2 Long-term Comparator-controlled Early Therapy Studies (regardless of the presence or absence of concomitant L-dopa)

	Three-year Study		Five-year Study	
	REQUIP (N=168) % occurrence	**Dopamine Agonist (N=167) % occurrence**	**REQUIP (N=179) % occurrence**	**L-dopa (N=89) % occurrence**
Arthrosis	—	—	3.9	5.6
Back Pain	11.9	11.4	17.9	16.9
Myalgia	—	—	4.5	6.7
Psychiatric				
Amnesia	—	—	3.4	9.0
Anxiety	4.8	9.0	11.7	9.0
Confusion	7.7	5.4	7.3	9.0
Depression	11.3	10.2	14.5	22.5
Dreaming Abnormal	—	—	5.0	3.4
Hallucination	9.5	9.0	17.3	5.6
Insomnia	12.5	10.8	25.1	23.6
Nervousness	6.0	2.4	–	—
Paronir ia	—	—	4.5	7.9
Somnolence	8.9	7.8	27.4	19.1
Yawning	—	—	5.0	1.1
Red Blood Cell				
Anemia	1.8	6.6	5.6	4.5
Resistance Mechanism				
Infection	—	—	5.6	0.0
Infection, Viral	14.3	14.4	8.4	13.5
Upper Respiratory Tract Infection	—	—	7.3	7.9
Respiratory System				
Bronchitis	4.8	7.2	4.5	7.9
Coughing	—	—	6.1	4.5
Dyspnea	6.5	3.0	7.3	10.1
Respiratory Disorder	—	—	7.8	5.6
Skin and Appendages				
Rash	—	—	7.8	6.7
Urinary System				
Urinary Incontinence	—	—	5.6	1.1
Urinary Tract Infection	—	—	10.6	12.4
Vision				
Vision Abnormal	—	—	3.9	5.6

[a] In the 5-year study, it was shown that initial treatment of early Parkinson's disease with REQUIP (without concomitant L-dopa) reduces the risk of developing abnormal involuntary movements (i.e. dyskinesias), compared to that associated with the administration of levodopa as initial therapy.

Impulse control symptoms and increased libido including hypersexuality have been reported (see Warnings and Precautions).
Psychotic reactions (other than hallucinations) including delusion, paranoia, and delirium have been reported.
Hypersensitivity reactions (including urticaria, angioedema, rash, pruritus) have been very rarely reported.

DRUG INTERACTIONS: Overview: CYP1A2 Interaction: In vitro metabolism studies showed that CYP1A2 was the major enzyme responsible for the metabolism of ropinirole. Inhibitors or inducers of this enzyme have been shown to alter its clearance when coadministered with ropinirole. Therefore, if therapy with a drug known to be a potent inhibitor of CYP1A2 is stopped or started during treatment with REQUIP, adjustment of the dose of REQUIP may be required.

Drug-Drug Interactions: Psychotropic Drugs: Neuroleptics and other centrally active dopamine antagonists may diminish the effectiveness of REQUIP. Therefore, concomitant use of these products is not recommended.

Based on population pharmacokinetic assessment, no interaction was seen between REQUIP and tricyclic antidepressants or benzodiazepines.

Anti-Parkinson Drugs: Based on population pharmacokinetic assessment, there were no interactions between REQUIP and drugs commonly used to treat Parkinson's disease, i.e., selegiline, amantadine, and anticholinergics.

Levodopa: The potential pharmacokinetic interaction of levodopa/carbidopa (100 mg/10 mg b.i.d.) and REQUIP (2 mg t.i.d.) was assessed in levodopa naive (de novo) male and female patients with Parkinson's disease (n=30, mean age 64 years). The rate and extent of availability of REQUIP at steady state were essentially the same with or without levodopa. Similarly, the rate and extent of availability of levodopa, as well as its elimination half-life, were essentially the same in the presence and absence of REQUIP.

Inhibitors of CYP1A2: Ciprofloxacin: The effect of ciprofloxacin (500 mg b.i.d.) on the pharmacokinetics of REQUIP (2 mg t.i.d.) was studied in male and female patients with Parkinson's disease (n=12, mean age 55 years). The extent of systemic availability of REQUIP was significantly increased when coadministered with ciprofloxacin (AUC increased by 1.84 fold). Thus, in patients already receiving CYP1A2 inhibitors such as ciprofloxacin, REQUIP therapy may be instituted in the recommended manner and the dose titrated according to clinical response. However, if therapy with a drug known to be an inhibitor of CYP1A2 is stopped or introduced during treatment with REQUIP, adjustment of the REQUIP dosage will be required.
Substrates of CYP1A2: Theophylline: The effect of oral theophylline (300 mg bid) on the pharmacokinetics of REQUIP (2 mg t.i.d.) was studied in male and female patients with Parkinson's disease (n=12, mean age 59 years). There was no marked change in the rate or extent of availability of REQUIP when coadministered with theophylline. Similarly, coadministration of REQUIP with intravenous theophylline (5 mg/kg) did not result in any marked change in the pharmacokinetics of theophylline. It is therefore unlikely that substrates of CYP1A2 would significantly alter the pharmacokinetics of REQUIP, and vice-versa.
Digoxin: The effect of REQUIP (2 mg t.i.d.) on the pharmacokinetics of digoxin (0.125-0.25 mg o.d.) was studied in male and female patients with Parkinson's disease (n=10, mean age 72 years). Coadministration at steady state with REQUIP resulted in a 10% decrease in digoxin AUC although mean trough digoxin plasma concentrations were unaltered. However, the effect of higher recommended doses of REQUIP on the pharmacokinetics of digoxin is not known.
Alcohol: No information is available on the potential for interaction between REQUIP and alcohol. As with other centrally active medications, patients should be cautioned against taking REQUIP with alcohol.
Drug-Lifestyle Interactions: Psycho-motor Performance: (See Warnings and Precautions, Sudden Onset of Sleep).

DOSAGE AND ADMINISTRATION:

Dosing Considerations: Renal Impairment: In patients with mild to moderate renal impairment, REQUIP may be titrated in the recommended manner according to clinical response. A study into the use of REQUIP in patients with end stage renal disease (patients on hemodialysis) has shown that a dose adjustment in these patients is required as follows:

The initial dose of REQUIP should be 0.25 mg three times a day. Further dose escalations should be based on tolerability and efficacy. The recommended maximum dose is 18 mg/day in patients receiving regular dialysis. Supplemental doses after dialysis are not required.

Patients with severe renal impairment (creatinine clearance less than 30 mL/min without regular dialysis) have not been studied and administration of REQUIP to such patients is not recommended.
Hepatic Impairment: Patients with hepatic impairment have not been studied and administration of REQUIP to such patients is not recommended.
Oestrogen Replacement Therapy: In patients already receiving oestrogen replacement therapy, REQUIP may be titrated in the recommended manner according to clinical response. However, if oestrogen replacement therapy is stopped or started during treatment with REQUIP, adjustment of the REQUIP dosage may be required.
Recommended Dose and Dosage Adjustment: REQUIP should be taken three times daily and may be taken with or without food (see Action and Clinical Pharmacology, Pharmacokinetics).

The recommended starting dosage is 0.25 mg three times daily. Based on individual patient response, dosage should then be titrated by weekly increments of 0.25 mg per dose as described in Table 4. After week 4, daily dosage may be increased by 0.5 to 1.0 mg per dose on a weekly basis until an optimal therapeutic response is established. Smaller dose increments are recommended for patients who may be at risk for orthostatic symptoms.

Table 4: REQUIP

Dosage Titration

	Week			
	1	2	3	4
Unit Dose (mg)	0.25	0.5	0.75	1.0
Total Daily Dose (mg)	0.75	1.5	2.25	3.0

In clinical trials, initial benefits were observed with 3 mg/day and higher doses. Doses greater than 24 mg/day have not been included in clinical trials.

In a 5-year, double-blind study of early therapy in Parkinson's disease patients, the average daily dose of REQUIP (based on the observed data set) was 10.1 mg at 6 months (median dose=9.0 mg), 14.4 mg at 3 years (median dose=15.0 mg), and 16.6 mg at 5 years (median dose=18.0 mg), regardless of levodopa supplementation.

When REQUIP is administered as adjunct therapy to levodopa, the dose of levodopa may be decreased gradually as tolerated once a therapeutic effect with REQUIP has been observed. A decrease in levodopa dosage may be necessary in order to avoid excessive dopamine stimulation.

REQUIP should be discontinued gradually over a 7-day period. The frequency of administration should be reduced from three times daily to twice daily for 4 days. For the remaining 3 days, the frequency should be reduced to once daily prior to complete withdrawal of REQUIP.
Missed Dose: Patients should be instructed that, if they miss a dose of REQUIP, they should wait and take the next dose as scheduled. There is no need to make up for the missed dose. Patients should not take two doses at once. If treatment is interrupted for one day or more, re-initiation by dose titration should be considered (see Dosage and Administration).

OVERDOSAGE:

Symptoms and Signs: There were no reports of intentional overdose of REQUIP in the premarketing clinical trials. A total of 27 patients accidentally took more than their prescribed dose of REQUIP, with 10 patients ingesting more than 24 mg/day. The largest overdose reported in premarketing clinical trials was 435 mg taken over a 7-day period (62.1 mg/day). Of patients who received a dose greater than 24 mg/day, one experienced mild oro-facial dyskinesia, another patient experienced intermittent nausea. Other symptoms reported with accidental overdoses were: agitation, increased dyskinesia, grogginess, sedation, orthostatic hypotension, chest pain, confusion, vomiting and nausea.
Recommended Management: It is anticipated that the symptoms of REQUIP overdose will be related to its dopaminergic activity. General supportive measures are recommended. Vital signs should be maintained, if necessary. Removal of any unabsorbed material (e.g. by gastric lavage) should be considered.

For management of a suspected drug overdose, contact your regional Poison Control Centre. See the *CPS* Directory section for a list of Poison Control Centres.

ACTION AND CLINICAL PHARMACOLOGY: Mechanism of Action: REQUIP is a non-ergoline dopamine agonist, which activates post-synaptic dopamine receptors.

In vitro studies have shown that ropinirole binds with high affinity to cloned human D_2, D_3, and D_4 receptors. The antiparkinson activity of ropinirole is believed to be due to its stimulatory effects on central post-synaptic dopamine D_2 receptors within the caudate-putamen.

Ropinirole is a potent agonist both in vitro and in vivo and restores motor function in animal models of Parkinson's disease. Ropinirole has been shown to reverse the motor deficits induced by the neurotoxin 1-methyl-4-phenyl-1,2,3,6- tetrahydropyridine (MPTP) in primates.

Neither ropinirole nor its metabolites bind with high affinity to dopamine D_1 receptors. Ropinirole also has very low affinity for 5-HT_1, 5-HT_2, benzodiazepine, $GABA_A$, muscarinic, alpha- or beta-adrenoreceptors. Ropinirole binds to opiate receptors with low affinity, however, studies show that this weak opiate activity has no consequences at pharmacological doses in vivo.

In rats, ropinirole binds to melanin-containing tissues (e.g. the eye) to a greater degree than non-pigmented tissues, and tissue levels decline with a half-life of 16-20 days. It is unknown whether or not ropinirole accumulates in these tissues over time.
Pharmacodynamics: In healthy normotensive subjects, single oral doses of REQUIP, in the range of 0.01 to 2.5 mg, had little or no effect on supine blood pressure and pulse rate. Upon standing, REQUIP caused decreases in systolic and mainly diastolic blood pressure at doses above 0.25 mg. In some subjects, these changes were associated with the emergence of orthostatic symptoms, bradycardia, and, in one case, transient sinus arrest in the context of a severe vasovagal syncope. The effect of repeat dosing and slow titration of REQUIP was not studied in healthy volunteers.

The mechanism of REQUIP-induced orthostatic symptoms probably relates to its dopamine D_2-mediated blunting of the noradrenergic response to standing and subsequent decrease in peripheral vascular resistance. Orthostatic signs and symptoms were often accompanied by nausea.

REQUIP had no dose-related effect on ECG wave form and rhythm in young healthy male volunteers.

At doses ≥0.8 mg REQUIP suppressed serum prolactin concentrations in healthy male volunteers.
Pharmacokinetics: Absorption, Bioavailability and Distribution: Ropinirole is rapidly absorbed with median peak concentrations occurring within 1.5 hours after oral dosing. Despite complete absorption, absolute bioavailability of ropinirole is reduced to approximately 50% as a result of first-pass metabolism. Relative bioavailability from a tablet compared to an oral solution is 85%. Over the therapeutic dose range, C_{max} and AUC values increase in proportion to the increase in dose (see Table 5).

The average oral clearance is approximately 47 L/h (range 17-113 L/h) and is constant over the entire dosage range. The terminal elimination half-life is approximately 6 h (range 2-27 h) and the volume of distribution at steady state is approximately 480 L (range 216-891 L) or 7.0 L/kg (range 3.1-12.9 L/kg).

Table 5: REQUIP

Steady-state Pharmacokinetic Parameters (mean and range) of Ropinirole in Patients with Parkinson's Disease Administered Ropinirole in a t.i.d. Regimen

Unit Dose (mg)	C_{max} (ng/mL)	C_{min} (ng/mL)	T_{max}[a] (h)	AUC_{0-8} (ng·h/mL)
1	5.3 (3.1–9.0)	2.6 (0.9–4.2)	2.0 (0.5–7.0)	27.5 (14.9–46.5)
2	9.8 (5.0–18.0)	4.8 (2.3–10.0)	1.0 (0.6–4.0)	53.8 (23.9–108)
4	23.7 (14.2–40.9)	13.1 (4.8–23.9)	1.0 (1.0–3.0)	136 (66.1–241)

[a] Median.

Steady state concentrations are expected to be achieved within 2 days of dosing. There is, on average, a two-fold higher steady-state plasma concentration of ropinirole following the recommended t.i.d. regimen compared to those observed following a single oral dose.

A high fat meal delayed the rate of absorption of ropinirole (median T_{max} was increased by 2.6 hours and C_{max} was decreased by 25%) in Parkinsonian patients. However, there was no marked change in the overall systemic availability of the drug. Ropinirole may be given with or without food. While administration of the drug with food may improve gastrointestinal tolerance, in severely fluctuating patients, the morning dose may be given without food in order to avoid a delay in time to switch "ON".

Population pharmacokinetic analyses have shown that frequently coadministered medications, such as levodopa, selegiline, amantadine, anticholinergic drugs, ibuprofen, benzodiazepines and antidepressants did not alter the pharmacokinetics of ropinirole.

Plasma protein binding is low (10 to 40%).

Ropinirole has a blood to plasma ratio of 1.2.
Metabolism: Ropinirole is extensively metabolized by the liver. The N-despropyl metabolite is the major metabolite circulating in the plasma. Based on AUC data, the plasma levels of the metabolite were consistently higher than those of the parent drug suggesting a nonsaturable conversion of ropinirole to the N-despropyl metabolite. The affinity of the N-despropyl metabolite for human cloned D_2 receptors is lower than the affinity of ropinirole. In addition the metabolite does not cross the blood-brain barrier; thus, it is unlikely to contribute to the therapeutic effects of ropinirole. The plasma concentrations of the hydroxylated metabolite are low and account for about 1-5% of the ropinirole concentrations. Although the hydroxylated metabolite was more active than ropinirole in in vitro D_2 receptor binding studies, at therapeutic doses it is not expected to contribute to the activity of ropinirole.

In vitro studies indicate that the major cytochrome P450 isozyme involved in the metabolism of ropinirole is CYP1A2. In patients with Parkinson's disease, ciprofloxacin, an inhibitor of CYP1A2, significantly increased the systemic availability of ropinirole, while theophylline, a substrate of CYP1A2, was devoid of such activity (see Drug Interactions).
Excretion: Recovery of radioactivity after oral and intravenous administration of ^{14}C-ropinirole was approximately 88% and 90% of the dose, respectively. Urinary excretion of unchanged ropinirole is low and represents approximately 5 to 10% of the dose. N-despropyl ropinirole is the predominant metabolite found in the urine (40%), followed by the glucuronide of the hydroxy metabolite (10%), and the carboxylic acid metabolite (10%) formed from N-despropyl ropinirole.
Special Populations and Conditions: Geriatrics: Population pharmacokinetic analysis revealed that the oral clearance of REQUIP, seen in patients under the age of 65 years (n=97), was reduced from 62.1 L/h to 45.5 L/h in patients between the ages of 65 and 75 years (n=63). In patients older than 75 years (n=11), oral clearance was similar to that seen in the 65 to 75 year age group (41.7 L/h). Dosage adjustment is not necessary in the elderly (65 years or above).
Gender: Population pharmacokinetic analysis indicated that the oral clearance and volume of distribution of REQUIP at steady state were similar in male patients (n=99, mean age 60 years) and female patients who were not taking concomitant estrogens (n=56, mean age 65 years).
Oestrogen Replacement Therapy: In women, on long-term treatment with conjugated estrogens (n=16, mean age 63 years), the oral clearance of REQUIP was decreased by an average of 36% compared to the oral clearance in women not receiving supplemental oestrogens (n=56, mean age 65 years). The average terminal elimination half-life was 9.0 hours in the oestrogen group and 6.5 hours in patients not taking oestrogens (see Warnings and Precautions and Dosage and Administration).
Renal/Hepatic Insufficiency: Based on population pharmacokinetics, no clinically significant differences were observed in the pharmacokinetics of REQUIP in Parkinsonian patients with mild to moderate renal impairment (creatinine clearance between 30 to 50 mL/min; n=18, mean age 74 years) compared to age-matched patients with creatinine clearance above 50 mL/min (n=44, mean age 70 years). Therefore, no dosage adjustment is necessary in Parkinsonian patients with mild to moderate renal impairment (see Warnings and Precautions and Dosage and Administration).

The use of REQUIP in patients with severe renal impairment (creatinine clearance less than 30 mL/min) without regular dialysis or with hepatic impairment has not been studied. Administration of REQUIP to such patients is not recommended (see Warnings and Precautions and Dosage and Administration).

In patients with end stage renal disease receiving regular dialysis, oral clearance of ropinirole is reduced by approximately 30%. Exposure to the N-despropyl inactive metabolite is increased 4.5-fold; there is no clinical experience with long-term exposure to high levels of this metabolite although exposure which is several-fold the maximum exposure in humans has been evaluated in toxicology studies with no apparent toxicity observed. The clinical relevance of these findings is unknown. The recommended maximum dose is limited to 18 mg/day in patients with Parkinson's disease (see Dosage and Administration, Renal Impairment).

STORAGE AND STABILITY: REQUIP tablets should be stored between 15-30°C. Protect from light and moisture. Close container tightly after each use.

INFORMATION FOR THE PATIENT: Published in e-CPS, available by subscription at www.e-cps.ca.

DOSAGE FORMS, COMPOSITION AND PACKAGING: 0.25 mg: Each white, pentagonal, film-coated, beveled-edged Tiltab tablet, imprinted with SB and 4890, contains: ropinirole 0.25 mg (as ropinirole hydrochloride). Nonmedicinal ingredients: croscarmellose sodium, hydrous lactose, hydroxypropyl methylcellulose, magnesium stearate, microcrystalline cellulose, polyethylene glycol, polysorbate 80 and titanium dioxide. Sucrose-, tartrazine- or any other azo dyes-free. Bottles of 100.
1 mg: Each green, pentagonal, film-coated, beveled-edged Tiltab tablet, imprinted with SB and 4892, contains: ropinirole 1 mg (as ropinirole hydrochloride). Nonmedicinal ingredients: croscarmellose sodium, FD&C Blue No. 2 aluminum lake, hydrous lactose, hydroxypropyl methylcellulose, iron oxide yellow, magnesium stearate, microcrystalline cellulose, polyethylene glycol and titanium dioxide. Sucrose-, tartrazine- or any other azo dyes-free. Bottles of 100.
2 mg: Each pale pink, pentagonal, film-coated, beveled-edged Tiltab tablet, imprinted with SB and 4893, contains: ropinirole 2 mg (as ropinirole hydrochloride). Nonmedicinal ingredients: croscarmellose sodium, hydrous lactose, hydroxypropyl methylcellulose, iron oxide red, iron oxide yellow, magnesium stearate, microcrystalline cellulose, polyethylene glycol and titanium dioxide. Sucrose-, tartrazine- or any other azo dyes-free. Bottles of 100.
5 mg: Each blue, pentagonal, film-coated, beveled-edged Tiltab tablet, imprinted with SB and 4894, contains: ropinirole 5 mg (as ropinirole hydrochloride). Nonmedicinal ingredients: croscarmellose sodium, FD&C Blue No. 2 aluminum lake, hydrous lactose, hydroxypropyl methylcellulose, magnesium stearate, microcrystalline cellulose, polyethylene glycol, polysorbate 80 and titanium dioxide. Sucrose-, tartrazine- or any other azo dyes-free. Bottles of 100.

(Shown in Product Identification Section)

Rescriptor®

delavirdine mesylate

Antiretroviral Agent

ViiV Healthcare ULC

Date of Preparation: April 23, 2010

PHARMACOLOGY: RESCRIPTOR (delavirdine mesylate) is a non-nucleoside reverse transcriptase inhibitor (NNRTI) of the human immunodeficiency virus-type 1 (HIV-1). Reverse transcriptase (RT) is located in the core of the HIV-1 virus and is released upon entry into the host cell. It uses the viral RNA as a template to form DNA. This is a pivotal step in the HIV-1 infection process.

Delavirdine mesylate (henceforth referred to as delavirdine) is a selective inhibitor of RT. It binds directly to RT and blocks RNA-dependent and DNA-dependent DNA polymerase activities. Delavirdine does not compete with template: primer or deoxynucleoside triphosphates. HIV-2 RT and human cellular DNA polymerases α, γ, or δ are not inhibited by delavirdine.

In vitro HIV-1 susceptibility: The antiviral activity of delavirdine in vitro has been demonstrated in both acute and chronic HIV infections in lymphoblastic and monocytic cell lines and peripheral blood lymphocytes with laboratory and clinical isolates of HIV-1. IC_{50} and IC_{90} values (50% and 90% inhibitory concentrations) for laboratory isolates (N=5) ranged from 0.005 to 0.030 μM and 0.04 to 0.10 μM, respectively. Mean IC_{50} of clinical isolates (N=74) was 0.038 μM (range 0.001 to 0.69 μM); 73 of 74 clinical isolates had an IC_{50} ≤0.18 μM. The IC_{90} of 24 of these clinical isolates ranged from 0.05 to 0.10 μM. In drug combination studies of delavirdine with zidovudine, didanosine, zalcitabine, lamivudine, interferon-α and protease inhibitors, additive to synergistic anti-HIV-1 activity was observed in cell culture. The relationship between the in vitro susceptibility of HIV-1 RT inhibitors and inhibition of HIV replication in humans has not been established.

Drug resistance: Phenotypic analysis of isolates from patients treated with delavirdine as monotherapy showed a 50-fold to 500-fold reduction in sensitivity in 14 of 15 patients by Week 8 of therapy. Genotypic analysis of HIV-1 isolates from patients receiving delavirdine plus zidovudine combination therapy (n=79) showed resistance conferring mutations in all isolates by Week 24 of therapy. In delavirdine treated patients the mutations in RT occurred predominantly at amino acid positions 103 and less frequently at position 181 and 236. In a separate study, an average of 86-fold increase in zidovudine susceptibility of patient isolates (n=24) was observed after 24-weeks of delavirdine and zidovudine combination therapy. The clinical relevance of the phenotypic and the genotypic changes associated with delavirdine therapy has not been established.

Cross-resistance: NNRTIs, when used alone or in combination, may confer cross-resistance to other NNRTIs.

Pharmacokinetics: The pharmacokinetic properties of delavirdine have been studied in healthy volunteers and in HIV 1-infected patients after single oral doses of delavirdine ranging from 10 mg to 400 mg and after multiple oral doses ranging from 20 mg tid to 850 mg tid.

Pharmacokinetic parameters of delavirdine after multiple dosing of delavirdine tablets 400 mg tid are shown in Table 1.

Table 1: RESCRIPTOR

Mean +/− Standard Deviation (Range) Steady-state Pharmacokinetic Parameters in HIV-1 Infected Patients (N=67) after 400 mg tid

Cmin (μM)	15±10 (0.1–45)
Cmax (μM)	35±20 (2–100)
AUC (μM·h)	180±100 (5–515)
Tmax (h)	1.3±0.7 (0.5–5)
T½ (h)	5.8±2.5[a] (2–13)

[a] n=54.

Special Populations: Hepatic or Renal Impairment: The pharmacokinetics of delavirdine in patients with hepatic or renal impairment have not been investigated (see Precautions).

Gender: Data from population pharmacokinetics suggest that the plasma concentrations of delavirdine tend to be higher in females than in males. However, this difference is not considered to be clinically significant.

Race: No significant differences in the pharmacokinetics of delavirdine were observed between different racial or ethnic groups.

Age: The pharmacokinetics of delavirdine have not been adequately studied in patients <16 years or >65 years of age.

Drug Interactions: Specific drug interaction studies were performed with delavirdine and a number of drugs. Table 2 summarizes the effect of delavirdine on the geometric mean AUC, Cmax and Cmin of coadministered drugs. Table 3 shows the effects of coadministered drugs on the geometric mean AUC, Cmax and Cmin of delavirdine.

For information regarding clinical recommendations, see Contraindications, Warnings, and Precautions, Drug Interactions.

Table 2: RESCRIPTOR

Pharmacokinetic Parameters for Coadministered Drugs in the Presence of Delavirdine

Coadministered Drug	Dose of Coadministered Drug	Dose of RESCRIPTOR	n	% Change in Pharmacokinetic Parameters of Coadministered Drug (90% CI): Cmax	AUC	Cmin
HIV-Protease Inhibitors						
Nelfinavir	750 mg tid × 14 days	400 mg tid × 7 days	12	↑88 (↑66 – ↑113)	↑107 (↑83 – ↑135)	↑136 (↑103 – ↑175)
	750 mg tid × 28 days	400 mg tid × 28 days	22	↑63[a] (↑28 – ↑106)	↑74[a] (↑38 – ↑120)	↑83[a] (↑40 – ↑138)
Indinavir	600 or 800 mg tid × 7 days	0 or 400 mg tid × 7 days	28	↔[b]	↑53[b] (↑7 – ↑120)	↑298[b] (↑104 – ↑678)
	600 mg Single-Dose	400 mg tid × 10 days	14	↓18[c] (↓25 – ↓10)	↑45[c] (↑30 – ↑62)	—
Saquinavir	Hard gel capsule 600 mg tid × 21 days	400 mg tid × 14 days	13	↑317 (↑187 – ↑504)	↑348 (↑215 – ↑535)	↑376 (↑256 – ↑535)
	Soft gel capsule 1000 or 1200 mg tid × 28 days	0 or 400 mg tid × 28 days	20	↑98[d] (↑4 – ↑277)	↑121[d] (↑14 – ↑340)	↑199[d] (↑37 – ↑553)
Ritonavir	600 mg bid for >35 days	400 mg tid × 21 days	12	↑54 (↑24 – ↑91)	↓51 (↓24 – ↓83)	↑76 (↑50 – ↑105)
Nucleoside Reverse Transcriptase Inhibitors						
Zidovudine	200 mg tid for >38 days	100 mg qid to 400 mg tid for 8–10 days	34	↔	↔	—
Didanosine (buffered tablets)	125 or 250 mg bid × 28 days	400 mg tid × 28 days	9	↓20[e] (↓44 – ↓15)	↓21[e] (↓40 – ↓5)	—
Anti-infective Agents						
Rifabutin	300 mg od for 15–99 days	400–1000 mg tid for 45–129 days	5	↑128 (↑71 – ↑203)	↑230 (↑199 – ↑396)	↑452 (↑246 – ↑781)
Clarithromycin	500 mg bid × 15 days	300 mg tid × 30 days	6	—	↑100	—

[a] Percent change based on a comparison to historical data.
[b] Indinavir 600 mg tid plus RESCRIPTOR 400 mg tid relative to indinavir 800 mg tid without RESCRIPTOR.
[c] Indinavir 600 mg single-dose plus RESCRIPTOR 400 mg tid relative to indinavir 800 mg single-dose alone.
[d] Saquinavir soft gel capsule 1000 mg tid plus RESCRIPTOR 400 mg tid relative to saquinavir soft gel capsule 1200 mg tid without RESCRIPTOR.
[e] RESCRIPTOR taken with didanosine (buffered tablets) relative to doses of RESCRIPTOR and didanosine separated by at least 1 h.
Legend: ↑Indicates increase; ↓Indicates decrease; ↔Indicates no significant change; —Indicates no data is available.

Table 3: RESCRIPTOR

Pharmacokinetic Parameters for Delavirdine in the Presence of Coadministered Drugs

Coadministered Drug	Dose of Coadministered Drug	Dose of RESCRIPTOR	n	% Change in Delavirdine Pharmacokinetic Parameters (90% CI): Cmax	AUC	Cmin
HIV-Protease Inhibitors						
Indinavir	600 mg Single-Dose	400 mg tid × 10 days	14	↔	↔	↔
	0 or 600 mg tid × 7 days	400 mg tid × 7 days	81	↔[a]	↔[a]	↔[a]
Nelfinavir	750 mg tid × 7 days	400 mg tid × 14 days	7	↓27 (↓49 – ↑4)	↓31 (↓57 – ↑10)	↓33 (↓70 – ↑49)
	750 mg tid × 28 days	400 mg tid × 28 days	77	↓38[a] (↓57 – ↓10)	↓35[a] (↓57 – ↓1)	49[a] (↓70 – ↓12)
Ritonavir	0 or 600 mg bid for >35 days	400 mg tid for 7–21 days	25	↔[a]	↔[a]	↔[a]
Saquinavir	Hard gel capsule 600 mg tid × 14 days	400 mg tid × 28 days	7	↔[a]	↔[a]	↔[a]
	Soft gel capsule 0 or 1000 mg tid × 28 days	400 mg tid for 7–28 days	23	↔[a]	↔[a]	↔[a]
Nucleoside Reverse Transcriptase Inhibitors						

(cont'd)

Table 3: RESCRIPTOR *(cont'd)*

Pharmacokinetic Parameters for Delavirdine in the Presence of Coadministered Drugs

Coadministered Drug	Dose of Coadministered Drug	Dose of RESCRIPTOR	n	% Change in Delavirdine Pharmacokinetic Parameters (90% CI) Cmax	AUC	Cmin
Zidovudine	0 or 200 mg tid for ≥7 days	400 mg tid for 7–14 days	42	↔[a]	↔[a]	↔[a]
Didanosine (buffered tablets)	125 or 250 mg bid × 28 days	400 mg tid × 28 days	9	↓32[b] (↓48 – ↓11)	↓19[b] (↓37 – ↑6)	↔[b]
Anti-infective Agents						
Clarithromycin	500 mg bid × 15 days	300 mg tid × 30 days	6	↔	↔	↔
Fluconazole	400 mg od × 15 days	300 mg tid × 30 days	8	↔	↔	↔
Ketoconazole	Various	200–400 mg tid	26	—	—	↑50[c]
Rifampin	600 mg od × 15 days	400 mg tid × 30 days	7	↓90 (↓94 – ↓83)	↓97 (↓98 – ↓95)	↓100
Rifabutin	300 mg od × 14 days	400 mg tid × 28 days	7	↓72 (↓61 – ↓80)	↓82 (↓74 – ↓88)	↓94 (↓90 – ↓96)
Sulfamethoxazole or Trimethoprim & Sulfamethoxazole	Various	200–400 mg tid	311	—	—	↔[c]
Other						
Antacid (Maalox TC)	20 mL	300 mg Single-Dose	12	↓52 (↓68 – ↓29)	↓44 (↓58 – ↓27)	—
Fluoxetine	Various	200–400 mg tid	36	—	—	↑50[c]
Phenytoin, Phenobarbital, Carbamazepine	Various	300–400 mg tid	8	—	—	↓90[c]

[a] Percent change based on a comparison to historical data.
[b] RESCRIPTOR taken with didanosine (buffered tablets) relative to doses of RESCRIPTOR and didanosine separated by at least 1 hr.
[c] Population pharmacokinetic data from efficacy studies.
Legend: ↑Indicates increase; ↓Indicates decrease; ↔Indicates no significant change; —Indicates no data is available.

INDICATIONS: RESCRIPTOR (delavirdine mesylate) is indicated for the treatment of HIV-1 infection in highly customized antiretroviral regimens, in patients who are likely to be intolerant to other non-nucleoside reverse transcriptase inhibitors (NNRTIs).

This indication is based on the modest antiretroviral efficacy shown in clinical trials in antiretroviral-naive patients, when RESCRIPTOR was used in combination with two other nucleoside reverse transcriptase inhibitors (NRTIs), compared to two NRTIs alone. There are insufficient data directly comparing RESCRIPTOR-containing antiretroviral regimens with currently preferred multi-drug regimens for treatment of HIV infection. There is no controlled clinical trial evidence for use of RESCRIPTOR in rescue-therapy regimens.

Resistant viruses emerge rapidly when RESCRIPTOR is used as monotherapy. Therefore, RESCRIPTOR should always be used in combination with at least two other appropriate antiretroviral agents. Non-nucleoside reverse transcriptase inhibitors, when used alone or in combination, may confer cross-resistance to other NNRTIs.

CONTRAINDICATIONS: RESCRIPTOR (delavirdine mesylate) is contraindicated in patients with previously demonstrated clinically significant hypersensitivity to any of the components of the formulation.

Coadministration of RESCRIPTOR is contraindicated with drugs that are highly dependent on CYP3A for clearance and for which elevated plasma concentrations are associated with serious and/or life-threatening events. These drugs are listed in Table 4. Also, see Precautions, Table 5, Drugs That Should Not Be Coadministered with RESCRIPTOR.

Table 4: RESCRIPTOR

Drugs That Are Contraindicated with RESCRIPTOR

Drug Class	Drugs Within Class That Are Contraindicated with RESCRIPTOR
Ergot derivatives	Dihydroergotamine, ergonovine, ergotamine, methylergonovine
Neuroleptic	Pimozide
Sedative/hypnotics	Alprazolam, midazolam, triazolam

WARNINGS: *Drug Interactions:* Delavirdine may inhibit the metabolism of many different drugs (eg, antiarrhythmics, calcium channel blockers, sedative hypnotics, and others), **serious and/or life threatening drug interactions could result from inappropriate coadministration of some drugs with delavirdine**. In addition, some drugs may markedly reduce delavirdine plasma concentrations, resulting in suboptimal antiviral activity and subsequent emergence of drug resistance. All prescribers should become familiar with the following tables in this monograph: Table 4, Drugs That Are Contraindicated with RESCRIPTOR; Table 6, Established and Other Potentially Significant Drug Interactions: Alteration in Dose or Regimen May Be Recommended Based on Drug Interaction Studies or Predicted Interaction. Additional details on drug interactions can be found in Table 2 and Table 3 under Pharmacology.

Concomitant use of lovastatin or simvastatin with RESCRIPTOR is not recommended. Caution should be exercised if RESCRIPTOR is used concurrently with other HMG-CoA reductase inhibitors (statins) that are also metabolized by the CYP3A4 pathway (e.g., atorvastatin) or CYP2C9 pathway (e.g., fluvastatin). The risk of myopathy including rhabdomyolysis may be increased when RESCRIPTOR is used in combination with these drugs.

Particular caution should be used when prescribing sildenafil in patients receiving RESCRIPTOR. Coadministration of sildenafil with RESCRIPTOR is expected to substantially increase sildenafil concentrations and may result in an increase in sildenafil-associated adverse events, including hypotension, visual changes and priapism (see Precautions, Drug Interactions and Information to Be Provided to the Patient, and the complete Prescribing Information for sildenafil).

Concomitant use of St. John's wort (hypericum perforatum) or St. John's wort containing products and RESCRIPTOR is not recommended. Coadministration of St. John's wort with non-nucleoside reverse transcriptase inhibitors (NNRTIs), including RESCRIPTOR, is expected to substantially decrease NNRTI concentrations and may result in suboptimal levels of RESCRIPTOR and lead to loss of virologic response and possible resistance to RESCRIPTOR or to the class of NNRTIs.

PRECAUTIONS: Hepatic Impairment: Delavirdine is metabolized primarily by the liver. Therefore, caution should be exercised when administering RESCRIPTOR (delavirdine mesylate) to patients with impaired hepatic function.

Resistance/Cross-Resistance: Non-nucleoside reverse transcriptase inhibitors, when used alone or in combination, may confer cross-resistance to other non-nucleoside reverse transcriptase inhibitors.

Skin Rash: Patients may experience a skin rash, which is usually temporary. Skin rash attributable to RESCRIPTOR has occurred in 18% of all patients on combination regimens in phase II and III controlled trials who received RESCRIPTOR 400 mg tid. Dose titration does not significantly reduce the incidence of rash. Skin rash is more common in patients with lower CD4 cell counts and typically occurs within 1 to 3 weeks of treatment.

Severe and life threatening skin reactions have occurred on rare occasions in patients treated with RESCRIPTOR, including Stevens-Johnson syndrome and erythema multiforme. None of them were associated with fatalities. RESCRIPTOR must be discontinued in patients developing a severe rash or a rash accompanied by symptoms such as fever, blistering, oral lesions, conjunctivitis, swelling, muscle or joint aches, or general malaise. As there are currently insufficient data on patients who have had a skin reaction to nevirapine or efavirenz and were further treated with RESCRIPTOR, close monitoring of these patients is recommended. Symptomatic relief has been obtained using diphenhydramine hydrochloride, hydroxyzine hydrochloride, and/or topical corticosteroids.

Fat Redistribution: Redistribution/accumulation of body fat including central obesity, dorsocervical fat enlargement (buffalo hump), peripheral wasting, facial wasting, breast enlargement, and "cushingoid appearance" have been observed in patients receiving antiretroviral therapy. The mechanism and long-term consequences of these events are currently unknown. A causal relationship has not been established.

Pregnancy: No adequate and well-controlled studies in pregnant women have been conducted. Since delavirdine has been shown to be teratogenic in rats, RESCRIPTOR should be used during pregnancy only if the potential benefit justifies the potential risk to the fetus. Of 9 pregnancies reported in premarketing clinical studies and postmarketing experience, a total of 10 infants were born (including 1 set of twins). Eight of the infants were born healthy. One infant was born HIV-positive but was otherwise healthy and with no congenital abnormalities detected, and 1 infant was born prematurely (34 to 35 weeks) with a small muscular ventricular septal defect that spontaneously resolved. The patient received approximately six weeks of treatment with delavirdine and zidovudine early in the course of pregnancy.

Antiretroviral Pregnancy Registry: To monitor maternal-fetal outcomes of pregnant women exposed to RESCRIPTOR and other antiretroviral agents, an Antiretroviral Pregnancy Registry has been established. Physicians are encouraged to register patients by calling ViiV Healthcare ULC's Drug Safety Department (1-877-393-8448).

Lactation: It is recommended that HIV-infected mothers not breast-feed their infants to avoid risking postnatal transmission of HIV. It is not known whether delavirdine is excreted in human milk. Since delavirdine has been found to be excreted in the milk of lactating rats, mothers should be instructed not to breast-feed their babies if they are receiving RESCRIPTOR.

Children: Safety and effectiveness of RESCRIPTOR has not been established in HIV-1-infected individuals younger than 16 years of age.

Geriatrics: Clinical studies of RESCRIPTOR did not include sufficient numbers of subjects aged 65 and over to determine whether they respond differently from younger subjects. In general, caution should be taken when dosing RESCRIPTOR in elderly patients due to the greater frequency of decreased hepatic, renal or cardiac function and of concomitant disease or other drug therapy.

Drug Interactions: (See also Contraindications, Warnings, and Pharmacology; Pharmacokinetics, Drug Interactions): Delavirdine is an inhibitor of CYP3A4 isoform and other isoforms to a lesser extent, including CYP2C9, CYP2D6 and CYP2C19. Coadministration of RESCRIPTOR and drugs primarily metabolized by CYP3A (e.g., HMG-CoA reductase inhibitors, and sildenafil) may result in increased plasma concentrations of the coadministered drug that could increase or prolong both its therapeutic effect or adverse effects.

Delavirdine is metabolized primarily by CYP3A, but in vitro data suggest that delavirdine may also be metabolized by CYP2D6. Coadministration of RESCRIPTOR and drugs that reduce CYP3A, such as rifampin, may decrease delavirdine plasma concentrations and reduce its therapeutic effect. Coadministration of RESCRIPTOR and drugs that inhibit CYP3A may increase delavirdine plasma concentrations (see Table 5, Drugs That Should Not Be Coadministered with RESCRIPTOR, and Table 6, Established and Other Potentially Significant Drug Interactions: Alteration in Dose or Regimen May Be Recommended Based on Drug Interaction Studies or Predicted Interaction).

Table 5: RESCRIPTOR

Drugs That Should Not Be Coadministered with RESCRIPTOR

Drug Class: Drug Name	Clinical Comment
Anticonvulsant Agents: phenytoin, phenobarbital, carbamazepine	May lead to loss of virologic response and possible resistance to RESCRIPTOR or to the class of non-nucleoside reverse transcriptase inhibitors.
Antimycobacterials: rifabutin[a], rifampin[a]	May lead to loss of virologic response and possible resistance to RESCRIPTOR or to the class of non-nucleoside reverse transcriptase inhibitors or other coadministered antiviral agents.
Ergot Derivatives: dihydroergotamine, ergonovine, ergotamine, methylergonovine	**Contraindicated** due to potential for serious and/or life-threatening reactions such as acute ergot toxicity characterized by peripheral vasospasm and ischemia of the extremities and other tissues.
Herbal Products: St. John's wort (hypericum perforatum)	May lead to loss of virologic response and possibly resistance to RESCRIPTOR or to the class of non-nucleoside reverse transcriptase inhibitors.
HMG-CoA Reductase Inhibitors: lovastatin, simvastatin	Potential for serious reactions such as risk of myopathy including rhabdomyolysis.

(cont'd)

Table 5: RESCRIPTOR *(cont'd)*

Drugs That Should Not Be Coadministered with RESCRIPTOR

Drug Class: Drug Name	Clinical Comment
Neuroleptic: pimozide	**Contraindicated** due to potential for serious and/or life-threatening reactions such as cardiac arrhythmias.
Sedative/hypnotics: alprazolam, midazolam, triazolam	**Contraindicated** due to potential for serious and/or life-threatening reactions such as prolonged or increased sedation or respiratory depression.

[a] For magnitude of interaction, see Pharmacology, Table 2 and Table 3.

Table 6: RESCRIPTOR

Established and Other Potentially Significant Drug Interactions: Alteration in Dose or Regimen May Be Recommended Based on Drug Interaction Studies or Predicted Interaction

Concomitant Drug Class: Drug Name	Effect on Concentration of Delavirdine or Concomitant Drug	Clinical Comment
HIV-Antiviral Agents		
Amprenavir	↑ Amprenavir	Appropriate doses of this combination, with respect to safety, efficacy and pharmacokinetics, have not been established.
Didanosine[a]	↓ Delavirdine ↓ Didanosine	Administration of didanosine (buffered tablets) and RESCRIPTOR should be separated by at least one hour.
Indinavir[a]	↑ Indinavir	A dose reduction of indinavir to 600 mg tid should be considered when RESCRIPTOR and indinavir are coadministered.
Lopinavir/Ritonavir	↑ Lopinavir ↑ Ritonavir	Appropriate doses of this combination, with respect to safety, efficacy and pharmacokinetics, have not been established.
Nelfinavir[a]	↑ Nelfinavir ↓ Delavirdine	Appropriate doses of this combination, with respect to safety, efficacy and pharmacokinetics, have not been established (see Pharmacology, Table 2 and Table 3).
Ritonavir	↑ Ritonavir	Appropriate doses of this combination, with respect to safety, efficacy and pharmacokinetics, have not been established.
Saquinavir[a]	↑ Saquinavir	A dose reduction of saquinavir (soft gelatin capsules) may be considered when RESCRIPTOR and saquinavir are coadministered (see Pharmacology, Table 2). Appropriate doses with respect to safety, efficacy and pharmacokinetics, have not been established.
Other Agents		
Acid Blockers: Antacids[a] H_2 Receptor Antagonists: cimetidine, famotidine, nizatidine, ranitidine Proton Pump Inhibitors: omeprazole, lansoprazole	↓ Delavirdine	Doses of an antacid and RESCRIPTOR should be separated by at least one hour, because the absorption of delavirdine is reduced when coadministered with antacids. These agents increase gastric pH and may reduce the absorption of delavirdine. Although the effect of these drugs on delavirdine absorption has not been evaluated, chronic use of these drugs with RESCRIPTOR is not recommended.
Amphetamines	↑ Amphetamine	Use with caution.
Amiodarone, lidocaine (systemic), quinidine, flecainide, propafenone		Caution is warranted and therapeutic concentration monitoring is recommended, if available, for antiarrhythmics when coadministered with RESCRIPTOR.
Anticoagulant: warfarin	↑ Warfarin	It is recommended that INR (international normalized ratio) be monitored.
Anti-infective: clarithromycin[a]	↑ Clarithromycin	When coadministered with RESCRIPTOR, clarithromycin should be adjusted in patients with impaired renal function: • For patients with CL_{CR} 30 to 60 mL/min the dose of clarithromycin should be reduced by 50%. • For patients with CL_{CR} <30 mL/min the dose of clarithromycin should be reduced by 75%.
Dihydropyridine Calcium Channel Blockers: amlodipine, diltiazem, felodipine, nifedipine, nimodipine, verapamil	↑ Dihydropyridine calcium channel blockers	Caution is warranted and clinical monitoring of patients is recommended.
Corticosteroid: dexamethasone	↓ Delavirdine	Use with caution. RESCRIPTOR may be less effective due to decreased delavirdine plasma concentrations in patients taking these agents concomitantly.

(cont'd)

Table 6: RESCRIPTOR *(cont'd)*

Established and Other Potentially Significant Drug Interactions: Alteration in Dose or Regimen May Be Recommended Based on Drug Interaction Studies or Predicted Interaction

Concomitant Drug Class: Drug Name	Effect on Concentration of Delavirdine or Concomitant Drug	Clinical Comment
Erectile Dysfunction Agent: sildenafil	↑ Sildenafil	Sildenafil should not exceed a maximum single dose of 25 mg in 48 hour period.
HMG-CoA Reductase Inhibitors: atorvastatin, fluvastatin	↑ Atorvastatin ↑ Cerivastatin ↑ Fluvastatin	Use lowest possible dose of atorvastatin or cerivastatin, or fluvastatin with careful monitoring, or consider other HMG-CoA reductase inhibitors such as pravastatin in combination with RESCRIPTOR.
Immunosuppressants: cyclosporine, tacrolimus	↑ Immunosuppressants	Therapeutic concentration monitoring is recommended for immunosuppressant agents when coadministered with RESCRIPTOR.
Narcotic Analgesic: methadone	↑ Methadone	Dosage of methadone may need to be decreased when coadministered with RESCRIPTOR.
Oral Contraceptives: ethinyl estradiol	↑ Ethinyl estradiol	Concentrations of ethinyl estradiol may increase. However, the clinical significance is unknown.

[a] For magnitude of interaction, see Pharmacology, Table 2 and Table 3.
Legend: ↑Indicates increase; ↓Indicates decrease.

Information to Be Provided to the Patient: Patients should be informed that RESCRIPTOR is not a cure for HIV-1 infection, and that they may continue to acquire illnesses associated with HIV-1 infection, including opportunistic infections. Treatment with RESCRIPTOR has not been shown to reduce the incidence or frequency of such illnesses, and patients should be advised to remain under the care of a physician when using RESCRIPTOR.

Patients should be advised that the use of RESCRIPTOR has not been shown to reduce the risk of transmission of HIV-1.

Patients should be instructed that the major toxicity of RESCRIPTOR is rash and should be advised to promptly notify their physician should a rash occur. The majority of rashes associated with RESCRIPTOR occur within 1 to 3 weeks after initiating treatment with RESCRIPTOR. The rash normally resolves in 3 to 14 days and may be treated symptomatically while therapy with RESCRIPTOR is continued. Any patient experiencing severe rash or rash accompanied by symptoms such as fever, blistering, oral lesions, conjunctivitis, swelling, muscle or joint aches should be advised to discontinue medication and consult a physician.

Patients should be informed that redistribution or accumulation of body fat may occur in patients receiving antiretroviral therapy and that the cause and long term health effects of these conditions are not known at this time.

Patients should be informed to take RESCRIPTOR every day as prescribed. Patients should not alter the dose of RESCRIPTOR without consulting their doctor. If a dose is missed, patients should take the next dose as soon as possible. However, if a dose is skipped, the patient should not double the next dose.

Patients with achlorhydria should take RESCRIPTOR with an acidic beverage (eg, orange or cranberry juice). However, the effect of an acidic beverage on the absorption of delavirdine in patients with achlorhydria has not been investigated.

Patients taking both RESCRIPTOR and antacids should be advised to take them at least one hour apart.

Because RESCRIPTOR may interact with certain drugs, patients should be advised to report to their doctor the use of any prescription and non-prescription medications or herbal products, particularly St. John's wort.

Patients receiving sildenafil and RESCRIPTOR should be advised that they may be at an increased risk of sildenafil-associated adverse events, including hypotension, visual changes, and prolonged penile erection, and should promptly report any symptoms to their doctor.

Patients taking RESCRIPTOR as a dispersion, should rinse the glass with water and swallow the rinse to ensure that the entire dose is consumed.

ADVERSE EFFECTS: The safety of RESCRIPTOR (delavirdine mesylate) alone and in combination with other antiretroviral therapies has been studied in patients in combination with nucleoside reverse transcriptase inhibitors (NRTIs) and protease inhibitors. The majority of adverse events were of mild or moderate intensity. The most frequently reported drug-related adverse event (i.e., an event considered by the investigator to be related to the blinded study medication, or an event with an unknown or missing causal relationship to the blinded medication) among patients receiving RESCRIPTOR was skin rash (see Table 7 and Precautions, Skin Rash).

Table 7: RESCRIPTOR

Percent of Patients with Treatment-emergent Rash in Pivotal Trials (Studies 21 Part II and 13C)[a]

Percent of Patients with:	Description of Rash Grade[b]	RESCRIPTOR 400 mg TID (N=412)	Control Group Patients (N=295)
Grade 1 Rash	Erythema, pruritus	69 (16.7%)	35 (11.9%)
Grade 2 Rash	Diffuse maculopapular rash, dry desquamation	59 (14.3%)	17 (5.8%)
Grade 3 Rash	Vesiculation, moist desquamation, ulceration	18 (4.4%)	0 (0.0%)
Grade 4 Rash	Erythema multiforme, Stevens-Johnson syndrome, toxic epidermal necrolysis, necrosis requiring surgery, exfoliative dermatitis	0 (0.0%)	0 (0.0%)
Rash of Any Grade		146 (35.4%)	52 (17.6%)
Treatment Discontinuation as a Result of Rash		13 (3.2%)	1 (0.3%)

[a] Includes rash reported regardless of causality.
[b] ACTG Toxicity Grading System; includes events reported as "rash", "maculopapular rash" and "urticaria".

Adverse events of moderate (ACTG grade 2) to severe (ACTG grade 3) intensity reported by at least 5% of evaluable patients in any treatment group in the pivotal trials, which includes patients receiving RESCRIPTOR in combination with zidovudine and/or lamivudine in Study 21 Part II for up to 98 weeks and in combination with zidovudine and either lamivudine, didanosine, or zalcitabine in Study 13C for up to 72 weeks are summarized in Table 8.

Other adverse events that occurred in patients receiving RESCRIPTOR (in combination treatment) in all phase II/III studies, and considered possibly related to treatment and of at least ACTG grade 2 (moderate) in intensity are listed below by body system.

Body as a Whole: abdominal cramps, abdominal distention, abdominal pain (localized), abscess, allergic reaction, chills, edema (generalized or localized), epidermal cyst, fever, infection, infection viral, lip edema, malaise, *M. tuberculosis* infection, neck rigidity, pain (generalized), redistribution/accumulation of body fat (see Precautions, Fat Redistribution) and sebaceous cyst.

Cardiovascular: abnormal cardiac rate and rhythm, cardiac insufficiency, cardiomyopathy, hypertension, migraine, pallor, peripheral vascular disorder, and postural hypotension.

Table 8: RESCRIPTOR

Treatment-emergent Adverse Events, Regardless of Causality, of Moderate-to-Severe or Life-threatening Intensity Reported by at Least 5% of Evaluable[a] Patients in Any Treatment Group

	Study 21 Part II			Study 13C	
Adverse Events	**ZDV + 3TC (N=123) % of pts (N)**	**400 mg tid RESCRIPTOR + ZDV (N=123) % of pts (N)**	**400 mg tid RESCRIPTOR + ZDV + 3TC (N=119) % of pts (N)**	**ZDV + ddI, ddC, or 3TC (N=172) % of pts (N)**	**400 mg tid RESCRIPTOR + ZDV + ddI, ddC or 3TC (N=170) % of pts (N)**
Body as a Whole					
Abdominal pain, generalized	2.4 (3)	3.3 (4)	5.0 (6)	1.7 (3)	2.4 (4)
Asthenia/ fatigue	16.3 (20)	15.4 (19)	16.0 (19)	8.1 (14)	5.3 (9)
Fever	2.4 (3)	1.6 (2)	3.4 (4)	6.4 (11)	7.1 (12)
Flu syndrome	4.9 (6)	7.3 (9)	5.0 (6)	5.2 (9)	2.4 (4)
Headache	14.6 (18)	12.2 (15)	16.8 (20)	12.8 (22)	11.2 (19)
Localized pain	4.9 (6)	5.7 (7)	5.0 (6)	2.9 (5)	1.8 (3)
Digestive					
Diarrhea	8.1 (10)	2.4 (3)	4.2 (5)	8.1 (14)	5.9 (10)
Nausea	17.1 (21)	20.3 (25)	16.8 (20)	9.3 (16)	14.7 (25)
Vomiting	8.9 (11)	4.9 (6)	2.5 (3)	4.1 (7)	6.5 (11)
Nervous					
Anxiety	1.6 (2)	2.4 (3)	6.7 (8)	4.1 (7)	3.5 (6)
Depressive symptoms	6.5 (8)	4.9 (6)	12.6 (15)	3.5 (6)	5.9 (10)
Insomnia	4.9 (6)	4.9 (6)	5.0 (6)	2.9 (5)	1.2 (2)
Respiratory					
Bronchitis	4.1 (5)	6.5 (8)	6.7 (8)	3.5 (6)	3.5 (6)
Cough	9.8 (12)	4.1 (5)	5.0 (6)	5.2 (9)	3.5 (6)
Pharyngitis	6.5 (8)	1.6 (2)	5.0 (6)	4.1 (7)	3.5 (6)
Sinusitis	8.9 (11)	7.3 (9)	5.0 (6)	2.3 (4)	1.2 (2)
Upper respiratory infection	11.4 (14)	6.5 (8)	7.6 (9)	8.7 (15)	4.7 (8)
Skin					
Rashes	3.3 (4)	19.5 (24)	13.4 (16)	7.6 (13)	18.8 (32)

[a] Evaluable patients in Study 21 Part II were those who received at least one dose of study medication and returned for at least one clinic study visit. Evaluable patients in Study 13C were those who received at least one dose of study medication.

Gastrointestinal: anorexia, bloody stool, colitis, constipation, decreased appetite, diarrhea (*C. difficile*), diverticulitis, dry mouth, dyspepsia, dysphagia, enteritis at all levels, eructation, fecal incontinence, flatulence, gagging, gastroenteritis, gastroesophageal reflux, gastrointestinal bleeding, gastrointestinal disorder, gingivitis, gum haemorrhage, hepatomegaly, increased appetite, increased saliva, increased thirst, jaundice, mouth or tongue inflammation or ulcers, nonspecific hepatitis, oral/enteric monilia, pancreatitis, rectal disorder, sialadenitis, tooth abscess, and toothache.

Hemic and Lymphatic: adenopathy, bruising, eosinophilia, granulocytosis, leukopenia, pancytopenia, purpura, spleen disorder, thrombocytopenia, and prolonged prothrombin time.

Metabolic and Nutritional Disorders: alcohol intolerance, amylase increased, bilirubinemia, hyperglycemia, hyperkalemia, hypertriglyceridemia, hyperuricemia, hypocalcemia, hyponatremia, hypophosphatemia, increased AST, increased gamma glutamyl transpeptidase, increased lipase, increased serum alkaline phosphatase, increased serum creatinine, and weight increase or decrease.

Musculoskeletal: arthralgia or arthritis of single and multiple joints, bone disorder, bone pain, myalgia, tendon disorder, tenosynovitis, tetany, and vertigo.

Nervous: abnormal coordination, agitation, amnesia, change in dreams, cognitive impairment, confusion, decreased libido, disorientation, dizziness, emotional lability, euphoria, hallucination, hyperesthesia, hyperreflexia, hypertonia, hypesthesia, impaired concentration, manic symptoms, muscle cramp, nervousness, neuropathy, nystagmus, paralysis, paranoid symptoms, restlessness, sleep cycle disorder, somnolence, tingling, tremor, vertigo, and weakness.

Respiratory: chest congestion, dyspnea, epistaxis, hiccups, laryngismus, pneumonia, and rhinitis.

Skin and Appendages: angioedema, dermal leukocytoclastic vasculitis, dermatitis, desquamation, diaphoresis, discoloured skin, dry skin, erythema, erythema multiforme, folliculitis, fungal dermatitis, hair loss, herpes zoster or simplex, maculopapular rash, nail disorder, petechiae, non-application site pruritus, seborrhea, skin disorder, skin hypertrophy, skin nodule, Stevens-Johnson syndrome, urticaria, vesiculobullous rash, and wart.

Special Senses: blepharitis, blurred vision, conjunctivitis, diplopia, dry eyes, ear pain, parosmia, photophobia, taste perversion, and tinnitus.

Urogenital: amenorrhea, breast enlargement, calculi of the kidney, chromaturia, epididymitis, hematuria, hemospermia, impaired urination, impotence, kidney pain, metrorrhagia, nocturia, polyuria, proteinuria, testicular pain, urinary tract infection, and vaginal moniliasis.

Postmarketing Experience: Adverse event terms reported from postmarketing surveillance that were not reported in the phase II and III trials are presented below by body system:
Digestive: hepatic failure.
Hemic and Lymphatic: hemolytic anemia.
Musculoskeletal: rhabdomyolysis.
Skin Rash: Stevens-Johnson syndrome and erythema multiforme.
Urogenital: acute kidney failure.

Laboratory Abnormalities: Marked laboratory abnormalities observed in at least 2% of patients during therapy in Studies 21 Part II and 13C are summarized in Table 9. Marked laboratory abnormalities are defined as a two-gradeshift from baseline to a Grade 3 and 4 abnormality in a patient at any time during study.

Table 9: RESCRIPTOR

Marked Laboratory Abnormalities Reported by ≥2% of Patients

		Study 21 Part II			Study 13C	
	Toxicity Limit	**ZDV + 3TC N=123 % pts**	**400 mg tid RESCRIPTOR N=123 % pts**	**400 mg tid RESCRIPTOR + ZDV + 3TC N=119 % pts**	**ZDV + ddI, ddC or 3TC N=172 % pts**	**400 mg tid RESCRIPTOR + ZDV + ddI, N=170 % pts**
Hematology						
Hemoglobin	<7 mg/dL	4.1	2.5	0.9	1.7	2.9
Neutrophils	<750/mm³	5.7	4.9	3.4	10.4	7.6
Prothrombin time (PT)	>1.5×ULN	0	0	1.7	2.9	2.4
Activated partial thromboplastin (APTT)	>2.33×ULN	0	0.8	0	5.8	2.4
Chemistry						
Alananine aminotransferase (ALT)	>5×ULN	2.5	4.1	5.1	3.5	4.1
Amylase	>2×ULN	0.8	2.5	2.6	3.5	2.9
Aspartate aminotransferase (AST)	>5×ULN	1.6	2.5	3.4	3.5	2.3
Bilirubin	>2.5×ULN	0.8	2.5	1.7	1.2	0
Gamma glutamyl transferase (GGT)	>5×ULN	N/A	N/A	N/A	4.1	1.8
Glucose (hypo/hyperglycemia)	<40 mg/dL >250 mg/dL	4.1	0.8	1.7	1.2	0.0

Legend: N/A=not applicable because no predose values were obtained for patients.

OVERDOSE:

Symptoms: Human experience of acute overdose with RESCRIPTOR is limited.

Treatment: Treatment of overdosage with RESCRIPTOR (delavirdine mesylate) should consist of general supportive measures, including monitoring of vital signs and observation of the clinical status of the patient. There is no specific antidote for overdosage with RESCRIPTOR. If indicated, elimination of unabsorbed drug should be achieved by emesis or gastric lavage. Since delavirdine is extensively metabolized by the liver and is highly protein bound, dialysis is unlikely to be beneficial in significant removal of the drug.

For management of a suspected drug overdose, CPhA recommends that you contact your **regional Poison Control Centre**. See the *CPS* Directory section for a list of Poison Control Centres.

DOSAGE: The recommended dosage for RESCRIPTOR (delavirdine mesylate) is 400 mg (four 100-mg tablets) three times daily administered in combination with other antiretroviral agents. The complete prescribing information for other antiretroviral agents should be consulted for information on dosage and administration.

RESCRIPTOR may be dispersed prior to consumption. To prepare a dispersion, add four tablets to at least 90 mL (3 ounces) of water, allow to stand for a few minutes, and then stir until a uniform dispersion occurs. The dispersion should be consumed promptly (see Pharmacology, Pharmacokinetics, Absorption and Bioavailability). The glass should be rinsed and the rinse swallowed to insure the entire dose is consumed.

RESCRIPTOR may be administered with or without food (see Pharmacology, Pharmacokinetics, Absorption and Bioavailability). Patients with achlorhydria should take RESCRIPTOR with an acidic beverage (eg. orange or cranberry juice). However, the effect of an acidic beverage on the absorption of delavirdine in patients with achlorhydria has not been investigated.

Patients taking both RESCRIPTOR and antacids should be advised to take them at least one hour apart.

INFORMATION FOR THE PATIENT: Published in e-CPS, available by subscription at www.e-cps.ca.

SUPPLIED: Each white, film-coated, capsule-shaped tablet marked with "U 3761", contains: delavirdine mesylate 100 mg. Nonmedicinal ingredients: carnauba wax, colloidal silicon dioxide, croscarmellose sodium, lactose, magnesium stearate, microcrystalline cellulose, propylene glycol and titanium dioxide. HDPE plastic, child resistant bottles of 360. Store at controlled room temperature (15 to 30°C). Keep container tightly closed. Protect from high humidity.

(Shown in Product Identification Section)

Resonium Calcium®

calcium polystyrene sulfonate

Ion-Exchange Resin

sanofi-aventis

SUPPLIED: Each jar contains: 300 g of the flavored calcium polystyrene sulfonate powdered resin. Also contains saccharin and vanillin. Sodium: <1 mmol (1 mg)/g. Alcohol-, gluten-, lactose-, parabens-, starch-, sucrose-, sulfite- and tartrazine-free. A plastic measure is included which holds 15 g of resin.

Restasis®

cyclosporine

Anti-Inflammatory—Immunomodulator

Allergan

Date of Preparation: August 12, 2010

SUMMARY PRODUCT INFORMATION:

Route of Administration	Dosage Form/ Strength	Clinically Relevant Nonmedicinal Ingredients
Ophthalmic	Emulsion, 0.05% w/v	Castor oil For a complete listing see Dosage Forms, Composition and Packaging.

INDICATIONS AND CLINICAL USE: RESTASIS (cyclosporine) ophthalmic emulsion, 0.05% w/v is indicated for the treatment of moderate to moderately severe (Level 2-3 severity by DEWS Guidelines)* aqueous deficient dry eye disease, characterized by moderate to moderately severe: ocular staining, reduction in tear production and fluctuating visual symptoms, such as blurred vision. This indication is based on a pooled analysis of a subpopulation of patients from three pivotal studies.

The efficacy of RESTASIS alone has not been demonstrated in patients with more severe disease (Level 4 DEWS Classification).

Geriatrics (>65 years of age): No overall difference in safety or effectiveness has been observed between elderly and younger subjects.

Pediatrics (<18 years of age): No pediatric data are available.

CONTRAINDICATIONS:

- Patients who are hypersensitive to this drug or to any ingredient in the formulation or component of the container. For a complete listing, see Dosage Forms, Composition and Packaging.
- Patients with active ocular infections.

WARNINGS AND PRECAUTIONS: General: For ophthalmic use only.

Ophthalmologic: RESTASIS (cyclosporine) ophthalmic emulsion, 0.05% w/v has not been studied in patients with a history of herpes keratitis, end stage lacrimal gland disease, keratoconjunctivitis sicca (KCS) secondary to the destruction of conjunctival goblet cells such as occurs with Vitamin A deficiency, or scarring, such as occurs with cicatricial pemphigoid, alkali burns, Stevens-Johnson syndrome, trachoma, or irradiation.

Patients should be advised to avoid touching the tip of the vial to the eye or any surface, as this may contaminate the emulsion. To avoid the potential for injury to the eye, patients should be advised to be careful not to touch the vial container to the eye.

RESTASIS should not be administered while the patient is wearing contact lenses. Patients with decreased tear production typically should not wear contact lenses. However, if contact lenses are worn, they should be removed prior to the administration of the emulsion. Lenses may be reinserted 15 minutes after the administration of RESTASIS.

Occupational Hazards: RESTASIS may cause transient blurred vision due to its emulsion formulation. If patients experience blurred vision, they should be advised not to drive or operate machinery until vision has cleared.

Special Populations: Pregnant Women: There are no adequate data from the use of RESTASIS in pregnant women. Studies in animals have shown reproductive toxicity at high maternotoxic doses.

RESTASIS should not be used during pregnancy unless the benefits outweigh the risks.

Nursing Women: Cyclosporine is known to be excreted in human milk following systemic administration, but excretion in human milk after topical administration has not been investigated. Although blood concentrations are undetectable after topical administration of RESTASIS, caution should be exercised when RESTASIS is administered to a nursing woman.

Pediatrics: The safety and efficacy of RESTASIS have only been studied in adults.

Geriatrics: No overall difference in safety or effectiveness has been observed between elderly and younger patients.

ADVERSE REACTIONS: Adverse Drug Reaction Overview: The most common adverse event following the use of RESTASIS (cyclosporine) ophthalmic emulsion, 0.05% w/v is ocular burning.

Clinical Trial Adverse Drug Reactions: Because clinical trials are conducted under very specific conditions, the adverse reaction rates observed in the clinical trials may not reflect the rates observed in practice and should not be compared to the rates in the clinical trials of another drug. Adverse drug reaction information from clinical trials is useful for identifying drug-related adverse events and for approximating rates.

In the combined data from the three key Phase 3 clinical studies, approximately 29% of treated patients experienced treatment-related adverse events (adverse reactions) in the first year. The majority were ocular, mild or moderate in severity, and none was serious. The most commonly reported adverse reaction was eye burning, which was reported in approximately 17% of patients in the first year; the incidence of new reports decreased to 5% at 2 years. The observed adverse drug reactions are provided in Table 1 for those events observed at an incidence of ≥1% in the three vehicle-controlled clinical trials.

Table 1: RESTASIS

Vehicle Controlled Clinical Trial Treatment-Related Adverse Drug Reactions Reported by ≥1% of Patients in the Cyclosporine 0.05% Treatment Group (ITT Population—Month 12 Pooled Data for Studies 192371-002, -003, -501)

		Vehicle/Cyclosporine 0.1%	
Reported Term	**Cyclosporine Ophthalmic Emulsion 0.05% N=436 (%)**	**6 month Controlled Phase—Vehicle N=442 (%)**	**6 month Extension Phase—Cyclosporine 0.1% N=323 (%)**
Special Senses			
Burning eye	74 (17.0%)	29 (6.6%)	21 (6.5%)
Irritation eye	13 (3.0%)	7 (1.6%)	5 (1.5%)
Foreign body sensation	12 (2.8%)	8 (1.8%)	2 (0.6%)
Hyperaemia conjunctival (NOS)	11 (2.5%)	9 (2.0%)	7 (2.2%)
Pain eye	10 (2.3%)	11 (2.5%)	5 (1.5%)
Stinging eye	10 (2.3%)	9 (2.0%)	7 (2.2%)
Discharge eye	9 (2.1%)	7 (1.6%)	1 (0.3%)
Photophobia	9 (2.1%)	3 (0.7%)	—
Pruritus eye	8 (1.8%)	7 (1.6%)	2 (0.6%)
Visual disturbance	8 (1.8%)	12 (2.7%)	1 (0.3%)
Dry eye	7 (1.6%)	2 (0.5%)	—
Body as a Whole			
Headache	7 (1.6%)	5 (1.1%)	2 (0.6%)

Note that active events are reported over 12 months; vehicle events are reported for 6 month exposure period.
Legend: NOS—not otherwise specified.

* Report of the International Dry Eye WorkShop (DEWS). The Ocular Surface, April 2007; 5(2):65-204.

The frequency of all adverse event reporting was generally highest shortly after initiation of RESTASIS treatment, but lessened as treatment continued.

Less Common Clinical Trial Adverse Drug Reactions (<1%): The observed adverse drug reactions are provided below for those events reported by <1% of patients in the cyclosporine 0.05% treatment group in the three vehicle-controlled clinical trials over 12 months.

Digestive System: dryness oral, nausea, salivary gland enlargement, stomatitis ulcer.

Musculoskeletal System: arthralgia.

Nervous System: dizziness.

Respiratory System: rhinitis, infection sinus.

Skin: rash, alopecia.

Special Senses: conjunctivitis (NOS), oedema eyelid, blepharitis, erythema eyelid, asthenopia, chalazion, conjunctivitis bacterial, corneal abrasion, corneal infiltrates, corneal neovascularisation, eczema eyelid, oedema eye, conjunctival haemorrhage, keratitis herpes simplex, keratitis superficial punctate, lacrimation increased, pain ear, ulcer corneal (NOS), ulcerative keratitis, vitreous floaters.

Post-Market Adverse Drug Reactions: Post-marketing reactions reported to date have been consistent with the events recorded during the vehicle-controlled clinical trials, with the majority of the reported events being ocular. Adverse reactions detected in post-marketing data but not seen with cyclosporine ophthalmic emulsion, 0.05% in clinical trials include eye swelling, hypersensitivity, urticaria.

DRUG INTERACTIONS: Overview: No interaction studies have been performed.

Drugs that affect cytochrome P-450 may alter cyclosporine metabolism. There is no detectable systemic absorption of RESTASIS (cyclosporine) ophthalmic emulsion, 0.05% w/v following ocular administration. Therefore, no interaction of topically applied RESTASIS with systemic drugs is expected to occur.

Drug-Drug Interactions: Interactions with other drugs have not been established.

Drug-Food Interactions: Interactions with food have not been established.

Drug-Herb Interactions: Interactions with herbal products have not been established.

Drug-Laboratory Test Interactions: Interactions with laboratory tests have not been established.

DOSAGE AND ADMINISTRATION: Dosing Considerations: There are no special dosing considerations which need to be taken into account prior to initiating therapy with RESTASIS (cyclosporine) ophthalmic emulsion, 0.05% w/v.

Recommended Dose and Dosage Adjustment: The recommended dose is one drop of RESTASIS, instilled twice a day in each eye approximately 12 hours apart.

This recommended dose is the maximum recommended dose, and should be used both as the starting dose and throughout long term treatment. Dosage adjustments should not be necessary based on any co-morbid conditions, given the low systemic availability of the product. Limited data from clinical studies exists for long term administration of RESTASIS (up to 40 months). It is expected that use of the product will continue long term.

Missed Dose: If a dose of this medication is missed, it should be taken as soon as possible. However, if it is almost time for the next dose, the missed dose should be skipped and the regular dosing schedule resumed. Doses should not be doubled. The dose should not exceed two drops in the affected eye(s) daily.

Administration: The vial should be inverted a few times to obtain a uniform, white, opaque emulsion before using.

The emulsion from one individual single-use vial is to be used immediately after opening for administration to one or both eyes, and the remaining contents should be discarded immediately after administration.

Patients should be advised to avoid touching the tip of the vial to the eye or any surface, as this may contaminate the emulsion.

RESTASIS should not be administered while the patient is wearing contact lenses. Patients with decreased tear production typically should not wear contact lenses. However, if contact lenses are worn, they should be removed prior to the administration of the emulsion. Lenses may be reinserted 15 minutes after the administration of RESTASIS.

RESTASIS may be used concomitantly with artificial tears. The patient should be advised to allow a 15 minute interval between administration of RESTASIS and the artificial tear product.

OVERDOSAGE:

There is no experience with overdose in humans using topical cyclosporine ophthalmic emulsion. Excessive topical use of cyclosporine ophthalmic emulsion would not be expected to contribute to any ocular toxicity. Due to low systemic concentrations of cyclosporine after topical treatment with the ophthalmic emulsion, the likelihood of systemic intoxication from topical overdose is remote.

A single vial of 0.05% cyclosporine emulsion contains 0.2 mg of cyclosporine. The recommended weight-normalized starting dose of NEORAL (cyclosporine), which is administered systemically for rheumatoid arthritis and plaque psoriasis, is 2.0 mg/kg/day. Therefore, the dose ingested by drinking the contents of an entire vial by a child weighing 14 kg (30 lb) would be approximately 140 times lower than the recommended starting dose of NEORAL.

> For management of a suspected drug overdose, contact your regional Poison Control Centre. See the *CPS* Directory section for a list of Poison Control Centres.

ACTION AND CLINICAL PHARMACOLOGY: Mechanism of Action: Cyclosporine is an immunosuppressive agent when administered systemically.

In patients whose tear production is presumed to be suppressed due to ocular inflammation associated with keratoconjunctivitis sicca (KCS), cyclosporine emulsion is thought to act as a partial immunomodulator. The exact mechanism of action is not known.

Pharmacodynamics: The administration of higher concentrations of cyclosporine emulsion was not found to improve the clinical response.

Pharmacokinetics: Blood cyclosporine A concentrations were measured using a specific high pressure liquid chromatography-mass spectrometry assay. Blood concentrations of cyclosporine A, in all the samples collected, after topical administration of cyclosporine ophthalmic emulsion 0.05% twice daily in humans for up to 12 months, were below the quantitation limit of 0.1 ng/mL. These levels are more than 6550 times lower than those measured during systemic cyclosporine treatment for non-life-threatening indications. There was no detectable drug accumulation in blood during 12 months of treatment with cyclosporine ophthalmic emulsion.

Special Populations and Conditions: Hepatic and Renal Insufficiency: Based on the low systemic availability of cyclosporine administered as ophthalmic emulsion, and as there was no detectable drug accumulation in blood during 12 months of treatment with RESTASIS (cyclosporine) ophthalmic emulsion, 0.05% w/v, no increased risk in patients with impaired renal or hepatic function would be expected to occur following the use of RESTASIS.

STORAGE AND STABILITY: RESTASIS (cyclosporine) ophthalmic emulsion, 0.05% w/v should be stored at 15-25°C. Patients should be instructed to keep unused vials within the resealable tray.

INFORMATION FOR THE PATIENT: Published in e-CPS, available by subscription at www.e-cps.ca.

DOSAGE FORMS, COMPOSITION AND PACKAGING: Each mL of sterile, preservative-free ophthalmic emulsion contains: cyclosporine 0.5 mg. Nonmedicinal ingredients: Carbomer Copolymer Type A, castor oil, glycerin, polysorbate 80, purified water and sodium hydroxide to adjust the pH. Low density polyethylene single use vials containing 0.4 mL each, trays of 30.

Restoril® ℞

temazepam
Hypnotic

Sepracor

Date of Preparation: June 26, 2009

PHARMACOLOGY: General: Temazepam is a benzodiazepine with hypnotic properties.

Benzodiazepines act as depressants of the CNS. It is believed that benzodiazepines enhance or facilitate the effects of the inhibitory neurotransmitter gamma-aminobutyric acid (GABA).

Benzodiazepines act as agonists at the benzodiazepine receptor sites. The benzodiazepine-GABA receptor-chloride ionophore complex functions mainly in the gating of the chloride channel. Benzodiazepines are thought to produce their pharmacological effects by facilitating GABA-mediated transmission in the CNS, which reportedly increase the frequency of the chloride channel opening.

In sleep laboratory studies, the effect of temazepam 15 and 30 mg, was compared to placebo over a 2-week period. There was a linear dose-response improvement in total sleep time and sleep latency with significant drug-placebo differences occurring for total sleep time at both doses, and for sleep latency at the higher dose. REM sleep was essentially unchanged and slow wave sleep was decreased.

Rebound Insomnia: A transient syndrome, known as "rebound insomnia", whereby the symptoms that led to treatment with a benzodiazepine recur in an enhanced form, may occur on withdrawal of hypnotic treatment. In the sleep laboratory studies, no measurable effects on daytime alertness or performance occurred following temazepam treatment or during the withdrawal period, even though a transient sleep disturbance in some sleep parameters was observed following the withdrawal of the higher doses.

The duration of hypnotic effect and the profile of unwanted effects may be influenced by the alpha (distribution) and beta (elimination) half-lives of the administered drug and any active metabolites formed. When half-lives are long, the drug or metabolite may accumulate during periods of nightly administration and be associated with impairments of cognitive and motor performance during waking hours. If half-lives are short, the drug and metabolites will be cleared before the next dose is ingested, and carry-over effects related to sedation or CNS depression should be minimal or absent. However, during nightly use and for an extended period, pharmacodynamic tolerance or adaptation to some effects of benzodiazepine hypnotics may develop.

If the drug has a very short elimination half-life, it is possible that a relative deficiency (i.e., in relation to the receptor site) may occur at some point in the interval between each night's use. This sequence of events may account for two clinical findings reported to occur after several weeks of nightly use of rapidly eliminated benzodiazepine hypnotics: 1) increased wakefulness during the last third of the night and 2) the appearance of increased daytime anxiety (see Warnings).

Pharmacokinetics: Orally administered temazepam is well absorbed in man. In a single and multiple dose absorption, distribution, metabolism and excretion (ADME) study, using ^3H labelled drug, temazepam was found to have minimal (8%) first-pass metabolism. There were no active metabolites formed and the only significant metabolite present in blood was the O-conjugate. Oral administration of 15 to 45 mg temazepam in man resulted in rapid absorption with significant blood levels achieved in 30 minutes and peak levels at 2 to 3 hours. Drug levels in blood declined in a biphasic manner with a short half-life ranging from 0.4 to 0.6 hours and a terminal half-life from 3.5 to 18 hours (mean 9 hours). The inactive O-conjugate metabolite was formed with a half-life of 10 hours and excreted with a half-life of approximately 2 hours. Thus, O-conjugation is the rate limiting step in the biodisposition. In a multiple dose study, steady-state was approximated after the second daily dose with no evidence of accumulation after 5 consecutive daily doses of 30 mg temazepam. Steady-state plasma levels at 2.5 hours were 382±192 ng/mL.

Approximately 96% of unchanged drug is bound to plasma protein.

Twenty-four hours after a single oral dose of temazepam approximately 80 to 90% of the drug was recovered in urine, primarily as the O-conjugate. Total recovery from feces and urine in single- and multiple-dose studies was approximately 95%, with only 3 to 13% of the radioactivity detectable in feces. Less than 1% of the dose was excreted as unchanged drug or N-desmethyltemazepam. A dose-proportional relationship has been established for the area under the plasma concentration/time curve over the 15 to 30 mg dose range.

At the dose of 30 mg once a day for 8 weeks, no evidence of enzyme induction was found in man.

INDICATIONS: Sleep disturbance may be the presenting manifestation of a physical and/or psychiatric disorder. Consequently, a decision to initiate symptomatic treatment of insomnia should only be made after the patient has been carefully evaluated.

Temazepam is indicated for the symptomatic relief of transient and short-term insomnia characterized by difficulty in falling asleep, frequent nocturnal awakenings and/or early morning awakenings.

Treatment with temazepam should usually not exceed 7 to 10 consecutive days. Use for more than 2 to 3 consecutive weeks requires complete re-evaluation of the patient. Prescriptions for temazepam should be written for short-term use (7 to 10 days) and it should not be prescribed in quantities exceeding a 1-month supply.

The use of hypnotics should be restricted for insomnia where disturbed sleep results in impaired daytime functioning.

CONTRAINDICATIONS: In patients with a known hypersensitivity to the drug, any component of its formulation, or to other benzodiazepines; myasthenia gravis; sleep apnea syndrome.

Temazepam is contraindicated in patients who in the past manifested paradoxical reactions to alcohol and/or sedative medications.

WARNINGS: General: Benzodiazepines should be used with extreme caution in patients with a history of substance or alcohol abuse.

The lowest possible effective dose should be prescribed for elderly patients. Inappropriate, heavy sedation in the elderly, may result in accidental events or falls.

The failure of insomnia to remit after 7 to 10 days of treatment may indicate the presence of a primary psychiatric and/or medical illness or the presence of sleep state misperception.

Worsening of insomnia or the emergence of new abnormalities of thinking or behavior may be the consequence of an unrecognized psychiatric or physical disorder. These have also been reported to occur in association with the use of drugs that act at the benzodiazepine receptors.

Pregnancy: The use of temazepam during pregnancy is not recommended.

Benzodiazepines may cause fetal damage when administered during pregnancy. During the first trimester of pregnancy, several studies have suggested an increased risk of congenital malformations associated with the use of benzodiazepines. During the last weeks of pregnancy, ingestion of therapeutic doses of a benzodiazepine hypnotic has resulted in neonatal CNS depression due to transplacental distribution.

If the drug is prescribed to a woman of childbearing potential, the patient should be warned of the potential risk to a fetus and advised to consult her physician regarding the discontinuation of the drug if she intends to become pregnant or suspects that she is pregnant.

Memory Disturbance: Anterograde amnesia of varying severity has been reported following therapeutic doses of benzodiazepines. The event is rare with temazepam. Anterograde amnesia is a dose-related phenomenon and elderly subjects may be at particular risk. Cases of transient global amnesia and "traveller's amnesia" have also been reported in association with benzodiazepines, the latter in individuals who have taken the drug, often in the middle of the night, to induce sleep while travelling.

Transient global amnesia and traveller's amnesia are unpredictable and not necessarily dose-related phenomena. Patients should be warned not to take temazepam under circumstances in which a full night's sleep and clearance of the drug from the body are not possible before they need again to resume full activity.

Abnormal thinking and psychotic behavioral changes have been reported to occur in association with the use of benzodiazepines including temazepam, although rarely. Some of the changes may be characterized by decreased inhibition, e.g., aggressiveness or extroversion that seem excessive, similar to that seen with alcohol and other CNS depressants (e.g., sedative/hypnotics). Particular caution is warranted in patients with a history of violent behavior and a history of unusual reactions to sedatives including alcohol and the benzodiazepines. Psychotic behavioral changes that have been reported with benzodiazepines include bizarre behavior, hallucinations, and depersonalization. Abnormal behaviors associated with the use of benzodiazepines have been reported more with chronic use and/or high doses but they may occur during the acute, maintenance or withdrawal phases of treatment.

It can rarely be determined with certainty whether a particular instance of abnormal behaviors listed above is drug induced, spontaneous in origin, or a result of an underlying psychiatric disorder. Nevertheless, the emergence of any new behavioral sign or symptom of concern requires careful and immediate evaluation.

Confusion: The benzodiazepines affect mental efficiency, e.g., concentration, attention and vigilance. The risk of confusion is greater in the elderly and in patients with cerebral impairment.

Anxiety, Restlessness: An increase in daytime anxiety and/or restlessness have been observed during treatment with temazepam. This may be a manifestation of interdose withdrawal due to the short elimination half-life of the drug.

Depression: Caution should be exercised if temazepam is prescribed to patients with signs or symptoms of depression that could be intensified by hypnotic drugs. The potential for self-harm (e.g., intentional overdose) is high in patients with depression and thus, the least amount of drug that is feasible should be available to them at any one time.

Potentiation of Drug Effects: Temazepam may potentiate the effects of other CNS depressant drugs such as alcohol, barbiturates, nonbarbiturate hypnotics, antihistamines, narcotics, antipsychotic and antidepressant drugs, and anticonvulsants. Therefore, different benzodiazepines should usually not be used simultaneously and careful consideration should be given if other CNS depressants are administered in combination with temazepam. Patients should be advised against the simultaneous use of other CNS depressant drugs and should be cautioned not to take alcohol because of the potentiation of effects that might occur.

Complex Sleep-Related Behaviours: Complex sleep-related behaviours such as "sleep-driving" (i.e., driving while not fully awake after ingestion of a sedative-hypnotic, with amnesia for the event) have been reported in patients who have taken temazepam. Other potentially dangerous behaviours have been reported in patients who got out of bed after taking a sedative-hypnotic and were not fully awake, including preparing and eating food, making phone calls, leaving the house, etc. As with "sleep-driving", patients usually do not remember these events. The use of alcohol and other CNS-depressants with temazepam appears to increase the risk of such behaviours, as does the use of temazepam at doses exceeding the maximum recommended dose. **Temazepam is not to be taken with alcohol.** Caution is needed with concomitant use of other CNS depressant drugs. Due to the risk to the patient and the community, discontinuation of temazepam should be strongly considered for patients who report any such complex sleep-related behaviours.

Severe Anaphylactic and Anaphylactoid Reactions: Rare cases of angioedema involving the tongue, glottis or larynx have been reported in patients after taking the first or subsequent doses of sedative-hypnotics, including temazepam. Some patients have had additional symptoms such as dyspnea, throat closing or nausea and vomiting that suggest anaphylaxis. Some patients have required medical therapy in the emergency department. If angioedema involves the throat, glottis or larynx, airway obstruction may occur and be fatal. Patients who develop angioedema after treatment with temazepam should not be rechallenged with the drug.

PRECAUTIONS: *Drug Interactions:* Temazepam may produce additive CNS depressant effects when coadministered with alcohol, sedative antihistamines, anticonvulsants, or psychotropic medications which themselves can produce CNS depression.

Compounds which inhibit certain hepatic enzymes (particularly cytochrome P450) may enhance the activity of benzodiazepines.

Drug Abuse, Dependence and Withdrawal: Withdrawal symptoms, similar in characteristic to those noted with barbiturates and alcohol (convulsions, tremor, abdominal and muscle cramps, vomiting, sweating dysphoria, perceptual disturbances and insomnia) have occurred following abrupt discontinuation of benzodiazepines, including temazepam.

The more severe symptoms are usually associated with higher dosages and longer usage, although patients given therapeutic dosages for as few as 1 to 2 weeks can also have withdrawal symptoms including daytime anxiety between nightly doses. Consequently, abrupt discontinuation should be avoided and a gradual dosage tapering schedule is recommended in any patient taking more than the lowest dose for more than a few weeks. The recommendation for tapering is particularly important in patients with a history of seizures.

The risk of dependence is increased in patients with a history of alcoholism, drug abuse, or in patients with marked personality disorders. Interdose daytime anxiety and rebound anxiety may increase the risk of dependency in temazepam treated patients. As with all hypnotics, repeat prescriptions should be limited to those who are under medical supervision.

Patients with Specific Conditions: Temazepam is O-conjugated in the liver and is primarily excreted by the kidney. Hence, temazepam should be given with caution to patients with impaired hepatic or renal function. Temazepam should also be given with caution to patients with severe pulmonary insufficiency: respiratory depression has been reported in patients with compromised respiratory function.

Temazepam should be used with caution in severely depressed patients or those in whom there is any evidence of latent depression; it should be recognized that suicidal tendencies may be present and protective measures may be necessary.

Patients Requiring Mental Alertness: Because of temazepam's CNS depressant effect, patients receiving the drug should be cautioned against engaging in hazardous occupations requiring complete mental alertness such as operating machinery or driving a motor vehicle. For the same reason, patients should be warned against the concomitant ingestion of temazepam and alcohol or CNS depressant drugs.

Lactation: It is not known whether or not temazepam is excreted in human milk. Therefore, it should not be given to nursing mothers.

Pregnancy: For teratogenic effects see Warnings. Nonteratogenic effects: a child born to a mother who is on benzodiazepines may be at risk for withdrawal symptoms from the drug during the postnatal period. Also, neonatal flaccidity has been reported in an infant born to a mother who had been receiving benzodiazepines.

Children: The safety and effectiveness of temazepam in children below the age of 18 have not been established.

Geriatrics and Debilitated Patients: Elderly patients are especially susceptible to dose-related adverse effects, such as drowsiness, dizziness, or impaired coordination. Inappropriate, heavy sedation may result in accidental events/falls. Therefore, the lowest possible dose should be used in these subjects.

Debilitated patients, or those with organic brain syndrome, are prone to CNS depression after even low doses of benzodiazepines and may experience paradoxical reactions to these drugs. Therefore, temazepam should be used only at the lowest possible dose and adjusted when necessary under careful observation, depending on the response of the patient.

Because temazepam is eliminated by O-conjugation, minimal accumulation occurs.

ADVERSE EFFECTS: During controlled clinical trials in which 1 076 patients received temazepam at bedtime, the adverse events occurring in 1% or more of patients are listed in Table 1.

Table 1: Restoril
Adverse Effects

	Restoril % incidence (n=1 076)	Placebo % incidence (n=783)
Drowsiness	9.1	5.6
Headache	8.5	9.1
Fatigue	4.8	4.7
Nervousness	4.6	8.2
Lethargy	4.5	3.4
Dizziness	4.5	3.3
Nausea	3.1	3.8
Hangover	2.5	1.1
Anxiety	2.0	1.5
Depression	1.7	1.8

(cont'd)

Table 1: Restoril *(cont'd)*

Adverse Effects

	Restoril % incidence (n=1 076)	Placebo % incidence (n=783)
Dry mouth	1.7	2.2
Diarrhea	1.7	1.1
Abdominal Discomfort	1.5	1.9
Euphoria	1.5	0.4
Weakness	1.4	0.9
Confusion	1.3	0.5
Blurred Vision	1.3	1.3
Nightmares	1.2	1.7
Vertigo	1.2	0.8

The following adverse events have been reported with an incidence of 0.5 to 0.9%:
Central Nervous System: anorexia, ataxia, equilibrium loss, tremor, increased dreaming.
Cardiovascular: dyspnea, palpitations.
Gastrointestinal: vomiting.
Muskuloskeletal: backache.
Special Senses: hyperhidrosis, burning eyes.

The following adverse events have been reported with an incidence of less than 0.5%: amnesia, hallucinations, horizontal nystagmus and paradoxical reactions including restlessness, overstimulation, and agitation.

OVERDOSE:

Symptoms: Manifestations of acute overdosage of temazepam, as with other benzodiazepines, can be expected to reflect the increasing CNS effects of the drug and include somnolence, confusion and coma, with reduced or absent reflexes. With large overdoses, respiratory depression, hypotension and finally coma will result.

Treatment: If the patient is conscious, vomiting should be induced mechanically or with emetics (e.g., syrup of ipecac 20 to 30 mL). Gastric lavage should be employed as soon as possible, utilizing concurrently a cuffed endotracheal tube if the patient is unconscious, in order to prevent aspiration and pulmonary complications. Maintenance of adequate pulmonary ventilation is essential and fluids should be administered i.v. to encourage diuresis. The use of pressor agents, such as norepinephrine bitartrate or metaraminol, i.v. may be necessary to combat hypotension but only if considered essential. The value of dialysis in emergency therapy for benzodiazepine overdosage has not been determined. If excitation occurs, barbiturates should not be used. It should be borne in mind that multiple agents may have been ingested.

The benzodiazepine antagonist, flumazenil, is a specific antidote in known or suspected benzodiazepine overdose. For conditions of use see flumazenil product monograph.

> For management of a suspected drug overdose, CPhA recommends that you contact your **regional Poison Control Centre**. See the *CPS* Directory section for a list of Poison Control Centres.

DOSAGE: The lowest effective dose should be used. Treatment should usually not exceed 7 to 10 consecutive days. Use of temazepam for more than 2 to 3 consecutive weeks requires complete re-evaluation of the patient.

An appropriate hypnotic dose should produce the desired hypnotic effect while avoiding oversedation and impairment of performance the next day.

Adults: The recommended adult dose is 30 mg before retiring, **15 mg may be sufficient for some patients.**

Geriatrics and Debilitated Patients: The initial dose should not exceed 15 mg before retiring (see Precautions).

Temazepam is intended only for short-term use and therefore, should not be prescribed in quantities exceeding those required for that cycle of administration. Prescription should not be renewed without further assessment of the patient's needs.

Children: Not indicated in children under 18 years of age.

INFORMATION FOR THE PATIENT: Published in e-CPS, available by subscription at www.e-cps.ca.

SUPPLIED: 15 mg: Each maroon and flesh, size 3 hard shell gelatin capsule, printed SANDOZ and RESTORIL 15 in white, contains: temazepam 15 mg. Nonmedicinal ingredients: colloidal silicon dioxide, D&C Red #28, D&C Yellow #10, FD&C Blue #1, gelatin, lactose, magnesium stearate, sodium lauryl sulfate and titanium dioxide. The agents used to polish the capsules are alcohol, canner special salt and Tween 60. Bottles of 100. Store at controlled room temperature (15 to 30°C). Protect from moisture and light.

30 mg: Each maroon and blue, size 3 hard shell gelatin capsule, printed SANDOZ and RESTORIL 30 in white, contains: temazepam 30 mg. Nonmedicinal ingredients: colloidal silicon dioxide, D&C Red #28, FD&C Blue #1, gelatin, lactose, magnesium stearate, sodium lauryl sulfate and titanium dioxide. The agents used to polish the capsules are alcohol, canner special salt and Tween 60. Bottles of 100. Store at controlled room temperature (15 to 30°C). Protect from moisture and light.

Resultz®

isopropyl myristate

Head Lice Treatment

Nycomed

Date of Revision: August 20, 2009

SUMMARY PRODUCT INFORMATION:

Route of Administration	Dosage Form/ Strength	Clinically Relevant Nonmedicinal Ingredients
Topical	Solution/50% isopropyl myristate	None For a complete listing see Dosage Forms, Composition and Packaging.

INDICATIONS AND CLINICAL USE: Resultz (isopropyl myristate) is indicated for:
- treatment of head lice in adults and children 2 years of age and older.

Resultz (isopropyl myristate) has been used in comparative clinical studies, in which Resultz has been shown to be both safe and effective in treating head lice infestations.

Pediatrics (2 years of age and older): Resultz has been used in children as young as 2 years old with no serious adverse effects. This age limit allows all members living in the same household to be treated with Resultz to more effectively avoid re-infestation.

WARNINGS AND PRECAUTIONS: General:
- For external use only.
- Do not use near the eyes. If product gets into eyes, immediately flush with water.
- Keep out of reach of children.
- If swallowed, patients should seek medical help or contact a Poison Control Centre (see Overdosage).
- If the infestation recurs or persists after the second application, patients should consult their doctor.

Sensitivity/Resistance: Resultz does not contain traditional insecticides or pesticides such as permethrin or pyrethrin which may cause allergic reactions in those sensitive to ragweed or chrysanthemum.

Resultz contains isopropyl myristate as the active ingredient a common ingredient in many cosmetic products, such as lipstick and sunscreen. It is not known to cause serious side effects or sensitivity reactions.

The resistance of lice to traditional lice products containing permethrin and pyrethrin has been reported. A resistance study harvested 82 lice from infested individuals in Southern Ontario in 2008. Genomic DNA (gDNA) was analyzed from these lice and found alleles known to confer resistance to permethrin and/or pyrethrin within the harvested population. These lice have shown a resistance allele frequency of 95%. The allele frequency is determined by counting the number of alleles (2) associated with resistance in the population. For example, 50 lice would have 100 alleles and if 45 of those lice had both alleles resistant to permethrin/pyrethrin, the gene frequency would be 90 divided by 100 which would be an allele frequency of 90%.

The mode of action of Resultz is physical—not neurotoxic—and therefore lice are unlikely to develop resistance to the product (see Action and Clinical Pharmacology, Mechanism of Action).

ADVERSE REACTIONS: Clinical Trial Adverse Drug Reactions: Because clinical trials are conducted under very specific conditions the adverse reaction rates observed in the clinical trials may not reflect the rates observed in practice and should not be compared to the rates in the clinical trials of another drug. Adverse drug reaction information from clinical trials is useful for identifying drug-related adverse events and for approximating rates.

Resultz has been demonstrated to be generally well tolerated in clinical studies and adverse events have been mild in nature. The following adverse events have been reported in phase III clinical studies and consist of a total of 655 patients treated with Resultz.

Common Clinical Trial Adverse Drug Reactions (≥1%-<10%): Clinical Study PP-06-0008 (total subjects=502): erythema (1.0%); hair disorder (1.0%).
Clinical Study PP-07-0004 (total subjects=153): erythema (2.0%); dry skin (3.3%); dandruff (7.8%).

Uncommon Clinical Trial Adverse Drug Reactions (≤0.1%-<1%): Clinical Study PP-06-0008 (total subjects=502): pruritus (0.2%); dandruff (0.6%); dry skin (0.8%).
Clinical Study PP-07-0004 (total subjects=153): burning at treatment site (0.5%); conjunctival hyperaemia (0.7%); pruritus (0.7%); rash (0.7%); urticaria (0.7%).

Post-Market Adverse Drug Reactions: The following adverse reactions have been reported in post-marketing use and causal relation to treatment with isopropyl myristate rinse could not be ruled out: abnormal hair texture (greasy and brittle); alopecia; dry skin; erythema; hypotrichosis; pruritis; rash; rash pruritic; swelling face.

DRUG INTERACTIONS: There have been no drug interaction studies performed with 50% isopropyl myristate rinse. Isopropyl myristate is found in many cosmetic products (>50% concentration) with daily exposures and combined usage with other cosmetics, as such there are no known product interaction concerns at this time.

DOSAGE AND ADMINISTRATION: Usage Guidelines: Approximate dosage for 1 adult/child 2 years of age and older (see Table 1).

Table 1: Resultz

Approximate Dosage for 1 Adult/Child 2 Years of Age and Older

Hair Length	Per Application	Total per Treatment (2 Applications)
Short	30–60 mL	60–120 mL
Shoulder length	60–90 mL	120–180 mL
Long	90–120 mL	180–240 mL

Administration: Head Lice Infestation : Day One:
- Use towels to protect the child/adult's eyes from treatment and prevent clothes from getting wet.
- Apply product to dry hair and massage into the hair until the scalp, especially the sides and nape (back underneath the hair) of the neck, are thoroughly wet with the product. This may take several minutes.
- Lice can crawl up and down the shaft of the hair quickly so it is important to apply the treatment to the scalp as well as from the roots to the ends of the hair. **See Usage Guidelines to estimate how much product you will need.**
- After completing application, allow product to remain on hair for 10 minutes.
- At the end of 10 minutes, rinse with warm water and wash hair, if desired. The feel of the product may remain on the hair following rinsing, this can assist with combing.
- If desired, nits and dead lice can be removed, following treatment, by combing with the fine tooth comb provided.
  - Comb wet hair with a regular comb to remove tangles.
  - Separate a section of hair not wider than the lice removal comb.
  - Using this comb tilted toward the scalp, comb section from scalp to end of hair.
  - Wipe comb with tissue and place tissue in a sealable plastic bag.
  - Repeat until all hair has been combed, to remove eggs, wiping comb with a tissue after each combing.
  - Dispose of all tissues in a sealed plastic bag, wash comb as described below (Daily Checking to Prevent Reinfestation).

Day Seven to Ten: Repeat Resultz application 7 to 10 days after the first treatment. A second treatment should be applied to kill any lice newly hatched from eggs.

Daily Checking to Prevent Reinfestation:
- Carefully inspect family members daily between treatments and for at least 2 weeks after treatment.
- Check all family members for head lice. If anyone in the family is infested, treat as soon as possible with Resultz.
- Soak all combs and brushes in hot water—at least 54°C for 10 minutes. Always inspect and rinse thoroughly before using. Avoid placing combs with plastic components in boiling water.
- All clothing, head gear, scarves, towels and bedding should be washed in very hot water and put in the dryer on the hottest setting for a minimum of 20 minutes. Dry cleaning should suffice for blankets, jackets and other non-washables. Mattresses which have been used by an infested person should not be used for 48 hours.

When Using Resultz:
- Keep out of eyes when rinsing hair.
- Close eyes tightly and do not open eyes until product is rinsed out.
- Protect eyes with washcloth, towel or other suitable method. If product gets into the eyes, flush with water.
- Care should be taken when applying this product since it will make hard surfaces such as floors and baths slippery.
- Protect clothing and upholstery with a towel as this product may stain fabric.
- **Patients should discontinue use and consult a physician if** skin irritation or infection is present or develops and/or if infestation of eyebrows or eyelashes occurs.

Caution: Keep away from any open flame or heat source which uses an open flame. Do not smoke while using this product.

OVERDOSAGE:

There has been no clinical or postmarketing experience with overdosage of 50% Isopropyl Myristate Rinse. Although 50% Isopropyl Myristate Rinse is intended for dermal administration only, a 28-Day repeat (every 3 days) oral dosing study in rats has been performed. The intent of the study was to simulate severe overexposure; the highest dose level (15 mL/kg) filled the animal's stomach. A 15 kg child would have to consume 225 mL of rinse every three days for 28 days to attain this dose level.

Animals exposed to high oral doses of 50% Isopropyl Myristate Rinse had histopathic findings in the lung (red discoloration involving multiple lobes), heart (cardiomyopathy), kidney (unilateral hydronephrosis and bilateral tubular mineralization), and liver (subacute inflammation). Other clinical findings included oily and sparse fur and scaling, dry and red discoloured skin. There were no deaths associated with overdosage. A lower incidence of these findings was seen at the end of the 14-day recovery period indicating some recovery once dosing had ceased.

Patients who ingest Isopropyl Myristate Rinse should seek immediate medical attention or contact the regional poison control centre.

For management of a suspected drug overdose, CPhA recommends that you contact your **regional Poison Control Centre**. See the *CPS* Directory section for a list of Poison Control Centres.

ACTION AND CLINICAL PHARMACOLOGY: Mechanism of Action: Head lice are insects which feed on human blood. They have an open circulatory system causing osmoregulation to be important in survival. Head lice lose water by evaporation from the general body surface, spiracles (breathing holes) and excretion of waste. Water loss from the general body surface is through the cuticle (outer layer of the insect exoskeleton) which is restricted by the epicuticular lipids of the outer layer of the cuticle. **This outer layer is primarily wax (cuticular hydrocarbons).** If a head louse is to survive, water loss must be kept to a minimum and must be offset by water gained (water balance). Food (human blood) is the louse's primary source of water. A net gain in water balance is necessary for normal growth; a net loss, if sustained, will ultimately lead to death.

Isopropyl myristate dissolves lanolin, cholesterol and many waxes. It is used in the cosmetic industry as an effective agent for solubilizing lanolin. The wax on the cuticle of insects, which is responsible for the retention of water, is made up of lanolin. Consequently, isopropyl myristate removes the wax layer from the cuticle of the lice and allows unchecked water loss and subsequent dehydration and death. This is an irreversible, physical process. Initial direct contact with isopropyl myristate induces rapid paralysis (100%) of lice within minutes. It is important that all of the lice on the affected persons head are in contact with isopropyl myristate rinse to ensure it will work effectively.

Resultz works differently from other commonly used head lice treatments; as such it may be an effective treatment in those cases where others have failed.

Pharmacokinetics: Absorption: In an open label study in children (aged 4 to 13), pharmacokinetic samples were collected for determination of plasma concentrations of isopropyl myristate (IPM) and cyclomethicone. Based on the results of the analyses, IPM showed no detectable absorption and cyclomethicone showed minimal absorption.

For a dermally applied compound, it is unlikely that differences in systemic exposure would be attributed to age-related differences in permeability. Barrier functions of the skin principally reside in the stratum corneum, which has been demonstrated in mammals to be fully functional at birth. Studies in rats and guinea pigs determined that at birth the ultrastructure of the stratum corneum, was indistinguishable from that of the adult. The data indicated that the development of the stratum corneum starts in the last quarter of gestation and is completed just before term. There may be differences in permeability expected in pre-term infants due to an undeveloped stratum corneum; however, full-term infants have been shown to have a completely functional stratum corneum with excellent barrier properties. Because there is no difference in dermal absorption between children 2 years of age or older, there should not be a concern of increased dermal absorption in this population.

STORAGE AND STABILITY: Store at 15-30°C. Do not store in direct sunlight.

INFORMATION FOR THE PATIENT: Published in e-CPS, available by subscription at www.e-cps.ca.

DOSAGE FORMS, COMPOSITION AND PACKAGING: Each bottle of a colourless solution for topical administration contains: isopropyl myristate 50% w/w. Nonmedicinal ingredients: cyclomethicone. Bottles of 120 and 240 mL.

Clinical Trials: Study Demographics and Trial Design: Approximately 870 subjects, ranging in age from 2 to 59 years, have been treated with isopropyl myristate rinse as part of the clinical development program. Most studies were investigator/evaluator blinded, some used permethrin (1%) or synergised pyrethrum (0.33% pyrethrin, 4% piperonyl butoxide) as an active control whereas others were open label using no comparator. Subjects with an active head lice infestation were included in these studies. Sentinel subjects, the youngest household member presenting with at least 3 live lice on the head, were included in the efficacy analysis. All subjects treated were included in the safety evaluation.

Study Results: In a Canadian Phase 2 open label study involving 29 patients, 96.5% of patients treated with isopropyl myristate rinse were lice free on Day 14.

In a US Phase 2 randomized, comparator study (0.33% pyrethrin, 4% piperonyl butoxide) involving 30 isopropyl myristate rinse treated patients, a significantly greater proportion of patients treated with isopropyl myristate rinse were lice free on Day 14.

A second US Phase 2 study was conducted in two stages. Stage 1, involving 27 isopropyl myristate rinse treated patients, was a randomized, comparator study (0.33% pyrethrin, 4% piperonyl butoxide), in which no combing was included. A greater proportion of patients treated with 50% Isopropyl Myristate Rinse were lice free on Day 24 than the comparator. However, there was no statistical difference between the two treatments. In Stage 2, an open label study, with combing, involving 20 isopropyl myristate rinse treated patients, 84% of patients treated with isopropyl myristate rinse were lice free on Day 24.

In a UK Phase 2 randomized, comparator study (1% permethrin) involving 37 isopropyl myristate rinse treated patients, a significantly greater proportion of patients treated with isopropyl myristate rinse were lice free on Day 14.

In a UK Phase 3 randomized, comparator study (1% permethrin) involving 74 isopropyl myristate rinse treated patients, a significantly greater proportion of patients treated with isopropyl myristate rinse were lice free on Day 14.

In a US Phase 3 multicenter, randomized, comparator study (0.33% pyrethrin, 4% piperonyl butoxide) involving 502 isopropyl myristate rinse treated patients, a greater proportion of patients treated with isopropyl myristate rinse were lice free on Day 24. However there was no statistical difference between the two.

In a second US Phase 3 multicenter, randomized, comparator study (0.33% pyrethrin, 4% piperonyl butoxide) involving 153 isopropyl myristate rinse treated patients, a significantly greater proportion of patients treated with isopropyl myristate rinse were lice free on Day 24.

The active comparator products used in the above clinical trials were sourced from the United Kingdom or the United States. Product formulations differ between countries despite having identical active ingredients.

Retin-A® Ⓟ

tretinoin

Comedolytic Agent

Johnson & Johnson

PHARMACOLOGY: Studies in animals have shown that tretinoin supplies all the physiologic requirements of Vitamin A except those needed for vision and reproduction. When animals were fed a diet in which Vitamin A was replaced by Vitamin A acid, there was no storage in the liver. This suggests that the acid may be the tissue-active form which is important for epithelial growth and general health, while the alcohol or ester form is necessary for vision and reproduction.

Repeated skin applications of Vitamin A acid over a period of days have produced detectable changes in the skin. Initially, the change is mild erythema, followed by flaking or peeling of the stratum corneum, which in itself is associated with a marked thinning of the stratum corneum and increased cellular turnover in the skin.

Local application of Vitamin A has been reported to have reduced abnormal cornification in follicular orifices, and Vitamin A acid was reported to be more potent than Vitamin A alcohol or its esters when applied locally in ointments to human skin.

Although the exact mode of action of tretinoin is unknown, current evidence suggests that topical tretinoin decreases cohesiveness of follicular cells with decreased microcomedo formation. Additionally, tretinoin stimulates mitotic activity and increased turnover of follicular epithelial cells, causing extrusion of the comedones.

INDICATIONS: For topical application in the treatment of acne vulgaris.

CONTRAINDICATIONS: Patients who have demonstrated a hypersensitivity to the drug.

WARNINGS: General: Excessive use of tretinoin should be avoided. In order to minimize the potential for additional skin irritation, care should be taken to avoid contact with the eyes, eyelids, angles of the nose, mouth, mucous membranes or other areas where treatment is not intended. Tretinoin may cause irritation of circumoral and other sensitive skin areas. Tretinoin should not be applied to severely inflamed skin or to open lesions.

Simultaneous use of harsh abrasives and other skin treatments, including sun lamp, should be avoided if possible.

In some patients temporary skin irritation may occur, especially in early weeks of treatment. Should these reactions occur to an excessive degree, and the skin becomes extremely red, swollen and crusted, use of tretinoin should be discontinued immediately.

An apparent exacerbation may develop due to the drug effect on previously seen deep lesions. This is an anticipated part of the therapeutic effect. Therapy should be continued.

Pregnancy: **Topical tretinoin should be used by women of childbearing years only after contraceptive counselling. It is recommended that topical tretinoin should not be used by pregnant women.**

There have been a few reports of birth defects among babies born to women exposed to **topical** tretinoin during pregnancy. To date, there have been no adequate and well-controlled prospective studies performed in pregnant women and the teratogenic blood level of tretinoin is not clear. However, a well-conducted retrospective cohort study of babies born to women exposed to topical tretinoin during the first trimester of pregnancy found no excess birth defects among these babies when compared with babies born to women in the same cohort who were not similarly exposed.

Oral tretinoin has been shown to be teratogenic and fetotoxic in rats when given in doses 1000 and 500 times the topical human dose, respectively.

In 9 out of 10 topical teratology studies of tretinoin conducted in rats and rabbits using several formulations, there has been no evidence of teratogenicity. In 1 out of 10 studies there was an increase in fetal malformations; however, a clear causal relationship of topical tretinoin in these findings could not be established. In a repeat of this study, there were no fetal malformations. Topical tretinoin can produce treatment-related fetal effects (delayed ossification of bones and an increase in supernumerary ribs). The fetal no-effect dose is 1 mg/kg/day (200 times the recommended clinical dose).

Lactation: It is not known whether tretinoin is excreted in human milk. Nevertheless, a decision should be made whether to discontinue nursing or to discontinue the drug taking into account the importance of the drug to the mother. Since many drugs are excreted in human milk, caution should be exercised when tretinoin is administered to a nursing mother.

PRECAUTIONS: General: For external use only.

Cosmetics may be used, but the areas to be treated should be cleansed thoroughly before the medication is applied. Astringent toiletries should be avoided.

Patients will be able to remove hair as usual (e.g., plucking, electrolysis, depilatories) but should avoid these procedures at night before applying tretinoin as they might result in skin irritation.

Permanent wave solutions, waxing preparations, medicated soaps and shampoos can sometimes irritate even normal skin. Caution should be used so that these products do not come into contact with skin treated with tretinoin.

Exposure to sunlight and sun lamps should be avoided or minimized during the use of tretinoin because of heightened susceptibility to UV radiation as a result of the use of tretinoin. A patient experiencing considerable sun exposure due to occupational duties, and/or any patient inherently sensitive to the sun, should exercise particular caution. When exposure to sunlight cannot be avoided use of sunburn protectant products with a SPF of at least 15 and protective clothing over treated areas is recommended when exposure cannot be avoided.

Hyper- or hypopigmentation has occasionally been reported when the product is used to the point of producing severe irritation. This is reversible when the medication is stopped.

Children: Safety and effectiveness have not been established in children.

Gels are flammable. Note: Keep away from heat and flame. Keep tube tightly closed.

Local Irritation: It is not recommended to initiate treatment with tretinoin or continue its use in the presence of skin irritation (e.g., erythema, peeling, pruritus, sunburn, etc.) until these symptoms subside.

In certain sensitive individuals, tretinoin may induce severe local erythema, swelling, pruritus, warmth, burning or stinging, blistering, crusting and/or peeling at the site of application. If the degree of local irritation warrants, the patient should be instructed to either apply the medication less frequently or discontinue its use temporarily.

Tretinoin has been reported to cause severe irritation on eczematous skin and should be used with utmost caution in patients with this condition. If a patient experiences severe or persistent irritation, the patient should be advised to discontinue application of tretinoin completely, and if necessary, consult a physician.

Weather extremes, such as wind, cold and low humidity may be irritating to skin treated with tretinoin and may increase its dryness.

Drug Interactions: Concomitant topical medication, medicated or abrasive soaps and cleansers, soaps and cosmetics that have a strong drying effect, and products with high concentrations of alcohol, astringents, spices or lime should be used with caution because of possible interaction with tretinoin. Particular caution should be exercised in using preparations containing sulfur, resorcinol, or salicylic acid with tretinoin. It is also advisable to "rest" a patient's skin until the effects of such preparations subside before use of tretinoin is begun.

ADVERSE EFFECTS: Some degree of local irritation is expected. The most commonly reported undesirable effects are dry skin, burning, stinging, warmth, erythema, pruritus, rash, peeling and temporary hypo- and hyperpigmentation. Rarely reported undesirable effects are blistering and crusting of the skin, eye irritation and edema. These reactions were usually mild to moderate in severity, generally well-tolerated and self-limiting, occurred early during the course of therapy and generally decreased over time with the exception of dry skin, which tended to persist.

True contact allergy to topical tretinoin is rarely encountered.

Changes in the skin may be anticipated, indicating an active effect of the medication. Expected changes include mild erythema and flaking or peeling of the stratum corneum. In certain very sensitive patients, the skin may become very erythematous, edematous, blistered or crusted. In such cases, application of tretinoin should be discontinued until the skin has fully recovered. Further applications should be at a level that the individual can tolerate. All adverse reactions observed are reversible when treatment is discontinued.

OVERDOSE:

Symptoms: If medication is applied excessively, no more rapid or better results will be obtained and marked redness, peeling, or discomfort may occur. Tretinoin is intended for topical use only. In the event of accidental ingestion, if the ingestion is recent, the stomach should be emptied immediately by gastric lavage or by induction of emesis. All other treatment should be appropriately supportive. Oral ingestion of the drug may lead to the same side effects as those associated with excessive oral intake of Vitamin A including teratogenesis in women of childbearing years. Therefore, in such cases pregnancy testing should be carried out in women of childbearing years. Reduce amount or frequency of application if undesirable reactions occur.

Treatment: See Symptoms.

For management of a suspected drug overdose, CPhA recommends that you contact your **regional Poison Control Centre**. See the *CPS* Directory section for a list of Poison Control Centres.

DOSAGE: Excessive use should be avoided.

Adults: Apply daily to the affected areas, preferably at bedtime, after cleansing with a mild, nonmedicated soap and water. The treated area should be washed no more than twice per day. After washing, the skin should be dried gently and completely without rubbing it. Allow at least 20 to 30 minutes to dry before applying medication. Only a sufficient quantity of medication should be applied to cover the affected areas lightly, using a gauze swab, cotton wool or the tips of clean fingers. Over-saturation should be avoided since excess medication could run into the eyes, angles of the nose or other areas where treatment is not intended.

Discontinue treatment if a severe local inflammatory response is experienced. Reinstitute therapy when the reaction has subsided and apply preparation every other day or less frequently. Should discomfort still be experienced, stop treatment completely.

Maintenance dose should be the least number of applications that will prevent recurrence of the condition. Maintenance therapy should be administered daily for best results.

Application of tretinoin may cause a transitory feeling of warmth or slight stinging. When administered according to recommended guidelines, tretinoin may produce a slight erythema similar to that of mild sunburn. In cases where it is necessary to temporarily discontinue therapy or reduce the frequency of application, therapy should be resumed or the frequency of application increased when the patient becomes able to tolerate the treatment.

Excess application of tretinoin does not provide more rapid or better results. In fact, marked redness, peeling or discomfort can occur. If excess application occurs accidentally or through over-enthusiastic use, tretinoin should be discontinued for several days before resuming therapy.

Therapeutic effects may be noticed after 2 to 3 weeks of use but more than 6 weeks of therapy may be required before definite beneficial effects are seen. During the early weeks of treatment, an apparent exacerbation of inflammatory lesions may occur. This is due to the action of the medication on deep, previously unseen lesions and should not be considered a reason to discontinue therapy. Once a satisfactory response has been obtained, it may be possible to maintain this improvement with less frequent applications.

Children: Safety and effectiveness have not been established in children.

INFORMATION FOR THE PATIENT: Published in e-CPS, available by subscription at www.e-cps.ca.

SUPPLIED: Cream: Each g of cream contains: tretinoin 0.01%, 0.025%, 0.05% or 0.1% in a bland, hydrophilic base. Nonmedicinal ingredients: butylated hydroxytoluene, isopropyl myristate, polyoxyl (40) stearate, purified water, sorbic acid, stearic acid, stearyl alcohol and xanthan gum. Tubes of 30 g.

Gel: Each g of gel contains: tretinoin 0.01% or 0.025%. Nonmedicinal ingredients: butylated hydroxytoluene, ethanol undenatured and hydroxypropyl cellulose. Tubes of 30 g.

Keep container closed when not in use. Store between 15 and 25°C.

Retin-A Micro® ℞

tretinoin

Comedolytic Agent

Johnson & Johnson

Date of Revision: March 31, 2008

PHARMACOLOGY: RETIN-A MICRO (tretinoin gel) (microsphere) is a novel formulation containing either 0.1% or 0.04% tretinoin by weight for the topical treatment of acne vulgaris.

Tretinoin is a member of the retinoid family of compounds, and an endogenous metabolite of vitamin A.

Tretinoin is highly effective in the treatment of acne, although the exact mode of action of tretinoin is unknown. Current evidence suggests that this efficacy is due primarily to the ability of tretinoin to modify abnormal follicular keratinization. Comedones form in follicles due to abnormal keratinization and intercellular cohesiveness, with an excess of keratin retained in the follicle. Tretinoin promotes detachment of cornified cells and the enhanced shedding of corneocytes from the follicle. By increasing the mitotic activity of follicular epithelia, tretinoin also increases the turnover rates of thin, loosely-adherent corneocytes. Through these actions, the comedo contents are extruded and the formation of the microcomedo, the precursor lesion of acne vulgaris, is reduced.

Additionally, tretinoin acts by modulating the proliferation and differentiation of epidermal cells. These effects are mediated by tretinoin's interaction with a family of nuclear retinoic acid receptors. Activation of these nuclear receptors causes changes in gene expression. The exact mechanisms whereby tretinoin-induced changes in gene expression regulate skin function are not understood.

This formulation uses patented methyl methacrylate/glycol dimethacrylate crosspolymer porous microspheres (MICROSPONGE System) to enable inclusion of the active ingredient, tretinoin, in an aqueous gel.

Irritation Potential: Although tretinoin is intrinsically irritating to the skin, RETIN-A MICRO (microsphere) 0.1%, was found to be significantly less irritating than RETIN-A Cream, 0.1%, in a cumulative 21 day irritation test in subjects with normal skin. In addition, a half-face comparative irritation trial conducted for up to 14 days in women with sensitive skin, without acne, RETIN-A MICRO (microsphere) 0.1%, was statistically less irritating than tretinoin cream, 0.1% (Table 1). There were no comparative studies conducted between RETIN-A MICRO (microsphere) 0.1% and 0.04% to assess comparative irritation potential.

Table 1: RETIN-A MICRO

RETIN-A MICRO 0.04% Overview of Cutaneous Treatment Effects. Percentage of Patients Experiencing Symptoms

Cutaneous Treatment Effect Response	Treatment	
	RETIN-A MICRO 0.04%	Vehicle
Erythema	64.0	53.5
Peeling	67.6	27.0
Dryness	59.6	31.9
Burning/Stinging	31.1	11.5
Itching	32.4	18.6

Pharmacokinetics: Tretinoin is an endogenous metabolite of vitamin A metabolism in man. Percutaneous absorption of RETIN-A MICRO (microsphere), as determined by the cumulative excretion of radio-labelled drug into urine and feces, was assessed in 44 healthy men and women. Estimates of in vivo bioavailability, mean (SD) %, following both single and multiple daily applications, for a period of 28 days, were 0.82 (0.11)% and 1.41 (0.54)%, respectively. The plasma concentrations of tretinoin and its metabolites, 13-cis-retinoic acid, all-trans-4-oxo-retinoic acid, and 13-cis-4-oxo-retinoic acid, generally ranged from 1 to 3 ng/mL and were essentially unaltered after either single or multiple daily applications relative to baseline levels.

Clinical Trials RETIN-A MICRO (microsphere) 0.04%: In two large vehicle-controlled clinical studies, RETIN-A MICRO (microsphere) 0.04%, applied once daily was significantly more effective than vehicle in reducing the severity of acne lesion counts. A total of 451 subjects with acne vulgaris were enrolled in the 2 controlled clinical studies. Of these 225 subjects applied RETIN-A MICRO (microsphere) 0.04%. The severity of acne experienced by patients enrolled in these studies is shown in Table 2.

Table 2: RETIN-A MICRO

Baseline Severity of Acne

Total facial lesion count	20–150
Comedones (open and closed)	10–100
Inflammatory lesions	10–50
No more than 2 nodules (deep inflammatory lesions of ≥1 cm)	

The mean reductions in lesion counts from baseline after treatment for 12 weeks are shown in Table 3.

Table 3: RETIN-A MICRO

Mean (LS Mean) Percent Reduction in Lesion Counts From BL to Week 12 RETIN-A MICRO 0.04% ITT/LOCF

Lesion Count	RETIN-A MICRO 0.04%		Vehicle	
	Study #1 N=108	Study #2 N=111	Study #1 N=110	Study #2 N=103
Non-inflammatory	-37.7	-28.5	1.8	-14.4
Inflammatory	-43.5	-40.7	-13.4	-28.3
Total	-39.7	-34.2	-8.0	-19.5

It takes 6-8 weeks to see significant clinical benefit from applying RETIN-A MICRO (microsphere) 0.04% to acne lesions. There are no comparative studies between RETIN-A MICRO (microsphere) 0.04% and 0.1%.

RETIN-A MICRO (microsphere) 0.04% was also significantly superior to the vehicle in the investigator's global evaluation of the clinical response. In study #1 14% of subjects using RETIN-A MICRO (microsphere) 0.04% achieved an excellent result compared to 5% (p<0.0001) of patients on vehicle control. In study #2, 19% of subjects using RETIN-A MICRO (microsphere) 0.04% achieved an excellent result compared to 9% (p=0.0052) of subjects on vehicle control.

Clinical Trials RETIN-A MICRO (microsphere) 0.1%: In two vehicle-controlled clinical studies, RETIN-A MICRO (microsphere) 0.1% applied once daily was significantly more effective than vehicle in reducing the severity of acne lesion counts. The mean reductions in lesion counts from baseline after treatment for 12 weeks are shown in Table 4.

Therapeutic results may be noticed after two weeks, but more than four weeks are required before consistent beneficial results are observed. In each study, at each return visit, there was a greater mean percent reduction in total lesion count with RETIN-A MICRO (microsphere) 0.1% than with vehicle (Table 5).

Table 4: RETIN-A MICRO

Mean Percent Reduction From BL to Week 12 RETIN-A MICRO 0.1% Studies

Lesion Count	RETIN-A MICRO 0.01%		Vehicle Gel	
	Study #1	Study #2	Study #1	Study #2
Non-inflammatory	−49	−32	−22%	−3%
Inflammatory	−37	−29	−18%	−24%
Total	−45	−32	−23%	−16%

Table 5: RETIN-A MICRO

Mean Percent Reduction From Baseline in Total Lesion Counts Over Time, Subjects Valid for Efficacy RETIN-A MICRO 0.1% Studies

Return Visit Week	RETIN-A MICRO 0.1%		Vehicle		
	N	Mean	N	Mean	p-value
Study #1					
2	77	18.3	80	6.3	0.006
4	77	22.3	78	14.4	0.127
7	75	38.9	77	18.2	<0.001
10	74	45.6	74	19.6	<0.001
12	72	44.5	72	22.8	<0.001
Study #2					
2	71	5.6	75	2.9	0.205
4	74	9.2	77	2.7	0.026
7	70	16.1	71	4.9	0.016
10	68	31.0	66	9.7	<0.001
12	71	32.3	67	16.2	0.002

RETIN-A MICRO (microsphere) 0.1% was also significantly superior to the vehicle in the investigator's global evaluation of the clinical response. In study #1, 35% of patients using RETIN-A MICRO (microsphere) 0.1% achieved an excellent result compared to 11% of patients on vehicle control. In study #2, 28% of patients using RETIN-A MICRO (microsphere) 0.1% achieved an excellent result compared to 9% of patients on vehicle control.

INDICATIONS: RETIN-A MICRO tretinoin gel (microsphere) is indicated for topical application in the treatment of acne vulgaris.

CONTRAINDICATIONS: RETIN-A MICRO tretinoin gel (microsphere) is contraindicated in individuals with a history of sensitivity reactions to any of its components. It should be discontinued if hypersensitivity to any of its ingredients is noted.

WARNINGS: General: The skin of certain sensitive individuals may become excessively dry, red, swollen, or blistered. If these effects occur, the medication should be either discontinued until the integrity of the skin is restored or the medication should be adjusted temporarily to a level the patient can tolerate. Excessive skin dryness may also be experienced; if so, use of an appropriate emollient during the day may be helpful.

RETIN-A MICRO tretinoin gel (microsphere) should be kept away from the eyes, the mouth, angles of the nose, and mucous membranes.

Tretinoin has been reported to cause severe irritation on eczematous skin and should be used with utmost caution in patients with this condition. If a reaction suggesting sensitivity or chemical irritation occurs, use of the medication should be discontinued (see Precautions, General).

Pregnancy: **Topical tretinoin should be used by women of childbearing years only after contraceptive counseling. It is recommended that topical tretinoin should not be used by pregnant women.**

There have been isolated reports of birth defects among babies born to women exposed to topical tretinoin during pregnancy. To date, there have been no adequate and well-controlled prospective studies performed in pregnant women and the teratogenic blood level of tretinoin is not known. However, a well-conducted retrospective cohort study of babies born to women exposed to topical tretinoin during the first trimester of pregnancy found no excess birth defects among these babies when compared with babies born to women in the same cohort who were not similarly exposed.

Oral tretinoin has been shown to be teratogenic and fetotoxic in rats when given in doses 1000 and 500 times the topical human dose, respectively.

In nine (9) out of ten (10) teratology studies of **topical** tretinoin conducted in rats and rabbits using several formulations, there has been no evidence of teratogenicity. In one (1) out of ten (10) studies there was an increase in fetal malformations; however, a clear causal relationship of topical tretinoin in these findings could not be established. In a repeat of this study, there were no fetal malformations. Topical tretinoin can produce treatment-related fetal effects (delayed ossification of bones and an increase in supernumerary ribs). The fetal no-effect dose is 1.0 mg/kg/day (200 times the recommended clinical dose).

Lactation: It is not known whether RETIN-A MICRO (microsphere) is excreted in human milk. Nevertheless, a decision should be made whether to discontinue nursing or to discontinue the drug, taking into account the importance of the drug to the mother. Since many drugs are excreted in human milk, caution should be exercised when tretinoin is administered to a nursing mother.

PRECAUTIONS: General: RETIN-A MICRO tretinoin gel (microsphere) is for external use only.

Although recent studies have shown that RETIN-A MICRO (microsphere) does not cause phototoxicity or photoallergy, unprotected exposure to sunlight, including sunlamps, should be minimized during the use of RETIN-A MICRO (microsphere).

Patients with sunburn should be advised not to use the product until fully recovered because of the possibility of a heightened susceptibility to sunlight as a result of the use of tretinoin. Patients who may be required to have considerable sun exposure due to their occupation and those with inherent sensitivity to the sun should exercise particular caution. Use of sunscreen products (at least SPF 15) and protective clothing over treated areas are recommended when exposure cannot be avoided (see Dosage).

Local Irritation: Excessive skin dryness may be experienced; if so, use of an appropriate emollient during the day may be helpful.

The skin of certain sensitive individuals may become excessively dry, red, swollen, or blistered. If these effects occur, the medication should be either discontinued until the integrity of the skin is restored or the medication should be adjusted temporarily to a level the patient can tolerate.

RETIN-A MICRO (microsphere) should be kept away from the eyes, the mouth, angles of the nose and mucous membranes. Tretinoin has been reported to cause severe irritation on eczematous skin and should be used with utmost caution in patients with this condition.

Medicated or abrasive soaps and cleansers, soaps and cosmetics that have a strong drying effect, and products with high concentrations of alcohol, astringents, spices or lime should be used with caution because of possible interaction with tretinoin. Avoid contact with the peel of limes.

Patients will be able to remove hair as usual (e.g. plucking, electrolysis, depilatories) but should avoid these procedures at night before applying RETIN-A MICRO (microsphere) as they might result in skin irritation.

Weather extremes, such as wind or cold, also may be irritating to patients being treated with tretinoin.

Drug Interactions: Caution should be exercised with the simultaneous use of topical over-the-counter acne preparations containing benzoyl peroxide, sulfur, resorcinol, or salicylic acid with RETIN-A MICRO (microsphere). It also is advisable to allow the effects of such preparations to subside before use of RETIN-A MICRO (microsphere) is begun.

Concomitant topical medication, medicated or abrasive soaps and cleansers, products that have a strong drying effect, products with high concentrations of alcohol, astringents, or spices should be used with caution because of possible interaction with tretinoin.

Avoid contact with the peel of limes.

Children: Safety and effectiveness in children below the age of 12 have not been established.

ADVERSE EFFECTS: The skin of certain sensitive individuals treated with RETIN-A MICRO tretinoin gel (microsphere) may become excessively red, edematous, blistered, or crusted. If these effects occur, the medication should be either discontinued until the integrity of the skin is restored, or the medication should be adjusted temporarily to a level the patient can tolerate. True contact allergy to topical tretinoin is rarely encountered. Temporary hyper- or hypopigmentation has been reported with repeated application of tretinoin. Some individuals have been reported to have heightened susceptibility to sunlight while under treatment with tretinoin. To date, all adverse effects of tretinoin have been reversible upon discontinuance of therapy (see Dosage).

OVERDOSE:

Symptoms: RETIN-A MICRO tretinoin gel (microsphere) is intended for topical use only. In the event of accidental ingestion, if the ingestion is recent, the stomach should be emptied immediately by gastric lavage or by induction of emesis. All other treatment should be appropriately supportive. Oral ingestion of the drug may lead to the same side effects as those associated with excessive oral intake of vitamin A including teratogenesis in women of childbearing years. Therefore, in such cases pregnancy testing should be carried out in females of childbearing age.

Treatment: See Symptoms.

> For management of a suspected drug overdose, CPhA recommends that you contact your **regional Poison Control Centre**. See the *CPS* Directory section for a list of Poison Control Centres.

DOSAGE: RETIN-A MICRO tretinoin gel (microsphere) should be applied once a day, to acne-prone skin areas, after washing with mild, non-medicated soap and dry skin gently. The gel may be applied at any time during the day or at bedtime. Use only a sufficient quantity of medication to cover the entire affected area lightly. Application of excessive amounts of gel may result in "caking" of the gel, and will not provide incremental efficacy.

A transitory feeling of warmth or slight stinging may be noted on application. In cases where it has been necessary to temporarily discontinue therapy or to reduce the frequency of application, therapy may be resumed or the frequency of application increased as the patient becomes able to tolerate the treatment. Frequency of application should be closely monitored by careful observation of the clinical therapeutic response and skin tolerance. RETIN-A MICRO (microsphere) applied once daily is effective in reducing the severity of acne and reducing the number of lesions. Efficacy has not been established for less than once daily dosing frequencies.

During the early weeks of therapy, an apparent exacerbation of inflammatory lesions may occur. This may be due to the action of the medication on deep, previously unseen lesions and should not be considered a reason to discontinue therapy.

Therapeutic results may be noticed after two weeks, but more than four weeks of therapy are required before consistent beneficial effects are observed. Patients in clinical trials were treated for 12 weeks.

Patients treated with RETIN-A MICRO (microsphere) may use cosmetics, but the areas to be treated should be cleansed thoroughly before the medication is applied.

Patients treated with RETIN-A MICRO (microsphere) should use effective sunscreens with a minimum SPF of 15 as well as protective clothing when exposure to sun cannot be avoided.

INFORMATION FOR THE PATIENT: Published in e-CPS, available by subscription at www.e-cps.ca.

SUPPLIED: 0.04%: Each g of gel contains: tretinoin microsphere 0.04%. Nonmedicinal ingredients: benzyl alcohol, butylated hydroxytoluene, carbomer 974P, cyclomethicone and dimethicone copolyol, disodium EDTA, glycerin, PPG-20 methyl glucose ether distearate, propylene glycol, propylene glycol dicaprylate/dicaprate, purified water, sorbic acid and trolamine. Tubes of 20 and 45 g. Pumps of 50 g. Keep container closed when not in use. Store between 15 and 25°C. Protect from heat.

0.1%: Each g of gel contains: tretinoin microsphere 0.1%. Nonmedicinal ingredients: benzyl alcohol, butylated hydroxytoluene, carbomer 934P, cyclomethicone and dimethicone copolyol, disodium EDTA, glycerin, PPG-20 methyl glucose ether distearate, propylene glycol dicaprylate/dicaprate, propylene glycol, purified water, sorbic acid and trolamine. Tubes of 20 and 45 g. Pumps of 50 g. Keep container closed when not in use. Store between 15 and 25°C. Protect from heat.

Retisol-A® Pr

tretinoin—parsol MCX—butyl methoxydibenzoylmethane

Acne Therapy

Stiefel, a GSK company

PHARMACOLOGY: The precise mechanism of action of tretinoin on the skin is not fully understood. It is known that tretinoin is both pharmacologically and structurally related to vitamin A which regulates epithelial cell growth and differentiation. Tretinoin itself is known to have an irritant and keratolytic effect on the skin. These 2 actions which occur simultaneously have been shown histologically in both animal and man to be associated with an increased growth rate and with a decrease in the cohesiveness of the epidermal cells. The result is a slightly thickened epidermis with an accelerated turnover rate and shedding of keratinized cells as very fine barely perceptible scales.

In acne vulgaris the induced fine scaling of the skin surface is accompanied by an increased production of less cohesive epidermal sebaceous cells which consequently flow out of the follicle at a more rapid rate. The thickened mass of sebaceous cellular debris, the comedones, appear to be initially extruded and then prevented from recurring by these actions. Histopathologically, acne is the impaction plus distention of the sebaceous follicles by tightly packed horny cells and disruption of the follicular epithelium. It has been postulated that tretinoin inhibits the synthesis or quality of the substance which binds the horny cells within the sebaceous follicle.

INDICATIONS: The treatment of acne vulgaris, primarily where comedones, papules and pustules predominate. Tretinoin is not effective in most cases of severe pustular and deep cystic nodular varieties (acne conglobata).

CONTRAINDICATIONS: Patients with known hypersensitivity to retinoids or to any ingredient contained in the preparation.

WARNINGS: Tretinoin is intended for external use only and should be kept away from eyes, nose, mouth, and other mucous membranes because of its irritant effect.

Do not apply to eyelids or to the skin at the corners of the eyes and mouth. Avoid the angles of the nose and nasolabial fold (if treatment in these areas is necessary, apply very sparingly). Topical use may induce severe local erythema and peeling at the site of application. If the degree of local irritation warrants, patients should be directed to use the medication less frequently, discontinue use temporarily or discontinue use altogether. Tretinoin has been reported to cause severe irritation of eczematous skin and tretinoin should only be used with utmost caution in patients with this condition.

Pregnancy: **Topical tretinoin should be used by women of childbearing years only after contraceptive counselling. It is recommended that topical tretinoin should not by used by pregnant women.**

There have been rare reports of birth defects among babies born to women exposed to **topical** tretinoin during pregnancy. However, there are no well controlled prospective studies of the use of topical tretinoin in pregnant women. A retrospective study of mothers exposed to topical tretinoin during the first trimester of pregnancy found no increase in the incidence of birth defects.

Topical retinoid teratology studies in rats and rabbits have been inconclusive. As with all retinoids, tretinoin administered **orally** at high doses is teratogenic.

Lactation: **It is not known whether tretinoin is excreted in human milk. Nevertheless, a decision should be made whether to discontinue nursing or to discontinue the drug taking into account the importance of the drug to the mother.**

PRECAUTIONS: Concomitant topical medications should be used with caution during therapy with tretinoin because of possible intensified reactions. Particular caution should be exercised when using preparations containing a peeling agent concomitantly (such as sulfur, resorcinol, benzoyl peroxide or salicylic acid) with tretinoin. It may be advisable to "rest" a patient's skin until the effects of previously used peeling agents subside before initiating tretinoin therapy.

Exposure to sunlight and sun lamps should be avoided or minimized during the use of tretinoin because of heightened susceptibility to UV radiation as a result of the use of tretinoin.

If a sunburn occurs, it is advisable to interrupt therapy until the severe erythema and peeling subside. Patients whose occupations require considerable exposure to the sun should exercise particular caution. Use of sunburn protectant products with a SPF of at least 15 and protective clothing over treated areas is recommended when exposure cannot be avoided.

ADVERSE EFFECTS: The skin of certain sensitive individuals, particularly those with fair complexion, may become excessively red, edematous, blistered or crusted when exposed to tretinoin. Pain, burning sensation, tenderness, irritation or pruritus have also been occasionally reported. If any of these effects occur, the medication should be discontinued until the integrity of the skin has been restored or the treatment schedule adjusted to the level the patient can tolerate. Temporary hyper- or hypopigmentation has been reported with repeated application of tretinoin. To date, all adverse clinical effects of tretinoin encountered have been reversible upon discontinuance of therapy. In many instances, reinstitution of therapy with tretinoin failed to produce the adverse effect previously experienced.

OVERDOSE:

Symptoms: Topical: If medication is applied excessively, marked redness, peeling or discomfort may occur.

Inadvertent oral ingestion of Retisol-A cream may lead to the same adverse effects as those associated with excessive oral intake of Vitamin A including teratogenesis in women of childbearing years. Therefore in such cases, pregnancy testing should be carried out in women of childbearing years

> For management of a suspected drug overdose, CPhA recommends that you contact your **regional Poison Control Centre**. See the *CPS* Directory section for a list of Poison Control Centres.

DOSAGE: Tretinoin should be applied to the affected area once a day. The area under treatment (not just clinical lesions) should be thoroughly cleansed with a mild soap, such as Acne-Aid Soap, and dried, followed by application of tretinoin with a gentle rubbing motion. Application may be accompanied by a transitory feeling of warmth or a stinging sensation. Treatment should be discontinued if a severe local inflammatory response is experienced.

In cases where it has been necessary to discontinue therapy or to reduce the frequency of applications, therapy may be resumed, when the adverse effects have ceased. In some patients, during the early weeks of therapy, an apparent exacerbation of the acne lesions may occur.

Therapeutic results may be noticed after 2 to 3 weeks of therapy; however, results may not be optimal until after 8 to 10 weeks of treatment. Once the acne lesions have responded satisfactorily, it may be possible to maintain the improved state with less frequent applications.

Patients being treated with tretinoin may continue to use water-based cosmetics; however, the area of skin to be treated should be thoroughly cleansed and dried before tretinoin application.

INFORMATION FOR THE PATIENT: Published in e-CPS, available by subscription at www.e-cps.ca.

SUPPLIED: Each g of cream contains: tretinoin USP 0.01%, 0.025%, 0.05% or 0.1% in a moisturizing cream base with 7.5% Parsol MCX and 2% Parsol 1789 (SPF 15). Nonmedicinal ingredients: butylated hydroxytoluene, carbomer 934, cyclomethicone, diisopropyl adipate, glycerin, imidurea/parabens, octyldodecyl neopentanoate, light mineral oil, phenyl trimethicone, polysorbate 60, purified water USP, sodium hydroxide 10%, sorbitan monostearate and stearyl alcohol. Tubes of 45 g. Store between 15 and 30°C.

Retrovir® (AZT™) Pr

zidovudine

Antiretroviral Agent

ViiV Healthcare ULC

Date of Revision: June 30, 2010

SUMMARY PRODUCT INFORMATION:

Route of Administration	Dosage Form/ Strength	Clinically Relevant Nonmedicinal Ingredients
Oral	Capsules/100 mg	None For a complete listing of ingredients for all dosage forms, see Dosage Forms, Composition and Packaging.
	Syrup/50 mg per 5 mL	
Intravenous Infusion	for Injection/10 mg per mL	

INDICATIONS AND CLINICAL USE: RETROVIR (AZT) (zidovudine) is indicated for:

- treatment of HIV infection when antiretroviral therapy is warranted.

Therapy with RETROVIR (AZT) has been shown to prolong survival and decrease the incidence of opportunistic infections in patients with advanced HIV disease at the initiation of therapy and to delay disease progression in asymptomatic HIV-infected patients.

RETROVIR (AZT) in combination with certain antiretroviral agents has been shown to be superior to monotherapy in one or more of the following: delaying death, delaying development of AIDS, increasing CD4 cell counts, and decreasing plasma HIV RNA. Use of RETROVIR (AZT) in some combinations is based on surrogate marker data. The complete prescribing information for each drug should be consulted before combination therapy which includes RETROVIR (AZT) is initiated.

The duration of clinical benefit from antiretroviral therapy may be limited. Alterations in antiretroviral therapy should be considered if disease progression occurs during treatment.

Maternal-Fetal HIV Transmission: RETROVIR (AZT) is also indicated for:

- the prevention of maternal-fetal HIV transmission as part of a regimen that includes oral RETROVIR (AZT) beginning between 14 and 34 weeks of gestation, intravenous RETROVIR (AZT) during labour, and administration of RETROVIR (AZT) Syrup to the newborn after birth.

However, transmission to infants may still occur in some cases despite the use of this regimen. The efficacy of this regimen for preventing HIV transmission in women who have received RETROVIR (AZT) for a prolonged period before pregnancy has not been evaluated. The safety of RETROVIR (AZT) for the mother or fetus during the first trimester of pregnancy has not been assessed.

The utility of RETROVIR (AZT) for the prevention of maternal-fetal HIV transmission was demonstrated in a randomized, double-blind, placebo-controlled trial (ACTG 076) conducted in HIV-infected pregnant women who had little or no previous exposure to RETROVIR (AZT) and CD4 cell counts of 200 to 1818 cells/mm^3 (median in the treated group: 560 cells/mm^3). Oral RETROVIR (AZT) was initiated between 14 and 34 weeks of gestation (median 11 weeks of therapy) followed by intravenous administration of RETROVIR (AZT) during labour and delivery. After birth, infants received oral RETROVIR (AZT) Syrup for 6 weeks. The study showed a statistically significant difference in the incidence of HIV infection in the infants (based on viral culture from peripheral blood) between the group receiving RETROVIR (AZT) and the group receiving placebo. Of 363 infants evaluated in the study, the estimated risk of HIV infection was 8.3% in the group receiving RETROVIR (AZT) and 25.5% in the placebo group, a relative reduction in transmission risk of 67.5%.

RETROVIR (AZT) was well tolerated by mothers and infants. There was no difference in pregnancy-related adverse events between the treatment groups. The mean difference in hemoglobin values was less than 1.0 g/dL for infants receiving RETROVIR (AZT) compared to infants receiving placebo. Infants did not require transfusion and hemoglobin values spontaneously returned to normal within 6 weeks after completion of therapy with RETROVIR (AZT). The long-term consequences of in utero and infant exposure to RETROVIR (AZT) are unknown.

CONTRAINDICATIONS:

- RETROVIR (AZT) (zidovudine) is contraindicated for patients who have potentially life-threatening allergic reactions to any of the components of the formulations (see Dosage Forms, Composition and Packaging).
- Due to the active ingredient zidovudine, RETROVIR (AZT) is contraindicated in patients with abnormally low neutrophil counts (<0.75×10^9/L) or abnormally low hemoglobin levels (<7.5 g/dL or 4.65 mmol/L).

WARNINGS AND PRECAUTIONS: Anaemia (usually not observed before six weeks of zidovudine therapy but occasionally occurring earlier), neutropenia (usually not observed before four weeks therapy but sometimes occurring earlier) and leucopenia (usually secondary to neutropenia) can be expected to occur in patients with advanced symptomatic HIV disease receiving zidovudine. These occurred more frequently at higher dosages (1200 to 1500 mg/day) and in patients with poor bone marrow reserve prior to treatment, particularly with advanced HIV disease.

Haematological parameters should be carefully monitored. For patients with advanced symptomatic HIV disease it is generally recommended that blood tests are performed at least every two weeks for the first three months of therapy and at least monthly thereafter. Blood tests should be performed at least weekly in patients receiving RETROVIR (AZT) intravenously.

Dosage reduction or interruption of zidovudine therapy may be necessary in patients whose haemoglobin level falls to between 7.5 g/dL (4.65 mmol/L) and 9 g/dL (5.59 mmol/L) or whose neutrophil count falls to between $0.75×10^9$/L and $1.0×10^9$/L.

General: Serious Adverse Reactions: Several serious adverse events have been reported with use of RETROVIR (AZT) (zidovudine) in clinical practice. Reports of pancreatitis, sensitization reactions (including anaphylaxis in one patient), vasculitis, and seizures have been rare. These adverse events, except for sensitization, have also been associated with HIV disease. Changes in skin and nail pigmentation have been associated with the use of RETROVIR (AZT).

Before combination therapy with RETROVIR (AZT) is initiated, consult the complete prescribing information for each drug. The safety profile of RETROVIR (AZT) plus other antiretroviral agents reflects the individual safety profiles of each component.

The incidence of adverse reactions appears to increase with disease progression, and patients should be monitored carefully, especially as disease progression occurs.

Endocrine and Metabolism: Fat Redistribution: Redistribution/accumulation of body fat including central obesity, dorsocervical fat enlargement ("buffalo hump"), peripheral wasting, facial wasting, breast enlargement, and "cushingoid appearance" have been observed in patients receiving antiretroviral therapy. The mechanism and long-term consequences of these events are currently unknown. A causal relationship has not been established.

Hematologic: Bone Marrow Suppression: RETROVIR (AZT) should be used with extreme caution in patients who have bone marrow compromise evidenced by granulocyte count <1000 cells/mm³ or hemoglobin <9.5 g/dL. In all of the placebo-controlled studies, but most frequently in patients with advanced symptomatic disease, anemia and granulocytopenia were the most significant adverse events observed (see Adverse Reactions). There have been reports of pancytopenia associated with the use of RETROVIR (AZT), which was reversible in most instances after discontinuation of the drug.

Hepatic/Biliary/Pancreatic: Lactic Acidosis/Severe Hepatomegaly with Steatosis: Rare occurrences of lactic acidosis in the absence of hypoxemia, and severe hepatomegaly with steatosis, (even in the absence of marked transaminase elevations) have been reported with the use of antiretroviral nucleoside analogues either alone or in combination, including RETROVIR (AZT) and zalcitabine, and are potentially fatal; it is not known whether these events are causally related to the use of these drugs. Lactic acidosis should be considered whenever a patient receiving therapy with RETROVIR (AZT) develops unexplained tachypnea, dyspnea, or fall in serum bicarbonate level. Under these circumstances, therapy with RETROVIR (AZT) should be suspended until the diagnosis of lactic acidosis has been excluded.

Clinical features which may be indicative of the development of lactic acidosis include generalized weakness, anorexia and sudden unexplained weight loss, gastrointestinal symptoms and respiratory symptoms (dyspnea and tachypnea).

Caution should be exercised when administering RETROVIR (AZT) to any patient, particularly obese women, with hepatomegaly, hepatitis, or other known risk factors for liver disease. These patients should be followed closely while on therapy with RETROVIR (AZT). The significance of elevated aminotransferase levels (suggesting hepatic injury) in HIV-infected patients prior to starting RETROVIR (AZT) or while on RETROVIR (AZT) is unclear. Treatment with RETROVIR (AZT) should be suspended in the setting of rapidly elevating aminotransferase levels, progressive hepatomegaly, or metabolic/lactic acidosis of unknown etiology.

Coadministration of zidovudine with other drugs metabolized by glucuronidation should be avoided because the toxicity of either drug may be potentiated (see Drug Interactions).

Data in patients with cirrhosis suggest that accumulation of zidovudine may occur in patients with hepatic impairment because of decreased glucuronidation. Dosage adjustments may be necessary, but as there is only limited data available precise recommendations cannot be made. If monitoring of plasma zidovudine levels is not feasible, physicians will need to monitor for signs of intolerance and adjust the dose and/or increase the interval between doses as appropriate.

Patients Co-infected with Hepatitis C Virus: Exacerbation of anaemia due to ribavirin has been reported when zidovudine is part of the regimen used to treat HIV although the exact mechanism remains to be elucidated. Therefore, the co-administration of ribavirin and zidovudine is not advised and consideration should be given to replacing zidovudine in a combination ART regimen if this is already established. This is particularly important in patients with a known history of zidovudine induced anaemia.

Use with Interferon- and Ribavirin-Based Regimens: In vitro studies have shown ribavirin can reduce the phosphorylation of pyrimidine nucleoside analogues such as zidovudine. Although no evidence of a pharmacokinetic or pharmacodynamic interaction (e.g., loss of HIV/HCV virologic suppression) was seen when ribavirin was coadministered with zidovudine in HIV/HCV co-infected patients, **hepatic decompensation (some fatal) has occurred in HIV/HCV co-infected patients receiving combination antiretroviral therapy for HIV and interferon alfa with or without ribavirin.** Patients receiving interferon alfa with or without ribavirin and RETROVIR should be closely monitored for treatment associated toxicities, especially hepatic decompensation, neutropenia, and anemia. Discontinuation of RETROVIR should be considered as medically appropriate. Dose reduction or discontinuation of interferon alfa, ribavirin, or both should also be considered if worsening clinical toxicities are observed, including hepatic decompensation (e.g., Child Pugh >6) (see the complete prescribing information for interferon and ribavirin).

Immune: Immune Reconstitution: During the initial phase of treatment, patients responding to antiretroviral therapy may develop an inflammatory response to indolent or residual opportunistic infections (such as MAC, CMV, PCP, and TB) which may necessitate further evaluation and treatment.

Ophthalmologic: Myopathy: Myopathy and myositis with pathological changes similar to that produced by HIV disease have been associated with prolonged use of RETROVIR (AZT).

Renal: Zidovudine is eliminated from the body primarily by renal excretion following metabolism in the liver (glucuronidation). In patients with severely impaired renal function, dosage reduction is recommended (see Dosage and Administration). Although very little data are available, patients with severely impaired hepatic function may be at greater risk of toxicity.

Very rare occurrences of pure red cell aplasia have been reported with zidovudine use. Discontinuation of zidovudine has resulted in normalization of hematological parameters in patients with suspected zidovudine-induced pure red cell aplasia.

Haemodialysis and peritoneal dialysis have no significant effect on zidovudine elimination whereas elimination of the glucuronide metabolite is increased. For patients with end-stage renal disease maintained on haemodialysis or peritoneal dialysis, the recommended dose is 100 mg every 6 to 8 h (see Action and Clinical Pharmacology, Pharmacokinetics).

Special Populations: Pregnant Women: A randomized, double-blind, placebo-controlled trial was conducted in HIV-infected pregnant women to determine the utility of RETROVIR (AZT) (zidovudine) for the prevention of maternal-fetal HIV-transmission. Congenital abnormalities occurred with similar frequency between infants born to mothers who received RETROVIR (AZT) and infants born to mothers who received placebo. Abnormalities were either problems in embryogenesis (prior to 14 weeks) or were recognized on ultrasound before or immediately after initiation of study drug.

Pregnant women considering the use of RETROVIR (AZT) during pregnancy for prevention of HIV-transmission to their infants should be advised that transmission may still occur in some cases despite therapy. The long-term consequences of in utero and infant exposure to RETROVIR (AZT) are unknown. The long-term effects of early or short-term use of RETROVIR (AZT) in pregnant women are also unknown.

There have been reports of mild, transient elevations in serum lactate levels, which may be due to mitochondrial dysfunction, in neonates and infants exposed in utero or peri-partum to nucleoside reverse transcriptase inhibitors (NRTIs). The clinical relevance of transient elevations in serum lactate is unknown. There have also been very rare reports of developmental delay, seizures and other neurological disease. However, a causal relationship between these events and NRTI exposure in utero or peri-partum has not been established. These findings do not affect current recommendations to use antiretroviral therapy in pregnant women to prevent vertical transmission of HIV.

Antiretroviral Pregnancy Registry: To monitor maternal-fetal outcomes of pregnant women exposed to RETROVIR (AZT), an Antiretroviral Pregnancy Registry has been established. Physicians are encouraged to register patients by calling ViiV Healthcare ULC's Drug Safety Department (1-877-393-8448).

Nursing Women: It is advisable to caution mothers against breastfeeding to avoid postnatal transmission of HIV to a child who may not yet be infected. Zidovudine is excreted in human milk at similar concentration to that found in serum.

Lactating mice administered zidovudine (200 mg/kg intraperitoneally) were found to have milk concentrations of zidovudine five times the corresponding serum zidovudine concentration. Milk concentrations of zidovudine declined at a slower rate than serum zidovudine concentrations.

Pediatrics: Use in Infancy: A positive test for HIV-antibody in children under 15 months of age may represent passively acquired maternal antibodies, rather than an active antibody response to infection in the infant. Thus, the presence of HIV-antibody in a child less than 15 months of age must be interpreted with caution, especially in the asymptomatic infant. Auxiliary diagnostic tests may be required to confirm infection in such children.

Use in Children: See Indications and Clinical Use; Adverse Reactions and Dosage and Administration. The pharmacokinetics of zidovudine in pediatric patients greater than 3 months of age is similar to that of zidovudine in adult patients.

Geriatrics: Zidovudine pharmacokinetics have not been studied in patients over 65 years of age and no specific data are available. However, since special care is advised in this age group due to age-associated changes such as the decrease in renal function and alterations in haematological parameters, appropriate monitoring of patients before and during use of zidovudine is advised.

ADVERSE REACTIONS: Adverse Drug Reaction Overview: Adults: The frequency and severity of adverse events associated with the use of RETROVIR (AZT) (zidovudine) in adults are greater in patients with more advanced infection at the time of initiation of therapy.

Clinical Trial Adverse Drug Reactions: Because clinical trials are conducted under very specific conditions the adverse reaction rates observed in the clinical trials may not reflect the rates observed in practice and should not be compared to the rates in the clinical trials of another drug. Adverse drug reaction information from clinical trials is useful for identifying drug-related adverse events and for approximating rates.

Adults: Anemia and Granulocytopenia: In all of the placebo-controlled studies, but most frequently in patients with advanced symptomatic HIV disease, anemia and granulocytopenia were the most significant adverse events observed.

Significant anemia most commonly occurred after 4 to 6 weeks of therapy and in many cases required dose adjustment, discontinuation of RETROVIR (AZT), and/or blood transfusions. Frequent blood counts are strongly recommended in patients with advanced HIV disease taking RETROVIR (AZT). For asymptomatic HIV-infected individuals and patients with early HIV disease, most of whom have better marrow reserve, blood counts may be obtained less frequently, depending upon the patient's overall status. If anemia or granulocytopenia develops, dosage adjustments may be necessary (see Dosage and Administration).

Table 1 summarizes the relative incidence of hematologic adverse events observed in clinical studies by severity of HIV disease present at the start of treatment.

Table 1: RETROVIR (AZT)

Relative Incidence of Hematologic Adverse Events Observed in Clinical Studies by Severity of HIV Disease Present at the Start of Treatment

	Granulocytopenia (<750 cells/mm³)			Anemia (Hgb <8 g/dL)		
Asymptomatic HIV Infection Study (n=1338)	**RETROVIR (AZT)**			**RETROVIR (AZT)**		
	1500 mg/day[a]	**500 mg/day**	**Placebo**	**1500 mg/day[a]**	**500 mg/day**	**Placebo**
CD4 ≤500	6.4% (n=457)	1.8%[b] (n=453)	1.6% (n=428)	6.4% (n=457)	1.1%[b] (n=453)	0.2% (n=428)
Early Symptomatic HIV Disease Study (n=713)	**Granulocytopenia (<750 cells/mm³)**			**Anemia (Hgb <8 g/dL)**		
	RETROVIR (AZT) 1200 mg/day[a]		**Placebo**	**RETROVIR (AZT) 1200 mg/day[a]**		**Placebo**
CD4 >200	4% (n=361)		1% (n=352)	4% (n=361)		0% (n=352)
Advanced Symptomatic HIV Disease Study (n=281)	**Granulocytopenia (<750 cells/mm³)**			**Anemia (Hgb <7.5 g/dL)**		
	RETROVIR (AZT) 1500 mg/day[a]		**Placebo**	**RETROVIR (AZT) 1500 mg/day[a]**		**Placebo**
CD4 >200	10% (n=30)[b]		3% (n=30)	3% (n=30)[b]		0% (n=30)
CD4 ≤200	47% (n=114)		10% (n=107)	29% (n=114)		5% (n=107)
Advanced Symptomatic HIV Disease Dose Comparison Study (n=524)	**Granulocytopenia (<750 cells/mm³)**			**Anemia (Hgb <7.5 g/dL)**		
	RETROVIR (AZT)			**RETROVIR (AZT)**		
	1200 mg/day[a]		**600 mg/day**	**1200 mg/day[a]**		**600 mg/day**
CD4 ≤200	51% (n=262)		37% (n=262)	39% (n=262)		29% (n=262)

[a] The currently recommended dose is 600 mg/day.
[b] Not statistically significant compared to placebo.

Other Adverse Events (Advanced HIV Disease): The anemia reported in patients with advanced HIV disease receiving RETROVIR (AZT) appeared to be the result of impaired erythrocyte maturation as evidenced by macrocytosis while on drug. Although mean platelet counts in patients receiving RETROVIR (AZT) were significantly increased compared to mean baseline values, thrombocytopenia did occur in some of these patients with advanced disease. Twelve percent of patients receiving RETROVIR (AZT) compared to 5% of patients receiving placebo had >50% decreases from baseline platelet count. Mild drug-associated elevations in total bilirubin levels have been reported as an uncommon occurrence in patients treated for asymptomatic HIV infection. The HIV-infected adults participating in these clinical trials often had baseline symptoms and signs of HIV disease and/or experienced adverse events at some time during the study. It was often difficult to distinguish adverse events possibly associated with administration of RETROVIR (AZT) from underlying signs of HIV disease or intercurrent illnesses.

Table 2 summarizes clinical adverse events or symptoms which occurred in at least 5% of all patients with advanced HIV disease treated with 1500 mg/day of RETROVIR (AZT) in the original placebo-controlled study. Of the items listed in the table, only severe headache, nausea, insomnia and myalgia were reported at a significantly greater rate in patients receiving RETROVIR (AZT).

Table 2: RETROVIR (AZT)

Percentage (%) of Patients with Clinical Events in Advanced HIV Disease

Adverse Event	RETROVIR (AZT) 1500 mg/day[a] (n=144) %	Placebo (n=137) %
Body as a Whole		
Asthenia	19	18
Diaphoresis	5	4
Fever	16	12
Headache	42	37
Malaise	8	7
Gastrointestinal		

(cont'd)

Table 2: RETROVIR (AZT) *(cont'd)*

Percentage (%) of Patients with Clinical Events in Advanced HIV Disease

Adverse Event	RETROVIR (AZT) 1500 mg/day[a] (n=144) %	Placebo (n=137) %
Anorexia	11	8
Diarrhea	12	18
Dyspepsia	5	4
Gastrointestinal Pain	20	19
Nausea	46	18
Vomiting	6	3
Musculoskeletal		
Myalgia	8	2
Nervous		
Dizziness	6	4
Insomnia	5	1
Paresthesia	6	3
Somnolence	8	9
Respiratory		
Dyspnea	5	3
Skin		
Rash	17	15
Special Senses		
Taste Perversion	5	8

[a] The currently recommended dose is 600 mg daily.

Clinical adverse events which occurred in less than 5% of all adult patients treated with 1500 mg/day of RETROVIR (AZT) in the advanced HIV study are listed below. Since many of these adverse events were seen in placebo-treated patients as well as patients treated with RETROVIR (AZT), their possible relationship to the drug is unknown.

Body as a Whole: back pain, body odour, chest pain, chills, edema of the lip, flu syndrome, hyperalgesia, lymphadenopathy.
Cardiovascular: vasodilation.
Gastrointestinal: bleeding gums, constipation, dysphagia, edema of the tongue, eructation, flatulence, mouth ulcer, rectal hemorrhage.
Musculoskeletal: arthralgia, muscle spasm, tremor, twitch.
Nervous: anxiety, confusion, depression, emotional lability, loss of mental acuity, nervousness, syncope, vertigo.
Respiratory: cough, epistaxis, hoarseness, pharyngitis, rhinitis, sinusitis.
Skin: acne, pruritus, urticaria.
Special senses: amblyopia, hearing loss, photophobia.
Urogenital: dysuria, polyuria, urinary frequency, urinary hesitancy.
Other Adverse Events (Early Symptomatic/Asymptomatic HIV Disease): All events of a severe or life-threatening nature were monitored for adults in the placebo-controlled studies in early HIV disease and asymptomatic HIV infection. Data concerning the occurrence of additional signs or symptoms were also collected. No distinction was made between events possibly associated with the administration of the study medication and those due to the underlying disease. Table 3 and Table 4 summarize all those events reported significantly more frequently by patients receiving RETROVIR (AZT) in these studies.

Table 3: RETROVIR (AZT)

Percentage (%) of Patients with Clinical Events in the Early Symptomatic HIV Disease Study

Adverse Event	RETROVIR (AZT) 1200 mg/day[a] (n=361) %	Placebo (n=352) %
Body as a Whole		
Asthenia	69	62
Gastrointestinal		
Dyspepsia	6	1
Nausea	61	41
Vomiting	25	13

[a] The currently recommended dose is 600 mg daily.

Table 4: RETROVIR (AZT)

Percentage (%) of Patients with Clinical Events[a] in an Asymptomatic HIV Infection Study

Adverse Event	RETROVIR (AZT) 1500 mg/day[b] (n=457) %	RETROVIR (AZT) 500 mg/day[b] (n=453) %	Placebo (n=428) %
Body as a Whole			
Asthenia	10.1	8.6[c]	5.8
Headache	58.0[c]	62.5	52.6
Malaise	55.6	53.2	44.9
Gastrointestinal			
Anorexia	19.3	20.1	10.5
Constipation	8.1	6.4[c]	3.5
Nausea	57.3	51.4	29.9
Vomiting	16.4	17.2	9.8
Nervous			
Dizziness	20.8	17.9[c]	15.2

[a] Reported in ≥5% of study population.
[b] The currently recommended dose is 600 mg/day.
[c] Not statistically significant versus placebo.

Several serious adverse events have been reported with the use of RETROVIR (AZT) in clinical practice. Myopathy and myositis with pathological changes similar to that produced by HIV disease have been associated with prolonged use of RETROVIR (AZT). Reports of hepatomegaly with steatosis, hepatitis, pancreatitis, lactic acidosis, sensitization reactions (including anaphylaxis in one patient), hyperbilirubinemia, vasculitis, and seizures have been rare. These adverse events, except for sensitization, have also been associated with HIV disease. A single case of macular edema has been reported with the use of RETROVIR (AZT). Changes in skin and nail pigmentation have been associated with the use of RETROVIR (AZT) (see Warnings and Precautions).

Combination Therapy with RETROVIR (AZT) and Zalcitabine: Only limited safety data are available on the combined use of RETROVIR (AZT) with zalcitabine. The major toxicities of zalcitabine are peripheral neuropathy and, less frequently, pancreatitis.

Table 5 includes clinical adverse events in the combination zalcitabine and zidovudine Protocol N3447/ACTG 106. Only eight patients were treated with the recommended combination regimen.

Table 5: RETROVIR (AZT)

Number and Percentage of Patients with Clinical Adverse Experiences Occurring in >3% of Patients Considered Possibly or Probably Related to Study Drug

HIVID + Zidovudine Combination Trial Pooled Concomitant Regimens	N3447/ACTG 106[a] No Prior Zidovudine n=47 (%)	
Body System/Adverse Event	**Mild/Moderate/Severe**	**Moderate/Severe**
Peripheral Neuropathy	12 (25.5)	2 (4.3)
Gastrointestinal		
Nausea	17 (36.2)	4 (8.5)
Oral Ulcers	13 (27.7)	2 (4.3)
Abdominal Pain	10 (21.3)	4 (8.5)
Diarrhea	7 (14.9)	5 (10.6)
Vomiting	7 (14.9)	1 (2.1)
Anorexia	6 (12.8)	3 (6.4)
Constipation	3 (6.4)	1 (2.1)
Skin and Appendages		
Pruritus	7 (14.9)	2 (4.3)
Rash	7 (14.9)	1 (2.1)
Erythematous Rash	3 (6.4)	1 (2.1)
Night Sweats	3 (6.4)	1 (2.1)
Maculopapular Rash	2 (4.3)	1 (2.1)
Follicular Rash	2 (4.3)	0 (0.0)
Central and Peripheral NS		
Headache	18 (38.3)	4 (8.5)
Musculoskeletal		
Myalgia	7 (14.9)	1 (2.1)
Arthralgia	4 (8.5)	1 (2.1)
Body as a Whole		
Fatigue	16 (34.0)	4 (8.5)
Fever	7 (14.9)	1 (2.1)
Rigors	4 (8.5)	1 (2.1)

(cont'd)

Table 5: RETROVIR (AZT) *(cont'd)*

Number and Percentage of Patients with Clinical Adverse Experiences Occurring in >3% of Patients Considered Possibly or Probably Related to Study Drug

HIVID + Zidovudine Combination Trial Pooled Concomitant Regimens	N3447/ACTG 106[a] No Prior Zidovudine n=47 (%)	
Body System/Adverse Event	**Mild/Moderate/Severe**	**Moderate/Severe**
Chest Pain	3 (6.4)	1 (2.1)
Weight Decrease	3 (6.4)	2 (4.3)
Respiratory		
Pharyngitis	4 (8.5)	1 (2.1)

[a] Median duration of treatment ranged from 22 to 92 weeks among the arms.

Children: Anemia and Granulocytopenia: The incidences of anemia and granulocytopenia among children with advanced HIV disease receiving RETROVIR (AZT) occurred with similar incidence to that reported for adults with AIDS or advanced ARC (see above). Table 6 summarizes the occurrence of anemia (Hgb <7.5 g/dL) and granulocytopenia (<750 cells/mm³) among 124 children receiving RETROVIR (AZT) for a mean of 267 days (range 3 to 855 days).

Table 6: RETROVIR (AZT)

The Occurrence of Anemia (Hgb <7.5 g/dL) and Granulocytopenia (<750 cells/mm³) Among 124 Children Receiving RETROVIR (AZT) for a Mean of 267 Days

	Granulocytopenia (<750 cells/mm³)		Anemia (Hgb <7.5 g/dL)	
	n	%	n	%
Advanced Pediatric HIV Disease (n=124)	48	39	28[a]	23

[a] Twenty-two children received one or more transfusions due to a decline in hemoglobin to <7.5 g/dL; an additional 15 children were transfused for hemoglobin levels >7.5 g/dL. Fifty-nine percent of the patients transfused had a pre-study history of anemia or transfusion requirement.

Management of neutropenia and anemia included, in some cases, dose modification and/or blood product transfusions. In the open-label studies, 17% had their dose modified (generally a reduction in dose by 30%) due to anemia, and 25% had their dose modified (temporary discontinuation or reduction by 30%) for neutropenia. Four children had RETROVIR (AZT) permanently discontinued because of neutropenia.

Macrocytosis was observed among the majority of children enrolled in the studies.

Other Adverse Events (Children): The clinical adverse events reported among adult recipients of RETROVIR (AZT) may also occur in children.

In the open-label studies involving 124 children, 16 different clinical adverse events were reported by 24 children. No event was reported by more than 5.6% of the study populations. Due to the open-label design of the studies, it was difficult to determine possible events related to the use of RETROVIR (AZT) versus disease-related events. Therefore, all clinical events reported as associated with therapy with RETROVIR (AZT) or of unknown relationship to therapy with RETROVIR (AZT) are presented in Table 7.

Table 7: RETROVIR (AZT)

Percentage (%) of Pediatric Patients with Clinical Events in Open-label Studies

Adverse Event	n	%
Body as a Whole		
Fever	4	3.2
Phlebitis[a]/Bacteremia	2	1.6
Headache	2	1.6
Gastrointestinal		
Nausea	1	0.8
Vomiting	6	4.8
Abdominal Pain	4	3.2
Diarrhea	1	0.8
Weight Loss	1	0.8
Nervous		
Insomnia	3	2.4
Nervousness/Irritability	2	1.6
Decreased Reflexes	7	5.6
Seizure	1	0.8
Cardiovascular		
Left Ventricular Dilation	1	0.8
Cardiomyopathy	1	0.8
S_3 Gallop	1	0.8
Congestive Heart Failure	1	0.8
Generalized Edema	1	0.8
ECG Abnormality	3	2.4

(cont'd)

Table 7: RETROVIR (AZT) *(cont'd)*

Percentage (%) of Pediatric Patients with Clinical Events in Open-label Studies

Adverse Event	n	%
Urogenital		
Hematuria/Viral Cystitis	1	0.8

[a] Peripheral vein i.v. catheter site.

Combination Therapy with RETROVIR (AZT) and 3TC (lamivudine): Pediatric Patients: Selected clinical adverse events and physical findings with a ≥5% frequency during therapy with 3TC 4 mg/kg twice daily plus RETROVIR (AZT) 160 mg/m² three times daily compared with didanosine in patients without, or with, minimal (≤56 days) prior antiretroviral therapy are listed in Table 8.

Table 8: RETROVIR (AZT)

Selected Clinical Adverse Events and Physical Findings (≥5% Frequency) in Pediatric Patients in Study ACTG300

Adverse Event	3TC Plus RETROVIR (AZT) (n=236)	Didanosine (n=235)
Body as a Whole		
Fever	25%	32%
Digestive		
Hepatomegaly	11%	11%
Nausea & vomiting	8%	7%
Diarrhea	8%	6%
Stomatitis	6%	12%
Splenomegaly	5%	8%
Respiratory		
Cough	15%	18%
Abnormal breath sounds/wheezing	7%	9%
Ear, Nose and Throat		
Signs or symptoms of ears[a]	7%	6%
Nasal discharge or congestion	8%	11%
Other		
Skin rashes	12%	14%
Lymphadenopathy	9%	11%

[a] Includes pain, discharge, erythema, or swelling of an ear.

Selected laboratory abnormalities experienced by patients without or minimal (≤56 days) prior antiretroviral therapy are listed in Table 9.

Table 9: RETROVIR (AZT)

Frequencies of Selected Laboratory Abnormalities in Pediatric Patients in Study ACTG300

Test (Abnormal Level)	3TC Plus RETROVIR (AZT)	Didanosine
Neutropenia (ANC <400/mm_3)	8%	3%
Anemia (Hgb <7.0 g/dL)	4%	2%
Thrombocytopenia (platelets <50 000/mm³)	1%	3%
ALT (>10×ULN)	1%	3%
AST (>10×ULN)	2%	4%
Lipase (>2.5×ULN)	3%	3%
Total amylase (>2.5×ULN)	3%	3%

Legend: ULN=upper limit of normal; ANC=absolute neutrophil count.

Use for the Prevention of Maternal-Fetal Transmission of HIV: In a randomized, double-blind, placebo-controlled trial in HIV-infected women and their infants conducted to determine the utility of RETROVIR (AZT) for the prevention of maternal-fetal HIV transmission, RETROVIR (AZT) Syrup at 2 mg/kg was administered every 6 hours for 6 weeks to infants beginning within 12 hours after birth. The most commonly reported adverse experiences were anemia (hemoglobin <9.0 g/dL) and neutropenia (<1000 cells/mm³). Anemia occurred in 22% of the infants who received RETROVIR (AZT) and in 12% of the infants who received placebo. The mean difference in hemoglobin values was less than 1.0 g/dL for infants receiving RETROVIR (AZT) compared to infants receiving placebo. No infants with anemia required transfusion and all hemoglobin values spontaneously returned to normal within 6 weeks after completion of therapy with RETROVIR (AZT). Neutropenia was reported with similar frequency in the group that received RETROVIR (AZT) (21%) and in the group that received placebo (27%). The long-term consequences of in utero and infant exposure to RETROVIR (AZT) are unknown.

Post-Market Adverse Drug Reactions: The following events have been reported in patients treated with RETROVIR (AZT) without regard to causality. Because they are reported voluntarily from a population of unknown size, estimates of frequency cannot be made. A reduction in dose or suspension of RETROVIR (AZT) therapy may be warranted in the management of these conditions.

Hematological: Anemia (which may require transfusions), neutropenia, leucopenia, aplastic anemia, thrombocytopenia, pancytopenia (with marrow hypoplasia) and pure red cell aplasia.

Anemia, neutropenia, leucopenia and aplastic anemia occur more frequently at higher dosages (1200-1500 mg/day) and in patients with advanced HIV disease (especially when there is poor bone marrow reserve prior to treatment), and particularly in patients with CD4 cell counts less than 100/mm³. Dosage reduction or cessation of therapy may become necessary (see Dosage and Administration). The incidence of neutropenia was also increased in those patients whose neutrophil counts, hemoglobin levels and serum vitamin B_{12} levels were low at the start of RETROVIR (AZT) therapy.

Body as a Whole: redistribution/accumulation of body fat (see Warnings and Precautions: Endocrine and Metabolism, Fat Redistribution). Convulsions, cardiomyopathy (thrombocytopenia, pancytopenia).

Gastrointestinal: oral mucosa pigmentation.

Liver/Pancreas: raised blood levels of liver enzymes and bilirubin.

Metabolism and Nutrition Disorders: anorexia, hyperlactatemia, lactic acidosis (see Warnings and Precautions: Hepatic/Biliary/Pancreatic, Lactic Acidosis/Severe Hepatomegaly with Steatosis).

Miscellaneous: gynecomastia, myopathy, hyperlactatemia.

Skin: sweating, nail and skin discoloration.

DRUG INTERACTIONS: Overview: Coadministration of RETROVIR (AZT) (zidovudine) with other drugs metabolized by glucuronidation should be avoided because the toxicity of either drug may be potentiated.

Drug-Drug Interactions: See Table 10.

Table 10: RETROVIR (AZT)
Established or Potential Drug-Drug Interactions

Proper name	Effect	Clinical comment
Atovaquone	Zidovudine does not appear to affect the pharmacokinetics of atovaquone.	Pharmacokinetic data have shown that atovaquone appears to decrease the rate of metabolism of zidovudine to its glucuronide metabolite (steady state AUC of zidovudine was increased by 33% and peak plasma concentration of the glucuronide was decreased by 19%). At zidovudine dosages of 500 or 600 mg/day it would seem unlikely that a three week, concomitant course of atovaquone for the treatment of acute PCP would result in an increased incidence of adverse reactions attributable to higher plasma concentrations of zidovudine. Extra care should be taken in monitoring patients receiving prolonged atovaquone therapy.
Bone Marrow Suppressive Agents/Cytotoxic Agents	Coadministration may increase risk of hematologic toxicity.	Coadministration of RETROVIR (AZT) with drugs that are cytotoxic or which interfere with RBC/WBC number or function (e.g. dapsone, flucytosine, vincristine, or adriamycin) may increase the risk of hematologic toxicity.
Clarithromycin	Clarithromycin tablets reduce the absorption of zidovudine.	This can be avoided by separating the administration of zidovudine and clarithromycin by at least two hours.
Fluconazole	Fluconazole interferes with the oral clearance and metabolism of RETROVIR (AZT).	Preliminary data suggests that fluconazole interferes with the oral clearance and metabolism of RETROVIR (AZT). In a pharmacokinetic interaction study in which 12 HIV-positive men received RETROVIR (AZT) alone and in combination with fluconazole, increases in the mean peak serum concentration (79%), AUC (70%) and half-life (38%) were observed at steady state. The clinical significance of this interaction is unknown.
Ganciclovir	Coadministration increases the risk of hematologic toxicities in some patients with advanced HIV disease.	Use of RETROVIR (AZT) in combination with ganciclovir increases the risk of hematologic toxicities in some patients with advanced HIV disease. Should the use of this combination become necessary in the treatment of patients with HIV disease, dose reduction or interruption of one or both agents may be necessary to minimize hematologic toxicity. Hematologic parameters, including hemoglobin, hematocrit, and white blood cell count with differential, should be monitored frequently in all patients receiving this combination.
Interferon-alpha	Hematologic toxicities have been seen when RETROVIR (AZT) is used concomitantly with interferon-alpha.	As with the concomitant use of RETROVIR (AZT) and ganciclovir, dose reduction or interruption of one or both agents may be necessary, and hematologic parameters should be monitored frequently.
Lamivudine	Coadministration resulted in an increase in C_{max} of zidovudine.	RETROVIR (AZT) and lamivudine were coadministered to 12 asymptomatic HIV-positive patients in a single-centre, open-label, randomized, crossover study. No significant differences were observed in AUC_{∞} or total clearance for lamivudine or zidovudine when the two drugs were administered together. Coadministration of RETROVIR (AZT) with lamivudine resulted in an increase of 39%±62% (mean±SD) in C_{max} of zidovudine.
Methadone	Plasma levels of zidovudine can be elevated in some patients while remaining unchanged in others.	In a pharmacokinetic study of 9 HIV-positive patients receiving methadone-maintenance (30 to 90 mg daily) concurrent with 200 mg of RETROVIR (AZT) every 4 hours, no changes were observed in the pharmacokinetics of methadone upon initiation of therapy with RETROVIR (AZT) and after 14 days of treatment with RETROVIR (AZT). No adjustments in methadone-maintenance requirements were reported. However, plasma levels of zidovudine were elevated in some patients while remaining unchanged in others. The exact mechanism and clinical significance of these data are unknown.
Phenytoin	A decrease in oral zidovudine clearance.	Phenytoin plasma levels have been reported to be low in some patients receiving RETROVIR (AZT), while in one case a high level was documented. However, in a pharmacokinetic interaction study in which 12 HIV-positive volunteers received a single 300 mg phenytoin dose alone and during steady-state zidovudine conditions (200 mg every 4 hours), no change in phenytoin kinetics was observed. Although not designed to optimally assess the effect of phenytoin on zidovudine kinetics, a 30% decrease in oral zidovudine clearance was observed.
Probenecid	May increase zidovudine levels.	Limited data suggest that probenecid may increase zidovudine levels by inhibiting glucuronidation and/or reducing renal excretion of zidovudine. Some patients who have used RETROVIR (AZT) concomitantly with probenecid have developed flu-like symptoms consisting of myalgia, malaise, and/or fever and maculopapular rash.

(cont'd)

Table 10: RETROVIR (AZT) *(cont'd)*
Established or Potential Drug-Drug Interactions

Proper name	Effect	Clinical comment
Ribavarin	Coadministration of ribavirin and zidovudine may lead to increased ribavirin levels and increased risk of anemia.	Preliminary data suggest that the use of ribavirin and zidovudine lead to increased ribavirin levels and increased risk of anemia. The use of ribavirin concomitantly with zidovudine in the treatment of HIV/Hep C co-infected patients is not advised. Consideration should be given to replacing zidovudine in a combination ART regimen if this is already established.
Stavudine	Zidovudine may inhibit intracellular phosphorylation of stavudine	Zidovudine may inhibit the intracellular phosphorylation of stavudine when the two medicinal products are used concurrently. Stavudine is therefore not recommended to be used in combination with zidovudine.
Valproic Acid	Increase in zidovudine AUC and a decrease in the plasma GZDV AUC.	The concomitant administration of valproic acid 250 mg (n=5) or 500 mg (n=1) every 8 hours and zidovudine 100 mg orally every 8 hours for 4 days to 6 HIV-infected, asymptomatic male volunteers resulted in a 79%±61% (mean±SD) increase in the plasma zidovudine AUC and a 22%±10% decrease in the plasma GZDV AUC as compared to the administration of zidovudine in the absence of valproic acid. The GZDV/zidovudine urinary excretion ratio decreased 58%±12%. Because no change in the zidovudine plasma half-life occurred, these results suggest that valproic acid may increase the oral bioavailability of zidovudine through inhibition of first-pass metabolism. Although the clinical signification of this interaction is unknown, patients should be monitored more closely for a possible increase in zidovudine-related adverse effects. The effect of zidovudine on the pharmacokinetics of valproic acid was not evaluated.
Other Agents		Some drugs such as trimethoprim-sulfamethoxazole, pyrimethamine, and acyclovir may be necessary for the management or prevention of opportunistic infections. In the placebo-controlled trial in patients with advanced HIV disease, increased toxicity was not detected with limited exposure to these drugs. However, there is one published report of neurotoxicity (profound lethargy) associated with concomitant use of RETROVIR (AZT) and acyclovir. Preliminary data from a drug interaction study (n=10) suggest that coadministration of 200 mg RETROVIR (AZT) and 600 mg rifampin decreases the area under the zidovudine plasma concentration curve by an average of 48%±34%. However, the effect of once daily dosing of rifampin on multiple daily doses of RETROVIR (AZT) is unknown. Other active substances including but not limited to acetylsalicylic acid, codeine, morphine, methadone, indomethacin, ketoprofen, naproxen, oxazepam, lorazepam, cimetidine, clofibrate, dapsone and isoprinosine may alter the metabolism of zidovudine by competitively inhibiting glucuronidation or directly inhibiting hepatic microsomal metabolism. Careful thought should be given to the possibilities of interactions before using such medicinal products, particularly for chronic therapy, in combination with zidovudine. Concomitant treatment, especially acute therapy, with potentially nephrotoxic or myelosuppressive medicinal products (for example systemic pentamidine, dapsone, pyrimethamine, co-trimoxazole, amphotericin, flucytosine, ganciclovir, interferon, vincristine, vinblastine and doxorubicin) may also increase the risk of adverse reactions to zidovudine. If concomitant therapy with any of these medicinal products is necessary then extra care should be taken in monitoring renal function and haematological parameters and, if required, the dosage of one or more agents should be adjusted.

DOSAGE AND ADMINISTRATION: Dosing Considerations: Monitoring of Patients: Hematologic toxicities appear to be related to pre-treatment bone marrow reserve and to dose and duration of therapy. In patients with poor bone marrow reserve, particularly in patients with advanced symptomatic HIV disease, frequent monitoring of hematologic indices is recommended to detect serious anemia or granulocytopenia (see Adverse Reactions). In patients who experience hematologic toxicity, reduction in hemoglobin may occur as early as 2 to 4 weeks, and granulocytopenia usually occurs after 6 to 8 weeks.

Patients treated with zidovudine should be under close clinical observation to manage potential opportunistic infections associated with HIV disease. Prompt recognition of infection or toxicities and appropriate management is required.

Recommended Dose and Dosage Adjustment: Oral Administration: Adults and Children 30 kg and Over: The recommended total oral daily dose of RETROVIR (AZT) (zidovudine) is 600 mg per day in divided doses in combination with other antiretroviral agents. The effectiveness of this dose compared to higher dosing regimens in improving neurologic dysfunction associated with HIV disease is unknown. A small randomized study found a greater effect of higher doses of RETROVIR (AZT) on improvement of neurological symptoms in patients with pre-existing neurological disease.

Suggested dosing regimens are listed in Table 11.

Table 11: RETROVIR (AZT)
Suggested Dosing Regimens

	Dosing Regimen	
Formulation	**Twice Daily (every 12 hours)**	**Three Times Daily (every 8 hours)**
Capsules	Three 100 mg RETROVIR (AZT) capsules	Two 100 mg RETROVIR (AZT) capsules
Syrup	6 teaspoonfuls (30 mL) RETROVIR (AZT) syrup	4 teaspoonfuls (20 mL) RETROVIR (AZT) syrup

Children: The recommended oral dose in children 3 months to 12 years of age, in combination with other antiretroviral agents, is provided in Table 12.

Available data are insufficient to propose specific dosing recommendations for children weighing <4 kg.

The appropriate dose of RETROVIR (AZT) for each child should be calculated based on body weight (kg) and should not exceed the recommended adult dose.

RETROVIR (AZT) Syrup should be used to provide accurate dosage when capsules are not appropriate.

RETROVIR (AZT) Syrup is available for dosing children who weigh less than 30 kg.

Children should be assessed for the ability to swallow capsules. If a child is unable to consistently swallow a RETROVIR (AZT) capsule, the RETROVIR (AZT) syrup formulation should be prescribed.

Table 12: RETROVIR (AZT)

Recommended Pediatric Dosage of RETROVIR (AZT)

Body Weight (kg)	Total Daily Dose	Dosage Regimen and Dose	
		Twice Daily (every 12 hours)	Three Times Daily (every 8 hours)
4 to <9	24 mg/kg/day	12 mg/kg	8 mg/kg
≥9 to <30	18 mg/kg/day	9 mg/kg	6 mg/kg
≥30	600 mg/day	300 mg	200 mg

Alternatively, dosing for RETROVIR (AZT) can be based on body surface area (BSA) for each child. The recommended oral dose of RETROVIR (AZT) is 480 mg/m²/day in divided doses (240 mg/m² twice daily or 160 mg/m² three times daily). In some cases the dose calculated by mg/kg will not be the same as that calculated by BSA.

Injection: Adults: The recommended dose is 1 to 2 mg/kg administered as a 1 hour infusion every 4 hours around the clock (6 times daily). Patients should receive intravenous RETROVIR (AZT) only until oral therapy can be administered.

The intravenous dosing regimen equivalent to the oral administration of 100 mg every 4 hours is approximately 1 mg/kg intravenously every 4 hours.

RETROVIR (AZT) injection is administered intravenously at a constant rate over 1 hour. Rapid infusion or bolus injection should be avoided. RETROVIR (AZT) injection should not be given intramuscularly.

The effectiveness of the intravenous dose compared to higher dosing regimens in improving the neurologic dysfunction associated with HIV disease is unknown. A small randomized study has found a greater effect of higher doses of RETROVIR (AZT) on improvement of neurological symptoms in patients with pre-existing neurological disease.

Children: The recommended dose of RETROVIR (AZT) I.V. injection in children 3 months to 12 years of age is 120 mg/m² every 6 hours, infused over 1 hour (480 mg/m² per day). Do not exceed 160 mg for any individual dose.

Prevention of Maternal-Fetal HIV Transmission: The recommended dosing regimen for administration to pregnant women (>14 weeks of pregnancy) and their newborn infant is:

- **Maternal Dosing.** 100 mg orally 5 times per day until the start of labour. During labour and delivery, intravenous RETROVIR (AZT) should be administered at 2 mg/kg (total body weight) over 1 hour followed by a continuous intravenous infusion at 1 mg/kg/h (total body weight) until clamping of the umbilical cord.
- **Infant Dosing.** 2 mg/kg of oral solution every 6 hours starting within 12 hours after birth and continuing through 6 weeks of age. Infants unable to receive oral dosing may be administered RETROVIR (AZT) intravenously at 1.5 mg/kg, infused over 30 minutes, every 6 hours. See Warnings and Precautions if hepatic disease or renal insufficiency is present.

Dose Adjustment: Significant anemia (haemoglobin of <7.5 g/dL or reduction of >25% of baseline) and/or significant granulocytopenia (granulocyte count of <750 cells/mm³ or reduction of >50% from baseline) may require a dose interruption until evidence of marrow recovery is observed (see Adverse Reactions). In patients who develop significant anemia, dose modification dose not necessarily eliminate the need for transfusion.

For less severe anemia or granulocytopenia, a reduction in daily dose may be adequate. If marrow recovery occurs following dose modification, gradual increases in dose may be appropriate depending on hematologic indices and patient tolerance.

In end-stage disease patients maintained on hemodialysis or peritoneal dialysis, recommended dosing is 100 mg every 6 to 8 hours for oral administration and 1 mg/kg every 6 to 8 hours for intravenous infusion.

There are insufficient data to recommend dose adjustment of RETROVIR (AZT) in patients with impaired hepatic function.

Administration: Method of Preparation of RETROVIR (AZT) Injection: RETROVIR (AZT) Injection must be diluted prior to administration. The calculated dose should be removed from the 20 mL vial and added to a recommended diluent to achieve a concentration no greater than 4 mg/mL. RETROVIR (AZT) Injection does not contain preservatives. Unused portion of the vial should be discarded. RETROVIR (AZT) must not be given intra-muscularly.

Recommended Diluents: 5% Dextrose Injection; 0.9% Sodium Chloride Injection; 5% Dextrose Injection and 0.45% Sodium Chloride Injection; Lactated Ringer's Injection; 5% Dextrose and Lactated Ringer's Injection.

The diluted solution should be administered within 8 hours if stored at 25°C or 24 hours if refrigerated at 2 to 8°C to minimize potential administration of a microbially contaminated solution.

Parenteral drug products should be inspected visually for particulate matter and discoloration prior to administration whenever solution and container permit. Should either be observed, the solution should be discarded and fresh solution prepared.

Incompatability: Admixture in biologic or colloidal fluids (e.g., blood products, protein solutions) is not recommended.

OVERDOSAGE:

Cases of acute overdose in both children and adults have been reported with doses up to 50 g. None were fatal.

The only consistent finding in these cases of overdose was spontaneous or induced nausea and vomiting. Hematologic changes were transient and not severe. Some patients experienced nonspecific CNS symptoms such as headache, dizziness, drowsiness, lethargy, and confusion. One report of a grand mal seizure possibly attributable to RETROVIR (AZT) (zidovudine) occurred in a 35-year-old male 3 hours after ingesting 36 g of RETROVIR (AZT). No other cause could be identified. All patients recovered without permanent sequelae. Hemodialysis and peritoneal dialysis appear to have a negligible effect on the removal of zidovudine while elimination of its primary metabolite, GZDV is enhanced.

Activated charcoal should be administered to aid in the removal of unabsorbed drug. General supportive measures are recommended.

Patients should be observed closely for evidence of toxicity (see Adverse Reactions) and given the necessary supportive therapy.

Hemodialysis and peritoneal dialysis appear to have a limited effect on elimination of zidovudine but enhance the elimination of the glucuronide metabolite.

> For management of a suspected drug overdose, contact your regional Poison Control Centre. See the *CPS* Directory section for a list of Poison Control Centres.

ACTION AND CLINICAL PHARMACOLOGY: Mechanism of Action: RETROVIR (AZT) (zidovudine) is a potent inhibitor of the in vitro replication of some retroviruses including human immunodeficiency virus, HIV. Zidovudine is a thymidine analogue in which the 3-hydroxy (-OH) group is replaced by an azido (-N_3) group. Cellular thymidine kinase converts zidovudine into zidovudine monophosphate. The monophosphate is further converted into the diphosphate by cellular thymidylate kinase and to the triphosphate derivative by other cellular enzymes. Zidovudine triphosphate interferes with the HIV viral RNA dependent DNA polymerase (reverse transcriptase) and thus inhibits viral replication. Zidovudine triphosphate also inhibits cellular α-DNA polymerase, but at concentrations 100-fold higher than those required to inhibit reverse transcriptase. In vitro, zidovudine triphosphate has been shown to be incorporated into growing chains of DNA by viral reverse transcriptase. When incorporation by the viral enzyme occurs, the DNA chain is terminated. Studies in cell culture suggest that zidovudine incorporation by cellular α-DNA polymerase may occur, but only to a very small extent and not in all test systems. Cellular γ-DNA polymerase shows some sensitivity to inhibition by the zidovudine triphosphate with 50% inhibitory concentration (IC_{50}) values 400 to 900 times greater than that for HIV reverse transcriptase.

Pharmacokinetics: Pharmacokinetic studies of RETROVIR (AZT) following intravenous dosing in adults indicate dose-independent kinetics over the range of 1 to 5 mg/kg with a mean zidovudine half-life of 1.1 hours. Zidovudine is rapidly metabolized in the liver to 3'-azido-3'-deoxy-5'-O-β-D- glucopyranuronosylthymidine (GZDV, formerly called GAZT), and both are rapidly eliminated by the kidney. A second metabolite, 3'-amino-3'-deoxythymidine (AMT) has been identified in the plasma following single dose intravenous administration of zidovudine. After oral dosing in adults, zidovudine is rapidly absorbed from the gastrointestinal tract with peak serum concentrations occurring within 0.5 to 1.5 hours, with an average oral bioavailability of 65%. RETROVIR (AZT) Capsules and Syrup are bioequivalent. In pediatric patients older than 3 months, the pharmacokinetics of zidovudine are similar to those in adult patients.

STORAGE AND STABILITY: RETROVIR (AZT) (zidovudine) Capsules should be stored at room temperature between 15 and 25°C and protected from light and moisture.

RETROVIR (AZT) Syrup should be stored at 15 to 25°C and protected from light.

RETROVIR (AZT) Injection should be stored at room temperature between 15 and 25°C and protected from light. Do not freeze.

SPECIAL HANDLING INSTRUCTIONS: Solution for infusion: Zidovudine i.v. for infusion must be diluted prior to administration.

Since no antimicrobial preservative is included, dilution must be carried out under full aseptic conditions, preferably immediately prior to administration, and any unused portion of the vial should be discarded.

The required dose should be added to and mixed with glucose i.v. infusion 5% w/v to give a final zidovudine concentration of either 2 mg/mL or 4 mg/mL. These dilutions are chemically and physically stable for up to 48 hours at both 5 and 25°C.

Should any visible turbidity appear in the product either before or after dilution or during infusion, the preparation should be discarded.

INFORMATION FOR THE PATIENT: Published in e-CPS, available by subscription at www.e-cps.ca.

DOSAGE FORMS, COMPOSITION AND PACKAGING: Capsules: Each gelatin capsule, with a white opaque cap and body, printed with "Wellcome" and a Unicorn logo on cap and "Y9C" and "100" on body, contains: zidovudine 100 mg. Nonmedicinal ingredients: cornstarch, magnesium stearate, microcrystalline cellulose and sodium starch glycolate; capsule shell: gelatin, titanium dioxide and imprinted with edible black ink. Bottles of 100.

I.V. Injection: Each mL of solution contains: zidovudine 10 mg in water for injection. Hydrochloric acid or sodium hydroxide may have been added to adjust pH to approximately 5.5. Preservative-free. Single use amber vials of 20 mL, boxes of 10.

Syrup: Each 5 mL of colorless to pale yellow, strawberry-flavored syrup contains: zidovudine 50 mg. Nonmedicinal ingredients: candied sugar flavor, citric acid, glycerin, strawberry flavor and sucrose. Sodium benzoate (0.2%) is added as a preservative and sodium hydroxide may have been added to adjust pH. Bottles of 240 mL.

(Shown in Product Identification Section)

Revatio™ Ⓟ

sildenafil citrate

cGMP-Specific Phosphodiesterase Type 5 Inhibitor—Treatment of Pulmonary Arterial Hypertension

Pfizer

Date of Revision: January 13, 2010

SUMMARY PRODUCT INFORMATION:

Route of Administration	Dosage Form/ Strength	All Nonmedicinal Ingredients
Oral	Film-coated tablet/20 mg sildenafil as sildenafil citrate	Tablet core: Anhydrous dibasic calcium phosphate, croscarmellose sodium, magnesium stearate, microcrystalline cellulose. Film coat: hypromellose, lactose, titanium dioxide (E-171), triacetin.

INDICATIONS AND CLINICAL USE: REVATIO (sildenafil citrate) is indicated for:

- treatment of primary pulmonary arterial hypertension (PPH) or pulmonary hypertension secondary to connective tissue disease, in patients with WHO functional class II or III who have not responded to conventional therapy.

CONTRAINDICATIONS: Sildenafil citrate has been shown to potentiate the hypotensive effects of nitrates in healthy volunteers and in patients, and is therefore contraindicated in patients who are taking any type of nitrate drug therapy, or who utilize short-acting nitrate-containing medications, due to the risk of developing potentially life-threatening hypotension. The use of organic nitrates, either regularly and/or intermittently, in any form (e.g. oral, sublingual, transdermal, by inhalation) is absolutely contraindicated (see Action and Clinical Pharmacology and Dosage and Administration).

REVATIO is contraindicated in patients who are hypersensitive to this drug or any ingredient in the formulation or component of the container. For a complete listing, see Dosage Forms, Composition and Packaging.

WARNINGS AND PRECAUTIONS:

> **Serious Warnings and Precautions**
> - Administration to patients with pulmonary veno-occlusive disease is not recommended.
> - There is evidence that patients at risk for NAION may have abnormal optic discs (e.g. crowded disc) prior to development of the condition. Causal association between the use of REVATIO (a PDE5 inhibitor) and NAION in patients with abnormal discs has not been established. If physicians are concerned about the overall risk of NAION, they should consider discussing these concerns with an ophthalmologist.
> - Administration of REVATIO (a PDE5 inhibitor) to patients with previously diagnosed NAION is not recommended. Physicians treating patients with previous NAION should consult an ophthalmologist prior to initiating REVATIO (see General).

General: REVATIO (sildenafil citrate) is not recommended in the following cases:

- Pulmonary vasodilators may significantly worsen the cardiovascular status of patients with pulmonary veno-occlusive disease. Since there are no clinical data on administration of REVATIO (sildenafil citrate) to patients with venous occlusive disease, administration of REVATIO to such patients is not recommended.
- The concomitant administration of the protease inhibitor ritonavir (a highly potent CYP3A4 inhibitor) substantially increases serum concentrations of sildenafil, therefore co-administration with REVATIO is not recommended (see Drug Interactions and Dosage and Administration).

Before prescribing REVATIO (sildenafil citrate), it is important to note the following:

- In clinical trials, sildenafil has been shown to have systemic vasodilatory properties that result in transient decreases in blood pressure (see Action and Clinical Pharmacology). Prior to prescribing REVATIO, physicians should carefully consider whether their patients with certain underlying conditions could be adversely affected by such vasodilatory effects, for example patients with resting hypotension (BP <90/50), or with fluid depletion, severe left ventricular outflow obstruction, or autonomic dysfunction.
- Sildenafil citrate is also marketed as VIAGRA for male erectile dysfunction.

When used to treat male erectile dysfunction, non-arteritic anterior ischaemic optic neuropathy (NAION) has been reported rarely post-marketing in temporal association with the use of all phosphodiesterase type-5 inhibitors. NAION can result in varying degrees of permanent loss of vision, for which there is no treatment. Most, but not all of these patients had underlying risk factors for the development of NAION, including but not necessarily limited to: low cup to optic disc ratio (the "crowded disc at risk"), age over 50, diabetes, hypertension, coronary artery disease, hyperlipidaemia and smoking. It is not possible to determine if NAION is related directly to the use of sildenafil or other PDE5 inhibitors, to the patient's underlying vascular risk factors or anatomical defects, to a combination of these, or to other factors.

- There is evidence that patients at risk for NAION may have abnormal optic discs (e.g. crowded disc) prior to development of the condition. Causal association between the use of PDE5 inhibitors and NAION in patients with abnormal discs has not been established. If physicians are concerned about the overall risk of NAION, they should consider discussing these concerns with an ophthalmologist.

Physicians should advise patients to stop use of REVATIO and seek medical attention in the event of a sudden loss of vision in one or both eyes.

A causal relationship has not been established between use of PDE5 inhibitors and NAION. However administration of REVATIO (a PDE5 inhibitor) to patients with previously diagnosed NAION is not recommended. Physicians treating patients with previous NAION should consult an ophthalmologist prior to initiating REVATIO.

- There are no controlled clinical data on the safety or efficacy of REVATIO in patients with retinitis pigmentosa (a minority of these patients have genetic disorders of retinal phosphodiesterases) (see Action and Clinical Pharmacology). If prescribed, this should be done with caution.
- Caution is advised when Phosphodiesterase Type 5 (PDE5) inhibitors are coadministered with alpha-blockers. PDE5 inhibitors, including sildenafil, and alpha-adrenergic blocking agents are both vasodilators with blood pressure lowering effects. When vasodilators are used in combination, an additive effect on blood pressure may be anticipated. In some patients, concomitant use of these two drug classes can lower blood pressure significantly, leading to symptomatic hypotension. In the sildenafil interaction studies with alpha-blockers (see Drug Interactions), cases of symptomatic hypotension consisting of dizziness and lightheadedness were reported. No cases of syncope or fainting were reported during these interaction studies. Consideration should be given to the fact that safety of combined use of PDE5 inhibitors and alpha-blockers may be affected by other variables, including intravascular volume depletion and concomitant use of anti-hypertensive drugs.
- REVATIO should be used with caution in patients with anatomical deformation of the penis (such as angulation, cavernosal fibrosis or Peyronie's disease) or in patients who have conditions, which may predispose them to priapism (such as sickle cell anemia, multiple myeloma or leukemia).
- In humans, sildenafil has no effect on bleeding time when taken alone or with acetylsalicylic acid. In vitro studies with human platelets indicate that sildenafil potentiates the anti-aggregatory effect of sodium nitroprusside (a nitric oxide donor). The combination of heparin and sildenafil had an additive effect on bleeding time in the anesthetized rabbit, but this interaction has not been studied in humans (see Drug Interactions and Action and Clinical Pharmacology).
- The incidence of epistaxis was higher in patients with pulmonary arterial hypertension (PAH) secondary to connective tissue disease (CTD) (sildenafil 12.9%, placebo 0%) than in primary pulmonary hypertension (PPH) patients (sildenafil 2.3%, placebo 2.4%). Incidence was also higher in sildenafil-treated patients with concomitant oral Vitamin K antagonist (8.8% versus 1.7% not treated with concomitant Vitamin K antagonist).
- There is no safety information on the administration of REVATIO to patients with bleeding disorders or active peptic ulceration. Therefore, REVATIO should be administered with caution to these patients.

Cardiovascular: There is no controlled clinical data on the safety or efficacy of REVATIO in the following groups, if prescribed, this should be done with caution:

- Patients who have suffered a myocardial infarction, stroke, or life-threatening arrhythmia within the last 6 months;
- Patients with coronary artery disease causing unstable angina;
- Patients with hypertension (BP >170/110);

Otologic: Sudden decrease or loss of hearing has been reported in a few numbers of postmarketing cases with the use of PDE5 inhibitors, including REVATIO. These events, which may be accompanied by tinnitus and dizziness, have been reported in temporal association to the intake of PDE5 inhibitors, including REVATIO. In some of the cases, medical conditions and other factors were reported that may have also played a role in the otologic adverse events. In many cases, medical follow-up information was limited. It is not possible to determine whether these events are related directly to the use of PDE5 inhibitors or to other factors (see Adverse Reactions, Post-Market Adverse Drug Reactions). Physicians should advise patients to seek prompt medical attention in case of sudden decrease or loss of hearing.

Special Populations: Pregnant Women: No evidence of teratogenicity, embryotoxicity or fetotoxicity was observed in rats and rabbits, which received up to 200 mg/kg/day during organogenesis. There are no adequate and well-controlled studies of sildenafil in pregnant women.

Nursing Women: It is not known if sildenafil citrate and/or metabolites are excreted in human breast milk. Since many drugs are excreted in human milk, caution should be used when REVATIO is administered to nursing women.

Pediatrics (<18 years): Safety and effectiveness in pediatric pulmonary hypertension patients has not been established.

Geriatrics (≥65 years): Healthy elderly volunteers had a reduced clearance of sildenafil, but studies did not include sufficient numbers of subjects to determine whether they respond differently from younger subjects. Other reported clinical experience has not identified differences in response between the elderly and younger pulmonary arterial hypertension patients. In general, dose selection for an elderly patient should be cautious, reflecting the greater frequency of decreased hepatic, renal, or cardiac function, and of concomitant disease or other drug therapy (see Action and Clinical Pharmacology and Dosage and Administration).

Combination Sildenafil Citrate + Epoprostenol: (See Adverse Reactions and Drug Interactions, Drug-Drug Interactions.)

Information to Be Provided to the Patient: Physicians should discuss with patients the contraindication of REVATIO with regular and/or intermittent use of organic nitrates.

Physicians should advise patients to stop use of REVATIO and seek immediate medical attention in the event of a sudden loss of vision in one or both eyes. Such an event may be a sign of non-arteritic anterior ischemic optic neuropathy (NAION), a cause of decreased vision including permanent loss of vision, that has been reported rarely post-marketing in temporal association with the use of all PDE5 inhibitors when used in the treatment of male erectile dysfunction. It is not possible to determine whether these events are related directly to the use of PDE5 inhibitors or to other factors. Should the vision loss be diagnosed as NAION, continued use of REVATIO is not recommended (see Warnings and Precautions, General).

ADVERSE REACTIONS: Adverse Drug Reaction Overview: Sildenafil Oral Administration: Safety data on REVATIO (sildenafil citrate) were obtained from a single pivotal study, consisting of 68 (25%) men and 209 (75%) women, and an open-label extension study in 277 treated patients with pulmonary arterial hypertension. 259 subjects who completed the pivotal study entered a long-term extension study. Doses up to 80 mg t.i.d. (4 times the recommended dose of 20 mg t.i.d.) were studied and exposure to REVATIO ranged from 68 to 614 days (N=149 patients treated for at least 1 year).

The overall frequency of discontinuation in REVATIO-treated patients at the recommended daily dose of 20 mg t.i.d. was low (2.9%) and the same as placebo (2.9%).

Clinical Trial Adverse Drug Reactions: Because clinical trials are conducted under very specific conditions the adverse reaction rates observed in the clinical trials may not reflect the rates observed in practice and should not be compared to the rates in the clinical trials of another drug. Adverse drug reaction information from clinical trials is useful for identifying drug-related adverse events and for approximating rates.

Sildenafil Oral Administration: In the pivotal placebo-controlled trial in pulmonary arterial hypertension, the adverse drug reactions that occurred in at least 3% of REVATIO-treated patients at any of the 20, 40, or 80 mg t.i.d. doses, and more commonly on REVATIO than on placebo, are shown in Table 1.

Table 1: REVATIO

Sildenafil Adverse Events More Frequent than Placebo in ≥3% of Patients (N≥2 Patients)

Adverse event (%)	Placebo (N=70)	Sildenafil Treatment Groups 20 mg (N=69)	40 mg (N=67)	80 mg (N=71)	Total (N=207)
Headache	39	46	42	49	46
Flushing	4	10	9	16	12
Dyspepsia	7	13	8	13	11
Back Pain	11	13	13	9	12
Diarrhea	6	9	12	10	10
Limb Pain	6	7	15	9	10
Myalgia	4	7	6	14	9
Cough	6	7	5	9	7
Epistaxis	1	9	8	4	7
Pyrexia	3	6	3	10	6

(cont'd)

Table 1: REVATIO *(cont'd)*

Sildenafil Adverse Events More Frequent than Placebo in ≥3% of Patients (N≥2 Patients)

Adverse event (%)	Placebo (N=70)	Sildenafil Treatment Groups 20 mg (N=69)	40 mg (N=67)	80 mg (N=71)	Total (N=207)
Influenza	3	6	6	4	5
Vertigo	1	1	5	3	3
Gastritis	0	3	3	4	3
Erythema	0	6	2	1	3
Insomnia	1	7	6	4	6
Visual disturbance	0	0	5	7	4
Dyspnea (exacerbated)	3	7	2	1	3
Sinusitis	0	3	5	1	3
Paresthesia	0	3	5	1	3
Rhinitis	0	4	2	3	3

In a placebo-controlled fixed dose titration study of REVATIO (starting with recommended dose of 20 mg TID and increased to 40 mg TID and then 80 mg TID) as an adjunct to intravenous epoprostenol in pulmonary arterial hypertension, the clinically meaningful adverse drug reactions that were reported by at least 2% of patients in the REVATIO arm are shown in Table 2.

Table 2: REVATIO

Sildenafil-Epoprostenol All Causality Adverse Events Reported by ≥2% of Sildenafil Treated Patients and More Frequent Than Placebo

Adverse Events	Percentage of Subjects Reporting Event: Placebo + epoprostenol (N=131)	Sildenafil + epoprostenol (N=134)
Blood and Lymphatic System Disorders		
Anaemia	3,1	4.5
Cardiac Disorders		
Palpitations	6.1	7.5
Endocrine Disorders		
Hyperthyroidism	0.8	2.2
Eye Disorders		
Chromatopsia	0	5.2
Ocular hyperaemia	0	2.2
Vision blurred	1.5	4.5
Gastrointestinal Disorders		
Abdominal distension	0.8	3
Diarrhoea	18.3	25.4
Dry mouth	0	3.7
Gastrooesophageal reflux disease	0.8	6
Nausea	18.3	34.3
Rectal haemorrhage	0	2.2
Vomiting	9.9	14.9
General Disorders and Administration Site Conditions		
Asthenia	20.6	23.9
Chest pain	9.9	14.2
Chills	0	5.2
Malaise	0.8	2.2
Oedema	13	24.6
Pain	2.3	4.5
Infections and Infestations		
Bronchitis	0.8	3.7
Cellulitis	1.5	3.7
Gastroentéritis	0.8	2.2

(cont'd)

Table 2: REVATIO *(cont'd)*

Sildenafil-Epoprostenol All Causality Adverse Events Reported by ≥2% of Sildenafil Treated Patients and More Frequent Than Placebo

Adverse Events	Percentage of Subjects Reporting Event	
	Placebo + epoprostenol (N=131)	Sildenafil + epoprostenol (N=134)
Upper respiratory tract infection	9.2	15.7
Investigations		
International normalised ratio increased	3.1	5.2
Metabolism and Nutrition Disorders		
Anorexia	1.5	4.5
Hypervolaemia	1.5	3.7
Musculoskeletal and Connective Tissue Disorders		
Arthralgia	2.3	6.7
Back pain	3.1	4.5
Myalgia	5.3	9.7
Pain in extremity	6.1	17.2
Pain in jaw	8.4	10.4
Shoulder pain	1.5	2.2
Nervous System Disorders		
Dizziness	19.1	20.9
Headache	33.6	56.7
Hypoaesthesia	1.5	3
Psychiatric Disorders		
Anxiety	1.5	3
Renal and Urinary Disorders		
Renal failure	1.5	2.2
Respiratory, Thoracic and Mediastinal Disorders		
Epistaxis	5.3	9
Haemoptysis	1.5	2.2
Hypoxia	1.5	3
Nasal congestion	2.3	9
Skin and Subcutaneous Tissue Disorders		
Rash	10.7	17.2
Vascular Disorders		
Flushing	13	19.4
Hypotension	6.1	9

Post-Market Adverse Drug Reactions: In post-marketing experience with sildenafil citrate at doses indicated for male erectile dysfunction (MED), serious cardiovascular, cerebrovascular, and vascular events, including myocardial infarction, sudden cardiac death, ventricular arrhythmia, cerebrovascular hemorrhage, transient ischemic attack, hypertension, pulmonary hemorrhage, and subarachnoid and intracerebral hemorrhages have been reported in temporal association with the use of the drug. Most, but not all, of these patients had preexisting cardiovascular risk factors. Many of these events were reported to occur during or shortly after sexual activity, and a few were reported to occur shortly after the use of sildenafil without sexual activity. Others were reported to have occurred hours to days after use concurrent with sexual activity. It is not possible to determine whether these events are related directly to sildenafil citrate, to sexual activity, to the patient's underlying cardiovascular disease, or to a combination of these or other factors.

Cases of sudden decrease or loss of hearing have been reported post-marketing in temporal association with the use of PDE5 inhibitors, including REVATIO. In some of the cases, medical conditions and other factors were reported that may have also played a role in the otologic adverse events. In many cases, medical follow-up information was limited. It is not possible to determine whether these events are related directly to the use of REVATIO, to the patient's underlying risk factors for hearing loss, a combination of these factors, or to other factors (see Warnings and Precautions and Information for the Patient).

DRUG INTERACTIONS:

Serious Drug Interactions
- Use of organic nitrates in any form is absolutely contraindicated (see Contraindications)

Overview: In vitro studies: Sildenafil metabolism is principally mediated by the cytochrome P-450 (CYP) isoforms 3A4 (major route) and 2C9 (minor route) (see Action and Clinical Pharmacology). Therefore drugs that affect these isoenzymes may affect sildenafil clearance.

Sildenafil is a weak inhibitor of the cytochrome P450 isoforms 1A2, 2C9, 2C19, 2D6, 2E1 and 3A4 (IC50>150 µM).

In vivo studies: Sildenafil (50 mg) did not potentiate the hypotensive effect of alcohol in healthy volunteers with mean maximum blood alcohol levels of 0.08%.

The drugs listed are based on either drug interaction case reports or studies, or predicted interactions due to the expected magnitude and seriousness of the interaction (ie. those identified as contraindicated).

Drug-Drug Interactions: Effects of Other Drugs on REVATIO Oral Administration: In vivo studies: Population pharmacokinetic analysis of clinical trial data indicated a reduction in sildenafil clearance and/or an increase of oral bioavailability when co-administered with CYP3A4 substrates and the combination of CYP3A4 substrates and beta-blockers. These were the only covariates with a statistically significant impact on sildenafil pharmacokinetics. The exposure to sildenafil in patients on CYP3A4 substrates and CYP3A4 substrates plus beta-blockers was 43% and 66% higher, respectively, compared to patients not receiving these drug classes.

Population data from patients in clinical trials indicated a reduction in sildenafil clearance when it was co-administered with CYP3A4 inhibitors. Sildenafil exposure without concomitant medication is shown to be 5-fold higher at a dose of 80 mg t.i.d. compared to the exposure at a dose of 20 mg t.i.d. This concentration range covers the same increased sildenafil exposure observed in specifically-designed drug interaction studies with CYP3A4 inhibitors (except for potent inhibitors such as ketoconazole, itraconazole, and ritonavir). Cimetidine (800 mg), a nonspecific CYP inhibitor, caused a 56% increase in plasma sildenafil concentrations when coadministered with sildenafil (50 mg) to healthy volunteers. When a single 100 mg dose of sildenafil was co-administered with erythromycin, a CYP3A4 inhibitor, at steady state (500 mg twice daily [b.i.d.] for 5 days), there was a 182% increase in sildenafil systemic exposure (AUC). In a study performed in healthy volunteers, co-administration of the HIV protease inhibitor saquinavir, a CYP3A4 inhibitor, at steady state (1200 mg t.i.d.) with sildenafil (100 mg single dose) resulted in a 140% increase in sildenafil C_{max} and a 210% increase in sildenafil AUC. Stronger CYP3A4 inhibitors such as ketoconazole or itraconazole will have still greater effects on plasma levels of sildenafil (see Dosage and Administration).

In another study in healthy volunteers, co-administration with the HIV protease inhibitor ritonavir (a highly potent P450 inhibitor) at steady state (500 mg b.i.d.) with sildenafil (100 mg single dose) resulted in a 300% (4-fold) increase in sildenafil C_{max} and a 1000% (11-fold) increase in sildenafil plasma AUC. At 24 hours, the plasma levels of sildenafil were still approximately 200 ng/mL, compared to approximately 5 ng/mL when sildenafil was dosed alone. This is consistent with ritonavir's marked effects on a broad range of P450 substrates (see Warnings and Precautions and Dosage and Administration). Although the interaction between other protease inhibitors and REVATIO has not been studied, their concomitant use is expected to increase sildenafil levels.

In a study of healthy male volunteers, co-administration of sildenafil at steady state (80 mg t.i.d.) with the endothelin antagonist bosentan (a moderate inducer of CYP3A4, CYP 2C9 and possibly of cytochrome P450 2C19) at steady state (125 mg b.i.d.) resulted in a 62.6% decrease of sildenafil AUC and a 55.4% decrease in sildenafil C_{max}. The combination of both drugs did not lead to clinically significant changes of blood pressure (supine and standing) and was well tolerated in healthy volunteers. Concomitant administration of potent CYP3A4 inducers is expected to cause greater decreases in plasma levels of sildenafil.

In drug-drug interaction studies, sildenafil (25 mg, 50 mg, or 100 mg) and the alpha-blocker doxazosin (4 mg or 8 mg) were administered simultaneously to patients with benign prostatic hyperplasia (BPH) stabilized on doxazosin therapy. In these study populations, mean additional reductions of supine systolic and diastolic blood pressure of 7/7 mmHg, 9/5 mmHg, and 8/4 mmHg, respectively, were observed. Mean additional reductions of standing blood pressure of 6/6 mmHg, 11/4 mmHg, and 4/5 mmHg, respectively, were also observed. There were infrequent reports of patients who experienced symptomatic postural hypotension. These reports included dizziness and light-headedness, but not syncope (see Warnings and Precautions).

Concomitant administration of single doses of doxazosin (4 or 8 mg) and sildenafil (25 or 50 mg) did not produce any clinically relevant effect on each other's pharmacokinetic parameters (AUC, C_{max}, T_{max}).

Concomitant administration of oral contraceptives (ethinyl estradiol 30 µg and levonorgestrel 150 µg) did not affect the pharmacokinetics of sildenafil.

Single doses of antacid (magnesium hydroxide/aluminum hydroxide) did not affect the bioavailability of sildenafil.

Effects of Oral REVATIO on Other Drugs: In vivo studies: When sildenafil 100 mg oral was co-administered with amlodipine, 5 mg or 10 mg oral, to hypertensive patients, the mean additional reduction on supine blood pressure was 8 mmHg systolic and 7 mmHg diastolic.

No significant interactions were shown with tolbutamide (single 250 mg dose) or warfarin (single 40 mg dose), both of which are metabolized by CYP2C9, when co-administered with 50 mg sildenafil.

No interactions were observed between sildenafil (100 mg single dose) and acenocoumarol.

Sildenafil (50 mg) did not potentiate the increase in bleeding time, measured using a standard simplate method, caused by acetylsalicylic acid (150 mg).

Sildenafil at steady state (80 mg t.i.d.) resulted in a 49.8% increase in AUC and a 42% increase in C_{max} of bosentan (125 mg b.i.d.).

In a study of healthy volunteers, sildenafil (100 mg did not affect the steady-state pharmacokinetics of the HIV protease inhibitors saquinavir (1200 mg t.i.d) and ritonavir (500 mg b.i.d), both of which are CYP3A4 substrates.

Sildenafil had no impact on the plasma levels of oral contraceptives (ethinyl estradiol 30 µg and levonorgestrel 150 µg).

Combination Oral Sildenafil Citrate + Epoprostenol: Based on the population pharmacokinetic analysis of Study A1481141 (sildenafil + epoprostenol), a 27% of decrease in sildenafil bioavailability was estimated. In the analysis of this study data, the inter-subject variability in the relative bioavailability of sildenafil was estimated at 48.2 %, and the effect of epoprostenol on sildenafil exposure was not considered as clinically relevant.

Drug-Food Interactions: Grapefruit juice is a weak inhibitor of CYP3A4 gut wall metabolism and may give rise to modest increases in plasma levels of oral sildenafil.

Drug-Herb Interactions: Interaction with herbal products has not been established.

Drug-Laboratory Test Interactions: Interaction with laboratory tests has not been established.

DOSAGE AND ADMINISTRATION: Dosing Considerations: Dosing of REVATIO (sildenafil citrate) may be affected by the following:
- concomitant administration of alpha-blockers
- concomitant administration of potent CYP3A4 inhibitors (e.g. ketoconazole, itraconazole, ritonavir) and weak CYP3A4 inhibitors (e.g. grapefruit juice)
- co-administration with CYP3A4 inducers (e.g. bosentan)

(See Warnings and Precautions and Drug Interactions.)

Recommended Dose and Dosage Adjustment: Adult Oral Dose: The recommended dose of REVATIO oral administration is 20 mg three times a day (t.i.d.).

No dose adjustments are required for renal impaired patients (including severe renal impairment, creatinine clearance <30 mL/min), and hepatic impaired patients (Child Pugh class A and B).

No dose adjustments are required for the co-administration of REVATIO with erythromycin and saquinavir.

Co-administration of REVATIO with CYP3A4 inducers (including bosentan; and more potent inducers such as barbiturates, carbamazepine, phenytoin, efavirenz, nevirapine, rifampin, rifabutin) may alter plasma levels of either or both medications. Dosage adjustments may be necessary (see Warnings and Precautions).

Co-administration of potent CYP3A4 inhibitors (e.g. ketoconazole, itraconazole, ritonavir) with REVATIO substantially increases serum concentrations of sildenafil and is therefore not recommended (see Warnings and Precautions and Drug Interactions).

Sildenafil was shown to potentiate the hypotensive effects of nitrates and its administration in patients who use nitric oxide donors, or nitrates in any form, is therefore contraindicated.

Geriatric Use: No dose adjustment is required. However, in general, dose selection for elderly patients should be cautious, reflecting the greater frequency of decreased hepatic, renal, or cardiac function, and of concomitant disease or other drug therapy (see Action and Clinical Pharmacology).

Oral Dose Administration: REVATIO (sildenafil citrate) should be taken approximately 6-8 hours apart, with or without food.

OVERDOSAGE:
In studies with healthy volunteers of single oral doses up to 800 mg, adverse events were similar to those seen at lower doses but incidence rates were increased.

In cases of overdose, standard supportive measures should be adopted as required. Renal dialysis is not expected to accelerate clearance as sildenafil is highly bound to plasma proteins and it is not eliminated in the urine.

For management of a suspected drug overdose, contact your regional Poison Control Centre. See the *CPS* Directory section for a list of Poison Control Centres.

ACTION AND CLINICAL PHARMACOLOGY: Mechanism of Action: Sildenafil is a potent and selective inhibitor of cGMP specific phosphodiesterase type-5 (PDE5) in the smooth muscle of the pulmonary vasculature, where PDE5 is responsible for degradation of cGMP. Sildenafil, therefore, increases cGMP within pulmonary vascular smooth muscle cells resulting in relaxation. In patients with pulmonary hypertension, this can lead to selective vasodilation of the pulmonary vascular bed and, to a lesser degree, vasodilatation in the systemic circulation.

Studies in vitro have shown that sildenafil has between 10 and 10 000-fold greater selectivity for PDE5 than for other phosphodiesterase isoforms namely PDEs 1, 2, 3, 4, and 6 and greater than 700-fold effect on PDE7-PDE11. In particular, sildenafil has greater than 4000-fold selectivity for PDE5 over PDE3, the cAMP-specific phosphodiesterase isoform involved in the control of cardiac contractility. Sildenafil is about 10-fold as potent for PDE5 compared to PDE6, an isoenzyme found in the retina; this lower selectivity is thought to be the basis for colour vision abnormalities observed with higher doses or plasma levels of sildenafil (see Warnings and Precautions).

In addition to pulmonary vascular smooth muscle and the corpus cavernosum, PDE5 is also found in other tissues including vascular and visceral smooth muscle and in platelets. The inhibition of PDE5 in these tissues by sildenafil may be the basis for the enhanced platelet antiaggregatory activity observed in vitro, and the mild peripheral arterial-venous dilatation in vivo.

Pharmacodynamics: Effects of REVATIO on Blood Pressure—Oral Administration: Single oral doses of sildenafil (100 mg) administered to healthy volunteers produced decreases in supine blood pressure (mean maximum decrease in systolic/diastolic blood pressure of 8.4/5.5 mmHg). The decrease in blood pressure was most notable approximately 1-2 hours after dosing, and was not different than placebo at 8 hours. Similar effects on blood pressure were noted with 25 mg, 50 mg and 100 mg doses of sildenafil, therefore the effects are not related to dose or plasma levels within this dosage range. Larger effects were recorded among patients receiving concomitant nitrates (see Contraindications).

Single oral doses of sildenafil up to 100 mg in healthy volunteers produced no clinically relevant effects on ECG. After chronic dosing of 80 mg t.i.d. to patients with pulmonary arterial hypertension, no clinically relevant effects on ECG were reported.

After chronic dosing of 80 mg t.i.d. sildenafil to healthy patients, the largest mean change from baseline in supine systolic and supine diastolic blood pressure was a decrease of 9.0 mmHg and 8.4 mmHg respectively.

After chronic oral dosing of 80 mg t.i.d. sildenafil to patients with systemic hypertension, the mean change from baseline in systolic and diastolic blood pressure was a decrease of 9.4 mmHg and 9.1 mmHg respectively.

After chronic oral dosing of 80 mg t.i.d. sildenafil to patients with pulmonary arterial hypertension, lesser effects in blood pressure reduction were observed (a reduction in both systolic and diastolic pressure of 2 mm Hg). This may be due to improvements in cardiac output secondary to the beneficial effects of sildenafil on pulmonary vascular resistance.

Pharmacokinetics: REVATIO (sildenafil citrate tablets) is rapidly absorbed after oral administration, with absolute bioavailability of about 40%. After oral three-times-daily (t.i.d.) dosing of REVATIO, AUC and C_{max} increase in proportion with dose over the dose range of 20-40 mg t.i.d. After 80 mg t.i.d., a slightly more than dose-proportional increase of sildenafil plasma levels has been observed. It is eliminated predominantly by hepatic metabolism (mainly cytochrome P450 3A4) and is converted to an active metabolite with properties similar to the parent, sildenafil. The concomitant use of potent cytochrome P450 3A4 (CYP3A4) inhibitors (e.g. ritonavir ketoconazole, itraconazole) as well as the nonspecific CYP inhibitor, cimetidine, is associated with increased plasma levels of sildenafil (see Drug Interactions and Dosage and Administration). Both sildenafil and the metabolite have terminal half-lives of about 4 hours.

Absorption: REVATIO is rapidly absorbed. Maximum observed plasma concentrations are reached within 30 to 120 minutes (median 60 minutes) of oral dosing in the fasted state. When REVATIO was administered with a high-fat meal, the rate of absorption was significantly decreased, with a 29% reduction in C_{max} and a 60-minute delay in T_{max}. This is not clinically relevant for chronic dosing in this patient population.

Distribution: The mean steady state volume of distribution (Vss) for sildenafil is 105 L, indicating distribution into the tissues. Sildenafil and its major circulating N-desmethyl metabolite are both approximately 96% bound to plasma proteins. Protein binding is independent of total drug concentrations.

Based upon measurements of sildenafil in semen of healthy volunteers 90 minutes after dosing, less than 0.0002% (average 188 ng) of the administered dose may appear in the semen of patients.

Metabolism: Sildenafil is cleared predominantly by the CYP3A4 (major route) and CYP2C9 (minor route) hepatic microsomal isoenzymes. The major circulating metabolite (UK-103,320) results from N-desmethylation of sildenafil at the N-methyl piperazine moiety. This metabolite has a phosphodiesterase selectivity profile similar to sildenafil and an in vitro potency for PDE5 approximately 50% of the parent drug. In healthy volunteers, plasma concentrations of this metabolite are approximately 40% of those seen for sildenafil, so that the metabolite accounts for about 20% of sildenafil's pharmacologic effects. In patients with pulmonary arterial hypertension, however, the ratio of UK-103,320 to sildenafil is higher. Plasma concentrations of UK-103,320 are approximately 72% those of sildenafil after 20 mg t.i.d. oral dosing (translating into a 36% contribution to sildenafil's pharmacological effects). The subsequent effect on efficacy is unknown.

Excretion: The total body clearance of sildenafil is 41 L/h with a resultant terminal phase halflife of 3-5 hours. After either oral or intravenous administration, sildenafil is excreted as metabolites predominantly in the feces (approximately 80% of administered dose) and to a lesser extent in the urine (approximately 13% of the administered dose).

Special Populations and Conditions: Pediatrics: Safety and effectiveness in pediatric pulmonary hypertension patients has not been established.

Geriatrics: Healthy elderly volunteers (65 years or over) had a reduced clearance of sildenafil, resulting in approximately 90 % higher plasma concentrations of sildenafil and the active N-desmethyl metabolite compared to those seen in healthy younger volunteers (18-45 years). Due to age differences in plasma protein binding, the corresponding increase in free sildenafil plasma concentration was approximately 40 %.

Gender: Comparison of the female PK data with historic control of male data resulted in ratios (90%CI) for C_{max} and AUC_t of 80% (65%;99%) and 103% (85%; 124%) respectively with a difference (90%CI) in T_{max} of 0.5 h (0.2 h;0.8 h). The average estimates for apparent oral clearance (CL/F) and volume of distribution (V/F) were similar for males (n=1335) and females (n=433). Therefore, there are no clinically significant gender differences in sildenafil pharmacokinetics.

Hepatic Insufficiency: In volunteers with hepatic cirrhosis (Child-Pugh A and B), sildenafil clearance was reduced, resulting in increases in AUC (84%) and C_{max} (47%) compared to agematched volunteers with no hepatic impairment. Patients with severe hepatic impairment (Child-Pugh class C) have not been studied.

Renal Insufficiency: In volunteers with mild (CLcr=50-80 mL/min) and moderate (CLcr=30-49 mL/min) renal impairment, the pharmacokinetics of a single oral dose of sildenafil (50 mg) were not altered. In volunteers with severe (CLcr <30 mL/min) renal impairment, sildenafil clearance was reduced, resulting in AUC (100%) and C_{max} (88%) compared to age-matched volunteers with no renal impairment. In addition, N-desmethyl metabolite AUC and C_{max} values were significantly increased 200 % and 79 % respectively in subjects with severe renal impairment compared to subjects with normal renal function.

Population Pharmacokinetics: Age, gender, race, and renal and hepatic function were included as covariates in the population pharmacokinetic model to evaluate sildenafil pharmacokinetics in pulmonary arterial hypertension patients. The data set available for the population pharmacokinetic evaluation contained a wide range of demographic data and laboratory parameters associated with hepatic and renal function. None of these factors had a statistically significant impact on sildenafil pharmacokinetics in patients with pulmonary hypertension. However, CYP3A4 substrates reduced the apparent clearance of sildenafil, alone and in combination, with beta-blockers (by 22.3% and 37.4%, respectively). No other factor had a statistically significant influence on sildenafil pharmacokinetics.

In patients with pulmonary hypertension, the average steady state concentrations were 20-50% higher over the investigated dose range of 20-80 mg t.i.d., when compared to those of healthy volunteers. There was a doubling of C_{min} levels compared to healthy volunteers. Both findings suggest a lower clearance and/or a higher oral bioavailability of sildenafil in patients with pulmonary hypertension compared to healthy volunteers.

STORAGE AND STABILITY: Store at 25°C; excursions permitted to 15-30°C [see USP Controlled Room Temperature].

SPECIAL HANDLING INSTRUCTIONS: Not applicable.

INFORMATION FOR THE PATIENT: Published in e-CPS, available by subscription at www.e-cps.ca.

DOSAGE FORMS, COMPOSITION AND PACKAGING: Each white, film-coated, round tablet marked RVT20 on one side and PFIZER on the other side, contains: sildenafil citrate equivalent to 20 mg of sildenafil. Nonmedicinal ingredients: anhydrous dibasic calcium phosphate, croscarmellose sodium, magnesium stearate and microcrystalline cellulose; film coat: hypromellose, lactose, titanium dioxide (E-171) and triacetin. Bottles of 90. Blisters of 90 (15 tablets per blister strip).

(Shown in Product Identification Section)

ReVia™ Ⓟ

naltrexone HCl

Opioid Antagonist

Apotex

Date of Preparation: May 9, 2003

PHARMACOLOGY: Pharmacodynamic Actions: REVIA (naltrexone hydrochloride) is a pure opioid antagonist. It markedly attenuates or completely blocks, reversibly, the subjective effects of intravenously administered opioids. [In this context, the term opioid is used to describe 1) classic morphine-like agonists and 2) analgesics possessing agonist and antagonist activity (eg, butorphanol, nalbuphine and pentazocine)].

When co-administered with morphine, on a chronic basis, REVIA blocks the physical dependence to morphine and presumably other opioids. REVIA has few, if any, intrinsic actions besides its opioid blocking properties. However, it does produce some pupillary constriction, by an unknown mechanism.

While the mechanism of action is not fully understood, the preponderance of evidence suggests that REVIA blocks the effects of opioids by competitive binding (ie, analogous to competitive inhibition of enzymes) at opioid receptors. This makes the blockade produced potentially surmountable, but overcoming full naltrexone blockade by administration of very high doses of opiates has resulted in excessive symptoms of histamine release in experimental subjects.

The mechanism of action of REVIA in the treatment of alcoholism is not understood; however, involvement of the endogenous opioid system is suggested by preclinical data. REVIA, an opioid receptor antagonist, competitively binds to such receptors and may block the effects of endogenous opioids. Opioid antagonists have been shown to reduce alcohol consumption by animals, and REVIA has been shown to reduce alcohol consumption in clinical studies.

REVIA is not aversive therapy and does not cause a disulfiram-like reaction either as a result of opiate use or ethanol ingestion. The administration of REVIA is not associated with the development of tolerance or dependence.

In subjects physically dependent on opioids, REVIA will precipitate withdrawal symptomatology.

Clinical studies indicate that 50 mg of REVIA will block the pharmacologic effects of 25 mg of intravenously administered heroin for periods as long as 24 hours. Other data suggest that doubling the dose of REVIA provides blockade for 48 hours, and tripling the dose of REVIA provides blockade for about 72 hours.

Pharmacokinetics/Bioavailability: Following oral administration, REVIA undergoes rapid and nearly complete absorption with approximately 96% of the dose absorbed from the gastrointestinal tract. Although well absorbed orally, naltrexone is subject to extensive "first-pass" hepatic metabolism with an oral bioavailability estimate ranging from 5 to 40%. The activity of naltrexone is believed to be due to both parent and the 6-β-naltrexol metabolite.

Following the administration of 50 mg REVIA tablets to 24 healthy adult male volunteers, the Cmax for REVIA and its major metabolite, 6-β-naltrexol were 8.6 ng/mL and 99.3 ng/mL, respectively. The maximum concentration (Cmax) and area under the curve (AUC), for both naltrexone and 6-β-naltrexol are dose proportional over the range of 50 to 200 mg. The time to maximum concentration (Tmax) is one hour for both naltrexone and 6-β-naltrexol. The mean elimination half-life ($t_{1/2}$) values for naltrexone and 6-β-naltrexol are 4 hours and 12.9 hours, respectively. The mean elimination half-life ($t_{1/2}$) and time to maximum concentration (Tmax) for REVIA and 6-β-naltrexol are independent of dose.

The volume of distribution for REVIA following intravenous administration is estimated to be 1350 litres. In vitro tests with human plasma show naltrexone to be 21% bound to plasma protein over the therapeutic dose range.

The systemic clearance (after intravenous administration) of REVIA approximates 3.5 L/min, which exceeds liver blood flow (~1.35 L/min), and suggests that REVIA is a highly extracted drug (>98% metabolized) and that extrahepatic sites of drug metabolism exist. The major metabolite of naltrexone is 6-β-naltrexol. Two other minor metabolites are 2-hydroxy-3-methoxy-6-β-naltrexol and 2-hydroxy-3-methyl-naltrexone. Naltrexone and its metabolites are also conjugated to form additional metabolic products. A renal clearance ranging from 30 to 127 mL/min for naltrexone suggests it is primarily cleared by glomerular filtration. A renal clearance of 230 to 369 mL/min for 6-β-naltrexol suggests an additional renal tubular secretory mechanism. REVIA and its metabolites are excreted primarily by the kidney (56% to 79% of the dose), with fecal excretion being a minor elimination pathway. The urinary excretion of unchanged REVIA accounts for less than 2% of an oral dose; urinary excretion of unchanged and conjugated 6-β-naltrexol accounts for approximately 43% of an oral dose. The pharmacokinetic profile of REVIA suggests that REVIA and its metabolites undergo enterohepatic recycling.

Adequate studies of naltrexone in patients with severe hepatic or renal impairment have not been conducted; however, a recent preliminary communication stated that naltrexone bioavailability is increased in patients with liver cirrhosis as compared to healthy subjects. (See Precautions, Special Risk Patients.)

Clinical Trials: Treatment of Opioid Addiction: REVIA has been shown to produce complete blockade of the euphoric effects of opioids in both volunteer and addict populations. When administered by means that enforce compliance, it will produce an effective opioid blockade, but has not been shown to affect the use of cocaine or other nonopioid drugs of abuse.

The drug is reported to be of greatest use in good prognosis opioid addicts who take the drug as part of a comprehensive occupational rehabilitative program, behavioural contract, or other compliance enhancing protocols.

Alcoholism: The efficacy of REVIA as an aid to the treatment of alcoholism was tested in placebo-controlled, outpatient, double-blind trials. These studies used a dose of REVIA 50 mg once daily for 12 weeks as an adjunct to social and psychotherapeutic methods. Patients with psychosis, dementia, and secondary psychiatric diagnosis were excluded from these studies.

In one of these studies, 104 alcohol-dependent patients were randomized to receive either REVIA 50 mg once daily or placebo. In this study, REVIA proved superior to placebo in measures of drinking including abstention rates (51% vs. 23%), number of drinking days, and relapse rates (31% vs. 60%). In a second study with 82 alcohol-dependent patients, the group of patients receiving REVIA were shown to have lower relapse rates (21% vs. 41%), less alcohol craving, and fewer drinking days compared with patients who received placebo.

The clinical use of REVIA as adjunctive pharmacotherapy for the treatment of alcoholism was also evaluated in a multicenter safety study. This study of 865 individuals with alcoholism included patients with comorbid psychiatric conditions, concomitant medications, polysubstance abuse and HIV disease. Results of this study demonstrated that the side-effect profile of REVIA appears to be similar in both alcoholic and opioid dependent populations.

REVIA was not uniformly helpful to all patients, and the expected effect of the drug is a modest improvement in the outcome of conventional treatment.

INDICATIONS: REVIA (naltrexone hydrochloride) is indicated to provide blockade of the pharmacologic effects of exogenously administered opioids as an adjunct to the maintenance of the opioid-free state in detoxified, formerly opioid-dependent individuals. There are no data that demonstrate an unequivocally beneficial effect of REVIA on the rates of recidivism among detoxified formerly opioid-dependent individuals, who self administer the drug. REVIA is expected to have a therapeutic effect only when given under conditions that support continued use of the medication.

REVIA is indicated in the treatment of alcohol dependence, as a component of a comprehensive psychotherapeutic or psychological alcoholism counselling program to support abstinence, and reduce the risk of relapse. The efficacy of REVIA beyond twelve weeks of treatment has not been established.

CONTRAINDICATIONS: REVIA (naltrexone hydrochloride) is contraindicated in: patients receiving opioid analgesics; patients currently dependent on opioids, including those currently maintained on opiate agonists [eg. Methadone or LAAM (levo-alpha-acetyl-methadol)]; patients in acute opioid withdrawal (see Warnings); any individual who has failed the NARCAN challenge (see Dosage); any individual who has a positive urine screen for opioids; any individual with a history of sensitivity to REVIA or any other components of this product. It is not known if there is any cross-sensitivity with naloxone or other phenanthrene containing opioids; any individual with acute hepatitis or liver failure.

WARNINGS: Unintended Precipitation of Withdrawal: **To prevent occurrence of an acute withdrawal syndrome, or exacerbation of a pre-existing sub-clinical withdrawal syndrome, patients should remain opioid-free for a minimum of 7-10 days before starting REVIA. Since the absence of an opioid drug in the urine often is not sufficient proof that the patient is opioid-free, a NARCAN challenge may be required to minimize the possibility of precipitating a withdrawal reaction following administration of REVIA. The NARCAN challenge test is described in Dosage.**

Hepatotoxicity: **REVIA (naltrexone hydrochloride) has the capacity to cause dose related hepatocellular injury. Prior to making a decision to initiate treatment with REVIA, the physician should establish whether the patient has subclinical liver injury or disease (see Precautions, Laboratory Tests). REVIA is contraindicated in acute hepatitis or liver failure, and its use even in patients with evidence of less severe liver disease or a history of recent liver disease must be carefully considered in light of its hepatotoxic potential.**

The evidence that identified REVIA as a hepatotoxin was not obtained in studies involving its use at the doses recommended for opiate blockade, or for treatment of alcohol dependence (50 mg/day). However, the margin of separation between the apparently safe and the hepatotoxic doses appears to be only five-fold or less.

Patients should be warned of the risk of hepatic injury and advised to stop the use of REVIA and seek medical attention if they experience symptoms of acute hepatitis.

Evidence of the hepatotoxic potential of REVIA is derived primarily from a placebo controlled study in which REVIA was administered to obese subjects at a dose approximately five-fold that recommended for the blockade of opiate receptors (300 mg/day). In the study, 5 of 26 REVIA recipients developed elevations of serum transaminases (ie, peak ALT values ranging from a low of 121 to a high of 532, or 3 to 19 times their baseline values) after three to eight weeks of treatment. Although the patients involved were generally clinically asymptomatic and the transaminase levels of all patients on whom follow-up was obtained returned to (or toward) baseline values in a matter of weeks, the lack of any transaminase elevations of similar magnitude in any of the 24 placebo patients in the same study is persuasive evidence that REVIA is a direct (ie, not an idiosyncratic) hepatotoxin. This conclusion is also supported by evidence from other placebo controlled studies in which exposure to REVIA at doses from one to two-fold the amount recommended for the treatment of alcoholism or opiate blockade (50 mg/day) consistently produced more numerous and more significant elevations of serum transaminase than did placebo, and reports of transaminase elevations in 3 of 9 patients with Alzheimer's Disease who received REVIA (up to 300 mg/day) for 5 to 8 weeks in an open clinical trial have been reported.

Although no cases of hepatic failure due to REVIA administration have ever been reported, physicians are advised to consider this as a possible risk of treatment and to use the same care in prescribing REVIA as they would other drugs with the potential for causing hepatic injury.

Attempt to Overcome Blockade: While REVIA is a potent antagonist with a prolonged pharmacologic effect (24 to 72 hours), the blockade produced by REVIA is surmountable. This is useful in patients who may require analgesia, but poses a potential risk to individuals who attempt, on their own, to overcome the blockade by administering large amounts of exogenous opioids. Indeed, any attempt by a patient to overcome the antagonism by taking opioids is very dangerous and may lead to a fatal overdose. Injury may arise because the plasma concentration of exogenous opioids attained immediately following their acute administration may be sufficient to overcome the competitive receptor blockade. As a consequence, the patient may be in immediate danger of suffering life endangering opioid intoxication (eg, respiratory arrest, circulatory collapse). **Patients should be told of the serious consequences of surmounting the opiate blockade. (See Information for the Patient.)**

There is also the possibility that a patient who had been treated with naltrexone will respond to lower doses of opioids than previously used, particularly if taken in such a manner that high plasma concentrations remain in the body beyond the time that naltrexone exerts its therapeutic effects. This could result in potentially life-threatening opioid intoxification (respiratory compromise or arrest, circulatory collapse, etc.). **Patients should be aware that they may be more sensitive to lower doses of opioids after naltrexone treatment is discontinued.**

PRECAUTIONS: General: Emergency Pain Management in Patients Receiving Fully Blocking Doses of REVIA: In an emergency situation in patients receiving fully blocking doses of REVIA, a suggested plan of management is regional analgesia, conscious sedation with a benzodiazepine, use of non-opioid analgesics or general anesthesia. In a situation requiring analgesia which can only be achieved with opioids, the amount of opioid required may be greater than usual, and the resulting respiratory depression may be deeper and more prolonged. In such circumstances, a rapidly acting opioid analgesic which minimizes the duration of respiratory depression is preferred. The amount of analgesic administered should be titrated to the needs of the patient. No methods to reverse opioid overdose in patient's receiving naltrexone have been established by clinical trials. However, the use of the opioid antagonist naloxone, should be considered when attempting reversal.

Additionally, non-receptor mediated actions may occur (e.g., facial swelling, itching, generalized erythema, presumably due to histamine release). Irrespective of the drug chosen to reverse REVIA blockade, the patient should be monitored closely by appropriately trained personnel in a hospital setting equipped and staffed for cardiopulmonary resuscitation.

Interference with the Action of Opioid Containing Drug Product: Patients taking REVIA may not benefit from opioid containing medicines, such as cough and cold preparations, antidiarrheal preparations, and opioid analgesics. Where a non-opioid containing alternative is available, it should be used.

Accidentally Precipitated Withdrawal: Severe opioid withdrawal syndromes precipitated by the accidental ingestion of REVIA have been reported in opioid-dependent individuals. Symptoms of withdrawal have usually appeared within five minutes of ingestion of REVIA and have lasted for up to 48 hours. Mental status changes including confusion, somnolence and visual hallucinations have occurred. Significant fluid losses from vomiting and diarrhea have required intravenous fluid administration. In all cases patients were closely monitored and therapy tailored to meet individual requirements.

Use of REVIA does not eliminate or diminish withdrawal symptoms. If REVIA is initiated early in the abstinence process, it will not preclude the patients's experience of the full range of signs and symptoms that would be experienced if REVIA had not been started. Numerous adverse events are known to be associated with withdrawal.

Special Risk Patients: Renal Impairment: REVIA and its primary metabolite are excreted primarily in the urine, and caution is recommended in administering the drug to patients with renal impairment.

Hepatic Impairment: Caution should be exercised when naltrexone hydrochloride is administered to patients with liver disease. An increase in naltrexone AUC of approximately 5- and 10-fold in patients with compensated and decompensated liver cirrhosis, respectively, compared with subjects with normal liver function has been reported. These data also suggest that alterations in naltrexone bioavailability are related to liver disease severity.

Drug Interactions: Studies to evaluate possible interactions between REVIA and drugs other than opiates have not been performed. Consequently, caution is advised if the concomitant administration of REVIA and other drugs is required.

The safety and efficacy of concomitant use of REVIA and disulfiram is unknown, and the concomitant use of two potentially hepatotoxic medications is not ordinarily recommended unless the probable benefits outweigh the known risks.

Lethargy and somnolence have been reported following doses of REVIA (naltrexone hydrochloride) and thioridazine.

Suicide: The risk of suicide is known to be increased in patients with substance abuse with or without concomitant depression. The risk is not abated by treatment with REVIA (see Adverse Effects).

Laboratory Tests: Tests designed to detect hepatic injury should be obtained prior to initiation of REVIA therapy and periodically thereafter (see Warnings, Hepatotoxicity).

Periodic testing of all patients after initiation of treatment is critical if the occurrence of REVIA induced liver damage is to be detected at the earliest possible time. Evaluations, using appropriate batteries of tests to detect liver injury are recommended on a monthly basis during the first six months of use; thereafter, clinical judgement about the frequency of monitoring must be relied upon.

Laboratory tests which may be used for the separation and detection of morphine, methadone, or quinine in the urine and with which REVIA does not interfere include thin-layer, gas-liquid, and high pressure liquid chromatographic methods.

Impairment of Fertility: REVIA (100 mg/kg, approximately 100 times the human therapeutic dose) caused a significant increase in pseudopregnancy in the rat. A decrease in the pregnancy rate of mated female rats also occurred. The relevance of these observations to human fertility is not known.

Pregnancy: There are no adequate and well-controlled studies in pregnant women. REVIA should be used in pregnancy only when the potential benefits justify the potential risk to the fetus. Naltrexone hydrochloride has been shown to have embryocidal and fetotoxic effects in rats and rabbits when given in dosages 30 and 60 times, respectively, the human dose.

Labour and Delivery: It is not known whether REVIA affects the duration of labour and delivery.

Lactation: It is not known whether REVIA is excreted in human milk. Because many drugs are excreted in human milk, REVIA should be administered to a nursing mother only when the potential benefits justify the potential risk to the infant.

Children: The safe use of REVIA in subjects younger than 18 years of age has not been established.

ADVERSE EFFECTS: While extensive clinical studies evaluating the use of REVIA (naltrexone hydrochloride) in detoxified, formerly opioid dependent individuals failed to identify any single, serious untoward risk of REVIA use, placebo controlled studies employing up to five-fold higher doses of REVIA (up to 300 mg/day) than that recommended for use in opiate receptor blockade have shown that REVIA caused hepatocellular injury in 5 of 26 patients exposed at this higher dose (see Warnings and Precautions, Laboratory Tests).

Aside from this finding, however, available evidence does not incriminate REVIA, used at any dose, as a cause of any other serious untoward event for the patient who is "opioid free". It is critical to recognize that REVIA can precipitate or exacerbate withdrawal signs and symptoms in any individual who is not completely free of exogenous opioids (see Contraindications, Warnings and Dosage).

Opioid Withdrawal-like Symptoms: Studies in alcoholic populations and in volunteers in clinical pharmacology studies have suggested that a small fraction of patients may experience an opioid withdrawal-like symptom complex consisting of tearfulness, mild nausea, abdominal cramps, restlessness, bone or joint pain, myalgia, and nasal symptoms. This may represent the unmasking of occult opioid use, or it may represent symptoms attributable to naltrexone. A number of alternative dosing patterns have been recommended to try to reduce the frequency of these complaints (see Individualization of Dosage).

Opioid Addiction: Events Other than Hepatocellular Injury Reported During Clinical Testing: The following adverse reactions have been reported both at baseline and during the REVIA clinical trials in opioid addiction at an incidence rate of more than 10%: Difficulty sleeping, anxiety, nervousness, abdominal pain/cramps, nausea and/or vomiting, low energy, joint and muscle pain, and headache.

The incidence was less than 10% for: Loss of appetite, constipation, increased thirst, increased energy, feeling down, irritability, dizziness, skin rash, delayed ejaculation, decreased potency, and chills.

The following events occurred in less than 1% of subjects:

Respiratory: nasal congestion, itching, rhinorrhea, sneezing, sore throat, excess mucus or phlegm, sinus trouble, heavy breathing, hoarseness, cough, shortness of breath.

Cardiovascular: nose bleeds, phlebitis, edema, increased blood pressure, non-specific ECG changes, palpitations, tachycardia.

Gastrointestinal: excessive gas, haemorrhoids, diarrhea, ulcer.

Musculoskeletal: painful shoulders, legs or knees, tremors, twitching.

Genitourinary: increased frequency of, or discomfort during urination, increased or decreased sexual interest.

Dermatologic: oily skin, pruritus, acne, athlete's foot, cold sore, alopecia.

Psychiatric: depression, paranoia, fatigue, restlessness, confusion, disorientation, hallucinations, nightmares, bad dreams.

Special Senses: eyes—blurred, burning, light sensitive, swollen, aching, strained; ears—"clogged", aching, tinnitus.

General: increased appetite, weight loss, weight gain, yawning, somnolence, fever, dry mouth, head "pounding", inguinal pain, swollen glands, "side" pains, cold feet, "hot spells".

Post-marketing Experience: Data collected from post-marketing use of REVIA show that most events usually occur early in the course of drug therapy and are transient. It is not always possible to distinguish these occurrences from those signs and symptoms that may result from a withdrawal syndrome. Events that have been reported include anorexia, asthenia, chest pain, fatigue, headache, hot flushes, malaise, changes in blood pressure, agitation, dizziness, hyperkinesia, nausea, vomiting, tremor, abdominal pain, diarrhea, elevations in liver enzymes or bilirubin, hepatic function abnormalities or hepatitis, palpitations, myalgia, anxiety, confusion, euphoria, hallucinations, insomnia, nervousness, somnolence, abnormal thinking, dyspnea, rash, increased sweating, and vision abnormalities.

Depression, suicide, attempted suicide and suicidal ideation have been reported in the post-marketing experience with REVIA used in the treatment of opioid dependence. No causal relationship has been demonstrated. In the literature, endogenous opioids have been theorized to contribute to a variety of conditions. In some individuals the use of opioid antagonists has been associated with a change in baseline levels of some hypothalamic, pituitary, or gonadal hormones. The clinical significance of such changes is not fully understood.

Laboratory Tests: With the exception of liver test abnormalities in investigator studies (see Warnings and Precautions), results of laboratory tests, like adverse reports, have not shown consistent patterns of abnormalities that can be attributed to treatment with REVIA.

In the trials evaluating REVIA for the blockade of opiate receptors, abnormal liver function tests and lymphocytosis were the two most common categories of abnormalities reported. These abnormalities are common among populations of parenteral opioid users and alcoholics. As is the case with the untoward events described above, a large proportion of patients had abnormal tests at baseline, further supporting the conclusion that the abnormalities observed are not attributable to REVIA.

Idiopathic thrombocytopenic purpura was reported in one patient who may have been sensitized to REVIA in a previous course of treatment with REVIA. The condition cleared without sequelae after discontinuation of REVIA and corticosteroid treatment.

Alcoholism: In two randomized, double-blind placebo controlled 12 week trials to evaluate the efficacy of REVIA as adjunctive treatment of alcohol dependence, a total of 93 patients received REVIA at a dose of 50 mg once daily. The most common (incidence greater than 10%) adverse events associated with the use of REVIA in these trials (incidence at least 5% greater than in patients receiving placebo) were: somnolence, nervousness, vomiting, weight decrease, dry mouth and decreased libido. The incidences of adverse events leading to discontinuation of REVIA in these trials were: vomiting (5%); agitation (2%); insomnia (2%); nervousness (1%); drowsiness (1%); and malaise (1%). Discontinuation rate for headache was 1% for patients on naltrexone and 2% for patients on placebo. No serious adverse events were reported during these two trials.

In an Open Label Safety Study with Approximately 570 Individuals with Alcoholism Receiving Naltrexone, the Following New Onset Adverse Reactions Occurred in 2% or More of the Patients		In an Open Label Safety Study with Approximately 570 Individuals with Alcoholism Receiving Naltrexone, the Following Adverse Events Were Responsible for Discontinuation in ≥1% of Patients	
Adverse Reaction	**Percent (%)**	**Adverse Reaction**	**Incidence of Discontinuation**
Nausea	10%	Nausea	6%
Headache	7%	Headache	3%
Dizziness	4%	Dizziness	3%
Nervousness	4%	Anxiety	2%
Fatigue	4%	Nervousness	2%
Insomnia	3%	Fatigue	1%
Vomiting	3%	Vomiting	1%
Anxiety	2%	Depression	1%
Somnolence	2%	Euphoria	1%
Dry Mouth	2%	Mouth Dry	1%
Dyspepsia	2%	Insomnia	1%

Depression, suicidal ideation, and suicidal attempts have been reported in all groups when comparing naltrexone, placebo, or controls undergoing treatment for alcoholism.

Rate Ranges of New Onset Events		
New Onset Event	**Naltrexone**	**Placebo**
Depression	0–15%	0–17%
Suicide Attempt/Ideation	0–1%	0–3%

Although no causal relationship with REVIA is suspected, physicians should be aware that treatment with REVIA does not reduce the risk of suicide in these patients (see Precautions).

Drug Abuse and Dependence: REVIA (naltrexone hydrochloride) is a pure opioid antagonist. It does not lead to physical or psychological dependence. Tolerance to the opioid antagonist effect is not known to occur.

OVERDOSE:

Symptoms: There is limited clinical experience with REVIA (naltrexone hydrochloride) overdosage in humans. In one study, subjects who received 800 mg daily REVIA for up to one week showed no evidence of toxicity.

Treatment: Consideration should be given to contacting a poison control center for the most up-to-date information. In view of the lack of actual experience in the treatment of REVIA overdose, patients should be treated symptomatically in a closely supervised environment.

For management of a suspected drug overdose, CPhA recommends that you contact your **regional Poison Control Centre**. See the *CPS* Directory section for a list of Poison Control Centres.

DOSAGE: Initiation of REVIA (naltrexone HCl) Therapy: **Do not attempt treatment with revia unless, in the medical judgement of the prescribing physician, there is no reasonable possibility of opioid use within the past 7-10 days. If there is any question of occult opioid dependence, perform a NARCAN challenge test and do not attempt to initiate revia therapy until NARCAN challenge is negative (see NARCAN Challenge Test).**

Treatment of Opioid Dependence: Initiate treatment with REVIA using the following guidelines:

Treatment should not be attempted until the patient has remained opioid-free for 7-10 days. Self-reporting of abstinence from opioids should be verified by analysis of the patient's urine for absence of opioids. The patient should not be manifesting withdrawal signs or reporting withdrawal symptoms.

If there is any question of occult opioid dependence perform a NARCAN challenge test (see below). If signs of opioid withdrawal are still observed following NARCAN challenge, treatment with REVIA should not be attempted. The NARCAN challenge can be repeated in 24 hours.

Treatment should be initiated carefully, slowly increasing the dose of REVIA administered. This can be accomplished by administration of 25 mg of REVIA initially. The patient should be observed for 1 hour. If no withdrawal signs occur, the patient may be given the rest of the daily dose.

Once the patient has been started on REVIA, 50 mg every 24 hours will produce adequate clinical blockade of the actions of parenterally administered opioids (i.e., this dose will block the effects of a 25 mg intravenous heroin challenge). A flexible approach to a dosing regimen may be employed in cases of supervised administration. Thus, patients may receive 50 mg of REVIA every weekday with a 100 mg dose on Saturday or patients may receive 100 mg every other day, or 150 mg every third day. While the degree of opioid blockade may be somewhat reduced by using higher doses at longer dosing intervals, improved patient compliance may result from dosing every 48-72 hours.

Several of the clinical studies reported in the literature have employed the following dosing regimen: 100 mg on Monday, 100 mg on Wednesday, and 150 mg on Friday. This dosing schedule appeared to be acceptable to many naltrexone patients successfully maintaining their opioid free state.

Treatment of Alcoholism: A dose of 50 mg once daily is recommended.

The placebo-controlled studies that demonstrated the efficacy of REVIA as an adjunctive treatment of alcoholism used a dose regimen of REVIA 50 mg once daily for up to 12 weeks. Other dose regimens or durations of therapy were not evaluated in these trials.

A patient is a candidate for treatment with REVIA if: the patient is willing to take a medicine to help with alcohol dependence; the patient is opioid free for 7-10 days; the patient does not have severe or active liver or kidney problems (typical guidelines suggest liver function tests no greater than three times the upper limits of normal, and bilirubin normal); and the patient is not allergic to REVIA, and no other contraindications are present.

Refer to Contraindications, Warnings, and Precautions for additional information.

REVIA should be used as part of a comprehensive treatment program for alcohol dependence. Factors associated with a good outcome include: appropriate management of comorbid conditions; use of community-based support groups; and good medication compliance. To achieve the best possible treatment outcome, appropriate compliance enhancing techniques should be implemented for all components of the treatment program, especially medication compliance.

The efficacy of REVIA beyond twelve weeks of treatment has not been established.

NARCAN Challenge Test: The NARCAN challenge test should not be performed in a patient showing clinical signs or symptoms of opioid withdrawal, or in a patient whose urine contains opioids. The NARCAN challenge test may be administered by either the intravenous or subcutaneous routes.

Intravenous: Inject 0.5 mL (0.2 mg) NARCAN (0.4 mg/mL). Observe patient for 30 seconds for signs or symptoms of withdrawal. If there is no evidence of withdrawal, inject another 1.5 mL (0.6 mg) of NARCAN. Observe patient for an additional 20 minutes.

Subcutaneous: Administer 2 mL (0.8 mg) NARCAN (0.4 mg/mL). Observe patient for 20 minutes for signs or symptoms of withdrawal.

Note: Individual patients, especially those with opioid dependence, may respond to lower doses of NARCAN. In some cases, 0.25 mL (0.1 mg) intravenous NARCAN (0.4 mg/mL) has produced a diagnostic response.

Interpretation of the Challenge: Monitor vital signs and observe the patient for signs and symptoms of opioid withdrawal. These may include, but are not limited to: nausea, vomiting, dysphoria, yawning, sweating, tearing, rhinorrhea, stuffy nose, craving for opioids, poor appetite, abdominal cramps, sense of fear, skin erythema, disrupted sleep patterns, fidgeting, uneasiness, poor ability to focus, mental lapses, muscle aches or cramps, pupillary dilation, piloerection, fever, changes in blood pressure, pulse or temperature, anxiety, depression, irritability, back ache, bone or joint pains, tremors, sensations of skin crawling or fasciculations. If signs or symptoms of withdrawal appear, the test is positive and no additional NARCAN should be administered.

Warning: If the test is positive, do not initiate REVIA therapy. Repeat the challenge in 24 hours (see Confirmatory Rechallenge (if necessary)). If the test is negative, REVIA therapy may be started if no other contraindications are present. If there is any doubt about the result of the test, withhold REVIA and repeat the challenge in 24 hours (see Confirmatory Rechallenge (if necessary)).

Confirmatory Rechallenge (if necessary): Four (4) mL (1.6 mg) of NARCAN (0.4 mg/mL) should be injected intravenously and the patient again observed for signs and symptoms of withdrawal. If none are present, REVIA may be administered. **If signs and symptoms of withdrawal are present, administration of REVIA should be delayed until repeated NARCAN challenge indicates the patient is no longer at risk.**

INFORMATION FOR THE PATIENT: Published in e-CPS, available by subscription at www.e-cps.ca.

SUPPLIED: Each pale yellow, film-coated, capsule-shaped tablet, engraved with "REVIA" on one side and with "177" and a bisect on the other side, contains: naltrexone HCl 50 mg. Nonmedicinal ingredients: colloidal silicon dioxide, crospovidone, lactose monohydrate, magnesium stearate, microcrystalline cellulose and Pale Yellow Opadry YS-1-6378-G. Bottles of 50. Store at controlled room temperature (15 to 30°C). Dispense in a tight container as defined in the USP.

Reyataz™ Ⓟ

atazanavir sulfate

Azapeptide Inhibitor of HIV-1 Protease

Bristol-Myers Squibb

Date of Preparation: December 3, 2003
Date of Revision: November 6, 2009

SUMMARY PRODUCT INFORMATION:

Route of Administration	Dosage Form/ Strength	Clinically Relevant Nonmedicinal Ingredients
Oral	Capsules, 150, 200 and 300 mg	Lactose monohydrate For a complete listing, see Dosage Forms, Composition and Packaging.

INDICATIONS AND CLINICAL USE: REYATAZ (atazanavir sulfate) is indicated in combination with other antiretroviral agents for the treatment of HIV-1 infection.

This indication is based on analyses of plasma HIV-1 RNA levels and CD4 cell counts from controlled studies of 96 weeks duration in antiretroviral-naive patients and 48 weeks duration in antiretroviral-treatment-experienced patients.

In antiretroviral-treatment experienced patients with prior virologic failure, coadministration of REYATAZ/ritonavir is recommended.

The number of baseline primary protease inhibitor mutations affects the virologic response to REYATAZ/ritonavir.

(See Warnings and Precautions and Dosage and Administration.)

Geriatrics (>65 years of age): Clinical studies of REYATAZ did not include sufficient numbers of patients aged 65 and over to determine whether they respond differently from younger patients. In general, dose selection for an elderly patient should reflect the greater frequency of decreased hepatic, renal, or cardiac function, and of concomitant disease or other drug therapy.

Pediatrics (from 6 to 18 years of age): Dosage is based on body weight not to exceed the adult dose (see Dosage and Administration). There are no dosing recommendations for pediatric patients less than 6 years of age.

CONTRAINDICATIONS: Patients with previously demonstrated clinically significant hypersensitivity (eg. Stevens-Johnson syndrome, erythema multiforme, or toxic skin eruptions) to any component of the product or container, including atazanavir. For a complete listing (see Dosage Forms, Composition and Packaging).

Coadministration of REYATAZ is contraindicated with drugs that are highly dependent on CYP3A4 and/or UGT1A for clearance and for which elevated plasma concentrations are associated with serious and/or life-threatening events. These drugs are listed in Table 1.

Table 1: REYATAZ

Drugs That Are Contraindicated with REYATAZ[a]

Drug Class	Drugs Within Class That Are Contraindicated with REYATAZ
Benzodiazepines	orally administered midazolam[b], triazolam
Ergot Derivatives	dihydroergotamine, ergotamine, ergonovine, methylergonovine
GI Motility Agent	cisapride[c]
HMG-CoA Reductase Inhibitors	lovastatin, simvastatin
Neuroleptic	pimozide
Antiarrhythmics	quinidine
Calcium Channel Blockers	bepridil[c]
Antimycobacterials	rifampin
Antineoplastics	irinotecan
Herbal Products	St. John's wort (Hypericum perforatum)
Protease Inhibitors	indinavir

[a] See Table 13 for more detailed information.
[b] Oral formulation of midazolam is not marketed in Canada. See Table 14 for parenterally administered midazolam.
[c] Not marketed in Canada.

WARNINGS AND PRECAUTIONS: General: Alert: Find out about medicines that should NOT be taken with REYATAZ. (See Contraindications and Drug Interactions.)

Atazanavir should always be used in combination with other antiretroviral agents. Atazanavir should not be added as a single agent when antiretrovirals are changed due to loss of virologic response.

Antiretroviral Treatment-Experienced Patients: Atazanavir 400 mg once daily has been shown to be inferior to lopinavir/ritonavir in antiretroviral experienced patients. There are limited safety data from controlled trials for REYATAZ plus ritonavir regimens without tenofovir. (See Drug Interactions and Dosage and Administration.)

Carcinogenesis and Mutagenesis: The incidence of benign hepatocellular adenomas was increased in high-dose female mice at systemic exposures approximately 7-fold higher than those in humans at the recommended 400 mg clinical dose. There was no increase in the incidence of tumors in male mice or in male or female rats at any dose tested. The clinical significance of the carcinogenic findings in female mice is unknown as the benign hepatic tumors occurred only at doses that induced liver toxicity.

Cardiovascular: Cardiac Conduction Abnormalities: Atazanavir has been shown to prolong the PR interval of the electrocardiogram in some patients. In healthy volunteers and in patients, abnormalities in atrioventricular (AV) conduction were asymptomatic and limited to first degree AV block with some exceptions (see Overdosage). There have been post-marketing reports of second-degree AV block, third-degree AV block, QTc prolongation, Torsades de Pointes and other conduction abnormalities in patients treated with REYATAZ (see Adverse Reactions, Post-Market Adverse Drug Reactions). In clinical trials, asymptomatic first degree AV block was observed in 5.9% of atazanavir-treated patients (n=920), 3.0% of efavirenz treated patients (n=329), 5.2% of lopinavir/ritonavir treated patients (n=252) and 10.4% of nelfinavir treated patients (n=48). In study AI424-045 asymptomatic first degree AV block was observed in 5% (6/118) of REYATAZ/ritonavir-treated patients and 5% (6/116) of lopinavir/ritonavir-treated patients who had on-study electrocardiogram measurements. Because of limited clinical experience, atazanavir should be used with caution in patients with preexisting conduction system disease (e.g., marked first-degree AV block or second or third-degree AV block).

Dose related asymptomatic prolongations in PR interval with REYATAZ have been observed in clinical studies. Caution should be used with medicinal products known to induce PR prolongations. In patients with pre-existing conduction problems (second degree or higher atrioventricular or complex bundle-branch block), REYATAZ should be used with caution and only if the benefits exceed the risk. Particular caution should be used when prescribing REYATAZ in association with medicinal products which have the potential to increase the QT interval and/or in patients with pre-existing risk factors (bradycardia, long congenital QT, electrolyte imbalances). (See Action and Clinical Pharmacology.)

In a pharmacokinetic study between atazanavir 400 mg once daily and diltiazem 180 mg once daily, a CYP3A substrate, there was a 2-fold increase in the diltiazem plasma concentration and an additive effect on the PR interval. When used in combination with atazanavir, a dose reduction of diltiazem by one half should be considered and ECG monitoring is recommended. In a pharmacokinetic study between atazanavir 400 mg once daily and atenolol 50 mg once daily, there was no substantial additive effect of atazanavir and atenolol on the PR interval. When used in combination with atazanavir, there is no need to adjust the dose of atenolol. (See Drug Interactions.)

Pharmacokinetic studies between atazanavir and other drugs that prolong the PR interval including beta blockers (other than atenolol), verapamil and digoxin have not been performed. An additive effect of atazanavir and these drugs cannot be excluded; therefore, caution should be exercised when atazanavir is given concurrently with these drugs, especially those that are metabolized by CYP3A4 (e.g., verapamil). (See Drug Interactions.)

Endocrine and Metabolism: Diabetes Mellitus/Hyperglycemia: New onset diabetes mellitus, exacerbation of pre-existing diabetes mellitus, and hyperglycemia have been reported during postmarketing surveillance in HIV-infected patients receiving protease inhibitor therapy. Some patients required either initiation or dose adjustments of insulin or oral hypoglycemic agents for treatment of these events. In some cases, diabetic ketoacidosis has occurred. In those patients who discontinued protease inhibitor therapy, hyperglycemia persisted in some cases. Because these events have been reported voluntarily during clinical practice, estimates of frequency cannot be made and a causal relationship between protease inhibitor therapy and these events has not been established.

Fat Redistribution: Redistribution/accumulation of body fat including central obesity, dorsocervical fat enlargement (buffalo hump), peripheral wasting, facial wasting, breast enlargement, and "cushingoid appearance" have been observed in patients receiving antiretroviral therapy. The mechanism and long-term consequences of these events are currently unknown. A causal relationship has not been established.

Hematologic: Hemophilia: There have been reports of increased bleeding, including spontaneous skin hematomas and hemarthrosis, in patients with hemophilia type A and B treated with protease inhibitors. In some patients additional factor VIII was given. In more than half of the reported cases, treatment with protease inhibitors was continued or reintroduced. A causal relationship between protease inhibitor therapy and these events has not been established.

Hepatic/Biliary/Pancreatic: Hepatic Impairment and Toxicity: REYATAZ is principally metabolized by the liver; caution should be exercised when administering this drug to patients with hepatic impairment because atazanavir concentrations may be increased (see Dosage and Administration). Patients with underlying hepatitis B or C viral infections or marked elevations in transaminases prior to treatment may be at increased risk for developing further transaminase elevations or hepatic decompensation. In these patients, test for liver enzymes before initiating therapy with REYATAZ and monitor liver enzymes during treatment. REYATAZ should not be administered to patients with severe hepatic impairment. REYATAZ/ritonavir is not recommended for use in patients with hepatic impairment.

Immune Reconstitution: Immune reconstitution syndrome has been reported in patients treated with combination antiretroviral therapy, including REYATAZ. During the initial phase of treatment, a patient whose immune system responds to therapy may develop an inflammatory response to indolent or residual opportunistic infections (such as MAC, CMV, PCP and TB), which may necessitate further evaluation and treatment.

Hyperbilirubinemia: Most patients taking atazanavir experience elevations in indirect (unconjugated) bilirubin related to inhibition of UDP-glucuronosyl transferase (UGT). This hyperbilirubinemia is generally reversible upon discontinuation of REYATAZ. If hepatic transaminase elevations occur with hyperbilirubinemia while a patient is receiving atazanavir, consideration should be given to also evaluating alternative etiologies. No long-term safety data are available for patients experiencing persistent elevations in total bilirubin >5×ULN. Alternative antiretroviral therapy to REYATAZ may be considered if jaundice or scleral icterus associated with bilirubin elevations present cosmetic concerns for patients. Dose reduction of atazanavir is not recommended since long-term efficacy of reduced doses has not been established (see Adverse Reactions).

There have been post-marketing reports of cholelithiasis, cholecystitis, and cholestasis in patients treated with atazanavir with ritonavir as part of their ART regimen (see Adverse Reactions, Post-Market Adverse Drug Reactions).

Renal: In healthy subjects, approximately 7% of the dose of atazanavir is eliminated unchanged in the urine. REYATAZ has been studied in adult subjects with severe renal impairment (n=20), including those on hemodialysis, at multiple doses of 400 mg once daily. The impact of renal impairment on atazanavir elimination for patients without hemodialysis is anticipated to be low. Moderate increases in atazanvir clearance and decreased exposure levels were seen in patients managed with hemodialysis. REYATAZ should not be administered to HIV-treatment-experienced patients with end stage renal disease managed with hemodialysis. (See Dosage and Administration and Action and Clinical Pharmacology.)

Cases of nephrolithiasis were reported during post-marketing surveillance in HIV-infected patients receiving atazanavir therapy. Because these events were reported voluntarily during clinical practice, estimates of frequency cannot be made. If signs or symptoms of nephrolithiasis occur, temporary interruption or discontinuation of therapy may be considered.

Resistance/Cross-Resistance: Resistance: In vitro HIV-1 isolates with a decreased susceptibility to ATV have been selected in vitro and obtained from patients treated with ATV or atazanavir/ritonavir (ATV/RTV). HIV-1 isolates that were 93- to 183-fold resistant to ATV from three different viral strains were selected in vitro by 5 months. The mutations in these HIV-1 viruses that contributed to ATV resistance included I50L, N88S, I84V, A71V, and M46I. Changes were also observed at the protease cleavage sites following drug selection. Recombinant viruses containing the I50L mutation were growth impaired and displayed increased in vitro susceptibility to other PIs (amprenavir, indinavir, lopinavir, nelfinavir, ritonavir, and saquinavir). The I50L and I50V substitutions yielded selective resistance to ATV and amprenavir, respectively, and did not appear to be cross-resistant.

Both genotypic and phenotypic resistances have developed during clinical studies.

Cross-Resistance: Cross-resistance among PIs has been observed. Baseline phenotypic and genotypic analyses of clinical isolates from ATV clinical trials of PI-experienced subjects showed that isolates cross-resistant to multiple PIs were cross-resistant to ATV. Greater than 90% of the isolates with mutations that included I84V or G48V were resistant to ATV. Greater than 60% of isolates containing L90M, G73S/T/C, A71V/T, I54V, M46I/L, or a change at V82 were resistant to ATV, and 38% of isolates containing a D30N mutation in addition to other changes were resistant to ATV. Isolates resistant to ATV were also cross-resistant to other PIs with >90% of the isolates resistant to indinavir, lopinavir, nelfinavir, ritonavir, and saquinavir, and 80% resistant to amprenavir. In treatment-experienced patients, PI-resistant viral isolates that developed the I50L mutation in addition to other PI resistance-associated mutations were also cross-resistant to other PIs.

Genotypic and/or phenotypic analysis of baseline virus may aid in determining ATV susceptibility before initiation of ATV/RTV therapy.

Overall, both the number and type of baseline PI mutations affected response rates in treatment-experienced patients.

Sexual Function/Reproduction: In a fertility and early embryonic development study in rats, atazanavir altered estrus cycling with no effects on mating, fertility or early embryonic development. Systemic drug exposure levels were equal (in male rats) or two times (in female rats) those at the human clinical dose (400 mg/day).

Skin: Rash: In controlled clinical trials, rash (all grades, regardless of causality) occurred in approximately 20% of patients treated with REYATAZ. The median time to onset of rash in clinical studies was 7.3 weeks and the median duration of rash was 1.4 weeks. Rashes were generally mild-to-moderate maculopapular skin eruptions. Treatment-emergent adverse reactions of moderate or severe rash (occurring at a rate of ≥2%) are presented for the individual clinical studies (see Adverse Reactions). Dosing with REYATAZ was often continued without interruption in patients who developed rash. The discontinuation rate for rash in clinical trials was <1%. REYATAZ should be discontinued if severe rash develops. Cases of Stevens-Johnson syndrome, erythema multiforme and toxic skin eruptions have been reported in patients receiving REYATAZ. (See Contraindications.)

Special Populations: Pregnant Women: There are no adequate and well-controlled studies in pregnant women. Cases of lactic acidosis, sometimes fatal, and symptomatic hyperlactatemia have been reported in patients (including pregnant women) receiving REYATAZ in combination with nucleoside analogues, which are known to be associated with increased risk of lactic acidosis. Female gender and obesity are also known risk factors for lactic acidosis syndrome. The contribution of REYATAZ to the risk of development of lactic acidosis syndrome has not been established.

Hyperbilirubinemia occurred frequently during treatment with REYATAZ. It is not known whether REYATAZ administered to the mother during pregnancy will exacerbate physiologic hyperbilirubinemia and lead to kernicterus in neonates and young infants. In the prepartum period, additional monitoring and alternative therapy should be considered. REYATAZ has been shown to cross the placenta.

No teratogenic effects were observed at maternally toxic doses in rats or rabbits. Systemic drug exposure levels were equal to (in rabbits) or two times (in rats) those at the human clinical dose (400 mg once daily). In the pre-and post-natal development assessment in rats, atazanavir produced a transient reduction in body weight in the offspring at maternally toxic drug exposure levels two times those at the human clinical dose.

REYATAZ should be used during pregnancy only if the potential benefit justifies the potential risk to the fetus (see Warnings and Precautions, Endocrine and Metabolism).

Antiretroviral Pregnancy Registry: To monitor maternal-fetal outcomes of pregnant women exposed to REYATAZ, an Antiretroviral Pregnancy Registry has been established. Physicians are encouraged to register patients by calling 1-800-258-4263.

Nursing Women: It is not known whether atazanavir is secreted in human milk. A study in lactating rats demonstrated that atazanavir is secreted in milk. It is recommended that HIV infected mothers not breast-feed their infants to avoid risking postnatal transmission of HIV. Because of both the potential for HIV transmission and the potential for serious adverse reactions in nursing infants, mothers should be instructed not to breast-feed if they are receiving REYATAZ.

Pediatrics (from 6 to 18 years of age): REYATAZ should not be administered in pediatric patients below the age of 3 months due to the risk of kernicterus. The safety, pharmacokinetic profile, and virologic response of REYATAZ were evaluated in pediatric patients in an open-label, multicenter clinical trial PACTG 1020A. The safety profile in pediatric patients was comparable to that observed in adults (see Adverse Reactions). The safety, activity, and pharmacokinetic profiles of REYATAZ in pediatric patients ages 3 months to less than 6 years have not been established.

Geriatrics (>65 years of age): Clinical studies of REYATAZ did not include sufficient numbers of patients aged 65 and over to determine whether they respond differently from younger patients. In general, appropriate caution should be exercised in the administration and monitoring of REYATAZ in elderly patients reflecting the greater frequency of decreased hepatic, renal, or cardiac function, and of concomitant disease or other drug therapy.

Lactose: Patients with rare hereditary problems of galactose intolerance, the Lapp lactase deficiency or glucose galactose malabsorption should not take this medicinal product.

Drug Interaction: Atazanavir is an inhibitor of CYP3A and UGT1A1. Coadministration of REYATAZ and drugs primarily metabolized by CYP3A [eg, calcium channel blockers, HMG-CoA reductase inhibitors, immunosuppressants, and phosphodiesterase (PDE5) inhibitors], or UGT1A1 (eg, irinotecan) may result in increased plasma concentrations of the other drug that could increase or prolong its therapeutic and adverse effects.

Atazanavir is a weak inhibitor of CYP2C8. Caution should be used when REYATAZ without ritonavir is coadministered with drugs highly dependent on CYP2C8 with narrow therapeutic indicies (eg, paclitaxel, repaglinide). When REYATAZ with ritonavir is coadministered with substrates of CYP2C8, clinically significant interactions are not expected. See the complete prescribing information for NORVIR for information on other potential drug interactions with ritonavir. Clinically significant interactions are not expected between atazanavir and substrates of CYP2C19, CYP2C9, CYP2D6, CYP2B6, CYP2A6, CYP1A2, or CYP2E1 (see Drug Interactions).

ADVERSE REACTIONS: Because clinical trials are conducted under very specific conditions, the adverse reaction rates observed in clinical trials may not reflect the rates observed in practice and should not be compared to the rates in the clinical trials of another drug. Adverse drug reaction information from clinical trials is useful for identifying drug-related adverse events and for approximate rates.

Clinical Trial Experience in Adults: REYATAZ has been evaluated for safety and tolerability in combination therapy with other antiretroviral medications in controlled clinical trials in 1806 adult patients receiving REYATAZ 400 mg once daily (1151 patients, 52 weeks median duration and 152 weeks maximum duration), or REYATAZ 300 mg once daily plus ritonavir 100 mg once daily (655 patients, 96 weeks median duration and 108 weeks maximum duration).

The more frequent adverse events of any severity with at least a possible relationship to regimens containing REYATAZ and one or more NRTIs were nausea (20%), diarrhea (10%) and jaundice (13%).

Jaundice was reported within a few days to a few months after the initiation of treatment and resulted in discontinuation of treatment in <1% of patients. Discontinuation of treatment due to adverse reactions was 5% in treatment-naïve patients and 5% in treatment-experienced patients.

Lipodystrophy, of moderate intensity or greater, was reported in regimens containing REYATAZ and one or more NRTIs as shown in Table 3 and Table 4 (see Warnings and Precautions).

Treatment-Emergent Adverse Events in Antiretroviral Treatment-Naive Patients: Drug-related clinical adverse events of moderate or severe intensity in ≥2% of treatment-naive patients receiving combination therapy including REYATAZ 300 mg with ritonavir 100 mg and REYATAZ 400 mg (without ritonavir) are presented in Table 2 and Table 3, respectively.

Table 2: REYATAZ

Selected Treatment-Emergent Adverse Events[a] of Moderate or Severe Intensity Reported in ≥2% of Adult Treatment-Naïve Patients[b], Study AI424-138

	Phase III Study AI424-138	
	96 Weeks[c] REYATAZ 300 mg Plus Ritonavir 100 mg (once daily) and Tenofovir Plus Emtricitabine[d] N=441	**96 Weeks[c] Lopinavir 400 mg Plus Ritonavir 100 mg (twice daily) and Tenofovir Plus Emtricitabine[d] N=437**
Digestive System		
Nausea	4%	8%
Jaundice/scleral icterus	5%	*
Diarrhea	2%	12%
Skin and Appendages		
Rash	3%	2%

[a] Includes events of possible, probable, certain, or unknown relationship to treatment regimen.
[b] Based on the regimen containing REYATAZ.
[c] Median time on therapy.
[d] As a fixed-dose combination: 300 mg tenofovir, 200 mg emtricitabine once daily.
* None reported in this treatment arm.

Table 3: REYATAZ

Treatment-Emergent Adverse Events[a] of Moderate or Severe Intensity Reported in ≥2% of Adult Treatment-Naive Patients[b], Studies AI424-034, AI424-007 and AI424-008

	Phase III Study AI424-034		Phase II Studies AI424-007, -008	
	64 Weeks[c] REYATAZ 400 mg Once Daily + Lamivudine + Zidovudine[e] N=404	**64 Weeks[c] Efavirenz 600 mg Once Daily + Lamivudine + Zidovudine[e] N=401**	**120 Weeks[c,d] REYATAZ 400 mg Once Daily + Stavudine/ Lamivudine or + Stavudine/ Didanosine N=279**	**73 Weeks[c,d] Nelfinavir 750 mg TID or 1250 mg BID + Stavudine + Lamivudine or + Stavudine + Didanosine N=191**
Body as a Whole				
Headache	6%	6%	1%	2%
Digestive System				
Diarrhea	1%	2%	3%	16%
Dyspepsia	2%	2%	<1%	<1%
Scleral icterus	2%	*	2%	*
Jaundice	5%	*	5%	*
Nausea	14%	12%	6%	4%
Abdominal pain	4%	4%	4%	2%
Vomiting	4%	7%	3%	3%
Metabolic and Nutritional System				
Lipodystrophy	1%	1%	7%	3%
Nervous System				
Insomnia	3%	3%	<1%	*
Dizziness	2%	7%	<1%	*
Peripheral neurologic symptoms	<1%	1%	4%	3%
Skin and Appendages				
Rash	7%	10%	5%	1%

[a] Includes adverse events of possible, probable, certain, or unknown relationship to treatment regimen. Assessments of relationship refer to regimens containing REYATAZ or comparator.
[b] Based on regimen(s) containing REYATAZ.
[c] Median time on therapy. In study AI424-034 efficacy analyses are based on 48 week data. Safety data are derived from a 64 week safety update report.
[d] Includes long-term follow-up.
[e] As a fixed dose combination: 150 mg lamivudine, 300 mg zidovudine twice daily.
* Not reported in this treatment arm.

Treatment-Emergent Adverse Events in Antiretroviral Treatment-Experienced Patients: Drug related clinical adverse events of moderate or severe intensity in ≥2% of treatment experienced patients receiving combination therapy including REYATAZ are presented in Table 4.

Table 4: REYATAZ

Treatment-Emergent Adverse Events[a] of Moderate or Severe Intensity Reported in ≥2% of Adult Treatment-Experienced Patients[b], Studies AI424-043 and AI424-045

	Phase III Study AI424-043		Phase III Study AI424-045**	
	48 Weeks[c] REYATAZ 400 mg Once Daily + 2 NRTIs N=144	48 Weeks[c] Lopinavir + Ritonavir (400/100 mg) b.i.d.[d] + 2 NRTIs N=146	48 Weeks[c] REYATAZ 300 mg Once Daily + Ritonavir 100 mg Once Daily + Tenofovir + NRTI N=119	48 Weeks[c] Lopinavir + Ritonavir (400/100 mg) b.i.d.[d] + Tenofovir + NRTI N=118
Body as a Whole				
Headache	4%	3%	<1%	<1%
Fever	—	—	2%	*
Digestive System				
Diarrhea	2%	4%	3%	11%
Scleral icterus	*	*	3%	*
Jaundice	3%	*	6%	*
Nausea	3%	4%	3%	2%
Vomiting	2%	2%	*	<1%
Pain abdomen	3%	2%	2%	2%
Metabolic and Nutritional System				
Lipodystrophy	6%	1%	5%	4%
Weight decreased	2%	<1%	*	2%
Musculoskeletal System				
Myalgia	*	*	4%	*
Nervous System				
Peripheral neurologic symptom	2%	5%	<1%	3%
Depression	—	—	2*	*
Skin and Appendages				
Rash	2%	*	*	<1%

a Includes adverse events of possible, probable, certain, or unknown relationship to treatment regimen. Assessments of relationship refer to regimens containing REYATAZ or comparator.
b Based on regimen(s) containing REYATAZ.
c Median time on therapy.
d As a fixed dose combination.
e Soft gelatin capsules.
* Not reported in this treatment arm.
** Note: There are limited safety data from controlled trials for REYATAZ plus ritonavir regimens without tenofovir (see Drug Interactions).

Less Common Clinical Trial Adverse Drug Reactions (<2%): Treatment-Emergent Adverse Events in all REYATAZ-Treated Patients: Treatment-emergent adverse events of at least moderate intensity occurring in less than 2% of adult patients receiving REYATAZ in all phase II/III clinical trials with at least a possible relationship to treatment with REYATAZ-containing regimens, and not listed in Table 2, Table 3 or Table 4 are listed below by body system.
Body as a Whole: allergic reaction, asthenia, chest pain, fatigue, malaise.
Cardiovascular System: hypertension, palpitation, syncope, edema.
Digestive System: abdominal distension, aphthous stomatitis, dysgeusia, flatulence, gastritis, hepatitis, hepatosplenomegaly, pancreatitis, dry mouth.
Immune System: allergic reaction.
Metabolic and Nutritional Disorders: weight gain, anorexia, appetite increased, weight decreased.
Musculoskeletal System: arthralgia, muscle atrophy, myopathy.
Nervous System: abnormal dream, abnormal gait, amnesia, anxiety, confusion, sleep disorder, somnolence.
Respiratory System: dyspnea.
Skin and Appendages: alopecia, eczema, pruritus, urticaria, vesiculobullous rash, vasodilatation.
Urogenital System: gynecomastia, hematuria, kidney pain, proteinuria, pollakiuria, nephrolithiasis.
Abnormal Hematologic and Clinical Chemistry Findings: Laboratory Abnormalities: The percentages of adult treatment-naive and treatment-experienced patients treated with combination therapy including REYATAZ 300 mg with ritonavir 100 mg and REYATAZ 400 mg (without ritonavir) with Grade 3-4 laboratory abnormalities are presented in Table 5, Table 6 and Table 7. The most frequently reported laboratory abnormality in patients receiving regimens containing REYATAZ and one or more NRTIs was elevated bilirubin. Elevations in bilirubin were reported predominantly as elevated indirect [unconjugated] bilirubin.

In clinical studies, the observed magnitude of dyslipidemia was less with REYATAZ than with comparators. However, the clinical impact of such findings has not been demonstrated.

Lipids—Treatment-Naïve Patients: Table 8 and Table 9 present the changes in lipids, insulin and glucose for the treatment-naive studies.

Lipids—Treatment-Experienced Patients: Table 10, Table 11 and Table 12 present the changes from baseline in lipids, insulin and glucose for the treatment-experienced studies.

Clinical Trial Experience in Pediatric Patients: The safety and tolerability of REYATAZ Capsules with and without ritonavir have been established in pediatric patients at least 6 years of age from the open-label, multicenter clinical trial PACTG 1020A. Use of REYATAZ in pediatric patients less than 6 years of age is under investigation.

The safety profile of REYATAZ in pediatric patients (6 to less than 18 years of age) was comparable to that observed in clinical studies of REYATAZ in adults. The most common Grade 2-4 adverse events (≥5%, regardless of causality) reported in pediatric patients were cough (21%), fever (19%), rash (14%), jaundice/scleral icterus (13%), diarrhea (8%), vomiting (8%), headache (7%), and rhinorrhea (6%). Asymptomatic second-degree atrioventricular block was reported in 2% of patients. The most common Grade 3-4 laboratory abnormality was elevation of total bilirubin (≥3.2 mg/dL) which occurred in 49% of pediatric patients. All other Grade 3-4 laboratory abnormalities occurred with a frequency of less than 3%. Both the frequency and severity of cardiac conduction abnormalities were greater in pediatric patients in this study than observed in clinical studies in adults.

Patients Co-infected with Hepatitis B and/or Hepatitis C Virus: Liver function tests should be monitored in patients with a history of hepatitis B or C.

In study AI424-138, 60 patients treated with REYATAZ/ritonavir 300 mg/100 mg once daily, and 51 patients treated with lopinavir/ritonavir 400 mg/100 mg twice daily, each with fixed dose tenofovir-emtricitabine were seropositive for hepatitis B and/or C at study entry. ALT levels >5 times ULN developed in 10% (6/60) of the REYATAZ/ritonavir-treated patients, and 8% (4/50) of the lopinavir/ritonavir-treated patients. AST levels >5 times ULN developed in 10% (6/60) of the REYATAZ/ritonavir-treated patients and none (0/50) of the lopinavir/ritonavir-treated patients.

In study AI424-045, 20 patients treated with REYATAZ/ritonavir 300 mg/100 mg once daily and 18 patients treated with lopinavir/ritonavir 400 mg/100 mg twice daily were seropositive for hepatitis B and/or C at study entry. ALT levels >5 times ULN developed in 25% (5/20) of the REYATAZ/ritonavir-treated patients and 6% (1/18) of the lopinavir/ritonavir-treated patients. AST levels >5 times ULN developed in 10% (2/20) of the REYATAZ/ritonavir-treated patients and 6% (1/18) of the lopinavir/ritonavir-treated patients (see Warnings and Precautions, Hepatic/Biliary/Pancreatic).

In studies AI424-008 and AI424-034, 74 patients treated with 400 mg of REYATAZ once daily, 58 who received efavirenz, and 12 who received nelfinavir were seropositive for hepatitis B and/or C at study entry. AST levels >5 times the upper limit of normal (ULN) developed in 9% of the REYATAZ-treated patients, 5% of the efavirenz-treated patients, and 17% of the nelfinavir-treated patients. ALT levels >5 times ULN developed in 15% of the REYATAZ-treated patients, 14% of the efavirenz-treated patients, and 17% of the nelfinavir-treated patients. Within atazanavir and control regimens, no difference in frequency of bilirubin elevations was noted between seropositive and seronegative patients.

Post-Market Adverse Drug Reactions: The following events have been identified during post approval use of REYATAZ. Because they are reported voluntarily from a population of unknown size, estimates of frequency cannot be made. These events have been chosen for inclusion due to their seriousness, frequency of reporting, or causal connection to REYATAZ, or a combination of these factors.
Body as a Whole: edema.
Cardiac Disorders and Vascular Disorders: second-degree AV block, third-degree AV block, QTc prolongation, Torsades de Pointes, left bundle branch block.
Gastrointestinal System: pancreatitis.
Hepatic System: hepatic function abnormalities.
Metabolism and Nutrition Disorders: hyperglycemia, diabetes mellitus.
Musculoskeletal System: arthralgia.
Renal System: nephrolithiasis.
Skin and Appendages: pruritus, alopecia, maculopapular rash.
Hepatobiliary Disorders: cholelithiasis, cholecystitis, cholestasis.

Table 5: REYATAZ

Grade 3-4 Laboratory Abnormalities Reported in ≥2% of Adult Treatment-Naïve Patients[a], Studies AI424-138

		Treatment-Naive Patients	
		Phase III Studies AI424-138	
Variable	Limit[c]	96 Weeks[b] REYATAZ 300 mg Plus Ritonavir 100 mg (once daily) and Tenofovir Plus Emtricitabine[d] N=441	96 Weeks[b] Lopinavir 400 mg Plus Ritonavir 100 mg (twice daily) and Tenofovir Plus Emtricitabine[d] N=437
Chemistry	**High**		
AST	≥5.1×ULN	3%	1%
ALT	≥5.1×ULN	3%	2%
Total Bilirubin	≥2.6×ULN	44%	<1%
Lipase	≥2.1×ULN	2%	2%
Creatine Kinase	≥5.1×ULN	8%	7%
Total Cholesterol	≥240 mg/dL	11%	25%
Hematology	**Low**		
Neutrophils	<750 cells/mm³	5%	2%
Prothrombin Time	≥1.51×ULN	2%	6%

a Based on the regimen containing REYATAZ.
b Median time on therapy.
c ULN=upper limit of normal.
d As a fixed-dose combination: 300 mg tenofovir, 200 mg emtricitabine once daily.

Table 6: REYATAZ

Selected Grade 3-4 Laboratory Abnormalities Reported in ≥2% of Adult Treatment-Naive Patients[a], Studies AI424-034, AI424-007 and AI424-008

		Treatment-Naive Patients			
		Phase III Study AI424-034		Phase II Studies AI424-007, 008	
Variable	Limit[d]	64 Weeks[b] REYATAZ 400 mg Once Daily + Lamivudine + Zidovudine[e] N=404	64 Weeks[b] Efavirenz 600 mg Once Daily + Lamivudine + Zidovudine[e] N=401	120 Weeks[b,c] REYATAZ 400 mg Once Daily + Stavudine + Lamivudine or + Stavudine + Didanosine N=279	73 Weeks[b,c] Nelfinavir 750 mg TID or 1250 mg BID + Stavudine + Lamivudine or + Stavudine + Didanosine N=191
Chemistry	**High**				
AST	≥5.1×ULN	2%	2%	7%	5%

(cont'd)

Table 6: REYATAZ *(cont'd)*

Selected Grade 3-4 Laboratory Abnormalities Reported in ≥2% of Adult Treatment-Naive Patients[a], Studies AI424-034, AI424-007 and AI424-008

		Treatment-Naive Patients			
		Phase III Study AI424-034		Phase II Studies AI424-007, 008	
Variable	**Limit[d]**	**64 Weeks[b] REYATAZ 400 mg Once Daily + Lamivudine + Zidovudine[e] N=404**	**64 Weeks[b] Efavirenz 600 mg Once Daily + Lamivudine + Zidovudine[e] N=401**	**120 Weeks[b,c] REYATAZ 400 mg Once Daily + Stavudine + Lamivudine or + Stavudine + Didanosine N=279**	**73 Weeks[b,c] Nelfinavir 750 mg TID or 1250 mg BID + Stavudine + Lamivudine or + Stavudine + Didanosine N=191**
ALT	≥5.1×ULN	4%	3%	9%	7%
Total Bilirubin	≥2.6×ULN	35%	<1%	47%	3%
Amylase	≥2.1×ULN	*	*	14%	10%
Lipase	≥2.1×ULN	<1%	1%	4%	5%
Creatine Kinase	≥5.1×ULN	6%	6%	11%	9%
Hematology	**Low**				
Hemoglobin	<8.0 g/L	5%	3%	<1%	4%
Neutrophils	<750 cells/mm[3]	7%	9%	3%	7%

[a] Based on regimen(s) containing REYATAZ.
[b] Median time on therapy. In Study AI424-034 efficacy analyses are based on 48 week data. Safety data are derived from a 64 week safety update report.
[c] Includes long term follow-up.
[d] ULN=upper limit of normal.
[e] As a fixed-dose combination: 150 mg lamivudine, 300 mg zidovudine twice daily.
* Not reported in this treatment arm.
** Note: There are limited safety data from controlled trials for REYATAZ plus ritonavir regimens without tenofovir (see Drug Interactions).

Table 7: REYATAZ

Selected Grade 3-4 Laboratory Abnormalities Reported in ≥2% of Adult Treatment-Experienced Patients[a], Studies AI424-043 and AI424-045

		Treatment-Experienced Patients			
		Phase III Study AI424-043		Phase III Studies AI424-045**	
		48 Weeks[b]		48 Weeks[b]	48 Weeks[b]
Variable	**Limit[c]**	**REYATAZ 400 mg Once Daily + 2NRTIs N=144**	**Lopinavir + Ritonavir (400/100 mg) BID[d] + 2NRTIs N=146**	**REYATAZ 300 mg Once Daily + Ritonavir 100 mg Once Daily + Tenofovir + NRTI N=119**	**Lopinavir + Ritonavir (400/100 mg) BID[d] + Tenofovir + NRTI N=118**
Chemistry	**High**				
AST	≥5.1×ULN	3%	3%	3%	3%
ALT	≥5.1×ULN	7%	3%	4%	3%
Total Bilirubin	≥2.6×ULN	25%	<1%	49%	<1%
Lipase	≥2.1×ULN	4%	3%	5%	6%
Creatine Kinase	≥5.1×ULN	8%	6%	8%	8%
Hematology	**Low**				
Platelets	<50 000/mm[3]	*	*	2%	3%
Neutrophils	<750 cells/mm[3]	6%	5%	7%	8%

(cont'd)

Table 7: REYATAZ *(cont'd)*

[a] Based on regimen(s) containing REYATAZ.
[b] Median time on therapy. In Study AI424-034 efficacy analyses are based on 48 week data. Safety data are derived from a 64 week safety update report.
[c] ULN=upper limit of normal.
[d] As a fixed dose combination.
* Not reported in this treatment arm.
** Note: There are limited safety data from controlled trials for REYATAZ plus ritonavir regimens without tenofovir. (See Drug Interactions.)

DRUG INTERACTIONS:

Serious Drug Interactions

Atazanavir is an inhibitor of CYP3A and UGT1A1. Coadministration of REYATAZ and drugs primarily metabolized by CYP3A or UGT1A1 may result in increased plasma concentrations of the other drug that could increase or prolong its therapeutic and adverse effects.

Atazanavir is a weak inhibitor of CYP2C8. Caution should be used when REYATAZ without ritonavir is coadministered with drugs highly dependent on CYP2C8 with narrow therapeutic indicies (eg, paclitaxel, repaglinide). When REYATAZ with ritonavir is coadministered with substrates of CYP2C8, clinically significant interactions are not expected.

The magnitude of CYP3A-mediated drug interactions on coadministered drug may change when REYATAZ is coadministered with ritonavir. See the complete prescribing information for NORVIR (ritonavir) for information on drug interactions with ritonavir.

- Refer to Contraindications.
- Refer to Table 13 for Drugs That Are Contraindicated or Not Recommended for Coadministration with REYATAZ.
- Refer to Table 14 for Established and Other Potentially Significant Drug Interactions.

Overview: Atazanavir is a metabolism-dependent CYP3A inhibitor, with a K_{inact} value of 0.05 to 0.06 min^{-1} and K_i value of 0.84 to 1.0 μM. Atazanavir is also a direct inhibitor for UGT1A1 (K_i=1.9 μM).

Coadministration of atazanavir and drugs primarily metabolized by CYP3A4 (e.g., calcium channel blockers, HMG CoA reductase inhibitors, immunosuppressants and phosphodiesterase (PDE5) inhibitors) or UGT1A1 (e.g., irinotecan) may result in increased plasma concentrations of the other drug that could increase or prolong both its therapeutic and adverse effects. Coadministration of atazanavir and drugs that induce CYP3A4, such as rifampin, may decrease atazanavir plasma concentrations and reduce its therapeutic effect. Coadministration of atazanavir and drugs that inhibit CYP3A4 may increase atazanavir plasma concentrations (see Table 13 and Table 14).

Clinically significant interactions are not expected between atazanavir and substrates of CYP2C19, CYP2C9, CYP2D6, CYP2B6, CYP2A6, CYP1A2, or CYP2E1. Atazanavir is a weak inhibitor of CYP2C8. Caution should be used when REYATAZ without ritonavir is coadministered with drugs highly dependent on CYP2C8 with narrow therapeutic indicies (eg. paclitaxel, repaglinide). When REYATAZ with ritonavir is coadministered with substrates of CYP2C8, clinically significant interactions are not expected.

Atazanavir should not be administered concurrently with medications with narrow therapeutic windows that are substrates of CYP3A or UGT1A1 (see Contraindications).

Atazanavir solubility decreases as pH increases. Reduced plasma concentrations of atazanavir are expected if antacids, buffered medications, H_2- receptor antagonists, and proton-pump inhibitors are administered with atazanavir.

Table 8: REYATAZ

Lipid, Glucose and Insulin Mean Values, Study AI424-138

	REYATAZ/Ritonavir[a,b]					Lopinavir/Ritonavir[b,c]				
	Baseline mmol/L[h] N=428[e]	**Week 48 mmol/L[h] N=372[e]**	**Week 48 Change[d,g] N=372[e]**	**Week 96 mmol/L[h] N=342[e]**	**Week 96 Change[d,g] N=342[e]**	**Baseline mmol/L[h] N=424[e]**	**Week 48 mmol/L[h] N=335[e]**	**Week 48 Change[d,g] N=335[e]**	**Week 96 mmol/L[h] N=291[e]**	**Week 96 Change[d,g] N=291[e]**
Total-Cholesterol[f]	3.86	4.36	+13%	4.38	+13%	3.88	4.84	+25%	4.81	+25%
HDL-Cholesterol[f]	0.95	1.2	+29%	1.14	+21%	0.93	1.24	+37%	1.19	+29%
LDL-Cholesterol[f]	2.38	2.70	+14%	2.72	+14%	2.4	2.87	+19%	2.84	+17%
Triglycerides[f]	1.42	1.63	+15%	1.58	+13%	1.46	2.2	+52%	2.08	+50%
Insulin	57.7	76.6	+18.1	58.9	+1.1	59.9	61.1	+1.2	51.8	–5.5
Glucose	4.77	4.86	+0.12	4.97	+0.22	4.88	4.9	+0.01	4.96	+0.05

[a] REYATAZ 300 mg plus ritonavir 100 mg once daily with the fixed-dose combination: 300 mg tenofovir, 200 mg emtricitabine once daily.
[b] Values obtained after initiation of serum lipid-reducing agents were not included in these analyses. Use of serum lipid-reducing agents was more common in the lopinavir/ritonavir treatment arm (8%) than in the REYATAZ/ritonavir arm (2%). Through Week 96, serum lipid-reducing agents were used in 10% in the lopinavir/ritonavir treatment arm and 3% in the REYATAZ/ritonavir arm.
[c] Lopinavir 400 mg plus ritonavir 100mg twice daily with the fixed-dose combination 300 mg tenofovir, 200 mg emtricitabine once daily.
[d] The change from baseline is the mean of within-patient changes from baseline for patients with both baseline and Week 48 or Week 96 values and is not a simple difference of the baseline and Week 48 or Week 96 mean values, respectively.
[e] Number of patients with LDL-cholesterol measured.
[f] Fasting.
[g] Absolute changes are reported for insulin and glucose levels.
[h] Units are pmol/L for insulin.

Table 9: REYATAZ

Lipid, Insulin, and Glucose Mean Values From Study AI424-034*

	REYATAZ[a]			Efavirenz[b]		
	Baseline	Week 48		Baseline	Week 48	
	mmol/L[c] (n=383[e])	mmol/L[c] (n=283[e])	% Change[c,f] (n=272[e])	mmol/L[c] (n=378[e])	mmol/L[c] (n=264[e])	% Change[c,f] (n=253[e])
Total Cholesterol	4.24	4.34	+2%	4.19	5.04	+21%
HDL-Cholesterol	1.01	1.11	+13%	0.98	1.19	+24%
LDL-Cholesterol[g]	2.53	2.53	+1%	2.53	2.95	+18%
Triglycerides[g]	1.56	1.4	−9%	1.46	1.9	+23%
Total-to-HDL Cholesterol Ratio <3	13%	17%	—	9%	14%	—
Insulin[d,g]	81.1	88.3	+9.3	71	82.5	+10.1
Glucose[d,g]	5	5.2	+0.17	5	5.2	+0.33

[a] REYATAZ 400 mg once daily with the fixed dose combination: 150 mg lamivudine, 300 mg zidovudine twice daily.
[b] Efavirenz 600 mg once daily with the fixed dose combination: 150 mg lamivudine, 300 mg zidovudine twice daily.
[c] Units are pmol/mL for insulin levels.
[d] Absolute changes are reported for insulin and glucose levels.
[e] Number of patients with LDL cholesterol measured.
[f] The change from baseline is the mean of within patient changes from baseline for patients with both baseline and Week 48 values and is not a simple difference of the baseline and Week 48 mean values.
[g] Fasting.
* No multivariate analyses were performed on these data.

Table 10: REYATAZ

Lipid, Insulin, and Glucose Mean Values From Study AI424-043*

	REYATAZ[a]			Lopinavir + Ritonavir[b]		
	Baseline	Week 48		Baseline	Week 48	
	mmol/L[c] (n=143[e])	mmol/L[c] (n=101[e])	% Change[d,g] (n=101[e])	mmol/L[c] (n=144[e])	mmol/L[c] (n=99[e])	% Change[d,g] (n=99[e])
Total Cholesterol	4.68	4.50	−2%	4.53	5.02	+12%
HDL-Cholesterol	1.01	1.06	+9%	0.96	1.11	+10%
LDL-Cholesterol[f,h]	2.74	2.56	−6%[f]	2.66	2.79	+3%
Triglycerides[h]	2.17	4.50	+1%	2.17	6.52	+53%
Total-to-HDL Cholesterol Ratio <3	7%	12%	—	7%	10%	—
Insulin[h]	76.1	86.1	+14.4	71.0	78.9	+7.9
Glucose[h]	4.9	5.1	+0.17	5	5.0	−0.6

[a] REYATAZ 400 mg once daily + 2 NRTIs.
[b] Lopinavir + ritonavir (400/100 mg) BID + 2 NRTIs.
[c] Units are pmol/mL for insulin levels.
[d] Absolute changes are reported for insulin and glucose levels.
[e] Number of patients with LDL cholesterol measured.
[f] Protocol-defined co-primary safety outcome measure.
[g] The change from baseline is the mean of within patient changes from baseline for patients with both baseline and Week 48 values and is not a simple difference of the baseline and Week 48 mean values.
[h] Fasting.
* No multivariate analyses were performed on these data.

Table 11: REYATAZ

Lipid and Glucose Mean Values from Study AI424-045*

	ATV 300/RTV[a]			LPV/RTV[b]		
	Baseline	Week 48		Baseline	Week 48	
	mmol/L (n=112[c])	mmol/L (n=75[c])	% Change (n=74)	mmol/L (n=108[c])	mmol/L (n=76[c])	% Change (n=73)
Total Cholesterol	4.86	4.40	−8%	4.68	4.83	6%
HDL-Cholesterol	1.03	1.00	−7%	1.01	1.06	2%
LDL-Cholesterol[e]	2.82	2.53	−10%	2.69	2.66	1%
Triglycerides	2.43	4.16	−4%	2.21	5.79	30%
Total-to-HDL Cholesterol Ratio <3	9%	13%	—	12%	13%	—
Glucose[d,e]	5.27	5.49	+0.22	5.00	5.10	+0.06

[a] REYATAZ 300 mg + ritonavir 100 mg once daily + tenofovir + 1 NRTI.
[b] Lopinavir + ritonavir (400/100 mg) BID + tenofovir + 1 NRTI.
[c] Number of patients with LDL cholesterol measured.
[d] Absolute changes are reported for glucose levels.
[e] Fasting.
* There are limited safety data from controlled trials for REYATAZ plus ritonavir regimens without tenofovir (see Drug Interactions). No multivariate analyses were performed on these data.

Table 12: REYATAZ

Lipid, Insulin and Glucose Values from Study AI424-044 (Nelfinavir Patients in Study AI424-008 Who Switched to REYATAZ[a] in the Long Term AI424-044 Study)*

	Baseline Study AI424-008	Entry Study AI424-044	Week 12 Study AI424-044	
	mmol/L[a] (n=54[b])	mmol/L[a] (n=33[b])	mmol/L[a] (n=41[b])	% Change[c] (n=29[b])
Total Cholesterol	4.34	5.53	4.53	−16%
HDL-Cholesterol	1.09	1.19	1.24	+5%
LDL-Cholesterol[d]	2.53	3.57	2.69	−21%
Triglycerides[d]	1.19	1.77	1.22	−28%
Insulin[d]	—	70.3	66.7	—
Glucose[d]	—	4.77	4.88	—

[a] Units are pmol/mL for insulin levels.
[b] Number of patients with LDL cholesterol measured.
[c] The change from entry is the mean of within patient changes from entry for patients with both entry and Week 12 values and is not a simple difference of the entry and Week 12 mean values.
[d] Fasting.
* No multivariate analyses were performed on these data.

Particular caution should be used when prescribing phosphodiesterase (PDE5) inhibitors for erectile dysfunction (eg, sildenafil, tadalafil) in patients receiving protease inhibitors, including REYATAZ. Coadministration of a protease inhibitor with a PDE5 inhibitor is expected to substantially increase PDE5 inhibitor concentrations and may result in an increase in PDE5 inhibitor-associated adverse events, including hypotension, visual changes, and priapism. (See the complete Product Monograph for sildenafil, and tadalafil.) Vardenafil should not be coadministered with REYATAZ (with and without ritonavir) (see Table 13 and Table 14).

Simvastatin and lovastatin are contraindicated with REYATAZ (see Table 13). Caution should be exercised if HIV protease inhibitors, including REYATAZ, are used concurrently with other HMG-CoA reductase inhibitors that are also metabolized by the CYP3A pathway. Use the lowest possible dose of atorvastatin or rosuvastatin with careful monitoring, or consider other HMG-CoA reductase inhibitors such as pravastatin or fluvastatin in combination with REYATAZ (with and without ritonavir). The risk of myopathy, including rhabdomyolysis, may be increased when HIV protease inhibitors, including REYATAZ, are used in combination with these drugs.

Midazolam is extensively metabolised by CYP3A4. Although not studied, coadministration of midazolam with REYATAZ may cause a large increase in the concentration of this benzodiazepine. Increases in benzodiazepine concentration are expected to be significantly higher with oral administration of the benzodiazepine, relative to parenteral. Therefore, REYATAZ should not be coadministered with orally administered midazolam, whereas caution should be used with coadministration of REYATAZ and parenteral midazolam. If REYATAZ is coadministered with parenteral midazolam, a close clinical monitoring for respiratory depression and/or prolonged sedation should be exercised and dosage adjustment should be considered.

Concomitant use of REYATAZ and St. John's wort (Hypericum perforatum), or products containing St. John's wort, is not recommended. Coadministration of protease inhibitors, including REYATAZ, with St. John's wort is expected to substantially decrease concentrations of the protease inhibitor and may result in suboptimal levels of atazanavir and lead to loss of virologic response and possible resistance to atazanavir or to the class of protease inhibitors.

The magnitude of CYP3A4-mediated drug interactions (effect on atazanavir or effect on coadministered drug) may change when REYATAZ is coadministered with ritonavir, a potent CYP3A4 inhibitor. The Product Monograph for ritonavir should be consulted for information on drug interactions with ritonavir.

Atazanavir has the potential to prolong the PR interval of the electrocardiogram in some patients. Caution should be used when coadministering REYATAZ with medicinal products known to induce PR interval prolongation (eg, atenolol, diltiazem).

The exposure to buprenorphine and the active metabolite, norbuprenorphine, were significantly increased when coadministered with atazanavir (with or without ritonavir), due to CYP3A4 and UGT1A1 inhibition. Coadministration of buprenorphine and REYATAZ/ritonavir warrants clinical monitoring for sedation and cognitive effects. A dose reduction of buprenorphine may be considered. There was no significant effect on atazanavir plasma concentration when REYATAZ plus ritonavir were coadministered with buprenorphine. Coadministration of buprenorphine and REYATAZ without ritonavir may substantially decrease atazanavir plasma concentrations. REYATAZ without ritonavir should not be coadministered with buprenorphine.

A drug interaction study in healthy subjects has shown that ritonavir significantly increases plasma fluticasone propionate exposures, resulting in significantly decreased serum cortisol concentrations. Concomitant use of REYATAZ with ritonavir and fluticasone propionate is expected to produce the same effects. Systemic corticosteroid effects, including Cushing's syndrome and adrenal suppression, have been reported during post-marketing use in patients receiving ritonavir and inhaled or intranasally administered fluticasone propionate. Therefore, coadministration of fluticasone propionate and REYATAZ/ritonavir is not recommended unless the potential benefit to the patient outweighs the risk of systemic corticosteroid side effects.

Exposure to rifabutin was significantly increased when coadministered with atazanavir (with or without ritonavir). Increased monitoring for neutropenia should be performed if these drugs are coadministered. Dosage reduction of rifabutin is recommended (see Table 14).

Drugs that are contraindicated or not recommended for coadministration with REYATAZ are included in Table 13. Drugs with established and other potentially significant drug interactions are included in Table 14. These recommendations are based on either drug interaction studies or predicted interactions due to the expected magnitude of interaction and potential for serious events or loss of efficacy.

Table 13: REYATAZ

Drugs That Are Contraindicated or Not Recommended for Coadministration with REYATAZ

Drug Class: Specific Drugs	Clinical Comment
Antiarrhythmics: quinidine	REYATAZ/ritonavir: **Contraindicated** if REYATAZ is coadministered with ritonavir due to potential for serious and/or life-threatening reactions such as cardiac arrhythmias.
Antineoplastics: irinotecan	Atazanavir inhibits UGT and may interfere with the metabolism of irinotecan resulting in increased irinotecan toxicities.
Antimycobacterials: rifampin	Rifampin substantially decreases plasma concentrations of atazanavir, which may result in loss of therapeutic effect and development of resistance.
Benzodiazepines: orally administered midazolam[a], triazolam	**Contraindicated** due to potential for serious and/or life-threatening events such as prolonged or increased sedation or respiratory depression.
Ergot Derivatives: dihydroergotamine, ergotamine, ergonovine, methylergonovine	**Contraindicated** due to potential for serious and/or life-threatening events such as acute ergot toxicity characterized by peripheral vasospasm and ischemia of the extremities and other tissues.
GI Motility Agent: cisapride[b]	**Contraindicated** due to potential for serious and/or life-threatening reactions such as cardiac arrhythmias.

(cont'd)

Table 13: REYATAZ *(cont'd)*

Drugs That Are Contraindicated or Not Recommended for Coadministration with REYATAZ

Drug Class: Specific Drugs	Clinical Comment
Proton Pump Inhibitors: omeprazole	Coadministration of omeprazole (40 mg once daily) with REYATAZ and ritonavir (300/100 mg once daily) resulted in a substantial reduction in atazanavir exposure (approximately 75% decrease in AUC, C_{max}, and C_{min}). Coadministration of omeprazole (20 mg once daily) with an increased dose of REYATAZ and ritonavir (400/100 mg once daily) in healthy volunteers resulted in a decrease of approximately 30% in the AUC, C_{max} and C_{min} of atazanavir relative to REYATAZ and ritonavir (300/100 mg once daily) without omeprazole. This decrease in AUC, C_{max} and C_{min} was not mitigated when an increased dose of REYATAZ and ritonavir (400/100 mg once daily) was temporally separated from omeprazole by 12 hours. Although not studied, similar results are expected with other proton pump inhibitors. This decrease in atazanavir exposure might negatively impact the efficacy of atazanavir. Coadministration of REYATAZ with proton pump inhibitors is not recommended. If the combination of REYATAZ with a proton pump inhibitor is judged unavoidable, close clinical monitoring is recommended in combination with an increase in the dose of REYATAZ to 400 mg with 100 mg of ritonavir; doses of proton pump inhibitors comparable to omeprazole 20 mg should not be exceeded.
HMG-CoA Reductase Inhibitors: lovastatin, simvastatin	**Contraindicated** due to potential for serious reactions such as myopathy including rhabdomyolysis.
Neuroleptic: pimozide	**Contraindicated** due to potential for serious and/or life-threatening reactions such as cardiac arrhythmias.
Protease Inhibitors: indinavir	Both REYATAZ and indinavir are associated with indirect (unconjugated) hyperbilirubinemia. Combinations of these drugs have not been studied and coadministration of REYATAZ and indinavir is not recommended.
Herbal Products: St. John's wort (Hypericum perforatum)	**Contraindicated** Patients taking REYATAZ should not use products containing St. John's wort (Hypericum perforatum) because coadministration may be expected to reduce plasma concentrations of atazanavir. This may result in loss of therapeutic effect and development of resistance.
Calcium Channel Blockers: bepridil[b]	Potential for serious and/or life-threatening adverse event. **Contraindicated** if REYATAZ is coadministered with ritonavir.
Erectile dysfunction agents (PDE5 inhibitors): Vardenafil	Vardenafil should not be coadministered with REYATAZ (with and without ritonavir).

[a] Oral formulation of midazolam is not marketed in Canada. See Table 14 for parenterally administered midazolam.
[b] Not marketed in Canada.

Table 14: REYATAZ

Established and Other Potentially Significant Drug Interactions: Alteration in Dose or Regimen May Be Recommended Based on Drug Interaction Studies or Predicted Interactions

Concomitant Drug Class: Specific Drugs	Effect on Concentration of REYATAZ or Concomitant Drug	Clinical Comment
	HIV Antiviral Agents	
Nucleoside Reverse Transcriptase Inhibitors (NRTIs):		
didanosine buffered formulations	↓ atazanavir	Coadministration with REYATAZ did not alter exposure to didanosine; however, exposure to atazanavir was markedly decreased by coadministration of REYATAZ with didanosine buffered tablets (presumably due to the increase in gastric pH caused by buffers in the didanosine tablets). Atazanavir should be given with food, 2 hours before or 1 hour after didanosine buffered formulations (which are given on an empty stomach).
didanosine EC formulation	↓ atazanavir ↓ didanosine	Due to the different food restrictions (didanosine EC given without food and atazanavir given with food) they should be administered at different times. Administration of the enteric-coated formulation of didanosine with atazanavir or atazanavir/ritonavir and a light meal decreased exposure to didanosine.
Nucleotide Reverse Transcriptase Inhibitors (NRTIs) :		
tenofovir DF	↓ atazanavir ↑ tenofovir	REYATAZ as a single PI, without ritonavir, may be less effective due to decreased atazanavir concentrations in patients taking REYATAZ and tenofovir DF. If REYATAZ is to be coadministered with tenofovir DF, it is recommended that REYATAZ 300 mg with ritonavir 100 mg be coadministered with tenofovir DF 300 mg (see Dosage and Administration). REYATAZ without ritonavir should not be coadministered with tenofovir. Atazanavir increases tenofovir concentrations. Higher tenofovir concentrations could potentiate tenofovir-associated adverse events, including renal disorders. Patients receiving atazanavir and tenofovir should be monitored for tenofovir-associated adverse events. No dose adjustment for tenofovir is recommended.
Non-nucleoside Reverse Transcriptase Inhibitors (NNRTIs):		

(cont'd)

Table 14: REYATAZ *(cont'd)*

Established and Other Potentially Significant Drug Interactions: Alteration in Dose or Regimen May Be Recommended Based on Drug Interaction Studies or Predicted Interactions

Concomitant Drug Class: Specific Drugs	Effect on Concentration of REYATAZ or Concomitant Drug	Clinical Comment
efavirenz	↓ atazanavir	Efavirenz decreases atazanavir exposure. **For treatment-naive patients:** If REYATAZ is combined with efavirenz, REYATAZ 400 mg (two 200-mg capsules) with ritonavir 100 mg should be administered once daily all as a single dose with food, and efavirenz should be administered on an empty stomach, preferably at bedtime. **For Treatment-experienced patients:** Do not coadminister REYATAZ with efavirenz in treatment-experienced patients due to decreased atazanavir exposure.
nevirapine	↓ atazanavir	Nevirapine, an inducer of CYP3A4, substantially decreases atazanavir exposure. There is a potential risk for nevirapine associated toxicity due to the increased nevirapine exposures. Do not coadminister REYATAZ with nevirapine.
Protease Inhibitor PIs:		
saquinavir (soft gelatin capsules)	↑ saquinavir	The safety and efficacy of this combination have not been established. In a clinicai study, saquinavir 1200 mg coadministered with REYATAZ 400 mg and tenofovir 300 mg (all given once daily) plus a nucleoside reverse transcriptase inhibitor did not provide adequate efficacy.
ritonavir	↑ atazanavir	If REYATAZ is coadministered with ritonavir, it is recommended that REYATAZ 300 mg once daily be given with ritonavir 100 mg once daily with food (see Dosage and Administration). See the complete product monograph for NORVIR (ritonavir) for information on drug interactions with ritonavir.
Other protease inhibitors	↑ Other PIs	Although not studied, the coadministration of REYATAZ plus ritonavir with other protease inhibitors would be expected to increase exposure to the other protease inhibitor and is not recommended.
	Other Agents	
Antacids and buffered medications:	↓ atazanavir	Reduced plasma concentrations of atazanavir are expected if antacids, including buffered medications, are administered with REYATAZ. REYATAZ should be administered 2 hours before or 1 hour after these medications.
Antiarrhythmics:	↑ amiodarone, lidocaine (systemic), quinidine	Coadministration with REYATAZ has the potential to produce serious and/or life-threatening adverse events and has not been studied. Caution is warranted and therapeutic concentration monitoring of these drugs is recommended if they are used concomitantly with REYATAZ. Quinidine is contraindicated when REYATAZ is coadministered with ritonavir.
Anticoagulants:	↑ warfarin	Coadministration with REYATAZ has the potential to produce serious and/or life-threatening bleeding and has not been studied. It is recommended that INR (International Normalized Ratio) be monitored.
Antidepressants:	↑ tricyclic antidepressants	Coadministration with REYATAZ has the potential to produce serious and/or life-threatening adverse events and has not been studied. Concentration monitoring of these drugs is recommended if they are used concomitantly with REYATAZ.
	↑ trazodone	Concomitant use of trazodone and REYATAZ with or without ritonavir may increase plasma concentrations of trazodone. Adverse events of nausea, dizziness, hypotension, and syncope have been observed following coadministration of trazodone and ritonavir. If trazodone is used with a CYP3A4 inhibitor such as REYATAZ, the combination should be used with caution and a lower dose of trazodone should be considered.
Antifungals:		
ketoconazole, itraconazole	↑ atazanavir ↑ ritonavir ↑ ketoconazole ↑ itraconazole	Coadministration of ketoconazole has only been studied with REYATAZ without ritonavir (negligible increase in atazanavir AUC and C_{max}). Due to the effect of ritonavir on ketoconazole, high doses of ketoconazole and itraconazole (>200 mg/day) should be used with caution with REYATAZ/ritonavir.

(cont'd)

Table 14: REYATAZ *(cont'd)*

Established and Other Potentially Significant Drug Interactions: Alteration in Dose or Regimen May Be Recommended Based on Drug Interaction Studies or Predicted Interactions

Concomitant Drug Class: Specific Drugs	Effect on Concentration of REYATAZ or Concomitant Drug	Clinical Comment
voriconazole	Effect is unknown	Coadministration of voriconazole with REYATAZ, with or without ritonavir has not been studied. However, administration of voriconazole with ritonavir 400 mg every 12 hours decreased voriconazole steady-state AUC by an average of 82%. The effect of lower ritonavir doses on voriconazole is not known at this time. Until data are available, voriconazole should not be administered to patients receiving REYATAZ/ritonavir. Coadministration of voriconazole with REYATAZ (without ritonavir) may increase atazanavir concentrations; however, no data are available.
Antimycobacterials:	↑ rifabutin	A rifabutin dose reduction of up to 75% (eg, 150 mg every other day or 3 times per week) is recommended. Concomitant use of REYATAZ with or without ritonavir and rifabutin may result in decreased neutrophil count or neutropenia. Increased monitoring for neutropenia should be performed if these drugs are coadministered. Further dosage reduction of rifabutin may be necessary.
Benzodiazepines: Parenterally administered midazolam[a]	↑ midazolam	If REYATAZ is coadministered with parenteral midazolam, close clinical monitoring for respiratory depression and/or prolonged sedation should be exercised and dosage adjustment should be considered.
Calcium channel blockers:	↑ diltiazem and desacetyl-diltiazem	A dose reduction of diltiazem by 50% should be considered. Caution is warranted. Coadministration of 400 mg atazanavir once daily and diltiazem 180 mg once daily had an added effect on the PR interval. ECG monitoring is recommended. Coadministration of REYATAZ/ritonavir with diltiazem has not been studied.
	↑ felodipine, nifedipine, nicardipine, and verapamil	Caution is warranted. Dose titration of the calcium channel blocker should be considered. ECG monitoring is recommended.
Erectile dysfunction agents (PDE5 inhibitors):	↑ sildenafil ↑ tadalafil ↑ vardenafil	Coadministration is expected to substantially increase the PDE5 inhibitor concentration and may result in an increase in PDE5 inhibitor-associated adverse events, including hypotension, visual changes and priapism. Reduced doses are recommended (sildenafil, 25 mg every 48 hours; tadalafil, 10 mg every 72 hours; with increased monitoring for adverse events. Vardenafil should not be coadministered with REYATAZ (with and without ritonavir).
H_2-Receptor Antagonists:	↓ atazanavir	Plasma concentrations of atazanavir were substantially decreased when REYATAZ 400 mg once daily was administered simultaneously with famotidine 40 mg twice daily, which may result in loss of therapeutic effect and development of resistance. Although not studied, similar results are expected with other H_2-receptor antagonists. **In treatment-naive patients:** The H_2-receptor antagonist dose should not exceed a 40 mg dose equivalent of famotidine twice daily. REYATAZ 300 mg with ritonavir 100 mg once daily (all as a single dose with food) should be administered simultaneously with, and/or at least 10 hours after, the dose of the H_2-receptor antagonist. **In treatment-experienced patients:** The H_2-receptor antagonist dose should not exceed a dose equivalent to famotidine 20 mg twice daily, and the REYATAZ and ritonavir doses should be administered simultaneously with, and/or at least 10 hours after, the dose of the H_2-receptor antagonist. • REYATAZ 300 mg with ritonavir 100 mg once daily (all as a single dose with food) if taken with an H_2-receptor • REYATAZ 400 mg with ritonavir 100 mg once daily (all as a single dose with food) if taken with both tenofovir and an H_2-receptor antagonist.
HMG-CoA Reductase Inhibitors:	↑ atorvastatin ↑ rosuvastatin	The risk of myopathy including rhabdomyolysis may be increased when protease inhibitors, including REYATAZ, are used in combination with these drugs. Caution should be exercised. Use the lowest possible dose with careful monitoring, or consider other HMG-CoA reductase inhibitors such as pravastatin or fluvastatin in combination with REYATAZ (with and without ritonavir).
Immunosuppressants:	↑cyclosporin, sirolimus, tacrolimus	Therapeutic concentration monitoring is recommended for immunosuppressant agents when coadministered with REYATAZ.

(cont'd)

Table 14: REYATAZ *(cont'd)*

Established and Other Potentially Significant Drug Interactions: Alteration in Dose or Regimen May Be Recommended Based on Drug Interaction Studies or Predicted Interactions

Concomitant Drug Class: Specific Drugs	Effect on Concentration of REYATAZ or Concomitant Drug	Clinical Comment
Inhaled/nasal corticosteroids (interaction with ritonavir):	↑ fluticasone propionate	In healthy volunteers, ritonavir significantly increased plasma fluticasone propionate exposures, resulting in significantly decreased serum cortisol concentrations. Concomitant use of REYATAZ/ritonavir with fluticasone propionate is expected to produce the same effects. Systemic corticosteroid effects including Cushing's syndrome and adrenal suppression have been reported when ritonavir was coadministered with inhaled or intranasally administered fluticasone propionate. These effects could also occur with other corticosteroids metabolized via the cytochrome P450 3A pathway, eg, budesonide. Therefore, concomitant use of REYATAZ/ritonavir and fluticasone propionate or other glucocorticoids that are metabolized by CYP3A4 is not recommended unless the potential benefit of treatment outweighs the risk of systemic corticosteroid effects. Concomitant use of fluticasone propionate and REYATAZ (without ritonavir) may increase plasma concentrations of fluticasone propionate. Use with Caution. Consider alternatives to fluticasone propionate, particularly for long-term use.
Macrolide Antibiotics:	↑ clarithromycin ↓ 14-OH clarithromycin ↑ atazanavir	Increased concentrations of clarithromycin may cause QTc prolongations; therefore, a dose reduction of clarithromycin by 50% should be considered when it is coadministered with REYATAZ. In addition, concentrations of the active metabolite 14-OH clarithromycin are significantly reduced; consider alternative therapy for indications other than infections due to *M. avium* complex. Caution is advised during coadministration as a high incidence of rash (20%) was observed in the pharmacokinetic trial in healthy volunteers. Coadministration of REYATAZ/ritonavir with clarithromycin has not been studied.
Oral Contraceptives: ethinyl estradiol and norgestimate or norethindrone	↑ ethinyl estradiol ↑ norethindrone[c] ↓ ethinyl estradiol ↑ norgestimate[b]	Mean concentrations of ethinyl estradiol and norethindrone, when coadministered with REYATAZ, are increased. Administration of REYATAZ/ritonavir with ethinyl estradiol and norgestimate decreases the mean concentration of ethinyl estradiol, and increases the mean concentration of 17- deacetyl norgestimate, the active metabolite of norgestimate. If an oral contraceptive is administered with REYATAZ plus ritonavir, it is recommended that the oral contraceptive contain at least 30 µg of ethinyl estradiol. If REYATAZ is administered without ritonavir, the oral contraceptive should contain no more that 30 µg of ethinyl estradiol. Use with caution as the effect of increases in concentration of the progestational agent are unknown and could increase the risk of acne, dyslipidemia, and insulin resistance. Coadministration of REYATAZ or REYATAZ /ritonavir with other hormonal contraceptives (eg, contraceptive patch, contraceptive vaginal ring, or injectable contraceptives) or oral contraceptives containing progestagens other than norethindrone or norgestimate, or less than 25 µg of ethinyl estradiol have not been studied; therefore alternative methods of contraception are recommended.

[a] See Table 13 for orally administered midazolam.
[b] In combination with atazanavir 300 mg and ritonavir 100 mg once daily.
[c] In combination with atazanavir 400 mg once daily.

Based on known metabolic profiles, clinically significant drug interactions are not expected between REYATAZ and fluvastatin, pravastatin, dapsone, trimethoprim/sulfamethoxazole, azithromycin or erythromycin. Coadministration of methadone and REYATAZ in subjects chronically treated with methadone did not result in clinically relevant interactions. REYATAZ does not interact with substrates of CYP2D6 (eg, nortriptyline, desipramine, metoprolol). Additionally, no clinically significant drug interaction was observed when REYATAZ was coadministered with fluconazole or acetaminophen.

Refer to Norvir Product Monograph for drug interaction of ritonavir with these drugs before prescribing REYATAZ 300 mg with ritonavir 100 mg.

DOSAGE AND ADMINISTRATION: Recommended Adult Dose: Therapy-Naïve Patients:

- REYATAZ 300 mg once daily taken with ritonavir 100 mg once daily taken with food.

or

- REYATAZ 400 mg (two 200-mg capsules) once daily (without ritonavir) taken with food, for patients who are unable to tolerate ritonavir.

Therapy-Experienced Patients:

- REYATAZ 300 mg once daily taken with ritonavir 100 mg once daily taken with food.

Capsules should not be opened, they should be swallowed whole with water.

Recommended Pediatric Dose (from 6 to 18 years of age): The recommended dosage of REYATAZ for pediatric patients (6 to less than 18 years of age) is based on body weight and should not exceed the recommended adult dosage. REYATAZ Capsules must be taken with food. The data are insufficient to recommend dosing of REYATAZ for any of the following: (1) patients less than 6 years of age, (2) **without ritonavir** in patients less than 13 years of age, and (3) treatment-experienced pediatric patients with body weight less than 25 kg.

Therapy-Naive Pediatric Patients: The recommended dosage of REYATAZ with ritonavir in treatment-naive patients at least 6 years of age is shown in Table 15.

For treatment-naive patients at least 13 years of age and at least 39 kg, who are unable to tolerate ritonavir, the recommended dose is REYATAZ 400 mg (without ritonavir) once daily with food.

Table 15: REYATAZ

Dosage for Treatment-Naive Pediatric Patients (6 to less than 18 years of age) for REYATAZ Capsules with Ritonavir

Body Weight		REYATAZ Dose[a,b]	Ritonavir Dose[b]
(kg)	(lbs)	(mg)	(mg)
15 to less than 25	33 to less than 55	150	80[c]
25 to less than 32	55 to less than 70	200	100[d]
32 to less than 39	70 to less than 86	250	100[d]
at least 39	at least 86	300	100[d]

a The recommended dosage of REYATAZ can be achieved using a combination of commercially available capsule strengths.
b The dosage of REYATAZ and ritonavir was calculated as follows:
• 15 kg to less than 20 kg: REYATAZ 8.5 mg/kg with ritonavir 4 mg/kg once daily with food.
• at least 20 kg: REYATAZ 7 mg/kg with ritonavir 4 mg/kg once daily with food not to exceed REYATAZ 300 mg and ritonavir 100 mg.
c Ritonavir liquid.
d Ritonavir capsule or liquid.

Therapy-Experienced Pediatric Patients: The recommended dosage of REYATAZ with ritonavir in treatment-experienced patients at least 6 years of age is shown in Table 16.

Table 16: REYATAZ

Dosage for Treatment-Experienced Pediatric Patients (6 to less than 18 years of age) for REYATAZ Capsules with Ritonavir

Body Weight		REYATAZ Dose[a,b]	Ritonavir Dose[b]
(kg)	(lbs)	(mg)	(mg)
25 to less than 32	55 to less than 70	200	100[c]
32 to less than 39	70 to less than 86	250	100[c]
at least 39	at least 86	300	100[c]

a The recommended dosage of REYATAZ can be achieved using a combination of commercially available capsule strengths.
b The dosage was calculated as REYATAZ 7 mg/kg with ritonavir 4 mg/kg once daily with food not to exceed REYATAZ 300 mg and ritonavir 100 mg.
c Ritonavir capsule or liquid.

Dosing Considerations: Concomitant Therapy: (See Warnings and Precautions and Drug Interactions.)
Ritonavir: There are limited safety data from controlled trials for REYATAZ plus ritonavir regimens without tenofovir. (See Warnings and Precautions and Drug Interactions.)
Efavirenz—Therapy-Naive Patients: If REYATAZ is combined with efavirenz, REYATAZ 400 mg (two 200 mg capsules) with ritonavir 100 mg should be administered once daily all as a single dose with food, and efavirenz should be administered on an empty stomach, preferably at bedtime.
Efavirenz—Therapy-Experienced Patients: Do not coadminister REYATAZ with efavirenz in treatment-experienced patients due to decreased atazanavir exposure.
Didanosine: When coadministered with didanosine buffered formulations, REYATAZ should be given (with food) two hours before or one hour after didanosine.
Tenofovir DF: If coadministered with tenofovir DF, it is recommended that 300 mg of REYATAZ and ritonavir 100 mg be given with tenofovir 300 mg (together as single daily doses with food). There are limited safety data from controlled trials for REYATAZ plus ritonavir regimens without tenofovir. REYATAZ without ritonavir should not be coadministered with tenofovir. (See Drug Interactions.)
Recommended Dose and Dosage Adjustment: Patients with Renal Impairment: For patients with renal impairment, including those with severe renal impairment who are not managed with hemodialysis, no dose adjustment is required for REYATAZ. Treatment-naive patients with end stage renal disease managed with hemodialysis should receive REYATAZ 300 mg with ritonavir 100 mg. REYATAZ, with or without ritonavir, **should not be used in antiretroviral-treatment experienced patients with end stage renal disease managed with hemodialysis**. REYATAZ without ritonavir should not be administered to patients managed with hemodialysis (see Warnings and Precautions and Action and Clinical Pharmacology, Special Populations and Conditions).
Patients with Hepatic Impairment: REYATAZ should be used with caution in patients with mild-to-moderate hepatic impairment. For patients with moderate hepatic impairment (Child-Pugh Class B) who have not experienced prior virologic failure, a dose reduction to 300 mg once daily should be considered. REYATAZ should not be used in patients with severe hepatic impairment (Child-Pugh Class C). REYATAZ/ritonavir has not been studied in subjects with hepatic impairment and is not recommended. (See Warnings and Precautions, Hepatic/Biliary/Pancreatic.)
Missed Dose: If a dose of REYATAZ is missed, patients should take the dose as soon as possible and then return to their normal schedule. However, if a dose is skipped, the patient should not double the next dose.

OVERDOSAGE:

Administration of activated charcoal may be used to aid in removal of unabsorbed drug. Treatment of overdosage with atazanavir should consist of general supportive measures, including monitoring of vital signs and ECG, and observations of the patient's clinical status. There is no specific antidote for overdose with atazanavir. Since atazanavir is extensively metabolized by the liver and is highly protein bound, dialysis is unlikely to be beneficial in significant removal of this medicine.

Human experience of acute overdose with atazanavir is limited. Single doses up to 1200 mg have been taken by healthy volunteers without symptomatic untoward effects. A single self-administered overdose of 58.4 g of atazanavir in an HIV-infected patient (146 times the 400 mg recommended dose) was associated with asymptomatic bilateral bundle branch block and PR interval prolongation. These events resolved spontaneously. At high doses that lead to high drug exposures, jaundice due to indirect (unconjugated) hyperbilirubinemia (without associated liver function test changes) or cardiac conduction abnormalities, including PR and/or QT interval prolongations, may be observed. (See Warnings and Precautions, Cardiovascular.)

For management of a suspected drug overdose, contact your regional Poison Control Centre. See the *CPS* Directory section for a list of Poison Control Centres.

ACTION AND CLINICAL PHARMACOLOGY: Mechanism of Action: REYATAZ (atazanavir) is an azapeptide HIV-1 protease inhibitor. The compound selectively inhibits the virus-specific processing of viral Gag and Gag-Pol polyproteins in HIV-1 infected cells, thus preventing formation of mature virions.
Pharmacokinetics: The pharmacokinetics of atazanavir were evaluated in healthy adult volunteers and in HIV-infected patients, after administration of REYATAZ 400 mg once daily and after administration of REYATAZ 300 mg with ritonavir 100 mg once daily (see Table 17).

Table 17: REYATAZ

Steady-State Pharmacokinetics of Atazanavir in Healthy Subjects or HIV-Infected Patients in the Fed State

Parameter	400 mg Once Daily		300 mg with Ritonavir 100 mg Once Daily	
	Healthy Subjects (n=14)	HIV-Infected Patients (n=13)	Healthy Subject (n=28)	HIV-Infected Patients (n=10)
C_{max} (ng/mL)				
Geometric mean (CV%)	5199 (26)	2298 (71)	6129 (31)	4422 (58)
Mean (SD)	5358 (1371)	3152 (2231)	6450 (2031)	5233 (3033)
T_{max} (h)				
Median	2.5	2.0	2.7	3.0
AUC (ng·h/mL)				
Geometric mean (CV%)	28132 (28)	14874 (91)	57039 (37)	46073 (66)
Mean (SD)	29303 (8263)	22262 (20159)	61435 (22911)	53761 (35294)
T-half (h)				
Mean (SD)	7.9 (2.9)	6.5 (2.6)	18.1 (6.2)[a]	8.6 (2.3)
C_{min} (ng/mL)				
Geometric mean (CV%)	159 (88)	120 (109)	1227 (53)	636 (97)
Mean (SD)	218 (191)	273 (298)[b]	1441 (757)	862 (838)

a n=26.
b n=12.

Absorption: Atazanavir is rapidly absorbed with a T_{max} of approximately 2.5 hours. Atazanavir demonstrates nonlinear pharmacokinetics with greater than dose-proportional increases in AUC and C_{max} values over the dose range of 200-800 mg once daily. Steady-state is achieved between Days 4 and 8, with an accumulation of approximately 2.3-fold.

Figure 1 displays the mean plasma concentrations of atazanavir on Day 29 (steady state) following atazanavir 400 mg once daily (as two 200-mg capsules) with a light meal and after atazanavir 300 mg (as two 150-mg capsules) with ritonavir 100 mg once daily with a light meal in HIV-infected adult patients.

Figure 1: REYATAZ

Mean (SD) Steady-state Plasma Concentrations of Atazanavir 400-mg (n=13) and 300 mg with Ritonavir (n=10) for HIV-infected Adult Patients

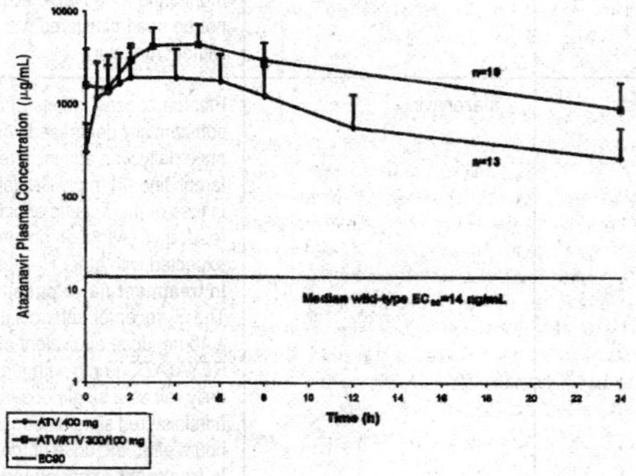

Food Effect: Administration of a single 400-mg dose of atazanavir with a light meal (357 kcal, 8.2 g fat, 10.6 g protein) resulted in a 70% increase in AUC and 57% increase in C_{max} relative to the fasting state. Administration of a single 400-mg dose of atazanavir with a high fat meal (721 kcal, 37.3 g fat, 29.4 g protein) resulted in a mean increase in AUC of 35% with no change in C_{max} relative to the fasting state. Administration of REYATAZ with either a light meal or high-fat meal decreased the coefficient of variation of AUC and C_{max} by approximately one half compared to the fasting state. Thus, REYATAZ is taken with food in order to enhance its bioavailability and reduce the pharmacokinetic variability.

Coadministration of REYATAZ and ritonavir with food optimizes the bioavailability of atazanavir. Coadministration of a single 300-mg dose of REYATAZ and a 100-mg dose of ritonavir with a light meal (336 total kcal, 5.1 g fat, 9.3 g protein and 63.3 g carbohydrates) resulted in a 33% increase in the AUC and a 40% increase in both the C_{max} and the 24-hour concentration of atazanavir relative to the fasting state. Coadministration with a high-fat meal (951 total kcal, 54.7 g fat, 35.9 g protein and 77.9 g carbohydrates) did not affect the AUC of atazanavir relative to fasting conditions and the C_{max} was within 11% of fasting values. The 24-hour concentration following a high-fat meal was increased by approximately 33% due to delayed absorption; the median T_{max} increased from 2.0 to 5.0 hours. Coadministration of REYATAZ with ritonavir with either a light or a high-fat meal decreased the coefficient of variation of AUC and C_{max} by approximately 25% compared to the fasting state.
Distribution: Atazanavir is 86% bound to human serum proteins and protein binding is independent of concentration. Atazanavir binds to both alpha-1-acid glycoprotein (AAG) and albumin to a similar extent (89% and 86%, respectively). In a multiple-dose study in HIV-infected patients dosed with atazanavir 400 mg once daily with a light meal for 12 weeks, atazanavir was detected in the cerebrospinal fluid and semen. The cerebrospinal fluid/plasma ratio for atazanavir (n=4) ranged between 0.0021 and 0.0226 and seminal fluid/plasma ratio (n=5) ranged between 0.11 and 4.42.
Metabolism: Studies in humans and in vitro studies using human liver microsomes have demonstrated that atazanavir is principally metabolized by CYP3A4 isozyme to oxygenated metabolites, which are then excreted in the bile as either free or glucuronidated metabolites. Additional minor metabolic pathways consist of N-dealkylation, hydrolysis and oxygenation with dehydrogenation.

Two minor metabolites of atazanavir in plasma have been characterized. Neither metabolite demonstrated in vitro antiviral activity.

Elimination: Following a single 400-mg dose of ^{14}C-atazanavir, 79% and 13% of the total radioactivity was recovered in the feces and urine, respectively. Unchanged drug accounted for approximately 20% and 7% of the administered dose in the feces and urine, respectively. The mean elimination half-life of atazanavir in healthy volunteers (n=214) and HIV-infected adult patients (n=13) was approximately 7 hours at steady state following a dose of 400 mg daily with a light meal.

Electrocardiogram: Effect on PR and QT Intervals: Concentration-and dose-dependent prolongation of the PR interval in the electrocardiogram has been observed in healthy volunteers receiving atazanavir. In a placebo-controlled study (AI424-076), the mean (+/−SD) maximum change in PR interval from the pre-dose value was 24 (+ /−15 msec) following oral dosing with 400 mg of atazanavir (n=65) compared to 13 (+11 msec) following dosing with placebo (n=67). The PR interval prolongations in this study were asymptomatic. There is limited information on the potential for pharmacodynamic interaction in humans between atazanavir and other drugs that prolong the PR interval of the electrocardiogram (see Warnings and Precautions).

Electrocardiographic effects of atazanavir were determined in a clinical pharmacology study of 72 healthy subjects. Oral doses of 400 mg and 800 mg were compared with placebo; there was no concentration-dependent effect of atazanavir on the QTc interval (using Fridericia's correction). In 1793 HIV-infected patients receiving antiretroviral regimens, QTc prolongation was comparable in the atazanavir and comparator regimens. No atazanavir-treated healthy subject or HIV-infected patient had a QTc interval >500 msec.

Special Populations and Conditions: Age/Gender/Race: A study of the pharmacokinetics of atazanavir was performed in young (n=29; 18-40 years) and elderly (n=30; ≥65 years) healthy subjects. There were no clinically important pharmacokinetic differences observed due to age or gender. There are insufficient data to determine whether there are any effects of race on the pharmacokinetics of atazanavir.

Pediatrics (from 6 to 18 years of age): The pharmacokinetic data from pediatric patients receiving REYATAZ Capsules with ritonavir based on body surface area are presented in Table 18.

Table 18: REYATAZ

Steady-State Pharmacokinetics of Atazanavir with Ritonavir in HIV Infected Pediatric Patients (6 to 18 years of age) in the Fed State

	205 mg/m² Atazanavir with 100 mg/m² Ritonavir Once Daily	
	Age Range (years)	
	At least 6 to 13 (n=17)	At least 13 to 18 (n=10)
Dose mg		
Median [min-max]	200 [150–400]	400 [250–500]
C_{max} ng/mL		
Geometric Mean (CV%)	4451 (33)	3711 (46)
AUC ng·h/mL		
Geometric Mean (CV%)	42 503 (36)	44 970 (34)
C_{min} ng/mL		
Geometric Mean (CV%)	535 (62)	1090 (60)

Renal Insufficiency: In healthy subjects, approximately 7% of the dose of atazanavir is eliminated unchanged in the urine. REYATAZ has been studied in adult subjects with severe renal impairment (n=20), including those on hemodialysis, at multiple doses of 400 mg once daily. The mean atazanavir C_{max} was 9% lower, AUC was 19% higher, and C_{min} was 96% higher in subjects with severe renal impairment not undergoing hemodialysis (n=10), than in age, weight, and gender matched subjects with normal renal function. Atazanavir was not appreciably cleared during hemodialysis. In a 4-hour dialysis session, 2.1% of the administered dose was removed. Subjects on hemodialysis appeared to display lower exposures as compared to healthy subjects and renally impaired subjects without hemodialysis. The geometric means for ATV AUC, C_{max} and C_{min}, for REYATAZ administered immediately following dialysis in subjects on hemodialysis (n=10) were 42%, 37% and 54% lower, respectively, relative to subjects with normal renal function. When REYATAZ was administered 2 hours before a 4 hour hemodialysis session, the geometric means for ATV AUC, C_{max} and C_{min} in hemodialysis subjects were 28%, 25% and 43% lower, respectively, than subjects with normal renal function. The mechanism of this decrease is unknown. (See Dosage and Administration.)

Hepatic Insufficiency: Atazanavir is metabolized and eliminated primarily by the liver. Atazanavir has been studied in adult patients with moderate to severe hepatic impairment (14 Child-Pugh B and 2 Child-Pugh C) after a single 400-mg dose. The mean AUC(0-∞) was 42% greater in patients with impaired hepatic function than in healthy volunteers. The mean half-life of atazanavir in hepatically impaired patients was 12.1 hours compared to 6.4 hours in healthy volunteers. Increased concentrations of atazanavir are expected in patients with moderately or severely impaired hepatic function. The pharmacokinetics of REYATAZ in combination with ritonavir have not been studied in subjects with hepatic impairment. REYATAZ should not be administered to patients with severe hepatic impairment. REYATAZ/ritonavir is not recommended for use in patients with hepatic impairment (see Warnings and Precautions and Dosage and Administration).

STORAGE AND STABILITY: REYATAZ capsules should be stored at 25°C excursions permitted to 15-30°C. Protect from moisture.

INFORMATION FOR THE PATIENT: Published in e-CPS, available by subscription at www.e-cps.ca.

DOSAGE FORMS, COMPOSITION AND PACKAGING: 150 mg: Each blue opaque cap and powder-blue opaque body, hard gelatin capsule, printed in white with "BMS", "150 mg", and in blue "3624", contains: atazanavir sulfate equivalent to 150 mg of atazanavir. Nonmedicinal ingredients: crospovidone, lactose monohydrate and magnesium stearate; capsule shell: FD&C Blue #2, gelatin and titanium dioxide. HDPE bottles of 60.

200 mg: Each blue opaque cap and body, hard gelatin capsule, printed in white with "BMS", "200 mg", and "3631", contains: atazanavir sulfate equivalent to 200 mg of atazanavir. Nonmedicinal ingredients: crospovidone, lactose monohydrate and magnesium stearate; capsule shell: FD&C Blue #2, gelatin and titanium dioxide. HDPE bottles of 60.

300 mg: Each red opaque cap and blue opaque body, hard gelatin capsule, printed in white with "BMS", "300 mg", and "3622", contains: atazanavir sulfate equivalent to 300 mg of atazanavir. Nonmedicinal ingredients: crospovidone, lactose monohydrate and magnesium stearate; capsule shell: black iron oxide, FD&C Blue #2, gelatin, red iron oxide, titanium dioxide and yellow iron oxide. HDPE bottles of 30.

(Shown in Product Identification Section)

Rhinaris® CS Anti-allergic

sodium cromoglycate

Seasonal Rhinitis Prophylaxis—Antiallergic

PendoPharm

Rhinaris® Lubricating Nasal Gel/Nasal Mist

polyethylene glycol—propylene glycol

Dry Nose—Rhinitis Therapy

PendoPharm

Rhinaris® Saline Pediatric Drops/Saline Spray—Daily Hygiene

sodium chloride

Nasal Lubricant

PendoPharm

Rhinaris® Sinus

sodium chloride

Nasal Rinse

PendoPharm

SUPPLIED: Anti-allergic Nasal Mist: The metered dose pump delivers approximately 0.13 mL of the 2% (w/v) solution or sodium cromoglycate 2.6 mg per spray mist. Nonmedicinal ingredients: benzalkonium chloride, edetate disodium and purified water. Plastic bottles of 13 and 26 mL with a metered dose pump attached to the bottle.

Lubricating Nasal Gel: Each g of gel contains: polyethylene glycol 15% and propylene glycol 20%. pH: 5.5. Nonmedicinal ingredients: benzalkonium chloride, carbopol 934P, carboxel X-395-F, potassium chloride, sodium chloride, sodium hydroxide and water. Tubes of 5 and 30 g.

Lubricating Nasal Mist: Each mL of solution contains: polyethylene glycol 15% and propylene glycol 5%. pH: 6. Nonmedicinal ingredients: benzalkonium chloride, dibasic sodium phosphate, monobasic potassium phosphate, potassium chloride, sodium chloride and water. Plastic bottles of 30 mL fitted with a metered pump (also available for pediatric purposes).

Saline Pediatric Drops: Each mL of solution contains: 0.9% sodium chloride solution. Nonmedicinal ingredients: benzalkonium chloride and water. Plastic bottles of 45 mL, dropper included.

Saline Spray: Each mL of solution contains: 0.9% sodium chloride solution. Nonmedicinal ingredients: benzalkonium chloride and water. Plastic squeeze bottles of 45 mL.

Saline Nasal Rinse: Solution contains: sodium chloride solution. Nonmedicinal ingredients : benzethonium chloride, phosphoric acid, purified water, sodium bicarbonate, sodium biphosphate and trisodium EDTA. Ready to use plastic bottles nasal wash systems of 420 mL and refill plastic bottles of 840 mL.

Rhinaris® Nozoil®

sesame oil

Nasal Lubricant

PendoPharm

SUPPLIED: Each bottle of nasal spray contains: purified sesame oil 100%. Bottles of 10 mL. Store at room temperature (15-25°C) and away from direct light.

Rhinaris® Sinomarin®

sea water

Nasal Cleanser

PendoPharm

SUPPLIED: Each nasal spray bottle contains: sterilized sea water (70%) and purified water (30%), equivalent to 2.3% sea salt. Inert propellant gas: nitrogen, which is not in contact with the product. Nasal spray bottles of 125 mL with anatomically designed nasal applicator, available in adult and children formats. Do not expose the bottle to temperatures above 50°C or to sunlight.

The reader is invited to consult CPhA's monograph **Corticosteroids: Eye, Ear, Nose**.

Rhinocort® Aqua™ Pr

budesonide

Glucocorticosteroid

AstraZeneca

Date of Preparation: January 19, 2000
Date of Revision: December 23, 2008

PHARMACOLOGY: RHINOCORT AQUA (budesonide) contains budesonide which is a potent synthetic glucocorticosteroid with strong topical and weak systemic effects.

RHINOCORT AQUA has a high topical anti-inflammatory potency and it is rapidly biotransformed in the liver. This favourable separation between topical anti-inflammatory activity and systemic effect is due to strong glucocorticosteroid receptor affinity and an effective first pass metabolism with a short half-life. The mechanism of action of intranasally administered budesonide has not yet been completely defined.

Pharmacokinetics: The systemic availability of oral budesonide in man is low (about 10%). With reference to the metered dose the systemic availability of budesonide from RHINOCORT AQUA is 33%. After application of budesonide in solution directly on the nasal mucosa, all the dose is systemically available, indicating that budesonide does not undergo local metabolism in the nose.

The maximal plasma concentration after administration of 256 µg budesonide from RHINOCORT AQUA is 0.64 nmol/L and is reached within 0.7 hours.

INDICATIONS: The treatment of seasonal allergic and allergic/non-allergic perennial and vasomotor rhinitis unresponsive to conventional therapy. Also indicated for the treatment of nasal polyps and in the prevention of nasal polyps after polypectomy.

CONTRAINDICATIONS: Hypersensitivity to any of the nasal spray's components. Active or quiescent tuberculosis. Untreated fungal, bacterial, or viral infections. Children under 6 years of age.

WARNINGS: In patients previously on prolonged periods or high doses of systemic steroids, withdrawal of steroids may cause symptoms such as tiredness, aches and pains, and depression. In severe cases, adrenal insufficiency may occur necessitating a temporary resumption of systemic steroids.

Careful attention must be given to patients with asthma or other clinical conditions in whom a rapid decrease in systemic steroids may cause a severe exacerbation of their symptoms.

Pregnancy: See Precautions.

PRECAUTIONS: Glucocorticosteroids may mask some signs of infection and new infections may appear during their use.

In transferring patients from a systemic steroid to RHINOCORT AQUA (budesonide), the reduction of the systemic steroid must be very gradual and carefully supervised by the physician since systemic withdrawal symptoms (e.g., joint and/or muscular pain, lassitude, depression) may occur in spite of maintenance or improvement of respiratory functions (see Dosage).

Patients should be informed that the full effect of RHINOCORT AQUA therapy is not achieved until 2 to 3 days of treatment have been completed. In rare cases the full effect of RHINOCORT AQUA therapy is not achieved until 2 weeks of treatment have been completed. Treatment of seasonal rhinitis should, if possible, start before the exposure to allergens.

Treatment with RHINOCORT AQUA should not be stopped abruptly but tapered off gradually.

Special care is needed in patients with fungal and viral nasal infections. Children who are on immunosuppressant drugs are more susceptible to infections than healthy children. Chicken pox and measles, for example, can have a more serious or fatal course in children on immunosuppressant corticosteroids. In such children, or in adults who have not had these diseases, particular care should be taken to avoid exposure. If exposed, therapy with varicella zoster immune globulin (VZIG) or pooled intravenous immunoglobulin (IVIG), as appropriate, may be indicated. If chicken pox develops, treatment with antiviral agents may be considered.

Concomitant treatment may sometimes be required to counteract eye symptoms caused by allergy.

The long term effects of budesonide in human subjects are still unknown, in particular, its local effects, and on developmental or immunologic processes. The nasal mucosa of those patients receiving long term, continuous therapy should be inspected at least twice a year. The possibility of atrophic rhinitis and/or pharyngeal candidiasis should be kept in mind.

Children: Until greater clinical experience has been gained, the continuous, long-term treatment of children is not recommended.

When budesonide is administered intranasally, the following should be kept in mind:

Glucocorticosteroid effects may be enhanced in patients with hypothyroidism and in those with cirrhosis. Reduced liver function may affect the elimination of corticosteroids. The intravenous pharmacokinetics of budesonide however, are similar in cirrhotic patients and in healthy subjects. The pharmacokinetics after oral ingestion of budesonide were affected by compromised liver function as evidenced by increased systemic availability. This is however, of limited clinical importance for RHINOCORT AQUA, as the oral contribution to the systemic availability is relatively small.

In hypoprothrombinemia, salicylates should be used cautiously in conjunction with glucocorticosteroids.

Because of the inhibitory effect of corticosteroids on wound healing in patients who have had recent nasal surgery or trauma, a nasal corticosteroid should be used with caution until healing has occurred.

Pregnancy: In experimental animal studies, budesonide was found to cross the placental barrier. Like other glucocorticosteroids, budesonide is teratogenic to rodent species. High doses of budesonide administered subcutaneously produced fetal malformations, primarily skeletal defects, in rabbits, rats, and in mice. Results from world-wide post marketing experience indicate inhaled budesonide during pregnancy has no adverse effects on the health of the fetus/new born child. Review of published literature of orally inhaled budesonide, including results from a large case control study performed with cases identified from 3 Swedish health registers showed that there was no association between exposure to inhaled budesonide and overall congenital malformations. Results from a similar study performed with intranasal budesonide, using the same 3 Swedish health registers showed that the use of intranasal budesonide was associated with a subgroup "less severe cardiovascular defects"; however there was no statistically significant association between the use of intranasal budesonide during pregnancy and overall congenital malformations, or overall frequency of cardiovascular defects in the offspring. Budesonide should be used during pregnancy only if the potential benefits clearly outweigh the risk to the fetus. Infants born of mothers who have received substantial doses of corticosteroids, especially oral steroids, during pregnancy should be carefully observed for hypoadrenalism.

Lactation: Budesonide is excreted in breast milk. The administration of RHINOCORT AQUA to women who are breastfeeding should only be considered if the expected benefit to the mother is greater than any possible risk to the child.

Children Under 6 Years of Age: RHINOCORT AQUA is not presently recommended for children younger than 6 years of age due to limited clinical data in this age group.

Glucocorticosteroids may mask some signs of infections and new infections may appear. A decreased resistance to localized infection has been observed during glucocorticosteroid therapy. During long-term therapy, pituitary-adrenal function, hematological status and height (in children) should be periodically assessed.

Patients should be advised to inform subsequent physicians of the prior use of glucocorticosteroids.

To ensure the proper dosage and administration of the drug, the patient should be instructed by a physician or other health professional in the use of RHINOCORT AQUA (see Information for the Patient).

Dose-related suppression of plasma and urinary cortisol has been observed in healthy volunteers after short-term administration of RHINOCORT AQUA. Although no important changes in basal plasma cortisol levels were manifested in patients with rhinitis using RHINOCORT AQUA at recommended doses, caution is advised.

Drug Interactions: To date budesonide has not been observed to interact with other drugs used for the treatment of rhinitis.

Cimetidine: The kinetics of budesonide were investigated in a study in healthy subjects without and with cimetidine, 1000 mg daily. After a 4 mg oral dose the values for C_{max} (nmol/L) and systemic availability (%) of budesonide without and with cimetidine (3.3 vs 5.1 nmol/L and 10 vs 12%, respectively) indicated a slight inhibitory effect on hepatic metabolism of budesonide, caused by cimetidine. This should be of little clinical importance.

Ketoconazole: The metabolism of budesonide is primarily mediated by CYP3A4, a subfamily of cytochrome P450. CYP3A4 inhibitors like ritonavir and azole antifungals (e.g. ketoconazole and itraconazole) increase the systemic exposure to budesonide. Therefore, concomitant use of budesonide and ritonavir or azole antifungals should be avoided unless the potential benefit outweighs the risk of systemic corticosteroids side-effects.

Omeprazole: At recommended doses, omeprazole has no effect on the pharmacokinetics of oral budesonide.

ADVERSE EFFECTS: The adverse reactions reported with RHINOCORT AQUA (budesonide) are consistent with what one would expect when applying a topical treatment to an already inflamed membrane. All side effects were transient. The most commonly reported side effects include: nasal and throat irritation, nasal bleeding and crusting. Other adverse events reported are itching throat, sore throat, cough, fatigue, nausea/dizziness, and headache. When patients are transferred to RHINOCORT AQUA from a systemic steroid, allergic conditions such as asthma or eczema may be unmasked. Uncommon side effects such as immediate and delayed hypersensitivity reactions (urticaria, rash, dermatitis, angioedema, pruritus etc.) may occur in association with local corticosteroid therapy. Very rare cases of anaphylactic reaction have been reported following the use of RHINOCORT AQUA. Additionally, very rare cases of ulcerations of the mucous membranes and nasal septal perforation have been reported following the use of intranasal corticosteroids.

OVERDOSE:

Symptoms: Like any other nasally administered corticosteroid, acute overdosing is unlikely in view of the total amount of active ingredient present. However, when used chronically in excessive doses or in conjunction with other corticosteroid formulations, systemic corticosteroid effects such as hypercorticism and adrenal suppression may appear. If such changes recur, the dosage of RHINOCORT AQUA (budesonide) should be discontinued slowly consistent with accepted procedures for discontinuation of chronic steroid therapy (see Dosage).

The restoration of the hypothalamic-pituitary-axis may be a slow process and during periods with pronounced physical stress such as severe infections, trauma, and surgical operations, a supplement with systemic steroids may be advisable.

Treatment: See Symptoms.

For management of a suspected drug overdose, CPhA recommends that you contact your **regional Poison Control Centre**. See the *CPS* Directory section for a list of Poison Control Centres.

DOSAGE: See Warnings.

Careful attention must be given to patients previously treated for prolonged periods with systemic corticosteroids when transferred to RHINOCORT AQUA (budesonide). Initially, RHINOCORT AQUA and the systemic corticosteroid must be given concomitantly, while the dose of the latter is gradually decreased. The usual rate of withdrawal of the systemic steroid is the equivalent of 2.5 mg of prednisone every four days if the patient is under close supervision. If continuous supervision is not feasible, the withdrawal of the systemic steroid should be slower, approximately 2.5 mg of prednisone (or equivalent) every ten days. If withdrawal symptoms appear, the previous dose of the systemic steroid should be resumed for a week before further decrease is attempted.

Rhinitis: Adults and Children Over 6 Years : Initially: The recommended starting dose is 256 µg daily. The dose can be administered once daily in the morning or divided into two administrations morning and evening. For example: 128 µg (2 sprays) into each nostril in the morning or, 64 µg (1 spray) into each nostril morning and evening.

Maintenance: After the desired clinical effect is obtained, the maintenance dose should be reduced to the smallest amount necessary to control the symptoms.

Treatment or Prevention of Nasal Polyps: The recommended dose is 64 µg (1 spray) into each nostril morning and evening (total daily dose is 256 µg).

Children Under 6 Years: Not recommended for children in this age group.

Patients should be informed that the full effect of RHINOCORT AQUA therapy may not become evident until 2 to 3 days of treatment have been completed. Full therapeutic benefit requires regular usage. Explain the absence of an immediate effect to the patient in order to ensure cooperation and continuation of the treatment with a regular dosage regime. Treatment of seasonal rhinitis should, if possible, start before exposure to the allergens. Concomitant treatment may sometimes be necessary to counteract eye symptoms caused by the allergy. In continuous long-term treatment, the nasal mucosa should be inspected regularly, e.g., every 6 months.

If the nasal passages are severely blocked, the drug may fail to reach the site of action. In such cases, a course of oral steroids or decongestants may be required before initiating RHINOCORT AQUA therapy.

Although systemic effects are negligible at recommended doses, RHINOCORT AQUA treatment should not be continued beyond three weeks in the absence of significant symptomatic improvement. RHINOCORT AQUA should not be used in the presence of untreated localized infections involving the nasal mucosa.

INFORMATION FOR THE PATIENT: Published in e-CPS, available by subscription at www.e-cps.ca.

SUPPLIED: Each dose of white to off-white, thixotropic suspension contains: budesonide 64 µg in water. Nonmedicinal ingredients: carboxymethylcellulose sodium, disodium edetate, glucose anhydrous, hydrochloric acid, microcrystalline cellulose, polysorbate 80, potassium sorbate and purified water. Amber glass bottles of 120 doses, provided with a pump spray mechanism, nasal adapter and patient instruction leaflet. Store at room temperature (15-30°C).

(Shown in Product Identification Section)

The reader is invited to consult CPhA's monograph **Corticosteroids: Eye, Ear, Nose**.

Rhinocort® Turbuhaler®

budesonide

Glucocorticosteroid

AstraZeneca

Date of Preparation: January 19, 2000
Date of Revision: December 23, 2008

PHARMACOLOGY: RHINOCORT TURBUHALER contains pure budesonide which is a potent synthetic glucocorticosteroid with strong topical and weak systemic effects.

RHINOCORT TURBUHALER has a high topical anti-inflammatory potency and it is rapidly biotransformed in the liver. This favourable separation between topical anti-inflammatory activity and systemic effect is due to strong glucocorticosteroid receptor affinity and an effective first-pass metabolism with a short half-life. The mechanism of action of intranasally administered budesonide has not yet been completely defined.

Pharmacokinetics: The systemic availability of oral budesonide in man is low (about 10%). With reference to the metered dose, the systemic availability of budesonide from RHINOCORT TURBUHALER is 22%. After application of budesonide in solution directly on the nasal mucosa, all the dose is systemically available, indicating that budesonide does not undergo local metabolism in the nose.

The maximal plasma concentration after administration of 800 µg budesonide from RHINOCORT TURBUHALER is 1.1 nmol/L and is reached within 0.4 hours.

INDICATIONS: The treatment of seasonal allergic and allergic/non-allergic perennial and vasomotor rhinitis unresponsive to conventional therapy. Also indicated for the treatment of nasal polyps and the prevention of nasal polyps after polypectomy.

CONTRAINDICATIONS: Hypersensitivity to budesonide. Active or quiescent tuberculosis. Untreated fungal, bacterial or viral infections. Children under 6 years of age.

WARNINGS: In patients previously on prolonged periods or high doses of systemic steroids, withdrawal of steroids may cause symptoms such as tiredness, aches and pains, and depression. In severe cases, adrenal insufficiency may occur necessitating a temporary resumption of systemic steroids.

Careful attention must be given to patients with asthma or other clinical conditions in whom a rapid decrease in systemic steroids may cause a severe exacerbation of their symptoms.

Pregnancy: See Precautions.

PRECAUTIONS: In transferring patients from a systemic steroid to RHINOCORT TURBUHALER, the reduction of the systemic steroid must be very gradual and carefully supervised by the physician since systemic withdrawal symptoms (e.g., joint and/or muscular pain, lassitude, depression) may occur in spite of maintenance or improvement of respiratory functions (see Dosage).

Patients should be informed that the full effect of RHINOCORT TURBUHALER therapy is not achieved until 2 to 3 days of treatment have been completed. In rare cases the full effect of RHINOCORT TURBUHALER therapy is not achieved until 2 weeks of treatment have been completed. Treatment of seasonal rhinitis should, if possible, start before the exposure to allergens.

During long-term therapy, pituitary-adrenal function, hematological status and height (in children) should be periodically assessed.

Treatment with RHINOCORT TURBUHALER should not be stopped abruptly but tapered off gradually.

Glucocorticosteroids may mask some signs of infection and new infections may appear during their use. A decreased resistance to localized infections has been observed during glucocorticosteroid therapy; this may require treatment with appropriate therapy or stopping the administration of RHINOCORT TURBUHALER.

Special care is needed in patients with fungal and viral nasal infections. Children who are on immunosuppressant drugs are more susceptible to infections than healthy children. Chicken pox and measles, for example, can have a more serious or fatal course in children on immunosuppressant corticosteroids. In such children, or in adults who have not had these diseases, particular care should be taken to avoid exposure. If exposed, therapy with varicella zoster immune globulin (VZIG) or pooled intravenous immunoglobulin (IVIG), as appropriate, may be indicated. If chicken pox develops, treatment with antiviral agents may be considered.

Concomitant treatment may sometimes be required to counteract eye symptoms caused by allergy.

The long-term effects of RHINOCORT TURBUHALER are still unknown, in particular, its local effects; the possibility of atrophic rhinitis and/or pharyngeal candidiasis should be kept in mind.

Children: Until greater clinical experience has been gained, the continuous, long-term treatment of children is not recommended.

When budesonide is administered intranasally, the following should be kept in mind: (a) Glucocorticosteroid effects may be enhanced in patients with hypothyroidism and in those with cirrhosis. Reduced liver function may affect the elimination of corticosteroids. The intravenous pharmacokinetics of budesonide however, are similar in cirrhotic patients and in healthy subjects. The pharmacokinetics after oral ingestion of budesonide were affected by compromised liver function as evidenced by increased systemic availability. This is however, of limited clinical importance for RHINOCORT TURBUHALER, as after inhalation, the oral contribution to the systemic availability is relatively small. (b) In hypoprothrombinemia, salicylates should be used cautiously in conjunction with glucocorticosteroids.

Because of the inhibitory effect of corticosteroids on wound healing in patients who have had recent nasal surgery or trauma, a nasal corticosteroid should be used with caution until healing has occurred.

Pregnancy: In experimental animal studies, budesonide was found to cross the blood-placenta barrier. Like other glucocorticosteroids, budesonide is teratogenic to rodent species. High doses of budesonide administered subcutaneously produced fetal malformations, primarily skeletal defects, in rabbits, rats, and in mice. Results from world-wide post marketing experience indicate inhaled budesonide during pregnancy has no adverse effects on the health of the fetus/new born child. Review of published literature of orally inhaled budesonide, including results from a large case control study performed with cases identified from 3 Swedish health registers showed that there was no association between exposure to inhaled budesonide and overall congenital malformations. Results from a similar study performed with intranasal budesonide, using the same 3 Swedish health registers showed that the use of intranasal budesonide was associated with a subgroup "less severe cardiovascular defects"; however there was no statistically significant association between the use of intranasal budesonide during pregnancy and overall congenital malformations, or overall frequency of cardiovascular defects in the offspring. Budesonide should be used during pregnancy only if the potential benefits clearly outweigh the risk to the fetus. Infants born of mothers who have received substantial doses of corticosteroids, especially oral steroids, during pregnancy should be carefully observed for hypoadrenalism.

Lactation: Budesonide is excreted in breast milk. The administration of RHINOCORT TURBUHALER to women who are breastfeeding should only be considered if the expected benefit to the mother is greater than any possible risk to the child.

Children Under 6 Years of Age: RHINOCORT TURBUHALER is not presently recommended for children younger than 6 years of age due to limited clinical data in this age group.

Patients should be advised to inform subsequent physicians of the prior use of glucocorticosteroids.

Dose-related suppression of plasma and urinary cortisol has been observed in healthy volunteers after short-term administration of RHINOCORT TURBUHALER. Although no important changes in basal plasma cortisol levels were manifested in patients with rhinitis using RHINOCORT TURBUHALER at recommended doses, caution is advised.

To ensure the proper dosage and administration of the drug, the patient should be instructed by a physician or other health professional in the use of RHINOCORT TURBUHALER (see Information for the Patient).

Drug Interactions: To date budesonide has not been observed to interact with other drugs used for the treatment of rhinitis.

Cimetidine: The kinetics of budesonide were investigated in a study in healthy subjects without and with cimetidine, 1000 mg daily. After a 4 mg oral dose the values for C_{max} (nmol/L) and systemic availability (%) of budesonide without and with cimetidine (3.3 vs 5.1 nmol/L and 10 vs 12%, respectively) indicated a slight inhibitory effect on hepatic metabolism of budesonide, caused by cimetidine. This should be of little clinical importance.

Ketoconazole: The metabolism of budesonide is primarily mediated by CYP3A4, a subfamily of cytochrome P450. CYP3A4 inhibitors like ritonavir and azole antifungals (e.g. ketoconazole and itraconazole) increase the systemic exposure to budesonide. Therefore, concomitant use of budesonide and ritonavir or azole antifungals should be avoided unless the potential benefit outweighs the risk of systemic corticosteroid side-effects.

Omeprazole: At recommended doses, omeprazole has no effect on the pharmacokinetics of oral budesonide.

ADVERSE EFFECTS: The adverse reactions reported with RHINOCORT TURBUHALER are consistent with what one would expect when applying a topical treatment to an already inflamed membrane. All side effects are transient. The most commonly reported side effects include: nasal and throat irritation, nasal bleeding and crusting. Other adverse events reported are itching throat, sore throat, cough, fatigue, nausea/dizziness, and headache. When patients are transferred to RHINOCORT TURBUHALER from a systemic steroid, allergic conditions such as asthma or eczema may be unmasked. Uncommon side effects such as immediate and delayed hypersensitivity reactions (urticaria, rash, dermatitis, angioedema, pruritus, etc.) may occur in association with local corticosteroid therapy. Very rare cases of anaphylactic reaction have been reported following the use of RHINOCORT TURBUHALER. Additionally, very rare cases of ulcerations of the mucous membranes and nasal septal perforation have been reported following the use of intranasal corticosteroids.

OVERDOSE:

Symptoms: Like any other nasally administered corticosteroid, acute overdosing is unlikely in view of the total amount of active ingredient present. However, when used chronically in excessive doses or in conjunction with other corticosteroid formulations, systemic corticosteroid effects such as hypercorticism and adrenal suppression may appear. If such changes recur, the dosage of RHINOCORT TURBUHALER should be discontinued slowly consistent with accepted procedures for discontinuation of chronic steroid therapy (see Dosage).

The restoration of the hypothalamic-pituitary-axis may be a slow process and during periods with pronounced physical stress such as severe infections, trauma, and surgical operations, a supplement with systemic steroids may be advisable.

Treatment: See Symptoms.

> For management of a suspected drug overdose, CPhA recommends that you contact your **regional Poison Control Centre**. See the *CPS* Directory section for a list of Poison Control Centres.

DOSAGE: See Warnings.

Careful attention must be given to patients previously treated for prolonged periods with systemic corticosteroids when transferred to RHINOCORT TURBUHALER. Initially, RHINOCORT TURBUHALER and the systemic corticosteroid must be given concomitantly, while the dose of the latter is gradually decreased. The usual rate of withdrawal of the systemic steroid is the equivalent of 2.5 mg of prednisone every four days if the patient is under close supervision. If continuous supervision is not feasible, the withdrawal of the systemic steroid should be slower, approximately 2.5 mg of prednisone (or equivalent) every ten days. If withdrawal symptoms appear, the previous dose of the systemic steroid should be resumed for a week before further decrease is attempted.

Rhinitis: Initial Dose: Adults: Two applications into each nostril in the morning (total daily dose: 400 µg).

Children (6 Years and Older): Two applications into each nostril in the morning (total daily dose: 400 µg). This dose should not be exceeded in children.

Maintenance Dose: Adults and Children (6 Years and Older): Use the lowest effective dose necessary to control symptoms.

Children Under 6 Years: Not recommended for children in this age group.

Treatment or Prevention of Nasal Polyps: Dose: One application (100 µg) into each nostril, morning and evening (total daily dose 400 µg).

Patients should be informed that the full effect of RHINOCORT TURBUHALER therapy may not become evident until 2 to 3 days of treatment have been completed. Full therapeutic benefit requires regular usage. Explain the absence of an immediate effect to the patient in order to ensure co-operation and continuation of the treatment with a regular dosage regime. Treatment of seasonal rhinitis should, if possible, start before exposure to the allergens. Concomitant treatment may sometimes be necessary to counteract eye symptoms caused by the allergy. In continuous long-term treatment, the nasal mucosa should be inspected regularly e.g. every six months.

If the nasal passages are severely blocked, the drug may fail to reach the site of action. In such cases, a course of oral steroids or decongestants may be required before initiating RHINOCORT TURBUHALER therapy.

The patient may not taste or feel any medication when using RHINOCORT TURBUHALER due to the small amount of drug dispensed.

Although systemic effects are negligible at recommended doses, RHINOCORT TURBUHALER treatment should not be continued beyond three weeks in the absence of significant symptomatic improvement. RHINOCORT TURBUHALER should not be used in the presence of untreated localized infections involving the nasal mucosa.

INFORMATION FOR THE PATIENT: Published in e-CPS, available by subscription at www.e-cps.ca.

SUPPLIED: Each dry powder inhaler contains: 200 doses of micronized budesonide 100 µg/dose. Each inhalation from TURBUHALER will provide 100 µg of budesonide active substance; no additives or carrier substances are included. Nonmedicinal ingredients: none. Store with the cover tightened, at room temperature (15-30°C).

(Shown in Product Identification Section)

Rho®-Nitro Pumpspray

nitroglycerin

Antianginal

sanofi-aventis

SUPPLIED: Each metered dose contains: nitroglycerin 0.4 mg in an aromatized oily solution. Nonmedicinal ingredients: ethanol anhydrous, medium chain partial glycerides, medium chain triglycerides and peppermint oil. Spray glass bottles delivering 75 (hospital trade packs) or 200 metered doses of 0.4 mg each.

Rhotral® 🄿

acebutolol HCl

Antihypertensive—Antianginal

sanofi-aventis

SUPPLIED: 100 mg: Each white to creamy white, shield-shaped, film-coated tablet, one side scored, debossed with "RH" above scoreline and with "100" below scoreline, other side debossed with "RHOTRAL", contains: acebutolol base 100 mg (as the HCl). Nonmedicinal ingredients: colloidal silicon dioxide, croscarmellose sodium, D&C Yellow No. 10 aluminum lake, dibasic calcium phosphate, magnesium stearate, microcrystalline cellulose, Opadry II White Y-22-7719, polyethylene glycol, povidone and talc. Bottles of 100 and 500.

200 mg: Each blue, shield-shaped, film-coated tablet, one side scored, debossed with "RH" above scoreline and with "200" below scoreline, other side debossed with "RHOTRAL", contains: acebutolol base 200 mg (as the HCl). Nonmedicinal ingredients: colloidal silicon dioxide, croscarmellose sodium, dibasic calcium phosphate, FD&C Blue No. 1 aluminum lake, magnesium stearate, microcrystalline cellulose, Opadry II White Y-22-7719, polyethylene glycol, povidone and talc. Bottles of 100 and 500.

400 mg: Each white to creamy white, shield-shaped, film-coated tablet, one side scored, debossed with "RH" above scoreline and with "400" below scoreline, other side debossed with "RHOTRAL", contains: acebutolol base 400 mg (as the HCl). Nonmedicinal ingredients: colloidal silicon dioxide, cornstarch, D&C Yellow No. 10 aluminum lake, lactose, magnesium stearate, methylcellulose, Opadry II White Y-22-7719, polyethylene glycol, povidone and talc. Bottles of 100.

Rhovane® 🄿

zopiclone

Hypnotic—Sedative

sanofi-aventis

SUPPLIED: Each oval, scored blue tablet, marked RHOVANE on one side and the logo RH on the other, contains: zopiclone 7.5 mg. The 7.5 mg tablet can be broken into two equal parts of 3.75 mg. Nonmedicinal ingredients: core: croscarmellose sodium, calcium phosphate dihydrate dibasic, magnesium stearate and microcrystalline cellulose; coating: carnauba wax, FD&C Blue #1, Opadry II White and polyethylene glycol. White high-density polyethylene bottles of 100 and 500. Store in a dry place, at room temperature (15-30°C). Protect from light. Keep in a safe place out of the reach of children.

Riboflavin

CPhA Monograph

see *Vitamin B2*

Rifadin® 🄿

rifampin

Antibiotic

sanofi-aventis

Date of Revision: July 23, 2010

PHARMACOLOGY: RIFADIN (rifampin) inhibits DNA-dependent RNA polymerase activity in susceptible cells. Specifically, it interacts with bacterial RNA polymerase, but does not inhibit the mammalian enzyme. Cross-resistance to rifampin has only been shown with other rifamycins. This is the probable mechanism of action by which rifampin exerts its therapeutic effects.

Pharmacokinetics: Absorption is more rapid when rifampin is administered 1 hour before meals. Peak blood levels in normal adults vary widely from individual to individual. Peak levels occur between 2 and 4 hours following the oral administration of a 600 mg dose with average peak values of 7 to 10 µg/mL.

Rifampin is distributed throughout the body and is detectable in many organs and body fluids, including the cerebrospinal fluid. The highest concentrations are present in the liver and bile.

In normal subjects, the biological half-life of rifampin in serum averages about 3 hours after a 600 mg oral dose, with increases up to 5.1 hours reported after 900 mg dose. Rifampin is eliminated from the blood equally in the urine and feces as unchanged drug and metabolites.

The principal metabolite in man is the biologically active desacetylrifampin. Desacetylation of rifampin in the body does not substantially modify its antimycobacterial activity. In Kirschner's medium, the MIC against *M. tuberculosis* varied from 0.1 to 2 µg/mL.

INDICATIONS: As a treatment of tuberculosis.

To achieve a complete kill of the bacillary population and to avoid selection of drug-resistant mutants, RIFADIN must be used concomitantly with at least one other active antituberculous drug. The selection of the specific drug for partner is determined by the in vitro sensitivity of the causative organisms, comparative safety and effectiveness, the patient's previous clinical history and the absorption/distribution pattern of the drug.

It is also indicated for the prophylaxis of bacterial meningitis or carriage of *N. meningitidis* or *H. influenza b* in persons exposed to a primary case.

CONTRAINDICATIONS:

- Jaundice associated with reduced bilirubin excretion.
- History of previous sensitivity to any of the rifamycins.
- Premature and newborn infants in whom the liver is not yet capable of functioning with full efficiency.
- RIFADIN passes into the breast milk and therefore should not be used during lactation.
- RIFADIN use is contraindicated when given concurrently with the combination of saquinavir/ritonavir (see Precautions).

WARNINGS: RIFADIN (rifampin) has been shown to produce liver dysfunction. There have been fatalities associated with jaundice in patients with liver disease or receiving RIFADIN concomitantly with other hepatotoxic agents. Since an increased risk may exist for individuals with liver disease, benefits must be weighed carefully against the risk of further liver damage. Patients with impaired liver function should only be given rifampin in case of necessity and then with caution and under strict medical supervision. In these patients, careful monitoring of liver function, especially serum alanine aminotransferase (ALT) and serum aspartate aminotransferase (AST) should be carried out prior to therapy and then every two to four weeks during therapy. If signs of hepatocellular damage occur, RIFADIN should be withdrawn.

In some cases, hyperbilirubinemia resulting from competition between rifampin and bilirubin for excretory pathways of the liver at the cell level can occur in the early days of treatment. An isolated report showing a moderate rise in bilirubin and/or transaminase level is not in itself an indication for interrupting treatment; rather, the decision should be made after repeating the tests, noting trends in the levels, and considering them in conjunction with the patient's clinical condition.

Rifampin has enzyme-inducing properties, including induction of delta aminolevulinic acid synthetase. Isolated reports have associated porphyria exacerbation with rifampin administration.

C. difficile-associated disease: *C. difficile*-associated disease (CDAD) has been reported with use of many antibacterial agents, including rifampin. CDAD may range in severity from mild diarrhea to fatal colitis. It is important to consider this diagnosis in patients who present with diarrhea, or symptoms of colitis, pseudomembranous colitis, toxic megacolon, or perforation of colon subsequent to the administration of any antibacterial agent. CDAD has been reported to occur over 2 months after the administration of antibacterial agents.

Treatment with antibacterial agents may alter the normal flora of the colon and may permit overgrowth of *C. difficile*. *C. difficile* produces toxins A and B, which contribute to the development of CDAD. CDAD may cause significant morbidity and mortality. CDAD can be refractory to antimicrobial therapy.

If the diagnosis of CDAD is suspected or confirmed, appropriate therapeutic measures should be initiated. Mild cases of CDAD usually respond to discontinuation of antibacterial agents not directed against *C. difficile*. In moderate to severe cases, consideration should be given to management with fluids and electrolytes, protein supplementation, and treatment with an antibacterial agent clinically effective against *C. difficile*. Surgical evaluation should be instituted as clinically indicated, as surgical intervention may be required in certain severe cases (see Adverse Effects).

PRECAUTIONS: General: A complete blood count (CBC), serum creatinine and liver function tests should be obtained prior to instituting therapy and periodically throughout the course of therapy. Because of a possible transient rise in transaminase and bilirubin values, blood for baseline clinical chemistries should be obtained before RIFADIN dosing.

RIFADIN (rifampin) increases the requirements for anticoagulant drugs of the coumarin type. This effect is not observed until the fifth day following initiation of treatment. The decrease in prothrombin time usually lasts between 5 and 7 days, and is the result of RIFADIN's ability to cause induction of drug metabolizing enzyme systems of the liver. As a result, the rate of metabolism of those drugs which are substrates for these enzymes can be altered, resulting in reduced pharmacological effects of the drugs involved. In patients receiving anticoagulants, it is recommended that daily prothrombin times be performed until the dose of the anticoagulant required has been established. This is particularly important when rifampin administration is either initiated or withdrawn.

The intermittent administration of high doses of RIFADIN >120 mg/dose has been reported to be associated with a hypersensitivity reaction, characterized by fever and myalgia. The incidence of this reaction is greater when RIFADIN is given on a once-a-week basis than on a twice or thrice weekly basis. It is recommended that when resuming treatment with RIFADIN after short or prolonged interruptions, it be given in small, gradually increasing doses. During the transitional period, the renal and hemapoietic systems should be closely monitored. The drug should be stopped immediately if renal failure, thrombocytopenia purpura or hemolytic anemia develop and should not be reinstituted.

Safe conditions for the use of ethambutol alone or in combination with RIFADIN have not been established for children under the age of 13 years. Although renal insufficiency does not alter blood levels of RIFADIN, marked increases in ethambutol levels are observed under similar conditions; this, therefore, should be taken into consideration in such patients receiving RIFADIN/ethambutol combination therapy. Caution is recommended when instituting therapeutic regimens in which isoniazid is to be used concurrently with RIFADIN, in patients with impaired liver function, the elderly and malnourished.

From experimental studies, it would appear that bromosulphalein (BSP) and RIFADIN compete with one another at the liver cell-bile canaliculus boundary. Clinically, this phenomenon can be reflected by spurious BSP levels. It is recommended that the BSP test be carried out at least 5 hours after the last dose of RIFADIN.

Urine, feces, saliva, sputum, sweat and tears may be colored red-orange by RIFADIN and its metabolites. Individuals to be treated should be made aware of these possibilities in order to prevent undue anxiety.

Patients should be advised that soft contact lenses may be permanently stained.

It has been reported that oral contraceptives have failed to prevent conception in some patients receiving RIFADIN in association with other antituberculosis drugs. It is therefore necessary that alternative or additional contraceptive measures be recommended.

Pregnancy: Teratogenic Effects: Although rifampin has been reported to cross the placental barrier and appear in the cord blood, the effect of combinations of RIFADIN with other anti-tuberculous drugs on the human fetus is not known. No obvious effect on the fetus was detected after the administration of RIFADIN to 15 pregnant patients. An increase in congenital malformations, primarily spinabifida and cleft palate, has been reported in the offspring of mice and rats given oral doses of RIFADIN 100 mg/kg/day during pregnancy.

RIFADIN should not be used in pregnant women or women with childbearing potential. If RIFADIN therapy is judged to be essential, such treatment should be implemented only after carefully weighing the potential benefits of therapy against the risks which may be involved. In women with childbearing potential, treatment with RIFADIN should be undertaken only when the possibility of pregnancy during therapy is judged to be remote.

Non-Teratogenic Effects: It is not known whether RIFADIN can affect reproduction capacity.

When administered during the last few weeks of pregnancy, rifampin can cause postnatal hemorrhages in the mother and infant. In this case, treatment with vitamin K may be indicated for postnatal hemorrhage.

Lactation: Rifampin is excreted in breast milk. Therefore, RIFADIN should be used in a nursing mother only if the potential benefit to the patient outweighs the potential risk to the infant.

Carcinogenesis, Mutagenesis, Impairment of Fertility: There are no known human data on long-term potential for carcinogenicity, mutagenicity, or impairment of fertility. A few cases of accelerated growth of lung carcinoma have been reported in man, but a causal relationship with the drug has not been established. An increase in the incidence of hepatomas in female mice (of a strain known to be particularly susceptible to the spontaneous development of hepatomas) was observed when rifampin was administered in doses two to ten times the average daily human dose for 60 weeks followed by an observation period of 46 weeks. No evidence of carcinogenicity was found in male mice of the same strain, mice of a different strain, or rats under similar experimental conditions.

Rifampin has been reported to possess immunosuppressive potential in rabbits, mice, rats, guinea pigs, human lymphocytes in vitro, and humans. Antitumor activity in vitro has been shown with rifampin.

There was no evidence of mutagenicity in bacteria, Drosophila melanogaster, or mice. An increase in chromatid breaks was noted when whole blood cell cultures were treated with rifampin.

Drug Interactions: Rifampin is a potent inducer of certain cytochrome P-450 enzymes. Coadministration of rifampin with other drugs that are metabolized through these cytochrome P-450 enzymes may accelerate the metabolism and reduce the activity of these other drugs. Therefore, caution should be used when prescribing rifampin with drugs metabolized by cytochrome P-450. To maintain optimum therapeutic blood levels, dosages of drugs metabolized by these enzymes may require adjustment when starting or stopping concomitantly administered rifampin.

Examples of drugs metabolized by cytochrome P-450 enzyme are: anticonvulsants (e.g., phenytoin), antiarrhythmics (e.g., disopyramide, mexiletine, quinidine, tocainide, propafenone), antiestrogens (e.g., tamoxifen, toremifen), antipsychotics (e.g., haloperidol), oral anticoagulants (e.g, warfarin) antifungals (e.g., fluconazole, itraconazole, ketoconazole), antiretroviral drugs (e.g., zidovudine, saquinavir, indinavir, efavirenz), barbiturates, beta-blockers, benzodiazepines (e.g., diazepam), benzodiazepine-related drugs (e.g. zopiclone, zolpidem), calcium channel blockers (e.g., diltiazem, nifedipine, verapamil), chloramphenicol, clarithromycin, corticosteroids, cardiac glycosides preparations, clofibrate, oral contraceptives, dapsone, doxycycline, estrogens, gestrinone, oral hypoglycemic agents (sulfonylureas), immunosuppressive agents (e.g., cyclosporine, tacrolimus), irinotecan, levothyroxine, losartan, narcotic analgesics, methadone, praziquantel, progestins, quinine, riluzole, selective 5-HT3 receptor antagonists (e.g., ondansetron), statins metabolized by CYP 3A4, telithromycin, theophylline, thiazolidinediones (e.g., rosiglitazone), tricyclic antidepressants (e.g., amitriptyline, nortriptyline).

Upon completion of the treatment with RIFADIN, a renewed readjustment of the dosage should be made.

Other Interactions: Atovaquone: When the two drugs are taken concomitantly, decreased concentrations of atovaquone and increased concentrations of rifampicin were observed.

Concurrent use of ketoconazole and rifampin has resulted in decreased serum concentration of both drugs. Concurrent use of rifampin and enalapril has resulted in decreased concentrations of enalaprilat, the active metabolite of enalapril. Dosage adjustments should be made if indicated by the patient's clinical condition.

Concomitant antacid administration may reduce the absorption of rifampin. Daily doses of rifampin should be given at least 1 hour before the ingestion of antacids.

Probenecid and cotrimoxazole have been reported to increase the blood level of rifampin.

When RIFADIN is given concomitantly with the combination saquinavir/ritonavir, the potential for hepatotoxicity is increased. Therefore, concomitant use of RIFADIN with saquinavir/ritonavir is contraindicated (see Contraindications).

When rifampin is given concomitantly with either halothane or isoniazid the potential for hepatotoxicity is increased. The concomitant use of RIFADIN, which contains rifampin, and halothane should be avoided. Patients receiving both rifampin and isoniazid should be monitored closely for hepatotoxicity (see Warnings).

Plasma concentration of sulfapyridine may be reduced following the concomitant administration of sulfasalazine and rifampin. This finding may be the result of alteration in the colonic bacteria responsible for the reduction of sulfasalazine to sulfapyridine and mesalamine.

Drug/Laboratory Tests Interactions: Therapeutic levels of rifampin have been shown to inhibit standard microbiological assays for serum folate and vitamin B_{12}. Therefore, alternate assay methods should be considered.

Transient abnormalities in liver function tests (e.g., elevation in serum bilirubin, abnormal bromsulphalein [BSP] excretion, alkaline phosphatase and serum transaminases), and reduced biliary excretion of contrast media used for visualization of the gallbladder have also been observed. Therefore, these tests should be performed before the morning dose of RIFADIN.

Rifampin has enzyme induction properties that can enhance the metabolism of endogenous substrates including adrenal hormones, thyroid hormones, and vitamin D.

Cross-reactivity and false-positive urine screening tests for opiates have been reported in patients receiving rifampicin when using the KIMS (Kinetic Interaction of Microparticles in Solution) method (e.g., Abuscreen OnLine opiates assay; Roche Diagnostic Systems). Confirmatory tests, such as gas chromatography/mass spectrometry, will distinguish rifampicin from opiates.

ADVERSE EFFECTS: RIFADIN (rifampin) is usually well tolerated at recommended dosage levels.

Gastrointestinal Disorders: heartburn, epigastric distress, anorexia, nausea, vomiting, gas, cramps, abdominal discomfort and diarrhea have been noted in some patients.

Occasionally, sore mouth, sore tongue associated with hypersensitivity reactions have been encountered.

Infection and Infestations: Although *C. difficile* has been shown in vitro to be sensitive to rifampin, pseudomembranous colitis has been reported with the use of rifampin (and other broad spectrum antibiotics). Therefore, it is important to consider this diagnosis in patients who develop diarrhea in association with antibiotic use (see Warnings).

Blood and Lymphatic System Disorders: Thrombocytopenia, purpura, leukopenia, hemolytic anaemia (may be related to hypersensitivity reactions) and decreased hemoglobin have been observed. Thrombocytopenia with or without purpura has occurred when RIFADIN and ethambutol were administered concomitantly according to an intermittent dose schedule twice weekly and in high doses. Thrombocytopenia has occurred primarily with high dose intermittent therapy, but has also been noted after resumption of interrupted treatment. It rarely occurs during well-supervised daily therapy. This effect is reversible if the drug is discontinued as soon as purpura occurs. Cerebral hemorrhage and fatalities have been reported when rifampin administration has been continued or resumed after the appearance of purpura.

Disseminated intravascular coagulation has also been rarely reported.

Agranulocytosis has been reported very rarely.

Occasionally, eosinophilia associated to hypersensitivity reactions has been encountered.

Nervous System Disorders: Headache, drowsiness, fatigue, ataxia, dizziness, inability to concentrate, mental confusion, psychoses, behavioral changes, muscular weakness, fever, pains in extremities and generalized numbness have also been noted.

Musculoskeletal and Connective Tissue Disorders: Rare reports of myopathy have also been observed. Bone pain (may be related to hypersensitivity reactions).

Eye Disorders: Visual disturbances have been observed.

Occasionally, conjunctivitis associated with hypersensitivity reactions has been encountered.

Endocrine Disorders: The following menstrual disturbances: breakthrough bleeding, spotting, amenorrhea, monthly prolongation of both menstrual interval and menses have been reported. Rare reports of adrenal insufficiency in patients with compromised adrenal function have been observed.

Renal and Urinary Disorders: Elevations in BUN and serum uric acid have been reported. Rarely, hemolysis, hemoglobinuria, hematuria, interstitial nephritis, renal insufficiency, acute tubular necrosis and acute renal failure have been noted.

These are generally considered to be hypersensitivity reactions. They usually occur during intermittent therapy or when treatment is resumed following intentional or accidental interruption of a daily dosage regimen, and are reversible when rifampin is discontinued and appropriate therapy instituted.

Skin and Subcutaneous Tissue Disorders: Cutaneous reactions are mild and self-limiting and do not appear to be hypersensitivity reactions. Typically, they consist of flushing and itching with or without a rash. More serious cutaneous reactions, which may be due to hypersensitivity, occur but are uncommon. Erythema multiforme including Stevens-Johnson syndrome, toxic epidermal necrolysis and vasculitis have been reported on rare occasions. Occasionally, pruritus, urticaria, skin rashes and pemphigoid reaction are associated with hypersensitivity reactions.

Hepatobiliary Disorders: Rarely, hepatitis or a shock-like syndrome with hepatic involvement and abnormal liver function tests has been reported. Transient abnormalities in liver function tests (elevations of serum bilirubin, BSP, alkaline phosphatase and serum transaminases) have been observed, particularly during the first few weeks of treatment (see Warnings).

A few cases of jaundice with evidence of hepatocellular damage have been reported in patients receiving RIFADIN. In some of them it was possible, under careful laboratory control, to resume treatment after an interval without recurrence of abnormalities.

Immune System Disorders: Immunological reactions (including anaphylaxis) with shortness of breath, wheezing, decrease in blood pressure and shock have occurred with intermittent dosage regimens. Other reactions which have occurred with intermittent dosage regimens include "flu" syndrome (such as episodes of fever, chills, headache, dizziness, bone pain and malaise).

The "flu" syndrome may also appear if rifampin is taken irregularly by the patient or if daily administration is resumed after a drug free interval. It rarely occurs during well-supervised daily therapy.

Occasionally, hypersensitivity reactions such as: pruritus, urticaria, skin rashes, pemphigoid reaction, eosinophilia, sore mouth, sore tongue, conjunctivitis, acute hemolytic anemia and acute renal failure (usually due to acute tubular necrosis or to acute interstitial nephritis) have been observed.

Investigations: decrease in blood pressure (associated with hypersensitivity reactions).

Respiratory, thoracic and mediastinal disorders: shortness of breath and wheezing are generally associated to hypersensitivity reactions.

Miscellaneous: Edema of the face and extremities has been reported.

Clinical trials have furnished no evidence to suggest that RIFADIN has any harmful effects on the cochleovestibular system.

OVERDOSE:

The minimum acute lethal or toxic dose is not well established. However, non fatal acute overdoses in adults have been reported with doses ranging from 9 to 12 g rifampicin. Fatal acute overdoses in adults have been reported with doses ranging from 14-60 g. Alcohol or a history of alcohol abuse was involved in some of the fatal and nonfatal reports.

Nonfatal overdoses, in pediatric patients aged 1 to 4 years old, of 100 mg/kg for one to two doses has been reported.

Symptoms: Nausea, vomiting, abdominal pain, pruritus, headache and increasing lethargy will probably occur within a short time after acute ingestion; unconsciousness may occur when there is severe hepatic disease. Brownish-red or orange discoloration of the skin, urine, sweat, saliva, tears, and feces will occur, and its intensity is proportional to the amount ingested. Facial or periorbital edema has also been reported in pediatric patients. Hypotension, sinus tachycardia, ventricular arrhythmias, seizures and cardiac arrest were reported in some fatal cases.

Liver enlargement, possibly with tenderness, can develop within a few hours after severe overdosage; bilirubin levels may increase and jaundice may develop rapidly. Hepatic involvement may be more marked in patients with prior impairment of hepatic function. Other physical findings remain essentially normal. A direct effect upon the hematopoietic system, electrolyte levels, or acid-base balance is unlikely.

Management: In the event of an acute oral overdose activated charcoal may be considered. General supportive measures are recommended and individual symptoms should be treated as they arise.

Antiemetic medication may be required to control severe nausea and vomiting. Active diuresis (with measured intake and output) will help promote excretion of the drug. Hemodyalisis may be of value in some patients. No specific antidote is known.

For management of a suspected drug overdose, contact your regional Poison Control Centre. See the *CPS* Directory section for a list of Poison Control Centres.

DOSAGE: Treatment of tuberculosis: Adults: 600 mg in a single daily dose. Should intolerance occur, the daily dosage may be reduced to 450 mg. In patients with impaired liver function, a daily dose of 8 mg/kg should not be exceeded. A daily dosage of 10 mg/kg is recommended for frail and elderly persons.

Children: 10 to 20 mg/kg not to exceed 600 mg/day. Data is not available for the determination of dosage for children under 5 years of age.

In treatment of pulmonary tuberculosis, RIFADIN (rifampin) must be used in conjunction with at least one other antituberculous agent. In general, therapy should be continued until bacterial conversion has been established and maximum clinical improvement has occurred.

To ensure optimum absorption, RIFADIN should be taken on an empty stomach (1 hour before breakfast).

Prophylaxis versus H. influenzae type b: Adults: 600 mg every 24 hours for 4 days.

Children (≥1 month): 20 mg/kg (up to 600 mg) every 24 hours for 4 days.

Neonates (<1 month): 10 mg/kg every 24 hours for 4 days.

Prophylaxis versus N. meningitidis: Adults: 600 mg every 12 hours for 2 days.

Children (≥1 month): 10 mg/kg (up to 600 mg) every 12 hours for 2 days.

Neonates (<1 month): 5 mg/kg every 12 hours for 2 days.

SUPPLIED: 150 mg: Each opaque maroon and opaque scarlet capsule contains: rifampin 150 mg. Nonmedicinal ingredients: cornstarch, D&C Red No. 28, FD&C Blue No. 1, FD&C Red No. 40, gelatin, magnesium stearate, titanium dioxide and white ink. Tartrazine-free. Bottles of 100.

300 mg: Each opaque maroon and opaque scarlet capsule contains: rifampin 300 mg. Nonmedicinal ingredients: cornstarch, D&C Red No. 28, FD&C Blue No. 1, FD&C Red No. 40, gelatin, magnesium stearate, titanium dioxide and white ink. Tartrazine-free. Bottles of 100.

(Shown in Product Identification Section)

Rifampin Ⓟ

Antibiotic

CPhA Monograph

Date of Revision: March 2008

This monograph has been compiled by CPhA and reviewed by experts. It may contain information different from that found in Health Canada-approved Product Monographs. The reader is referred to the *CPS* Editorial Policy for more information.

SUMMARY PRODUCT INFORMATION:

Drug	Route of Administration	Dosage Form	Product Strength
Rifampin	Oral	Capsule	150 mg, 300 mg
	IV[a]	Solution	600 mg/vial
Rifampin/Isoniazid/ Pyrazinamide	Oral	Tablet	300 mg/120 mg/50 mg

[a] Available through Health Canada's Special Access Programme.

INDICATIONS AND CLINICAL USE: Rifampin is used in the following clinical settings to treat or prevent infections caused by susceptible organisms:

- Treatment of respiratory and nonrespiratory tuberculosis in a regimen with other antituberculosis drugs. First-line drugs are rifampin, isoniazid, ethambutol and pyrazinamide [*Canadian tuberculosis standards*. 6th ed. http://www.phac-aspc.gc.ca/tbpc-latb/pubs/pdf/tbstand07_e.pdf]. To prevent or delay the emergence of drug resistance, rifampin must be used in combination with at least one other effective antituberculosis drug. Choice of appropriate drug combinations should be based on local epidemiology, in vitro sensitivity and comparative safety as well as the patient's clinical history.
- Alternative treatment of latent tuberculous infection. Isoniazid monotherapy is first-line in this setting [*Canadian tuberculosis standards*. 6th ed. http://www.phac-aspc.gc.ca/tbpc-latb/pubs/pdf/tbstand07_e.pdf].
- Prophylaxis of selected individuals exposed to persons with invasive disease due to meningococcus (*N. meningitidis*) [*Guidelines for the prevention and control of meningococcal disease*. http://www.phac-aspc.gc.ca/publicat/ccdr-rmtc/05pdf/31s1_e.pdf] and *H. influenzae* type b (Hib). Chemoprophylaxis for invasive Hib is not required for household contacts of cases when they are completely immunized against Hib [*Canada immunization guide*. 7th ed. http://www.phac-aspc.gc.ca/publicat/cig-gci/pdf/cig-gci-2006_e.pdf].
- Treatment of prosthetic valve endocarditis caused by staphylococci. Rifampin is used in a multiple-drug regimen [Infective endocarditis: diagnosis, antimicrobial therapy, and management of complications. *Circulation* 2005;111(23):e394-434].

Rifampin is sometimes used in multiple-drug regimens for the treatment of infections caused by susceptible strains of *M. avium* complex, *M. kansasii*, *M. marinum*, *M. leprae* (leprosy), *L. pneumophila* (Legionnaires' disease), brucellosis, Rhodococcus equi, *B. anthracis*.

Geriatrics: Older patients receiving multiple medications may be at an increased risk for drug-drug interactions due to the ability of rifampin to induce hepatic microsomal enzymes. The effectiveness of medications may be compromised with concomitant rifampin.

CONTRAINDICATIONS:

- Patients who develop severe hypersensitivity reactions to rifamycins including rifampin.
- Patients who have jaundice associated with reduced bilirubin excretion.
- Premature and newborn infants in whom the liver is not yet capable of functioning with full efficiency.

WARNINGS AND PRECAUTIONS: Warnings: Rifampin has been shown to produce liver dysfunction. There have been fatalities associated with jaundice in patients with preexisting liver disease or in patients receiving rifampin in combination with other hepatotoxic agents. Therefore, the benefits must be weighed carefully against the risk in individuals with impaired liver function. Perform serum aminotransferases levels in these patients at baseline and every 2 to 4 weeks while on therapy. Monitor clinical symptoms of gastrointestinal toxicity (e.g., nausea, vomiting) and hypersensitivity reactions (e.g., fever, rash). Monitor clinical status and appropriate levels of interacting drugs, if possible. Monitor platelet count if indicated.

Precautions: Urine, feces, saliva, sputum, sweat and tears may be colored reddish orange by rifampin and its metabolites but this is not harmful to the patient. To prevent undue anxiety, patients should be made aware of this possibility (see Adverse Reactions).

Soft contact lenses should not be worn during rifampin therapy and for several days after completing therapy as they may become permanently stained.

For prophylaxis of individuals exposed to persons with invasive disease due to *N. meningitidis* and *H. influenzae* type b, rifampin should be given only to selected individuals. Contact the local public health unit or refer to specific guidelines (e.g., Guidelines for control of meningococcal disease. *Can Commun Dis Rep* 2005;31S1:1-20 at http://www.phac-aspc.gc.ca/publicat/ccdr-rmtc/05pdf/31s1_e.pdf) for further recommendations on which contacts should receive prophylaxis.

Daily treatment with rifampin is often better tolerated than intermittent therapy, since rare hypersensitivity reactions are more likely to occur during intermittent therapy. Resumption of treatment after termination of a course of long-term therapy with the drug involves risks and therefore should, if possible, be avoided. If this is unavoidable, the risk of adverse reactions may be minimized if the drug-free interval or rest period is less than or closely resembles the interval of the previous drug treatment period. When resuming treatment with rifampin, the drug should be reintroduced gradually, beginning with a daily dose of 75 mg and increasing the dose by 75 mg daily until the required dosage is reached (see Dosage and Administration). During the transitional period, renal and hepatic function should be closely monitored. Corticosteroids may be useful in preventing adverse reactions since antigen-antibody complexes are suspected causes. If, as may happen in exceptional cases, the patient develops thrombocytopenia, purpura, hemolytic anemia or renal failure, treatment should be stopped at once and not reinstituted at a later date.

The 2-month regimen of rifampin and pyrazinamide for the treatment of latent tuberculosis infection is associated with increased risk of severe liver injury and death. As a result, the IDSA and CDC now recommend that this regimen not be offered as first-line therapy to persons with latent tuberculosis infection. If this regimen is to be used, a TB expert should be consulted.

Baseline measurements of bilirubin, hepatic enzymes, serum creatinine and a complete blood count are recommended for adults treated for tuberculosis with rifampin. Routine laboratory monitoring for toxicity in people with normal baseline results is generally not necessary. Baseline testing is generally not necessary for children unless a complicating condition is known or clinically suspected.

All patients, including children, should be clinically evaluated for adverse reactions at least monthly during therapy. Patients should also be instructed to report signs of adverse reactions such as hepatitis immediately (e.g., fatigue, weakness, malaise, anorexia, nausea or vomiting, dark urine, yellowing of the skin).

Rifampin should be used with caution in patients with porphyria as it could induce delta-aminolevulinic acid synthetase activity.

Special Populations: Pregnant Women: Rifampin crosses the placenta. Reproductive and fetal toxicity studies in rats and mice with rifampin alone have indicated teratogenic effects, most commonly spina bifida and cleft palate, at doses of 100 mg/kg and above. Although the effect of rifampin alone or in combination with other antituberculosis drugs on the human fetus is not known, the drug has been used in combination with isoniazid and/or ethambutol to treat active tuberculosis disease in pregnant women. The Canadian Thoracic Society (CTS), the American Thoracic Society (ATS), the US Centers for Disease Control and Prevention (CDC) and the Infectious Diseases Society of America (IDSA) consider rifampin to be safe for use in pregnancy.

When administered during the last few weeks of pregnancy, rifampin has been shown to cause postnatal hemorrhage in the mother and infant; therefore, vitamin K_1 should be given during labor to mothers receiving rifampin and to their offspring immediately after birth. In the newborn, careful surveillance for bleeding symptoms and decrease of coagulation factors is mandatory.

Nursing Women: Rifampin transfers into breast milk in limited amounts and is thought to represent a low risk to the nursing infant. Rifampin is compatible with breast-feeding according to the American Academy of Pediatrics.

ADVERSE REACTIONS: CNS: headache, drowsiness, fatigue, ataxia, dizziness, inability to concentrate, mental confusion, visual disturbances.

Dermatologic: Pruritus, urticaria, skin rashes have occasionally been encountered.

Gastrointestinal: Sore mouth, sore tongue, dyspepsia, epigastric distress, anorexia, nausea, vomiting, gas, cramps and diarrhea have been noted. Isolated cases of pseudomembranous colitis have been reported.

Hematologic: Thrombocytopenia, eosinophilia, hemolytic anemia, purpura, transient leukopenia and decreased hemoglobin have been observed. Thrombocytopenia has occurred when rifampin and ethambutol were administered concomitantly according to an intermittent dose schedule twice weekly and in high doses.

Hepatic: Transient elevations of serum bilirubin and alkaline phosphatase have been observed. Severe cholestatic hepatitis is rare. In isolated cases, induction of porphyria has been noted.

A few cases of jaundice with evidence of hepatocellular damage have been reported in patients receiving rifampin. In some of them it was possible to resume rifampin treatment without recurrence of abnormalities. However, hepatitis and fatalities associated with jaundice have also been reported (see Warnings).

Hypersensitivity: Hypersensitivity reactions, especially a flu-like syndrome (fever, chills, dizziness, pain in extremities, dyspnea), have been noted. Hematuria, renal insufficiency and acute renal failure have also occurred infrequently. These hypersensitivity reactions are usually associated with high-dose intermittent rifampin therapy (900 to 1200 mg twice weekly) or resumption of treatment after termination of a course of long-term therapy (see Precautions). True hypersensitivity reactions are rare (may occur in 0.07-0.3% of patients) [American Thoracic Society/Centers for Disease Control and Prevention/Infectious Diseases Society of America: treatment of tuberculosis. *Am J Resp Crit Care Med* 2003;167(4):603-62].

Immunologic reactions such as thrombocytopenia, hemolytic anemia, acute renal failure and thrombotic thrombocytopenia purpura have been reported.

Renal: Acute tubular necrosis, renal insufficiency, interstitial nephritis, increased blood urea nitrogen and serum uric acid concentrations, light chain proteinuria, hematuria, and acute renal failure have occurred infrequently with rifampin.

Miscellaneous: All secretions (sweat, urine, sputum, tears) may be colored reddish orange by rifampin and its metabolites (see Precautions).

Disturbances of menstruation including breakthrough bleeding, spotting, amenorrhea, and prolongation of both the menstrual interval and menses have been reported in women taking rifampin either alone or in conjunction with oral contraceptives.

A few patients receiving rifampin experienced a drug-induced lupus-like syndrome consisting principally of malaise, myalgias, arthritis, and peripheral edema and accompanied by positive antinuclear antibody test results.

Monitor for signs and symptoms of immune reconstitution inflammatory syndrome (fever, malaise, local reactions in organs) during tuberculosis therapy after initiation of antiretroviral therapy in patients co-infected with HIV [*Canadian tuberculosis standards*. 6th ed. http://www.phac-aspc.gc.ca/tbpc-latb/pubs/pdf/tbstand07_e.pdf].

DRUG INTERACTIONS: Overview: Since the chemotherapy of tuberculosis involves the use of at least two drugs, the possible adverse reactions of each drug should be borne in mind, as well as the interactions that may occur. Caution is recommended when instituting therapeutic regimens in which isoniazid is to be used concurrently with rifampin, in patients with impaired liver function, the elderly and in malnourished patients.

Drug-Drug Interactions:

Table 1: Rifampin

Summary of Drug Interactions

Drugs whose plasma concentrations may be decreased by rifampin			
Alfentanil	Contraceptive, oral or other systemic hormonal[a]	Lamotrigine	Sirolimus
Amiodarone	Corticosteroids	Losartan	Sulfonylureas
Anticoagulants, oral[b]	Cyclosporine[c]	Macrolide antibiotics (i.e, clarithromycin, erythromycin)	Sunitinib
Atovaquone	Dapsone	Methadone	Tacrolimus
Barbiturates	Digoxin	Morphine	Tamoxifen
Benzodiazepines[d] (i.e., midazolam, diazepam, triazolam)	Disopyramide	Non-nucleoside reverse transcriptase inhibitors (e.g., delavirdine, efavirenz)	Telithromycin
Beta-blockers[e]	Dolasetron	Ondansetron	Terbinafine
Buspirone	Erlotinib	Phenytoin	Theophyllines
Calcium channel blockers (e.g., diltiazem, nifedipine, verapamil)	HMG-CoA reductase inhibitors[f]	Propafenone	Tocainide
Caspofungin	Imidazoles (i.e., fluconazole, itraconazole, ketoconazole)	Protease inhibitors	Tricyclic antidepressants
Chloramphenicol		Quinidine	Zaleplon

Drugs that may reduce the metabolism of rifampin leading to increased rifampin plasma concentrations and toxicity			
Clarithromycin		Erythromycin	
Delavirdine		Protease inhibitors	

Drugs that may decrease plasma concentrations of rifampin (e.g., by impaired absorption)

Drug	Comments
Aminosalicylic acid	Give the combination of these two agents at an interval of 8 to 12 hours apart.
Antacids	Daily doses of rifampin should be given at least 1 hour before ingestion of an antacid.

Drug that can increase risk of hepatotoxicity if used concomitantly with rifampin

Drug	Comments
Isoniazid	The incidence of hepatotoxicity may be higher in slow isoniazid acetylators, those receiving high doses of isoniazid, prior general anesthesia and those with pre-existing liver disease.
Pyrazinamide	See Precautions.

[a] Unplanned pregnancies and menstrual irregularities may occur. Patients receiving rifampin should use contraceptive methods other than oral contraceptives or use additional contraceptive methods during and for at least one cycle after rifampin administration is completed.
[b] Avoid unless benefit outweighs risks. Rifampin and oral anticoagulants should not be coadministered unless no alternative is available. If coadministered, monitor INR frequently after rifampin is withdrawn.
[c] The addition of rifampin to cyclosporine regimens may require a 2- to 4-fold increase in cyclosporine dose to maintain therapeutic blood concentrations.
[d] Benzodiazepines that do not interact with rifampin include temazepam and oxazepam.
[e] Rifampin is likely to increase clearance of all beta-blockers that are oxidatively metabolized by the liver, such as propranolol, bisoprolol and metoprolol. Atenolol and other renally excreted beta-blockers are less likely to interact.
[f] Because pravastatin is not significantly metabolized by the CYP system, rifampin may have limited effect on its pharmacokinetics.

Rifampin is a known inducer of cytochrome P450 isoenzymes CYP1A2, CYP2C9, CYP2C19, CYP2D6 and CYP3A4. As a consequence, the rate of metabolism of numerous drugs can be accelerated, which can result in reduced pharmacologic effects of the drugs involved or toxicity when rifampin is discontinued. Adjustments in the dose and monitoring of the effects of these drugs is necessary when they are used concomitantly with rifampin. This is particularly important when rifampin administration is either initiated or withdrawn. The effect on enzyme induction may develop gradually over several days after starting rifampin and may take even longer to dissipate after withdrawal of rifampin. See Table 1.

Drug-Laboratory Interactions: Cross-reactivity and false positive results may occur with urine screening tests for opiates that use Kinetic Interaction of Microparticles in Solution (KIMS) methods when the patient tested is taking rifampin. If opiate abuse is suspected, the results should be confirmed by other diagnostic tests (e.g., gas chromatography/mass spectrometry).

DOSAGE AND ADMINISTRATION: Rifampin injection is available through the Special Access Programme, Health Canada (see Appendix 2). The iv dose is equivalent to the oral dose.

To ensure optimal absorption after oral administration, rifampin should be taken on an empty stomach (1 hour before a meal or 2 hours after a meal with a full glass of water). Should gastric intolerance occur, the daily dosage may be taken after meals and/or reduced. Dosage adjustment is necessary for patients with hepatic dysfunction but not those with renal failure. Consult an expert for patients with severe liver disease.

Treatment of Active Tuberculosis Disease (in combination with at least one other antituberculosis drug): Adults: 10 mg/kg once daily (maximum 600 mg daily) or by directly observed drug administration, 10 mg/kg (maximum 600 mg/day) two or three times weekly. Children: 10 to 20 mg/kg once daily (maximum 600 mg daily) or by directly observed drug administration, 10 to 20 mg/kg (maximum 600 mg per dose) twice weekly.

Treatment of Latent Tuberculous Infection: Rifampin is used alone (for isoniazid-resistant infection or intolerance to isoniazid) for a period of 4 months in adults. The adult dose is 10 mg/kg daily (maximum 600 mg per dose). The pediatric dose is 10 to 20 mg/kg daily (maximum of 600 mg per dose) for 6 months.

Prophylaxis of *N. meningitidis*: Adults: 600 mg every 12 hours for 2 days. Children: ≥1 month: 10 mg/kg (maximum 600 mg) every 12 hours for 2 days; <1 month: 5 mg/kg every 12 hours for 2 days [*Guidelines for the prevention and control of meningococcal disease*. http://www.phac-aspc.gc.ca/publicat/ccdr-rmtc/05pdf/31s1_e.pdf].

Prophylaxis of *H. influenzae* type b: Adults and children ≥12 y: 600 mg every 24 hours for 4 days. Children: >1 month: 20 mg/kg (maximum 600 mg) every 24 hours for 4 days; <1 month: 10 mg/kg every 24 hours for 4 days.

Treatment of *M. avium* Complex Nodular or Bronchiectatic Pulmonary Disease: In combination with clarithromycin 1000 mg or azithromycin 500 mg, rifampin 600 mg and ethambutol 25 mg/kg thrice weekly [An official ATS/IDSA statement: diagnosis, treatment, and prevention of nontuberculous mycobacterial diseases. *Am J Resp Crit Care Med* 2007;175(4):367-416].

Treatment of Fibrocavitary *M. avium* Complex Lung Disease or Severe Nodular or Bronchiectatic Pulmonary Disease: In combination with clarithromycin 500 to 1000 mg daily or azithromycin 250 mg daily, rifampin 600 mg daily and ethambutol 15 mg/kg daily. Continue treatment until culture-negative for 1 year [An official ATS/IDSA statement: diagnosis, treatment, and prevention of nontuberculous mycobacterial diseases. *Am J Resp Crit Care Med* 2007;175(4):367-416].

Treatment of *M. kansasii* Pulmonary Disease: Routine susceptibility testing for *M. kansasii* isolates is necessary for rifampin. In combination with other antituberculosis agents (isoniazid 300 mg daily and ethambutol 15 mg/kg daily [An official ATS/IDSA statement: diagnosis, treatment, and prevention of nontuberculous mycobacterial diseases. *Am J Resp Crit Care Med* 2007;175(4):367-416]), the adult dose is 600 mg daily. Continue treatment until culture-negative for 1 year.

Treatment of *M. leprae* (leprosy) Infection: Paucibacillary: In combination with dapsone 100 mg po daily, the adult dose is 600 mg once monthly for 6 months. Multibacillary: In combination with other drugs, the adult dose of rifampin is 600 mg once monthly for 12 months. Single lesion: In combination with ofloxacin 400 mg and minocycline 100 mg, the adult dose of rifampin is 600 mg as a single dose.

Treatment of *M. marinum* Infection: In combination with ethambutol, the adult dose is 600 mg daily for at least 3 months.

Prosthetic Valve Endocarditis Caused by Staphylococci: In combination with other agents, the adult dose is 300 mg po/iv every 8 hours for ≥6 weeks. The pediatric dose is 20 mg/kg po/iv divided three times daily in combination with other agents [Infective endocarditis: diagnosis, antimicrobial therapy, and management of complications. *Circulation* 2005;111(23):e394-433].

OVERDOSAGE:

Signs and Symptoms: Common side effects of acute overdose of rifampin include gastrointestinal symptoms, e.g., epigastric pain, nausea, vomiting and diarrhea. Other side effects include flushing, angioedema and obtundation. Anterior uveitis and neurologic effects consisting of generalized numbness, extremity pain, ataxia and muscular weakness are occasionally observed. Children who have received an overdose of rifampin have developed facial or periorbital edema. Brownish-red or orange discoloration of the skin, urine, sweat, saliva, tears, and feces is proportional to amount ingested.

Following a massive overdose of rifampin, liver involvement, manifested by enlargement (possibly with tenderness), jaundice and increased bilirubin levels and liver enzymes, can develop within a few hours. Hepatotoxicity may be more marked in patients with prior hepatic impairment such as patients with chronic liver disease, and in the elderly.

Recommended Management: General management of acute overdose of rifampin includes supportive measures. Closely observe vital signs. Single-dose activated charcoal may be administered soon after ingestion to reduce further absorption. Severe nausea and vomiting can be relieved by the administration of antiemetic medication.

For management of a suspected drug overdose, CPhA recommends that you contact your **regional Poison Control Centre**. See the *CPS* Directory section for a list of Poison Control Centres.

ACTION AND CLINICAL PHARMACOLOGY: Rifampin is a semisynthetic derivative of rifamycin B, an antibiotic produced by *Streptomyces mediterranei*. Rifampin is active against microorganisms of the genus Mycobacterium, including *M. tuberculosis, M. kansasii, M. marinum, M. avium, M. intracellulare* and *M. leprae*. Rifampin is also active against some gram-negative bacteria including *N. meningitidis, H. influenzae* type b, *Brucella melitensis* and *L. pneumophila*, in addition to some gram-positive bacteria including *S. aureus, S. epidermidis* and *B. anthracis*. Because of rapid emergence of resistant strains, it is generally recommended that rifampin be used in combination with other antibacterial agents.

Rifampin inhibits bacterial DNA-dependent RNA polymerase which leads to suppression of RNA synthesis in susceptible bacteria. The site of action appears to be the β-subunit of the enzyme. Rifampin does not affect mammalian RNA polymerase.

Rifampin may be bacteriostatic or bactericidal, depending on the concentration of the drug and the relative susceptibility of the organism. Rifampin is most effective when cell division is occurring. Rifampin is effective against both intracellular and extracellular *M. tuberculosis* organisms.

Pharmacokinetics: Rifampin is readily absorbed and peak plasma concentrations are reached between 2 and 4 hours following a single oral administration of a 600 mg dose. Absorption of rifampin can be reduced by up to 30% if the drug is taken after food (see Dosage and Administration) and is delayed.

Rifampin is distributed throughout the body and is detectable in many organs and body fluids, including the cerebrospinal fluid, where concentrations are increased if the meninges are inflamed (CSF concentrations are reported to be 10 to 20% of plasma rifampin concentrations). High concentrations are found in the liver, bile and urine. Approximately 80% of rifampin in the serum is bound to protein. Rifampin crosses the placenta and is excreted in breast milk (see Warnings and Precautions, Special Populations, Nursing Women).

The half-life of rifampin is initially 2 to 5 hours, but because of enhanced biliary excretion, it decreases by 40% during the first two weeks of therapy. Neither the peak concentration nor the half-life of rifampin is significantly altered in patients with impaired or absent renal function; these parameters are, however, increased in patients with impaired liver function or bile flow obstruction.

The principal metabolite of rifampin is desacetylated rifampin. To a large extent, desacetylated rifampin retains the antimycobacterial properties of rifampin, and is detectable in the blood, bile and urine following an oral dose of rifampin. Rifampin undergoes enterohepatic circulation, but the metabolite does not. Rifampin and its metabolite are excreted principally by the liver into the bile; however, the maximum excretory capacity of the liver is surpassed at doses larger than 5 mg/kg. In contrast, the amount of rifampin excreted by the kidney in the urine is proportional to the concentration of the drug in the blood, and high urinary concentrations result with recommended doses. From 6 to 30% of a dose is excreted in the urine. Hemodialysis and peritoneal dialysis do not significantly reduce plasma concentrations of rifampin.

Rifater® Ⓟ

rifampin—isoniazid—pyrazinamide

Antituberculous Antibiotic

sanofi-aventis

Date of Revision: March 11, 2009

PHARMACOLOGY: RIFATER (rifampin/isoniazid/pyrazinamide) is an antibacterial fixed combination product containing 120 mg rifampin, 50 mg isoniazid and 300 mg pyrazinamide used for the treatment of tuberculosis. Rifampin, isoniazid and pyrazinamide are bactericidal agents active against both intracellular and extracellular tuberculosis organisms.

Rifampin inhibits DNA-dependent RNA polymerase activity in susceptible cells. Specifically, it interacts with bacterial RNA polymerase, but does not inhibit the mammalian enzyme. Cross-resistance to rifampin has only been shown with other rifamycins. Isoniazid kills actively growing tubercle bacilli by inhibition of mycolic acid synthesis. The mechanism of action of pyrazinamide is unknown. In vitro and in vivo the drug is active only at a slightly acidic pH.

Pharmacokinetics: Pharmacokinetic studies in normal volunteers have shown that the 3 ingredients in RIFATER have comparable bioavailability whether they are given together as individual dose forms or as RIFATER.

Once daily doses of 4 to 7 tablets in tuberculosis patients resulted in the following steady-state pharmacokinetics: See Table 1.

Table 1: RIFATER

Steady State Pharmacokinetic Parameters of Isoniazid, Rifampin and Pyrazinamide

	Half-Life (h)	C_{max} (mg/L)	T_{max} (h)	AUC (mg/L·h)
Isoniazid	2.5	7.6	1.5	34.2
Rifampin	2.0	9.5	2.2	47.9
Pyrazinamide	7.7	41.7	1.8	509.4

INDICATIONS: RIFATER (rifampin/isoniazid/pyrazinamide) is indicated in the initial phase of the short-course treatment of pulmonary tuberculosis. During this phase, which should last 2 months, RIFATER should be administered on a daily, continuous basis. When indicated, the addition of other antituberculosis drugs, such as streptomycin and/or ethambutol, should be considered.

Following the initial phase and treatment with RIFATER, treatment should be continued with rifampin and isoniazid for at least 4 months. Treatment should be continued for longer if the patient is still sputum or culture positive, if resistant organisms are present, or if the patient is HIV positive. Susceptibility tests should be performed in the event of persistent positive cultures during the course of treatment.

In the treatment of tuberculosis, the small number of resistant cells present within large populations of susceptible cells can rapidly become the predominant type. Since resistance can emerge rapidly, susceptibility tests should be performed in the event of persistent positive cultures during the course of treatment. Bacteriologic smears or cultures should be obtained before the start of therapy to confirm the susceptibility of the organism to rifampin, isoniazid, and pyrazinamide and they should be repeated throughout therapy to monitor response to the treatment. If test results show resistance to any of the components of RIFATER and the patient is not responding to therapy, the drug regimen should be modified.

RIFATER is not recommended for pediatric use (see Precautions and Dosage).

CONTRAINDICATIONS: RIFATER (rifampin/isoniazid/pyrazinamide) is contraindicated in patients with a history of hypersensitivity to rifampin, isoniazid, pyrazinamide, or any of the components of the product.

Other contraindications include patients with severe hepatic damage; severe adverse reactions to isoniazid, such as drug fever, chills, and arthritis; patients with acute liver disease of any etiology; and patients with acute gout.

RIFATER use is also contraindicated when given concurrently with the combination of saquinavir/ritonavir (see Precautions, Drug Interactions).

WARNINGS: RIFATER (rifampin/isoniazid/pyrazinamide) is a combination of 3 drugs, each of which has been associated with liver dysfunction.

C. difficile-associated Disease: *C. difficile*-associated disease (CDAD) has been reported with use of many antibacterial agents, (including RIFATER). CDAD may range in severity from mild diarrhea to fatal colitis. It is important to consider this diagnosis in patients who present with diarrhea, or symptoms of colitis, pseudomembranous colitis, toxic megacolon, or perforation of colon subsequent to the administration of any antibacterial agent. CDAD has been reported to occur over 2 months after the administration of antibacterial agents.

Treatment with antibacterial agents may alter the normal flora of the colon and may permit overgrowth of *C. difficile. C. difficile* produces toxins A and B, which contribute to the development of CDAD. CDAD may cause significant morbidity and mortality. CDAD can be refractory to antimicrobial therapy.

If the diagnosis of CDAD is suspected or confirmed, appropriate therapeutic measures should be initiated. Mild cases of CDAD usually respond to discontinuation of antibacterial agents not directed against *C. difficile*. In moderate to severe cases, consideration should be given to management with fluids and electrolytes, protein supplementation, and treatment with an antibacterial agent clinically effective against *C. difficile*. Surgical evaluation should be instituted as clinically indicated, as surgical intervention may be required in certain severe cases (see Adverse Effects).

Isoniazid: Severe and sometimes fatal hepatitis associated with isoniazid therapy may occur and may develop even after many months of treatment. The risk of developing hepatitis is age related. Approximate case rates by age are: 0/1000 for persons under 20 years of age, 3/1000 for persons in the 20 to 34 year age group, 12/1000 for persons in the 35 to 49 year age group, 23/1000 for persons in the 50 to 64 year age group, and 8/1000 for persons over 65 years of age. The risk of hepatitis is increased with daily consumption of alcohol. Precise data to provide a fatality rate for isoniazid-related hepatitis is not available; however, in a U.S. Public Health Service Surveillance Study of 13 838 persons taking isoniazid, there were 8 deaths among 174 cases of hepatitis.

Therefore, patients given isoniazid should be carefully monitored and interviewed at monthly intervals. Serum transaminase concentration becomes elevated in about 10 to 20% of patients, usually during the first few months of therapy, but it can occur at any time. Usually enzyme levels return to normal despite continuance of the drug, but in some cases progressive liver dysfunction occurs. Patients should be instructed to report immediately any of the prodromal symptoms of hepatitis, such as fatigue, weakness, malaise, anorexia, nausea, or vomiting. If these symptoms appear or if signs suggestive of hepatic damage are detected, isoniazid should be discontinued promptly since continued use of the drug in these cases has been reported to cause a more severe form of liver damage.

Patients with tuberculosis should be given appropriate treatment with alternative drugs. If isoniazid must be reinstituted, it should be reinstituted only after symptoms and laboratory abnormalities have cleared. The drug should be restarted in very small and gradually increasing doses and should be withdrawn immediately if there is any indication of recurrent liver involvement. Treatment should be deferred in persons with acute hepatic diseases.

Ophthalmologic examinations (including ophthalmoscopy) should be done before isoniazid is started and periodically thereafter, even without occurrence of visual symptoms.

Rifampin: Rifampin has been shown to produce liver dysfunction. Fatalities associated with jaundice have occurred in patients with liver disease and in patients taking rifampin with other hepatotoxic agents. Since an increased risk may exist for individuals with liver disease, benefits must be weighed carefully against the risk of further liver damage. Patients with impaired liver function should only be given rifampin in cases of necessity and then with caution and under strict medical supervision. In these patients, careful monitoring of liver function, especially serum ALT and serum AST should be carried out prior to therapy and then every 2 to 4 weeks during therapy. If signs of hepatocellular damage occur, RIFATER, because it contains rifampin should be withdrawn.

In some cases, hyperbilirubinemia resulting from competition between rifampin and bilirubin for excretory pathways of the liver at the cell levels can occur in the early days of treatment. An isolated report showing a moderate rise in bilirubin and/or transaminase level is not in itself an indication for interrupting treatment; rather, the decision should be made after repeating the tests, noting trends in the levels, and considering them in conjunction with the patient's clinical condition.

High rifampin dose (greater than 600 mg), non-daily and interrupted therapy are associated with a higher incidence of immunological reactions including anaphylaxis; shock and renal failure; hematopoietic reactions (thrombocytopenia, leukopenia or acute haemolytic anemia); "flu syndrome" (fever, chills, headache, dizziness, bone pain and malaise); shortness of breath; cutaneous, gastrointestinal, and hepatic reactions. Patients at increased risk of immunological reactions should be closely monitored. Patients should be advised of the importance of following the prescribed dosage regimen and should be cautioned against interruption of therapy (see Adverse Effects and Information for the Patient).

Rifampin has enzyme-inducing properties, including induction of delta aminolevulinic acid synthetase. Isolated reports have associated porphyria exacerbation with rifampin administration.

Pyrazinamide: Patients started on pyrazinamide should have baseline serum uric acid and liver function determinations. Patients with pre-existing liver disease or those patients at increased risk for drug-related hepatitis (e.g., alcohol abusers) should be followed closely.

Because it contains pyrazinamide, RIFATER should be discontinued and not be resumed if signs of hepatocellular damage or hyperuricemia accompanied by an acute gouty arthritis appear. RIFATER should be used with caution in patients with renal impairment (increased risk of hyperuricemia) or with a history of gout. If hyperuricemia accompanied by an acute gouty arthritis occurs without liver dysfunction, patient should be transferred to a regimen not containing pyrazinamide (see Contraindications).

PRECAUTIONS: General: RIFATER should be used with caution in patients with a history of diabetes mellitus, as management may be more difficult.

A complete blood count (CBC), liver function tests (serum bilirubin, bromsulphalein [BSP] excretion, alkaline phosphatase and serum transaminases), and blood uric acid determinations should be obtained prior to instituting therapy and periodically throughout the course of therapy. Because of a possible transient rise in transaminase and bilirubin values, blood for baseline clinical chemistries should be obtained before RIFATER dosing (see Drug Interactions, Drug/Laboratory Tests Interactions).

RIFATER, because it contains rifampin, may produce a red-orange coloration of the urine, sweat, sputum, and tears. Individuals to be treated should be made aware of these possibilities in order to prevent undue anxiety. Patients should be advised that soft contact lenses may be permanently stained.

Isoniazid: All drugs should be stopped and an evaluation of the patient should be made at the first sign of a hypersensitivity reaction.

Predisposition to peripheral neuropathy (polyneuritis, presenting as paresthesia, muscle weakness, loss of reflexes, etc.) is increased in susceptible populations/conditions such as in adolescence, pregnancy and breastfeeding, elderly, malnutrition, slow acetylator status, alcohol abuse, diabetes, HIV infection, renal failure or seizure disorders. Care should be exercised in the treatment of those predisposed populations/conditions who may also require pyridoxine (vitamin B_6) supplementation with the isoniazid therapy to help prevent neuropathy (see Adverse Effects and Dosage).

Use of isoniazid should be carefully monitored in the following:

1. Patients who are receiving phenytoin concurrently. Isoniazid may decrease the excretion of phenytoin or may enhance its effects. To avoid phenytoin intoxication, appropriate adjustment of the anticonvulsant dose should be made.
2. Daily users of alcohol. Daily ingestion of alcohol may be associated with a higher incidence of isoniazid hepatitis.
3. Patients with current chronic liver disease or severe renal dysfunction.
4. Intravenous drug use is a factor associated with an increased risk of hepatitis.
5. Being a Black or Hispanic woman is a factor associated with an increased risk of hepatitis.
6. Because there is a higher frequency of isoniazid-associated hepatitis among persons older than 35 years of age, a transaminase measurement should be obtained at baseline and at least monthly during therapy in this age group (see Warnings).
7. Data suggests that the risk of isoniazid-associated hepatitis may be increased during postpartum period.
8. HIV-infected population has a greater risk of isoniazid-associated adverse reactions. They should be closely monitored by the physician taking into account any underlying conditions, such as hepatic disease.

Rifampin: Rifampin has been observed to increase the requirements for anticoagulant drugs of the coumarin type. This effect is not observed until the fifth day following initiation of treatment. The decrease in prothrombin time usually lasts between 5 and 7 days. In patients receiving anticoagulants and rifampin concurrently, it is recommended that the prothrombin time be performed daily or as necessary to establish and maintain the required dose of anticoagulant. This is particularly important when rifampin administration is either initiated or withdrawn.

The patient should be advised that the reliability of oral contraceptives may be affected; consideration should be given to using alternative contraceptive measures.

Pyrazinamide: Pyrazinamide inhibits renal excretion of urates, frequently resulting in hyperuricemia which is usually asymptomatic. If hyperuricemia is accompanied by acute gouty arthritis, RIFATER, because it contains pyrazinamide, should be discontinued.

Pregnancy: Teratogenic Effects: Animal reproduction studies have not been conducted with RIFATER. It is also not known whether RIFATER can cause fetal harm when administered to a pregnant woman. RIFATER should be given to a pregnant woman only if clearly needed.

Isoniazid: It has been reported that in both rats and rabbits, isoniazid may exert an embryocidal effect when administered orally during pregnancy, although no isoniazid-related congenital anomalies have been found in reproduction studies in mammalian species (mice, rats, and rabbits). RIFATER, because it contains isoniazid, should be prescribed during pregnancy only when therapeutically necessary. The benefit of preventive therapy should be weighed against a possible risk to the fetus. Preventive treatment generally should be started after delivery because of the increased risk of tuberculosis for new mothers.

Rifampin: Although rifampin has been reported to cross the placental barrier and appear in cord blood, the effect of rifampin, alone or in combination with other antituberculosis drugs, on the human fetus is not known. An increase in congenital malformations, primarily spina bifida and cleft palate, has been reported in the offspring of rodents given oral doses of 150 to 250 mg/kg/day of rifampin during pregnancy. The possible teratogenic potential in women capable of bearing children should be carefully weighed against the benefits of RIFATER therapy.

Pyrazinamide: Animal reproductive studies have not been conducted with pyrazinamide. It is also not known whether pyrazinamide can cause fetal harm when administered to a pregnant woman. RIFATER, because it contains pyrazinamide, should be given to a pregnant woman only if clearly needed.

Non-Teratogenic Effects: It is not known whether RIFATER can affect reproduction capacity.

Rifampin: When administered during the last few weeks of pregnancy, rifampin can cause postnatal hemorrhages in the mother and infant. In this case, treatment with vitamin K may be indicated for postnatal hemorrhage.

Lactation: Since rifampin, isoniazid, and pyrazinamide are known to pass into maternal breast milk, a decision should be made whether to discontinue nursing or to discontinue RIFATER, taking into account the importance of the drug to the mother.

Children: Safety and effectiveness in children have not been established.

Carcinogenesis, Mutagenesis, Impairment of Fertility: Increased frequency of chromosomal aberrations was observed in vitro in lymphocytes obtained from patients treated with combinations of rifampin, isoniazid, and pyrazinamide and combinations of streptomycin, rifampin, isoniazid, and pyrazinamide.

Isoniazid: Isoniazid has been reported to induce pulmonary tumors in a number of strains of mice.

Rifampin: There are no known human data on long-term potential for carcinogenicity, mutagenicity, or impairment of fertility. A few cases of accelerated growth of lung carcinoma have been reported in man, but a causal relationship with the drug has not been established. An increase in the incidence of hepatomas in female mice (of a strain known to be particularly susceptible to the spontaneous development of hepatomas) was observed when rifampin was administered in doses 2 to 10 times the average daily human dose for 60 weeks followed by an observation period of 46 weeks. No evidence of carcinogenicity was found in male mice of the same strain, mice of a different strain, or rats under similar experimental conditions.

Rifampin has been reported to possess immunosuppressive potential in rabbits, mice, rats, guinea pigs, human lymphocytes in vitro, and humans. Antitumor activity in vitro has been shown with rifampin.

There was no evidence of mutagenicity in bacteria, *Drosophila melanogaster*, or mice. An increase in chromatid breaks was noted when whole blood cell cultures were treated with rifampin.

Pyrazinamide: In lifetime bioassays in rats and mice, pyrazinamide was administered in the diet at concentrations of up to 10 000 ppm. This resulted in estimated daily doses of 2 g/kg for the mouse, or 40 times the maximum human dose, and 0.5 g/kg for the rat, or 10 times the maximum human dose. Pyrazinamide was not carcinogenic in rats or male mice and no conclusion was possible for female mice.

Pyrazinamide was not mutagenic in the Ames bacterial test, but induced chromosomal aberrations in human lymphocyte cell cultures.

Drug Interactions: Isoniazid: Enzyme Inhibition: Isoniazid is known to inhibit certain cytochrome P450 enzymes. Administration of RIFATER, because it contains isoniazid, with drugs that undergo biotransformation through these metabolic pathways may decrease elimination of coadministered drugs. Therefore, caution should be used when prescribing RIFATER with drugs metabolized by cytochrome P450. Dosages of drugs metabolized by these enzymes may require adjustment when starting or stopping concomitantly administered RIFATER to maintain optimum therapeutic blood levels.

Isoniazid has been reported to inhibit the metabolism of the following drugs: anticonvulsants (e.g., carbamazepine, phenytoin, primidone, valproic acid), benzodiazepines (e.g., diazepam), haloperidol, ketoconazole, theophylline, and warfarin. It may be necessary to adjust the dosages of these drugs if they are given currently with RIFATER because it contains isoniazid. The impact of the competing effects of rifampin and isoniazid on the metabolism of these drugs is unknown.

Other Interactions: Concomitant antacid administration may reduce the absorption of isoniazid. Ingestion with food may also reduce the absorption of isoniazid. Daily doses of isoniazid should be given on an empty stomach at least 1 hour before the ingestion of antacids or food.

Corticosteroids (e.g., prednisolone) may decrease the serum concentration of isoniazid by increasing acetylation rate and/or renal clearance. Para-aminosalicylic acid may increase the plasma concentration and elimination half-life of isoniazid by competing for acetylating enzymes.

Pharmacodynamic Interactions: Daily ingestion of alcohol may be associated with a higher incidence of isoniazid hepatitis. Isoniazid, when given concomitantly with rifampin, has been reported to increase the hepatotoxicity of both drugs. Patients receiving both rifampin and isoniazid as in RIFATER should be monitored closely for hepatotoxicity.

In case reports, the CNS effects of meperidine (drowsiness), cycloserine (dizziness, drowsiness), and disulfiram (acute behavioral and coordination changes) may be exaggerated when concomitant isoniazid is given. Concurrent isoniazid and levodopa administration may produce symptoms of excess catecholamine stimulation (agitation, flushing, palpitations) or lack of levodopa effect.

Isoniazid may produce hyperglycemia and lead to loss of glucose control in patients on oral hypoglycemics.

Fast acetylation of isoniazid may produce high concentrations of hydrazine which facilitates deflorination of enflurane. Renal function should be monitored in patients receiving this drug combination.

Food Interactions: Because isoniazid has some monoamine oxidase inhibiting activity, an interaction with tyramine-containing foods (cheese, red wine) may occur. Diamine oxidase may also be inhibited, causing exaggerated response (e.g., headache, sweating, palpitations, flushing, hypotension) to foods containing histamine (e.g., skipjack, tuna, other tropical fish). Tyramine- and histamine-containing foods should be avoided.

Rifampin: Enzyme Induction: Rifampin is a potent inducer of certain cytochrome P450 enzymes. Administration of RIFATER, because it contains rifampin, with drugs that undergo biotransformation through these metabolic pathways may accelerate elimination of coadministered drugs. Therefore, caution should be used when prescribing RIFATER with drugs metabolized by cytochrome P450. To maintain optimum therapeutic blood levels, dosages of drugs metabolized by these enzymes may require adjustment when starting or stopping concomitantly administered RIFATER.

Examples of drugs metabolized by cytochrome P450 enzyme are: anticonvulsants (e.g., phenytoin), antiarrhythmics (e.g., disopyramide, mexiletine, quinidine, tocainide, propafenone), antiestrogens (e.g., tamoxifen, toremifen), antipsychotics (e.g., haloperidol), oral anticoagulants (e.g., warfarin), antifungals (e.g., fluconazole, itraconazole, ketoconazole), antiretroviral drugs (e.g., zidovudine, saquinavir, indinavir, efavirenz), barbiturates, beta-blockers, benzodiazepines (e.g., diazepam), benzodiazepine-related drugs (e.g., zopiclone, zolpidem), calcium channel blockers (e.g., diltiazem, nifedipine, verapamil), chloramphenicol, clarithromycin, corticosteroids, cardiac glycoside preparations, clofibrate, oral contraceptives, dapsone, doxycycline, estrogens, gestrinone, oral hypoglycemic agents (sulfonylureas), immunosuppressive agents (e.g., cyclosporine, tacrolimus), irinotecan, levothyroxine, losartan, methadone, narcotic analgesics, praziquantel, progestins, quinine, riluzole, selective 5-HT3 receptor antagonists (e.g., ondansetron), statins metabolized by CYP 3A4, telithromycin, theophylline, thiazolidinediones (e.g., rosiglitazone) and tricyclic antidepressants (e.g., amitryptyline, nortriptyline). It may be necessary to adjust the dosages of these drugs if they are given concurrently with RIFATER since it contains rifampin.

Other Interactions: Atovaquone: When the two drugs are taken concomitantly, decreased concentrations of atovaquone and increased concentrations of rifampin were observed.

Concurrent use of ketoconazole and rifampin has resulted in decreased serum concentration of both drugs. Concurrent use of rifampin and enalapril has resulted in decreased concentrations of enalaprilat, the active metabolite of enalapril. Dosage adjustments should be made if indicated by the patient's clinical condition.

Concomitant antacid administration may reduce the absorption of rifampin. Daily doses of rifampin should be given at least 1 hour before the ingestion of antacids.

Probenecid and cotrimoxazole have been reported to increase the blood level of rifampin.

When RIFATER is given concomitantly with the combination saquinavir/ritonavir, the potential for hepatotoxicity is increased. Therefore, concomitant use of RIFATER with saquinavir/ritonavir is contraindicated (see Contraindications).

When rifampin is given concomitantly with either halothane or isoniazid the potential for hepatotoxicity is increased. The concomitant use of RIFATER and halothane should be avoided. Patients receiving both rifampin and isoniazid as in RIFATER should be monitored closely for hepatotoxicity (see Warnings).

Plasma concentrations of sulfapyridine may be reduced following the concomitant administration of sulfasalazine and rifampin. This finding may be the result of alteration in the colonic bacteria responsible for the reduction of sulfasalazine to sulfapyridine and mesalamine.

The patient should be advised that the reliability of oral contraceptives may be affected; consideration should be given to using alternative contraceptive measures.

Drug/Laboratory Tests Interactions: Rifampin: Therapeutic levels of rifampin have been shown to inhibit standard microbiological assays for serum folate and vitamin B_{12}. Therefore, alternate assay methods should be considered.

Transient abnormalities in liver function tests (e.g., elevation in serum bilirubin, abnormal bromsulphalein [BSP] excretion, alkaline phosphatase and serum transaminases), and reduced biliary excretion of contrast media used for visualization of the gallbladder have also been observed. Therefore, these tests should be performed before the morning dose of RIFATER.

Rifampin and isoniazid have been reported to alter vitamin D metabolism. In some cases, reduced levels of circulating 25-hydroxy vitamin D and 1,25-dihydroxy vitamin D have been accompanied by reduced serum calcium and phosphate, and elevated parathyroid hormone. Rifampin can also enhance the metabolism of adrenal hormones.

Cross-reactivity and false-positive urine screening tests for opiates have been reported in patients receiving rifampin when using the KIMS (Kinetic Interaction of Microparticles in Solution) method (e.g., Abuscreen OnLine opiates assay; Roche Diagnostic Systems). Confirmatory tests, such as gas chromatography/mass spectrometry, will distinguish rifampin from opiates.

Pyrazinamide: Pyrazinamide has been reported to interfere with Acetest and Ketostix urine tests to produce a pink-brown colour.

ADVERSE EFFECTS: The adverse reactions reported during therapy with RIFATER are consistent with reactions described or listed below for the individual components.

Isoniazid: The most frequent reactions are those affecting the nervous system and the liver (see Warnings).

Blood and Lymphatic System Disorders: agranulocytosis; hemolytic, sideroblastic, or aplastic anemia; thrombocytopenia, eosinophilia. Lymphadenopathy (associated with hypersensitivity reactions).

Gastrointestinal Disorders: nausea, vomiting, epigastric distress and pancreatitis.

General Disorders and Administration Site Conditions: fever (associated with hypersensitivity reactions).

Hepatobiliary Disorders: elevated serum transaminases (ALT, AST), bilirubinemia, bilirubinuria, jaundice, and occasionally severe and sometimes fatal hepatitis. The common prodromal symptoms are anorexia, nausea, vomiting, fatigue, malaise, and weakness. Mild and transient elevation of serum transaminase levels occurs in 10 to 20% of persons taking isoniazid. The abnormality usually occurs in the first 4 to 6 months of treatment but can occur at any time during therapy. In most instances, enzyme levels return to normal with no necessity to discontinue medication. In occasional instances, progressive liver damage occurs, with accompanying symptoms. In these cases, the drug should be discontinued immediately. The frequency of progressive liver damage increases with age. It is rare in persons under 20, but occurs in up to 2.3% of those over 50 years of age.

Immune System Disorders: hypersensitivity reactions including fever, skin eruptions (morbilliform, maculopapular, purpuric, or exfoliative), acne, pemphigus, rash, exfoliative dermatitis, Stevens-Johnson syndrome, systemic lupus erythematosus-like syndrome, lymphadenopathy, vasculitis and anaphylactic reactions.

Metabolism and Nutrition Disorders: pyridoxine deficiency, pellagra, hyperglycemia and metabolic acidosis.

Musculoskeletal and Connective Tissue Disorders: rheumatic syndrome and systemic lupus erythematosus-like syndrome (associated with hypersensitivity reactions).

Nervous System Disorders: peripheral neuropathy (polyneuritis, presenting as paresthesia, muscle weakness, loss of reflexes, etc.) is the most common toxic effect. It is dose-related, occurs most often in those predisposed to neuritis or pyridoxine deficiency (e.g., adolescents, pregnant and nursing women, elderly, malnourished, slow acetylators, alcoholics, diabetics, HIV-infected patients, renal failure or seizure disorders), and is usually preceded by paresthesias of the feet and hands. The incidence is higher in "slow inactivators" (see Precautions and Dosage).

Other neurotoxic effects, which are uncommon with conventional doses, are convulsions (see Overdose, Symptoms and Treatment), toxic encephalopathy, optic neuritis and atrophy, memory impairment, and toxic psychosis.

Reproductive System and Breast Disorders: gynecomastia.

Skin and Subcutaneous Tissue Disorders: acne, Stevens-Johnson syndrome, pemphigus, rash, exfoliative dermatitis, and skin eruptions (morbilliform, maculopapular, purpuric, or exfoliative) are generally associated with hypersensitivity reactions.

Vascular Disorders: vasculitis (associated with hypersensitivity reactions).

Rifampin:

Blood and Lymphatic System Disorders: Thrombocytopenia with or without purpura has occurred primarily with high dose intermittent therapy, but has also been noted after resumption of interrupted treatment. It rarely occurs during well-supervised daily therapy. This effect is reversible if the drug is discontinued as soon as purpura occurs. Cerebral hemorrhage and fatalities have been reported when rifampin administration has been continued or resumed after the appearance of purpura.

Leukopenia, eosinophilia (associated to hypersensitivity reactions), hemolytic anemia (may be related to hypersensitivity reactions), and decreased hemoglobin have been observed.

Disseminated intravascular coagulation and hemolysis has also been rarely reported.

Agranulocytosis has been reported very rarely.

Endocrine Disorders: Menstrual disturbances have been observed. Rare reports of adrenal insufficiency in patients with compromised adrenal function have been observed.

Eye Disorders: Visual disturbances and conjunctivitis (associated to hypersensitivity reactions) have been observed.

Gastrointestinal Disorders: heartburn, epigastric distress, anorexia, nausea, vomiting, flatulence, cramps, abdominal discomfort, and diarrhea have been noted in some patients. Occasionally, sore mouth, sore tongue associated to hypersensitivity reactions have been encountered.

General Disorders and Administration Site Conditions: Edema of the face and extremities has been reported.

Hepatobiliary Disorders: Rarely, hepatitis or a shock-like syndrome with hepatic involvement and abnormal liver function tests has been reported. Transient abnormalities in liver function tests (e.g., elevation in serum bilirubin, abnormal bromsulphalein [BSP] excretion, alkaline phosphatase and serum transaminases) have been observed (see Warnings and Drug/Laboratory Tests Interactions). A few cases of jaundice with evidence of hepatocellular damage have been reported in patients receiving rifampin. In some of them it was possible, under careful laboratory control, to resume treatment after an interval without recurrence of abnormalities.

Immune System Disorders: Reactions, which usually occurred with intermittent dosage regimens, include "flu" syndrome (such as episodes of fever, chills, headache, dizziness, bone pain and malaise) and immunological reactions (including anaphylaxis) with shortness of breath, wheezing, decrease in blood pressure and shock. The "flu" syndrome may also appear if rifampin is taken irregularly by the patient or if daily administration is resumed after a drug free interval. It rarely occurs during well-supervised daily therapy. Occasionally, pruritus, urticaria, skin rash, pemphigoid reaction, eosinophilia, sore mouth, sore tongue, conjunctivitis, acute hemolytic anemia and acute renal failure (usually due to acute tubular necrosis or to acute interstitial nephritis) have been observed as hypersensitivity reactions.

Infections and Infestations: Although *C. difficile* has been shown in vitro to be sensitive to rifampin, pseudomembranous colitis has been reported with the use of rifampin (and other broad spectrum antibiotics). Therefore, it is important to consider this diagnosis in patients who develop diarrhea in association with antibiotic use (see Warnings).

Investigations: decrease in blood pressure (associated with hypersensitivity reactions).

Musculoskeletal and Connective Tissue Disorders: Rare reports of myopathy have also been observed. Bone pain (may be related to hypersensitivity reactions).

Nervous System Disorders: headache, fever, drowsiness, fatigue, ataxia, dizziness, inability to concentrate, mental confusion, psychoses, behavioral changes, muscular weakness, pains in extremities, and generalized numbness have been observed.

Renal and Urinary Disorders: Elevations in BUN and serum uric acid have been reported. Rarely, hemoglobinuria, hematuria, interstitial nephritis, renal insufficiency, acute tubular necrosis and acute renal failure have been noted. These are generally considered to be hypersensitivity reactions. They usually occur during intermittent therapy or when treatment is resumed following intentional or accidental interruption of a daily dosage regimen, and are reversible when rifampin is discontinued and appropriate therapy instituted.

Respiratory, Thoracic and Mediastinal Disorders: Shortness of breath and wheezing are generally associated to hypersensitivity reactions.

Skin and Subcutaneous Tissue Disorders: Cutaneous reactions are mild and self-limiting and do not appear to be hypersensitivity reactions. Typically, they consist of flushing and itching with or without a rash. More serious cutaneous reactions which may be due to hypersensitivity occur but are uncommon. Erythema multiforme including Stevens-Johnson syndrome, toxic epidermal necrolysis and vasculitis have been reported on rare occasions. Occasionally, pruritus, urticaria, skin rash and pemphigoid reaction are associated to hypersensitivity reactions.

Pyrazinamide:

Blood and Lymphatic System Disorders: Thrombocytopenia with our without purpura and sideroblastic anemia with erythroid hyperplasia, vacuolation of erythrocytes and increased serum concentration have occurred rarely with this drug. Adverse effects on blood clotting mechanisms have also been rarely reported.

Congenital, Familial and Genetic Disorders: Porphyria has been reported rarely.

Gastrointestinal Disorders: GI disturbances including aggravation of peptic ulcer, nausea, vomiting, and anorexia have also been reported.

General Disorders and Administration Site Condition: Fever has been reported rarely. Malaise has also been reported.

Hepatobiliary Disorders: The principal adverse effect is a hepatic reaction (see Warnings). Hepatotoxicity appears to be dose related, and may appear at any time during therapy. The hepatic reaction can vary from a symptomless abnormality of hepatic cell function (detected only through laboratory liver function tests) through a mild syndrome of fever, malaise and liver tenderness, to more serious reactions as clinical jaundice and rare cases of acute yellow atrophy and death.

Immune System Disorders: Hypersensitivity reactions including rashes, urticaria, and pruritus have been reported.

Metabolism and Nutrition Disorders: Pyrazinamide can cause hyperuricemia and gout (see Precautions).

Musculoskeletal and Connective Tissue Disorders: Mild arthralgia and myalgia have been reported frequently.

Renal and Urinary Disorders: Dysuria and interstitial nephritis have been reported rarely.

Skin and Subcutaneous Tissue Disorders: Very rarely, angioedema has been reported. Acne and photosensitivity have been reported rarely. Occasionally, rashes, erythema, urticaria, and pruritus associated with hypersensitivity reactions have been encountered.

OVERDOSE: General:

There is no human experience with RIFATER overdosage.

Isoniazid: Untreated or inadequately treated cases of gross isoniazid overdosage can be fatal, but good response has been reported in most patients treated within the first few hours after drug ingestion.

Ingested acutely, as little as 1.5 g isoniazid may cause toxicity in adults. Doses of 35 to 40 mg/kg have resulted in seizures.

Ingestion of 80 to 150 mg/kg isoniazid has been associated with severe toxicity and, if untreated, significant mortality.

Rifampin: The minimum acute lethal or toxic dose is not well established. However, non fatal acute overdoses in adults have been reported with doses ranging from 9 to 12 g rifampin. Fatal acute overdoses in adults have been reported with doses ranging from 14-60 g, including one case of fatal overdose: a 26-year-old man died after self-administering 60 g of rifampin. Alcohol or a history of alcohol abuse was involved in some of the fatal and non-fatal reports. Nonfatal overdoses in pediatric patients ages 1 to 4 years old of 100 mg/kg for one to two doses has been reported.

Pyrazinamide: Overdosage experience with pyrazinamide is limited.

Symptoms: The following signs and symptoms have been seen with each individual component in an overdosage situation.

Isoniazid: Isoniazid overdosage produces signs and symptoms within 30 minutes to 3 hours after ingestion. Nausea, vomiting, dizziness, slurring of speech, blurring of vision, visual hallucinations (including bright colors and strange designs) are among the early manifestations. With marked overdosage, respiratory distress and CNS depression, progressing rapidly from stupor to profound coma, are to be expected, along with severe, intractable seizures. Severe metabolic acidosis, acetonuria, and hyperglycemia are typical laboratory findings.

Rifampin: Nausea, vomiting, abdominal pain, pruritus, headache and increasing lethargy will probably occur within a short time after rifampin overdosage; unconsciousness may occur when there is severe hepatic disease. Brownish-red or orange discoloration of the skin, urine, sweat, saliva, tears, and feces will occur, and its intensity is proportional to the amount ingested. Facial or periorbital edema has also been reported in pediatric patients. Hypotension, sinus tachycardia, ventricular arrhythmias, seizures and cardiac arrest were reported in some fatal cases.

Liver enlargement, possibly with tenderness, can develop within a few hours after severe overdosage; bilirubin levels may increase and jaundice may develop rapidly. Hepatic involvement may be more marked in patients with prior impairment of hepatic function. Other physical findings remain essentially normal. A direct effect upon the hematopoietic system, electrolyte levels, or acid-base balance is unlikely.

Pyrazinamide: In 1 case of pyrazinamide overdosage, abnormal liver function tests developed. These spontaneously reverted to normal when the drug was stopped.

Treatment: The airway should be secured and adequate respiratory exchange should be established in cases of overdosage with RIFATER.

Seizures may be controlled with i.v. diazepam or short-acting barbiturates, and i.v. pyridoxine (dose equivalent to the amount of isoniazid ingested).

Obtain blood samples for immediate determination of gases, electrolytes, BUN, glucose, etc.; type and cross-match blood in preparation for possible hemodialysis.

Gastric lavage as soon as possible within the first 2 to 3 hours after ingestion is advised, but it should not be attempted until convulsions are under control. Following evacuation of gastric contents, the instillation of activated charcoal slurry into the stomach may help absorb any remaining drug from the gastrointestinal tract. Antiemetic medication may be required to control severe nausea and vomiting.

Rapid control of metabolic acidosis is fundamental to management. Give i.v. sodium bicarbonate at once and repeat as needed, adjusting subsequent dosage on the basis of laboratory findings (e.g., serum sodium, pH, etc).

Forced osmotic diuresis must be started early and should be continued for some hours after clinical improvement to hasten renal clearance of drug and help prevent relapse; monitor fluid intake and output.

Hemodialysis is advised for severe cases; if this is not available, peritoneal dialysis can be used along with forced diuresis.

Along with measures based on initial and repeated determination of blood gases and other laboratory tests as needed, utilize meticulous respiratory and other intensive care to protect against hypoxia, hypotension, aspiration pneumonitis, etc.

> For management of a suspected drug overdose, contact your **regional Poison Control Centre**. See the *CPS* Directory section for a list of Poison Control Centres.

DOSAGE: Adults: Patients should be given the following single daily dose either 1 hour before or 2 hours after a meal with a full glass of water: Patients weighing 44 kg or less: 4 tablets; patients weighing between 45 to 54 kg: 5 tablets; patients weighing 55 kg or greater: 6 tablets.

RIFATER is recommended in the initial phase of short-course therapy which is usually continued for 2 months. When indicated, the addition of other antituberculosis drugs, such as streptomycin and/or ethambutol, should be considered.

Following the initial phase, treatment should be continued with rifampin and isoniazid for at least 4 months. Treatment should be continued for longer if the patient is still sputum or culture positive, if resistant organisms are present, or if the patient is HIV positive.

Concomitant administration of pyridoxine (B_6) is recommended in those predisposed to neuropathy (e.g., adolescents, pregnant and nursing women, elderly, malnourished, slow acetylators, alcoholics, diabetics, HIV-infected patients, renal failure or seizure disorders).

The maximum daily dose for adults, regardless of weight, is: rifampin: up to 720 mg/day (see Warnings); isoniazid: up to 300 mg/day; pyrazinamide: up to 1800 mg/day.

Children: The ratio of the drugs in RIFATER may not be appropriate in children (e.g., higher mg/kg doses of isoniazid are usually given in children than adults). RIFATER is therefore not recommended for pediatric use (see Precautions).

INFORMATION FOR THE PATIENT: Published in e-CPS, available by subscription at www.e-cps.ca.

SUPPLIED: Each light pinky-beige, round, sugar-coated tablet contains: rifampin 120 mg, isoniazid 50 mg and pyrazinamide 300 mg. Nonmedicinal ingredients: acacia, aluminum hydroxide gel, black ink, calcium stearate, carnauba wax, colophony, kaolin, magnesium carbonate, paraffin, povidone, red ferric oxide, silicon dioxide, sodium carboxymethylcellulose, sodium lauryl sulfate, sucrose, talc, titanium dioxide and white beeswax. Bottles of 60. Store at controlled room temperature (15 to 30°C). Protect from moisture.

(Shown in Product Identification Section)

Rilutek® Ⓟ

riluzole

Antiglutamate

sanofi-aventis

Date of Revision: May 11, 2010

SUMMARY PRODUCT INFORMATION:

Route of Administration	Dosage Form/Strength	Nonmedicinal Ingredients
Oral	Film-Coated Tablet/50 mg	Core: anhydrous colloidal silica, anhydrous dibasic calcium phosphate, croscarmellose sodium, magnesium stearate, microcrystalline cellulose. Film-coating: hydroxypropyl methylcellulose, polyethylene glycol, titanium dioxide.

INDICATIONS AND CLINICAL USE: RILUTEK (riluzole):

- may extend survival and/or time to tracheostomy in some patients with amyotrophic lateral sclerosis (ALS).

There is no evidence that RILUTEK exerts a therapeutic effect on motor function, lung function, fasciculations, muscle strength and motor symptoms.

RILUTEK has not been shown to be effective in the late stage of ALS.

Initially, RILUTEK should be prescribed only by physicians experienced in the diagnosis and management of ALS. If necessary, subsequent follow up and continuing treatment of the patient may be undertaken by non-specialized physicians, under the supervision of a specialist.

The symptomatic management of patients with ALS is not changed by the addition of RILUTEK. Knowledge of the disease natural history and use of management strategies that assist the patient in coping with complications of the inevitable decline in motor power, such as non-invasive positive pressure ventilation (NIPPV), remain the most effective means to prolonging quality survival.

RILUTEK is not a cure for ALS, but a modest prolongation of survival represents a first step forward in treating ALS patients. No data exist to help predict how any individual patient will benefit from RILUTEK treatment. No evidence exists to define the duration of the benefit of continued RILUTEK use. Similarly, there is no evidence of additional benefit if RILUTEK were continued after tracheostomy is performed for ventilation.

The following advisory recommendations are made:

- ALS patients for whom Class I evidence suggests RILUTEK may prolong survival includes those who have:
  - definite or probable ALS by World Federation of Neurology (WFN) criteria (other causes for progressive muscle atrophy have been excluded)
  - symptoms present for less than 5 years
  - FVC >60% predicted
  - no tracheostomy
- ALS patients for whom no Class I evidence supports the use of RILUTEK, but for whom there may be potential benefit includes those who have:
  - suspected or possible ALS by WFN criteria
  - symptoms present for more than 5 years
  - FVC <60% predicted
  - tracheostomy for prevention of aspiration only (ventilator independent)
- RILUTEK is of uncertain benefit in patients with:
  - tracheostomy required for ventilation
  - other incurable life-threatening disorders
  - other forms of anterior horn cell disease

The safety and efficacy of RILUTEK have not been studied in motor neuron diseases other than ALS. Therefore, RILUTEK should not be used in any other form of motor neuron disease.

Geriatrics (>65 years): In controlled clinical trials, about 30% of patients were over 65. There were no differences in adverse effects between younger and older patients. A brief discussion can be found in the appropriate sections (see Warnings and Precautions, Special Populations, Geriatrics (>65 years) and Action and Clinical Pharmacology, Special Populations and Conditions, Geriatrics).

Pediatrics (<18 years of age): The safety and efficacy of RILUTEK in any neurodegenerative disease occurring in children or adolescents have not been established.

CONTRAINDICATIONS: RILUTEK is contraindicated in:

- Patients who have a history of hypersensitivity reactions to riluzole or any of the tablet components. For a complete listing of the tablet components, see the Dosage Forms, Composition and Packaging.
- Patients who have hepatic disease or who have baseline transaminases greater than 3 times the ULN (upper limit of normal) (see Warnings and Precautions, General, Liver Injury/Monitoring Liver Chemistries; Action and Clinical Pharmacology, Special Populations and Conditions, Hepatic Insufficiency; Dosage and Administration, Special Populations, Hepatic Insufficiency).
- Patients who are pregnant or breast-feeding

WARNINGS AND PRECAUTIONS: General: Liver Injury/Monitoring Liver Chemistries: RILUTEK is contraindicated in patients who have hepatic disease or who have baseline transaminases greater than 3 times the ULN (upper limit of normal) (see Contraindications).

RILUTEK should be used with caution in patients with a history of abnormal liver function, with known concomitant liver insufficiency or in patients with elevations in any of serum transaminase (ALT; AST), bilirubin, or gamma-glutamyl transferase (GGT) levels. Baseline elevations of several liver function tests (especially including elevated bilirubin) should preclude the use of RILUTEK (see Contraindications; Dosage and Administration, Special Populations, Hepatic Insufficiency; Adverse Reactions, Abnormal Hematologic and Clinical Chemistry Findings).

Liver chemistries should be monitored in all patients on RILUTEK as the drug can increase serum aminotransferase, even in patients without a prior history of liver abnormality. Serum ALT levels should be measured every month during the first 3 months of treatment, every 3 months during the remainder of the first year, and periodically thereafter (see Warnings and Precautions, Monitoring and Laboratory Tests).

There were uncommon instances of jaundice and hepatitis.

RILUTEK should be discontinued if the ALT levels increase to 5× the ULN. There is no experience with dose reduction or rechallenge in patients who have developed an increase of ALT to 5 × ULN. Readministration of RILUTEK to patients in this situation cannot be recommended. In cases of RILUTEK-induced hepatic injury manifested by elevated liver enzymes, the effect of the hepatic injury on RILUTEK metabolism is unknown (see Action and Clinical Pharmacology, Special Populations and Conditions, Hepatic Insufficiency).

Findings from Clinical Trials: Experience in almost 800 ALS patients indicates that about 50% of RILUTEK-treated patients will experience at least one ALT level above the ULN, about 8% will have elevations >3×ULN, and about 2% of patients will have elevations >5×ULN. A single non-ALS patient with epilepsy treated with concomitant carbamazepine and phenobarbital experienced marked, rapid elevations of liver enzymes with jaundice (ALT 26×ULN, AST 17×ULN, and bilirubin 11×ULN) four months after starting RILUTEK; these returned to normal 7 weeks after treatment discontinuation.

Maximum increases in serum ALT usually occurred within 3 months after the start of RILUTEK therapy and were usually transient when <5×ULN. In trials, if ALT levels were <5×ULN, treatment continued and ALT levels usually returned to below 2×ULN within 2 to 6 months. However, treatment in studies was discontinued if ALT levels exceeded 5×ULN; in these cases, the levels generally returned to less than 2×ULN within 2 to 6 months.

Hematologic: Patients should be warned to report any febrile illness to their physicians. The report of a febrile illness should prompt treating physicians to check white blood cell counts and to discontinue RILUTEK in case of neutropenia (see Adverse Reactions, Abnormal Hematologic and Clinical Chemistry Findings).

Among approximately 5000 patients given RILUTEK for ALS, there were three cases of marked neutropenia (absolute neutrophil count less than 500/mm³), all seen within the first 2 months of RILUTEK treatment. In one case, neutrophil counts rose on continued treatment. In a second case, counts rose after therapy was stopped. A third case was more complex, with marked anemia as well as neutropenia and the etiology of both is uncertain.

Respiratory, Thoracic and Mediastinal Disorders : Interstitial lung disease: Cases of interstitial lung disease have been reported in patients treated with RILUTEK, some of them were severe (see Adverse Reactions). If respiratory symptoms develop such as dry cough and/or dyspnea, chest radiography should be performed, and in case of findings suggestive of interstitial lung disease (e.g. bilateral diffuse lung opacities), RILUTEK should be discontinued immediately. In the majority of the reported cases, symptoms resolved after drug discontinuation and symptomatic treatment.

Hepatic/Biliary/Pancreatic: See Contraindications, Warnings and Precautions, General, Liver Injury/Monitoring Liver Chemistries and Special Populations, Hepatic Insufficiency, Action and Clinical Pharmacology, Special Populations and Conditions, Hepatic Insufficiency; Dosage and Administration, Special Populations, Hepatic Insufficiency.

Special Populations: Pregnant Women: There are no adequate and well-controlled studies in pregnant women and RILUTEK is known to cross the placental barrier in rats. RILUTEK must not be used in pregnant women (see Contraindications).

In the pregnant rat, the transfer of ^{14}C-riluzole across the placenta to the foetus has been detected. Oral administration of riluzole to pregnant animals during the period of organogenesis caused embryotoxicity in rats and rabbits at doses of 27 mg/kg and 60 mg/kg, respectively, or 2.6 and 11.5 times, respectively, the recommended maximum human daily dose on a mg/m² basis. Evidence of maternal toxicity was also observed at these doses.

When administered to rats prior to and during mating (males and females) and throughout gestation and lactation (females), RILUTEK produced adverse effects on pregnancy (decreased implantations, increased intrauterine death) and offspring viability and growth at an oral dose of 15 mg/kg or 1.5 times the maximum daily dose on a mg/m² basis.

Nursing Women: In rat studies, ^{14}C-riluzole was detected in maternal milk. It is not known whether riluzole is excreted in human breast milk. Because many drugs are excreted in human milk, and because of the potential for serious adverse reactions in nursing infants from RILUTEK, RILUTEK must not be used in nursing women (see Contraindications).

Pediatrics (<18 years of age): The safety and efficacy of RILUTEK in any neurodegenerative disease occurring in children or adolescents have not been established.

Geriatrics (>65 years): In controlled clinical trials, about 30% of patients were over 65. There were no differences in adverse effects between younger and older patients. Based on pharmacokinetic data, there are no special instructions for the use of RILUTEK in this population (see Action and Clinical Pharmacology, Special Populations and Conditions, Geriatrics).

Gender: See Action and Clinical Pharmacology, Special Populations and Conditions, Gender.

Race: See Action and Clinical Pharmacology, Special Populations and Conditions, Race.

Hepatic Insufficiency: See Contraindications; Warnings and Precautions, General, Liver Injury/Monitoring Liver Chemistries; Action and Clinical Pharmacology, Special Populations and Conditions, Hepatic Insufficiency; Dosage and Administration, Special Populations, Hepatic Insufficiency.

Renal Insufficiency: RILUTEK is not recommended for use in patients with impaired renal function, as studies at repeated doses have not been conducted in this population (see Dosage and Administration, Special Populations, Renal Insufficiency; Action and Clinical Pharmacology, Special Populations and Conditions, Renal Insufficiency).

Monitoring and Laboratory Tests: Hepatic: Because of risks of hepatitis and jaundice, serum transaminases, including ALT levels, should be measured before and during therapy with RILUTEK. Serum ALT levels should be measured every month during the first 3 months of treatment, every 3 months during the remainder of the first year, and periodically thereafter. Serum ALT levels should be measured more frequently in patients who develop elevated ALT levels (see Warnings and Precautions, General, Liver Injury/Monitoring Liver Chemistries).

As noted in the Warnings and Precautions, General, Liver Injury/Monitoring Liver Chemistries, there is no experience with continued treatment of patients once ALT exceeds 5×ULN. If a decision is made to continue to treat these patients, frequent monitoring (at least weekly) of complete liver function is recommended. Treatment should be discontinued if ALT exceeds 10×ULN or if clinical jaundice develops. Because there is no experience with rechallenge of patients who have had RILUTEK discontinued for ALT >5×ULN, no recommendations about restarting RILUTEK can be made.

Blood Counts: In the two controlled trials in patients with ALS, the frequency with which values for hemoglobin, hematocrit, and erythrocyte counts fell below the lower limit of normal was greater in RILUTEK-treated patients than in placebo-treated patients; however, these changes were mild and transient. The proportions of patients observed with abnormally low values for these parameters showed a dose-response relationship. Only one patient was discontinued from treatment because of severe anemia. The significance of this finding is unknown.

ADVERSE REACTIONS: Adverse Drug Reaction Overview: The most commonly observed adverse events associated with the use of RILUTEK, more frequently than with placebo treatment were: asthenia, nausea, elevations in liver function tests, dizziness, decreased lung function, diarrhea, abdominal pain, pneumonia, vomiting, vertigo, circumoral paresthesia, anorexia and somnolence.

Approximately 14% (n=199) of the 1396 individuals with ALS who received RILUTEK in clinical trials discontinued treatment because of an adverse event. Of those patients who discontinued due to adverse events, the most commonly reported associated adverse events were nausea, abdominal pain, constipation and ALT elevations.

Hepatitis, anaphylactoid reaction, angioedema and pancreatitis have been reported in isolated cases.

Clinical Trial Adverse Drug Reactions: Because clinical trials are conducted under very specific conditions the adverse drug reaction rates observed in the clinical trials may not reflect the rates observed in practice and should not be compared to the rates in the clinical trials of another drug. Adverse drug reaction information from clinical trials is useful for identifying drug-related adverse events and for approximating rates.

The events cited in Table 1 reflect all adverse experiences of ALS patients in placebo-controlled trials, treated with either RILUTEK at the recommended daily dosage of 100 mg/day or placebo, where the incidence with RILUTEK was numerically greater than placebo by at least 1%.

Confirmatory Phase IV trial (study 401): Study 401 is an open-label Phase IV confirmatory trial conducted in Canada, consisting of a prospective treatment arm of n=414 ALS patients treated with RILUTEK at the recommended daily dosage of 100 mg/day and a historical control arm for which there are no safety data. Patients treated with RILUTEK were instructed to report any events that occurred during the study. However, the investigators had to report only a) any events which required discontinuation of study drug and b) all serious adverse events, with the exception of events due to the progression of ALS, hospitalization for permanently assisted ventilation or tracheostomy (primary efficacy endpoints). In addition, the investigators were to assess causality as either possibly related, or not related, to RILUTEK.

Study medication was permanently discontinued in response to an adverse reaction considered **possibly related to study medication** in 35/414 (8.5%) of the patients. Within this subset, there were only two patients with serious adverse reactions: one patient presented with vomiting and diarrhea of moderate intensity and another patient presented with increased alanine aminotransferase rated as severe in intensity.

Table 2 shows the most common treatment-emergent adverse reactions (TEAR) considered possibly related to study medication and for which the incidence was ≥1%.

Table 1: RILUTEK

Adverse Events Occurring in Placebo-controlled Clinical Trials, for Which the Incidence With RILUTEK Was ≥1% Than Placebo

System Organ Class	Preferred Term	Rilutek (100 mg/day) Studies 216, 301, 302 (N=395) %	Placebo Studies 216, 301, 302 (N=406) %
General Disorders and Administration Site Conditions	Asthenia	17	11
	Pain	5	2
Gastrointestinal Disorders	Nausea	14	9
	Abdominal pain	5	4
	Vomiting	4	2
	Paraesthesia oral	1	0
Nervous System Disorder	Headache	7	6
	Dizziness	3	2
	Somnolence	2	1
Cardiac Disorders	Tachycardia	3	2
Hepatobiliary Disorders	Alanine aminotransferase (ALT) abnormal	29	14
	Aspartate aminotransferase (AST) abnormal	23	19
	Gamma-glutamyltransferase (GGT) abnormal	15	11
	Blood bilirubin abnormal	12	8

Table 2: RILUTEK

The Most Common Treatment-emergent Adverse Reactions (TEAR) Considered Possibly Related to Study Medication Occurring in Study 401 and for Which the Incidence Was ≥1%

System Organ Class	Preferred Term	Studies 401 (N=414) %
Gastrointestinal disorders	Nausea	6
	Stomach discomfort	3
	Diarrhea	2
	Dyspepsia	1
	Constipation	1
	Hypoaesthesia oral	1
General Disorders and Administration Site Conditions	Fatigue	4
Nervous System Disorder	Dizziness	4
	Headache	1
	Dysgeusia	1
Psychiatric Disorders	Insomnia	1
Skin and Subcutaneous Tissue Disorders	Rash	1
	Pruritus	1
Hepatobiliary Disorders[a]	Alanine aminotransferase (ALT) abnormal	1

[a] Alert terms (ALT and/or AST values >10 times the upper limit of normal) or abnormal values that led to study drug termination.

Other Events Observed During the Clinical Development of RILUTEK: RILUTEK has been administered to 1713 individuals during all clinical trials, some of which were placebo-controlled (safety data from Study 401 are not included due to differences in data collection process). All reported adverse events are included below except those already listed in the previous tables, those too general to be informative, and those events where a drug cause was remote. For the placebo-controlled trials, events are included if the incidence rate for RILUTEK is numerically greater than the rate for placebo. It is important to emphasize that although the events reported occurred during treatment with RILUTEK, they were not necessarily caused by it.

Events are classified within body system categories and enumerated in order of decreasing frequency using the following definitions: common (≥1%), uncommon (≥0.1% and <1%); rare (≥0.01% and <0.1%), very rare <0.01%).

Blood and Lymphatic System Disorders: Uncommon: leucocytosis, leucopenia. Rare: aplastic anemia, hypochromic anemia, iron deficiency anemia, lymphadenopathy, neutropenia.

Cardiac Disorders: Uncommon: bundle branch block, congestive heart failure, heart failure, pericarditis, ventricular extrasystoles. Rare: bradycardia, cyanosis, ventricular fibrillation, ventricular tachycardia.

Endocrine Disorders: Rare: diabetes insipidus, parathyroid disorder.

Ear and Labyrinth Disorders: Rare: deafness, ear pain, hyperacusis, vestibular disorder.

Eye Disorders: Uncommon: amblyopia, ophthalmitis. Rare: blepharitis, cataract, glaucoma, photophobia.

Gastrointestinal Disorders: Uncommon: enlarged abdomen, esophageal stenosis, fecal impaction, fecal incontinence, gastrointestinal haemorrhage, gastrointestinal ulceration, glossitis, pancreatitis, peritonitis, tenesmus. Rare: hematemesis, proctitis, enlarged salivary gland, tongue discoloration.

General Disorders and Administration Site Conditions: Uncommon: abnormal gait, edema, hernia, injection site reaction. Rare: generalized edema, hypothermia.
Hepatobiliary Disorders: Uncommon: jaundice, hepatitis. Rare: cholecystitis, biliary pain.
Immune System Disorders: Uncommon: anaphylactoid reaction. Rare: angioedema.
Infections and Infestations: Uncommon: cellulitis, flu syndrome, laryngitis, respiratory moniliasis. Rare: breast abscess, cutaneous moniliasis, pseudomembranous enterocolitis, pyelonephritis, tooth caries, vaginal moniliasis.
Injury, Poisoning and Procedural Complications: Uncommon: intentional injury, subdural hematoma.
Metabolism and Nutrition: Uncommon: diabetes mellitus, hypokalemia, hyponatremia, increased appetite. Rare: hypercalcemia, hypercholesteremia, tetany.
Musculoskeletal and Connective Tissue Disorders: Uncommon: arthrosis, leg cramps. Rare: bone necrosis, osteoporosis, rheumatoid arthritis, trismus.
Neoplasm Benign, Malignant and Unspecified (Including Cysts and Polyps): Uncommon: bone neoplasm, lung carcinoma, neoplasm, prostate carcinoma, thyroid neoplasia. Rare: enlarged uterine fibroids.
Nervous System Disorders: Common: tremor. Uncommon: amnesia, ataxia, cerebral hemorrhage, coma, convulsion, dysarthria, extrapyramidal syndrome, facial paralysis, hypokinesia, hypesthesia, incoordination, hemiplegia, migraine, myoclonus, stupor. Rare: acrodynia, cerebral embolism, cerebral ischemia, CNS depression, dementia, hypotonia, peripheral neuritis, subarachnoid hemorrhage, taste loss, wrist drop.
Psychiatric Disorders: Uncommon: apathy, attempted suicide, libido decreased, delirium, delusions, depersonalization, emotional lability, hallucinations, increased libido, manic reaction. Rare: abnormal dreams, acute brain syndrome, psychotic depression, schizophrenic reaction.
Renal and Urinary Disorders: Uncommon: hematuria, kidney calculus, kidney pain, urinary incontinence, urinary retention, urinary urgency, urine abnormality. Rare: nocturia.
Reproductive System and Breast Disorders: Uncommon: impotence, metrorrhagia, priapism. Rare: amenorrhea, breast pain, uterine hemorrhage.
Respiratory, Thoracic and Mediastinal Disorders: Uncommon: asthma, epistaxis, hemoptysis, hiccup, hypoxia, pleural effusion, respiratory acidosis, stridor, yawn, interstitial lung disease (see Warnings and Precautions).
Skin and Subcutaneous Tissue Disorders: Uncommon: ecchymosis, psoriasis, skin disorder, skin ulceration, urticaria. Rare: contact dermatitis, erythema multiforme, purpura, skin granuloma, skin nodule.
Vascular Disorders: Uncommon: hypotension, lower extremity embolus, peripheral vascular disease. Rare: hemorrhage, mesenteric artery occlusion, thrombosis.
Abnormal Hematologic and Clinical Chemistry Findings: Table 3 shows number of patients treated with RILUTEK at the recommended daily dosage of 100 mg/day or placebo who had values for investigational parameters that were above the ULN at any time during the studies and the incidence was numerically greater than placebo by at least 1% (see also Contraindications and Warnings and Precautions, General, Liver Injury/Monitoring Liver Chemistries).

Table 3: RILUTEK

Abnormal Hematologic and Clinical Chemistry Occurring in Placebo-controlled Clinical Trials, for Which the Incidence With RILUTEK Was ≥1% Than Placebo

System Organ Class	Preferred Term	Rilutek (100 mg/day) Studies 216, 301, 302 (N=395) %	Placebo Studies 216, 301, 302 (N=406) %
Investigations	Alanine aminotransferase (ALT) abnormal	29	14
	Aspartate aminotransferase (AST) abnormal	23	19
	Gamma-glutamyltransferase (GGT) abnormal	15	11
	Blood creatine phosphokinase (CPK) abnormal	13	11
	Blood bilirubin abnormal	12	8

Very common: abnormal liver function test. Uncommon: increased gamma glutamyl transferase, increased alkaline phosphatase, positive direct Coombs test, increased gamma globulins. Rare: increased lactic dehydrogenase.
Post-Market Adverse Drug Reactions: Post-Market Spontaneous Adverse Drug Reactions: This section provides the adverse drug reactions not listed above which have been reported through post-market surveillance. Although a causal relationship with RILUTEK may be suspected, other causes can not be excluded. The adverse drug reactions (ADRs) have been classified as per the MEDRA terminology. In some cases, the ADRs have been re-classified so that like-reactions are grouped together.
Blood and Lymphatic System Disorders: disseminated intravascular coagulation, granulocytopenia, lymphopenia, methaemoglobinaemia, normochromic normocytic anaemia, pancytopenia, platelet count decreased, prothrombin time shortened, red blood cell count decreased, thrombocytopenia, thrombocytopenic purpura, white blood cell count decreased, white blood cell count increased.
Cardiac Disorders: atrial fibrillation, cardiac failure, cardiac murmur, congestive cardiomyopathy, cor pulmonale, heart rate decreased, myocardial infarction, myocardial ischaemia.
Congenital, Familial and Genetic Disorders: congenital central nervous system anomaly, congenital foot malformation, exomphalos, talipes.
Drug Interactions: cardioactive drug level increased.
Endocrine Disorders: inappropriate antidiuretic hormone selection.
Eye Disorders: blindness.
Gastrointestinal Disorders: abdominal pain lower, abdominal pain upper, dysphagia, gastrointestinal disorders, gastrointestinal dysplasia, illeus, illeus paralytic, intestinal functional disorder, intestinal obstruction, mouth ulceration, oesophagitis, pancreatitis acute.
General Disorders and Administration Site Conditions: chest pain, condition aggravated, death, disease progression, general physical health deterioration, inflammation, influenza like illness, malaise, pyrexia, sudden death.
Hepatobiliary Disorders: cholestasis, cytolytic hepatitis, hepatitis cholestatic, hepatitis fulminant, hepatocellular damage, hepatotoxicity.
Infections and Infestations: hepatitis B, herpes zoster infection neurological, lobar pneumonia, urinary tract infection.
Injury, Poisoning and Procedural Complications: accidental overdose, extradural haematoma, post procedural haemorrhage.
Metabolism and Nutrition Disorders: blood methaemoglobin present, blood potassium decreased, decreased appetite, dehydration, diabetic ketoacidosis, hyperamylasaemia, hyperlipidaemia, lactic acidosis.
Musculoskeletal and Connective Tissue Disorders: amyotrophy, arthralgia, back pain, muscle rigidity, myalgia, pain in extremity, rhabdomyolysis, shoulder pain.
Neoplasms Benign, Malignant and Unspecified (Incl Cysts and Polyps): gastric cancer, lung neoplasm malignant, non-Hodgkin's lymphoma.
Nervous System Disorders: cerebral hematoma, depressed level of consciousness, disturbance in attention, dystonia, hypoaesthesia, intercostal neuralgia, intracranial pressure increased, lethargy, loss of consciousness, motor neurone disease, myasthenia gravis, neuropathy peripheral, poor quality sleep, radiculopathy, sedation, sensory disturbance, somnolence.
Pregnancy, Puerperium and Perinatal Conditions: intra-uterine death.
Psychiatric Disorders: anxiety, completed suicide, depression, mental disorder, mental status change, psychiatric symptom, psychiatric disorder, restlessness.
Renal and Urinary Disorders: anuria, blood creatinine increased, dysuria, pancreatorenal syndrome, renal failure, renal failure acute, renal impairment.
Reproductive System and Breast Disorders: postmenopausal haemorrhage.
Respiratory, Thoracic and Mediastinal Disorders: alveolitis, alveolitis allergic, aspiration, choking, cough, dyspnoea, eosinophilic pneumonia, interstitial lung disease, Mendelson's syndrome, nasal congestion, pneumonitis, pulmonary embolism, pulmonary toxicity, respiratory disorder, respiratory distress, respiratory failure.
Skin and Subcutaneous Tissue Disorders: alopecia, drug eruption, hyperhidrosis, pemphigoid, pruritus, rash, rash popular, skin discolouration, skin exfoliation, skin nodule.
Vascular Disorders: blood pressure increased, flushing.

DRUG INTERACTIONS: Overview: There have been no clinical studies to evaluate the interaction of RILUTEK with other drugs As with all drugs, the potential for interaction by a variety of mechanisms is a possibility.
Hepatotoxic Drugs: The clinical trials in ALS excluded patients on concomitant medications which were potentially hepatotoxic, (e.g., allopurinol, methyldopa, sulfasalazine). Accordingly, there is no information about the safety of administering RILUTEK in conjunction with such medications. If the practitioner chooses to prescribe such a combination, caution should be exercised.
Drugs Highly Bound to Plasma Proteins: RILUTEK is highly bound (96%) to plasma proteins, binding mainly to serum albumin and to lipoproteins. The effect of RILUTEK (up to 5 µg/mL) on warfarin (5 µg/mL) binding did not show any displacement of warfarin. Conversely, RILUTEK binding was unaffected by the addition of warfarin, digoxin, imipramine and quinine at high therapeutic concentrations.
Effect of Other Drugs on RILUTEK Metabolism: In vitro studies using human liver microsomal preparations suggest that CYP 1A2 is the principal isozyme involved in the initial oxidative metabolism of RILUTEK, and, therefore, potential interactions may occur when RILUTEK is given concurrently with agents that affect CYP 1A2 activity. Potential inhibitors of CYP 1A2 (e.g., caffeine, phenacetin, theophylline, amitriptyline, and quinolones) could decrease the rate of RILUTEK elimination, while inducers of CYP 1A2 (e.g., cigarette smoke, charcoal-broiled food, rifampicin, and omeprazole) could increase the rate of RILUTEK elimination.
Effect of RILUTEK on the Metabolism of Other Drugs: CYP 1A2 is the principal isoenzyme involved in the initial oxidative metabolism of RILUTEK; potential interactions may occur when RILUTEK is given concurrently with other agents which are also metabolized primarily by CYP 1A2 (e.g. theophylline, caffeine and tacrine). Currently, it is not known whether RILUTEK has any potential for enzyme induction in humans.
Drug-Drug Interactions: There have been no clinical studies to evaluate the interaction of RILUTEK with other drugs. As CYP 1A2 is the principal isoenzyme involved in the initial oxidative metabolism of RILUTEK, it appears that CYP 1A2 inhibition or induction is the major source of potential drug interaction.
Drug-Food Interactions: A high fat meal decreases absorption (see Action and Clinical Pharmacology, Pharmacokinetics, Absorption). RILUTEK tablets should be taken at least 1 hour before, or 2 hours after, a meal to avoid a food-related decrease in bioavailability (see Dosage and Administration).
Drug-Herb Interactions: Interactions with herbal products have not been established.
Drug-Laboratory Test Interactions: Interactions with laboratory tests have not been established.

DOSAGE AND ADMINISTRATION: Initially, RILUTEK should be prescribed only by physicians experienced in the diagnosis and management of ALS. If necessary, subsequent follow up and continuing treatment of the patient may be undertaken by non-specialized physicians, under the supervision of a specialist.
Dosing Considerations: RILUTEK tablets should be taken at least 1 hour before, or 2 hours after, a meal to avoid a food-related decrease in bioavailability.
Recommended Dose and Dosage Adjustment: The dose at which survival benefit is seen in clinical trials is 50 mg every 12 hours.
No evidence exists to define the duration of the benefit of continued RILUTEK use. Similarly, there is no evidence of additional benefit if RILUTEK is continued after tracheostomy is performed for ventilation.
Special Populations : Pediatrics (<18 years of age): RILUTEK is not recommended for use in children, as the safety and efficacy of RILUTEK in any neurodegenerative disease occurring in children or adolescents have not been established.
Geriatrics (>65 years): Based on pharmacokinetic data from a dedicated PK study and from the efficacy trials, there are no special instructions for the use of RILUTEK in this population (see Action and Clinical Pharmacology, Special Populations and Conditions, Geriatrics).
Hepatic Insufficiency: RILUTEK is contraindicated in patients who have hepatic disease or who have baseline transaminases greater than 3 times the ULN (upper limit of normal). Liver chemistries should be monitored in all patients on RILUTEK regularly for the first year of treatment, and periodically thereafter (see Contraindications, Warnings and Precautions, General, Liver Injury/Monitoring Liver Chemistries; Action and Clinical Pharmacology, Special Populations and Conditions, Hepatic Insufficiency).
Renal Insufficiency: RILUTEK is not recommended for use in patients with impaired renal function, as studies at repeated doses have not been conducted in this population (see Warnings and Precautions, Special Populations, Renal Insufficiency; Action and Clinical Pharmacology, Special Populations and Conditions, Renal Insufficiency).
Missed Dose: If a dose of RILUTEK is missed, the next dose should be taken at the next scheduled time. Extra tablets should not be taken to make up for the missed dose.

OVERDOSAGE:
Experience with RILUTEK overdose in humans is limited. Neurological and psychiatric symptoms, acute toxic encephalopathy with stupor, coma, and methemoglobinemia have been observed in isolated cases. No specific antidote or information on treatment of overdosage with RILUTEK is available. In the event of overdose, RILUTEK therapy should be discontinued immediately. Treatment should be supportive and directed toward alleviating symptoms. Severe methemoglobinemia may be rapidly reversible after treatment with methylene blue.
The estimated oral median lethal dose is 94 mg/kg and 39 mg/kg for male mice and rats, respectively.

> For management of a suspected drug overdose, contact your regional Poison Control Centre. See the *CPS* Directory section for a list of Poison Control Centres.

ACTION AND CLINICAL PHARMACOLOGY: Mechanism of Action: The etiology and pathogenesis of ALS are not known, although a number of hypotheses have been advanced. One hypothesis is that motor neurons, made vulnerable through either genetic predisposition or environmental factors, are injured by glutamate. In some cases of familial ALS the enzyme superoxide dismutase has been found to be defective.
The mode of action of RILUTEK is unknown. Its pharmacological properties include the following, some of which may be related to its effect: 1) an inhibitory effect on glutamate release, 2) inactivation of voltage-dependent sodium channels, and 3) ability to interfere with intracellular events that follow transmitter binding at excitatory amino acid receptor.
Pharmacodynamics: RILUTEK has also been shown, in a single study, to delay median time to death in a transgenic mouse model of ALS. These mice express human superoxide dismutase bearing one of the mutations found in one of the familial forms of human ALS.
It is also neuroprotective in various in vivo experimental models of neural injury involving excitotoxic mechanisms. In vitro, riluzole protected cultured rat motor neurons from the excitotoxic effects of glutamic acid and prevented the death of cortical neurons induced by anoxia.
Due to its blockade of glutamatergic neuro-transmission, riluzole also exhibits myorelaxant and sedative properties in animal models at doses of 30 mg/kg (about 20 times the recommended human daily dose) and anticonvulsant properties at a dose of 2.5 mg/kg (about 2 times the recommended human daily dose).
Pharmacokinetics: Absorption: Pharmacokinetics are linear over a dose range of 25-100 mg given every 12 hours.
Riluzole is rapidly absorbed after oral administration with maximal plasma concentrations occurring within 60 to 90 minutes. Riluzole is well absorbed (approximately 90%), with average absolute oral bioavailability of about 60% (CV=30%). A high fat meal decreases absorption, reducing AUC by about 20% and peak blood levels by about 45%.
With multiple-dose administration, riluzole accumulates in plasma by about 2 fold and steady-state is reached in less than 5 days.
The 50 mg market tablet was equivalent, with respect to AUC, to the tablet used in the dose ranging clinical trials, while the C_{max} was approximately 30% higher. Both tablets have been used in clinical trials. However, if doses greater than those recommended are given, it is likely that higher plasma levels will be achieved, the safety of which has not been established (see Dosage and Administration).
Distribution: Riluzole is extensively distributed throughout the body and has been shown to cross the blood brain barrier. The volume of distribution of riluzole is about 3.4 L/kg.
Riluzole is 96% bound to plasma proteins, mainly to albumin and lipoproteins over the clinical concentration range.
Metabolism: Riluzole is extensively metabolized to six major and a number of minor metabolites, not all of which have been identified. Some metabolites appear pharmacologically active in in vitro assays. The metabolism of riluzole is mostly hepatic and consists of cytochrome P450-dependent hydroxylation and glucuronidation.

There is marked inter-individual variability in the clearance of riluzole, probably attributable to variability of CYP 1A2 activity, the principal isozyme involved in N-hydroxylation.

In vitro studies using liver microsomes show that hydroxylation of the primary amine group producing N-hydroxyriluzole (RPR 112512), is the main metabolic pathway in human, monkey, dog and rabbit. In humans, cytochrome P450 1A2 is the principal isozyme involved in N-hydroxylation. In vitro studies predict that CYP 2D6, CYP 2C19, CYP 3A4 and CYP 2E1 are unlikely to contribute significantly to riluzole metabolism in humans. Whereas direct glucuroconjugation of riluzole (involving the glucurotransferase isoform UGT-HP4) is very slow in human liver microsomes, N-hydroxyriluzole is readily conjugated at the hydroxylamine group resulting in the formation of O-(>90%) and N-glucuronides.

Excretion: Following a single 150 mg dose of ^{14}C-riluzole to 6 healthy males, 90% and 5% of the radioactivity was recovered in the urine and feces respectively over a period of 7 days. Glucuronides accounted for more than 85% of the metabolites in urine. Only 2% of a riluzole dose was recovered in the urine as unchanged drug.

The mean elimination half-life of riluzole is 12 hours (CV=35%) after repeated doses.

Special Populations and Conditions: Geriatrics: The pharmacokinetic parameters of riluzole after multiple dose administration (4.5 days of treatment at 50 mg riluzole BID) in n=18 elderly and n=18 young subjects are not affected in the elderly (>70 years). (See Warnings and Precautions, Special Populations, Geriatrics (>65 years).)

Gender: In one placebo-controlled clinical trial with population pharmacokinetics, RILUTEK mean clearance was found to be 30% lower in female patients (corresponding to an approximate increase in AUC of 45%). CYP 1A2 activity has been reported to be lower in women than in men. Therefore, a gender effect on riluzole kinetics may be expected in women, resulting in higher blood concentrations of riluzole and its metabolites. However, regarding benefits or adverse events of riluzole, no gender effect was seen in controlled trials.

Smoking: Cigarette smoking is known to induce CYP 1A2. Patients who smoke cigarettes would be expected to eliminate riluzole faster. There is no information, however on the effect of, or need for, dosage adjustment in these patients.

Race: A clinical study was conducted in Germany to evaluate the pharmacokinetics of riluzole and its metabolite N-hydroxyriluzole following repeated oral administration twice daily for 8 days in n=16 healthy Japanese and n=16 Caucasian adult males, with the former having Japanese citizenship, and resident in North America or Europe for <10 years. Results showed no difference in mean pharmacokinetic parameters between the two groups, either for RILUTEK or the major metabolite.

Hepatic Insufficiency: The AUC of riluzole after single oral dose of 50 mg increases by about 1.7 fold in n=6 subjects with mild chronic liver insufficiency and by about 3 fold in n=6 subjects with moderate chronic liver insufficiency, compared to n=12 healthy subjects. The pharmacokinetics of RILUTEK have not been studied in patient with severe hepatic impairment (see Contraindications; Warnings and Precautions, General, Liver Injury/Monitoring Liver Chemistries; Dosage and Administration, Recommended Dose and Dosage Adjustment, Special Populations, Hepatic Insufficiency).

Renal Insufficiency: After a single oral dose of riluzole 50 mg, no significant difference in mean pharmacokinetic parameters between n=12 subjects with moderate or severe chronic renal insufficiency (10 to 50 mL/min) and n=12 healthy volunteers were observed. (See Warnings and Precautions, Special Populations, Renal Insufficiency, Dosage and Administration, Recommended Dose and Dosage Adjustment, Special Populations, Renal Insufficiency.)

STORAGE AND STABILITY: RILUTEK should be stored at room temperature (15 to 30°C) and protected from bright light.

Keep in a safe place out of the reach of children.

INFORMATION FOR THE PATIENT: Published in e-CPS, available by subscription at www.e-cps.ca.

DOSAGE FORMS, COMPOSITION AND PACKAGING: Each white, film-coated, capsule-shaped tablet, engraved with "RPR 202" on one side, contains: riluzole 50 mg. Nonmedicinal ingredients: core: anhydrous colloidal silica, anhydrous dibasic calcium phosphate, croscarmellose sodium, magnesium stearate and microcrystalline cellulose; film-coating: hydroxypropyl methylcellulose, polyethylene glycol and titanium dioxide. Bottles of 60, designed with a child-resistant closure.

(Shown in Product Identification Section)

Rimexolone ℞

CPhA Monograph

see *Corticosteroids: Eye Ear Nose*

Rimso®-50 ℞

dimethyl sulfoxide

Intravesical Instillation for the Treatment of Interstitial Cystitis

Alveda

PHARMACOLOGY: The mode of action of Rimso-50 (dimethyl sulfoxide 50%) as a treatment for interstitial cystitis is speculative at this time. Hypotheses center around the following: anti-inflammation, analgesic, improvement of blood supply, softening of collagen due to action on cross-linking.

Pharmacokinetics: Dimethyl sulfoxide is metabolized in man by oxidation to dimethyl sulfone or by the reduction to dimethyl sulfide. Dimethyl sulfoxide and dimethyl sulfone are excreted in the urine and feces. Dimethyl sulfide is eliminated through the breath and skin and is responsible for the characteristic odor from patients on dimethyl sulfoxide medication. Dimethyl sulfone can persist in serum for longer than 2 weeks after a single intravesical instillation. No residual accumulation of dimethyl sulfoxide has occurred in man or lower animals who have received treatment for protracted periods of time. Following topical application dimethyl sulfoxide is absorbed and generally distributed in the tissues and body fluids.

INDICATIONS: Rimso-50 (dimethyl sulfoxide 50%) is indicated for the symptomatic relief of patients with interstitial cystitis. Rimso-50 has not been approved as being safe and effective for any other indication. There is no clinical evidence of effectiveness of dimethyl sulfoxide in the treatment of bacterial infections of the urinary tract.

CONTRAINDICATIONS: None.

WARNINGS: Dimethyl sulfoxide can initiate the liberation of histamine and there has been an occasional hypersensitivity reaction with topical administration of dimethyl sulfoxide. This hypersensitivity has been reported in some patients receiving intravesical Rimso-50 (dimethyl sulfoxide 50%); The physician should be cognizant of this possibility in prescribing Rimso-50. If anaphylactoid symptoms develop, appropriate therapy should be instituted.

PRECAUTIONS: Changes in the refractive index and lens opacities have been seen in monkeys, dogs and rabbits given dimethyl sulfoxide chronically. No ophthalmic changes attributable to intravesical instillation of dimethyl sulfoxide were reported in patients carefully followed for up to 17 months; nevertheless, full eye evaluations, including slit lamp examinations are recommended prior to and at 6 month intervals during treatment with Rimso-50 (dimethyl sulfoxide 50%).

Along with the ophthalmic examinations, patients should be investigated with respect to biochemical parameters, particularly renal and hepatic function and complete blood count at approximately 6 month intervals.

Intravesical instillation Rimso-50 may be harmful to patients with urinary tract malignancy because of dimethyl sulfoxide-induced vasodilation.

Pediatrics: The safety and effectiveness of Rimso-50 in children have not been established.

Pregnancy: The safety of dimethyl sulfoxide for the human fetus has not been established, hence it should be given to pregnant women only when the potential benefits to the mother have been weighed against possible hazards to the child.

Dimethyl sulfoxide caused teratogenic responses in hamsters, rats and mice when administered intraperitoneally at high doses (2.5-12 g/kg). Oral or topical doses of dimethyl sulfoxide did not cause problems of reproduction in rats, mice or hamsters. Topical doses (5 g/kg – first two days, then 2.5 g/kg – last eight days) produced terata in rabbits, but in another study, topical doses of 1.1 g/kg days three through sixteen of gestation failed to produce any abnormalities.

Lactation: It is not known whether dimethyl sulfoxide is excreted in human milk. Because many drugs are excreted in human milk, mothers receiving dimethyl sulfoxide should refrain from nursing.

ADVERSE EFFECTS: A garlic like taste may be noted by the patient within a few minutes after instillation of Rimso-50 (dimethyl sulfoxide 50%). This taste may last several hours and because of the presence of metabolites, an odor on the breath and skin may remain for 72 hours.

Transient chemical cystitis has been noted following instillation of 100% dimethyl sulfoxide.

The patient may experience moderately severe discomfort on administration. Usually this becomes less prominent with repeated administration.

OVERDOSE:

The oral LD50 of dimethyl sulfoxide in the dog is greater than 10 g/kg. It is improbable that this dosage level could be obtained with intravesical instillation of Rimso-50 (dimethyl sulfoxide 50%) in patients.

Treatment: In case of accidental oral ingestion, specific measures should be taken to induce emesis. Additional measures which may be considered are gastric lavage, activated charcoal and force diuresis.

> For management of a suspected drug overdose, CPhA recommends that you contact your **regional Poison Control Centre**. See the *CPS* Directory section for a list of Poison Control Centres.

DOSAGE: Instillation of 50 mL of Rimso-50 (dimethyl sulfoxide 50%) directly into the bladder may be accomplished by catheter or aseptic syringe and allowed to remain for 15 minutes. Application of an analgesic lubricant gel such as lidocaine jelly to the urethra is suggested prior to the insertion of the catheter to avoid spasm. The medication is expelled by spontaneous voiding. It is recommended that treatment be repeated every two weeks until maximum symptomatic relief is obtained. Thereafter, time intervals between therapy may be increased appropriately.

In selected cases where symptomatic relief is not complete, the bladder may be gently distended by gravity instillation with up to 500 mL of a solution prepared immediately prior to instillation in a glass vial, with one part Rimso-50 and one part sterile water prior to the instillation of the standard dose of Rimso-50. After retention of Rimso-50 for 15 minutes the medication is again expelled by spontaneous voiding.

Administration of oral analgesic medication or suppositories containing belladonna and opium prior to the instillation of Rimso-50 can reduce bladder spasm in particularly sensitive patients.

In patients with severe interstitial cystitis and very sensitive bladders, the initial treatment, and possibly the second and third (depending on patient response) should be done under anesthesia (preferably saddle block type).

Rimso-50 is recommended for bladder instillation only.

SUPPLIED: Each bottle contains: 50 mL (54 g) of sterile and non-pyrogenic 50% w/w dimethyl sulfoxide aqueous solution. Store at room temperature (15 to 30°C). Protect from light.

Risedronate ℞

CPhA Monograph

see *Bisphosphonates: Oral*

Risperdal® Consta® ℞

risperidone

Antipsychotic

Janssen-Ortho

Date of Preparation: July 8, 2004
Date of Revision: December 1, 2009

SUMMARY PRODUCT INFORMATION:

Route of Administration	Dosage Form/Strength	Nonmedicinal Ingredients
Intramuscular Injection	Powder for injectable prolonged-release suspension 12.5 mg, 25 mg, 37.5 mg and 50 mg	Citric acid anhydrous, disodium hydrogen phosphate dihydrate, polylactide-co-glycolide (PLG), polysorbate 20, sodium carboxymethylcellulose, sodium chloride, sodium hydroxide, water for injection

INDICATIONS AND CLINICAL USE: Adults: Schizophrenia and Related Disorders: RISPERDAL CONSTA (risperidone) powder for injectable prolonged-release suspension is indicated for the management of the manifestations of schizophrenia and related psychotic disorders. RISPERDAL CONSTA was found to improve both positive and negative symptoms of schizophrenia.

The efficacy of RISPERDAL CONSTA is based in part on a 12-week, placebo-controlled trial in schizophrenic inpatients or outpatients, along with extrapolation from the established efficacy of oral RISPERDAL in this population.

The effectiveness of RISPERDAL CONSTA in longer-term use, that is, more than 12 weeks, has not been systematically evaluated in controlled trials. However, oral RISPERDAL has been shown to be effective in maintaining clinical improvement during long-term therapy (1 year).

Patients should be periodically reassessed to determine the need for continued treatment (see Dosage and Administration).

Bipolar Disorder: RISPERDAL CONSTA is indicated as monotherapy maintenance treatment in patients with bipolar I disorder, who have previously responded to oral antipsychotics or other anti-manic treatment, to delay occurrence of manic episodes.

For patients who have never taken oral risperidone, it is recommended to establish tolerability with oral risperidone prior to initiating treatment with RISPERDAL CONSTA.

Geriatrics (>65 years of age): See Warnings and Precautions, Serious Warnings and Precautions Box and Special Populations.

Pediatrics (<18 years of age): No data available. See Warnings and Precautions, Special Populations.

CONTRAINDICATIONS: RISPERDAL CONSTA is contraindicated in patients who are hypersensitive to this drug or to any ingredient in the formulation or component of the container.

WARNINGS AND PRECAUTIONS:

> **Serious Warnings and Precautions**
> **Increased Mortality in Elderly Patients with Dementia: Elderly patients with dementia treated with atypical antipsychotic drugs are at an increased risk of death compared to placebo. Analyses of thirteen placebo-controlled trials with various atypical antipsychotics (modal duration of 10 weeks) in these patients showed a mean 1.6-fold increase in death rate in the drug-treated patients. Although the causes of death were varied, most of the deaths appeared to be either cardiovascular (e.g., heart failure, sudden death) or infectious (e.g., pneumonia) in nature (see Warnings and Precautions, Special Populations, Use in Geriatric Patients with Dementia).**

General: Administration: RISPERDAL CONSTA should be injected into the gluteal or deltoid muscle, and care must be taken to avoid inadvertent injection of RISPERDAL CONSTA into a blood vessel (see Dosage and Administration and Adverse Reactions, Post-Market Adverse Drug Reactions [retinal artery occlusion]).

Potential for Cognitive and Motor Impairment: Somnolence was reported by 5% of patients treated with RISPERDAL CONSTA in repeated-dose trials. Since risperidone has the potential to impair judgment, thinking, or motor skills, patients should be cautioned about operating hazardous machinery, including automobiles, until they are reasonably certain that treatment with RISPERDAL CONSTA does not affect them adversely.

QT Interval: As with other antipsychotics, caution should be exercised when RISPERDAL CONSTA is prescribed in patients with a history of cardiac arrhythmias, in patients with congenital long QT syndrome, and in concomitant use with drugs known to prolong the QT interval.

Carcinogenesis and Mutagenesis: Osteodystrophy and Tumours in Animals: RISPERDAL CONSTA produced osteodystrophy in male and female rats in a 1-year toxicity study and a 2-year carcinogenicity study at a dose of 40 mg/kg administered IM every 2 weeks.

RISPERDAL CONSTA produced renal tubular tumours (adenoma, adenocarcinoma) and adrenomedullary pheochromocytomas in male rats in the 2-year carcinogenicity study at 40 mg/kg administered IM every 2 weeks. In addition, RISPERDAL CONSTA produced an increase in a marker of cellular proliferation in renal tissue in males in the 1-year toxicity study and in renal tumour-bearing males in the 2-year carcinogenicity study at 40 mg/kg administered IM every 2 weeks. (Cellular proliferation was not measured at the low dose or in females in either study.)

The effect dose for osteodystrophy and the tumour findings is 8 times the IM maximum recommended human dose (MRHD) (50 mg) on a mg/m² basis and is associated with a plasma exposure (AUC) 2 times the expected plasma exposure (AUC) at the IM MRHD. The no-effect dose for these findings was 5 mg/kg (equal to the IM MRHD on a mg/m² basis). Plasma exposure (AUC) at the no-effect dose was one-third the expected plasma exposure (AUC) at the IM MRHD.

Neither the renal or adrenal tumours, nor osteodystrophy, was seen in studies of orally administered risperidone. Osteodystrophy was not observed in dogs at doses up to 14 times (based on AUC) the IM MRHD in a 1-year toxicity study.

The renal tubular and adrenomedullary tumours in male rats and other tumour findings are described in more detail under Warnings and Precautions, Carcinogenesis, Mutagenesis, Impairment of Fertility.

The relevance of these findings to human risk is unknown.

Carcinogenesis, Mutagenesis, Impairment of Fertility: Carcinogenesis—Oral: Carcinogenicity studies were conducted in Swiss albino mice and Wistar rats. Risperidone was administered in the diet at doses of 0.63, 2.5, and 10 mg/kg for 18 months to mice and for 25 months to rats. These doses are equivalent to 2.4, 9.4, and 37.5 times the oral maximum recommended human dose (MRHD) (16 mg/day) on a mg/kg basis, or 0.2, 0.75, and 3 times the oral MRHD (mice) or 0.4, 1.5, and 6 times the oral MRHD (rats) on a mg/m² basis. A maximum tolerated dose was not achieved in male mice. There was a significant increase in pituitary gland adenomas in female mice at doses 0.75 and 3 times the oral MRHD on a mg/m² basis. There was a significant increase in endocrine pancreatic adenomas in male rats at doses 1.5 and 6 times the oral MRHD on a mg/m² basis. Mammary gland adenocarcinomas were significantly increased in female mice at all doses tested (0.2, 0.75, and 3 times the oral MRHD on a mg/m² basis), in female rats at all doses tested (0.4, 1.5, and 6 times the oral MRHD on a mg/m² basis), and in male rats at a dose 6 times the oral MRHD on a mg/m² basis.

Carcinogenesis—IM: RISPERDAL CONSTA was evaluated in a 24-month carcinogenicity study in which SPF Wistar rats were treated every 2 weeks with IM injections of either 5 mg/kg or 40 mg/kg of risperidone. These doses are 1 and 8 times the MRHD (50 mg) on a mg/m² basis. A control group received injections of 0.9% NaCl, and a vehicle control group was injected with placebo microspheres. There was a significant increase in pituitary gland adenomas, endocrine pancreas adenomas, and adrenomedullary pheochromocytomas at 8 times the IM MRHD on a mg/m² basis. The incidence of mammary gland adenocarcinomas was significantly increased in female rats at both doses (1 and 8 times the IM MRHD on a mg/m² basis). A significant increase in renal tubular tumours (adenomas, adenocarcinomas) was observed in male rats at 8 times the IM MRHD on a mg/m² basis. Plasma exposures (AUC) in rats were 0.3 and 2 times (at 5 and 40 mg/kg, respectively) the expected plasma exposure (AUC) at the IM MRHD.

Dopamine D_2 receptor antagonists have been shown to chronically elevate prolactin levels in rodents. Serum prolactin levels were not measured during the carcinogenicity studies of oral risperidone; however, measurements taken during subchronic toxicity studies showed that oral risperidone elevated serum prolactin levels 5- to 6-fold in mice and rats at the same doses used in the oral carcinogenicity studies. Serum prolactin levels increased in a dose-dependent manner up to 6- and 1.5-fold in male and female rats, respectively, at the end of the 24-month treatment with RISPERDAL CONSTA every 2 weeks. Increases in the incidence of pituitary gland, endocrine pancreas, and mammary gland neoplasms have been found in rodents after chronic administration of other antipsychotic drugs and may be prolactin-mediated.

The relevance for human risk of the findings of prolactin-mediated endocrine tumours in rodents is unknown (see Warnings and Precautions, Hyperprolactinemia).

Mutagenesis: No evidence of mutagenic potential for oral risperidone was found in the in vitro Ames reverse mutation test, in vitro mouse lymphoma assay, in vitro rat hepatocyte DNA-repair assay, in vivo oral micronucleus test in mice, the sex-linked recessive lethal test in Drosophila, or the in vitro chromosomal aberration test in human lymphocytes or in Chinese hamster cells.

In addition, no evidence of mutagenic potential was found in the in vitro Ames reverse mutation test for RISPERDAL CONSTA.

Impairment of Fertility: Oral risperidone (0.16 to 5 mg/kg) was shown to impair mating, but not fertility, in Wistar rats in three reproductive studies (two mating and fertility studies and a multigenerational study) at doses 0.1 to 3 times the oral maximum recommended human dose (MRHD) (16 mg/day) on a mg/m² basis. The effect appeared to be in females, since impaired mating behaviour was not noted in the mating and fertility study in which males only were treated. In a subchronic study in Beagle dogs in which oral risperidone was administered at doses of 0.31 to 5 mg/kg, sperm motility and concentration were decreased at doses 0.6 to 10 times the oral MRHD on a mg/m² basis. Dose-related decreases were also noted in serum testosterone at the same doses. Serum testosterone and sperm values partially recovered, but remained decreased after treatment was discontinued. No no-effect doses were noted in either rat or dog.

No mating and fertility studies were conducted with RISPERDAL CONSTA.

Cardiovascular: RISPERDAL CONSTA may induce orthostatic hypotension associated with dizziness, tachycardia, and in some patients, syncope, probably reflecting its alpha-adrenergic antagonistic properties. Syncope was reported in 0.8% (12/1499) of patients treated with RISPERDAL CONSTA in repeated-dose studies. Clinically significant hypotension has been observed postmarketing with concomitant use of risperidone and antihypertensive treatment.

RISPERDAL CONSTA has not been evaluated or used to any appreciable extent in patients with a recent history of myocardial infarction or unstable heart disease. Patients with these diagnoses were excluded from clinical studies during the product's premarket testing. The electrocardiograms of 202 schizophrenic patients treated with 25 mg or 50 mg RISPERDAL CONSTA and 98 schizophrenic patients treated with placebo in a double-blind, placebo-controlled trial were evaluated. Compared with placebo, there were no statistically significant differences in QTc intervals (using Fridericia's and linear correction factors) during treatment with RISPERDAL CONSTA.

The electrocardiograms of 227 patients were evaluated in the 24-month double-blind, placebo-controlled treatment period of a trial assessing the efficacy and safety of RISPERDAL CONSTA when administered as monotherapy for maintenance treatment in patients with bipolar I disorder. There were no clinically relevant differences in QTc intervals (using Fridericia's and linear correction factors) during treatment with RISPERDAL CONSTA compared to placebo.

RISPERDAL CONSTA should be used with caution in the elderly and patients with renal or hepatic impairment, as well as those with cardiovascular disease (e.g. heart failure, history of myocardial infarction or ischemia, cerebrovascular disease, conduction abnormalities), and conditions such as dehydration and hypovolemia. Special care should be taken to avoid hypotension in patients with a history of cerebrovascular insufficiency or ischemic heart disease, and in patients taking medications to lower blood pressure. Monitoring of cardiovascular signs should be considered in all such patients.

Endocrine and Metabolism: Body Temperature Regulation: Disruption of the body's ability to reduce core body temperature has been attributed to antipsychotic drugs. Appropriate care is advised when prescribing RISPERDAL CONSTA for patients who will be experiencing conditions which may contribute to an elevation or reduction of core temperature, e.g. exercising strenuously, exposure to extreme heat or cold, receiving concomitant medication with anticholinergic activity, or being subject to dehydration.

Hyperglycemia: As with some other antipsychotics, hyperglycemia and exacerbation of pre-existing diabetes have been reported very rarely during the use of oral RISPERDAL (see Adverse Reactions, Post-Market Adverse Drug Reactions). Diabetic ketoacidosis has also been reported.

Assessment of the relationship between atypical antipsychotic use and glucose abnormalities is complicated by the possibility of an increased background risk of diabetes mellitus in patients with schizophrenia and the increasing incidence of diabetes mellitus in the general population. Given these confounders, the relationship between atypical antipsychotic use and hyperglycemia-related adverse events is not completely understood. However, epidemiological studies suggest an increased risk of treatment-emergent hyperglycemia-related adverse events in patients treated with the atypical antipsychotics. Precise risk estimates for hyperglycemia-related adverse events in patients treated with atypical antipsychotics are not available.

Any patient treated with atypical antipsychotics should be monitored for symptoms of hyperglycemia including polydipsia, polyuria, polyphagia, and weakness. Patients who develop symptoms of hyperglycemia during treatment with atypical antipsychotics should undergo fasting blood glucose testing. In some cases, hyperglycemia has resolved when the atypical antipsychotic was discontinued; however, some patients required continuation of antidiabetic treatment despite discontinuation of the suspect drug. Patients with risk factors for diabetes mellitus (e.g., obesity, family history of diabetes) who are starting treatment with atypical antipsychotics should undergo fasting blood glucose testing at the beginning of treatment and periodically during treatment. Patients with an established diagnosis of diabetes mellitus who are started on atypical antipsychotics should be monitored regularly for worsening of glucose control.

Hyperprolactinemia: Antipsychotic drugs elevate prolactin levels with the effect persisting during chronic administration. Since tissue culture experiments indicate that approximately one-third of human breast cancers are prolactin dependent in vitro, RISPERDAL CONSTA should only be administered to patients with previously detected breast cancer if the benefits outweigh the potential risks. Caution should also be exercised when considering RISPERDAL CONSTA treatment in patients with pituitary tumours. Possible manifestations associated with elevated prolactin levels are nonpuerperal lactation, amenorrhea, abnormal sexual function, ejaculation failure, decreased libido, and impotence.

As is common with compounds that increase prolactin release, increases in pituitary gland, mammary gland, and adrenal medullary neoplasia, as well as endocrine pancreatic islet cell hyperplasia and/or neoplasia, were observed with oral RISPERDAL and RISPERDAL CONSTA in carcinogenicity studies conducted in mice and rats. Neither clinical studies nor epidemiologic studies conducted to date have shown an association between chronic administration of this class of drugs and tumorigenesis in humans. The available evidence is considered too limited to be conclusive at this time.

Weight Gain: In the 12-week, placebo-controlled study in patients with schizophrenia, 9% of patients treated with RISPERDAL CONSTA (25 mg or 50 mg) and 6% of placebo-treated patients met a weight gain criterion of >7%. With continued treatment, weight gain (mean: 2.6 kg in the long-term study) has been seen.

In the 24-month, double-blind, placebo-controlled treatment period of the trial assessing the efficacy and safety of RISPERDAL CONSTA when administered as monotherapy for maintenance treatment in patients with bipolar I disorder, 11.6% of patients treated with RISPERDAL CONSTA compared with 2.8% of patients treated with placebo experienced a weight gain of >7% of body weight at endpoint.

Gastrointestinal: Antiemetic Effect: Consistent with its dopamine antagonistic effects, RISPERDAL CONSTA may have an antiemetic effect. Such an effect may mask signs of toxicity due to overdosage with other drugs, or may mask symptoms of disease such as brain tumour, intestinal obstruction or Reye's syndrome.

Genitourinary: Priapism: Rare cases of priapism have been reported. This adverse reaction, as with other psychotropic drugs, did not appear to be dose-dependent and did not correlate with the duration of treatment. The most likely mechanism of priapism is a relative decrease in sympathetic tone.

Hepatic/Biliary/Pancreatic: Use in Patients with Hepatic Impairment: Whereas the pharmacokinetics of oral RISPERDAL in patients with hepatic impairment were comparable to those in young volunteers, the mean free fraction of risperidone was increased by about 35%. Although patients with hepatic impairment were not studied with RISPERDAL CONSTA, it is recommended that patients with any degree of hepatic impairment be carefully titrated on oral RISPERDAL/RISPERDAL M-TAB before treatment with RISPERDAL CONSTA is initiated at a dose of 25 mg. Alternatively, a starting dose of 12.5 mg RISPERDAL CONSTA may be appropriate (see Dosage and Administration).

Neurologic: Neuroleptic Malignant Syndrome (NMS): Neuroleptic malignant syndrome is a potentially fatal symptom complex that has been reported in association with antipsychotic drugs, including oral RISPERDAL.

Clinical manifestations of NMS are hyperthermia, muscle rigidity, altered mental status (including catatonic signs) and evidence of autonomic instability (irregular blood pressure, tachycardia, cardiac arrhythmias, and diaphoresis). Additional signs may include elevated creatine phosphokinase, myoglobinuria (rhabdomyolysis), and acute renal failure.

In arriving at a diagnosis, it is important to identify cases where the clinical presentation includes both serious medical illness (e.g., pneumonia, systemic infection, etc.) and untreated or inadequately treated extrapyramidal signs and symptoms. Other important considerations in the differential diagnosis include central anticholinergic toxicity, heat stroke, drug fever, and primary central nervous system pathology.

The management of NMS should include: 1) immediate discontinuation of all antipsychotic drugs including RISPERDAL CONSTA, and other drugs not essential to concurrent therapy; 2) intensive symptomatic treatment and medical monitoring; and 3) treatment of any concomitant serious medical problems for which specific treatments are available. There is no general agreement about specific pharmacological treatment regimens for uncomplicated NMS. After the last administration of RISPERDAL CONSTA, plasma levels of risperidone are present for up to a minimum of 6 weeks.

If a patient requires antipsychotic drug treatment after recovery from NMS, the potential reintroduction of drug therapy should be carefully considered. The patient should be carefully monitored, since recurrence of NMS has been reported.

Tardive Dyskinesia (TD): A syndrome consisting of potentially irreversible, involuntary, dyskinetic movements may develop in patients treated with conventional antipsychotic drugs. Although TD appears to be most prevalent in the elderly, especially elderly females, it is impossible to predict at the onset of treatment which patients are likely to develop TD. It has been suggested that the occurrence of parkinsonian side effects is a predictor for the development of TD. In clinical studies with oral RISPERDAL, the observed incidence of drug-induced parkinsonism was lower with RISPERDAL than with haloperidol. In the optimal clinical dose range, the difference between risperidone and haloperidol was significant. The risk of developing TD may be less with RISPERDAL and RISPERDAL CONSTA.

The risk of developing TD and the likelihood that it will become irreversible are believed to increase as the duration of treatment and the total cumulative dose of antipsychotic drugs administered to the patient increase. However, the syndrome can develop, although less commonly, after relatively brief periods of treatment at low doses. There is no known treatment for established cases of TD. The syndrome may remit, partially or completely, if antipsychotic drug treatment is withdrawn. However, antipsychotic drug treatment itself may suppress the signs and symptoms of TD, thereby masking the underlying process. The effect of symptom suppression upon the long-term course of TD is unknown.

In view of these considerations, RISPERDAL CONSTA should be prescribed in a manner that is most likely to minimize the risk of TD. As with any antipsychotic drug, RISPERDAL CONSTA should be reserved for patients who appear to be obtaining substantial benefit from the drug. In such patients, the smallest dose and the shortest duration of treatment should be sought. The need for continued treatment should be reassessed periodically.

If signs and symptoms of TD develop during treatment with RISPERDAL CONSTA, withdrawal of the drug should be considered. However, some patients may require treatment with RISPERDAL CONSTA despite the presence of the syndrome.

Seizures: During premarketing testing, seizures occurred in 0.3% (5/1499) of patients treated with RISPERDAL CONSTA. Therefore, RISPERDAL CONSTA should be used cautiously in patients with a history of seizures.

Use in Patients with Parkinson's Disease or Dementia with Lewy Bodies (DLB): Physicians should weigh the risks versus the benefits when prescribing antipsychotics, including RISPERDAL CONSTA, to patients with Parkinson's Disease or Dementia with Lewy Bodies (DLB) since both groups may be at increased risk of Neuroleptic Malignant Syndrome as well as having an increased sensitivity to antipsychotic medications. Manifestation of this increased sensitivity can include confusion, obtundation, postural instability with frequent falls, in addition to extrapyramidal symptoms.

Psychiatric: Suicide: The possibility of suicide or attempted suicide is inherent in psychosis and bipolar disorder, and thus, close supervision and appropriate clinical management of high-risk patients should accompany drug therapy. RISPERDAL CONSTA is to be administered by a healthcare professional (see Dosage and Administration); therefore, suicide due to an overdose is unlikely.

Renal: Use in Patients with Renal Impairment: The pharmacokinetics of oral RISPERDAL were significantly altered in patients with renal disease. In a study with oral risperidone in patients with moderate to severe renal disease, clearance of risperidone and its active metabolite 9-hydroxyrisperidone combined decreased by 60% compared to young healthy subjects (see Action and Clinical Pharmacology, Pharmacokinetics). Although patients with renal impairment were not studied with RISPERDAL CONSTA, it is recommended that patients with any degree of renal impairment be carefully titrated on oral RISPERDAL/RISPERDAL M-TAB with lower starting doses and lower maximal doses, before treatment with RISPERDAL CONSTA is initiated at a dose of 25 mg. Alternatively, a starting dose of 12.5 mg RISPERDAL CONSTA may be appropriate. It may also be useful to monitor renal function in these patients (see Dosage and Administration).

Special Populations: Pregnant Women: The safety of RISPERDAL CONSTA during pregnancy has not been established. No clinical studies have been conducted with RISPERDAL CONSTA. In animal studies, risperidone did not show direct reproductive toxicity. However, due to its prolactin-elevating and CNS-depressant activities, reproductive performance and pup survival were adversely affected in rats. Risperidone was not teratogenic in either rats or rabbits. The microspheres are hydrolyzed to the endogenous components of lactic acid and hydroxyacetic acid, which are not teratogenic.

Placental transfer of risperidone occurs in rat pups. There are no adequate and well-controlled studies in pregnant women. However, there was one report of a case of agenesis of the corpus callosum in an infant exposed to risperidone in utero. The causal relationship to risperidone therapy is unknown.

Reversible extrapyramidal symptoms in the neonate were observed following post-marketing use of risperidone during the last trimester of pregnancy.

RISPERDAL CONSTA should not be used during pregnancy unless the expected benefits to the patient markedly outweigh the potential risks to the fetus.

Nursing Women: Risperidone appeared in the milk of lactating dogs. The concentration of risperidone was similar in milk and plasma, while that of 9-hydroxyrisperidone was higher in milk than in plasma. It has been demonstrated that risperidone and 9-hydroxyrisperidone are also excreted in human breast milk.

Nursing should not be undertaken while a patient is receiving RISPERDAL CONSTA and for at least 12 weeks after the last injection.

Pediatrics (<18 years of age): The safety and efficacy of RISPERDAL CONSTA in children under the age of 18 have not been established.

Geriatrics (>65 years of age): Geriatric patients generally have decreased renal, hepatic and cardiac function, and an increased tendency to postural hypotension. Therefore, lower starting doses, lower rates of dose adjustment and lower maximal doses are recommended in these patients.

Risperidone is substantially excreted by the kidneys. Thus, the risk of toxic reactions to this drug may be greater in patients with impaired renal function. Because elderly patients are more likely to have decreased renal function, caution should be taken in dose selection and titration. It may also be useful to monitor renal function in these patients (see Dosage and Administration and Action and Clinical Pharmacology, Pharmacokinetics).

In an open-label study, 57 clinically stable elderly patients with schizophrenia (≥65 years old) received RISPERDAL CONSTA every 2 weeks for up to 12 months. In general, no differences in the tolerability of RISPERDAL CONSTA were observed between otherwise healthy elderly and nonelderly patients. RISPERDAL CONSTA has not been studied in elderly patients with bipolar disorder. Dosing recommendations for otherwise healthy elderly patients are the same as for nonelderly patients. Because elderly patients exhibit a greater tendency to orthostatic hypotension than nonelderly patients, elderly patients should be instructed in nonpharmacologic interventions that help to reduce the occurrence of orthostatic hypotension (e.g., sitting on the edge of the bed for several minutes before attempting to stand in the morning and slowly rising from a seated position). In addition, monitoring of orthostatic vital signs should be considered in elderly patients for whom orthostatic hypotension is of concern (see Warnings and Precautions, Cardiovascular; Dosage and Administration and Action and Clinical Pharmacology).

Use in Geriatric Patients with Dementia: Overall Mortality: Elderly patients with dementia treated with atypical antipsychotic drugs have an increased mortality compared to placebo in a meta-analysis of 13 controlled trials of various atypical antipsychotic drugs. In six placebo-controlled trials with oral RISPERDAL in this population, the incidence of mortality was 4.0% for RISPERDAL-treated patients compared to 3.1% for placebo-treated patients.

Concomitant Use with Furosemide: In the oral RISPERDAL placebo-controlled trials in elderly patients with dementia, a higher incidence of mortality was observed in patients treated with furosemide plus risperidone (7.3%; mean age 89 years, range 75-97) when compared to patients treated with risperidone alone (3.1%; mean age 84 years, range 70-96), furosemide alone (4.1%; mean age 80 years, range 67-90) or placebo without furosemide (2.9%; mean age 88 years, range 71-100). The increase in mortality in patients treated with furosemide plus risperidone was observed in two of the four clinical trials.

No pathophysiological mechanism has been identified to explain this finding, and no consistent pattern for cause of death has been observed. Nevertheless, caution should be exercised and the risks and benefits of this combination should be considered prior to the decision to use. There was no increased incidence of mortality among patients taking other diuretics as concomitant medication with risperidone. Irrespective of treatment, dehydration was an overall risk factor for mortality and should therefore be carefully avoided in elderly patients with dementia.

Cerebrovascular Adverse Events (CVAEs) in Elderly Patients with Dementia: In placebo-controlled trials in elderly patients with dementia, there was a significantly higher incidence of cerebrovascular adverse events (stroke and transient ischemic attacks) including fatalities in patients (mean age 85 years; range 73-97) treated with oral RISPERDAL compared to patients receiving placebo. There is insufficient information to determine whether CVAEs in elderly patients with dementia are associated specifically with RISPERDAL or other antipsychotic agents.

Dysphagia: Esophageal dysmotility and aspiration have been associated with antipsychotic drug use. Aspiration pneumonia is a common cause of morbidity and mortality in patients with advanced Alzheimer's dementia. RISPERDAL CONSTA and other antipsychotic drugs should be used cautiously in patients at risk for aspiration pneumonia.

ADVERSE REACTIONS: Clinical Trial Adverse Drug Reactions: Because clinical trials are conducted under very specific conditions the adverse reaction rates observed in the clinical trials may not reflect the rates observed in practice and should not be compared to the rates in the clinical trials of another drug. Adverse drug reaction information from clinical trials is useful for identifying drug-related adverse events and for approximating rates.

The prescriber should be aware that the numbers in the tables and tabulations cannot be used to predict the incidence of side effects in the course of usual medical practice where patient characteristics and other factors differ from those which prevailed in the clinical trial. Similarly, the cited frequencies cannot be compared with figures obtained from other clinical investigations involving different treatments, uses, and investigators. The cited figures, however, do provide the prescribing physician with some basis for estimating the relative contribution of drug and non-drug factors to the side effect incidence rate in the population studied.

Schizophrenia: The safety of RISPERDAL CONSTA was evaluated from a clinical trial database consisting of 1499 patients exposed to one or more doses of RISPERDAL CONSTA for the treatment of schizophrenia. Of these 1499 patients, 332 were patients who received RISPERDAL CONSTA while participating in a 12-week, double-blind, placebo-controlled trial. A total of 202 of the 332 were patients with schizophrenia who received 25 mg or 50 mg RISPERDAL CONSTA. The conditions and duration of treatment with RISPERDAL CONSTA in the other clinical trials varied greatly and included (in overlapping categories) double-blind, fixed- and flexible-dose, placebo- or active-controlled studies and open-label phases of studies, inpatients and outpatients, and short-term (up to 12 weeks) and longer-term (up to 4 years) exposures.

Adverse findings were assessed by spontaneous reports of adverse events, laboratory tests, vital signs, body weight, and ECGs. Adverse events were classified using the World Health Organization preferred terms. Treatment-emergent adverse events were defined as those events with an onset between the first dose and 49 days after the last dose.

Adverse Events Associated with Discontinuation of Treatment: RISPERDAL CONSTA is generally well tolerated at doses of 12.5 mg to 50 mg. In the 12-week, placebo-controlled trial in patients with schizophrenia who received 25 mg or 50 mg, the incidence of patients who discontinued treatment due to an adverse event was lower with RISPERDAL CONSTA (11%; 22/202 patients) than with placebo (13%; 13/98 patients). The more common adverse events causing discontinuation included: psychiatric (17% vs. 11% placebo): primarily psychosis, hallucination, agitation, suicide attempt, and anxiety; neurological (1.4% vs. 1% placebo): primarily hyperkinesia. No adverse events leading to discontinuation were found to be unexpected nor were considered to be clinically relevant to RISPERDAL CONSTA.

Commonly Observed Adverse Events in the Controlled Clinical Trial: Table 1 enumerates adverse events that occurred at an incidence of 2% or more, and were at least as frequent among schizophrenic patients treated with 25 mg or 50 mg RISPERDAL CONSTA as patients treated with placebo in the 12-week, placebo-controlled trial. This table shows the percentage of patients in each dose group who spontaneously reported at least one episode of an event at some time during double-blind treatment. All patients were titrated to a dose of 4 mg oral RISPERDAL during a one-week run-in period. Patients who received RISPERDAL CONSTA were given doses of oral RISPERDAL (2 mg for patients in the 25 mg group, and 4 mg for patients in the 50 mg group) during the 3 weeks after the first injection to provide therapeutic levels until the main release phase of risperidone from the injection site had begun. Patients who received placebo injections were given placebo tablets.

Serious Adverse Events: In the 12-week, placebo-controlled trial, the most frequently reported serious adverse events during the double-blind period among schizophrenic patients were psychosis, hallucination, agitation, suicide attempt, and anxiety. No serious adverse events were found to be unexpected nor were considered to be clinically relevant to RISPERDAL CONSTA.

Table 1: RISPERDAL CONSTA

Treatment-Emergent Adverse Events Reported by ≥2% of Patients with Schizophrenia Treated with RISPERDAL CONSTA and Equal or Greater than Placebo in a 12-Week, Double-Blind, Placebo-Controlled Clinical Trial

	Percentage of Patients Reporting Event		
		RISPERDAL CONSTA	
WHO Body System Disorder/ Preferred Term	**Placebo (n=98)**	**25 mg (n=99)**	**50 mg (n=103)**
Psychiatric			
Insomnia	14	16	13
Hallucination	5	7	6
Somnolence	3	5	6
Suicide attempt	3	1	4
Abnormal thinking	2	0	3
Abnormal dreaming	0	2	0
Central & Peripheral Nervous System			
Headache	12	15	22
Dizziness	6	8	11
Akathisia	4	2	9
Parkinsonism[a]	3	4	10
Tremor	0	0	3
Hypoesthesia	0	2	0
Gastrointestinal			
Dyspepsia	2	7	7
Constipation	1	5	7
Mouth dry	1	0	7
Toothache	0	1	3
Saliva increased	1	6	2
Tooth disorder	0	4	2
Diarrhea	3	5	1
Body as a Whole–General			
Fatigue	0	3	7
Pain	4	10	3
Peripheral edema	1	2	3
Leg pain	1	4	1
Fever	0	2	1
Syncope	0	2	0
Respiratory System			
Rhinitis	8	14	4
Coughing	4	5	2
Sinusitis	0	3	1
Upper respiratory tract infection	1	2	0
Metabolic & Nutritional			
Weight increase	2	5	4
Weight decrease	1	4	1
Cardiovascular			
Hypertension	2	3	3
Hearing & Vestibular			
Ear disorder (NOS)[b]	0	0	3
Vision			
Vision abnormal	0	2	3
Skin & Appendage			
Acne	0	2	2
Skin dry	0	2	0
Musculoskeletal			
Myalgia	1	4	2

[a] Includes adverse events of bradykinesia, extrapyramidal disorder, and hypokinesia.
[b] Not Otherwise Specified.

Adverse Reactions during Long-Term Treatment: The long-term safety of RISPERDAL CONSTA was evaluated in 615 patients with schizophrenia treated up to one year with 25 mg, 50 mg, or 75 mg in an open trial. A total of 400 patients completed the one-year trial. The most frequently reported adverse events (>10%) for all dose groups combined were anxiety, psychosis, insomnia, depression, headache, hyperkinesia and rhinitis.

Less Common Clinical Trial Adverse Drug Reactions (≤1%): During its premarketing assessment, RISPERDAL CONSTA was administered to 1499 patients in multiple-dose studies. The conditions and duration of exposure to RISPERDAL CONSTA varied greatly, and included (in overlapping categories) open-label and double-blind studies, uncontrolled and controlled studies, inpatient and outpatient studies, fixed-dose and titration studies, and short-term and long-term exposure studies. In all studies, untoward events associated with this exposure were obtained by spontaneous report and were recorded by clinical investigators using terminology of their own choosing. Consequently, it is not possible to provide a meaningful estimate of the proportion of individuals experiencing adverse events without first grouping similar types of untoward events into a smaller number of standardized event categories.

In the listings that follow, spontaneously reported adverse events were classified using World Health Organization (WHO) preferred terms. The frequencies presented, therefore, represent the proportion of the 1499 patients exposed to multiple doses of RISPERDAL CONSTA who experienced an event of the type cited on at least one occasion while receiving RISPERDAL CONSTA. All reported events are included except those already listed in Table 1, those events for which a drug cause was remote, those event terms which were so general as to be uninformative, and those events reported only once which did not have a substantial probability of being acutely life-threatening. It is important to emphasize that, although the reported events occurred during treatment with RISPERDAL CONSTA, they were not necessarily caused by it.

Events are further categorized by body system and listed in order of decreasing frequency according to the following definitions: frequent adverse events are those occurring in at least 1/100 patients (only those not already listed in the tabulated results from the placebo-controlled trial appear in this listing); infrequent adverse events are those occurring in 1/100 to 1/1000 patients; and rare events are those occurring in fewer than 1/1000 patients.

Psychiatric Disorders: Frequent: anxiety, psychosis, depression, agitation, nervousness, paranoid reaction, delusion, apathy. Infrequent: anorexia, impaired concentration, impotence, emotional lability, manic reaction, decreased libido, increased appetite, amnesia, confusion, euphoria, depersonalization, paroniria, delirium, psychotic depression.

Central and Peripheral Nervous Systems Disorders: Frequent: hypertonia, dystonia. Infrequent: dyskinesia, vertigo, leg cramps, tardive dyskinesia*, involuntary muscle contractions, paresthesia, abnormal gait, bradykinesia, convulsions, hypokinesia, ataxia, fecal incontinence, oculogyric crisis, tetany, apraxia, dementia, migraine. Rare: neuroleptic malignant syndrome.

Body as a Whole/General Disorders: Frequent: back pain, chest pain, asthenia. Infrequent: malaise, choking.

Gastrointestinal Disorders: Frequent: nausea, vomiting, abdominal pain. Infrequent: gastritis, gastroesophageal reflux, flatulence, hemorrhoids, melena, dysphagia, rectal hemorrhage, stomatitis, colitis, gastric ulcer, gingivitis, irritable bowel syndrome, ulcerative stomatitis.

Respiratory System Disorders: Frequent: dyspnea. Infrequent: pneumonia, stridor, hemoptysis. Rare: pulmonary edema.

Skin and Appendage Disorders: Frequent: rash. Infrequent: eczema, pruritus, erythematous rash, dermatitis, alopecia, seborrhea, photosensitivity reaction, increased sweating.

Metabolic and Nutritional Disorders: Infrequent: hyperuricemia, hyperglycemia, hyperlipemia, hypokalemia, glycosuria, hypercholesterolemia, obesity, dehydration, diabetes mellitus, hyponatremia.

Musculoskeletal System Disorders: Frequent: arthralgia, skeletal pain. Infrequent: torticollis, arthrosis, muscle weakness, tendinitis, arthritis, arthropathy.

Heart Rate and Rhythm Disorders: Frequent: tachycardia. Infrequent: bradycardia, AV block, palpitation, bundle branch block. Rare: T-wave inversion.

Cardiovascular Disorders: Frequent: hypotension. Infrequent: postural hypotension.

Urinary System Disorders: Frequent: urinary incontinence. Infrequent: hematuria, micturition frequency, renal pain, urinary retention.

Vision Disorders: Infrequent: conjunctivitis, eye pain, abnormal accommodation.

Reproductive Disorders, Female: Frequent: amenorrhea. Infrequent: nonpuerperal lactation, vaginitis, dysmenorrhea, breast pain, leukorrhea.

Resistance Mechanism Disorders: Infrequent: abscess.

Liver and Biliary System Disorders: Frequent: increased hepatic enzymes. Infrequent: hepatomegaly, increased ALT. Rare: bilirubinemia, increased GGT, hepatitis, hepatocellular damage, jaundice, fatty liver, increased AST.

Reproductive Disorders, Male: Infrequent: ejaculation failure.

Application Site Disorders: Frequent: injection site pain. Infrequent: injection site reaction.

Hearing and Vestibular Disorders: Infrequent: earache, deafness, hearing decreased.

Red Blood Cell Disorders: Frequent: anemia.

White Cell and Resistance Disorders: Infrequent: lymphadenopathy, leukopenia, cervical lymphadenopathy. Rare: granulocytopenia, leukocytosis, lymphopenia.

Endocrine Disorders: Infrequent: hyperprolactinemia, gynecomastia, hypothyroidism.

Platelet, Bleeding and Clotting Disorders: Infrequent: purpura, epistaxis. Rare: pulmonary embolism, hematoma, thrombocytopenia.

Myo-, Endo-, and Pericardial and Valve Disorders: Infrequent: myocardial ischemia, angina pectoris, myocardial infarction.

Vascular (Extracardiac) Disorders: Infrequent: phlebitis. Rare: intermittent claudication, flushing, thrombophlebitis.

Bipolar Disorder: Safety data are presented from a clinical trial assessing the efficacy and safety of RISPERDAL CONSTA as monotherapy maintenance treatment in patients with bipolar I disorder. Patients who met criteria for a stable response to treatment with RISPERDAL CONSTA during a 26-week open label stabilization period were randomized into a 24-month double-blind placebo-controlled period in which they received RISPERDAL CONSTA (n=154) or placebo (n=149) as monotherapy. The majority of patients were treated with the 25 mg dose of RISPERDAL CONSTA.

Safety data are also presented from a clinical trial assessing the efficacy and safety of RISPERDAL CONSTA when administered as adjunctive maintenance treatment in patients with bipolar disorder. In this study, patients who met criteria for stable remission following 16 weeks of open label treatment with RISPERDAL CONSTA, while continuing treatment as usual (mood stabilizers, antidepressants, and/or anxiolytics), were randomized to RISPERDAL CONSTA or placebo, as adjunct to their treatment as usual, for up to 52 weeks. RISPERDAL CONSTA is not indicated as adjunctive maintenance treatment in bipolar disorder.

Adverse events during exposure to study treatment were obtained by general inquiry and recorded by clinical investigators using their own terminology. Consequently, to provide a meaningful estimate of the proportion of individuals experiencing adverse events, events were grouped into standardized categories using MedDRA terminology.

Monotherapy: Adverse Events Associated with Discontinuation of Treatment : In the 24-month, double-blind, placebo-controlled trial evaluating RISPERDAL CONSTA as monotherapy maintenance treatment in patients with bipolar I disorder per study protocol, an adverse event was not recorded as the reason for discontinuation when a patient experienced a mood-related adverse event in association with relapse. One patient (0.6%) in the RISPERDAL CONSTA group experienced an adverse event, hyperglycemia, that led to discontinuation and was not associated with relapse. Thirty-three patients (22%) in the placebo group and 15 patients (9.7%) in the RISPERDAL CONSTA group who discontinued double-blind treatment due to relapse had adverse events with action taken of permanent stop. For the majority of patients in both treatment groups these adverse events were psychiatric. Depression was the only psychiatric adverse event associated with discontinuation of more relapsed patients in the RISPERDAL CONSTA group than in the placebo group (5% RISPERDAL CONSTA versus 2% placebo).

Commonly Observed Adverse Events in the Controlled Clinical Trial: Table 2 enumerates adverse events that occurred at an incidence of 2% or more, and were at least as frequent among bipolar patients treated with RISPERDAL CONSTA as patients treated with placebo in the 24-month, double-blind treatment period of the trial assessing the efficacy and safety of RISPERDAL CONSTA when administered as monotherapy for maintenance treatment in patients with bipolar I disorder.

Serious Adverse Events: In the 24-month, placebo-controlled monotherapy trial, the most frequently reported serious adverse events in the RISPERDAL CONSTA group during the double-blind period were psychiatric disorders: depression (3% RISPERDAL CONSTA versus 1% placebo), Bipolar I disorder (2% RISPERDAL CONSTA versus 6% placebo), and mania (2% RISPERDAL CONSTA versus 7% placebo).

Less Common Clinical Trial Adverse Events (≤1%): All reported events in the RISPERDAL CONSTA group during the double-blind treatment period of the monotherapy trial reported at least as frequently in the placebo group are listed below except those already listed in Table 2.

Psychiatric Disorders: depressed mood, libido decreased, drug dependence.

Nervous System Disorders: akathisia, dyskinesia, parkinsonism, hypoaesthesia, radiculitis, sedation, sinus headache, somnolence, tremor.

Infections and Infestations: bronchitis, anogenital warts, bacteriuria, ear infection, fungal infection , furuncle, gastroenteritis viral, influenza, onychomycosis, papilloma viral infection, paronychia, pharyngitis streptococcal, sinusitis, tinea infection, urinary tract infection, viral upper respiratory tract infection.

General Disorders and Administration Site Conditions: pyrexia, feeling cold, pain, thirst.

Gastrointestinal Disorders: abdominal pain, constipation, dry mouth, duodenal ulcer, gastritis, gingival bleeding, hemorrhoids, mouth ulceration, salivary hypersecretion, tooth loss, vomiting.

Investigations: electrocardiogram QT prolonged, electrocardiogram T-wave abnormal, alanine aminotransferase increased, gamma-glutamyltransferase increased, hepatic enzyme increased.

* In the integrated database of multiple-dose studies (1499 patients with schizophrenia or schizoaffective disorder), 9 patients (0.6%) treated with RISPERDAL CONSTA (all dosages combined) experienced an adverse event of tardive dyskinesia.

Metabolism and Nutrition Disorders: decreased appetite, dehydration, hyperglycemia, anorexia, diabetes mellitus, hypertriglyceridemia, increased appetite, obesity, type 2 diabetes mellitus.

Musculoskeletal and Connective Tissue Disorders: musculoskeletal pain, myalgia.

Reproductive System and Breast Disorders: erectile dysfunction, sexual dysfunction, ejaculation disorder.

Table 2: RISPERDAL CONSTA

Treatment-Emergent Adverse Events Reported by ≥2% of Patients with Bipolar I Disorder Treated with RISPERDAL CONSTA and Equal or Greater than Placebo as Monotherapy in a 24-Month, Double-Blind, Placebo-Controlled Clinical Trial

MedDRA Body System or Organ Class/ Dictionary-Derived Term	Percentage of Patients Reporting Event	
	Placebo (N=149)	RISPERDAL CONSTA (N=154)
Psychiatric Disorders		
Insomnia	6	8
Depression	2	6
Nervous System Disorders		
Headache	7	7
Dizziness	1	3
Infections and Infestations		
Nasopharyngitis	3	4
Viral infection	1	2
General Disorders and Administration Site Conditions		
Fatigue	3	4
Asthenia	1	2
Gastrointestinal Disorders		
Diarrhea	1	2
Nausea	1	2
Investigations		
Weight increased	1	5
Musculoskeletal and Connective Tissue Disorders		
Back pain	3	3
Vascular Disorders		
Hypertension	1	3

Cardiac Disorders: bundle branch block right, myocardial ischemia.

Respiratory, Thoracic and Mediastinal Disorders: cough, nasal congestion, nasal polyps, pharyngolaryngeal pain, sinus congestion.

Blood and Lymphatic Disorders: anemia, lymphadenitis.

Eye Disorders: conjunctivitis, visual disturbance.

Skin and Subcutaneous Tissue Disorders: dermatitis, dermatitis contact.

Ear and Labyrinth Disorders: ear pain.

Immune System Disorders: hypersensitivity.

Renal and Urinary Disorders: stress urinary incontinence.

Adjunctive Therapy: Adverse Events Associated with Discontinuation of Treatment: In the 52-week, double-blind phase of the placebo-controlled trial in which RISPERDAL CONSTA was administered as adjunctive therapy to patients with bipolar disorder in addition to their treatment as usual, approximately 4% (3/72) of patients treated with RISPERDAL CONSTA discontinued due to an adverse event, compared with 1.5% (1/67) of placebo-treated patients. Adverse events that led to discontinuation that occurred more frequently in the RISPERDAL CONSTA group were hypokinesia, tardive dyskinesia and hypertensive heart disease (1.4%, one patient each).

Commonly Observed Adverse Events in the Controlled Clinical Trial: Table 3 enumerates adverse events that occurred at an incidence of 2% or more, and were at least as frequent among bipolar patients treated with RISPERDAL CONSTA as patients treated with placebo in the 52-week trial in which RISPERDAL CONSTA was administered as adjunctive therapy to patients with bipolar disorder in addition to continuing with their treatment as usual. RISPERDAL CONSTA is not indicated as adjunctive maintenance treatment in bipolar disorder.

Table 3: RISPERDAL CONSTA

Treatment-Emergent Adverse Events Reported by ≥2% of Patients with Bipolar Disorder Treated with RISPERDAL CONSTA and Equal or Greater than Placebo as Adjunctive Therapy in a 52-Week, Double-Blind, Placebo-Controlled Clinical Trial

MedDRA Body System or Organ Class/ Dictionary-Derived Term	Percentage of Patients Reporting Event	
	Placebo (N=67)	RISPERDAL CONSTA (N=72)
Nervous System Disorders		
Tremor	16	24
Parkinsonism[a]	6	15

(cont'd)

Table 3: RISPERDAL CONSTA *(cont'd)*

Treatment-Emergent Adverse Events Reported by ≥2% of Patients with Bipolar Disorder Treated with RISPERDAL CONSTA and Equal or Greater than Placebo as Adjunctive Therapy in a 52-Week, Double-Blind, Placebo-Controlled Clinical Trial

MedDRA Body System or Organ Class/ Dictionary-Derived Term	Percentage of Patients Reporting Event	
	Placebo (N=67)	RISPERDAL CONSTA (N=72)
Akathisia	6	6
Dyskinesia[b]	3	6
Sedation	0	6
Memory impairment	3	4
Disturbance in attention	0	4
Psychiatric Disorders		
Irritability	3	3
Sleep disorder	3	3
Musculoskeletal and Connective Tissue Disorders		
Arthralgia	3	4
Musculoskeletal stiffness	0	3
General Disorders and Administration Site Conditions		
Gait abnormal	0	4
Infections and Infestations		
Upper respiratory tract infection	3	6
Nasopharyngitis	3	3
Urinary tract infection	2	3
Metabolism and Nutrition Disorders		
Decreaced appetite	2	6
Increased appetite	0	3
Gastrointestinal Disorders		
Loose stools	2	4
Salivary hypersecretion	3	3
Investigations		
Weight increased	2	7
Reproductive System and Breast Disorders		
Amenorrhea	2	4
Respiratory, Thoracic and Mediastinal Disorders		
Cough	2	4
Dyspnea exertional	0	3
Skin and Subcutaneous Tissue Disorders		
Alopecia	0	3
Eye Disorders		
Visual acuity reduced	0	3
Vascular Disorders		
Orthostatic hypotension	0	3

a Parkinsonism includes muscle rigidity, hypokinesia, cogwheel rigidity, and bradykinesia.
b Dyskinesia includes muscle twitching and dyskinesia.

Serious Adverse Events: In the 52-week, placebo-controlled adjunctive therapy trial, the most frequently reported serious adverse events in the RISPERDAL CONSTA group during the double-blind period was mania (4% RISPERDAL CONSTA versus 6% placebo).

Less Common Clinical Trial Adverse Events (≤1%): All reported events in the RISPERDAL CONSTA group during the double-blind treatment period of the adjunctive therapy trial reported at least as frequently in the placebo group are listed below except those already listed in Table 3.

Nervous System Disorders: cogwheel rigidity, drooling, neuritis, tardive dyskinesia.

Psychiatric Disorders: anxiety, libido decreased, middle insomnia, panic attack, suicide attempt.

Musculoskeletal and Connective Tissue Disorders: pain in extremity, posture abnormal.

General Disorders and Administration Site Conditions: chest pain, malaise, pain.

Infections and Infestations: fungal infection, furuncle, pneumonia, sinusitis, tuberculosis.

Metabolism and Nutrition Disorders: anorexia, hyperlipidemia.

Gastrointestinal Disorders: hemorrhoidal hemorrhage, hemorrhoids, halitosis, tongue disorder.

Investigations: corneal reflex decreased, urine analysis abnormal.

Reproductive System and Breast Disorders: menorrhagia, menstrual disorder.

Respiratory, Thoracic and Mediastinal Disorders: dyspnoea.

Skin and Subcutaneous Tissue Disorders: alopecia areata, dry skin, face edema, pain of skin, seborrhoeic dermatitis.

Eye Disorders: cataract.

Vascular Disorders: hypotension.

Blood and Lymphatic Disorders: anemia.

Cardiac Disorders: hypertensive heart disease.

Endocrine Disorders: hypothyroidism.

Injury, Poisoning and Procedural Complications: blister.

Renal and Urinary Disorders: enuresis.

Adverse Events Observed Across Indications: Extrapyramidal Symptoms: Schizophrenia: Two methods were used to measure extrapyramidal symptoms (EPS) in the 12-week, placebo-controlled trial comparing three doses of RISPERDAL CONSTA (25 mg, 50 mg, and 75 mg) with placebo including: 1) the incidence of spontaneous reports of EPS symptoms; and 2) the change from baseline to endpoint on the total score (sum of the subscale scores for parkinsonism, dystonia, and dyskinesia) of the Extrapyramidal Symptom Rating Scale (ESRS).

As shown in Table 1, the overall incidence of EPS related adverse events (akathisia, dystonia, parkinsonism, and tremor) in patients treated with 25 mg RISPERDAL CONSTA was comparable to that of patients treated with placebo; the incidence of EPS-related adverse events was higher in patients treated with 50 mg RISPERDAL CONSTA.

The median change from baseline to endpoint in total ESRS score showed no worsening in patients treated with RISPERDAL CONSTA compared with patients treated with placebo: 0 (placebo group); −1 (25 mg group, significantly less than the placebo group); and 0 (50 mg group).

Bipolar Disorder: There were no clinically meaningful changes from baseline to study endpoint for mean ESRS total score during any phase of the monotherapy study. Similarly, there were no meaningful changes from baseline to study endpoint on dyskinetic symptoms (measured using the Abnormal Involuntary Movement Scale), akathisia symptoms (Barnes Akathisia Scale) or Parkinsonian symptoms (Simpson-Angus Rating Scale) during any phase of the adjunctive therapy study. As shown in Table 3, a higher incidence of EPS-related adverse events was noted in the adjunctive therapy study, predominantly tremor.

Vital Sign Changes: Hypotension (including orthostatic) and tachycardia have been observed following the administration of RISPERDAL CONSTA. In the placebo controlled trial in patients with schizophrenia, orthostatic hypotension was observed in 2% of patients treated with 25 mg or 50 mg RISPERDAL CONSTA (see Warnings and Precautions, Cardiovascular).

Weight Changes: In the 12-week, placebo-controlled trial, 9% of patients with schizophrenia treated with RISPERDAL CONSTA (25 or 50 mg), compared with 6% of patients treated with placebo, experienced a weight gain of >7% of body weight at endpoint.

In the 24-month, double-blind, placebo-controlled treatment period of the trial assessing the efficacy and safety of RISPERDAL CONSTA when administered as monotherapy for maintenance treatment in patients with bipolar I disorder, 11.6% of patients treated with RISPERDAL CONSTA compared with 2.8% of patients treated with placebo experienced a weight gain of >7% of body weight at endpoint (see Warnings and Precautions, Endocrine and Metabolism).

ECG Changes: Compared with placebo, there were no statistically significant differences in QTc intervals (using Fridericia's and linear correction factors) during treatment with RISPERDAL CONSTA in the 12-week, placebo-controlled trial in patients with schizophrenia (see Warnings and Precautions, General, QT Interval).

The electrocardiograms of 227 patients were evaluated in the 24-month double-blind, placebo-controlled treatment period of a trial assessing the efficacy and safety of RISPERDAL CONSTA when administered as monotherapy for maintenance treatment in patients with bipolar I disorder. There were no clinically relevant differences in QTc intervals (using Fridericia's and linear correction factors) during treatment with RISPERDAL CONSTA compared to placebo (see Warnings and Precautions, General, QT Interval).

Pain Assessment and Local Injection Site Reactions: Gluteal: The mean intensity of injection pain reported by patients with schizophrenia using a visual analog scale (0=no pain to 100=unbearably painful) decreased in all treatment groups from the first to the last injection (placebo: 16.7 to 12.6; 25 mg: 12.0 to 9.0; 50 mg: 18.2 to 11.8). After the sixth injection (Week 10), investigator ratings indicated that 1% of patients treated with 25 mg or 50 mg RISPERDAL CONSTA experienced redness, swelling, or induration at the injection site.

Deltoid: In a separate study to observe local-site tolerability, RISPERDAL CONSTA was administered into the deltoid muscle every 2 weeks over a period of 8 weeks, (patients received up to 2 injections per arm as alternate arms were injected). No patient discontinued treatment due to local injection site pain or reaction. Clinician ratings indicated that only mild redness, swelling, or induration at the injection site was observed in subjects treated with 37.5 mg or 50 mg RISPERDAL CONSTA at 2 hours after deltoid injection. All ratings returned to baseline at the predose assessment of the next injection 2 weeks later. No moderate or severe reactions were observed in any subject.

The tolerability of repeated injections of RISPERDAL CONSTA in the deltoid muscle for more than 8 weeks has not been systematically studied.

Hyperprolactinemia: RISPERDAL CONSTA elevated plasma prolactin levels. Possible manifestations associated with elevated prolactin levels are nonpuerperal lactation, amenorrhea, abnormal sexual function, ejaculation failure, decreased libido, and impotence.

Other Adverse Events: As with other antipsychotics, cases of water intoxication, either due to polydipsia or to syndrome of inappropriate secretion of antidiuretic hormone (SIADH), have occasionally been reported during treatment with oral RISPERDAL.

Abnormal Hematologic and Clinical Chemistry Findings: Laboratory Changes: The percentage of patients treated with RISPERDAL CONSTA who experienced potentially important changes in routine serum chemistry, hematology, or urinalysis parameters was similar to or less than that of placebo patients. Additionally, no patients discontinued treatment due to changes in serum chemistry, hematology, or urinalysis parameters.

In one study with oral RISPERDAL in which testosterone levels were measured, testosterone decreased below the normal range in 6 out of 85 patients.

Post-Market Adverse Drug Reactions: In addition, adverse events reported with risperidone treatment since market introduction which were temporally related to risperidone therapy include the following: agitation, abdominal pain, edema, angioedema, skin manifestations of allergy including cases of Stevens-Johnson syndrome, systemic manifestations of allergy including a case of anaphylactic shock, urinary incontinence, gynecomastia, agranulocytosis, neutropenia, thrombopenia, apnea, atrial fibrillation, benign pituitary adenomas, intestinal obstruction, jaundice, mania, pancreatitis, Parkinson's disease aggravated, pulmonary embolism, alopecia and hypothermia. Cerebrovascular adverse events, including cerebrovascular accidents and transient ischemic attacks, have been reported during treatment with oral RISPERDAL (see Warnings and Precautions, Special Populations, Use in Geriatric Patients with Dementia, Cerebrovascular Adverse Events (CVAEs) in Elderly Patients with Dementia). Hyperglycemia and exacerbation of pre-existing diabetes have been reported in very rare cases during treatment with risperidone (see Warnings and Precautions, Endocrine and Metabolism). Diabetic ketoacidosis has also been reported. As with other neuroleptics, sudden deaths have been reported during treatment with risperidone. Most of the patients had pre-existing cardiovascular disease or were morbidly obese. A relationship to risperidone has not been established at this time.

Retinal artery occlusion after injection of RISPERDAL CONSTA has been reported very rarely during post-marketing surveillance. RISPERDAL CONSTA should be injected into the gluteal or deltoid muscle, and care must be taken to avoid inadvertent injection of RISPERDAL CONSTA into a blood vessel (see Dosage and Administration).

Injection site reactions including injection site abscess, cellulitis, cyst, hematoma, necrosis, nodule, and ulcer have been reported with RISPERDAL CONSTA. These events were reported as serious. Isolated cases required surgical intervention.

As with other neuroleptics, sudden death, torsades de pointes, ventricular tachycardia, arrhythmia, cardiopulmonary arrest and QT prolongation have been reported during treatment with risperidone. Many of the patients had pre-existing cardiovascular disease, were on concomitant medications known to prolong the QT interval, had risk factors for QT prolongation, took an overdose of risperidone, and/or were morbidly obese. Very rarely, QT prolongation has been reported in the absence of confounding factors.

DRUG INTERACTIONS: Overview: Given the primary central nervous system effects of RISPERDAL CONSTA, caution should be used when it is taken in combination with other centrally acting drugs and alcohol.

Because of its potential for inducing hypotension, RISPERDAL CONSTA may enhance the hypotensive effects of other therapeutic agents. RISPERDAL CONSTA may antagonize the effects of levodopa and dopamine agonists.

Clinically significant hypotension has been observed postmarketing with concomitant use of risperidone and antihypertensive medications.

Caution is advised when prescribing RISPERDAL CONSTA with drugs known to prolong the QT interval.

Drug-Drug Interactions: Concomitant Use with Furosemide: See Warnings and Precautions regarding increased mortality in elderly patients with dementia concomitantly receiving furosemide and oral RISPERDAL.

Carbamazepine and Other CYP 3A4 Enzyme Inducers: Carbamazepine has been shown to decrease substantially the plasma levels of risperidone and its active metabolite 9-hydroxyrisperidone (n=11). Similar effects may be observed with other CYP 3A4 hepatic enzyme inducers. Consequently, in the presence of carbamazepine or other CYP 3A4 hepatic enzyme inducers the dose of RISPERDAL CONSTA may have to be adjusted. At the initiation of therapy with carbamazepine or other known CYP 3A4 hepatic enzyme inducers, patients should be closely monitored for the first 4-8 weeks, since the dose of RISPERDAL CONSTA may need to be adjusted. A dose increase, or additional oral RISPERDAL, may need to be considered. On discontinuation of carbamazepine or other CYP 3A4 hepatic inducers, the dosage of RISPERDAL CONSTA should be re-evaluated and, if necessary, decreased. Patients may be placed on a lower dose of RISPERDAL CONSTA between 2 and 4 weeks before the planned discontinuation of carbamazepine or other CYP 3A4 inducers to adjust for the expected increase in plasma concentrations of risperidone plus 9-hydroxyrisperidone. For patients treated with the recommended dose (25 mg) of RISPERDAL CONSTA, it is recommended to continue treatment with the 25 mg dose unless clinical judgment necessitates lowering the RISPERDAL CONSTA dose to 12.5 mg or necessitates interruption of RISPERDAL CONSTA treatment (see also Dosage and Administration). The efficacy of the 12.5 mg dose has not been investigated in clinical trials.

Drugs That Inhibit CYP 2D6 and Other CYP Isozymes: The metabolism of risperidone, a substrate of the hepatic cytochrome P450 isozyme 2D6 (CYP 2D6), is affected by the debrisoquine hydroxylation polymorphism (see Action and Clinical Pharmacology, Pharmacokinetics). CYP 2D6 is also responsible for the metabolism of a variety of drugs, including phenothiazines, antidepressants (tricyclics and SSRIs), antiarrhythmics and some β-blockers. Consequently, potential interaction between RISPERDAL CONSTA and drugs that are also substrates of CYP 2D6 should also be considered.

Fluoxetine and Paroxetine: Fluoxetine and paroxetine, CYP 2D6 inhibitors, increase the plasma concentration of risperidone but less so of risperidone and 9-hydroxyrisperidone combined. Pharmacokinetic interaction with fluoxetine was examined in a study which measured steady-state plasma levels of oral risperidone and its metabolites before and following 3 weeks of co-treatment with fluoxetine (n=10). The addition of fluoxetine resulted in about a 2- to 3-fold increase in peak and AUC levels of risperidone and about a 50% increase in peak and AUC levels for risperidone and 9-hydroxyrisperidone combined. Similarly, pharmacokinetic interaction with paroxetine was examined in a study which measured steady-state plasma levels of risperidone and its metabolites before and following 4 weeks of co-treatment with paroxetine (n=10). After 4 weeks of paroxetine treatment, the sum of the concentrations of risperidone and 9-hydroxyrisperidone increased significantly by 45% over baseline. When fluoxetine or paroxetine is initiated in patients receiving the recommended dose of 25 mg of RISPERDAL CONSTA, it is recommended to continue treatment with the 25 mg dose unless clinical judgment necessitates lowering the RISPERDAL CONSTA dose to 12.5 mg or necessitates interruption of treatment with RISPERDAL CONSTA. When RISPERDAL CONSTA is initiated in patients already receiving fluoxetine or paroxetine, a starting dose of 12.5 mg can be considered. The efficacy of the 12.5 mg dose has not been investigated in clinical trials (see also Dosage and Administration).

Erythromycin: Erythromycin, a CYP 3A4 inhibitor, did not change the pharmacokinetics of risperidone or risperidone and 9-hydroxyrisperidone combined. Risperidone was administered as a single dose of 1 mg with multiple doses of erythromycin (500 mg q.i.d.) in healthy volunteers (n=18).

The Effect of Other Drugs on the Metabolism of Risperidone: Galantamine and Donepezil: The cholinesterase inhibitors galantamine (n=15) and donepezil (n=24) did not show an effect on the pharmacokinetics of risperidone or risperidone and 9-hydroxyrisperidone combined. Galantamine 12 mg o.d. was co-administered with risperidone 0.5 mg o.d. in healthy elderly volunteers. Donepezil 5 mg o.d. was co-administered with risperidone 0.5 mg b.i.d. in healthy male volunteers.

Cimetidine and Ranitidine: Risperidone was administered as a single dose of 1 mg with multiple doses of either cimetidine (400 mg b.i.d.) or ranitidine (150 mg b.i.d.) in healthy young volunteers (n=12). The effect of the drug interaction of cimetidine and ranitidine on risperidone and 9-hydroxyrisperidone combined was minimal.

Clozapine: Chronic administration of clozapine with risperidone may decrease the clearance of risperidone.

Topiramate: Healthy Volunteers: A drug-drug interaction study between risperidone and topiramate was conducted in 12 healthy volunteers (6 males, 6 females), ages 28-40 years, with single-dose administration of risperidone (2 mg) and multiple doses of topiramate (titrated up to 200 mg/day). In the presence of topiramate, systemic exposure of risperidone and 9-hydroxyrisperidone combined was reduced such that mean $AUC_{0-\infty}$ was 11% lower and mean C_{max} was statistically significantly (18%) lower. In the presence of topiramate, systemic exposure of risperidone was statistically significantly reduced such that mean C_{max} and $AUC_{0-\infty}$ were 29% and 23% lower, respectively. The pharmacokinetics of 9-hydroxyrisperidone were unaffected. The effects of a single dose (2 mg/day) of risperidone on the pharmacokinetics of multiple doses of topiramate have not been studied.

Patients with Bipolar Disorder: A drug-drug interaction study conducted in 52 patients with various types of bipolar disorder (24 males, 28 females), ages 19-56 years, evaluated the steady-state pharmacokinetics of risperidone and topiramate when administered concomitantly. Eligible subjects were stabilized on a risperidone dose of 1-6 mg/day for 2 to 3 weeks. Topiramate was then titrated up to escalating doses of 100, 250 and 400 mg/day along with risperidone for up to 6 weeks. Risperidone was then tapered and discontinued over 4 weeks while maintaining topiramate (up to 400 mg/day). There was a statistically significant reduction in risperidone systemic exposure (16% and 33% for AUC_{12} and 13% and 34% for C_{max} at the 250 and 400 mg/day doses, respectively). Minimal alterations were observed in the pharmacokinetics of risperidone and 9-hydroxyrisperidone combined and 9-hydroxyrisperidone. Topiramate systemic exposure was slightly reduced (12.5% for mean C_{max} and 11% for mean AUC_{12}) in the presence of risperidone, which achieved statistical significance. There were no clinically significant changes in the systemic exposure of risperidone and 9-hydroxyrisperidone combined or of topiramate. The effects of higher doses of topiramate (>400 mg/day) are unknown. Therefore, if combination therapy is chosen, patients receiving both risperidone and topiramate should be closely monitored.

Effects of Risperidone on the Metabolism of Other Drugs: Lithium: Oral risperidone (3 mg b.i.d.) did not show an effect on the pharmacokinetics of lithium (400, 450, or 560 b.i.d.) (n=13).

Valproate: Oral risperidone (4 mg o.d.) did not show an effect on the pharmacokinetics of valproate (1000 mg/day) (n=9). However, more subjects reported adverse events with the risperidone-valproate therapy compared to the placebo-valproate group in the clinical trial.

Digoxin: The effect of oral risperidone (0.5 mg/day administered b.i.d.) on the steady-state plasma concentrations of digoxin (0.125 mg/day) was examined in a double-blind, two-way crossover trial in 19 healthy elderly volunteers (median age 68 years, range 61 to 75 years). Risperidone did not affect the steady-state pharmacokinetics of digoxin, and concurrent administration of the two drugs was well tolerated.

In vitro studies, in which risperidone was given in the presence of various highly protein-bound agents, indicated that clinically relevant changes in protein binding would not occur either for RISPERDAL CONSTA or for any of the drugs tested.

Drug-Food Interactions: Interactions with food have not been established.

Drug-Herb Interactions: Interactions with herbal products have not been established.

Drug-Laboratory Test Interactions: Interactions with laboratory tests have not been established.

DOSAGE AND ADMINISTRATION

Dosing Considerations: RISPERDAL CONSTA is a treatment option for patients where the risk of relapse requires intervention according to clinical judgment. For patients who have never taken oral RISPERDAL/RISPERDAL M-TAB, it is recommended to establish tolerability with oral RISPERDAL/RISPERDAL M-TAB prior to initiating treatment with RISPERDAL CONSTA.

- Patients prone to hypotension
- Geriatrics
- Patients with renal impairment
- Patients with hepatic impairment

Administration: RISPERDAL CONSTA should be administered every 2 weeks by deep intramuscular gluteal or deltoid injection. Each injection should be administered by a healthcare professional using the appropriate enclosed safety needle (see Instructions for Use). When selecting an intramuscular site for injection, it is recommended that the healthcare professional conduct an assessment of the patient and site characteristics considering such factors as age, physical condition, skin integrity and size of the muscle.

For gluteal administration, use the 2-inch needle alternating injections between the two buttocks. For deltoid administration, use the 1-inch needle alternating injections between the two arms. Prior to each administration, the site of injection should be examined for any signs of clinically significant or persistent local reaction. If such signs are present, an alternate site should be chosen for injection. Care must be taken to avoid inadvertent injection of RISPERDAL CONSTA into a blood vessel. Do **not** administer intravenously (see Warnings and Precautions, General and Instructions for Use).

While gluteal and deltoid injections of RISPERDAL CONSTA have demonstrated bioequivalence under the recommended injection parameters, the tolerability of repeated injections of RISPERDAL CONSTA in the deltoid muscle for more than 8 weeks has not been systematically studied.

Recommended Dose and Dosage Adjustment: Schizophrenia: The recommended dose is 25 mg IM every 2 weeks. Although dose response for effectiveness has not been established for RISPERDAL CONSTA, some patients not responding to 25 mg may benefit from a higher dose of 37.5 mg or 50 mg. The maximum dose should not exceed 50 mg RISPERDAL CONSTA every 2 weeks. No additional benefit was observed with dosages greater than 50 mg RISPERDAL CONSTA in clinical trials in patients with schizophrenia; however, a higher incidence of adverse effects was observed.

Although no controlled studies have been conducted to answer the question of how long patients should be treated with RISPERDAL CONSTA, oral RISPERDAL/RISPERDAL M-TAB has been shown to be effective in maintaining clinical improvement during long-term therapy (1 year) in patients with schizophrenia. It is recommended that responding patients be continued on treatment with RISPERDAL CONSTA at the lowest dose needed. Patients should be periodically reassessed to determine the need for continued treatment.

Bipolar Disorder: The recommended dose is 25 mg IM every 2 weeks. Although dose response for effectiveness has not been established for RISPERDAL CONSTA, some patients not responding to 25 mg may benefit from a higher dose of 37.5 mg or 50 mg. In clinical trials the majority of patients were treated with the 25 mg dose. The maximum dose should not exceed 50 mg RISPERDAL CONSTA every 2 weeks. Doses above 50 mg have not been studied in this population. It is recommended that responding patients be continued with the lowest dose needed and reassessed periodically to determine the need for continued treatment.

RISPERDAL CONSTA is not indicated as adjunctive treatment in patients with bipolar disorder.

General Dosing Information: A lower initial dose of 12.5 mg may be appropriate when clinical factors warrant dose adjustment, such as in patients with hepatic or renal impairment (see below), for certain drug interactions that increase risperidone plasma concentrations (see Drug Interactions), or in patients who have a history of poor tolerability to psychotropic medications. The efficacy of the 12.5 mg dose has not been investigated in clinical trials.

Oral RISPERDAL/RISPERDAL M-TAB (or another antipsychotic medication) should be given with the first injection of RISPERDAL CONSTA and continued for 3 weeks to ensure that adequate therapeutic plasma concentrations are maintained prior to the main release phase of risperidone from the injection site (see Action and Clinical Pharmacology).

Upward dose adjustment should not be made more frequently than every 4 weeks. The clinical effects of this dose adjustment should not be anticipated earlier than 3 weeks after the first injection with the higher dose.

In patients with clinical factors such as hepatic or renal impairment, or for certain drug interactions that increase risperidone plasma concentrations (see Drug Interactions), dose reduction as low as 12.5 mg may be appropriate. The efficacy of the 12.5 mg dose has not been investigated in clinical trials.

Two different dose strengths of RISPERDAL CONSTA should not be combined in a single administration.

Pediatrics: RISPERDAL CONSTA has not been studied in children younger than 18 years old.

Geriatrics: For elderly patients treated with RISPERDAL CONSTA, the recommended dosage is 25 mg IM every 2 weeks. Oral RISPERDAL/RISPERDAL M-TAB (or another antipsychotic medication) should be given with the first injection of RISPERDAL CONSTA and should be continued for 3 weeks to ensure that adequate therapeutic plasma concentrations are maintained prior to the main release phase of risperidone from the injection site (see Action and Clinical Pharmacology). RISPERDAL CONSTA has not been studied in elderly patients with bipolar disorder. Elderly patients and patients with a predisposition to hypotensive reactions or for whom such reactions would pose a particular risk should be instructed in nonpharmacologic interventions that help to reduce the occurrence of orthostatic hypotension (e.g., sitting on the edge of the bed for several minutes before attempting to stand in the morning and slowly rising from a seated position). These patients should avoid sodium depletion or dehydration, and circumstances that accentuate hypotension (alcohol intake, high ambient temperature, etc.). Monitoring of orthostatic vital signs should be considered (see Warnings and Precautions, Cardiovascular).

Patients with Hepatic Impairment: RISPERDAL CONSTA has not been studied in hepatically impaired patients.

RISPERDAL CONSTA should be used with caution in patients with hepatic impairment.

Patients with impaired hepatic function have increases in plasma concentration of the free fraction of risperidone and this may result in an enhanced effect. If hepatically impaired patients require treatment with RISPERDAL CONSTA, a starting dose of 0.5 mg b.i.d. oral risperidone (e.g., RISPERDAL M-TAB) is recommended during the first week. In the second week, 1 mg b.i.d. or 2 mg q.d. can be given. If an oral dose of at least 2 mg is well tolerated, an injection of 25 mg RISPERDAL CONSTA can be administered every 2 weeks. Alternatively, a starting dose of 12.5 mg RISPERDAL CONSTA may be appropriate (see Warnings and Precautions, Hepatic/Biliary/Pancreatic and Action and Clinical Pharmacology, Pharmacokinetics). The efficacy of the 12.5 mg dose has not been investigated in clinical trials.

Oral supplementation should be continued for 3 weeks after the first injection until the main release of risperidone from the injection site has begun. In some patients, slower titration may be medically appropriate.

Patients with Renal Impairment: RISPERDAL CONSTA has not been studied in renally impaired patients.

RISPERDAL CONSTA should be used with caution in patients with renal impairment.

Patients with renal impairment have less ability to eliminate the active antipsychotic fraction than normal adults. If renally impaired patients require treatment with RISPERDAL CONSTA, a starting dose of 0.5 mg b.i.d. oral risperidone (e.g., RISPERDAL M-TAB) is recommended during the first week. In the second week, 1 mg b.i.d. or 2 mg q.d. can be given. If an oral dose of at least 2 mg is well tolerated, an injection of 25 mg RISPERDAL CONSTA can be administered every 2 weeks. Alternatively, a starting dose of 12.5 mg RISPERDAL CONSTA may be appropriate (see Warnings and Precautions, Renal and Action and Clinical Pharmacology, Pharmacokinetics). The efficacy of the 12.5 mg dose has not been investigated in clinical trials.

Oral supplementation should be continued for 3 weeks after the first injection until the main release of risperidone from the injection site has begun. In some patients, slower titration may be medically appropriate.

Switching from Other Antipsychotics: There are no systematically collected data to specifically address switching patients from other antipsychotics to RISPERDAL CONSTA, or concerning concomitant administration with other antipsychotics. Previous antipsychotics should be gradually discontinued to ensure that therapeutic concentrations are maintained during the 3 weeks after the first injection of RISPERDAL CONSTA until the main release phase of risperidone from the injection site has begun. For patients who have never taken oral RISPERDAL/RISPERDAL M-TAB, it is recommended to establish tolerability with oral RISPERDAL/RISPERDAL M-TAB prior to initiating treatment with RISPERDAL CONSTA. As recommended with other antipsychotic medications, the need for continuing existing EPS medication should be re-evaluated periodically.

Reinitiation of Treatment in Patients Previously Discontinued: There are no data to specifically address reinitiation of treatment. When restarting patients who have had an interval off treatment with RISPERDAL CONSTA, supplementation with oral RISPERDAL (or another antipsychotic medication) should be administered.

Instructions for Use: RISPERDAL CONSTA:

> RISPERDAL CONSTA prolonged-release microspheres in the vial must be reconstituted **only** in the diluent in the syringe supplied in the dose pack and must be administered with **only** the appropriate needle supplied in the dose pack for gluteal (2-inch needle) or deltoid (1-inch needle) administration. Do not substitute any components in the dose pack. To assure that the intended dose of risperidone is delivered, the full contents from the vial must be administered. Administration of partial contents may not deliver the intended dose of risperidone.

Remove the dose pack of RISPERDAL CONSTA from the refrigerator and allow it to come to room temperature prior to reconstitution.

Contents of the dose pack:

- One vial containing RISPERDAL CONSTA prolonged-release microspheres
- One prefilled syringe containing the diluent for RISPERDAL CONSTA
- One inner carton containing the following components for reconstitution and administration:
  - One ALARIS SmartSite needle-free vial access device for reconstitution
  - Two needles for intramuscular injection (a 20G TW 2-inch safety needle with Needle-Pro safety device for gluteal administration and a 21G UTW 1-inch safety needle with Needle-Pro safety device for deltoid administration)

1. Flip off the coloured plastic cap from the vial.
2. Peel back the blister pouch and remove the vial access device by holding the white luer cap.
   Do not touch the spike tip of the access device at any time.
3. Place vial on a hard surface. With a straight push-down movement, press the spike tip of the vial access device through the centre of the vial's rubber stopper until the device securely snaps onto the vial top.
4. Swab the syringe connection point (blue circle) of the vial access device with preferred antiseptic prior to attaching the syringe to the vial access device.
5. The prefilled syringe has a white tip consisting of 2 parts: a white collar and a smooth white cap. To open the syringe, hold the syringe by the white collar and **snap** off the smooth white cap (**do not twist off the white cap**). Remove the white cap together with the rubber tip cap inside.
   For all assembly steps, hold the syringe only by the white collar located at the tip of the syringe. Be careful not to overtighten components when assembling. Overtightening connections may cause syringe component parts to loosen from the syringe body.
6. While holding the **white collar** of the syringe, insert and **press** the syringe tip into the blue circle of the vial access device and **twist** in a clockwise motion to secure the connection of the syringe to the vial access device (avoid over-twisting).
   Hold the skirt of the vial access device during attachment to prevent it from spinning.
   Keep the syringe and the vial access device aligned.
7. Inject the entire contents of the syringe containing the diluent into the vial.
8. Shake the vial vigorously while holding the plunger rod down with the thumb for a minimum of 10 seconds to ensure a homogeneous suspension.
   When properly mixed, the suspension appears uniform, thick, and milky in colour. The microspheres will be visible in liquid, but no dry microspheres remain.

9.

Do not store the vial after reconstitution or the suspension may settle.

10. Invert the vial completely and slowly withdraw the entire contents of the suspension from the vial into the syringe.
11. Tear the section of the vial label at the perforation and apply detached label to syringe for identification purposes.
12. While holding the **white collar** of the syringe, unscrew the syringe from the vial access device. Discard both the vial and vial access device appropriately.
13. Open the needle pack and select the appropriate needle. Do **not** touch the connection part of the needle; only touch the transparent sheath of the needle.
    For **gluteal** injection, select the **20G** TW **2-inch** needle (longer needle with **yellow** coloured hub). For **deltoid** injection, select the **21G** UTW **1-inch** needle (shorter needle with **green** coloured hub).
14. While holding the white collar of the syringe, attach the Luer connection of the orange Needle-Pro safety device to the syringe with an easy clockwise twisting motion.
15. While continuing to hold the **white collar** of the syringe, grasp the transparent needle sheath and seat the needle firmly on the orange Needle-Pro safety device with a push and a clockwise twist.
16.

Resuspension of RISPERDAL CONSTA will be necessary prior to administration as settling will occur over time once product is reconstituted. Resuspend the microspheres in the syringe by shaking vigorously.

17. While holding the **white** collar of the syringe, pull the transparent needle sheath straight away from the needle. **Do not twist** the sheath as the Luer connections may be loosened.
18. Tap the syringe gently to make any air bubbles rise to the top.
    Remove air in syringe by depressing the plunger rod while holding the needle in an upright position. Inject the entire contents of the syringe intramuscularly into the selected gluteal or deltoid muscle of the patient. Gluteal injection should be made into the upper-outer quadrant of the gluteal area.
    Do not administer intravenously.

Warning: To avoid a needle stick injury with a contaminated needle:
- Do not use free hand to press the Needle-Pro safety device over the needle.
- Do not intentionally disengage the Needle-Pro safety device.
- Do not attempt to straighten the needle or engage Needle-Pro safety device if the needle is bent or damaged.
- Do not mishandle the Needle-Pro safety device as it may cause the needle to protrude from the Needle-Pro safety device.

19. After injection is complete, press the needle into the orange Needle-Pro safety device using a one-handed technique. Perform a one-handed technique by **gently** pressing the orange Needle-Pro safety device against a table top or other hard, flat surface. **As the orange Needle-Pro safety device is pressed, the needle will firmly engage into the orange Needle-Pro safety device.** Visually confirm that the needle is fully engaged into the orange Needle-Pro safety device before discarding. Discard needle into an appropriate sharps container. Also discard the other (unused) needle provided in the dose pack in the same way.
    Parenteral drug products should be inspected visually for particulate matter and discoloration prior to administration whenever solution and container permit.
    Syringes should be inspected visually for discoloration and leakage prior to administration. Those showing discoloration or leakage should not be used.

Reconstitution:

Vial Size	Volume of Diluent to be Added to Vial	Approximate Available Volume	Nominal Concentration per mL
12.5 mg			
5 mL	2 mL	2 mL	6.25 mg/mL
25 mg			
5 mL	2 mL	2 mL	12.5 mg/mL
37.5 mg			
5 mL	2 mL	2 mL	18.75 mg/mL
50 mg			
5 mL	2 mL	2 mL	25 mg/mL

RISPERDAL CONSTA must be suspended **only** in the diluent supplied in the dose pack. The entire volume of diluent (2 mL) must be used for suspension of the microspheres.

Upon suspension in the diluent, it is recommended to use RISPERDAL CONSTA immediately. RISPERDAL CONSTA must be used within 6 hours of suspension. Resuspension of RISPERDAL CONSTA will be necessary prior to administration as settling will occur over time since the product is in suspension. Keeping the vial upright, shake vigorously back and forth for as long as it takes to resuspend the microspheres. Reconstituted product in syringe must be resuspended by shaking vigorously if 2 minutes elapse prior to injection. Once in suspension, the product should not be exposed to temperatures above 25°C.

OVERDOSAGE:

Human Experience: No cases of overdose were reported in premarketing studies with RISPERDAL CONSTA. Because RISPERDAL CONSTA is to be administered by healthcare professionals, the potential for overdosage by patients is low.

Cases of overdose have been reported with oral RISPERDAL; the estimated doses were between 20 and 360 mg. In general, reported signs and symptoms were those resulting from an exaggeration of the drug's known pharmacological effects, namely drowsiness, sedation, tachycardia, hypotension, and extrapyramidal symptoms. In overdose, QT-prolongation, widened QRS complex, convulsions, hyponatremia and hypokalemia were also reported.

Torsade de pointes has been reported in association with combined overdose of oral RISPERDAL and paroxetine.

Treatment of Overdosage: In case of acute overdosage, establish and maintain an airway to ensure adequate oxygenation and ventilation. Cardiovascular monitoring should commence immediately and should include continuous electrocardiographic monitoring to detect possible arrhythmias.

There is no specific antidote to RISPERDAL CONSTA. Therefore, appropriate supportive measures should be instituted. The possibility of multiple drug involvement should be considered. Hypotension and circulatory collapse should be treated with appropriate measures such as intravenous fluids and/or sympathomimetic agents (epinephrine and dopamine should not be used, since beta stimulation may worsen hypotension in the setting of risperidone-induced alpha blockade). In cases of severe extrapyramidal symptoms, anticholinergic medication should be administered. Close medical supervision and monitoring should continue until the patient recovers.

For management of a suspected drug overdose, contact your regional Poison Control Centre. See the *CPS Directory* section for a list of Poison Control Centres.

ACTION AND CLINICAL PHARMACOLOGY: Mechanism of Action: Risperidone, a benzisoxazole derivative, is a novel antipsychotic drug which binds with high affinity to serotonin type 2 ($5-HT_2$), dopamine type 2 (D_2), and α_1-adrenergic receptors. Risperidone binds with a lower affinity to the α_2-adrenergic and histamine H_1 receptors. Risperidone does not bind to dopamine D_1 receptors and has no affinity (when tested at concentrations $>10^{-5}$ M) for muscarinic cholinergic receptors. Due to the lack of muscarinic receptor binding, risperidone is not expected to produce anticholinergic adverse effects.

Receptor occupancy was also demonstrated in vivo in humans. Using positron emission tomography, risperidone was shown to block both $5-HT_{2A}$ and dopamine D_2 receptors in three healthy volunteers. Although risperidone is a potent D_2 antagonist, which is considered to improve the positive symptoms of schizophrenia, it causes less depression of motor activity and induction of catalepsy in animal models than classical antipsychotics. Risperidone has also been found to be one of the most potent known antagonists of $5-HT_{2A}$ (cloned human receptor); $5-HT_{2A}$ antagonism has been shown to reverse deficits in several in vivo animal models predictive of novel antipsychotic activity (PCP-induced social deficit, microdialysis assessment of dopamine output in prefrontal cortex, glutamate antagonist-induced hyperlocomotion). Balanced central serotonin and dopamine antagonism may reduce extrapyramidal side effect liability.

Pharmacokinetics: Risperidone is well absorbed, as illustrated by a mass balance study of a single, 1 mg oral dose of ^{14}C-risperidone administered as solution to three healthy male volunteers. Total recovery of radioactivity at 1 week was 84%, including 70% in urine and 14% in feces.

Absorption: After a single intramuscular injection of RISPERDAL CONSTA, there is a small initial release of the drug (<1% of the dose), followed by a lag time of 3 weeks. The main release of the drug starts from week 3 onward, is maintained from 4 to 6 weeks, and subsides by 7 weeks following the intramuscular (IM) injection. Therefore, oral antipsychotic supplementation should be given during the first 3 weeks of treatment with RISPERDAL CONSTA to maintain therapeutic levels until the main release of risperidone from the injection site has begun (see Dosage and Administration). Following single doses of RISPERDAL CONSTA, the pharmacokinetics of risperidone, 9-hydroxyrisperidone (the major metabolite), and risperidone plus 9-hydroxyrisperidone were linear in the dosing range of 12.5 mg to 50 mg.

The combination of the release profile and the dosage regimen (IM injections every 2 weeks) of RISPERDAL CONSTA results in sustained therapeutic concentrations. Steady-state plasma concentrations are reached after 4 injections and are maintained for 4 to 6 weeks after the last injection. Following multiple doses of 25 mg to 50 mg RISPERDAL CONSTA, plasma concentrations of risperidone, 9-hydroxyrisperidone, and risperidone plus 9-hydroxyrisperidone are linear. The half-life of risperidone plus 9-hydroxyrisperidone is 3 to 6 days, and is associated with a monoexponential decline in plasma concentrations. This half-life of 3 to 6 days is related to the erosion of the microspheres and subsequent absorption of risperidone. The elimination phase is complete approximately 7 to 8 weeks after the last injection.

After repeated IM injections of 25 mg or 50 mg RISPERDAL CONSTA every 2 weeks, median trough and peak plasma concentrations of risperidone plus 9-hydroxyrisperidone fluctuated between 9.9 ng/mL to 19.2 ng/mL and 17.9 ng/mL to 45.5 ng/mL, respectively. Fluctuations in plasma concentrations were lower with RISPERDAL CONSTA than with risperidone oral tablets. Median C_{max}/C_{min} ratios for risperidone were approximately 2 after IM injection and 20-30 after oral intake; median C_{max}/C_{min} ratios for risperidone plus 9-hydroxyrisperidone were approximately 2 after IM injection and 3-4 after oral intake.

Gluteal and deltoid intramuscular injections at the same doses are bioequivalent and, therefore, interchangeable.

Distribution: Once absorbed, risperidone is rapidly distributed. The volume of distribution is 1-2 L/kg. In plasma, risperidone is bound to albumin and α_1-acid glycoprotein. The plasma protein binding of risperidone is approximately 88%, and that of 9-hydroxyrisperidone is 77%. Neither risperidone nor 9-hydroxyrisperidone displaces each other from plasma binding sites.

Metabolism: Risperidone is extensively metabolized in the liver. The main metabolic pathway is through hydroxylation of risperidone to 9-hydroxyrisperidone by the enzyme, cytochrome $P450IID_6$ (CYP 2D6). A minor metabolic pathway is through N-dealkylation. The main metabolite, 9-hydroxyrisperidone, has similar pharmacological activity to risperidone. Consequently, the clinical effect of the drug results from the combined concentrations of risperidone plus 9-hydroxyrisperidone. The hydroxylation of risperidone is dependent upon debrisoquine 4-hydroxylase, i.e. the metabolism of risperidone is sensitive to debrisoquine hydroxylation type genetic polymorphism. Consequently, the concentrations of parent drug and active metabolite differ substantially in extensive and poor metabolizers. However, the concentration of risperidone and 9-hydroxyrisperidone combined did not differ substantially between extensive and poor metabolizers, and elimination half-lives were similar in all subjects (approximately 20 to 24 hours).

Excretion: The clearance of risperidone and risperidone plus 9-hydroxyrisperidone was 13.7 L/h and 5.0 L/h in extensive CYP 2D6 metabolizers, and 3.3 L/h and 3.2 L/h in poor CYP 2D6 metabolizers, respectively. No accumulation of risperidone was observed during long-term use (up to 12 months) in patients treated every 2 weeks with 25 mg or 50 mg of RISPERDAL CONSTA.

Special Populations and Conditions: Pediatrics: No data available.

Geriatrics: In an open-label trial, steady-state concentrations of risperidone plus 9-hydroxyrisperidone in otherwise healthy elderly patients (≥65 years old) treated with risperidone powder for injectable prolonged-release suspension for up to 12 months fell within the range of values observed in otherwise healthy non-elderly patients. For these reasons, dosing recommendations are the same for otherwise healthy elderly patients and nonelderly patients (see Dosage and Administration).

Gender: No specific pharmacokinetic study was conducted to investigate gender effects, but a population pharmacokinetic analysis did not identify important differences in the disposition of risperidone due to gender (with or without correction for body weight).

Race: No specific pharmacokinetic study was conducted to investigate race effects, but a population pharmacokinetic analysis did not identify important differences in the disposition of risperidone due to race.

Hepatic Insufficiency: Whereas the pharmacokinetics of oral risperidone in subjects with liver disease were comparable to those in young healthy subjects, the mean free fraction of risperidone in plasma was increased by about 35% because of the diminished concentration of both albumin and α_1-acid glycoprotein. Although patients with hepatic impairment were not studied with risperidone powder for injectable prolonged-release suspension, it is recommended that patients with hepatic impairment be carefully titrated on oral risperidone before treatment with RISPERDAL CONSTA is initiated at a dose of 25 mg. Alternatively, a starting dose of 12.5 mg RISPERDAL CONSTA may be appropriate (see Warnings and Precautions, Hepatic/Biliary/Pancreatic and Dosage and Administration).

Renal Insufficiency: In patients with moderate to severe renal disease treated with oral risperidone, clearance of risperidone and 9-hydroxyrisperidone combined was decreased by about 60%, C_{max} and AUC were increased by about 40% and 160% respectively, and half-life was prolonged by about 60% compared with young healthy subjects. Although patients with renal impairment were not studied with risperidone powder for injectable prolonged-release suspension, it is recommended that patients with renal impairment be carefully titrated on oral risperidone before treatment with RISPERDAL CONSTA is initiated at a dose of 25 mg. Alternatively, a starting dose of 12.5 mg RISPERDAL CONSTA may be appropriate (see Warnings and Precautions, Renal and Dosage and Administration).

STORAGE AND STABILITY: The entire kit should be stored in the refrigerator (2-8°C) and protected from light.

If refrigeration is unavailable, kit can be stored at temperatures not exceeding 25°C for no more than 7 days prior to administration. Do not expose unrefrigerated product to temperatures above 25°C. Protect from light.

RISPERDAL CONSTA must be suspended **only** in the diluent supplied in the dose pack. The entire volume of diluent (2 mL) must be used for suspension of the microspheres.

Upon suspension in the diluent, it is recommended to use RISPERDAL CONSTA immediately. RISPERDAL CONSTA must be used within 6 hours of suspension. Resuspension of RISPERDAL CONSTA will be necessary prior to administration as settling will occur over time since the product is in suspension. Keeping the vial upright, shake vigorously back and forth for as long as it takes to resuspend the microspheres. Reconstituted product in syringe must be resuspended by shaking vigorously if 2 minutes elapse prior to injection. Once in suspension, the product should not be exposed to temperatures above 25°C.

RISPERDAL CONSTA should be kept out of the reach of children.

INFORMATION FOR THE PATIENT: Published in e-CPS, available by subscription at www.e-cps.ca.

DOSAGE FORMS, COMPOSITION AND PACKAGING: 12.5 mg: Each vial of white to off-white, free-flowing powder contains: risperidone 12.5 mg. Risperidone is micro-encapsulated in 7525 polylactide-co-glycolide (PLG) at a concentration of 381 mg risperidone per g of microspheres. The diluent for parenteral use is a clear, colorless solution in a prefilled syringe. Composition of the diluent includes polysorbate 20, sodium carboxymethylcellulose, disodium hydrogen phosphate dihydrate, citric acid anhydrous, sodium chloride, sodium hydroxide, and water for injection. The microspheres are suspended in the diluent prior to injection.

25 mg: Each vial of white to off-white, free-flowing powder contains: risperidone 25 mg. Risperidone is micro-encapsulated in 7525 polylactide-co-glycolide (PLG) at a concentration of 381 mg risperidone per g of microspheres. The diluent for parenteral use is a clear, colorless solution in a prefilled syringe. Composition of the diluent includes polysorbate 20, sodium carboxymethylcellulose, disodium hydrogen phosphate dihydrate, citric acid anhydrous, sodium chloride, sodium hydroxide, and water for injection. The microspheres are suspended in the diluent prior to injection.

37.5 mg: Each vial of white to off-white, free-flowing powder contains: risperidone 37.5 mg. Risperidone is micro-encapsulated in 7525 polylactide-co-glycolide (PLG) at a concentration of 381 mg risperidone per g of microspheres. The diluent for parenteral use is a clear, colourless solution in a prefilled syringe. Composition of the diluent includes polysorbate 20, sodium carboxymethylcellulose, disodium hydrogen phosphate dihydrate, citric acid anhydrous, sodium chloride, sodium hydroxide, and water for injection. The microspheres are suspended in the diluent prior to injection.

50 mg: Each vial of white to off-white, free-flowing powder contains: risperidone 50 mg. Risperidone is micro-encapsulated in 7525 polylactide-co-glycolide (PLG) at a concentration of 381 mg risperidone per g of microspheres. The diluent for parenteral use is a clear, colourless solution in a prefilled syringe. Composition of the diluent includes polysorbate 20, sodium carboxymethylcellulose, disodium hydrogen phosphate dihydrate, citric acid anhydrous, sodium chloride, sodium hydroxide, and water for injection. The microspheres are suspended in the diluent prior to injection.

It is provided as a kit, and includes: a vial containing the risperidone microspheres, a prefilled syringe containing 2 mL of diluent for RISPERDAL CONSTA, one ALARIS SmartSite Needle-Free Vial Access Device, and two Needle-Pro safety needles for intramuscular injection (a 20G TW 2-inch needle with Needle-Pro safety device for gluteal administration and a 21G UTW 1-inch needle with Needle-Pro safety device for deltoid administration). The colour of the vial cap varies by dosage strength: violet (12.5 mg), pink (25 mg), green (37.5 mg) or blue (50 mg). The syringe barrel has a green band.

(Shown in Product Identification Section)

Risperdal® Tablets

risperidone

Antipsychotic

Janssen-Ortho

Risperdal® Oral Solution

risperidone tartrate

Antipsychotic

Janssen-Ortho

Risperdal® M-Tab®

risperidone

Antipsychotic

Janssen-Ortho

Date of Preparation: April 14, 1993
Date of Revision: June 30, 2008

SUMMARY PRODUCT INFORMATION:

Route of Administration	Dosage Form/Strength	Clinically Relevant Nonmedicinal Ingredients
Oral	Tablet 0.25, 0.5, 1, 2, 3 and 4 mg	Lactose
	Solution 1 mg/mL	None
	Orally disintegrating tablets 0.5, 1, 2, 3 and 4 mg	Aspartame For a complete listing see Dosage Forms, Composition and Packaging.

INDICATIONS AND CLINICAL USE: Adults: Schizophrenia: RISPERDAL (risperidone) is indicated for the acute treatment and maintenance treatment of schizophrenia and related psychotic disorders. In controlled clinical trials, RISPERDAL was found to improve both positive and negative symptoms of schizophrenia.

RISPERDAL has been shown to be effective in maintaining clinical improvement during long-term therapy (1 year).

Severe Dementia—Symptomatic Management of Inappropriate Behaviour: RISPERDAL may be useful in severe dementia for the short-term symptomatic management of inappropriate behaviour due to aggression and/or psychosis. Other behavioural disturbances seen in this patient population as well as disease stage remained unaffected by RISPERDAL treatment.

Physicians are advised to assess the risks and benefits of the use of RISPERDAL in elderly patients with dementia, taking into account risk predictors for stroke or existing cardiovascular comorbidities in the individual patient (see Warnings and Precautions; Adverse Reactions and Dosage and Administration).

Bipolar Disorder—Mania: RISPERDAL is indicated as monotherapy for the acute management of manic episodes associated with Bipolar I disorder.

The efficacy of RISPERDAL in the treatment of acute bipolar mania was established in three 3-week, placebo-controlled trials. The safety and effectiveness of RISPERDAL for long-term use, and for prophylactic use in bipolar disorder have not been evaluated. Physicians who elect to use RISPERDAL for extended periods should periodically re-evaluate the long-term risks and benefits of the drug for the individual patient (see Dosage and Administration).

Geriatrics (>65 years of age): See Warnings and Precautions, Serious Warnings and Precautions Box and Special Populations.

Pediatrics (<18 years of age): The safety and efficacy of RISPERDAL in children under the age of 18 have not been established.

CONTRAINDICATIONS: RISPERDAL is contraindicated in patients who are hypersensitive to this drug or to any ingredients in the formulation or component of the container. For a complete listing, see Dosage Forms, Composition and Packaging.

WARNINGS AND PRECAUTIONS:

> **Serious Warnings and Precautions**
> **Increased Mortality in Elderly Patients with Dementia: Elderly patients with dementia treated with atypical antipsychotic drugs are at an increased risk of death compared to placebo. Analyses of thirteen placebo-controlled trials with various atypical antipsychotics (modal duration of 10 weeks) in these patients showed a mean 1.6-fold increase in the death rate in the drug-treated patients. Although the causes of death were varied, most of the deaths appeared to be either cardiovascular (e.g., heart failure, sudden death) or infectious (e.g., pneumonia) in nature (see Warnings and Precautions, Special Populations, Use in Geriatric Patients with Dementia).**

General: Body Temperature Regulation: Disruption of the body's ability to reduce core body temperature has been attributed to antipsychotic drugs. Appropriate care is advised when prescribing RISPERDAL for patients who will be experiencing conditions which may contribute to an elevation or reduction of core temperature, e.g., exercising strenuously, exposure to extreme heat or cold, receiving concomitant medication with anticholinergic activity, or being subject to dehydration (see Adverse Reactions, Post-Market Adverse Drug Reactions).

Phenylketonurics: Phenylalanine is a component of aspartame. RISPERDAL M-TAB tablets contain phenylalanine (0.14, 0.28, 0.42-0.56, 0.63 and 0.84 mg) per 0.5, 1, 2, 3 and 4 mg tablets, respectively.

QT Interval: As with other antipsychotics, caution should be exercised when RISPERDAL is prescribed in patients with a history of cardiac arrhythmias, in patients with congenital long QT syndrome, and in concomitant use with drugs known to prolong the QT interval.

Carcinogenesis and Mutagenesis: Carcinogenesis: Carcinogenicity studies were conducted in Swiss albino mice and Wistar rats. Risperidone was administered in the diet at doses of 0.63, 2.5 and 10 mg/kg for 18 months to mice and for 25 months to rats. These doses are equivalent to 2.4, 9.4 and 37.5 times the maximum recommended human dose (MRHD) (16 mg/day) on a mg/kg basis or 0.2, 0.75 and 3 times the MRHD (mice) or 0.4, 1.5 and 6 times the MRHD (rats) on a mg/m² basis. A maximum tolerated dose was not achieved in male mice. There were statistically significant increases in pituitary gland adenomas, endocrine pancreas adenomas, and mammary gland adenocarcinomas. Table 1 summarizes the multiples of the human dose on a mg/m² (mg/kg) basis at which these tumours occurred.

Antipsychotic drugs have been shown to chronically elevate prolactin levels in rodents. Serum prolactin levels were not measured during the risperidone carcinogenicity studies; however, measurements during subchronic toxicity studies showed that risperidone elevated serum prolactin levels 5- to 6-fold in mice and rats at the same doses used in the carcinogenicity studies. An increase in mammary, pituitary, and endocrine neoplasms has been found in rodents after chronic administration of other antipsychotic drugs and is considered to be prolactin-mediated. The relevance for human risk of the findings of prolactin-mediated endocrine tumours is unknown (see Warnings and Precautions, Endocrine and Metabolism).

Table 1: RISPERDAL

Summary of Carcinogenicity Studies in Mice and Rats

Tumour Type	Species	Sex	Multiples of Maximum Human Dose in mg/m² (mg/kg): Lowest Effect Level	Highest No-Effect Level
Pituitary adenomas	mouse	female	0.75 (9.4)	0.2 (2.4)
Endocrine pancreas adenomas	rat	male	1.5 (9.4)	0.4 (2.4)
Mammary gland adenocarcinomas	mouse	female	0.2 (2.4)	none
	rat	female	0.4 (2.4)	none
	rat	male	6.0 (37.5)	1.5 (9.4)
Mammary gland neoplasm, Total	rat	male	1.5 (9.4)	0.4 (2.4)

Mutagenicity: Risperidone had no mutagenic effects when tested by the DNA-repair test in rat hepatocytes, the Ames reverse mutation test in *S. typhimurium* and *E. coli*, the mammalian cell gene mutation test in mouse lymphoma cells, the sex-linked recessive lethal test in *D. melanogaster*, the chromosome aberration test in human lymphocytes and Chinese hamster lung cells, and the micronucleus test in the mouse bone marrow cells.

Impairment of Fertility: Risperidone (0.16 to 5 mg/kg) was shown to impair mating, but not fertility, in Wistar rats in three reproductive studies (two Segment I and a multigenerational study) at doses 0.1 to 3 times the maximum recommended human dose (MRHD) on a mg/m² basis. The effect appeared to be in females, since impaired mating behaviour was not noted in the Segment I study in which males only were treated. In a subchronic study in Beagle dogs in which risperidone was administered at doses of 0.31 to 5 mg/kg, sperm motility and concentration were decreased at doses 0.6 to 10 times the MRHD on a mg/m² basis. Dose-related decreases were also noted in serum testosterone at the same doses. Serum testosterone and sperm parameters partially recovered, but remained decreased after treatment was discontinued. No no-effect doses were noted in either rat or dog.

Cardiovascular: During clinical trials, RISPERDAL has been observed to cause orthostatic hypotension and tachycardia, especially during the initial dose titration period and the first few weeks of treatment. Rare cases of syncope, cardiac arrhythmias and first degree AV-block have been reported. Clinically significant hypotension has also been observed postmarketing with concomitant use of risperidone and antihypertensive treatment. The likelihood of excessive hypotension or syncope can be minimized by limiting the initial dose of the drug to 1-2 mg per day, q.d. or b.i.d., in adult patients and to 0.25 to 0.5 mg b.i.d. in special patient populations, and by increasing the dose slowly (see Dosage and Administration). A dose reduction should be considered if hypotension occurs.

Patients with a history of clinically significant cardiac disorders were excluded from clinical trials. Therefore, RISPERDAL should be used with caution in patients with cardiovascular diseases (e.g., heart failure, history of myocardial infarction or ischemia, cerebrovascular disease, conduction abnormalities) and other conditions such as dehydration and hypovolemia. Special care should be taken to avoid hypotension in patients with a history of cerebrovascular insufficiency or ischemic heart disease, and in patients taking medications to lower blood pressure. Monitoring of orthostatic vital signs should be considered in all such patients.

Endocrine and Metabolism: Hyperglycemia: As with some other antipsychotics, hyperglycemia and exacerbation of pre-existing diabetes have been reported very rarely during the use of RISPERDAL (see Adverse Reactions, Post-Market Adverse Drug Reactions). Diabetic ketoacidosis has also been reported.

Assessment of the relationship between atypical antipsychotic use and glucose abnormalities is complicated by the possibility of an increased background risk of diabetes mellitus in patients with schizophrenia and the increasing incidence of diabetes mellitus in the general population. Given these confounders, the relationship between atypical antipsychotic use and hyperglycemia-related adverse events is not completely understood. However, epidemiological studies suggest an increased risk of treatment-emergent hyperglycemia-related adverse events in patients treated with the atypical antipsychotics. Precise risk estimates for hyperglycemia-related adverse events in patients treated with atypical antipsychotics are not available.

Any patient treated with atypical antipsychotics should be monitored for symptoms of hyperglycemia including polydipsia, polyuria, polyphagia, and weakness. Patients who develop symptoms of hyperglycemia during treatment with atypical antipsychotics should undergo fasting blood glucose testing. In some cases, hyperglycemia has resolved when the atypical antipsychotic was discontinued; however, some patients required continuation of antidiabetic treatment despite discontinuation of the suspect drug. Patients with risk factors for diabetes mellitus (e.g., obesity, family history of diabetes) who are starting treatment with atypical antipsychotics should undergo fasting blood glucose testing at the beginning of treatment and periodically during treatment. Patients with an established diagnosis of diabetes mellitus who are started on atypical antipsychotics should be monitored regularly for worsening of glucose control.

Hyperprolactinemia: Antipsychotic drugs elevate prolactin levels with the effect persisting during chronic administration.

Schizophrenia: In controlled clinical trials, prolactin levels were higher in patients treated with RISPERDAL than in haloperidol-treated patients; however, the incidence of solicited adverse events considered to be possibly prolactin-related in patients treated with RISPERDAL (≤10 mg/day) was low (<6%), and similar to that in haloperidol-treated patients (see Adverse Reactions, Table 2).

Bipolar Disorder: In controlled clinical trials, patients treated with RISPERDAL had higher prolactin levels than patients treated with haloperidol. The incidence of potentially prolactin-related adverse events in patients treated with 1-6 mg/day RISPERDAL was 2.3%, and greater than what was reported for patients on placebo (0.5%) or haloperidol (0%) (see Adverse Reactions).

Since tissue culture experiments indicate that approximately one-third of human breast cancers are prolactin-dependent in vitro, RISPERDAL should only be administered to patients with previously detected breast cancer if the benefits outweigh the potential risks. Caution should also be exercised when considering RISPERDAL treatment in patients with pituitary tumours. Possible manifestations associated with elevated prolactin levels are amenorrhea, galactorrhea, and menorrhagia (see Adverse Reactions).

In carcinogenicity studies, the administration of risperidone resulted in an increase in the incidence of mammary neoplasms in both rats and mice. In addition, adenomas of the endocrine pancreas in male rats and pituitary adenomas in female mice have been noted. These changes have been attributed to elevated prolactin levels and have also been observed with other dopamine receptor antagonists. The physiological differences between rats and humans with regard to prolactin make the clinical significance of these findings unclear. To date, neither clinical studies nor epidemiological studies have shown an association between chronic administration of these drugs and mammary tumorigenesis.

Weight Gain: Schizophrenia: In pooled 6- to 8-week placebo-controlled clinical trials, which compared RISPERDAL and placebo in the treatment of schizophrenia, 18% of patients treated with RISPERDAL and 9% of placebo-treated patients met a weight gain criterion of ≥7% of baseline body weight. This difference was statistically significant. With continued treatment, weight gain (mean: 2.3 kg in long-term studies) has been seen.

Bipolar Disorder: In the 3-week controlled clinical trials, the incidence of weight increases of ≥7% was similar among patients treated with placebo, risperidone and haloperidol (2.5%, 2.6% and 3.5%, respectively). The incidence of patients with weight increases of ≥7% was higher with longer treatment duration: 16.7% in patients who received an additional 9 weeks of risperidone during open-label treatment extensions and 15% and 11% in patients treated for a total of 12 weeks with risperidone and haloperidol, respectively.

Gastrointestinal: Antiemetic Effect: Consistent with its dopamine antagonistic effects, RISPERDAL may have an antiemetic effect. Such an effect may mask signs of toxicity due to overdosage with other drugs, or may mask symptoms of disease such as brain tumour or intestinal obstruction or Reye's syndrome.

Genitourinary: Priapism: Rare cases of priapism have been reported with RISPERDAL. This adverse reaction, as with other psychotropic drugs, did not appear to be dose-dependent and did not correlate with the duration of treatment. The most likely mechanism of priapism is a relative decrease in sympathetic tone.

Hepatic/Biliary/Pancreatic: Although the pharmacokinetics of RISPERDAL in patients with hepatic impairment were comparable to those in young volunteers, the free fraction of risperidone was increased by about 35% (see Action and Clinical Pharmacology, Pharmacokinetics and Table 8). Since this may lead to a more pronounced pharmacological effect, lower starting doses and lower maximal doses are recommended in patients with any degree of hepatic impairment (see Dosage and Administration).

Neurologic: Neuroleptic Malignant Syndrome (NMS): Neuroleptic malignant syndrome is a potentially fatal symptom complex that has been reported in association with antipsychotic drugs, including RISPERDAL.

Clinical manifestations of NMS are hyperthermia, muscle rigidity, altered mental status (including catatonic signs) and evidence of autonomic instability (irregular blood pressure, tachycardia, cardiac arrhythmias, and diaphoresis). Additional signs may include elevated creatine phosphokinase, myoglobinuria (rhabdomyolysis) and acute renal failure.

In arriving at a diagnosis, it is important to identify cases where the clinical presentation includes both serious medical illness (e.g., pneumonia, systemic infection, etc.) and untreated or inadequately treated extrapyramidal signs and symptoms. Other important considerations in the differential diagnosis include central anticholinergic toxicity, heat stroke, drug fever, and primary central nervous system pathology.

The management of NMS should include: 1) immediate discontinuation of all antipsychotic drugs including RISPERDAL, and other drugs not essential to concurrent therapy; 2) intensive symptomatic treatment and medical monitoring; and 3) treatment of any concomitant serious medical problems for which specific treatments are available. There is no general agreement about specific pharmacological treatment regimens for uncomplicated NMS.

If a patient requires antipsychotic drug treatment after recovery from NMS, the potential reintroduction of drug therapy should be carefully considered. The patient should be carefully monitored, since recurrence of NMS has been reported.

Tardive Dyskinesia (TD): A syndrome consisting of potentially irreversible, involuntary, dyskinetic movements may develop in patients treated with conventional antipsychotic drugs. Although TD appears to be most prevalent in the elderly, especially elderly females, it is impossible to predict at the onset of treatment which patients are likely to develop TD. It has been suggested that the occurrence of parkinsonian side effects is a predictor for the development of TD. In clinical studies, the observed incidence of drug-induced parkinsonism was lower with RISPERDAL than with haloperidol. In the optimal clinical dose range, the difference between risperidone and haloperidol was significant. The risk of developing TD may be less with RISPERDAL. In longer-term clinical studies, RISPERDAL was associated with a lower incidence of treatment-emergent dyskinesia compared to haloperidol.

The risk of developing TD and the likelihood that it will become irreversible are believed to increase as the duration of treatment and the total cumulative dose of antipsychotic drugs administered to the patient increase. However, the syndrome can develop, although less commonly, after relatively brief periods of treatment at low doses. There is no known treatment for established cases of TD. The syndrome may remit, partially or completely, if antipsychotic drug treatment is withdrawn. However, antipsychotic drug treatment itself may suppress the signs and symptoms of TD, thereby masking the underlying process. The effect of symptom suppression upon the long-term course of TD is unknown.

In view of these considerations, RISPERDAL should be prescribed in a manner that is most likely to minimize the risk of TD. As with any antipsychotic drug, RISPERDAL should be reserved for patients who appear to be obtaining substantial benefit from the drug. In such patients, the smallest dose and the shortest duration of treatment should be sought. The need for continued treatment should be reassessed periodically.

If signs and symptoms of TD develop during treatment with RISPERDAL, withdrawal of the drug should be considered. However, some patients may require treatment with RISPERDAL despite the presence of the syndrome.

Potential Effect on Cognitive and Motor Performance: Since RISPERDAL may cause somnolence, patients should be cautioned against driving a car or operating hazardous machinery until they are reasonably certain that RISPERDAL does not affect them adversely.

Schizophrenia: In controlled clinical trials (see Adverse Reactions, Table 3 and Table 4), the incidence of somnolence in patients on RISPERDAL was clinically similar to placebo (3-4% of patients on RISPERDAL ≤10 mg versus 1% of patients on placebo).

Bipolar Disorder: In controlled clinical trials for the acute management of manic episodes (see Adverse Reactions, Table 7), the incidence of somnolence was higher in patients treated with RISPERDAL compared to placebo or haloperidol (12% of patients on RISPERDAL 1-6 mg/day versus 4% of patients on placebo and 4% of patients on haloperidol).

Seizures: Antipsychotic drugs are known to lower the seizure threshold. In clinical trials, seizures have occurred in a few patients treated with RISPERDAL. Therefore, caution should be used in administering RISPERDAL to patients having a history of seizures or other predisposing factors.

Use in Patients with Parkinson's Disease or Dementia with Lewy Bodies (DLB): Physicians should weigh the risks versus the benefits when prescribing antipsychotics, including RISPERDAL, to patients with Parkinson's Disease or Dementia with Lewy Bodies (DLB) since both groups may be at increased risk of Neuroleptic Malignant Syndrome as well as having an increased sensitivity to antipsychotic medications. Manifestation of this increased sensitivity can include confusion, obtundation, postural instability with frequent falls, in addition to extrapyramidal symptoms.

Psychiatric: Suicide: The possibility of suicide or attempted suicide is inherent in psychosis and bipolar mania, and thus, close supervision and appropriate clinical management of high-risk patients should accompany drug therapy.

Renal: The pharmacokinetics of RISPERDAL were significantly altered in patients with renal disease. In patients with moderate to severe renal disease, clearance of risperidone and its active metabolite 9-hydroxyrisperidone, combined, decreased by 60%, compared to young, healthy subjects (see Action and Clinical Pharmacology, Pharmacokinetics and Table 8). Therefore, lower starting doses and lower maximal doses of risperidone are recommended in patients with any degree of renal impairment. It may also be useful to monitor renal function in these patients (see Dosage and Administration).

Special Populations: Pregnant Women: The safety of RISPERDAL during pregnancy has not been established. In animal studies, risperidone did not show direct reproductive toxicity. However, due to its prolactin-elevating and CNS-depressant activities, reproductive performance and pup survival were adversely affected in rats. Risperidone was not teratogenic in either rats or rabbits.

Placental transfer of risperidone occurs in rat pups. There are no adequate and well-controlled studies in pregnant women. However, there was one report of a case of agenesis of the corpus callosum in an infant exposed to risperidone in utero. The causal relationship to risperidone therapy is unknown.

Reversible extrapyramidal symptoms in the neonate were observed following post-marketing use of risperidone during the last trimester of pregnancy.

RISPERDAL should not be used during pregnancy unless the expected benefits to the patient markedly outweigh the potential risks to the fetus.

Nursing Women: Risperidone appeared in the milk of lactating dogs. The concentration of risperidone was similar in milk and plasma, while that of 9-hydroxyrisperidone was higher in the milk than in plasma. It has been demonstrated that risperidone and 9-hydroxyrisperidone are also excreted in human breast milk.

Nursing should not be undertaken while a patient is receiving RISPERDAL.

Pediatrics (<18 years of age): The safety and efficacy of RISPERDAL in children under the age of 18 have not been established.

Geriatrics (>65 years of age): Geriatric patients generally have decreased renal, hepatic and cardiac function, and an increased tendency to postural hypotension. Therefore, lower starting doses, lower rates of dose adjustment and lower maximal doses are recommended in these patients.

Risperidone is substantially excreted by the kidneys. Thus, the risk of toxic reactions to this drug may be greater in patients with impaired renal function. Because elderly patients are more likely to have decreased renal function, caution should be taken in dose selection and titration. It may also be useful to monitor renal function in these patients (see Dosage and Administration, Action and Clinical Pharmacology, Pharmacokinetics and Table 8).

In schizophrenic patients, doses exceeding 3 mg per day are not recommended. In patients with behavioural disturbances due to severe dementia, the optimal dose is 0.5 mg b.i.d. (1.0 mg per day) and the maximal dose is 1 mg b.i.d. (2.0 mg per day).

Use in Geriatric Patients with Dementia: See Indications and Clinical Use.

Overall Mortality: Elderly patients with dementia treated with atypical antipsychotic drugs have an increased mortality compared to placebo in a meta-analysis of 13 controlled trials of various atypical antipsychotic drugs. In six placebo-controlled trials with RISPERDAL in this population, the incidence of mortality was 4.0% for RISPERDAL-treated patients compared to 3.1% for placebo-treated patients.

Concomitant Use with Furosemide: In risperidone placebo-controlled trials in elderly patients with dementia, a higher incidence of mortality was observed in patients treated with furosemide plus risperidone (7.3%; mean age 89 years, range 75-97) when compared to patients treated with risperidone alone (3.1%; mean age 84 years, range 70-96), furosemide alone (4.1%; mean age 80 years, range 67-90) or placebo without furosemide (2.9%; mean age 88 years, range 71-100). The increase in mortality in patients treated with furosemide plus risperidone was observed in two of the four clinical trials.

No pathophysiological mechanism has been identified to explain this finding, and no consistent pattern for cause of death observed. Nevertheless, caution should be exercised and the risks and benefits of this combination should be considered prior to the decision to use. There was no increased incidence of mortality among patients taking other diuretics as concomitant medication with risperidone. Irrespective of treatment, dehydration was an overall risk factor for mortality and should therefore be carefully avoided in elderly patients with dementia.

Cerebrovascular Adverse Events (CVAEs) in Elderly Patients with Dementia: Analysis of clinical trials in elderly patients with dementia suggests that the use of RISPERDAL in dementia patients may be associated with an increased incidence of reports of CVAEs such as stroke and transient ischemic attacks, including fatalities. In placebo-controlled trials, there was a significantly higher incidence of CVAEs in patients treated with RISPERDAL compared to placebo-treated patients (see Adverse Reactions). There is insufficient information to determine whether CVAEs in elderly patients with dementia are associated specifically with RISPERDAL or other antipsychotic agents.

Therefore, physicians are advised to assess risks and benefits of the use of RISPERDAL in elderly patients with dementia taking into account risk predictors for stroke in the individual patient. Patients/caregivers should be advised to immediately report signs and symptoms of potential CVAEs such as sudden weakness or numbness in the face, arms or legs, and speech or vision problems (see Indications and Clinical Use, Adverse Reactions and Dosage and Administration).

All treatment options should be considered without delay, including discontinuation. Furthermore, caution should be exercised in prescribing RISPERDAL to patients with vascular comorbidities, such as hypertension and cardiovascular disease (see Warnings and Precautions, Cardiovascular).

Dysphagia: Esophageal dysmotility and aspiration have been associated with antipsychotic drug use. Aspiration pneumonia is a common cause of morbidity and mortality in patients with advanced Alzheimer's dementia. RISPERDAL and other antipsychotic drugs should be used cautiously in patients at risk for aspiration pneumonia.

ADVERSE REACTIONS: Clinical Trial Adverse Drug Reactions: Because clinical trials are conducted under very specific conditions the adverse reaction rates observed in the clinical trials may not reflect the rates observed in practice and should not be compared to the rates in the clinical trials of another drug. Adverse drug reaction information from clinical trials is useful for identifying drug-related adverse events and for approximating rates.

Schizophrenia and Related Psychotic Disorders: Adverse Events Associated with Discontinuation of Treatment: An estimated 9% of approximately 1800 patients who received RISPERDAL (risperidone) in controlled clinical trials discontinued treatment due to adverse reactions. The more common events causing discontinuation included: **Psychiatric** (4.1%): primarily psychosis, agitation, suicide attempt, somnolence; **Neurological** (3.2%): primarily extrapyramidal disorder, dizziness; and **Cardiovascular** (1.2%): primarily hypotension. Other events leading to discontinuation included: tachycardia/palpitations (0.6%), nervousness (0.4%), nausea (0.3%) and insomnia (0.3%).

Commonly Observed Adverse Events in Short-term Clinical Trials: The most frequent adverse reactions reported during clinical trials with RISPERDAL were insomnia, agitation, extrapyramidal disorder, anxiety, headache and rhinitis (see Table 3 and Table 4). In some instances, it has been difficult to differentiate adverse events from symptoms of the underlying psychosis.

Serious Adverse Events: The most serious adverse reactions reported were rare cases of syncope, cardiac arrhythmias, first degree AV-block, and seizures.

Extrapyramidal Symptoms: Parkinsonian side effects reported were usually mild but dose-related; they were reversible upon dose reduction and/or administration of antiparkinson medication.

Vital Sign Changes: Hypotension (including orthostatic) and tachycardia (including reflex tachycardia) have been observed following the administration of RISPERDAL (see Warnings and Precautions, Cardiovascular).

ECG Changes: Electrocardiograms were evaluated in patients treated with RISPERDAL (N=380), haloperidol (N=126) and placebo (N=120). In the RISPERDAL group, eight patients had a slight increase in QTc intervals from less than 450 msec at baseline to intervals ranging from 450 to 474 msec during treatment. Changes of this type were not seen in placebo-treated patients but were observed in three haloperidol-treated subjects.

Hyperprolactinemia: RISPERDAL elevated plasma prolactin levels. Associated manifestations, namely amenorrhea, galactorrhea, and menorrhagia, have occurred.

In controlled clinical trials prolactin levels were higher in patients treated with RISPERDAL than in haloperidol-treated patients; however, the incidence of solicited adverse events considered to be possibly prolactin-related in patients treated with RISPERDAL (≤10 mg/day) was low (<6%), and similar to that in haloperidol-treated patients.

Table 2: RISPERDAL

Prolactin-related Adverse Events Solicited From Women and Men in the Two Fixed-dose Schizophrenia Trials

	RISPERDAL (mg/day)			
	1–2	**4–6**	**8–10**	**Placebo**
Women	**N=78**	**N=90**	**N=98**	**N=14**
Amenorrhea	5 (6%)	4 (4%)	6 (6%)	1 (7%)
Galactorrhea	1 (1%)	2 (2%)	2 (2%)	0
Men	**N=238**	**N=223**	**N=219**	**N=74**
Ejaculatory dysfunction	7 (3%)	6 (3%)	9 (4%)	2 (3%)
Erectile dysfunction	6 (2%)	9 (4%)	6 (3%)	1 (1%)
Gynecomastia	2 (1%)	0	1 (<1%)	1 (1%)

Note: Adverse events were solicited using the UKU questionnaire. See Kleinberg DL, Davis JM, De Coster R, Van Baelen B, Brecher M. Prolactin levels and adverse events in patients treated with risperidone. J Clin Psychopharmacol 1999;19(1):57-61.

Weight Gain: In a pool of 6- to 8-week placebo-controlled clinical trials, which compared RISPERDAL and placebo in the treatment of schizophrenia, 18% of patients treated with RISPERDAL and 9% of placebo-treated patients met a weight gain criterion of ≥7% of baseline body weight. This difference was statistically significant. With continued treatment, weight gain (mean: 2.3 kg in long-term studies) has been seen.

Other Adverse Events: Erectile dysfunction, ejaculatory dysfunction, orgastic dysfunction, and rash have also been reported during treatment with RISPERDAL. As with other antipsychotics, cases of water intoxication, either due to polydipsia or to syndrome of inappropriate secretion of antidiuretic hormone (SIADH), have occasionally been reported during treatment with RISPERDAL.

Adverse Events in North American Studies: Table 3 enumerates adverse events that occurred at an incidence of 1% or more, and were at least as frequent among patients treated with RISPERDAL receiving doses of ≤10 mg/day as among placebo-treated patients in the pooled results of two 6- to 8-week controlled trials. Patients received RISPERDAL at fixed doses of 2, 6, 10, or 16 mg/day in the dose comparison trial, or up to a maximum dose of 10 mg/day in the flexible dose study. Table 3 shows the percentage of patients in each dose group (≤10 mg/day or 16 mg/day) who spontaneously reported at least one episode of an event at some time during their treatment. Patients given doses of 2, 6, or 10 mg did not differ substantially in these rates. Reported adverse events were classified using the World Health Organization preferred terms.

Table 3: RISPERDAL

Treatment-emergent Adverse Experience Incidence in 6- to 8-Week Controlled Clinical Trials in Schizophrenia[a]

	RISPERDAL		
Body System/ Preferred Term	**≤10 mg/day (N=324) %**	**16 mg/day (N=77) %**	**Placebo (N=142) %**
Psychiatric			
Insomnia	26	23	19

(cont'd)

Table 3: RISPERDAL *(cont'd)*

Treatment-emergent Adverse Experience Incidence in 6- to 8-Week Controlled Clinical Trials in Schizophrenia[a]

Body System/ Preferred Term	RISPERDAL ≤10 mg/day (N=324) %	RISPERDAL 16 mg/day (N=77) %	Placebo (N=142) %
Agitation	22	26	20
Anxiety	12	20	9
Somnolence	3	8	1
Aggressive reaction	1	3	1
Neurological			
Extrapyramidal symptoms[b]	17	34	16
Headache	14	12	12
Dizziness	4	7	1
Gastrointestinal			
Constipation	7	13	3
Nausea	6	4	3
Dyspepsia	5	10	4
Vomiting	5	7	4
Abdominal pain	4	1	0
Saliva increased	2	0	1
Toothache	2	0	0
Respiratory			
Rhinitis	10	8	4
Coughing	3	3	1
Sinusitis	2	1	1
Pharyngitis	2	3	0
Dyspnea	1	0	0
Body as a Whole			
Back pain	2	0	1
Chest pain	2	3	1
Fever	2	3	0
Dermatological			
Rash	2	5	1
Dry skin	2	4	0
Seborrhea	1	0	0
Infections			
Upper respiratory	3	3	1
Visual			
Abnormal vision	2	1	1
Musculoskeletal			
Arthralgia	2	3	0
Cardiovascular			
Tachycardia	3	5	0

[a] Events reported by at least 1% of patients treated with RISPERDAL ≤10 mg/day are included, and are rounded to the nearest %. Comparative rates for RISPERDAL 16 mg/day and placebo are provided as well. Events for which the RISPERDAL incidence (in both dose groups) was equal to or less than placebo are not listed in the table, but included the following: nervousness, injury, and fungal infection.

[b] Includes tremor, dystonia, hypokinesia, hypertonia, hyperkinesia, oculogyric crisis, ataxia, abnormal gait, involuntary muscle contractions, hyporeflexia, akathisia, and extrapyramidal disorders. Although the incidence of 'extrapyramidal symptoms' does not appear to differ for the "≤10 mg/day" group and placebo, the data for individual dose groups in fixed-dose trials do suggest a dose/response relationship.

Adverse Events in All International Trials: Table 4 lists the overall incidence of adverse reactions noted for all international controlled clinical trials including the North American trials. Some adverse events were reported at a higher incidence in the North American trials than appear in Table 3, due to differences in reporting practices and/or methodology.

Table 4: RISPERDAL

Adverse Reactions Reported at a Frequency of ≥1% in All International Trials in Schizophrenia[a]

Body System/Preferred Term	RISPERDAL ≤10 mg/day (N=1202) %	RISPERDAL >10 mg/day (N=535) %	Placebo (N=176) %
Psychiatric			
Insomnia	13	10	16
Agitation	9	7	16
Anxiety	7	6	7
Somnolence	4	2	1
Nervousness	2	2	3
Impaired concentration	1	0	0
Aggressive reaction	1	1	3
Suicide attempt	1	2	1
Psychosis	1	1	0
Neurological			
Extrapyramidal disorder	7	13	7
Headache	6	3	10
Dizziness	3	2	1
Hyperkinesia (includes akathisia)	2	3	2
Tremor	1	2	2
Rigidity	1	2	2
Hypokinesia	1	1	1
Dystonia	1	2	1
Oculogyric crisis	1	1	1
Dyskinesia	1	1	1
Gastrointestinal			
Constipation	3	2	2
Nausea	3	1	2
Vomiting	2	2	3
Increased salivation	2	2	1
Dyspepsia	1	2	3
Anorexia	1	0	1
Abdominal pain	1	0	1
Respiratory			
Rhinitis	3	1	3
Coughing	1	1	1
Special Senses			
Abnormal vision	2	0	1
Cardiovascular			
Tachycardia	1	2	0
Other			
Fatigue	2	1	1

[a] Events reported by at least 1% of patients treated with RISPERDAL are rounded to the nearest %.

Adverse Reactions During Long-Term Treatment: Long-term clinical trials with RISPERDAL were carried out in 1235 chronic schizophrenic patients, with 671 patients receiving the drug for at least one year. The pattern of adverse events observed in patients receiving RISPERDAL in long-term clinical trials is consistent with those observed in short-term trials.

Adverse events were collected through spontaneous reporting, open questioning or utilization of the UKU side effect rating scale. Listed (in decreasing order) are those events which developed or showed deterioration during treatment compared to baseline in at least 10% of patients. **Psychic:** asthenia/lassitude/increased fatiguability, concentration difficulties, sleepiness/sedation, reduced duration of sleep, increased duration of sleep, failing memory, increased dream activity, insomnia; **Autonomic:** orthostatic dizziness, constipation, nausea/vomiting, polyuria/polydipsia, palpitations/tachycardia, reduced salivation, accommodation disturbances, increased tendency to sweating, diarrhea, micturition disturbances; **Other:** weight gain, weight loss, amenorrhea, ejaculatory dysfunction, erectile dysfunction, diminished sexual desire, tension headache, headache, increased sexual desire, orgastic dysfunction, pruritus.

Behavioural Disturbances in Severe Dementia: Adverse Events Associated with Discontinuation of Treatment: In the fixed-dose, dose-response study, 95/617 patients discontinued treatment due to an adverse event. The most frequently reported adverse events were somnolence, extrapyramidal symptoms (EPS), and agitation, with somnolence and EPS being dose-related. See Table 5.

Table 5: RISPERDAL

Adverse Events Leading to Discontinuation in Trials in Elderly Patients with Dementia

		RISPERDAL		
Adverse Event	**Placebo (N=161) %**	**0.5 mg/day (N=147) %**	**1 mg/day (N=147) %**	**2 mg/day (N=162) %**
Somnolence	1.9	0	4.8	6.8
Extrapyramidal symptoms (EPS)	1.2	1.4	3.4	3.7
Agitation	2.5	2	1.4	3.7

Incidence of Adverse Events: Table 6 enumerates adverse events from the fixed-dose, dose-response study that were more frequent in the RISPERDAL groups than in the placebo group and/or were dose-related.

Table 6: RISPERDAL

Treatment-emergent Adverse Events in the Fixed-dose Study in Elderly Patients with Dementia

		RISPERDAL		
Body System/Preferred Term	**Placebo (N=161) %**	**0.5 mg/day (N=147) %**	**1 mg/day (N=147) %**	**2 mg/day (N=162) %**
Body as a Whole				
Edema peripheral	6	16	13	18
Psychiatric				
Somnolence	8	10	17	27
Neurological				
Extrapyramidal symptoms (EPS)	8	7	13	22
Respiratory				
Rhinitis	5	5	6	10
Dyspnea	1	1	1	5
Cardiovascular				
Hypotension	3	2	3	5
Tachycardia	1	1	0	2

Events are rounded to the nearest %.

Other adverse events which occurred with a high incidence but with similar frequencies in the patients treated with RISPERDAL and placebo included injury (28 to 38%), falls (13 to 25%), urinary tract infection (13 to 21%), and purpura (10 to 17%).

Cerebrovascular Adverse Events (CVAEs) in Elderly Patients with Dementia: In 6 placebo-controlled dementia trials for elderly patients taking RISPERDAL for 4 to 12 weeks within the approved dosage range, the pooled incidence rate of CVAEs was 3%, compared to 1% for age-matched patients taking placebo. Five patients died in the RISPERDAL group (5/1009) versus 1 patient in the placebo group (1/712) (see Indications and Clinical Use, Warnings and Precautions and Dosage and Administration).

Postmarketing for the Elderly Dementia Population: Review of the global post-marketing database for the elderly dementia patient population (over 2.4 million patient-years as of October 2002) identified approximately 37 cases of cerebrovascular adverse events such as strokes and transient ischemic attacks. Of these cases, 16 were fatal.

There is insufficient information to determine whether CVAEs in elderly patients with dementia are associated specifically with RISPERDAL or other antipsychotic agents.

Bipolar Disorder—Mania: Adverse Events Associated with Discontinuation of Treatment: In the 3-week placebo-controlled trials, a total of 4.2% of patients discontinued from the studies because of an adverse event: 4.1% for placebo, 4.8% for RISPERDAL and 2.8% for haloperidol. The most common adverse event leading to discontinuation was manic reaction: 1.0% for placebo and 1.6% for RISPERDAL.

Incidence of Adverse Events: In the 3-week placebo-controlled trials, in which patients received dosages of 1-6 mg/day risperidone, the most commonly observed adverse events associated with the use of RISPERDAL (incidence of ≥5% and at least twice placebo) included extrapyramidal disorder, hyperkinesia, dystonia and somnolence. Adverse events that occurred in these trials with an incidence of ≥1% and more frequently in patients treated with risperidone than placebo are shown in Table 7.

Table 7: RISPERDAL

Treatment-emergent Adverse Events Reported in Double-blind Monotherapy Trials in Bipolar Disorder (≥1% and More Frequent Than Placebo)

Adverse Event System Organ Class **Adverse Event Preferred Term**	**Placebo (N=409) n (%)**	**RISPERDAL (N=434) n (%)**
Total No. Subjects with Emerging Adverse Event	232 (56.7)	305 (70.3)
Central & Peripheral Nervous System Disorders	99 (24.2)	200 (46.1)
Extrapyramidal disorder	25 (6.1)	85 (19.6)
Headache	30 (7.3)	39 (9.0)
Hyperkinesia	10 (2.4)	37 (8.5)
Tremor	15 (3.7)	28 (6.5)
Dizziness	20 (4.9)	24 (5.5)
Dystonia	2 (0.5)	22 (5.1)
Hypertonia	4 (1.0)	16 (3.7)
Muscle contractions involuntary	1 (0.2)	5 (1.2)
Psychiatric Disorders	78 (19.1)	103 (23.7)
Somnolence	15 (3.7)	53 (12.2)
Manic reaction	11 (2.7)	13 (3.0)
Gastrointestinal System Disorders	63 (15.4)	82 (18.9)
Nausea	4 (1.0)	18 (4.1)
Dyspepsia	9 (2.2)	16 (3.7)
Saliva increased	2 (0.5)	13 (3.0)
Mouth dry	4 (1.0)	5 (1.2)
Body as a Whole—General Disorders	44 (10.8)	51 (11.8)
Fatigue	3 (0.7)	8 (1.8)
Pain	6 (1.5)	8 (1.8)
Fever	3 (0.7)	6 (1.4)
Asthenia	3 (0.7)	5 (1.2)
Edema	1 (0.2)	5 (1.2)
Respiratory System Disorders	30 (7.3)	33 (7.6)
Rhinitis	5 (1.2)	6 (1.4)
Sinusitis	1 (0.2)	6 (1.4)
Skin and Appendages Disorders	15 (3.7)	23 (5.3)
Acne	0	5 (1.2)
Musculoskeletal System Disorders	14 (3.4)	16 (3.7)
Myalgia	7 (1.7)	8 (1.8)
Cardiovascular Disorders, General	12 (2.9)	14 (3.2)
Hypertension	8 (2.0)	9 (2.1)
Vision Disorders	6 (1.5)	11 (2.5)
Vision abnormal	3 (0.7)	8 (1.8)
Heart Rate and Rhythm Disorders	5 (1.2)	10 (2.3)
Tachycardia	2 (0.5)	6 (1.4)
Reproductive Disorders, Female	5 (2.8)	8 (4.4)
Lactation nonpuerperal	0	5 (2.8)
Liver and Biliary System Disorders	2 (0.5)	6 (1.4)
AST increased	1 (0.2)	5 (1.2)

Note: Incidence is based on the number of subjects, not the number of events.
Note: Incidence for female reproductive disorders is based on the number of female subjects (placebo, N=181; risperidone, N=180).

Suicide: In the 3-week double-blind phase of controlled clinical trials, suicide-related adverse events occurred at an incidence of 0.45% for patients treated with risperidone (2 patients/448) compared to 0 for patients treated with placebo (0 patients/424). Suicide attempt and completed suicide occurred in one patient each.

The incidence of suicide-related adverse events was 0.67% (3 patients/446) during 9 weeks of open-label risperidone treatment. Suicide attempts were reported for two patients and completed suicide occurred in one patient.

Hyperprolactinemia: In controlled clinical trials, patients treated with RISPERDAL had higher prolactin levels than patients treated with placebo or haloperidol. Associated manifestations that occurred in fewer than 1% of patients treated with RISPERDAL during the bipolar clinical trials, which are not listed in Table 7, included ejaculation failure, abnormal sexual function, decreased libido, and impotence.

Extrapyramidal Symptoms in Bipolar Disorder Clinical Trials: Adverse events related to extrapyramidal symptoms (EPS) were reported more frequently in all clinical trials for bipolar disorder than schizophrenia, regardless of study population demographics, and this may be consistent with a greater susceptibility to EPS-related adverse reactions in bipolar patients that has been observed in clinical practice. The lower mean body weight and body mass index (BMI) of an Indian study population (RIS-IND-2) and a higher mean risperidone dose may have contributed to a higher incidence of EPS-related AEs in this trial (45%, mean modal dose 5.6 mg/day; mean modal dose is the average of individual subjects' most frequent daily dose) compared to the US (36.6%, mean modal dose 4.0 mg/day) and international (31.2%, mean modal dose 4.2 mg/day) trials. EPS-related adverse events in all studies were usually mild, dose-related and reversible upon dose reduction and/or administration of antiparkinsonian medication.

Abnormal Hematologic and Clinical Chemistry Findings: In one study in which testosterone levels were measured, testosterone decreased below the normal range in 6 out of 85 patients.

Post-Market Adverse Drug Reactions: Adverse events reported since market introduction of RISPERDAL, which were temporally (but not necessarily causally) related to RISPERDAL therapy, include the following: edema, angioedema, increased hepatic enzyme levels, skin manifestations of allergy including cases of Stevens-Johnson syndrome, systemic manifestations of allergy including a case of anaphylactic shock, neuroleptic malignant syndrome, body temperature dysregulation, urinary incontinence, gynecomastia, seizures, tardive dyskinesia, hypertension, leukopenia, priapism, neutropenia, thrombopenia, apnea, atrial fibrillation, benign pituitary adenomas, cerebrovascular disorder including cerebrovascular accident, intestinal obstruction, jaundice, mania, pancreatitis, Parkinson's disease aggravated and pulmonary embolism.

Hyperglycemia and exacerbation of pre-existing diabetes have been reported in very rare cases during RISPERDAL treatment. Diabetic ketoacidosis has also been reported (see Warnings and Precautions, Endocrine and Metabolism).

As with other neuroleptics, sudden death, Torsades de Pointe, ventricular tachycardia, arrhythmia, cardiopulmonary arrest and QT prolongation have been reported during RISPERDAL treatment. Many of the patients had pre-existing cardiovascular disease, were on concomitant medications known to prolong the QT interval, had risk factors for QT prolongation, took an overdose of risperidone, and/or were morbidly obese. Very rarely, QT prolongation has been reported in the absence of confounding factors.

DRUG INTERACTIONS: Overview: Given the primary central nervous system effects of RISPERDAL, caution should be used when it is taken in combination with other centrally acting drugs and alcohol. Because of its potential for inducing hypotension, RISPERDAL may enhance the hypotensive effects of other therapeutic agents. RISPERDAL may antagonize the effects of levodopa and dopamine agonists.

Clinically significant hypotension has been observed postmarketing with concomitant use of risperidone and antihypertensive medications.

Caution is advised when prescribing RISPERDAL with drugs known to prolong the QT interval.

Drug-Drug Interactions: Concomitant Use with Furosemide: See Warnings and Precautions, Special Populations regarding increased mortality in elderly patients with dementia concomitantly receiving furosemide.

Carbamazepine and Other CYP 3A4 Enzyme Inducers: Carbamazepine has been shown to decrease substantially the plasma levels of risperidone and its active metabolite, 9-hydroxyrisperidone (n=11). Similar effects may be observed with other CYP 3A4 hepatic enzyme inducers. Consequently, in the presence of carbamazepine or other CYP 3A4 hepatic enzyme inducers, the dose of RISPERDAL may have to be adjusted. On discontinuation of these drugs, the dosage of RISPERDAL should be re-evaluated and, if necessary, decreased.

Drugs That Inhibit CYP 2D6 and Other CYP Isozymes: The metabolism of RISPERDAL, a substrate of the hepatic cytochrome P450 isozyme 2D6 (CYP 2D6), is affected by the debrisoquine hydroxylation polymorphism (see Action and Clinical Pharmacology, Pharmacokinetics). CYP 2D6 is also responsible for the metabolism of a variety of drugs, including phenothiazines, antidepressants (tricyclics and SSRIs), antiarrhythmics and some β-blockers. Consequently, potential interaction between RISPERDAL and drugs that are also substrates of CYP 2D6, should also be considered.

Fluoxetine and Paroxetine: Fluoxetine and paroxetine, CYP 2D6 inhibitors, increase the plasma concentration of risperidone but less so of risperidone and 9-hydroxyrisperidone combined. Pharmacokinetic interaction with fluoxetine was examined in a study which measured steady-state plasma levels of risperidone and its metabolites before and following 3 weeks of co-treatment with fluoxetine (n=10). The addition of fluoxetine resulted in about a 2- to 3-fold increase in peak and AUC levels of risperidone and about a 50% increase in peak and AUC levels for risperidone and 9-hydroxyrisperidone combined. Similarly, pharmacokinetic interaction with paroxetine was examined in a study which measured steady-state plasma levels of risperidone and its metabolites before and following 4 weeks of co-treatment with paroxetine (n=10). After 4 weeks of paroxetine treatment, the sum of the concentrations of risperidone and 9-hydroxyrisperidone increased significantly by 45% over baseline. When concomitant fluoxetine or paroxetine is initiated or discontinued, the physician should re-evaluate the dosing of RISPERDAL.

Erythromycin: Erythromycin, a CYP 3A4 inhibitor, did not change the pharmacokinetics of risperidone or risperidone and 9-hydroxyrisperidone combined. Risperidone was administered as a single dose of 1 mg with multiple doses of erythromycin (500 mg q.i.d.) in healthy volunteers (n=18).

The Effect of Other Drugs on the Metabolism of Risperidone: Galantamine and Donepezil: The cholinesterase inhibitors, galantamine (n=15) and donepezil (n=24), did not show an effect on the pharmacokinetics of risperidone or risperidone and 9-hydroxyrisperidone combined. Galantamine 12 mg o.d. was co-administered with risperidone 0.5 mg o.d. in healthy elderly volunteers. Donepezil 5 mg o.d. was co-administered with risperidone 0.5 mg b.i.d. in healthy male volunteers.

Cimetidine and Ranitidine: Risperidone was administered as a single dose of 1 mg with multiple doses of either cimetidine (400 mg b.i.d.) or ranitidine (150 mg b.i.d.) in healthy young adult volunteers (n=12). The effect of the drug interaction of cimetidine and ranitidine on risperidone and 9-hydroxyrisperidone combined was minimal.

Clozapine: Chronic administration of clozapine with risperidone may decrease the clearance of risperidone.

Topiramate: Healthy Volunteers: A drug-drug interaction study between risperidone and topiramate was conducted in 12 healthy volunteers (6 males, 6 females), ages 28-40 years, with single-dose administration of risperidone (2 mg) and multiple doses of topiramate (titrated up to 200 mg/day). In the presence of topiramate, systemic exposure of risperidone and 9-hydroxyrisperidone combined was reduced such that mean $AUC_{0-\infty}$ was 11% lower and mean C_{max} was statistically significantly (18%) lower. In the presence of topiramate, systemic exposure of risperidone was statistically significantly reduced such that mean C_{max} and $AUC_{0-\infty}$ were 29% and 23% lower, respectively. The pharmacokinetics of 9-hydroxyrisperidone were unaffected. The effects of a single dose (2 mg/day) of risperidone on the pharmacokinetics of multiple doses of topiramate have not been studied.

Patients with Bipolar Disorder: A drug-drug interaction study conducted in 52 patients with various types of bipolar disorder (24 males, 28 females), ages 19-56 years, evaluated the steady-state pharmacokinetics of risperidone and topiramate when administered concomitantly. Eligible subjects were stabilized on a risperidone dose of 1-6 mg/day for 2 to 3 weeks. Topiramate was then titrated up to escalating doses of 100, 250 and 400 mg/day along with risperidone for up to 6 weeks. Risperidone was then tapered and discontinued over 4 weeks while maintaining topiramate (up to 400 mg/day). There was a statistically significant reduction in risperidone systemic exposure (16% and 33% for AUC_{12} and 13% and 34% for C_{max} at the 250 and 400 mg/day doses, respectively). Minimal alterations were observed in the pharmacokinetics of risperidone and 9-hydroxyrisperidone combined and of 9-hydroxyrisperidone. Topiramate systemic exposure was slightly reduced (12.5% for mean C_{max} and 11% for mean AUC_{12}) in the presence of risperidone, which achieved statistical significance. There were no clinically significant changes in the systemic exposure of risperidone and 9-hydroxyrisperidone combined or of topiramate. The effects of higher doses of topiramate (>400 mg/day) are unknown. Therefore, if combination therapy is chosen, patients receiving both risperidone and topiramate should be closely monitored.

Effects of Risperidone on the Metabolism of Other Drugs: Lithium: RISPERDAL (3 mg b.i.d.) did not show an effect on the pharmacokinetics of lithium (400, 450 or 560 mg b.i.d.) (n=13).

Valproate: RISPERDAL (4 mg o.d.) did not show an effect on the pharmacokinetics of valproate (1000 mg/day) (n=9). However, more subjects reported adverse events with the risperidone-valproate therapy compared to the placebo-valproate group in the clinical trial.

Digoxin: The effect of RISPERDAL (0.5 mg/day administered b.i.d.) on the steady-state plasma concentrations of digoxin (0.125 mg/day) was examined in a double-blind, two-way, crossover trial in healthy elderly volunteers (median age 68 years, range 61 to 75 years, n=19). RISPERDAL did not affect the steady-state pharmacokinetics of digoxin, and concurrent administration of the two drugs was well tolerated.

In vitro studies, in which risperidone was given in the presence of various, highly protein-bound agents, indicated that clinically relevant changes in protein binding would not occur either for RISPERDAL or for any of the drugs tested.

Drug-Food Interactions: RISPERDAL oral solution is compatible with the following beverages: water, coffee, orange juice and low-fat milk. However, it is not compatible with cola or tea. Also see Dosage and Administration.

Drug-Herb Interactions: Interactions with herbal products have not been established.

Drug-Laboratory Test Interactions: Interactions with laboratory tests have not been established.

DOSAGE AND ADMINISTRATION: Dosing Considerations: Refer to Special Populations for dosing recommendations in the following patients: patients prone to hypotension; geriatrics; patients with renal impairment; patients with hepatic impairment.

Recommended Dose and Dosage Adjustment: Adults: Schizophrenia and Related Psychotic Disorders: RISPERDAL can be administered on either a o.d. or b.i.d. schedule, generally beginning with 1 to 2 mg per day. The dose should be adjusted gradually over several days based on clinical response to a target dose of 4 to 6 mg per day. Some patients may benefit from lower initial doses and/or a slower adjustment schedule.

Further dosage adjustments, if indicated, should generally occur at intervals of not less than one week since steady state for the active metabolite would not be achieved for approximately one week in the typical patient. When dosage adjustments are necessary, small increments/decrements of 1 mg are recommended.

In controlled clinical trials, optimal therapeutic effects were seen in the 4 to 8 mg per day dose range. However, clinical experience indicates that in the majority of patients adequate therapeutic effect is achieved at the 6 mg per day dose. Doses above 10 mg per day have not been shown to be more efficacious than lower doses and were associated with more extrapyramidal symptoms and other adverse events.

The safety of RISPERDAL has not been established above 16 mg total daily dose, administered twice daily. If administered once daily, safety has not been established beyond a single dose of 8 mg.

Switching from Other Antipsychotics: When medically appropriate, gradual discontinuation of the previous treatment, while RISPERDAL therapy is initiated, is recommended. In all cases, the period of overlapping antipsychotic administration should be minimized. When switching patients from depot antipsychotics, initiate RISPERDAL therapy in place of the next scheduled injection. The need for continuing existing antiparkinsonian medications should be re-evaluated periodically.

Maintenance Therapy: It is recommended that responding patients be continued on RISPERDAL at the lowest dose needed to maintain remission. Patients should be reassessed periodically to determine the need for maintenance treatment. While there is no body of evidence available to answer the question of how long the patient should be treated with RISPERDAL, the effectiveness of maintenance treatment is well established for many other antipsychotic drugs.

Behavioural Disturbances in Severe Dementia: Physicians are advised to assess the risks and benefits of the use of RISPERDAL in elderly patients with dementia, taking into account risk predictors for stroke or existing cardiovascular comorbidities in the individual patient (see Indications and Clinical Use, Warnings and Precautions and Adverse Reactions).

Discontinuation should be considered if signs and symptoms of cerebrovascular adverse events occur.

A starting dose of RISPERDAL 0.25 mg b.i.d. is recommended. This dosage should be adjusted by increments of 0.25 mg per day approximately every 2 to 4 days. The optimal dose is 0.5 mg b.i.d. (1.0 mg per day) for most patients. Some patients, however, may benefit from higher doses up to a maximum of 1.0 mg b.i.d. (2.0 mg per day).

Periodic dosage adjustments (increase or decrease) or discontinuation of treatment should be considered because of the instability of the symptoms treated.

Since there is no experience in younger patients, dosage recommendations cannot be made.

Bipolar Mania: RISPERDAL should be administered on a once-daily schedule, starting with 2 mg to 3 mg per day. Dosage adjustments, based on clinical response and tolerability, should occur at intervals of not less than 24 hours and in dosage increments or decrements of 1 mg per day. RISPERDAL doses higher than 6 mg per day were not studied in patients with bipolar disorder.

In two controlled trials, the most common daily dose was 1-4 mg/day. In each of the three controlled trials, RISPERDAL was effective across the dose range used, although the effect size in the 3-4 mg/day mean modal dose group was larger than in the 5-6 mg/day mean modal dose group (mean modal dose is the average of the most frequent daily dose across the three trials).

The safety and effectiveness of RISPERDAL for long-term use and for prophylactic use in bipolar disorder have not been evaluated. Physicians who elect to use RISPERDAL for extended periods should periodically re-evaluate the long-term risks and benefits of the drug for the individual patient.

Special Populations: Geriatrics: Risperidone is substantially excreted by the kidneys. Thus, the risk of toxic reactions to this drug may be greater in patients with impaired renal function. Because elderly patients are more likely to have decreased renal function, caution should be taken in dose selection and titration. It may also be useful to monitor renal function in these patients (see Warnings and Precautions, Special Populations, Action and Clinical Pharmacology, Pharmacokinetics and Table 8).

In elderly schizophrenic patients, the doses of RISPERDAL should be adjusted slowly from a 0.25 mg b.i.d. starting dose to a maximum daily dose of 3 mg. Since the elimination of RISPERDAL is somewhat slower in these patients, the potential for accumulation should be considered (see Action and Clinical Pharmacology, Pharmacokinetics and Table 8).

Patients Prone to Hypotension: Caution should be exercised in patients prone to hypotension and the use of lower starting doses of 0.25 to 0.5 mg b.i.d. should be considered.

Patients with Impaired Liver Function: RISPERDAL should be used with caution in patients with hepatic impairment.

Patients with impaired hepatic function have increases in plasma concentration of the free fraction of risperidone and this may result in an enhanced effect. In general, starting and consecutive dosing should be halved, and dose titration should be slower for patients with hepatic impairment, administered on a b.i.d. schedule.

In patients with schizophrenia and related psychotic disorders with impaired liver function, the starting dose should be 0.25 to 0.5 mg b.i.d. This dosage can be individually adjusted in 0.5 mg b.i.d. increments to 1 to 2 mg b.i.d. Increases to dosages above 1.5 mg b.i.d. should generally occur at intervals of at least 1 week (see Warnings and Precautions, Hepatic/Biliary/Pancreatic, Action and Clinical Pharmacology, Pharmacokinetics and Table 8).

Patients with Impaired Kidney Function: RISPERDAL should be used with caution in patients with renal impairment.

Patients with renal impairment have less ability to eliminate the active antipsychotic fraction than normal adults. In general, starting and consecutive dosing should be halved, and dose titration should be slower for patients with renal impairment, administered on a b.i.d. schedule. The recommended initial dose is 0.5 mg b.i.d. and dosage increases should be in increments of no more than 0.5 mg b.i.d. Increases to dosages above 1.5 mg b.i.d. should generally occur at intervals of at least 1 week. In some patients, slower titration may be medically appropriate (see Warnings and Precautions, Renal, Action and Clinical Pharmacology, Pharmacokinetics and Table 8).

Missed Dose: The missed dose should be taken at the next scheduled dose. Doses should not be doubled.

Administration: RISPERDAL may be given as tablets or oral solution. RISPERDAL M-TAB is given as orally disintegrating tablets. All may be taken with or without meals. In order to avoid orthostatic hypotension, the dose of RISPERDAL should be adjusted gradually.

RISPERDAL M-TAB tablets should not be split into halves.

OVERDOSAGE:

Cases of overdose have been reported with RISPERDAL; the estimated doses were between 20 and 360 mg. In general, reported signs and symptoms were those resulting from an exaggeration of the drug's known pharmacological effects, namely drowsiness, sedation, tachycardia, hypotension and extrapyramidal symptoms. In overdose, QT-prolongation, widened QRS complex, convulsions, hyponatremia and hypokalemia were also reported. Torsades de pointes has been reported in association with combined overdose of oral RISPERDAL and paroxetine.

Treatment of Overdosage: Since there is no specific antidote to RISPERDAL, treatment is primarily supportive. A patent airway must be established and maintained to ensure adequate ventilation and oxygenation. Gastric lavage (after intubation, if the patient is unconscious) and administration of activated charcoal together with a laxative should be considered.

Cardiovascular monitoring should commence immediately and should include continuous electrocardiographic monitoring to detect possible arrhythmias. Hypotension and circulatory collapse should be treated with appropriate measures such as intravenous fluids. Epinephrine should not be used since beta stimulation may worsen hypotension in the setting of RISPERDAL-induced alpha blockade. In cases of severe extrapyramidal reactions, anticholinergic medication should be administered. Close medical supervision and monitoring should continue until the patient recovers.

In managing overdosage, the physician should consider the possibility of multiple drug involvement.

For management of a suspected drug overdose, CPhA recommends that you contact your **regional Poison Control Centre**. See the *CPS* Directory section for a list of Poison Control Centres.

ACTION AND CLINICAL PHARMACOLOGY: Mechanism of Action: Risperidone, a benzisoxazole derivative, is a novel antipsychotic drug which binds with high affinity to serotonin type 2 ($5\text{-}HT_2$), dopamine type 2 (D_2), and α_1-adrenergic receptors. Risperidone binds with a lower affinity to the α_2-adrenergic and histamine H_1 receptors. Risperidone does not bind to dopamine D_1 receptors and has no affinity (when tested at concentrations $>10^{-5}$ M) for muscarinic cholinergic receptors. Due to the lack of muscarinic receptor binding, risperidone is not expected to produce anticholinergic adverse effects.

Receptor occupancy was also demonstrated in vivo in humans. Using positron emission tomography, risperidone was shown to block both $5\text{-}HT_{2A}$ and dopamine D_2 receptors in three healthy volunteers. Although risperidone is a potent D_2 antagonist, which is considered to improve the positive symptoms of schizophrenia, it causes less depression of motor activity and induction of catalepsy in animal models than classical antipsychotics. Risperidone has also been found to be one of the most potent known antagonists of $5\text{-}HT_{2A}$ (cloned human receptor); $5\text{-}HT_{2A}$ antagonism has been shown to reverse deficits in several in vivo animal models predictive of novel antipsychotic activity (PCP-induced social deficit, microdialysis assessment of dopamine output in prefrontal cortex, glutamate antagonist-induced hyperlocomotion). Balanced central serotonin and dopamine antagonism may reduce extrapyramidal side-effect liability.

Pharmacokinetics: Absorption: Risperidone was well absorbed after oral administration, had high bioavailability, and showed dose-proportionality in the therapeutic dose range, although inter-individual plasma concentrations varied considerably. Mean peak plasma concentrations of risperidone and 9-hydroxyrisperidone were reached at about 1 hour and 3 hours, respectively, after drug administration. Food did not affect the extent of absorption; thus, risperidone can be given with or without meals.

Distribution: Risperidone is rapidly distributed. The volume of distribution is 1-2 L/kg. Steady-state concentrations of risperidone and 9-hydroxyrisperidone were reached within 1-2 days and 5-6 days, respectively. In plasma, risperidone is bound to albumin and alpha$_1$-acid glycoprotein (AGP). The plasma protein binding of risperidone is approximately 88%, that of the metabolite 77%.

Metabolism: Risperidone is extensively metabolized in the liver by CYP 2D6 to a major active metabolite, 9-hydroxyrisperidone, which appears approximately equi-effective with risperidone with respect to receptor-binding activity. (A second minor pathway is N-dealkylation.) Consequently, the clinical effect of the drug likely results from the combined concentrations of risperidone plus 9-hydroxyrisperidone. The hydroxylation of risperidone is dependent upon debrisoquine 4-hydroxylase, i.e., the metabolism of risperidone is sensitive to the debrisoquine hydroxylation type genetic polymorphism. Consequently, the concentrations of parent drug and active metabolite differ substantially in extensive and poor metabolizers. However, the concentration of risperidone and 9-hydroxyrisperidone combined did not differ substantially between extensive and poor metabolizers, and elimination half-lives were similar in all subjects (approximately 20 to 24 hours).

Excretion: One week after administration, 70% of the dose is excreted in the urine and 14% in the faeces. In urine, risperidone plus 9-hydroxyrisperidone represents 35-45% of the dose. The remainder is inactive metabolites.

Special Populations and Conditions: Table 8 summarizes the pharmacokinetic parameters observed in various subpopulations:

Table 8: RISPERDAL

Median Pharmacokinetic Parameters of Risperidone and 9-hydroxyrisperidone Combined Following a Single, 1 mg Oral Dose of Risperidone in Different Patient Populations

Parameters	Young	Elderly	Liver Disease	Renal Disease	
				Moderate	Severe
N	8	12	8	7	7
age (yr)	30	69	51	57	52
range	25–35	65–78	35–73	34–68	29–66
T_{max}, h	2	1.5	1	1	2
C_{max}, ng/mL	9.1	10.2	8.5	13	13.3
$t_{½}$, h	17	23	16	25	29
$AUC_{0-\infty}$, ng·h/mL	132	189	145	272	417
Cl_{ren}, mL/min/1.73 m²	55	41	57	17	9.5
Risperidone, % unbound	16	14	22	14	16
Cl_{oral}, mL/min	127	89	119	61	40

Legend: N=number of subjects; T_{max}=time to peak plasma concentration; C_{max}=peak plasma concentration; $t_{½}$=elimination half-life; $AUC_{0-\infty}$=area under plasma concentration time curve; Cl_{ren}=renal clearance; Cl_{oral}=oral clearance.

The results indicate that a 1 mg dose of risperidone produced modest pharmacokinetic changes in elderly subjects, including reduced clearance of the active antipsychotic fraction by about 30%. In patients with impaired liver function, the unbound fraction of risperidone was increased by about 35% due to diminished concentrations of both α_1-AGP and albumin. In patients with impaired renal function, the changes were substantial; C_{max} and AUC of risperidone and 9-hydroxyrisperidone combined were increased by about 40% and 160% respectively, half-life was prolonged by about 60% and clearance decreased by about 60%.

Plasma Levels in Patients with Severe Dementia: The plasma levels of risperidone and its major metabolite, 9-hydroxyrisperidone, were determined at steady state. Blood samples were obtained from 85% of all trial patients receiving risperidone. Blood samples were drawn prior to the morning dose. Thus, the plasma levels shown in Table 9 represent trough levels.

Table 9: RISPERDAL

Median Trough Plasma Levels of Risperidone and 9-hydroxyrisperidone Combined at Steady State in Patients with Severe Dementia

Dose (mg/day) (b.i.d. dosing)	Median Trough Plasma Levels (ng/mL)
0.5	5.8
1	14.3
2	24

The plasma concentration of risperidone and 9-hydroxyrisperidone combined was dose proportional over the dosing range of 0.5 to 2 mg daily dose (0.25 to 1 mg b.i.d.).

STORAGE AND STABILITY: RISPERDAL tablets and RISPERDAL M-TAB orally disintegrating tablets should be stored between 15-30°C. Protect from light and moisture.

RISPERDAL oral solution should be stored between 15-30°C. Protect from light and freezing.

RISPERDAL should be kept out of the reach of children.

INFORMATION FOR THE PATIENT: Published in e-CPS, available by subscription at www.e-cps.ca.

DOSAGE FORMS, COMPOSITION AND PACKAGING: Film-coated Tablets: 0.25 mg: Each yellow, oblong, biconvex tablet, marked "JANSSEN" on one side and "Ris 0.25" on the other side, contains: risperidone 0.25 mg. Nonmedicinal ingredients: colloidal silicon dioxide, cornstarch, hydroxypropyl methylcellulose, lactose, magnesium stearate, microcrystalline cellulose, propylene glycol, sodium lauryl sulfate, talc, titanium dioxide and yellow ferric oxide. Bottles of 100.

0.5 mg: Each brownish-red, half-scored, oblong, biconvex tablet, marked "JANSSEN" on one side and "Ris 0.5" on the other side, contains: risperidone 0.5 mg. Nonmedicinal ingredients: colloidal silicon dioxide, cornstarch, hydroxypropyl methylcellulose, lactose, magnesium stearate, microcrystalline cellulose, propylene glycol, red ferric oxide, sodium lauryl sulfate, talc and titanium dioxide. Bottles of 100.

1 mg: Each white, oblong, biconvex tablet, marked "Ris" and "1" on one side, contains: risperidone 1 mg. Tablets may be scored. Nonmedicinal ingredients: colloidal silicon dioxide, cornstarch, hydroxypropyl methylcellulose, lactose, magnesium stearate, microcrystalline cellulose, propylene glycol and sodium lauryl sulfate. Blisters of 60. Bottles of 500.

2 mg: Each orange, scored, oblong, biconvex tablet, marked "Ris" and "2" on one side, contains: risperidone 2 mg. Nonmedicinal ingredients: colloidal silicon dioxide, cornstarch, FD&C Yellow #6 Aluminum Lake, hydroxypropyl methylcellulose, lactose, magnesium stearate, microcrystalline cellulose, propylene glycol, sodium lauryl sulfate, talc and titanium dioxide. Blisters of 60. Bottles of 500.

3 mg: Each yellow, scored, oblong, biconvex tablet, marked "Ris" and "3" on one side, contains: risperidone 3 mg. Nonmedicinal ingredients: colloidal silicon dioxide, cornstarch, D&C Yellow #10, hydroxypropyl methylcellulose, lactose, magnesium stearate, microcrystalline cellulose, propylene glycol, sodium lauryl sulfate, talc and titanium dioxide. Blisters of 60. Bottles of 250.

4 mg: Each green, scored, oblong, biconvex tablet, marked "Ris" and "4" on one side, contains: risperidone 4 mg. Nonmedicinal ingredients: colloidal silicon dioxide, cornstarch, D&C Yellow #10, FD&C Blue #2 Aluminum Lake, hydroxypropyl methylcellulose, lactose, magnesium stearate, microcrystalline cellulose, propylene glycol, sodium lauryl sulfate, talc and titanium dioxide. Bottles of 60.

M-Tab: 0.5 mg: Each orally disintegrating, light coral, round, biconvex tablet, marked "R0.5", contains: risperidone 0.5 mg. Nonmedicinal ingredients: aspartame, carbomer 934P, gelatin, glycine, mannitol, peppermint oil, polacrilex resin, red ferric oxide, simethicone and sodium hydroxide. Blisters of 28 per carton.

1 mg: Each orally disintegrating, light coral, square, biconvex tablet, marked "R1", contains: risperidone 1 mg. Nonmedicinal ingredients: aspartame, carbomer 934P, gelatin, glycine, mannitol, peppermint oil, polacrilex resin, red ferric oxide, simethicone and sodium hydroxide. Blisters of 28 per carton.

2 mg: Each orally disintegrating biconvex tablet, marked "R2", contains: risperidone 2 mg. Tablets manufactured prior to 2006 are light coral and round. Tablets manufactured from 2006 onwards are coral and square. Nonmedicinal ingredients: aspartame, carbomer 934P, gelatin, glycine, mannitol, peppermint oil, polacrilex resin, red ferric oxide, simethicone, sodium hydroxide and xanthan gum. Blisters of 28 per carton.

3 mg: Each orally disintegrating, coral, round, biconvex tablet, marked "R3", contains: risperidone 3 mg. Nonmedicinal ingredients: aspartame, carbomer 934P, gelatin, glycine, mannitol, peppermint oil, polacrilex resin, red ferric oxide, simethicone, sodium hydroxide and xanthan gum. Blisters of 28 per carton.

4 mg: Each orally disintegrating, coral, round, biconvex tablet, marked "R4", contains: risperidone 4 mg. Nonmedicinal ingredients: aspartame, carbomer 934P, gelatin, glycine, mannitol, peppermint oil, polacrilex resin, red ferric oxide, simethicone, sodium hydroxide and xanthan gum. Blisters of 28 per carton.

Oral Solution: Each mL of oral solution contains: risperidone 1 mg as risperidone tartrate. Nonmedicinal ingredients: benzoic acid, purified water, sodium hydroxide and tartaric acid. Bottles of 30 mL with a plastic child-resistant closure and a calibrated (in mg and in mL) pipette. The minimum calibrated volume is 0.25 mL, while the maximum calibrated volume is 3 mL. Calibration marks every 0.25 mL up to 3 mL are printed on this pipette. Patient Instructions (including illustrations) for using the RISPERDAL calibrated dispensing pipette are provided (see Information for the Patient). Tests indicate that RISPERDAL oral solution is compatible with the following beverages: water, coffee, orange juice and low-fat milk. However, it is **not** compatible with cola or tea.

(Shown in Product Identification Section)

Ritalin® Ⓒ

methylphenidate HCl

CNS Stimulant

Novartis Pharmaceuticals

Ritalin® SR Ⓒ

methylphenidate HCl

CNS Stimulant

Novartis Pharmaceuticals

Date of Preparation: August 31, 1984
Date of Revision: December 10, 2007

PHARMACOLOGY: RITALIN (methylphenidate hydrochloride) is a racemate consisting of a 1:1 mixture of d-methylphenidate (d-MPH) and l-methylphenydate (l-MPH).

RITALIN is a mild CNS stimulant with more prominent effects on mental than motor activities.

The mode of action in man is not completely understood, but its stimulant effects are thought to be due to cortical stimulation and possibly to stimulation of the reticular activating system.

There is neither specific evidence which clearly establishes the mechanism whereby methylphenidate produces its mental and behavioral effects in children, nor conclusive evidence regarding how these effects relate to the condition of the CNS.

Pharmacokinetics: Methylphenidate is rapidly and extensively absorbed from the tablets following oral administration; however, owing to extensive first-pass metabolism, bioavailability is low (approximately 30%) and large individual differences exist (11 to 52%). In one study, the administration of methylphenidate with food accelerated absorption, but had no effect on the amount absorbed.

Peak plasma concentrations of 10.8 and 7.8 ng/mL were observed, on average, 2 hours after administration of 0.30 mg/kg in children and adults, respectively. Peak plasma concentrations showed marked variability between subjects. Both the area under the concentration-time curve (AUC), and the peak plasma concentrations (C_{max}) showed dose-proportionality.

Methylphenidate is eliminated from the plasma with a mean half-life of 2.4 hours in children and 2.1 hours in adults. The apparent mean systemic clearance after an oral dose is 10.2 and 10.5 L/h/kg in children and adults, respectively for a 0.3 mg/kg dose, and 0.565 L/h/kg after an intravenous dose of the racemate in healthy adult volunteers. These data indicate that the pharmacokinetics of methylphenidate in hyperactive children is similar to that in healthy adult volunteers. The apparent distribution volume of methylphenidate in children was approximately 20 L/kg, with substantial variability (11 to 33 L/kg). The volume of distribution after an intravenous dose (V_{ss}) is 2.23 L/kg for the racemate in healthy adult volunteers.

Following oral administration of methylphenidate, 78 to 97% of the dose is excreted in the urine and 1 to 3% in the feces in the form of metabolites within 48 to 96 hours. The main urinary metabolite is ritalinic acid (α-phenyl-2-piperidine acetic acid, PPAA); unchanged methylphenidate is excreted in the urine in small quantities (<1%). Peak PPAA plasma concentrations occurred at approximately the same time as peak methylphenidate concentrations, however, levels were several-fold greater than those of the unchanged drug. The half-life of PPAA was approximately twice that of methylphenidate.

In blood, methylphenidate and its metabolites are distributed between plasma (57%) and erythrocytes (43%). Methylphenidate and its metabolites exhibit low plasma protein binding (approximately 15%).

Methylphenidate in the extended-release tablets is more slowly but as extensively absorbed as in the regular tablets. Relative bioavailability of the RITALIN SR tablet, compared to the RITALIN tablet, measured by the urinary excretion of the methylphenidate major metabolite (PPAA), was 105% (49 to 168%) in children and 101% (85 to 152%) in adults. The time to peak rate in children was 4.7 hours (1.3 to 8.2 hours) for the extended-release tablets and 1.9 hours (0.3 to 4.4 hours) for the regular tablets. The elimination half-life and the cumulative urinary excretion of PPAA are not significantly different between the two dosage forms. An average of 67% of the extended-release tablet dose was excreted in children as compared to 86% in adults.

INDICATIONS: RITALIN (methylphenidate hydrochloride) is indicated for the treatment of Attention Deficit Hyperactivity Disorder (ADHD).

A diagnosis of ADHD (DSM-IV) implies the presence of hyperactive-impulsive or inattentive symptoms that caused impairment and that were present before age 7 years. The symptoms must be persistent, must be more severe than is typically observed in individuals at a comparable level of development, must cause clinically significant impairment, e.g., in social, academic, or occupational functioning, and must be present in 2 or more settings, e.g., school (or work) and at home. The symptoms must not be better accounted for by another mental disorder. For the Inattentive Type, at least 6 of the following symptoms must have persisted for at least 6 months: lack of attention to details/careless mistakes, lack of sustained attention, poor listener, failure to follow through on tasks, poor organization, avoids tasks requiring sustained mental effort, loses things, easily distracted, forgetful. For the Hyperactive-Impulsive Type, at least 6 of the following symptoms must have persisted for at least 6 months: fidgeting/squirming, leaving seat, inappropriate running/climbing, difficulty with quiet activities, "on the go," excessive talking, blurting answers, can't wait turn, intrusive. For a Combined Type diagnosis, both inattentive and hyperactive-impulsive criteria must be met.

Special Diagnostic Considerations: The specific etiology of ADHD is unknown, and there is no single diagnostic test. Adequate diagnosis requires the use not only of medical but of special psychological, educational, and social resources. Learning may or may not be impaired. The diagnosis must be based upon a complete history and evaluation of the patient and not solely on the presence of the required number of DSM-IV characteristics.

Need for Comprehensive Treatment Program: RITALIN is indicated as an integral part of a total treatment program for ADHD that may include other measures (psychological, educational, social) for patients with this syndrome. Drug treatment may not be indicated for all patients with this syndrome. Drug treatment is not intended for use in the patient who exhibits symptoms secondary to environmental factors and/or other primary psychiatric disorders, including psychosis. Appropriate educational placement is essential in children and adolescents with this diagnosis and psychosocial intervention is often helpful. When remedial measures alone are insufficient, the decision to prescribe drug treatment medication will depend upon the physician's assessment of the chronicity and severity of the patient's symptoms.

Long-Term Use: The effectiveness of RITALIN for long-term use, i.e. for more than 4 weeks has not been systematically evaluated in placebo-controlled trials. Therefore, the physician who elects to use RITALIN for extended periods should periodically re-evaluate the long-term usefulness of the drug for the individual patient (see Dosage).

Narcolepsy.

CONTRAINDICATIONS: Anxiety, tension, agitation, thyrotoxicosis, advanced arteriosclerosis, symptomatic cardiovascular disease, moderate to severe hypertension, glaucoma and pheochromocytoma. Known or suspected hypersensitivity to the drug or its excipients. Also contraindicated in patients with motor tics or with a family history or diagnosis of Tourette's syndrome.

Monoamine Oxidase Inhibitors: RITALIN is contraindicated during treatment with monoamine oxidase inhibitors, and also within a minimum of 14 days following discontinuation of a monoamine oxidase inhibitor (hypertensive crises may result).

WARNINGS: Cardiovascular: Sudden Death and Pre-existing Structural Cardiac Abnormalities or Other Serious Heart Problems: Children and Adolescents: Sudden death has been reported in association with stimulant drugs used for ADHD treatment at usual doses in children and adolescents with structural cardiac abnormalities or other serious cardiac problems. Although some serious heart problems alone carry an increased risk of sudden death, RITALIN and RITALIN SR generally should not be used in children, adolescents, or adults with known structural cardiac abnormalities, cardiomyopathy, serious heart rhythm abnormalities, or other serious cardiac problems that may place them at increased vulnerability to the sympathomimetic effects of a stimulant drug.

Adults: Sudden deaths, stroke, and myocardial infarction have been reported in adults taking stimulant drugs at usual doses for ADHD. Although the role of stimulants in these adult cases is also unknown, adults have a greater likelihood than children of having serious structural cardiac abnormalities, cardiomyopathy, serious heart rhythm abnormalities, coronary artery disease, or other serious cardiac problems. Adults with such abnormalities should also generally not be treated with stimulant drugs (see Contraindications).

Misuse and Cardiovascular Events: Misuse of stimulants of the central nervous system may be associated with sudden death and other serious cardiovascular adverse events.

Hypertension and Other Cardiovascular Conditions: Sympathomimetic medications can cause a modest increase in average blood pressure and average heart rate and individuals may have larger increases. While the mean changes alone would not be expected to have short-term consequences, all patients should be monitored for larger changes in heart rate and blood pressure. Caution is indicated in treating patients whose underlying medical conditions might be compromised by increases in blood pressure or heart rate, e.g., those with pre-existing hypertension, heart failure, recent myocardial infarction, or ventricular arrhythmia (see also Warnings and Contraindications).

General: Children: Theoretically there exists a pharmacological potential for all ADHD drugs to increase the risk of sudden/cardiac death. Although confirmation of an incremental risk for adverse cardiac events arising from treatment with ADHD medications is lacking, prescribers should consider this potential risk.

All drugs with sympathomimetic effects prescribed in the management of ADHD should be used with caution in patients who: a) are involved in strenuous exercise or activities, b) use ADHD drugs or c) have a family history of sudden/cardiac death. Prior to the initiation of treatment with sympathomimetic medications, a personal and family history (including assessment for a family history of sudden death or ventricular arrhythmia) and physical exam should be obtained to assess for the presence of cardiac disease. In patients with relevant risk factors and based on the clinician's judgment, further cardiovascular evaluation may be considered (e.g., electrocardiogram and echocardiogram). Patients who develop symptoms such as exertional chest pain, unexplained syncope, or other symptoms suggestive of cardiac disease during ADHD treatment should undergo a prompt cardiac evaluation.

Cerebrovascular: Cerebrovascular Conditions: Patients with pre-existing CNS abnormalities, e.g., cerebral aneurysm and/or other vascular abnormalities such as vasculitis or pre-existing stroke should not be treated with RITALIN. Patients with additional risk factors (history of cardiovascular disease, concomitant medications that elevate blood pressure) should be assessed regularly for neurological/psychiatric signs and symptoms after initiating treatment with RITALIN (see Cardiovascular and Precautions, Drug Interactions).

Psychiatric Conditions: Co-morbidity of psychiatric disorders in ADHD is common and should be taken into account when prescribing stimulant products. Treatment of ADHD with stimulant products including RITALIN should not be initiated in patients with acute psychosis, acute mania or acute suicidality. These acute conditions should be treated and controlled before ADHD treatment is considered.

In the case of emergent psychiatric symptoms or exacerbation of pre-existing psychiatric symptoms, RITALIN should not be given to patients unless the benefit outweighs the potential risk.

Psychotic Symptoms: Psychotic symptoms, including visual and tactile hallucinations have been reported in patients administered usual prescribed doses of stimulant products, including RITALIN (see Adverse Effects). Physicians should consider treatment discontinuation.

Bipolar Illness: Particular care should be taken in using stimulants to treat ADHD in patients with comorbid bipolar disorder because of concern for possible induction of a mixed/manic episode in such patients. Prior to initiating treatment with a stimulant, patients with comorbid depressive symptoms should be adequately screened to determine if they are at risk for bipolar disorder; such screening should include a detailed psychiatric history, including a family history of suicide, bipolar disorder, and depression.

Aggressive Behaviour: Emergent aggressive behaviour or an exacerbation of baseline aggressive behaviour has been reported during stimulant therapy, including RITALIN. However, patients with ADHD may experience aggression as part of their medical condition. Therefore causal association with treatment is difficult to assess. Physicians should evaluate the need for adjustment of treatment regimen in patients experiencing these behavioural changes, bearing in mind that upwards or downwards titration may be appropriate. Treatment interruption can be considered.

Suicidal Tendency: Patients with emergent suicidal ideation and behaviour during treatment for ADHD should be evaluated immediately by their physician. The physician should initiate appropriate treatment of the underlying psychiatric condition and consider a possible change in the ADHD treatment regimen.

Depression: RITALIN should not be used to treat severe exogenous or endogenous depression.

Use in Children Under Six Years of Age: RITALIN should not be used in children under 6 years of age, since safety and efficacy in this age group have not been established.

Endocrine and Metabolism: Long-Term Suppression of Growth: Although a causal relationship has not been established, suppression of growth (i.e., weight gain and/or height) has been reported with the long-term use of stimulants in children. Therefore, patients requiring long-term therapy should be carefully monitored. In addition, the use of "Drug Holidays" is recommended, that is, withholding the drug on weekends and during school holidays inasmuch as the clinical situation permits.

Fatigue: RITALIN should not be used for the prevention or treatment of normal fatigue states.

Neurologic: Seizures: There is some clinical evidence that RITALIN may lower the convulsive threshold in patients with prior history of seizures, with prior EEG abnormalities in absence of seizures and, very rarely, in patients with no prior EEG evidence or history of seizures. Clinical experience has shown that a small number of patients may experience an increase in seizure frequency when treated with RITALIN. If seizure frequency rises, the drug should be discontinued.

Ophthalmologic: Visual Disturbance: Symptoms of visual disturbances have been encountered in rare cases. Difficulties with accommodation and blurring of vision have been reported.

Pregnancy: Studies to establish safe use of methylphenidate in pregnant women have not been conducted. Methylphenidate hydrochloride has been shown to have teratogenic effects in rabbits when given in doses of 200 mg/kg/day. The systemic exposure in rabbit at this dose is 5.1 times that in humans at the maximum recommended human dose (60 mg).

Therefore, RITALIN should not be given to pregnant women unless the potential benefit outweighs the risk to fetus.

Lactation: It is not known whether the active substance of RITALIN and/or its metabolites pass into the breast milk. For safety reasons, the physician should assess the patient's medical condition and advise one of the following options: refrain from breast-feeding their infants while taking RITALIN, or discontinue the drug while nursing.

Drug Dependence: RITALIN should be given cautiously to emotionally unstable patients, such as those with a history of drug dependence or alcoholism, because such patients may increase dosage on their own initiative.

Chronically abusive use can lead to marked tolerance and psychological dependence with varying degrees of abnormal behavior. Frank psychotic episodes can occur, especially with parenteral abuse. Careful supervision is required during drug withdrawal, since severe depression as well as the effects of chronic overactivity can be unmasked. Long-term follow-up may be required because of the patient's basic personality disturbances.

Clinical data indicate that treatment with RITALIN during childhood and/or adolescence does not seem to result in increased predisposition for addiction.

PRECAUTIONS: Patients with an element of agitation may react adversely; discontinue therapy if necessary.

Periodic CBC, differential, and platelet counts are advised during prolonged therapy.

Drug treatment is not indicated in all cases of Attention-Deficit Hyperactivity Disorder and should be considered only in light of the complete history and evaluation of the child. The decision to prescribe RITALIN (methylphenidate hydrochloride) should depend on the physician's assessment of the chronicity and severity of the child's symptoms and their appropriateness for his/her age. Prescription should not depend solely on the presence of one or more abnormal behavioral characteristics. Where these symptoms are associated with acute stress reactions, treatment with RITALIN is usually not indicated.

Long-term effects of RITALIN in children have not been well established.

Occupational Hazards: Because RITALIN may affect performance, patients should be cautioned against engaging in hazardous activities (i.e., operation of automobiles or dangerous machinery).

Drug Interactions: Pharmacodynamic Interactions: RITALIN may decrease the effectiveness of drugs used to treat hypertension. Use with caution in patients being treated with drugs that elevate blood pressure and including MAO inhibitors (see also Warnings, Cerebrovascular, Cerebrovascular Conditions).

As an inhibitor of dopamine reuptake, RITALIN may be associated with pharmacodynamic interactions when coadministered with direct and indirect dopamine agonists (including DOPA and tricyclic antidepressants) as well as dopamine antagonists (antipsychotics, e.g. haloperidol). The coadministration of RITALIN with antipsychotics is not recommended because of the counteracting mechanism of action.

Case reports suggested a potential interaction of RITALIN with coumarin anticoagulants, some anticonvulsants (e.g. phenobarbital, diphenylhydantoin, primidone), phenylbutazone and tricyclic antidepressants but pharmacokinetic interactions were not confirmed when explored at higher sample sizes. Downward dosage adjustments of these drugs might be required when given concomitantly with RITALIN.

Alcohol may exacerbate the adverse CNS effect of psychoactive drugs, including RITALIN. Therefore, patients should be advised to abstain from alcohol during treatment.

Pharmacokinetic Interactions: RITALIN is not metabolized by cytochrome P450 to a clinically relevant extent. Inducers or inhibitors of cytochrome P450 are not expected to have any relevant impact on RITALIN pharmacokinetics. Conversely, the d- and l-enantiomers of methylphenidate in RITALIN did not relevantly inhibit cytochrome P450 1A2, 2C8, 2C9, 2C19, 2D6, 2E1 or 3A.

RITALIN coadministration did not increase plasma concentrations of the CYP2D6 substrate desipramine.

An interaction with the anticoagulant ethylbiscoumacetate in 4 subjects was not confirmed in a subsequent study with a higher sample size (n=12).

Other specific drug-drug interaction studies with RITALIN have not been performed in vivo.

Other: Methylphenidate may induce false positive laboratory tests for amphetamines, particularly with immunoassays screen test.

Clonidine: Serious adverse events have been reported in concomitant racemic methylphenidate use with clonidine, although no causality for the combination has been established. The safety of using methylphenidate in combination with clonidine or other centrally acting alpha 2 agonists has not been systematically evaluated.

ADVERSE EFFECTS: Frequency estimate: very common ≥10%; common ≥1% to <10%; uncommon ≥0.1% to <1%; rare ≥0.01% to <0.1%; very rare <0.01%.

Nervousness and insomnia are very common adverse reactions which occur at the beginning of RITALIN treatment, but can usually be controlled by reducing dosage and/or omitting the afternoon or evening dose. Decreased appetite is also common but usually transient.

Central and Peripheral Nervous Systems: Common: dizziness, drowsiness, headache, dyskinesia. Rare: Symptoms of visual disturbances, difficulties in visual accommodation and blurred vision. Very rare: hyperactivity, convulsions, muscle cramps, choreoathetoid movements, tics, or exacerbation of existing tics, transient depressed moods, cerebrovascular disorders including vasculitis, cerebral haemorrhages and cerebrovascular accidents, Tourette's syndrome, psychosis (sometimes with visual and tactile hallucinations).

Very rare reports of poorly documented neuroleptic malignant syndrome (NMS) have been received. In most of these reports patients were also receiving other medications. It is uncertain what role methylphenidate played in these cases.

Gastrointestinal: Common: nausea, vomiting and abdominal pain may occur at the start of treatment and may be alleviated if taken with food. Dry mouth. Very rare: abnormal liver function, ranging from transaminase elevation to hepatic coma.

Cardiovascular: Common: palpitations, changes in blood pressure and heart rate (usually an increase), tachycardia, cardiac arrhythmias. Rare: angina pectoris.

Skin and/or Hypersensitivity Reactions: Common: rash, pruritus, urticaria, fever, arthralgia, scalp hair loss. Very rare: exfoliative dermatitis, erythema multiforme, thrombocytopenic purpura, hypersensitivity reactions.

Hematologic: Very rare: leukopenia, thrombocytopenia, anemia.

Miscellaneous: Rare: moderately reduced weight gain and slight growth retardation during prolonged use in children.

In children, loss of appetite, abdominal pain, insomnia, and tachycardia may occur more frequently; however, any of the other adverse reactions listed above may also occur.

Post-Market Adverse Events: Adverse events reported since market introduction in patients taking RITALIN include sudden cardiac death, suicide, suicidal ideation, suicide attempt, Stevens-Johnson Syndrome, pancreatitis, aplastic anaemia, hypoglycaemia, and transient pancytopenia. No causal relationship between RITALIN and these events has been established.

Adverse Events with Other Methylphenidate Hydrochloride Products: Nervousness and insomnia are the most common adverse reactions reported with other methylphenidate products. Other reactions include hypersensitivity (including skin rash, urticaria, fever, arthralgia, exfoliative dermatitis, erythema multiforme with histopathological findings of necrotizing vasculitis, and thrombocytopenic purpura); anorexia; nausea; dizziness; headache; dyskinesia; drowsiness; blood pressure and pulse changes, both up and down; tachycardia; angina; abdominal pain; weight loss during prolonged therapy. There have been rare reports of Tourette's syndrome. Toxic psychosis has been reported. Although a definite causal relationship has not been established, the following have been reported in patients taking this drug: instances of abnormal liver function, e.g., hepatic coma; isolated cases of cerebral arteritis and/or occlusion; leukopenia and/or anaemia; transient depressed mood; a few instances of scalp hair loss. Very rare reports of neuroleptic malignant syndrome (NMS) have been received, and in most of these, patients were concurrently receiving therapies associated with NMS. In a single report, a ten-year-old boy who had been taking methylphenidate for approximately 18 months experienced an NMS-like event within 45 minutes of ingesting his first dose of venlafaxine. It is uncertain whether this case represented a drug-drug interaction, a response to either drug alone, or some other cause.

OVERDOSE:

Symptoms: Signs and symptoms of acute overdosage, resulting principally from overstimulation of the CNS and from excessive sympathomimetic effects, may include the following: vomiting, agitation, tremors, hyperreflexia, muscle twitching, convulsions (may be followed by coma), euphoria, confusion, hallucinations, delirium, sweating, flushing, headache, hyperpyrexia, tachycardia, palpitations, cardiac arrhythmias, hypertension, mydriasis and dryness of mucous membranes.

Treatment: Management consists of providing supportive measures and symptomatic treatment of life-threatening events, e.g., hypertensive crisis, cardiac arrhythmias, convulsions. For the most current guidance for treatment of symptoms of overdose, the practitioner should consult a certified Poison Control Centre or current toxicological publication.

Supporting measures include preventing self-injury and protecting the patient from external stimuli that would exacerbate the overstimulation already present. If the overdose is oral and the patient is conscious, gastric contents could be evacuated by induction of emesis, followed by administration of activated charcoal. Airway protected gastric lavage is necessary in hyperactive or unconscious patients, or those with depressed respiration.

Intensive care must be provided to maintain adequate circulation and respiratory exchange; external cooling procedures may be required to reduce hyperpyrexia.

Efficacy of peritoneal dialysis or extracorporeal hemodialysis for methylphenidate overdosage has not been established.

For management of a suspected drug overdose, CPhA recommends that you contact your **regional Poison Control Centre**. See the *CPS* Directory section for a list of Poison Control Centres.

DOSAGE: RITALIN should be administered starting at the lowest possible dose; dosage should then be individually and slowly adjusted to the lowest effective dosage since individual patient response to methylphenidate varies widely.

RITALIN should not be used in patients with symptomatic cardiovascular disease and should generally not be used in patients with known structural cardiac abnormalities (see Contraindications and Warnings).

Children: Theoretically there exists a pharmacological potential for all ADHD drugs to increase the risk of sudden/cardiac death. Although confirmation of an incremental risk for adverse cardiac events arising from treatment with ADHD medications is lacking, prescribers should consider this potential risk.

All drugs with sympathomimetic effects prescribed in the management of ADHD should be used with caution in patients who: a) are involved in strenuous exercise or activities b) use stimulants or c) have a family history of sudden/cardiac death. Prior to the initiation of treatment with sympathomimetic medications, a personal and family history (including assessment for a family history of sudden death or ventricular arrhythmia) and physical exam should be obtained to assess for the presence of cardiac disease. In patients with relevant risk factors and based on the clinician's judgment, further cardiovascular evaluation may be considered (e.g., electrocardiogram and echocardiogram). Patients who develop symptoms such as exertional chest pain, unexplained syncope, or other symptoms suggestive of cardiac disease during ADHD treatment should undergo a prompt cardiac evaluation.

Patients who are considered to need extended treatment with methylphenidate should undergo periodic evaluation of their cardiovascular status (see Warnings).

Caution should be exercised in prescribing concomitant drugs.

Dosage of RITALIN (methylphenidate hydrochloride) should be individualized according to the needs and responses of the patient.

Children (6 years and over): RITALIN: RITALIN should be initiated in small doses, (e.g., 5 to 10 mg t.i.d.) with weekly increments of 5 to 10 mg in the daily dosage. Dosage should be individualized on the basis of factors such as age, body weight and individual response. Timing of drug administration should be aimed to coincide with periods of greatest academic, behavioral and social stress.

Daily dosage above 60 mg is not recommended.

If symptoms do not improve after dose titration over a one-month period, the drug should be discontinued.

If symptoms worsen or other adverse events occur, the dosage should be reduced or, if necessary, the drug discontinued.

RITALIN SR: RITALIN SR tablets have a duration of action of approximately 8 hours. Therefore, RITALIN SR tablets may be used in place of RITALIN tablets when the 8-hour dosage of RITALIN SR corresponds to the titrated 8-hour dosage of RITALIN. RITALIN SR tablets must be swallowed whole and never be crushed or chewed.

If paradoxical aggravation of symptoms or other adverse effects occur, reduce dosage, or if necessary, discontinue the drug.

Methylphenidate should be periodically discontinued to assess the child's condition. Improvement may be sustained when the drug is either temporarily or permanently discontinued.

Drug treatment should not and need not be indefinite and usually may be discontinued after puberty.

Adults: RITALIN: Administer in divided doses 2 or 3 times daily. Average daily dosage is 20 to 30 mg. Some patients may require 40 to 60 mg daily. In others, 10 to 15 mg daily will be adequate. Patients who are unable to sleep if medication is taken late in the day should take the last dose before 6 p.m.

RITALIN SR: RITALIN SR tablets have a duration of action of approximately 8 hours. Therefore, RITALIN SR tablets may be used in place of RITALIN tablets when the 8-hour dosage of RITALIN SR corresponds to the titrated 8-hour dosage of RITALIN. RITALIN SR tablets must be swallowed whole and never be crushed or chewed.

INFORMATION FOR THE PATIENT: Published in e-CPS, available by subscription at www.e-cps.ca.

SUPPLIED: RITALIN: 10 mg: Each pale blue, round, flat-faced, beveled-edged tablet, scored and imprinted "AB" on one side with "CIBA" on the other, contains: methylphenidate HCl 10 mg. Nonmedicinal ingredients: cornstarch, FD&C Green No. 3, lactose, magnesium stearate, polyethylene glycol, sugar and talc. Bottles of 100 and 500.

20 mg: Each pale yellow, round, flat-faced, beveled-edged tablet, scored and imprinted "PN" on one side with "CIBA" on the other, contains: methylphenidate HCl 20 mg. Nonmedicinal ingredients: D&C Yellow No. 10, lactose, magnesium stearate, polyethylene glycol, sugar, tragacanth and talc. Bottles of 100 and 500.

RITALIN SR: Each white, round, biconvex, film-coated, extended release tablet, "16" printed on one side with "CIBA" printed on the other in black ink, contains: methylphenidate HCl 20 mg. Nonmedicinal ingredients: cellulose compounds, cetostearyl alcohol, castor oil compounds, lactose, magnesium stearate, talc and titanium dioxide. Bottles of 100.

Protect from heat (store between 2 and 30°C) and humidity. Keep out of reach and sight of children.

(Shown in Product Identification Section)

Rituxan® Ⓟ

rituximab

Antineoplastic

Roche

Date of Preparation: March 17, 2000
Date of Revision: July 29, 2010

SUMMARY PRODUCT INFORMATION:

Route of Administration	Dosage Form/ Strength	Clinically Relevant Nonmedicinal Ingredients
Intravenous	Injection–10 mg/mL	Not applicable For a complete listing see Dosage Forms, Composition and Packaging.

DESCRIPTION: RITUXAN is a chimeric mouse/human monoclonal antibody that binds specifically to the transmembrane antigen CD20.

INDICATIONS AND CLINICAL USE: Non-Hodgkin's Lymphoma (NHL): RITUXAN (rituximab) is indicated for:

- the treatment of patients with relapsed or refractory low-grade or follicular, CD20 positive, B-cell non-Hodgkin's lymphoma.
- the treatment of patients with CD20 positive, diffuse large B-cell non-Hodgkin's lymphoma in combination with CHOP (cyclophosphamide, doxorubicin, vincristine, and prednisone) chemotherapy.
- the treatment of patients with previously untreated Stage III/IV follicular, CD20 positive, B-cell non-Hodgkin's lymphoma in combination with CVP (cyclophosphamide, vincristine and prednisolone) chemotherapy.
- the maintenance treatment of patients with follicular non-Hodgkin's lymphoma who have responded to induction therapy with either CHOP or CHOP plus rituximab.

Chronic Lymphocytic Leukemia (CLL) : RITUXAN (rituximab) is indicated for:

- The treatment of patients with previously untreated B-cell chronic lymphocytic leukemia (B-CLL), stage B or C, in combination with fludarabine and cyclophosphamide.

The use of RITUXAN in CLL is based on an improvement in progression-free survival. Overall survival benefit has not been demonstrated in patients with or without previous treatment for CLL. The efficacy of treatment with R-FC in CLL patients who were previously treated with Rituxan in combination with fludarabine and cyclophosphamide has not been studied.

Geriatrics (≥ 65 years of age): In the CLL setting, exploratory subgroup analysis indicates that use in the geriatric population is associated with differences in efficacy and safety.

Rheumatoid Arthritis (RA): RITUXAN in combination with methotrexate is indicated in adult patients:

- to reduce signs and symptoms in adult patients with moderately to severely active rheumatoid arthritis who have had an inadequate response or intolerance to one or more tumour necrosis factor (TNF) inhibitor therapies.

RITUXAN in combination with methotrexate has been shown to reduce the rate of progression of joint damage as measured by x-ray.

CONTRAINDICATIONS: RITUXAN (rituximab) is contraindicated in patients with known Type I hypersensitivity or anaphylactic reactions to murine proteins, Chinese Hamster Ovary (CHO) cell proteins, or to any component of this product (see Warnings and Precautions).

RITUXAN is also contraindicated in patients who have or have had progressive multifocal leukoencephalopathy (PML).

WARNINGS AND PRECAUTIONS:

Serious Warnings and Precautions

Progressive Multifocal Leukoencephalopathy: Patients with Rheumatoid Arthritis, Non-Hodgkin's Lymphoma and Chronic Lymphocytic Leukemia who received treatment with RITUXAN may have an increased risk of Progressive Multifocal Leukoencephalopathy (PML). PML can cause disability or death. Healthcare professionals should monitor patients on RITUXAN for any new sign or symptom that may be suggestive of PML. Further treatment with RITUXAN should be withheld immediately at the first sign or symptom suggestive of PML (see Warnings and Precautions, Progressive Multifocal Leukoencephalopathy).

Non-Hodgkin's Lymphoma and Chronic Lymphocytic Leukemia: RITUXAN (rituximab) is a potent drug. Several adverse reactions are associated with RITUXAN, some of which are severe and life-threatening. This drug should only be used by health professionals experienced in treating cancer in a setting where full resuscitation facilities are immediately available (see Dosage and Administration and Warnings and Precautions).

Deaths within 24 hours of RITUXAN infusion have occurred. Approximately 80% of fatal infusion reactions occurred in association with the first infusion. Carefully monitor patients during infusions. Discontinue RITUXAN infusion and provide medical treatment for Grade 3 or 4 infusion reactions (see Warnings and Precautions).

Severe, including fatal, adverse reactions have occurred in patients receiving RITUXAN including: Acute renal failure and Tumor Lysis Syndrome (TLS); mucocutaneous reactions; hepatitis reactivation and JC virus infection resulting in Progressive Multifocal Leukoencephalopathy (PML). Patients should be screened for infectious disease history (see Warnings and Precautions).

Rheumatoid Arthritis: Several adverse reactions are associated with RITUXAN, some of which are severe and life-threatening (see Warnings and Precautions, Rheumatoid Arthritis). This drug should only be used by health professionals experienced in treating rheumatoid arthritis in a setting where medications and supportive care measures for the treatment of hypersensitivity reactions, (e.g., epinephrine, antihistamines, glucocorticoids) are immediately available in the event of an allergic reaction during administration (see Dosage and Administration).

Non-Hodgkin's Lymphoma and Chronic Lymphocytic Leukemia: Infusion-Related Events: RITUXAN is associated with infusion-related reactions, which may be related to release of cytokines and/or other chemical mediators. Severe infusion-related reactions might be clinically indistinguishable from hypersensitivity reactions or cytokine release syndrome. Severe infusion-related reactions with fatal outcome have been reported during post-marketing use. Severe infusion-related reactions usually manifested within 30 minutes to 2 hours after starting the first infusion with RITUXAN. These reactions were characterized by pulmonary events, and included, in some cases, rapid tumour lysis and features of tumour lysis syndrome in addition to fever, chills, rigors, hypotension, urticaria, bronchospasm, acute respiratory distress syndrome, angioedema and other symptoms (see Adverse Reactions, Experience From Clinical Trials in Hemato-Oncology).

Infusion related deaths (death within 24 hours of infusion) have been reported at a rate of approximately 0.04-0.07% (4-7 per 10 000 patients treated). Nearly all fatal events occurred in association with the first infusion.

Patients with a high number (>25×10^9/L) of circulating malignant cells or high tumour burden such as patients with CLL and mantle cell lymphoma, who may be at higher risk of especially severe cytokine release syndrome, should only be treated with extreme caution and when other therapeutic alternatives have been exhausted. These patients should be very closely monitored throughout the first infusion. Consideration should be given to the use of a reduced infusion rate for the first infusion in these patients or a split dosing over two days during the first cycle and any subsequent cycles if the lymphocyte count is still >25 x 10^9/L; in the CLL ML17102 trial, 47% of patients required a delayed and/or slowed infusion, and 17% of patients required split dosing.

Premedication consisting of an anti-pyretic and an antihistaminic (e.g. acetaminophen and diphenhydramine) should always be administered before each infusion of RITUXAN. Medications for the treatment of hypersensitivity reactions, e.g., epinephrine, antihistamines and glucocorticoids should be available for immediate use in the event of a reaction during administration. In the CLL clinicals trial, most patients received high-dose boluses intravenous corticosteroids [100 mg Prednisone IV] before each RITUXAN infusion.

Patients should be monitored closely throughout the infusion. Patients with a high tumour burden or with a high number (>25×10^9/L) of circulating malignant cells such as patients with CLL and mantle cell lymphoma may be at higher risk of developing severe infusion-related reactions. If mild, the symptoms are usually reversible with interruption of RITUXAN infusion. Treatment of infusion-related symptoms with diphenhydramine and acetaminophen is recommended. Additional treatment with bronchodilators or IV saline or IV corticosteroids may be indicated and should be immediately available. In patients with severe reaction, the infusion should be interrupted immediately (see Dosage and Administration) and they should receive aggressive symptomatic treatment. Since initial improvement may be followed by deterioration, these patients should be closely monitored until tumour lysis syndrome and pulmonary infiltration have been ruled out. In most cases, the infusion can be resumed at a 50% reduction in rate (e.g., from 100 mg/h to 50 mg/h) when symptoms have completely resolved. Most patients who have experienced non-life-threatening reactions have been able to complete the full course of therapy (see Dosage and Administration). Further treatment of patients after complete resolution of signs and symptoms has rarely resulted in repeated severe infusion-related reactions. In the patients with a severe reaction, the decision to administer further infusions should be made by the treating physician on a case-by-case basis after assessing the risk versus benefit to the patient.

Pulmonary Events: Pulmonary events have included hypoxia, pulmonary infiltrates, and acute respiratory failure. Some of these events have been preceded by severe bronchospasm and dyspnea. Patients with a history of pulmonary insufficiency or those with pulmonary tumour infiltration may be at greater risk of poor outcome and should be treated with increased caution.

Acute respiratory failure may be accompanied by events such as pulmonary interstitial infiltration or edema, visible on a chest x-ray. The syndrome usually manifests itself within one or two hours of initiating the first infusion. Patients who experience severe pulmonary events should have their infusion interrupted immediately (see Dosage and Administration) and should receive aggressive symptomatic treatment. In some cases, symptoms worsened over time, while in others initial improvement was followed by clinical deterioration. Therefore, patients experiencing pulmonary events or other severe infusion-related symptoms should be closely monitored until complete resolution of their symptoms occur.

Tumour Lysis Syndrome: RITUXAN mediates the rapid lysis of benign and malignant CD20 positive cells. Signs and symptoms (e.g., hyperuricemia, hyperkalemia, hypocalcemia, hyperphosphatemia, acute renal failure, elevated LDH, high fevers) consistent with tumour lysis syndrome (TLS) have been reported to occur within 1 to 2 hours though initial reports of TLS were not diagnosed until 12-24 hours after the first infusion in NHL patients with high numbers of circulating malignant lymphocytes. Acute renal failure requiring dialysis with instances of fatal outcome has been reported in the setting of TLS in NHL patients. Prophylaxis for TLS should be considered for patients at risk of developing rapid tumour lysis (e.g. patients with a high tumour burden or with a high number (>25×10^9/L) of circulating malignant cells such as patients with CLL and mantle cell lymphoma). These patients should be followed closely and appropriate laboratory monitoring performed. Appropriate medical therapy should be provided for patients who develop signs and symptoms consistent with rapid tumour lysis. Following treatment for and complete resolution of signs and symptoms, subsequent RITUXAN therapy has been administered in conjunction with prophylactic therapy for TLS in a limited number of cases.

Anaphylaxis: Anaphylactic reactions, including fatalities, have been reported in patients treated with RITUXAN. These reactions may be clinically indistinguishable from severe infusion-related reactions, other hypersensitivity reactions or cytokine release syndrome. True hypersensitivity reactions typically occur after starting the second or subsequent infusion of RITUXAN. Epinephrine, antihistamines and glucocorticoids should be available for immediate use in the event of a hypersensitivity reaction to RITUXAN.

Carcinogenesis and Mutagenesis: No long-term animal studies have been performed to establish the carcinogenic or mutagenic potential of RITUXAN, or to determine its effects on fertility in males or females. Individuals of childbearing potential should use effective contraceptive methods during treatment and for up to 12 months following therapy with RITUXAN.

Cardiovascular: Since transient hypotension may occur during infusion with RITUXAN, consideration should be given to withholding anti-hypertensive medications 12 hours prior to and throughout infusion with RITUXAN. Serious and potentially fatal cardiovascular events have been reported rarely following administration of RITUXAN. These events included: cardiac arrhythmias such as atrial flutter and fibrillation, cardiac failure and cardiogenic shock. Infusions with RITUXAN should be discontinued in the event of serious or life-threatening cardio-pulmonary events. Patients who develop clinically significant cardiovascular events should undergo cardiac monitoring during and after subsequent infusions of RITUXAN. Patients with preexisting cardiac conditions including arrhythmias and angina have had recurrences of these events during therapy with RITUXAN and should be monitored throughout the infusion and immediate post-infusion period.

Effects on Ability to Drive and Use Machines: It is not known whether RITUXAN has an effect on the ability to drive and operate machines, though the pharmacologic activity and adverse events reported to date do not indicate that such an effect is to be expected.

Gastrointestinal: Abdominal pain, bowel obstruction and perforation, in some cases leading to death, were observed in patients receiving RITUXAN in combination with chemotherapy for DLBCL. A causal association with rituximab has not been established.

In post-marketing reports, which include both patients with low-grade or follicular NHL and DLBCL, the mean time to onset of symptoms was 6 days (range 1-77) in patients with documented gastrointestinal perforation. Complaints of abdominal pain, especially early in the course of treatment, should prompt a thorough diagnostic evaluation and appropriate treatment.

Hematologic: Myelosuppression: Although RITUXAN is not myelosuppressive in monotherapy, caution should be exercised when considering treatment of patients with neutrophil counts <1.5×10^9/L and/or platelet counts of <75×10^9/L, as clinical experience with such patients is limited. RITUXAN has been used in patients who underwent autologous bone marrow transplantation and in other risk groups with a presumable reduced bone marrow function without inducing myelotoxicity.

Grade 3-4 neutropenia and decreased white blood cell counts were very common in ML17102 with combination therapy of RITUXAN with Fludarabine and Cyclophosphamide. Grade 4 lymphopenia was not captured. Neutropenia and febrile neutropenia occurred in higher frequencies in the R-FC arm. This increase did not result in a statistically significant increase in hospitalization rates.

Immune: HAMA/HACA Formation: Human anti-murine antibody (HAMA) was not detected in 67 patients evaluated. Of 356 patients evaluated for human anti-chimeric antibody (HACA), 1.1% (4 patients) were positive. Patients who develop HAMA/HACA titers may have allergic or hypersensitivity reactions when treated with this or other murine or chimeric monoclonal antibodies.

Immunization: The safety of immunization with any vaccine, particularly live viral vaccines, following therapy with RITUXAN has not been studied. The ability to generate a primary or anamnestic humoral response to any vaccine has also not been studied.

Infections: Hepatitis B Reactivation with Related Fulminant Hepatitis: Cases of Hepatitis B virus (HBV) reactivation, occasionally with fulminant hepatitis, hepatic failure, and death has been reported in some patients with hematologic malignancies treated with RITUXAN. The majority of patients received RITUXAN in combination with chemotherapy. Isolated cases have been reported in patients who either had evidence of antibodies against Hepatitis B surface antigen before treatment or did not have any such antibodies. The median time to diagnosis of hepatitis was approximately 4 months after the initiation of RITUXAN and approximately one month after the last dose (see Adverse Reactions).

Hepatitis B reactivation can occur in oncology patients even if Hepatitis B surface antigen status is normal. HBV screening should be considered for patients before initiation of treatment with RITUXAN. Reactivation of HBV infection is a well-known complication in patients with chronic hepatitis B, especially in those receiving cytotoxic or immunosuppressive therapy. In addition, non-Hodgkin's lymphoma of itself may be an independent risk factor for HBV reactivation. Carriers of hepatitis B, and patients with evidence of having recovered from hepatitis B, should be closely monitored for clinical and laboratory signs of active HBV infection and for signs of hepatitis during and up to one year following therapy with RITUXAN.

In patients who develop reactivation of viral hepatitis B, RITUXAN and any concomitant chemotherapy should be discontinued and appropriate treatment including antiviral therapy initiated. There are insufficient data regarding the safety of resuming therapy with RITUXAN in patients who develop hepatitis subsequent to HBV reactivation.

Additional Serious Viral Infections: The following additional serious viral infections, either new, reactivated or exacerbated, have been identified in clinical studies or postmarketing reports. The majority of patients were profoundly immune-suppressed. These viral infections included JC virus [progressive multifocal leukoencephalopathy (PML)] (see Warnings and Precautions, Non-Hodgkin's Lymphoma and Chronic Lymphocytic Leukemia, Progressive Multifocal Leukoencephalopathy), cytomegalovirus, herpes simplex virus, parvovirus B19, varicella zoster virus, West Nile virus, and hepatitis C. In some cases, the viral infections occurred up to one year following discontinuation of RITUXAN and have resulted in death. RITUXAN treatment should not be initiated in patients with severe active infections.

Tuberculosis Reactivation: In the CLL clinical trial ML17102, one patient treated with RITUXAN plus Fludarabine and Cyclophosphamide experienced reactivation of tuberculosis. Patients who develop reactivation of tuberculosis should be treated as per current medical practice and RITUXAN should be discontinued. There are no data regarding the safety of resuming therapy with RITUXAN in patients who develop tuberculosis reactivation.

Pneumocystis Jiroveci Pneumonia: Cases of *Pneumocystis Jiroveci* Pneumonia (PJP) have been reported in patients receiving RITUXAN in combination with chemotherapy. These cases included patients with multiple risk factors for PJP, including the underlying disease state and other immunosuppressive therapies. The use of PJP prophylaxis should be considered according to local guidelines.

Monitoring and Laboratory Tests: Complete blood counts (CBC) and platelet counts should be obtained at regular intervals in patients with hematologic malignancies during therapy with RITUXAN and more frequently in patients who develop cytopenias (see Adverse Reactions).

Neurologic: Four cases of stroke or cerebral ischemia originated from a clinical study (GELA, LNH98-5) and concerned patients from 72 to 79 years of age, who had received rituximab in combination with CHOP chemotherapy, all with a history of cardiovascular disease or cardiovascular risk factors. In particular, lacunar lesions were seen in two patients, both of whom had a medical history of hypertension, the major risk factor of such small vessel disease. In 2 of these reports, the events were fatal and in the other two, the events were reported to have resolved. Furthermore, if the accepted definition of TIA (duration of signs/symptoms <24 hours) is applied, then one of the four patients with reported stroke experienced a TIA.

Progressive Multifocal Leukoencephalopathy: Very rare cases of Progressive Multifocal Leukoencephalopathy have been reported during post-marketing use of RITUXAN in NHL. The majority of patients had received RITUXAN in combination with chemotherapy or as part of a hematopoietic stem cell transplant.

Patients being treated with RITUXAN should be instructed to report any new neurological signs or symptoms to their physician. Physicians treating patients with non-Hodgkin's lymphoma and chronic lymphocytic leukemia should be alert to any new signs or symptoms that may be suggestive of PML and consider PML in the differential diagnosis of patients reporting new-onset neurological symptoms. Consultation with a neurologist should be considered as clinically indicated. Symptoms of PML are diverse, progress over days to weeks, and can include progressive weakness on one side of the body or clumsiness of limbs, disturbance of vision, and changes in thinking, memory and orientation leading to confusion and personality changes. Further treatment with RITUXAN should be withheld immediately at the first sign or symptom suggestive of PML and an evaluation that includes a magnetic resonance imaging (MRI) scan without and, where clinically indicated, with gadolinium-enhancement of the brain should be performed. Cerebrospinal fluid analysis for JC viral DNA is recommended to confirm a diagnosis of PML. Discontinue RITUXAN and consider discontinuation or reduction of any concomitant chemotherapy or immunosuppressive therapy in patients with confirmed PML.

The absolute risk for PML in patients treated with RITUXAN cannot be precisely estimated and factors that might increase an individual patient's risk for PML have not been identified. There are no known interventions that can reliably prevent or adequately treat PML if it occurs. It is not known whether early detection of PML and discontinuation of RITUXAN will mitigate the disease. The relationship between the risk of PML and the duration of treatment is unknown.

Skin: Severe mucocutaneous reactions including Stevens Johnson Syndrome, lichenoid dermatitis, vesiculobullous dermatitis, toxic epidermal necrolysis and paraneoplastic pemphigus have been reported rarely. Some of these cases were fatal. The onset varied from days to several months following exposure to RITUXAN. Patients experiencing a severe mucocutaneous reaction should interrupt treatment with RITUXAN and seek prompt medical evaluation. Skin biopsy may help to establish a diagnosis and guide subsequent treatment. The safety of re-administration of RITUXAN in these patients has not been determined.

Rheumatoid Arthritis: Infusion-Related Events: RITUXAN is associated with infusion-related reactions, which may be related to release of cytokines and/or other chemical mediators. Premedication with IV glucocorticoid significantly reduced the incidence and severity of these events (see Adverse Reactions, Rheumatoid Arthritis).

RITUXAN has caused severe infusion reactions. In spontaneous reports, fatal infusion reactions were reported very rarely in patients with autoimmune diseases and other co-morbidities (e.g. pulmonary fibrosis and SLE). The co- morbidities may have contributed to the fatal outcome (see Warnings and Precautions, Non-Hodgkin's Lymphoma and Chronic Lymphocytic Leukemia).

In clinical studies, 10/990 (1 %) patients with rheumatoid arthritis who received a first infusion of RITUXAN at any dose experienced a serious reaction during the infusion. Four out of 10 patients that experienced serious infusion reactions did not receive premedication with i.v. steroids. No infusion reactions in the RA population were fatal. Most infusion events reported were mild to moderate in severity. The most common symptoms were headache, pruritus, throat irritation, flushing, rash, urticaria, hypertension, and pyrexia. In general, the proportion of patients experiencing any infusion reaction was higher following the first infusion of any treatment course than following the second infusion. Subsequent RITUXAN infusions were better tolerated by patients than the initial infusion. Fewer than 1% of patients experienced serious IRRs, with most of these reported during the first infusion of the first course. (See Adverse Reactions, Rheumatoid Arthritis.) The infusion-related reactions reported with RITUXAN were usually reversible with a reduction in rate, or interruption, of the infusion and administration of appropriate symptomatic treatment, if required. In most cases, the infusion can be resumed at a 50% reduction in rate (e.g. from 100 mg/h to 50 mg/h) when symptoms have completely resolved.

Anaphylaxis: Anaphylactic and other hypersensitivity reactions have been reported following the IV administration of proteins to patients. Medicinal products for the treatment of hypersensitivity reactions, e.g., epinephrine, antihistamines and glucocorticoids, should be available for immediate use in the event of an allergic reaction during administration of RITUXAN.

In clinical studies 10/990 (1%) patients with rheumatoid arthritis who received a first infusion of RITUXAN at any dose experienced a serious reaction during the infusion. Four out of 10 patients that experienced serious infusion reactions did not receive premedication with i.v. steroids. Infusions with RITUXAN should be administered in an environment where full resuscitation facilities (see Serious Warnings and Precautions) are immediately available, and under the close supervision of an experienced health-professional.

Carcinogenesis and Mutagenesis: See Warnings and Precautions, Non-Hodgkin's Lymphoma and Chronic Lymphocytic Leukemia.

Cardiovascular: Since hypotension may occur during infusion with RITUXAN, consideration should be given to withholding anti-hypertensive medications 12 hours prior to the infusion of RITUXAN.

Angina pectoris, or cardiac arrhythmias such as atrial flutter and fibrillation heart failure have occurred in patients treated with RITUXAN. Patients who develop clinically significant arrythmias should undergo cardiac monitoring during and after subsequent infusions of RITUXAN. Patients with a history of cardiac disease such as angina and arrhythmias should be monitored during and after infusions (see Dosage and Administration).

Concomitant Use with Biologic Agents and DMARDs Other than Methotrexate in RA: Limited data are available on the safety of the use of biologic agents or DMARDs other than methotrexate in patients exhibiting peripheral B-cell depletion following treatment with rituximab. Patients should be closely observed for signs of infection if biologic agents and/or DMARDs are used concomitantly.

Effects on Ability to Drive and Use Machines: See Warnings and Precautions, Non-Hodgkin's Lymphoma and Chronic Lymphocytic Leukemia.

Immune: A total of 96/1039 (9.2%) patients with rheumatoid arthritis tested positive for HACA in clinical studies. The emergence of HACA was not associated with clinical deterioration or with an increased risk of reactions to subsequent infusions in the majority of patients. The presence of HACA could be associated with worsening of infusion or allergic reactions after the second infusion of subsequent courses. Such events could include hypersensitivity or anaphylactic reactions or anaphylactic shock. Failure to deplete B-cells after receipt of further treatment courses has also been observed rarely.

Immunization: Physicians should review the patient's vaccination status and follow current immunization guidelines prior to RITUXAN therapy. Vaccination should be completed at least 4 weeks prior to first administration of RITUXAN.

The safety of immunization with live viral vaccines following RITUXAN therapy has not been studied. Therefore vaccination with live virus vaccines is not recommended while on RITUXAN or while peripherally B cell depleted.

Patients treated with RITUXAN may receive non-live vaccinations. However, response rates to non-live vaccines may be reduced. In a randomized study, patients with RA treated with RITUXAN and methotrexate had comparable response rates to tetanus recall antigen (39% vs 42%), reduced rates to pneumococcal polysaccharide vaccine (43% vs 82% to at least 2 pneumococcal antibody serotypes), and KLH neoantigen (47% vs 93%), when given at least 6 months after RITUXAN as compared to patients only receiving methotrexate. Should non-live vaccinations be required while receiving RITUXAN therapy, these should be completed at least 4 weeks prior to commencing the next course of RITUXAN.

In the overall experience of RITUXAN repeat treatment over one year, the proportions of patients with positive antibody titers against *S. pneumoniae*, influenza, mumps, rubella, varicella and tetanus toxoid were generally similar to the proportions at baseline.

Infections: Serious infections can occur during therapy with RITUXAN. RITUXAN should not be administered to patients with an active and/or severe infection or severely immuno-compromised patients (e.g. in hypogammaglobulinemia or AIDS where levels of CD4 or CD8 are very low). Physicians should exercise caution when considering the use of RITUXAN in patients with a history of recurring or chronic infections or with underlying conditions which may further predispose patients to serious infection (see Adverse Reactions, Rheumatoid Arthritis). Patients who develop infection following therapy with RITUXAN should be promptly evaluated and treated appropriately.

Hepatitis B Reactivation: In patients with NHL receiving rituximab in combination with cytotoxic chemotherapy, very rare cases of hepatitis B reactivation have been reported (see Warnings and Precautions, Non-Hodgkin's Lymphoma and Chronic Lymphocytic Leukemia).

HBV screening should be considered for patients before initiation of treatment with RITUXAN.

Progressive Multifocal Leukoencephalopathy: Cases of fatal progressive multifocal leukoencephalopathy have been reported following use of RITUXAN for the treatment of autoimmune diseases (including RA). Several, but not all of the reported cases had multiple risk factors for PML, including the underlying disease, long-term immunosuppressive therapy or chemotherapy. PML has also been reported in patients with autoimmune disease not treated with RITUXAN.

Patients being treated with RITUXAN should be instructed to report any new neurological signs or symptoms to their physician. Physicians treating patients with autoimmune diseases should be alert to any new signs or symptoms that may be suggestive of PML and consider PML in the differential diagnosis of patients reporting new-onset neurological symptoms. Consultation with a neurologist should be considered as clinically indicated. Symptoms of PML are diverse, progress over days to weeks, and can include progressive weakness on one side of the body or clumsiness of limbs, disturbance of vision, and changes in thinking, memory and orientation leading to confusion and personality changes. Further treatment with RITUXAN should be withheld immediately at the first sign or symptom suggestive of PML and an evaluation that includes a magnetic resonance imaging (MRI) scan without and, where clinically indicated, with gadolinium-enhancement of the brain should be performed. Cerebrospinal fluid analysis for JC viral DNA is recommended to confirm a diagnosis of PML. Discontinue RITUXAN and consider discontinuation or reduction of any concomitant chemotherapy or immunosuppressive therapy in patients with confirmed PML.

The absolute risk for PML in patients treated with RITUXAN cannot be precisely estimated and factors that might increase an individual patient's risk for PML have not been identified. There are no known interventions that can reliably prevent or adequately treat PML if it occurs. It is not known whether early detection of PML and discontinuation of RITUXAN will mitigate the disease. The relationship between the risk of PML and the duration of treatment is unknown.

The efficacy and safety of RITUXAN for the treatment of autoimmune diseases other than rheumatoid arthritis has not been established.

Retreatment in Patients with RA: Safety and efficacy of retreatment have not been established in controlled trials. A limited number of patients have received two to five courses (two infusions per course) of treatment in an uncontrolled setting. In clinical trials in patients with RA, most of the patients who received additional courses did so 24 weeks after the previous course and none were retreated sooner than 16 weeks.

Use in Patients with RA Who Had no Prior Inadequate Response to TNF Antagonists: A favourable benefit-risk relationship has not been established in patients with RA with prior inadequate responses to non-biologic DMARDs, and in MTX-naïve patients. The use of RITUXAN in patients with RA who have no prior inadequate response to one or more TNF antagonists is not recommended.

Special Populations: Pregnant Women: IgG immunoglobulins are known to pass the placental barrier. Developmental toxicity studies performed in cynomolgus monkeys revealed no evidence of embryotoxicity in utero. Newborn offspring of maternal animals exposed to RITUXAN were noted to have depleted B-cell populations during the postnatal phase. B-cell levels in human neonates following maternal exposure to RITUXAN have not been studied in clinical trials. There are no adequate and well-controlled data from studies in pregnant women, however, transient B-cell depletion and lymphocytopenia have been reported in some infants born to mothers exposed to rituximab during pregnancy. For these reasons, RITUXAN should not be administered to pregnant women unless the possible benefit outweighs the potential risk. Women of childbearing age should employ effective contraceptive methods during and for up to 12 months after treatment with RITUXAN.

The potential risk of transmissible maternal infections either recently acquired or reactivated through the use of rituximab should also be considered when prescribing RITUXAN to pregnant women.

Nursing Women: It is not known whether RITUXAN is excreted in human milk. Because human IgG is excreted in human milk and the potential for absorption and immunosuppression in the infant is unknown, women should be advised to discontinue nursing until circulating drug levels are no longer detectable (see Action and Clinical Pharmacology).

Pediatrics: The safety and effectiveness of RITUXAN in pediatric patients have not been established.

Geriatrics: No dose adjustment is required in geriatric patients (aged >65 years). In diffuse large B-cell lymphoma clinical studies, no overall differences in effectiveness were observed between elderly and younger subjects. However, geriatric patients were more likely to experience cardiac adverse events, mostly supraventricular arrhythmias. Serious pulmonary adverse events were also more common among the elderly, including pneumonia and pneumonitis.

In low-grade or follicular lymphoma clinical studies, no over-all differences in safety or effectiveness were observed between geriatric and younger subjects.

In the trial of previously untreated CLL patients, patients over the age of 65 had, in general, more grade 3/4 AEs with increasing age, and more AEs were recorded in the R-FC arm compared with FC alone. Similar patterns were observed for SAEs (see Adverse Reactions). The effect of rituximab when added to FC seems to be most pronounced with younger age. Due to the small size of the subgroup of patients over the age of 70 (FC n=25, R-FC n=33), no meaningful conclusion can be drawn for the effect rituximab might have in this age category.

In RA clinical studies, adverse reactions, including incidence, severity and type of adverse reaction were similar between older and younger patients.

Safety findings were similar in the BO17072 trial in previously treated CLL patients. Grade 3/4 AEs and SAEs generally increased with age in both arms of the study and were more frequently reported in the R-FC arm than the FC arm. However, the incidence of grade 3/4 AEs was the same in R-FC and FC-treated patients over the age of 70 years.

ADVERSE REACTIONS: Adverse Drug Reaction Overview—Hemato-Oncology: Clinical trials have been conducted in patients with various malignancies and benign disorders in hematology treated with RITUXAN, predominantly in combination with chemotherapy. Across all hematologic indications, the most frequently observed serious adverse drug reactions were:

- bacterial infections, viral infections, bronchitis
- neutropenia, leucopenia, febrile neutropenia, thrombocytopenia
- infusion related reactions, angioedema.

The majority of serious infusion-related reactions occurred during the first infusion of RITUXAN.

Clinical Trial Adverse Drug Reactions: Because clinical trials are conducted under very specific conditions the adverse reaction rates observed in the clinical trials may not reflect the rates observed in practice and should not be compared to the rates in the clinical trials of another drug. Adverse drug reaction information from clinical trials is useful for identifying drug-related adverse events and for approximating rates.

Experience From Clinical Trials in Hemato-Oncology: The frequencies of adverse drug reactions (ADRs) reported with RITUXAN alone or in combination with chemotherapy are summarised in the tables below and are based on data from clinical trials. These ADRs had either occurred in single arm studies or had occurred with at least a 2% difference compared to the control arm in at least one of the major randomized clinical trials. ADRs are added to the appropriate category in the tables below according to the highest incidence seen in any of the major clinical trials. Within each frequency grouping ADRs are listed in descending order of severity. Frequencies are defined as very common ≥1/10, common ≥1/100 to <1/10 and uncommon ≥1/1000 to <1/100.

RITUXAN Monotherapy/Maintenance Therapy: The ADRs in Table 1 are based on data from single-arm studies including 356 patients with low-grade or follicular lymphoma treated with RITUXAN weekly as single-agent for the treatment or re-treatment of non-Hodgkin's lymphoma up to 4 weeks in most patients and from 25 patients who received doses other than 375 mg/m² for four doses and up to 500 mg/m² single dose in the Phase I setting. Table 1 also contains ADRs based on data from 166 patients with follicular lymphoma who received RITUXAN as maintenance therapy for up to 2 years following response to initial induction with CHOP or R-CHOP. The ADRs were reported up to 12 months after treatment with monotherapy and up to 1 month after treatment with RITUXAN maintenance.

Table 1: RITUXAN

Summary of ADRs Reported in Patients with Low-Grade or Follicular Lymphoma Receiving RITUXAN Monotherapy (N=356) or RITUXAN Maintenance Treatment (N=166) in Clinical Trials

System Organ Class	Very Common (≥10%)	Common (≥1%–<10%)	Uncommon (≥0.1%–<1%)
Infections and Infestations	bacterial infections, viral infections	sepsis, +pneumonia, +febrile infection, +herpes zoster, +respiratory tract infection, fungal infections, infections of unknown etiology	
Blood and the Lymphatic System Disorders	neutropenia, leucopenia	anemia, thrombocytopenia	coagulation disorders, transient aplastic anemia, hemolytic anemia, lymphadenopathy
Immune System Disorders	angioedema	hypersensitivity	
Metabolism and Nutrition Disorders		hyperglycemia, weight decrease, peripheral edema, face edema, increased LDH, hypocalcemia	
Psychiatric Disorders			depression, nervousness,
Nervous System Disorders		paresthesia, hypoesthesia, agitation, insomnia, vasodilatation, dizziness, anxiety	dysgeusia
Eye Disorders		lacrimation disorder, conjunctivitis	
Ear and Labyrinth Disorders		tinnitus, ear pain	
Cardiac Disorders		+myocardial infarction, arrhythmia, +atrial fibrillation, tachycardia, +cardiac disorder	+left ventricular failure, +supraventricular tachycardia, +ventricular tachycardia, +angina, +myocardial ischemia, bradycardia
Vascular Disorders		hypertension, orthostatic hypotension, hypotension	
Respiratory, Thoracic and Mediastinal Disorders		bronchospasm, respiratory disease, chest pain, dyspnea, cough, rhinitis	asthma, bronchiolitis obliterans, lung disorder, hypoxia
Gastrointestinal Disorders	nausea	vomiting, diarrhea, abdominal pain, dysphagia, stomatitis, constipation dyspepsia, anorexia, throat irritation	abdominal enlargement
Skin and Subcutaneous Tissue Disorders	pruritus, rash	urticaria, +alopecia, sweating, night sweats	
Musculoskeletal, Connective Tissue and Bone Disorders		hypertonia, myalgia, arthralgia, back pain, neck pain, pain	
General Disorders and Administration Site Conditions	fever, chills, asthenia, headache	tumour pain, flushing, malaise, cold syndrome	pain at the infusion site
Investigations	decreased IgG levels		

For each term, the frequency count was based on reactions of all grades (from mild to severe), except for terms marked with "+" where the frequency count was based only on severe (≥grade 3 NCI common toxicity criteria) reactions. Only the highest frequency observed in either trial is reported.

RITUXAN as Monotherapy: The adverse events listed below were considered by the investigator to be related or of unknown relationship to RITUXAN and were reported during or up to 12 months after treatment. Adverse events were graded according to the four scale National Cancer Institute (NCI) Common Toxicity Criteria. (See Table 2.)

Table 2: RITUXAN

Summary of Adverse Events Reported in ≥1% of 356 NHL Patients Receiving RITUXAN Monotherapy in Clinical Trials

Body System Adverse Event	All Grades		Grade 3 and 4	
	N	%	N	%
Any Adverse Event	324	91.0	63	17.7
Blood and Lymphatic Systems				
Leukopenia	44	12.4	10	2.8
Neutropenia	40	11.2	15	4.2
Thrombocytopenia	34	9.6	6	1.7
Anemia	13	3.7	4	1.1
Body as a Whole				
Fever	172	48.3	2	0.6
Chills	113	31.7	8	2.2
Asthenia	64	18.0	1	0.3
Headache	45	12.6	2	0.6
Throat irritation	27	7.6	—	—
Abdominal pain	25	7.0	2	0.6
Back pain	16	4.5	1	0.3
Flushing	15	4.2	—	—
Pain	15	4.2	—	—
Chest pain	8	2.2	—	—
Infection	7	2.0	2	0.6
Malaise	7	2.0	—	—
Tumour pain	6	1.7	—	—
Cold syndrome	5	1.4	—	—
Neck pain	4	1.1	—	—
Cardiovascular System				
Hypotension	35	9.8	3	0.8
Hypertension	16	4.5	1	0.3
Arrhythmia	5	1.4	2	0.6
Tachycardia	5	1.4	—	—
Hypotension orthostatic	4	1.1	—	—
Digestive System				
Nausea	61	17.1	1	0.3
Vomiting	24	6.7	1	0.3
Diarrhea	15	4.2	—	—
Anorexia	10	2.8	—	—
Dyspepsia	10	2.8	—	—
Dysphagia	5	1.4	1	0.3
Stomatitis	5	1.4	—	—
Constipation	4	1.1	—	—
Metabolic and Nutritional Disorders				
Angioedema	38	10.7	1	0.3
Hyperglycemia	19	5.3	1	0.3
Peripheral edema	17	4.8	—	—
Hypocalcemia	8	2.2	—	—
Increased lactate-dehydrogenase	8	2.2	—	—
Face edema	4	1.1	—	—
Decreased weight	4	1.1	—	—
Musculoskeletal System				
Myalgia	29	8.1	1	0.3
Arthralgia	21	5.9	2	0.6
Hypertonia	5	1.4	—	—
Pain	4	1.1	1	0.3

(cont'd)

Table 2: RITUXAN *(cont'd)*

Summary of Adverse Events Reported in ≥1% of 356 NHL Patients Receiving RITUXAN Monotherapy in Clinical Trials

Body System Adverse Event	All Grades		Grade 3 and 4	
	N	%	N	%
Nervous System				
Dizziness	26	7.3	—	—
Paresthesia	9	2.5	—	—
Anxiety	8	2.2	—	—
Insomnia	8	2.2	—	—
Vasodilatation	6	1.7	—	—
Agitation	5	1.4	—	—
Hypesthesia	5	1.4	—	—
Respiratory System				
Bronchospasm	28	7.9	5	1.4
Rhinitis	26	7.3	1	0.3
Increased cough	18	5.1	1	0.3
Dyspnea	8	2.2	3	0.8
Pneumonia	7	2.0	1	0.3
Infection	6	1.7	1	0.3
Sinusitis	6	1.7	—	—
Pharyngitis	5	1.4	—	—
Bronchitis	4	1.1	—	—
Chest pain	4	1.1	—	—
Respiratory disease	4	1.1	—	—
Skin and Appendages				
Pruritus	44	12.4	1	0.3
Rash	40	11.2	1	0.3
Urticaria	26	7.3	3	0.8
Sweat	10	2.8	—	—
Night sweat	10	2.8	—	—
Herpes zoster	8	2.2	1	0.3
Herpes simplex	5	1.4	1	0.3
Special Senses				
Lacrimation disorder	11	3.1	—	—
Conjunctivitis	5	1.4	—	—
Ear pain	4	1.1	—	—
Tinnitus	4	1.1	—	—

Less Common Clinical Trial Adverse Drug Reactions (<1%): The following adverse events were also reported: coagulation disorders, asthma, lung disorder, bronchiolitis obliterans, hypoxia, abdominal enlargement, pain at the infusion site, bradycardia, lymphadenopathy, nervousness, depression, dysgeusia.

Subpopulations: Elderly Patients (≥65 years): The incidence of any adverse event and of grade 3 and 4 adverse events was similar in elderly (N=94) and younger (N=237) patients (88.3% versus 92.0% for any adverse event and 16.0% versus 18.1% for grade 3 and 4 adverse events).

Bulky Disease: Patients with bulky disease (N=39) had a higher incidence of grade 3 and 4 adverse events than patients without bulky disease (N=195; 25.6% versus 15.4%). The incidence of any adverse event was similar in these two groups (92.3% in bulky disease versus 89.2% in non-bulky disease).

Retreatment: The percentage of patients reporting any adverse event and grade 3 and 4 adverse events upon re-treatment (N=60) with further courses of RITUXAN was similar to the percentage of patients reporting any adverse event and grade 3 and 4 adverse events upon initial exposure (N=203; 95.0% versus 89.7% for any adverse event and 13.3% versus 14.8% for grade 3 and 4 adverse events).

RITUXAN Maintenance Treatment: The following data are from a phase III clinical trial where patients with relapsed or refractory follicular non-Hodgkin's lymphoma were randomized in a first phase to induction treatment with CHOP (cyclophosphamide, doxorubicin, vincristine, prednisone) or RITUXAN plus CHOP (R-CHOP). Patients who responded to induction treatment with CHOP or R-CHOP were randomized in a second phase to receive no further treatment (observation) or maintenance treatment with RITUXAN.

In the induction phase of the trial, a total of 462 patients (228 on CHOP, 234 on R-CHOP) contributed to the safety evaluation of the two induction regimens. (See Table 3.)

Table 3: RITUXAN

Induction Phase: Summary of NCIC-CTC Grade 3 and 4 Adverse Events Reported in ≥1% of 462 Patients in Either Treatment Group (CHOP or R-CHOP)

	Incidence N (%)	
System Organ Class	**CHOP**	**R-CHOP**
Adverse Event	**152 (67)**	**185 (79)**
Blood and Lymphatic System Disorders		
Neutropenia[a]	108 (47)	129 (55)
Leucopenia	106 (46)	111 (47)
Thrombocytopenia	18 (8)	17 (7)
Febrile neutropenia[a]	8 (4)	14 (6)
Hematotoxicity	12 (5)	9 (4)
Anemia	5 (2)	6 (3)
Lymphopenia	3 (1)	2 (<1)
Cardiac Disorders		
Cardiac disorder	6 (3)	2 (<1)
Gastrointestinal Disorders		
Nausea[a]	9 (4)	13 (6)
Vomiting	8 (4)	7 (3)
Diarrhea	5 (2)	6 (3)
Abdominal pain	6 (3)	4 (2)
Constipation[a]	1 (<1)	7 (3)
Stomatitis[a]	1 (<1)	4 (2)
General Disorders and Administration Site Conditions		
Asthenia	10 (4)	5 (2)
Pyrexia	6 (3)	7 (3)
Pain	1 (<1)	3 (1)
Immune System Disorders		
Hypersensitivity[a]	—	10 (4)
Infections and Infestations		
Neutropenic infection	18 (8)	15 (6)
Sepsis	5 (2)	3 (1)
Urinary tract infection	4 (2)	3 (1)
Pneumonia	—	3 (1)
Metabolism and Nutrition Disorders		
Hyperglycemia	5 (2)	4 (2)
Musculoskeletal and Connective Tissue Disorders		
Back pain[a]	1 (<1)	4 (2)
Pain in extremity	3 (1)	—
Nervous System Disorders		
Sensory disturbance	4 (2)	7 (3)
Respiratory, Thoracic and Mediastinal Disorders		
Dyspnea	6 (3)	3 (1)
Skin and Subcutaneous Tissue Disorders		
Alopecia[a]	15 (7)	30 (13)
Skin disorder[a]	2 (<1)	4 (2)
Vascular Disorders		
Deep vein thrombosis	3 (1)	2 (<1)

[a] Adverse events that were reported at a higher incidence (≥2% difference) in the R-CHOP group compared to the CHOP group and, therefore, may be attributable to RITUXAN.

A total of 333 patients (167 observation, 166 rituximab) were included in the safety evaluation of the maintenance phase of the study. Maintenance treatment with RITUXAN consisted of a single infusion of RITUXAN at 375 mg/m² body surface area administered every 3 months for a maximum period of 2 years or until disease progression. (See Table 4.)

Table 4: RITUXAN

Maintenance Phase: Summary of NCIC-CTC Adverse Events (Grades 1-4 and Grades 3-4) Reported in ≥1% of 333 Patients in Either Treatment Group (observation or RITUXAN maintenance)

	Incidence			
	Observation		RITUXAN	
	N=167		N=166	
System Organ Class	**Grades 1–4 N (%)**	**Grades 3–4 N (%)**	**Grades 1–4 N (%)**	**Grades 3–4 N (%)**
Adverse Event **Total Patients with at Least One Adverse Event**	**138 (83)**	**41 (25)**	**151 (91)**	**64 (39)**
Blood and Lymphatic System Disorders				
Leukopenia[a,b]	37 (22)	4 (2)	50 (30)	9 (5)
Neutropenia[a,b]	22 (13)	8 (5)	40 (24)	18 (11)
Thrombocytopenia	23 (14)	2 (1)	20 (12)	1 (<1)
Hematotoxicity	4 (2)	4 (2)	2 (1)	2 (1)
Lymphopenia	2 (1)	—	2 (1)	—
Cardiac Disorders				
Cardiac disorder[b]	9 (5)	4 (2)	10 (6)	6 (4)
Palpitations[a]	—	—	3 (2)	—
Angina pectoris	2 (1)	2 (1)	—	—
Arrhythmia	—	—	2 (1)	—
Ear and Labyrinth Disorders				
Hearing impaired	1 (<1)	—	2 (1)	—
Eye Disorders				
Conjunctivitis[a]	—	—	3 (2)	—
Gastrointestinal Disorders				
Diarrhea[a]	14 (8)	2 (1)	17 (10)	2 (1)
Abdominal pain[a]	11 (7)	—	17 (10)	—
Nausea	14 (8)	—	14 (8)	—
Stomatitis[a]	2 (1)	—	14 (8)	—
Dyspepsia	6 (4)	—	8 (5)	—
Vomiting[a]	4 (2)	—	9 (5)	—
Constipation[a]	2 (1)	—	8 (5)	—
Abdominal pain upper	3 (2)	—	4 (2)	—
Abdominal distension	3 (2)	—	2 (1)	—
Dry mouth	3 (2)	—	2 (1)	—
Reflux esophagitis	3 (2)	—	—	—
Gastric ulcer	2 (1)	—	—	—
Gastrointestinal ulcer	—	—	2 (1)	—
Intestinal obstruction	—	—	2 (1)	2 (1)
General Disorders and Administration Site Conditions				
Asthenia[a]	43 (26)	4 (2)	50 (30)	1 (<1)
Pyrexia[a]	6 (4)	1 (<1)	12 (7)	2 (1)
Influenza like illness[a]	6 (4)	—	10 (6)	—
Pain[a]	2 (1)	—	7 (4)	—
Chest pain	5 (3)	—	3 (2)	—
Edema due to cardiac disease	3 (2)	—	4 (2)	—

(cont'd)

Table 4: RITUXAN *(cont'd)*

Maintenance Phase: Summary of NCIC-CTC Adverse Events (Grades 1-4 and Grades 3-4) Reported in ≥1% of 333 Patients in Either Treatment Group (observation or RITUXAN maintenance)

	Incidence			
	Observation		RITUXAN	
	N=167		N=166	
System Organ Class	Grades 1–4 N (%)	Grades 3–4 N (%)	Grades 1–4 N (%)	Grades 3–4 N (%)
Edema peripheral	3 (2)	—	3 (2)	—
Chills[a]	—	—	5 (3)	—
Chest discomfort	1 (<1)	—	2 (1)	—
Immune System Disorders				
Hypersensitivity[a]	1 (<1)	—	12 (7)	—
Infections and Infestations				
Nasopharyngitis[a]	5 (3)	—	14 (8)	—
Upper respiratory tract infection[a]	4 (2)	—	13 (8)	—
Sinusitis[a]	2 (1)	—	10 (6)	—
Herpes zoster[a]	4 (2)	—	7 (4)	2 (1)
Bronchitis	6 (4)	—	4 (2)	—
Lower respiratory tract infection[a]	2 (1)	—	7 (4)	—
Urinary tract infection	4 (2)	—	5 (3)	—
Herpes simplex[a]	2 (1)	—	6 (4)	—
Influenza	3 (2)	—	5 (3)	—
Pharyngitis[a]	1 (<1)	—	6 (4)	—
Pneumonia[a]	2 (1)	1 (<1)	5 (3)	4 (2)
Respiratory tract infection[a]	—	—	7 (4)	3 (2)
Candidiasis	1 (<1)		3 (2)	
Gastroenteritis	2 (1)	—	2 (1)	—
Lung infection	1 (<1)	—	3 (2)	—
Rhinitis	1 (<1)	—	3 (2)	—
Cystitis	1 (<1)	—	2 (1)	—
Diverticulitis	1 (<1)	—	2 (1)	—
Ear infection	1 (<1)	—	2 (1)	—
Eye infection[a]	—	—	3 (2)	—
Localized infection	1 (<1)	—	2 (1)	—
Onychomycosis	1 (<1)	—	2 (1)	—
Oral infection	1 (<1)		2 (1)	
Vaginal candidiasis	1 (<1)	—	2 (1)	—
Viral infection[a]	—	—	3 (2)	—
Cellulitis	2 (1)		—	
Febrile infection	—	—	2 (1)	2 (1)
Infection	2 (1)	—	—	—
Otitis externa	—	—	2 (1)	—
Investigations				
Weight decreased	6 (4)	—	8 (5)	—
Weight increased[a]	3 (2)	—	7 (4)	—
Blood lactate dehydrogenase increased	1 (<1)	—	3 (2)	—

(cont'd)

Table 4: RITUXAN *(cont'd)*

Maintenance Phase: Summary of NCIC-CTC Adverse Events (Grades 1-4 and Grades 3-4) Reported in ≥1% of 333 Patients in Either Treatment Group (observation or RITUXAN maintenance)

	Incidence			
	Observation		RITUXAN	
	N=167		N=166	
System Organ Class	**Grades 1–4 N (%)**	**Grades 3–4 N (%)**	**Grades 1–4 N (%)**	**Grades 3–4 N (%)**
Blood alkaline phosphatase increased	—	—	2 (1)	—
Metabolism and Nutrition Disorders				
Anorexia	8 (5)	—	5 (3)	—
Hyperglycemia	3 (2)	—	2 (1)	—
Hypokalemia	2 (1)	—	1 (<1)	—
Diabetes mellitus	2 (1)	—	—	—
Gout	—	—	2 (1)	—
Musculoskeletal and Connective Tissue Disorders				
Arthralgia[a]	13 (8)	—	20 (12)	—
Myalgia[a]	12 (7)	—	17 (10)	—
Back pain	8 (5)	—	12 (7)	—
Pain in extremity[a]	2 (1)	—	11 (7)	—
Bone pain	5 (3)	—	7 (4)	—
Shoulder pain	2 (1)	—	5 (3)	—
Groin pain	2 (1)	—	4 (2)	—
Musculoskeletal pain	3 (2)	—	1 (<1)	—
Neck pain	1 (<1)	—	2 (1)	—
Flank pain	—	—	2 (1)	—
Muscle spasms	—	—	2 (1)	—
Muscular weakness	—	—	2 (1)	—
Neoplasms Benign, Malignant and Unspecified (including Cysts and Polyps)				
Cancer pain	1 (<1)	—	2 (1)	—
Nervous System Disorders				
Sensory disturbance	40 (24)	2 (1)	38 (23)	3 (2)
Headache	8 (5)	—	9 (5)	—
Dizziness	6 (4)	—	3 (2)	—
Insomnia	5 (3)	—	4 (2)	—
Dysgeusia	2 (1)	—	1 (<1)	—
Vertigo	1 (<1)	—	2 (1)	—
Syncope	2 (1)	—	—	—
Psychiatric Disorders				
Anxiety	6 (4)	—	6 (4)	—
Depression	4 (2)	—	4 (2)	—
Mood altered	1 (<1)	—	2 (1)	—
Renal and Urinary Disorders				
Dysuria	3 (2)	—	4 (2)	—
Pollakisuria	1 (<1)	—	4 (2)	—
Nephrolithiasis	2 (1)	—	1 (<1)	—
Nocturia	1 (<1)	—	2 (1)	—

(cont'd)

Table 4: RITUXAN *(cont'd)*

Maintenance Phase: Summary of NCIC-CTC Adverse Events (Grades 1-4 and Grades 3-4) Reported in ≥1% of 333 Patients in Either Treatment Group (observation or RITUXAN maintenance)

	Incidence			
	Observation		RITUXAN	
	N=167		N=166	
System Organ Class	**Grades 1–4 N (%)**	**Grades 3–4 N (%)**	**Grades 1–4 N (%)**	**Grades 3–4 N (%)**
Hematuria	—	—	2 (1)	—
Renal colic	—	—	2 (1)	—
Urinary incontinence	2 (1)	—	—	—
Reproductive System and Breast Disorders				
Amenorrhea	—	—	2 (1)	—
Testicular pain	2 (1)	—	—	—
Respiratory, Thoracic and Mediastinal Disorders				
Cough[a]	15 (9)	—	22 (13)	2 (1)
Dyspnea	7 (4)	—	5 (3)	—
Dyspnea exertional	2 (1)	—	4 (2)	—
Rhinitis allergic	2 (1)	—	2 (1)	—
Nasal congestion	—	—	3 (2)	—
Pharyngolaryngeal pain	—	—	3 (2)	—
Lung disorder	—	—	2 (1)	—
Pleural effusion	2 (1)	—	—	—
Pleuritic pain	—	—	2 (1)	—
Skin and Subcutaneous Tissue Disorders				
Alopecia	12 (7)	—	12 (7)	3 (2)
Rash	11 (7)	—	10 (6)	—
Hyperhidrosis	10 (6)	2 (1)	7 (4)	—
Night sweats	10 (6)	—	6 (4)	—
Pruritus	6 (4)	—	6 (4)	—
Skin disorder	4 (2)	—	3 (2)	—
Rash pruritic	3 (2)	—	3 (2)	—
Nail disorder	2 (1)	—	2 (1)	—
Dermatitis	1 (<1)	—	2 (1)	—
Psoriasis	3 (2)	—	—	—
Rash erythematous	1 (<1)	—	2 (1)	—
Periorbital edema	2 (1)	—	—	—
Vascular Disorders				
Hot flush[a]	3 (2)	—	7 (4)	—
Hemorrhage	3 (2)	—	3 (2)	—
Hypertension	3 (2)	2 (1)	3 (2)	3 (2)
Lymphedema	—	—	2 (1)	—

[a] Adverse events (Grades 1-4) that were reported at a higher incidence (≥2% difference) in the RITUXAN maintenance group compared to observation and, therefore, may be attributable to RITUXAN.

[b] Adverse events (Grades 3-4) that were reported at a higher incidence (≥2% difference) in the RITUXAN maintenance group compared to observation and, therefore, may be attributable to RITUXAN.

RITUXAN in Combination with Chemotherapy in NHL and CLL: The ADRs listed in Table 5 are based on rituximab-arm data from controlled clinical trials that occurred in addition to those seen with monotherapy/maintenance therapy and/or at a higher frequency grouping: 202 patients with diffuse large B-cell lymphoma (DLBCL) treated with R-CHOP, and from 234 and 162 patients with follicular lymphoma treated with R-CHOP or R-CVP, respectively, and from 397 previously untreated CLL patients and 274 previously treated patients, treated with RITUXAN in combination with fludarabine and cyclophosphamide (R-FC).

Table 5: RITUXAN

Summary of Severe ADRs Reported in Patients Receiving R-CHOP in DLBCL (N=202), R-CHOP in Follicular Lymphoma (N=234) and R-CVP in Follicular Lymphoma (N=162) and R-FC in Previously Untreated CLL (N=397) or Previously Treated CLL (N=274)

System Organ Class	Very Common (≥10%)	Common (≥1%–<10%)
Infections and Infestations	bronchitis	acute bronchitis, sinusitis,hepatitis B[a]
Blood and the Lymphatic System Disorders	febrile neutropenia thrombocytopenia	pancytopenia granulocytopenia
Skin and Subcutaneous Tissue Disorders	alopecia	skin disorder
General Disorders and Administration Site Conditions		fatigue, shivering

[a] Includes reactivation and primary infections; frequency based on R-FC regimen in previously treated CLL.
Frequency count was based on only severe reactions defined in clinical trials as ≥ grade 3 NCI common toxicity criteria.
Only the highest frequency observed in any trial is reported.

RITUXAN in Combination with CVP Chemotherapy: The following data are based on 321 patients from a randomized phase III clinical trial comparing RITUXAN plus CVP (R-CVP) to CVP alone (162 R-CVP, 159 CVP). Differences between the treatment groups with respect to the type and incidence of adverse event were mainly accounted for by typical adverse events associated with RITUXAN monotherapy. (See Table 6.)

Table 6: RITUXAN

Summary of Adverse Events (all intensities) Reported in ≥1% of 321 Patients in Either Treatment Group (CVP or R-CVP)

Body System	Incidence: CVP N=159 N (%)	R-CVP N=162 N (%)
Blood and Lymphatic System Disorders		
Neutropenia	3 (1.9)	13 (8.0)
Anemia NOS	4 (2.5)	4 (2.5)
Leukopenia NOS	—	2 (1.2)
Lymphadenopathy	2 (1.3)	—
Cardiac Disorders		
Palpitations	2 (1.3)	2 (1.2)
Tachycardia NOS	1 (0.6)	2 (1.2)
Ear and Labyrinth Disorders		
Ear pain	3 (1.9)	4 (2.5)
Tinnitus	1 (0.6)	2 (1.2)
Vertigo	2 (1.3)	—
Eye Disorders		
Vision blurred	4 (2.5)	5 (3.1)
Eye pain	1 (0.6)	4 (2.5)
Dry eye NOS	1 (0.6)	2 (1.2)
Eye irritation	2 (1.3)	1 (0.6)
Gastrointestinal Disorders		
Nausea	56 (35.2)	55 (24.0)
Constipation	43 (27.0)	42 (25.9)
Abdominal pain NOS	21 (13.2)	23 (14.2)
Vomiting NOS	25 (15.7)	19 (11.7)
Dyspepsia	16 (10.1)	23 (14.2)
Diarrhea NOS	19 (11.9)	19 (11.7)
Abdominal pain upper	10 (6.3)	11 (6.8)
Stomatitis	11 (6.9)	7 (4.3)
Oral pain	3 (1.9)	9 (5.6)
Abdominal distension	3 (1.9)	4 (2.5)
Abdominal discomfort	2 (1.3)	4 (2.5)
Flatulence	2 (1.3)	4 (2.5)
Mouth ulceration	3 (1.9)	3 (1.9)
Ascites	3 (1.9)	1 (0.6)

(cont'd)

Table 6: RITUXAN *(cont'd)*

Summary of Adverse Events (all intensities) Reported in ≥1% of 321 Patients in Either Treatment Group (CVP or R-CVP)

Body System	Incidence: CVP N=159 N (%)	R-CVP N=162 N (%)
Gastritis NOS	1 (0.6)	3 (1.9)
Abdominal pain lower	2 (1.3)	1 (0.6)
Aphthous stomatitis	1 (0.6)	2 (1.2)
Gastroesophageal reflux disease	1 (0.6)	2 (1.2)
Rectal hemorrhage	2 (1.3)	1 (0.6)
Toothache	2 (1.3)	1 (0.6)
Dysphagia	—	2 (1.2)
Hypoesthesia oral	—	2 (1.2)
Loose stools	2 (1.3)	—
Tongue ulceration	2 (1.3)	—
General Disorders and Administration Site Conditions		
Fatigue	39 (24.5)	38 (23.5)
Pyrexia	14 (8.8)	21 (13.0)
Asthenia	14 (8.8)	8 (4.9)
Lethargy	9 (5.7)	12 (7.4)
Influenza like illness	7 (4.4)	13 (8.0)
Rigors	3 (1.9)	16 (9.9)
Pain NOS	5 (3.1)	12 (7.4)
Chest pain	5 (3.1)	11 (6.8)
Chest tightness	2 (1.3)	11 (6.8)
Edema peripheral	8 (5.0)	5 (3.1)
Mucosal inflammation NOS	4 (2.5)	5 (3.1)
Axillary pain	4 (2.5)	—
Feeling hot	1 (0.6)	2 (1.2)
Malaise	1 (0.6)	2 (1.2)
Chest discomfort	—	2 (1.2)
Hyperpyrexia	—	2 (1.2)
Immune System Disorders		
Hypersensitivity NOS	1 (0.6)	5 (3.1)
Seasonal allergy	1 (0.6)	2 (1.2)
Infections and Infestations		
Nasopharyngitis	11 (6.9)	15 (9.3)
Upper respiratory tract infection NOS	9 (5.7)	4 (2.5)
Urinary tract infection NOS	6 (3.8)	6 (3.7)
Herpes simplex	4 (2.5)	4 (2.5)
Pneumonia NOS	2 (1.3)	6 (3.7)
Lower respiratory tract infection NOS	1 (0.6)	6 (3.7)
Influenza	4 (2.5)	2 (1. 2)
Pharyngitis	3 (1.9)	1 (0.6)
Viral infection NOS	—	4 (2.5)
Gastroenteritis viral NOS	1 (0.6)	2 (1.2)
Herpes zoster	2 (1.3)	1 (0.6)
Oral candidiasis	1 (0.6)	2 (1.2)
Tooth abscess	2 (1.3)	1 (0.6)
Infection NOS	—	2 (1.2)
Neutropenic sepsis	2 (1.3)	

(cont'd)

Table 6: RITUXAN *(cont'd)*

Summary of Adverse Events (all intensities) Reported in ≥1% of 321 Patients in Either Treatment Group (CVP or R-CVP)

Body System	Incidence CVP N=159 N (%)	Incidence R-CVP N=162 N (%)
Respiratory tract infection NOS	—	2 (1.2)
Sinusitis NOS	2 (1.3)	—
Injury, Poisoning and Procedural Complications		
Excoriation	3 (1.9)	1 (0.6)
Joint sprain	2 (1.3)	1 (0.6)
Investigations		
Weight increased	2 (1.3)	6 (3.7)
Weight decreased	4 (2.5)	3 (1.9)
Blood glucose increased	2 (1.3)	—
Blood lactate dehydrogenase increased	2 (1.3)	—
Metabolism and Nutrition Disorders		
Anorexia	5 (3.1)	2 (1.2)
Appetite increased NOS	2 (1.3)	2 (1.2)
Hyperglycemia NOS	—	2 (1.2)
Musculoskeletal and Connective Tissue Disorders		
Back pain	16 (10.1)	13 (8.0)
Arthralgia	11 (6.9)	14 (8.6)
Pain in extremity	9 (5.7)	10 (6.2)
Myalgia	7 (4.4)	9 (5.6)
Muscle cramp	3 (1.9)	10 (6.2)
Bone pain	5 (3.1)	5 (3.1)
Groin pain	5 (3.1)	2 (1.2)
Pain in jaw	3 (1.9)	4 (2.5)
Neck pain	6 (3.8)	—
Chest wall pain	2 (1.3)	3 (1.9)
Joint swelling	3 (1.9)	2 (1.2)
Buttock pain	2 (1.3)	—
Facial pain	—	2 (1.2)
Nervous System Disorders		
Headache	30 (18.9)	29 (17.9)
Peripheral neuropathy NOS	25 (15.7)	30 (18.5)
Paresthesia	25 (15.7)	28 (17.3)
Hypoesthesia	11 (6.9)	14 (8.6)
Dizziness	13 (8.2)	9 (5.6)
Dysgeusia	8 (5.0)	11 (6.8)
Peripheral sensory neuropathy	5 (3.1)	1 (0.6)
Polyneuropathy NOS	3 (1.9)	2 (1.2)
Neuropathy NOS	2 (1.3)	2 (1.2)
Parosmia	4 (2.5)	—
Dysphonia	2 (1.3)	1 (0.6)
Hyperesthesia	1 (0.6)	2 (1.2)
Paresthesia oral	—	3 (1.9)
Tremor	1 (0.6)	2 (1.2)
Burning sensation NOS	—	2 (1.2)
Sinus headache	2 (1.3)	—
Psychiatric Disorders		

(cont'd)

Table 6: RITUXAN *(cont'd)*

Summary of Adverse Events (all intensities) Reported in ≥1% of 321 Patients in Either Treatment Group (CVP or R-CVP)

Body System	Incidence CVP N=159 N (%)	Incidence R-CVP N=162 N (%)
Insomnia	16 (10.1)	20 (12.3)
Depression	7 (4.4)	4 (2.5)
Anxiety	4 (2.5)	3 (1.9)
Mood alteration NOS	1 (0.6)	3 (1.9)
Sleep disorder NOS	1 (0.6)	2 (1.2)
Irritability	—	2 (1.2)
Renal and Urinary Disorders		
Dysuria	4 (2.5)	2 (1.2)
Pollakiuria	2 (1.3)	4 (2.5)
Micturition urgency	2 (1.3)	3 (1.9)
Cystitis NOS	2 (1.3)	2 (1.2)
Hematuria	—	2 (1.2)
Renal failure acute	—	2 (1.2)
Urinary retention	—	2 (1.2)
Reproductive System and Breast Disorders		
Breast pain	1 (0.6)	2 (1.2)
Vaginal hemorrhage	2 (1.3)	1 (0.6)
Amenorrhea NOS	—	2 (1.2)
Respiratory, Thoracic and Mediastinal Disorders		
Cough	8 (5.0)	25 (15.4)
Pharyngolaryngeal pain	15 (9.4)	17 (10.5)
Dyspnea	9 (5.7)	14 (8.6)
Bronchitis NOS	3 (1.9)	6 (3.7)
Nasal congestion	3 (1.9)	4 (2.5)
Throat irritation	—	6 (3.7)
Asthma NOS	3 (1.9)	1 (0.6)
Dyspnea exertional	3 (1.9)	1 (0.6)
Pleural effusion	2 (1.3)	2 (1.2)
Rhinitis NOS	3 (1.9)	1 (0.6)
Throat tightness	—	4 (2.5)
Bronchospasm NOS	—	3 (1.9)
Hiccups	2 (1.3)	1 (0.6)
Hoarseness	2 (1.3)	1 (0.6)
Productive cough	1 (0.6)	2 (1.2)
Respiratory tract congestion	1 (0.6)	2 (1.2)
Wheezing	1 (0.6)	2 (1.2)
Sinus pain	2 (1.3)	—
Skin and Subcutaneous Tissue Disorders		
Alopecia	21 (13.2)	22 (13.6)
Rash NOS	7 (4.4)	22 (13.6)
Pruritus	1 (0.6)	15 (9.3)
Night sweats	8 (5.0)	5 (3.1)
Sweating increased	5 (3.1)	6 (3.7)
Urticaria NOS	—	9 (5.6)
Erythema	—	5 (3.1)
Acne NOS	—	4 (2.5)

(cont'd)

Table 6: RITUXAN *(cont'd)*

Summary of Adverse Events (all intensities) Reported in ≥1% of 321 Patients in Either Treatment Group (CVP or R-CVP)

Body System	Incidence	
	CVP N=159 N (%)	**R-CVP N=162 N (%)**
Dry skin	1 (0.6)	3 (1.9)
Hypotrichosis	1 (0.6)	3 (1.9)
Rash generalized	2 (1.3)	2 (1.2)
Contusion	2 (1.3)	1 (0.6)
Psoriasis	2 (1.3)	1 (0.6)
Rash pruritic	1 (0.6)	2 (1.2)
Skin lesion NOS	—	3 (1.9)
Pain of skin	2 (1.3)	
Vascular Disorders		
Flushing	4 (2.5)	21 (13.0)
Hypertension NOS	3 (1.9)	8 (4.9)
Hypotension NOS	1 (0.6)	6 (3.7)
Lymphedema NOS	2 (1.3)	—
Phlebitis NOS	—	2 (1.2)

RITUXAN in Combination with CHOP Chemotherapy: Table 7 shows all grade 3 to 4 clinical adverse events, including grade 2 infections, reported in ≥1% of patients in either treatment group (CHOP and RITUXAN plus CHOP [R-CHOP]) in a randomized phase III clinical trial in the total safety population (n=398). Adverse events were graded according to the four-scale National Cancer Institute of Canada (NCIC) Common Toxicity Criteria.

Table 7: RITUXAN

Summary of Grade 3 and 4 Adverse Events (including Grade 2 infections) Reported in ≥1% of 398 Patients in Either Treatment Group (CHOP or R-CHOP)

Any Grade 3 and 4 Adverse Event (including Grade 2 infections)	Incidence	
	CHOP N=196	**R-CHOP N=202**
	N (%)	**N (%)**
Body System	**148 (75.5)**	**164 (81.2)**
Blood and Lymphatic System Disorders		
Febrile neutropenia[b]	47 (24.0)	46 (22.8)
Neutropenia	10 (5.1)	11 (5.4)
Anemia	10 (5.1)	9 (4.5)
Pancytopenia	2 (1.0)	2 (1.0)
Thrombocytopenia	2 (1.0)	2 (1.0)
Cardiac Disorders		
Cardiac failure	11 (5.6)	9 (4.5)
Atrial fibrillation[a]	1 (0.5)	5 (2.5)
Pulmonary edema	2 (1.0)	4 (2.0)
Tachycardia	1 (0.5)	3 (1.5)
Cardiomyopathy	3 (1.5)	—
Left ventricular dysfunction	2 (1.0)	—
Endocrine Disorders		
Diabetes mellitus inadequate control	4 (2.0)	2 (1.0)
Gastrointestinal Disorders		
Vomiting	13 (6.6)	8 (4.0)
Abdominal pain[a]	9 (4.6)	13 (6.4)
Constipation	8 (4.1)	6 (3.0)
Nausea	9 (4.6)	4 (2.0)
Diarrhea	5 (2.6)	5 (2.5)
Gastrointestinal disorder	3 (1.5)	2 (1.0)

(cont'd)

Table 7: RITUXAN *(cont'd)*

Summary of Grade 3 and 4 Adverse Events (including Grade 2 infections) Reported in ≥1% of 398 Patients in Either Treatment Group (CHOP or R-CHOP)

Any Grade 3 and 4 Adverse Event (including Grade 2 infections)	Incidence	
	CHOP N=196	**R-CHOP N=202**
	N (%)	**N (%)**
Abdominal pain upper	2 (1.0)	—
Dysphagia	2 (1.0)	—
Gastritis	2 (1.0)	—
Ileus paralytic	2 (1.0)	—
Melaena	2 (1.0)	—
General Disorders and Administration Site Conditions		
Pyrexia	34 (17.3)	26 (12.9)
Fatigue	14 (7.1)	9 (4.5)
General physical health deterioration	10 (5.1)	10 (5.0)
Mucosal inflammation	5 (2.6)	8 (4.0)
Shivering[a]	2 (1.0)	7 (3.5)
Chest pain	4 (2.0)	4 (2.0)
Influenza-like illness	3 (1.5)	4 (2.0)
Fall	4 (2.0)	3 (1.5)
Malaise	4 (2.0)	2 (1.0)
Multi-organ failure	4 (2.0)	2 (1.0)
Asthenia	1 (0.5)	4 (2.0)
Edema lower limb	1 (0.5)	4 (2.0)
Edema	—	3 (1.5)
Ulcer	2 (1.0)	1 (0.5)
Hepato-Billiary Disorders		
Cholestasis	1 (0.5)	3 (1.5)
Infections and Infestations		
Bronchitis[a]	16 (8.2)	24 (11.9)
Urinary tract infection	18 (9.2)	20 (9.9)
Pneumonia	15 (7.7)	11 (5.4)
Sepsis	7 (3.6)	4 (2.0)
Septic shock	7 (3.6)	4 (2.0)
Herpes zoster[a]	3 (1.5)	8 (4.0)
Implant infection	5 (2.6)	4 (2.0)
Staphylococcal septicemia	3 (1.5)	5 (2.5)
Superinfection lung	4 (2.0)	5 (2.5)
Acute bronchitis[a]	1 (0.5)	5 (2.5)
Lung infection	4 (2.0)	2 (1.0)
Sinusitis[a]	—	5 (2.5)
Herpes simplex	3 (1.5)	3 (1.5)
Tonsillitis	3 (1.5)	3 (1.5)
Infection	3 (1.5)	2 (1.0)
Nasopharyngitis	3 (1.5)	2 (1.0)
Cystitis	2 (1.0)	1 (0.5)
Erysipelas	2 (1.0)	1 (0.5)
Gastroenteritis helicobacter	2 (1.0)	—
Septicemia escherichial	2 (1.0)	—
Tooth infection	2 (1.0)	—
Injury and Poisoning		

(cont'd)

Table 7: RITUXAN *(cont'd)*

Summary of Grade 3 and 4 Adverse Events (including Grade 2 infections) Reported in ≥1% of 398 Patients in Either Treatment Group (CHOP or R-CHOP)

	Incidence	
	CHOP N=196	R-CHOP N=202
Any Grade 3 and 4 Adverse Event (including Grade 2 infections)	**N (%)**	**N (%)**
Femoral neck fracture	2 (1.0)	2 (1.0)
Investigations		
Abnormal ejection fraction	4 (2.0)	4 (2.0)
Positive blood cultures	4 (2.0)	1 (0.5)
Metabolism and Nutrition Disorders		
Anorexia	5 (2.6)	4 (2.0)
Dehydration	2 (1.0)	—
Hyperglycemia	2 (1.0)	—
Musculoskeletal, Connective Tissue and Bone Disorders		
Back pain[a]	2 (1.0)	5 (2.5)
Sciatica	2 (1.0)	2 (1.0)
Nervous System Disorders		
Paresthesia	2 (1.0)	5 (2.5)
Dizziness (exc vertigo)	3 (1.5)	2 (1.0)
Cerebrovascular accident	1 (0.5)	3 (1.5)
Polyneuropathy	2 (1.0)	2 (1.0)
Depressed level of consciousness	2 (1.0)	—
Psychiatric Disorders		
Confusion	5 (2.6)	—
Depression	2 (1.0)	2 (1.0)
Renal and Urinary Disorders		
Renal colic	2 (1.0)	2 (1.0)
Urinary retention	2 (1.0)	1 (0.5)
Renal failure	2 (1.0)	—
Respiratory, Thoracic and Mediastinal Disorders		
Dyspnea[a]	7 (3.6)	18 (8.9)
Cough	7 (3.6)	8 (4.0)
Rhinitis	5 (2.6)	2 (1.0)
Rhinorrhea	4 (2.0)	1 (0.5)
Skin and Subcutaneous Tissue Disorders		
Pruritus	3 (1.5)	3 (1.5)
Vascular Disorders		
Venous thrombosis deep limb	6 (3.1)	6 (3.0)
Hypotension	3 (1.5)	5 (2.5)
Hypertension[a]	1 (0.5)	5 (2.5)
Pulmonary embolism	3 (1.5)	2 (1.0)
Venous thrombosis	1 (0.5)	4 (2.0)
Peripheral ischemia	2 (1.0)	—
Phlebitis	2 (1.0)	—

[a] Adverse events that were reported at a higher incidence (≥2% difference) in the R-CHOP group as compared to the CHOP group and, therefore, may be attributable to R-CHOP.
[b] Febrile neutropenia as reported by investigators: fever and neutropenia with or without documented infection (see Infections).

The following terms have been reported as adverse events, however, were reported at a similar (<2% difference between the groups) or lower incidence in the RITUXAN-arms compared to control arms: hematotoxicity, neutropenic infection, urinary tract infection, septic shock, superinfection lung, implant infection, septicemia staphylococcal, lung infection, rhinorrhea, pulmonary edema, cardiac failure, sensory disturbance, venous thrombosis, mucosal inflammation NOS, influenza-like illness, edema lower limb, abnormal ejection fraction, pyrexia, general physical health deterioration, fall, multi-organ failure, venous thrombosis deep limb, abnormal ejection fraction, positive blood culture, anorexia, diabetes mellitus inadequate control.

The safety profile for RITUXAN in combination with other chemotherapies (e.g. MCP, CHVP-IFN) is comparable to the safety profile as described for the combination of RITUXAN and CVP, CHOP or FC in equivalent populations.

RITUXAN in Combination with FC Chemotherapy: Table 8 shows all grade 3 to 4 clinical adverse events and serious adverse events reported with a ≥2% difference in frequency between either treatment group (R-FC and FC) in ML17102 and BO17072. Grade 1 and 2 adverse events and grade 4 lymphocytopenia were not captured in the study ML17102. A total of 550 SAEs in 344 patients were reported across the two arms in ML17102. Infections and infestations (15% in FC vs 18% in R-FC) and blood and lymphatic system disorders (11% in FC vs 17% in R-FC) were reported at higher frequencies, as expected, for the rituximab-containing arm. One case of tuberculosis was recorded as an adverse event in the R-FC arm.

Table 8: RITUXAN

Summary of Grade 3 & 4 Adverse Events and Serious Adverse Events that Occurred with a Difference in Incidence of ≥2% Between Either the R-FC Arm or the FC Arm

	Incidence			
	ML17102 (previously untreated CLL)		BO17072 (previously treated CLL)	
	FC N=396 N (%)	R-FC N=397 N (%)	FC N=272 N (%)	R-FC N =274 N (%)
Any Grade 3 and 4 Adverse Event[a]				
Blood and Lymphatic System Disorders				
Neutropenia	75 (18.9)	119 (30.0)	108 (39.7)	116 (42.3)
Leukopenia	46 (11.6)	93 (23.4)		
Thrombocytopenia	39 (9.8)	26 (6.5)		
Febrile neutropenia	22 (5.6)	37 (9.3)	32 (11.8)	40 (14.6)
Anemia	26 (6.6)	16 (4.0)		
Pancytopenia	5 (1.3)	13 (3.3)		
Granulocytopenia			12 (4.4)	18 (6.6)
General Disorders and Administration Site Conditions				
Pyrexia	21 (5.3)	12 (3.0)		
Infections and infestations				
Hepatitis B				6 (2.2)
Any Serious Adverse Event[a]				
Blood and Lymphatic System Disorders				
Febrile neutropenia	22 (5.6)	30 (7.6)	21 (7.7)	29 (10.6)
Anemia			11 (4.0)	3 (1.1)

[a] Grade 1 and 2 adverse events and grade 4 lymphocytopenia were not captured in ML17102.

Table 9: RITUXAN

Summary of Grade 3 or 4 Adverse Events and Deaths by Binet Stage in ML17102

Binet Stage	FC	R-FC
Overall Incidence	246 (62%)	304 (77%)
Binet Stage A		
N	20	18
Total pts with at least one AE (%)	14 (70%)	13 (72%)
Deaths (%)	3 (15%)	1 (6%)
Binet Stage B		
N	253	256
Total pts with at least one AE (%)	144 (57%)	189 (74%)
Deaths (%)	32 (13%)	13 (5%)
Binet Stage C		
N	122	123
Total pts with at least one AE (%)	87 (71%)	102 (83%)
Deaths (%)	12 (10%)	19 (15%)

In the subgroup analysis of Binet stage, in both arms of ML17102, the rate of Grade 3 or 4 AEs slightly increased from Binet stage B to Binet stage C. In the Binet stage A subgroup, there was no difference in the incidence of Grade 3 or 4 AEs between the FC and R-FC arms. In Binet stage B and C patients, the rates of Grade 3 or 4 AEs were higher in the R-FC arm compared to the FC arm. Similar patterns were observed for SAEs. See Table 10.

Table 10: RITUXAN

Summary of Grade 3 or 4 Adverse Events and Fatal AEs by Binet Stage in BO17072

Binet Stage	FC	R-FC
Binet Stage A		
N	31	24
Total pts with at least one grade 3/4 AE (%)	20 (65%)	18 (75%)
Fatal AEs (%)	4 (13%)	4 (17%)
Binet Stage B		
N	157	164
Total pts with at least one grade 3/4 AE (%)	109 (69%)	127 (77%)
Fatal AEs (%)	12 (8%)	16 (10%)
Binet Stage C		
N	84	86
Total pts with at least one grade 3/4 AE (%)	71 (85%)	74 (86%)
Fatal AEs (%)	10 (12%)	16 (19%)

Table 11: RITUXAN

Summary of Grade 3 or 4 Adverse Events and Deaths by Age in ML17102

Age (years old)	FC	R-FC
<65		
N	280	275
Total pts with at least one AE (%)	168 (60%)	203 (74%)
Deaths (%)	31 (11%)	26 (9%)
≥65–≤70		
N	91	90
Total pts with at least one AE (%)	59 (65%)	72 (80%)
Deaths (%)	15 (16%)	6 (7%)
>70		
N	25	32
Total pts with at least one AE (%)	19 (76%)	29 (91%)
Deaths (%)	1 (4%)	1 (3%)

In the subgroup analysis of age in ML17102, Grade 3 or 4 AEs tended to increase with increasing age >65 years, especially for >70 yrs and more AEs were recorded in the R-FC arm compared with FC alone. Similar patterns were observed for SAEs.

Table 12: RITUXAN

Summary of Grade 3 or 4 Adverse Events and Fatal AEs by Age in BO17072

Age (years old)	FC	R-FC
<65		
N	159	154
Total pts with at least one grade 3/4 AE (%)	105 (66%)	109 (71%)
Fatal AEs (%)	12 (8%)	5 (3%)
≥65–≤70		
N	68	74
Total pts with at least one grade 3/4 AE (%)	53 (78%)	67 (91%)
Fatal AEs (%)	6 (9%)	19 (26%)
>70		
N	45	46
Total pts with at least one grade 3/4 AE (%)	42 (93%)	43 (93%)
Fatal AEs (%)	8 (18%)	12 (26%)

Further Information on Selected, Serious Adverse Drug Reactions: Infusion-Related Reactions: (See Warnings and Precautions.)

Monotherapy—4 Weeks Treatment: Hypotension, fever, chills, rigors, urticaria, bronchospasm, sensation of tongue or throat swelling (angioedema), nausea, fatigue, headache, pruritus, dyspnea, rhinitis, vomiting, flushing, and pain at disease sites have occurred in association with RITUXAN infusion as part of an infusion-related symptom complex. Such infusion-related symptoms occurred in the majority of patients during the first infusion with RITUXAN. The incidence of infusion-related symptoms decreased from 77% (7% Grade 3/4) with the first infusion to approximately 30% (2% Grade 3/4) with the fourth infusion and to 14% (no Grade 3/4 events) with the eighth infusion.

Maintenance Treatment (NHL) Up to 2 Years: Non-serious signs and symptoms suggestive of an infusion-related reaction were reported in 41% of patients under general disorders (mainly asthenia, pyrexia, influenza like illness, pain) and in 7% of patients for immune system disorders (hypersensitivity). Serious infusion-related reactions occurred in <1% of patients.

Combination Therapy (R-CVP in NHL; R-CHOP in DLBCL, R-FC in CLL): Severe infusion-related reactions occurred in up to 12% of all patients at the time of the first treatment cycle with rituximab in combination with chemotherapy. The incidence of severe infusion-related reactions decreased to less than 1% by the eighth cycle of therapy. The signs and symptoms were consistent with those observed during monotherapy (see Warnings and Precautions), but also included dyspepsia, rash, hypertension, tachycardia, features of tumour lysis syndrome. Additional reactions reported in isolated cases at the time of R-CHOP therapy were myocardial infarction, atrial fibrillation and pulmonary edema and acute reversible thrombocytopenia.

Infections: Monotherapy—4 Weeks Treatment: These were usually common, non-opportunistic and mild. RITUXAN induced B-cell depletion in 70 to 80% of patients but was associated with decreased serum immunoglobulins in only a minority of patients. Infectious events, irrespective of causal assessment, occurred in 30.3% of 356 patients: 18.8% of patients had bacterial infections, 10.4% had viral infections, 1.4% had fungal infections, and 5.9% had infections of unknown etiology. Severe infectious events (grade 3 or 4), including sepsis occurred in 3.9% of patients; in 1.4% during the treatment period and in 2.5% during the follow up period.

Maintenance Treatment (NHL) Up to 2 Years: The proportion of patients with grade 1 to 4 infections was 26% in the observation group and 47% in the RITUXAN group with severe (grade 3/4) infections in 2% of patients on observation and 11% receiving RITUXAN maintenance treatment. Severe infections reported in ≥1% of patients in the RITUXAN arm were pneumonia (2%), respiratory tract infection (2%), febrile infection (1%), and herpes zoster (1%). In a large proportion of infections (all grades), the infectious agent was not specified or isolated, however, where an infectious agent was specified, the most frequently reported underlying agents were bacterial (observation 2%, RITUXAN 11%), viruses (observation 8%, RITUXAN 11 %) and fungi (observation 3%, RITUXAN 4%). There was no cumulative toxicity in terms of infections reported over the 2-year maintenance period.

Combination Therapy (R-CVP in NHL; R-CHOP in DLBCL, R-FC in CLL): In the R-CVP study the overall proportion of patients with infections or infestations during treatment and for 28 days after trial treatment end was comparable between the treatment groups (33% R-CVP, 32% CVP). The most common infections were upper respiratory tract infections which were reported for 12.3% patients on R-CVP and 16.4% patients receiving CVP; most of these infections were nasopharyngitis. Serious infections were reported in 4.3% of the patients receiving R-CVP and 4.4% of the patients receiving CVP. No life-threatening infections were reported during this study.

In the R-CHOP study the overall incidence of grade 2 to 4 infections was 45.5% in the R-CHOP group and 42.3% in the CHOP group. Grade 2 to 4 fungal infections were more frequent in the R-CHOP group (4.5% vs 2.6% in the CHOP group); this difference was due to a higher incidence of localized Candida infections during the treatment period. The incidence of grade 2 to 4 herpes zoster, including ophthalmic herpes zoster, was higher in the R-CHOP group (4.5%) than in the CHOP group (1.5%), with 7 of a total of 9 cases in the R-CHOP group occurring during the treatment phase. The proportion of patients with grade 2 to 4 infections and/or febrile neutropenia was 55.4% in the R-CHOP group and 51.5% in the CHOP group. Febrile neutropenia (i.e. no report of concomitant documented infection) was reported only during the treatment period, in 20.8% in the R-CHOP group and 15.3% in the CHOP group.

In patients with CLL, the overall incidence of grade 3 or 4 infections during treatment and for 28 days after the end of trial treatment was comparable between the treatment groups both in previously untreated (18% R-FC, 17% FC) and in the previously treated setting (19% R-FC, 18% FC). The incidence of grade 3 or 4 hepatitis B infection (reactivation and primary infection) was 2% R-FC vs. 0% FC.

Hematologic Events: Monotherapy—4 Weeks: Hematologic adverse events occur in a minority of patients and are usually mild and reversible. Severe neutropenia was reported in 4.2% of patients, severe anemia was reported in 1.1% of patients and severe thrombocytopenia was reported in 1.7% of patients. A single occurrence of transient aplastic anemia (pure red cell aplasia) and two occurrences of hemolytic anemia following therapy with RITUXAN were reported.

Maintenance Treatment (NHL) Up to 2 Years: Leucopenia (all grades) occurred in 26% of patients on observation vs 32% of patients in the RITUXAN arm, and neutropenia was reported in 14% of patients on observation and in 25% of patients on RITUXAN. There was a higher incidence of grade 3-4 leucopenia (observation 2%, RITUXAN 5%) and neutropenia (observation 5%, RITUXAN 11%) in the RITUXAN arm compared to the observation arm. The incidence of grade 3 to 4 thrombocytopenia (observation 1%, RITUXAN <1%) was low.

Combination Therapy (R-CVP in NHL; R-CHOP in DLBCL, R-FC in CLL): Severe (grade 3/4) Adverse Events Neutropenia: There was a higher incidence of grade 3-4 neutropenia in the RITUXAN containing study arms compared to the chemotherapy arms. In the R-CVP study, the incidence of neutropenia was 24% in the R-CVP arm versus 14% in the CVP arm. These laboratory findings were reported as adverse events and resulted in medical intervention in 3.1% of patients on R-CVP and 0.6% of patients on CVP. The higher incidence of neutropenia in the R-CVP group was not associated with a higher incidence of infections and infestations. In the R-CHOP study, the incidence of severe neutropenia was 97% in the R-CHOP arm versus 88% in the CHOP arm. In CLL patients, grade 3 or 4 neutropenia was reported in 30% of patients in the R-FC arm and in 19% of patients in the FC arm. In previously untreated patients with CLL, grade 3/4 neutropenia was reported as an adverse event in 30% of patients in the R-FC arm and in 19% of patients in the FC arm. In patients with previously treated CLL, the incidence of grade 3/4 neutropenia adverse events was slightly higher in the R-FC arm (42% R-FC) compared to FC arm (40%).

Severe (grade 3/4) Adverse Events Leucopenia: In the R-CHOP study, the incidence of severe leucopenia was 88% in the R-CHOP arm versus 79% in the CHOP arm. In previously untreated CLL, more patients receiving R-FC experienced grade 3/4 adverse events of leucopenia (23%) compared with patients receiving FC (12%). In patients with previously treated CLL, the overall incidence of grade 3/4 leucopenia adverse events was comparable between the treatment arms (4% R-FC, 3% FC).

Severe (grade 3/4) Adverse Events Anemia and Thrombocytopenia: No relevant difference between the treatment arms was observed with respect to grade 3 and 4 anemia or thrombocytopenia. In the R-CVP study, the incidence of anemia was 0.6% in the R-CVP arm versus 1.9% in the CVP arm. The incidence of thrombocytopenia was 1.2% in the R-CVP arm versus 0% in the CVP arm. In the R-CHOP study, the incidence of anemia was 14% in the R-CHOP arm versus 19% in the CHOP arm. The incidence of thrombocytopenia was 15% in the R-CHOP arm versus 16% in the CHOP arm. The time to recovery from all hematological abnormalities was comparable in the two treatment groups. In the CLL first-line study, grade 3/4 anemia was reported by 4% of patients treated with R-FC compared to 7% of patients receiving FC, and grade 3 or 4 thrombocytopenia was reported by 7% of patients in the R-FC group compared to 10% of patients in the FC group. In the previously treated CLL study, adverse events of grade 3/4 anemia were reported in 12% of patients treated with R-FC compared to 13% of patients receiving FC and grade 3/4 thrombocytopenia was reported by 11% of patients in the R-FC group compared to 9% of patients in the FC group.

Cardiovascular Events: (See Warnings and Precautions.)

Monotherapy—4 Weeks Treatment: Cardiovascular events were reported in 18.8% of patients during the treatment period. The most frequently reported events were hypotension and hypertension. Two patients (0.6%) experienced grade 3 or 4 arrhythmia (including ventricular and supraventricular tachycardia) during an infusion with RITUXAN and one patient with a history of myocardial infarction experienced angina pectoris, evolving into myocardial infarction 4 days later.

Maintenance Treatment (NHL) Up to 2 Years: The incidence of grade 3 to 4 cardiac disorders was comparable between the two treatment groups (5% in observation, 7% in RITUXAN). Cardiac events were reported as serious adverse event in <1% of patients on observation and in 3% of patients on RITUXAN: atrial fibrillation (1%), myocardial infarction (1%), left ventricular failure (<1%), myocardial ischemia (<1%).

Combination Therapy (R-CVP in NHL; R-CHOP inDLBCL, R-FC in CLL): In the R-CVP study the overall incidence of cardiac disorders in the safety population was low (4% R-CVP, 5% CVP), with no relevant differences between the treatment groups.

In the R-CHOP study the incidence of grade 3 and 4 cardiac arrhythmias, predominantly supraventricular arrhythmias such as tachycardia and atrial flutter/fibrillation, was higher in the R-CHOP group (14 patients, 6.9%) as compared to the CHOP group (3 patients, 1.5%). All of these arrhythmias either occurred in the context of a RITUXAN infusion or were associated with predisposing conditions such as fever, infection, acute myocardial infarction or pre-existing respiratory and cardiovascular disease (see Warnings and Precautions). No difference between the R-CHOP and CHOP group was observed in the incidence of other grade 3 and 4 cardiac events including heart failure, myocardial disease and manifestations of coronary artery disease.

In CLL, the overall incidence of grade 3 or 4 cardiac disorders was low both in previously untreated patients (4% R-FC, 3% FC) and in previously treated patients (4% R-FC, 4% FC).

IgG Levels: Maintenance Treatment (NHL) Up to 2 Years: After induction treatment, median IgG levels were below the lower limit of normal (LLN) (<7 g/L) in both the observation and the RITUXAN groups. In the observation group, the median IgG level subsequently increased to above the LLN, but remained constant during RITUXAN treatment. The proportion of patients with IgG levels below the LLN was about 60% in the RITUXAN group throughout the 2 year treatment period, while it decreased in the observation group (36% after 2 years).

Neurologic Events: Combination Therapy (R-CVP in NHL; R-CHOP in DLBCL, R-FC in CLL): During the treatment period, four patients (2%) in the R-CHOP group, all with cardiovascular risk factors, experienced thromboembolic cerebrovascular accidents during the first treatment cycle. There was no difference between the treatment group in the incidence of other thromboembolic events. In contrast, three patients (1.5%) had cerebrovascular events in the CHOP group, all of which occurred during the follow-up period.

In CLL, the overall incidence of grade 3 or 4 nervous system disorders was low both in previously untreated patients (4% R-FC, 4% FC) and in previously treated patients (3% R-FC, 3% FC).

Pulmonary Events: (See Warnings and Precautions.)

Three pulmonary events have been reported in temporal association with RITUXAN infusion as a single agent: acute, infusion-related bronchospasm, an acute pneumonitis presenting 1-4 weeks post infusion with RITUXAN, and bronchiolitis obliterans. The bronchiolitis obliterans was associated with progressive pulmonary symptoms and culminated in death several months following the last infusion with RITUXAN. The safety of resumption or continued administration of RITUXAN in patients with pneumonitis or bronchiolitis obliterans is unknown.

Malignancy: In the CLL previously untreated study, the incidence of malignancy following exposure to RITUXAN was 4.5% compared to 3.8% in patients not exposed to RITUXAN.

Subpopulations: Monotherapy—4 Weeks Treatment: Elderly Patients (≥65 Years): The incidence of any ADR and of grade 3 and 4 ADRs was similar in elderly (N=94) and younger (N=237) patients (88.3% versus 92.0% for any ADR and 16.0% versus 18.1% for grade 3 and 4 ADRs).

Bulky Disease: Patients with bulky disease (N=39) had a higher incidence of grade 3 and 4 ADRs than patients without bulky disease (N=195; 25.6% versus 15.4%). The incidence of any ADR was similar in these two groups (92.3% in bulky disease versus 89.2% in non-bulky disease).

Retreatment with Monotherapy: The percentage of patients reporting any ADR and grade 3 and 4 ADRs upon re-treatment (N=60) with further courses of RITUXAN was similar to the percentage of patients reporting any ADR and grade 3 and 4 ADRs upon initial exposure (N=203; 95.0% versus 89.7% for any ADR and 13.3% versus 14.8% for grade 3 and 4 ADRs).

RITUXAN in Combination with FC Chemotherapy: Table 13 shows all serious clinical adverse events reported in ≥1% of patients in either treatment group (R-FC and FC) in ML17102. Grade 1 and 2 adverse events and grade 4 lymphocytopenia were not captured in the study.

Table 13: RITUXAN

Summary of Serious Adverse Events that Occurred with an Incidence of ≥1%

	Incidence			
	ML17102[a] (previously untreated CLL)		BO17072 (previously treated CLL)	
	FC N=396 N (%)	R-FC N=397 N (%)	FC N=272 N (%)	R-FC N=274 N (%)
Blood and Lymphatic System Disorders[b]				
Febrile neutropenia	22 (6)	30 (8)	21 (8)	29 (11)
Anemia	9 (2)	6 (2)	11 (4)	3 (1)
Anemia hemolytic autoimmune			5 (2)	2 (<1)
Hemolytic anemia			3 (1)	2 (<1)
Leukopenia	3 (<1)	9 (2)	1 (<1)	3 (1)
Neutropenia	3 (<1)	8 (2)	7 (3)	8 (3)
Thrombocytopenia	5 (1)	6 (2)		
Autoimmune thrombocytopenia			4 (1)	2 (<1)
Pancytopenia	3 (<1)	6 (2)	5[c] (2)	5 (2)
Febrile bone marrow aplasia			2 (<1)	3 (1)
Infections and Infestations				
Pneumonia	20 (5)	18 (5)	18 (7)	15 (5)
Herpes Zoster	6 (2)	8 (2)	3 (1)	1 (<1)
Sepsis	8 (2)	5 (1)	3 (1)	4 (1)
Bronchitis	5 (1)	5 (1)	2 (<1)	6 (2)
Infection	2 (<1)	5 (1)		
Sinusitis	1 (<1)	4 (1)		
Septic shock			2 (<1)	5 (2)
Neutropenic sepsis			4 (1)	2 (<1)
Hepatitis B			0	5 (2)
Respiratory tract infection			3 (1)	2 (<1)
P. jiroveci pneumonia			3 (1)	1 (<1)
General Disorders and Administration Site Conditions				
Pyrexia	20 (5)	18 (5)	9 (3)	14 (5)
Cardiac Disorders				
Angina Pectoris	2 (<1)	5 (1)		
Gastrointestinal Disorders				
Diarrhea	2 (<1)	5 (1)		
Vomiting			3 (1)	1 (<1)

(cont'd)

Table 13: RITUXAN *(cont'd)*

Summary of Serious Adverse Events that Occurred with an Incidence of ≥1%

	Incidence			
	ML17102[a] (previously untreated CLL)		BO17072 (previously treated CLL)	
	FC N=396 N (%)	R-FC N=397 N (%)	FC N=272 N (%)	R-FC N=274 N (%)
Neoplasms, benign, malignant and unspecified (including cysts and polyps)				
Squamous cell carcinoma of skin			4[c] (1)	1(<1)
Tumor lysis syndrome			3 (1)	1 (<1)
Basal cell carcinoma			3 (1)	–

[a] Grade 1 and 2 adverse events and grade 4 lymphocytopenia were not captured in the study.
[b] Grade 4 lymphocytopenia was not captured in ML17102.
[c] Onset in one patient before starting study medication.

Combination Therapy: Elderly patients (≥65 years): The incidence of grade 3/4 blood and lymphatic adverse events was higher in elderly patients (≥65 years of age) compared to younger patients, with previously untreated or previously treated CLL.

Post-Market Adverse Drug Reactions: The reporting frequencies in this section (rare, very rare) are based on estimated marketed exposures and largely data derived from spontaneous reports.

Additional cases of severe infusion-related reactions have been reported during post-marketing use of RITUXAN (see Warnings and Precautions). As part of the continuing post-marketing surveillance of the safety of RITUXAN, the following serious adverse reactions have been observed:

Blood and Lymphatic System: Neutropenia: Rarely, the onset of neutropenia has occurred more than four weeks after the last infusion of RITUXAN. Cases of infusion-related acute reversible thrombocytopenia have been reported.

In post-marketing studies of RITUXAN in patients with Waldenstrom's macroglobulinemia, transient increases in serum IgM levels have been observed following treatment initiation, which may be associated with hyperviscosity and related symptoms. The transient IgM increase usually returned to at least baseline level within 4 months from the administration/start of RITUXAN treatment.

Body as a Whole: Anaphylaxis; mucositis and serum sickness-like reactions have been reported rarely.

Cardiovascular System: Severe cardiac events, including congestive heart failure and myocardial infarction have been observed, mainly in patients with prior cardiac condition and/or cardiotoxic chemotherapy and mostly associated with infusion-related reactions. Vasculitis, predominantly cutaneous, such as leukocytoclastic vasculitis and fatal cardiac failure have been reported very rarely.

Infections and Infestations: Very rare cases of HBV reactivation, occasionally with fulminant hepatitis, hepatic failure, and death has been reported in some patients with hematologic malignancies treated with RITUXAN. The majority of patients received RITUXAN in combination with chemotherapy (see Warnings and Precautions).

Progression of Kaposi's sarcoma has been observed in rituximab-exposed patients with pre-existing Kaposi's sarcoma. These cases occurred in non-approved indications and the majority of patients were HIV positive.

Increase in fatal infections in HIV lymphoma has been reported very rarely when RITUXAN is used with chemotherapy.

Immune Phenomena: Paraneoplastic neuropathy, encephalomyelitis, polymyositis, have been rarely reported. Other possible rare adverse events include: optic neuritis, uveitis, vasculitis, serum sickness or a lupus-like syndrome, pleuritis and arthritis. Systemic vasculitis has been reported very rarely.

Nervous System: Cases of cranial neuropathy with or without peripheral neuropathy have been rarely reported. Signs and symptoms of cranial neuropathy, such as severe vision loss, hearing loss, loss of other senses and facial nerve palsy, occurred at various times up to several months after completion of rituximab therapy.

Respiratory System: Respiratory failure/insufficiency and pulmonary infiltrates in the context of infusion-related reactions (see Warnings and Precautions). In addition to pulmonary events associated with infusions interstitial lung disease, some with fatal outcome, has been reported; pleural effusions, and pneumonia.

Skin and Appendages: Severe bullous skin reactions (including toxic epidermal necrolysis) and pemphigus, some with fatal outcome, have been reported rarely.

Urogenital System: renal insufficiency/failure.

Rheumatoid Arthritis: The clinical efficacy of RITUXAN, given together with methotrexate was studied in three double blind controlled clinical trials (one phase III trial and two phase II trials) in patients with rheumatoid arthritis. More than 1000 patients received at least one treatment course and were followed for periods ranging from 6 months to over 3 years; approximately 600 patients received two or more courses of treatment during the follow up period.

Patients received 2×1000 mg of RITUXAN separated by an interval of two weeks; in addition to methotrexate (10-25 mg/week). Infusions of RITUXAN were administered after an IV infusion of 100 mg methylprednisolone; patients also received treatment with oral prednisolone for 15 days. Listed in Table 14 are ADRs that occurred with at least a 2% difference compared to the control arm and more frequently by patients who had received at least one infusion of RITUXAN than among patients that had received placebo in the phase III trial and the combined population included in phase II studies. In these studies, adverse reactions were more frequent in patients treated with RITUXAN than in patients treated with placebo. Frequencies are defined as very common (≥1/10) and common (≥1/100 to <1/10).

The most frequent ADRs considered due to receipt of 2×1000 mg RITUXAN in Phase II and III studies were acute infusion reactions. Infusion reactions occurred in 15% of patients following the first infusion of rituximab and 5% in placebo patients. Infusion reactions decreased to 2% following the second infusion in both rituximab and placebo groups.

Table 14: RITUXAN

Summary of Adverse Drug Reactions Occurring in Patients with Rheumatoid Arthritis Receiving RITUXAN During Phase II and III Clinical Studies

	Pooled Phase II Study Population		Phase III Study Population	
	Very Common (≥10%)	Common (≥1 %–<10%)	Very Common (≥10%)	Common (≥1%–<10%)
Acute Infusion Reactions[a]		Hypertension, rash, pruritus, chills, pyrexia, rhinitis, throat irritation, tachycardia, oropharyngeal pain		Hypertension, nausea, rash, pyrexia, pruritus, urticaria, throat irritation, hot flush, hypotension
Gastrointestinal Disorders		Dyspepsia		Dyspepsia
Infections and Infestations	Any Infection	Urinary tract infections	Any infection, upper respiratory tract infection	
Metabolism and Nutritional Disorders				Hypercholesterolemia

(cont'd)

Table 14: RITUXAN *(cont'd)*

Summary of Adverse Drug Reactions Occurring in Patients with Rheumatoid Arthritis Receiving RITUXAN During Phase II and III Clinical Studies

	Pooled Phase II Study Population		Phase III Study Population	
	Very Common (≥10%)	Common (≥1 %–<10%)	Very Common (≥10%)	Common (≥1%–<10%)
Musculoskeletal Disorders		Arthralgia/ musculoskeletal pain		Arthralgia/musculoskeletal pain, osteoarthritis, bursitis
Nervous System Disorders		Migraine		Paraesthesia, sciatica

[a] Reactions occurring during or within 24 hours of infusion.
This table include all events with an incidence difference of ≥2 % for rituximab compared to placebo.

Table 15: RITUXAN

Adverse Reactions Occurring in at Least 1% of Patients and More Frequently in Rheumatoid Arthritis Patients Receiving RITUXAN During Phase II and III Clinical Studies

	Pooled Phase II Study Population		Phase III Study Population	
	MTX + Placebo N=189 n (%)	RITUXAN + MTX N=232 n (%)	MTX + Placebo N=209 n (%)	RITUXAN + MTX N=308 n (%)
Acute Infusion Reactions[a]				
Hypertension	10 (5%)	22 (9%)	11 (5%)	21 (7%)
Nausea	14 (7%)	19 (8%)	5 (2%)	22 (7%)
Rash	6 (3%)	18 (8%)	9 (4%)	17 (6%)
Pyrexia	1 (<1%)	12 (5%)	7 (3%)	15 (5%)
Pruritus	1 (<1%)	14 (6%)	4 (2%)	12 (4%)
Urticaria	0	2 (<1%)	3 (1%)	10 (3%)
Rhinitis	2 (1%)	6 (3%)	4 (2%)	8 (3%)
Throat irritation	0	5 (2%)	0	6 (2%)
Hot flush	4 (2%)	2 (<1%)	0	6 (2%)
Hypotension	11 (6%)	10 (4%)	1 (<1%)	5 (2%)
Chills	3 (2%)	13 (6%)	6 (3%)	3 (<1%)
Gastrointestinal Disorders				
Dyspepsia	3 (2%)	9 (4%)	0	7 (2%)
Abdominal pain upper	3 (2%)	7 (3%)	1 (<1%)	4 (1%)
General Disorders				
Asthenia	0	3 (1%)	1 (<1%)	6 (2%)
Infections and Infestations				
Any infection	56 (30%)	85 (37%)	78 (37%)	127 (41%)
Urinary tract Infections	8 (4%)	14 (6%)	17 (8%)	15 (5%)
Upper respiratory tract	28 (15%)	31 (13%)	26 (12%)	48 (16%)
Lower respiratory tract infection/pneumonia	10 (5%)	9 (4%)	5 (2%)	8 (3%)
Metabolism and Nutritional Disorders				
Hypercholesterolemia	1 (<1%)	3 (1%)	0	6 (2%)
Musculoskeletal Disorders				
Arthralgia/musculoskeletal pain	8 (4%)	18 (7%)	6 (3%)	17 (7%)
Muscle spasms	0	1 (<1%)	2 (1%)	7 (2%)
Osteoarthritis	1 (<1%)	4 (2%)	0	6 (2%)
Nervous System				
Paresthesia	2 (1%)	4 (2%)	1 (<1%)	8 (3%)
Migraine	0	4 (2%)	2 (1%)	5 (2%)

[a] Reactions occurring within 24 hours of infusion.

The following adverse events were reported at a frequency between 1% and 2% greater in the RITUXAN arms compared to the control arms: lower respiratory tract infections/pneumonia, abdominal pain upper, muscle spasms, asthenia, anxiety.

In addition to the events tabulated above, medically significant events reported rarely in the population treated with rituximab and considered potential reactions to treatment include the following:

General Disorders: generalized edema.

Immune System Disorders: anaphylaxis, anaphylactoid reaction.

Respiratory Disorders: bronchospasm, wheezing, laryngeal edema.

Skin and Subcutaneous Disorders: angioneurotic edema, generalized pruritus.

The following serious adverse events were reported with a incidence rate of at least 1% :

rheumatoid Arthritis and osteoarthritis (Pooled Phase II Study Population).
rheumatoid Arthritis (Phase III Study Population).

Multiple Courses: Multiple courses of treatment are associated with a similar ADR profile to that observed following first exposure. The safety profile improved with subsequent courses due to a decrease in IRRs, RA exacerbation and infections, all of which were more frequent in the first 6 months of treatment.

In a study where all patients initially received RITUXAN followed by retreatment with either RITUXAN or placebo, the safety profile was similar to placebo. The proportion of patients who experienced any AEs, SAEs infections or serious infections was comparable between the placebo and RITUXAN retreatment arms.

Adverse Reactions Reported in RA Patients who had no Prior Inadequate Response to TNF Antagonists: Listed below are additional ADRs reported in Phase III placebo-controlled RA trials in either DMARD-IR or MTX Naive patients. These ADRs occurred with at least a 2% greater difference compared to control arm:

Very Common (≥10%): headache.

Common (≥1%-<10%): diarrhea, dizziness, bronchitis, sinusitis, gastroenteritis, fatigue, alopecia, mouth ulceration, gastro-esophageal reflux, peripheral edema, erythema, depression anxiety, tinea pedis (listed in decreasing order of frequency).

Further Information on Selected Adverse Drug Reactions: Please note that the information presented below includes the all exposure population of more than 3000 RA patients who have received at least one treatment course and were followed for periods ranging from 6 months to over 5 years with an overall exposure equivalent to 7198 patient years. The patient populations receiving RITUXAN differed between studies, ranging from early active RA patients who were methotrexate (MTX) naïve, through MTX inadequate responders (MTX-IR) to patients who had inadequate response to anti-TNF therapies (TNF-IR).

Infusion-related Reactions: The most frequent ADRs following receipt of RITUXAN in clinical studies were infusion-related reactions. Among the 3095 patients treated with RITUXAN, 1077 (35%) experienced at least one IRR. The vast majority of IRRs were CTC Grade 1 or 2. In clinical studies fewer than 1% (14/3095 patients) of patients with RA who received an infusion of RITUXAN at any dose experienced a serious infusion-related reaction. There were no CTC Grade 4 IRRs and no deaths due to IRRs. The proportion of CTC Grade 3 events, and of IRRs leading to withdrawal decreased by course and were rare from course 3 onwards.

Signs and or symptoms suggesting an infusion-related reaction (nausea, pruritus, fever, urticaria/rash, chills, pyrexia, rigors, sneezing, angioneurotic oedema, throat irritation, cough and bronchospasm, with or without associated hypotension or hypertension) were observed in 720/3095 (23%) patients with rheumatoid arthritis following first infusion of the first exposure to RITUXAN. Premedication with IV glucocorticoid significantly reduced the incidence and severity of these events (see Warnings and Precautions, Rheumatoid Arthritis).

Infections: The overall rate of infection was approximately 97 per 100 patient years in patients treated with RITUXAN. The infections were predominately mild to moderate and consisted mostly of upper respiratory tract infections and urinary tract infections. In the all-exposure population the rate of serious infections, was approximately 4 per 100 patient years, some of which were fatal, including *C. difficile* colitis, pneumonia, progressive multifocal leukoencephalopathy (PML), neutropenic sepsis, septic shock and abdominal sepsis. In addition to the ADRs in Table 14, medically serious events reported also included pneumonia (including atypical pneumonia) at a frequency of 1.9%.

Malignancies: In RA clinical studies, the incidence of malignancy following exposure to rituximab is 0.8 per 100 patient years, which is within the range expected for an age- and gender- matched population. The rate of melanoma in RA clinical studies was 0.06 per 100 patient years (95% CI 0.02-0.14 per 100 patient years), which is similar to the rate expected for an age and gender matched population. This overall rate includes 3 patients of 431 in the Study 2 extension.

On the basis of limited experience with RITUXAN in rheumatoid arthritis patients, a possible risk for the development of solid tumours cannot be excluded at this time, although present data do not seem to suggest any increased risk.

Post-Market Adverse Drug Reactions: In addition to ADRs seen in RA clinical trials for rituximab, progressive multifocal leukoencephalopathy (PML) and serum sickness-like reaction have been reported during post marketing experience.

DRUG INTERACTIONS: Overview: There have been no formal drug interaction studies performed with RITUXAN (rituximab). However, the existing data suggest that rituximab does not affect the pharmacokinetics of drugs which are used in combination with RITUXAN.

Drug-Drug Interactions: There have been no formal drug interaction studies performed with RITUXAN (rituximab). The tolerability of simultaneous or sequential combination of RITUXAN with chemotherapy other than CHOP and CVP or agents which are liable to cause depletion of normal B-cells is not well defined.

Renal failure requiring dialysis has been observed in patients treated with the combination of RITUXAN and cisplatin. If this combination is used, extreme caution should be exercised and renal function should be monitored closely.

Based on information from the limited number of previously treated CLL patients in study BO17072, coadministration with RITUXAN did not appear to have an effect on the pharmacokinetics of fludarabine or cyclophosphamide.

Coadministration with methotrexate had no effect on the pharmacokinetics of RITUXAN in rheumatoid arthritis patients.

Concomitant Use with Biologic Agents and DMARDs Other than Methotrexate in RA: Limited data are available on the safety of the use of biologic agents or DMARDs other than methotrexate in patients exhibiting peripheral B-cell depletion following treatment with rituximab. Patients should be closely observed for signs of infection if biologic agents and/or DMARDs are used concomitantly.

In the RA clinical trial program, 373 RITUXAN-treated patients received subsequent therapy with other DMARDs, of whom 240 received a biologic DMARD. In these patients the rate of serious infection while on RITUXAN (prior to receiving a biologic DMARD) was 6.1 per 100 patient years compared to 4.9 per 100 patient years following subsequent treatment with the biologic DMARD.

Drug-Food Interactions: There have been no formal drug-food interaction studies performed with RITUXAN.

Drug-Herb Interactions: There have been no formal drug-herb interaction studies performed with RITUXAN.

Drug-Laboratory Test Interactions: There have been no formal drug-laboratory interaction studies performed with RITUXAN.

DOSAGE AND ADMINISTRATION:

RITUXAN (rituximab) infusions should be administered in a setting where full resuscitation facilities (see Boxed Serious Warnings and Precautions) are immediately available, and under the close supervision of someone experienced and capable of dealing with severe infusion-related reactions. RITUXAN should be administered as an IV infusion through a dedicated line. **Do not administer as an intravenous push or bolus (see Administration).**

Hypersensitivity reactions and severe infusion-related reaction may occur with administration of RITUXAN (see Warnings and Precautions). Since transient hypotension may occur during infusion with RITUXAN, consideration should be given to withholding anti-hypertensive medications 12 hours prior to and throughout infusion with RITUXAN. Premedication consisting of an analgesic/anti-pyretic (e.g. acetaminophen) and an antihistamine drug (e.g. diphenhydramine) should always be administered before each infusion of RITUXAN. In the clinical trial for CLL ML17102, most patients also received high-dose IV corticosteroids before each dose.

Patients who develop clinically significant arrhythmias should undergo cardiac monitoring during and after subsequent infusions of RITUXAN. Patients with pre-existing cardiac conditions such as angina and arrhythmias should be monitored during and after the infusion of RITUXAN.

Preparation for Administration: Use appropriate aseptic technique. RITUXAN does not contain any preservative or bacteriostatic agent. Withdraw the necessary amount of RITUXAN and dilute to a final concentration of 1 to 4 mg/mL into an infusion bag containing either 0.9% Sodium Chloride Injection USP or 5% Dextrose Injection USP. To avoid foaming, gently invert the bag to mix the solution. Discard any unused portion left in the vial. Parenteral drug products should be inspected visually for particulate matter and discoloration prior to administration.

Non-Hodgkin's Lymphoma: Usual Dose: Low Grade or Follicular Non-Hodgkin's Lymphoma: Initial Treatment: The recommended dosage of RITUXAN as a single agent, is 375 mg/m^2 given as an IV infusion once weekly for four doses (days 1, 8, 15, and 22).

The recommended dosage of RITUXAN in combination with CVP chemotherapy is 375 mg/m^2 for 8 cycles (21 days/cycle), administered as an IV infusion on day 1 of each chemotherapy cycle after IV administration of the corticosteroid component of CVP.

Maintenance Treatment: The recommended dose of RITUXAN for patients who have responded to induction treatment, is 375 mg/m^2 every 3 months until disease progression or for a maximum period of two years.

Diffuse Large B-cell Non-Hodgkin's Lymphoma: RITUXAN should be used in combination with CHOP chemotherapy. The recommended dosage of RITUXAN is 375 mg/m^2 administered on day 1 of each chemotherapy cycle after i.v. administration of the glucocorticoid component of CHOP. The other components of CHOP (cyclophosphamide, doxorubicin, vincristine) should be given after the administration of RITUXAN.

Chronic Lymphocytic Leukemia: The recommended dosage of RITUXAN in combination with chemotherapy for previously untreated and previously treated patients is 375 mg/m^2 body surface area administered on day 1 of the first treatment cycle followed by 500 mg/m^2 body surface area administered on day 1 of each subsequent cycle for 6 cycles in total. The chemotherapy should be given after RITUXAN infusion.

Prophylaxis with adequate hydration and administration of uricostatics (such as allopurinol) starting 48 hours prior to start of therapy is recommended for CLL patients to reduce the risk of tumour lysis syndrome. For CLL patients whose lymphocyte counts are >25×10⁹/L it is recommended to administer methylprednisolone IV shortly before infusion with RITUXAN to decrease the rate and severity of acute infusion reactions and/or cytokine release syndrome. In ML17102 an equivalent of 80 mg of methylprednisolone (100 mg prednisone IV) was given prior to infusions with RITUXAN. Seventy-four percent (74%) of patients in the R-FC arms of ML17102 received at least one dose of corticosteroids, with 27% receiving two or more doses.

Dosage Adjustments During Treatment: No dose reductions of RITUXAN are recommended but 47% of patients in the clinical trial for CLL ML17102 required a delayed and/or slowed infusion, and 17% required their first dose split over two days. When RITUXAN is given in combination with CHOP chemotherapy, standard dose reductions for the chemotherapeutic drugs should be applied. When RITUXAN is given as maintenance treatment, treatment should be delayed in case of significant clinical toxicity according to standard practice.

RITUXAN as a Component of Zevalin (ibritumomab tiuxetan) Therapeutic Regimen: As a required component of the Zevalin therapeutic regimen, RITUXAN is administered twice. The first administration of RITUXAN is a single infusion of 250 mg/m² and should precede the second administration by 7-9 days. At the second administration, RITUXAN 250 mg/m² should be infused within 4 hours prior to the administration of ⁹⁰Y-ibritumomab tiuxetan. Refer to the Zevalin product monograph for full prescribing information.

Administration: Do not administer as an intravenous push or bolus. Premedication with glucocorticoids should be considered, particularly if RITUXAN is not given in combination with steroid-containing chemotherapy. Premedication may attenuate infusion-related events. In the clinical trial for CLL ML17102, the equivalent of 80 mg methylprednisolone (100 mg prednisone IV) was given to most patients prior to each infusion.

First Infusion: The RITUXAN solution for infusion should be administered intravenously at an initial rate of 50 mg/h. RITUXAN should not be mixed or diluted with other drugs. If hypersensitivity or infusion-related events do not occur, escalate the infusion rate in 50 mg/h increments every 30 minutes, to a maximum of 400 mg/h. If hypersensitivity or an infusion related event develops, the infusion should be temporarily slowed or interrupted (see Warnings and Precautions). The infusion can continue at one-half the previous rate upon improvement of patient symptoms.

Subsequent Infusions: Subsequent infusions of RITUXAN can be administered at an initial rate of 100 mg/h, and increased by 100 mg/h increments at 30-minute intervals, to a maximum of 400 mg/h as tolerated.

Missed Dose: Missed or delayed doses should not be omitted but administered at a later time point, based on professional judgment observing the total number of planned cycles and the planned interval between doses.

Rheumatoid Arthritis: Usual Dose: A course of RITUXAN consists of two 1000 mg IV infusions. The recommended dosage of RITUXAN is 1000 mg by IV infusion followed two weeks later by the second 1000 mg IV infusion.

Patients should receive 100 mg IV methylprednisolone to be completed 30 minutes prior to both RITUXAN infusions to decrease the incidence and severity of infusion-related reactions (see Warnings and Precautions).

Retreatment in Patients with RA: The need for further courses should be evaluated 24 weeks following the previous course with retreatment given based on residual or disease activity returning to a level above a DAS28-ESR of 2.6 (treatment to remission). Patients may receive further courses no sooner than 16 weeks following the previous course.

Administration: First Infusion of Each Course: The recommended initial rate for infusion is 50 mg/h; after the first 30 minutes, it can be escalated in 50 mg/h increments every 30 minutes, to a maximum of 400 mg/h.

Second Infusion of Each Course: Subsequent doses of RITUXAN can be infused at an initial rate of 100 mg/h, and increased by 100 mg/h increments at 30 minutes intervals, to a maximum of 400 mg/h.

OVERDOSAGE:

There has been no experience with overdosage in human clinical trials. Single doses higher than 1000 mg have not been tested in controlled clinical studies. The highest dose tested to date is 5 g in patients with chronic lymphocytic leukemia. No additional safety signals were identified. Patients who experience overdose should have immediate interruption or reduction of their infusion and be closely supervised. Consideration should be given to the need for regular monitoring of blood cell count and for increased risk of infections while patients are B-cell-depleted.

For management of a suspected drug overdose, contact your regional Poison Control Centre. See the *CPS* Directory section for a list of Poison Control Centres.

ACTION AND CLINICAL PHARMACOLOGY: Rituximab binds specifically to the antigen CD20 (human B-lymphocyte-restricted differentiation antigen, Bp35), a hydrophobic transmembrane protein with a molecular weight of approximately 35 kD located on pre-B and mature B lymphocytes. The antigen is also expressed on >90% of B-cell non-Hodgkin's lymphomas (NHL) but is not found on hematopoietic stem cells, pro-B-cells, normal plasma cells or other normal tissues. CD20 regulates an early step(s) in the activation process for cell cycle initiation and differentiation, and possibly functions as a calcium ion channel. CD20 is not shed from the cell surface and does not internalize upon antibody binding. Free CD20 antigen is not found in the circulation.

Type B lymphocytes are believed to play a central role in the pathogenesis of rheumatoid arthritis (RA) and associated chronic synovitis. In this setting, B-cells may be acting at multiple sites in the autoimmune/inflammatory process, including through production of rheumatoid factor (RF) and other autoantibodies, antigen presentation, T cell activation, and/or pro-inflammatory cytokine production. Depletion of CD 20 surface antigen positive B-cells was associated with reduction of pro-inflammatory cytokines in rheumatoid synovial tissue.

Mechanism of Action: The Fab domain of rituximab binds to the CD20 antigen on B-lymphocytes and the Fc domain recruits immune effector functions to mediate B-cell lysis in vitro. Possible mechanisms of cell lysis include complement-dependent cytotoxicity (CDC) and antibody-dependent cell-mediated cytotoxicity (ADCC). The antibody has been shown to induce apoptosis in the DHL-4 human B-cell lymphoma line.

Pharmacodynamics: Normal Tissue Cross-Reactivity: Rituximab binding was observed on lymphoid cells in the thymus, the white pulp of the spleen, and a majority of B-lymphocytes in peripheral blood and lymph nodes. Little or no binding was observed in non-lymphoid tissues examined.

Pharmacokinetics: Non-Hodgkin's Lymphoma: In patients given single doses at 10, 50, 100, 250 or 500 mg/m² as an IV infusion, serum levels and the half-life of rituximab were proportional to dose. In 9 patients given 375 mg/m² as an IV infusion for four doses, the mean serum half-life was 59.8 hours (range 11.1 to 104.6 hours) after the first infusion and 174 hours (range 26 to 442 hours) after the fourth infusion. The wide range of half-lives may reflect the variable tumour burden among patients and the changes in CD20 positive (normal and malignant) B-cell populations upon repeated administrations.

Rituximab at a dose of 375 mg/m² was administered as an IV infusion at weekly intervals for four doses to 166 patients. The peak and trough serum levels of rituximab were inversely correlated with baseline values for the number of circulating CD20 positive B-cells and measures of disease burden. Median steady-state serum levels were higher for responders compared to nonresponders; however, no difference was found in the rate of elimination as measured by serum half-life. Serum levels were higher in patients with International Working Formulation (IWF) subtypes B, C, and D as compared to those with subtype A. Rituximab was detectable in the serum of patients three to six months after completion of treatment.

The pharmacokinetic profile of rituximab when administered as six infusions of 375 mg/m² in combination with six cycles of CHOP chemotherapy was similar to that seen with rituximab alone.

Administration of RITUXAN (rituximab) resulted in a rapid and sustained depletion of circulating and tissue-based B-cells. Lymph node biopsies performed 14 days after therapy showed a decrease in the percentage of B-cells in seven of eight patients who had received single doses of rituximab ≥100 mg/m². Among the 166 patients in the pivotal study, circulating B-cells (measured as CD19+ cells) were depleted within the first three doses with sustained depletion for up to 6 to 9 months post-treatment in 83% of patients. One of the responding patients (1%), failed to show significant depletion of CD19+ cells after the third infusion of rituximab as compared to 19% of the nonresponding patients. B-cell recovery began at approximately six months following completion of treatment. Median B-cell levels returned to normal by twelve months following completion of treatment.

There were sustained and statistically significant reductions in both IgM and IgG serum levels observed from 5 through 11 months following rituximab administration. However, only 14 % of patients had reductions in IgG and/or IgM serum levels, resulting in values below the normal range.

Peripheral B-cell counts declined to levels below normal following the first dose of RITUXAN. In patients treated for hematological malignancies, B-cell repletion began within 6 months of treatment returning to normal levels between 9 and 12 months after completion of therapy. In rheumatoid arthritis patients, immediate depletion of B-cells in the peripheral blood was observed following two infusions of 1000 mg of RITUXAN separated by a 14 day interval. Peripheral blood B-cell counts begin to increase from week 24 and evidence of repopulation is observed in the majority of patients by week 40, whether RITUXAN was administered as monotherapy or in combination with methotrexate.

Diffuse Large B-cell Non-Hodgkin's Lymphoma (DLCL): Elimination and distribution have not been extensively studied in patients with diffuse large B-cell non-Hodgkin's lymphoma, but available data indicate that serum levels of rituximab in DLCL patients are comparable to those in patients with low-grade or follicular NHL following treatment with similar doses.

Chronic Lymphocytic Leukemia (CLL): No pharmacokinetic information in the untreated CLL population is available. Rituximab was administered as an IV infusion at a first-cycle dose of 375 mg/m² increased to 500 mg/m² each cycle for 5 doses in combination with fludarabine and cyclophosphamide in the previously treated, low tumor burden CLL patients (absolute lymphocytes <25×10⁹ cells/L). The mean (± SD) C_{max} and $AUC_{0-\tau}$ was 175±76 µg/mL and 728±488 µg·d/mL, respectively, after the first-cycle dose (N=21). The mean (± SD) C_{max} and $AUC_{0-\tau}$ was 408±199 µg/mL and 4080±2400 µg·d/mL, respectively, after the fifth 500 mg/m² infusion (N=15).

Rheumatoid Arthritis: Following two intravenous infusions of rituximab at a dose of 1000 mg, two weeks apart, the mean terminal half-life was 20.8 days (range, 8.58 to 35.9 days), mean systemic clearance was 0.23 L/day (range, 0.091 to 0.67 L/day), and mean steady-state distribution volume was 4.6 L (range, 1.7 to 7.51 L). Population pharmacokinetic analysis of the same data gave similar mean values for systemic clearance and half-life, 0.26 L/day and 20.4 days, respectively. Population pharmacokinetic analysis revealed that BSA and gender were the most significant covariates to explain inter individual variability in pharmacokinetic parameters. After adjusting for BSA, male subjects had a larger volume of distribution and a faster clearance than female subjects. The gender-related pharmacokinetic differences are not considered to be clinically relevant and dose adjustment is not required.

The pharmacokinetics of rituximab were assessed following two IV doses of 500 mg and 1000 mg on Days 1 and 15 in four studies (WA17047, WA17045, WA17044, U3384G). In all these studies, rituximab pharmacokinetics were dose proportional over the limited dose range studied. See Table 16.

Table 16: RITUXAN

Mean PK Parameters for Rituximab

	C_{first} (µg/mL)	C_{second} (µg/mL)	$t_{½}$ (days)
2×0.5 g in Course 1			
WA17047	171±54 (32)	198±58 (29)	14.83±5.78 (39)
WA17045	157±45.9 (29)	183±54.7 (30)	15.65±5.12 (33)
WA17044	164±41 (25)	193±61 (32)	16.38±6.06 (37)
2×0.5 g in Course 2			
WA17047	170±38 (22)	ND	ND
WA17045	ND	ND	ND
WA17044	175±41 (24)	207±69 (33)	19.37±5.97 (31)
2×1 g in Course 1			
WA17047	341±84 (25)	404±102 (25)	16.89±5.36 (32)
WA17045	318±85.8 (27)	381±98.3 (26)	18.50 ± 5.82 (31)
WA17044	312±103 (33)	365±126 (34)	17.95±6.21 (35)
U3384G	298±91.2 (30.6)	355±112 (31.4)	21.2±8.2 (38.7)
2×1 g in Course 2			
WA17047	370±101 (27%)	ND	ND
WA17045	ND	ND	ND
WA17044	348±89 (26)	386±132 (34)	21.82±6.39 (29)
U3384G	317±107 (33.8)	377±120 (31.8)	20.9±5.77 (27.6)

Legend: C_{first}=post-infusion concentration after first infusion; C_{second}=post-infusion concentration after second infusion; Values are mean ± SD (CV%); ND=not determined.

The PK parameters in the anti-TNF inadequate responder population, following the same dosage regimen (2×1000 mg, iv, 2 weeks apart), were similar with a mean maximum serum concentration of 369 µg/mL and a mean terminal half-life of 19.2 days.

In patients with rheumatoid arthritis, the duration of peripheral B-cell depletion was variable. The majority of patients received further treatment prior to full B-cell repletion.

Special Populations and Conditions: Pediatrics: The safety and effectiveness of RITUXAN in pediatric patients have not been established. Please see Warnings and Precautions, Special Populations, Pediatrics.

Geriatrics: Age had no effect on the pharmacokinetics of rituximab. Please see Warnings and Precautions, Special Populations, Geriatrics.

Gender: Gender had no effect on the pharmacokinetics of rituximab.

Hepatic Insufficiency: No pharmacokinetic data are available in patients with hepatic impairment.

Renal Insufficiency: No pharmacokinetic data are available in patients with renal impairment.

STORAGE AND STABILITY: RITUXAN (rituximab) vials are stable at 2 to 8°C. Do not use beyond expiration date stamped on carton. Keep the vial in the outer carton to protect it from light.

As RITUXAN for infusion does not contain any antimicrobial preservative, it is essential to ensure that prepared solutions for infusion are not microbiologically compromised. RITUXAN solutions for infusion are stable at 2 to 8°C for 24 hours and at room temperature for an additional 12 hours. However, administration should take place as per standard practices after the aseptic preparation of intravenous admixtures.

Incompatibilities: No incompatibilities between RITUXAN and polyvinylchloride or polyethylene bags have been observed.

INFORMATION FOR THE PATIENT: Published in e-CPS, available by subscription at www.e-cps.ca.

DOSAGE FORMS, COMPOSITION AND PACKAGING: Each mL of sterile, clear, colorless liquid concentrate for i.v. administration contains: rituximab 10 mg. Nonmedicinal ingredients: hydrochloric acid, polysorbate 80, sodium chloride, sodium citrate, sodium hydroxide and water for injection. Single-use vials of 10 and 50 mL, cartons of 2 and 1, respectively.

Riva-Dicyclomine

dicyclomine HCl

Antispasmodic

Riva

SUPPLIED: Each blue capsule contains: dicyclomine HCl 10 mg, USP. Nonmedicinal ingredients: colloidal silicon dioxide, lactose and magnesium stearate. Bottles of 500.

Riva-Loperamide
loperamide HCl
Antidiarrheal

Riva

PHARMACOLOGY: Diarrhea may be defined as a failure or imbalance of one or a combination of activities in the gut which include secretion, absorption and motility. Loperamide has been shown to act on all of these functions via cholinergic, noncholinergic, opiate and nonopiate receptor-mediated mechanisms. In this way, loperamide effectively reduces fecal output and frequency, improves stool consistency and relieves symptoms of abdominal cramping and fecal incontinence.

INDICATIONS: As an adjunct to rehydration therapy for the symptomatic control of acute nonspecific diarrhea; for chronic diarrhea associated with inflammatory bowel disease; and for reducing the volume of discharge for ileostomies, colostomies and other intestinal resections.

CONTRAINDICATIONS: In children under 2 years of age.

Loperamide is contraindicated in patients with known hypersensitivity to loperamide or any of the other components; cases in which constipation must be avoided.

WARNINGS: Loperamide should not be used in the case of acute dysentery which is characterized by blood in stools and elevated temperature. Fluid and electrolyte depletion may occur in patients who have diarrhea. The use of loperamide does not preclude the administration of appropriate fluid and electrolyte therapy.

In some patients with acute ulcerative colitis and in pseudomembranous colitis associated with broad spectrum antibiotics, agents which inhibit intestinal motility or delay intestinal transit time have been reported to induce toxic megacolon. Loperamide therapy should be discontinued promptly if abdominal distention occurs or if other untoward symptoms develop.

Children: The use of loperamide is not recommended for children under 12 years of age except on the advice of a physician (see Dosage).

Use loperamide with special caution in young children and those with compromised blood brain barrier (e.g., meningitis) because of the greater variability of response in these groups. Dehydration, particularly in young children, may further influence the variability of response to loperamide.

In case of accidental ingestion of loperamide by children, see Overdose: Symptoms and Treatment.

PRECAUTIONS: *Pregnancy:* Safe use of loperamide during pregnancy has not been established. Reproduction studies performed in the rat and the rabbit revealed no evidence of impaired fertility or harm to the fetus at dosage levels up to 30-fold the therapeutic dose for man.

Patients with hepatic dysfunction should be monitored for signs of CNS toxicity due to the extensive first pass metabolism of loperamide in the liver.

If improvement in symptoms of acute diarrhea is not observed within 48 hours, the use of loperamide should be discontinued.

Dependence Liability: Physical dependence to loperamide in humans has not been observed. However studies in morphine-dependent monkeys demonstrated that loperamide at doses above those recommended for humans prevented signs of morphine withdrawal. However, in humans, the naloxone challenge pupil test, which when positive indicates opiate-like effects, performed after a single high dose, or after more than 2 years of therapeutic use of loperamide, was negative.

ADVERSE EFFECTS: The adverse effects reported in adults during clinical trials are difficult to distinguish from symptoms associated with the diarrheal syndrome. In adults, they were generally of a minor and self-limiting nature, e.g., abdominal pain or discomfort; drowsiness or dizziness; dry mouth; nausea and vomiting; hypersensitivity, including skin rash. Opiate-like effects (CNS) have been observed in young children (under 3 years of age).

OVERDOSE:

Symptoms: In clinical trials, an adult who took three 20 mg doses within a 24-hour period was nauseated after the second dose and vomited after the third dose. In studies designed to examine the potential for side effects, intentional ingestion of up to 60 mg of loperamide in a single dose to healthy subjects resulted in no significant adverse effects.

Treatment: Clinical trials have demonstrated that a slurry of activated charcoal administered promptly after ingestion of loperamide can reduce the amount of drug which is absorbed into the systemic circulation by as much as 9-fold. If vomiting occurs spontaneously upon ingestion, a slurry of 100 g of activated charcoal should be administered orally as soon as fluids can be retained.

If vomiting has not occurred, gastric lavage should be performed followed by administration of 100 g of the activated charcoal slurry through the gastric tube. In the event of overdosage, patients should be monitored for signs of CNS depression for at least 24 hours. If CNS depression is observed, naloxone may be administered. If responsive to naloxone, vital signs must be monitored carefully for recurrence of symptoms of drug overdose for at least 24 hours after the last dose of naloxone.

In view of the prolonged action of loperamide and the short duration (1 to 3 hours) of naloxone, the patient must be monitored closely and treated repeatedly with naloxone as indicated. Since relatively little drug is excreted in the urine, forced diuresis is not expected to be effective for loperamide overdosage.

> For management of a suspected drug overdose, CPhA recommends that you contact your **regional Poison Control Centre**. See the *CPS* Directory section for a list of Poison Control Centres.

DOSAGE: Adults: Acute Diarrhea: The recommended initial dose is 4 mg followed by 2 mg after each unformed stool. Daily dosage should not exceed 16 mg.

Chronic Diarrhea: The recommended initial dose is 4 mg followed by 2 mg after each unformed stool until diarrhea is controlled; thereafter the dosage should be reduced to meet individual requirements. When the optimal daily dosage has thus been established, this amount can be administered as a single daily dose or in divided doses.

The average daily maintenance dosage used in clinical trials has been 4 to 8 mg. If improvement is not observed after treatment with 16 mg/day for 10 days, symptoms are unlikely to be controlled by further administration.

Children: Acute or Chronic Diarrhea: Loperamide should be used in children only on the advice of a physician. For children up to but not including 12 years of age, the following schedule will usually fulfill initial dosage requirements. See Table 1.

Table 1: Riva-Loperamide

Recommended First-Day Dosage Schedule

2–5 years: (10–20 kg)	1 mg t.i.d. (3 mg daily dose)
5–8 years: (20–30 kg)	2 mg b.i.d. (4 mg daily dose)
8–12 years: (greater than 30 kg)	2 mg t.i.d. (6 mg daily dose)

Following the first treatment day, it is recommended that subsequent doses (1 mg/10 kg body weight) be administered only after a loose stool.

Duration of Treatment: Loperamide may be administered for prolonged periods of time. Blood, urine, liver and kidney function, ECG and ophthalmological examinations have revealed no significant abnormalities after several years of administration. No tolerance to the antidiarrheal effect has been observed. Naloxone pupil challenge studies in patients with chronic diarrhea who have received loperamide orally for prolonged periods indicate a lack of CNS effects.

SUPPLIED: Each light green, cylindrical caplet, inscribed "R" and "2 mg" on the scored side and "Loperamide" on the other side, contains: loperamide HCl 2mg. Nonmedicinal ingredients: croscarmellose sodium, D&C Yellow No. 10 aluminum lake, FD&C Blue No. 1 aluminum lake, lactose, magnesium stearate, microcrystalline cellulose and povidone. HDPE bottles of 100 and 500. Store between 15 and 30°C.

> The reader is invited to consult CPhA's monograph **Corticosteroids: Eye, Ear, Nose.**

Rivanase AQ.
beclomethasone dipropionate
Corticosteroid

Riva

SUPPLIED: Each spray of suspension delivered by the nasal applicator contains: beclomethasone dipropionate 50 µg. Nonmedicinal ingredients: benzalkonium chloride, cellulose, dextrose, phenyl ethanol, polysorbate and sodium carboxymethyl cellulose. Glass bottles of 200 doses fitted with a metering atomizing pump and a nasal applicator. Store between 15 and 30°C and protect from light. Discard 3 months after first use.

Rivasol
zinc sulfate monohydrate
Anorectal Therapy

Riva

Rivasol HC
zinc sulfate monohydrate—hydrocortisone acetate
Anorectal Therapy

Riva

SUPPLIED: Rivasol: Each tube contains: zinc sulfate monohydrate 0.5% in a petroleum base. Nonmedicinal ingredients: methyl- and propylparaben. Tubes of 15 and 30 g with applicator.

Rivasol HC: Each tube contains: zinc sulfate monohydrate 0.5% and hydrocortisone acetate 0.5% in a petroleum base. Nonmedicinal ingredients: methyl- and propylparaben. Tubes of 15 and 30 g with applicator.

Store in a cool place under 22°C.

Rivotril®
clonazepam
Anticonvulsant

Roche

SUPPLIED: 0.5 mg: Each pale orange, cylindrical, biplane, scored tablet, edges bevelled, with "ROCHE 0.5" engraved on one face, scored on the other, contains: clonazepam 0.5 mg. Nonmedicinal ingredients: cornstarch, iron oxide red, iron oxide yellow, lactose, magnesium stearate, potato starch and talc. Energy: 2.4 kJ (0.6 kcal). Gluten-, paraben-, sodium-, sulfite- and tartrazine-free. Bottles of 100 and 500. Keep in a tightly closed, light-resistant container. Store at 15 to 30°C.

2 mg: Each white, cylindrical, biplane, scored tablet, edges bevelled, with "ROCHE -2-" on one side, cross-scored on the other, contains: clonazepam 2 mg. Nonmedicinal ingredients: cornstarch, lactose, magnesium stearate and microcrystalline cellulose. Energy: 2.4 kJ (0.6 kcal). Gluten-, paraben-, sodium-, sulfite- and tartrazine-free. Bottles of 100 and 500. Keep in a tightly closed, light-resistant container. Store at 15 to 30°C.

Robaxacet®
methocarbamol—acetaminophen
Muscle Relaxant—Analgesic

Pfizer Consumer Healthcare

Robaxacet® Extra Strength
methocarbamol—acetaminophen
Muscle Relaxant—Analgesic

Pfizer Consumer Healthcare

Robaxacet®-8 Ⓝ
methocarbamol—acetaminophen—codeine phosphate
Muscle Relaxant—Analgesic

Pfizer Consumer Healthcare

PHARMACOLOGY: The precise mechanism of action of methocarbamol is not known. Methocarbamol is thought to act on the CNS, perhaps depressing polysynaptic reflexes. It has no direct action on the contractile mechanism of striated muscle, the motor end plate or the nerve fiber. Methocarbamol is metabolized to yield a dealkylated and a hydroxylated product. These 2 metabolites are found primarily as glucuronide and sulfate conjugates. Based on elimination of radioactivity, the half-life of methocarbamol and its metabolites is about 2 hours. Animal studies reveal that methocarbamol crosses the placental barrier and blood-brain barrier.

Acetaminophen is a nonopiate, nonsalicylate analgesic and antipyretic. Acetaminophen is conjugated in the liver to form glucuronide and sulfate conjugates. Its plasma half-life has been reported to be from 1 to 2 hours.

Codeine is readily absorbed from the gastrointestinal tract, and a therapeutic dose reaches peak analgesic effectiveness in about 2 hours and persists for 4 to 6 hours. Oral codeine (60 mg) given to healthy males has been shown to achieve peak blood levels of 0.016 mg/100 mL at approximately 1 hour post-dose. The codeine plasma half-life for a 60 mg oral dose is about 2.9 hours. Blood levels causing CNS depression begin at 0.05 to 0.19 mg/100 mL.

The single lethal dose of codeine in adults is estimated to be approximately 0.5 to 1.0 g. Codeine is rapidly distributed from blood to body tissues and taken up preferentially by parenchymatous organs such as liver, spleen and kidney. It passes the blood-brain barrier and is found in fetal tissue and breast milk. The drug is not bound by plasma protein nor is it accumulated in body tissues. Codeine is metabolized in the liver to morphine and norcodeine, each representing about 10% of the administered dose of codeine. About 90% of the dose is excreted within 24 hours, primarily through the kidneys. Urinary excretion products are free and glucuronide-conjugated codeine (about 70%), free and conjugated norcodeine (about 10%), free and conjugated morphine (about 10%), normorphine (under 4%) and hydrocodone (1%). The remainder of the dose appears in the feces.

INDICATIONS: Pain due to or associated with skeletal muscle spasm: acute torticollis, acute strains and sprains, acute low back pain, acute tenosynovitis, ankle sprain, fracture, trauma, acute bursitis, acute myositis, whiplash injury.

Robaxacet-8 may be used when the pain is more severe.

CONTRAINDICATIONS: Hypersensitivity to methocarbamol, acetaminophen or codeine.

Robaxacet-8: Patients allergic to codeine or other opioids, have suffered head injury, are at risk of blocked intestines or suffer from seizures.

WARNINGS: Do not exceed recommended dosage as severe liver damage due to acetaminophen toxicity may occur. Avoid alcohol.

Do not use with other products containing acetaminophen.

This package contains enough drug to seriously harm a child.

Do not take if allergic to acetaminophen or any of the listed ingredients. Stop use and consult a doctor if you develop allergic reactions such as wheezing, rash or itching, if symptoms last more than 5 days or fever lasts more than 3 days. Do not use without consulting a doctor if you suffer from chronic alcoholism, serious liver or kidney disease, are pregnant, nursing or under a physician's care. Consult a physician prior to combining with sedating drugs, tranquilizers, other depressants, any other medications including prescription drugs.

Robaxacet-8: Do not use without consulting a doctor if you have difficulty breathing, asthma, chronic lung disease.

PRECAUTIONS: May cause drowsiness or dizziness. Sedatives and tranquilizers may increase drowsiness.

Keep out of reach of children.

Talk to your doctor if you still have symptoms after 5 days or if fever lasts more than 3 days.

Robaxacet-8: Consult your physician if you feel sedated or drowsy, confused, have shallow breathing or have severe constipation.

Occupational Hazards: Methocarbamol and codeine may impair the mental and/or physical abilities required for the performance of potentially hazardous tasks such as driving a car or operating machinery. The patient using this drug should be cautioned accordingly. Since methocarbamol may possess a general CNS depressant effect, patients receiving Robaxacet products should be cautioned about combined effects with alcohol and other CNS depressants.

The administration of Robaxacet-8 or other narcotics may obscure the diagnosis or clinical course in patients with acute abdominal conditions. In the presence of head injury, other intracranial lesions or a pre-existing increase in intracranial pressure, the respiratory depressant effects of narcotics and their capacity to elevate cerebrospinal fluid pressure may be markedly exaggerated. Furthermore, narcotics produce adverse reactions which may obscure the clinical course of patients with head injuries.

Robaxacet-8 should be given with caution to certain patients such as the elderly or debilitated, and those with severe impairment of hepatic or renal function, hypothyroidism, Addison's disease and prostatic hypertrophy or urethral stricture.

Drug Interactions: Methocarbamol may cause a color interference in certain screening tests for 5-hydroxyindoleacetic acid (5-HIAA) and vanillylmandelic acid (VMA).

Patients receiving other narcotic analgesics, general anesthetics, phenothiazines, tranquilizers, sedative-hypnotics or other CNS depressants (including alcohol) concomitantly with Robaxacet-8 may exhibit an additive CNS depression. When such combined therapy is contemplated, the dose of one or both agents should be reduced.

The use of MAO inhibitors or tricyclic antidepressants with codeine preparations may increase the effect of either the antidepressant or codeine. The concurrent use of anticholinergics with codeine may produce paralytic ileus.

Pregnancy: There are no adequate and well-controlled studies of this product in pregnant women. This product should be used during pregnancy only when in the judgment of the physician the potential benefits outweigh the potential hazards.

The effects of Robaxacet products on the mother and fetus, on the duration of labor and delivery, or on later growth, development and functional maturation of the child is unknown.

Lactation: It is not known whether methocarbamol or its metabolites are secreted in human milk; however, there are indications small quantities of acetaminophen and codeine have been found in breast milk.

Robaxacet-8: Codeine may cause harm to a breast fed baby. Contact your physician immediately if you are breastfeeding and your baby is having difficulty breathing or feeding, or is very sleepy or limp.

Children: Safety and effectiveness of this product in children 12 years of age or younger have not been established.

ADVERSE EFFECTS: The most common complaints to methocarbamol are drowsiness, nausea and dizziness or lightheadedness (seen in approximately 4 to 5% of patients). The following reactions have been associated with the drug, some of them rarely; in some instances, causal relationships have not been established: headache, nasal congestion, blurred vision, rash, pruritus and urticaria.

Adverse reactions that have been associated with the use of acetaminophen include: nausea, vomiting or diarrhea. Rarely, hypersensitivity reactions have been reported, as manifested by thrombocytopenic purpura, hemolytic anemia and agranulocytosis.

The most frequently observed adverse reactions to codeine include lightheadedness, dizziness, drowsiness, nausea, vomiting, constipation and depression of respiration. Less common reactions to codeine include euphoria, dysphoria, pruritus and skin rashes.

Gastrointestinal discomfort may be minimized by taking this product with food.

Drug Abuse and Dependence: Codeine (present in Robaxacet-8) can produce drug dependence of the morphine type, and therefore has the potential for being abused. Psychic dependence, physical dependence and tolerance may develop upon repeated administration of this drug, and it should be prescribed and administered with the same degree of caution appropriate to the use of other oral narcotic-containing medications.

OVERDOSE:

In case of accidental overdose: Contact a physician or poison control centre immediately, even if you do not notice any possible signs or symptoms such as increased sweating, nausea, vomiting, stomach pain, blurred vision and loss of appetite.

Symptoms: Methocarbamol: No deaths or major toxicity have been reported from overdosage with methocarbamol, administered parenterally or orally. One adult survived the deliberate ingestion of 22 to 30 g of methocarbamol without serious toxicity. Another survived 30 to 50 g. The principal symptom was drowsiness in both cases.

Acetaminophen and Codeine: Serious overdose with acetaminophen and codeine is characterized by respiratory depression (a decrease in respiratory rate and/or tidal volume; Cheyne-Stokes respiration; cyanosis), extreme somnolence progressing to stupor or coma, skeletal muscle flaccidity, cold and clammy skin, and sometimes bradycardia and hypotension. In severe overdosage, apnea, circulatory collapse, cardiac arrest and death may occur. The ingestion of very large amounts of this drug may, in addition, result in acute hepatic toxicity from acetaminophen.

Treatment: Methocarbamol: Supportive measures include maintenance of an adequate airway, monitoring urinary output and vital signs, and the administration of i.v. fluids, if necessary. There is no experience with forced diuresis or with dialysis in the treatment of methocarbamol overdosage. Likewise, the usefulness of hemodialysis in managing methocarbamol overdose is unknown.

Acetaminophen and Codeine: Primary attention should be given to reestablishment of adequate respiratory exchange through provision of a patent airway and the institution of assisted or controlled ventilation. The narcotic antagonist naloxone is a specific antidote against respiratory depression which may result from overdosage or unusual sensitivity to narcotics, including codeine. Therefore, an appropriate dose of naloxone (usual initial adult dose: 0.4 mg) should be administered, preferably by the i.v. route, and simultaneously with efforts at respiratory resuscitation. Since the duration of action of codeine may exceed that of the antagonist, the patient should be kept under continued surveillance and repeated doses of the antagonist should be administered as needed to maintain adequate respiration. An antagonist should not be administered in the absence of clinically significant respiratory or cardiovascular depression. Oxygen, i.v. fluids, vasopressors and other supportive measures should be employed as indicated. Gastric emptying may be useful in removing unabsorbed drug.

Acetaminophen in massive overdosage may cause hepatotoxicity in some patients. Clinical and laboratory evidence of hepatotoxicity may be delayed for up to 1 week. Close clinical monitoring and serial hepatic enzyme determinations are therefore recommended.

The antidote, N-acetylcysteine, should be administered as early as possible, and within 16 hours of the overdose ingestion for optimal results. Following recovery, there are no residual, structural or functional hepatic abnormalities.

> For management of a suspected drug overdose, CPhA recommends that you contact your **regional Poison Control Centre**. See the *CPS* Directory section for a list of Poison Control Centres.

DOSAGE: Regular Strength: Adult Dosage: Adults and Children over 12 years: 2 caplets every 6 hours. Not to exceed 8 caplets daily. These dosage recommendations provide 3.2 and 4.8 g, respectively, methocarbamol and 2.6 and 3.9 g, respectively, acetaminophen/day.

Extra Strength: Adult Dosage: Adults and Children over 12 years: 2 caplets every 6 hours. Not to exceed 8 caplets daily. This recommended dosage provides 3.2 g methocarbamol and 4 g acetaminophen/day. Use only on the advice of a physician.

Robaxacet-8: Adults Dosage: 1 or 2 caplets every 6-8 hours. Do not exceed 8 caplets in 24 hours.

SUPPLIED: Robaxacet: Each green and white caplet, green layer scored and white layer engraved "RO", contains: methocarbamol 400 mg and acetaminophen 325 mg. Nonmedicinal ingredients: celluloses, cornstarch, crospovidone, D&C Yellow No. 10, FD&C Blue No. 1, magnesium stearate, polyethylene glycol, povidone, pregelatinized starch, sodium lauryl sulfate, sodium starch glycolate and stearic acid. Energy: <1 kJ (<1 kcal). Sodium: <1 mmol (0.82 mg). Bottles of 40. Blisters of 18. Store at room temperature (15 to 30°C).

Robaxacet Extra Strength: Each green and white caplet, green layer scored and engraved "EX", and white layer engraved "RO", contains: methocarbamol 400 mg and acetaminophen 500 mg. Nonmedicinal ingredients: celluloses, cornstarch, crospovidone, D&C Yellow No. 10, FD&C Blue No. 1, magnesium stearate, polyethylene glycol, povidone, pregelatinized starch, sodium lauryl sulfate, sodium starch glycolate and stearic acid. Energy: <1 kJ (<1 kcal). Sodium: <1 mmol (0.46 mg). Bottles of 40. Blisters of 18. Store at room temperature (15 to 30°C).

Robaxacet-8: Each coated, blue and white caplet, white layer engraved "RO", blue layer scored, contains: methocarbamol 400 mg, acetaminophen 325 mg and codeine phosphate 8 mg. Nonmedicinal ingredients: celluloses, cornstarch, crospovidone, FD&C Blue No. 1, magnesium stearate, polyethylene glycol, povidone, pregelatinized starch, silicon dioxide, sodium lauryl sulfate, sodium starch glycolate and stearic acid. Energy: <1 kJ (<1 kcal). Sodium: <1 mmol (0.9 mg). Bottles of 100. Blisters of 18. Store at room temperature (15 to 30°C).

Robaxin®
methocarbamol
Skeletal Muscle Relaxant

Pfizer Consumer Healthcare

Robaxin®-750
methocarbamol
Skeletal Muscle Relaxant

Pfizer Consumer Healthcare

PHARMACOLOGY: The precise mechanism of action of methocarbamol is not known. Methocarbamol is thought to act on the CNS, perhaps depressing polysynaptic reflexes. It has no direct action on the contractile mechanism of striated muscle, the motor end plate or the nerve fiber. Methocarbamol is metabolized to yield a dealkylated and a hydroxylated product. These 2 metabolites are found primarily as glucuronide and sulfate conjugates. Based on elimination of radioactivity, the half-life of methocarbamol and its metabolites is about 2 hours. Animal studies reveal that methocarbamol crosses the placental barrier and blood-brain barrier.

INDICATIONS: An adjunct to rest, physical therapy and other measures for the relief of discomforts associated with acute, painful musculoskeletal conditions.

CONTRAINDICATIONS: Hypersensitivity to methocarbamol.

PRECAUTIONS: Keep all medicine safely away from children.

Talk to your doctor before taking this medication if you are pregnant or nursing.

May cause drowsiness or dizziness.

Do not drink alcohol.

Do not take more than the recommended dose unless under the direction of a physician.

Talk to your doctor if you still have symptoms after 5 days

Occupational Hazards: Methocarbamol may impair the ability of the patient to engage in potentially hazardous activities such as operating machinery or driving a motor vehicle; ambulatory patients should therefore be cautioned accordingly. Patients should be cautioned about combined effects of methocarbamol with alcohol and with other CNS depressants.

Methocarbamol may cause a color interference in screening tests for 5-hydroxyindoleacetic acid (5-HIAA) and vanillylmandelic acid (VMA).

Pregnancy: Safe use in pregnancy has not been established with regard to possible adverse effects in fetal development.

Lactation: It is not known whether methocarbamol is excreted in human milk.

Children: Safety and effectiveness in children 12 years of age and less have not been established.

ADVERSE EFFECTS: Following oral administration, minor untoward effects such as lightheadedness, dizziness, drowsiness and mild nausea occasionally occur, and frequently disappear on reduction of dosage (seen in approximately 4 to 5% of patients). Allergic manifestations such as urticaria, pruritus, rash or conjunctivitis with nasal congestion have been reported in a few hypersensitive patients.

OVERDOSE:

In case of accidental over dose contact a physician or poison control center immediately, even if there are no symptoms.

Symptoms: No deaths or major toxicity have been reported from overdosage with methocarbamol, administered parenterally or orally. One adult survived the deliberate ingestion of 22 to 30 g of methocarbamol without serious toxicity. Another survived 30 to 50 g. The principal symptom was drowsiness in both cases. However, 3 deaths have been reported when methocarbamol was combined with alcohol and other drugs.

Treatment: Supportive measures include maintenance of an adequate airway, monitoring urinary output and vital signs and the administration of i.v. fluids, if necessary. There is no experience with forced diuresis or with dialysis in the treatment of methocarbamol overdose. Likewise, the usefulness of hemodialysis in managing methocarbamol overdose is unknown.

> For management of a suspected drug overdose, CPhA recommends that you contact your **regional Poison Control Centre**. See the *CPS* Directory section for a list of Poison Control Centres.

DOSAGE: Adults: 6 g daily for first 48 to 72 hours of acute skeletal muscle spasm. Severe conditions: 8 g daily. Thereafter reduce dosage to 4 g daily.

SUPPLIED: Robaxin: Each white, scored, compressed tablet, engraved "RO", contains: methocarbamol 500 mg. Nonmedicinal ingredients: cornstarch, magnesium stearate, povidone, sodium lauryl sulfate, sodium starch glycolate and stearic acid. Energy: <1 kJ (<1 kcal). Sodium: <1 mmol (0.4 mg). Bottles of 50.

Robaxin-750: Each white, scored, capsule-shaped tablet, monogrammed "RO", contains: methocarbamol 750 mg. Nonmedicinal ingredients: cornstarch, magnesium stearate, povidone, sodium lauryl sulfate, sodium starch glycolate and stearic acid. Energy: <1 kJ (<1 kcal). Sodium: <1 mmol (0.59 mg). Bottles of 50.

Robaxisal® Extra Strength
methocarbamol—ASA
Skeletal Muscle Relaxant—Analgesic

Pfizer Consumer Healthcare

Robaxisal®-C Ⓝ
methocarbamol—ASA—codeine phosphate
Skeletal Muscle Relaxant—Analgesic

Pfizer Consumer Healthcare

PHARMACOLOGY: The precise mechanism of action of methocarbamol is not known. Methocarbamol is thought to act on the CNS, perhaps depressing polysynaptic reflexes. It has no direct action on the contractile mechanism of striated muscle, the motor end plate or the nerve fibre. Methocarbamol is metabolized to yield a dealkylated and a hydroxylated product. These 2 metabolites are found primarily as glucuronide and sulfate conjugates. Based on elimination of radioactivity, the half-life of methocarbamol and its metabolites is about 2 hours. Animal studies reveal that methocarbamol crosses the placental barrier and blood-brain barrier.

ASA interferes with the production of prostaglandins in various organs and tissues through acetylation and inactivation of the enzyme cyclooxygenase. The main action of the drug is thought to be peripheral; however, it may have similar activity in the CNS. The reduction in tissue levels of prostaglandins may be responsible for the analgesic and anti-inflammatory effects of the drug. ASA is most effective against pain of low to moderate intensity associated with inflammation.

Codeine is readily absorbed from the gastrointestinal tract, and a therapeutic dose reaches peak analgesic effectiveness in about 2 hours and persists for 4 to 6 hours. Oral codeine (60 mg) given to healthy males has been shown to achieve peak blood levels of 0.016 mg/100 mL at approximately 1 hour post-dose. The codeine plasma half-life for a 60 mg oral dose is about 2.9 hours. Blood levels causing CNS depression begin at 0.05 to 0.19 mg/100 mL.

INDICATIONS: Pain due to or associated with skeletal muscle spasm: acute torticollis, acute strains and sprains, acute low back pain, acute tenosynovitis, ankle sprain, fracture, trauma, acute bursitis, acute myositis, whiplash injury.

Robaxisal-C may be used when the pain is more severe.

CONTRAINDICATIONS: Hypersensitivity to methocarbamol, ASA, or codeine.

Patients who have had a bronchospastic reaction, generalized urticaria, angioedema, severe rhinitis, laryngeal edema or shock precipitated by ASA or nonsteroidal anti-inflammatory drugs. Some patients sensitive to ASA, may be cross-sensitive to other nonsteroidal anti-inflammatory drugs as well as tartrazine dye. Patients with asthma associated nasal polyps have an increased risk of sensitivity to ASA.

Do not use in patients with active peptic ulcer.

This product should not be used in children, teenagers, and young adults with varicella or influenza, unless directed by a physician.

Robaxisal-C: Patients allergic to codeine or other opioids, have suffered head injury, are at risk of blocked intestines or suffer from seizures.

PRECAUTIONS: Keep all medicine safely away from children.

Ask your doctor about Reye's Syndrome before giving this medication to a child who has chicken pox or flu symptoms.

May cause drowsiness or dizziness.

Do not drink alcohol.

Do not take more than the recommended dose unless under the direction of a physician.

Talk to your doctor if you still have symptoms after 5 days.

Consult your doctor if you feel sedated or drowsy, confused, have shallow breathing or have severe constipation.

Do not use without consulting a doctor if you have difficulty breathing, asthma, chronic lung disease.

Occupational Hazards: Methocarbamol and codeine may impair the ability of the patient to engage in potentially hazardous activities such as operating machinery or driving a motor vehicle; ambulatory patients should therefore be cautioned accordingly. Patients should be cautioned about combined effects of methocarbamol and codeine with alcohol and with other CNS depressants.

The administration of opioids may obscure the diagnosis or clinical course in patients with acute abdominal conditions. In the presence of head injury, other intracranial lesions or a pre-existing increase in intracranial pressure, the respiratory depressant effects of opioids and their capacity to elevate cerebrospinal fluid pressure may be markedly exaggerated. Furthermore, narcotics produce adverse reactions which may obscure the clinical course of patients with head injuries.

Drug Interactions: Methocarbamol may cause a color interference in certain screening tests for 5-hydroxyindoleacetic acid (5-HIAA) and vanillylmandelic acid (VMA).

Patients receiving other opioid analgesics, general anesthetics, phenothiazines, tranquilizers, sedative-hypnotics or other CNS depressants concomitantly with Robaxisal-C may exhibit an additive CNS depression. When such combined therapy is contemplated, the dose of one or both agents should be reduced.

The use of MAO inhibitors or tricyclic antidepressants with codeine preparations may increase the effect of either the antidepressant or codeine. The concurrent use of anticholinergics with codeine may produce paralytic ileus.

Pregnancy: There are no adequate and well-controlled studies in pregnant women. This product should be used during pregnancy only when in the judgment of the physician the potential benefits outweigh the potential hazards.

Lactation: Codeine may cause harm to a breast fed baby. Contact your physician immediately if you are breastfeeding and your baby is having difficulty breathing or feeding, or is very sleepy or limp.

ADVERSE EFFECTS: Methocarbamol: The most common complaints to methocarbamol are drowsiness, nausea and dizziness or lightheadedness (seen in approximately 4 to 5 % of patients). The following reactions have been associated with the drug, some of them rarely; in some instances, causal relationships have not been established: headache, nasal congestion, blurred vision, rash, pruritus and urticaria.

ASA:

Gastrointestinal: ulcer, hemorrhage, dyspepsia, heartburn, epigastric distress, nausea, vomiting, diarrhea, abdominal pain may occur with increasing incidence at higher dosages.

Hepatic: Reversible hepatotoxicity particularly in patients with juvenile rheumatoid arthritis and systemic lupus erythematosus has been reported rarely.

Otic: Tinnitus and hearing loss, usually completely reversible, may occur in patients receiving large doses of ASA or with long-term use and are dose related.

Skin: Skin eruptions and lesions have been reported. Stevens-Johnson's syndrome has rarely been associated with ASA.

Chronic salicylate intoxication may result from high doses or from prolonged therapy with high doses. Tinnitus and hearing loss are the most frequent signs of chronic intoxication. Other manifestations such as dimness of vision, headache, dizziness, mental confusion, drowsiness, sweating, thirst, hyperventilation, tachycardia, nausea, vomiting and sometimes diarrhea may occur.

Codeine: Drug Abuse and Dependence: Codeine can produce drug dependence of the morphine type, and therefore has the potential for being abused. Psychic dependence, physical dependence and tolerance may develop upon repeated administration of this drug, and it should be prescribed and administered with the same degree of caution appropriate to the use of other oral opioid-containing medications.

OVERDOSE:

In case of accidental overdose, contact a physician or poison control centre immediately, even if there are no symptoms.

Symptoms: Methocarbamol: No deaths or major toxicity have been reported from overdosage with methocarbamol, administered parenterally or orally. One adult survived the deliberate ingestion of 22 to 30 g of methocarbamol without serious toxicity. Another survived 30 to 50 g. The principal symptom was drowsiness in both cases.

Codeine: Respiratory depression (reduced respiratory rate and/or tidal volume; Cheyne-Stokes respiration; cyanosis), extreme somnolence progressing to stupor or coma, skeletal muscle flaccidity, cold or clammy skin, and sometimes hypotension and bradycardia. Severe overdosage may result in apnea, circulatory collapse, cardiac arrest and death. Miosis can be one characteristic of morphine derivative overdose. Mydriasis can take place in terminal narcosis, severe hypoxia or as a toxic effect of pethidine or its congeners.

ASA: Symptoms of acute toxicity with ASA may occur with doses greater than 150 mg/kg. Doses greater than 500 mg/kg are potentially fatal. Acid-base and electrolyte disturbances, dehydration, hyperpyrexia, hyperglycemia or hypoglycemia are the principal physiologic manifestations of acute ASA toxicity. Other symptoms of toxicity include burning pain in the mouth or throat, dizziness, tinnitus and sweating. In more severe cases, presence of CNS symptoms such as lethargy, disorientation, or confusion may be a predictor for the development of pulmonary edema. Coma and convulsions may be delayed for 24 to 48 hours. Cardiac arrhythmias have been reported. Bleeding disorders, cerebral edema, oliguria are also possible.

Treatment: Gastric lavage, administration of activated charcoal. If respiratory depression occurs, give attention to the re-establishment of respiratory exchange by ventilation and administration of a narcotic antagonist, e.g., naloxone.

For management of a suspected drug overdose, CPhA recommends that you contact your **regional Poison Control Centre**. See the *CPS* Directory section for a list of Poison Control Centres.

DOSAGE: Robaxisal Extra Strength: Adults: 2 caplets, 4 times a day.

Robaxisal-C: Adults: 1 or 2 caplets 3 or 4 times a day.

SUPPLIED: Robaxisal Extra Strength: Each pink and white, coated caplet, white layer monogrammed "RO", pink layer scored and engraved "EX", contains: methocarbamol 400 mg and ASA 500 mg. Nonmedicinal ingredients: cellulose, cornstarch, FD&C Red No. 3, magnesium stearate, polyethylene glycol, povidone, sodium lauryl sulfate, sodium starch glycolate and stearic acid. Energy: <1 kJ (<1 kcal). Sodium: <1 mmol (0.36 mg). Bottles of 40. Blisters of 18. Store at room temperature (15 to 30°C).

Robaxisal-C ¼: Each orange and white caplet, orange layer monogrammed "RO", contains: methocarbamol 400 mg, ASA 325 mg and codeine phosphate 16.2 mg. Nonmedicinal ingredients: cornstarch, FD&C Yellow No. 6, magnesium stearate, povidone, sodium starch glycolate and stearic acid. Energy: <1 kJ (<1 kcal). Bottles of 24. Store at room temperature (15 to 30°C).

Robaxisal-C ½: Each coral and white caplet, white layer monogrammed "RO", contains: methocarbamol 400 mg, ASA 325 mg, codeine phosphate 32.4 mg. Nonmedicinal ingredients: cellulose, cornstarch, FD&C Blue No. 1, FD&C Red No. 40, FD&C Yellow No. 6, magnesium stearate, polyethylene glycol, povidone, sodium starch glycolate and stearic acid. Energy: <1 kJ (<1 kcal). Bottles of 24 and 250. Store at room temperature (15 to 30°C).

Robax Platinum®

methocarbamol—ibuprofen

Muscle Relaxant—Analgesic

Pfizer Consumer Healthcare

PHARMACOLOGY: A bioavailability study has demonstrated that methocarbamol and ibuprofen when taken (orally) in combination, are bioequivalent to methocarbamol and ibuprofen when taken individually. This indicates that the absorption and bioavailability of these drugs is independent of each other's presence. There is no pharmacological interaction between methocarbamol and ibuprofen. Methocarbamol is a muscle relaxant and ibuprofen is an analgesic with antipyretic and anti-inflammatory properties.

Methocarbamol: Methocarbamol is effective in reducing muscle spasm and pain in acute musculoskeletal disorders secondary to trauma and inflammation. Each drug of the combination of methocarbamol and aspirin contributed to the therapeutic effects against acute painful skeletal muscle problems of spasm, pain and tenderness.

Orally administered methocarbamol is well absorbed from the gastrointestinal tract. Animal studies indicate that absorption occurs in the small intestine. Studies in humans dosed with radio-labelled (C^{14}) methocarbamol indicated that 97-99% of the administered radioactivity was recovered in the urine over 3 days. In a comparative bioavailability study, following oral administration peak plasma concentration was reached in approximately 45 minutes when methocarbamol was administered in combination with ibuprofen. The plasma half life of methocarbamol administered alone was 1.25±0.27 hours and 1.30±0.29 hours when administered in combination.

In a dose proportionality study of single doses of 500 mg, 1500 mg and 3000 mg, it was shown that kinetics of methocarbamol are not linear. However, rates of elimination suggest that no accumulation is expected with chronic dosing every 6 hours.

Methocarbamol has been shown to be metabolized in humans by dealkylation, hydroxylation and conjugation with glucuronic acid and sulfate, presumably in the liver. Two metabolites identified are: 3-(2-hydroxyphenoxy),1,2-propanediol-1-carbamate and 3-(4-hydroxy-2-methoxyphenoxy)-1,2-propanediol-1-carbamate.

Extremely small amounts of unchanged methocarbamol have also been recovered in the feces.

The precise mechanism of action is not known. Methocarbamol is thought to act on the central nervous system, perhaps depressing polysynaptic reflexes.

Ibuprofen: Ibuprofen, like all nonsteroidal anti-inflammatory drugs (NSAIDs), is an analgesic, antipyretic, and anti-inflammatory medication. There is strong evidence to support the view that the main mechanism of action of ibuprofen (like other NSAIDs) is related to decreasing prostaglandin biosynthesis.

Prostaglandins are naturally-occurring fatty acid derivatives that are widely distributed in the tissues. They are believed to be a common factor in the production of pain, fever, and inflammation. Prostaglandins are believed to sensitise tissues to pain- and inflammation-producing mediators such as histamine, 5-hydroxytryptamine, and kinins. The enzyme catalysing the committed step in prostaglandin biosynthesis is prostaglandin endoperoxide synthase, also known as cyclooxygenase. There is significant evidence that the main mechanism of analgesic/antipyretic action of NSAIDs is prostaglandin biosynthesis inhibition. Other pharmacologic effects such as lysosome and plasma membrane stabilization have been observed, but the potential relevance of these effects to ibuprofen-induced analgesia and antipyresis is unclear.

Ibuprofen is rapidly and almost completely absorbed. Peak serum concentration occurs within 1-2 hours in adults. In a comparative bioavailability study, following oral administration peak plasma concentration was reached in approximately 1.6 hours for ibuprofen alone and in approximately 1.3 hours when ibuprofen was administered in combination with methocarbamol. The plasma half-life of ibuprofen administered alone was 2.11±0.43 hours, and 2.08±0.37 hours when administered in combination. Food decreases the rate but not the extent of absorption.

The volume of distribution in adults after oral administration is 0.1-0.2 L/kg.

At therapeutic concentrations ibuprofen is highly bound to whole human plasma and to site II of purified albumin. There is no appreciable plasma accumulation of ibuprofen or its metabolites with repeated doses.

In humans, drug concentrations have been found in the synovial fluid of inflamed tissue approximately 5-12 hours after oral administration. In children (mean age 11 years), synovial fluid peak levels were reached within 5-6 hours of oral administration.

Cytochrome P450 (CYP) 2C9 has been identified as the most important catalyst for formation of all oxidative metabolites of R-(−) and S-(+) ibuprofen. Approximately 80% of a dose is recovered in urine, primarily as carboxymetabolites and conjugated hydroxymetabolites. Ibuprofen does not appear to induce the formation of drug metabolising enzymes in the rat.

There is no evidence of a differential metabolism or elimination of ibuprofen in the elderly. A pharmacokinetic evaluation of ibuprofen in geriatric subjects (65 to 78 years) compared with young adult subjects (22 to 35 years) found that there was no clinically significant difference in the kinetic profiles of ibuprofen for these age groups. Furthermore, there was no statistically significant difference between the two populations in the urinary excretion pattern of the drug and its major metabolites.

Breast Milk and Placental Transport: The high protein binding and lower pH of breast milk versus plasma tend to inhibit the excretion of ibuprofen into breast milk.

Ibuprofen excretion in breast milk following ingestion of one 400 mg ibuprofen tablet every 6 hours for five doses was below the level (i.e. 1 µg/mL) of detection. However, a later study using a more sensitive assay showed ibuprofen to be rapidly excreted in breast milk 30 minutes following oral ingestion of 400 mg of ibuprofen at a concentration of 13 ng/mL. A milk:plasma ratio of 1:126 was determined and the exposure of a suckling infant was calculated to be approximately 0.0008% of the maternal dose. It is not known whether ibuprofen crosses the placenta. Animal studies have shown that methocarbamol crosses the placenta.

In a comparative bioavailability study in humans after a single dose of combination (methocarbamol 500 mg and ibuprofen 200 mg) drug product, and single-drug methocarbamol 500 mg or ibuprofen 200 mg, the following pharmacological parameters were determined: see Table 1.

Table 1: Robax Platinum
Pharmacological Parameters

Parameter	Orally Administered Combination Drug Product	Orally Administered Single Drug
Methocarbamol mean t_{max}	0.72±0.35 hours	1.01±0.52 hours
Ibuprofen mean t_{max}	1.36±1.04 hours	1.65±0.96 hours
Methocarbamol mean $t_{½}$	1.30±0.29 hours	1.25±0.27 hours
Ibuprofen mean $t_{½}$	2.08±0.37 hours	2.11±0.43 hours
Methocarbamol mean C_{max}	8686.37±2635.47 ng/mL	7698.73±2657.59 ng/mL
Ibuprofen mean C_{max}	20 376.2±5592.44 ng/mL	18 435.6±4582.87 ng/mL
Methocarbamol k_{el}/hr	0.556±0.116	0.579±0.116
Ibuprofen k_{el}/hr	0.344±0.065	0.342±0.067

The results of this study show that methocarbamol 500 mg and ibuprofen 200 mg administered as a combination drug product are bioequivalent to methocarbamol 500 mg and ibuprofen 200 mg when administered individually.

INDICATIONS: If symptoms worsen or persist for more than 5 days, contact a physician or healthcare professional.

Adults and Children over 12 years: For effective relief of pain associated with muscle spasm such as back pain, tense neck muscles, strains and sprains.

A double-blind, randomized study showed that ibuprofen 400 mg every 4 hours for a total of 3 doses relieved muscle soreness following exercise significantly better than acetaminophen 1000 mg and placebo.

A double-blind, randomized study showed that ibuprofen 400 mg relieved headache pain significantly better than acetaminophen 1000 mg and placebo. Another double-blind, placebo-controlled, randomized study showed that ibuprofen 400 mg began to exert a significant analgesic effect on headache within 30 minutes after dosing. A recent study confirmed that ibuprofen 400 mg provided a significantly faster onset of relief as measured by first perceptible relief, meaningful relief, per cent attaining complete relief, and superior overall analgesic efficacy compared to acetaminophen 1000 mg for relief of episodic tension-type headache.

Ibuprofen has been studied in other pain models including dental, muscle contraction headache, soft tissue injury, post surgery, dysmenorrhea, and migraine, with equally effective pain relief results.

Methocarbamol has been studied in muscle relaxation models including tetanus therapy, muscle spasms, painful muscle conditions, and in combination with analgesics, with positive results. In gynecological postoperative patients, methocarbamol reduced the use of narcotics and other sedatives for pain and discomfort.

CONTRAINDICATIONS: The following are contraindications to the use of methocarbamol/ibuprofen combination drug product.

Known hypersensitivity to methocarbamol or ibuprofen. There is a potential for cross-reactivity between different NSAIDs and ibuprofen, and patients sensitive to other carbamate derivatives and methocarbamol.

Active peptic ulcer, a history of recurrent ulceration or active inflammatory disease of the GI system.

The combination drug product should not be used in patients who have significant hepatic impairment or active liver disease.

Severely impaired or deteriorating renal function (creatinine clearance <30 mL/min). Individuals with lesser degrees of renal impairment are at risk of deterioration of their renal function when prescribed NSAIDs and must be monitored.

Patients with the complete or partial syndrome of nasal polyps, or in whom asthma, anaphylaxis, urticaria, rhinitis or other allergic manifestations are precipitated by ASA or other nonsteroidal anti-inflammatory agents. Fatal anaphylactoid reactions have occurred in such individuals. As well, individuals with the above medical problems are at risk of a severe reaction even if they have taken NSAIDs in the past without any adverse effects.

Not recommended for use with other NSAIDs because of the absence of any evidence demonstrating synergistic benefits and the potential for additive side effects.

Serious GI toxicity, such as peptic ulceration, perforation and gastrointestinal bleeding, **sometimes severe and occasionally fatal**, can occur at any time, with or without symptoms in patients treated with NSAIDs including ibuprofen.

Do not use in the third trimester of pregnancy, because of risk of premature closure of the ductus arteriosus and prolonged parturition.

WARNINGS: General: Patients with heart disease, high blood pressure, diabetes, thyroid disease, narrow angle glaucoma, or difficulty in urination due to enlargement of the prostate gland should not take this drug unless directed by a physician.

Side effects may be minimized by using the smallest dose for the shortest duration of time.

As with other anti-inflammatory drugs, ibuprofen may mask the usual signs of infection.

Do not use if taking other acetylsalicylic acid (ASA) or other products containing ibuprofen or if allergic to ASA, salicylates or anti-inflammatory drugs.

If nervousness, dizziness, or sleeplessness occurs, use of Advil should be discontinued and a physician should be consulted. If symptoms do not improve within 5 days or are accompanied by fever, a physician should be consulted.

Contact your physician if pregnant or nursing or taking any prescription drug before using.

May cause drowsiness or dizziness.

Avoid alcohol.

Exercise caution when driving a motor vehicle or operating machinery.

Gastrointestinal (GI) System: Serious GI toxicity, such as peptic ulceration, perforation and gastrointestinal bleeding, **sometimes severe and occasionally fatal**, can occur at any time, with or without symptoms in patients treated with NSAIDs including ibuprofen.

Minor upper GI problems, such as dyspepsia, are common, usually developing early in therapy. Physicians should remain alert for ulceration and bleeding in patients treated with nonsteroidal anti-inflammatory drugs, even in the absence of previous GI tract symptoms.

In patients observed in clinical trials of such agents, symptomatic upper GI ulcers, gross bleeding, or perforation appear to occur in approximately 1% of patients treated for 3-6 months and in about 2-4% of patients treated for one year. The risk continues beyond one year and possibly increases. The incidence of these complications increases with increasing dose.

Combination methocarbamol/ibuprofen should be given under close medical supervision to patients prone to gastrointestinal irritation, particularly those with history of peptic ulcer, diverticulosis or ulcerative colitis and Crohn's Disease. In these cases the physician must weigh the benefits of treatment against the possible hazards.

Physicians should inform patients about the signs and/or symptoms of serious GI toxicity and instruct them to contact a physician immediately if they experience persistent dyspepsia or other symptoms or signs suggestive of gastrointestinal ulceration or bleeding. Because serious GI tract ulceration and bleeding can occur without warning symptoms, physicians should follow chronically treated patients by checking their haemoglobin periodically and by being vigilant for the signs and symptoms of ulceration and bleeding and should inform the patients of the importance of this follow-up.

If ulceration is suspected or confirmed, or if GI bleeding occurs, Robax Platinum should be discontinued immediately, appropriate treatment instituted and the patient monitored closely.

No studies, to date, have identified any group of patients not at risk of developing ulceration and bleeding. A prior history of serious GI events and other factors such as excess alcohol intake, smoking, age, female gender and concomitant oral steroid and anticoagulant use have been associated with increased risk. Studies to date show that all NSAIDs can cause GI tract adverse events. Although existing data does not clearly identify differences in risk between various NSAIDs, this may be shown in the future.

Aseptic Meningitis: In occasional cases with some NSAIDs (ibuprofen) the symptoms of aseptic meningitis (stiff neck, severe headaches, nausea, vomiting, fever, or clouding of consciousness) have been observed. Patients with autoimmune disorders (systemic lupus erythematosus, mixed connective tissue disease etc.) seem to be pre-disposed. Therefore, in such patients, the physician must be vigilant to the development of this complication.

Pregnancy: There are no adequate data regarding use of methocarbamol/ibuprofen in pregnant women. Use during late pregnancy should be avoided.

Reproductive studies conducted in rats and rabbits have not demonstrated evidence of developmental abnormalities. However, animal reproduction studies are not always predictive of human response. Because of the known effects of NSAIDs on the fetal cardiovascular system, use of ibuprofen during late pregnancy should be avoided. As with other drugs known to inhibit prostaglandin synthesis, an increased incidence of dystocia and delayed parturition occurred in rats. Administration of ibuprofen is not recommended during pregnancy.

Renal Function: Long-term administration of nonsteroidal anti-inflammatory drugs to animals has resulted in renal papillary necrosis and other abnormal renal pathology. In humans, there have been reports of acute interstitial nephritis with hematuria, proteinuria, and occasionally nephrotic syndrome.

A second form of renal toxicity has been seen in patients with prerenal conditions leading to the reduction in renal blood flow or blood volume, where the renal prostaglandins have a supportive role in the maintenance of renal perfusion. In these patients, administration of an NSAID may cause a dose-dependent reduction in prostaglandin formation and may precipitate overt renal decompensation. Patients at greatest risk of this reaction are those with impaired renal function, heart failure, liver dysfunction, those taking diuretics, and the elderly. Discontinuation of nonsteroidal anti-inflammatory therapy is usually followed by recovery to the pre-treatment state.

Like other NSAIDs, ibuprofen inhibits renal prostaglandin synthesis, which may decrease renal function and cause sodium retention. Renal blood flow and glomerular filtration rate decreased in patients with mild impairment of renal function who took 1200 mg/day of ibuprofen for one week. Renal papillary necrosis has been reported. A number of factors appear to increase the risk of renal toxicity. In comparative clinical trials involving 7624 ibuprofen-treated, 2822 ASA-treated and 2843 placebo-treated patients, adverse reactions involving renal function were reported by 0.6% of the ibuprofen group, 0.3% of the ASA group and 0.1% of the placebo group. The analysis included data from trials which employed doses greater than 1200 mg, used for longer periods than OTC recommendations and by patients being treated for serious conditions. Ibuprofen and its metabolites are eliminated primarily by the kidneys; therefore the drug should be used with great caution in patients with impaired renal function. In these cases, utilisation of lower doses of Robax Platinum should be considered and patients carefully monitored. Methocarbamol may also affect renal function if therapy lasts 5 days or more.

During long-term therapy kidney function should be monitored periodically.

Genitourinary Tract: Some NSAIDs are known to cause persistent urinary symptoms (bladder pain, dysuria, urinary frequency), hematuria or cystitis. The onset of these symptoms may occur at any time after the initiation of therapy with an NSAID. Some cases have become severe on continued treatment. Should urinary symptoms occur, treatment with ibuprofen/methocarbamol combination **must be stopped immediately** to obtain recovery. This should be done before any urological investigations of treatments are carried out.

Hepatic Function: As with other nonsteroidal anti-inflammatory drugs, borderline elevations of one or more liver function tests may occur in up to 15% of patients. These abnormalities may progress, may remain essentially unchanged, or may be transient with continued therapy. A patient with symptoms and/or signs suggesting liver dysfunction, or in whom an abnormal liver test has occurred, should be evaluated for evidence of the development of more severe hepatic reaction while on therapy with this drug. Severe hepatic reactions including jaundice and cases of fatal hepatitis have been reported with nonsteroidal anti-inflammatory drugs.

Although such reactions are rare, if abnormal liver tests persist or worsen, if clinical signs and symptoms consistent with liver disease develop, or if systemic manifestations occur (e.g. eosinophilia, rash, etc.), this drug should be discontinued.

During long-term therapy, liver function tests should be monitored periodically. If there is a need to prescribe this drug in the presence of impaired liver function, it must be done under strict observation.

The frequency of acute liver injury among 311 716 patients who were prescribed ibuprofen was 1.6/100 000. For NSAID users as a group, the only factors that had an independent effect on the occurrence of acute liver injury were the simultaneous use of hepatotoxic medication or the presence of rheumatoid arthritis. Based on these data, the short-term use of ibuprofen as an analgesic/antipyretic should not be of concern regarding the development of liver disease.

Geriatrics: Patients older than 65 years and frail or debilitated patients are most susceptible to a variety of adverse reactions from NSAIDs: the incidence of these adverse reactions increases with dose and duration of treatment. In addition, these patients are less tolerant to ulceration and bleeding. Most reports of fatal GI events are in this population. Older patients are also at risk of lower esophageal ulceration and bleeding.

For such patients, consideration should be given to a starting dose lower than the one usually recommended, with individual adjustment when necessary and under close supervision.

The OTC dose of 1200 mg ibuprofen per day for up to 7 days is reported to be safe for the over 65 years of age group.

Children: The combination methocarbamol/ibuprofen has not been studied in children. Furthermore, the safety and efficacy of methocarbamol (other than in the management of tetanus) in children younger than 12 years of age also have not been established; therefore, Robax Platinum should not be administered to children in this age group.

Fluid and Electrolyte Balance: Fluid retention and edema have been observed in patients treated with ibuprofen. Therefore, as with many other NSAIDs, the possibility of precipitating congestive heart failure in elderly patients or those with compromised cardiac function should be borne in mind. Ibuprofen should be used with caution in patients with heart failure, hypertension or other conditions predisposing to fluid retention. With NSAID treatment there is a potential risk of hyperkalemia, particularly in patients with conditions such as diabetes mellitus or renal failure; elderly patients; or in patients receiving concomitant therapy with β-adrenergic blockers, angiotensin converting enzyme inhibitors or some diuretics.

Serum electrolytes should be monitored periodically during long-term therapy, especially in those who are at risk.

Special Warnings: Skin: In rare cases, serious skin reactions such as Stevens-Johnson syndrome, toxic epidermal necrolysis, exfoliative dermatitis and erythema multiforme have been associated with the use of some NSAIDs. Because the rate of these reactions is low, they have usually been noted during post-marketing surveillance in patients taking other medications also associated with the potential development of these serious skin reactions. Thus, causality is **not** clear. These reactions are potentially life threatening but may be reversible if the causative agent is discontinued and appropriate treatment instituted. Patients should be advised that if they experience a skin rash, reddening or blisters they should discontinue their NSAID and contact their physician for assessment and advice, including which additional therapies to discontinue.

Other: Stop use and check with your physician if you vomit blood, have bloody or black stools, or experience any weakness.

Use with caution in the elderly.

PRECAUTIONS: Cardiovascular Function: Congestive heart failure in patients with marginal cardiac function, elevated blood pressure and palpitations have been reported following ibuprofen administration.

Ophthalmology: Blurred and/or diminished vision has been reported with the use of ibuprofen. If such symptoms develop this drug product should be discontinued and an ophthalmologic examination performed; ophthalmic examination should be carried out at periodic intervals in any patient receiving this drug product for an extended period of time.

Central Nervous System: Some patients may experience drowsiness, dizziness, vertigo, insomnia or depression with the use of this product. If patients experience these side effects, they should exercise caution in carrying out activities that require alertness.

Anticoagulants: A study reported lack of change in hypoprothrombinemia caused by warfarin when administered with ibuprofen. Other studies have shown that the concomitant use of NSAIDs and anticoagulants increases the risk of GI adverse events such as ulceration and bleeding. Because prostaglandins play an important role in hemostasis, and NSAIDs affect platelet function, concurrent therapy of Robax Platinum with warfarin requires close monitoring to be certain that no change in anticoagulant dosage is necessary.

Oral Hypoglycemics: Ibuprofen may increase hypoglycemic effects of oral antidiabetic agents and insulin.

Infection: In common with other anti-inflammatory drugs, ibuprofen may mask the usual signs of infection.

CNS Depressants: Methocarbamol has potential to cause drowsiness and dizziness. The patient should be cautioned against the operation of motor vehicles or machinery. Since methocarbamol may possess a general CNS depressant effect, patients taking Robax Platinum should be cautioned about combined effects with alcohol and other CNS depressants.

Methocarbamol may produce false positive tests for urinary 5-hydroxyindoleacetic acid (5-HIAA) and vanillylmandelic acid (VMA).

Lactation: Methocarbamol was detected in the breast milk of dogs. Assuming small amounts of methocarbamol are also excreted in human breast milk, it is doubtful any adverse clinical effects would be seen in the nursing infant. Newborns with neonatal tetanus have been treated with larger doses of intravenous or oral methocarbamol without ill effects from the drug. One study showed an ibuprofen concentration of 13 ng/mL 30 minutes after ingesting 400 mg. The milk:plasma ratio was 1:126. This translates to an infant exposure of 0.0008% of the maternal dose. It is not known to what extent, if any, ibuprofen crosses the human placenta. No adverse effect has been detected in children 6 months of age who were administered ibuprofen.

Hematology: Drugs inhibiting prostaglandin biosynthesis do interfere with platelet function to varying degrees; therefore, patients who may be adversely affected by such an action should be carefully observed when ibuprofen is administered. Blood dyscrasias (such as neutropenia, leukopenia, thrombocytopenia, aplastic anemia and agranulocytosis) associated with the use of NSAIDs are rare, but could occur with severe consequences.

Drug Interactions: Methotrexate: Ibuprofen and other NSAIDs have been reported to reduce renal tubular secretion of methotrexate in-vitro. This may enhance the toxicity of methotrexate. Caution should be used when ibuprofen is administered concomitantly with methotrexate.

Lithium: Plasma lithium levels should be carefully monitored in patients taking combination therapy of ibuprofen and lithium. Ibuprofen has been shown to decrease the renal lithium clearance and increase plasma lithium levels.

Acetylsalicylic Acid (ASA) or Other NSAIDs: The use of ibuprofen in addition to any other NSAID, including ASA, is not recommended due to the possibility of additive side effects. Animal studies show that aspirin given with NSAIDs including ibuprofen, yields a net decrease in anti-inflammatory activity with lowered blood levels of the non-aspirin drug. Single dose bioavailability studies in normal volunteers have failed to show an effect of aspirin on ibuprofen blood levels. Correlation clinical studies have not been conducted.

Acetaminophen: Although interactions have not been reported, concurrent use with ibuprofen is not advisable; it may increase the risk of adverse renal effect.

Digoxin: Ibuprofen has been shown to increase serum digoxin concentration. Increased monitoring and dosage adjustments of digitalis glycoside may be necessary during concurrent ibuprofen therapy and following discontinuation of ibuprofen therapy.

Antihypertensives: Ibuprofen can interfere with blood pressure control in certain patients under treatment for mild to moderate hypertension.

Prostaglandins are an important factor in cardiovascular homeostasis and inhibition of their synthesis by NSAIDs may interfere with circulatory control. NSAIDs may elevate blood pressure in patients receiving antihypertensive medication. Two meta analyses, have observed this relationship for NSAIDs as a class and for certain NSAIDs in particular, but ibuprofen did not significantly affect blood pressure in either meta analysis. Consistent with this lack of effect, a study showed that ibuprofen 1600 mg/day for 14 days did not attenuate the antihypertensive effect of two β-adrenergic blockers. Another study showed no effect of three weeks' therapy with ibuprofen on the antihypertensive efficacy of verapamil, but it is not known whether this lack of interaction extends to other classes of calcium channel blockers.

When renal perfusion pressure is reduced both prostaglandins and angiotensin II are important mediators of renal autoregulation. As a class, the combination of an NSAID and angiotensin converting enzyme inhibitor theoretically may have the potential to decrease renal function. One study found a clinically significant decrease in renal function in 4 of 17 patients treated with hydrochlorothiazide and fosinopril who received ibuprofen 2400 mg/day for one month. In contrast, another study found no effect on the antihypertensive effect of enalapril or on plasma renin or aldosterone following two days' treatment with ibuprofen 1200 mg/day.

The relationship of ibuprofen and antihypertensives is clearly not well defined. The benefits of concomitant medication should be analysed and compared to the potential risks before being prescribed. If ibuprofen is being recommended for long-term use, then periodic monitoring of blood pressure may be useful. Blood pressure monitoring is not necessary if ibuprofen is being recommended for short-term use as an analgesic.

Diuretics: Because of its fluid retention properties, high doses of ibuprofen can decrease the diuretic and antihypertensive effects of diuretics, and increased diuretic dosage may be required. Patients with impaired renal function who are taking potassium-sparing diuretics should not take ibuprofen.

Clinical studies, as well as random observations, have shown that ibuprofen can reduce the natriuretic effect of furosemide and thiazides in some patients. This response has been attributed to inhibition of renal prostaglandin synthesis. During concomitant therapy with ibuprofen, the patient should be observed closely for signs of renal failure as well as to assure diuretic efficacy.
Antacids: A bioavailability study has shown that there was no interference with the absorption of ibuprofen when given in conjunction with an antacid containing aluminum hydroxide and magnesium hydroxide.
H-2 Antagonists: In studies with human volunteers, coadministration of cimetidine or ranitidine with ibuprofen had no substantive effect on ibuprofen serum concentrations.
Coumarin-type: Numerous studies have shown that the concomitant use of NSAIDs and anticoagulants increases the risk of GI adverse events such as ulceration and bleeding. Because prostaglandins play an important role in hemostasis, and NSAIDs affect platelet function, concurrent therapy of ibuprofen with warfarin requires close monitoring to be certain that no change in anticoagulant dosage is necessary. Several short-term controlled studies failed to show that ibuprofen significantly affected prothrombin time or a variety of other clotting factors when administered to individuals on coumarin-type anticoagulants. Nevertheless, the physician should be cautious when administering ibuprofen to patients on anticoagulants.
Other Drugs: Although ibuprofen binds extensively to plasma proteins, interactions with other protein-bound drugs occur rarely. Nevertheless, caution should be observed when other drugs, also having a high affinity for protein binding sites, are used concurrently. Some observations have suggested a potential for ibuprofen to interact with furosemide, pindolol, digoxin, and phenytoin. However, the mechanisms and clinical significance of these observations are presently not known. No interactions have been reported when ibuprofen has been used in conjunction with probenecid, thyroxine, steroids, antibiotics or benzodiazepines.

ADVERSE EFFECTS: Ibuprofen:
Gastrointestinal: The adverse reactions most frequently seen with prescribed ibuprofen therapy involve the gastrointestinal system. 3 to 9%: nausea, epigastric pain, heartburn. 1 to 3%: diarrhea, abdominal distress, nausea and vomiting, indigestion, constipation, abdominal cramps or pain, fullness of the gastrointestinal tract (bloating or flatulence). Less than 1%: gastric or duodenal ulcer with bleeding and/or perforation, gastrointestinal hemorrhage, melena, hepatitis, jaundice, abnormal liver function, AST, serum bilirubin and alkaline phosphatase.
Allergic: Less than 1%: anaphylaxis. Causal relationship unknown: fever, serum sickness, lupus erythematosus.
Central Nervous System: 3 to 9%: dizziness. 1 to 3%: headache, nervousness. Less than 1%: depression, insomnia. Causal relationship unknown: paresthesias, hallucinations, dream abnormalities. Aseptic meningitis and meningoencephalitis, in one case accompanied by eosinophilia in the cerebrospinal fluid, have been reported in patients who took ibuprofen intermittently and did not have any connective tissue disease.
Dermatologic: 3 to 9%: rash (including maculopapular type). 1 to 3%: pruritus. Less than 1%: vesiculobullous eruptions, urticaria, erythema multiforme. Causal relationship unknown: alopecia, Stevens-Johnson syndrome.
Cardiovascular: Less than 1%: congestive heart failure in patients with marginal cardiac function, elevated blood pressure. Causal relationship unknown: arrhythmias (sinus tachycardia, sinus bradycardia, palpitations).
Special Senses: 1 to 3%: tinnitus. Less than 1%: amblyopia (blurred and/or diminished vision, scotomata and/or changes in colour vision). Any patient with eye complaints during ibuprofen therapy should have an ophthalmological examination. Causal relationship unknown: conjunctivitis, diplopia, optic neuritis.
Hematologic: 1 to 20%: leukopenia and decreases in hemoglobin and hematocrit. Causal relationship unknown: hemolytic anemia, thrombocytopenia, granulocytopenia, bleeding episodes (e.g. purpura, epistaxis, hematuria, menorrhagia).
Renal: 3 to 9%: decreased creatinine clearance, polyuria, azotemia.
Hepatic: 3 to 9%: hepatitis, jaundice, abnormal liver function, AST, serum bilirubin, and alkaline phosphatase.
Endocrine: Causal relationship unknown: gynecomastia, hypoglycemic reaction. Menstrual delays of up to two weeks and dysfunctional uterine bleeding occurred in nine patients taking ibuprofen, 400 mg t.i.d., for three days before menses.
Metabolic: 1 to 3%: decreased appetite, edema, fluid retention. Fluid retention generally responds to drug discontinuation.
Methocarbamol: May cause drowsiness, dizziness, blurred vision, lightheadedness, somnolence, vertigo, anorexia, headache, fever, nausea, allergic reactions such as urticaria, pruritus, rash, skin eruptions, conjunctivitis with nasal congestion.

Oral administration of methocarbamol may cause the urine in some patients, following elimination from the body, to turn brown, black, blue or green after a period of time.
Other Ibuprofen Adverse Events: Health professionals should keep in mind other potential adverse events associated with ibuprofen use including: Crohn's disease, colitis, gastritis, hematemesis, mouth ulceration, abdominal distension, dyspepsia, abdominal pain upper, hypersensitivity, cerebrovascular accident, angioneurotic edema, dermatitis bullous, face edema, purpura, cardiac failure, myocardial infarction, angina pectoris, vertigo, visual disturbance, agranulocytosis, anemia, aplastic anemia, hematuria, interstitial nephritis, renal failure, nephrotic syndrome, proteinuria, and renal papillary necrosis, liver disorder, asthma, bronchospasm, dyspnea, wheezing, meningitis aseptic, meningitis, edema, swelling, and peripheral edema.

OVERDOSE:
In case of accidental overdose, contact a physician or poison control centre immediately, even if there are no symptoms.
Symptoms: Methocarbamol overdose toxicity or death has not been reported. One adult survived the deliberate ingestion of 22 to 30 g of methocarbamol without serious toxicity. Another survived 30 to 50 g. The principal symptom was drowsiness in both cases. However, 3 deaths have been reported when methocarbamol was combined with alcohol and other drugs.

Clinical findings associated with major ibuprofen overdose include abdominal pain, nausea, vomiting, lethargy and drowsiness. Other CNS symptoms include headache, tinnitus, CNS depression, dizziness, drowsiness, seizures, apnea and stupor, rarely progressing to coma. Examination may reveal hyper- or hypothermia, abnormal respiration ranging from hyperventilation to respiratory depression, hypotension, sinus tachycardia or bradycardia, and abnormal neurological and neuromuscular activity with ataxia, nystagmus, and seizure activity. Subsequently, renal dysfunction with oliguria or anuria may supervene, and clinical evidence of bleeding due to hypoprothrombinemia and thrombocytopenia may occur later. An elevated anion gap metabolic acidosis can be seen following large ingestions.

The toxicity of ibuprofen overdose is dependent upon the amount of drug ingested and the time elapsed since ingestion; individual responses may vary, thus making it necessary to evaluate each case separately. Although uncommon, serious toxicity and death have been reported with ibuprofen overdosage. The most frequently reported symptoms of ibuprofen overdose include abdominal pain, nausea, vomiting, lethargy, vertigo, drowsiness (somnolence), dizziness and insomnia. Other CNS symptoms include headache, loss of consciousness, tinnitus, CNS depression, convulsions and seizures. Metabolic acidosis, abnormal hepatic function, hyperkalemia, renal failure, dyspnea, respiratory depressions coma, acute renal failure, and apnea (primarily in very young pediatric patients) may rarely occur. Cardiovascular toxicity, including hypotension, bradycardia, tachycardia and atrial fibrillation, also have been reported.
Treatment: Acute ibuprofen overdose does not normally result in significant morbidity or mortality, although serious toxicity has been reported following very large overdoses. Deaths have been rare. Treatment is directed towards specific clinical signs and symptoms, and is generally supportive.

Adverse effects associated with ibuprofen overdose usually depend on the amount of drug ingested and time elapsed; however, because each individual response may vary, each occurrence of overdose has to be evaluated individually. In general, ingestion of up to 200 mg/kg will not cause symptoms of toxicity, and observation at home is recommended. If symptoms are to appear, they will occur within 4 hours of poisoning, and the patient should be taken to a medical facility.

For overdoses >200 mg/kg (ibuprofen), the patient should be referred to a medical facility and gastrointestinal decontamination with administration of activated charcoal (1 g/kg) should be instituted. However, little drug is likely to be captured if the time elapsed after ingestion is greater than 1 hour. Because seizures can occur in children with ibuprofen overdose, emesis should not be induced at this level of overdose. The onset of symptoms is usually within 4 hours of ingestion so the patient should be observed for at least this period of time.

For overdoses greater than 400 mg/kg (ibuprofen), in-hospital observation is indicated. Initial laboratory tests should include arterial blood gases, electrolyte levels, blood urea nitrogen (BUN), creatinine, and liver function studies.

In pediatric patients, the estimated amount of ibuprofen ingested per body weight may be helpful to predict the potential for development of toxicity although each case must be evaluated. Ingestion of less than 100 mg/kg is unlikely to produce toxicity. Pediatric patients ingesting 100 to 200 mg/kg may be managed with induced emesis and a minimal observation time of at least four hours. Pediatric patients ingesting 200 to 400 mg/kg of ibuprofen should have immediate gastric emptying and at least four hours observation. Pediatric patients ingesting greater than 400 mg/kg require immediate medical referral, careful observation and appropriate supportive therapy. Ipecac-induced emesis is not recommended in overdoses greater than 400 mg/kg because of the risk for convulsions and the potential for aspiration of gastric contents.
Methocarbamol Overdose Treatment: Within ½ to 1 hour of ingestion, gastric lavage and/or emesis may reduce absorption. Supportive measures include maintenance of an adequate airway, monitoring urinary output and vital signs and the administration of i.v. fluids, if necessary. There is no experience with forced diuresis or with dialysis in the treatment of methocarbamol overdose. Likewise, the usefulness of hemodialysis in managing methocarbamol overdose is unknown.

For management of a suspected drug overdose, CPhA recommends that you contact your **regional Poison Control Centre**. See the *CPS* Directory section for a list of Poison Control Centres.

DOSAGE: Adult Dosage: Adults and Children over 12 years: 1 to 2 caplets every 4-6 hours. Do not exceed 6 caplets in 24 hours, unless recommended by a physician.

SUPPLIED: Each biconvex, bilayer blue-grey and white caplet with "RO" on one side contains: methocarbamol 500 mg and ibuprofen 200 mg. Nonmedicinal ingredients: FD&C Blue No. 2, ferric oxide (red), hypromellose, magnesium stearate, methylcellulose, microcrystalline cellulose, polyethylene glycol, povidone, sodium lauryl sulfate and sodium starch glycolate. Blisters of 18. Bottles of 40 and 60. Store in closed containers under room temperature (15 to 30°C) conditions. Protect from light.

Robitussin®
guaifenesin
Expectorant

Pfizer Consumer Healthcare

Robitussin® DM
guaifenesin—dextromethorphan HBr
Expectorant—Antitussive

Pfizer Consumer Healthcare

Robitussin® DM Cough Control
guaifenesin—dextromethorphan HBr
Expectorant—Antitussive

Pfizer Consumer Healthcare

Robitussin® DM CoughGels™
dextromethorphan HBr
Antitussive

Pfizer Consumer Healthcare

Robitussin® Cough & Cold
guaifenesin—dextromethorphan HBr—pseudoephedrine HCl
Expectorant—Antitussive—Decongestant

Pfizer Consumer Healthcare

Robitussin® Extra Strength
guaifenesin
Expectorant

Pfizer Consumer Healthcare

Robitussin® Extra Strength DM Cough Control
guaifenesin—dextromethorphan HBr
Expectorant—Antitussive

Pfizer Consumer Healthcare

Robitussin® Extra Strength Cough & Cold
guaifenesin—dextromethorphan HBr—pseudoephedrine HCl
Expectorant—Antitussive—Decongestant

Pfizer Consumer Healthcare

Robitussin® Children's Cough & Cold
dextromethorphan HBr—pseudoephedrine HCl
Antitussive—Decongestant

Pfizer Consumer Healthcare

Robitussin® Total Cough Cold and Flu
acetaminophen—dextromethorphan HBr—pseudoephedrine HCl
Pain Reliever—Antitussive—Decongestant

Pfizer Consumer Healthcare

Robitussin® Total Extra Strength Nighttime, Cough Cold and Flu
acetaminophen—dextromethorphan HBr—pseudoephedrine HCl—chlorpheniramine maleate
Pain Reliever—Antitussive—Decongestant

Pfizer Consumer Healthcare

PHARMACOLOGY: Guaifenesin, as the expectorant, enhances the output of lower respiratory tract fluid. The enhanced flow of less viscid secretions promotes ciliary action, and facilitates the removal of inspissated mucus. As a result, dry, unproductive coughs become more productive and less frequent.

Dextromethorphan is a synthetic, non-narcotic, centrally-acting cough suppressant. The antitussive effectiveness of dextromethorphan has been demonstrated in both animal and human clinical studies, and the incidence of toxic effects has been remarkably low.

Pseudoephedrine produces vasoconstriction resulting in a nasal decongestant effect.

Acetaminophen has analgesic and antipyretic properties. It will reduce aches, pains and fever associated with cough, cold and flu symptoms.

Chlorpheniramine is an orally effective antihistamine (H_1-receptor antagonist) when administered in doses of 2 to 4 mg/dose, up to 24 mg/day. Chlorpheniramine has antihistaminic and anticholinergic properties.
INDICATIONS: For the management of coughs associated with cold, bronchitis, laryngitis, tracheitis, pharyngitis and influenza.

CONTRAINDICATIONS: Hypersensitivity to guaifenesin, dextromethorphan or sympathomimetic amines; marked hypertension; patients who are receiving MAO inhibitors should not take Robitussin DM, DM Cough Control, DM Coughgels, Cough & Cold, Extra Strength DM, Extra Strength Cough & Cold, Children's Cough & Cold or Robitussin Total Cough Cold and Flu and Robitussin Total Extra Strength Nighttime Cough Cold and Flu.

Patients with diabetes, heart or thyroid disease, high blood pressure, glaucoma or difficulty in urination due to prostate enlargement should not take Robitussin Cough & Cold, Extra Strength Cough & Cold, Children's Cough & Cold or Robitussin Total Cough Cold and Flu and Robitussin Total Extra Strength Nighttime Cough Cold and Flu.

PRECAUTIONS: Before prescribing medication to suppress or modify cough, it is important to ascertain that the underlying cause of the cough is identified, that modification of the cough does not increase the risk of clinical or physiologic complications, and that appropriate therapy for the primary disease is provided.

If cough worsens, lasts for more than 5 days or is accompanied by high fever, rash or persistent headache (as these could be signs of a serious condition), or in patients with hypertension, consult a physician.

Do not exceed recommended dosage. Keep safely out of reach of children.

This package contains enough medication to seriously harm a child.

Do not use if you have an allergy to any of the listed ingredients.

Robitussin Total Cough Cold and Flu and Robitussin Total Extra Strength Nighttime Cough Cold and Flu: Do not use with other products containing acetaminophen. Taking more than the maximum daily dose may cause severe or possibly fatal liver damage. Stop use and consult a doctor if you develop allergic reactions such as wheezing, rash or itching, if symptoms last more than 5 days or fever lasts more than 3 days.

Consult a healthcare professional before using this product if you suffer from persistent/chronic cough (as occurs with smoking), breathing problems, shortness of breath or chronic lung disease (e.g. chronic bronchitis, asthma or emphysema), if you are pregnant, nursing, or if you have taken a drug for high blood pressure or depression in the past 14 days, including monoamine oxidase inhibitors (MAOIs). Or if you suffer from chronic alcoholism, serious liver or kidney disease, diabetes, heart or thyroid disease, high blood pressure, glaucoma or difficulty urinating due to an enlarged prostate, consult a physician before taking.

Robitussin Children's Cough and Cold: Do not use longer than 7 days. Do not give with other antitussives, nasal decongestants or any other cough and cold medications since harm may occur. Stop use and consult a physician if cough or symptoms worsen or persist for more than 7 days or are accompanied by a high fever (>38°C), rash, persistent headache or the production of thick yellow/green phlegm as these could be signs of a serious condition.

ADVERSE EFFECTS: The following may possibly occur: Robitussin, Robitussin Extra-Strength: nausea, gastrointestinal upset, drowsiness.

Robitussin Cough & Cold, Robitussin Extra-Strength Cough & Cold: nausea, vomiting, dry mouth, nervousness, insomnia.

Robitussin DM, Robitussin DM Cough Control, Robitussin Extra Strength DM: drowsiness, dizziness, nausea, vomiting, confusion.

Robitussin DM CoughGels, Robitussin Children's: drowsiness, dizziness, nausea, vomiting, stomach ache.

Robitussin Children's Cough & Cold: drowsiness, dizziness, nausea, vomiting, stomach ache, insomnia, confusion, CNS stimulation, muscular weakness, dry mouth, palpitation, difficulty in micturition, wheezing, rash, itching, breathing difficulties, convulsions, drowsiness, hallucinations, rapid heart rate.

Robitussin Total Cough Cold & Flu: drowsiness, dizziness, nausea, vomiting, stomach ache, insomnia, confusion, CNS stimulation, muscular weakness, dry mouth, palpitation, difficulty in micturition, abdominal pain, rash, urticaria.

Robitussin Total Extra Strength Nighttime Cough and Cold: drowsiness, dizziness, nausea, vomiting, stomach ache, insomnia, confusion, CNS stimulation, muscular weakness, dry mouth, palpitation, difficulty in micturition, excitability, abdominal pain, rash, urticaria.

OVERDOSE:

In case of accidental overdose, contact a physician or poison control centre immediately, even if there are no symptoms.

> For management of a suspected drug overdose, CPhA recommends that you contact your **regional Poison Control Centre**. See the *CPS* Directory section for a list of Poison Control Centres.

DOSAGE: **Robitussin:** Take every 6-8 hours as follows: Maximum 4 doses/day. Adults and children 12 years and over: 10 to 20 mL. Children under 12 years: **Do not use.**

Robitussin DM and Cough & Cold: Take every 6 to 8 hours as follows: Maximum 4 doses/day. Adults and children 12 years and over: 10 mL. Children under 12 years: **Do not use.**

Robitussin DM Cough Control: Take every 6-8 hours or as directed by a physician. Maximum 4 doses/day. Adults and children 12 years and over: 15 mL. Children under 12 years: **Do not use.**

Robitussin DM CoughGels: Take every 6-8 hours as follows: Adults and children 12 years and over: 2 capsules. Children 6 to 11: 1 capsule. Maximum 4 doses/day. Children under 12 years: **Do not use.**

Robitussin Extra Strength, Extra Strength DM and Extra Strength Cough & Cold: Take every 6 to 8 hours as follows: Adults and children 12 years and over: 10 mL. Children under 12 years: **Do not use.**

Robitussin Children's Cough & Cold: Take every 6 to 8 hours as follows: Children 6 to under 12 years: 2 tsp, 10 mL. Children under 6 years: **Do not use.**

Robitussin Total Cough Cold & Flu: Take every 6 hours or as directed by a physician: Adults (12 years and over): 2 tablespoons (30 mL). Children under 12 years: **Do not use.**

Robitussin Total Extra Strength Nighttime Cough and Cold: Take every 6 hours or as directed by a physician: Adults (12 years and over): 2 tablespoons (30 mL). Children under 12 years: **Do not use.**

SUPPLIED: **Robitussin:** Each 5 mL of red, cherry-flavored syrup contains: guaifenesin 100 mg. Nonmedicinal ingredients: alcohol, caramel color, citric acid, flavor, glycerin, invert sugar, FD&C Red No. 40, sodium benzoate, sodium chloride and water. Energy: 15.3 kJ (3.7 kcal). Sodium: <1 mmol (2.8 mg). Bottles of 100 and 250 mL. Store at room temperature (15 to 30°C).

Robitussin DM: Each 5 mL of red, cherry-flavored syrup contains: guaifenesin 100 mg and dextromethorphan HBr 15 mg. Nonmedicinal ingredients: alcohol, citric acid, flavors, FD&C Red No. 40, FD&C Yellow No. 6, glycerin, invert sugar, sodium benzoate and water. Energy: 12.4 kJ (3.0 kcal). Sodium: <1 mmol (0.8 mg). Bottles of 100 and 250 mL. Store at room temperature (15 to 30°C).

Robitussin DM Cough Control: Each 5 mL of clear, colorless to slightly yellow, cherry-flavored syrup contains: guaifenesin 100 mg and dextromethorphan HBr 10 mg. Nonmedicinal ingredients: acesulfame potassium, citric acid, flavors, glycerin, methylparaben, polyethylene glycol, povidone, saccharin sodium, sodium benzoate and water. Low sodium. Alcohol-, dye- and sugar-free. Bottles of 115 mL. Store at room temperature (15 to 30°C).

Robitussin DM CoughGels: Each red colored, liquid-filled capsule contains: dextromethorphan HBr 15 mg. Nonmedicinal ingredients: coconut oil, FD&C Blue No. 1, FD&C Red No. 40, gelatin, glycerin, mannitol, polyethylene glycol, polyvinyl acetate phthalate, povidone, propyl gallate, propylene glycol, sorbitol, sorbitol anhydrides, titanium dioxide and water. Energy: <4.2 kJ (1 kcal). Sodium: <1 mmol (0.78 mg). Alcohol- and sucrose-free. Blister packs of 20. Store at room temperature (15 to 30°C).

Robitussin Cough & Cold: Each 5 mL of pink, cherry-flavored syrup contains: guaifenesin 100 mg, pseudoephedrine HCl 30 mg and dextromethorphan HBr 15 mg. Nonmedicinal ingredients: alcohol, citric acid, flavors, D&C Red No. 33, FD&C Red No. 40, glycerin, invert sugar, sodium benzoate and water. Energy: 17.6 kJ (4.2 kcal). Sodium: <1 mmol (0.8 mg). Bottles of 100 and 250 mL. Store at room temperature (15 to 30°C).

Robitussin Extra Strength: Each 5 mL of red, cherry-flavored syrup contains: guaifenesin 200 mg. Nonmedicinal ingredients: citric acid, corn syrup, FD&C Red No. 40, flavors, glycerin, polyethylene glycol, propylene glycol, sodium benzoate, sodium carboxymethylcellulose, sodium saccharin, sorbitol and water. Energy: 49 kJ (11.7 kcal). Sodium: <1 mmol (4.1 mg). Bottles of 100 and 250 mL. Store at room temperature (15 to 30°C).

Robitussin Extra Strength Cough & Cold: Each 5 mL of red, cherry-flavored syrup contains: guaifenesin 200 mg, dextromethorphan HBr 15 mg, pseudoephedrine HCl 30 mg. Nonmedicinal ingredients: citric acid, corn syrup, FD&C Red No. 40, flavors, glycerin, polyethylene glycol, propylene glycol, sodium benzoate, sodium carboxymethylcellulose, sodium saccharin, sorbitol and water. Energy: 49 kJ (11.7 kcal). Sodium: <1 mmol (4.1 mg). Bottles of 100 and 250 mL. Store at room temperature (15 to 30°C).

Robitussin Extra Strength DM: Each 5 mL of red, cherry-flavored syrup contains: guaifenesin 200 mg, dextromethorphan HBr 15 mg. Nonmedicinal ingredients: citric acid, corn syrup, FD&C Red No. 40, flavors, glycerin, polyethylene glycol, propylene glycol, sodium benzoate, sodium carboxymethylcellulose, sodium saccharin, sorbitol and water. Energy: 49 kJ (11.7 kcal). Sodium: <1 mmol (4.1 mg). Bottles of 100 and 250 mL. Store at room temperature (15 to 30°C).

Robitussin Children's Cough & Cold: Each 5 mL of red, grape-flavored syrup contains: dextromethorphan HBr 7.5 mg and pseudoephedrine HCl 15 mg. Nonmedicinal ingredients: citric acid, D&C Red No. 33, FD&C Blue No. 1, FD&C Red No. 40, flavors, glycerin, maltol, sodium saccharin, sodium benzoate, sodium chloride, sodium cyclamate, sorbitol and water. Energy: 5.02 kJ (1.2 kcal). Sodium: <1 mmol (1.7 mg). Bottles of 100 mL. Store at room temperature (15 to 30°C).

Robitussin Total Cough Cold and Flu: Each 30 mL of red, cherry flavoured syrup contains: acetaminophen 650 mg, dextromethorphan HBr 30 mg and pseudoephedrine HCl 30 mg. Nonmedicinal ingredients: citric acid, D&C Red No. 33, FD&C Red No. 40, flavours, glycerin, polyethylene glycol, propylene glycol, sodium benzoate, sodium carboxymethylcellulose, sodium citrate dihydrate, sorbitol, sucralose and water. Energy: 6.7 kcal/5 mL. Sodium: 60 mg/30 mL. Bottles of 115 mL and 240 mL. Store at room temperature (15 to 30°C).

Robitussin Total Extra Strength Nighttime, Cough Cold and Flu: Each 30 mL of red, cherry flavoured syrup contains: acetaminophen 1000 mg, dextromethorphan HBr 30 mg, pseudoephedrine HCl 60 mg and chlorpheniramine maleate 4 mg. Nonmedicinal Ingredients: citric acid, D&C Red No. 33, FD&C Red No. 40, flavours, glycerin, polyethylene glycol, propylene glycol, sodium benzoate, sodium carboxymethylcellulose, sodium citrate dihydrate, sorbitol, sucralose and water. Energy: 6.7 kcal/5 mL. Sodium: 60 mg/30 mL. Bottles of 115 mL and 240 mL. Store at room temperature (15 to 30°C).

Robitussin® AC Ⓝ

guaifenesin—codeine phosphate—pheniramine maleate

Expectorant—Antitussive—Antihistamine

Pfizer Consumer Healthcare

INDICATIONS: To facilitate expectoration and control cough associated with inflamed mucosa temporarily.

CONTRAINDICATIONS: Hypersensitivity to codeine, guaifenesin or pheniramine, or pre-existing respiratory depression.

Patients allergic to codeine or other opioids, have suffered head injury, are at risk of blocked intestines or suffer from seizures.

PRECAUTIONS: Keep out of reach of children.

Do not exceed recommended dosage.

This package contains sufficient medication to seriously harm a child.

Stop use and consult a doctor if symptoms worsen or persist for more than 7 days or if high fever, rash or persistent headache is present, as these may be signs of a serious condition.

Patients should be advised to use under the direction of a physician if medication has been taken in the last 14 days for high blood pressure or depression, including monoamine oxidase inhibitors (MAOIs), or if taking other antihistamines, decongestants, tranquilizers or sedating drugs.

Sedatives and tranquilizers may increase drowsiness.

Administer with caution to patients with cardiac or peripheral vascular disease, glaucoma, hyperthyroidism, diabetes mellitus or hypertension, persistent chronic cough (as occurs with smoking), breathing problems or shortness of breath, chronic lung disease (e.g., chronic bronchitis, asthma or emphysema), prostate enlargement and bladder neck obstruction and in pregnancy or lactation.

Product may cause drowsiness or excitability. Avoid alcohol, driving a motor vehicle or operating machinery.

Before prescribing medication to suppress or modify cough, it is important to ascertain that the underlying cause of the cough is identified, that modification of the cough does not increase the risk of clinical or physiologic complications, and that appropriate therapy for the primary disease is provided.

In young children the respiratory centre is especially susceptible to the depressant action of narcotics. Benefit to risk ratio should be carefully considered especially in children with respiratory embarrassment, e.g., croup. Estimation of dosage relative to the child's age and weight is of great importance.

Tolerance, psychological dependence and physical dependence may develop in patients receiving codeine phosphate over a prolonged period.

Use with extreme caution in patients having an acute asthmatic attack, patients with chronic obstructive pulmonary disease or cor pulmonale, patients having a substantially decreased respiratory reserve and patients with pre-existing respiratory depression, hypoxia or hypercapnia. Usual therapeutic doses may decrease respiratory drive while simultaneously increasing airway resistance to the point of apnea. In patients with asthma or pulmonary emphysema, codeine may, due to its drying action on the respiratory mucosa, increase viscosity of bronchial secretions and suppress the cough reflex.

Use with caution in sedated or debilitated patients, in patients who have undergone thoracotomies or laparotomies, since suppression of the cough reflex may lead to retention of secretions postoperatively in these patients.

The respiratory depressant effects of codeine and its capacity to elevate cerebrospinal fluid pressure may be markedly exaggerated in the presence of head injury or intracranial lesions or pre-existing increase in intracranial pressure. Narcotics produce adverse reactions which may obscure the clinical course of a patient with head injuries. In such patients, codeine must be used with extreme caution and only if its use is deemed essential.

Use with caution in patients with seizures as the seizures may be exacerbated or induced by opioids.

Use with caution in patients with cardiac arrhythmias due to the cholinergic effects of the drug.

Codeine should be given with caution and the initial dose should be reduced in certain patients such as the debilitated and those with severe impairment of hepatic or renal function, hypothyroidism, Addison's disease, prostatic hypertrophy or urethral stricture.

Geriatrics: Elderly patients may be more susceptible to the adverse effects of codeine, especially respiratory depression. Use with caution; the initial dose should be reduced and the effects monitored.

The administration of codeine or other narcotics may obscure the diagnosis or clinical course in patients with acute abdominal conditions.

Codeine should not be used in patients with diarrhea associated with pseudomembranous colitis.

Use with caution in patients with acute ulcerative colitis or other severe inflammatory bowel disease due to the risk of toxic megacolon.

Caution should be exercised and dosage may need to be reduced when administered with other drugs that depress the CNS (including alcohol), with MAO inhibitors, phenothiazines or tricyclic antidepressants.

Consult your doctor if you feel sedated or drowsy, confused, have shallow breathing or have severe constipation.

Do not administer to patients with glaucoma or prostate enlargement.

Occupational Hazards: Warn patients against driving or operating machinery if they become drowsy or show impaired mental and/or physical abilities while taking codeine.

Pregnancy: Since codeine phosphate crosses the placental barrier, its use in pregnancy is not recommended.

Codeine may cause harm to a breast fed baby. Contact your physician immediately if you are breastfeeding and your baby is having difficulty breathing or feeding, or is very sleepy or limp.

Lactation: Codeine is excreted in small amounts which are probably insignificant with usual analgesic or antitussive doses.

ADVERSE EFFECTS: Adverse reactions due to codeine phosphate may include drowsiness, nausea, vomiting and constipation. Infrequent adverse effects include palpitation, dry mouth, skin rash, pruritus and, rarely, hyperhidrosis and agitation have been reported. Respiratory depression is seen in higher dosage, and there is a potential for tolerance, psychological dependence or physical dependence to occur.

OVERDOSE:

In case of accidental overdose, contact a physician or poison control centre immediately, even if there are no symptoms.

Symptoms: May result in euphoria, dysphoria, visual disturbances, hypotension and coma or death from respiratory depression.

Treatment: Symptomatic and supportive therapy. Maintain ventilation and administer oxygen as needed. The narcotic antagonist naloxone should be administered. If the patient is conscious and has not lost the gag reflex, empty the stomach by inducing emesis with ipecac syrup. If the patient is extremely drowsy, unconscious, convulsing or has no gag reflex, perform gastric lavage. Follow with activated charcoal (50 to 100 g in adults) and a cathartic.

> For management of a suspected drug overdose, CPhA recommends that you contact your **regional Poison Control Centre**. See the *CPS* Directory section for a list of Poison Control Centres.

DOSAGE: Take every 4 to 6 hours as follows: Adults 12 years and over: 10 mL (2 tsp). Children under 12: **Do not use.** Maximum 6 doses daily.

SUPPLIED: Each 5 mL of orange, cherry-flavored syrup contains: guaifenesin 100 mg, codeine phosphate 10 mg and pheniramine maleate 7.5 mg. Nonmedicinal ingredients: alcohol, caramel, citric acid, FD&C Red No. 40, FD&C yellow No. 6, flavors, glycerin, invert sugar, purified water and sodium benzoate. Energy: 48 kJ (11.48 kcal)/5 mL. Sodium: <1 mmol (0.8 mg). Bottles of 1 L. Store at room temperature (15 to 30°C).

Rocaltrol® Pr

calcitriol

Vitamin D3 Metabolite

Roche

Date of Preparation: June 6, 1979
Date of Revision: January 26, 2009

PHARMACOLOGY: The supply of vitamin D in man depends on dietary intake and/or exposure to the ultraviolet rays of the sun for conversion of 7-dehydrocholesterol to vitamin D_3 (cholecalciferol). Vitamin D_3 must be metabolized in the liver and the kidney before it is fully active on its target tissues. The initial transformation is catalyzed by a vitamin D_3-25-hydroxylase enzyme (25-OHase) present in the liver, and the product of this reaction is 25-hydroxy-vitamin D_3 (25-OH-D_3). The latter undergoes hydroxylation in the mitochondria of kidney tissue. This reaction is activated by the renal 25-hydroxy-vitamin D_3-1 alphahydroxylase (alpha-OHase) to produce 1,25-$(OH)_2D_3$ (calcitriol).

The 2 known sites of action of calcitriol are intestine and bone, but additional evidence suggests that it also acts on the kidney and the parathyroid gland.

In acutely uremic rats, calcitriol has been shown to stimulate calcium absorption. It is the most active known form of vitamin D_3 in stimulating intestinal calcium transport. This agent also promotes the intestinal absorption of phosphorus through stimulation of an active transport system distinct from the calcium transport process.

Calcitriol stimulates bone resorption which serves to mobilize calcium for the circulation, when an intestinal source of calcium is absent. This effect is related to the role of vitamin D in maintaining the homeostasis of calcium and phosphorus in plasma. In addition, calcitriol may interact directly with osteoblasts.

Calcitriol's effects on the renal transport of calcium and phosphate appear to be influenced by the presence or absence of the parathyroid glands, vitamin D status, volume expansion and the dose of vitamin D metabolite used. With the available information it is not possible to determine which vitamin D metabolite, if any, influences divalent ion transport by the renal tubule under physiologic conditions or if so, whether an interaction with parathyroid hormone is required.

The presence of a direct negative feedback effect of calcitriol on the parathyroid gland has been suspected. Some investigators have postulated that calcitriol may exert a direct influence on the parathyroids. Although inhibition of PTH secretion by calcitriol has been demonstrated in vitro, the data obtained from in vivo studies are more equivocal.

INDICATIONS: Rocaltrol (calcitriol) is indicated in the management of:
- Hypocalcemia and osteodystrophy in patients with chronic renal failure undergoing dialysis.
- Hypocalcemia and its clinical manifestations associated with:
  - Post surgical hypoparathyroidism
  - Idiopathic hypoparathyroidism
  - Pseudohypoparathyroidism
- Vitamin D resistant rickets (familial hypophosphatemia).

CONTRAINDICATIONS: Rocaltrol (calcitriol) should not be given to patients with hypercalcemia or with a known hypersensitivity to calcitriol, vitamin D or its analogues and derivatives. It should not be administered if there is evidence of vitamin D overdosage.

WARNINGS: Since Rocaltrol (calcitriol) is a potent cholecalciferol derivative with profound effects on intestinal absorption of dietary calcium and inorganic phosphate, it should not be used concomitantly with other vitamin D products or their derivatives.

Therapy with Rocaltrol should only be considered when adequate laboratory facilities for monitoring of blood and urine chemistries are available. During treatment progressive hypercalcemia either due to hyper-responsiveness or overdosage may become so severe as to require emergency treatment.

Chronic hypercalcemia can lead to generalized vascular calcification, nephrocalcinosis, calcifications of the cornea or other soft tissues. During treatment with Rocaltrol **the serum total calcium (mg/dL) times serum inorganic phosphate product (Ca x P) should not exceed 70 mg^2/dL^2.**

Dialysate calcium level of 7 mg % or above in addition to excessive dietary calcium supplements may lead to frequent episodes of hypercalcemia.

In patients on digitalis, hypercalcemia may precipitate cardiac arrhythmias; in such patients, Rocaltrol should be used with extreme caution.

To control serum inorganic phosphate levels and dietary phosphate absorption in patients undergoing dialysis, oral aluminum carbonate or aluminum hydroxide gel must be used. Magnesium containing antacids may contribute towards hypermagnesemia in patients on chronic renal dialysis and should be avoided during therapy with Rocaltrol.

Pregnancy: The safety of Rocaltrol in women who are or may become pregnant has not been established; use of Rocaltrol in these cases may be considered only when the potential benefits have been weighed against possible hazards to mother and fetus.

Lactation: Rocaltrol may be excreted in human milk. In view of the potential for hypercalcemia in the mother and for adverse reactions from Rocaltrol in nursing infants, mothers may breastfeed while taking Rocaltrol, provided that the serum calcium levels of the mother and infant are monitored.

PRECAUTIONS: Patient Selection and Follow-up: Patients with renal osteodystrophy and hypocalcemia, poorly managed by conventional vitamin D therapy are likely to respond to Rocaltrol (calcitriol). The desired therapeutic margin of Rocaltrol is narrow; therefore, the optimal daily dose must be carefully determined for each patient by dose titration to obtain satisfactory response in the biochemical parameters and clinical manifestations (see Dosage).

Excessive dosage of Rocaltrol induces hypercalcemia and hypercalciuria; therefore, early in treatment during dosage adjustment serum calcium should be determined at least twice weekly. A fall in serum alkaline phosphatase values may indicate impending hypercalcemia. Should hypercalcemia develop, the drug should be discontinued immediately until the serum calcium has normalized. This may take several days to a week.

In patients with normal renal function, chronic hypercalcemia may be associated with an increase in serum creatinine. While the elevation of serum creatinine is usually reversible, it is important in such patients to pay careful attention to those factors which may lead to hypercalcemia. Rocaltrol therapy should always be started at the lowest possible dose and increased with careful monitoring of serum calcium concentrations. An estimate of daily dietary calcium intake should be made and the intake adjusted when indicated.

Patients with normal renal function taking Rocaltrol should avoid dehydration. Adequate fluid intake should be maintained.

Patients with vitamin D resistant rickets (familial hypophosphatemia) should pursue their oral phosphate therapy. However, the possible stimulation of intestinal phosphate absorption by Rocaltrol should be taken into account since this effect may modify the requirement for phosphate supplements.

Essential Laboratory Tests: Serum calcium, inorganic phosphorus, magnesium, alkaline phosphatase as well as 24-hour urinary calcium and phosphorus should be determined periodically during maintenance therapy with Rocaltrol. During the initial phase of the medication, serum calcium should be determined more frequently (at least twice weekly). Periodic ophthalmological examinations and radiological evaluation of suspected anatomical regions for early detection of ectopic calcifications are advisable.

Drug Interactions: Hypercalcemia in patients on digitalis may precipitate cardiac arrhythmias. Intestinal absorption of Rocaltrol may be impaired by resins such as cholestyramine and by use of mineral oil as a laxative. Although the precise mechanism involved is unknown, there is evidence that long-term anticonvulsant treatment, particularly with diphenylhydantoin and barbiturates, may interfere with the actions of vitamin D. Patients under concurrent treatment with such agents may require slightly higher doses of Rocaltrol.

Information to Be Provided to the Patient: The patient and his or her immediate relatives should be informed about the need for compliance with dosage instructions, strict adherence to prescribed calcium intake, dietary and supplementary, and avoidance of unapproved non-prescription drugs or medications. Patients should also be made aware of the symptoms of hypercalcemia and should seek medical attention if such symptoms are noted (see Adverse Effects).

ADVERSE EFFECTS: The following adverse reactions, based on clinical studies, have been reported in association with Rocaltrol treatment:

1. Most frequent: hypercalcemia (20-30%).
2. Less frequent: headache, nausea, vomiting, constipation, abdominal cramp, pruritis, conjunctivitis, agitation, extremity pain, apprehension, polyuria, insomnia, elevated AST and/or ALT, elevated alkaline phosphatase, hypercalciuria, hypermagnesemia, hyperphosphatemia, elevated lymphocytes, elevated hematocrit, elevated neutrophils, elevated hemoglobin.

The number of adverse effects reported from clinical use of Rocaltrol over a period of 15 years in all indications is very low with each individual effect, including hypercalcemia, occurring at a rate of 0.001% or less.

Hypersensitivity reactions (pruritus, rash, urticaria, and very rarely severe erythematous skin disorders) may occur in susceptible individuals. The adverse effects of Rocaltrol (calcitriol) are, in general, similar to those encountered with excessive vitamin D intake. The early and late signs and symptoms associated with vitamin D intoxication and hypercalcemia are:

1. Early: weakness, headache, somnolence, nausea, cardiac arrhythmias, excessive thirst, vomiting, dry mouth, constipation, muscle pain, bone pain, metallic taste, abdominal pain or stomach ache.
2. Late: polyuria, polydipsia, urinary tract infections, anorexia, weight loss, nocturia, conjunctivitis (calcific), pancreatitis, photophobia, rhinorrhea, pruritus, hyperthermia, decreased libido, elevated BUN, albuminuria, hypercholesterolemia, elevated AST and ALT, ectopic calcification, hypertension, cardiac arrhythmias, and rarely, overt psychosis.

OVERDOSE:

Symptoms: Administration of Rocaltrol (calcitriol) to patients in excess of their daily requirements can cause hypercalcemia, hypercalciuria and hyperphosphatemia. Conversely, high intake of calcium and phosphate concomitantly with therapeutic doses of Rocaltrol may cause similar abnormalities. In dialysis patients, high levels of calcium in the dialysis bath may contribute to hypercalcemia. The serum calcium times phosphate (Ca x P) product should not be allowed to exceed 70 mg^2/dL^2.

Treatment: Treatment of Hypercalcemia and Overdosage: General treatment of hypercalcemia (more than 1 mg/dL or 0.25 mmol/L above the upper limit of the normal range) or serum creatinine more than 120 µmol/L consists of immediate discontinuation of Rocaltrol therapy, institution of a low calcium diet and withdrawal of calcium supplements. Serum calcium and phosphate levels should be determined daily until normocalcemia ensues. Hypercalcemia frequently resolves in 2 to 7 days. When serum calcium concentrations have returned to within normal limits, 'Rocaltrol' therapy may be reinstituted at a dose of 0.25 µg/day less than prior therapy. Serum calcium levels should be carefully monitored (at least twice weekly) during this period of dosage adjustment and subsequent dosage titration. In dialysis patients, persistent or markedly elevated serum calcium levels may be corrected by dialysis against a calcium-free dialysate.

Treatment of Accidental Overdosage: The treatment of acute accidental overdosage with Rocaltrol should consist of general supportive measures. If drug ingestion is discovered within a relatively short time, induction of emesis or gastric lavage may be of benefit in preventing further absorption. If the drug has passed through the stomach, the administration of mineral oil may promote its fecal elimination. Serial serum electrolyte determinations (especially calcium ion) rate of urinary calcium excretion and assessment of electrocardiographic abnormalities due to hypercalcemia should be obtained. Such monitoring is critical in patients receiving digitalis. Discontinuation of supplemental calcium and low calcium diet are also indicated in accidental overdosage. Due to the relatively short pharmacological action of calcitriol, further measures are probably unnecessary. Should, however, persistent and markedly elevated serum calcium levels occur, there are a variety of therapeutic alternatives which may be considered, depending on the patient's underlying condition. These include the use of drugs such as phosphates and corticosteroids as well as measures to induce an appropriate forced diuresis. The use of peritoneal dialysis against a calcium-free dialysate has also been reported.

For management of a suspected drug overdose, CPhA recommends that you contact your **regional Poison Control Centre**. See the *CPS* Directory section for a list of Poison Control Centres.

DOSAGE: The optimal daily dose of Rocaltrol (calcitriol) must be carefully determined for each patient. The effectiveness of calcitriol therapy is predicated on the assumption that each patient is receiving an adequate daily intake of calcium. The recommended daily intake for calcium is in the order of 800 mg for adults and 350 mg for infants during the first 6 months of life.

To ensure that each patient receives an adequate daily intake of calcium, the physician should either prescribe a calcium supplement or instruct the patient in appropriate dietary measures.

However, because of improved calcium absorption from the gastrointestinal tract, some patients on Rocaltrol may be maintained on a lower calcium intake or no supplementation at all.

Dialysis Patients: Adults: Titration: The recommended initial dose of Rocaltrol is 0.25 µg/day. If a satisfactory response in the biochemical parameters and clinical manifestations of the disease state are not observed, dosage may be increased by 0.25 µg/day at 2- to 4-week intervals. During this titration period, serum calcium levels should be obtained at least twice weekly, and if hypercalcemia is noted, the drug should be immediately discontinued until normocalcemia ensues.

Maintenance: Patients with normal or only slightly reduced serum calcium levels may respond to Rocaltrol doses of 0.25 µg every other day. Most patients undergoing hemodialysis respond to between 0.5 and 1 µg/day.

In order to decrease the risk of hypercalcemic episodes, a downward adjustment of the dose of Rocaltrol may be advisable once a reduction in serum alkaline phosphatase has been achieved.

Hypoparathyroidism and Vitamin D Resistant Rickets: Adults: The recommended initial dose of Rocaltrol is 0.25 µg/day. If a satisfactory response in the biochemical parameters and clinical manifestations of the disease are not observed, the dose may be increased by 0.25 µg/day at 2- to 4-week intervals. During the dosage titration period, serum calcium levels should be measured at least twice weekly and, if hypercalcemia is present, Rocaltrol should be immediately discontinued until normocalcemia ensues. Consideration should also be given to lowering the calcium intake.

Malabsorption is occasionally noted in patients with hypoparathyroidism; hence, larger doses of Rocaltrol may be needed.

Children: Initiation of Treatment: X linked hypophosphatemic rickets: 0.01 to 0.02 µg/kg/day (mean 0.018 µg/kg/day).
Vitamin D dependency rickets type 1: 0.010 to 0.025 µg/kg/day (mean 0.017 µg/kg/day).
Hypoparathyroidism: 0.03 to 0.05 µg/kg/day (mean 0.04 µg/kg/day).

Response is checked after 2 weeks to ascertain that the dose has not produced hypercalcemia. Biochemical evaluation should include serum calcium (total and ionized if available), phosphate, alkaline phosphatase, and creatinine. If satisfactory biochemical improvement has not occurred, the dose is increased by about 25% and the effect re-evaluated in 2 weeks. Until the desired response to treatment is achieved, the dose is gradually increased or decreased in this manner. Improvement in the radiographic lesions of rickets takes several weeks to become apparent.

For severely hypocalcemic or symptomatic patients, an initial dose as high as 0.05 µg/kg/day may be used to treat the hypocalcemia. In this situation, the serum calcium concentration should be monitored very closely (hospitalization recommended) and, as soon as the patient is out of danger from hypocalcemia, the dose reduced.

Maintenance: X linked hypophosphatemic rickets: 0.01 to 0.05 µg/kg/day (mean 0.022 µg/kg/day).
Vitamin D dependency rickets type 1: 0.0046 to 0.015 µg/kg/day.
Hypoparathyroidism: 0.014 to 0.040 µg/kg/day (mean 0.025 µg/kg/day).

Assessment of serum calcium (total and ionized), phosphate, alkaline phosphatase and creatinine should be made at 3 to 4 month intervals once treatment has been established and for as long as the medication is administered.

Hypercalcemia can occur at any time while the patient is treated with Rocaltrol (even if the dose has not been changed). Patients with rachitic or osteomalacic bone changes may become hypercalcemic as the bones become remineralized and therefore take up less calcium from the blood. To decrease the risk of hypercalcemia, a downward adjustment of the Rocaltrol dose may be advisable once a reduction in serum alkaline phosphatase has been achieved.

The single most important indicator of calcitriol overdose appears to be hypercalcemia as determined by accurate and frequent measurement of the serum calcium concentration. Signs of hypercalcemia such as polyuria, nocturia, polydipsia, nausea, vomiting, anorexia, weight loss, and constipation should be watched for but are less sensitive indicators of toxicity. Most hypercalcemic patients are asymptomatic.

If hypercalcemia occurs, Rocaltrol is discontinued for 1 to 2 weeks or until hypercalcemia disappears. Hypercalcemia frequently resolves in 2 to 7 days. Therapy is then resumed with a dose about 25% lower than that which caused intoxication. If the dose has been increased or decreased for any reason, the calcium level should be re-evaluated at 2-week intervals.

Fasting urine samples for measurement of calcium/creatinine ratio may be used to monitor the development of hypercalciuria.

Kidney ultrasounds may be indicated yearly during Rocaltrol therapy. However, the clinical significance of the finding of nephrocalcinosis is not known.

Rocaltrol solution must be measured accurately and can be administered directly into the mouth of the infant. The bottle should be closed tightly each time after use, and when stored between 15 and 30°C and protected from light, the solution is stable for 6 weeks after opening.

Intermittent (pulse) Therapy: Oral intermittent (pulse) therapy with Rocaltrol 2 or 3 times weekly has been shown to be effective even in patients refractory to continuous therapy. Serum calcium levels should be monitored during therapy.

SUPPLIED: Capsules: 0.25 µg: Each brown-orange to red-orange, opaque (first-half)/white to grey-yellow or grey-orange, opaque (second half), oval soft gelatin capsule contains: calcitriol 0.25 µg. Nonmedicinal ingredients: butylhydroxyanisole, butylhydroxytoluene, fractioned coconut oil, gelatin, glycerol 85%, hydrogenated products of partially hydrolysed starch, red iron oxide, titanium dioxide E 171 and yellow iron oxide. Blister cards of 20 capsules, cartons of 5 blister cards, for a total of 100 capsules per unit. Store at 15-25°C in the original container. Protect from light and moisture. Keep blister in the outer carton.

0.50 µg: Each brown-orange to red-orange, opaque, oval soft gelatin capsule contains: calcitriol 0.50 µg. Nonmedicinal ingredients: butylhydroxyanisole, butylhydroxytoluene, fractioned coconut oil, gelatin, glycerol 85%, hydrogenated products of partially hydrolysed starch, red iron oxide, titanium dioxide E 171 and yellow iron oxide. Blister cards of 20 capsules, cartons of 5 blister cards, for a total of 100 capsules per unit. Store at 15-25°C in the original container. Protect from light and moisture. Keep blister in the outer carton.

Solution: Each mL of clear, colourless oily solution contains: calcitriol 1.0 µg. Nonmedicinal ingredients: butylated hydroxyanisole, butylated hydroxytoluene and medium chain triglyceride. Bottles of 10 mL. Store at 15-30°C in the original container. Protect from light.

(Shown in Product Identification Section)

Rocephin® Ⓟ
ceftriaxone sodium
Antibiotic

Roche

SUPPLIED: Each vial of sterile white to pale yellow crystalline powder contains: ceftriaxone sodium (expressed as anhydrous free acid), equivalent to ceftriaxone 0.25 g or 1 g; and as a pharmacy bulk vial containing the equivalent of ceftriaxone 10 g (not for direct administration). **The availability of the pharmacy bulk vial is restricted to hospitals with a recognized i.v. admixture program.** No added excipients. Sodium content of each gram of Rocephin is approximately 83 mg (3.6 mEq sodium ion). pH 6 to 8. Solutions are yellowish in color.

Sterile powder should be stored at a controlled room temperature (between 15 and 30°C) and protected from light.

Rocuronium Bromide Injection Ⓟ
rocuronium bromide
Nondepolarizing Skeletal Neuromuscular Blocking Agent

Hospira

SUPPLIED: Each mL of sterile nonpyrogenic solution for i.v. injection only contains: rocuronium bromide 10 mg, sodium acetate, anhydrous 1.2 mg and sodium chloride approx. 3.1 mg. May contain: sodium hydroxide and/or glacial acetic acid to adjust the pH to approximately 4.0. Boxes of 10. Store under refrigeration (2-8°C) until ready to use. To facilitate use in the operating room, the unopened vials may be stored up to 90 days at room temperature (15-30°C). Use punctured vials within 30 days.

Rocuronium Bromide Injection Ⓟ
rocuronium bromide
Nondepolarizing Skeletal Neuromuscular Blocking Agent

Sandoz

SUPPLIED: Each mL of sterile solution contains: rocuronium bromide 10 mg. Nonmedicinal ingredients: glacial acetic acid and sodium hydroxide to adjust pH, sodium acetate trihydrate, sodium chloride and water for injection. Clear multidose vials of 5 mL, boxes of 10. Store between 2 and 8°C until ready to use. To facilitate use in the operating room, the unopened vials may be stored up to 90 days at room temperature between 15 and 30°C. Use punctured vials within 30 days.

Rofact® Ⓟ
rifampin
Antituberculosis Agent

Valeant

PHARMACOLOGY: Rifampin may be bacteriostatic or bactericidal in action, depending on the concentration of the drug attained at the side of infection and the susceptibility of the infecting organism. Rifampin usually is rapidly bactericidal against *M. leprae* in vivo.

Rifampin suppresses initiation of chain formation for RNA synthesis in susceptible bacteria by inhibiting DNA-depending RNA polymerase. The β subunit of the enzyme appears to be the site of action. Rifampin is most active against susceptible bacteria when they are undergoing cell division; however, the drug also has some effect when bacteria are in the metabolic resting state.

Pharmacokinetics: Absorption: Rifampin is well absorbed from the gastrointestinal tract.

Distribution: Rifampin diffuses well to most body tissues and fluids, including the cerebrospinal fluid, where concentrations are increased if the meninges are inflamed; concentrations in the liver, gallbladder, bile, and urine are higher than those found in the blood; therapeutic concentrations are achieved in the saliva, reaching 20% of serum concentrations; crosses the placenta, with fetal serum concentrations at birth found to be approximately 33% of the maternal serum concentration; penetrates into aqueous humor; and is distributed into breast milk. Being lipid-soluble, rifampin may reach and kill susceptible intracellular, as well as extracellular, bacteria and *Mycobacteria* species.

Volume of Distribution: 1.6 L/kg.

Protein binding: high to very high (89%).

Biotransformation: hepatic.

Metabolism: Rifampin is eliminated principally by the liver into bile but the maximum excretory capacity of the liver is surpassed at doses higher than 5 mg/kg body weight. The concentration of rifampin in the blood is dose-related. Metabolism of rifampin takes place by desacetylation at position 25 of the molecule resulting in desacetyl rifampin as the major metabolite in man. The antimycobacterial properties of rifampin are retained by desacetylated rifampin and they are detectable in the blood, bile and urine of man following an oral dose of rifampin. Six hours following administration of rifampin, the ratio of desacetylated rifampin to rifampin is up to 50% in serum, 30 to 60% in urine and 100% in bile.

Half-life: Absorption half-life approximately 0.6 hour. Elimination half-life initially 3 to 5 hours; with repeated administration half-life decreases to 2 to 3 hours.

Time to Peak Plasma Concentration: 1.5 to 4 hours after oral administration; peak concentration may be decreased and delayed following administration with food.

Peak Plasma Concentration: Adults: 7 to 9 µg/mL after 600 mg. Children (6 months to 5 years): approximately 11 µg/mL after a dose of 10 mg/kg of body weight (mg/kg) mixed in applesauce or simple syrup.

Elimination: biliary/fecal; enterohepatic recirculation of rifampin, but not of its deacetylated active metabolite; 60 to 65% of dose appear in feces; renal 6 to 15% excreted as unchanged drug, and 15% excreted as active metabolite in urine; 7% excreted as inactive 3-formyl derivative.

Rifampin does not accumulate in patients with impaired renal function; its rate of excretion is increased during the first 6 to 10 days of therapy, probably because of auto-induction of hepatic microsomal oxidative enzymes; after high doses, excretion may be slower because of saturation of its biliary excretory mechanism.

In dialysis: Rifampin is not removed from the blood by either hemodialysis or peritoneal dialysis.

INDICATIONS: Treatment of pulmonary tuberculosis. In order to avoid emergence of resistance, rifampin must be administered concomitantly with at least one other effective antituberculosis drug. Selection of the appropriate drug combinations should be determined on the basis of in vitro sensitivity tests, comparative safety as well as the patient's previous clinical history.

The following are the most frequently used treatment regimens for previously untreated patients: rifampin with isoniazid; with ethambutol; with isoniazid and ethambutol.

The possibility of a drug interaction as well as the individual properties and special precautions relating to drugs used in concomitant therapy should be taken into consideration, e.g., PAS is known to delay the absorption of rifampin. When such concomitant medication is employed, it is recommended that an interval of 8 to 12 hours between each drug be observed.

CONTRAINDICATIONS: In patients with a history of previous sensitivity or hypersensitivity to any other ingredient in the formulation. Rifampin is contraindicated in hepatic function impairment since rifampin is metabolized in the liver and may also be hepatotoxic. Rifampin is contraindicated in premature and newborn infants in whom the liver is not yet capable of functioning with full efficiency. Rifampin passes into breast milk and therefore should not be given during lactation.

WARNINGS:

> Rifampin should not be administered to patients also receiving saquinavir/ritonavir (ritonavir boosted saquinavir) as part of their combination antiretroviral therapy (ART) for HIV infection.

Hepatic dysfunction has been produced by rifampin. In patients with existing liver impairment the incidence of clinically evident hepatic adverse reactions is significantly increased. The incidence of hepatic adverse reactions and fatalities is much greater in patients given combination therapy as compared to monotherapy. Factors such as alcoholism, liver cirrhosis, extensive liver tuberculosis, adenocarcinoma of the liver and neoplasm of the biliary tract predispose the patient to the increased hepatic risk. Risks in such patients should be carefully evaluated against benefits. Assessment of liver function on a regular basis is essential. Periodic blood counts should also be carried out in patients receiving long-term treatment.

Tumorigenicity: Studies in female mice of a strain known to be particularly susceptible to the spontaneous development of hepatomas have shown that rifampin, given in doses of 2 to 10 times the maximum human dose for 1 year, causes a significant increase in the development of hepatomas. However, studies in male mice of the same strain, in other strains of mice or female mice, or in rats have not shown that rifampin is tumorigenic.

Pregnancy: Pregnancy/Reproduction: Rifampin crosses the placenta. It is recommended that pregnant women with tuberculosis be treated for a minimum of 9 months with multidrug therapy, including rifampin. It has rarely caused postnatal hemorrhages in the mother and infant when administered during the last few weeks of pregnancy; vitamin K may be indicated. Neonates should be carefully observed for evidence of adverse effects.

PRECAUTIONS: Daily treatment with rifampin is often better tolerated than intermittent therapy, since rare hypersensitivity reactions may occur. Therefore, when resuming treatment with rifampin after short or prolonged interruptions, the drug should be given in small, gradually increasing doses. During the transitional period, renal function should be closely monitored.

If as may happen in exceptional cases, the patient develops thrombocytopenia, purpura, hemolytic anemia or renal failure, treatment with rifampin should be stopped immediately and not be reinstituted at a later date.

Since rifampin has been observed to increase the requirements for anticoagulant drugs of the coumarin type, the same can be expected for Rofact. This effect was not observed until the fifth day following the initiation of treatment. The decrease in prothrombin time lasts 5 to 7 days on the average. The cause of this phenomenon is unknown. In patients receiving anticoagulants it is recommended that daily prothrombin times be performed until the required dose of the anticoagulant has been established.

Safe conditions for the use of ethambutol alone or in combination with rifampin have not been as yet established for children under the age of 13 years. Although renal insufficiency does not alter blood levels of rifampin, marked increases in ethambutol levels are observed under similar conditions; this should be taken into consideration in such patients receiving rifampin/ethambutol concomitantly. If in the opinion of the physician, ethambutol therapy is to be used in combination with rifampin, the possible visual deterioration associated with ethambutol should be carefully considered.

When instituting therapy with a combination of rifampin and isoniazid, caution is recommended in the elderly, the malnourished and in patients with impaired liver function.

Elevation of sulfobromophthalein (BSP) following administration of rifampin has been reported. Experimental studies indicate that rifampin and BSP compete with one another at the liver cell-bile boundary. Therefore, the BSP test should be performed prior to the daily dose of rifampin to avoid false-positive test results.

When rifampin is used concomitantly with other antituberculosis agents the possible adverse effects of each drug as well as the interaction between the different drugs should be taken into consideration.

In order to prevent undue anxiety, patients should be made aware of the possibility that urine, feces, saliva, sputum, sweat and tears may be colored red/orange by rifampin and its metabolites. Patients should be advised that soft contact lenses may be permanently stained.

Concurrent use of estrogen-containing contraceptives with rifampin may decrease the effectiveness of the contraceptive because of stimulation of estrogen metabolism or reduction in enterohepatic circulation of estrogens, resulting in menstrual irregularities, intermenstrual bleeding, and unplanned pregnancies. Patients should be advised to use an additional method of contraception throughout the whole cycle while taking rifampin and estrogen-containing oral contraceptives concurrently.

Both in the laboratory animal and man, the administration of rifampin has been associated with evidence of induction of drug metabolizing enzyme systems of the liver. As a consequence, the rate of metabolism of those compounds which are substrates of such enzymes can be altered and in some instances accelerated, a phenomenon which can result in a reduced pharmacological effect of the drug involved. Changes of possible clinical significance have been reported for the following: oral anticoagulants, hypoglycemic agents, dapsone, digitalis compounds and corticosteroids as well as oral contraceptives and ethambutol. Appropriate adjustment in the dosage and monitoring of effects of these drugs is therefore necessary when they are used concomitantly with rifampin. This is particularly important when rifampin administration is both initiated and withdrawn.

Microbiological techniques for assaying the serum concentrations of folic acid and vitamin B_{12} are not suitable for use during treatment with rifampin.

Upon completion of the treatment with rifampin, a renewed evaluation and readjustment of the dosage of any concomitantly administered drug should be made.

ADVERSE EFFECTS: Gastrointestinal disturbances including dyspepsia, epigastric distress, anorexia, nausea, vomiting, gas, cramps and diarrhea have been reported. Headache, drowsiness, fatigue, ataxia, dizziness, inability to concentrate, mental confusion, visual disturbances, muscular weakness, fever, pain in extremities and generalized numbness have also been noted. Pruritus, urticaria, skin rashes, eosinophilia, sore mouth and/or tongue, dyspnea and acute renal failure have occasionally been encountered. Thrombocytopenia, purpura, leukopenia, hemolytic anemia and decreased hemoglobin have been observed. Thrombocytopenia has been reported to occur in patients given ethambutol and rifampin concomitantly on an intermittent dose schedule twice weekly and in high doses. Elevations in blood urea nitrogen (BUN) and serum uric acid have been reported.

Transient abnormalities in liver function tests such as elevations of serum bilirubin and BSP, elevation of alkaline phosphatase and serum transaminases have been reported particularly during the first few weeks of treatment. The following menstrual disturbances, breakthrough bleeding, spotting, amenorrhea and prolongation of both the menstrual interval and menses have been reported to occur in women taking rifampin.

A few cases of jaundice with evidence of hepato-cellular damage have been reported in patients receiving rifampin. In some of them it was possible, under careful laboratory control, to resume treatment after an interval without recurrence of abnormalities.

Clinical trials have not shown any harmful effects on the cochleovestibular system caused by rifampin.

OVERDOSE:

The LD_{50} of rifampin in mice, rats, and rabbits is 0.885; 1.72; and 2.12 g/kg, respectively. In humans, acute overdosage with rifampin doses up to 12 g have not been fatal. However, at least 1 fatality has been reported following ingestion of a single 60 g dose of rifampin.

Symptoms: Overdosage of rifampin produces symptoms that are principally extensions of common adverse reactions. These include nausea, vomiting, lethargy, and brownish-red or orange discoloration of skin, urine, sweat, saliva, tears, and feces in proportion to the amount of drug ingested. Following massive overdosage of rifampin, hepatic involvement can develop within a few hours and is manifested by liver enlargement, possibly with tenderness, jaundice, rapid increases in total and direct serum bilirubin and liver enzymes, and loss of consciousness.

Treatment: In acute rifampin overdosage, the stomach should be emptied by gastric lavage. Activated charcoal slurry then may be instilled into the stomach to adsorb any drug remaining in the gastrointestinal tract. An antiemetic may be required to control severe nausea and vomiting. Active diuresis, with measured intake and output, may promote excretion of the drug. If serious hepatic impairment occurs which lasts more than 24 to 48 hours, bile drainage or hemodialysis may be indicated. Reversal of liver enlargement and improvement of impaired hepatic function usually occur within 72 hours in patients with previously adequate hepatic function.

> For management of a suspected drug overdose, CPhA recommends that you contact your **regional Poison Control Centre**. See the *CPS* Directory section for a list of Poison Control Centres.

DOSAGE: It is recommended that rifampin be administered once daily on an empty stomach (1 hour before a meal) to ensure optimum absorption.

In the treatment of pulmonary tuberculosis, rifampin must be given in conjunction with at least one other antituberculosis agent. In general, therapy should be continued until bacterial conversion has been established and maximum clinical improvement has occurred.

If a rifampin-PAS combination therapy is employed, it is recommended that the two drugs be administered at intervals of 8 to 12 hours.

Usual Adult and Adolescent Dose: Tuberculosis: in combination with other antituberculosis medications: oral, 600 mg once a day for the entire treatment period; or 10 mg/kg of body weight, up to 600 mg, 2 or 3 times a week, depending on the treatment regimen. Meningococcal infection (prophylaxis): oral, 600 mg 2 times a day for 2 days.

In patients with impaired liver function, a daily dose of 8 mg/kg should not be exceeded. A daily dosage of 10 mg/kg of body weight is recommended for frail and elderly persons.

Usual Pediatric Dose: Infants up to 1 month of age: Tuberculosis: in combination with other antituberculosis medications: oral, 10 to 20 mg/kg of body weight once a day; or 10 to 20 mg/kg of body weight, 2 or 3 times a week, depending on the treatment regimen. Meningococcal infection (prophylaxis): oral, 5 mg/kg of body weight every 12 hours for 2 days.

Children 1 month of age and over: Tuberculosis: in combination with other antituberculosis medications: oral, 10 to 20 mg/kg of body weight, up to 600 mg, once a day; or 10 to 20 mg/kg of body weight, up to 600 mg, 2 or 3 times a week, depending on the treatment regimen. Meningococcal infection (prophylaxis): oral, 10 mg/kg of body weight every 12 hours for 2 days. The maximum daily dose should not exceed 600 mg.

SUPPLIED: 150 mg: Each coni-snap #4 elongated, maroon opaque colored capsule, branded radial "ICN R11" contains: rifampin USP 150 mg. Nonmedicinal ingredients: croscarmellose sodium, magnesium stearate and talc. Bottles of 100.

300 mg: Each lok-type #1 capsule with brown opaque cap and scarlet opaque body branded "ICN R12" contains: rifampin USP 300 mg. Nonmedicinal ingredients: croscarmellose sodium, magnesium stearate, sodium lauryl sulfate and talc. Bottles of 100.

Rogaine®

minoxidil

Hair Regrowth Treatment

Johnson & Johnson

PHARMACOLOGY: When applied topically, minoxidil topical solution has been shown to stimulate hair growth in individuals with androgenetic alopecia (male pattern baldness). The basic change in androgenetic alopecia is the conversion of terminal, non-vellus hair to vellus hair, i.e., hair which is thinner, shorter, and less pigmented. Although the exact mechanism of action of minoxidil in the treatment of androgenetic alopecia is not known, there may be more than one mechanism by which minoxidil topical solution stimulates hair growth; they include: vasodilation of the micro circulation around the hair follicles which may stimulate hair growth; and direct stimulation of the hair follicle cells to enter into a proliferative phase: resting phase (telogen) follicles being stimulated to pass into growth phase (anagen) follicles.

The failure to detect evidence of systemic effects during treatment with topical minoxidil reflects the poor absorption of topical minoxidil, which averages about 1.4% (range 0.3 to 4.5%) from normal intact scalp. Absorption is about 2% when applied topically to shaved scalps of hypertensive patients. Increasing the amount of drug applied or increasing the frequency of application of topical minoxidil also results in increased absorption. The use of minoxidil in conjunction with occlusion (plastic dressing) application to sunburn areas, and increasing the surface area of application has minimal to no effect on the absorption of topical minoxidil.

Results of extensive pharmacokinetic studies indicate that the 3 major factors by which topical minoxidil absorption is increased are: increasing the magnitude of the dose applied; increasing the frequency of dosing; and decreasing the barrier function of the stratum corneum.

Serum minoxidil levels and systemic effects resulting from administration of topical minoxidil are governed by the drug's absorption rate through the skin. Following cessation of topical dosing of minoxidil, approximately 95% of systemically absorbed drug is eliminated within 4 days. Minoxidil and its metabolites are excreted principally in the urine.

Although the percutaneous drug absorption data are highly variable, clinical studies show that greater than 99% of the patients had serum minoxidil concentrations below 5 ng/mL, and fewer than 0.2% had concentrations greater than 12 ng/mL after using 1 mL of minoxidil topical solution twice per day for up to 54 months.

Absorption from the gastrointestinal tract following oral administration of minoxidil tablets is essentially complete (at least 95%). Approximately 90% of orally administered minoxidil is metabolized, predominantly by conjugation with glucuronic acid at the N-oxide position in the pyrimidine ring and by conversion to more polar products.

The hemodynamic effects of minoxidil do not correlate directly with serum levels. There is a delay in onset relative to observable serum concentrations, peak hemodynamic effects lag 1 hour behind peak serum concentrations, and hemodynamic effects persist long after nearly all the minoxidil has disappeared from the circulation. It appears that minoxidil requires bioactivation before exerting its hemodynamic activity. The active metabolite is considered to be minoxidil sulfate. Sulfotransferase enzyme which converts minoxidil to minoxidil sulfate has been isolated from various human tissues including liver, platelets, scalp skin, hair follicles and epidermal keratinocytes. Possibly the effects of minoxidil on hair regrowth is mediated by this active metabolite as well. In clinical studies, no correlation between serum or tissue minoxidil concentrations and hair regrowth was established.

Minoxidil does not bind to plasma proteins; its renal clearance corresponds to glomerular filtration rate and it does not cross the blood brain barrier. Minoxidil and its metabolites are hemodialyzable, although this does not rapidly reverse its pharmacological effect.

Minoxidil topical solution is not effective in all individuals. After 4 months of treatment with minoxidil topical solution, only 26% of individuals reported moderate (defined as new individual hairs that covered all or some of the thinning areas but not as close together as hairs on the rest of the head) to dense hair regrowth (new hairs that cover or almost completely cover the thinning area and are as close together as hairs on the non-thinning areas of the head). A similar response was obtained in 11% of the subjects using the vehicle control. Thirty-one percent of the vehicle users and 33% of the minoxidil topical solution users reported minimal regrowth at 4 months. The net increase of non-vellus hair attributable to minoxidil was a mean of 33 hairs in a circle 2.5 cm in diameter. The investigator's global improvement rating showed no statistically significant difference in terminal hair growth between treatment groups.

After further 8 months of treatment, the 2% group had an additional 112 non-vellus hairs. Based on the investigator's assessment, 39% of the subjects achieved moderate to dense terminal hair while 40% of the users rated their regrowth as moderate and 8% as dense; 36% reported minimal regrowth (some new hairs which do not grow as close together as hairs on non-thinning areas and not enough to cover the thinning areas) while 16% had no regrowth.

A temporary hair loss may occur upon initiation of therapy; this increase in shedding generally occurs 2 to 6 weeks after beginning of treatment and subsides within a few weeks. This shedding upon initiation of therapy is due to hair shifting from resting phase (telogen) to growth phase (anagen).

The response time differs greatly between individuals. It takes at least 4 months of twice daily applications. Compliance with the twice daily regimen must be fastidious for optimal success.

The effect is maintained only for as long as the product is used. Cessation of treatment will result in loss of the newly regrown hair within about 3 months and progressive hair loss will resume.

It is not known which individuals may show a satisfactory response, but younger men who have been balding for a shorter period of time (less than 10 years) or who have a smaller area of hair loss (less than a diameter of 10 cm) tend to respond better than older men who have been balding for longer periods of time and/or have a large area of hair loss or in those with an area of baldness that is devoid of all hair.

INDICATIONS: For the treatment of androgenetic alopecia (male pattern baldness) on the top of the scalp (vertex). Minoxidil topical solution's effectiveness in the treatment of receding hairlines has not been demonstrated in clinical trials. Minoxidil topical solution is not approved for use in women.

CONTRAINDICATIONS: In those consumers with a history of hypersensitivity to minoxidil, propylene glycol or ethanol.

Minoxidil topical solution should not be used by pregnant or nursing women.

Minoxidil topical solution should not be used if the skin of the scalp is shaved, broken, inflamed, irritated, infected or severely sunburned (using minoxidil topical solution on mildly sunburned scalp is not harmful) or if prescription medications for treating disorders of the skin are being used that could possibly be applied to the scalp.

Minoxidil topical solution is not for use by individuals whose baldness is not due to hereditary factors. Minoxidil topical solution is effective in treating only vertex male pattern baldness (alopecia androgenetica). Certain prescription and non-prescription medications, certain treatments, such as cancer chemotherapy, or certain diseases, such as iron deficiency, thyroid disorders or secondary syphilis, as well as severe nutritional problems and poor grooming habits, may also cause temporary hair loss none of which should be treated with minoxidil topical solution.

WARNINGS: Although the following systemic effects have not been associated with the topical use of minoxidil topical solution, there is some absorption of minoxidil from the skin and the potential exists for systemic effects such as salt and water retention, tachycardia, angina and edema. Consumers should be made aware of and monitor themselves for signs of systemic effects of minoxidil. In the event of systemic side effects discontinue the drug and seek a physicians care. Consumers should discontinue use of minoxidil topical solution and contact their physician in the event of systemic effects and/or severe dermatologic reactions.

Pregnancy: The safety for use of minoxidil topical solution in pregnancy has not been established.

Lactation: The safety for use of minoxidil topical solution in lactating women has not been established. Systemically absorbed minoxidil is secreted in human milk.

Children: Safety and effectiveness of minoxidil topical solution in patients under 18 years of age have not been established.

Information to Be Provided to the Patient: Do not apply to other parts of the body except the scalp.

Do not use if skin on scalp is diseased, irritated, or inflamed.

Do not use in conjunction with any other topical prescription medications.

Discontinue use if skin irritations or lesions develop.

Do not apply more than the recommended dose.

Accidental ingestion of minoxidil topical solution can cause serious adverse effects. Contact Poison Control Centre immediately.

PRECAUTIONS: General: Minoxidil topical solution will cause burning and irritation of the eye. In the event of accidental contact with sensitive surfaces (eye, abraded skin, mucous membranes), the area should be bathed with copious amounts of cool tap water. Hands should be washed thoroughly after use.

Patients with known cardiovascular disease or cardiac arrhythmia should contact a physician before using minoxidil topical solution. Some patients have experienced changes in hair colour and/or texture with minoxidil topical solution use.

Inhalation of the spray mist should be avoided.

Drug Interactions: There are currently no known drug interactions associated with concomitant use of systemic drugs and topical minoxidil. Absorption of topical minoxidil is controlled and rate-limited by the stratum corneum. Topical drugs, e.g., tretinoin and anthralin, which alter the stratum corneum barrier, could result in increased absorption of topical minoxidil if applied concurrently.

ADVERSE EFFECTS: The most frequently encountered adverse reactions in clinical trials with minoxidil topical solution were minor respiratory reactions. These included colds and respiratory infections, rhinitis, sinusitis, coughing and bronchitis. Dermatological reactions were the second most frequent adverse reactions seen. These included local irritation, scaling, erythema, dermatitis, dry skin, itching, burning sensation and rash. In light of the findings that systemic levels of minoxidil from topical application are low in relation to systemic levels from oral dosing, the prevalence of effects which are commonly associated with the oral use of minoxidil are quite low.

Infrequent adverse reactions included sore throat, backache, strain and spasm, flu-like illness, dental problems, and infection. Rarely reported adverse reactions included headache, diarrhea, hypertrichosis, muscle pull or sprain, tendon, bursae, fascia and ligament disorders, hay fever, aches and pain, and physical injuries.

The occurrence rates for adverse reactions seen in greater than 1% of patients were obtained from placebo-controlled clinical studies involving 2386 patients (1188 minoxidil topical solution and 1198 placebo) and are listed in Table 1.

Table 1: Rogaine

Adverse Reactions >1% Seen with Rogaine Treatment in Males as Compared to Placebo

Body System	Treatment %	Placebo %
Dermatological		
Rash	1.43	0.42
Itching	1.94	1.25
Scaling	1.35	1.09
Respiratory		
Rhinitis	1.26	1.34
Coughing	1.09	0.50
Colds/Upper Resp. Inf.	3.37	4.34
Sinusitis	1.18	0.92
Gastrointestinal		
Sore Throat	1.77	2.34
Dental Problems	1.01	0.58
Musculoskeletal		
Backache/Strain/Spasm	1.09	0.58
Miscellaneous		
Infections	2.02	1.92

Adverse Reactions Seen in Less Than 1% of Males:

Dermatological: eczema, hypertrichosis, seborrhea, folliculitis, dry skin, dermatitis, erythema, and burning and irritation.

Cardiovascular: hypotension, increased blood pressure, chest discomfort, tachycardia, and pulse changes.

Metabolic/Nutritional: edema and weight gain.

Allergic: allergic reactions, hay fever, flu-like illness, and urticaria.

Neurological: dizziness/lightheadedness, fever, asthenia, headache, insomnia, tingling, and sciatica.

Special Senses: ear infections, ear inflammation and conjunctivitis.

Gastrointestinal: abdominal pain, nausea, diarrhea, vomiting, tonsillitis, gastroenteritis, hemorrhoids, hepatitis, and oral ulcers.

Urinary Tract: kidney calculi and urethritis.

Psychiatric: tiredness/fatigue.

Genital Tract: prostatic inflammation and epididymal disorders.

Musculoskeletal: aches and pain, fracture, joint pain, stiffness and inflammation, muscle pull and sprain, and tendon, bursae, fascia, and ligament disorders.

Respiratory: lung congestion, sneezing, pharyngitis and bronchitis.

Miscellaneous: (not otherwise specified or not elsewhere classified): aches/pains, physical injury, flu-like illness and cellulitis.

OVERDOSE:

Symptoms: Because of the high concentration of minoxidil in minoxidil topical solution, accidental oral ingestion could result in systemic absorption sufficient to cause the predictable cardiovascular effects of minoxidil (e.g., reduced blood pressure, reflex tachycardia, fluid retention).

Signs and symptoms of overdosage would most likely include cardiovascular effects associated with fluid retention, sudden weight gain, lowered blood pressure, tachycardia, faintness and dizziness. Fluid retention can be managed with appropriate diuretic therapy. Tachycardia can be controlled by administration of beta-adrenergic blocking agent.

Minoxidil and its metabolites are hemodialyzable, although this does not rapidly reverse its pharmacological effect.

Intentional Oral Ingestion: Significant toxicity after minoxidil exposure, whether tablet or topical formulations, was associated with oral route, intentional reason, and coingestion of other products. A male who ingested 60 mL (1 bottle) of 2% minoxidil with 360 mL of cognac experienced tachycardia, hypotension and a non-Q wave myocardial infarction. In another report, a patient who inadvertently drank minoxidil solution; he ingested 600 mg and developed syncope, hypotension, and acute renal failure.

Unintentional Oral Exposure: There have been 27 spontaneous reports of unintentional oral exposure to minoxidil solution involving 12 pediatric patients and 15 adults. No adverse events were associated with 17 of the reports. Of the remaining 10 cases, 1 pediatric patient experienced lethargy, 1 pediatric patient had flushed cheeks, and 1 pediatric patient was more active and had diarrhea. One adult patient had tachycardia in addition to nausea and vomiting. No report of unintentional oral exposure was associated with hospitalization or death.

One additional unintentional oral exposure involved a 3-year old child who swallowed a 1 to 2 mL of 3% topical minoxidil solution. After vomiting, he was treated in an emergency room. The child was alert and active with no obvious signs of distress. His temperature was 37°C, pulse rate was 152 bpm, respiration rate was 32 rpm, and systolic blood pressure 110 by palpation. Cardiovascular, chest, lungs, abdomen, head, skin, and neurologic examinations were normal. Blood levels taken indicated a total minoxidil level (glucuronide and unchanged) of 320.6 ng/mL. The child was discharged without sequelae.

Reports in which patients exceeded the recommended topical dose of 1 mL twice daily of minoxidil topical solution, side effects observed are similar to those previously reported at recommended doses.

If exaggerated hypotension is encountered, it is most likely to occur in association with residual sympathetic nervous system blockade from previous therapy (guanethidine-like effects or α-adrenergic blockade). The recommended treatment is i.v. administration of normal saline. Sympathomimetic drugs, such as norepinephrine or epinephrine, should be avoided because of their excessive cardiac-stimulating action. Phenylephrine, angiotensin II, vasopressin and dopamine, which reverse the effects of orally administered minoxidil, should only be used if inadequate perfusion of a vital organ is evident.

Treatment: See Symptoms.

> For management of a suspected drug overdose, CPhA recommends that you contact your **regional Poison Control Centre**. See the *CPS* Directory section for a list of Poison Control Centres.

DOSAGE: For external use only. Use minoxidil topical solution only as directed.

A total dose of 1 mL minoxidil topical solution should be applied twice per day to the scalp, beginning at the centre of the affected area. This dose should be used regardless of the size of the affected area. The total daily dose should not exceed 2 mL. The method of application varies according to the disposable applicator used, as indicated below. After applying minoxidil topical solution, wash hands thoroughly. Do not apply minoxidil topical solution to any other area of the body.

Apply minoxidil topical solution when the hair and scalp are thoroughly dry.

A. **Pump-Spray Applicator:** Works best for applying minoxidil topical solution to large areas of the scalp. 1) Remove large outer cap and keep it. 2) Remove inner Child-Resistant cap by pushing down while turning the cap counterclockwise. Retain Child-Resistant cap. 3) Insert the pump spray applicator into the bottle and screw on tightly. 4) After aiming the pump at the centre of the thinning or bald area of the scalp, press the pump once and spread minoxidil topical solution with fingertips to cover all the thinning or bald area. Repeat for a total of 6 squirts, to apply a total dose of 1 mL. **Avoid breathing spray mist.** 5) To retain Child-Resistant feature, remove Pump-Spray applicator and retain for next application. Replace Child-Resistant cap by tightly screwing on in a clockwise direction.

B. **Child-Resistant Dropper:** Works best for applying minoxidil topical solution to small areas of the scalp or under hair. 1) Remove large outer cap and keep it. 2) Remove inner Child-Resistant cap by pushing down while turning the cap counterclockwise. Throw this cap away. 3) Squeeze the rubber bulb and insert the dropper into the bottle. 4) Release the bulb, allowing the dropper to fill to the 1 mL line. If the level of the solution is above the 1 mL level, squeeze the extra amount back into the bottle. 5) Place the tip near the part of the scalp you want to treat and gently squeeze the bulb to gradually release the solution. To prevent the solution from running off the scalp, apply a small amount at a time. 6) Replace the dropper in the bottle and screw on tightly. 7) Replace large outer cap over the dropper applicator when not in use. 8) For future use, the dropper can be removed by pushing down while turning the dropper cap counterclockwise.

Clinical experience with minoxidil topical solution indicates that twice daily application for 4 or more months may be required before evidence of hair growth stimulation can be expected. Onset and degree of effect may be variable among consumers. Relapse to pretreatment appearance following discontinuation of minoxidil topical solution occurs within 3 to 4 months.

A contact time of at least 4 hours is necessary to ensure optimal results. Activities such as swimming, showering or physical activity involving excessive perspiration should be avoided for at least 4 hours after application.

If a dose is missed, minoxidil topical solution should be applied as soon as remembered if within a few hours of the time usually applied; do not apply if it is almost time for the next dose. If a dose is missed, the amount used in the next regular dose should not be doubled.

INFORMATION FOR THE PATIENT: Published in e-CPS, available by subscription at www.e-cps.ca.

SUPPLIED: Each mL of clear, colorless to slightly yellow solution contains: minoxidil 20 mg (2%), in alcohol (63%), propylene glycol (20%) and water. Bottles containing 60 mL of solution with the following metered disposable applicators: pump spray and child-resistant dropper assemblies. For external use only. Store at controlled room temperature (15 to 30°C).

Rogitine® Ⓟ

phentolamine mesylate

Alpha-adrenoreceptor Blocker

Paladin

SUPPLIED: Each ampul contains: phentolamine mesylate 10 mg, sodium metabisulfite 0.5 mg to adjust pH, glucose 35 mg and water up to 1 mL. Boxes of 5. Incompatible with alkaline solutions. Store at 2 to 8°C. Do not freeze. Protect from heat and light.

Rosasol® Ⓟ

metronidazole

Antirosacea Agent

Stiefel, a GSK company

PHARMACOLOGY: Metronidazole is a nitroimidazole with antiprotozoal and antibacterial activity. The exact mechanism of action of metronidazole in the reduction of inflammatory lesions, erythema and telangiectasia associated with rosacea is not known but may involve antibacterial and/or anti-inflammatory effects. In rosacea patients treated with 1% metronidazole cream once or twice a day, for 1 and 2 months, metronidazole serum level ranged between 20 - 45 ng/mL. This degree of transcutaneous absorption of metronidazole from a 1% cream corresponds to at most 1% of the level reached when the minimum oral metronidazole dose (200 mg/day) necessary for improvement of rosacea was administered.

ROSASOL (metronidazole 1%) topical cream with sunscreens also contains the sunscreens octyl methoxycinnamate, 7.5% and butyl methoxydibenzoyl methane, 2%, which help reduce the worsening of rosacea usually observed following exposure to the sun.

INDICATIONS: ROSASOL (metronidazole 1%) topical cream with sunscreens is indicated for the treatment of inflammatory lesions (papules and pustules), erythema and telangiectasia associated with rosacea.

CONTRAINDICATIONS: ROSASOL (metronidazole 1%) topical cream with sunscreens is contraindicated in patients with a prior history of hypersensitivity to metronidazole or other nitroimidazoles or to Parsol MCX, Parsol 1789 or to any other components contained in the preparation.

WARNINGS: ROSASOL (metronidazole 1%) topical cream with sunscreens should not be used in or near the eyes. In case of contact with the eyes, rinse thoroughly with copious amounts of water. If irritation persists a physician should be consulted.

As excessive sunlight will worsen rosacea, excessive exposure to sunlight should be avoided.

Pregnancy: The safety of ROSASOL during pregnancy has not been established. It is known that metronidazole crosses the placental barrier and penetrates rapidly into the fetal circulation. No teratogenic effects were observed in mice, rabbits or in rats receiving oral dose levels considerably higher than the human dose level. However, ROSASOL should only be used during pregnancy if the potential benefits to the mother justify the potential risks to the fetus.

Lactation: Following oral administration, metronidazole is secreted in human milk in a concentration similar to the plasma concentrations. Although metronidazole blood levels are much lower following topical application than after oral administration, ROSASOL should be used in nursing mothers only if the benefits justify the potential risks to the baby.

Pediatrics: The safety and effectiveness of ROSASOL has not been established in children.

PRECAUTIONS: Following topical administration, the absorption of metronidazole is minimal which yields much smaller plasma concentrations than following oral or I.V. route. Consequently, the adverse reactions observed following oral or I.V. administration of the drug were not reported with ROSASOL (metronidazole 1%) topical cream with sunscreens.

General: Although rosacea is a chronic disease, there is no information available on the long term use of ROSASOL for the treatment of rosacea. In controlled clinical trials, patients were treated for 12 weeks (see Dosage).

If irritation or hypersensitivity reactions develop, ROSASOL should be applied less often or should be discontinued and appropriate therapy initiated.

Metronidazole is a nitroimidazole and should be used with caution in patients who have or have had any evidence of dyscrasia.

Drug Interactions: Metronidazole has been reported to potentiate the anticoagulant effect of warfarin and other coumarin anticoagulants, resulting in a prolongation of prothrombin time. This interaction is probably much less following topical administration but must not be neglected if ROSASOL is prescribed to a patient on this type of anticoagulant therapy.

Dermatological Sensitivity: During the course of clinical trials, contact dermatitis was not observed in patients treated with ROSASOL nor in patients receiving the vehicle. Nevertheless, physicians should be aware of the possibility of skin sensitivity reactions to metronidazole and/or of cross-sensitization with other imidazole preparations, such as clotrimazole and tioconazole.

ADVERSE EFFECTS: Mild to moderate and rarely severe stinging (burning), erythema or itching have been reported with ROSASOL (metronidazole 1%) topical cream with sunscreens. These sensations were self-limiting and of short duration. Watering of the eyes if applied close to the ocular region, temporary redness and mild dryness has been reported with topical metronidazole.

Table 1 provides a listing of the related adverse events reported during controlled clinical studies in which 60 patients received ROSASOL. All these adverse events occurred at the site of application. Related adverse events were not observed in other body systems.

Table 1: ROSASOL

Adverse Events

Adverse Event	Severity	Incidence (No of patients)	Follow-up Treatment
Brown spot on cheek	Mild	1	None
Burning /Stinging	Mild	8	None
	Moderate	4	Thinner application in one patient
	Severe	1	Stopped drug for 3 days
Dryness	Mild	1	None
	Moderate	2	None
	Severe	1	None
Edema	Mild	1	None
Erythema	Mild	4	None
	Moderate	2	Ice application in one patient
	Severe	2	Thinner application in one patient
Irritation	Mild	1	Patient voluntarily withdrew from study
Oiliness	Mild	1	None
	Moderate	1	None
Pink crust on the cheek	Mild	1	None
Pruritus	Mild	4	None
	Moderate	1	None
Small comedones	Mild	1	None

OVERDOSE:

Symptoms: A large ingestion of metronidazole may produce vomiting, nausea and slight disorientation.

Treatment: There is no specific antidote. Give ipecac syrup or do gastric lavage; then, activated charcoal followed by a saline cathartic.

> For management of a suspected drug overdose, CPhA recommends that you contact your **regional Poison Control Centre**. See the *CPS* Directory section for a list of Poison Control Centres.

DOSAGE: ROSASOL (metronidazole 1%) topical cream with sunscreens should be applied to the areas affected by rosacea twice daily, once in the morning and once in the evening. The areas should be washed with a mild soap, rinsed well with lukewarm water and patted dry before application. Care should be taken to avoid eyes, nostrils, mouth and other mucous membranes.

Significant therapeutic results should be evident within the first month of treatment and controlled clinical studies have demonstrated continuing improvement through 12 weeks of therapy. The dosage for long-term administration is uncertain.

The method of application to affected areas only may not lead to a full sun protection (SPF 15). The patient should be instructed to use a regular sunscreen for areas not covered by ROSASOL.

INFORMATION FOR THE PATIENT: Published in e-CPS, available by subscription at www.e-cps.ca.

SUPPLIED: Each tube of cream (SPF15) contains: 1 % metronidazole USP with 7.5% Parsol MCX and 2% Parsol 1789. Nonmedicinal ingredients: Arlacel 60, DC Fluid 344, DC Fluid 556, diisopropyl adipate, dimethyl isosorbide, EDTA, emulsifying wax, glycerin, light mineral oil, octyl dodecyl neopentanoate, Phenonip (as preservative), polysorbate 60, purified stearic acid, purified water and sodium hydroxide. Tubes of 30 g. Store at 15 to 30°C.

Rosuvastatin Ⓟ

CPhA Monograph

see ***HMG-CoA Reductase Inhibitors***

Rotarix™

rotavirus vaccine, human, live, attenuated, oral

Active Immunizing Agent

GlaxoSmithKline

Date of Revision: February 17, 2010

SUMMARY PRODUCT INFORMATION:

Route of Administration	Dosage Form/ Strength	Clinically Relevant Nonmedicinal Ingredients
Oral	Suspension/not less than $10^{6.0}$ $CCID_{50}$ of human rotavirus RIX4414 strain, per 1.5 mL dose.	Dulbecco's Modified Eagle Medium (DMEM), sucrose, di-sodium adipate, sterile water. For a complete listing see Dosage Forms, Composition and Packaging.

DESCRIPTION: ROTARIX (human rotavirus, live, attenuated, oral vaccine) is a suspension presented in monodose oral applicators for oral administration. The vaccine includes an antacid component to protect the vaccine during passage through the stomach and prevent its inactivation due to acidic environment.

INDICATIONS AND CLINICAL USE: ROTARIX is indicated for active immunization of infants from the age of 6 weeks for the prevention of gastroenteritis caused by rotavirus types G1P[8], G2P[4], G3P[8], G4P[8] and G9P[8].

The results from the clinical trials suggest that the vaccine's efficacy may vary with the type of rotavirus causing the infection.

CONTRAINDICATIONS: ROTARIX should not be administered in:

- Infants who are hypersensitive to this drug or to any ingredient in the formulation or component of the container. For a complete listing, see Dosage Forms, Composition and Packaging.
- Infants who experienced hypersensitivity after previous administration of rotavirus vaccines.
- Infants with uncorrected congenital malformation (such as Meckel's diverticulum) of the gastrointestinal tract that would predispose for intussusception.

WARNINGS AND PRECAUTIONS: General: It is good clinical practice that vaccination should be preceded by a review of the medical history (especially with regard to previous vaccination and possible occurrence of undesirable events) and a clinical examination.

As with other vaccines, administration of ROTARIX should be postponed in infants suffering from acute severe febrile illness. However, the presence of a minor infection such as a cold should not result in the deferral of vaccination.

No safety or efficacy data are available for the administration of ROTARIX to:

- Individuals who have received a blood transfusion or blood products, including immunoglobulins, within 42 days.

No efficacy data are available for the administration of ROTARIX to:

- Immunocompromised patients such as individuals with malignancies receiving immunosuppressive therapy or who are otherwise immunocompromised.

The administration of ROTARIX should be postponed in infants suffering from diarrhea or vomiting.

Excretion of the vaccine virus in the stools is known to occur after vaccination with peak excretion around the 7th day. Viral antigen particles detected by ELISA were found in 50% (at day 7) of stools after the first dose and 17.4% (at day 3) and 4% (at day 7) of stools after the second dose. When these stools were tested for the presence of live vaccine strain, only 17% were positive.

Contacts of recent vaccinees should be advised to observe personal hygiene (e.g. wash their hands after changing child's diapers).

As with any vaccine, a protective immune response may not be elicited in all vaccinees.

ROTARIX does not protect against gastroenteritis due to other pathogens than rotavirus.

No data are available on the use of ROTARIX for post-exposure prophylaxis.

Under no circumstances should ROTARIX be injected.

Gastrointestinal: There are no data on the safety and efficacy of ROTARIX in infants with gastrointestinal illnesses. Administration of ROTARIX may be considered with caution in such infants when, in the opinion of the physician, withholding the vaccine entails a greater risk.

Immune: In some clinical trials, ROTARIX was not administered to infants known to have immunodeficient household members. There is a theoretical risk that the live virus vaccine can be transmitted to non-vaccinate contacts. Therefore, ROTARIX should be administered with caution to individuals known to have immunodeficient close contacts such as:

- Individuals with malignancies or who are otherwise immunocompromised; or
- Individuals receiving immunosuppressive therapy.

However, because nearly all children are infected with naturally occurring rotavirus by the age of 5 years, vaccination of infants may decrease the risk of exposure of immunodeficient household contacts to naturally occurring rotavirus. The health care provider should assess the potential risks and benefits of administering ROTARIX to infants known to have immunodeficient close contacts.

Asymptomatic and mildly symptomatic HIV infections are not expected to affect the safety or efficacy of ROTARIX. A clinical study in a limited number of asymptomatic or mildly symptomatic HIV positive infants showed no apparent safety problems (see Adverse Reactions, Safety in Infants with Human Immunodeficiency (HIV) Infection). Administration of ROTARIX in immunosuppressed infants, including infants on immunosuppressive therapy, should be based on careful consideration of potential benefits and risks.

Sensitivity/Resistance: The vaccine contains 1073 mg of sucrose as an excipient. This amount is too low to cause adverse events in patients with rare hereditary problems such as fructose intolerance, glucose-galactose malabsorption or sucrase-isomaltase insufficiency.

Special Populations: Pregnant Women: ROTARIX is not intended for use in adults. Thus, human data on use during pregnancy are not available and animal reproduction studies have not been performed.

Breastfeeding Infants: Evidence from some clinical trials with ROTARIX suggests breastfeeding does not reduce the protection against rotavirus gastroenteritis afforded by ROTARIX. Therefore breast feeding may be continued during the vaccination schedule.

ADVERSE REACTIONS: Adverse Drug Reaction Overview:

- **Clinical trials for the lyophilized formulation**

In a total of eleven placebo controlled clinical trials, approximately 80 000 doses of ROTARIX were administered to approximately 40 200 infants.

In two clinical trials (Finland), ROTARIX lyophilized formulation was administered alone (administration of routine pediatric vaccines was staggered). The incidence and severity of diarrhea, vomiting, loss of appetite, fever and irritability was not different in the group receiving ROTARIX when compared to the group receiving placebo. No increase in the incidence or severity of these reactions was seen with the second dose.

In the remaining nine trials (Europe, Canada, USA, Latin America, Singapore, South Africa), ROTARIX lyophilized formulation was coadministered with routine paediatric vaccines (see Drug Interactions). The adverse reaction profile observed in these subjects was similar to the adverse reaction profile observed in subjects receiving the same pediatric vaccines and placebo.

Clinical Trial Adverse Drug Reactions: Because clinical trials are conducted under very specific conditions the adverse reaction rates observed in the clinical trials may not reflect the rates observed in practice and should not be compared to the rates in the clinical trials of another drug. Adverse drug reaction information from clinical trials is useful for identifying drug-related adverse events and for approximating rates.

Intussusception: The risk of intussusception has been evaluated in a large safety trial conducted in Latin America and Finland where 63 225 subjects were enrolled. No increased risk of intussusception in the ROTARIX group was observed and observed rates were comparable to the placebo group. Data are shown in Table 1 and Table 2.

* Up to the data lock point.

Table 1: ROTARIX

Rate of Intussusception within 31 Days After Administration

Intussusception	ROTARIX N=31 673	Placebo N=31 552	Relative Risk (95% CI)
First dose	1	2	0.50 (0.07;3.80)
Second dose	5	5	0.99 (0.31;3.21)

Legend: CI=Confidence Interval.

Table 2: ROTARIX

Rate of Intussusception Up to One Year of Age

Intussusception	ROTARIX N=10 159	Placebo N=10 010	Relative Risk (95% CI)
First dose up to one year	4	14	0.28 (0.10;0.81)

Legend: CI: Confidence Interval.

In 11 other clinical studies (N=12 220) there were 7 cases of intussusception reported, 5 IS cases in HRV vaccinees and 2 cases in placebo recipient. It is to be highlighted that none of these studies were powered to compare the incidence of intussusception in the ROTARIX and placebo groups.

Solicited Adverse Reactions: In study Rota-036, detailed safety information was collected by parents/guardians for 8 consecutive days following vaccination with ROTARIX (i.e. day of vaccination and the next 7 days). A diary card was completed to record irritability, cough/runny nose, the infant's temperature, loss of appetite, vomiting, or diarrhea on a daily basis during the first week following each dose of ROTARIX or placebo. Adverse reactions among recipients of ROTARIX and placebo occurred at similar rates. See Table 3.

Table 3: ROTARIX

Percentage of Subjects with Each Solicited General Symptom Assessed as Causally Related to Vaccination, Reported From Day 0 to Day 7 After Each HRV Vaccine/Placebo Dose—Rota-036 Pooled Countries (Czech Republic, Finland, France, Germany, Italy and Spain)

	ROTARIX					Placebo				
				95 % CI					95 % CI	
Symptom	N	n	%	LL	UL	N	n	%	LL	UL
Dose 1										
Cough/Runny nose	914	58	6.3	4.9	8.1	490	29	5.9	4.0	8.4
Diarrhea	914	18	2.0	1.2	3.1	490	7	1.4	0.6	2.9
Fever	914	133	14.6	12.3	17.0	490	67	13.7	10.8	17.0
Irritability/Fussiness	914	299	32.7	29.7	35.9	490	171	34.9	30.7	39.3
Loss of appetite	914	126	13.8	11.6	16.2	490	71	14.5	11.5	17.9
Vomiting	914	44	4.8	3.5	6.4	490	24	4.9	3.2	7.2
Dose 2										
Cough/Runny nose	905	53	5.9	4.4	7.6	486	34	7.0	4.9	9.6
Diarrhea	905	6	0.7	0.2	1.4	486	8	1.6	0.7	3.2
Fever	905	164	18.1	15.7	20.8	486	95	19.5	16.1	23.4
Irritability/Fussiness	905	238	26.3	23.5	29.3	486	123	25.3	21.5	29.4
Loss of appetite	905	118	13.0	10.9	15.4	486	57	11.7	9.0	14.9
Vomiting	905	18	2.0	1.2	3.1	486	23	4.7	3.0	7.0

Legend: N=number of subjects having received the considered dose of HRV vaccine/placebo; n/%=number/percentage of subjects with the specified symptom reported for the considered dose; 95% CI: exact 95% confidence interval, LL=Lower Limit, UL=Upper Limit.

Statistically significant differences were not detected between groups for the comparison between ROTARIX and Placebo groups for the percentage of subjects with each specified solicited symptom (any, grade 3 and related) reported from Day 0 to Day 7 after any ROTARIX/placebo doses (P-value >0.05 for each comparison).

Unsolicited Adverse Events (pooled analysis): Infants were monitored for unsolicited adverse reactions that occurred in the 31 day period following vaccination in 8 clinical studies. The following adverse reactions occurred at a statistically higher incidence (P-value <0.05) among recipients of ROTARIX (N=5543) as compared with placebo recipients (N=1852): Rhinorrhea (ROTARIX 1.55%, placebo 3.02%), Pharyngitis (ROTARIX 1.86%, placebo 2.00%) and Bronchitis (ROTARIX 1.95%, placebo 1.03%). In another study (Rota-036: ROTARIX N=2646, placebo N=1348) the incidence of rhinorrhea, pharyngitis and bronchitis was similar between the ROTARIX and placebo groups.

Serious Adverse Events (SAEs): Study Rota-023: Among the total vaccinated cohort of 63 225 infants in study Rota-023 (31,673 in the HRV group and 31 552 in the placebo group), a total of 1975 subjects (948 infants in the HRV vaccine group and 1047 infants in the placebo group) reported at least one SAE (up to 30-90 days post Dose 2). No imbalance was observed between treatment groups for SAEs assessed as related to vaccination by the investigators. The overall SAE profile was in favour of the HRV vaccine with significantly fewer SAEs/hospitalizations reported in the HRV vaccine group compared to the placebo group, especially with respect to preventing GE related SAEs.

In study Rota-023, a potential imbalance between groups was noted for Convulsions reported cases: 16 subjects in ROTARIX group (5.1/10 000) versus 6 subjects in the placebo group (1.9/10 000). However, no potential imbalance was noted between groups when SAEs related to "Convulsive disorders" were pooled ('Convulsions', 'Epilepsy', 'Grand mal convulsion', 'Status epilepticus' and 'Tonic convulsion'): 20 subjects in the ROTARIX group versus 12 in the placebo group.

Other Clinical Trials: Infants were monitored for serious adverse events that occurred in the 31 day period following vaccination in 8 clinical studies. In these eight trials, 608 subjects reported at least one SAE (450 in vaccinees and 158 in placebo recipients). The incidence of subjects reporting at least one SAE in the group receiving ROTARIX (8.12%, 95% CI: 7.41%; 8.87%) was similar to the incidence in the placebo group (8.53%, 95% CI: 7.30%; 9.90%).

Deaths: In 8262 infants enrolled and vaccinated in 10 completed trials, a total of 18 deaths were reported: 12 deaths in ROTARIX (0.19%, N=6290) and 6 in placebo (0.30%, N=1972). In the large safety study (Rota-023), 99 deaths occurred during the study*: 56 in ROTARIX group (N=31 673) and 43 in the placebo group (N=31 552). None of the cases were assessed as related to vaccination and no potential imbalance was detected for the 99 fatal cases in terms of overall mortality (P-value=0.198).

Safety in Preterm Infants: In a clinical study, 1009 preterm infants were administered ROTARIX or placebo (198 were 27-30 weeks gestational age and 801 were 31-36 weeks gestational age). The first dose was administered from 6 weeks after birth. SAEs were observed in 5.1% of recipients of ROTARIX as compared to 6.8% of placebo recipients. Similar rates of solicited and unsolicited symptoms were observed in ROTARIX and placebo recipients. No cases of intussusception were reported. For premature infants born less than 36 weeks of gestation, and who remain hospitalized at the time of recommended administration, close monitoring for at least 48 hours after vaccination could be considered.
Safety in Infants with Human Immunodeficiency (HIV) Infection: In a clinical study, 100 infants with HIV infection were administered three doses of ROTARIX or placebo. The safety profile was similar between ROTARIX and placebo recipients.

Table 4: ROTARIX

Adverse Reactions Considered by the Investigator as Being at Least Possibly Related to ROTARIX Vaccination

Frequency	Adverse Event	System/Organ Class
Very Common ≥10%	irritability	Psychiatric Disorders
	loss of appetite	Gastrointestinal disorders
Common ≥1% and <10%	diarrhea, vomiting, flatulence, abdominal pain,	Gastrointestinal disorders
	regurgitation of food	
	fever, fatigue	General disorders and administration site conditions
Uncommon ≥0.1% and <1%	crying, sleep disorder	Psychiatric Disorders
	somnolence	Nervous system disorders
	constipation	Gastrointestinal disorders
Rare ≥0.01% and <0.1%	upper respiratory tract infection	Infections and infestations
	hoarseness, rhinorrhea	Respiratory, thoracic and mediastinal disorders
	dermatitis, rash	Skin and subcutaneous tissue disorders
	muscle cramp	Musculoskeletal and connective tissue disorders

- **Clinical trials for the liquid formulation**

In a total of 4 clinical trials, approximately 3800 doses of ROTARIX liquid formulation were administered to approximately 1930 infants. Those trials have shown that the safety and reactogenicity profile of the liquid formulation is comparable to the lyophilized formulation.
Post-Market Adverse Drug Reactions: The following events have been spontaneously reported during post-approval use of ROTARIX. Because these events were reported voluntarily from a population of uncertain size, it is not possible to reliably estimate their frequency or to establish a causal relationship to vaccine exposure.
Gastrointestinal Disorders: hematochezia, intussusception.
Infections and Infestations: Kawasaki disease.
DRUG INTERACTIONS: Overview: Immunosuppressive therapies may reduce the immune response to vaccines. The potential interaction of these therapies with ROTARIX is not known.
Use with Other Vaccines: ROTARIX can be given concomitantly with any of the following monovalent or combination vaccines [including hexavalent vaccines (DTPa-HBV-IPV/Hib)]: diphtheria-tetanus-whole cell pertussis vaccine (DTPw), diphtheria-tetanus-acellular pertussis vaccine (DTPa), *H. influenzae* type b vaccine (Hib), inactivated polio vaccine (IPV), hepatitis B vaccine (HBV), pneumococcal conjugate vaccine and meningococcal serogroup C conjugate vaccine. Clinical studies demonstrated that the immune responses to and the safety profiles of the administered vaccines were unaffected.

Concomitant administration of ROTARIX and oral polio vaccine (OPV) does not affect the immune response to the polio antigens but may reduce that to ROTARIX vaccine. The immune response to ROTARIX is unaffected when OPV is administered two weeks apart from ROTARIX.

DOSAGE AND ADMINISTRATION: Dosing Considerations:
- ROTARIX is for **oral** use only.
- **Under no circumstances should ROTARIX be injected.**

Recommended Dose and Dosage Adjustment: The vaccination course consists of two doses. The first dose can be administered from the age of 6 weeks. There should be an interval of at least 4 weeks between doses. ROTARIX may be given to preterm infants following the same vaccination course. This could be incorporated into the Canadian Immunization Schedule (2 and 4 months). Other immunization schedules have also been evaluated. The administration of the 2 doses should be completed by the age of 24 weeks.

In particular circumstances, if the vaccine is given at an earlier age, and that the second dose is given within the shortest interval of 4 weeks, a lower immune response might be induced.

It is strongly recommended that infants who receive a first dose of ROTARIX complete the 2 dose regimen with ROTARIX. There are no data on safety, immunogenicity or efficacy when ROTARIX is administered for the first dose and another rotavirus vaccine is administered for the second dose or vice versa.

In clinical trials, spitting or regurgitation of the vaccine has rarely been observed and, under such circumstances, a replacement dose was not given. However, in the unlikely event that an infant spits out or regurgitates most of the vaccine dose, a single replacement dose may be given at the same vaccination visit.

There are no restrictions on the infant's consumption of food or liquid, including breastmilk, either before or after vaccination.

There is no evidence available to suggest that breastfeeding would reduce the protection against rotavirus gastroenteritis afforded by ROTARIX. Therefore, breastfeeding may be continued during the vaccination schedule.

The number of doses that would provide sufficient protection in immune compromised subjects has not been determined.
Administration: See Special Handling Instructions.

OVERDOSAGE:
No case of overdose has been reported.

For management of a suspected drug overdose, CPhA recommends that you contact your **regional Poison Control Centre**. See the *CPS* Directory section for a list of Poison Control Centres.

ACTION AND CLINICAL PHARMACOLOGY: Rotavirus infection is the leading cause of severe acute gastroenteritis in infants and young children throughout the world. Rotavirus is transmitted mainly by the fecal-oral route, through close person-to-person contact, and through fomites. Ingested virus particles infect the cells in the villi of the small intestine, typically leading to villous atrophy. Characteristic clinical features include diarrhea, vomiting, fever and abdominal discomfort, occasionally leading to fatal dehydrating illness. Improvements or increased efforts in hygiene and sanitation are known to be of limited efficacy.

Rotavirus infection affects 95% of children by the age of 3 to 5 years worldwide. The incidence of rotavirus infections is highest in children between 6 and 24 months of age. Primary infection after 3 months of age usually causes the most severe disease. Subsequent infections are possible but typically cause much milder symptoms.

The mortality rate associated with rotavirus is estimated to be 611 000 (range 454 000-705 000) annual deaths worldwide. Although the number of deaths due to rotavirus may be underestimated because testing for rotavirus is not routine, the mortality for Canada is proportionally compatible with estimated numbers from the US of 20 to 102 deaths per year. Rotavirus is estimated to cause 39% (range 29% to 45%) of childhood diarrhea hospitalizations.

Morbidity due to hospitalizations for diarrhea caused by rotavirus is high in industrialized countries. Nearly every child in the US is infected with rotavirus by the age of 5 years and the majority will have gastroenteritis, resulting in approximately 410 000 physician visits, 205 000-272 000 emergency department visits and 55 000-70 000 hospitalizations each year.

In Canada, rotavirus gastroenteritis during the winter and spring seasons have been estimated as representing between 37% (Greater Toronto) to 71% (Quebec) of community acquired gastroenteritis cases resulting in hospitalization, in children aged less than 5 years. In Quebec, the annual number of hospitalizations for rotavirus gastroenteritis in 0-4 year olds was estimated as 2000-2500, representing 40-50% of the annual number of its hospitalizations for gastroenteritis in this age range within the province. Hospital-acquired rotavirus infection among children also results in significant burden, both by prolonging the affected child's hospital stay and act as a reservoir that can propagate additional cases of nosocomial rotavirus. Globally, the incidence rates of nosocomial rotavirus infection vary, ranging from 0.97 to 27.7 per 100 hospital admissions. A surveillance study conducted in the Halifax regional municipality over the period of 1991-1999 observed that rotavirus infection accounted for 31% of nosocomial diarrhea episodes with an identified pathogen in children <18 years of age. The incidence of circulating rotavirus strains documented in recent Canadian reports has indicated that the distribution of rotavirus strains identified is similar to other developed countries, with G1 as the predominant strain, with only sporadic isolations of other serotypes.

Worldwide, circulating strains of G serotypes 1 to 4, associated with P genotypes P[8] and P[4] (G1P[8], G2P[4], G3P[8], and G4P[8]) predominate. Based on a recent review of the global distribution of rotavirus serotypes/genotypes, these strains were responsible for 88.5% of rotavirus diarrhea among children worldwide, with G1P[8] type being the predominant strain accounting for 64.7% of rotavirus infections.

Based on the distribution of P and G combinations, G1P[8], G2P[4], G3P[8] and G4P[8] represent over 90% of the rotavirus infections in North America, Europe and Australia.
Mechanism of Action: ROTARIX contains a live, attenuated human rotavirus that replicates in the small intestine and induces immunity. ROTARIX vaccine is derived from the human 89-12 strain which belongs to G1 serotype and P[8] genotype. G1 is the most prevalent strain worldwide. It is known that the genotype P[8] is shared by most other circulating strains, including serotypes G3, G4 and G9.

The immunologic mechanism by which ROTARIX protects against rotavirus gastro-enteritis is not completely understood. A relationship between antibody responses to rotavirus vaccination and protection against rotavirus gastroenteritis has not been established.

STORAGE AND STABILITY: Store in a refrigerator (2 to 8°C). Do not freeze.

In order to protect the vaccine from light it is recommended that the vaccine is stored in the original package.

The expiry date of the vaccine is indicated on the label and packaging.

SPECIAL HANDLING INSTRUCTIONS: The vaccine is presented as a clear, colorless liquid, free of visible particles, for oral administration.

The vaccine is ready to use (no reconstitution or dilution is required).

The vaccine is to be administered orally without mixing with any other vaccines or solutions.

The vaccine should also be inspected visually for any foreign particulate matter and/or abnormal physical appearance prior to administration. In the event of either being observed, discard the vaccine. Any unused vaccine or waste material should be disposed of in accordance with local requirements.

This medicinal product must not be mixed with other medicinal products.
Administration of the Vaccine:
1. Remove the protective tip cap from the **oral** applicator.
2. This vaccine is for **oral administration only**. The child should be seated in a reclining position. Administer **orally** (i.e. into the child's mouth towards the inner cheek) the entire content of the **oral** applicator.
3. **Do not inject.**

INFORMATION FOR THE PATIENT: Published in e-CPS, available by subscription at www.e-cps.ca.

DOSAGE FORMS, COMPOSITION AND PACKAGING: Each 1.5 mL dose of oral suspension is formulated to contain not less than $10^{6.0}$ $CCID_{50}$ of human rotavirus RIX4414 strain (live, attenuated), produced on Vero cells. Each dose also contains Dulbecco's Modified Eagle Medium (DMEM), sucrose, di-sodium adipate and sterile water. Oral applicators (Type 1, Ph. Eur.) with a plunger stopper (butyl rubber), pack sizes of 1, 5, 10, 25, 50 and 100.

RotaTeq®

rotavirus vaccine, live, oral, pentavalent

Live, Oral Pentavalent Vaccine Against Rotavirus Gastroenteritis

Merck Frosst

Date of Revision: June 4, 2010

SUMMARY PRODUCT INFORMATION:

Route of Administration	Dosage Form/ Strength	Clinically Relevant Nonmedicinal Ingredients
Oral	Solution Minimum dose levels of reassortants: G1 2.2×10^6 infectious units G2 2.8×10^6 infectious units G3 2.2×10^6 infectious units G4 2.0×10^6 infectious units P1A[8] 2.3×10^6 infectious units	For a complete listing see Dosage Forms, Composition and Packaging.

INDICATIONS AND CLINICAL USE: RotaTeq (rotavirus vaccine, live, oral, pentavalent) is indicated for the prevention of rotavirus gastroenteritis caused by the serotypes G1, G2, G3, G4, and G-serotypes that contain P1A[8], when administered to infants (see Dosage and Administration).

CONTRAINDICATIONS:
- Patients who are hypersensitive to this vaccine or to any ingredient in the formulation or component of the container. For a complete listing, see Dosage Forms, Composition and Packaging.
- Individuals who develop symptoms suggestive of hypersensitivity after receiving a dose of RotaTeq should not receive further doses of RotaTeq.
- Individuals with Severe Combined Immunodeficiency Disease (SCID). Cases of gastroenteritis associated with vaccine virus have been reported post-marketing in infants with SCID.

WARNINGS AND PRECAUTIONS: General: No safety or efficacy data are available from clinical trials regarding the administration of RotaTeq to:
1. immunocompromised patients such as
   - individuals with malignancies or who are otherwise immunocompromised;
   - individuals receiving immunosuppressive therapy;
2. individuals infected with HIV; or
3. individuals who have received a blood transfusion or blood products, including immunoglobulins within 42 days.

Infants with serious medical conditions were excluded from the trials. However, a small subset of infants with such conditions (e.g., cystic fibrosis, failure to thrive, cancer, congenital heart disease, and neutropenia) were diagnosed after enrollment in the study. No fecal shedding of vaccine strains was seen in this group. Health care providers must consider the benefits and potential risks of administering RotaTeq to infants with serious medical conditions while keeping in mind nearly all children are infected with naturally occurring rotavirus by age 5 years.

In clinical trials, RotaTeq was not administered to infants known to have immunodeficient household members. In these trials, RotaTeq was shed in the stools of 8.9% of vaccine recipients almost exclusively in the week after dose 1, in no vaccine recipient after dose 2, and in only one vaccine recipient (0.3%) after dose 3. Transmission of vaccine virus strains to non-vaccinated contacts has been observed post-marketing. RotaTeq should be administered with caution to individuals with immunodeficient close contacts such as:

- individuals with malignancies or who are otherwise immunocompromised; or
- individuals receiving immunosuppressive therapy.

However, because nearly all children are infected with naturally occurring rotavirus by the age of 5 years, vaccination of infants may decrease the risk of exposure of immunodeficient household contacts to naturally occurring rotavirus. The health care provider should assess the potential risks and benefits of administering RotaTeq to infants known to have immunodeficient close contacts.

Infants with active gastrointestinal illness, chronic diarrhea or growth retardation, or a history of congenital abdominal disorders or intussusception were not to be included in the clinical studies. Administration of RotaTeq may be considered with caution in such infants when, in the opinion of the physician, withholding the vaccine entails a greater risk.

Any acute infection or febrile illness may be reason for delaying use of RotaTeq except when, in the opinion of the physician, withholding the vaccine entails a greater risk. Low-grade fever itself and mild upper respiratory infection are not contraindications to vaccination with RotaTeq.

As with any vaccine, vaccination with RotaTeq may not result in complete protection in all recipients.

The clinical studies were not designed to assess the level of protection provided by only 1 or 2 doses of RotaTeq. Post hoc analyses of data from a large clinical study suggest that RotaTeq provides protection against hospitalizations and emergency department visits for rotavirus gastroenteritis during administration of the 3-dose vaccination series starting from 14 days post dose 1. However, to provide the level and duration of protection against rotavirus gastroenteritis that was observed in the clinical studies, infants should receive all 3 doses.

No clinical data are available for RotaTeq when administered after exposure to rotavirus.

Carcinogenesis and Mutagenesis: RotaTeq has not been evaluated for its carcinogenic or mutagenic potential or its potential to impair fertility.

Special Populations: Pregnant Women: RotaTeq is a pediatric vaccine and is not indicated for use in adults. There have been no studies in women or any developmental and reproductive toxicity studies in animals.

Nursing Women: As RotaTeq is a pediatric vaccine and is not indicated for use in adults, information on the safety of the vaccine when used during lactation is not available.

Pediatrics (6 weeks of age or above): RotaTeq has been shown to be generally well tolerated and efficacious in preventing rotavirus gastroenteritis when administered to infants 6 weeks through 32 weeks of age (see Dosage and Administration for the recommended dosage schedule).

RotaTeq may be given to pre-term infants according to their chronological age. Safety and efficacy have not been established in infants less than 6 weeks or more than 32 weeks of age.

Geriatrics: RotaTeq is not indicated for use in adult populations.

ADVERSE REACTIONS: Adverse Drug Reaction Overview: 71 725 infants were evaluated in 3 placebo-controlled clinical trials (Study 006, Study 007, and Study 009) including 36 165 infants who received RotaTeq and 35 560 infants who received placebo. Parents/guardians were contacted on days 7, 14, and 42 after each dose regarding intussusception and any other serious adverse events.

The vaccine is generally well tolerated.

Clinical Trial Adverse Drug Reactions: Because clinical trials are conducted under very specific conditions the adverse reaction rates observed in the clinical trials may not reflect the rates observed in practice and should not be compared to the rates in the clinical trials of another vaccine. Adverse drug reaction information from clinical trials is useful for identifying vaccine-related adverse events and for approximating rates.

Intussusception: In the large-scale (34 837 vaccine recipients and 34 788 placebo recipients), placebo-controlled Rotavirus Efficacy and Safety Trial (REST, Study 006), RotaTeq did not increase the risk of intussusception relative to placebo (see Table 1). Active surveillance was employed to identify potential cases of intussusception at days 7, 14, and 42 after each dose and every 6 weeks thereafter for 1 year after dose one. There were no confirmed cases of intussusception during the 42-day period after dose one, and there was no clustering of cases among vaccine recipients at any time period after any dose. Following the 1-year safety follow-up period, 4 cases of intussusception were reported in children who had received placebo during the study.

Table 1: RotaTeq

Confirmed Cases of Intussusception in Recipients of RotaTeq as Compared with Placebo Recipients During REST

	RotaTeq (n=34 837)	Placebo (n=34 788)	Relative Risk (95% CI)
Confirmed intussusception cases within 42 days after each dose[a]	6	5	1.6 (0.4, 6.4)
Confirmed intussusception cases within 365 days after dose one	13	15	0.9 (0.4, 1.9)

[a] Relative Risk and 95% Confidence Interval based upon group sequential design stopping criteria employed in REST.

Hematochezia: Hematochezia reported as an adverse experience occurred in 0.6% (39/6,130) of vaccine and 0.6% (34/5560) of placebo recipients within 42 days of any dose. Hematochezia reported as a serious adverse experience occurred in <0.1% (4/36 150) of vaccine and <0.1% (7/35 536) of placebo recipients within 42 days of any dose.

Serious Adverse Events: Serious adverse events occurred in 2.4% of recipients of RotaTeq when compared to 2.6% of placebo recipients within the 42-day period of a dose in the phase 3 clinical studies of RotaTeq. The most frequently reported serious adverse events for RotaTeq compared to placebo were: bronchiolitis (0.6% RotaTeq vs. 0.7% Placebo), gastroenteritis (0.2% RotaTeq vs. 0.3% Placebo), pneumonia (0.2% RotaTeq vs. 0.2% Placebo), fever (0.1% RotaTeq vs. 0.1% Placebo), and urinary tract infection (0.1% RotaTeq vs. 0.1% Placebo).

Deaths: Across the clinical studies, 52 deaths were reported. There were 25 deaths in the RotaTeq recipients compared to 27 deaths in the placebo recipients. The most commonly reported cause of death was sudden infant death syndrome (SIDS), which was observed in 8 recipients of RotaTeq and 9 placebo recipients.

Seizures: All seizures reported in the phase 3 trials of RotaTeq (by vaccination group and interval after dose) are shown in Table 2.

Table 2: RotaTeq

Seizures Reported by Day Range in Relation to Any Dose in the Phase 3 Trials of RotaTeq

Day Range	1–7	1–14	1–42
RotaTeq	10	15	33
Placebo	5	8	24

Seizures reported as serious adverse experiences occurred in <0.1% (27/36 150) of vaccine and <0.1% (18/35 536) of placebo recipients (not significant). Ten febrile seizures were reported as serious adverse experiences, 5 were observed in vaccine recipients and 5 in placebo recipients.

Kawasaki Disease: Kawasaki disease was reported in the phase III clinical trials in <0.1% (5/36 150) of vaccine recipients and <0.1% (1/35 536) of placebo recipients within 42 days of any dose (not statistically significant).

Solicited Adverse Experiences Regardless of Causality: In 11 711 infants (6138 recipients of RotaTeq) from the 3 studies, a Vaccination Report Card was used by parents/guardians to record the child's temperature and any episodes of diarrhea and vomiting on a daily basis during the first week following each vaccination. Table 3 summarizes the frequencies of these adverse events, regardless of cause.

Although an increase in elevated temperature among vaccine recipients compared to placebo recipients was observed in Study 007, the incidences of elevated temperature for the combined data from Studies 006, 007, and 009 were comparable as shown in Table 3.

Table 3: RotaTeq

Solicited Adverse Experiences Within the First Week After Doses 1, 2, and 3 (Detailed Safety Cohort)

	Dose 1		Dose 2		Dose 3	
Adverse Experience	RotaTeq	Placebo	RotaTeq	Placebo	RotaTeq	Placebo
	n=5616	n=5077	n=5215	n=4725	n=4865	n=4382
Elevated temperature[a]	17.1%	16.2%	20.0%	19.4%	18.2%	17.6%
	n=6130	n=5560	n=5703	n=5173	n=5496	n=4989
Vomiting	6.7%	5.4%	5.0%	4.4%	3.6%	3.2%
Diarrhea	10.4%	9.1%	8.6%	6.4%	6.1%	5.4%

[a] Temperature ≥100.5°F [38.1°C] rectal equivalent obtained by adding 1 degree F to otic and oral temperatures and 2 degrees F to axillary temperatures.

Vaccine-Related Adverse Experiences Compared to Placebo: Parents/guardians of the 11 711 infants were also asked to report the presence of other events on the Vaccination Report Card for 42 days after each dose. Overall, 47% of infants given RotaTeq experienced a vaccine-related adverse experience compared with 45.8% of infants given placebo. The most commonly reported adverse experiences that occurred more frequently with vaccine than with placebo were pyrexia (20.9%), diarrhea (17.6%) and vomiting (10.1%).

The following vaccine-related adverse experiences were observed among recipients of RotaTeq at a frequency at least 0.3% greater than that observed among placebo recipients (see Table 4).

Table 4: RotaTeq

Adverse Experiences (Incidence ≥1%) Observed in Recipients of RotaTeq at a Frequency at Least 0.3% Greater Than the Frequency Among Placebo Recipients

Adverse Experiences	Vaccine (%)	Placebo (%)
Gastrointestinal Disorders		
Diarrhea	17.6	15.1
Vomiting	10.1	8.2
General Disorders and Administration—Site Conditions		
Pyrexia	20.9	18.7

Administration of other licensed vaccines was permitted in all studies. The safety of RotaTeq when administered concomitantly with prespecified licensed vaccines including *H. influenzae* type b and hepatitis B vaccine, diphtheria and tetanus toxoids and acellular pertussis (DTaP) vaccine, inactivated poliovirus vaccine (IPV), pneumococcal conjugate vaccine, and hexavalent vaccines was evaluated in all 3 phase III, placebo-controlled studies. In a subsequent controlled study, the safety of RotaTeq when administered concomitantly with oral poliovirus vaccine was evaluated. RotaTeq was well tolerated; the frequency of adverse experiences observed was generally similar to that seen when the concomitant vaccines were administered with placebo.

Other Adverse Events: Otitis media and bronchospasm occurred in more vaccine than placebo recipients (14.5% versus 13.0% and 1.1% versus 0.7%, respectively) overall; however, among cases that were considered to be vaccine-related in the opinion of the study investigator, the incidence was the same for vaccine and placebo recipients for otitis media (0.3%) and bronchospasm (<0.1%).

Safety in Pre-Term Infants: RotaTeq or placebo was administered to 2070 pre-term infants (25 to 36 weeks gestational age, median 34 weeks) according to their age in weeks since birth in REST. All pre-term infants were followed for serious adverse experiences; a subset of 308 infants was monitored for all adverse experiences. There were 4 deaths throughout the study, 2 among vaccine recipients (1 SIDS and 1 motor vehicle accident) and 2 among placebo recipients (1 SIDS and 1 unknown cause). No cases of intussusception were reported. Serious adverse experiences occurred in 5.5% of vaccine and 5.8% of placebo recipients. The most common serious adverse experience was bronchiolitis, which occurred in 1.4% of vaccine and 2.0% of placebo recipients. Parents/guardians were asked to record the child's temperature and any episodes of vomiting and diarrhea daily for the first week following vaccination. The frequencies of these adverse experiences and irritability within one week after each of the three doses are summarized in Table 5.

Table 5: RotaTeq

Solicited Adverse Experiences Within the First Week of Doses 1, 2, and 3 Among Pre-term Infants

	Dose 1		Dose 2		Dose 3	
Adverse Event	RotaTeq	Placebo	RotaTeq	Placebo	RotaTeq	Placebo
	n=127	n=133	n=124	n=121	n=115	n=108
Elevated temperature[a]	18.1%	17.3%	25.0%	28.1%	14.8%	20.4%
	n=154	n=154	n=137	n=137	n=135	n=129
Vomiting	5.8%	7.8%	2.9%	2.2%	4.4%	4.7%
Diarrhea	6.5%	5.8%	7.3%	7.3%	3.7%	3.9%
Irritability	3.9%	5.2%	2.9%	4.4%	8.1%	5.4%

[a] Temperature ≥100.5°F [38.1°C] rectal equivalent obtained by adding 1 degree F to otic and oral temperatures and 2 degrees F to axillary temperatures.

Less Common Clinical Trial Adverse Drug Reactions: Nasopharyngitis occurred in 0.6% of vaccine recipients and 0.3% of placebo recipients; this is the only less common (incidence <1%) vaccine-related adverse experience that occurred at a frequency that was at least 0.3% greater among vaccine recipients than among placebo recipients.

Abnormal Hematologic and Clinical Chemistry Findings: Routine laboratory evaluations were not performed during the conduct of clinical trials; therefore, no laboratory adverse experiences were reported.

Post-Market Adverse Drug Reactions: The following adverse experiences have been spontaneously reported during post-approval use of RotaTeq. Because these experiences were reported voluntarily from a population of uncertain size, it is not possible to reliably estimate their frequency or to establish a causal relationship to vaccine exposure.

Skin and Subcutaneous Tissue Disorders: urticaria.

Infections and Infestations: Kawasaki disease.

Gastrointestinal Disorders: gastroenteritis with vaccine viral shedding in infants with Severe Combined Immunodeficiency Disease (SCID).

DRUG INTERACTIONS: Overview: There are no known drug interactions (see Dosage and Administration, Use with Other Vaccines).

Immunosuppressive therapies may reduce the immune response to vaccines. The potential interaction of these therapies with RotaTeq is not known.

Use with Other Vaccines: RotaTeq was administered with other routine infant vaccines in the clinical trials. The immune response following concomitant administration of RotaTeq with diphtheria and tetanus toxoids and acellular pertussis (DTaP) vaccine, inactivated poliovirus vaccine (IPV), *H. influenzae* type b conjugate vaccine, hepatitis B vaccine and pneumococcal conjugate vaccine was formally examined in a subset of Study 006. The immune responses to the specified vaccines were unaffected by RotaTeq. The results of a separate study indicate that concomitant administration of RotaTeq and oral poliovirus vaccine (OPV) does not affect the immune response to the poliovirus antigens, but may reduce that to RotaTeq. The immune responses to RotaTeq are unaffected when OPV is administered two weeks after RotaTeq. Concomitant administration of RotaTeq with these infant vaccines was well tolerated.

DOSAGE AND ADMINISTRATION: Dosing Considerations: For oral use only. Not for injection.

Recommended Dose and Dosage Adjustment: The vaccination series consists of three ready-to-use liquid doses of RotaTeq administered orally to infants.

The first dose of RotaTeq should be administered at 6 to 12 weeks of age; the subsequent doses should be administered at an interval of 4 to 10 weeks between each dose, which includes a 2, 4 and 6 months immunization schedule.

There are no restrictions on the infant's consumption of food or liquid, including breast milk, either before or after vaccination with RotaTeq.

RotaTeq may be given to pre-term infants according to their chronological age.

If for any reason an incomplete dose is administered (e.g., infant spits or regurgitates the vaccine), a replacement dose is not recommended. The infant should continue to receive any remaining doses in the recommended series.

Administration: Each dose is supplied in a container consisting of a squeezable plastic, latex-free dosing tube with a twist-off cap, allowing for direct oral administration. The dosing tube is contained in a pouch.

To administer the vaccine:

Tear open the pouch and remove the dosing tube.

Clear the fluid from the dispensing tip by holding tube vertically and tapping cap.

Open the dosing tube in 2 easy motions:

1. Puncture the dispensing tip by screwing cap clockwise **clockwise** until it becomes tight.
2. Remove cap by turning it **counterclockwise**.

Administer dose by gently squeezing liquid into infant's mouth toward the inner cheek until dosing tube is empty. (A residual drop may remain in the tip of the tube.)

Discard the empty tube and cap in approved biological waste containers according to local regulations.

Use with Other Vaccines: For concomitant use with other licensed pediatric vaccines, see Drug Interactions, Use with Other Vaccines.

Reconstitution: The vaccine is to be administered orally without mixing with any other vaccines or solutions. Do not reconstitute or dilute.

OVERDOSAGE:

There are no data with regard to overdose.

> For management of a suspected drug overdose, CPhA recommends that you contact your **regional Poison Control Centre**. See the *CPS* Directory section for a list of Poison Control Centres.

ACTION AND CLINICAL PHARMACOLOGY: Rotavirus is the leading cause of severe acute gastroenteritis in infants and young children in industrialized and developing countries. If left untreated without prompt oral or intravenous administration of fluids, rotavirus gastroenteritis may cause dehydration that can be fatal. Although other viral agents cause gastroenteritis, rotavirus has been demonstrated to be the etiologic virus directly responsible for the majority of gastroenteritis cases requiring medical care.

Rotavirus gastroenteritis is a universal disease affecting over 95% of infants and young children by the time they are 5 years old, regardless of their socioeconomic status or environmental conditions. Because nearly every child is infected with rotavirus early in life, the number of physician office visits and hospitalizations caused by this pathogen has a significant impact on public health resources. Rotavirus gastroenteritis is a seasonal illness in temperate climates with epidemics occurring in the winter months and is generally endemic in tropical and subtropical climates.

Rotavirus is a physically robust virus that can survive on objects for more than 60 minutes. The fecal-oral route is considered as the primary mode of rotavirus transmission; although, other modes may be involved as indicated by widespread infection and the lack of documented oral-fecal transmission for all cases.

Globally, it is estimated that 138 million children develop rotavirus gastroenteritis each year which results in 25 million clinic visits, 2.1 million hospitalizations and 352 000 to 592 000 deaths. In the US it is estimated that 3.5 million children develop rotavirus gastroenteritis each year which results in 500 000 physician office visits, 55 000 hospitalizations, and 20 to 102 deaths. The greatest proportion of hospitalizations occurs among infants and young children between 6 months and 35 months of age.

Rotavirus is responsible for approximately 28% to 78% of all hospitalizations for diarrhea in young children worldwide, regardless of geographic region and season. One out of every 8 children will seek care from a physician and one out of every 73 children will be hospitalized for rotavirus gastroenteritis in the US by the time they are 5 years old.

Similarly, in Canada, rotavirus-associated diarrhea represents an important cause of health care resource utilization including hospitalization. In a population based prospective Toronto-area study, between 1 in 106 and 1 in 160 children are hospitalized for rotavirus by age 5 years of age. The true hospitalization rate may be greater than these estimates since emergency department visits and hospital visits of short duration were not completely evaluated in this study.

Two separate studies conducted over different rotavirus seasons found approximately 78% of gastroenteritis episodes in young hospitalized children during the peak winter-spring months were attributable to rotavirus. Among those hospitalized, children who tested positive for rotavirus presented with vomiting more frequently upon admission and a greater proportion required intravenous fluids as compared with children who tested negative for rotavirus. Other than hospitalization, rotavirus is also responsible for pediatric office visits, over 20% of which may still require further hospital care.

A recent Toronto-area study measuring rotavirus associated diarrhea seen in emergency departments, pediatric practices and child care centres found that the illness presented with a mean duration of 5.8 to 6.1 days.

Although the number of deaths due to rotavirus may be underestimated because testing for rotavirus is not routine, the mortality for Canada is proportionally compatible with estimated numbers from the US of 20 to 102 deaths per year.

Adults who are in contact with infected infants are at particular high risk of rotavirus infection. Data from two recent Canadian studies showed that diarrhea rates in household members in the 2-week period before and after exposure to rotavirus-associated diarrhea in children <3 years of age were: 65-74% in contacts with other children less than 3 years of age; 38-43% in contacts with those 3 to 18 years of age; and 29-35% in those older than 18.

Mechanism of Action: Protection from natural rotavirus infection is largely serotype specific. The human rotavirus serotypes (G1, G2, G3, G4, and P1A[8]) have been selected for RotaTeq because these strains caused nearly 90% of rotavirus disease in North America, Europe and Australia and over 88% of rotavirus disease worldwide between 1973 and 2003. In the Toronto area, most strains observed in stool samples collected from November 1997 to June 1998 were G1 (65%) and G2 (31%) with sporadic occurrences of G3, G4, and G9. The exact immunologic mechanism by which RotaTeq protects against rotavirus gastroenteritis is unknown. Studies suggest a combination of factors is important in rotavirus immunity including neutralizing antibodies to the outer capsid G proteins, serum and secretory IgA, and other local mucosal responses (see Immunogenicity).

Immunogenicity: A relationship between antibody responses to RotaTeq and protection against rotavirus gastroenteritis has not yet been established. However, RotaTeq induces antibodies that neutralize human serotypes G1, G2, G3, G4 and P1A[8]. In phase III clinical studies, 92.9% to 100% of recipients of RotaTeq achieved a significant rise in serum anti-rotavirus IgA after a three-dose regimen.

STORAGE AND STABILITY: Store and transport refrigerated at 2 to 8°C. Protect from light. The product must be used before the expiration date.

RotaTeq should be administered as soon as possible after being removed from refrigeration. When out of refrigeration, vaccine should not be exposed to freezing temperatures and should be stored at temperatures at or below 25°C. Under these conditions, administration may be delayed for up to 4 hours. For additional information regarding stability under conditions other than recommended, call at: 1-800-567-2594. Vaccine not administered should be discarded in approved biological waste containers according to local regulations.

INFORMATION FOR THE PATIENT: Published in e-CPS, available by subscription at www.e-cps.ca.

DOSAGE FORMS, COMPOSITION AND PACKAGING: RotaTeq (rotavirus vaccine, live, oral, pentavalent) is supplied as a sterile solution for oral use in a single-dose tube. It is a pale yellow, clear liquid that may have a pink tint. Each single dose (2 mL) contains: human-bovine rotavirus reassortants: G1, G2, G3, G4, and P1A[8]. The minimum dose levels at the end of shelf life of the reassortants are as follows: G1 2.2×10^6 infectious units, G2 2.8×10^6 infectious units, G3 2.2×10^6 infectious units, G4 2.0×10^6 infectious units, P1A[8] 2.3×10^6 infectious units. Nonmedicinal ingredients: cell culture media, diluent, polysorbate 80, sodium citrate dihydrate, sodium hydroxide, sodium phosphate monobasic monohydrate and sucrose. The reassortants are suspended in a buffered stabilizer solution. There are no preservatives or thimerosal present. Manufacturing process residuals: The reassortants are propagated in Vero cells using standard tissue culture techniques in the absence of antifungal agents. Residual cell DNA content per dose of vaccine is below the World Health Organization (WHO) recommended upper limit of 100 µg/dose for orally administered vaccines. Trace amounts of fetal bovine serum may also be present. Single, pre-filled 2 mL unit dose in a 4-mL squeezable plastic (low density polyethylene) oral dosing tube with a plastic (high density polyethylene) twist-off cap. The dosing tube is contained in a pouch. The container and delivery system are latex-free. Packages of one single-dose tube.

Rougier Clean Derm
chlorhexidine gluconate
Antiseptic

Rougier Pharma

SUPPLIED: Each mL of red limpid liquid, slightly viscous, contains: chlorhexidine gluconate 4% w/v. Nonmedicinal ingredients: cocamidopropylamine oxide, FD&C red #40, glycerin, hydroxyethyl cellulose, isopropyl alcohol, purified water, sodium hydroxide and sorbitan monolaurate. Bottles of 300 mL. Keep bottle tightly closed below 25°C and protected from light. Keep out of the reach of children.

Rougier Magnesium
magnesium glucoheptonate
Magnesium Supplement

Rougier Pharma

INDICATIONS: In hypomagnesemic states: malnutrition, excessive gastrointestinal losses due to severe diarrhea or prolonged vomiting, malabsorption syndrome, liver cirrhosis, diabetic acidosis, chronic alcoholism, electrolyte abnormalities following the use of potent diuretics.

CONTRAINDICATIONS: Renal insufficiency.

WARNINGS: No data supplied by the manufacturer.

PRECAUTIONS: Magnesium forms insoluble chelates with tetracyclines, thus inhibiting antibiotic absorption. Therefore, concomitant administration of magnesium and tetracyclines should be avoided.

Administer magnesium cautiously in conjunction with drugs which affect electrolyte balance: diuretics, corticosteroids, cardiovascular agents.

When barbiturates, narcotics or other CNS depressants are administered concomitantly with magnesium, their dosage should be adjusted carefully because of the additive central depressive effects of magnesium.

Prolonged administration should be conducted under close medical supervision.

ADVERSE EFFECTS: No data supplied by the manufacturer.

OVERDOSE:

Symptoms: The absence or depression of deep tendon reflexes; drowsiness, heart block and respiratory paralysis may also occur.

Treatment: I.V. administration of 5 to 10 mEq of calcium as gluconate (10 to 20 mL of 10% calcium gluconate) is usually adequate for reversal of heart block or respiratory depression. In extreme cases, peritoneal dialysis using a dialysate free of magnesium or hemodialysis may be necessary.

> For management of a suspected drug overdose, CPhA recommends that you contact your **regional Poison Control Centre**. See the *CPS* Directory section for a list of Poison Control Centres.

DOSAGE: Adults: 15 to 30 mL 1 to 3 times per day, with meals. Average dose: 15 mL 4 times per day.

SUPPLIED: Each mL of clear orange liquid, contains: magnesium glucoheptonate 100 mg (5 mg elemental magnesium). Nonmedicinal ingredients: artificial flavouring, caramel, citric acid, potassium sorbate, purified water, sodium benzoate and sucrose. Energy: 23.12 kJ (5.44 kcal)/5 mL. Bottles of 500 mL and 2 L.

Rougier Vap
chlorhexidine gluconate
Local Antiseptic

Rougier Pharma

SUPPLIED: Each mL of reddish-pink limpid liquid contains: chlorhexidine gluconate 2% w/v. Nonmedicinal ingredients: 4% v/v isopropyl alcohol, FD&C red #40 and purified water. Vaporizing pumps of 300 mL. Keep bottle tightly closed below 25°C and protected from light. Keep out of the reach of children.

Rovamycine® Pr
spiramycin
Antibiotic

Odan

PHARMACOLOGY: Rovamycine (spiramycin) is a macrolide antibiotic produced by *S. ambofaciens*.

It is active against the following Gram-positive organisms: *S. aureus* (including penicillin-resistant strains), β-haemolytic streptococci, *S. viridans*, *S. faecalis* and *S. pneumoniae*, *C. diphteriae*, clostridia.

Except for *B. pertussis*, *H. influenzae* (approximately 50% of strains) and Neisseria, Gram-negative organisms are generally considered as resistant to spiramycin.

Bacterial resistance to spiramycin has been reported to develop, including cross-resistance between spiramycin and erythromycin. However, most of the erythromycin-resistant strains of *S. aureus* are still sensitive to spiramycin.

The mechanism of action of spiramycin has not been elucidated.

INDICATIONS: The treatment of infections of the respiratory tract, buccal cavity, skin and soft tissues due to susceptible organisms.

N. gonorrhoeae: as an alternate choice of treatment for gonorrhea in patients allergic to the penicillins. Before treatment of gonorrhea, the possibility of concomitant infection due to *T. pallidum* should be excluded.

CONTRAINDICATIONS: Rovamycine (spiramycin) is contraindicated in patients with known hypersensitivity to the drug.

The levels of spiramycin attained in the cerebrospinal fluid are much lower than those in the blood and are too low to be clinically useful. Therefore Rovamycine must not be used in patients with meningitis.

PRECAUTIONS: Administer antibiotics, including Rovamycine (spiramycin) cautiously to any patient who has demonstrated some form of allergy, particularly to drugs.

The possibility of superinfection caused by overgrowth of nonsusceptible organisms should be kept in mind during prolonged or repeated therapy. If superinfection occurs, discontinue the drug and take appropriate measures.

Safety of this product for use during pregnancy has not been established.

Spiramycin has been reported to inhibit the absorption of carbidopa and decrease levodopa plasma levels. When necessary, patients should be closely monitored and the levodopa dosage levels adjusted.

ADVERSE EFFECTS: Gastrointestinal: nausea, vomiting, diarrhea and very rare cases of pseudo-membranous colitis.
Liver System: very rare cases of liver tests function abnormalities.
Hypersensitivity Reactions: rash, urticaria, pruritus, very rarely angioedema and anaphylactic shocks. Isolated cases of vasculitis, including Henoch-Schonlein purpura.
Peripheral and CNS: occasional cases of transient paresthesia.
Hematologic: Very rare cases of acute hemolysis have been reported.

OVERDOSE:
Symptoms: No case of accidental overdosage has been reported. In oral doses over 4 g (16 400 000 I.U.) per day, abdominal discomfort, nausea or diarrhea may occur.
Treatment: No specific treatment has been proposed. Management should be symptomatic.

For management of a suspected drug overdose, CPhA recommends that you contact your **regional Poison Control Centre**. See the *CPS* Directory section for a list of Poison Control Centres.

DOSAGE: Adults: 6 000 000 to 9 000 000 International Units per 24 hours, in 2 divided doses (2 to 3 capsules of Rovamycine 500, twice a day).

In severe infections, the daily dosage may be increased to 12 000 000 to 15 000 000 International Units per day (4 to 5 capsules of Rovamycine 500, twice a day).

Gonorrhea: 12 000 000 to 13 500 000 International Units (8 to 9 capsules of Rovamycine 500) in a single dose.
Children: The use of Rovamycine 250 is recommended in children. The usual daily dosage is based on 150 000 I.U./kg body weight per 24 hours, in 2 or 3 divided doses; the following calculated dosages are given as a guide.

Child Body Weight	Dosage in Capsules of Rovamycine 250 (750 000 I.U. Spiramycin/Capsule)
15 kg	3 capsules/day
20 kg	4 capsules/day
30 kg	6 capsules/day

Spiramycin is stable in gastric juices and absorption is not affected by food. In severe infections, the daily dosage may be increased by one half.

In the treatment of beta hemolytic streptococcal infections, adequate Rovamycine dosage should be administered for 10 days.

SUPPLIED: Rovamycine 250: Each orange and red capsule, imprinted "ODAN 250" in black ink, contains: spiramycin 750 000 I.U. Nonmedicinal ingredients: D&C Red No. 28, FD&C Blue No. 1, FD&C Red No. 40, FD&C Yellow No. 6, gelatin, lactose, magnesium stearate, sodium croscarmellose and titanium dioxide. Tartrazine-free. Bottles of 50. Store in a dry place between 15 and 30°C.
Rovamycine 500: Each blue and violet capsule, imprinted "ODAN 500" in black ink, contains: spiramycin 1 500 000 I.U. Nonmedicinal ingredients: colloidal silicon dioxide, D&C Red No. 28, D&C Red No. 33, FD&C Blue No. 1, FD&C Red No. 40, gelatin, lactose, magnesium stearate, microcrystalline cellulose, povidone, sodium croscarmellose, talc and titanium dioxide. Tartrazine-free. Bottles of 50. Store in a dry place between 15 and 30°C.

Rub A-535 Antiphlogistine

methyl salicylate—camphor—menthol—eucalyptus oil

Topical Analgesic

Church & Dwight

INDICATIONS: External counterirritant cream for temporary pain relief of stiff and sore muscles, backache, strains, arthritic and rheumatic pain, sciatica, lumbago and bursitis.

CONTRAINDICATIONS: Salicylate hypersensitivity.

WARNINGS: No data supplied by the manufacturer.

PRECAUTIONS: For external use only. Do not apply to wounds or damaged skin and avoid contact with eyes and mucous membranes. Discontinue use if rash or irritation occurs. If condition persists for more than 7 days, consult physician. Do not bandage after application and avoid external sources of heat such as heating pads. Do not use if you are allergic to salicylates or are taking anticoagulant medications. Keep out of reach of children. Store in a cool place.

ADVERSE EFFECTS: No data supplied by the manufacturer.

OVERDOSE:
No data supplied by the manufacturer.

For management of a suspected drug overdose, CPhA recommends that you contact your **regional Poison Control Centre**. See the *CPS* Directory section for a list of Poison Control Centres.

DOSAGE: Adults and Children over 2 years of age: Massage into affected area until completely absorbed, not more than 3 or 4 times daily.

SUPPLIED: Ancient Secret—Natural Source: Each g contains: methyl salicylate 15% (extracted from teaberry leaves of Gaultheria procumbens), l-menthol 3.0% (from Mint Oil extracted from the leaves of Menthae piperitae), d- camphor 3.0% (extracted from the wood of Cinnamomum camphora), eucalyptus oil 1.5% (extracted from eucalyptus leaves of Eucalyptus globulus, E. fructicetorum and E. smithii) w/w. Nonmedicinal ingredients: carbomer, polyethylene glycol, polysorbate, propylene glycol, purified water and trolamine. Tubes of 85 g.
Dual Action: Each g contains: methyl salicylate 15%, menthol 3.0%, camphor 3.0%, eucalyptus oil 1.5% w/w. Nonmedicinal ingredients: carbomer, polyethylene glycol, polysorbate, propylene glycol, purified water and trolamine. Tubes of 100 g.
Extra Strength: Each g contains: methyl salicylate 18%, camphor 1%, menthol 0.75% and eucalyptus oil 0.5% w/w. Nonmedicinal ingredients: anhydrous lanolin, beeswax, glycerin, isobornyl acetate, light mineral oil, paraffin, propylene glycol stearate, salicylic acid, stearic acid, trolamine, purified water and white petrolatum. Tubes of 100 g. Jars of 160 g.
Rub Heat: Each g contains: methyl salicylate 12.5%, camphor 1%, menthol 0.75% and eucalyptus oil 0.5% w/w. Nonmedicinal ingredients: anhydrous lanolin, beeswax, glycerin, isobornyl acetate, light mineral oil, paraffin, propylene glycol stearate, purified water, salicylic acid, stearic acid, trolamine and white petrolatum. Tubes of 50 and 100 g. Jars of 450 g.
Sport Ultra Heat: Each g contains: methyl salicylate 30%, eucalyptus oil 3% w/w. Nonmedicinal ingredients: carbomer, polyethylene glycol 400, polysorbate, propylene glycol, purified water and trolamine. Glide-on applicator containers of 100 g.

RUB A-535® Antiphlogistine Capsaicin

capsaicin

Topical Analgesic

Church & Dwight

Date of Revision: June 11, 2009

INDICATIONS: RUB A-535 Antiphlogistine Capsaicin cream is indicated for the temporary relief of muscle and joint pain associated with rheumatoid arthritis and osteoarthritis, backache, lumbago, strains and sprains, pain of tendons and ligaments. The product is specially formulated to combine capsaicin, a proven natural arthritis pain reliever and natural skin conditioners and moisturizers, glucosamine, chondroitin, aloe vera and vitamin E. It provides an effective, odourless pain relief without drying out skin.

CONTRAINDICATIONS: Patients who are hypersensitive to capsaicin or the fruits of capsicum plants, ingredients in the formulation or components in the container. This product should not be used on raw, broken or irritated skin.

WARNINGS: This product is for external use only. If rash or irritation occurs, discontinue use. If condition worsens or symptoms persist or clear up and occur again within a few days, discontinue use of this product and consult a doctor. Avoid contact with eyes. After application wash hands thoroughly to prevent spreading the product to eyes and mucous membranes. Flush with water if contact does occur. The application of external heat such as an electric heating pad, a hot water bottle, or sweating through exercise may result in excessive skin irritation or burn.

PRECAUTIONS: *Drug Interactions:* This product contains chondroitin which can cause bleeding in individuals with bleeding disorders or are taking anticoagulants.
Pregnancy: Safety in pregnancy has not been established; however, no problems in humans were documented.
Lactation: It has not been determined if capsaicin is excreted in breast milk. However, problems in human have not been documented.

ADVERSE EFFECTS: Transient skin irritation, local burning, stinging or erythema may be most prominent during the first week of treatment, which diminishes or disappears with continued use at the recommended dose. If this product is applied less frequently than recommended or used intermittently, the burning effect may persist.

OVERDOSE:
Keep out of reach of children.

For management of a suspected drug overdose, CPhA recommends that you contact your **regional Poison Control Centre**. See the *CPS* Directory section for a list of Poison Control Centres.

DOSAGE: Adults and Children 12 Years and Older: Apply an amount just enough to cover the affected area and massage gently until completely absorbed, not more that 3 to 4 times daily. **Do not bandage.** Wash hands immediately after use. If used on arthritic hands, avoid contact with eyes and mucous membranes and wash hands 30 minutes after application. Use this product for 1-4 weeks to see beneficial effect.

SUPPLIED: Each container contains: capsaicin 0.05% w/w. Nonmedicinal ingredients: aloe barbadensis leaf extract, butylated hydroxytoluene, calcium disodium EDTA, cetyl alcohol, chondroitin sulfate sodium, citric acid, diazolidinyl urea, dimethicone, glucosamine sulfate potassium chloride, glycerin, glyceryl stearate and peg-75 stearate, lanolin, light mineral oil, menthyl lactate, methyl paraben, propylene glycol, propyl paraben, purified water, sodium phosphate dibasic, vitamin E and xanthan gum. Containers with sponge applicator of 65 mL. Store at room temperature not exceeding 27°C.

Rub A-535 Antiphlogistine Ice

menthol

Topical Analgesic

Church & Dwight

SUPPLIED: Regular: Each g of penetrating gel contains: menthol 4% w/w. Nonmedicinal ingredients: carbomer 934, FD&C Blue #1, isopropyl alcohol, polyethylene glycol, polysorbate 20, propylene glycol, purified water and trolamine. Tubes of 100 g. Jars of 250 g. Glide-on applicator containers of 100 g.
Sport: Each g of penetrating gel contains: menthol 5% w/w. Nonmedicinal ingredients: carbomer 934, FD&C Blue #1, isopropyl alcohol, polyethylene glycol, polysorbate 20, propylene glycol, purified water and trolamine. Glide-on applicator containers of 100 g.

Rub A-535 Antiphlogistine No Odour

triethanolamine salicylate

Topical Analgesic

Church & Dwight

SUPPLIED: Each g contains: triethanolamine salicylate 13.3% w/w. Nonmedicinal ingredients: acetylated lanolin alcohol, caprylic/capric triglyceride, carbomer 980, cetyl alcohol, diazolidinyl urea, diethanolamine cetyl phosphate, isopropylpalmitate, methylparaben, perfume, propylene glycol, propylparaben, purified water, stearic acid and trolamine. Tubes of 50 and 100 g.

Rub A-535® Extra Strength Arthritis Roll-On Lotion

triethanolamine salicylate—menthol—capsaicin

Topical Analgesic

Church & Dwight

INDICATIONS: Specially formulated for the temporary relief of muscle and joint pain associated with rheumatoid arthritis and osteoarthritis, backache, lumbago, strains and sprains, pain of tendons and ligaments. Mild, pleasantly scented, non-greasy.

CONTRAINDICATIONS: Known hypersensitivity to salicylates, capsaicin or the fruits of capsicum plant, menthol or to any of the non-medicinal ingredients. This product should not be used on raw, broken or irritated skin.

WARNINGS: This product is for external use only. If rash or irritation occurs, discontinue use. If condition worsens or symptoms persist for more than 7 days, or clear up and occur again within a few days, discontinue use of this product and consult a doctor. Avoid contact with eyes. After application wash hands thoroughly to prevent spreading the product to eyes and mucous membranes. Flush eyes with water if contact does occur. The application of external heat such as an electric heating pad, a hot water bottle, or sweating through exercise may result in excessive skin irritation or burn.

PRECAUTIONS: *Drug Interactions:* When administered concomitantly with anti-coagulant drugs possible additive effect on blood thinning may occur and may increase the risk of bleeding.
Pregnancy: Do not use this product if pregnant unless directed by a physician. Safety in pregnancy has not been established; however, if absolutely needed, the product should be used with caution and application should be limited to a small area.
Lactation: Use during breast feeding should be avoided as small amounts of salicylates are distributed in breast milk. It is not known whether capsaicin, topically applied, is distributed in breast milk.

ADVERSE EFFECTS: Transient skin irritation, local burning, stinging or erythema may be most prominent during the first week of treatment, which diminishes or disappears with continued use at the recommended dose. If this product is applied less frequently than recommended or used intermittently, the burning effect may persist.

OVERDOSE:
Keep out of reach of children.

For management of a suspected drug overdose, CPhA recommends that you contact your **regional Poison Control Centre**. See the *CPS* Directory section for a list of Poison Control Centres.

DOSAGE: Adults and children 12 years and older: Apply an amount just enough to cover the affected area and massage gently until completely absorbed, not more that 3 to 4 times daily. **Do not bandage.** Wash hands immediately after use. If used on arthritic hands, avoid contact with eyes and mucous membranes and wash hands 30 minutes after application.

SUPPLIED: Each container contains (w/w): triethanolamine salicylate 10%, menthol 1.25%, capsaicin 0.035%. Nonmedicinal ingredients: alcohol, allantoin, butylated hydroxytoluene, calcium disodium EDTA, caprylic/capric triglyceride, carbomer, Chamomilla recutita (Matricaria) flower extract, diazolidinyl urea, dimethicone, isobornyl acetate, propylene glycol, purified water and triethanolamine. Containers with roll-on applicator of 88 mL. Store at room temperature not exceeding 27°C.

Rythmodan® Ⓟ

disopyramide

Antiarrhythmic

sanofi-aventis

Date of Revision: February 22, 2008

PHARMACOLOGY: In both animal and man the electrophysiological and hemodynamic effects of disopyramide are qualitatively similar to those of quinidine and procainamide.

Although the exact mechanism of action has not been completely elucidated, it would appear from animal studies that disopyramide exerts its antiarrhythmic activity in the following manner: 1) Reduces automaticity in cardiac Purkinje fibers by depressing the slope of Phase 4 diastolic depolarization. The action manifests itself both in normal Purkinje fibers and in fibers damaged by either ischemia or infarction. 2) Depresses conduction velocity in atria, AV node, Purkinje fibers and ventricular muscle by decreasing the rate of rise of phase 0 depolarization in these fibers. 3) Prolongs action potential duration and effective refractory period in atria, Purkinje fibers and ventricular muscle. 4) Depresses excitability of both atrial and ventricular muscles by its direct effect on the myocardium. 5) Although the anticholinergic action of disopyramide may cause an increase in the sinus rate of normal hearts, the usual effect on the rapid cardiac rate associated with an arrhythmia is a decrease with possibly a reduction in blood pressure. Disopyramide exerts a negative inotropic action on cardiac muscle.

Disopyramide is rapidly absorbed after oral administration and reaches peak levels in about 1 to 2 hours. Absorption is slower with the long acting form, peak levels being reached in 4.5 to 6.2 hours.

Serum levels of disopyramide are correlated with antiarrhythmic activity. Usual therapeutic plasma levels are 2 to 4 μg/mL. At these concentrations, disopyramide in the blood is about equally distributed between plasma and erythrocytes. Plasma protein binding of disopyramide in humans varies with drug concentration. At therapeutic concentrations, protein binding is about 50%. Toxic plasma levels have not been defined in man, but are thought to exceed 10.5 μg/mL.

Mean plasma half-life of disopyramide in healthy humans is 6.7 hours (range of 4 to 10 hours) while with the long acting form it is 14.5 hours, and even longer in ill, hospitalized patients. Patients with impaired renal function (creatinine clearance less than 40 mL/minute), have demonstrated disopyramide half-lives of 10 to 18 hours. Hepatic impairment may also prolong the half-life. Little or no tissue accumulation occurs.

In healthy humans, urinary and fecal excretion of disopyramide and its metabolites account for about 80% and 10% of the dose, respectively. Forty percent (40%) to 60% of a given dose is excreted in the urine as the unchanged drug and 15% to 25% as the mono-N-dealkylated metabolite. The remainder of a given dose is excreted via the bile into the feces. The plasma concentration of this metabolite is about 1/10th that of disopyramide.

INDICATIONS:

> No antiarrhythmic drug has been shown to reduce the incidence of sudden death in patients with asymptomatic ventricular arrhythmias. Most antiarrhythmic drugs have the potential to cause dangerous arrhythmias; some have been shown to be associated with an increased incidence of sudden death. In light of the above, physicians should carefully consider the risks and benefits of antiarrhythmic therapy for all patients with ventricular arrhythmias.

Disopyramide is indicated for the treatment of documented life-threatening ventricular arrhythmias, such as sustained ventricular tachycardia. Disopyramide may also be used for the treatment of patients with documented symptomatic ventricular arrhythmias when the symptoms are of sufficient severity to require treatment. Because of the proarrhythmic effects of disopyramide its use should be reserved for patients in whom, in the opinion of the physician, the benefit of treatment clearly outweighs the risks.

For patients with sustained ventricular tachycardia, disopyramide therapy should be initiated in the hospital. Hospitalization may also be required for certain other patients depending on their cardiac status and underlying cardiac disease.

The effects of disopyramide in patients with recent myocardial infarction have not been adequately studied and, therefore, its use in this condition cannot be recommended.

CONTRAINDICATIONS: Disopyramide is contraindicated in the presence of shock, renal failure, severe intraventricular conduction defects (i.e. bundle-branch block associated with first-degree atrioventricular block, double block [left posterior or anterior hemiblock and right bundle-branch block]), pre-existing second and third degree A-V block (if no pacemaker is present), known hypersensitivity to the drug or to any ingredient in the formulation (for a complete list, see Supplied).

Disopyramide is contraindicated in patients with a pre-existing long QT (see Warnings, Other Cardiac Effects, Q-T Prolongation).

Disopyramide is contraindicated in patients with severe sinus node dysfunction (see Precautions, Patients with Special Disease or Conditions, Conductions Abnormalities).

Disopyramide should not be used in the presence of uncompensated or inadequately compensated congestive heart failure (see Warnings).

Disopyramide is contraindicated in most patients with extensive myocardial disease, but may on occasion be used in these patients under the close supervision of a cardiologist if in their opinion the patient's condition justifies it. When used in these patients continuous ECG monitoring in a CCU facility is mandatory.

Due to its anticholinergic activity, disopyramide is contraindicated in most patients with glaucoma or in patients in whom urinary retention is present (see Precautions).

Rythmodan-LA is contraindicated in children or in patients with cardiomyopathies, severe renal or hepatic insufficiency.

Concomitant administration of disopyramide with other antiarrhythmics or other drugs liable to provoke ventricular arrhythmias and especially torsade de pointes is contraindicated (see Precautions, Drug Interactions, Concomitant Antiarrhythmic Therapy and Drugs Associated with Risk of «torsade de pointes»).

WARNINGS: General: All antiarrhythmic drugs can produce unwanted effects when they are used to treat symptomatic but not life threatening arrhythmia; the expected benefit should be balanced against their risks.

Proarrhythmia and cardiac decompensation are special risks associated with the use of antiarrhythmic drugs in patients with structural heart disease. Special caution should be exercised when prescribing in this context (see Precautions, Drug Interactions, Concomitant Antiarrhythmic Therapy).

Life threatening and haemodynamically significant arrhythmia are difficult to treat and affected patients are at high risk. Treatment of these arrhythmias, whatever modality, must be initiated in the hospital.

Mortality: The results of Cardiac Arrhythmia Suppression Trial (CAST) in post-myocardial infarction patients with asymptomatic ventricular arrhythmias showed a significant increase in mortality and in non-fatal cardiac arrest rate in patients treated with encainide or flecainide compared with a matched placebo-treated group. CAST was continued using a revised protocol with the moricizine and placebo arms only. The trial was prematurely terminated because of a trend towards an increase in mortality in the moricizine treated group.

The applicability of these results to other populations or other antiarrhythmic agents is uncertain, but at present it is prudent to consider these results when using any antiarrhythmic agent.

Negative Inotropic Properties: Heart Failure: Because of its negative inotropic effect disopyramide may cause or worsen congestive heart failure. Therefore, this drug should not be used in patients with heart failure, and should be especially avoided in patients with a previous history of heart failure except in the very special circumstances described below:

In patients in whom the failure is exacerbated or caused by an arrhythmia, disopyramide may be used to suppress the ectopy but it must be borne in mind that any such benefit on cardiac function may be overcome by the depressant effect on cardiac output, and thereby result in even worse failure even though routine methods of anti-failure therapy including optimal digitalization are attempted. Careful monitoring is essential under these circumstances.

Patients with compensated heart failure may be treated with disopyramide, but careful attention must be given to the maintenance of cardiac function including optimal digitalization. Close observation is mandatory, as any benefit of disopyramide either therapeutic or prophylactic could be accompanied by an unacceptable lowering of cardiac output.

For most patients the encroachment on their cardiac reserve may be of minimal clinical consequence, but in patients with a limited reserve as a result of pump dysfunction and/or imbalanced work load, even a minor encroachment on reserve can precipitate clinically evident failure or make its control more difficult, and even result in a gross low output congestive cardiac failure state.

Hypotension: On rare occasions disopyramide has caused syncope with sudden loss of consciousness. In the cases reported, this was believed to be due to an excessive hypotensive action of the drug or, in some cases, due to concomitant use with other hypotensive or negative inotropic agents.

Severe hypotension following disopyramide administration has been observed usually in patients with primary myocardial disease (cardiomyopathy), and also in inadequately compensated congestive heart failure or advanced myocardial disease with low output state, or in patients on other hypotensive medication e.g., beta-adrenergic blockers or verapamil. An oral loading dose of disopyramide should not be given to such patients; initial dosage and subsequent dosage adjustments should be made under close supervision.

If severe hypotension develops, disopyramide should be discontinued promptly (see Precautions, Drug Interactions).

Other Cardiac Effects: QRS Widening: Significant widening (greater than 25%) of the QRS complex may occur during disopyramide administration; in such cases disopyramide should be discontinued.

Q-T Prolongation: As with other quinidine-like antiarrhythmic drugs, prolongation of the Q-T interval (corrected) and worsening of the arrhythmia may occur with disopyramide, particularly in response to higher doses. Patients who have evidenced prolongation of the Q-T interval in response to quinidine may be at particular risk. If a Q-T prolongation greater than 25% is observed and if ectopy continues, the patient should be monitored closely, and consideration be given to discontinuing disopyramide.

Disopyramide, as with other quinidine-like antiarrhythmic drugs, has been associated with torsades de pointes.

Heart Block: If first degree heart block develops in a patient receiving disopyramide, the dosage should be reduced. If the block persists despite reduction of dosage, continuation of the drug must depend upon weighing the benefit being obtained against the risk of higher degree of heart block. Development of second or third degree AV block or unifascicular or trifascicular block requires discontinuation of disopyramide therapy, unless the ventricular rate is adequately controlled by a temporary or implanted ventricular pacemaker (see Contraindications).

PRECAUTIONS: Patients with Special Diseases or Conditions: Atrial Tachyarrhythmias: Disopyramide is usually ineffective in atrial flutter and its usefulness in atrial fibrillation is not proven. If atrial flutter or fibrillation is present, the patient should be fully digitalized prior to disopyramide use so that drug-induced changes in AV conduction do not result in an increase of ventricular rate beyond physiologically acceptable limits.

Conduction Abnormalities: Disopyramide therapy in patients with sick sinus syndrome (including bradycardia-tachycardia syndrome), Wolff-Parkinson White (WPW) syndrome or bundle branch block requires care, since the effect of disopyramide in these conditions is difficult to predict. Sinoatrial node function deterioration has been reported in sick sinus syndrome patients treated with disopyramide (see Contraindications).

Digitalis Intoxication: Since disopyramide has not been studied in patients with digitalis intoxication, it should be used with caution in these patients.

Anticholinergic Activity: Glaucoma: In patients with a family history of angle-closure glaucoma, intraocular pressure should be measured before initiating disopyramide therapy. Disopyramide should not be administered to patients with angle-closure glaucoma unless topical application of miotics (e.g. pilocarpine ophthalmic drops) is used to counteract the anticholinergic effects of the drug (see Contraindications).

Urinary Retention: Urinary retention may occur in patients of either sex, but males with benign prostatic hypertrophy are at particular risk. If acute urinary retention develops, disopyramide therapy should be temporarily discontinued, except in occasional instances, in which continued control of the arrhythmia with disopyramide is considered mandatory. In such cases, overriding measures should be taken (e.g., catheter drainage or operative relief). If disopyramide is discontinued, and later reintroduced, a lower dose should be used (see Contraindications).

Myasthenia Gravis: Disopyramide should be used with special care in myasthenia gravis since its anticholinergic properties could precipitate a myasthenic crisis.

Renal Impairment: More than 50% of disopyramide is excreted unchanged in urine. Therefore, in impaired renal function reduce the dose and increase the dosing interval (see Dosage); ECG should be carefully monitored for prolongation of PR interval, QRS widening, or other signs of overdosage (see Pharmacology and Overdose). Rythmodan-LA tablets should not be used in patients with severe renal impairment.

Hepatic Impairment: Hepatic impairment also increases disopyramide plasma half-life; reduce dosage for patients with such impairment. The ECG should be carefully monitored for signs of overdosage.

Rythmodan-LA tablets should not be used in severe hepatic impairment.

Hypokalemia: Although there is no experience with disopyramide in severe hypokalemia, other antiarrhythmic agents are frequently ineffective or may be hazardous in such patients, as potassium abnormalities can by themselves induce arrhythmia; a significant potassium deficit should be corrected before instituting disopyramide therapy.

Patients having concomitant treatment with diuretics, stimulant laxatives or other hypokalemia inducing drugs are at particular risk of hypokalemia (see Precautions, Drug Interactions, Hypokalemia Inducing Drugs).

During treatment with disopyramide, potassium imbalance should be checked and corrected if necessary.

Hypoglycemia: Significant lowering of blood glucose has occasionally been reported during disopyramide administration. The physician should be alert to this possibility, especially in patients with congestive heart failure, the elderly, treated diabetics, chronic malnutrition, hepatic, renal or other diseases, or who are taking drugs (e.g., β-adrenergic blockers, alcohol) which could compromise preservation of the normal gluco-regulatory mechanisms in the absence of food.

In these patients blood glucose levels should be carefully monitored (see Drug Interactions).

Pregnancy: Animal studies have not demonstrated any teratogenic effect and only minimal evidence of impaired fertility.

Disopyramide has been reported to stimulate contraction of the pregnant uterus.

Disopyramide should be used in pregnant women only when it is clearly indicated and the benefit/risk ratio has been carefully evaluated.

Lactation: Disopyramide is excreted in human milk. Therefore, if use of the drug is deemed essential in lactating women, an alternative method of infant feeding should be instituted.

Children: The safety and effectiveness of Rythmodan or Rythmodan-LA in children have not been established and are therefore not recommended in this population.

Occupational Hazards: Driving a Vehicle or Performing Other Hazardous Tasks: Some adverse reactions may impair the patient's ability to concentrate and react, and hence the ability to drive or operate machinery (see Adverse Effects).

Drug Interactions: Concomitant Antiarrhythmic Therapy: The concomitant use of disopyramide with other Class I antiarrhythmic agent and/or β-adrenergic blockers should be reserved for patients with life-threatening arrhythmias who are demonstrably unresponsive to single agent antiarrhythmic therapy. Such use may produce serious negative inotropic effects, or may excessively prolong conduction. This should be considered particularly in patients with any degree of cardiac decompensation or those with a prior history, thereof. Patients receiving more than one antiarrhythmic drug must be carefully monitored.

Proarrhythmia and cardiac decompensation are special risks associated with the use of antiarrhythmic drugs in patients with structural heart disease. Special caution should be exercised when prescribing in this context (see Warnings, General).

Administer disopyramide cautiously to patients who have recently received other antiarrhythmic drugs. Disopyramide should not be started until at least one half-life after stopping the other antiarrhythmic agent. (Half-life of quinidine is about 6 hours. Half-life of procainamide is about 3 hours.) In these cases loading dose of disopyramide should not be used. Excessive widening of QRS or excessive negative inotropic effect may occur.

Quinidine: Concomitant administration of disopyramide and quinidine resulted in slight increases in plasma disopyramide levels and slight decreases in plasma quinidine levels.

Verapamil: Although the interaction is poorly documented, the concurrent use of verapamil and disopyramide may aggravate or precipitate congestive heart failure or result in excessive hypotension (see Warnings).

Digoxin: Concomitant digoxin and disopyramide therapy has not resulted in changes in serum digoxin levels.

Drugs Associated with Risk of "torsade de pointes": Combination with drugs associated with risk of "torsade de pointes" is not recommended (see Warnings, Other Cardiac Effects, Q-T Prolongation).

Anticholinergic Agents: The anticholinergic effect of disopyramide may be additive with that of other agents having anticholinergic properties (i.e. atropine).

Phosphodiesterase Type 5 Inhibitors: There is evidence that phosphodiesterase Type 5 inhibitors may be potentially associated with a risk of QT prolongation. Concomitant administration of disopyramide with such drugs may potentially enhance this QT prolongation effect and is not recommended.

Drugs Affecting Hepatic Microsomal Enzymes: There is some evidence that disopyramide is metabolized by hepatic CYP3A.

Drugs (e.g.: phenobarbital, rifampin, phenytoin) that induce hepatic microsomal enzymes may accelerate the metabolism of disopyramide, resulting in lower plasma concentrations. When microsomal enzymes inducers are used concomitantly with disopyramide, serum concentrations of disopyramide should be closely monitored to avoid subtherapeutic concentrations.

When prescribing a drug metabolized by CYP3A (such as theophylline, H.I.V. protease inhibitors [e.g. ritonavir, indinavir, saquinavir], cyclosporin A, warfarin), it should be kept in mind that disopyramide is probably also a substrate of this isoenzyme and thus competitive inhibition of metabolism might occur, possibly increasing serum levels of these drugs.
Erythromycin: There are reported cases of patients with clinically stable cardiac condition under disopyramide therapy where the addition of erythromycin resulted in polymorphic ventricular tachycardia, QTc prolongation, and elevation of disopyramide serum levels. Erythromycin appears to inhibit disopyramide metabolism in the liver. Additional documentation is needed to substantiate this possible interaction. However closer monitoring is advised when the two drugs are combined.
Ethanol: In healthy subjects, ethanol did not affect the half-life or total body clearance of disopyramide. However, combination could result in hypoglycemia in patients at risk (see Precautions, Hypoglycemia).
Insulin: There have been reports of potentiation of the hypoglycemic effect of insulin by disopyramide (see Precautions, Hypoglycemia).
Warfarin: Potentiation of the hypoprothrombinemic effect of warfarin has been reported in several patients receiving disopyramide and warfarin. However, in a study in several patients receiving disopyramide and warfarin concomitantly, the hypoprothrombinemic effect of warfarin was not increased and, in 2 patients, actually was decreased slightly. Further study is needed to determine whether a potential interaction exists.
Hypokalemia Inducing Drugs: The concomitant use of stimulant laxatives is not recommended, as patients are at particular risk of hypokalemia. The use of another type of laxative is more appropriate (see Precautions, Patients with Special Diseases or Conditions, Hypokalemia).

Precaution should also be exercised in case of association with other hypokalemia inducing drugs, such as: potassium-depleting diuretics (e.g. thiazides, furosemide, ethacrinic acid), amphotericin B, cosyntropin (corticotrophin analogue), gluco and mineralo-corticoids (see Precautions, Patients with Special Diseases or Conditions, Hypokalemia).

ADVERSE EFFECTS: Rare occurrence of congestive heart failure, hypotension, widening QRS, sinus arrest, nodal rhythm dissociation, cardiac arrest and cardiovascular collapse have been reported. An occasional paradoxical ventricular tachycardia evolving sometimes to fibrillation has been observed. A definite relationship to the drug was not always established in the above cardiovascular effects.

Intra-cardiac conduction abnormalities may occur: QT interval prolongation, atrioventricular block and bundle-branch block.

Other types of arrhythmia have been reported: bradycardia, sinus block.

The most common adverse reactions which are dose dependent are associated with the anticholinergic properties of the drug. These may be transitory, but may be persistent and can be severe. Urinary retention is the most serious anticholinergic effect.

The following reactions were reported in more than 10% of patients:
Anticholinergic: dry mouth (16 to 30%), urinary retention (7 to 13%), constipation.
Gastrointestinal: nausea, indigestion, vomiting, diarrhea, flatulence, bad taste in the mouth, anorexia.

The following reactions were reported in 1 to 10% of patients:
Anticholinergic: blurred vision, dry eyes/nose/throat.
Cardiovascular: hypotension with or without CHF, increased CHF, cardiac conduction disturbances, proarrhythmic effects (6%), edema, dyspnea, cyanosis, chest pain.
Dermatologic: skin reactions including pruritus, urticaria, morbilliform eruption, abdominal rash, photosensitization.
General: dizziness, vertigo, drowsiness, profuse sweating.
Genitourinary: urinary hesitancy and frequency.
Other: raised AST levels.

The following were reported in less than 1% of patients: dysuria, headache, feeling of warmth, pallor, peripheral paresthesia, fatigue, malaise, insomnia, confusion, transitory psychosis, elevated BUN, elevated creatinine, decreased hemoglobin/hematocrit, hypoglycemia, neutropenia, idiosyncratic reaction to drug. In a few instances cholestatic jaundice has been reported. A definite causal relationship has not been established.

A high plasma concentration has been associated with impotence.

Other atropine-like ocular adverse reactions were reported: disorders of accommodation, diplopia.

Epigastralgia has been also reported.
Skin Reactions: very rarely, rashes; isolated reports of anaphylactic-type reactions (e.g. angioedema) possibly culminating in shock (essentially reported in association with the injectable formulation).

OVERDOSE:

Symptoms: Patients who took deliberate overdoses of oral disopyramide presented with an early loss of consciousness after an apneic period, cardiac arrhythmias and loss of spontaneous respiration, leading to death. Serum levels in these patients were as high as 114 mg/L taken at various times after ingestion, including post-mortem.

The clinical signs of overdose may also include: bilateral mydriasis (suggestive of overdose); syncope, hypotension or shock; cardiac arrest due to intraventricular block or asystole; respiratory symptoms; coma (with bilateral mydriasis) in cases of massive intoxication.

Toxic plasma levels of disopyramide produce excessive widening of QRS complex and QT interval as a premonitory sign of other arrhythmias, in particular torsade de pointes which can result in repeated syncopes, worsening of CHF, hypotension, varying kinds and degrees of conduction disturbance, bradycardia and finally asystole. Obvious anticholinergic effects are also observed.

Treatment: Discontinue drug and initiate gastric lavage; no specific antidote has been identified: treatment of overdosage should be symptomatic and may include the administration of isoproterenol, dopamine, intra-aortic balloon counterpulsation, mechanically assisted respiration and hemoperfusion with charcoal.

Hemodialysis may be employed to rapidly lower serum concentration of drug. In vitro studies with human blood have demonstrated good dialyzability. Its clearance was 33 mL/minute at a blood flow 250 mL/minute when an initial plasma concentration of 22 µg/mL was dialyzed using an artificial kidney (Cordis-DOW-4).

The ECG should be monitored and supportive therapy with vasopressors, sympathomimetics, cardiac glycosides and diuretics should be given, as required.

Should progressive heart block develop, endocardial pacing should be implemented. In case of any impaired renal function, measures to increase glomerular filtration rate may reduce the toxicity (disopyramide is excreted primarily by the kidney). Altering the urinary pH in man does not affect plasma half-life or the amount of disopyramide excreted in urine.

The anticholinergic effects could be reversed with neostigmine, at the discretion of the physician.

For management of a suspected drug overdose, CPhA recommends that you contact your **regional Poison Control Centre**. See the *CPS* Directory section for a list of Poison Control Centres.

DOSAGE: The dosage should be individualized for each patient based upon response and tolerance and patient weight.
Capsules: Usual daily dose: 400 to 800 mg given in 4 divided doses. Rarely, control may be maintained on daily doses of less than 400 mg.

If rapid control of arrhythmia is essential, an initial dosage schedule for most adults is a single loading dose of 300 mg followed by 100 mg every 6 hours. If satisfactory control of the arrhythmias is not obtained with the maintenance dose of 100 mg every 6 hours, increase to 150 mg or subsequently to 200 mg every 6 hours if necessary.

For patients with cardiomyopathy or possible cardiac decompensation, loading doses should not be given, an initial dosage should be limited to 100 mg every 6 hours. Subsequent dosage adjustments should be made gradually with close monitoring for possible development of hypotension and/or congestive heart failure (see Warnings).

For patients of small stature (body weight less than 50 kg) and for patients with mild hepatic or renal insufficiency (creatinine clearance above 60 mL/minute) a loading dose of 200 mg is recommended followed by 100 mg every 6 hours. The recommended maintenance dose of these patients is 400 mg/day given in doses of 100 mg every 6 hours.

In patients with severe hepatic or renal insufficiency (creatinine clearance below 50 mL/minute) an initial loading dose of 100 mg is recommended. These patients are best managed with repeated plasma disopyramide determinations and subsequent dosage and frequency of administration (see Table 1) should be based on the results of these determinations (see Precautions).

Table 1: Rythmodan

Dosage Interval for Patients with Renal Insufficiency (Rythmodan Capsules)

Creatinine clearance (mL/min)	40–30	30–15	<15
Approximate maintenance-dosing interval	q8h	q12h	q24h

No loading dose should be given to patients who are being transferred from other oral antiarrhythmic agents such as quinidine or procainamide (see Precautions, Drug Interactions).

SUPPLIED: 100 mg: Each green/yellow, hard gelatin capsule, marked RY RL contains: disopyramide 100 mg. Nonmedicinal ingredients: cornstarch, magnesium stearate, pregelatinized starch and talc; capsule body and head : FD&C Blue #2, gelatin, titanium dioxide and yellow iron oxide. Blister packs of 84 (6×14).
150 mg: Each opaque, white, hard gelatin capsule, marked RY 150, contains: disopyramide 150 mg. Nonmedicinal ingredients: cornstarch, magnesium stearate, pregelatinized starch and talc; capsule body and head: gelatin and titanium dioxide. Blister packs of 84 (6×14).

(Shown in Product Identification Section)

Rythmol® Ⓟ
propafenone HCl
Antiarrhythmic

Abbott

Date of Preparation: October 21, 1987
Date of Revision: August 6, 2009

SUMMARY PRODUCT INFORMATION:

Route of Administration	Dosage Form/ Strength	Clinically Relevant Nonmedicinal Ingredients
Oral	Film-coated tablets/150 mg and 300 mg	Croscarmellose sodium, hypromellose, magnesium stearate, maize starch, microcrystalline cellulose, macrogol 400 and 6000, purified water, titanium dioxide This is a complete listing of nonmedicinal ingredients.

INDICATIONS AND CLINICAL USE: RYTHMOL (propafenone hydrochloride) is indicated for:
- the treatment of documented life-threatening ventricular arrhythmias, such as sustained ventricular tachycardia prevention.

RYTHMOL may also be used for the treatment of patients with documented symptomatic ventricular arrhythmias when the symptoms are of sufficient severity to require treatment. Because of the proarrhythmic effects of RYTHMOL, its use should be reserved for patients in whom, in the opinion of the physician, the benefit of treatment clearly outweighs the risks.

For patients with sustained ventricular tachycardia, RYTHMOL therapy should be initiated in the hospital. Initiation in hospital may also be required for certain other patients depending on their cardiac status and underlying cardiac disease.

The effects of RYTHMOL in patients with recent myocardial infarction have not been adequately studied and, therefore, its use in this condition cannot be recommended.

There is no evidence from controlled clinical trials that the use of RYTHMOL favourably affects survival or the incidence of sudden death.
Geriatrics (>65 years of age): Evidence from clinical trials and experience showed that use in elderly patients is associated with differences in safety. See Warnings and Precautions.
Pediatrics (<18 years of age): RYTHMOL has not been studied in children in controlled clinical trials and therefore use in this age group is not recommended.
CONTRAINDICATIONS:
- Patients who are hypersensitive to this drug or to any ingredient in the formulation or component of the container. For a complete listing, see Dosage Forms, Composition and Packaging.
- Severe or uncontrolled congestive heart failure. See Warnings and Precautions.
- Cardiogenic shock.
- Sinoatrial, atrioventricular and intraventricular disorders of impulse conduction and sinus node dysfunction (e.g. sick sinus syndrome) in the absence of an artificial pacemaker.
- Severe bradycardia (less than 50 beats/min).
- Marked hypotension.
- Bronchospastic disorders.
- Severe disorders of electrolyte balance.
- Severe hepatic failure. See Warnings and Precautions.

WARNINGS AND PRECAUTIONS:

Serious Warnings and Precautions
- No antiarrhythmic drug has been shown to reduce the incidence of sudden death in patients with asymptomatic ventricular arrhythmias. Most antiarrhythmic drugs have the potential to cause dangerous arrhythmias; some have been shown to be associated with an increased incidence of sudden death. In light of the above, physicians should carefully consider the risks and benefits of antiarrhythmic therapy for all patients with ventricular arrhythmias.

Cardiovascular: Mortality: The results of the Cardiac Arrhythmia Suppression Trials (CAST) in post-myocardial infarction patients with asymptomatic ventricular arrhythmias showed a significant increase in mortality and in the non-fatal cardiac arrest rate in patients treated with flecainide or encainide compared with a matched placebo-treated group. CAST was continued using a revised protocol with the moricizine and placebo arms only. The trial was prematurely terminated because of a trend towards an increase in mortality in the moricizine treated group.

The applicability of these results to other populations or other antiarrhythmic agents is uncertain, but at present it is prudent to consider these results when using any antiarrhythmic agent in patients with structural heart disease.
Proarrhythmic Effects: RYTHMOL (propafenone hydrochloride) may cause new or worsen existing arrhythmias. Such proarrhythmic effects range from an increase in frequency of premature ventricular contractions (PVCs) to the development of more severe ventricular tachycardia, ventricular fibrillation or torsades de pointes. It is therefore essential that each patient administered propafenone hydrochloride be evaluated clinically and electrocardiographically prior to, and during therapy to determine whether the response to propafenone supports continued treatment.

Overall in clinical trials with RYTHMOL, 4.7% of all patients had new or worsened ventricular arrhythmia possibly representing a proarrhythmic event [0.7% was an increase in PVCs, 4.0% a worsening, or new appearance, of ventricular tachycardia (VT) or ventricular fibrillation (VF)]. Of the patients who had worsening of VT (4%), 92% had a history of VT and/or VT/VF, 71% had coronary artery disease, and 68% had a prior myocardial infarction. The incidence of proarrhythmia in patients with less serious or benign arrhythmias which include patients with an increase in frequency of PVCs, was 1.6%. Although most proarrhythmic events occurred during the first week of therapy, late events also were seen and the CAST study suggests that a risk is present throughout treatment. See Warnings and Precautions, Cardiovascular, Mortality.
Congestive Heart Failure: During treatment with oral RYTHMOL in patients with depressed baseline function (mean Ef=33.5%), no significant decreases in ejection fraction (Ef) were seen. In clinical trial experience, new or worsened congestive heart failure (CHF) has been reported in 3.7% of patients; of those 0.9% were considered probably or definitely related to RYTHMOL. Of the patients with CHF probably related to RYTHMOL, 80% had preexisting heart failure and 85% had coronary artery disease. CHF attributable to RYTHMOL developed rarely (<0.2%) in patients who had no previous history of CHF.

Propafenone hydrochloride exerts both beta blockade and a dose related direct negative inotropic effect on myocardium. Therefore, RYTHMOL should not be prescribed in patients with uncontrolled congestive heart failure where left ventricular output is less than 35%.

Caution should be exercised when using RYTHMOL in patients with minimal cardiac reserve or in those who are receiving other drugs with negative inotropic potential.
Effects on Cardiac Conduction: Propafenone hydrochloride slows cardiac conduction which may result in a dose-related prolongation of PR interval and QRS complex, development of first or higher degree AV block, bundle branch block and intraventricular conduction delay. See Adverse Reactions. Therefore, development of signs of increasing depression of cardiac conductivity during RYTHMOL therapy requires a reduction in dosage or a discontinuation of RYTHMOL unless the ventricular rate is adequately controlled by a pacemaker.

Effects on Pacemaker Threshold: Patients with permanent pacemakers should have their existing thresholds re-evaluated after initiation of or change in RYTHMOL therapy because of a possible increase in endocardial stimulation threshold.

Hematologic: Hematologic Disturbances: Agranulocytosis has been reported infrequently in patients taking RYTHMOL. The onset is generally within four to six weeks and presenting symptoms have included fever, fatigue, and malaise. Agranulocytosis occurs in less than 0.1% of patients taking RYTHMOL. Patients should be instructed to immediately report fever, fatigue, malaise or any signs of infection, especially in the first three months of therapy. Prompt discontinuation of RYTHMOL therapy is recommended when a decreased white blood cell count or other signs and symptoms warrant consideration of agranulocytosis/granulocytopenia. Cessation of RYTHMOL therapy is usually followed by recovery of blood counts within two weeks.

Hepatic/Biliary/Pancreatic: Use in Patients with Impaired Hepatic Function: Since propafenone hydrochloride is highly metabolized by the liver it should be administered cautiously to patients with impaired hepatic function. See Contraindications. Administration of RYTHMOL to these patients results in an increase in bioavailability to approximately 70% compared to 3 to 40% for patients with normal liver function, prolongation of the half-life, a decrease in the systemic clearance, and a reduction in the serum protein binding of the drug. As a result, the dose of RYTHMOL given to patients with impaired hepatic function should be reduced. See Dosage and Administration. It is important to monitor electrocardiographic intervals for signs of excessive pharmacological effects. See Overdosage and/or adverse reactions, until an individualized dosage regimen has been determined.

A number of patients with liver abnormalities associated with RYTHMOL therapy have been reported in foreign post-marketing experience. Some appeared due to be hepatocellular injury, some were cholestatic and some showed a mixed picture. Some of these reports were simply discovered through clinical chemistries, others because of clinical symptoms. One case was rechallenged with a positive outcome.

Increased hepatic enzymes (alkaline phosphatase, serum transaminases) (0.2%), hepatitis (0.03%) and cholestasis (0.1%) have also been observed. See Adverse Reactions, Less Common Clinical Trial Adverse Drug Reactions (<1%).

Immune: Elevated ANA Titres: In long-term studies, positive antinuclear antibody (ANA) titres have been reported in 21% of patients receiving RYTHMOL. However, it is impossible to determine what exact percentage of patients had a new positive ANA titre as a result of RYTHMOL therapy. This laboratory finding has not been associated with clinical symptoms. One case of Lupus-like syndrome has been reported which resolved upon discontinuation of therapy. Laboratory evaluation for antinuclear antibodies should be performed initially and at regular intervals. It is recommended that patients in whom an abnormal ANA test has occurred be evaluated regularly. If worsening elevation of ANA titres or clinical symptoms are detected, RYTHMOL should be discontinued.

Neurologic: Exacerbation of myasthenia gravis has been reported during RYTHMOL therapy.

Renal: There is limited experience with use of oral propafenone hydrochloride in patients with impaired renal function. In patients whose kidney function is impaired, there may be drug accumulation after standard therapeutic doses. Since a considerable percentage of propafenone metabolites are excreted in the urine (18.5 to 38% of the dose/48 hours), RYTHMOL should be used cautiously in patients with renal impairment and only after consideration of the benefit/risk ratio. These patients should be carefully monitored for signs of toxicity. See Overdosage. The dose in these patients has not been determined.

Respiratory: Nonallergic Bronchospasm (e.g. chronic bronchitis, emphysema): Patients with bronchospastic disease should, in general, not receive RYTHMOL or other agents with beta-adrenergic blocking activity. See Contraindications.

Sexual Function/Reproduction: Impaired Spermatogenesis: Clinical evaluation of spermatogenesis was undertaken in 11 normal subjects, given oral RYTHMOL 300 mg twice daily for four days which was then increased to 300 mg three times daily for an additional four days. Patients were followed for 128 days post-treatment and demonstrated a 28% reduction in semen sample volume following the last dose (Day 8) and a 27% reduction in sperm count, on Day 72. Follicle-stimulating hormone (FSH) and testosterone levels were also slightly decreased. Neither the decrease in sperm count nor the decrease in sample volume were sustained beyond the single visit in which they occurred, and both values remained within the laboratories normal reference range. Reduced spermatogenesis was also observed in animal experiments. The significance of these findings is uncertain.

Special Populations: Pregnant Women: Propafenone hydrochloride has been shown to be embryotoxic in the rat when given in doses of 600 mg/kg (about six times the maximum recommended human dose on a mg/m² basis) and in the rabbit when given in doses of 150 mg/kg (about three times the maximum recommended human dose on a mg/m² basis). In a perinatal and postnatal study in rats, propafenone hydrochloride produced dose-dependent increases in maternal and neonatal mortality, decreased maternal and pup body weight gain and reduced neonatal physiological development.

There are no adequate and well controlled studies in pregnant women. RYTHMOL should be used during pregnancy only when the potential benefit outweighs the risk to the fetus. Propafenone hydrochloride is known to pass the placental barrier in humans. The concentration of propafenone hydrochloride in the umbilical cord has been reported to be about 30% of that in the maternal blood.

Labour and Delivery: It is not known whether the use of RYTHMOL during labour or delivery has immediate or delayed adverse effects on the fetus, or whether it prolongs the duration of labour or increases the need for forceps delivery or other obstetrical intervention.

Nursing Women: Propafenone and 5-hydroxypropafenone are excreted in human milk. Because of possible serious adverse reactions in nursing infants, an alternative method of infant feeding should be considered when the use of RYTHMOL is considered essential.

Pediatrics (<18 years of age): The use of RYTHMOL in children is not recommended, since safety and efficacy have not been established.

Geriatrics (>65 years of age): A slight increase in the incidence of dizziness was observed in elderly patients. Because of the possible increased risk of impaired hepatic or renal function in this age group, RYTHMOL should be used with caution. The effective dose may be lower in these patients.

Gender: The effect of gender on propafenone hydrochloride, when administered as RYTHMOL, has not been investigated.

Race: The effect of different races on propafenone hydrochloride, when administered as RYTHMOL, has not been investigated.

ADVERSE REACTIONS: Adverse Drug Reaction Overview: In 2127 patients treated with RYTHMOL (propafenone hydrochloride) in North American controlled and open clinical trials, the most common adverse reactions reported were dizziness (12.5%), nausea and/or vomiting (10.7%), unusual taste (8.8%) and constipation (7.2%). The adverse effects judged to be most severe were aggravation or induction of arrhythmia (4.7%), congestive heart failure (3.7%) and ventricular tachycardia (3.4%). The incidences for these three adverse reactions in patients with a previous history of myocardial infarction (MI) were 6.9, 5.3 and 5.5%, respectively, while in patients without a history of MI the incidences were 3.0, 2.4 and 1.8%, respectively. Approximately 20% of patients had RYTHMOL discontinued due to adverse reactions.

Adverse reactions were dose related and occurred most frequently during the first month of therapy.

Clinical Trial Adverse Drug Reactions: Because clinical trials are conducted under very specific conditions the adverse reaction rates observed in the clinical trials may not reflect the rates observed in practice and should not be compared to the rates in the clinical trials of another drug. Adverse drug reaction information from clinical trials is useful for identifying drug-related adverse events and for approximating rates.

The adverse events listed in Table 1 were observed in greater than one percent of patients.

Table 1: RYTHMOL

Adverse Events Observed in Greater than 1% of Patients Treated with RYTHMOL (propafenone hydrochloride) Tablets

	Incidence by Total Daily Dose (%)			Overall Incidence at Any Dose (%) (N=2127)	% of Patients who Discontinued
	450 mg	600 mg	900 mg		
Cardiovascular System					
Dyspnea	2.2	2.3	3.6	5.3	1.6
Proarrhythmia	2	2.1	2.9	4.7	4.7
Angina	1.7	2.1	3.2	4.6	0.5
Congestive Heart Failure	0.8	2.2	2.6	3.7	1.4
Ventricular Tachycardia	1.4	1.6	2.9	3.4	1.2
Palpitations	0.6	1.6	2.6	3.4	0.5
First Degree AV Block	0.8	1.2	2.1	2.5	0.3
Syncope	0.8	1.3	1.4	2.2	0.7
QRS Duration, Increased	0.5	0.9	1.7	1.9	0.5
Bradycardia	0.5	0.8	1.1	1.5	0.5
PVC's	0.6	0.6	1.1	1.5	0.1
Edema	0.6	0.4	1	1.4	0.2
Bundle Branch Block	0.3	0.7	1	1.2	0.5
Atrial Fibrillation	0.7	0.7	0.5	1.2	0.4
Intraventricular Conduction Delay	0.2	0.7	0.9	1.1	0.1
Hypotension	0.1	0.5	1	1.1	0.4
Central Nervous System					
Dizziness	3.6	6.6	11	12.5	2.4
Headaches	1.5	2.5	2.8	4.5	1
Blurred Vision	0.6	2.4	3.1	3.8	0.8
Ataxia	0.3	0.6	1.5	1.6	0.2
Insomnia	0.3	1.3	0.7	1.5	0.3
Tremor(s)	0.3	0.8	1.1	1.4	0.3
Drowsiness	0.6	0.5	0.7	1.2	0.2
Gastrointestinal System					
Nausea and/or Vomiting	2.4	6.1	8.9	10.7	3.4
Unusual Taste	2.5	4.9	6.3	8.8	0.7
Constipation	2	4.1	5.3	7.2	0.5
Dyspepsia	1.3	1.7	2.5	3.4	0.9
Diarrhea	0.5	1.6	1.7	2.5	0.6
Dry Mouth	0.9	1	1.4	2.4	0.2
Anorexia	0.5	0.7	1.6	1.7	0.4
Abdominal Pain/Cramping	0.8	0.9	1.1	1.7	0.4
Flatulence	0.3	0.7	0.9	1.2	0.1
Other					
Fatigue	1.8	2.8	4.1	6	1
Rash	0.6	1.4	1.9	2.6	0.8
Weakness	0.6	1.6	1.7	2.4	0.7
Atypical Chest Pain	0.5	0.7	1.4	1.8	0.2
Anxiety	0.7	0.5	0.9	1.5	0.6
Diaphoresis	0.6	0.4	1.1	1.4	0.3
Pain, Joints	0.2	0.4	0.9	1	0.1

(cont'd)

Table 1: RYTHMOL (cont'd)
Adverse Events Observed in Greater than 1% of Patients Treated with RYTHMOL (propafenone hydrochloride) Tablets

Less Common Clinical Trial Adverse Drug Reactions (<1%): The following adverse reactions were reported less frequently than 1% in clinical trials. Causality and relationship to propafenone hydrochloride therapy cannot necessarily be judged from these events.

Cardiovascular: atrial flutter, AV dissociation, cardiac arrest, flushing, hot flashes, sick sinus syndrome, sinus pause or arrest, supraventricular tachycardia, torsades de pointes, ventricular fibrillation.

Gastrointestinal: gastroenteritis.

Hepatic: A number of patients with liver abnormalities associated with propafenone hydrochloride therapy have been reported in foreign post-marketing experience. Some appeared due to hepatocellular injury, some were cholestatic and some showed a mixed picture. Some of these reports were simply discovered through clinical chemistries, others because of clinical symptoms. One case was rechallenged with a positive outcome.

Cholestasis (0.1%), elevated liver enzymes (alkaline phosphatase, serum transaminases) (0.2%), hepatitis (0.03%).

Immune System: allergic reactions.

Nervous System: abnormal dreams, abnormal speech, abnormal vision, confusion, depression, memory loss, numbness, paresthesias, psychosis/mania, seizures (0.3%), tinnitus, unusual smell sensation, vertigo.

Other: alopecia, eye irritation, impotence, increased glucose, positive ANA (0.7%), muscle cramps, muscle weakness, nephrotic syndrome, pain, pruritus, reddening of the skin.

Abnormal Hematologic and Clinical Chemistry Findings: Hematologic: agranulocytosis (see Warnings and Precautions), anemia, bruising, granulocytopenia, leukopenia, purpura, thrombocytopenia.

Post-Market Adverse Drug Reactions: Cardiovascular: ventricular fibrillation.

Gastrointestinal: jaundice.

Hematologic: increased bleeding time.
Nervous System: apnea, coma.
Other: hyponatremia/inappropriate ADH secretion, lupus erythematosis, chest pain, urticaria, kidney failure.

There have been post-marketing reports of patients experiencing conversion of paroxysmal atrial fibrillation to atrial flutter with accompanying 2:1 or 1:1 conduction block. However, the clinical significance has not been established.

DRUG INTERACTIONS: Overview: Drugs that inhibit CYP2D6 (e.g. quinidine), CYP1A2 (e.g. cimetidine) and CYP3A4 (e.g. ketoconazole, cimetidine, erythromycin and grapefruit juice) might lead to increased plasma levels of propafenone. When RYTHMOL (propafenone hydrochloride) is administered with inhibitors of these enzymes, the patients should be closely monitored and the dose adjusted accordingly.

Co-administration of RYTHMOL with drugs metabolized by CYP2D6 (e.g. venlafaxine) might lead to increased levels of these drugs and/or of propafenone.

Drug-Drug Interactions: (See Table 2.)

Table 2: RYTHMOL

Established or Potential Drug-Drug Interactions

Proper Name	Ref	Effect	Clinical Comment
Digitalis	CT, T	Propafenone hydrochloride has been shown to produce dose-related increases in serum digoxin levels ranging from approximately 35% at 450 mg/day to 85% at 900 mg/day of propafenone hydrochloride without affecting digoxin renal clearance. Elevations of digoxin levels were maintained for up to 16 months during concomitant administration.	Plasma digoxin levels of patients on concomitant therapy should be measured, and digoxin dosage should ordinarily be reduced when propafenone hydrochloride is started, especially if a relatively large digoxin dose is used or if plasma concentrations are relatively high.
Beta-agonists	CT, T	In a study involving healthy subjects, concomitant administration of propafenone hydrochloride and propranolol resulted in substantial increases in propranolol plasma concentration and elimination $t_{½}$ with no change in propafenone plasma levels from control values. Similar observations have been reported with metoprolol. Propafenone appears to inhibit the hydroxylation pathway for the two beta-antagonists (just as quinidine inhibits propafenone metabolism). Increased plasma concentrations of metoprolol could overcome its relative cardioselectivity. In propafenone hydrochloride clinical trials, patients who were receiving beta-blockers concurrently did not experience an increased incidence of side effects.	While the therapeutic range for beta-blockers is wide, a reduction in dosage may be necessary during concomitant administration with propafenone hydrochloride.
Anticoagulants	CT	In a study of eight healthy subjects receiving propafenone hydrochloride and concomitant warfarin, mean steady-state warfarin plasma concentrations increased 39% with a corresponding prolongation in prothrombin times of approximately 25%.	It is therefore recommended that in patients treated with propafenone hydrochloride and anticoagulants (e.g. warfarin, acenocoumarol) concomitantly, prothrombin time should be carefully monitored and the dose of anticoagulant adjusted as necessary.
Cimetidine	CT	Concomitant administration of propafenone hydrochloride tablets and cimetidine resulted in a 20% increase in steady-state plasma concentrations of propafenone with no detectable changes in electrocardiographic parameters beyond that measured on propafenone hydrochloride alone.	Therefore, patients should be carefully monitored and the dose of propafenone hydrochloride adjusted when appropriate.
Lidocaine	T	No clinically significant effects on the pharmacokinetics of propafenone or lidocaine have been seen following their concomitant use in healthy volunteers. However, the concomitant use of propafenone hydrochloride and intravenous lidocaine has been reported to increase the frequency and severity of central nervous system side effects of lidocaine.	Therefore, the combination of propafenone hydrochloride and lidocaine should be used with caution.
Desipramine	C, T	Concomitant administration of propafenone hydrochloride and desipramine may result in elevated serum desipramine levels.	Both desipramine, a tricyclic antidepressant, and propafenone are cleared by oxidative pathways of demethylation and hydroxylation carried out by the hepatic P-450 cytochrome.
Cyclosporin	C, T	Propafenone hydrochloride therapy may increase levels of cyclosporin.	
Theophylline	C, T	Propafenone hydrochloride may increase theophylline concentration during concomitant therapy with the development of theophylline toxicity.	
Rifampin	T	Rifampin may accelerate the metabolism and decrease the plasma levels and antiarrhythmic efficacy of propafenone.	
Ritonavir, Lopinavir/ritonavir	T		Due to the potential for increased plasma concentrations, co-administration of 800-1200 mg/day doses of ritonavir and propafenone hydrochloride is contraindicated. Furthermore, based on results of a desipramine interaction study, lopinavir/ritonavir does not inhibit CYP2D6-mediated metabolism at clinically relevant concentrations. However, caution should be used when co-administering propafenone with any ritonavir-boosted protease inhibitors.
Amiodarone	T	Combination therapy of amiodarone and propafenone hydrochloride can affect conduction and repolarization and lead to abnormalities that have the potential to be proarrhythmic.	Dose adjustments of both compounds based on therapeutic response may be required.
Phenobarbital	T	Phenobarbital is a known inducer of CYP3A4.	Response to propafenone hydrochloride therapy should be monitored during concomitant chronic phenobarbital use.
Fluoxetine, Paroxetine and Fluvoxamine	C, T	Concomitant administration of propafenone hydrochloride and fluoxetine in extensive metabolizers increased the S propafenone C_{max} and AUC by 39 and 50% and the R propafenone C_{max} and AUC by 71 and 50%. Elevated levels of plasma propafenone may occur when propafenone hydrochloride is used concomitantly with paroxetine.	Lower doses of propafenone may be sufficient to achieve the desired therapeutic response. In poor metabolizers, concomitant administration of propafenone hydrochloride and fluvoxamine may require a dose reduction of propafenone.

Legend: C=case study; CT=clinical trial; T=theoretical.

Drug-Food Interactions: Co-administration of RYTHMOL with grapefruit juice might lead to increased plasma levels of propafenone. Bioavailability is enhanced by administration of the drug with food.
Drug-Herb Interactions: Caution should be exercised when administering RYTHMOL with cytochrome P450 modulating herbal products such as St. John's wort.
Drug-Lifestyle Interactions: Driving and Using Machines: Blurred vision, dizziness, fatigue and postural hypotension may affect the patient's speed of reaction and impair the individual's ability to operate machinery and motor vehicles.

DOSAGE AND ADMINISTRATION: Dosing Considerations:

- The dose of RYTHMOL (propafenone hydrochloride) must be individually determined on the basis of patient's response and tolerance. The usefulness of monitoring plasma levels for optimization of therapy has not been established. The recommended dose titration regimen can be used for both fast and slow metabolizers. See Action and Clinical Pharmacology.

Recommended Dose and Dosage Adjustment: The initial dose of RYTHMOL is 150 mg given every 8 hours (450 mg/day). Dosage may be increased at three to four day intervals to 300 mg every 12 hours (600 mg/day). Should a further increase in dosage be necessary a maximum dose of 300 mg every 8 hours (900 mg/day) may be given.

In those patients in whom widening of the QRS complex (>0.12 seconds) or prolongation of PR interval (>0.24 seconds) occurs, the dosage of RYTHMOL should be reduced.

In patients with mild to moderate hepatic insufficiency RYTHMOL therapy should be initiated with 150 mg given once daily (150 mg/day). See Warnings and Precautions. The dosage may be increased at a minimum of 4 day intervals to 150 mg twice daily (300 mg/day) then to 150 mg every 8 hours (450 mg/day) and, if necessary, to 300 mg every 12 hours (600 mg/day).

There is no information on dosing with RYTHMOL in patients with renal impairment. RYTHMOL should be used cautiously in these patients and only after consideration of the benefit/risk ratio. These patients should be carefully monitored for signs of toxicity. Lower doses may be required. See Warnings and Precautions.

In elderly patients, the effective dose of RYTHMOL may be lower. See Warnings and Precautions.

There is no information on the appropriate regimen for the transfer from lidocaine to RYTHMOL .

Missed Dose: If you forget to take one tablet, take another as soon as you remember, unless it is almost time for your next dose. If it is, do not take the missed tablet at all. Never double-up on a missed dose.
Administration: Administration of RYTHMOL with food is recommended.

OVERDOSAGE:
The symptoms of overdose may include hypotension, somnolence, convulsions, bradycardia, conduction disturbances, ventricular tachycardia and/or ventricular fibrillation. Death may occur.

If ingestion is recent, perform gastric lavage or induce emesis. Supportive measures such as mechanical respiratory assistance and cardiac massage may be necessary.

Defibrillation and the use of a temporary pacemaker, as well as infusion of isoproterenol and dopamine have been effective in controlling cardiac rhythm and blood pressure. Convulsions have been alleviated with intravenous diazepam.

Detoxification measures such as forced diuresis, hemoperfusion and hemodialysis have not proven useful.

Treatment: Owing to high protein binding (>95%) and the large volume of distribution, hemodialysis is ineffective and attempts to achieve elimination via hemoperfusion are of limited efficacy.

For management of a suspected drug overdose, contact your regional Poison Control Centre. See the *CPS* Directory section for a list of Poison Control Centres.

ACTION AND CLINICAL PHARMACOLOGY: Mechanism of Action: RYTHMOL (propafenone hydrochloride) is an antiarrhythmic agent which possesses class 1C properties in the modified electrophysiological classification of Vaughan-Williams. Propafenone hydrochloride has a direct stabilizing action on myocardial cell membranes. The electrophysiological effect of propafenone hydrochloride manifests itself as a reduction of the upstroke velocity (Phase 0) of the monophasic action potential, while Phase 4 spontaneous automaticity is depressed. Diastolic excitability threshold is increased and effective refractory period prolonged. In Purkinje fibers, and to a lesser extent myocardial fibers, propafenone hydrochloride reduces the fast inward sodium current.

In addition to a local anesthetic effect, approximately equal to procaine, propafenone hydrochloride has weak beta-blocking activity. Clinical trials employing isoproterenol challenge and exercise testing suggest that the affinity of propafenone hydrochloride for beta-adrenergic receptors, as calculated from dose ratios and drug concentrations, is about 1/40 that of propranolol. Propafenone hydrochloride also inhibits the slow calcium influx at high concentrations, however, this action is weak (approximately 1/100 of verapamil) and does not contribute to its antiarrhythmic effect.

Pharmacodynamics: Electrophysiology: Electrophysiology studies have shown that propafenone hydrochloride prolongs atrioventricular conduction and in some instances significantly lengthens sinus nodal recovery times with a non-significant effect on sinus cycle length. Both atrioventricular (AV) nodal conduction time (AH interval) and His-Purkinje conduction time (HV interval) are prolonged. Propafenone hydrochloride increases atrial, AV nodal and ventricular effective refractory periods. Propafenone hydrochloride causes a dose-dependent increase in the PR interval and QRS complex duration. Non-significant increases in the QTc interval and occasional slowing of the heart rate have also been observed.

(cont'd)

Hemodynamics: Propafenone hydrochloride can exert a negative inotropic effect on the myocardium. Increases in pulmonary capillary wedge pressure and systemic and pulmonary vascular resistance, with a concurrent mild depression of cardiac output and cardiac index, have occurred following RYTHMOL (propafenone hydrochloride) administration. Decreases in left ventricular function have been recorded in patients with depressed baseline function.

Pharmacokinetics: Absorption: Due to a genetically determined presence or deficiency of one metabolizing pathway (CYP2D6), patients may be categorized into fast (over 90% of all patients) or slow metabolizers of propafenone hydrochloride, resulting in low or high plasma concentrations respectively. Following oral administration in fast metabolizers, propafenone hydrochloride is nearly completely absorbed and undergoes extensive first-pass hepatic metabolism resulting in a dose-dependent absolute bioavailability ranging from 3 to 40%. Peak plasma concentrations occur within three hours. For fast metabolizers of propafenone hydrochloride, the elimination $t_{½}$ is 5.5±2.1 hours; for slow metabolizers, the elimination $t_{½}$ is 17.2±8.0 hours. In fast metabolizers, there is a non-linear increase in drug plasma concentration and bioavailability with increase in dosage, presumably due to saturation of first pass hepatic metabolism. This departure from dose linearity occurs when single doses above 150 mg are given. A 300 mg dose gives plasma levels six times that of a 150 mg dose. Similarly, for a 3-fold increase in daily dose from 300 to 900 mg/day there is a 10-fold increase in steady-state plasma concentration. In slow metabolizers, as opposed to fast metabolizers, a linear relationship between propafenone hydrochloride dose and plasma concentration was observed.

Slow metabolizers had higher propafenone plasma concentrations which they required for suppression of arrhythmia since they did not produce the active metabolite 5-hydroxypropafenone (5-OHP). These higher propafenone plasma concentrations may lead to clinically evident beta-blockade.

Despite these differences in pharmacokinetics, steady-state conditions are achieved after three to four days in all patients. Therapeutic plasma levels of propafenone appear to be in the range of 0.5 to 2.0 μg/mL.

Metabolism: In fast metabolizers, propafenone undergoes extensive hepatic metabolism with less than 1% excreted as unchanged drug. The major active metabolites are 5-hydroxypropafenone (5-OHP) which is formed by CYP2D6 and N-depropylpropafenone (NDPP) which is formed by CYP3A4 and CYP1A2; both metabolites occurring in concentrations less than 20% of the parent compound. In vitro preparations and animal studies have shown that the 5-OHP metabolite possesses antiarrhythmic and beta-adrenoreceptor blocking activity comparable to propafenone.

Propafenone is 97% bound to plasma proteins.

Influence of Food: Bioavailability is enhanced by administration of the drug with food.

Special Populations and Conditions: Pediatrics: Propafenone hydrochloride pharmacokinetics have not been evaluated in patients less than 18 years of age.

Geriatrics: Propafenone hydrochloride pharmacokinetics have not been evaluated in elderly patients greater than 65 years of age. However, a slight increase in the incidence of dizziness was observed in elderly patients. Because of the possible increased risk of impaired hepatic or renal function in this age group, propafenone hydrochloride should be used with caution. The effective dose may be lower in these patients.

STORAGE AND STABILITY: Store RYTHMOL (propafenone hydrochloride) at controlled room temperature, between 15 to 25°C. Do not use beyond the expiry date indicated on the label.

INFORMATION FOR THE PATIENT: Published in e-CPS, available by subscription at www.e-cps.ca.

DOSAGE FORMS, COMPOSITION AND PACKAGING: 150 mg: Each white, biconvex, film-coated tablet, embossed with "150" over a triangle of arched sides on one side contains: propafenone HCl 150 mg. Nonmedicinal ingredients: croscarmellose sodium, hypromellose, macrogol 400 and 6000, magnesium stearate, maize starch, microcrystalline cellulose and titanium dioxide. Bottles of 100.

300 mg: Each white, biconvex, film-coated tablet, embossed with a score on both sides with a triangle of arched side above and "300" below the score on one side contains: propafenone HCl 300 mg. Nonmedicinal ingredients: croscarmellose sodium, hypromellose, macrogol 400 and 6000, magnesium stearate, maize starch, microcrystalline cellulose and titanium dioxide. Bottles of 100.

(Shown in Product Identification Section)

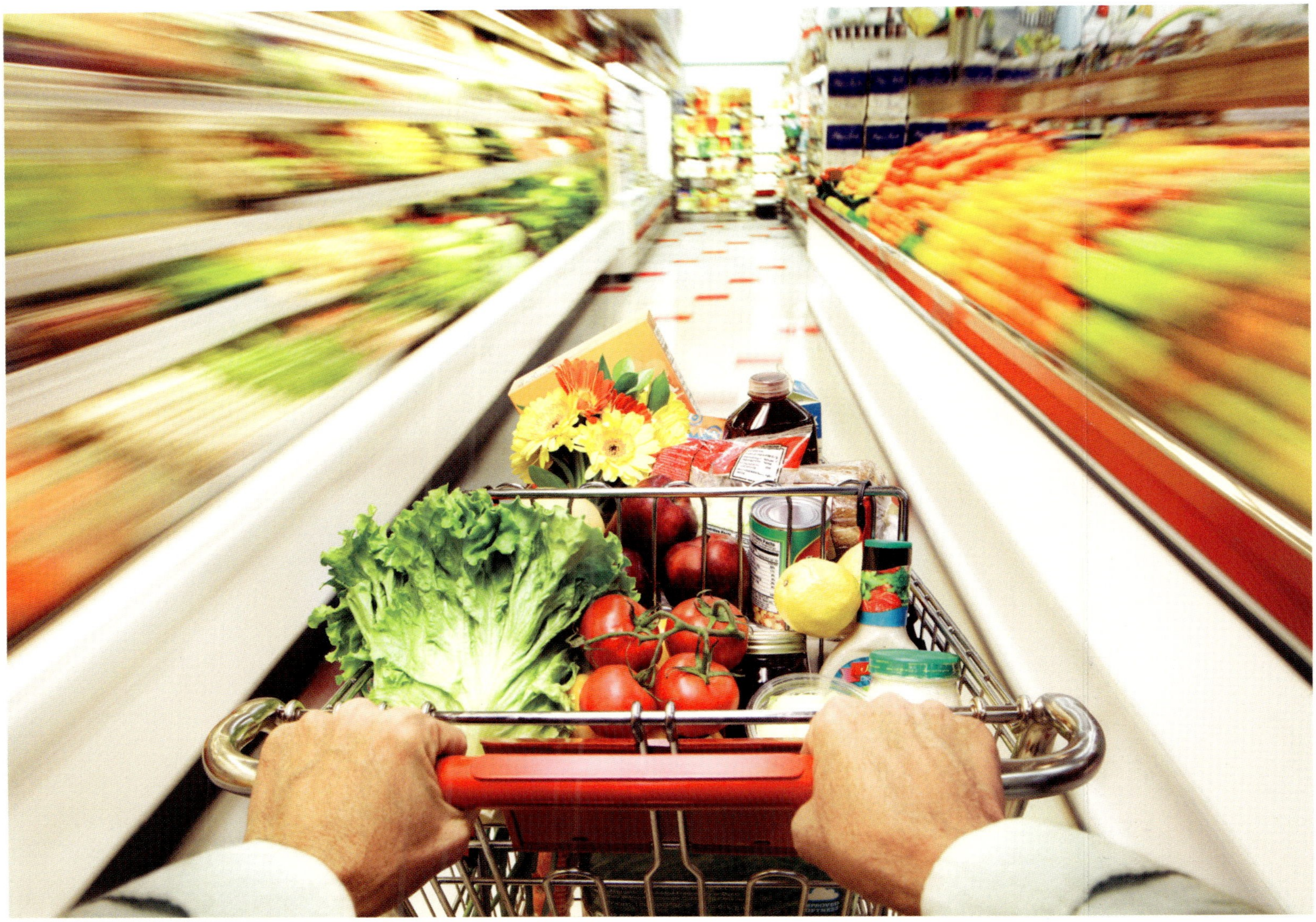

S

LIFE HAPPENS

Symbicort® is indicated for regular treatment of asthma in patients 12 years and older with reversible obstructive airways disease, where the use of a combination product is appropriate. This may include patients on effective maintenance doses of long-acting beta$_2$-agonists and inhaled corticosteroids and patients who are symptomatic on current inhaled corticosteroid therapy. In patients with asthma, Symbicort Maintenance and Reliever Therapy **(SMART)** is taken as regular maintenance treatment and as needed in response to symptoms.

The dosage should be individualized according to disease severity. Asthma patients should be regularly reassessed so that the dosage of SYMBICORT they are receiving remains optimal.

To relieve acute asthmatic symptoms while taking SYMBICORT on a regular basis, a fast-acting inhaled bronchodilator or fast-acting ICS/LABA combination should be used.

SYMBICORT is also indicated for the maintenance treatment of moderate to severe COPD, including chronic bronchitis and emphysema in patients with persistent symptoms and a history of exacerbations, where the use of a combination product is considered appropriate.

SYMBICORT is not indicated for the relief of acute bronchospasm in COPD patients.

Adverse reactions that have been associated with budesonide or formoterol (1-10%) include palpitations, candida infections in the oropharynx, headache, tremor, mild irritation in the throat, coughing and hoarseness. In clinical trials the most commonly occurring side effect in COPD patients was nasopharyngitis (9%).

HPA-axis function status should be assessed periodically.

WARNING for asthma patients:

Data from a large placebo-controlled US study (Salmeterol Multi-center Asthma Research Trial) comparing the safety of the long-acting beta$_2$-adrenergic agonist salmeterol to that of a placebo added to the original asthma therapy showed an increase in asthma-related deaths in patients receiving salmeterol. Although the trial results were specific to salmeterol, one of the conclusions derived from this study is that long-acting beta$_2$-adrenergic agonists may increase the risk of asthma exacerbation and possibly asthma-related death. Post-hoc analysis of the trial data suggests that the risks may be lower in those patients who were using inhaled corticosteroids (ICS) at study entry. However, these post-hoc analysis results are not conclusive. The actual ICS dosage used by these patients was not assessed in the study. Available data for formoterol fumarate dihydrate do not suggest increased risk, however it can not be excluded that the findings with salmeterol may apply to all long-acting beta$_2$-adrenergic agonists including formoterol fumarate dihydrate, one of the active ingredients in SYMBICORT. SYMBICORT contains a combination of formoterol fumarate dihydrate and budesonide (an inhaled corticosteroid). Given that the actual ICS dosage used by patients in the salmeterol trial was not assessed, it is not known whether the potential risk associated with long-acting beta$_2$-adrenergic agonists would apply to SYMBICORT. When treating asthma patients, SYMBICORT should be used only in patients whose conditions are not adequately controlled using low-to-medium dose inhaled corticosteroids or whose disease severity clearly warrants the initiation of treatment with two maintenance therapies.[1]

WE GET IT

Pr Symbicort®
budesonide/formoterol fumarate dihydrate

AstraZeneca

Member
R&D PAAB
SY943E 06/11

Reference: 1. Symbicort® Turbuhaler® Product Monograph. AstraZeneca Canada Inc. July 29, 2009.

S

Pr TORISEL™

(temsirolimus) Injection

Pfizer Oncology

A FIRST-LINE STANDARD FOR THE MANAGEMENT OF mRCC[1,2]

Pr SUTENT® capsules
sunitinib malate

PrSUTENT®: AN ORAL MULTITARGETED RECEPTOR TYROSINE KINASE INHIBITOR[3]

Sunitinib (SUTENT) is the first-line standard of care for mRCC patients with good or intermediate prognosis.[1]

DEMONSTRATED MORE THAN DOUBLE MEDIAN PFS vs. IFN-α[3,4,*]

Significantly longer progression-free survival: 47.3 weeks with SUTENT compared to 22.0 weeks with IFN-α (95% CI: 42.6–50.7 and 16.4–24.0, respectively; $p<0.000001$).[3,*]

➤ **Four-fold higher objective response rate**
38.7% with SUTENT vs. 7.7% with IFN-α (95% CI: 33.7–43.8 and 5.2–10.9, respectively; $p<0.001$)[3,*]

TREND FOR OVERALL SURVIVAL ADVANTAGE vs. IFN-α[3,4,*]

Overall Survival in Treatment-naïve Metastatic RCC Study[3,*]

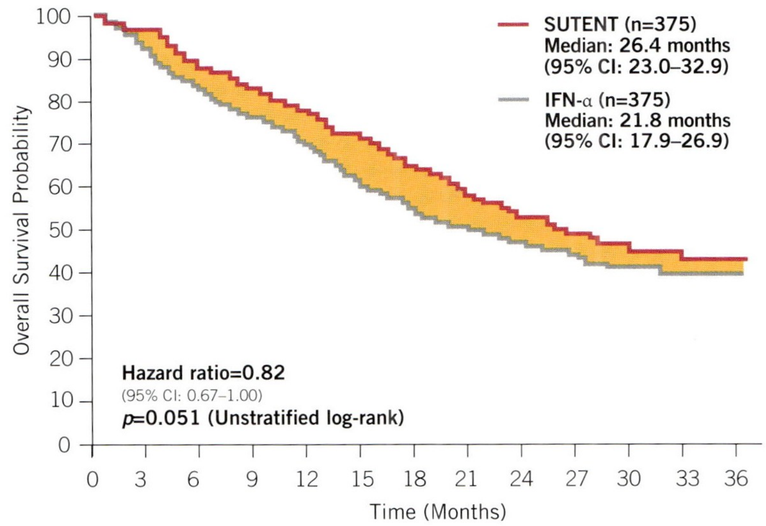

Number of subjects at risk:

	0	6	12	18	24	30	36
SUTENT	375	326	283	229	180	61	2
IFN-α	375	295	242	187	149	53	1

* OS results represent a final analysis and PFS results represent an interim analysis from a Phase III, randomized, multi-centre, international trial. Overall survival was defined as the time from randomization to date of death due to any cause. Median OS was 26.4 months for SUTENT (95% CI: 23.0–32.9 months) and 21.8 months for IFN-α (95% CI: 17.9–26.9. HR=0.821; 95% CI: 0.673–1.001; p=0.051). Patients were treated with either 50 mg SUTENT once daily in cycles of 4 weeks on/2 weeks off (n=375) or 9 MIU IFN-α 3 times per week, administered subcutaneously (n=375) until disease progression or study withdrawal. Primary endpoint was PFS and secondary endpoints included objective response rate (ORR) by Response Evaluation Criteria in Solid Tumours (RECIST), overall survival (OS) and safety.

➤ **The primary analysis showed a trend towards improved outcomes vs. IFN-α**

26.4 months for SUTENT arm vs. 21.8 months for IFN-α (95% CI: 0.67–1.00; p=0.051).[3]

➤ **Manageable adverse event profile**

The most common adverse events (all grades) reported in ≥10% of patients receiving SUTENT for treatment-naïve mRCC (n=375) vs. IFN-α (n=360) were fatigue (54.9% vs. 51.7%), diarrhea (61.1% vs. 13.6%), nausea (52.0% vs. 34.4%), dysgeusia (46.7% vs. 13.9%), dyspepsia (31.5% vs. 3.6%), stomatitis (29.3% vs. 2.8%), anorexia (34.4% vs. 28.1%), hypertension (30.1% vs. 1.7%), vomiting (31.2% vs. 11.4%), rash (30.7% vs. 9.2%), mucosal inflammation (26.1% vs. 1.7%) and hand-foot syndrome (30.0% vs. 0.6%). The most common grade 3/4 adverse events (occurring in ≥10% of SUTENT patients) were hypertension (12.3% vs. 0.3%), fatigue (11.5% vs. 13.3%), thrombocytopenia (8.8% vs. 0.6%), neutropenia (10.7% vs. 3.3%) and hand-foot syndrome (8.5% vs. 0%).[3]

SUTENT is indicated for the treatment of metastatic renal cell carcinoma (mRCC) of clear cell histology. Approval for mRCC is based on statistically significant progression-free survival in patients with good performance status (ECOG 0–1). There was a trend for overall survival advantage.

Important safety information[3]

- Treatment-related tumour hemorrhage has been observed in patients receiving SUTENT.
- Decreases in left ventricular ejection fraction of ≥20% and below the LLN have been reported. Baseline and periodic evaluations of LVEF should be considered.
- Patients should be monitored for hypertension and treated as appropriate. Those with uncontrolled hypertension should not be treated with SUTENT.
- SUTENT has not been studied in patients with severe hepatic or renal impairment.
- Rare cases of myopathy and/or rhabdomyolysis (some with acute renal failure), cardiomyopathy (in some cases with fatal outcome), and pulmonary embolism (including fatal cases) have been reported.
- Contraindicated in pregnant women and patients with hypersensitivity to sunitinib malate or other components of SUTENT.

Please refer to the Prescribing Summary for complete information.

SEROQUEL XR (quetiapine fumarate extended-release) is indicated for the symptomatic relief of major depressive disorder (MDD) when currently available approved antidepressant drugs have failed either due to lack of efficacy and/or lack of tolerability.

While there is no evidence that the efficacy of SEROQUEL XR is superior to other antidepressants, it provides a treatment option for patients who have failed on previous antidepressant treatments. Clinicians must take into account the safety concerns associated with antipsychotic drugs, a class of drugs to which SEROQUEL XR belongs. Safety concerns of this class include: weight gain, hyperlipidemia, hyperglycaemia, tardive dyskinesia and neuroleptic malignant syndrome (see WARNINGS AND PRECAUTIONS). SEROQUEL XR should only be prescribed in patients with MDD by clinicians who are aware of the importance and are experienced in the early detection and management of the above-mentioned safety issues associated with this class.

Long-term safety of SEROQUEL XR in MDD has not been systematically evaluated. Thus, the physician who elects to use SEROQUEL XR in the treatment of MDD should use SEROQUEL XR for the shortest time that is clinically indicated. When lengthier treatment is indicated, the physician must periodically re-evaluate the long-term usefulness of the drug for the individual patient keeping in mind the long-term risks.

SEROQUEL XR is also indicated for the management of the manifestations of schizophrenia, as monotherapy for the acute management of manic episodes associated with bipolar disorder and as monotherapy for the acute management of depressive episodes associated with bipolar I and bipolar II disorder. Please consult the Product Monograph for complete prescribing information.

SEROQUEL XR (quetiapine fumarate extended-release) is contraindicated in patients with a known hypersensitivity to this medication or any of its ingredients.

During acute MDD therapy with SEROQUEL XR, the most commonly observed adverse events associated with the use of SEROQUEL XR (incidence of at least 5% and an incidence at least 5% higher than that observed with placebo) were as follows: *Adults:* dry mouth (35%), sedation (28%), somnolence (24%), dizziness (14%) and fatigue (7%). *Elderly:* somnolence (33%), dry mouth (20%), headache (19%) and fatigue (8%).

Increases in blood glucose and hyperglycaemia, and occasional reports of diabetes have been observed in clinical trials.

Eye examinations are recommended prior to, or shortly after, initiation of treatment and at 6-month intervals thereafter. Caution should be used in the elderly and those with known hepatic and renal impairment.

Serious Warnings and Precautions

Increased Mortality in Elderly Patients With Dementia

Elderly patients with dementia treated with atypical antipsychotic drugs are at an increased risk of death compared to placebo. Analyses of thirteen placebo-controlled trials with various atypical antipsychotics (modal duration of 10 weeks) in these patients showed a mean 1.6-fold increase in death rate in the drug-related patients. Although the causes of death were varied, most of the deaths appeared to be either cardiovascular (e.g., heart failure, sudden death) or infectious (e.g., pneumonia) in nature.

Please consult the Product Monograph for warnings, precautions and adverse events.

Reference: 1. SEROQUEL XR® Product Monograph. AstraZeneca Canada Inc. February 17, 2010.

SeroquelXR.ca

AstraZeneca

Member R&D PAAB

SE10-1120E 11/11

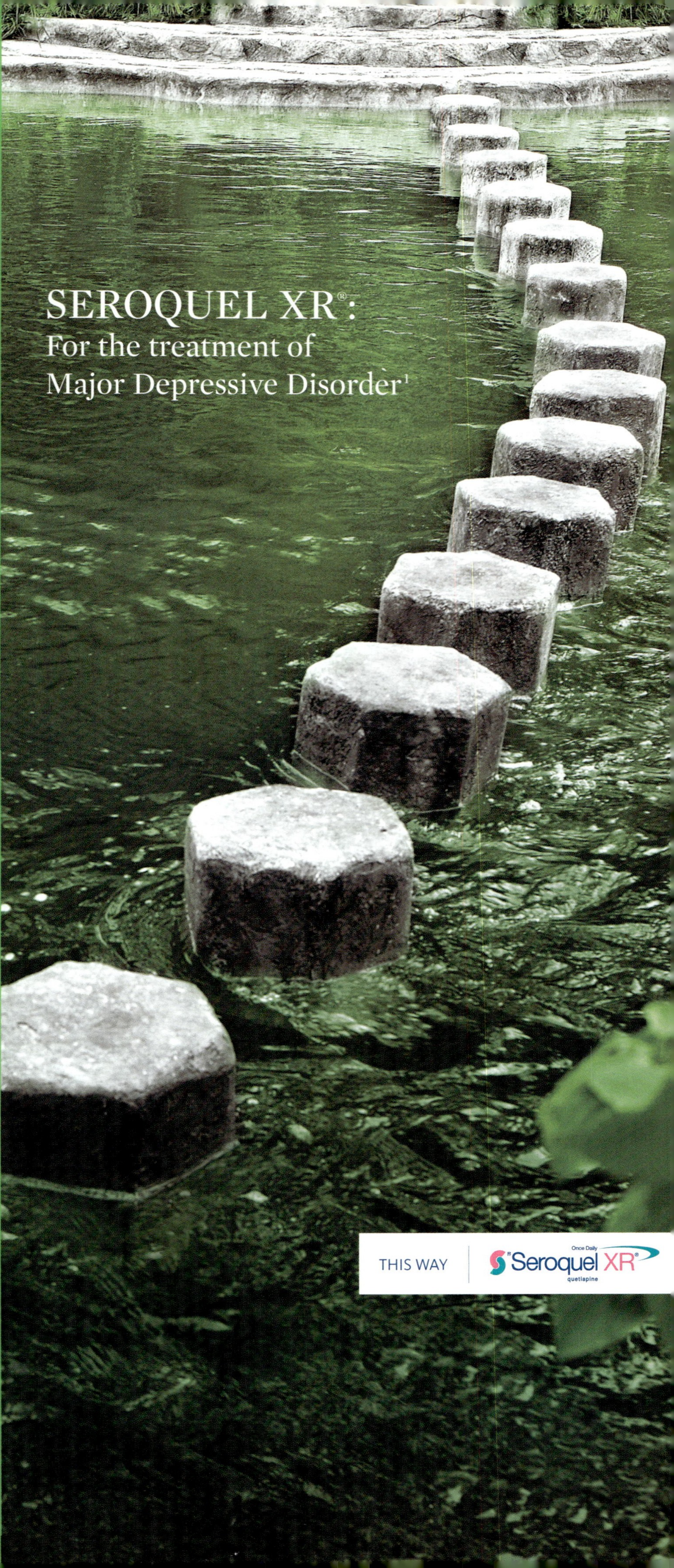

S

Saizen® Ⓟ

somatropin

Human Growth Hormone

EMD Canada

Saizen® click.easy® Ⓟ

somatropin

Human Growth Hormone

EMD Canada

Date of Revision: December 18, 2007

SUMMARY PRODUCT INFORMATION:

Route of Administration	Dosage Form/ Strength	Clinically Relevant Nonmedicinal Ingredients
Subcutaneous injection, Intramuscular injection	Lyophilized powder for reconstitution/ 3.33 mg/vial, 5 mg/vial	For a complete listing see Dosage Forms, Composition and Packaging.
Subcutaneous injection	Lyophilized powder for reconstitution/ 8.8 mg (5.83 mg/mL) click.easy,	

DESCRIPTION: SAIZEN (somatropin for injection) is available in 3.33 mg and 5 mg doses.

SAIZEN 8.8 mg (5.83 mg/mL) click.easy (somatropin for injection) is new presentations of SAIZEN pre-assembled with a bacteriostatic solvent cartridge (0.3% (w/v) metacresol in water for injection) in a reconstitution device click.easy.

Somatropin is a polypeptide hormone consisting of 191 amino acid residues and its structure is identical to that of growth hormone extracted from human pituitary glands. A large loop is formed by a disulfide bond between Cys^{53} and Cys^{165}. A second, smaller loop is formed by a disulfide bond near the carboxyl-terminal between Cys^{182} and Cys^{189}. The solution is a slightly opalescent liquid. It is produced by recombinant (rDNA) technology in a mammalian cell expression system. SAIZEN is also therapeutically equivalent to human growth hormone of pituitary origin.

INDICATIONS AND CLINICAL USE: SAIZEN is indicated for:

Pediatric Indications: Growth Hormone Insufficiency or Deficiency: SAIZEN is indicated for the long-term treatment of children with growth failure due to inadequate secretion of normal endogenous growth hormone. Other causes for growth failure should be ruled out.

Turner's Syndrome: SAIZEN is indicated for the treatment of short stature in girls with gonadal dysgenesis (Turner's Syndrome) when epiphyses are not closed.

Chronic Renal Failure: SAIZEN is indicated for the treatment of growth failure in children due to Chronic Renal Failure.

Small for Gestational Age (SGA): SAIZEN is indicated for growth disturbance (current height Standard Deviation Score (SDS) <−2) in short children born small for gestational age (SGA) with a birth weight and/or length below −2 standard deviations (SD), who failed to show catch-up growth (Height Velocity SDS <0 during the last year) by 2 years of age or later.

Adult Indication: Adult Growth Hormone Deficiency: SAIZEN is indicated for the replacement therapy in adult patients with acquired or idiopathic growth hormone deficiency (GHD) as diagnosed by a single dynamic test for growth hormone deficiency (peak GH ≤5 µg/L). Patients with a growth hormone deficiency with onset in childhood should be retested before treatment starts.

CONTRAINDICATIONS: SAIZEN is contraindicated and should not be administered in the following cases:

- Acute critical illness with complications following cardiac surgery, abdominal surgery, multiple trauma or acute respiratory failure. Clinical studies demonstrated that high doses of another somatropin, were associated with a significantly increased morbidity and mortality in those patients (see Warnings and Precautions).
- In patients with closed epiphyses, SAIZEN has no effect on cartilaginous growth areas of the long bone. Treatment of pediatric growth disorders with SAIZEN should be discontinued when the patient has reached satisfactory adult height, or the epiphyses are fused.
- In the presence of progression of an underlying intracranial tumour. An intracranial tumour should be inactive prior to instituting therapy, and SAIZEN should be discontinued if there is evidence of recurrent activity. Patients should be examined frequently for progression or recurrence of the underlying disease process.
- Patients known to be hypersensitive to somatropin and any of the excipients in powder for solution for injection or the solvent.
- Active neoplasia (either newly diagnosed or recurrent). Any pre-existing neoplasia should be inactive.
- Proliferative or preproliferative diabetic retinopathy.
- In patients with Prader-Willi syndrome who are severely obese or have severe respiratory impairment (see Warnings and Precautions). Unless patients with Prader-Willi syndrome also have a diagnosis of growth hormone deficiency, SAIZEN is not indicated for long-term treatment of pediatric patients who have growth failure due to genetically confirmed Prader-Will syndrome.

SAIZEN treatment should be discontinued in critically ill patients.

SAIZEN is not recommended for use during pregnancy and lactation.

SAIZEN is not recommended for use in patients who have undergone renal transplant until one year post-transplant.

SAIZEN reconstituted with bacteriostatic diluent should not be administered to patients sensitive to benzyl alcohol.

WARNINGS AND PRECAUTIONS: General: SAIZEN treatment should be carried out under regular guidance of a physician experienced in the diagnosis and management of growth disorders.

In clinical studies in non-growth hormone deficient adult patients, a significant increase in mortality has been reported among somatropin treated patients with acute critical illness in intensive care units due to complications following cardiac surgery, abdominal surgery, multiple accident trauma or acute respiratory failure (see Contraindications). In 2 clinical studies with another somatropin and in published articles, where growth hormone was given at doses much higher than those used in the SAIZEN trials (approximately double to triple the dosage), the death rate in this patient population doubled (41.9%) relative to placebo (19.3%). The safety of continuing somatropin treatment in patients receiving replacement doses for approved indications who concurrently develop acute or critical illnesses has not been established. Therefore, the potential benefit of treatment continuation with growth hormone in patients having such an illness should be weighted against the potential risks.

Slipped capital femoral epiphysis is often associated with endocrine disorders such as GHD and hypothyroidism, and growth spurts. In children treated with growth hormone, slipped capital femoral epiphysis may either be due to underlying endocrine disorders or to the increased growth velocity caused by treatment. Physicians and parents should be alert to the development of a limp or complaints of hip or knee pain in children treated with SAIZEN.

Concomitant glucocorticoid therapy may inhibit the response to SAIZEN and should not exceed 10-15 mg hydrocortisone equivalent/m^2 body surface area during SAIZEN treatment.

Injection sites should be varied to prevent localized lipoatrophy, in particular in the case of long-term, subcutaneous administrations of SAIZEN.

Scoliosis has also been reported in patients treated with growth hormone.

Carcinogenesis and Mutagenesis: Carcinogenicity studies have not been conducted. Mutagenicity studies showed no mutagenic activity with SAIZEN.

Leukemia has been reported in a small number of growth hormone deficient patients, treated with growth hormone. Based on the current evidence, experts cannot conclude that growth hormone therapy is responsible for these occurrences.

Endocrine and Metabolism: Because human growth hormone may induce a state of insulin-resistance, SAIZEN patients should be monitored for evidence of glucose intolerance. SAIZEN should be used with caution in patients with diabetes mellitus (adjustment of their antidiabetic therapy may be required) or a family history of diabetes mellitus. SGA patients are a subgroup of patients at higher risk of developing diabetes in whom fasting insulin and blood glucose should be closely monitored before initiating and during treatment with SAIZEN. SAIZEN administration is followed by a transient phase of hypoglycemia of approximately 2 hours, then from 2-4 hours onward by an increase in blood glucose levels despite high insulin concentrations. To detect insulin resistance, patients should be monitored for evidence of glucose intolerance.

Hypothyroidism may develop during SAIZEN therapy. Growth hormone can affect the metabolism of thyroid hormones by increasing the extrathyroidal conversion of T4 to T3 and this lowering effect on T4 may unmask incipient central hypothyroidism in hypopituitary patients. Therefore, thyroid function should be evaluated before starting SAIZEN therapy and regularly assessed during treatment, not less frequently than annually. If hypothyroidism is diagnosed in the course of SAIZEN therapy, it should be corrected because untreated hypothyroidism will jeopardize the response to growth hormone.

There have been reports of fatalities after initiating therapy with growth hormone in pediatric patients with Prader-Willi syndrome who had one or more of the following risk factors: severe obesity, history of upper airway obstruction or sleep apnea, or unidentified respiratory infection. Male patients with one or more of these factors may be at greater risk than females. Patients with Prader Willi syndrome should be evaluated for signs of upper airway obstruction and sleep apnea before initiation of treatment with growth hormone. If during treatment with growth hormone, patients show signs of upper airway obstruction (including onset of or increased snoring) and/or new onset of sleep apnea, treatment should also be interrupted. All patients with Prader-Willi syndrome treated growth hormone should also have effective weight control and be monitored for signs of respiratory infection, which should be diagnosed as early as possible and treated aggressively (see Contraindications). Unless patients with Prader-Willi syndrome also have a diagnosis of growth hormone deficiency, SAIZEN is not indicated for the long-term treatment of pediatric patients who have growth failure due to genetically-confirmed Prader-Willi syndrome.

Hematologic: Serum levels of inorganic phosphorus, alkaline phosphatase, and IGF-1 may increase with SAIZEN therapy.

Sensitivity/Resistance: Patients who are sensitive to the preservative metacresol, found in the diluent, should consider using SAIZEN supplied with bacteriostatic diluent containing benzyl alcohol as preservative.

Special Populations: Pregnant Women: Reproduction studies have not been conducted. It is not known whether somatropin can cause fetal harm when administered to a pregnant woman or can affect reproduction capacity. Somatropin should only be given to a pregnant woman if the benefits outweigh the risks.

Nursing Women: It is not known whether this drug is excreted in human milk. Due to the large molecular weight, it is unlikely that it would be passed intact into the maternal milk and absorption of intact protein from the gastrointestinal tract of the infant is also unlikely. However, secretion of breakdown products of the drug in breast milk has not been studied. Because many drugs are excreted in human milk, caution should be exercised when somatropin is administered to a nursing mother.

Pediatrics: SAIZEN is indicated for use in children (see Indications and Clinical Use).

Geriatrics: Not indicated for treatment in the geriatric population.

Monitoring and Laboratory Tests: Patients with growth failure due to chronic renal failure should be regularly examined and monitored for progression of renal osteodystrophy. Slipped capital femoral epiphysis or avascular necrosis of the femoral head may occur in children with advanced renal osteodystrophy and it is uncertain whether these complications are affected by growth hormone therapy. In these patients, radiograms of the hips and laboratory exams (serum calcium, phosphorus, alkaline phosphatase and PTH) should be made prior to initiating growth hormone therapy and regularly followed subsequently. Physicians and parents should be alert to the development of a limp or complaints of hip or knee pain (as knee pain may be referred hip pain) in patients treated with growth hormone therapy.

Bone age should be monitored periodically during SAIZEN administration especially in patients who are pubertal and/or receiving concomitant thyroid replacement therapy. Under these circumstances, epiphyseal maturation may progress rapidly.

Patients with growth hormone deficiency secondary to an intracranial lesion should be examined frequently for progression or recurrence of the underlying disease process.

Patients with an intra or extracranial neoplasia in remission who are receiving treatment with growth hormone should be examined carefully and at regular intervals by the physician. Patients developing neoplasia should be reported to Health Canada by the treating physician.

In short children born SGA other medical reasons or treatments that could explain growth disturbance should be ruled out before starting treatment.

For SGA patients, it is recommended to measure IGF-I level before start of treatment and twice a year thereafter. If on repeated measurements IFG-I levels exceed +2 SD compared to references for age and pubertal status, the IGF-I/GFBP-3 ratio could be taken into account to consider dose adjustment.

Experience in initiating treatment in SGA patients near onset of puberty is limited. It is therefore not recommended to initiate treatment near onset of puberty. Experience with SGA patients with Silver-Russel syndrome is limited.

Some of the height gain obtained with treating short children born SGA with somatropin may be lost if treatment is stopped before final height is reached.

In case of persistent oedema or severe paraesthesia the dosage should be decreased in order to avoid the development of carpal tunnel syndrome. Growth hormone deficiency in the Adult is a lifelong condition and should be treated accordingly, however experience with patients over sixty years and experience with prolonged treatment is limited.

Growth hormone administration is followed by a transient phase of hypoglycemia of approximately 2 hours, then from 2-4 hours onward by an increase in blood glucose levels despite high insulin concentrations. To detect insulin resistance, patients should be monitored for evidence of glucose intolerance.

Idiopathic intracranial hypertension has been recognized as a complication (early in treatment usually) of growth hormone treatment. The diagnosis is made on the basis of clinical symptoms such as severe, persistent or recurrent headache, visual problems, nausea and/or vomiting, papilloedema and temporal relationship to growth hormone. Physicians and parents should be attentive to relevant symptoms such as headache and visual problems in patients under SAIZEN therapy. Fundoscopic examination should be performed routinely before initiating treatment with SAIZEN to exclude pre-existent papilloedema and repeated if there is any clinical suspicion. If papilloedema is confirmed by fundoscopy, SAIZEN treatment should be stopped. It can be restarted at a lower dose after idiopathic-intracranial hypertension has resolved which occurs rapidly when treatment is withdrawn. If growth hormone treatment is restarted, careful monitoring for symptoms of intracranial hypertension is necessary, and treatment should be discontinued if intracranial hypertension recurs. At present, there is insufficient evidence to guide clinical decision making in patients with resolved intracranial hypertension.

Occupational Hazards: SAIZEN does not interfere with the patient's ability to drive or use machinery.

ADVERSE REACTIONS: Adverse Drug Reaction Overview: Application Site Disorders: Common: Injection site reactions: Some patients may experience redness and itching at the site of injection, particularly when the subcutaneous route is used.

Localized lipoatrophy, which can be avoided by varying the site of injection.

Body as a Whole—General Disorders: Uncommon (in children): Fluid retention: peripheral oedema, stiffness, arthralgia, myalgia, paresthesia.

CNS: Uncommon: idiopathic intracranial hypertension.

Endocrine Disorders: hypothyroidism (frequency not determined).

Musculoskeletal Disorders: slipped capital femoral epiphysis (frequency not determined).

Metabolism Disorders: hyperglycemia (frequency not determined).

In a few children, the use of SAIZEN has resulted in the transient formation of antibodies. The clinical significance of these antibodies is unknown, though to date the antibodies have been of low binding capacity and have not been associated with growth attenuation except in patients with gene deletions. In very rare instances, where short stature is due to deletion of the growth-hormone gene complex, treatment with growth hormone, may induce growth attenuating antibodies.

Intermittent dosage has been associated with the appearance of hypoglycaemia.

Slipped capital femoral epiphysis at the site of the hip joint may occur. A child with an unexplained limp should be examined.

Some cases of acute leukemia have been reported in growth hormone deficient children, untreated as well as treated with growth hormone, and might possibly represent a slightly increased incidence compared with non-growth hormone deficient children. A causal relationship to growth hormone therapy has not yet been established.

Toxicity in newborns has been associated with benzyl alcohol as a preservative (see Warnings and Precautions).

Clinical Trial Adverse Drug Reactions: Because clinical trials are conducted under very specific conditions the adverse reaction rates observed in the clinical trials may not reflect the rates observed in practice and should not be compared to the rates in the clinical trials of another drug. Adverse drug reactions information from clinical trials is useful for identifying drug-related adverse events and for approximating rates.

Pediatric Indications: Growth Hormone Deficiency: See Table 1.

Table 1: SAIZEN

Percentage of Patients with Adverse Events by System Organ Class, Preferred Term (whether on or off treatment with SAIZEN)

System Organ Class	Preferred Term	On Treatment (N=224)	Off Treatment (N=15)
Infections and Infestations	Nasopharyngitis	21.4%	
	Upper respiratory tract infection	17.9%	
	Influenza	17.0%	
	Bronchitis	12.5%	
	Otitis media	9.4%	
	Ear infection	8.9%	
	Varicella	7.6%	6.7%
	Pharyngitis streptococcal	7.1%	
	Pharyngitis	6.7%	
	Tonsillitis	6.7%	
	Viral infection	6.7%	
	Rhinitis	6.3%	
	Sinusitis	5.8%	6.7%
	Gastroenteritis viral	6.3%	
	Urinary tract infection	5.4%	
	Gastroenteritis	5.4%	
	Acute tonsillitis	4.0%	6.7%
	Scarlet fever	4.5%	
	Pneumonia	4.0%	
	Herpes simplex	1.8%	
	Rubella	1.8%	
	Mumps	1.3%	
	Impetigo	1.3%	
	Respiratory tract infection	1.3%	
	Viral pharyngitis	1.3%	
General Disorders and Administration Site Conditions	Pyrexia	38.4%	6.7%
	Injection site pain	6.7%	
	Fatigue	6.3%	
	Asthenia	1.8%	
	Chest pain	1.3%	
	Injection site bruising	1.3%	
	Injection site reaction	1.3%	
Respiratory, Thoracic and Mediastinal Disorders	Pharyngolaryngeal pain	32.6%	
	Cough	30.4%	
	Nasal congestion	7.6%	
	Epistaxis	6.7%	
	Rhinorrhoea	4.9%	
	Asthma	3.1%	
	Rhinitis allergic	3.1%	
	Paranasal sinus hypersecretion	1.3%	
	Wheezing	1.3%	
	Dysphonia	1.3%	
	Sinus congestion	1.3%	
Nervous System Disorders	Headache	37.5%	
	Convulsion	3.6%	
	Dizziness	2.7%	
	Epilepsy	2.2%	
	Disturbance in attention	1.8%	
	Lethargy	1.3%	
Gastrointestinal Disorders	Vomiting	17.4%	
	Diarrhoea	11.6%	
	Abdominal pain upper	9.8%	
	Gastrointestinal disorder	7.6%	
	Abdominal pain	5.4%	
	Nausea	4.5%	
	Stomach discomfort	4.0%	
	Constipation	2.7%	
	Toothache	1.3%	
	Dental discomfort	1.3%	
Investigations	Thyroxine decreased	19.2%	
	Hormone level abnormal	2.2%	
	Blood triglycerides increased	1.8%	6.7%
	Body temperature increased	1.8%	
	Weight increased	1.3%	
	Cardiac murmur	1.3%	
	Drug specific antibody present	1.3%	
Surgical and Medical Procedures	Substitution therapy	12.9%	
	Tooth extraction	2.7%	
	Appendicectomy	1.8%	
	Myringotomy	1.8%	
	Tonsillectomy	1.3%	
Musculoskeletal and Connective Tissue Disorders	Arthralgia	12.9%	
	Pain in extremity	9.4%	
	Muscle spasms	2.7%	
	Back pain	1.8%	
	Bone pain	1.3%	
	Myalgia	1.3%	
Skin and Subcutaneous Tissue Disorders	Rash	7.1%	
	Eczema	2.7%	
	Pruritus	2.7%	
	Psoriasis	1.8%	13.3%
	Erythema	2.2%	
	Urticaria	1.8%	
	Acne	1.3%	
Injury, Poisoning and Procedural Complications	Treatment noncompliance	3.6%	
	Joint injury	2.2%	
	Hand fracture	2.2%	
	Road traffic accident	1.8%	6.7%
	Fall	1.8%	

(cont'd)

Table 1: SAIZEN *(cont'd)*

Percentage of Patients with Adverse Events by System Organ Class, Preferred Term (whether on or off treatment with SAIZEN)

System Organ Class	Preferred Term	On Treatment (N=224)	Off Treatment (N=15)
	Skin laceration	1.8%	
	Arthropod bite	1.3%	
	Joint sprain	1.3%	
	Foot fracture	1.3%	
Endocrine Disorders	Delayed puberty	6.3%	
	Hypothyroidism	5.8%	6.7%
	Hypogonadism	2.2%	
	Hypopituitarism	1.8%	
	Diabetes insipidus	1.3%	
	Secondary hypogonadism	1.3%	
Ear and Labyrinth Disorders	Ear pain	11.6%	
	Hypoacusis	1.3%	
	Middle ear effusion	1.3%	
	Otorrhoea	1.3%	
Metabolism and Nutrition Disorders	Hypoglycaemia	3.1%	
	Iron deficiency	2.2%	
	Obesity	2.2%	
	Insulin resistance	1.3%	
Reproductive System and Breast Disorders	Varicocele	2.2%	
	Gynaecomastia	1.8%	
Immune System Disorders	Hypersensitivity	4.5%	
	Seasonal allergy	4.5%	
Psychiatric Disorders	Mental disorder	1.8%	
	Nervousness	1.8%	
	Depression	1.3%	
Blood and Lymphatic System Disorders	Lymphadenopathy	2.7%	
	Anaemia	2.2%	
Renal and Urinary Disorders	Enuresis	2.7%	
Eye Disorders	Conjunctivitis	2.2%	
Congenital, Familial and Genetic Disorders	Cryptorchism	2.7%	13.3%
Neoplasms Benign, Malignant and Unspecified (incl cysts and polyps)	Craniopharyngioma	1.8%	

The most frequently reported AEs were those commonly reported in any paediatric patient population, with pharyngolaryngeal pain (32.6%), pyrexia (38.4%), cough (30.4%), headache (37.5%), nasopharyngitits (21.4%), upper respiratory tract infection (17.9%) and influenza (17.0%) being the most frequently reported. These events were well tolerated without the need for hospitalisation. In addition to the treatment related adverse events reported above, two patients developed anti-hGH antibodies. In both cases, the antibodies did not have any growth inhibiting effect. None of the patients developed antibodies to host cell protein. Three transfer patients who had anti-hGH antibodies prior to treatment became negative within 6 months of treatment with SAIZEN. Hypothyroidism (5.8%) and decreased thyroxine (19.2%) were seen in several patients. One patient died of recurrent craniopharyngioma and one patient experienced lipoatrophy.

Turner's Syndrome: See Table 2.

A clinical study was conducted in 91 girls with Turner's syndrome to receive either SAIZEN alone or in conjunction with oxandrolone.

In girls treated with SAIZEN alone the percentage of patients who experienced specific adverse events were: skin reaction at injection site (13%), pain at injection site (7%), deepening/hoarseness of voice (7%), pain in limbs (7%), pigmented naevi (4%), clitorimegaly (3%), hypercholesterolaemia (3%), and 1% each for edema, hair loss, increased ephelides and seborrhea.

For the group treated with SAIZEN and oxandrolone the percentage of patients who experienced adverse events were: clitoromegaly (30%), pain in limbs (11%), deepening/hoarseness of voice (9%), pain at injection site (9%), skin reaction at injection site (8%), elevated creatinine kinase (4%), hypercholesterolaemia (4%), and 2% each for virilization, exanthem, hyperlipidemia, pigmented naevi, edema, lipodystrophy, haematoma, muscle cramps, increased freckles and hair loss. Thus, the addition of oxandrolone was associated with some virilizing effects, especially at doses of more than 0.05 mg/kg daily.

A total of 18 (20%) patients exhibited a treatment emergent abnormality in the response to glucose loading at some time during the study, of whom only 7 patients (7.7%) had detectable glucose intolerance on two or more occasions. Four patients discontinued treatment in association with these abnormalities. It should be noted that impaired glucose tolerance is commonly found in Turner's syndrome patients.

Table 2: SAIZEN

Percentage of Patients with Adverse Events by System Organ Class, Preferred Term (whether on or off treatment with SAIZEN)

System Organ Class	Preferred Term	On Treatment (N=81)	Off Treatment (N=0)
Respiratory, Thoracic and Mediastinal Disorders	Cough	51.9%	
	Pharyngolaryngeal pain	45.7%	
	Epistaxis	14.8%	
	Dysphonia	11.1%	
	Rhinorrhoea	8.6%	
	Vocal cord thickening	1.2%	
General Disorders and Administration Site Conditions	Pyrexia	46.9%	
	Injection site reaction	16.0%	
	Injection site pain	12.3%	
	Oedema	2.5%	
	Localised oedema	1.2%	
Infections and Infestations	Rhinitis	17.3%	
	Influenza	9.9%	
	Ear infection	6.2%	
	Otitis media	6.2%	
	Bronchitis	4.9%	
	Sinusitis	4.9%	
	Fungal infection	3.7%	
	Nasopharyngitis	3.7%	
	Urinary tract infection	3.7%	
	Varicella	3.7%	
	Fungal skin infection	2.5%	
	Scarlet fever	2.5%	
	Tonsillitis	2.5%	
	Pneumonia	1.2%	
	Candidiasis	1.2%	
	Acute tonsillitis	1.2%	
	Gastroenteritis	1.2%	
	Helminthic infection	1.2%	
	Herpes zoster	1.2%	
	Measles	1.2%	
	Meningitis viral	1.2%	
	Mumps	1.2%	
	Otitis media chronic	1.2%	
	Paronychia	1.2%	
	Pertussis	1.2%	
	Pharyngitis	1.2%	
	Respiratory tract infection	1.2%	
	Viral infection	1.2%	
	Vulvitis	1.2%	
	Rhinitis	17.3%	
	Influenza	9.9%	
	Ear infection	6.2%	
	Otitis media	6.2%	
Nervous System Disorders	Headache	44.4%	
	Petit mal epilepsy	1.2%	

(cont'd)

Table 2: **SAIZEN** *(cont'd)*

Percentage of Patients with Adverse Events by System Organ Class, Preferred Term (whether on or off treatment with SAIZEN)

System Organ Class	Preferred Term	On Treatment (N=81)	Off Treatment (N=0)
	Convulsion	1.2%	
	Dizziness	1.2%	
	Epilepsy	1.2%	
	Febrile convulsion	1.2%	
	Hypertonia	1.2%	
Ear and Labyrinth Disorders	Ear pain	28.4%	
	Hearing impaired	2.5%	

Chronic Renal Failure: See Table 3.

Table 3: **SAIZEN**

Percentage of Patients with Adverse Events by System Organ Class, Preferred Term (whether on or off treatment with SAIZEN)

System Organ Class	Preferred Term	On Treatment (N=65)	Off Treatment (N=11)
Infections and Infestations	Upper respiratory tract infection	26.2%	
	Otitis media	20.0%	
	Viral infection	20.0%	
	Catheter related infection	18.5%	9.1%
	Rhinitis	16.9%	
	Urinary tract infection	13.8%	
	Influenza	13.8%	
	Gastroenteritis	10.8%	
	Nasopharyngitis	9.2%	
	Herpes simplex	7.7%	
	Bronchitis	7.7%	
	Pharyngitis	7.7%	
	Tonsillitis	7.7%	
	Varicella	7.7%	
	Staphylococcal infection	6.2%	
	Pyelonephritis	4.6%	
	Sinusitis	4.6%	
	Tonsillitis streptococcal	4.6%	
	Sepsis	3.1%	
	Cytomegalovirus infection	3.1%	
	Infection parasitic	3.1%	
	Hepatitis C	3.1%	
	Localised infection	3.1%	
	Pharyngitis streptococcal	3.1%	
	Respiratory tract infection viral	3.1%	
	Streptococcal infection	3.1%	
	Ear infection	1.5%	
	Fungal infection	1.5%	
	Abscess	1.5%	
	Appendicitis	1.5%	
	Cystitis	1.5%	
	Dental caries	1.5%	
	Endotoxic shock	1.5%	
	Gastroenteritis viral	1.5%	
	Hepatitis B	1.5%	

(cont'd)

Table 3: **SAIZEN** *(cont'd)*

Percentage of Patients with Adverse Events by System Organ Class, Preferred Term (whether on or off treatment with SAIZEN)

System Organ Class	Preferred Term	On Treatment (N=65)	Off Treatment (N=11)
	Herpes zoster	1.5%	
	Infection	1.5%	
	Injection site abscess	1.5%	
	Laryngitis	1.5%	
	Onychomycosis	1.5%	
	Paronychia	1.5%	
	Pseudomonas infection	1.5%	
	Scarlet fever	1.5%	
	Skin infection	1.5%	
	Staphylococcal sepsis	1.5%	
	Vaginal candidiasis	1.5%	
	Vaginal infection	1.5%	
	Viral rash	1.5%	
Gastrointestinal Disorders	Peritonitis	20.0%	
	Vomiting	20.0%	
	Diarrhoea	15.4%	
	Abdominal pain	7.7%	
	Inguinal hernia	7.7%	
	Gingival hyperplasia	7.7%	
	Constipation	6.2%	
	Nausea	6.2%	
	Abdominal pain upper	4.6%	
	Tooth disorder	3.1%	
	Dysphagia	3.1%	
	Abdominal hernia	1.5%	
	Breath odour	1.5%	
	Colonic polyp	1.5%	
	Dyspepsia	1.5%	
	Enteritis	1.5%	
	Faecal incontinence	1.5%	
	Food poisoning	1.5%	
	Frequent bowel movements	1.5%	
	Gastritis	1.5%	
	Gingival hypertrophy	1.5%	
	Intestinal obstruction	1.5%	
	Salivary gland enlargement	1.5%	
	Stomach discomfort	1.5%	
	Umbilical hernia	1.5%	
General Disorders and Administration Site Conditions	Pyrexia	23.1%	9.1%
	Fatigue	4.6%	
	Face oedema	4.6%	
	Oedema peripheral	3.1%	
	Chest pain	3.1%	
	Gait disturbance	3.1%	
	Injection site haemorrhage	3.1%	
	Injection site pain	3.1%	
	Local swelling	1.5%	

(cont'd)

Table 3: SAIZEN *(cont'd)*

Percentage of Patients with Adverse Events by System Organ Class, Preferred Term (whether on or off treatment with SAIZEN)

System Organ Class	Preferred Term	On Treatment (N=65)	Off Treatment (N=11)
	Asthenia	1.5%	
	Catheter site inflammation	1.5%	
	Chills	1.5%	
	Difficulty in walking	1.5%	
	Generalised oedema	1.5%	
	Inflammation	1.5%	
	Influenza like illness	1.5%	
	Injection site reaction	1.5%	
	Oedema	1.5%	
Nervous System Disorders	Headache	23.1%	
	Dizziness	4.6%	
	Convulsion	3.1%	
	Psychomotor hyperactivity	1.5%	
	Benign intracranial hypertension	1.5%	
	Paraesthesia	1.5%	
	Petit mal epilepsy	1.5%	
	Balance disorder	1.5%	
	Brain oedema	1.5%	
	Cerebral infarction	1.5%	
	Coordination abnormal	1.5%	
	Hypertonia	1.5%	
	Mental retardation severity unspecified	1.5%	
	Nervous system disorder	1.5%	
	Optic neuritis	1.5%	
Surgical and Medical Procedures	Renal transplant	27.7%	45.5%
Renal and Urinary Disorders	Renal failure	12.3%	9.1%
	Dysuria	4.6%	
	Renal impairment	4.6%	
	Proteinuria	3.1%	
	Enuresis	3.1%	
	Hydronephrosis	1.5%	
	Renal disorder	1.5%	
	Bladder disorder	1.5%	
	Haematuria	1.5%	
	Micturition disorder	1.5%	
	Neurogenic bladder	1.5%	
	Pyuria	1.5%	
	Urethral disorder	1.5%	
	Urinary retention	1.5%	
Respiratory, Thoracic and Mediastinal Disorders	Pharyngolaryngeal pain	15.4%	
	Cough	13.8%	
	Rhinitis allergic	6.2%	9.1%
	Rhinorrhoea	4.6%	
	Epistaxis	3.1%	
	Adenoidal hypertrophy	3.1%	
	Pulmonary oedema	3.1%	

(cont'd)

Table 3: SAIZEN *(cont'd)*

Percentage of Patients with Adverse Events by System Organ Class, Preferred Term (whether on or off treatment with SAIZEN)

System Organ Class	Preferred Term	On Treatment (N=65)	Off Treatment (N=11)
	Wheezing	3.1%	
	Asthma	1.5%	
	Pharyngeal erythema	1.5%	
	Respiratory tract congestion	1.5%	
	Atelectasis	1.5%	
	Dyspnoea	1.5%	
	Mediastinal disorder	1.5%	
	Nasal congestion	1.5%	
	Nasal discomfort	1.5%	
	Rales	1.5%	
	Sneezing	1.5%	
	Throat irritation	1.5%	
Musculoskeletal and Connective Tissue Disorders	Pain in extremity	13.8%	
	Arthralgia	10.8%	
	Neck pain	4.6%	
	Back pain	4.6%	
	Renal osteodystrophy	3.1%	
	Bone pain	3.1%	
	Groin pain	1.5%	
	Aseptic necrosis bone	1.5%	
	Muscle spasms	1.5%	
	Musculoskeletal discomfort	1.5%	
	Osteochondrosis	1.5%	
	Arthropathy	1.5%	
	Epiphysiolysis	1.5%	
	Knee deformity	1.5%	
	Lower limb deformity	1.5%	
	Myalgia	1.5%	
	Rickets	1.5%	
	Shoulder pain	1.5%	
Metabolism and Nutrition Disorders	Hypercalcaemia	7.7%	
	Hyperkalaemia	6.2%	
	Glucose tolerance impaired	3.1%	
	Fluid overload	3.1%	
	Hyperphosphataemia	3.1%	
	Decreased appetite	3.1%	
	Hyperuricaemia	1.5%	9.1%
	Anorexia	1.5%	
	Diabetes mellitus	1.5%	
	Fluid retention	1.5%	
	Hyperglycaemia	1.5%	
	Hyperlipidaemia	1.5%	
	Hypermagnesaemia	1.5%	
	Hypervolaemia	1.5%	
	Hypokalaemia	1.5%	
	Malnutrition	1.5%	
	Metabolic acidosis	1.5%	

(cont'd)

Table 3: SAIZEN *(cont'd)*

Percentage of Patients with Adverse Events by System Organ Class, Preferred Term (whether on or off treatment with SAIZEN)

System Organ Class	Preferred Term	On Treatment (N=65)	Off Treatment (N=11)
Injury, Poisoning and Procedural Complications	Injury	13.8%	
	Accidental overdose	3.1%	
	Fall	3.1%	
	Arthropod bite	1.5%	
	Excoriation	1.5%	
	Post procedural vomiting	1.5%	
Investigations	Blood creatinine increased	7.7%	
	Weight decreased	3.1%	
	Aspartate aminotransferase increased	1.5%	
	Blood parathyroid hormone increased	1.5%	
	Blood pressure decreased	1.5%	
	Blood urea increased	1.5%	
	Blood urine present	1.5%	
	Body temperature increased	1.5%	
	Liver function test abnormal	1.5%	
	Metabolic function test	1.5%	
	Urine output decreased	1.5%	
Skin and Subcutaneous Tissue Disorders	Acne	4.6%	
	Rash	1.5%	
	Onychorrhexis	1.5%	
	Rash pruritic	1.5%	
	Skin depigmentation	1.5%	
	Skin hypertrophy	1.5%	
	Skin nodule	1.5%	
	Urticaria	1.5%	
	Alopecia	1.5%	
	Angioneurotic oedema	1.5%	
	Dermatitis contact	1.5%	
	Ecchymosis	1.5%	
	Eczema	1.5%	
	Nail dystrophy	1.5%	
	Psoriasis	1.5%	
	Rash papular	1.5%	
	Skin discolouration	1.5%	
	Skin inflammation	1.5%	
	Skin reaction	1.5%	
Immune System Disorders	Transplant rejection	6.2%	9.1%
	Hypersensitivity	4.6%	
	Kidney transplant rejection	4.6%	
	Drug hypersensitivity	1.5%	
Blood and Lymphatic System Disorders	Anaemia	9.2%	
	Lymphadenopathy	7.7%	
	Nephrogenic anaemia	4.6%	
	Neutropenia	1.5%	
	Coagulopathy	1.5%	
	Leukocytosis	1.5%	

(cont'd)

Table 3: SAIZEN *(cont'd)*

Percentage of Patients with Adverse Events by System Organ Class, Preferred Term (whether on or off treatment with SAIZEN)

System Organ Class	Preferred Term	On Treatment (N=65)	Off Treatment (N=11)
Vascular Disorders	Hypertension	9.2%	
	Hypotension	6.2%	
	Haemorrhage	3.1%	
	Hypertensive crisis	1.5%	
	Haematoma	1.5%	
	Hot flush	1.5%	
	Peripheral coldness	1.5%	
	Vasculitis	1.5%	
	Vasospasm	1.5%	
Reproductive System and Breast Disorders	Gynaecomastia	3.1%	
	Testicular torsion	3.1%	
	Balanitis	1.5%	
	Breast disorder	1.5%	
	Epididymitis	1.5%	
	Testicular disorder	1.5%	
Eye Disorders	Eyelid oedema	3.1%	
	Eye pain	1.5%	
	Optic atrophy	1.5%	
	Optic discs blurred	1.5%	
	Papilloedema	1.5%	
	Vision blurred	1.5%	
Ear and Labyrinth Disorders	Ear pain	4.6%	
	Ear disorder	1.5%	
	Hypoacusis	1.5%	
	Ear discomfort	1.5%	
Endocrine Disorders	Hyperparathyroidism	4.6%	
	Hypoparathyroidism	1.5%	
	Hypothyroidism	1.5%	
Cardiac Disorders	Cyanosis	1.5%	
	Cardiac disorder	1.5%	
	Cardiac failure	1.5%	
	Pericarditis	1.5%	
Congenital, Familial and Genetic Disorders	Hydrocele	3.1%	
	Congenital foot malformation	1.5%	
Neoplasms Benign, Malignant and Unspecified (incl cysts and polyps)	Skin papilloma	3.1%	
	Parathyroid tumour benign	1.5%	
Psychiatric Disorders	Attention deficit/hyperactivity disorder	1.5%	
	Insomnia	1.5%	

In clinical studies with SAIZEN in Chronic Renal Failure, the following adverse events were considered possibly related to treatment by the investigator: pseudotumor cerebri, deterioration of renal function, hyperthyroidism, injection site infection, renal transplant rejection, papilloedema, hypothyroidism, impaired OGTT and abnormal AST.

Small for Gestational Age: Common and very common adverse reactions (frequency ≥1%) are tabulated in Table 4.

The most common (incidence >5%) adverse events observed in clinical trials with SGA patients were mild to moderate in severity. The most frequently reported AEs were those commonly reported in any paediatric patient population, with ear infection, bronchitis, nasopharyngitis, gastroenteritis, varicella and pharyngolaryngeal pain being the most frequently reported. These events were well tolerated without the need for drug discontinuation. The number, type and severity of events did not differ between periods with r-hGH treatment and periods with observation without treatment, or between the first and second and third year of r-hGH treatment.

Oral glucose tolerance tests (OGTT) were used during the treatment and observation periods in studies GF 4001 and GF 6283. Increased insulin levels were observed after 18 months of r-hGH treatment in study GF 4001 and this increase was sustained during the 3-year treatment period but were normalised during the follow-up period. Similar results were observed for the children who received continuous treatment (Group TTOO), but were less apparent for children who received intermittent treatment (Group TOTO) in study GF 6283. Abnormal glucose levels during the OGTT indicative of impaired glucose tolerance were observed in a few patients in both studies, and more often during continuous treatment (study GF 4001 and Group TTOO in study GF 6283) than during intermittent treatment (Group TOTO in study GF 6283). There was no report on diabetes mellitus in any of the studies but in one child (patient no. 6283102003) in study GF 6283, who had received r-hGH treatment continuously for 2 years, a fasting glucose value of 11.2 mmol/L was observed after 2 years of observation without treatment. There was no withdrawal in any of the studies due to change in glucose tolerance. These results are similar to those reported in the literature.

Table 4: SAIZEN

Percentage of Patients with Adverse Events by System Organ Class, Preferred Term (whether on or off treatment with SAIZEN—pooling of GF 4001 and GF 6283)

System Organ Class	Preferred Term	On Treatment (N=100)	Off Treatment (N=34)
Infections and Infestations	Ear infection	19.0%	14.7%
	Bronchitis	19.0%	8.8%
	Nasopharyngitis	14.0%	20.6%
	Gastroenteritis	14.0%	5.9%
	Varicella	13.0%	11.8%
	Otitis media	7.0%	11.8%
	Otitis media acute	4.0%	2.9%
	Tonsillitis	4.0%	
	Laryngitis	4.0%	
	Lung infection	3.0%	2.9%
	Pharyngitis	2.0%	5.9%
	Influenza	2.0%	2.9%
	Urinary tract infection	2.0%	2.9%
	Upper respiratory tract infection	2.0%	
	Viral infection	2.0%	
	Acute tonsillitis		2.9%
	Tooth abscess	1.0%	2.9%
	Cystitis	1.0%	
	Furuncle	1.0%	
	Helicobacter gastritis		2.9%
	Infectious mononucleosis	1.0%	
	Paronychia	1.0%	
	Pneumonia viral	1.0%	
	Respiratory tract infection	1.0%	
	Rubella	1.0%	
	Sepsis	1.0%	
	Sinusitis	1.0%	
	Tracheobronchitis	1.0%	
	Viral rash	1.0%	
Respiratory, Thoracic and Mediastinal Disorders	Pharyngolaryngeal pain	17.0%	8.8%
	Rhinitis	5.0%	5.9%
	Asthma	5.0%	
	Maxillary sinusitis	3.0%	
	Epistaxis	2.0%	
	Lung disorder	1.0%	
	Nasal congestion	1.0%	
	Rales	1.0%	
Gastrointestinal Disorders	Diarrhoea	2.0%	5.9%
	Constipation	2.0%	2.9%
	Abdominal pain	1.0%	2.9%
	Vomiting	1.0%	2.9%
	Food poisoning	1.0%	
	Gastrooesophageal reflux disease	1.0%	

(cont'd)

Table 4: SAIZEN *(cont'd)*

Percentage of Patients with Adverse Events by System Organ Class, Preferred Term (whether on or off treatment with SAIZEN—pooling of GF 4001 and GF 6283)

System Organ Class	Preferred Term	On Treatment (N=100)	Off Treatment (N=34)
	Inguinal hernia	1.0%	
	Irritable bowel syndrome	1.0%	
	Peritonitis	1.0%	
	Toothache		2.9%
Injury, Poisoning and Procedural Complications	Head injury	2.0%	
	Upper limb fracture	1.0%	2.9%
	Arthropod sting	1.0%	
	Burns second degree		2.9%
	Cervical vertebral fracture	1.0%	
	Contusion	1.0%	
	Fall	1.0%	
	Foreign body trauma	1.0%	
	Joint sprain	1.0%	
	Thermal burn	1.0%	
	Traumatic haematoma	1.0%	
	Wrist fracture	1.0%	
Surgical and Medical Procedures	Tonsillectomy	4.0%	
	Appendicectomy	3.0%	
	Ear tube insertion	3.0%	
	Myringoplasty	1.0%	
	Gastric operation	1.0%	
	Otorhinolaryngological surgery	1.0%	
	Skin neoplasm excision	1.0%	
Nervous System Disorders	Headache	5.0%	5.9%
	Coma	1.0%	
	Dizziness	1.0%	
	Febrile convulsion	1.0%	
	Tremor	1.0%	
Blood and Lymphatic System Disorders	Anaemia	3.0%	
	Hypochromic anaemia	2.0%	2.9%
	Eosinophilia	2.0%	2.9%
	Thrombocytopenia	2.0%	2.9%
	Pancytopenia	1.0%	
	Granulocytopenia	1.0%	
	Iron deficiency anaemia	1.0%	
Musculoskeletal and Connective Tissue Disorders	Arthralgia	3.0%	2.9%
	Muscle hypertrophy	1.0%	
	Myalgia	1.0%	
	Osteoarthritis	1.0%	
	Osteochondrosis	1.0%	
General Disorders and Administration Site Conditions	Pyrexia	4.0%	
	Injection site inflammation	1.0%	
	Difficulty in walking	1.0%	
Skin and Subcutaneous Tissue Disorders	Urticaria	1.0%	2.9%
	Acne	1.0%	
	Henoch-Schonlein purpura	1.0%	

(cont'd)

Table 4: SAIZEN *(cont'd)*

Percentage of Patients with Adverse Events by System Organ Class, Preferred Term (whether on or off treatment with SAIZEN—pooling of GF 4001 and GF 6283)

System Organ Class	Preferred Term	On Treatment (N=100)	Off Treatment (N=34)
	Pruritus generalised	1.0%	
	Rash	1.0%	
Investigations	Aspartate aminotransferase increased	1.0%	
	Blood glucose increased	1.0%	
	Body temperature increased	1.0%	
	Glycosylated haemoglobin increased	1.0%	
	Haemoglobin decreased	1.0%	
Renal and Urinary Disorders	Haematuria	1.0%	
	Polyuria		2.9%
	Renal insufficiency	1.0%	
	Ureteric stenosis	1.0%	
Psychiatric Disorders	Sleep disorder	2.0%	
	Aggression	1.0%	
	Polydipsia psychogenic	1.0%	
Congenital, Familial and Genetic Disorders	Cryptorchism		2.9%
	Eyelid ptosis congenital	1.0%	
	Pigmented naevus		2.9%
Cardiac Disorders	Cardiac disorder	1.0%	
	Cardiac failure	1.0%	
Endocrine Disorders	Autoimmune thyroiditis	1.0%	
	Hypothyroidism		2.9%
Immune System Disorders	Allergy to animal	1.0%	
	Drug hypersensitivity	1.0%	
Eye Disorders	Conjunctivitis		2.9%
Metabolism and Nutrition Disorders	Glucose tolerance impaired	1.0%	
Neoplasms Benign, Malignant and Unspecified (incl cysts and polyps)	Cyst	1.0%	
Reproductive System and Breast Disorders	Hypertrophy breast		2.9%

Adult Indications: Adult Growth Hormone Deficiency: See Table 5 and Table 6.

Table 5: SAIZEN

Percentage of Patients with Adverse Events by System Organ Class, Preferred Term (whether on or off treatment with SAIZEN)

System Organ Class	Preferred Term	On Treatment (N=107)	Off Treatment (N=44)
Musculoskeletal and Connective Tissue Disorders	Arthralgia	35.5%	18.2%
	Back pain	13.1%	6.8%
	Myalgia	9.3%	2.3%
	Pain in extremity	9.3%	2.3%
	Joint swelling	6.5%	6.8%
	Joint stiffness	6.5%	
	Musculoskeletal stiffness	4.7%	2.3%
	Tendonitis	4.7%	
	Groin pain	1.9%	4.5%

(cont'd)

Table 5: SAIZEN *(cont'd)*

Percentage of Patients with Adverse Events by System Organ Class, Preferred Term (whether on or off treatment with SAIZEN)

System Organ Class	Preferred Term	On Treatment (N=107)	Off Treatment (N=44)
	Shoulder pain	3.7%	
	Muscle spasms	1.9%	2.3%
	Pain in jaw	1.9%	2.3%
	Chest wall pain	1.9%	
	Dupuytren's contracture	1.9%	
	Musculoskeletal discomfort	1.9%	
Nervous System Disorders	Headache	20.6%	18.2%
	Paraesthesia	9.3%	2.3%
	Dizziness	7.5%	6.8%
	Carpal tunnel syndrome	7.5%	4.5%
	Hypoaesthesia	6.5%	
	Sinus headache	3.7%	2.3%
	Sciatica	1.9%	4.5%
	Memory impairment	2.8%	
	Loss of consciousness	1.9%	
Infections and Infestations	Influenza	17.8%	4.5%
	Nasopharyngitis	14.0%	2.3%
	Lower respiratory tract infection	9.3%	6.8%
	Urinary tract infection	4.7%	2.3%
	Bronchitis	3.7%	4.5%
	Upper respiratory tract infection	4.7%	
	Tooth abscess	4.7%	
	Ear infection	1.9%	2.3%
	Gastroenteritis	2.8%	
	Otitis externa	1.9%	
	Tonsillitis	1.9%	
General Disorders and Administration Site Conditions	Oedema peripheral	16.8%	9.1%
	Fatigue	10.3%	4.5%
	Influenza like illness	6.5%	2.3%
	Injection site bruising	1.9%	6.8%
	Asthenia	2.8%	4.5%
	Chest pain	2.8%	
	Oedema	1.9%	2.3%
	Pyrexia	2.8%	
	Chills	1.9%	
	Pain	1.9%	
Investigations	Free fatty acids increased	10.3%	4.5%
	Insulin-like growth factor increased	7.5%	
	Blood cholesterol increased	2.8%	2.3%
	Thyroxine free decreased	3.7%	
	Alanine aminotransferase increased	2.8%	

(cont'd)

Table 5: SAIZEN *(cont'd)*

Percentage of Patients with Adverse Events by System Organ Class, Preferred Term (whether on or off treatment with SAIZEN)

System Organ Class	Preferred Term	On Treatment (N=107)	Off Treatment (N=44)
	Glycosylated haemoglobin increased	2.8%	
	Weight decreased	2.8%	
	Neutrophil count increased	1.9%	
	White blood cell count increased	1.9%	
	Blood urine present	1.9%	
	Lymphocyte count decreased	1.9%	
Gastrointestinal Disorders	Nausea	6.5%	6.8%
	Diarrhoea	7.5%	2.3%
	Abdominal pain upper	7.5%	
	Vomiting	4.7%	
	Abdominal distension	2.8%	
	Abdominal pain	2.8%	
	Stomach discomfort	2.8%	
	Abdominal discomfort	1.9%	
	Frequent bowel movements	1.9%	
	Gastrooesophageal reflux disease	1.9%	
Metabolism and Nutrition Disorders	Fluid retention	8.4%	
	Hyperglycaemia	3.7%	2.3%
	Dehydration	2.8%	
	Dyslipidaemia	2.8%	
Skin and Subcutaneous Tissue Disorders	Hyperhidrosis	4.7%	
	Rash	2.8%	2.3%
	Skin disorder	2.8%	
	Pruritus	1.9%	
	Nail pigmentation	1.9%	
Respiratory, Thoracic and Mediastinal Disorders	Pharyngolaryngeal pain	4.7%	4.5%
	Cough	2.8%	6.8%
	Dyspnoea	1.9%	4.5%
	Nasal congestion	2.8%	2.3%
Psychiatric Disorders	Insomnia	7.5%	
	Depression	4.7%	
	Depressive delusion	2.8%	
	Anxiety	1.9%	
	Depressed mood	1.9%	
Eye Disorders	Conjunctivitis	2.8%	
	Vision blurred	2.8%	
	Eye pain	1.9%	2.3%
Renal and Urinary Disorders	Haematuria	8.4%	4.5%
	Nephrolithiasis	1.9%	

(cont'd)

Table 5: SAIZEN *(cont'd)*

Percentage of Patients with Adverse Events by System Organ Class, Preferred Term (whether on or off treatment with SAIZEN)

System Organ Class	Preferred Term	On Treatment (N=107)	Off Treatment (N=44)
Injury, Poisoning and Procedural Complications	Fall	1.9%	
	Joint dislocation	1.9%	
	Joint sprain	1.9%	
Vascular Disorders	Hypertension	3.7%	6.8%
	Hypotension	1.9%	
Endocrine Disorders	Hypothyroidism	6.5%	
	Hyperthyroidism	1.9%	
Reproductive System and Breast Disorders	Metrorrhagia	2.8%	
	Dysmenorrhoea	1.9%	
Blood and Lymphatic System Disorders	Anaemia	1.9%	
	Lymphadenopathy	1.9%	
Neoplasms Benign, Malignant and Unspecified (incl cysts and polyps)	Pituitary tumour	1.9%	
Ear and Labyrinth Disorders	Ear discomfort	1.9%	2.3%
	Ear pain	1.9%	

Table 6: SAIZEN

SAIZEN Adult GHD

Month From Start of Study	Number of Patients Still on Treatment by Visit Since Study Start		
	Total # of Patients	Patient Still on Treatment	
		r-hGH	Placebo[b]
DBPC start	115	60 (100%)	55 (100%)
DBPC end	115	53 (88%)	51 (93%)
Month 12	115	49 (82%)	48 (87%)
Month 18	115	34 (57%)	34 (62%)
Month 24[a]	42	15 (68%)	13 (65%)
Month 30[a]	42	11 (50%)	11 (55%)
Month 36[a]	42	6 (27%)	6 (30%)

[a] Only 2 of the 6 sites scheduled treatment beyond 18 months.
[b] Treatment with SAIZEN started in month 6.
2 patients had their last visit before one of the presented month and the last after that month.

Withdrawals for this study during both the double-blind, placebo controlled phase and the open-label phase were due to patient decision (7%), protocol violation (0.9%), adverse events (12.2%), lost to follow-up (0.9%) and other (2.6%).

Edema, muscle pain, joint pain, and joint disorders were reported to occur in up to 10% of adult patients receiving growth hormone replacement therapy. These side effects occurred primarily early in therapy and tended to be transient.

Adult patients with growth hormone deficiency, following diagnosis of growth hormone deficiency in childhood, reported side effects less frequently than those with adult onset growth hormone deficiency.

Less Common Clinical Trial Adverse Drug Reactions: Clinical trial adverse drug reactions with a frequency of less than 1% are presented in Table 7.

DRUG INTERACTIONS: Concomitant glucorticoid therapy may reduce the growth promoting effect of somatropin. If glucocorticoid replacement is required, the dose should be carefully adjusted. Published in vitro data indicate that growth hormone may be an inducer of cytochrome P450 34A.

When SAIZEN is administered in combination with drugs known to be metabolized by CYP P450 3A4 hepatic enzymes, it is advisable to monitor clinical effectiveness of such drugs.

Interactions with food, herbal products or laboratory tests have not been established.

DOSAGE AND ADMINISTRATION: Dosing Considerations: Before initiating a patient on SAIZEN therapy, please review completely the Contraindications and Warnings and Precautions sections.

SAIZEN dosage should be individualized for each patient according to body weight.

SAIZEN treatment should be carried out under regular guidance of a physician experienced in the diagnosis and management of growth disorders.

For SAIZEN 3.33 mg and 5 mg, once the appropriate dose for a patient has been determined, reconstitute each vial of SAIZEN with the diluent supplied. For use in patients sensitive to benzyl alcohol, see Warnings and Precautions.

Recommended Dose and Dosage Adjustment: Growth Failure Due to Inadequate Endogenous Growth Hormone Secretion: It is recommended that SAIZEN be administered subcutaneously at a dose of 0.2 mg/kg body weight per week. The dosage can be increased to 0.27 mg/kg per week if there is insufficient response to treatment.

Growth Failure in Girls Due to Gonadal Dysgenesis (Turner's Syndrome): It is recommended that SAIZEN be administered subcutaneously at a dose of 0.375 mg/kg body weight per week (optimal dosing 0.32-0.375 mg/kg/week).

Concomitant therapy with non-androgenic anabolic steroids in patients with Turner's syndrome can enhance the growth response.

Growth Failure in Children with Chronic Renal Failure: It is recommended that SAIZEN be administered subcutaneously at a dose of 0.35 mg/kg body weight per week.

Growth Disturbance in Short Children Born Small for Gestational Age (SGA): It is recommended that SAIZEN be administered subcutaneously at a dose of 0.47 mg/kg body weight/week.

Adult Growth Hormone Deficiency: It is recommended that SAIZEN be administered subcutaneously at a dose of 0.005 mg/kg/day at the start of therapy. This dose may be increased after 4 weeks to 0.01 mg/kg/day if well tolerated. The minimum effective dose should be used and dose requirements may decline with age.

Table 7: SAIZEN

List of Adverse Events with a Frequency of Less Than 1% in Clinical Trials Performed with SAIZEN in Registered Indications

Indication	System Organ Class	Preferred Terms: Pediatric	Preferred Terms: Adult
GHD	Blood and Lymphatic System Disorders	Iron deficiency anaemia, neutrophilia, plasmacytosis	Microcytic anaemia, neutropenia, neutrophilia
	Cardiac Disorders	Angina pectoris, aortic valve stenosis, palpitations	Atrial fibrillation, coronary artery disease, left ventricular failure
	Congenital, Familial and Genetic Disorders	Atrial septal defect, epidermal naevus, facial dysmorphism, foetal alcohol sindrome, lymphangioma, pigmented naevus, turner's syndrome	—
	Ear and Labyrinth Disorders	Deafness, deafness bilateral, ear congestion, ear discomfort, motion sickness, tinnitus, tympanic membrane hyperaemia, tympanic membrane perforation	—
	Endocrine Disorders	Adrenocortical insufficiency chronic, empty sella syndrome, hyperthyroidism	Adrenocortical insufficiency acute, pituitary cyst, toxic nodular goitre
	Eye Disorders	Blepharitis, blindness, diplopia, eye haemorrhage, eye irritation, eyelid oedema, eyelid ptosis, lacrimal cyst, optic atrophy, papilloedema, vision blurred, visual acuity reduced, visual disturbance	Accommodation disorder, asthenopia, cataract, conjunctivitis allergic, dry eye, eyelid cyst, eyelid oedema, optic discs blurred
	Gastrointestinal Disorders	Abdominal pain lower, aphthous stomatitis, dyspepsia, faeces hard, flatulence, gingival bleeding, gingival hypertrophy, irritable bowel syndrome, mouth ulceration, oral mucosal blistering, pancreatitis, salivary gland hypertrophy, tooth disorder	Anal fissure, colitis ulcerative, constipation, diverticulum, dysphagia, food poisoning, gastritis, gastrointestinal haemorrhage, haemorrhoids, intestinal polyp, tooth disorder, toothache
	General Disorders and Administration Site Conditions	Adverse drug reaction, adverse event, application site pain, chills, cyst rupture, feeling cold, feeling hot, hernia, influenza like illness, infusion site bruising, injection site atrophy, injection site haemorrhage, injection site hypertrophy, injection site induration, injection site irritation, injection site mass, injection site rash, injection site scar, injection site swelling, instillation site pruritus, irritability, local swelling, malaise, mucosal ulceration, no adverse effect, oedema peripheral, pain	Application site reaction, chest discomfort, discomfort, facial pain, injection site pain, injection site reaction, malaise
	Hepatobiliary Disorders	Liver disorder	Cholelithiasis, gallbladder polyp, hepatic function abnormal
	Immune System Disorders	Drug hypersensitivity, multiple allergies, selective IgG subclass deficiency	Hypersensitivity, seasonal allergy
	Infections and Infestations	Acarodermatitis, appendicitis, bacteriuria body tinea, conjunctivitis infective, cystitis, enterobiasis, erythema infectiosum, eye infection, febrile infection, fungal infection, furuncle, gastric infection, genital infection, hepatitis b, herpes zoster, herpetic stomatitis, infectious mononucleosis, injection site infection, kidney infection, lice infestation, localised infection, lower respiratory tract infection, lymph gland infection, measles, meningitis viral, molluscum contagiosum, nail infection, oral candidiasis, orchitis, otitis externa, paronychia, pertussis, pharyngotonsillitis, postoperative wound infection, pyelonephritis, skin infection, staphylococcal infection, streptococcal infection, tinea capitis, tinea infection, tooth abscess, tooth infection, vaginal infection, viraemia, viral upper respiratory tract infection, vulvitis, vulvovaginal mycotic infection, wound infection	Breast infection, cystitis, eye infection, gastroenteritis viral, gingival infection, helicobacter infection, herpes zoster oticus, hordeolum, infected sebaceous cyst, labyrinthitis, pharyngitis, sinusitis, viral infection, vulvovaginal mycotic infection
	Injury, Poisoning and Procedural Complications	Animal scratch, arthropod sting, concussion, confusion postoperative, contusion, exposure to toxic agent, fibula fracture, head injury, heat exhaustion, humerus fracture, joint ligament rupture, limb injury, lower limb fracture, medical device discomfort, mouth injury, multiple fractures, muscle strain, soft tissue injury, splinter, sunburn, superficial injury of eye, thermal burn, tibia fracture, vaccination complication, wound	Ankle fracture, back injury, contusion, laceration, muscle strain, procedural pain, wrist fracture

(cont'd)

Table 7: SAIZEN *(cont'd)*

List of Adverse Events with a Frequency of Less Than 1% in Clinical Trials Performed with SAIZEN in Registered Indications

Indication	System Organ Class	Preferred Terms: Pediatric	Preferred Terms: Adult
	Investigations	Blood corticotrophin decreased, blood cortisol decreased, blood gonadotrophin decreased, blood iron decreased, blood sodium decreased, catheterisation cardiac, diagnostic procedure, glucose tolerance test abnormal, glucose urine, head circumference abnormal, hepatic enzyme increased, iodine uptake abnormal, lipids increased, platelet count decreased, transaminases increased, weight decreased, white blood cell count decreased, white blood cells urine positive	Blood calcium increased, blood creatinine increased, blood glucose decreased, blood potassium decreased, body temperature decreased, gamma-glutamyltransferase increased, haemoglobin increased, heart rate increased, hepatic enzyme increased, high density lipoprotein decreased, liver function test abnormal, low density lipoprotein increased, lymph node palpable, monocyte count decreased, prostate examination abnormal, semen volume decreased, weight increased
	Metabolism and Nutrition Disorders	Anorexia, decreased appetite dehydration, fluid overload fluid retention, glucose tolerance impaired, hypercholesterolaemia, hyperinsulinaemia, hyponatraemia, increased appetite, polydipsia, weight gain poor	Decreased appetite, diabetes mellitus, hypercholesterolaemia, hyperkalaemia, hypertriglyceridaemia, hypoglycaemia, increased appetite, iron deficiency, polydipsia
	Musculoskeletal and Connective Tissue Disorders	Arthropathy, chondropathy flank pain, groin pain, growth retardation, joint effusion, joint range of motion decreased, juvenile arthritis, limb discomfort, muscle contracture, musculoskeletal pain, myopathy, neck pain, osteochondrosis, rickets, scoliosis, shoulder pain, spinal disorder, temporomandibular joint syndrome, torticollis	Arthritis, arthropathy, axillary mass, bone pain, bursitis, ganglion, limb deformity, muscle fatigue, muscle tightness, musculoskeletal chest pain, musculoskeletal pain, myopathy, sacral pain, synovitis, tendon disorder
	Neoplasms Benign, Malignant and Unspecified (incl. cysts and polyps)	Astrocytoma, glioma, metastases to spine, neoplasm progression, pinealoma, pituitary tumour, skin papilloma, tumour flare	Acrochordon, basal cell carcinoma, glioma, haemangioma, uterine leiomyoma
	Nervous System Disorders	Amnesia, brain oedema, carpal tunnel syndrome, cerebral atrophy, clonus, coordination abnormal, depressed level of consciousness, encephalitis, grand mal convulsion, hemiparesis, hyperreflexia, hypoaesthesia, hipotonia, intracranial pressure increased, memory impairment, mental retardation severity unspecified, migraine, paraesthesia, psychomotor hyperactivity, reflexes abnormal, somnolence, status epilepticus, syncope tonic convulsion, transient ischaemic attack, tremor	Cerebellar infarction, cerebrovascular accident, disturbance in attention, drooling, hyperaesthesia, lethargy, syncope, syncope vasovagal, tremor, trigeminal neuralgia, visual field defect
	Psychiatric Disorders	Abnormal behaviour, aggression, attention deficit/hyperactivity disorder, crying, emotional disorder, personality change, personality disorder, restlessness, stress, tic	Aggression, early morning awakening, mood altered, mood swings, stress
	Renal and Urinary Disorders	Bladder spasm, dysuria, glycosuria, haematuria, leukocyturia, nocturia, polyuria, proteinuria	Micturition urgency, proteinuria, renal colic, urinary incontinence
	Reproductive System and Breast Disorders	Bilateral breast buds, breast pain, breast swelling, dysmenorrhoea, epididymal cyst, female genital-digestive tract fistula, menstruation irregular, metrorrhagia, priapism, pruritus genital, testicular retraction, testicular swelling, vaginal erythema, vaginal haemorrhage, vaginal ulceration	Breast pain, breast tenderness, gynaecomastia menorrhagia, menstruation irregular, withdrawal bleed, withdrawal bleeding irregular
	Respiratory, Thoracic and Mediastinal Disorders	Dyspnoea, dyspnoea exertional, hyperventilation, pharyngeal erythema, pharyngeal ulceration, rhinalgia, tonsillar hypertrophy	Asthma, nasal dryness, rhinitis allergic, sinus disorder, sleep apnoea syndrome
	Skin and Subcutaneous Tissue Disorders	Alopecia, angioneurotic oedema, dandruff, dermatitis dermatitis allergic, dermatitis contact, dry skin, hair growth abnormal, hyperhidrosis, hyperkeratosis, keloid scar, lipoatrophy, lipodystrophy acquired, neurodermatitis, periorbital oedema, pigmentation disorder, rash erythematous, rash maculo-papular, rash papular, rash pruritic, scar, seborrhoea, skin discolouration, skin hyperpigmentation, skin hypopigmentation, skin lesion	Acne, alopecia, dermatitis, dermatitis contact, erythema, hypertrichosis, parapsoriasis, petechiae, photosensitivity reaction, rash generalised, rash pruritic, scar, seborrhoeic dermatitis, skin inflammation, skin nodule, sweat gland disorder, urticaria
	Social Circumstances	Family stress	—

(cont'd)

Table 7: SAIZEN *(cont'd)*

List of Adverse Events with a Frequency of Less Than 1% in Clinical Trials Performed with SAIZEN in Registered Indications

Indica-tion	System Organ Class	Preferred Terms	
		Pediatric	Adult
	Surgical and Medical Procedures	Abscess drainage, adenoidectomy, adenotonsillectomy, adhesiolysis, allergenic desensitisation procedure, astrocytoma surgery, brain tumour operation, dental disorder prophylaxis, dental treatment, drug therapy, ear operation, ear tube insertion, explorative laparotomy, eye muscle tenotomy, foot operation, hernia repair, hormone replacement therapy, intra-aortic balloon placement, medical device implantation, mineral supplementation, mole excision, orchidopexy, surgery, testicular operation, urethral operation, urethral repair, wart excision	—
	Vascular Disorders	Flushing, poor peripheral circulation	Hot flush, lymphoedema, orthostatic hypotension
TS, CRF, SGA		No patients experienced AEs on treatment with a frequency of less than 1%.[a]	

[a] CRF, TS, SGA: clinical trials included a subject number inferior or equal to 100 patients.

Missed Dose: For patients who miss a dose, it is not recommended to double the next dose. Administer the regular dose at the next scheduled dosage time.

Administration: SAIZEN 8.8 mg (5.83 mg/mL) click.easy: SAIZEN, once reconstituted, should be administered using the one.click auto-injector or the easypod electromechanical auto-injector. The route of injection, using either device, is subcutaneous.

The calculated dose should be set on the one.click device. Follow the instructions given in Information for the Patient.

Although SAIZEN in the click.easy device is intended for the one.click auto-injector or the easypod electromechanical auto-injector, SAIZEN, once reconstituted, can also be accessed with a conventional syringe for a subcutaneous injection.

SAIZEN 3.33 mg, 5 mg: SAIZEN should be administered using sterile, disposable syringes and needles. The syringe used should be of appropriately small volume to ensure the accurate dose withdrawal. The calculated dose should be withdrawn for either subcutaneous or intramuscular injection.

Paediatric Indications: Growth Failure Due to Inadequate Endogenous Growth Hormone Secretion:

a. Subcutaneous injection: The weekly dose can be divided into 3 single doses (corresponding to 0.067 mg/kg per injection) or into 6 or 7 single daily doses (corresponding to 0.033 or 0.028 mg/kg per injection, respectively). The injection site should be altered to prevent lipoatrophy. For subcutaneous injections, the use of a needle which is 1.25 cm long is recommended.
b. Intramuscular injection: The weekly dose should be divided into 3 single injections (corresponding to 0.0067 mg/kg). For intramuscular injections, the use of a needle which is at least 2.5 cm long is recommended to ensure the injection reaches the intramuscular layer.

Growth Failure in Girls Due to Gonadal Dysgenesis (Turner's Syndrome): The weekly dose can be divided into 3 single doses (corresponding to 0.137-0.161 mg/kg per injection) or into 7 single daily doses (corresponding to 0.045-0.054 mg/kg per injection).

Growth Failure in Children with Chronic Renal Failure: The daily subcutaneous injection consists of a single injection of 0.05 mg/kg body weight. The injection site should be altered to prevent lipoatrophy. A needle 1.25 cm long should be used for subcutaneous injections.

Growth Disturbance in Short Children Born Small for Gestational Age (SGA): For SGA patients, SAIZEN should be administered as a daily subcutaneous injection consisting of a single injection of 0.067 mg/kg body weight. The injection site should be altered to prevent lipoatrophy. A needle 1.25 cm long should be used for subcutaneous injections.

Adult Indication: Adult Growth Hormone Deficiency: At the start of somatropin therapy, a low dose of 0.005 mg/kg/day is recommended, given as a daily subcutaneous injection. The dose should be adjusted stepwise, controlled by Insulin-like Growth Factor 1 (IGF-1) age-adjusted normal values, to 0.01 mg/kg/day if well tolerated. The recommended final GH dose seldom exceeds 1.0 mg/day. In general, the lowest efficacious dose should be administered. In older or overweight patients, lower doses may be necessary.

Reconstitution: See Information for the Patient/Proper use of this Medication for reconstitution instructions.

OVERDOSAGE:

No cases of acute overdosage have been reported. However, exceeding the recommended doses can cause side effects. Overdosage can lead to hypoglycemia followed by hyperglycemia. Long- term overdosage could result in signs and symptoms of gigantism and/or acromegaly consistent with the known effects of excess human growth hormone. If any signs of overdosage occur, treatment should be discontinued.

For management of a suspected drug overdose, CPhA recommends that you contact your **regional Poison Control Centre**. See the *CPS* Directory section for a list of Poison Control Centres.

ACTION AND CLINICAL PHARMACOLOGY: General: Somatropin is a polypeptide hormone consisting of 191 amino acid residues and its structure is identical to that of growth hormone extracted from human pituitary glands. It is produced by recombinant (rDNA) technology in a mammalian cell expression system. Somatropin is also therapeutically equivalent to human growth hormone of pituitary origin.

SAIZEN provides an exogenous supply of human growth hormone for those patients lacking the ability to produce adequate endogenous supplies.

Pharmacology: Linear Growth: Somatropin stimulates linear growth in patients with pituitary growth hormone deficiency, Turner's syndrome and chronic renal failure. Treatment of these patients with SAIZEN results in increased growth rates and IGF-1 levels similar to those seen for children treated with growth hormone of pituitary origin.

Skeletal Growth: The measurable increase in growth (body length) after somatropin treatment results from its effect on cartilaginous growth areas of the long bones. It is known that somatropin's effect is mediated by a sulfation factor, IGF-1, which permits the incorporation of sulfate into cartilage. IGF-1 is present in low concentration in the serum of growth hormone deficient patients and increases during somatropin therapy.

Cell Growth: Somatropin brings about cellular growth as demonstrated by an increase in the muscular, visceral and red cell mass. In muscle tissue, the increase in mass is associated with a corresponding increase in both number and dimension of muscular fibre cells.

Carbohydrate Metabolism: Somatropin has an effect on carbohydrate metabolism. The diabetogenic effect of somatropin is well-known in clinical medicine. Acromegalic patients often suffer from diabetes mellitus while hypopituitary children experience hypoglycemia. In healthy patients, very large doses of somatropin may interfere with glucose tolerance. A simultaneous increase in the plasma insulin level is observed upon somatropin administration.

The diabetogenic activity of somatropin is perhaps due to several concomitant factors:

a. Reduced transport of glucose into peripheral tissues.
b. Increased release of glucose from the liver.
c. Reduced concentration of insulin at the muscular level.
d. Reduced glycolysis from the block of the enzyme triose phosphate dehydrogenase, mediated by non-esterified fatty acids.

Protein Metabolism: Somatropin has an effect on protein metabolism. Somatropin is an anabolic agent that stimulates intracellular transport of amino acids, net retention of nitrogen and protein synthesis which can be quantified by observing the decline in urinary nitrogen excretion and BUN.

Lipid Metabolism: Lipid metabolism is also affected by somatropin. This occurs when intracellular lipolysis is stimulated, thus increasing the plasma concentration of free fatty acids and stimulating the oxidation of fatty acids. In the diabetic patient, somatropin has been shown to accentuate ketogenesis.

Connective Tissue Metabolism: Connective tissue metabolism is affected by somatropin's ability to stimulate the synthesis of chondroitin sulfate and collagen as well as the urinary excretion of hydroxyproline.

Mineral Metabolism: Somatropin affects mineral metabolism by inducing the net retention of phosphorus and potassium and to a lesser degree sodium. Somatropin induces the increased intestinal absorption of calcium and the increased renal tubular reabsorption of phosphorus with increased serum and inorganic phosphate. Increased serum alkaline phosphatase may also be observed during somatropin therapy.

Pharmacokinetics: The pharmacokinetics of SAIZEN are linear at least up to doses of 8 IU (2.67 mg). At higher doses (60 IU/20 mg) some degree of non-linearity cannot be ruled out, however with no clinical relevance.

Following IV administration in healthy volunteers the volume of distribution at steady-state is around 7 L, total metabolic clearance is around 15 L/h while the renal clearance is negligible, and the drug exhibits an elimination half-life of 20 to 35 min.

Following single-dose SC and IM administration of SAIZEN, the apparent terminal half-life is much longer, around 1 to 6 hours (median 2.7 hours). This is due to a rate limiting absorption process.

Maximum serum growth hormone (GH) concentrations following injection are reached after approximately 4 hours (range 2 to 7 hours) and serum GH levels return to baseline within 24 hours, indicating that no accumulation of injected GH will occur during repeated administrations.

The absolute bioavailability of both routes is 70-90 %.

Table 8: SAIZEN

Summary of Somatropin's Pharmaceutical Parameters

	Distribution Steady State	Metabolic Clearance	Terminal Half-life (range)	Time to C_{max}	Bioavailability
Single dose	7 L	15 L/h	4 hours (1 to 6 hours)	4 hours	70-90%

Special Populations and Conditions: SAIZEN is indicated for children with chronic renal failure (see Indications and Clinical Use). No other studies have been conducted with special populations and conditions.

STORAGE AND STABILITY: SAIZEN 3.33 mg/vial, 5 mg/vial: 3.33 mg Vial: Store SAIZEN lyophilized product under refrigeration at 2-8°C.

5 mg Vial: Store SAIZEN lyophilized product at room temperature.

Do not use SAIZEN after the expiry date shown on label.

Reconstitution: The recommended diluents for reconstitution are:

3.33 mg Vial: Sodium Chloride Injection, USP and Bacteriostatic Sodium Chloride Injection, USP.

5 mg Vial: Water for Injection, USP and Bacteriostatic Water for Injection, USP.

Incompatibility: SAIZEN should not be mixed with other drugs.

Preparation of Solution: To prevent possible contamination of the vial, wipe the rubber stopper with an antiseptic solution before puncturing it with the needle.

After determining appropriate patient dose, reconstitute each 5 mg vial of SAIZEN with 1-3 mL of Bacteriostatic Water for Injection, USP (Benzyl Alcohol preserved), each 3.33 mg vial of SAIZEN with up to 5 mL of Bacteriostatic Sodium Chloride Injection, USP (Benzyl Alcohol preserved).

To reconstitute SAIZEN, inject the diluent into the vial of SAIZEN aiming the liquid against the glass vial wall. Swirl the vial with a **gentle** rotary motion until contents are dissolved completely. **Do not shake.** If shaken, the solution will appear opalescent; however, this opalescence does not indicate any decrease in potency. Parenteral drug products should be inspected visually prior to administration. Do not inject if the reconstituted product contains particulate matter or is discoloured. For use in patients sensitive to the diluent see Warnings and Precautions.

Stability of Solution and Storage: SAIZEN 3.33 mg/Vial: When reconstituted with Bacteriostatic Sodium Chloride Injection, USP, the reconstituted solution may be stored at 2-8°C for up to 21 days.

When reconstituted with Sodium Chloride Injection, USP, the reconstituted solution should be administered immediately (within 3 hours). Any unused solution should be discarded.

SAIZEN 5 mg/Vial: When reconstituted with 1 mL to 5 mL Bacteriostatic Water for Injection, USP, the reconstituted solution may be stored at 2-8°C for up to 14 days.

When reconstituted with Water for Injection, USP, the reconstituted solution should be administered immediately (within 3 hours). Any unused solution should be discarded.

SAIZEN 8.8 mg (5.83 mg/mL) click.easy: Store at room temperature (25°C or below) in original package. Do not freeze. Store reconstituted product at 2-8°C in the cartridge for up to 28 days. Keep in a safe place out of the reach of children. Do not use after expiry date.

SPECIAL HANDLING INSTRUCTIONS: SAIZEN solution should not be administered if it contains particles or is not clear.

Any unused product or waste material should be disposed of in accordance with local requirements.

INFORMATION FOR THE PATIENT: Published in e-CPS, available by subscription at www.e-cps.ca.

DOSAGE FORMS, COMPOSITION AND PACKAGING: SAIZEN: 3.33 mg: Each vial of sterile, nonpyrogenic, lyophilized powder contains: somatropin 3.33 mg. Nonmedicinal ingredients: disodium phosphate dihydrate, mannitol and sodium dihydrogen phosphate monohydrate. Cartons of 1 and 10 vials with diluent (5 mL Bacteriostatic Sodium Chloride Injection, USP).

5 mg: Each vial of sterile, nonpyrogenic, lyophilized powder contains: somatropin 5 mg. Nonmedicinal ingredients: phosphoric acid, sodium hydroxide and sucrose. Cartons of 1 and 2 vials with diluent (10 mL Bacteriostatic Water for Injection, USP).

SAIZEN 8.8 mg (5.83 mg/mL) click.easy: Each vial of sterile, nonpyrogenic, lyophilized powder for reconstitution contains: somatropin 8.8 mg. Nonmedicinal ingredients: phosphoric acid, sodium hydroxide and sucrose. 1 vial of SAIZEN product and 1 cartridge of bacteriostatic solvent pre-assembled in 1 reconstitution device (click.easy) comprising of the main body, the cap assembly and the sterile transfer cannula. 5 vials of SAIZEN product and 5 cartridges of bacteriostatic solvent pre-assembled in 5 reconstitution devices (click.easy) comprising each of the main body, the cap assembly and sterile transfer cannula. The DIN 2R 3 mL vials of SAIZEN and the cartridges of the solvent are of neutral glass (Type I). There is no latex in the components of the vial, cartridge or reconstitution device.

Salagen® Ⓟ
pilocarpine HCl
Cholinomimetic Agent

Pfizer

PHARMACOLOGY: Pilocarpine tablets are made from the naturally occurring alkaloid pilocarpine which is obtained from the leaflets of the South American shrub Pilocarpus jaborandi. Pilocarpine is a cholinomimetic (cholinergic parasympathomimetic) agent capable of exerting a broad spectrum of pharmacologic effects with predominant muscarinic action. Dependent upon the dosage and the individual, oral pilocarpine will increase secretion by the exocrine glands (e.g., sweat, salivary, lacrimal, gastric, pancreatic, intestinal and respiratory mucous cells) and stimulate smooth muscle (e.g., gastrointestinal tract, bronchi, ureters, urinary bladder, gallbladder and biliary tract). Pilocarpine may also produce arrhythmias and/or paradoxical effects on the cardiovascular system manifest by hypertension after a brief episode of hypotension.

The bioavailability of oral multiple-dose pilocarpine tablets has been determined in 19 healthy male volunteers. Pilocarpine tablets 5 mg and 10 mg were administered orally for 2 days, at 8 a.m., noon, and 6 p.m. for a total of 6 doses. The results are presented in Table 1.

Table 1: Salagen

Bioavailability Parameters Following Multiple-Dose Oral Pilocarpine Tablets[a]

Dose	T_{max} (h)	C_{max} (ng/mL)	AUC[b] h(ng/mL)	$t_{1/2}$ (h)
5 mg (n=10)	1.25	14.61	33.04	0.76
10 mg (n=9)	0.85	41.35	107.96	1.35

[a] Pilocarpine tablets given orally, 3 times daily, for 2 days; the results determined after the final dose.
[b] Trapezoidal values.

Pharmacokinetics: Special Populations: Geriatrics: Pharmacokinetics in elderly male volunteers (n=11) were comparable to those in younger men. In 5 healthy elderly female volunteers, the mean C_{max} and AUC were approximately twice that of elderly males and young normal male volunteers.

Hepatic Impairment: In (n=12) cirrhotic subjects with mild to moderate hepatic impairment (Child-Pugh Grades A, mild (n=9) & B, moderate (n=3)), administration of a single 5 mg oral dose resulted in decreased apparent plasma clearance. Relative to normal volunteers, subjects with mild and moderate hepatic impairment had 1.4- and 3.3-fold lower apparent plasma clearance, respectively. Compared to normal subjects, C_{max} values were 20-40% higher in subjects with mild and moderate hepatic impairment. AUC values were 1.4- and 3.3-fold higher in subjects with mild and moderate impairment, respectively. The plasma elimination half-life of pilocarpine was increased by 30% in subjects with mild hepatic impairment but was at least 2-fold higher in subjects with moderate impairment. Moderate hepatic impairment produced markedly different pharmacokinetic profiles and AUC was positively correlated (r^2 = 0.669) with Child-Pugh score. Thus, in patients with mild and moderate hepatic impairment, treatment initiation should employ a reduced daily dosage. No pharmacokinetic data are available for any dose of pilocarpine in patients with severe hepatic impairment (Child-Pugh Grade C; see Precautions and Dosage).

Renal Impairment: There is no reliable data for the pharmacokinetics of orally administered pilocarpine in patients with renal disease (see Precautions and Dosage).

Absorption and Distribution: When taken with a high fat meal by 12 healthy male volunteers, there was a decrease in the rate of absorption of pilocarpine from pilocarpine tablets. Mean T_{max}'s were 1.47 and 0.87 hours, and mean C_{max}'s were 51.8 and 59.2 ng/mL for fed and fasted, respectively.

The results of an in vitro protein binding study indicate ^{3}H-pilocarpine HCl is not bound to plasma proteins as determined in either rat or human plasma.

Biotransformation and Elimination: Limited information is available about the metabolism and elimination of pilocarpine in humans. Inactivation of pilocarpine is thought to occur at neuronal synapses and probably in plasma. Pilocarpine and its minimally-active or inactive degradation products, which include pilocarpic acid, are excreted in the urine.

INDICATIONS: For the treatment of the symptoms of xerostomia (dry mouth) due to salivary gland hypofunction caused by radiotherapy for cancer of the head and neck.

For the treatment of the symptoms of xerostomia (dry mouth) and xerophthalmia (dry eyes) in patients with Sjögren's syndrome.

CONTRAINDICATIONS: In patients with uncontrolled asthma; when miosis is undesirable (e.g., acute iritis and in narrow-angle [angle closure] glaucoma); in patients with known sensitivity to pilocarpine, or to any of the tablet's excipients.

WARNINGS: Cardiovascular Disease: Patients with significant cardiovascular disease may be unable to compensate for transient changes in hemodynamics or rhythm induced by pilocarpine. Pulmonary edema has been reported as a complication of pilocarpine toxicity. Pilocarpine tablets should be administered with caution and under close medical supervision to patients with significant cardiovascular disease.

Pulmonary Disease: Pilocarpine has been reported to increase airway resistance, bronchial smooth muscle tone, and bronchial secretions. Pilocarpine tablets should be administered with caution and under close medical supervision to patients with significant pulmonary disease (e.g., controlled asthma, chronic bronchitis, or chronic obstructive pulmonary disease).

Should any adverse changes in the patient's cardiopulmonary condition occur, or be suspected, therapy with pilocarpine tablets should be discontinued immediately.

PRECAUTIONS: General: Pilocarpine toxicity is characterized by an exaggeration of its parasympathomimetic effects.

The dose-related cardiovascular pharmacologic effects of pilocarpine include hypotension, hypertension, bradycardia, and tachycardia (see also Warnings).

Occupational Hazards: Ocular administration of pilocarpine has been reported to cause visual blurring and impairment of depth perception which may result in decreased visual acuity, especially at night and in patients with central lens changes. Patients should be cautioned about driving at night or performing hazardous activities in reduced lighting while receiving therapy with pilocarpine tablets.

Special Diseases and Conditions: Gastrointestinal Disease: Pilocarpine tablets should be administered with caution to patients with known or suspected cholelithiasis or biliary tract disease. Contractions of the gallbladder and biliary smooth muscle could precipitate complications including cholecystitis, cholangitis, and biliary obstruction.

Cholinergic agonists, like pilocarpine, may cause increased acid secretion. This possibility should be considered when treating patients with active peptic ulcer disease.

Renal Disease: Pilocarpine may increase ureteral smooth muscle tone and could theoretically precipitate renal colic or "ureteral reflux" in patients with renal dysfunction (eg. nephrolithiasis).

There is no reliable data for the pharmacokinetics of orally administered pilocarpine in patients with renal disease. Thus, caution should be observed if pilocarpine is to be administered to patients with renal disease (see Dosage).

Hepatic Impairment: Decreased pilocarpine plasma clearance was observed in patients with mild to moderate hepatic impairment (see Pharmacology). Patients with mild and moderate hepatic impairment should begin treatment at a reduced daily dose, gradually increasing the dosage up to 5 mg three to four times daily as safety and tolerability allow. (See Dosage.) No pharmacokinetic data are available for any dose of pilocarpine in patients with severe hepatic impairment (Childs-Pugh Grade C). Therefore, pilocarpine is not recommended for use in patients with severe hepatic impairment. However, should clinical judgement deem it necessary, the drug should be used with extreme caution (see Dosage).

CNS Disorders: Cholinergic agonists, like pilocarpine HCl, may have dose-related central nervous system effects. This should be considered when treating patients with underlying cognitive or psychiatric disturbances.

Drug Interactions: Pilocarpine tablets should be administered with caution to patients taking beta-adrenergic antagonists because of the possibility of conduction disturbances. Drugs with parasympathomimetic effects administered concurrently with pilocarpine tablets would be expected to result in additive pharmacologic effects. Pilocarpine tablets might antagonize the anticholinergic effects of drugs used concomitantly. These effects should be considered when anticholinergic properties may be contributing to the therapeutic effect of concomitant medication (e.g., atropine, inhaled ipratropium).

While no formal drug interaction studies have been performed, the following concomitant drugs were used in at least 10% of patients in either or both Sjögren's pivotal studies: acetaminophen, ASA, artificial tears, calcium, conjugated estrogens, hydroxychloroquine sulfate, ibuprofen, levothyroxine sodium, medroxyprogesterone acetate, methotrexate, multivitamins, naproxen, omeprazole and prednisone. There were no reports of drug toxicities during either trial.

Children: Safety and effectiveness of pilocarpine tablets have not been studied in children under 18 years of age.

Impairment of Fertility: The data obtained from a study in rats suggest that pilocarpine may impair the fertility of male and female humans. Therefore, pilocarpine tablets should be administered to individuals who are attempting to conceive a child only if the potential benefit justifies potential impairment of fertility.

Pregnancy: The safety of pilocarpine tablets has not been established in human pregnancy. Therefore, pilocarpine tablets should only be used during pregnancy if the potential benefit to the mother justifies the potential risk to the fetus.

Lactation: It is not presently known whether this drug is excreted in human milk. Because many drugs are excreted in human milk and because of the potential for serious adverse reactions in nursing infants from pilocarpine tablets, a decision should be made whether to discontinue nursing or to discontinue the drug.

Dependence Liability: Pilocarpine does not have the potential for addiction; consequently, there have been no reports of addiction with the use of pilocarpine. There are no known withdrawal effects associated with pilocarpine either in animals or in humans. The pharmacologic effects, other than salivation, are not pleasurable, thus, there is no reason to suspect it will be abused.

ADVERSE EFFECTS: Head and Neck Cancer Patients: In the controlled clinical studies, 217 patients of whom 147 (68%) were male and 70 (32%) were female were administered pilocarpine tablets. The mean age of the patients was approximately 58 years; the majority of patients were between 50 and 64 years (51%), 33% were 65 years and older, and 16% were younger than 50 years.

No serious drug-related adverse events were reported with use of pilocarpine tablets in these controlled clinical trials.

Table 2 presents the adverse events observed during treatment with pilocarpine tablets which were considered to be a consequence of the expected pharmacologic effects of pilocarpine. These adverse events were dose-dependent and generally of mild or moderate intensity. Such adverse events usually subside within 6 hours of discontinuation of therapy.

Table 2: Salagen

The Most Frequent Adverse Events, by Dose, Associated with Salagen Tablets (% of Patients Reporting)

Adverse Event	Placebo t.i.d. (n=152) %	5 mg t.i.d. (15 mg/day) (n=141) %	10 mg t.i.d. (30 mg/day) (n=121) %
Sweating	9	29	68
Nausea	4	6	15
Rhinitis	7	5	14
Chills	<1	3	14
Vasodilatation (Flushing)	3	8	13
Urinary Frequency	7	9	12
Dizziness	4	5	12
Asthenia	3	6	12

Table 3 presents additional adverse events (incidence ≥ 3%) reported at dosages of 15 to 30 mg/day in the controlled clinical trials.

Table 3: Salagen

Adverse Events (Incidence ≥3%) Reported at Dosages of 15-30 mg/day Salagen Tablets (% of Patients Reporting)

Adverse Event	Placebo t.i.d. (n=152) %	5–10 mg t.i.d. (15–30 mg/day) (n=217) %
Headache	8	13
Dyspepsia	5	7
Lacrimation	8	6
Diarrhea	5	6
Edema	4	5
Abdominal Pain	4	4
Amblyopia	2	4
Vomiting	1	4
Pharyngitis	8	3
Hypertension	1	3

The following events were reported by head and neck cancer patients at incidences of 1 to 2% at dosages of 15 to 30 mg/day:
Cardiovascular: tachycardia.
Digestive: dysphagia, taste perversion.
Musculoskeletal: myalgias.
Nervous: tremor.
Respiratory: epistaxis, sinusitis, voice alteration.
Skin: pruritus, rash.
Special Senses: abnormal vision, conjunctivitis.

In long-term treatment were 2 patients with underlying cardiovascular disease of whom 1 experienced a myocardial infarct and another an episode of syncope. The association with drug is uncertain.

Sjögren's Syndrome Patients: In the controlled clinical studies, 376 patients of whom 19 (5%) were male and 357 (95%) were female were administered pilocarpine tablets. The mean age of the patients was approximately 55 years; the majority of patients were between 40 and 69 years (70%), 16% were 70 years and older, and 14% were younger than 40 years of age.

No serious drug-related adverse events were reported with use of pilocarpine tablets in these controlled clinical trials.

Table 4 presents the adverse events observed during treatment with pilocarpine tablets which were considered to be a consequence of the expected pharmacologic effects of pilocarpine. These adverse events were dose-dependent and generally of mild or moderate intensity.

Table 5 presents additional adverse events (incidence ≥3%) reported at dosages of 10 to 30 mg/day in the controlled clinical trials.

The following events were reported by Sjögren's patients at incidences of 1 to 2% at dosages of 10 to 30 mg/day:
Body as a Whole: accidental injury, allergic reaction, fever, abnormal lab test.
Cardiovascular: palpitation, tachycardia.
Digestive: constipation, flatulence, glossitis, stomatitis.
Metabolic and Nutritional: edema, face edema.
Musculoskeletal: back pain, myalgia.
Nervous: somnolence.
Respiratory: cough increased, epistaxis.
Skin: pruritus.
Special Senses: blurred vision, tinnitus.
Urogenital: urinary incontinence, urinary tract infection, vaginitis.

OVERDOSE:

Symptoms: Toxicity from pilocarpine is characterized chiefly by exaggeration of parasympathomimetic effects and resembles "muscarinic poisoning" (e.g., consumption of mushrooms of the genus Inocybe). Dose-dependent symptoms include salivation, sweating, vomiting, respiratory distress, hypotension, diarrhea, nausea and shock. Mental confusion and cardiac arrhythmias can also occur.

A fatal overdose with oral administration of ocular pilocarpine, resulting from poisoning, has been reported in the literature. The symptoms included: salivation, pinpoint pupils, sweating, dyspnea, tachypnea, tachycardia, and pulmonary edema.

There are several reports of pilocarpine overdosage reported with the treatment of angle-closure glaucoma. Cardiovascular decompensation has been noted in patients with acute closed-angle glaucoma who have received intraocular instillation of pilocarpine in excess of 60 to 100 mg over short periods prior to eye surgery. Other reported symptoms occurring in this situation include nausea, vomiting, profuse sweating, tremor, hypotension, sinus bradycardia, AV block, changes in mental state, and shock.

Table 4: Salagen

Most Frequent Adverse Events, by Dose, Associated with Salagen Tablets (% of Patients Reporting)

Adverse Event	Placebo q.i.d. (n=253) %	2.5 mg q.i.d. (10 mg/day) (n=121) %	5 mg q.i.d. (20 mg/day) (n=255) %	5–7.5 mg q.i.d. (20–30 mg/day) (n=114) %
Sweating	7	11	40	47
Urinary Frequency	4	11	10	6
Chills	2	1	4	6
Vasodilatation (Flushing)	2	2	9	3
Increased Salivation	0	0	3	4

Table 5: Salagen

Adverse Events (Incidence ≥3%) Reported at Dosages of 10-30 mg/day Salagen Tablets (% of Patients Reporting)

Adverse Event	Placebo q.i.d. (n=253) %	2.5–7.5 mg q.i.d. (10–30 mg/day) (n=376) %
Headache	19	18
Flu Syndrome	9	12
Nausea	9	12
Dyspepsia	7	8
Rhinitis	8	8
Diarrhea	7	7
Dizziness	7	6
Pain	2	4
Abdominal Pain	4	5
Pharyngitis	5	4
Sinusitis	5	4
Vomiting	3	1
Asthenia	2	4
Rash	3	3
Infection	6	3

Treatment: Overdosage with pilocarpine should be treated with atropine titration (0.5 to 1 mg given s.c. or i.v.) and supportive measures to maintain respiration and circulation. Epinephrine (0.3 to 1 mg, s.c. or i.m.) may also be of value in the presence of severe cardiovascular depression or bronchoconstriction. It is not known if pilocarpine is dialyzable.

For management of a suspected drug overdose, CPhA recommends that you contact your **regional Poison Control Centre**. See the *CPS* Directory section for a list of Poison Control Centres.

DOSAGE: The usual dose for initiation of treatment is 5 mg 3 or 4 times daily. Titration up to 10 mg (2 tablets)/dose, not to exceed a total of 30 mg (6 tablets)/day, may be considered for patients who have not responded adequately and who can tolerate the lower doses. The lowest dose that is tolerated and effective should be used for maintenance.

Treatment should begin at the first signs of xerostomia. Clinical experience indicates that the relief of xerostomia and/or xerophthalmia improves over time with the administration of pilocarpine tablets. Administration at the above recommended dosage, for 12 or more weeks may be required before relief can be expected. Onset and degree of relief may vary among patients.

Hepatic impairment: Patients with mild and moderate hepatic impairment should begin treatment at a reduced daily dosage, gradually increasing the dosage up to 5 mg three to four times daily as safety and tolerability allow. No pharmacokinetic data are available for any dose of pilocarpine in patients with severe hepatic impairment (Child-Pugh Grade C). Therefore, pilocarpine is not recommended for use in patients with severe hepatic impairment. However, should clinical judgment deem it necessary, the drug should be used with extreme caution (see Precautions and Pharmacology).

Renal Impairment: There is no reliable data for the pharmacokinetics of orally administered pilocarpine in patients with renal disease. Thus, caution should be observed if pilocarpine is to be administered to patients with renal disease (see Precautions).

INFORMATION FOR THE PATIENT: Published in e-CPS, available by subscription at www.e-cps.ca.

SUPPLIED: Each white, round, biconvex, film-coated unscored tablet, printed with "SAL" on one side and "5" on the other side, contains: pilocarpine HCl 5 mg. Nonmedicinal ingredients: microcrystalline cellulose and stearic acid; coating: hydroxypropyl methylcellulose, polyethylene glycol, polysorbate 80 and titanium dioxide; ink: ethanol, ethylene glycol monoethyl ether, lecithin, methyl alcohol, N-butyl alcohol, propylene glycol, shellac and synthetic black iron oxide. Polish: carnauba wax. Bottles of 100. Store at room temperature (15 to 30°C).

(Shown in Product Identification Section)

Salazopyrin®

sulfasalazine

Anti-inflammatory

Pfizer

Salazopyrin EN-tabs®

sulfasalazine

Anti-inflammatory

Pfizer

Date of Revision: July 6, 2009

PHARMACOLOGY: About 20% of sulfasalazine is absorbed in the small intestine after oral administration. A small percentage of the absorbed sulfasalazine is excreted in the urine and the rest via the bile into the small intestine (enterohepatic circulation). This portion together with the unabsorbed sulfasalazine enters the colon where it is split by bacteria into two main metabolites, sulfapyridine and 5-aminosalicylic acid (5-ASA). The peak serum concentration is reached after 3 to 5 hours. The mean serum half-life after a single dose is about 6 hours; after repeated doses it is about 8 hours. After intake of SALAZOPYRIN EN-tabs (sulfasalazine delayed-release tablets), sulfasalazine has been detected in serum somewhat later than after intake of plain tablets, as expected, the peak serum concentration being observed between 3 and 12 hours.

Sulfapyridine is absorbed, partially acetylated and/or hydroxylated in the liver and/or conjugated with glucuronic acid. In patients who are slow acetylators, the serum concentration of free sulfapyridine is higher than in fast acetylators. The major part is excreted in the urine. Nonacetylated sulfapyridine is bound to serum proteins and reaches a maximum serum concentration after 12 hours. Sulfapyridine has a tendency towards accumulation. It does not disappear completely from the serum until 3 days after withdrawal of the drug.

The total urinary recovery of sulfasalazine and its sulfapyridine metabolites in healthy subjects during 3 days after the administration of a single 2 g dose of sulfasalazine averaged 91%.

The absorbed **5-aminosalicylic acid** is partly excreted in the urine, mainly as acetyl-5-aminosalicylic acid. A larger portion of 5-aminosalicylic acid is excreted in the feces.

The mode of action of sulfasalazine is unclear, suggested as being: anti-inflammatory, immunosuppressive and bacteriostatic.

In clinical cases of inflammatory bowel disease (IBD), the anti-inflammatory effects seem to relieve the acute symptoms of diarrhea, gut inflammation, mucosal edema and bleeding. The long-term protection afforded by therapy with sulfasalazine may be due to immunosuppressive properties of the drug.

Anti-inflammatory Effects: Sulfasalazine inhibits superoxide production by granulocytes stimulated with immune complexes or formyl peptides. In addition 5-ASA is a powerful scavenger of oxygen free radicals. Other granulocyte functions inhibited by sulfasalazine include degranulation, chemotaxis and random migration. These inhibitory effects on inflammatory cell functions may contribute to the beneficial clinical activity of sulfasalazine.

Sulfasalazine is a relatively weak inhibitor of the cyclo-oxygenase enzyme, but a potent inhibitor of 15-prostaglandin dehydrogenase (PGDH), the main metabolic pathway for the prostaglandins.

On the lipoxygenase side of the arachidonic acid cascade, sulfasalazine has been shown to exert an inhibitory effect on several enzymes including 5-LO and LTC_4 synthetase. In line with this effect, sulfasalazine has been shown to inhibit the release of lipoxygenase product from inflammatory cells and tissue.

Taken together, these effects of sulfasalazine on arachidonic acid metabolizing enzymes would lead to a decrease in pro-inflammatory lipoxygenase products with a simultaneous increase in immunosuppressive, anti-inflammatory prostaglandins, which may have a bearing on the clinical activity.

Effects on Immunological Functions: Since the disorders in which sulfasalazine has clinical activity are considered to be of autoimmune nature, the effect of sulfasalazine on immune competent cells is of interest. Both natural killer cell activity and T-cell proliferation are inhibited by sulfasalazine in in vitro systems.

Antibacterial Effects: In vitro studies have shown that both sulfasalazine and its main metabolites inhibit bacterial growth. A reduction in several bacterial species of the gut flora has also been observed after clinical treatment with sulfasalazine.

Pharmacokinetics: Patients with Rheumatoid Arthritis: The pharmacokinetics of sulfasalazine and its metabolites after a 2 g single oral dose were compared in patients with rheumatoid arthritis and patients with ulcerative colitis. The study showed a large individual variability, which is also found in studies in healthy volunteers, but no difference between the two patient groups was observed, except for a significantly higher peak concentration of sulfapyridine in rheumatoid arthritis patients. The area under the plasma concentration curve (AUC) for sulfapyridine was also increased, but the difference was not significant.

Bioavailability in Elderly Patients with Rheumatoid Arthritis: The pharmacokinetics of sulfasalazine and its metabolites were compared in young (mean age 40.5 years) and elderly (mean age 74.4 years) rheumatoid arthritis patients after a single oral (2 g) dose taken fasting and at steady state. The only difference found between the two age groups was a prolonged half-life ($t_{½}$) in the elderly, but no significant difference in either the plasma concentration at steady state and the renal clearance. For sulfapyridine both T_{max} and volume of distribution were significantly increased in the elderly after the single doses, but this difference with age disappeared at chronic dosing. The data indicates that there is no major age dependent difference in the pharmacokinetics of sulfasalazine. However, the effect of acetylation phenotype is much more important.

INDICATIONS: Adjunctive therapy in the treatment of severe ulcerative colitis, proctitis or distal ulcerative colitis and Crohn's disease. It is especially useful for chronic administration.

The EN-tabs are indicated for the treatment of active rheumatoid arthritis, when treatment with an adequate conventional first line therapy has failed.

CONTRAINDICATIONS: In patients with hypersensitivity to sulfasalazine, its metabolites, or any other component of the product, sulfonamides, or salicylates.

In infants under 2 years of age.

In patients with intestinal and urinary obstructions.

In patients with porphyria, as these drugs have been reported to precipitate an acute attack.

In patients in whom acute asthmatic attacks, urticaria, rhinitis or other allergic manifestations are precipitated by ASA or other nonsteroidal anti-inflammatory agents. Fatal anaphylactic reactions have occurred in such individuals.

WARNINGS: Complete blood counts (including differential white cell count), liver function test, and assessment of renal function (including urinalysis) should be performed in all patients before starting therapy with sulfasalazine, and frequently during the first 3 months of therapy. Thereafter, monitoring should be performed as clinically indicated (see Precautions, Laboratory Tests).

Sulfasalazine should be used only after critical appraisal of the risk to benefit in patients with hepatic or renal damage, blood dyscrasias, severe allergy or bronchial asthma. Pancreatitis has been observed in some susceptible individuals.

Deaths associated with the administration of sulfasalazine have been reported from hypersensitivity reactions, agranulocytosis, aplastic anemia, other blood dyscrasias, renal and liver damage, irreversible neuromuscular and CNS changes and fibrosing alveolitis. The presence of clinical signs such as sore throat, fever, pallor, purpura, or jaundice during sulfasalazine treatment may indicate myelosuppression, hemolysis, or hepatotoxicity. Discontinue treatment with sulfasalazine while awaiting the results of blood tests.

Oligospermia with infertility have been observed in men treated with sulfasalazine. Withdrawal of the drug appears to reverse these effects within 2 to 3 months.

Patients, especially those with glucose-6-phosphate dehydrogenase deficiency, should be observed closely for signs of hemolytic anemia. This reaction is frequently dose related. If toxic or hypersensitivity reactions occur, the drug should be discontinued immediately.

PRECAUTIONS: Patients hypersensitive to furosemide, thiazide diuretics, carbonic anhydrase inhibitors, may also be hypersensitive to this medication.

Sulfasalazine should be administered under medical supervision. Sulfasalazine shares the potential toxic effects of other sulfonamides, especially sulfapyridine and the usual precautions of sulfonamide therapy should be observed.

Bone marrow depression (most often expressed as leukopenia) has been reported, usually within the first 3 months of starting treatment. In the majority of patients this has been reversible upon stopping the drug. A full blood count, including differential white blood cell count, should be carried out before starting treatment and monitored closely during the first 3 months of treatment.

Afterwards, patients should be screened if their condition changes or if they present with any symptoms of infection. A falling trend in the blood count is a better indicator than a single value.

Red cell and platelet counts should be carried out before and periodically during therapy.

Sulfasalazine should be used with caution in patients with reduced kidney or liver function. Liver function tests and urinalysis should be carried out before and periodically during therapy (see Warnings).

When concurrent therapy with other drugs is administered, as in rheumatoid arthritis, the recommended frequency of monitoring is as follows: initially, every second week during first 3 months after onset of treatment, every 6 months thereafter.

Sulfasalazine may produce an orange-yellow color of the urine. Similar discoloration of the skin and yellow staining of soft contact lenses have occasionally been reported.

Isolated instances have been reported when the EN-tabs have passed undisintegrated through the digestive tract. This may be due, in part, to a lack of intestinal esterase in these patients. If this is observed, the administration of EN-tabs should be discontinued.

Adequate fluid intake must be maintained in order to prevent crystalluria and kidney stone formation.

Children: Use in children with systemic onset juvenile rheumatoid arthritis may result in a serum sickness-like reaction; therefore, sulfasalazine is not recommended in these patients.

Pregnancy: Pregnancy and Reproduction: Teratogenic Effects: Reproduction studies have been performed in rats and rabbits at doses up to 6 times the human dose and have revealed no evidence of impaired female fertility or harm to the fetus due to sulfasalazine.

The outcome of pregnancy in a group of pregnant women with intestinal bowel disease (IBD) treated with sulfasalazine alone or sulfasalazine and concomitant steroid therapy was compared with untreated IBD pregnancies. The incidence of fetal morbidity and mortality was comparable between the groups and to the expected outcome in the general population.

Oral sulfasalazine inhibits the absorption and metabolism of folic acid and may cause folic acid deficiency.

Because the possibility of harm cannot be completely ruled out, sulfasalazine should be used during pregnancy only if clearly needed.

Nonteratogenic Effects: Sulfasalazine and sulfapyridine pass the placental barrier. Although sulfapyridine has been shown to have a poor bilirubin displacing capacity, the potential for kernicterus in newborns should be kept in mind.

A case of agranulocytosis has been reported in an infant whose mother was taking both sulfasalazine and prednisone throughout pregnancy.

Lactation: Caution should be exercised when sulfasalazine is administered to a nursing woman, since it is excreted in the milk. The concentration of sulfapyridine in milk is about 30 to 60% of that in serum. However, since sulfapyridine has a poor bilirubin displacing capacity, the risk for kernicterus in healthy suckling children may be low with therapeutic doses. Sulfasalazine and sulfapyridine are found in low levels in breast milk. Caution should be used, particularly if breastfeeding premature infants or those deficient in glucose-6-phosphate dehydrogenase (G6PD).

Drug Interactions: The following drug interactions and/or related problems have been selected on the basis of their potential clinical significance (possible mechanism in parentheses where appropriate):

Note: Combinations containing any of the following medications, depending on the amount present, may also interact with this medication.

Antibiotics, or

Anticoagulants, coumarin or indandione derivatives, or

Anticonvulsants, hydantoin, or

Antidiabetic agents, oral, or

Digitalis glycosides or folic acid, (sulfasalazine may inhibit absorption and lower the serum concentrations of these medications; folic acid requirements may be increased in patients receiving sulfasalazine); (patients taking digitalis glycosides should be monitored closely for evidence of altered digitalis effect. Reduced absorption of digoxin resulting in non-therapeutic serum levels, has been reported in patients taking digoxin concomitantly with oral sulfasalazine).

Methenamine (in acid urine methenamine breaks down into formaldehyde which may form an insoluble precipitate with certain sulfonamides and may also increase the danger of crystalluria; concomitant use is not recommended).

Methotrexate (may be displaced from protein binding sites and/or metabolism may be inhibited by sulfonamides, resulting in increased or prolonged effects and/or toxicity; dosage adjustments may be necessary during and after sulfonamide therapy; co-administration of oral sulfasalazine and methotrexate to rheumatoid arthritis patients did not alter the pharmacokinetic disposition of the drugs; however, an increased incidence of gastrointestinal adverse events, especially nausea, was reported).

Oxyphenbutazone or phenylbutazone (effects may be potentiated when used concomitantly with sulfonamides because of displacement from plasma protein binding sites).

Photosensitizing medications, other (caution in concomitant use of sulfasalazine with these medications is recommended because of possible additive photosensitizing effects).

Probenecid (decreases renal tubular secretion of sulfonamides when used concomitantly, resulting in increased and more prolonged sulfonamide concentrations and/or toxicity; sulfonamide dosage adjustments may be necessary during and after probenecid therapy and sulfonamide serum determinations may be useful in prolonged probenecid therapy).

Sulfinpyrazone (concomitant use may displace sulfonamides from protein binding sites and may decrease renal excretion, resulting in increased sulfonamide concentrations and/or toxicity; sulfonamide dosage adjustments may be necessary during and after sulfinpyrazone therapy).

Thiopurine methyltransferase (TPMT) (Due to inhibition of thiopurine methyltransferase (TPMT) by sulfasalazine, bone marrow suppression and leukopenia have been reported when thiopurine 6-mercaptopurine or its prodrug, azathioprine, and oral sulfasalazine were used concomitantly).

Medical Problems: Use of this medication should be carefully considered when the following medical problems exist: blood dyscrasias, G6PD deficiency, hepatic function impairment, intestinal and urinary tract obstruction, porphyria or renal function impairment.

Laboratory Tests: The following may be especially important in patient monitoring (other tests may be warranted in some patients, depending on their condition): Complete blood count, including differential white blood cell count, liver function test, and assessment of renal function (including urinalysis) should be performed in all patients before starting therapy with sulfasalazine, and frequently during the first 3 months of therapy. Thereafter, monitoring should be performed as clinically indicated or if patients present with any symptom of infection. A falling trend in the blood count is a better indicator than a single value (see Warnings).

Proctoscopy and sigmoidoscopy may be required periodically during treatment to determine patient response and dosage adjustments.

ADVERSE EFFECTS: Adverse reactions with sulfasalazine may be more frequent and more severe in patients who are slow acetylators.

Most side effects are dose dependent, and the symptoms can be alleviated by reducing the dosage. Increased incidences of adverse reactions are seen with the daily dosage of 4 g or more, or total serum sulfapyridine levels above 50 µg/mL. Hypersensitivity reactions have been noted, in which a dose reduction is irrelevant.

It has been shown that the frequency and severity of the rather common dyspeptic manifestations experienced by patients with gastric intolerance to sulfasalazine tablets are markedly reduced when using EN-tabs.

The most commonly reported adverse reactions are: nausea, vomiting, gastric distress, methemoglobinemia, anorexia, headache and apparently reversible oligospermia. These occur in about one-third of patients. Less frequent adverse reactions are skin rash, erythema, pruritus, urticaria, fever, Heinz-body anemia, hemolytic anemia, leukopenia, megaloblastic (macrocytic) anemia, and cyanosis, which may occur in a frequency of 1 in every 30 patients or less.

Although the listing which follows includes a few adverse reactions which have not been reported with this specific drug, the pharmacological similarities among the sulfonamides require that each of these reactions be considered when sulfasalazine is administered.

Other adverse reactions which occur rarely, in approximately 1 in 1000 patients or less are:

Blood Dyscrasias: aplastic anemia, agranulocytosis, purpura, thrombocytopenia and hypoprothrombinemia, pancytopenia, macrocytosis, congenital neutropenia, and myelodysplastic syndrome.

Hypersensitivity: erythema multiforme (Stevens-Johnson syndrome), exfoliative dermatitis, epidermal necrolysis (Lyell's syndrome) with corneal damage, anaphylaxis, serum sickness syndrome, pneumonitis with or without eosinophilia, vasculitis, fibrosing alveolitis, pleuritis, pericarditis with or without tamponade, allergic myocarditis, polyarteritis nodosa, hepatitis and hepatic necrosis with or without immune complexes, parapsoriasis varioliformis acuta (Mucha Habermann syndrome), rhabdomyolysis, photosensitization, arthralgia, periorbital edema, conjunctival and scleral injection, alopecia and induction of autoantibodies.

Skin: facial edema, exanthema, lichens planus, toxic pustuloderma, drug rash with eosinophilia and systemic symptoms (DRESS).

Gastrointestinal: hepatitis, pancreatitis, bloody diarrhea, impaired folic acid absorption, impaired digoxin absorption, stomatitis, mouth ulceration, diarrhea, abdominal pain, aggravation of ulcerative colitis, pseudomembranous colitis, and neutropenic enterocolitis.

Respiratory: cough, dyspnea, interstitial lung disease (some with fatal outcome).

Central Nervous System: transverse myelitis, convulsions, transient lesions of the posterior spinal column, cauda equina syndrome, Guillain-Barré syndrome, peripheral neuropathy, encephalopathy, mental depression, vertigo, hearing loss, insomnia, ataxia, hallucinations, tinnitus and drowsiness. Three cases of aseptic meningitis have been reported during the use of delayed-release sulfasalazine in the treatment of rheumatic diseases.

Nervous System: smell and taste disorders.

Hepatic: elevation of liver enzymes, hepatic failure, hepatitis fulminant, sometimes leading to liver transplantation, jaundice, cholestatic jaundice, cirrhosis, and possible hepatocellular damage including liver necrosis and liver failure.

Renal: toxic nephrosis with oliguria and anuria, nephrotic syndrome, hematuria, crystalluria proteinuria, interstitial nephritis, and hemolytic-uretic syndrome.

Musculoskeletal/Connective Tissue: Sjögren's syndrome, systemic lupus erythematosis.

Other: urine discoloration and skin discoloration. The sulfonamides bear certain chemical similarities to some goitrogens, diuretics, acetazolamide and the thiazides, and oral hypoglycemic agents. Goiter production, diuresis, and hypoglycemia have occurred rarely in patients receiving sulfonamides. Cross-sensitivity may exist with these agents. Rats appear to be especially susceptible to the goitrogenic effects of sulfonamides and long-term administration has produced thyroid malignancies in this species.

OVERDOSE:

Symptoms: Similar to those of any sulfonamide, the most likely symptoms would be gastrointestinal disturbances (nausea and vomiting), drowsiness, convulsions, hematuria, crystalluria or anuria. Patients with impaired renal function are at increased risk of serious toxicity. Patients should be observed for development of methemoglobinemia or sulfahemoglobinemia. If these occur, treat appropriately. Serum sulfapyridine concentrations may be used to monitor progress of recovery from overdosage.

Treatment: Gastric lavage or emesis plus catharsis as indicated. Alkalinize urine. If kidney function is normal, force fluids. If anuria is present, restrict fluids and salt, and treat appropriately. Catheterization of the ureters may be indicated for complete renal blockage by crystals. The low molecular weight of sulfasalazine and its metabolites may facilitate their removal by dialysis. For agranulocytosis, discontinue the drug immediately, hospitalize the patient and institute appropriate therapy.

For hypersensitivity reactions, discontinue treatment immediately. Such reactions may be controlled with antihistamines and, if necessary, systemic corticosteroids.

For management of a suspected drug overdose, CPhA recommends that you contact your **regional Poison Control Centre**. See the *CPS* Directory section for a list of Poison Control Centres.

DOSAGE: The dosage should be adjusted according to the response to the treatment and the patient's tolerance to the drug. The tablets/delayed-release tablets should be taken at regular and even intervals over the 24-hour period. The tablets should preferably be taken with a meal. For intestinal inflammatory diseases the nighttime dose interval should not exceed 8 hours.

Patients not previously treated with sulfasalazine should increase the dose gradually during the first few weeks. The incidence of adverse reactions tends to increase with daily dosages of 4 g or more; patients receiving these doses should be advised of this possibility and should be carefully observed for the appearance of adverse reactions.

Geriatrics: Based on pharmacokinetic studies, no special dosage instructions are required for elderly patients.

Renal Deficiency: Sulfasalazine should be used with caution in patients with renal deficiency.

Inflammatory Bowel Disease, Ulcerative Colitis, Crohn's Disease: **Acute attacks:** Adults: Severe attacks: 2 to 4 tablets, 3 to 4 times daily. Moderate and mild attacks: 2 tablets 3 to 4 times daily.

Children: 25 to 35 kg body weight: 1 tablet 3 times daily; 35 to 50 kg body weight: 2 tablets 2 to 3 times daily.

Prophylaxis: Adults: In the state of remission in ulcerative colitis the maintenance dose recommended for keeping the patient free from symptoms is 2 tablets 2 to 3 times a day. Treatment with this dosage should continue indefinitely, unless adverse effects are observed. In case of deterioration, raise the dosage to 2 to 4 tablets, 3 to 4 times a day.

Children: 25 to 35 kg body weight: 1 tablet twice daily; 35 to 50 kg body weight: 1 tablet 2 to 3 times daily.

Patients experiencing gastrointestinal side effects with the uncoated tablet should use the EN-tabs or a lower dose.

Rheumatoid Arthritis: Adults: 2 delayed-release tablets, 2 times daily.

When starting therapy, it is suggested to increase the daily dose as follows: 1st week: 1 delayed-release tablet in the evening. 2nd week: 1 delayed-release tablet in the morning and 1 delayed-release tablet in the evening. 3rd week: 1 delayed-release tablet in the morning and 2 delayed-release tablets in the evening. 4th week and after: 2 delayed-release tablets in the morning and 2 delayed-release tablets in the evening.

If no response has been seen after 2 months treatment, the dose may be increased to 3 g/day. Some patients may do well with 1.5 g/day.

A clinical effect generally appears 1 to 2 months after initiation of treatment. Concurrent therapy with analgesics and/or anti-inflammatory agents is recommended until the therapeutic effect of the EN-tabs is apparent. The EN-tabs are effective and well tolerated in long-term treatment.

Children: The use of sulfasalazine in Juvenile Rheumatoid Arthritis is not recommended since its efficacy/safety has not been established.

INFORMATION FOR THE PATIENT: Published in e-CPS, available by subscription at www.e-cps.ca.

SUPPLIED: Tablets: Each yellow-orange, round, convex tablet, engraved with "KPh" on one side and "101" and a score on the other side, contains: sulfasalazine USP 500 mg. Nonmedicinal ingredients: silicon dioxide, starch and magnesium stearate. Tartrazine-free. Bottles of 100 and 300.

EN-tabs: Each yellow-orange, elliptical, convex, enteric-coated, delayed-release tablet, engraved with "KPh" on one side and "102" on the other side, contains: sulfasalazine USP 500 mg. Nonmedicinal ingredients: beeswax, carnauba wax, cellulose acetate phthalate, glyceryl monostearate, polyethylene glycol, propylene glycol and talc. Tartrazine-free. Bottles of 100 and 300.

(Shown in Product Identification Section)

Salinex® Nasal Spray/Nasal Drops/Nasal Mist

sodium chloride

Nasal Cleanser

Sandoz

Salinex® Nasal Lubricant/Nasal Lubricant Gel

sodium chloride—polyethylene glycol—propylene glycol

Rhinitis Therapy—Nasal Lubricant

Sandoz

SUPPLIED: Adult's Nasal Spray: Each mL of aqueous solution contains: sodium chloride 9 mg. Nonmedicinal ingredients: benzalkonium chloride, glycerin and purified water. Bottles of 30 mL fitted with metered pump. Store between 15 and 30°C.

Children's Nasal Spray: Each mL of aqueous solution contains: sodium chloride 9 mg. Nonmedicinal ingredients: benzalkonium chloride, glycerin and purified water. Bottles of 30 mL fitted with metered pump. Store between 15 and 30°C.

Infants'/Children's Nasal Drops: Each mL of aqueous solution contains: sodium chloride 9 mg. Nonmedicinal ingredients: benzalkonium chloride, glycerin and purified water. Bottles of 30 mL, dropper included. Store between 15 and 30°C.

Nasal Mist: Each mL of aqueous solution contains: sodium chloride 9 mg. Nonmedicinal ingredients: benzalkonium chloride, glycerin and purified water. Squeeze bottles of 30 mL. Store between 15 and 30°C.

Nasal Lubricant: Each mL of solution contains: sodium chloride 9 mg, polyethylene glycol 160 mg and propylene glycol 50 mg. Bottles of 30 mL fitted with metered pump. Store between 15 and 30°C.

Nasal Lubricant Gel: Each g contains: sodium chloride 9 mg, polyethylene glycol 152 mg and propylene glycol 200 mg. Tubes of 30 g. Store between 15 and 30°C.

Salofalk®, Rectal Suspension ℞

5-ASA

Lower Gastrointestinal Tract Anti-inflammatory

Axcan Pharma

Date of Revision: March 14, 2008

SUMMARY PRODUCT INFORMATION:

Route of Administration	Dosage Form/ Strength	Clinically Relevant Nonmedicinal Ingredients
Rectal	Suspension 2 g/60 g and 4 g/60 g	Potassium metabisulfite

INDICATIONS AND CLINICAL USE: SALOFALK (mesalamine, 5-aminosalicylic acid, 5-ASA) rectal suspension, 4 g/60 g is indicated:
- in the management of distal ulcerative colitis (DUC) extending to the splenic flexure including refractory DUC defined to include patients who are difficult to manage with conventional therapies and patients who are allergic to sulfasalazine (SAS).
- as adjunctive therapy in more extensive disease as well as for the prevention of relapse in distal ulcerative colitis.

SALOFALK rectal suspension, 2 g/60 g is indicated:
- for the prevention of relapse in distal ulcerative colitis.

Geriatrics: Clinical studies with SALOFALK rectal suspension, 2 g/60 g and 4 g/60 g, have not been performed in the geriatric population.
Pediatrics (2-12 years of age): In children between the ages of 2 and 12 years, information on the safety and efficacy of SALOFALK 2 g and 4 g rectal suspensions is limited. Use of the drug should be limited to situations where a clear benefit is expected.

CONTRAINDICATIONS: SALOFALK (mesalamine, 5-aminosalicylic acid, 5-ASA) is contraindicated in:
- patients who are hypersensitive to this drug or to any ingredient in the formulation or component of the container. For a complete listing, see Dosage Forms, Composition and Packaging.
- cases of existing gastric or duodenal ulcer.
- in patients with urinary tract obstructions.
- infants under two years of age.

Patients hypersensitive to salicylates, including Aspirin, may also be hypersensitive to this medication.

WARNINGS AND PRECAUTIONS: General: SALOFALK should be used only if the benefits clearly outweigh the risks in patients with underlying liver or kidney disease, bleeding or clotting disorders as well as during pregnancy and lactation.

Patients with renal dysfunction, or elevated Blood Urea Nitrogen (BUN), or elevated serum creatinine, or with proteinuria, should be carefully monitored while receiving SALOFALK.

Concomitant treatment with mesalamine can increase the risk of myelosuppression in patients receiving azathioprine or 6-mercaptopurine.
Carcinogenesis and Mutagenesis: Carcinogenicity studies in animals and mutagenicity tests were negative.
Cardiovascular: Cardiac side effects, including pericarditis and myocarditis were uncommonly reported with the use of mesalamine.
Gastrointestinal: Epigastric pain, also commonly associated with inflammatory bowel disease (IBD) and prednisone or SAS therapy (18%), should be investigated in order to exclude pericarditis and pancreatitis either as adverse drug reactions to 5-ASA or secondary manifestations of IBD.
Renal: Initial assessment and periodic monitoring of the renal function is recommended since mesalamine is substantially excreted by the kidney, and prolonged mesalamine therapy may damage the kidneys.

Because elderly patients are more likely to have decreased renal function, closer monitoring of the renal function may be needed.
Sensitivity/Resistance: Caution should be exercised when mesalamine (5-aminosalicylic acid, 5-ASA) is first used in patients known to be allergic to sulfasalazine. These patients should be instructed to discontinue therapy at the first sign of rash or fever.
Special Populations: Pregnant Women: SALOFALK should be used during pregnancy only if the benefits clearly outweigh the risks to the fetus. 5-ASA is known to cross the placental barrier, and no clinical studies have been performed in pregnant women.

Animal studies did not show evidence of impaired fertility or harm to the fetus due to mesalamine, however, because animal reproduction studies are not always predictive of human response, SALOFALK should be used during pregnancy only if clearly needed.
Nursing Women: There are no clinical trial studies in nursing women. SALOFALK should be used in nursing women only if the benefits to the mother clearly outweigh the risks to the child. Mesalamine and its main metabolite N-acetyl-5-ASA are excreted in breast milk. The concentration of mesalamine is much lower than in maternal blood, but the metabolite N-acetyl-5-ASA appears in similar concentrations.

When SALOFALK is used in nursing women, infants should be monitored for changes in stool consistency as hypersensitivity reactions like diarrhea in the infants have been reported.
Pediatrics (2-12 years of age): In children between the ages of 2 and 12 years, information on the safety and efficacy of SALOFALK 2 g and 4 g rectal suspensions is limited. Use of the drug should be limited to situations where a clear benefit is expected.

SALOFALK should not be used in infants/toddlers aged less than 24 months.
Geriatrics: Clinical studies with SALOFALK rectal suspension, 2 g/60 g and 4 g/60 g, have not been performed in geriatric populations.

Mesalamine is substantially excreted by the kidney, and the risk of toxic reactions to this drug may be greater in patients with impaired renal function. Because elderly patients are more likely to have decreased renal function, it may be useful to monitor renal function.

ADVERSE REACTIONS: Adverse Drug Reaction Overview: Hypersensitivity reactions have been reported in a sub-group of patients known to be allergic to sulfasalazine including rash, fever, and dizziness. The apparent frequency is estimated at 3-4%, with reactions occurring at the onset of therapy and resolving promptly following discontinuation.

In rare cases, following 5-ASA administration, exacerbations of ulcerative colitis characterized by cramping, acute abdominal pain and diarrhea have been reported. Acute pancreatitis, hepatitis, pericarditis, interstitial nephritis, and pleural effusion, have also been reported in association with 5-ASA. Both pancreatitis and pericarditis have also been reported as manifestations of IBD.

Other reported side effects include headache, flatulence, nausea, and alopecia, but do not appear to be common.
Clinical Trial Adverse Drug Reactions: Because clinical trials are conducted under very specific conditions the adverse reaction rates observed in the clinical trials may not reflect the rates observed in practice and should not be compared to the rates in the clinical trials of another drug. Adverse drug reaction information from clinical trials is useful for identifying drug-related adverse events and for approximating rates. See Table 1.

Table 1: SALOFALK, Rectal Suspension
Clinical Trial Adverse Events Reported in >0.1% of Patients

Body System Preferred Term	SALOFALK n=841 %	Placebo n=176 %
Cardiac Disorders		
Pericarditis	0.1	0
Gastrointestinal Disorders		
Abdominal pain	7.9	7.9
Flatulence	6.0	4.5
Nausea	5.6	6.8
Diarrhea	2.1	3.9
Abdominal distension	1.4	1.1
Hemorrhoids	1.3	0

(cont'd)

Table 1: SALOFALK, Rectal Suspension *(cont'd)*
Clinical Trial Adverse Events Reported in >0.1% of Patients

Body System Preferred Term	SALOFALK n=841 %	Placebo n=176 %
Proctalgia	1.1	0
Constipation	0.9	2.2
Anal discomfort	0.5	1.7
Pancreatitis	0.1	0
Condition aggravated	0.1	0
General Disorders and Administration Site Conditions		
Fatigue	3.3	4.5
Pyrexia	3.0	0
Administration site reactions	1.3	0.5
Edema peripheral	0.5	6.2
Asthenia	0.1	2.2
Infections and Infestations		
Influenza	5.2	0.5
Urinary tract infection	0.5	2.2
Upper respiratory tract infection	0.1	0.5
Musculoskeletal, Connective Tissue and Bone Disorders		
Arthralgia	2.0	1.1
Back pain	1.3	0.5
Nervous System Disorders		
Headache	6.7	11.3
Dizziness	1.7	2.8
Insomnia	0.1	1.7
Respiratory, Thoracic and Mediastinal Disorders		
Pharyngolaryngeal pain	2.0	2.8
Skin and Subcutaneous Tissue Disorders		
Rash	2.8	2.2
Spots	2.2	5.1
Pruritus	1.1	0.5
Alopecia	0.8	1.1

Post-Market Adverse Drug Reactions: This section discusses adverse reactions that have been reported during marketed use of SALOFALK and other 5-ASA products. Because these reactions are reported voluntarily from a population of uncertain size, it is not always possible to reliably estimate their frequency or to establish a causal relationship to drug exposure.

The following adverse events have been reported more frequently with the use of rectal mesalamine (suppository and rectal suspension): Abdominal pain, abdominal pain upper, anorectal disorder, diarrhea, feces discoloured, flatulence, gastrointestinal pain, rectal discharge, rectal haemorrhage, vomiting, and condition aggravated. Chest pain, alopecia, dizziness, headache, insomnia, nausea, pruritus, pyrexia, rash. Interstitial nephritis, chromaturia, back pain, fatigue, and glossodynia, were also observed with rectal and/or oral mesalamine.

In addition, isolated cases of the following events were reported: Renal failure acute, renal failure chronic, kidney fibrosis, blood creatinine abnormal, BUN increased. In breast-fed infants whose mothers were receiving oral mesalamine: weight decrease, diarrhea, and thrombosis of the superior sagittal sinus. Fetal nephropathy in pregnant women who were receiving oral mesalamine has been reported. One death due to acute toxic hepatitis or to a Reye's syndrome. One death associated with agranulocytosis (and grade 4 neutropenia) with infection. Pericarditis constrictive, myocarditis, angina pectoris, atrial fibrillation, cardiac flutter, sinus tachycardia, palpitations, edema peripheral, and hypotension. Dyspnea, eosinophilic pneumonia, lung infiltration, pneumonia aspiration, and cough. Tongue edema, tongue discoloration, rash generalized, rash pustular, erythema, rash erythematous, skin discoloration, skin necrosis, urticaria, acute febrile neutrophilic dermatosis, lichenoid keratosis, and hyperhidrosis. Arthralgia, arthritis, muscle spasms, musculoskeletal pain/stiffness, tremor, myalgia, neck pain, and pain. Abdominal cramps, abdominal discomfort, abdominal distension, anal discomfort, burning sensation (rectal), constipation, defecation urgency, painful defecation, diarrhea haemorrhagic, haematochezia, proctalgia, rectal cramps, malabsorption, steatorrhea, vomiting, and medication residue in stools. Asthenia, delirium, coma, insomnia, vision blurred, eating disorder symptoms, feeling hot, dysgeusia, and parosmia. Hypocalcaemia, hypomagnesaemia, hypothyroidism, rhinorrhea, infection, influenza like illness, weight loss.

DRUG INTERACTIONS: Overview: Interaction between azathioprine, 6-mercaptopurine and aminosalicylates (including mesalamine) can increase the risk of leucopenia. Other potential interactions with a number of drugs could occur (see Drug-Drug Interactions).
Drug-Drug Interactions: Interaction between azathioprine, 6-mercaptopurine and aminosalicylates including mesalamine, has been reported. Concomitant treatment with mesalamine can increase the risk of myelosuppression in patients receiving azathioprine or 6-mercaptopurine. An increase in whole blood 6-thioguanine nucleotide (6-TGN) concentrations has been reported although the mechanism of this interaction remains unclear.

The hypoglycemic effect of sulfonylureas may be enhanced. Interactions with coumarin, methotrexate, probenecid, sulfinpyrazone, spironolactone, furosemide and rifampicin cannot be excluded. Potentiation of undesirable glucocorticoid effects on the stomach is possible.

A theoretical interaction of salicylates with Varicella Virus Vaccine might increase the risk of Reye's syndrome; as a result, the use of salicylates (including mesalamine) is discouraged for six weeks following varicella vaccination.

Drug-food, drug-herb, or drug-laboratory interactions have not been studied.

DOSAGE AND ADMINISTRATION: Dosing Considerations: In children between the ages of 2 and 12 years, information on the safety and efficacy of SALOFALK 2 g and 4 g rectal suspensions is limited. Use of the drug should be limited to situations where a clear benefit is expected.

Recommended Dose and Dosage Adjustment: Acute Episodes: SALOFALK (mesalamine, 5-aminosalicylic acid, 5-ASA) rectal suspension, 4 g/60 g is self-administered on a daily basis during acute episodes of disease. Usually one unit-dose rectal suspension (4 g 5-ASA) is taken upon retiring and retained during the entire rest period. Best results are expected with prolonged retention.

The usual course of therapy is one unit daily at bedtime. Response to treatment and adjustment in dosing frequency should be determined by periodic examination, including endoscopy and the assessment of symptomatology including rectal bleeding, stool frequency, and general well-being.

Daily dosing is continued until a significant response is achieved or the patient achieves remission.

Prevention of Relapses: SALOFALK rectal suspension, 2 g/60 g is self-administered in the same manner on a daily basis to prevent relapse.

If, alternatively, the 4 g/60 g preparation is used to prevent relapse, the dose can usually be reduced to alternate days or every third day, depending upon disease activity. Abrupt discontinuation of 5-ASA is not recommended. Dose tapering is recommended and each patient should be titrated to meet individual needs. Maintenance therapy is recommended to assure continued remission. However, should symptoms of diarrhea and rectal bleeding recur, dosage should be increased to 4 g/60 g/day.

Missed Dose: If a dose of SALOFALK is missed, it should be used as soon as possible, unless it is almost time for the next dose. A patient should not use two SALOFALK doses at the same time to make up for a missed dose.

Administration: SALOFALK (mesalamine, 5-ASA) rectal suspension, 4 g/60 g is self-administered on a daily basis during acute episodes of disease.

SALOFALK rectal suspension, 2 g/60 g is self-administered in the same manner on a daily basis to prevent relapse.

OVERDOSAGE:
Reports of overdose are not available.

> For management of a suspected drug overdose, contact your regional Poison Control Centre. See the *CPS* Directory section for a list of Poison Control Centres.

ACTION AND CLINICAL PHARMACOLOGY: Mechanism of Action: The mechanism of action of 5-ASA is multi-factorial and is still under investigation with several proposed biochemical mechanisms. Inflammatory intestinal disease is often accompanied by diffuse tissue reactions including ulceration and cellular infiltration of lymphocytes, plasma cells, eosinophils, polymorphonuclear cells and activated phagocytic cells.

The interference of 5-ASA with either leukotriene or prostaglandin metabolism may play a major role in suppressing the inflammatory response mechanism. 5-ASA prevents accumulation of thromboxane B2 and 6-keto-prostaglandin F1. Both 5-ASA and SAS reverse H_2O, and Cl-secretion and increase Na+ secretion in experimentally-induced colitis in guinea pigs. SAS and 5-ASA are known to inhibit polymorphonuclear cell migration possibly via lipoxygenase inhibition at concentrations lower than those required to inhibit prostaglandin synthesis. It is thus possible that both SAS and 5-ASA are capable of inhibiting both pathways via lipoxygenase inhibition.

Intestinal secretion is stimulated not only by prostaglandins but also by the metabolites of arachidonic acid generated via the lipoxygenase pathway. Upon phagocytic activation and arachidonic acid metabolism activation, reactive oxygen metabolites are generated. 5-ASA acts as a dose dependent antioxidant which scavenges oxygen derived free radicals produced by activated phagocytes. In addition, 5-ASA associates with the membrane surface, allowing chain breaking anti-oxidant activity when peroxidation is initiated within the membrane. 5-ASA is able to block initiation of oxidation from solution as well as propagation within the membrane. 5-ASA also inhibits the formation of both eicosanoids and cytokines.

Pharmacodynamics: SALOFALK rectal suspension contains mesalamine (5-aminosalicylic acid, 5-ASA), the active principle of the prodrug sulfasalazine. Although the 5-ASA mode of action is not clear, it appears to be multi-factorial. 5-ASA is thought to affect the inflammatory process through its ability to inhibit prostaglandin synthesis, interfere with leukotriene synthesis and consequent leukocyte migration as well as act as a potent scavenger of free radicals. Regardless of the mode of action, 5-ASA appears to be active mainly topically rather than systemically.

Pharmacokinetics: Absorption: Systemic absorption of rectally administered 5-ASA is low as shown by urinary recoveries which range from 5 to 35% of the amount given. In contrast, oral administration of free 5-ASA leads to high systemic absorption with rapid absorption from the small intestine; however, this route of administration provides for a reduced chance of topical effectiveness in the distal bowel. Rectally administered 5-ASA thus acts locally on the recto-sigmoidal colon. Satisfactory dosages (4 g 5-ASA rectal suspension) have reached the splenic flexure.

Distribution: Rectal administration allows for direct targeting of free 5-ASA to the sites of inflammation along the mucosal lumen of the rectum, sigmoid and distal large bowel. Free intraluminal 5-ASA is taken up by mucosal cells, where it is acetylated and inactivated as N-Ac-5-ASA. Following rectal dosing, both free 5-ASA and its inactive metabolite, N-Ac-5-ASA, can be found within 1-2 hours post administration in plasma.

Metabolism: 5-ASA metabolism is metabolised by acetylation. The only major metabolite of 5-ASA identified in man is N-acetyl-5-aminosalicylic acid (N-Ac-5-ASA). Following rectal dosing, both free and acetylated forms can be found in plasma within 1-2 hours post administration. Usually plasma concentrations are low and do not exceed a maximum serum level of about 10 µg/mL at rectal daily doses of up to 4 grams. Peak plasma levels of rectally administered 5-ASA (4 g rectal suspension) are reached within 3 to 6 hours, with a value of 2.6±2.3 µg/mL. Plasma levels are therefore negligible approximately 24 hours after dosing. Following mucosal absorption, passage through the liver results in further acetylation. These results are consistent with pharmacokinetic parameters as measured for 5-ASA and its metabolites determined in studies with solid oral dosage forms. In solid oral dosage studies, it has been determined that 5-ASA and its metabolite N-Ac-5-ASA are short lived in the serum with a half-life reported between 0.5-1.5 hours and 5-10 hours respectively; 5-ASA is partially absorbed rapidly ($t_{½}$=0.4-2.4 hours) and partially recovered unchanged in the feces.

Excretion: The kidneys excrete both free 5-ASA and acetylated forms (N-Ac-5-ASA) into the urine. Urinary clearance of absorbed drug occurs rapidly, mainly as the acetylated metabolite. The recovery rate in urine varies between 8 and 17 percent of the administered dose. Unabsorbed drug is excreted as the free and acetylated forms via feces.

STORAGE AND STABILITY: SALOFALK rectal suspensions, packaged in aluminum foil, are stable for 24 months at room temperature, preferably under 25°C. Without aluminum foil packaging, the suspension is stable for 18 months. Product expiration date and lot number are printed on the bottle base.

SPECIAL HANDLING INSTRUCTIONS: SALOFALK rectal suspension will cause staining of direct contact surfaces, including but not limited to fabrics, flooring, painted surfaces, marble, granite, vinyl, and enamel.

INFORMATION FOR THE PATIENT: Published in e-CPS, available by subscription at www.e-cps.ca.

DOSAGE FORMS, COMPOSITION AND PACKAGING: 2 g/60 g: Each unit of use rectal retention enema contains: 5-ASA 2 g/60 g. Nonmedicinal ingredients: carbomer, edetate disodium, potassium acetate, potassium metabisulfite, purified water, sodium benzoate and xanthan gum. Each unit consists of a rectal dosing package designed for self-administration and disposal. A removable protective sheath covers the pre-lubricated enema nozzle until ready for use. A one-way valve allows the suspension to flow from the bottle through the applicator nozzle and into the rectal vault as the patient squeezes the thin-walled collapsible bottle. Boxes of 7 bottles.

4 g/60 g: Each unit of use rectal retention enema contains: 5-ASA 4 g/60 g. Nonmedicinal ingredients: carbomer, edetate disodium, potassium acetate, potassium metabisulfite, purified water, sodium benzoate and xanthan gum. Each unit consists of a rectal dosing package designed for self-administration and disposal. A removable protective sheath covers the pre-lubricated enema nozzle until ready for use. A one-way valve allows the suspension to flow from the bottle through the applicator nozzle and into the rectal vault as the patient squeezes the thin-walled collapsible bottle. Boxes of 7 bottles.

(Shown in Product Identification Section)

Salofalk®, Suppositories Ⓟ

5-ASA

Lower Gastrointestinal Tract Anti-inflammatory

Axcan Pharma

Date of Preparation: July 15, 1994
Date of Revision: September 10, 2004

PHARMACOLOGY: SALOFALK suppositories contain mesalamine (5-aminosalicylic acid, 5-ASA), the active principle of the prodrug sulfasalazine (SAS). Although its mode of action is not clear, 5-ASA is thought to affect the inflammatory process through its ability to inhibit prostaglandin synthesis, interfere with leukotriene synthesis and consequent leukocyte migration as well as act as a potent scavenger of free radicals. Regardless of the mode of action, 5-ASA appears to be active only topically. SALOFALK suppositories are inserted into the rectum thus providing topical application to the affected area.

Rectal administration, either as 500 or 1000 mg suppositories or as 4 g/60 g or 2 g/60 g rectal suspension of mesalamine (5-aminosalicylic acid) allows for direct targeting of free 5-ASA to the sites of inflammation along the mucosal lumen of the rectum, sigmoid and distal large bowel. Systemic absorption of rectally administered 5-ASA is low as shown by urinary and rectal recoveries which range from 5 to 35% of the amount given. Rectally administered 5-ASA with minimal systemic absorption thus acts locally on the recto-sigmoidal colon. Plasma concentrations are low, peaking at about 10 µg/mL for daily rectal dosing of 4 grams and are negligible 24 hours after administration.

Pharmacokinetics: 5-ASA and its major metabolite N-acetyl-5-aminosalicylic acid (N-Ac-5-ASA) are short lived in the serum with a half-life reported at between 5-10 hours and 24 hours. N-acetyl-5-ASA exhibits a half life reported at 5-10 hours and 24 hours. In patients with active ulcerative colitis or Crohn's disease receiving 500 mg of 5-ASA t.i.d. orally, mean steady state plasma levels of 5-ASA and N-acetyl-5-ASA averaged 0.7 and 1.2 µg/mL respectively and were reached within 4-6 hours after administration. Treatment with a smaller dose (250 mg t.i.d.) achieved levels of 0.4 and 1.0 µg/mL respectively. The elimination half life thus appears to be dose dependent (1.4±0.6 hour at 500 mg t.i.d. vs 0.6±0.2 hour at 250 mg t.i.d.).

Regardless of the mode of administration, 5-aminosalicylic acid appears to be only effective topically.

INDICATIONS: SALOFALK mesalamine (5-aminosalicylic acid) suppositories, 500 or 1000 mg are indicated in the management of ulcerative proctitis and as adjunctive therapy in more extensive distal ulcerative colitis (DUC).

CONTRAINDICATIONS: SALOFALK mesalamine (5-aminosalicylic acid) is contraindicated in patients with urinary tract obstructions and in infants under two years of age. Patients hypersensitive to salicylates including Aspirin may also be hypersensitive to this medication.

WARNINGS: Mesalamine (5-aminosalicylic acid, 5-ASA) should be used only after critical appraisal of the risk to benefit ratio in patients with underlying liver of kidney disease, bleeding or clotting disorders as well as during pregnancy and lactation. Caution should be exercised in patients with elevated BUN.

PRECAUTIONS: Periodic urinalysis to assess kidney function is recommended since prolonged mesalamine (5-aminosalicylic acid) therapy may damage the kidneys. Caution should be exercised when mesalamine is first used in patients known to be allergic to sulfasalazine (SAS). These patients should be instructed to discontinue therapy at the first sign of rash or fever.

Epigastric pain, also commonly associated with I.B.D. and prednisone or SAS therapy (18%, Singleton et al N.C.D.S., 1983), should be investigated in order to exclude pericarditis and pancreatitis or hepatitis either as adverse drug reactions to 5-ASA or secondary manifestations of inflammatory bowel disease.

Drug Interactions: No known drug interaction exist. The hypoglycemic effect of sulfonylureas may be enhanced. Interactions with coumarin, methotrexate, probenecid, sulfinpyrazone, spironolactone, furosemide and rifampicin can not be excluded.

ADVERSE EFFECTS: Hypersensitivity reactions have been reported in a sub-group of patients known to be allergic to SAS including rash, fever, and dizziness. The apparent frequency is estimated at 3-4%, with reactions occurring at the onset of therapy and resolving promptly following discontinuation.

In rare cases, following mesalamine (5-aminosalicylic acid) administration, exacerbation of ulcerative colitis characterized by cramping, acute abdominal pain and diarrhea has been reported. Acute pancreatitis, hepatitis and pleural effusion have also been reported in association both with mesalamine and SAS, as have rare instances of pericarditis. Both pancreatitis and pericarditis have also been reported as manifestations of inflammatory bowel disease. Finally, acute or chronic interstitial nephritis has been reported in association with orally-administered mesalamine.

Other reported side effects include headache, flatulence, nausea, and alopecia, but do not appear to be common. During controlled clinical trials involving the administration of either rectal mesalamine or placebo, the following adverse reactions were reported in more than 0.1% of cases: see Table 1.

Table 1: SALOFALK, Suppositories
Adverse Reactions Reported in More Than 0.1% of Cases

Symptom	% (N) SALOFALK (N=841)	% (N) Placebo (N=176)
Abdominal pain, cramps & discomfort	7.9 (67)	7.9 (14)
Headache	6.7 (57)	11.3 (20)
Gas or flatulence	6.0 (51)	4.5 (8)
Nausea	5.6 (47)	6.8 (12)
Flu	5.2 (44)	0.5 (1)
Tired, weak, malaise or fatigue	3.3 (28)	4.5 (8)
Fever	3.0 (26)	0
Rash	2.8 (24)	2.2 (4)
Spots	2.2 (19)	5.1 (9)
Cold, sore throat	2.0 (17)	2.8 (5)
Diarrhea	2.1 (18)	3.9 (7)
Leg, joint pain	2.0 (17)	1.1 (2)
Dizziness	1.7 (15)	2.8 (5)
Bloating	1.4 (12)	1.1 (2)
Back pain	1.3 (11)	0.5 (1)
Pain on insertion of tip (enema)	1.3 (11)	0.5 (1)
Hemorrhoids	1.3 (11)	0
Itching	1.1 (10)	0.5 (1)
Rectal pain	1.1 (10)	0
Constipation	0.9 (8)	2.2 (4)

(cont'd)

Table 1: SALOFALK, Suppositories *(cont'd)*
Adverse Reactions Reported in More Than 0.1% of Cases

Symptom	% (N) SALOFALK (N=841)	Placebo (N=176)
Hair loss	0.8 (7)	1.1 (2)
Peripheral edema	0.5 (5)	6.2 (11)
UTI, urinary burning	0.5 (5)	2.2 (4)
Rectal pain, soreness or burning	0.5 (5)	1.7 (3)
Asthenia	0.1 (1)	2.2 (4)
Insomnia	0.1 (1)	1.7 (3)
Upper respiratory tract infection	0.1 (1)	0.5 (1)
Pericarditis	0.1 (1)	0
Pancreatitis	0.1 (1)	0
Exacerbation of IBD	0.1 (1)	0

OVERDOSE:
There is no experience with acute overdosage in humans. The drug is not metabolized to salicylate. There is no specific antidote and treatment is symptomatic and supportive.

For management of a suspected drug overdose, CPhA recommends that you contact your **regional Poison Control Centre**. See the *CPS* Directory section for a list of Poison Control Centres.

DOSAGE: One 500 mg SALOFALK mesalamine (5-aminosalicylic acid) suppositories are self-administered on a daily t.i.d. or b.i.d. basis. One 1000 mg SALOFALK suppository is self-administered on a once daily basis. The usual adult dose is 1.0-1.5 g/day and dosing is continued until a significant response is achieved or until the patient achieves remission. Dose tapering is recommended. Abrupt discontinuation is not recommended. Best results are expected with prolonged retention.

In children between the ages of 2 and 12, information on the safety and efficacy of SALOFALK suppositories is limited. Therefore, use should be limited to situations where a clear benefit is expected.

SUPPLIED: 500 mg: Each suppository contains: 5-ASA 500 mg. Nonmedicinal ingredients: Witepsol H-15 (suppository wax base). Strips of 5 suppositories; boxes of 30 suppositories. Store in a cool place, preferably between 20 and 25°C. SALOFALK mesalamine suppositories will cause staining of direct contact surfaces, including but not limited to fabrics, flooring, painted surfaces, marble, granite, vinyl, and enamel.
1000 mg: Each suppository contains: 5-ASA 1000 mg. Nonmedicinal ingredients: Witepsol H-15 (suppository wax base). Strips of 5 suppositories; boxes of 30 suppositories. Store in a cool place, preferably between 20 and 25°C. SALOFALK mesalamine suppositories will cause staining of direct contact surfaces, including but not limited to fabrics, flooring, painted surfaces, marble, granite, vinyl, and enamel.

Salofalk®, Tablets ℞

5-ASA

Lower Gastrointestinal Tract Anti-inflammatory

Axcan Pharma

Date of Preparation: July 15, 1994
Date of Revision: September 10, 2004

PHARMACOLOGY: SALOFALK enteric-coated tablets contain 5-aminosalicylic acid (5-ASA), the active principle of the prodrug sulfasalazine. Although its mode of action is not clear, 5-ASA is thought to affect the inflammatory process through its ability to inhibit prostaglandin synthesis, interfere with leukotriene synthesis and consequent leukocyte migration as well as act as a potent scavenger of free radicals. Regardless of the mode of action, 5-ASA appears to be active only topically. SALOFALK enteric-coated tablets are coated to allow passage through the stomach intact, delivering 5-ASA above pH 6 to the distal small bowel and proximal colon thus providing 5-ASA throughout the terminal ileum and colon.
Pharmacokinetics: 5-ASA and its major metabolite N-acetyl-5-aminosalicylic acid (N-Ac-5-ASA) are short lived in the serum with a half-life reported at between 5-10 hours and 24 hours. It is partially absorbed rapidly ($t_{1/2}$=0.4-2.4 hours) and partially recovered unchanged in the feces. Urinary (44%) and fecal (35%) recovery rates are similar to those achieved when 5-ASA is administered as sulfasalazine.

INDICATIONS: SALOFALK (5-aminosalicylic acid) enteric-coated tablets are indicated in the treatment of acute ulcerative colitis and in the prevention of relapse of Crohn's disease in patients following bowel resection.

CONTRAINDICATIONS: SALOFALK is contraindicated in cases of existing gastric or duodenal ulcer, in patients with urinary tract obstructions and in infants under two years of age. Patients hypersensitive to salicylates including Aspirin may also be hypersensitive to this medication.

WARNINGS: 5-aminosalicylic acid (5-ASA, mesalazine) should be used only after critical appraisal of the risk to benefit ratio in patients with underlying liver or kidney disease, bleeding or clotting disorders as well as during pregnancy and lactation. Caution should be exercised in patients with elevated BUN. Patients with pyloric stenosis may have prolonged retention of SALOFALK enteric-coated tablets.

PRECAUTIONS: Periodic urinalysis to assess kidney function is recommended since prolonged 5-aminosalicylic acid therapy may damage the kidneys. Caution should be exercised when 5-aminosalicylic acid is first used in patients known to be allergic to sulfasalazine. These patients should be instructed to discontinue therapy at the first sign of rash or fever.

Epigastric pain, also commonly associated with Inflammatory Bowel Disease (I.B.D.) and prednisone or sulfasalazine therapy (18%, Singleton et al. N.C.D.S., 1983-), should be investigated in order to exclude pericarditis, pancreatitis or hepatitis either as adverse drug reactions to 5-ASA or secondary manifestations of I.B.D.
Drug Interactions: No known drug interactions exist. The hypoglycemic effect of sulfonylureas may be enhanced. Interactions with coumarins, methotrexate, probenecid, sulfinpyrazone, spironolactone, furosemide and rifampicin cannot be excluded. Potentiation of undesirable glucocorticoid effects on the stomach is possible.

ADVERSE EFFECTS: Hypersensitivity reactions have been reported in a sub-group of patients known to be allergic to sulfasalazine including rash, fever, and dizziness. The apparent frequency is estimated at 3-4%, with reactions occurring at the onset of therapy and resolving promptly following discontinuation.

In rare cases, following 5-ASA administration, exacerbation of ulcerative colitis, characterized by cramping, acute abdominal pain and diarrhea, has been reported. Acute pancreatitis, hepatitis and pleural effusion have also been reported in association both with 5-ASA and sulfasalazine, as have rare instances of pericarditis. Both pancreatitis and pericarditis have also been reported as manifestations of inflammatory bowel disease. Finally, acute or chronic interstitial nephritis has been reported in association with orally administered 5-ASA.

Other reported side effects include headache, flatulence, nausea, and alopecia, but do not appear to be common.

During controlled clinical trials involving the administration of either 5-ASA or placebo, the following adverse reactions were reported in more than 0.1% of cases: see Table 1.

Table 1: SALOFALK, Tablets
Adverse Reactions Reported in More Than 0.1% of Cases

Symptom	N (%) SALOFALK (N=841)	Placebo (N=176)
Abdominal pain, cramps & discomfort	67 (7.9)	14 (7.9)
Headache	57 (6.7)	20 (11.3)
Gas or flatulence	51 (6.0)	8 (4.5)
Nausea	47 (5.6)	12 (6.8)
Flu	44 (5.2)	1 (0.5)
Tired, weak, malaise or fatigue	28 (3.3)	8 (4.5)
Fever	26 (3.0)	0
Rash	24 (2.8)	4 (2.2)
Spots	19 (2.2)	9 (5.1)
Cold, sore throat	17 (2.0)	5 (2.8)
Diarrhea	18 (2.1)	7 (3.9)
Leg, joint pain	17 (2.0)	2 (1.1)
Dizziness	15 (1.7)	5 (2.8)
Bloating	12 (1.4)	2 (1.1)
Back pain	11 (1.3)	1 (0.5)
Pain on insertion of tip (enema)	11 (1.3)	1 (0.5)
Hemorrhoids	11 (1.3)	0
Itching	10 (1.1)	1 (0.5)
Rectal pain	10 (1.1)	0
Constipation	8 (0.9)	4 (2.2)
Hair loss	7 (0.8)	2 (1.1)
Peripheral edema	5 (0.5)	11 (6.2)
UTI, urinary burning	5 (0.5)	4 (2.2)
Rectal pain, soreness or burning	5 (0.5)	3 (1.7)
Asthenia	1 (0.1)	4 (2.2)
Insomnia	1 (0.1)	3 (1.7)
Upper respiratory tract infection	1 (0.1)	1 (0.5)
Pericarditis	1 (0.1)	0
Pancreatitis	1 (0.1)	0
Exacerbation of IBD	1 (0.1)	0

OVERDOSE:
There is no experience with acute overdosage in humans. The drug is not metabolized to salicylate. If the amount ingested is considered dangerous or excessive, vomiting should be induced with ipecac syrup unless the patient is convulsing, comatose or has lost the gag reflex, in which case gastric lavage using a large bore tube should be performed. If indicated, activated charcoal and a saline cathartic should follow. There is no specific antidote and treatment is symptomatic and supportive.

For management of a suspected drug overdose, CPhA recommends that you contact your **regional Poison Control Centre**. See the *CPS* Directory section for a list of Poison Control Centres.

DOSAGE: In the acute ulcerative colitis inflammatory stage, and in the prevention of recurrence of Crohn's disease, SALOFALK (5-aminosalicylic acid) enteric-coated tablets must be taken reliably and consistently by the patient in order to ensure therapeutic success. Tablets should be swallowed whole before meals with plenty of fluid.
Adults: For the treatment of acute ulcerative colitis, two 500 mg SALOFALK (5- aminosalicylic acid) enteric-coated tablets, three or four times per day (total adult dose: 3 g/day-4 g/day). Abrupt discontinuation is not recommended. Prolonged treatment may be required.

For the prevention of recurrence of Crohn's disease in patients following bowel resection, the total adult dose is 3 g/day in divided doses. Prolonged treatment is required.

SUPPLIED: Each ochre, oblong, enteric-coated tablet contains: 5-ASA 500 mg. Nonmedicinal ingredients: colloidal silicon dioxide, glycine, magnesium stearate, microcrystalline cellulose, povidone and sodium carbonate; coating: carnauba wax, hydroxypropyl methylcellulose, iron oxide, methacrylic acid copolymer, polydimethyl siloxane, polysorbate, sodium hydroxide, talc, titanium dioxide and triethyl citrate. Bottles of 150 and 500. Store at controlled room temperature (15 to 30°C). Protect from light.

(Shown in Product Identification Section)

Sandomigran® Ⓟ
pizotifen malate
Vascular Headache Prophylaxis

Paladin

Sandomigran DS® Ⓟ
pizotifen malate
Vascular Headache Prophylaxis

Paladin

SUPPLIED: Sandomigran: Each biconvex, ivory-colored, sugar-coated tablet contains: pizotifen 0.5 mg as derived from 0.73 mg of pizotifen malate. Nonmedicinal ingredients: cornstarch, lactose, magnesium stearate, povidone and talc. Bottles of 100.
Sandomigran DS: Each circular, flat, white compressed, tablet bevelled edge, scored on one side, contains: pizotifen 1 mg as derived from 1.46 mg of pizotifen malate. Nonmedicinal ingredients: lactose, magnesium stearate and microcrystalline cellulose. Bottles of 100.

Sandostatin® Ⓟ
octreotide acetate
Synthetic Octapeptide Analogue of Somatostatin

Novartis Pharmaceuticals

Sandostatin® LAR® Ⓟ
octreotide acetate
Synthetic Octapeptide Analogue of Somatostatin

Novartis Pharmaceuticals

Date of Preparation: June 6, 1989
Date of Revision: September 3, 2009

SUMMARY PRODUCT INFORMATION:

Route of Administration	Dosage Form/ Strength	Clinically Relevant Nonmedicinal Ingredients
SANDOSTATIN: Subcutaneous and intravenous infusion	Solution in ampoules (1 mL): 50 µg/ mL, 100 µg/ mL, 500 µg/ mL or Multidose Vials (5 mL): 200 µg/ mL	Lactic acid, phenol and mannitol For a complete listing see Dosage Forms, Composition and Packaging.
SANDOSTATIN LAR: Intramuscular	Powder for slow release suspension: 10, 20 or 30 mg octreotide per vial (5 mL) [supplied with one pre-filled syringe with 2.5 mL diluent and two needles] Single dose vial (5 mL)	Poly (DL-lactide-co-glycolide), carboxymethylcellulose sodium and mannitol. For a complete listing see Dosage Forms, Composition and Packaging.

INDICATIONS AND CLINICAL USE: SANDOSTATIN s.c. Ampoules and Multidose Vials: General: SANDOSTATIN (octreotide acetate) therapy is indicated for control of symptoms in patients with metastatic carcinoid and vasoactive intestinal peptide-secreting tumors (VIPomas) as well as in patients with acromegaly.

Data are insufficient to determine whether SANDOSTATIN decreases the size, rate of growth, or development of metastases in patients with these tumors.

SANDOSTATIN is also indicated for the prevention of complications following pancreatic surgery in patients undergoing high risk procedures.

SANDOSTATIN is also indicated for the emergency management of bleeding gastro-oesophageal varices in patients with cirrhosis and as protection from rebleeding. SANDOSTATIN is used in association with specific intervention such as endoscopic sclerotherapy.

Carcinoid Tumors: SANDOSTATIN is indicated for the symptomatic treatment of metastatic carcinoid tumors where it suppresses or inhibits the severe diarrhea and flushing episodes associated with the disease.

Vasoactive Intestinal Peptide Tumors (VIPomas): SANDOSTATIN is indicated for the treatment of the profuse watery diarrhea associated with VIP-secreting tumors. Significant improvement has been noted in the overall condition of these otherwise therapeutically unresponsive patients. Therapy with SANDOSTATIN results in improvement in electrolyte abnormalities, e.g., hypokalemia, often enabling reduction of fluid and electrolyte support.

Acromegaly: SANDOSTATIN is indicated to reduce blood levels of growth hormone and IGF-1 (somatomedin C) including acromegalic patients who have had inadequate response to, or cannot be treated with surgical resection, pituitary irradiation and/or bromocriptine mesylate at maximally tolerated doses.

Since the effects of pituitary irradiation may not become maximal for several years, adjunctive therapy with SANDOSTATIN to reduce blood levels of GH and IGF-1 offers potential benefit before the effects of irradiation are manifested.

A clinically relevant growth hormone (GH) reduction (by 50% or more) occurs in almost all patients, and normalisation (plasma GH <5 µg/L) can be achieved in about half of the cases.

In most patients, SANDOSTATIN markedly reduces the clinical symptoms of the disease such as headache, skin and soft tissue swelling, hyperhydrosis, arthralgia, paresthesia. In patients with a large pituitary adenoma, SANDOSTATIN treatment may result in some shrinkage of the tumour mass.

Prevention of Complications Following Pancreatic Surgery: SANDOSTATIN inhibits basal and stimulated exocrine pancreatic secretion and when administered peri- and post-operatively in patients undergoing high risk pancreatic surgery, reduces the incidence and severity of typical post-operative complications (e.g. pancreatic fistula, abscess and subsequent sepsis and post-operative acute pancreatitis).

Bleeding Gastro-oesophageal Varices: In patients presenting with bleeding gastro-oesophageal varices due to underlying cirrhosis, SANDOSTATIN administration in combination with specific intervention (e.g. sclerotherapy) provides better control of bleeding and early rebleeding, reduces transfusion requirements and improves 5-day survival).

SANDOSTATIN LAR (Octreotide [as acetate] for Injectable Suspension): Acromegaly: SANDOSTATIN LAR is indicated for acromegalic patients who are adequately controlled with SANDOSTATIN administered subcutaneously, including those in whom surgery, radiotherapy or dopamine agonist treatment is inappropriate or ineffective, or in the interim period until radiotherapy becomes fully effective (see Dosage and Administration).

In most patients, SANDOSTATIN LAR markedly reduces the clinical symptoms of the disease, such as headache, perspiration, paresthesia, fatigue, osteoarthralagia and carpel tunnel syndrome.

Carcinoid Tumors: SANDOSTATIN LAR is indicated for the treatment of the severe diarrhea and flushing episodes associated with carcinoid tumors in patients in whom symptoms are adequately controlled on s.c. treatment with SANDOSTATIN.

Vasoactive Intestinal Peptide Tumors (VIPomas): SANDOSTATIN LAR is indicated for the treatment of the profuse watery diarrhea associated with VIP-secreting tumors in patients in whom symptoms are adequately controlled on s.c. treatment with SANDOSTATIN.

In patients with carcinoid syndrome and VIPomas, the effect of SANDOSTATIN LAR on tumor size and rate of growth has not been determined. In patients with carcinoid syndrome and VIPomas, the effect of SANDOSTATIN LAR on development of metastases has not been determined.

CONTRAINDICATIONS: SANDOSTATIN and SANDOSTATIN LAR (octreotide acetate) are contraindicated in patients with a known hypersensitivity to octreotide or to any of the excipients.

WARNINGS AND PRECAUTIONS: General: Sudden escape from symptomatic control by SANDOSTATIN (octreotide acetate) may occur infrequently, with rapid recurrence of severe symptoms. Dosage adjustment therefore may be required.

As GH-secreting pituitary tumors may sometimes expand, causing serious complications (e.g. visual field defects), it is essential that all patients treated with SANDOSTATIN s.c. or SANDOSTATIN LAR be carefully monitored. If evidence of tumour expansion appears, alternative procedures may be advisable.

Octreotide alters the balance between the counter-regulatory hormones, insulin, glucagon and growth hormone, which may result in hypoglycemia or hyperglycemia. Octreotide also suppresses secretion of thyroid stimulating hormone, which may result in hypothyroidism. Cardiac conduction abnormalities have also occurred during treatment with octreotide.

Carcinogenesis and Mutagenesis: Studies in laboratory animals have demonstrated no mutagenic potential of octreotide acetate. No long-term studies in animals to assess carcinogenicity have been completed. SANDOSTATIN s.c. did not impair fertility in rats at doses up to 1000 µg/kg/day.

Cardiovascular: In both acromegalic and carcinoid syndrome patients, bradycardia, arrhythmias and conduction abnormalities have been reported during octreotide therapy. Dose adjustments of drugs such as beta-blockers, calcium channel blockers, or agents to control fluid and electrolyte balance, may be necessary. Other EKG changes were observed such as QT prolongation, axis shifts, early repolarization, low voltage, R/S transition, early R wave progression, and non-specific ST-T wave changes. The relationship of these events to octreotide acetate is not established because many of these patients have underlying cardiac disease (see Warnings and Precautions). In one acromegalic patient with severe congestive heart failure, initiation of SANDOSTATIN Injection therapy resulted in worsening of CHF with improvement when drug was discontinued. Confirmation of a drug effect was obtained with a positive rechallenge (see Adverse Reactions).

Endocrine and Metabolism: Glucose Metabolism: SANDOSTATIN therapy is occasionally associated with mild transient hypo- or hyperglycemia but may also result in overt diabetes due to alterations in the balance between the counter-regulatory hormones, insulin, glucagon and growth hormone. Patients should be closely observed on introduction of SANDOSTATIN therapy and at each change of dosage for symptomatic evidence of hyper- and hypoglycemia. Insulin requirement of patients with type I diabetes mellitus may be reduced by administration of SANDOSTATIN. In non-diabetics and type II diabetics with partially intact insulin reserves, SANDOSTATIN administration can result in prandial increases in glycemia. Severe hyperglycemia, subsequent pneumonia, and death following initiation of SANDOSTATIN (octreotide acetate) Injection therapy was reported in one patient with no history of hyperglycemia.

Predicting the effect of SANDOSTATIN on glucose tolerance in any given patients is not possible at this time. It is recommended that all acromegalic patients have their serum glucose carefully monitored during initiation and titration of therapy with SANDOSTATIN s.c. or SANDOSTATIN LAR.

Since following bleeding episodes from esophageal varices, there is an increased risk for the development of insulin-dependent diabetes or for changes in insulin requirement in patients with pre-existing diabetes, an appropriate monitoring of blood glucose is required.

It is therefore recommended that glucose tolerance and antidiabetic treatment be periodically monitored during therapy with SANDOSTATIN s.c. or SANDOSTATIN LAR.

Thyroid Function: Data on the effect of chronic therapy with SANDOSTATIN on hypothalamic/pituitary function have not been obtained. A progressive drop in T_4 levels has been reported, culminating in clinical and biochemical hypothyroidism after 19 months of therapy in one clinical trial patient (carcinoid) receiving 1500 µg of SANDOSTATIN s.c. daily. Minimal impairment of thyroid function was recorded in some acromegalic patients following treatment with SANDOSTATIN LAR. Therefore, baseline and periodic assessment of thyroid function (TSH, total and/or free T_4) should be monitored during chronic therapy with octreotide acetate.

Gastrointestinal: Nutrition: There is evidence that SANDOSTATIN therapy may alter absorption of dietary fats in some patients. It is suggested that periodic quantitative 72-hour fecal fat and serum carotene determinations be performed to aid in the assessment of possible drug-induced aggravation of fat malabsorption.

Depressed vitamin B12 levels and abnormal Schilling's tests have been observed in some patients receiving octreotide therapy, and monitoring of vitamin B12 levels is recommended during therapy with SANDOSTATIN LAR (octreotide acetate for injectable suspension).

Octreotide has been investigated for the reduction of excessive fluid loss from the G.I. tract in patients with conditions producing such a loss. If such patients are receiving total parenteral nutrition (TPN), serum zinc may rise excessively when the fluid loss is reversed. Patients on TPN and octreotide should have periodic monitoring of zinc levels.

Hepatic/Biliary/Pancreatic: Gallbladder and Related Events: Single doses of SANDOSTATIN Injection have been shown to inhibit gallbladder contractility and decrease bile secretion in normal volunteers. In clinical trials with SANDOSTATIN Injection (primarily patients with acromegaly or psoriasis) in patients who had not previously received octreotide, the incidence of biliary tract abnormalities was 63% (27% gallstones, 24% sludge without stones, 12% biliary duct dilatation). The incidence of stones or sludge in patients who received SANDOSTATIN Injection for 12 months or longer was 52%. The incidence of gallbladder abnormalities did not appear to be related to age, sex or dose but was related to duration of exposure.

In clinical trials 52% of acromegalic patients, most of whom received SANDOSTATIN LAR for 12 months or longer, developed new biliary abnormalities including gallstones, microlithiasis, sediment, sludge and dilatation. The incidence of new cholelithiasis was 22%, of which 7% were microstones.

In clinical trials 62% of malignant carcinoid patients who received SANDOSTATIN LAR for up to 18 months developed new biliary abnormalities including gallstones, sludge and dilatation. New gallstones occurred in a total of 24% of patients.

Across all trials, a few patients developed acute cholecystitis, ascending cholangitis, biliary obstruction, cholestatic hepatitis, or pancreatitis during octreotide therapy or following its withdrawal. One patient developed ascending cholangitis during SANDOSTATIN Injection therapy and died. Despite the high incidence of new gallstones in patients receiving octreotide, 1% of patients developed acute symptoms requiring cholecystectomy.

It is recommended that patients on extended therapy with SANDOSTATIN or SANDOSTATIN LAR be evaluated periodically (at about 6 to 12-month intervals) using ultrasound evaluations of the gallbladder and bile ducts.

Baseline and periodic (at about 6 to 12-month intervals) ultrasonography is recommended during therapy with SANDOSTATIN and SANDOSTATIN LAR to assess the presence of gallstones. If gallstones do occur, they are usually asymptomatic. Symptomatic gallstones should receive medical attention.

Liver Impairment: In patients with liver cirrhosis, the half-life of the drug may be increased, necessitating adjustment of the maintenance dosage.

Information to Be Provided to the Patient : Careful instruction in sterile subcutaneous and intramuscular injection techniques should be given to the patients and to other persons who may administer SANDOSTATIN or SANDOSTATIN LAR injections (see Information for the Patient).

Patients with carcinoid tumors and VIPomas should be advised to adhere closely to their scheduled return visits for reinjection in order to minimize exacerbation of symptoms.

Patients with acromegaly should also be urged to adhere to their return visit schedule to help assure steady control of GH and IGF-1 levels.

Renal: Renal Impairment: In patients with severe renal failure requiring dialysis, the half-life of the drug may be increased, necessitating adjustment of the maintenance dosage.

Sexual Function/Reproduction: The therapeutic benefits of a reduction in growth hormone (GH) levels and normalization of insulin-like growth factor 1 (IGF-1) concentration in female acromegalic patients could potentially restore fertility. Pregnancy in acromegalic patients may increase the risk of gestational diabetes, hypertension and exacerbation of the underlying cardiac disease, therefore female patients of childbearing potential should be advised to use adequate contraception during treatment with octreotide.

Special Populations: Pregnant Women: There are no adequate and well-controlled studies in pregnant women. In the postmarketing experience, data on a limited number of pregnancies have been reported in patients on octreotide therapy.

Nursing Women: It is not known whether octreotide is excreted in human breast milk. Animal studies have shown excretion of octreotide in breast milk. Patients should not breast-feed during SANDOSTATIN treatment.

Pediatrics: Experience with SANDOSTATIN s.c. and SANDOSTATIN LAR in the pediatric population is limited.

SANDOSTATIN Injection has been primarily used in patients with congenital hyperinsulinism (also called nesidioblastosis). The youngest patient to receive the drug was 1 month old. At doses of 1-40 µg/kg body weight/day, the majority of side effects observed were gastrointestinal-steatorrhea, diarrhea, vomiting and abdominal distension. Poor growth has been reported in several patients treated with SANDOSTATIN Injection for more than 1 year; catch-up growth occurred after SANDOSTATIN Injection was discontinued. A 16-month-old male with enterocutaneous fistula developed sudden abdominal pain and increased nasogastric drainage and died 8 hours after receiving a single 100 µg subcutaneous dose of SANDOSTATIN Injection.

Monitoring and Laboratory Tests: Laboratory tests that may be helpful as biochemical markers in determining and following patient response depend on the specific tumor. Based on diagnosis, measurement of the following substances may be useful in monitoring the progress of therapy:
Carcinoid: 5-HIAA (urinary 5-hydroxyindole acetic acid), plasma serotonin, plasma Substance P.
VIPoma: VIP (plasma vasoactive intestinal peptide).

Acromegaly: Growth hormone—IGF-1 (somatomedin C).

Responsiveness to octreotide may be evaluated by determining growth hormone levels at 1-4 hour intervals for 8-12 hours after subcutaneous injection of SANDOSTATIN Injection (not SANDOSTATIN LAR). Alternatively, a single measurement of IGF-1 (somatomedin C) level may be made two weeks after initiation of SANDOSTATIN Injection or dosage change. After patients are switched from SANDOSTATIN Injection to SANDOSTATIN LAR, GH and IGF-1 determinations may be made after 3 monthly injections of SANDOSTATIN LAR. (Steady-state serum levels of octreotide are reached only after a period of 3 months of monthly injections.) Growth hormone can be determined using the mean of 4 assays taken at 1 hour intervals. Somatomedin C can be determined with a single assay. All GH and IGF-1 determinations should be made 4 weeks after the previous SANDOSTATIN LAR.

Baseline and periodic total and/or free T_4 measurements should be performed during chronic therapy (see information under Warnings and Precautions).

ADVERSE REACTIONS: Adverse Drug Reaction Overview: The most frequent adverse reactions reported with SANDOSTATIN (octreotide as acetate) and SANDOSTATIN LAR (octreotide as acetate) include gastrointestinal disorders, nervous system disorders, hepatobiliary disorders, and metabolism and nutritional disorders.

Clinical Trial Adverse Drug Reactions: Because clinical trials are conducted under very specific conditions the adverse reaction rates observed in the clinical trials may not reflect the rates observed in practice and should not be compared to the rates in the clinical trials of another drug. Adverse drug reaction information from clinical trials is useful for identifying drug-related adverse events and for approximating rates.

SANDOSTATIN s.c. Ampoules and Multidose Vials in GEP and Acromegaly: See Table 1.

Table 1: SANDOSTATIN

Composite Listing of Adverse Reactions in 196 GEP Endocrine Tumor Patients and 114 Acromegalic Patients Treated with SANDOSTATIN

Adverse Reaction Profile According to Body System	GEP Endocrine Tumor Patients (n=196) %	Acromegalic Patients (n=114) %
Gastrointestinal		
Diarrhea	6.6	57.9
Abdominal Discomfort	4.1	43.9
Stools (Loose)	3.1	36.0
Nausea	8.7	29.8
Flatulence	0.5	13.2
Constipation	1.0	8.8
Abdominal Distention	—	7.9
Stools (Abnormal)	0.5	6.1
Cholelithiasis	<1.0	4.4
Rectal Gas	—	4.4
Vomiting	2.6	4.4
Fatty Stools	3.6	—
Gastrointestinal Bleeding	0.5	—
Rectal Disorders	0.5	—
Hemorrhoids	—	1.8
Cholecystitis	—	1.8
Eructations	—	1.8
Integumentary		
Pain at Injection Site	8.2	9.6
Acne	—	4.4
Bruise	0.5	4.4
Pruritus	—	4.4
Alopecia/Baldness/Hair Loss	1.0	3.5
Musculoskeletal		
Backache/Pain	0.5	4.4
Joint Pain	—	4.4
Arthritis	—	2.6
Arm/Leg Heavy-tired	—	2.6
Leg Ache/Pain	—	2.6
Osteoarthritis	—	1.8
Vertebral Disk Disorder	—	1.8
Twitching	—	1.8
Respiratory		
Throat Pain	0.5	2.6
Flu Symptoms	—	6.1
Cold Symptoms	—	6.1
Sinusitis	—	3.5
Nasal Congestion	—	1.8
Cardiovascular		
Leg Cramps	—	3.5
Dyspnea	—	1.8
Epistaxis	—	1.8
Chest Pain	0.5	—
Edema	1.0	2.6
Ischemic Attack	0.5	—
Hypertension	0.5	—
Thrombophlebitis	0.5	—
Cramps		2.6
Autonomic		
Visual Disturbances	0.5	2.6
Mouth Dry/Furry/Xerostomia	0.5	1.8
Flushing	0.5	1.8
Numbness	—	1.8
Hot Flash	—	1.8
CNS		
Headache	1.5	18.4
Dizziness	1.5	14.9
Fatigue	1.0	9.6
Anxiety/Nervousness	0.5	2.6
Asthenia	0.5	—
Bell's Palsy	0.5	—
Seizure	0.5	—
Depression	0.5	2.6
Sleepiness/Insomnia	0.5	1.8
Weakness	1.0	—
Moody	—	2.6
Appetite Loss	—	1.8
Irritability	—	1.8
Tinnitus	—	1.8
Urogenital		
Urinary Tract Infection	—	6.1
Pollakiuria	—	3.5
Vaginal Infection	—	2.6
Vaginal Itch	—	1.8
Breast Lump	—	1.8
Dysuria	—	1.8
Kidneys, pain in	—	1.8
Polyuria	—	1.8
Prostatitis	—	1.8
Tumor Breast	—	1.8
Hematologic		
Hematoma, injection site	—	9.6
Endocrine		

(cont'd)

Table 1: SANDOSTATIN *(cont'd)*

Composite Listing of Adverse Reactions in 196 GEP Endocrine Tumor Patients and 114 Acromegalic Patients Treated with SANDOSTATIN

Adverse Reaction Profile According to Body System	GEP Endocrine Tumor Patients (n=196) %	Acromegalic Patients (n=114) %
Hypoadrenalism	—	2.6
Hypothyroidism	—	1.8
Hypogonadism	—	1.8
Hypoglycemia	—	1.8
Miscellaneous		
Foot Pain	—	1.8
Fever	—	1.8
Otitis	—	1.8
Weight Gain	—	1.8

Local reactions after s.c. administration of SANDOSTATIN include pain and sensations of stinging, tingling or burning at the site of injection, with redness and swelling. These rarely last more than fifteen minutes. Local discomfort may be reduced by allowing the solution to reach room temperature before injection and by slowly injecting SANDOSTATIN.

In clinical trials, acromegalic patients had a higher incidence of diarrhea, abdominal pain/discomfort, nausea and loose stools than patients treated with SANDOSTATIN s.c. for other indications. It is believed that the primary reason for this observation is that patients who received SANDOSTATIN s.c. for carcinoid syndrome, VIPoma and other gastroenteropancreatic tumors had these gastrointestinal symptoms at baseline and would only report them as adverse events if they became more frequent or severe during SANDOSTATIN s.c. treatment.

The adverse event rate for SANDOSTATIN during study B301 is presented in comparison to placebo (see Table 2). This comparison more accurately reflects the difference in adverse event rates between SANDOSTATIN and placebo.

Table 2: SANDOSTATIN

Number % Patients in U.S. Studies B301, B302, B303 with Adverse Events by Treatment and by Body System. Events Occurring in ≥3%

Specific Adverse Event by Body System	Placebo B301 n=55 (%)	SANDOSTATIN B301 n=60 (%)	SANDOSTATIN B301, B302 & B303 n=114 (%)
Skin			
Pain at injection site	2 (3.6)	5 (8.3)	11 (9.6)
Acne	—	2 (3.3)	5 (4.4)
Bruise	1 (1.1)	2 (3.3)	5 (4.4)
Pruritus	—	—	5 (4.4)
Alopecia/Baldness/Hair Loss	—	—	4 (3.5)
Musculoskeletal			
Backache/Pain	—	—	5 (4.4)
Joint Pain	2 (3.6)	1 (1.7)	5 (4.4)
Respiratory			
Flu Symptoms	—	2 (3.3)	7 (6.1)
Cold Symptoms	—	2 (3.3)	7 (6.1)
Sinusitis	—	—	4 (3.5)
Cardiovascular			
Leg Cramps	—	—	4 (3.5)
Hematologic			
Hematoma, injection site	6 (10.9)	1 (1.7)	11 (9.6)
Gastrointestinal			
Diarrhea	6 (10.9)	32 (53.3)	66 (57.9)
Abdominal Discomfort	7 (12.7)	14 (23.3)	50 (43.9)
Stools (Loose)	8 (14.5)	16 (26.7)	41 (36.0)
Nausea	6 (10.9)	17 (28.3)	34 (29.8)
Flatulence	2 (3.6)	6 (10.0)	15 (13.2)
Constipation	—	1 (1.7)	10 (8.8)
Abdominal Distention	—	2 (3.3)	9 (7.9)
Stools (Abnormal)	—	3 (5.0)	7 (6.1)
Cholelithiasis	—	—	5 (4.4)

(cont'd)

Table 2: SANDOSTATIN *(cont'd)*

Number % Patients in U.S. Studies B301, B302, B303 with Adverse Events by Treatment and by Body System. Events Occurring in ≥3%

Specific Adverse Event by Body System	Placebo B301 n=55 (%)	SANDOSTATIN B301 n=60 (%)	SANDOSTATIN B301, B302 & B303 n=114 (%)
Rectal Gas	—	—	5 (4.4)
Vomiting	1 (1.8)	3 (5.0)	5 (4.4)
Urogenital			
Urinary Tract Infection	—	3 (5.0)	7 (6.1)
Pollakiuria	2 (3.6)	1 (1.7)	4 (3.5)
Central Nervous			
Headache	6 (10.9)	8 (13.3)	21 (18.4)
Dizziness	6 (10.9)	5 (8.3)	17 (14.9)
Fatigue	2 (3.6)	3 (5.0)	11 (9.6)

Gastrointestinal side effects include anorexia, nausea, vomiting, crampy abdominal pain, abdominal bloating, flatulence, loose stools, diarrhea and steatorrhea. Although measured fecal fat excretion may increase, there is no evidence to date that long-term treatment with SANDOSTATIN s.c. has led to nutritional deficiency due to malabsorption. In rare instances, gastrointestinal side effects may resemble acute intestinal obstruction with progressive abdominal distention, severe epigastric pain, abdominal tenderness and guarding. Occurrence of gastrointestinal side effects may be reduced by avoiding meals around the time of SANDOSTATIN s.c. administration, that is, by timing injections between meals or at bedtime.

SANDOSTATIN s.c. Ampoules and Multidose Vials in the Prevention of Complications Following Pancreatic Surgery: Local reactions at the site of injection were the most frequently reported side effects in 247 patients undergoing pancreatic surgery treated with SANDOSTATIN s.c. for 7 consecutive days starting on the day of the operation, at least 1 hour before laparatomy. Pruritus, exanthema, vomiting, biliary sludge and fever were each reported in 0.4 % of patients and flushes and rash occurred in 0.8% of patients.

SANDOSTATIN Ampoules and Multidose Vials in Bleeding Gastro-oesophageal Varices: Raised blood glucose levels were reported in 23 of 98 cirrhotic patients treated with SANDOSTATIN 25 µg/hour administered by i.v. infusion over 5 days for the emergency management of bleeding oesophageal varices. Diarrhea occurred in 5% of patients.

SANDOSTATIN LAR (Octreotide for Injectable Suspension) in Acromegaly: No clinical studies have been performed which compare SANDOSTATIN LAR to placebo. However, the profile of adverse reactions recorded in acromegalic patients treated with SANDOSTATIN LAR was similar to that known for SANDOSTATIN s.c., administration. Local injection site reactions to SANDOSTATIN may occur and are usually mild and of short duration. These reactions include pain, and rarely swelling and rash. In the double blind studies, gastrointestinal side effects following administration of SANDOSTATIN LAR were the most frequent adverse events and included abdominal pain, diarrhea (loose stools), flatulence and steatorrheic stools.

Adverse events occurring in ≥2% of patients who participated in the major studies in acromegaly (including their long-term extensions of up to 30 months duration) are listed in Table 3, by dose group. It should be noted that some patients may appear under multiple dose levels since some patients switched dose levels.

Table 3: SANDOSTATIN LAR

Adverse Events Occurring in ≥2% of Patients Treated with SANDOSTATIN LAR

Adverse Event	Dose Level		
	10 mg n=57 (%)	20 mg n=233 (%)	30 mg n=129 (%)
Application Site			
Injection Site Pain	1.8	9.0	10.9
Injection Site Reaction	—	2.1	3.9
Body as a Whole			
Influenza-like Symptoms	8.8	10.3	17.8
Fatigue	3.5	5.2	11.6
Pain	1.8	5.6	2.3
Surgery	3.5	2.1	6.2
Back Pain	1.8	3.4	2.3
Asthenia	3.5	1.3	4.7
Edema	1.8	3.0	1.6
Malaise	1.8	1.3	3.9
Accidental Trauma	3.5	1.3	2.3
Hot Flushes	—	2.6	1.6
Tumor nos.	—	0.9	3.1
Fever	—	0.9	3.1
Cardiovascular			
Hypertension	1.8	9.9	7.0

(cont'd)

Table 3: SANDOSTATIN LAR *(cont'd)*

Adverse Events Occurring in ≥2% of Patients Treated with SANDOSTATIN LAR

	Dose Level		
Adverse Event	**10 mg n=57 (%)**	**20 mg n=233 (%)**	**30 mg n=129 (%)**
CNS and Peripheral			
Headache	7.0	8.6	12.4
Dizziness	5.3	6.0	10.1
Paresthesia	1.8	3.4	7.0
Cramps	1.8	3.4	3.9
Vertigo	3.5	1.7	1.6
Gastrointestinal			
Diarrhea	7.0	21.5	30.2
Abdominal Pain	12.3	15.0	25.6
Flatulence	12.3	12.4	23.3
Constipation	14.0	8.2	14.7
Nausea	3.5	4.3	7.8
Vomiting	1.8	3.0	6.2
Dyspepsia	1.8	3.0	3.9
Steatorrhea	5.3	1.3	4.7
Feces Discolored	—	2.6	3.9
Tenesmus	—	0.9	3.9
Liver and Biliary			
Cholelithiasis	3.5	7.3	12.4
Gallbladder Disorder	—	3.9	7.0
Musculoskeletal			
Arthralgia	—	2.6	6.2
Arthropathy	—	3.0	4.7
Myalgia	1.8	2.1	3.9
Back Pain	—	3.0	0.8
Pain Leg(s)	3.5	0.9	0.8
Psychiatric Disorder			
Insomnia	3.5	3.9	1.6
Anxiety	—	1.3	4.7
Depression	—	2.1	1.6
Somnolence	1.8	0.4	2.3
Nervousness	1.8	0.4	2.3
Resistance Mechanism			
Infection Viral	1.8	2.6	3.9
Abscess	—	2.1	1.6
Infection	1.8	1.7	2.3
Respiratory			
URTI	3.5	3.4	4.7
Coughing	1.8	4.3	3.1
Pharyngitis	1.8	4.3	3.1
Rhinitis	—	—	5.4

(cont'd)

Table 3: SANDOSTATIN LAR *(cont'd)*

Adverse Events Occurring in ≥2% of Patients Treated with SANDOSTATIN LAR

	Dose Level		
Adverse Event	**10 mg n=57 (%)**	**20 mg n=233 (%)**	**30 mg n=129 (%)**
Bronchitis	1.8	3.0	1.6
Respiratory Disorder	1.8	1.3	3.1
Sinusitis	1.8	0.9	2.3
Urinary			
UTI	1.8	2.1	3.1
Cystitis	—	0.9	2.3
Dysuria	—	0.4	2.3
Micturition Frequency	—	—	2.3
Skin and Appendages			
Sweating Increased	1.8	3.4	4.7
Pruritus	1.8	1.3	4.7
Alopecia	1.8	0.9	3.9
Rash Erythematosus	—	2.6	0.8
Rash	3.5	—	—
Other			
Anemia	5.3	6.4	17.1
Conjunctivitis	—	2.1	3.1
Ear Disorder	—	—	2.3
Menstrual Disorder	—	1.3	2.3
Neoplasm, surgery	—	—	2.3

Other Adverse Events (regardless of relationship) Occurring at an 1% ≥ Incidence <2% Reported in the Major Studies in Acromegaly (all doses combined): Body as a Whole: edema peripheral, syncope.
Cardiovascular: hypertension aggravated.
Central and Peripheral Nervous Systems: cramps, vertigo, neuralgia, cramps legs, neuropathy, hyperkinesia.
Endocrine: growth hormone overproduction, hypothyroidism, goiter.
Gastrointestinal System: gastritis, hemorrhoids, gastroenteritis, hemorrhage rectum, hernia, eructation, gastrointestinal disorder, stomatitis ulcerative.
Hearing and Vestibular: deafness, ear discharge.
Heart Rate and Rhythm: tachycardia.
Liver and Biliary: hepatitis, liver fatty.
Metabolic and Nutritional: weight increase, hypoglycemia.
Musculoskeletal System: arthrosis, surgery, bone fracture, osteonecrosis.
Platelet, Bleeding and Clotting: epistaxis.
Psychiatric: amnesia, sleep disorder.
Red Blood Cell: anemia hypochromic.
Reproductive Disorders: Female: breast pain female, intermenstrual bleeding, lactation non purperal. Male: prostate disorder.
Resistance Mechanism: moniliasis, otitis media, pharyngitis, tonsillitis, herpes simplex, herpes zoster.
Respiratory System: dyspnea, pneumonia.
Skin and Appendages: skin disorder, skin dry, acne, nail disorder.
Urinary System: urinary tract infection, cystitis, dysuria, micturition frequency.
Vascular (Extracardiac): phlebitis, cerebrovascular, vein varicose.
Carcinoid Tumors: No clinical studies have been performed which compare SANDOSTATIN LAR to placebo. However, the profile of adverse reactions recorded in patients with carcinoid tumors treated with SANDOSTATIN LAR was similar to that known for SANDOSTATIN s.c. administration. In a 6-month study during which patients with carcinoid tumors were treated with either SANDOSTATIN LAR i.m. at 4-week intervals or SANDOSTATIN s.c. t.i.d., gastrointestinal side effects were the most frequently reported adverse events in both groups and included abdominal pain, diarrhea (loose stools), constipation, flatulence nausea and vomiting. The incidences of these adverse events were similar between the 10, 20 and 30 mg dosages of SANDOSTATIN LAR.

Local injection site reactions to SANDOSTATIN may occur and are usually mild and of short duration. These reactions include pain, and rarely swelling and rash.

General: Prolonged use of SANDOSTATIN s.c. or SANDOSTATIN LAR may result in gallstone formation (see Warnings and Precautions). Pancreatitis may develop in patients on long-term treatment with SANDOSTATIN who develop cholelithiasis.

Because of its inhibitory action on growth hormone, glucagon and insulin, SANDOSTATIN s.c. or SANDOSTATIN LAR may impair glucose regulation. Postprandial glucose tolerance may be impaired and in some instances, with chronic administration, a state of persistent hyperglycemia may be induced. Hypoglycemia has also been observed.

Acute pancreatitis has been reported in rare instances. Generally, this effect is seen within the first hours or days of SANDOSTATIN s.c. treatment and resolves on withdrawal of the drug.

Rarely, hair loss has been reported in patients receiving SANDOSTATIN s.c. and SANDOSTATIN LAR treatment.

Rarely, hypersensitivity reactions have been reported.

Isolated reports of anaphylactic reactions have been reported. SANDOSTATIN administered s.c. and to a much lesser degree by i.v. infusion, can lead to hypersensitivity reaction that may range from generalized pruritus to cardiovascular shock or bronchospasm, with one case of death having been reported.

Isolated reports of bradycardia have been reported. In patients who are predisposed by having relatively low pretreatment heart rates or whose cardiovascular system is already compromised, as in cirrhotic patients with bleeding esophageal varices, it is of importance that physicians be alerted to the possible undesirable effect of bradycardia. Tachycardia has also been observed.

There have been isolated reports of hepatic dysfunctions associated with SANDOSTATIN s.c. and SANDOSTATIN LAR administration. These consist of the following:

- acute hepatitis without cholestasis and normalization of transaminase values on withdrawal of SANDOSTATIN s.c. has occurred;
- the slow development of hyperbilirubinemia in association with elevation of alkaline phosphatase, gamma glutamyl transferase and, to a lesser extent, transaminases.

Rarely, dehydration has been reported.

Post-Market Adverse Drug Reactions: Spontaneously reported adverse drug reactions are presented below. Because these events are reported voluntarily from a population of uncertain size, it is not always possible to reliably estimate their frequency or clearly establish a causal relationship to SANDOSTATIN or SANDOSTATIN LAR exposure.

Cardiac Disorders: arrhythmias.

Hepato-biliary Disorders: acute pancreatitis, acute hepatitis without cholestasis, cholestatic hepatitis, cholestasis, jaundice, cholestatic jaundice.

Hypersensitivity: anaphylaxis, allergy/hypersensitivity reactions.

Investigations: increased alkaline phosphatase levels, increased gamma glutamyl transferase level.

Skin and Subcutaneous Tissue Disorders: urticaria.

Gastrointestinal Motility Disorder: ileus, intestinal obstruction.

DRUG INTERACTIONS: Drug-Drug Interactions: Many patients with carcinoid syndrome or VIPomas being treated with SANDOSTATIN s.c. have also been, or are being, treated with many other drugs to control the symptomatology or progression of the disease, generally without serious drug interaction. Included are chemotherapeutic agents, H_2 antagonists, antimotility agents, drugs affecting glycemic states, solutions for electrolyte and fluid support or hyperalimentation, antihypertensive diuretics and anti-diarrheal agents.

Where symptoms are severe and SANDOSTATIN therapy is added to other therapies used to control glycemic states, such as sulfonylureas, insulin and diazoxide, to beta blockers, calcium channel blockers or to agents for the control of fluid and electrolyte balance, patients must be monitored closely and adjustment made in the other therapies as the symptoms of the disease are controlled. Evidence currently available suggests these imbalances in fluid and electrolytes or glycemic states are secondary to correction of pre-existing abnormalities and not to a direct metabolic action of SANDOSTATIN. Adjustment of the dosage of drugs, such as insulin, affecting glucose metabolism may be required following initiation of SANDOSTATIN therapy in patients with diabetes.

Since SANDOSTATIN has been associated with alterations in nutrient absorption, its effect on absorption of any orally administered drugs should be carefully considered. A single case of transplant rejection episode (renal/whole pancreas) in a patient immunosuppressed with cyclosporine has been reported. SANDOSTATIN treatment to reduce exocrine secretion and close a fistula in this patient resulted in decreases in blood levels of cyclosporine and may have contributed to the rejection episode. SANDOSTATIN has also been found to delay the intestinal absorption of cyclosporine or cimetidine.

Concomitant administration of octreotide and bromocriptine increases the bioavailability of bromocriptine.

Limited published data indicate that somatostatin analogs might decrease the metabolic clearance of compounds known to be metabolized by cytochrome P450 enzymes, which may be due to the suppression of growth hormone. Since it cannot be excluded that octreotide may have this effect, other drugs mainly metabolized by the CYP 3A4 and which have a low therapeutic index should therefore be used with caution (e.g. terfenadine, quinidine).

Drug-Food Interactions: Interactions with food have not been established.

Drug-Herb Interactions: Interactions with herbal products have not been established.

Drug-Laboratory Test Interactions: No known interference exists with clinical laboratory tests, including amine or peptide determinations.

DOSAGE AND ADMINISTRATION:

Dosing Considerations: Parenteral drug products should be inspected visually for particulate matter and discoloration prior to administration. **Do not use if particulates and/or discoloration are observed.**

Recommended Dose and Dosage Adjustment: SANDOSTATIN s.c. Ampoules and Multidose Vials: Subcutaneous injection is the recommended route of administration of SANDOSTATIN (octreotide acetate) for control of symptoms in most instances. Intravenous bolus injections have been used under emergency conditions. Multiple injections at the same site within short periods of time should be avoided. The initial dosage is 50 µg, administered subcutaneously, once or twice daily. Thereafter, the number of injections and dosage may be increased gradually based on patient tolerability, clinical response and effects on levels of tumour-produced hormones (in cases of carcinoid tumors on the urinary excretion of 5-hydroxyindole-acetic acid). Dosage information for patients with specific tumors is listed below. The drug is usually given in a b.i.d or t.i.d schedule.

Carcinoid Tumors: The suggested daily dosage of SANDOSTATIN during the first two weeks of therapy ranges from 100 to 600 µg per day in two to four divided doses (mean daily dosage is 300 µg). In the clinical studies, the **median** daily maintenance dosage was approximately 450 µg, but clinical and biochemical benefits were obtained in some patients with as little as 50 µg, while others required doses up to 1500 µg per day. However, experience with doses above 750 µg per day is limited.

VIPomas: Daily dosages of 200 to 300 µg in two to four divided doses are recommended during the initial 2 weeks of therapy (range 150 to 750 µg) to control symptoms of the disease. On an individual basis, dosage may be adjusted to achieve a therapeutic response, but usually doses above 450 µg per day are not required.

Acromegaly: Daily dosages of 100 µg to 300 µg b.i.d. or t.i.d. are recommended at the beginning of treatment. Dosage adjustment should be based on monthly assessment of GH levels and clinical symptoms, and on tolerability. In most patients, the optimal daily dose will be 200 to 300 µg per day. A maximum dose of 1500 µg should not be exceeded.

If no relevant reduction of GH levels and no improvement of clinical symptoms have been achieved within 3 months of starting treatment with SANDOSTATIN, therapy should be discontinued.

Prevention of Complications Following Pancreatic Surgery: Daily dosage of 100 µg t.i.d., administered subcutaneously, for 7 consecutive days starting on the day of the operation at least one hour before laparatomy.

Bleeding Gastro-oesophageal Varices in Patients with Cirrhosis: The recommended dose of SANDOSTATIN is 25 µg/hour by continuous i.v. infusion for 48 hours. In patients with high risk of rebleeding, infusion should be maintained up to a maximum of 5 days.

Immediately prior to use, the contents of the ampoule or multidose vial should be diluted in physiological saline. The volume of dilution will depend on the infusion system used and should be adjusted to ensure a continuous infusion of SANDOSTATIN at the recommended rate. Once diluted, the solution should be used within 24 hours. Discard unused portion.

As with all parenteral drugs, i.v. admixtures should be inspected visually for clarity, particulate matter, precipitation, discoloration and leakage prior to administration, whenever solution and container permit.

SANDOSTATIN LAR (Octreotide For Injectable Suspension): SANDOSTATIN LAR may only be administered by deep intragluteal injection. The site of repeat intragluteal injection should be alternated between the left and right gluteal muscle.

SANDOSTATIN LAR (octreotide acetate for injectable suspension) must be administered under the supervision of a physician. **Do not directly inject diluent without preparing suspension.** It is important to closely follow the mixing instructions included in the packaging. SANDOSTATIN LAR must be administered immediately after mixing. SANDOSTATIN LAR should be administered intragluteally at four week intervals. Administration of SANDOSTATIN LAR at intervals greater than 4 weeks is not recommended because there is no adequate information on whether such patients could be satisfactorily controlled. Deltoid injections are to be avoided because of significant discomfort at the injection site when given in that area. **SANDOSTATIN LAR should never be administered by the IV or S.C. routes.** The following dosage regimens are recommended.

Acromegaly: For patients who are adequately controlled with SANDOSTATIN s.c., it is recommended to start treatment with the administration of 20 mg SANDOSTATIN LAR at four week intervals for three months. Treatment with SANDOSTATIN LAR can be started the day after the last dose of s.c. SANDOSTATIN. Subsequent dosage adjustments should be based upon serum growth hormone (GH) and insulin-like growth factor 1/somatomedin C (IGF 1) concentrations and clinical symptoms.

For patients in whom, within this three month period, clinical symptoms and biochemical parameters (GH, IGF 1) are not fully controlled (GH concentrations still above 2.5 µg/L) the dose may be increased to 30 mg every four weeks.

For patients whose serum GH concentrations are consistently below 1 µg/L, whose IGF 1 serum concentrations normalized, and in whom most reversible signs/symptoms of acromegaly have disappeared after three months of treatment with 20 mg, 10 mg SANDOSTATIN LAR may be administered every four weeks. However, particularly in this group of patients, it is recommended to closely monitor adequate control of serum GH and IGF 1 concentrations and clinical signs/symptoms at this low dose of SANDOSTATIN LAR.

For patients in whom surgery, radiotherapy or dopamine agonist treatment is inappropriate, or in the interim period until radiotherapy becomes fully effective, a short test dosing of SANDOSTATIN s.c. is recommended to assess the response and systemic tolerability of octreotide prior to initiating treatment with SANDOSTATIN LAR as described above.

Carcinoid Tumors and VIPomas: Patients not currently treated with SANDOSTATIN s.c. should begin therapy with SANDOSTATIN s.c. The suggested daily dose during the first two weeks of therapy ranges from 100-600 µg/day in 2-4 divided doses (mean daily dose is 300 µg). Some patients may require doses up to 1500 µg/day. The suggested daily dose for VIPomas is 200-300 µg in 2-4 divided doses (range 150-750 µg); dosage may be adjusted on an individual basis to control symptoms but usually doses above 450 µg/day are not required.

SANDOSTATIN s.c. should be continued for at least 2 weeks. Thereafter, patients who are considered "responders" to octreotide acetate and who tolerate the drug may be switched to SANDOSTATIN LAR in the dosage regimen described below.

Patients currently receiving SANDOSTATIN s.c. can be switched to SANDOSTATIN LAR in a dosage of 20 mg i.m. intragluteally at 4-week intervals for 2 months. Gluteal injection sites should be alternated to avoid irritation. Because of the need for serum octreotide to reach therapeutically effective levels following initial injection of SANDOSTATIN LAR, carcinoid tumor and VIPoma patients should continue to receive SANDOSTATIN s.c. for at least two weeks in the same dosage they were taking before the switch. Failure to continue s.c. injections for this period may result in exacerbation of symptoms. Some patients may require 3 or 4 weeks of such therapy.

After two months of a 20 mg dosage of SANDOSTATIN LAR, dosage may be increased to 30 mg every 4 weeks if symptoms are not adequately controlled. Patients who achieve good control on a 20 mg dose may have their dose lowered to 10 mg for a trial period. If symptoms recur, dosage should then be increased to 20 mg every 4 weeks. A dose of 10 mg is not recommended as a starting dose, however, because therapeutically effective levels of octreotide are reached more rapidly with a 20 mg dose.

Dosages higher than 30 mg are not recommended because there is no information on their usefulness.

Despite good overall control of symptoms, patients with carcinoid tumors and VIPomas often experience periodic exacerbation of symptoms (regardless of whether they are being maintained on SANDOSTATIN s.c. or SANDOSTATIN LAR). During these periods they may be given SANDOSTATIN s.c. for a few days at the dosage they were receiving prior to switch to SANDOSTATIN LAR. When symptoms are again controlled, SANDOSTATIN s.c. can be discontinued.

Administration: Preparation of SANDOSTATIN LAR (Octreotide [as acetate] for Injectable Suspension): SANDOSTATIN LAR is supplied in kits containing: One vial of SANDOSTATIN LAR 10 mg, 20 mg or 30 mg octreotide [as acetate] for injectable suspension (microspheres for depot suspension). One prefilled syringe containing the diluent. One 19G×1.5" (40 mm) standard needle for transfer and drug product reconstitution. One 19G×1.5" (38.1 mm) safety injection needle. And one instruction booklet.

Follow the instructions below carefully to ensure complete saturation of the powder and its uniform suspension before i.m. injection.

SANDOSTATIN LAR suspension must only be prepared **immediately** before administration. SANDOSTATIN LAR should only be administered by a trained health professional.

1. Before handling the component, allow the SANDOSTATIN LAR vial and pre-filled syringe with diluent to **reach room temperature** (approximately 30 to 60 minutes) and wash your hands with soap and hot water.
   Place the package on a clean and flat surface.
   Remove the flip off cap from the vial containing SANDOSTATIN LAR.
   Assure that the powder is settled at the bottom of the vial by lightly tapping the vial.
2. Remove the cap from the pre-filled syringe with diluent. Attach the **standard needle "c"** supplied for reconstitution to the pre-filled syringe with diluent.
   Note: **Make sure NOT to use the safety injection needle** at this stage.
3. Clean the rubber stopper of the vial with an alcohol swab.
   Insert the needle through the centre of the rubber stopper of the Sandostatin LAR vial.
4. Without disturbing the SANDOSTATIN LAR powder, **gently inject the diluent into the vial by running the diluent down the inside wall of the vial.** Do not inject the diluent directly into the powder.
   Withdraw the needle from the vial. To avoid contamination please make sure not to expose the needle to surfaces.
5. **Do not disturb the vial** until the diluent has totally wetted the SANDOSTATIN LAR powder (approximately 2-5 minutes). **Without inverting the vial**, check the powder on the walls and bottom of the vial. If dry spots exist, allow undisturbed wetting to continue. At this stage, prepare the patient for injection.
6. Once complete wetting has occurred, the vial should be moderately swirled for a minimum of 30 seconds **until a uniform milky suspension is achieved. Do not vigorously shake the vial** as this may cause the suspension to flocculate, making it unusable.
7. Immediately re-insert the needle through the rubber stopper and then, with the bevel down and the vial tipped at approximately 45 degree angle, slowly draw the contents of the vial into the syringe. **Do not invert the vial** when filling the syringe as this may affect the amount withdrawn.
   It is normal for a small amount of residual suspension to remain on the walls and bottom of the vial. This is a calculated overfill.
8. Remove the needle for transfer from the syringe and immediately attach the safety injection needle to the syringe.
9. Remove the protective needle cover, gently invert the syringe as needed to maintain a uniform suspension and expel any air from the syringe.
   The drug is now ready for administration. The administration must occur immediately after the suspension has been prepared.
10. Clean the injection site with an alcohol swab. Insert needle into the right or left gluteus and draw back to ensure that no blood vessel has been penetrated. Inject slowly i.m. by deep intragluteal injection with steady pressure.
    SANDOSTATIN LAR must be given only by deep intragluteal injection, never i.v.
11. Using a single handed operation, activate the safety system of the needle
    - either with help of a rigid surface, e.g. table
    - or with a finger, e.g. forefinger making sure always to keep all fingers behind the needle tip.

    An audible "clic" confirms the proper activation of the safety mechanism.
    Immediately dispose of properly all packaging and devices implemented for the preparation and administration of the drug product into an approved sharp container.

SANDOSTATIN LAR must be given only by deep intragluteal injection, never intravenously. If a blood vessel has been penetrated, another injection site must be selected. The site of repeat intragluteal injection should be alternated between the left and right gluteal muscle. Do not use the same gluteal region each time (every 4 weeks).

As with all parenteral admixtures, the constituted product should be examined for the presence of foreign particulate matter, agglomeration or discolouration. Any defective units should be discarded.

Reconstitution: Parenteral Products: Solution for continuous i.v. infusion: Immediately prior to use, the contents of the ampoule or multidose vial should be diluted in physiological saline. The volume of dilution will depend on the infusion system used and should be adjusted to ensure a continuous infusion of SANDOSTATIN at a rate of 25 µg/hour. The following are examples of dilutions which may be used: see Table 4.

Table 4: SANDOSTATIN

Examples of Dilutions

SANDOSTATIN			Volume of Physiological Saline	Approximate Available Volume mL	Nominal Concentration µg/mL	Infusion Rate mL/h (µg/h)
Concentration µg/mL	Size mL	Volume mL				
500	1	1	49	50	10	2.5 (25)
200	5	2.5	47.5	50	10	2.5 (25)
200	5	3	93	96	6.25	4 (25)

As with all parenteral drugs, i.v. admixtures should be inspected visually for clarity, particulate matter, precipitation, discoloration and leakage prior to administration, whenever solution and container permit.

SANDOSTATIN diluted in physiological saline is stable for 24 hours when stored at room temperature. Discard unused portion.

Octreotide acetate is not stable in Total Parenteral Nutrition (TPN) solutions.

OVERDOSAGE:

SANDOSTATIN s.c. Ampoules and Multidose Vials: A limited number of accidental overdoses of SANDOSTATIN in adults and children have been reported. In adults, the doses ranged from 2400-6000 µg/day administered by continuous infusion (100-250 µg/hour) or subcutaneously (1500 µg t.i.d.). The adverse events reported were arrhythmia, hypotension, cardiac arrest, brain hypoxia, pancreatitis, hepatitis steatosis, diarrhoea, weakness, lethargy, weight loss, hepatomegaly, and lactic acidosis.

In children, the doses ranged from 50-3000 µg/day administered by continuous infusion (2.1-500 µg/hour) or subcutaneously (50-100 µg). The only adverse event reported was mild hyperglycaemia.

No unexpected adverse events have been reported in cancer patients receiving SANDOSTATIN at doses of 3000-30 000 µg/day in divided doses subcutaneously.

The management of overdosage is symptomatic.

SANDOSTATIN LAR (Octreotide for Injectable Suspension): A limited number of accidental overdoses of SANDOSTATIN LAR have been reported. The doses ranged from 100 mg to 163 mg/month of SANDOSTATIN LAR. The only adverse event reported was hot flushes.

Cancer patients receiving doses of SANDOSTATIN LAR up to 60 mg/month and up to 90 mg/2 weeks have been reported. These doses were in general well tolerated; however, the following adverse events have been reported: frequent urination, fatigue, depression, anxiety, and lack of concentration.

The management of overdosage is symptomatic.

For management of a suspected drug overdose, CPhA recommends that you contact your **regional Poison Control Centre**. See the *CPS* Directory section for a list of Poison Control Centres.

ACTION AND CLINICAL PHARMACOLOGY: Mechanism of Action: General: Octreotide acetate is a synthetic octapeptide analogue of naturally occurring somatostatin with similar pharmacological effects, but with a prolonged duration of action. It inhibits pathologically increased secretion of growth hormone (GH) and of peptides and serotonin produced within the gastro-entero-pancreatic (GEP) endocrine system.

In normal healthy subjects, octreotide acetate has been shown to inhibit:

- Release of growth hormone (GH) stimulated by arginine infusion, exercise and insulin-induced hypoglycemia.
- Postprandial release of insulin, glucagon, gastrin, other peptides of the GEP endocrine system, and arginine-stimulated release of insulin and glucagon.
- Thyrotropin releasing hormone (TRH) stimulated release of thyroid stimulating hormone (TSH). The precise mode of action of octreotide acetate on portal hypertension is still unclear. It is thought to reduce splanchnic blood flow primarily by inhibiting vasoactive gastrointestinal hormone secretion and exerting a direct vasomotor effect on splanchnic vessels, thus reducing portal blood flow. Using human sephanous veins, it has been shown that vasoconstriction is mediated by type 2 somatostatin receptors.

Pharmacokinetics: SANDOSTATIN s.c. Ampoules and Multidose Vials: After subcutaneous (s.c.) injection of SANDOSTATIN, octreotide acetate is rapidly and completely absorbed. Peak plasma concentrations are reached within 30 minutes. The half-life after subcutaneous administration is 100 minutes. After intravenous injection the elimination is biphasic with α and β half-lives of approximately 10 and 90 minutes, respectively. The volume of distribution is 0.4 L/Kg body weight and the total body clearance is 160 mL/min. Plasma protein binding amounts to 65% with only negligible amounts bound to red blood cells.

SANDOSTATIN LAR (Octreotide as acetate for Injectable Suspension): In patients with acromegaly, SANDOSTATIN LAR, a galenical formulation of octreotide consisting of microspheres for depot suspension suitable for repeat intramuscular administration at intervals of four weeks, delivers consistent and therapeutic octreotide serum concentrations thus consistently lowering GH and normalizing IGF-1 serum concentrations in the majority of patients.

In patients with carcinoid tumors and Vasoactive Intestinal Peptide Tumors (VIPomas), treatment with SANDOSTATIN LAR provides continuous control of symptoms related to the underlying disease.

The pharmacokinetic profile of octreotide acetate after injection of SANDOSTATIN LAR reflects the release profile from the polymer matrix and its biodegradation. Once released into the systemic circulation, octreotide distributes according to its known pharmacokinetic properties as described above for SANDOSTATIN administered subcutaneously.

After single intramuscular injections of SANDOSTATIN LAR, the serum octreotide concentration reaches a transient initial peak within one hour after administration followed by progressive decrease to a low undetectable octreotide level within 24 hours. After this initial peak on the first day, octreotide remains at sub-therapeutic levels in the majority of patients for the following seven days. Thereafter, octreotide concentrations increase again, and reach plateau concentrations around day 14 and remain relatively constant during the following three to four weeks. The peak level during day 1 is lower than levels during the plateau phase and no more than 0.5% of the total drug release occurs during day 1. After about day 42, the octreotide concentration decreases slowly, concomitantly with the terminal degradation phase of the polymer matrix dosage form.

In patients with acromegaly, plateau octreotide concentrations after single doses of 10 mg, 20 mg and 30 mg of SANDOSTATIN LAR are 358, 926 and 1710 pg/mL, respectively. Steady state octreotide concentrations reached after three injections at four week intervals, are higher by a factor of approximately 1.6 to 1.8 reaching 1557 and 2384 pg/mL after multiple injections of 20 and 30 mg SANDOSTATIN LAR, respectively.

In patients with carcinoid tumors, the mean octreotide serum concentrations after six doses of 10 mg, 20 mg and 30 mg of SANDOSTATIN LAR administered by intramuscular injection every four weeks were 1231 pg/mL, 2620 pg/mL and 3928 pg/mL, respectively. Concentrations were dose proportional and steady-state concentrations were reached after two injections of 20 and 30 mg and after three injections of 10 mg.

In patients with acromegaly, no accumulation of octreotide beyond that expected from overlapping release profiles occurred over a period of up to 28 monthly SANDOSTATIN LAR injections.

STORAGE AND STABILITY: SANDOSTATIN s.c. Ampoules and Multidose Vials: Ampoules: For prolonged storage, SANDOSTATIN ampoules must be stored at 2 to 8°C.

Keep container in the outer carton in order to protect from light. Do not freeze.

Keep in a safe place out of the reach of children and pets.

Multidose Vials: For prolonged storage, SANDOSTATIN multidose vials must be stored at 2 to 8°C.

Keep container in the outer carton in order to protect from light. Do not freeze.

For day-to-day use, both the ampoules and the multidose vials may be stored at room temperature for up to 2 weeks; they must be protected from light. The ampoules should be opened just prior to administration and any unused portion discarded.

Keep in a safe place out of the reach of children and pets.

SANDOSTATIN LAR (Octreotide for Injectable Suspension): The SANDOSTATIN LAR vials must be stored at 2 to 8°C. Keep vial in the outer carton in order to protect it from light. The vials can remain at room temperature on the day of the injection. However the suspension must only be prepared immediately prior to i.m. injection.

Store the pre-filled syringe with 2.5 mL diluent at 2 to 8°C.

The SANDOSTATIN LAR powder, once suspended in the diluent, should be used immediately.

Keep in a safe place out of the reach of children and pets.

INFORMATION FOR THE PATIENT: Published in e-CPS, available by subscription at www.e-cps.ca.

DOSAGE FORMS, COMPOSITION AND PACKAGING: SANDOSTATIN: Ampoules: Each ampoule contains: octreotide (as acetate) 50 µg, 100 µg or 500 µg. Nonmedicinal ingredients: lactic acid and mannitol. Sodium hydrogen carbonate is added to provide a buffered solution pH 4.2±0.2. Ampoules of 1 mL, boxes of 5.

Multidose Vials: Each multidose vial contains: octreotide (as acetate) 1000 µg (200 µg/mL). Nonmedicinal ingredients: lactic acid, mannitol and phenol. Sodium hydrogen carbonate is added to provide a buffered solution pH 4.2±0.2. Vials of 5 mL.

SANDOSTATIN LAR: Each kit contains: 1 single dose vial of octreotide (as acetate) slow release 10, 20 or 30 mg; 1 glass pre-filled syringe containing 2.5 mL of diluent; one 19G×1.5" (40 mm) standard needle for transfer and drug product reconstitution, one 19G×1.5" (38.1 mm) safety injection needle; and an instruction booklet. Nonmedicinal ingredients: mannitol and poly (DL-actide-co-glycolide); diluent: mannitol, sodium carboxymethylcellulose and water for injection.

(Shown in Product Identification Section)

Sandoz® Alfuzosin ℞

alfuzosin HCl

Symptomatic Treatment of Benign Prostatic Hyperplasia (BPH)—Adjunctive Therapy in Acute Urinary Retention (AUR)

Sandoz

SUPPLIED: Each once-daily, prolonged-release, three-layer, round and biconvex tablet, contains: alfuzosin hydrochloride 10 mg in a white matrix layer between two inactive yellow layers. Nonmedicinal ingredients: colloidal hydrated silica, ethylcellulose, hydrogenated castor oil, hydroxypropyl methylcellulose (hypromellose), magnesium stearate, mannitol, microcrystalline cellulose, povidone and yellow ferric oxide. High density polyethylene (HDPE) bottles of 100. Store between 15 and 30°C.

Sandoz® Amiodarone ℞

amiodarone HCl

Antiarrhythmic

Sandoz

SUPPLIED: Each pink, round, biconvex tablet, embossed with "R-200" on one side and scored on the other side, contains: amiodarone HCl 200 mg. Nonmedicinal ingredients: anhydrous colloidal silica, colloidal silicon dioxide, corn starch, erythrosine, lactose, magnesium stearate and polyvidone. HDPE bottles of 100. Store at room temperature (15 to 30°C). Protect from light.

Sandoz® Amlodipine ℞

amlodipine besylate

Antihypertensive—Antianginal

Sandoz

SUPPLIED: 2.5 mg: Each white or almost white, oblong, beveled tablet, with "2.5" coded on one tablet face, contains: amlodipine besylate equivalent to amlodipine 2.5 mg. Nonmedicinal ingredients: calcium hydrogen phosphate anhydrous, magnesium stearate, microcrystalline cellulose and sodium starch glycolate. HDPE bottles of 100. Store between 15 and 30°C. Protect from light.

5 mg: Each white or almost white, octagonal, scored tablet, debossed on one tablet face as "AML 5", contains: amlodipine besylate equivalent to amlodipine 5 mg. Nonmedicinal ingredients: calcium hydrogen phosphate anhydrous, magnesium stearate, microcrystalline cellulose and sodium starch glycolate. HDPE bottles of 100 and 500. Store between 15 and 30°C. Protect from light.

10 mg: Each white or almost white, octagonal, scored tablet, debossed on one tablet face as "AML 10", contains: amlodipine besylate equivalent to amlodipine 10 mg. Nonmedicinal ingredients: calcium hydrogen phosphate anhydrous, magnesium stearate, microcrystalline cellulose and sodium starch glycolate. HDPE bottles of 100 and 500. Store between 15 and 30°C. Protect from light.

Sandoz® Anagrelide ℞

anagrelide HCl

Platelet-reducing Agent

Sandoz

SUPPLIED: Each white, opaque capsule and body imprinted with "E155" in black ink, contains: anagrelide HCl equivalent to anagrelide base 0.5 mg. Nonmedicinal ingredients: black iron oxide, crospovidone, gelatin, lactose monohydrate, magnesium stearate, microcrystalline cellulose, pregelatinized starch and titanium dioxide. Bottles of 100. Store between 15 and 25°C, in a light-resistant container.

Sandoz® Anuzinc

zinc sulfate monohydrate

Anorectal Therapy

Sandoz

Sandoz® Anuzinc HC ℞

hydrocortisone acetate—zinc sulfate monohydrate

Anorectal Therapy

Sandoz

Sandoz® Anuzinc HC Plus ℞

pramoxine HCl—hydrocortisone acetate—zinc sulfate monohydrate

Anorectal Therapy

Sandoz

SUPPLIED: Sandoz Anuzinc: Ointment: Each tube contains: zinc sulfate monohydrate 0.5%. Nonmedicinal ingredients: light mineral oil and petrolatum. Tubes of 30 g with applicator. Store in a cool place under 22°C.

Suppositories: Each suppository contains: zinc sulfate monohydrate 10 mg. Nonmedicinal ingredients: triglyceride base. Boxes of 12 and 24. Store in a cool place under 22°C.

Sandoz Anuzinc HC: Ointment: Each g contains: hydrocortisone acetate 5 mg and zinc sulfate monohydrate 5 mg. Nonmedicinal ingredients: methylparaben, mineral oil (petrolatum) and propylparaben. Tubes of 15 g and 30 g with applicator. Store between 15 and 30°C.

Suppositories: Each suppository contains: hydrocortisone acetate 10 mg and zinc sulfate monohydrate 10 mg. Nonmedicinal ingredients: methylparaben, propylparaben and triglyceride base. Boxes of 12 and 24. Store between 15 and 30°C.

Sandoz Anuzinc HC Plus: Ointment: Each g contains: pramoxine HCl 10 mg, hydrocortisone acetate 5 mg and zinc sulfate monohydrate 5 mg. Nonmedicinal ingredients: methylparaben, mineral oil (petrolatum) and propylparaben. Tubes of 15 g and 30 g with applicator. Store between 15 and 30°C.

Suppositories: Each suppository contains: pramoxine HCl 20 mg, hydrocortisone acetate 10 mg and zinc sulfate monohydrate 10 mg. Nonmedicinal ingredients: methylparaben, propylparaben and triglyceride base. Boxes of 12. Store between 15 and 30°C.

The reader is invited to consult CPhA's monograph **HMG-CoA Reductase Inhibitors**.

Sandoz® Atorvastatin ℞

atorvastatin calcium

Lipid Metabolism Regulator

Sandoz

SUPPLIED: 10 mg: Each white to off-white, oval, biconvex, film-coated tablet, debossed with "SZ 10" on one side, contains: atorvastatin 10 mg (as atorvastatin calcium). Nonmedicinal ingredients: carboxymethylcellulose sodium, colloidal silicon dioxide, glycerin, hypromellose, lactose monohydrate, magnesium stearate, microcrystalline cellulose, polyethylene glycol, pregelatinised starch, sodium lauryl sulfate, sodium starch glycolate, talc, titanium dioxide, triacetin and trometthamine. Store between 15 and 30°C. Blisters of 30. Bottles of 100 and 500.

20 mg: Each white to off-white, oval, biconvex, film-coated tablet, debossed with "SZ 20" on one side, contains: atorvastatin 20 mg (as atorvastatin calcium). Nonmedicinal ingredients: carboxymethylcellulose sodium, colloidal silicon dioxide, glycerin, hypromellose, lactose monohydrate, magnesium stearate, microcrystalline cellulose, polyethylene glycol, pregelatinised starch, sodium lauryl sulfate, sodium starch glycolate, talc, titanium dioxide, triacetin and tromethamine. Store between 15 and 30°C. Blisters of 30. Bottles of 100 and 500.
40 mg: Each white to off-white, oval, biconvex, film-coated tablet, debossed with "SZ 40" on one side, contains: atorvastatin 40 mg (as atorvastatin calcium). Nonmedicinal ingredients: carboxymethylcellulose sodium, colloidal silicon dioxide, glycerin, hypromellose, lactose monohydrate, magnesium stearate, microcrystalline cellulose, polyethylene glycol, pregelatinised starch, sodium lauryl sulfate, sodium starch glycolate, talc, titanium dioxide, triacetin and tromethamine. Store between 15 and 30°C. Blisters of 30. Bottles of 100 and 500.
80 mg: Each white to off-white, oval, biconvex, film-coated tablet, debossed with "SZ 80" on one side, contains: atorvastatin 80 mg (as atorvastatin calcium). Nonmedicinal ingredients: carboxymethylcellulose sodium, colloidal silicon dioxide, glycerin, hydroxyethyl cellulose, hypromellose, lactose monohydrate, magnesium stearate, microcrystalline cellulose, polyethylene glycol, pregelatinised starch, sodium lauryl sulfate, sodium starch glycolate, talc, titanium dioxide, triacetin and tromethamine. Store between 15 and 30°C. Blisters of 30. Bottles of 100.

Sandoz® Azithromycin Powder for Oral Suspension Ⓟ
azithromycin monohydrate
Antibiotic

Sandoz

SUPPLIED: After reconstitution, each bottle of caramel-flavored suspension contains: azithromycin monohydrate equivalent to 300 mg/15 mL (100 mg/5 mL); 600 mg/15 mL (200 mg/5 mL); 900 mg/22.5 mL (200 mg/5 mL); or 1500 mg/37.5 mL (200 mg/5 mL) of azithromycin. Nonmedicinal ingredients: aspartame, colloidal anhydrous silica, cream caramel, hydroxypropylcellulose, sucrose, titanium dioxide, trisodium phosphate anhydrous and xanthan gum. Store the dry powder at controlled room temperature (15-30°C). Protect from light. Store the reconstitute suspension between 5 and 30°C. Discard unused portion after 10 days. A graduated syringe is included in the package.

Sandoz® Azithromycin Tablets Ⓟ
azithromycin monohydrate hemiethanolate
Antibiotic

Sandoz

SUPPLIED: Each pink, oval-shaped, film-coated tablet, scored on both sides and engraved "A250" on one side, contains: azithromycin monohydrate hemiethanolate equivalent to azithromycin 250 mg. Nonmedicinal ingredients: cellulose microcrystalline, colloidal anhydrous silica, D&C Red # 30 aluminum lake, hydroxypropylcellulose, hydroxypropyl methylcellulose, lactose monohydrate, magnesium stearate, maize starch, polyethylene glycol, sodium lauryl sulfate, sodium starch glycolate, talc and titanium dioxide. Aluminum-backed blister strips of 6. Bottles of 100. Store at room temperature (15 to 30°C).

Sandoz® Bicalutamide Ⓟ
bicalutamide
Nonsteroidal Antiandrogen

Sandoz

SUPPLIED: Each white, or almost white, round, biconvex film-coated tablet, with a sign "B" on one side and "50" on the other side contains: bicalutamide 50 mg. Nonmedicinal ingredients: colloidal anhydrous silica, hydroxypropyl methylcellulose, lactose monohydrate, magnesium stearate, polyethylene glycol, povidone, sodium starch glycolate, titanium dioxide and triacetin. Blister packs of 30. Store at room temperature (15 to 30°C).

Sandoz® Bisoprolol Ⓟ
bisoprolol fumarate
Beta-adrenoceptor Blocking Agent

Sandoz

PHARMACOLOGY: Sandoz Bisoprolol (bisoprolol fumarate) is a synthetic β_1-selective (cardioselective) adrenoceptor blocking agent without significant membrane stabilizing activity or intrinsic sympathomimetic activity in its therapeutic dosage range. This preferential effect is not absolute, however, and at higher dose bisoprolol may also inhibit β_2-adrenoceptors, located chiefly in the bronchial and vascular musculature.
Pharmacodynamics: The most prominent effect of bisoprolol fumarate is the negative chronotropic effect, resulting in a reduction in resting and exercise heart rate. There is a fall in resting and exercise cardiac output with little observed change in stroke volume, and only a small increase in right atrial pressure, or pulmonary capillary wedge pressure at rest or during exercise.
Mechanism of Action: The mechanism of action of its antihypertensive effects has not been completely established. Factors which may be involved include: antagonism of β-adrenoceptors to decreased cardiac output; inhibition of renin release by the kidneys; diminution of tonic sympathetic outflow from the vasomotor centers in the brain.
In normal volunteers, bisoprolol fumarate therapy resulted in a reduction of exercise and isoproterenol-induced tachycardia. The maximal effect occurred with 1-4 hours post-dosing. Effects persisted for 24 hours at doses equal to or greater than 5 mg.
Electrophysiology studies in man have demonstrated that bisoprolol fumarate significantly decreases heart rate, increases sinus node recovery time, prolongs AV node refractory periods, and with rapid atrial stimulation, prolongs AV nodal conduction.
Bisoprolol fumarate is well absorbed following oral administration. The absolute bioavailability after a 10 mg dose is greater than 80%. Absorption is not affected by the presence of food. The first pass metabolism of bisoprolol fumarate is less than 20%.
Binding to serum proteins is approximately 30%. Peak plasma concentrations occur within 2-4 hours of dosing with 5 to 20 mg and mean peak values range from 16 ng/mL at 5 mg to 70 ng/mL at 20 mg. Once daily dosing with bisoprolol fumarate results in less than two fold intersubject variation in peak plasma levels. The plasma elimination half-life is 9-12 hours and is slightly longer in elderly patients in part because of decreased renal function in that population. Steady-state is attained within 5 days with once-daily dosing. In both young and elderly populations, plasma accumulation is low; the accumulation factor ranges from 1.1 to 1.3, and is what would be expected from the first order kinetics and once-daily dosing. Plasma concentrations are proportional to administered dose in the range of 5 to 20 mg. Pharmacokinetic characteristics of the 2 enantiomers are similar.
Bisoprolol fumarate is eliminated equally by renal and non renal pathways with about 50% of the dose appearing unchanged in the urine and the remainder appearing in the form of inactive metabolites. In humans, the known metabolites are labile or have no known pharmacologic activity. Less than 2% of the dose is excreted in the faeces. Bisoprolol fumarate is not metabolized by cytochrome P450 II D6 (debrisoquin hydroxylase).
In subjects with creatinine clearance less than 40 mL/min, the plasma half-life is increased approximately three-fold compared to healthy subjects.
In patients with liver cirrhosis, the rate of elimination of bisoprolol fumarate is more variable and significantly slower than that in healthy subjects, with plasma half-life ranges from 8.3 to 21.7 hours.
A comparative, randomized, single-dose, 2-way crossover bioavailability study of Sandoz Bisoprolol 10 mg tablets was performed vs the Canadian reference in healthy adult males under fasting conditions. The summary of the comparative bioavailability study carried out by Sandoz Canada Inc. is presented in Table 1.

Table 1: Sandoz Bisoprolol
Summary Table of the Comparative Bioavailability Data (1×10 mg) Sandoz Bisoprolol From Measured Data

Parameter	Geometric Mean Arithmetic Mean (CV %)		% Ratio of Geometric Means
	Test	Reference[a]	
AUC_{0-T} (ng·h/mL)	609.80 615.79 (14.33)	618.42 625.50 (15.17)	98.61
AUC_I (ng·h/mL)	642.87 650.16 (15.29)	652.76 661.07 (15.95)	98.48
C_{max} (ng/mL)	40.37 40.78 (15.27)	38.20 39.20 (16.48)	104.32
T_{max} (h)[b]	2.80 (44.26)	3.47 (46.71)	
$T_{½}$ (h)[b]	11.07 (13.40)	11.13 (13.47)	

[a] Monocor, Crystaal a Division of Biovail Corporation, Canada.
[b] The T_{max} and $T_{½}$ parameters are to be expressed as the arithmetic means (CV %).

INDICATIONS: Sandoz Bisoprolol (bisoprolol fumarate) is indicated in the management of patients with mild to moderate hypertension. It may be used alone or in combination with other antihypertensive agents, particularly thiazide diuretics.
Sandoz Bisoprolol is not recommended for the emergency treatment of hypertensive crisis.

CONTRAINDICATIONS: Sandoz Bisoprolol (bisoprolol fumarate) is contraindicated in patients with cardiogenic shock, overt heart failure, second or third degree A-V block, right ventricular failure secondary to pulmonary hypertension, and sinus bradycardia.

WARNINGS: Cardiac Failure: Special caution should be exercised when administering bisoprolol fumarate to patients with a history of severe heart failure. Safety and effectiveness of bisoprolol doses higher than 10 mg/day in patients with heart failure have not been established. Sympathetic stimulation is a vital component supporting circulatory function in congestive heart failure and inhibition with beta-blockade always carries the potential hazard of further depressing myocardial contractility and precipitating cardiac failure. In general β-blocking agents should be avoided in patients with overt congestive heart failure.
However, in some patients with compensated cardiac failure, it may be necessary to utilize them. In such a situation, they must be used cautiously. Bisoprolol fumarate acts selectively without abolishing the effects of digitalis. However, the positive inotropic effect of digitalis may be reduced by the negative inotropic effect of bisoprolol fumarate when the two drugs are used concomitantly. The effects of β-blockers and digitalis are additive in depressing A-V conduction.
Patients without a History of Cardiac Failure: In patients without a history of cardiac failure continued depression of the myocardium with β-blockers in some cases lead to cardiac failure. At the first sign or symptom of impending cardiac failure, patients should be treated appropriately and the response observed closely. If cardiac failure continues, bisoprolol fumarate therapy should be immediately withdrawn.
Abrupt Cessation of Therapy with Bisoprolol: Exacerbation of angina pectoris and, in some instances, myocardial infarction or ventricular arrhythmia, have been observed in patients with coronary artery disease following abrupt cessation of therapy with β-blockers. Patients should, therefore, be cautioned against interruption or discontinuation of therapy without the physician's advice. Even in patients without overt coronary artery disease, it may be advisable to taper therapy with bisoprolol fumarate over approximately two weeks and the patient should be carefully observed. The same frequency of administration should be maintained. If withdrawal symptoms occur, therapy with bisoprolol fumarate should be reinstituted, at least temporarily.
Peripheral Vascular Disease: Beta-blockers can precipitate or aggravate symptoms of arterial insufficiency in patients with peripheral vascular disease. Caution should be exercised in such individuals.
Oculomucocutaneous Syndrome: Various skin rashes have been reported with β-blockers, including bisoprolol fumarate. A severe syndrome (oculomucocutaneous syndrome), whose signs include conjunctivitis sicca and psoriasiform rashes, otitis, and sclerosing serositis, has occurred with the chronic use of one β-adrenoceptor blocking agent (practolol). This syndrome has not been observed with bisoprolol fumarate or any other such agent. However, physicians should be alert to the possibility of such reactions and should discontinue treatment in the event that they occur.
Sinus Bradycardia: Severe sinus bradycardia, resulting from unopposed vagal activity following β-blockade, may occur with the use of bisoprolol fumarate. In such cases, the dosage should be reduced or bisoprolol fumarate discontinued.
Thyrotoxicosis: In patients with thyrotoxicosis, possible deleterious effects from long-term use of bisoprolol fumarate have not been adequately appraised.
β-adrenoceptor blockade may mask clinical signs of hyperthyroidism, such as tachycardia or its complications, and gives a false impression of improvement. Abrupt withdrawal of β blockade may be followed by an exacerbation of the symptoms of hyperthyroidism or precipitate thyroid storm.
Therefore, in such patient from whom bisoprolol fumarate is to be discontinued, withdrawal should be gradual and the patient monitored closely.

PRECAUTIONS: Appropriate laboratory tests for monitoring renal, hepatic, and hematopoietic function should be performed at regular intervals during long-term treatment with bisoprolol fumarate.
Bronchospastic Disease: In general, patients with bronchospastic pulmonary disease should not receive β-blockers. However, because bisoprolol fumarate is relative β_1-selective, it may be used cautiously in patients with bronchospastic disease who do not respond to, or who cannot tolerate other antihypertensive treatment. Since β_1-selectivity is not absolute, the lowest possible dose should be employed, a β_2-agonist (bronchodilator) should be made available, and the patient should be monitored closely. In patients already on bronchodilators therapy, the dose may have to be increased.
Anaesthesia: It is not advisable to withdraw β-adrenoceptor blocking drugs prior to surgery in the majority of patients. However, care should be taken when using bisoprolol fumarate with anaesthetic agents such as those which may depress the myocardium. Vagal dominance, if it occurs, may be corrected with atropine (1 to 2 mg IV).
Some patients receiving beta-adrenoceptor blocking agents have been subject to protracted severe hypotension during anaesthesia. Difficulty in restarting the heart and maintaining the heart beat has also been reported (see also Overdose).
In emergency surgery, since bisoprolol fumarate is a competitive antagonist at beta-adrenoceptor sites, its effects may be reversed, if required, by sufficient doses of such agonists as isoproterenol or noradrenaline.
Allergic Type Reaction: There may be increased difficulty in treating an allergic type reaction in patients on beta-blockers. In these patients, the reaction may be more severe due to pharmacologic effects of the beta-blockers and the problems with fluid changes. Epinephrine should be administered with caution since it may not have its usual effects in the treatment of anaphylaxis. On the one hand, larger doses of epinephrine may be needed to overcome the bronchospasm, while on the other, these doses can be associated with excessive alpha-adrenergic stimulation with consequent hypertension, reflex bradycardia and heart block and possible potentiation of bronchospasm. Alternatives to the use of large doses of epinephrine include vigorous supportive care such as fluids and the use of a beta-agonist including parenteral salbutamol or isoproterenol to overcome bronchospasm or norepinephrine to overcome hypotension.
Risk of Anaphylactic Reaction: While taking β-blockers, patients with a history of severe anaphylactic reaction to a variety of allergens may be more reactive to repeated challenge, either accidental, diagnostic, or therapeutic. Such patients may be unresponsive to the usual doses of epinephrine used to treat allergic reactions.
Diabetes Mellitus and Hypoglycemia: Beta-blockers may mask some of the manifestations of hypoglycemia, particularly tachycardia. Non-selective beta-blockers may potentiate insulin-induced hypoglycemia and delay recovery of serum glucose levels. Therefore, bisoprolol fumarate should be used with caution in patients subject to spontaneous hypoglycemia, or in diabetic patients (especially those with labile diabetes) receiving insulin or oral hypoglycemic agents.
Impaired Renal or Hepatic Function: Appropriate laboratory tests for monitoring renal, hepatic and hematopoietic function should be performed at regular intervals during long-term treatment. Use caution in adjusting dose in hepatic and renal impaired patients (see Dosage).
Geriatrics: Bisoprolol fumarate has been used in elderly patients with essential hypertension. Although the response rates and mean decreases in diastolic blood pressure were similar to that in younger patients, there was a tendency for older patients to be maintained on higher doses of bisoprolol fumarate. Observed reductions in heart rate were slightly greater in the elderly than in the young and tended to increase with increasing dose.

Pregnancy: Bisoprolol fumarate was not teratogenic in rats at doses up to 150 mg/kg/day, which is 375 times the maximum recommended human daily dose. Bisoprolol fumarate was fetotoxic (increased late resorptions) at 50 mg/kg/day and maternotoxic (decreased food intake and body-weight gain) at 150 mg/kg/day. Bisoprolol fumarate was not teratogenic in rabbits at doses up to 12.5 mg/kg/day, which is 31 times the maximum recommended human daily dose, but was embryolethal (increased early resorptions) at 12.5 mg/kg/day.

There are no studies in pregnant women. Bisoprolol fumarate should be used during pregnancy only if the potential benefit justifies the potential risk to the fetus.

Lactation: Small amounts of bisoprolol fumarate (<2% of the dose) have been detected in the milk of lactating rats. It is not known whether this drug is excreted in human milk. If use of bisoprolol fumarate is considered essential, then mothers should stop nursing.

Children: Safety and effectiveness in children have not been established.

Drug Interactions: Other β-blocking Agents: Bisoprolol fumarate should not be combined with other β-blocking agents.

Catecholamine-Depleting Drugs: Patients receiving catecholamine-depleting drugs, such as reserpine or guanethidine, should be monitored closely because the added β-adrenergic blocking action of bisoprolol fumarate may produce excessive reduction of sympathetic activity.

Centrally Active Antihypertensive Agents: β-blockers may exacerbate the rebound hypertension which can follow the withdrawal of clonidine. If the two drugs are coadministered, the β-blocker should be withdrawn several days before discontinuing clonidine. If replacing clonidine by β-blocker therapy, the introduction of β-blockers should be delayed for several days after clonidine administration has stopped (see also prescribing information for clonidine).

Antiarrhythmic Agents: Bisoprolol fumarate should be used with care when myocardial depressants or inhibitors of A-V conduction, such as certain calcium antagonists (particularly of the phenylalkylamine (verapamil) and benzothiazepine (diltiazem) classes), or antiarrhythmic agents, such as disopyramide, are used concurrently.

Calcium Channel Blockers: Combined use of β-blockers and calcium channel blockers with negative inotropic effects can lead to prolongation of S-A and A-V conduction, particularly in patients with impaired ventricular function or conduction abnormalities. This may result in severe hypotension, bradycardia and cardiac failure.

Pharmacokinetic Interactions: Concurrent use of rifampin increases the metabolic clearance of bisoprolol fumarate, resulting in a shortened elimination half-life of bisoprolol fumarate. Therefore, compounds with enzymatic induction potential should be administered with caution to patients receiving bisoprolol fumarate therapy. Pharmacokinetic studies document no clinically relevant adverse interactions with other agents given concomitantly, including thiazide diuretics, digoxin, and cimetidine. There was no effect of bisoprolol fumarate on prothrombin time in patients on stable doses of warfarin.

Exaggerated hypertensive responses have been reported from the combined use of beta-adrenergic antagonist and alpha-adrenergic stimulants including those contained in proprietary cold remedies and vasoconstrictive nasal drops. Patients receiving beta-blockers should be warned of this potential hazard.

Information to Be Provided to the Patient: Patients, especially those with coronary artery disease should be warned against discontinuing use of bisoprolol fumarate without a physician's supervision. Patients should also be advised to consult a physician if any difficulty in breathing occurs or if they develop signs or symptoms of congestive heart failure or excessive bradycardia.

Patients subject to spontaneous hypoglycemia, or diabetic patients receiving insulin or oral hypoglycemic agents, should be cautioned that the β-blockers may mask some of the manifestations of hypoglycemia, particularly tachycardia, and bisoprolol fumarate should be used with caution.

ADVERSE EFFECTS: In two multi-centre, placebo-controlled clinical trials involving 404 mild-to-moderate hypertensive patients, the most frequently reported adverse reactions (>2%), whether or not drug related, were: arthralgia (2.7%), dizziness (3.5%), headache (10.9%), insomnia (2.5%), diarrhea (3.5%), nausea (2.2%), coughing (2.5%), pharyngitis (2.2%), rhinitis (4.0%), sinusitis (2.2%), URT infection (5.0%), fatigue (8.2%), and peripheral edema (3%).

In total, 187 out of 404 patients (46.3%) reported at least one adverse event. Overall, the events reported were mild to moderate in severity.

Twenty-seven out of 404 patients (6.7%) discontinued therapy due to an adverse event or an intercurrent illness.

Table 2 presents the adverse experiences, whether or not drug related, reported by >1% of all patients (n=404) enrolled in the two placebo-controlled trials of bisoprolol fumarate given in single daily doses of 2.5-40 mg. The adverse drug reactions that appear to be dose related are bradycardia, diarrhea, asthenia, fatigue and sinusitis. As the incidence of bradycardia is 0.5%, it is the only dose related adverse experience not listed below. (See Table 2).

Table 2: Sandoz Bisoprolol

Adverse Experience (>1%): Placebo-Controlled Trials (n=404)

Body System/Adverse Experience	All Adverse Experiences n (%)
Musculoskeletal	
Arthralgia	11 (2.7)
Myalgia	7 (1.7)
Muscle cramps	6 (1.5)
CNS	
Dizziness	14 (3.5)
Headache	44 (10.9)
Paresthesia	5 (1.2)
Hypoesthesia	6 (1.5)
Autonomic Nervous System	
Dry mouth	5 (1.2)
Hearing and Vestibular	
Earache	5 (1.2)
Psychiatric	
Impotence	5 (1.2)
Insomnia	10 (2.5)
Somnolence	5 (1.2)
Gastrointestinal	
Diarrhea	14 (3.4)
Dyspepsia	5 (1.2)
Nausea	9 (2.2)
Vomiting	6 (1.5)
Respiratory	
Coughing	10 (2.5)
Dyspnea	6 (1.5)
Pharyngitis	9 (2.2)
Rhinitis	16 (4.0)
Sinusitis	9 (2.2)
URT infection	20 (5.0)
Body as a Whole	
Asthenia	6 (1.5)
Chest pain	6 (1.5)
Fatigue	33 (8.2)
Edema peripheral	12 (3.0)

In one long-term, open-label, extension study involving 144 hypertensive patients, the most frequently reported adverse experiences (>2%), whether or not drug related were: arthralgia (4.2%), myalgia (2.1%), muscle cramps (2.1%), dizziness (4.9%), headache (8.3%), earache (2.1%), impotence (2.1%), libido decrease (2.1%), abdominal pain (2.1%), diarrhea (2.8%), bronchitis (2.8%) coughing (4.2%), pharyngitis (4.2%), rhinitis (8.3%), sinusitis (4.9%), URT infection (6.9%), back pain (2.1%), chest pain (2.1%), fatigue (6.9%), fever (2.1%), peripheral edema (3.5%), pain (2.1%) and traumatic injury (2.1%).

The adverse experiences reported were generally mild to moderate in severity. Seventy-nine out of 144 patients (54.9%) reported at least one adverse experience. Out of the total number of patients enrolled, 12 (8.3%) discontinued therapy due to an adverse experience or an intercurrent illness.

Table 3 presents the adverse experiences reported by at least 1% of all patients (n=144) enrolled in the long-term, open-label, extension study in which patients received doses of bisoprolol fumarate ranging from 5 to 20 mg daily.

Table 3: Sandoz Bisoprolol

Adverse Experience (>1%): Long-Term, Open-label, Extension Study (n=144)

Body System/Adverse Experience	All Adverse Experiences n (%)
Musculoskeletal	
Arthralgia	6 (4.2)
Myalgia	3 (2.1)
Muscle cramps	3 (2.1)
CNS	
Dizziness	7 (4.9)
Headache	12 (8.3)
Neuralgia	2 (1.4)
Vision	
Eye abnormality	2 (1.4)
Vision abnormal	2 (1.4)
Hearing and Vestibular	
Earache	3 (2.1)
Tinnitus	2 (1.4)
Psychiatric	
Depression	2 (1.4)
Impotence	3 (2.1)
Libido decreased	3 (2.1)
Insomnia	2 (1.4)
Paroniria	2 (1.4)
Gastrointestinal	
Abdominal pain	3 (2.1)
Diarrhea	4 (2.8)
Dyspepsia	2 (1.4)

(cont'd)

Table 3: Sandoz Bisoprolol *(cont'd)*

Adverse Experience (>1%): Long-Term, Open-label, Extension Study (n=144)

Body System/Adverse Experience	All Adverse Experiences n (%)
Respiratory	
Bronchitis	4 (2.8)
Bronchospasm	2 (1.4)
Coughing	6 (4.2)
Pharyngitis	6 (4.2)
Rhinitis	12 (8.3)
Sinusitis	7 (4.9)
URT infection	10 (6.9)
Body as a Whole	
Allergy	2 (1.4)
Back pain	3 (2.1)
Chest pain	3 (2.1)
Fatigue	10 (6.9)
Fever	3 (2.1)
Hot flushes	2 (1.4)
Malaise	2 (1.4)
Edema generalized	2 (1.4)
Edema peripheral	5 (3.5)
Pain	3 (2.1)
Traumatic injury	3 (2.1)

The following is a list of spontaneous adverse experience reported with bisoprolol fumarate since its entry into the US market and the markets of some European countries. In these cases, an incidence of causal relationship cannot be accurately determined. The adverse experiences are listed according to body system and are as follows:

CNS (Central Nervous System): dizziness, vertigo, headache, paraesthesia, somnolence, decreased concentration/memory, aphasia, insomnia, muscle contractions (involuntary), paresis, sleep disturbances, sleepiness, syncope, tingling sensation, coma, encephalopathy, speech disorder, hallucination, confusion.

Autonomic Nervous System: dry mouth.

Cardiovascular: bradycardia, palpitations and other rhythm disturbances, hypotension, dyspnea on exertion, embolism, extrasystoles, atrial fibrillation, left cardiac failure, myocardial infarction, Raynaud-like disorder, hypertension, cardiac failure, circulatory failure, A-V block, cardiac arrest, tachycardia, ventricular fibrillation, arrhythmia.

Skin: rash, pruritus, alopecia, angioedema, exfoliative dermatitis, hyperpigmentation, psoriaform rash, skin photosensitivity, epidermal necrolysis, erythema multiforme, scleroderma, skin discolouration, urticaria.

Special Senses: ocular pain/pressure, abnormal lacrimation, taste abnormalities, ageusia, anosmia, conjunctivitis, visual disturbances.

Metabolic: hypoglycemia.

Respiratory: asthma/bronchopasm, dyspnea, shortness of breath, pulmonary edema, pneumonitis, respiratory insufficiency.

Hematologic: purpura vasculitis and peripheral ischemia.

Gastrointestinal: vomiting and diarrhea.

Musculoskeletal: muscle cramps, twitching/tremor, arthralgia and myalgia.

Genitourinary: Peyronie's disease, galactorrhea, mastalgia, still-birth.

General: fatigue, asthenia, malaise, edema, weight gain, death, scleroderma, overdose effect, asthenia.

Laboratory Abnormalities: In clinical trials, the most frequently reported laboratory change was an increase in serum triglycerides, but this was not a consistent finding.

Sporadic liver abnormalities have been reported. In two U.S. well-controlled studies versus placebo with bisoprolol fumarate treatment for 4-12 weeks, the incidence of concomitant elevations in AST and ALT of between 1-2 times normal was 3.9% for bisoprolol fumarate compared to 2.5% for placebo. No patient had concomitant elevations greater than twice normal.

Experience from long-term, uncontrolled studies with bisoprolol fumarate treatment for 6 to 18 months, the incidence of one or more concomitant elevations in AST and ALT of between 1 to 2 times normal was 6.2%. The incidence of multiple occurrences was 1.9%. For concomitant elevations in AST and ALT of greater than twice normal, the incidence was 1.5%. The incidence of multiple occurrences was 0.3%. In many cases these elevations were attributed to underlying disorders, or resolved during continued treatment with bisoprolol fumarate.

Other laboratory changes include small increases in uric acid, creatinine, BUN, serum potassium, glucose, and phosphorus and decreased in WBC and platelets. These were generally not of clinical importance and rarely resulted in discontinuation of bisoprolol fumarate.

As with other β-blockers, ANA conversions have also been reported on bisoprolol fumarate. About 15% of patients in long-term studies converted to a positive titre, although about one-third of these patients subsequently reconverted to a negative titre while on continued therapy.

OVERDOSE:

The most common signs expected with overdosage of β-blockers are bradycardia, hypotension, congestive heart failure, bronchospasm and hypoglycemia. To date, a few cases of overdose with bisoprolol fumarate have been reported. Bradycardia and/or hypotension were noted. Sympathomimetic agents were given in some cases, and all patients recovered. In general, if overdose occurs, therapy with bisoprolol fumarate should be stopped and supportive, symptomatic treatment should be provided. Patients should be monitored closely. Limited data suggest that bisoprolol fumarate is not dialysable.

Based on the expected pharmacologic actions and recommendations for other β-blockers, the following general measures should be considered when clinically warranted:

Bradycardia: Administer IV atropine. If the response is inadequate, isoproterenol or another agent with positive chronotropic properties may be given cautiously. Under some circumstances, transvenous pacemaker insertion may be necessary. Intravenous glucagon has been described to be useful.

Hypotension: IV fluids and vasopressors such as dopamine or norepinephrine should be administered. Monitor blood pressure continuously. Intravenous glucagon may be useful.

Heart Block (second or third degree): Patients should be carefully monitored and treated with isoproterenol infusion or transvenous cardiac pacemaker insertion, as appropriate.

Congestive Heart Failure: Initiate conventional therapy (i.e. digitalis, diuretics, inotropic agents, vasodilating agents). Glucagon has been reported to be useful.

Bronchospasm: Administer bronchodilator therapy such as isoproterenol or terbutaline (β_2 stimulants) and/or IV aminophylline.

Hypoglycemia: Administer IV glucose.

Based on the severity of symptoms, management may require intensive support care and facilities for administering cardiac and respiratory support.

It should be remembered that bisoprolol fumarate is a competitive antagonist of isoproterenol and hence large doses of isoproterenol can be expected to reverse many of the effects of excessive doses of bisoprolol fumarate. However, complications of excess isoproterenol should not be overlooked.

For management of a suspected drug overdose, CPhA recommends that you contact your **regional Poison Control Centre**. See the *CPS* Directory section for a list of Poison Control Centres.

DOSAGE: In the treatment of mild to moderate hypertension, Sandoz Bisoprolol (bisoprolol fumarate) must be individualized to the needs of the patient. The usual starting dose is 5 mg once daily either added to a diuretic or alone. If the response to 5 mg is inadequate, the dose may be increased to 10 mg and then, if necessary, to 20 mg once daily. An appropriate interval for dose titration is 2 weeks.

Increasing the dose beyond 20 mg once daily produces only a small incremental benefit.

Patients with Renal or Hepatic Impairment: In patients with hepatic impairment (hepatitis or cirrhosis) or renal dysfunction (creatinine clearance less than 40 mL/min) as in other patients, the initial daily dose should be 5 mg. Because of the possibility of accumulation, caution must be used in dose titration. Since limited data suggest that bisoprolol fumarate is not dialysable, drug replacement is not necessary in patients undergoing dialysis.

Geriatrics: In the elderly, it is not usually necessary to adjust the dose, unless there is also significant renal or hepatic dysfunction (see Precautions).

Children: There is no pediatric experience with bisoprolol fumarate, therefore, its use cannot be recommended for children.

SUPPLIED: 5 mg: Each pink, film-coated, round, biconvex tablet, imprinted "E" over "771" on one side and bisected on the other side, contains: bisoprolol fumarate 5 mg. Nonmedicinal ingredients: colloidal silicon dioxide, corn starch, dibasic calcium phosphate anhydrous, FD&C red #40 aluminum lake, FD&C yellow #6 aluminum lake, hydroxypropyl methylcellulose, magnesium stearate, microcrystalline cellulose, polyethylene glycol, polysorbate 80 and titanium dioxide. Bottles of 30 and 100. Store between 15 and 30°C. No other special storage conditions are necessary.

10 mg: Each white, film-coated, round, biconvex tablet, imprinted "E" over "774" on one side and plain on the other side, contains: bisoprolol fumarate 10 mg. Nonmedicinal ingredients: colloidal silicon dioxide, corn starch, dibasic calcium phosphate anhydrous, hydroxypropyl methylcellulose, magnesium stearate, microcrystalline cellulose, polyethylene glycol, polysorbate 80 and titanium dioxide. Bottles of 30 and 100. Store between 15 and 30°C. No other special storage conditions are necessary.

Sandoz® Bupropion SR Ⓟ

bupropion HCl

Antidepressant

Sandoz

SUPPLIED: 100 mg: Each aquamarine, round, biconvex, film-coated, sustained-release tablet, imprinted "E" over "410" on one side and plain on the other, contains: bupropion HCl 100 mg. Nonmedicinal ingredients: carnauba wax, FD&C blue #1, hydrochloric acid, hydroxypropyl cellulose, hydroxypropyl methylcellulose, magnesium stearate, microcrystalline cellulose, polyethylene glycol, polysorbate, titanium dioxide and water. Bottles of 30 and 60.

150 mg: Each plum, round, biconvex, film-coated, sustained-release tablet, imprinted "E" over "415" one one side and plain on the other, contains: bupropion HCl 150 mg. Nonmedicinal ingredients: carnauba wax, FD&C blue #2, FD&C red #40, hydrochloric acid, hydroxypropyl cellulose, hydroxypropyl methylcellulose, magnesium stearate, microcrystalline cellulose, polyethylene glycol, polysorbate, titanium dioxide and water. Bottles of 30 and 60.

Store at room temperature (between 15 and 25°C), in a dry place and protect from light. Keep tightly closed.

Sandoz® Calcitonin NS Ⓟ

calcitonin salmon

Bone Metabolism Regulator

Sandoz

SUPPLIED: Each actuation contains: synthetic calcitonin (salmon) 200 IU. Nonmedicinal ingredients: benzalkonium chloride (as a preservative), hydrochloric acid (for pH adjustment), purified water and sodium chloride. Unopened Sandoz Calcitonin Nasal Spray should be stored in the refrigerator between 2 and 8°C and protected from freezing. After priming, Sandoz Calcitonin Nasal Spray should be stored at room temperature (below 25°C) and used within 4 weeks. To ensure correct delivery, the bottle should be kept in an upright position.

Sandoz® Carbamazepine Ⓟ

carbamazepine

Anticonvulsant—Symptomatic Relief of Trigeminal Neuralgia—Antimanic

Sandoz

SUPPLIED: Chewtabs: 100 mg : Each white with red specks, round, flat-faced, beveled-edge, chewable tablet, engraved on one side and engraved with bisect on the other, contains: carbamazepine 100 mg. Nonmedicinal ingredients: cherry-mint flavour, cornstarch, erythrosine, gelatin, glycerin, magnesium stearate, silicon dioxide, sodium starch glycolate, stearic acid and sugar. Bottles of 100. Store at room temperature (below 30°C). Protect from humidity and light.

200 mg: Each white with red specks, oval, biconvex, chewable tablet, engraved on one side and engraved with bisect on the other, contains: carbamazepine 200 mg. Nonmedicinal ingredients: cherry-mint flavour, cornstarch, erythrosine, gelatin, glycerin, magnesium stearate, silicon dioxide, sodium starch glycolate, stearic acid and sugar. Bottles of 100. Store at room temperature (below 30°C). Protect from humidity and light.

CR: 200 mg : Each beige-orange, oval, slightly biconvex, controlled-release tablet, engraved on both sides, fully bisected on both sides, contains: carbamazepine 200 mg. Nonmedicinal ingredients: acrylic esters, castor oil derivative, cellulose compounds, iron oxides, magnesium stearate, silicon dioxide, talc and titanium dioxide. Bottles of 100. Store at room temperature (below 25°C). Protect from humidity.

400 mg: Each brown-orange, oval, slightly biconvex, controlled-release tablet, engraved on both sides, fully bisected on both sides, contains: carbamazepine 400 mg. Nonmedicinal ingredients: acrylic esters, castor oil derivative, cellulose compounds, iron oxides, magnesium stearate, silicon dioxide, talc and titanium dioxide. Bottles of 100. Store at room temperature (below 25°C). Protect from humidity.

Sandoz® Cefprozil ℞
cefprozil
Antibiotic

Sandoz

SUPPLIED: Oral Suspension: 125 mg/5 mL: Each 5 mL of reconstituted orange-flavoured suspension contains: cefprozil 125 mg. Nonmedicinal ingredients: aspartame, citric acid, colloidal silicon dioxide, FD&C Yellow No. 6, flavours (natural and artificial), glycine, microcrystalline cellulose, polysorbate 80, sodium benzoate, sodium carboxymethylcellulose, sodium chloride, simethicone and sucrose. Bottles of 75 and 100 mL. Store dry powder between 15 and 30°C. The reconstituted oral suspension must be refrigerated between 2 and 8°C for up to 14 days. Keep container tightly closed. Discard unused portion after 14 days.
250 mg/5 mL: Each 5 mL of reconstituted orange-flavoured suspension contains: cefprozil 250 mg. Nonmedicinal ingredients: aspartame, citric acid, colloidal silicon dioxide, FD&C Yellow No. 6, flavours (natural and artificial), glycine, microcrystalline cellulose, polysorbate 80, sodium benzoate, sodium carboxymethylcellulose, sodium chloride, simethicone and sucrose. Bottles of 75 and 100 mL. Store dry powder between 15 and 30°C. The reconstituted oral suspension must be refrigerated between 2 and 8°C for up to 14 days. Keep container tightly closed. Discard unused portion after 14 days.
Tablets: 250 mg: Each white to cream tinged, oval, unscored tablet, embossed "347" on one side and "250" on the other side, contains: cefprozil 250 mg. Nonmedicinal ingredients: hypromellose, magnesium stearate, methylcellulose, microcrystalline cellulose, polyethylene glycol, polysorbate 80, sodium starch glycolate and titanium dioxide. Bottles of 100. Store between 15 and 30°C.
500 mg: Each beige, oval, unscored tablet, embossed "348" on one side and "500" on the other side, contains: cefprozil 500 mg. Nonmedicinal ingredients: ferric oxide yellow, hypromellose, magnesium stearate, methylcellulose, microcrystalline cellulose, polyethylene glycol, polysorbate 80, sodium starch glycolate and titanium dioxide. Bottles of 100. Store between 15 and 30°C.

Sandoz® Clarithromycin ℞
clarithromycin
Antibiotic

Sandoz

SUPPLIED: 250 mg: Each yellow, oblong, convex, film-coated tablet, scored on both sides, contains: clarithromycin 250 mg. Nonmedicinal ingredients: colloidal silica anhydrous, croscarmellose sodium, magnesium stearate, microcrystalline cellulose, Opadry yellow and powdered cellulose. HDPE bottles of 100 and 250. Store between 15 and 30°C in a tightly closed container.
500 mg: Each yellow, oblong, convex, film-coated tablet, scored on both sides, contains: clarithromycin 500 mg. Nonmedicinal ingredients: colloidal silica anhydrous, croscarmellose sodium, magnesium stearate, microcrystalline cellulose, Opadry yellow and powdered cellulose. HDPE bottles of 100 and 250. Store between 15 and 30°C in a tightly closed container.

Sandoz® Clonazepam T/C
clonazepam
Anticonvulsant

Sandoz

SUPPLIED: 0.5 mg: Each orange, round tablet, scored on one side and debossed "RHO" over "0.5" on the other side, contains: clonazepam 0.5 mg, USP. Nonmedicinal ingredients: corn starch, D&C Yellow No. 6 aluminum lake, lactose anhydrous, magnesium stearate and microcrystalline cellulose. Bottles of 100 and 500.
1 mg: Each green, round tablet, scored on one side and debossed "RHO" over "1" on the other side, contains: clonazepam 1 mg, USP. Nonmedicinal ingredients: corn starch, FD&C Blue No. 2 aluminum lake, lactose anhydrous, magnesium stearate and microcrystalline cellulose. Bottles of 100.
2 mg: Each white, round tablet, scored on one side and debossed "RHO" over "2" on the other side, contains: clonazepam 2 mg, USP. Nonmedicinal ingredients: corn starch, lactose anhydrous, magnesium stearate and microcrystalline cellulose. Bottles of 100 and 500.
Store in air-tight, light-resistant containers at room temperature (15 to 30°C).

Sandoz® Cortimyxin Ophthalmic Ointment ℞
hydrocortisone—neomycin sulfate—polymyxin B sulfate—bacitracin zinc
Anti-inflammatory—Antibacterial

Sandoz

Sandoz® Cortimyxin Otic Solution ℞
hydrocortisone—neomycin sulfate—polymyxin B sulfate
Anti-inflammatory—Antibacterial

Sandoz

SUPPLIED: Ophthalmic Ointment: Each g of sterile ophthalmic ointment contains: polymyxin B sulfate 10 000 units, bacitracin zinc 400 units, neomycin 3.5 mg (as sulfate) and hydrocortisone 10 mg. Nonmedicinal ingredients: petrolatum. Tubes of 3.5 g. Store between 15 and 25°C.
Otic Solution: Each mL of sterile otic solution contains: polymyxin B sulfate 10 000 units, neomycin 3.5 mg (as sulfate) and hydrocortisone 10 mg. Nonmedicinal ingredients: copper sulfate pentahydrate, glycerin, polysorbate 80, potassium metabisulfite, propylene glycol, sulfuric acid and/or potassium hydroxide to adjust pH and water for injection. Dropper bottles of 10 mL. Store between 15 and 30°C.

Sandoz® Cyclosporine ℞
cyclosporine
Immunosuppressant

Sandoz

SUPPLIED: 25 mg: Each clear, oblong soft gelatin capsule, imprinted E0932 and filled with a clear, yellowish oil-like liquid, contains: cyclosporine 25 mg. Nonmedicinal ingredients: D-alpha-tocopheryl, ethanol, macrogol-glycerol hydroxystearate, polyethylene glycol and polyethylene glycol 400; shell: gelatin, glycerol and sorbitol. Packs of 30 (3 full aluminum blister strips of 10 capsules each). Store at temperatures between 15 and 25°C and do not remove from the blister packs until required for use. Occasional increases in temperature up to 30°C do not affect the quality of the product.
50 mg: Each clear, oblong soft gelatin capsule, imprinted E0934 and filled with a clear, yellowish oil-like liquid, contains: cyclosporine 50 mg. Nonmedicinal ingredients: D-alpha-tocopheryl, ethanol, macrogol-glycerol hydroxystearate, polyethylene glycol and polyethylene glycol 400; shell: gelatin, glycerol and sorbitol. Packs of 30 (3 full aluminum blister strips of 10 capsules each). Store at temperatures between 15 and 25°C and do not remove from the blister packs until required for use. Occasional increases in temperature up to 30°C do not affect the quality of the product.
100 mg: Each clear, oblong soft gelatin capsule, imprinted E0933 and filled with a clear, yellowish oil-like liquid, contains: cyclosporine 100 mg. Nonmedicinal ingredients: D-alpha-tocopheryl, ethanol, macrogol-glycerol hydroxystearate, polyethylene glycol and polyethylene glycol 400; shell: gelatin, glycerol and sorbitol. Packs of 30 (3 full aluminum blister strips of 10 capsules each). Store at temperatures between 15 and 25°C and do not remove from the blister packs until required for use. Occasional increases in temperature up to 30°C do not affect the quality of the product.

Sandoz® Diclofenac Rapide ℞
diclofenac potassium
Anti-inflammatory—Analgesic

Sandoz

Sandoz® Diclofenac ℞
diclofenac sodium
Anti-inflammatory—Analgesic

Sandoz

Sandoz® Diclofenac SR ℞
diclofenac sodium
Anti-inflammatory —Analgesic

Sandoz

SUPPLIED: Sandoz Diclofenac Rapide: Each reddish-brown, round, biconvex, sugar-coated tablet, with "S" printed on one side and "50-K" printed on the other side in white ink, contains: diclofenac potassium 50 mg. Nonmedicinal ingredients: carnauba wax, cellulose, colloidal silicon dioxide, corn starch, ferric oxide, magnesium stearate, polyethylene glycol, povidone, sodium carboxymethyl starch, sucrose, talc, titanium dioxide, tribasic calcium phosphate and white ink. Bottles of 100. Protect from heat (i.e., store between 15-30°C) and humidity.
Sandoz Diclofenac: Suppositories: 50 mg: Each bullet shaped suppository, white to yellowish white in colour, with a smooth surface and a fat-like odour, contains: diclofenac sodium 50 mg. Nonmedicinal ingredients: semi-synthetic glycerides. Cartons of 30. Store between 15 and 30°C. Protect from heat.
100 mg: Each bullet shaped suppository, white to yellowish white in colour, with a smooth surface and a fat-like odour, contains: diclofenac sodium 100 mg. Nonmedicinal ingredients: semi-synthetic glycerides. Cartons of 30. Store between 15 and 30°C. Protect from heat.
Tablets: 25 mg: Each yellow, round, slightly biconvex, enteric-coated tablet, with "S" printed on one side and "25" on the other side in black ink, contains: diclofenac sodium 25 mg. Nonmedicinal ingredients: black ink, castor oil derivatives, cellulose compound, colloidal silicon dioxide, corn starch, hypromellose, iron oxides, lactose, magnesium stearate, microcrystalline cellulose, polyethylene glycol, povidone, sodium starch glycolate, talc and titanium dioxide. Bottles of 100. Protect from heat (i.e., store between 15-30°C) and humidity.
50 mg: Each light brown, round, slightly biconvex, enteric-coated tablet, with "S" printed on one side and "50" on the other side in black ink, contains: diclofenac sodium 50 mg. Nonmedicinal ingredients: black ink, castor oil derivatives, colloidal silicon dioxide, corn starch, hypromellose, iron oxides, lactose, magnesium stearate, microcrystalline cellulose, polyethylene glycol, povidone, sodium starch glycolate, talc and titanium dioxide. Bottles of 100. Protect from heat (i.e., store between 15-30°C) and humidity.
Sandoz Diclofenac SR: 75 mg: Each light pink, triangular, biconvex, film-coated, slow-release tablet, with "S" printed on one side and "SR 75" on the other side in black ink, contains: diclofenac sodium 75 mg. Nonmedicinal ingredients: black ink, carnauba wax, cellulose compounds, cetyl alcohol, colloidal silicon dioxide, hypromellose, magnesium stearate, polysorbate 80, povidone, red iron oxide, sucrose, talc and titanium dioxide. Bottles of 100. Protect from heat (i.e., store between 15-30°C) and humidity.
100 mg: Each pink, round, biconvex, film-coated, slow-release tablet, with "S" printed on one side and "SR 100" on the other side in black ink, contains: diclofenac sodium 100 mg. Nonmedicinal ingredients: black ink, carnauba wax, cellulose compounds, cetyl alcohol, colloidal silicon dioxide, hypromellose, magnesium stearate, polysorbate 80, povidone, red iron oxide, sucrose, talc and titanium dioxide. Bottles of 100. Protect from heat (i.e., store between 15-30°C) and humidity.

The reader is invited to consult CPhA's monograph **Calcium Channel Blockers**.

Sandoz® Diltiazem CD ℞
diltiazem HCl
Antihypertensive—Antianginal

Sandoz

SUPPLIED: 120 mg: Each light turquoise blue opaque controlled delivery capsule, filled with off-white round pellets and imprinted RXP 120 mg, contains: diltiazem HCl 120 mg. Nonmedicinal ingredients: acetyl tributyl citrate, ethylcellulose, magnesium stearate, methylacrylic acid copolymer Type B, polysorbate, sugar spheres and talc; capsule: FD&C Blue #1, gelatin and titanium dioxide. Bottles of 100 and 500. Preserve in tight containers between 15 and 30°C.
180 mg: Each light turquoise blue opaque/light blue opaque controlled delivery capsule, filled with off-white round pellets and imprinted RXP 180 mg, contains: diltiazem HCl 180 mg. Nonmedicinal ingredients: acetyl tributyl citrate, ethylcellulose, magnesium stearate, methylacrylic acid copolymer Type B, polysorbate, sugar spheres and talc; capsule: FD&C Blue #1, gelatin and titanium dioxide. Bottles of 100 and 500. Preserve in tight containers between 15 and 30°C.
240 mg: Each light blue opaque controlled delivery capsule, filled with off-white round pellets and imprinted RXP 240 mg, contains: diltiazem HCl 240 mg. Nonmedicinal ingredients: acetyl tributyl citrate, ethylcellulose, magnesium stearate, methylacrylic acid copolymer Type B, polysorbate, sugar spheres and talc; capsule: FD&C Blue #1, gelatin and titanium dioxide. Bottles of 100 and 500. Preserve in tight containers between 15 and 30°C.
300 mg: Each light grey opaque/light blue opaque controlled delivery capsule, filled with off-white round pellets and imprinted RXP 300 mg, contains: diltiazem HCl 300 mg. Nonmedicinal ingredients: acetyl tributyl citrate, ethylcellulose, magnesium stearate, methylacrylic acid copolymer Type B, polysorbate, sugar spheres and talc; capsule: black iron oxide, FD&C Blue #1, gelatin and titanium dioxide. Bottles of 100. Preserve in tight containers between 15 and 30°C.

Sandoz® Diltiazem T ℞
diltiazem HCl
Antihypertensive—Antianginal

Sandoz

SUPPLIED: 120 mg: Each purple opaque extended release capsule, filled with off-white round pellets and imprinted RXP 120 mg in white, contains: diltiazem HCl 120 mg. Nonmedicinal ingredients: D&C Red #28, ethylcellulose, eudragit, FD&C Blue #1, gelatin, hydroxypropylmethyl cellulose, magnesium stearate, polysorbate, povidone, sugar spheres, talc and titanium dioxide. Bottles of 100. Store in a tight container between 15 and 30°C. Protect from light.
180 mg: Each green opaque/white opaque extended release capsule, filled with off-white round pellets and imprinted RXP 180 mg in black, contains: diltiazem HCl 180 mg. Nonmedicinal ingredients: black iron oxide, ethylcellulose, eudragit, FD&C Green #3, gelatin, hydroxypropylmethyl cellulose, magnesium stearate, polysorbate, povidone, sugar spheres, talc and titanium dioxide. Bottles of 100. Store in a tight container between 15 and 30°C. Protect from light.

240 mg: Each purple opaque/green opaque extended release capsule, filled with off-white round pellets and imprinted RXP 240 mg in white, contains: diltiazem HCl 240 mg. Nonmedicinal ingredients: D&C Red #28, ethylcellulose, eudragit, FD&C Blue #1, FD&C Green #3, gelatin, hydroxypropylmethyl cellulose, magnesium stearate, polysorbate, povidone, sugar spheres, talc and titanium dioxide. Bottles of 100. Store in a tight container between 15 and 30°C. Protect from light.
300 mg: Each purple opaque/white opaque extended release capsule, filled with off-white round pellets and imprinted RXP 300 mg in black, contains: diltiazem HCl 300 mg. Nonmedicinal ingredients: black iron oxide, D&C Red #28, ethylcellulose, eudragit, FD&C Blue #1, gelatin, hydroxypropylmethyl cellulose, magnesium stearate, polysorbate, povidone, sugar spheres, talc and titanium dioxide. Bottles of 100. Store in a tight container between 15 and 30°C. Protect from light.
360 mg: Each green opaque extended release capsule, filled with off-white round pellets and imprinted RXP 360 mgin white, contains: diltiazem HCl 360 mg. Nonmedicinal ingredients: ethylcellulose, eudragit, FD&C Green #3, gelatin, hydroxypropylmethyl cellulose, magnesium stearate, polysorbate, povidone, sugar spheres, talc and titanium dioxide. Bottles of 100. Store capsules in a tight container between 15 and 30°C. Protect from light.

Sandoz® Estradiol Derm ℞
estradiol-17β
Estrogen

Sandoz

SUPPLIED: 50 µg: Each thin, oval, multilayer, transparent, 20 cm² transdermal therapeutic system contains: estradiol hemihydrate 4.1 mg equivalent to 4 mg of estradiol-17β for continuous delivery of 50 µg/day. Nonmedicinal ingredients: acrylic copolymer and d-α-tocopherol. Patient packs of 8 patches. Store patches between 15 to 30°C. Protect from freezing. Each patch is individually sealed in a separate pouch. Do not store out of the pouch. Apply immediately upon removal from the protective pouch. Keep out of the reach of children and pets both before use and when disposing of used patches.
75 µg: Each thin, oval, multilayer, transparent, 30 cm² transdermal therapeutic system contains: estradiol hemihydrate 6.2 mg equivalent to 6 mg of estradiol-17β for continuous delivery of 75 µg/day. Nonmedicinal ingredients: acrylic copolymer and d-α-tocopherol. Patient packs of 8 patches. Store patches between 15 to 30°C. Protect from freezing. Each patch is individually sealed in a separate pouch. Do not store out of the pouch. Apply immediately upon removal from the protective pouch. Keep out of the reach of children and pets both before use and when disposing of used patches.
100 µg: Each thin, oval, multilayer, transparent, 40 cm² transdermal therapeutic system contains: estradiol hemihydrate 8.3 mg equivalent to 8 mg of estradiol-17β for continuous delivery of 100 µg/day. Nonmedicinal ingredients: acrylic copolymer and d-α-tocopherol. Patient packs of 8 patches. Store patches between 15 to 30°C. Protect from freezing. Each patch is individually sealed in a separate pouch. Do not store out of the pouch. Apply immediately upon removal from the protective pouch. Keep out of the reach of children and pets both before use and when disposing of used patches.

Sandoz® Famciclovir ℞
famciclovir
Antiviral Agent

Sandoz

SUPPLIED: 125 mg: Each white, round, biconvex, film-coated tablet with bevelled edges, debossed with "FV" on one side and "125" on the other, contains: famciclovir 125 mg. Nonmedicinal ingredients: hydroxypropyl cellulose, hydroxypropyl methylcellulose, lactose, magnesium stearate, polyethylene glycols, sodium starch glycolate and titanium dioxide. Blister packages of 10. Store between 15 and 30°C.
250 mg: Each white, round, biconvex, film-coated tablet with bevelled edges, debossed with "FV" on one side and "250" on the other, contains: famciclovir 250 mg. Nonmedicinal ingredients: hydroxypropyl cellulose, hydroxypropyl methylcellulose, lactose, magnesium stearate, polyethylene glycols, sodium starch glycolate and titanium dioxide. Bottles of 100. Blister packages of 30. Store between 15 and 30°C.
500 mg: Each white, oval, biconvex, film-coated tablet with bevelled edges, debossed with "FV" on one side and "500" on the other, contains: famciclovir 500 mg. Nonmedicinal ingredients: hydroxypropyl cellulose, hydroxypropyl methylcellulose, lactose, magnesium stearate, polyethylene glycols, sodium starch glycolate and titanium dioxide. Bottles of 100. Blister packages of 21. Store between 15 and 30°C.

The reader is invited to consult CPhA's monograph **Calcium Channel Blockers**.

Sandoz® Felodipine ℞
felodipine
Antihypertensive

Sandoz

SUPPLIED: 5 mg: Each pale red to gray-red, round, biconvex, film-coated, extended release tablet, embossed "F5" on one side contains: felodipine 5 mg. Nonmedicinal ingredients: ferric oxide (yellow), ferric oxide (red), hydroxypropyl methylcellulose, lactose monohydrate, magnesium stearate, microcrystalline cellulose, polyethylene glycol, sodium lauryl sulphate and titanium dioxide. Blister packs of 30. Bottles of 100. Keep at room temperature (15 to 30°C) in a dry place and protect from light.
10 mg: Each pale red to gray-red, biconvex, film-coated, extended release tablet, embossed "F10" on one side contains: felodipine 10 mg. Nonmedicinal ingredients: ferric oxide (yellow), ferric oxide (red), hydroxypropyl methylcellulose, lactose monohydrate, magnesium stearate, microcrystalline cellulose, polyethylene glycol, sodium lauryl sulphate and titanium dioxide. Blister packs of 30. Bottles of 100. Keep at room temperature (15 to 30°C) in a dry place and protect from light.

Sandoz® Fenofibrate S ℞
fenofibrate
Lipid Metabolism Regulator

Sandoz

SUPPLIED: 100 mg: Each white, oval, biconvex, film-coated tablet, engraved «SDZ» on one side and «F100» on the other contains: fenofibrate 100 mg. Nonmedicinal ingredients: croscarmellose sodium, hydroxypropylcellulose, hydroxypropyl methylcellulose, polyethylene glycol, purified water and titanium dioxide. Bottles of 90. Store between 15 and 30°C. Protect from light and moisture.
160 mg: Each white, oval, biconvex, film-coated tablet, engraved «SDZ» on one side and «F160» on the other contains: fenofibrate 160 mg. Nonmedicinal ingredients: croscarmellose sodium, hydroxypropylcellulose, hydroxypropyl methylcellulose, polyethylene glycol, purified water and titanium dioxide. Bottles of 90. Store between 15 and 30°C. Protect from light and moisture.

Sandoz® Fentanyl Patch Ⓝ
fentanyl
Opioid Analgesic

Sandoz

SUPPLIED: 12 µg/h: Each matrix-based transdermal patch contains: fentanyl 2.1 mg. Nonmedicinal ingredients: acrylic-vinylacetate copolymer adhesive, polyethyleneterephthalate backing foil and siliconized polyethyleneterephthalate release liner. Cartons containing 5 individually packaged systems. Each patch system is packaged in foil paper/PE/AL/PE sachets. Store in sealed pouch between 15 and 25°C. Do not refrigerate. Protect from freezing.
25 µg/h: Each matrix-based transdermal patch contains: fentanyl 4.2 mg. Nonmedicinal ingredients: acrylic-vinylacetate copolymer adhesive, polyethyleneterephthalate backing foil and siliconized polyethyleneterephthalate release liner. Cartons containing 5 individually packaged systems. Each patch system is packaged in foil paper/PE/AL/PE sachets. Store in sealed pouch between 15 and 25°C. Do not refrigerate. Protect from freezing.
37 µg/h: Each matrix-based transdermal patch contains: fentanyl 6.3 mg. Nonmedicinal ingredients: acrylic-vinylacetate copolymer adhesive, polyethyleneterephthalate backing foil and siliconized polyethyleneterephthalate release liner. Cartons containing 5 individually packaged systems. Each patch system is packaged in foil paper/PE/AL/PE sachets. Store in sealed pouch between 15 and 25°C. Do not refrigerate. Protect from freezing.
50 µg/h: Each matrix-based transdermal patch contains: fentanyl 8.4 mg. Nonmedicinal ingredients: acrylic-vinylacetate copolymer adhesive, polyethyleneterephthalate backing foil and siliconized polyethyleneterephthalate release liner. Cartons containing 5 individually packaged systems. Each patch system is packaged in foil paper/PE/AL/PE sachets. Store in sealed pouch between 15 and 25°C. Do not refrigerate. Protect from freezing.
75 µg/h: Each matrix-based transdermal patch contains: fentanyl 12.6 mg. Nonmedicinal ingredients: acrylic-vinylacetate copolymer adhesive, polyethyleneterephthalate backing foil and siliconized polyethyleneterephthalate release liner. Cartons containing 5 individually packaged systems. Each patch system is packaged in foil paper/PE/AL/PE sachets. Store in sealed pouch between 15 and 25°C. Do not refrigerate. Protect from freezing.
100 µg/h: Each matrix-based transdermal patch contains: fentanyl 16.8 mg. Nonmedicinal ingredients: acrylic-vinylacetate copolymer adhesive, polyethyleneterephthalate backing foil and siliconized polyethyleneterephthalate release liner. Cartons containing 5 individually packaged systems. Each patch system is packaged in foil paper/PE/AL/PE sachets. Store in sealed pouch between 15 and 25°C. Do not refrigerate. Protect from freezing.

Sandoz® Finasteride ℞
finasteride
Type II 5 Alpha-reductase Inhibitor

Sandoz

SUPPLIED: Each blue, biconvex, apple-shaped, film-coated tablet, embossed "SZ" on one side and "5" on the other side, contains: finasteride 5 mg. Nonmedicinal ingredients: docusate sodium, hypromellose, indigotine lake, lactose monohydrate, magnesium stearate, microcrystalline cellulose, povidone, propylene glycol, sodium starch glycolate, talc and titanium dioxide. Blisters of 30 (3×10). Bottles of 100 and 500. Blisters: Store at room temperature between 15 and 30°C, protect from light and humidity. Bottles: Store at room temperature between 15 and 30°C, protect from light.

The reader is invited to consult CPhA's monograph **Sulfonylureas**.

Sandoz® Glimepiride ℞
glimepiride
Oral Hypoglycemic Agent (Sulfonylurea)

Sandoz

SUPPLIED: 1 mg: Each light red, flat, modified oblong tablet, scored on both sides, and on one side of the tablet debossed "G" on the left side of the score and "1" on the right side, contains: glimepiride 1 mg. Nonmedicinal ingredients: ferric oxide red, lactose monohydrate, magnesium stearate, microcrystalline cellulose, povidone and sodium starch glycolate. Blister packs of 30. Store between 15 and 30°C, away from heat, moisture and direct light.
2 mg: Each light green, flat, modified oblong tablet, scored on both sides, and on one side of the tablet debossed "G" on the left side of the score and "2" on the right side, contains: glimepiride 2 mg. Nonmedicinal ingredients: ferric oxide yellow, indigotine (FD&C Blue No. 2 Aluminum Lake), lactose monohydrate, magnesium stearate, microcrystalline cellulose, povidone and sodium starch glycolate. Blister packs of 30. Store between 15 and 30°C, away from heat, moisture and direct light.
4 mg: Each light blue, flat, modified oblong tablet, scored on both sides, and on one side of the tablet debossed "G" on the left side of the score and "4" on the right side, contains: glimepiride 4 mg. Nonmedicinal ingredients: indigotine (FD&C Blue No. 2 Aluminum Lake), lactose monohydrate, magnesium stearate, microcrystalline cellulose, povidone and sodium starch glycolate. Blister packs of 30. Store between 15 and 30°C, away from heat, moisture and direct light.

The reader is invited to consult CPhA's monograph **Sulfonylureas**.

Sandoz® Glyburide ℞
glyburide
Oral Hypoglycemic

Sandoz

SUPPLIED: 2.5 mg: Each white, round, flat-faced, beveled-edge tablet, scored and engraved "GLY" over "2.5" on one side and plain on the other, contains: glyburide 2.5 mg. Nonmedicinal ingredients: croscarmellose sodium, lactose, magnesium stearate and microcrystalline cellulose. Bottles of 500. Store at room temperature (15 to 30°C).
5 mg: Each white, capsule-shaped, flat-faced, beveled-edge tablet, scored on one side and engraved "GLY 5" on the other, contains: glyburide 5 mg. Nonmedicinal ingredients: croscarmellose sodium, lactose, magnesium stearate and microcrystalline cellulose. Bottles of 100 and 500. Store at room temperature (15 to 30°).

Sandoz® Leflunomide ℞
leflunomide
Antirheumatic—Immunomodulator Agent

Sandoz

SUPPLIED: 10 mg: Each white, circular, biconvex, film-coated tablet, plain on one side and debossed «L10» on the other side, contains: leflunomide 10 mg. Nonmedicinal ingredients: cornstarch, colloidal silicon dioxide, hydroxypropyl cellulose, hydroxypropyl methylcellulose, lactose anhydrous, lactose monohydrate, magnesium stearate, polyethylene glycol, povidone and titanium dioxide. HDPE Bottles of 30. Store between 15 and 30°C. Protect from light and moisture.
20 mg: Each light yellow, triangular, biconvex, film-coated tablet, plain on one side and debossed «L20» on the other side, contains: leflunomide 20 mg. Nonmedicinal ingredients: cornstarch, colloidal silicon dioxide, hydroxypropyl cellulose, hydroxypropyl methylcellulose, lactose anhydrous, lactose monohydrate, magnesium stearate, polyethylene glycol, povidone, titanium dioxide and yellow ferric oxide. HDPE Bottles of 30. Store between 15 and 30°C. Protect from light or moisture.

Sandoz® Letrozole

letrozole

Nonsteroidal Aromatase Inhibitor—Inhibitor of Estrogen Biosynthesis—Antitumour Agent

Sandoz

SUPPLIED: Each dark yellow, round, slightly biconvex tablet with bevelled edges, bearing the imprint "FV" on one side and "CG" on the other, contains: letrozole 2.5 mg. Nonmedicinal ingredients: cellulose compounds (microcrystalline cellulose and methylhydroxypropylcellulose), corn starch, iron oxide, lactose, magnesium stearate, polyethylene glycol, sodium starch glycolate, silicon dioxide, talc and titanium dioxide. Blister packages of 30. Protect from heat (store at room temperature 15 to 30°C). Protect from moisture.

Sandoz® Levofloxacin

levofloxacin

Antibacterial

Sandoz

SUPPLIED: 250 mg: Each terra cotta pink-coloured, octagonal, biconvex, film-coated tablet, with imprint "LVF 250" on one side, contains: levofloxacin hemihydrate equivalent to levofloxacin (anhydrous) 250 mg. Nonmedicinal ingredients: colloidal silicon dioxide, croscarmellose sodium, ferric oxide red, ferric oxide yellow, glycerol dibehenate, hypromellose, hydroxypropyl cellulose, lactose monohydrate, polyethylene glycol, povidone, sodium starch glycolate, talc and titanium dioxide. Bottles of 50. Store between 15 and 30°C in well closed containers. Protect from moisture.

500 mg: Each peach-coloured, octagonal, biconvex, film-coated tablet, with imprint "LVF 500" on one side, contains: levofloxacin hemihydrate equivalent to levofloxacin (anhydrous) 500 mg. Nonmedicinal ingredients: colloidal silicon dioxide, croscarmellose sodium, ferric oxide red, ferric oxide yellow, glycerol dibehenate, hypromellose, hydroxypropyl cellulose, lactose monohydrate, polyethylene glycol, povidone, sodium starch glycolate, talc and titanium dioxide. Bottles of 100. Store between 15 and 30°C in well closed containers. Protect from moisture.

750 mg: Each white, octagonal, biconvex, film-coated tablet, with imprint "LVF 750" on one side, contains: levofloxacin hemihydrate equivalent to levofloxacin (anhydrous) 750 mg. Nonmedicinal ingredients: colloidal silicon dioxide, croscarmellose sodium, glycerol dibehenate, hypromellose, hydroxypropyl cellulose, lactose monohydrate, polyethylene glycol, povidone, sodium starch glycolate, talc and titanium dioxide. Bottles of 50. Store between 15 and 30°C in well closed containers. Protect from moisture.

The reader is invited to consult CPhA's monograph **ACE Inhibitors**.

Sandoz® Lisinopril

lisinopril

Angiotensin Converting Enzyme Inhibitor

Sandoz

SUPPLIED: 5 mg: Each pink, round, convex, uncoated tablet, scored on one side and plain on the other side, contains: lisinopril 5 mg. Nonmedicinal ingredients: calcium hydrogen phosphate dihydrate, croscarmellose sodium, ferric oxide, magnesium stearate, maize starch and mannitol. Blisters of 30 (2×15). Bottles of 100 and 500. Store between 15 and 30°C.

10 mg: Each pink, round, convex, uncoated tablet, plain on either side, contains: lisinopril 10 mg. Nonmedicinal ingredients: calcium hydrogen phosphate dihydrate, croscarmellose sodium, ferric oxide, magnesium stearate, maize starch and mannitol. Blisters of 30 (2×15). Bottles of 100 and 500. Store between 15 and 30°C.

20 mg: Each pink, round, convex, uncoated tablet, plain on either side, contains: lisinopril 20 mg. Nonmedicinal ingredients: calcium hydrogen phosphate dihydrate, croscarmellose sodium, ferric oxide, magnesium stearate, maize starch and mannitol. Blisters of 30 (2×15). Bottles of 100 and 500. Store between 15 and 30°C.

The reader is invited to consult CPhA's monograph **ACE Inhibitors** and **Thiazide Diuretics**.

Sandoz® Lisinopril HCT

lisinopril—hydrochlorothiazide

Angiotensin Converting Enzyme Inhibitor—Diuretic

Sandoz

SUPPLIED: 10/12.5 mg: Each orange, round, biconvex, uncoated tablet contains: lisinopril 10 mg and hydrochlorothiazide 12.5 mg. Nonmedicinal ingredients: calcium hydrogen phosphate dihydrate, croscarmellose sodium, ferric oxide, magnesium stearate, maize starch and mannitol. Blisters of 30 (2×15). Bottles of 100. Store between 15 and 30°C. Keep container tightly closed. Protect from light.

20/12.5 mg: Each white, oblong, biconvex, uncoated tablet contains: lisinopril 20 mg and hydrochlorothiazide 12.5 mg. Nonmedicinal ingredients: calcium hydrogen phosphate dihydrate, croscarmellose sodium, magnesium stearate, maize starch and mannitol. Blisters of 30 (2×15). Bottles of 100. Store between 15 and 30°C. Keep container tightly closed. Protect from light.

20/25 mg: Each orange, round, biconvex, uncoated tablet contains: lisinopril 20 mg and hydrochlorothiazide 25 mg. Nonmedicinal ingredients: calcium hydrogen phosphate dihydrate, croscarmellose sodium, ferric oxide, magnesium stearate, maize starch and mannitol. Blisters of 30 (2×15). Bottles of 100. Store between 15 and 30°C. Keep container tightly closed. Protect from light.

Sandoz® Metformin FC

metformin HCl

Antihyperglycemic

Sandoz

SUPPLIED: 500 mg: Each white, round, biconvex, film-coated tablet, debossed "RXP" on top of "500" on one side, and scored on the other side, contains: metformin HCl 500 mg. Nonmedicinal ingredients: colloidal anhydrous silica, magnesium stearate, microcrystalline cellulose, polyvinylpyrrolidone and sodium starch glycolate; film-coating: hydroxypropyl methylcellulose, lactose monohydrate, polyethylene glycol and titanium oxide. Bottles of 100 and 500. Store at room temperature (15 to 30°C) in well-closed containers.

850 mg: Each white, oblong, biconvex, film-coated tablet, with both sides score notched and debossed on one side "M" on one half and "850" on the other half, contains: metformin HCl 850 mg. Nonmedicinal ingredients: colloidal anhydrous silica, magnesium stearate, microcrystalline cellulose, polyvinylpyrrolidone and sodium starch glycolate; film-coating: hydroxypropyl methylcellulose, lactose monohydrate, polyethylene glycol and titanium oxide. Bottles of 100 and 500. Store at room temperature (15 to 30°C) in well-closed containers.

Sandoz® Methylphenidate SR

methylphenidate HCl

CNS Stimulant

Sandoz

SUPPLIED: Each white, round, biconvex, film-coated, extended-release tablet, with "20" printed on one side and "SZ" printed on the other side in black ink, contains: methylphenidate hydrochloride 20 mg. Nonmedicinal ingredients: castor oil compounds, cellulose compounds, cetostearyl alcohol, lactose, magnesium stearate, talc and titanium dioxide. Bottles of 100. Protect from heat (store between 2 and 30°C) and humidity.

Sandoz® Metoprolol SR

metoprolol tartrate

β-Adrenergic Receptor Blocking Agent

Sandoz

SUPPLIED: 100 mg: Each orange-brown, film-coated, round, slow-release tablet, imprinted with "SZ 100" on one side, contains: metoprolol tartrate 100 mg. Nonmedicinal ingredients: carnauba wax, castor oil compounds, cellulose compounds, iron oxides, magnesium stearate, phosphates polysorbate, talc and titanium dioxide. Bottles of 100. Store between 2 and 30°C. Protect from heat, light and humidity.

200 mg: Each light yellow, film-coated, round, slow-release tablet, imprinted with "SZ 200" on one side, contains: metoprolol tartrate 200 mg. Nonmedicinal ingredients: carnauba wax, castor oil compounds, cellulose compounds, iron oxides, magnesium stearate, phosphates polysorbate, talc and titanium dioxide. Bottles of 100. Store between 2 and 30°C. Protect from heat, light and humidity.

Sandoz® Metoprolol (Type L)

metoprolol tartrate

β-adrenergic Receptor Blocking Agent

Sandoz

SUPPLIED: 50 mg: Each pink, film-coated, capsule-shaped, biconvex tablet, scored on one side and engraved "50" on the other side, contains: metoprolol tartrate 50 mg. Nonmedicinal ingredients: carnauba wax, colloidal silicon dioxide, croscarmellose sodium, D&C Red #30 Aluminum Lake 30%, hydroxypropyl methylcellulose, lactose monohydrate, magnesium stearate, microcrystalline cellulose, polyethylene glycol, Sunset Yellow Aluminum Lake 40% and titanium dioxide. Bottles of 100 and 500. Store at room temperature (15 to 30°C). Protect from light.

100 mg: Each blue, film-coated, capsule-shaped, biconvex tablet, scored on one side and engraved "100" on the other side, contains: metoprolol tartrate 100 mg. Nonmedicinal ingredients: carnauba wax, colloidal silicon dioxide, croscarmellose sodium, hydroxypropyl methylcellulose, Indigotine Aluminum Lake 12-14% (Blue #2), lactose monohydrate, magnesium stearate, microcrystalline cellulose, polydextrose, polyethylene glycol and titanium dioxide. Bottles of 100 and 500. Store at room temperature (15 to 30°C). Protect from light.

The reader is invited to consult CPhA's monograph **Tetracyclines**.

Sandoz® Minocycline

minocycline HCl

Antibiotic

Sandoz

SUPPLIED: 50 mg: Each orange-colored, hard gelatin capsule, imprinted with «RXP-50» on body and cap, contains: minocycline HCl equivalent to minocycline base 50 mg. Nonmedicinal ingredients: corn starch, FD&C Yellow #6, gelatin, magnesium stearate and titanium dioxide. Tartrazine-free. Bottles of 100. Store at room temperature (15 to 30°C). Protect from light.

100 mg: Each orange- and purple-colored, hard gelatin capsule, imprinted with «RXP-100» on body and cap, contains: minocycline HCl equivalent to minocycline base 100 mg. Nonmedicinal ingredients: corn starch, FD&C Blue #1, FD&C Red #3, FD&C Yellow #6, gelatin, magnesium stearate and titanium dioxide. Tartrazine-free. Bottles of 100. Store at room temperature (15 to 30°C). Protect from light.

Sandoz® Mirtazapine

mirtazapine

Antidepressant

Sandoz

SUPPLIED: 15 mg: Each yellow, round, biconvex, bevelled-edge, film-coated tablet, debossed "E" over "20" on one side and bisected on the other side, contains: mirtazapine 15 mg. Nonmedicinal ingredients: colloidal silicon dioxide, hydroxypropyl methylcellulose, iron oxide yellow, lactose monohydrate, magnesium stearate, polyethylene glycol 400, polysorbate 80, pregelatinized starch and titanium dioxide. HDPE bottles of 50. Store at room temperature between 15 and 30°C. Dispense in a tight, light resistant container.

30 mg: Each red-brown, round, biconvex, film-coated tablet, debossed "E" over "212" on one side and bisected on the other side, contains: mirtazapine 30 mg. Nonmedicinal ingredients: colloidal silicon dioxide, FD&C yellow #6, hydroxypropyl methylcellulose, iron oxide red, lactose monohydrate, magnesium stearate, polyethylene glycol 400, polysorbate 80, pregelatinized starch and titanium dioxide. HDPE bottles of 100. Store at room temperature between 15 and 30°C. Dispense in a tight, light resistant container.

Sandoz® Naratriptan

naratriptan HCl

5-HT1 Receptor Agonist—Migraine Therapy

Sandoz

SUPPLIED: Each green coloured, "D" shaped film-coated tablet, with "SZ" debossed on one side and "248" on the other side, contains: naratriptan 2.5 mg (as naratriptan HCl). Nonmedicinal ingredients: Aluminum Lake FD&C Blue #2, cellulose microcrystalline, croscarmellose sodium, hypromellose, iron oxide yellow, lactose anhydrous, lactose monohydrate, magnesium stearate, titanium dioxide and triacetin. Blister packs of 2 and 6 (4 blister packs inserted into a carton). Store between 15 and 30°C.

Sandoz® Nitrazepam

nitrazepam

Hypnotic—Anticonvulsant

Sandoz

SUPPLIED: 5 mg: Each white, round, flat-faced, bevelled-edge tablet, engraved "RHO" on top and "5" underneath on one side and scored on the other side, contains: nitrazepam 5 mg. Nonmedicinal ingredients: croscarmellose sodium, lactose, magnesium stearate and microcrystalline cellulose. Bottles of 100 and 500.

10 mg: Each white, round, flat-faced, bevelled-edge tablet, engraved "RHO" on top and "10" underneath on one side and scored on the other side, contains: nitrazepam 10 mg. Nonmedicinal ingredients: croscarmellose sodium, lactose, magnesium stearate and microcrystalline cellulose. Bottles of 100 and 500.

Store at room temperature (15 to 30°C). Protect from light.

Sandoz® Olanzapine ODT

olanzapine

Antipsychotic

Sandoz

SUPPLIED: 5 mg: Each yellow, round, biconvex, oral disintegrating tablet, engraved with an "S" on one side and "5" on the other, contains: olanzapine 5 mg (16 µmol). Nonmedicinal ingredients: colloidal silicon dioxide, crospovidone, flavouring mint powder, hydroxypropyl cellulose, lactose monohydrate, magnesium stearate and talc. Blister strips in cartons of 30 tablets per carton. Store between 15 and 30°C in original container. Protect from light and moisture.

10 mg: Each yellow, round, flat, oral disintegrating tablet, engraved with an "S" on one side and "10" on the other, contains: olanzapine 10 mg (32 µmol). Nonmedicinal ingredients: colloidal silicon dioxide, crospovidone, flavouring mint powder, hydroxypropyl cellulose, lactose monohydrate, magnesium stearate and talc. Blister strips in cartons of 30 tablets per carton. Store between 15 and 30°C in original container. Protect from light and moisture.

15 mg: Each yellow, round, biconvex, oral disintegrating tablet, engraved with an "S" on one side and "15" on the other, contains: olanzapine 15 mg (48 µmol). Nonmedicinal ingredients: colloidal silicon dioxide, crospovidone, flavouring mint powder, hydroxypropyl cellulose, lactose monohydrate, magnesium stearate and talc. Blister strips in cartons of 30 tablets per carton. Store between 15 and 30°C in original container. Protect from light and moisture.

20 mg: Each yellow, round, flat, oral disintegrating tablet, engraved with an "S" on one side and "20" on the other, contains: olanzapine 20 mg (64 µmol). Nonmedicinal ingredients: colloidal silicon dioxide, crospovidone, flavouring mint powder, hydroxypropyl cellulose, lactose monohydrate, magnesium stearate and talc. Blister strips in cartons of 30 tablets per carton. Store between 15 and 30°C in original container. Protect from light and moisture.

Sandoz® Omeprazole

omeprazole

H+, K+-ATPase Inhibitor

Sandoz

SUPPLIED: 10 mg: Each two-piece HPMC capsule filled with pellets, consisting of a pink cap imprinted with OME 10 and a pink body imprinted with OME 10, contains: omeprazole 10 mg. Nonmedicinal ingredients: carrageenan, croscarmellose sodium, dibutyl sebacate, hypromellose, hypromellose phthalate, iron oxide red, lactose anhydrous, low-substituted hydroxypropyl cellulose, microcrystalline cellulose, polysorbate 80, potassium chloride, povidone, talc, titanium dioxide and water. HDPE child-resistant cap bottles of 30. Store bottle tightly capped between 15 and 30°C. Protect from moisture.

20 mg: Each two-piece HPMC capsule filled with pellets, consisting of a dark pink cap imprinted with OME 20 and a pink body imprinted with OME 20, contains: omeprazole 20 mg. Nonmedicinal ingredients: carrageenan, croscarmellose sodium, dibutyl sebacate, hypromellose, hypromellose phthalate, iron oxide red, lactose anhydrous, low-substituted hydroxypropyl cellulose, microcrystalline cellulose, polysorbate 80, potassium chloride, povidone, talc, titanium dioxide and water. HDPE child-resistant cap bottles of 30, 100 and 500. Store bottle tightly capped between 15 and 30°C. Protect from moisture.

Sandoz® Orphenadrine

orphenadrine citrate

Skeletal Muscle Relaxant

Sandoz

SUPPLIED: Each white, round-shaped, extended-release tablet, debossed "E" over "22" on one side and plain on the other side, contains: orphenadrine citrate 100 mg. Nonmedicinal ingredients: calcium stearate, ethylcellulose and lactose monohydrate. Bottles of 100. Store at room temperature (15 to 30°C). Protect from heat and moisture. Dispense in tight, light-resistant containers. Keep tightly closed.

Sandoz® Pantoprazole

pantoprazole sodium

H+, K+-ATPase Inhibitor

Sandoz

SUPPLIED: 20 mg: Each yellow, oval, enteric-coated tablet, imprinted "20" in black on one side, contains: pantoprazole 20 mg (as pantoprazole sodium sesquihydrate). Nonmedicinal ingredients: calcium stearate, cellulose microcrystalline, crospovidone, ferric oxide black, ferric oxide red, ferric oxide yellow, hydroxypropylcellulose, hypromellose, macrogol, methacrylic acid–ethyl acrylate copolymer, polysorbate 80, ponceau 4R aluminum lake, povidone, quinoline yellow aluminum lake, shellac, silica-colloidal anhydrous, sodium carbonate anhydrous, sodium lauryl sulfate, titanium dioxide and triethyl citrate. HDPE bottles of 100. Store between 15 and 30°C.

40 mg: Each yellow, oval, enteric-coated tablet, imprinted "S40" in black on one side, contains: pantoprazole 40 mg (as pantoprazole sodium sesquihydrate). Nonmedicinal ingredients: calcium stearate, cellulose microcrystalline, crospovidone, ferric oxide black, ferric oxide red, ferric oxide yellow, hydroxypropylcellulose, hypromellose, macrogol, methacrylic acid–ethyl acrylate copolymer, polysorbate 80, ponceau 4R aluminum lake, povidone, quinoline yellow aluminum lake, shellac, silica-colloidal anhydrous, sodium carbonate anhydrous, sodium lauryl sulfate, titanium dioxide and triethyl citrate. HDPE bottles of 100 and 500. Aluminum blister packs of 30. Store between 15 and 30°C.

Sandoz® Pioglitazone

pioglitazone HCl

Antidiabetic—Insulin Resistance Reducing Agent

Sandoz

SUPPLIED: 15 mg: Each white, round tablet with imprint "PGT" on one side, and "15" on the other side, contains: pioglitazone HCl equivalent to pioglitazone 15 mg. Nonmedicinal ingredients: carboxymethylcellulose calcium, hydroxypropylcellulose, lactose monohydrate and magnesium stearate. HDPE bottles of 100. Store between 15 and 30°C. Keep container tightly closed and protect from moisture and humidity.

30 mg: Each white, round tablet with imprint "PGT" on one side, and "30" on the other side, contains: pioglitazone HCl equivalent to pioglitazone 30 mg. Nonmedicinal ingredients: carboxymethylcellulose calcium, hydroxypropylcellulose, lactose monohydrate and magnesium stearate. HDPE bottles of 100. Store between 15 and 30°C. Keep container tightly closed and protect from moisture and humidity.

45 mg: Each white, round tablet with imprint "PGT" on one side, and "45" on the other side, contains: pioglitazone HCl equivalent to pioglitazone 45 mg. Nonmedicinal ingredients: carboxymethylcellulose calcium, hydroxypropylcellulose, lactose monohydrate and magnesium stearate. HDPE bottles of 100. Store between 15 and 30°C. Keep container tightly closed and protect from moisture and humidity.

Sandoz® Pramipexole

pramipexole dihydrochloride

Antiparkinsonian Agent—Dopamine Agonist

Sandoz

SUPPLIED: 0.25 mg: Each white to off-white, oval-shaped tablet, with break line on both sides and debossed with "P", ".25" on one side, contains: pramipexole dihydrochloride monohydrate 0.25 mg. Nonmedicinal ingredients: Betacyclodextrin-Kleptose, cellulose microcrystalline, corn starch, magnesium stearate, povidone and silicon dioxide colloidal. Bottles of 100. Store between 15 and 30°C. Protect from light.

0.5 mg: Each white to off-white, oval-shaped tablet, with break line on both sides and debossed with "P", ".5" on one side, contains: pramipexole dihydrochloride monohydrate 0.5 mg. Nonmedicinal ingredients: Betacyclodextrin-Kleptose, cellulose microcrystalline, corn starch, magnesium stearate, povidone and silicon dioxide colloidal. Bottles of 100. Store between 15 and 30°C. Protect from light.

1 mg: Each white to off-white, circular-shaped tablet, with break line on both sides and debossed with "P", "1" on one side, contains: pramipexole dihydrochloride monohydrate 1 mg. Nonmedicinal ingredients: Betacyclodextrin-Kleptose, cellulose microcrystalline, corn starch, magnesium stearate, povidone and silicon dioxide colloidal. Bottles of 100. Store between 15 and 30°C. Protect from light.

1.5 mg: Each white to off-white, circular-shaped tablet, with break line on both sides and debossed with "P", "1.5" on one side, contains: pramipexole dihydrochloride monohydrate 1.5 mg. Nonmedicinal ingredients: Betacyclodextrin-Kleptose, cellulose microcrystalline, corn starch, magnesium stearate, povidone and silicon dioxide colloidal. Bottles of 100. Store between 15 and 30°C. Protect from light.

The reader is invited to consult CPhA's monograph **HMG-CoA Reductase Inhibitors**.

Sandoz® Pravastatin

pravastatin sodium

Lipid Metabolism Regulator

Sandoz

SUPPLIED: 10 mg: Each rounded rectangular-shaped, pink to peach, biconvex tablet, engraved "PRA" over "10" on one side and plain on the other side, contains: pravastatin sodium 10 mg. Nonmedicinal ingredients: croscarmellose sodium, lactose monohydrate, magnesium stearate, microcrystalline cellulose and red ferric oxide. Bottles of 100. Unit dose blister packages of 30. Store at room temperature (15 to 30°C). Protect from moisture and light.

20 mg: Each rounded rectangular-shaped, yellow, biconvex tablet engraved "PRA" over "20" on one side and plain on the other side, contains: pravastatin sodium 20 mg. Nonmedicinal ingredients: croscarmellose sodium, lactose monohydrate, magnesium stearate, microcrystalline cellulose and yellow ferric oxide. Bottles of 100. Unit dose blister packages of 30. Store at room temperature (15 to 30°C). Protect from moisture and light.

40 mg: Each rounded rectangular-shaped, green, biconvex tablet, engraved "PRA" over "40" on one side and plain on the other side, contains: pravastatin sodium 40 mg. Nonmedicinal ingredients: croscarmellose sodium, D&C Yellow #10, FD&C Blue #1, lactose monohydrate, magnesium stearate and microcrystalline cellulose. Bottles of 100. Unit dose blister packages of 30. Store at room temperature (15 to 30°C). Protect from moisture and light.

Sandoz® Prednisolone

prednisolone acetate

Ophthalmic Corticosteroid

Sandoz

SUPPLIED: 0.12%: Each mL of sterile ophthalmic suspension contains: prednisolone acetate 1.2 mg (0.12%). Nonmedicinal ingredients: benzalkonium chloride 0.01% as preservative, citric acid to adjust pH, dibasic sodium phosphate, edetate disodium, glycerine, hypromellose, polysorbate 80 and water for injection. Plastic dropper bottles of 10 mL. Store between 15 and 30°C. Do not freeze. Shake well before use.

1%: Each mL of sterile ophthalmic suspension contains: prednisolone acetate 10 mg (1%). Nonmedicinal ingredients: benzalkonium chloride 0.01% as preservative, citric acid to adjust pH, dibasic sodium phosphate, edetate disodium, glycerine, hypromellose, polysorbate 80 and water for injection. Plastic dropper bottles of 5 and 10 mL. Store between 15 and 30°C. Do not freeze. Shake well before use.

Sandoz® Proctomyxin HC

hydrocortisone—framycetin sulfate—cinchocaine HCl—esculin

Antibacterial—Corticosteroid—Anorectal Therapy

Sandoz

SUPPLIED: Ointment: Each g of ointment contains: hydrocortisone 5 mg, cinchocaine HCl 5 mg, framycetin sulfate 10 mg and esculin 10 mg. Nonmedicinal ingredients: lanolin, mineral oil and petroleum jelly. Tubes of 15 and 30 g, boxes of 1. Store between 15 and 30°C.

Suppositories: Each suppository contains: hydrocortisone 5 mg, cinchocaine HCl 5 mg, framycetin sulfate 10 mg and esculin 10 mg. Boxes of 12 and 24. Store between 15 and 30°C.

Sandoz® Quetiapine ℞
quetiapine fumarate
Antipsychotic

Sandoz

SUPPLIED: 25 mg: Each peach-coloured, round, biconvex, film-coated tablet, debossed with "SZ" on one side and "25" on the other side, contains: quetiapine fumarate equivalent to quetiapine free base 25 mg. Nonmedicinal ingredients: anhydrous calcium hydrogen phosphate, hypromellose, iron oxide red, iron oxide yellow, lactose monohydrate, magnesium stearate, microcrystalline cellulose, polyethylene glycol 400, povidone, sodium starch glycolate and titanium dioxide. Blisters of 60. HDPE bottles of 100 and 500. Store between 15 and 30°C.
100 mg: Each yellow-coloured, round, biconvex, film-coated tablet, debossed with "SZ" on one side and "100" on the other side, contains: quetiapine fumarate equivalent to quetiapine free base 100 mg. Nonmedicinal ingredients: anhydrous calcium hydrogen phosphate, hypromellose, iron oxide yellow, lactose monohydrate, magnesium stearate, microcrystalline cellulose, polyethylene glycol 400, povidone, sodium starch glycolate and titanium dioxide. HDPE bottles of 100 and 500. Store between 15 and 30°C.
200 mg: Each white to off-white, round, biconvex, film-coated tablet, debossed with "SZ" on one side and "200" on the other side, contains: quetiapine fumarate equivalent to quetiapine free base 200 mg. Nonmedicinal ingredients: anhydrous calcium hydrogen phosphate, hypromellose, lactose monohydrate, magnesium stearate, microcrystalline cellulose, polyethylene glycol 400, povidone, sodium starch glycolate and titanium dioxide. HDPE bottles of 100. Store between 15 and 30°C.
300 mg: Each white to off-white, capsule-shaped, film-coated tablet, debossed with "SZ" on one side and "300" on the other side, contains: quetiapine fumarate equivalent to quetiapine free base 300 mg. Nonmedicinal ingredients: anhydrous calcium hydrogen phosphate, hypromellose, lactose monohydrate, magnesium stearate, microcrystalline cellulose, polyethylene glycol 400, povidone, sodium starch glycolate and titanium dioxide. HDPE bottles of 100. Store between 15 and 30°C.

Sandoz® Rabeprazole ℞
rabeprazole sodium
H+, K+-ATPase Inhibitor

Sandoz

SUPPLIED: 10 mg: Each pink, round, biconvex, enteric-coated tablet, with "R10" printed on one side, contains: rabeprazole sodium 10 mg. Nonmedicinal ingredients: calcium hydroxide, dibutyl sebacate, ferric oxide red, ferric oxide yellow, hypromellose, hypromellose phthalate, low-substituted hydroxypropyl cellulose, mannitol, sodium stearyl fumarate, talc and titanium dioxide. Unit dose blister packages of 30 (3×10). Bottles of 100. Store between 15 and 25°C, protected from moisture and heat.
20 mg: Each yellow, round, biconvex, enteric-coated tablet, with "R20" printed on one side, contains: rabeprazole sodium 20 mg. Nonmedicinal ingredients: calcium hydroxide, dibutyl sebacate, ferric oxide yellow, hypromellose, hypromellose phthalate, low-substituted hydroxypropyl cellulose, mannitol, sodium stearyl fumarate, talc and titanium dioxide. Unit dose blister packages of 30 (3×10). Bottles of 100. Store between 15 and 25°C, protected from moisture and heat.

Sandoz® Rivastigmine ℞
rivastigmine hydrogen tartrate
Cholinesterase Inhibitor

Sandoz

SUPPLIED: 1.5 mg: Each yellow, hard-gelatin capsule, with "ENA713 1.5 mg" printed in red on the body, contains: rivastigmine hydrogen tartrate equivalent to rivastigmine base 1.5 mg. Nonmedicinal ingredients: hydroxypropyl methylcellulose, magnesium stearate, microcrystalline cellulose and silicon dioxide; hard gelatin capsule: gelatin, red and/or yellow iron oxides and titanium dioxide. Bottles of 100. Blister strips of 14, cartons of 4. Store at room temperature (15-30°C).
3 mg: Each orange, hard-gelatin capsule, with "ENA713 3 mg" printed in red on the body, contains: rivastigmine hydrogen tartrate equivalent to rivastigmine base 3 mg. Nonmedicinal ingredients: hydroxypropyl methylcellulose, magnesium stearate, microcrystalline cellulose and silicon dioxide; hard gelatin capsule: gelatin, red and/or yellow iron oxides and titanium dioxide. Bottles of 100. Blister strips of 14, cartons of 4. Store at room temperature (15-30°C).
4.5 mg: Each red, hard-gelatin capsule, with "ENA713 4.5 mg" printed in white on the body, contains: rivastigmine hydrogen tartrate equivalent to rivastigmine base 4.5 mg. Nonmedicinal ingredients: hydroxypropyl methylcellulose, magnesium stearate, microcrystalline cellulose and silicon dioxide; hard gelatin capsule: gelatin, red and/or yellow iron oxides and titanium dioxide. Bottles of 100. Blister strips of 14, cartons of 4. Store at room temperature (15-30°C).
6 mg: Each orange and red, hard-gelatin capsule, with "ENA713 6 mg" printed in red on the body, contains: rivastigmine hydrogen tartrate equivalent to rivastigmine base 6 mg. Nonmedicinal ingredients: hydroxypropyl methylcellulose, magnesium stearate, microcrystalline cellulose and silicon dioxide; hard gelatin capsule: gelatin, red and/or yellow iron oxides and titanium dioxide. Bottles of 100. Blister strips of 14, cartons of 4. Store at room temperature (15-30°C).

Sandoz® Sotalol ℞
sotalol HCl
Antiarrhythmic

Sandoz

SUPPLIED: 80 mg: Each blue, capsule-shaped, biconvex tablet, scored on one side, debossed "RXP-80" on the other side, contains: sotalol HCl 80 mg. Nonmedicinal ingredients: colloidal silicon dioxide, dextrates, indigotine (Blue #2), magnesium stearate and methylcellulose. Bottles of 100.
160 mg: Each blue, capsule-shaped, biconvex tablet, scored on one side, debossed "RXP-160"on the other side, contains: sotalol HCl 160 mg. Nonmedicinal ingredients: colloidal silicon dioxide, dextrates, indigotine (Blue #2), magnesium stearate and methylcellulose. Bottles of 100.
Store at room temperature (15 to 30°C). Protect from light.

Sandoz® Sumatriptan ℞
sumatriptan succinate
5-HT1 Receptor Agonist—Migraine Therapy

Sandoz

SUPPLIED: 50 mg: Each white, triangular, biconvex tablet, debossed "RXP" on one side and plain on the other, contains: sumatriptan succinate equivalent to sumatriptan base 50 mg. Nonmedicinal ingredients: ammonio methacrylate copolymer type A, carboxymethylcellulose sodium, croscarmellose sodium, grapefruit flavour (contains maltodextrin and natural and artificial flavours), lactose monohydrate, magnesium stearate and microcrystalline cellulose. Blister packs of 6. Store between 15 and 30°C.
100 mg: Each pink, triangular, biconvex tablet, debossed "RXP" on one side and plain on the other, contains: sumatriptan succinate equivalent to sumatriptan base 100 mg. Nonmedicinal ingredients: ammonio methacrylate copolymer type A, carboxymethylcellulose sodium, croscarmellose sodium, ferric oxide red, ferric oxide yellow, grapefruit flavour (contains maltodextrin and natural and artificial flavours), lactose monohydrate, magnesium stearate and microcrystalline cellulose. Blister packs of 6. Store between 15 and 30°C.

Sandoz® Tamsulosin ℞
tamsulosin HCl
Selective Antagonist of Alpha1A Adrenoreceptor Subtype in the Prostate

Sandoz

SUPPLIED: Each hard gelatin, sustained-release capsule, with an orange body and olive green cap, with a black line at each end of the capsule and "TSL 0.4" printed in black ink on the capsule, contains: tamsulosin HCl 0.4 mg. Nonmedicinal ingredients: methacrylic acid-ethyl acrylate copolymer (polysorbate 80, sodium lauryl sulfate), microcrystalline cellulose, talc and triethylcitrate; capsule shell: black iron oxide, FD&C Blue No. 2, gelatin, red iron oxide, titanium dioxide and yellow iron oxide; capsule imprinting ink: antifoam, black iron oxide, shellac glaze and soya lecithin. Bottles of 100. Store between 15 and 30°C.

Sandoz® Terbinafine ℞
terbinafine HCl
Antifungal Agent

Sandoz

SUPPLIED: Each whitish to yellow tinged white, circular, biconvex, with beveled edges tablet, scored on one side and embossed "T" on the other side, contains: terbinafine HCl equivalent to terbinafine base 250 mg. Nonmedicinal ingredients: cellulose microcrystalline granulate, colloidal anhydrous silica, hypromellose, magnesium stearate and sodium starch glycolate. Blister packs of 28. Bottles of 100. Store between 15 and 30°C. Protect from light.

Sandoz® Topiramate ℞
topiramate
Antiepileptic—Migraine Prophylaxis

Sandoz

SUPPLIED: 25 mg: Each white, round, biconvex, film-coated tablet, debossed "RXP" on one side and "25" on the other side, contains: topiramate 25 mg. Nonmedicinal ingredients: hydroxypropyl methylcellulose, lactose monohydrate, magnesium stearate, microcrystalline cellulose, polyethylene glycol, polysorbate 80, pregelatinized starch, purified water, sodium starch glycolate and titanium dioxide. Bottles of 100. Store between 15 and 30°C in a tightly closed container. Protect from moisture.
100 mg: Each yellow, round, biconvex, film-coated tablet, debossed "RXP" on one side and "100" on the other side, contains: topiramate 100 mg. Nonmedicinal ingredients: hydroxypropyl methylcellulose, lactose monohydrate, magnesium stearate, microcrystalline cellulose, polyethylene glycol, polysorbate 80, pregelatinized starch, purified water, sodium starch glycolate, titanium dioxide and yellow iron oxide. Bottles of 100. Store between 15 and 30°C in a tightly closed container. Protect from moisture.
200 mg: Each salmon-coloured, round, biconvex, film-coated tablet, debossed "RXP" on one side and "200" on the other side, contains: topiramate 200 mg. Nonmedicinal ingredients: hydroxypropyl methylcellulose, lactose monohydrate, magnesium stearate, microcrystalline cellulose, polyethylene glycol, polysorbate 80, pregelatinized starch, purified water, red iron oxide, sodium starch glycolate and titanium dioxide. Bottles of 100. Store between 15 and 30°C in a tightly closed container. Protect from moisture.

Sandoz® Venlafaxine XR ℞
venlafaxine HCl
Antidepressant—Anxiolytic

Sandoz

SUPPLIED: 37.5 mg: Each extended-release, hard gelatin capsule, with grey cap and flesh pink body, with "37.5 mg" printed in red ink, contains: venlafaxine HCl equivalent to venlafaxine base 37.5 mg. Nonmedicinal ingredients: ammonia, gelatin, hypromellose, iron oxide black, iron oxide red, magnesium stearate, poly(ethyl acrylate, methyl methacrylate, trimethylammonioethyl methacrylate chloride), poly(butyl methacrylate, (2-dimethylaminoethyl) methacrylate, methyl methacrylate), potassium hydroxide, propylene glycol, shellac, sodium lauryl sulfate and titanium dioxide. Bottles of 100. Store between 15 and 30°C, in a dry place.
75 mg: Each extended-release, hard gelatin capsule, with flesh pink cap and body, with "75 mg" printed in red ink, contains: venlafaxine HCl equivalent to venlafaxine base 75 mg. Nonmedicinal ingredients: ammonia, gelatin, hypromellose, iron oxide red, magnesium stearate, poly(ethyl acrylate, methyl methacrylate, trimethylammonioethyl methacrylate chloride), poly(butyl methacrylate, (2-dimethylaminoethyl) methacrylate, methyl methacrylate), potassium hydroxide, propylene glycol, shellac, sodium lauryl sulfate and titanium dioxide. Bottles of 100 and 250. Store between 15 and 30°C, in a dry place.
150 mg: Each extended-release, hard gelatin capsule, with dark Swedish orange cap and body, with "150 mg" printed in white ink, contains: venlafaxine HCl equivalent to venlafaxine base 150 mg. Nonmedicinal ingredients: gelatin, hypromellose, iron oxide black, iron oxide red, iron oxide yellow, magnesium stearate, poly(ethyl acrylate, methyl methacrylate, trimethylammonioethyl methacrylate chloride), poly(butyl methacrylate, (2-dimethylaminoethyl) methacrylate, methyl methacrylate), povidone, propylene glycol, shellac, sodium hydroxide, sodium lauryl sulfate and titanium dioxide. Bottles of 100 and 250. Store between 15 and 30°C, in a dry place.

Sandoz® Zopiclone ℞
zopiclone
Hypnotic

Sandoz

SUPPLIED: 5 mg: Each round, white, biconvex, film-coated tablet, engraved "5" on one side and "RXP" on the other side, contains: zopiclone 5 mg. Nonmedicinal ingredients: calcium phosphate dihydrate, cornstarch, hydroxypropyl methylcellulose, lactose, magnesium stearate, maltodextrin, polydextrose, polyethylene glycol, sodium croscarmellose, titanium dioxide and triacetin. Bottles of 100. Store in a dry place between 15 and 30°C. Protect from light.
7.5 mg: Each oval, blue, film-coated tablet, scored on one side and engraved "RXP 7.5" on the other side, contains: zopiclone 7.5 mg. Nonmedicinal ingredients: calcium phosphate dihydrate, cornstarch, D&C Yellow #10 aluminum lake, FD&C Blue #1 aluminum lake, FD&C Blue #2 aluminum lake, hydroxypropyl methylcellulose, lactose, magnesium stearate, maltodextrin, polydextrose, polyethylene glycol, sodium croscarmellose, titanium dioxide and triacetin. Bottles of 100 and 500. Store in a dry place between 15 and 30°C. Protect from light.

Sarna® HC ℞
hydrocortisone
Topical Corticosteroid

Stiefel, a GSK company

SUPPLIED: 1.0%: Each mL of lotion contains: hydrocortisone USP 1.0% in a soothing emollient base. Nonmedicinal ingredients: camphor, cetyl alcohol, citric acid anhydrous, colloidal silicone dioxide, DMDM hydantoin, edetate disodium, fragrance, glyceryl stearate blend, isopropyl myristate, menthol crystals, PEG 400 monostearate, purified water, stearic acid, white petrolatum and xanthan gum. Plastic bottles of 150 mL with flip-top.
2.5%: Each mL of lotion contains: hydrocortisone USP 2.5% in a soothing emollient base. Nonmedicinal ingredients: camphor, cetyl alcohol, citric acid anhydrous, colloidal silicone dioxide, DMDM hydantoin, edetate disodium, fragrance, glyceryl stearate blend, isopropyl myristate, menthol crystals, PEG 400 monostearate, purified water, stearic acid, white petrolatum and xanthan gum. Plastic tubes of 75 mL.

Sarna-P®
camphor—menthol—pramoxine HCl
Antipruritic—Surface Anesthetic

Stiefel, a GSK company

SUPPLIED: Each mL of lotion contains: pramoxine HCl 1%, camphor 0.5% and menthol 0.5% in a soothing, moisturizing emollient base. Nonmedicinal ingredients: carbomer 1342, cetyl alcohol, DMDM hydantoin, fragrance, glyceryl stearate blend, isopropyl myristate, polyethylene glycol, purified water, sodium hydroxide, stearic acid and white petrolatum. Plastic bottles of 150 mL with flip-top.

Sativex® Ⓝ
delta-9-tetrahydrocannabinol—cannabidiol
Cannabinoid Analgesic

GW Pharma/Bayer

Date of Revision: December 18, 2008

SATIVEX buccal spray is indicated as adjunctive treatment for the symptomatic relief of neuropathic pain in multiple sclerosis in adults. SATIVEX buccal spray is also indicated as adjunctive analgesic treatment in adult patients with advanced cancer who experience moderate to severe pain during the highest tolerated dose of strong opioid therapy for persistent background pain. SATIVEX has been issued a marketing authorization with conditions, to reflect the promising nature of the clinical evidence and the need for confirmatory studies to verify the clinical benefit. Patients should be advised of the conditional nature of the authorization.

SUMMARY PRODUCT INFORMATION:

Route of Administration	Dosage Form/ Strength	All Nonmedicinal Ingredients
Buccal	Buccal spray delta-9-tetrahydrocannabinol 27 mg/mL (from Tetranabinex—Cannabis sativa L. extract) and cannabidiol 25 mg/mL (from Nabidiolex—Cannabis sativa L. extract)	Ethanol anhydrous, propylene glycol, peppermint oil This is a full listing of all nonmedicinal ingredients.

INDICATIONS AND CLINICAL USE: SATIVEX buccal spray may be useful as adjunctive treatment for the symptomatic relief of neuropathic pain in multiple sclerosis (MS) in adults.

The effectiveness of SATIVEX in long-term use (i.e. more than 4-6 weeks) has not been evaluated in placebo-controlled clinical trials. The physician who elects to use SATIVEX for extended periods in the treatment of neuropathic pain in MS should periodically re-evaluate the long-term usefulness of the drug for the individual patient.

SATIVEX may be useful as adjunctive analgesic treatment in adult patients with advanced cancer who experience moderate to severe pain during the highest tolerated dose of strong opioid therapy for persistent background pain.

Delta-9-tetrahydrocannabinol (THC) and cannabidiol (CBD) are the principal active components in SATIVEX. THC is a psychotropic agent which may produce physical and psychological dependence and has the potential to be abused. Both active components, THC and CBD, are scheduled under the Controlled Drugs and Substances Act.

Geriatrics: There are limited data available on the use of SATIVEX in elderly patients, therefore, the drug should be prescribed cautiously and carefully monitored in this patient population.

Pediatrics (<18 years of age): The safety and efficacy of SATIVEX have not been established in adolescents or children under 18 years of age, therefore SATIVEX should not be used in adolescents or children.

CONTRAINDICATIONS: SATIVEX is contraindicated in:
- patients with known or suspected allergy to cannabinoids, propylene glycol, ethanol or peppermint oil
- patients with serious cardiovascular disease, such as ischemic heart disease, arrhythmias, poorly controlled hypertension or severe heart failure
- patients with a history of schizophrenia or any other psychotic disorder
- children under 18 years of age
- women of child-bearing potential not on a reliable contraceptive or men intending to start a family (see Warnings and Precautions, Use in Women of Child-bearing Potential)
- pregnant or nursing women (see Warnings and Precautions, Use in Women of Child-bearing Potential)

WARNINGS AND PRECAUTIONS:

Serious Warnings and Precautions
THC and CBD are the principal active components in SATIVEX. THC can produce physical and psychological dependence and has the potential for being abused.

THC has complex effects on the central nervous system (CNS). These can result in changes of mood, decrease in cognitive performances and memory, decrease in ability to control drives and impulses, and alteration of the perception of reality, particularly altered time sense. Fainting episodes have been observed with use of SATIVEX. CNS effects, with dizziness being the most frequent (see Table 2), appear to be dose-related, increasing in frequency with higher dosages, and subject to great inter-patient variability. They usually resolve on reduction of doses, increasing the interval between doses or interruption of SATIVEX (see Overdosage). Because of the potential of THC to alter the mental state, SATIVEX should be used only as indicated and prescriptions should be limited to the amount necessary for the period between clinic visits. Drug administration should be discontinued in patients experiencing a psychotic reaction or a suicidal ideation and the patient should be closely observed in an appropriate setting until his/her mental state returns to normal. Patients should stop taking SATIVEX if they become confused or disorientated. Patients should be warned not to drive or engage in activities requiring unimpaired judgement and coordination.

Cannabinoids have cardiovascular effects that include tachycardia, and transient changes in blood pressure, including episodes of postural hypotension. Use of SATIVEX is not recommended in patients with pre-existing cardiovascular disease, such as ischaemic heart disease, arrhythmias, poorly controlled hypertension or severe heart failure.

Published reports on cannabinoids are equivocal with regard to the effects of THC on seizure threshold. Until further information is available, caution should be used when treating patients with a history of epilepsy or recurrent seizures.

General: During the initial self-titration period, patients may experience unacceptable adverse events, including dizziness. These should resolve with down-titration or interruption of treatment (see Overdosage, Signs and Symptoms).

Careful dose titration and monitoring are advised if SATIVEX is used in patients on a drug product containing fentanyl, or its analogues such as alfentanil and sufentanil (PK interaction).

Care should be taken with sedatives, drugs with sedating or psychotropic effects and hypnotics as coadministration with SATIVEX may have an additive effect.

Buccal Mucosa: Regular inspection of the oral mucosa is advised. Patients should be advised not to continue spraying on to sore or inflamed mucosa.

Administration site irritation was common both during short-term and long-term use of SATIVEX.

Cardiovascular: See Serious Warnings and Precautions.

CNS Effects: See Serious Warnings and Precautions, Overdosage and Adverse Reactions.

Driving and Operating Machinery: SATIVEX may impair the mental and/or physical abilities required for certain potentially hazardous activities such as driving a car or operating machinery. Patients should be warned not to drive or engage in activities requiring unimpaired judgement and coordination. Patients should also be cautioned about the additive/synergistic effects of SATIVEX with other CNS depressants, including opioids, GABA inhibitors, sedative/hypnotics and alcohol.

Genitourinary: See Use in Women of Child-bearing Potential.

Hematologic: Clinical laboratory investigations did not reveal any trends of clinical significance in hematological parameters.

Hepatic/Biliary/Pancreatic: No consistent effect of SATIVEX on clinical chemistry parameters has been observed.

No specific studies have been carried out in patients with significant hepatic or renal impairment, therefore SATIVEX should be used with caution in such patients. Frequent review by the clinician is recommended.

SATIVEX contains approximately 50% v/v of ethanol. Each dose contains up to 0.04 g of ethanol. The median daily dose of 5 sprays would be up to 0.2 g ethanol. Ethanol may be harmful for those suffering from alcoholism. This should also be taken into account in high-risk groups such as patients with liver disease.

Immune: No clinically significant abnormalities of immune function have been observed in clinical trials with SATIVEX.

Neurologic: In clinical studies with SATIVEX, an increase in the number of falls has been observed. Whether this is due to dizziness, orthostatic hypotension or reduced spasticity has not been established. Patients should be made aware that care should be taken to avoid falls.

There is not sufficient information to characterize the effect of SATIVEX on the seizure threshold. Caution should be used in treating patients with a history of epilepsy or recurrent seizures.

Peri-Operative Considerations: SATIVEX may produce transient minor changes in blood pressure and heart rate. The central and peripheral effects of SATIVEX should be taken into consideration in peri-operative situations.

Psychiatric: SATIVEX should not be used in patients with a personal or strong family history of psychosis (including schizophrenia and affective psychosis) as symptoms may be aggravated by cannabinoids. SATIVEX should be used with caution, if at all, in patients receiving other psychoactive drugs because of the potential for additive or synergistic CNS effects. In cases of disorientation (or confusion), hallucinations, delusional beliefs, or psychotic reaction, SATIVEX should be stopped immediately and the patient monitored until the symptom has completely resolved (see Contraindications).

Suicidal ideations and other symptoms associated with depression have been reported. A causal association between SATIVEX administration and suicidal ideation cannot be ruled out. The reported incidences of depression symptoms are consistent with that observed in populations of MS patients followed for a prolonged period of time. In case of a suicidal ideation, SATIVEX should be stopped immediately and the patient monitored until the symptom has completely resolved.

In acute studies with SATIVEX, disorientation (5.0%), depression including depressed mood (3.6%), dissociation (3.0%), euphoric mood (2.4%), anxiety (1.1%) and paranoia (0.9%) have been reported. Auditory hallucination was reported by 0.3% of patients receiving SATIVEX in acute studies (placebo 0%). In long-term Phase III extension studies (n=662), the following additional adverse events, with a plausible causal relationship to SATIVEX, have also been reported by patients: hallucination (0.9%), illusion (0.6%), visual hallucination (0.5%) and delusional perception (0.2%).

Sensitivity/Resistance: SATIVEX is contraindicated in patients with known or suspected allergy to cannabinoids, propylene glycol, ethanol or peppermint oil (see Contraindications).

Use in Women of Child-bearing Potential: Independent research in laboratory species has found that cannabinoids have been associated with evidence of reproductive toxicity in early gestation and have been found to affect spermatogenesis. Therefore, women of child-bearing potential should take reliable contraceptive precautions for the duration of treatment and for three months after discontinuation of therapy. Male patients with a partner of childbearing potential should ensure that reliable contraceptive precautions are maintained for the duration of therapy and for three months after discontinuation of therapy.

Special Populations: Pregnant Women: Animal studies have indicated that cannabinoids may have detrimental effects on fetal development. SATIVEX is contraindicated in pregnant women. SATIVEX should not be used in women who intend to start a family.

In clinical trials with SATIVEX, all female participants had to use a reliable contraceptive and all male participants had to ensure contraception with their partner. If a female participant became pregnant, she had to discontinue from the trial.

Nursing Women: In studies in laboratory species, due to the lipophilic nature of cannabinoids, considerable levels of cannabinoids were found in the maternal breast milk. Even at 1 mg/kg/day there were 40-60 times the plasma level of cannabinoids in the breast milk.

SATIVEX is contraindicated in nursing women.

Pediatrics (<18 years of age): Animal data have indicated that cannabinoids interfere with the development of neonatal and adolescent rodents. SATIVEX is contraindicated in children under 18 years of age.

Geriatrics: There are limited data available on the use of SATIVEX in elderly patients, therefore, the drug should be prescribed cautiously and carefully monitored in this patient population.

Hepatic and Renal Impairment: No specific studies have been carried out in patients with significant hepatic or renal impairment. (See Warnings and Precautions.)

Monitoring and Laboratory Tests: Routine laboratory monitoring, appropriate for the patient's disease condition and concomitant medication, is recommended. Due to accumulation of cannabinoids in the body fat, trace amount of cannabinoids may be detected in the blood and urine for some weeks after SATIVEX is discontinued.

Drug Dependence/Abuse Liability: Recreational cannabis is known to produce dependence in some users. THC is a psychotropic agent which may produce physical and psychological dependence and has the potential to be abused.

SATIVEX contains THC and should be used with caution in patients with a history of substance abuse, including alcohol abuse or dependence. Multiple substance abuse is common and marijuana, which contains the same active compounds, is a frequently abused substance. Therefore, SATIVEX is not recommended in patients with addiction and drug abuse liability. In long-term open-label studies with SATIVEX, no increase in the dosing level of SATIVEX was observed.

ADVERSE REACTIONS: Adverse Drug Reaction Overview: SATIVEX has been administered to 662 patients during Phase III long-term open-extension studies in various neurological conditions (excluding pain in cancer studies). More than 420 patients have received more than six months treatment with SATIVEX, and over 310 patients have received SATIVEX for more than one year.

In addition to the adverse events (all-causality) reported in the controlled acute studies (refer to Table 1 and Table 2) the following adverse events observed in patients (n=662) on long-term treatment with SATIVEX were considered to have a plausible causal relationship to SATIVEX: tooth discolouration (3.8%), oral mucosal disorder (3.5%), oral mucosal discolouration (1.5%), oral mucosal exfoliation (1.1%), stomatitis (1.1%), anxiety (1.8%), hypotension (1.8%), appetite decreased (1.4%) and syncope (1.2%).

Clinical Trial Adverse Drug Reactions: The following data summarize the adverse events in patients in clinical trials with various neurological conditions. Patients in clinical trials for relief of pain in cancer are described separately.

In all placebo-controlled trials in various indications (brachial plexus injury, MS symptoms, other defects of neurological function) adverse events have usually been mild or moderate in severity with discontinuation rates from treatment due to undesirable effects of 10.7% of patients on SATIVEX compared to 3.2% on placebo. In most patients, adverse events have resolved without treatment, and some on a reduction of dosage of SATIVEX. The studies from which these figures are derived incorporate a period of titration to optimal therapeutic and/or maximum tolerated dose during which unwanted effects are likely to be maximal. Because SATIVEX is self-titrated to effect, patients are likely to experience a higher incidence of adverse events during the titration period than when the optimal dose is established.

Because clinical trials are conducted under very specific conditions, the adverse reaction rates observed in the clinical trials may not reflect the rates observed in practice and should not be compared to the rates in the clinical trials of another drug. Adverse drug reaction information from clinical trials is useful for identifying drug-related adverse events and for approximating rates.

Treatment-emergent adverse events that occurred in 1% or more of patients treated with SATIVEX, and at an incidence greater than 1% more frequently than placebo, in the acute phase in all Phase III trials are given below in Table 1 and Table 2. Table 1 includes all adverse events related to the application site, as the placebo used in studies contained the same excipients (ethanol and propylene glycol) as used in SATIVEX.

Table 1 excludes CNS effects, while Table 2 lists only CNS effects.

Table 1: SATIVEX

Treatment-Emergent Adverse Events for SATIVEX in Placebo-controlled Studies in Various Neurological Conditions Occurring at 1% or Above and at >1% More Frequently Than in Placebo (excluding CNS effects)

	SATIVEX n=921 (%)	Placebo n=853 (%)
Ear and Labyrinth Disorders		
Vertigo	4.2	1.3
Eye Disorders		
Vision blurred	2.2	0.8
Gastrointestinal Disorders		
Abdominal pain upper	2.1	0.8
Abdominal pain[b]	1.0	0.8
Constipation	2.9	1.4
Diarrhoea	5.9	4.7
Dry mouth	8.1	2.7
Glossodynia[a]	1.0	0.9
Mouth ulceration[a]	1.8	1.4
Nausea	13.4	8.3
Oral discomfort[a]	2.6	2.8
Oral pain[a]	3.5	3.0
Vomiting	5.9	3.5
General Disorders and Administration Site Conditions		
Application site irritation[a]	1.5	2.0
Application site pain[a]	3.1	2.8
Asthenia	4.8	2.2
Fatigue	13.0	7.7
Thirst	1.0	0.2
Infections and Infestations		
Pharyngitis[a]	1.4	1.3
Injury, Poisoning and Procedural Complications		
Fall	1.5	1.2
Metabolism and Nutrition Disorders		
Anorexia	1.7	0.4
Appetite increased	2.3	0.5
Musculoskeletal and Connective Tissue Disorders		
Sensation of heaviness	1.2	0.1
Nervous System Disorders		
Dysgeusia (abnormal taste)[a]	5.3	1.5
Respiratory, Thoracic and Mediastinal Disorders		
Throat irritation[a]	1.1	0.1
Vascular Disorders		
Flushing	1.0	0.2

[a] Application site reaction.
[b] Included as there is a plausible relationship with SATIVEX.

Table 2: SATIVEX

Treatment-Emergent CNS Adverse Events for Sativex in Placebo-controlled Studies in Various Neurological Conditions Occurring at 1% or Above and at >1% More Frequently Than in Placebo

	SATIVEX n=921 (%)	Placebo n=853 (%)
General Disorders and Administration Site Conditions		
Feeling abnormal	2.4	0.5
Feeling drunk	4.5	0.6

(cont'd)

Table 2: SATIVEX *(cont'd)*

Treatment-Emergent CNS Adverse Events for Sativex in Placebo-controlled Studies in Various Neurological Conditions Occurring at 1% or Above and at >1% More Frequently Than in Placebo

	SATIVEX n=921 (%)	Placebo n=853 (%)
Nervous System Disorders		
Amnesia (includes short term memory loss)	1.2	0.4
Balance disorder (balance impaired)	2.4	1.2
Disturbance in attention	4.1	0.4
Dizziness	32.6	9.7
Dysarthria	1.6	0.2
Lethargy	2.5	0.8
Memory impairment	1.6	0.5
Somnolence	7.9	3.0
Psychiatric Disorders		
Anxiety[a]	1.1	0.8
Depression (includes depressed mood)	3.6	1.6
Disorientation (includes confusion)	5.0	0.7
Dissociation	3.0	0.2
Euphoric mood	2.4	0.8
Paranoia[a]	0.9	0.1

[a] Included as there is a plausible relationship with SATIVEX.

Application Site: Application site type events were reported by approximately 20% of patients receiving SATIVEX or placebo. These included glossodynia, mouth ulceration, oral discomfort, oral pain, application site irritation, application site pain and dysgeusia. The incidences were similar for SATIVEX treated patients and placebo appearing to indicate that some application site type reactions may be due to the excipients (50% ethanol and 50% propylene glycol). The majority of these reactions consisted of mild to moderate stinging at the time of application. Mouth ulceration was observed in 1.8% of patients using SATIVEX, and 1.4% in placebo. Two cases of possible leukoplakia were observed but neither was confirmed histologically; a third case was unrelated.

Patients who complain of discomfort should be advised to vary the site of application within the mouth, and should not continue spraying onto sore or inflamed mucus membranes. Regular inspection of the oral mucosa is strongly recommended in long-term administration. If lesions are observed or persistent soreness reported, treatment should be interrupted until complete resolution occurs.

Cardiovascular: THC may cause tachycardia. Its effects on blood pressure are inconsistent, but occasionally patients may experience orthostatic hypotension and/or syncope upon abrupt standing, particularly during initial dose titration when caution is essential. SATIVEX is not recommended in patients with pre-existing cardiovascular disease, such as ischemic heart disease, arrhythmias, poorly controlled hypertension or severe heart failure.

Adverse Events in Patients with Pain in Cancer: Treatment-emergent adverse events that occurred in 3% or more of patients given SATIVEX or placebo in a trial for patients with pain in cancer are given in Table 3.

Table 3: SATIVEX

Treatment-Emergent Adverse Events for SATIVEX in a Placebo-Controlled Study in Patients with Pain in Cancer

	SATIVEX n=60 (%)	Placebo n=59 (%)
Blood and Lymphatic System Disorders		
Anaemia nos	0	5
Cardiac Disorders		
Cardio-respiratory arrest	0	3
Ear and Labyrinth Disorders		
Vertigo	5	2
Gastrointestinal Disorders		
Nausea	12	10
Vomiting	8	7
Constipation	5	10
Oral pain	2	5
Diarrhoea	7	3
Glossodynia	3	0
Abdominal pain upper	2	3
Dry mouth	0	3

(cont'd)

Table 3: SATIVEX *(cont'd)*

Treatment-Emergent Adverse Events for SATIVEX in a Placebo-Controlled Study in Patients with Pain in Cancer

	SATIVEX n=60 (%)	Placebo n=59 (%)
Stomatitis	2	3
General Disorders and Administration Site Conditions		
Pain exacerbated	0	3
Pyrexia	0	3
Weakness	5	0
Disease progression	3	0
Hepatobiliary Disorders		
Hepatic cytolysis	0	3
Infections and Infestations		
Oral candidiasis	3	2
Urinary tract infection	0	7
Lower respiratory tract infection	0	5
Investigations		
GGT increased	3	5
Blood urea increased	2	5
Liver function tests abnormal	5	3
Blood creatinine increased	2	3
Blood calcium increased	0	5
Musculoskeletal and Connective Tissue Disorders		
Pain in limb	2	3
Buttock pain	0	3
Neoplasms Benign, Malignant and Unspecified (incl. Cysts and Polyps)		
Neoplasm progression	10	5
Malignant neoplasm progression	2	5
Nervous System Disorders		
Somnolence	15	14
Dizziness	12	5
Disturbance in attention	3	0
Dysgeusia	3	0
Headache	3	0
Psychiatric Disorders		
Confusion	7	3
Hallucination	3	2
Insomnia	3	2
Panic attack	3	0
Euphoric mood	3	0
Renal and Urinary Disorders		
Urinary retention	5	0
Haematuria	3	0
Respiratory, Thoracic and Mediastinal Disorders		
Dyspnoea	2	3
Vascular Disorders		

(cont'd)

Table 3: SATIVEX *(cont'd)*

Treatment-Emergent Adverse Events for SATIVEX in a Placebo-Controlled Study in Patients with Pain in Cancer

	SATIVEX n=60 (%)	Placebo n=59 (%)
Hypotension	5	0

Urinary Retention and Infections: The combined incidence of urinary retention and urinary infections appear to be increased in the cancer patients taking SATIVEX over those on placebo. Caution is advised in the urinary care of the cancer patients who are using SATIVEX.

Abnormal Hematologic and Clinical Chemistry Findings: No consistent effect of SATIVEX on haematologic and clinical chemistry parameters has been observed.

Post-Market Adverse Drug Reactions: There are no data available yet.

DRUG INTERACTIONS:

> **Serious Drug Interactions**
> - Care should be taken with sedatives, drugs with sedating or psychotropic effects and hypnotics as coadministration with SATIVEX may have an additive effect.
> - Alcohol may interact with SATIVEX, particularly in affecting coordination, concentration and ability to respond quickly.

Overview: The two main components of SATIVEX, delta-9-tetrahydrocannabinol (THC) and cannabidiol (CBD), are metabolized by the Cytochrome P450 enzyme system, including CYP1A2, CYP2C9, CYP2D6, CYP2C19 and CYP3A4. The inhibitory effects seen in vitro and in animal models were only seen at exposures significantly higher than the maximum observed in clinical trials. In clinical trials where SATIVEX has been taken concomitantly with other drugs metabolized by the Cytochrome P450 enzyme system, no clinically apparent drug-drug interactions have been seen in these trials at clinical doses.

In an in vitro study with 1:1% (v/v) THC botanical drug substance (BDS) and CBD BDS, no relevant induction of Cytochrome P450 enzymes was seen for human CYP1A2, CYP2C9, CYP2C19 and CYP3A4 enzymes in human hepatocytes, at doses of up to 1 μM (314 ng/mL).

Drug-Drug Interactions: There may be a potential risk of drug-drug interactions due to CYP450 inhibition by SATIVEX. Caution should be exercised in patients taking drugs known to be substrates for CYP450 2D6 and/or CYP450 3A4, in particular fentanyl and the related opioids sufentanil and alfentanil.

Amitriptyline is metabolized by CYP2C19, CYP1A2, CYP2C9, CYP3A4 and CYP2D6, and there is thus a potential risk of an interaction with SATIVEX, leading to raised plasma levels of amitriptyline. In clinical trials with SATIVEX, patients have been restricted to a maximum of 75 mg amitriptyline daily. No difference in the adverse event profile between patients taking amitriptyline and the general population of MS patients was noted.

Protein Binding: THC is highly bound to plasma proteins, and therefore might displace other protein-bound drugs. Although this displacement has not been confirmed in vivo, practitioners should monitor patients for a change in dosage requirements when administering SATIVEX to patients who are receiving other drugs which are tightly protein-bound.

Drug-Food Interactions: No interactions with food have been established.

Drug-Herb Interactions: Interactions with herbal products have not been established.

Drug-Laboratory Test Interactions: No laboratory interactions have been established. Cannabinoids may be detected in the plasma and urine several weeks after SATIVEX is discontinued (see Warnings and Precautions, Monitoring and Laboratory Tests).

Drug-Lifestyle Interactions: Effects of smoked or other forms of cannabis would be additive to those of SATIVEX with a likelihood of producing intoxication or other unwanted effects and are not recommended while using this product.

DOSAGE AND ADMINISTRATION:

Adults: Dosing Considerations: SATIVEX is for buccal use only. The spray should be directed to below the tongue, or towards the inside of the cheeks. The site should be varied. The patient should be advised not to direct the spray towards the pharynx and not to inhale the spray. It must not be sprayed into the nose.

In the extension phase of Study GWMS0107 in MS, the median daily dosage of SATIVEX in the 63 patients was 5 actuations (sprays) after dose titration was completed. The majority of patients required 12 sprays or less; dosage should be adjusted as needed and tolerated. There is limited experience with doses higher than 12 sprays per day. Some patients may require and may tolerate a higher number of sprays.

In study GWCA0101, in patients with pain in cancer, the median daily dosage of SATIVEX was 8 actuations (sprays).

Treatment Initiation and Stabilization:
- On day one of treatment, patients should take one spray during the morning and one spray during the afternoon/evening. The morning dose can be taken at any time between waking up and 12 noon and the afternoon dose can be taken at any time between 4 pm and bedtime
- On subsequent days the patient may gradually increase the total number of sprays, by one spray each day, as needed and tolerated. There should be at least a 15 minute gap between sprays. During initial titration, sprays should be evenly spread out over the day.
- If unacceptable adverse reactions such as dizziness or other CNS-type reactions develop at any time, dosing should be suspended until they have resolved. Some patients may be able to continue therapy at the dose reached by increasing the interval between doses; others may require their subsequent doses reduced. Patients should then carefully re-titrate to a tolerated dosage regimen that gives acceptable pain relief.

Following the titration period, patients are advised to maintain the optimal dose achieved. Re-titration upwards or downwards may be appropriate if there are any changes in the severity of the patient's conditions, changes in his/her concomitant medication or if unacceptable side effects develop.

Missed Dose: SATIVEX is a self-titration regime to be used "as required" for relief of pain, therefore "missed dose" is not applicable.

Administration: Priming:
1. Shake the vial gently before use.
2. Remove the protective cap.
3. Holding the vial in an upright position, prime the SATIVEX vial by pressing on the actuator two or three times firmly and quickly, directing into a tissue until a fine spray appears.

Important: Point the spray safely away when priming it into a tissue. Do not prime it near children, pets or an open flame.

Normal Use:
1. Shake the vial gently before use.
2. Remove the protective cap.
3. Hold the vial in the upright position and direct into the mouth. Press firmly and quickly towards the buccal surface in the following regions: below the tongue or towards the inside of the cheeks. The site should be varied. Never aim at the throat, as SATIVEX can cause irritation.
4. Replace the protective cap.
5. Keep away from sources of heat and direct sunlight.

OVERDOSAGE:

Sativex: Signs and Symptoms: There is no experience of deliberate overdose with SATIVEX. Signs and symptoms of overdose were reported from a thorough QT study conducted according to international standards. After receiving 18 sprays in 20 minutes, some subjects showed serious psychiatric signs and symptoms. The initial adverse reactions appeared within one to two hours and were consistent with the intoxication effects of cannabis and THC. In four patients out of 257, the intoxication symptoms developed into major psychiatric symptoms such as depression, anxiety, paranoia, delusions, hallucinations, and/or psychosis. These serious symptoms reached a plateau after two to three hours and lasted for nine to 24 hours.

Management: Recommended treatments include counselling and interventions to prevent injury. Additional treatments should be symptomatic and supportive. Benzodiazepines may be used in patients with severe agitation. The recovering patient must be followed up until all clinical symptoms dissipate. The possibility of multiple drug involvement should be considered. The nearest local Poison Control Centre must be contacted for current information.

Experience with oral THC overdose is as follows: Signs and Symptoms: Following **mild** THC intoxication, symptoms include drowsiness, euphoria, heightened sensory awareness, altered time perception, reddened conjunctiva, dry mouth and tachycardia; following **moderate** THC intoxication, symptoms include memory impairment, depersonalization, mood alteration, urinary retention, and reduced bowel motility; and following **severe** THC intoxication, symptoms include decreased motor coordination, lethargy, slurred speech, and postural hypotension. Apprehensive patients may experience panic reactions and seizures may occur in patients with existing seizure disorders.

The estimated lethal human dose of intravenous THC is 30 mg/kg (2100 mg/70 kg).

Management: An overdose severe enough to cause depression of consciousness should be treated with the normal precautions for dealing with an unconscious patient by securing the airway and monitoring vital signs. Patients experiencing depressive, hallucinatory or psychotic reactions should be placed in a quiet area and offered reassurance. Benzodiazepines (5 to 10 mg diazepam per oral) may be used for treatment of extreme agitation. In the case of hypotension, patients should be placed in the Trendelenburg position (head lower than feet) or modified Trendelenburg position (only the legs elevated) until the condition remits. Intravenous fluids or pressors are rarely required.

For management of a suspected drug overdose, CPhA recommends that you contact your **regional Poison Control Centre**. See the *CPS* Directory section for a list of Poison Control Centres.

ACTION AND CLINICAL PHARMACOLOGY: Mechanism of Action: Mammalian tissues contain at least two types of cannabinoid (CB) receptor, CB_1 and CB_2. CB_1 receptors are present at nerve terminals in the CNS and also in some peripheral tissues including dorsal root ganglia, sympathetic ganglia, adrenal gland, heart, lung, reproductive tissues, urinary bladder, gastrointestinal tissues, and immune cells. Within the brain, the distribution of CB_1 receptors is heterogeneous, with a pattern consistent with the demonstrated effects of cannabinoids on motor function, cognition and memory. Relevant for pain modulation, CB_1 receptors are found on pain pathways in the brain and spinal cord, as well as on terminals of peripheral nervous system primary afferent neurons where they may mediate cannabinoid-induced analgesia. CB_2 receptors are present primarily on peripheral and central immune cells, where they may modulate immune function through release of cytokines. Cannabidiol (CBD) is an agonist of TRPV-1 (vanilloid) receptor with an inhibitory action on adenosine uptake.

Pharmacodynamics: Animal Data: The principal pharmacological effects of THC include analgesic, muscle relaxant, antiemetic, appetite stimulant and psychoactive effects. CBD has analgesic, anticonvulsant, muscle relaxant, anxiolytic, neuroprotective, anti-oxidant and anti-psychotic activity. THC is metabolised to 11-hydroxy-tetrahydrocannabinol (11-OH-THC), a psycho-active metabolite. The main primary metabolite of CBD is 7-hydroxy-cannabidiol.

Pharmacokinetics: Human Data: Summary of pharmacokinetic parameters for SATIVEX in healthy volunteers—Single dose PK in two studies. The differences seen in the PK data may reflect the inter-subject variability and the conduct of the study (see Table 4, Table 5 and Table 6).

Table 4: SATIVEX

Mean Pharmacokinetic Parameters (GWPK0112)[a]

Treatment	Analyte	T_{max} (h) (n=12)	C_{max} (ng/mL) (n=12)	$t_{1/2}$ (h) (n=12)	AUC_{0-t} (min[b]ng/mL) (n=12)	AUC_{inf} (min[b]ng/mL) (n=12)
SATIVEX[b] (Under the tongue)	CBD	1.63	2.50	1.44	408.53	427.33
	THC	1.63	5.54	1.76	808.78	837.25
	11-OH-THC	1.58	6.24	2.15	1522.09	1632.46
SATIVEX[b] (Inside the cheek)	CBD	2.80	3.02	1.81	384.13	407.79
	THC	2.40	6.14	1.34	751.23	770.62
	11-OH-THC	2.40	6.13	1.91	1293.14	1362.12

[a] The pharmacokinetic data show great inter-subject variability. THC, CBD, and 11-OH-THC appear in the plasma from about 30 minutes after dosing.

[b] 4 sprays (total 10.8 mg THC+10 mg CBD).

Table 5: SATIVEX

Mean Pharmacokinetic Parameters (GWPK0215)

Treatment	Analyte	T_{max}[b] (h) (n=24)	C_{max} (ng/mL) (n=24)	$t_{1/2}$ (h) (n=24)	AUC_{0-t} (min[a]ng/mL) (n=24)	AUC_{inf} (min[a]ng/mL) (n=24)
SATIVEX[a] (Under the tongue)	CBD	4.22	3.33	1.81	680.61	718.46
	THC	4.38	4.90	1.40	894.80	918.81
	11-OH-THC	3.83	4.49	2.17	1423.20	1463.67

[a] 4 sprays (total 10.8 mg THC+10 mg CBD).

[b] As the data here represent more than one peak, T_{max} may represent an early buccal absorption and later gastrointestinal absorption.

Individual subject plasma concentration data and pharmacokinetic parameters show a high degree of inter-subject variability.

Table 6: SATIVEX

Summary of Pharmacokinetic Parameters for SATIVEX in MS Patients—Steady-state PK

Parameters	Cannabinoid (Analyte)	Visit A (n=13)	Visit B (n=7)
Pre-dose trough (ng/mL)	CBD	0.12–4.41	0.75–4.19
	THC	0.16–4.64	0.47–5.67
	11-OH-THC	0.05–5.41	1.02–5.67
C_{max} (ng/mL)	CBD	1.09–16.97	3.83–13.69
	THC	2.30–28.66	2.86–33.63
	11-OH-THC	2.76–20.45	3.74–14.22
T_{max} (hours)	CBD	1–6	3.0–6
	THC	1–6	2.5–6
	11-OH-THC	1–6	1.5–6

Note: Visit A took place after at least 20 weeks on SATIVEX. Visit B occurred 8 weeks after Visit A. All patients were using at least 5 sprays daily.

Plasma levels have been studied in a limited number of patients on stable self-titrated doses during chronic therapy in the extension phase of study GWMS0001EXT. Most patients apparently had self-titrated their dosing to a level at which plasma concentrations for both THC and CBD were generally in the range of 5-10 ng/mL or less. Sampling of plasma concentration levels during chronic dosing suggests that significant accumulation of cannabinoids does not occur.

Absorption: Following a single buccal administration, maximum plasma concentrations of both CBD and THC typically occur within two to four hours. When administered buccally, blood levels of THC and other cannabinoids are lower compared with inhalation of smoked cannabis. The resultant concentrations in the blood are lower than those obtained by inhaling the same dose because absorption is slower, redistribution into fatty tissues is rapid and additionally some of the THC undergoes hepatic first pass metabolism to 11-OH-THC, a psycho-active metabolite.

Distribution: Cannabinoids are distributed throughout the body; they are highly lipid soluble and accumulate in fatty tissue. The release of cannabinoids from fatty tissue is responsible for the prolonged terminal elimination half-life.

Metabolism: THC and CBD are metabolized in the liver by a number of cytochrome P450 isoenzymes, including CYP2C9, CYP2C19, CYP2D6 and CYP3A4. They may be stored for as long as four weeks in the fatty tissues from which they are slowly released at sub-therapeutic levels back into the blood stream and metabolized via the renal and biliary systems.

Excretion: Elimination from plasma is bi-exponential with an initial half-life of one to two hours. The terminal elimination half-lives are of the order of 24 to 36 hours or longer. SATIVEX is excreted in the urine and faeces.

Special Populations and Conditions: No pharmacokinetic studies were done in any special population.

STORAGE AND STABILITY: SATIVEX should not be used beyond its expiry date, and should be used within 28 days once it has been opened and is in use.

Prior to opening, SATIVEX should be stored upright in a refrigerator (2-8°C). Do not freeze. Once opened, the spray may be stored at room temperature (15-25°C) and should be used within 28 days.

Keep away from sources of heat and direct sunlight. Keep away from reach of children.

SPECIAL HANDLING INSTRUCTIONS: None.

INFORMATION FOR THE PATIENT: Published in e-CPS, available by subscription at www.e-cps.ca.

DOSAGE FORMS, COMPOSITION AND PACKAGING: Each buccal spray contains: delta-9-tetrahydrocannabinol 27 mg/mL (from Tetranabinex—Cannabis sativa L. extract) and cannabidiol 25 mg/mL (from Nabidiolex—Cannabis sativa L. extract). Non-medicinal ingredients: ethanol anhydrous, peppermint oil and propylene glycol. Amber glass vials of 5.5 mL (51 metered sprays), cartons of 4. Vials fitted with a metering pump possessing a polypropylene dip tube and elastomer neck, covered with a polyethylene cap. The metering pump delivers 100 μL per actuation (spray).

Scopolamine

Anticholinergic

CPhA Monograph

Scopolamine HBr

Anticholinergic

CPhA Monograph

Date of Revision: October 2007

This monograph has been compiled by CPhA and reviewed by experts. It may contain information different from that found in Health Canada-approved Product Monographs. The reader is referred to the *CPS* Editorial Policy for more information.

SUMMARY PRODUCT INFORMATION:

Route of Administration[a]	Dosage Form[a]	Strength[a]
Parenteral	Injectable solution	0.4 mg/mL, 0.6 mg/mL
Transdermal	Disc	1.5 mg/disc

[a] For specific product information consult Health Canada's Drug Product Database http://www.hc-sc.gc.ca/dhp-mps/prodpharma/databasdon/index_e.html

PHARMACOLOGY: Scopolamine is one of the major active alkaloids found in the belladonna leaf. Scopolamine hydrobromide is the trihydrate hydrobromide salt of scopolamine. The butylbromide salt is also available in Canada, under the generic name hyoscine butylbromide, and is not discussed in this monograph.

Scopolamine, like atropine, is an antimuscarinic agent producing competitive antagonism of the actions of acetylcholine at muscarinic receptors. The anticholinergic properties of scopolamine and atropine differ in that scopolamine has more potent activity on the iris, ciliary body and certain secretory (salivary, bronchial and sweat) glands. Atropine has more potent activity on the heart, intestine and bronchial muscle and a more prolonged duration of action.

Scopolamine, at usual dosages, produces CNS depression. However, excitement, restlessness, hallucinations or delirium may paradoxically occur, especially in the presence of severe pain.

In addition to its systemic anticholinergic effects, scopolamine is effective in the prevention of motion sickness. The ability of scopolamine to prevent motion-induced nausea is believed to be associated with inhibition of vestibular input to the CNS, which results in inhibition of the vomiting reflex. In addition, scopolamine may have a direct action on the vomiting centre within the reticular formation of the brain stem.

Scopolamine is not effective as a single agent for the prophylaxis of chemotherapy-induced nausea and vomiting.

Pharmacokinetics: Scopolamine is rapidly absorbed following im or sc injection. It is well absorbed from the gastrointestinal tract as well as percutaneously, following topical application of a transdermal disc behind the ear. Scopolamine is believed to be metabolized in the liver and excreted in the urine. The duration of action of the parenteral formulation is 4 hours while that of the transdermal system is up to 72 hours.

INDICATIONS: Scopolamine is used mainly for the prevention of nausea and vomiting associated with motion sickness in adults (transdermal application). Scopolamine hydrobromide is used as an adjunct to anesthesia to inhibit salivation and excessive respiratory secretions and to produce sedation and amnesia.

CONTRAINDICATIONS: Hypersensitivity to scopolamine or to any ingredient or component in the formulation or administration system; angle-closure glaucoma; prostatic hyperplasia; pyloric obstruction; tachycardia secondary to cardiac insufficiency or thyrotoxicosis; paralytic ileus.

WARNINGS: Occupational Hazards: Since drowsiness, disorientation and confusion may occasionally occur with the use of scopolamine, patients should be cautioned about engaging in activities that require mental alertness, such as driving a motor vehicle or operating dangerous machinery.

Children: Children are particularly susceptible to the side effects of belladonna alkaloids. The manufacturer of the transdermal discs recommends they not be used in children.

PRECAUTIONS: Use with caution in patients taking drugs which act on the CNS, or patients with urinary bladder neck obstruction.

Caution should be exercised when administering an antiemetic or antimuscarinic drug to patients suspected of having intestinal obstruction, or to patients with gastroparesis, constipation or tachyarrhythmias.

The transdermal disc should be used with special caution in the elderly or in individuals with impaired metabolic, liver or kidney function; they should also be used with caution in patients with fever or during exposure to high environmental temperatures, because of the risk of hyperthermia.

Drug Interactions: Scopolamine should be used with caution in patients taking drugs acting on the CNS. This applies particularly to patients taking medications with anticholinergic properties, e.g., oxybutynin, tolterodine, belladonna alkaloids, antihistamines, antidepressants (tricyclics and MAO inhibitors), phenothiazines, amantadine and quinidine. These combinations should be avoided whenever possible; if they are used concomitantly, the lowest effective dose of each agent should be used.

Parasympatholytic or sympathomimetic agents or barbiturates should be administered with caution to persons wearing scopolamine transdermal discs.

Pregnancy: Scopolamine readily crosses the placenta. The use of scopolamine in women of childbearing potential requires that the potential benefit of the drug be weighed against the possible risk to the mother and fetus.
Lactation: Scopolamine appears in minute quantities in milk. Since neonates are particularly sensitive to anticholinergic agents, caution is indicated. The American Academy of Pediatrics considers scopolamine to be compatible with breastfeeding.
Children: See Warnings.
Geriatrics: Elderly patients are at increased risk of CNS effects such as confusion and hallucinations when using scopolamine transdermal discs. If these effects occur, the disc should be removed immediately and the site washed thoroughly to remove unabsorbed scopolamine. If symptoms persist, appropriate measures should be taken (see Overdose).

ADVERSE EFFECTS: The most frequently reported adverse effects of transdermal scopolamine are dry mouth and drowsiness, occurring in 29% and 17% of patients, respectively. Other less frequent side effects include: ocular effects such as blurred vision, mydriasis and cycloplegia (may be unilateral if caused by hand-to-eye contact after handling the transdermal disc) and acute angle-closure glaucoma in predisposed patients; CNS effects such as disorientation, hallucinations and delirium (elderly are more susceptible); dermatologic effects such as rash and erythema (rare) and allergic contact dermatitis that may be delayed in onset during long-term therapy.
Withdrawal: Symptoms such as nausea, vomiting, dizziness and headache have occurred following discontinuation of the transdermal system.

OVERDOSE:
Symptoms: Systemic effects resulting from scopolamine overdose include: mydriasis, blurred vision, photophobia, acute angle-closure glaucomoa in predisposed individuals; thirst; decreased gastointestinal motility; flushed, hot, dry skin; drowsiness, nervousness or light-headedness progressing to confusion and acute toxic psychosis; seizures or coma in severe cases; respiratory depression, hyperthermia, urinary retention; tachycardia and rarely, hypertension and arrhythmias.
Treatment: Treatment generally involves symptomatic and supportive care including maintenance of fluid and electrolyte balance, monitoring of bowel sounds, urine output and vital signs, and in severe cases, ECG monitoring. Following oral ingestions, vomiting should not be induced; activated charcoal should be administered. Agitation and seizures can be treated with iv benzodiazepines such as diazepam. Propranolol can be used to manage tachyarrhythmias. Hyperpyrexia can be relieved with the use of fans or cool mist.

> For management of a suspected drug overdose, CPhA recommends that you contact your **regional Poison Control Centre**. See the *CPS* Directory section for a list of Poison Control Centres.

DOSAGE: **Parenteral (Scopolamine Hydrobromide):** Adults: 0.3 to 0.6 mg im, iv or sc; if necessary, the dose may be repeated 3 or 4 times daily.
Children: 0.006 mg/kg/dose or 0.2 mg/m² im, iv or sc.
Transdermal (Scopolamine): Adults: To obtain optimum effect, one transdermal scopolamine disc should be applied to the dry, hairless skin behind the ear approximately 12 hours before the antiemetic effect is required. A disc can be left in place for up to 72 hours as needed but should be removed when travel is complete.
The hands should be washed and dried thoroughly following application. Only 1 disc should be worn at a time. Once the disc has been affixed, it should not be touched again while it is being worn. Upon removal, the disc should be discarded and the hands and application site washed thoroughly to prevent any traces of scopolamine from coming into direct contact with the eyes (see Precautions and Adverse Effects).
If a disc becomes displaced, it should be removed and replaced with a second disc on a different skin site in the postauricular area. If scopolamine administration is required for longer than 72 hours, the first disc should be removed and a second disc placed behind the opposite ear to minimize skin irritation. When a disc is removed, the skin should be washed to remove unabsorbed scopolamine.
Children: The transdermal system is not recommended for use in children.

Scopolamine Hydrobromide
scopolamine HBr
Anticholinergic

Hospira

SUPPLIED: Each mL contains: scopolamine hydrobromide 0.4 or 0.6 mg. Nonmedicinal ingredients: hydrobromic acid and water for injection. Ampuls of 1 mL, boxes of 10.

Seasonale™ Ⓟ
levonorgestrel—ethinyl estradiol
Oral Contraceptive

Paladin

Date of Preparation: June 26, 2007
Date of Revision: June 10, 2010

SUMMARY PRODUCT INFORMATION:

Route of Administration	Dosage Form/ Strength	Clinically Relevant Nonmedicinal Ingredients
Oral	Tablet 0.15 mg levonorgestrel and 0.03 mg ethinyl estradiol	Anhydrous lactose For a complete listing see Dosage Forms, Composition and Packaging.

INDICATIONS AND CLINICAL USE: Seasonale (levonorgestrel and ethinyl estradiol, USP) tablets are indicated for:
- The prevention of pregnancy.

CONTRAINDICATIONS: Oral contraceptives should not be used in women who have the following conditions:
- Patients who are hypersensitive to this drug or to any ingredient in the formulation or component of the container. For a complete listing, see Dosage Forms, Composition and Packaging.
- History of or actual thrombophlebitis or thromboembolic disorders.
- History of or actual cerebrovascular disorders.
- History of or actual myocardial infarction or coronary artery disease.
- Valvular heart disease with complications.
- Active liver disease or history of or actual benign or malignant liver tumours.
- Steroid-dependent jaundice, cholestatic jaundice, history of jaundice in pregnancy.
- Known or suspected carcinoma of the breast.
- Carcinoma of the endometrium or other known or suspected estrogen-dependent neoplasia.
- Undiagnosed abnormal vaginal bleeding.
- Any ocular lesion arising from ophthalmic vascular disease, such as partial or complete loss of vision or defect in visual fields.
- Known or suspected pregnancy.
- Presence of severe or multiple risk factor(s) for arterial or venous thrombosis:
  - diabetes mellitus with vascular symptoms
  - severe hypertension (persistent values of ≥160/100mm Hg)
  - severe dyslipoproteinemia
  - hereditary or acquired predisposition for venous or arterial thrombosis, such as Factor V Leiden mutation and activated protein C (APC-) resistance, antithrombin-III-deficiency, protein C deficiency, protein S deficiency, hyperhomocysteinaemia (e.g. due to MTHFR C677 T, A1298 mutations), prothrombin mutation G20210A and antiphospholipid-antibodies (anticardiclipin-antibodies, lupus anticoagulant).
  - major surgery associated with an increased risk of post-operative thromboembolism
  - prolonged immobilization
  - heavy smoking (>15 cigarettes per day) and over age 35
- Current or history of migraine with focal neurological symptoms.

WARNINGS AND PRECAUTIONS:

> **Serious Warnings and Precautions**
> Cigarette smoking increases the risk of serious adverse effects on the heart and blood vessels. This risk increases with age and becomes significant in oral contraceptive users older than 35 years of age. Women should be counselled not to smoke (see Cardiovascular).
> Birth control pills **do not protect** against sexually transmitted diseases including HIV/AIDS. For protection against STDs, it is advisable to use latex condoms **in combination with** birth control pills.
> Use of Seasonale provides women with more hormonal exposure on a yearly basis than conventional monthly oral contraceptives containing similar strength synthetic estrogens and progestins (9 additional weeks of hormonal exposure per year). While this added exposure may pose an additional risk of thrombotic and thromboembolic diseases, studies to date with Seasonale have not suggested, nor can exclude, this additional risk.

General: Discontinue Medication at the Earliest Manifestation of:
A. **Thromboembolic and cardiovascular disorders** such as thrombophlebitis, pulmonary embolism, cerebrovascular disorders, myocardial ischemia, mesenteric thrombosis, and retinal thrombosis.
B. **Conditions that predispose to venous stasis and vascular thrombosis** (e.g., immobilization after accidents or confinement to bed during long-term illness). Other non-hormonal methods of contraception should be used until regular activities are resumed. For use of oral contraceptives when surgery is contemplated, see Peri-Operative Considerations.
C. **Visual defects—partial or complete**
D. **Papilledema or ophthalmic vascular lesions**
E. **Severe headache of unknown etiology or worsening of pre-existing migraine headache.**

Seasonale Oral Contraceptive: Seasonale is a 91-day cyclic dosing regimen (84 days with active oral tablets of 0.15 mg levonorgestrel and 0.03 mg ethinyl estradiol, followed by 7 days with placebo tablets). Pregnancy should be ruled out in cases of unanticipated bleeding/spotting, missed withdrawal bleeding/amenorrhea or signs and symptoms of pregnancy.
The following information is provided from studies of combination oral contraceptives. The use of combination hormonal contraceptives is associated with increased risks of several serious conditions including myocardial infarction, thromboembolism, stroke, hepatic neoplasia and gallbladder disease, although the risk of serious morbidity and mortality is small in healthy women without underlying risk factors. The risk of morbidity and mortality increases significantly if associated with the presence of other risk factors such as hypertension, hyperlipidemias, obesity and diabetes.
The information contained in this section is principally from studies carried out in women who used combination oral contraceptives with higher formulations of estrogens and progestogens than those in common use today. The effect of long-term use of combination hormonal contraceptives with lower doses of both estrogen and progestogen administered orally remains to be determined.

Carcinogenesis and Mutagenesis: Breast Cancer: Increasing age and a strong family history are the most significant risk factors for the development of breast cancer. Other established risk factors include obesity, nulliparity, and late age for first full-term pregnancy. The identified groups of women that may be at increased risk of developing breast cancer before menopause are long-term users of oral contraceptives (more than eight years) and starters at early age. In a few women, the use of oral contraceptives may accelerate the growth of an existing but undiagnosed breast cancer. Since any potential increased risk related to oral contraceptive use is small, there is no reason to change prescribing habits at present.
Women receiving oral contraceptives should be instructed in self-examination of their breasts. Their physicians should be notified whenever any masses are detected. A yearly clinical breast examination is also recommended, because, if a breast cancer should develop, drugs that contain estrogen may cause a rapid progression.

Cervical Cancer: Some studies suggest that oral contraceptive use has been associated with an increase in risk of cervical intraepithelial neoplasia or invasive cervical cancer in some populations of women. However, there continues to be controversy about the extent to which the findings may be due to differences in sexual behaviours and other factors.

Hepatocellular Carcinoma: Hepatocellular carcinoma may be associated with oral contraceptives. The risk appears to increase with duration of hormonal contraceptive use. However, the attributable risk (the excess incidence) of liver cancers in oral contraceptive users is extremely small.

Cardiovascular: See also Contraindications; Warnings and Precautions, Boxed Warning, General, Hematologic, Ophthalmologic.
Use of Seasonale provides women with more hormonal exposure on a yearly basis than conventional monthly oral contraceptives containing similar strength synthetic estrogens and progestins (9 additional weeks of hormonal exposure per year). While this added exposure may pose an additional risk of thrombotic and thromboembolic diseases, studies to date with Seasonale have not suggested, nor can exclude, this additional risk. Two subjects had pulmonary embolism and one subject had myocardial infarction while on Seasonale in clinical studies. Coagulation profile has not been studied with Seasonale.
In the post-market period, there have been cases of myocardial infarction, stroke, deep vein thrombosis and pulmonary embolism reported with the use of Seasonale.
Prescribers are advised to carefully assess a patient's baseline and cumulative risk of thromboembolism and discuss the risk of thromboembolism with all patients before prescribing Seasonale.

Predisposing Factors for Coronary Artery Disease: Cigarette smoking increases the risk of serious cardiovascular side effects and mortality. Birth control pills increase this risk, especially with increasing age. Convincing data are available to support an upper age limit of 35 years for oral contraceptive use by women who smoke.
Other women who are independently at high risk for cardiovascular disease include those with diabetes, hypertension, abnormal lipid profile, or a family history of these. Whether oral contraceptives accentuate this risk is unclear.
In low-risk, non-smoking women of any age, the benefits of oral contraceptive use outweigh the possible cardiovascular risks associated with low-dose formulations. Consequently, oral contraceptives may be prescribed for these women up to the age of menopause.

Thromboembolism: See Hematologic.

Hypertension: Patients with essential hypertension whose blood pressure is well-controlled may be given oral contraceptives but only under close supervision. If a significant elevation of blood pressure in previously normotensive or hypertensive subjects occurs at any time during the administration of the drug, cessation of medication is necessary.

Endocrine and Metabolism: Diabetes: Current low-dose oral contraceptives exert minimal impact on glucose metabolism. Diabetic patients, or those with a family history of diabetes, should be observed closely to detect any worsening of carbohydrate metabolism. Patients predisposed to diabetes who can be kept under close supervision may be given oral contraceptives. Young diabetic patients whose disease is of recent origin, well-controlled, and not associated with hypertension or other signs of vascular disease such as ocular fundal changes, should be monitored more frequently while using oral contraceptives.

Lipid and Other Metabolic Effects: A small proportion of women will have adverse lipid changes while on oral contraceptives. Alternative contraception should be used in women with uncontrolled dyslipidemias (see also Contraindications). Elevations of plasma triglycerides may lead to pancreatitis and other complications.

Genitourinary: Vaginal Bleeding and Bleeding Irregularities: In the pivotal, controlled clinical study 7.7% of subjects on Seasonale discontinued medication prematurely due to unacceptable bleeding vs. 1.8% of subjects on the 28-day cycle regimen.
Table 1 shows the percentage of subjects with inter-menstrual bleeding and/or spotting.
Persistent irregular vaginal bleeding requires assessment to exclude underlying pathology.

Fibroids: Patients with fibroids (leiomyomata) should be carefully observed. Sudden enlargement, pain, or tenderness requires discontinuation of the use of oral contraceptives.

Hematologic: Epidemiological studies have shown that the incidence of VTE in users of oral contraceptives with low estrogen content (<50 µg ethinyl estradiol) ranges from about 20 to 40 cases per 100 000 women-years, but this risk estimate varies according to the progestogen. This compares with 5 to 10 cases per 100 000 women-years for non-users.
The use of any combined oral contraceptive carries an increased risk of venous thromboembolism (VTE) compared with no use. The excess risk of VTE is highest during the first year a woman ever uses a combined oral contraceptive. The increased risk is less than the risk of VTE associated with pregnancy, which is estimated as 60 cases per 100 000 pregnancies. VTE is fatal in 1-2% of cases.

Other Risk Factors for Venous Thromboembolism: Other generalized risk factors for venous thromboembolism include, but are not limited to, a personal history, obesity, a family history (the occurrence of VTE in a direct relative at a relatively early age may indicate genetic predisposition), severe obesity (body mass index >30 kg/m²) and systemic lupus erythematosus. The risk of VTE also increases with age and smoking. The risk of VTE may be temporarily increased with prolonged immobilization, major surgery or trauma. Also patients with varicose veins and leg cast should be closely supervised.

If a hereditary or acquired predisposition to venous thromboembolism is suspected, the woman should be referred to a specialist for advice before deciding on any COC use.

Table 1: Seasonale

Percentage of Subjects with Inter-menstrual Bleeding and/or Spotting

Days of Inter-menstrual Bleeding and/or Spotting	Percentage of Subjects[a]	
Seasonale	Cycle 1 (N=385)	Cycle 4 (N=261)
≥7 days	65%	42%
≥20 days	35%	15%
28-day regimen	Cycles 1–4 (N=194)	Cycles 10–13 (N=158)
≥7 days	38%	39%
≥20 days	6%	4%

[a] Based on spotting and/or bleeding on days 1-84 of a 91-day cycle in the Seasonale subjects and days 1–21 of a 28-day cycle over 4 cycles in the 28-day dosing regimen.

Hepatic/Biliary/Pancreatic: Jaundice: Patients who have had jaundice should be given oral contraceptives only with great care and under close observation. Oral contraceptive-related cholestasis has been described in women with a history of pregnancy-related cholestasis. Women with a history of cholestasis may have the condition recur with subsequent hormonal contraceptive use.

The development of severe generalized pruritus or icterus requires that the medication be withdrawn until the problem is resolved.

If a patient develops jaundice that proves to be cholestatic in type, the use of oral contraceptives should not be resumed. In patients taking oral contraceptives, changes in the composition of the bile may occur and an increased incidence of gallstones has been reported.

Hepatic Nodules: Hepatic nodules (adenoma and focal nodular hyperplasia) have been reported, particularly in long-term users of oral contraceptives. Although these lesions are extremely rare, they have caused fatal intra-abdominal hemorrhage and should be considered in women presenting with an abdominal mass, acute abdominal pain, or evidence of intra-abdominal bleeding.

Gallbladder Disease: Users of oral contraceptives have a greater risk of developing gallbladder disease requiring surgery within the first year of use. The risk may double after four or five years of use.

Neurologic: Migraine and Headache: The onset or exacerbation of migraine or the development of headache of a new pattern that is recurrent, persistent or severe, requires discontinuation of oral contraceptives and evaluation of the cause. Women with migraine (particularly migraine with aura) who take combination oral contraceptives may be at an increased risk of stroke (see Contraindications).

Ophthalmologic: Patients who are pregnant or are taking oral contraceptives may experience corneal edema that may cause visual disturbances and changes in tolerance to contact lenses, especially of the rigid type. Soft contact lenses usually do not cause disturbances. If visual changes or alterations in tolerance to contact lenses occur, temporary or permanent cessation of wear may be advised.

Peri-Operative Considerations: There is an increased risk of thromboembolic complications in oral contraceptive users after major surgery. If feasible, oral contraceptives should be discontinued and an alternative method substituted at least one month prior to **major** elective surgery. Oral contraceptive use should not be resumed until the first menstrual period after hospital discharge following surgery.

Psychiatric: Emotional Disorders: Patients with a history of emotional disturbances, especially the depressive type, may be more prone to have a recurrence of depression while taking oral contraceptives. In case of a serious recurrence, a trial of an alternate method of contraception should be made, which may help to clarify the possible relationship. Women with premenstrual syndrome (PMS) may have a varied response to oral contraceptives, ranging from symptomatic improvement to worsening of the condition.

Renal: Fluid Retention: Hormonal contraceptives may cause some degree of fluid retention. They should be prescribed with caution, and only with careful monitoring, in patients with conditions which might be aggravated by fluid retention.

Sexual Function/Reproduction: Return to Fertility: After discontinuing oral contraceptive therapy, the patient should delay pregnancy until at least one normal spontaneous menstrual cycle has occurred in order to date the pregnancy. An alternative contraceptive method should be used during this time.

Amenorrhea: Seasonale is a 91-day cyclic dosing regimen (84 days with active oral tablets of 0.15 mg levonorgestrel and 0.03 mg ethinyl estradiol, followed by 7 days with placebo tablets). In the case of unanticipated bleeding/spotting, missed withdrawal bleeding or amenorrhea, the possibility of pregnancy must be considered.

Women with a history of oligomenorrhea, secondary amenorrhea, or irregular cycles may remain anovulatory or become amenorrheic following discontinuation of estrogen-progestin combination therapy.

Amenorrhea, especially if associated with breast secretion, which continues for six months or more after withdrawal, warrants a careful assessment of hypothalamic-pituitary function.

Special Populations: Pregnant Women: Oral contraceptive use should be discontinued if pregnancy is confirmed. Oral contraceptives should not be taken by pregnant women. However, if conception accidentally occurs while taking the pill, there is no conclusive evidence that the estrogen and progestin contained in the oral contraceptive will damage the developing child.

Nursing Women: In breast-feeding women, the use of hormonal contraceptives results in the hormonal components being excreted in breast milk and may reduce its quantity and quality. If the use of oral contraceptives is initiated after the establishment of lactation, there does not appear to be any effect on the quantity and quality of the milk.

A few adverse effects on the child have been reported, including jaundice and breast enlargement. The nursing mother should be advised not to use combination hormonal contraceptives, but to use other forms of contraception until she has completely weaned her child.

Pediatrics: The safety and efficacy of Seasonale has not been established in women under the age of 18 years.

Use of this product before menarche is not indicated.

Geriatrics: Seasonale is not indicated for use in post-menopausal women.

Monitoring and Laboratory Tests: Physical Examination and Follow-up: Before hormonal contraceptives are used, a thorough history and physical examination should be performed, including a blood pressure determination. Breasts, liver, extremities and pelvic organs should be examined. A Papanicolaou smear should be taken if the patient has been sexually active.

The first follow-up visit should be three months after the initiation of hormonal contraceptive therapy. Thereafter, examinations should be performed at least once a year, or more frequently if indicated. Women with a strong family history of breast cancer or who have breast nodules should be monitored with particular care. At each annual visit, examination should include those procedures that were done at the initial visit, as outlined above or as per the recommendations of the Canadian Task Force on the Periodic Health Examination.

ADVERSE REACTIONS: Adverse Drug Reaction Overview: An increased risk of the following serious adverse reactions has been associated with the use of oral contraceptives: thrombophlebitis; pulmonary embolism; mesenteric thrombosis; neuro-ocular lesions (e.g., retinal thrombosis); myocardial infarction; cerebral thrombosis; cerebral hemorrhage; hypertension; benign hepatic tumours; gallbladder disease; congenital anomalies.

The following adverse reactions also have been reported in patients receiving oral contraceptives: Nausea and vomiting, usually the most common adverse reaction, occurs in approximately 10 % or fewer of patients during the first cycle. The following other reactions, as a general rule, are seen less frequently or only occasionally: gastrointestinal symptoms (such as abdominal cramps and bloating); breakthrough bleeding; spotting; change in menstrual flow; dysmenorrhea; amenorrhea during and after treatment; temporary infertility after discontinuation of treatment; edema; chloasma or melasma which may persist; breast changes (tenderness, enlargement, secretion); change in weight (increase or decrease); endocervical hyperplasia; possible diminution in lactation when given immediately postpartum; cholestatic jaundice; migraine; increase in size of uterine leiomyomata; rash (allergic); mental depression; reduced tolerance to carbohydrates; vaginal candidiasis; premenstrual like syndrome; intolerance to contact lenses; change in corneal curvature (steepening); cataracts; optic neuritis; retinal thrombosis; changes in libido; chorea; changes in appetite; cystitis-like syndrome; rhinitis; headache; nervousness; dizziness; hirsutism; loss of scalp hair; erythema multiforme; erythema nodosum; hemorrhagic eruption; vaginitis; porphyria; impaired renal function; Raynaud's phenomenon; auditory disturbances; hemolytic uremic syndrome; pancreatitis.

Clinical Trial Adverse Drug Reactions: Because clinical trials are conducted under very specific conditions the adverse reaction rates observed in the clinical trials may not reflect the rates observed in practice and should not be compared to the rates in the clinical trials of another drug. Adverse drug reaction information from clinical trials is useful for identifying drug-related adverse events and for approximating rates.

Seasonale included 15 027 28-day equivalent cycles for the safety ITT data. Across studies SEA-301, SEA-301A and SEA 303, 609 subjects completed 1 year treatment, 123 subjects completed 18 months treatment and 108 subjects completed 2 years treatment.

Two subjects had pulmonary embolism and one subject had myocardial infarction while on Seasonale in clinical studies.

The comparative safety data with a conventional monthly oral contraceptive containing similar strength synthetic estrogens and progestins on lipids profile, liver functions and endometrial biopsies (50 subjects only) is available for one year only.

Study SEA-301: (A Phase III, Parallel, Randomized, Multicenter, Open-Label Clinical Study to Evaluate the Efficacy and Safety of Seasonale Extended Oral Contraceptive Therapy—84-Day Active Cycle.)

Table 2 shows the incidence rates for the most frequently reported adverse events for all treated patients. The table displays results where the 5% or greater criterion was observed within any treatment group.

Table 2: Seasonale

Study SEA-301: Incidence of Most Frequently Reported Adverse Events Occurring in 5% or More Patients—All Treated Patients (ITT)

MedDRA System Organ Class	Seasonale (N=456)		Control (N=226)	
	N	%	N	%
Infections and Infestations				
Nasopharyngitis	100	21.93	67	29.65
Sinusitis NOS	45	9.87	25	11.06
Influenza	32	7.02	15	6.64
Fungal infection NOS	27	5.92	11	4.87
Upper respiratory tract infection NOS	25	5.48	22	9.73
Urinary tract infection NOS	20	4.39	14	6.19
Nervous System Disorders				
Headache NOS	94	20.61	64	28.32
Reproductive System and Breast Disorders				
Menorrhagia	53	11.62	6	2.65
Dysmenorrhoea	26	5.70	9	3.98
Gastrointestinal Disorders				
Pharyngolaryngeal pain	37	8.11	12	5.31
Nausea	34	7.46	20	8.85
Musculoskeletal and Connective Tissue Disorders				
Back pain	29	6.36	19	8.41
Psychiatric Disorders				
Depression NOS	10	2.19	13	5.75

Study SEA-301A: (A Phase IIb, Parallel, Multicenter, Open-Label Clinical Study To Evaluate The Safety Of Seasonale Extended Oral Contraceptive Therapy—84-Day Active Cycle.)

Table 3 shows the incidence rates for the most frequently reported adverse events for all treated patients. The table displays results where the 5% or greater criterion was observed within any treatment group.

Table 3: Seasonale

Study SEA-301A: Incidence of Treatment—Emergent Adverse Events Occurring in 5% or More of All Treated Patients

MedDRA System Organ Class and Preferred Term	Seasonale (N=189)	
	N	%
Infections and Infestations		
Sinusitis NOS	36	19.05
Nasopharyngitis	31	16.40
Upper respiratory tract infection NOS	31	16.40
Urinary tract infection NOS	19	10.05
Vaginosis fungal NOS	12	6.35
Nervous System Disorders		
Headache NOS	32	16.93
Reproductive System and Breast Disorders		

(cont'd)

Table 3: Seasonale *(cont'd)*

Study SEA-301A: Incidence of Treatment—Emergent Adverse Events Occurring in 5% or More of All Treated Patients

	Seasonale (N=189)	
MedDRA System Organ Class and Preferred Term	**N**	**%**
Dysmenorrhoea	18	9.52
Menorrhagia[a]	15	7.94
General Disorders and Administration Site Conditions		
Influenza like illness	17	8.99
Investigations		
Smear cervix abnormal	17	8.99
Musculoskeletal and Connective Tissue Disorders		
Back pain	15	7.94
Gastrointestinal Disorders		
Nausea	12	6.35
Pharyngolaryngeal pain	11	5.82
Abdominal pain NOS	10	5.29
Immune System Disorders		
Seasonal allergy	10	5.29

[a] Due to coding differences between studies SEA-301 and SEA-301A, "intermenstrual bleeding" should be combined with "menorrhagia" in study SEA-301A for comparison with "menorrhagia" in study SEA-301.

Study SEA-303: (A Phase IIIb, Multicenter, Double-Blind Clinical Study to Evaluate the Safety and Tolerability of Seasonale Ultra-Lo Following a Run-In of Seasonale Extended Regimen Oral Contraceptive Therapy.)

Table 4 and Table 5 show the incidence rates for the most frequently reported adverse events for all treated patients. The tables display results where the 5% or greater criterion was observed within any treatment group.

Table 4: Seasonale

Study SEA-303: Incidence of Treatment Emergent Adverse Events During the 6-Month Run-In Period Occurring in 5% or More of Treated Patients

	All Patients[b] (N=1070)	
MedDRA System Organ Class and Preferred Term	**N**	**%**
Nervous System Disorders		
Headache NOS	248	23.18
Infections and Infestations		
Nasopharyngitis	98	9.16
Upper respiratory tract infection NOS	70	6.54
Sinusitis NOS	61	5.70
Reproductive System and Breast Disorders		
Dysmenorrhoea	75	7.01
Intermenstrual bleeding	89	8.32
Menorrhagia[a]	43	4.02
Musculoskeletal and Connective Tissue Disorders		
Back pain	81	7.57
Gastrointestinal Disorders		
Nausea	91	8.50
Investigations		
Weight increased	57	5.33

[a] Menorrhagia is listed even though the incidence is <5% for all treatment groups for completeness when looking at bleeding and/or spotting related AEs.

[b] All patients (N=1070) entered a 6-month Seasonale Run-in period. Characteristics of those discontinuing during the run-in period can be found in the SEA-303 study report. Those completing the run-in period were randomized 1:2 to Seasonale (N=229) or Seasonale Lo (N=465).

Less Common Clinical Trial Adverse Drug Reactions (≥1% to <5%): Study SEA-301: Infections and Infestations: urinary tract infection, bronchitis, pharyngitis streptococcal, ear infection, vaginitis bacterial, vaginosis fungal, bladder infection, pharyngitis, vaginal candidiasis.
Gastrointestinal Disorders: abdominal pain upper, vomiting, dyspepsia, toothache, abdominal pain, diarrhoea, abdominal distension, constipation.
Nervous System: migraine, dizziness (excl. vertigo), sinus headache.
Musculoskeletal and Connective Tissue Disorders: muscle cramps, arthralgia, pain in limb, myalgia, neck pain, muscle spasms, tendonitis.
Reproductive System and Breast Disorders: breast tenderness.
Skin and Subcutaneous Tissue Disorders: acne, acne aggravated, rash.
General Disorders and Administration Site Conditions: influenza like illness, fatigue, pain, pyrexia, chest pain.
Respiratory, Thoracic and Mediastinal Disorders: sinus congestion, cough, nasal congestion, asthma.
Psychiatric Disorders: depression, insomnia, mood swings, libido decreased.
Injury, Poisoning and Procedural Complications: muscle strain, post procedural pain, accident, road traffic accident.
Investigations: weight increased.

Table 5: Seasonale

Study SEA-303: Incidence of Treatment-Emergent Adverse Events During the 9-Month Randomized Double-Blind Period Occurring in 5% or More of All Treated Patients

	Seasonale Randomized (N=229)	
MedDRA System Organ Class and Preferred Term	**N**	**%**
Nervous System Disorders		
Headache NOS	58	25.33
Infections and Infestations		
Nasopharyngitis	30	13.10
Upper respiratory tract infection NOS	22	9.61
Sinusitis NOS	27	11.79
Urinary tract infection NOS	13	5.68
Reproductive System and Breast Disorders		
Intermenstrual bleeding	8	3.49
Dysmenorrhoea	15	6.55
Musculoskeletal and Connective tissue disorders		
Back pain	22	9.61

Menorrhagia is listed even though the incidence is <5% for all treatment groups for completeness when looking at bleeding and/or spotting related AEs.

Immune System Disorders: hypersensitivity, seasonal allergy.
Ear and Labyrinth Disorders: ear pain.
Study SEA-301A: Infections and Infestations: bronchitis, Candidal infection, cervicitis, ear infection, folliculitis, fungal infection, gastroenteritis viral, gingivitis infection, herpes simplex infection, influenza, laryngitis, nail infection, otitis media, papilloma viral infection, pharyngitis streptococcal, pneumonia, post-operative wound infection, tooth caries, tooth infection, vaginitis bacterial.
Gastrointestinal Disorders: abdominal pain upper, constipation, diarrhoea, dyspepsia, food poisoning, gastro-oesophageal reflux disease, toothache, vomiting.
Nervous System Disorders: dizziness (excl. vertigo), hypoaesthesia, migraine, sinus headache, vasovagal attack.
Reproductive System and Breast Disorders: breast cyst, breast tenderness, intermenstrual bleeding, premenstrual syndrome, vaginal discharge.
Musculoskeletal and Connective Tissue Disorders: arthralgia, joint swelling, muscle spasms, myalgia, neck pain, pain in limb.
Investigations: alanine aminotransferase increased, blood pressure increased, liver function tests abnormal, weight increased.
General Disorders and Administration Site Conditions: chest tightness, fall, fatigue, pain, pyrexia.
Skin and Subcutaneous Tissue Disorders: acne, contusion, dermatitis atopic, erythema, rash, urticaria.
Injury, Poisoning and Procedural Complications: arthropod bite, post procedural pain, road traffic accident, animal bite, muscle strain, burns, laceration, sunburn.
Psychiatric Disorders: anxiety, depression, insomnia, libido decreased, stress symptoms.
Respiratory, Thoracic and Mediastinal Disorders: cough, nasal congestion, sinus congestion.
Immune Systems Disorders: allergy aggravated, hypersensitivity.
Neoplasms Benign, Malignant and Unspecified (Incl. Cysts and Polyps): breast lump, uterine fibroids.
Vascular Disorders: hypertension.
Cardiac Disorders: arrhythmia.
Ear and Labyrinth Disorders: vertigo.
Renal and Urinary Disorders: calculus renal.
Hepatobiliary Disorders: cholelithiasis.
Eye Disorders: dry eye.
Study SEA-303: Incidence of Treatment-Emergent Adverse Events During 6-Month Seasonale Run-In—All Treated Patients (Safety): Infections and Infestations: bronchitis, ear infection, fungal infection, influenza, pharyngitis streptococcal, urinary tract infection, vaginitis bacterial, vaginosis fungal.
Nervous System Disorders: dizziness (excl. vertigo), headache aggravated, migraine, sinus headache.
Gastrointestinal Disorders: abdominal distension, abdominal pain, diarrhoea, dyspepsia, pharyngolaryngeal pain, toothache, vomiting.
Musculoskeletal and Connective Tissue Disorders: arthralgia, muscle cramps, myalgia, neck pain, pain in limb.
Reproductive System and Breast Disorders: breast tenderness, menorrhagia.
General Disorders and Administration Site Conditions: fatigue, pain, pyrexia.
Skin and Subcutaneous Tissue Disorders: acne, rash.
Psychiatric Disorders: anxiety, depression, insomnia, irritability, mood swings.
Injury, Poisoning and Procedural Complications: muscle strain, post procedural pain.
Respiratory, Thoracic and Mediastinal Disorders: cough, nasal congestion, sinus congestion.
Ear and Labyrinth Disorders: ear pain.
Study SEA-303: Incidence of Treatment-Emergent Adverse Events During 9-Month Double Blind Period—All Treated Patients (Safety): Infections and Infestations: bladder infection, bronchitis, ear infection, fungal infection, gastroenteritis viral, influenza, pharyngitis, pharyngitis streptococcal, vaginitis bacterial, vaginosis fungal.
Nervous System Disorders: dizziness (excl. vertigo), headache aggravated, migraine, sinus headache.
Musculoskeletal and Connective Tissue Disorders: arthralgia, muscle cramps, myalgia, neck pain, pain in limb.
Reproductive System and Breast Disorders: intermenstrual bleeding, menorrhagia.
Gastrointestinal Disorders: abdominal distension, abdominal pain, abdominal pain upper, constipation, diarrhoea, dyspepsia, nausea, pharyngolaryngeal pain, toothache, vomiting.
Respiratory, Thoracic and Mediastinal Disorders: cough, nasal congestion, sinus congestion, sinus pain.
Psychiatric Disorders: anxiety, depression, insomnia, mood swings, stress symptoms.
Injury, Poisoning and Procedural Complications: back injury, concussion, joint sprain, muscle strain, post procedural pain.
General Disorders and Administration Site Conditions: chest pain, influenza like illness, pain, pyrexia.
Skin and Subcutaneous Tissue Disorders: acne.
Immune System Disorders: hypersensitivity.
Investigations: weight increased.
Less Common Clinical Trial Adverse Drug Reactions (<1%): Study SEA-301: Infections and Infestations: tonsillitis, tooth abscess, cervicitis, gastroenteritis viral, cystitis, gastroenteritis, herpes simplex, herpes viral infection, herpes zoster, lice infestation, lower respiratory tract infection, meningitis viral, pneumonia, staphylococcal infection, tooth infection, upper respiratory tract infection viral, bacterial infection, eye infection, furuncle (excl. genital), genital warts, gingival abscess, kidney infection, laryngitis, localised infection, Lyme disease, malaria, nail fungal infection, oral candidiasis, otitis media, pertussis, respiratory tract infection, sinusitis acute, skin bacterial infection, stye, upper respiratory tract infection, vaginal infection, vaginitis, viral infection, vulvitis, wound infection.

Gastrointestinal Disorders: flatulence, gastro-oesophageal reflux disease, abdominal pain lower, gastric ulcer, tooth disorder, abdominal discomfort, colitis, colon spastic, constipation aggravated, dry mouth, gastrointestinal upset, hemorrhoidal bleeding, hiatus hernia, inguinal hernia, irritable bowel syndrome, oral pain, rectal haemorrhage, salivary gland calculus.
Nervous System: tension headaches, hypoaesthesia, headache aggravated, migraine aggravated, Cluster headaches, disturbance in attention, facial palsy, paraesthesia, sciatica, syncope, vasovagal attack.
Musculoskeletal and Connective Tissue Disorders: bursitis, joint swelling, arthritis, bone disorder, plantar fasciitis, bone spur, intervertebral disc herniation, musculoskeletal chest pain, neck stiffness, rotator cuff syndrome, swelling, temporomandibular joint disorder.
Reproductive System and Breast Disorders: breast enlargement, dyspareunia, premenstrual syndrome, oligomenorrhoea, pelvic pain, uterine cervix ulcer, vaginal discharge, vulvovaginal dryness, breast discharge, breast fibrosis, cervical cyst, genital rash, ovarian cyst, ovarian pain, post-coital bleeding, uterine cervical disorder, uterine cyst , vaginal irritation, vaginal odour, vulval disorder.
Skin and Subcutaneous Tissue Disorders: genital pruritus female, night sweats, pruritus, contusion, dermatitis atopic, skin cysts, urticaria, alopecia, dermatitis contact, eczema, erythema, onychoclasis, rash papular, skin disorder, skin lesion, skin ulcer, solar urticaria, sweating increased.
General Disorders and Administration Site Conditions: facial pain, analgesic effect, fatigue aggravated, feeling hot, groin pain, injection site pain, limb discomfort, oedema lower limb, thirst.
Respiratory, Thoracic and Mediastinal Disorders: rhinitis, upper respiratory tract congestion, asthma aggravated, nasal sinus drainage, pulmonary congestion, rhinitis allergic, sinus pain, chest wall pain, dyspnoea, postnasal drip, rhinitis atrophic, rhinitis seasonal, sinus disorder.
Psychiatric Disorders: anxiety, irritability, mood alteration, attention deficit/hyperactivity disorder, bipolar I disorder, emotional disturbance, loss of libido, nervousness, obsessive-compulsive disorder, panic attack, sleep disorder, stammering.
Injury, Poisoning and Procedural Complications: arthropod bite, joint sprain, back injury, limb injury, animal bite, bite, burns, burns second degree, caustic injury, concussion, ear canal abrasion, facial bones fracture, foot fracture, gun shot wound, hand fracture, laceration, ligament injury, ligament sprain, nerve injury, post-traumatic wound, infection, sunburn, whiplash injury.
Investigations: smear cervix abnormal, weight decreased, blood cholesterol increased, blood pressure increased, blood urine present, colonoscopy, heart rate increased, *H. pylori*, antibody positive, lipids increased, liver function tests abnormal, white blood cell count increase.
Immune System Disorders: allergy aggravated, drug hypersensitivity, allergy to insect sting, food allergy.
Ear and Labyrinth Disorders: motion sickness, ear congestion, Eustachian tube disorder, labyrinthitis, sensation of block in ear, vertigo.
Surgical and Medical Procedures: tooth extraction, eye operation, breast operation, cervical cautery, cholecystectomy, dental operation, knee operation, ligament repair.
Blood and Lymphatic System Disorders: ABO haemolytic disease of newborn, anaemia, lymphadenopathy, iron deficiency anaemia, mononucleosis syndrome.
Vascular Disorders: carotid artery occlusion, hot flushes, hypertension.
Eye Disorders: conjunctivitis, vision blurred, conjunctival hyperaemia, corneal ulcer, eye irritation, lacrimal disorder, pterygium, retinal detachment.
Metabolism and Nutrition Disorders: appetite increased, fluid retention, hunger.
Neoplasms Benign, Malignant and Unspecified (Incl. Cysts and Polyps): breast lump, basal cell carcinoma, fibrocystic breast disease.
Renal and Urinary Disorders: loin pain, urinary frequency, urine odour foul.
Cardiac Disorders: palpitations, palpitations aggravated.
Endocrine Disorders: goitre.
Hepatobiliary Disorders: cholecystitis.
Study SEA-301A: Infections and Infestations: bacterial infection, bladder infection, carbuncle (excl. genital), dry socket, eye infection, folliculitis, gingivitis infection, kidney infection, oral infection, pelvic inflammatory disease, pharyngitis, pyelonephritis, respiratory tract infection, stye, tooth abscess, viral infection, vulvitis.
Gastrointestinal Disorders: abdominal distension, abdominal pain lower, Crohn's disease, gastrointestinal upset, gingivitis, irritable bowel syndrome, oral pain, tooth impacted.
Nervous System Disorders: carpal tunnel syndrome, headache aggravated, hypertonia, migraine aggravated, sciatica, sleep apnoea syndrome, tension headaches.
Reproductive System and Breast Disorders: amenorrhoea, breast pain, cervical dysplasia, cervical friability, cervical polyp, ovarian cyst, vaginal cyst, vaginal pain, vulvovaginal discomfort.
Musculoskeletal and Connective Tissue Disorders: back disorder, back pain aggravated, fibromyalgia, foot deformity, muscle cramps, myositis, neck stiffness, tendonitis.
Investigations: arthroscopy, aspartate aminotransferase increased, cardiac murmur, urine analysis abnormal, white blood cell count increased.
General Disorders and Administration Site Conditions: axillary pain, chest pain, injection site pain, oedema, rigors.
Skin and Subcutaneous Tissue Disorders: acne aggravated, alopecia, dermatitis contact, dermatitis, erythema nodosum, genital pruritus female, milia, pruritus, psoriasis, rash generalised, rash papular, sebaceous cyst, skin discolouration, skin lesion, sweating increased.
Injury, Poisoning and Procedural Complications: accident, arthropod sting, heat stroke, joint dislocation, joint sprain, limb injury, muscle injury, neck injury, tendon injury.
Psychiatric Disorders: anxiety aggravated, depression aggravated, emotional disturbance, insomnia exacerbated, mood swings, panic attack.
Respiratory, Thoracic and Mediastinal Disorders: asthma aggravated, asthma, dyspnoea, epistaxis, nasal sinus drainage, postnasal drip, upper respiratory tract congestion.
Immune Systems Disorders: drug hypersensitivity, food allergy.
Neoplasms Benign, Malignant and Unspecified (Incl Cysts and Polyps): benign breast neoplasm, benign neoplasm, breast mass, cyst, hepatic noeplasm, vulval cancer.
Vascular Disorders: hot flushes.
Cardiac Disorders: palpitations.
Ear and Labyrinth Disorders: ear pain, motion sickness, tinnitus.
Renal and Urinary Disorders: haematuria, polyuria, urinary frequency.
Surgical and Medical Procedures: carpal tunnel decompression, ear operation, lump excision, oral surgery, scar excision, wisdom teeth removal.
Hepatobiliary Disorders: cholecystitis.
Blood and Lymphatic System Disorders: anaemia, mononucleosis syndrome.
Congenital, Familial and Genetic Disorders: dentofacial anomaly.
Endocrine Disorders: hypothroidism.
Metabolism and Nutrition Disorders: appetite increased.
Study SEA-303: Incidence of Treatment-Emergent Adverse Events During 6-Month Seasonale Run-In—All Treated Patients (Safety): Infections and Infestations: bacterial infection, Bartholin's abscess, bladder infection, bronchitis acute, Candidal infection, cellulitis, chlamydial infection, cystitis, endometritis, eye infection, furuncle (excl. genital), gastroenteritis, gastroenteritis bacterial, gastroenteritis viral, gingivitis infection, herpes simplex, herpes zoster, infection, kidney infection, meningitis viral, nail fungal infection, otitis externa, otitis media, papilloma viral infection, pharyngitis, pleurisy viral, pneumonia, rash pustular, respiratory tract infection, skin infection, stye, tonsillitis, tooth abscess, tooth caries, tooth infection, upper respiratory tract infection, upper respiratory tract infection viral, vaginal candidiasis, vaginitis, viral infection.
Nervous System Disorders: amnesia, carpal tunnel syndrome, head discomfort, hypertonia, hypoaesthesia, migraine aggravated, multiple sclerosis, nerve compression, somnolence, syncope, tension headaches.
Gastrointestinal Disorders: abdominal discomfort, abdominal pain lower, abdominal pain upper, constipation, flatulence, food poisoning, gastric ulcer, gastric ulcer Helicobacter, gastritis, gastro-oesophageal reflux disease, gingival oedema, gingival recession, haemorrhoids, irritable bowel syndrome aggravated, lip disorder, mouth ulceration, oral pain, stomach discomfort, throat irritation.
Musculoskeletal and Connective Tissue Disorders: arthritis, back pain aggravated, bunion, bursitis, costochondritis, jaw disorder, muscle atrophy, muscle spasms, muscle stiffness, muscle tightness, myalgia aggravated, neck stiffness, nodule on extremity, pain in jaw, peripheral swelling, plantar fasciitis, swelling, temporomandibular joint disorder, tendonitis exacerbated.
Reproductive System and Breast Disorders: amenorrhoea, breast discharge, breast enlargement, breast oedema, breast pain, cervical dysplasia, dyspareunia, hypomenorrhoea, pelvic pain, premenstrual syndrome, post-coital bleeding, uterine haemorrhage, vaginal discharge, vaginal irritation, vulvovaginal disorder, vulvovaginal discomfort, vulvovaginal dryness.
General Disorders and Administration Site Conditions: axillary pain, chest pain, chest pressure sensation, chest tightness, fall, fatigue aggravated, inflammation, influenza like illness, injection site pain, injection site reaction, mucous membrane disorder, oedema lower limb, oedema, oedema peripheral, pain exacerbated, ulcer.
Skin and Subcutaneous Tissue Disorders: acne aggravated, alopecia, contusion, dermatitis contact, dermatitis, dry skin, eczema, erythema nodosum, genital pruritus female, ingrown hair, ingrowing nail, night sweats, photosensitivity allergic reaction, pigmentation disorder, pruritus, pruritus breast, psoriasis, rash erythematous, rosacea, seborrhoea, skin irritation, skin lesion, sweat gland disorder, urticaria.
Psychiatric Disorders: alcoholic hangover, anxiety disorder, bipolar disorder, depression aggravated, emotional disturbance, libido decreased, libido increased, mood alteration, panic attack, sleep disorder, stress symptoms.
Injury, Poisoning and Procedural Complications: abrasion, animal bite, ankle fracture, arthropod bite, arthropod sting, back injury, bite, foot fracture, headache postoperative, heat stroke, injury, joint sprain, laceration, ligament injury, limb injury, mouth injury, muscle injury, nausea postoperative, neck injury, postoperative wound complication, post vaccination syndrome, road traffic accident, sunburn, tooth injury.
Respiratory, Thoracic and Mediastinal Disorders: asthma exercise induced, asthma, dyspnoea, epistaxis, laryngeal oedema, lung disorder, nasal polyps, respiratory disorder, rhinitis allergic, rhinorrhoea, sinus pain.
Investigations: antinuclear antibody, blood cholesterol increased, blood in stool, blood pressure increased, blood triglycerides increased, heart rate increased, liver function tests abnormal, smear cervix abnormal, weight increased.
Ear and Labyrinth Disorders: motion sickness.
Surgical and Medical Procedures: breast cosmetic surgery, dental operation, endodontic procedure, hernia repair, oral surgery, septoplasty, tooth extraction, tooth repair.
Immune System Disorders: allergy aggravated, drug hypersensitivity, hypersensitivity, seasonal allergy.
Renal and Urinary Disorders: bladder discomfort, bladder irritability, bladder pain, dysuria, haematuria, urinary frequency, urine odour foul.
Vascular Disorders: hot flushes, hypertension, pulmonary embolism, varicose veins.
Eye Disorders: conjunctivitis, conjunctivitis hyperaemia, dry eye, eye disorder, eye irritation, eye swelling, vision blurred.
Metabolism and Nutrition Disorders: appetite increased, dehydration, hunger, hyponatraemia ketoacidosis.
Neoplasms Benign, Malignant and Unspecified (Incl. Cysts and Polyps): cervical carcinoma stage III, cyst, fibromatosis, papilloma, uterine fibroids.
Blood and Lymphatic System Disorders: lymphadenopathy, mononucleosis syndrome.
Cardiac Disorders: angina pectoris, palpitations, tachycardia.
Endocrine Disorders: hyperthyroidism aggravated, thyroiditis.
Hepatobiliary Disorders: fatty liver alcoholic.
Pregnancy, Puerperium and Perinatal Conditions: ectopic pregnancy.
Study SEA-303: Incidence of Treatment-Emergent Adverse Events During 9-Month Double Blind Period—All Treated Patients (Safety): Infections and Infestations: cellulitis, eye infection, gastroenteritis Salmonella, herpes simplex, oral candidiasis, pharyngitis viral, pneumonia, pyelonephritis, respiratory tract infection, skin infection, tonsillitis, trichomoniasis.
Nervous System Disorders: carpal tunnel syndrome, hypoaesthesia, multiple sclerosis aggravated, nerve compression, tension headaches.
Musculoskeletal and Connective Tissue Disorders: intervertebral disc herniation, muscle spasms, neck stiffness, pain in jaw, peripheral swelling, shoulder blade pain, tendonitis.
Reproductive System and Breast Disorders: breast discharge, breast pain, breast tenderness, endometrial atrophy, endometriosis, hypomenorrhoea, ovarian pain, pelvic pain, premenstrual syndrome, vaginal irritation.
Gastrointestinal Disorders: food poisoning, gastric ulcer, gastritis, gastro-oesophageal reflux disease, irritable bowel syndrome, rectal haemorrhage.
Respiratory, Thoracic and Mediastinal Disorders: asthma aggravated, asthma, pulmonary congestion, rhinitis allergic, rhinorrhoea, sinus disorder.
Psychiatric Disorders: alcoholic hangover, anxiety aggravated, confusion, depression aggravated, irritability, libido decreased, mood alteration, panic disorder.
Injury, Poisoning and Procedural Complications: animal bite, arthropod bite, arthropod sting, corneal abrasion, foot fracture, laceration, limb injury, nausea postoperative, road traffic accident, sunburn.
General Disorders and Administration Site Conditions: chest tightness, fatigue, fatigue aggravated, inflammation localised.
Skin and Subcutaneous Tissue Disorders: acne aggravated, contusion, dermatitis, eczema, hair growth abnormal, pruritus, rash, urticaria.
Immune System Disorders: allergy aggravated, drug hypersensitivity, seasonal allergy.
Investigations: blood cholesterol increased, skin test positive, smear cervix abnormal, x-ray chest abnormal.
Ear and Labyrinth Disorders: ear disorder, ear pain.
Neoplasms Benign, Malignant and Unspecified (Incl. Cysts and Polyps): cyst, fibrocystic breast disease, skin papilloma.
Surgical and Medical Procedures: breast cosmetic surgery, eye operation, meniscectomy (knee), rotator cuff repair, tooth extraction, wisdom teeth removal.
Metabolism and Nutrition Disorders: dehydration, diabetes mellitus, fluid retention, hypercholesterolaemia.
Vascular Disorders: hot flushes.
Blood and Lymphatic System Disorders: anaemia, lymphadenopathy, mononucleosis syndrome.
Renal and Urinary Disorders: bladder pain, calculus renal, cystitis interstitial.
Cardiac Disorders: palpitations.
Hepatobiliary Disorders: cholecystitis.
Abnormal Hematologic and Clinical Chemistry Findings: In study SEA-301 (1-year trial), for triglycerides, the percentage of patients on Seasonale going from normal to high was 6.2% compared to that of 1.9% for patients on control (median increase of 136 (43.6%) for Seasonale patients compared to 206 (63.1%) for control patients). For LDL, 17.9% of patients on Seasonale shifted from normal to high values, compared to that of 14.6% for patients on control (median increase in LDL of 40 (27.2%) for Seasonale patients compared to an increase of 37 (22.8%) for control patients). The percentage of Seasonale patients who went from normal to high for total cholesterol was 22.1% compared to that of 23.4% for patients on control (median increase of 37 (17.2%) for Seasonale patients compared to 29 (13.3%) for control patients).

In study SEA-301A (2-year extension trial of SEA-301 with no control), 5 subjects had increase in cholesterol/LDL or triglycerides above the normal ranges among 173 tested Seasonale subjects. Seven subjects had increase in liver enzymes above the normal range excluding the subject with large common bile duct stone.

The coagulation profile was not studied with this Seasonale regimen.

Post-Market Adverse Drug Reactions: The following other serious and unexpected adverse events have been reported in users of Seasonale in the post marketing period. These adverse events are compiled from spontaneous reports and are listed regardless of frequency and whether or not a causal relationship with Seasonale has been established.
Blood and Lymphatic System Disorders: anaemia.
Cardiac Disorders: cardiac arrest, supraventricular tachycardia.
Congenital, Familial and Genetic Disorders: Arnold-Chiari malformation, bicuspid aortic valve, brain malformation, patent ductus arteriosus, spina bifida, talipes.
Endocrine Disorders: hyperprolactinaemia.
Gastrointestinal Disorders: colitis ischemic.
Musculoskeletal and Connective Tissue Disorders: acquired macrocephaly, muscle mass.
Neoplasms Benign, Malignant and Unspecified (Incl. Cysts and Polyps): renal neoplasm.
Nervous System Disorders: brain damage, convulsion, epilepsy, hydrocephalus, hypotonia.
Pregnancy, Puerperium and Perinatal Conditions: abortion spontaneous, intra-uterine death.
Psychiatric Disorders: suicidal ideation.
Renal and Urinary Disorders: neurogenic bladder.
Reproductive System and Breast Disorders: cervical polyp, dysfunctional uterine bleeding, pelvic pain, vaginal haemorrhage.
Skin and Subcutaneous Tissue Disorders: acute febrile neutrophilic dermatosis, leukocytoclastic vasculitis, skin lesion.

In the post-market period, there have been cases of myocardial infarction, stroke, deep vein thrombosis and pulmonary embolism reported with the use of Seasonale.

DRUG INTERACTIONS: Overview: The concurrent administration of oral contraceptives with other drugs may result in an altered response to either agent (see Table 6 and Table 7). Reduced effectiveness of the oral contraceptive, should it occur, is more likely with the low-dose formulations. It is important to ascertain all drugs that a patient is taking, both prescription and non-prescription, before oral contraceptives are prescribed.

Drug-Drug Interactions: Refer to *Oral Contraceptives 1994* (Chapter 8), Health Canada, for possible drug interactions with hormonal contraceptives.

Table 6: Seasonale

Drugs Which May Decrease the Efficacy of Oral Contraceptives

Class of Compound	Drug	Proposed Mechanism	Suggested Management
Anticonvulsants	Carbamazepine Ethosuximide Phenobarbital Phenytoin Primidone Lamotrigine	Induction of hepatic microsomal enzymes. Rapid metabolism of estrogen and increased binding of progestin and ethinyl estradiol to SHBG.	Use higher dose oral contraceptives (50 µg ethinyl estradiol), another drug or another method.
Antibiotics	Ampicillin Cotrimoxazole Penicillin	Enterohepatic circulation disturbance, intestinal hurry.	For short course, use additional method or use another drug. For long course, use another method.
	Rifampin	Increased metabolism of progestin. Suspected acceleration of estrogen metabolism.	Use another method.
	Chloramphenicol Metronidazole Neomycin Nitrofurantoin Sulfonamides Tetracyclines	Induction of hepatic microsomal enzymes. Also disturbance of enterohepatic circulation.	For short course, use additional method or use another drug. For long course, use another method.
	Troleandomycin	May retard metabolism of oral contraceptives, increasing the risk of cholestatic jaundice.	
Antifungals	Griseofulvin	Stimulation of hepatic metabolism of contraceptive steroids may occur.	Use another method.
Cholesterol Lowering Agents	Clofibrate	Reduces elevated serum triglycerides and cholesterol; this reduces oral contraceptive efficacy.	Use another method.
Sedatives and Hypnotics	Benzodiazepines Barbiturates Chloral hydrate Glutethimide Meprobamate	Induction of hepatic microsomal enzymes.	For short course, use additional method or another drug. For long course, use another method or higher dose oral contraceptives.
Antacids		Decreased intestinal absorption of progestin	Dose two hours apart.
Other Drugs	Phenylbutazone Antihistamines Analgesics Antimigraine preparations Vitamin E	Reduced oral contraceptive efficacy has been reported. Remains to be confirmed.	

Table 7: Seasonale

Modification of Other Drug Action by Oral Contraceptives

Class of Compound	Drug	Modification of Drug Action	Suggested Management
Alcohol		Possible increased levels of ethanol or acetaldehyde.	Use with caution.
Alpha-II adrenoreceptor agents	Clonidine	Sedation effect increased.	Use with caution.
Anticoagulants	All	Oral contraceptives increase clotting factors, decrease efficacy. However, oral contraceptives may potentiate action in some patients.	Use another method.
Anticonvulsants	All	Estrogens may increase risk of seizures.	Use another method.
	Lamotrigine	Combination oral contraceptives have been shown to significantly decrease plasma concentrations of lamotrigine likely due to induction of lamotrigine glucoronidation. Decreased lamotrigine levels may lead to breakthrough seizures.	Use another method.
Antidiabetic drugs	Oral hypoglycaemic and insulin	Oral contraceptives may impair glucose tolerance and increase blood glucose.	Use low-dose estrogen and progestin oral contraceptive or another method. Monitor blood glucose.

(cont'd)

Table 7: Seasonale *(cont'd)*

Modification of Other Drug Action by Oral Contraceptives

Class of Compound	Drug	Modification of Drug Action	Suggested Management
Antihypertensive agents	Guanethidine and methyldopa	Estrogen component causes sodium retention, progestin has no effect.	Use low-dose estrogen oral contraceptive or use another method.
	Beta blockers	Increased drug effect (decreased metabolism).	Adjust dose of drug if necessary. Monitor cardiovascular status.
Antipyretics	Acetaminophen	Increased metabolism and renal clearance.	Dose of drug may have to be increased.
	Antipyrine	Impaired metabolism.	Decrease dose of drug.
	ASA	Effects of ASA may be decreased by the short-term use of oral contraceptives.	Patients on chronic ASA therapy may require an increase in ASA dosage.
Aminocaproic acid		Theoretically, a hypercoagulable state may occur because oral contraceptives augment clotting factors.	Avoid concomitant use.
Betamimetic agents	Isoproterenol	Estrogen causes decreased response to these drugs.	Adjust dose of drug as necessary. Discontinuing oral contraceptives can result in excessive drug activity.
Caffeine		The actions of caffeine may be enhanced as oral contraceptives may impair the hepatic metabolism of caffeine.	Use with caution.
Cholesterol lowering agents	Clofibrate	Their action may be antagonized by oral contraceptives. Oral contraceptives may also increase metabolism of clofibrate.	May need to increase dose of clofibrate.
Corticosteroids	Prednisone	Markedly increased serum levels.	Possible need for decrease in dose.
Cyclosporine		May lead to an increase in cyclosporine levels and hepatotoxicity.	Monitor hepatic function. The cyclosporine dose may have to be decreased.
Folic acid		Oral contraceptives have been reported to impair folate metabolism.	May need to increase dietary intake, or supplement.
Meperidine		Possible increased analgesia and CNS depression due to decreased metabolism of meperidine.	Use combination with caution.
Phenothiazine tranquilizers	All phenothiazines, reserpine and similar drugs	Estrogen potentiates the hyperprolactinemia effect of these drugs.	Use other drugs or lower dose oral contraceptives. If galactorrhea or hyperprolactinemia occurs, use other method.
Sedatives and hypnotics	Chlordiazepoxide Lorazepam Oxazepam Diazepam	Increased effect (increased metabolism).	Use with caution.
Theophylline	All	Decreased oxidation, leading to possible toxicity.	Use with caution. Monitor theophylline levels.
Tricyclic antidepressants	Clomipramine (possibly others)	Increased side effects: i.e., depression	Use with caution.
Vitamin B_{12}		Oral contraceptives have been reported to reduce serum levels of Vitamin B_{12}	May need to increase dietary intake, or supplement.

Several of the anti-HIV protease inhibitors have been studied with co-administration of combination oral hormonal contraceptives; significant changes (increase and decrease) in the mean AUC of the estrogen and progestogen have been noted in some cases. The efficacy and safety of oral contraceptive products may be affected. Healthcare providers should refer to the label of the individual anti-HIV protease inhibitor for further drug-drug interaction information.

Drug-Food Interactions: Interactions with food have not been established.

Drug-Herb Interactions: Herbal products containing St. John's Wort (hypericum perforatum) may induce hepatic enzymes (cytochrome P450) and p-glycoprotein transporter and may reduce the effectiveness of contraceptive steroids. This may also result in breakthrough bleeding.

Drug-Laboratory Test Interactions: Laboratory Tests: Results of laboratory tests should be interpreted with the knowledge that the patient is taking an oral contraceptive. The following laboratory tests are modified:

A. **Liver Function Tests:** Aspartate serum transaminase (AST)—variously reported elevations Alkaline phosphatase and gamma-glutamyl transferase (GGT)—slightly elevated.
B. **Coagulation Tests:** Minimal elevation of test values reported for such parameters as prothrombin and Factors VII, VIII, IX and X.
C. **Thyroid Function Tests:** Protein binding of thyroxine is increased as indicated by increased total serum thyroxine concentrations and decreased T3 resin uptake.
D. **Lipoproteins:** Small changes of unproven clinical significance may occur in lipoprotein cholesterol fractions.

E. **Gonadotropins:** LH and FSH levels are suppressed by the use of oral contraceptives. Wait two weeks after discontinuing the use of oral contraceptives before measurements are made.
F. **Glucose tolerance:** Oral glucose tolerance remained unchanged or was slightly decreased.

Tissue Specimens: Pathologists should be advised of hormonal contraceptive use when specimens from surgical procedures and/or Pap smears are submitted for examination.

Drug-Lifestyle Interactions: Cigarette smoking increases the risk of serious cardiovascular side effects from oral contraceptive use. This risk increases with age and heavy smoking (15 or more cigarettes per day) and is quite marked in women over 35 years of age. Women who use oral contraceptives should be strongly advised not to smoke.

Several health advantages other than contraception have been reported.

1. Combination oral contraceptives reduce the incidence of cancer of the endometrium and ovaries.
2. Oral contraceptives reduce the likelihood of developing benign breast disease and, as a result, decrease the incidence of breast biopsies.
3. Oral contraceptives reduce the likelihood of development of functional ovarian cysts.
4. Pill users have less menstrual blood loss and have more regular cycles, thereby reducing the chance of developing iron-deficiency anemia.
5. The use of oral contraceptives may decrease the severity of dysmenorrhea and premenstrual syndrome, and may improve acne vulgaris, hirsutism, and other androgen-mediated disorders.
6. Oral contraceptives decrease the incidence of acute pelvic inflammatory disease and, thereby, reduce as well the incidence of ectopic pregnancy.
7. Oral contraceptives have potential beneficial effects on endometriosis.

DOSAGE AND ADMINISTRATION: Dosing Considerations: Correct use of contraceptives can result in lower failure rates. If withdrawal bleeding does not occur while taking white (inactive) tablets, the possibility of pregnancy must be considered. Appropriate diagnostic measures to rule out pregnancy should be taken at the time of any missed menstrual period. Seasonale should be discontinued if pregnancy is confirmed.

The tablets should not be removed from the protective blister packaging to avoid damage to the product. The plastic dispenser should be kept in the foil pouch until dispensed to the patient.

Recommended Dose and Dosage Adjustment: The dosage of Seasonale is one pink (active) tablet taken daily for 84 consecutive days followed by 7 days of white (inert) tablets. To achieve maximum contraceptive effectiveness, Seasonale must be taken exactly as directed and at intervals not exceeding 24 hours. Ideally, the tablets should be taken at the same time of the day on each day of active treatment.

During the first cycle of medication, the patient is instructed to begin taking Seasonale on the first Sunday after the onset of menstruation. If menstruation begins on a Sunday, the first tablet (pink) is taken that day. One pink tablet should be taken daily for 84 consecutive days, followed by 7 days on which a white (inert) tablet is taken. Withdrawal bleeding should occur during the 7 days following discontinuation of pink active tablets. During the first cycle, contraceptive reliance should not be placed on Seasonale until a pink (active) tablet has been taken daily for 7 consecutive days and a non-hormonal back-up method of birth control (such as condoms or spermicide) should be used during those 7 days. The possibility of ovulation and conception prior to initiation of medication should be considered.

The patient begins her next and all subsequent 91-day course of tablets without interruption on the same day of the week (Sunday) on which she began her first course, following the same schedule: 84 days on which pink tablets are taken followed by 7 days on which white tablets are taken. If in any cycle the patient starts the tablets later than the proper day, she should protect herself against pregnancy by using a non-hormonal back-up method of birth control until she has taken a pink tablet daily for 7 consecutive days.

If spotting or breakthrough bleeding occurs, the patient is instructed to continue on the same regimen. This type of bleeding is usually transient and without significance; however, if the bleeding is persistent or prolonged, the patient is advised to consult her healthcare provider.

In the non-lactating mother, Seasonale may be initiated no earlier than Day 28 of postpartum for contraception due to the increased risk for thromboembolism. When the tablets are administered in the postpartum period, the increased risk of thromboembolic disease associated with the postpartum period must be considered (see also Contraindications and Warnings and Precautions).

The patient should be advised to use a non-hormonal back-up method for the first 7 days of tablet-taking. However, if intercourse has already occurred, the possibility of ovulation and conception prior to initiation of medication should be considered. Seasonale may be initiated immediately after a first-trimester abortion; if the patient starts Seasonale immediately, additional contraceptive measures are not needed.

This product (like all oral contraceptives) is intended to prevent pregnancy. Oral contraceptives do not protect against transmission of HIV (AIDS) and other sexually transmitted diseases such as chlamydia, genital herpes, genital warts, gonorrhea, hepatitis B and syphilis.

Missed Dose: Detailed patient instructions regarding missed pills are presented in the "How to take Seasonale", Missed Dose section of Information for the Patient. If a patient misses one pink tablet, she should take it as soon as possible, meaning she can take two tablets in one day. If a patient misses two pink tablets, she should take 2 tablets on the day she remembers and 2 tablets on the following day. Should three or more tablets be missed, the regular dosing schedule should be resumed, that is one pink tablet per day. Any time the patient misses two or more pink tablets, she should also use another method of non-hormonal back-up contraception until she has taken a pink tablet daily for seven consecutive days. If the patient misses one or more white tablets, she is still protected against pregnancy provided she begins taking pink tablets again on the appropriate day. The possibility of ovulation increases with each successive day that scheduled pink tablets are missed. The risk of pregnancy increases with each active (pink) tablet missed.

OVERDOSAGE:

Serious ill effects have not been reported following acute ingestion of large doses of oral contraceptives by young children. Overdosage may cause nausea, and withdrawal bleeding may occur in females. There is no antidote and further treatment should be symptomatic.

For management of a suspected drug overdose, CPhA recommends that you contact your **regional Poison Control Centre**. See the *CPS* Directory section for a list of Poison Control Centres.

ACTION AND CLINICAL PHARMACOLOGY: Mechanism of Action: Combination oral contraceptives act by suppression of gonadotropins. Although the primary mechanism of this action is inhibition of ovulation, other alterations include changes in the cervical mucus (which increase the difficulty of sperm entry into the uterus) and changes in the endometrium (which reduce the likelihood of implantation).

Pharmacodynamics: Norgestrel is a racemate containing equal parts of D- and L- enantiomers. The L-enantiomer has been tested in a broad range of biological assays and its inactivity has been confirmed. The D-enantiomer (named levonorgestrel) accounts for all the biological activity found in norgestrel, as levonorgestrel was twice as potent as the racemate in experiments in which norgestrel was effective.

Pharmacokinetics: Absorption: No specific investigation of the absolute bioavailability of Seasonale in humans has been conducted. However, published literature indicates that levonorgestrel is rapidly and completely absorbed after oral administration (bioavailability nearly 100%) and is not subject to first-pass metabolism. Ethinyl estradiol is rapidly and almost completely absorbed from the gastrointestinal tract but, due to first-pass metabolism in gut mucosa and liver, the bioavailability of ethinyl estradiol is approximately 43%.

The effect of food on the rate and extent of absorption of levonorgestrel and ethinyl estradiol following oral administration of Seasonale has not been evaluated.

The mean plasma pharmacokinetic parameters of Seasonale following a single dose of two tablets in normal healthy women under fasting conditions are reported in Table 8.

Distribution: The apparent volume of distribution of levonorgestrel and ethinyl estradiol are reported to be approximately 1.8 L/kg and 4.3 L/kg, respectively. Levonorgestrel is about 97.5-99% protein-bound, principally to the sex hormone binding globulin (SHBG) and, to a lesser extent, serum albumin. Ethinyl estradiol is about 95-97% bound to serum albumin. Ethinyl estradiol does not bind to SHBG, but induces SHBG synthesis, which leads to decreased levonorgestrel clearance. Following repeated daily dosing of combination levonorgestrel and ethinyl estradiol oral contraceptives, levonorgestrel plasma concentrations accumulate more than when predicted based on single-dose kinetics, due in part, to increased SHBG levels that are induced by ethinyl estradiol and a possible reduction in hepatic metabolic capacity.

Table 8: Seasonale

Summary of Mean±SD Pharmacokinetic Parameters Following a Single Dose Administration of Seasonale in Healthy Female Subjects Under Fasting Conditions

Analyte	C_{max} (mean±SD)	$t_{½}$ (mean±SD)	$AUC_{0-\infty}$ (mean±SD)	T_{max}
Levonorgestrel	5.6±1.5 ng/mL	29.8±8.3 hours	60.8±25.6 ng·h/mL	1.4±0.3 hrs
Ethinyl Estradiol	145±45 pg/mL	15.4±3.2 hours	1307±361 pg·h/mL	1.6±0.5 hrs

Metabolism: Following absorption, levonorgestrel is conjugated at the 17β-OH position to form sulfate and to a lesser extent, glucuronide conjugates in plasma. Significant amounts of conjugated and unconjugated 3α,5β-tetrahydrolevonorgestrel are also present in plasma, along with much smaller amounts of 3α,5α-tetrahydrolevonorgestrel and 16β-hydroxylevonorgestrel. Levonorgestrel and its Phase I metabolites are excreted primarily as glucuronide conjugates. Metabolic clearance rates may differ among individuals by several-fold, and this may account in part for the wide variation observed in levonorgestrel concentrations among users.

First-pass metabolism of ethinyl estradiol involves formation of ethinyl estradiol-3-sulfate in the gut wall followed by 2-hydroxylation of a portion of the remaining untransformed ethinyl estradiol by hepatic CYP3A4. Levels of CYP3A4 vary widely among individuals and can explain the variation in rates of ethinyl estradiol hydroxylation. Hydroxylation at the 4-, 6- and 16- positions may also occur, although to a much lesser extent than 2-hydroxylation. The various hydroxylated metabolites are subject to further methylation and/or conjugation.

Excretion: About 45% of levonorgestrel and its metabolites are excreted in the urine and about 32% are excreted in feces, mostly as glucuronide conjugates. The terminal elimination half-life for levonorgestrel after a single dose of Seasonale was found to be about 30 hours.

Ethinyl estradiol is excreted in the urine and feces as glucuronide and sulfate conjugates and it undergoes enterohepatic recirculation. The terminal elimination half-life of ethinyl estradiol after a single dose of Seasonale was found to be about 15 hours.

Special Populations and Conditions: Pediatrics: The safety and efficacy of Seasonale has not been established in women under the age of 18 years. Use of this product before menarche is not indicated.

Geriatrics: Seasonale is not indicated for use in post-menopausal women.

Race: No formal studies on the effect of race on the pharmacokinetics of Seasonale have been conducted.

Hepatic Insufficiency: No formal studies have been conducted to evaluate the effect of hepatic disease on the pharmacokinetics of Seasonale. However, steroid hormones may be poorly metabolized in patients with impaired liver function.

Renal Insufficiency: No formal studies have been conducted to evaluate the effect of renal disease on the pharmacokinetics of Seasonale.

Genetic Polymorphism: No data are available.

STORAGE AND STABILITY: Store at room temperature (15 to 30°C). Keep out of the reach of children and pets.

SPECIAL HANDLING INSTRUCTIONS: Not applicable.

INFORMATION FOR THE PATIENT: Published in e-CPS, available by subscription at www.e-cps.ca.

DOSAGE FORMS, COMPOSITION AND PACKAGING: Seasonale (levonorgestrel and ethinyl estradiol, USP) tablets are available in Extended-Cycle Tablet Dispensers. The Tablet Dispenser consists of three plastic leaves in a booklet configuration where individual blister cards are inserted and held in place. Each of these leaves contains either 28 or 35 holes for tablets to be pushed out of the blister cards through the aluminum foil. The first two blister cards contain 28 active pink tablets and the third blister card contains 28 active pink tablets and 7 inert white tablets for a total of 35 tablets. Altogether, the 3 blister cards hold 91 tablets consisting of 84 active pink tablets (each containing 0.15 mg of levonorgestrel and 0.03 mg ethinyl estradiol) and 7 inert white tablets. The compact is then packaged in a foil pouch with a desiccant. Three foil pouches are packaged in each carton. The active pink tablets are round, film-coated, biconvex, unscored tablets with a debossed S on one side and **62** on the other side. The inert tablets are white, round, biconvex, unscored tablets debossed with S on one side and **197** on the other side.

Nonmedicinal ingredients: pink tablets: anhydrous lactose, FD&C Blue No. 1, FD&C Red No. 40, hydroxypropyl methylcellulose, magnesium stearate, microcrystalline cellulose, polyethylene glycol, polysorbate 80 and titanium dioxide; white tablets: anhydrous lactose, hydroxypropyl methylcellulose, magnesium stearate and microcrystalline cellulose.

(Shown in Product Identification Section)

Sebivo® Ⓟ

telbivudine

Antiviral Agent

Novartis Pharmaceuticals

Date of Preparation: November 20, 2006
Date of Revision: May 6, 2009

SUMMARY PRODUCT INFORMATION:

Route of Administration	Dosage Form/ Strength	Clinically Relevant Nonmedicinal Ingredients
Oral	Film-coated tablet 600 mg	None. For a complete listing, please see Dosage Forms, Composition and Packaging.

INDICATIONS AND CLINICAL USE: SEBIVO is indicated for the treatment of chronic hepatitis B in adults of 16 years and older with compensated liver disease with evidence of viral replication and active liver inflammation.

This indication is based on a single Phase 3 intent-to-treat trial for 104 weeks in nucleoside-naive patients with HB e Ag positive or HB e Ag negative chronic HBV infection with compensated liver disease. The primary endpoint was based on virological, serological and biochemical data. There are no available data on telbivudine in patients harbouring lamivudine resistant virus nor in patients with decompensated chronic hepatitis B, co-infected patients (co-infected with HIV or Hepatitis C or D) or in patients in the liver transplant setting.

Geriatrics (>65 years of age): Available data are insufficient to support a specific dose recommendation for patients over the age of 65 years (see Warnings and Precautions).

Pediatrics (<16 years of age): No studies have been performed in children under the age of 16 years.

CONTRAINDICATIONS: SEBIVO is contraindicated in patients with previously demonstrated hypersensitivity to telbivudine or any component of the product. For a complete listing, see Dosage Forms, Composition and Packaging.

WARNINGS AND PRECAUTIONS:

Serious Warnings and Precautions
Severe acute exacerbations of hepatitis B have been reported in patients who have discontinued anti-hepatitis B therapy. Hepatic function must be monitored closely, with both clinical and laboratory follow-up for at least several months in patients who discontinue anti-hepatitis B therapy. If appropriate, re-initiation of anti-hepatitis B therapy may be warranted.

Lactic acidosis and severe hepatomegaly with steatosis, including fatal cases, have been reported with the use of nucleoside analogues alone or in combination with antiretrovirals.

Musculoskeletal: Cases of myopathy have been reported with telbivudine use several weeks to months after starting therapy. Myopathy has also been reported with some other drugs in this class.

Uncomplicated myalgia has been reported in telbivudine-treated patients (see Adverse Reactions). Myopathy, defined as persistent unexplained muscle aches and/or muscle weakness in conjunction with increases in creatine kinase (CK) values, should be considered in any patient with diffuse myalgias, muscle tenderness or muscle weakness. Among patients with telbivudine-associated myopathy, there has not been a uniform pattern with regard to the degree or timing of CK elevations. In addition, the predisposing factors for the development of myopathy among telbivudine recipients are unknown. Patients should be advised to report promptly unexplained muscle aches, pain, tenderness or weakness. Telbivudine therapy should be interrupted if myopathy is suspected, and discontinued if myopathy is diagnosed. It is not known if the risk of myopathy during treatment with drugs in this class is increased with concurrent administration of other drugs associated with myopathy, including corticosteroids, chloroquine, hydroxychloroquine, certain HMGCoA reductase inhibitors, fibric acid derivatives, penicillamine, zidovudine, cyclosporine, erythromycin, niacin and/or azole antifungals. Physicians considering concomitant treatment with these or other agents associated with myopathy should weigh carefully the potential benefits and risks and should monitor patients for any signs or symptoms of unexplained muscle pain, tenderness or weakness, particularly during periods of upward dosage titration.

Neurologic: An increased risk of developing peripheral neuropathy has been observed with the combination use of telbivudine and pegylated interferon alfa-2a (see Drug Interactions). In a pilot trial of telbivudine and pegylated interferon alfa-2a used in combination, peripheral neuropathy has been a common serious event in 10% of patients. Additionally, non-serious peripheral neuropathy cases were also reported. Symptoms of these cases included weakness and paresthesias and pain in the legs, with the time to onset in most cases being 3 months. An increased risk can not be ruled out for combination treatment with other interferon products (pegylated or standard). The benefit of the combination of telbivudine with interferon alfa (pegylated or standard) is not currently established.

Peripheral neuropathy has also occurred uncommonly in clinical trial patients receiving telbivudine monotherapy (0.3%; 5/2000) and in post marketing reports. If peripheral neuropathy is suspected in a patient receiving telbivudine, treatment with telbivudine should be reconsidered.

Use of Telbivudine in Lamivudine Resistant Patients: Available evidence does not support the use of telbivudine in patients with established lamivudine resistant Hepatitis B virus infection. In vitro, telbivudine was not active against the single mutant M204V hepatitis B virus (HBV) strains containing double mutant rtM204V/rtL180M or single mutant rtM204I. (See Action and Clinical Pharmacology, Pharmacodynamics and Resistance, In Vitro.) There have been no clinical studies in these patients.

Use of Telbivudine in Adefovir Resistant Patients: There are no adequate and well controlled studies of telbivudine treatment in patients with established adefovir-resistant Hepatitis B virus infection. HBV encoding the adefovir resistance-associated substitution rtN236T and rtA181V remain fully susceptible to telbivudine, with 0.5- and 1.0-fold susceptibility in cell culture, respectively.

Patients with Renal Impairment: Telbivudine is eliminated primarily by renal excretion, therefore dose interval adjustment is recommended in patients with creatinine clearance <50 mL/min (<0.835 mL/s), including patients on hemodialysis (see Dosage and Administration). In addition, co-administration of SEBIVO with substances that affect renal function may alter plasma concentrations of telbivudine and/or the co-administered substance (see Drug Interactions).

Telbivudine has not been studied in patients on CAPD (continuous ambulatory peritoneal dialysis).

Liver Transplant Recipients: The safety and efficacy of telbivudine in liver transplant recipients are unknown. The steady state pharmacokinetics of telbivudine were not altered following multiple dose administration in combination with cyclosporine (4 mg/kg/day, given in two divided doses). There is no information at higher doses of cyclosporine. If telbivudine treatment is considered necessary in a liver transplant recipient who has received or is receiving an immunosuppressant that may affect renal function, such as cyclosporine or tacrolimus, renal function must be monitored both before and during treatment with SEBIVO (see Drug Interactions).

Cardiovascular: There is no evidence of cardiotoxicity for telbivudine. In an in vitro hERG model, telbivudine was negative at concentrations up to 10 000 μM. In a thorough QTc prolongation clinical study in healthy subjects, telbivudine was not observed to have an effect on QT intervals or other electrocardiographic parameters after multiple daily doses up to 1800 mg.

Sexual Function/Reproduction: There are no clinical data on the effects of telbivudine on male or female fertility. In reproductive toxicology studies, no evidence of impaired fertility was seen when either male or female rats were treated with telbivudine at doses up to 2000 mg/kg/day (systemic exposures approximately 14 times those achieved in humans at the therapeutic dose) and mated with untreated rats.

Special Populations: Co-infected Patients: SEBIVO has not been investigated in co-infected hepatitis B patients (e.g. patients co-infected with HIV, HCV or HDV).

Pregnant Women: There are no adequate and well-controlled studies of telbivudine in pregnant women. Animal studies do not indicate direct or indirect harmful effects with respect to pregnancy, embryonic/foetal development, parturition or postnatal development. SEBIVO should be used during pregnancy only if the benefit to the mother outweighs the potential risk to the foetus.

Telbivudine is not teratogenic and has shown no adverse effects in developing embryos and foetuses in preclinical studies. Studies in pregnant rats and rabbits showed that telbivudine crosses the placenta. Developmental toxicity studies revealed no evidence of harm to the foetus in rats and rabbits at doses up to 1000 mg/kg/day, providing exposure levels 6- to 37-times higher, respectively, than those observed with the therapeutic dose (600 mg/day) in humans.

Pregnancy Registry: To monitor fetal outcomes of pregnant women exposed to telbivudine, healthcare providers are encouraged to register such patients in the AntiRetroviral Pregnancy Registry by calling 1-800-258-4263.

Labour and Delivery: There are no studies in pregnant women and no data on the effect of telbivudine on transmission of HBV from mother to infant. Therefore, appropriate interventions should be used to prevent neonatal acquisition of HBV infection.

Nursing Women: Telbivudine is excreted in the milk of rats. It is not known whether telbivudine is excreted in human milk. Women should not breast-feed if they are taking SEBIVO.

Pediatrics (<16 years of age): The safety and effectiveness of SEBIVO in pediatric patients below the age of 16 have not been established.

Geriatrics (>65 years of age): Clinical studies of telbivudine did not include sufficient numbers of patients ≥65 years of age to determine whether they respond differently from younger subjects. In general, caution must be exercised when prescribing SEBIVO to elderly patients in view of the greater frequency of decreased renal function due to concomitant disease or concomitant use of other medicinal products (see Action and Clinical Pharmacology, Special Populations and Conditions, Renal Insufficiency). It may be useful to monitor renal function in this population.

ADVERSE REACTIONS: Adverse Drug Reaction Overview: Assessment of adverse reactions is primarily based on 2 studies (007 GLOBE study and NV-02B-015) in which 1699 patients received either double-blind treatment with telbivudine 600 mg/day (n=847) or with lamivudine 100 mg/day (n-8952) for 104 weeks. The most common telbivudine related adverse event was CK elevation. There were also several cases of myopathy and uncomplicated myalgia in patients with CK elevations beyond week 52 in the 007 study (see Warnings and Precautions, Musculoskeletal). Median duration of treatment in the 007 GLOBE study was 60 weeks for telbivudine- and lamivudine-treated patients.

Clinical Trial Adverse Drug Reactions: Because clinical trials are conducted under very specific conditions the adverse reaction rates observed in the clinical trials may not reflect the rates observed in practice and should not be compared to the rates in the clinical trials of another drug. Adverse drug reaction information from clinical trials is useful for identifying drug-related adverse events and for approximating rates.

In clinical studies telbivudine was generally well tolerated, with most adverse experiences classified as mild or moderate in severity. Frequently occurring adverse events regardless of attributability to telbivudine were upper respiratory tract infection (15%), nasopharyngitis (19%), fatigue (13%), headache (10%), dizziness (4%) and myalgia (3%). Frequently occurring adverse events regardless of attributability to lamivudine were headache (11%), upper respiratory tract infection (14%), nasopharyngitis (16%), fatigue (11%), dizziness (5%), and myalgia (2%).

In the 007 GLOBE study, discontinuation from the study due to any adverse event in the first 52 weeks was 0.3% for the telbivudine arm, and 0.7% for the lamivudine arm. In the telbivudine arm, there were more study drug discontinuations and interruptions due to musculoskeletal events associated with CK elevations than were in the lamivudine arm (see Warnings and Precautions, Musculoskeletal, and Abnormal Hematologic and Clinical Chemistry Findings).

Clinical adverse events of moderate to severe intensity and considered at least possibly related to treatment during the pivotal 007 GLOBE study clinical trial are presented in Table 1.

Less common (<1%) Clinical Trial Adverse Drug Reactions: Peripheral neuropathy.

Abnormal Hematologic and Clinical Chemistry Findings: The most common lab abnormality associated with telbivudine treatment was CK (creatinine kinase) elevation. The majority of CK elevations were asymptomatic and decreased by the next visit while remaining on treatment. Grade 3-4 CK elevation occurred in 9% of telbivudine-treated patients and 3% of lamivudine-treated patients in Study 007 (including data on all patients to Week 52 and some patients from the ongoing second year of this study). In Study 007, 0.7% (5/680) of patients receiving telbivudine and 0% (0/687) of patients receiving lamivudine discontinued or dose interrupted due to CK elevations (see Table 3 for more details). Most CK elevations were asymptomatic but the mean recovery time was longer for subjects in telbivudine than subjects on lamivudine. Additional patients also discontinued or dose interrupted due to CK elevations in the ongoing second year of the GLOBE study. Some of these CK elevations were associated with myopathy and muscle weakness (see Warnings and Precautions, Musculoskeletal).

Table 1: SEBIVO

Clinical Adverse Events Attributed to Study Drug in ≥1% of Patients with Chronic Hepatitis B Reported in the Pooled 104 Week in the 007 GLOBE and NV-02B-015 Studies

	Telbivudine 600 mg n=847 (%)	Lamivudine 100 mg n=852 (%)
General		
Fatigue	4.4	2.6
Gastrointestinal		
Nausea	2.6	2.0
Diarrhea	1.3	0.7
Abdominal Pain	0.7	1.3
Nervous System		
Headache	3.0	2.9
Dizziness	1.4	0.8
Dermatological		
Rash	1.2	0.7
Respiratory System		
Nasopharyngitis	0.9	0.6
Cough	0.7	0.6

In the pooled analysis (study 007 and NV-02B-015), by 104 weeks of treatment, Grade 3/4 CK elevations occurred in 12.6% of telbivudine-treated patients and 4.0% of lamivudine-treated patients.

Table 2: SEBIVO

Treatment-Emergent Grade 3-4[a] Laboratory Abnormalities[b] in Patients with Chronic Hepatitis B by Week in the 104-Week Pooled 007 GLOBE and NV02B-015 Studies

Test	Telbivudine 600 mg n=847 (%)	Lamivudine 100 mg n=852 (%)
Creatine Kinase (CK) ≥7.0×ULN	13	4
ALT >3.0×baseline	5	8
AST >3.0×baseline	6	10
Lipase >2.5×ULN	2	4
Amylase >3.0×ULN	<1	<1
Total Bilirubin >5.0×ULN	<1	<1
Neutropenia[b] (ANC ≤749/mm^3)	2	2
Thrombocytopenia[b] (Platelets ≤49 999/mm^3)	<1	<1

[a] Grading system corresponds to the 1992 version of the DAIDS AE grading table.
[b] Confirmed on next laboratory value.

Table 3: SEBIVO

Treatment-Emergent New Onset CK Abnormalities[a] in Patients with Chronic Hepatitis B in Studies 007 (GLOBE) and 015 Pooled 104 Weeks

CK Toxicity Grade[e,b]	Telbivudine 600 mg n=847 (%)	Lamivudine 100 mg n=852 (%)
Grade 1 (1 to 3.0×ULN)	38.8	35.0
Grade 2 (>3.0 to 7.0×ULN)	28.0	7.9
Grade 3 (>7.0 to 10.0×ULN)	5.3	1.2
Grade 4 (>10×ULN)	7.3	2.8
Total of Grades 1-4 (≥1×ULN)	79.5	46.8
Discontinuation/Interruption due to CK[c]	0.9[d]	0.1

[a] On-treatment value worsened from baseline to Grade 1 to 4 during therapy up to Week 52.
[b] 22% of patients had pre-treatment Grade 1-4 CK elevations.
[c] Discontinuation/interruption due to adverse events with preferred terms "BIOOD CREATINE PHOSPHOKINASE INCREASED" Additional discontinuations/dose interruptions have occurred after week 52 in this study.
[d] One patient discontinued in each treatment group and 5 patients in telbivudine group had study drug interrupted.
[e] CK toxicity grade corresponds to the 1992 version of the DAIDS AE grading table.

The incidence of ALT flares was similar in the two treatment arms in the first six months. ALT flares occurred less frequently in both arms after Week 24, with a lower incidence in the telbivudine arm (2.0%) compared to the lamivudine arm (5.3%). Periodic monitoring of hepatic function is recommended during treatment. See Table 4.

Exacerbations of Hepatitis After Discontinuation of Treatment: There are insufficient data in patients who have discontinued telbivudine treatment to determine the effects on post-treatment exacerbations of hepatitis after discontinuation of telbivudine treatment (see Warnings and Precautions). However severe acute exacerbations of hepatitis B may occur in patients who have discontinued anti-hepatitis B therapy and hepatic function must therefore be closely monitored in those patients, with both clinical and laboratory follow-up for at least several months.

Table 4: SEBIVO

Analysis of Categories of ALT Flares After Week 24 in Patients with Chronic Hepatitis B in the 007 GLOBE Study

ALT Flare Category[a]	Telbivudine 600 mg n=680 (%)	Lamivudine 100 mg n=687 (%)
ALT ≥2×Baseline and ≥2×ULN[b]	0.3	1.0
ALT ≥3×Baseline and ≥3×ULN	0.1	1.9
ALT ≥500 IU/L and ≥2×Baseline	0.1	1.2
ALT ≥2×Baseline and bilirubin ≥2×Baseline and ≥2×ULN	0	0.4
Total Week 24 to Week 52	0.6	4.5

[a] Each patient can only be represented in one category.
[b] Upper Limit of Normal.

Drug Abuse and Dependence: Telbivudine is not a controlled substance and no potential for dependence has been observed.
Post-Market Adverse Drug Reactons: The following adverse drug reactions have been identified based on post-marketing spontaneous reports and are organized by system organ classes. Because these reactions are reported voluntarily from a population of uncertain size, it is not always possible to reliably estimate their frequency.
Musculoskeletal, Connective Tissue and Bone Disorders: rhabdomyolysis.

DRUG INTERACTIONS: Overview: Since telbivudine is eliminated primarily by renal excretion (see Action and Clinical Pharmacology, Excretion), co-administration of SEBIVO with substances that affect renal function may affect clinical plasma concentrations of telbivudine and/or the co-administered substance. Drug-drug interaction studies were performed with the co-administration of telbivudine with lamivudine, adefovir dipivoxil, pegylated interferon alfa-2a and cyclosporine A.
Telbivudine and peginteferon alfa-2a: A pilot clinical trial investigating the combination of telbivudine 600 mg daily, with pegylated interferon alfa-2a, 180 micrograms once weekly by subcutaneous administration, indicates that this combination is associated with an increased risk for developing **serious peripheral neuropathy** at the rate of 10%. (See Warnings and Precautions.) An increased risk can not be ruled out for combination treatment with other interferon products (pegylated or standard). The benefit of telbivudine in combination with interferon alfa (pegylated or standard) is not currently established.

There appeared to be no statistically significant effect of a single 180 subcutaneous dose of peginterferon (180 µg) on the steady state pharmacokinetics of telbivudine. In the presence of high inter-individual variability, the mean C_{max} and $AUC_{0\ to\ 168\ h}$ of peginterferon were increased by approximately 64% and 40% respectively, when co-administered with multiple doses of telbivudine (600 mg) in healthy subjects.
Telbivudine and lamivudine: The steady-state pharmacokinetics of telbivudine and lamivudine were not clinically significantly altered following multiple dose administration of a subtherapeutic dose of telbivudine (200 mg) in combination with lamivudine (100 mg) in healthy subjects. There is no information at a clinical dose of telbivudine.
Telbivudine and adefovir dipivoxil: The steady-state pharmacokinetics of telbivudine and adefovir dipivoxil appeared to be unaltered following multiple dose administration of telbivudine (600 mg) in combination with multiple dose adefovir dipivoxil (10 mg) in healthy subjects.
Telbivudine and cyclosporine A: The steady-state pharmacokinetics of telbivudine and cyclosporine A appeared to be unaltered following multiple dose administration of telbivudine in combination with multiple doses of cyclosporine A (4 mg/kg/day given in two divided doses) in healthy subjects. There is no information at higher doses of cyclosporine A.
Telbivudine and tenofovir disoproxil fumarate: The steady-state pharmacokinetics of telbivudine were unaltered following multiple dose administration in combination with tenofovir disoproxil fumarate.
Telbivudine effect on the pharmacokinetics of other drugs: Telbivudine does not alter the pharmacokinetics of lamivudine, adefovir dipivoxil, cyclosporine A or tenofovir disoproxil fumarate. No definitive conclusion could be drawn regarding the effects of telbivudine on the pharmacokinetics of pegylated interferon-alfa 2a due to the high inter-individual variability of pegylated interferon-alfa 2a concentrations (see Drug Interaction between Telbivudine and peginteferon alfa-2a).

The effects of co-administration of SEBIVO with other drugs that are renally eliminated or are known to affect renal function have not been evaluated and patients should be monitored closely for adverse events when SEBIVO is co-administered with such drugs.

At concentrations up to 12 times that used in humans, telbivudine did not inhibit in vitro metabolism mediated by any of the following human hepatic microsomal cytochrome P450 (CYP) isoenzymes known to be involved in human drug metabolism: 1A2, 2C9, 2C19, 2D6, 2E1, and 3A4. Telbivudine does not induce cytochrome P450 isoenzymes in animals. Based on the above results and the known elimination pathway of telbivudine, the potential for CYP450-mediated interactions involving SEBIVO with other medicinal products is low.

DOSAGE AND ADMINISTRATION: Dosing Considerations: Dose interval adjustment is recommended in patients with moderate to severe renal impairment (creatinine clearance <50 mL/min) (see Renal Impairment/Insufficiency).
Recommended Dose and Dosage Adjustment: The recommended dose of SEBIVO for the treatment of chronic hepatitis B is 600 mg once daily, taken orally, with or without food.

The optimal treatment duration has not been established.
Renal Impairment/Insufficiency: (See Warnings and Precautions, Special Populations and Action and Clinical Pharmacology, Special Populations and Conditions, Renal Insufficiency).

SEBIVO may be used for the treatment of chronic hepatitis B in patients with impaired renal function. No adjustment of the recommended dose of telbivudine is necessary in patients whose creatinine clearance is ≥50 mL/min (≥0.835 mL/s). Adjustment of the dose interval is required in patients with creatinine clearance <50 mL/min (<0.835 mL/s) including those with end stage renal disease (ESRD) on haemodialysis, as shown in Table 5.

Table 5: SEBIVO

Dose Interval Adjustment of SEBIVO in Patients with Renal Impairment

Creatinine clearance (mL/min)	Dose of SEBIVO
≥50	600 mg once daily
30–49	600 mg once every 48 hours
<30 (not requiring dialysis)	600 mg once every 72 hours
ESRD[a]	600 mg once every 96 hours

[a] End stage renal disease.

End Stage Renal Disease (ESRD) Patients: For patients with ESRD, SEBIVO should be administered after haemodialysis (see Action and Clinical Pharmacology, Special Populations and Conditions, Renally Impaired Patients on Haemodialysis). Telbivudine has not been studied in CAPD patients.
Hepatic Impairment: No adjustment of the recommended dose of SEBIVO is necessary in patients with hepatic impairment (see Action and Clinical Pharmacology, Special Populations and Conditions, Hepatic Insufficiency).
Pediatric Patients (age below 16 years): No studies have been performed in children under the age of 16 years (see Warnings and Precautions).
Elderly Patients (age above 65 years): Available data are insufficient to support a specific dose recommendation for patients over the age of 65 years (see Warnings and Precautions).

OVERDOSAGE:
Activated charcoal should be administered to aid in the removal of unabsorbed drug. General supportive measures are recommended.

Tested doses of up to 1800 mg/day for four days (three times greater than the recommended daily dose) have been well tolerated. A maximum tolerated dose of telbivudine has not been determined.

For management of a suspected drug overdose, contact your **regional Poison Control Centre**. See the *CPS* Directory section for a list of Poison Control Centres.

ACTION AND CLINICAL PHARMACOLOGY: Mechanism of Action: Telbivudine is a synthetic thymidine nucleoside analogue with activity against HBV DNA polymerase.
Pharmacodynamics: Telbivudine is efficiently phosphorylated by cellular kinases to the active triphosphate form, which has an intracellular half-life of 14 hours. Telbivudine-5'-triphosphate inhibits HBV DNA polymerase (reverse transcriptase) by competing with the natural substrate, thymidine 5'-triphosphate. Incorporation of telbivudine-5'-triphosphate into viral DNA causes DNA chain termination, resulting in inhibition of HBV replication. Telbivudine is an inhibitor of both HBV first-strand (EC_{50}=0.4-1.3 µM) and second-strand (EC_{50}=0.12-0.24 µM) synthesis, and shows a distinct preference for inhibiting second-strand production. By contrast, telbivudine-5'-triphosphate at concentrations up to 100 µM did not inhibit human cellular DNA polymerases alpha, beta, or gamma. In assays relating to human mitochondrial structure, function and DNA content, telbivudine lacked an appreciable toxic effect at concentrations up to 10 µM and did not increase lactic acid production in vitro.
Pharmacokinetics: The single- and multiple-dose pharmacokinetics of telbivudine were evaluated in healthy subjects and in patients with chronic hepatitis B. Telbivudine pharmacokinetics are similar between both populations.
Absorption: Following oral administration of a 600 mg single dose of telbivudine to healthy subjects (n=12), steady state peak plasma concentration (C_{max}) of telbivudine was 3.69±1.25 µg/mL (Mean±SD) which occurred between 1 and 4 hours (median 2.0 hours). The telbivudine area under the plasma concentration-time curve (AUC_{0-INF}) was 26.1±7.2 µg·h/mL (Mean±SD), and trough plasma concentrations (C_{trough}) were approximately 0.2-0.3 µg/mL. Steady state was achieved after approximately 5 to 7 days of once-daily administration with approximately 1.5-fold accumulation, suggesting an effective half-life of approximately 15 hours. The pharmacokinetics of telbivudine are dose-related in the 25 to 1800 mg dose range.
Effect of Food on Oral Absorption: Telbivudine absorption and exposure were unaffected when a single 600 mg dose was administered with food. SEBIVO may be taken with or without food.
Distribution: In vitro binding of telbivudine to human plasma proteins is low (3.3%). After oral dosing, the estimated apparent volume of distribution is in excess of total body water, suggesting that telbivudine is widely distributed into tissues.
Metabolism: No metabolites of telbivudine were detected following administration of ^{14}C-telbivudine in humans. Telbivudine is not a substrate, inhibitor or inducer of the cytochrome P450 (CYP450) enzyme system (see Drug Interactions).
Excretion: After reaching peak concentration, plasma disposition of telbivudine declined in a bi-exponential manner with a terminal elimination half-life ($t_{1/2}$) of 41.8±11.8 hours. Telbivudine is eliminated primarily by urinary excretion of unchanged substance. The renal clearance of telbivudine approaches normal glomerular filtration rate, suggesting that passive diffusion is the main mechanism of excretion. Approximately 42% of the dose is recovered in the urine over 7 days following a single 600 mg oral dose of telbivudine. Because renal excretion is the predominant route of elimination, patients with moderate to severe renal dysfunction and those undergoing haemodialysis require a dose interval adjustment (see Dosage and Administration).
Resistance: In Vitro: The activity of telbivudine was assessed in cell-based assays against a number of HBV genomic variants associated with lamivudine and adefovir resistance in HBV-infected patients. The M204V mutant is a key intermediate leading to the emergence of the L180M/M204V lamivudine resistant strain. Telbivudine failed to exhibit antiviral activity against the M204I and L180M/M204V mutants as indicated by the fold changes to wild type of >1360+/262, and demonstrated only marginal activity against the L180M/M204I double mutant (fold change of >1049+/226).

In cell culture, telbivudine showed a 2-fold enhanced activity against HBV containing the N236T mutation and wild type activity against HBV containing the A181T mutation, the most common form of adefovir-resistance mutations seen in HBV-infected patients. HBV encoding an A181V amino acid substitution showed 3- to 5-fold reduced susceptibility to telbivudine in cell culture. In HIV-1 infected patients, nucleoside analogues such as lamivudine and entecavir can induce YMDD-based (M184V) HIV drug resistant strains. Telbivudine does not demonstrate activity against HIV-1 in cell culture. The presence or absence of telbivudine activity against HIV has not been evaluated in clinical trials.
Clinical Resistance: The safety and efficacy of long term (104 week) telbivudine treatment SEBIVO were evaluated in two established international active-controlled clinical studies that included 1699 patients with chronic hepatitis B (007 GLOBE and NV-02B-015).
Week 52: In an as-treated analysis of the Phase 3 global registration trial (007 GLOBE study), 59% (252/430) of treatment-naïve HBeAg-positive and 89% (202/227) of treatment-naïve HBeAg-negative patients receiving telbivudine 600 mg once daily achieved nondetectable serum HBV DNA levels (<300 copies/mL) by Week 52. At Week 52, 145/430 (34%) and 19/227 (8%) of HBeAg-positive and HBeAg-negative telbivudine recipients, respectively, had evaluable HBV DNA (≥1000 copies/mL). Genotypic analysis detected one or more amino acid substitutions associated with virologic failure (rtM204I, rtL80I/V, rtA181T, rtL180M, rtL229W/V) in 49 of 103 HBeAg-positive and 12 of 12 HBeAg-negative patients with amplifiable HBV DNA and ≥16 weeks of treatment. The rtM204I substitution was the most frequent mutation and was associated with virologic rebound (≥1 log_{10} increase above nadir) in 34 of 46 patients with this mutation. The clinical resistance data indicate negligible selection of YMDD mutant HBV by the M204V pathway. No L180M/M204V double mutant was seen in patients treated with telbivudine in the 007 GLOBE study. No novel or telbivudine-specific resistance mutations were identified.
Week 104: In the (007 GLOBE study), 55.7% (255/458) of treatment-naïve HBeAg-positive and 82.0% (182/222) of treatment-naïve HBeAg-negative patients receiving telbivudine 600 mg/day once daily achieved nondetectable serum HBV DNA levels (<300 copies/mL) by Week 104. Genotypic analysis of 203 evaluable sample pairs with HBV DNA ≥1000 copies/mL demonstrated that the primary mutation associated with telbivudine resistance was rtM204I often associated with mutations rtL180M and rtL80I/V and infrequently with rtV27A, rtL82M, rtV173L, rtT184I, and rtA200V. Baseline factors associated with development of genotypic drug resistance included: lamivudine treatment, higher baseline HBV DNA, lower baseline serum ALT, and increased body weight/BMI. On treatment response parameters at Week 24 that predicted emergence of drug resistant virus by Week 104 were HBV DNA >300 copies/mL and elevation of serum ALT.
Cross-Resistance: Cross-resistance has been observed among HBV nucleoside analogues. In cell-based assays, lamivudine-resistant HBV strains containing either the rtM204I mutation or the rtL180M/rtM204V double mutation had ≥1000-fold reduced susceptibility to telbivudine. HBV encoding the adefovir resistance-associated substitutions at rtN236T and A181V had 0.5- and 1.0-fold change in susceptibility to telbivudine in cell culture, respectively. Substitution at rtA194T had 0.99-fold shift in susceptibility to telbivudine in cell culture.

In cell culture testing, telbivudine retains full activity against an M204V single mutant strain that is an intermediate in the lamivudine resistance pathway. However, telbivudine showed reduced activity against recombinant HBV variants containing the YMDD mutations associated with lamivudine resistance (L180M/M204V or M204I). Based on the very similar IC_{50} values for telbivudine and lamivudine against these mutants in in vitro studies, efficacy in patients with established lamivudine resistance is not expected. The use of telbivudine in these patients should therefore only be considered in well controlled clinical trials until availability of further clinical data. Clinical data indicate that telbivudine-resistant HBV strains are likely to carry the M204I mutation which is known to be resistant to lamivudine but remains sensitive to PMEA the active component of adefovir. HBV encoding the adefovir resistance-associated substitutions rtN236T or rtA181 remained susceptible to telbivudine.
Special Populations and Conditions: Pediatrics and Geriatrics: Pharmacokinetic studies have not been conducted in paediatric or elderly subjects.
Gender: There are no significant gender-related differences in telbivudine pharmacokinetics.
Race: There are no significant race-related differences in telbivudine pharmacokinetics.
Hepatic Insufficiency: The pharmacokinetics of telbivudine following a single 600 mg dose have been studied in patients (without chronic hepatitis B) with various degrees of hepatic impairment. There were no changes in telbivudine pharmacokinetics in hepatically impaired subjects compared to unimpaired subjects. Results of these studies indicate that no dosage adjustment is necessary for patients with hepatic impairment (see Dosage and Administration).
Renal Insufficiency: The single-dose pharmacokinetics of telbivudine have been evaluated in patients (without chronic hepatitis B) with various degrees of renal impairment (as assessed by creatinine clearance). Based on the results shown in Table 6, adjustment of the dose interval for telbivudine is recommended in patients with creatinine clearance of <50 mL/min (<0.835 mL/s) (see Dosage and Administration).

Table 6: SEBIVO

Pharmacokinetic Parameters (Mean±SD) of Telbivudine in Subjects with Various Degrees of Renal Function After a Single Dose

	Renal function (creatinine clearance in mL/min)				
	Normal (>80) (n=8) 600 mg	**Mild (50–80) (n=8) 600 mg**	**Moderate (30–49) (n=8) 400 mg**	**Severe (<30) (n=6) 200 mg**	**ESRD/Post-Haemodialysis (n=6) 200 mg**
C_{max} (µg/mL)	3.4±0.9	3.2±0.9	2.8±1.3	1.6±0.8	2.1±0.9
$AUC_{0\text{-}INF}$ (µg·h/mL)	28.5±9.6	32.5±10.1	36.0±13.2	32.5±13.2	67.4±36.9
CL_{RENAL} (L/h)	7.6±2.9	5.0±1.2	2.6±1.2	0.7±0.4	

Renally Impaired Patients on Haemodialysis: Haemodialysis (up to 4 hours) reduces systemic telbivudine exposure by approximately 23%. Following dose interval adjustment for creatinine clearance, no additional dose modification is necessary during routine haemodialysis (see Dosage and Administration). SEBIVO should be administered after haemodialysis.

STORAGE AND STABILITY: SEBIVO film-coated tablets should be stored at a temperature between 15-30°C.

SPECIAL HANDLING INSTRUCTIONS: Not applicable.

INFORMATION FOR THE PATIENT: Published in e-CPS, available by subscription at www.e-cps.ca.

DOSAGE FORMS, COMPOSITION AND PACKAGING: Each white to slightly yellowish film-coated, ovaloid-shaped tablet, imprinted with "LDT" on one side contains: telbivudine 600 mg. Nonmedicinal ingredients: colloidal silicon dioxide, magnesium stearate, microcrystalline cellulose, povidone and sodium starch glycolate; coating: hypromellose, polyethylene glycol, talc and titanium dioxide. PVC/aluminum blisters of 28.

(Shown in Product Identification Section)

Secaris®
polyethylene glycol—propylene glycol
Rhinitis Therapy

PendoPharm

SUPPLIED: Each g of lubricant nasal gel contains: polyethylene glycol 15% and propylene glycol 20%, adjusted to pH 5.5. Nonmedicinal ingredients: benzalkonium chloride, carbomer 934P, potassium chloride, sodium carboxymethylcellulose, sodium chloride and water. Tubes of 5 and 30 g.

Sectral® Ⓟ
acebutolol HCl
Antihypertensive—Antianginal

sanofi-aventis

SUPPLIED: 100 mg: Each white to off-white, shield-shaped, film-coated tablet, one side scored, debossed with "SECTRAL" above scoreline and with "100" below scoreline, other side debossed with "rPr" in a heart, contains: acebutolol base 100 mg (as the hydrochloride). Nonmedicinal ingredients: colloidal silicon dioxide, croscarmellose sodium, D&C Yellow #10 Aluminum Lake, dibasic calcium phosphate (dihydrate), magnesium stearate, microcrystalline cellulose, Opadry II White Y-22-7719, polyethylene glycol, povidone and talc. Gluten-, lactose- and tartrazine-free. Bottles of 100 and 500.

200 mg: Each blue, shield-shaped, film-coated tablet, one side scored, debossed with "SECTRAL" above scoreline and with "200" below scoreline, other side debossed with "rPr" in a heart, contains: acebutolol base 200 mg (as the hydrochloride). Nonmedicinal ingredients: colloidal silicon dioxide, croscarmellose sodium, dibasic calcium phosphate (dihydrate), FD&C Blue #1 Aluminum Lake, magnesium stearate, microcrystalline cellulose, Opadry II White Y-22-7719, polyethylene glycol, povidone and talc. Gluten-, lactose-, and tartrazine-free. Bottles of 100 and 500.

400 mg: Each white to off-white, shield-shaped, film-coated tablet, one side scored, debossed with "SECTRAL" above scoreline and with "400" below scoreline, other side debossed with "rPr" in a heart, contains: acebutolol base 400 mg (as the hydrochloride). Nonmedicinal ingredients: colloidal silicon dioxide, D&C Yellow No. 10 Aluminum Lake, lactose monohydrate, magnesium stearate, methylcellulose, Opadry II White Y-22-7719, polyethylene glycol, povidone, starch and talc. Gluten- and tartrazine-free. Bottles of 100.

(Shown in Product Identification Section)

Selax™
docusate sodium
Stool Softener

Odan

SUPPLIED: Capsules: Each light red soft gelatin capsule contains: docusate sodium USP 100 mg. Nonmedicinal ingredients: FD&C Red #40, FD&C Yellow #6, gelatin, glycerin, methylparaben, polyethylene glycol, propylene glycol, propylparaben, purified water and sorbitol. Gluten- and tartrazine-free. Bottles of 100 and 1000. Unidose of 100. Store between 15 and 30°C.

Syrup: Each 5 mL of clear red syrup, with peppermint-cherry flavor contains: docusate sodium USP 20 mg. Nonmedicinal ingredients: amaranth FD&C Red #2, flavor (cherry, orange, peppermint), methylparaben, propylene glycol, propylparaben, purified water and sucrose. Alcohol-, gluten- and tartrazine-free. Bottles of 250 and 500 mL.

Select™ 1/35 Ⓟ
norethindrone—ethinyl estradiol
Oral Contraceptive

Pfizer

PHARMACOLOGY: Estrogen-progestogen combinations act primarily through the mechanism of gonadotropin suppression due to the estrogenic and progestational activity of their components. Although the primary mechanism of action is inhibition of ovulation, alterations in the cervical mucus and the endometrium may also contribute to effectiveness.

INDICATIONS: Prevention of pregnancy.

CONTRAINDICATIONS: History of or actual thrombophlebitis or thromboembolic disorders; history of or actual cerebrovascular disorders; history of or actual myocardial infarction or coronary arterial disease; active liver disease or history of or actual benign or malignant liver tumors; history of or known or suspected carcinoma of the breast; history of or known or suspected estrogen-dependent neoplasia; undiagnosed abnormal vaginal bleeding; any ocular lesion arising from ophthalmic vascular disease, such as partial or complete loss of vision or defect in visual fields; when pregnancy is suspected or diagnosed.

WARNINGS: Predisposing Factors for Coronary Artery Disease: Cigarette smoking increases the risk of serious cardiovascular side effects and mortality. Birth control pills increase this risk, especially with increasing age. Convincing data are available to support an upper age limit of 35 years for oral contraceptive use by women who smoke.

Other women who are independently at high risk for cardiovascular disease include those with diabetes, hypertension, abnormal lipid profile, or a family history of these. Whether oral contraceptives accentuate this risk is unclear.

In low-risk, nonsmoking women of any age, the benefits of oral contraceptive use outweigh the possible cardiovascular risks associated with low dose formulations. Consequently, oral contraceptives may be prescribed for these women up to the age of menopause.

> Cigarette smoking increases the risk of serious adverse effects on the heart and blood vessels. This risk increases with age and becomes significant in oral contraceptive users over 35 years of age. Women should be counseled not to smoke.

Discontinue Medication at the Earliest Manifestation of the Following:
A. Thromboembolic and cardiovascular disorders such as: thrombophlebitis, pulmonary embolism, cerebrovascular disorders, myocardial ischemia, mesenteric thrombosis, and retinal thrombosis.
B. Conditions that predispose to venous stasis and to vascular thrombosis, e.g., immobilization after accidents or confinement to bed during long-term illness. Other nonhormonal methods of contraception should be used until regular activities are resumed. For use of oral contraceptives when surgery is contemplated, see Precautions.
C. Visual defects, partial or complete.
D. Papilledema or ophthalmic vascular lesions.
E. Severe headache of unknown etiology or worsening of pre-existing migraine headache.

PRECAUTIONS: Physical Examination and Follow-up: Before oral contraceptives are used, a thorough history and physical examination should be performed, including a blood pressure determination. Breasts, liver, extremities and pelvic organs should be examined and a Papanicolaou smear should be taken if the patient has been sexually active.

The first follow-up visit should be done 3 months after oral contraceptives are prescribed. Thereafter, examinations should be performed at least once a year or more frequently if indicated. At each annual visit, examination should include those procedures that were done at the initial visit as outlined above or per recommendations of the Canadian Workshop on Screening for Cancer of the Cervix. Its suggestion was that, for women who had 2 consecutive negative Pap smears, screening could be continued every 3 years up to the age of 69.

Pregnancy: Fetal abnormalities have been reported to occur in the offspring of women who have taken estrogen-progestogen combinations in early pregnancy. Rule out pregnancy as soon as it is suspected.

Lactation: The use of oral contraceptives during the period a mother is breast-feeding her infant may not be advisable. The hormonal components are excreted in breast milk and may reduce its quantity and quality. The long-term effects on the developing child are not known.

Hepatic Function: Patients who have had jaundice including a history of cholestatic jaundice during pregnancy should be given oral contraceptives with great care and under close observation.

The development of severe generalized pruritus or icterus requires that the medication be withdrawn until the problem is resolved.

If a patient develops jaundice that proves to be cholestatic in type, the use of oral contraceptives should not be resumed. In patients taking oral contraceptives, changes in the composition of the bile may occur and an increased incidence of gallstones has been reported.

Hepatic nodules have been reported to be associated with use of oral contraceptives, particularly in long-term users of oral contraceptives. These nodules include benign hepatic adenomas, focal nodular hyperplasia and other hepatic lesions. In addition, hepatocellular carcinoma has been reported. Although these lesions are extremely rare, they have caused fatal intra-abdominal hemorrhage and should be considered in women presenting with an abdominal mass, acute abdominal pain, or evidence of intra-abdominal bleeding.

Hypertension: Patients with essential hypertension whose blood pressure is well-controlled may be given oral contraceptives but only under close supervision. If a significant elevation of blood pressure in previously normotensive or hypertensive subjects occurs at any time during the administration of the drug, cessation of medication is necessary.

Migraine and Headache: The onset or exacerbation of migraine or the development of headache of a new pattern which is recurrent, persistent or severe, requires discontinuation of oral contraceptives and evaluation of the cause.

Diabetes: Current low dose oral contraceptives exert minimal impact on glucose metabolism. Diabetic patients, or those with a family history of diabetes, should be observed closely to detect any worsening of carbohydrate metabolism. Patients predisposed to diabetes who can be kept under close supervision may be given oral contraceptives. Young diabetic patients whose disease is of recent origin, well-controlled, and not associated with hypertension or other signs of vascular disease such as ocular fundal changes, should be monitored more frequently while using oral contraceptives.

Ocular Disease: Patients who are pregnant or are taking oral contraceptives, may experience corneal edema that may cause visual disturbances and changes in tolerance to contact lenses, especially of the rigid type. Soft contact lenses usually do not cause disturbances. If visual changes or alterations in tolerance to contact lenses occur, temporary or permanent cessation of wear may be advised.

Breasts: Increasing age and a strong family history are the most significant risk factors for the development of breast cancer. Other established risk factors include obesity, nulliparity and late age at first full-term pregnancy. The identified groups of women that may be at increased risk of developing breast cancer before menopause are long-term users of oral contraceptives (more than 8 years) and starters at early age. In a few women, the use of oral contraceptives may accelerate the growth of an existing but undiagnosed breast cancer. Since any potential increased risk related to oral contraceptive use is small, there is no reason to change prescribing habits at present.

Women receiving oral contraceptives should be instructed in self-examination of their breasts. Their physicians should be notified whenever any masses are detected. A yearly clinical breast examination is also recommended because, if a breast cancer should develop, drugs that contain estrogen may cause a rapid progression.

Vaginal Bleeding: Persistent irregular vaginal bleeding requires assessment to exclude underlying pathology.

Fibroids: Patients with fibroids (leiomyomata) should be carefully observed. Sudden enlargement, pain, or tenderness require discontinuation of the use of oral contraceptives.

Emotional Disorders: Patients with a history of emotional disturbances, especially the depressive type, may be more prone to have a recurrence of depression while taking oral contraceptives. In cases of a serious recurrence, a trial of an alternate method of contraception should be made which may help to clarify the possible relationship. Women with premenstrual syndrome (PMS) may have a varied response to oral contraceptives, ranging from symptomatic improvement to worsening of the condition.

Metabolic and Endocrine Diseases: In metabolic or endocrine diseases and when metabolism of calcium and phosphorus is abnormal, careful clinical evaluation should precede medication and a regular follow-up is recommended.

Connective Tissue Disease: The use of oral contraceptives in some women has been associated with positive lupus erythematous cell tests and with clinical lupus erythematous. In some instances exacerbation of rheumatoid arthritis and synovitis has been observed.

Laboratory Tests: Results of laboratory tests should be interpreted in the light of the fact that the patient is on oral contraceptives. The laboratory tests listed below are modified.
A. Liver Function Tests: Aspartate serum transaminase (AST): variously reported elevations. Alkaline phosphatase and gamma glutamine transaminase (GGT): slightly elevated.
B. Coagulation Tests: Minimal elevation of test values reported for such parameters as Factors VII, VIII, IX and X. Increased platelet aggregation, decreased antithrombin III.
C. Thyroid Function Tests: Protein binding of thyroxine is increased as indicated by increased total serum thyroxine concentrations and decreased T_3 resin uptake.
D. Lipoproteins: Small changes of unproven clinical significance may occur in lipoprotein cholesterol fractions.
E. Gonadotropins: LH and FSH levels are suppressed by the use of oral contraceptives. Wait 2 weeks after discontinuing the use of oral contraceptives before measurements are made.

Tissue Specimens: Pathologists should be advised of oral contraceptive therapy when specimens obtained from surgical procedures and Pap smears are submitted for examination.

Return to Fertility: After discontinuing oral contraceptive therapy, the patient should delay pregnancy until at least 1 normal spontaneous cycle has occurred in order to date the pregnancy. An alternate contraceptive method should be used during this time.

Amenorrhea: Women having a history of oligomenorrhea, secondary amenorrhea, or irregular cycles may remain anovulatory or become amenorrheic following discontinuation of estrogen-progestin combination therapy.

Amenorrhea, especially if associated with breast secretion, that continues for 6 months or more after withdrawal, warrants a careful assessment of hypothalamic-pituitary function.

Thromboembolic Complications—Postsurgery: There is an increased risk of postsurgery thromboembolic complications in oral contraceptive users after major surgery. If feasible, oral contraceptives should be discontinued and an alternative method substituted at least 1 month prior to **major** elective surgery. Oral contraceptives should not be resumed until the first menstrual period after hospital discharge following surgery.

Drug Interactions: The concurrent administration of oral contraceptives with other drugs may result in an altered response to either agent. Reduced effectiveness of the oral contraceptive, should it occur, is more likely with the low dose formulations. It is important to ascertain all drugs that a patient is taking, both prescription and nonprescription, before oral contraceptives are prescribed.

Refer to the revised 1994 Report on Oral Contraceptives, Health Canada, for possible drug interactions with oral contraceptives.

Noncontraceptive Benefits of Oral Contraceptives: Several health advantages other than contraception have been reported.

Effects on Menses: increased menstrual cycle regularity; decreased menstrual blood loss; decreased incidence of iron deficiency anemia secondary to reduced menstrual blood loss; decreased incidence of dysmenorrhea.

Effects Related to Ovulation Inhibition: decreased incidence of functional ovarian cysts; decreased incidence of ectopic pregnancy.

Effects on Other Organs of the Reproductive Tract: decreased incidence of acute salpingitis; decreased incidence of endometrial cancer (50%); decreased incidence of ovarian cancer (40%); potential beneficial effects on endometriosis; improvement of acne vulgaris, hirsutism, and other androgen-mediated disorders.

Effects on Breasts: decreased incidence of benign breast disease (fibroadenomas and fibrocystic breast disease); decreased incidence of breast biopsies.

The noncontraceptive benefits of oral contraceptives should be considered in addition to the efficacy of these preparations when counselling patients regarding contraceptive method selection.

> Oral contraceptives **do not protect** against sexually transmitted diseases including HIV/AIDS. For protection against STDs, it is advisable to use latex condoms **in combination with** oral contraceptives.

ADVERSE EFFECTS: An increased risk of the following serious adverse reactions has been associated with the use of oral contraceptives: thrombophlebitis; pulmonary embolism; mesenteric thrombosis; neuro-ocular lesions, (e.g., retinal thrombosis); myocardial infarction; cerebral thrombosis; cerebral hemorrhage; hypertension; benign hepatic tumors; gallbladder disease.

The following adverse reactions also have been reported in patients receiving oral contraceptives: nausea and vomiting, usually the most common adverse reaction, occurs in approximately 10% or less of patients during the first cycle. Other reactions, as a general rule, are seen less frequently or only occasionally.

Other adverse reactions: gastrointestinal symptoms (such as abdominal cramps and bloating); breakthrough bleeding; spotting; change in menstrual flow; dysmenorrhea; amenorrhea during and after treatment; infertility after discontinuance of treatment; edema; chloasma or melasma which may persist; breast changes: tenderness, enlargement, and secretion; change in weight (increase or decrease); endocervical hyperplasias; possible diminution in lactation when given immediately postpartum; cholestatic jaundice; migraine; increase in size of uterine leiomyomata; rash (allergic); mental depression; reduced tolerance to carbohydrates; vaginal candidiasis; premenstrual-like syndrome; intolerance to contact lenses; change in corneal curvature (steepening); cataracts; optic neuritis; retinal thrombosis; changes in libido; chorea; changes in appetite; cystitis-like syndrome; rhinitis; headache; nervousness; dizziness; hirsutism; loss of scalp hair; erythema multiforme; erythema nodosum; hemorrhagic eruption; vaginitis; porphyria; impaired renal function; Raynaud's phenomenon; auditory disturbances; hemolytic uremic syndrome; pancreatitis; arterial thromboembolism.

OVERDOSE:

Symptoms: Numerous cases of the ingestion, by children, of estrogen-progestogen combinations have been reported. Although mild nausea may occur, there appears to be no other reaction.

Treatment: Treatment should be limited to a laxative such as citrate of magnesia with the aim of removing unabsorbed material as rapidly as possible.

> For management of a suspected drug overdose, CPhA recommends that you contact your **regional Poison Control Centre**. See the *CPS* Directory section for a list of Poison Control Centres.

DOSAGE: Information for the Patient on How to Take the Birth Control Pill:

1. **Read these directions:**
   - before you start taking your pills, and
   - any time you are not sure what to do.
2. **Look at your pill pack** to see if it has 21 or 28 pills:
   - 21-Pill Pack: 21 active pills (with hormones) taken daily for 3 weeks, and then no pills taken for 1 week

     or
   - 28-Pill Pack: 21 active pills (with hormones) taken daily for 3 weeks, and then 7 "reminder" pills (no hormones) taken daily for 1 week.
3. It is recommended that you use a second method of birth control (e.g., latex condoms and spermicidal foam or gel) for the first 7 days of the first cycle of pill use. This will provide a back-up in case pills are forgotten while you are getting used to taking them.
4. **When receiving any medical treatment, be sure to tell your doctor that you are using birth control pills.**
5. **Many women have spotting or light bleeding, or may feel sick to their stomach during the first 3 months on the pill.** If you do feel sick, do not stop taking the pill. The problem will usually go away. If it does not go away, check with your doctor or clinic.
6. **Missing pills also can cause some spotting or light bleeding,** even if you make up the missed pills. You also could feel a little sick to your stomach on the days you take 2 pills to make up for missed pills.
7. **If you miss pills at any time, you could get pregnant. The greatest risks for pregnancy are:**
   - when you start a pack late, or
   - when you miss pills at the beginning or at the very end of the pack.
8. **Always be sure you have ready:**
   - **another kind of birth control** (such as latex condoms and spermicidal foam or gel) to use as a back-up in case you miss pills, and
   - **an extra, full pack of pills.**
9. **If you experience vomiting or diarrhea, or if you take certain medicines,** such as antibiotics, your pills may not work as well. Use a back-up method, such as latex condoms and spermicidal foam or gel, until you can check with your doctor or clinic.
10. **If you forget more than 1 pill 2 months in a row,** talk to your doctor or clinic about how to make pill-taking easier or about using another method of birth control.
11. **If your questions are not answered here, call your doctor or clinic.**

When to start the first pack of pills: Be sure to read these instructions:
- before you start taking your pills, and
- any time you are not sure what to do.

Decide with your doctor or clinic what is the best day for you to start taking your first pack of pills. Your pills may be either a 21-day or a 28-day type.

A. 21-Day Combination: With this type of birth control pill, you are on pills for 21 days and off pills for 7 days. You must not be off the pills for more than 7 days in a row.

1. **The first day of your menstrual period (bleeding) is Day 1 of your cycle.** Your doctor may advise you to start taking the pills on Day 1, on Day 5, or on the first Sunday after your period begins. If your period starts on Sunday, start that same day.
2. Take 1 pill at approximately the same time every day for 21 days; **then take no pills for 7 days.** Start a new pack on the eighth day. You will probably have a period during the 7 days off the pill. (This bleeding may be lighter and shorter than your usual period.)

B. 28-Day Combination: With this type of birth control pill, you take 21 pills that contain hormones and seven pills that contain no hormones.

1. **The first day of your menstrual period (bleeding) is Day 1 of your cycle.** Your doctor may advise you to start taking the pills on Day 1, on Day 5, or on the first Sunday after your period begins. If your period starts on Sunday, start that same day.
2. Take 1 pill at approximately the same time every day for 28 days. Begin a new pack the next day, **not missing any days.** Your period should occur during the last 7 days of using that pill pack.

What to do during the month:

1. **Take a pill at approximately the same time every day until the pack is empty.**
   - Try to associate taking your pill with some regular activity such as eating a meal or going to bed.
   - Do not skip pills even if you have bleeding between monthly periods or feel sick to your stomach (nausea).
   - Do not skip pills even if you do not have sex very often.
2. **When you finish a pack:**
   - **21 pills: Wait 7 days** to start the next pack. You will have your period during that week.
   - **28 pills:** Start the next pack **on the next day**. Take one pill every day. Do not wait any days between packs.

What to do if you miss pills: Table 1 outlines the actions you should take if you miss 1 or more of your birth control pills. Match the number of pills missed with the appropriate starting time for your type of pill pack.

Table 1: Select 1/35

What to Do if You Miss Pills

Sunday Start	**Other Than Sunday Start**
Miss 1 pill	**Miss 1 pill**
Take it as soon as you remember, and take the next pill at the usual time. This means that you might take 2 pills in one day.	Take it as soon as you remember, and take the next pill at the usual time. This means that you might take 2 pills in one day.
Miss 2 pills in a row	**Miss 2 pills in a row**
First 2 Weeks: 1. Take 2 pills the day you remember and 2 pills the next day. 2. Then take 1 pill a day until you finish the pack. 3. Use a back-up method of birth control if you have sex in the 7 days after you miss the pills. **Third Week:** 1. Keep taking 1 pill a day until Sunday. 2. On Sunday, safely discard the rest of the pack and start a new pack that day. 3. Use a back-up method of birth control if you have sex in the 7 days after you miss the pills. 4. You may not have a period this month. **If you miss 2 periods in a row, call your doctor or clinic.**	**First 2 Weeks:** 1. Take 2 pills the day you remember and 2 pills the next day. 2. Then take 1 pill a day until you finish the pack. 3. Use a back-up method of birth control if you have sex in the 7 days after you miss the pills. **Third Week:** 1. Safely dispose of the rest of the pill pack and start a new pack that same day. 2. Use a back-up method of birth control if you have sex in the 7 days after you miss the pills. 3. You may not have a period this month. **If you miss 2 periods in a row, call your doctor or clinic.**
Miss 3 or more pills in a row	**Miss 3 or more pills in a row**
Anytime in the Cycle: 1. Keep taking 1 pill a day until Sunday. 2. On Sunday, safely discard the rest of the pack and start a new pack that day. 3. Use a back-up method of birth control if you have sex in the 7 days after you miss the pills. 4. You may not have a period this month. **If you miss 2 periods in a row, call your doctor or clinic.**	**Anytime in the Cycle:** 1. Safely dispose of the rest of the pill pack and start a new pack that same day. 2. Use a back-up method of birth control if you have sex in the 7 days after you miss the pills. 3. You may not have a period this month. **If you miss 2 periods in a row, call your doctor or clinic.**

Note: 28-Day Pack: If you forget any of the 7 "reminder" pills (without hormones) in Week 4, just safely dispose of the pills you missed. Then keep taking 1 pill each day until the pack is empty. You do not need to use a back-up method.

Always be sure you have on hand:
- a back-up method of birth control (such as latex condoms and spermicidal foam or gel) in case you miss pills, and
- an extra, full pack of pills.

If you forget more than 1 pill 2 months in a row, talk to your doctor or clinic, about ways to make pill-taking easier or about using another method of birth control.

Dosage: A. **21-Day Pack:** With this type of birth control pill, the patient is 21 days on pills with 7 days off pills. The patient must not be off the pills for more than 7 days in a row.

1. **The first day of the patient's menstrual period (bleeding) is Day 1 of a cycle.** The doctor may advise the patient to start taking the pills on Day 1, on Day 5, or on the first Sunday after a period begins. If a period starts on Sunday, the patient starts that same day.
2. The pack must be labeled correctly before starting. The pack is preprinted with a Sunday starting day. If the patient is starting on a day other than a Sunday, she should use the Flexi-start sticker labels provided. The patient peels off the label with the chosen starting day and applies it over the preprinted days on top of the card.
3. The patient takes 1 pill at approximately the same time every day for 21 days; **then she takes no pills for 7 days.** She starts a new pack on the eighth day. She will probably have a period during the 7 days off the pill. (This bleeding may be lighter and shorter than a usual period.)

B. **28-Day Pack:** With this type of birth control pill, the patient takes 21 pills which contain hormones and 7 pills which contain no hormones.

1. **The first day of the patient's menstrual period (bleeding) is Day 1 of a cycle.** The doctor may advise the patient to start taking the pills on Day 1, on Day 5, or on the first Sunday after a period begins. If a period starts on Sunday, the patient starts that same day.
2. The pack must be labeled correctly before starting. The pack is preprinted with a Sunday starting day. If the patient is starting on a day other than a Sunday, she should use the Flexi-start sticker labels provided. The patient peels off the label with the chosen starting day and applies it over the preprinted days on top of the card.
3. The patient takes 1 pill at approximately the same time every day for 28 days. She begins a new pack the next day, **not missing any days on the pills.** The patient's period should occur during the last 7 days of using that pill pack.

What to do during the month:

1. **The patient takes a pill at approximately the same time every day until the pack is empty.**
   - The patient should try to associate taking the pill with some regular activity like eating a meal or going to bed.
   - The patient must not skip pills even if she has bleeding between monthly periods or feels sick to her stomach (nausea).
   - The patient must not skip pills even if she does not have sex very often.
2. **When a pack is finished:**
   - **21 pills: The patient must wait 7 days** to start the next pack. A period will begin during that week.
   - **28 pills:** The patient starts the next pack **on the next day**. She takes 1 pill every day. She does not wait any days between packs.

INFORMATION FOR THE PATIENT: Published in e-CPS, available by subscription at www.e-cps.ca.

SUPPLIED: Each white circular tablet, impressed "SEARLE" on one side and "BX" on the other contains: norethindrone 1 mg and ethinyl estradiol 0.035 mg. Inert orange-colored tablets are impressed "SEARLE" on one side and "P" on the other. Nonmedicinal ingredients: Active tablets: cornstarch, lactose, magnesium stearate and povidone. Placebo tablets: FD&C Yellow No. 6 lake, lactose hydrous, magnesium stearate and microcrystalline cellulose. Dispensers of 21 days (21 active tablets) and 28 days (21 active and 7 inert tablets).

(Shown in Product Identification Section)

Selective Serotonin Reuptake Inhibitors

citalopram HBr
escitalopram oxalate
fluoxetine HCl
fluvoxamine maleate
paroxetine HCl
sertraline HCl

Antidepressant—Antiobsessional—Antibulimic—Antipanic—Anxiolytic—Post-traumatic Stress Disorder Therapy—Premenstrual Dysphoric Disorder Therapy

CPhA Monograph

Date of Revision: February 2010

This monograph has been compiled by CPhA and reviewed by experts. It may contain information different from that found in Health Canada-approved Product Monographs. The reader is referred to the *CPS* Editorial Policy for more information.

SUMMARY PRODUCT INFORMATION:

Drug	Route of Administration	Dosage Form	Strength
Citalopram	Oral	Tablet	10 mg, 20 mg, 40 mg
Escitalopram	Oral	Tablet	10 mg, 20 mg
Fluoxetine	Oral	Capsule	10 mg, 20 mg
		Solution	20 mg/5 mL
Fluvoxamine	Oral	Tablet	50 mg, 100 mg
Paroxetine	Oral	Immediate-release tablet	10 mg, 20 mg, 30 mg, 40 mg
		Controlled-release tablet	12.5 mg, 25 mg
Sertraline	Oral	Tablet	25 mg, 50 mg, 100 mg

PHARMACOLOGY: Selective serotonin reuptake inhibitors (SSRIs) are potent and highly selective inhibitors of the reuptake of serotonin at the presynaptic neuronal membrane. This results in increased serotonin concentrations in the synapse, leading to altered serotonergic transmission. SSRIs have little effect on the reuptake of norepinephrine or dopamine and exhibit low to negligible binding affinity for adrenergic, histaminergic, muscarinergic, GABA or benzodiazepine receptors.

The SSRIs do not resemble each other structurally. Although 2 of these agents possess 3 rings, the structures of the SSRIs differ significantly from those of tricyclics and all other antidepressants currently available.

Although the precise mechanism of action of SSRIs cannot be unequivocally stated, their known effects on serotonin transmission, combined with their clinical effectiveness in depressive disorders and other conditions, have contributed to many of the current theories of the pathophysiology of these disorders.

Pharmacokinetics: SSRIs are well absorbed after oral administration. With the exception of sertraline, whose bioavailability appears to be moderately increased in the presence of food, the absorption of SSRIs is not significantly altered when they are taken with meals. As with other classes of antidepressants, clinical improvement is gradual, occurring over 6 to 12 weeks.

The SSRIs are metabolized in the liver and eliminated in the urine and feces to varying degrees. These agents should be used cautiously in patients with significant hepatic or renal impairment. Only fluoxetine and sertraline form active metabolites (see Table 1).

The pharmacokinetics of these agents have been shown not to be significantly altered in healthy elderly patients; however, caution is advised with respect to initial dosage.

Table 1 lists various pharmacokinetic properties of the SSRIs.

INDICATIONS: Table 2 lists the current labeled indications for the available SSRIs. Various SSRIs have also been used in the management of bulimia nervosa, chronic fatigue syndrome, fibromyalgia and premature ejaculation.

CONTRAINDICATIONS: Patients with known hypersensitivity to the respective agents.

Because of reports of serious and sometimes fatal reactions such as serotonin syndrome in patients taking an MAO inhibitor either with or shortly after discontinuation of an SSRI, a strict washout period is recommended between therapy with these classes of drugs (see Warnings). In the case of fluoxetine, which has a long elimination half-life, a minimum 5-week period is recommended between discontinuation of fluoxetine and initiation of therapy with an MAO inhibitor (see Warnings and Precautions). For all other SSRIs a minimum 2-week washout period is recommended between SSRI and MAO inhibitor therapy.

WARNINGS: Self-harm/Harm to Others: There have been clinical trial and post-marketing reports with SSRIs, in both children and adults, of severe agitation-type adverse events associated with self-harm or harm to others. The agitation-type adverse events include akathisia, agitation, disinhibition, emotional lability, hostility, aggression and depersonalization, occurring within several weeks of initiating therapy in some cases.

Systematic monitoring is advised, especially during the acute phase of treatment, for suicidal ideation or any other indicators of potential suicidality or self-harm in patients of all ages taking SSRIs.

Table 1: SSRIs

Pharmacokinetic Properties (based on multiple-dosing[a])

SSRI (active metabolite)	Protein Binding (%)	Time to Steady-state (days)	Elimination Half-life	Comments
Citalopram	80	7 to 14	37 hours	Racemic mixture of r and s-enantiomers
Escitalopram	55	7 to 10	27 to 33 hours	S-enantiomer of racemic citalopram
Fluoxetine (norfluoxetine[b])	94.5	14 to 28	4 to 6 days (9 days)	Will be present in the body for several weeks after discontinuation.
Fluvoxamine	80	10 to 14	17 to 22 hours	—
Paroxetine immediate-release	95	7 to 14	24 hours	—
Paroxetine controlled-release	95	14	15 to 20 hours	—
Sertraline (N-desmethyl-sertraline[c])	98	7	25 to 26 hours (62 to 104 hours)	Presence of food increases the peak serum concentration by 30% and the AUC by 39%.

[a] The pharmacokinetics of some agents become nonlinear with multiple-dosing, due to partial saturation of the specific cytochrome P450 system believed to be involved; therefore, the half-lives expressed in the table are those seen with multiple-dosing, which more closely reflects clinical use.

[b] Norfluoxetine is believed to be as potent and effective as the parent compound.

[c] N-desmethylsertraline is considered to be 5 to 10 times **less** potent than the parent compound and exerts a negligible pharmacologic effect.

Serotonin Syndrome: A potentially fatal reaction known as serotonin syndrome may result from the combination of serotonergic agents with different mechanisms of action (see Precautions, Drug Interactions). The greatest risk occurs when SSRIs and MAO inhibitors are combined or when there is an inadequate washout between therapies. Combining SSRIs with other types of serotonergic agents generally leads to no or mild symptoms of a serotonin syndrome. However, in rare cases two non-MAO inhibitor serotonergic drugs can lead to a severe serotonin syndrome.

The signs and symptoms of serotonin syndrome may develop rapidly (within 24 hours of initiation of drug or dosage increase) and can include mental status changes, agitation, myoclonus, hyperreflexia, tremor and diarrhea. Severe cases may progress to malignant hyperthermia, rhabdomyolysis, seizures, respiratory arrest, disseminated intravascular coagulation and ventricular arrhythmias. The syndrome may be mild and may remit within 12 to 24 hours following discontinuation of the serotonergic agents and with supportive therapy. However, it may be associated with severe hyperthermia and serious or fatal complications. A washout period is recommended between therapy with SSRIs and other serotonergic agents, especially MAO inhibitors (see Contraindications).

Management of serotonin syndrome includes discontinuation of the serotonergic agents and initiation of supportive care, which will lead to symptom resolution in mild cases. For more severe reactions, serotonin antagonists (e.g., cyproheptadine), benzodiazepines and dantrolene have been used, as well as other symptomatic and supportive measures such as external cooling.

Suicide: See also Self-harm/Harm to Others. Although SSRIs are considerably less toxic in single drug overdose than many other antidepressants, they should be prescribed in the smallest quantity consistent with good patient care, given the potential for attempted suicide in depressed patients. Because of the known comorbidity between depression and many anxiety disorders, the same precaution is recommended when SSRIs are used to treat these conditions.

Other: Because of the long elimination half-life of fluoxetine and its active metabolite, it is important to consider that these compounds will be present in the body for weeks after discontinuation.

Rash (e.g., maculopapular, purpuric, pustular, vesiculobullous, follicular, urticaria, erythema multiforme) has occurred in 2 to 4% of patients treated with SSRIs. Dermatologic reactions usually occur within the first few weeks of therapy. In a small number of patients, systemic signs and symptoms have accompanied dermatologic reactions. Anaphylactoid reactions (e.g., bronchospasm, urticaria, angioedema) and serious systemic illness have been reported rarely. Cases of cross-sensitivity among SSRIs have been reported. It is generally recommended that SSRIs be discontinued if rash, urticaria or any signs of hypersensitivity occur during therapy.

PRECAUTIONS: Concomitant Illness: Diabetes: Fluoxetine may affect glycemic control. Hypoglycemia has occurred during therapy, as has hyperglycemia upon its discontinuation. It may be necessary to make adjustments to the dosage of insulin or oral antihyperglycemic agents when fluoxetine is initiated or discontinued.

Hematologic: SSRIs have been associated with an increased risk of bleeding, particularly in combination with other drugs that affect platelet function such as ASA or other NSAIDs, and in patients with a history of bleeding disorders.

Table 2: SSRIs

Labeled Indications

SSRI	Depressive Illness	Bulimia Nervosa	Obsessive-Compulsive Disorder	Panic Disorder	Social Phobia (Social Anxiety Disorder)	Generalized Anxiety Disorder	Post-traumatic Stress Disorder	Premenstrual Dysphoric Disorder
Citalopram	Yes	—	—	—	—	—	—	—
Escitalopram	Yes	—	Yes	—	—	Yes	—	—
Fluoxetine	Yes	Yes	Yes	—	—	—	—	—
Fluvoxamine	Yes	—	Yes	—	—	—	—	—
Paroxetine immediate-release	Yes	—	Yes	Yes	Yes	Yes	Yes	—
Paroxetine controlled-release	Yes	—	—	Yes	Yes	—	—	Yes
Sertraline	Yes	—	Yes	Yes	—	—	—	—

Hepatic Disease: The clearance of SSRIs is significantly reduced in patients with liver disease because of their extensive hepatic metabolism. SSRIs should be used with caution in these patients, with lower and less frequent dosing.

Hyponatremia: Hyponatremia has occurred in patients receiving SSRIs. In most cases it occurred in older patients who were on diuretic therapy or who were otherwise volume depleted. There is a possible association between hyponatremia during SSRI therapy and the syndrome of inappropriate antidiuretic hormone secretion (SIADH). The hyponatremia appears to be reversible on discontinuation of the SSRI. It has been recommended that electrolytes be monitored throughout therapy, especially in older individuals and those at increased risk of hyponatremia/SIADH.

Mania/Hypomania: Precipitation of a manic or hypomanic state has occurred in patients treated with SSRIs. This effect may be dose-related and may occur more frequently in patients with bipolar disorder. SSRIs should be used with caution in patients with a history of mania. If mania or hypomania occur during SSRI therapy, the dosage should be decreased or the drug discontinued.

Renal Impairment: Although renal excretion is considered to be a minor route of elimination of SSRIs and their active metabolites, caution is prudent when SSRIs are used in patients with significant renal impairment.

Seizures: Seizures have occurred in patients receiving therapeutic doses of SSRIs. The overall incidence (0.1 to 0.2%) appears to be similar to, or less than, the incidence of seizures in patients receiving other antidepressants; however, patients with a history of seizures were excluded from many of the clinical trials. SSRIs should be used with caution in patients with a history of seizures and discontinued if seizures occur.

Self-harm/Harm to Others: See Warnings.

Sexual Dysfunction: SSRIs commonly cause sexual dysfunction (see Adverse Effects), which can affect adherence to therapy. The reported incidence of sexual dysfunction with SSRIs ranges from 30 to 60% and is dose-dependent. Sexual function should be assessed at baseline, and monitored during therapy. Management of treatment emergent sexual dysfunction is challenging. Dosage reduction or drug holidays could lead to relapse of symptoms. Switching to an antidepressant with a lower propensity to cause sexual dysfunction may be helpful. Add-on therapy with drugs such as bupropion or sildenafil has been of modest benefit in some studies.

Suicide: See Warnings.

Withdrawal: A syndrome has been described following discontinuation or dosage reduction of SSRIs with the exception of fluoxetine because of its long half-life. It is generally recommended that SSRIs be gradually tapered prior to discontinuation, although this may not always prevent the withdrawal syndrome. Symptoms usually begin within 1 to 7 days following discontinuation and most commonly include dizziness, nausea, fatigue, headache and insomnia. Less commonly, shock-like sensations, paresthesias and visual disturbances have been reported. Without intervention, symptoms usually resolve within 1 to 3 weeks. Severe cases are infrequent but can be protracted and disabling. Reinstatement of the SSRI results in resolution of symptoms within hours. If severe withdrawal symptoms recur, consider switching to fluoxetine and tapering gradually.

Pregnancy: Both untreated maternal depression and SSRI use during pregnancy may pose risks to a developing fetus. SSRIs as a group have not been associated with an increased risk of major birth defects. Paroxetine use during the first trimester may be associated with a slightly increased risk of congenital heart defects, primarily involving the ventricular or atrial septum.

Use of SSRIs after the 20th week of pregnancy may be associated with an increased risk of persistent pulmonary hypertension of the newborn.

Further study of the use of SSRIs in pregnancy is needed to address concerns about a possible increased incidence of early delivery or low birth weight, and about potential long-term neurodevelopmental toxicity or behavioral teratology. Neonates exposed to SSRIs in the third trimester may experience withdrawal symptoms including tremors, shivering, increased muscle tone, feeding or digestive problems or respiratory distress.

The decision whether to continue SSRI therapy during pregnancy should be made on a case-by-case basis, balancing the risk of discontinuing antidepressant therapy with that of fetal exposure to the SSRI.

Lactation: SSRIs are excreted in breast milk. Fluoxetine reaches higher concentrations in breast milk than other SSRIs. Fluvoxamine, paroxetine and sertraline reach very low levels in breast milk. If the decision is made to continue breast feeding during SSRI therapy, the infant should be closely monitored for signs of adverse effects such as increased somnolence or difficulty feeding.

Children: See Warnings, Self-harm/Harm to Others. SSRIs have not been approved in Canada for use in children.

Geriatric: SSRIs are generally well tolerated in the elderly. Lower initial dosages may be indicated in some elderly patients (e.g., those who are frail or malnourished).

Occupational Hazards: Because SSRIs can sometimes cause sedation, patients should be advised not to drive or operate hazardous machinery until they know how the drug affects them.

Drug Interactions: SSRIs have the potential to interact with other drugs by many different mechanisms, given that they are hepatically metabolized, inhibit several microsomal isoenzymes and because they are among the many classes of drugs that affect serotonin transmission. Because of their long elimination half-lives, they have the potential to interact with other drugs even after they have been discontinued. Table 3 illustrates many of the interactions that have occurred with SSRIs. Not every interaction has been reported with each of the SSRIs.

Table 3: SSRIs

Drug Interactions

Interacting Drug(s)	Outcome	Proposed Mechanism	Recommendations
Clopidogrel	Decreased clinical effects of clopidogrel	Decreased conversion of clopidogrel to active metabolite due to inhibition of CYP2C19 (fluoxetine, fluvoxamine, sertraline)	Avoid concurrent therapy.
Codeine	Reduced analgesia	Moderate to strong CYP2D6 inhibitors (fluoxetine, paroxetine, sertraline) markedly reduce the conversion of codeine to morphine.	Monitor for changes in pain control and adjust therapy as required.
Cyproheptadine	Decreased SSRI effects (e.g., worsening of depressive symptoms)	Serotonin antagonism by cyproheptadine	Watch for reduced antidepressant response to SSRI if cyproheptadine started during therapy.
Drugs metabolized (or activated) by cytochrome P450 system, especially CYP1A2, CYP2C9, CYP2C19, CYP2D6 and CYP3A4.	Increased serum levels and potentiated clinical and adverse effects of interacting drug (e.g., atomoxetine, carbamazepine, clozapine, dextromethorphan and many others) or decreased efficacy due to inhibition of enzymatic conversion of prodrug to active form (e.g., codeine, tamoxifen)	Inhibition of cytochrome P450 enzymes by SSRIs, specifically: CYP1A2 (fluvoxamine),[a] CYP2C9 (fluoxetine, fluvoxamine), CYP2C19 (fluoxetine, fluvoxamine,[a] sertraline), CYP2D6 (fluoxetine,[a] paroxetine,[a] sertraline) and CYP3A4 (fluoxetine, fluvoxamine)	Be aware of the possible interaction and appropriately monitor and/or adjust drug dosages when an SSRI or interacting drug is added to or discontinued from a patient's regimen.
NSAIDs, including low-dose ASA	Increased risk of gastrointestinal bleeding	Additive effects on platelet function, possibly involving serotonin	Avoid combination if possible[b]; consider acetaminophen for pain; consider antidepressant with less effect on serotonin.

(cont'd)

Table 3: SSRIs *(cont'd)*

Drug Interactions

Interacting Drug(s)	Outcome	Proposed Mechanism	Recommendations
Pimozide, quinine, sibutramine, ziprasidone	Increased risk of QTc prolongation	May involve increased concentration of interacting drug or an unknown pharmacodynamic mechanism	Avoid combination.
Serotonergic agents (e.g., MAO inhibitors, amphetamine derivatives, dextromethorphan, dihydroergotamine, lithium, meperidine, pentazocine, selegiline, St. John's wort, TCAs, trazodone, triptans, tryptophan).	Serotonin syndrome (see Warnings)	Additive serotonin effects	Concurrent use of SSRIs and MAO inhibitors is contraindicated. Sequential use could be hazardous as well (see Contraindications, Warnings). Clinicians should be aware of the possibility of serious reactions arising from concurrent use of SSRIs and other serotonergic drugs. If possible, avoid concurrent use of 2 or more agents with serotonergic activity.
Tamoxifen	Decreased effectiveness of tamoxifen	Inhibitors of CYP2D6 (fluoxetine, paroxetine, sertraline) may decrease conversion of prodrug tamoxifen to its active metabolites [*BMJ* 2010;340:c693].	Avoid combination.
Warfarin	Increased hypoprothrombinemic response	The mechanism of this effect is unclear. SSRIs may possess an intrinsic inhibitory effect on hemostasis.	Monitor patients on warfarin more closely when an SSRI is initiated or discontinued. Note that there might be an increased risk of bleeding even when the hypoprothrombinemic response is in the desired range.

[a] Potent inhibitor.
[b] It is not known whether COX-2 selective NSAIDs are less likely to cause bleeding in combination with SSRIs.

ADVERSE EFFECTS: (See also Warnings, Precautions.) SSRIs have been associated with numerous adverse effects, some of which occur frequently; however, some of these effects mimic symptoms of the condition being treated, and often subside with continued therapy. The incidences of some adverse effects have been similar or higher in placebo groups and have varied among the different SSRIs and indeed when the same drug is used for different indications. Please refer to individual product monographs for detailed accounts of the incidences of adverse effects when used for various indications.

The following is a listing of the adverse effects of SSRIs in general. Within each frequency category, the adverse effects are presented in alphabetical order.

Most common (overall incidence >10%): diarrhea, headache, insomnia, nausea, nervousness, sexual dysfunction (males: mainly ejaculatory delay; females: decreased libido, anorgasmia), somnolence.

Relatively common (overall incidence 1 to 10%): abnormal dreams, abdominal pain, anorexia, dizziness, dysmenorrhea, dyspnea, excessive sweating, excessive yawning, flatulence, flu-like symptoms, hot flushes, joint and muscle pain, lymphadenopathy, palpitations, rash, taste perception changes, tremor, visual disturbances, upper respiratory tract infection, weight gain.

Relatively rare (overall incidence <1%): abnormal bleeding, anemia, hypoglycemia, orthostatic hypotension, platelet function changes.

OVERDOSE:

Symptoms: Most cases of overdose of SSRIs have involved multiple drug ingestions, including tricyclic antidepressants, benzodiazepines and/or alcohol. Most fatalities involved combined ingestions; however, there have been a few reported cases of fatal overdose attributable to an SSRI alone. Some of the symptoms of SSRI overdose are believed to be extensions of their pharmacologic effects. The symptoms of overdose include somnolence, nausea and vomiting, ECG changes, nystagmus, dilated pupils, coma.

Treatment: Although SSRIs have exhibited a fairly wide margin of safety, it is recommended that SSRI overdose be observed closely since fatalities have occasionally occurred with both multiple and single ingestions.

There is no specific treatment or antidote for SSRI overdose. Management should involve symptomatic and supportive care. The possibility of multiple drug involvement should be considered.

The first priority should be to establish and maintain a patent airway, with adequate ventilation and oxygenation. Vital signs and ECG should be monitored. Administration of activated charcoal, with or without sorbitol, should be considered. If the patient has a significantly decreased level of consciousness, clinicians should consider whether it is necessary to intubate the patient with a cuffed tube prior to administering charcoal.

Agitation, myoclonus or seizures can be treated with iv benzodiazepines. For information on management of serotonin syndrome, see Warnings.

Hemodialysis, forced diuresis, peritoneal dialysis and exchange transfusion are not reported to be of benefit in the treatment of SSRI overdose.

For management of a suspected drug overdose, CPhA recommends that you contact your **regional Poison Control Centre**. See the *CPS* Directory section for a list of Poison Control Centres.

DOSAGE: As with other antidepressants, it may take several weeks to realize the full clinical benefit of SSRI therapy for any indication. It is generally recommended that therapy for depression be continued for at least 6 months following marked resolution of symptoms for first episodes and for at least two years for subsequent episodes. Some experts recommend lifelong therapy for patients who have had more than two episodes.

To avoid a possible withdrawal reaction, SSRIs should be gradually tapered rather than abruptly discontinued. A 2-week washout period is recommended between therapy with SSRIs and other serotonergic drugs, especially MAO inhibitors. In the case of fluoxetine, a 5-week washout period is advised between discontinuation of fluoxetine and commencement of therapy with MAO inhibitors (see Contraindications, Warnings and Precautions, Drug Interactions).

The absorption of SSRIs is not significantly altered in the presence of food, with the exception of sertraline, whose peak serum level and AUC are significantly increased. It is recommended that sertraline be taken with meals and that the other SSRIs may be taken with food as desired, especially if this helps reduce stomach upset caused by the drug.

Since SSRIs can cause either somnolence or insomnia, the timing of daily doses can be tailored depending on the individual patient's response (e.g., patients who experience somnolence may take their SSRI at bedtime).

SSRIs should be used with caution and at a lower and less frequent dosage in patients with hepatic disease. Caution is also advised when they are used in patients with severe renal impairment.

Patients should be informed that many of the side effects of SSRIs are transient in nature and can mimic the signs and symptoms of the condition being treated.

Children (see Warnings, Self-harm/Harm to Others): When off-label use in children has been deemed necessary, it has been suggested that SSRI therapy be initiated in children and adolescents at one-quarter to one-half the usual initial adult dose and that dosage increases be made at intervals of at least a week. Smaller dosage increments than are recommended for adults should be considered. The adult guidelines for maximum daily dose should be followed in adolescents. Lower maximum doses should be used in children.

Table 4 lists the adult dosages of the SSRIs for their labeled indications.

Table 4: SSRIs

Adult Dosage[a]

SSRI	Indication	Dose
Citalopram	Depression	Initial: 20 mg daily, morning or evening. May be taken with food to lessen stomach irritation. Usual effective dose: 20 to 40 mg once daily. Maximum: 60 mg daily. Dosage increases in increments of 20 mg daily should occur at intervals of no less than 1 wk.
Escitalopram	Depression, Generalized Anxiety Disorder, Obsessive-compulsive Disorder	Initial: 5 to 10 mg daily. May be taken with food to lessen stomach irritation. Usual effective dose: 10 to 20 mg daily. Maximum: 20 mg daily.
Fluoxetine	Depression	Initial: 10 to 20 mg daily in the morning. May be taken with food to lessen stomach irritation. If sedation occurs, dose may be taken at bedtime. After several weeks, dose may be increased by 20 mg daily at weekly (or longer) intervals. Usual effective dose: 20 mg daily. Usual maximum: 80 mg daily.[b]
	Bulimia Nervosa	Usual effective dose: 60 mg daily.[c] Lower dose might be effective.
	Obsessive-compulsive Disorder	Initial: 20 mg daily in the morning. May be taken with food to lessen stomach irritation. If sedation occurs, dose may be taken at bedtime. After several weeks, dose may be increased by 20 mg daily at weekly (or longer) intervals. Usual effective dose: 20 to 60 mg daily. Usual maximum: 80 mg daily.[b]
Fluvoxamine	Depression	Initial: 50 mg daily at bedtime. Dosage may be increased every few days by 50 mg daily if necessary. Usual effective dose: 100 to 200 mg daily. Doses higher than 150 mg daily should be divided so that the maximum bedtime dose is 150 mg. Usual maximum: 300 mg daily.
	Obsessive-compulsive Disorder	Initial: 50 mg daily at bedtime. Dosage may be increased every few days by 50 mg daily if necessary. Usual effective dose: 100 to 300 mg daily. Doses higher than 150 mg daily should be divided so that the maximum bedtime dose is 150 mg. Usual maximum: 300 mg daily.
Paroxetine immediate-release	Depression	Initial: 20 mg daily in the morning. If necessary, may be gradually increased by 10 mg daily at 1- to 2-wk intervals, to 40 mg daily. Usual effective dose: 20 mg daily. Usual maximum: 50 mg daily.
	Obsessive-compulsive Disorder	Initial: 20 mg daily in the morning. If necessary, may be gradually increased by 10 mg daily at 1- to 2-wk intervals, to 40 mg daily. Usual effective dose: 40 mg daily. Usual maximum: 60 mg daily.
	Panic Disorder	Initial: 10 mg daily in the morning. Usual effective dose: 40 mg daily. Usual maximum: 60 mg daily.
	Social Phobia (Social Anxiety Disorder), Generalized Anxiety Disorder or Post-traumatic Stress Disorder	Initial: 20 mg daily in the morning. May increase gradually in 10 mg/day increments to a maximum of 50 mg daily.
Paroxetine controlled-release	Depression	Initial: 12.5–25 mg daily. If necessary, may increase by 12.5 mg daily at intervals of at least 1 wk. Usual effective dose: 25 to 62.5 mg daily. Maximum: 62.5 mg daily.
	Panic Disorder	Initial: 12.5 mg daily. If necessary, may increase by 12.5 mg daily at intervals of at least 1 wk. Usual effective dose: 12.5 to 75 mg. Maximum: 75 mg daily.
	Premenstrual Dysphoric Disorder	Initial: 12.5 mg daily during the luteal phase of the menstrual cycle (beginning 14 days before expected onset of menses and terminating on the first day of menses. Some patients not responding to 12.5 daily may benefit from a dose of 25 mg daily. Continuous use throughout the menstrual cycle may be considered if suboptimal response to luteal phase therapy. Dosage increases should occur at intervals of at least 1 wk. Maximum: 25 mg daily.
	Social Phobia (Social Anxiety Disorder)	Initial: 12.5 mg. If necessary, may increase by 12.5 mg daily at intervals of at least 1 wk. Usual effective dose: 12.5 to 37.5 mg. Maximum: 37.5 mg

(cont'd)

Table 4: SSRIs *(cont'd)*

Adult Dosage[a]

SSRI	Indication	Dose
Sertraline	Depression or Obsessive-compulsive Disorder	Initial: 50 mg daily with evening meal, or with breakfast. If necessary, dosage may be increased at intervals of at least 1 wk. Usual effective dose: 50 to 100 mg daily. Usual maximum: 200 mg daily.
	Panic Disorder	Initial: 25 mg daily. If necessary, dosage may be increased at intervals of at least 1 wk. Usual effective dose: 50 to 200 mg daily. Usual maximum: 200 mg daily.

[a] SSRIs are generally well tolerated in older patients. Lower initial dosages may be indicated in some elderly patients (e.g., the very old or those with comorbid conditions or malnutrition).

[b] Higher doses have been used in some patients with refractory depression.

[c] Because SSRIs can cause hyponatremia, which may further complicate the electrolyte changes associated with purging behaviors, it may be advisable to assess electrolyte levels prior to initiation of SSRI therapy.

Selegiline

Selective Irreversible Monoamine Oxidase (MAO) B Inhibitor

CPhA Monograph

Date of Preparation: October 2006

This monograph has been compiled by CPhA and reviewed by experts. It may contain information different from that found in Health Canada-approved Product Monographs. The reader is referred to the *CPS* Editorial Policy for more information.

SUMMARY PRODUCT INFORMATION:

Route of Administration	Dosage Form	Strength
Oral	Tablet	5 mg

INDICATIONS AND CLINICAL USE: Selegiline is indicated for:
- Treatment of idiopathic Parkinson's disease as adjunctive therapy in patients with a diminished response to levodopa/carbidopa. Selegiline has also been used as monotherapy for initial treatment of Parkinson's disease.

When selegiline is added to ongoing levodopa/carbidopa therapy for Parkinson's disease, it decreases the amount of "off" time, reduces the required dose of levodopa and has other beneficial effects such as reduced end-of-dose akinesia, tremor and sialorrhea, and improved speech and dressing ability.

Selegiline may provide additional benefit in terms of control of motor symptoms of Parkinson's disease in patients who are currently maintained on optimal doses of levodopa, in those exhibiting signs of tolerance to levodopa and those with end-of dose phenomena while on levodopa.

Some patients may experience an exacerbation of levodopa-related adverse effects after starting therapy with selegiline, presumably due to the increased availability of levodopa at the site of action in the CNS. This phenomenon should be anticipated, generally occurs within two weeks of initiating therapy with selegiline, and may be managed by reducing the dose of levodopa by 10 to 30%.

Selegiline has also been evaluated as therapy for depression and for mild-to-moderate Alzheimer's disease.

Geriatrics: Parkinson's disease occurs principally in patients aged >50 years, therefore it is expected that selegiline will be used primarily in geriatric patients.

CONTRAINDICATIONS:
- Hypersensitivity to selegiline or to any ingredient in the formulation.
- Extrapyramidal disorders other than Parkinson's disease, such as excessive tremor or tardive dyskinesia, or in patients with severe psychosis or profound dementia.
- Concurrent use of pethidine (meperidine).
- Active peptic ulcer.

WARNINGS AND PRECAUTIONS:

Serious Warnings and Precautions
- Selegiline should not be used at dosages >10 mg/day because of the risks associated with nonselective MAO inhibition, i.e., potential for hypertensive crisis precipitated by ingestion of particular foods, beverages or medications.
- Serious adverse events (serotonin syndrome) may occur when selegiline is combined with tricyclic antidepressants (TCAs) or selective serotonin reuptake inhibitors (SSRIs).

General: Serotonin Syndrome: Combined use of selegiline and TCAs has been associated with a syndrome comprised of agitation, diaphoresis, changes in behaviour and in mental status, hyperpyrexia, hypertension, muscular rigidity or myoclonus, altered consciousness, restlessness, syncope, tremors, and rarely, fatalities. Similar reactions have been reported in patients receiving selegiline in combination with SSRIs (e.g., fluoxetine, paroxetine, sertraline). As it is not possible to identify patients at risk of such reactions, it seems prudent to avoid use of TCAs or SSRIs in patients receiving selegiline. If these combinations are used, patients should be counseled accordingly and monitored closely. At least 14 days should elapse between discontinuation of selegiline and initiation of treatment with a TCA or an SSRI other than fluoxetine. Fluoxetine and its active metabolite, norfluoxetine, have very long half-lives; thus, the interval between discontinuation of fluoxetine and initiation of selegiline therapy should be five weeks.

Cardiovascular: Hypertensive reactions, including hypertensive crisis, have been associated with selegiline and consumption of tyramine-rich foods (see Drug Interactions, Drug-Food Interactions). Patients should be counseled on the need to avoid or minimize consumption of tyramine-rich foods.

Neurologic: Exacerbation of levodopa-associated dyskinesias can occur (e.g., blepharospasm, bradykinesia, dystonic manifestations, facial grimacing, festination, "freezing", tremor, involuntary movements, loss of balance, speech problems, stiff neck, tardive dyskinesia), presumably as the result of increased dopamine availability in the CNS.

Psychiatric: Apathy, anxiety, depression, delusions, hallucinations, insomnia, irritability, psychosis/behaviour/mood changes, overstimulation, restlessness, sleep disturbances and vivid dreams may occur, presumably as the result of increased dopamine availability in the CNS and the presence of the amphetamine metabolites of selegiline.

ADVERSE REACTIONS: More Common Adverse Drug Reactions: See Table 1.

Less Common Adverse Drug Reactions (<1%): Cardiovascular: Cardiac arrhythmias (including tachycardia and sinus bradycardia), palpitations, hypertension, hypotension, orthostatic hypotension, syncope, peripheral edema, angina pectoris and exacerbation of angina pectoris have been reported in patients receiving selegiline.

Central Nervous System: anxiety, lethargy, malaise.

Endocrine and Metabolism: weight loss.

Dermatologic: hair loss.

Gastrointestinal: diarrhea.

Genitourinary: urinary retention.

Hematologic: anemia.

Musculoskeletal: generalized aches, leg pain, lower back pain.

Table 1: Selegiline
More Common Adverse Drug Reactions (≥1%)

Body System	Effect	Clinical Comment
CNS	Confusion, dizziness/light headedness/fainting, insomnia, hallucinations, headache, vivid dreams.	May be related to increased availability of dopamine. Reducing the dose of levodopa may ameliorate these effects.
Gastrointestinal	Nausea, abdominal pain, dry mouth.	May be related to increased availability of dopamine. Reducing the dose of levodopa may ameliorate these effects; domperidone 10 mg QID, before meals and at bedtime, may also be helpful.
Movement disorders	Dyskinesias.	May be related to increased availability of dopamine. Reducing the dose of levodopa may ameliorate these effects.

DRUG INTERACTIONS:

Serious Drug Interactions
- The combination of pethidine (meperidine) and selegiline can provoke serious systemic reactions (serotonin syndrome). Use of this combination is contraindicated.

Selegiline does not significantly alter the distribution or elimination of levodopa or cabergoline.

Drug-Drug Interactions: See Table 2.

Table 2: Selegiline
Drug-Drug Interactions

Interacting Drug	Effect	Clinical Comment
Alpha/beta agonists (e.g., pseudoephedrine, ephedrine), alpha$_1$ agonists (e.g., midodrine, phenylephrine), amphetamines (e.g., dextroamphetamine, phentermine), buspirone, methylphenidate, reserpine	Possible increased hypertensive effect of interacting drug.	Avoid combination.
Atomoxetine, bupropion	Potential increased neurotoxicity of interacting drug.	Avoid combination; mechanism may involve increased dopaminergic activity.
Levodopa	Increased adverse effects of levodopa (e.g., headache insomnia, nausea).	Monitor for adverse effects of levodopa, including hypertension.
Oral contraceptives	Exposure to selegiline is 20-fold greater in women taking oral contraceptives than in those not taking oral contraceptives, presumably due to an increased oral bioavailability of selegiline. In contrast, hormone replacement therapy with estradiol and levonorgestrel did not significantly affect the pharmacokinetics of selegiline.	It may be necessary to reduce the dose of selegiline in women taking oral contraceptives. As selectivity of MAO inhibition is lost at higher plasma levels, these women may be more susceptible to adverse effects related to MAO-A inhibition (i.e., acute reactions precipitated by tyramine ingestion and adrenergic agents) and should be counseled accordingly. This advice does not appear to apply to women taking hormone replacement therapy.
Serotonergic drugs such as dextromethorphan, ergotamine, L-tryptophan, methadone, mirtazapine, pethidine (meperidine), sibutramine, SSRIs, venlafaxine, TCAs, tramadol, triptans (except eletriptan, naratriptan) (See Contraindications and Warnings and Precautions.)	Increased serotonergic effect of interacting drug (possible serotonin syndrome).	Avoid combination; allow 2-week wash out period between drugs, 5 weeks after discontinuing fluoxetine; combination with pethidine (meperidine) is contraindicated.

Drug-Food Interactions: At high doses, selegiline is a nonselective inhibitor of MAO. Patients receiving high doses of selegiline are susceptible to hypertensive reactions induced by tyramine-rich foods and beverages (e.g., cheese, red wine, beer, pickled fish, caviar, smoked or cured meats, liver, yeast extract, or meat extracts such as Bovril, Oxo or Marmite). Do not exceed the recommended daily dose.

Administration with a high-fat meal increases the bioavailability of selegiline.

DOSAGE AND ADMINISTRATION: **Recommended Dose and Dosage Adjustment: Adults and Geriatrics:** See Table 3.

Table 3: Selegiline
Dose in Adult Patients Including Geriatric Patients

Indication	Route	Maximum Dose	Clinical Comment
Idiopathic Parkinson's disease	Oral	5 mg BID	Usually administered with breakfast and lunch to minimize interference with sleep.

Genetic Polymorphism: The pharmacokinetics and pharmacodynamics of selegiline are not affected by polymorphisms in the gene coding for CYP2D6, as defined by the debrisoquine metabolic ratio, or CYP2C19, as determined by the mephenytoin hydroxylator phenotype.

OVERDOSAGE:
Signs and Symptoms: The MAO-B selectivity of selegiline is lost at doses above 10 mg daily. The information presented here pertains to MAO inhibitors in general, as there is limited experience with selegiline in overdose.

Clinical effects of excessive MAO inhibition result from accumulation of amines such as serotonin and norepinephrine. Initial symptoms include hypertension, drowsiness, dizziness, confusion, tremors and headache, which may progress to agitation, muscle rigidity and seizures. Dysrhythmias, sweating, chills and hyperthermia can also occur. Late phase symptoms include hypotension, bradycardia, cardiovascular collapse, respiratory depression, pulmonary edema and coma. Potential complications include rhabdomyolysis, hemolysis, disseminated intravascular coagulation, acute renal failure (secondary to hypotension or rhabdomyolysis) and hypertensive crisis.

The risk of hypertensive crisis is increased in the presence of drugs such as amphetamines, cocaine, decongestants (e.g., pseudoephedrine, phenylephrine) or foods containing tyramine (see Drug Interactions, Drug-Food Interactions). Other overdose symptoms may be exacerbated by co-ingestion of serotonergic drugs such as dextromethorphan, ergotamine, L-tryptophan, mirtazapine, pethidine (meperidine), sibutramine, SSRIs, SNRIs (duloxetine, venlafaxine), TCAs, triptans (except eletriptan, naratriptan).

Recommended Management: Initial management of MAO inhibitor overdose should focus first on establishing the airway and stabilizing the heart rate and blood pressure, and subsequently on management of rhabdomyolysis, hyperthermia, seizures and muscle rigidity. Gut decontamination with activated charcoal can be considered within 2 hours of overdose once the patient is stabilized.

Because severe hypertension is often short-lived, it is important to use agents with a shorter duration of action such as nitroprusside, nitroglycerin or phentolamine. These drugs should be titrated to response. Beta-blockers, including labetalol, should not be used.

Hyperthermia should be aggressively managed using ice packs, evaporative cooling, cooling blankets, or extracorporeal cooling methods. Benzodiazepines are useful for muscle rigidity, seizures and agitation. Dysrhythmias can be treated with lidocaine. Once the patient is stable, a dose of activated charcoal 1 g/kg may be given if overdose occurred within the previous 2 hours. Gastric lavage can be considered within 1 hour of massive ingestions; consultation with a regional poison control centre is advised.

Consideration should be given to the possibility of mixed overdose and its potential medical implications.

For management of a suspected drug overdose, CPhA recommends that you contact your **regional Poison Control Centre**. See the *CPS* Directory section for a list of Poison Control Centres.

ACTION AND CLINICAL PHARMACOLOGY: Mechanism of Action: Selegiline is a selective and irreversible inhibitor of monoamine oxidase type B. The principal site of action for selegiline in the treatment of Parkinson's disease is the nigrostriatal pathway in the CNS. Inhibition of MAO-B in the striatum slows breakdown of dopamine.

At doses used for the treatment of Parkinson's disease, selegiline does not inhibit peripheral metabolism of catecholamines. At doses higher than those used for the treatment of Parkinson's disease (i.e., >10 mg/day) selegiline does inhibit MAO-A.

Pharmacokinetics: Adults: Absorption: Selegiline is rapidly absorbed after oral administration. Peak plasma concentrations ranging from 0.9 to 2.7 ng/mL were detected within 0.5 to 0.9 hours after oral administration in the fasting state. Because of extensive first-pass metabolism, the oral bioavailability of the drug is approximately 10% after administration of a 10 mg oral dose. Administration with a high-fat meal increases the bioavailability of selegiline.

Distribution: Selegiline is rapidly distributed throughout the body and has a large volume of distribution (Vd). The apparent Vd was 508 L after administration of a 10 mg iv dose. The drug is highly bound to plasma proteins. Despite the relatively short half-lives of selegiline and desmethylselegiline, the AUC of both compounds increases significantly during multiple dosing, a phenomenon that has been interpreted as an indication of saturable tissue binding.

Metabolism and Excretion: Selegiline undergoes extensive first-pass metabolism in the gut wall and liver after absorption from the gastrointestinal tract.

The terminal elimination half-life of selegiline is 1.6 hours after administration of a 10 mg iv dose and 1.2 to 1.8 hours after administration of a single oral 10 mg dose. Total body clearance of selegiline is estimated to occur at a rate of 240 L/hour.

Three metabolites of selegiline have been identified, all of which are pharmacologically active. N-desmethylselegiline ($t_{1/2}$ 2.0 hours), the major metabolite of selegiline, is also an irreversible inhibitor of MAO in humans. The other metabolites are L-amphetamine ($t_{1/2}$ 17.7 hours) and L-methamphetamine ($t_{1/2}$ 20.5 hours), both of which have CNS stimulant properties.

Metabolism of selegiline is mediated mainly by CYP2B6 and CYP1A2. CYP3A4 and CYP2D6 do not appear to be involved in its metabolism. Whether CYP2C19 plays a role is not clear.

Senna Tablets Peristaltic Stimulant
sennosides
Peristaltic Stimulant

Tanta

Senna Laxative Pills Regular Strength Peristaltic Stimulant
sennosides
Peristaltic Stimulant

Tanta

Senna Laxative Pills Extra Strength Peristaltic Stimulant
sennosides
Peristaltic Stimulant

Tanta

Senna-S Tablets Peristaltic Stimulant-Surfactant
sennosides—docusate sodium
Peristaltic Stimulant-Surfactant

Tanta

SUPPLIED: Senna Tablets: Each brown, convex tablet contains: 8.6 mg of standardized sennosides, a natural vegetable derivative. Bottles of 100.

Senna Laxative Pills Regular Strength Peristaltic Stimulant: Each light beige, round tablet, contains: 15 mg of standardized sennosides, a natural vegetable derivative. Blister packs of 30.

Senna Laxative Pills Extra Strength Peristaltic Stimulant: Each blue, round tablet, contains: 25 mg of standardized sennosides, a natural vegetable derivative. Blister packs of 24.

Senna-S Tablets Peristaltic Stimulant-Surfactant: Each orange, round, convex tablet, contains: 8.6 mg of standardized sennosides, a natural vegetable derivative in combination with 50 mg of docusate sodium as a stool softener. Bottles of 60.

Senokot® Preparations
senna (standardized sennosides)
Peristaltic Stimulant

Purdue Pharma

Date of Revision: November 23, 2009

INDICATIONS: For relief of functional constipation (occasional). The natural source senna in all Senokot products provides comfortable, overnight relief from occasional constipation.

CONTRAINDICATIONS: The "acute abdomen". Do not use if you have intestinal obstructions and/or stenosis, atony, appendicitis, inflammatory colon disease (e.g. Crohn's disease, ulcerative colitis), abdominal pain of unknown origin, and/or a severe dehydration state with water and electrolyte depletion.

WARNINGS: If griping occurs, reduce dosage. Administer with caution to nursing mothers.

Do not use in the presence of abdominal pain, nausea, fever or vomiting unless directed by a physician.

Overuse or extended use may cause dependence for bowel function. Consult a health care practitioner if symptoms persist or worsen.

Do not take any type of laxative for more than 1 week, unless your physician has ordered a special schedule.

Laxatives should not be taken within 2 hours of another medicine because the desired effect of the other medicine may be reduced.

Rectal bleeding or failure to have a bowel movement after use of a laxative may indicate a serious condition. Discontinue use and consult a physician.

If there has been a sudden change in bowel movements that persists over a period of 2 weeks, consult a physician before using a laxative. Laxative products should not be used for a period longer than 1 week unless directed by a physician.

If pregnant or nursing, seek the advice of a health care practitioner before using this product. Consult a health care practitioner prior to use if you are taking heart medications, diuretics, adrenocorticosteroids, licorice root or other health products that may aggravate electrolyte imbalance. In case of overdose: Call a Regional Poison Control Centre and/or your physician and/or your local emergency number immediately, or go to your local hospital emergency, even if you do not notice any signs or symptoms. Keep all medicines out of the reach of children.

PRECAUTIONS: _Drug Interactions:_ There are no known drug interactions with sennosides.

ADVERSE EFFECTS: In clinical trials, adverse effects were seen in approximately 4% of the cases; in about one-third of these, the effects were ascribed to dose being too high. Most frequently, these consisted of cramps and/or griping, usually described as "mild" or "slight", or "occasional", which are extensions of the activities associated with bowel evacuation. Only 0.21% of cases were reported as severe cramping; in some cases this resulted in cessation of treatment. Nausea and vomiting may also occur. Hypersensitivity skin reactions are an uncommon occurrence; very rarely anaphylactoid reactions have been reported.

Due to the presence of chrysophanic acid in natural senna, Senokot laxatives may cause discolouration of breast milk, urine, or feces depending on the acidity (yellow-brown discolouration) or alkalinity (red-violet discolouration) of the substance. There is no pathologic significance to this discolouration. Urine discolouration, if present may interfere with the interpretation of laboratory tests. Prolonged use or misuse of these products may also result in the development of atonic colon. Reversible pigmentation of the colon, i.e., melanosis coli, may also result from prolonged use of senna containing preparations; this effect is considered benign.

OVERDOSE:

Symptoms: Prolonged use or overdosage with any stimulant laxative including those containing senna may cause diarrhea, leading to excessive water loss and possible electrolyte imbalance.

Treatment: In case of accidental overdosage, seek professional assistance.

> For management of a suspected drug overdose, CPhA recommends that you contact your **regional Poison Control Centre**. See the *CPS* Directory section for a list of Poison Control Centres.

DOSAGE: Syrup: Adults: 10-15 mL (2-3 teaspoons) 1-2 times per day. Take at bedtime, as required. Maximum, 15 mL twice a day. Administer preferably at bedtime. Evacuation generally occurs within 6-12 hours following ingestion. The correct dose of the sennosides-containing laxatives is the smallest required to produce comfortable soft-formed stool and varies between individuals.

Adults (Pregnant): 5-10 mL (1-2 teaspoons) 1-2 times per day. Take at bedtime, not to exceed 10 mL twice a day. Adjust dosage as necessary. Administer preferably at bedtime. Evacuation generally occurs within 6-12 hours following ingestion. The correct dose of the sennosides-containing laxatives is the smallest required to produce comfortable soft-formed stool and varies between individuals.

Children (6 to 12 years): 5-10 mL (1-2 teaspoons) 1-2 times per day. Take at bedtime, not to exceed 10 mL twice a day. Adjust dosage as necessary. Administer preferably at bedtime. Evacuation generally occurs within 6-12 hours following ingestion. The correct dose of the sennosides-containing laxatives is the smallest required to produce comfortable soft-formed stool and varies between individuals.

Children (2 to 5 years): 3-5 mL (1/2-1 teaspoon) 1-2 times per day. Adjust dosage as necessary. Maximum 5 mL twice a day. Administer preferably at bedtime. Evacuation generally occurs within 6-12 hours following ingestion. The correct dose of the sennosides-containing laxatives is the smallest required to produce comfortable soft-formed stool and varies between individuals.

Infants (less than 2 years): Consult physician.

Tablets: Adults: Take 2-4 tablets 1-2 times per day. Take at bedtime, as required. Maximum, 4 tablets twice a day. Administer preferably at bedtime. Evacuation generally occurs within 6-12 hours following ingestion. The correct dose of the sennosides-containing laxatives is the smallest required to produce comfortable soft-formed stool and varies between individuals.

Adults (Pregnant): Take 1-2 tablets 1-2 times per day. Take at bedtime, not to exceed 2 tablets twice a day. Administer preferably at bedtime. Evacuation generally occurs within 6-12 hours following ingestion. The correct dose of the sennosides-containing laxatives is the smallest required to produce comfortable soft-formed stool and varies between individuals.

Children (6 to 12 years): Take 1-2 tablets 1-2 times per day. Take at bedtime, not to exceed 2 tablets twice a day. Administer preferably at bedtime. Evacuation generally occurs within 6-12 hours following ingestion. The correct dose of the sennosides-containing laxatives is the smallest required to produce comfortable soft-formed stool and varies between individuals.

SUPPLIED: Syrup: Each mL contains: standardized sennosides 1.7 mg. Nonmedicinal ingredients: alcohol (7%), chocolate flavour, cocoa flavour, methylparaben, propylparaben, sodium hydroxide, sucrose (66 g/100 mL) and water. Bottles of 100, 250 and 500 mL. Store at 15-25°C.

Tablets: Each tablet contains: standardized sennosides 8.6 mg. Nonmedicinal ingredients: corn starch, magnesium stearate and microcrystalline cellulose. Packages of 10. Bottles of 30, 100 and 1000. Unit dose, boxes of 1000. Store at 15-25°C.

(Shown in Product Identification Section)

Senokot®•S

senna (standardized sennosides from senna concentrate CG)—docusate sodium

Peristaltic Stimulant—Stool Softener

Purdue Pharma

Date of Revision: December 5, 2008

PHARMACOLOGY: The laxative agent in Senokot•S is a natural vegetable derivative (senna), standardized for predictable results. The principal constituents of Senokot•S are senna glycosides. These include sennosides A & B, and the glycoside derivatives of rhein and chrysophanic acid. These glycosides, when converted into aglycones in the colon, function as laxative agents.

Only minimal amounts of the metabolites of senna (aglycones) are absorbed systemically. The actual extent to which such metabolites are distributed to body tissues and fluids is unknown; they may be excreted in the bile, and have been detected in small amounts in breast milk.

Docusate sodium is a surface active agent useful in the medical management of certain types of constipation and fecal impaction.

Pharmacodynamic Properties: The laxative principles of the senna plant have been identified as sennosides (senna glycosides). Enzymatic action by colonic bacteria converts the glycosides into aglycones, which induce colonic peristalsis through stimulation of the intrinsic peristaltic mechanism in the colonic wall. This action is virtually colon-specific, since these compounds have little or no action in the stomach and small intestine. The stimulant effect on the Myenteric (Auerbach's) plexus in the colonic wall is reportedly free of mucosal injury. Senna also has effects on electrolyte and water transport.

Preclinical Safety Data: Results from published acute, subchronic and chronic toxicology studies as well as genotoxicity and reproductive studies with senna or docusate sodium indicate that these ingredients are safe when used as recommended. In a GLP compliant carcinogenicity study, lifetime exposure to senna did not result in any evidence of carcinogenicity in rats dosed at levels as high as 300 mg/kg/day. Finally, in a published (non-GLP compliant) two-year carcinogenicity study, rats fed diets containing as high as 1% docusate sodium (about 200 mg/day) showed no treatment-related lesions.

INDICATIONS: Relief of functional constipation through combined stool softening and peristaltic stimulation. Specifically indicated for postpartum patients, for use by patients with heart disease where straining at stool must be avoided, and in constipation in the presence of hemorrhoids, anal fissures or other conditions where hard, dry stools may cause discomfort.

CONTRAINDICATIONS: The "acute abdomen".

WARNINGS: See Precautions.

PRECAUTIONS: If griping occurs, subsequent dosage should be reduced. Administer with caution to nursing mothers.

Do not use in the presence of abdominal pain, nausea, fever or vomiting.

Overuse or extended use may cause dependence for bowel function.

Do not take any type of laxative for more than 1 week, unless your physician has ordered a special schedule.

Laxatives should not be taken within 2 hours of another medicine because the desired effect of the other medicine may be reduced.

Do not administer concomitantly with mineral oil since the docusate sodium component of Senokot•S may increase absorption of oil.

Rectal bleeding or failure to have a bowel movement after use of a laxative may indicate a serious condition. Discontinue use and consult a physician.

If there has been a sudden change in bowel movements that persists over a period of 2 weeks, consult a physician before using a laxative. Laxative products should not be used for a period longer than 1 week unless directed by a doctor.

If pregnant or nursing, seek the advice of a health care professional before using this product.

Drug Interactions: There are no known drug interactions with sennosides.

ADVERSE EFFECTS: In clinical trials, adverse effects were seen in approximately 4% of the cases; in about one-third of these, the effects were ascribed to dose being too high. Most frequently these consisted of cramps and/or griping, usually described as "mild" or "slight", or "occasional", which are extensions of the activities associated with bowel evacuation. Only 0.21% of cases were reported as severe cramping; in some cases this resulted in cessation of treatment. Nausea and vomiting may also occur. Hypersensitivity skin reactions are an uncommon occurrence; very rarely anaphylactoid reactions have been reported.

Due to the presence of chrysophanic acid in natural senna, Senokot laxatives may cause discolouration of breast milk, urine, or feces depending on the acidity (yellow-brown discolouration) or alkalinity (red-violet discolouration) of the substance. There is no pathologic significance to this discolouration. Urine discolouration, if present may interfere with the interpretation of laboratory test. Prolonged use of these products may also result in the development of atonic colon. Reversible pigmentation of the colon, i.e., melanosis coli, may also result from prolonged use of senna containing preparations; this effect is considered benign.

OVERDOSE:

Symptoms: Prolonged use or overdosage with any stimulant laxative including those containing senna may cause diarrhea, leading to excessive water loss and possible electrolyte imbalance.

Treatment: In case of accidental overdosage, seek professional assistance.

> For management of a suspected drug overdose, CPhA recommends that you contact your **regional Poison Control Centre**. See the *CPS* Directory section for a list of Poison Control Centres.

DOSAGE: Evacuation generally occurs within 6 to 12 hours following ingestion. The correct dose of the sennosides-containing laxatives is the smallest required to produce comfortable soft-formed stool and varies between individuals.

Tablets: Adults: 1 to 2 tablets at bedtime, as required. Maximum, 4 tablets twice a day.

Pregnancy and Children (6 to 12 years): ½ to 1 tablet at bedtime, not to exceed 2 tablets twice a day.

SUPPLIED: Each orange, film-coated tablet, stamped S/S on one side, contains: standardized sennosides 8.6 mg and docusate sodium 50 mg. Nonmedicinal ingredients: corn starch, guar gum, magnesium stearate, microcrystalline cellulose and silicon dioxide; film coating: D&C Yellow No. 10 Aluminum Lake, FD&C Yellow No. 6 Aluminum Lake, lecithin, polyethylene glycol, polyvinyl alcohol, talc and titanium dioxide. Sodium: <1 mmol (2.6 mg). Tartrazine-free. Packages of 10. Bottles of 20, 60 and 1000. Store at room temperature (15-25°C).

(Shown in Product Identification Section)

Sensipar® Pr

cinacalcet HCl

Calcimimetic Agent

Amgen

Date of Revision: September 16, 2009

SUMMARY PRODUCT INFORMATION:

Route of Administration	Dosage Form/ Strength	Clinically Relevant Nonmedicinal Ingredients
Oral	Tablet/30 mg, 60 mg, 90 mg	For a complete listing of the nonmedicinal ingredients see Dosage Forms, Composition and Packaging.

INDICATIONS AND CLINICAL USE: SENSIPAR (cinacalcet hydrochloride) is indicated for the treatment of secondary hyperparathyroidism (HPT) in patients with Chronic Kidney Disease (CKD) receiving dialysis.

SENSIPAR controls parathyroid hormone levels, calcium and phosphorous levels, and the serum calcium-phosphorous product (Ca×P), in patients with CKD receiving dialysis.

SENSIPAR is indicated for the reduction of hypercalcemia in patients with parathyroid carcinoma.

SENSIPAR is indicated for the reduction of clinically significant hypercalcemia, as defined by relevant treatment guidelines, in patients with primary HPT for whom parathyroidectomy is not clinically appropriate or is contraindicated.

CONTRAINDICATIONS: SENSIPAR (cinacalcet hydrochloride) is contraindicated in patients with hypersensitivity to any of the components of this product.

For a complete listing of the nonmedicinal ingredients see Dosage Forms, Composition and Packaging.

WARNINGS AND PRECAUTIONS: Seizures: In three clinical studies of CKD patients receiving dialysis, 5% of the patients in both the SENSIPAR (cinacalcet hydrochloride) and placebo groups reported a history of seizure disorder at baseline. During the trials, seizures (primarily generalized or tonic-clonic) were observed in 1.4% (9/656) of SENSIPAR-treated patients and 0.4% (2/470) of placebo-treated patients. Five of the nine SENSIPAR-treated patients had a history of a seizure disorder and two were receiving anti-seizure medication at the time of their seizure. Both placebo-treated patients had a history of seizure disorder and were receiving anti-seizure medication at the time of their seizure. While the basis for the reported difference in seizure rate is not clear, the threshold for seizures is lowered by significant reductions in serum calcium levels. Therefore, serum calcium levels should be closely monitored in patients receiving SENSIPAR, particularly in patients with a history of a seizure disorder.

Cardiovascular: Hypotension and/or Worsening Heart Failure: In postmarketing safety surveillance, isolated, idiosyncratic cases of hypotension and/or worsening heart failure have been reported in patients with impaired cardiac function, in which a causal relationship to SENSIPAR could not be completely excluded and may be mediated by reductions in serum calcium levels. Clinical trial data showed hypotension occurred in 7% of SENSIPAR-treated patients, 12% of placebo-treated patients, and heart failure occurred in 2% of patients receiving SENSIPAR or placebo.

Hypocalcemia: SENSIPAR lowers serum calcium, and therefore patients should be carefully monitored for the occurrence of hypocalcemia. Potential manifestations of hypocalcemia include paresthesias, myalgias, cramping, tetany, and convulsions.

Serum Calcium: In clinical trials of CKD patients receiving dialysis, SENSIPAR treatment was not initiated in patients with a serum calcium (corrected for albumin) less than the lower limit of the normal range. Since SENSIPAR lowers serum calcium, patients should be monitored for the occurrence of hypocalcemia.

In CKD patients receiving dialysis who were administered SENSIPAR, 4% of serum calcium values were less than 1.875 mmol/L (see Adverse Reactions). In the event of hypocalcemia, calcium-containing phosphate binders and/or vitamin D sterols can be used to raise serum calcium. If hypocalcemia persists, reduce the dose or discontinue administration of SENSIPAR (see Dosage and Administration). Potential manifestations of hypocalcemia may include paresthesias, myalgias, cramping, tetany, and convulsions.

Cinacalcet is not indicated for CKD patients not receiving dialysis. Investigational studies have shown that cinacalcet-treated CKD patients not receiving dialysis have an increased risk for hypocalcemia (serum calcium levels <8.4 mg/dL [2.1 mmol/L]) compared with cinacalcet-treated CKD patients receiving dialysis, which may be due to lower baseline calcium levels and/or the presence of residual kidney function.

General: Adynamic bone disease may develop if intact parathyroid hormone (iPTH) levels are suppressed below 100 pg/mL. If iPTH levels decrease below the current National Kidney Foundation-Kidney/Disease Outcomes Quality Initiative (NKF-K/DOQI) recommended target range (150-300 pg/mL) in patients receiving dialysis treated with SENSIPAR, the dose of SENSIPAR and/or vitamin D sterols should be reduced or therapy discontinued.

Hepatic Insufficiency: Due to the potential for 2- to 4-fold higher plasma levels of SENSIPAR, patients with moderate to severe hepatic impairment should be closely monitored when initiating treatment (see Action and Clinical Pharmacology).

Testosterone Levels: Testosterone levels are often below the normal range in patients with end stage renal disease. In a clinical study of CKD patients receiving dialysis, free testosterone levels decreased by a median of 31.3% in the SENSIPAR-treated patients and by 16.3% in the placebo-treated patients after 6 months of treatment. The clinical significance of these reductions in serum testosterone is unknown. An open label extension of this study showed no further reductions in free and total testosterone concentrations over a period of 3 years in SENSIPAR-treated patients.

Impairment of Fertility: SENSIPAR had no effect on fertility in animal studies.

Special Populations: Pregnant Women: There are no studies on the use of SENSIPAR in pregnant women. SENSIPAR was not teratogenic in rabbits when given a dose of 0.4 times, on an area under the curve (AUC) basis, the maximum human dose for secondary HPT (180 mg once daily). There were no effects on fertility in males or females at exposures up to 4 times a human dose of 180 mg/day. In pregnant rats, there were slight decreases in body weight and food consumption at the highest dose. The non-teratogenic dose in rats was 4.4 times, on an AUC basis, the maximum dose for patients with secondary HPT (180 mg once daily). Decreased fetal weights were seen in rats at doses where dams had severe hypocalcemia. SENSIPAR has been shown to cross the placental barrier in rabbits. Although animal studies have shown no evidence of teratogenicity, SENSIPAR should be used during pregnancy only if the potential benefit justifies the potential risk to the fetus.

Nursing Women: It is not known whether SENSIPAR is excreted in human milk. Studies in rats have shown that SENSIPAR is excreted in the milk with a high milk to plasma ratio. A decision should be made whether to discontinue nursing or discontinue SENSIPAR, taking into account the importance of SENSIPAR to the mother.

Pediatrics: The safety and efficacy of SENSIPAR in pediatric patients have not been established.

Geriatrics: Of the 1136 patients enrolled in the SENSIPAR phase 3 clinical program, 26% were >65 years old, while 9% were >75 years old. No overall differences in safety and efficacy of SENSIPAR were observed in patients greater or less than 65 years of age (see Dosage and Administration).

Carcinogenicity: SENSIPAR, administered orally for 104 weeks, showed no evidence of carcinogenic potential in mice and rats. Doses administered to mice and rats resulted in total systemic exposure (AUCs) 2 times the exposures observed in humans. The nature, incidence, and distribution of tumours in rats and mice of both sexes did not indicate any SENSIPAR-induced carcinogenesis. A decreased incidence of thyroid C-cell adenomas was observed in rats treated with SENSIPAR.

Mutagenicity: SENSIPAR was negative in the Ames assay, chromosomal aberration assay, Chinese Hamster Ovary HGPRT forward mutation assay, and in the mouse micronucleus assay. These tests indicate that SENSIPAR has no genetic toxicity either with respect to DNA damage, including gene mutations, large scale chromosomal damage, recombinations or numerical changes.

Effect on the Ability to Drive and Use Machines: No effects on the ability to drive or operate machinery have been observed.

Monitoring and Laboratory Tests: Patients with CKD and Secondary Hyperparathyroidism: Serum calcium should be measured within 1 week and iPTH should be measured 1 to 4 weeks after initiation or dose adjustment of SENSIPAR. Once the maintenance dose levels have been established, serum calcium and serum phosphorus should be measured approximately monthly, and PTH (iPTH) every 1 to 3 months (see Dosage and Administration). Either the intact PTH (iPTH) or bio-active PTH (biPTH) may be used to measure plasma PTH levels. Treatment with SENSIPAR does not alter the relationship between iPTH and biPTH.

ADVERSE REACTIONS: Adverse Drug Reaction Overview: Studies were conducted in patients with CKD receiving dialysis. SENSIPAR (cinacalcet hydrochloride) was safe and generally well tolerated.

Hypocalcemia: SENSIPAR lowers serum calcium, and therefore patients should be carefully monitored for the occurrence of hypocalcemia. Potential manifestations of hypocalcemia include paresthesias, myalgias, cramping, tetany, and convulsions (see Warnings and Precautions).

Clinical Trial Adverse Drug Reactions: Because clinical trials are conducted under very specific conditions the adverse reaction rates observed in the clinical trials may not reflect the rates observed in practice and should not be compared to the rates in the clinical trials of another drug. Adverse drug reaction information from clinical trials is useful for identifying drug-related adverse events and for approximating rates.

Secondary Hyperparathyroidism in Patients with Chronic Kidney Disease Receiving Dialysis: In three double-blind placebo-controlled clinical trials, 1126 CKD patients receiving dialysis received study drug (656 SENSIPAR, 470 placebo) for up to six months. Adverse events reported during the studies were typical for the dialysis patient population. The most frequently reported adverse events (incidence of at least 5% in the SENSIPAR-treated group) are provided in Table 1. The most frequently reported events in the SENSIPAR group were nausea and vomiting which were generally mild to moderate in severity, brief in duration, and infrequently led to discontinuation of study drug.

Table 1: SENSIPAR

Adverse Event Incidence (≥5%) in Patients Receiving Dialysis

Preferred Term	Placebo (N=470) %	Cinacalcet (N=656) %
Nausea	19	31
Vomiting	15	27
Diarrhea	20	21
Headache	17	16
Myalgia	14	15
Pain Abdominal	14	12
Infection Upper Respiratory	13	12
Dizziness	8	10
Dyspnea	9	9
Pain Limb	10	9
Dyspepsia	8	8
Arthralgia	9	7
Fever	10	7
Fatigue	7	7
Hypertension	5	7
Hypotension	12	7
Edema Peripheral	7	7
Asthenia	4	7
Cough	7	6
Pruritus	7	6
Anorexia	4	6
Thrombosis Vascular Access	7	6
Pain Chest, Non-Cardiac	4	6
Access Infection	4	5

The incidence of serious adverse events (29% vs 31%) and deaths (2% vs 3%) was similar in the SENSIPAR and placebo groups, respectively.

12-Month Experience with SENSIPAR: Two hundred sixty-six patients from the two pivotal phase 3 studies continued to receive SENSIPAR or placebo treatment in a 6-month double-blind extension study (12-month total treatment duration). The incidence and nature of adverse events in this study were similar in the two treatment groups, and comparable to those observed in the pivotal phase 3 studies.

Parathyroid Carcinoma and Primary Hyperparathyroidism: One hundred sixty patients with primary HPT or parathyroid carcinoma participated in SENSIPAR clinical trials with exposure for up to 5.5 years.

The safety profile of SENSIPAR in these patient populations is generally consistent with that seen in patients with CKD receiving dialysis. The most frequent adverse drug reactions in these patient populations were nausea and vomiting.

Laboratory Values: Serum calcium levels should be monitored in patients receiving SENSIPAR (see Warnings and Precautions and Dosage and Administration). In the three phase 3 studies in patients with CKD receiving dialysis, 4% of all serum calcium values in patients receiving SENSIPAR were <1.875 mmol/L, compared with <1% in the placebo group.

Post-Market Adverse Drug Reactions: There have been reports of diarrhea, myalgia, rash, and hypersensitivity reactions, including angioedema and urticaria, associated with SENSIPAR therapy.

Isolated cases of severe hypersensitivity reactions have been reported.

Isolated, idiosyncratic cases of hypotension and/or worsening heart failure have been reported in SENSIPAR-treated patients with impaired cardiac function in postmarketing safety surveillance.

DRUG INTERACTIONS: Drug-Drug Interactions: Effect of SENSIPAR on Other Drugs: Drugs Metabolized by CYP450 2D6: SENSIPAR (cinacalcet hydrochloride) is an inhibitor of CYP2D6. Therefore, dose adjustments of concomitant medications that are predominantly metabolized by CYP2D6 (e.g., metoprolol) and particularly those with a narrow therapeutic index (e.g., flecainide, vinblastine, thioridazine and most tricyclic antidepressants) may be required.

Desipramine: Concurrent administration of 90 mg SENSIPAR with 50 mg desipramine, a tricyclic antidepressant metabolized primarily by CYP2D6, increased desipramine exposure by approximately 3.6-fold in CYP2D6 extensive metabolizers.

Amitriptyline: Concurrent administration of 25 mg or 100 mg SENSIPAR with 50 mg amitriptyline, a tricyclic antidepressant metabolized in part by CYP2D6, increased exposure to amitriptyline and its active metabolite nortriptyline by approximately 20% in extensive metabolizers of CYP2D6 enzymes. Dose reductions of amitriptyline may be required in some subjects receiving SENSIPAR concurrently.

Drugs Metabolized by Other CYP Enzymes: Based on in vitro data, SENSIPAR is not an inhibitor of other CYP enzymes at concentrations achieved clinically, including CYP1A2, CYP2C9, CYP2C19, and CYP3A4. In vitro studies indicate that SENSIPAR is not an inducer of CYP1A2, CYP2C19 and CYP3A4.

Midazolam: Co-administration of SENSIPAR (90 mg) with orally administered midazolam (2 mg), a CYP3A4 and CYP3A5 substrate, did not alter the pharmacokinetics of midazolam. These data suggest that SENSIPAR would not affect the pharmacokinetics of those classes of drugs that are metabolized by CYP3A4 and CYP3A5, such as certain immunosuppressants, including cyclosporine and tacrolimus.

Warfarin: SENSIPAR does not affect the pharmacokinetics or pharmacodynamics (as measured by prothrombin time and clotting factor VII) of warfarin.

The lack of effect of cinacalcet on the pharmacokinetics of R and S warfarin and the absence of auto induction upon multiple dosing in patients indicates that cinacalcet is not an inducer of CYP3A4, CYP1A2 or CYP2C9 in humans.

Effect of Other Drugs on SENSIPAR: SENSIPAR is metabolized by multiple cytochrome P450 enzymes, primarily CYP3A4 and CYP1A2, which limits the potential for other drugs to increase cinacalcet concentrations.

Ketoconazole: SENSIPAR is metabolized in part by the enzyme CYP3A4. Co-administration of 200 mg bid of ketoconazole, a strong inhibitor of CYP3A4, caused an approximate 2-fold increase in cinacalcet exposure. Dose adjustment of SENSIPAR may be required if a patient initiates or discontinues therapy with a strong CYP3A4 inhibitor (e.g., ketoconazole, erythromycin, itraconazole) or inducer (e.g., rifampin, phenytoin) of this enzyme.

Calcium Carbonate: Co-administration of calcium carbonate (single 1500 mg dose) did not alter the pharmacokinetics of SENSIPAR.

Pantoprazole: Co-administration of pantoprazole (80 mg qd) did not alter the pharmacokinetics of SENSIPAR.

Sevelamer HCl: Co-administration of sevelamer HCl (2400 mg tid) did not alter the pharmacokinetics of SENSIPAR.

Drug-Food Interactions: After oral administration of SENSIPAR (cinacalcet hydrochloride), maximum plasma concentration is achieved in approximately 2 to 6 hours. Administration of SENSIPAR with food results in an approximate 50 to 80% increase in bioavailability. Increases in plasma concentration are similar, regardless of the fat content of the meal.

Drug-Herb Interactions: Interactions with herbal products have not been established.

Drug-Laboratory Test Interactions: Interactions with laboratory tests have not been established.

DOSAGE AND ADMINISTRATION:

SENSIPAR (cinacalcet hydrochloride) is administered orally. Tablets should be taken whole and should not be divided. Take SENSIPAR with food or shortly after a meal (see Drug Interactions).

Secondary Hyperparathyroidism in Patients with Chronic Kidney Disease Receiving Dialysis: The recommended starting oral dose of SENSIPAR is 30 mg once daily. SENSIPAR should be titrated every 2 to 4 weeks to a maximum dose of 180 mg once daily to achieve a target PTH between 1.5 to 5 times the upper limit of normal:

In CKD patients, PTH levels should be assessed at least 12 hours after dosing with cinacalcet.

Current NKF/KDOQI Bone Metabolism Guidelines for the iPTH, Ca×P, serum phosphorus, and serum calcium targets should be considered. See Table 2.

Table 2: SENSIPAR

NKF-K/DOQI Bone Metabolism Guidelines for Patients Receiving Dialysis[a]

Parameter	Target Range
iPTH	16.5–33.0 pmol/L [150–300 pg/mL]
Ca×P	<4.51 $mmol^2/L^2$ [<55 mg^2/dL^2]

(cont'd)

Table 2: SENSIPAR *(cont'd)*

NKF-K/DOQI Bone Metabolism Guidelines for Patients Receiving Dialysis[a]

Parameter	Target Range
Phosphorus	1.13–1.78 mmol/L [3.5–5.5 mg/dL]
'Corrected' calcium	2.10–2.37 mmol/L [8.4–9.5 mg/dL]

[a] Adapted from National Kidney Foundation: K/DOQI clinical practice guidelines: bone metabolism and disease in chronic kidney disease. *American Journal of Kidney Disease* 42:S1-S201, 2003.

During dose titration, serum calcium levels should be monitored frequently and if serum calcium levels decrease below the normal range, appropriate steps should be taken to increase serum calcium levels (see Warnings and Precautions). Calcium levels should be corrected for albumin or ionized calcium levels should be measured.

Parathyroid Carcinoma and Primary Hyperparathyroidism: The recommended starting dose of SENSIPAR for adults is 30 mg twice per day.

The dosage of SENSIPAR should be titrated sequentially every 2 to 4 weeks through dosages of 30 mg twice daily, 60 mg twice daily, and 90 mg twice daily to reduce serum calcium levels. For further information on higher dosages (90 mg 3 or 4 times daily).

Special Populations: Geriatric Patients: Age does not alter the pharmacokinetics of SENSIPAR; no dose adjustment is required for geriatric patients.

Patients with Renal Impairment: Renal impairment does not alter the pharmacokinetics of SENSIPAR; no dosage adjustment is necessary for renal impairment.

Patients with Hepatic Impairment: Moderate to severe hepatic impairment (Child-Pugh classification) increases SENSIPAR drug concentrations by approximately 2- to 4-fold. In patients with moderate-severe hepatic impairment, PTH and serum calcium concentrations should be closely monitored during dose titration of SENSIPAR.

OVERDOSAGE:
Doses titrated up to 300 mg once daily have been safely administered to patients receiving dialysis. Overdosage of SENSIPAR (cinacalcet hydrochloride) may lead to hypocalcemia. In the event of overdosage, patients should be monitored for signs and symptoms of hypocalcemia and appropriate measures taken to correct serum calcium levels (see Warnings and Precautions).

Since SENSIPAR is highly protein bound, hemodialysis is not an effective treatment for overdosage of SENSIPAR.

> For management of a suspected drug overdose, CPhA recommends that you contact your **regional Poison Control Centre**. See the *CPS* Directory section for a list of Poison Control Centres.

ACTION AND CLINICAL PHARMACOLOGY: Mechanism of Action: Secondary hyperparathyroidism is a progressive disease, which occurs in patients with chronic kidney disease and manifests as increases in parathyroid hormone levels and derangements in calcium and phosphorous metabolism. Increased PTH stimulates osteoclastic activity resulting in cortical bone resorption and marrow fibrosis. The calcium-sensing receptor on the surface of the chief cell of the parathyroid gland is the principal regulator of PTH secretion. SENSIPAR (cinacalcet hydrochloride) directly lowers PTH levels by increasing the sensitivity of the calcium sensing receptor to extracellular calcium. The reduction in PTH is associated with a concomitant decrease in serum calcium levels.

Pharmacodynamics: Reduction in iPTH levels is correlated with cinacalcet concentration. The nadir in iPTH level occurs approximately 2 to 6 hours post dose, corresponding with the C_{max} of cinacalcet. After steady state is reached, serum calcium concentrations remain constant over the dosing interval.

Pharmacokinetics: Absorption and Distribution: After oral administration of SENSIPAR, maximum plasma concentration is achieved in approximately 2 to 6 hours. The absolute bioavailability of cinacalcet is approximately 25%. Administration of SENSIPAR with food results in an approximate 50 to 80% increase in bioavailability. Increases in plasma concentrations are similar regardless of the fat content of the meal.

After absorption, cinacalcet concentrations decline in a biphasic fashion with an initial half-life of approximately 6 hours and a terminal half-life of 30 to 40 hours. Steady state drug levels are achieved within 7 days with minimal accumulation. The AUC and C_{max} of cinacalcet increase linearly over the dose range of 30 to 180 mg once daily. The pharmacokinetics of cinacalcet does not change over time. The volume of distribution is high (approximately 1000 L), indicating extensive distribution. Cinacalcet is approximately 97% bound to plasma proteins and distributes minimally into red blood cells.

Metabolism and Excretion: Cinacalcet is metabolized by multiple enzymes, primarily CYP3A4 and CYP1A2. The major circulating metabolites are inactive. After administration of a 75 mg radio-labeled dose to healthy volunteers, cinacalcet was rapidly and extensively metabolized by oxidation followed by conjugation. Renal excretion of metabolites was the prevalent route of elimination of radioactivity. Approximately 80% of the dose was recovered in the urine and 15% in the feces.

Special Populations and Conditions: Pediatrics: The pharmacokinetics of SENSIPAR have not been studied in patients <18 years of age (see Warnings and Precautions).

Geriatrics: The pharmacokinetics of SENSIPAR are similar in patients greater than, or less than, 65 years of age. No dosage adjustment based on age is necessary.

Hepatic Insufficiency: Mild hepatic impairment did not notably affect the pharmacokinetics of SENSIPAR. Compared to subjects with normal liver function, average AUC of cinacalcet was approximately 2-fold higher in subjects with moderate impairment and approximately 4-fold higher in subjects with severe impairment (see Warnings and Precautions). Because doses are titrated for each subject based on safety and efficacy parameters, no additional dose adjustment is necessary for subjects with hepatic impairment.

Renal Insufficiency: The pharmacokinetic profile of SENSIPAR in patients with mild, moderate, and severe renal insufficiency, and those on hemodialysis or peritoneal dialysis is comparable to that in healthy volunteers. No dosage adjustment based on renal function is necessary.

STORAGE AND STABILITY: Store at 15°C to 30°C.
Shelf-life: Tablets stored in bottles: 48 months.

INFORMATION FOR THE PATIENT: Published in e-CPS, available by subscription at www.e-cps.ca.

DOSAGE FORMS, COMPOSITION AND PACKAGING: 30 mg: Each light green, film-coated, oval-shaped tablet, marked with "AMG" on one side and "30" on the opposite side, contains: cinacalcet HCl 30 mg. Nonmedicinal ingredients: colloidal silicon dioxide, crospovidone, magnesium stearate, microcrystalline cellulose, povidone, pre-gelatinized starch and water. Tablets are coated with colour (Opadry II green), clear film-coat (Opadry clear), and carnauba wax. Bottles of 30.

60 mg: Each light green, film-coated, oval-shaped tablet, marked with "AMG" on one side and "60" on the opposite side, contains: cinacalcet HCl 60 mg. Nonmedicinal ingredients: colloidal silicon dioxide, crospovidone, magnesium stearate, microcrystalline cellulose, povidone, pre-gelatinized starch and water. Tablets are coated with colour (Opadry II green), clear film-coat (Opadry clear), and carnauba wax. Bottles of 30.

90 mg: Each light green, film-coated, oval-shaped tablet, marked with "AMG" on one side and "90" on the opposite side, contains: cinacalcet HCl 90 mg. Nonmedicinal ingredients: colloidal silicon dioxide, crospovidone, magnesium stearate, microcrystalline cellulose, povidone, pre-gelatinized starch and water. Tablets are coated with colour (Opadry II green), clear film-coat (Opadry clear), and carnauba wax. Bottles of 30.

Sensodyne®
potassium nitrate—sodium fluoride
Desensitizing Toothpaste with Fluoride

GlaxoSmithKline Consumer Healthcare

INDICATIONS: Specially formulated to relieve the pain of tooth sensitivity to hot, cold, sweet or sour foods or beverages as well as tactile stimulae like the bristles of a toothbrush.
Antibacterial Action: Helps remove odour-causing bacteria that can cause bad breath, with brushing.

OVERDOSE:

> For management of a suspected drug overdose, CPhA recommends that you contact your **regional Poison Control Centre**. See the *CPS* Directory section for a list of Poison Control Centres.

DOSAGE: Brush teeth thoroughly twice a day, every day. Sensodyne helps prevent the pain of dental hypersensitivity by building up a protective barrier and insulating the nerve within the tooth. With consistent use, decreased sensitivity should occur within 2 weeks. Sensodyne offers the benefits of a daily toothpaste including cavity protection, plaque removal with brushing, and a fresh mouth feeling.

SUPPLIED: Sensodyne Baking Soda Clean Toothpaste with Fluoride: Each mL of white toothpaste contains: potassium nitrate 5% and sodium fluoride 0.243% (delivers approximately 1100 ppm fluoride). Also contains baking soda and mint flavoring. Alcohol-free. Tubes of 100 mL.

Sensodyne Brilliant Whitening Toothpaste with Fluoride: Each mL of white toothpaste contains: potassium nitrate 5% and sodium fluoride 0.243% (delivers approximately 1100 ppm fluoride). Also contains mint flavoring. Alcohol-free. Tubes of 100 mL.

Sensodyne Cool Mint Gel Toothpaste with Fluoride: Each mL of blue gel contains: potassium nitrate 5% and sodium fluoride 0.24% (delivers approximately 1100 ppm fluoride). Also contains mint flavoring. Alcohol-free. Tubes of 100 mL.

Sensodyne Fresh Mint Toothpaste with Fluoride: Each mL of green toothpaste contains: potassium nitrate 5% and sodium fluoride 0.243% (delivers approximately 1100 ppm fluoride). Also contains mint flavoring. Alcohol-free. Tubes of 100 and 135 mL.

Sensodyne Ultra Fresh Toothpaste with Fluoride: Each mL of blue gel and white toothpaste contains: potassium nitrate 5% and sodium fluoride 0.243% (delivers approximately 1100 ppm fluoride). Also contains mint flavoring. Alcohol-free. Tubes of 100 mL.

Sensodyne Whitening Plus Tartar Fighting Mint Toothpaste with Fluoride: Each mL of white toothpaste contains: potassium nitrate 5% and sodium fluoride 0.243% (delivers approximately 1100 ppm fluoride). Also contains tetrapotassium pyrophosphate and mint flavoring. Alcohol-free. Tubes of 18, 100 and 135 mL.

Sensodyne-F® Iso-Active™
potassium nitrate—sodium fluoride
Desensitizing Toothpaste with Fluoride

GlaxoSmithKline Consumer Healthcare

INDICATIONS: Specially formulated to relieve the pain of tooth sensitivity to hot, cold, sweet or sour foods or beverages as well as tactile stimulae like the bristles of a toothbrush.
Antibacterial Action: Helps remove odour-causing bacteria that can cause bad breath, with brushing.

OVERDOSE:

> For management of a suspected drug overdose, CPhA recommends that you contact your **regional Poison Control Centre**. See the *CPS* Directory section for a list of Poison Control Centres.

DOSAGE: Brush teeth thoroughly twice a day, every day, as with any regular toothpaste. Sensodyne iso-active helps prevent the pain of dental hypersensitivity by building up a protective barrier and insulating the nerve within the tooth. With consistent use, decreased sensitivity should occur within 2 weeks. Sensodyne iso-active unique gel-to-foam formula penetrates hard to reach areas in between teeth and along the gum line. Sensodyne iso-active offers the benefits of a daily toothpaste including cavity protection, plaque removal with brushing, and a fresh mouth feeling.

SUPPLIED: Sensodyne iso-active Multi Action: Each mL of blue gel toothpaste contains: potassium nitrate 5% and sodium fluoride 0.254% (delivers approximately 1150 ppm fluoride). Contains mint flavoring and iso-pentane. Sodium-lauryl sulphate-, and alcohol-free. Canisters of 100 mL.

Sensodyne iso-active Whitening: Each mL of blue gel toothpaste contains: potassium nitrate 5% and sodium fluoride 0.254% (delivers approximately 1150 ppm fluoride). Contains mint flavoring, isopentane, and pentasodium triphosphate. Sodium-lauryl sulphate-, and alcohol-free. Canisters of 100 mL.

Sensodyne® Original
strontium chloride
Desensitizing Toothpaste

GlaxoSmithKline Consumer Healthcare

INDICATIONS: Specially formulated to relieve the pain of tooth sensitivity to hot, cold, sweet or sour foods or beverages as well as tactile stimulae like the bristles of a toothbrush.
Antibacterial Action: Helps remove odour-causing bacteria that can cause bad breath, with brushing.

OVERDOSE:

> For management of a suspected drug overdose, CPhA recommends that you contact your **regional Poison Control Centre**. See the *CPS* Directory section for a list of Poison Control Centres.

DOSAGE: Brush teeth thoroughly twice a day, every day. Sensodyne Original helps prevent the pain of dental hypersensitivity by forming an occlusive barrier in dentine tubules, preventing painful stimuli from reaching the nerve. Sensodyne Original offers the benefits of a daily toothpaste including fighting plaque build-up with brushing and providing a fresh mouth feeling.

SUPPLIED: Each mL of low abrasion, pink toothpaste contains: strontium chloride. Also contains mint flavouring. Alcohol-free. Tubes of 100 mL.

Sensodyne® ProNamel®
sodium fluoride—potassium nitrate
Daily Anti-cavity Toothpaste to Help Protect Enamel Against Acid Wear

GlaxoSmithKline Consumer Healthcare

INDICATIONS: To help protect teeth from the growing concern of acid wear. Everyday foods such as fruit, soft drinks, orange juice and wine contain acids that soften the enamel surface, which is then more easily worn away by brushing. As the enamel becomes thinner, teeth can visibly become less white, weaker and can become sensitive. Once enamel is worn away, it is gone for good. ProNamel from Sensodyne is specially formulated to protect enamel against acid wear. Because it contains fluoride, it also provides all the benefits of a regular daily toothpaste.

OVERDOSE:

> For management of a suspected drug overdose, CPhA recommends that you contact your **regional Poison Control Centre**. See the *CPS* Directory section for a list of Poison Control Centres.

DOSAGE: Use as your regular toothpaste, brush twice daily.
Protects teeth against acid wear.

Rehardens tooth enamel.
Suitable for people with sensitive teeth.

SUPPLIED: Sensodyne ProNamel Fresh Wave Daily Anti-cavity Toothpaste: Each mL of white toothpaste contains: potassium nitrate 5% w/w and sodium fluoride 0.254% w/w (fluoride 0.115% w/w). Also contains cocamidopropyl betaine, flavour, glycerin, hydrated silica, PEG-8, sodium hydroxide, sodium saccharin, sorbitol, titanium dioxide, water and xanthan gum. Tubes of 75 mL.
Sensodyne ProNamel Mint Essence Daily Anti-cavity Toothpaste: Each mL of white toothpaste contains: potassium nitrate 5% w/w and sodium fluoride 0.254% w/w (fluoride 0.115% w/w). Also contains cocamidopropyl betaine, flavour, glycerin, hydrated silica, PEG-8, sodium hydroxide, sodium saccharin, sorbitol, titanium dioxide, water and xanthan gum. Tubes of 75 mL.
Sensodyne ProNamel Mint Breeze Gentle Whitening Daily Anti-cavity Toothpaste: Each mL of white toothpaste contains: potassium nitrate 5% w/w and sodium fluoride 0.254% w/w (fluoride 0.115% w/w). Also contains cocamidopropyl betaine, flavour, glycerin, hydrated silica, PEG-8, sodium hydroxide, sodium saccharin, sorbitol, sucralose, titanium dioxide, water and xanthan gum. Tubes of 75 mL.

Sensodyne® ProNamel® for Children

sodium fluoride

Daily Anti-cavity Toothpaste to Help Protect Against Acid Wear and Cavities

GlaxoSmithKline Consumer Healthcare

INDICATIONS: Developed with dentists to help protect children's teeth from the growing problem of acid wear.

Everyone recognizes sugar-related tooth decay as a major issue in children's oral health. However, dentists are increasingly concerned about acid wear, caused by acids found in fruits, juices, soft drinks and other items in today's diet. Most children's permanent teeth come through between the ages of 6-13. These new teeth, as well as their baby teeth, are vulnerable to attack from acids. These acids soften the enamel, allowing it to be slowly worn away. Once enamel is gone, it is gone forever. ProNamel for Children by Sensodyne was developed in collaboration with dentists. It is a daily anti-cavity toothpaste specially formulated to strengthen the tooth enamel, and to help protect your children's teeth from acid wear as well as tooth decay. Ask your dentist.

OVERDOSE:

For management of a suspected drug overdose, CPhA recommends that you contact your **regional Poison Control Centre**. See the *CPS* Directory section for a list of Poison Control Centres.

DOSAGE: Children over 6 years of age: Brush teeth thoroughly twice daily for 2 minutes. Avoid swallowing.

Should be used as part of an oral health program that includes regular flossing, and dental check-ups. Instruct children in good brushing and rinsing habits.

Children under 6 years should use a pea-sized amount and be supervised while brushing to prevent swallowing. Speak to your dentist before using with children younger than 6 years of age.

As with all toothpastes containing fluoride, keep out of reach of children under 6 years of age. If large quantity of toothpaste is accidentally swallowed, get medical advice right away.

ProNamel for Children is specially formulated for children and does not contain an anti-sensitivity ingredient.

SUPPLIED: Each mL of white toothpaste contains: sodium fluoride 0.254% w/w (fluoride 0.115% w/w). Also contains cocamidopropyl betaine, flavour, glycerin, hydrated silica, PEG-8, sodium hydroxide, sodium saccharin, sorbitol, sucralose, titanium dioxide, water and xanthan gum. Tubes of 75 mL.

Sensorcaine®

bupivacaine HCl

Local Anesthetic

AstraZeneca

Sensorcaine® with Epinephrine

bupivacaine HCl—epinephrine

Local Anesthetic

AstraZeneca

Date of Preparation: March 2, 2000
Date of Revision: February 25, 2008

SUMMARY PRODUCT INFORMATION:

Route of Administration	Dosage Form/ Strength	Clinically Relevant Nonmedicinal Ingredients
Parenteral	Sterile Solution: 2.5 and 5 mg/mL bupivacaine HCl Solutions with epinephrine contain 5 µg/mL (1:200 000) epinephrine as bitartrate	SENSORCAINE with Epinephrine: sodium metabisulfite and citric acid (certain vial presentations, please refer to the product label) For a complete listing see Dosage Forms, Composition and Packaging.

INDICATIONS AND CLINICAL USE: Adults (>18 years of age): SENSORCAINE (bupivacaine hydrochloride) and SENSORCAINE with Epinephrine (bupivacaine hydrochloride and epinephrine) are indicated for the production of local or regional anaesthesia or analgesia with the following procedures:

- Local infiltration
- Peripheral minor or major nerve blocks
- Epidural block for surgery
- Epidural block by continuous infusion or intermittent bolus for postoperative or labour pain relief

Standard procedures for local infiltration, minor and major nerve blocks, retrobulbar block or epidural block should be observed.
Geriatrics (>65 years of age): Elderly patients should be given reduced doses commensurate with their age and physical condition.
Pediatrics (<2 years of age): Until further experience is gained in children younger than two years, administration of any presentation of bupivacaine injection in this age group is not recommended.

CONTRAINDICATIONS: SENSORCAINE (bupivacaine hydrochloride) and SENSORCAINE with Epinephrine are contraindicated:

- In patients with a hypersensitivity to bupivacaine, or to any local anaesthetic agent of the amide type, or to other components of bupivacaine injections.
- For intravenous regional anaesthesia (Bier block) since unintentional leakage of bupivacaine over the tourniquet may cause systemic toxic reactions. Cardiac arrest and death have occurred (see Dosage and Administration).
- In obstetric paracervical block anaesthesia. Use of other local anaesthetics in this technique has resulted in foetal bradycardia and death.

SENSORCAINE with Epinephrine is contraindicated in patients with a hypersensitivity to sodium metabisulfite (see Dosage Forms, Composition and Packaging).

WARNINGS AND PRECAUTIONS: General: Local anaesthetics should only be used by clinicians who are well versed in diagnosis and management of dose-related toxicity and other acute emergencies which may arise from the block to be performed, and then only after ensuring the immediate availability of cardiopulmonary resuscitative equipment, resuscitative drugs, including oxygen, and the personnel resources needed for proper management of toxic reactions and related emergencies (see Adverse Reactions and Overdosage). Delay in proper management of dose-related toxicity, underventilation from any cause and/or altered sensitivity may lead to the development of acidosis, cardiac arrest and, possibly, death.

An intravenous cannula must be inserted before the local anaesthetic is injected for nerve blocks which may result in hypotension or bradycardia, or where acute systemic toxicity may develop following inadvertent intravascular injection.

The lowest dosage of local anaesthetic that results in effective anaesthesia or analgesia should be used to avoid high plasma levels and serious adverse reactions. Injections should be made slowly or in incremental doses, with frequent aspirations before and during the injection to avoid intravascular injection.

Injection of repeated doses of local anaesthetics may cause significant increases in plasma levels with each repeated dose due to slow accumulation of the drug, or its metabolites, or to slow metabolic degradation. Tolerance to elevated blood levels varies with the physical condition of the patient.

Major peripheral nerve blocks may imply the administration of a large volume of local anaesthetic in areas of high vascularity, often close to large vessels where there is an increased risk of intravascular injection and/or rapid systemic absorption which can lead to high plasma concentrations.

SENSORCAINE with Epinephrine should not be used in areas of the body supplied by end arteries, such as digits, nose, ears or penis, or otherwise having compromised blood supply.

Local anaesthetic procedures should be carried out sufficiently away from an inflamed region. Injections should not be performed through inflamed tissue or when there is sepsis at or near the injection site.

Cardiovascular: There have been reports of cardiac arrest or death during use of bupivacaine for epidural anaesthesia or peripheral nerve blockade. In some instances, resuscitation has been difficult or impossible despite apparently adequate preparation and management.

Ventricular arrhythmia, ventricular fibrillation, sudden cardiovascular collapse and death have been reported when bupivacaine was utilized for local anaesthetic procedures that may have resulted in high systemic concentrations of bupivacaine.

Epidural anaesthesia or analgesia may lead to hypotension and bradycardia. The risk of such effects can be reduced either by preloading the circulation with crystalloidal or colloidal solutions or by injecting a vasopressor such as ephedrine 20-40 mg i.m. Hypotension should be treated promptly, e.g., with ephedrine 5-10 mg intravenously and repeated as necessary. Children should be given ephedrine doses commensurate with their age and weight.

SENSORCAINE with Epinephrine should be used with caution in patients who may have severe or untreated hypertension, ischemic heart disease, cerebral vascular insufficiency, heart block, peripheral vascular disorder and any other pathological condition that might be aggravated by the effects of epinephrine.

Local anaesthetics should be used with caution in patients with impaired cardiovascular function because they may be less able to compensate for functional changes associated with the prolongation of A-V conduction produced by amide-type local anaesthetics.

Patients with partial or complete heart block require special attention since local anaesthetics may depress myocardial conduction. To reduce the risk of potentially serious adverse reactions, attempts should be made to optimize the patient's condition before major blocks are performed. Dosage should be adjusted accordingly.

Central nerve blocks may cause cardiovascular depression, especially in the presence of hypovolemia. Epidural anaesthesia should be used with caution in patients with impaired cardiovascular function.

Endocrine and Metabolism: SENSORCAINE with Epinephrine should be used with caution in patients whose medical history and physical evaluation suggest the existence of poorly controlled hyperthyroidism or advanced diabetes.

Epidural Anaesthesia: It is recommended that a test dose be administered initially and the effects monitored before the full dose is given (see Dosage and Administration). When clinical conditions permit, the test dose should contain epinephrine (15 to 25 µg) as this amount of epinephrine, if injected into a blood vessel, is likely to produce a transient response within 45 seconds consisting of an increase in heart rate and systolic blood pressure. Patients on beta-blockers may not manifest changes in heart rate, but blood pressure monitoring can detect an evanescent rise in systolic blood pressure.

During epidural administration, bupivacaine should be administered in incremental doses of 3 to 5 mL with sufficient time between doses to detect toxic manifestations of unintentional intravascular or intrathecal injection. Frequent aspirations for blood or cerebrospinal fluid (where applicable, i.e., when using a "continuous" intermittent catheter technique), should be performed before and during each supplemental injection because plastic tubing in the epidural space can migrate into a blood vessel or through the dura. A negative aspiration, however, does not ensure against an intravascular or intrathecal injection.

Injection in Head and Neck Area: Inadvertent intravascular or subarachnoid injection of small doses of local anaesthetics injected into the head and neck area, including retrobulbar, dental and stellate ganglion blocks, may produce adverse reactions similar to systemic toxicity seen with unintentional intravascular injections of larger doses. The injection procedures require the utmost care. Confusion, convulsions, respiratory depression and/or respiratory arrest, and cardiovascular stimulation or depression leading to cardiac arrest, have been reported. These reactions may be due to intra-arterial injection of the local anaesthetic with retrograde flow to the cerebral circulation. Patients receiving these blocks should remain under constant observation and monitoring for their cardiac and pulmonary functions. Resuscitative equipment and personnel for treating adverse reactions should be immediately available. Dosage recommendations should not be exceeded (see Dosage and Administration).

Ophthalmic Surgery: Retrobulbar injections may very occasionally reach the cranial subarachnoid space causing temporary blindness, cardiovascular collapse, apnoea, convulsions, etc. These reactions, which may be due to intra-arterial injection or direct injection into the central nervous system via the sheaths of the optic nerve, must be diagnosed and treated promptly.

Clinicians who perform retrobulbar blocks should be aware that there have been reports of respiratory arrest following local anaesthetic injection. Prior to retrobulbar block, as with all other regional procedures, the immediate availability of equipment, drugs, and personnel to manage respiratory arrest or depression, convulsions, and cardiac stimulation or depression should be assured (see Warnings and precautions, Injection in Head and Neck Area).

Retrobulbar injections of local anaesthetics carry a low risk of persistent ocular muscle dysfunction. The primary causes include trauma and/or local toxic effects on muscles and/or nerves. The severity of such tissue reactions is related to the degree of trauma, the concentration of the local anaesthetic and the duration of exposure of the tissue to the local anaesthetic. For this reason, as with all local anaesthetics, the lowest effective concentration and dose of local anaesthetic should be used. Vasoconstrictors, and other additives may aggravate tissue reactions and should be used only when indicated.

Hepatic/Biliary/Pancreatic: Because amide-type local anaesthetics such as bupivacaine are metabolized by the liver, these drugs, especially repeat doses, should be used cautiously in patients with hepatic disease. Patients with severe hepatic disease, because of their inability to metabolize local anaesthetics normally, are at a greater risk of developing toxic plasma concentrations.

Peri-Operative Considerations: It is essential that aspiration for blood or cerebrospinal fluid (where applicable) be done prior to injecting any local anaesthetic, for both the original dose and all subsequent doses, to avoid intravascular or subarachnoid injection. However, a negative aspiration does not ensure against an intravascular or subarachnoid injection.

The safety and effectiveness of local anaesthetics depend on proper dosage, correct technique, adequate precautions and readiness for emergencies. Regional or local anaesthetic procedures should always be performed in a properly equipped and staffed area.

Resuscitative equipment and resuscitative drugs, including oxygen, should be available for immediate use (see Warnings and Precautions; Adverse Reactions and Overdosage).

During major regional nerve blocks, the patients should be in an optimal condition and have i.v. fluids running via an indwelling catheter to assure a functioning intravenous pathway. The clinician responsible should have adequate and appropriate training in the procedure to be performed, should take the necessary precautions to avoid intravascular injection (see Dosage and Administration), and should be familiar with the diagnosis and treatment of side effects, systemic toxicity and other complications (see Adverse Reactions and Overdosage).

Careful and constant monitoring of cardiovascular and respiratory vital signs (adequacy of ventilation) and the patient's state of consciousness should be performed after each local anaesthetic injection. It should be kept in mind at such times that restlessness, anxiety, incoherent speech, lightheadedness, numbness and tingling of the mouth and lips, metallic taste, tinnitus, dizziness, blurred vision, tremors, twitching, depression, or drowsiness may be early warning signs of central nervous system toxicity.

Renal: Local anaesthetics should be used with caution in patients in poor general condition due to severe renal dysfunction although regional anaesthesia is frequently indicated in these patients.

Hyper-Sensitivity: SENSORCAINE with Epinephrine contains sodium metabisulfite, that may cause allergic reactions including anaphylactic or anaphylactoid reactions or asthmatic episodes in susceptible people. The overall prevalence of sulfite sensitivity in the general population is unknown and probably low. Sulfite sensitivity is seen more frequently in asthmatic than in non-asthmatic people.

Special Populations: Debilitated and acutely ill patients should be given reduced doses commensurate with their age and physical condition.

Pregnant Women: There are no adequate and well-controlled studies in pregnant women of the effect of bupivacaine on the developing foetus.

Bupivacaine has been used in a large number of pregnant women and women of childbearing age for surgical, gynaecological, or obstetric procedures. No specific disturbances to the reproductive process have so far been reported, e.g., no increased incidence of malformations.

However, bupivacaine should be used during pregnancy only if the potential benefit justifies the potential risk to the foetus. This does not exclude the use of bupivacaine at term for obstetrical anaesthesia or analgesia.

Labour and Delivery: SENSORCAINE/SENSORCAINE with Epinephrine 0.25% and 0.5% can be used at term for obstetrical anaesthesia or analgesia.

Local anaesthetics rapidly cross the placenta, and when used for epidural block anaesthesia, can cause varying degrees of maternal, foetal and neonatal toxicity (see Action and Clinical Pharmacology). The incidence and degree of toxicity depend upon the procedure performed, the type and amount of drug used, and the technique of drug administration. Adverse reactions in the parturient, foetus and neonate involve alterations of the central nervous system, peripheral vascular tone and cardiac function.

Maternal hypotension has resulted from regional anaesthesia (see Warnings and Precautions, Cardiovascular). Local anaesthetics produce vasodilation by blocking sympathetic nerves. It is extremely important to avoid aortocaval compression by the gravid uterus during administration of regional block to parturients. Elevating the patient's legs and positioning her on her left side will help prevent decreases in blood pressure. The foetal heart rate also should be monitored continuously, and electronic foetal monitoring is highly advisable.

Epidural anaesthesia may alter the forces of parturition through changes in uterine contractility or maternal expulsive efforts. Epidural anaesthesia has been reported to prolong the second stage of labour by removing the parturient's urge to bear down or by interfering with motor function. The use of SENSORCAINE 0.25% has been shown to interfere less than the 0.5% solution. Obstetrical anaesthesia may increase the need for forceps assistance.

The addition of epinephrine may potentially decrease uterine blood flow and contractility, especially after inadvertent injection into maternal blood vessels.

Nursing Women: Bupivacaine is excreted in the breast milk, but in such small quantities that there is generally no risk of affecting the infant at therapeutic doses. It is not known whether epinephrine enters breast milk or not, but it is unlikely to affect the breast-fed infant.

Pediatrics: Until further experience is gained in children younger than two years, administration of any presentation of bupivacaine injection in this age group is not recommended.

Geriatrics: Elderly patients should be given reduced doses commensurate with their age and physical condition.

ADVERSE REACTIONS: Reactions to bupivacaine bupivacaine are characteristic of those associated with other local-acting anaesthetics of the amide type.

Adverse reactions to local anaesthetics are very rare in the absence of overdose or inadvertent intravascular injection. The effects of systemic overdose and unintentional intravascular injections can be serious, but should be distinguished from the physiological effects of the nerve block itself (e.g. a decrease in blood pressure and bradycardia during epidural anaesthesia). Neurological damage, caused directly (e.g. nerve trauma) or indirectly (e.g. epidural abscess) by the needle puncture, is a rare but well recognized consequence of regional, and particularly epidural anaesthesia.

The most commonly encountered acute adverse experiences that demand immediate management are related to the central nervous system and the cardiovascular system. These adverse experiences are generally dose-related and due to high plasma levels which may result from overdosage (see Overdosage), rapid absorption from the injection site, diminished tolerance or from inadvertent intravascular injection. In addition to systemic dose-related toxicity, unintentional subarachnoid injection of drug during the intended performance of caudal or lumbar epidural block or nerve blocks near the vertebral column (especially in the head and neck region) may result in underventilation or apnoea ("Total or High Spinal"). Also, hypotension due to loss of sympathetic tone and respiratory paralysis or underventilation due to cephalad extension of the motor level of anaesthesia may occur. This may lead to secondary cardiac arrest if untreated.

Central Nervous System: These are characterized by excitation and/or depression. Restlessness, anxiety, dizziness, tinnitus, blurred vision or tremors may occur, possibly proceeding to convulsions. However, excitement may be transient or absent, with depression being the first manifestation of an adverse reaction. This may quickly be followed by drowsiness merging into unconsciousness and respiratory arrest. Other central nervous system effects may be nausea, vomiting, chills, paraesthesia, numbness of the tongue, hyperacousis, lightheadedness, dysarthria and constriction of the pupils.

Cardiovascular System: High doses or unintentional intravascular injection may lead to high plasma levels and related depression of the myocardium, decreased cardiac output, heart block, hypotension, bradycardia, hypertension, ventricular arrhythmias, including ventricular tachycardia and ventricular fibrillation, and cardiac arrest. Reactions due to systemic absorption may be either slow or rapid in onset. Cardiovascular collapse and cardiac arrest can occur rapidly (see Warnings and Precautions, Cardiovascular and Overdosage).

Allergic: Allergic type reactions are rare (<0.1%) and may occur as a result of sensitivity to local anaesthetics of the amide type. These reactions are characterized by signs such as urticaria, pruritus, erythema, angioneurotic oedema (including laryngeal oedema), tachycardia, sneezing, nausea, vomiting, dizziness, syncope, excessive sweating, elevated temperature, and in the most severe instances, anaphylactic shock.

Neurologic: The incidence of adverse neurologic reactions may be related to the total dose of local anaesthetic administered but is also dependent upon the particular drug used, the route of administration and the physical condition of the patient. Nerve trauma, neuropathy, urinary retention, diplopia and spinal cord dysfunction (e.g., anterior spinal artery syndrome, arachnoiditis, cauda equina syndrome, in rare cases paresis and paraplegia), have been associated with regional anaesthesia. Neurological effects may be related to local anaesthetic techniques, with or without a contribution from the drug.

High or Total Spinal Blockade: In the practice of caudal or lumbar epidural block, occasional unintentional penetration of the subarachnoid space by the catheter may occur, resulting in High or Total Spinal Blockage. Subsequent adverse effects may depend partially on the amount of drug administered subdurally.

Extensive loss of motor and sensory functions, loss of consciousness, and cardiovascular and respiratory depression may happen. The cardiovascular depression is caused by extensive sympathetic blockade which may result in profound hypotension and bradycardia, or even cardiac arrest. Respiratory depression is caused by blockade of the innervation of the respiratory muscles, including the diaphragm.

DRUG INTERACTIONS: Drug-Drug Interactions: See Warnings and Precautions concerning solutions containing a vasoconstrictor.

Bupivacaine should be used cautiously in persons with known drug allergies or sensitivities.

Local Anaesthetics and Agents Structurally Related to Amide-type Local Anaesthetics: Bupivacaine should be used with caution in patients receiving other amide-type local anaesthetics such as lidocaine, ropivacaine, mepivicaine and prilocaine since the toxic effects are additive.

Antiarrhythmic Drugs: Bupivacaine should also be used with caution with structurally related agents such as the antiarrhythmics, procainamide, disopyramide, tocainide, mexiletine and flecainide.

Class III Antiarrhythmic Drugs: Specific interaction studies with bupivacaine and class III anti-arrhythmic drugs (e.g. amiodarone) have not been performed, but caution is advised. Patients being treated with class III anti-arrhythmic drugs should be under close surveillance and ECG monitoring since cardiac affects may be additive.

Ergot-containing Drugs: Bupivacaine with epinephrine or other vasopressors or vasoconstrictors should not be used concomitantly with ergot-type oxytocic drugs, because a severe persistent hypertension may occur and cerebrovascular and cardiac accidents are possible.

Monoamine Oxidase (MAO) Inhibitors : Bupivacaine with epinephrine or other vasopressors or vasoconstrictors should be used with extreme caution in patients receiving monoamine oxidase inhibitors (MAO) because severe prolonged hypertension may result. In situations when concurrent therapy is necessary, careful patient monitoring is essential.

Antidepressants (triptyline, imipramine): Bupivacaine with epinephrine or other vasopressors or vasoconstrictors should be used with extreme caution in patients receiving antidepressants of the triptyline or imipramine types because severe prolonged hypertension may result. In situations when concurrent therapy is necessary, careful patient monitoring is essential.

Neuroleptics (phenothiazines) : Neuroleptics such as phenothiazines may oppose the vasoconstrictor effects of epinephrine resulting in hypotensive responses and tachycardia.

Sedatives: If sedatives are used to reduce patient apprehension, they should be used in reduced doses, since local anaesthetic agents, like sedatives, are central nervous system depressants which in combination may have an additive effect.

General Anaesthetics-inhalation Agents (halothane, enflurane): Solutions containing epinephrine should be used with caution in patients undergoing general anaesthesia with inhalation agents such as halothane and enflurane, due to the risk of serious dose-related cardiac arrhythmias. In deciding whether to use these products concurrently in the same patient, the combined action of both agents upon the myocardium, the concentration and volume of vasoconstrictor used, and the time since injection, when applicable, should be taken into account.

Prior use of chloroprocaine, or any other local anaesthetic, may interfere with subsequent use of bupivacaine. Because of this, and because safety of intercurrent use with bupivacaine and other local anaesthetics has not been established, such use is not recommended.

H_2-antagonists: The H_2-antagonists cimetidine and ranitidine have been shown to reduce the clearance of bupivacaine; ranitidine to a lesser degree than cimetidine. Concomitant administration may increase likelihood of toxicity of bupivacaine.

Non-selective Beta-blockers: Non-selective beta-blockers such as propranolol enhance the pressor effects of epinephrine, which may lead to severe hypertension and bradycardia.

Drug-Food Interactions: Interactions of bupivicaine with food have not been established.

Drug-Herb Interactions: Interactions of bupivicaine with herbal products have not been established.

Drug-Laboratory Test Interactions: Interactions of bupivicaine with laboratory tests have not been established.

Drug-Lifestyle Interactions: Interactions of bupivacaine with lifestyle have not been established.

DOSAGE AND ADMINISTRATION:

Dosing Considerations: General: The dosage varies and depends upon the area to be anaesthetized, the number of neuronal segments to be blocked, the depth of anaesthesia and degree of muscle relaxation required, individual tolerance, tissue vascularity, and the technique of anaesthesia. The lowest concentration of anaesthetic and the lowest dosage needed to provide effective anaesthesia should be administered. The rapid injection of a large volume of local anaesthetic solution should be avoided and fractional doses should be used when feasible. In general, complete block of all nerve fibres in large nerves requires the higher concentrations of drug. In smaller nerves, or when a less intense block is required (e.g., in the relief of labour pain), the lower concentrations are indicated. The volume of drug used will affect the extent of spread of anaesthesia.

The use of bupivacaine with epinephrine will prolong the anaesthetic action.

Special Populations: Local anaesthetics should be used with caution in patients in poor general condition due to aging or other compromising factors such as advanced liver disease or severe renal dysfunction although regional anaesthesia is frequently indicated in these patients.

Debilitated, elderly patients and acutely ill patients should be given reduced doses commensurate with their age and physical condition.

Recommended Dose and Dosage Adjustment: Adults: The dosages in Table 1 are recommended as a guide for use in the average adult for the more commonly used techniques. The clinician's experience and knowledge of the patient's physical condition are of importance in calculating the required dose.

When prolonged blocks are used, the risks of reaching a toxic plasma concentration or inducing a local neural injury must be considered. The maximum dosage limit must be determined by evaluating the size and physical condition of the patient and considering the usual rate of systemic absorption from a specific injection site. Experience to date indicates that 400 mg administered over 24 hours is well tolerated in average adults. Until further experience is gained, this dose should not be exceeded in 24 hours.

In order to avoid intravascular injection, aspiration should be repeated prior to and during administration of the main dose, which should be injected slowly or in incremental doses, at a rate of 25-50 mg/min, while closely observing the patient's vital functions and maintaining verbal contact. An inadvertent intravascular injection may be recognized by a temporary increase in heart rate and an accidental intrathecal injection by signs of a spinal block. If toxic symptoms occur, the injection should be stopped immediately.

Children: Until further experience is gained, bupivacaine is not recommended for children younger than two years of age.

For bolus administration or intermittent injections, unless stated otherwise (see Table 2), a dose of up to 2 mg/kg of SENSORCAINE or SENSORCAINE with Epinephrine is recommended. The dose administered will depend on the age and body weight of the patient, the site of surgery, and the condition of the patient. The addition of epinephrine will prolong the duration of the block by 50-100%.

Use in Epidural Anaesthesia: When an epidural dose is to be injected, a test dose of a local anaesthetic is recommended (see Warnings and Precautions). SENSORCAINE 0.5% with Epinephrine (Table 1), or 3-5 mL lidocaine (Xylocaine 1-2%) with epinephrine, can be used if a vasoconstrictor is not contraindicated. Verbal contact and repeated monitoring of heart rate and blood pressure should be maintained for five minutes after the test dose. In the absence of signs of subarachnoid or intravascular injection, the main dose may be given.

During epidural administration, bupivacaine should be administered slowly in incremental doses of 3 to 5 mL, with sufficient time between doses to detect toxic manifestations of unintentional intravascular or intrathecal injection.

OVERDOSAGE:

Acute systemic toxicity from local anaesthetics is generally related to high plasma levels encountered during therapeutic use, or to unintended subarachnoid or intravascular injection, exceptionally rapid absorption from highly vascularized areas or overdosage and originates mainly in the central nervous and the cardiovascular systems (see Adverse Reactions and Warnings and Precautions). Central nervous system reactions are similar for all amide local anaesthetics, while cardiac reactions are more dependent on the drug, both quantitatively and qualitatively.

Table 1: SENSORCAINE/SENSORCAINE with Epinephrine

Dosage Recommendations in Adults for SENSORCAINE/SENSORCAINE with Epinephrine Isotonic Solutions

Type of Block	Conc. (%)	Each Dose[a] (mL)	(mg)	Onset (min)	Duration (h) Without Epinephrine	Indication
Local Infiltration	0.25	up to 60[b]	up to 150[b]	1–3	3–4	Surgical operations and postoperative analgesia
	0.5	up to 30[b]	up to 150[b]	1–3	4–8	
Epidural	0.5[c]	3–5	15–25			Test dose
Lumbar Epidural	0.25	6–15	15–37.5	2–5	1–2	Labor and postoperative pain relief
	0.5	15–30	75–150	15–30	2–3	Surgical operations including Cesarean Section
Thoracic Epidural	0.25	5–15	12.5–37.5	10–15	1.5–2	Surgical operations
	0.5	5–10	25–50	10–15	2–3	
Caudal Epidural	0.25	20–30	50–75	20–30	1–2	Pain relief and diagnostic use
	0.5	20–30	100–150	15–30	2–3	Surgical operations and postoperative analgesia
Intercostal (per nerve)	0.5	2–3	10–15	3–5	4–8	Pain relief for surgery, postoperative and trauma
Brachial Plexus	0.5	30	150	15–30	4–8	Surgical operations
Sciatic	0.5	10–20	50–100	15–30	4–8	Surgical operations
Digital[d]	0.25	1–5	2.5–12.5	2–5	3–4	Surgical operations

(cont'd)

Table 1: SENSORCAINE/SENSORCAINE with Epinephrine *(cont'd)*

Dosage Recommendations in Adults for SENSORCAINE/SENSORCAINE with Epinephrine Isotonic Solutions

Type of Block	Conc. (%)	Each Dose[a] (mL)	(mg)	Onset (min)	Duration (h) Without Epinephrine	Indication
Peripheral Nerves	0.25	up to 40[b]	up to 100[b]	10–20	3–5	Therapeutic (pain relief)
	0.5	up to 30[b]	up to 150[b]	5–10	4–8	Surgical operations
Sympathetic[e]						Ischemic conditions or sympathetic maintained pains e.g., visceral pain conditions such as pancreatitis or cancer, pain of herpes zoster
Stellate Block	0.25	5–15	12.5–37.5	10–20	3–6	
Lumbar	0.25	10–20	25–50	10–20	3–6	
Paravertebral Block						
Coeliac Plexus Block	0.25	20–40	50–100	10–20	3–6	

[a] For epidural blocks, dose includes test dose.
[b] No more than 400 mg in 24 hours.
[c] With epinephrine 1:200 000 (5 µg/mL).
[d] Without epinephrine.
[e] See Warnings and Precautions.

Table 2: SENSORCAINE/SENSORCAINE with Epinephrine

Dosage Recommendations in Children (Over 2 Years of Age) for SENSORCAINE/SENSORCAINE with Epinephrine Isotonic Solutions

Type of Block	Conc. (%)	Each Dose mL/kg	Each Dose mg/kg
Local Infiltration	0.25 0.5	up to 0.8 up to 0.4	up to 2 up to 2
Caudal Epidural[c]			
Lumbosacral	0.25	0.5	1.25[d]
Thoracolumbar	0.25	0.6–1.0	1.5–2.5[d]
Lumbar Epidural	0.25 0.5	0.5–1.0 0.3–0.5	1.25–2.5 1.5–2.5
Dorsal (Penile)	0.25[a] 0.5[a]	0.1–0.2 0.1–0.2	0.25–0.5 0.5–1.0
Intercostal	0.25[b] 0.5[b]	0.8–1.2 0.4–0.6	2–3 2–3

[a] Without epinephrine.
[b] With epinephrine 1:200 000 (5 µg/mL).
[c] Consider both age and weight for calculation of dosages.
[d] Onset: 20–30 minutes, Duration: 2–6 hours.
Note: The use of SENSORCAINE/SENSORCAINE with Epinephrine for anaesthesia and/or analgesia may be supplementary to light general anaesthesia.

Symptoms: Accidental intravascular injections of local anaesthetics may cause immediate (within seconds to a few minutes) systemic toxic reactions. In the event of overdose, systemic toxicity appears later (15-60 minutes after injection) due to the slower increase in local anaesthetic blood concentration.

Central nervous system toxicity is a graded response with symptoms and signs of escalating severity. The first symptoms are usually circumoral paresthesia, numbness of the tongue, lightheadedness, hyperacousis, tinnitus and visual disturbances. Dysarthria, muscular twitching or tremors are more serious and precede the onset of generalized convulsions. These signs must not be mistaken for a neurotic behaviour. Unconsciousness and grand mal convulsions may follow which may last from a few seconds to several minutes. Hypoxia and hypercarbia occur rapidly following convulsions due to the increased muscular activity, together with the interference with normal respiration and loss of the airway. In severe cases apnoea may occur. Acidosis, hyperkalaemia, hypocalcaemia and hypoxia increase and extend the toxic effects of local anaesthetics.

Recovery is due to redistribution and subsequent metabolism and excretion of the local anaesthetic drug. Recovery may be rapid unless large amounts of the drug have been administered.

Cardiovascular system toxicity may be seen in severe cases and is generally preceded by signs of toxicity in the central nervous system. In patients under heavy sedation or receiving a general anaesthetic, prodromal CNS symptoms may be absent. Hypotension, bradycardia, arrhythmia and even cardiac arrest may occur as a result of high systemic concentrations of local anaesthetics, but in rare cases cardiac arrest has occurred without prodromal CNS effects.

Cardiovascular toxic reactions are usually related to depression of the conduction system of the heart and myocardium, leading to decreased cardiac output, hypotension, heart block, bradycardia and sometimes ventricular arrhythmias, including ventricular tachycardia, ventricular fibrillation and cardiac arrest.

In children, early signs of local anaesthetic toxicity may be difficult to detect in cases where the block is given during general anaesthesia.

Treatment: The first consideration is prevention, best accomplished by careful and constant monitoring of cardiovascular and respiratory vital signs and the patient's state of consciousness after each local anaesthetic injection. At the first sign of change, oxygen should be administered. If signs of acute systemic toxicity appear, injection of the local anaesthetic should be immediately stopped.

The first step in the management of systemic toxic reactions, as well as underventilation or apnoea due to unintentional subarachnoid injection of drug solution, consists of immediate attention to the establishment and maintenance of a patent airway and assisted or controlled ventilation with 100% oxygen and a delivery system capable of permitting immediate positive airway pressure by mask or endotracheal intubation. This may prevent convulsions if they have not already occurred.

If necessary, use drugs to control the convulsions. An anticonvulsant should be given i.v. if the convulsions do not stop spontaneously in 15-20 seconds. Thiopental 1-3 mg/kg i.v. will control the convulsions rapidly. Alternatively diazepam 0.1 mg/kg body weight (bw) i.v. may be used, although its action will be slower. Prolonged convulsions may jeopardize the patient's ventilation and oxygenation. Therefore, early endotracheal intubation must be considered in such situations. Injection of a muscle relaxant (e.g. succinylcholine 1 mg/kg bw) will facilitate endotracheal intubation, controlled ventilation, and secure optimal oxygenation.

If cardiovascular depression is evident (hypotension, bradycardia), ephedrine 5-10 mg i.v. should be given and may be repeated, if necessary, after 2-3 minutes. Children should be given ephedrine doses commensurate with their age and weight.

Should circulatory arrest occur, immediate cardiopulmonary resuscitation should be instituted. Optimal oxygenation and ventilation and circulatory support as well as treatment of acidosis are of vital importance, since hypoxia and acidosis will increase the systemic toxicity of local anaesthetics. Epinephrine (0.1-0.2 mg intravenous or intracardial injections) should be given as soon as possible and repeated, if necessary. A successful resuscitation may require prolonged efforts.

The supine position is dangerous in pregnant women at term because of aortocaval compression by the gravid uterus. Therefore, during treatment of systemic toxicity, maternal hypotension or foetal bradycardia following regional block, the parturient should be maintained in the left lateral decubitus position if possible, or manual displacement of the uterus off the great vessels should be accomplished. Resuscitation of obstetrical patients may take longer than resuscitation of nonpregnant patients and closed-chest cardiac compression may be ineffective. Rapid delivery of the foetus may improve the response to resuscitative efforts.

If cardiac arrest should occur, a successful outcome may require prolonged resuscitative efforts.

For management of a suspected drug overdose, CPhA recommends that you contact your **regional Poison Control Centre**. See the *CPS* Directory section for a list of Poison Control Centres.

ACTION AND CLINICAL PHARMACOLOGY: Bupivacaine is a long-acting, amide-type local anaesthetic with both anaesthetic and analgesic effects. At high doses it produces surgical anaesthesia, while at lower doses it produces sensory block (analgesia) with less pronounced motor block.

Mechanism of Action: As with other local anaesthetics, bupivacaine causes a reversible blockade of impulse propagation along nerve fibres by preventing the inward movement of sodium ions through the cell membrane of the nerve fibres. The sodium channel of the nerve membrane is considered a receptor for local anaesthetic molecules.

Onset and Duration of Action: As with other local anaesthetics, the onset and duration of action depends on the injection site, the route of administration and the concentration and volume of anaesthetic (see Dosage and Administration, Recommended Dose and Dosage Adjustment, Adults, Table 1). It has also been noted that there is a period of analgesia that persists after the return of sensation, during which time the need for potent analgesics is reduced. The presence of epinephrine may prolong the duration of action for infiltration and peripheral nerve blocks but has less marked effect on epidural blocks.

SENSORCAINE 0.5% has a long duration of action of 2-5 hours following a single epidural injection and up to 12 hours after peripheral nerve blocks. The onset of blockade is slower than with lidocaine, especially when anaesthetizing large nerves. When used in low concentrations, i.e., 0.25%, there is less effect on motor nerve fibres and the duration of action is shorter.

Hemodynamics: Bupivacaine, like other local anaesthetics, may also have effects on other excitable membranes e.g. in the brain and myocardium. If excessive amounts of drug reach the systemic circulation rapidly, symptoms and signs of toxicity will appear, emanating mainly from the central nervous and cardiovascular systems.

Central nervous system toxicity (see Overdosage) usually precedes the cardiovascular effects as central nervous system toxicity occurs at lower plasma concentrations. Direct effects of local anaesthetics on the heart include slow conduction, negative inotropism and eventually cardiac arrest.

Indirect cardiovascular effects (hypotension, bradycardia) may occur after epidural administration depending on the extent of the concomitant sympathetic block.

Pharmacokinetics: Absorption: The plasma concentration of local anaesthetics is dependent upon the dose, the route of administration, the patient's hemodynamic/circulatory condition, and the vascularity of the injection site. The addition of epinephrine to bupivacaine may decrease the peak plasma concentration, whereas the time to peak plasma concentration usually is little affected. The effect varies with the type of block, dose and concentration.

Peak levels of bupivacaine in the blood are reached in 20 to 45 minutes, depending on injection site and type of block. A decline to insignificant levels is achieved during the next three to six hours. Intercostal blocks give the highest peak plasma concentration due to a rapid absorption (maximum plasma concentrations in the order of 1-4 mg/L after a 400 mg dose), while subcutaneous abdominal injections give the lowest plasma concentration. Epidural and major plexus blocks are intermediate. In children, rapid absorption and high plasma concentrations (in the order of 1-1.5 mg/L after a dose of 3 mg/kg) are seen with caudal block.

Bupivacaine shows complete, biphasic absorption from the epidural space with plasma half-lives in the order of seven minutes after initial administration, slowing to six hours over time. The slow absorption is rate-limiting in the elimination of bupivacaine, which explains why the apparent elimination half-life after epidural administration is longer than after intravenous administration.

Distribution: Bupivacaine has a total plasma clearance of 0.58 L/min a volume of distribution at steady state of 73 L.

Bupivacaine readily crosses the placenta and equilibrium in regard to the unbound concentration is rapidly reached. The degree of plasma protein binding in the foetus is less than in the mother, which results in lower total plasma concentrations in the foetus than in the mother. The free concentration, however, is the same in both mother and foetus.

In adults the protein-binding capacity of bupivacaine is high at 96%. Generally, the lower the plasma concentration of drug, the higher the percentage of drug bound to plasma proteins. Bupivacaine is mainly bound to alpha-1-acid glycoprotein.

An increase in total plasma concentration has been observed during continuous epidural infusion for postoperative pain relief. This is related to a postoperative increase in alpha-1-acid glycoprotein. The unbound, i.e. pharmacologically active, concentration is similar before and after surgery.

Metabolism: Bupivacaine is extensively metabolized in the liver predominantly by aromatic hydroxylation to 4-hydroxy-bupivacaine and N-dealkylation to 2,6-pipecoloxylidine (PPX), both mediated by cytochrome P450 3A4.

Excretion: The terminal half-life of bupivacaine in adults is 2.7 hours, and in neonates it is prolonged up to eight hours. Bupivacaine has an intermediate hepatic extraction ratio of 0.38 after i.v. administration. In children between 1 to 7 years the pharmacokinetics are similar to those in adults. The elderly may have a prolonged half-life.

The kidney is the main excretory organ for most local anaesthetics and their metabolites. About 1% of bupivacaine is excreted in the urine as unchanged drug in 24 h and approximately 5% as PPX. The plasma concentrations of PPX and 4-hydroxy-bupivacaine during and after continuous administration of bupivacaine are low as compared to the parent drug.

Clearance of bupivacaine is almost entirely due to liver metabolism and more sensitive to changes in intrinsic hepatic enzyme function than to liver perfusion.

STORAGE AND STABILITY: Store SENSORCAINE (bupivacaine hydrochloride) and SENSORCAINE with Epinephrine at 15-30°C. Do not freeze. Protect SENSORCAINE with Epinephrine from light. Do not use if solution is coloured or contains a precipitate.

SPECIAL HANDLING INSTRUCTIONS: SENSORCAINE (bupivacaine hydrochloride) solutions in glass vials may be autoclaved for 15-20 minutes at 121°C. Due to the nature of the Polyamp system, the plastic ampoules must not be autoclaved.

Due to the heat sensitivity of epinephrine, products containing epinephrine must not be autoclaved.

SENSORCAINE/SENSORCAINE with Epinephrine are without preservative and are for single use only. Discard unused portion.

Adequate precautions should be taken to avoid prolonged contact between local anaesthetic solutions containing epinephrine (low pH) and metal surfaces (e.g., needles or metal parts of syringes), since dissolved metal ions, particularly copper ions, may cause severe local irritation (swelling, oedema) at the site of injection and accelerate the degradation of epinephrine.

INFORMATION FOR THE PATIENT: Published in e-CPS, available by subscription at www.e-cps.ca.

DOSAGE FORMS, COMPOSITION AND PACKAGING: SENSORCAINE: Each mL of sterile, isotonic solution contains: bupivacaine HCl 2.5 mg (0.25%) or 5 mg (0.5%). Nonmedicinal ingredients: sodium chloride, sodium hydroxide and/or hydrochloric acid and water for injection. pH is 4.0 to 6.5. Single use vials of 20 mL. Polyamp Duofit (plastic ampoules suitable for Luer fit and Luer lock syringes) of 10 mL.

SENSORCAINE with Epinephrine (1:200 000): Each mL of sterile, isotonic solution contains: bupivacaine HCl 2.5 mg (0.25%) or 5 mg (0.5%) and epinephrine 5 µg (1:200 000). Nonmedicinal ingredients: citric acid (certain vial presentations), sodium chloride, sodium hydroxide and/or hydrochloric acid, sodium metabisulfite and water for injection. pH is 3.3. to 5.5. Single use vials of 20 mL.

SENSORCAINE and SENSORCAINE with Epinephrine are sterile isotonic solutions (see Table 3 for availability).

The pK_a of bupivacaine (8.1) is similar to that of lidocaine. However, bupivacaine possesses a greater degree of lipid solubility and is protein bound (95%) to a greater extent than lidocaine (64%).

The solubility of bupivacaine is limited at pH >6.5. This must be taken into consideration when alkaline solutions, i.e., carbonates, are added since precipitation might occur. In the case of epinephrine-containing solutions, mixing with alkaline solutions may cause rapid degradation of epinephrine.

Table 3: SENSORCAINE/SENSORCAINE with Epinephrine
Availability of SENSORCAINE and SENSORCAINE with Epinephrine

SENSORCAINE (bupivacaine hydrochloride) Concentration	Epinephrine Dilution (if present)	Polyamp Duofit (plastic ampoules)[a] (mL) 10	Single-Use Vials (mL) 20
0.25%			•
0.25%	1:200 000[b]		•
0.5%		•	
0.5%	1:200 000[b]		•

[a] Plastic ampoules suitable for Luer fit and Luer lock syringes.
[b] Contains sodium metabisulfite as an antioxidant.

Vials are supplied in units of 10 and polyethylene Polyamp Duofit in units of 50.

Septra® Injection ℞

sulfamethoxazole—trimethoprim

Antibacterial

GlaxoSmithKline

Date of Revision: November 27, 2008

PHARMACOLOGY: SEPTRA (sulfamethoxazole and trimethoprim) is an antibacterial agent with a wide spectrum of activity. It contains two active antibacterial components, sulfamethoxazole and trimethoprim, which act synergistically on many species of bacteria.

Sulfamethoxazole and trimethoprim act sequentially in two successive steps in the biosynthesis of nucleic acids. Trimethoprim is an inhibitor of dihydrofolate reductase, the enzyme which reduces dihydrofolic acid to its tetrahydro form. This biochemical step is essential in the production of the folate coenzymes which are involved in the biosynthesis of thymine, purine, serine and methionine. Sulfamethoxazole exerts its antibacterial activity by competing with para-aminobenzoic acid.

Most pathogenic bacteria meet their need for dihydrofolic acid by synthesizing it from para-aminobenzoic acid, pteridine and glutamic acid. Animals, in contrast, depend on exogenous sources for their needs of folic acid and do not rely upon intracellular synthesis.

Under usual circumstances, sulfamethoxazole or trimethoprim acting alone do not produce complete block in this biosynthesis of nucleic acids. Instead, they cause sufficient reduction in the synthesis of folate coenzymes to produce bacteriostasis. When the two agents act together, the superimposition of their effects produces a complete block in the synthesis, leading to death of the organism. Thus the effect of the dual action is to reduce the minimum inhibitory concentrations (MIC) of each agent (synergism) and to convert a bacteriostatic action to a bactericidal action.

The activity of SEPTRA therefore depends upon the ability of both sulfamethoxazole and trimethoprim to affect the folate metabolism of the bacterium; however, for SEPTRA to be therapeutic it must not affect the folate metabolism of the host. Since sulfamethoxazole affects only the de novo synthesis of dihydrofolic acid by bacteria, it does not affect folate metabolism of animals. Since in animals, as in bacteria, the folates have to be recycled to the active form by dihydrofolate reductase, trimethoprim could be expected to affect mammalian folate metabolism. Trimethoprim, however, was especially selected from similar folate inhibitors because of its low toxicity for animals and high toxicity for bacteria. This difference has since been shown to be due to the fact that the affinity of trimethoprim for the dihydrofolate reductase of bacteria is some 40 000 times greater than for the corresponding mammalian enzyme.

Pharmacokinetics: Peak plasma levels of trimethoprim and sulfamethoxazole are higher and achieved more rapidly after one hour of intravenous infusion of SEPTRA for infusion than after oral administration of an equivalent dose of a trimethoprim-sulfamethoxazole oral presentation. Plasma concentration, elimination half-life and urinary excretion rates show no significant differences following either the oral or intravenous route of administration.

Absorption: Both trimethoprim and sulfamethoxazole are rapidly absorbed following oral administration. Detectable levels of both drugs appear in the blood in about five minutes with significant levels being reached within an hour. Peak blood levels for both compounds are attained usually in two to four hours, are maintained for about seven hours, and detectable amounts are still present after 24 hours. When the two drugs are administered together, the individual blood levels are similar to those achieved when the drugs are administered separately, thus indicating no effect in absorption of one drug by the other.

Distribution: The ratio of one part trimethoprim to five parts sulfamethoxazole achieves drug concentrations in the blood in the ratio of approximately 1:20, a ratio considered to be optimal against a wide range of bacteria. Unlike sulfamethoxazole, trimethoprim concentrates in tissues; biopsy material from a small number of patients taking trimethoprim preoperatively indicated that the concentration of trimethoprim in the tissues exceeded that of the plasma sampled at the same time—most significant in the lung (by 10 times). A similar pattern occurs in animals. Levels of trimethoprim in the sputum were also found to be higher than in the plasma following oral administration of trimethoprim-sulfamethoxazole. The concentrations of both drugs have also been found to be well-maintained in lymph and tissue fluids.

In serum, the degree of protein-binding by trimethoprim varies with the concentration, but it normally is about 44% bound to plasma protein. Sulfamethoxazole was found to be about 70% bound to plasma protein. Addition of sulfamethoxazole reduced the binding of trimethoprim by 3 to 4%, but there was no change in the protein-binding of sulfamethoxazole (about 66%) at therapeutically attainable concentrations of the two drugs.

Metabolism and Excretion: Studies conducted on the individual components administered separately, indicate that in the presence of a high fluid intake, approximately 50%, and in the presence of a low fluid intake, approximately 40% of the orally ingested trimethoprim is excreted unchanged in the urine within 24 hours. Approximately 10% of the excreted drug is in the form of metabolites with little or no antibacterial activity. Some trimethoprim is excreted in the bile, where concentrations twice those of plasma are obtained, but as it is almost completely reabsorbed; very little appears in the feces. Studies with radio-labelled trimethoprim indicated that it is almost completely absorbed following oral administration in man; less than 4% of the radioactivity appeared in the feces over a period of six days. Radioactivity was eliminated from the plasma and urine at almost identical rates; almost all of an oral dose being excreted in the urine within 48 hours. The biological half-life of trimethoprim was calculated to be 10 hours (range of 6.2 to 12 hours in four patients), which corresponds well to the half-life of 9 to 11 hours determined in man for sulfamethoxazole.

About 60% of the orally ingested sulfamethoxazole is excreted in the urine within 48 hours. Of the excreted drug, approximately half is the N^4 acetylated derivative, a fifth is the N^4 conjugate, a sixth is the unchanged parent compound, and about a tenth is another N^4 free compound.

Although the amount of each drug excreted is similar when given separately or in combination, the method of excretion by the kidney is quite different. Sharpstone demonstrated that there is net tubular reabsorption of filtered sulfamethoxazole, at least in patients with normal renal function, whereas with trimethoprim there is a tubular secretory mechanism of excretion in patients with normal or impaired renal function.

Renal clearance of sulfamethoxazole increased with rising urine flow-rate, was independent of urine pH when this was less than 7, but increased with alkalinization of the urine above a pH of 7. The clearance of trimethoprim was unaffected by alteration in urine flow-rate but increased sharply with falling urine pH.

In patients with impaired renal function, sulfamethoxazole excretion was only slightly decreased, whereas trimethoprim excretion decreased markedly in severe renal impairment.

INDICATIONS: SEPTRA (sulfamethoxazole and trimethoprim) has been effective in the treatment of infections against the following gram-positive and gram-negative organisms:

Gram-Negative Organisms: *H. influenzae, N. gonorrhoeae, E. coli,* Klebsiella species, *E. aerogenes, P. mirabilis, P. vulgaris,* Salmonella species, Shigella species, *V. cholerae.*

Gram-Positive Organisms: *S. pyogenes, S. viridans, S. albus, S. aureus, D. pneumoniae.*

Other Organisms: *B. melitensis, N. asteroides, N. brasiliensis, P. brasiliensis, P. jiroveci, S. somaliensis.*

Sensitivity tests should be performed whenever possible to determine choice of therapy. These tests should be repeated if there is a failure to respond, relapse or early recurrence.

SEPTRA may be indicated for the following infections when caused by susceptible strains of the above organisms.

Urinary Tract Infections: Treatment of acute uncomplicated urinary tract infections*. It is recommended that initial episodes of uncomplicated urinary tract infections be treated with a single effective antibacterial agent rather than the combination.

Upper and Lower Respiratory Tract Infections: Treatment of acute exacerbations of chronic bronchitis.

Treatment of *P. jiroveci* pneumonia*. SEPTRA is also indicated in the treatment of infants and children with a diagnosis of *P. jiroveci* pneumonitis, especially if they are immunosuppressed.

Gastrointestinal Tract Infections: Treatment of cholera, as an adjunct to fluid and electrolyte replacement, when the organism has been shown to be sensitive in vitro.

Treatment of bacillary dysentry*.

Other Infections: Treatment of nocardiosis*. Brucellosis (second line therapy), when used in combination with gentamicin or rifampicin.

SEPTRA is not indicated in infections associated with Pseudomonas, Mycoplasma, nor when the infection is caused by a virus.

This drug has not yet been fully evaluated in streptococcal infections.

* SEPTRA Injection has been investigated clinically in these indications.

CONTRAINDICATIONS: SEPTRA (sulfamethoxazole and trimethoprim) is contraindicated in patients with a known hypersensitivity to trimethoprim or sulfonamides, co-trimoxazole or any excipients of SEPTRA and in patients with documented megaloblastic anemia due to folate deficiency, evidence of marked liver parenchymal damage, or blood dyscrasias.

SEPTRA is contraindicated in patients with marked renal impairment where repeated serum assays cannot be carried out (see also Precautions).

Pregnancy: SEPTRA is contraindicated in pregnant patients and in nursing mothers, because sulfonamides pass the placenta and are excreted in the milk and may cause kernicterus.

Lactation: See Pregnancy.

Children: SEPTRA is contraindicated in infants less than two months of age.

WARNINGS: Fatalities associated with the administration of sulfonamides and SEPTRA, although rare, have occurred due to severe reactions, including Stevens-Johnson syndrome, toxic epidermal necrolysis (Lyell's syndrome), fulminant hepatic necrosis, agranulocytosis, aplastic anemia, other blood dyscrasias, and hypersensitivity of the respiratory tract.

SEPTRA (sulfamethoxazole and trimethoprim) should be discontinued at the first appearance of skin rash or any sign of adverse reaction. Clinical signs, such as rash, sore throat, fever, arthralgia, cough, shortness of breath, pallor, purpura, or jaundice may be early indications of serious reactions. Cough, shortness of breath, and/or pulmonary infiltrates may be indicators of pulmonary hypersensitivity to sulfonamides which while rare, has been fatal. In rare instances a skin rash may be followed by more severe reactions, such as Stevens-Johnson syndrome, toxic epidermal necrolysis, hepatic necrosis, or serious blood disorder. Complete blood counts should be done frequently in patients receiving sulfonamides.

SEPTRA should not be used in the treatment of streptococcal pharyngitis. Clinical studies have documented that patients with group A β-hemolytic streptococcal tonsillopharyngitis have a greater incidence of bacteriologic failure when treated with SEPTRA than to those patients treated with penicillin, as evidenced by failure to eradicate this organism from the tonsillopharyngeal area.

SEPTRA Injection contains sodium metabisulfite, a sulfite that may cause allergic-type reactions including anaphylactic symptoms and life-threatening or less severe asthmatic episodes in certain susceptible people. The overall prevalence of sulfite sensitivity in the general population is unknown and probably low. Sulfite sensitivity is seen more frequently in asthmatic than in nonasthmatic people.

PRECAUTIONS: General: SEPTRA should only be used where, in the judgement of the physician, the benefit of treatment outweighs any possible risks; consideration should be given to the use of a single effective antibacterial agent.

Clinicians should be aware that first line therapy in the management of all patients with diarrheal disease in the maintenance of adequate hydration.

SEPTRA should be given with caution to patients with impaired renal or hepatic function, to those with possible folate deficiency (e.g., the elderly, chronic alcoholics, rheumatoid arthritics, patients receiving anticonvulsant therapy, patients with malabsorption syndrome, and patients in malnutrition states), and to those with severe allergy or bronchial asthma. Because of possible interference with folate metabolism, regular blood counts are advisable in these patients as well as patients who are on long term therapy. Changes indicative of folic acid impairment have, in certain specific situations, been reversed by folinic acid therapy.

A folate supplement should also be considered with prolonged high dosage of SEPTRA (see Adverse Effects).

In glucose-6-phosphate dehydrogenase-deficient individuals, hemolysis may occur. This reaction is frequently dose-related.

The administration of SEPTRA to patients known or suspected to be at risk of acute porphyria should be avoided. Both trimethoprim and sulfonamides (although not specifically sulfamethoxazole) have been associated with clinical exacerbation of porphyria.

Caution should be exercised in administering trimethoprim to patients at risk of hyperkalemia and hyponatremia. Serum potassium and sodium and renal function should be closely monitored, and dosage should be adjusted for renal function (see Precautions, Renal Impairment and Dosage).

The risk factors for hyperkalemia are high trimethoprim dosage (20 mg/kg/day), renal insufficiency (serum creatinine ≥1.2 mg/dL), hypoaldosteronism, older age, dietary potassium and other drugs that impair potassium excretion. The likely mechanism is via trimethoprim inhibition of sodium channels in the distal nephron, similar to that of the potassium-sparing diuretic amiloride.

Hyperkalemia is generally reversible on discontinuation of trimethoprim. In patients presented with hyperkalemia due to SEPTRA, SEPTRA can be discontinued and appropriate standard potassium-lowering therapy instituted.

Except under careful supervision trimethoprim-sulfamethoxazole should not be given to patients with serious hematological disorders (see Adverse Effects).

Functional inhibition of the renal tubular secretion of creatinine may produce a spurious fall in the estimated rate of creatinine clearance.

SEPTRA may affect the results of thyroid function tests but this is probably of little or no clinical significance.

The possibility of superinfection with a non-sensitive organism should be borne in mind.

Local irritation and inflammation due to extravascular infiltration of the infusion has been observed with SEPTRA Injection. If these occur, the infusion should be discontinued and restarted at another site.

Fluid Overload is possible, especially when very high doses are being administered to patients with underlying cardio-pulmonary disease.

An adequate urinary output should be maintained at all times. Evidence of crystalluria in vivo is rare, although sulfonamide crystals have been noted in cooled urine from treated patients. In patients suffering from hypoalbuminaemia the risk may be increased.

Gastrointestinal: *C. difficile*—Associated Disease (CDAD): *C. difficile*-associated disease (CDAD) has been reported with use of many antibacterial agents, including SEPTRA. CDAD may range in severity from mild diarrhea to fatal colitis. It is important to consider this diagnosis in patients who present with diarrhea, or symptoms of colitis, pseudomembranous colitis, toxic megacolon, or perforation of colon subsequent to the administration of any antibacterial agent. CDAD has been reported to occur over 2 months after the administration of antibacterial agents.

Treatment with antibacterial agents may alter the normal flora of the colon and may permit overgrowth of *C. difficile*. *C. difficile* produces toxins A and B, which contribute to the development of CDAD. CDAD may cause significant morbidity and mortality. CDAD can be refractory to antimicrobial therapy.

If the diagnosis of CDAD is suspected or confirmed, appropriate therapeutic measures should be initiated. Mild cases of CDAD usually respond to discontinuation of antibacterial agents not directed against *C. difficile*. In moderate to severe cases, consideration should be given to management with fluids and electrolytes, protein supplementation, and treatment with an antibacterial agent clinically effective against *C. difficile*. Surgical evaluation should be instituted as clinically indicated, as surgical intervention may be required in certain severe cases. (See Adverse Effects.)

Renal Impairment: In patients with renal impairment, a reduced or less frequent dosage is recommended in order to avoid accumulation of trimethoprim in the blood (see Dosage). Non-ionic diffusion is the main factor in the renal handling of trimethoprim, and as renal failure advances, trimethoprim excretion decreases. For such patients, serum assays are necessary. SEPTRA should not be used when the serum creatinine level is above 2 mg per 100 mL, in order to avoid possible permanent impairment of renal function.

Geriatrics: There may be an increased risk of severe adverse reactions in elderly patients, particularly when complicating conditions exist, e.g., impaired kidney and/or liver function, or concomitant use of other drugs. Severe skin reactions, or generalized bone marrow suppression (see Warnings and Adverse Effects), or a specific decrease in platelets (with or without purpura) are the most frequently reported severe adverse reactions in elderly patients. In those concurrently receiving certain diuretics, primarily thiazides, an increased incidence of thrombocytopenia with or without purpura has been reported. Appropriate dosage adjustments should be made for patients with impaired kidney function (see Dosage).

Close supervision is recommended when SEPTRA is used in elderly patients or in patients taking high doses of SEPTRA as these patients may be more susceptible to hyperkalemia and hyponatremia.

Special care should be exercised when treating the elderly or suspected folate-deficient patients; folate supplementation should be considered.

Children: SEPTRA is not recommended for pediatric patients younger than 2 months of age (see Contraindications).

Pregnancy: Trimethoprim and sulfamethoxazole cross the placenta and their safety in human pregnancy has not been established. Trimethoprim is a folate antagonist and, in animal studies, both agents have been shown to cause fetal abnormalities. At doses in excess of the recommended human therapeutic dose, trimethoprim and sulfamethoxazole have been reported to cause cleft palate and other fetal abnormalities in rats, findings typical of a folate antagonist. Effects with trimethoprim were preventable by administration of dietary folate. In rabbits, fetal loss was seen at doses of trimethoprim in excess of human therapeutic doses. Case-control studies have shown that there may be an association between exposure to folate antagonists and birth defects in humans. Therefore, SEPTRA should be avoided in pregnancy, particularly in the first trimester, unless the potential benefit to the mother outweighs the potential risk to the fetus; folate supplementation should be considered if SEPTRA is used in pregnancy.

Sulfamethoxazole competes with bilirubin for binding to plasma albumin. As significant maternally derived drug levels persist for several days in the newborn, there may be a risk of precipitating or exacerbating neonatal hyperbilirubinaemia, with an associated theoretical risk of kernicterus, when SEPTRA is administered to the mother near the time of delivery. This theoretical risk is particularly relevant in infants at increased risk of hyperbilirubinaemia, such as those who are preterm and those with glucose-6-phosphate dehydrogenase deficiency.

Lactation: Trimethoprim and sulfamethoxazole are excreted in breast milk. Administration of SEPTRA should be avoided in late pregnancy and in lactating mothers where the mother or infant has, or is at particular risk of developing hyperbilirubinaemia. Additionally, administration of SEPTRA should be avoided in infants younger than eight weeks in view of predisposition of young infants to hyperbilirubinaemia.

Patients with Special Diseases and Conditions: **Use in the Treatment of and Prophylaxis for *P. jiroveci* Pneumonia in Patients with Acquired Immunodeficiency Syndrome (AIDS):** The incidence of side effects, particularly rash, severe hypersensitivity reactions, fever, leukopenia, neutropenia, thrombocytopenia and elevated aminotransferase (transaminase) values in AIDS patients who are being treated with SEPTRA for *P. jiroveci* pneumonia (PJP) has been reported to be greatly increased compared with the incidence normally associated with the use of SEPTRA in non-AIDS patients. If signs of bone marrow depression occur, the patient should be given calcium folinate supplementation (5-10 mg/day). The incidence of hyperkalemia and hyponatremia appears to be increased in AIDS patients receiving SEPTRA. Adverse effects are generally less severe in patients receiving SEPTRA for prophylaxis. A history of mild intolerance to SEPTRA in AIDS patients does not appear to predict intolerance of subsequent secondary prophylaxis. However, if a patient develops skin rash or any sign of adverse reaction, therapy with SEPTRA should be re-evaluated (see Warnings). Rhabdomyolysis has been reported in HIV positive patients receiving trimethoprim-sulfamethoxazole for prophylaxis or treatment of PJP. In some cases, rhabdomyolysis led to acute renal failure requiring emergency dialysis.

Severe hypersensitivity reactions have also been reported in HIV-infected patients on re-exposure to SEPTRA, sometimes after a dosage interval of a few days. Concomitant administration of intravenous diphenhydramine may permit continued infusion.

The concomitant use of leucovorin with SEPTRA for the acute treatment of *P. jiroveci* pneumonia in patients with HIV infection was associated with increased rates of treatment failure and morbidity in a placebo-controlled study.

Phenylketonuric Patients: Trimethoprim has been noted to impair phenylalanine metabolism but this is of no significance in phenylketonuric patients on appropriate dietary restriction.

Drug-Food Interactions: Caution should be excercised in patients following potassium enriched dietary regimens.

Drug Interactions: In elderly patients concurrently receiving certain diuretics, primarily thiazides, an increased incidence of thrombocytopenia with or without purpura has been reported.

Occasional reports suggest that patients receiving pyrimethamine at doses in excess of 25 mg weekly may develop megaloblastic anemia should SEPTRA be prescribed concurrently.

In some situations, concomitant treatment with zidovudine may increase risk of hematological adverse reactions to SEPTRA. If concomitant treatment is necessary, consideration should be given to monitoring of hematological parameters.

Administration of SEPTRA 160 mg/800 mg causes a 40% increase in lamivudine exposure because of the trimethoprim component. Lamivudine has no effect on the pharmacokinetics of trimethoprim or sulfamethoxazole.

It has been reported that SEPTRA may prolong the prothrombin time in patients who are receiving the anticoagulant warfarin. This interaction should be kept in mind when SEPTRA is given to patients already on anticoagulant therapy, and the coagulation time should be reassessed.

SEPTRA may inhibit the hepatic metabolism of phenytoin. SEPTRA, given at a common clinical dosage, increased the phenytoin half-life by 39% and decreased the phenytoin metabolic clearance rate by 27%. When administering these drugs concurrently, one should be alert for possible excessive phenytoin effect. Close monitoring of the patient's condition and serum phenytoin levels is advisable.

Sulfonamides can also displace methotrexate from plasma protein binding sites, thus increasing free methotrexate concentrations. Folate supplementation should be considered.

If SEPTRA is considered appropriate therapy in patients receiving other anti-folate drugs, a folate supplementation should be considered.

Concomitant use of trimethoprim with digoxin has been shown to increase plasma digoxin levels in a proportion of elderly patients.

Caution should be exercised in patients taking any other drugs that can cause hyperkalemia.

Reversible deterioration in renal function has been observed in patients treated with SEPTRA and cyclosporin following renal transplantation. When trimethoprim is administered simultaneously with drugs that form cations at physiological pH, and are also partly excreted by active renal secretion (e.g. procainamide, amantadine), there is the possibility of competitive inhibition of this process which may lead to an increase in plasma concentration of one or both of the drugs.

Interaction with sulphonylurea hypoglycemic agents is uncommon but potentiation has been reported.

Concurrent use of rifampicin and SEPTRA results in a shortening of the plasma half life of trimethoprim after a period of about one week. This is not thought to be of clinical significance.

Trimethoprim is an inhibitor of cytochrome P450 2C8 enzyme and may interact with other drugs that are primarily metabolized by the 2C8 isoform. Sulfamethoxazole is an inhibitor of cytochrome P450 2C9 and may interact with other drugs that are primarily metabolized by the 2C9 isoform.

Laboratory Tests: Drug/Laboratory Test Interactions: SEPTRA, specifically the trimethoprim component, can interfere with a serum methotrexate assay as determined by the competitive binding protein technique (CBPA) when a bacterial dihydrofolate reductase is used as the binding protein. No interference occurs, however, if methotrexate is measured by a radioimmunoassay (RIA).

The presence of trimethoprim and sulfamethoxazole may also interfere with the Jaffé alkaline picrate reaction assay for creatinine, resulting in overestimations of about 10% in the range of normal values.

Information to Be Provided to the Patient: Patients should be instructed to maintain an adequate fluid intake in order to prevent crystalluria and stone formation.

Patients should tell their physician of all dietary regimens and supplements.

ADVERSE EFFECTS: The most common adverse effects are hyperkalemia, anorexia, monilial overgrowth, headache, local thrombophlebitis at the site of injection, gastrointestinal disturbances (nausea, vomiting, diarrhea) and allergic skin reactions (such as rash and urticaria). **Fatalities associated with the administration of sulfonamides and SEPTRA although rare, have occurred due to severe reactions, including Stevens-Johnson syndrome, toxic epidermal necrolysis (Lyell's syndrome), fulminant hepatic necrosis, agranulocytosis, aplastic anemia, other blood dyscrasias, and hypersensitivity of the respiratory tract** (see Warnings).

General: weakness, fatigue, insomnia, vision troubles, alopecia, epistaxis, local thrombophlebitis at the site of injection, edema. Monilial overgrowth is common.

Allergic: Stevens-Johnson syndrome, toxic epidermal necrolysis (Lyell's syndrome), anaphylaxis, allergic myocarditis, erythema multiforme, toxicoderma, exfoliative dermatitis, angioedema, drug fever, chills, allergic vasculitis resembling Henoch-Schönlein purpura, serum sickness, serum sickness-like syndrome, generalized allergic reactions, generalized skin eruptions, fixed drug eruption, photosensitivity, conjunctival and scleral injection, pruritus, urticaria, and rash. In addition, periarteritis nodosa and systemic lupus erythematosus and anaphylactoid reactions (sweating and collapse) have been reported.

Cardiovascular: QT prolongation.

Endocrine and Metabolism: The sulfonamides bear certain chemical similarities to some goitrogens, diuretics (acetazolamide and the thiazides), and oral hypoglycemic agents. Cross-sensitivity may exist with these agents. Diuresis and hypoglycemia have occurred rarely in patients receiving sulfonamides.

Anorexia, hyperkalemia, hyponatremia, hypoglycemia (see also Precautions).

Gastrointestinal: pseudomembranous enterocolitis, pancreatitis, stomatitis, glossitis, dry mouth, nausea, vomiting, pyrosis, gastric intolerance, gastritis or gastroenteritis, dyspepsia emesis, abdominal pain, constipation, flatulence, diarrhea.

Genitourinary: impaired renal function (sometimes reported as renal failure), interstitial nephritis, kidney changes (as indicated by abnormal elevations in blood urea nitrogen, blood non-protein nitrogen, serum creatinine and urine protein levels), toxic nephrosis with oliguria and anuria, crystalluria, hematuria, urgency, and dysuria.

Hematologic: leukopenia, neutropenia, thrombocytopenia, megaloblastic anaemia, aplastic and hemolytic anemia, methemoglobinemia, purpura, agranulocytosis, hypoprothrombinemia, eosinophilia, haemolysis in certain susceptible G-6-PD deficient patients and bone marrow depression.

Hepatic/Biliary/Pancreatic: hepatitis, including cholestatic jaundice and hepatic necrosis, jaundice, elevation of serum transaminase, alkaline phosphatase and bilirubin.

Hepatic changes including fatalities have been recorded in at-risk patients. Cholestatic jaundice and hepatic necrosis may be fatal.

Musculoskeletal: arthralgia, rhabdomyolysis and myalgia.

Neurologic: aseptic meningitis, convulsions, peripheral neuritis, ataxia, tremor, vertigo, tinnitus, headache.

Aseptic meningitis was rapidly reversible on withdrawal of the drug, but recurred in a number of cases on re-exposure to either SEPTRA or to trimethoprim alone.

Ophthalmologic: uveitis.

Psychiatric: hallucinations, depression, apathy, nervousness, dizziness.

Respiratory: pulmonary infiltrates, cough, shortness of breath, dyspnea.

OVERDOSE:

Symptoms: Acute: The amount of a single dose of SEPTRA (sulfamethoxazole and trimethoprim) that is either associated with symptoms of overdosage or is likely to be life-threatening has not been reported. Signs and symptoms of overdosage reported with sulfonamides include anorexia, colic, nausea, vomiting, dizziness, headache, drowsiness, and unconsciousness. Pyrexia, hematuria, and crystalluria may be noted. Blood dyscrasias and jaundice are potential late manifestations of overdosage. Signs of acute overdosage with trimethoprim include nausea, vomiting, dizziness, headache, mental depression, confusion, and bone marrow depression.

General principles of treatment include the forcing oral fluids; and the administration of intravenous fluids if urine output is low and renal function is normal. Acidification of the urine will increase renal elimination of trimethoprim. Inducing diuresis plus alkalinisation of urine will enhance the elimination of sulfamethoxazole. Alkalinisation will reduce the rate of elimination of trimethoprim. The patient should be monitored with blood counts and appropriate blood chemistries, including electrolytes. If a significant blood dyscrasia or jaundice occurs, specific therapy should be instituted for these complications. Peritoneal dialysis is not effective and hemodialysis is only moderately effective in eliminating trimethoprim and sulfamethoxazole.

There is no known antidote for sulfonamide poisoning; however, calcium folinate (leucovorin), 3 to 6 mg im for 5 to 7 days, is an effective antidote for adverse effects in the hemopoietic system caused by trimethoprim.

Chronic: Use of SEPTRA at high doses and/or for extended periods of time may cause confusion and bone marrow depression manifested as thrombocytopenia, leukopenia, and/or megaloblastic anemia. If signs of bone marrow depression occur, the patient should be given leucovorin; 5 to 15 mg leucovorin daily has been recommended by some investigators.

Treatment: See Symptoms.

For management of a suspected drug overdose, contact your **regional Poison Control Centre**. See the *CPS* Directory section for a list of Poison Control Centres.

DOSAGE: **IV:** SEPTRA Injection may be used only in patients who are unable to take oral medication or where there is a need for rapid attainment of high serum concentrations. Oral treatment should be substituted as soon as possible.

Serious Systemic Infections: Adults: The intravenous dosage of SEPTRA Injection depends on the severity of the infection. A dose of 160 to 240 mg trimethoprim + 800 to 1200 mg sulfamethoxazole may be given every 6, 8 or 12 hours. This dose must be properly diluted (see Parenteral Products) and infused over a period of one-half to one hour.

Children: The recommended daily dosage for children is 5 to 10 mg trimethoprim/kg body weight/day and 25 to 50 mg sulfamethoxazole/kg body weight/day. This daily dosage must be properly diluted and administered in equally divided doses by infusion over a period of one-half to one hour (see Table 1).

Table 1: SEPTRA

Serious Systemic Infections—Dosage IV in Children and Adults

Volume of Undiluted SEPTRA Injection per Body Weight[a] (conversion factor 0.31 to 0.63 mL/kg)				
Body Weight (kg)	Volume of Undiluted SEPTRA for Infusion (mL)			
	Total Daily Dose	Dose Every 12 Hours (b.i.d.)	Dose Every 8 Hours (t.i.d.)	Dose Every 6 Hours (q.i.d.)
5	1.6–3.2	0.8–1.6	0.5–1.1	0.4–0.8
10	3.1–6.3	1.6–3.2	1.0–2.1	0.8–1.6
20	6.2–12.6	3.1–6.3	2.1–4.2	1.6–3.2
40	12.4–25.2	6.2–12.6	4.1–8.4	3.1–6.3
60	18.6–37.8	9.3–18.9	6.2–12.6	4.7–9.5

[a] SEPTRA Injection must be properly diluted (see Parenteral Products) and administered in equally divided doses.

Treatment should be continued until the patient has been symptom free for two days; the majority will require treatment for at least five days.

Other diseases, including certain tropical diseases rarely seen in Canada have also been successfully treated with SEPTRA. The duration of treatment is as follows: cholera: 7 days; nocardiosis: 12 weeks; brucellosis: 2 weeks to 3 months

P. jiroveci Pneumonitis: Children and Adults: The recommended daily intravenous dosage is 20 mg trimethoprim/kg body weight + 100 mg sulfamethoxazole/kg body weight. This daily dosage is to be divided into four equal doses infused over a period of one-half to one hour, at six-hour intervals, until oral therapy can be instituted (see Table 2).

Table 2: SEPTRA

***P. jiroveci* Pneumonitis—Dosage IV in Children and Adults**

Volume of Undiluted SEPTRA Injection per Body Weight[a] (conversion factor 1.25 mL/kg)		
Body Weight (kg)	Volume of Undiluted SEPTRA Injection (mL)	
	Total Daily Dose	Dose Every 6 Hours (q.i.d.)
5	6.3	1.6
10	12.5	3.1
20	25.0	6.3
40	50.0	12.5

(cont'd)

Table 2: SEPTRA *(cont'd)*

***P. jiroveci* Pneumonitis—Dosage IV in Children and Adults**

Volume of Undiluted SEPTRA Injection per Body Weight[a] (conversion factor 1.25 mL/kg)		
Body Weight (kg)	**Volume of Undiluted SEPTRA Injection (mL)**	
	Total Daily Dose	**Dose Every 6 Hours (q.i.d.)**
60	75.0	18.8
80	100.0	25.0

[a] SEPTRA Injection must be properly diluted (see Parenteral Products) and administered at six-hour intervals.

Therapy should be continued for a total treatment period of at least two weeks. The aim is to obtain peak plasma or serum levels of trimethoprim of greater than or equal to 5 µg/mL (see Adverse Effects).

Patients with Impaired Renal Function: When renal function is impaired, a reduced dosage should be employed using Table 3.

Table 3: SEPTRA

Recommended Dose Regimen in Patients with Impaired Renal Function

Creatinine Clearance (mL/min)	Recommended Dose Regimen
Above 25	Usual standard regimen
15 to 25	Half the usual regimen
Below 15	Use not recommended

Parenteral Products: **Caution:** Direct iv injection is not recommended. SEPTRA Injection must be diluted in one of the following diluents: Ringer's solution; sodium chloride 0.9% solution; sodium chloride 0.18% + dextrose 4% solution; dextrose 5% solution; dextrose 10% solution; 10% Dextran 40 in sodium chloride 0.9% solution; 10% Dextran 40 in dextrose 5% solution; 6% Dextran 70 in sodium chloride 0.9% solution; 6% Dextran 70 in dextrose 5% solution.

	Volume of Diluent (mL)	Approx. Available Volume (mL)	Nominal Concentration (mg/mL)	
			Trimethoprim	Sulfamethoxazole
5 mL ampoule	125	130	0.62	3.1

The prepared solution must be kept at room temperature and administration started within five hours. Do not mix the prepared infusion solution with other drugs or solutions. If, upon visual inspection, there is cloudiness or evidence of precipitation after mixing, the solution should be discarded and a fresh solution prepared.

SUPPLIED: Each mL of solution for injection contains: trimethoprim 16 mg and sulfamethoxazole 80 mg. Nonmedicinal ingredients: ethanol, propylene glycol, sodium hydroxide (for pH adjustment), sodium metabisulfite, tromethamine and water for injection. Ampoules of 5 mL, packages of 10. Store at room temperature between 15 to 30°C and protected from light.

Serc® ℞

betahistine dihydrochloride

Antivertigo Agent

Abbott Products

Date of Preparation: October 15, 1996

Date of Revision: May 26, 2010

PHARMACOLOGY: Betahistine is a histamine H_1-agonist with an intrinsic activity equal to that of histamine and an H_1-agonistic activity of about 0.07 times that of histamine. This H_1-agonist activity has been confirmed in in vivo studies where, like histamine, the hypotensive response produced by betahistine could be blocked by H_1-receptor antagonists. Betahistine also induces bronchoconstriction and increased vasopermeability after parenteral administration, further confirming its H_1-agonistic properties. In contrast to histamine, betahistine is virtually inactive at the H_2-receptor. Only marginal increases in gastric acid secretion are produced following very high parenteral doses of betahistine. The compound did not produce relaxation in the rat uterus, and no H_2-agonist activity was noted in heart muscle. Receptor binding studies have shown that betahistine is a potent H_3-receptor antagonist.

Orally administered doses of betahistine dihydrochloride are rapidly and completely absorbed from the gastrointestinal tract. The drug is rapidly metabolized to one primary metabolite—2-pyridylacetic acid and excreted in the urine. Studies with radio-labelled betahistine have demonstrated a plasma half-life of 3.4 hours and a urinary half-life of 3.5 hours for the radio-label. Urinary excretion of the label was about 90% complete within 24 hours of administration.

INDICATIONS: SERC (betahistine dihydrochloride) tablets are indicated for reducing the episodes of recurrent vertigo associated with Ménière's disease.

CONTRAINDICATIONS: The use of SERC (betahistine dihydrochloride) tablets is contraindicated in patients with known hypersensitivity to betahistine or to any of the tablet constituents.

Several patients with a history of peptic ulcer have experienced an exacerbation of symptoms while using SERC. Although experiments in animals and in humans have shown that the gastrointestinal side effects associated with betahistine dihydrochloride are not related to gastric acid production, SERC is contraindicated in the presence of peptic ulcer and in patients with a history of this condition.

SERC is also contraindicated in patients with pheochromocytoma.

PRECAUTIONS: General: Although clinical intolerance to SERC (betahistine dihydrochloride) tablets has not been demonstrated in patients with bronchial asthma, caution should be exercised when giving the product to asthmatic patients.

Children: SERC is not recommended for use in children.

Pregnancy: The safety of SERC in human pregnancy has not been established. Animal studies are insufficient with respect to effects on pregnancy, embryonal/foetal development, parturition and postnatal development. The potential risk for humans is unknown. Betahistine should not be used during pregnancy unless clearly necessary.

Lactation: It is not known whether betahistine is excreted in human milk. There are no animal studies on the excretion of betahistine in milk. The importance of the drug to the mother should be weighed against the benefits of nursing and the potential risks for the child.

Drug Interactions: No in vivo interaction studies have been performed. In vitro data revealed no inhibition of Cytochrome P450 enzymes.

ADVERSE EFFECTS: The following undesirable effects have been experienced with the below indicated frequencies in betahistine-treated patients in placebo-controlled clinical trials.

Gastrointestinal Disorders: Common (≥1/100 to <1/10): nausea and dyspepsia.

In addition to those events reported during clinical trials, the following undesirable effects have been reported spontaneously during post-marketing use and in scientific literature. A frequency cannot be estimated from the available data and is therefore classified as 'not known'.

Immune System Disorders: Hypersensitivity reactions, e.g. anaphylaxis have been reported.

Nervous System Disorders: headache.

Somnolence occurred during treatment with betahistine dihydrochloride, but a causal relationship has not been established.

Cardiac Disorders: Ventricular extrasystoles occurred during treatment with betahistine dihydrochloride, but a causal relationship has not been established.

Gastrointestinal Disorders: Mild gastric complaints (e.g. vomiting, gastrointestinal pain, abdominal distension and bloating) have been observed. These can normally be minimized or eliminated by taking the dose during meals or by lowering the dose.

Skin and Subcutaneous Tissue Disorders: Cutaneous and subcutaneous hypersensitivity reactions have been reported, in particular angioneurotic oedema, urticaria, skin rashes of various types, and pruritus.

OVERDOSE:

Symptoms: A few overdose cases (up to 640 mg), with mild to moderate symptoms of nausea, dry mouth, dyspepsia, abdominal pain and somnolence have been reported. Presumably, more serious complications (e.g. convulsion, pulmonary or cardiac complications) may occur in cases of intentional overdose of betahistine above 640 mg, especially in combination with other overdosed drugs.

Treatment: Standard overdose protocol/supportive measures should be followed.

> For management of a suspected drug overdose, CPhA recommends that you contact your **regional Poison Control Centre**. See the *CPS* Directory section for a list of Poison Control Centres.

DOSAGE: The usual adult daily dosage range is 24 to 48 mg administered orally in divided doses.

BID Dosing: 24 mg tablets: 1 tablet twice daily.

TID Dosing: 16 mg tablets: ½ to 1 tablet 3 times daily.

As SERC (betahistine dihydrochloride) can cause gastrointestinal upset in some patients, it is recommended that doses be taken with a meal.

INFORMATION FOR THE PATIENT: Published in e-CPS, available by subscription at www.e-cps.ca.

SUPPLIED: 16 mg: Each round, biconvex, scored, white to almost white tablet, with beveled edges, one side inscribed "S", the other side with "267" on either side of the score, contains: betahistine dihydrochloride 16 mg. Nonmedicinal ingredients: citric acid, colloidal anhydrous silica, mannitol, microcrystalline cellulose and talc. The diameter of the tablet is 8.5 mm. Individual blister packages, boxes of 100. Store at controlled room temperature (15 to 30°C) and protect from exposure to moisture.

24 mg: Each round, biconvex, scored, white to almost white tablet, with beveled edges, one side inscribed with "S", the other side with "289" on either side of the score, contains: betahistine dihydrochloride 24 mg. Nonmedicinal ingredients: citric acid, colloidal anhydrous silica, mannitol, microcrystalline cellulose and talc. The diameter of the tablet is 10 mm. Individual blister packages, boxes of 100. Store at controlled room temperature (15 to 30°C) and protect from exposure to moisture.

(Shown in Product Identification Section)

Serevent® Diskhaler® Disk ℞

salmeterol xinafoate

Bronchodilator

GlaxoSmithKline

Serevent® Diskus® ℞

salmeterol xinafoate

Bronchodilator

GlaxoSmithKline

Date of Revision: August 8, 2008

SUMMARY PRODUCT INFORMATION:

Route of Administration	Dosage Form/ Strength	Clinically Relevant Nonmedicinal Ingredients
Oral Inhalation	Dry powder for inhalation/ 50 µg salmeterol/blister	Lactose and milk protein For a complete listing see Dosage Forms, Composition and Packaging.

INDICATIONS AND CLINICAL USE: Asthma: SEREVENT (salmeterol xinafoate) is indicated for:

- long-term, twice-daily (morning and evening) administration in the maintenance treatment of asthma in patients 4 years of age and older with reversible obstructive airway disease, including patients with nocturnal asthma, who are using optimal corticosteroid treatment and experiencing breakthrough symptoms requiring regular use of a rapid onset, short duration bronchodilator.

Corticosteroids should not be stopped because salmeterol is prescribed.

When treating asthma patients, SEREVENT should be used only as additional therapy for patients whose conditions are not adequately controlled using low- to medium-dose inhaled corticosteroids or the severity of whose disease clearly warrants the initiation of treatment with two maintenance therapies, including SEREVENT. It is **not** indicated for patients whose asthma can be managed by occasional use of a rapid onset, short duration, inhaled β_2-agonist or for patients whose asthma can be successfully managed by inhaled corticosteroids along with occasional use of a rapid onset, short duration, inhaled β_2-agonist.

SEREVENT is a slow onset, long-acting, β_2-agonist and should not be used as a rescue medication. To relieve acute asthmatic symptoms, a rapid onset, short duration inhaled bronchodilator (e.g. salbutamol) should be used.

Chronic Obstructive Pulmonary Disease (COPD): SEREVENT is indicated for:

- long term, twice daily (morning and evening) administration in the maintenance treatment of bronchospasm and relief of dyspnea associated with COPD, including chronic bronchitis and emphysema.

Geriatrics: There is no need to adjust the dose in otherwise healthy elderly patients.

Pediatrics (<4 years of age): At present, there is insufficient clinical data to recommend the use of salmeterol xinafoate in children younger than 4 years of age.

CONTRAINDICATIONS:

- Patients who are hypersensitive to this drug or to any ingredient in the formulation or component of the container and to adrenergic compounds. For a complete listing, see Dosage Forms, Composition and Packaging.
- Patients with cardiac tachyarrhythmias.
- SEREVENT (salmeterol xinafoate) dry powder for inhalation (SEREVENT DISKHALER Disk and SEREVENT DISKUS) formulations contain lactose (which contains milk protein) and is therefore contraindicated in patients with an allergy to lactose or milk.
- Patients with a history of anaphylactic shock, anaphylactic reaction or angioedema associated with sameterol xinafoate or any component of this drug.

WARNINGS AND PRECAUTIONS:

> **Warning:** Long-acting β_2-adrenergic agonists, such as salmeterol, the active ingredient in SEREVENT, may increase the risk of asthma-related death. When treating asthma patients, SEREVENT should be used only as additional therapy for patients whose conditions are not adequately controlled using low- to medium-dose inhaled corticosteroids or the severity of whose disease clearly warrants the initiation of treatment with two maintenance therapies, including SEREVENT. Data from a large placebo-controlled US study (Salmeterol Multi-center Asthma Research Trial, also known as "SMART") comparing the safety of salmeterol (SEREVENT Inhalation Aerosol) to that of a placebo added to the original asthma therapy showed an increase in asthma-related deaths in patients receiving salmeterol (13 deaths out of 13,176 patients treated for 28 weeks on salmeterol versus 3 deaths out of 13,179 patients on placebo). Data from this study also suggested that African American patients may be at greater risk of serious respiratory-related events or deaths when using salmeterol compared to placebo. It is not known if this was due to pharmacogenetic or other factors (see Dosage and Administration).

Use in Asthma: Important Information: SEREVENT (salmeterol xinafoate) should not be initiated in patients with significantly worsening or acutely deteriorating asthma, which may be a life-threatening condition. Serious acute respiratory events, including fatalities, have been reported worldwide, when SEREVENT has been initiated in this situation.

Although it is not possible from these reports to determine whether SEREVENT contributed to these events or simply failed to relieve the deteriorating asthma, the use of SEREVENT in this setting is inappropriate.

In most cases these reports have occurred in patients with severe asthma (e.g., patients with a history of corticosteroid dependence, low pulmonary function, intubation, mechanical ventilation, frequent hospitalizations, or previous life-threatening acute asthma exacerbations) and/or in some patients in whom asthma has been acutely deteriorating (e.g., unresponsive to usual medications, increasing need for inhaled rapid onset, short duration $β_2$-agonists, increasing need for systemic corticosteroids, significant increase in symptoms, recent emergency room visits, sudden or progressive deterioration in pulmonary function). However, they have occurred in a few patients with less severe asthma as well. There are no data demonstrating that SEREVENT provides greater efficacy than or additional efficacy to rapid onset, short duration, inhaled $β_2$-agonists in patients with worsening asthma.

General: SEREVENT is not a substitute for inhaled or oral corticosteroids. All asthma patients should be advised that they must also use corticosteroids if they are taking SEREVENT. Corticosteroid therapy should not be stopped or reduced when SEREVENT is initiated.

There are no data demonstrating that SEREVENT has a clinical anti-inflammatory effect and could be expected to take the place of, or reduce the dose of, corticosteroids. Asthmatic patients must be warned not to stop or reduce corticosteroid therapy even if they feel better as a result of initiating SEREVENT. Any change in corticosteroid dosage should be made **only** after clinical evaluation

In the treatment of COPD, the role of inhaled corticosteroid therapy is less well established and SEREVENT could be used with or without concomitant corticosteroids. The use of oral or inhaled corticosteroids should be determined by the treating physician.

SEREVENT should not be used to treat acute asthma or COPD symptoms. It is crucial to inform patients of this and prescribe a rapid onset, short duration, inhaled bronchodilator to relieve acute symptoms. The use of bronchodilator should be determined by the treating physician.

The role of long-acting $β_2$-agonists in the management of asthma and COPD: The management of asthma should normally follow a stepwise program, and **patient response should be monitored clinically and by lung function tests.** Sudden or progressive deterioration in asthma control is potentially life-threatening; treatment plan must be re-evaluated, and consideration be given to increasing corticosteroid therapy. **In patients at risk, daily peak flow monitoring with precise instructions for acceptable variation limits should be considered.**

Increased use of inhaled, rapid onset, short duration $β_2$-agonists is a marker of destabilization of asthma and requires re-evaluation of the patient and consideration of alternative treatment regimens, especially inhaled or systemic corticosteroids.

Long-acting $β_2$-agonists are an alternative additional therapy for patients with moderate asthma with unsatisfactory symptom control despite an optimal dose of inhaled steroids particularly when there are nocturnal symptoms.

Before introducing long-acting $β_2$-agonists, adequate education should be provided to the patient on how to use the drug and what to do if asthma flares up.

Long-acting $β_2$-agonists are an additional therapy for COPD patients requiring long acting control of symptoms.

Use with rapid onset, short duration bronchodilators: When asthmatic patients begin treatment with SEREVENT, those who have been taking rapid onset, short duration, inhaled $β_2$-agonists on a regular daily basis should be advised to discontinue their regular daily-dosing regimen and should be clearly instructed to use rapid onset, short duration, inhaled $β_2$-agonists only for symptomatic relief if they develop asthma symptoms while taking SEREVENT.

When beginning treatment with SEREVENT, COPD patients should be instructed to use their rapid onset, short duration bronchodilators as determined by their treating physician, at the lowest dose to relieve their symptoms. The regular twice daily administration of SEREVENT should reduce the excessive use of rapid onset, short duration inhaled bronchodilators.

Cardiovascular and Other Effects: Although clinically not significant, a small increase in QTc interval has been reported at therapeutic doses. It is not known if this becomes clinically significant when concomitant medications causing similar effects are prescribed and/or in the presence of heart diseases, hypokalemia, or hypoxia.

Fatalities have been reported in association with excessive use of inhaled sympathomimetic drugs. Large doses of inhaled or oral salmeterol (12 to 20 times the recommended dose) have been associated with clinically significant prolongation of the QTc interval, which has the potential for producing ventricular arrhythmias. Fatalities have been reported following excessive use of aerosol preparations containing sympathomimetic amines, the exact cause of which is unknown. Cardiac arrest was reported in several instances.

In a very large scale post-marketing surveillance study in the UK, involving over twenty-four thousand patients comparing safety of salmeterol and salbutamol in the treatment of asthma, the overall cardiovascular deaths on salmeterol treatment were 0.17% vs. 0.12% on salbutamol (p=0.308). The subdivision of these deaths into groups dependent on asthma severity was as follows: See Table 1.

Table 1: SEREVENT

Investigator Assessment of Severity of Asthma

	Mild (%)	Moderate (%)	Severe (%)
Salmeterol	0.04	0.11	0.55
Salbutamol	0.14	0.07	0.27

Test for interaction p=0.233.

In individual patients any $β_2$-adrenergic agonist may have a clinically significant cardiac effect.

No clinically significant effect on the cardiovascular system is usually seen after the administration of inhaled salmeterol in recommended doses. Cardiovascular effects such as increased blood pressure and heart rate may occasionally be seen with all sympathomimetic drugs, especially at higher than therapeutic doses. Central nervous system effects (increased excitement) can occur after the use of SEREVENT. Occurrence of cardiovascular or central nervous system effects may require discontinuation of the drug.

Salmeterol, like all sympathomimetic amines, should be used with caution in patients with cardiovascular disorders, especially coronary insufficiency, cardiac arrhythmias, and hypertension; in patients with convulsive disorders or thyrotoxicosis; and in patients who are unusually responsive to sympathomimetic amines.

As has been described with other β-adrenergic agonist bronchodilators, clinically significant changes in systolic and/or diastolic blood pressure, pulse rate, and electrocardiograms have been seen infrequently in individual patients in controlled clinical studies with salmeterol.

Ear/Nose/Throat: Symptoms of laryngeal spasm, irritation, or swelling, such as stridor and choking, have been reported rarely in patients receiving SEREVENT.

Systemic Effects: The results of a drug interaction study conducted in healthy subjects indicated that concomitant use of systemic ketoconazole (a strong cytochrome P450 3A4 inhibitor) increased exposure to salmeterol in some subjects. This increase in plasma salmeterol exposure may lead to prolongation in the QTc interval. Due to the potential increased risk of cardiovascular adverse events, the concomitant use of salmeterol with ketoconazole is not recommended (see Drug Interactions and Action and Clinical Pharmacology, Pharmacokinetics). Caution should also be exercised when other CYP3A4 inhibitors are coadministered with salmeterol (e.g. ritonavir, atazanavir, clarithromycin, indinavir, itraconazole, nefazodone, nelfinavir, saquinavir, telithromycin).

Endocrine and Metabolism: Metabolic Effects: In common with other β-adrenergic agents, salmeterol can induce reversible metabolic changes (e.g. hyperglycemia, hypokalemia).

There have been very rare reports of increases in blood glucose levels (see Adverse Reactions, Post-Market Adverse Drug Reactions) and this should be considered when prescribing to patients with a history of diabetes mellitus.

Doses of the related $β_2$-adrenoceptor agonist salbutamol, when administered intravenously, have been reported to aggravate pre-existing diabetes mellitus and ketoacidosis. Administration of $β_2$-adrenoceptor agonists may cause a decrease in serum potassium, possibly through intracellular shunting, which has the potential to increase the likelihood of arrythmias. The effect is usually seen at higher therapeutic doses and the decrease is usually transient, not requiring supplementation. Therefore, salmeterol should be used with caution in patients predisposed to low levels of serum potassium.

Hypersensitivity: Immediate hypersensitivity reactions may occur after administration of SEREVENT, as demonstrated by rare cases of urticaria, angioedema, rash, bronchospasm and very rare cases of anaphylactic shock, or anaphylactic reaction.

Respiratory: As with other inhaled medications, paradoxical bronchospasm (which can be life-threatening) has been reported following the use of SEREVENT. If it occurs, treatment with SEREVENT should be discontinued immediately and alternative therapy instituted.

Special Populations: Pregnant Women: In animal studies, some effects on the fetus, typical for a β-agonist occurred at exposure levels substantially higher than those that occur with therapeutic use. Extensive use of other β-agonists has provided no evidence that effects in animals are relevant to human use.

There are no adequate and well-controlled studies with SEREVENT in pregnant women. SEREVENT should be used during pregnancy only if the potential benefit justifies the potential risk to the fetus.

Use in Labour and Delivery: There are no well-controlled human studies that have investigated effects of salmeterol on preterm labour or labour at term. Because of the potential for β-agonist interference with uterine contractility, use of SEREVENT during labour should be restricted to those patients in whom the benefits clearly outweigh the risks.

Nursing Women: Plasma levels of salmeterol after inhaled therapeutic doses are very low (85 to 200 pg/mL) in humans and therefore levels in milk should be correspondingly low. Studies in lactating animals indicate that salmeterol is likely to be secreted in only very small amounts in breast milk. However, since there is no experience with use of SEREVENT by nursing mothers, a decision should be made whether to discontinue nursing or to discontinue the drug, taking into account the importance of the drug to the mother. Caution should be exercised when salmeterol xinafoate is administered to a nursing woman.

Pediatrics: (<4 years of age): The safety and efficacy of SEREVENT in children younger than 4 years of age have not been established.

(4-11 years of age): The safety and efficacy of salmeterol in children 4-11 years old with asthma have been evaluated in controlled clinical trials for up to 1 year.

Geriatrics: No apparent differences in the efficacy and safety of SEREVENT were observed when geriatric patients were compared with younger patients in asthma and COPD clinical trials. As with other $β_2$-agonists, however, special caution should be observed when using SEREVENT in elderly patients who have concomitant cardiovascular disease that could be adversely affected by this class of drug.

Monitoring and Laboratory Tests: Monitoring Control of Asthma: Asthma may deteriorate acutely over a period of hours or chronically over several days or longer. If the patient's rapid onset, short duration inhaled $β_2$-agonist becomes less effective or the patient needs more inhalation than usual, this may be a marker of destabilization of asthma. In this setting, the patient requires immediate re-evaluation with reassessment of the treatment regimen. Increasing the daily dosage of SEREVENT in this situation is not appropriate. SEREVENT should not be used more frequently than twice daily (morning and evening) at the recommended dose.

Use in Adolescents/Children and Asthma Severity Reassessment: In adolescents and children, the severity of asthma may be variable with age and periodic reassessment should be considered to determine if continued maintenance therapy with SEREVENT is still indicated. Compliance, especially neglect of anti-inflammatory therapy and overuse of rapid onset, short duration $β_2$-agonists, should be carefully followed in adolescents/children receiving long-acting $β_2$-agonists.

ADVERSE REACTIONS: Adverse Drug Reaction Overview: As with other inhalation therapy, the potential for paradoxical bronchospasm should be kept in mind. If it occurs, the preparation should be discontinued immediately and alternative therapy instituted.

Adverse reactions to SEREVENT (salmeterol xinafoate) are similar in nature to reactions to other selective $β_2$-adrenoceptor agonists, i.e. palpitation; immediate hypersensitivity reactions, including urticaria, rash, bronchospasm, edema, angioedema, and anaphylactic shock or anaphylactic reaction; headache; tremor; nervousness and paradoxical bronchospasm. There have also been reports of arthralgia and muscle cramps.

Cardiac arrhythmias (including atrial fibrillation, supraventricular tachycardia and extrasystoles) have been reported, usually in susceptible patients.

Clinically significant changes in blood glucose and/or serum potassium were seen rarely during clinical studies with long-term administration of SEREVENT at recommended doses.

Asthma: Data from a large placebo-controlled US study comparing the safety of salmeterol to that of a placebo added to the original asthma therapy showed an increase in asthma-related deaths in patients receiving salmeterol. Data from this study also suggested that African American patients may be at greater risk of serious respiratory-related events or deaths when using salmeterol compared to placebo. It is not known if this was due to pharmacogenetic or other factors.

Clinical Trial Adverse Drug Reactions: Because clinical trials are conducted under very specific conditions the adverse reaction rates observed in the clinical trials may not reflect the rates observed in practice and should not be compared to the rates in the clinical trials of another drug. Adverse drug reaction information from clinical trials is useful for identifying drug-related adverse events and for approximating rates.

Use in Adolescents and Adults: In controlled, multidose clinical trials involving almost 2000 patients, the most frequently occurring adverse events were headache, tremor and palpitations (see Table 2), which are pharmacologically predictable effects of $β_2$-adrenoceptor agonists. Tremor tended to be transient, dose-related and reduced with regular therapy. Headache and palpitations were reported but the incidence was not significantly different from placebo.

Table 2: SEREVENT

Number (and percentage) of Patients with Adverse Events

Adverse Event	SEREVENT (50 µg b.i.d.) n=1462 (%)	Placebo n=195 (%)
Headache	62 (4.2)	5 (2.6)
Palpitations	22 (1.5)	4 (2.1)
Tremor	20 (1.4)	4 (2.1)

In a subsequent controlled clinical trial patients received either salmeterol in combination with beclomethasone dipropionate (BDP) or BDP alone. A rapid onset, short duration inhaled $β_2$-adrenergic drug was also provided to all patients for use on an as-needed basis. The incidence of pharmacologically predictable adverse events was similar in all groups except for tremor which was significantly higher in the salmeterol 100 µg group compared with the other two groups (see Table 3).

Table 3: SEREVENT

Number (and percentage) of Patients with Drug-related Adverse Events

Adverse Event	Salmeterol 50 µg b.i.d. + BDP[a] 500 µg b.i.d. n=243 (%)	Salmeterol 100 µg b.i.d.[b] + BDP[a] 500 µg b.i.d. n=244 (%)	BDP[a] 1000 µg n=251 (%)
Headache	26 (11)	38 (16)	42 (17)
Tremors	6 (2)	19 (8)	2 (<1)
Palpitations	4 (2)	6 (2)	4 (2)
Tachycardia	4 (2)	5 (2)	2 (<1)

[a] BDP=Beclomethasone dipropionate.
[b] 100 µg b.i.d. is not a recommended dose.

Use in Children: Two multicenter, randomized, double-blind studies have compared twice daily administration of SEREVENT 25 µg and 50 µg versus salbutamol in patients aged 4 to 16 years with asthma. Adverse events that occurred with an incidence of ≥3 in the salmeterol groups, irrespective of the relationship to treatment, are summarized in Table 4.

The studies did not reveal any unexpected or clinically important differences between treatment with salmeterol 25 µg bid or 50 µg bid and salbutamol 200 µg bid. There was no evidence to suggest that children of a younger age were more at risk than those in the older age groups.

Other Asthma Clinical Trial Adverse Drug Reactions: In US clinical trials, other events occurring in the SEREVENT treatment group at a frequency of 1% to 3% were:

Table 4: SEREVENT

Number (and percentage) of Patients with Adverse Events (incidence ≥3%) in 2 Large 12-month Pediatric Clinical Trials

Adverse Event	SEREVENT 25 µg b.i.d. (n=251) (%)	SEREVENT 50 µg b.i.d. (n=277) (%)	Salbutamol 200 µg b.i.d. (n=255) (%)
Ear, Nose and Throat			
Upper Respiratory Tract Infection (URTI)	48	49	53
Sore Throat	23	19	20
Ear Infection	10	19	5
Nasal Symptoms	5	3	4
Eye			
Conjunctivitis	7	6	5
Eye Infection	3	0	1
Gastrointestinal			
Nausea and Vomiting	6	6	5
Gastric Upset	4	4	3
Gastroenteritis	4	5	1
Abdominal Pain	3	4	4
Hypersensitivity			
Allergic Rhinitis	8	10	7
Miscellaneous			
Fever	8	12	10
Influenza	10	6	9
Viral Infections	5	5	3
Chickenpox	3	1	3
Injuries	3	2	2
Neurological			
Headaches	14	14	13
Respiratory			
Asthma	50	56	47
Cough	18	23	18
Chest Infection	10	12	13
Bronchitis	7	10	9
Skin			
Eczema	5	7	3

Ear/Nose/Throat: laryngitis, rhinitis.
Gastrointestinal: abdominal pain, dental pain, diarrhea, nausea and vomiting, viral gastroenteritis.
Hypersensitivity: urticaria.
Musculoskeletal: back pain, muscle cramp/contraction, muscular soreness, myalgia/myositis, pain in joints.
Neurological: malaise/fatigue, nervousness.
Respiratory: bronchitis/tracheitis.
Skin: rash/skin eruption.
Urogenital: dysmenorrhea.

In small dose-response studies, tremor, nervousness, and palpitations appeared to be dose related.

COPD: Two multicenter, 12-week, controlled studies have evaluated twice-daily doses of SEREVENT inhalation aerosol in patients with COPD. In clinical trials, SEREVENT was generally well tolerated over chronic dosing periods. The most frequently reported adverse events with SEREVENT 50 µg twice daily were headache, upper respiratory tract infection and sore throat. Table 5 includes all events (whether considered drug-related or non-drug-related by the investigator) that occurred at a rate of over 3% in the SEREVENT inhalation aerosol treatment group and were more common in the SEREVENT inhalation aerosol group than in the placebo group.

Table 5: SEREVENT

Adverse Experience Incidence (>3%) in 2 Large 12-week COPD Clinical Trials

Adverse Event	SEREVENT 50 µg b.i.d. n=267 (%)	Placebo n=278 (%)	Ipratropium 40 µg q.i.d. n=271 (%)
Ear, Nose and Throat			
Upper Respiratory Tract Infection (URTI)	9	7	9
Sore Throat	8	3	6
Nasal Sinus Infection	4	1	2
Gastrointestinal			
Diarrhea	5	3	4
Musculoskeletal			
Back Pain	4	3	3
Neurological			
Headache	12	10	8
Respiratory			
Chest Congestion	4	3	3

Common cold, rhinorrhea, bronchitis, cough, exacerbation of chest congestion, chest pain, and dizziness occurred at 3% or more but were equally common on placebo.

Electrocardiographic Monitoring in Patients with COPD: Continuous electrocardiographic (Holter) monitoring was performed on 284 patients in two large COPD clinical trials during five 24-hour periods. No significant increase in the incidence of ventricular and supraventricular ectopic events was observed between SEREVENT and placebo. No cases of sustained ventricular tachycardia were observed. At baseline, non-sustained, asymptomatic ventricular tachycardia was recorded for 7 (7.1%), 8 (9.4%), and 3 (3.0%) patients in the placebo, SEREVENT, and ipratropium groups, respectively. During treatment, non-sustained, asymptomatic ventricular tachycardia that represented a clinically significant change from baseline was reported for 11 (11.6%), 15 (18.3%), and 20 (20.8%) patients receiving placebo, SEREVENT, and ipratropium, respectively. Four of these cases of ventricular tachycardia were reported as adverse events (1 placebo, 3 SEREVENT) by one investigator based upon review of Holter data. One case of ventricular tachycardia was observed during ECG evaluation of chest pain (ipratropium) and reported as an adverse event.

Other COPD Clinical Trial Adverse Drug Reactions: Other events occurring in the SEREVENT inhalation aerosol treatment group at a frequency of 1% to 3% were:
Ear/Nose/Throat: cold symptoms, earache, epistaxis, nasal congestion, nasal sinus congestion, sinus headache, sneezing.
Gastrointestinal: abdominal pain, constipation, dyspepsia, gastric pain, gastric upset, heartburn, nausea, oral candidiasis, surgical removal of tooth, vomiting, xerostomia.
Musculoskeletal: leg cramps, muscle injury of neck, myalgia, neck pain, pain in arm, shoulder pain.
Neurological: insomnia.
Non Site Specific: discomfort in chest, fatigue, fever, pain in body.
Respiratory: acute bronchitis, dyspnea, influenza, lower respiratory tract infection, pneumonia, respiratory tract infection, shortness of breath.
Urogenital: urinary tract infection.

Post-Market Adverse Drug Reactions: In extensive worldwide postmarketing experience, serious exacerbations of asthma, including some that have been fatal, have been reported. In most cases, these have occurred in patients with severe asthma and/or in some patients in whom asthma has been acutely deteriorating (see Warnings and Precautions), but they have occurred in a few patients with less severe asthma as well. It was not possible from these reports to determine whether SEREVENT contributed to these events or simply failed to relieve the deteriorating asthma.

Postmarketing experience includes rare reports of upper airway symptoms of laryngeal spasm, irritation, or swelling, such as stridor and choking. Hypertension and arrhythmias (including atrial fibrillation, supraventricular tachycardia, and extrasystoles) have been reported. There have also been reports of oropharyneal irritation and very rare reports of hyperglycemia. Immediate hypersensitivity reactions have also been reported after administration of SEREVENT, as demonstrated by rare cases of urticaria, angiodema, rash, and bronchospasm, and very rare cases of anaphylactic shock or anaphylactic reaction. Because these events are voluntarily reported from a population of unknown size, estimates of frequency cannot be made.

DRUG INTERACTIONS: Overview: Use SEREVENT (salmeterol xinafoate)with caution in patients receiving other medications causing hypokalemia and/or increased QTc interval (diuretics, high dose steroids, antiarrhythmics, astemizole, terfenadine) and monoamine oxidase inhibitors or tricyclic antidepressants, since cardiac and vascular effects may be potentiated.

Inhibitors of Cytochrome P450 3A4: Coadministration of repeat dose ketoconazole (a cytochrome P450 3A4 inhibitor) and salmeterol in healthy subjects resulted in a significant increase in plasma salmeterol exposure (1.4-fold increase in C_{max} and 15-fold increase in AUC). This increase in plasma salmeterol exposure may cause a prolongation of the QTc interval (see Warnings and Precautions and Action and Clinical Pharmacology, Pharmacokinetics).

Cromoglycate: In clinical trials, inhaled cromolyn sodium did not alter the safety profile of SEREVENT when administered concurrently.

Ipratropium Bromide: In COPD trials, ipratropium bromide did not alter the safety profile of SEREVENT when administered concurrently.

Drug-Drug Interactions: See Table 6.

Table 6: SEREVENT

Established or Potential Drug-Drug Interactions

Proper Name	Ref	Effect	Clinical Comment
Sympathomimetic Agents	CT	May lead to deleterious cardiovascular effects.	Aerosol bronchodilators of the rapid onset, short duration adrenergic stimulant type may be used for relief of breakthrough symptoms while using salmeterol for asthma. However, increasing use of such preparations to control symptoms indicates deterioration of asthma control and the patient's therapy plan should be reassessed. The regular, concomitant use of salmeterol and other sympathomimetic agents is not recommended.
Monoamine Oxidase Inhibitors or Tricyclic Antidepressants	CS	Action of salmeterol on vascular system may be potentiated.	Salmeterol should be administered with extreme caution to patients being treated with monoamine oxidase inhibitors or tricyclic antidepressants, or within 2 weeks of discontinuation of such agents.
Methylxanthines	CT	Unknown	The concurrent use of intravenously or orally administered methylxanthines (e.g., aminophylline, theophylline) by patients receiving salmeterol has not been completely evaluated.

(cont'd)

Table 6: SEREVENT *(cont'd)*

Established or Potential Drug-Drug Interactions

Proper Name	Ref	Effect	Clinical Comment
Beta-blockers	CS	May antagonize the bronchodilating action of salmeterol.	Non-selective beta-blocking drugs, should never be prescribed in combination with salmeterol. Cardioselective beta-blocking drugs should be used with caution in patients using medications for bronchodilation.
Inhibitors of cytochrome P450 3A4	CT	Increased systemic exposure to salmeterol xinafoate.	Caution is advised when coadministering potent cytochrome P450 3A4 inhibitors (e.g. ketoconazole) (See Drug Interactions, Warnings and Precautions and Action and Clinical Pharmacology, Pharmacokinetics.)

Legend: C=Case Study; CT=Clinical Trial; CS=Class Statements; T=Theoretical.

DOSAGE AND ADMINISTRATION: Dosing Considerations: When treating asthma patients, SEREVENT should be used only as additional therapy for patients whose conditions are not adequately controlled using low- to medium-dose inhaled corticosteroids or the severity of whose disease clearly warrants the initiation of treatment with two maintenance therapies, including SEREVENT. It is **not** indicated for patients whose asthma can be managed by occasional use of a rapid onset, short duration, inhaled β_2-agonist or for patients whose asthma can be successfully managed by inhaled corticosteroids along with occasional use of a rapid onset, short duration, inhaled β_2-agonist.

General Considerations for Asthma and COPD: The dosage or frequency of SEREVENT administration should not be increased since there may be serious adverse effects associated with excessive dosing. SEREVENT should not be used more than twice daily.

Elderly and Patients with Impaired Renal or Hepatic Function: There is no need to adjust the dose in the otherwise healthy elderly or in patients with impaired renal function. Because salmeterol is predominantly cleared by hepatic metabolism, patients with hepatic disease should be closely monitored.

Asthma: SEREVENT (salmeterol xinafoate) should not be initiated in patients with significantly worsening or acutely deteriorating asthma, which may be a life-threatening condition (see Warnings and Precautions).

SEREVENT is not a replacement for inhaled or oral corticosteroid therapy; its use is complementary to it. Patients must be warned not to stop or reduce anti-inflammatory therapy without medical advice, even if they feel better on SEREVENT.

SEREVENT should not be used to treat acute symptoms. It is crucial to inform patients of this and prescribe a rapid onset, short duration β_2-agonist for this purpose. The need for additional symptomatic bronchodilator therapy is usually reduced with SEREVENT (see Warnings and Precautions). Medical attention should be sought if patients find that rapid onset, short duration relief bronchodilator treatment becomes less effective or if they need more inhalations than usual.

Bronchodilators should not be the only or the main treatment in patients with moderate to severe or unstable asthma. Patients with severe asthma require regular medical assessment since death may occur. These patients will require high dose inhaled or oral corticosteroid therapy. Sudden worsening of symptoms may require increased corticosteroid dosage which should be administered under medical supervision.

As twice-daily regular treatment, SEREVENT provides 24-hour bronchodilation and can replace regular use of a rapid onset, short duration (4 hour) inhaled or oral bronchodilator (e.g. salbutamol) when optimum corticosteroid therapy is being used.

For full therapeutic benefit, regular usage of SEREVENT is recommended in the treatment of reversible airways obstruction.

Adolescents/Children: At present, there are insufficient clinical data to recommend the use of salmeterol xinafoate in children younger than 4 years of age. Based on available data, no adjustment of salmeterol dosage in pediatric patients is warranted. In adolescents/children the severity of asthma may be variable with age and periodic reassessment should be considered to determine if continued maintenance therapy with SEREVENT is still indicated.

COPD: Counselling on smoking cessation should be the first step in treating patients with chronic obstructive pulmonary disease. Smoking cessation produces symptomatic benefits and has been shown to confer a survival advantage by slowing or stopping the progression of chronic bronchitis and emphysema.

Use with Rapid Onset, Short Duration Bronchodilators: When beginning treatment with SEREVENT, COPD patients should be instructed to use their rapid onset, short duration bronchodilators as determined by their treating physician, at the lowest dose to relieve their symptoms. The regular twice-daily administration of SEREVENT should reduce the excessive use of rapid onset, short duration, inhaled bronchodilators.

Recommended Dose and Dosage Adjustment: Asthma: Maintenance Therapy: SEREVENT DISKHALER Disk: SEREVENT DISKHALER Disks are for use with a SEREVENT DISKHALER device only.

Patients 4 years of Age and Older: One blister [50 µg of salmeterol (as the xinafoate)] twice daily.

SEREVENT DISKUS: Patients 4 years of Age and Older: One blister [50 µg of salmeterol (as the xinafoate)] twice daily.

Recommended Dose—COPD: For maintenance treatment of bronchospasm and relief of dyspnea associated with COPD (including chronic bronchitis and emphysema), the usual dosage is 50 µg of salmeterol (as the xinafoate) twice daily.

SEREVENT DISKHALER Disk: One blister [50 µg of salmeterol (as the xinafoate)] twice daily.

SEREVENT DISKUS: One blister [50 µg of salmeterol (as the xinafoate)] twice daily.

Missed Dose: If a patient forgets to inhale a dose, instruct the patient to inhale another as soon as they remember **unless** it is near the time for their next dose. If so the patient should wait until the next dose and resume the regular dosing schedule. Do not double dose.

Administration: SEREVENT is administered by the inhaled route only.

OVERDOSAGE:

Do Not Exceed Recommended Dosage: As with other inhaled β_2-adrenergic drugs, SEREVENT should not be used more often or at higher doses than recommended. Fatalities have been reported in association with excessive use of inhaled sympathomimetic drugs. Large doses of inhaled or oral salmeterol (12 to 20 times the recommended dose) have been associated with clinically significant prolongation of the QTc interval, which has the potential for producing ventricular arrhythmias (see Warning and Precautions, Cardiovascular and Other Effects).

The expected signs and symptoms of salmeterol overdosage are those typical of excessive β_2 adrenergic stimulation including tremor, headache, tachycardia, increases in systolic blood pressure, cardiac arrhythmias, hypokalemia, hypertension, or hypotension, metabolic acidosis (in rare cases) and, in extreme cases, sudden death. Treatment should be symptomatic; cardiac and respiratory function should be monitored and support provided if necessary. The preferred antidote for overdosage with salmeterol is the judicious use of a cardioselective β-blocking agent. Cardioselective β-blocking drugs should be used with caution, bearing in mind the danger of inducing an asthmatic attack. Serum potassium level should be monitored.

Fatalities have been reported following excessive use of aerosol preparations containing sympathomimetic amines, the exact cause of which is unknown. Cardiac arrest was reported in several instances.

For management of a suspected drug overdose, contact your **regional Poison Control Centre**. See the *CPS* Directory section for a list of Poison Control Centres.

ACTION AND CLINICAL PHARMACOLOGY: Mechanism of Action: SEREVENT (salmeterol xinafoate) is a selective, long-acting (12 hours), slow onset (10-20 minutes) β_2-adrenoceptor agonist with a long side-chain which binds to the exo-site of the receptor.

Salmeterol offers more effective protection against histamine-induced bronchoconstriction and produces a longer duration of bronchodilation, lasting for at least 12 hours, than recommended doses of conventional rapid onset, short duration β_2-agonists.

In contrast to conventional rapid onset, short duration β_2-agonists, the onset of the bronchodilator effect of salmeterol usually occurs in 10-20 minutes. However, the full benefits only become apparent after the first or second dose of the drug. Regular dosing produces sustained improvement in lung function thereby reducing symptoms of airways obstruction.

In vitro tests on human lung, have shown salmeterol is a potent and long-lasting inhibitor of the release of mast cell mediators, such as histamine, leukotrienes and prostaglandin D_2.

In man, salmeterol inhibits the early and late phase response to inhaled allergen. The late phase response is inhibited for over 30 hours after a single dose, when the bronchodilator effect is no longer evident. The full clinical significance of these findings is not yet clear. The mechanism is different from the anti-inflammatory effect of corticosteroids.

Pharmacodynamics: In patients, salmeterol by both pressurised and powder inhalers in single doses of 25 µg or greater has been shown to produce bronchodilation lasting for approximately 12 hours. This long duration of action has been confirmed by challenge studies using exercise, histamine and methacholine as bronchoconstrictor agents. Salmeterol has also been shown to abolish both the early and late phase bronchoconstrictor response to inhaled allergen, the clinical significance of which has not been established.

Pharmacokinetics: Salmeterol acts locally in the lung; plasma levels therefore do not predict therapeutic effect. Because of the low therapeutic dose, systemic levels of salmeterol are low or undetectable after inhalation of recommended doses (50 µg twice daily).

Salmeterol is predominantly cleared by hepatic metabolism; liver function impairment may lead to accumulation of salmeterol in plasma. Therefore, patients with hepatic disease should be closely monitored.

An in vitro study showed that salmeterol is extensively metabolised to α-hydroxysalmeterol (aliphatic oxidation) by cytochrome P450 3A4 (CYP3A4). A repeat dose study with salmeterol and erythromycin in healthy volunteers showed no clinically significant changes in pharmacodynamic effects at 500 mg three times daily doses of erythromycin. However, a salmeterol-ketoconazole interaction study resulted in a significant increase in plasma salmeterol exposure (see Warnings and Precautions and Drug Interactions).

In a placebo-controlled, crossover drug interaction study in 15 healthy subjects, coadministration of salmeterol (50 µg twice daily inhaled) and the cytochrome P450 3A4 (CYP3A4) inhibitor, ketoconazole (400 mg once daily orally), for 7 days, resulted in a significant increase in plasma salmeterol exposure (1.4-fold C_{max} and 15-fold AUC). There was no increase in salmeterol accumulation with repeat dosing. Three subjects were withdrawn from salmeterol and ketoconazole coadministration due to QTc prolongation or palpitations with sinus tachycardia. In the remaining 12 subjects, coadministration of salmeterol and ketoconazole did not result in a clinically significant effect on heart rate, blood potassium or QTc duration (see Warnings and Precautions and Drug Interactions).

STORAGE AND STABILITY: SEREVENT DISKHALER Disk should not be exposed to extremes of temperature, and should be stored below 25°C and protected from humidity.

A SEREVENT DISKHALER Disk may be kept in the DISKHALER at all times but a blister should only be pierced immediately prior to use. Failure to observe this instruction will affect operation of the DISKHALER.

SEREVENT DISKUS should be stored below 30°C and in a dry place.

INFORMATION FOR THE PATIENT: Published in e-CPS, available by subscription at www.e-cps.ca.

DOSAGE FORMS, COMPOSITION AND PACKAGING: DISKHALER Disks: Each circular, double-foil blister pack contains: 4 regularly distributed blisters, each containing a dry powder blend of microfine salmeterol (as the xinafoate salt). Each blister contains: salmeterol 50 µg. Nonmedicinal ingredients: lactose (which contains milk protein). Cartons of 15 disks (4 blisters/disk). DISKHALER Disks are available individually.

DISKUS: Each dose of dry powder of microfine salmeterol (as the xinafoate salt) for inhalation contains: the equivalent of salmeterol 50 µg. Nonmedicinal ingredients: lactose (milk sugar), including milk protein, which acts as the "carrier". Formats of 60 doses.

(Shown in Product Identification Section)

Serophene® 🄿

clomiphene citrate

Ovulatory Agent

EMD Canada

Date of Preparation: August 25, 1998
Date of Revision: April 2007

PHARMACOLOGY: Serophene (clomiphene citrate) is an orally-administered, non-steroidal agent which may induce ovulation in anovulatory women in appropriately selected cases.

Mechanism of Action: The stimulation of an ovulatory response to cyclic Serophene therapy is believed to be related to its antiestrogenic properties; by competing with estrogen for binding sites at the hypothalamic level, it may cause increased secretion of luteinizing hormone (LH) and follicle-stimulating hormone (FSH), with subsequent ovarian stimulation and preovulatory LH surge, resulting in maturation of the ovarian follicle and development of the corpus luteum.

The involvement of the pituitary is indicated by increased urinary excretion of gonadotropins and by the response of the ovary as manifested by increased urinary estrogen excretion.

Following therapy with Serophene, presumptive signs of ovulation resemble those associated with normal menstrual cycle. It should be noted, however, that during drug administration and for several days thereafter, the effects of endogenous estrogen on the vaginal mucosa and cervical mucus are inhibited.

Suggested criteria for ovulation following Serophene may include the ovulatory peak of estrogen excretion, a biphasic basal body temperature curve, urinary excretion of pregnanediol at postovulatory of higher levels, and endometrial histologic findings characteristic of the luteal phase. In most patients, ovulation appears to occur from 6 to 12 days after completion of therapy at recommended dosage.

A review of fourteen publications appearing between 1964 and 1983 showed that an ovulatory response occurred in 74% of 8228 patients with ovulatory dysfunction who received clomiphene citrate. Successful therapy characterized by pregnancy occurred in 31% of the 8228 patients. (See Table 1.)

Table 1: Serophene

Pregnancies Following Clomiphene Citrate USP[a]

Author		No. of Patients	Ovulation Rate	Pregnancy Rate
Gysler et al.	(1982)	428	85.3	42.8
Hummond et al.	(1983)	159	86.0	49.0
Kase et al.	(1967)	81	60.5	25.9
Kistner	(1965)	50	96.0	26.0
MacGregor et al.	(1968)	6714	70.0	32.7
Murray & Osmond-Clarke	(1971)	328	66.5	25.0
O'Herlity et al.	(1981)	30	70.0	27.0
Pildes	(1965)	36	50.0	11.1
Rabau et al.	(1967)	101	62.6	33.6
Rust et al.	(1974)	105	91.4	38.1
Seegar-Jones & Moraes-Ruehsen	(1967)	73	83.0	30.1
Spellacy & Cohen	(1967)	35	80.0	20.0
Sutaria et al.	(1980)	51	64.7	31.4

(cont'd)

Table 1: Serophene *(cont'd)*

Pregnancies Following Clomiphene Citrate USP[a]

Author		No. of Patients	Ovulation Rate	Pregnancy Rate
Whitelow et al.	(1964)	37	72.9	45.9
Total		8828	74.21	31.33

[a] The reported data included patients receiving other than recommended dosage regimen.

INDICATIONS: Serophene (clomiphene citrate) is indicated in the treatment of ovulatory failure in patients desiring pregnancy, whose partners have adequate sperm and who have potentially functional hypothalamic-hypophyseal ovarian systems and adequate endogenous estrogens. Impediments to this goal must be excluded or adequately treated before beginning therapy. The workup and treatment of candidates for Serophene therapy should be supervised by physicians experienced in management of gynecologic or endocrine disorders. The workup of the patient must begin with a careful and detailed history of menstrual and reproductive function, and a complete physical examination. It should be followed by a selective and careful laboratory investigation, based on historical and physical findings.

The following considerations are appropriate for selection of patients:

1. If any doubt exists as to the presence of early pregnancy, Serophene therapy should be withheld until a diagnosis of pregnancy has been excluded.
2. The partner's potential fertility and potency should be ascertained by semen analysis and other indicated examinations.
3. Mechanical impediments to conception, such as tubal obstruction, should be excluded or adequately treated before undertaking Serophene therapy.
4. The diagnosis of ovulatory dysfunction should be established by such standard techniques as basal body temperature curves, serial vaginal smears, cervical mucus, endometrial biopsy, and pregnanediol determination.
5. Appropriate diagnostic measures should be undertaken to exclude primary pituitary failure or primary ovarian failure. Intact pituitary and ovaries are required for successful therapy. Ovulatory dysfunction in the presence of abnormally high levels of pituitary gonadotropins is indicative of ovarian failure, and patients in this category cannot be expected to respond to Serophene. Adequacy of endogenous estrogen, as estimated by vaginal smears, cervical mucus, endometrial biopsy, or urinary estrogen determination, furnishes a measure of ovarian function and indirectly of pituitary function. Bleeding after progesterone administration (progesterone alone, not combined with estrogen) furnishes evidence of an adequate level of endogenous estrogen. A good level of endogenous estrogen provides a favourable prognosis for treatment with Serophene. A reduced estrogen level, although less favourable, does not always preclude successful therapy.
6. Patients with abnormal or excessive bleeding should have particularly careful evaluation prior to Serophene therapy. It is most important to ensure that neoplastic lesions are not overlooked.
7. Clinical evaluation of liver function should always precede Serophene therapy.
8. When disorders such as diabetes, adrenal disease, or thyroid disease are identified during investigation, specific treatment should be undertaken and subfertility therapy reconsidered only after the underlying disorder has been adequately treated. Serophene cannot be expected to be a substitute for specific therapy of these conditions.

CONTRAINDICATIONS: *Pregnancy:* Serophene (clomiphene citrate) should not be administered during pregnancy since studies in rats and rabbits have shown clomiphene to be teratogenic. Studies in humans have not been done. However, there have been reports of congenital malformations and fetal death associated with clomiphene administration in humans, although a direct causal relationship has not been established. To prevent inadvertent Serophene administration during early pregnancy, careful pelvic examination must be done prior to each course of therapy, the basal body temperature must be recorded throughout all treatment cycles, and the patient should be carefully observed to determine whether ovulation has occurred. If the basal body temperature following Serophene is biphasic and is not followed by menses, the patient should be examined carefully for the presence of an ovarian cyst and should have a pregnancy test. The next course of therapy should be delayed until the possibility of pregnancy has been excluded.

Medical Problems: Serophene should not be used when the following medical problems exist (reasons given where appropriate):

Liver disease: Serophene therapy is contraindicated in patients with active liver disease of history of hepatic function impairment.

Abnormal bleeding: Serophene is contraindicated in patients with abnormal bleeding of undetermined origin. (Careful evaluation is recommended; neoplastic lesions should not be overlooked). Serophene is not indicated for the management of menstrual disorders.

Fibroid tumours of the uterus.

Ovarian cyst: Serophene should not be given in the presence of an ovarian cyst, since further enlargement of the ovary may occur.

Mental depression.

Thrombophlebitis.

WARNINGS: Visual Symptoms: Patients should be advised that blurring or other visual symptoms, dizziness or light-headedness may occasionally occur during therapy with Serophene (clomiphene citrate). Patients should be warned that visual symptoms may render such activities as driving a car or operating machinery more hazardous than usual, particularly under conditions of variable lighting. The significance of these visual symptoms is not yet understood (see Adverse Effects). If the patient has any visual symptoms, treatment should be discontinued and complete ophthalmologic evaluation carried out.

PRECAUTIONS: Diagnosis prior to Serophene therapy: Careful attention should be given to diagnosis in candidates for Serophene (clomiphene citrate) therapy. Complete pelvic examination including cervical cytology is mandatory prior to treatment, and pelvic examination should be repeated before each subsequent course. Serophene should not be given in the presence of an ovarian cyst, since further enlargement of the ovary may occur.

Patients in later reproductive life have a greater tendency to endometrial carcinoma as well as a higher incidence of anovulatory disorders. Dilation and curettage should always be done for diagnosis before starting Serophene therapy in such patients. If abnormal bleeding is present, full diagnostic measures are mandatory.

Overstimulation of the ovary during Serophene therapy: In order to minimize the hazard associated with the occasional abnormal ovarian enlargement associated with Serophene (clomiphene citrate) therapy (see Adverse Effects), the lowest dose consistent with expectation of good results should be used. The patient should be advised of the possibility of ovarian cyst formation and should be instructed to return for repeat pelvic examination between 2 and 3 weeks after starting each course of treatment. Some patients with polycystic ovarian syndrome who are unusually sensitive to gonadotropin may have an exaggerated response to usual doses of Serophene. It should be borne in mind that maximal enlargement of the ovary, whether physiologic or abnormal, does not occur until several days after discontinuation of the recommended dose of Serophene. The patient who complains of pelvic pain after receiving Serophene should be examined with care. If enlargement of the ovary occurs, additional Serophene therapy should not be given until the ovaries have returned to pretreatment size, and the dosage or duration of the next course should be reduced. Experience has shown that the ovarian enlargement and cyst formation associated with Serophene therapy regress spontaneously within a few days or weeks after discontinuing treatment. Unless surgical indication for laparotomy exists, such cystic enlargement should always be managed conservatively.

Multiple Pregnancy: The incidence of multiple pregnancy (including triplets, quadruplets and quintuplets) has been increased up to tenfold when conception takes place during a cycle in which clomiphene citrate therapy is given. During clinical studies, 353 infants were born of 163 multiple pregnancies. Of these infants, 293 survived, including 27 of 62 infants from triplet, quadruplet and quintuplet pregnancies. The patient and her partner should be advised of the frequency and potential hazards of multiple pregnancy before starting treatment.

Diagnostic Interference: Plasma desmosterol concentrations (only with long-term use, possibly indicating interference with cholesterol synthesis). Plasma transcortin concentrations. Serum thyroxine concentrations. Sex hormone-binding globulin concentrations. Sulfobromophthalein (BSP) retention (indicating hepatotoxicity) and thyroxine-binding globulin (TBG) concentrations (may be increased).

Carcinogenicity: Two cases of bilateral breast carcinoma in women treated with clomiphene have been reported.

Patient check-ups: The following procedures may be especially important in patient monitoring (other tests may be warranted in some patients, depending on condition): Complete pelvic examination for evaluation of ovarian size (recommended prior to each course of treatment with clomiphene). Daily basal body temperature. Estrogen excretion determinations. Histological studies of luteal phase endometrium. Serum progesterone concentrations. Urinary excretion of pregnanediol (recommended during or after a cycle of clomiphene treatment to determine whether ovulation has occurred). Endometrial biopsy (recommended prior to initiation of clomiphene treatment in older patients to rule out the presence of endometrial carcinoma). Liver function tests (recommended prior to initiation of therapy with clomiphene). Ophthalmologic, including slit-lamp, examination (recommended if treatment with clomiphene is continued for more than 1 year).

ADVERSE EFFECTS: Note: At recommended dosage, adverse reactions are usually rare. Incidence and severity of adverse reactions tend to be related to dose and duration of treatment and are usually reversible after clomiphene therapy is discontinued.

Use of clomiphene is associated with an increased incidence of multiple pregnancies and, therefore, possible premature deliveries.

Clomiphene may cause a decrease in cervical mucus which may interfere with response.

The following adverse reactions have been selected on the basis of their potential clinical significance (possible cause in parentheses where appropriate—not necessarily inclusive).

Those indicating need for medical attention: Incidence more frequent than 5%.

Abdominal discomfort (bloating, stomach or pelvic pain) may be most often related to ovulatory or premenstrual phenomena, to ovarian enlargement or to enlargement of fibroids.

At recommended dosage, abnormal ovarian enlargement (see Precautions) is infrequent, although the usual cyclic variations in ovarian size may be exaggerated. Similarly, cyclic ovarian pain (mittelschmerz) may be accentuated. With higher or prolonged dosage, more frequent ovarian enlargement and cyst formation (usually luteal) may occur, and the luteal phase of the cycle may be prolonged. Rare instances of massive ovarian enlargement are on record. Southam and Janovski described such an instance in a patient with polycystic ovarian syndrome whose clomiphene citrate therapy consisted of 100 mg daily for 14 days. Abnormal ovarian enlargement usually regresses spontaneously, and while laparotomy was performed on several such patients, investigators believe most of these patients should have been treated conservatively.

Note: Maximum ovarian enlargement occurs several days after clomiphene therapy is discontinued.

Blurred vision (ocular toxicity): Visual symptoms (see Warnings for further recommendations) described usually as "blurring" or spots or flashes, disappear within a few days or weeks after Serophene (clomiphene citrate) is discontinued. These symptoms appear to be due to intensification and prolongation of after-images. Symptoms often first appear or are accentuated with exposure to a more brightly lit environment. While measured visual acuity has not generally been affected, one patient taking 200 mg daily developed visual blurring on the seventh day of treatment, which progressed to severe diminution of visual acuity by the tenth day. No other abnormality was found and the visual acuity returned to normal on the third day after treatment was stopped. Another patient treated during the clinical studies developed scotomata during prolonged Serophene administration, which disappeared on placebo. Monolateral exophthalmos associated with laboratory evidence of hyperthyroidism was observed in one patient concomitant with completion of the third course of clomiphene citrate. In a 34 year-old patient who had taken 3 courses of clomiphene citrate, slit-lamp microscopic examination showed a mild amount of posterior cortical subcapsular opacity in each eye. Ophthalmoscopic examination revealed normal findings. The ocular diagnosis was posterior cortical senile cataracts.

Yellowing of eyes and skin (hepatotoxicity).

Those indicating need for medical attention only if they continue or are bothersome: Incidence more frequent than 10%: Hot flashes: The vasomotor symptoms resemble long menopausal "hot flashes" are not usually severe and disappear promptly after treatment is discontinued.

Incidence less frequent or rare: 1 to 2%.

Breast discomfort; dizziness or lightheadedness; headache; heavy menstrual periods or bleeding between periods; mental depression, nervousness, restlessness, sleeplessness, or tiredness; nausea or vomiting.

Other less frequently reported symptoms during therapy have included: urticaria or allergic dermatitis, weight gain, increased urinary frequency or volume, constipation or diarrhea; moderate, reversible hair loss has been reported in a few patients, primarily on continuous therapy.

Serophene has not been reported to cause significant abnormality in the hematologic or renal systems, in protein bound iodine, or in serum cholesterol. Analysis by gas liquid chromatography (GLC) of serum sterols from patients on prolonged, continuous administration of Serophene yields a peak compatible with an elevated level of desmosterol. This peak is indicative of an interference with cholesterol synthesis. However, the serum sterol GLC pattern from patients receiving recommended doses of Serophene is not significantly altered.

Sulfobromophthalein (BSP) retention of greater than 5% has been reported in 32 of 141 patients in whom it was measured, including 5 of 43 patients who received approximately the dose of clomiphene citrate now recommended. Retention was usually minimal unless associated with prolonged continuous clomiphene citrate administration or with apparently unrelated live disease. In some patients, pre-existing BSP retention decreased even though clomiphene citrate therapy was continued. Other liver function tests were usually normal. In a later study in which patients were given 6 consecutive monthly courses of clomiphene citrate (100 mg daily for 3 days) or matching placebo, BSP tests were done on 94 patients. Values in excess of 5% retention were recorded in 11 patients, 6 of whom had received drug and 5 placebo. One patient developed jaundice on the nineteenth day of treatment (50 mg/day); liver biopsy revealed bile stasis without evidence of hepatitis. A male prison subject who received 200 mg daily for 77 days developed the clinical picture of infectious hepatitis; his cellmate was discovered to have had infectious hepatitis four months earlier.

Ovarian cancer has been reported in a very small number of infertile women who have been treated with fertility drugs. A causal relationship between treatment with fertility drugs and ovarian cancer has not been established.

Birth Defects: From 2339 completed pregnancies associated with clomiphene citrate administration, 58 birth defects have been reported, for a cumulative rate of 2.5%. They have been reported in 4 conceptions in the abortion/stillbirth category, 14 of 353 infants from multiple pregnancies, and 39 of 1676 infants from single pregnancies. Three live-born infants failed to survive.

Reported defects were congenital heart lesions (8 infants), Down's syndrome (5 infants), club foot (4 infants), congenital gut lesions (4 infants), hypospadias (3 infants), microcephaly (2 infants), harelip and cleft palate (2 infants), congenital hip (2 infants), polydactyly (both twins), conjoined twins with teratomatous malformation, patent ductus arteriosus, amaurosis (blindness), arteriovenous fistula, inguinal hernia, umbilical hernia, syndactyly, pectus excavatum, myopathy, dermoid cyst of scalp, omphalocele, spina bifida occulta, ichthyosis, persistent lingual frenulum, and 7 infants with multiple somatic defects.

Eight of the entire group of 58 infants were born to 7 of 153 mothers who received a course of clomiphene citrate during the first 6 weeks after conception.

An interval of 4, 4, and 10 months respectively elapsed between the last clomiphene citrate therapy and conception in 3 mothers. In a fourth mother, conception occurred during a subsequent ovulation induced by gonadotropin therapy.

The cumulative rate of congenital abnormalities does not exceed that reported in the general population.

OVERDOSE:

Treatment: There is no known antidote, but gastric lavage should be performed.

> For management of a suspected drug overdose, CPhA recommends that you contact your **regional Poison Control Centre**. See the *CPS* Directory section for a list of Poison Control Centres.

DOSAGE: Patients receiving clomiphene should be under supervision of a physician experienced in the treatment of gynecologic or endocrine disorders. Patients should be chosen for therapy with Serophene (clomiphene citrate) only after careful diagnostic evaluation (see Indications).

The plan of therapy should be outlined in advance. Impediments to achieving the goal of therapy must be excluded or adequately treated before beginning Serophene.

Patients who have been hypoestrogenic for prolonged periods may require pretreatment with estrogen to provide a more normal endometrium for ovum implantation. Estrogen therapy should be discontinued immediately before initiation of clomiphene citrate.

In some patients, a single injection of 5000 to 10 000 USP units of human chorionic gonadotropin (hCG) is given 3 to 7 days after the last dose of clomiphene to stimulate the midcycle LH surge which results in ovulation.

Many patients will respond to 50 mg of Serophene (clomiphene citrate) daily for 5 days (see Recommended Dosage). In the determination of a recommended starting dose schedule, efficacy must be balanced against potential adverse reactions. For example, the data available so far suggest that ovulation and pregnancy are slightly more attainable on 100 mg/day for 5 days than on 50 mg/day for 5 days. As the dosage is increased, however, ovarian overstimulation and other adverse reactions may be expected to increase. Furthermore, although the data does not yet establish a relationship between dosage and multiple births, it would seem reasonable on pharmacologic grounds that such a relationship does exist. For these reasons, it would seem prudent to begin the treatment of the usual patient with a lower dose, 50 mg daily for 5 days, and to increase the dose only in those patients who do not respond to the first course (see Recommended Dosage).

Patients with unusual sensitivity to pituitary gonadotropins (for example, those with polycystic ovarian syndrome) may require a lower dosage or shorter duration of clomiphene therapy. Use of clomiphene is not recommended in patients with ovarian cysts because further enlargement may occur. A patient's report of abdominal pain during clomiphene therapy indicates immediate pelvic examination. If ovarian enlargement or cyst formation has occurred, it is recommended that clomiphene therapy be withdrawn until the ovaries have returned to pretreatment size, usually within a few days or weeks. Dosage and duration of the next course of clomiphene should be reduced. If the patient receiving clomiphene experiences any visual disturbances, it is recommended that clomiphene therapy be withdrawn and a complete ophthalmologic examination performed. Ocular adverse reactions usually disappear within a few days or weeks after the last dose of clomiphene.

The majority of patients who are going to respond will respond to the first course of therapy, and 3 courses should constitute an adequate therapeutic trial. Treatment beyond this is not recommended in the patient who does not exhibit evidence of ovulation. If ovulatory menses does not occur after 3 to 4 cycles of clomiphene therapy at the maximum dose, or pregnancy after a treatment-free interval of 3 to 6 months, the diagnosis should be reevaluated.

Pregnancy: In most patients, ovulation appears to occur from 6 to 12 days after completion of therapy. For regularity of cyclic ovulatory response, it is also important that each course of Serophene be started on or about the fifth cycle day, once ovulation has been established. The importance of properly timed coitus cannot be over-emphasized. Conception should be attempted by having intercourse every other day, starting within 48 hours before ovulation.

If a cycle of Serophene is followed by a biphasic course of basal body temperature and menses do not ensue, the next cycle of Serophene should be delayed until it is confirmed that the patient is not pregnant.

In common with other therapeutic modalities, Serophene therapy follows the rule of diminishing returns, such that likelihood of conception diminishes with each succeeding course of therapy. If pregnancy has not been achieved after 3 ovulatory responses to Serophene, further treatment is not recommended. Patients should be advised of the possibility of multiple pregnancy and its potential hazards if conception occurs during a cycle in which Serophene is given.

Recommended Dosage: Serophene (clomiphene citrate) tablets.

Usual adult dose: Oral, 50 mg (1 tablet) a day for five days, starting on the fifth day of the menstrual cycle, if bleeding occurs or at any time in the patient who has had no recent uterine bleeding. If ovulation without conception occurs, this cycle is repeated until conception or for three or four cycles. When ovulation occurs at the regimen of 50 mg daily for 5 days, there is no advantage to increasing the dose in subsequent cycles of treatment. If ovulation does not occur, the dose is increased to 100 mg a day for five days (starting as early as 30 days after the previous course), repeated if ovulation without conception occurs. Some patients require up to 250 mg/day to induce ovulation.

Note: The majority of patients who are going to respond will respond to the first course of therapy, and 3 courses should constitute an adequate therapeutic trial. If ovulatory menses do not occur after 3 cycles of clomiphene therapy at the maximum dose, or pregnancy after a treatment-free interval of 3 to 6 months, the diagnosis should be reevaluated. Treatment beyond this is not recommended in the patient who does not exhibit evidence of ovulation.

Usual adult prescribing limits: Doses over 100 mg a day for five days have been associated with a higher incidence of adverse reactions, and patients receiving these doses should be carefully monitored.

INFORMATION FOR THE PATIENT: Published in e-CPS, available by subscription at www.e-cps.ca.

SUPPLIED: Each round, white, flat, beveled-edge scored tablet, identified S on one side, contains: clomiphene citrate USP 50 mg. Bottles of 50. Blister packs of 10. Store in well-closed containers, protected from light, between 15 to 30°C.

(Shown in Product Identification Section)

Seroquel® Pr

quetiapine fumarate

Antipsychotic

AstraZeneca

Date of Revision: February 17, 2010

SUMMARY PRODUCT INFORMATION:

Route of Administration	Dosage Form/Strength	Nonmedicinal Ingredients
Oral	Immediate-release tablet/ 25, 100, 200 and 300 mg	The core of the tablet contains the excipients calcium hydrogen phosphate dihydrate, lactose monohydrate, magnesium stearate, microcrystalline cellulose, povidone, and sodium starch glycolate type A. The coating of the tablet contains hydroxypropyl methylcellulose 2910, polyethylene glycol 400, red ferric oxide (25 mg tablets), titanium dioxide, and yellow ferric oxide (25 mg and 100 mg tablets).

INDICATIONS AND CLINICAL USE: Adults: Schizophrenia: SEROQUEL (quetiapine fumarate immediate-release) is indicated for the management of the manifestations of schizophrenia. The antipsychotic efficacy of SEROQUEL was established in short-term (6-week) controlled inpatient trials. The efficacy of SEROQUEL in long-term use, that is, for more than 6 weeks, has not been systematically evaluated in controlled trials of patients with manifestations of schizophrenia.

Bipolar Disorder: SEROQUEL is indicated as monotherapy for the:

- Acute management of manic episodes associated with bipolar disorder.
- Acute management of depressive episodes associated with bipolar I and bipolar II disorder.

The efficacy of SEROQUEL in bipolar mania was established in two 12-week clinical trials of bipolar patients. The safety and effectiveness of SEROQUEL for long-term use, and for prophylactic use in bipolar mania has not been evaluated.

The efficacy of SEROQUEL in bipolar depression was established in four 8-week clinical trials that included either bipolar I or bipolar II patients.

Geriatrics (>65 years of age): SEROQUEL is not indicated in elderly patients with dementia. See Warnings and Precautions, Serious Warnings and Precautions Box and Special Populations.

Pediatrics (<18 years of age): The safety and efficacy of SEROQUEL in children under the age of 18 years have not been established.

CONTRAINDICATIONS: SEROQUEL (quetiapine fumarate immediate-release) is contraindicated in patients with a known hypersensitivity to this medication or any of its ingredients. For a complete listing, see Dosage Forms, Composition and Packaging.

WARNINGS AND PRECAUTIONS:

Serious Warnings and Precautions

Increased Mortality in Elderly Patients with Dementia: Elderly patients with dementia treated with atypical antipsychotic drugs are at an increased risk of death compared to placebo. Analyses of thirteen placebo controlled trials with various atypical antipsychotics (modal duration of 10 weeks) in these patients showed a mean 1.6 fold increase in death rate in the drug-related patients. Although the causes of death were varied, most of the deaths appeared to be either cardiovascular (e.g., heart failure, sudden death) or infectious (e.g., pneumonia) in nature (see Warnings and Precautions, Special Populations, Use in Geriatric Patients with Dementia).

General: Body Temperature Regulation: Although not reported with SEROQUEL (quetiapine fumarate immediate-release) disruption of the body's ability to reduce core body temperature has been attributed to antipsychotic agents. Appropriate care is advised when prescribing SEROQUEL for patients who will be experiencing conditions which may contribute to an elevation of core temperature, e.g., exercising strenuously, exposure to extreme heat, receiving concomitant medication with anticholinergic activity, or being subject to dehydration.

Acute Withdrawal (discontinuation) Symptoms: Acute discontinuation symptoms such as insomnia, nausea, headache, diarrhea, vomiting, dizziness and irritability, have been described after abrupt cessation of antipsychotic drugs including SEROQUEL. Gradual withdrawal over a period of at least one to two weeks is advisable. Symptoms usually resolved after 1 week post-discontinuation.

Cardiovascular: Hypotension and Syncope: As with other drugs that have high α1 adrenergic receptor blocking activity, SEROQUEL may induce orthostatic hypotension, dizziness, and sometimes syncope, especially during the initial dose titration period. These events may lead to falls.

Syncope was reported in 1% (35/4083) of patients treated with SEROQUEL, compared with 0.3% (3/1006) on placebo, and 0.4% (2/527) on active control drugs. The risk of hypotension and syncope may be reduced by more gradual titration to the target dose (see Dosage and Administration). SEROQUEL should be used with caution in patients with known cardiovascular disease (e.g., history of myocardial infarction or ischemic heart disease, heart failure or conduction abnormalities), cerebrovascular disease, or other conditions predisposing to hypotension (e.g., dehydration, hypovolemia and treatment with antihypertensive medications) (see Overdosage).

Cholesterol and Triglyceride Elevations: Very common (≥10%) cases of elevations in serum triglyceride levels (≥2.258 mmol/L on at least one occasion), elevations in total cholesterol (predominantly LDL cholesterol) (≥6.2064 mmol/L on at least one occasion), and decreases in HDL cholesterol (<1.025 mmol/L males; <1.282 mmol/L females at any time) have been observed during treatment with quetiapine in clinical trials (see Adverse Reactions). Lipid changes should be managed as clinically appropriate.

In short-term placebo-controlled schizophrenia trials, SEROQUEL-treated patients showed mean increases from baseline in cholesterol and triglyceride of 11% and 17%, respectively, compared to mean decreases in the placebo-treated patients. LDL cholesterol was not measured in these trials.

In short-term placebo-controlled bipolar depression trials, SEROQUEL-treated patients had decreases from baseline in mean cholesterol and increases from baseline in mean triglyceride of 0.7% and 12%, respectively, compared to decreases in mean cholesterol and increases in mean triglyceride of 1.8% and 2% respectively for placebo-treated patients.

QT Prolongation: In clinical trials, quetiapine was not associated with a persistent increase in absolute QT intervals. However, in post-marketing experience, there were cases reported of QT prolongation with overdose (see Overdosage). As with other antipsychotics, caution should be exercised when quetiapine is prescribed in patients with cardiovascular disease or family history of QT prolongation. Also caution should be exercised when quetiapine is prescribed either with medicines known to increase QT interval or with concomitant neuroleptics, especially for patients with increased risk of QT prolongation, i.e., the elderly, patients with congenital long QT syndrome, congestive heart failure, heart hypertrophy, hypokalemia, or hypomagnesemia (see Drug Interactions).

Endocrine and Metabolism: Hyperglycaemia: As with some other antipsychotics, hyperglycaemia and diabetes mellitus (including exacerbation of pre-existing diabetes, diabetic ketoacidosis, and diabetic coma including some fatal cases) in the aggregate have been reported rarely (≥0.01%-<0.1%) during the use of SEROQUEL in post-marketing experience, sometimes in patients with no reported history of hyperglycaemia (see Adverse Reactions, Post-Market Adverse Drug Reactions).

Increases in blood glucose and hyperglycaemia, and occasional reports of diabetes, have been observed in clinical trials with quetiapine (see Adverse Reactions, Abnormal Hematologic and Clinical Chemistry Findings).

Assessment of the relationship between atypical antipsychotic use and glucose abnormalities is complicated by the possibility of an increased background risk of diabetes mellitus in patients with schizophrenia and the increasing incidence of diabetes mellitus in the general population. Given these confounders, the relationship between atypical antipsychotic use and hyperglycaemia-related adverse events is not completely understood. However, epidemiological studies suggest an increased risk of treatment-emergent hyperglycaemia-related adverse events in patients treated with the atypical antipsychotics. Precise risk estimates for hyperglycaemia-related adverse events in patients treated with atypical antipsychotics are not available.

Any patient treated with atypical antipsychotics should be monitored for symptoms of hyperglycaemia including polydipsia, polyuria, polyphagia, and weakness. Patients who develop symptoms of hyperglycaemia during treatment with atypical antipsychotics should undergo fasting blood glucose testing. In some cases, hyperglycaemia has resolved when the atypical antipsychotic was discontinued; however, some patients required continuation of anti-diabetic treatment despite discontinuation of the suspect drug. Patients with risk factors for diabetes mellitus (e.g., obesity, family history of diabetes) who are starting treatment with atypical antipsychotics should undergo fasting blood glucose testing at the beginning of treatment and periodically during treatment. Patients with an established diagnosis of diabetes mellitus who are started on atypical antipsychotics should be monitored regularly for worsening of glucose control.

Hyperprolactinemia: During clinical trials with quetiapine, elevation in prolactin levels occurred in 3.6% (158/4416) of patients treated with quetiapine compared to 2.6% (51/1968) on placebo (see Adverse Reactions).

Increased prolactin levels with quetiapine were observed in rat studies. As is common with compounds which stimulate prolactin release, the administration of SEROQUEL resulted in an increase in the incidence of mammary neoplasms in rats. The physiological differences between rats and humans with regard to prolactin make the clinical significance of these findings unclear. To date, neither clinical nor epidemiological studies have shown an association between chronic administration of drugs that stimulate prolactin release, and mammary tumourigenesis. Tissue culture experiments, however, indicate that approximately one third of human breast cancers are prolactin dependent in vitro; a factor of potential importance if prescription of these drugs is contemplated in a patient with previously detected breast cancer.

Possible manifestations associated with elevated prolactin levels are amenorrhea, galactorrhea, and menorrhagia.

In the multiple fixed-dose schizophrenia clinical trial there were no differences in prolactin levels at study completion for SEROQUEL, across the recommended dose range, and placebo.

Hypothyroidism: Clinical trials in schizophrenia demonstrated that SEROQUEL is associated with a dose-related decrease in total and free thyroxine (T_4). On average SEROQUEL was associated with about a 20% mean reduction in thyroxine levels (both total and free). Forty-two percent of SEROQUEL-treated patients showed at least a 30% reduction in total T_4 and 7% showed at least a 50% reduction. Maximum reduction of thyroxine levels generally occurred during the first two to four weeks of treatment with SEROQUEL. These reductions were maintained without adaptation or progression during longer term treatment. Decreases in T_4 were not associated with systematic changes in TSH or clinical signs or symptoms of hypothyroidism. Approximately 0.4% (12/2595) of patients treated with SEROQUEL (schizophrenia and bipolar mania studies combined) experienced persistent increases in TSH, and 0.25% of patients were treated with thyroid replacement.

Weight Gain: In controlled schizophrenia clinical trials (up to 6 weeks), mean weight gain was approximately 2.3 kg compared to a mean weight gain of 0.1 kilograms in patients taking placebo (n=427). In open-label extension trials, after 9 to 13 weeks of SEROQUEL monotherapy, the mean weight increase was 1.58 kg (n=170). After 53 to 78 weeks of treatment, the mean weight increase was 1.98 kg (n=137). These data are obtained from uncontrolled, open-label trials; the relevance of these findings to clinical practice is unknown. Weight change over time appeared to be independent of quetiapine dose (see Adverse Reactions).

In the acute placebo-controlled bipolar mania clinical trials (up to 12 weeks) mean weight gain in patients taking SEROQUEL was 1.8 kg compared to a mean weight loss of 0.1 kg in patients taking placebo. In patients completing the entire 12 weeks of treatment mean weight gain in patients taking SEROQUEL was 2.8 kg.

In the acute placebo-controlled bipolar depression clinical trials (8 weeks) mean weight gain in patients taking SEROQUEL was 1.15 kg compared to a mean weight gain of 0.1 kg in patients taking placebo. During maintenance treatment, patients treated with SEROQUEL 300 mg or placebo lost on average 0.1 kg and 0.6 kg, respectively, while patients treated with SEROQUEL 600 mg gained on average 0.8 kg. In patients who completed 40 and 54 weeks of maintenance treatment a small mean decrease was seen in the SEROQUEL 300 mg group (−0.2 kg) and placebo group (−0.8 kg) while patients in the SEROQUEL 600 mg group showed a mean weight gain of 1.2 kg (see Adverse Reactions).

Based on the cumulative acute placebo-controlled clinical trial database, weight gain (based on ≥7% increase in body weight from baseline) was reported in 9.6% in quetiapine-treated patients and 3.8% in placebo-treated patients, which occurs predominantly during the early weeks of treatment in adults (see Adverse Reactions).

Gastrointestinal: Antiemetic Effect: Consistent with its dopamine antagonist effects, SEROQUEL may have an antiemetic effect. Such an effect may mask signs of toxicity due to overdosage of other drugs, or may mask symptoms of disease such as brain tumour or intestinal obstruction.

Dysphagia and Aspiration Pneumonia: Dysphagia and aspiration have been reported with quetiapine. Although a causal relationship with aspiration pneumonia has not been established, SEROQUEL should be used with caution in patients at risk for aspiration pneumonia. See Warnings and Precautions, Special Populations and Adverse Reactions.

Hematologic: Neutropenia: Severe neutropenia ($<0.5\times10^9$/L) has been uncommonly reported in quetiapine clinical trials. There was no apparent dose relationship. Possible risk factors for leucopenia and/or neutropenia include pre-existing low white cell count (WBC) and history of drug induced leucopenia and/or neutropenia. SEROQUEL should be discontinued in patients with a neutrophil count $<1.0\times10^9$/L. These patients should be observed for signs and symptoms of infection and neutrophil counts followed (until they exceed 1.5×10^9/L). See Adverse Reactions, Abnormal Hematologic and Clinical Chemistry Findings and Post-Market Adverse Drug Reactions.

Hepatic/Biliary/Pancreatic: Hepatic Impairment: Decreased clearance of SEROQUEL was observed in patients with mild hepatic impairment (see Action and Clinical Pharmacology, Special Populations and Conditions). Patients with mild hepatic impairment should be started on 25 mg/day. The dose should be increased daily in increments of 25 to 50 mg/day to an effective dose, depending on the clinical response and tolerability in the individual patient. No pharmacokinetic data are available for any dose of SEROQUEL in patients with moderate or severe hepatic impairment. However, should clinical judgement deem treatment with SEROQUEL necessary, the drug should be used with great caution in patients with moderate or severe hepatic impairment (see Action and Clinical Pharmacology, Special Populations and Conditions and Dosage and Administration).

Transaminase Elevations: During premarketing clinical trials, therapy with SEROQUEL was associated with elevation of hepatic transaminases, primarily ALT. Within a clinical trial database of 1892 SEROQUEL-treated schizophrenia patients, with baseline ALT levels <60 IU/L, 5.3% (101/1892) had treatment-emergent ALT elevations to >120 IU/L, 1.5% (29/1892) had elevations to >200 IU/L, and 0.2% (3/1892) had elevations to >400 IU/L. No patients had values in excess of 800 IU/L. None of the SEROQUEL-treated patients who had elevated transaminase values manifested clinical symptomatology associated with liver impairment. The majority of transaminase elevations were seen during the first two months of treatment. Most elevations were transient (80%) while patients continued on SEROQUEL therapy. Of the 101 SEROQUEL-treated patients whose enzyme levels increased to >120 IU/L, 40 discontinued treatment while their ALT values were still raised. In 114 SEROQUEL-treated patients whose baseline ALT was >90 IU/L, only 1 experienced an elevation to >400 IU/L.

In the bipolar disorder trials, the proportions of patients with transaminase elevations of >3 times the upper limits of the normal reference range, was approximately 1% for both SEROQUEL-treated and placebo-treated patients.

Precautions should be exercised when using SEROQUEL in patients with pre-existing hepatic disorders, in patients who are being treated with potentially hepatotoxic drugs, or if treatment-emergent signs or symptoms of hepatic impairment appear.

For patients who have known or suspected abnormal hepatic function prior to starting SEROQUEL, standard clinical assessment, including measurement of transaminase levels is recommended. Periodic clinical reassessment with transaminase levels is recommended for such patients, as well as for patients who develop any signs and symptoms suggestive of a new onset liver disorder during SEROQUEL therapy.

Neurologic: Neuroleptic Malignant Syndrome (NMS): Neuroleptic Malignant Syndrome is a potentially fatal symptom complex that has been reported in association with antipsychotic drugs, including SEROQUEL.

The clinical manifestations of NMS are hyperthermia, muscle rigidity, altered mental status, and evidence of autonomic instability (irregular pulse or blood pressure, tachycardia, diaphoresis, and cardiac dysrhythmia). Additional signs may include elevated creatine phosphokinase, myoglobinuria (rhabdomyolysis) and acute renal failure.

In arriving at a diagnosis, it is important to identify cases where the clinical presentation includes both serious medical illness (e.g., pneumonia, systemic infection, etc.) and untreated or inadequately treated extrapyramidal signs and symptoms. Other important considerations in the differential diagnosis include central anticholinergic toxicity, heat stroke, drug fever and primary central nervous system pathology.

The management of NMS should include immediate discontinuation of antipsychotic drugs, including SEROQUEL, and other drugs not essential to concurrent therapy; intensive symptomatic treatment and medical monitoring; and treatment of any concomitant serious medical problems for which specific treatments are available. There is no general agreement about specific pharmacological treatment regimens for uncomplicated NMS.

If a patient requires antipsychotic drug treatment after recovery from NMS, the potential reintroduction of drug therapy should be carefully considered. The patient should be carefully monitored since recurrences of NMS have been reported.

Tardive Dyskinesia (TD) and Extrapyramidal Symptoms (EPS): Tardive Dyskinesia is a syndrome of potentially irreversible, involuntary, dyskinetic movements that may develop in patients treated with antipsychotic drugs including quetiapine. Although the prevalence of the syndrome appears to be highest among the elderly, especially elderly women, it is impossible to rely upon estimates to predict which patients are likely to develop the syndrome.

In placebo-controlled clinical trials for schizophrenia and bipolar mania the incidence of EPS was no different from that of placebo across the recommended therapeutic dose range. It has been hypothesized that agents with a lower EPS liability may also have a lower liability to produce TD. This relationship predicts that quetiapine should have less potential than typical antipsychotic agents to induce TD in schizophrenia and bipolar mania patients. In short-term, placebo-controlled clinical trials for bipolar depression, the incidence of EPS was higher in quetiapine treated patients than in placebo treated patients. See Adverse Reactions.

The risk of developing TD and the likelihood that it will become irreversible are believed to increase as the duration of treatment and the total cumulative dose of antipsychotic drugs administered to the patient increase. However, the syndrome can develop, although much less commonly, after relatively brief treatment periods at low doses.

There is no known treatment for established cases of TD, although the syndrome may remit, partially or completely, if antipsychotic treatment is withdrawn. Antipsychotic treatment, itself, however, may suppress (or partially suppress) the signs and symptoms of the syndrome and thereby may possibly mask the underlying process. The effect that symptomatic suppression has upon the long-term course of the syndrome is unknown.

Given these considerations, SEROQUEL should be prescribed in a manner that is most likely to minimize the occurrence of TD. Chronic antipsychotic treatment should generally be reserved for patients who appear to suffer from a chronic illness that is known to respond to antipsychotic drugs, and for whom alternative, equally effective, but potentially less harmful treatments are not available or appropriate. In patients who do require chronic treatment, the smallest dose and the shortest duration of treatment producing a satisfactory clinical response should be sought. The need for continued treatment should be reassessed periodically.

If signs and symptoms of TD appear in a patient on SEROQUEL, dose reduction or drug discontinuation should be considered. Some patients may require treatment with SEROQUEL despite the presence of the syndrome. The symptoms of TD can worsen or even arise after discontinuation of treatment (see Adverse Reactions).

Seizures: In controlled schizophrenia clinical trials, there was no difference in the incidence of seizures in patients treated with SEROQUEL or placebo (incidence of 0.4% or 3 events per 100 patient years in patients given SEROQUEL, compared with 0.5% or 6.9 events per 100 patient years for placebo). Nevertheless, as with other antipsychotics, caution is recommended when treating patients with a history of seizures or with conditions associated with a lowered seizure threshold (see Adverse Reactions).

Potential Effect on Cognitive and Motor Performance: Somnolence was a very commonly reported adverse event in patients treated with SEROQUEL, especially during the initial dose titration period. Since SEROQUEL may cause sedation and impair motor skill, patients should be cautioned about performing activities requiring mental alertness, such as operating a motor vehicle or hazardous machinery, until they are reasonably certain that SEROQUEL therapy does not affect them adversely. Somnolence may lead to falls.

Ophthalmologic: Cataracts: The development of cataracts was observed in association with quetiapine treatment in chronic dog studies at 4 times the recommended human dose. Lens changes have also been observed in patients during long-term SEROQUEL treatment, but a causal relationship to SEROQUEL use has not been established. The possibility of lenticular changes during long-term use of SEROQUEL in man, thus can not be excluded at this time. Eye examinations (e.g., slit lamp exam) prior to or shortly after initiation of treatment with SEROQUEL and at 6 month intervals thereafter, are recommended. If clinically significant lens changes associated with SEROQUEL use are observed, discontinuation of SEROQUEL should be considered.

Psychiatric: Suicide/Suicidal Thoughts or Clinical Worsening: Depressive episodes are associated with an increased risk of suicidal thoughts, self-harm and suicide (suicide-related events). This risk persists until significant remission of depression occurs. As improvement may not occur during the first few weeks or more of treatment, patients should be closely monitored until such improvement occurs. It is general clinical experience that the risk of suicide may increase in the early stages of recovery. In addition to depressive episodes associated with bipolar disorder, depression may be co-morbid with schizophrenia.

Schizophrenia as well as manic episodes associated bipolar disorder, can also be associated with an increased risk of suicide-related events, and thus close supervision and appropriate clinical management of high risk patients should accompany drug therapy.

Patients with a history of suicide-related events are also known to be at a greater risk of suicidal thoughts or suicide attempts, and should receive careful monitoring during treatment.

In placebo-controlled bipolar depression clinical trials with SEROQUEL, the incidence of treatment emergent suicidal ideation or suicidal behaviour, as measured by the Columbia Analysis of Suicidal Behaviour, was 1.5% for SEROQUEL-treated patients and 2.0% for placebo-treated patients.

Renal: There is little experience with SEROQUEL in patients with renal impairment, except in a low (subclinical) single dose study (see Action and Clinical Pharmacology, Special Populations and Conditions). SEROQUEL should thus be used with caution in patients with known renal impairment, especially during the initial dosing period (see Dosage and Administration).

Special Populations: Pregnant Women: Patients should be advised to notify their physician if they become pregnant or intend to become pregnant during treatment with SEROQUEL. The safety and efficacy of SEROQUEL during human pregnancy have not been established. Therefore, SEROQUEL should only be used during pregnancy if the expected benefits justify the potential risks.

Nursing Women: The degree to which quetiapine is excreted into human milk is unknown. Women who are breast-feeding should therefore be advised to avoid breast-feeding while taking SEROQUEL.

Pediatrics (<18 years of age): The safety and efficacy of SEROQUEL in children under the age of 18 years have not been established.

Geriatrics (≥65 years of age): The number of patients 65 years of age or over, with schizophrenia or related disorders, exposed to SEROQUEL, during clinical trials was limited (n=38). When compared to younger patients the mean plasma clearance of quetiapine was reduced by 30% to 50% in elderly subjects. In addition, as this population has more frequent hepatic, renal, central nervous system, and cardiovascular dysfunctions, and more frequent use of concomitant medication, caution should be exercised with the use of SEROQUEL in the elderly patient (see Dosage and Administration).

Use in Geriatric Patients with Dementia: Overall Mortality: Elderly patients with dementia treated with atypical antipsychotic drugs showed increased mortality compared to placebo in a meta-analysis of 13 controlled trials of various atypical antipsychotic drugs. In two placebo-controlled trials with oral SEROQUEL in this population, the incidence of mortality was 5.5% for SEROQUEL-treated patients compared to 3.2% for placebo-treated patients. SEROQUEL is not indicated in elderly patients with dementia.

Cerebrovascular Adverse Events: An increased risk of cerebrovascular adverse events has been seen in the dementia population with some atypical antipsychotics. The mechanism for this increased risk is not known. There is insufficient data with quetiapine to know if there is an increased risk of cerebrovascular events associated with quetiapine. An increased risk, however, cannot be excluded. SEROQUEL is not indicated in patients with dementia.

Vascular Disease: SEROQUEL should be used with caution in patients with risk factors for stroke or with a history of stroke.

Dysphagia: Esophageal dysmotility and aspiration have been associated with antipsychotic drug use. Aspiration pneumonia is a common cause of morbidity and mortality in elderly patients, in particular those with advanced Alzheimer's dementia. SEROQUEL and other antipsychotic drugs should be used cautiously in patients at risk for aspiration pneumonia. See Warnings and Precautions, Gastrointestinal and Adverse Reactions.

ADVERSE REACTIONS: The stated frequencies of adverse events represent the proportion of individuals who experienced, at least once, a treatment-emergent adverse event of the type listed. An event was considered treatment-emergent if it occurred for the first time or worsened while receiving therapy following baseline evaluation.

Clinical Trial Adverse Drug Reactions: The prescriber should be aware that the figures in the tables and tabulations cannot be used to predict the incidence of side effects in the course of usual medical practice where patient characteristics and other factors differ from those that prevailed in the clinical trials. Similarly, the cited frequencies cannot be compared with figures obtained from other clinical investigations involving different treatments, uses, and investigators. The figures cited, however, do provide the prescribing physician with some basis for estimating the relative contribution of drug and nondrug factors to the side effect incidence in the populations studied.

Adverse Events Associated with Discontinuation: Short-Term Placebo-Controlled Clinical Trials: Schizophrenia: Overall, 3.9% of SEROQUEL (quetiapine fumarate immediate-release) treated patients (n=510) discontinued treatment due to adverse events compared with 2.9% of placebo-treated patients (n=206). Somnolence, the single most common adverse event leading to withdrawal from quetiapine treatment, led to the withdrawal of four quetiapine-treated patients and no placebo-treated patients. Postural hypotension, hypotension, and/or tachycardia led to withdrawal of 1.8% of quetiapine-treated subjects, compared to 0.5% of placebo-treated subjects.

Bipolar Disorder: Bipolar Mania: Discontinuations due to adverse events were similar for SEROQUEL (5.7%) and placebo (5.1%).

Bipolar Depression: Discontinuations due to adverse events were 13.1% for SEROQUEL and 6.3% for placebo. Sedation, somnolence and dizziness were the most common adverse events leading to discontinuation in the SEROQUEL treatment groups.

Combined Short- and Long-Term Controlled Trial Database in Schizophrenia: In a premarketing controlled clinical trial database of 1710 SEROQUEL-treated patients, 5% discontinued due to an adverse event. Somnolence was the single most common adverse event leading to withdrawal of 24 patients from SEROQUEL, and was the only adverse event leading to withdrawal that occurred in more than 1% of patients. Cardiovascular adverse events (e.g., postural hypotension, hypotension, tachycardia, dizziness) accounted for 20% of all subject withdrawals from quetiapine treatment. Sixteen (0.9%) quetiapine-treated subjects were withdrawn due to elevated liver enzymes. Four quetiapine-treated subjects were withdrawn because of leucopenia. Two of these subjects had at least one clinically significant, non-baseline low neutrophil count. Two quetiapine-treated subjects were withdrawn from the trial because of suspected neuroleptic malignant syndrome (NMS).

Commonly Observed Adverse Events in Short-Term Placebo-Controlled Clinical Trials: Schizophrenia: The following treatment-emergent adverse events, derived from Table 1, commonly occurred during acute therapy with SEROQUEL (incidence of at least 5%, and an incidence at least 5% higher than that observed with placebo): somnolence, dizziness, dry mouth, postural hypotension, and elevated ALT levels.

Bipolar Disorder: Bipolar Mania: In the bipolar mania studies, the following treatment-emergent adverse events commonly occurred during acute therapy with SEROQUEL (incidence of at least 5%, and an incidence at least 5% higher than that observed with placebo): somnolence, dry mouth, and weight gain.

Bipolar Depression: In the bipolar depression studies, the following treatment-emergent adverse events commonly occurred during acute therapy with SEROQUEL (incidence of at least 5%, and an incidence at least 5% higher than that observed with placebo): dry mouth, somnolence, sedation, dizziness and constipation.

Incidence of Adverse Events in Placebo-Controlled Clinical Trials: Certain portions of the discussion below relating to objective or numeric safety parameters are derived from studies in patients with schizophrenia and have not been duplicated for bipolar mania trials. However, this information is also generally applicable to bipolar mania. Table 1 enumerates the incidence, rounded to the nearest percent, of treatment-emergent adverse events that occurred during acute therapy (up to 6 weeks) of schizophrenia in 1% or more of patients treated with SEROQUEL (doses of 150 mg/day or more) where the incidence in patients treated with SEROQUEL was greater than the incidence in placebo-treated patients.

Table 1: SEROQUEL

Adverse Events Reported for at Least 1% of SEROQUEL-Treated Subjects (doses ≥150 mg/day) and for a Higher Percentage of SEROQUEL-Treated Subjects than Subjects who Received Placebo in Short-Term, Placebo-Controlled Schizophrenia Phase II-III Trials

Body System and COSTART Term	Percentage of Subjects with Adverse Events[a] SEROQUEL (n=449)	Placebo (n=202)
Whole Body		
Headache	20	17
Abdominal Pain	4	1
Back Pain	2	1
Fever	2	1
Nervous System		
Somnolence	18	11
Dizziness	10	4
Digestive System		
Constipation	9	5
Dry Mouth	7	2
Dyspepsia	6	2
Gamma Glutamyl Transpeptidase Increased	2	1
Cardiovascular System		
Postural Hypotension	8	2
Tachycardia	7	5
Palpitation	1	0
Metabolic and Nutritional Disorders		
ALT Increased	7	2

(cont'd)

Table 1: SEROQUEL *(cont'd)*

Adverse Events Reported for at Least 1% of SEROQUEL-Treated Subjects (doses ≥150 mg/day) and for a Higher Percentage of SEROQUEL-Treated Subjects than Subjects who Received Placebo in Short-Term, Placebo-Controlled Schizophrenia Phase II-III Trials

Body System and COSTART Term	Percentage of Subjects with Adverse Events[a] SEROQUEL (n=449)	Placebo (n=202)
AST Increased	4	1
Weight Gain	2	0
Endocrine System		
Hypothyroidism	1	0
Skin and Appendages		
Rash	4	3
Respiratory System		
Rhinitis	3	1
Hemic and Lymphatic Systems		
Leucopenia	2	0
Special Senses		
Ear Pain	1	0

[a] Subjects may have had more than one adverse event.

Table 2 enumerates the incidence, rounded to the nearest percent, of treatment-emergent adverse events that occurred during acute therapy (8 weeks) of bipolar depression in ≥1% of patients treated with SEROQUEL (doses of 300 or 600 mg/day) where the incidence in patients treated with SEROQUEL was greater than the incidence in placebo-treated patients.

Table 2: SEROQUEL

Adverse Events Reported for at Least 1% of SEROQUEL-Treated Subjects (doses of 300 or 600 mg/day) and for a Higher Percentage of SEROQUEL-Treated Subjects than Subjects Who Received Placebo in 8-Week Placebo-Controlled Bipolar Depression Phase III Trials

Body System and MedDRA Preferred Term[b]	Percentage of Subjects with Adverse Events[a] SEROQUEL (n=1712)	Placebo (n=602)
General Disorders		
Fatigue	7	5
Irritability	2	1
Asthenia	2	1
Nervous System Disorders		
Somnolence	22	6
Sedation	18	6
Dizziness	14	6
Akathisia	3	1
Lethargy	3	1
Tremor	2	1
Paraesthesia	2	1
Hypersomnia	2	0
Extrapyramidal Disorder	2	1
Dysarthria	2	0
Restless Legs Syndrome	1	0
Dysgeusia	1	0
Gastrointestinal Disorders		
Dry Mouth	29	9
Constipation	8	3
Dyspepsia	4	3
Dysphagia	1	0
Cardiac Disorders		
Palpitations	3	1
Tachycardia	2	0

(cont'd)

Table 2: SEROQUEL *(cont'd)*

Adverse Events Reported for at Least 1% of SEROQUEL-Treated Subjects (doses of 300 or 600 mg/day) and for a Higher Percentage of SEROQUEL-Treated Subjects than Subjects Who Received Placebo in 8-Week Placebo-Controlled Bipolar Depression Phase III Trials

Body System and MedDRA Preferred Term[b]	Percentage of Subjects with Adverse Events[a] SEROQUEL (n=1712)	Placebo (n=602)
Orthostatic Hypotension	2	1
Metabolism and Nutritional Disorders		
Increased Appetite	4	2
Weight Increased	3	1
Musculoskeletal and Connective Tissue Disorders		
Arthralgia	2	1
Respiratory Disorders		
Nasal Congestion	3	1
Cough	2	1
Special Senses		
Vision Blurred	3	1

[a] Events for which SEROQUEL incidence was equal to or less than placebo are not listed in the table. Table reports percentage rounded to the nearest integer.

[b] Patients with multiple events falling under the same preferred term are counted only once in that term.

Other Adverse Drug Reactions: Weight Gain: During acute therapy (up to 6 weeks) in placebo-controlled schizophrenia clinical trials, mean weight gain in patients taking SEROQUEL was 2.3 kilograms compared to a mean weight gain of 0.1 kilograms in patients taking placebo. In open-label extension trials with SEROQUEL monotherapy, mean weight gain after 9 to 13 weeks was 1.58 kg, after 14 to 26 weeks, 0.26 kg, after 27 to 39 weeks, 1.66 kg, after 40 to 52 weeks, −1.53 kg and after 53 to 78 weeks, 1.98 kg (see Warnings and Precautions, Endocrine and Metabolism). In the acute placebo-controlled bipolar mania clinical trials (up to 12 weeks) mean weight gain in patients taking SEROQUEL was 1.8 kg compared to a mean weight loss of 0.1 kg in patients taking placebo. In patients completing the entire 12 weeks of treatment mean weight gain in patients taking SEROQUEL was 2.8 kg.

In the acute placebo-controlled bipolar depression clinical trials (8 weeks) mean weight gain in patients taking SEROQUEL was 1.15 kg compared to a mean weight gain of 0.1 kg in patients taking placebo. During maintenance treatment, patients treated with SEROQUEL 300 mg or placebo lost on average 0.1 kg and 0.6 kg, respectively, while patients treated with SEROQUEL 600 mg gained on average 0.8 kg. In patients who completed 40 and 54 weeks of maintenance treatment a small mean decrease was seen in the SEROQUEL 300 mg group (-0.2 kg) and placebo group (-0.8 kg) while patients in the SEROQUEL 600 mg group showed a mean weight gain of 1.2 kg. See Warnings and Precautions.

Based on the cumulative acute placebo-controlled clinical trial database, weight gain (based on ≥7% increase in body weight from baseline) was reported in 9.6% in quetiapine-treated patients and 3.8% in placebo-treated patients, which occurs predominantly during the early weeks of treatment in adults (see Warnings and Precautions).

Seizures: There have been uncommon reports (≥0.1%-<1%) of seizures in patients administered quetiapine, although the frequency was no greater than that observed in patients administered placebo in controlled clinical trials (see Warnings and Precautions, Neurologic).

Restless Legs Syndrome: There have been uncommon cases of restless legs syndrome in patients administered quetiapine.

Priapism: There have been rare reports (≥0.01%-<0.1%) of priapism in patients administered quetiapine.

Somnolence: Somnolence may occur, usually during the first two weeks of treatment, which generally resolves with the continued administration of SEROQUEL.

Neuroleptic Malignant Syndrome: As with other antipsychotics, rare cases of neuroleptic malignant syndrome have been reported in patients treated with SEROQUEL (see Warnings and Precautions, Neurologic).

Vital Signs: As with other antipsychotics with α1 adrenergic blocking activity, SEROQUEL may induce postural hypotension, associated with dizziness, tachycardia and, in some patients, syncope, especially during the initial dose titration period (see Warnings and Precautions, Cardiovascular). In placebo-controlled clinical trials in schizophrenia, postural hypotension was reported with an incidence of 8% in SEROQUEL-treated patients compared to 2% in placebo-treated patients. SEROQUEL was associated with a mean baseline to endpoint increase in heart rate of 3.9 beats per minute, compared to 1.6 beats per minute among placebo-treated patients.

Peripheral Edema: As with other antipsychotic agents, common cases (≥1%-<10%) of peripheral edema have been reported in patients treated with quetiapine.

Mild Asthenia: As with other antipsychotic agents, common cases of mild asthenia have been reported in patients treated with quetiapine.

Hypersensitivity: Uncommon cases of hypersensitivity including angioedema have been reported.

ECG Changes: Between group comparisons for pooled placebo-controlled trials revealed no statistically significant SEROQUEL/placebo differences in the proportions of patients experiencing potentially important changes in ECG parameters, including QT, QTc, and PR intervals. However, the proportions of patients meeting the criteria for tachycardia were compared in four 3- to 6-week-placebo-controlled clinical trials for the treatment of schizophrenia revealing a 1% (4/399) incidence for SEROQUEL compared to 0.6% (1/156) incidence for placebo. SEROQUEL use was associated with a mean increase in heart rate, assessed by ECG, of 7 beats per minute compared to a mean increase of 1 beat per minute among placebo patients. This slight tendency to tachycardia may be related to SEROQUEL's potential for inducing orthostatic changes (see Warnings and Precautions, Cardiovascular). In bipolar mania trials, the proportion of patients meeting the criteria for tachycardia was 0.5% (1/192) for SEROQUEL compared to 0% (0/178) for placebo. In bipolar depression trials, the proportion of patients meeting the criteria for tachycardia in the acute phase was 0.06% (1/1704) for SEROQUEL compared to 0% (0/598) for placebo. During maintenance treatment, the proportion was 0.4% (1/278) compared to 0.4% (0/284) for placebo.

Tardive Dyskinesia: There have been uncommon cases of tardive dyskinesia reported in patients administered quetiapine (see Warnings and Precautions, Neurologic).

Extrapyramidal Symptoms (EPS): Table 3 enumerates the percentage of patients with treatment-emergent extrapyramidal symptoms in a short-term acute phase clinical trial in patients with schizophrenia comparing five fixed doses of SEROQUEL with placebo (n=~50 patients per group), as assessed by: 1) spontaneous complaints of parkinsonism (extrapyramidal syndrome, hypertonia, tremor and cogwheel rigidity), or akathisia; 2) Simpson-Angus scores (mean change from baseline); and 3) use of anticholinergic medication to treat emergent EPS.

There were no differences between the SEROQUEL and placebo treatment groups in the incidence of EPS or concomitant use of anticholinergics and no evidence of dose-related increase in EPS or in the use of concomitant anticholinergics across the dose range of 75-750 mg/day.

In 2 bipolar mania placebo-controlled clinical trials using variable doses of SEROQUEL, there were no differences between the SEROQUEL and placebo treatment groups in the incidence of EPS, as assessed by Simpson-Angus total scores and Barnes Akathisia rating scale, spontaneous complaints of EPS and the use of concomitant anticholinergic medications to treat EPS.

In short-term placebo-controlled clinical trials in schizophrenia and bipolar mania, the aggregated incidence of EPS-related adverse events was similar to placebo (schizophrenia: 7.8% for quetiapine and 8.0% for placebo; bipolar mania: 11.2% for quetiapine and 11.4% for placebo). In short-term placebo-controlled clinical trials in bipolar depression, the aggregated incidence of EPS-related adverse events was 8.9% for quetiapine compared to 3.8% for placebo. The incidence of individual EPS-related adverse events (e.g., akathisia, extrapyramidal disorder, tremor, dyskinesia, dystonia, restlessness, muscle contractions involuntary, psychomotor hyperactivity and muscle rigidity), however was generally low and did not exceed 4% for any individual adverse event. In long-term studies of schizophrenia and bipolar disorder the aggregated exposure adjusted incidence of treatment-emergent EPS was similar between quetiapine and placebo. See Warnings and Precautions, Neurologic.

Table 3: SEROQUEL

Treatment-Emergent Extrapyramidal Symptoms, Assessed by Spontaneous Reports, Simpson Scale, and Incidence of Anticholinergic Use

		SEROQUEL				
	Placebo	**75 mg**	**150 mg**	**300 mg**	**600 mg**	**750 mg**
Spontaneous Reports of Parkinsonian Symptoms[a]	10%	6%	4%	4%	8%	4%
Spontaneous Reports of Akathisia	8%	2%	2%	0%	0%	2%
Simpson Scale	−0.6	−1.0	−1.2	−1.6	−1.8	−1.8
Incidence of Anticholinergic Use	14%	11%	10%	8%	12%	11%

[a] Patients may have had more than one Parkinsonism adverse event.

Blurred Vision: There have been common cases of blurred vision in patients administered quetiapine.
Dysphagia: There have been uncommon cases of dysphagia in patients administered quetiapine. In clinical trials an increase in the rate of dysphagia with quetiapine versus placebo was only observed in bipolar depression. See Warnings and Precautions, Gastrointestinal and Special Populations.
Dysarthria: There have been common cases of dysarthria in patients administered quetiapine.
Acute Withdrawal (discontinuation) Symptoms: Acute discontinuation symptoms such as insomnia, nausea, headache, diarrhea, vomiting, dizziness and irritability, have been described after abrupt cessation of antipsychotic drugs including SEROQUEL. Gradual withdrawal over a period of at least one to two weeks is advisable. Symptoms usually resolved after 1 week post-discontinuation.
Abnormal Dreams and Nightmares: There have been common cases of abnormal dreams and nightmares in patients administered quetiapine.
Suicide-Related Events: In short-term placebo-controlled clinical trials across all indications and ages, the incidence of suicide-related events (suicidal thoughts, self-harm and suicide) was 0.9% for both quetiapine (61/6270) and for placebo (27/3047). In these trials of patients with schizophrenia the incidence of suicide-related events was 1.4% (3/212) for quetiapine and 1.6% (1/62) for placebo in patients 18-24 years of age, 0.8% (13/1663) for quetiapine and 1.1% (5/463) for placebo in patients ≥25 years of age.

In these trials of patients with bipolar mania the incidence of suicide-related events was 0% for both quetiapine (0/60) and placebo (0/58) in patients 18-24 years of age, 1.2% for both quetiapine (6/496) and placebo (6/503) in patients ≥25 years of age.

In these trials of patients with bipolar depression the incidence of suicide-related events was 3.0% (7/233) for quetiapine and 0% (0/120) for placebo in patients 18-24 and 1.8% for both quetiapine (19/1616) and placebo (11/622) in patients ≥25 years of age. (See Warnings and Precautions.)
Irritability: There have been common cases of irritability in patients administered quetiapine.
Increased Appetite: There have been common cases of increased appetite in patients administered quetiapine.
Abnormal Hematologic and Clinical Chemistry Findings: As with other antipsychotics, common cases of leucopenia and/or neutropenia have been observed in patients administered SEROQUEL. Uncommon cases of eosinophilia and thrombocytopenia (platelet count decreased, ≤100×10⁹/L on at least one occasion) have been observed.

Based on clinical trial adverse event reports not associated with neuroleptic malignant syndrome, rare cases of elevations in blood creatine phosphokinase have been reported in patients administered quetiapine.

Common cases of elevations in serum prolactin levels have been observed (>20 µg/L in males and >30 µg/L in females) (see Warnings and Precautions, Endocrine and Metabolism, Hyperprolactinemia).

In all placebo-controlled monotherapy clinical trials among patients with a baseline neutrophil count $\geq 1.5\times10^9$/L, the incidence of at least one occurrence of neutrophil count $<1.5\times10^9$/L was 1.72% in patients treated with SEROQUEL, compared to 0.73% in placebo-treated patients. In clinical trials conducted prior to a protocol amendment for discontinuation of patients with treatment-emergent neutrophil count $<1.0\times10^9$/L, among patients with a baseline neutrophil count $\geq 1.5\times10^9$/L, the incidence of at least one occurrence of neutrophil count $<0.5\times10^9$/L was 0.21% in patients treated with SEROQUEL and 0% in placebo treated patients and the incidence ≥ 0.5-$<1.0\times10^9$/L was 0.75% in patients treated with SEROQUEL and 0.11% in placebo-treated patients. (See Warnings and Precautions, Hematologic.)

Asymptomatic elevations in serum transaminases (AST, ALT) or gamma-GT levels have been observed in some patients administered SEROQUEL. These elevations were usually reversible on continued SEROQUEL treatment (see Warnings and Precautions, Hepatic/Biliary/Pancreatic).

SEROQUEL treatment was associated with small dose-related decreases in thyroid hormone levels, particularly total T_4 and free T_4. The reduction in total and free T_4 was maximal within the first 2 to 4 weeks of quetiapine treatment, with no further reduction during long-term treatment. There was no evidence of clinically significant changes in TSH concentration over time. In nearly all cases, cessation of quetiapine treatment was associated with a reversal of the effects on total and free T_4, irrespective of the duration of treatment (see Warnings and Precautions, Endocrine and Metabolism). Smaller decreases in total T_3 and reverse T_3 were seen only at higher doses. Levels of TBG were unchanged and in general reciprocal increases in TSH were not observed and there was no indication that SEROQUEL causes clinically relevant hypothyroidism.
Hyperglycaemia: Blood glucose increases to hyperglycaemic levels (fasting blood glucose ≥7.0 mmol/L or a non fasting blood glucose ≥11.1 mmol/L on at least one occasion) have been observed commonly (≥1%-<10%) with quetiapine in clinical trials.

In 2 long-term bipolar maintenance placebo-controlled adjunct clinical trials, mean exposure 213 days for SEROQUEL (646 patients) and 152 days for placebo (680 patients), the exposure-adjusted rate of any increased blood glucose level (≥7.0 mmol/L) for patients more than 8 hours since a meal was 18.0 per 100 patient years for SEROQUEL (10.7% of patients) and 9.5 for placebo per 100 patient years (4.6% of patients).

In short-term (12 weeks duration or less) placebo-controlled clinical trials (3342 treated with quetiapine and 1490 treated with placebo), the percent of patients who had a fasting blood glucose ≥7.0 mmol/L or a non fasting blood glucose ≥11.1 mmol/L was 3.5% for quetiapine and 2.1% for placebo.

In a 24-week trial (active-controlled, 115 patients treated with SEROQUEL) designed to evaluate glycemic status with oral glucose tolerance testing of all patients, at week 24 the incidence of a treatment-emergent post-glucose challenge glucose level ≥11.1 mmol/L was 1.7% and the incidence of a fasting treatment-emergent blood glucose level ≥7.0 mmol/L was 2.6%. (See Warnings and Precautions, Endocrine and Metabolism.)
Cholesterol and Triglyceride Elevations: Very common (≥10%) cases of elevations in serum triglyceride levels (≥2.258 mmol/L on at least one occasion), elevations in total cholesterol (predominantly LDL cholesterol) (≥6.2064 mmol/L on at least one occasion), and decreases in HDL cholesterol levels (<1.025 mmol/L males; <1.282 mmol/L females at any time) have been observed during treatment with quetiapine in clinical trials (see Warnings and Precautions, Cardiovascular). Lipid changes should be managed as clinically appropriate.

In one 24 week clinical trial, where LDL cholesterol was directly measured as opposed to calculated, there was a slight mean increase in total cholesterol in patients administered SEROQUEL, which was driven by increases in LDL cholesterol. The mean LDL level increased at Week 24 by 10% in patients administered SEROQUEL, which was statistically significant. The total cholesterol/HDL ratio did not change significantly during therapy with SEROQUEL. Furthermore, triglycerides did not increase significantly nor did HDL cholesterol decrease during therapy. (See Warnings and Precautions, Cardiovascular.)
Post-Market Adverse Drug Reactions: During post-marketing experience, leucopenia and/or neutropenia have been reported during SEROQUEL treatment. Resolution of leucopenia and/or neutropenia has followed cessation of therapy with SEROQUEL. Possible risk factors for leucopenia and/or neutropenia include pre-existing low white cell count and history of drug induced leucopenia and/or neutropenia. (See Warnings and Precautions, Hematologic.)

As with some other antipsychotics, hyperglycaemia and diabetes mellitus (including exacerbation of pre-existing diabetes, diabetic ketoacidosis, and diabetic coma including some fatal cases) in the aggregate have been reported rarely (≥0.01%-<0.1%) during the use of SEROQUEL, sometimes in patients with no reported history of hyperglycaemia. (See Warnings and Precautions, Endocrine and Metabolism.)

Anaphylactic reactions have been reported very rarely in post-marketing reports, including a case with a fatal outcome, possibly related to SEROQUEL treatment. The reporting rate of anaphylaxis associated with SEROQUEL use, which is generally accepted to be an underestimate due to underreporting, does not exceed the background incidence rate estimates. Estimates of the background incidence rate (all cause) of severe life-threatening anaphylaxis in the general population range between 80 and 210 cases per million person-years, and the incidence rate of drug-induced anaphylaxis is reported to be 16 cases per million person-years. In addition, the all cause fatal anaphylaxis rate is reported to be one case per million person-years while the drug-induced fatal anaphylaxis is estimated to be 0.3 cases per million person-years. If a patient develops anaphylaxis after treatment with SEROQUEL, the drug should be discontinued and an alternative treatment started.

Based on post-marketing reports, galactorrhea has been reported rarely.

DRUG INTERACTIONS: Drug-Drug Interactions: Given the primary central nervous system effects of quetiapine, SEROQUEL (quetiapine fumarate immediate-release) should be used with caution in combination with other centrally acting drugs.

Caution should be exercised when quetiapine is used concomitantly with drugs known to cause electrolyte imbalance or to increase QT interval (see Warnings and Precautions, Cardiovascular).
The Effect of SEROQUEL on Other Drugs: Alcohol: SEROQUEL potentiated the cognitive and motor effects of alcohol in a clinical trial in subjects with psychotic disorders. Alcoholic beverages should be avoided while taking SEROQUEL.
Antihypertensive Agents: Because of its potential for inducing hypotension, SEROQUEL may enhance the effects of certain antihypertensive agents.
Levodopa and Dopamine Agonists: As it exhibits in vitro dopamine antagonism, SEROQUEL may antagonize the effects of levodopa and dopamine agonists.
Lithium: The single dose pharmacokinetics of lithium were not altered when coadministered with SEROQUEL.
Antipyrine: SEROQUEL did not induce the hepatic enzyme systems involved in the metabolism of antipyrine.
Lorazepam: SEROQUEL did not affect the single dose pharmacokinetics of lorazepam.
Divalproex: Coadministration of SEROQUEL (150 mg bid) and divalproex (500 mg bid) increased the mean oral clearance and the mean maximum plasma concentration of total valproic acid (administered as divalproex) by 11%. These changes were not clinically relevant.
The Effect of Other Drugs on SEROQUEL: Hepatic Enzyme Inducers: Concomitant use of SEROQUEL with hepatic enzyme inducers such as carbamazepine may substantially decrease systemic exposure to quetiapine. In a multiple dose trial in patients to assess the pharmacokinetics of quetiapine given before and during treatment with carbamazepine (a known hepatic enzyme inducer), coadministration of carbamazepine significantly increased the clearance of quetiapine. This increase in clearance reduced systemic quetiapine exposure (as measured by AUC) to an average of 13% of the exposure during administration of quetiapine alone; although a greater effect was seen in some patients. As a consequence of this interaction, lower plasma concentrations can occur, and hence, in each patient, consideration for a higher dose of SEROQUEL, depending on clinical response, should be considered. It should be noted that the recommended maximum daily dose of SEROQUEL is 800 mg/day and continued treatment at higher doses should only be considered as a result of careful consideration of the benefit risk assessment for an individual patient.

Coadministration of SEROQUEL and another microsomal enzyme inducer, phenytoin, caused five-fold increases in the clearance of quetiapine. Increased doses of SEROQUEL may be required to maintain control of psychotic symptoms in patients coadministered SEROQUEL and phenytoin and other hepatic enzyme inducers (e.g, barbiturates, rifampicin, etc.).

The dose of SEROQUEL may need to be reduced if phenytoin or carbamazepine or other hepatic enzyme inducers are withdrawn and replaced with a non-inducer (e.g., sodium valproate).
CYP 3A4 Inhibitors: CYP 3A4 is the primary enzyme responsible for cytochrome P450-mediated metabolism of quetiapine. Thus, coadministration of compounds (such as ketoconazole, erythromycin, clarithromycin, diltiazem, verapamil, or nefazodone), which inhibit CYP 3A4, may increase the concentration of quetiapine. In a multiple-dose trial in healthy volunteers to assess the pharmacokinetics of quetiapine given before and during treatment with ketoconazole, coadministration of ketoconazole resulted in an increase in mean C_{max} and AUC of quetiapine of 235% and 522%, respectively, with a corresponding decrease in mean oral clearance of 84%. The mean half-life of quetiapine increased from 2.6 to 6.8 hours, but the mean t_{max} was unchanged. Due to the potential for an interaction of a similar magnitude in a clinical setting, the dosage of SEROQUEL should be reduced during concomitant use of quetiapine and potent CYP 3A4 inhibitors (such as azole antifungals, macrolide antibiotics, and protease inhibitors). Special consideration should be given in elderly and debilitated patients. The risk-benefit ratio needs to be considered on an individual basis in all patients.
Divalproex: Coadministration of SEROQUEL (150 mg bid) and divalproex (500 mg bid) increased the mean maximum plasma concentration of quetiapine by 17% without changing the mean oral clearance.
Cimetidine: In a clinical study examining the pharmacokinetics of SEROQUEL following coadministration with cimetidine, (a non-specific P450 enzyme inhibitor), no clinically significant interaction was observed.
Thioridazine: Coadministration of thioridazine (200 mg b.i.d.) with SEROQUEL (300 mg b.i.d.), increased the clearance of SEROQUEL by 65%.
Fluoxetine, Imipramine, Haloperidol, and Risperidone: Fluoxetine (60 mg daily), imipramine (75 mg b.i.d.), haloperidol (7.5 mg b.i.d.), and risperidone (3 mg b.i.d.) did not significantly alter the steady state pharmacokinetics of SEROQUEL.
Drug-Food Interactions: SEROQUEL can be administered with or without food.
Drug-Herb Interactions: Interactions with herbal products have not been established.
Drug-Laboratory Test Interactions: Interactions with laboratory tests have not been established.

DOSAGE AND ADMINISTRATION: Recommended Dose and Dosage Adjustment: SEROQUEL (quetiapine fumarate immediate-release) can be administered with or without food (see Action and Clinical Pharmacology, Pharmacokinetics).
Schizophrenia: The usual starting dose of SEROQUEL is 25 mg b.i.d., titrated with increments of 25-50 mg b.i.d. per day, as tolerated, to a target dose of 300 mg/day given b.i.d. within four to seven days.

Further dosage adjustments may be indicated depending on the clinical response and tolerability in the individual patient. Dosage adjustments should generally occur at intervals of not less than 2 days, as steady state for SEROQUEL would not be achieved for approximately 1-2 days in the typical patient. When adjustments are necessary, dose increments/decrements of 25-50 mg b.i.d. are recommended.

Clinical trials suggest that the usual effective treatment dose will be in the range of 300-600 mg/day. However, some patients may require as little as 150 mg/day. In schizophrenia, the safety of doses above 800 mg/day has not been evaluated.

The need for continuing existing EPS medications should be re-evaluated periodically as SEROQUEL has not been associated with treatment-emergent EPS across the clinical dose range.
Bipolar Disorder: Bipolar Mania: Usual Dose: The titration rate, based on the clinical trials is shown in Table 4.

Table 4: SEROQUEL

Titration Rate

Day	1	2	3	4	5	6
BID	100 mg/day	200 mg/day	300 mg/day	400 mg/day	Up to 600 mg/day	Up to 800 mg/day

Dosage adjustments should be made depending on the clinical response and tolerability in the individual patient.

Approximately 85% of patients responded between 400 and 800 mg/day, while over 50% of patients responded between 600 and 800 mg/day (the average median dose for responders during the last week of treatment was approximately 600 mg/day). In bipolar mania, the safety of doses above 800 mg/day has not been evaluated.
Bipolar Depression : Usual Dose: The titration rate, based on the clinical trials is shown in Table 5.

Table 5: SEROQUEL

Titration Rate

Day	1	2	3	4
Once Daily	50 mg/day	100 mg/day	200 mg/day	300 mg/day

Patients in 300 mg fixed dosage arms were continued on SEROQUEL 300 mg/day, from day 4 onward. In clinical trials that had a fixed 600 mg dosage arm, SEROQUEL was further titrated to 400 mg on Day 5 and up to 600 mg by Day 8, depending on clinical response and tolerability of individual patients. Antidepressant efficacy was demonstrated with SEROQUEL at both 300 mg/day and 600 mg/day, however no additional benefit was seen in the 600 mg group during short-term treatment. Thus, a usual target dose of 300 mg/day is recommended.

In bipolar depression, the safety of doses above 600 mg/day has not been evaluated.

SEROQUEL should be administered once daily at bedtime.

Dosing Considerations in Special Populations: Elderly: In clinical trials, 38 patients with schizophrenia or related disorders, 65 years of age or over, were treated with SEROQUEL (see Warnings and Precautions, Special Populations). Given the limited experience with SEROQUEL in the elderly, and the higher incidence of concomitant illness and concomitant medication in this population, SEROQUEL should be used with caution. The mean plasma clearance of SEROQUEL was reduced by 30% to 50% in elderly subjects when compared to younger patients. The rate of dose titration may thus need to be slower, and the daily therapeutic target dose lower, than that used in younger patients.

Hepatic Impairment: Quetiapine is extensively metabolized by the liver (see Actions and Pharmacology, Special Populations and Conditions). Therefore, SEROQUEL should be used with caution in patients with mild hepatic impairment, especially during the initial dosing period. Patients with mild hepatic impairment should be started on 25 mg/day. The dose should be increased daily in increments of 25 to 50 mg/day to an effective dose, depending on the clinical response and tolerance in the individual patient. No pharmacokinetic data are available for any dose of SEROQUEL in patients with moderate to severe hepatic impairment. However, should clinical judgement deem treatment with SEROQUEL necessary, the drug should be used with great caution in patients with moderate or severe hepatic impairment (see Warnings and Precautions, Hepatic/Biliary/Pancreatic and Action and Clinical Pharmacology, Special Populations and Conditions).

Renal Impairment: As clinical experience is lacking, caution is advised (see Warnings and Precautions, Renal).

Missed Dose: If a dose is missed by only a few hours, take it as soon as possible. If most of the day has passed since the missed dose, skip that dose and wait until next scheduled dose. Never take two doses at once.

OVERDOSAGE:

Experience: Clinical Trials: One death has been reported in a clinical trial following an overdose of 13 600 mg of quetiapine alone, however, survival has also been reported in acute overdoses of up to 30 000 mg of quetiapine. Most patients who overdosed reported no adverse events or recovered fully from the reported events.

Post-Marketing: In post-marketing experience, there have been cases of coma and death in patients taking a SEROQUEL overdose. The lowest reported dose associated with coma has been in a patient who took 5000 mg and had a full recovery within 3 days. The lowest reported dose associated with a death was in a patient who took 6000 mg.

In post-marketing experience, there were cases reported of QT prolongation with overdose.

Patients with pre-existing severe cardiovascular disease may be at an increased risk of the effects of overdose (see Warnings and Precautions, Cardiovascular, Hypotension and Syncope).

Symptoms: In general, reported signs and symptoms were those resulting from an exaggeration of the drug's known pharmacological effects (e.g., drowsiness and sedation, tachycardia and hypotension).

Treatment: There is no specific antidote to quetiapine. In cases of severe intoxication, the possibility of multiple drug involvement should be considered, and intensive care procedures are recommended, including establishing and maintaining a patent airway, ensuring adequate oxygenation and ventilation, and monitoring and support of the cardiovascular system.

Close medical supervision and monitoring should be continued until the patient recovers.

> For management of a suspected drug overdose, contact your regional Poison Control Centre. See the *CPS* Directory section for a list of Poison Control Centres.

ACTION AND CLINICAL PHARMACOLOGY: Mechanism of Action and Pharmacodynamics: SEROQUEL (quetiapine fumarate immediate-release), a dibenzothiazepine derivative, is an antipsychotic agent. Quetiapine and the active plasma metabolite, N-desalkyl quetiapine interact with a broad range of neurotransmitter receptors. The extent to which the N-desalkyl quetiapine metabolite contributes to the pharmacological activity of SEROQUEL is not known.

Quetiapine: Quetiapine exhibits affinity for brain serotonin $5HT_2$ and $5HT_{1A}$ receptors (in vitro, Ki=288 and 557 nM, respectively), and dopamine D_1 and D_2 receptors (in vitro, Ki=558 and 531 nM, respectively). It is this combination of receptor antagonism with a higher selectivity for $5HT_2$ relative to D_2 receptors, which is believed to contribute to the clinical antipsychotic properties and low extrapyramidal symptoms (EPS) liability of quetiapine compared to typical antipsychotics. Quetiapine also has high affinity for histamine H_1 receptors (in vitro, Ki=10 nM) and adrenergic α_1 receptors (in vitro, Ki=13 nM), with a lower affinity for adrenergic α_2 receptors (in vitro, Ki=782 nM), but no appreciable affinity at cholinergic muscarinic and benzodiazepine receptors.

N-desalkyl Quetiapine: N-desalkyl quetiapine, similar to quetiapine, exhibits affinity for brain serotonin $5HT_2$ and dopamine D_1 and D_2 receptors. Additionally, like quetiapine, N-desalkyl quetiapine has high affinity at serotonin $5HT_1$ receptors, and histaminergic and adrenergic α_1 receptors, with a lower affinity at adrenergic α_2 receptors.

Pharmacokinetics: The pharmacokinetics of quetiapine and N-desalkyl quetiapine are linear within the clinical dose range. The kinetics of quetiapine are similar in men and women, and smokers and non-smokers.

Absorption: Quetiapine is well absorbed following oral administration. In studies with radiolabelled drug, approximately 73% of the total radioactivity is recovered in the urine and 21% in the faeces over a period of one week. The bioavailability of quetiapine is marginally affected by administration with food, with C_{max} and AUC values increased by 25% and 15%, respectively. Peak plasma concentrations of quetiapine generally occur within 2 hours after oral administration. Steady-state peak molar concentrations of the active metabolite N-desalkyl quetiapine are 35% of that observed for quetiapine.

Distribution: Quetiapine has a mean apparent volume of distribution of 10±4 L/kg, and is approximately 83% bound to plasma proteins.

Elimination and Metabolism: The elimination half-life of quetiapine is approximately 6-7 hours upon multiple dosing within the proposed clinical dosage range. The elimination half-life of N-desalkyl quetiapine is approximately 12 hours. The average molar dose fraction of free quetiapine and the active human plasma metabolite N-desalkyl quetiapine is <5% excreted in the urine.

Quetiapine is extensively metabolized by the liver, with parent compound accounting for less than 5% of the dose in the urine and faeces, one week following the administration of radiolabelled quetiapine. Since quetiapine is extensively metabolised by the liver, higher plasma levels are expected in the hepatically impaired population, and dosage adjustment may be needed in these patients.

Major routes of metabolism of quetiapine involve oxidation of the alkyl side chain, hydroxylation of the dibenzothiazepine ring, sulphoxidation, and phase 2 conjugation. The principal human plasma metabolites are the sulfoxide, and the parent acid metabolite, neither of which are pharmacologically active.

In vitro investigations established that CYP 3A4 is the primary enzyme responsible for cytochrome P450-mediated metabolism of quetiapine. N-desalkyl quetiapine is primarily formed and eliminated via CYP 3A4.

Quetiapine and several of its metabolites (including N-desalkyl quetiapine) were found to be weak inhibitors of human cytochrome P450 1A2, 2C9, 2C19, 2D6 and 3A4 activities in vitro. In vitro CYP inhibition is observed only at concentrations approximately 5 to 50-fold higher than those observed at a dose range of 300 to 800 mg/day in humans.

Special Populations and Conditions: Geriatrics (≥65 years of age): The mean clearance of quetiapine in the elderly is approximately 30 to 50% of that seen in adults aged 18-65 years (see Warnings and Precautions, Special Populations and Dosage and Administration).

Hepatic Insufficiency: In 8 cirrhotic subjects with mild hepatic impairment, administration of a single 25 mg (sub-clinical) oral dose of SEROQUEL resulted in a 40% increase in both AUC and C_{max}. Clearance of the drug decreased by 25% whereas t½ was elevated by nearly 45%. Therefore, SEROQUEL should be used with caution in patients with mild hepatic impairment, especially during the initial dosing period. No pharmacokinetic data are available for any dose of SEROQUEL in patients with moderate or severe hepatic impairment (see Warnings and Precautions, Hepatic/Biliary/Pancreatic and Dosage and Administration).

Renal Insufficiency: At single low (sub-clinical) doses, the mean plasma clearance of quetiapine was reduced by approximately 25% in subjects with severe renal impairment (creatinine clearance less than 30 mL/min/1.73 m²). However, the individual clearance values remained within the range observed for healthy subjects (see Warnings and Precautions, Renal and Dosage and Administration).

STORAGE AND STABILITY: SEROQUEL (quetiapine fumarate immediate-release) should be stored between 15-30°C.

INFORMATION FOR THE PATIENT: Published in e-CPS, available by subscription at www.e-cps.ca.

DOSAGE FORMS, COMPOSITION AND PACKAGING: 25 mg: Each peach coloured, round, biconvex, film-coated, immediate-release tablet, intagliated with "SEROQUEL" and "25" on one side and plain on the other, contains: quetiapine fumarate equivalent to quetiapine free base 25 mg. Nonmedicinal ingredients: tablet core: calcium hydrogen phosphate dihydrate, lactose monohydrate, magnesium stearate, microcrystalline cellulose, povidone and sodium starch glycolate type A; coating: hydroxypropyl methylcellulose 2910, polyethylene glycol 400, red ferric oxide, titanium dioxide and yellow ferric oxide. Blister packages of 60. High density polyethylene (HDPE) bottles of 100.

100 mg: Each yellow coloured, round, biconvex, film-coated, immediate-release tablet, intagliated with "SEROQUEL" and "100" on one side and plain on the other, contains: quetiapine fumarate equivalent to quetiapine free base 100 mg. Nonmedicinal ingredients: tablet core: calcium hydrogen phosphate dihydrate, lactose monohydrate, magnesium stearate, microcrystalline cellulose, povidone and sodium starch glycolate type A; coating: hydroxypropyl methylcellulose 2910, polyethylene glycol 400, titanium dioxide and yellow ferric oxide. Blister packages of 60. High density polyethylene (HDPE) bottles of 100.

200 mg: Each white, round, biconvex, film-coated, immediate-release tablet, intagliated with "SEROQUEL" and "200" on one side and plain on the other, contains: quetiapine fumarate equivalent to quetiapine free base 200 mg. Nonmedicinal ingredients: tablet core: calcium hydrogen phosphate dihydrate, lactose monohydrate, magnesium stearate, microcrystalline cellulose, povidone and sodium starch glycolate type A; coating: hydroxypropyl methylcellulose 2910, polyethylene glycol 400 and titanium dioxide. Blister packages of 90. High density polyethylene (HDPE) bottles of 100.

300 mg: Each white, capsule-shaped, biconvex, film-coated, immediate-release tablet, intagliated with "SEROQUEL" on one side and "300" on the other, contains: quetiapine fumarate equivalent to quetiapine free base 300 mg. Nonmedicinal ingredients: tablet core: calcium hydrogen phosphate dihydrate, lactose monohydrate, magnesium stearate, microcrystalline cellulose, povidone and sodium starch glycolate type A; coating: hydroxypropyl methylcellulose 2910, polyethylene glycol 400 and titanium dioxide. High density polyethylene (HDPE) bottles of 100.

(Shown in Product Identification Section)

Seroquel XR® Ⓟ

quetiapine fumarate

Antipsychotic—Antidepressant Agent

AstraZeneca

Date of Revision: February 17, 2010

SUMMARY PRODUCT INFORMATION:

Route of Administration	Dosage Form/Strength	Nonmedicinal Ingredients
Oral	Extended-release tablet/50, 150, 200, 300 and 400 mg	The core of the tablet contains the excipients hydroxypropyl methylcellulose, lactose monohydrate, magnesium stearate, microcrystalline cellulose and sodium citrate. The coating of the tablet contains hydroxypropyl methylcellulose, polyethylene glycol 400, red ferric oxide (50 mg tablets), titanium dioxide, and yellow ferric oxide (50, 200 and 300 mg tablets).

INDICATIONS AND CLINICAL USE: Adults: Schizophrenia: SEROQUEL XR (quetiapine fumarate extended-release) is indicated for the management of the manifestations of schizophrenia.

Bipolar Disorder: SEROQUEL XR is indicated as monotherapy for the:

- Acute management of manic episodes associated with bipolar disorder.
- Acute management of depressive episodes associated with bipolar I and bipolar II disorder.

Major Depressive Disorder: SEROQUEL XR is indicated for the symptomatic relief of major depressive disorder (MDD) when currently available approved antidepressant drugs have failed either due to lack of efficacy and/or lack of tolerability. While there is no evidence that the efficacy of SEROQUEL XR is superior to other antidepressants, it provides a treatment option for patients who have failed on previous antidepressant treatments.

Clinicians must take into account the safety concerns associated with antipsychotic drugs, a class of drugs to which SEROQUEL XR belongs. Safety concerns of this class include: weight gain; hyperlipidemia; hyperglycaemia; Tardive Dyskinesia; and Neuroleptic Malignant Syndrome (see Warnings and Precautions). SEROQUEL XR should only be prescribed in patients with MDD by clinicians who are aware of the importance and are experienced in the early detection and management of the above-mentioned safety issues associated with this class.

Long-term safety of SEROQUEL XR in MDD has not been systematically evaluated. Thus, the physician who elects to use SEROQUEL XR in the treatment of MDD should use SEROQUEL XR for the shortest time that is clinically indicated. When lengthier treatment is indicated, the physician must periodically re-evaluate the long-term usefulness of the drug for the individual patient keeping in mind the long-term risks.

Geriatrics (>65 years of age): SEROQUEL XR is not indicated in elderly patients with dementia. See Warnings and Precautions, Boxed Serious Warnings and Precautions and Special Populations.

Pediatrics (<18 years of age): The safety and efficacy of SEROQUEL XR in children under the age of 18 years have not been established.

CONTRAINDICATIONS: SEROQUEL XR (quetiapine fumarate extended-release) is contraindicated in patients with a known hypersensitivity to this medication or any of its ingredients. For a complete listing, see Dosage Forms, Composition and Packaging.

WARNINGS AND PRECAUTIONS:

> **Serious Warnings and Precautions**
> **Increased Mortality in Elderly Patients with Dementia: Elderly patients with dementia treated with atypical antipsychotic drugs are at an increased risk of death compared to placebo. Analyses of thirteen placebo controlled trials with various atypical antipsychotics (modal duration of 10 weeks) in these patients showed a mean 1.6 fold increase in death rate in the drug-related patients. Although the causes of death were varied, most of the deaths appeared to be either cardiovascular (e.g., heart failure, sudden death) or infectious (e.g., pneumonia) in nature (see Warnings and Precautions, Special Populations, Use in Geriatric Patients with Dementia).**

General: Body Temperature Regulation: Disruption of the body's ability to reduce core body temperature has been attributed to antipsychotic agents. Appropriate care is advised when prescribing SEROQUEL XR (quetiapine fumarate extended-release) for patients who will be experiencing conditions which may contribute to an elevation of core temperature, e.g., exercising strenuously, exposure to extreme heat, receiving concomitant medication with anticholinergic activity or being subject to dehydration.

Acute Withdrawal (discontinuation) Symptoms: Acute discontinuation symptoms, such as insomnia, nausea, headache, diarrhea, vomiting, dizziness and irritability have been described after abrupt cessation of antipsychotic drugs, including SEROQUEL XR. Gradual withdrawal over a period of at least one to two weeks is advisable. Symptoms usually resolved after 1 week post-discontinuation. See Adverse Reactions.

Cardiovascular: Hypotension and Syncope: As with other drugs that have high α_1 adrenergic receptor blocking activity, SEROQUEL XR may induce orthostatic hypotension, dizziness and sometimes syncope, especially during the initial dose titration period. These events may lead to falls.

In placebo-controlled SEROQUEL XR trials, there was little difference in the adverse reaction reporting rate of syncope in patients treated with SEROQUEL XR (0.5%, 11/2388) compared to patients on placebo (0.3%, 4/1267).

Syncope was reported in 1% (35/4083) of patients treated with SEROQUEL (quetiapine, immediate release formulation), compared with 0.3% (3/1006) on placebo and 0.4% (2/527) on active control drugs.

SEROQUEL XR should be used with caution in patients with known cardiovascular disease (e.g., history of myocardial infarction or ischemic heart disease, heart failure or conduction abnormalities), cerebrovascular disease or other conditions predisposing to hypotension (e.g., dehydration, hypovolemia and treatment with antihypertensive medications) (see Overdosage).

Cholesterol and Triglyceride Elevations: Very common (≥10%) cases of elevations in serum triglyceride levels (≥2.258 mmol/L on at least one occasion), elevations in total cholesterol (predominantly LDL cholesterol) (≥6.2064 mmol/L on at least one occasion), and decreases in HDL cholesterol (<1.025 mmol/L males; <1.282 mmol/L females at any time) have been observed during treatment with quetiapine in clinical trials (see Adverse Reactions). Lipid changes should be managed as clinically appropriate.

In schizophrenia clinical trials, SEROQUEL XR-treated patients had increases from baseline in mean cholesterol and triglycerides of 4% and 14%, respectively, compared to decreases from baseline in mean cholesterol and triglycerides of 2% and 6% for placebo-treated patients. In a 3-week bipolar mania clinical trial, SEROQUEL XR-treated patients had increases from baseline in mean cholesterol and triglycerides of 2% and 20%, respectively, compared to decreases in mean cholesterol and triglycerides of 2% and 5% for placebo-treated patients. In a bipolar depression clinical trial, SEROQUEL XR-treated patients had decreases from baseline in mean cholesterol and increases from baseline in mean triglycerides of 2% and 11%, respectively, compared to decreases in mean cholesterol and triglycerides of 3% and 2% for placebo-treated patients. In 6-week MDD monotherapy clinical trials, SEROQUEL XR treated patients had increases from baseline in mean triglycerides of 8%, compared to a mean decrease of 1% for placebo-treated patients. In the same trials, both SEROQUEL XR- and placebo-treated patients had decreases from baseline in mean cholesterol of 1% and 3%, respectively. In a longer-term randomized withdrawal MDD trial, patients who completed at least 158 days of SEROQUEL XR treatment (n=196), showed mean increases from baseline in triglycerides of approximately 5% and mean decreases from baseline in cholesterol of approximately 4%.

QT Prolongation: In clinical trials, quetiapine was not associated with a persistent increase in absolute QT intervals. However, in post-marketing experience, there were cases reported of QT prolongation with overdose (see Overdosage). As with other antipsychotics, caution should be exercised when quetiapine is prescribed in patients with cardiovascular disease or family history of QT prolongation. Also caution should be exercised when quetiapine is prescribed either with medicines known to increase QT interval or with concomitant neuroleptics, especially for patients with increased risk of QT prolongation, i.e., the elderly, patients with congenital long QT syndrome, congestive heart failure, heart hypertrophy, hypokalemia, or hypomagnesemia (see Drug Interactions).

Endocrine and Metabolism: Hyperglycemia: As with some other antipsychotics, hyperglycaemia and diabetes mellitus (including exacerbation of pre-existing diabetes, diabetic ketoacidosis, and diabetic coma including some fatal cases) in the aggregate have been reported rarely (≥0.01%-<0.1%) during the use of quetiapine in post-marketing experience, sometimes in patients with no reported history of hyperglycaemia (see Adverse Reactions, Post-Market Adverse Drug Reactions).

Blood glucose increases to hyperglycaemic levels (fasting blood glucose ≥7.0 mmol/L or a non fasting blood glucose ≥11.1 mmol/L on at least one occasion) have been observed commonly (≥1%-<10%) with quetiapine in clinical trials. Occasional reports of diabetes have also been observed in clinical trials with quetiapine (see Adverse Reactions, Abnormal Hematologic and Clinical Chemistry Findings).

Assessment of the relationship between atypical antipsychotic use and glucose abnormalities is complicated by the possibility of an increased background risk of diabetes mellitus in patients with schizophrenia and the increasing incidence of diabetes mellitus in the general population. Given these confounders, the relationship between atypical antipsychotic use and hyperglycemia-related adverse events is not completely understood. However, epidemiological studies suggest an increased risk of treatment-emergent hyperglycemia-related adverse events in patients treated with the atypical antipsychotics. Precise risk estimates for hyperglycemia-related adverse events in patients treated with atypical antipsychotics are not available.

Any patient treated with atypical antipsychotics should be monitored for symptoms of hyperglycemia including polydipsia, polyuria, polyphagia, and weakness. Patients who develop symptoms of hyperglycemia during treatment with atypical antipsychotics should undergo fasting blood glucose testing. In some cases, hyperglycemia has resolved when the atypical antipsychotic was discontinued; however, some patients required continuation of anti-diabetic treatment despite discontinuation of the suspect drug. Patients with risk factors for diabetes mellitus (e.g., obesity, family history of diabetes) who are starting treatment with atypical antipsychotics should undergo fasting blood glucose testing at the beginning of treatment and periodically during treatment. Patients with an established diagnosis of diabetes mellitus who are started on atypical antipsychotics should be monitored regularly for worsening of glucose control.

Hyperprolactinemia: During clinical trials with quetiapine, elevation in prolactin levels occurred in 3.6% (158/4416) of patients treated with quetiapine compared to 2.6% (51/1968) on placebo (see Adverse Reactions).

Increased prolactin levels with quetiapine were observed in rat studies. As is common with compounds which stimulate prolactin release, the administration of quetiapine resulted in an increase in the incidence of mammary neoplasms in rats. The physiological differences between rats and humans with regard to prolactin make the clinical significance of these findings unclear. To date, neither clinical nor epidemiological studies have shown an association between chronic administration of drugs that stimulate prolactin release, and mammary tumourigenesis. Tissue culture experiments, however, indicate that approximately one third of human breast cancers are prolactin dependent in vitro; a factor of potential importance if prescription of these drugs is contemplated in a patient with previously detected breast cancer.

Possible manifestations associated with elevated prolactin levels are amenorrhea, galactorrhea, and menorrhagia.

In the multiple fixed-dose schizophrenia clinical trial there were no differences in prolactin levels at study completion for SEROQUEL, across the recommended dose range, and placebo.

Hypothyroidism: In SEROQUEL XR clinical trials, 0.2% (4/1755) of patients on SEROQUEL XR compared to 0% (0/796) on placebo experienced decreased free thyroxine and 2.7% (46/1716) on SEROQUEL XR compared to 1.4% (11/785) on placebo experienced increased TSH; however, no patients experienced a combination of clinically significant decreased free thyroxine and increased TSH. In schizophrenia trials, no patients had events of hypothyroidism.

In clinical trials, on average SEROQUEL was associated with about a 20% mean reduction in thyroxine levels (both total and free). Forty-two percent of SEROQUEL-treated patients showed at least a 30% reduction in total T_4 and 7% showed at least a 50% reduction. Maximum reduction of thyroxine levels generally occurred during the first two to four weeks of treatment with SEROQUEL. These reductions were maintained without adaptation or progression during longer term treatment. Decreases in T_4 were not associated with systematic changes in TSH or clinical signs or symptoms of hypothyroidism. Approximately 0.4% (12/2595) of patients treated with SEROQUEL experienced persistent increases in TSH, and 0.25% of patients were treated with thyroid replacement.

Weight Gain: In 6-week placebo-controlled schizophrenia clinical trials, for patients treated with SEROQUEL XR mean weight gain was 1.77 kg (n=951) compared to 2.19 kg (n=414) in patients treated with SEROQUEL. For patients treated with placebo the mean weight gain was 0.26 kg (n=319). In a 3-week placebo-controlled bipolar mania clinical trial, for patients treated with SEROQUEL XR mean weight gain was 1.3 kg (n=151) compared to 0.1 kg (n=160) in patients treated with placebo. In an 8-week placebo-controlled bipolar depression clinical trial, for patients treated with SEROQUEL XR mean weight gain was 1.3 kg (n=137) compared to −0.2 kg (n=140) in patients treated with placebo. In 6-week placebo-controlled MDD acute monotherapy clinical trials, for patients treated with SEROQUEL XR mean weight gain was 0.87 kg (n=1149) compared to 0.31 kg (n=648) in patients treated with placebo. In a longer-term randomized withdrawal MDD trial, patients who completed at least 158 days of SEROQUEL XR treatment (n=196), mean weight gain for patients in SEROQUEL XR 50, 150 and 300 mg/day groups was 1.0 kg, 2.5 kg, and 3.0 kg respectively. In these same patients the percentage of patients experiencing a weight increase of ≥7% by 158 days in SEROQUEL XR 50, 150, and 300 mg/day groups was 13%, 24%, and 33% respectively.

Based on the cumulative acute placebo-controlled clinical trial database, weight gain (based on ≥7% increase in body weight from baseline) was reported in 9.6% in quetiapine-treated patients and 3.8% in placebo-treated patients, which occurs predominantly during the early weeks of treatment in adults (see Adverse Reactions).

Gastrointestinal: Antiemetic Effect: Consistent with its dopamine antagonist effects, SEROQUEL XR may have an antiemetic effect. Such an effect may mask signs of toxicity due to overdosage of other drugs, or may mask symptoms of disease such as brain tumour or intestinal obstruction.

Dysphagia and Aspiration Pneumonia: Dysphagia and aspiration have been reported with quetiapine. Although a causal relationship with aspiration pneumonia has not been established, SEROQUEL XR should be used with caution in patients at risk for aspiration pneumonia. See Warnings and Precautions, Special Populations and Adverse Reactions.

Hematologic: Neutropenia: Severe neutropenia (<0.5×10⁹/L) has been uncommonly reported in quetiapine clinical trials. There was no apparent dose relationship. Possible risk factors for leucopenia and/or neutropenia include pre-existing low white cell count (WBC) and history of drug induced leucopenia and/or neutropenia. SEROQUEL XR should be discontinued in patients with a neutrophil count <1.0×10⁹/L. These patients should be observed for signs and symptoms of infection and neutrophil counts followed (until they exceed 1.5×10⁹/L). (See Adverse Reactions, Abnormal Hematologic and Clinical Chemistry Findings and Post-Market Adverse Drug Reactions.)

Hepatic/Biliary/Pancreatic: Hepatic Impairment: Decreased clearance of SEROQUEL was observed in patients with mild hepatic impairment (see Action and Clinical Pharmacology, Special Populations and Conditions). No pharmacokinetic data are available for quetiapine in patients with moderate or severe hepatic impairment. However, should clinical judgement deem treatment with SEROQUEL XR necessary, the drug should be used with great caution in patients with moderate or severe hepatic impairment (see Action and Clinical Pharmacology, Special Populations and Conditions and Dosage and Administration).

Transaminase Elevations: Asymptomatic, transient and reversible elevations in serum transaminases (primarily ALT) associated with SEROQUEL XR have been reported. The proportions of patients with transaminase elevations of >3 times the upper limits of the normal reference range in a pool of placebo-controlled trials were approximately 1% for both SEROQUEL XR and placebo.

During premarketing clinical trials, therapy with SEROQUEL was associated with elevation of hepatic transaminases, primarily ALT. Within a clinical trial database of 1892 SEROQUEL-treated schizophrenia patients, with baseline ALT levels <60 IU/L, 5.3% (101/1892) had treatment-emergent ALT elevations to >120 IU/L, 1.5% (29/1892) had elevations to >200 IU/L, and 0.2% (3/1892) had elevations to >400 IU/L. No patients had values in excess of 800 IU/L. None of the SEROQUEL-treated patients who had elevated transaminase values manifested clinical symptomatology associated with liver impairment. The majority of transaminase elevations were seen during the first two months of treatment. Most elevations were transient (80%) while patients continued on SEROQUEL therapy. Of the 101 SEROQUEL-treated patients whose enzyme levels increased to >120 IU/L, 40 discontinued treatment while their ALT values were still raised. In 114 SEROQUEL-treated patients whose baseline ALT was >90 IU/L, only 1 experienced an elevation to >400 IU/L.

Precautions should be exercised when using SEROQUEL XR in patients with pre-existing hepatic disorders, in patients who are being treated with potentially hepatotoxic drugs, or if treatment-emergent signs or symptoms of hepatic impairment appear.

For patients who have known or suspected abnormal hepatic function prior to starting SEROQUEL XR, standard clinical assessment, including measurement of transaminase levels is recommended. Periodic clinical reassessment with transaminase levels is recommended for such patients, as well as for patients who develop any signs and symptoms suggestive of a new onset liver disorder during SEROQUEL XR therapy.

Neurologic: Neuroleptic Malignant Syndrome (NMS): Neuroleptic Malignant Syndrome is a potentially fatal symptom complex that has been reported in association with antipsychotic drugs, including SEROQUEL XR.

The clinical manifestations of NMS are hyperthermia, muscle rigidity, altered mental status, and evidence of autonomic instability (irregular pulse or blood pressure, tachycardia, diaphoresis, and cardiac dysrhythmia). Additional signs may include elevated creatine phosphokinase, myoglobinuria (rhabdomyolysis) and acute renal failure.

In arriving at a diagnosis, it is important to identify cases where the clinical presentation includes both serious medical illness (e.g., pneumonia, systemic infection, etc.) and untreated or inadequately treated extrapyramidal signs and symptoms. Other important considerations in the differential diagnosis include central anticholinergic toxicity, heat stroke, drug fever and primary central nervous system pathology.

The management of NMS should include immediate discontinuation of antipsychotic drugs, including SEROQUEL XR, and other drugs not essential to concurrent therapy; intensive symptomatic treatment and medical monitoring; and treatment of any concomitant serious medical problems for which specific treatments are available. There is no general agreement about specific pharmacological treatment regimens for uncomplicated NMS.

If a patient requires antipsychotic drug treatment after recovery from NMS, the potential reintroduction of drug therapy should be carefully considered. The patient should be carefully monitored since recurrences of NMS have been reported.

Tardive Dyskinesia (TD) and Extrapyramidal Symptoms (EPS): Tardive dyskinesia is a syndrome of potentially irreversible, involuntary, dyskinetic movements that may develop in patients treated with antipsychotic drugs including quetiapine. Although the prevalence of the syndrome appears to be highest among the elderly, especially elderly women, it is impossible to rely upon estimates to predict which patients are likely to develop the syndrome.

In placebo-controlled clinical trials for schizophrenia and bipolar mania the incidence of EPS was no different from that of placebo across the recommended therapeutic dose range. It has been hypothesized that agents with a lower EPS liability may also have a lower liability to produce TD. This relationship predicts that quetiapine should have less potential than typical antipsychotic agents to induce TD in schizophrenia and bipolar mania patients. In short-term, placebo-controlled clinical trials for bipolar depression and major depressive disorder, the incidence of EPS was higher in quetiapine treated patients than in placebo treated patients. See Adverse Reactions.

The risk of developing TD and the likelihood that it will become irreversible are believed to increase as the duration of treatment and the total cumulative dose of antipsychotic drugs administered to the patient increase. However, the syndrome can develop, although much less commonly, after relatively brief treatment periods at low doses.

There is no known treatment for established cases of TD, although the syndrome may remit, partially or completely, if antipsychotic treatment is withdrawn. Antipsychotic treatment, itself, however, may suppress (or partially suppress) the signs and symptoms of the syndrome and thereby may possibly mask the underlying process. The effect that symptomatic suppression has upon the long-term course of the syndrome is unknown.

Given these considerations, SEROQUEL XR should be prescribed in a manner that is most likely to minimize the occurrence of TD. Chronic antipsychotic treatment should generally be reserved for patients who appear to suffer from a chronic illness that is known to respond to antipsychotic drugs, and for whom alternative, equally effective, but potentially less harmful treatments are not available or appropriate. In patients who do require chronic treatment, the smallest dose and the shortest duration of treatment producing a satisfactory clinical response should be sought. The need for continued treatment should be reassessed periodically.

If signs and symptoms of TD appear in a patient on SEROQUEL XR, dose reduction or drug discontinuation should be considered. Some patients may require treatment with SEROQUEL XR despite the presence of the syndrome. The symptoms of TD can worsen or even arise after discontinuation of treatment (see Adverse Reactions).

Seizures: In controlled clinical trials with SEROQUEL XR, there was no difference in the incidence of seizures in patients treated with SEROQUEL XR (0.04%, 1/2388) or placebo (0.2%, 3/1267). Nevertheless, as with other antipsychotics, caution is recommended when treating patients with a history of seizures or with conditions associated with a lowered seizure threshold (see Adverse Reactions).

Potential Effect on Cognitive and Motor Performance: Somnolence was a very commonly reported adverse event in patients treated with SEROQUEL XR, especially during the initial dose titration period. Since SEROQUEL XR may cause sedation and impair motor skill, patients should be cautioned about performing activities requiring mental alertness, such as operating a motor vehicle or hazardous machinery, until they are reasonably certain that SEROQUEL XR does not affect them adversely. Somnolence may lead to falls.

Ophthalmologic: Cataracts: The development of cataracts was observed in association with quetiapine treatment in chronic dog studies at 4 times the recommended human dose. Lens changes have also been observed in patients during long-term SEROQUEL treatment, but a causal relationship to SEROQUEL use has not been established. The possibility of lenticular changes during long-term use of SEROQUEL XR in man, thus can not be excluded at this time. Eye examinations (e.g., slit lamp exam) prior to or shortly after initiation of treatment with SEROQUEL XR and at 6 month intervals thereafter, are recommended. If clinically significant lens changes associated with SEROQUEL XR use are observed, discontinuation of SEROQUEL XR should be considered.

Psychiatric: Suicide/Suicidal Thoughts or Clinical Worsening: Depressive episodes are associated with an increased risk of suicidal thoughts, self-harm and suicide (suicide-related events). This risk persists until significant remission of depression occurs. As improvement may not occur during the first few weeks or more of treatment, patients should be closely monitored until such improvement occurs. It is general clinical experience that the risk of suicide may increase in the early stages of recovery. In addition to depressive episodes associated with bipolar disorder and MDD, depression may be co-morbid with schizophrenia.

Schizophrenia as well as manic episodes associated bipolar disorder, can also be associated with an increased risk of suicide-related events, and thus close supervision and appropriate clinical management of high risk patients should accompany drug therapy.

Patients with a history of suicide-related events are also known to be at a greater risk of suicidal thoughts or suicide attempts, and should receive careful monitoring during treatment.

In a bipolar mania clinical trial with SEROQUEL XR, the incidence of treatment-emergent suicidal ideation or suicidal behaviour, as measured by the Columbia Analysis of Suicidal Behaviour, was 1.3% for SEROQUEL XR-treated patients and 3.8% for placebo-treated patients.

In a bipolar depression clinical trial with SEROQUEL XR, the incidence of treatment-emergent suicidal ideation or suicidal behaviour, as measured by the Columbia Analysis of Suicidal Behaviour, was 0.7% for SEROQUEL XR-treated patients and 1.4% for placebo-treated patients.

In MDD acute clinical trials, the incidence of treatment emergent suicidal ideation or suicide attempt was 0.7% in SEROQUEL XR treated patients and 0.7% in placebo-treated patients. In a longer-term randomized withdrawal study in patients with MDD, the incidence during randomized treatment was 0.3% for SEROQUEL XR and 0.5% for placebo.

Renal: There is little experience with SEROQUEL XR in patients with renal impairment, except in a low (subclinical) single dose study with SEROQUEL (see Action and Clinical Pharmacology, Special Populations and Conditions). SEROQUEL XR should thus be used with caution in patients with known renal impairment, especially during the initial dosing period (see Dosage and Administration).

Special Populations: Pregnant Women: Patients should be advised to notify their physician if they become pregnant or intend to become pregnant during treatment with SEROQUEL XR. The safety and efficacy of SEROQUEL XR during human pregnancy have not been established. Therefore, SEROQUEL XR should only be used during pregnancy if the expected benefits justify the potential risks.

Nursing Women: The degree to which quetiapine is excreted into human milk is unknown. Women who are breast-feeding should therefore be advised to avoid breast-feeding while taking SEROQUEL XR.

Pediatrics (<18 years of age): The safety and efficacy of SEROQUEL XR in children under the age of 18 years have not been established.

Geriatrics (≥65 years of age): The number of patients 65 years of age or over exposed to SEROQUEL XR during clinical trials was limited (n=68). When compared to younger patients the mean plasma clearance of quetiapine was reduced by 30% to 50% in elderly subjects. In addition, as this population has more frequent hepatic, renal, central nervous system, and cardiovascular dysfunctions, and more frequent use of concomitant medication, caution should be exercised with the use of SEROQUEL XR in the elderly patient (see Dosage and Administration).

In a clinical trial that evaluated non-demented elderly patients (aged 66 to 89 years) with MDD, the tolerability of SEROQUEL XR once daily was comparable to that seen in adults (aged 18-65 years) other than the incidence of extrapyramidal symptoms. See Warnings and Precautions, Neurologic, Tardive Dyskinesia (TD) and Extrapyramidal Symptoms (EPS); Adverse Reactions.

Use in Geriatric Patients with Dementia: Overall Mortality: Elderly patients with dementia treated with atypical antipsychotic drugs showed increased mortality compared to placebo in a meta-analysis of 13 controlled trials of various atypical antipsychotic drugs. In two placebo-controlled trials with oral SEROQUEL in this population, the incidence of mortality was 5.5% for SEROQUEL-treated patients compared to 3.2% for placebo-treated patients. SEROQUEL XR is not indicated in elderly patients with dementia.

Cerebrovascular adverse events: An increased risk of cerebrovascular adverse events has been seen in the dementia population with some atypical antipsychotics. The mechanism for this increased risk is not known. There is insufficient data with quetiapine to know if there is an increased risk of cerebrovascular events associated with quetiapine. An increased risk, however, cannot be excluded. SEROQUEL XR is not indicated in patients with dementia.

Vascular disease: SEROQUEL XR should be used with caution in patients with risk factors for stroke or with a history of stroke.

Dysphagia: Esophageal dysmotility and aspiration have been associated with antipsychotic drug use. Aspiration pneumonia is a common cause of morbidity and mortality in elderly patients, in particular those with advanced Alzheimer's dementia. SEROQUEL XR and other antipsychotic drugs should be used cautiously in patients at risk for aspiration pneumonia. See Warnings and Precautions, Gastrointestinal and Adverse Reactions.

ADVERSE REACTIONS: The stated frequencies of adverse events represent the proportion of individuals who experienced, at least once, a treatment-emergent adverse event of the type listed. An event was considered treatment-emergent if it occurred for the first time or worsened while receiving therapy following baseline evaluation.

Clinical Trial Adverse Drug Reactions: The prescriber should be aware that the figures in the tables and tabulations cannot be used to predict the incidence of side effects in the course of usual medical practice where patient characteristics and other factors differ from those that prevailed in the clinical trials. Similarly, the cited frequencies cannot be compared with figures obtained from other clinical investigations involving different treatments, uses, and investigators. The figures cited, however, do provide the prescribing physician with some basis for estimating the relative contribution of drug and nondrug factors to the side effect incidence in the populations studied.

Adverse Events Associated with Discontinuation: Short-Term Placebo-Controlled Clinical Trials: Schizophrenia: In short-term, placebo-controlled schizophrenia trials, there was no difference in the incidence of adverse events associated with discontinuation of SEROQUEL XR or placebo. Overall, 6.4% of SEROQUEL XR-treated patients discontinued treatment due to adverse events compared to 7.5% of placebo-treated patients.

Bipolar Disorder: Bipolar Mania: In a 3-week placebo-controlled bipolar mania trial, 4.6% of patients on SEROQUEL XR discontinued due to adverse events compared to 8.1% on placebo.

Bipolar Depression: In an 8-week placebo-controlled bipolar depression trial, 13.1% of patients on SEROQUEL XR discontinued due to adverse events compared to 3.6% on placebo. Sedation (6.6%) and somnolence (3.6%) were the most common adverse events leading to discontinuation in the SEROQUEL XR treatment group.

Major Depressive Disorder: In placebo-controlled monotherapy MDD trials, 14.3% of patients on SEROQUEL XR discontinued due to adverse events compared to 4.5% on placebo. In a placebo-controlled monotherapy trial in elderly patients with MDD, 9.6% of patients on SEROQUEL XR discontinued due to adverse events compared to 4.1% on placebo.

Commonly Observed Adverse Events in Short-Term Placebo-Controlled Clinical Trials: Schizophrenia: During acute therapy with SEROQUEL XR, the most commonly observed adverse events associated with the use of SEROQUEL XR (incidence of at least 5%, and an incidence at least 5% higher than that observed with placebo) were sedation, dry mouth, somnolence, and dizziness.

Bipolar Disorder: Bipolar Mania: During acute therapy with SEROQUEL XR, the most commonly observed adverse events associated with the use of SEROQUEL XR (incidence of at least 5%, and an incidence at least 5% higher than that observed with placebo) were sedation, dry mouth, somnolence, constipation, dizziness, weight gain and dysarthria.

Bipolar Depression: During acute therapy with SEROQUEL XR, the most commonly observed adverse events associated with the use of SEROQUEL XR (incidence of at least 5%, and an incidence at least 5% higher than that observed with placebo) were dry mouth, somnolence, sedation, increased appetite, weight gain and dyspepsia.

Major Depressive Disorder: The most commonly observed adverse events associated with the use of SEROQUEL XR (incidence of at least 5%, and an incidence at least 5% higher than that observed with placebo) during acute monotherapy with SEROQUEL XR were dry mouth, sedation, somnolence dizziness and fatigue.

Incidence of Adverse Events in Placebo-Controlled Clinical Trials: Table 1 enumerates the incidence, rounded to the nearest percent, of treatment-emergent adverse events that occurred during acute therapy (up to 6 weeks) of schizophrenia in ≥1% of patients treated with SEROQUEL XR (doses ranging from 300 to 800 mg/day) where the incidence in patients treated with SEROQUEL XR was greater than the incidence in placebo-treated patients.

Table 1: SEROQUEL XR

Adverse Events Reported for at Least 1% of SEROQUEL XR-Treated Subjects (doses ranging from 300 to 800 mg/day) and for a Higher Percentage of SEROQUEL XR-Treated Subjects Than Subjects Who Received Placebo in Short-Term, Placebo-Controlled Schizophrenia Phase III Trials

	Percentage of Subjects with Adverse Events[b]	
Body System and MedDRA Term[a]	**SEROQUEL XR (n=951)**	**Placebo (n=319)**
Whole Body		
Fatigue	3	2
Anxiety	2	1
Irritability	1	0
Pyrexia	1	0
Nervous System		
Sedation	13	7
Somnolence	12	4
Dizziness	10	4
Tremor	2	1
Restlessness	2	1
Gastrointestinal System		
Dry Mouth	12	1
Constipation	6	5
Dyspepsia	5	2
Cardiovascular System		
Orthostatic Hypotension	7	5
Hypotension	3	1
Tachycardia	3	1
Heart Rate Increased	4	1
Metabolic and Nutritional Disorders		
Increased Appetite	2	0
Special Senses		
Vision Blurred	2	1

(cont'd) **Table 1: SEROQUEL XR** *(cont'd)*

[a] Patients with multiple events falling under the same preferred term are counted only once in that term.
[b] Events for which SEROQUEL XR incidence was equal to or less than placebo are not listed in the table, but included the following: headache, insomnia, and nausea.

Table 2 enumerates the incidence, rounded to the nearest percent, of treatment-emergent adverse events that occurred during acute therapy (3 weeks) of bipolar mania in ≥1% of patients treated with SEROQUEL XR (300-800 mg/day) where the incidence in patients treated with SEROQUEL XR was greater than the incidence in placebo-treated patients.

Table 2: SEROQUEL XR

Adverse Events Reported for at Least 1% of SEROQUEL XR-Treated Subjects (doses ranging from 300 to 800 mg/day) and for a Higher Percentage of SEROQUEL XR-Treated Subjects Than Subjects Who Received Placebo in a Short-Term (3-week), Placebo-Controlled Bipolar Mania Phase III Trial

	Percentage of Subjects with Adverse Events[b]	
Body System and MedDRA Term[a]	**SEROQUEL XR (n=151)**	**Placebo (n=160)**
General Disorders and Administration Site Conditions		
Fatigue	7	4
Contusion	1	0
Pain	1	0
Nervous System Disorders		
Sedation	34	8
Somnolence	17	4
Dizziness	10	4
Dysarthria	5	0
Lethargy	2	1
Sluggishness	2	1
Dizziness Postural	1	0
Gastrointestinal Disorders		
Dry Mouth	34	7
Constipation	10	3
Dyspepsia	7	4
Toothache	3	1
Cardiovascular Disorders		
Heart Rate Increased	3	0
Orthostatic Hypotension	3	0
Tachycardia	2	1
Metabolic and Nutritional Disorders		
Weight Increased	7	1
Increased Appetite	4	2
Musculoskeletal and Connective Tissue Disorders		
Back Pain	3	2
Arthralgia	1	0
Psychiatric Disorders		
Abnormal Dreams	3	0

(cont'd)

Table 2: SEROQUEL XR *(cont'd)*

Adverse Events Reported for at Least 1% of SEROQUEL XR-Treated Subjects (doses ranging from 300 to 800 mg/day) and for a Higher Percentage of SEROQUEL XR-Treated Subjects Than Subjects Who Received Placebo in a Short-Term (3-week), Placebo-Controlled Bipolar Mania Phase III Trial

Body System and MedDRA Term[a]	Percentage of Subjects with Adverse Events[b]	
	SEROQUEL XR (n=151)	Placebo (n=160)
Bipolar I Disorder	1	0
Respiratory Disorders		
Nasal Congestion	5	1
Dry Throat	1	0
Special Senses		
Vision Blurred	2	1

[a] Patients with multiple events falling under the same preferred term are counted only once in that term.
[b] Events for which SEROQUEL XR incidence was equal to or less than placebo are not listed in the table. Table reports percentage rounded to the nearest integer.

Table 3 enumerates the incidence, rounded to the nearest percent, of treatment-emergent adverse events that occurred during acute therapy (8 weeks) of bipolar depression in ≥1% of patients treated with SEROQUEL XR (300 mg/day) where the incidence in patients treated with SEROQUEL XR was greater than the incidence in placebo-treated patients.

Table 3: SEROQUEL XR

Adverse Events Reported for at Least 1% of SEROQUEL XR-Treated Subjects (dose of 300 mg/day) and for a Higher Percentage of SEROQUEL XR-Treated Subjects Than Subjects Who Received Placebo in a Short-Term (8-week), Placebo-Controlled Bipolar Depression Phase III Trial

Body System and MedDRA Term[a]	Percentage of Subjects with Adverse Events[b]	
	SEROQUEL XR (n=137)	Placebo (n=140)
General Disorders		
Fatigue	6	2
Irritability	4	3
Anxiety	2	1
Nervous System Disorders		
Somnolence	29	6
Sedation	23	7
Dizziness	13	11
Paraesthesia	3	2
Dysarthria	2	0
Disturbance in Attention	2	1
Hypersomnia	1	0
Akathisia	1	0
Mental Impairment	1	0
Gastrointestinal Disorders		
Dry Mouth	37	7
Constipation	8	6
Dyspepsia	7	1
Toothache	3	0
Cardiovascular Disorders		
Heart Rate Increased	1	0
Infection and Infestations		
Gastroenteritis Viral	4	1
Urinary Tract Infection	2	0
Metabolic and Nutritional Disorders		
Increased Appetite	12	6
Weight Increased	7	1
Decreased Appetite	2	1
Musculoskeletal and Connective Tissue Disorders		
Arthralgia	4	1

(cont'd)

Table 3: SEROQUEL XR *(cont'd)*

Adverse Events Reported for at Least 1% of SEROQUEL XR-Treated Subjects (dose of 300 mg/day) and for a Higher Percentage of SEROQUEL XR-Treated Subjects Than Subjects Who Received Placebo in a Short-Term (8-week), Placebo-Controlled Bipolar Depression Phase III Trial

Body System and MedDRA Term[a]	Percentage of Subjects with Adverse Events[b]	
	SEROQUEL XR (n=137)	Placebo (n=140)
Back Pain	3	1
Muscle Spasm	3	1
Neck Pain	1	0
Psychiatric Disorders		
Abnormal Dreams	3	0
Confusional State	1	0
Disorientation	1	0
Skin and Subcutaneous Tissue Disorders		
Hyperhidrosis	2	1

[a] Patients with multiple events falling under the same preferred term are counted only once in that term.
[b] Events for which SEROQUEL XR incidence was equal to or less than placebo are not listed in the table. Table reports percentage rounded to the nearest integer.

Table 4 enumerates the incidence, rounded to the nearest percent, of treatment-emergent adverse events that occurred during acute monotherapy (up to 8 weeks) of MDD in ≥1% of patients treated with SEROQUEL XR (50-300 mg/day) where the incidence in patients treated with SEROQUEL XR was greater than the incidence in placebo-treated patients.

Table 4: SEROQUEL XR

Adverse Events Reported for at Least 1% of SEROQUEL XR-Treated Subjects (Doses Ranging From 50 to 300 mg/day) and for a Higher Percentage of SEROQUEL XR-Treated Subjects Than Subjects Who Received Placebo in Short-Term, Placebo-Controlled MDD Monotherapy Phase III Trials

Body System and MedDRA Term[a, b]	Percentage of Subjects with Adverse Events[c]	
	SEROQUEL XR (n=1149)	Placebo (n=648)
General Disorders and Administration Site Conditions		
Fatigue	7	2
Irritability	4	3
Nervous System Disorders		
Sedation	28	4
Somnolence	24	7
Dizziness	14	8
Disturbance in attention	2	<1
Hypersomnia	2	<1
Lethargy	2	1
Gastrointestinal System Disorders		
Dry mouth	35	8
Constipation	8	4
Vomiting	3	1
Dyspepsia	4	3
Metabolic and Nutritional Disorders		
Increased appetite	5	3
Weight increased	3	<1
Musculoskeletal and Connective Tissue Disorders		
Back pain	3	2
Myalgia	3	2
Musculoskeletal stiffness	2	1
Psychiatric Disorders		
Abnormal dreams	2	1
Respiratory Disorders		
Nasal congestion	2	1
Special senses		

(cont'd)

Table 4: SEROQUEL XR *(cont'd)*

Adverse Events Reported for at Least 1% of SEROQUEL XR-Treated Subjects (Doses Ranging From 50 to 300 mg/day) and for a Higher Percentage of SEROQUEL XR-Treated Subjects Than Subjects Who Received Placebo in Short-Term, Placebo-Controlled MDD Monotherapy Phase III Trials

Body System and MedDRA Term[a, b]	Percentage of Subjects with Adverse Events[c]	
	SEROQUEL XR (n=1149)	Placebo (n=648)
Vision blurred	3	2

[a] Patients with multiple events falling under the same preferred term are counted only once in that term.
[b] The following adverse events occurred in 1% of patients treated with SEROQUEL XR compared to <1% in placebo: chills, dysarthria, dysgeusia, sluggishness, akathisia, dizziness postural, tachycardia, restless legs syndrome, gastroesophageal reflux disease, pharyngolaryngeal pain and restlessness.
[c] Events for which SEROQUEL XR incidence was equal to or less than placebo are not listed in the table. Table reports percentage rounded to the nearest integer.

Table 5 enumerates the incidence of treatment-emergent adverse events that are dose related that occurred during acute monotherapy fixed dose studies (6-weeks) in ≥1% of patients treated with SEROQUEL XR (50-300 mg/day) where the incidence of the adverse events in patients treated with SEROQUEL XR 150 mg and/or 300 mg was greater than the incidence in SEROQUEL XR 50 mg and placebo-treated patients.

Table 5: SEROQUEL XR

Dose Related Adverse Events in ≥1% of Patients Treated with SEROQUEL XR (Doses 50, 150 and 300 mg/day) Where the Incidence of the Adverse Events in Patients Treated with SEROQUEL XR 150 mg and/or 300 mg was Greater than the Incidence in SEROQUEL XR 50 mg and Placebo-Treated Patients in Short-Term Fixed Dose, Placebo-Controlled MDD Monotherapy Phase III Trials

Body System and MedDRA Term[a]	Percentage of Subjects with Adverse Events[b]			
	Placebo (n=338)	SEROQUEL XR 50 mg (n=181)	SEROQUEL XR 150 mg (n=328)	SEROQUEL XR 300 mg (n=331)
General Disorders and Administration Site Conditions				
Pain	0	1	1	2
Chills	0	1	0	2
Nervous System Disorders				
Sedation	6	27	37	34
Somnolence	9	18	22	28
Dizziness	8	9	13	15
Dysarthria	0	1	1	3
Disturbance in attention	0	1	2	2
Hypoaesthesia	1	0	1	2
Akathisia	1	0	2	1
Lethargy	1	2	3	1
Paraesthesia	1	1	2	1
Hypersomnia	0	1	2	1
Gastrointestinal System Disorders				
Dry mouth	9	22	36	40
Constipation	4	7	7	9
Nausea	8	8	12	9
Vomiting	2	2	4	5
Dyspepsia	3	2	5	4
Gastrooesophageal reflux disease	0	0	1	2
Abdominal distension	1	0	0	2
Abdominal pain	1	1	2	1
Cardiovascular Disorders				
Tachycardia	0	1	2	1
Metabolic and Nutritional Disorders				
Increased appetite	3	4	5	4
Weight increased	1	1	2	3

(cont'd)

Table 5: SEROQUEL XR *(cont'd)*

Dose Related Adverse Events in ≥1% of Patients Treated with SEROQUEL XR (Doses 50, 150 and 300 mg/day) Where the Incidence of the Adverse Events in Patients Treated with SEROQUEL XR 150 mg and/or 300 mg was Greater than the Incidence in SEROQUEL XR 50 mg and Placebo-Treated Patients in Short-Term Fixed Dose, Placebo-Controlled MDD Monotherapy Phase III Trials

Body System and MedDRA Term[a]	Percentage of Subjects with Adverse Events[b]			
	Placebo (n=338)	SEROQUEL XR 50 mg (n=181)	SEROQUEL XR 150 mg (n=328)	SEROQUEL XR 300 mg (n=331)
Musculoskeletal and Connective Tissue Disorders				
Back pain	2	2	5	5
Arthralgia	2	2	3	3
Myalgia	2	4	5	3
Muscle tightness	1	1	0	2
Psychiatric Disorders				
Anxiety	2	1	2	3
Abnormal dreams	3	2	4	2
Restlessness	0	0	1	2
Nightmare	1	1	1	2
Infections and Infestations				
Nasopharyngitis	3	2	4	3
Gastroenteritis	0	1	2	1
Respiratory Disorders				
Nasal congestion	2	1	2	3
Sinus congestion	1	1	2	2
Dyspnoea	1	1	1	2
Epistaxis	0	1	0	2
Nasal dryness	0	0	1	1
Special Senses				
Vision blurred	1	2	3	5

[a] Patients with multiple events falling under the same preferred term are counted only once in that term.
[b] Events for which SEROQUEL XR incidence was equal to or less than placebo are not listed in the table.

Table 6 enumerates the incidence, rounded to the nearest percent, of treatment-emergent adverse events that occurred during acute monotherapy (9 weeks) of elderly patients with MDD in ≥1% of patients treated with SEROQUEL XR (50-300 mg/day) where the incidence in patients treated with SEROQUEL XR was greater than the incidence in placebo-treated patients.

Table 6: SEROQUEL XR

Adverse Events Reported for at Least 1% of SEROQUEL XR-Treated Subjects (Doses ranging from 50 to 300 mg/day) and for a Higher Percentage of SEROQUEL XR-Treated Subjects Than Subjects Who Received Placebo in a Short-Term, Placebo-Controlled Elderly MDD Monotherapy Phase III Trial

Body System and MedDRA Term[a,b]	Percentage of Subjects with Adverse Events[c]	
	SEROQUEL XR (n=166)	Placebo (n=172)
General Disorders and Administration Site Conditions		
Fatigue	8	3
Asthenia	4	1
Nervous System Disorders		
Somnolence	33	8
Headache	19	14
Dizziness	18	15
Sedation	5	1
Dysgeusia	2	1
Balance disorder	2	1
Dizziness postural	2	1

(cont'd)

Table 6: SEROQUEL XR *(cont'd)*

Adverse Events Reported for at Least 1% of SEROQUEL XR-Treated Subjects (Doses ranging from 50 to 300 mg/day) and for a Higher Percentage of SEROQUEL XR-Treated Subjects Than Subjects Who Received Placebo in a Short-Term, Placebo-Controlled Elderly MDD Monotherapy Phase III Trial

Body System and MedDRA Term[a,b]	Percentage of Subjects with Adverse Events[c]	
	SEROQUEL XR (n=166)	Placebo (n=172)
Akathisia	2	1
Gastrointestinal System Disorders		
Dry mouth	20	10
Constipation	5	2
Abdominal pain upper	3	2
Dyspepsia	2	1
Cardiovascular System Disorders		
Hypotension	2	0
Metabolic and Nutritional Disorders		
Weight increased	5	4
Weight decreased	2	1
Musculoskeletal and Connective Tissue Disorders		
Back pain	2	1
Extrapyramidal disorder	4	1
Pain in extremity	2	1
Respiratory Disorders		
Nasal congestion	2	0

a Patients with multiple events falling under the same preferred term are counted only once in that term.
b The following adverse events occurred in 1% of patients treated with SEROQUEL XR compared to <1% in placebo: hypersomnia, restless legs syndrome, joint sprain, muscular weakness, pharyngolaryngeal pain and vision blurred.
c Events for which SEROQUEL XR incidence was equal to or less than placebo are not listed in the table. Table reports percentage rounded to the nearest integer.

Other Adverse Events: Weight Gain: In 6-week placebo-controlled schizophrenia clinical trials, for patients treated with SEROQUEL XR mean weight gain was 1.77 kg (n=951) compared to 2.19 kg (n=414) in patients treated with SEROQUEL (quetiapine, immediate release formulation). For patients treated with placebo the mean weight gain was 0.26 kg (n=319). In a 3-week placebo-controlled bipolar mania clinical trial, for patients treated with SEROQUEL XR mean weight gain was 1.3 kg (n=151) compared to 0.1 kg (n=160) in patients treated with placebo. In an 8-week placebo-controlled bipolar depression clinical trial, for patients treated with SEROQUEL XR mean weight gain was 1.3 kg (n=137) compared to −0.2 kg (n=140) in patients treated with placebo. In placebo-controlled MDD acute monotherapy clinical trials, for patients treated with SEROQUEL XR mean weight gain was 0.87 kg (n=1149) compared to 0.31 kg (n=648) in patients treated with placebo. In a longer-term randomized withdrawal MDD trial, patients who completed at least 158 days of SEROQUEL XR treatment (n=196), mean weight gain for patients in SEROQUEL XR 50, 150 and 300 mg/day groups was 1.0 kg, 2.5 kg, and 3.0 kg respectively. In these same patients the percentage of patients experiencing a weight increase of ≥7% by 158 days in SEROQUEL XR 50, 150, and 300 mg/day groups was 13%, 24%, and 33% respectively. See Warnings and Precautions.

Based on the cumulative acute placebo-controlled clinical trial database, weight gain (based on ≥7% increase in body weight from baseline) was reported in 9.6% in quetiapine-treated patients and 3.8% in placebo-treated patients, which occurs predominantly during the early weeks of treatment in adults (see Warnings and Precautions).

Seizures: There have been uncommon reports (≥0.1%-<1%) of seizures in patients administered quetiapine, although the frequency was no greater than that observed in patients administered placebo in controlled clinical trials (see Warnings and Precautions, Neurologic).

Restless Legs Syndrome: There have been uncommon cases of restless legs syndrome in patients administered quetiapine.

Priapism: There have been rare reports (≥0.01%-<0.1%) of priapism in patients administered quetiapine.

Somnolence: Somnolence may occur, usually during the first two weeks of treatment, which generally resolves with the continued administration of SEROQUEL XR.

Neuroleptic Malignant Syndrome: As with other antipsychotics, rare cases of neuroleptic malignant syndrome have been reported in patients treated with quetiapine (see Warnings and Precautions, Neurologic).

Vital Signs: As with other antipsychotics with α1 adrenergic blocking activity, SEROQUEL XR may induce postural hypotension, associated with dizziness, tachycardia and, in some patients, syncope, especially during the initial dose titration period (see Warnings and Precautions, Cardiovascular). In placebo-controlled clinical trials in schizophrenia, postural hypotension was reported with an incidence of 8% in SEROQUEL (quetiapine, immediate release formulation)-treated patients compared to 2% in placebo-treated patients. SEROQUEL was associated with a mean baseline to endpoint increase in heart rate of 3.9 beats per minute, compared to 1.6 beats per minute among placebo-treated patients.

Peripheral Edema: As with other antipsychotics, common cases (≥1%-<10%) of peripheral edema have been reported in patients treated with quetiapine.

Mild Asthenia: As with other antipsychotic agents, common cases of mild asthenia have been reported in patients treated with quetiapine.

Rhinitis: There have been common reports of rhinitis in patients administered quetiapine.

Hypersensitivity: Uncommon cases of hypersensitivity including angioedema have been reported.

ECG Changes: In schizophrenia trials, 0.8% of SEROQUEL XR patients, and no placebo patients, had tachycardia (>120 bpm) at any time during the trials. In MDD monotherapy trials, 0.2% of SEROQUEL XR patients, and no placebo patients, had tachycardia (>120 bpm) at any time during the trials. SEROQUEL XR was associated with a mean increase in heart rate, assessed by ECG, of 7 beats per minute compared to a mean decrease of 1 beat per minute for placebo. This is consistent with the rates of SEROQUEL.

This slight tendency to tachycardia may be related to the potential of SEROQUEL XR for inducing orthostatic changes (see Warnings and Precautions, Cardiovascular).

Tardive Dyskinesia: There have been uncommon cases of tardive dyskinesia reported in patients administered quetiapine (see Warnings and Precautions, Neurologic).

Extrapyramidal Symptoms (EPS): In three-arm, placebo-controlled clinical trials for the treatment of schizophrenia, utilizing doses between 300 mg and 800 mg of SEROQUEL XR, the incidence of any adverse events potentially related to EPS was 7.5% for SEROQUEL XR, 7.7% for SEROQUEL, and 4.7% in the placebo group and without evidence of dose response. In these studies, the incidence rates of the individual adverse events (e.g., akathisia, extrapyramidal disorder, tremor, dyskinesia, dystonia, restlessness, and muscle rigidity) were generally low and did not exceed 3% for any treatment group.

At the end of treatment, the mean change from baseline in SAS total score and BARS Global Assessment score was similar across the treatment groups. The use of concomitant anticholinergic medications was infrequent and similar across the treatment groups.

The incidence of EPS was consistent with that seen with the profile of SEROQUEL in schizophrenia patients. The incidence of EPS did not increase with the dose of SEROQUEL XR.

In short-term placebo-controlled clinical trials in schizophrenia and bipolar mania, the aggregated incidence of EPS-related adverse events was similar to placebo (schizophrenia: 7.8% for quetiapine and 8.0% for placebo; bipolar mania: 11.2% for quetiapine and 11.4% for placebo). In short-term placebo-controlled clinical trials in bipolar depression, the aggregated incidence of EPS-related adverse events was 8.9% for quetiapine compared to 3.8% for placebo. The incidence of individual EPS-related adverse events (e.g., akathisia, extrapyramidal disorder, tremor, dyskinesia, dystonia, restlessness, muscle contractions involuntary, psychomotor hyperactivity and muscle rigidity), however was generally low and did not exceed 4% for any individual adverse event. In short-term, placebo-controlled monotherapy clinical trials in MDD the aggregated incidence of EPS was 5.4% for SEROQUEL XR and 3.2% for placebo. In a short-term placebo-controlled monotherapy trial in elderly patients with MDD, the aggregated incidence of EPS was 9.0% for SEROQUEL XR and 2.3% for placebo. In long-term studies of schizophrenia, bipolar disorder and MDD the aggregated exposure adjusted incidence of treatment-emergent EPS was similar between quetiapine and placebo. See Warnings and Precautions, Neurologic.

Dysphagia: There have been uncommon cases of dysphagia in patients administered quetiapine. In clinical trials, an increase in the rate of dysphagia with quetiapine versus placebo was only observed in bipolar depression. See Warnings and Precautions, Gastrointestinal and Special Populations.

Dysarthria: There have been common cases of dysarthria in patients administered quetiapine.

Acute Withdrawal (discontinuation) Symptoms: In acute placebo-controlled, monotherapy clinical trials, which evaluated discontinuation symptoms, the aggregated incidence of discontinuation symptoms after abrupt cessation was 12.1% for quetiapine and 6.7% for placebo. The aggregated incidence of the individual adverse events (e.g., insomnia, nausea, headache, diarrhea, vomiting, dizziness and irritability) did not exceed 5.3% in any treatment group and usually resolved 1 week after discontinuation. See Warnings and Precautions.

Abnormal Dreams and Nightmares: There have been common cases of abnormal dreams and nightmares in patients administered quetiapine.

Suicide-Related Events: In short-term placebo-controlled clinical trials across all indications and ages, the incidence of suicide-related events (suicidal thoughts, self-harm and suicide) was 0.9% for both quetiapine (61/6270) and for placebo (27/3047).

In these trials of patients with schizophrenia the incidence of suicide-related events was 1.4% (3/212) for quetiapine and 1.6% (1/62) for placebo in patients 18-24 years of age, 0.8% (13/1663) for quetiapine and 1.1% (5/463) for placebo in patients ≥25 years of age.

In these trials of patients with bipolar mania the incidence of suicide-related events was 0% for both quetiapine (0/60) and placebo (0/58) in patients 18-24 years of age, 1.2% for both quetiapine (6/496) and placebo (6/503) in patients ≥25 years of age.

In these trials of patients with bipolar depression the incidence of suicide-related events was 3.0% (7/233) for quetiapine and 0% (0/120) for placebo in patients 18-24 years of age and 1.8% for both quetiapine (19/1616) and placebo (11/622) in patients ≥25 years of age. (See Warnings and Precautions.)

In these trials of patients with MDD the incidence of suicide related events was 2.1% (3/144) for quetiapine and 1.3% (1/75) for placebo in patients 18-24 and 0.6% (11/1798) for quetiapine and 0.7% for placebo (7/1054) in patients ≥25 years of age.

Irritability: There have been common cases of irritability in patients administered quetiapine.

Increased Appetite: There have been common cases of increased appetite in patients administered quetiapine.

Abnormal Hematologic and Clinical Chemistry Findings: As with other antipsychotics, common cases of leucopenia and/or neutropenia have been observed in patients administered quetiapine. Uncommon cases of eosinophilia and thrombocytopenia (platelet count decreased, $\leq 100\times10^9$/L on at least one occasion) have been observed.

Based on clinical trial adverse event reports not associated with neuroleptic malignant syndrome, rare cases of elevations in blood creatine phosphokinase have been reported in patients administered quetiapine.

Common cases of elevations in serum prolactin levels have been observed (>20 µg/L in males and >30 µg/L in females) (see Warnings and Precautions, Endocrine and Metabolism, Hyperprolactinemia).

In three-arm, SEROQUEL XR placebo-controlled monotherapy clinical trials, among patients with a baseline neutrophil count $\geq 1.5\times10^9$/L, the incidence of at least one occurrence of neutrophil count $<1.5\times10^9$/L was 1.5% in patients treated with SEROQUEL XR and 1.5% for SEROQUEL, compared to 0.8% in placebo-treated patients.

In all placebo-controlled monotherapy clinical trials among patients with a baseline neutrophil count $\geq 1.5\times10^9$/L, the incidence of at least one occurrence of neutrophil count $<1.5\times10^9$/L was 1.72% in patients treated with SEROQUEL, compared to 0.73% in placebo-treated patients. In clinical trials conducted prior to a protocol amendment for discontinuation of patients with treatment-emergent neutrophil count $<1.0\times10^9$/L, among patients with a baseline neutrophil count $\geq 1.5\times10^9$/L, the incidence of at least one occurrence of neutrophil count $<0.5\times10^9$/L was 0.21% in patients treated with SEROQUEL and 0% in placebo-treated patients and the incidence ≥ 0.5-$<1.0\times10^9$/L was 0.75% in patients treated with SEROQUEL and 0.11% in placebo-treated patients. (See Warnings and Precautions, Hematologic.)

Common cases of asymptomatic elevations in serum transaminases [AST, ALT] or uncommon cases of γ-GT levels have been observed in some patients administered quetiapine. These elevations were usually reversible on continued quetiapine treatment (see Warnings and Precautions, Hepatic/Biliary/Pancreatic).

SEROQUEL treatment was associated with small dose-related decreases in thyroid hormone levels, particularly total T_4 and free T_4. The reduction in total and free T_4 was maximal within the first 2 to 4 weeks of quetiapine treatment, with no further reduction during long-term treatment. There was no evidence of clinically significant changes in TSH concentration over time. In nearly all cases, cessation of quetiapine treatment was associated with a reversal of the effects on total and free T_4, irrespective of the duration of treatment. Smaller decreases in total T_3 and reverse T_3 were seen only at higher doses. Levels of TBG were unchanged and in general reciprocal increases in TSH were not observed and there was no indication that SEROQUEL causes clinically relevant hypothyroidism (see Warnings and Precautions, Endocrine and Metabolism).

Hyperglycaemia: Blood glucose increases to hyperglycaemic levels (fasting blood glucose ≥7.0 mmol/L or a non fasting blood glucose ≥11.1 mmol/L on at least one occasion) have been observed commonly (≥1%-<10%) with quetiapine in clinical trials.

In two long-term bipolar maintenance placebo-controlled adjunct clinical trials, mean exposure 213 days for SEROQUEL (646 patients) and 152 days for placebo (680 patients), the exposure-adjusted rate of any increased blood glucose level (≥7.0 mmol/L) for patients more than 8 hours since a meal was 18.0 per 100 patient years for SEROQUEL (10.7% of patients) and 9.5 for placebo per 100 patient-years (4.6% of patients).

In short-term (12 weeks duration or less) placebo-controlled clinical trials (3342 treated with quetiapine and 1490 treated with placebo), the percent of patients who had a fasting blood glucose ≥7.0 mmol/L or a non fasting blood glucose ≥11.1 mmol/L was 3.5% for quetiapine and 2.1% for placebo.

In a 24-week trial (active-controlled, 115 patients treated with SEROQUEL) designed to evaluate glycemic status with oral glucose tolerance testing of all patients, at week 24 the incidence of a treatment-emergent post-glucose challenge glucose level ≥11.1 mmol/L was 1.7% and the incidence of a fasting treatment-emergent blood glucose level ≥7.0 mmol/L was 2.6%. (See Warnings and Precautions, Endocrine and Metabolism.)

Cholesterol and Triglyceride Elevations: Very common (≥10%) cases of elevations in serum triglyceride levels (≥2.258 mmol/L on at least one occasion), elevations in total cholesterol (predominantly LDL cholesterol) (≥6.2064 mmol/L on at least one occasion), and decreases in HDL cholesterol levels (<1.025 mmol/L males; <1.282 mmol/L females at any time) have been observed during treatment with quetiapine in clinical trials (see Warnings and Precautions, Cardiovascular). Lipid changes should be managed as clinically appropriate.

In one 24-week clinical trial, where LDL cholesterol was directly measured as opposed to calculated, there was a slight mean increase in total cholesterol in patients administered SEROQUEL, which was driven by increases in LDL cholesterol. The mean LDL level increased at Week 24 by 10% in patients administered SEROQUEL, which was statistically significant. The total cholesterol/HDL ratio did not change significantly during therapy with SEROQUEL. Furthermore, triglycerides did not increase significantly nor did HDL cholesterol decrease during therapy. (See Warnings and Precautions, Cardiovascular.)

Post-Market Adverse Drug Reactions: During post-marketing experience, leucopenia and/or neutropenia have been reported during SEROQUEL treatment. Resolution of leucopenia and/or neutropenia has followed cessation of therapy with SEROQUEL. Possible risk factors for leucopenia and/or neutropenia include pre-existing low white cell count and history of drug-induced leucopenia and/or neutropenia. (See Warnings and Precautions, Hematologic.)

As with some other antipsychotics, hyperglycaemia and diabetes mellitus (including exacerbation of pre-existing diabetes, diabetic ketoacidosis, and diabetic coma including some fatal cases) in the aggregate have been reported rarely (≥0.01%-<0.1%) during the use of SEROQUEL, sometimes in patients with no reported history of hyperglycaemia. (See Warnings and Precautions, Endocrine and Metabolism.)

Anaphylactic reactions have been reported very rarely in post-marketing reports, including a case with a fatal outcome, possibly related to SEROQUEL treatment. The reporting rate of anaphylaxis associated with SEROQUEL use, which is generally accepted to be an underestimate due to underreporting, does not exceed the background incidence rate estimates. Estimates of the background incidence rate (all cause) of severe life-threatening anaphylaxis in the general population range between 80 and 210 cases per million person-years, and the incidence rate of drug-induced anaphylaxis is reported to be 16 cases per million person-years. In addition, the all cause fatal anaphylaxis rate is reported to be one case per million person-years while the drug-induced fatal anaphylaxis is estimated to be 0.3 cases per million person-years. If a patient develops anaphylaxis after treatment with SEROQUEL XR, the drug should be discontinued and an alternative treatment started.

Based on post-marketing reports, galactorrhea has been reported rarely.

DRUG INTERACTIONS: Drug-Drug Interactions: Given the primary central nervous system effects of quetiapine, SEROQUEL XR (quetiapine fumarate extended-release) should be used with caution in combination with other centrally acting drugs.

Caution should be exercised when quetiapine is used concomitantly with drugs known to cause electrolyte imbalance or to increase QT interval (see Warnings and Precautions, Cardiovascular).

The Effect of SEROQUEL XR on Other Drugs: Alcohol: SEROQUEL (quetiapine, immediate-release formulation) potentiated the cognitive and motor effects of alcohol in a clinical trial in subjects with psychotic disorders. Alcoholic beverages should be avoided while taking SEROQUEL XR.

Antihypertensive Agents: Because of its potential for inducing hypotension, SEROQUEL XR may enhance the effects of certain antihypertensive agents.

Levodopa and Dopamine Agonists: As it exhibits in vitro dopamine antagonism, SEROQUEL XR may antagonize the effects of levodopa and dopamine agonists.

Lithium: The single dose pharmacokinetics of lithium were not altered when coadministered with SEROQUEL.

Antipyrine: SEROQUEL did not induce the hepatic enzyme systems involved in the metabolism of antipyrine.

Lorazepam: SEROQUEL did not affect the single dose pharmacokinetics of lorazepam.

Divalproex: Coadministration of SEROQUEL (150 mg bid) and divalproex (500 mg bid) increased the mean oral clearance and the mean maximum plasma concentration of total valproic acid (administered as divalproex) by 11%. These changes were not clinically relevant.

The Effect of Other Drugs on SEROQUEL XR: Hepatic Enzyme Inducers: Concomitant use of SEROQUEL XR with hepatic enzyme inducers such as carbamazepine may substantially decrease systemic exposure to quetiapine. In a multiple dose trial in patients to assess the pharmacokinetics of SEROQUEL given before and during treatment with carbamazepine (a known hepatic enzyme inducer), coadministration of carbamazepine significantly increased the clearance of quetiapine. This increase in clearance reduced systemic quetiapine exposure (as measured by AUC) to an average of 13% of the exposure during administration of quetiapine alone; although a greater effect was seen in some patients. As a consequence of this interaction, lower plasma concentrations can occur, and hence, in each patient, consideration for a higher dose of SEROQUEL XR, depending on clinical response, should be considered. It should be noted that the recommended maximum daily dose of SEROQUEL XR is 800 mg/day and continued treatment at higher doses should only be considered as a result of careful consideration of the benefit risk assessment for an individual patient.

Coadministration of SEROQUEL and another microsomal enzyme inducer, phenytoin, caused five-fold increases in the clearance of quetiapine. Increased doses of SEROQUEL XR may be required to maintain control of psychotic symptoms in patients coadministered SEROQUEL XR and phenytoin and other hepatic enzyme inducers (e.g., barbiturates, rifampicin, etc.).

The dose of SEROQUEL XR may need to be reduced if phenytoin or carbamazepine or other hepatic enzyme inducers are withdrawn and replaced with a non-inducer (e.g., sodium valproate).

CYP 3A4 Inhibitors: CYP 3A4 is the primary enzyme responsible for cytochrome P450-mediated metabolism of quetiapine. Thus, coadministration of compounds (such as ketoconazole, erythromycin, clarithromycin, diltiazem, verapamil, or nefazodone), which inhibit CYP 3A4, may increase the concentration of SEROQUEL XR. In a multiple-dose trial in healthy volunteers to assess the pharmacokinetics of SEROQUEL given before and during treatment with ketoconazole, coadministration of ketoconazole resulted in an increase in mean C_{max} and AUC of quetiapine of 235% and 522%, respectively, with a corresponding decrease in mean oral clearance of 84%. The mean half-life of quetiapine increased from 2.6 to 6.8 hours, but the mean t_{max} was unchanged. Due to the potential for an interaction of a similar magnitude in a clinical setting, the dosage of SEROQUEL XR should be reduced during concomitant use of quetiapine and potent CYP3A4 inhibitors (such as azole antifungals, macrolide antibiotics, and protease inhibitors). Special consideration should be given in elderly and debilitated patients. The risk-benefit ratio needs to be considered on an individual basis in all patients.

Divalproex: Coadministration of SEROQUEL (150 mg bid) and divalproex (500 mg bid) increased the mean maximum plasma concentration of quetiapine by 17% without changing the mean oral clearance.

Cimetidine: In a clinical study examining the pharmacokinetics of SEROQUEL following coadministration with cimetidine, (a non-specific P450 enzyme inhibitor), no clinically significant interaction was observed.

Thioridazine: Coadministration of thioridazine (200 mg b.i.d.) with SEROQUEL (300 mg b.i.d.), increased the clearance of SEROQUEL by 65%.

Fluoxetine, Imipramine, Haloperidol, and Risperidone: Fluoxetine (60 mg daily), imipramine (75 mg b.i.d.), haloperidol (7.5 mg b.i.d.), and risperidone (3 mg b.i.d.) did not significantly alter the steady state pharmacokinetics of SEROQUEL.

In Patients Taking the Following Antidepressants: Amitriptyline, bupropion, citalopram, duloxetine, escitalopram, fluoxetine, paroxetine, sertraline and venlafaxine, addition of SEROQUEL XR (150 mg or 300 mg/day; for up to 4 weeks) did not appear to have a consistent overall effect on the trough or pre-dose plasma concentrations of the antidepressant.

Drug-Food Interactions: SEROQUEL XR can be taken with or without food (see Action and Clinical Pharmacology, Pharmacokinetics).

Drug-Herb Interactions: Interactions with herbal products have not been established.

Drug-Laboratory Test Interactions: Interactions with laboratory tests have not been established.

DOSAGE AND ADMINISTRATION:

Recommended Dose and Dosage Adjustment: SEROQUEL XR (quetiapine fumarate extended-release) tablets should be swallowed whole and not split, chewed or crushed.

SEROQUEL XR can be administered with or without food (see Action and Clinical Pharmacology, Pharmacokinetics).

SEROQUEL XR should be administered once daily, generally in the evening.

Schizophrenia: Usual Dose: The titration rate, based on the clinical trials is shown in Table 7.

Table 7: SEROQUEL XR

Titration Rate

	Day 1	Day 2	After Day 2
Once Daily Dosing	300 mg	600 mg	Up to 800 mg

The dose should be adjusted within the effective dose range of 400 mg to 800 mg per day, depending on the clinical response and tolerability of the patient. In a controlled clinical trial, the treatment effect size of 600 mg and 800 mg doses of SEROQUEL XR was greater than that of the 400 mg dose.

In schizophrenia, the safety of doses above 800 mg/day has not been evaluated.

The need for continuing existing EPS medications should be re-evaluated periodically as SEROQUEL XR has not been associated with treatment-emergent EPS across the clinical dose range.

Bipolar Disorder : Bipolar Mania: Usual Dose: The titration rate, based on the clinical trial is shown in Table 8.

Table 8: SEROQUEL XR

Titration Rate

	Day 1	Day 2	After Day 2
Once Daily Dosing	300 mg	600 mg	Up to 800 mg

The dose should be adjusted within the effective dose range of 400 mg to 800 mg per day, depending on the clinical response and tolerability of the patient.

In bipolar mania, the safety of doses above 800 mg/day has not been evaluated.

Bipolar Depression: Usual Dose: The titration rate, based on the clinical trial is shown in Table 9.

Table 9: SEROQUEL XR

Titration Rate

	Day 1	Day 2	Day 3	Day 4 and Thereafter
Once Daily Dosing	50 mg/day	100 mg/day	200 mg/day	300 mg/day

The usual target dose is 300 mg/day. The dose may be further increased depending on the response and tolerability of the patient. The maximum dose is 600 mg/day.

In SEROQUEL clinical trials antidepressant efficacy was demonstrated with SEROQUEL at both 300 mg/day and 600 mg/day, however no additional benefit was seen in the 600 mg group during short-term treatment.

In bipolar depression, the safety of doses of quetiapine above 600 mg/day has not been evaluated.

Major Depressive Disorder : SEROQUEL XR is indicated for the symptomatic relief of major depressive disorder (MDD) when currently available approved antidepressant drugs have failed either due to lack of efficacy and/or lack of tolerability. While there is no evidence that the efficacy of SEROQUEL XR is superior to other antidepressants, it provides a treatment option for patients who have failed on previous antidepressant treatments.

Clinicians must take into account the safety concerns associated with antipsychotic drugs, a class of drugs to which SEROQUEL XR belongs. Safety concerns of this class include: weight gain; hyperlipidemia; hyperglycaemia; Tardive Dyskinesia; and Neuroleptic Malignant Syndrome (see Warnings and Precautions). SEROQUEL XR should only be prescribed in patients with MDD by clinicians who are aware of the importance and are experienced in the early detection and management of the above-mentioned safety issues associated with this class.

Usual Dose: The titration rate, based on the clinical trials is shown in Table 10.

Table 10: SEROQUEL XR

Titration Rate

	Day 1	Day 2	Day 3
Once daily dosing	50 mg	50 mg	150 mg

The usual target dose is 150 mg. Some patients may respond to doses as low as 50 mg/day and where clinically indicated dose may be increased to 300 mg/day after Day 4. In clinical trials, doses between 50-300 mg/day were shown to be efficacious, however, the incidence of certain adverse events increased with dose (see Adverse Reactions).

In MDD, the safety of doses above 300 mg/day has not been evaluated.

Some of the safety concerns associated with SEROQUEL XR and this class of agents (i.e., antipsychotics), may be dose-related (see Warnings and Precautions, Adverse Reactions). The SEROQUEL XR dose should thus be periodically reassessed to achieve and maintain the lowest effective dose. Furthermore, as the long-term safety of SEROQUEL XR in MDD has not been systematically evaluated, the physician who elects to use SEROQUEL XR in the treatment of MDD should use SEROQUEL XR for the shortest time that is clinically indicated. When long-term treatment is believed to be indicated, the physician must periodically re-evaluate the long-term usefulness of the drug for the individual patient keeping in mind the long-term risks.

Switching Patients from SEROQUEL Tablets to SEROQUEL XR Tablets: For more convenient dosing, patients who are currently being treated with divided doses of SEROQUEL (quetiapine, immediate release formulation) may be switched to SEROQUEL XR at the equivalent total daily dose taken once daily. Individual dosage adjustments may be necessary.

Switching Patients From Other Antidepressants: For many antidepressants a gradual taper is recommended prior to complete discontinuation of the drug (physicians should refer to the approved Product Monograph of the specific antidepressant). There are no systematically collected data to address switching patients from other antidepressants to SEROQUEL XR. Generally there should be no need for a wash-out period between stopping an antidepressant and starting SEROQUEL XR. The physician may elect to initiate SEROQUEL XR treatment while tapering the antidepressant, however patients may experience additive side effects during the overlap period.

Switching Patients From Other Antipsychotics: There are no systematically collected data to specifically address switching patients from other antipsychotics to SEROQUEL XR, or concerning concomitant administration with other antipsychotics. While immediate discontinuation of the previous antipsychotic treatment may be acceptable for some patients, more gradual discontinuation may be most appropriate for others. In all cases, the period of overlapping antipsychotic administration should be minimized. When switching patients from depot antipsychotics, if medically appropriate, initiate SEROQUEL XR therapy in place of next scheduled injection. The need for continuing existing EPS medication should be re-evaluated periodically.

The following cross-titration schedule has been used in clinical trials with schizophrenia: See Table 11.

Table 11: SEROQUEL XR

Cross-titration Schedule

	Day 1	Day 2	Day 3
SEROQUEL XR	300 mg	600 mg	Up to 800 mg
% Reduction of ongoing antipsychotic treatment	75%	50%	25%

Dosing Considerations in Special Populations: Elderly: As with other antipsychotics, SEROQUEL XR should be used with caution in the elderly, especially during the initial dosing period. The rate of dose titration of SEROQUEL XR may need to be slower, and the daily therapeutic target dose lower, than that used in younger patients. In clinical trials, 68 patients, 65 years of age or over, were treated with SEROQUEL XR (see Warnings and Precautions, Special Populations). Given the limited experience with SEROQUEL XR in the elderly, and the higher incidence of concomitant illness and concomitant medication in this population, SEROQUEL XR should be used with caution. The mean plasma clearance of SEROQUEL was reduced by 30% to 50% in elderly subjects when compared to younger patients. Elderly patients should be started on the lowest available dose (i.e., 50 mg/day) of SEROQUEL XR. The dose can be increased in increments of 50 mg/day to an effective dose, depending on the clinical response and tolerance of the individual patient.

In elderly patients with MDD, initial dosing should begin at 50 mg on Days 1-3, the dose can be increased to 100 mg on Day 4, and 150 mg on Day 8.

Hepatic Impairment: Quetiapine is extensively metabolized by the liver (see Action and Clinical Pharmacology, Special Populations and Conditions). Therefore, SEROQUEL XR should be used with caution in patients with mild hepatic impairment, especially during the initial dosing period. Patients with mild hepatic impairment should be started on the lowest available dose (i.e., 50 mg/day) of SEROQUEL XR. The dose should be increased daily in increments of 50 mg/day to an effective dose, depending on the clinical response and tolerance in the individual patient. No pharmacokinetic data are available for quetiapine in patients with moderate to severe hepatic impairment. However, should clinical judgement deem treatment with SEROQUEL XR necessary, the drug should be used with great caution in patients with moderate or severe hepatic impairment (see Warnings and Precautions, Hepatic/Biliary/Pancreatic and Action and Clinical Pharmacology, Special Populations and Conditions).

Renal Impairment: As clinical experience is lacking, caution is advised (see Warnings and Precautions, Renal).

Missed Dose: SEROQUEL XR should be taken at the same time each day. If a previous day's dose has been missed, administration should be resumed the next day at the normal administration time.

OVERDOSAGE:

Experience: Clinical Trials: One death has been reported in a clinical trial following an overdose of 13 600 mg of quetiapine alone, however, survival has also been reported in acute overdoses of up to 30 000 mg of quetiapine. Most patients who overdosed reported no adverse events or recovered fully from the reported events.

Post-Marketing: In post-marketing experience, there have been cases of coma and death in patients taking a SEROQUEL (quetiapine, immediate-release formulation) overdose. The lowest reported dose associated with coma has been in a patient who took 5000 mg and had a full recovery within 3 days. The lowest reported dose associated with a death was in a patient who took 6000 mg.

In post-marketing experience, there were cases reported of QT prolongation with overdose.

Patients with pre-existing severe cardiovascular disease may be at an increased risk of the effects of overdose (see Warnings and Precautions, Cardiovascular, Hypotension and Syncope).

Symptoms: In general, reported signs and symptoms were those resulting from an exaggeration of the drug's known pharmacological effects e.g., drowsiness and sedation, tachycardia and hypotension.

Treatment: There is no specific antidote to quetiapine. In cases of severe intoxication, the possibility of multiple drug involvement should be considered, and intensive care procedures are recommended, including establishing and maintaining a patent airway, ensuring adequate oxygenation and ventilation, and monitoring and support of the cardiovascular system.

Close medical supervision and monitoring should be continued until the patient recovers.

> For management of a suspected drug overdose, contact your regional Poison Control Centre. See the *CPS* Directory section for a list of Poison Control Centres.

ACTION AND CLINICAL PHARMACOLOGY: Mechanism of Action and Pharmacodynamics: SEROQUEL XR (quetiapine fumarate extended-release), a dibenzothiazepine derivative, is a psychotropic agent. Quetiapine and the active plasma metabolite, norquetiapine interact with a broad range of neurotransmitter receptors. It is the direct and indirect effects of quetiapine and norquetiapine that contribute to the pharmacological activity of SEROQUEL XR.

Quetiapine: Quetiapine exhibits affinity for brain serotonin $5HT_2$ and $5HT_{1A}$ receptors (in vitro, Ki=288 and 557 nM, respectively), and dopamine D_1 and D_2 receptors (in vitro, Ki=558 and 531 nM, respectively). It is this combination of receptor antagonism with a higher selectivity for $5HT_2$ relative to D_2 receptors, which is believed to contribute to the clinical psychotropic properties and low extrapyramidal symptoms (EPS) liability of quetiapine compared to typical antipsychotics. Quetiapine also has high affinity for histamine H_1 receptors (in vitro, Ki=10 nM) and adrenergic α_1 receptors (in vitro, Ki=13 nM), with a lower affinity for adrenergic α_2 receptors (in vitro, Ki=782 nM), but no appreciable affinity at cholinergic muscarinic and benzodiazepine receptors.

Norquetiapine: Norquetiapine, similar to quetiapine, exhibits affinity for brain serotonin $5HT_2$ and dopamine D_1 and D_2 receptors. Norquetiapine also has high affinity at histaminergic and adrenergic α1 receptors, with a lower affinity at adrenergic α2 and serotonin $5HT_{1A}$ receptors. Additionally norquetiapine has high affinity for the norepinephrine transporter (NET).

Quetiapine differs from norquetiapine in having no appreciable affinity for muscarinic M_1 receptors whereas norquetiapine has high affinity.

Pharmacokinetics: The pharmacokinetics of quetiapine and norquetiapine are linear within the clinical dose range. The kinetics of quetiapine are similar in men and women, and smokers and non-smokers.

Absorption: Quetiapine is well absorbed following oral administration. SEROQUEL XR achieves peak plasma concentrations at approximately 6 hours after administration (T_{max}). SEROQUEL XR displays dose-proportional pharmacokinetics for doses of up to 800 mg administered once daily. The maximum plasma concentration (C_{max}) and the area under the plasma concentration-time curve (AUC) for SEROQUEL XR administered once daily are comparable to those achieved for the same total daily dose of SEROQUEL (quetiapine, immediate-release formulation) administered twice daily. The mean plasma concentrations for each dose of SEROQUEL XR versus 300 mg of SEROQUEL over a 24-hour dosing interval under fasting conditions are shown in Figure 1. Steady-state peak molar concentrations of the active metabolite norquetiapine are 35% of that observed for quetiapine.

Figure 1: SEROQUEL XR

Mean Quetiapine Plasma Concentrations (ng/mL) for Each Dose of Quetiapine Under Fasted Conditions Versus Time

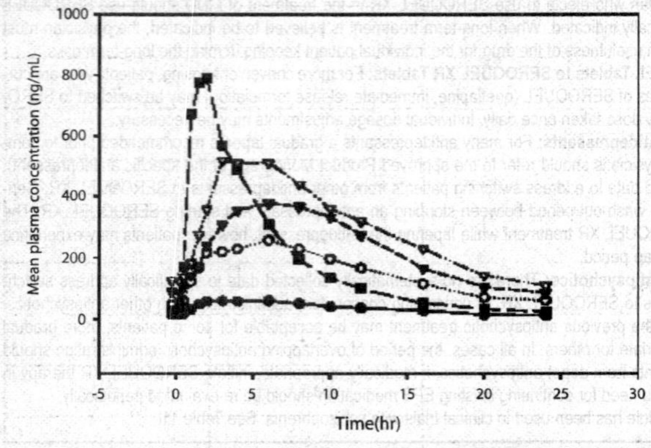

In a study (n=10) examining the effects of food on the bioavailability of quetiapine, a high-fat meal was found to produce statistically significant increases in the SEROQUEL XR C_{max} and AUC of 44% to 52% and 20% to 22%, respectively, for the 50-mg and 300-mg tablets. In comparison, a light meal had no significant effect on the C_{max} or AUC of quetiapine. This increase in exposure is not clinically significant, and therefore SEROQUEL XR can be taken with or without food.

Distribution: Quetiapine has a mean apparent volume of distribution of 10±4 L/kg, and is approximately 83% bound to plasma proteins.

Excretion and Metabolism: The elimination half-life of quetiapine is approximately 6-7 hours upon multiple dosing within the proposed clinical dosage range. Quetiapine is extensively metabolized by the liver, with the parent compound accounting for less than 5% of the dose in the urine and faeces, one week following the administration of radiolabelled quetiapine. Since quetiapine is extensively metabolized by the liver, higher plasma levels are expected in the hepatically impaired population, and dosage adjustment may be needed in these patients. The elimination half-life of norquetiapine is approximately 12 hours. The average molar dose fraction of free quetiapine and the active human plasma metabolite norquetiapine is <5% excreted in the urine.

Major routes of metabolism of quetiapine involve oxidation of the alkyl side chain, hydroxylation of the dibenzothiazepine ring, sulphoxidation, and phase 2 conjugation. The principal human plasma metabolites are the sulfoxide, and the parent acid metabolite, neither of which are pharmacologically active.

In vitro investigations established that CYP 3A4 is the primary enzyme responsible for cytochrome P450-mediated metabolism of quetiapine. Norquetiapine is primarily formed and eliminated via CYP3A4.

Quetiapine and several of its metabolites (including norquetiapine) were found to be weak inhibitors of human cytochrome P450 1A2, 2C9, 2C19, 2D6 and 3A4 activities in vitro. In vitro CYP inhibition is observed only at concentrations approximately 5 to 50-fold higher than those observed at a dose range of 300 to 800 mg/day in humans.

Special Populations and Conditions: Geriatrics (≥65 years of age): The mean clearance of quetiapine in the elderly is approximately 30 to 50% of that seen in adults aged 18-65 years (see Warnings and Precautions, Special Populations and Dosage and Administration).

Hepatic Insufficiency: In 8 cirrhotic subjects with mild hepatic impairment, administration of a single 25 mg (sub-clinical) oral dose of SEROQUEL resulted in a 40% increase in both AUC and C_{max}. Clearance of the drug decreased by 25% whereas $t_{1/2}$ was elevated by nearly 45%. Therefore, SEROQUEL XR should be used with caution in patients with mild hepatic impairment, especially during the initial dosing period. No pharmacokinetic data are available for quetiapine in patients with moderate or severe hepatic impairment (see Warnings and Precautions, Hepatic/Biliary/Pancreatic and Dosage and Administration).

Renal Insufficiency: At single low (sub-clinical) doses, the mean plasma clearance of quetiapine was reduced by approximately 25% in subjects with severe renal impairment (creatinine clearance less than 30 mL/min/1.73 m^2). However, the individual clearance values remained within the range observed for healthy subjects (see Warnings and Precautions, Renal and Dosage and Administration).

STORAGE AND STABILITY: SEROQUEL XR (quetiapine fumarate extended-release) should be stored between 15-30°C.

INFORMATION FOR THE PATIENT: Published in e-CPS, available by subscription at www.e-cps.ca.

DOSAGE FORMS, COMPOSITION AND PACKAGING: 50 mg: Each peach coloured, capsule-shaped, biconvex, film-coated, extended-release tablet, intagliated with "XR 50" on one side and plain on the other, contains: quetiapine fumarate equivalent to quetiapine free base 50 mg. Nonmedicinal ingredients: tablet core: hydroxypropyl methylcellulose, lactose monohydrate, magnesium stearate, microcrystalline cellulose and sodium citrate; coating: hydroxypropyl methylcellulose, polyethylene glycol 400, red ferric oxide, titanium dioxide and yellow ferric oxide. High-density polyethylene (HDPE) bottles of 60.

150 mg: Each white, capsule-shaped, biconvex, film-coated, extended-release tablet, intagliated with 'XR 150' on one side and plain on the other, contains: quetiapine fumarate equivalent to quetiapine free base 150 mg. Nonmedicinal ingredients: tablet core: hydroxypropyl methylcellulose, lactose monohydrate, magnesium stearate, microcrystalline cellulose and sodium citrate; coating: hydroxypropyl methylcellulose, polyethylene glycol 400 and titanium dioxide. HDPE bottles of 60.

200 mg: Each yellow, capsule-shaped, biconvex, film-coated, extended-release tablet, intagliated with "XR 200" on one side and plain on the other, contains: quetiapine fumarate equivalent to quetiapine free base 200 mg. Nonmedicinal ingredients: tablet core: hydroxypropyl methylcellulose, lactose monohydrate, magnesium stearate, microcrystalline cellulose and sodium citrate; coating: hydroxypropyl methylcellulose, polyethylene glycol 400, titanium dioxide and yellow ferric oxide. HDPE bottles of 60.

300 mg : Each pale yellow, capsule-shaped, biconvex, film-coated, extended-release tablet, intagliated with "XR 300" on one side and plain on the other, contains: quetiapine fumarate equivalent to quetiapine free base 300 mg. Nonmedicinal ingredients: tablet core: hydroxypropyl methylcellulose, lactose monohydrate, magnesium stearate, microcrystalline cellulose and sodium citrate; coating: hydroxypropyl methylcellulose, polyethylene glycol 400, titanium dioxide and yellow ferric oxide. HDPE bottles of 60.

400 mg : Each white, capsule-shaped, biconvex, film-coated, extended-release tablet, intagliated with "XR 400" on one side and plain on the other, contains: quetiapine fumarate equivalent to quetiapine free base 400 mg. Nonmedicinal ingredients: tablet core: hydroxypropyl methylcellulose, lactose monohydrate, magnesium stearate, microcrystalline cellulose and sodium citrate; coating: hydroxypropyl methylcellulose, polyethylene glycol 400 and titanium dioxide. HDPE bottles of 60.

(Shown in Product Identification Section)

Serostim® Ⓟ

somatropin

Human Growth Hormone

EMD Canada

Date of Revision: December 2007

SUMMARY PRODUCT INFORMATION:

Route of Administration	Dosage Form/ Strength	Clinically Relevant Nonmedicinal Ingredients
Subcutaneous injection	Lyophilized powder for reconstitution/ 5 mg/vial, 6 mg/vial	For a complete listing, see Dosage Forms, Composition and Packaging.

DESCRIPTION: SEROSTIM (somatropin for injection) is available in 5 mg/vial and 6 mg/vial.

Somatropin is a polypeptide hormone consisting of 191 amino acid residues and its structure is identical to that of growth hormone extracted from human pituitary glands. It is produced by recombinant (rDNA) technology in a mammalian cell expression system.

SEROSTIM is an anabolic and anti-catabolic agent which exerts its influence by interacting with specific receptors on a variety of cell types including myocytes, hepatocytes, adipocytes, lymphocytes and hematopoietic cells. Some, but not all of its effects are mediated by another class of hormones known as somatomedins (IGF-I and IGF-II).

INDICATIONS AND CLINICAL USE: SEROSTIM (somatropin for injection) is indicated for the treatment of HIV wasting associated with catabolism, weight loss or cachexia.

Geriatrics: The dosage and administration schedule in the elderly should be the same as for adults (see also Warnings and Precautions).

Pediatrics: There is limited experience with SEROSTIM in patients under 18 years of age. SEROSTIM should not be used in the pediatric age group until further data becomes available.

CONTRAINDICATIONS: SEROSTIM (somatropin for injection) is contraindicated and should not be administered in the following cases:

- In patients with acute critical illness due to complications following open heart or abdominal surgery, multiple accidental trauma or patients having acute respiratory failure.
- In the presence of any progression of underlying intracranial tumour. Intracranial tumour should be inactive prior to instituting therapy and SEROSTIM should be discontinued if there is evidence of recurrent activity. Patients should be examined frequently for progression or recurrence of the underlying disease process.
- In patients who are hypersensitive to or have a history of previous allergic reaction to somatropin or to any of the excipients.
- In patients with active neoplasia (either newly diagnosed or recurrent). Any anti-tumour therapy should be completed prior to starting therapy with SEROSTIM.
- In patients with diabetes mellitus.
- In patients with proliferative or preproliferative diabetic retinopathy.

WARNINGS AND PRECAUTIONS: General: SEROSTIM (somatropin for injection) therapy should be carried out under the regular guidance of a physician who is experienced in the diagnosis and management of AIDS. Inadequate nutritional intake and hypogonadism, which are common in individuals with AIDS and which may contribute to catabolism and weight loss, should be corrected prior to initiation of SEROSTIM therapy.

Information to Be Provided to the Patient: Patients being treated with SEROSTIM should be informed of the potential benefits and risks associated with treatment. Patients should be instructed to contact their physician should they experience any side effects or discomfort during treatment with SEROSTIM.

It is recommended that SEROSTIM 5 mg/vial and 6 mg/vial be administered using sterile, disposable syringes and needles. Patients should be thoroughly instructed in the importance of proper disposal and cautioned against any reuse of needles and syringes. An appropriate container for the disposal of used needles and syringes should be used.

When SEROSTIM is administered subcutaneously at the same site over a long period, local tissue atrophy may result. This can be avoided by rotating the injection site daily.

Carcinogenesis and Mutagenesis: Carcinogenicity studies have not been conducted. There is no evidence from animal studies to date of SEROSTIM-induced mutagenicity.

Kaposi's sarcoma, lymphoma, cervical cancer in women and other malignancies are common in AIDS patients. In clinical studies, the risk of developing new Kaposi sarcoma lesions and lymphomas were not found to be increased. The effect of SEROSTIM on the incidence of cervical cancer has not been assessed in clinical trials since the majority of patients included were male. The potential effects of growth hormone on other malignancies are unknown. Evidence is available suggesting the possibility that growth hormone might increase the risk of development of cancers other than lymphoma, in particular colorectal cancer. Although this evidence is not conclusive, the advisability of a regular screening program for colorectal cancer should be discussed with patients having known risk factors for this malignancy.

Cardiovascular: No cases of intracranial hypertension (IH) have been observed among patients with AIDS wasting treated with SEROSTIM. The syndrome of IH, with papilledema, visual changes, headache, nausea and/or vomiting has been reported in a small number of children with growth failure treated with growth hormone products. Nevertheless, funduscopic evaluation of patients is recommended at the initiation and periodically during the course of SEROSTIM therapy.

Endocrine and Metabolism: Hyperglycemia may occur in HIV-infected individuals due to a variety of reasons. SEROSTIM use was associated with a minimal increase of mean blood glucose concentration. Patients with other risk factors for glucose intolerance should be monitored closely during SEROSTIM therapy.

Growth hormone can affect the metabolism of thyroid hormones by increasing the extrathyroidal conversion of T4 to T3. Thyroid function should be evaluated before starting SEROSTIM therapy and regularly assessed during treatment.

Immune: As for any recombinant product, SEROSTIM is potentially immunogenic. Consequently, if any serious hypersensitivity or allergic reaction occurs, SEROSTIM should be discontinued immediately and appropriate therapy initiated. None of the study participants with AIDS wasting who were treated with SEROSTIM for the first time developed detectable antibodies to SEROSTIM.

Musculoskeletal: Increased tissue turgor (non-edematous swelling, particularly in the hands and feet) and musculoskeletal discomfort (pain, swelling and/or stiffness) may occur during treatment with SEROSTIM, but may resolve spontaneously, with analgesic therapy, or after reducing the frequency of dosing (see Dosage and Administration).

Carpal tunnel syndrome may occur during treatment with SEROSTIM. If the symptoms of carpal tunnel syndrome do not resolve by decreasing the weekly number of doses of SEROSTIM, it is recommended that treatment be discontinued.

Sexual Function/Reproduction: Reproduction studies have been performed in rats and rabbits. Doses up to 5 to 10 times the human dose, based on body surface area, have revealed no evidence of impaired fertility or harm to the fetus due to SEROSTIM.

Special Populations: Pregnant Women: Reproduction studies have been performed in rats and rabbits. Doses up to 5 to 10 times the human dose, based on body surface area, have revealed no evidence of impaired fertility or harm to the fetus due to SEROSTIM. There are, however, no adequate and well-controlled studies in pregnant women. Because animal reproduction studies are not always predictive of human response, this drug should be used during pregnancy only if clearly needed.

Nursing Women: It is not known whether this drug is excreted in human milk. However, a study done on lactating rats showed that the concentration in milk 24 h after administration were 30 times higher than blood concentration at the same time point. Because many drugs are excreted in human milk, caution should be exercised when somatropin is administered to a nursing mother. SEROSTIM is not recommended for use during lactation.

Pediatrics: There is limited experience with SEROSTIM in patients under 18 years of age. SEROSTIM should not be used in the pediatric group until further data becomes available.

Geriatrics: Clinical studies with SEROSTIM did not include sufficient numbers of subjects aged 65 and over to determine whether they respond differently from younger subjects. Elderly patients may be more sensitive to growth hormone action, and may be more prone to develop adverse reactions. Thus, dose selection for an elderly patient should be cautious, usually starting at the low end of the dosing range.

Monitoring and Laboratory Tests: SEROSTIM therapy should be carried out under the regular guidance of a physician who is experienced in the diagnosis and management of AIDS. Monitoring is advisable when SEROSTIM is administered in combination with drugs known to be metabolised by cytochrome 3A4 hepatic enzymes, such as some anti-retroviral drugs.

Thyroid function should be evaluated before starting SEROSTIM therapy and regularly assessed during treatment.

Patients on SEROSTIM therapy should be monitored for the emergence of any new malignancy and the treatment discontinued if a new tumour or signs of relapse are detected.

Glucose levels should be determined before starting SEROSTIM therapy and closely monitored during therapy.

Occupational Hazards: SEROSTIM is not expected to interfere with the patient's ability to drive or use machinery. No formal studies on the effects on the ability to drive and use machinery have been performed.

ADVERSE REACTIONS: Adverse Drug Reaction Overview: The most commonly reported adverse events reported in clinical studies conducted with SEROSTIM (somatropin for injection) were: musculoskeletal discomfort, fever, increased tissue turgor, diarrhoea, neuropathy, nausea, headache, abdominal pain, fatigue, leucopenia and albuminuria. Among these, increased tissue turgor, nausea and musculoskeletal discomfort were more frequent in the SEROSTIM group as compared to the placebo group (statistically significant, $p \leq 0.05$).

The most frequently reported adverse reactions resulting in clinical intervention (e.g., discontinuation of SEROSTIM, adjustment in dosage, or the need for concomitant medication to treat an adverse reaction symptom) were increased tissue turgor and musculoskeletal discomfort.

Clinical Trial Adverse Drug Reactions: Because clinical trials are conducted under widely varying conditions, adverse reaction rates observed in the clinical trials of a drug cannot be directly compared with rates in the clinical trials of another drug and may not reflect the rates observed in practice. The adverse reaction information from clinical trials does, however, provide a basis for identifying the adverse events that appear to be related to drug use and for approximating rates.

In two placebo-controlled clinical trials in which 205 patients were treated with SEROSTIM the most common adverse reactions felt to be associated with SEROSTIM were musculoskeletal discomfort and increased tissue turgor (non-edematous swelling, particularly of the hands or feet) (see Warnings and Precautions). These symptoms were generally rated by investigators as mild to moderate in severity and usually subsided with continued treatment. Discontinuations as a result of these events were rare.

Because of the diverse clinical manifestations of AIDS, and the frequent occurrence of adverse events associated with underlying disease process, it was often difficult to distinguish adverse events possibly associated with the administration of SEROSTIM from underlying signs or symptoms of AIDS or associated intercurrent illnesses.

In two small studies, 11 children with HIV-associated failure to thrive were treated subcutaneously with human growth hormone. In one study, five children (age range, 6 to 17 years) were treated with 0.04 mg/kg/day for 26 weeks. In a second study, six children (age range, 8 to 14 years) were treated with 0.07 mg/kg/day for 4 weeks. Treatment appeared to be well tolerated in both studies. These preliminary data collected on a limited number of patients with HIV-associated failure to thrive appear to be consistent with safety observations in growth hormone treated adults with HIV wasting.

Common Clinical Trial Adverse Events: Clinical adverse events which occurred during the first 12 weeks of study in at least 1% of those who received SEROSTIM during the two placebo-controlled trials are listed in Table 1 by treatment group.

Table 1: SEROSTIM

Clinical Adverse Events in at Least 1% of Patients

Body System/Preferred Term	SEROSTIM (n=205) %	Placebo (n=150) %
Body as a Whole, General		
Fever	31.2	29.3
Increased Tissue Turgor[a]	27.3	2.7
Fatigue	17.1	16.0
Rigors	9.3	6.7
Influenza-like Symptoms	5.4	8.0
Malaise	4.9	3.3
Asthenia	3.9	4.0
Carpal Tunnel Syndrome	2.9	0.0
Tolerance Increased	2.9	0.0
Death	2.4	2.0
Chest Pain	2.4	0.7
Pain	1.0	2.7
Hot Flashes	1.0	0.7
Allergic Reaction	1.0	0.0
Gastrointestinal System		
Diarrhoea	25.9	20.0
Nausea[a]	25.9	16.0
Abdominal Pain	17.1	18.7
Vomiting	11.7	12.0
Flatulence	5.9	2.7
Leukoplakia Oral	5.4	4.0
Mouth Dry	4.4	1.3
Constipation	2.9	2.7
Dyspepsia	2.4	4.7
Dysphagia	2.0	1.3
Oesophagitis	2.0	0.7
Pancreatitis	1.5	0.7
Stomatitis Ulcerative	1.0	3.3
Colitis	1.0	1.3
Rectal Disorder	1.0	1.3
Gastritis	1.0	0.7
Tongue Ulceration	1.0	0.7
Gingivitis	1.0	0.0
Tongue Disorder	1.0	0.0
Musculoskeletal System		
Musculoskeletal Discomfort[a]	53.7	33.3
Muscle Weakness	2.4	0.7
Central and Peripheral Nervous Systems		
Neuropathy	25.9	17.3
Headache	19.0	20.7
Dizziness	3.4	4.7
Convulsions	1.5	1.3
Encephalopathy	1.5	0.0
Tremor	1.0	1.3
Nystagmus	1.0	0.7
Meningism	1.0	0.0
Respiratory System		
Dyspnoea	9.8	6.0
Coughing	9.3	13.3
Sinusitis	8.8	10.0
Upper Resp Tract Infection	7.8	6.0
Pharyngitis	5.9	4.7
Rhinitis	3.9	6.0
Pneumonia	3.9	2.7
Bronchitis	2.4	4.0
Sputum Increased	2.4	0.0
Respiratory Disorder	2.0	0.7

(cont'd)

Table 1: SEROSTIM *(cont'd)*

Clinical Adverse Events in at Least 1% of Patients

Body System/Preferred Term	SEROSTIM (n=205) %	Placebo (n=150) %
Bronchospasm	1.5	2.0
Pneumonitis	1.5	0.7
Pleurisy	1.5	0.0
White Cell and Reticuloendothelial System Disorders		
Lymphadenopathy	14.1	16.0
Lymphadenopathy Cervical	2.0	3.3
Eosinophilia	1.0	2.7
Skin and Appendages		
Sweating Increased	14.1	8.7
Rash[a]	5.9	13.3
Skin Disorder	5.9	6.0
Folliculitis	4.9	2.7
Alopecia	2.0	0.7
Photosensitivity Reaction	2.0	0.7
Pigmentation Abnormal	1.5	1.3
Seborrhoea	1.5	0.7
Dermatitis	1.0	1.3
Skin Ulceration	1.0	1.3
Acne	1.0	0.0
Skin Discolouration	1.0	0.0
Verruca	1.0	0.0
Psychiatric		
Anorexia	12.2	9.3
Insomnia	11.2	9.3
Depression	8.8	6.0
Anxiety	5.4	6.0
Somnolence	2.4	0.7
Nervousness	2.0	0.7
Appetite Increased	1,5	2.0
Amnesia	1,0	0.7
Thinking Abnormal	1.0	0.0
Metabolic and Nutritional		
Hyperglycaemia	10.2	6.0
Hypertriglyceridaemia	9.3	7.3
Dehydration	3.4	4.0
Cachexia	1.5	2.7
Hypokalaemia	1.5	0.7
Glycosuria	1.0	2.0
Thirst	1.0	0.7
Acidosis	1.0	0.0
Resistance Mechanism Disorders		
Moniliasis	9.3	8.0

(cont'd)

Table 1: SEROSTIM *(cont'd)*

Clinical Adverse Events in at Least 1% of Patients

Body System/Preferred Term	SEROSTIM (n=205) %	Placebo (n=150) %
Infection Bacterial	6.8	2.0
P. Carinii Infection	4.4	5.3
Infection Viral	4.4	1.3
Infection	2.9	2.0
Herpes Simplex	2.4	5.3
Sepsis	1.5	2.0
Abscess	1.5	1.3
Infection Fungal	1.5	0.7
Herpes Zoster	1.0	0.7
Urinary System		
Albuminuria	15.1	9.3
Haematuria	6.8	4.7
Urinary Tract Infection	1.0	0.7
Nocturia	1.0	0.0
Liver and Biliary System		
Hepatic Function Abnormal	2.0	0.7
Hepatomegaly	1.5	2.7
Hepatitis	1.0	0.0
Red Blood Cell		
Anaemia	12.2	8.7
Heart Rate and Rhythm		
Tachycardia	11.2	6.0
Vision		
Retinitis	3.4	2.7
Vision Abnormal	2.9	3.3
Photophobia	1.0	0.0
Platelet, Bleeding and Clotting		
Thrombocytopenia	5.9	6.0
Purpura	1.0	4.7
Cardiovascular, General		
ECG Abnormal	1.5	2.7
Heart Murmur	1.5	1.3
Hypertension	1.5	0.7
Hypotension	1.0	1.3
Application Site		
Injection Site Pain	2.9	1.3
Injection Site Reaction	2.0	2.7
Neoplasms		
Sarcoma	3.4	2.7
Reproductive, Male		
Epididymitis	1.0	0.7
Penis Disorder	1.0	0.7

(cont'd)

Table 1: SEROSTIM *(cont'd)*

Clinical Adverse Events in at Least 1% of Patients

Body System/Preferred Term	SEROSTIM (n=205) %	Placebo (n=150) %
Hernia Inguinal	1.0	0.0
Hearing and Vestibular		
Ear Disorder	2.0	2.0
Earache	2.0	1.3
Hearing Decreased	1.0	0.0
Endocrine		
Gynaecomastia	2.4	0.7
Breast Pain Male	1.5	0.0

[a] Statistically significant difference, p<0.05.

Table 1 displays all adverse events reported in clinical studies, regardless of causality assessment and severity. Among the adverse events, several can be considered as adverse reactions to SEROSTIM, either by analyzing the difference in frequency as compared to placebo, or by evaluating their plausibility in relationship to the known mechanism of action of SEROSTIM. Carpal tunnel syndrome, peripheral neuropathies and hyperglycaemia were more frequent than in the placebo group and are known effects of somatropin (see Warnings and Precautions).

Less Common Clinical Trial Adverse Drug Reactions: Adverse events which occurred in less than 1% of study participants receiving SEROSTIM in the two placebo-controlled clinical efficacy studies are listed below by body system (see Table 2). The list of adverse events has been compiled regardless of causal relationship to SEROSTIM.

Table 2: SEROSTIM

Adverse Events Which Occurred in Less Than 1% of Patients

Body as a Whole, General	Syncope, chest pain substernal, hypovolaemia
Gastrointestinal System	Abdomen enlarged, eructation, haemorrhoids, melaena, oesophageal ulceration, duodenitis, enanthema, gastric ulcer, gastrointestinal disorder, haemorrhage rectum, haemorrhoids thrombosed, hiccup, intestinal obstruction, peptic ulcer, periodontal destruction, stomatitis aphthous, tooth disorder
Musculoskeletal System	Bursitis
Central and Peripheral Nervous Systems	Cerebral atrophy, migraine, gait abnormal, neuritis cranial, sensory disturbance, dysphonia, hyperkinesias, hyperreflexia, vertigo
Respiratory System	Chest x-ray abnormal, hypoxia, pneumothorax, respiratory insufficiency
White Cell and Reticuloendothelial System Disorders	Leukocytosis
Skin and Appendages	Skin dry, eczema, rash maculo-papular, hypertrichosis, psoriasis
Psychiatric	Agitation, confusion, concentration impaired, libido decreased, libido increased, neurosis
Metabolic and Nutritional	Hypoglycaemia, hyperkalaemia, hypophosphataemia, serum iron decreased, diabetes mellitus, hyperglobulinaemia, hypocalcaemia, hyponatraemia, oedema pharynx, serum iron increased
Resistance Mechanism Disorders	Toxoplasmosis
Urinary System	Dysuria, nephropathy toxic, renal calculus, urine abnormal, polyuria, renal cyst
Liver and Biliary System	Cholecystitis, hepatitis cholestatic, hepatosplenomegaly, jaundice
Red Blood Cell	Splenomegaly
Heart Rate and Rhythm	Bradycardia, qt prolonged, palpitation
Vision	Conjunctivitis, conjunctival discolouration, glaucoma, miosis, retinal oedema
Platelet, Bleeding and Clotting	Prothrombin increased
Cardiovascular, General	Hypotension postural, cardiomegaly, cyanosis
Application Site	Otitis externa
Neoplasms	Lymphoma malignant
Reproductive, Male	Prostatic disorder, genital eruption male, orchitis
Hearing and Vestibular	Tinnitus
Endocrine	Adrenal hypercorticism, hypothyroidism
Vascular (extracardiac)	Peripheral ischaemia, atherosclerosis, flushing, purpura, telangiectasis

The types and incidences of adverse events reported in an open-label, extension trial and in a single, foreign trial, for up to one year, were not different from, or greater in frequency, than those observed in the primary, placebo-controlled, clinical trials.

Abnormal Hematologic and Clinical Chemistry Findings: See Table 3.

Table 3: SEROSTIM

Abnormal Hematologic and Clinical Chemistry Findings

Adverse Event	SEROSTIM (n=205) %	Placebo (n=150) %
Leukopenia[a]	15.1	24.7
Albuminuria	15.1	9.3
Granulocytopenia	14.1	21.3
Lymphadenopathy	14.1	16.0
Anemia	12.2	8.7
AST increased	11.7	6.0
Tachycardia	11.2	6.0
Hyperglycemia	10.2	6.0
ALT increased	10.2	5.3
Phosphatase alkaline increased	7.3	4.7
Creatinine phosphokinase increased	2.0	0.7
LDH increased	2.0	0.7
Amylase increased	1.5	2.0

[a] Statistically significant difference, p<0.05.

Post-Market Adverse Drug Reactions: During post-marketing surveillance, the following adverse reactions have been reported. The indicated frequency is an estimate based on reporting rates.

Reactions Reported at Frequency >1% : Body as a Whole, General Disorders: oedema (mainly peripheral), carpal tunnel syndrome.

Musculoskeletal Disorders: arthralgia, myalgia.

Central and Peripheral Nervous Systems Disorders: paresthesia, hypoesthesia.

Metabolism Disorders: increase in blood glucose levels.

Reactions Reported at Frequency <1%: Central and Peripheral Nervous Systems Disorders: Idiopathic intracranial hypertension has been reported with somatropin in children.

Diabetes: During post-marketing surveillance, cases of new onset glucose intolerance, diabetes mellitus and exacerbation of pre-existing diabetes mellitus have been reported in patients receiving SEROSTIM. Some patients developed diabetic ketoacidosis. In some patients, these conditions improved when SEROSTIM was discontinued while in others the glucose intolerance persisted.

Neoplasms: Some cases of malignancies (mainly lymphoma) have been reported in post-marketing surveillance (see Warnings and Precautions).

DRUG INTERACTIONS: During clinical trials in which all patients received concomitant anti-retroviral therapy there were no detectable increases in plasma viral load following SEROSTIM (somatropin for injection) therapy, as measured by quantitative HIV-RNA analysis. Patients with AIDS wasting considered for treatment with SEROSTIM should also receive concomitant approved anti-retroviral therapy.

No formal interaction studies have been performed in patients treated with SEROSTIM. Published in vitro data indicate that growth hormone treatment may increase cytochrome P450 3A4 mediated antipyrine clearance in man.

Interactions with food, herbal products and laboratory tests have not been established.

DOSAGE AND ADMINISTRATION:

Dosing Considerations: Before initiating a patient on SEROSTIM (somatropin for injection) therapy, please review completely the Contraindications and Warnings and Precautions.

SEROSTIM treatment should be carried out under regular guidance of a physician experienced in the diagnosis and management of HIV and wasting.

SEROSTIM dosage should be individualized for each patient according to body weight.

Recommended Dose and Dosage Adjustment: SEROSTIM should be administered subcutaneously daily at bedtime according to the following dosage recommendations:

Weight Range	Dose[a]
>55 kg	6 mg sc daily
45–55 kg	5 mg sc daily
35–45 kg	4 mg sc daily

[a] Based on an approximate daily dosage of 0.1 mg/kg.

In patients who weigh less than 35 kg, SEROSTIM should be administered at a dose of 0.1 mg/kg subcutaneously daily at bedtime.

Missed Dose: For patients who miss a dose, it is not recommended to double the next dose. The patients should be reminded to contact the physician monitoring their treatment.

Administration: Administer subcutaneously daily at bedtime. Dose reductions for side effects felt to be related to treatment with SEROSTIM, which are unresponsive to symptomatic treatment, may be effected by reducing the number of doses given per week. In controlled trials, dose reductions were accomplished by reducing the frequency of dosing to five or three times a week.

Injection sites should be rotated.

SEROSTIM 5 mg/vial and 6 mg/vial: SEROSTIM once reconstituted should be administered using sterile, disposable syringes and needles. The syringe used should be of appropriately small volume to ensure accurate dose withdrawal. The calculated dose should be withdrawn for subcutaneous administration.

Reconstitution: See Information for the Patient/Proper use of this Medication for reconstitution instructions.

SEROSTIM 5 mg/vial and 6 mg/vial: Once the appropriate dose for a patient has been determined, reconstitute each vial of SEROSTIM with the diluent supplied.

Once SEROSTIM 5 mg/vial or 6 mg/vial is reconstituted with the diluent supplied (Sterile Water for Injection, USP), the reconstituted solution should be used immediately (within 3 hours). Although not recommended, it may be stored for up to 24 hours at 2-8°C. As there is no preservative in this reconstituted solution, any unused solution should be discarded once the dose is given.

OVERDOSAGE:

Glucose intolerance can occur with overdosage. Long-term overdosage with growth hormone could results in signs and symptoms of acromegaly.

For management of a suspected drug overdose, CPhA recommends that you contact your **regional Poison Control Centre**. See the *CPS* Directory section for a list of Poison Control Centres.

ACTION AND CLINICAL PHARMACOLOGY: Mechanism of Action: HIV-associated wasting is a metabolic disorder characterized by specific abnormalities of intermediary metabolism resulting in weight loss, inappropriate depletion of lean body mass (LBM), and paradoxical preservation of body fat. LBM includes primarily skeletal muscle, organ tissue, blood and blood constituents. LBM depletion results in muscle weakness, organ failure, immune deficiency, general inanition and death. Unlike nutritional intervention for HIV-associated wasting, in which supplemental calories are converted predominantly to body fat which is essentially inert in day-to-day metabolic balance, the anabolic and anti-catabolic effects of somatropin treatment resulted in a prompt and sustained increase in LBM and a decrease in body fat with a significant increase in body weight due to the dominant effect of LBM gain.

Pharmacodynamics: Effects on Protein, Lipid, and Carbohydrate Metabolism: A one-week study in 6 patients with HIV-associated wasting has shown that treatment with somatropin improves nitrogen balance, increases protein-sparing lipid oxidation, and has little effect on overall carbohydrate metabolism.

Lean Body Mass Accrual: In the same study, treatment with somatropin resulted in the retention of phosphorous, potassium, nitrogen, and sodium. The ratio of retained potassium and nitrogen during somatropin therapy was consistent with retention of these elements in lean tissue. In clinical studies (12 weeks), somatropin significantly increased lean body mass. There was also a proportionate increase in intracellular and extracellular fluid during somatropin therapy suggesting accretion of normally hydrated lean body tissue.

Physical Performance: Treadmill performance was examined in a 12-week placebo-controlled study. Work output improved significantly in the somatropin-treated group after 12 weeks of therapy and was correlated with LBM. No such correlation was seen with body fat. Isometric muscle performance, as measured by grip strength dynamometry, declined, probably as a result of a transient increase in tissue turgor known to occur with r-hGH therapy.

Pharmacokinetics: Subcutaneous Absorption: The absolute bioavailability of somatropin after subcutaneous administration of a formulation not equivalent to the marketed formulation was determined to be 70-90%. The $t_{1/2}$ (Mean±SD) after subcutaneous administration is significantly longer than that seen after intravenous administration to normal male volunteers, down-regulated with somatostatin (3.94±3.44 h vs. 0.58±0.08 h), indicating that the subcutaneous absorption of the clinically tested formulation of the compound is slow and rate-limiting.

Distribution: The steady-state volume of distribution (Mean±SD) following IV administration of somatropin in healthy volunteers is 12.0±1.08 L.

Metabolism: Although the liver plays a role in the metabolism of growth hormone (GH), GH is primarily cleaved in the kidney. GH undergoes glomerular filtration and after cleavage within the renal cells, the peptides and amino acids are returned to the systemic circulation.

Excretion: The $t_{1/2}$ (Mean±SD) in nine patients with AIDS-related wasting with an average weight of 56.7±6.8 kg, given a fixed dose of 6.0 mg r-hGH subcutaneously was 4.28±2.15 h. The renal clearance of r-hGH after subcutaneous administration in nine patients with AIDS-related wasting was 0.0015±0.0037 L/h. No significant accumulation of r-hGH appears to occur after 6 weeks of dosing as indicated.

Table 4: SEROSTIM

Summary of SEROSTIM Pharmacokinetics Parameters in Healthy Volunteers

Parameters		C_{max} (mIU/mL)	AUC_{last} (mIU/mL)	AUC (mIU/mL)	AUC extrapolated (%)	t_{max} (h) median values
SEROSTIM	Mean (Min-max)	146 (92–244)	1090 (706–1440)	1150 (867–1490)	4.37 (0.9–12.2)	3.05 (2.00–6.00)

Legend: 1 mg=approx. 3 IU.

Special Populations and Conditions: Pediatrics: Available evidence suggests that r-hGH clearances are similar in adults and children, but no clinical studies were conducted in children with acquired immune deficiency syndrome or AIDS-related complex.

Gender: Biomedical literature indicates that a gender-related difference in the mean clearance of r-hGH could exist (clearance of r-hGH in males >clearance of r-hGH in females). However, no gender-based analysis is available on SEROSTIM (somatropin for injection) in normal volunteers or patients infected with HIV.

Renal Insufficiency: It has been reported that individuals with chronic renal failure tend to have decreased hGH clearance compared to normals, but there are no data on SEROSTIM use in the presence of renal insufficiency.

Hepatic Insufficiency: A reduction in r-hGH clearance has been noted in patients with severe liver dysfunction. However, the clinical significance of this in HIV+ patients is unknown.

STORAGE AND STABILITY: SEROSTIM: Storage Recommendations: SEROSTIM 5 mg and 6 mg Vials: Store SEROSTIM (somatropin for injection) lyophilized product at or below 25°C. Do not use SEROSTIM after the expiry date shown on the label.

Diluents for Reconstitution: The recommended diluents for reconstitution are:

SEROSTIM 5 mg and 6 mg Vials: Sterile Water for Injection, USP.

Incompatibility: SEROSTIM should not be mixed with other drugs.

Preparation of Solution: To prevent possible contamination of the vial, wipe the rubber stopper with an antiseptic solution before puncturing it with the needle.

To reconstitute SEROSTIM, inject 1 mL of diluent into the vial of SEROSTIM, aiming the liquid against the vial wall. Swirl the vial with a **gentle** rotary motion until the contents are dissolved completely. **Do not shake.** Because SEROSTIM is a protein, shaking can result in a cloudy solution; however, this opalescence does not indicate any decrease in potency.

Parenteral drug products should be inspected visually prior to administration. Do not inject if the reconstituted product contains particulate matter or is discoloured.

Stability and Storage of Solution: SEROSTIM 5mg and 6 mg Vials: When reconstituted with the diluent provided (Sterile Water for Injection, USP), the reconstituted solution should be used immediately (within 3 hours). Although not recommended, it may be stored for up to 24 hours at 2-8°C. As there is no preservative in this reconstituted solution, any unused solution should be discarded once the dose is given.

SPECIAL HANDLING INSTRUCTIONS: The SEROSTIM (somatropin for injection) solution should not be administered if it contains particles or is not clear.

Any unused product or waste material should be disposed of in accordance with local requirements.

INFORMATION FOR THE PATIENT: Published in e-CPS, available by subscription at www.e-cps.ca.

DOSAGE FORMS, COMPOSITION AND PACKAGING: 5 mg: Each vial of sterile, non-pyrogenic, lyophilized powder contains: somatropin 5 mg. Nonmedicinal ingredients: phosphoric acid, sodium hydroxide and sucrose. Sodium hydroxide and/or phosphoric acid for pH adjustment to pH 7.5±0.1. Cartons of 1 and 7 vials with diluent (Water for Injection).

6 mg: Each vial of sterile, non-pyrogenic, lyophilized powder contains: somatropin 6 mg. Nonmedicinal ingredients: phosphoric acid, sodium hydroxide and sucrose. Sodium hydroxide and/or phosphoric acid for pH adjustment to pH 7.5±0.1. Cartons of 1 and 7 vials with diluent (Water for Injection).

Serotonin Reuptake Inhibitors

CPhA Monograph

see *Selective Serotonin Reuptake Inhibitors*

Sertraline

CPhA Monograph

see *Selective Serotonin Reuptake Inhibitors*

Sevorane® AF

sevoflurane

Inhalation Anesthetic

Abbott

Date of Preparation: September 18, 1995
Date of Revision: April 14, 2009

SUMMARY PRODUCT INFORMATION:

Route of Administration	Dosage Form/ Strength	Nonmedicinal Ingredients
Inhalation	Volatile Liquid/99.9875% w/w sevoflurane (on anhydrous basis)	None.

INDICATIONS AND CLINICAL USE: SEVORANE AF (sevoflurane) is indicated for:

- induction and maintenance of general anesthesia in adult and pediatric patients for inpatient and outpatient surgery.

Geriatrics (>65 years of age): For a brief discussion, see Warnings and Precautions, Special Populations, Geriatrics (>65 years of age).

Pediatrics (<18 years of age): For a brief discussion, see Warnings and Precautions, Special Populations, Pediatrics (<18 years of age).

CONTRAINDICATIONS:

- SEVORANE AF (sevoflurane) is contraindicated in patients with known sensitivity to sevoflurane or to other halogenated agents.
- Sevoflurane is contraindicated in patients in whom liver dysfunction, jaundice or unexplained fever, leucocytosis, or eosinophilia has occurred after a previous halogenated anesthetic administration (see Warnings and Precautions).
- Sevoflurane is contraindicated in patients with known or suspected genetic susceptibility to malignant hyperthermia, or in patients with a known or suspected history of malignant hyperthermia.
- Sevoflurane should not be used when general anesthesia is contraindicated.

WARNINGS AND PRECAUTIONS: General: SEVORANE AF (sevoflurane) should be administered only by persons trained in the administration of general anesthesia. Facilities for maintenance of a patent airway, artificial ventilation, oxygen enrichment, and circulatory resuscitation must be immediately available. Since levels of anesthesia may be altered rapidly, only vaporizers producing predictable concentrations of sevoflurane should be used.

Because clinical experience in administering sevoflurane to patients with renal insufficiency (creatinine >1.5 mg/dL) is limited, its safety in these patients has not been established. (See Action and Clinical Pharmacology.)

Fresh gas flow rates of less than 2 L/min in a circle absorber system are not recommended, as safety at lower rates has not yet been established.

Compound A is produced when sevoflurane interacts with soda lime and BARALYME (see Action and Clinical Pharmacology). Its concentration in a circle absorber system increases with increasing absorber temperature and increasing sevoflurane concentrations and with decreasing fresh gas flow rates. It has been reported that the concentration of Compound A increases significantly with prolonged dehydration of BARALYME. Although Compound A is a dose-dependent nephrotoxin in rats, there have been no cases of renal toxicity reported in humans, when sevoflurane is used as recommended.

During the maintenance of anesthesia, increasing the concentration of sevoflurane produces dose-dependent decreases in blood pressure. Due to sevoflurane's insolubility in blood, these hemodynamic changes may occur more rapidly than with other volatile anesthetics. Excessive decreases in blood pressure or respiratory depression may be related to depth of anesthesia and may be corrected by decreasing the inspired concentration of sevoflurane.

The recovery from general anesthesia should be assessed carefully before patient is discharged from the post-anesthesia care unit.

Safe Use of CO_2 Absorbents: Carbon dioxide absorbents containing potassium hydroxide should not be used, as safe limits for its level of hydration have not been established.

Care should be taken to avoid using dried out (i.e., desiccated) CO_2 absorbents. The color indicator of most CO_2 absorbents does not necessarily change as a result of desiccation. Therefore, the lack of significant color change should not be taken as an assurance of adequate hydration. CO_2 absorbents should be replaced routinely regardless of the state of the color indicator.

Rare cases of extreme heat, smoke, and/or spontaneous fire in the anesthesia machine have been reported during sevoflurane use in conjunction with the use of desiccated CO_2 absorbent, specifically those containing potassium hydroxide (e.g. BARALYME). An unusually delayed rise or unexpected decline of inspired sevoflurane concentration compared to the vaporizer setting may be associated with excessive heating of the CO_2 absorbent canister.

An exothermic reaction, enhanced sevoflurane degradation, and production of degradation products (see Storage and Stability) can occur when the CO_2 absorbent becomes desiccated, such as after an extended period of dry gas flow through the CO_2 absorbent canisters. Sevoflurane degradants (methanol, formaldehyde, carbon monoxide, and Compounds A, B, C, and D) were observed in the respiratory circuit of an experimental anesthesia machine using desiccated CO_2 absorbents and maximum sevoflurane concentrations (8%) for extended periods of time (≥2 hours). Concentrations of formaldehyde observed at the anesthesia respiratory circuit (using sodium hydroxide containing absorbents) were consistent with levels known to cause respiratory irritation.

Carcinogenesis and Mutagenesis: Studies on carcinogenesis have not been performed. No mutagenic effect was noted in the Ames test.

Endocrine and Metabolism: Malignant Hyperthermia: In susceptible individuals, potent inhalation anesthetic agents, including sevoflurane, may trigger a skeletal muscle hypermetabolic state leading to high oxygen demand and the clinical syndrome known as malignant hyperthermia.

In clinical trials, one case of malignant hyperthermia was reported. In genetically susceptible pigs, sevoflurane induced malignant hyperthermia. The clinical syndrome is signaled by hypercapnia, and may include muscle rigidity, tachycardia, tachypnea, cyanosis, arrhythmias, and/or unstable blood pressure. Some of these non-specific signs may also appear during light anesthesia, acute hypoxia, hypercapnia and hypovolemia.

Treatment of malignant hyperthermia includes discontinuation of triggering agents, administration of intravenous dantrolene sodium, and application of supportive therapy. (Consult information for intravenous dantrolene sodium for additional information on patient management.) Renal failure may appear later, and urine flow should be monitored and sustained if possible.

Use of inhaled anesthetic agents has been associated with rare increases in serum potassium levels that have resulted in cardiac arrhythmias and death in pediatric patients during the postoperative period. Patients with latent as well as overt neuromuscular disease, particularly Duchenne muscular dystrophy, appear to be most vulnerable. Concomitant use of succinylcholine has been associated with most, but not all, of these cases. These patients also experienced significant elevations in serum creatine kinase levels and, in some cases, changes in urine consistent with myoglobinuria. Despite the similarity in presentation to malignant hyperthermia, none of these patients exhibited signs or symptoms of muscle rigidity or hypermetabolic state. Early and aggressive intervention to treat the hyperkalemia and resistant arrhythmias is recommended, as is subsequent evaluation for latent neuromuscular disease.

Hepatic/Biliary/Pancreatic: It has been reported that previous exposure to halogenated hydrocarbon anesthetics, especially if the interval is less than 3 months, may increase the potential for hepatic injury.

Hepatitis: As with other halogenated anesthetics, sevoflurane may cause sensitivity hepatitis in patients who have been sensitized by previous exposure to halogenated anesthetics (see Contraindications and Adverse Reactions). Therefore, appropriate alternative anesthetic agent(s) should be considered, this is especially important in patients with pre-existing hepatic conditions.

Hepatic Impairment: In a limited number of patients with mild-to-moderate hepatic impairment (N=16), the hepatic function was not affected by sevoflurane. The safety of sevoflurane in patients with severe hepatic impairment has not been established; therefore, sevoflurane should be used with caution in these patients.

Renal Impairment: Because clinical experience in administering sevoflurane in patients with renal insufficiencies (creatinine >1.5 mg/dL) is limited (N=35), its safety in these patients has not been established. Therefore, sevoflurane should be used with caution in patients with renal insufficiency. Limited pharmacokinetic data in these patients appear to suggest that the half-life of sevoflurane may be increased. The clinical significance is unknown at this time (see Action and Clinical Pharmacology).

Neurologic: Although recovery of consciousness following sevoflurane administration generally occurs within minutes, the impact on intellectual function for two or three days following anesthesia has not been studied. As with other anesthetics, small changes in moods may persist for several days following administration. Patients should be advised that performance of activities requiring mental alertness, such as operating a motor vehicle or hazardous machinery, may be impaired for some time after general anesthesia.

Peri-Operative Considerations: Neurosurgery: Due to the limited number of patients who received sevoflurane during neurosurgical procedures (N=22), safety in neurosurgery has not been fully established at this time and sevoflurane should be used with caution. In a study of 20 patients, there was no difference between sevoflurane and isoflurane with regard to recovery from anesthesia. In 2 studies, a total of 22 patients with intracranial pressure (ICP) monitors received either sevoflurane or isoflurane. There was no difference between sevoflurane and isoflurane with regard to ICP response to inhalation of 0.5, 1.0, and 1.5 MAC inspired concentrations of volatile agent during N_2O-O_2-fentanyl anesthesia. During progressive hyperventilation from $PaCO_2$=40 to $PaCO_2$=30, ICP response to hypocarbia was preserved with sevoflurane at both 0.5 and 1.0 MAC concentrations. In patients at risk for elevations of ICP, sevoflurane should be administered cautiously in conjunction with ICP-reducing maneuvers such as hyperventilation.

Special Populations: Pregnant Women: There are no adequate and well-controlled studies in pregnant women. Sevoflurane should be used during pregnancy only if clearly needed.

Cesarean Section: Due to the limited number of patients studied, safety in cesarean section has not been fully established at this time and sevoflurane should be used with caution. Sevoflurane has been used as part of general anesthesia for elective cesarean section in 29 women. There were no untoward effects in mother or neonate.

Labour, Delivery: See Nursing Women.

Nursing Women: The safety of sevoflurane in labour, delivery and nursing mothers has not yet been demonstrated; therefore, sevoflurane should be used with caution in these patients.

Pediatrics (<18 years of age): The concentration of sevoflurane required for maintenance of general anesthesia is age-dependent (see Dosage and Administration). Incidences of bradycardia (more than 20 beats/min less than normal) is lower for sevoflurane (3%) than for halothane (7%). Emergence times for sevoflurane are faster than with halothane (12 vs 19 minutes, respectively). A higher incidence of agitation occurs with sevoflurane (208/837 patients or 25%) when compared with halothane (114/661 patients or 17%).

Geriatrics (>65 years of age): MAC decreases with increasing age. The average concentration of sevoflurane to achieve MAC in an 80 year old is approximately 50% of that required in a 20 year old. In adults, the incidence of bradycardia is greater with sevoflurane than with isoflurane.

ADVERSE REACTIONS: Adverse Drug Reaction Overview: Adverse events are derived from controlled clinical trials conducted in the United States, Canada and Europe. The reference drugs were isoflurane, enflurane, and propofol in adults and halothane in pediatric patients. The studies were conducted using a variety of premedications, other anesthetics, and surgical procedures of varying length. Most adverse events reported were mild and transient, and may reflect the surgical procedures, patient characteristics (including disease) and/or medications administered.

Clinical Trial Adverse Drug Reactions: Because clinical trials are conducted under very specific conditions the adverse reaction rates observed in the clinical trials may not reflect the rates observed in practice and should not be compared to the rates in the clinical trials of another drug. Adverse drug reaction information from clinical trials is useful for identifying drug-related adverse events and for approximating rates.

Of the 5182 patients enrolled in the clinical trials, 2906 were exposed to sevoflurane, including 118 adults and 507 pediatric patients who underwent mask induction. Each patient was counted once for each type of adverse event. Adverse events reported in patients in clinical trials are presented within each body system in order of decreasing frequency in the following listings (see Table 1, Table 2, Table 3 and Table 4). One case of malignant hyperthermia was reported in pre-registration clinical trials.

Less Common Clinical Trial Adverse Drug Reactions (<1%): See Warnings and Precautions for information regarding malignant hyperthermia.

Abnormal Hematologic and Clinical Chemistry Findings: Transient elevations in glucose, liver function tests, and white blood cell count may occur as with use of other anesthetic agents.

Post-Market Adverse Drug Reactions: There have been post-marketing reports of rare events of malignant hyperthermia (see Contraindications and Warnings and Precautions). Rare events of allergic reactions, such as rash, urticaria, pruritus, bronchospasm, anaphylactic or anaphylactoid reactions have also been reported (see Contraindications). Cases of dystonic movement with spontaneous resolution have been reported in children receiving sevoflurane for induction of anesthesia. Seizure-like activity may occur on extremely rare occasions following sevoflurane administration. Reported events were of short duration and there was no evidence of any abnormality during emergence from anesthesia or in the postoperative period. There have also been reports of post-operative hepatitis. In addition, there have been rare post-marketing reports of hepatic failure and hepatic necrosis associated with the use of potent volatile anesthetic agents, including sevoflurane. Due to the uncontrolled nature of these spontaneous reports, a causal relationship to sevoflurane has not been established.

Rare reports of hypersensitivity (including dermatitis contact, rash, dyspnoea, wheezing, chest discomfort, swelling face, or anaphylactic reaction) have been received, particularly in association with long-term occupational exposure to inhaled anesthetic agents, including sevoflurane.

Table 1: SEVORANE AF

Adverse Events During the Induction Period (from onset of anesthesia by mask induction to surgical incision) Possibly or Probably Related Incidence >1%

Body System	Adverse Event	Incidence
Adult Patients (N=118)		
Cardiovascular	Bradycardia	5%
	Hypotension	4%
	Tachycardia	2%
Nervous System	Agitation	7%
Respiratory System	Laryngospasm	8%
	Airway Obstruction	8%
	Breathholding	5%
	Cough Increased	5%
Pediatric Patients (N=507)		
Cardiovascular	Tachycardia	6%
	Hypotension	4%
Nervous System	Agitation	15%
	Increased Salivation	2%
Respiratory System	Breathholding	5%
	Cough Increased	5%
	Laryngospasm	3%
	Apnea	2%

Note: Similar incidence of adverse events was noted when all adverse reactions were recorded, not only possibly or probably related.

Table 2: SEVORANE AF

Adverse Events for All Patients During All Anesthetic Periods Possibly or Probably Related Incidence >1% (N=2906)

Body System	Adverse Event	Incidence
Body as a Whole	Fever	1%
	Shivering	6%
	Hypothermia	1%
	Movement	1%
	Headache	1%
Cardiovascular	Hypotension	11%
	Hypertension	2%
	Bradycardia	5%
	Tachycardia	2%
Nervous System	Somnolence	9%
	Agitation	9%
	Dizziness	4%
	Increased Salivation	4%
Digestive System	Nausea	25%
	Vomiting	18%
Respiratory System	Cough Increased	11%
	Breathholding	2%
	Laryngospasm	2%

Table 3: SEVORANE AF

All Adverse Events for All Patients During All Anesthetic Periods Incidence >1%

Body System	Adverse Event	Incidence Sevorane AF (n=2906)	Incidence Ref. Agent (n=2276)
Body as a Whole	Fever	11%	12%
	Shivering	7%	8%
	Hypothermia	2%	2%
	Movement	1%	1%
	Headache	2%	3%
Cardiovascular	Hypotension	15%	16%
	Hypertension	10%	9%
	Bradycardia	7%	8%
	Tachycardia	4%	4%
Nervous System	Somnolence	14%	17%
	Agitation	11%	9%
	Dizziness	8%	9%
	Increased Salivation	7%	11%
Digestive System	Nausea	37%	36%
	Vomiting	25%	27%
Respiratory System	Cough Increased	24%	29%
	Breathholding	3%	3%
	Laryngospasm	2%	3%

Table 4: SEVORANE AF

All Adverse Events For All Patients During All Anesthetic Periods Incidence <1% (reported in 3 or more patients)—(N=2906)

Body System	Adverse Event
Body as a Whole	Asthenia, pain
Cardiovascular	Arrhythmia, ventricular extrasystoles, supraventricular extrasystoles, complete AV block, bigeminy, hemorrhage, inverted T wave, atrial fibrillation, atrial arrhythmia, second degree AV block, syncope, S-T depressed
Nervous System	Crying, nervousness, confusion, hypertonia, dry mouth, insomnia

(cont'd)

Table 4: SEVORANE AF *(cont'd)*

All Adverse Events For All Patients During All Anesthetic Periods Incidence <1% (reported in 3 or more patients)—(N=2906)

Body System	Adverse Event
Respiratory System	Sputum increased, apnea, hypoxia, wheezing, bronchospasm, hyperventilation, pharyngitis, hiccup, hypoventilation, dyspnea, stridor
Metabolism and Nutrition	Increases in LDH, AST, ALT, BUN, alkaline phosphatase, creatinine, bilirubinemia, glycosuria, fluorosis, albuminuria, hypophosphatemia, acidosis, hyperglycemia
Hemic and Lymphatic System	Leucocytosis, thrombocytopenia
Skin and Special Senses	Pruritus, taste perversion, rash, conjunctivitis
Urogenital	Urination impaired, urine abnormality, urinary retention, oliguria

DRUG INTERACTIONS: Overview: In clinical trials, no significant adverse reactions occurred with other drugs commonly used in the perioperative period, including: central nervous system depressants, autonomic drugs, skeletal muscle relaxants, anti-infective agents, hormones and synthetic substitutes, blood derivatives, and cardiovascular drugs, including epinephrine.
Drug-Drug Interactions: Intravenous anesthetics: Sevoflurane administration is compatible with barbiturates, non-barbiturates (such as propofol) and benzodiazepines.
Benzodiazepines and Opioids: Benzodiazepines and opioids would be expected to decrease the MAC of sevoflurane in the same manner as with other inhalational anesthetics. Sevoflurane administration is compatible with benzodiazepines and opioids as commonly used in surgical practice.
Nitrous oxide: As with other halogenated volatile anesthetics, the anesthetic requirement for sevoflurane is decreased when administered in combination with nitrous oxide. Using 50% N_2O, the MAC equivalent dose requirement is reduced approximately 50% in adults, and approximately 25% in pediatric patients (see Dosage and Administration).
Neuromuscular Blocking Agents: As is the case with other volatile anesthetics, sevoflurane increases both the intensity and duration of neuromuscular blockade induced by non-depolarizing muscle relaxants. The effect of sevoflurane on succinylcholine and the duration of depolarizing neuromuscular blockade has not been studied.
Drug-Laboratory Test Interactions: Interactions with laboratory tests have not been established.
Drug-Lifestyle Interactions: Performance of activities requiring mental alertness, such as operating a motor vehicle or hazardous machinery, may be impaired for some time after general anesthesia (see Warnings and Precautions, Neurologic).

DOSAGE AND ADMINISTRATION: Dosing Considerations: Fresh gas flow rates of less than 2 L/min in a circle absorber system are not recommended, as safety at lower rates has not yet been established.

The concentration of SEVORANE AF (sevoflurane) being delivered from a vaporizer during anesthesia should be known. This may be accomplished by using a vaporizer calibrated specifically for sevoflurane. The administration of general anesthesia must be individualized based on the patient's response.
Pre-anesthetic medication: No specific premedication is either indicated or contraindicated with sevoflurane. The decision as to whether or not to premedicate and the choice of premedication is left to the discretion of the anesthesiologist.
Induction: Sevoflurane has a non-pungent odour and does not cause respiratory irritability; therefore, it is suitable for mask induction in pediatrics and adults.
Maintenance: Surgical levels of anesthesia can usually be achieved with concentrations of 0.5 to 3% sevoflurane with or without the concomitant use of nitrous oxide. Sevoflurane can be administered with any type of anesthesia circuit.
Recommended Dose and Dosage Adjustment: MAC values according to age are presented in Table 5.

Table 5: SEVORANE AF

MAC Values According to Age

Age of Patient	Number of Patients	MAC in Oxygen	MAC in 65% N_2O/ 35% O_2
Infants	26		
1–<6 months		3.0%	—
6–<12 months		2.8%	—
Children	39		
1–<3 years		2.6%	2.0%
3–12 years		2.5%	—
Adults	41		
25 years		2.5%	1.4%
40 years		2.1%	1.1%
60 years		1.6%	0.9%
80 years		1.4%	0.7%

Note 1: In 12 neonates of full-term gestational age, MAC was determined to be 3.3%.
Note 2: In 1-<3 yrs old pediatric patients, 60% N_2O/40% O_2 was used.

Administration: SEVORANE AF (sevoflurane) should be administered only by persons trained in the administration of general anesthesia (see Warnings and Precautions).

OVERDOSAGE:
In the event of overdosage, or what may appear to be overdosage, the following action should be taken: discontinue administration of sevoflurane, maintain a patent airway, initiate assisted or controlled ventilation with oxygen and maintain adequate cardiovascular function.

For management of a suspected drug overdose, CPhA recommends that you contact your **regional Poison Control Centre**. See the *CPS* Directory section for a list of Poison Control Centres.

ACTION AND CLINICAL PHARMACOLOGY: Pharmacodynamics: SEVORANE AF (sevoflurane) is an inhalational anesthetic agent for use in induction and maintenance of general anesthesia. Sevoflurane has a non-pungent odour and does not cause respiratory irritability. Sevoflurane is suitable for mask induction in adults and pediatric. Minimum alveolar concentration (MAC) of sevoflurane in oxygen for a 40 year old adult is 2.1%. The MAC of sevoflurane decreases with age. (See Dosage and Administration for details).

Emergence times in pediatric patients are faster for sevoflurane (12 minutes) than for halothane (19 minutes). Time to first analgesia in pediatric patients is earlier in sevoflurane (approx. 52 minutes) than with halothane (approx. 68 minutes). The facts should be taken into account in cases where post-anesthesia pain is anticipated.

Pharmacokinetics: Solubility: Because of the low solubility of sevoflurane in blood (blood/gas partition coefficient at 37°C = 0.63 to 0.69), a minimal amount of sevoflurane is required to be dissolved in the blood before the alveolar partial pressure is in equilibrium with the arterial partial pressure. Therefore there is a rapid rate of increase in the alveolar (end-tidal) concentration (F_A) toward the inspired concentration (F_I) during induction and rapid elimination via the lungs when it is discontinued.
Distribution: The effects of sevoflurane on the displacement of drugs from serum and tissue proteins have not been investigated. Other fluorinated volatile anesthetics have been shown to displace drugs from serum and tissue proteins in vitro. The clinical significance of this is unknown. Clinical studies have shown no untoward effects when sevoflurane is administered to patients taking drugs that are highly bound and have a small volume of distribution (e.g. phenytoin).
Metabolism: Sevoflurane is metabolized by cytochrome P450 2E1, to hexafluoroisopropanol (HFIP) with the release of inorganic fluoride and CO_2. Once formed, HFIP is rapidly conjugated with glucuronic acid and eliminated as a urinary metabolite. No other metabolite pathways for sevoflurane have been identified. In vivo metabolism studies suggest that approximately 5% of the sevoflurane dose may be metabolized.

Cytochrome P450 2E1 is the principal isoform identified for sevoflurane metabolism and this may be induced by chronic exposure to isoniazide and ethanol. This is similar to the metabolism of isoflurane and enflurane and is distinct from that of methoxyflurane which is metabolized via a variety of cytochrome P450 isoforms. The metabolism of sevoflurane is not inducible by barbiturates. Inorganic fluoride concentrations peak within 2 hours of the end of sevoflurane anesthesia and return to baseline concentrations within 48 hours post-anesthesia in the majority of cases (67%). The rapid and extensive pulmonary elimination of sevoflurane minimizes the amount of anesthetic available for metabolism.

In 12 clinical trials with sevoflurane, approximately 7% (55 out of 886) of adults evaluated for inorganic fluoride had serum concentrations greater than 50 µM; there were no reports of toxicity associated with elevated fluoride ion levels.
Excretion: Up to 3.5% of the sevoflurane dose appears in the urine as inorganic fluoride. Studies on fluoride indicate that up to 50% of fluoride clearance is non-renal (via fluoride being taken up into bone).
Compound A Production in Anesthesia Circuit: The only known degradation reaction in the clinical setting is through direct contact with CO_2 absorbents (soda lime and BARALYME) producing Compound A (pentafluoroisopropenyl fluoromethyl ether).

The concentrations of Compound A measured in the anesthesia circuit when sevoflurane is used as indicated are not known to be deleterious to humans. Fresh gas flow rates below 2 L/min in a circle absorber system are not recommended, as safety at lower rates has not yet been established.
Special Populations and Conditions: Pediatrics: Sevoflurane pharmacokinetics have not been investigated in pediatric population.
Geriatrics: Sevoflurane pharmacokinetics have not been investigated in geriatric population.
Gender: No gender related pharmacokinetic differences have been observed in adult patients studied.
Race: Pharmacokinetic differences due to race have not been identified.
Hepatic Insufficiency: Limited pharmacokinetic data in these patients appear to suggest that the half-life of sevoflurane may be increased. The clinical significance is unknown at this time.
Renal Insufficiency: Limited pharmacokinetic data in these patients appear to suggest that the half-life of sevoflurane may be increased. The clinical significance is unknown at this time.
STORAGE AND STABILITY: Sevoflurane is stable when stored under normal room lighting conditions. No discernible degradation of sevoflurane occurs in the presence of strong acids or heat. Sevoflurane is not corrosive to stainless steel, brass, aluminum, nickel-plated brass, chrome-plated brass, or copper beryllium alloy.

Chemical degradation can occur upon exposure of inhaled anesthetics to CO_2 absorbent within the anesthesia machine. When used as directed with fresh absorbents, degradation of sevoflurane is minimal, and degradants are undetectable or non-toxic. Sevoflurane degradation and subsequent degradant formation are enhanced by increasing absorbent temperature, desiccated CO_2 absorbent (especially potassium hydroxide-containing, e.g. BARALYME), increased sevoflurane concentration and decreased fresh gas flow. Sevoflurane can undergo alkaline degradation by two pathways. The first results from the loss of hydrogen fluoride with the formation of pentafluoroisopropanyl fluoromethyl ether (PIFE or more commonly known as Compound A). The second occurs only in the presence of desiccated CO_2 absorbents and leads to the dissociation of sevoflurane into hexafluoroisopropanol (HFIP) and formaldehyde. HFIP is inactive, non-genotoxic, rapidly glucoronidated, cleared, and has toxicity comparable to sevoflurane. Formaldehyde is present during normal metabolic processes. Upon exposure to a highly desiccated absorbent, formaldehyde can further degrade into methanol and formate. Formate can contribute to the formation of carbon monoxide, in the presence of high temperature. Methanol can react with Compound A to form the methoxy addition product Compound B. Compound B can undergo further HF elimination to form Compounds C, D, and E. With highly desiccated absorbents, especially those containing potassium hydroxide (e.g. BARALYME), the formation of formaldehyde, methanol, carbon monoxide, Compound A and perhaps some of its degradants, Compounds B, C, and D may occur.

The interaction with CO_2 absorbents is not unique to sevoflurane. The production of degradants in the anesthesia circuit results from the extraction of the acidic proton in the presence of a strong base (KOH and/or NaOH) forming an alkene (Compound A) from sevoflurane similar to formation of 2-bromo-2-chloro-1,1-difluoro ethylene (BCDFE) from halothane.
Lewis Acid Degradation: At least 300 ppm of water is present as a Lewis Acid inhibitor. No other additives or chemical stabilizers are utilized.
Storage Conditions: Sevoflurane should be stored between 15 and 25°C.

INFORMATION FOR THE PATIENT: Published in e-CPS, available by subscription at www.e-cps.ca.

DOSAGE FORMS, COMPOSITION AND PACKAGING: Each bottle of clear, colorless liquid contains only: sevoflurane (about 99.9875% w/w on anhydrous basis). PEN (polyethylene naphthalate) plastic bottles of 250 mL with ROPP and with QUIK-FIL closures.

Silkis™ Ⓟ
calcitriol
Topical Nonsteroidal Antipsoriatic Agent

Galderma

Date of Preparation: November 26, 2009
Date of Revision: March 9, 2010

SUMMARY PRODUCT INFORMATION:

Route of Administration	Dosage Form/ Strength	Clinically Relevant Nonmedicinal Ingredients
Topical	Ointment 3 µg/g	None For a complete listing see Dosage Forms, Composition and Packaging.

INDICATIONS AND CLINICAL USE: Silkis (calcitriol) ointment 3 µg/g is indicated for:
- Topical treatment of mild to moderate plaque type psoriasis (psoriasis vulgaris) with up to 35% body surface area involvement.

Geriatrics (>65 years of age): Clinical studies of Silkis ointment did not include sufficient numbers of subjects 65 years and older to determine whether they respond differently from younger subjects. See Warnings and Precautions.
Pediatrics (<18 years of age): Silkis is not recommended for pediatric use. Safety and effectiveness in pediatric patients have not been established.

CONTRAINDICATIONS:
- Patients who are hypersensitive to this drug or to any ingredient in the formulation or component of the container. For a complete listing, see Dosage Forms, Composition and Packaging.
- **Not for ophthalmic or internal use.**
- Patients with hypercalcemia and patients known to suffer from abnormal calcium metabolism.
- Patients on systemic treatment of calcium homeostasis.
- Patients with severe renal impairment or end-stage renal disease.

WARNINGS AND PRECAUTIONS: General: Serum calcium levels should be monitored at regular intervals if risk factors for hypercalcemia are present. If the serum calcium level becomes elevated, calcitriol therapy should be discontinued and the serum calcium level monitored in these patients until it returns to normal.

Due to the potential effect of Vitamin D and its metabolites on calcium metabolism, substances that may increase the absorption of calcitriol must not be added to the ointment or used concomitantly with the ointment.

Silkis ointment must not be covered with an occlusive dressing.

Silkis is not recommended for severe, extensive psoriasis (i.e., involvement of more than 35% of the body surface).

Silkis should not be applied to the eyes, lips or facial skin.

Silkis is not approved for use in other clinical forms of psoriasis.

No more than 30 g of Silkis ointment should be used per day.

Carcinogenesis and Mutagenesis: Animal data suggest that the vehicle of Silkis ointment may enhance the ability of ultraviolet radiation (UVR) to induce skin tumours. Patients who apply Silkis ointment to exposed skin should avoid excessive exposure of the treated areas to either natural or artificial sunlight, including tanning booths and sun lamps. Physicians may wish to limit or avoid using phototherapy in patients who use Silkis ointment.

Endocrine and Metabolism: If abnormal serum calcium levels are observed, treatment with calcitriol should be discontinued.

Hepatic/Biliary/Pancreatic: Silkis is not recommended in patients with reduced liver function.

Renal: Silkis is not recommended in patients with mild to moderate renal impairment.

Skin: Hands should be washed after applying Silkis in order to avoid unintentional application to other areas. In case of severe irritation or a contact allergic reaction, treatment with Silkis should be discontinued.

Special Populations: Pregnant Women: There are no adequate and well-controlled studies in pregnant women, although studies in experimental animals have not shown teratogenic effects. Silkis should be used during pregnancy only if the anticipated benefit clearly outweighs the potential risk.

Nursing Women: It is not known whether calcitriol is excreted in human milk. Silkis has been found in the milk of lactating rats. Calcitriol should be used by nursing women only if the anticipated benefit clearly outweighs the potential risk.

Geriatrics (>65 years of age): Of the total number of subjects in clinical studies of Silkis, 14% were 65 and over. The incidence of drug-related adverse events, serious adverse events, and adverse events leading to discontinuation were higher in subjects 65 or older than in subjects 18 to <65. In general, use in elderly patients should be cautious, reflecting the greater frequency of decreased hepatic, renal, or cardiac function, and of concomitant disease or other drug therapy.

Pediatrics (<18 years of age): There are insufficient data in patients under 18 years of age to determine the safety and efficacy in this population. Silkis is not recommended in pediatric patients.

Monitoring and Laboratory Tests: Serum calcium levels should be monitored at regular intervals if risk factors for hypercalcemia are present. If serum calcium becomes elevated, treatment with calcitriol should be discontinued.

ADVERSE REACTIONS: Adverse Drug Reaction Overview: The clinical trial adverse reaction data for Silkis is largely based on two 8-week randomized, vehicle-controlled trials as well as one long term (1 year) safety study. These data provide information on twice daily exposure in 743 patients, including 239 exposed for 6 months and 116 exposed for at least one year. The most common adverse reactions experienced were laboratory test abnormality, skin discomfort, pruritus, and psoriasis.

Clinical Trial Adverse Drug Reactions: Because clinical trials are conducted under very specific conditions the adverse reaction rates observed in the clinical trials may not reflect the rates observed in practice and should not be compared to the rates in the clinical trials of another drug. Adverse drug reaction information from clinical trials is useful for identifying drug-related adverse events and for approximating rates.

Silkis was studied in two vehicle-controlled 8 week studies with 419 patients treated with Silkis twice daily. Drug-related adverse reactions that occurred in at least 1% of patients in the Silkis group are shown in Table 1.

Table 1: Silkis

Summary of Drug-related Adverse Events (at least 1%) of the Two Pooled Vehicle-controlled Studies

	Calcitriol Ointment 3 µg/g (n=419)	Calcitriol Vehicle Ointment (n=420)
Total number of AEs	58	71
Total number of subjects with AEs	36 (8.6%)	45 (10.7%)
Skin and Appendages		
Discomfort skin	11 (2.6%)	9 (2.1%)
Pruritus	6 (1.4%)	4 (1%)
Lab Test Abnormal		
Lab test abnormality	14 (3.3%)	15 (3.6%)

In these two studies, among subjects having laboratory monitoring, hypercalcemia (albumin-adjusted calcium above the upper limit of normal) at any post-baseline point during the 8 week trials, was observed in 24% (18/74) of calcitriol-exposed subjects compared to 16% (13/79) of vehicle-exposed subjects. No subject had an albumin-adjusted calcium result over the alert level (10% above the upper limit of the normal range) at any time-point throughout the study. Hypercalcemia was not reported as an adverse event during either study.

A one-year multi-center, open-label, non-comparative study enrolled 324 patients with psoriasis. Silkis was applied twice daily for up to 52 weeks. The most common adverse events were laboratory test abnormality (8%), urine test abnormality (4%), psoriasis (4%), flu syndrome (4%), hypercalciuria (3%), pruritus (3%) and skin infection (3%). There were 10 cases (3%) of hypercalcemia (defined as an albumin-adjusted serum total calcium concentration above the upper limit of the reference range (2.15 to 2.55 mmol/L). With one exception (2.72 mmol/L), all other albumin-adjusted serum total calcium concentrations were less than 5% above the upper limit of normal. There were 3 subjects with reported kidney stones.

Less Common Clinical Trial Adverse Drug Reactions (<1%): Skin and Appendages: psoriasis (0.2%).

Post-Market Adverse Drug Reactions: Because post-market adverse drug reactions are reported voluntarily from a population of uncertain size, it is not always possible to reliably estimate their frequency or establish a causal relationship to drug exposure.

The following post-market adverse reactions have been reported with the use of Silkis ointment: acute blistering dermatitis, erythema, pruritus, skin burning sensation, and skin discomfort. Two serious, unexpected related reports have been received which describe skin atrophy and blisters over the body, burning sensation and extensive flare-up of weepy eczema.

DRUG INTERACTIONS: Overview: Silkis (calcitriol) ointment 3 µg/g must be used with caution in patients receiving medications known to increase serum calcium levels, such as thiazide diuretics, or medications with pharmacological effects impacted by a change in calcium levels, such as digoxin. Caution must also be exercised in patients receiving calcium supplements or high doses of vitamin D.

Silkis has a slight irritant potential, and therefore it is possible that concomitant use of peeling agents, astringents, or irritant products may produce an additive irritant effect.

Drug-Food Interactions: Interactions with food have not been established.

Drug-Herb Interactions: Interactions with herbal products have not been established.

Drug-Laboratory Test Interactions: Interactions with laboratory tests have not been established.

DOSAGE AND ADMINISTRATION: Dosing Considerations:

- Silkis is for **topical use only** and not for oral, ophthalmic or intravaginal use.
- There is no clinical trial experience with the use of Silkis in children and there is limited experience with the use of Silkis in the elderly (see Warnings and Precautions).
- Silkis should be used in pregnant or nursing women only if the benefit versus risk is favourable (see Warnings and Precautions).
- Silkis is contraindicated in patients with severe renal impairment or end-stage renal disease.
- Silkis is not recommended in patients with mild to moderate renal impairment or in patients with liver dysfunction (see Warnings and Precautions).

Recommended Dose and Dosage Adjustment: Silkis (calcitriol) ointment 3 µg/g should be applied to the areas affected with psoriasis twice daily, morning and evening, after washing and gentle drying. No more than 30 g of Silkis ointment should be used daily. No more than 35% of the body can be treated.

No additional therapeutic benefit has been demonstrated with higher doses or more frequent application.

Missed Dose: If a dose of Silkis is missed, it should be applied as soon as the patient remembers and further dosing resumed as usual.

Administration: The affected area should be washed and dried gently. The ointment should be applied and rubbed in gently until the medication is no longer visible. The treated area should not be bandaged or occluded in any way.

Hands should be washed thoroughly with soap and water after each application.

After satisfactory improvement has occurred, the drug should be discontinued. If recurrence takes place after discontinuation, the treatment may be reinstituted.

OVERDOSAGE:

The accidental ingestion of Silkis (calcitriol) ointment 3 µg/g may produce symptoms that are consistent with vitamin D toxicity and hypercalcemia. The initial clinical signs (polyuria, polydypsia, dyspepsia) should be confirmed with a serum analysis of calcium levels prior to initiating treatment for hypercalcemia.

Topically applied calcitriol can be absorbed in sufficient amounts to produce systemic effects. If signs of hypercalcemia occur with the prescribed use of Silkis, treatment should be discontinued.

For management of a suspected drug overdose, CPhA recommends that you contact your **regional Poison Control Centre**. See the *CPS* Directory section for a list of Poison Control Centres.

ACTION AND CLINICAL PHARMACOLOGY: Mechanism of Action: Calcitriol (1α-25-dihydroxyvitamin D_3) is the naturally occurring and biologically active metabolite of vitamin D_3, primarily produced in the skin by exposure to the ultraviolet rays of the sun. Vitamin D_3 must be metabolically activated in the liver and the kidney before it is fully active at target tissues as calcitriol.

Calcitriol primarily regulates systemic calcium and phosphate homeostasis by effects on the gastrointestinal tract, bone, and kidney. The mechanism of action of calcitriol in the treatment of psoriasis has not been established.

Pharmacokinetics: The systemic exposure of calcitriol ointment 3 µg/g was assessed in 23 patients with chronic plaque psoriasis over 21 days with a total of 30 g/day application to 35% body surface area. At Day 21, the geometric mean plasma concentration values of C_{max} increased by 36% over baseline and the geometric mean value of $AUC_{(0-12\,hr)}$ increased by 44%. There was no correlation between the observed elevated calcitriol levels and the pharmacodynamic parameters of serum albumin adjusted calcium, serum phosphorus, urinary calcium and urinary phosphorus.

Absorption: Considerable inter-subject variability in calcitriol permeation through the skin is observed.

STORAGE AND STABILITY: Store at room temperature (15-30°C).

INFORMATION FOR THE PATIENT: Published in e-CPS, available by subscription at www.e-cps.ca.

DOSAGE FORMS, COMPOSITION AND PACKAGING: Each g of a white, translucent, ointment contains: 3 µg (0.0003% w/w) of calcitriol. Other components of the ointment are vitamin E (dl-α tocopherol) added as an antioxidant, mineral oil, and white petrolatum. Collapsible aluminium tubes of 5 and 60 g coated internally with an epoxy-phenolic resin and fitted with a white high density polyethylene or polypropylene screw cap.

Simponi™ Ⓟ

golimumab

Tumour Necrosis Factor Alpha (TNFα) Inhibitor

Schering-Plough

Date of Preparation: April 7, 2009
Date of Revision: March 18, 2010

SIMPONI should be prescribed by physicians who have sufficient knowledge of rheumatoid arthritis and/or ankylosing spondylitis and/or psoriatic arthritis and who have fully familiarized themselves with the efficacy/safety profile of SIMPONI.

SUMMARY PRODUCT INFORMATION:

Route of Administration	Dosage Form/ Strength	Clinically Relevant Nonmedicinal Ingredients
Subcutaneous injection (SC)	50 mg/0.5 mL SmartJect Autoinjector 50 mg/0.5 mL pre-filled syringe	Sorbitol, L-histidine, L-histidine hydrochloride, polysorbate 80, water for injection For a complete listing, see Dosage Forms, Composition and Packaging.

DESCRIPTION: SIMPONI (golimumab) is a human IgG1κ monoclonal antibody that exhibits multiple glycoforms with predicted molecular masses ranging from 149 802 daltons to 151 064 daltons. Golimumab is produced by a recombinant cell line cultured by continuous perfusion and is purified by a series of steps that includes measures to inactivate and remove viruses. Golimumab forms high affinity, stable complexes with both the soluble and transmembrane bioactive forms of human TNF, which prevents the binding of TNF to its receptors. Golimumab does not bind or neutralize human lymphotoxin. Golimumab inhibits TNF-induced activation of human endothelial cells and human diploid fibroblasts, and significantly reduces clinical symptoms and joint degradation in a human TNF transgenic mouse model of arthritis.

Autoinjector/Pre-filled Syringe: SIMPONI is supplied as a single-use sterile solution in a Type 1 glass syringe with a fixed stainless steel needle. The syringe is fitted with a passive safety guard or contained in a single-use autoinjector. SIMPONI does not contain preservatives.

INDICATIONS AND CLINICAL USE: Rheumatoid Arthritis (RA): SIMPONI, in combination with methotrexate (MTX), is indicated for:

- Reducing signs and symptoms in adult patients with moderately to severely active rheumatoid arthritis.

Psoriatic Arthritis (PsA): SIMPONI, is indicated for:

- Reducing signs and symptoms in adult patients with moderately to severely active psoriatic arthritis, alone or in combination with MTX. SIMPONI can be used in combination with MTX in patients who do not respond adequately to MTX alone.

Ankylosing Spondylitis (AS): SIMPONI is indicated for:

- Reducing signs and symptoms in adult patients with active ankylosing spondylitis who have had an inadequate response to conventional therapies.

Geriatrics (≥65 years of age): See Warnings and Precautions, Special Populations, Geriatrics (≥65 years of age) and Action and Clinical Pharmacology, Special Populations and Conditions, Geriatrics.

Pediatrics (<18 years of age): No studies with SIMPONI have been performed in pediatric patients.

CONTRAINDICATIONS:

- Patients with severe infections such as sepsis, tuberculosis and opportunistic infections (see Warnings and Precautions, Infections).
- Patients who are hypersensitive to golimumab, latex or any other ingredient in the formulation or component of the container. For a complete listing, see Dosage Forms, Composition and Packaging.

WARNINGS AND PRECAUTIONS:

Serious Warnings and Precautions

Infections

- **Serious infections leading to hospitalization or death, including sepsis, tuberculosis (TB), invasive fungal, and other opportunistic infections have been observed with the use of TNF antagonists including SIMPONI. Administration of SIMPONI should be discontinued if a patient develops a serious infection or sepsis. Treatment with SIMPONI should not be initiated in patients with active infections including chronic or localized infections (see Infections).**
- **Physicians should exercise caution when considering the use of SIMPONI in patients with a history of recurring or latent infections, including TB, or with underlying conditions, which may predispose patients to infections, who have resided in regions where TB and invasive fungal infections such as histoplasmosis, coccidioidomycosis, or blastomycosis are endemic.**

- Tuberculosis (frequently disseminated or extrapulmonary at clinical presentation) has been observed in patients receiving TNF-blocking agents, including SIMPONI. Tuberculosis may be due to reactivation of latent tuberculosis infection or to new infection.
- Before starting treatment with SIMPONI, all patients should be evaluated for both active and latent tuberculosis.
- If latent tuberculosis is diagnosed, treatment for latent tuberculosis should be started with anti-tuberculosis therapy before initiation of SIMPONI.
- Physicians should monitor patients receiving SIMPONI for signs and symptoms of active tuberculosis, including patients who tested negative for latent tuberculosis infection.

Malignancy

- Lymphoma and other malignancies, some fatal, have been reported in children and adolescent patients treated with TNF blockers, of which SIMPONI is a member.

Infections: Bacterial (including sepsis and pneumonia), mycobacterial (tuberculosis), invasive fungal and opportunistic infections, including fatalities, have been reported in patients receiving TNF-blocking agents, including SIMPONI. Some of these serious infections have occurred in patients on concomitant immunosuppressive therapy that, in addition to their underlying disease could predispose them to infections.

SIMPONI should not be given to patients with a clinically important, active infection. Caution should be exercised when considering the use of SIMPONI in patients with a chronic infection or a history of recurrent infection. Patients should be advised of and avoid exposure to potential risk factors for infection as appropriate.

Tuberculosis: Patients should be evaluated for tuberculosis risk factors (including close contact with a person with active tuberculosis) and tested for latent tuberculosis infection prior to treatment with SIMPONI. Treatment of latent tuberculosis infection should be initiated prior to therapy with SIMPONI.

Anti-tuberculosis therapy should be considered prior to initiation of SIMPONI in patients with a past history of latent or active tuberculosis in whom an adequate course of treatment cannot be confirmed.

Tests for latent tuberculosis may yield false negative results, especially in patients who are immunocompromised or severely ill. Prior to initiating SIMPONI, treatment for latent TB should be considered in patients who have significant risk factors for TB despite a negative test for latent tuberculosis. The decision to initiate anti-tuberculosis therapy in these patients should only be made following consultation with a physician with expertise in the treatment of tuberculosis and taking into account both the risk for latent tuberculosis infection and the risks of anti-tuberculosis therapy.

Patients receiving SIMPONI should be monitored closely for signs and symptoms of active tuberculosis during and after treatment, including patients who tested negative for latent tuberculosis infections.

Opportunistic Infections: Cases of histoplasmosis, coccidioidomycosis and pneumocystosis have been observed in patients receiving SIMPONI. For patients who have resided in or travelled to regions where invasive fungal infections such as histoplasmosis, coccidioidomycosis, or blastomycosis are endemic, the benefits and risks of SIMPONI treatment should be carefully considered before initiation of SIMPONI therapy.

In at risk patients treated with SIMPONI, an invasive fungal infection should be suspected if they develop a serious systemic illness. Invasive fungal infections may present as disseminated rather than localized disease, and antigen and antibody testing may be negative in some patients with active infection. Appropriate empiric antifungal therapy should be considered while a diagnostic workup is being performed. The decision to administer empiric antifungal therapy should be made in consultation with a physician with expertise in the diagnosis and treatment of invasive fungal infections and should take into account both the risk for severe fungal infection and the risks of antifungal therapy.

Hepatitis B Virus (HBV) Reactivation: As observed with the use of other immunosuppressive drugs, the use of TNF blocking agents has been associated with reactivation of hepatitis B virus in patients who are chronic carriers of the virus (i.e., surface antigen positive). Chronic carriers of hepatitis B should be appropriately evaluated and monitored prior to the initiation of, during treatment with, and for several months following discontinuation of SIMPONI.

Malignancies: The potential role of TNF-blocking therapy in the development of malignancies is not known. Caution should be exercised when considering TNF-blocking therapy for patients with a history of malignancy or when considering continuing treatment in patients who develop malignancy.

Pediatric Malignancy: Malignancies, some fatal, have been reported among children, adolescents, and young adults who received treatment with TNF-blocking agents (initiation of therapy ≤18 years of age), of which SIMPONI is a member. Approximately half the cases were lymphomas, including Hodgkin's and non-Hodgkin's lymphoma. The other cases represented a variety of malignancies, including rare malignancies that are usually associated with immunosuppression, and malignancies that are not usually observed in children and adolescents. The malignancies occurred after a median of 30 months (range 1 to 84 months) after the first dose of TNF blocker therapy. Most of the patients were receiving concomitant immunosuppressants. These cases were reported post-marketing and are derived from a variety of sources, including registries and spontaneous post-marketing reports.

Lymphoma: In the controlled portions of clinical trials of all the TNF-blocking agents including SIMPONI, more cases of lymphoma have been observed among patients receiving anti-TNF treatment compared with control patients. During the SIMPONI Phase 2 and Phase 3 clinical trials, the incidence of lymphoma in SIMPONI-treated patients was higher than expected in the general population. Patients with rheumatoid arthritis and other chronic inflammatory diseases, particularly patients with highly active disease and/or chronic exposure to immunosuppressant therapies, may be at higher risk (up to several fold) than the general population for the development of lymphoma, even in the absence of TNF-blocking therapy.

Leukemia: Cases of acute and chronic leukemia have been reported with post-marketing TNF-blocker use in rheumatoid arthritis and other indications. Even in the absence of TNF blocker therapy, patients with rheumatoid arthritis may be at a higher risk (approximately 2-fold) than the general population for the development of leukemia.

Non-lymphoma Malignancy: In the controlled portions of the SIMPONI Phase 2 and Phase 3 clinical trials in RA, PsA, and AS, the incidence of non-lymphoma malignancies (excluding non-melanoma skin cancer) was similar between the SIMPONI and the control groups.

In an exploratory clinical trial evaluating the use of SIMPONI in patients with severe persistent asthma, more patients treated with SIMPONI reported malignancies compared with control patients. The significance of this finding is unknown.

Cardiovascular: Congestive Heart Failure (CHF): Cases of worsening congestive heart failure (CHF) and new onset CHF have been reported with TNF blockers. Cases of CHF in patients with known cardiovascular risk factors have been observed with SIMPONI. SIMPONI has not been studied in patients with CHF. SIMPONI should be used with caution in patients with heart failure. If a decision is made to administer SIMPONI to patients with heart failure, they should be closely monitored during therapy, and SIMPONI should be discontinued if new or worsening symptoms of heart failure appear.

Use with Anakinra: Serious infections were seen in clinical studies with concurrent use of anakinra (an interleukin-1 antagonist) and another TNF-blocking agent, etanercept, with an increased risk of neutropenia and no added clinical benefit. Because of the nature of the adverse events seen with this combination therapy, similar toxicities may also result from the combination of anakinra and other TNF-blocking agents. Therefore, the combination of SIMPONI and anakinra is not recommended (see Drug Interactions, Drug-Drug Interactions).

Concurrent Administration of SIMPONI with Abatacept: In clinical studies, concurrent administration of TNF-blocking agents and abatacept have been associated with an increased risk of infections including serious infections compared with TNF-blocking agents alone, without increased clinical benefit. Because of the nature of the adverse events seen with the combination of TNF-blocking agents and abatacept therapy, the combination of SIMPONI and abatacept is not recommended (see Drug Interactions, Drug-Drug Interactions).

Switching between Biological DMARDS: When switching from one biologic to another, patients should continue to be monitored for signs of infection.

Hematologic: There have been reports of pancytopenia, leukopenia, neutropenia, and thrombocytopenia in patients receiving TNF blockers, including SIMPONI. Caution should be exercised in patients treated with SIMPONI who have a current or past history of significant cytopenias.

Immune: Immunosuppression: The possibility exists for TNF-blocking agents, including SIMPONI, to affect host defences against infections and malignancies since TNF mediates inflammation and modulates cellular immune responses. In Phase I RA studies, in 81 patients evaluated, there were no substantial differences between subjects receiving golimumab and placebo with respect to responses to delayed-type hypersensitivity antigens. The impact of treatment with golimumab on the development and course of malignancies, as well as active and/or chronic infections, is not fully understood (see Warnings and Precautions and Adverse Reactions).

Immunizations: Patients treated with SIMPONI may receive concurrent vaccinations, except for live vaccines. Live vaccines should not be administered concurrently.

No data are available on the response to vaccination, risk of infection or transmission of infection with the administration of live vaccines to patients receiving SIMPONI. Psoriatic arthritis patients treated with SIMPONI in one Phase 3 PsA study were able to mount effective B-cell immune responses to pneumococcal polysaccharide vaccine. Similar numbers of psoriatic arthritis patients receiving SIMPONI and not receiving SIMPONI had at least a 2-fold increase in antibody titers. The proportions of patients with response to pneumococcal vaccine were lower among SIMPONI and control-treated patients receiving MTX compared with patients not receiving MTX. Overall, the data indicate that SIMPONI does not suppress the humoral immune response to this vaccine.

Hypersensitivity: Allergic reactions (e.g., rash, urticaria, and rarely anaphylaxis and serum sickness like reactions) have been observed in patients treated with TNF-blocking agents. If any serious allergic or anaphylactic reaction occurs, administration of SIMPONI should be discontinued immediately and appropriate therapy initiated.

Immunogenicity: Allergic Reactions: Latex Sensitivity: The needle cover on the pre-filled syringe as well as the pre-filled syringe in the autoinjector contains dry natural rubber (a derivative of latex), which may cause allergic reactions in individuals sensitive to latex.

Autoimmunity: Treatment with SIMPONI may result in the formation of autoantibodies and, rarely, in the development of a lupus-like syndrome. If a patient develops symptoms of a lupus-like syndrome following treatment with golimumab, treatment should be discontinued (see Adverse Reactions, Immune, Autoantibodies).

Neurologic: Use of TNF-blocking agents, including SIMPONI, have been associated in rare cases with new onset or exacerbation of clinical symptoms and/or radiographic evidence of central nervous system demyelinating disorders, including multiple sclerosis. In patients with pre-existing or recent onset of demyelinating disorders, the benefits and risks of anti-TNF treatment should be carefully considered before initiation of SIMPONI therapy.

Sexual Function/Reproduction: It is not known whether golimumab can impair fertility in humans. No impairment of fertility was observed in a fertility and general reproduction toxicity study conducted in mice using the analogous anti-mouse TNFα antibody.

Special Populations: Pregnant Women: An embryofetal developmental toxicology study was performed in which pregnant cynomolgus monkeys were treated with golimumab during the first trimester at dosages up to 50 mg/kg twice weekly (over 500-fold higher in terms of dose/body weight ratio than the proposed clinical dose of 50 mg every 4 weeks). The mean peak maternal serum concentration obtained in this study (1576 µg/mL) is over 900-fold higher than median steady-state C_{max} value (1.71 µg/mL) following 50 mg every 4-week SC dosing in patients with RA, PsA, and AS. Umbilical cord blood samples collected at the end of the second trimester showed that fetuses were exposed to golimumab during gestation. Fetal serum concentrations were approximately 50% of the maternal serum concentrations. In this study, in utero exposure to golimumab produced no developmental defects to the fetus.

A pre- and post-natal developmental study was performed in which pregnant cynomolgus monkeys were treated with golimumab during the second and third trimesters, and during lactation. Golimumab was present in the neonatal serum from the time of birth and for up to six months postpartum. The mean peak maternal serum concentration obtained in this study (1482 µg/mL) is over 860-fold higher than median steady-state C_{max} value (1.71 µg/mL) following 50 mg every 4-week SC dosing in patients with RA, PsA, and AS. Golimumab was detected in the breast milk at concentrations that were approximately 350-fold lower than the maternal serum concentrations. Exposure to golimumab during gestation and during the postnatal period caused no developmental defects in the infants.

There have been no studies in pregnant women. It is not known whether SIMPONI can cause fetal harm when administered to a pregnant woman or can affect reproduction capacity. SIMPONI should be given to a pregnant woman only if clearly needed.

Nursing Women: In a pre- and post-natal developmental toxicology study in cynomolgus monkeys golimumab was detected in the breast milk at concentrations that were approximately 350-fold lower than the maternal serum concentrations.

It is not known whether golimumab is excreted in human milk or absorbed systemically after ingestion. Because many drugs and immunoglobulins are excreted in human milk, and because of the potential for adverse reactions in nursing infants from SIMPONI, a decision should be made whether to discontinue nursing or to discontinue the drug, taking into account the importance of the drug to the mother.

Pediatrics (<18 years of age): Specific studies of SIMPONI in pediatric patients have not been conducted.

Geriatrics (≥65 years of age): In the Phase 3 studies in RA, PsA, and AS, no overall differences in AEs, SAEs, and serious infections in patients age 65 or older (N=155:132 in RA, 16 in PsA, 7 in AS) who received SIMPONI were observed compared with younger patients. Because there is a higher incidence of infections in the elderly population in general, caution should be used in treating the elderly.

Renally and Hepatically Impaired: Specific studies of SIMPONI have not been conducted in these patient populations.

Monitoring and Laboratory Tests: There is no known interference between SIMPONI and laboratory tests.

ADVERSE REACTIONS: Adverse Drug Reaction Overview: Safety data from Phase 2 and 3 clinical trials are available from 2578 SIMPONI-treated patients including 1600 with rheumatoid arthritis, 394 with psoriatic arthritis, 353 with ankylosing spondylitis, and 231 with severe persistent asthma. Adverse Drug Reactions (ADRs) observed with SIMPONI are summarized in Table 1 (RA, PsA, and AS).

Upper respiratory tract infection was the most common adverse reaction reported in the combined Phase 3 RA, PsA and AS studies through Week 16, occurring in 7.2% of SIMPONI-treated patients as compared with 5.8% of control-treated patients.

Clinical Trial Adverse Drug Reactions: Because clinical trials are conducted under very specific conditions the adverse reaction rates observed in the clinical trials may not reflect the rates observed in practice and should not be compared to the rates in the clinical trials of another drug. Adverse drug reaction information from clinical trials is useful for identifying drug-related adverse events and for approximating rates.

Table 1 summarizes the adverse drug reactions that occurred at a rate equal to or higher than 1% in SIMPONI groups and at a frequency higher than the placebo group during the placebo-controlled period of the Phase 3 studies in RA, AS and PsA, respectively.

Table 1: SIMPONI

Adverse Drug Reactions Reported by ≥ 1% of Patients in the Phase 3 Trials of RA, PsA, and AS through Week 16[a]

	Placebo ± DMARDs	SIMPONI ± DMARDs
Patients treated	639	1659
Adverse Reaction		
Upper respiratory tract infection (nasopharyngitis, pharyngitis, laryngitis, and rhinitis)	84 (13.1%)	258 (15.6%)
Injection site reaction (injection site erythema, urticaria, induration, pain, bruising, pruritus, irritation, paresthesia)	14 (2.2%)	97 (5.8%)
Viral infections (such as influenza and herpes)	20 (3.1%)	75 (4.5%)
Alanine aminotransferase increased	18 (2.8%)	58 (3.5%)
Hypertension	10 (1.6%)	51 (3.1%)
Aspartate aminotransferase increased	10 (1.6%)	44 (2.7%)
Dizziness	7 (1.1%)	32 (1.9%)
Bronchitis	9 (1.4%)	31 (1.9%)
Superficial fungal infections	8 (1.3%)	31 (1.9%)
Sinusitis	8 (1.3%)	27 (1.6%)
Paraesthesia	3 (0.5%)	27 (1.6%)

(cont'd)

Table 1: SIMPONI *(cont'd)*

Adverse Drug Reactions Reported by ≥ 1% of Patients in the Phase 3 Trials of RA, PsA, and AS through Week 16[a]

	Placebo ± DMARDs	SIMPONI ± DMARDs
Non-serious Allergic reactions	7 (1.1%)	24 (1.4%)
Bacterial infections (such as cellulitis)	6 (0.9%)	24 (1.4%)
Anemia	6 (0.9%)	20 (1.2%)
Pyrexia	4 (0.6%)	20 (1.2%)
Alopecia	4 (0.6%)	18 (1.1%)
Constipation	2 (0.3%)	18 (1.1%)

a Patients may have taken concomitant MTX, sulfasalazine, hydroxychloroquine, low dose corticosteroids (≤10 mg of prednisone/day or equivalent), and/or NSAIDs during the trials).

Less Common Clinical Trial Adverse Drug Reactions (<1%): Adverse drug reactions that occurred at rates less than 1% during the SIMPONI clinical trials included the following events listed by system organ class:
Blood and Lymphatic Disorders: leucopenia, thrombocytopenia, pancytopenia.
Cardiac Disorders: congestive heart failure (new onset or worsening).
Investigations: neutrophil count decreased.
Infections and Infestations: septic shock, sepsis, tuberculosis, histoplasmosis, coccidioidomycosis, pneumocystosis, lower respiratory tract infection (pneumonia), opportunistic infections (invasive fungal infections, bacterial, atypical mycobacterial and protozoal), arthritis bacterial, pyelonephritis, bursitis infective, abscess, and hepatitis B reactivation.
Musculoskeletal and Connective Tissue Disorders: lupus-like syndrome.
Neoplasm Begnign and Malignant: lymphoma, pediatric malignancy*, leukemia*.
Nervous System Disorders: demyelinating disorders.
Skin and Subcutaneous Tissue Disorders: psoriasis: new onset, palmar/plantar, and pustular.
Deaths: During the placebo-controlled Phase 2 and Phase 3 trials in RA, PsA, AS and severe, persistent asthma, there was 1 (0.13%) death among 753 patients in the placebo group and 5 deaths (0.25%) among 2024 patients in the combined SIMPONI group. The most common cause of death among SIMPONI-treated patients (2 out of 5 patients) was sepsis. In the controlled and uncontrolled Phase 2 and 3 RA, PsA, and AS studies, there were 11 deaths among 2347 patients treated with at least one dose of SIMPONI over an exposure period of 3101 patient years (0.35 per 100 patient years), and one death among placebo patients over an exposure period of 344 patient years (0.29 per 100 patient years).
Injection Site Reactions:
- In controlled Phase 3 trials through Week 16 in RA, PsA and AS, 5.8% of SIMPONI-treated patients had injection site reactions compared with 2.2% in control-treated patients. The majority of the injection site reactions were mild and moderate and the most frequent manifestation was injection site erythema. There were no serious injection site reactions.
- In controlled phase 2 and 3 trials in RA, PsA, AS and severe persistent asthma, no patients treated with SIMPONI developed anaphylactic reactions.

Malignancies: (See Warnings and Precautions, Malignancies.)
- Lymphoma: In the controlled portions of clinical trials of TNF-blocking agents including SIMPONI, more cases of lymphoma has been observed among patients receiving anti-TNF treatment compared with patients in the control groups. The incidence of lymphoma per 100 patient-years of follow up in patients with RA, PsA and AS during the controlled portions of Phase 2 and 3 clinical trials was 0.21 (95% CI: 0.03, 0.77) in SIMPONI-treated patients compared with an incidence of 0 (95% CI: 0.00, 0.96) in the control group. In the controlled and uncontrolled portions of these clinical trials, in 2347 SIMPONI-treated patients with a median follow up of 1.4 years, the incidence of lymphoma was 3.8 higher than expected in the general population. Patients with RA and other chronic inflammatory diseases, particularly patients with highly active disease and/or chronic exposure to immunosuppressant therapies, may be at higher risk (up to several fold) than the general population for the development of lymphoma, even in the absence of TNF-blocking therapy.
- Malignancies other than lymphoma: In the controlled portions of the SIMPONI Phase 2 and Phase 3 clinical trials in RA, PsA and AS, the incidence of non-lymphoma malignancies and non-melanoma skin cancer per 100-patient years was not elevated in the SIMPONI group compared with the control group. In the controlled and uncontrolled portions of these trials, the incidence of malignancies other than lymphoma (excluding non-melanoma skin cancer) in SIMPONI-treated patients was similar to that expected in the general population and the most frequently observed malignancies in SIMPONI-treated patients were breast cancer and lung cancer.
- In an exploratory clinical trial involving patients with severe persistent asthma, more patients treated with SIMPONI had malignancies compared with control patients. The significance of this finding in the asthma population is unknown.
- The potential role of TNF-blocking therapy in the development of malignancies is unknown.

Hepatic:
- In controlled Phase 3 trials through Week 16, mild ALT elevations (>1 and <3×ULN) occurred in similar proportions of SIMPONI-treated and control patients in the RA and PsA studies (22.1% to 27.4% of patients); in the AS study, more SIMPONI-treated patients (25.6%) than control patients (3.9%) had mild ALT elevations. Through 1 year of follow-up, the incidence of mild ALT elevations was similar in SIMPONI-treated and control patients in the RA and PsA studies. In the AS study, the incidence of mild ALT elevations was higher in SIMPONI-treated patients than in control patients.
- In the RA and AS studies through Week 16, ALT elevations ≥5×ULN were uncommon and seen in more SIMPONI-treated patients (0.4% to 0.9%) than control patients (0.0%). This trend was not observed in the PsA population. Through 1 year of follow-up, the incidence of ALT elevations ≥5×ULN was similar in both SIMPONI-treated and control patients in the Phase 3 RA, PsA and AS studies. The majority of these elevations were asymptomatic.
- In the controlled Phase 3 trials in RA, PsA and AS through Week 16, the proportions of patients with hepatobiliary adverse events were 0.9% (SIMPONI 50 mg), 0.7% (SIMPONI 100 mg) and 0.6% (placebo). At Week 24, the proportions of patients with hepatobiliary adverse events were 0.9% (SIMPONI 50 mg), 1.3% (SIMPONI 100 mg) and 0.6% (placebo).

Infections: (See Warnings and Precautions, Infections.)
- Upper respiratory tract infection was the most common adverse reaction reported in the combined Phase 3 RA, PsA and AS studies through Week 16, occurring in 7.2% of SIMPONI-treated patients (incidence per patient-year: 0.26; 95% confidence interval; CI: 0.22, 0.31) as compared with 5.8% of control patients (incidence per patient-year: 0.23; 95% CI: 0.17, 0.31). The incidence per patient year (95% CI) of upper respiratory tract infections through 1 year of follow up was 0.23 events (0.21, 0.25) for SIMPONI-treated patients and 0.25 events (0.20, 0.31) for control patients.
- In controlled Phase 3 trials through Week 16 in RA, PsA, and AS, infections were observed in 28.3% of SIMPONI-treated patients (incidence per patient-year: 1.28; 95% CI: 1.18, 1.38) compared with 24.7% of control patients (incidence per patient-year: 1.17; 95% CI: 1.02, 1.33). The incidence per patient year (95% CI) of infections through 1 year of follow up was 1.32 events (1.27, 1.38) for SIMPONI-treated patients and 1.31 events (1.18, 1.44) for control patients.
- In controlled Phase 3 trials through Week 16 in RA, PsA, and AS, serious infections were observed in 1.4% of SIMPONI-treated patients (incidence per patient-year: 0.06; 95% CI: 0.04, 0.08) and 1.3% of control-treated patients (incidence per patient-year: 0.04; 95% CI: 0.02, 0.08). Serious infections observed in SIMPONI-treated patients included sepsis, pneumonia, cellulitis, abscess, and tuberculosis. The incidence per patient year (95% CI) of serious infections through 1 year of follow up was 0.05 events (0.04, 0.06) for SIMPONI-treated patients and 0.06 events (0.04, 0.09) for control patients.

Immune: Autoantibodies:
- Use of TNF-blocking agents has been associated with the formation of autoantibodies and, rarely, in the development of a lupus-like syndrome.
- In Phase 3 trials in RA, PsA, and AS through 1 year of follow up, 4.0% of SIMPONI-treated patients and 2.6% of control patients were newly ANA-positive (at titers of 1:160 or greater). The frequency of anti-dsDNA antibodies at 1 year of follow up in patients anti-dsDNA negative at baseline was uncommon.

Immunogenicity: Antibodies to SIMPONI, nearly all neutralizing in vitro, were detected in 4.3% of SIMPONI-treated patients across the Phase 3 RA, PsA, and AS studies through Week 24. Similar rates were shown across rheumatologic indications. Treatment with concomitant MTX resulted in a lower proportion of patients with antibodies to SIMPONI than patients receiving SIMPONI without MTX (approximately 2% versus 7%, respectively).

* Observed with other TNF blockers, but not observed in clinical studies with golimumab.

The small number of patients positive for antibodies to SIMPONI limits the ability to draw definitive conclusions regarding the relationship between antibodies to SIMPONI and clinical efficacy or safety measures.

DRUG INTERACTIONS: Overview: SIMPONI can be used in combination with methotrexate in adult patients with RA, AS or PsA. Specific drug interaction studies have not been conducted with SIMPONI.
Drug-Drug Interactions: Concurrent Use of SIMPONI with Anakinra or Abatacept: The combination of SIMPONI and anakinra or abatacept is not recommended (see Warnings and Precautions).
Vaccinations: Live vaccines should not be given concurrently with SIMPONI (see Warnings and Precautions, Immunizations).
Methotrexate: Although concomitant use of methotrexate results in higher steady-state trough concentrations of SIMPONI and reduction of its apparent clearance (approximately by 17%) in patients with RA, PsA, or AS, the data do not suggest the need for dose adjustment of either SIMPONI or methotrexate (see Action and Clinical Pharmacology, Pharmacokinetics).
Drug-Herb Interactions: Interactions with herbal products have not been established.

DOSAGE AND ADMINISTRATION: Dosing Considerations: SIMPONI is intended for use under the guidance and supervision of a physician. After an initial training in proper subcutaneous injection technique, an adult patient with rheumatoid arthritis, psoriatic arthritis, or ankylosing spondylitis may self-inject with SIMPONI if a physician determines that it is appropriate and with medical follow-up as necessary.

Comprehensive instructions for the administration of SIMPONI are given in Information for the Patient, Proper Use of This Medication for preparation and giving an injection of SIMPONI. Patients should be instructed to inject the full amount of SIMPONI according to the directions provided in Information for the Patient.
Recommended Dose and Dosage Adjustment: SIMPONI is administered by subcutaneous injection.
Adult Rheumatoid Arthritis Patients: 50 mg of SIMPONI given as a subcutaneous injection once a month, on the same date each month.
Adult Psoriatic Arthritis Patients: 50 mg of SIMPONI given as a subcutaneous injection once a month, on the same date each month.
Adult Ankylosing Spondylitis Patients: 50 mg of SIMPONI given as a subcutaneous injection once a month, on the same date each month.

Available data from RA, PsA, and AS clinical trials suggest that clinical response is usually achieved within 14-16 weeks of treatment (after 4 doses). Continued therapy should be carefully reconsidered in a patient not responding within this time period.
Geriatrics: Pharmacokinetic parameters including apparent clearance were not influenced by age in SIMPONI clinical trials.
Missed Dose: Patients who miss a dose of SIMPONI, should be advised to inject this missed dose as soon as they become aware of it, and then follow with their next scheduled dose (see Information for the Patient, Proper Use of This Medication, autoinjector and pre-filled syringe).
Administration: SIMPONI is supplied as a single-use, sterile solution in a pre-filled syringe and single-use autoinjector administered by subcutaneous injection (see Dosing Considerations).

OVERDOSAGE:
The maximum tolerated dose of SIMPONI has not been established in humans. Single doses up to 10 mg/kg intravenously have been administered in a clinical study without dose-limiting toxicity. In case of overdosage, it is recommended that the patient be monitored for any signs or symptoms of adverse effects and appropriate symptomatic treatment be instituted immediately.

For management of a suspected drug overdose, CPhA recommends that you contact your **regional Poison Control Centre**. See the *CPS* Directory section for a list of Poison Control Centres.

ACTION AND CLINICAL PHARMACOLOGY: Mechanism of Action: Golimumab is a human monoclonal antibody that forms high affinity, stable complexes with both the soluble and transmembrane bioactive forms of human TNF, which prevents the binding of TNF to its receptors. No binding to other TNF superfamily ligands was observed; in particular, golimumab does not bind or neutralize human lymphotoxin. TNFα is synthesized primarily by activated monocytes, macrophages and T-cells as a transmembrane protein that self-associates to form the bioactive homotrimer and is rapidly released from the cell surface by proteolysis. The binding of TNF to either the p55 or p75 TNF receptors leads to the clustering of the receptor cytoplasmic domains and initiates signaling. TNF has been identified as a key sentinel cytokine that is produced in response to various stimuli and subsequently promotes the inflammatory response through activation of the caspase-dependent apoptosis pathway and the transcription factors nuclear factor (NF)-κB and activator protein-1 (AP-1). TNF also modulates the immune response through its role in the organization of immune cells in germinal centers. Elevated expression of TNF has been linked to chronic inflammatory diseases such as rheumatoid arthritis, as well as spondyloarthropathies such as psoriatic arthritis and ankylosing spondylitis, and is an important mediator of the articular inflammation and structural damage that are characteristic of these diseases.
Pharmacodynamics: Nonclinical: The binding of human TNF by golimumab was shown to neutralize TNF-induced cell-surface expression of the adhesion molecules E-selectin, vascular cell adhesion molecule (VCAM)-1 and intercellular adhesion molecule (ICAM)-1 by human endothelial cells. TNF-induced secretion of interleukin (IL)-6, IL-8 and granulocyte-macrophage colony stimulating factor (GM-CSF) by human endothelial cells was also inhibited by golimumab. Consistent with other human IgG1 antibodies, golimumab is capable of binding to Fc receptors and activating complement. However, no golimumab-mediated cell lysis was seen with lipopolysaccharide (LPS)-stimulated human monocytes upon addition of complement or effector cells. In addition, no golimumab-induced apoptosis was detected with LPS-stimulated human peripheral blood mononuclear cells. The effect of golimumab in vivo was tested in a human TNF transgenic mouse model of experimental arthritis. Golimumab treatment produced a statistically significant delay in the onset of clinical symptoms compared with untreated mice, as well as a significant reduction in joint pathology.
Clinical: SIMPONI was effective in modulating select markers of inflammation and bone metabolism across indications. Improvement in C-reactive protein (CRP) levels were observed relative to placebo groups and treatment with SIMPONI resulted in significant reductions from baseline in serum levels of IL-6, ICAM-1, matrix metalloproteinase-3 (MMP-3) and vascular endothelial growth factor (VEGF) compared to control treatment. In addition, levels of TNFα were significantly reduced in RA and AS patients and levels of IL-8 were reduced in PsA patients. These changes were observed at the first assessment (Week 4) after the initial SIMPONI administration and were generally sustained through Weeks 14 and/or 24. SIMPONI with or without methotrexate (MTX) resulted in significant changes in serum levels of select markers of bone metabolism [increases in osteocalcin and procollagen type I N-terminal propeptide (PINP) and decreases in deoxy-pyridinolin (DPD) levels] at Week 4. All of these biomarker changes are consistent with an improvement in the disease processes with reduced inflammation, increased bone growth and decreased bone resorption.
Pharmacokinetics: Following SC administration of SIMPONI to healthy subjects or patients with RA, the median time to reach maximum serum concentrations (T_{max}) ranged from 2 to 6 days. SIMPONI exhibited dose-proportional pharmacokinetics in patients with RA over the dose range of 0.1 to 10.0 mg/kg following single intravenous (IV) dose. Following a single IV administration over the same dose range in patients with RA, mean systemic clearance of SIMPONI was estimated to be 4.9 to 6.7 mL/day/kg, and mean volume of distribution ranged from 58 to 126 mL/kg. The volume of distribution for SIMPONI indicates that SIMPONI is distributed primarily in the circulatory system with limited extravascular distribution. Median terminal half-life values were estimated to be approximately 2 weeks in healthy subjects and patients with RA, PsA, or AS. Following SC administration of SIMPONI in healthy subjects, the following PK parameters were obtained as shown in Table 2.

Table 2: SIMPONI

Pharmacokinetic Parameters of SIMPONI Following a Single Subcutaneous Injection of 50 mg SIMPONI in Healthy Subjects

Pharmacokinetic Parameter	SIMPONI 50 mg (n=26)	SIMPONI 100 mg (n=211)
Maximum observed serum concentration (C_{max}, μg/mL)	2.7±0.9	6.2±2.9
Time to reach C_{max} (T_{max}, day)[a]	5 (2, 10)	4 (1, 10)
Area under the curve from time 0 to infinity (AUC_{inf}, μg·day/mL)	49.4±15.3	99.6±42.5

(cont'd)

Table 2: SIMPONI *(cont'd)*

Pharmacokinetic Parameters of SIMPONI Following a Single Subcutaneous Injection of 50 mg SIMPONI in Healthy Subjects

Pharmacokinetic Parameter	SIMPONI 50 mg (n=26)	SIMPONI 100 mg (n=211)
Terminal half-life ($T_{1/2}$, day)	11±3	12±3
Apparent systemic clearance (CL/F, mL/day/kg)	17.1±9.0	15.1±6.3
Apparent volume of distribution (V_z/F, mL/kg)	252±71	247±106

[a] Mean±SD values are shown for all PK parameters except for T_{max} which is presented as the median value with the range of minimum and maximum.

By cross-study comparisons of mean AUC_{inf} values following an IV or SC administration of SIMPONI, the absolute bioavailability of SC SIMPONI was estimated to be 44% to 58%.

When 50 mg SIMPONI was administered SC to patients with RA, PsA or AS every 4 weeks, serum concentrations reached steady state by Week 12. With concomitant use of methotrexate, treatment with 50 mg SIMPONI SC every 4 weeks resulted in a median steady-state trough serum concentration of approximately 0.6 µg/mL in patients with active RA despite methotrexate therapy, and approximately 0.5 µg/mL in patients with active PsA and approximately 0.6 µg/mL in patients with AS. Patients with RA, PsA or AS who did not receive concomitant use of methotrexate had approximately 30% lower steady-state trough concentrations of SIMPONI than those who received SIMPONI with methotrexate. Population pharmacokinetic analysis in patients with RA also indicated that concomitant use of methotrexate could reduce the apparent clearance of SIMPONI by 17.1%. However, concomitant use of nonsteroidal anti-inflammatory drugs, oral corticosteroids or sulfasalazine was not found to influence the apparent clearance of SIMPONI.

Population pharmacokinetic analyses showed there was a trend toward higher apparent clearance of SIMPONI with increasing weight. As a result, patients with heavier weight tend to have lower steady-state trough concentrations of SIMPONI. However, across the RA, PsA, and AS populations, a treatment benefit of golimumab 50 mg and 100 mg was observed for all subgroups by weight quartiles with no meaningful differences in clinical efficacy among these subgroups. Therefore, there is no need to adjust the dosage of SIMPONI based on a patient's weight. No gender-related pharmacokinetic differences were observed with SIMPONI after correction for patients' body weights. Pharmacokinetic parameters of SIMPONI were not influenced by age in adult patients. Patients with age ≥65 years had apparent clearance of SIMPONI similar to patients with age <65 years. No ethnicity-related pharmacokinetic differences were observed between Caucasians and Asians.

Patients who developed anti-SIMPONI antibodies generally had low trough steady-state serum concentrations of SIMPONI.

Special Populations and Conditions: Pediatrics: Specific studies of SIMPONI in pediatric patients have not been conducted.

Geriatrics: Pharmacokinetic parameters of SIMPONI were not influenced by age in adult patients. Patients with age ≥65 years had apparent clearance of SIMPONI similar to patients with age <65 years.

Gender: No gender-related pharmacokinetic differences were observed with SIMPONI after correction for patients' body weights.

Race: No ethnicity-related pharmacokinetic differences were observed between Caucasians and Asians.

Hepatic Insufficiency: SIMPONI has not been studied in this patient population. No dose recommendation can be made.

Renal Insufficiency: SIMPONI has not been studied in this patient population. No dose recommendation can be made.

STORAGE AND STABILITY: The shelf-life of SIMPONI is 24 months.

Store SIMPONI refrigerated at 2 to 8°C. Keep the product in original carton until time of use to protect from light. Do not freeze. Do not shake.

Keep out of reach of children.

SPECIAL HANDLING INSTRUCTIONS: See Information for the Patient, Proper Use of This Medication for comprehensive instructions for the use, handling, and disposal of the autoinjector and the pre-filled syringe.

INFORMATION FOR THE PATIENT: Published in e-CPS, available by subscription at www.e-cps.ca.

DOSAGE FORMS, COMPOSITION AND PACKAGING: SIMPONI is supplied as a single-use, sterile solution in a Type 1 glass syringe with a fixed stainless steel needle. The syringe is contained in a single-use autoinjector or fitted with a passive safety guard. The syringe is stoppered with a coated stopper and the needle is covered with a needle shield to prevent leakage of the solution through the needle and to protect the needle during handling prior to administration. The fixed needle is a 5-bevel, 27G, half-inch stainless steel needle. The needle shields are manufactured using a dry natural rubber containing latex (see Warnings and Precautions, Immunogenicity, Allergic Reactions, Latex Sensitivity).

Each mL of SIMPONI contains 100 mg of golimumab, 0.87 mg L-histidine and L-histidine hydrochloride, 41.0 mg sorbitol, 0.15 mg polysorbate 80, and Water for Injection. There is one strength of SIMPONI available: 50 mg of golimumab in 0.5 mL.

Autoinjector: Each single-use autoinjector contains 50 mg golimumab per 0.5 mL in an autoinjector. SIMPONI is supplied as a sterile solution in a Type 1 glass syringe with a fixed stainless steel needle. This syringe is contained in a single-use autoinjector. The needle shields are manufactured from dry natural rubber containing latex (see Warnings and Precautions, Immunogenicity, Allergic Reactions, Latex Sensitivity). Packs of 1 autoinjector.

Pre-Filled Syringes: Each single-use pre-filled syringe of sterile solution contains 50 mg golimumab per 0.5 mL syringe. SIMPONI is supplied as a sterile solution in a Type 1 glass syringe with a fixed stainless steel needle. The needle shields are manufactured from dry natural rubber containing latex (see Warnings and Precautions, Immunogenicity, Allergic Reactions, Latex Sensitivity). Packs of 1 pre-filled syringe.

SIMPONI is packaged in a single-use outer carton.

Simulect® ℞
basiliximab
Immunosuppressant

Novartis Pharmaceuticals

Date of Preparation: September 1, 2000
Date of Revision: May 17, 2006

SUMMARY PRODUCT INFORMATION:

Route of Administration	Dosage Form/ Strength	Clinically Relevant Nonmedicinal Ingredients
Injection	20 mg sterile lyophilized powder	None

SIMULECT is a potent drug. This drug should only be used by physicians experienced in immunosuppression therapy and management of organ transplantation patients in a setting where full resuscitation facilities are immediately available.

INDICATIONS AND CLINICAL USE: SIMULECT (basiliximab) is indicated for the prophylaxis of acute organ rejection in de novo renal transplantation and is to be used concomitantly with Neoral (cyclosporine for microemulsion) and corticosteroid-based immunosuppression.

CONTRAINDICATIONS: SIMULECT (basiliximab) is contraindicated in patients with known hypersensitivity to basiliximab, mouse cell proteins or any other component of the formulation.

WARNINGS AND PRECAUTIONS: General: SIMULECT (basiliximab) should be prescribed only by physicians who are experienced in the use of immunosuppressive therapy following organ transplantation.

Patients receiving SIMULECT should be managed in facilities equipped and staffed with adequate laboratory and supportive medical resources including medications for the treatment of severe hypersensitivity reactions.

The addition of agents other than Neoral (cyclosporine for microemulsion) and corticosteroids to SIMULECT therapy may increase the risk of overimmunosuppression.

Please note that following initiation of treatment with NEORAL, due to the different bioavailabilities of the different oral cyclosporine formulations, patients should not be converted to any other oral formulation of cyclosporine without appropriate monitoring of cyclosporine blood concentrations, serum creatinine levels and blood pressure. This does not apply to the conversion between NEORAL soft gelatine capsule and NEORAL oral solution as these two dosage forms are bioequivalent.

It is therefore important that prescribers, pharmacists and patients be aware that substitution of NEORAL with any other oral formulation of cyclosporine is not recommended as this may lead to alterations in cyclosporine blood concentrations. For this reason, it might be appropriate to prescribe by brand.

Immune: Severe acute (less than 24 hours) hypersensitivity reactions have been observed both on initial exposure to SIMULECT and on reexposure to a subsequent course of therapy. These included anaphylactoid type reactions such as urticaria, pruritus, sneezing, hypotension, tachycardia, dyspnea, bronchospasm, pulmonary edema, and respiratory failure (<1/1000 patients). If severe hypersensitivity occurs, therapy with SIMULECT should be permanently discontinued and no further dose should be administered.

Therefore, physicians prescribing SIMULECT for a second course of therapy should be fully aware of the risks of anaphylactic reaction and should exercise caution. There is accumulating evidence that a subgroup of patients is at increased risk of developing hypersensitivity reactions. These are patients in whom, following the initial administration of SIMULECT, the concomitant immunosuppression was discontinued prematurely, for example, due to abandoned transplantation or due to early loss of the graft. Acute hypersensitivity reactions were observed on re-administration of SIMULECT for a subsequent transplantation in some of these patients.

Individual cases of suspected cytokine release syndrome (CRS) have been reported during post-marketing experience with SIMULECT (see Adverse Reactions, Post-Market Adverse Drug Reactions). Review of the clinical symptoms for each of the cases does not support the diagnosis of CRS. However, the contribution of SIMULECT could not be excluded.

Special Populations: Pregnant Women: There are no data in pregnant women. SIMULECT (basiliximab) should not be given to pregnant women except in cases where the potential benefit for the mother outweighs the potential risk for the fetus.

Nursing Women: There are no data in lactating women. Since basiliximab is an immunoglobulin G ($IgG_{1\kappa}$) antibody, it may cross the human placenta and may be excreted in human milk. Women receiving SIMULECT should not breast feed for 4 months following the last dose.

Pediatrics: No adequate and well-controlled studies have been completed in pediatric patients. Safety and efficacy in pediatric patients have not been established and pharmacokinetic data is very limited (see Action and Clinical Pharmacology, Pharmacokinetics). No studies have been performed in neonates or children aged less than two years.

Geriatrics: Controlled clinical trials of SIMULECT have included a small number of patients 65 years and older (SIMULECT 15; placebo 19). From the available data comparing SIMULECT and placebo-treated patients, the adverse event profile in patients ≥65 years of age is not different from patients <65 years of age and no initial age-related dosing adjustment is required. Caution must be used in giving immunosuppressive drugs to elderly patients.

Use in Women of Childbearing Potential: Women of childbearing potential should use effective contraception before beginning SIMULECT therapy, during therapy and for 4 months after completion of SIMULECT therapy.

ADVERSE REACTIONS: Clinical Trial Adverse Drug Reactions: Because clinical trials are conducted under very specific conditions the adverse reaction rates observed in the clinical trials may not reflect the rates observed in practice and should not be compared to the rates in the clinical trials of another drug. Adverse drug reaction information from clinical trials is useful for identifying drug-related adverse events and for approximating rates.

SIMULECT (basiliximab) does not appear to add to the background of adverse events seen in organ transplant patients as a consequence of their underlying disease and the concurrent administration of immunosuppressants and other medications. In two controlled, double-blind, multicenter trials, the pattern of adverse events in 363 SIMULECT-treated patients was indistinguishable from that of 359 placebo-treated patients.

The cumulative incidence of adverse events which occurred in ≥6% in either treatment group during the first 12 months post-transplantation for the pooled studies is summarized in Table 1.

Serious adverse events occurred with similar incidence and profile in both the SIMULECT and placebo treatment groups (SIMULECT 59%, placebo 63% overall).

The rates of malignancies, reported infections, serious infections and infectious organisms were similar in the SIMULECT and placebo treatment groups. No specific SIMULECT-related risk was identified.

Incidence of Malignant Neoplasms: The incidence of malignancies among the 722 patients in the two 12-month controlled trials was not significantly different between the SIMULECT and placebo-treatment groups, and compared to the incidence reported in the literature for renal allograft recipients. Overall, lymphoma/lymphoproliferative disease occurred in 1 patient (0.3%) in the SIMULECT group compared with 2 patients (0.6%) in the placebo group. Other malignancies were reported among 5 patients (1.4%) in the SIMULECT group compared with 7 patients (1.9%) in patients treated with placebo. No differences were found in the incidence of malignancies and lymphoproliferative disease between SIMULECT 7% (21/295) and placebo 7% (21/291) in a pooled analysis of two five-year extension studies.

Incidence of Infectious Episodes: Cytomegalovirus infection was reported in 14% of SIMULECT-treated patients and 18% of placebo-treated patients. The rates of infections (SIMULECT 81%, placebo 81%), serious infections (SIMULECT 27.5%, placebo 27.3%) and infectious organisms were similar in the SIMULECT and placebo treatment groups.

In a pooled analysis of two five-year extension studies, the incidence and cause of death remained similar in both treatment groups (SIMULECT 15%, placebo 11%). The primary cause of death being cardiac-related disorders (SIMULECT 5%, placebo 4%).

Table 1: SIMULECT

Adverse Events in Controlled Clinical Trials (≥6%)

Organ System/ Adverse Experience	SIMULECT (N=363) %	PLACEBO (N=359) %
Body as a Whole		
Asthenia	35 (10%)	28 (8%)
Chest Pain	25 (7%)	27 (8%)
Drug Level Increased	21 (6%)	26 (7%)
Fatigue	30 (8%)	29 (8%)
Infection Viral	44 (12%)	54 (15%)
Edema	78 (21%)	71 (20%)
Edema Generalised	25 (7%)	24 (7%)
Edema—Legs	40 (11%)	29 (8%)
Edema—Peripheral	104 (29%)	109 (30%)
Pain	152 (42%)	141 (39%)
Pyrexia	73 (20%)	87 (24%)
Cardiovascular		
Hypertension	97 (27%)	93 (26%)

(cont'd)

Table 1: SIMULECT *(cont'd)*
Adverse Events in Controlled Clinical Trials (≥6%)

Organ System/ Adverse Experience	SIMULECT (N=363) %	PLACEBO (N=359) %
Hypotension	30 (8%)	38 (11%)
Nervous System		
Dizziness	40 (11%)	33 (9%)
Headache	87 (24%)	80 (22%)
Paraesthesia	27 (7%)	31 (9%)
Tremor	52 (14%)	66 (18%)
Gastro-Intestinal System		
Addomen Enlarged	28 (8%)	27 (8%)
Abdominal Pain	76 (21%)	97 (27%)
Constipation	175 (48%)	177 (49%)
Diarrhea	75 (21%)	68 (19%)
Dyspepsia	50 (14%)	64 (18%)
Moniliasis	36 (10%)	29 (8%)
Nausea	123 (34%)	143 (40%)
Vomiting	73 (20%)	79 (22%)
Heart Rate and Rhythm Disorders		
Tachycardia	28 (8%)	21 (6%)
Metabolic and Nutritional		
Acidosis	37 (10%)	46 (13%)
Dehydration	22 (6%)	20 (6%)
Hypercholesterolemia	41 (11%)	38 (11%)
Hyperglycemia	58 (16%)	43 (12%)
Hyperkalemia	80 (22%)	85 (24%)
Hyperlipaemia	31 (9%)	25 (7%)
Hyperuricemia	49 (13%)	52 (14%)
Hypocalcemia	39 (11%)	41 (11%)
Hypokalemia	66 (18%)	85 (24%)
Hypomagnesemia	34 (9%)	43 (12%)
Hypophosphatemia	45 (12%)	46 (13%)
Weight Increase	40 (11%)	46 (13%)
Musculo-Skeletal		
Arthralgia	21 (6%)	23 (6%)
Back Pain	36 (10%)	48 (13%)
Cramps	33 (9%)	28 (8%)
Pain Leg(s)	46 (13%)	40 (11%)
Psychiatric		
Insomnia	86 (24%)	102 (28%)
Red Blood Cell		
Anemia	93 (26%)	101 (28%)
Polycythaemia	24 (7%)	16 (4%)
Respiratory System		
Chest Sounds Abnormal	29 (8%)	25 (7%)
Coughing	41 (11%)	37 (10%)
Dyspnea	59 (16%)	50 (14%)
Pharyngitis	35 (10%)	29 (8%)
Rhinitis	38 (10%)	39 (11%)
Sinusitis	26 (7%)	23 (6%)

(cont'd)

Table 1: SIMULECT *(cont'd)*
Adverse Events in Controlled Clinical Trials (≥6%)

Organ System/ Adverse Experience	SIMULECT (N=363) %	PLACEBO (N=359) %
Upper Respiratory Tract Infection	71 (20%)	64 (18%)
Skin and Appendages Disorders		
Acne	53 (15%)	56 (16%)
Herpes Simplex	30 (8%)	32 (9%)
Post-operative Wound Complication	58 (16%)	63 (18%)
Pruritus	29 (8%)	31 (9%)
Rash	24 (7%)	30 (8%)
Skin Disorder	29 (8%)	25 (7%)
Urinary System		
Bladder Disorders	34 (9%)	38 (11%)
Dysuria	36 (10%)	30 (8%)
Hematuria	33 (9%)	41 (11%)
NPN Increased	36 (10%)	23 (6%)
Oliguria	25 (7%)	25 (7%)
Surgery	21 (6%)	27 (8%)
Urinary Tract Infection	168 (46%)	166 (46%)

Post-Market Adverse Drug Reactions: During post-marketing experience with SIMULECT very rare cases (1/10 000) of suspected cytokine release syndrome have been reported.

Recent reports of anaphylaxis and other infusion-related adverse events suggest that patients receiving subsequent courses of therapy with SIMULECT (for example, among those receiving a second transplant) are at higher risk of these events.

DRUG INTERACTIONS: Overview: Because SIMULECT is an immunoglobulin, no metabolic interactions are to be expected. Therefore, no formal drug-drug interaction studies have been conducted.

In controlled clinical trials a limited number of patients, treated with the recommended doses of SIMULECT, have also been administered azathioprine, mycophenolate mofetil, tacrolimus or antibody therapy such as OKT_3 or ATG/ALG with no increase in adverse events in SIMULECT patients as compared to placebo patients.

Azathioprine and Mycophenolate Mofetil: During the first 3 months post-transplantation, 10.5% of patients in the SIMULECT group and 21.7% of patients in the placebo group were treated with azathioprine or mycophenolate mofetil for at least one month. There was no increase in adverse events or infections in the SIMULECT group compared to the placebo group, and no patients in the SIMULECT group experienced lymphoma or any other malignancy during the first 12 months post-transplantation.

Antibody Therapy: During the first 3 months post-transplantation, 14% of patients in the SIMULECT group and 27% of patients in the placebo group received augmented immunosuppression with antibody therapy (Orthoclone OKT_3 or ATG/ALG) with no increase in adverse events or infections in the SIMULECT group compared to the placebo group. No patients in the SIMULECT group who received antibody therapy experienced lymphoma or any other malignancy during the first 12 months post-transplantation.

Of 172 renal transplantation patients treated with SIMULECT in one clinical trial, the incidence of human anti-murine antibody (HAMA) was 3.5% (6/172); since 4 of the 6 patients positive for HAMA also received Orthoclone OKT_3, the incidence may be as low as 1.2% (2/172). Analysis of rejection outcome in patients treated with Orthoclone OKT_3 demonstrates a lower rate of graft loss in the SIMULECT (7/47=15%) than placebo-treated patients (16/71=23%), indicating the use of SIMULECT has no deleterious effect upon the subsequent efficacy of Orthoclone OKT_3. The available clinical data on the use of Orthoclone OKT_3 in patients previously treated with SIMULECT suggests that subsequent use of Orthoclone OKT_3 or other murine anti-lymphocyte antibody preparations is not precluded.

The use of SIMULECT does not preclude subsequent treatment with murine anti-lymphocytic antibody preparations.

DOSAGE AND ADMINISTRATION: Reconstituted SIMULECT (basiliximab) can be administered either as an intravenous infusion over 20 to 30 minutes or as a bolus injection.

Recommended Dose and Dosage Adjustment: The recommended total dose is 40 mg, given in two doses of 20 mg each. The first 20 mg dose should be given within 2 hours prior to transplantation surgery. The second 20 mg dose should be given 4 days after transplantation.

Administration: Reconstitution: Instructions for Use and Handling:

Reconstitution Table

Vial Size	Diluent Volume to be Added to Vial	Approximate Available Volume	Actual Concentration
20 mg	5 mL	5 mL	4 mg/mL

To prepare the infusion/injection solution add 5 mL of Sterile Water for Injection to the vial containing the SIMULECT lyophilized powder. **Care must be taken during reconstitution to maintain sterility because the formulation contains no antimicrobial preservatives.** Shake the vial gently to dissolve the powder. The sterile product is stable at 2-8°C for 24 hours or at room temperature for 4 hours. Discard the reconstituted solution if not used within 24 hours.

OVERDOSAGE:
In clinical studies SIMULECT (basiliximab) has been administered to humans in single doses of up to 60 mg and multiple doses of up to 150 mg over 24 days with no untoward acute effects.

In a 39-week study in rhesus monkeys followed by a 13-week recovery period, the no observable effect level was set at the highest dose level of 24 mg/kg week, leading to exposure values greater than 1000-times the systemic exposure (AUC) in renal transplant patients given the recommended clinical dose together with concomitant immunosuppressive therapy.

For management of a suspected drug overdose, CPhA recommends that you contact your **regional Poison Control Centre**. See the *CPS* Directory section for a list of Poison Control Centres.

ACTION AND CLINICAL PHARMACOLOGY: Mechanism of Action: SIMULECT (basiliximab) is a chimeric murine/human monoclonal antibody (IgG_{1k}) that is selectively directed against the interleukin-2 receptor alpha-chain (IL-2R alpha, also known as CD25 antigen), which is expressed on the surface of T-lymphocytes in response to antigenic challenge. SIMULECT specifically binds to the CD25 antigen on activated T-lymphocytes expressing the high affinity interleukin-2 receptor and thereby prevents binding of interleukin-2, the signal for T-cell proliferation.

Complete and consistent blocking of the interleukin-2 receptor is maintained as long as serum basiliximab levels exceed 0.2 μg/mL. As concentration falls below this level, expression of the CD25 antigen returns to pretherapy values within 1-2 weeks. Cytokine release syndrome or myelosuppression was not observed during SIMULECT administration in the pivotal transplantation trials.

Pharmacokinetics: See Table 2.

Table 2: SIMULECT

Summary of Basiliximab's Pharmacokinetic Parameters in Patients Undergoing Kidney Transplantation

	C_{max}	$t_{½}$ (h)	Clearance	Volume of distribution
Single dose mean	7.1±5.1 mg/L	7.2±3.2 days	41±19 mL/h	8.6±4.1 L

Single-dose and multiple-dose pharmacokinetic studies have been conducted in patients undergoing kidney transplantation. Cumulative doses have ranged from 15 mg up to 150 mg.

Peak serum concentration following intravenous infusion of 20 mg over 30 minutes is 7.1±5.1 mg/L. There is a dose-proportional increase in C_{max} and AUC up to the highest tested single dose of 60 mg.

The volume of distribution at steady state is 8.6±4.1 L. The extent and degree of distribution to various body compartments has not been fully studied. In vitro studies using human tissues indicate that SIMULECT binds only to lymphocytes and macrophages/monocytes. The terminal half-life is 7.2±3.2 days. Total body clearance is 41±19 mL/h.

No clinically relevant influence of body weight or gender on distribution volume or clearance has been observed in adult patients. Elimination half-life was not influenced by age (20-69 years), gender or race.

In a clinical trial with 23 adult liver transplant patients, the disposition of SIMULECT was characterized by a steady-state distribution volume of 7.5±2.5 L, half-life of 4.1±2.1 days and clearance of 75±24 mL/h. Contributing to clearance were drug loss via drained ascites fluid and post-operative bleeding. Offsetting the faster drug clearance was a lower receptor-saturating-concentration threshold of 0.1 μg/mL in this population. Hence, the duration of IL-2R alpha blockade at a given SIMULECT dose level is similar to that seen in adult renal transplant patients.

Special Populations and Conditions: Pediatrics: Safety and efficacy in pediatric patients have not been established and pharmacokinetic data is very limited (see Warnings and Precautions). No data exist on the use of SIMULECT (basiliximab) in neonates or infants aged less than 2 years. In one clinical study in 12 pediatric de novo renal transplant patients aged 2-11 years (n=8), the volume of distribution at steady state was 5.2±2.8 L, half-life was 11.5±6.3 days and clearance was 17±6 mL/h.

Clearance and volume were not influenced by age (2-11 years), body weight (9-37 kg) or body surface area (0.44-1.20 m²) in this age group. The disposition of SIMULECT in pediatric renal transplant patients was characterized by an average 50% lower clearance compared to adult patients. In adolescents aged 12-15 (n=4), the volume of distribution at steady-state was 10.1±7.6L, half-life was 7.2±3.6 days and clearance was 45±25 mL/h. Disposition in adolescents was similar to that in adult renal transplant patients. The relationship between serum concentration and receptor saturation was assessed in two patients (2 and 12 years) and was similar to that characterized in adult renal transplant patients. No adequate and well-controlled studies have been completed in pediatric patients.

STORAGE AND STABILITY: Store in its original container at 2-8°C. It is recommended that after reconstitution the colourless, clear to opalescent solution should be used immediately. If not used immediately, it is stable at 2-8°C for 24 hours or at room temperature for 4 hours. Discard the reconstituted solution if not used within 24 hours.

Shipping and storage should be under refrigerated conditions (2-8°C).

SPECIAL HANDLING INSTRUCTIONS: Instructions for Use and Handling:

Reconstitution Table			
Vial Size	Diluent Volume to be Added to Vial	Approximate available Volume	Actual Concentration
20 mg	5 mL	5 mL	4 mg/mL

To prepare the infusion/injection solution add 5 mL of Sterile Water for Injection to the vial containing the SIMULECT lyophilized powder. **Care must be taken during reconstitution to maintain sterility because the formulation contains no antimicrobial preservatives.** Shake the vial gently to dissolve the powder. The sterile product is stable at 2-8°C for 24 hours or at room temperature for 4 hours. Discard the reconstituted solution if not used within 24 hours.

The reconstituted solution is isotonic and may be given as a bolus injection or diluted to a volume of 50 mL or greater with normal saline or dextrose 5 % for infusion.

Since no data are available on the compatibility of SIMULECT with other intravenous substances, SIMULECT should not be mixed with other medications/substances and should always be given through a separate infusion line.

Compatibility with the following infusion sets has been verified:

Infusion Bag: Baxter minibag NaC1 0.9%.

Infusion Sets: Luer Lock, H. Noolens; Sterile vented i.v. set, Abbott; Infusion set, Codan; Infusomat, Braun; Infusionsgerat R 87 plus, Ohmeda; Lifecare 5000 Plumset Microdrip, Abbott; Vented basic set, Baxter; Flashball device, Baxter; Vented primary administration set, Imed.

Compatibility with other commercial devices has not been tested.

DOSAGE FORMS, COMPOSITION AND PACKAGING: Each vial of sterile, lyophilized powder for injection/infusion contains: basiliximab 20 mg (after reconstitution with 5 mL of Sterile Water for Injection). Nonmedicinal ingredients: disodium hydrogen phosphate, glycine, mannitol, potassium dihydrogen phosphate, sodium chloride and sucrose. Preservative-free. Glass vials, packages of 1. Sterile Water for Injection is not supplied.

(Shown in Product Identification Section)

Simvastatin ℞

CPhA Monograph

see *HMG-CoA Reductase Inhibitors*

Sinemet® ℞

levodopa—carbidopa

Antiparkinson Agent

Merck Frosst

Date of Revision: July 1, 2010

SUMMARY PRODUCT INFORMATION:

Route of Administration	Dosage Form/ Strength	Clinically Relevant Nonmedicinal Ingredients
Oral	Tablet 100 mg/10 mg, 100 mg/25 mg, 250 mg/25 mg	Pregelatinized starch For a complete listing, see Dosage Forms, Composition and Packaging.

INDICATIONS AND CLINICAL USE: SINEMET (levodopa and carbidopa) is indicated for the treatment of Parkinson's disease.

SINEMET is not recommended for the treatment of drug-induced extrapyramidal reactions.

Although the administration of carbidopa permits control of Parkinson's disease with much lower doses of levodopa, there is no conclusive evidence at present that this is beneficial other than reducing nausea and vomiting, permitting more rapid titration, and providing a somewhat smoother response to levodopa. Carbidopa does not decrease adverse reactions due to central effects of levodopa. By permitting more levodopa to reach the brain, particularly when nausea and vomiting is not a dose-limiting factor, certain adverse CNS effects, e.g., dyskinesias, may occur at lower dosages and sooner during therapy with SINEMET than with levodopa.

Pediatrics (<18 years of age): The safety and effectiveness of SINEMET in patients under 18 years of age has not been established.

CONTRAINDICATIONS:

- Patients who are hypersensitive to this drug or to any ingredient in the formulation. For a complete listing, see Dosage Forms, Composition and Packaging.
- Nonselective monoamine oxidase (MAO) inhibitors are contraindicated for use with SINEMET (levodopa and carbidopa). These inhibitors must be discontinued at least two weeks prior to initiating therapy with SINEMET. SINEMET may be administered concomitantly with a MAO inhibitor with selectivity for MAO type B (e.g. selegiline HCl) (see Drug Interactions, Drug-Drug Interactions, Psychoactive Drugs) at the manufacturer's recommended dose which maintains selectivity for MAO type B.
- SINEMET should not be administered to patients with clinical or laboratory evidence of uncompensated cardiovascular, endocrine, hematologic, hepatic, pulmonary (including bronchial asthma), or renal disease; or to patients with narrow angle glaucoma.
- As with levodopa, SINEMET should not be given when administration of a sympathomimetic amine is contraindicated (e.g., epinephrine, norepinephrine or isoproterenol).
- Because levodopa may activate a malignant melanoma, SINEMET should not be used in patients with suspicious, undiagnosed skin lesions or a history of melanoma.

WARNINGS AND PRECAUTIONS:

Serious Warnings and Precautions

Sudden Onset of Sleep

Patients receiving treatment with SINEMET (levodopa and carbidopa) and other dopaminergic agents have reported suddenly falling asleep while engaged in activities of daily living, including the driving of a car, which has sometimes resulted in accidents. Although some of the patients reported somnolence while on SINEMET, others perceived that they had no warning signs, such as excessive drowsiness, and believed that they were alert immediately prior to the event.

Physicians should alert patients of the reported cases of sudden onset of sleep, bearing in mind that these events are **not** limited to initiation of therapy. Patients should also be advised that sudden onset of sleep has occurred without warning signs and should be specifically asked about factors that may increase the risk with SINEMET such as concomitant medications or the presence of sleep disorders. Given the reported cases of somnolence and sudden onset of sleep (not necessarily preceded by somnolence), physicians should caution patients about the risk of operating hazardous machinery, including driving motor vehicles, while taking SINEMET. If drowsiness or sudden onset of sleep should occur, patients should be informed to refrain from driving or operating machines and to immediately contact their physician.

Episodes of falling asleep while engaged in activities of daily living have also been reported in patients taking other dopaminergic agents, therefore, symptoms may not be alleviated by substituting these products.

While dose reduction clearly reduces the degree of somnolence, there is insufficient information to establish that dose reduction will eliminate episodes of falling asleep while engaged in activities of daily living.

Currently, the precise cause of this event is unknown. It is known that many Parkinson's disease patients experience alterations in sleep architecture, which results in excessive daytime sleepiness or spontaneous dozing, and that dopaminergic agents can also induce sleepiness.

General: When patients already receiving levodopa are switched to SINEMET, levodopa must be discontinued for at least 12 hours or more before SINEMET is started. SINEMET should be substituted at a dosage that will provide approximately 20% of the previous levodopa dosage (see Dosage and Administration).

Patients who are taking SINEMET should be instructed not to take additional levodopa unless it is prescribed by the physician.

Periodic evaluations of hepatic, hematopoietic, cardiovascular and renal function are recommended during extended therapy with SINEMET (levodopa and carbidopa).

Physical Activity: Patients who improve while on therapy with SINEMET should increase physical activities gradually, with caution, consistent with other medical considerations such as the presence of osteoporosis or phlebothrombosis.

Cardiovascular: Care should be exercised in administering SINEMET to patients with a history of myocardial infarction or who have atrial, nodal, or ventricular arrhythmias. In such patients, cardiac function should be monitored with particular care during the period of initial dosage adjustment in a facility with provisions for intensive cardiac care.

Gastrointestinal: SINEMET should be administered cautiously to patients with a history of peptic ulcer disease due to the possibility of upper gastrointestinal hemorrhage.

Neurologic: The levodopa induced involuntary movements and "on and off" phenomenon may appear earlier with combination therapy.

As with levodopa, SINEMET may cause involuntary movements and mental disturbances. These reactions are thought to be due to increased brain dopamine following administration of levodopa. Because carbidopa permits more levodopa to reach the brain and thus, more dopamine to be formed, dyskinesias may occur at lower dosages and sooner with SINEMET than with levodopa. The occurrence of dyskinesias may require dosage reduction.

SINEMET should be used cautiously in patients who have a history of seizures or have conditions associated with seizure or have a lowered seizure threshold.

Neuroleptic Malignant Syndrome: A symptom complex resembling the neuroleptic malignant syndrome including muscular rigidity, elevated body temperature, altered consciousness, mental changes, autonomic instability and increased serum creatine phosphokinase has been reported in association with rapid dose reduction, withdrawal of, or changes in antiparkinsonian therapy. Therefore, patients should be observed carefully when the dosage of SINEMET is reduced abruptly or discontinued, especially if the patient is receiving neuroleptics.

Psychomotor Performance: Certain side effects that have been reported with SINEMET may affect some patients' ability to drive or operate machinery.

Given the reported cases of somnolence and sudden onset of sleep (not necessarily preceded by somnolence), physicians should caution patients about the risk of operating hazardous machinery, including driving motor vehicles, while taking SINEMET. If drowsiness or sudden onset of sleep should occur, patients should be informed to refrain from driving or operating machines and to immediately contact their physician (see Warnings and Precautions, Boxed Serious Warnings and Precautions, Sudden Onset of Sleep).

Ophthalmologic: Use in Patients with Glaucoma: Pupillary dilatation and activation of latent Horner's syndrome have been reported during levodopa treatment. Patients with chronic wide angle glaucoma should therefore be treated cautiously with SINEMET. The intraocular pressure should be well controlled and the patient monitored carefully for changes in intraocular pressure during therapy.

Peri-Operative Considerations: If general anesthesia is required, therapy with SINEMET may be continued as long as the patient is permitted to take fluids and medication by mouth. If therapy is interrupted temporarily, the usual daily dosage may be administered as soon as the patient is able to take oral medication (see Dosage and Administration, Adjustment and Maintenance of Therapy).

Psychiatric: Patients should be monitored carefully for the development of depression with suicidal tendencies. Patients with past or current psychoses should be treated with caution.

Behavioural Changes: Pathological (compulsive) gambling, hypersexuality, and increased libido have been reported in patients treated with dopaminergic agents, including SINEMET (see Adverse Reactions). Dose reduction/taper discontinuation should be considered.

Hallucinations: Hallucinations and confusion are known side effects of treatment with dopaminergic agents, including levodopa. Patients should be aware of the fact that hallucinations (mostly visual) can occur.

Skin: Melanoma: Epidemiological studies have shown that patients with Parkinson's disease have a higher risk (2- to approximately 6-fold higher) of developing melanoma than the general population. Whether the increased risk observed was due to Parkinson's disease or other factors, such as drugs used to treat Parkinson's disease, is unclear. For the reasons stated above, patients and healthcare providers are advised to monitor for melanomas frequently and on a regular basis when using SINEMET for **any** indication. Ideally, periodic skin examinations should be performed by appropriately qualified individuals (e.g., dermatologists).

Special Populations: Pregnant Women: Although the effects of SINEMET on human pregnancy and lactation are unknown, both levodopa and combinations of carbidopa and levodopa have caused visceral and skeletal malformations in rabbits. Therefore, use of SINEMET in women of child-bearing potential requires that the anticipated benefits of the drug be weighed against possible hazards to the mother and to the fetus.

Nursing Women: It is not known whether carbidopa is excreted in human milk. In a study of one nursing mother with Parkinson's disease, excretion of levodopa in breast milk was reported. SINEMET should not be given to nursing mothers unless the anticipated benefits to the mother outweigh the potential hazards to the infant.

Pediatrics (<18 years of age): The safety of SINEMET in patients under 18 years of age has not been established.

Monitoring and Laboratory Tests: Periodic evaluations of hepatic, hematopoietic, cardiovascular and renal function are recommended during extended therapy with SINEMET (levodopa and carbidopa).

SINEMET may cause a false-positive reaction for urinary ketone bodies when a tape test is used for determination of ketonuria. False-negative tests may result with the use of glucose-oxidase methods of testing for glucosuria. Caution should be exercised when interpreting the plasma and urine levels of catecholamines and their metabolites in patients on levodopa or levodopa-carbidopa therapy (see Drug Interactions, Drug-Laboratory Test Interactions).

ADVERSE REACTIONS: Clinical Trial and Post-Market Adverse Drug Reactions: The most common serious adverse reactions occurring with SINEMET (levodopa and carbidopa) are dyskinesias, including choreiform, dystonic and other involuntary movements, and nausea. Other serious adverse reactions are mental changes including paranoid ideation and psychotic episodes, depression with or without development of suicidal tendencies, and dementia. Convulsions also have occurred; however, a causal relationship with SINEMET has not been established.

Other adverse reactions reported in clinical trials or in post-marketing experience include:

Body as a Whole: syncope, chest pain, anorexia, asthenia.

Cardiovascular: cardiac irregularities and/or palpitation, hypotension, orthostatic effects including hypotensive episodes, hypertension, phlebitis.

Gastrointestinal: vomiting, gastrointestinal bleeding, development of duodenal ulcer, diarrhea, dark saliva, constipation, dyspepsia, dry mouth, taste alterations.

Hematologic: leukopenia, hemolytic and non-hemolytic anemia, thrombocytopenia, agranulocytosis.

Hypersensitivity: angioedema, urticaria, pruritus, Henoch-Schönlein purpura, bullous lesions (including pemphigus-like reactions).

Musculoskeletal: back pain, shoulder pain, muscle cramps.

Nervous System/Psychiatric: neuroleptic malignant syndrome (see Warnings and Precautions), bradykinetic episodes (the "on-off" phenomenon), dizziness, somnolence including very rarely excessive daytime somnolence and sudden sleep onset episodes, paresthesia, psychotic episodes including delusions, hallucinations and paranoid ideation, dream abnormalities including nightmares, insomnia, headache, depression with or without development of suicidal tendencies, dementia, agitation, confusion, increased libido including hypersexuality.

Pathological (compulsive) Gambling: Pathological (compulsive) gambling has been reported in post-market data, including those in the literature, for antiparkinson drugs. Sporadic cases of pathological (compulsive) gambling have been reported in patients treated with dopaminergic agents, including levodopa. Dosage adjustment should be considered in the management of this behaviour.

Respiratory: dyspnea, upper respiratory infection.

Skin: alopecia, rash, increased sweating, dark sweat, malignant melanoma (see Contraindications and Warnings and Precautions, Skin).

Urogenital: dark urine, urinary frequency, urinary tract infection.

Other adverse reactions that have been reported with levodopa alone and with various levodopa-carbidopa formulations, and may occur with SINEMET are:

Body as a Whole: fatigue.

Cardiovascular: myocardial infarction.

Gastrointestinal: sialorrhea, dysphagia, bruxism, hiccups, abdominal pain and distress, flatulence, burning sensation of tongue, gastrointestinal pain, heart burn.

Metabolic: weight gain or loss, edema.

Musculoskeletal: leg pain.

Nervous System/Psychiatric: decreased mental acuity, disorientation, ataxia, numbness, increased hand tremor, muscle twitching, blepharospasm (which may be taken as an early sign of excess dosage, consideration of dosage reduction may be made at this time), trismus, activation of latent Horner's syndrome, anxiety, euphoria, falling and gait abnormalities, extrapyramidal disorder, nervousness, memory impairment, peripheral neuropathy.

Respiratory: pharyngeal pain, cough.

Skin: flushing.

Special Senses: diplopia, blurred vision, dilated pupils, and oculogyric crises.

Urogenital: urinary retention, urinary incontinence, priapism.

Miscellaneous: faintness, hoarseness, malaise, hot flashes, sense of stimulation, bizarre breathing patterns.

Abnormal Hematologic and Clinical Chemistry Findings: Laboratory tests which have been reported to be abnormal are alkaline phosphatase, AST, ALT, lactic dehydrogenase, bilirubin, blood urea nitrogen, creatinine, uric acid, and positive Coomb's test.

Decreased hemoglobin, hematocrit, elevated serum glucose, and white blood cells, bacteria and blood in the urine have been reported.

Decreased white blood cell count and serum potassium; protein and glucose in urine have been reported with levodopa alone and with various levodopa-carbidopa formulations, and may occur with SINEMET.

DRUG INTERACTIONS: Drug-Drug Interactions: Caution should be exercised when the following drugs are administered concomitantly with SINEMET:

Antihypertensive Drugs: Symptomatic postural hypotension can occur when SINEMET is added to the treatment of a patient receiving antihypertensive drugs. Therefore, when therapy with SINEMET is started, dosage adjustment of the antihypertensive drug may be required.

Psychoactive Drugs: Dopamine D2 receptor antagonists (e.g. phenothiazines, butyrophenones, and risperidone) may reduce the therapeutic effects of levodopa. The beneficial effects of levodopa in Parkinson's disease have been reported to be reversed by phenytoin and papaverine. Patients taking these drugs with SINEMET should be carefully observed for loss of antiparkinsonian effect.

Concomitant therapy with selegiline and levodopa-carbidopa preparations may be associated with severe orthostatic hypotension not attributable to levodopa-carbidopa alone (see Contraindications).

There have been rare reports of adverse reactions, including hypertension and dyskinesia, resulting from the concomitant use of tricyclic antidepressants and SINEMET. For patients receiving monoamine oxidase inhibitors, see Contraindications.

Isoniazid: Isoniazid may reduce the therapeutic effects of levodopa.

Anesthetics: When general anesthesia is required, SINEMET should be discontinued the night before. Therapy with SINEMET may be continued as soon as the patient is able to take medication by mouth.

Iron: Studies have demonstrated that ferrous sulphate decreases the bioavailability of carbidopa and/or levodopa. Because this interaction may be due to the formation of drug-iron complexes, other iron supplement formulations and iron-containing multivitamins may have similar effects.

Metoclopramide: Although metoclopramide may increase the bioavailability of levodopa by increasing gastric emptying, metoclopramide may also adversely affect disease control by its dopamine receptor antagonistic properties.

Drug-Food Interactions: Since levodopa competes with certain amino acids, the absorption of levodopa may be impaired in some patients on a high protein diet.

Drug-Laboratory Test Interactions: SINEMET may cause a false-positive reaction for urinary ketone bodies when a tape test is used for determination of ketonuria. This reaction will not be altered by boiling the urine specimen. False-negative tests may result with the use of glucose-oxidase methods of testing for glucosuria.

Cases of falsely diagnosed pheochromocytoma in patients with levodopa-carbidopa therapy have been reported very rarely. Caution should be exercised when interpreting the plasma and urine levels of catecholamines and their metabolites in patients on levodopa or levodopa-carbidopa therapy.

DOSAGE AND ADMINISTRATION: Dosing Considerations: In order to reduce the incidence of adverse reactions and achieve maximal benefit, therapy with SINEMET (levodopa and carbidopa) must be individualized and drug administration must be continuously matched to the needs and tolerance of the patient. It should be borne in mind that the therapeutic range of SINEMET is narrower than that of levodopa alone because of its greater milligram potency. Therefore, titration and adjustment of dosage should be made in small steps and the dosage ranges recommended should usually not be exceeded. The appearance of involuntary movements should be regarded as a sign of levodopa toxicity and as an indication of overdosage, requiring dose reduction. Treatment should, therefore, aim at maximal benefit without dyskinesias.

If a patient being treated with levodopa is switched to therapy with SINEMET, levodopa must be discontinued at least twelve hours or more before therapy with SINEMET is initiated.

SINEMET tablets are available in a 4:1 ratio (SINEMET 100/25) and in a 10:1 ratio of levodopa to carbidopa (SINEMET 100/10 and SINEMET 250/25). Tablets of the two ratios may be given separately or combined as needed to provide the optimal dosage.

Studies have shown that peripheral dopa decarboxylase is saturated by carbidopa at doses between 70 to 150 mg per day. Patients receiving less than 70 mg per day of carbidopa are more likely to experience nausea and vomiting. Experience with total daily dosages of carbidopa greater than 200 mg is limited.

For patients who require only low doses of levodopa, e.g., less than 700 mg, SINEMET 100/25 may be helpful.

Recommended Dose and Dosage Adjustment: Induction of Therapy in Patients Not Receiving Levodopa: Dosage is best initiated with one tablet of SINEMET 100/25 three times a day. This dosage schedule provides 75 mg of carbidopa per day. Dosage may be carefully increased by one tablet every three days until the optimal dosage has been reached which does not produce dyskinesias.

While increasing the dosage during the induction period, the doses should be divided, aiming at a frequency of dosing of at least four times a day. If further titration is necessary after a daily dosage level of six tablets of SINEMET 100/25 has been reached, tablets of SINEMET 100/10 or SINEMET 250/25 may be used as needed to provide the optimal dosage.

Usually no patient should receive more than 1500 mg of levodopa a day. Some patients, including those with postencephalitic parkinsonism, are more sensitive to levodopa and require specially careful dosage adjustment.

Induction of Therapy in Patient Receiving Levodopa: Levodopa must be discontinued at least twelve hours or more before SINEMET is started. A dosage of SINEMET should be used that will provide approximately 20% of the previous levodopa daily dosage; this can be started in the morning after the day in which the treatment with levodopa has been stopped. For example, if a patient is receiving 4000 mg of levodopa per day, the dosage of SINEMET should not provide more than 750 mg of levodopa per day divided into four to six doses.

Tablets of SINEMET 100/25 should be used to start medication for patients requiring lower dosages of levodopa.

Adjustment and Maintenance of Therapy: Therapy should be individualized and adjusted according to the desired therapeutic response. At least 70 to 100 mg of carbidopa per day should be provided. When a greater proportion of carbidopa is required, one tablet of SINEMET 100/25 may be substituted for each tablet of SINEMET 100/10. When more levodopa is required, SINEMET 250/25 should be substituted for SINEMET 100/25 or 100/10. If necessary, the dosage of SINEMET 250/25 may be increased by one-half or one tablet every day or every other day to a maximum of eight tablets a day. Experience with total daily dosages of carbidopa greater than 200 mg is limited.

Because both therapeutic and adverse responses occur more rapidly with SINEMET than with levodopa alone, patients should be monitored closely during the dose adjustment period. Specifically, involuntary movements will occur more rapidly with SINEMET than with levodopa. The occurrence of involuntary movements may require dosage reduction. Blepharospasm may be a useful early sign of excess dosage in some patients.

Current evidence indicates that other standard antiparkinsonian drugs may be continued while SINEMET is being administered although their dosage may have to be adjusted.

If general anesthesia is required, therapy with SINEMET may be continued as long as the patient is permitted to take fluids and medication by mouth. If therapy is interrupted temporarily, the usual daily dosage may be administered as soon as the patient is able to take oral medication.

Missed Dose: If a tablet is missed, it should be taken as soon as possible. If it is almost time to take the next tablet, the missed tablet should not be taken, and the normal schedule should be resumed.

OVERDOSAGE:

Management of acute overdosage with SINEMET (levodopa and carbidopa) is basically the same as management of acute overdosage with levodopa alone. However, pyridoxine is not effective in reversing the actions of SINEMET.

General supportive measures should be employed, along with immediate gastric lavage. Intravenous fluids should be administered judiciously and an adequate airway maintained. Electrocardiographic monitoring should be instituted and the patient carefully observed for the possible development of arrhythmias; if required, appropriate antiarrhythmic therapy should be given. The possibility that the patient may have taken other drugs as well as SINEMET should be taken into consideration. To date, no experience has been reported with dialysis; hence, its value in overdosage is not known.

For up-to-date information on the management of a suspected drug overdose, the physician should consider contacting a regional Poison Control Centre.

For management of a suspected drug overdose, CPhA recommends that you contact your **regional Poison Control Centre**. See the *CPS* Directory section for a list of Poison Control Centres.

ACTION AND CLINICAL PHARMACOLOGY: Mechanism of Action: The symptoms of Parkinson's disease are related to depletion of dopamine in the corpus striatum. Administration of dopamine is ineffective in the treatment of Parkinson's disease because it does not cross the blood-brain barrier. However, levodopa, the metabolic precursor of dopamine, does cross the blood-brain barrier, and is converted to dopamine in the basal ganglia. This is thought to be the mechanism whereby levodopa relieves the symptoms of Parkinson's disease.

Pharmacodynamics: When levodopa is administered orally it is rapidly converted to dopamine by decarboxylation in peripheral tissues so that only a small portion of a given dose is transported unchanged to the central nervous system. For this reason, large doses of levodopa are required for adequate therapeutic effect and these may often be attended by nausea and other adverse reactions, some of which are attributable to dopamine formed in peripheral tissues.

Carbidopa inhibits decarboxylation of peripheral levodopa. It does not cross the blood-brain barrier and does not affect the metabolism of levodopa within the central nervous system. Since its decarboxylase inhibiting activity is limited to peripheral tissues, administration of carbidopa with levodopa makes more levodopa available for transport to the brain. Combined therapy with levodopa and carbidopa reduces the amount of levodopa required for optimum therapeutic benefit by about 75-80%, permits an earlier response to therapy, and also reduces the incidence of nausea, vomiting and cardiac arrhythmias. Combined therapy, however, does not decrease adverse reactions due to central effects of levodopa.

Pharmacokinetics: At steady state, the bioavailability of carbidopa from SINEMET tablets is approximately 99% relative to the concomitant administration of carbidopa and levodopa. Since levodopa competes with certain aminoacids, the absorption of levodopa may be impaired in some patients on a high protein diet.

Following simultaneous administration of carbidopa and levodopa in man, both plasma levels and plasma half-life of levodopa are markedly increased over those found when the same dosage of levodopa is given alone, while plasma levels of dopamine and homovanillic acid are reduced or do not change. Nevertheless, the plasma levels vary greatly between patients.

The plasma half-life of levodopa is about 50 minutes, without carbidopa. When carbidopa and levodopa are administered together, the half-life of levodopa is increased to about 1.5 hours.

In clinical pharmacologic studies, simultaneous administration of carbidopa and levodopa produced greater urinary excretion of levodopa in proportion to the excretion of dopamine than administration of the two drugs at separate times.

Pyridoxine hydrochloride (vitamin B_6), in oral doses of 10 mg to 25 mg, may reverse the effects of levodopa by increasing the rate of aromatic amino acid decarboxylation. Carbidopa inhibits this action of pyridoxine.

STORAGE AND STABILITY: Store your tablets at 15-30°C in a tightly closed container. Protect from sunlight.

INFORMATION FOR THE PATIENT: Published in e-CPS, available by subscription at www.e-cps.ca.

DOSAGE FORMS, COMPOSITION AND PACKAGING: SINEMET 100/10: Each dark dapple-blue, oval, scored, uncoated tablet, engraved "647" on one side and "SINEMET" on the other, contains: levodopa 100 mg and carbidopa 10 mg expressed as anhydrous carbidopa. Nonmedicinal ingredients: cornstarch, FD&C Blue #2, magnesium stearate, microcrystalline cellulose and pregelatinized starch. Bottles of 100.

SINEMET 100/25: Each yellow, oval, scored, uncoated tablet, engraved "SINEMET" on one side and "650" on the other, contains: levodopa 100 mg and carbidopa 25 mg expressed as anhydrous carbidopa. Nonmedicinal ingredients: cornstarch, D&C Yellow #10, FD&C Yellow #6, magnesium stearate, microcrystalline cellulose and pregelatinized starch. Bottles of 100 and 500.

SINEMET 250/25: Each light dapple-blue, oval, scored, uncoated tablet, engraved "SINEMET" on one side, and "654" on the other, contains: levodopa 250 mg and carbidopa 25 mg expressed as anhydrous carbidopa. Nonmedicinal ingredients: cornstarch, FD&C Blue #2, magnesium stearate, microcrystalline cellulose and pregelatinized starch. Bottles of 100.

(Shown in Product Identification Section)

Sinemet® CR ℞

levodopa—carbidopa

Antiparkinson Agent

Merck Frosst

Date of Revision: July 1, 2010

SUMMARY PRODUCT INFORMATION:

Route of Administration	Dosage Form/ Strength	Clinically Relevant Nonmedicinal Ingredients
Oral	Tablet 100 mg/25 mg, 200 mg/50 mg	For a complete listing, see Dosage Forms, Composition and Packaging.

INDICATIONS AND CLINICAL USE: SINEMET CR (levodopa and carbidopa) is indicated for the treatment of Parkinson's disease.

SINEMET CR is not recommended for the treatment of drug-induced extrapyramidal reactions.

Pediatrics (<18 years of age): The safety and effectiveness of SINEMET CR in patients under 18 years of age has not been established.

CONTRAINDICATIONS:

- Patients who are hypersensitive to this drug or to any ingredient in the formulation. For a complete listing, see Dosage Forms, Composition and Packaging.
- Nonselective monoamine oxidase (MAO) inhibitors are contraindicated for use with SINEMET CR. These inhibitors must be discontinued at least two weeks prior to initiating therapy with SINEMET CR. SINEMET CR may be administered concomitantly with a MAO inhibitor with selectivity for MAO type B (e.g. selegiline HCl) (see Drug Interactions, Drug-Drug Interactions, Psychoactive Drugs) at the manufacturer's recommended dose which maintains selectivity for MAO type B.
- SINEMET CR should not be administered to patients with clinical or laboratory evidence of uncompensated cardiovascular, endocrine, hematologic, hepatic, pulmonary (including bronchial asthma), or renal disease; or to patients with narrow angle glaucoma.
- As with levodopa, SINEMET CR should not be given when administration of a sympathomimetic amine is contraindicated (e.g., epinephrine, norepinephrine or isoproterenol).
- Because levodopa may activate a malignant melanoma, SINEMET CR should not be used in patients with suspicious undiagnosed skin lesions or a history of melanoma.

WARNINGS AND PRECAUTIONS:

Serious Warnings and Precautions

Sudden Onset of Sleep: Patients receiving treatment with SINEMET CR (levodopa and carbidopa) and other dopaminergic agents have reported suddenly falling asleep while engaged in activities of daily living, including the driving of a car, which has sometimes resulted in accidents. Although some of the patients reported somnolence while on SINEMET CR, others perceived that they had no warning signs, such as excessive drowsiness, and believed that they were alert immediately prior to the event.

Physicians should alert patients of the reported cases of sudden onset of sleep, bearing in mind that these events are **not** limited to initiation of therapy. Patients should also be advised that sudden onset of sleep has occurred without warning signs and should be specifically asked about factors that may increase the risk with SINEMET CR such as concomitant medications or the presence of sleep disorders. Given the reported cases of somnolence and sudden onset of sleep (not necessarily preceded by somnolence), physicians should caution patients about the risk of operating hazardous machinery, including driving motor vehicles, while taking SINEMET CR. If drowsiness or sudden onset of sleep should occur, patients should be informed to refrain from driving or operating machines and to immediately contact their physician.

While dose reduction clearly reduces the degree of somnolence, there is insufficient information to establish that dose reduction will eliminate episodes of falling asleep while engaged in activities of daily living.

Episodes of falling asleep while engaged in activities of daily living have also been reported in patients taking other dopaminergic agents, therefore, symptoms may not be alleviated by substituting these products.

Currently, the precise cause of this event is unknown. It is known that many Parkinson's disease patients experience alterations in sleep architecture, which results in excessive daytime sleepiness or spontaneous dozing, and that dopaminergic agents can also induce sleepiness.

General: When patients are receiving levodopa monotherapy or SINEMET (levodopa and carbidopa), this medication must be discontinued at least 8 hours before therapy with SINEMET CR is started. (For appropriate dosage substitutions, see Dosage and Administration.)

Periodic evaluations of hepatic, hematopoietic, cardiovascular and renal function are recommended during extended therapy (see Adverse Reactions).

Physical Activity: Patients who improve while on therapy with SINEMET CR should increase physical activities gradually, with caution, consistent with other medical considerations such as the presence of osteoporosis or phlebothrombosis.

Cardiovascular: Care should be exercised in administering SINEMET CR to patients with a history of recent myocardial infarction who have residual atrial, nodal, or ventricular arrhythmias. In such patients, cardiac function should be monitored with particular care during the period of initial dosage administration and titration, in a facility with provisions for intensive cardiac care.

Gastrointestinal: SINEMET CR should be administered cautiously to patients with a history of peptic ulcer disease due to the possibility of upper gastrointestinal hemorrhage.

Neurologic: As with levodopa or SINEMET, SINEMET CR may cause involuntary movements and mental disturbances. These reactions are thought to be due to increased brain dopamine following administration of levodopa. These adverse reactions may be more prolonged with SINEMET CR than with SINEMET.

SINEMET CR should be used cautiously in patients who have a history of seizures or have conditions associated with seizure or have a lowered seizure threshold.

Neuroleptic Malignant Syndrome: A symptom complex resembling the neuroleptic malignant syndrome including muscular rigidity, elevated body temperature, altered consciousness, mental changes, autonomic instability and increased serum creatine phosphokinase has been reported in association with rapid dose reduction, withdrawal of, or changes in antiparkinsonian therapy. Therefore, patients should be observed carefully when the dosage of SINEMET CR is reduced abruptly or discontinued, especially if the patient is receiving neuroleptics.

Psychomotor Performance: Certain side effects that have been reported with SINEMET CR may affect some patients' ability to drive or operate machinery.

Given the reported cases of somnolence and sudden onset of sleep (not necessarily preceded by somnolence), physicians should caution patients about the risk of operating hazardous machinery, including driving motor vehicles, while taking SINEMET CR. If drowsiness or sudden onset of sleep should occur, patients should be informed to refrain from driving or operating machines and to immediately contact their physician (see Warnings and Precautions, Boxed Serious Warnings and Precautions, Sudden Onset of Sleep).

Ophthalmologic: Patients with chronic wide angle glaucoma may be treated cautiously with SINEMET CR (levodopa and carbidopa), provided the intraocular pressure is well controlled and the patient monitored carefully for changes in intraocular pressure during therapy.

Peri-Operative Considerations: If general anesthesia is required, SINEMET CR may be continued as long as the patient is permitted to take oral medication. If therapy is interrupted temporarily, the usual dosage should be administered as soon as the patient is able to take oral medication (see Dosage and Administration, Recommended Dose and Dosage Adjustment, Interruption of Therapy).

Psychiatric: All patients should be observed carefully for the development of depression with concomitant suicidal tendencies. Patients with past or current psychoses should be treated with caution.

Behavioural Changes: Pathological (compulsive) gambling, hypersexuality, and increased libido have been reported in patients treated with dopaminergic agents including SINEMET CR (see Adverse Reactions). Dose reduction/taper discontinuation should be considered.

Hallucinations: Hallucinations and confusion are known side effects of treatment with dopaminergic agents, including levodopa. Patients should be aware of the fact that hallucinations (mostly visual) can occur.

Skin: Melanoma: Epidemiological studies have shown that patients with Parkinson's disease have a higher risk (2- to approximately 6-fold higher) of developing melanoma than the general population. Whether the increased risk observed was due to Parkinson's disease or other factors, such as drugs used to treat Parkinson's disease, is unclear. For the reasons stated above, patients and healthcare providers are advised to monitor for melanomas frequently and on a regular basis when using SINEMET CR for **any** indication. Ideally, periodic skin examinations should be performed by appropriately qualified individuals (e.g., dermatologists).

Special Populations: Pregnant Women: Although the effects of SINEMET CR on human pregnancy and lactation are unknown, both levodopa and combinations of carbidopa and levodopa have caused visceral and skeletal malformations in rabbits. Therefore, use of SINEMET CR in women of child-bearing potential requires that the anticipated benefits of the drug be weighed against possible hazards to the mother and to the fetus.

Nursing Women: It is not known whether carbidopa is excreted in human milk. In a study of one nursing mother with Parkinson's disease, excretion of levodopa in breast milk was reported. SINEMET CR should not be given to nursing mothers unless the anticipated benefits to the mother outweigh the potential hazards to the infant.

Pediatrics (<18 years of age): Safety of SINEMET CR in patients under 18 years of age has not been established.

Monitoring and Laboratory Tests: Periodic evaluations of hepatic, hematopoietic, cardiovascular and renal function are recommended during extended therapy (see Adverse Reactions).

SINEMET CR may cause a false-positive reaction for urinary ketone bodies when a tape test is used for determination of ketonuria. False-negative tests may result with the use of glucose-oxidase methods of testing for glucosuria. Caution should be exercised when interpreting the plasma and urine levels of catecholamines and their metabolites in patients on levodopa or levodopa-carbidopa therapy. (See Drug Interactions, Drug-Laboratory Test Interactions.)

ADVERSE REACTIONS: Clinical Trial Adverse Drug Reactions: In controlled clinical trials involving 748 patients with moderate to severe motor fluctuations, SINEMET CR (levodopa and carbidopa) did not produce side effects which were unique to the controlled release formulation.

The adverse reaction reported most frequently was dyskinesia (12.8%). Occasionally, prolonged, and at times, severe afternoon dyskinesias have occurred in some patients.

Other adverse reactions that were reported frequently were: nausea (5.5%), hallucinations (5.3%), confusion (4.9%), dizziness (3.5%), headache (2.5%), depression (2.5%), chorea (2.5%), dry mouth (2.3%), somnolence (2.1%), including very rarely excessive daytime somnolence and sudden sleep onset episodes, dream abnormalities (2.1%), dystonia (2.0%) and asthenia (2.0%).

Adverse reactions occurring less frequently (less than 2%) were:

System	%
Body as a Whole	
Chest pain	1.7
Fatigue	0.9
Weight loss	0.8
Cardiovascular	
Orthostatic hypotension	0.8
Palpitation	0.8
Hypotension	0.5
Nervous System/Psychiatric	
Insomnia	1.7
Falling	1.6
On-off phenomenon	1.2
Paresthesia	0.9
Disorientation	0.8
Anxiety disorders	0.8
Decreased mental acuity	0.7
Extrapyramidal disorder	0.7
Gait abnormalities	0.7
Agitation	0.5
Memory impairment	0.5
Gastrointestinal	
Anorexia	1.9
Constipation	1.5
Vomiting	1.3
Diarrhea	1.2
Gastrointestinal pain	0.9
Dyspepsia	0.8
Musculoskeletal	

System	%
Muscle cramps	0.9
Respiratory	
Dyspnea	1.6
Special Senses	
Blurred vision	1.1

Other adverse reactions reported in clinical trials or in post-marketing experience include: orthostatic effects, hypertension, myocardial infarction, cardiac irregularities, syncope, hypotensive episodes, dysphagia, heartburn, taste alterations, dark saliva, leg pain, shoulder pain, back pain, angioedema, urticaria, pruritus, bullous lesions (including pemphigus-like reactions), nervousness, sleep disorders, neuroleptic malignant syndrome (see Warnings and Precautions), increased tremor, peripheral neuropathy, increased libido including hypersexuality, psychotic episodes including delusions and paranoid ideation, cough, pharyngeal pain, common cold, upper respiratory infection, blurred vision, flushing, alopecia, rash, dark sweat, dark urine, urinary incontinence, urinary frequency, urinary tract infection, malignant melanoma (see Contraindications and Warnings and Precautions, Skin).

Pathological (compulsive) Gambling: Pathological (compulsive) gambling has been reported in post-market data, including those in the literature, for antiparkinson drugs. Sporadic cases of pathological (compulsive) gambling have been reported in patients treated with dopaminergic agents, including levodopa. Dosage adjustment should be considered in the management of this behaviour.

Post-Market Adverse Drug Reactions: Other adverse reactions that have been reported with levodopa or SINEMET and may be potential side effects with SINEMET CR are listed below.

Cardiovascular: arrhythmias, non-specific ECG changes, phlebitis.

Gastrointestinal: sialorrhea, bruxism, hiccups, gastrointestinal bleeding, flatulence, burning sensation of tongue, development of duodenal ulcer.

Genitourinary: urinary retention, hematuria, and priapism.

Hematologic: leukopenia, hemolytic and non-hemolytic anemia, thrombocytopenia, agranulocytosis.

Hypersensitivity: Henoch-Schoenlein purpura.

Nervous System/Psychiatric: ataxia, numbness, increased hand tremor, muscle twitching, blepharospasm (which may be taken as an early sign of excess dosage, consideration of dosage reduction may be needed at this time), trismus, activation of latent Horner's syndrome, euphoria and dementia, depression with suicidal tendencies, bradykinetic episodes.

Skin: increased sweating.

Special Senses: diplopia, dilated pupils, oculogyric crises.

Miscellaneous: weight gain, edema, faintness, hoarseness, malaise, hot flashes, sense of stimulation, bizarre breathing patterns.

Convulsions have occurred; however, a causal relationship with levodopa or levodopa/carbidopa combinations has not been established.

Abnormal Hematologic and Clinical Chemistry Findings: Laboratory tests which have been reported to be abnormal are creatinine, uric acid, alkaline phosphatase, AST, ALT, lactic dehydrogenase, bilirubin, and blood urea nitrogen, and Coomb's test.

Decreased hemoglobin, hematocrit, white blood cell count and serum potassium have been reported as well as bacteria, blood, protein and glucose in the urine.

Abnormalities in various laboratory tests have occurred with SINEMET and may also occur with SINEMET CR.

DRUG INTERACTIONS: Drug-Drug Interactions: Caution should be exercised when the following drugs are administered concomitantly with SINEMET CR:

Antihypertensive Drugs: Symptomatic postural hypotension has occurred when levodopa/decarboxylase inhibitor combinations were added to the treatment of patients receiving antihypertensive drugs. Therefore, when therapy with SINEMET CR is started, dosage adjustment of the antihypertensive drug may be required.

Psychoactive Drugs: Dopamine D_2 receptor antagonists (e.g., phenothiazines, butyrophenones, and risperidone) may reduce the therapeutic effects of levodopa. The beneficial effects of levodopa in Parkinson's disease have been reported to be reversed by phenytoin and papaverine. Patients taking these drugs with SINEMET CR should be observed carefully for loss of therapeutic response.

Concomitant therapy with selegiline and levodopa-carbidopa preparations may be associated with severe orthostatic hypotension not attributable to levodopa-carbidopa alone (see Contraindications).

There have been rare reports of adverse reactions, including hypertension and dyskinesia, resulting from the concomitant use of tricyclic antidepressants and carbidopa-levodopa preparations. (For patients receiving monoamine oxidase inhibitors, see Contraindications.)

Isoniazid: Isoniazid may reduce the therapeutic effects of levodopa.

Anesthetics: When general anesthesia is required, SINEMET CR should be discontinued the night before. Therapy with SINEMET CR may be continued as soon as the patient is able to take medication by mouth.

Iron: Studies have demonstrated that ferrous sulphate decreases the bioavailability of carbidopa and/or levodopa. Because this interaction may be due to the formation of drug-iron complexes, other iron supplement formulations and iron-containing multivitamins may have similar effects.

Metoclopramide: Although metoclopramide may increase the bioavailability of levodopa by increasing gastric emptying, metoclopramide may also adversely affect disease control by its dopamine receptor antagonistic properties.

Other Drugs: Although specific interaction studies were not performed with other concomitant drugs, in clinical trials of SINEMET CR patients were allowed to receive tricyclic antidepressants, benzodiazepines, propranolol, thiazides, angiotensin converting enzyme inhibitors, calcium channel blockers, digoxin, H_2 antagonists, salicylates and other nonsteroidal anti-inflammatory drugs. SINEMET CR was also used with other antiparkinson agents (see Dosage and Administration).

Drug-Food Interactions: Since levodopa competes with certain amino acids, the absorption of levodopa may be impaired in some patients on a high protein diet.

Drug-Laboratory Test Interactions: SINEMET CR may cause a false-positive reaction for urinary ketone bodies when a tape test is used for determination of ketonuria. This reaction will not be altered by boiling the urine specimen. False-negative tests may result with the use of glucose-oxidase methods of testing for glucosuria.

Cases of falsely diagnosed pheochromocytoma in patients with levodopa-carbidopa therapy have been reported very rarely. Caution should be exercised when interpreting the plasma and urine levels of catecholamines and their metabolites in patients on levodopa or levodopa-carbidopa therapy.

DOSAGE AND ADMINISTRATION: Dosing Considerations: SINEMET CR (levodopa and carbidopa) tablets contain a 4:1 ratio of levodopa to carbidopa. SINEMET CR 200/50 contains levodopa 200 mg/carbidopa 50 mg (anhydrous equivalent) per tablet. SINEMET CR 100/25 contains levodopa 100 mg/carbidopa 25 mg (anhydrous equivalent) per tablet. The daily dosage of SINEMET CR must be determined by careful titration. Patients should be monitored closely during the dose adjustment period, particularly with regard to appearance or worsening of nausea or abnormal involuntary movements, including dyskinesias, chorea and dystonia.

SINEMET CR 200/50 may be administered as whole or as half tablets. **SINEMET CR 100/25 should only be administered as whole tablets. To maintain the controlled release properties of the product, tablets should not be chewed or crushed.**

Standard antiparkinson drugs, other than levodopa alone, may be continued while SINEMET CR is being administered, although their dosage may have to be adjusted. The delayed onset of action with SINEMET CR may require the supplemental use of conventional SINEMET tablets for optimal control in the mornings.

Recommended Dose and Dosage Adjustment: Initial Dosage and Titration for Patients Currently Treated with Conventional Levodopa/Decarboxylase Inhibitor Combinations: Dosage with SINEMET CR 200/50 should be substituted at an amount that eventually provides approximately 10 to 30 percent more levodopa per day. The interval between doses should be prolonged by 30 to 50 percent. Initially, patients should receive SINEMET CR 200/50 at a dosage that provides the same amount of levodopa, but with a longer dosing interval. Depending on clinical response, the dosage may be increased.

A guide for the initiation of treatment with SINEMET CR 200/50 is shown in Table 1.

Table 1: SINEMET CR

Guideline for Initial Conversion from SINEMET to SINEMET CR 200/50

SINEMET Total Daily Dose[a] Levodopa (mg)	SINEMET CR 200/50 (levodopa 200 mg/carbidopa 50 mg) Suggested Dosage Regimen
300–400	1 tablet b.i.d.
500–600	1½ tablets b.i.d. or 1 tablet t.i.d.
700–800	a total of 4 tablets in 3 or more divided doses (e.g., 1½ tablets a.m., 1½ tablets early p.m., and 1 tablet later p.m.)
900–1000	a total of 5 tablets in 3 or more divided doses (e.g., 2 tablets a.m., 2 tablets early p.m., and 1 tablet later p.m.)

[a] For dosing ranges not shown in the table, see Dosage and Administration.

SINEMET CR 100/25 is available to facilitate titration when 100 mg steps are required and as an alternative to the half tablet of SINEMET CR 200/50.

Initial Dosage for Patients Currently Treated with Levodopa Alone: Levodopa or SINEMET (levodopa and carbidopa) must be discontinued at least eight hours before therapy with SINEMET CR 200/50 is started. SINEMET CR should be substituted at a dosage that will provide approximately 25% of the previous levodopa dosage. In patients with mild to moderate disease, the initial dose is usually 1 tablet of SINEMET CR 200/50 two times daily.

Patients Without Prior Levodopa Therapy: SINEMET CR 100/25 may be used in early stage patients who have not had prior levodopa therapy or to facilitate titration when necessary in patients receiving SINEMET CR 200/50. The initial recommended dose is 1 tablet of SINEMET CR 100/25 twice daily. For patients who require more levodopa, a daily dose of 1 to 4 tablets of SINEMET CR 100/25 twice a day is generally well-tolerated.

When appropriate, levodopa therapy may also be initiated with SINEMET CR 200/50. The initial recommended dose in patients with mild to moderate disease is 1 tablet of SINEMET CR 200/50 two times daily. Initial dosages should not exceed 600 mg per day of levodopa or be given at intervals of less than 6 hours.

Titration: Doses and dosing intervals must be adjusted on an individual basis, depending upon therapeutic response. An interval of at least 3 days between dosage adjustments is recommended. Most patients have been adequately treated with 2 to 8 tablets of SINEMET CR 200/50 per day, administered as divided doses at intervals ranging from 4 to 12 hours during the waking day.

If the divided doses of SINEMET CR 200/50 are not equal, it is recommended that the smaller doses be given at the end of the day.

Maintenance: Because Parkinson's disease is progressive, periodic clinical evaluations are recommended and adjustment of the dosage regimen of SINEMET CR may be required.

Addition of Other Antiparkinson Medications: Anticholinergic agents, dopamine agonists, amantadine and lower doses of selective MAO-B inhibitors can be given with SINEMET CR. When combining therapies, dosage adjustments may be necessary.

Interruption of Therapy: Patients should be observed carefully if abrupt reduction or discontinuation of SINEMET CR is required, especially if the patient is receiving neuroleptics (see Warnings and Precautions).

If general anesthesia is required, SINEMET CR may be continued as long as the patient is permitted to take oral medication. If therapy is interrupted temporarily, the usual dosage should be administered as soon as the patient is able to take oral medication.

Missed Dose: If a tablet is missed, it should be taken as soon as possible. If it is almost time to take the next tablet, the missed tablet should not be taken, and the normal schedule should be resumed.

OVERDOSAGE:

Management of acute overdosage with SINEMET CR (levodopa and carbidopa) is basically the same as management of acute overdosage with levodopa; however, pyridoxine is not effective in reversing the actions of SINEMET CR.

Electrocardiographic monitoring should be instituted and the patient observed carefully for the development of arrhythmias; if required, appropriate antiarrhythmic therapy should be given. The possibility that the patient may have taken other drugs as well as SINEMET CR should be taken into consideration. To date, no experience has been reported with dialysis; hence, its value in overdosage is not known.

For up-to-date information on the management of a suspected drug overdose, the physician should consider contacting a regional Poison Control Centre.

> For management of a suspected drug overdose, CPhA recommends that you contact your **regional Poison Control Centre**. See the *CPS* Directory section for a list of Poison Control Centres.

ACTION AND CLINICAL PHARMACOLOGY: Mechanism of Action: SINEMET CR (levodopa and carbidopa), a combination of levodopa, the metabolic precursor of dopamine, and carbidopa, an aromatic amino acid decarboxylase inhibitor, is available in a polymer-based controlled-release tablet formulation. SINEMET CR can be useful in reducing "off" time in patients treated previously with a conventional levodopa/decarboxylase inhibitor combination who have had predictable peak dose dyskinesias and unpredictable motor fluctuations.

The symptoms of Parkinson's disease are related to depletion of dopamine in the corpus striatum. While the administration of dopamine is ineffective in the treatment of Parkinson's disease because it does not cross the blood-brain barrier, levodopa, the metabolic precursor of dopamine, does cross the blood-brain barrier and is converted to dopamine in the basal ganglia. This is thought to be the mechanism whereby levodopa relieves the symptoms of Parkinson's disease.

Pharmacodynamics: Levodopa is rapidly decarboxylated to dopamine in peripheral tissues so that only a small portion of a given dose is transported unchanged to the central nervous system. For this reason, large doses of levodopa are required for adequate therapeutic effect and these may often be attended by nausea and other adverse reactions, some of which are attributable to dopamine formed in peripheral tissues.

Carbidopa, a decarboxylase inhibitor, does not cross the blood-brain barrier and does not affect the metabolism of levodopa within the central nervous system. Since its decarboxylase inhibiting activity is limited to peripheral tissues, administration of carbidopa with levodopa makes more levodopa available for transport to the brain. Combined therapy with levodopa and carbidopa reduces the amount of levodopa required for optimum therapeutic benefit by about 75-80%, permits an earlier response to therapy, and also reduces the incidence of nausea, vomiting and cardiac arrhythmias. Combined therapy, however, does not decrease adverse reactions due to central effects of levodopa.

Following years of treatment with preparations containing levodopa, an increasing number of parkinsonian patients develop fluctuations in motor performance and dyskinesias. The advanced form of motor fluctuations ("on-off" phenomenon) is characterized by unpredictable swings from mobility to immobility. Although the causes of the motor fluctuations are not completely understood, it has been demonstrated that they can be attenuated by treatment regimens that produce steady plasma levels of levodopa.

In clinical trials, patients with motor fluctuations experienced reduced "off" time with SINEMET CR when compared with SINEMET. Global ratings of improvement and activities of daily living in the "on" and "off" states, as assessed by both patient and physician, were slightly better in some patients during therapy with SINEMET CR than with SINEMET. In patients without motor fluctuations, SINEMET CR provided therapeutic benefit similar to SINEMET but with less frequent dosing.

Pyridoxine hydrochloride (vitamin B_6), in oral doses of 10 mg to 25 mg, may reverse the effects of levodopa by increasing the rate of aromatic amino acid decarboxylation. Carbidopa inhibits this action of pyridoxine.

Pharmacokinetics: SINEMET CR 200/50 contains levodopa, 200 mg and carbidopa, 50 mg (anhydrous equivalent), per tablet, in a controlled-release formulation designed to release the active ingredients over a 4- to 6-hour period.

The absorption of levodopa following SINEMET CR 200/50 is gradual and continuous for 4 to 5 hours although the majority of the dose is absorbed in 2 to 3 hours. With conventional SINEMET Tablets, absorption is rapid and is virtually complete in 2 to 3 hours. The pharmacokinetic parameters of levodopa, following the administration of SINEMET CR 200/50 and conventional SINEMET Tablets to healthy elderly volunteers, are presented in Table 2.

Table 2: SINEMET CR

Mean Pharmacokinetic Parameters of Levodopa Following the Administration of Two SINEMET 100/25 Tablets or One SINEMET CR 200/50 Tablet in Healthy Elderly Volunteers

	Single Dose		Steady-state	
	SINEMET	SINEMET CR 200/50	SINEMET	SINEMET CR 200/50
Bioavailability[a] %	—	—	99	71
C_{max}, µg/mL	3.26	1.15	3.20	1.14
Trough Cp at 8 h, µg/mL	0.048	0.090	0.074	0.163
Peak time, h	0.5	2.1	0.7	2.4
AUC, µg· h/mL	5.31	4.01	5.62	4.19

[a] Relative to an intravenous dose.

In general, peak levodopa plasma levels are lower, bioavailability is less and time to reach peak levels is delayed when using SINEMET CR. Levodopa plasma levels following a single dose are essentially identical to those following repeated administration. However, with SINEMET CR, levodopa plasma concentrations fluctuate less, namely peak plasma levels are lower and end of dose levels (trough concentrations) higher than after conventional therapy.

The bioavailability of 2 half tablets of SINEMET CR 200/50 is approximately 20% greater than that of one intact tablet. The bioavailability of SINEMET CR is somewhat increased in the presence of food. Dose-proportionality has been demonstrated over the dose range of one and two SINEMET CR 200/50 Tablets.

The pharmacokinetics of levodopa following administration of SINEMET CR 100/25 were studied in patients with Parkinson's disease. Chronic three month, open-label, twice daily dosing with SINEMET CR 100/25 (range: 200 mg levodopa, 50 mg carbidopa up to 600 mg levodopa, 150 mg carbidopa per day) did not result in accumulation of plasma levodopa. The dose-adjusted bioavailability for one SINEMET CR 100/25 tablet was equivalent to that for one SINEMET CR 200/50 tablet. The mean peak concentration of levodopa following the administration of one SINEMET CR 100/25 tablet was greater than 50% of that following one SINEMET CR 200/50 tablet. Mean time-to-peak plasma levels may be slightly less for SINEMET CR 100/25 than for SINEMET CR 200/50.

Elimination half-life of levodopa in the presence of carbidopa is about 1.5 hours. Following SINEMET CR, the apparent half-life of levodopa may be prolonged because of continuous absorption.

STORAGE AND STABILITY: Store your tablets between 15 and 30°C in a tightly closed container. Protect from sunlight.

INFORMATION FOR THE PATIENT: Published in e-CPS, available by subscription at www.e-cps.ca.

DOSAGE FORMS, COMPOSITION AND PACKAGING: SINEMET CR 100/25: Each pink-colored, oval-shaped, biconvex, compressed tablet, engraved 601 with bar on one side and SINEMET CR on the other, contains: levodopa 100 mg and carbidopa 25 mg (anhydrous equivalent). Nonmedicinal ingredients: hydroxypropyl cellulose, magnesium stearate, polyvinyl acetate-crotonic acid copolymer and red ferric oxide. Bottles of 100.

SINEMET CR 200/50: Each peach-colored, oval-shaped, biconvex, scored compressed tablet, engraved 521 on one side and SINEMET CR on the other, contains: levodopa 200 mg and carbidopa 50 mg (anhydrous equivalent). Nonmedicinal ingredients: D&C yellow No. 10 Aluminum Lake, hydroxypropyl cellulose, magnesium stearate, polyvinyl acetate-crotonic acid copolymer and red ferric oxide. Bottles of 100, 250 and 500.

SINEMET CR is a controlled-release formulation of levodopa and carbidopa, in a ratio of 4:1. The tablet contains a polymer-based drug delivery system which controls the release of levodopa and carbidopa as it slowly erodes.

(Shown in Product Identification Section)

Singulair® Pr

montelukast sodium

Leukotriene Receptor Antagonist

Merck Frosst

Date of Revision: June 3, 2010

SUMMARY PRODUCT INFORMATION:

Route of Administration	Dosage Form/Strength	All Nonmedicinal Ingredients
Oral	Tablet 10 mg Chewable tablets 4 mg, 5 mg Granules 4 mg	For a complete listing see Dosage Forms, Composition and Packaging.

INDICATIONS AND CLINICAL USE: SINGULAIR (montelukast sodium) is indicated in adult and pediatric patients 2 years of age and older for the prophylaxis and chronic treatment of asthma, including prevention of day- and night-time symptoms, the treatment of acetylsalicylic acid (ASA)-sensitive asthmatic patients, and the prevention of exercise-induced bronchoconstriction.

SINGULAIR is effective alone or in combination with other agents used in the maintenance treatment of chronic asthma. SINGULAIR and inhaled corticosteroids may be used concomitantly with additive effects to control asthma or to reduce the inhaled corticosteroid dose while maintaining clinical stability.

In patients who continue to experience asthma symptoms, SINGULAIR can be an additional treatment option following initial management with an "as needed" short-acting beta-agonist (SABA), an inhaled corticosteroid, or inhaled corticosteroid together with a long-acting beta agonist.

In adults, SINGULAIR can be a treatment option after "as needed" SABAs if patients remain symptomatic and cannot or will not use an inhaler device or would prefer not to be treated with an inhaled corticosteroid.

In children, SINGULAIR can be a treatment option after "as needed" SABAs if patients remain symptomatic and cannot appropriately use an inhaler device.

SINGULAIR can be a treatment option in patients who experience exercise-induced bronchoconstriction.

SINGULAIR is indicated for the relief of symptoms of seasonal allergic rhinitis in patients 15 years old or older. SINGULAIR should be considered when other treatments are not effective or not tolerated.

CONTRAINDICATIONS:

- Patients who are hypersensitive to this drug or to any ingredient in the formulation. For a complete listing, see Dosage Forms, Composition and Packaging.

WARNINGS AND PRECAUTIONS: Information to Be Provided to the Patient: Patients should be advised to take SINGULAIR daily as prescribed, even when they are asymptomatic as well as during periods of asthma worsening, and to contact their physicians if their asthma is not well-controlled. Patients should be advised that SINGULAIR is not for the treatment of acute asthma attacks. They should have appropriate rescue medication available.

Chewable Tablets: Phenylketonurics: Phenylketonuric patients should be informed that the 4 mg and the 5 mg chewable tablets contains phenylalanine (a component of aspartame) 0.674 and 0.842 mg per 4 mg and 5 mg chewable tablet.

General: The efficacy of oral SINGULAIR for the treatment of acute asthma attacks has not been established. Therefore, SINGULAIR should not be used to treat acute asthma attacks. Patients should be advised to have appropriate rescue medication available.

While the dose of concomitant inhaled corticosteroid may be reduced gradually under medical supervision, SINGULAIR should not be abruptly substituted for inhaled or oral corticosteroids.

When SINGULAIR is prescribed for the prevention of exercise-induced bronchoconstriction, patients should be advised to always have readily available appropriate rescue medication.

Patients with known acetylsalicylic acid (ASA) sensitivity should continue avoidance of ASA or non-steroidal anti-inflammatory agents while taking SINGULAIR. Although SINGULAIR is effective in improving airway function in asthmatic patients with documented ASA sensitivity, it has not been shown to truncate bronchoconstrictor response to ASA and other non-steroidal anti-inflammatory drugs in ASA-sensitive asthmatic patients.

Neuropsychiatric Post-marketing Events: Neuropsychiatric events have been reported in patients taking SINGULAIR (see Adverse Reactions, Post-Market Adverse Drug Reactions). While other factors may have contributed to some of these events, the clinical details of some post-marketing reports involving SINGULAIR appear consistent with a drug-induced effect.

Physicians should discuss these adverse experiences with their patients and/or caregivers. Patients and/or caregivers should be instructed to notify their physician if these changes occur. Physicians should carefully evaluate the risks and benefits of continuing treatment with SINGULAIR if such events occur.

Eosinophilic Conditions: In rare cases, patients with asthma on therapy with SINGULAIR may present with systemic eosinophilia, sometimes presenting with clinical features of vasculitis consistent with Churg-Strauss syndrome, a condition which is often treated with systemic corticosteroid therapy. These events usually, but not always, have been associated with the reduction of oral corticosteroid therapy. Although there is insufficient evidence to suggest a direct pathological role of SINGULAIR in the development of Churg-Strauss syndrome, the association appears to be due to either unmasking (through a reduction or discontinuation of steroids) or progression of previous disease. Physicians should be alert to eosinophilia, vasculitic rash, arthralgia, worsening pulmonary symptoms, cardiac complications, and/or neuropathy presenting in their patients. A causal association between SINGULAIR and these underlying conditions has not been established (see Adverse Reactions).

Hepatic/Biliary: Hepatic Insufficiency: Patients with mild-to-moderate hepatic insufficiency and clinical evidence of cirrhosis had evidence of decreased metabolism of montelukast resulting in approximately 41% higher mean montelukast area under the plasma concentration curve (AUC) following a single 10 mg dose. The elimination of montelukast is slightly prolonged compared with that in healthy subjects (mean half-life, 7.4 hours). No dosage adjustment is required in patients with mild-to-moderate hepatic insufficiency. There are no clinical data in patients with severe hepatic insufficiency (Child-Pugh score >9).

Post-Marketing Surveillance: In post-marketing surveillance, elevations in serum transaminases have been reported in patients who were treated with SINGULAIR. These events were usually asymptomatic and transient. Serious hepatic adverse events such as jaundice have been reported although no deaths or liver transplantations have been attributed to the use of SINGULAIR (see Adverse Reactions).

Special Populations: Pregnant Women: SINGULAIR has not been studied in pregnant women. SINGULAIR should be used during pregnancy only if clearly needed.

During worldwide marketing experience, congenital limb defects have been rarely reported in the offspring of women being treated with SINGULAIR during pregnancy. Most of these women were also taking other asthma medications during their pregnancy. A causal relationship between these events and SINGULAIR has not been established.

Nursing Women: It is not known if SINGULAIR is excreted in human milk. Because many drugs are excreted in human milk, caution should be exercised when SINGULAIR is given to a nursing mother.

Pediatrics (<15 years): Safety and efficacy of SINGULAIR have been established in adequate and well-controlled studies in pediatric patients with asthma 6 to 14 years of age. Safety and efficacy profiles in this age group are similar to that seen in adults (see Adverse Reactions, Clinical Trial Adverse Drug Reactions).

The safety of SINGULAIR 4 mg chewable tablets in pediatric patients 2 to 5 years of age has been demonstrated in a 12-week double-blind, placebo-controlled study in 689 patients (see Action and Clinical Pharmacology and also Adverse Reactions). Efficacy of SINGULAIR in this age group is based on extrapolation of the demonstrated efficacy in adults 15 years of age and older and pediatric patients 6 to 14 years of age with asthma, and that the disease course, pathophysiology and the drug's effect are substantially similar among these populations. The findings of the exploratory efficacy evaluations along with pharmacokinetics and extrapolation of data from older patients, support the overall conclusion that SINGULAIR is efficacious in the maintenance treatment of asthma in patients 2 to 5 years of age (see Action and Clinical Pharmacology).

SINGULAIR has been evaluated for safety in a 6-week, placebo-controlled clinical study in 175 asthma patients 6 months to 2 years of age receiving 4 mg as oral granules daily in the evening. There were no safety concerns compared to older pediatric patients (see Adverse Reactions, Pediatric Patients 6 Months to 2 Years of Age with Asthma). Since this study was not powered to detect between group differences in efficacy endpoints, the efficacy of SINGULAIR could not be determined in this age group.

Geriatrics (>65 years of age): In clinical studies, there were no age-related differences in the efficacy or safety profiles of SINGULAIR.

Effects on Ability to Drive and Use Machines: There is no evidence that SINGULAIR affects the ability to drive and use machines.

ADVERSE REACTIONS: Adverse Drug Reaction Overview: SINGULAIR has been generally well tolerated. Side effects, which usually were mild, generally did not require discontinuation of therapy. The overall incidence of side effects reported with SINGULAIR was comparable to placebo.

Clinical Trial Adverse Drug Reactions: Adults 15 Years of Age and Older with Asthma: SINGULAIR has been evaluated for safety in approximately 2600 adult patients 15 years of age and older in clinical studies. In two similarly designed, 12-week placebo-controlled clinical studies, the only adverse experiences reported as drug-related in ≥1% of patients treated with SINGULAIR and at a greater incidence than in patients treated with placebo were abdominal pain and headache. The incidences of these events were not significantly different in the two treatment groups.

In placebo-controlled clinical trials, the following adverse experiences reported with SINGULAIR occurred in ≥1% of patients and at an incidence greater than or equal to that in patients treated with placebo, regardless of drug relationship (see Table 1).

Table 1: SINGULAIR

Adverse Experiences Occurring in ≥1% of Patients with an Incidence ≥ to that in Patients Treated with Placebo, Regardless of Drug Relationship

	SINGULAIR 10 mg/day (n=1955) (%)	Placebo (n=1180) (%)
Body as a Whole		
Asthenia/Fatigue	1.8	1.2
Fever	1.5	0.9
Pain, Abdominal	2.9	2.5
Trauma	1.0	0.8
Digestive System Disorders		
Diarrhea	3.1	3.1
Dyspepsia	2.1	1.1
Gastroenteritis, Infectious	1.5	0.5
Pain, Dental	1.7	1.0
Nervous System/Psychiatric		
Dizziness	1.9	1.4
Headache	18.4	18.1
Insomnia	1.3	1.3
Respiratory System Disorders		

(cont'd)

Table 1: SINGULAIR *(cont'd)*

Adverse Experiences Occurring in ≥1% of Patients with an Incidence ≥ to that in Patients Treated with Placebo, Regardless of Drug Relationship

	SINGULAIR 10 mg/day (n=1955) (%)	Placebo (n=1180) (%)
Congestion, Nasal	1.6	1.3
Cough	2.7	2.4
Influenza	4.2	3.9
Skin/Skin Appendages Disorder		
Rash	1.6	1.2
Laboratory Adverse Experiences[a]		
ALT Increased	2.1	2.0
AST Increased	1.6	1.2
Pyuria	1.0	0.9

[a] Number of patients tested (SINGULAIR and placebo, respectively): ALT and AST, 1935, 1170; pyuria, 1924, 1159.

Cumulatively, 544 patients were treated with SINGULAIR for at least 6 months, 253 for one year and 21 for two years in clinical trials. With prolonged treatment, the adverse experience profile did not change.

Pediatric Patients 6 to 14 Years of Age with Asthma: SINGULAIR has been evaluated for safety in approximately 475 pediatric patients 6 to 14 years of age. Cumulatively, 263 pediatric patients 6 to 14 years of age were treated with SINGULAIR for at least 3 months, 164 for 6 months or longer in clinical trials. The safety profile in pediatric patients is generally similar to the adult safety profile and to placebo. With prolonged treatment, the adverse experience profile did not change.

In a 56-week double-blind study evaluating growth rate in pediatric patients 6 to 8 years of age receiving SINGULAIR, the following events not previously observed with the use of SINGULAIR occurred with a frequency ≥2% and more frequently than in pediatric patients who received placebo, regardless of causality assessment: atopic dermatitis, myopia, rhinitis (infective), skin infection, tooth infection, headache, varicella, gastroenteritis and acute bronchitis.

Pediatric Patients 2 to 5 Years of Age with Asthma: SINGULAIR has been evaluated for safety in 573 pediatric patients 2 to 5 years of age. In a 12-week, placebo-controlled clinical study, the only adverse experience reported as drug-related in >1% of patients treated with SINGULAIR and at a greater incidence than in patients treated with placebo was thirst. The incidence of thirst was not significantly different in the two treatment groups. Cumulatively, 363 patients 2 to 5 years of age were treated with SINGULAIR. Of these, 338 were continuously treated for at least 6 months and 256 for >1 year. The safety profile of SINGULAIR in pediatric patients 2 to 5 years of age is generally similar to the safety profiles in adults 15 years of age and older in pediatric patients 6 to 14 years of age, and to placebo. With prolonged treatment, the adverse experience profile did not change.

Pediatric Patients 6 Months to 2 Years of Age with Asthma: SINGULAIR has been evaluated in 175 pediatric patients 6 months to 2 years of age. In a 6-week, placebo-controlled clinical study, the adverse experiences reported as drug related in >1% of patients treated with SINGULAIR and at a greater incidence than in patients treated with placebo were diarrhea, hyperkinesia, asthma, eczematous dermatitis and rash. The incidences of these adverse experiences were not significantly different in the two treatment groups.

Adults 15 Years of Age and Older with Seasonal Allergic Rhinitis: SINGULAIR has been evaluated in 1751 adult patients 15 years of age and older for the treatment of seasonal allergic rhinitis in clinical studies. SINGULAIR administered once daily at bedtime was generally well tolerated with a safety profile similar to that of placebo. In similar designed, 2-week, placebo-controlled, clinical studies, no adverse experience reported as drug related in ≥1% of patients treated with SINGULAIR and at a greater incidence than in patients treated with placebo were observed. The incidence of somnolence was similar to that of placebo.

Post-Market Adverse Drug Reactions: The following adverse drug reactions have been reported very rarely (<1/10 000) in post-marketing use of SINGULAIR. Because these reactions are reported voluntarily from a population of uncertain size, it is not always possible to reliably estimate their frequency or establish a causal relationship to drug exposure.

Infections and Infestations: upper respiratory infection.

Blood and Lymphatic System Disorders: increased bleeding tendency.

Immune System Disorders: hypersensitivity reactions including anaphylaxis, and very rarely, hepatic eosinophilic infiltration.

Psychiatric Disorders: agitation including aggressive behavior or hostility (including temper tantrums in pediatric patients), very rarely reported as serious; anxiousness, depression, irritability, restlessness, somnambulism, sleep disorders including dream abnormalities and insomnia, suicidal thinking and behavior (suicidality), tremor, visual hallucinations.

Nervous System Disorders: dizziness, drowsiness, paraesthesia/hypoesthesia, and very rarely seizure.

Cardiac Disorders: palpitations.

Gastrointestinal Disorders: diarrhea, dyspepsia, nausea, vomiting.

Skin and Subcutaneous Tissue Disorders: angioedema, bruising, erythema nodosum, pruritus, rash, urticaria.

Musculoskeletal, Connective Tissue and Bone Disorders: arthralgia, myalgia including muscle cramps.

Hepato-biliary Disorders: increased ALT, AST, and isolated cases of hepatitis (including cholestatic, hepatocellular, and mixed-pattern liver injury). In post-marketing surveillance, elevations in serum transaminases have been reported in patients who were treated with SINGULAIR. These events were usually asymptomatic and transient. Serious hepatic adverse events such as jaundice have been reported although no deaths or liver transplantations have been attributed to the use of SINGULAIR (see Warnings and Precautions).

General Disorders: edema.

Eosinophilic Conditions: In rare cases, patients with asthma on therapy with SINGULAIR may present with systemic eosinophilia, sometimes presenting with clinical features of vasculitis consistent with Churg-Strauss syndrome, a condition which is often treated with systemic corticosteroid therapy. These events usually, but not always, have been associated with the reduction of oral corticosteroid therapy. Physicians should be alert to eosinophilia, vasculitic rash, arthralgia, worsening pulmonary symptoms, cardiac complications, and/or neuropathy presenting in their patients. A causal association between SINGULAIR and these underlying conditions has not been established. The Churg-Strauss syndrome complicating antileukotriene therapy is thought to relate to unmasking of an underlying vasculitic syndrome associated with moderate or severe asthma treated with corticosteroids (see Warnings and Precautions, Eosinophilic Conditions).

DRUG INTERACTIONS: Overview: SINGULAIR may be administered with other therapies routinely used in the prophylaxis and chronic treatment of asthma, and in the treatment of allergic rhinitis (see Drug-Drug Interactions).

Although additional specific interaction studies were not performed, SINGULAIR was used concomitantly with a wide range of commonly prescribed drugs in clinical studies without evidence of clinical adverse interactions. These medications included thyroid hormones, sedative hypnotics, nonsteroidal anti-inflammatory agents, benzodiazepines and decongestants.

In vitro studies have shown that montelukast is an inhibitor of CYP 2C8. However, data from a clinical drug-drug interaction study involving montelukast and rosiglitazone (a probe substrate representative of drugs primarily metabolized by CYP 2C8) in 12 healthy individuals demonstrated that the pharmacokinetics of rosiglitazone are not altered when the drugs are coadministered, indicating that montelukast does not inhibit CYP 2C8 in vivo. Therefore, montelukast is not anticipated to alter the metabolism of drugs metabolized by this enzyme (e.g., paclitaxel, rosiglitazone, repaglinide).

Drug-Drug Interactions: Montelukast 10 mg once daily to pharmacokinetic steady state:

- did not cause clinically significant changes in the kinetics of an intravenous dose of theophylline.
- did not change the pharmacokinetic profile of warfarin or influence the effect of a single 30 mg oral dose of warfarin on prothrombin time or INR (International Normalized Ratio).
- did not change the pharmacokinetic profile or urinary excretion of immunoreactive digoxin.
- did not change the plasma concentration profile of terfenadine or its carboxylated metabolite and does not prolong the QTc interval following coadministration with terfenadine 60 mg twice daily.

Montelukast at doses of ≥100 mg daily to pharmacokinetic steady state:

- did not significantly alter the plasma concentrations of either component of an oral contraceptive containing norethindrone 1 mg/ethinyl estradiol 35 μg.
- did not cause any clinically significant change in plasma profiles of either prednisone and prednisolone following administration of either oral prednisone or IV prednisolone.

Phenobarbital, which induces hepatic metabolism, decreased the AUC of montelukast approximately 40% following a single 10 mg dose of montelukast; no dosage adjustment for SINGULAIR is recommended.

DOSAGE AND ADMINISTRATION: Dosing Considerations: The safety and efficacy of SINGULAIR was demonstrated in clinical trials where it was administered in the evening without regard to the time of food ingestion. There have been no clinical trials evaluating the relative efficacy of morning versus evening dosing. However, no difference in pharmacokinetics was noted between morning and evening dosing.

General Recommendations: The therapeutic effect of SINGULAIR on parameters of asthma occurs within one day. SINGULAIR tablets, chewable tablets, and oral granules can be taken with or without food. Patients should be advised to continue taking SINGULAIR while their asthma is controlled, as well as during periods of worsening asthma.

Therapy with SINGULAIR in Relation to Other Treatments for Asthma: SINGULAIR can also be added to a patient's existing treatment regimen.

Bronchodilator Treatments: SINGULAIR can be added to the treatment regimen of patients who are not adequately controlled on bronchodilator alone. When a clinical response is evident (usually after the first dose), the patient's bronchodilator therapy can be reduced as tolerated.

Inhaled Corticosteroids: Treatment with SINGULAIR provides additional clinical benefit to patients treated with inhaled corticosteroids. A reduction in the corticosteroid dose can be made as tolerated. The dose should be reduced gradually with medical supervision. In some patients, the dose of inhaled corticosteroids can be tapered off completely. It remains to be determined whether the withdrawal from inhaled corticosteroids can be maintained for extended periods, or possibly indefinitely. SINGULAIR should not be abruptly substituted for inhaled corticosteroids.

Oral Corticosteroids: Limited data suggest that SINGULAIR may provide additional clinical benefit in patients currently treated with oral corticosteroids.

Recommended Dose and Dosage Adjustment: Adults 15 Years of Age and Older with Asthma and/or Seasonal Allergic Rhinitis: The dosage for adults 15 years of age and older is one 10 mg tablet daily to be taken in the evening.

Pediatric Patients 6 to 14 Years of Age with Asthma: The dosage for pediatric patients 6 to 14 years of age is one 5 mg chewable tablet daily to be taken in the evening. No dosage adjustment within this age group is necessary.

Pediatric Patients 2 to 5 Years of Age with Asthma: The dosage for pediatric patients 2 to 5 years of age is one 4 mg chewable tablet daily to be taken in the evening or one packet of 4 mg granules to be taken orally once a day in the evening. No dosage adjustment within this age group is necessary.

Special Population: No dosage adjustment is necessary for the elderly, for patients with renal insufficiency, or mild to moderate hepatic impairment, or for patients of either gender.

Administration of Oral Granules: SINGULAIR oral granules can be administered either directly in the mouth, or mixed with a spoonful of cold or room temperature soft food (e.g., applesauce). The packet should not be opened until ready to use. After opening the packet, the full dose of SINGULAIR oral granules must be administered immediately (within 15 minutes). If mixed with food, SINGULAIR oral granules must not be stored for future use. SINGULAIR oral granules are not intended to be dissolved in liquid for administration. However, liquids may be taken subsequent to administration.

Missed Dose: SINGULAIR should be taken as prescribed. However, if a dose is missed, the usual schedule should be resumed as prescribed.

OVERDOSAGE:

No specific information is available on the treatment of overdosage with SINGULAIR. In chronic asthma studies, SINGULAIR has been administered at doses up to 200 mg/day to adult patients for 22 weeks and in short-term studies, up to 900 mg/day to patients for approximately one week without clinically important adverse experiences.

There have been reports of acute overdosage in post-marketing experience and clinical studies with SINGULAIR. These include reports in adults and children with a dose as high as 1000 mg. The clinical and laboratory findings observed were consistent with the safety profile in adults and pediatric patients. There were no adverse experiences in the majority of overdosage reports. The adverse experiences were consistent with the safety profile of SINGULAIR and most frequently included abdominal pain, somnolence, thirst, headache, vomiting, psychomotor hyperactivity, and less frequently convulsion.

It is not known whether montelukast is dialyzable by peritoneal dialysis or hemodialysis.

For management of a suspected drug overdose, contact your regional Poison Control Centre. See the *CPS* Directory section for a list of Poison Control Centres.

ACTION AND CLINICAL PHARMACOLOGY: Mechanism of Action: The cysteinyl leukotrienes (LTC_4, LTD_4, LTE_4), are potent inflammatory eicosanoids released from various cells including mast cells and eosinophils. These important proasthmatic mediators bind to cysteinyl leukotriene (CysLT) receptors. The CysLT type-1 ($CysLT_1$) receptor is found in the human airway (including airway smooth muscle cells and airway macrophages) and on other pro-inflammatory cells (including eosinophils and certain myeloid stem cells). CysLTs have been correlated with the pathophysiology of asthma and allergic rhinitis. In asthma, leukotriene-mediated effects include a number of airway actions, including bronchoconstriction, mucous secretion, vascular permeability, and eosinophil recruitment. In allergic rhinitis, CysLTs are released from the nasal mucosa after allergen exposure during both early- and late-phase reactions and are associated with symptoms of allergic rhinitis. Intranasal challenge with CysLTs has been shown to increase nasal airway resistance and symptoms of nasal obstruction.

SINGULAIR has not been assessed in intranasal challenge studies. The clinical relevance of intranasal challenge studies is unknown.

Montelukast is an orally active compound that significantly improves parameters of asthmatic inflammation. Based on biochemical and pharmacological bioassays, it binds with high affinity and selectivity to the $CysLT_1$ receptor (in preference to other pharmacologically important airway receptors such as the prostanoid, cholinergic, or β-adrenergic receptor). Montelukast potently inhibits physiologic actions of LTC_4, LTD_4, and LTE_4 at the $CysLT_1$ receptor without any agonist activity.

Pharmacodynamics: Montelukast causes inhibition of airway cysteinyl leukotriene receptors as demonstrated by the ability to inhibit bronchoconstriction due to inhaled LTD_4 in asthmatic patients. Doses as low as 5 mg cause substantial blockage of LTD_4-induced bronchoconstriction. In a placebo-controlled, crossover study (n=12), SINGULAIR inhibited early- and late-phase bronchoconstriction due to antigen challenge by 75% and 57% respectively.

Montelukast causes bronchodilation within 2 hours of oral administration; these effects were additive to the bronchodilation caused by a β-agonist.

Clinical studies in adults 15 years of age and older demonstrated there is no additional clinical benefit to montelukast doses above 10 mg once daily. This was shown in two chronic asthma studies using doses up to 200 mg once daily and in one exercise challenge study using doses up to 50 mg, evaluated at the end of the once daily dosing interval.

The effect of SINGULAIR on eosinophils in the peripheral blood was examined in clinical trials in adults and pediatric (6 to 14 years of age) asthmatic patients. SINGULAIR decreased mean peripheral blood eosinophils approximately 13% to 15% from baseline compared with placebo over the double-blind treatment periods.

In patients with seasonal allergic rhinitis aged 15 years and older who received SINGULAIR, a median decrease of 13% in peripheral blood eosinophil counts was noted, compared with placebo, over the double-blind treatment periods.

There have been no clinical trials evaluating the relative efficacy of morning versus evening dosing. Although the pharmacokinetics of montelukast are similar whether dosed in the morning or the evening, efficacy was demonstrated in clinical trials in adults and pediatric patients in which montelukast was administered in the evening without regard to the time of food ingestion.

Pharmacokinetics: Absorption: Montelukast is rapidly absorbed following oral administration. For the 10 mg film-coated tablet, the mean peak plasma concentration (C_{max}) is achieved 3 to 4 hours (T_{max}) after administration in adults in the fasted state. The mean oral bioavailability is 64%. The oral bioavailability and C_{max} are neither influenced by a standard meal in the morning nor by a high fat snack in the evening. Safety and efficacy were demonstrated in clinical trials where the 4 mg chewable tablet, the 5 mg chewable tablet, and the 10 mg film-coated tablet were administered in the evening without regard to the timing of food ingestion. The safety of SINGULAIR was also demonstrated in a clinical study in which the 4 mg oral granules were administered in the evening without regard to the timing of food ingestion.

For the 5 mg chewable tablet, the C_{max} is achieved 2 hours after administration in adults in the fasted state. The mean oral bioavailability is 73% in the fasted state versus 63% when administered with a standard meal in the morning. However, food does not have a clinically important influence with chronic administration of the chewable tablet. The comparative pharmacokinetics of montelukast when administered as two 5 mg chewable tablets versus one 10 mg film-coated tablet has not been evaluated.

For the 4 mg chewable tablet, C_{max} is achieved 2 hours after administration in pediatric patients 2 to 5 years of age in the fasted state.

The 4 mg oral granule formulation was shown to be bioequivalent to the 4 mg chewable tablet when administered to healthy adults in the fasted state. Bioequivalence was also demonstrated when the granules were administered with applesauce. The coadministration of a high fat meal decreased the rate of absorption (C_{max} 112.8 versus 175.4 ng/mL with and without a high fat meal, respectively), although the extent of absorption was not affected by food (AUC_T 1133.8 versus 1119.2 ng·h/mL with and without a high fat meal, respectively).

Distribution: Montelukast is more than 99% bound to plasma proteins. The steady-state volume of distribution of montelukast averages 8 to 11 L. Studies in rats with radiolabeled montelukast indicate minimal distribution across the blood-brain barrier. In addition, concentrations of radiolabeled material at 24 hours post-dose were minimal in all other tissues.

Metabolism: Montelukast is extensively metabolized. In studies with therapeutic doses, plasma concentrations of metabolites of montelukast are undetectable at steady state in adults and pediatric patients.

In vitro studies using human liver microsomes indicate that cytochrome P450 3A4 and 2C9 are involved in the metabolism of montelukast. Clinical studies investigating the effect of known inhibitors of cytochrome P450 3A4 (e.g. ketoconazole, erythromycin) or 2C9 (e.g. fluconazole) on montelukast pharmacokinetics have not been conducted. Based on further in vitro results in human liver microsomes, therapeutic plasma concentrations of montelukast do not inhibit cytochromes P450 3A4, 2C9, 1A2, 2A6, 2C19, or 2D6 (see Drug Interactions).

Excretion: The plasma clearance of montelukast averages 45 mL/min in healthy adults. Following an oral dose of radiolabeled montelukast, 86% of the radioactivity was recovered in 5-day fecal collections and <0.2% was recovered in urine. Coupled with estimates of montelukast oral bioavailability, this indicates montelukast and its metabolites are excreted almost exclusively via the bile.

In several studies, the mean plasma half-life of montelukast ranged from 2.7 to 5.5 hours in healthy young adults. The pharmacokinetics of montelukast are nearly linear for oral doses up to 50 mg. No difference in pharmacokinetics was noted between dosing in the morning or in the evening. During once-daily dosing with 10 mg montelukast, there is little accumulation of the parent drug in plasma (~14%).

Special Populations and Conditions: Pediatrics: The plasma concentration profile of montelukast following the administration of 10 mg film-coated tablet is similar in adolescents ≥15 years old and young adults. The 10 mg film-coated tablet is recommended for use in patients ≥15 years old.

Pharmacokinetic studies show that the plasma profiles of the 4 mg oral granule formulation in pediatric patients 6 months to 2 years of age, the 4 mg chewable tablet in pediatric patients 2 to 5 years of age, and the 5 mg chewable tablets in pediatric patients 6 to 14 years of age were similar to the plasma profile of the 10 mg film-coated tablet in adults. The 5 mg chewable tablet should be used in pediatric patients 6 to 14 years of age and the 4 mg chewable tablet should be used in pediatric patients 2 to 5 years of age. Since the 4 mg oral granule formulation is bioequivalent to the 4 mg chewable tablet, it can also be used as an alternative formulation to the 4 mg chewable tablet in pediatric patients 2 to 5 years of age.

Geriatrics: The pharmacokinetic profile and the oral bioavailability of a single 10 mg oral dose of montelukast are similar in elderly and younger adults. The plasma half-life of montelukast is slightly longer in the elderly. No dosage adjustment in the elderly is required.

Gender: The pharmacokinetics of montelukast are similar in males and females.

Race: Pharmacokinetic differences due to race have not been studied. In clinical studies, there do not appear to be any differences in clinically important effects.

Hepatic Insufficiency: Patients with mild to moderate hepatic insufficiency and clinical evidence of cirrhosis had evidence of decreased metabolism of montelukast resulting in approximately 41% higher mean montelukast area under the plasma concentration curve (AUC) following a single 10 mg dose. The elimination of montelukast is slightly prolonged compared with that in healthy subjects (mean half-life, 7.4 hours). No dosage adjustment is required in patients with mild to moderate hepatic insufficiency. There are no clinical data in patients with hepatitis or severe hepatic insufficiency (Child-Pugh score >9).

Renal Insufficiency: Since montelukast and its metabolites are not excreted in the urine, the pharmacokinetics of montelukast were not evaluated in patients with renal insufficiency. No dosage adjustment is recommended in these patients.

STORAGE AND STABILITY: Store the 10 mg film-coated tablets, and the 4 mg and 5 mg chewable tablets at room temperature (15-30°C), protected from moisture and light.

Store the 4 mg oral granules at room temperature (15-30°C), in the original package.

INFORMATION FOR THE PATIENT: Published in e-CPS, available by subscription at www.e-cps.ca.

DOSAGE FORMS, COMPOSITION AND PACKAGING: Chewable Tablets: 4 mg: Each pink, oval, biconvex-shaped, chewable tablet, with the code MSD 711 on one side and SINGULAIR on the other, contains: montelukast sodium 4.2 mg, which is the molar equivalent to free acid 4 mg. Nonmedicinal ingredients: aspartame, cherry flavor, croscarmellose sodium, hydroxypropyl cellulose, magnesium stearate, mannitol, microcrystalline cellulose and red ferric oxide. Blister packages of 30.

5 mg: Each pink, round, biconvex-shaped, chewable tablet, with the code MSD 275 on one side and SINGULAIR on the other, contains: montelukast sodium 5.2 mg, which is the molar equivalent to free acid 5 mg. Nonmedicinal ingredients: aspartame, cherry flavor, croscarmellose sodium, hydroxypropyl cellulose, magnesium stearate, mannitol, microcrystalline cellulose and red ferric oxide. Blister packages of 30.

Tablets: Each beige, rounded square-shaped, film-coated tablet, with the code MSD 117 on one side and SINGULAIR on the other, contains: montelukast sodium 10.4 mg, which is the molar equivalent of free acid 10 mg. Nonmedicinal ingredients: croscarmellose sodium, hydroxypropyl cellulose, lactose monohydrate, magnesium stearate and microcrystalline cellulose; film-coating: carnauba wax, hydroxypropyl cellulose, hydroxypropyl methylcellulose, red ferric oxide, titanium dioxide and yellow ferric oxide. Blister packages of 30 and 50.

Oral Granules: Each 4 mg packet of oral granules (presented as a white, coarse, granular, free-flowing homogeneous solid in a foil packet) contains: montelukast sodium 4.2 mg, which is the molar equivalent to 4 mg of free acid. Nonmedicinal ingredients: hydroxypropyl cellulose, magnesium stearate and mannitol. Packages of 30.

(Shown in Product Identification Section)

Sintrom® Ⓟ

acenocoumarol

Oral Anticoagulant

Paladin

SUPPLIED: 1 mg: Each peach colored, biconvex round tablet contains: acenocoumarol 1 mg. Nonmedicinal ingredients: alcohol, colloidal silicon dioxide, cornstarch, FD&C Yellow No. 6, gelatin, glycerin, lactose, magnesium stearate and talc. Energy: 0.67 kJ (0.16 kcal). Bisulfite-, gluten-, parabens-, sodium- and tartrazine-free. Bottles of 100.

4 mg: Each white, flat-faced tablet, debossed with Paladin shield on one side and double scored on the other, contains: acenocoumarol 4 mg. Nonmedicinal ingredients: colloidal silicon dioxide, cornstarch, lactose, magnesium stearate and talc. Energy: 1.76 kJ (0.42 kcal). Alcohol-, bisulfite-, gluten-, parabens-, sodium- and tartrazine-free. Bottles of 100.

(Shown in Product Identification Section)

Sinutab® Sinus and Allergy

acetaminophen—pseudoephedrine HCl—chlorpheniramine maleate

Analgesic—Decongestant—Antihistamine

McNeil Consumer Healthcare

Sinutab® with Codeine Ⓝ

acetaminophen—pseudoephedrine HCl—chlorpheniramine maleate—codeine phosphate

Analgesic—Decongestant—Antihistamine

McNeil Consumer Healthcare

Sinutab® Sinus Non Drowsy

acetaminophen—pseudoephedrine HCl

Analgesic—Decongestant

McNeil Consumer Healthcare

Sinutab® Nightime

acetaminophen—pseudoephedrine HCl—diphenhydramine HCl

Analgesic—Decongestant—Antihistamine

McNeil Consumer Healthcare

INDICATIONS: Symptomatic relief of headache, facial pain, malaise, fever, nasal and sinus congestion often associated with acute and chronic sinusitis, allergic rhinitis, vasomotor rhinitis and the common cold.

CONTRAINDICATIONS: Sensitivity to any of the components. Patients receiving or having received MAOIs in the preceding 3 weeks.

WARNINGS: Massive acetaminophen overdose can be toxic and potentially fatal. In adults, hepatotoxicity from acetaminophen is unlikely to occur with overdoses of less than 10 g ingested at one time and fatalities are unlikely to occur with overdoses of less than 15 g ingested at one time.

PRECAUTIONS: Recommended dose should not be exceeded without consulting a physician. Since the depressant effects of antihistamines are additive to those of other drugs affecting the CNS, patients should be cautioned against drinking alcoholic beverages or taking hypnotics, sedatives, psychotherapeutic agents or other drugs with CNS depressant effects during antihistamine therapy.

Occupational Hazards: Patients should be cautioned not to operate vehicles or hazardous machinery until their response to the drug has been determined.

Pregnancy: Safety in pregnancy not yet established.

Use with caution in elderly, pregnant or nursing patients and patients with hyperthyroidism, hypertension, glaucoma, asthma, chronic lung disease, prostatic hypertrophy, diabetes mellitus, cardiovascular diseases, chronic alcoholism, serious kidney or liver disease, in patients taking a drug for depression, including MAOIs.

Sinutab with Codeine: Codeine may be habit forming.

ADVERSE EFFECTS: Acetaminophen may occasionally cause gastric upset. The incidence and severity of this adverse effect is less than that after ASA administration.

Pseudoephedrine may cause mild stimulation, particularly in patients sensitive to sympathomimetic drugs.

Excitement may occur in children. Nausea, diarrhea, mild stimulation, and abdominal pain from sympathomimetic agents may occur.

Drowsiness, confusion and gastrointestinal upset may occur with antihistamines.

OVERDOSE:

Symptoms: Symptoms of massive overdosage include gastric irritation, nausea and vomiting, chills, hyperthermia, tinnitus, hypotension, circulatory collapse, cyanosis, methemoglobinemia, jaundice, coma, disorientation, hallucinations, hyperreflexia, tremors, convulsions, respiratory failure and renal damage.

Treatment: Evacuate the stomach by emesis or gastric lavage and administer activated charcoal.

For management of a suspected drug overdose, CPhA recommends that you contact your **regional Poison Control Centre**. See the *CPS* Directory section for a list of Poison Control Centres.

DOSAGE: Sinutab Sinus and Allergy: Regular Strength: Adults: 2 caplets every 4 to 6 hours. Maximum 8 caplets/day. Children 6 to 12 years: 1 caplet every 4 to 6 hours, not to exceed 4 caplets/day.

Extra Strength: Adults: 1 to 2 caplets every 4 to 6 hours. Maximum 8 caplets/day.

Sinutab with Codeine: Adults: 1 to 2 tablets every 4 to 6 hours. Maximum 8 tablets/day.

Sinutab Sinus Non Drowsy: Regular Strength: Adults: 2 caplets every 4 to 6 hours. Maximum 8 caplets/day. Children 6 to 12 years: 1 caplet every 4 to 6 hours. Maximum 4 caplets/day.

Extra Strength (Daytime): Adults: 1 to 2 caplets every 4 to 6 hours. Do not exceed 8 caplets/day.

Sinutab Nightime: Extra Strength: Adults and children over 12 years of age: 2 caplets at bedtime. Do not exceed 2 caplets/day.

SUPPLIED: Sinutab Sinus and Allergy: Regular Strength: Each yellow caplet imprinted "Sinutab" on both sides contains: acetaminophen 325 mg, pseudoephedrine HCl 30 mg and chlorpheniramine maleate 2 mg. Nonmedicinal ingredients: cellulose, croscarmellose sodium, D&C Yellow No. 10, FD&C Yellow No. 6, hypromellose, polyethylene glycol, polysorbate, starch, titanium dioxide, wax and zinc stearate. Energy: 0.76 kJ (0.18 kcal). Boxes of 12, 24 and 36 in blister packages.

Extra Strength: Each yellow caplet imprinted "Sinutab" on both sides contains: acetaminophen 500 mg, pseudoephedrine HCl 30 mg and chlorpheniramine maleate 2 mg. Nonmedicinal ingredients: cellulose, croscarmellose sodium, D&C Yellow No. 10, FD&C Yellow No. 6, hypromellose, polyethylene glycol, polysorbate, starch, titanium dioxide, wax and zinc stearate. Energy: 0.76 kJ (0.18 kcal). Boxes of 24 and 48 in blister packages.

Sinutab with Codeine: Each blue, biconvex tablet contains: acetaminophen 325 mg, pseudoephedrine HCl 30 mg, chlorpheniramine maleate 2 mg and codeine phosphate 8 mg. Nonmedicinal ingredients: cornstarch, FD&C Blue No. 1, gelatin (pork), guar gum, hydrogenated vegetable oil, isopropyl alcohol, lactose, magnesium stearate and stearic acid. Energy: 4.7 kJ (1.13 kcal). Sodium-free. Bottles of 16.

Sinutab Sinus Non Drowsy: Regular Strength: Each orange caplet imprinted "Sinutab" on both sides contains: acetaminophen 325 mg and pseudoephedrine HCl 30 mg. Nonmedicinal ingredients: cellulose, croscarmellose sodium, FD&C Yellow No. 6, polyethylene glycol, hypromellose, polysorbate, starch, titanium dioxide, wax and zinc stearate. Energy: 0.8 kJ (0.19 kcal). Sodium: <1 mmol (0.01 mg). Boxes of 24 in blister packages.

Extra Strength (Daytime): Each orange caplet imprinted "Sinutab" on both sides contains: acetaminophen 500 mg and pseudoephedrine HCl 30 mg. Nonmedicinal ingredients: croscarmellose sodium, FD&C Yellow No. 6, hypromellose, polyethylene glycol, polysorbate, starch, titanium dioxide, wax and zinc stearate. Energy: 1.05 kJ (0.25 kcal). Sodium: 0.02 mg. Boxes of 12 and 24 in a blister package.

Sinutab Nightime: Extra Strength: Each white caplet, printed "NIGHT/NUIT" on both sides, contains: acetaminophen 500 mg, pseudoephedrine HCl 30 mg and diphenhydramine HCl 25 mg. Nonmedicinal ingredients: cellulose, croscarmellose sodium, hypromellose, propylene glycol, silicon dioxide, titanium dioxide, wax and zinc stearate. Available as part of Sinutab Extra Strength Daytime/Nightime Combo Pack.

Combo Pack: Each box contains: 18 caplets of Sinutab Non Drowsy Extra Strength (Daytime) and 6 caplets of Sinutab Nightime Extra Strength.

All preparations are gluten-, paraben-, sulfite- and tartrazine-free. Sinutab with Codeine also contain lactose; others are lactose-free.

Slow-K®

potassium chloride

Potassium Supplement

Novartis Pharmaceuticals

Date of Preparation: January 28, 1970
Date of Revision: September 16, 2008

SUMMARY PRODUCT INFORMATION:

Route of Administration	Dosage Form/ Strength	Clinically Relevant Nonmedicinal Ingredients
Oral	600 mg sugar-coated tablet	Cetostearyl alcohol, gelatine, magnesium stearate For a complete listing see Dosage Forms, Composition and Packaging.

INDICATIONS AND CLINICAL USE: SLOW-K is indicated for:

- treatment of potassium depletion in patients with hypokalemia and metabolic alkalosis.
- prevention of potassium depletion when the dietary intake of potassium is inadequate for this purpose. The prophylactic administration of potassium ion may be indicated in patients receiving digitalis and/or diuretics for the treatment of congestive heart failure, and hepatic cirrhosis with ascites. SLOW-K may be indicated in selected patients with hypertension on long-term diuretic therapy, hyperaldosteronism states with normal renal function, the nephrotic syndrome, and certain diarrheal states.

Potassium ions participate in a number of essential physiological processes (see Action and Clinical Pharmacology). Depletion may occur whenever the rate of potassium loss through renal excretion and/or loss from the gastrointestinal tract exceeds the rate of potassium intake. Although there is no uniform correlation between plasma concentrations of potassium and total body stores, clinical signs of potassium deficiency are usually observed whenever the plasma potassium concentration falls below 3.5 mEq/Litre (hypokalemia).

Hypokalemia can be prevented and/or corrected by giving supplementary potassium. Administration of potassium salts is an alternative to increasing dietary intake of potassium-rich foods, which may not always be practical. In view of the frequency with which deficits of K+ and Cl− coexist, potassium chloride is the preferred salt for most of the clinical conditions associated with hypokalemia (see Warnings and Precautions).

SLOW-K (slow-release potassium chloride) is a sugar-coated (not enteric-coated) tablet containing 600 mg potassium chloride in a wax matrix. This formulation is intended to provide a controlled release of potassium chloride from the matrix, thereby minimizing the likelihood of producing high localized concentration of potassium within the gastrointestinal tract. The release of potassium chloride is largely pH- independent and occurs at a rate sufficient to permit complete absorption during its transit through the gastrointestinal tract.

Geriatrics: As renal function, and hence the potential for maintaining potassium balance may decrease with age, serum potassium levels should be monitored regularly and dosage adjusted as appropriate. As gastrointestinal motility may also be affected by age, elderly patients should be reminded to swallow solid oral potassium salts with adequate amounts of fluid. (See Warnings and Precautions, Special Populations.)

Pediatrics: Safety and effectiveness in children have not been established. SLOW-K is therefore not recommended for pediatric use (see Warnings and Precautions, Special Populations).

CONTRAINDICATIONS:

- Hypersensitivity to potassium administration, e.g., in adynamia episodica hereditaria or congenital paramyotonia or patients who are hypersensitive to any ingredient in the formulation or component of the container. For a complete listing, see Dosage Forms, Composition and Packaging.
- Hyperkalemia of any etiology, since a further increase in the serum potassium concentration in such patients can produce cardiac arrhythmia and cardiac arrest. Hyperkalemia may complicate any of the following conditions: marked renal failure, untreated Addison's disease, hyperadrenalism associated with adrenogenital syndrome, hyporeninemic hypoaldosteronism, extensive tissue breakdown (as in severe burns, trauma, massive hemolysis, rhabdomyolysis, tumour lysis), acute dehydration, heat cramps, metabolic acidosis.
- Renal impairment with oliguria or azotemia.
- Concomitant administration of SLOW-K and potassium-sparing diuretics (e.g. spironolactone, triamterene or amiloride) (see Drug Interactions).
- Patients in whom there is cause for arrest or delay in tablet passage through the gastrointestinal tract. These states include:
  - Partial or complete esophageal obstruction, for example by carcinomas (esophageal, post-cricoidal, thyroidal), aortic aneurysm, left-atrial enlargement, inflammatory stricture due to reflux esophagitis, and esophageal displacement due to cardiac surgery (e.g. valve replacement).
  - Stenosis or atony in any part of the gastrointestinal tract (e.g. pyloric stenosis, intestinal strictures).

  In these instances, potassium supplementation should be with a liquid preparation.

WARNINGS AND PRECAUTIONS: Cardiovascular: Potassium supplements should be used with caution in diseases associated with heart block since increased serum potassium may increase the degree of block.

Endocrine and Metabolism: In patients with impaired mechanisms for excreting potassium, the administration of potassium salts can produce hyperkalemia and cardiac arrest. This occurs most commonly in patients given potassium by the intravenous route but may also occur in patients given potassium orally. Potentially fatal hyperkalemia can develop rapidly and be asymptomatic. The use of potassium salts in patients with chronic renal disease, or any other condition which impairs potassium excretion, requires particularly careful monitoring of the serum potassium concentration and appropriate dosage adjustment.

SLOW-K should be used with caution in patients receiving any drug known to have a potential for hyperkalemia, such as ACE inhibitors, angiotensin-II-receptor-antagonists, NSAIDs (e.g. indomethacin), beta-blockers, heparin, digoxin and cyclosporine. (See Drug Interactions.)

Hypokalemia in patients with metabolic acidosis should be treated with an alkalinizing potassium salt such as potassium acetate, potassium bicarbonate or potassium citrate.

Clinical signs of hypokalemia (plasma potassium concentrations less than 3.5 mEq/Litre) include impaired neuromuscular function, which may vary from minimal weakness to frank paralysis; intestinal dilatation and ileus; and, more frequently, abnormalities of myocardial function with disturbed ECG patterns characterized by an exaggerated U wave, a broad and flat T wave, and a depressed ST segment.

In some patients, diuretic-induced magnesium deficiency will prevent the restoration of intracellular deficits of potassium, so that hypomagnesemia should be corrected at the same time as hypokalemia.

Gastrointestinal: Since anticholinergic agents have the potential to reduce gastrointestinal motility, they should be prescribed with caution when given concomitantly with solid oral potassium preparations, particularly in high doses.

A probable association exists between the use of coated tablets containing potassium salts, with or without thiazide diuretics, and the incidence of serious small bowel ulceration. Such preparations should be used only when adequate dietary supplementation is not practical, and should be discontinued if abdominal pain, distention, nausea, vomiting or gastrointestinal bleeding occurs.

SLOW-K is a wax matrix tablet formulated to provide a controlled rate of release of potassium chloride and thus to minimize the possibility of a high local concentration of potassium near the bowel wall. While the reported frequency of small bowel lesions is very much less with wax matrix tablets (less than one per 100 000 patient years) than with enteric-coated potassium chloride tablets (40-50 per 100 000 patient years), a few cases associated with wax matrix tablets have been reported.

SLOW-K should be discontinued immediately and the possibility of bowel obstruction or perforation considered if pronounced nausea, severe vomiting, diarrhea, abdominal pain, distention or gastrointestinal bleeding occurs.

Such risks may be increased in patients with esophageal stasis, known peptic and/or gastric ulcers, delayed intestinal transit, or intestinal ischemia due to generalized atherosclerotic vascular disease.

Patients with ostomies may have an altered intestinal transit time and are better treated with other forms of potassium salt.

Sensitivity/Resistance: SLOW-K contains sucrose (=saccharose). Patients with rare hereditary disorders like fructose-intolerance, glucose-galactose malabsorption, or sucrase-isomaltase insufficiency should not use this medicine.

Special Populations: Pregnant Women: For SLOW-K, no clinical data on exposed pregnancies are available. There is no indication in animal studies of direct or indirect harmful effects with respect to pregnancy, embryonal/foetal development, parturition or postnatal development.

In general, no drug should be taken during the first trimester, and the benefits and risks of drug administration should be carefully considered throughout pregnancy.

Pregnancy is associated with gastrointestinal hypomotility. Solid oral potassium supplements should therefore only be given to pregnant women if such therapy is considered essential.

Nursing Women: The excretion of potassium in milk has not been studied in animals or human. The normal K+ content of human milk is approximately 13 mEq/Litre. Since oral potassium becomes part of the body's potassium pool, provided the body potassium is not excessive, the contribution of SLOW-K can be expected to have little or no effect on the potassium level in human milk.

SLOW-K should only be given during breast-feeding when the expected benefit to the mother outweighs the potential risk to the baby.

Pediatrics: Safety and effectiveness in children have not been established. SLOW-K is therefore not recommended for pediatric use.

Geriatrics: As renal function, and hence the potential for maintaining potassium balance may decrease with age, serum potassium levels should be monitored regularly and dosage adjusted as appropriate. As gastrointestinal motility may also be affected by age, elderly patients should be reminded to swallow solid oral potassium salts with adequate amounts of fluid.

Monitoring and Laboratory Tests: Periodic serum potassium determinations are recommended during long-term potassium supplementation. When blood samples are taken for the analysis of plasma potassium, it is important to remember that artifactual elevations can occur after an improper venipuncture technique or as a result of in-vitro hemolysis of the sample.

The correction of hypokalemia, particularly in the presence of cardiac disease, renal disease or acidosis requires careful attention to acid-base balance and appropriate monitoring of serum electrolytes, the electrocardiogram and the clinical status of the patient.

ADVERSE REACTIONS: Adverse Drug Reaction Overview: Gastrointestinal: The most common adverse reactions to oral potassium salts are nausea, vomiting, flatulence, abdominal discomfort and diarrhea.

There have also been reports of esophageal and gastrointestinal obstruction, haemorrhage ulceration with or without perforation of the upper or lower gastrointestinal tract (see Warnings and Precautions). Small bowel lesions have been reported following the administration of SLOW-K (slow-release potassium chloride). The incidence is much lower than that reported for enteric-coated potassium chloride tablets (see Warnings and Precautions).

Electrolytes: One of the most severe adverse effects is hyperkalemia (see Warnings and Precautions).

Skin: Pruritus and/or skin rash, as well as urticaria, have been reported rarely.

DRUG INTERACTIONS: Overview: Concomitant treatment with potassium sparing diuretics (spironolactone, triamterene, amiloride) is contraindicated.

SLOW-K should be used with caution in patients receiving agents known to have a potential for hyperkalemia, such as ACE inhibitors (e.g. captopril, enalapril; see Warnings and Precautions), angiotensin-II receptor antagonists, NSAID's (e.g. indomethacin), beta-blockers, heparin, digoxin and cyclosporine.

Since anticholinergic agents have the potential to reduce gastrointestinal motility, they should be prescribed with caution when given concomitantly with solid oral potassium preparations, particularly in high doses.

Drug-Drug Interactions: See Table 1.

Table 1: SLOW-K

Established or Potential Drug-Drug Interactions

SLOW-K	Ref	Clinical Comment
ACE inhibitors	T	increase risk of hyperkalemia
Angiotensin-II receptor antagonists	T	increase risk of hyperkalemia
NSAID's	T	increase risk of hyperkalemia
Beta-blockers	T	increase risk of hyperkalemia
Heparin	T	increase risk of hyperkalemia
Digoxin	T	increase risk of hyperkalemia
Cyclosporine	T	increase risk of hyperkalemia
Anticholinergic agents	T	Reduce gastrointestinal motility

Legend: C=case study; CT=clinical trial; T=theoretical.

Drug-Food Interactions: The interaction of SLOW-K has not been studied with regards to food.

Drug-Herb Interactions: The interaction of SLOW-K with herbal medications on supplements has not been studied.

Drug-Laboratory Test Interactions: Specific drug laboratory interaction studies have not been conducted with SLOW-K.

Drug-Lifestyle Interactions: Specific drug lifestyle interaction studies have not been conducted with SLOW-K.

DOSAGE AND ADMINISTRATION: Dosing Considerations: The usual dietary intake of potassium by the average adult is 50 to 100 mEq per day. Potassium depletion sufficient to cause hypokalemia usually requires the loss of 200 or more mEq of potassium from the total body store.

Recommended Dose and Dosage Adjustment: Dosage must be adjusted to the individual needs of each patient, and to the cause and degree of the manifest or potential hypokalemic state. Where intermittent diuretic therapy is being used, SLOW-K (slow-release potassium chloride) should preferably be given on days other than those on which diuretic is administered.

- **Prevention of hypokalemia:** Typically in the range of 20 mEq per day.
- **Correction of hypokalemia:** Typically in the range of 40 to a maximum of 100 mEq per day, depending on initial plasma K+ concentrations. The response to treatment should preferably be monitored by repeated plasma K+ determinations, and SLOW-K continued until the hypokalemia has been corrected.

The usual dosage range is 2 to 6 SLOW-K tablets daily. It is recommended not to exceed 12 tablets daily. If the daily requirement exceeds 20 mEq K+, it should be taken in divided doses, so that not more than 20 mEq K+ is given in a single dose.

SLOW-K is preferably administered after meals. The tablets must not be crushed, chewed or sucked but should be swallowed whole with fluids while the patient is upright.

The insoluble wax matrix is excreted in a softened form and may be found in the feces.

OVERDOSAGE:

Overdosage from therapeutic doses of solid oral potassium salts in persons with normal excretory mechanisms rarely occurs. However, if excretory mechanisms are impaired, potentially fatal hyperkalemia may occur. Acute (accidental or intentional) overdosages of solid oral potassium salts have resulted in severe and/or fatal hyperkalemia.

Symptoms: Overdosage with potassium is characterized chiefly by cardiovascular, neuromuscular and gastrointestinal disturbances.

Cardiovascular: ECG changes, hypotension and shock, bundle-branch block, ventricular arrhythmias, ventricular fibrillation leading, possibly, to cardiac arrest.

Neuromuscular: paresthesia, areflexia, convulsions, flaccid paralysis of striated muscle leading possibly to respiratory paralysis.

Gastrointestinal: nausea, vomiting, diarrhea and abdominal cramp.

It is important to recognize that hyperkalemia is usually asymptomatic and may be manifested only by an increased serum potassium concentration and characteristic electrocardiographic changes which include increased amplitude and peaking of the T-wave, and flattening or absence of P-wave. As hyperkalemia worsens prolongation of the P-R interval, widening of the QRS complex with ST segment depression, and arrhythmias may develop.

Widening of the QRS complex is one of the most ominous signs and indicates the need for aggressive treatment.

Treatment: The plasma concentration and electrocardiogram must be monitored in every case of potassium overdosage, as well as serum electrolytes, BUN, glucose and arterial blood gases.

Electrocardiographic signs of hyperkalemia (tall peaked T waves, P-R prolongation, disappearance of P waves, QRS widening, heart block) are indications for immediate treatment.

In severe hyperkalemia (plasma potassium exceeds 8 mEq/L or ECG abnormalities include absence of P wave, presence of widened QRS complex or ventricular arrhythmia):

- Administer intravenously 300 to 500 mL/hour of 10% dextrose solution containing 10-20 units of insulin per 1000 mL.
- Correct acidosis, if present, with intravenous sodium bicarbonate (44 to 132 mEq per Litre of glucose solution).
- Administer 10 to 30 mL of 10% calcium gluconate intravenously over 1 to 5 minutes under continuous ECG monitoring.
- Administer cation exchange resin by high retention enema. 30 to 50 g sodium polystyrene sulfonate suspended in 100 mL warm aqueous sorbitol solution should be kept in the sigmoid colon for several hours, if possible. The colon is then irrigated with a non-sodium containing solution to remove the resin. Repeated enemas can be administered, or the resin given repeatedly by mouth to maintain a physiologic potassium concentration.
- Hemodialysis or peritoneal dialysis may be of use, particularly in patients with renal failure.

In moderately severe hyperkalemia (plasma potassium between 6.5 and 8 mEq/L or ECG peaking of T wave):

- Administer intravenously 300 to 500 mL/hour of 10% dextrose solution containing 10-20 units of insulin per 1000 mL.
- Correct acidosis, if present, with intravenous sodium bicarbonate (44 to 132 mEq per Litre of glucose solution).
- Correct hyponatremia and hypovolemia, if present.

Once the patient's cardiac state has been stabilized, in the case of a recent acute ingestion of SLOW-K (slow-release potassium chloride), consideration should be given to the evacuation of the stomach. When overdosage is the result of chronic therapeutic ingestion, SLOW-K should be discontinued immediately as well as potassium containing foods and medications and also potassium-sparing diuretics.

In treating hyperkalemia, it should be recalled that in patients who have been stabilized on digitalis, lowering the serum potassium concentration too rapidly can produce digitalis toxicity.

> For management of a suspected drug overdose, contact your **regional Poison Control Centre**. See the *CPS* Directory section for a list of Poison Control Centres.

ACTION AND CLINICAL PHARMACOLOGY: Mechanism of Action: Potassium ion is the principal intracellular ion of most body tissues. Potassium ions are involved in a number of essential physiological processes, including the maintenance of intracellular tonicity, the transmission of nerve impulses, the contraction of cardiac, skeletal, and smooth muscle, the maintenance of normal renal function and the regulation of the acid-base balance.

Pharmacokinetics: Absorption: Concentrations of potassium ions range in intracellular fluid from 130-150 up to 160 mEq/Litre and in plasma from 3.5 to 5.0 mEq/Litre.

KCl is gradually released from SLOW-K over a period of approximately 4 hours during its transit through the gastrointestinal tract. Absorption of potassium from the bowel is complete.

Excretion: Normally any amount given in excess of intracellular requirements is rapidly eliminated with approximately 90% excreted via the kidneys within 8 hours, and more than 98% within 24 hours.

Special Populations and Conditions: Pediatrics: Safety and effectiveness in children have not been established. SLOW-K is therefore not recommended for pediatric use. (See Warnings and Precautions, Special Populations.)

Geriatrics: As renal function, and hence the potential for maintaining potassium balance may decrease with age, serum potassium levels should be monitored regularly and dosage adjusted as appropriate. As gastrointestinal motility may also be affected by age, elderly patients should be reminded to swallow solid oral potassium salts with adequate amounts of fluid. (See Warnings and Precautions, Special Populations.)

STORAGE AND STABILITY: Protect tablets from heat (i.e. store below 30°C) and humidity.

Keep out of reach of children.

INFORMATION FOR THE PATIENT: Published in e-CPS, available by subscription at www.e-cps.ca.

DOSAGE FORMS, COMPOSITION AND PACKAGING: Each light-orange, round, biconvex, sugar-coated tablet, contains: potassium chloride 600 mg (equivalent to 8 mEq of potassium) in a slow-release wax matrix core. Nonmedicinal ingredients: cetostearyl alcohol, gelatin and magnesium stearate; coating: carnauba wax, gelatin, purified talc, red iron oxide, spray dried Acacia, sucrose (granulated), titanium dioxide and yellow iron oxide. Bottles of 100 and 500.

(Shown in Product Identification Section)

Sodium Bicarbonate

Alkalinizer

CPhA Monograph

Date of Preparation: November 2004
Date of Revision: August 2009

> This monograph has been compiled by CPhA and reviewed by experts. It may contain information different from that found in Health Canada-approved Product Monographs. The reader is referred to the *CPS* Editorial Policy for more information.

SUMMARY PRODUCT INFORMATION:

Route of Administration	Dosage Form	Strength
Oral	Powder	Various
Oral	Tablet	325 mg, 500 mg
IV	Solution	42 mg/mL (10 mL syringe), 75 mg/mL (50 mL syringe), 84 mg/mL (50 mL syringe and vial)

PHARMACOLOGY: Sodium bicarbonate is an alkalinizing agent. It increases plasma bicarbonate, buffers excess hydrogen ions, raises blood pH and reverses the clinical signs of acidemia. Sodium bicarbonate can alter the effect of certain drugs on sodium channels in cardiac tissue. Sodium bicarbonate dissociates to sodium and bicarbonate ions in water. Sodium is the principal cation of the extracellular fluid. Bicarbonate is found in body fluids and plasma. The normal plasma level of bicarbonate ranges from 22 to 28 mmol/L. Bicarbonate is a component of the principal extracellular buffer in the body, the bicarbonate-carbonic acid buffer. Bicarbonate buffers excess hydrogen ions by converting to carbonic acid or carbon dioxide and water. Plasma bicarbonate is regulated by the kidney. In a healthy adult with normal renal function, less than 1% of bicarbonate is excreted in the urine; most of the filtered bicarbonate ion is reabsorbed.

INDICATIONS: Oral: Sodium bicarbonate is given as a gastric, systemic and urinary alkalinizer. It can be used in conditions (e.g., chronic renal failure) requiring prolonged therapy with an alkalinizing agent.

Parenteral: Sodium bicarbonate iv is indicated for the treatment of metabolic acidosis which may occur in severe renal disease, uncontrolled diabetes (see Precautions), shock or severe dehydration, extracorporeal circulation of blood, cardiac arrest and severe lactic acidosis. The underlying cause of the acidemia should also be addressed.

Urine alkalinization in the treatment of drug overdose, to diminish nephrotoxicity of heme pigments and reduce the frequency of contrast medium-induced nephrotoxicity.

Drug overdose with agents that produce cardiotoxic effects involving sodium channel blockade.

Sodium bicarbonate is used in severe diarrhea when loss of bicarbonate has been significant and as an adjunct in the treatment of hyperkalemia.

CONTRAINDICATIONS: Patients with: metabolic or respiratory alkalosis, hypocalcemia (because of an increased risk of alkalosis-induced tetany), excessive chloride loss from vomiting or from continuous gastrointestinal suction, states of hypoventilation or a risk of developing diuretic-induced hypochloremic alkalosis. Sodium bicarbonate should not be used as an antidote in the treatment of acute ingestion of strong acids.

PRECAUTIONS: Routine use during cardiopulmonary resuscitation (CPR) is not recommended. In certain circumstances such as pre-existing metabolic acidosis, hyperkalemia, tricyclic antidepressant overdose or prolonged cardiac arrest, bicarbonate may be useful in CPR.

Sodium bicarbonate should be used with caution, due to the potentially large sodium load, in edematous or sodium-retaining conditions (e.g., heart failure), in renal insufficiency (e.g., oliguria or anuria), in patients receiving corticosteroids or corticotropin.

Administration of iv sodium bicarbonate may cause fluid or solute overload. This results in the dilution of serum electrolytes, overhydration, congestive states or pulmonary edema. Hypertonic solutions may cause phlebitis. Avoid extravasation.

Metabolic alkalosis from excessive sodium bicarbonate therapy may cause hypokalemia (due to an intracellular potassium shift) and decreased ionized serum calcium concentrations (which may result in tetany and carpopedal spasm as the plasma pH rises). To minimize the risks of bicarbonate administration in preexisting hypokalemia and/or hypocalcemia, these electrolyte disturbances should be corrected before or during sodium bicarbonate therapy.

The use of sodium bicarbonate in the treatment of diabetic ketoacidosis is controversial. Sodium bicarbonate may produce a paradoxical decrease in cerebrospinal fluid pH which may result in decreased CNS function and increased stupor. Severe hypokalemia may result due to an intracellular shift of potassium mediated by both insulin and bicarbonate therapy. In addition, sodium bicarbonate has the potential of causing rebound alkalosis, impaired oxygen delivery to tissues, lactic acidosis and sodium overload. In general, sodium bicarbonate should be reserved for severe acidemia (e.g., arterial pH <7), and its benefits in the management of diabetic ketoacidosis must be weighed against the potential complications of bicarbonate therapy.

Children Under 2 Years: IV administration of sodium bicarbonate in neonates and children under 2 years should not exceed 8 mmol/kg/day. Slow administration rates using less concentrated solutions (e.g., 0.5 mmol/mL or 4.2%) are recommended to reduce the possibility of producing hypernatremia, decreasing cerebrospinal fluid pressure or inducing intracranial hemorrhage.

Drug Interactions: Sodium bicarbonate is physically and/or chemically incompatible with many drugs. Specialized references should be consulted for specific compatibility information.

Alkalinization of the urine can decrease the clearance of amphetamines, quinidine, pseudoephedrine and possibly other sympathomimetics. Urinary alkalinization can increase the clearance of chlorpropamide, lithium, salicylates and tetracyclines.

Pregnancy: It is not known whether sodium bicarbonate can cause fetal harm when administered during pregnancy.

Lactation: It is not known to what extent sodium bicarbonate distributes into breast milk.

ADVERSE EFFECTS: Oral sodium bicarbonate may cause gastric distention and flatulence.

Extravasation of hypertonic solutions of sodium bicarbonate has been reported to cause chemical cellulitis resulting in tissue necrosis, ulceration, and/or sloughing at the site of injection.

Excessive parenteral doses may cause hypokalemia, accompanied by dry mouth, increased thirst, irregular heart beat, mood or mental changes, muscle cramps or pain, or weak pulse.

Administration of large doses or administration to patients with renal impairment may cause metabolic alkalosis which may be accompanied by hyperirritability or tetany.

Rapid alkalinization with sodium bicarbonate, in patients with ketoacidosis, may result in cerebral dysfunction, obtundation, seizures, and peripheral tissue hypoxia and lactic acidosis.

Hypernatremia, hyperosmolality and peripheral or pulmonary edema may occur when sodium bicarbonate is administered in large doses or in patients with renal insufficiency, heart failure or those predisposed to sodium retention and edema.

OVERDOSE:

Symptoms: See Adverse Effects.

Treatment: Sodium bicarbonate should be stopped and the patient managed according to the degree of alkalemia present. Sodium chloride 0.9% injection may be given iv. Potassium chloride may also be indicated if hypokalemia is present. Severe alkalemia may be accompanied by hyperirritability or tetany and these symptoms may be controlled by calcium gluconate. An acidifying agent such as ammonium chloride may also be indicated in severe alkalemia, except in patients with hepatic disease.

> For management of a suspected drug overdose, CPhA recommends that you contact your **regional Poison Control Centre**. See the *CPS* Directory section for a list of Poison Control Centres.

DOSAGE: To aid in converting: 84 mg of sodium bicarbonate = 1 mmol (1 mEq) of sodium bicarbonate = 1 mmol (1 mEq) each of sodium and bicarbonate ions. An 8.4% sodium bicarbonate solution = 84 mg/mL of sodium bicarbonate = 1 mmol (1 mEq)/mL of sodium bicarbonate.

Oral: Acidosis Associated with Chronic Renal Failure: Adults: Initial dose is 1.7 to 3 g daily in divided doses, with subsequent adjustment according to plasma bicarbonate concentration; fluid and electrolyte balance must be carefully monitored in these patients because of the potentially large sodium load associated with bicarbonate therapy.

Antacid: Adults: 325 mg to 2 g given 1 to 4 times daily for short term use.

Urinary Alkalinizer: Adults: 4 g initially, then 1 to 2 g every 4 hours. Some patients may require up to 16 g daily. Dosage should be titrated to maintain desired urinary pH.

Parenteral: Acidosis: Adults and Children Over 2 Years: The dosage of sodium bicarbonate can be based on the severity of the condition, laboratory values and the patient's weight.

Frequent evaluations of the patient are required during therapy to monitor acid-base and fluid and electrolyte balance. Full correction of acid-base balance should not be attempted during the first 24 hours because of the risk of delayed compensation and alkalosis. The initial dose is usually 2 to 5 mmol/kg administered as an iv infusion over 4 to 8 hours. Repeated dosage will be dependent on response to the initial dose and the clinical condition of the patient with respect to the cause of acidosis. Generally, the magnitude and frequency of subsequent doses should decrease once symptoms of severe acidosis have ameliorated.

Children ≤2 Years: The initial dose for infants and children under 2 years is usually 1 mmol/kg administered slowly in a concentration of 0.5 mmol/mL (see Precautions). Subsequent dosage will depend on the clinical status of the patient. A maximum daily dose of 8 mmol/kg has been recommended.

Cardiac Arrest: Sodium bicarbonate is not recommended for routine use during CPR. It is only used when clearly indicated and where adequate ventilation can be ensured (see Precautions).

Adults: An initial dose of 1 mmol/kg (1 mL of sodium bicarbonate 8.4% solution per kg body weight) may be given by rapid iv injection with repeated doses of 0.5 mmol/kg (0.5 mL/kg sodium bicarbonate 8.4%) every 10 minutes during continued cardiac arrest.

Children: An initial dose of 1 mmol/kg may be given slowly iv in a concentration of 1 mmol/mL (8.4% solution) to children 2 years of age and older. Subsequent doses of 1 mmol/kg may be considered at 10 minute intervals during continued cardiac arrest. Infants and children under 2 years may receive the above dosage, but a lower solution concentration is recommended (e.g., 0.5 mmol/mL or 4.2%).

Cardiotoxic Effects of Drug Overdose: An iv bolus of 1 to 2 mmol/kg over 1 to 2 minutes. This can be repeated as needed to maintain a blood pH of 7.45 to 7.55. Bolus dosing can be followed by a continuous infusion of sodium bicarbonate if required.

Contrast Medium-Induced Nephrotoxicity: Sodium bicarbonate can be administered to patients at risk for contrast medium-induced nephrotoxicity to help avoid this complication. In one suggested regimen add 150 mmol of sodium bicarbonate to 850 mL D5W. Administer at 3 mL/kg/h for 1 hour before contrast administration then 1 mL/kg/h for 6 hours after.

Urinary Alkalinization: In the presence of adequate urine output, urine alkalinization can be achieved by infusing 100 to 150 mmol sodium bicarbonate in 1 litre D5W at 150-200 mL/h. The infusion rate should be adjusted to a target urinary pH of 7.0 to 8.0.

Sodium Bicarbonate Injection

sodium bicarbonate

Alkalizer

Hospira

SUPPLIED: 4.2%: Each mL contains: sodium bicarbonate 42 mg (0.5 mEq) in water for injection. Abboject syringes of 10 mL, boxes of 10.

7.5%: Each mL contains: sodium bicarbonate 75 mg (0.9 mEq) in water for injection. Abboject syringes of 50 mL, boxes of 10.

8.4%: Each mL contains: sodium bicarbonate 84 mg (1 mEq) in water for injection. Vials of 50 mL, trays of 25. Abboject syringes of 10 and 50 mL, boxes of 10.

The solution contains no bacteriostat, antimicrobial agent or added buffer and is intended only for use as a single dose injection. When smaller doses are required, the unused portion should be discarded with the entire unit.

Store between 15 and 25°C. Protect from freezing and avoid excessive heat.

Sodium Chloride Injection, USP
sodium chloride
Isotonic Vehicle—Electrolyte Replenisher

Hospira

SUPPLIED: Bacteriostatic with Preservative: Each mL contains: sodium chloride 9 mg. Also contains benzyl alcohol, hydrochloric acid and water for injection. Fliptop plastic vials of 10, 20 and 30 mL. Boxes of 25.
Preservative-free: Each mL contains: sodium chloride 9 mg. Also contains hydrochloric acid and/or sodium hydroxide and water for injection. Osmolarity: 0.3 mOsmol/mL. Fliptop plastic vials of 10 and 20 mL. Boxes of 25.

Sodium Sulamyd® Ⓟ
sulfacetamide sodium
Ophthalmic Antibacterial

Sandoz

PHARMACOLOGY: Sodium sulfacetamide, a bacteriostatic sulfonamide, is effective against a wide range of microorganisms, commonly associated with external ocular infections. Sodium sulfacetamide inhibits the growth of susceptible strains of *P. aeruginosa*, *S. aureus*, *S. albus*, *K. pneumoniae*, *E. coli* and *E. aerogenes*. Sodium sulfacetamide penetrates into ocular fluids and tissues in high concentration.

INDICATIONS: The treatment of conjunctivitis, corneal ulcer, and other superficial ocular infections due to susceptible microorganisms, and as adjunctive treatment in systemic therapy of trachoma.

CONTRAINDICATIONS: Hypersensitivity to sulfonamide preparations.

PRECAUTIONS: The solutions are incompatible with silver preparations. Do not use solutions if coloured. Sulfonamides may be inactivated by the para-aminobenzoic acid present in purulent exudates. If sensitivity reactions occur, discontinue treatment.

Topical anesthetics derived from aminobenzoic acid may antagonize the antibacterial effect of topical sulfonamides if applied concurrently.

If prompt clinical response is not obtained with Ophthalmic Solution 10%, further evaluation is advised.

Prolonged use of topical antibiotics may give rise to overgrowth of nonsusceptible microorganisms and fungi.

Cross-sensitivity among sulfonamides may occur.

Safety and effectiveness for use in children below the age of 6 years have not been established.

The solution 10% is intended for topical application only and not for injection.

Pregnancy: Safety during pregnancy has not been established.

ADVERSE EFFECTS: Sodium sulfacetamide may cause local irritation. Most often the reactions result from allergic sensitization. Although sensitivity reactions to sodium sulfacetamide are rare, instances of Stevens-Johnson syndrome and systemic lupus erythematosus (in one case producing a fatal outcome) have been reported following the use of ophthalmic sulfonamide preparations.

OVERDOSE:
Symptoms: A single overdose of ophthalmic sodium sulfacetamide would not be expected to produce symptoms.

> For management of a suspected drug overdose, CPhA recommends that you contact your **regional Poison Control Centre**. See the *CPS* Directory section for a list of Poison Control Centres.

DOSAGE: 10% Solution with Methylcellulose: 1 or 2 drops into the lower conjunctival sac every 2 or 3 hours during the day and less often at night.

SUPPLIED: Each mL of sterile ophthalmic solution contains: sulfacetamide sodium USP 100 mg (10%) with methylcellulose USP. Nonmedicinal ingredients: hydroxypropyl methylcellulose, methylparaben, monobasic sodium phosphate, propylparaben, sodium thiosulfate and water. Plastic dropper bottles of 15 mL. Store between 2 and 30°C. Protect from light.

Sodium Thiosulfate Injection USP
sodium thiosulfate
Antidote

Hospira

SUPPLIED: Each mL of sterile aqueous solution contains: 250 mg sodium thiosulfate. Nonmedicinal ingredients: 10.5 mg disodium hydrogen phosphate and 1 mg sodium metabisulfite. May contain sulfuric acid or sodium hydroxide as pH adjusters. Preservative-free. Single use vials of 10 mL, cartons of 5. Store between 15 and 25°C. Protect from light. Discard unused portion.

Soflax™
docusate sodium
Stool Softener

Pharmascience

SUPPLIED: Capsules: 100 mg: Each orange, oval, soft gelatin capsule, ink-printed in white with "PMS" on one side and "100" on the other, contains: docusate sodium USP 100 mg. Unit dose packages of 30 and 100. Bottles of 100 and 1000. Store between 15 and 30°C in a tight, light-resistant container in a dry area. Protect from freezing.
200 mg: Each orange, oblong, soft gelatin capsule, ink-printed in white with "PMS" on one side and "200" on the other, contains: docusate sodium USP 200 mg. Bottles of 1000. Store between 15 and 30°C in a tight, light-resistant container in a dry area. Protect from freezing.
Syrup: Each mL of a clear, dark pink syrup, contains: docusate sodium USP 4 mg. Bottles of 500 mL. Store between 15 and 30°C in a tight, light resistant container in a dry area. Protect from freezing.

Soflax™
docusate sodium
Stool Softener

PendoPharm

Soflax C™
docusate calcium
Stool Softener

PendoPharm

SUPPLIED: Soflax: Pediatric Drops: Each mL of a clear, red, vanilla-flavored solution contains: docusate sodium USP 10 mg. Bottles of 25 mL with calibrated dropper. Store between 15 and 30°C in a dry area. Protect from freezing.
Syrup: Each mL of a clear, dark pink syrup, contains: docusate sodium USP 4 mg. Bottles of 250 mL. Store between 15 and 30°C in a dry area. Protect from freezing.
Soflax C: Each red, oblong softgel capsule filled with clear liquid, ink-printed with "PMS" on one side of the capsule and "240" on the other side, contains: docusate calcium 240 mg. Unit dose packages of 30. Store between 15 and 30°C in a dry area.

Sofracort® Ⓟ
framycetin sulfate—gramicidin—dexamethasone
Antibiotic—Corticosteroid

sanofi-aventis

Date of Revision: April 21, 2006

INDICATIONS: Ear: Otitis externa (acute and chronic) and other inflammatory and seborrheic conditions of the external ear.
Eye: Blepharitis and infected eczema of the eyelid; allergic, infective and rosacea conjunctivitis; rosacea keratitis; scleritis and episcleritis; iridocyclitis, and other inflammatory conditions of the anterior segment of the eye.

CONTRAINDICATIONS: Ear: Viral and fungal infections; acute purulent, untreated infections; perforation of the eardrum and known hypersensitivity to any of the ingredients.
Eye: Herpes simplex and other viral diseases of the cornea and conjunctiva; tuberculosis and fungal diseases of the eye; trachoma. Acute purulent, untreated infections of the eye, which, like other diseases caused by microorganisms, may be masked or enhanced by the presence of the steroid. Known hypersensitivity to any of the ingredients.

WARNINGS: No data supplied by the manufacturer.

PRECAUTIONS: Extended ophthalmic use of corticosteroids may increase intraocular pressure in some individuals in such cases, intraocular pressure should be checked regularly. In conditions causing thinning of the cornea, topical steroids may cause perforation. Cataract has occurred after prolonged treatment with topical steroids.

Pregnancy: The safety of prolonged use of topical steroids during pregnancy has not been substantiated. The benefits of use should be weighed against possible adverse effects on the fetus.

The drug should be discontinued if there are signs of sensitivity to any of its ingredients.

Patients are advised to inform the physicians of the prior use of corticosteroids.

Children: Although it is unlikely that infants will be treated with Sofracort for prolonged periods, there is a risk of adrenal suppression, even without occlusive dressings, after prolonged treatment of these patients with topical steroids.

ADVERSE EFFECTS: See Precautions. Increased intraocular pressure; perforation of the cornea; hypersensitivity; burning or stinging of the eye.

OVERDOSE:
No data supplied by the manufacturer.

> For management of a suspected drug overdose, CPhA recommends that you contact your **regional Poison Control Centre**. See the *CPS* Directory section for a list of Poison Control Centres.

DOSAGE: Ear: Instill 2 or 3 drops in the ear canal 3 or 4 times daily by tilting head to one side. Squeeze bottle carefully. To avoid possibility of reinfection later, do not touch ear with dropper. Alternatively, a saturated gauze wick may be inserted by the physician into the external auditory meatus.
Eye: In acute conditions, 1 or 2 drops every 1 to 2 hours may be instilled (generally for 2 or 3 days). Subsequently, 1 or 2 drops 3 or 4 times daily.

SUPPLIED: Each mL of sterile drops contains: framycetin sulfate BP 5 mg, gramicidin 0.05 mg and dexamethasone 0.5 mg. pH is 4.5 to 5.0. Calibrated dropper bottles of 8 mL. Store at controlled room temperature. Use within 4 weeks of opening.

Soliris™ Ⓟ
eculizumab
Humanized Monoclonal Antibody

Alexion

Date of Preparation: June 29, 2009

SUMMARY PRODUCT INFORMATION:

Route of Administration	Dosage Form/ Strength	Clinically Relevant Nonmedicinal Ingredients
Intravenous (IV) infusion	300 mg single-use vial	Polysorbate 80 (vegetable origin) For a complete listing, see Dosage Forms, Composition and Packaging.

DESCRIPTION: Soliris is a formulation of eculizumab which is a recombinant humanized monoclonal IgG2/4$_{\kappa}$ antibody that binds to the human C5 complement protein and inhibits the activation of terminal complement. Eculizumab contains human constant regions and murine complementarity-determining regions grafted onto the human framework light- and heavy-chain variable regions. Eculizumab is composed of two 448 amino acid heavy chains and two 214 amino acid light chains and has a molecular weight of approximately 148 kDa.

Eculizumab is produced in a murine myeloma (NS0 cell line) expression system and purified by affinity and ion exchange chromatography. The bulk drug substance manufacturing process also includes specific viral inactivation and removal steps.

Soliris is a sterile, clear, colorless, preservative-free 10 mg/mL solution for intravenous (IV) infusion and is supplied in 30-mL single-use vials. The product is formulated at pH 7.0 and each vial contains 300 mg of eculizumab, 13.8 mg sodium phosphate monobasic, 53.4 mg sodium phosphate dibasic, 263.1 mg sodium chloride, 6.6 mg polysorbate 80 (vegetable origin) and Water for Injection, USP.

INDICATIONS AND CLINICAL USE: Soliris is indicated for: the treatment of patients with paroxysmal nocturnal hemoglobinuria (PNH) to reduce hemolysis.

Soliris was studied in clinical trials in patients with a history of at least one transfusion during the past two years.

Geriatrics: No data are available.
Pediatrics: No data are available.
Distribution Restrictions: Soliris should be administered under the supervision of a qualified health professional.

CONTRAINDICATIONS: Patients treated with Soliris have increased susceptibility to infection with encapsulated organisms. Do not initiate Soliris therapy in patients:
- with unresolved serious infections such as *N. meningitidis*;
- who are not currently vaccinated against *N. meningitidis*;
- who are hypersensitive to this drug or to any ingredient in the formulation or component of the container.

WARNINGS AND PRECAUTIONS:

> **Serious Warnings and Precautions:**
> **SERIOUS MENINGOCOCCAL INFECTIONS: Soliris increases the risk of meningococcal infections.**
> - **All patients must be vaccinated with a meningococcal vaccine at least 2 weeks prior to receiving the first dose of Soliris; revaccinate according to current medical guidelines for vaccine use.**

- **All patients must be monitored for early signs of meningococcal infections, evaluated immediately if infection is suspected, and treated with antibiotics, if necessary.**
- **Vaccination may not prevent all meningococcal infections.**

Meningococcal Infection: The use of Soliris increases a patient's susceptibility to serious meningococcal infections (septicemia and/or meningitis). All patients without proof of prior meningococcal vaccination must receive the meningococcal vaccine at least 2 weeks prior to receiving the first dose of Soliris. All patients should be monitored and revaccinated according to current medical guidelines for vaccine use. Quadravalent, conjugated meningococcal vaccines against serotypes A, C, Y and W135 are strongly recommended, if available.

Vaccination may not prevent all meningococcal infections. All patients must be monitored for early signs and symptoms of meningococcal infections and evaluated and treated immediately if an infection is suspected. Patients should be informed of these signs and symptoms and steps to take to seek medical care immediately. There have been 3 reported cases of **serious** meningococcal infection in Soliris treated patients in clinical trials: two in vaccinated PNH patients and one in an unvaccinated patient with idiopathic membranous glomerulonephropathy.

Other Systemic Infections: Soliris blocks terminal complement; therefore patients may have increased susceptibility to infections, especially with encapsulated bacteria, such as *H. influenza* and *S. pneumoniae*. **Vaccinating patients against these organisms was not assessed in clinical trials.** Use caution when administering Soliris to patients with any systemic infection.

Serious infections, infectious agents and subsequent treatments for these infections should be documented for all patients treated with Soliris.

General: As with all protein products, administration of Soliris may result in infusion reactions, including anaphylaxis or other hypersensitivity reactions. In clinical trials, no PNH patients experienced an infusion reaction which required discontinuation of Soliris. Soliris administration should be interrupted in all patients experiencing severe infusion reactions and appropriate medical therapy administered.

Monitoring after Soliris Discontinuation: Since Soliris therapy increases the number of PNH cells (e.g., in the double-blind, placebo-controlled C04-001 study, the proportion of PNH RBCs increased among Soliris-treated patients by a median of 28% from baseline (range from −25% to 69%), patients who discontinue treatment with Soliris may be at increased risk for serious hemolysis. Serious hemolysis is identified by serum LDH levels greater than the pre-treatment level, along with any of the following: greater than 25% absolute decrease in PNH clone size (in the absence of dilution due to transfusion) in one week or less; a hemoglobin level of <5 gm/dL or a decrease of >4 gm/dL in one week or less; angina; change in mental status; a 50% increase in serum creatinine level; or thrombosis. Monitor any patient who discontinues Soliris for at least 8 weeks to detect serious hemolysis and other reactions.

If serious hemolysis occurs after Soliris discontinuation, consider the following procedures/treatments: blood transfusion (packed RBCs), or exchange transfusion if the PNH RBCs are >50% of the total RBCs by flow cytometry, anticoagulation, corticosteroids, or reinstitution of Soliris, but this was not tested in clinical trials.

In clinical studies, 16 of 196 PNH patients discontinued treatment with Soliris. Patients were followed for evidence of worsening hemolysis and no serious hemolysis was observed.

Thrombosis Prevention and Management: In clinical studies of patients with PNH, there were fewer thrombotic events with Soliris treatment than during the same period of time prior to treatment. The effect of withdrawal of anticoagulant therapy during Soliris treatment has not been established. Therefore, treatment with Soliris should not alter anticoagulant management.

Laboratory Monitoring: Serum LDH levels increase during hemolysis and may assist in monitoring Soliris effects, including the response to discontinuation of therapy. PNH patients receiving Soliris therapy should be monitored for intravascular hemolysis by measuring LDH levels, and may require dose adjustment within the recommended 14±2 day dosing schedule during the maintenance phase (up to every 12 days). In clinical studies, six patients achieved a reduction in serum LDH levels only after a decrease in the Soliris dosing interval from 14 to 12 days. All other patients achieved a reduction in serum LDH levels with the 14 day dosing interval.

In the two studies in PNH patients (C04-001 and C04-002), the LDH value rapidly decreased. These decreases were sustained over the Soliris treatment duration. A reduction in LDH from baseline can be used to assess therapeutic response.

Table 1: Soliris

LDH Values During the First 26 Weeks in Soliris-Treated Patients

Study Week	Mean (Standard Deviation) LDH[a]	
	C04-001 (N=43)	C04-002 (N=97)
Baseline	2200 (157.7)	2201 (104.9)
Week 1	700 (59.2)	688 (40.6)
Week 2	393 (28.1)	406 (24.9)
Week 4	292 (25.8)	301 (15.5)
Week 12	413 (142.7)	408 (57.6)
Week 26	327 (67.6)	346 (33.2)

[a] LDH reference range: 103-223 U/L.

Immunization: Prior to initiating Soliris therapy, it is recommended that PNH patients should receive immunizations according to current immunization guidelines. Additionally, all patients must receive a meningococcal vaccine at least 2 weeks prior to receiving Soliris. If available, tetravalent, conjugated vaccines are recommended (see Warnings and Precautions).

Carcinogenesis and Mutagenesis: Carcinogenesis and mutagenesis studies have not been performed. There is no evidence to suggest that the use of Soliris is associated with carcinogenesis.

Cardiovascular: There were no serious cardiovascular adverse events.

Dependence/Tolerance: There is no evidence to suggest that the use of Soliris is associated with drug abuse or dependence.

Ear/Nose/Throat: There were no serious ENT adverse events.

Endocrine and Metabolism: There were no serious endocrine or metabolic adverse events.

Gastrointestinal: Rare episodes of severe abdominal pain were reported.

Genitourinary: There were no serious genitourinary adverse events.

Hematologic: The safety and efficacy of Soliris has not been established in patients with underlying hematologic diseases (e.g., hemolytic anemia, sickle cell anemia, thalassemia, porphyria). In clinical trials, analysis by history of bone marrow failure showed that eculizumab was effective in reducing the burden of hemolysis (as measured by hemolysis indicator LDH AUC) and reduced transfusion requirements in subjects with both PNH and history of bone marrow failure (e.g., aplastic anemia, myelodysplasias).

Hepatic/Biliary/Pancreatic: There were no serious hepatic dysfunctions after Soliris therapy. The safety and efficacy of Soliris have not been assessed in patients with hepatic disease.

Immune: Infrequent, low titer antibody responses have been detected in Soliris-treated patients across all PNH and non-PNH studies with a frequency (3.4%) similar to that of placebo (4.8%). No patients have developed neutralizing antibodies following therapy with Soliris and there has been no observed correlation of antibody development to clinical response or adverse events.

Soliris blocks terminal complement; therefore patients may have increased susceptibility to *N. meningitis* (see Boxed Serious Warnings and Precautions, Serious Meningococcal Infections).

Neurologic: Transient severe headaches were reported.

Ophthalmologic: There were no serious ophthalmologic adverse events.

Peri-Operative Considerations: There is no data on continuing or discontinuing Soliris or adjusting dose for Peri-Operative considerations.

Psychiatric: There were no serious psychiatric adverse events.

Renal: There was no serious evidence of serious renal impairment after Soliris therapy. The safety and efficacy of Soliris have not been assessed in patients with renal disease.

Respiratory: There were no serious respiratory adverse events.

Sensitivity/Resistance: As with all infusions with biologic agents, there is a risk of infusion reactions and anaphylaxis.

Sexual Function/Reproduction: The safety of Soliris during pregnancy and breastfeeding has not been established. See Special Populations, Pregnant Women.

Skin: There were no serious skin (photosensitivity, photoallergic or phototoxic) adverse events.

Special Populations: Formal studies have not been conducted to evaluate the pharmacokinetics of Soliris administration in special patient populations based on gender, race, age (pediatric or geriatric), or metabolic status (renal or hepatic impairment).

Pregnant Women: PNH is a serious illness. Pregnant women with PNH and their fetuses have high rates of morbidity and mortality during pregnancy and the postpartum period. There are no adequate and well-controlled studies of Soliris in pregnant women. Animal reproduction studies have not been conducted with Soliris. Soliris, a recombinant IgG molecule (humanized anti-C5 antibody), is expected to cross the placenta. Soliris should not be used during pregnancy unless the potential benefit justifies the potential risk to the mother and the fetus.

Labor and Delivery: It is not known whether Soliris has an effect on the mother and the fetus during labor and delivery.

Nursing Women: It is not known whether Soliris is secreted into human milk. IgG is excreted in human milk, so it is expected that Soliris will be present in human milk. However, published data suggest that breast milk antibodies do not enter the neonatal and infant circulation in substantial amounts. Caution should be exercised when Soliris is administered to a nursing woman. The unknown risks to the infant from gastrointestinal or limited systemic exposure to Soliris should be weighed against the known benefits of breastfeeding.

Pediatrics (<18 years of age): The safety and effectiveness of Soliris therapy in pediatric patients below the age of 18 have not been established.

Geriatrics (>65 years of age): In PNH studies, 15 patients 65 years of age or older were treated with Soliris. Although there were no apparent age-related differences observed in these studies, the number of patients aged 65 and over is not sufficient to determine whether they respond differently from younger patients.

Monitoring and Laboratory Tests: PNH patients receiving Soliris therapy should be monitored for intravascular hemolysis by measuring LDH levels and may require dose adjustment within the recommended 14±2 day dosing schedule during the maintenance phase (up to every 12 days).

ADVERSE REACTIONS: Adverse Drug Reaction Overview: Soliris for the treatment of PNH was studied in three clinical studies that included 195 eculizumab-treated patients and most of these patients have been enrolled in the E05-001 extension study. There was one pivotal trial (C04-001) comparing the eculizumab-treatment arm to a placebo-treatment arm. Meningococcal infections are the most important adverse reactions experienced by patients receiving Soliris therapy. In PNH clinical studies, two patients experienced serious meningococcal sepsis. Both patients had previously received a meningococcal vaccine. In clinical studies among patients without PNH, meningococcal meningitis and septicaemia occurred in one unvaccinated patient (see Warnings and Precautions).

The most commonly reported adverse events regardless of causality are headache, nasopharyngitis, upper respiratory infections, nausea, diarrhea and arthralgia, each occurring in at least 20 percent of patients, and pyrexia, myalgia, fatigue, and herpes simplex, each occurring in ≥5/100 patients.

Adverse events reported at a very common (>10%) or common incidence (>1 to <10%) with eculizumab in a total of 140 patients in C04-001 and C04-002 are listed by system organ class and preferred term in Table 2, Table 3 and Table 4. Adverse events were mostly mild to moderate in severity. Incidence of uncommon or rare events cannot be accurately estimated due to limited patient exposure (195 PNH patients); see also: Uncommon Clinical Trial Adverse Drug Reactions (<1%).

Supportive safety data were obtained in 11 clinical studies that included 716 patients exposed to eculizumab in six disease populations other than PNH. There was an un-vaccinated patient in a study for idiopathic membranous glomerulonephropathy who experienced severe meningococcal meningitis and septicaemia. In double-blind, placebo-controlled studies for patients with diseases other than PNH (N=526 patients with Soliris; N=221 patients with placebo), adverse events reported with Soliris at an incidence of 2% or greater than the incidence reported with placebo were: upper respiratory tract infection, rash, and injury.

Clinical Trial Adverse Drug Reactions: Because clinical trials are conducted under very specific conditions the adverse reaction rates observed in the clinical trials may not reflect the rates observed in practice and should not be compared to the rates in the clinical trials of another drug. Adverse drug reaction information from clinical trials is useful for identifying drug-related adverse events and for approximating rates.

In the double blind randomized phase III trial for PNH (C04-001), 43 patients received Soliris and 44 received placebo. The duration of treatment was 6 months in both treatment groups. Drug-related adverse events occurring in more than 2 Soliris-treated patients are summarized in Table 2. The most frequent were headaches and fatigue. Most headaches were mild and did not persist after the initial administration phase of Soliris and resolved within 24-48 hours after Soliris infusion.

Headaches were observed in 44.2% (19/43 patients) of patients treated with Soliris and 27.3% (12/44 patients) in placebo-treated patients and were mild/moderate in all but 1 Soliris-treated and 1 placebo-treated patients. Most headaches did not persist after the initial administration phase of Soliris. In addition, the following adverse event incidence was increased by 5% or more with Soliris as compared to placebo: nasopharyngitis (25.0%), nausea (17.1%), pyrexia (14.3%), myalgia (7.9%), fatigue (7.9%), and herpes simplex (5.7%).

Among 193 patients with PNH treated with Soliris in the single arm, clinical study (C04-002) or the follow-up study, the adverse reactions were similar to those reported in the placebo-controlled clinical study. Serious adverse reactions occurred among 16% of the patients in these studies. The most common serious adverse reactions were: viral infection (2%), headache (2%), anemia (2%), and pyrexia (2%).

There was no evidence of an increased incidence of infection across PNH studies with Soliris as compared to placebo, including serious infections, severe infections or multiple infections.

Overall serious adverse event (SAE) rates were similar between patients treated with Soliris (16.4%) versus placebo (20.5%) in the combined C04-001 and C04-002 phase 3 PNH studies.

A total of 28 drug-related Serious Adverse events were reported by 20 (10.3%) of the 195 PNH patients enrolled in clinical trials (C02-001, C04-001, C04-002, and E05-001). The most common drug-related SAEs were pyrexia (5), headache (3), septic shock (2), and viral infection (2). The only SAE in more than one patient considered related to Soliris was pyrexia (1.4%). SAEs that occurred in more than one patient were anemia (2.9%), pyrexia (2.1%), headache (1.4%), hemolysis (1.4%), and intervertebral disc protrusion (1.4%).

In PNH studies, 2 patients died of adverse events. The causes of death were chronic myelomonocytic leukemia, and cerebral herniation. In non-PNH trials, there were 3 deaths, 2 in eculizumab-treated patients (complications post cholecystectomy; electrocution); and one in a placebo-treated patient (pulmonary embolism). None of the deaths was considered to be treatment-related.

In the C04-001 study there was a single adverse event that led to study discontinuation with Soliris treatment due to pregnancy. There were no other adverse events leading to discontinuation in the Soliris or placebo treatment groups in that study. In the C04-002 PNH study, there was one patient who discontinued study participation due to a fatal cerebral herniation adverse event that was considered unrelated to study medication.

Table 2: Soliris

Adverse Reactions[a] Reported in ≥2 Patients in Study C04-001

	C04-001	
	Soliris (N=43)	Placebo (N=44)
Gastrointestinal		
Nausea	2 (4.7%)	1 (2.3%)
Abdominal pain	2 (4.7%)	1 (2.3%)
General		
Fatigue	3 (7.0%)	0 (0.0%)
Infections and Infestations		
Upper respiratory tract infection	2 (4.7%)	0 (0.0%)
Oral herpes	2 (4.7%)	0 (0.0%)

(cont'd)

Table 2: Soliris *(cont'd)*

Adverse Reactions[a] Reported in ≥2 Patients in Study C04-001

	C04-001	
	Soliris (N=43)	Placebo (N=44)
Nervous System		
Headache	15 (34.9%)	2 (4.5%)
Skin and Subcutaneous Tissue		
Dry skin	2 (4.7%)	0 (0.0%)

[a] Drug-related Adverse Events occurring at a higher frequency (1 or more patients) in the Soliris-treated patients relative to placebo.

Table 3 summarizes adverse reactions occurring in Soliris-treated patients for study C04-001, study C04-002, and all Soliris-treated patients in clinical trials (C02-001, C04-001, C04-002, and E05-001). They were mostly mild to moderate in severity. There were minimal differences between study C04-001, study C04-002 and the total Soliris experience. The most common drug related adverse event was headache; all others were reported with a frequency of 6.7% or lower.

Table 3: Soliris

Adverse Reactions Reported in ≥2 Patients in Soliris Clinical Studies

	C04-001 (N=43)	C04-002 (N=97)	Total Soliris Patients (N=195)
Gastrointestinal Disorders			
Nausea	2 (4.7%)	7 (7.2%)	12 (6.2%)
Vomiting	1 (2.3%)	4 (4.1%)	8 (4.1%)
Diarrhea	0 (0.0%)	1 (1.0%)	6 (3.1%)
Constipation	0 (0.0%)	3 (3.1%)	5 (2.6%)
Abdominal pain	2 (4.7%)	2 (2.1%)	4 (2.1%)
Dyspepsia	0 (0.0%)	1 (1.0%)	2 (1.0%)
General Disorders and Administration Site Conditions			
Pyrexia	1 (2.3%)	6 (6.2%)	12 (6.2%)
Fatigue	3 (7.0%)	3 (3.1%)	9 (4.6%)
Chills	0 (0.0%)	0 (0.0%)	3 (1.5%)
Infections and Infestations			
Upper respiratory tract infection	2 (4.7%)	2 (2.1%)	4 (2.1%)
Urinary tract infection	0 (0.0%)	3 (3.1%)	4 (2.1%)
Nasopharynitis	0 (0.0%)	1 (1.0%)	3 (1.5%)
Oral herpes	2 (4.7%)	1 (1.0%)	3 (1.5%)
Viral infection	0 (0.0%)	1 (1.0%)	3 (1.5%)
Musculoskeletal and Connective Tissue Disorders			
Myalgia	0 (0.0%)	4 (4.1%)	7 (3.6%)
Arthralgia	0 (0.0%)	4 (4.1%)	6 (3.1%)
Pain in extremity	1 (2.3%)	2 (2.1%)	6 (3.1%)
Neck pain	1 (2.3%)	2 (2.1%)	3 (1.5%)
Nervous System Disorders			
Headache	15 (34.9%)	42 (43.3%)	71 (36.4%)
Dizziness	0 (0.0%)	8 (8.2%)	13 (6.7%)
Dysgeusia	0 (0.0%)	1 (1.0%)	3 (1.5%)
Migraine	Not listed	Not listed	5 (2.6%)
Respiratory, Thoracic and Mediastinal Disorders			
Cough	1 (2.3%)	0 (0.0%)	5 (2.6%)
Pharyngolaryngeal pain	0 (0.0%)	1 (1.0%)	3 (1.5%)
Skin and Subcutaneous Tissue Disorders			
Pruritus	1 (2.3%)	3 (3.1%)	8 (4.1%)
Alopecia	0 (0.0%)	1 (1.0%)	3 (1.5%)

Adverse events of all causes (drug related and non-drug related) are summarized in Table 4 for all 195 patients included in all PNH trials (C02-001, C04-001, C04-002, and E05-001).

Table 4: Soliris

Adverse Events Regardless of Causality Reported in ≥5% of PNH Patients in all Clinical Studies

	No (%) of Patients (N=195)
Gastrointestinal Disorders	
Nausea	49 (25.1)
Diarrhea	43 (22.1)
Vomiting	32 (16.4)
Abdominal pain	25 (12.8)
Constipation	23 (11.8)
Abdominal pain upper	16 (8.2)
Dyspepsia	10 (5.1)
General	
Pyrexia	33 (16.9)
Influenza-like illness	22 (11.3)
Fatigue	19 (9.7)
Peripheral edema	12 (6.2)
Chest pain	12 (6.2)
Infections and Infestations	
Upper respiratory tract infections	60 (30.80)
Nasopharyngitis	82 (42.1)
Viral infections	22 (11.3)
Urinary tract infection	22 (11.3)
Oral herpes	15 (7.7)
Influenza	14 (7.2)
Sinusitis	12 (6.2)
Respiratory tract infections	12 (6.2)
Rhinitis	11 (5.6)
Bronchitis	10 (5.1)
Injury Poisoning	
Contusion	22 (11.3)
Musculoskeletal and Connective Tissue Disorders	
Back pain	39 (20)
Arthralgia	31 (15.9)
Pain in extremities	28 (14.4)
Myalgia	21 (10.8)
Muscle spasm	14 (7.2)
Musculoskeletal pain	12 (6.2)
Neck pain	10 (5.1)
Joint swelling	10 (5.1)
Nervous System Disorders	
Headache	100 (51.3)
Dizziness	30 (15.4)
Psychiatric Disorders	
Insomnia	23 (11.8)
Respiratory, Thoracic and Mediastinal Disorders	
Cough	31 (15.9)
Pharyngolaryngeal pain	28 (14.4)
Epistaxis	19 (9.7)
Dyspnea	12 (6.2)
Nasal congestion	10 (5.1)

(cont'd)

Table 4: Soliris *(cont'd)*

Adverse Events Regardless of Causality Reported in ≥5% of PNH Patients in all Clinical Studies

	No (%) of Patients (N=195)
Skin and Subcutaneous Tissue Disorders	
Pruritus	15 (7.7)
Rash	13 (6.7)
Vascular Disorders	
Hematoma	11 (5.6)

Uncommon Clinical Trial Adverse Drug Reactions (<1%): The following Adverse Reactions were reported by 2 patients or less in the Soliris clinical trials (195 PNH patients). These reactions are presented by frequency category: common reactions are those reported in 2 patients (1%), uncommon reactions are those occurring in 1 patient (<1%).
Blood and Lymphatic Disorders: Common: thrombocytopenia; Uncommon: coagulopathy.
Cardiac Disorder: Uncommon: palpitation.
Ear and Labyrinth Disorders: Uncommon: tinnitus, vertigo.
Endocrine Disorders: Uncommon: Basedow's disease.
Eye Disorders: Uncommon: conjunctival irritation, blurred vision.
Gastrointestinal Disorders: Uncommon: abdominal distension, gastroesophageal reflux disease, gingival pain, infrequent bowel movements.
General Disorders and Administration Site Conditions: Common: chest discomfort, infusion reaction; uncommon: peripheral edema, chest pain, face edema, physical health deterioration, influenza-like illness.
Hepatobiliary Disorders: Uncommon: jaundice.
Immune System Disorders: Uncommon: hypersensitivity.
Infections and Infestations: Common: bronchitis, gastrointestinal infection, sepsis, septic shock; Uncommon: influenza, abscess, cellulitis, fungal infection, gingival infection, hemophilus infection, lower respiratory tract infection, meningococcal sepsis, Neisseria infection, sinusitis.
Investigation: Uncommon: alanine aminotransferase increase, aspartate aminotransferase increase, gamma glutamyltransferase increase.
Metabolism and Nutrition Disorders: Uncommon: anorexia, decreased appetite.
Musculoskeletal and Connective Tissue Disorders: Common: back pain, musculoskeletal pain; Uncommon: bone pain, joint swelling, muscle spasms, trismus.
Neoplasm benign, malignant and unspecified: Uncommon: malignant melanoma, myelodysplastic syndrome.
Nervous System Disorders: Common: paresthesia; uncommon: syncope.
Psychiatric Disorders: Common: depression; Uncommon: anxiety, insomnia, mood swings, sleep disorder.
Renal and Urinary Disorders: Common: dysuria; Uncommon: renal impairment.
Reproductive System and Breast Disorders: Uncommon: menstrual disorder.
Respiratory, Thoracic and Mediastinal Disorders: Common: nasal congestion, throat irritation; Uncommon: rhinorrhea, epistaxis.
Skin and Subcutaneous Tissue Disorders: Common: dry skin, rash; Uncommon: hyperhydrosis, petechiae, skin depigmentation, urticaria.
Vascular Disorders: Uncommon: hematoma, hot flush, hypotension.

During clinical trials, three patients became pregnant while being treated with Soliris; all discontinued treatment as per protocol. One pregnancy was continued to term and a healthy baby was delivered. Effective methods of contraception are recommended for patients being actively treated with Soliris and for at least the two-month follow-up period after discontinuation.

Abnormal Hematologic and Clinical Chemistry Findings: CTC Grades 3 and 4 laboratory abnormalities were tabulated for PNH patients who had normal values at baseline. Laboratory abnormalities were seen in 0% (creatinine) to 15.6% (direct bilirubin) of Soliris-treated patients and they occurred at similar or slightly lower frequency in placebo-treated patients.

Table 5: Soliris

CTC Grade 3/4 Laboratory Abnormalities in Clinical Studies of Soliris in PNH Patients

	Percent of Patients[a]	
	Soliris (N=195)	Placebo (N=44)
Neutropenia	14.8	3.8
Thrombocytopenia	0.8	6.4
Elevated ALT	1.1	2.5
Elevated AST	11.1	N/A[b]
Elevated Direct Bilirubin	15.6	8.3
Elevated total Bilirubin	3.6	0
Elevated BUN	5.5	0
Elevated Creatinine	0	0

[a] Worst on-study values in patients with normal baseline.
CTC grades: neutropenia (Grade 3 ≥0.5-1.0×10⁹/L, Grade 4 <0.5×10⁹/L); thrombocytopenia (Grade 3 ≥10-50×10⁹/L, Grade 4 <10×10⁹/L); Elevated AST and ALT (Grade 3 >3-10×ULN, Grade 4 >10×ULN); Elevated Bilirubin (Grade 3 >3-10×ULN, Grade 4 >10×ULN); Elevated BUN; Elevated Creatinine (Grade 3 >3-6×ULN, Grade 4 >6×ULN).
[b] All placebo-treated patients had elevated AST at baseline.

Low titer human anti-human antibodies were detected in 3/140 (2.1%) PNH patients treated with Soliris and in 1/44 (2.3%) placebo-treated PNH patients. These low titer antibodies occurred transiently and with no apparent correlation between antibody development and either clinical response (i.e., reduction in hemolysis) or adverse events to Soliris; these responses in the placebo group were therefore considered as false positive.

In the rheumatoid arthritis clinical trial of Soliris, one patient exhibited an increase in anti-DNA antibody titer from 1:40 to 1:80 that was deemed an adverse drug reaction. Nine Soliris- and one placebo-treated patient had anti-DNA antibody titers of >1:80 at the end of 26 weeks of treatment. The clinical significance of these observations is unknown.

Post-Market Adverse Drug Reactions: There has been limited post-marketing experience with Soliris. Overall, safety data from post-marketing spontaneous reports is consistent with the known safety profile observed in clinical studies. Infrequent cases of serious or fatal meningococcal infections have been reported.

DRUG INTERACTIONS: Overview: Drug interaction studies have not been performed with Soliris. In clinical trials, Soliris has been administered to patients treated concomitantly with medications commonly used in patients with PNH including erythropoietin stimulating agents, corticosteroids, anabolic steroids, anticoagulants, and immunosuppressants. An increased incidence of adverse events was not observed.
Drug-Drug Interactions: There are no drug-drug interactions known at this time.
Drug-Food Interactions: There are no drug-food interactions known at this time.
Drug-Herb Interactions: There are no drug-herb interactions known at this time.
Drug-Laboratory Test Interactions: There are no drug-laboratory interactions known at this time.
Drug-Lifestyle Interactions: There are no drug-lifestyle interactions known at this time.

DOSAGE AND ADMINISTRATION: Recommended Dose and Dosage Adjustment: Recommended Dosage Regimen: Soliris therapy consists of:

- 600 mg every 7 days for the first 4 weeks, followed by
- 900 mg for the fifth dose 7 days later, then
- 900 mg every 14 days thereafter.

Soliris should be administered at the recommended dosage regimen time points, or within two days of these time points (see Warnings and Precautions).
Dose Modifications/Discontinuations: A fixed dosage regimen was studied in clinical studies in PNH. There are no recommended modifications to the dosing regimen for Soliris. In case of a missed dose, resume the regular schedule as soon as possible.
Discontinuation: Please refer to Warnings and Precautions, General, Monitoring after Soliris Discontinuation.
Administration: DO NOT ADMINISTER AS AN IV PUSH OR BOLUS INJECTION.

The Soliris admixture should be administered by intravenous infusion over 35 minutes via gravity feed, a syringe-type pump, or an infusion pump. Admixed solutions of Soliris are stable for 24 hours at 2-8°C and at room temperature. However, Soliris contains no preservative so infusion of the admixture should begin as soon as possible after mixing.

If an adverse reaction occurs during the administration of Soliris, the infusion may be slowed or stopped at the discretion of the physician. If the infusion is slowed, the total infusion time should not exceed two hours. Monitor the patient for at least one hour following completion of the infusion for signs or symptoms of an infusion reaction.
Reconstitution: Soliris must be diluted to a final admixture concentration of 5 mg/mL using the following steps:

- Withdraw the required amount of Soliris from the vial into a sterile syringe.
- Transfer the recommended dose to an infusion bag.
- Dilute Soliris to a final concentration of 5 mg/mL by adding the appropriate amount (equal volume of diluent to drug volume) of 0.9% Sodium Chloride Injection, USP; 0.45% Sodium Chloride Injection, USP; 5% Dextrose in Water Injection, USP; or Ringer's Injection, USP to the infusion bag.
- The final admixed Soliris 5 mg/mL infusion volume is 120 mL for 600 mg doses or 180 mL for 900 mg doses. Gently invert the infusion bag containing the diluted Soliris solution to ensure thorough mixing of the product and diluent. Discard any unused portion left in a vial, as the product contains no preservatives.
- Prior to administration, the admixture should be allowed to adjust to room temperature (18-25°C). The admixture must not be heated in a microwave or with any heat source other than ambient air temperature. The Soliris admixture should be inspected visually prior to administration, and discarded if there is any particulate matter and/or discoloration.

Table 6: Soliris

Reconstitution

Dose	Vial Size	Volume of Diluent	Approximate Available Volume	Nominal Concentration per mL
600 mg	30 mL×2	60 mL	120 mL	5 mg/mL
900 mg	30 mL×3	90 mL	180 mL	5 mg/mL

OVERDOSAGE:
Soliris is to be administered under the supervision of a healthcare professional which minimizes the potential of a significant overdose. No cases of overdose have been reported during clinical studies.

> For management of a suspected drug overdose, CPhA recommends that you contact your **regional Poison Control Centre**. See the *CPS* Directory section for a list of Poison Control Centres.

ACTION AND CLINICAL PHARMACOLOGY: Mechanism of Action: A genetic mutation in PNH patients leads to the generation of populations of abnormal blood cells that are deficient in terminal complement inhibitors (known as PNH cells), rendering PNH red blood cells sensitive to persistent terminal complement-mediated destruction. The subsequent intravascular hemolysis is the primary disease manifestation in PNH patients. The destruction and loss of these PNH cells results in low blood counts (anemia), and also fatigue, difficulty in functioning, pain, dark urine, shortness of breath, and blood clots.

Eculizumab, the active ingredient in Soliris, is a monoclonal antibody that specifically binds to the complement protein C5 with high affinity, thereby inhibiting its cleavage to C5a and C5b and preventing the generation of the terminal complement complex C5b-9. Soliris inhibits terminal complement mediated intravascular hemolysis in PNH patients.
Pharmacodynamics: Pharmacotherapeutic group: Immunomodulators, ATC code: L04AA25. Soliris is a recombinant humanized monoclonal IgG2/4$_\kappa$ antibody that binds to the human C5 complement protein and inhibits the activation of terminal complement. The Soliris antibody contains human constant regions and murine complementarity determining regions grafted onto the human framework light- and heavy-chain variable regions. Soliris is composed of two 448 amino acid heavy chains and two 214 amino acid light chains and has a molecular weight of approximately 148kDa.

Soliris is produced in a murine myeloma (NS0 cell line) expression system and purified by affinity and ion exchange chromatography. The bulk drug substance manufacturing process also includes specific viral inactivation and removal steps.
Pharmacokinetics: In 40 patients with PNH, **the pharmacokinetic parameters were estimated with a 1-compartmental model as an approximation to the complex disposition of monoclonal antibodies** after multiple doses. Mean clearance was 0.28±0.12 mL/hr/kg, mean volume of distribution was 110.3±17.9 mL/kg, and mean elimination half-life was 11.3±3.4 days. Based on these approximations, the onset of steady state is predicted to be approximately 49-56 days with the proposed dosing regimen. Pharmacodynamic activity correlates directly with eculizumab serum concentrations and maintenance of trough levels above ≥35 µg/mL results in essentially complete blockade of hemolytic activity in the majority of patients.

Figure 1: Soliris

Serum Profile of IV Infusion of Soliris Estimated with a One Compartment Model (PK Parameters: Vdist=110.3 mL/kg; Half-life=11.3 days, Body Weight=75±11.8kg)

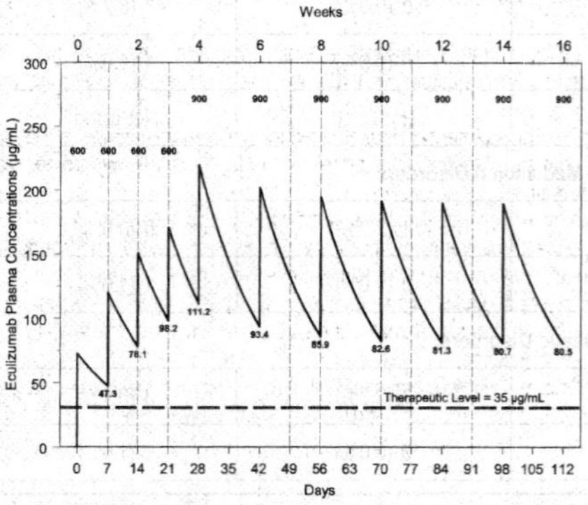

Trough serum concentrations of Soliris progressively increase during the 5-week induction period with 600 mg of Soliris dosed every week for 4 weeks from approximately 47.3 µg/mL one week after the first dose to 111.2 µg/mL one week after the fourth 600 mg dose. The last induction dose of 900mg of Soliris is given one week later. Trough serum concentrations of Soliris then slowly decrease to approximately 80 µg/mL during the maintenance phase of dosing (steady-state) with 900 mg of Soliris administered every 2 weeks.

In clinical trials, patients in the lowest weight quartile had the highest median serum trough levels of Soliris. Although analysis of safety data by weight quartile demonstrates that patients in the lowest weight quartile do not appear to be at an increased safety risk, the results must be interpreted with caution. As with all patients treated with Soliris, low weight patients should be closely monitored.

The recommended dosage regimen for Soliris was designed to maintain threshold concentrations of Soliris in plasma greater than approximately 35 µg/mL to inhibit terminal complement activation in treated patients.

Absorption, Distribution, Metabolism, and Excretion: No specific human studies have been performed with Soliris to evaluate ADME in humans.

Absorption: Soliris is administered intravenously; therefore, eculizumab bioavailability is assumed to be 100% with immediate absorption into the vascular space.

Distribution: Soliris is a humanized antibody and is expected to have distribution similar to native human antibodies, primarily limited to the vascular space.

Metabolism: Human antibodies undergo endocytotic digestion in the cells of the reticuloendo-thelial system. Eculizumab contains only naturally occurring amino acids and has no known active metabolites. Human antibodies are predominately catabolized by lysosomal enzymes to small peptides and amino acids.

Excretion: No specific studies have been performed to evaluate the hepatic, renal, lung, or gastrointestinal routes of excretion/elimination for Soliris. In normal kidneys, antibodies are not excreted and are excluded from filtration by their size.

STORAGE AND STABILITY: Soliris vials must be stored in the original carton until time of use under refrigerated conditions at 2-8°C and protected from light. Do not use beyond the expiration date stamped on the carton. Refer to Dosage and Administration, Reconstitution for information on the stability and storage of diluted solutions of Soliris.

DO NOT FREEZE. DO NOT SHAKE.

INFORMATION FOR THE PATIENT: Published in e-CPS, available by subscription at www.e-cps.ca.

DOSAGE FORMS, COMPOSITION AND PACKAGING: Each mL of sterile, clear, colorless, preservative-free solution for intravenous (IV) infusion contains: eculizumab 10 mg. The product is formulated at pH 7.0 and each vial contains 300 mg of eculizumab, 13.8 mg sodium phosphate monobasic, 53.4 mg sodium phosphate dibasic, 263.1 mg sodium chloride, 6.6 mg polysorbate 80 (vegetable origin) and Water for Injection, USP. Single-use vials of 30 mL, cartons of one vial.

The reader is invited to consult CPhA's monograph **Corticosteroids: Systemic**.

Solu-Cortef®

hydrocortisone sodium succinate

Glucocorticoid

Pfizer

PHARMACOLOGY: Sterile Solu-Cortef, the highly water-soluble sodium succinate ester of hydrocortisone, permits the immediate i.v. administration of high doses of hydrocortisone in a small volume of diluent and is, therefore, particularly useful in situations where high blood levels of hydrocortisone are required rapidly.

Solu-Cortef has the same metabolic and anti-inflammatory actions as hydrocortisone. When given parenterally and in equimolar quantities, the 2 compounds are equivalent in biologic activity. Following the i.v. injection of hydrocortisone sodium succinate, experimental evidence of its effects has been noted within a few minutes and persists for a variable period. Excretion of the administered dose is nearly complete within 12 hours. Thus, if constantly high blood levels are required, hydrocortisone sodium succinate should be injected every 4 to 6 hours. Hydrocortisone sodium succinate may also be administered by i.v. infusion, or by i.m. injection. The preferred method for initial emergency use is i.v. injection.

INDICATIONS: Endocrine Disorders: Primary or secondary adrenocortical insufficiency (hydrocortisone or cortisone is the drug of choice; synthetic analogs may be used in conjunction with mineralocorticoids where applicable; in infancy, mineralocorticoid supplementation is of particular importance).

Acute adrenocortical insufficiency (hydrocortisone or cortisone is the drug of choice; mineralocorticoid supplementation may be necessary, particularly when synthetic analogs are used).

Preoperatively and in the event of serious trauma or illness, in patients with known adrenal insufficiency or when adrenocortical reserve is doubtful. Shock unresponsive to conventional therapy, if adrenocortical insufficiency exists or is suspected.

Congenital adrenal hyperplasia.

Nonsuppurative thyroiditis.

Hypercalcemia associated with cancer.

Rheumatic Disorders: As adjunctive therapy for short-term administration (to tide the patient over an acute episode or exacerbation) in: post-traumatic osteoarthritis, synovitis or osteoarthritis, rheumatoid arthritis, including juvenile rheumatoid arthritis, (selected cases may require low dose maintenance therapy), acute and subacute bursitis, epicondylitis, acute nonspecific tenosynovitis, acute gouty arthritis, psoriatic arthritis, ankylosing spondylitis.

Collagen Diseases: During an exacerbation or as maintenance therapy in selected cases of: systemic lupus erythematosus, acute rheumatic carditis, systemic dermatomyositis (polymyositis).

Dermatologic Diseases: pemphigus, severe erythema multiforme (Stevens-Johnson syndrome), exfoliative dermatitis, bullous dermatitis herpetiformis, severe seborrheic dermatitis, severe psoriasis, mycosis fungoides.

Allergic States: Control of severe or incapacitating allergic conditions intractable to adequate trials of conventional treatment in: bronchial asthma, contact dermatitis, atopic dermatitis, serum sickness, seasonal or perennial allergic rhinitis, drug hypersensitivity reactions, urticarial transfusion reactions, acute noninfectious laryngeal edema (epinephrine is the drug of first choice).

Ophthalmic Diseases: Severe acute and chronic allergic and inflammatory processes involving the eye, such as: herpes zoster ophthalmicus, iritis, iridocyclitis, chorioretinitis, diffuse posterior uveitis and choroiditis, optic neuritis, sympathetic ophthalmia, anterior segment inflammation, allergic conjunctivitis, allergic corneal marginal ulcers, keratitis.

Gastrointestinal Diseases: To tide the patient over a critical period of the disease in: ulcerative colitis (systemic therapy), regional enteritis (systemic therapy).

Respiratory Diseases: symptomatic sarcoidosis, berylliosis, fulminating or disseminated pulmonary tuberculosis when used concurrently with appropriate antituberculous chemotherapy, Loeffler's syndrome not manageable by other means, aspiration pneumonitis.

Hematologic Disorders: acquired (autoimmune) hemolytic anemia, idiopathic thrombocytopenia purpura in adults (i.v. only; i.m. administration is contraindicated), erythroblastopenia (RBC anemia), congenital (erythroid) hypoplastic anemia, secondary thrombocytopenia in adults.

Neoplastic Diseases: for palliative management of: leukemias and lymphomas in adults, acute leukemia of childhood.

Edematous States: To induce diuresis or remission of proteinuria in the nephrotic syndrome, without uremia, or the idiopathic type or that due to lupus erythematosus.

Medical Emergencies: Hydrocortisone sodium succinate is indicated in the treatment of 1) shock secondary to adrenocortical insufficiency or shock unresponsive to conventional therapy when adrenal cortical insufficiency may be present; and 2) acute allergic disorders (status asthmaticus, anaphylactic reactions, insect stings, etc.) following epinephrine.

Although there are no well-controlled (double-blind, placebo) clinical trials, data from experimental animal models indicate that corticosteroids may be useful in hemorrhagic, traumatic and surgical shock in which standard therapy (e.g., fluid replacement, etc.) has not been effective (see Warnings).

Miscellaneous: Tuberculous meningitis with subarachnoid block or impending block when used concurrently with appropriate antituberculous chemotherapy. Trichinosis with neurologic or myocardial involvement.

CONTRAINDICATIONS: In patients with known hypersensitivity to any components of the product and in patients with systemic fungal infections.

WARNINGS: In patients on corticosteroid therapy subjected to unusual stress, increased dosage or rapidly acting corticosteroids before, during and after the stressful situation is indicated.

Corticosteroids may mask some signs of infection, and new infections may appear during their use. There may be decreased resistance and inability to localize infection when corticosteroids are used. Infections with any pathogen including viral, bacterial, fungal, protozoan or helminthic infections, in any location in the body, may be associated with the use of corticosteroids alone or in combination with other immunosuppressive agents that affect cellular immunity, humoral immunity or neutrophil function. These infections may be mild, but can be severe and at times fatal. With increasing doses of corticosteroids, the rate of occurrence of infectious complications increases.

Average and large doses of hydrocortisone can cause elevation of blood pressure, salt and water retention, and increased excretion of potassium. These effects are less likely to occur with synthetic derivatives except when used in large doses. Dietary salt restriction and potassium supplementation may be necessary. All corticosteroids increase calcium excretion.

Administration of live or live, attenuated vaccines is contraindicated in patients receiving immunosuppressive doses of corticosteroids. Killed or inactivated vaccines may be administered to patients receiving immunosuppressive doses of corticosteroids; however, the response to such vaccines may be diminished. Indicated immunization procedures may be undertaken in patients receiving non-immunosuppressive doses of corticosteroids.

The use of hydrocortisone sodium succinate in active tuberculosis should be restricted to those cases of fulminating or disseminated tuberculosis in which the corticosteroid is used for the management of the disease in conjunction with appropriate antituberculosis regimen.

If corticosteroids are indicated in patients with latent tuberculosis or tuberculin reactivity, close observation is necessary as reactivation of the disease may occur. During prolonged corticosteroid therapy, these patients should receive chemoprophylaxis.

Because rare instances of anaphylactoid reactions (e.g., bronchospasm) have occurred in patients receiving parenteral corticosteroid therapy, appropriate precautionary measures should be taken prior to administration, especially when the patient has a history of allergy to any drug.

This product contains benzyl alcohol. Benzyl alcohol has been reported to be associated with a fatal "Gasping Syndrome" in premature infants.

Although recent studies have not been conducted with hydrocortisone or other corticosteroids, studies of methylprednisolone sodium succinate in septic shock suggest that increased mortality may occur in some subgroups of patients at higher risk (i.e., elevated creatinine greater than 2.0 mg/dL or with secondary infections).

Pregnancy: Some animal studies have shown that corticosteroids, when administered to the mother at high doses, may cause fetal malformations. Adequate human reproductive studies have not been done with corticosteroids. Therefore the use of this drug in pregnancy, nursing mothers, or women of childbearing potential requires that the benefits of the drug be carefully weighed against the potential risk to the mother and embryo or fetus. Since there is inadequate evidence of safety in human pregnancy, this drug should be used in pregnancy only if clearly needed.

Corticosteroids readily cross the placenta. Infants born of mothers who have received substantial doses of corticosteroids during pregnancy must be carefully observed and evaluated for signs of adrenal insufficiency. There are no known effects of corticosteroids on labor and delivery. Corticosteroids are excreted in breast milk.

Lactation: See Pregnancy.

PRECAUTIONS: Corticosteroids should be used cautiously in patients with ocular herpes simplex for fear of corneal perforation.

Psychic derangements may appear when corticosteroids are used, ranging from euphoria, insomnia, mood swings, personality changes, and severe depression to frank psychotic manifestations. Also, existing emotional instability or psychotic tendencies may be aggravated by corticosteroids.

Steroids should be used with caution in nonspecific ulcerative colitis, if there is a probability of impending perforation, abscess or other pyogenic infections, also in diverticulitis, fresh intestinal anastomoses, active or latent peptic ulcer, renal insufficiency, hypertension, osteoporosis, and myasthenia gravis.

Although controlled clinical trials have shown corticosteroids to be effective in speeding the resolution of acute exacerbations of multiple sclerosis, they do not show that corticosteroids affect the ultimate outcome or natural history of the disease. The studies do show that relatively high doses of corticosteroids are necessary to demonstrate a significant effect (see Dosage).

An acute myopathy has been described with the use of high doses of corticosteroids, most often occurring in patients with disorders of neuromuscular transmission (e.g., myasthenia gravis), or in patients receiving concomitant therapy with neuromuscular blocking drugs (e.g., pancuronium). This acute myopathy is generalized, may involve ocular and respiratory muscles, and may result in quadriparesis. Elevations of creatine kinase may occur. Clinical improvement or recovery after stopping corticosteroids may require weeks to years.

Kaposi's sarcoma has been reported to occur in patients receiving corticosteroid therapy. Discontinuation of corticosteroids may result in clinical remission.

Carcinogenesis, Mutagenesis, Impairment of Fertility: There is no evidence that corticosteroids are carcinogenic, mutagenic or impair fertility.

Labor and Delivery: No effect known.

Lactation: Because prednisone is excreted in breast milk, it is reasonable to assume that all corticoids are. No data is known for hydrocortisone sodium succinate.

Children: Growth may be supressed in children receiving long-term, daily-divided dose glucocorticoid therapy. The use of such a regimen should be restricted to the most serious indications.

Drug Interactions: The pharmacokinetic interactions listed below are potentially clinically important.

Drugs that induce hepatic enzymes such as phenobarbital, phenytoin and rifampin may increase the clearance of corticosteroids and may require increases in corticosteroid dose to achieve the desired response.

Drugs such as troleandomycin and ketoconazole may inhibit the metabolism of corticosteroids and thus decrease their clearance. Therefore the dose of corticosteroid should be titrated to avoid steroid toxicity.

Corticosteroids may increase the clearance of chronic high dose ASA. This could lead to decreased salicylate serum levels or increase the risk of salicylate toxicity when corticosteroid is withdrawn. ASA should be used cautiously in conjunction with corticosteroids in patients suffering from hypoprothrombinemia.

The effect of corticosteroids on oral anticoagulants is variable. There are reports of enhanced as well as diminished effects of anticoagulant when given concurrently with corticosteroids. Therefore coagulation indices should be monitored to maintain the desired anticoagulant effect.

ADVERSE EFFECTS: Note: The following are typical for all systemic corticosteroids. Their inclusion in this list does not necessarily indicate that the specific event has been observed with this particular formulation.

Fluid and Electrolyte Disturbances: congestive heart failure in susceptible patients, hypertension, hypokalemic alkalosis. Sodium retention, fluid retention and potassium loss which are correctable and largely preventable by restricting sodium intake to 500 mg/day and supplementing potassium intake, and increased calcium excretion.

Musculoskeletal: steroid myopathy, muscle weakness, osteoporosis, pathologic fractures, vertebral compression fractures, aseptic necrosis, loss of muscle mass, tendon rupture (particularly of the Achilles tendon).

Gastrointestinal: peptic ulceration with possible perforation and hemorrhage, gastric hemorrhage, pancreatitis, esophagitis, ulcerative esophagitis, perforation of the bowel, abdominal distention.

Increases in ALT, AST and alkaline phosphatase have been observed following corticosteroid treatment. These changes are usually small, not associated with any clinical syndrome and are reversible upon discontinuation.

Dermatologic: impaired wound healing (usually at high doses), petechiae and ecchymoses, thin fragile skin, facial erythema, increased sweating.

Metabolic: negative nitrogen balance due to protein catabolism.

Neurological: increased intracranial pressure, pseudotumor cerebri, psychic derangements/psychotic, manifestations including euphoria, insomnia, mood swings, personality changes, depression; exacerbation of pre-existing emotional instability or psychotic tendencies, seizures, headache, vertigo.

Endocrine: menstrual irregularities, development of Cushingoid state, suppression of pituitary-adrenal axis leading to secondary adrenocortical and pituitary unresponsiveness, decreased carbohydrate tolerance, manifestation of latent diabetes mellitus, increased requirements for insulin or oral hypoglycemic agents in diabetics, suppression of growth in children.

Ophthalmic: posterior subcapsular cataracts (associated with prolonged, high dose systemic therapy), glaucoma, increased intraocular pressure, exophthalmos.

Immune System: masking of infections, latent infections becoming active, opportunistic infections, hypersensitivity reactions including anaphylaxis, may suppress reactions to skin tests.

The following additional reactions are related to parenteral corticosteroid therapy: hyperpigmentation or hypopigmentation, s.c. and cutaneous atrophy, sterile abscess, anaphylactoid reaction (e.g., bronchospasm, laryngeal edema, urticaria).

Miscellaneous: This product contains benzyl alcohol that has been associated with fatal "Gasping Syndrome" in premature infants.

OVERDOSE:

Symptoms: There is no clinical syndrome of acute overdosage with hydrocortisone. Hydrocortisone is dialyzable.

Treatment: See Symptoms.

For management of a suspected drug overdose, CPhA recommends that you contact your **regional Poison Control Centre**. See the *CPS* Directory section for a list of Poison Control Centres.

DOSAGE: This preparation may be administered by i.v. injection, by i.v. infusion, or by i.m. injection; the preferred method for initial emergency use being i.v. injection. Following the initial emergency period, consideration should be given to employing a longer-acting injectable preparation or an oral preparation.

Therapy is initiated by administering hydrocortisone sodium succinate i.v. over a period of 30 seconds (e.g., 100 mg) to 10 minutes (e.g., 500 mg or more). In general, high-dose corticosteroid therapy should be continued only until the patient's condition has stabilized, usually not beyond 48 to 72 hours. Although adverse effects associated with high dose, short-term corticoid therapy are uncommon, peptic ulceration may occur. Prophylactic antacid therapy may be indicated. When high-dose hydrocortisone therapy must be continued beyond 48 to 72 hours, hypernatremia may occur. Under such circumstances it may be desirable to replace hydrocortisone sodium succinate with a corticosteroid product such as methylprednisolone sodium succinate which causes little or no sodium retention.

The initial dose of hydrocortisone sodium succinate is 100 to 500 mg or more depending on the severity of the condition. This dose may be repeated at intervals of 2, 4, or 6 hours as indicated by the patient's response and clinical condition. While the dose may be reduced for infants and children, it is governed more by the severity of the condition and response of the patient than by age or body weight but should not be less than 25 mg daily.

Patients subjected to severe stress following corticosteroid therapy should be observed closely for signs and symptoms of adrenocortical insufficiency.

Corticosteroid therapy is an adjunct to, and not a replacement for, conventional therapy.

Preparation of Solutions: Parenteral drug products should be inspected visually for particulate matter and discoloration prior to administration, whenever solution and container permit.

I.V./I.M. Injection: To use Solu-Cortef Act-O-Vial reconstitute Act-O-Vial according to Directions For Using The Act-O-Vial System. Further dilution is not necessary for i.v. or i.m. injection.

I.V. Infusion: For i.v. infusion, first reconstitute Act-O-Vials according to instructions. The **100 mg** solution may then be added to 100 to 1 000 mL of 5% Dextrose in Water (or isotonic saline solution or 5% dextrose in isotonic saline solution if patient is not on sodium restriction). The **250 mg** solution may be added to 250 to 1 000 mL, the **500 mg** solution may be added to 500 to 1 000 mL and the **1 000 mg** solution to 1 000 mL of the same diluents. In cases, where administration of a small volume of fluid is desirable, 100 mg to 3 000 mg of Solu-Cortef may be added to 50 mL of the above diluents. The resulting solutions are stable for at least 4 hours and may be administered either directly or by i.v. piggy back.

Table 1 provides the stability data of hydrocortisone in 5% Dextrose in Water, USP (D5W) or 0.9% Sodium Chloride Injection, UPS (NS), at room temperature.

Table 1: Solu-Cortef

Solu-Cortef Stability

Concentration	Stability (time)
≤1 mg/mL	24 hours
1 mg/mL < x <25 mg/mL[a]	unpredictable, 4 to 6 hours
≥25 mg/mL	3 days

[a] "x" is the concentration of Solu-Cortef prepared that is above 1 mg/mL but below 25 mg/mL.

Freezing: In-house studies have shown reconstituted hydrocortisone sodium succinate 50 mg/mL and 125 mg/mL to be physically and chemically stable after 1 month of freezing. Once thawed, the above guidelines should be followed for hydrocortisone sodium succinate.

Directions for Using the Act-O-Vial System: Press down on plastic activator to force diluent into the lower compartment. Gently agitate to effect solution. Remove plastic tab covering center of stopper. Sterilize top of stopper with a suitable germicide. Insert needle squarely through center of stopper until tip is just visible. Invert vial and withdraw dose.

Storage: Store unreconstituted product at controlled room temperature 15 to 30°C. Store solution at controlled room temperature 15 to 30°C and protect from light. Use solution only if it is clear. Discard unused solutions after 3 days. The Act-O-Vial is a single dose vial and once reconstituted solution is used, any remaining portion should be discarded.

SUPPLIED: Act-O-Vials: 100 mg: Each 2 mL (when mixed) contains: hydrocortisone (as hydrocortisone sodium succinate) 100 mg, monobasic sodium phosphate anhydrous 0.8 mg, dibasic sodium phosphate dried 8.76 mg, benzyl alcohol 18.1 mg and sterile water for injection q.s. Sodium: <0.5 mmol/mL. Vial packs of 10.

250 mg: Each 2 mL (when mixed) contains: hydrocortisone (as hydrocortisone sodium succinate) 250 mg, monobasic sodium phosphate anhydrous 2 mg, dibasic sodium phosphate dried 21.8 mg, benzyl alcohol 16.4 mg and sterile water for injection q.s. Sodium: <1 mmol/mL. Vial packs of 10.

500 mg: Each 4 mL (when mixed) contains: hydrocortisone (as hydrocortisone sodium succinate) 500 mg, monobasic sodium phosphate anhydrous 4 mg, dibasic sodium phosphate dried 44 mg, benzyl alcohol 33.4 mg and sterile water for injection q.s. Sodium: <0.5002 mmol/mL. Vial packs of 5.

1 g: Each 8 mL (when mixed) contains: hydrocortisone (as hydrocortisone sodium succinate) 1 g, monobasic sodium phosphate anhydrous 8 mg, dibasic sodium phosphate dried 87.32 mg, benzyl alcohol 66.9 mg and sterile water for injection q.s. Sodium: <0.4978 mmol/mL. Vial packs of 5.

Solugel® 4
benzoyl peroxide
Acne Therapy

Stiefel, a GSK company

Solugel® 8 ℞
benzoyl peroxide
Acne Therapy

Stiefel, a GSK company

PHARMACOLOGY: The topical use of benzoyl peroxide provides therapeutic control of acne through drying and desquamative action as well as antibacterial activity.

INDICATIONS: Acne vulgaris.

CONTRAINDICATIONS: Patients with a known sensitivity to benzoyl peroxide or any of the components should not use this medication.

PRECAUTIONS: For external use only. Do not permit product to come in contact with the eyes or mucous membranes. Very fair individuals should always be started with a single application. Benzoyl peroxide may bleach colored fabrics.

OVERDOSE:

For management of a suspected drug overdose, CPhA recommends that you contact your **regional Poison Control Centre**. See the *CPS* Directory section for a list of Poison Control Centres.

DOSAGE: Wash thoroughly with a non-medicated soap such as Acne-Aid and water. Apply once or twice daily to affected areas or according to the instructions of a physician.

SUPPLIED: Each g of gel contains: benzoyl peroxide 4% (Solugel 4), or 8% (Solugel 8) in a unique patented hydrophase gel base. Nonmedicinal ingredients: cetyl alcohol, dimethyl isosorbide, fragrance, promulgen G, purified water and simethicone. Tubes of 45 g. Store below 27°C.

Solu-Medrol™ ℞
methylprednisolone sodium succinate
Glucocorticoid

Pfizer

Date of Preparation: September 23, 2003
Date of Revision: May 15, 2006

SUMMARY PRODUCT INFORMATION:

Route of Administration	Dosage Form/Strength	Clinically Relevant Nonmedicinal Ingredients
Intravenous or intramuscular injection or by intravenous infusion	Sterile powder 40 mg, 125 mg, 500 mg, 1 g	Lactose hydrous For a complete listing see Dosage Forms, Composition and Packaging.

INDICATIONS AND CLINICAL USE: Intravenous administration of SOLU-MEDROL (methylprednisolone sodium succinate) is indicated in situations in which a rapid and intense hormonal effect is required. These include the following:

Hypersensitivity and dermatologic conditions:

- Status asthmaticus
- Anaphylactic reactions (see text)
- Drug reactions
- Contact dermatitis
- Urticaria
- Generalized neurodermatitis
- Reactions to insect bites
- Pemphigus foliaceous and vulgaris
- Exfoliative dermatitis
- Erythema multiforme

As Adjunctive therapy in:

- Acute systemic lupus erythematosus
- Acute rheumatic fever
- Acute gout

Ulcerative Colitis: In addition to the above conditions, colonic instillation of SOLU-MEDROL in retention enemas or by continuous drip, have been shown to be a useful adjunct in the treatment of patients with ulcerative colitis.

In anaphylactic reactions: epinephrine or norepinephrine should be administered first for an immediate hemodynamic effect followed by intravenous injection of SOLU-MEDROL and other accepted procedures. There is evidence that the corticoids through their prolonged hemodynamic effect are of value in preventing recurrent attacks of acute anaphylactic reactions.

In sensitivity reactions: such as in serum sickness, allergic dermatosis (urticaria) and reactions to insect bites, SOLU-MEDROL is capable of providing relief within ½ to 2 hours. In some asthmatic patients it may be advantageous to administer SOLU-MEDROL by slow intravenous drip over a period of hours.

As adjunctive therapy in fulminating acute systemic lupus erythematosus and acute rheumatic fever, and to relieve pain during the acute manifestations of gout: SOLU-MEDROL may be given by slow intravenous administration over a period of several minutes. Thereafter, the patient should be placed on intramuscular or oral therapy as required for continued relief of symptoms. In these conditions, other accepted measures of therapy should also be instituted.

Shock: In severe hemorrhagic or traumatic shock, adjunctive use of intravenous methylprednisolone sodium succinate (SOLU-MEDROL) may aid in achieving hemodynamic restoration. Corticoid therapy should not replace standard methods of combating shock, but present evidence indicates that concurrent use of large doses of corticoids with other measures may improve survival rates.

Organ Transplants: Corticosteroids both, parenterally and orally, in high doses have been used following organ transplantation as part of multi-faceted attempts to reduce the rejection phenomenon. SOLU-MEDROL is suitable for such indications.

Cerebral Edema of Non Traumatic Origin: Administration of SOLU-MEDROL immediately prior to intracranial surgery and in the immediate post-operative period has reduced the duration of post-operative complications related to cerebral edema.

CONTRAINDICATIONS: Except when used for short-term or emergency therapy as in acute sensitivity reactions, SOLU-MEDROL (methylprednisolone sodium succinate) is contraindicated in patients with arrested tuberculosis, herpes simplex keratitis, acute psychoses, Cushing's syndrome, peptic ulcer, markedly elevated serum creatinine, vaccinia and varicella. SOLU-MEDROL is also contraindicated for systemic fungal infections and known hypersensitivity to the ingredients.

WARNINGS AND PRECAUTIONS: General: SOLU-MEDROL (methylprednisolone sodium succinate) should not be used to treat head injury as demonstrated by the results of a multicenter study. The study results revealed an increased mortality in the 2 weeks after injury in patients administered methylprednisolone sodium succinate compared to placebo (1.18 relative risk).

Recent studies do not establish the efficacy of SOLU-MEDROL in septic shock, and suggest that increased mortality may occur in some subgroups at higher risk (i.e. elevated serum creatinine greater than 2.0 mg/dL or secondary infections).

Since complications of treatment with glucocorticoids are dependent on the size of the dose and the duration of treatment, a risk/benefit decision must be made in each individual case as to dose and duration of treatment and as to whether daily or intermittent therapy should be used.

In patients on corticosteroid therapy subjected to unusual stress, increased dosage of rapidly acting corticosteroids before, during and after the stressful situation is indicated.

Dosage must be decreased or discontinued gradually when the drug has been administered for more than a few days.

Patients should be advised to inform subsequent physicians of the prior use of SOLU-MEDROL.

The diluent for reconstitution of the vials is Bacteriostatic Water for Injection (included in the Act-O-Vials), which contains benzyl alcohol. Benzyl alcohol has been reported to be associated with fatal "Gasping Syndrome" in premature infants.

Cardiovascular: There are reports of cardiac arrhythmias and/or circulatory collapse and/or cardiac arrest following the rapid administration of large intravenous doses of methylprednisolone sodium succinate (greater than 0.5 g administered over a period of less than 10 minutes). Bradycardia has been reported during or after the administration of large doses of methylprednisolone sodium succinate, and may be unrelated to the speed or duration of infusion.

Endocrine and Metabolism: Since methylprednisolone, like prednisolone, suppresses endogenous adrenocortical activity, it is highly important that the patient receiving SOLU-MEDROL be under careful observation, not only during the course of treatment but for some time after treatment is terminated.

Gastrointestinal: The existence of diabetes, osteoporosis, renal insufficiency, chronic psychosis, diverticulitis, fresh intestinal anastomoses, active or latent peptic ulcer, hypertension, myasthenia gravis or predisposition to thrombophlebitis requires that SOLU-MEDROL (methylprednisolone sodium succinate) be administered with extreme caution. The same caution should also be used in non-specific ulcerative colitis, if there is a probability of impending perforation, abscess or other pyogenic infections.

Immune: Corticosteroids may mask some signs of infection, and new infections may appear during their use. There may be decreased resistance and inability to localize infection when corticosteroids are used. Infections with any pathogen including viral, bacterial, fungal, protozoan or helminthic infections, in any location in the body, may be associated with the use of corticosteroids alone or in combination with other immunosuppressive agents that affect cellular immunity, humoral immunity, or neutrophil function. These infections may be mild, but can be severe and at times fatal. With increasing doses of corticosteroids, the rate of occurrence of infectious complications increases.

Administration of live or live, attenuated vaccines is contraindicated in patients receiving immunosuppressive doses of corticosteroids. Killed or inactivated vaccines may be administered to patients receiving immunosuppressive doses of corticosteroids; however, the response to such vaccines may be diminished. Indicated immunization procedures may be undertaken in patients receiving non immunosuppressive doses of corticosteroids.

The use of methylprednisolone sodium succinate in active tuberculosis should be restricted to those cases of fulminating or disseminated tuberculosis in which the corticosteroid is used for the management of the disease in conjunction with appropriate anti-tuberculosis regimen.

If corticosteroids are indicated in patients with latent tuberculosis or tuberculin reactivity, close observation is necessary as reactivation of the disease may occur. During prolonged corticosteroid therapy, these patients should receive chemoprophylaxis.

Because rare instances of anaphylactoid (e.g. bronchospasm) reactions have occurred in patients receiving parenteral corticosteroid therapy, appropriate precautionary measures should be taken prior to administration, especially when the patient has a history of allergy to any drug.

Neurologic: Convulsions have been reported with concurrent use of methylprednisolone and cyclosporine. Since concurrent administration of these agents results in a mutual inhibition of metabolism, it is possible that convulsions and other adverse events associated with the individual use of either drug may be more apt to occur.

An acute myopathy has been described with the use of high doses of corticosteroids, most often occurring in patients with disorders of neuromuscular transmission (e.g. myasthenia gravis), or in patients receiving concomitant therapy with neuromuscular blocking drugs (e.g. pancuronium). This acute myopathy is generalized, may involve ocular and respiratory muscles, and may result in quadriparesis. Elevations of creatine kinase may occur. Clinical improvement or recovery after stopping corticosteroids may require weeks to years.

Ophthalmologic: Corticosteroids should be used cautiously in patients with ocular herpes simplex because of possible corneal perforation.

Psychiatric: Psychic derangements may appear when corticosteroids are used, ranging from euphoria, insomnia, mood swings, personality changes, and severe depression to frank psychotic manifestations. Also, existing emotional instability or psychotic tendencies may be aggravated by corticosteroids, and therefore these patients should be treated with caution.

Skin: Kaposi's sarcoma has been reported to occur in patients receiving corticosteroid therapy. Discontinuation of corticosteroids may result in clinical remission.

Special Populations: Pregnant Women: Some animal studies have shown that corticosteroids, when administered to the mother at high doses, may cause fetal malformations. There are, however, no adequate and well-controlled studies in pregnant women. Because animal reproduction studies are not always predictive of human response, the use of this drug during pregnancy, in nursing mothers and women of child-bearing potential, requires that the benefits of the drug be carefully weighed against the potential risk to the mother and embryo or fetus. Newborn infants of mothers who received such therapy during pregnancy should be observed for signs of hypoadrenalism and appropriate measures instituted if such signs are present. No effect is known upon labour and delivery.

Nursing Women: Because prednisolone is excreted in breast milk it is reasonable to assume that all corticosteroids are. No specific data are available for methylprednisolone sodium succinate.

ADVERSE REACTIONS: The following Adverse Reactions have been reported with the systemic use of corticosteroid preparations (e.g. SOLU-MEDROL (methylprednisolone sodium succinate)). Their inclusion in this list does not necessarily indicate that the specific event has been observed with SOLU-MEDROL:

Infections and Infestations: masking of infections, latent infections becoming active, opportunistic infections.

Immune System Disorders: hypersensitivity reactions, including anaphylaxis with or without circulatory collapse, cardiac arrest, bronchospasm, may suppress reactions to skin tests.

Endocrine Disorders: development of Cushingoid state, suppression of pituitary-adrenal axis, suppression of growth in children.

Metabolism and Nutrition Disorders: sodium retention, sodium excretion, fluid retention, diuresis, decreased carbohydrate tolerance, manifestation of latent diabetes mellitus, increased requirements for insulin or oral hypoglycemic agents in diabetics, negative nitrogen balance due to protein catabolism.

Psychiatric Disorders: psychic derangements.

Nervous System Disorders: increased intracranial pressure with papilloedema (pseudotumor cerebri), seizures.

Eye Disorders: posterior subcapsular cataracts, exophthalmos, increased intraocular pressure.

Cardiac Disorders: congestive heart failure in susceptible patients, myocardial rupture following a myocardial infarction, arrhythmia, hypertension, hypotension.

Vascular Disorders: ecchymosis, petechiae.

Gastrointestinal Disorders: peptic ulceration with possible perforation and hemorrhage, gastric hemorrhage, pancreatitis, esophagitis, perforation of the bowel, transient nausea, vomiting or dysgeusia (with rapid administration of large doses).

Skin and Subcutaneous Tissue Disorders: thin fragile skin, impaired wound healing.

Musculoskeletal and Connective Tissue Disorders: steroid myopathy, muscle weakness, osteoporosis, aseptic necrosis, pathologic fractures, vertebral compression fractures, tendon rupture, particularly of the Achilles tendon.

Reproductive System and Breast Disorders: menstrual irregularities.

Abnormal Hematologic and Clinical Chemistry Findings: potassium loss with resulting hypokalemic alkalosis, sodium and fluid retention, increases in alanine transaminase (ALT), aspartate transaminase (AST) and alkaline phosphatase.

DRUG INTERACTIONS: Overview: CYP3A4 inhibitors (such as macrolides, triazole antifungals, and some calcium channel blockers) may inhibit the metabolism of methylprednisolone and thus decrease its clearance. Therefore the dose of methylprednisolone should be titrated to avoid steroid toxicity.

Drug-Drug Interactions: Table 1 includes the common interactions seen with Solu-Medrol and other drug products. Methylprednisolone, like all glucocorticoids, can cause the following effects when administered in combination with these products. Table 1 is meant to serve as a guide to professionals when considering a rational course of therapy.

Drug-Food Interactions: Interactions with food have not been established.

Drug-Herb Interactions: Interactions with herbal products have not been established.

Drug-Laboratory Test Interactions: Interactions with laboratory tests have not been established.

DOSAGE AND ADMINISTRATION:

Recommended Dose and Dosage Adjustment: As adjunctive therapy in life threatening conditions (e.g., shock states), the recommended dose of SOLU-MEDROL (methylprednisolone sodium succinate) is 30 mg per kg, given intravenously over a period of at least 30 minutes. The large doses may be repeated every 4-6 hours for up to 48 hours.

In other indications, initial dosage will vary from 10 to 500 mg depending on the clinical problem being treated. Larger doses may be required for short-term management of severe, acute conditions. Therapy may be initiated by administering SOLU-MEDROL intravenously over a period of at least 5 minutes (e.g., doses up to 250 mg) to at least 30 minutes (e.g., doses greater than 250 mg). Subsequent doses may be given intravenously or intramuscularly at intervals dictated by the patient's response and clinical condition. Corticosteroid therapy is an adjunct to, and not replacement for, conventional therapy.

SOLU-MEDROL in doses of 40 to 120 mg administered as retention enemas or by continuous drip three to seven times weekly for periods of two or more weeks have been shown to be a useful adjunct in the treatment of some patients with ulcerative colitis. Many patients can be controlled with 40 mg of SOLU-MEDROL administered in from 1 to 10 fluid ounces of water depending on the degree of involvement of the inflamed colonic mucosa. Other accepted therapeutic measures should, of course, be instituted.

Administration: SOLU-MEDROL may be administered by intravenous or intramuscular injection or by intravenous infusion, the preferred method for initial emergency use being intravenous injection. To administer intravenous (or intramuscular) injection, prepare solution as directed.

Reconstitution: Directions for Using the ACT-O-VIAL System:

1. Press down on plastic activator to force diluent into the lower compartment.
2. Gently agitate to effect solution.
3. Remove plastic tab covering center of stopper.
4. Sterilize top of stopper with suitable germicide.
5. Insert needle **squarely through center** of stopper until tip is just visible. Invert vial and withdraw dose.

Parenteral drug products should be inspected visually for particulate matter and discolouration prior to administration, whenever solution and container permit. See Table 2.

SOLU-MEDROL 40 mg Vial: Reconstitute with 1 mL Bacteriostatic Water for Injection USP (benzyl alcohol as preservative).
SOLU-MEDROL 125 mg Vial: Reconstitute with 2 mL Bacteriostatic Water for Injection USP (benzyl alcohol as preservative).
SOLU-MEDROL 500 mg Vial: Reconstitute with 8 mL Bacteriostatic Water for Injection USP (benzyl alcohol as preservative).
SOLU-MEDROL 1 g Vial: Reconstitute with 16 mL Bacteriostatic Water for Injection USP (benzyl alcohol as preservative).

Store powder or reconstituted solution at room temperature (between 15 and 30°C). Use reconstituted solution within 48 hours. SOLU-MEDROL Vials and Act-O-Vials are single dose vials. Discard unused portion.

To prepare solutions for intravenous infusion, first reconstitute SOLU-MEDROL as directed. The medication may be administered in dilute solutions by admixing the reconstituted product with: Dextrose 5% Water (D5W) or 0.9% Sodium Chloride (NS) or Dextrose 5% in 0.45% Sodium Chloride.

Dilute solution concentrations of 0.25 mg/mL or greater are physically and chemically stable for 48 hours.

Table 1: SOLU-MEDROL
Common Interactions Seen with Solu-Medrol and Other Drug Products

Class of Drug	Drug(s) Involved	Affects Therapy of Drugs	Clinical Implication	Mechanism
Antibiotic/Antifungal Therapy	Troleandomycin Erythromycin Ketoconazole	Methylprednisolone	Enhanced clinical effects and side effects of methylprednisolone.	Enzyme inhibition: Reduced MP elimination.
	Rifampin	Methylprednisolone	May reduce efficacy; dosage adjustment may be required.	Enzyme induction, increased clearance.
Anticholinesterase	Neostigmine, pyridostigmine	Anticholinesterase	Precipitation of myasthenic crisis.	
Anticoagulants	Oral anticoagulants or heparin	Anticoagulant	Increased **or** decreased clotting. Monitor response. Adjust dose.	
Anticonvulsants	e.g., phenolbarbitone, phenytoin	Methylprednisolone	May reduce methylprednisolone efficacy. Monitor clinical response. Adjust dose if necessary.	Enzyme induction: increased clearance of methylprednisolone
Antidiabetic Drugs	e.g., insulin, glibenclamide, metformin	Antidiabetic	May impair glucose control. Monitor glucose levels and adjust dose of antidiabetic therapy.	Diabetogenic effects of corticosteroid.
Antihypertensive Agents	All antihypertensives	Antihypertensive	May result in partial loss of hypertensive control.	Mineralocorticoid effect of corticosteroid leading to raised blood pressure.
Diuretics	All potassium losing diuretics e.g., furosemide		Enhanced toxicity. Monitor K^+ levels and supplement if necessary.	Potassium loss
Cardioactive Drugs	Digoxin and related glycosides	Digoxin	Potentiation of digoxin toxicity	Corticosteroid-induced potassium loss (mineralocorticoid effect)
Immunizing Agents	Live vaccine: poliomyelitis, BCG, mumps, measles, rubella, smallpox	Vaccine	May see increased toxicity from vaccine. Disseminated viral disease may occur.	Corticosteroid induced immunosuppression
	Killed virulent vaccines	Vaccine	Reduced response to vaccine	Impaired immune response
Immuno-suppressants	Methotrexate Azathioprine	Methylprednisolone	May allow reduced dose of corticosteroid.	Synergistic effect on disease state
	Cyclosporin (CYA)	Both	Monitor cyclosporine A levels. Adjust dose as necessary.	Mutual inhibition of metabolism
Neuromuscular Blocking Agents	Pancuronium	Pancuronium	Partial reversal of neuromuscular block	
Psychotherapeutic	Anxiolytics Antipsychotics	CNS active drug	Recurrence or poor control of CNS symptoms. May require dose adjustment.	CNS effects of corticosteroid
Salicylates		Salicylate	Apparent decrease in salicylate efficacy or salicylate toxicity upon reduction of corticosteroid dose.	Increased clearance and decreased plasma level.
Sympathomimetic Agents	e.g., salbutamol		Increased efficacy and potentially increased toxicity.	Increased response to sympathetic agents.

Table 2: SOLU-MEDROL

Parenteral Drug Products

Size	Volume of Diluent to be Added	Nominal Concentration per mL
40 mg AOV	Entire contents supplied	40 mg/mL
125 mg AOV	Entire contents supplied	62.5 mg/mL
500 mg AOV	Entire contents supplied	125 mg/mL
1 g AOV	Entire contents supplied	125 mg/mL
40 mg Vial	1 mL	40 mg/mL
125 mg Vial	2 mL	62.5 mg/mL
500 mg Vial	8 mL	62.5 mg/mL
1 g Vial	16 mL	62.5 mg/mL

Compatibility: The compatibility and stability of SOLU-MEDROL, in solutions and with other drugs in intravenous admixtures is dependent on admixture pH, concentration, time, temperature, and the ability of methylprednisolone to solubilize itself. Thus, to avoid compatibility and stability problems, whenever possible it is recommended that SOLU-MEDROL be administered separate from other drugs and as either I.V. push, through an I.V. medication chamber, or as an I.V. "piggy-back" solution. If desired, reconstituted methylprednisolone sodium succinate may be diluted with dextrose 5% in water, normal saline, or dextrose 5% in 0.45% or 0.9% sodium chloride. The resulting solutions are physically and chemically stable for 48 hours.

OVERDOSAGE:

There is no clinical symptom of acute overdosage with SOLU-MEDROL (methylprednisolone sodium succinate). Methylprednisolone is dialyzable. Continuous overdosage would require careful gradual reduction of dosage in order to prevent the occurrence of acute adrenal insufficiency.

For management of a suspected drug overdose, CPhA recommends that you contact your **regional Poison Control Centre**. See the *CPS* Directory section for a list of Poison Control Centres.

ACTION AND CLINICAL PHARMACOLOGY: Pharmacodynamics: Methylprednisolone is a potent anti-inflammatory steroid. It has a greater anti-inflammatory potency than prednisolone and has less tendency than prednisolone to induce sodium and water retention.

Methylprednisolone sodium succinate has the same metabolic and anti-inflammatory actions as methylprednisolone. When given parenterally and in equimolar quantities, the two compounds are equivalent in biologic activity. The relative potency of methylprednisolone sodium succinate and hydrocortisone sodium succinate, following intravenous administration, is at least four to one. This is in good agreement with the relative oral potency of methylprednisolone and hydrocortisone.

Pharmacokinetics: The metabolism and excretion of methylprednisolone sodium succinate is similar to that of other corticosteroids. It influences carbohydrate, protein, fat and purine metabolism, electrolyte and water balance, and the functional capacities of the cardiovascular system, the kidney, skeletal muscle, the nervous system and other organs and tissues. Like other corticosteroids, methylprednisolone sodium succinate endows the organism with the capacity to resist not a few but all types of noxious stimuli and environmental change.

Exceeding prednisolone in anti-inflammatory potency and having even less tendency than prednisolone to induce retention of sodium and water, methylprednisolone sodium succinate offers the use of lower doses with an enhanced split between anti-inflammatory and mineralocorticoid activities. Thus methylprednisolone sodium succinate may be indicated for emergency use in patients in whom increased sodium retention would be hazardous.

The relative potency of methylprednisolone sodium succinate (SOLU-MEDROL) and hydrocortisone sodium succinate (SOLU-CORTEF), as indicated by depression of eosinophil count, following intravenous administration, is at least four to one. This is in good agreement with the relative oral potency of methylprednisolone (MEDROL) and hydrocortisone (CORTEF). Studies indicate that the administration of methylprednisolone results in an appreciable prolongation of plasma steroid levels over those obtained following equivalent doses of hydrocortisone or prednisolone. Table 3 illustrates this prolongation of blood levels expressed as the half-life in minutes of the 17-hydroxy-corticosteroid levels obtained following intravenous administration of methylprednisolone, prednisolone and hydrocortisone.

Table 3: SOLU-MEDROL

Prolongation of Blood Levels

Compound	Dose	Half-life (minutes)
Methylprednisolone	25 mg	188
Prednisolone	25 mg	69
Hydrocortisone	25 mg	57

STORAGE AND STABILITY: Store unreconstituted SOLU-MEDROL Sterile Powder at room temperature (15-30°C). Store reconstituted solution at room temperature (15-30°C). Use reconstituted solution within 48 hours after mixing. Protect unreconstituted sterile powder and reconstituted solution from light.

INFORMATION FOR THE PATIENT: Published in e-CPS, available by subscription at www.e-cps.ca.

DOSAGE FORMS, COMPOSITION AND PACKAGING: Act-O-Vials: 40 mg: Each 1 mL (when mixed) contains: methylprednisolone (as methylprednisolone sodium succinate) 40 mg, monobasic sodium phosphate anhydrous 1.6 mg, dibasic sodium phosphate dried 17.5 mg, lactose hydrous 25 mg and bacteriostatic water for injection q.s. In diluent, benzyl alcohol 8.8 mg with sterile water for injection q.s. Vial packs of 10.

125 mg: Each 2 mL (when mixed) contains: methylprednisolone (as methylprednisolone sodium succinate) 125 mg, monobasic sodium phosphate 1.6 mg, dibasic sodium phosphate dried 17.4 mg, and bacteriostatic water for injection q.s. In diluent benzyl alcohol 17.6 mg with sterile water for injection q.s. Vial packs of 10.

500 mg: Each 4 mL (when mixed) contains: methylprednisolone (as methylprednisolone sodium succinate) 500 mg, monobasic sodium phosphate anhydrous 6.4 mg, dibasic sodium phosphate dried 69.6 mg and bacteriostatic water for injection q.s. In diluent benzyl alcohol 33.7 mg with sterile water for injection q.s. Vial packs of 5.

1 g: Each 8 mL (when mixed) contains: methylprednisolone (as methylprednisolone sodium succinate) 1 g, monobasic sodium phosphate anhydrous 12.8 mg, dibasic sodium phosphate dried 139.2 mg and bacteriostatic water for injection q.s. In diluent benzyl alcohol 66.8 mg with sterile water for injection q.s. Single vials.

Vials: 500 mg: Each 8 mL (when mixed) contains: methylprednisolone (as methylprednisolone sodium succinate) 500 mg, monobasic sodium phosphate anhydrous 6.4 mg, dibasic sodium phosphate dried 69.6 mg and diluent q.s. Vial packs of 5.

1 g: Each 16 mL (when mixed) contains: methylprednisolone (as methylprednisolone sodium succinate) 1 g, monobasic sodium phosphate anhydrous 12.8 mg, dibasic sodium phosphate dried 139.2 mg and diluent q.s. Single vials.

Somavert™ Ⓟ

pegvisomant

GH Receptor Antagonist

Pfizer

Date of Revision: November 9, 2009

SUMMARY PRODUCT INFORMATION:

Route of Administration	Dosage Form/ Strength	Clinically Relevant Nonmedicinal Ingredients
Subcutaneous Injection	Lyophilized powder 10, 15 and 20 mg per vial	None For a complete listing see Dosage Forms, Composition and Packaging.

INDICATIONS AND CLINICAL USE: SOMAVERT (pegvisomant for injection) is indicated for the treatment of acromegaly in patients who have had an inadequate response to surgery, and/or radiation therapy, and other medical therapies, or for whom these therapies are not appropriate. The goal of treatment is to normalize serum IGF-I levels and to improve clinical signs and symptoms.

Geriatrics: There is limited information in patients over 65 years of age (see Warnings and Precautions, Special Populations, Geriatrics).

Pediatrics: The safety and effectiveness of SOMAVERT in pediatric patients have not been established.

CONTRAINDICATIONS: SOMAVERT (pegvisomant for injection) is contraindicated in patients with a history of hypersensitivity to any of its components. The stopper on the vial of SOMAVERT may contain latex.

WARNINGS AND PRECAUTIONS: General: In clinical studies, patients on opioids often needed higher serum pegvisomant concentrations to achieve appropriate IGF-I suppression compared with patients not receiving opioids (see Drug Interactions, Drug-Drug Interactions and Dosage and Administration, Recommended Dose and Dosage Adjustment).

Tumor Growth: Tumors that secrete growth hormone (GH) may expand and cause serious complications. Therefore, all patients with these tumors, including those who are receiving SOMAVERT (pegvisomant for injection), should be carefully monitored with periodic imaging scans of the sella turcica. During clinical studies of SOMAVERT, two patients manifested progressive tumor growth. Both patients had, at baseline, large globular tumors impinging on the optic chiasm, which had been relatively resistant to previous anti-acromegalic therapies. Overall, mean tumor size was unchanged during the course of treatment with SOMAVERT in the clinical studies.

Information to Be Provided to the Patient: Patients and any other persons who may administer SOMAVERT should be carefully instructed by a health care professional on how to properly reconstitute and inject the product (see Information for the Patient). No studies on the effect on the ability to drive and use machines have been performed.

Patients should be informed about the need for serial monitoring of liver enzyme tests, and told to discontinue therapy and contact their physician if they become jaundiced immediately. In addition, patients should be made aware that serial IGF-I levels will need to be obtained to allow their physician to properly adjust the dose of SOMAVERT.

Endocrine and Metabolism: Glucose Metabolism: GH opposes the effects of insulin on carbohydrate metabolism by decreasing insulin sensitivity; thus, glucose tolerance may increase in some patients treated with SOMAVERT. Although no clinically relevant hypoglycemia was observed during clinical trials among acromegalic patients with diabetes treated with SOMAVERT, these patients should be carefully monitored and doses of anti-diabetic drugs reduced as necessary (see Drug Interactions, Drug-Drug Interactions and Dosage and Administration, Recommended Dose and Dosage Adjustment).

GH Deficiency: SOMAVERT is a potent antagonist of GH action. A state of functional GH deficiency may result from administration of SOMAVERT, despite the presence of elevated serum GH levels. During treatment with SOMAVERT, patients should be carefully observed for clinical signs and symptoms of a GH-deficient state. Dose adjustments of SOMAVERT should be made to maintain serum IGF-I concentrations within the age-adjusted normal range.

Hepatic/Biliary/Pancreatic: Liver Tests (LTs): Elevations of serum concentrations of alanine aminotransferase (ALT) and aspartate aminotransferase (AST) greater than 10 times the upper limit of normal (ULN) were reported in two patients (0.8%) treated with SOMAVERT during pre-marketing clinical studies. One patient was rechallenged with SOMAVERT, and the recurrence of elevated transaminase levels suggested a probable causal relationship between administration of the drug and the elevation in liver enzymes. A liver biopsy performed on the second patient was consistent with chronic hepatitis of unknown etiology. In both patients, the transaminase elevations normalized after discontinuation of the drug.

During the pre-marketing clinical studies, the incidence of elevations in ALT greater than 3 times but less than or equal to 10 times the ULN in patients treated with SOMAVERT and placebo were 1.2% and 2.1%, respectively.

Elevations in ALT and AST levels were not associated with increased levels of serum total bilirubin (TBIL) and alkaline phosphatase (ALP), with the exception of two patients with minimal associated increases in ALP levels (i.e., less than 3 times ULN). The transaminase elevations did not appear to be related to the dose of SOMAVERT administered, generally occurred within 4 to 12 weeks of initiation of therapy, and were not associated with any identifiable biochemical, phenotypic, or genetic predictors.

In a global post-marketing combination study with a somatostatin analogue, one out of 25 patients in the pegvisomant group and 1 out of 27 in the octreotide acetate group had transaminases greater than three or more times the upper limit of normal (ULN). Three patients out of 26 (approximately 10%) treated with the combination were found to have serum concentrations of alanine aminotransferase (ALT) and aspartate aminotransferase (AST) ranging from 13 to 45 times the ULN within 3 months of starting this treatment. Two of these patients received supratherapeutic doses of octreotide acetate (30 mg every 2 weeks) combined with a normal dose of SOMAVERT (10 mg daily). All three patients completely recovered after discontinuation of treatment. The safety and efficacy of pegvisomant in combination with other medicinal products, including somatostatin analogues, in the treatment of acromegaly have not been established and, therefore, the combination of somatostatin analogues with pegvisomant is not recommended.

Baseline serum ALT, AST, TBIL, and ALP levels should be obtained prior to initiating therapy with SOMAVERT. Table 1 lists recommendations regarding initiation of treatment with SOMAVERT, based on the results of these liver tests (LTs).

If a patient develops LT elevations, or any other signs or symptoms of liver dysfunction while receiving SOMAVERT, the following patient management is recommended (see Table 2).

Table 1: SOMAVERT

Initiation of Treatment with SOMAVERT Based on Results of Liver Tests

Baseline LT Levels	Recommendations
Normal	May treat with SOMAVERT. Monitor LTs at monthly intervals during the first 6 months of treatment, quarterly for the next 6 months, and then biannually for the next year.
Elevated, but less than or equal to 3 times ULN	May treat with SOMAVERT; however, monitor LTs monthly for at least one year after initiation of therapy and then biannually for the next year.
Greater than 3 times ULN	Do not treat with SOMAVERT until a comprehensive workup establishes the cause of the patient's liver dysfunction. Determine if cholelithiasis or choledocholithiasis is present, particularly in patients with a history of prior therapy with somatostatin analogs. Based on the workup, consider initiation of therapy with SOMAVERT. If the decision is to treat, LTs and clinical symptoms should be monitored very closely.

Immune: Immunogenicity: In pre-marketing clinical studies, approximately 17% of the patients had low titer, non-neutralizing anti-GH antibodies. These antibodies do not appear to have clinical significance. An assay for anti-pegvisomant antibodies in a patient receiving SOMAVERT is not commercially available.

Table 2: SOMAVERT

Continuation of Treatment with SOMAVERT Based on Results of Liver Tests

LT Levels and Clinical Signs/Symptoms	Recommendations
Greater than or equal to 3 but less than 5 times ULN (without signs/symptoms of hepatitis or other liver injury, or increase in serum TBIL)	May continue therapy with SOMAVERT. However, monitor LTs weekly to determine if further increases occur (see below). In addition, perform a comprehensive hepatic workup to discern if an alternative cause of liver dysfunction is present.
At least 5 times ULN, or transaminase elevations at least 3 times ULN associated with any increase in serum TBIL (with or without signs/symptoms of hepatitis or other liver injury)	Discontinue SOMAVERT immediately. Perform a comprehensive hepatic workup, including serial LTs, to determine if and when serum levels return to normal. If LTs normalize (regardless of whether an alternative cause of the liver dysfunction is discovered), consider cautious reinitiation of therapy with SOMAVERT, with frequent LT monitoring.
Signs or symptoms suggestive of hepatitis or other liver injury (e.g., jaundice, bilirubinuria, fatigue, nausea, vomiting, right upper quadrant pain, ascites, unexplained edema, easy bruisability)	Discontinue SOMAVERT immediately. Immediately perform a comprehensive hepatic workup. If liver injury is confirmed, the drug should be discontinued permanently.

Special Populations: Pregnant Women: There are no adequate and well-controlled studies in pregnant women. SOMAVERT should be used during pregnancy only if the potential benefit justifies the potential risk to the patient.

Nursing Women: It is not known whether pegvisomant is excreted in human milk. Because many drugs are excreted in human milk, caution should be exercised when SOMAVERT is administered to a nursing woman.

Pediatrics: The safety and effectiveness of SOMAVERT in pediatric patients have not been established.

Geriatrics: Clinical studies of SOMAVERT did not include sufficient numbers of subjects aged 65 and over to determine whether these subjects respond differently from younger subjects. In general, dose selection for an elderly patient should be cautious, usually starting at the low end of the dosing range, reflecting the greater frequency of decreased hepatic, renal, or cardiac function, and of concomitant disease or other drug therapy.

Monitoring and Laboratory Tests: Liver Tests: Recommendations for monitoring liver function are stated above (see Warnings and Precautions, Hepatic/Biliary/Pancreatic, Liver Tests (LTs)).

IGF-I Levels: Treatment with SOMAVERT should be evaluated by monitoring serum IGF-I concentrations four to six weeks after therapy is initiated or any dose adjustments are made, and at least every six months after IGF-I levels have normalized. The goals of treatment should be to maintain a patient's serum IGF-I concentration within the age-adjusted normal range and to control the signs and symptoms of acromegaly.

GH Levels: Pegvisomant interferes with the measurement of serum GH concentrations by commercially available GH assays (see Drug Interactions, Drug-Laboratory Test Interactions). Furthermore, even when accurately determined, GH levels usually increase during therapy with SOMAVERT. Therefore, treatment with SOMAVERT should not be monitored or adjusted based on serum GH concentrations.

ADVERSE REACTIONS: Adverse Drug Reaction Overview: Safety was evaluated in a randomized, multicenter, placebo-controlled, 12 week study, of patients treated with 10 mg/day (n=26), 15 mg/day (n=26), or 20 mg/day (n=28) of SOMAVERT (pegvisomant for injection) or placebo (n=32).

Table 3 shows the incidence of treatment-emergent adverse events reported in at least two patients treated with SOMAVERT and at frequencies greater than placebo during the 12-week, placebo-controlled study. The majority of reported adverse events were of mild to moderate intensity and limited duration. Adverse events did not appear to be dose dependent.

Clinical Trial Adverse Drug Reactions: Because clinical trials are conducted under very specific conditions the adverse reaction rates observed in the clinical trials may not reflect the rates observed in practice and should not be compared to the rates in the clinical trials of another drug. Adverse drug reaction information from clinical trials is useful for identifying drug-related adverse events and for approximating rates.

Table 3: SOMAVERT

Number of Patients with Acromegaly (Incidence) Reporting Adverse Events in a 12-week Placebo-controlled Study with SOMAVERT[a]

	SOMAVERT			
Event	**10 mg/day n=26**	**15 mg/day n=26**	**20 mg/day n=28**	**Placebo n=32**
Body as a Whole				
Infection[c]	6 (23%)	0	0	2 (6%)
Pain	2 (8%)	1 (4%)	4 (14%)	2 (6%)
Injection Site Reaction[b]	2 (8%)	1 (4%)	3 (11%)	0
Accidental Injury	2 (8%)	1 (4%)	0	1 (3%)
Back Pain	2 (8%)	0	1 (4%)	1 (3%)
Flu Syndrome	1 (4%)	3 (12%)	2 (7%)	0
Chest Pain	1 (4%)	2 (8%)	0	0
Digestive				
Abnormal Liver Function Tests	3 (12%)	1 (4%)	1 (4%)	1 (3%)
Diarrhea	1 (4%)	0	4 (14%)	1 (3%)
Nausea	0	2 (8%)	4 (14%)	1 (3%)
Nervous				
Dizziness	2 (8%)	1 (4%)	1 (4%)	2 (6%)
Paresthesia	0	0	2 (7%)	2 (6%)
Metabolic and Nutritional Disorders				
Peripheral Edema	2 (8%)	0	1 (4%)	0
Cardiovascular				
Hypertension	0	2 (8%)	0	0
Respiratory				
Sinusitis	2 (8%)	0	1 (4%)	1 (3%)

(cont'd)

Table 3: SOMAVERT (cont'd)

[a] Table includes only those events that were reported in at least 2 patients and at a higher incidence in patients treated with SOMAVERT than in patients treated with placebo.

[b] Including injection site hypersensitivity and/or injection site hypertrophy (e.g. lipohypertrophy).

[c] The 6 events coded as "infection" in the group treated with SOMAVERT 10 mg were reported as cold symptoms (3), upper respiratory infection (1), blister (1), and ear infection (1). The 2 events in the placebo group were reported as cold symptoms (1) and chest infection (1).

Nine acromegalic patients (5.6%) withdrew from pre-marketing clinical studies because of adverse events, including two patients with marked transaminase elevations (see Warnings and Precautions, Hepatic/Biliary/Pancreatic, Liver Tests (LTs)), one patient with lipohypertrophy at the injection sites, and one patient with substantial weight gain.

Abnormal Hematologic and Clinical Chemistry Findings: Laboratory Changes: Elevations of serum concentrations of ALT and AST greater than ten times the ULN were reported in two subjects (0.8%) exposed to SOMAVERT in pre-marketing clinical studies (see Warnings and Precautions, Hepatic/Biliary/Pancreatic, Liver Tests (LTs)).

Immunogenicity: In pre-marketing clinical studies, approximately 17% of the patients had low titer, non-neutralizing anti-GH antibodies. These antibodies do not appear to have clinical significance. An assay for anti-pegvisomant antibodies in a patient receiving SOMAVERT is not commercially available.

DRUG INTERACTIONS: Drug-Drug Interactions: Acromegalic patients with diabetes mellitus being treated with insulin and/or oral hypoglycemic agents may require dose reductions of these therapeutic agents after the initiation of therapy with SOMAVERT (pegvisomant for injection) (see Warnings and Precautions, Endocrine and Metabolism, Glucose Metabolism and Dosage and Administration, Recommended Dose and Dosage Adjustment).

Some patients concomitantly receiving opioids required higher serum concentrations of pegvisomant to achieve appropriate IGF-I suppression as compared to patients not receiving opioids, suggesting opioids may confer a resistance to the clinical effects of pegvisomant. The mechanism of action and their clinical relevance is unclear (or unknown) (see Warnings and Precautions, General and Dosage and Administration, Recommended Dose and Dosage Adjustment).

Pegvisomant in Combination with Somatostatin Analogues: Hepatic enzyme elevations (greater than 10 times upper limit of normal [ULN]) have been reported in patients treated with the combination of SOMAVERT and octreotide acetate particularly when higher than recommended doses of octreotide acetate were used. The safety and efficacy of pegvisomant in combination with other medicinal products, including somatostatin analogues, in the treatment of acromegaly have not been established and, therefore, the combination of somatostatin analogues with pegvisomant is not recommended (see Warnings and Precautions, Hepatic/Biliary/Pancreatic).

Drug-Laboratory Test Interactions: Pegvisomant has significant structural similarity to GH, which causes it to cross-react in commercially available GH assays. Because serum concentrations of pegvisomant at therapeutically effective doses are generally 100 to 1000 times higher than endogenous serum GH levels seen in patients with acromegaly, commercially available GH assays will overestimate true GH levels. Treatment with SOMAVERT should therefore not be monitored or adjusted based on serum GH concentrations reported from these assays. Instead, monitoring and dose adjustments should only be based on serum IGF-I levels.

DOSAGE AND ADMINISTRATION: Recommended Dose and Dosage Adjustment: A loading dose of 40 mg of SOMAVERT (pegvisomant for injection) should be administered subcutaneously under physician supervision. The patient should then be instructed to begin daily subcutaneous injections of 10 mg of SOMAVERT. Serum IGF-I concentrations should be measured every four to six weeks and appropriate dose adjustments made accordingly in increments of 5 mg/day (or decrements of 5 mg/day if IGF-I levels have decreased below normal range) in order to maintain the serum IGF-I concentration within the age-adjusted normal range and alleviate the signs and symptoms of acromegaly. It is unknown whether patients who remain symptomatic while achieving normalized IGF-I levels would benefit from increased dosing with SOMAVERT. The maximum dose should not exceed 30 mg/day.

Acromegalic patients with diabetes mellitus being treated with insulin and/or oral hypoglycemic agents may require dose reductions of these therapeutic agents after the initiation of therapy with SOMAVERT (pegvisomant for injection) (see Warnings and Precautions, Endocrine and Metabolism and Drug Interactions, Drug-Drug Interactions).

Some patients concomitantly receiving opioids may require higher serum concentrations of pegvisomant to achieve appropriate IGF-I suppression (see Warnings and Precautions, General and Drug Interactions, Drug-Drug Interactions).

Administration: SOMAVERT is supplied as a lyophilized powder. Each vial of SOMAVERT should be reconstituted with 1 mL of the diluent provided in the package (Sterile Water for Injection, Ph. Eur). Detailed instructions regarding reconstitution and administration are included in the package of SOMAVERT and should be closely followed. To prepare the solution, withdraw 1 mL of Sterile Water for Injection, Ph. Eur. and inject it into the vial of SOMAVERT, aiming the stream of liquid against the glass wall. Hold the vial between the palms of both hands and gently roll it to dissolve the powder. **Do not shake the vial**, as this may cause denaturation of pegvisomant. After reconstitution, each vial of SOMAVERT contains 10, 15, or 20 mg of pegvisomant protein in 1 mL of solution. Parenteral drug products should be inspected visually for particulate matter and discoloration prior to administration. The solution should be clear after reconstitution. If the solution is cloudy, do not inject it. Only one dose should be administered from each vial. SOMAVERT should be administered within three hours after reconstitution. The site of injection should be rotated daily to help prevent lipohypertrophy.

Reconstitution: Parenteral Products:

Vial Size	Volume of Diluent to Be Added to Vial	Approximate Available Volume	Nominal Concentration per mL
6 mL	1 mL of Sterile Water for Injection, Ph. Eur	1 mL	10, 15, or 20 mg of pegvisomant protein in 1 mL of solution

OVERDOSAGE:

There was one reported incident of acute overdosage with SOMAVERT (pegvisomant for injection) during pre-marketing clinical studies in which a patient self-administered 80 mg/day for seven days. The patient experienced a slight increase in fatigue, had no other complaints, and demonstrated no significant clinical laboratory abnormalities.

In cases of overdose, administration of SOMAVERT should be discontinued and not resumed until IGF-I levels return to within or above the normal range.

For management of a suspected drug overdose, contact your **regional Poison Control Centre**. See the *CPS* Directory section for a list of Poison Control Centres.

ACTION AND CLINICAL PHARMACOLOGY: Pharmacodynamics: SOMAVERT (pegvisomant for injection) contains pegvisomant for injection, an analog of human growth hormone (GH) that has been structurally altered to act as a GH receptor antagonist.

Pegvisomant selectively binds to GH receptors on cell surfaces, where it blocks the binding of endogenous GH, and thus interferes with GH signal transduction. Pegvisomant is highly selective for the GH receptor, and does not cross-react with other cytokine receptors, including prolactin. Inhibition of GH action results in decreased serum concentrations of insulin-like growth factor-I (IGF-I), as well as other GH-responsive serum proteins, including IGFBP-3 (IGF binding protein-3), and the acid-labile subunit (ALS).

Pharmacokinetics: Absorption: Following subcutaneous administration, peak serum pegvisomant concentrations are not generally attained until 33 to 77 hours after administration. The mean extent of absorption of a 20-mg subcutaneous dose was 57%, relative to a 10-mg intravenous dose.

Distribution: The mean apparent volume of distribution of pegvisomant is 7 L (12% coefficient of variation), suggesting that pegvisomant does not distribute extensively into tissues. Proportional increases in C_{max} and AUC are not observed when pegvisomant is given in single, escalating doses; however, approximate dose linear pharmacokinetics are observed at steady state following multiple doses. Mean±SD serum pegvisomant concentrations after long term therapy with daily doses of 10, 15, and 20 mg were 9300±6300; 14 300±7500; and 18 100±10 100 ng/mL, respectively.

Studies in rats show that radiolabeled pegvisomant does not cross the blood-brain barrier.

Metabolism and Excretion: The pegvisomant molecule contains covalently bound polyethylene glycol polymers in order to reduce the clearance rate. The mean total body systemic clearance of pegvisomant following multiple doses is estimated to be 28 mL/h (95% CI: 23.8, 32.4 mL/h) for subcutaneous doses ranging from 10 to 20 mg/day. Clearance of pegvisomant was found to increase by 0.6 mL/h for each kilogram of body weight above 94 kg. Pegvisomant had a mean serum half-life of 138±68 hours following a 20 mg subcutaneous dose. Less than 1% of administered drug is recovered in the urine over 96 hours, suggesting that renal excretion is not the primary route of elimination. The elimination route of pegvisomant has not been studied in humans.

Special Populations and Conditions: Pediatrics: Differences in the pharmacokinetics of SOMAVERT in these populations has not been studied.

Geriatrics: Differences in the pharmacokinetics of SOMAVERT in these populations has not been studied.

Gender: No gender effect on the pharmacokinetics of SOMAVERT was found in a population pharmacokinetic analysis.

Race: Differences in the pharmacokinetics of SOMAVERT in these populations has not been studied.

Hepatic Insufficiency: No pharmacokinetic studies have been conducted in patients with hepatic insufficiency.

Renal Insufficiency: No pharmacokinetic studies have been conducted in patients with renal insufficiency.

STORAGE AND STABILITY: Prior to reconstitution, SOMAVERT (pegvisomant for injection) should be stored in a refrigerator at 2 to 8°C. Protect from freezing.

Reconstituted Solutions: SOMAVERT should be administered within three hours of reconstitution. Only one dose should be administered from each vial.

INFORMATION FOR THE PATIENT: Published in e-CPS, available by subscription at www.e-cps.ca.

DOSAGE FORMS, COMPOSITION AND PACKAGING: 10 mg: Each single-dose vial of sterile, white lyophilized powder for subcutaneous injection after reconstitution with 1 mL of Sterile Water for Injection, contains: pegvisomant protein 10 mg. Nonmedicinal ingredients: glycine, mannitol, sodium phosphate dibasic anhydrous and sodium phosphate monobasic monohydrate. Package of 1 single-dose vials and one 8 mL vial of Sterile Water for Injection, Ph. Eur. The stopper in the vial may contain latex.

15 mg: Each single-dose vial of sterile, white lyophilized powder for subcutaneous injection after reconstitution with 1 mL of Sterile Water for Injection, contains: pegvisomant protein 15 mg. Nonmedicinal ingredients: glycine, mannitol, sodium phosphate dibasic anhydrous and sodium phosphate monobasic monohydrate. Package of 1 single-dose vials and one 8 mL vial of Sterile Water for Injection, Ph. Eur. The stopper in the vial may contain latex.

20 mg: Each single-dose vial of sterile, white lyophilized powder for subcutaneous injection after reconstitution with 1 mL of Sterile Water for Injection, contains: pegvisomant protein 20 mg. Nonmedicinal ingredients: glycine, mannitol, sodium phosphate dibasic anhydrous and sodium phosphate monobasic monohydrate. Package of 1 single-dose vials and one 8 mL vial of Sterile Water for Injection, Ph. Eur. The stopper in the vial may contain latex.

Soriatane® ℞

acitretin

Keratinization Disorder Therapy

Actavis

Date of Preparation: May 16, 2008
Date of Revision: August 4, 2010

PHARMACOLOGY: SORIATANE (acitretin) is a retinoid, an aromatic analog of vitamin A. The mechanism of action of SORIATANE is unknown, however, evidence exists for a wide range of actions at various cellular and subcellular levels. These include: regulation of RNA/DNA synthesis, modulation of factors which influence epidermal proliferation, modification of glycoprotein synthesis and modulation of the immune response. Whatever the exact mechanism of action, the most prominent effect of acitretin is a modulation of cellular differentiation in the epidermis, which re establishes a more normal pattern of cell growth.

Use of acitretin in psoriatic patients results in improvement manifested by a decrease in scale, erythema and thickness of lesions, and decreased inflammation in the epidermis and dermis.

Oral absorption of SORIATANE was optimal when given with food. Following administration of a single oral dose of 50 mg SORIATANE to healthy volunteers, maximum plasma acitretin concentrations ranged from 196 to 728 ng/mL (mean 416 ng/mL) and were achieved in two to five hours (mean 2.7 hours). Following multiple doses, acitretin plasma concentrations reached steady-state conditions within two weeks. In psoriatic patients who received SORIATANE (10 to 50 mg/day) for eight weeks, mean steady state trough concentrations of acitretin ranged between 6 and 25 ng/mL in a dose-dependent manner. In patients administered multiple oral doses of SORIATANE for up to nine months, the range of elimination half life ($t_{½}$) values observed was 33-92 hours for acitretin (harmonic mean=48 hours) and 28-123 hours for cis-acitretin (harmonic mean=64 hours).

In a multiple-dose study in healthy young and elderly subjects, increased acitretin plasma concentrations were seen in elderly subjects. The range of terminal elimination half-lives observed for acitretin were 37-96 hours (harmonic mean=54 hours) in elderly and 39-70 hours (harmonic mean=53 hours) in young subjects.

Following oral absorption, acitretin undergoes metabolism and interconversion by simple isomerization to its 13-cis form. Both acitretin and its 13-cis isomer are eliminated from the body primarily by metabolism to chain-shortened breakdown products and conjugates. Acitretin is more than 98% bound to plasma proteins, primarily albumin.

Measurable levels of etretinate (TEGISON), of which acitretin is the active metabolite, have been detected in plasma samples of patients administered SORIATANE. The use of alcohol may have been a factor contributing to the presence of etretinate in these patients. In a two-way crossover study in healthy volunteers, all 10 subjects formed etretinate following the ingestion of a single 100 mg oral dose of acitretin in the presence of alcohol (1.4 g/kg ethanol over approximately 3 hours). Peak concentrations of etretinate measured in these subjects ranged from 22 ng/mL to 105 ng/mL (mean: 55 ng/mL). When acitretin was administered in the absence of ethanol in this study, etretinate was not measurable. However, the formation of etretinate from acitretin in the absence of ethanol cannot be excluded. Etretinate has a long elimination phase. When etretinate has been used as primary therapy, etretinate has been found in the blood of some patients up to 2.9 years after discontinuation of treatment. Of 240 evaluated psoriatic patients who received treatment with SORIATANE (5-60 mg/day) with no restrictions on alcohol use, 7.5% were found to have measurable concentrations of etretinate (range: 5-62 ng/mL) and a further 27% had a trace of etretinate in the plasma which was not measurable.

INDICATIONS: SORIATANE (acitretin) may be indicated for the treatment of: severe psoriasis (includes erythrodermic and pustular types) and other disorders of keratinization.

Severe psoriasis is a condition that involves more than 10% of body surface area or is physically, occupationally or psychologically disabling.

Because of significant adverse effects associated with its use, SORIATANE should be reserved for patients with the diseases listed above when these are unresponsive to or intolerant of standard treatment. SORIATANE should only be prescribed by physicians knowledgeable in the use of systemic retinoids. It is recommended that each SORIATANE prescription is limited to preferably a one-month supply in order to encourage patients to return for their regular appointments.

Most patients experience a relapse after discontinuing therapy. Subsequent courses, when clinically indicated, have produced similar therapeutic results.

CONTRAINDICATIONS: *Pregnancy:* SORIATANE (acitretin) is contraindicated in pregnancy. Retinoids are known to cause severe birth defects in a very high percentage of infants exposed to them in utero (see Warnings, Pregnancy).

Females must not become pregnant while taking SORIATANE and effective contraception must be practised for an undetermined period of time of at least two years following discontinuation of SORIATANE. Thereafter, the patient and physician should assess the risks and desirability of discontinuing effective contraception, based on the most current information available. Measurable levels of etretinate (TEGISON), the prodrug of acitretin, have been detected in plasma samples of patients administered SORIATANE. The use of alcohol appears to be a factor contributing to the interconversion of acitretin back to etretinate. Ethanol must not be ingested during treatment with SORIATANE as clinical evidence has shown that etretinate can be formed with concurrent ingestion of acitretin and alcohol. Ethanol should be avoided for two months after cessation of therapy. The length of time necessary to wait after termination of SORIATANE treatment to ensure that no etretinate will be detectable in the blood has not been determined. Etretinate has a long elimination phase. When etretinate has been used as primary therapy, etretinate has been found in the blood of some patients up to 2.9 years after discontinuation of treatment.

SORIATANE is contraindicated in females of childbearing potential unless **all** of the following conditions apply:

1. The patient has severe psoriasis or other severe disorders of keratinization which are resistant to standard therapies.
2. The patient is reliable in understanding and carrying out instructions.
3. The patient is able to comply with mandatory contraceptive measures.
4. The patient has received, and acknowledged understanding of, a careful oral and printed explanation of the hazards of fetal exposure to SORIATANE and the risk of possible contraception failure. This explanation may include showing a line drawing to the patient of an infant with the characteristic external deformities resulting from retinoid exposure during pregnancy.
5. The patient has had a serum or urine pregnancy test with a sensitivity of at least 50 mIU/mL with a negative result, performed in a licensed laboratory, within two weeks prior to initiating therapy. The patient has had two or three days of the next normal menstrual period before SORIATANE therapy is initiated.
6. The same effective and uninterrupted contraceptive measures must be taken every time therapy is repeated, however long the intervening period may have been and must be continued for 2 years afterwards.

(Regarding items 2 to 5, see Warnings, Pregnancy.)

SORIATANE is also contraindicated in patients with severely impaired hepatic or renal function, intractable hyperlipidemia, hypervitaminosis A or hypersensitivity to vitamin A or its metabolites.

SORIATANE should not be administered in cases of hypersensitivity to any excipients of the drug product (see Supplied).

WARNINGS: *Pregnancy:* Pregnancy, Pregnancy Testing and Contraception: The use of systemic retinoids in humans has been associated with congenital abnormalities. There is an extremely high risk that major human fetal abnormalities will occur if pregnancy occurs during treatment with SORIATANE (acetretin). Potentially any exposed fetus can be affected. Major fetal abnormalities associated with retinoid administration during pregnancy have been reported; including meningomyelocoele, meningoencephalocoele, multiple synostosis, facial dysmorphia, anophthalmia, syndactyly, absences of terminal phalanges, malformations of hip, ankle and forearm, low set ears, high palate, decreased cranial volume and alterations of the skull and cervical vertebrae on X-ray.

Female patients of childbearing potential must not be given SORIATANE until pregnancy is excluded. A serum or urine pregnancy test with a sensitivity of at least 50 mIU/mL must be performed within two weeks prior to starting SORIATANE treatment. SORIATANE treatment should start on the second or third day of the next normal menstrual period following this negative pregnancy test.

Effective contraception must be used for at least one month before starting SORIATANE treatment, during treatment and for an undetermined period of time of at least two years duration after discontinuation of treatment (see Contraindications). Thereafter, the patient and physician should assess the risks and desirability of discontinuing effective contraception, based on the most current information available. It is recommended that two reliable forms of contraception be used simultaneously unless abstinence is the chosen method.

Pregnancy occurring during treatment with SORIATANE and for an undetermined period of time of at least two years duration after its discontinuation carries the risk of fetal malformation (see Warnings above). Females must be fully counselled on the serious risks to the fetus should they become pregnant whilst undergoing SORIATANE treatment or after discontinuation of SORIATANE treatment. If pregnancy does occur during this time the physician and patient should discuss the desirability of continuing the pregnancy.

It is strongly recommended that all female patients of childbearing potential treated with SORIATANE have monthly pregnancy tests during treatment and at regular intervals for an undetermined period of time of at least 2 years duration after the discontinuation of treatment. These pregnancy tests will: a) Serve primarily to reinforce to the patient the necessity of avoiding pregnancy. b) In the event of accidental pregnancy, provide the physician and patient an immediate opportunity to discuss the serious risk to the fetus from this exposure to SORIATANE and the desirability of continuing the pregnancy in view of the potential teratogenic effect of SORIATANE (see Warnings above).

Women of childbearing potential who have switched from TEGISON (etretinate) therapy to SORIATANE must continue to follow the contraceptive recommendations for TEGISON when on SORIATANE therapy.

Lactation: Clinical data indicate that acitretin is excreted in human milk. Therefore, nursing mothers should not receive SORIATANE because of the potential for serious adverse reactions in nursing infants. Women should not breast-feed for an undetermined period of time of at least two years following discontinuation of SORIATANE.

Hyperostosis: In clinical trials with SORIATANE, patients were prospectively evaluated for evidence of development or change in bony abnormalities of the vertebral column following six months of treatment. Of 262 patients treated with SORIATANE, 7% had pre-existing abnormalities of the spine which showed new changes or progression of pre-existing findings. Changes included degenerative spurs, anterior bridging of spinal vertebrae, diffuse idiopathic skeletal hyperostosis, and narrowing and destruction of cervical disc space. These existing abnormalities may be in some part attributable to the underlying psoriasis and/or the patient's age. During the six-month period of observation, no bone changes were seen in patients who had normal pretreatment X-rays. Other retinoids including TEGISON (etretinate), of which SORIATANE is the active metabolite, have been associated with the development of extraosseous calcification and/or hyperostosis. Calcification of the ligaments of the spine, tendon insertions of the arms and legs, and intraosseous membranes of the arms and legs, have been reported. Hyperostotic changes of the vertebrae, forearms, hips, acetabula, legs and calcanei have also been reported. It is not clear whether the extraosseous calcification and/or hyperostosis are progressive. Pre-treatment radiographs of the cervical, thoracic and lumbar spine may be useful when monitoring patients on long-term SORIATANE therapy. Early recognition of musculoskeletal symptoms associated with SORIATANE therapy may be important. There is some evidence that scintigraphic changes appear before radiographic findings. Scintigraphic changes may disappear after discontinuation of SORIATANE treatment, however, radiographic changes may persist. Bone scintigraphy may be important in monitoring patients on SORIATANE therapy since scintigraphic changes seem to precede radiographic changes.

In adults receiving long-term treatment with SORIATANE, appropriate examinations should be periodically performed in view of possible ossification abnormalities. If such disorders arise, the continuation of therapy should be discussed with the patient on the basis of a careful risk/benefit analysis. In one patient, spinal hyperostosis and calcification of spinal ligaments, resulting in compression of the spinal chord, appeared after several years' therapy with TEGISON.

Hepatotoxicity: Hepatic function should be checked before starting treatment with SORIATANE every 1-2 weeks for the first 2 months after commencement and then every 3 months during treatment. If abnormal results are obtained, weekly checks should be instituted. If hepatic function fails to return to normal or deteriorates further, SORIATANE must be withdrawn. In such cases it is advisable to continue monitoring hepatic function for at least 3 months. Elevations of AST, ALT or LDH have occurred in 20-28% of patients treated with SORIATANE. One of the 329 patients treated in clinical trials had clinical jaundice with elevated serum bilirubin and transaminases considered possibly related to SORIATANE treatment. Liver function test results in this patient returned to normal after SORIATANE was discontinued.

If hepatotoxicity is suspected during treatment with SORIATANE, the drug should be discontinued and the etiology further investigated.

Ten of 652 patients treated in clinical trials of etretinate, of which acitretin is the active metabolite, had clinical or histologic hepatitis considered to be possibly or probably related to etretinate treatment. There have been four reports of hepatitis-related deaths worldwide; two of these patients had received etretinate for a month or less before presenting with hepatic symptoms.

PRECAUTIONS: General: Patients should be advised that a transient worsening of their psoriasis may occur during the initial SORIATANE (acitretin) treatment period.

Benign Intracranial Hypertension (Pseudotumor Cerebri): SORIATANE and other retinoids have been associated with cases of pseudotumour cerebri (benign intracranial hypertension). Early symptoms and signs of benign intracranial hypertension include headache, nausea and vomiting and, visual disturbances. Patients with these symptoms should be examined for papilledema and if present, they should discontinue SORIATANE immediately and be referred for neurological diagnosis and care.

As tetracyclines can also cause an increase in intracranial pressure, their combination with SORIATANE should be avoided.

Ophthalmic Effects: Drug related ophthalmic effects (dry eyes, irritation of eyes, brow and lash loss, blepharitis and/or crusting of lids, photophobia, redness, recurrent styes, pannus and subepithelial corneal lesions) were noted during treatment with SORIATANE in 29% of 252 patients who were followed with ophthalmic examinations. Patients should be advised that they may experience decreased tolerance to contact lenses during the initial treatment period.

Occupational Hazards: Overall in clinical studies, decreased night vision was reported by two patients and blurring of vision by three patients. Patients should be advised of these potential problems and warned to be cautious when driving or operating any vehicle at night.

The following additional ophthalmic effects have occurred in patients taking etretinate, of which SORIATANE is the active metabolite: decreased visual acuity, minimal posterior subcapsular cataract, iritis, blot retinal hemorrhage and scotoma.

Any patient receiving SORIATANE therapy, experiencing visual difficulties should discontinue this drug and undergo ophthalmic evaluation.

Lipids: Blood lipid determinations should be performed before SORIATANE is administered and again at intervals of one or two weeks until the lipid response to the drug is established, which is usually within four to eight weeks. Approximately 65% of patients receiving SORIATANE during clinical trials experienced an elevation in serum triglycerides. Approximately 30% developed a decrease in high density lipoproteins (HDL). Approximately 9% experienced elevated serum cholesterol levels. These effects of SORIATANE were reversible upon cessation of therapy.

Patients with an increased tendency to develop hypertriglyceridemia include those with diabetes mellitus, obesity, increased alcohol intake or a familial history of these conditions.

Hypertriglyceridemia and lowered HDL may increase a patient's cardiovascular risk status. In addition, elevation of serum triglycerides to greater than 800 mg/dL has been associated with acute pancreatitis. Therefore, every attempt should be made to control significant elevations of triglycerides or HDL decreases by reduction of weight or restriction of dietary fat and alcohol intake while continuing SORIATANE therapy.

If, despite these measures, hypertriglyceridemia and low HDL levels persist, the discontinuation of SORIATANE should be considered. An associated risk of atherogenesis cannot be ruled out if these conditions persist.

Glucose Tolerance: In diabetics, retinoids can either improve or worsen glucose tolerance. Blood-sugar levels must therefore be checked more frequently than usual in the early stages of treatment (see Drug Interactions).

Vitamin A: SORIATANE is a derivative of vitamin A. To avoid the risk of additive toxic effects, patients should be advised against taking other systemic retinoids or vitamin supplements containing vitamin A.

Methotrexate: Due to an increased hepatitis risk, the combined use of SORIATANE and methotrexate should be avoided.

Children: Safety and efficacy of SORIATANE in children have not been established. Ossification of interosseous ligaments and tendons of the extremities, skeletal hyperostosis and premature epiphyseal closure have been reported with other systemic retinoids, including TEGISON (etretinate) of which SORIATANE is the active metabolite. Due to the uncertain effect of long term SORIATANE therapy on growth and skeletal development, SORIATANE should only be used in pediatric patients with the most severe forms of keratinization disorders for which there are no effective alternative therapies. Pretreatment X-rays for bone age including X-rays of the knees are advised. Bone scans (scintigraphs) and/or X-rays should be considered at yearly intervals when monitoring children on long-term therapy. In addition pain or limitation of movement should be evaluated by appropriate radiological examination.

Blood Donation: It is recommended that blood donation for transfusion purposes be deferred during therapy with SORIATANE and for an undetermined period of time of at least two years duration after discontinuation of treatment. Theoretically, blood from such donors could present a small risk to the fetus if transfused to a pregnant mother during the first trimester of pregnancy (see Contraindications).

Drug Interactions: Concomitant administration of vitamin A and other systemic retinoids must be avoided due to the risk of possible additive toxic effects.

The concomitant administration of methotrexate and etretinate has been associated with hepatitis, a similar increased hepatitis risk may be expected with the combined use of SORIATANE and methotrexate.

Concomitant use of SORIATANE and tetracyclines should be avoided due to the risk of possible additive effects (see Precautions, Benign Intracranial Hypertension (Pseudotumor Cerebri)).

If SORIATANE is given concurrently with phenytoin, it must be remembered that SORIATANE partially reduces phenytoin's protein binding.

Preliminary studies indicated that SORIATANE does not influence the endogenous progesterone plasma concentrations induced by oral contraceptives. Microdosed progesterone preparations (minipills) may be an inadequate method of contraception during SORIATANE therapy.

Concomitant administration of phenprocoumon and SORIATANE does not alter the hypothrombinemic effect of phenprocoumon or the plasma disposition of SORIATANE.

The pharmacokinetics of SORIATANE and digoxin are not altered by concomitant multiple dose regimens of these two drugs.

Concomitant administration of cimetidine did not alter the oral bioavailability of SORIATANE or the isomerization to its 13-cis form. Single oral doses of SORIATANE did not affect the steady state plasma concentration or renal clearance of cimetidine.

Limited data which could not be duplicated, indicated that SORIATANE treatment either increased insulin sensitivity directly or interacted with glyburide to do so. Careful supervision of diabetic patients under treatment with SORIATANE is recommended.

ADVERSE EFFECTS: Hypervitaminosis A produces a wide spectrum of signs and symptoms primarily of the mucocutaneous, musculoskeletal, hepatic and central nervous systems. Nearly all of the clinical adverse events reported to date with SORIATANE (acitretin) administration resemble those of the hypervitaminosis A syndrome. Table 1 and Table 2 list, grouped by frequency, the adverse reactions reported during clinical trials in which patients were treated with SORIATANE for psoriasis.

Table 1: SORIATANE

Adverse Events

Body System	Most Frequent >10%	Less Frequent[a] 1–10%	Rare[a] <1%
Skin and Appendages	Skin peeling/scaling Alopecia Pruritus Sticky skin Nail disorder Dry skin Erythematous rash Erythema Skin atrophy Hyperesthesia	Paronychia Paresthesia Psoriaform rash Rash Photosensitivity reaction Pyogenic granuloma Bullous eruption Skin ulceration Cold/clammy skin Increased sweating Purpura Abnormal hair texture Skin fissures Hypoesthesia Infection Seborrhea	Dermatitis Abnormal skin odour Skin nodule Skin hypertrophy Skin disorder Impaired healing Eczema Otitis externa Flushing Acne
Mucous Membranes	Cheilitis/dry lips Rhinitis Dry mouth	Thirst Stomatitis Gingivitis Increased saliva Gingival bleeding Epistaxis Rhagades (corner of mouth)	Ulcerative stomatitis Pharyngitis Anal disorder Nose bleeds Altered saliva
Eye Disorders	Xerophthalmia	Conjunctivitis/irritation Abnormal/blurred vision Blepharitis[b] Eye pain Photophobia	Abnormal lacrimation Decreased night vision Cataract Eye abnormality Pannus[b] Recurrent styes[b] Subepithelial corneal lesions[b]
Musculoskeletal	Arthralgia	Myalgia Bone pain Spinal hyperostosis[c] Back pain Hypertonia Arthritis	Arthrosis Leg cramps Olecranon bursitis
CNS	Rigors	Headache Pain	Abnormal gait Pseudotumor cerebri

(cont'd)

Table 1: SORIATANE *(cont'd)*

Adverse Events

Body System	Most Frequent >10%	Less Frequent[a] 1–10%	Rare[a] <1%
Gastrointestinal		Nausea Abdominal pain	Constipation Diarrhea Tenesmus Dyspepsia Glossitis Melena Tongue ulceration Pancreatitis
Special Senses/Other		Tinnitus Taste perversion Earache Ceruminosis	Deafness Taste loss
Psychiatric		Insomnia Nervousness	Depression Somnolence Dysphonia
Respiratory			Coughing Laryngitis Sinusitis Increased sputum
Urinary			Dysuria Abnormal urine Balanoposthitis
Reproductive			Leukorrhea
Cardiovascular			Increased bleeding time Chest pain Angioedema Vasculitis[d]
Body as a Whole		Fatigue Anorexia Increased appetite Impotence Edema	Malaise Fever Moniliasis[e] Muscle weakness Alcohol intolerance Hot flashes Hepatitis[f] Icterus[f]

[a] Some may bear no relationship to therapy.
[b] Based on review of eye examination forms by consulting ophthalmologist (n=252).
[c] Incidence of 7% based on review of films by consulting radiologist (n=262).
[d] Vasculitis has not been documented with acitretin but has been seen with other retinoids.
[e] Increased incidence of vulvovaginitis due to *C. albicans* has been noted during treatment with SORIATANE.
[f] Events observed and reported rarely.

Table 2: SORIATANE

Laboratory Abnormalities

Body System	Laboratory Abnormality (%)		Comments
Hepatic	**Increased**		—In most patients, elevations were slight to moderate and returned to normal either during continuation of therapy or after cessation of treatment. —**If hepatotoxicity is suspected, therapy should be discontinued (see Contraindications and Warnings).**
	ALT	(28%)	
	AST	(23%)	
	LDH	(21%)	
	Alkaline Phosphatase	(16%)	
	GGTP	(14%)	
	Direct Bilirubin	(11%)	
	Increased		—These changes are more common in patients who are predisposed to hypertriglyceridemia (see Precautions).
	Triglycerides	(65%)	
	Cholesterol	(9%)	
	Decreased		—The effects on triglycerides, cholesterol and HDL were reversible upon cessation of SORIATANE therapy.
	HDL	(30%)	
	Increased		
	Total Bilirubin	(2%)	
	Globulin	(2%)	
	Decreased		
	Serum Albumin	(1%)	
Renal	**Increased**		
	Uric Acid	(17%)	

(cont'd)

Table 2: **SORIATANE** *(cont'd)*

Laboratory Abnormalities

Body System	Laboratory Abnormality (%)			Comments
	Creatinine		(5%)	
	BUN		(2%)	
Hematologic	**Increased**			
	Reticulocytes		(38%)	
	WBC		(11%)	
	Eosinophils		(8%)	
	Monocytes		(7%)	
	Bands		(4%)	
	Basophils		(3%)	
	Decreased			
	WBC		(7%)	
	Increased		**Decreased**	
	(16%)	Neutrophils	(5%)	
	(2%)	Lymphocytes	(11%)	
	(4%)	Hemoglobin	(9%)	
	(2%)	Platelets	(6%)	
	(3%)	Hematocrit	(5%)	
	(2%)	RBC	(3%)	
Urinary	RBC in urine		(10%)	
	WBC in urine		(7%)	
	Glycosuria		(4%)	
	Acetonuria		(3%)	
	Proteinuria		(2%)	
Electrolytes	**Increased**		**Decreased**	
	(16%)	Phosphorus	(3%)	
	(12%)	Potassium	(3%)	
	(12%)	Magnesium	(12%)	
	(2%)	Sodium	(1%)	
	(4%)	Calcium	(2%)	
	(2%)	Chloride	(3%)	

Other reported laboratory abnormalities include: increased creatinine phosphokinase (37%), increased (21%) or decreased (7%) fasting blood sugar and increased (7%) or decreased (3%) iron.

OVERDOSE:

Symptoms: To date, there has been no experience with acute overdose of SORIATANE (acitretin). In the event of acute overdosage, evacuation of the stomach should be considered during the first few hours after this overdose. Signs and symptoms of overdosage with SORIATANE would probably be similar to acute vitamin A toxicity, i.e., severe headache, nausea or vomiting, drowsiness, irritability, and pruritus. Elevated intracranial pressure has been reported with both acute and chronic vitamin A overdoses as well as in patients treated with therapeutic doses of SORIATANE. Patients with a SORIATANE overdose should be monitored closely for signs of increased intracranial pressure. If overdosage occurs in patients already receiving therapeutic doses of SORIATANE, the drug must be discontinued immediately.

All female patients of childbearing potential who have taken an overdose of SORIATANE must:

1. Have a pregnancy test at the time of the overdose.
2. Use an effective form of contraception for an undetermined period of time of at least two years duration after the overdose.

If the pregnancy test is positive, the patient should be fully counselled on the serious risk to the fetus from this exposure to SORIATANE and the physician and patient should discuss the desirability of continuing the pregnancy (see Contraindications and Warnings).

Treatment: See Symptoms.

For management of a suspected drug overdose, CPhA recommends that you contact your **regional Poison Control Centre**. See the *CPS* Directory section for a list of Poison Control Centres.

DOSAGE: There is intersubject variation in the pharmacokinetics, clinical efficacy, and incidence of side effects with SORIATANE (acitretin). Individualization of dosage is required to achieve maximum therapeutic response while minimizing side effects.

Initial Therapy: SORIATANE therapy should be initiated at 25 mg per day, given as a single dose with the main meal. If by four weeks the response is unsatisfactory, and in the absence of toxicity, the daily dose may be gradually increased to a maximum of 75 mg per day. The dose may be reduced if necessary to minimize side effects.

Maintenance Therapy: Psoriasis: Maintenance doses of 25 to 50 mg per day may be given after initial response to treatment. The maintenance dose should be based on clinical efficacy and tolerability. It may be necessary in some cases to increase the dose to a maximum of 75 mg per day.

In general, therapy should be terminated when lesions have resolved sufficiently. Relapses may be treated as outlined for initial therapy.

Other Keratinization Disorders: Maintenance doses of 10 mg to a maximum of 50 mg per day may be given for disorders of keratinization.

INFORMATION FOR THE PATIENT: Published in e-CPS, available by subscription at www.e-cps.ca.

SUPPLIED: 10 mg: Each brown and white, hard gelatin capsule (No. 4) with "ACTAVIS" in black lettering contains: acitretin 10 mg. Nonmedicinal ingredients: gelatin, glucose, liquid, spray-dried, microcrystalline cellulose and sodium ascorbate; gelatin capsule shell: iron oxide (yellow, black and red) and titanium dioxide. Push-through blister packages of 30. Store at 15-25°C. Protect from heat and light. The product is sensitive to moisture. Therefore store in original package. Keep out of reach of children. The medicine should not be used after the expiry date (EXP) shown on the package.

25 mg: Each brown and yellow, hard gelatin capsule (No. 1) with "ACTAVIS" in black lettering contains: acitretin 25 mg. Nonmedicinal ingredients: gelatin, glucose, liquid, spray-dried, microcrystalline cellulose and sodium ascorbate; gelatin capsule shell: iron oxide (yellow, black and red) and titanium dioxide. Push-through blister packages of 30. Store at 15-25°C. Protect from heat and light. The product is sensitive to moisture. Therefore store in original package. Keep out of reach of children. The medicine should not be used after the expiry date (EXP) shown on the package.

(Shown in Product Identification Section)

The reader is invited to consult CPhA's monograph **Corticosteroids: Topical**.

Spectro® EczemaCare Medicated Cream

clobetasone 17-butyrate

Topical Corticosteroid

GlaxoSmithKline Consumer Healthcare

PHARMACOLOGY: Spectro EczemaCare Medicated Cream (0.05% clobetasone butyrate) is a moderately potent fluorinated topical corticosteroid. The corticosteroids are a class of compounds comprising steroid hormones secreted by the adrenal cortex and their synthetic analogs which are effective when applied locally to control many types of inflammatory, allergic and pruritic dermatoses. Clobetasone butyrate has been shown to have topical and systemic pharmacologic and metabolic effects characteristic of the corticosteroid class of drugs. Topical corticosteroids such as clobetasone 17-butyrate are effective in the treatment of corticosteroid-responsive dermatoses primarily because of their anti-inflammatory, anti-pruritic, and vasoconstrictive actions. However, while the physiologic, pharmacologic and clinical effects of the corticosteroids are well known, the exact mechanisms of their actions in each disease are uncertain.

Corticosteroids suppress inflammation by acting on multiple factors that are critical in generating the inflammatory responses. Corticosteroids are thought to induce a protein (lipocortin) that inhibits phopholipase A2, which results in decreased release of arachidonic acid and its derivatives (prostaglandins and leukotrienes). Due to decreased production of a number of lipolytic and proteolytic enzymes, migration of leukocytes to the area of injury is inhibited. Similarly, corticosteroids inhibit adhesion of leukocytes to the vascular walls in the inflamed area by suppressing the activity of endothelial adhesion molecule-1 (ELAM-1) and intracellular adhesion molecule-1 (ICAM-1). Corticosteroids also act upon the host immune responses by suppressing the production and release of cytokines such as interleukins, interferon-gamma, and tumor necrosis factor-alpha. Although the biological effects by corticosteroids are not fully elucidated, the net effect of these multiple actions is the marked reduction of the inflammatory responses.

INDICATIONS: Spectro EczemaCare Medicated Cream (clobetasone butyrate) is indicated in the treatment and control of small patches of eczema and dermatitis including atopic eczema and irritant and allergic contact dermatitis. To be applied to itchy, red, dry and inflamed skin to clear the flare-up and to break the itch-scratch cycle of eczema and dermatitis.

CONTRAINDICATIONS: If no anti-infective agent is used simultaneously, clobetasone butyrate is not indicated for the treatment of primarily infected skin lesions caused by infection with fungi (e.g. Candidiasis, Tinea) or bacteria (e.g. Impetigo), primary cutaneous viral infections (i.e., herpes simplex, vaccinia and varicella), syphilitic skin infections or tuberculous skin lesions. Clobetasone butyrate is contraindicated in patients with a hypersensitivity to any of the components of the preparation. Clobetasone butyrate is also contraindicated in patients with acne vulgaris and rosacea.

WARNINGS: If topical corticosteroids are used, over extensive areas, in large quantities, or on the face, scalp, axillae and scrotum, sufficient absorption may occur, giving rise to adrenal suppression and other systemic effects. Similarly absorption can be increased by the use of occlusion, which can lead to adrenal suppression especially in infants and children. The management of eczema and dermatitis in infants and young children requires the supervision of a physician. Treatment without the management of a physician is therefore limited to adults and children aged 12 years and over.

Use in children under 12 years only on the advice of a physician.

Use for no more than 7 days continuous treatment.

Patients are warned in product labelling against letting the cream get into the eye.

Patients are warned in product labelling not to use other topical corticosteroids, either prescribed or obtained over-the-counter (such as hydrocortisone), at the same time as Spectro EczemaCare Medicated Cream as this may increase the risk of unwanted effects.

PRECAUTIONS: General: Spectro EczemaCare Medicated Cream should be used with caution in patients with stasis dermatitis and other skin diseases associated with impaired circulation.

If a symptomatic response is not noted within a few days to a week, the local application of Spectro EczemaCare Medicated Cream should be discontinued and the patient re-evaluated. The safety and effectiveness of Spectro EczemaCare Medicated Cream when used under occlusive dressings has not been determined.

Although hypersensitivity reactions are rare with topically applied corticosteroids, the drug should be discontinued and appropriate therapy initiated if there are signs of hypersensitivity. If irritation develops, Spectro EczemaCare Medicated Cream should be discontinued and appropriate therapy instituted. Allergic contact dermatitis from corticosteroids, although uncommon, can be diagnosed by observing 'failure to heal' rather than clinical exacerbation as with most topical products not containing corticosteroids. Such an observation should be corroborated with appropriate diagnostic patch testing.

Patients are advised in product labelling to use Spectro EczemaCare Medicated Cream only for the treatment of eczema or dermatitis and not to use it on the groins, genitals, on axilla or between the toes or on the face or scalp unless such use is conducted under medical supervision.

Patients are advised in product labelling that they should not use clobetasone butyrate for the treatment of psoriasis as there are no adequate studies that support the efficacy of clobetasone butyrate in the treatment of psoriasis.

Effect on Infection: In case of bacterial infections of the skin, appropriate anti-bacterial agents should be used as primary therapy. If it is considered necessary, the topical corticosteroid may be used as an adjunct to control inflammation, erythema and itching. If a symptomatic response is not noted within a few days to a week, the local application of corticosteroid should be discontinued until the infection is brought under control.

During the use of topical corticosteroids, secondary infections may occur. Appropriate antimicrobial therapy should be used whenever treating inflammatory lesions which have become infected. Any spread of infection requires withdrawal of topical corticosteroid therapy, and systemic administration of antimicrobial agents. Bacterial infection is encouraged by the warm, moist conditions induced by occlusive dressings, and so the skin should be cleansed before a fresh dressing is applied.

Systemic Effects: Significant systemic absorption may result when corticosteroids are applied over large areas of the body, used for prolonged periods or under occlusive dressings. To minimise this possibility, treatment should be interrupted periodically or one area of the body should be treated at a time when long-term therapy is anticipated. In infants, the diaper may act as an occlusive dressing and increase absorption. Further, children may be more susceptible to systemic toxicity due to larger skin surface to body mass ratios.

Patients are advised in product labelling to inform subsequent physicians of the prior use of corticosteroids.

Drug Interactions: There have been no reported interactions with other medicinal products or other forms of interaction.

Long Term Effects: Prolonged or extensive use of topical corticosteroid products may produce atrophy of the skin and subcutaneous tissue, particularly on flexor surfaces and on the face. If this is noted, the use of Spectro EczemaCare Medicated Cream should be discontinued.

Spectro EczemaCare Medicated Cream should be applied to the face only if in the estimation of a physician it is necessary and the benefits of application to the face outweigh the risks.

Pregnancy: Topical administration of corticosteroids to pregnant animals can cause abnormalities of fetal development. The relevance of this finding to human beings has not been established. However, the administration of clobetasone butyrate topical preparations during pregnancy and lactation should only be considered if the expected benefit to the mother is greater than any possible risk to the fetus.

Women, who are pregnant or breast feeding, are advised in product labelling not to use Spectro EczemaCare Medicated Cream without medical advice.

Drugs of this class should not be used extensively in pregnant patients in large amounts or for prolonged periods of time.
Lactation: See Pregnancy.
Children: Spectro EczemaCare Medicated Cream is suitable for use in adults and children aged 12 years or older. Use in children under 12 years only on the advice of a physician.

Because of the higher ratio of skin surface area to body mass, children are at greater risk than adults for HPA axis suppression when treated with topical corticosteroids. They are also at greater risk of glucocorticosteroid insufficiency after withdrawal of treatment and of Cushing's syndrome while on treatment. Adverse effects including striae have been reported with use of topical corticosteroids in infants and children. HPA axis suppression and Cushing's syndrome have been reported in children receiving topical corticosteroids. Manifestations of adrenal suppression in children include: linear growth retardation, delayed weight gain, low plasma cortisol levels and absence of response to ACT stimulation.

In clinical practice, a substantial proportion of the use of Spectro EczemaCare Medicated Cream has been in children. There have been no published reports of significant untoward effects.

ADVERSE EFFECTS: Side effects associated with short-term (up to 14 days) use include:
Hypersensitivity: Local hypersensitivity reactions such as erythema, rash, pruritus, urticaria, local skin burning and allergic contact dermatitis may occur at the site of application and may resemble symptoms of the condition under treatment. In the unlikely event of signs of hypersensitivity appearing, application should stop immediately.

Exacerbation of symptoms may occur.

Local burning, irritation, itching, skin atrophy, dryness of the skin, atrophy of subcutaneous tissues, telangiectasia, striae, change in pigmentation, secondary infection and hypertrichosis have been observed following topical corticosteroid therapy.

Local atrophic changes could possibly occur in situations where moisture increases absorption of clobetasone butyrate, but only after prolonged use.

When large areas of the body are being treated with Spectro EczemaCare Medicated Cream (clobetasone butyrate) it is possible that some patients will absorb sufficient steroid to cause transient adrenal suppression despite the low degree of systemic activity associated with clobetasone butyrate.

OVERDOSE:

Symptoms: Acute overdosage is very unlikely to occur. Chronic overdosage requires continuous use of large quantities for long periods of time. In the case of chronic overdosage or misuse, the features of hypercortisolism may appear. As with any corticosteroid, treatment should be discontinued gradually if the symptoms of hypercortisolism appear. However, because of the risk of acute adrenal suppression in such cases, drug withdrawal should be carried out under medical supervision.
Treatment: See Symptoms.

> For management of a suspected drug overdose, CPhA recommends that you contact your **regional Poison Control Centre**. See the *CPS* Directory section for a list of Poison Control Centres.

DOSAGE: Spectro EczemaCare Medicated Cream is suitable for use in adults and children aged 12 years or older. Use in children under 12 years only on the advice of a physician.

Spectro EczemaCare Medicated Cream should be applied sparingly to the affected area twice a day for up to 7 days using fingertip units.

A single streak of cream from the top crease in the finger to the fingertip is one "fingertip unit". This is enough to treat a patch area equal to the front and back of one hand. For smaller areas, squeeze out half a fingertip unit—enough to cover a patch of skin the same size as the palm of one hand.

If the condition resolves within 7 days, treatment with Spectro EczemaCare Medicated Cream should be stopped. If the condition does not improve in the first 7 days or becomes worse the patient is advised in product labelling to see a physician. If, after the recommended maximum duration of treatment, improvement is seen but further treatment is required, the patient is advised in product labelling to see a physician.

Under conditions of nonprescription use, the total dose of Spectro EczemaCare Medicated Cream applied should not exceed 15 g/week in adults.

SUPPLIED: Each tube of cream contains: clobetasone butyrate 0.05%. Nonmedicinal ingredients: arlacel, beeswax substitute, cetostearyl alcohol, chlorocresol, citric acid monohydrate, dimethicone, glycerin, glyceryl monostearate, purified water and sodium citrate dihydrate. Tubes of 30 g. Store between 15-25°C.

Spectro Jel®

dermatological preparation
Non-irritating Everyday Cleanser For Sensitive/Problem Prone Skin

GlaxoSmithKline Consumer Healthcare

DESCRIPTION: A gentle, soap-free, non-foaming, deep pore cleanser made with purified water. Spectro Jel is a non-irritating cleanser, formulated to the natural pH of skin, specifically for sensitive, problem prone skin. Spectro Jel washes away surface skin bacteria and dead skin cells. Gently removes dirt, oil and make-up. It is suitable for everyday use on face, hands and entire body. Spectro Jel is formulated for minimal disruption of your natural moisture barrier. It will not dry out sensitive problem prone skin even with repeated washings. Contains 3 moisturizers to moisturize and condition sensitive, problem prone skin. Ingredients include moisturizing emollients and humectants to help hydrate the skin. Unlike some other cleansers, it does not contain known skin irritants such as alcohol, parabens, propylene glycol, lanolin, or sodium lauryl sulfate.

INDICATIONS: Indicated for use on all skin types whenever a gentle daily skin cleanser is required. It is especially useful for sensitive problem prone skin or when frequent skin washing is required. In the management of problem prone skin, it can be used as an adjunctive gentle cleanser or as a gentle cleansing agent after diaper changes in pediatrics or geriatrics.

CONTRAINDICATIONS: Hypersensitivity to any of the ingredients.

WARNINGS: No data supplied by the manufacturer.

PRECAUTIONS: No data supplied by the manufacturer.

ADVERSE EFFECTS: No data supplied by the manufacturer.

OVERDOSE:
No data supplied by the manufacturer.

> For management of a suspected drug overdose, CPhA recommends that you contact your **regional Poison Control Centre**. See the *CPS* Directory section for a list of Poison Control Centres.

DOSAGE: Use as frequently as needed. Massage gently into wet or dry skin with clean hands for at least 30 seconds. Rinse off with cold or lukewarm water, or it may be wiped off without rinsing. Dry the skin with a clean soft towel.

SUPPLIED: Squeeze bottles of 200 mL and pump bottles of 500 mL in either fragrance or fragrance free formulations.

Spiriva® Pr

tiotropium bromide monohydrate
Bronchodilator

Boehringer Ingelheim

Date of Preparation: November 6, 2002
Date of Revision: June 29, 2010

SUMMARY PRODUCT INFORMATION:

Route of Administration	Dosage Form/Strength	Nonmedicinal Ingredients
Oral Inhalation	Capsule /18 μg	Lactose monohydrate (which contains milk protein)

INDICATIONS AND CLINICAL USE: SPIRIVA (tiotropium bromide monohydrate) is indicated for:
- long term, once daily, maintenance treatment of bronchospasm associated with chronic obstructive pulmonary disease (COPD), including chronic bronchitis and emphysema.

Relief of dyspnea was evaluated using the Transition Dyspnea Index (TDI). A TDI score of ≥1 unit was considered clinically significant, and patients with this score were considered responders. In the one-year and six-month trials, there was a statistically significant higher percentage of responders treated with SPIRIVA than placebo.

Geriatrics (>65 years of age): As expected for all predominantly renally excreted drugs, advanced age (≥65 years) was associated with a decrease of tiotropium renal clearance which may be explained by decreased renal function. Tiotropium excretion in urine after inhalation decreased from 14% in young healthy volunteers to about 7% in the older COPD patients. However, plasma concentrations did not change significantly with advancing age within COPD patients (≥69 years vs ≤58 years) if compared to inter- and intra-individual variability (43% increase in AUC_{0-4} after dry powder inhalation). Consequently, geriatric patients can use tiotropium at the recommended dose.

Pediatrics: Safety and effectiveness of SPIRIVA in patients less than 18 years of age were not studied.

CONTRAINDICATIONS: SPIRIVA (tiotropium bromide monohydrate) is contraindicated in:
- patients with a history of hypersensitivity to atropine or its derivatives (e.g. ipratropium or oxitropium), or to any component of this product (see Dosage Forms, Composition and Packaging).

WARNINGS AND PRECAUTIONS: General: SPIRIVA (tiotropium bromide monohydrate) should not be used more frequently than once daily.

SPIRIVA, as a once daily maintenance bronchodilator, should not be used for the initial treatment of acute episodes of bronchospasm, i.e. rescue therapy.

Immediate hypersensitivity reactions such as skin rash, urticaria, angioedema of the lip, tongue and face, bronchospasm, and oropharyngeal edema may occur after administration of SPIRIVA.

As with other anticholinergic drugs, SPIRIVA should be used with caution in patients with narrow-angle glaucoma, prostatic hyperplasia or bladder-neck obstruction.

No studies on the effects on the ability to drive and use machines have been performed. The occurrence of dizziness or blurred vision may influence the ability to drive and use machinery.

This product contains 5.5 mg of lactose monohydrate per capsule.

Carcinogenesis and Mutagenesis: Animal data only.

Ophthalmologic: Patients should be cautioned to avoid getting the drug powder into their eyes. They should be advised that this may result in precipitation or worsening of narrow-angle glaucoma, eye pain or discomfort, temporary blurring of vision, visual halos or colored images in association with red eyes from conjunctival congestion and corneal oedema. Should any combination of these symptoms develop, they should consult a doctor immediately. Miotic drops alone are not considered to be effective treatment.

Renal: As plasma concentration increases with decreased renal function in patients with moderately to severe renal impairment (creatinine clearance ≤50 mL/min), SPIRIVA should be used only if the expected benefit outweighs the potential risk. There is no long term experience in patients with severe renal impairment (see Pharmacokinetics).

Respiratory: Inhaled medicines may cause inhalation-induced bronchospasm. If this occurs, treatment with SPIRIVA should be discontinued immediately.

Special Populations: Pregnant Women: There are no studies of SPIRIVA in pregnant women. Because animal reproduction studies are not always predictive of human response, SPIRIVA should be used during pregnancy only if the benefits outweigh any possible risk to the unborn child.

Oral reproduction studies with tiotropium were performed at doses up to 500 mg/kg in rats and 100 mg/kg in rabbits. These doses correspond, in each species, to about 215 000 and 86 000 times the Maximum Recommended Human Dose (MRHD) respectively, on a mg/m² basis. Inhalation reproduction studies with tiotropium were conducted in rats and rabbits at doses of 2 and 0.5 mg/kg/day (about 860 and 430 times the MRHD on a mg/m² basis). These studies demonstrated no evidence of teratogenic effects as a result of tiotropium administration.

Labour and Delivery: The safety and effectiveness of SPIRIVA have not been studied during labor and delivery.

Nursing Women: Based on lactating rodent studies, a small amount of tiotropium (1.9%) is excreted in milk over two days. Clinical data from nursing women exposed to SPIRIVA are not available. SPIRIVA should not be used in nursing women unless the expected benefit outweighs any possible risk to the infant.

Pediatrics (<18 years of age): Safety and effectiveness of SPIRIVA in patients less than 18 years of age were not studied.

ADVERSE REACTIONS: Adverse Drug Reaction Overview: Adverse reactions to SPIRIVA are similar in nature to reactions to other anticholinergic bronchodilators. Many of the listed undesirable effects can be assigned to the anticholinergic properties of SPIRIVA.

In controlled clinical studies, the commonly observed undesirable effects were anticholinergic undesirable effects such as dry mouth which occurred in approximately 4% of patients. In 26 clinical trials, dry mouth led to discontinuation in 18 of 9,149 tiotropium treated patients (0.2 %).

Other undesirable effects consistent with anticholinergic effects include palpitations, supraventricular tachycardia, atrial fibrillation, blurred vision, glaucoma, constipation and intestinal obstruction including ileus paralytic as well as urinary retention.

An increase in anticholinergic effects may occur with increasing age.

Clinical Trial Adverse Drug Reactions: Because clinical trials are conducted under very specific conditions the adverse reaction rates observed in the clinical trials may not reflect the rates observed in practice and should not be compared to the rates in the clinical trials of another drug. Adverse drug reaction information from clinical trials is useful for identifying drug-related adverse events and for approximating rates.

Of the 1456 patients in the four one-year controlled clinical trials and the 1207 patients in the two six-month controlled clinical trials, 906 and 402 patients, respectively, were treated with SPIRIVA at the recommended dose of 18 μg once a day.

One-Year Studies: Four multi-center, one-year, controlled studies have evaluated once daily doses of SPIRIVA in patients with COPD. Table 1 shows adverse events that occurred with a frequency of ≥3% in the SPIRIVA group in the placebo-controlled trials, and where the rates in the SPIRIVA group exceeded placebo by ≥1%. The frequency of corresponding events in the ipratropium-controlled trials are included for comparison.

Table 1: SPIRIVA

Adverse Event Incidence (% Patients) in One-Year COPD Clinical Trials

	Placebo Controlled Studies		Ipratropium Controlled Studies	
Body System Event	**SPIRIVA [n=550]**	**Placebo [n=371]**	**SPIRIVA [n=356]**	**Ipratropium [n=179]**
Body as a Whole				
Accidents	13	11	5	8
Chest Pain (non-specific)	7	5	5	2
Edema, Dependent	5	4	3	5
Gastrointestinal System Disorders				
Abdominal Pain	5	3	6	6
Constipation	4	2	1	1
Dry Mouth[a]	16	3	12	6

(cont'd)

Table 1: SPIRIVA *(cont'd)*

Adverse Event Incidence (% Patients) in One-Year COPD Clinical Trials

Body System Event	Placebo Controlled Studies SPIRIVA [n=550]	Placebo Controlled Studies Placebo [n=371]	Ipratropium Controlled Studies SPIRIVA [n=356]	Ipratropium Controlled Studies Ipratropium [n=179]
Dyspepsia	6	5	1	1
Vomiting	4	2	1	2
Musculoskeletal System				
Myalgia	4	3	4	3
Resistance Mechanism Disorders				
Infection	4	3	1	3
Moniliasis	4	2	3	2
Respiratory System (upper)				
Epistaxis	4	2	1	1
Pharyngitis	9	7	7	3
Rhinitis	6	5	3	2
Sinusitis	11	9	3	2
Upper Respiratory Tract Infection	41	37	43	35
Skin and Appendage Disorders				
Rash	4	2	2	2
Urinary System				
Urinary Tract Infection	7	5	4	2

[a] Dry mouth was usually mild and led to discontinuation of therapy in 0.3% of SPIRIVA treated patients.

Arthritis, coughing and influenza-like symptoms occurred at a rate of ≥3% in the SPIRIVA treatment group, but were <1% in excess of the placebo groups.

Other events that occurred in the SPIRIVA group at a frequency of 1-3% in the placebo-controlled trials and where the rates exceeded that in the placebo group include:

Body as a Whole: allergic reaction, leg pain.
Central and Peripheral Nervous System: dysphonia, paraesthesia.
Gastrointestinal System Disorders: gastrointestinal disorder not otherwise specified (NOS), gastroesophageal reflux, stomatitis (including ulcerative stomatitis).
Metabolic and Nutritional Disorders: hypercholesterolemia, hyperglycemia.
Musculoskeletal System Disorders: skeletal pain.
Myo-Endo Pericardial and Valve Disorders: angina pectoris (including aggravated angina pectoris).
Psychiatric Disorder: depression.
Resistance Mechanism Disorders: herpes zoster.
Respiratory System Disorder (upper): laryngitis.
Vision Disorder: cataract.

Adverse reactions with incidences >0.1% and <1% in excess of placebo include:

Cardiovascular System: tachycardia.
Urinary System: difficulty urinating and urinary retention (in men with predisposing factors).
Hypersensitivity Reactions: angio-oedema (1 of 906 patients in the four one-year trials).

As with other orally inhaled drugs, pharyngo-oral irritation and paradoxical bronchospasm were observed.

Six Month Studies: Two multi-center, six-month, salmeterol and placebo-controlled studies have evaluated once daily doses of SPIRIVA in patients with COPD. Table 2 shows adverse events where the frequency was ≥3% in the SPIRIVA 18 µg once daily group and where the rates in the SPIRIVA group exceeded placebo by at least 1%.

Table 2: SPIRIVA

Adverse Event Incidence (% Patients[a]) in Six-Month COPD Clinical Trials

Body System Event	Combined Data (Trials 205.130 & 205.137) SPIRIVA [n=402]	Salmeterol [n=405]	Placebo [n=400]
Body as a Whole			
Accidents	4.2	5.2	2.5
Back Pain	4.0	4.0	3.0
Headache	6.5	6.9	4.5
Influenza Like Symptoms	6.7	5.2	4.0
Gastrointestinal System Disorders			
Dry Mouth	8.2	1.7	2.3
Respiratory System (upper)			
Pharyngitis	4.5	3.5	3.0
Upper Respiratory Tract Infection	19.4	17.0	16.0
Respiratory System (lower)			
Coughing	5.2	5.9	3.5

[a] Percentages are calculated using total number of patients treated as the denominator.

Long-Term (4-year) Study: The long term effects of treatment with SPIRIVA was assessesd in a four-year, multinational, placebo-controlled trial (205.235) involving 5993 patients with COPD, during which all patients were permitted to use all respiratory medications as prescribed by their health care providers other than inhaled anticholinergics. In total, there were 9468 person-years of exposure to tiotropium and 8746 person-years of exposure to placebo, which includes the 30 day follow-up period.

Adverse events were experienced by 93% of the tiotropium group and 92% of the placebo group. The proportion of patients who experienced serious adverse events was 52% in the tiotropium group and 50% in the placebo group. Fatal events during the treatment period occurred in 381 patients (12.8%) in the tiotropium group and 411 (13.7%) in the placebo group.

Given the duration of the trial and differences in discontinuation rates, comparisons between study drugs are most appropriately assessed by examination of exposure adjusted rates (i.e. incidence rates). Incidence rates of selected events are computed as the number of patients experiencing an event divided by the person years at risk. Time at risk is time of exposure + 30 days for subjects who did not experience a specific event, and time from start of treatment to onset of a specific event for subjects who experienced this event. Rates are presented per 100 person-years of time at risk to tiotropium or placebo.

The most common adverse events were COPD exacerbations (65% of patients), pneumonia (14% of patients), and dyspnea (14% of patients). The incidence rate per 100 person years for COPD exacerbation was 45.5 and 38.1 for placebo and tiotropium, respectively. The rate per 100 person years for pneumonia was 5.14 in placebo and 4.94 in tiotropium group (Table 3).

Table 3: SPIRIVA

Frequency [N (%)] of Patients with Adverse Events Occurring with Incidence of Preferred Term >3% – Using Collapsed Tiotropium Preferred Terms[a] - treated Set

	Tiotropium N=2986 N (%)	Tiotropium N=2986 IR[b]	Placebo N=3006 N (%)	Placebo N=3006 IR[b]
Total with Adverse Events	2764 (92.6)		2774 (92.3)	
COPD Exacerbations	1934 (64.8)	38.1	1986 (66.1)	45.5
Pneumonia	433 (14.5)	4.94	418 (13.9)	5.14
Dyspnoea	364 (12.2)	4.09	443 (14.7)	5.49
Nasopharyngitis	373 (12.5)	4.33	324 (10.8)	4.06
Upper Respiratory Tract Infection	298 (10.0)	3.38	290 (9.6)	3.57
Hypertension	275 (9.2)	3.08	284 (9.4)	3.45
Bronchitis	232 (7.8)	2.57	233 (7.8)	2.82
Cough	238 (8.0)	2.64	213 (7.1)	2.57
Back Pain	198 (6.6)	2.18	188 (6.3)	2.25
Urinary Tract Infections	190 (6.4)	2.08	169 (5.6)	2.00
Sinusitis	194 (6.5)	2.14	160 (5.3)	1.90
Influenza	158 (5.3)	1.73	158 (5.3)	1.87
Headache	171 (5.7)	1.88	136 (4.5)	1.61
Oedema	145 (4.9)	1.57	130 (4.3)	1.52
Constipation	151 (5.1)	1.63	111 (3.7)	1.29
Diarrhoea	138 (4.6)	1.50	122 (4.1)	1.43
Cataract	120 (4.0)	1.30	123 (4.1)	1.45
Atrial Fibrillation	119 (4.0)	1.28	113 (3.8)	1.32
Mouth Dry	152 (5.1)	1.68	80 (2.7)	0.93
Depression	131 (4.4)	1.42	98 (3.3)	1.14
Insomnia	131 (4.4)	1.42	91 (3.0)	1.06
Arthralgia	125 (4.2)	1.36	94 (3.1)	1.10
Benign Prostatic Hyperplasia	122 (4.1)	1.32	96 (3.2)	1.12
Rhinitis	101 (3.4)	1.09	112 (3.7)	1.32
Abdominal Pain	113 (3.8)	1.22	96 (3.2)	1.12
Respiratory Failure	88 (2.9)	0.94	120 (4.0)	1.39
Hypercholesterolaemia	104 (3.5)	1.12	97 (3.2)	1.13
Nausea	93 (3.1)	1.00	94 (3.1)	1.09
Dizziness	103 (3.4)	1.11	81 (2.7)	0.94

[a] Tiotropium preferred terms include multiple MedDRA preferred terms.
[b] Incidence rate per 100 person years.

Other than lung cancer, serious adverse events reported by >1% of patients in either treatment group were either cardiac or respiratory in nature and are displayed in Table 4.

The most common reason for discontinuation from treatment was due to an exacerbation of a patient's underlying respiratory disease.

Table 4: SPIRIVA

Frequency [n (%)] and Incidence Rate (per 100 person years) of Patients Experiencing Serious Adverse Events[a] Reported by >1% of Patients in Any Treatment Group According to System Organ Class (SOC) During the Treatment Period (from first to last day of study drug + 30 days)

	Tiotropium N=2986		Placebo N=3006	
	N (%)	IR[b]	N (%)	IR[b]
Cardiac SOC	322 (10.8)	3.56	350 (11.6)	4.22
Angina	48 (1.6)	0.51	31 (1.0)	0.36
Atrial Fibrillation	69 (2.3)	0.74	67 (2.2)	0.77
Cardiac Failure	57 (1.9)	0.61	42 (1.4)	0.48
Cardiac Failure Congestive	27 (0.9)	0.29	42 (1.4)	0.48
Coronary Artery Disease	20 (0.7)	0.21	32 (1.1)	0.37
Myocardial Infarction	65 (2.2)	0.69	84 (2.8)	0.97
Respiratory (lower) SOC	911 (30.5)	11.32	985 (32.8)	13.47
Bronchitis	35 (1.2)	0.37	27 (0.9)	0.31
COPD Exacerbation	688 (23.0)	8.19	742 (24.7)	9.70
Dyspnea	36 (1.2)	0.38	54 (1.8)	0.62
Pneumonia	296 (9.9)	3.28	290 (9.6)	3.46
Respiratory Failure	85 (2.8)	0.90	113 (3.8)	1.31

[a] Excluding lung cancer (multiple different terms).

Consolidated Safety Database: Pooled Analysis of Tiotropium/HandiHaler (Tio/HH) vs Placebo Studies: Clinical Trial Evidence: All Trial Participants: Data included in this section are based on pooled data from 26 randomized placebo-controlled parallel group clinical trials in phase III and IV with treatment periods ranging between four weeks and four years. The cutoff date for these analyses was June 2008. Adverse drug reactions were identified from data obtained in clinical trials and spontaneous reporting during post approval use of the drug. The clinical trial database includes 9149 tiotropium patients, contributing 11 958 person years of exposure to tiotropium. Under each treatment, 'N with event' is the number of patients with the selected adverse drug reaction or adverse event.

The frequencies assigned to the undesirable effects listed below are based on crude incidence rates of adverse drug reactions (i.e. events attributed to tiotropium) observed in the tiotropium group (9149 patients) from 26 pooled placebo-controlled clinical trials with treatment periods ranging from four weeks to four years.

Frequency is defined using the following convention:

Very common (≥1/10); common (≥1/100 to <1/10); uncommon (≥1/1000 to <1/100); rare (≥1/10 000 to <1/1000); very rare (<1/10 000), not known (cannot be estimated from the available data).

Table 5: SPIRIVA

Adverse Drug Reactions

MedDRA Preferred Term	Frequency
Metabolism and Nutrition Disorders	
Dehydration	Not known[a]
Nervous System Disorders	
Dizziness	Uncommon
Insomnia	Rare
Eye Disorders	
Vision Blurred	Uncommon
Glaucoma	Rare
Intraocular Pressure Increased	Rare
Cardiac Disorders	
Atrial Fibrillation	Uncommon
Supraventricular Tachycardia	Rare
Tachycardia	Rare
Palpitations	Rare
Respiratory, Thoracic and Mediastinal Disorders	
Pharyngitis	Uncommon
Dysphonia	Uncommon
Cough	Uncommon
Bronchospasm	Rare
Epistaxis	Rare
Laryngitis	Rare
Sinusitis	Rare

(cont'd)

Table 5: SPIRIVA *(cont'd)*

Adverse Drug Reactions

MedDRA Preferred Term	Frequency
Gastrointestinal Disorders	
Dry Mouth, Usually Mild	Common
Stomatitis	Uncommon
Gastroesophageal Reflux Disease	Uncommon
Constipation	Uncommon
Intestinal Obstruction, Including Ileus Paralytic	Rare
Gingivitis	Rare
Glossitis	Rare
Oropharyngeal Candidiasis	Rare
Dysphagia	Rare
Skin and Subcutaneous Tissue Disorders, Immune System Disorders	
Rash	Uncommon
Urticaria	Rare
Pruritus	Rare
Hypersensitivity (including immediate reactions)	Rare
Angioneurotic Oedema	Not known[a]
Skin Infection, Skin Ulcer	Not known[a]
Dry Skin	Not known[a]
Musculoskeletal and Connective Tissue Disorders	
Joint Swelling	Not known[a]
Renal and Urinary Disorders	
Dysuria	Uncommon
Urinary Retention (usually in men with predisposing factors)	Uncommon
Urinary Tract Infection	Rare

[a] No events attributed to tiotropium in 9149 tiotropium treated patients; however, events are considered adverse drug reactions associated with tiotropium.

Post-Market Adverse Drug Reactions: The following adverse reactions have been identified primarily by reporting in the world-wide post-marketing experience of SPIRIVA HandiHaler: dysphonia, epistaxis, palpitations, dizziness, rash, urticaria, pruritus, atrial fibrillation, tachycardia.

Post-marketing adverse experiences also include rare reports of syncope/loss of consciousness, chest pain, myocardial infarction, anginal pectoris, arrhythmia, and cardiac failure. Because these reactions are reported voluntarily from a population of uncertain size, it is not always possible to reliably estimate their frequency or establish a causal relationship to drug exposure.

DRUG INTERACTIONS: Overview: Although no formal drug interaction studies have been performed, SPIRIVA has been used concomitantly with other drugs without additional adverse drug reactions. These include sympathomimetic bronchodilators, methylxanthines, and oral and inhaled steroids commonly used in the treatment of COPD.

The co-administration of SPIRIVA with other anticholinergic containing drugs has not been studied and is, therefore, not recommended.

Tiotropium does not inhibit cytochrome P450 1A1, 1A2, 2B6, 2C9, 2C19, 2D6, 2E1, 3A4 even in supratherapeutic concentrations of 1 µMol/L (=0.4 µg/mL), which makes clinically relevant metabolic interactions by tiotropium extremely unlikely.

Drug-Drug Interactions: Interactions with drugs administered concomitantly with tiotropium are not expected due to the low dose and low steady state plasma concentration of tiotropium (18 µg, C_{ss} 2-20 pg/mL) and the lack of cytochrome P450 inhibition by tiotropium. Similarly, effects of concomitantly administered drugs on tiotropium metabolism are not expected due to the minor contribution of enzymatic metabolism of tiotropium.

DOSAGE AND ADMINISTRATION: Dosing Considerations:

- Counselling by doctors on smoking cessation should be the first step in treating patients with COPD, who smoke, independent of the clinical presentation i.e. chronic bronchitis (with or without airflow limitation) or emphysema. Cessation of smoking produces dramatic symptomatic benefits and has been shown to confer a survival advantage.
- Elderly patients, hepatically impaired patients, and renally impaired patients can use SPIRIVA at the recommended dose. However, as with all renally excreted drugs, SPIRIVA use should be monitored closely in patients with moderate to severe renal impairment.
- There is no experience with SPIRIVA in infants and children and therefore should not be used in the age group.

Recommended Dose and Dosage Adjustment: The recommended dosage of SPIRIVA (tiotropium bromide monohydrate) is inhalation of the contents of one capsule (18 µg) once daily. **The capsule must not be swallowed.**

Missed Dose: Patients should be advised that if they forget to take a dose, they should take one as soon as they remember but do not take two doses at the same time or on the same day. Then take the next dose as usual.

Patients should be advised that if they take more SPIRIVA 18 microgram than they should—talk to their doctor immediately.

Administration: SPIRIVA should be administered once daily, at the same time of day, by inhalation only through the HandiHaler inhalation device. To ensure proper administration of SPIRIVA, the doctor or other qualified health care professional should teach the patient how to operate the HandiHaler inhalation device (see Information for the Patient).

OVERDOSAGE:

Acute intoxication by inadvertent oral ingestion of SPIRIVA (tiotropium bromide monohydrate) capsules is unlikely since the drug has a low oral bioavailability. Should signs of serious anticholinergic toxicity appear, vital signs should be carefully monitored and appropriate therapy should be initiated.

There were no systemic anticholinergic adverse effects following a single inhaled dose of up to 282 µg tiotropium in healthy volunteers. Additionally, no relevant adverse effects, beyond bilateral conjunctivitis and dry mouth were observed following 7 day dosing with up to 141 µg tiotropium/day in healthy volunteers, (which resolved while still under treatment). In a multiple dose study in COPD patients with a maximum daily dose of 36 µg tiotropium over four weeks, dry mouth was the only observed adverse event attributable to tiotropium.

For management of a suspected drug overdose, contact your regional Poison Control Centre. See the *CPS* Directory section for a list of Poison Control Centres.

ACTION AND CLINICAL PHARMACOLOGY: Mechanism of Action: SPIRIVA (tiotropium bromide monohydrate) is a long acting, muscarinic receptor antagonist that is used as a once-daily inhaled bronchodilator for the treatment of bronchospasm associated with Chronic Obstructive Pulmonary Disease (COPD). SPIRIVA is a quaternary ammonium molecule with a duration of action sufficient to provide 24 hours of bronchoprotection with once-a-day inhalational administration. In vitro studies using recombinant human receptors as well as animal and human tissue preparations, showed that tiotropium is a potent, reversible, M_3-selective muscarinic receptor antagonist, with no other receptor interactions detected at clinically relevant concentrations.

Muscarinic acetylcholine receptors are widely distributed throughout the body and serve a variety of important functions. Stimulation of muscarinic receptors in response to the activation of the parasympathetic nervous system is the dominant neural bronchoconstrictor pathway in all mammals, including humans. In fact, the reversal of chronic obstructive disease with antimuscarinic agents is a well established therapeutic approach.

There are five subtypes (M_1-M_5) of muscarinic receptors which exhibit distinct pharmacology and tissue distribution. M_3 receptors predominate in visceral smooth muscles and typically mediate the direct contractile effects of acetylcholine. In addition, M_3, as well as M_1 receptors, are also found in the central nervous system and autonomic ganglia. M_2 receptors predominate in the heart and mediate the bradycardic effects of acetylcholine. They are also found on parasympathetic nerve terminals where their activation inhibits the release of acetylcholine. The physiological roles of M_4 and M_5 receptors are still uncertain.

The long duration of action of tiotropium is thought to be due to its high affinity to, and slow dissociation kinetics from, the muscarinic M_3-receptor subtype. Tiotropium has a higher affinity for human muscarinic 3 (hM_3)-receptors (KD value:8.89 pmol/L) than for hM_2-receptors (KD value:31.96 pmol/L). In addition, and most importantly, tiotropium dissociates very slowly from hM_3-receptors. Dissociation half-lives of the receptor-ligand complex are 27.1 hours for hM_3-receptors and 3.6 hours for hM_2-receptors. For comparison, dissociation half-lives of ipratropium are 0.22 and 0.04 hours for hM_3- and hM_2-receptors, respectively. As an N-quaternary anticholinergic, tiotropium is broncho-selective when administered by inhalation, demonstrating an acceptable therapeutic range before giving rise to systemic anticholinergic effects.

Pharmacodynamics: The clinical pharmacology studies confirmed the intended pharmacodynamic effect of bronchodilation in subjects with COPD. The bronchodilation following inhalation of tiotropium is primarily a site-specific effect, rather than a systemic effect. Trough forced expiratory volume in one second (FEV_1), 24 hours after a previous dose, (i.e. prior to subsequent dosing) remained significantly increased over baseline relative to placebo; the majority of the maintenance bronchodilation was achieved within a few days of treatment. Pharmacodynamic steady state was attained within the first week of once-daily dosing. Repeated inhalation of SPIRIVA has not been linked with tolerance towards bronchodilatory effects of the drug. Bronchodilatory effects gradually returned to baseline levels upon cessation of treatment with no evidence of rebound. Multiple dose studies supported the once daily dosing regimen for tiotropium administered by inhalation of a dry powder formulation. Studies with supratherapeutic doses have confirmed that reduced salivation is among the most sensitive effects. This clinical physiologic effect is mirrored by reports of dry mouth.

The clinical development program included four one-year and two six-month randomized, double-blind studies in 2663 patients, 1308 receiving SPIRIVA. The one-year program consisted of two placebo-controlled and two ipratropium-controlled trials. The six-month trials were salmeterol and placebo-controlled. All studies included measurements of lung function as well as health outcome measures of dyspnea, exacerbations and health-related quality of life.

SPIRIVA administered once daily provided significant improvement in lung function (forced expiratory volume in one second, FEV_1; and forced vital capacity, FVC) within 30 minutes following the first dose and was maintained for 24 hours whether SPIRIVA was administered in the morning or in the evening. Pharmacodynamic steady state was reached within one week with the majority of bronchodilation observed by the third day. The bronchodilator effects of SPIRIVA were maintained throughout the one-year period of administration with no evidence of tolerance.

Pharmacokinetics: Absorption: The pharmacokinetic profile of SPIRIVA (tiotropium bromide monohydrate) supports that plasma concentrations are very low following inhalation of an 18 µg dose; although the terminal elimination half life is between 5-7 days, there is only moderate accumulation upon repeated once daily dosing.

Absorption and Bioavailability: For tiotropium, absolute bioavailability was most reliably estimated from the total urinary excretion values in healthy volunteers rather than plasma concentrations. The absolute oral bioavailability of tiotropium is 2-3% for a 64 µg dose. The low extent of absorption and low oral bioavailability is expected based on animal experiments with radiolabeled drug. The absolute bioavailability of tiotropium after an inhaled dose of 108 µg (three 36 µg inhalation capsules) is 19.5%. Low oral bioavailability is a definite advantage in limiting systemic absorption following obligate ingestion of a portion of an orally-inhaled drug.

Pharmacokinetics After Inhalation: After chronic, once-daily inhalation of tiotropium (18 µg) by COPD patients, pharmacokinetic steady state was reached after 2-3 weeks with no accumulation thereafter. Maximum steady state tiotropium plasma concentrations (17-19 pg/mL) were observed 5 minutes after inhalation and decreased to approximately 3-4 pg/mL at trough. At steady state, urinary excretion of unchanged tiotropium during the first 4 hours following administration accounted for 1.42% (88.7% gCV) and 1.97% (74.4% gCV) in older and younger patients, respectively.

Onset of Pharmacodynamic Steady State: Study results supported that pharmacodynamic steady state was attained within the first week of dosing; additionally, the multiple dose studies supported the once daily dosing regimen for tiotropium administered by inhalation of a dry powder formulation.

Distribution: The absolute bioavailability of SPIRIVA after dry powder inhalation is 19.5% and is negligible after oral administration (2-3%). The apparent volume of distribution is 32 L/kg suggesting extensive tissue binding.

Tiotropium is moderately bound to human plasma proteins (72%). This binding is not of the restrictive type considering the high renal clearance of 669 mL/min.

Metabolism: The drug is not metabolized to a great extent; the majority of the drug is excreted as the parent compound.

Tiotropium is predominantly eliminated via renal secretion of unchanged drug. Seventy-four percent of an intravenous dose was recovered in urine ($Ae_{0-\infty}$) after intravenous infusion in healthy young male subjects. The indication of active renal secretion is based on a renal clearance of 669 mL/min after intravenous infusion and 486 mL/min after inhalation, while calculated creatinine clearance was 118 mL/min and 113 mL/min, respectively.

The tiotropium ester was shown to be non-enzymatically cleaved and enzymatically metabolized in animals. In humans, a small part (up to 20%) might also be metabolized in the liver. Tiotropium does not inhibit cytochrome P450 1A1, 1A2, 2B6, 2C9, 2C19, 2D6, 2E1, 3A4 even in supratherapeutic concentrations of 1 µMol/L (=0.4 µg/mL), which makes clinically relevant metabolic interactions by tiotropium extremely unlikely.

Excretion: Urinary data in healthy subjects demonstrate that tiotropium was excreted with a geometric mean elimination half-life of 5.7 days (3.2-7.3 days) after intravenous, and 4.8 days (3.6-6.2 days) after inhalation. The long elimination half-life indicates a slow redistribution process, and it is likely that the slow dissociation from muscarinic receptors contributes to the slow redistribution. Indication of active renal secretion is based on a renal clearance of 669 mL/min after intravenous infusion and 486 mL/min after inhalation, while calculated creatinine clearance was 118 mL/min and 113 mL/min, respectively. Urinary recovery was approximately 74% as unchanged substance. Total clearance was 880 mL/min.

Special Populations and Conditions: Pediatrics: Pharmacokinetics in children were not investigated as tiotropium development is currently restricted to therapy for COPD in adults.

Geriatrics: As expected for all predominantly renally excreted drugs, advanced age (≥65 years) was associated with a decrease of tiotropium renal clearance which may be explained by decreased renal function. Tiotropium excretion in urine after inhalation decreased from 14% in young healthy volunteers to about 7% in the older COPD patients. However, plasma concentrations did not change significantly with advancing age within COPD patients (≥69 years vs ≤58 years) if compared to inter- and intra-individual variability (43% increase in AUC_{0-4} after dry powder inhalation). Consequently, geriatric patients can use tiotropium at the recommended dose.

The high renal clearance of tiotropium suggests the possibility of a decreased renal elimination in the elderly (≥69 years) as a result of decreased renal function with age. To investigate this, pharmacokinetic parameters were determined for different age groups.

Although highly variable, the results suggested that tiotropium plasma concentrations were moderately increased in the elderly COPD patients for both C_{5min} and C_{2hr}. There is an age dependent decrease in the fraction of tiotropium excreted in the urine. Total urinary excretion decreases from about 14% in young healthy volunteers to about 7% in the older COPD patients, corresponding to decreased renal clearance with age from 326 mL/min to 163 mL/min, respectively. This decrease in tiotropium renal clearance with advanced age exceeded the change in creatinine clearance; creatinine clearance was approximately 113 mL/min in young healthy volunteers and 61 mL/min in elderly COPD patients. This suggested that the renal secretion of tiotropium was more sensitive to age than glomerular filtration.

Gender: To assess potential sex-related effects on tiotropium pharmacokinetics, plasma and urine samples were collected from a subset of COPD patients at selected centres for assessment of tiotropium concentrations. Although there was a slight trend to higher plasma concentrations in females, it is considered that male and female COPD patients showed no significant differences in drug plasma concentrations or urinary excretion of tiotropium.

Hepatic Insufficiency: Impaired liver function is not expected to have any clinically relevant influence on tiotropium pharmacokinetics. Tiotropium is predominantly cleared by renal elimination (74% in young healthy volunteers) and by simple non-enzymatic ester cleavage to products that do not bind to muscarinic receptors.

Renal Insufficiency: In common with all other drugs that undergo predominantly renal excretion, renal impairment was associated with reduced renal drug clearance and increased plasma drug concentrations. Mild renal impairment (CL_{CR} 50-80 mL/min) which is often seen in elderly patients did not lead to a clinically significant change in tiotropium pharmacokinetics. However, in COPD patients with moderate to severe renal impairment (CL_{CR} <50 mL/min), the intravenous administration of tiotropium resulted in doubling of the plasma concentrations seen in patients with normal renal function (82% increase in AUC_{0-4h}), which was confirmed by plasma concentrations after dry powder inhalation.

In a study conducted to investigate the pharmacokinetics of tiotropium in patients with varying degrees of renal impairment in comparison to healthy volunteers, a single dose of tiotropium (4.8 µg) was administered as an intravenous infusion over 15 minutes. The results indicate that renal tiotropium clearance decreased with creatinine clearance. Tiotropium plasma concentrations (AUC_{0-4h}) were 39, 81 and 94% higher in mild, moderate and severe renal impairment when compared to control subjects. SPIRIVA should be used in patients with moderate to severe renal impairment only if the expected benefit outweighs the potential risk.

STORAGE AND STABILITY: After opening a strip, the in-use shelf life of the remaining capsules in the strip is 5 days. If more than one capsule is exposed to air inadvertently, the exposed unused capsules must be discarded.

SPECIAL HANDLING INSTRUCTIONS: Temperature: Store capsules and HandiHaler device between 15-25°C. Do not freeze. Moisture: Protect from moisture.

INFORMATION FOR THE PATIENT: Published in e-CPS, available by subscription at www.e-cps.ca.

DOSAGE FORMS, COMPOSITION AND PACKAGING: Each light green, hard gelatin capsule, with T1 01 printed on one side of the capsule and the Boehringer Ingelheim company logo on the other side, contains a dry powder blend of 18 µg tiotropium (equivalent to 22.5 µg tiotropium bromide monohydrate) with lactose monohydrate (which contains milk protein) as a carrier. The dry powder within the capsule is intended for oral inhalation only. SPIRIVA capsules are partially filled but contain exact amount of medication as declared on the label. Ten SPIRIVA capsules are packaged in an aluminum /PVC/aluminum blister card. One blister card consists of two 5-cavity strips joined along a perforated line. Cartons of 30 SPIRIVA capsules (3 blister cards) and one HandiHaler device; cartons of 10 SPIRIVA capsules (1 blister card) and one HandiHaler device. Refill packs: cartons of 30 SPIRIVA capsules (3 blister cards).

Inhalation Device: The HandiHaler inhalation device is a reusable plastic device used for the administration of SPIRIVA capsules. It is gray coloured with "HandiHaler", "Boehringer Ingelheim", and the Boehringer Ingelheim company logo, printed on the front face.

The HandiHaler operates with flow rates as low as 20 L/min. All patients, regardless of their disease severity, achieved sufficient flows through the HandiHaler. To use the delivery system, a SPIRIVA capsule is placed in the center chamber of the HandiHaler inhalation device and the capsule is pierced by pressing and releasing the green piercing button on the side of the device. The tiotropium formulation is dispersed into the air stream when the patient inhales slowly and deeply through the mouthpiece. The HandiHaler inhalation devices are available individually.

(Shown in Product Identification Section)

Sporanox® Capsules Ⓟ

itraconazole

Antifungal

Janssen-Ortho

Date of Preparation: June 19, 2002

Date of Revision: May 13, 2010

SUMMARY PRODUCT INFORMATION:

Route of Administration	Dosage Form/Strength	Clinically Relevant Nonmedicinal Ingredients
Oral	Capsule 100 mg	None For a complete listing see Dosage Forms, Composition and Packaging.

INDICATIONS AND CLINICAL USE: SPORANOX (itraconazole) capsules are indicated for the treatment of the following systemic fungal infections in normal, predisposed or immunocompromised patients:

1. Invasive and non-invasive pulmonary aspergillosis.
2. Oral and/or esophageal candidiasis.
3. Chronic pulmonary histoplasmosis.
4. Cutaneous and lymphatic sporotrichosis.
5. Paracoccidioidomycosis.
6. Chromomycosis.
7. Blastomycosis.

The type of organism responsible for the infection should be isolated and identified and other relevant laboratory studies (wet mount, histopathology, serology) should be undertaken as appropriate to confirm diagnosis. Therapy may be initiated prior to obtaining these results when clinically warranted; however, once these results become available, antifungal therapy should be adjusted accordingly.

SPORANOX capsules are also indicated for the treatment of the following topical fungal infections in normal, predisposed or immunocompromised patients:

8. Dermatomycoses due to tinea corporis, tinea cruris, tinea pedis, and pityriasis versicolor, where oral therapy is considered appropriate.
9. Onychomycosis.

Prior to initiating treatment with SPORANOX capsules, appropriate nail or skin specimens should be obtained for laboratory testing (KOH preparation, fungal culture, or nail biopsy) in order to confirm the diagnosis of onychomycosis or dermatomycoses.

Since elimination of itraconazole from skin and nail tissues is slower than from plasma, optimal clinical and mycological responses are thus reached 2 to 4 weeks after the cessation of treatment for skin infections and 6 to 9 months after the cessation of treatment for nail infections.

Geriatrics (>65 years of age): See Warnings and Precautions, Special Populations, Geriatrics (>65 years of age).

Pediatrics (<18 years of age): No data available. See Warnings and Precautions, Special Populations, Pediatrics (<18 years of age).

CONTRAINDICATIONS:

- **Congestive Heart Failure:** SPORANOX capsules should not be administered to patients with evidence of ventricular dysfunction such as congestive heart failure (CHF) or a history of CHF except for the treatment of life-threatening or other serious infections (see Warnings and Precautions, Serious Warnings and Precautions and Cardiovascular, Use in Patients with Underlying Cardiac Disease; Adverse Reactions, Post-Market Adverse Drug Reactions and Drug Interactions, Drug-Drug Interactions, Calcium Channel Blockers).
- **Drug Interactions:** Coadministration of the following drugs is contraindicated with SPORANOX capsules (see Warnings and Precautions, Serious Warnings and Precautions and Drug Interactions, Serious Drug Interactions):
  - CYP3A4 metabolized substrates that can prolong the QT-interval e.g., cisapride, dofetilide, levacetylmethadol (levomethadyl), pimozide, and quinidine are contraindicated with SPORANOX capsules. Coadministration may result in increased plasma concentrations of these substrates, which can lead to QT prolongation and serious cardiac arrhythmias
  - CYP3A4 metabolized HMG-CoA reductase inhibitors such as lovastatin and simvastatin
  - Triazolam and oral midazolam
  - Ergot alkaloids such as dihydroergotamine, ergometrine (ergonovine), ergotamine and methylergometrine (methylergonovine)
  - Eletriptan
  - Nisoldipine

- SPORANOX capsules are contraindicated in patients with a known hypersensitivity to itraconazole or its excipients. For a complete listing, see Dosage Forms, Composition and Packaging. There is no information regarding cross-hypersensitivity between itraconazole and other azole antifungal agents. Caution should be used in prescribing SPORANOX capsules to patients with hypersensitivity to other azoles.
- SPORANOX capsules should not be administered for the treatment of onychomycosis or dermatomycoses (tinea corporis, tinea cruris, tinea pedis, pityriasis versicolor) to pregnant patients or to women contemplating pregnancy.

WARNINGS AND PRECAUTIONS:

Serious Warnings and Precautions

- **Congestive Heart Failure: SPORANOX capsules should not be administered to patients with evidence of ventricular dysfunction such as congestive heart failure (CHF) or a history of CHF except for the treatment of life-threatening or other serious infections.** If signs or symptoms of congestive heart failure occur during administration of SPORANOX capsules, discontinue administration. When itraconazole was administered intravenously to dogs and healthy human volunteers, negative inotropic effects were seen (see Contraindications; Warnings and Precautions, Cardiovascular, Use in Patients with Underlying Cardiac Disease; Adverse Reactions, Post-Market Adverse Drug Reactions and Drug Interactions, Drug-Drug Interactions, Calcium Channel Blockers).
- **Drug Interactions: Coadministration of cisapride, pimozide, quinidine, dofetilide or levacetylmethadol (levomethadyl) with SPORANOX (itraconazole) capsules or oral solution is contraindicated.** SPORANOX, a potent cytochrome P450 3A4 isoenzyme system (CYP3A4) inhibitor, may increase plasma concentrations of drugs metabolized by this pathway. Serious cardiovascular events, including QT prolongation, torsades de pointes, ventricular tachycardia, cardiac arrest, and/or sudden death have occurred in patients using cisapride, pimozide, levacetylmethadol (levomethadyl), or quinidine concomitantly with SPORANOX and/or other CYP3A4 inhibitors (see Contraindications and Drug Interactions, Serious Drug Interactions; Overview and Drug-Drug Interactions).
- **Liver Toxicity:** SPORANOX capsules have been associated with rare cases of serious hepatotoxicity, including liver failure and death. Some of these cases had neither pre-existing liver disease nor a serious underlying medical condition and some of these cases developed within the first week of treatment. It is advisable to monitor liver function. If clinical signs or symptoms develop that are consistent with liver disease, such as anorexia, nausea, vomiting, jaundice, fatigue, abdominal pain, dark urine, or pale stools, treatment should be discontinued and liver function testing performed. Continued use of SPORANOX capsules or reinstitution of treatment with SPORANOX capsules is strongly discouraged unless there is a serious or life-threatening situation where the expected benefit exceeds the risk (see Warnings and Precautions, General, Hepatic/Biliary/Pancreatic, Hepatic Effects/Use in Patients with Hepatic Impairment and Adverse Reactions).

General: SPORANOX capsules and SPORANOX oral solution should not be used interchangeably. This is because drug exposure is greater with the oral solution than with the capsules when the same dose of drug is given. In addition, the topical effects of mucosal exposure may be different between the two formulations. SPORANOX oral solution is indicated only for the treatment of oral and/or esophageal candidiasis. Due to the pharmacokinetic properties, SPORANOX capsules are not recommended for initiation of treatment in patients with immediately life-threatening systemic fungal infections.

Cardiovascular: Cardiac Dysrhythmias: Life-threatening cardiac dysrhythmias and/or sudden death have occurred in patients using cisapride, pimozide, levacetylmethadol (levomethadyl) or quinidine concomitantly with itraconazole and/or other CYP3A4 inhibitors. Concomitant administration of these drugs with itraconazole is contraindicated (see Contraindications and Drug Interactions, Serious Drug Interactions and Drug-Drug Interactions).

Use in Patients with Underlying Cardiac Disease: SPORANOX has been associated with reports of CHF. In post-marketing experience, heart failure was more frequently reported in patients receiving a total daily dose of 400 mg than among those receiving lower total daily doses. This suggests that the risk of heart failure might increase with the total daily dose of itraconazole.

SPORANOX capsules should not be administered for the treatment of onychomycosis or dermatomycoses in patients with evidence of ventricular dysfunction such as CHF or a history of CHF. SPORANOX capsules should not be used for other indications in patients with evidence of ventricular dysfunction unless the benefit clearly outweighs the risk.

The benefit/risk assessment should take into consideration factors such as the severity of the indication, the dosing regimen (e.g. total daily dose), and the individual risk factors for congestive heart failure. These risk factors include cardiac disease, such as ischemic and valvular disease; significant pulmonary disease, such as chronic obstructive pulmonary disease; renal failure and other edematous disorders. Such patients should be informed of the signs and symptoms of congestive heart failure, treated with caution, and monitored for signs and symptoms of congestive heart failure during treatment; if such signs or symptoms do occur during treatment, SPORANOX capsules should be discontinued (see Drug Interactions and Adverse Reactions, Post-Market Adverse Drug Reactions).

Itraconazole has been shown to have a negative inotropic effect. When itraconazole was administered intravenously to anesthetized dogs, a dose-related negative inotropic effect was documented. In a healthy volunteer study (n=8) of SPORANOX for injection, a transient asymptomatic decrease of the left ventricular ejection fraction was observed using gated SPECT imaging; this resolved before the next infusion, 12 hours later.

Calcium channel blockers can have negative inotropic effects which may be additive to those of itraconazole. In addition, itraconazole can inhibit the metabolism of calcium channel blockers. Therefore, caution should be used when coadministering itraconazole and calcium channel blockers due to an increased risk of CHF. Concomitant administration of SPORANOX and nisoldipine is contraindicated.

Cases of CHF, peripheral edema, and pulmonary edema have been reported in the post-marketing period among patients being treated for onychomycosis and/or systemic fungal infections (see Adverse Reactions, Post-Market Adverse Drug Reactions).

Ear/Nose/Throat: Hearing Loss: Transient or permanent hearing loss has been reported in patients receiving treatment with itraconazole. Several of these reports included concurrent administration of quinidine, which is contraindicated (see Contraindications and Drug Interactions). The hearing loss usually resolves when treatment is stopped, but can persist in some patients.

Gastrointestinal: Use in Patients with Decreased Gastric Acidity: Absorption of itraconazole from SPORANOX capsules is impaired when gastric acidity is decreased. In patients also receiving acid-neutralizing medicines (e.g. aluminum hydroxide), these should be administered at least 2 hours after the intake of SPORANOX capsules. In patients with achlorhydria, such as certain AIDS patients on acid secretion suppressors (e.g. H_2-antagonists, proton pump inhibitors), it is advisable to administer SPORANOX capsules with a cola beverage.

Hepatic/Biliary/Pancreatic: Hepatic Effects/Use in Patients with Hepatic Impairment: Rare cases of serious hepatotoxicity (including liver failure and death) have been observed with SPORANOX treatment. Some of these cases had neither pre-existing liver disease nor a serious underlying medical condition and some of these cases developed within the first week of treatment.

In patients with elevated or abnormal liver enzymes or active liver disease, or who have experienced liver toxicity with other drugs, treatment with SPORANOX capsules is strongly discouraged unless there is a serious or life-threatening situation where the expected benefit exceeds the risk. Liver function monitoring should be done in patients with pre-existing hepatic function abnormalities or those who have experienced liver toxicity with other medications and should be considered in all patients receiving SPORANOX capsules. Treatment should be stopped immediately and liver function testing should be conducted in patients who develop signs and symptoms suggestive of liver dysfunction. Such signs and symptoms include unusual fatigue, anorexia, nausea and/or vomiting, jaundice, abdominal pain, dark urine or pale stools (see Warnings and Precautions, Serious Warnings and Precautions, General and Adverse Reactions).

Itraconazole binds extensively to plasma proteins.

Limited data are available on the use of oral itraconazole in patients with hepatic impairment. In cirrhotic patients, the mean terminal half-life of itraconazole was increased by 131% and its mean C_{max} decreased by 47% (see Action and Clinical Pharmacology, Special Populations and Conditions, Hepatic Insufficiency). Caution should be exercised when this drug is administered in this patient population.

Immune: Use in Acquired Immunodeficiency Syndrome (AIDS) and Neutropenic Patients: Studies with itraconazole in neutropenic and AIDS patients have indicated that itraconazole plasma concentrations are lower than those in healthy subjects (particularly in those patients who are achlorhydric); therefore, monitoring of the itraconazole plasma concentrations and a dose adjustment, if necessary, are recommended. In one study, adequate plasma concentrations of itraconazole (measured by HPLC) for antifungal prophylaxis in neutropenic patients were greater than 250 ng/mL.

Inadequate plasma concentrations were frequently found in patients whose antineoplastic therapy predisposed them to very poor oral absorption and frequent vomiting. In this case, antiemetics can be coadministered and it is particularly important that SPORANOX capsules be administered with meals.

There has been one report of reduced itraconazole absorption when taken with didanosine. Since the excipients in the didanosine formulation are known to have an acid-neutralizing effect, and since the absorption of itraconazole can be affected by the level of acidity in the stomach, it is recommended that didanosine be administered at least 2 hours after dosing with SPORANOX capsules.

The results from a study in which 8 HIV-infected individuals were treated with zidovudine, 8±0.4 mg/kg/day with or without SPORANOX capsules 100 mg b.i.d., showed that the pharmacokinetics of zidovudine were not affected during concomitant administration of SPORANOX capsules.

In patients with AIDS having received treatment for a systemic fungal infection such as sporotrichosis, blastomycosis or histoplasmosis and who are considered at risk for relapse, the treating physician should evaluate the need for a maintenance treatment.

Neurologic: If neuropathy occurs that may be attributable to SPORANOX capsules, the treatment should be discontinued.

Renal: Use in Patients with Renal Insufficiency: Limited data are available on the use of oral itraconazole in patients with renal impairment. Caution should be exercised when this drug is administered in this patient population (see Action and Clinical Pharmacology, Special Populations and Conditions, Renal Insufficiency).

In a few patients, hypokalemia has been reported. Consequently, serum potassium should be monitored in patients at risk during high-dose itraconazole therapy.

Itraconazole cannot be removed by dialysis.

Special Populations: Women of Child-Bearing Age: In women of child-bearing potential, an effective form of contraception must be used during therapy. SPORANOX should not be administered to women of child-bearing potential for the treatment of onychomycosis or dermatomycoses unless they are using effective measures to prevent pregnancy and they begin therapy on the second or third day following the onset of menses. Effective contraception should be continued throughout SPORANOX therapy and for 2 months following the end of treatment.

Pregnant Women: There are no studies available on the use of itraconazole in pregnant women; therefore, SPORANOX capsules should be used in pregnancy only if the benefit outweighs the potential risk. Itraconazole has been shown to produce teratogenic effects (major skeletal and secondary soft tissue defects) when administered at high doses (40 mg/kg/day, 5 times MRHD or higher) to pregnant rats. When administered to pregnant mice at high doses (80 mg/kg/day, 10 times MRHD or higher) itraconazole has been shown to produce encephaloceles and/or macroglossia. SPORANOX capsules should not be used for the treatment of onychomycosis or dermatomycoses in pregnant patients or in women contemplating pregnancy (see Contraindications).

There is limited information on the use of itraconazole during pregnancy. During post-marketing experience, cases of congenital abnormalities have been reported. These cases included skeletal, genitourinary tract, cardiovascular and ophthalmic malformations, as well as chromosomal and multiple malformations. A causal relationship with SPORANOX capsules has not been established.

Nursing Women: Itraconazole is excreted in human milk; therefore, the patient should be advised to discontinue nursing while taking SPORANOX capsules.

Pediatrics (<18 years of age): The efficacy and safety of SPORANOX capsules have not been established in children. No pharmacokinetic data are available in children. A small number of patients from age 3 to 16 years have been treated with 100 mg/day of itraconazole for systemic fungal infections and no serious adverse events have been reported. Toxicological studies have shown that itraconazole, when administered to rats, can produce bone toxicity. While no such toxicity has been reported in adult patients, the long-term effect of itraconazole in children is unknown.

Since clinical data on the use of SPORANOX capsules in pediatric patients is limited, SPORANOX capsules should not be used in children unless the potential benefit outweighs the potential risks.

Geriatrics (>65 years of age): The pharmacokinetics of SPORANOX capsules after single and repeated dosing of 100 mg once daily in 12 elderly subjects were found to be similar to those in young and middle-aged adults. Therefore, no dose adjustments are required in elderly patients.

Monitoring and Laboratory Tests: Plasma levels 3 to 4 hours after dosing with itraconazole should be monitored in patients requiring treatment for more than one month, in patients with systemic mycoses who have factors predisposing to poor absorption (such as achlorhydria, renal insufficiency, neutropenia, AIDS) or in those who are taking drugs which may alter itraconazole absorption or metabolism (such as rifampicin and phenytoin).

Due to the presence of an active metabolite, monitoring of plasma levels by bioassay will indicate plasma levels roughly 3 times higher than will monitoring by high-performance liquid chromatography, unless solvent conditions for the HPLC assay are adjusted to allow simultaneous detection of both the parent drug and this metabolite (hydroxy-itraconazole).

Liver function monitoring should be done in patients with pre-existing hepatic abnormalities, or those who have experienced liver toxicity with other medications and should also be considered in all patients receiving treatment with SPORANOX capsules.

Hypokalemia has been reported in a few patients. Therefore, serum potassium should be monitored in patients at risk during high-dose itraconazole therapy.

ADVERSE REACTIONS: Adverse Drug Reaction Overview: SPORANOX has been associated with rare cases of serious hepatotoxicity, including liver failure and death. Some of these cases had neither pre-existing liver disease nor a serious underlying medical condition. If clinical signs or symptoms develop that are consistent with liver disease, treatment should be discontinued and liver function testing performed. Before consideration is given to reinstituting therapy, the risks and benefits of SPORANOX use should be reassessed (see Warnings and Precautions, Hepatic/Biliary/Pancreatic and General).

The most frequently reported adverse experiences in association with the use of SPORANOX were of gastrointestinal origin, such as dyspepsia, nausea, vomiting, diarrhea, abdominal pain and constipation. Other adverse experiences reported very rarely (<1/10 000) include reversible increases in hepatic enzymes, hepatitis, menstrual disorder, dizziness and allergic reactions (such as pruritus, rash, urticaria and angioedema), peripheral neuropathy, Stevens-Johnson syndrome, alopecia, hypokalemia, edema, congestive heart failure and pulmonary edema.

Clinical Trial Adverse Drug Reactions: Because clinical trials are conducted under very specific conditions the adverse reaction rates observed in the clinical trials may not reflect the rates observed in practice and should not be compared to the rates in the clinical trials of another drug. Adverse drug reaction information from clinical trials is useful for identifying drug-related adverse events and for approximating rates.

Adverse experiences during short-term therapy with SPORANOX capsules occurred in 7.8% of patients. During long-term therapy in patients, most of whom had underlying pathology and received multiple concomitant treatments, the incidence of adverse experiences was higher (20.6%). The most common adverse experiences (reported by at least 1% of patients) during short-term or long-term therapy with SPORANOX capsules are presented in Table 1.

Table 1: SPORANOX Capsules

Most Common Adverse Experiences (≥1%) During Long-term Therapy with SPORANOX Capsules in Comparison with Short-term Therapy

	Short-term Therapy	Long-term Therapy
Total Number of Patients	**12 889**	**916**
Body System[a]/Adverse Event	**Incidence (%)**	
Gastrointestinal[a]	4.4	9.1
Nausea	1.6	2.9
Dermatological[a]	0.8	4.5
Rash	<1.0	1.6
Pruritus	<1.0	1.3
Central Nervous Systems[a]	2.1	4.3

(cont'd)

Table 1: SPORANOX Capsules *(cont'd)*

Most Common Adverse Experiences (≥1%) During Long-term Therapy with SPORANOX Capsules in Comparison with Short-term Therapy

	Short-term Therapy	Long-term Therapy
Total Number of Patients	**12 889**	**916**
Body System[a]/Adverse Event	**Incidence (%)**	
Headache	1.0	1.1
Respiratory System[a]	<1.0	3.9
Liver and Biliary System[a]	0.11	2.7
Miscellaneous[a]	0.7	5.6
Edema	<1.0	1.0

[a] Rates represent summary of all types of adverse events recorded for the body system.

For 834 clinical trial patients receiving 2-4 cycles of one week therapy, the most frequently reported adverse events during the treatment and follow-up period were abdominal pain (1.9%), nausea (1.6%) and headache (1.3%).

Less Common Clinical Trial Adverse Drug Reactions (<1%): The following adverse experiences have been reported at an incidence greater than 0.5% and less than 1% during short-term therapy with SPORANOX capsules:
Central and Peripheral Nervous Systems: dizziness/faintness; vertigo.
Gastrointestinal: dyspepsia/epigastric pain/upset stomach; abdominal pain/discomfort; vomiting; pyrosis; diarrhea; gastritis; flatulence/meteorism; constipation; decreased appetite; other gastric complaints.
General: edema; pain; fatigue; fever.
Immune: allergic reaction.
Psychiatric: sleepiness/somnolence.
Skin: pruritus; rash.

The following adverse experiences have been reported at an incidence of greater than 0.5% but less than 1% of patients during long-term therapy with SPORANOX capsules:
Cardiovascular: chest pain; hypertension.
Central and Peripheral Nervous Systems: dizziness.
Gastrointestinal: vomiting; dyspepsia/epigastralgia; diarrhea; abdominal pain.
General: pain; fatigue; fever.
Liver and Biliary System: increase in liver enzymes; abnormal liver function tests; jaundice; hepatitis; cirrhosis; hepatocellular damage; abnormal hepatic function.
Metabolic and Nutritional: hypokalemia.
Respiratory System: bronchitis/bronchospasm; dyspnea; coughing; rhinitis; sinusitis.
Abnormal Hematologic and Clinical Chemistry Findings: An increase in liver enzymes and abnormal liver function tests have been reported infrequently in patients treated with SPORANOX. In post-marketing experience, high triglyceride levels have been reported very rarely.
Post-Market Adverse Drug Reactions: Worldwide post-marketing experiences with the use of SPORANOX (across all three SPORANOX formulations: SPORANOX capsules, SPORANOX oral solution and SPORANOX IV) include reports of the adverse events listed below.
Blood and Lymphatic System Disorders: leukopenia, neutropenia, thrombocytopenia.
Immune System Disorders: serum sickness, angioneurotic edema, anaphylactic, anaphylactoid and allergic reactions.
Metabolism and Nutrition Disorders: hypertriglyceridemia, hypokalemia.
Nervous System Disorders: peripheral neuropathy, paresthesia, hypoesthesia, headache, dizziness.
Eye Disorders: visual disturbances, including vision blurred and diplopia.
Ear and Labyrinth Disorders: tinnitus, transient or permanent hearing loss.
Cardiac Disorders: congestive heart failure.
Respiratory, Thoracic and Mediastinal Disorders: pulmonary edema.
Gastrointestinal Disorders: pancreatitis, abdominal pain, vomiting, dyspepsia, nausea, diarrhea, constipation, dysgeusia.
Hepatobiliary Disorders: serious hepatotoxicity (including some cases of fatal acute liver failure), hepatitis, reversible increases in hepatic enzymes.
Skin and Subcutaneous Tissue Disorders: toxic epidermal necrolysis, Stevens-Johnson syndrome, erythema multiforme, exfoliative dermatitis, leukocytoclastic vasculitis, urticaria, alopecia, photosensitivity, rash, pruritus.
Musculoskeletal and Connective Tissue Disorders: myalgia, arthralgia.
Renal and Urinary Disorders: pollakiuria, urinary incontinence.
Reproductive System and Breast Disorders: menstrual disorders, erectile dysfunction.
General Disorders and Administration Site Conditions: edema, pyrexia.

DRUG INTERACTIONS:

Serious Drug Interactions
- Concomitant administration of SPORANOX with levacetylmethadol (levomethadyl), dofetilide, quinidine, cisapride and pimozide may result in serious cardiovascular events.
- Concomitant administration of SPORANOX with ergot alkaloids, such as dihydroergotamine, ergometrine, ergotamine and methylergometrine (methylergonovine) may result in serious and/or life-threatening ischemia.
- Concomitant administration of SPORANOX with HMG-CoA reductase inhibitors, such as lovastatin and simvastatin, may increase the risk of skeletal muscle toxicity including rhabdomyolysis.
- Concomitant administration of SPORANOX with benzodiazepines, such as midazolam and triazolam, could potentiate and prolong hypnotic and sedative effects.
- Concomitant administration of SPORANOX with fentanyl could increase or prolong fentanyl plasma concentrations and may cause potentially fatal respiratory depression.
- Concomitant administration of eletriptan with SPORANOX can elevate plasma eletriptan concentrations which could result in serious adverse events.
- Concomitant administration of SPORANOX and nisoldipine is contraindicated.

(See Contraindications, Warnings and Precautions, and Drug-Drug Interactions.)

Overview: Itraconazole and its major metabolite, hydroxy-itraconazole, are inhibitors of CYP3A4. Therefore, the following drug interactions may occur (see Table 2 and the following drug class subheadings):

1. SPORANOX may decrease the elimination of drugs metabolized by CYP3A4, resulting in increased plasma concentrations of these drugs when they are administered with SPORANOX. These elevated plasma concentrations may increase or prolong both therapeutic and adverse effects of these drugs. Whenever possible, plasma concentrations of these drugs should be monitored, and dosage adjustments made after concomitant SPORANOX therapy is initiated. When appropriate, clinical monitoring for signs or symptoms of increased or prolonged pharmacologic effects is advised. Upon discontinuation, depending on the dose and duration of treatment, itraconazole plasma concentrations decline gradually (especially in patients with hepatic cirrhosis or in those receiving CYP3A4 inhibitors). This is particularly important when initiating therapy with drugs whose metabolism is affected by itraconazole.
2. Inducers of CYP3A4 may decrease the plasma concentrations of itraconazole. SPORANOX may not be effective in patients concomitantly taking SPORANOX and one of these drugs. Therefore, administration of these drugs with SPORANOX is not recommended.
3. Other inhibitors of CYP3A4 may increase the plasma concentrations of itraconazole. Patients who must take SPORANOX concomitantly with one of these drugs should be monitored closely for signs or symptoms of increased or prolonged pharmacologic effects of SPORANOX.

Drug-Drug Interactions: See Table 2.

Table 2: SPORANOX Capsules

Selected Drugs That Are Predicted to Alter the Plasma Concentration of Itraconazole or Have Their Plasma Concentration Altered by Itraconazole[a]

Drug plasma concentration increased by itraconazole	
Antiarrhythmics	digoxin, dofetilide[b], quinidine[b], disopyramide
Anticonvulsants	carbamazepine
Antimycobacterials	rifabutin
Antineoplastics	busulfan, docetaxel, vinca alkaloids
Antipsychotics	pimozide[b]
Benzodiazepines	alprazolam, diazepam, midazolam[b,c], triazolam[b]
Calcium Channel Blockers	dihydropyridines (including nisoldipine[b]), verapamil
Ergot Alkaloids	dihydroergotamine[b], ergometrine (ergonovine)[b], ergotamine[b], methylergometrine (methylergonovine)[b]
Gastrointestinal Motility Agents	cisapride[b]
Glucocorticosteroids	budesonide, dexamethasone, methylprednisolone, fluticasone
HMG-CoA Reductase Inhibitors	atorvastatin, cerivastatin, lovastatin[b], simvastatin[b]
5-HT_1 Receptor Agonists	eletriptan[b]
Immunosuppressants	cyclosporine, tacrolimus, sirolimus
Oral Hypoglycemics	oral hypoglycemics (i.e. repaglinide)
Protease Inhibitors	indinavir, ritonavir, saquinavir
Oral Anticoagulants	warfarin
Other	alfentanil, buspirone, trimetrexate, trazodone, fentanyl, levacetylmethadol (levomethadyl)[b], halofantrine, cilostazol
Decrease plasma concentration of itraconazole	
Anticonvulsants	carbamazepine, phenobarbital, phenytoin
Antimycobacterials	isoniazid, rifabutin, rifampin
Gastric Acid Suppressors/Neutralizers	antacids, H_2-receptor antagonists, proton pump inhibitors
Non-nucleoside Reverse Transcriptase Inhibitors	nevirapine
Increase plasma concentration of itraconazole	
Macrolide Antibiotics	clarithromycin, erythromycin
Protease Inhibitors	indinavir, lopinavir/ritonavir, ritonavir

[a] This list is not all-inclusive.
[b] Contraindicated with SPORANOX based on clinical and/or pharmacokinetic studies (see Warnings and Precautions and below).
[c] For information on parenterally administered midazolam, see the benzodiazepine paragraph below.

Antiarrhythmics: The class IA antiarrhythmics quinidine and disopyramide, and class III antiarrhythmics, such as dofetilide, are known to prolong the QT interval. Coadministration of quinidine or dofetilide with SPORANOX may increase plasma concentrations of quinidine or dofetilide, which could result in serious cardiovascular events. Therefore, concomitant administration of SPORANOX and quinidine or dofetilide is contraindicated (see Contraindications and Warnings and Precautions).

Concomitant administration of digoxin or disopyramide and SPORANOX has led to increased plasma concentrations of digoxin (likely via inhibition of P-glycoprotein) or disopyramide. Patients should be carefully monitored if SPORANOX is coadministered with either of these drugs.

Anticonvulsants: Reduced plasma concentrations of itraconazole were reported when SPORANOX was administered concomitantly with phenytoin. Carbamazepine, phenobarbital, and phenytoin are all inducers of CYP3A4. Although interactions with carbamazepine and phenobarbital have not been studied, concomitant administration of SPORANOX and these drugs would be expected to result in decreased plasma concentrations of itraconazole. In addition, in vivo studies have demonstrated an increase in plasma carbamazepine concentrations in subjects concomitantly receiving ketoconazole. Although there are no data regarding the effect of itraconazole on carbamazepine metabolism, because of the similarities between ketoconazole and itraconazole, concomitant administration of SPORANOX and carbamazepine may inhibit the metabolism of carbamazepine.

Antimycobacterials: Drug interaction studies have demonstrated that plasma concentrations of azole antifungal agents and their metabolites, including itraconazole and hydroxyitraconazole, were significantly decreased when these agents were given concomitantly with rifabutin or rifampin. In vivo data suggest that rifabutin is metabolized in part by CYP3A4. SPORANOX may inhibit the metabolism of rifabutin. Although no formal study data are available for isoniazid, similar effects should be anticipated. Therefore, the efficacy of SPORANOX could be substantially reduced if given concomitantly with one of these agents. Coadministration is not recommended.

Antineoplastics: SPORANOX may inhibit the metabolism of busulfan, docetaxel, and vinca alkaloids, which could lead to increased plasma concentration of these antineoplastic agents.

Antipsychotics: Pimozide is known to prolong the QT interval and is partially metabolized by CYP3A4. Coadministration of pimozide with SPORANOX could result in serious cardiovascular events. Therefore, concomitant administration of SPORANOX and pimozide is contraindicated (see Contraindications and Warnings and Precautions).

Benzodiazepines: Concomitant administration of SPORANOX and alprazolam, diazepam, oral midazolam, or triazolam could lead to increased plasma concentrations of these benzodiazepines. Increased plasma concentrations could potentiate and prolong hypnotic and sedative effects. Concomitant administration of SPORANOX and oral midazolam or triazolam is contraindicated (see Contraindications and Warnings and Precautions). If midazolam is administered parenterally, special precaution and patient monitoring is required since the sedative effect may be prolonged.

Calcium Channel Blockers: Edema has been reported in patients concomitantly receiving SPORANOX and dihydropyridine calcium channel blockers. Appropriate dosage adjustment may be necessary.

Calcium channel blockers can have a negative inotropic effect which may be additive to those of itraconazole; itraconazole can inhibit the metabolism of calcium channel blockers such as dihydropyridines (e.g. nifedipine and felodipine) and verapamil. Therefore, caution should be used when coadministering itraconazole and calcium channel blockers due to an increased risk of CHF. Concomitant administration of SPORANOX and nisoldipine is contraindicated (see Contraindications; Warnings and Precautions and Adverse Reactions, Post-Market Adverse Drug Reactions).

Ergot Alkaloids: Concomitant administration of SPORANOX with ergot alkaloids, such as dihydroergotamine, ergometrine (ergonovine), ergotamine and methylergometrine (methylergonovine) is contraindicated due to the risk of serious and/or peripheral ischemia (see Contraindications). In some cases, concomitant use of potent CYP3A4 inhibitors (protease inhibitors, macrolide antibiotics and antifungal agents) with ergot alkaloids has resulted in serious and/or life-threatening ischemia, including fatalities and cases of gangrene.

Gastric Acid Suppressors/Neutralizers: Reduced plasma concentrations of itraconazole were reported when SPORANOX capsules were administered concomitantly with H_2-receptor antagonists. Studies have shown that absorption of itraconazole is impaired when gastric acid production is decreased. Therefore, SPORANOX should be administered with a cola beverage if the patient has achlorhydria or is taking H_2-receptor antagonists or other gastric acid suppressors. Antacids should be administered at least 1 hour before or 2 hours after administration of SPORANOX capsules. In a clinical study, when SPORANOX capsules were administered with omeprazole (a proton pump inhibitor), the bioavailability of itraconazole was significantly reduced.

Gastrointestinal Motility Agents: Coadministration of SPORANOX with cisapride can elevate plasma cisapride concentrations which could result in serious cardiovascular events. Therefore, concomitant administration of SPORANOX with cisapride is contraindicated (see Contraindications and Warnings and Precautions).

Glucocorticosteroids: SPORANOX markedly increased systemic exposure to oral and intravenous dexamethasone (3.7-fold and 3.3-fold increases, respectively), inhaled budesonide (4.2-fold increase), fluticasone and methylprednisolone, and enhanced their adrenal-suppressant effect. Careful follow-up is recommended when itraconazole is coadministered with these drugs.

HMG-CoA Reductase Inhibitors: Human pharmacokinetic data suggest that SPORANOX inhibits the metabolism of atorvastatin, cerivastatin, lovastatin, and simvastatin, which may increase the risk of skeletal muscle toxicity, including rhabdomyolysis. Concomitant administration of SPORANOX with HMG-CoA reductase inhibitors, such as lovastatin and simvastatin, is contraindicated (see Contraindications and Warnings and Precautions).

5-HT_1 Receptor Agonists: Coadministration of eletriptan with SPORANOX can elevate plasma eletriptan concentrations which could result in serious adverse events. Therefore, concomitant use of eletriptan with SPORANOX is contraindicated (see Contraindications).

Immunosuppressants: Concomitant administration of SPORANOX and cyclosporine, tacrolimus or sirolimus has led to increased plasma concentrations of these immunosuppressants.

Macrolide Antibiotics: Erythromycin and clarithromycin are known inhibitors of CYP3A4 (see Table 2) and may increase plasma concentrations of itraconazole. In a small pharmacokinetic study involving HIV-infected patients, clarithromycin was shown to increase plasma concentrations of itraconazole. Similarly, following administration of 1 gram of erythromycin ethyl succinate and 200 mg itraconazole as single doses, the mean C_{max} and $AUC_{0-\infty}$ of itraconazole increased by 44% (90% CI: 119-175%) and 36% (90% CI: 108-171%), respectively.

Non-nucleoside Reverse Transcriptase Inhibitors: Nevirapine is an inducer of CYP3A4. In vivo studies have shown that nevirapine induces the metabolism of ketoconazole, significantly reducing the bioavailability of ketoconazole. Studies involving nevirapine and itraconazole have not been conducted. However, because of the similarities between ketoconazole and itraconazole, concomitant administration of SPORANOX and nevirapine is not recommended.

Nucleoside Reverse Transcriptase Inhibitors: In a clinical study, when 8 HIV-infected subjects were treated concomitantly with SPORANOX capsules 100 mg twice daily and the nucleoside reverse transcriptase inhibitor zidovudine 8±0.4 mg/kg/day, the pharmacokinetics of zidovudine were not affected. Other nucleoside reverse transcriptase inhibitors have not been studied.

Oral Anticoagulants: SPORANOX enhances the anticoagulant effect of coumarin-like drugs, such as warfarin.

Oral Hypoglycemic Agents: Severe hypoglycemia has been reported in patients concomitantly receiving azole antifungal agents and oral hypoglycemic agents. Blood glucose concentrations should be carefully monitored when SPORANOX and oral hypoglycemic agents are co-administered.

Polyenes: Prior treatment with itraconazole, like other azoles, may reduce or inhibit the activity of polyenes such as amphotericin B. However, the clinical significance of this drug effect has not been clearly defined.

Protease Inhibitors: Concomitant administration of SPORANOX and protease inhibitors metabolized by CYP3A4, such as indinavir, ritonavir, and saquinavir, may increase plasma concentrations of these protease inhibitors. In addition, concomitant administration of SPORANOX and indinavir and ritonavir (but not saquinavir) may increase plasma concentrations of itraconazole. Coadministration of lopinavir/ritonavir and itraconazole leads to significant increase of itraconazole concentrations. Caution is advised when SPORANOX and protease inhibitors must be given concomitantly.

Other:

- Levacetylmethadol (levomethadyl) is known to prolong the QT interval and is metabolized by CYP3A4. Coadministration of levacetylmethadol with SPORANOX could result in serious cardiovascular events. Therefore, concomitant administration of SPORANOX and levacetylmethadol is contraindicated.
- Halofantrine has the potential to prolong the QT interval at high plasma concentrations. Caution is advised when SPORANOX and halofantrine are administered concomitantly.
- In vitro data suggest that alfentanil is metabolized by CYP3A4. Administration with SPORANOX may increase plasma concentrations of alfentanil.
- Human pharmacokinetic data suggest that concomitant administration of SPORANOX and buspirone results in significant increases in plasma concentrations of buspirone.
- Itraconazole may lead to substantial increases in trazodone plasma concentrations with the potential for adverse effects. A lower dose of trazodone should be considered.
- In vitro data suggest that trimetrexate is extensively metabolized by CYP3A4. An in vitro rat liver model demonstrated that ketoconazole potently inhibits the metabolism of trimetrexate. Although there are no data regarding the effect of itraconazole on trimetrexate metabolism, because of the similarities between ketoconazole and itraconazole, concomitant administration of SPORANOX and trimetrexate may inhibit the metabolism of trimetrexate.
- Cilostazol is a CYP 3A4 metabolized drug that should be used with caution when co-administered with SPORANOX.
- Fentanyl plasma concentrations could be increased or prolonged by concomitant use of SPORANOX and may cause potentially fatal respiratory depression.

Drug-Food Interactions: For optimal absorption, SPORANOX capsules should be taken immediately after a full meal (see Action and Clinical Pharmacology, Pharmacokinetics).

Drug-Herb Interactions: Interactions with herbal products have not been established.

Drug-Laboratory Interactions: Interactions with laboratory tests have not been established.

DOSAGE AND ADMINISTRATION:

Dosing Considerations: When SPORANOX therapy is indicated, the type of organism responsible for the infection should be isolated and identified; however, therapy may be initiated prior to obtaining these results when clinically warranted.

SPORANOX capsules is a different preparation than SPORANOX oral solution and should not be used interchangeably.

For maximal absorption, it is essential to administer SPORANOX capsules immediately after a full meal (see Action and Clinical Pharmacology). See Warnings and Precautions for treatment of patients with decreased gastric acidity.

Concomitant administration of SPORANOX with certain medications may require a dose adjustment for either SPORANOX or for the other medication (see Drug Interactions).

Patients with Hepatic Impairment: Limited data are available on the use of oral itraconazole in patients with hepatic impairment. Caution should be exercised when this drug is administered in this patient population (see Warnings and Precautions, Hepatic/Biliary/Pancreatic, Hepatic Effects/Use in Patients with Hepatic Impairment; Action and Clinical Pharmacology, Special Populations and Conditions, Hepatic Insufficiency).

Patients with Renal Impairment: Limited data are available on the use of oral itraconazole in patients with renal impairment. Caution should be exercised when this drug is administered in this patient population (see Warnings and Precautions, Renal, Use in Patients with Renal Insufficiency; Action and Clinical Pharmacology, Special Populations and Conditions, Renal Insufficiency).

Recommended Dose and Dosage Adjustment: SPORANOX capsules should be administered at a dose of 100-400 mg/day. Dosage recommendations vary according to the infection treated.

Oral Candidiasis: The recommended dose is 100 mg daily for 2 weeks. The dose should be increased to 200 mg/day in patients with AIDS and neutropenic patients.

Esophageal Candidiasis: The recommended dose is 100 mg daily for 4 weeks. The dose should be increased to 200 mg/day in patients with AIDS and neutropenic patients.

Blastomycosis and Chronic Pulmonary Histoplasmosis: The recommended dose is 200 mg once daily. If there is no obvious improvement or there is evidence of progressive fungal disease, the dose should be increased in 100 mg increments to a maximum of 400 mg daily. Doses above 200 mg per day should be given in 2 divided doses.

Treatment should be continued for a minimum of 3 months and until clinical parameters and laboratory tests indicate that the active fungal infection has subsided. An inadequate period of treatment may lead to recurrence of active infection.

Other Systemic Mycoses: See Table 3.

Table 3: SPORANOX Capsules

Dosing Recommendations for Other Systemic Mycoses

Indication	Dose	Median Duration
Aspergillosis		
Pulmonary	200 mg o.d.	3–4 months
Invasive pulmonary	200 mg b.i.d.	3–4 months
Sporotrichosis	100 mg o.d.	3 months
Paracoccidioidomycosis	100 mg o.d.	6 months
Chromomycosis		
due to *Fonsecaea pedrosoi*	200 mg o.d.	6 months
due to *Cladosporium carrioni*	100 mg o.d.	3 months

Dermatomycoses: Standard Dosages: Tinea corporis/Tinea cruris: The recommended dose is 100 mg once daily for 14 consecutive days.

Tinea pedis: The recommended dose is 100 mg once daily for 28 consecutive days.

Pityriasis versicolor: The recommended dose is 200 mg once daily for 7 consecutive days.

Alternative Dosages: Shorter dosing schedules have also been found to be effective in the treatment of tinea corporis/tinea cruris and tinea pedis. The shorter dosages are:

Tinea corporis/tinea cruris: 200 mg o.d. for 7 consecutive days;

Tinea pedis: 200 mg b.i.d. for 7 consecutive days.

Equivalency between standard and alternative dosages was not established. Patients with chronic recalcitrant tinea pedis may benefit from the standard dosage of a lower daily dose (100 mg) for a longer period of time (4 weeks).

Onychomycosis: The recommended clinical dose for onychomycosis is: A one-week treatment course consists of 200 mg twice daily for 7 days. Treatment with 2 one-week courses is recommended for fingernail infections and 3 one-week courses for toenail infections. The one-week courses are always separated by a 3-week drug-free interval. Clinical response will become evident as the nail regrows, following discontinuation of the treatment. See Table 4.

Table 4: SPORANOX Capsules

Recommended Clinical Dose for Onychomycosis

Site of onychomycosis	Pulse[a] 1 Week 1	Week 2	Week 3	Week 4	Pulse[a] 2 Week 5	Week 6	Week 7	Week 8	Pulse[a] 3 Week 9
Toenails with or without fingernail involvement	200 mg b.i.d. for 7 days	itraconazole-free weeks			200 mg b.i.d. for 7 days	itraconazole-free weeks			200 mg b.i.d. for 7 days
Fingernails only	200 mg b.i.d. for 7 days	itraconazole-free weeks			200 mg b.i.d. for 7 days				

[a] A pulse equals a one-week course of treatment.

Tissue Elimination of itraconazole: Elimination of itraconazole from skin and nail tissues is slower than from plasma. Optimal clinical and mycological responses are reached 2 to 4 weeks after the cessation of treatment for skin infections and 6 to 9 months after the cessation of treatment for nail infections.

Missed Dose: Physicians should use clinical judgment based on the type and severity of the infection.

Administration: SPORANOX capsules must be swallowed whole.

OVERDOSAGE:

There is no experience of overdosage with itraconazole; however, based on animal toxicity data, symptoms of a gastrointestinal or central nervous system nature may be expected to occur.

Although no data are available for SPORANOX, administration of activated charcoal absorbs almost all commonly ingested drugs, and should be administered as quickly as possible to most patients who ingest potentially toxic amounts. Standard supportive treatment should be applied as necessary.

It has been reported that itraconazole cannot be removed by dialysis. No specific antidote is available.

> For management of a suspected drug overdose, contact your regional Poison Control Centre. See the *CPS* Directory section for a list of Poison Control Centres.

ACTION AND CLINICAL PHARMACOLOGY: Mechanism of Action: In vitro studies have demonstrated that itraconazole inhibits the cytochrome P450-dependent synthesis of ergosterol, which is a vital component of fungal and yeast cell membranes. This inhibition leads to deteriorated membranes, disturbed enzyme activities, and an uncoordinated synthesis of chitin, all together contributing to the antifungal activity. The inhibition of ergosterol synthesis has been attributed to interference with the reactions involved in the removal of the 14-α-methyl group of the precursor of ergosterol, lanosterol. Itraconazole has a very low affinity for mammalian P450 enzymes in contrast to fungal P450 enzymes. Itraconazole is fungitoxic to dermatophytes and yeasts.

Pharmacodynamics: In vitro: A 50% inhibition of the cholesterol biosynthesis is obtained in vitro in human lymphocytes with itraconazole at a concentration of 4×10^{-7}M, which is more than 100 times the concentration of itraconazole needed to produce a 50% inhibition of the ergosterol synthesis in *C. albicans*.

Up to a concentration of 10^{-5}M, itraconazole did not inhibit the cytochrome P450 dependent aromatization of androstenedione to estrogens by human placental microsomes.

In vivo: In male volunteers, basal serum levels of cholesterol remained similar to the control values obtained before itraconazole treatment of 100 mg o.d. for one month.

Long-term administration of itraconazole (up to 400 mg/day for up to a maximum of 2 years) indicated a slight decrease in plasma cholesterol in 67 patients who had a baseline cholesterol plasma level higher than 200 mg/dL. Only 9.5% of patients showed a shift to a somewhat higher plasma cholesterol level. Similar results were observed in 29 patients with baseline cholesterol levels of at least 250 mg/dL and itraconazole therapy (50-400 mg/day) for a minimum of 3 months. Twenty-three patients showed a reduction and 6 patients had an increased cholesterol level. In this study, the overall decrease in cholesterol did not coincide with alterations in the triglyceride levels.

There was no significant effect of itraconazole 100 or 200 mg taken daily for 35 days on the serum levels of 25-hydroxycholecalciferol and 1,25-dihydroxycholecalciferol in 12 volunteers. In volunteers receiving single or multiple doses of itraconazole for up to 30 days, no effect on serum levels of the following hormones were observed: basal plasma cortisol, testosterone, aldosterone, cortisol response to cosyntropin (ACTH) and plasma prolactin and response of plasma prolactin, follicle-stimulating hormone (FSH) and luteinizing hormone (LH) to an intravenous luteinizing hormone-releasing hormone (LHRH) challenge.

Plasma progesterone and estradiol levels measured once weekly (before, during and for 2 weeks after a 5-week administration period of itraconazole 200 mg/day) and saliva progesterone concentrations measured daily during the 5-week administration reflected a totally normal hormonal profile throughout the menstrual cycle.

In healthy female volunteers with normal, regular menstrual cycles, a single 300 mg dose of itraconazole taken during the late follicular phase did not modify the circadian variation in plasma 17β-estradiol levels. The same dose taken during the luteal phase had no effects on 17β-estradiol and progesterone levels.

Male patients with superficial mycoses who received 50 or 100 mg itraconazole for up to 2 months showed no change in levels of testosterone, sex hormone-binding globulin (SHBG), luteinizing hormone (LH), follicle-stimulating hormone (FSH) and estradiol.

In 15 patients with systemic mycoses receiving 200 to 400 mg/day itraconazole, adrenal function was studied before and after 12.4±5 (7-24) months of treatment. No change in the response of plasma cortisol to ACTH stimulation was observed. Average testosterone values measured in these patients before and after itraconazole were not statistically significantly different. However, one of eight patients treated with itraconazole 600 mg/day for severe or refractory systemic fungal infection, demonstrated a blunted cortisol response after one month of treatment. Reduction of the dose to 400 mg/day was associated with resolution of the symptoms associated with adrenal insufficiency and an improved cortisol response.

The administration of 200 mg itraconazole daily for 5 weeks had no significant influence on the heart rate, blood pressure, ECG-intervals and systolic time intervals in volunteers. This finding was confirmed in cancer patients who received 50 mg itraconazole daily for 48 weeks.

In 6 healthy volunteers, itraconazole 200 mg daily did not seem to have a negative influence on immune functions. After 5 weeks of itraconazole treatment, only values for OKT4 positive lymphocyte showed a significant shift from 42±3.3% to 53±3.3%. This increase, as well as shifts in the other immunological parameters, remained within the normal ranges.

Pharmacokinetics: Absorption: The pharmacokinetics of itraconazole after intravenous administration and its absolute oral bioavailability from an oral solution were studied in a randomized crossover study using 6 healthy male volunteers. The total plasma clearance averaged 381±95 mL/min and the apparent volume of distribution averaged 796±185 L. The observed absolute oral bioavailability of itraconazole was 55%.

The oral bioavailability of itraconazole capsules is maximal when the capsules are given immediately after a full meal. The pharmacokinetics of itraconazole were studied using 6 healthy male volunteers who received, in a cross-over design, single 100 mg doses of itraconazole as a polyethylene glycol capsule, with or without food. The same 6 volunteers also received 50 mg or 200 mg with food in a crossover design. In this study, only itraconazole plasma concentrations were measured. (See Table 5.)

Table 5: SPORANOX Capsules

Pharmacokinetic Parameters for Itraconazole

	50 mg (fed)	100 mg (fed)	100 mg (fasted)	200 mg (fed)
C_{max} (ng/mL)	45±16	132±67	38±20	289±100
T_{max} (hours)	3.2±1.3	4.0±1.1	3.3±1.0	4.7±1.4
$AUC_{0-\infty}$ (ng·h/mL)	567±264	1899±838	722±289	5211±2116

Values are means±standard deviation.

Doubling the SPORANOX dose results in approximately a 3-fold increase in the itraconazole plasma concentrations.

Values given in Table 6 represent data from a crossover pharmacokinetic study in which 27 healthy male volunteers each took a single 200 mg dose of SPORANOX capsules with or without food.

Table 6: SPORANOX Capsules

Crossover Pharmacokinetic Study of Itraconazole in Healthy Male Volunteers

	Itraconazole		Hydroxy-itraconazole	
	Fed	Fasted	Fed	Fasted
C_{max} (ng/mL)	239±85	140±65	397±103	286±101
T_{max} (hours)	4.5±1.1	3.9±1.0	5.1±1.6	4.5±1.1
$AUC_{0-\infty}$ (ng·h/mL)	3423±1154	2094±905	7978±2648	5191±2489
$t_{½}$ (hours)	21±5	21±7	12±3	12±3

Values are means±standard deviation.

Steady-state concentrations were reached within 15 days following oral doses of 50-400 mg daily. Values given in Table 7 are data at steady-state from a pharmacokinetic study in which 27 healthy male volunteers took 200 mg SPORANOX capsules b.i.d. (with food) for 15 days.

Table 7: SPORANOX Capsules

Steady-state Pharmacokinetic Study of Itraconazole in Healthy Male Volunteers

	Itraconazole	Hydroxy-itraconazole
C_{max} (ng/mL)	2282±514	3488±742
C_{min} (ng/mL)	1855±535	3349±761
T_{max} (hours)	4.6±1.8	3.4±3.4
AUC_{0-12h} (ng·h/mL)	22 569±5375	38 572±8450
$t_{½}$ (hours)	64±32	56±24

Values are means±standard deviation.

Results of the pharmacokinetic study suggest that itraconazole may undergo saturation metabolism with multiple dosing.

Distribution: The plasma protein binding of itraconazole is 99.8% and that of hydroxy-itraconazole is 99.5%.

Concentrations of itraconazole in whole blood are 60% of those in plasma. Uptake in keratinous tissues, especially the skin, is up to 5 times higher than in plasma, and elimination of itraconazole is related to epidermal regeneration. Therefore, therapeutic levels in the skin persist for 2 to 4 weeks after discontinuation of a 4-week treatment. Therapeutic levels of itraconazole in nails persist for 6 to 9 months after cessation of treatment. Itraconazole is also present in sebum and to a lesser extent in sweat. Itraconazole is extensively distributed into tissues which are prone to fungal invasion. Concentrations in lung, kidney, liver, bone, stomach, spleen and muscle were found to be 2 to 3 times higher than the corresponding plasma concentration.

Metabolism: Itraconazole is extensively metabolized by the liver into a large number of metabolites. One of the metabolites is hydroxy-itraconazole, which has antifungal activity comparable to itraconazole in vitro. Antifungal drug levels measured by bioassay were about 3 times those of itraconazole assayed by high-performance liquid chromatography. The main metabolic pathways were oxidative scission of the dioxolane ring, aliphatic oxidation at the 1-methylpropyl substituent, N-dealkylation of this 1-methylpropyl substituent, oxidative degradation of the piperazine ring and triazolone scission.

Excretion: Fecal excretion of the parent drug varies between 3-18% of the dose. Renal excretion of the parent drug is less than 0.03% of the dose. After one week, urinary excretion amounted to 35% of the dose and fecal excretion represented 54% of the dose.

Special Populations and Conditions: Pediatrics: No data available. See Warnings and Precautions, Special Populations, Pediatrics (<18 years of age).

Geriatrics: See Warnings and Precautions, Special Populations, Geriatrics (>65 years of age).

Hepatic Insufficiency: Itraconazole is predominantly metabolized in the liver. Pharmacokinetic data for patients with hepatic insufficiency is limited to subjects who received a single 100 mg dose of SPORANOX capsules. A pharmacokinetic study using a single 100 mg dose of itraconazole (one 100 mg capsule) was conducted in 6 healthy and 12 cirrhotic subjects. A statistically significant reduction in mean C_{max} (47%; mean cirrhotic C_{max} 87±18 ng/mL, mean healthy C_{max} 164±34 ng/mL) and a twofold increase in the elimination half-life (37±7 hrs and 16±5 hrs, respectively) of itraconazole were noted in cirrhotic subjects compared with healthy subjects. However, overall exposure to itraconazole, based on AUC was similar in cirrhotic patients and in healthy subjects (mean cirrhotic AUC 1449±207 ng.h/mL, mean healthy AUC 1856±388 ng.h/mL). Data are not available in cirrhotic patients during long-term use of itraconazole. Patients with impaired hepatic function should be carefully monitored when taking itraconazole. The prolonged elimination half-life of itraconazole observed in cirrhotic patients should be considered when deciding to initiate therapy with other medicines metabolized by CYP3A4. (See Warnings and Precautions, Hepatic/Biliary/Pancreatic.)

Renal Insufficiency: Limited data are available on the use of itraconazole in patients with renal insufficiency. Caution should be exercised when the drug is administered in this patient population (see Warnings and Precautions, Renal). Pharmacokinetic data in renally impaired patients is limited to subjects who received a single 200 mg dose of SPORANOX capsules. A pharmacokinetic study using a single 200 mg dose of itraconazole (four 50 mg capsules) was conducted in three groups of patients with renal impairment (uremia: n=7; hemodialysis: n=7; continuous ambulatory peritoneal dialysis: n=5). Mean±SD pharmacokinetic parameters are summarized in Table 8.

Table 8: SPORANOX Capsules

Mean Pharmacokinetic Parameters in Renally Impaired Patients Receiving a Single 200 mg Oral Dose of Itraconazole

Patient Group (n)	T_{max} (h)	C_{max} (ng/mL)	AUC_{0-8h} (ng·h/mL)
Uremic (7)	4.0±1.2	213±178	1026±819
Hemodialysis			
Off dialysis (7)	4.7±1.4	140±119	634±507
On dialysis (7)	4.1±0.9	113±83	507±371
CAPD (5)	4.4±2.2	77±29	325±107

Plasma concentration vs. time profiles showed wide inter-subject variation in all three groups. In uremic subjects (mean CrCl 13 mL/min/1.73 m²), mean plasma concentrations and overall exposure, based on AUC_{∞}, were slightly reduced compared with healthy subject in a previous study (AUC_{∞} values of 3454±3132 vs. 4161±1949 ng hr/mL in uremic patients and healthy subjects, respectively). C_{max} and AUC_{0-8h} values were reduced 30-40% in hemodialysis patients on non-dialysis days, compared to uremic patients (see Table 8), and further reduced 10-20% on dialysis days. In CAPD patients, C_{max} and AUC_{0-8h} values were reduced to one-third the values seen in non-dialyzed uremic patients.

STORAGE AND STABILITY: SPORANOX capsules should be stored at room temperature (15-30°C). They should be protected from light and moisture. Keep out of the reach of children.

INFORMATION FOR THE PATIENT: Published in e-CPS, available by subscription at www.e-cps.ca.

DOSAGE FORMS, COMPOSITION AND PACKAGING: Each pink and blue capsule, imprinted in white with "JANSSEN" on the cap and "[logo]" on the body, contains: itraconazole 100 mg in a pellet formulation. Nonmedicinal ingredients: D&C Red No. 22, D&C Red No. 28, FD&C Blue No. 1, FD&C Blue No. 2, gelatin, hydroxypropylmethylcellulose, polyethylene glycol, sugar spheres (NF) and titanium dioxide. HDPE bottles of 30. Pulsepak cartons of 7 blister cards containing 4 capsules. The pulsepak is specifically designed for use in the treatment of onychomycosis.

(Shown in Product Identification Section)

Sporanox® Oral Solution ℞

itraconazole

Antifungal

Janssen-Ortho

Date of Preparation: June 6, 2002
Date of Revision: May 13, 2010

SUMMARY PRODUCT INFORMATION:

Route of Administration	Dosage Form/ Strength	Clinically Relevant Nonmedicinal Ingredients
Oral	Solution 10 mg/mL	None For a complete listing see Dosage Forms, Composition and Packaging.

INDICATIONS AND CLINICAL USE: SPORANOX (itraconazole) oral solution 10 mg/mL is indicated for the treatment of oral and/or esophageal candidiasis in adult HIV-positive or other immunocompromised patients.

SPORANOX oral solution as treatment for oral and/or esophageal candidiasis was not investigated in neutropenic patients. Due to the pharmacokinetic properties, SPORANOX oral solution is not recommended for initiation of treatment in patients at immediate risk of systemic candidiasis.

Note: SPORANOX oral solution and SPORANOX capsules should not be used interchangeably.

Geriatrics (>65 years of age): The efficacy and safety of SPORANOX oral solution have not been established in geriatric patients (see Warnings and Precautions, Special Populations, Geriatrics (>65 years of age)).

Pediatrics (<18 years of age): The efficacy and safety of SPORANOX oral solution have not been established in pediatric patients (see Warnings and Precautions, Special Populations, Pediatrics (<18 years of age)).

CONTRAINDICATIONS:

- **Congestive Heart Failure:** SPORANOX oral solution should not be administered to patients with evidence of ventricular dysfunction, such as congestive heart failure (CHF) or a history of CHF except for the treatment of life-threatening or other serious infections (see Warnings and Precautions, Serious Warnings and Precautions and Cardiovascular, Use in Patients with Underlying Cardiac Disease; Adverse Reactions, Post-Market Adverse Drug Reactions and Drug Interactions, Drug-Drug Interactions, Calcium Channel Blockers).
- **Drug Interactions:** Coadministration of the following drugs is contraindicated with SPORANOX oral solution (see Warnings and Precautions, Serious Warnings and Precautions and Drug Interactions, Serious Drug Interactions):
  - CYP3A4 metabolized substrates that can prolong the QT-interval e.g., cisapride, dofetilide, levacetylmethadol (levomethadyl), pimozide, and quinidine are contraindicated with SPORANOX oral solution. Co-administration may result in increased plasma concentrations of these substrates, which can lead to QT prolongation and serious cardiac arrhythmias
  - CYP3A4 metabolized HMG-CoA reductase inhibitors such as lovastatin and simvastatin
  - Triazolam and oral midazolam
  - Ergot alkaloids such as dihydroergotamine, ergometrine (ergonovine), ergotamine and methylergometrine (methylergonovine)

- Eletriptan
- Nisoldipine
- SPORANOX oral solution is contraindicated in patients with a known hypersensitivity to itraconazole or its excipients. For a complete listing, see Dosage Forms, Composition and Packaging. There is no information regarding cross-hypersensitivity between itraconazole and other azole antifungal agents. Caution should be used in prescribing SPORANOX oral solution to patients with hypersensitivity to other azoles.

WARNINGS AND PRECAUTIONS:

Serious Warnings and Precautions

- **Congestive Heart Failure: SPORANOX oral solution should not be administered to patients with evidence of ventricular dysfunction such as congestive heart failure (CHF) or a history of CHF except for the treatment of life-threatening or other serious infections.** If signs or symptoms of congestive heart failure occur during administration of SPORANOX oral solution, discontinue administration. When itraconazole was administered intravenously to dogs and healthy human volunteers, negative inotropic effects were seen (see Contraindications; Warnings and Precautions, Cardiovascular, Use in Patients with Underlying Cardiac Disease; Adverse Reactions, Post-Market Adverse Drug Reactions and Drug Interactions, Drug-Drug Interactions, Calcium Channel Blockers).
- **Drug Interactions: Coadministration of cisapride, pimozide, quinidine, dofetilide or levacetylmethadol (levomethadyl) with SPORANOX (itraconazole) capsules or oral solution is contraindicated.** SPORANOX, a potent cytochrome P450 3A4 isoenzyme system (CYP3A4) inhibitor, may increase plasma concentrations of drugs metabolized by this pathway. Serious cardiovascular events, including QT prolongation, torsades de pointes, ventricular tachycardia, cardiac arrest, and/or sudden death have occurred in patients using cisapride, pimozide, levacetylmethadol (levomethadyl), or quinidine concomitantly with SPORANOX and/or other CYP3A4 inhibitors (see Contraindications and Drug Interactions, Serious Drug Interactions; Overview and Drug-Drug Interactions).
- **Liver Toxicity:** SPORANOX oral solution has been associated with rare cases of serious hepatotoxicity, including liver failure and death. Some of these cases had neither pre-existing liver disease nor a serious underlying medical condition and some of these cases developed within the first week of treatment. It is advisable to monitor liver function. If clinical signs or symptoms develop that are consistent with liver disease, such as anorexia, nausea, vomiting, jaundice, fatigue, abdominal pain, dark urine, or pale stools, treatment should be discontinued and liver function testing performed. Continued use of SPORANOX oral solution or reinstitution of treatment with SPORANOX oral solution is strongly discouraged unless there is a serious or life-threatening situation where the expected benefit exceeds the risk (see Warnings and Precautions, General, Hepatic/Biliary/Pancreatic, Hepatic Effects/Use in Patients with Hepatic Impairment and Adverse Reactions).

General: SPORANOX oral solution and SPORANOX capsules should not be used interchangeably. SPORANOX oral solution is indicated only for the treatment of oropharyngeal and/or esophageal candidiasis. The efficacy of SPORANOX oral solution for other indications is unknown. The two dosage forms have different absorption profiles. SPORANOX oral solution contains the excipient hydroxypropyl-β-cyclodextrin, which produced adenocarcinomas of the exocrine pancreas in a rat but not in a similar mouse carcinogenicity study. The clinical relevance of these findings is unknown.

Patients on Continuous Treatment: In patients receiving continuous treatment of more than one month and in patients developing symptoms such as anorexia, nausea, vomiting, fatigue, abdominal pain or dark urine, it is advisable to monitor liver function. If tests are abnormal, treatment should be terminated.

Cardiovascular: Cardiac Dysrhythmias: Life-threatening cardiac dysrhythmias and/or sudden death have occurred in patients using cisapride, pimozide, levacetylmethadol (levomethadyl) or quinidine concomitantly with itraconazole and/or other CYP3A4 inhibitors. Concomitant administration of these drugs with itraconazole is contraindicated (see Contraindications and Drug Interactions, Serious Drug Interactions and Drug-Drug Interactions).

Use in Patients with Underlying Cardiac Disease: SPORANOX has been associated with reports of CHF. In post-marketing experience, heart failure was more frequently reported in patients receiving a total daily dose of 400 mg than among those receiving lower total daily doses. This suggests that the risk of heart failure might increase with the total daily dose of itraconazole.

SPORANOX oral solution should not be used in patients with evidence of ventricular dysfunction such as CHF or a history of CHF unless the benefit clearly outweighs the risk.

The benefit/risk assessment should take into consideration factors such as the severity of the indication, the dosing regimen (e.g., total daily dose), and the individual risk factors for congestive heart failure.

These risk factors include cardiac disease, such as ischemic and valvular disease; significant pulmonary disease, such as chronic obstructive pulmonary disease; and renal failure and other edematous disorders. Such patients should be informed of the signs and symptoms of congestive heart failure, treated with caution, and monitored for signs and symptoms of congestive heart failure during treatment; if such signs or symptoms do occur during treatment, itraconazole should be discontinued (see Adverse Reactions, Post-Market Adverse Drug Reactions and Drug Interactions).

Itraconazole has been shown to have a negative inotropic effect. When itraconazole was administered intravenously to anesthetized dogs, a dose-related negative inotropic effect was documented. In a healthy volunteer study (n=8) of SPORANOX for injection, a transient asymptomatic decrease of the left ventricular ejection fraction was observed using gated SPECT imaging; this resolved before the next infusion, 12 hours later.

Calcium channel blockers can have negative inotropic effects which may be additive to those of itraconazole. In addition, itraconazole can inhibit the metabolism of calcium channel blockers. Therefore, caution should be used when coadministering itraconazole and calcium channel blockers due to an increased risk of CHF. Concomitant administration of SPORANOX and nisoldipine is contraindicated.

Cases of congestive heart failure (CHF), peripheral edema, and pulmonary edema have been reported in the post-marketing period among patients being treated for onychomycosis and/or systemic fungal infections (see Adverse Reactions, Post-Market Adverse Drug Reactions).

Ear/Nose/Throat: Hearing Loss: Transient or permanent hearing loss has been reported in patients receiving treatment with itraconazole. Several of these reports included concurrent administration of quinidine, which is contraindicated (see Contraindications and Drug Interactions). The hearing loss usually resolves when treatment is stopped, but can persist in some patients.

Hepatic/Biliary/Pancreatic: Hepatic Effects/Use in Patients with Hepatic Impairment: Rare cases of serious hepatotoxicity (including liver failure and death) have been observed with SPORANOX treatment. Some of these cases had neither pre-existing liver disease nor a serious underlying medical condition and some of these cases developed within the first week of treatment. In patients with elevated or abnormal liver enzymes or active liver disease, or who have experienced liver toxicity with other drugs, treatment with SPORANOX oral solution is strongly discouraged unless there is a serious or life-threatening situation where the expected benefit exceeds the risk. Liver function monitoring should be done in patients with pre-existing hepatic function abnormalities or those who have experienced liver toxicity with other medications and should be considered in all patients receiving SPORANOX oral solution. Treatment should be stopped immediately and liver function testing should be conducted in patients who develop signs and symptoms suggestive of liver dysfunction. Such signs and symptoms include unusual fatigue, anorexia, nausea and/or vomiting, jaundice, abdominal pain, dark urine or pale stools (see Warnings and Precautions, Serious Warnings and Precautions, General and Adverse Reactions, Post-Market Adverse Drug Reactions).

Itraconazole binds extensively to plasma proteins.

Limited data are available on the use of oral itraconazole in patients with hepatic impairment. In cirrhotic patients, the mean terminal half-life of itraconazole was increased by 131% and its mean C_{max} decreased by 47% (see Action and Clinical Pharmacology, Special Populations and Conditions, Hepatic Insufficiency). Caution should be exercised when this drug is administered in this patient population.

Neurologic: If neuropathy occurs that may be attributable to SPORANOX oral solution, the treatment should be discontinued.

Renal: Use in Patients with Renal Insufficiency: Limited data are available on the use of oral itraconazole in patients with renal impairment. Caution should be exercised when this drug is administered in this patient population (see Action and Clinical Pharmacology, Special Populations and Conditions, Renal Insufficiency).

In a few patients, hypokalemia has been reported. Consequently serum potassium should be monitored in patients at risk during high-dose itraconazole therapy.

Itraconazole cannot be removed by dialysis.

Special Populations: Women of Child-Bearing Age: In women of child-bearing potential, an effective form of contraception must be used during therapy. Effective contraception should be continued throughout SPORANOX therapy and for 2 months following the end of treatment.

Pregnant Women: There are no studies available on the use of itraconazole in pregnant women. SPORANOX oral solution should only be given to pregnant women in life-threatening cases and when in these cases the potential benefit outweighs the potential harm to the fetus. Itraconazole has been shown to produce teratogenic effects (major skeletal and secondary soft tissue defects) when administered at high doses (40 mg/kg/day, 5 times the maximum recommended human dose (MRHD) or higher) to pregnant rats. When administered to pregnant mice at high doses (80 mg/kg/day, 10 times MRHD or higher), itraconazole has been shown to produce encephaloceles and/or macroglossia.

There is limited information on the use of itraconazole during pregnancy. During post-marketing experience, cases of congenital abnormalities have been reported. These cases included skeletal, genitourinary tract, cardiovascular and ophthalmic malformations, as well as chromosomal and multiple malformations. A causal relationship with SPORANOX oral solution has not been established.

Nursing Women: Itraconazole is excreted in human milk; therefore, the patient should be advised to discontinue nursing while taking SPORANOX oral solution.

Pediatrics (<18 years of age): The efficacy and safety of SPORANOX oral solution have not been established in pediatric patients. A pharmacokinetic study was conducted with SPORANOX oral solution in 26 pediatric patients, ages 6 months to 12 years, requiring systemic antifungal treatment. Itraconazole was dosed at 5 mg/kg once daily for 2 weeks and no serious unexpected adverse events were reported.

Toxicological studies have shown that itraconazole, when administered to rats, can produce bone toxicity. While no such toxicity has been reported in adult patients, the long-term effect of itraconazole in children is unknown.

Since clinical data on the use of SPORANOX oral solution in pediatric patients is limited, SPORANOX oral solution should not be used in children unless the potential benefit outweighs the potential risks.

Geriatrics (>65 years of age): Since clinical data on the use of SPORANOX oral solution in elderly patients is limited, it is advised to use SPORANOX oral solution in these patients only if the potential benefit outweighs the potential risks.

Cystic Fibrosis: In cystic fibrosis patients, variability in therapeutic levels of itraconazole was observed with steady-state dosing of oral solution using 2.5 mg/kg b.i.d. Steady-state concentrations of >250 ng/mL were achieved in approximately 50% of subjects greater than 16 years of age, but in none of the patients less than 16 years of age. If a patient does not respond to SPORANOX oral solution, consideration should be given to switching to alternative therapy.

Use in Acquired Immunodeficiency Syndrome (AIDS) and Neutropenic Patients: Studies with SPORANOX capsules in neutropenic and AIDS patients have indicated that itraconazole plasma concentrations are lower than those in healthy subjects (particularly in those patients who are achlorhydric). However, the bioavailability of itraconazole oral solution, when tested in AIDS patients, was found satisfactory and not altered by the stage of HIV infection.

The results from a study in which 8 HIV-infected individuals were treated with zidovudine, 8±0.4 mg/kg/day with or without SPORANOX capsules 100 mg b.i.d., showed that the pharmacokinetics of zidovudine were not affected during concomitant administration of SPORANOX capsules.

Monitoring and Laboratory Tests: Due to the presence of an active metabolite, hydroxy-itraconazole, plasma levels monitored by bioassay will yield plasma levels roughly three times higher than that obtained by high-pressure liquid chromatography (HPLC), unless solvent conditions for the HPLC assay are adjusted to allow simultaneous detection of both the parent drug and the metabolite.

Liver function monitoring should be done in patients with pre-existing hepatic abnormalities, or those who have experienced liver toxicity with other medications and should also be considered in all patients receiving treatment with SPORANOX oral solution.

Hypokalemia has been reported in a few patients. Therefore, serum potassium should be monitored in patients at risk during high-dose itraconazole therapy.

ADVERSE REACTIONS: Adverse Drug Reaction Overview: SPORANOX has been associated with rare cases of serious hepatotoxicity, including liver failure and death. Some of these cases had neither pre-existing liver disease nor a serious underlying medical condition. If clinical signs or symptoms develop that are consistent with liver disease, treatment should be discontinued and liver function testing performed. Before consideration is given to reinstituting therapy, the risks and benefits of SPORANOX use should be reassessed (see Warnings and Precautions, General and Hepatic/Biliary/Pancreatic).

Clinical Trial Adverse Drug Reactions: Because clinical trials are conducted under very specific conditions the adverse reaction rates observed in the clinical trials may not reflect the rates observed in practice and should not be compared to the rates in the clinical trials of another drug. Adverse drug reaction information from clinical trials is useful for identifying drug-related adverse events and for approximating rates.

SPORANOX Oral Solution: The adverse event profile was analyzed for 889 HIV-positive and other immunocompromised patients receiving SPORANOX oral solution for the treatment of oral and esophageal candidiasis. The most frequently reported adverse events were of gastrointestinal origin. The total observed incidence of adverse events that are possibly or directly drug related, during treatment or within 14 days post-treatment for itraconazole oral solution is 18.2%. A listing of adverse events reported with a frequency ≥1% for itraconazole in all worldwide studies of oropharyngeal and esophageal candidiasis is presented in Table 1.

Table 1: SPORANOX Oral Solution

Adverse Experience Incidence ≥1.0% in Worldwide Trials of Oropharyngeal and Esophageal Candidiasis, by Body System

Body System/Adverse Event	Itraconazole n=889
Gastrointestinal System Disorder	12.3%
Nausea	5.3%
Diarrhea	4.5%
Vomiting	3.4%
Abdominal Pain	2.5%
Skin and Appendages Disorders	2.4%
Rash	1.3%
Central and Peripheral Nervous Systems	1.7%
Headache	1.1%
Liver and Biliary System Disorders	1.3%
Special Senses	1.1%
Taste Perversion	1.0%
Body as a Whole	1.0%

Post-Market Adverse Drug Reactions: Worldwide post-marketing experiences with the use of SPORANOX (across all three SPORANOX formulations: SPORANOX capsules, SPORANOX oral solution and SPORANOX IV) include the adverse events listed below.

Blood and Lymphatic System Disorders: leukopenia, neutropenia, thrombocytopenia.
Immune System Disorders: serum sickness, angioneurotic edema, anaphylactic, anaphylactoid and allergic reactions.
Metabolism and Nutrition Disorders: hypertriglyceridemia, hypokalemia.
Nervous System Disorders: peripheral neuropathy, paresthesia, hypoesthesia, headache, dizziness.
Eye Disorders: visual disturbances, including vision blurred and diplopia.
Ear and Labyrinth Disorders: tinnitus, transient or permanent hearing loss.
Cardiac Disorders: congestive heart failure.
Respiratory, Thoracic and Mediastinal Disorders: pulmonary edema.
Gastrointestinal Disorders: pancreatitis, abdominal pain, vomiting, dyspepsia, nausea, diarrhea, constipation, dysgeusia.

Hepatobiliary Disorders: serious hepatotoxicity (including some cases of fatal acute liver failure), hepatitis, reversible increases in hepatic enzymes.
Skin and Subcutaneous Tissue Disorders: toxic epidermal necrolysis, Stevens-Johnson syndrome, erythema multiforme, exfoliative dermatitis, leukocytoclastic vasculitis, urticaria, alopecia, photosensitivity, rash, pruritus.
Musculoskeletal and Connective Tissue Disorders: myalgia, arthralgia.
Renal and Urinary Disorders: pollakiuria, urinary incontinence.
Reproductive System and Breast Disorders: menstrual disorders, erectile dysfunction.
General Disorders and Administration Site Conditions: edema, pyrexia.

DRUG INTERACTIONS:

Serious Drug Interactions

- Concomitant administration of SPORANOX oral solution with levacetylmethadol (levomethadyl), dofetilide, quinidine, cisapride and pimozide may result in serious cardiovascular events.
- Concomitant administration of SPORANOX oral solution with ergot alkaloids, such as dihydroergotamine, ergometrine, ergotamine and methylergometrine (methylergonovine) may result in serious and/or life-threatening ischemia.
- Concomitant administration of SPORANOX oral solution with HMG-CoA reductase inhibitors, such as lovastatin and simvastatin, may increase the risk of skeletal muscle toxicity including rhabdomyolysis.
- Concomitant administration of SPORANOX oral solution with benzodiazepines, such as midazolam and triazolam, could potentiate and prolong hypnotic and sedative effects.
- Concomitant administration of SPORANOX with fentanyl could increase or prolong fentanyl plasma concentrations and may cause potentially fatal respiratory depression.
- Concomitant administration of eletriptan with SPORANOX can elevate plasma eletriptan concentrations which could result in serious adverse events.
- Concomitant administration of SPORANOX and nisoldipine is contraindicated.

(See Contraindications; Warnings and Precautions, and Drug-Drug Interactions.)

Overview: Itraconazole and its major metabolite, hydroxy-itraconazole, are inhibitors of CYP3A4. Therefore, the following drug interactions may occur (see Table 2 and the drug class subheadings that follow):

1. SPORANOX may decrease the elimination of drugs metabolized by CYP3A4, resulting in increased plasma concentrations of these drugs when they are administered with SPORANOX. These elevated plasma concentrations may increase or prolong both therapeutic and adverse effects of these drugs. Whenever possible, plasma concentrations of these drugs should be monitored, and dosage adjustments made after concomitant SPORANOX therapy is initiated. When appropriate, clinical monitoring for signs or symptoms of increased or prolonged pharmacologic effects is advised. Upon discontinuation, depending on the dose and duration of treatment, itraconazole plasma concentrations decline gradually (especially in patients with hepatic cirrhosis or in those receiving CYP3A4 inhibitors). This is particularly important when initiating therapy with drugs whose metabolism is affected by itraconazole.
2. Inducers of CYP3A4 may decrease the plasma concentrations of itraconazole. SPORANOX may not be effective in patients concomitantly taking SPORANOX and one of these drugs. Therefore, administration of these drugs with SPORANOX is not recommended.
3. Other inhibitors of CYP3A4 may increase the plasma concentrations of itraconazole. Patients who must take SPORANOX concomitantly with one of these drugs should be monitored closely for signs or symptoms of increased or prolonged pharmacologic effects of SPORANOX.

Drug-Drug Interactions: See Table 2.

Table 2: SPORANOX Oral Solution

Selected Drugs That Are Predicted to Alter the Plasma Concentration of Itraconazole or Have Their Plasma Concentration Altered by Itraconazole[a]

Drug plasma concentration increased by itraconazole	
Antiarrhythmics	digoxin, dofetilide[b], quinidine[b], disopyramide
Anticonvulsants	carbamazepine
Antimycobacterials	rifabutin
Antineoplastics	busulfan, docetaxel, vinca alkaloids
Antipsychotics	pimozide[b]
Benzodiazepines	alprazolam, diazepam, midazolam[b,c], triazolam[b]
Calcium Channel Blockers	dihydropyridines (including nisoldipine[b]), verapamil
Ergot Alkaloids	dihydroergotamine[b], ergometrine (ergonovine)[b], ergotamine[b], methylergometrine (methylergonovine)[b]
Gastrointestinal Motility Agents	cisapride[b]
Glucocorticosteroids	budesonide, dexamethasone, methylprednisolone, fluticasone
HMG-CoA Reductase Inhibitors	atorvastatin, cerivastatin, lovastatin[b], simvastatin[b]
5-HT_1 Receptor Agonists	eletriptan[b]
Immunosuppressants	cyclosporine, tacrolimus, sirolimus
Oral Hypoglycemics	oral hypoglycemics (i.e. repaglinide)
Protease Inhibitors	indinavir, ritonavir, saquinavir
Oral Anticoagulants	warfarin
Other	alfentanil, buspirone, trazodone, trimetrexate, fentanyl, levacetylmethadol (levomethadyl)[b], halofantrine, cilostazol
Decrease plasma concentration of itraconazole	
Anticonvulsants	carbamazepine, phenobarbital, phenytoin
Antimycobacterials	isoniazid, rifabutin, rifampin
Gastric Acid Suppressors/Neutralizers	antacids, H_2-receptor antagonists, proton pump inhibitors
Non-nucleoside Reverse Transcriptase Inhibitors	nevirapine
Increase plasma concentration of itraconazole	
Macrolide Antibiotics	clarithromycin, erythromycin
Protease Inhibitors	indinavir, lopinavir/ritonavir, ritonavir

(cont'd)

Table 2: SPORANOX Oral Solution *(cont'd)*

a This list is not all-inclusive.
b Contraindicated with SPORANOX based on clinical and/or pharmacokinetic studies (see Warnings and Precautions and below).
c For information on parenterally administered midazolam, see the benzodiazepine paragraph below.

Antiarrhythmics: The class IA antiarrhythmics quinidine and disopyramide and class III antiarrhythmics, such as dofetilide, are known to prolong the QT interval. Coadministration of quinidine or dofetilide with SPORANOX may increase plasma concentrations of quinidine or dofetilide which could result in serious cardiovascular events. Therefore, concomitant administration of SPORANOX and quinidine or dofetilide is contraindicated (see Contraindications and Warnings and Precautions).

Concomitant administration of digoxin or disopyramide and SPORANOX has led to clinically significant increases in plasma concentrations of digoxin (likely via inhibition of P-glycoprotein) or disopyramide. Patients should be carefully monitored if SPORANOX is coadministered with either of these drugs.

Anticonvulsants: Reduced plasma concentrations of itraconazole were reported when SPORANOX was administered concomitantly with phenytoin. Carbamazepine, phenobarbital, and phenytoin are all inducers of CYP3A4. Although interactions with carbamazepine and phenobarbital have not been studied, concomitant administration of SPORANOX and these drugs would be expected to result in decreased plasma concentrations of itraconazole. In addition, in vivo studies have demonstrated an increase in plasma carbamazepine concentrations in subjects concomitantly receiving ketoconazole. Although there are no data regarding the effect of itraconazole on carbamazepine metabolism, because of the similarities between ketoconazole and itraconazole, concomitant administration of SPORANOX and carbamazepine may inhibit the metabolism of carbamazepine.

Antimycobacterials: Drug interaction studies have demonstrated that plasma concentrations of azole antifungal agents and their metabolites, including itraconazole and hydroxy-itraconazole, were significantly decreased when these agents were given concomitantly with rifabutin or rifampin. In vivo data suggest that rifabutin is metabolized in part by CYP3A4. SPORANOX may inhibit the metabolism of rifabutin. Although no formal study data are available for isoniazid, similar effects should be anticipated. Therefore, the efficacy of SPORANOX could be substantially reduced if given concomitantly with one of these agents. Coadministration is not recommended.

Antineoplastics: SPORANOX may inhibit the metabolism of busulfan, docetaxel, and vinca alkaloids.

Antipsychotics: Pimozide is known to prolong the QT interval and is partially metabolized by CYP3A4. Coadministration of pimozide with SPORANOX could result in serious cardiovascular events. Therefore, concomitant administration of SPORANOX and pimozide is contraindicated (see Contraindications and Warnings and Precautions).

Benzodiazepines: Concomitant administration of SPORANOX and alprazolam, diazepam, oral midazolam, or triazolam could lead to increased plasma concentrations of these benzodiazepines. Increased plasma concentrations could potentiate and prolong hypnotic and sedative effects. Concomitant administration of SPORANOX and oral midazolam or triazolam is contraindicated (see Contraindications and Warnings and Precautions). If midazolam is administered parenterally, special precaution and patient monitoring is required since the sedative effect may be prolonged.

Calcium Channel Blockers: Edema has been reported in patients concomitantly receiving SPORANOX and dihydropyridine calcium channel blockers. Appropriate dosage adjustment may be necessary.

Calcium channel blockers can have a negative inotropic effect which may be additive to those of itraconazole; itraconazole can inhibit the metabolism of calcium channel blockers such as dihydropyridines (e.g., nifedipine and felodipine) and verapamil. Therefore, caution should be used when coadministering itraconazole and calcium channel blockers due to an increased risk of CHF. Concomitant administration of SPORANOX and nisoldipine is contraindicated (see Warnings and Precautions and Adverse Reactions, Post-Market Adverse Drug Reactions for more information).

Ergot Alkaloids: Concomitant administration of SPORANOX with ergot alkaloids, such as dihydroergotamine, ergometrine (ergonovine), ergotamine and methylergometrine (methylergonovine) is contraindicated due to the risk of cerebral and/or peripheral ischemia (see Contraindications). In some cases, concomitant use of potent CYP3A4 inhibitors (protease inhibitors, macrolide antibiotics and antifungal agents) with ergot alkaloids has resulted in serious and/or life-threatening ischemia, including fatalities and cases of gangrene.

Gastric Acid Suppressors/Neutralizers: Reduced plasma concentrations of itraconazole were reported when SPORANOX capsules were administered concomitantly with H_2-receptor antagonists. Studies have shown that absorption of itraconazole is impaired when gastric acid production is decreased. Therefore, SPORANOX should be administered with a cola beverage if the patient has achlorhydria or is taking H_2-receptor antagonists or other gastric acid suppressors. Antacids should be administered at least 1 hour before or 2 hours after administration of SPORANOX capsules. In a clinical study, when SPORANOX capsules were administered with omeprazole (a proton pump inhibitor), the bioavailability of itraconazole was significantly reduced. However, as itraconazole is already dissolved in SPORANOX oral solution, the effect of H_2-receptor antagonists is expected to be substantially less than the capsules. Nevertheless, caution is advised when the two drugs are coadministered.

Gastrointestinal Motility Agents: Coadministration of SPORANOX with cisapride can elevate plasma cisapride concentrations which could result in serious cardiovascular events. Therefore, concomitant administration of SPORANOX with cisapride is contraindicated (see Contraindications and Warnings and Precautions).

Glucocorticosteroids: SPORANOX markedly increased systemic exposure to oral and intravenous dexamethasone (3.7-fold and 3.3-fold increases, respectively), inhaled budesonide (4.2-fold increase), fluticasone and methylprednisolone, and enhanced their adrenal-suppressant effect. Careful follow-up is recommended when itraconazole is coadministered with these drugs.

HMG-CoA Reductase Inhibitors: Human pharmacokinetic data suggest that SPORANOX inhibits the metabolism of atorvastatin, cerivastatin, lovastatin, and simvastatin, which may increase the risk of skeletal muscle toxicity, including rhabdomyolysis. Concomitant administration of SPORANOX with HMG-CoA reductase inhibitors, such as lovastatin and simvastatin, is contraindicated (see Contraindications and Warnings and Precautions).

5-HT_1 Receptor Agonists: Coadministration of eletriptan with SPORANOX can elevate plasma eletriptan concentrations which could result in serious adverse events. Therefore, concomitant use of eletriptan with SPORANOX is contraindicated (see Contraindications).

Immunosuppressants: Concomitant administration of SPORANOX and cyclosporine, tacrolimus or sirolimus has led to increased plasma concentrations of these immunosuppressants.

Macrolide Antibiotics: Erythromycin and clarithromycin are known inhibitors of CYP3A4 (see Table 2) and may increase plasma concentrations of itraconazole. In a small pharmacokinetic study involving HIV-infected patients, clarithromycin was shown to increase plasma concentrations of itraconazole. Similarly, following administration of 1 gram of erythromycin ethyl succinate and 200 mg itraconazole as single doses, the mean C_{max} and $AUC_{0-\infty}$ of itraconazole increased by 44% (90% CI: 119-175%) and 36% (90% CI: 108-171%), respectively.

Non-nucleoside Reverse Transcriptase Inhibitors: Nevirapine is an inducer of CYP3A4. In vivo studies have shown that nevirapine induces the metabolism of ketoconazole, significantly reducing the bioavailability of ketoconazole. Studies involving nevirapine and itraconazole have not been conducted. However, because of the similarities between ketoconazole and itraconazole, concomitant administration of SPORANOX and nevirapine is not recommended.

Nucleoside Reverse Transcriptase Inhibitors: In a clinical study, when 8 HIV-infected subjects were treated concomitantly with SPORANOX capsules 100 mg twice daily and the nucleoside reverse transcriptase inhibitor zidovudine 8±0.4 mg/kg/day, the pharmacokinetics of zidovudine were not affected. Other nucleoside reverse transcriptase inhibitors have not been studied.

Oral Anticoagulants: SPORANOX enhances the anticoagulant effect of coumarin-like drugs, such as warfarin.

Oral Hypoglycemic Agents: Severe hypoglycemia has been reported in patients concomitantly receiving azole antifungal agents and oral hypoglycemic agents. Blood glucose concentrations should be carefully monitored when SPORANOX and oral hypoglycemic agents are coadministered.

Polyenes: Prior treatment with itraconazole, like other azoles, may reduce or inhibit the activity of polyenes such as amphotericin B. However, the clinical significance of this drug effect has not been clearly defined.

Protease Inhibitors: Concomitant administration of SPORANOX and protease inhibitors metabolized by CYP3A4, such as indinavir, ritonavir, and saquinavir, may increase plasma concentrations of these protease inhibitors. In addition, concomitant administration of SPORANOX and indinavir and ritonavir (but not saquinavir) may increase plasma concentrations of itraconazole. Coadministration of lopinavir/ritonavir and itraconazole leads to significant increase of itraconazole concentrations. Caution is advised when SPORANOX and protease inhibitors must be given concomitantly.

Other:

- Levacetylmethadol (levomethadyl) is known to prolong the QT interval and is metabolized by CYP3A4. Co-administration of levacetylmethadol with SPORANOX could result in serious cardiovascular events. Therefore, concomitant administration of SPORANOX and levacetylmethadol is contraindicated.

- Halofantrine has the potential to prolong the QT interval at high plasma concentrations. Caution is advised when SPORANOX and halofantrine are administered concomitantly.
- In vitro data suggest that alfentanil is metabolized by CYP3A4. Administration with SPORANOX may increase plasma concentrations of alfentanil.
- Human pharmacokinetic data suggest that concomitant administration of SPORANOX and buspirone results in significant increases in plasma concentrations of buspirone.
- Itraconazole may lead to substantial increases in trazodone plasma concentrations with the potential for adverse effects. A lower dose of trazodone should be considered.
- In vitro data suggest that trimetrexate is extensively metabolized by CYP3A4. An in vitro rat liver model demonstrated that ketoconazole potently inhibits the metabolism of trimetrexate. Although there are no data regarding the effect of itraconazole on trimetrexate metabolism, because of the similarities between ketoconazole and itraconazole, concomitant administration of SPORANOX and trimetrexate may inhibit the metabolism of trimetrexate.
- Cilostazol is a CYP 3A4 metabolized drug that should be used with caution when co-administered with SPORANOX.
- Fentanyl plasma concentrations could be increased or prolonged by concomitant use of SPORANOX and may cause potentially fatal respiratory depression.

Drug-Food Interactions: For optimal absorption, SPORANOX oral solution should be taken without food.
Drug-Herb Interactions: Interactions with herbal products have not been established.
Drug-Laboratory Interactions: Interactions with laboratory tests have not been established.

DOSAGE AND ADMINISTRATION: Dosing Considerations: When SPORANOX oral solution may be indicated, the type of organism responsible for the infection should be isolated and identified; however, therapy may be initiated prior to obtaining these results, when clinically warranted.

For optimal absorption, itraconazole oral solution should be taken without food.

Patients with Hepatic Impairment: Limited data are available on the use of oral itraconazole in patients with hepatic impairment. Caution should be exercised when this drug is administered in this patient population (see Warnings and Precautions, Hepatic/Biliary/Pancreatic, Hepatic Effects/Use in Patients with Hepatic Impairment; Action and Clinical Pharmacology, Special Populations and Conditions, Hepatic Insufficiency).

Patients with Renal Impairment: Limited data are available on the use of oral itraconazole in patients with renal impairment. Caution should be exercised when this drug is administered in this patient population (see Warnings and Precautions, Renal, Use in Patients with Renal Insufficiency; Action and Clinical Pharmacology, Special Populations and Conditions, Renal Insufficiency).

Recommended Dose and Dosage Adjustment: Oral Candidiasis: The recommended dosage of itraconazole oral solution for oral candidiasis is 200 mg daily in a single dose or divided doses; treatment should continue for 1-2 weeks to decrease the likelihood of relapse.

Esophageal Candidiasis: The recommended dosage for esophageal candidiasis is 100 mg daily for a minimum treatment of three weeks. Treatment should continue for two weeks following resolution of symptoms. Doses of up to 200 mg per day may be used based on medical assessment of the patient's response to therapy.

Administration: The solution should be swished in the oral cavity and swallowed. There should be no rinsing after swallowing.

OVERDOSAGE:
There is no experience of overdosage with SPORANOX oral solution; however, based on animal toxicity data, symptoms of a gastrointestinal or central nervous system nature may be expected to occur.

Although no data are available for SPORANOX, administration of activated charcoal absorbs almost all commonly ingested drugs, and should be administered as quickly as possible to most patients who ingest potentially toxic amounts. Standard supportive treatment should be applied as necessary.

It has been reported that itraconazole cannot be removed by dialysis. No specific antidote is available.

> For management of a suspected drug overdose, contact your regional Poison Control Centre. See the *CPS Directory* section for a list of Poison Control Centres.

ACTION AND CLINICAL PHARMACOLOGY: Mechanism of Action: Itraconazole, a triazole derivative, has a broad-spectrum activity; with respect to Candida spp., its activity includes *C. albicans*, *C. glabrata* and *C. krusei*.

In vitro studies have demonstrated that itraconazole impairs the synthesis of ergosterol in fungal cells. Ergosterol is a vital cell membrane component in fungi. Impairment of its synthesis ultimately results in an antifungal effect.

Pharmacokinetics: Absorption: The oral bioavailability of itraconazole is maximal when SPORANOX oral solution is taken without food. During chronic administration, steady-state is reached after 1-2 weeks. Peak plasma levels are observed 2 hours (fasting) to 5 hours (with food) following oral administration. After repeated once-a-day administration of itraconazole 200 mg in fasting condition, steady-state plasma concentrations of itraconazole fluctuate between 1 and 2 µg/mL (trough to peak). When the oral solution is taken with food, steady-state plasma concentrations of itraconazole are about 25% lower.

Distribution: The plasma protein binding of itraconazole is 99.8%. Itraconazole is extensively distributed into tissues that are prone to fungal invasion. Concentrations in human lung, kidney, liver, bone, stomach, spleen and muscle were found to be two to three times higher than the corresponding plasma concentration.

Metabolism: Itraconazole is extensively metabolized by the liver into a large number of metabolites. One of the metabolites is hydroxy-itraconazole, which has in vitro a comparable antifungal activity to itraconazole. Plasma levels of hydroxy-itraconazole are about two times higher than those of itraconazole.

Excretion: After repeated oral administration, elimination of itraconazole from plasma is biphasic with a terminal half-life of 1.5 days. Fecal excretion of the parent drug varies between 3%-18% of the dose. Renal excretion of the parent drug is less than 0.03% of the dose. About 35% of the dose is excreted as metabolites in the urine within one week.

Special Populations and Conditions: Pediatrics: Limited pharmacokinetic data are available in pediatric patients.
Geriatrics: No data are available in geriatric patients.
Hepatic Insufficiency: Itraconazole is predominantly metabolized in the liver. Pharmacokinetic data for patients with hepatic insufficiency is limited to subjects who received a single 100 mg dose of SPORANOX capsules. A pharmacokinetic study using a single 100 mg dose of itraconazole (one 100 mg capsule) was conducted in 6 healthy and 12 cirrhotic subjects. A statistically significant reduction in mean C_{max} (47%; mean cirrhotic C_{max} 87±18ng/mL, mean healthy C_{max} 164±34 ng/mL) and a twofold increase in the elimination half-life (37±7 hrs and 16±5 hrs, respectively) of itraconazole were noted in cirrhotic subjects compared with healthy subjects. However, overall exposure to itraconazole, based on AUC was similar in cirrhotic patients and in healthy subjects (mean cirrhotic AUC 1449±207 ng·h/mL, mean healthy AUC 1856±388 ng·h/mL). Data are not available in cirrhotic patients during long-term use of itraconazole Patients with impaired hepatic function should be carefully monitored when taking itraconazole. The prolonged elimination half-life of itraconazole observed in cirrhotic patients should be considered when deciding to initiate therapy with other medicines metabolized by CYP3A4 (see Warnings and Precautions, Hepatic/Biliary/Pancreatic).

Renal Insufficiency: Limited data are available on the use of itraconazole in patients with renal insufficiency. Caution should be exercised when the drug is administered in this patient population (see Warnings and Precautions, Renal). Pharmacokinetic data in renally impaired patients is limited to subjects who received a single 200 mg dose of SPORANOX capsules. A pharmacokinetic study using a single 200 mg dose of itraconazole (four 50 mg capsules) was conducted in three groups of patients with renal impairment (uremia: n=7; hemodialysis: n=7; continuous ambulatory peritoneal dialysis: n=5). Mean±SD pharmacokinetic parameters are summarized in Table 3.

Table 3: SPORANOX Oral Solution

Mean Pharmacokinetic Parameters in Renally Impaired Patients Receiving a Single 200 mg Oral Dose of Itraconazole

Patient Group (n)	T_{max} (h)	C_{max} (ng/mL)	$AUC_{0\text{-}8h}$ (ng·h/mL)
Uremic (7)	4.0±1.2	213±178	1026±819
Hemodialysis			
Off dialysis (7)	4.7±1.4	140±119	634±507
On dialysis (7)	4.1±0.9	113±83	507±371
CAPD (5)	4.4±2.2	77±29	325±107

Plasma concentration vs. time profiles showed wide inter-subject variation in all three groups. In uremic subjects (mean CrCl 13 mL/min/1.73 m²), mean plasma concentrations and overall exposure, based on AUC_{∞}, were slightly reduced compared with healthy subject in a previous study (AUC_{∞} values of 3454±3132 vs. 4161±1949 ng hr/mL in uremic patients and healthy subjects, respectively). C_{max} and $AUC_{0\text{-}8h}$ values were reduced 30-40% in hemodialysis patients on non-dialysis days, compared to uremic patients (see Table 3), and further reduced 10-20% on dialysis days. In CAPD patients, C_{max} and $AUC_{0\text{-}8h}$ values were reduced to one-third the values seen in non-dialyzed uremic patients.

Cystic Fibrosis: In cystic fibrosis patients, variability in therapeutic levels of itraconazole was observed with steady-state dosing of oral solution using 2.5 mg/kg b.i.d. Steady-state concentrations of >250 ng/mL were achieved in approximately 50% of subjects greater than 16 years of age, but in none of the patients less than 16 years of age. If a patient does not respond to SPORANOX oral solution, consideration should be given to switching to alternative therapy.

STORAGE AND STABILITY: SPORANOX oral solution should be stored at 15-25°C. Discard remaining unused product three months after opening bottle. Keep out of the reach of children.

INFORMATION FOR THE PATIENT: Published in e-CPS, available by subscription at www.e-cps.ca.

DOSAGE FORMS, COMPOSITION AND PACKAGING: Each mL of oral solution contains: itraconazole 10 mg. Nonmedicinal ingredients: caramel flavour, cherry flavour 1 and 2, hydrochloric acid, hydroxypropyl-β-cyclodextrin, propylene glycol, purified water, sodium hydroxide, sodium saccharin and sorbitol. Amber glass bottles of 150 mL.

(Shown in Product Identification Section)

Sprycel™ Ⓟ
dasatinib
Protein-tyrosine Kinase Inhibitor

Bristol-Myers Squibb

Date of Preparation: March 22, 2007
Date of Revision: May 12, 2010

SUMMARY PRODUCT INFORMATION:

Route of Administration	Dosage Form/ Strength	Clinically Relevant Nonmedicinal Ingredients
Oral	Tablet 20 mg, 50 mg, 70 mg and 100 mg	Lactose monohydrate For a complete listing see Dosage Forms, Composition and Packaging.

INDICATIONS AND CLINICAL USE: SPRYCEL (dasatinib) is indicated for the treatment of adults with Philadelphia chromosome positive (Ph+) chronic, accelerated, or blast phase chronic myeloid leukemia (CML) with resistance or intolerance to prior therapy including imatinib mesylate.

Approval of SPRYCEL in CML is based on the rates of hematologic and cytogenetic responses in clinical trials with a minimum of 24 months of follow-up.

SPRYCEL is also indicated for the treatment of adults with Ph+ acute lymphoblastic leukemia (ALL) with resistance or intolerance to prior therapy.

Approval in Ph+ ALL is based on the rates of hematologic and cytogenetic responses in clinical trials with a minimum of 24 months of follow-up.

Geriatrics (>65 years of age): While the safety profile of SPRYCEL in the geriatric population was similar to that in the younger population, patients aged 65 years and older are more likely to experience fluid retention, congestive heart failure, gastrointestinal bleeding and dyspnea events and should be monitored closely. No differences in efficacy were observed between older and younger patients. However, in the two randomized studies in patients with chronic phase CML, the rates of major cytogenetic response (MCyR) were lower among patients aged 65 years and older (42% MCyR in patients ≥65 years versus 56% MCyR in the rest of the study population and 47% MCyR in patients ≥65 years versus 68% MCyR in the rest of the study population in studies CA180017 and CA180034, respectively).

Pediatrics (<18 years of age): The safety and efficacy of SPRYCEL in patients <18 years of age have not been established (see Warnings and Precautions, Special Populations).

CONTRAINDICATIONS: Use of SPRYCEL is contraindicated in patients with hypersensitivity to dasatinib or to any other component of SPRYCEL.

WARNINGS AND PRECAUTIONS:

> **Serious Warnings and Precautions**
> - SPRYCEL (dasatinib) should only be prescribed by a qualified physician who is experienced in the use of antineoplastic therapy.
> - Myelosuppression (thrombocytopenia, neutropenia, and anemia (see Warnings and Precautions, Myelosuppression).
> - Hemorrhage, including fatal outcomes (see Warnings and Precautions, Hemorrhage).
> - Fluid retention, pleural effusion, pericardial effusion (see Warnings and Precautions, Fluid Retention).
> - Congestive heart failure, pulmonary edema (see Warnings and Precautions, Fluid Retention and Cardiovascular).

Myelosuppression: Treatment with SPRYCEL (dasatinib) is associated with thrombocytopenia, neutropenia, and anemia. Their occurrence is more frequent in patients with advanced phase CML or Ph+ ALL than in chronic phase CML. Complete blood counts should be performed weekly for the first 2 months and then monthly thereafter, or as clinically indicated. Myelosuppression was generally reversible and usually managed by withholding SPRYCEL temporarily or dose reduction (see Dosage and Administration and Adverse Reactions, Abnormal Hematologic and Clinical Chemistry Findings). Severe (CTC Grade 3 or 4) cases of anemia were managed with blood transfusions. Packed red blood cells were transfused in 30% of chronic phase CML patients and 79% of myeloid blast phase CML patients. Platelet transfusions were required in 17% of chronic phase CML patients and 66% of myeloid blast phase CML patients.

In a Phase III dose-optimization study in patients with chronic phase CML, Grade 3 or 4 myelosuppression was reported less frequently in patients treated with 100 mg once daily (neutropenia 35%, thrombocytopenia 23% and anemia 13%) than in patients treated with 70 mg twice daily (neutropenia 45%, thrombocytopenia 38% and anemia 18%) (see Adverse Reactions).

Hemorrhage: Patients were excluded from participation in initial SPRYCEL (dasatinib) clinical studies if they took medications that inhibit platelet function or anticoagulants. In subsequent trials, the use of anticoagulants, aspirin, and non-steroidal anti-inflammatory drugs (NSAIDs) was allowed concurrently with SPRYCEL if the platelet count was >50 000.

Overall, 198 (9.1%) patients experienced Grade 3-4 bleeding. Fifty (2%) patients experienced fatal bleeding.

Intracranial hemorrhage occurred in 48 (2.2%) of patients, of which 21 (0.96%) cases were considered related to SPRYCEL. Intracranial hemorrhage was fatal in 19 (0.9%) patients, of which nine (0.4%) were considered related to SPRYCEL.

Gastrointestinal hemorrhage regardless of relationship to SPRYCEL occurred in 13% of patients. The bleeding was severe in 6% of patients and generally required treatment interruptions and packed cell transfusions. Other episodes of severe bleeding occurred in 3% of patients.

Fluid Retention: SPRYCEL is associated with fluid retention, which was severe in 11% of patients, including severe pleural and pericardial effusion reported in 7% and 2% of patients, respectively (see Adverse Reactions). Severe ascites and generalized edema were each reported in ≤1% of patients. Other manifestations of fluid retention included pulmonary edema (3%), congestive heart failure/cardiac dysfunction (4%), and pericardial effusion (5%). Nineteen patients had severe pulmonary edema. Patients who develop symptoms suggestive of pleural effusion such as dyspnea or dry cough should be evaluated by chest X-ray.

Fluid retention events were typically managed by supportive care measures that include diuretics or short courses of steroids. Pleural effusion required oxygen in some cases and at least one thoracentesis in 64 (3%) patients.

In the Phase III dose-optimization study in patients with chronic phase CML, Grade 3 or 4 fluid retention events were reported less frequently in patients treated with 100 mg once daily (5%) than in patients treated with 70 mg twice daily (11%) (see Adverse Reactions).

Cardiovascular: Patients were excluded from enrolment of dasatinib trials for a broad range of cardiac events or conditions. A significantly abnormal ECG at screening was also an exclusion criterion. No prospective evaluation of cardiac function was carried out.

Congestive heart failure/cardiac dysfunction was reported in 96 (4%) of subjects during the study, of which 49 (2%) were considered to be severe. In some cases, the event was triggered by an acute volume load, including transfusion of blood products.

QT Prolongation: In vitro data suggest that dasatinib and its N-dealkylated metabolite, BMS-582691 have the potential to prolong cardiac ventricular repolarization (QT interval, see Safety Pharmacology). In 865 patients with leukemia treated with SPRYCEL in Phase II clinical studies, the mean changes from baseline in QTcF interval were 4-6 msec; the upper 95% confidence intervals for all mean changes from baseline were <7 msec and lower 95% confidence interval for all mean changes from baseline were >−2 msec. Of the 2182 patients who received SPRYCEL in clinical studies, 21 patients (<1%) experienced a QTcF >500 msec.

SPRYCEL should be administered with caution in patients who have or may develop prolongation of QTc. These include patients with hypokalemia or hypomagnesemia, patients with congenital long QT syndrome, patients taking anti arrhythmic medicines or other medicinal products that lead to QT prolongation, and cumulative high-dose anthracycline therapy.

Hypokalemia or hypomagnesemia should be corrected prior to administration of SPRYCEL. (See Drug-Drug Interactions and Action and Clinical Pharmacology, Electrocardiogram.)

Hepatic Impairment: The effect of hepatic impairment on the single-dose pharmacokinetics of dasatinib was assessed in 8 moderately hepatic impaired subjects who received a 50-mg dose and 5 severely hepatic-impaired subjects who received a 20-mg dose compared to matched healthy subjects who received a 70-mg dose of SPRYCEL. Hepatic impairment did not result in clinically meaningful change in dasatinib exposure at the doses studied. However no pharmacokinetic information is available from patients with hepatic impairment treated with a 70-100 mg dose of SPRYCEL (see Action and Clinical Pharmacology, Pharmacokinetics, Special Populations and Conditions). Due to the limitations of this clinical study, caution is recommended in patients with hepatic impairment.

In nonclinical studies, increased liver weight and foci of hepatocellular alteration were observed in rats, and hepatocellular vacuolation was observed in monkeys following repeat dose administration of dasatinib (6 to 9 months). Increased ALT was observed in monkeys, and increased AST and/or decreased albumin were observed in rats and monkeys.

In clinical studies, 4 cases of hepatotoxicity, 2 cases of cytolytic hepatitis, 1 case of hepatic steatosis and 1 case of hepatitis were observed.

Renal Impairment: There are currently no clinical studies with SPRYCEL in patients with impaired renal function (clinical studies have excluded patients with serum creatinine concentration >1.5 times the upper limit of the normal range). Dasatinib and its metabolites are minimally excreted via the kidney. Since the renal excretion of unchanged dasatinib and its metabolites is <4%, a decrease in total body clearance is not expected in patients with renal insufficiency. The effect of dialysis on dasatinib pharmacokinetics has not been studied.

Rhabdomyolysis: Cases of rhabdomyolysis with acute renal failure have been reported. Patients with muscle symptoms (muscle aches/pains) should be investigated to rule out rhabdomyolysis (elevated creatine kinase, elevated serum creatinine, hyperkalemia, hyperphosphatemia, brown urine, elevated ALT and AST).

Carcinogenesis and Mutagenesis: Carcinogenicity studies were not performed with dasatinib.

Dasatinib was clastogenic in vitro to dividing Chinese hamster ovary cells with and without metabolic activation at concentrations ranging from 5 to 60 μg/mL. Dasatinib was not mutagenic when tested in in vitro bacterial cell assays (Ames test) and was not genotoxic in an in vivo rat micronucleus study.

Drug-Drug Interactions: CYP3A4 Inhibitors: Concomitant use of dasatinib and medicinal products that potently inhibit CYP3A4 (e.g. ketoconazole, itraconazole, erythromycin, clarithromycin, ritonavir, atazanavir, lopinavir, grapefruit juice) may increase exposure to dasatinib. Therefore, in patients receiving SPRYCEL, coadministration of a potent CYP3A4 inhibitor is not recommended. Selection of an alternate concomitant medication with no or minimal CYP3A4 inhibition potential is recommended. If systemic administration of a potent CYP3A4 inhibitor cannot be avoided, close monitoring for toxicity and a SPRYCEL dose reduction to 20 or 40 mg daily should be considered (see Drug Interactions and Dosage and Administration).

CYP3A4 Inducers: Concomitant use of dasatinib and medicinal products that induce CYP3A4 (e.g. dexamethasone, phenytoin, carbamazepine, rifampicin, phenobarbital or Hypericum perforatum, also known as St. John's Wort) may substantially reduce exposure to dasatinib, potentially increasing the risk of therapeutic failure. In addition, more healthy male subjects experienced increases in QTcF of >30 msec from the baseline ECG recordings when dasatinib and rifampicin were administered 12 hours apart compared to when dasatinib was administered alone (25% vs. 10%). No subject experienced QTcF >450 msec or a change from baseline >60 msec (see Drug Interactions). Therefore, concomitant use of potent CYP3A4 inducers with dasatinib is not recommended. In patients in whom rifampicin or other CYP3A4 inducers are indicated, alternative agents with less enzyme induction potential should be used.

CYP3A4 Substrates: Concomitant use of dasatinib and a CYP3A4 substrate may increase exposure to the CYP3A4 substrate. In addition, three healthy subjects (n=48) experienced increases in QTcF of >30 msec from the baseline ECG recordings following concomitant use of a single dose of dasatinib and simvastatin. No subject experienced QTcF >450 msec or a change from baseline >60 msec (see Drug Interactions). Therefore, caution is warranted when SPRYCEL is co-administered with a drug that potentially alters CYP3A4 activity, a QTc prolonger, or CYP3A4 substrates of narrow therapeutic index such as macrolide antibiotics, benzodiazepine, pimozide, quinidine, or ergot alkaloids (ergotamine, dihydroergotamine). The effect of a CYP3A4 substrate on the pharmacokinetic parameters of dasatinib has not been studied.

H2 Antagonists or Proton Pump Inhibitors: Long-term suppression of gastric acid secretion by H2 antagonists or proton pump inhibitors (e.g. famotidine and omeprazole) is likely to reduce dasatinib exposure (see Drug Interactions). **The use of antacids should be considered in place of H2 antagonists or proton pump inhibitors in patients receiving SPRYCEL therapy.**

Antacids: Concomitant use of dasatinib and aluminum hydroxide/magnesium hydroxide may reduce exposure to dasatinib. However, **aluminum hydroxide/magnesium hydroxide products may be administered up to 2 hours prior to, or 2 hours following the administration of dasatinib** (see Drug Interactions).

Antiemetics: No information is available on the safety of concomitant use of dasatanib with antiemetics (prochlorperazine, metochlopramide, 5-HT3 inhibitors).

Lactose: SPRYCEL tablets 20 mg, 50 mg, 70 mg and 100 mg contain lactose in proportional amounts of 27 mg, 67.5 mg, 94.5 mg and 135 mg, respectively. SPRYCEL therefore contains 189 mg of lactose in the 140 mg daily dose of dasatinib and 135 mg in the 100 mg daily dose. Patients with rare hereditary problems of galactose intolerance, the Lapp lactase deficiency or glucose-galactose malabsorption should not take dasatinib.

Special Populations: Pregnant Women: There are no adequate data from the use of dasatinib in pregnant women. Studies in animals have shown that at concentrations which are readily achievable in humans receiving therapeutic doses of SPRYCEL, fetal toxicity was observed in both pregnant rats and rabbits. Fetal death was observed in rats. The potential risk for humans is unknown.

SPRYCEL is, therefore, not recommended for use in women who are pregnant or contemplating pregnancy. If SPRYCEL is used during pregnancy, or if the patient becomes pregnant while taking SPRYCEL, the patient should be apprised of the potential hazard to the fetus.

Nursing Women: It is unknown whether SPRYCEL is excreted in human milk. Women who are taking SPRYCEL should not breastfeed.

Pediatrics (<18 years of age): The safety and efficacy of SPRYCEL in patients <18 years of age have not been established.

Geriatrics (>65 years of age): Of the 2182 patients in clinical studies of SPRYCEL, 547 (25%) were 65 years of age and older and 105 (5%) were 75 years of age and older. While the safety profile of SPRYCEL in the geriatric population was similar to that in the younger population, patients aged 65 years and older are more likely to experience fluid retention, congestive heart failure, gastrointestinal bleeding and dyspnea events and should be monitored closely. No differences in efficacy were observed between older and younger patients. However, in the two randomized studies in patients with chronic phase CML, the rates of major cytogenetic response (MCyR) were lower among patients aged 65 years and older (42% MCyR in patients ≥65 years versus 56% MCyR in the rest of the study population and 47% MCyR in patients ≥65 years versus 68% MCyR in the rest of the study population in studies CA180017 and CA180034, respectively).

Sexual Function/Reproduction: The effects of SPRYCEL on male and female fertility are not known. The potential effects of SPRYCEL on sperm have not been studied. Sexually active male or female patients taking SPRYCEL should use adequate contraception.

Monitoring and Laboratory Tests: Complete blood counts should be performed weekly for the first 2 months and then monthly thereafter, or as clinically indicated (see Warnings and Precautions, Myelosuppression). Hepatic function tests (AST, ALT and bilirubin), CK and renal function tests should be performed every two weeks for the first 2 months and then monthly thereafter or as clinically indicated (see Warnings and Precautions, Hepatic Impairment and Rhabdomyolysis).

ADVERSE REACTIONS: Adverse Drug Reaction Overview: The data described below reflect exposure to SPRYCEL in 2182 patients with leukemia in clinical studies (1850 patients treated with 140 mg once daily or 70 mg twice daily and 332 patients treated with 50 mg twice daily or 100 mg once daily. The median duration of therapy was 15 months (range <1-31 months).

The majority of SPRYCEL-treated patients experienced adverse reactions at some time. Most reactions were mild to moderate. SPRYCEL was discontinued due to study drug toxicity in 8-15% of patients in all stages of CML or Ph+ ALL.

The most frequently reported adverse events, in the pooled safety data of 2182 patients, regardless of causality or severity, were diarrhea, fluid retention, headache, musculoskeletal pain, hemorrhage, pyrexia, fatigue, infection, skin rash, nausea, dyspnea, cough, upper respiratory tract infection/inflammation, vomiting, pain and abdominal pain.

Clinical Trial Adverse Drug Reactions in Patients Treated with SPRYCEL: All treatment-emergent adverse events (excluding laboratory abnormalities), regardless of relationship to study drug, that were reported in at least 5% of the patients treated with SPRYCEL in clinical studies are shown in Table 1 for chronic phase CML and Table 2 for advanced phase CML and Ph+ALL.

In the Phase III dose-optimization study exploring lower doses of SPRYCEL (100 mg/day) in patients with chronic phase CML, the median duration of therapy was approximately 22 months (range <1-30 months). In the Phase III dose-optimization study exploring the once daily schedule of SPRYCEL (140 mg once daily) in patients with advanced diseases, the median duration of therapy was 13.62 months (range .03-31.15 months) for accelerated phase CML, 3.19 months (range .03-27.73 months) for myeloid blast CML, 3.55 months (range .10-22.08 months) for lymphoid blast CML, and 2.99 months (range .16-23.46 months) for Ph+ ALL.

Table 1: SPRYCEL

Adverse Events Reported in ≥5% of Patients in Clinical Studies of Chronic Phase CML (Recommended Starting Dose: 100 mg Once Daily)

	Phase III								All Other	
	100 mg QD n=165		50 mg BID[a] n=167		140 mg QD[a] n=163		70 mg BID[a] n=167		70 mg BID[a] n=488	
	Percent (%) of Patients									
Preferred Term	All Grades	Grade 3/4	All Grades	Grade 3/4	All Grades	Grade 3/4	All Grades	Grade 3/4	All Grades	Grade 3/4
Headache	45	1	35	1	45	4	46	4	46	2
Musculoskeletal pain	45	3	31	2	44	2	35	5	46	3
Infection (including bacterial, viral, fungal, non-specified)	42	5	36	2	39	4	37	4	47	7
Upper respiratory tract infection/inflammation	40	1	47	2	31	0	32	1	47	2
Diarrhea	38	3	42	5	43	4	46	7	51	4
Fluid Retention	33	5	38	5	45	9	43	11	57	14
Superficial edema	21	0	24	0	21	1	26	1	36	<1
Pleural effusion	14	2	23	4	26	5	25	6	34	9
Generalized edema	4	1	0	0	6	0	1	0	6	1
Congestive heart failure/cardiac dysfunction[b]	2	1	1	1	5	2	7	3	6	4

(cont'd)

Table 1: SPRYCEL *(cont'd)*

Adverse Events Reported in ≥5% of Patients in Clinical Studies of Chronic Phase CML (Recommended Starting Dose: 100 mg Once Daily)

	Phase III								All Other	
	100 mg QD n=165		50 mg BID[a] n=167		140 mg QD[a] n=163		70 mg BID[a] n=167		70 mg BID[a] n=488	
	Percent (%) of Patients									
Preferred Term	**All Grades**	**Grade 3/4**	**All Grades**	**Grade 3/4**	**All Grades**	**Grade 3/4**	**All Grades**	**Grade 3/4**	**All Grades**	**Grade 3/4**
Pericardial effusion	2	1	6	2	6	2	2	1	5	1
Pulmonary edema	1	0	1	1	0	0	3	1	3	1
Ascites	0	0	0	0	0	0	0	0	<1	0
Pulmonary hypertension	0	0	1	0	1	0	2	1	2	1
Fatigue	34	2	31	0	37	2	25	4	47	4
Cough	30	1	30	0	26	1	31	0	37	1
Skin rash	29	2	32	2	37	1	31	2	44	1
Arthralgia	27	2	22	2	25	1	20	4	28	2
Dyspnea	27	2	29	7	31	8	28	6	44	7
Pain	25	1	22	2	24	1	23	1	30	1
Hemorrhage	23	3	23	4	29	2	26	2	33	3
Gastrointestinal bleeding	5	1	8	4	5	1	6	2	7	2
CNS bleeding	0	0	1	0	1	0	0	0	1	0
Nausea	22	1	29	1	32	1	39	2	37	1
Abdominal pain	19	1	24	1	26	4	20	2	29	2
Pyrexia	18	1	26	1	26	0	25	1	37	2
Constipation	16	2	14	1	12	0	10	0	15	<1
Myalgia	16	0	11	0	17	1	12	1	17	1
Chest pain	15	2	14	4	14	1	13	1	17	1
Dizziness	14	1	12	0	15	1	14	2	19	<1
Pruritus	14	1	10	0	13	0	11	0	14	0
Vomiting	14	1	18	2	20	2	29	1	20	1
Neuropathy (including peripheral neuropathy)	12	1	14	1	14	0	10	1	19	1
Pneumonia (including bacterial, viral, and fungal)	11	4	11	4	10	6	14	6	11	5
Hyperhidrosis	10	0	8	0	7	0	5	0	13	0
Insomnia	10	0	6	0	12	0	6	0	11	0
Mucosal inflammation (including mucositis/stomatitis)	10	0	14	0	10	1	11	1	14	<1
Weight increased	10	1	7	0	5	0	6	1	11	<1
Abdominal distension	10	0	8	0	7	0	5	0	13	0
Arrhythmia (including tachycardia)	8	0	6	1	9	1	7	2	11	2
Asthenia	8	1	13	1	9	1	14	0	20	1
Dyspepsia	8	0	7	1	16	0	12	0	11	0
Palpitations	8	0	4	0	2	0	7	0	5	0
Anorexia	7	0	11	2	9	0	13	1	19	<1
Chills	7	0	10	0	7	0	7	0	10	0
Depression	7	1	8	2	7	1	5	1	8	1
Visual disorder	7	0	4	0	4	0	5	0	7	0
Weight decreased	7	0	10	0	12	1	14	1	16	1
Alopecia	6	0	3	0	4	0	7	0	10	0
Enterocolitis infection	6	1	7	1	4	1	8	1	6	1
Hypertension	6	0	6	1	6	1	9	2	8	<1
Urinary frequency	6	1	5	0	7	0	5	0	5	<1
Dry skin	5	0	2	0	3	0	3	0	7	0

(cont'd)

Table 1: SPRYCEL *(cont'd)*

Adverse Events Reported in ≥5% of Patients in Clinical Studies of Chronic Phase CML (Recommended Starting Dose: 100 mg Once Daily)

	Phase III								All Other	
	100 mg QD n=165		50 mg BID[a] n=167		140 mg QD[a] n=163		70 mg BID[a] n=167		70 mg BID[a] n=488	
	Percent (%) of Patients									
Preferred Term	**All Grades**	**Grade 3/4**	**All Grades**	**Grade 3/4**	**All Grades**	**Grade 3/4**	**All Grades**	**Grade 3/4**	**All Grades**	**Grade 3/4**
Muscle inflammation	5	0	10	1	3	0	5	0	10	<1
Acne	5	0	8	1	9	0	10	0	9	<1
Flushing	4	0	4	0	6	0	7	0	9	0
Hypersensitivity (including erythema nodosum)	4	1	1	0	7	2	3	1	4	1
Anxiety	4	0	8	2	6	0	7	0	7	0
Herpes virus infection	4	1	2	0	6	0	5	1	5	<1
Contusion	2	0	7	0	6	0	2	0	7	0
Gastritis	2	0	5	1	7	1	5	1	6	1
Musculoskeletal stiffness	1	0	5	0	2	0	2	0	4	0

[a] Not a recommended starting dosage of SPRYCEL for chronic phase CML. Data provided for context with the dose optimization trial.
[b] Includes ventricular dysfunction, cardiac failure, cardiac failure congestive, cardiomyopathy, congestive cardiomyopathy, diastolic dysfunction, ejection fraction decreased and ventricular failure.

Table 2: SPRYCEL

Adverse Events Reported in ≥5% of Patients in Clinical Studies of Advanced Phase CML and Ph+ALL (Recommended Starting Dose: 140 mg Once Daily)

	Phase III				All Other	
	140 mg QD n=304		70 mg BID[a] n=305		70 mg BID[a] n=423	
	All Grades	**Grade 3/4**	**All Grades**	**Grade 3/4**	**All Grades**	**Grade 3/4**
Preferred Term	Percent (%) of Patients					
Infection	45	14	38	12	51	13
Diarrhea	44	6	49	6	63	10
Hemorrhage	43	12	39	12	59	21
Gastrointestinal bleeding	16	8	18	9	26	13
CNS bleeding	4	1	4	1	4	2
Fluid Retention	42	8	50	12	65	16
Superficial oedema	25	<1	26	2	48	2
Pleural Effusion	24	7	36	8	37	10
Generalised oedema	2	0	5	1	10	1
Congestive heart failure/cardiac dysfunction[b]	3	1	4	2	5	3
Pericardial effusion	2	1	7	2	10	2
Pulmonary oedema	2	1	4	2	6	1
Ascites	<1	<1	1	0	4	1
Pulmonary hypertension	<1	0	2	<1	3	1
Pyrexia	38	3	37	3	59	10
Headache	37	4	33	4	43	4
Musculoskeletal pain	36	7	34	6	50	8
Nausea	33	2	30	3	42	2
Fatigue	29	5	30	5	42	6
Vomiting	27	1	27	3	37	3
Dyspnea	27	6	32	9	40	11
Cough	27	0	30	0	37	1
Skin rash	26	<1	27	2	41	2
Upper respiratory tract infection/inflammation	24	1	24	1	31	3
Pain	23	2	19	1	36	4

(cont'd)

Table 2: SPRYCEL *(cont'd)*

Adverse Events Reported in ≥5% of Patients in Clinical Studies of Advanced Phase CML and Ph+ALL (Recommended Starting Dose: 140 mg Once Daily)

	Phase III				All Other	
	140 mg QD n=304		70 mg BID[a] n=305		70 mg BID[a] n=423	
	All Grades	**Grade 3/4**	**All Grades**	**Grade 3/4**	**All Grades**	**Grade 3/4**
Preferred Term	Percent (%) of Patients					
Arthralgia	21	2	17	2	23	2
Abdominal pain	19	4	18	3	35	4
Weight decreased	16	1	16	2	22	2
Mucosal inflammation (including mucositis/stomatitis)	16	1	16	1	26	2
Pneumonia (including bacterial, viral, and fungal)	15	9	17	8	21	11
Constipation	15	1	12	0	20	<1
Anorexia	14	1	21	2	26	2
Neuropathy (including peripheral neuropathy)	13	1	10	<1	16	<1
Arrhythmia (including tachycardia)	13	1	10	1	16	2
Asthenia	12	2	11	3	22	5
Chest pain	12	1	9	1	16	2
Febrile neutropenia	11	11	13	13	17	16
Myalgia	11	1	10	1	16	1
Weight increased	10	1	10	1	22	2
Hyperhidrosis	9	0	7	0	12	0
Pruritus	9	0	9	1	13	0
Dizziness	8	1	9	<1	17	0
Dyspepsia	8	0	5	0	12	<1
Depression	7	0	8	<1	10	<1
Hypertension	7	1	7	2	8	1
Hypotension	6	2	5	1	9	3
Insomnia	6	0	7	0	11	<1
Sepsis (including fatal outcomes)	6	4	10	7	12	9

(cont'd)

Table 2: SPRYCEL *(cont'd)*

Adverse Events Reported in ≥5% of Patients in Clinical Studies of Advanced Phase CML and Ph+ALL (Recommended Starting Dose: 140 mg Once Daily)

	Phase III				All Other	
	140 mg QD n=304		70 mg BID[a] n=305		70 mg BID[a] n=423	
	All Grades	Grade 3/4	All Grades	Grade 3/4	All Grades	Grade 3/4
Preferred Term	Percent (%) of Patients					
Anxiety	6	1	6	<1	10	<1
Contusion	6	<1	2	0	8	0
Dry skin	6	0	4	0	7	0
Lung infiltration	5	2	3	1	6	3
Renal failure	5	4	2	1	5	4
Abdominal distension	5	<1	8	0	16	0
Colitis (including neutropenic colitis)	5	3	6	2	8	3
Enterocolitis infection	5	1	3	2	7	2
Visual disorder	4	<1	4	<1	7	1
Chills	4	0	7	<1	16	<1
Herpes virus infection	4	1	2	<1	8	1
Oral soft tissue disorder	4	0	1	0	8	0
Somnolence	4	1	6	1	4	<1
Urinary frequency	4	0	4	<1	6	<1
Gastritis	4	1	4	1	5	<1
Pneumonitis	4	2	3	1	6	2
Acne	3	0	2	0	6	0
Flushing	3	0	5	0	10	0
Alopecia	2	0	6	0	6	0

[a] Not a recommended starting dosage of SPRYCEL for advanced phase CML and Ph+ALL. Data provided for context with the dose optimization trial.

[b] Includes ventricular dysfunction, cardiac failure, cardiac failure congestive, cardiomyopathy, congestive cardiomyopathy, diastolic dysfunction, ejection fraction decreased, and ventricular failure.

In a Phase II randomized study of chronic phase CML, 101 patients received SPRYCEL (starting dosage 70 mg twice daily) and 49 patients received imatinib (starting dosage 800 mg daily). Crossover to the alternate therapy was permitted in this study. The median duration of therapy prior to crossover was longer for SPRYCEL than for imatinib. Selected adverse events, regardless of relationship to study drug, are presented in Table 3.

Table 3: SPRYCEL

Selected Adverse Events in Phase II Randomized Study (Chronic Phase CML)

	SPRYCEL[a] n=101		Imatinib[a] n=49	
	All Grades	Grade 3/4	All Grades	Grade 3/4
Preferred Term	Percent (%) of Patients			
Nausea	32	0	39	0
Pleural Effusion	26	5	0	0
Superficial Edema	26	1	47	0
Vomiting	18	0	27	0
Congestive Heart Failure/Cardiac Dysfunction[b]	3	2	0	0

[a] Starting dosage: SPRYCEL 70 mg twice daily; imatinib 800 mg daily.

[b] Includes ventricular dysfunction, cardiac failure, cardiac failure congestive, cardiomyopathy, congestive cardiomyopathy, diastolic dysfunction, ejection fraction decreased, and ventricular failure.

Less Common Clinical Trial Adverse Drug Reactions (<5% all grades) Reported in Clinical Trials in Patients Treated with SPRYCEL: The following adverse reactions, regardless of relationship to therapy or dosing regimen, were reported in patients in the SPRYCEL clinical studies (1850 patients treated with 140 mg once daily or 70 mg twice daily) at a frequency of <5%. These reactions are presented by frequency category. Frequent reactions are those occurring in ≥1% of patients, infrequent reactions are those occurring in 0.1%-<1% of patients and rare reactions are those occurring in <0.1% of patients. These events are included based on clinical relevance.

Gastrointestinal Disorders: Frequent: dysphagia; Infrequent: anal fissure, esophagitis, upper gastrointestinal ulcer, pancreatitis, ileus.

General Disorders and Administration Site Conditions: Frequent: malaise; Infrequent: temperature intolerance.

Musculoskeletal and Connective Tissue Disorders: Frequent: muscular weakness; Infrequent: tendonitis, rhabdomyolysis.

Nervous System Disorders: Frequent: dysgeusia, syncope, amnesia, tremor, convulsion; Infrequent: cerebrovascular accident, transient ischemic attack; Rare: reversible posterior leukoencephalopathy syndrome.

Respiratory, Thoracic, and Mediastinal Disorders: Frequent: asthma; Infrequent: bronchospasm, acute respiratory distress syndrome.

Skin and Subcutaneous Tissue Disorders: Frequent: dermatitis including eczema, urticaria, skin ulcer, pigmentation disorder, photosensitivity; Infrequent: bullous conditions, nail disorder, acute febrile neutrophilic dermatosis, palmar-plantar erythrodysaesthesia syndrome, panniculitis.

Vascular Disorders: Frequent: thrombophlebitis; Rare: livedo reticularis.

Investigations: Frequent: Infrequent: blood creatine phosphokinase increased; Rare: platelet aggregation abnormal.

Metabolism and Nutrition Disorders: Frequent: appetite disturbances, hyperuricemia; Infrequent: hypoalbuminemia.

Cardiac Disorders: Frequent: angina pectoris, cardiomegaly; Infrequent: electrocardiogram QT prolonged, myocardial infarction, pericarditis, ventricular arrhythmia (including ventricular tachycardia), myocarditis; Rare: acute coronary syndrome, cor pulmonale.

Psychiatric Disorders: Frequent: confusional state, affect lability; Infrequent: libido decreased.

Blood and Lymphatic System Disorders: Frequent: pancytopenia; Infrequent: coagulopathy; Rare: aplasia pure red cell.

Eye Disorders: Frequent: conjunctivitis, dry eye.

Renal and Urinary Disorders: Infrequent: proteinuria.

Ear and Labyrinth Disorders: Frequent: tinnitus, vertigo.

Reproductive System and Breast Disorders: Frequent: gynecomastia; Infrequent: menstruation irregular.

Hepatobiliary Disorders: Infrequent: cholecystitis, cholestasis, hepatitis.

Neoplasms Benign, Malignant and Unspecified: Infrequent: tumor lysis syndrome.

Abnormal Hematologic and Clinical Chemistry Findings: Myelosuppression was commonly reported in all studies. However, the frequency of Grade 3 or 4 neutropenia, thrombocytopenia, and anemia was higher in patients with advanced phase CML or Ph+ ALL than in chronic phase CML. Most patients continued treatment without further progressive myelosuppression.

In patients who experienced severe myelosuppression, recovery generally occurred following brief dose interruptions and/or reductions. Occasionally permanent discontinuation of treatment was required.

Elevations of transaminases or bilirubin were reported in all disease phases, but were more common in patients with advanced disease. The numbers of patients who developed three or more simultaneous significant elevations of transaminases or bilirubin suggestive of hepatic toxicity were as follows: Chronic phase, 4; accelerated, 13; myeloid blast, 13; lymphoid blast, 7. Most events were managed with dose reduction or interruption. One patient required discontinuation of treatment due to abnormalities of liver function tests. Although causality has not been established, the occurrence of abnormal liver function tests on treatment should be followed closely and consideration given to discontinuing SPRYCEL.

Hypocalcemia: Between 48% and 76% of patients experienced hypocalcemia at least once during this period. Grade 3 or 4 abnormalities were reported in 2, 7, 16, 13 and 9% of the patients in the chronic phase CML (n=1150), accelerated phase CML (n=502), myeloid blast phase CML (n=280), lymphoid blast phase CML (n=115) and Ph+ ALL (n=135), respectively. The percentage of patients with hypocalcemia who were treated with calcium supplements is 7% for chronic phase CML, 16% for accelerated phase CML, 28% for myeloid blast CML, 20% for lymphoid blast CML and 20% for Ph+ALL.

Hypophosphatemia: Between 41% and 50% of patients experienced hypophosphatemia at least once during this period. Grade 3 or 4 abnormalities were reported in 10, 13, 20, 19 and 21% of the patients in the chronic phase CML (n=1150), accelerated phase CML (n=502), myeloid blast phase CML (n=280), lymphoid blast phase CML (n=115) and Ph+ ALL (n=135), respectively.

In the Phase II randomized study, the frequency of Grade 3 or 4 neutropenia, thrombocytopenia, and anemia was 63%, 57%, and 20%, respectively, in the SPRYCEL group and 39%, 14%, and 8%, respectively, in the imatinib group. The frequency of Grade 3 or 4 hypocalcemia was 5% in the SPRYCEL group and 0% in the imatinib group. Laboratory abnormalities are shown in Table 4 for chronic phase CML and in Table 5 for advanced phase CML and Ph+ALL.

Table 4: SPRYCEL

CTC Grades 3/4 Laboratory Abnormalities in Clinical Studies of Chronic Phase CML (Recommended Starting Dose: 100 mg Once Daily)

	Phase III				All Other
	100 mg QD n=165	50 mg BID[a] n=167	140 mg QD[a] n=163	70 mg BID[a] n=167	70 mg BID[a] n=488
Preferred Term	Percent (%) of Patients				
Hematology Parameters					
Neutropenia	35	47	44	45	53
Thrombocytopenia	23	36	41	38	51
Anemia	13	18	19	18	22
Biochemistry Parameters					
Hypophosphatemia	10	8	6	9	13
Hypokalemia	2	2	4	4	4
Hypocalcemia	1	0	2	3	3
Elevated ALT	0	1	1	1	1
Elevated AST	1	1	1	0	1
Elevated Bilirubin	1	0	1	1	1
Elevated Creatinine	0	0	1	1	1

[a] Not a recommended starting dosage of SPRYCEL for chronic phase CML. Data provided for context with dose optimization trial.

CTC grades: neutropenia (Grade 3 ≥0.5-<1.0×10⁹/L, Grade 4 <0.5×10⁹/L); thrombocytopenia (Grade 3 ≥25-<50×10⁹/L, Grade 4 <25×10⁹/L); anemia (hemoglobin Grade 3 ≥65-<80 g/L, Grade 4 <65 g/L); elevated creatinine (Grade 3 >3-6×upper limit of normal range (ULN), Grade 4 >6×ULN); elevated bilirubin (Grade 3 >3-10×ULN, Grade 4 >10×ULN); elevated AST or ALT (Grade 3 >5-20×ULN, Grade 4 >20×ULN); hypocalcemia (Grade 3 <7.0-6.0 mg/dL, Grade 4 <6.0 mg/dL); hypophosphatemia (Grade 3 <2.0-1.0 mg/dL, Grade 4 <1.0 mg/dL); hypokalemia (Grade 3 <3.0-2.5 mmol/L, Grade 4 <2.5 mmol/L).

Table 5: SPRYCEL

CTC Grades 3/4 Laboratory Abnormalities in Clinical Studies of Advanced Phase CML and Ph+ALL (Recommended Starting Dose: 140 mg Once Daily)

	Phase III		All Other
	140 mg QD n=304	70 mg BID[a] n=305	70 mg BID[a] n=423
Preferred Term	Percent (%) of Patients		
Hematology Parameters			
Neutropenia	67	72	81
Thrombocytopenia	71	71	83

(cont'd)

Table 5: SPRYCEL *(cont'd)*

CTC Grades 3/4 Laboratory Abnormalities in Clinical Studies of Advanced Phase CML and Ph+ALL (Recommended Starting Dose: 140 mg Once Daily)

	Phase III		All Other
	140 mg QD n=304	70 mg BID[a] n=305	70 mg BID[a] n=423
Preferred Term	**Percent (%) of Patients**		
Anemia	54	51	67
Biochemistry Parameters			
Hypophosphatemia	14	14	21
Hypokalemia	9	14	17
Hypocalcemia	6	9	14
Elevated ALT	4	3	8
Elevated AST	2	1	5
Elevated Bilirubin	3	2	4
Elevated Creatinine	3	1	1

[a] Not a recommended starting dosage of SPRYCEL for advanced phase CML and Ph+ALL. Data provided for context with dose optimization trial.

CTC grades: neutropenia (Grade 3 ≥0.5-<1.0×10⁹/L, Grade 4 <0.5×10⁹/L); thrombocytopenia (Grade 3 ≥25-<50×10⁹/L, Grade 4 <25×10⁹/L); anemia (hemoglobin Grade 3 ≥65-<80 g/L, Grade 4 <65 g/L); elevated creatinine (Grade 3 >3-6×upper limit of normal range (ULN), Grade 4 >6×ULN); elevated bilirubin (Grade 3 >3-10×ULN, Grade 4 >10×ULN); elevated AST or ALT (Grade 3 >5-20×ULN, Grade 4 >20×ULN); hypocalcemia (Grade 3 <7.0-6.0 mg/dL, Grade 4 <6.0 mg/dL); hypophosphatemia (Grade 3 <2.0-1.0 mg/dL, Grade 4 <1.0 mg/dL); hypokalemia (Grade 3 <3.0-2.5 mmol/L, Grade 4 <2.5 mmol/L).

The following additional adverse reactions have been identified during post approval use of SPRYCEL. Because these reactions are reported voluntarily from a population of uncertain size, it is not always possible to reliably estimate their frequency or establish a causal relationship to drug exposure.

Cardiac Disorders	atrial fibrillation/atrial flutter[a]
Vascular Disorders	thrombosis/embolism (including pulmonary embolism, deep vein thrombosis)[b]
Respiratory, Thoracic and Mediastinal Disorders	interstitial lung disease
Gastrointestinal Disorders	fatal gastrointestinal hemorrhage[c]

[a] Typically reported in elderly patients or in patients with confounding factors including significant underlying or concurrent cardiac or cardiovascular disorders, or other significant comorbidities (eg, severe infection/sepsis, electrolyte abnormalities).

[b] Typically reported in patients with underlying malignancies or other confounding or risk factors, including cardiovascular disorders, history of surgery, or other comorbidities.

[c] Typically reported in patients with progressive underlying malignancies (eg, advanced phase of CML or Ph+ ALL) or severe or life-threatening comorbidities (eg, severe gastrointestinal disorders, infection or sepsis, thrombocytopenia).

DRUG INTERACTIONS: Overview: Dasatinib is not an inducer of human CYP enzymes. Dasatinib is an inhibitor of CYP3A4 and may decrease the metabolic clearance of drugs that are primarily metabolized by CYP3A4. At clinically relevant concentrations, dasatinib does not inhibit CYP 1A2, 2A6, 2B6, 2C8, 2C9, 2C19, 2D6, or 2E1.

Drug-Drug Interactions: Drugs That May Increase Dasatinib Plasma Concentrations: CYP3A4 Inhibitors: In vitro studies indicate that dasatinib is a CYP3A4 substrate. In a study of 18 patients with solid tumors, 20-mg SPRYCEL once daily coadministered with 200 mg of ketoconazole BID increased the dasatinib C_{max} and AUC by four- and five-fold, respectively. Substances that inhibit CYP3A4 activity (eg, ketoconazole, itraconazole, erythromycin, clarithromycin, grape fruit juice) may decrease metabolism and increase concentrations of dasatinib (see Warnings and Precautions, Drug-Drug Interactions and Dosage and Administration).

Drugs That May Decrease Dasatinib Plasma Concentrations: CYP3A4 Inducers: Data from a study of 20 healthy subjects indicate that when a single morning dose of SPRYCEL was administered following 8 days of continuous evening administration of 600 mg of rifampicin, a potent CYP3A4 inducer, the mean C_{max} and AUC of dasatinib were decreased by 81% and 82%, respectively. In addition, more healthy male subjects experienced increases in QTcF of >30 msec from the baseline recordings when a single dose of dasatinib was administered 12 hours following rifampicin compared to when dasatinib was given alone (25% vs. 10%, n=20). No subject experienced QTcF >450 msec or a change from baseline >60 msec (see Warnings and Precautions, Cardiovascular and Drug-Drug Interactions).

Antacids: Nonclinical data indicate that dasatinib has pH dependent solubility. In a study of 24 healthy subjects, administration of 30 mL of aluminum hydroxide/magnesium hydroxide 2 hours prior to a single 50 mg dose of SPRYCEL was associated with no relevant change in dasatinib AUC or C_{max}. On the contrary, when 30 mL of aluminum hydroxide/magnesium hydroxide was administered to the same subjects concomitantly with a 50 mg dose of SPRYCEL, a 55% reduction in dasatinib AUC and a 58% reduction in C_{max} were observed (see Warnings and Precautions, Drug-Drug Interactions).

Famotidine: In a study of 24 healthy subjects, administration of a single 50 mg dose of SPRYCEL 10 hours following famotidine reduced the AUC and C_{max} of SPRYCEL by 61% and 63%, respectively (see Warnings and Precautions, Drug-Drug Interactions).

Drugs That May Have Their Plasma Concentration Altered by Dasatinib: CYP3A4 Substrates: Single dose data from a study of 54 healthy subjects indicate that the mean C_{max} and AUC of simvastatin, a prototypical CYP3A4 substrate, were increased by 37% and 20%, respectively, when simvastatin (80 mg) was administered in combination with a single 100 mg dose of SPRYCEL. In addition, three healthy subjects (n=48) experienced QTcF of >30 msec from the baseline ECG recordings following the concomitant use of a single dose of simvastatin and dasatinib. No subject experienced QTcF >450 msec or a change from baseline >60 msec. The effect of CYP3A4 substrates on the pharmacokinetics of dasatinib has not been studied (see Warnings and Precautions, Cardiovascular and Drug-Drug Interactions).

DOSAGE AND ADMINISTRATION: Current dosing recommendations are based on the results of two randomized Phase III dose-optimization studies in patients with chronic and advanced phases CML and Ph+ALL.

- The recommended starting dosage of SPRYCEL (dasatinib) for chronic phase CML is 100 mg administered orally once daily (OD), either in the morning or in the evening.
- The recommended starting dosage of SPRYCEL for accelerated phase CML, or myeloid or lymphoid blast CML, is 140 mg/day administered orally once daily (140 mg QD) either in the morning or in the evening.
- The recommended starting dosage of SPRYCEL for Ph+ALL is 140 mg administered orally once daily (140 mg QD) either in the morning or in the evening.

SPRYCEL can be taken with or without food. Tablets should not be crushed or cut; they should be swallowed as a whole.

In clinical studies, treatment with SPRYCEL was continued until disease progression or until no longer tolerated by the patient. The effect of stopping treatment after the achievement of a complete cytogenetic response (CCyR) has not been investigated.

CYP3A4 inhibitors such as ketoconazole may **increase** SPRYCEL plasma concentrations. Selection of an alternate concomitant medication with no or minimal enzyme inhibition potential is recommended. If SPRYCEL must be administered with a strong CYP3A4 inhibitor, a dose decrease to 20 or 40 mg daily should be considered (see Warnings and Precautions, Drug-Drug Interactions and Drug Interactions).

Dose Escalation: In clinical studies of adult CML and Ph+ ALL patients, dose escalation to 140 mg once daily (chronic phase CML) or 180 mg once daily (advanced phase CML and Ph+ ALL) was allowed in patients who did not achieve a hematologic or cytogenetic response at the recommended dosage.

Dose Adjustment for Adverse Reactions: Myelosuppression: In clinical studies, myelosuppression was managed by dose interruption, dose reduction, or discontinuation of study therapy. Hematopoietic growth factor has been used in patients with resistant myelosuppression. Guidelines for dose modifications are summarized in Table 6.

Table 6: SPRYCEL

Dose Adjustments for Neutropenia and Thrombocytopenia

Chronic Phase CML (starting dose 100 mg once daily)	ANC[a] <0.5×10⁹/L and/or Platelets <50×10⁹/L	1. Stop SPRYCEL until ANC ≥1.0×10⁹/L and platelets ≥50×10⁹/L. 2. Resume treatment with SPRYCEL at the original starting dose. 3. If platelets <25×10⁹/L and/or recurrence of ANC <0.5×10⁹/L for >7 days, repeat Step 1 and resume SPRYCEL at a reduced dose of 80 mg once daily (second episode) or discontinue (third episode).
Accelerated Phase CML, Blast Phase CML and Ph+ ALL (starting dose 140 mg once daily)	ANC <0.5×10⁹/L and/or Platelets <10×10⁹/L	1. Check if cytopenia is related to leukemia (marrow aspirate or biopsy). 2. If cytopenia is unrelated to leukemia, stop SPRYCEL until ANC ≥1.0×10⁹/L and platelets ≥20×10⁹/L and resume at the original starting dose. 3. If recurrence of cytopenia, repeat Step 1 and resume SPRYCEL at a reduced dose of 100 mg once daily (second episode) or 80 mg once daily (third episode). 4. If cytopenia is related to leukemia, consider dose escalation to 180 mg once daily.

[a] ANC=absolute neutrophil count.

Non-Hematological Adverse Reactions: If a severe non-hematological adverse reaction develops with SPRYCEL use, treatment must be withheld until the event has resolved or improved. Thereafter, treatment can be resumed as appropriate at a reduced dose depending on the initial severity of the event.

Pediatrics (<18 years of age): SPRYCEL is not recommended for use in children below 18 years of age due to a lack of data on safety and efficacy.

Hepatic Impairment: No clinical pharmacokinetic trials were conducted with a 70-100 mg dose of SPRYCEL in patients with decreased liver function. SPRYCEL should be used with caution in patients with moderate to severe hepatic impairment (see Warnings and Precautions).

Renal Impairment: No clinical trials were conducted with SPRYCEL in patients with decreased renal function (trials excluded patients with serum creatinine concentration >1.5 times the upper limit of the normal range). Since the renal clearance of dasatinib and its metabolites is <4%, a decrease in total body clearance is not expected in patients with renal insufficiency.

OVERDOSAGE:
Experience with overdose of SPRYCEL in clinical studies is limited to isolated cases. The highest reported dosage ingested was 280 mg per day for 1 week in two patients and both developed a significant decrease in platelet counts. Since SPRYCEL is associated with severe myelosuppression (see Warnings and Precautions and Adverse Reactions), patients who ingested more than the recommended dosage should be closely monitored for myelosuppression and appropriate supportive treatment given.

For management of a suspected drug overdose, CPhA recommends that you contact your **regional Poison Control Centre**. See the *CPS* Directory section for a list of Poison Control Centres.

ACTION AND CLINICAL PHARMACOLOGY: Mechanism of Action: Dasatinib inhibits the activity of the BCR-ABL kinase and SRC family kinases (LYN, HCK), along with a number of other kinases including c-KIT, ephrin (EPH) receptor kinases, and PDGFβ receptor. Dasatinib is a potent inhibitor of the BCR-ABL and SRC family kinases with potency at sub nanomolar concentrations It binds not only to the inactive but also to the active conformation of the enzyme.

Pharmacodynamics: In vitro, dasatinib is active in leukemic cell lines representing variants of imatinib sensitive and resistant disease. These nonclinical studies show that dasatinib can overcome imatinib resistance resulting from BCR-ABL overexpression, BCR-ABL kinase domain mutations (14/15 mutations with exception of T315I), activation of alternate signaling pathways involving the SRC family kinases (LYN, HCK), and multidrug resistance gene, MDR1, overexpression.

In vivo, in separate experiments using murine models of CML, dasatinib prevented the progression of chronic CML to blast phase and prolonged the survival of mice bearing patient-derived CML cell lines.

Pharmacokinetics: The pharmacokinetics of SPRYCEL (dasatinib) were evaluated in 229 healthy subjects and in 84 patients with leukemia.

Absorption: Dasatinib is rapidly absorbed in patients following oral administration. Peak concentrations were observed between 0.5-3 hours. The overall mean terminal half-life of dasatinib is approximately 5-6 hours.

Distribution: In patients, SPRYCEL has a large apparent volume of distribution (2505 L) suggesting that the drug is extensively distributed in the extravascular space.

Metabolism: Dasatinib is extensively metabolized in humans. In a study of 8 healthy subjects administered 100 mg of [^{14}C]-labeled dasatinib, unchanged dasatinib represented 29% of circulating radioactivity in plasma. Plasma concentration and measured in vitro activity indicate that metabolites of dasatinib are unlikely to play a major role in the observed pharmacology of the drug. CYP3A4 is a major enzyme responsible for the metabolism of dasatinib.

Excretion: Elimination is predominantly in the feces, mostly as metabolites. Following a single oral dose of [^{14}C]-labeled dasatinib, approximately 89% of the dose was eliminated within 10 days, with 4% and 85% of the administered radioactivity recovered in the urine and feces, respectively. Unchanged dasatinib accounted for 0.1% and 19% of the administered dose in urine and feces, respectively, with the remainder of the dose being metabolites.

Special Populations and Conditions: Pediatrics: No clinical studies were conducted with SPRYCEL in pediatric populations.

Hepatic Insufficiency: The effect of hepatic impairment on the single-dose pharmacokinetics of dasatinib was assessed in 8 moderately hepatic impaired subjects who received a 50-mg dose and 5 severely hepatic-impaired subjects who received a 20-mg dose compared to matched healthy subjects who received a 70-mg dose of SPRYCEL. The mean C_{max} and AUC of dasatinib adjusted for the 70-mg dose was decreased by 47% and 8%, respectively, in moderate hepatic impairment compared to subjects with normal hepatic function. In severe hepatic impaired subjects, the mean C_{max} and AUC adjusted for the 70-mg dose was decreased by 43% and 28%, respectively, compared to subjects with normal hepatic function. Hepatic impairment did not result in clinically meaningful change in dasatinib exposure at the doses studied. However no pharmacokinetic information is available from patients with hepatic impairment treated with a 70-100 mg dose of SPRYCEL. Due to limitations of this clinical study, caution is recommended in patients with hepatic impairment (see Warnings and Precautions and Dosage and Administration).

Renal Insufficiency: No clinical studies were conducted with SPRYCEL in patients with decreased renal function. Less than 4% of SPRYCEL and its metabolites are excreted via the kidney. (See Warnings and Precautions.)

Electrocardiogram: In five Phase II clinical studies in patients with leukemia, repeated baseline and on-treatment ECGs were obtained at pre-specified time points and read centrally for 865 patients receiving SPRYCEL 70 mg BID. QT interval was corrected for heart rate by Fridericia's method. At all post-dose time points on day 8, the mean changes from baseline in QTcF interval were 4-6 msec, with associated upper 95% confidence intervals <7 msec and lower 95% confidence intervals >−2 msec. Of the 2182 patients who received SPRYCEL in clinical trials, 21 patients (<1%) experienced a QTcF >500 msec. (See Warnings and Precautions.)

Drug-Drug Interactions: See Drug Interactions.

Drug-Food Interactions: Data from a study of 54 healthy subjects administered a single, 100-mg dose of dasatinib 30 minutes following consumption of a high-fat meal indicated a 14% increase in the mean AUC of dasatinib. Consumption of a low-fat meal 30 minutes prior to dasatinib resulted in a 21% increase in the mean AUC of dasatinib. The observed food effects do not represent clinically relevant changes in exposure.

STORAGE AND STABILITY: SPRYCEL (dasatinib) tablets should be stored at room temperature between 15-30°C.

SPECIAL HANDLING INSTRUCTIONS: Procedures for proper handling and disposal of anticancer drugs should be considered. Several guidelines on this subject have been published. There is no general agreement that all of the procedures recommended in the guidelines are necessary or appropriate.

SPRYCEL (dasatinib) tablets consist of a core tablet (containing the active drug substance), surrounded by a film coating to prevent exposure of pharmacy and clinical personnel to the active drug substance. However, if tablets are crushed or broken, pharmacy and clinical personnel should wear disposable chemotherapy gloves. Personnel who are pregnant should avoid exposure to crushed and/or broken tablets.

INFORMATION FOR THE PATIENT: Published in e-CPS, available by subscription at www.e-cps.ca.

DOSAGE FORMS, COMPOSITION AND PACKAGING: 20 mg: Each white to off-white, biconvex, round, film-coated tablet with "BMS" debossed on one side and "527" on the other side, contains: dasatinib (as monohydrate) 20 mg. Nonmedicinal ingredients: croscarmellose sodium, hydroxypropyl cellulose, lactose monohydrate, magnesium stearate and microcrystalline cellulose; film-coating: hypromellose, polyethylene glycol and titanium dioxide. HDPE bottles of 60.

50 mg: Each white to off-white, biconvex, oval, film-coated tablet with "BMS" debossed on one side and "528" on the other side, contains: dasatinib (as monohydrate) 50 mg. Nonmedicinal ingredients: croscarmellose sodium, hydroxypropyl cellulose, lactose monohydrate, magnesium stearate and microcrystalline cellulose; film-coating: hypromellose, polyethylene glycol and titanium dioxide. HDPE bottles of 60.

70 mg: Each white to off-white, biconvex, round, film-coated tablet with "BMS" debossed on one side and "524" on the other side, contains: dasatinib (as monohydrate) 70 mg. Nonmedicinal ingredients: croscarmellose sodium, hydroxypropyl cellulose, lactose monohydrate, magnesium stearate and microcrystalline cellulose; film-coating: hypromellose, polyethylene glycol and titanium dioxide. HDPE bottles of 60.

100 mg: Each white to off-white, biconvex, oval, film-coated tablet with "BMS 100" debossed on one side and "852" on the other side, contains: dasatinib (as monohydrate) 100 mg. Nonmedicinal ingredients: croscarmellose sodium, hydroxypropyl cellulose, lactose monohydrate, magnesium stearate and microcrystalline cellulose; film-coating: hypromellose, polyethylene glycol and titanium dioxide. HDPE bottles of 30.

(Shown in Product Identification Section)

SSRIs 🅿

CPhA Monograph

see *Selective Serotonin Reuptake Inhibitors*

Stalevo™ 🅿

levodopa—carbidopa—entacapone

Antiparkinsonian Dopaminergic Agent

Novartis Pharmaceuticals

Date of Revision: November 19, 2009

SUMMARY PRODUCT INFORMATION:

Route of Administration	Dosage Form/ Strength	Nonmedicinal Ingredients
Oral	Tablets 50/12.5/200 mg, 75/18.75/200 mg, 100/25/200 mg, 125/31.25/200 mg, 150/37.5/200 mg	Croscarmellose sodium, glycerol 85%, hypromellose, magnesium stearate, maize starch, mannitol, polysorbate 80, povidone, red iron oxide (E 172), sucrose, titanium dioxide (E 171), yellow iron oxide (E 172) (note: yellow iron oxide is not used in 75/18.75/200 mg and 125/31.25/200 mg tablets).

INDICATIONS AND CLINICAL USE: STALEVO (levodopa, carbidopa and entacapone) is indicated to treat patients with idiopathic Parkinson's disease:

- To substitute for immediate-release levodopa/carbidopa and entacapone previously administered as individual products.
- To replace immediate-release levodopa/carbidopa therapy (without entacapone) when patients experience the signs and symptoms of end of dose "wearing off" (only recommended when patients are taking a total daily dose of levodopa of 600 mg or less and not experiencing dyskinesias, see Dosage and Administration).

Geriatrics: No adjustment of STALEVO dosage is necessary in elderly patients.

Pediatrics (<18 years of age): Safety and effectiveness in pediatric patients have not been established. Therefore, the use of STALEVO is not recommended in children under 18 years of age.

CONTRAINDICATIONS:

- Patients with known hypersensitivity to STALEVO (levodopa, carbidopa and entacapone) or to the excipients of the drug product. For a complete listing, see Dosage Forms, Composition and Packaging.
- Concomitant use with non-selective monoamine oxidase (MAO) inhibitors (e.g. phenelzine and tranylcypromine). The combination of selective MAO-A and selective MAO-B inhibitors is equivalent to non-selective MAO-inhibition, therefore, they should not both be given concomitantly with STALEVO. As with levodopa/carbidopa non-selective MAO inhibitors must be discontinued at least two weeks prior to initiating therapy with STALEVO. Selective MAO-B inhibitors should not be used at higher than recommended doses (e.g. selegiline 10 mg/day) when co-administered with STALEVO (see Drug Interactions, Selegiline).
- Patients with clinical or laboratory evidence of uncompensated cardiovascular, endocrine, hematologic, pulmonary (including bronchial asthma), or renal disease.
- Patients with a previous history of Neuroleptic Malignant Syndrome (NMS) and/or non-traumatic rhabdomyolysis.
- Patients with liver impairment (see Warnings and Precautions, Hepatic Impairment).
- As with levodopa, STALEVO should not be given when administration of a sympathomimetic amine is contraindicated.
- Patients with pheochromocytoma due to the increased risk of hypertensive crisis.
- Patients with narrow angle glaucoma.
- Because levodopa may activate a malignant melanoma, STALEVO should not be used in patients with suspicious, undiagnosed skin lesions or a history of melanoma.

WARNINGS AND PRECAUTIONS:

Sudden Onset of Sleep

Patients receiving treatment with entacapone in combination with levodopa/decarboxylase inhibitor and/or other dopaminergic agents have reported suddenly falling asleep while engaged in activities of daily living, including the driving of a car, which sometimes resulted in accidents. Although some of the patients reported somnolence while treated with levodopa/dopa decarboxylase inhibitor and entacapone, others perceived that they had no warning signs, such as excessive drowsiness, and believed that they were alert immediately prior to the event.

Physicians should alert patients of the reported cases of sudden onset of sleep, bearing in mind that these events are **not** limited to initiation of therapy. Patients should also be advised that sudden onset of sleep has occurred without warning signs and should be specifically asked about factors that may increase the risk with STALEVO (levodopa, carbidopa and entacapone), such as concomitant medications or the presence of sleep disorders. Given the reported cases of somnolence and sudden onset of sleep (not necessarily preceded by somnolence), physicians should caution patients about the risk of operating hazardous machinery, including driving motor vehicles, while taking STALEVO. If drowsiness or sudden onset of sleep should occur, patients should be informed to refrain from driving or operating machines and to immediately contact their physician.

Episodes of falling asleep while engaged in activities of daily living have also been reported in patients taking other dopaminergic agents, therefore, symptoms may not be alleviated by substituting these products.

While dose reduction clearly reduces the degree of somnolence, there is insufficient information to establish that dose reduction will eliminate episodes of falling asleep while engaged in activities of daily living.

Currently, the precise cause of this event is unknown. It is known that many Parkinson's disease patients experience alterations in sleep architecture, which results in excessive daytime sleepiness or spontaneous dozing, and that dopaminergic agents can also induce sleepiness.

Skin: Melanoma: Epidemiological studies have shown that patients with Parkinson's disease have a higher risk (2- to approximately 6-fold higher) of developing melanoma than the general population. Whether the increased risk observed was due to Parkinson's disease or other factors, such as drugs used to treat Parkinson's disease, is unclear. For the reasons stated above, patients and healthcare providers are advised to monitor for melanomas frequently and on a regular basis when using STALEVO for **any** indication. Ideally, periodic skin examinations should be performed by appropriately qualified individuals (e.g., dermatologists).

General: STALEVO is not recommended for the treatment of drug-induced extrapyramidal reactions.

Periodic evaluation of hepatic, haematopoietic, cardiovascular and renal function is recommended during extended therapy with STALEVO.

Because carbidopa and entacapone permit more levodopa to reach the brain and more dopamine to be formed, certain dopaminergic adverse effects, e.g. dyskinesias, "on-off" phenomenon, nausea, vomiting and hallucinations may occur at lower doses and earlier with levodopa preparations containing carbidopa and entacapone than with levodopa alone. Therefore, a direct switch from levodopa or levodopa/dopa decarboxylase inhibitor is not recommended for patients who have dyskinesias or whose daily levodopa dose is above 600 mg. In such patients it is recommended that entacapone tablets be introduced as adjunctive therapy to levodopa/dopa decarboxylase inhibitor and the dose of levodopa be adjusted, prior to switching to STALEVO (see Dosage and Administration).

Because STALEVO contains entacapone, it should not be used concurrently with COMTAN (entacapone).

If STALEVO treatment is discontinued and the patient is switched to levodopa/DDC inhibitor therapy without entacapone, it is necessary to adjust the dosing of other antiparkinsonian treatments, especially levodopa, to achieve a sufficient level of control of the parkinsonian symptoms (see Dosage and Administration).

Drugs Metabolized by Catechol-O-Methyltransferase (COMT): When a single 400 mg dose of entacapone was given together with intravenous isoprenaline (isoproterenol) and epinephrine without coadministered levodopa/dopa decarboxylase inhibitor, the overall mean maximal changes in heart rate during infusion were about 50% and 80% higher than with placebo, for isoprenaline and epinephrine, respectively.

Therefore, drugs known to be metabolized by COMT, such as isoproterenol, epinephrine, norepinephrine, dopamine, dobutamine, alpha-methyldopa, apomorphine, isoetherine and bitolterol should be administered with caution in patients receiving entacapone regardless of the route of administration (including inhalation), as their interaction may result in increased heart rates, possibly arrhythmias, and excessive changes in blood pressure.

Ventricular tachycardia was noted in a 32 year old healthy male volunteer in an interaction study after epinephrine infusion and oral entacapone administration. Treatment with propranolol was required. A causal relationship to entacapone administration appears probable but cannot be attributed with certainty.

Cardiovascular: In patients with a history of myocardial infarction or who have residual atrial nodal, or ventricular arrhythmias, cardiac function should be monitored with particular care during the period of initial dosage adjustments in a facility with provisions for intensive cardiac care.

Orthostatic Hypotension/Syncope: Entacapone may aggravate levodopa-induced orthostatic hypotension. STALEVO should be given with caution to patients who are treated with drugs which may cause orthostatic hypotension. In controlled clinical trials approximately 1.2% of patients who received 200 mg entacapone and 0.8% of patients treated with placebo as adjunct to levodopa/dopa decarboxylase inhibitor reported at least one episode of syncope. Reports of syncope were generally more frequent in patients in both treatment groups who had an episode of documented hypotension.

Endocrine and Metabolism: Patients with Fructose Intolerance: STALEVO tablets contain sucrose. Therefore, patients with rare hereditary problems of fructose intolerance, glucose-galactose malabsorption or sucrase-isomaltase insufficiency should not take this medicine.

Hormone Levels: Of the ingredients in STALEVO, levodopa is known to depress prolactin secretion and increase growth hormone levels.

Gastrointestinal: As with levodopa, treatment with STALEVO may increase the possibility of upper gastrointestinal hemorrhage in patients with a history of peptic ulcer. STALEVO should be administered with caution to these patients.

Since levodopa competes with certain amino acids, the absorption of levodopa may be impaired in some patients on a high protein diet. Excessive acidity also delays stomach emptying, thus delaying absorption of levodopa.

Diarrhea: In clinical trials, diarrhea was reported as an adverse event in 60 of 603 (10.0%) and 16 of 400 (4.0%) of patients treated with 200 mg of entacapone or placebo as adjunct to levodopa/dopa decarboxylase inhibitor, respectively. In patients treated with entacapone, diarrhea was generally mild to moderate in severity (8.6%) but was reported as severe in 1.3%. Diarrhea resulted in withdrawal in 10 of 603 (1.7%) patients (1.2% with mild to moderate diarrhea and 0.3% with severe diarrhea). Diarrhea generally resolved after discontinuation of entacapone. Two patients with diarrhea required hospitalization. Typically, diarrhea presents within 4 to 12 weeks after entacapone is started, but it may appear as early as the first week and as late as many months after the initiation of treatment.

For patients experiencing diarrhea, close monitoring of weight is recommended in order to assess the need for treatment discontinuation to avoid excessive weight loss (see also Warnings and Precautions, Hepatic/Biliary/Pancreatic). Some patients who experienced diarrhea and weight loss during entacapone treatment were subsequently diagnosed with colitis, following colonoscopy and biopsy.

Hepatic/Biliary/Pancreatic: Abnormal Weight Decrease: In isolated cases, combined progressive anorexia, asthenia and weight decrease within a relatively short period of time have been reported prior to elevations in liver enzymes and serious hepatic adverse events. For patients who experience progressive anorexia, asthenia and weight decrease within a relatively short period of time, a general medical evaluation including assessment of liver function should be considered.

Hepatic Impairment: The metabolism of entacapone is slowed in patients with mild to moderate (Child-Pugh grading Class A and B) hepatic insufficiency caused by cirrhotic disease. In these patients, the AUC and C_{max} values were approximately two-fold greater than those in demographically-matched healthy volunteers. As there are no clinical trial data to establish a safe and effective dosing regimen for hepatically impaired patients, STALEVO should be not be administered to patients with hepatic impairment (see Contraindications).

Biliary Excretion: Caution should be exercised when administering STALEVO to patients with biliary obstruction, as entacapone is excreted mostly via the bile (see Drug Interactions, Drugs Interfering with Biliary Excretion).

Musculoskeletal: Rhabdomyolysis: Rhabdomyolysis secondary to severe dyskinesias or Neuroleptic Malignant Syndrome (NMS) has been observed rarely in patients with Parkinson's disease. Very rare cases of rhabdomyolysis have been reported with entacapone treatment.

Symptoms associated with rhabdomyolysis can include muscle pain, muscle tenderness and weakness, bruising, elevated temperature, urinary retention, confusion, and elevated CPK. Acute renal failure is serious complication associated rhabdomyolysis and has been reported in some cases of rhabdomyolysis that have occurred during entacapone treatment.

Neurologic: STALEVO should be used cautiously in patients who have a history of seizures or have conditions associated with seizure or have a lowered seizure threshold.

Neuroleptic Malignant Syndrome: A symptom complex resembling the neuroleptic malignant syndrome (NMS), characterized by elevated temperature, muscular rigidity, altered consciousness (e.g., agitation, confusion, coma), autonomic instability (tachycardia, labile blood pressure) and elevated CPK has been reported in association with the rapid dose reduction, or withdrawal of, or changes in antiparkinsonian therapy, including levodopa/carbidopa and entacapone. In individual cases, only some of these symptoms and/or findings may be evident. This, uncommon but life-threatening, syndrome should be considered in the differential diagnosis for any patient who develops a high fever or severe rigidity.

Cases with similar signs and symptoms have been reported in association with entacapone therapy, especially following abrupt reduction or discontinuation of entacapone and other dopaminergic medications. The complicated nature of these cases makes it difficult to determine what role, if any, entacapone may have played in their pathogenesis. No cases have been reported following abrupt withdrawal or dose reduction of entacapone treatment during clinical studies.

Prescribers should exercise caution when discontinuing STALEVO. If a decision is made to discontinue treatment with STALEVO, withdrawal should proceed slowly. The patient should be monitored closely for signs and/or symptoms and other dopaminergic treatments should be adjusted as needed. If signs and/or symptoms occur despite a slow withdrawal of STALEVO, an increase in levodopa dosage may be necessary. Tapering discontinuation of STALEVO has not been systematically evaluated.

Dyskinesia: Entacapone may potentiate the dopaminergic side effects of levodopa and may cause and/or exacerbate pre-existing dyskinesia. Although decreasing the dose of levodopa may ameliorate this side effect, many patients in controlled trials who received entacapone or placebo as adjunct to levodopa/dopa decarboxylase inhibitor therapy continued to experience frequent dyskinesias despite a reduction in their dose of levodopa. The rates of withdrawal for dyskinesia were 1.5% and 0.8% for 200 mg entacapone and placebo, respectively.

Occupational Hazards: Psychomotor Performance: Entacapone together with levodopa may cause dizziness and symptomatic orthostatism. Therefore, patients should be cautioned about operating machinery, including automobiles, until they are reasonably certain that the drug treatment does not affect them adversely.

STALEVO may have a major influence on the ability to drive and use machines. Patients being treated with STALEVO and presenting with somnolence and/or sudden sleep onset episodes must be instructed to refrain from driving or engaging in activities where impaired alertness may put themselves or others at risk of serious injury or death (e.g. operating machines) until such recurrent episodes have resolved (see Warnings and Precautions, Sudden Onset of Sleep).

Ophthalmologic: Patients with chronic wide angle glaucoma may be treated cautiously with STALEVO provided the intraocular pressure is well controlled and the patient is monitored carefully for changes in intraocular pressure during therapy.

Peri-Operative Considerations: If general anaesthesia is required, therapy with STALEVO may be continued for as long as the patient is permitted to take fluids and medication by mouth. If therapy has to be stopped temporarily, STALEVO may be restarted as soon as oral medication can be taken at the same daily dosage as before (see Drug Interactions).

Psychiatric: As with levodopa, STALEVO may cause mental disturbances. All patients treated with STALEVO should be monitored carefully for the development of mental changes (e.g. hallucinations and psychoses), depression with suicidal tendencies, and serious antisocial behaviour. Patients with past or current psychosis should be treated with caution.

Pathological gambling, increased libido and hypersexuality have been reported in Parkinson's disease patients treated with dopamine agonists and other dopaminergic treatments including STALEVO, and were generally reversible upon dose reduction or treatment discontinuation (see Adverse Reactions).

Hallucinations: Dopaminergic therapy in Parkinson's disease patients has been associated with hallucinations. In clinical trials, hallucinations developed in approximately 4% of patients treated with 200 mg entacapone or placebo, as adjunct to levodopa/dopadacrboxylase inhibitor. Hallucinations led to drug discontinuation and premature withdrawal from clinical trials in 0.8% and 0% of patients treated with 200 mg entacapone and placebo, respectively. Hallucinations led to hospitalization in 1.0% and 0.3% of patients in the 200 mg entacapone and placebo groups, respectively.

Renal: Renal Impairment: The pharmacokinetics of entacapone were not significantly changed in patients with moderate to severe renal insufficiency. STALEVO should be administered cautiously to patients with severe renal disease (see Pharmacokinetics, Special Populations and Conditions). There is no experience with entacapone in patients receiving dialysis.

Urine, Sweat and Saliva Discoloration: STALEVO may cause a harmless intensification in the color of the patient's urine to brownish-orange. STALEVO may also cause darkening of sweat and saliva.

Respiratory: Fibrotic Complications: Cases of retroperitoneal fibrosis, pulmonary infiltrates, pleural effusion, and pleural thickening have been reported in some patients treated with ergot derived dopaminergic agents. These complications may resolve when the drug is discontinued, but complete resolution does not always occur. Although these adverse events are believed to be related to the ergoline structure of these compounds, it is unknown whether other, non-ergot derived drugs (e.g., entacapone, levodopa) that increase dopaminergic activity can cause them. It should be noted that the expected incidence of fibrotic complications is so low that even if entacapone caused these complications at rates similar to those attributable to other dopaminergic therapies, it is unlikely that it would have been detected in a cohort of the size exposed to entacapone. Four cases of pulmonary fibrosis were reported during clinical development of entacapone; three of these patients were also treated with pergolide and one with bromocriptine. The duration of treatment with entacapone ranged from 7 to 17 months.

Special Populations: Pregnant Women: There are no studies or clinical experience of the use of STALEVO in pregnant women. Use of STALEVO in women of child-bearing potential requires that the anticipated benefits of the drug be weighed against possible hazards to mother and child.

It has been reported from individual cases that levodopa crosses the human placental barrier, enters the fetus, and is metabolized. Carbidopa concentrations in fetal tissue appeared to be minimal.

Although the effects on human pregnancy are unknown, both levodopa and combinations of carbidopa and levodopa have caused visceral and skeletal malformations in rabbits. Regarding reproduction toxicity of entacapone, decreased fetal weight and a slightly delayed bone development were noticed in rabbits treated at systemic exposure levels in the therapeutic range.

Nursing Women: Levodopa is excreted in human breast milk. There is evidence that lactation is suppressed during treatment with levodopa. Carbidopa and entacapone were excreted in milk in animals but it is not known whether they are excreted in human breast milk. The safety of levodopa, carbidopa or entacapone in the infant is not known. Women should not breast-feed during treatment with STALEVO.

Pediatrics: The safety and efficacy of STALEVO in pediatric patients has not been established and use in patients below the age of 18 is not recommended.

Geriatrics: No adjustment of STALEVO dosage is necessary in elderly patients.

Monitoring and Laboratory Tests: The laboratory tests required during extended levodopa therapy should normally be conducted during STALEVO treatment also.

Commonly, levels of blood urea nitrogen, creatinine, and uric acid are lower during administration of levodopa/carbidopa than with levodopa alone. Transient abnormalities include elevated values of blood urea, AST, ALT, LDH, bilirubin, and alkaline phosphatase.

Decreased hemoglobin, hematocrit, elevated serum glucose and white blood cells, bacteria and blood in the urine have been reported during levodopa/carbidopa treatment.

Positive Coombs' tests have been reported, both for levodopa/carbidopa and for levodopa alone, but hemolytic anemia is extremely rare.

Levodopa/carbidopa may cause a false positive result when a dipstick is used to test for urinary ketone; this reaction is not altered by boiling the urine sample. The use of glucose oxidase methods may give false negative results for glycosuria.

Entacapone is a chelator of iron. The impact of entacapone on the body's iron stores is unknown; however, a tendency towards decreased serum iron concentrations was noted in a clinical trial. In a controlled clinical study serum ferritin levels (as marker of iron deficiency and subclinical anemia) were not changed with entacapone compared to placebo after one year of treatment and there was no difference in the rates of anemia or decreased hemoglobin levels.

Cases of falsely diagnosed pheochromocytoma in patients on levodopa/carbidopa therapy have been reported very rarely. Caution should be exercised when interpreting plasma and urine levels of catecholamines and their metabolites in patients on levodopa or levodopa/carbidopa therapy.

ADVERSE REACTIONS: The following section describes the undesirable effects reported for levodopa/carbidopa and for entacapone used in combination with levodopa/DDC inhibitor.

Levodopa/carbidopa: Adverse Drug Reaction Overview: The most common serious adverse reactions occurring with levodopa/carbidopa are dyskinesias, including choreiform, dystonic and other involuntary movements, and nausea.

Other serious adverse reactions are mental changes including paranoid ideation and psychotic episodes, depression with or without development of suicidal tendencies, and dementia. Convulsions also have occurred; however, a causal relationship with levodopa/carbidopa therapy has not been established.

Other adverse reactions reported in clinical trials or in post-marketing experience include:

Body as a Whole: chest pain, asthenia.

Cardiovascular: cardiac irregularities and/or palpitation, syncope, hypotension, orthostatic effects including hypotensive episodes, hypertension, phlebitis.

Gastrointestinal: vomiting, anorexia, gastrointestinal bleeding, development of duodenal ulcer, diarrhea, dark saliva, constipation, dyspepsia, dry mouth, taste alterations.

Hematologic: leukopenia, hemolytic and non-hemolytic anemia, thrombocytopenia, agranulocytosis.

Hypersensitivity: angioedema, urticaria, pruritus, Henoch-Schönlein purpura, bullous lesions (including pemphigus-like reactions).

Musculoskeletal: back pain, shoulder pain, muscle cramps.

Nervous System/Psychiatric: neuroleptic malignant syndrome (see Warnings and Precautions), bradykinetic episodes ("on-off" phenomenon), dizziness, somnolence including very rarely excessive daytime somnolence and sudden sleep onset episodes, paresthesia, psychotic episodes including delusions, hallucinations and paranoid ideation, dream abnormalities including nightmares, insomnia, headache, depression with or without development of suicidal tendencies, dementia, agitation, confusion, increased libido including hypersexuality. Convulsions have also occurred, but a causal relationship with levodopa/carbidopa has not been established.

Respiratory: dyspnea, upper respiratory infection.

Skin: alopecia, rash, increased sweating, dark sweat.

Urogenital: dark urine, urinary frequency, urinary tract infection.

Abnormal Hematologic and Clinical Chemistry Findings: Decreased hemoglobin and hematocrit; abnormalities in alkaline phosphatase, AST, ALT, lactic dehydrogenase, bilirubin, blood urea nitrogen (BUN), Coombs' test; elevated serum glucose; white blood cells, bacteria, and blood in the urine.

Other adverse reactions that have been reported with levodopa alone and with various levodopa-carbidopa formulations, and may occur with STALEVO (levodopa, carbidopa and entacapone) are:

Body as a Whole: fatigue.

Cardiovascular: myocardial infarction.

Gastrointestinal: sialorrhea, dysphagia, bruxism, hiccups, abdominal pain and distress, flatulence, burning sensation of tongue, gastrointestinal pain, heart burn.

Metabolic: weight gain or loss, edema.

Musculoskeletal: leg pain.

Nervous System/Psychiatric: decreased mental acuity, disorientation, ataxia, numbness, increased hand tremor, muscle twitching, blepharospasm (which may be taken as an early sign of excess dosage, consideration of dosage reduction may be made at this time), trismus, activation of latent Horner's syndrome, anxiety, euphoria, falling and gait abnormalities, extrapyramidal disorder, nervousness, memory impairment, peripheral neuropathy.

Respiratory: pharyngeal pain, cough.

Skin: flushing, malignant melanoma (see Contraindications and Warnings and Precautions).

Special Senses: diplopia, blurred vision, dilated pupils, and oculogyric crises.

Urogenital: urinary retention, urinary incontinence, priapism.

Miscellaneous: faintness, hoarseness, malaise, hot flashes, sense of stimulation, bizarre breathing patterns.

Abnormal Hematologic and Clinical Chemistry Findings: decreased white blood cell count and serum potassium; increased serum creatinine and uric acid; protein and glucose in urine.

Entacapone: Adverse Drug Reaction Overview: Clinical Trial Adverse Drug Reactions: Because clinical trials are conducted under very specific conditions the adverse reaction rates observed in the clinical trials may not reflect the rates observed in practice and should not be compared to the rates in the clinical trials of another drug. Adverse drug reaction information from clinical trials is useful for identifying drug-related adverse events and for approximating rates.

A total of 1450 patients with Parkinson's disease received entacapone during the pre-marketing clinical trials. Patients treated in double-blind placebo controlled trials received entacapone or placebo as adjunct to levodopa/dopa decarboxylase inhibitor. Approximately 14% of the 603 patients given entacapone in the double-blind placebo-controlled trials discontinued treatment due to adverse events compared to 9% of the 400 patients who received placebo. The most frequent causes of discontinuation in decreasing order for entacapone vs placebo are: psychiatric reasons (2% vs 1%), diarrhea (2 % vs 0%), dyskinesia/hyperkinesia (2% vs 1%), nausea (2% vs 1%), abdominal pain (1% vs 0%), and aggravation of Parkinson's disease symptoms (1% vs 1%).

Incidence of Adverse Events in Placebo Controlled Trials: The most frequently observed adverse events reported with entacapone were dyskinesias/hyperkinesia (29%/10%), nausea (14%), abnormal urine (intensification of the color of urine, 13%), diarrhea (10%), dizziness (10%) and abdominal pain (9%). Dyskinesia, nausea and abdominal pain, may be more common with higher doses (>1400 mg/day) than with lower doses of entacapone.

Adverse events related to the treatment with entacapone are usually mild to moderate in severity, leading only rarely to discontinuation of the treatment. See Table 1.

Table 1: STALEVO

Adverse Events, Irrespective of Causal Relationship to Study Drug, Occurring in ≥1% of Entacapone Patients During Controlled Phase 3 Studies

Adverse Events by Body System	Entacapone N=603 % of patients	Placebo N=400 % of patients
Autonomic Nervous System Disorders		
Hypotension postural	4.3	4.0
Body as a Whole—General Disorders		
Fatigue	6.1	3.5
Pain	6.0	4.5
Back pain	5.0	3.0
Sweating increased	3.6	3.0
Asthenia	1.8	1.3
Weight decrease	1.7	0.5
Fever	1.3	0.5
Syncope	1.0	0.8
Central & Peripheral Nervous System Disorders		
Dyskinesia	25.2	14.8
Hyperkinesia	9.5	5.0
Hypokinesia	8.6	7.5
Dizziness	7.5	6.0
Ataxia	1.2	0.5
Speech disorder	1.2	0.8
Gastrointestinal System Disorders		
Nausea	13.8	7.5
Diarrhea	10.0	4.0
Abdominal pain	8.1	4.5
Constipation	6.3	4.3
Vomiting	4.0	1.0
Mouth dry	3.0	0.3
Dyspepsia	2.3	0.8
Flatulence	1.5	0.3

(cont'd)

Table 1: STALEVO *(cont'd)*

Adverse Events, Irrespective of Causal Relationship to Study Drug, Occurring in ≥1% of Entacapone Patients During Controlled Phase 3 Studies

Adverse Events by Body System	Entacapone N=603 % of patients	Placebo N=400 % of patients
Anorexia	1.5	1.3
Gastrointestinal disorders	1.0	0.3
Gastritis	1.0	0.3
Musculoskeletal System Disorders		
Arthralgia	1.8	1.5
Platelet, Bleeding & Clotting Disorders		
Purpura	1.5	0.8
Psychiatric Disorders		
Hallucinations	4.1	4.0
Paroniria	2.2	1.8
Anxiety	2.0	1.3
Agitation	1.7	0.3
Confusion	1.7	1.5
Somnolence	1.7	0.3
Amnesia	1.3	0.8
Sleep disorder	1.3	0.8
Reproductive Disorders, Male		
Prostatic disorder	1.0	0.3
Resistance Mechanism Disorders		
Infection bacterial	1.3	0.0
Respiratory System Disorders		
Dyspnoea	2.7	1.3
Bronchitis	1.2	1.0
Skin and Appendages Disorders		
Rash	3.6	3.0
Special Senses Other, Disorders		
Taste perversion	1.0	0.3
Urinary System Disorders		
Urine abnormal	9.5	0.0
Cystitis	1.2	0.5

Less Common Clinical Trial Adverse Drug Reactions (<1%): Body as a Whole—General Disorders: malaise, hot flushes, temperature changed sensation, aspiration, oedema generalised, carpal tunnel syndrome, leg pain.
Cardiovascular Disorders, General: hypertension, heart valve disorders.
Central and Peripheral Nervous System Disorders: hypoaesthesia, muscle contractions involuntary, eye abnormality, hypotonia.
Endocrine Disorders: hyperthyroidism.
Gastrointestinal System Disorders: gastroenteritis, oesophagitis, tooth disorder, saliva increased, dysphagia, feces discoloured, diverticulitis, change in bowel habits, fecal abnormality.
Heart Rate and Rhythm Disorders: extrasystoles, bradycardia, bundle branch block, fibrillation atrial.
Liver and Biliary System Disorders: gamma-GT increased, cholelithiasis, bilirubinemia, cholangitis.
Metabolic and Nutritional Disorders: hyperglycemia, hypoglycemia, phosphatase alkaline increased, hypercholesterolemia.
Musculoskeletal System Disorders: bursitis, arthritis, tendinitis.
Myo-, Endo-, Pericardial and Valve Disorders: angina pectoris.
Platelet, Bleeding and Clotting Disorders: epistaxis, thrombocytopenia.
Psychiatric Disorders: nervousness, thinking abnormal, concentration impaired, dreaming abnormal, delusion, paranoid reaction.
Reproductive Disorders, Female: breast fibroadenosis.
Reproductive Disorders, Male: impotence, sexual function abnormal.
Resistance Mechanism Disorders: herpes simplex.
Respiratory System Disorders: pneumonia, pharyngitis, sinusitis.
Secondary Terms—Events: inflicted injury.
Skin and Appendages Disorders: pruritus, skin disorder, dermatitis, eczema, dermatitis fungal.
Special Senses Other, Disorders: taste loss.
Urinary System Disorders: urinary incontinence, hematuria, albuminuria, dysuria, nocturia, renal pain.
Vascular (Extracardiac) Disorders: skin cold clammy, claudication intermittent.
Vision Disorders: diplopia, conjunctivitis, cataract, photopsia.
White Cell and Res Disorders: leucopenia.
The following adverse events were reported only once but are considered clinically important: hepatic function abnormal, hepatic enzymes increased (>3 times ULN), cholecystitis and allergic reaction.
Abnormal Hematologic and Clinical Chemistry Findings: Slight decreases in hemoglobin, erythrocyte count and hematocrit have been reported during entacapone treatment. The underlying mechanism may involve decreased absorption of iron from the gastrointestinal tract. During long-term treatment (6 months) with entacapone a clinically significant decrease in hemoglobin has been observed in 1.5% of patients.

Post-Market Adverse Drug Reactions: The cumulative exposure of entacapone during the period September 1998 to February 2006 is estimated as 710 877 patient years. Voluntary reports of adverse events that have been received since market introduction that are not listed above, are listed in Table 2. Because these reactions are reported voluntarily from a population of uncertain size, it is not always possible to reliably estimate their frequency or establish a causal relationship to drug exposure.

Table 2: STALEVO

Entacapone Post-Market Spontaneous Adverse Event Report

Adverse Event	Frequency: Common (≥1%)	Uncommon (<1% and ≥0.1%)	Rare (<0.1% and ≥0.01%)	Very rare (<0.01%)
Liver and Biliary System Disorders				
Hepatitis with mainly cholestatic features				X
Clinically significant increases in liver enzymes			X	
Central and Peripheral Nervous System Disorders				
Neuroleptic Malignant Syndrome				X
Gastrointestinal Disorders				
Colitis				X
Musculoskeletal System Disorders				
Rhabdomyolysis				X
Skin and Appendage Disorders				
Erythematous/maculopapular rash			X	
Urticaria				X
Skin, hair, beard and nail discoloration				X

Isolated cases of hepatic failure and severe, serious skin reactions resembling erythema multiforme and toxic epidermal necrolysis have been reported in patients treated with entacapone.

Patients treated with entacapone in combination with levodopa/dopa decarboxylase inhibitor have very rarely reported falling asleep while engaged in activities of daily living, including operation of motor vehicles, which has sometimes resulted in accidents (see Warnings and Precautions).

Pathological (compulsive) gambling has been reported in post-market data, including those in the literature, for antiparkinson drugs. Parkinson's disease patients treated with dopamine agonists and other dopaminergic treatments including STALEVO, especially at high doses, have been reported as exhibiting signs of pathological gambling, increased libido and hypersexuality. Pathological gambling, increased libido and hypersexuality were generally reversible upon reduction of the dose or treatment discontinuation.

DRUG INTERACTIONS: Overview: Protein Binding: Entacapone is highly protein bound (98%). In vitro studies have shown that entacapone, at therapeutic concentrations, does not displace drugs of which a large proportion is bound to plasma proteins (e.g. warfarin, salicylic acid, phenylbutazone and diazepam). Entacapone is not markedly displaced by any of these drugs at therapeutic concentrations (see Action and Clinical Pharmacology).

Drugs Metabolized by Cytochrome P450: Data from in vitro studies using human liver microsomal preparations indicate that entacapone inhibits cytochrome P450 2C9 (IC50 ~4 μM).

Other P450 isoenzymes (CYP1A2, CYP2A6, CYP2D6, CYP2E1, CYP3A and CYP2C19) were inhibited only by very high concentrations of entacapone (IC50 from 200 to greater than 1000 μM). The highest concentration of entacapone achieved with an oral 200 mg dose is approximately 5 μM and is not expected to inhibit these enzymes.

Drugs Metabolized by Cytochrome P450 (CYP2C9): Entacapone has been shown to inhibit the activity of cytochrome P450 2C9 in vitro and may potentially interfere with drugs whose metabolism is dependent on this isoenzyme, such as S-warfarin. However, in an interaction study in healthy volunteers, entacapone did not change the plasma levels of S-warfarin, while the AUC for R-warfarin increased on average by 18% [CI90 11-26%]. The INR values increased on average by 13% [CI90 6-19%]. Thus, control of INR is recommended when entacapone treatment is initiated for patients receiving warfarin.

Drugs Interfering with Biliary Excretion: As most entacapone excretion is via the bile, caution should be exercised when drugs known to interfere with biliary excretion, glucuronidation, and intestinal beta-glucuronidase are given concurrently with STALEVO (levodopa, carbidopa and entacapone). These include probenicid, cholestyramine, and some antibiotics (e.g. erythromycin, rifampicin, ampicillin and chloramphenicol).

Drug-Drug Interactions: Drugs Metabolized by the Catechol-O-Methyltransferase (COMT): The experience of the clinical use of entacapone with medicinal products that are metabolized by COMT (e.g. catechol-structured compounds: rimiterole, isoprenaline, adrenaline, noradrenaline, dopamine, dobutamine, alpha-methyldopa, apomorphine, and paroxetine) is still limited (see Warnings and Precautions). Regardless of their route of administration, including inhalation, drugs known to be metabolized by COMT should be used with caution in patients treated concomitantly with entacapone, as their interaction may result in increased heart rates, possible arrhythmias and excessive changes in blood pressure (see Warnings and Precautions).

Non-Selective MAO Inhibitors: STALEVO should not be given concomitantly with non-selective monoamine oxidase (MAO) inhibitors (e.g. phenelzine and tranylcypromine). The combination of selective MAO-A and selective MAO-B inhibitors is equivalent to non-selective MAO-inhibition, therefore, they should not both be given concomitantly with STALEVO preparations. Non-selective MAO inhibitors must be discontinued at least two weeks prior to initiating therapy with entacapone (see Contraindications).

Selegiline: In two multiple-dose interaction studies in patients with Parkinson's disease, no interactions between entacapone and selegiline (10 mg) were observed in the presence of coadministered levodopa/dopa decarboxylase inhibitor. More than 400 parkinsonian patients in phase 2 and 3 studies used selegiline in combination with entacapone and levodopa/DDC inhibitor without any apparent interactions. Selegiline should not be used at higher than recommended doses (10 mg/day) when co-administered with STALEVO (also see Contraindications).

Antihypertensives: Symptomatic postural hypotension may occur when levodopa is initiated in patients already receiving antihypertensives. Dosage adjustment of the antihypertensive agent may be required when STALEVO therapy is started.

Dopamine D2 Receptor Antagonists (e.g., phenothiazines, butyrophenones, risperidone) and Isoniazid: Dopamine D2 receptor antagonists (e.g., phenothiazines, butyrophenones, risperidone) and isoniazid may reduce the therapeutic effects of levodopa.

Phenytoin and Papaverine: The beneficial effects of levodopa in Parkinson's disease have been reported to be reversed by phenytoin and papaverine. Patients taking these drugs with levodopa/carbidopa should be carefully observed for loss of therapeutic response.

Metoclopramide: Although metoclopramide may increase the bioavailability of levodopa by increasing gastric emptying, metoclopramide may also adversely affect disease control by its dopamine receptor antagonistic properties.

Tricyclic Antidepressants and Noradrenaline Re-Uptake Inhibitors: There have been rare reports of adverse reactions, including hypertension and dyskinesia, resulting from the concomitant use of tricyclic antidepressants and levodopa/carbidopa.

In a single-dose study in healthy volunteers, no interactions between entacapone and imipramine were observed in the absence of coadministration of levodopa/dopa decarboxylase inhibitor.

The potential for interactions between entacapone and tricyclic antidepressants or noradrenaline re-uptake inhibitors has not been systematically evaluated in patients with Parkinson's disease. The experience on the clinical use of entacapone with tricyclic antidepressants and noradrenaline reuptake inhibitors (desipramine, maprotiline and venlafaxine) is limited. Therefore, patients should be carefully monitored when STALEVO is administered in combination with these drugs.

Iron: Studies have demonstrated that ferrous sulphate decreases the bioavailability of levodopa and/or carbidopa. Also, entacapone may impair the absorption of iron from the gastrointestinal tract. Therefore, STALEVO and iron-containing supplements or multivitamins should be ingested at least 2 to 3 hours apart.

Pyridoxine: STALEVO may be given to patients with Parkinson's disease who are taking vitamin preparations that contain pyridoxine hydrochloride (Vitamin B6).

Anesthetics: When general anesthetics are required STALEVO may be continued for as long as the patient is permitted to take fluids and medication by mouth. If therapy has to be stopped temporarily, STALEVO may be restarted as soon as oral medication can be taken at the same daily dosage as before.

Drug-Food Interactions: Since levodopa competes with certain amino acids, the absorption of STALEVO may be impaired in some patients on a high protein diet.

DOSAGE AND ADMINISTRATION: Dosing Considerations:

- As with levodopa/carbidopa, non-selective monoamine oxidase (MAO) inhibitors are contraindicated for use with STALEVO (levodopa, carbidopa and entacapone). These inhibitors must be discontinued at least two weeks prior to initiating therapy with STALEVO. STALEVO may be administered concomitantly with the manufacturer's recommended dose of MAO inhibitors with selectivity for MAO type B (e.g., selegiline HCl).
- For special patient populations see Contraindications, Warnings and Precautions, Gastrointestinal, Neurologic and Renal.
- STALEVO tablets should not be divided. The tablets should always be swallowed whole.
- STALEVO may be taken with or without food. As with levodopa/dopa decarboxylase inhibitor, taking STALEVO with a small snack (e.g., biscuits) or liquid may help control gastrointestinal side effects.

Recommended Dose and Dosage Adjustment: The daily dosage must be titrated for each patient to achieve optimal therapeutic response to levodopa. The daily dose should preferably be optimized using one of the five available tablet strengths (50/12.5/200 mg, 75/18.75/200 mg, 100/25/200 mg, 125/31.25/200 mg or 150/37.5/200 mg levodopa/carbidopa/entacapone).

Patients should be instructed to take only one STALEVO tablet at each dosing time. Patients receiving less than 70-100 mg carbidopa a day are more likely to experience nausea and vomiting. The experience with total daily dosage greater than 200 mg carbidopa is limited, the maximum recommended daily dose of entacapone is 1600 mg and therefore the maximum STALEVO dose is 8 tablets per day.

STALEVO is intended mainly for use in patients already receiving treatment with corresponding doses of standard-release levodopa/DDC inhibitor and entacapone.

Starting STALEVO Therapy: Switching from Levodopa/DDC Inhibitor (carbidopa or benserazide) Preparations and Entacapone to STALEVO:

a. Patients who are currently receiving treatment with entacapone and standard-release levodopa/carbidopa in doses equal to STALEVO tablet strengths can be directly switched to the corresponding STALEVO tablets. For example, patients taking one tablet of 100/25 mg levodopa/carbidopa with one tablet of entacapone 200 mg four times daily can be switched to one 100/25/200 mg STALEVO tablet four times daily.
b. When initiating STALEVO therapy in patients currently receiving treatment with entacapone and levodopa/carbidopa in doses not equal to the available STALEVO tablet strengths (50/12.5/200 mg, 75/18.75/200 mg, 100/25/200 mg, 125/31.25/200 mg or 150/37.5/200 mg), STALEVO dosing should be carefully titrated for optimal clinical response. At the start of therapy, STALEVO should be adjusted to correspond as closely as possible to the total daily dose of levodopa currently used.
c. When initiating STALEVO in patients currently treated with entacapone and levodopa/benserazide in a standard-release formulation, treatment should be stopped for one night and STALEVO therapy started the next morning. The therapy should begin with a dosage of STALEVO that will provide either the same amount of levodopa or slightly (5-10%) more.

Switching in Patients not Currently Treated with Entacapone to STALEVO: Initiation of STALEVO at a dosage corresponding to current treatment may be considered in some patients with Parkinson's disease and end-of-dose "wearing-off" who are not stabilised on their current standard-release levodopa/DDC inhibitor treatment. However, a direct switch from levodopa/DDC inhibitor to STALEVO is not recommended for patients who have dyskinesias or whose daily levodopa dose is above 600 mg. In such patients it is advisable to introduce entacapone treatment as a separate medication (entacapone tablets) and adjust the levodopa dose if necessary, before switching to STALEVO.

Entacapone enhances the effects of levodopa, which may cause certain dopaminergic adverse effects e.g., dyskinesias, "on-off" phenomenon, nausea, vomiting, and hallucinations to occur at lower doses and earlier than with preparations containing levodopa alone. It may therefore be necessary, particularly in patients with dyskinesia, to reduce levodopa dosage by 10-30% within the first days to first weeks after initiating STALEVO treatment. The daily dose of levodopa can be reduced by extending the dosing intervals and/or by reducing the amount of levodopa per dose, according to the clinical condition of the patient.

Dosage Adjustment During the Course of the Treatment: When more levodopa is required, an increase in the frequency of doses and/or the use of an alternative strength of STALEVO should be considered, within the dosage recommendations.

When less levodopa is required, the total daily dosage of STALEVO should be reduced either by decreasing the frequency of administration by extending the time between doses, or by decreasing the strength of STALEVO at an administration.

If other levodopa products are used concomitantly with a STALEVO tablet, the maximum dosage recommendations should be followed.

Discontinuation of STALEVO Therapy: If STALEVO treatment (levodopa/carbidopa/entacapone) is discontinued and the patient is switched to levodopa/DDC inhibitor therapy without entacapone, it is necessary to adjust the dosing of other antiparkinsonian treatments, especially levodopa, to achieve a sufficient level of control of the parkinsonian symptoms (see Warnings and Precautions).

Missed Dose: If there is more than an hour left until the next dose, the missed dose should be taken immediately and the next tablet at the next scheduled dose. If there is less than an hour until the next dose, the missed dose should be taken immediately and an hour must elapse until the next dose is taken, following which the patient can go back to the normal schedule.

Doses should not be doubled. Always leave at least an hour between STALEVO tablets, to avoid possible side effects.

Administration: Each tablet is to be taken orally either with or without food (see Actions and Clinical Pharmacology, Pharmacokinetics). One tablet contains one treatment dose. The tablets should always be swallowed whole.

OVERDOSAGE:

Symptoms: There are very few cases of overdosage with levodopa reported in the published literature. Based on the limited available information, the acute symptoms of levodopa/dopa decarboxylase inhibitor overdosage can be expected to arise from dopaminergic overstimulation. Doses of a few grams may result in CNS disturbances, with an increasing likelihood of cardiovascular disturbance (e.g., hypotension, tachycardia) and more severe psychiatric problems at higher doses. An isolated report of rhabdomyolysis and another of transient renal insufficiency suggest that levodopa overdosage may give rise to systemic complications, secondary to dopaminergic overstimulation.

The COMT inhibition by entacapone is dose-dependent. Therefore, a massive overdose of entacapone may produce a 100 % inhibition of COMT enzyme in man, and prevent the metabolism of endogenous and exogenous catechols. The post-marketing data includes isolated cases of accidental and intentional overdose in which the reported highest daily dose of entacapone has been 16 000 mg. The acute symptoms and signs in these cases of overdose included confusion, mydriasis, decreased activity, somnolence, hypotonia, skin discoloration and urticaria.

Treatment: Management of acute overdose with STALEVO (levodopa, carbidopa and entacapone) is the same as management of acute overdosage with levodopa and entacapone. Pyridoxine is not effective in reversing the actions of STALEVO.

Hospitalization is advised and general supportive measures should be employed, along with immediate gastric lavage and repeated doses of charcoal over time. This may hasten the elimination of entacapone in particular by decreasing its absorption/reabsorption from GI tract. Intravenous fluids should be administered judiciously and an adequate airway maintained.

The adequacy of the respiratory, circulatory and renal systems should be carefully monitored and appropriate supportive measures employed. Electrocardiographic monitoring should be instituted and the patient carefully observed for the possible development of arrhythmias; if required, appropriate antiarrhythmic therapy should be given. The possibility that the patient may have taken other drugs, increasing the risk of drug interations (especially catechol-structured drugs should be taken into consideration). To date, no experience has been reported with dialysis in management of levodopa/carbidopa overdose; hence, its value in overdosage is not known. Hemodialysis or hemoperfusion is unlikely to reduce entacapone levels due to its high binding to plasma protein.

> For management of a suspected drug overdose, contact your regional Poison Control Centre. See the *CPS* Directory section for a list of Poison Control Centres.

ACTION AND CLINICAL PHARMACOLOGY: Mechanism of Action: Levodopa: Current evidence indicates that symptoms of Parkinson's disease are related to depletion of dopamine in the corpus striatum. Administration of dopamine is ineffective in the treatment of Parkinson's disease apparently because it does not cross the blood-brain barrier. However, levodopa, the metabolic precursor of dopamine, does cross the blood-brain barrier, and presumably is converted to dopamine in the brain. This is thought to be the mechanism whereby levodopa relieves symptoms of Parkinson's disease.

Carbidopa: When levodopa is administered orally it is rapidly decarboxylated to dopamine in extracerebral tissues so that only a small portion of a given dose is transported unchanged to the central nervous system. Carbidopa does not cross the blood-brain barrier and does not affect the metabolism of levodopa within the central nervous system. Since its decarboxylase inhibiting activity is limited to peripheral tissues, administration of carbidopa with levodopa makes more levodopa available for transport to the brain.

When coadministered with levodopa, carbidopa increases plasma levels of levodopa and reduces the amount of levodopa required to produce a given response by about 75%. Carbidopa prolongs the plasma half-life of levodopa from 50 minutes to 1.5 hours and decreases plasma and urinary dopamine and its major metabolite, homovanillic acid. The T_{max} of levodopa, however, was unaffected by the coadministration.

Entacapone: Entacapone is a reversible, selective and mainly peripherally acting inhibitor of catechol-O-methyltransferase (COMT). Entacapone has no antiparkinsonian effect of its own and is designed for concomitant administration with levodopa preparations.

COMT catalyzes the transfer of the methyl group of S-adenosyl-L-methionine to the phenolic group of substrates that contain a cathecol structure. Physiological substrates of COMT include dopa, catecholamines (dopamine, norepinephrine, epinephrine) and their hydroxylated metabolites. In the presence of a decarboxylase inhibitor, COMT becomes the major enzyme which is responsible for the metabolism of levodopa to 3-methoxy-4-hydroxy-l-phenylalanine (3-OMD).

The mechanism of action of entacapone is believed to be related to its ability to inhibit COMT and thereby alter the plasma pharmacokinetics of levodopa. When administered with levodopa and carbidopa, entacapone decreases the degradation of levodopa in the peripheral tissues further by inhibiting the metabolism of levodopa to 3-OMD through the COMT pathway. This leads to more sustained plasma concentrations of levodopa. It is believed that at a given frequency of levodopa administration, these more sustained plasma levels of levodopa result in more constant dopaminergic stimulation in the brain leading to greater effects on the signs and symptoms of Parkinson's disease. The higher levodopa levels also lead to increased levodopa adverse effects, sometimes requiring a decrease in the dose of levodopa.

When 200 mg entacapone is administered together with levodopa/carbidopa, it increases the area under the curve (AUC) of levodopa by approximately 35% and the elimination half-life of levodopa is prolonged from 1.3 h to 2.4 h. Studies in healthy volunteers and in patients with Parkinson's disease show that entacapone dose-dependently decreases the formation of 3-OMD from levodopa. The chronic use of entacapone (200 mg, 3 to 10 times daily) in patients with Parkinson's disease, decreases the AUC of 3-OMD by 42 to 61%.

Pharmacodynamics: In animals, while entacapone enters the CNS to a minimal extent, it has been shown to inhibit central COMT activity. In humans, entacapone inhibits the COMT enzyme in peripheral tissues. The effects of entacapone on central COMT activity in humans have not been studied.

Pharmacokinetics: Pharmacokinetics of STALEVO (levodopa, carbidopa and entacapone) : The pharmacokinetics of levodopa, carbidopa and entacapone following administration of STALEVO tablets have been studied in comparative bioavailability studies in healthy volunteers.

Pharmacokinetics of Levodopa, Carbidopa and Entacapone: Entacapone pharmacokinetics are linear over a dose range of 5 to 200 mg. A slight non linearity in AUC was seen at doses greater than or equal to 400 mg in a single dose, dose-response, study in patients with Parkinson's disease. The pharmacokinetics of entacapone are independent of levodopa/carbidopa.

Absorption: There are large intra- and interindividual variations in the absorption of levodopa, carbidopa and entacapone. Both levodopa and entacapone are rapidly absorbed and eliminated.

Entacapone is rapidly absorbed from the GI tract, reaching peak concentrations (C_{max}) in the plasma in approximately one hour. Carbidopa is absorbed and eliminated slightly more slowly than levodopa. When given separately without the other two active substances, the bioavailability of levodopa is 15-33%, that of carbidopa 40-70%, and that of entacapone 35% after a 200 mg oral dose. C_{max}, after a single 200 mg dose of entacapone, is approximately 1.2 µg/mL. Meals rich in large neutral amino acids may delay and reduce the absorption of levodopa. Food does not affect the absorption of entacapone to any significant extent.

Distribution: The distribution volume of levodopa (Vd 0.36-1.6 L/kg) is moderately small; no data are available for carbidopa. The volume of distribution of entacapone at steady state after i.v. injection is small (20 L).

Levodopa is bound to plasma proteins only to a minor extent (about 10-30%), while carbidopa is bound approximately 36%, and while entacapone is extensively bound (about 98% over the concentration range of 0.4 to 50 µg/mL), mainly to serum albumin. Entacapone does not distribute widely into tissues due to its high plasma protein binding.

Metabolism: Levodopa is extensively metabolized to various metabolites, decarboxylation by dopa decarboxylase (DDC) and O-methylation by catechol-O-methyltransferase (COMT) being the most important pathways.

Carbidopa is metabolised to two main metabolites which are excreted in the urine as glucuronides and unconjugated compounds. Unchanged carbidopa accounts for 30% of the total urinary excretion.

Entacapone undergoes extensive metabolism, mainly in the liver. The main metabolic pathway of entacapone in humans is the isomerization to the cis-isomer, followed by direct glucuronidation of the parent and cis-isomer; the glucuronide conjugate is inactive. The elimination of entacapone occurs mainly by non-renal metabolic pathways. It is estimated that 80-90% of the dose is excreted in feces, although this has not been confirmed in man. Approximately 10-20% is excreted in urine. Only traces of entacapone are found as unchanged drug in urine. The major part (95 %) of the drug excreted in urine is conjugated with glucuronic acid. Of the metabolites found in urine only about 1 % have been formed through oxidation.

Excretion: Total clearance of levodopa is in the range of 0.55-1.38 L/kg/h. The elimination half-life is ($t_{1/2}$) 0.6-1.3 hours for levodopa and 2-3 hours for carbidopa, each given separately.

The total body clearance of entacapone, after i.v. administration, is about 800 mL/min. It is eliminated with a short elimination half-life; the half-life for β-phase being about 0.5 hours and for the γ-phase about 2.5 hours. The β-phase is predominant, and the γ-phase accounts for approximately 8% of the plasma-time-concentration curve (AUC) following i.v. administration.

Due to short elimination half-lives, no true accumulation of levodopa or entacapone occurs on repeated administration.

Special Populations and Conditions: Pediatrics: Safety and effectiveness in pediatric patients have not been established.

Geriatrics: The pharmacokinetics of STALEVO were not studied in Parkinson's disease patients or in healthy volunteers older than 55 years of age in the comparative bioavailability studies.

In elderly patients given levodopa without carbidopa and entacapone, absorption is greater and elimination is slower than in young subjects. However, when combined with carbidopa, the absorption of levodopa is similar in both elderly and the young patients, although the AUC is still 1.5 times greater in the elderly due to decreased DDC activity and lower clearance caused by aging. Entacapone pharmacokinetics are independent of age.

Gender: The bioavailability of levodopa is significantly higher in women than in men when given with or without carbidopa and/or entacapone (on average, 40% for AUC and 30% for C_{max}). No formal gender studies have been conducted with entacapone.

Hepatic Insufficiency: As there are no clinical trial data to establish a safe and effective dosing regimen for hepatically impaired patients, STALEVO should be not be administered to patients with hepatic impairment (see Contraindications).

The metabolism of entacapone is slowed in patients with mild to moderate (Child-Pugh grading Class A and B) hepatic insufficiency caused by cirrhotic disease. In these patients, the AUC and C_{max} values were approximately two-fold greater than those in demographically-matched healthy volunteers.

Renal Insufficiency: STALEVO should be administered cautiously to patients with severe renal disease. There are no studies on the pharmacokinetics of levodopa and carbidopa in patients with renal impairment (see Warnings and Precautions).

The pharmacokinetics of entacapone were evaluated in healthy volunteers and in patients with moderately (Cl_{cr} 0.60-0.89 mL/sec/1.73 m^2) and severely (Cl_{cr} 0.20-0.44 mL/sec/1.73 m^2) impaired renal function. After a single oral dose of 200 mg, the pharmacokinetics of entacapone were not significantly changed in patients with moderate to severe renal insufficiency.

Concurrent Diseases: STALEVO is contraindicated for patients with clinical or laboratory evidence of uncompensated cardiovascular, endocrine, hematologic, pulmonary (including bronchial asthma), or renal disease (see Contraindications).

STALEVO should be administered cautiously to patients with biliary obstruction, or history of peptic ulcer disease or convulsions (see Warnings and Precautions).

STORAGE AND STABILITY: Store at room temperature (15-30°C).

INFORMATION FOR THE PATIENT: Published in e-CPS, available by subscription at www.e-cps.ca.

DOSAGE FORMS, COMPOSITION AND PACKAGING: 50 mg/12.5 mg/200 mg: Each brownish- or greyish-red, round, convex, unscored, film-coated tablet, marked with "LCE 50" on one side, contains: levodopa 50 mg, carbidopa 12.5 mg and entacapone 200 mg. Bottles of 100.

75 mg/18.75 mg/200 mg: Each light brownish red, oval-shaped, unscored, film-coated tablet, marked with "LCE 75" on one side, contains: levodopa 75 mg, carbidopa 18.75 mg and entacapone 200 mg. Bottles of 100.

100 mg/25 mg/200 mg : Each brownish- or greyish-red, oval-shaped, unscored, film-coated tablet, marked with "LCE 100" on one side, contains: levodopa 100 mg, carbidopa 25 mg and entacapone 200 mg. Bottles of 100.
125 mg/31.25 mg/200 mg: Each light brownish red, oval-shaped, unscored, film-coated tablet, marked with "LCE 125" on one side, contains: levodopa 125 mg, carbidopa 31.25 mg and entacapone 200 mg. Bottles of 100.
150 mg/37.5 mg/200 mg : Each brownish- or greyish-red, elongated-ellipse shaped, unscored, film-coated tablet, marked with "LCE 150" on one side, contains: levodopa 150 mg, carbidopa 37.5 mg and entacapone 200 mg. Bottles of 100.

(Shown in Product Identification Section)

Starlix®

nateglinide
Oral Antidiabetic

Novartis Pharmaceuticals

Date of Preparation: February 6, 2002
Date of Revision: November 25, 2009

PHARMACOLOGY: Nateglinide is an amino acid derivative that improves glycemic control by restoring early insulin secretion. Nateglinide induces significant insulin secretion within the first 15 minutes following a meal. Early insulin secretion results in suppression of hepatic glucose production, reducing meal-related glucose excursions and post-meal hyperinsulinemia which has been associated with delayed hypoglycemia.

Early insulin secretion is an essential mechanism to maintain normal glycemic control. The loss of early insulin secretion characterizes Type 2 diabetes. Nateglinide when taken just before meals restores early insulin secretion through a rapid and transient interaction with the ATP-sensitive potassium (K^+ATP) channel on pancreatic β-cells. Electrophysiologic studies demonstrate that nateglinide has >300-fold selectivity for pancreatic β-cell versus cardiovascular K^+ATP channels. The extent of insulin release is dependent on ambient glucose concentrations such that less insulin is secreted as glucose levels fall. The action of nateglinide is dependent upon functioning beta cells in the pancreatic islets.

Pharmacokinetics: Absorption: Following oral administration prior to a meal, nateglinide is rapidly absorbed with mean peak plasma drug concentrations (C_{max}) generally occurring within 1 hour to peak plasma concentration (T_{max}) after dosing. When administered to patients with Type 2 diabetes over the dosage range of 60 to 240 mg 3 times a day for 1 week, nateglinide demonstrated linear pharmacokinetics for both AUC (area under the time/plasma concentration curve) and C_{max}. T_{max} was found to be independent of dose in this patient population. Absolute bioavailability is estimated to be 73%. When given with meals, the extent of nateglinide absorption (AUC) remains unaffected. However, there is a delay in the rate of absorption characterized by a decrease in C_{max} and a delay in time to T_{max}. Nateglinide is usually taken immediately (1 minute) before a meal but may be taken up to 30 minutes before meals (see Dosage).

Distribution: Based on i.v. data, the steady-state volume of distribution of nateglinide is estimated to be approximately 10 L. Nateglinide is extensively bound (98%) to serum proteins, primarily serum albumin and to a lesser extent α_1 acid glycoprotein. The extent of serum protein binding is independent of drug concentration over the test range of 0.1 to 10 μg/mL.

Metabolism: Nateglinide is extensively metabolized by the mixed-function oxidase system prior to elimination. The major routes of metabolism are hydroxylation followed by glucuronide conjugation. The major metabolites are less potent than nateglinide. The isoprene minor metabolite possesses similar potency as the parent compound nateglinide.

Data available from both in vitro and in vivo experiments indicate that nateglinide is predominantly metabolized by cytochrome P450 isoenzyme CYP2C9 (70%) and to a lesser extent by CYP3A4 (30%) (see Precautions, Drug Interactions).

Excretion: Nateglinide and its metabolites are rapidly and completely eliminated following oral administration. Within 6 hours after dosing, approximately 75% of the administered ^{14}C-nateglinide is recovered in the urine. Most of the ^{14}C-nateglinide (83%) is excreted in the urine with an additional 10% eliminated in the feces. Approximately 16% of the ^{14}C-nateglinide is excreted in the urine as parent compound. In all studies of healthy volunteers and patients with Type 2 diabetes, nateglinide plasma concentrations declined rapidly with an average elimination half-life of 1.5 hours. Consistent with this short elimination half-life, there is no apparent accumulation of nateglinide upon multiple dosing of up to 240 mg 3 times daily for 7 days.

Special Populations: Geriatrics: There was no difference in the safety and efficacy profile of nateglinide between the elderly and the general population. In addition, age did not influence the pharmacokinetic properties of nateglinide. Therefore, no special dose adjustments are necessary for elderly patients.

Gender: No clinically significant differences in nateglinide pharmacokinetics were observed between men and women. Therefore, no dose adjustment based on gender is needed.

Race: Results of a population pharmacokinetic analysis included subjects of Caucasian (n=255), black (n=12) and other ethnic origins (n=45). The results did not indicate any influence of race on the pharmacokinetics of nateglinide, but the numbers are small.

Renal Impairment: The systemic availability and the half-life of nateglinide in diabetic subjects with moderate to severe renal insufficiency (CrCl: 0.25 to 0.83 mL/sec/1.73 m^2 or 15 to 50 mL/min/1.73 m^2), whether or not on dialysis, do not differ to a clinically significant extent from those in healthy subjects, therefore no dose adjustment is necessary.

Hepatic Impairment: The systemic availability and the half-life of nateglinide in non-diabetic subjects with mild to moderate hepatic insufficiency do not differ to a clinically significant extent from those in healthy subjects. Consequently, dose adjustment for patients with mild to moderate hepatic disease is not required. Since patients with moderate to severe hepatic disease were not studied, nateglinide should be used with caution in such patients.

Pharmacodynamics and Clinical Effects: In clinical studies, treatment with nateglinide resulted in an improvement in glycemic control, as measured by glycosylated hemoglobin A1c (HbA_{1C}) and post-meal glucose. Fasting plasma glucose (FPG) levels were also reduced. This is consistent with the mechanism of action of nateglinide which is to restore early insulin secretion and thereby reduce post-meal glucose. The improvement in glycemic control was durable, with maintenance of effect compared to baseline for at least 52 weeks. In the 24-week, placebo-controlled, clinical trials, the mean weight gain in patients treated with nateglinide was 1 kg or less.

Clinical Studies: Compared to repaglinide in healthy subjects, nateglinide was associated with a faster rise of insulin concentrations (within 30 minutes) and a shorter duration (return to placebo levels in 1.5 versus 4 hours) resulting in less total insulin exposure. Nateglinide was also more effective in blunting the post-meal plasma glucose excursion compared to repaglinide (89% vs 56%) without inducing prolonged hypoglycemia.

The loss of first phase insulin secretion is a hallmark of Type 2 diabetes. Nateglinide restores this response in patients with Type 2 diabetes.

The United Kingdom Prospective Diabetes Study (UKPDS) demonstrated in patients with Type 2 diabetes that improved glycemic control, as reflected in HbA_{1C} and fasting glucose levels, was associated with a reduction in the diabetic complications retinopathy, neuropathy and nephropathy.

The DECODE study (Diabetes Epidemiology Collaborative Analysis of Diagnostic Criteria in Europe study published in 1999) and the Diabetes Intervention Study demonstrated the role of 2-hour plasma glucose as an independent risk factor for total and cardiovascular mortality whereas FPG did not significantly contribute to the prediction of mortality.

A total of 2122 patients with Type 2 diabetes were treated with nateglinide in double-blind, placebo or active controlled studies. These studies included two 24-week placebo controlled studies, two 24-week active controlled studies, and five additional efficacy studies with treatment durations of 8 weeks (2 studies), 12 weeks (2 studies) or 16 weeks. In addition, 3 controlled extension studies were carried out to 52 weeks. All 9 studies were characterized by a lengthy washout period of prior therapy so as to adequately evaluate the treatment effect of nateglinide by minimizing confounding effects of previous antidiabetic medications. In these studies, nateglinide was administered before main meals, usually breakfast, lunch and dinner.

Effect on Post-meal (prandial) Plasma Glucose: Restoration of early insulin release during meals, resulting in reduced post-meal plasma glucose, is an important component of optimal therapy in Type 2 diabetes.

In an 8-week study that compared the effect of nateglinide 120 mg taken with meals, glyburide 10 mg once daily, and placebo on daytime glucose and insulin profiles, treatment with nateglinide was associated with a greater reduction of the post-meal glucose excursion and less total insulin exposure.

The rapid rise and short duration of insulin release associated with nateglinide results in a reduction in glucose fluctuations throughout the day. Nateglinide significantly reduced the standard deviation of the plasma glucose levels compared to glyburide. The results illustrated in Figure 1 suggest that the postprandial insulin pattern in response to nateglinide approximates the physiological pattern.

After a liquid (Sustacal, Mead Johnson) meal, both nateglinide and glyburide reduced the incremental glucose exposure over 4 hours. This reduction was statistically significantly greater for nateglinide compared to glyburide (i.e., the percent change from baseline AUC_{0-4} was -64%, -32% and -1% for nateglinide, glyburide and placebo respectively).

Figure 1: Starlix

Unadjusted Insulin Levels—Change from Baseline (Pretreatment)

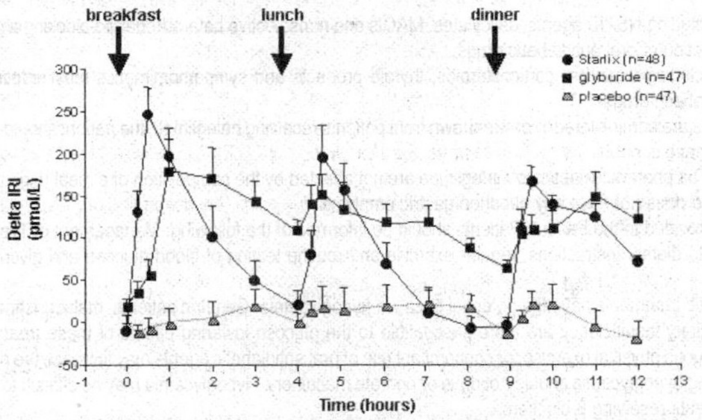

In a 24-week, placebo-controlled study conducted to evaluate the effect of nateglinide as monotherapy and in combination with metformin, there was a statistically significant reduction in incremental mealtime plasma glucose $AUC_{(0\text{-}130\ min)}$. The post-meal glycemic excursion was reduced by 16% with metformin, 34% with nateglinide 120 mg before meals and by 40% with the combination of nateglinide 120 mg before meals plus metformin 500 mg t.i.d. These data confirm that the efficacy of nateglinide in lowering post-meal glucose is maintained when administered with a drug with a complementary mode of action.

Monotherapy: Two 24-week, placebo-controlled studies were conducted in patients with Type 2 diabetes that were inadequately controlled on diet alone. In Study A, statistically significant reductions in HbA_{1C} occurred in a dose-dependent manner over the range of 60 to 180 mg when nateglinide was administered just before breakfast, lunch, and dinner as monotherapy. The mean change from baseline for reduction of HbA_{1C} was 0.004 to 0.006 (0.4 to 0.6%). The difference from placebo was 0.006 to 0.01 (0.6 to 1.0%) for 120 mg nateglinide before breakfast, lunch, and dinner. Statistically significant reductions in fasting plasma glucose (FPG) over the range of 0.61 to 0.93 mmol/L were also observed.

In a second 24-week study (Study B) conducted to evaluate the effect of nateglinide monotherapy, the mean change from baseline for reduction of HbA_{1C} was 0.005 (0.5%). The difference from placebo was 0.009 (0.9%) for 120 mg nateglinide before breakfast, lunch, and dinner, which was statistically significant.

Combination with Metformin: The results of above study (Study B) suggest that nateglinide and metformin are synergistic when used in combination, due to complementary modes of action. The combination of the 2 drugs demonstrated an 84% responder rate based on a reduction of >10% from pretreatment baseline HbA_{1C}. The effect on HbA_{1C} and FPG was greater with nateglinide plus metformin combination therapy than with either agent alone. Virtually all of the post-meal glucose effect was due to nateglinide. Metformin had a greater effect on HbA_{1C} than nateglinide.

Other: In a 24-week active controlled study, patients who were stabilized on high dose sulfonylurea for at least 3 months and directly switched to monotherapy with nateglinide 60 or 120 mg before meals experienced reduced glycemic control as evidenced by increases in FPG and HbA_{1C}.

In a 12-week study of patients inadequately controlled on glyburide 10 mg once daily, the addition of nateglinide 120 mg before meals did not produce any additional benefit.

INDICATIONS: Nateglinide is indicated as monotherapy in addition to diet and exercise to lower the blood sugar in patients with Type 2 diabetes mellitus who are not controlled satisfactorily by diet and exercise alone.

Nateglinide is indicated also in combination with metformin in patients not controlled satisfactorily on diet, exercise, and either nateglinide or metformin alone.

Management of Type 2 diabetes should include diet control. Caloric restriction, weight loss, and exercise are essential for the proper treatment of the diabetic patient. This is important not only in the primary treatment of Type 2 diabetes, but also in maintaining the efficacy of drug therapy. Prior to initiation of therapy with nateglinide, secondary causes of poor glycemic control, e.g., infection, should be investigated and treated.

CONTRAINDICATIONS: In patients with: known hypersensitivity to the drug or its inactive ingredients; type 1 diabetes; diabetic ketoacidosis.

PRECAUTIONS: Hypoglycemia: Hypoglycemia has been observed in patients with Type 2 diabetes treated with oral antidiabetic agents. Geriatric patients, malnourished patients and those with adrenal or pituitary insufficiency or severe renal impairment are more susceptible to the glucose lowering effect of these treatments. The risk of hypoglycemia may be increased by strenuous physical exercise, ingestion of alcohol, and/or insufficient caloric intake.

Combination with other oral antidiabetic agents may increase the risk of hypoglycemia.

Hypoglycemia may be difficult to recognize in elderly subjects and in subjects receiving β-blockers.

Nateglinide should be used with caution in patients with moderate to severe hepatic impairment because such patients have not been studied.

Pregnancy: Nateglinide was not teratogenic in rats at doses up to 1000 mg/kg (20 times the maximum daily human dose when compared on the basis of body surface area). In the rabbit, embryonic development was adversely affected and the incidence of gallbladder agenesis or small gallbladder was increased at a dose which also resulted in maternal toxicity (i.e., 500 mg/kg, which is 21 times the maximum daily human dose based on body surface area).

There are no adequate and well-controlled studies in pregnant women. Nateglinide is not recommended for use in pregnancy.

Because current information strongly suggests that abnormal blood glucose levels during pregnancy are associated with a higher incidence of congenital anomalies as well as increased neonatal morbidity and mortality, most experts recommend that insulin be used during pregnancy to maintain blood glucose levels as close to normal as possible.

Lactation: Studies in lactating rats showed that nateglinide is excreted in the milk; the $AUC_{0\text{-}48h}$ ratio in milk to plasma was about 1.4. Body weights were lower in offspring of rats administered nateglinide at 1000 mg/kg during the peri- and postnatal period. It is not known whether nateglinide is excreted in human milk. Because many drugs are excreted in human milk, nateglinide should not be administered to a nursing woman.

Children: The safety and effectiveness of nateglinide in pediatric patients have not been established.

Geriatrics: Among patients receiving nateglinide as monotherapy in controlled clinical studies ranging from 8 weeks to 1 year in duration, 436 patients (30%) were 65 or older and 80 patients (5.4%) were 75 or older. No differences in safety or efficacy between these subjects and those less than 65 were observed for nateglinide. There was no increase in frequency of hypoglycemia in patients over the age of 65. However, greater sensitivity of some older individuals to nateglinide therapy cannot be ruled out.

Drug Interactions: Data available from both in vitro and in vivo drug metabolism experiments indicate that nateglinide is predominantly metabolized by the cytochrome P450 isoenzyme CYP2C9 (70%) and to a lesser extent by CYP3A4 (30%). Nateglinide has the ability to inhibit the in vitro metabolism of tolbutamide, a CYP2C9 substrate. No inhibition of CYP 3A4 metabolic reactions is expected based on in vitro experiments, suggesting a low potential for clinically significant pharmacokinetic drug interactions.

Glyburide: Concomitant administration of nateglinide (120 mg t.i.d.) and glyburide (10 mg/day) to healthy volunteers had no clinically relevant effect on the pharmacokinetics of either agent.

Metformin: In healthy volunteers, nateglinide (120 mg t.i.d.) taken with metformin (500 mg/day) did not alter the pharmacokinetics of either agent.

Digoxin: Nateglinide (120 mg t.i.d.) when administered with digoxin (1 mg/day) to healthy volunteers, did not alter the steady-state pharmacokinetic properties of either agent.

Warfarin: Nateglinide (120 mg t.i.d.) taken with warfarin (30 mg/day) by healthy volunteers had no clinically relevant effect on the pharmacokinetics of either agent.

Diclofenac: Administration of nateglinide (120 mg b.i.d.) with diclofenac (75 mg/day) to healthy volunteers did not alter the pharmacokinetics of either agent.

In an interaction trial with sulfinpyrazone, a potent and selective CYP2C9 inhibitor, a modest increase in nateglinide AUC (28%) was observed in healthy volunteers, with no changes in the mean C_{max} and elimination half-life. A more prolonged effect and possibly a risk of hypoglycemia cannot be excluded in patients when nateglinide is co-administered with CYP2C9 inhibitors.

Nateglinide is highly bound to plasma proteins (98%), mainly albumin. In an in vitro displacement study with highly protein-bound drugs such as furosemide, propranolol, captopril, nicardipine, pravastatin, glyburide, warfarin, phenytoin, ASA, tolbutamide, and metformin, there was no influence by these drugs on the extent of nateglinide protein binding. In a separate in vitro study, nateglinide had no influence on the serum protein binding of propranolol, glyburide, nicardipine, warfarin, phenytoin, ASA and tolbutamide.

Certain drugs, including NSAID agents, salicylates, MAOIs and nonselective beta-adrenergic-blocking agents may potentiate the hypoglycemic action of oral antidiabetic drugs.

Certain drugs including thiazides, corticosteroids, thyroid products and sympathomimetics may reduce the hypoglycemic action of oral antidiabetic drugs.

When these drugs are administered to or withdrawn from patients receiving nateglinide, the patient should be observed closely for changes in glycemic control.

Food Interactions: The pharmacokinetics of nateglinide are not affected by the composition of a meal (high protein, fat or carbohydrate). Nateglinide does not have any effect on gastric emptying.

Information to Be Provided to the Patient: Patients should be informed of the following: Management of Type 2 diabetes should include adherence to dietary instructions, regular exercise and routine testing of blood glucose and glycosylated hemoglobin (HbA_{1C}).

All oral antidiabetic treatments have the potential to cause hypoglycemia. Geriatric patients, malnourished patients and those with adrenal or pituitary insufficiency are more susceptible to the glucose lowering effects of these treatments. A missed or delayed meal, strenuous physical exercise, or concomitant use of oral antidiabetic agents may increase the risk of hypoglycemia. Patients experiencing hypoglycemia should not drive or operate machinery. Hypoglycemia may be difficult to recognize in elderly patients and in patients receiving β-blockers.

Nateglinide should be taken before meals and is usually taken immediately (1 minute) before meals but may be taken up to 30 minutes before meals. Patients who skip a meal should be instructed to skip a dose for that meal.

Laboratory Tests: Since the primary mechanism of action for nateglinide is reducing post-meal glucose (an essential contributor to HbA_{1C}), the therapeutic response to nateglinide may be monitored with 1 to 2 hour post-meal glucose measurements. In addition, glycosylated hemoglobin (HbA_{1C}) should also be measured periodically.

ADVERSE EFFECTS: Nateglinide was administered either as monotherapy or combination therapy to 2122 patients with Type 2 diabetes including 1791 exposed for at least 12 weeks, 1224 for at least 24 weeks and 190 for 52 weeks. Of these, 1136, 789 and 113 patients were exposed to nateglinide monotherapy for 12, 24 and 52 weeks respectively.

Discontinuation due to adverse events occurred in 4.9% of nateglinide-treated patients vs 5.5% in patients receiving placebo. Among nateglinide-treated patients, the most common reasons for discontinuation were fatigue (0.8%), thirst (0.7%), and polyuria (0.5). Only 0.3% of nateglinide-treated patients discontinued due to hypoglycemia.

Table 1 lists common adverse events for nateglinide patients, regardless of attribution, in placebo controlled studies and active controlled studies (i.e. metformin and glyburide) of up to 24 weeks in duration.

Table 1: Starlix

Commonly Reported Adverse Events (% of Patients)[a]

Event	Placebo controlled studies		Active controlled studies		
	Starlix N=973	Placebo N=458	Starlix N=378	Metformin N=194	Glyburide N=243
Body as a Whole—General Disorders					
Accidental Trauma	2.7	1.7	1.9	1.0	5.3
Central and Peripheral Nervous System Disorders					
Dizziness	3.6	2.2	3.7	1.5	3.7
Gastrointestinal					
Abdominal Pain	3.1	3.1	2.1	0.5	0.8
Dyspepsia	2.5	2.2	0.5	2.1	1.2
Metabolic					
Hypoglycemia (confirmed)[b]	2.8	0.4	0.3	0.5	5.3
Musculoskeletal					
Arthropathy	2.7	2.2	1.3	3.1	2.5
Respiratory					
Coughing	2.2	2.2	0.5	2.6	2.5
Upper Respiratory Tract Infection	10.4	8.1	6.9	3.6	10.3

[a] Events ≥2% for the Starlix group in the placebo controlled studies and = events in the placebo group.
[b] Any symptomatic event confirmed by a plasma glucose equivalent of ≤3.3 mmol/L.

The most frequently occurring symptoms of hypoglycemia among patients who received nateglinide were tremor, increased sweating, dizziness and asthenia. These events were generally mild; most events took place during the day, within 4 hours of the previous meal and drug intake.

Rare cases of elevations in liver enzymes were reported.

Rare cases of hypersensitivity reactions such as rash, itching and urticaria were reported.

In all completed clinical studies there was no relation of dose on the overall incidence of adverse experiences.

OVERDOSE:

Symptoms: In a clinical study in patients with Type 2 diabetes, nateglinide was administered in increasing doses up to 720 mg a day for 7 days and there were no clinically significant adverse events reported. There have been no instances of overdose with nateglinide in clinical trials. However, an overdose may result in an exaggerated glucose lowering effect with the development of hypoglycemic symptoms.

Treatment: Hypoglycemic symptoms without loss of consciousness or neurological findings should be treated with oral glucose and adjustments in dosage and/or meal patterns. Severe hypoglycemic reactions with coma, seizure or other neurological symptoms should be treated with i.v. glucose. As nateglinide is highly protein bound, dialysis is not an efficient means of removing it from the blood.

> For management of a suspected drug overdose, CPhA recommends that you contact your **regional Poison Control Centre**. See the *CPS* Directory section for a list of Poison Control Centres.

DOSAGE: Nateglinide should be taken prior to meals. It is usually taken immediately (1 minute) before a meal but may be taken up to 30 minutes before meals.

Monotherapy: The usual starting and maintenance dose is 120 mg before meals.

If an adequate response is not achieved, a dose of 180 mg before meals may be used or metformin may be added to the current dose (see Dosage, Combination Therapy with Metformin). The 60 mg dose of nateglinide may be used in patients who are near goal HbA_{1c} (e.g. HbA_{1c} <0.075), when treatment is initiated.

Since the primary mechanism of nateglinide is reducing mealtime glucose (an essential contributor to HbA_{1C}), the therapeutic response to nateglinide may be monitored with 1 to 2 hour post-meal glucose. In addition, glycosylated hemoglobin (HbA_{1C}) should be measured periodically.

Combination Therapy with Metformin: For patients on nateglinide monotherapy who require additional therapy, metformin may be added to the maintenance dose.

For patients on metformin monotherapy who require additional therapy, the usual dose of nateglinide is 120 mg before meals. For some patients who are close to their therapeutic target (e.g., HbA_{1C} <0.075), nateglinide 60 mg before meals may be sufficient.

Elderly: No special dose adjustments are usually necessary.

Renal and Hepatic Impairment: No dosage adjustment is necessary in patients with mild to severe renal insufficiency or in patients with mild hepatic insufficiency. Dosing of patients with moderate to severe hepatic dysfunction has not been studied. Therefore, nateglinide should be used with caution in patients with moderate to severe liver disease.

INFORMATION FOR THE PATIENT: Published in e-CPS, available by subscription at www.e-cps.ca.

SUPPLIED: 60 mg: Each pink, round, beveled-edged, film-coated tablet with "Starlix" debossed on one side and "60" on the other side, contains: nateglinide 60 mg. Nonmedicinal ingredients: colloidal silicon dioxide, croscarmellose sodium, hydroxypropyl methylcellulose, iron oxide (red or yellow), lactose (hydrous), magnesium stearate, microcrystalline cellulose, polyethylene glycol, povidone, talc and titanium dioxide. Cartons of 7 blister strips of 12 tablets. Store between 15 and 30°C. Keep bottles tightly closed.

120 mg: Each yellow, ovaloid, film-coated tablet, with "Starlix" debossed on one side and "120" on the other side, contains: nateglinide 120 mg. Nonmedicinal ingredients: colloidal silicon dioxide, croscarmellose sodium, hydroxypropyl methylcellulose, iron oxide (red or yellow), lactose (hydrous), magnesium stearate, microcrystalline cellulose, polyethylene glycol, povidone, talc and titanium dioxide. Cartons of 7 blister strips of 12 tablets. Store between 15 and 30°C. Keep bottles tightly closed.

(Shown in Product Identification Section)

Statex Ⓝ

morphine sulfate

Opioid Analgesic

Paladin

SUPPLIED: Drops: 20 mg/mL: Each mL of clear unflavored and colorless liquid contains: morphine sulfate 20 mg. Graduated bottles of 25 and 100 mL with calibrated dropper, filled to deliver 1 mL (20 mg of morphine sulfate). Calorie content: 160 kcal/100 mL. Store between 15-30°C in a well closed light resistant container.

50 mg/mL: Each mL of clear unflavored and colorless liquid contains: morphine sulfate 50 mg. Graduated bottles of 50 mL with calibrated dropper, filled to deliver 1 mL (50 mg of morphine sulfate). Calorie content: 160 kcal/100 mL. Store between 15-30°C in a well closed light resistant container.

Suppositories: 5 mg: Each white cone-shape suppository contains: morphine sulfate 5 mg. Boxes of 10. The suppository should be placed against the rectal mucosa. The drug is not absorbed if pushed into a mass of stool or if it is placed in the anal canal. Store between 15-30°C in a well closed light resistant container.

20 mg: Each white cone-shape suppository contains: morphine sulfate 20 mg. Boxes of 10. The suppository should be placed against the rectal mucosa. The drug is not absorbed if pushed into a mass of stool or if it is placed in the anal canal. Store between 15-30°C in a well closed light resistant container.

30 mg: Each white cone-shape suppository contains: morphine sulfate 30 mg. Boxes of 10. The suppository should be placed against the rectal mucosa. The drug is not absorbed if pushed into a mass of stool or if it is placed in the anal canal. Store between 15-30°C in a well closed light resistant container.

Syrup: 1 mg/mL: Each mL of unflavored (clear) or orange flavored syrup contains: morphine sulfate 1 mg. Graduated bottles of 250 and 500 mL in plastic bottles. Uni-dose of 5, 10 and 15 mL (unflavoured) in amber glass bottles. Store between 15-30°C in a well closed light resistant container.

5 mg/mL: Each mL of unflavored (clear) or orange flavored syrup contains: morphine sulfate 5 mg. Graduated bottles of 250 and 500 mL in plastic bottles. Uni-dose of 5 and 10 mL (unflavoured) in amber glass bottles. Store between 15-30°C in a well closed light resistant container.

10 mg/mL: Each mL of unflavoured syrup contains: morphine sulfate 10 mg. Graduated bottles of 250 mL in plastic bottles. Store between 15-30°C in a well closed light resistant container.

TABLETS: 5 mg: Each green, round tablet, scored on one side, identified with Paladin logo on the other side, contains: morphine sulfate 5 mg. Bottles of 100. Control packs of 100 (4×25 tablets in blister). Store between 15-30°C in a well closed light resistant container.

10 mg: Each blue, round tablet, scored on one side, identified with Paladin logo on the other side, contains: morphine sulfate 10 mg. Bottles of 100. Control packs of 100 (4×25 tablets in blister). Store between 15-30°C in a well closed light resistant container.

25 mg: Each pink, round tablet, scored on one side, identified with Paladin logo on the other side, contains: morphine sulfate 25 mg. Bottles of 100. Control packs of 100 (4×25 tablets in blister). Store between 15-30°C in a well closed light resistant container.

50 mg: Each orange, round tablet, scored on one side, identified with Paladin logo on the other side, contains: morphine sulfate 50 mg. Bottles of 100. Control packs of 100 (4×25 tablets in blister). Store between 15-30°C in a well closed light resistant container.

Statins Ⓟ

CPhA Monograph

see *HMG-CoA Reductase Inhibitors*

Stelara™ Ⓟ

ustekinumab

Selective Immunomodulating Agent

Janssen-Ortho

Date of Preparation: December 12, 2008
Date of Revision: June 18, 2010

SUMMARY PRODUCT INFORMATION:

Route of Administration	Dosage Form/ Strength	Clinically Relevant Nonmedicinal Ingredients
Subcutaneous injection	Sterile solution in single-use vial or pre-filled syringe: 45 mg/0.5 mL	None For a complete listing see Dosage Forms, Composition and Packaging.

DESCRIPTION: STELARA (ustekinumab) is a fully human IgG1k monoclonal antibody with an approximate molecular weight of 148 600 daltons. STELARA (ustekinumab) is produced by a recombinant cell line cultured by continuous perfusion and is purified by a series of steps that includes measures to inactivate and remove viruses.

STELARA is supplied as a sterile solution of ustekinumab for subcutaneous administration in a single-use glass vial. The vial is stoppered with a coated stopper. STELARA does not contain preservatives. STELARA contains 90 mg ustekinumab per mL.

STELARA is also supplied as a single-use, sterile solution in a glass syringe with a fixed 27G, half-inch needle and needle cover. The needle cover is manufactured using a dry natural rubber (a derivative of latex) (see Warnings and Precautions, Hypersensitivity Reactions). The syringe is fitted with a passive safety guard.

INDICATIONS AND CLINICAL USE: STELARA (ustekinumab) is indicated in adult patients for the treatment of chronic moderate to severe plaque psoriasis who are candidates for phototherapy or systemic therapy.

CONTRAINDICATIONS:
- Patients with known hypersensitivity to STELARA or any of its components.
- Patients with severe infections such as sepsis, tuberculosis and opportunistic infections (see Warnings and Precautions, Infections).

WARNINGS AND PRECAUTIONS: Carcinogenesis and Mutagenesis: STELARA (ustekinumab) is a selective immunomodulator. Immunomodulating agents have the potential to increase the risk of malignancy. Some patients who received ustekinumab in clinical studies developed malignancies (see Adverse Reactions). In the controlled and non-controlled portions of psoriasis clinical studies, the incidence of malignancies excluding nonmelanoma skin cancers was 0.36 per 100 patient-years of follow-up for ustekinumab-treated patients (8 patients in 2249 patient-years of follow-up) and included breast, colon, head and neck, kidney, prostate, and thyroid cancers. The rate of malignancies reported in ustekinumab-treated patients was comparable to the rate expected in the general population (standardized incidence ratio=0.68 [95% confidence interval: 0.29, 1.34]. The incidence of nonmelanoma skin cancer was 0.80 per 100 patient-years of follow-up for ustekinumab-treated patients (18 patients in 2245 patient-years of follow-up).

STELARA (ustekinumab) has not been studied in patients with a history of malignancy. Caution should be exercised when considering the use of STELARA in patients with a history of malignancy or when considering continuing treatment in patients who develop a malignancy.

Hepatic/Biliary/Pancreatic: Specific studies have not been conducted in patients with hepatic insufficiency.

Hypersensitivity Reactions: In post-marketing experience, serious allergic reactions, including possible anaphylaxis, have been reported. If an anaphylactic or other serious allergic reaction occurs, administration of STELARA (ustekinumab) should be discontinued immediately and appropriate therapy instituted (see Adverse Reactions).

The needle cover on the pre-filled syringe contains dry natural rubber (a derivative of latex), which may cause allergic reactions in individuals sensitive to latex.

Immune: Immunization: It is recommended that live viral or bacterial vaccines not be given concurrently with STELARA (ustekinumab). No data are available on the secondary transmission of infection by live vaccines in patients receiving STELARA. Caution is advised when administering some live vaccines to household contacts of patients receiving STELARA because of the potential risk for shedding from the household contact and transmission to the patient. Patients receiving STELARA may receive concurrent inactivated or non-live vaccinations (see Drug Interactions).

Immunosuppression: The safety and efficacy of STELARA (ustekinumab) in combination with immunosuppressive agents or phototherapy have not been evaluated. Caution should be exercised when considering concomitant use of immunosuppressive agents and STELARA.

Immunotherapy: STELARA (ustekinumab) has not been evaluated in patients who have undergone allergy immunotherapy. STELARA may affect allergy immunotherapy. Caution should be exercised in patients receiving or who have received allergy immunotherapy particularly for anaphylaxis.

Infections: STELARA (ustekinumab) is a selective immunomodulator and may have the potential to increase the risk of infections and reactivate latent infections.

In clinical studies, serious bacterial, fungal, and viral infections have been observed infrequently in patients receiving ustekinumab. STELARA (ustekinumab) should not be given to patients with an existing clinically important, active infection.Caution should be exercised when considering the use of STELARA in patients with a chronic infection or a history of recurrent infection.

Prior to initiating treatment with STELARA (ustekinumab), patients should be evaluated for tuberculosis infection. STELARA should not be given to patients with active tuberculosis. Treatment of latent tuberculosis infection should be initiated prior to administering STELARA. Anti-tuberculosis therapy should also be considered prior to initiation of STELARA in patients with a past history of latent or active tuberculosis in whom an adequate course of treatment cannot be confirmed. In clinical studies, patients with latent tuberculosis who were concurrently treated with isoniazid did not develop tuberculosis. Patients receiving STELARA should be monitored closely for signs and symptoms of active tuberculosis during and after treatment.

Patients should be instructed to seek medical advice if signs or symptoms suggestive of an infection occur. If a patient develops a serious infection, they should be closely monitored and STELARA (ustekinumab) should not be administered until the infection resolves (see Adverse Reactions).

Neurologic: Reversible Posterior Leukoencephalopathy Syndrome: One case of reversible posterior leukoencephalopathy syndrome (RPLS) was observed during the clinical development program which included 3523 STELARA-treated subjects. The subject, who had received 12 doses of STELARA over approximately two and a half years, presented with headache, seizures and confusion in the setting of alcohol abuse. No additional STELARA injections were administered and the subject fully recovered with appropriate treatment.

RPLS is a neurological disorder, which is not caused by demyelination or a known infectious agent. RPLS can present with headache, seizures, confusion and visual disturbances. Conditions with which it has been associated include preeclampsia, acute hypertension, cytotoxic agents, immunosuppressive therapy and alcohol abuse. Fatal outcomes have been reported.

If RPLS is suspected, STELARA should be discontinued and appropriate treatment administered.

Renal: Specific studies have not been conducted in patients with renal insufficiency.

Special Populations: Pregnant Women: There is no evidence from animal studies of teratogenicity, birth defects or developmental delays at dose levels up to approximately 45-fold higher than the highest equivalent dose intended to be administered to psoriasis patients. However, animal reproductive and developmental studies are not always predictive of human response.

It is not known whether STELARA (ustekinumab) can cause fetal harm when administered to a pregnant woman or whether it can affect reproductive capacity. While it is known that human IgG antibodies, like ustekinumab, cross the placenta, no adequate and well-controlled studies have been conducted to evaluate if ustekinumab can cross the human placenta in pregnant women. In developmental toxicity studies in monkeys, ustekinumab was detected in fetal serum following repeated dosing of pregnant monkeys during the period of organogenesis. Although ustekinumab crossed the monkey placenta there was no evidence of teratogenicity in these studies. STELARA should be given to a pregnant woman only if the benefit clearly outweighs the risk.

Nursing Women: Ustekinumab is excreted in the milk of lactating monkeys administered ustekinumab. It is not known if ustekinumab is absorbed systemically after ingestion. Because many drugs and immunoglobulins are excreted in human milk, and because of the potential for adverse reactions in nursing infants from ustekinumab, a decision should be made whether to discontinue nursing or to discontinue the drug.

Pediatrics (<18 years of age): Specific studies of STELARA (ustekinumab) in pediatric patients have not been conducted.

Geriatrics (>65 years of age): No major age-related differences in clearance or volume of distribution were observed in clinical studies. While the experience in the elderly is limited, no overall differences in efficacy or safety in patients age 65 and older [N=131] who received ustekinumab were observed compared with younger patients.

ADVERSE REACTIONS: Adverse Drug Reaction Overview: The following serious adverse reactions were reported:
- Serious infections
- Malignancies

The most common adverse reactions (>10%) in controlled and uncontrolled portions of the psoriasis clinical studies with STELARA (ustekinumab) were nasopharyngitis and upper respiratory tract infection. Most were considered to be mild and did not necessitate drug discontinuation.

Clinical Trial Adverse Drug Reactions: Because clinical trials are conducted under very specific conditions the adverse reaction rates observed in the clinical trials may not reflect the rates observed in practice and should not be compared to the rates in the clinical trials of another drug. Adverse drug reaction information from clinical trials is useful for identifying drug-related adverse events and for approximating rates.

The safety data described below reflect exposure to STELARA (ustekinumab) in 3 placebo-controlled studies of 2266 patients, including 1970 exposed for at least 6 months, 1285 exposed for at least 1 year and 373 for at least 18 months.

Table 1 summarizes the adverse drug reactions that occurred at a rate of at least 1% and at a higher rate by preferred term in the STELARA (ustekinumab) group during the placebo-controlled period of the Phase 3 studies (PHOENIX 1 and PHOENIX 2).

Table 2 presents the rates at which the STELARA ADRs occurred in treatment groups in the ACCEPT trial.

Infections: In placebo-controlled studies of psoriasis patients, the rates of infection or serious infection were similar between ustekinumab-treated patients and those treated with placebo. In the placebo-controlled period of clinical studies of psoriasis patients, the rate of infection was 1.39 per patient-year of follow-up in ustekinumab-treated patients, and 1.21 per patient-year of follow-up in placebo-treated patients. Serious infections occurred in 0.01 per patient-year of follow-up in ustekinumab-treated patients (5 serious infections in 407 patient-years of follow-up) and 0.02 per patient-year of follow-up in placebo-treated patients (3 serious infections in 177 patient-years of follow-up) (see Warnings and Precautions).

In the controlled and non-controlled portions of placebo-controlled psoriasis clinical studies, the rate of infection was 1.24 per patient-year of follow-up in ustekinumab-treated patients. The incidence of serious infections was 0.01 per patient-year of follow-up in ustekinumab-treated patients (24 serious infections in 2251 patient-years of follow-up) and included cellulitis, diverticulitis, osteomyelitis, viral infections, gastroenteritis, pneumonia, and urinary tract infections.

Table 1: STELARA

Adverse Drug Reactions Reported by ≥1% of Patients Through Week 12 in PHOENIX I and 2

		STELARA (ustekinumab)	
	Placebo	**45 mg**	**90 mg**
Patients treated	665	664	666
Nasopharyngitis	51 (7.7%)	56 (8.4%)	49 (7.4%)
Upper respiratory tract infection	30 (4.5%)	36 (5.4%)	28 (4.2%)
Headache	23 (3.5%)	33 (5.0%)	32 (4.8%)
Fatigue	14 (2.1%)	18 (2.7%)	17 (2.6%)
Diarrhea	12 (1.8%)	13 (2.0%)	13 (2.0%)
Back pain	8 (1.2%)	9 (1.4%)	14 (2.1%)
Dizziness	8 (1.2%)	8 (1.2%)	14 (2.1%)
Pharyngolaryngeal pain	7 (1.1%)	9 (1.4%)	12 (1.8%)
Pruritus	9 (1.4%)	10 (1.5%)	9 (1.4%)
Injection site erythema	3 (0.5%)	6 (0.9%)	13 (2.0%)
Myalgia	4 (0.6%)	7 (1.1%)	8 (1.2%)
Depression	3 (0.5%)	8 (1.2%)	4 (0.6%)

Table 2: STELARA

Adverse Drug Reactions Reported by ≥1% of Patients Through Week 12 in ACCEPT

		STELARA (ustekinumab)	
	ENBREL (etanercept)	**45 mg**	**90 mg**
Patients treated	347	209	347
Nasopharyngitis	29 (8.4%)	21 (10.0%)	34 (9.8%)
Upper respiratory tract infection	20 (5.8%)	13 (6.2%)	22 (6.3%)
Headache	38 (11.0%)	31 (14.8%)	41 (11.8%)
Fatigue	13 (3.7%)	8 (3.8%)	19 (5.5%)
Diarrhea	9 (2.6%)	8 (3.8%)	9 (2.6%)
Back pain	7 (2.0%)	14 (6.7%)	15 (4.3%)
Dizziness	8 (2.3%)	3 (1.4%)	6 (1.7%)
Pharyngolaryngeal pain	14 (4.0%)	5 (2.4%)	14 (4.0%)
Pruritus	14 (4.0%)	12 (5.7%)	16 (4.6%)
Injection site erythema	51 (14.7%)	2 (1.0%)	2 (0.6%)
Myalgia	7 (2.0%)	3 (1.4%)	7 (2.0%)

Malignancies: In the placebo-controlled period of the psoriasis clinical studies, the incidence of non-melanoma skin cancer was 0.74 per 100 patient-years of follow-up for ustekinumab-treated patients (3 patients in 406 patient-years of follow-up) compared with 1.13 per 100 patient-years of follow-up for placebo-treated patients (2 patient in 176 patient-years of follow-up) during the placebo-controlled periods. In a Phase 3 clinical trial (ACCEPT) comparing ustekinumab and etanercept for the treatment of moderate to severe plaque psoriasis, 209 patients received ustekinumab 45mg, 347 patients received ustekinumab 90 mg, and 347 patients received etanercept. Through Week 12, three (0.5%) subjects in the ustekinumab groups had a non-melanoma skin cancer detected in areas of psoriasis that had cleared with treatment. No skin cancers were observed in the etanercept group but due to the short treatment period, the possible pre-existing malignancies and the differences in efficacy, the clinical relevance has not been established.

The incidence of malignancies excluding non-melanoma skin cancer was 0.25 per 100 patient-years of follow-up for ustekinumab-treated patients (1 patient in 406 patient-years of follow-up) compared with 0.57 per 100 patient-years of follow-up for placebo-treated patients (1 patient in 177 patient-years of follow-up) during the placebo-controlled periods. In the ACCEPT trial, through Week 12, one subject (0.2%) with a familial history of breast cancer was diagnosed with breast cancer versus no malignancies in the etanercept group.

In the controlled and non-controlled portions of the placebo-controlled psoriasis clinical trials, the incidence of malignancies excluding non-melanoma skin cancers was 0.36 per 100 patient-years of follow-up for ustekinumab-treated patients (8 patients in 2249 patient-years of follow-up) and included breast, colon, head and neck, kidney, prostate, and thyroid cancers. The rate of malignancies reported in ustekinumab-treated patients was comparable to the rate expected in the general population (standardized incidence ratio=0.68 [95% confidence interval: 0.29, 1.34]). The incidence of non-melanoma skin cancer was 0.80 per 100 patient-years of follow-up for ustekinumab-treated patients (18 patients in 2245 patient-years of follow-up).

Hypersensitivity Reactions: In clinical studies of ustekinumab, rash and urticaria have each been observed in <2% of patients.

Immunogenicity: Approximately 5% of patients treated with ustekinumab developed antibodies to ustekinumab, which were generally low-titer. No apparent correlation of antibody development to injection site reactions was seen. Patients positive for antibodies to ustekinumab exhibited median serum levels of ustekinumab that were consistently lower than those in patients negative or undetectable for antibodies to ustekinumab and tended to have lower efficacy; however, antibody positivity does not preclude a clinical response.

Less Common Clinical Trial Adverse Drug Reactions (<1%): The following adverse drug reactions occurred at rates less than 1% during the psoriasis clinical trials:

Infections and Infestations: cellulitis.

General Disorders and Administration Site Conditions: injection site reactions (including pain, swelling, pruritus, induration, hemorrhage, bruising and irritation).

Abnormal Hematologic and Clinical Chemistry Findings: During the placebo-controlled period of the Phase 2 and Phase 3 studies (through week 12), an increase in non-fasting blood glucose levels was observed, as follows: Subjects with any abnormal value: 49 (6.7%) placebo vs. 83 (5.3%) in the combined ustekinumab group; Subjects with >1 abnormal value: 9 (1.2%) placebo vs 35 (2.2%) in the combined ustekinumab group. The clinical significance of these changes in glucose is unknown. No such increase in fasting blood glucose levels was observed in the same subjects.

Post-Market Adverse Drug Reactions : Immune system disorders: Common - Hypersensitivity reactions (including rash, urticaria); Rare - Serious allergic reactions.

DRUG INTERACTIONS: Overview: Specific drug interaction studies have not been conducted with STELARA (ustekinumab).

In population pharmacokinetic analysis, the effect of the most frequently used concomitant medications in patients with psoriasis (including paracetamol/acetaminophen, ibuprofen, acetylsalicylic acid, metformin, atorvastatin, naproxen, levothyroxine, hydrochlorothiazide, and influenza vaccine) on pharmacokinetics of ustekinumab was explored and none of the concomitant medications exerted significant impact. The pharmacokinetics of ustekinumab was not impacted by the prior use of methotrexate, cyclosporine, or other biological therapeutics for the treatment of psoriasis.

Drug-Drug Interactions: Live Vaccines: Live vaccines should not be given concurrently with STELARA (ustekinumab) (see Warnings and Precautions).

Immunosuppressants: The safety and efficacy of STELARA (ustekinumab) in combination with immunosuppressive agents or phototherapy have not been evaluated (see Warnings and Precautions).

Drug-Food Interactions: Interactions with food have not been established.

Drug-Herb Interactions: Interactions with herbal products have not been established.

Drug-Laboratory Test Interactions: Interactions with laboratory tests have not been established.

Drug-Lifestyle Interactions: The pharmacokinetics of ustekinumab were not impacted by the use of tobacco or alcohol.

DOSAGE AND ADMINISTRATION: STELARA (ustekinumab) is administered by subcutaneous injection.

Dosing Considerations: STELARA (ustekinumab) is intended for use under the guidance and supervision of a physician. A patient may self-inject with STELARA (ustekinumab) if a physician determines that it is appropriate after proper training in subcutaneous injection technique.

Prior to subcutaneous administration, visually inspect the solution for particulate matter and discoloration. The product is colourless to light yellow and may contain a few small translucent or white particles of protein. This appearance is not unusual for proteinaceous solutions. The product should not be used if solution is discolored or cloudy, or if other particulate matter is present. STELARA (ustekinumab) does not contain preservatives; therefore, any unused product remaining in the vial or syringe should not be used.

The needle cover on the pre-filled syringe contains dry natural rubber (a derivative of latex), which may cause allergic reactions in individuals sensitive to latex.

Patients should be instructed to inject the full amount of STELARA (ustekinumab) according to the directions provided in the Information for the Patient (see Information for the Patient).

Recommended Dose and Dosage Adjustment: The recommended dose of STELARA (ustekinumab) is 45 mg administered at Weeks 0 and 4, then every 12 weeks thereafter. Alternatively, 90 mg may be used in patients with a body weight greater than 100 kg.

In patients weighing >100 kg, both 45 mg and 90 mg were shown to be efficacious. However, 90 mg was efficacious in a higher percentage of these patients than the 45 mg dose.

For patients who inadequately respond to dosing every 12 weeks, consideration may be given to treating as often as every 8 weeks.

Consideration should be given to discontinuing treatment in patients who have shown no response up to 12 weeks of treatment.

Re-treatment: Re-treatment with a dosing regimen of Weeks 0 and 4 followed by 12 week dosing after interruption of therapy has been shown to be safe and effective.

OVERDOSAGE:

Single doses up to 4.5 mg/kg intravenously have been administered in clinical studies without dose limiting toxicity. In case of overdosage, it is recommended that the patient be monitored for any signs or symptoms of adverse reactions or effects and appropriate symptomatic treatment be instituted immediately.

> For management of a suspected drug overdose, contact your regional Poison Control Centre. See the *CPS* Directory section for a list of Poison Control Centres.

ACTION AND CLINICAL PHARMACOLOGY: Mechanism of Action: STELARA (ustekinumab) is a fully human IgG1k monoclonal antibody, a first-in-class agent that binds with high affinity and specificity to the p40 protein subunit of the human cytokines interleukin IL-12 and IL-23. STELARA inhibits the bioactivity of human IL-12 and IL-23 by preventing these cytokines from binding to their IL-12Rβ1 receptor protein expressed on the surface of immune cells. STELARA cannot bind to IL-12 or IL-23 that is pre-bound to IL-12Rβ1 cell surface receptors. Thus, STELARA is not likely to contribute to complement or antibody- mediated cytotoxicity of the receptor-bearing cell.

IL-12 and IL-23 are heterodimeric cytokines secreted by activated antigen-presenting cells, such as macrophages and dendritic cells. IL-12 and IL-23 participate in immune function by contributing to NK cell activation and CD4+T-cell differentiation and activation. However, abnormal regulation of IL-12 and IL-23 has been associated with immune-mediated diseases, such as psoriasis. STELARA (ustekinumab) prevents IL-12 and IL-23 contributions to immune cell activation, such as intracellular signaling and cytokine secretion. Thus, STELARA is believed to interrupt signalling and cytokine cascades that are central to psoriasis pathology.

Pharmacodynamics: Treatment with ustekinumab resulted in significant improvement in histological measures of psoriasis including epidermal hyperplasia and cell proliferation. These results are consistent with the clinical efficacy observed. STELARA (ustekinumab) had no apparent effect on the percentages of circulating immune cell populations including memory and naive T-cell subsets or circulating cytokine levels.

Treatment with ustekinumab resulted in a decrease in the gene expression of its molecular targets IL-12 and IL-23 as shown by analyses of mRNA obtained from lesional skin biopsies of psoriatic patients at baseline and up to two weeks post-treatment. In addition, ustekinumab down-regulated the gene expression of inflammatory cytokines and chemokines such as MCP-1, TNF-alpha, IP-10 and IL-8 in lesional skin biopsies. These results are consistent with the significant clinical benefit observed with ustekinumab treatment.

Clinical response (improvement in PASI) appeared to be related to serum ustekinumab levels. Patients with psoriasis with higher clinical responses as measured by PASI response had higher median serum concentrations of ustekinumab than those with lower clinical responses. Overall, the proportion of patients with psoriasis who achieved PASI 75 response increased with increasing serum levels of ustekinumab. The proportion of patients who achieved PASI 75 response at Week 28 increased with increasing serum ustekinumab trough levels at Week 28.

Pharmacokinetics: The median pharmacokinetic parameters of ustekinumab following a single SC administration in adult patients with psoriasis are shown in Table 3. The pharmacokinetic parameters of ustekinumab (CL/F, Vz/F, and $t_{1/2}$) were generally comparable between 45 mg and 90 mg subcutaneous doses.

Table 3: STELARA

Summary of Pharmacokinetic Parameters of Ustekinumab Following a Single 45 or 90 mg Subcutaneous Administration in Adult Patients with Psoriasis

Dose	45 mg			90 mg		
PK Parameter	**N**	**Median (Range)**	**Mean (± SD)**	**N**	**Median (Range)**	**Mean (± SD)**
C_{max} (µg/mL)	22	2.4 (1.0, 5.4)	2.7 (±1.2)	24	5.3 (1.2, 12.3)	6.1 (±3.6)
t_{max} (day)	22	13.5 (1.9, 58.2)	15.3 (±13.5)	24	7 (2.9, 27.1)	9.9 (±7.4)

(cont'd)

Table 3: STELARA *(cont'd)*

Summary of Pharmacokinetic Parameters of Ustekinumab Following a Single 45 or 90 mg Subcutaneous Administration in Adult Patients with Psoriasis

Dose	45 mg			90 mg		
PK Parameter	**N**	**Median (Range)**	**Mean (± SD)**	**N**	**Median (Range)**	**Mean (± SD)**
AUC (µg·day/mL)	18	84.9 (31.2, 1261.9)	196.7 (±298.2)	21	226.9 (57.1, 755.5)	274.9 (±206.5)
$t_{1/2}$ (day)	18	19.8 (5.0, 353.6)	45.6 (±80.2)	21	21.2 (13.6, 85.8)	26.7 (±19.3)
CL/F (mL/day/kg)	18	5.3 (0.2, 12.9)	5.8 (±3.5)	21	4.5 (1.5, 14.9)	5.7 (±3.6)
Vz/F (mL/kg)	18	154.2 (32.6, 280.5)	160.5 (±64.5)	21	160.5 (37.3, 354.1)	178.7 (±85.2)

Source data: C0379T04 CSR.

Absorption: The median time to reach the maximum serum concentration (t_{max}) was 8.5 days after a single 90 mg subcutaneous administration in healthy subjects (n=30). The median t_{max} values of ustekinumab following a single subcutaneous administration of either 45 mg or 90 mg in patients with psoriasis were comparable to that observed in healthy subjects.

The absolute bioavailability (F) of ustekinumab following a single subcutaneous administration was estimated to be 57.2% in patients with psoriasis (n=17).

Distribution: The median apparent volume of distribution during the terminal phase (Vz/F) following a single subcutaneous administration to patients with psoriasis ranged from 76 to 161 mL/kg (n=4 to 21).

Metabolism: The exact metabolic pathway for ustekinumab is unknown.

Excretion: The median apparent clearance (CL/F) following a single subcutaneous administration to patients with psoriasis ranged from 2.7 to 5.3 mL/day/kg. The median half-life ($t_{1/2}$) of ustekinumab was approximately 3 weeks in patients with psoriasis, ranging from 15 to 32 days across all psoriasis studies (n=4 to 21).

Dose Linearity: The systemic exposure of ustekinumab (C_{max} and AUC) increased in a linear manner following a single subcutaneous administration at doses ranging from approximately 24 mg to 240 mg in patients with psoriasis.

Single Dose vs. Multiple Doses: Serum concentration-time profiles of ustekinumab were generally predictable after single or multiple subcutaneous dose administrations on the basis of a one-compartment model. Steady-state serum concentrations of ustekinumab were achieved by Week 28 after initial subcutaneous doses at Weeks 0 and 4 followed by doses every 12 weeks. The median steady-state trough concentration ranged from 0.21 µg/mL to 0.26 µg/mL (45 mg; n=242 to 390) and from 0.47 µg/mL to 0.49 µg/mL (90 mg; n=236 to 386). There was no apparent accumulation in serum ustekinumab concentration over time when given subcutaneously every 12 weeks.

Impact of Weight on Pharmacokinetics: Serum ustekinumab concentrations were affected by patient weight. When given the same dose, patients of higher weight (>100 kg) had lower median serum ustekinumab concentrations compared with those in patients of lower weight (≤100 kg). However, across doses, the median trough serum concentrations of ustekinumab in patients with higher weight (>100 kg) in the 90 mg group were comparable to those in patients with lower weight (≤100 kg) in the 45 mg group.

Of the demographic factors (e.g., gender, race, age, body size), baseline patient physical or biochemical characteristics, or medical or medication history, or concomitant medications evaluated in a population pharmacokinetic analysis, only body weight, diabetes comorbidity, and positive immune response to ustekinumab were found to be important covariates affecting the systemic exposure to ustekinumab in patients with moderate to severe psoriasis. Clinical relevance of the effects of these important covariates, however, needs to be evaluated concurrently with clinical efficacy and safety data.

The effect of the most frequently used concomitant medications in patients with psoriasis (including paracetamol/acetaminophen, ibuprofen, acetylsalicylic acid, metformin, atorvastatin, naproxen, levothyroxine, hydrochlorothiazide, and influenza vaccine) on pharmacokinetics of ustekinumab was explored and none of the concomitant medications exerted significant impact. The pharmacokinetics of ustekinumab was not impacted by the prior use of methotrexate, cyclosporine, or other biological therapeutics for the treatment of psoriasis.

Special Populations and Conditions: Pediatrics (<18 years of age): Specific studies of STELARA (ustekinumab) in pediatric patients have not been conducted.

Geriatrics (>65 years of age): No specific studies have been conducted in elderly patients.

Gender, Race and Genetic Polymorphism: The apparent clearance of ustekinumab was not impacted by sex, age, or race.

Hepatic Insufficiency: No pharmacokinetic data are available in patients with impaired hepatic function.

Renal Insufficiency: No pharmacokinetic data are available in patients with renal insufficiency.

STORAGE AND STABILITY: STELARA (ustekinumab) must be refrigerated at 2 to 8°C and protected from light. Keep the product in the original carton to protect from light until the time of use. Do not freeze. Do not shake.

SPECIAL HANDLING INSTRUCTIONS: Following administration of STELARA (ustekinumab), the syringe should be disposed of in a puncture-resistant container for syringes and needles. Patients or caregivers should be instructed in the technique as well as proper syringe and needle disposal, and not to reuse these items.

INFORMATION FOR THE PATIENT: Published in e-CPS, available by subscription at www.e-cps.ca.

DOSAGE FORMS, COMPOSITION AND PACKAGING: Pre-filled Syringes: Each mL of sterile solution contains: ustekinumab 90 mg. Nonmedicinal ingredients: L-histidine, L-histidine monohydrochloride monohydrate, polysorbate 80, sucrose and water for injection. Preservative-free. Single-use Type 1 glass syringes with a fixed 27G, half-inch needle and needle cover, packages of 1. The needle cover is manufactured using a dry natural rubber (a derivative of latex) (see Warnings and Precautions, Hypersensitivity Reactions). The syringe is fitted with a passive safety guard.

Vials: Each mL of sterile solution contains: ustekinumab 90 mg. Nonmedicinal ingredients: L-histidine, L-histidine monohydrochloride monohydrate, polysorbate 80, sucrose and water for injection. Preservative-free. Single-use (Type 1) glass vials of 0.5 mL with a coated stopper, packages of 1.

(Shown in Product Identification Section)

Stieprox® Ⓟ

ciclopirox olamine

Topical Antifungal

Stiefel, a GSK company

Date of Preparation: March 13, 2003
Date of Revision: February 15, 2006

SUMMARY PRODUCT INFORMATION:

Route of Administration	Dosage Form/ Strength	Clinically Relevant Nonmedicinal Ingredients
Topical	Shampoo 1.5%	Coconut diethanolamide and Sodium lauryl ether sulphate For a complete listing see Dosage Forms, Composition and Packaging.

INDICATIONS AND CLINICAL USE: STIEPROX (ciclopirox olamine 1.5%) shampoo is indicated for:

- topical treatment and prophylaxis of dandruff or the treatment of seborrhoeic dermatitis in which the yeast *M. furfur* is involved.

Geriatrics: No data is available.

Pediatrics: No data is available.

CONTRAINDICATIONS:

- Patients who are hypersensitive to this drug or to any ingredient in the formulation or component of the container. For a complete listing, see Dosage Forms, Composition and Packaging.

WARNINGS AND PRECAUTIONS: General: STIEPROX (ciclopirox olamine 1.5%) shampoo is for external use only. Avoid contact with eyes. In case of contact with the eyes, rinse thoroughly with copious amounts of water. If irritation persists, a physician should be consulted.
Skin: If a reaction suggesting hypersensitivity or chemical irritation should occur with the use of STIEPROX shampoo, treatment should be applied less often or should be discontinued and appropriate therapy instituted.
Special Populations: Pregnant Women: The safety of STIEPROX shampoo during pregnancy has not been established. There is evidence that ciclopirox olamine crosses the placental barrier. Reproductive studies in mice, rats, rabbits and monkeys, at doses of ciclopirox olamine 10 times that of a topical human dose, have revealed no significant evidence of impaired fertility or harm to the fetus. STIEPROX should only be used during pregnancy if the potential benefits to the mother justify the potential risks to the fetus.

No pregnant women were enrolled during clinical trials with STIEPROX.
Nursing Women: It is unknown if ciclopirox olamine is excreted in human milk. Because many drugs are excreted in human milk precaution should be exercised.
Pediatrics: The safety and effectiveness of STIEPROX has not been established in children.
Geriatrics: The safety and effectiveness of STIEPROX has not been established in a geriatric population.

ADVERSE REACTIONS: Adverse Drug Reaction Overview: STIEPROX (ciclopirox olamine 1.5%) shampoo is well tolerated with a low incidence of adverse reactions.
Clinical Trial Adverse Drug Reactions: Because clinical trials are conducted under very specific conditions, the adverse reaction rates observed in the clinical trials may not reflect the rates observed in practice and should not be compared to the rates in the clinical trials of another drug. Adverse Drug Reaction information from clinical trials is useful for identifying drug-related adverse events and for approximating rates.

Table 1 provides the list of the Common Adverse Drug Reactions (>1%) observed with STIEPROX (ciclopirox olamine 1.5%) shampoo during the controlled clinical trials.

Table 1: STIEPROX

Common Adverse Drug Reaction to STIEPROX or its Vehicle

	STIEPROX n=216	Placebo n=238
Administration site conditions		
Scalp Pruritus	4 (2%)	4 (2%)

Less Common Clinical Trial Adverse Drug Reactions: Administration Site Conditions: Uncommon: erythema, erosion of scalp.
Eye Disorders: Uncommon: stinging, watering, infection.
Nervous System Disorders: Uncommon: headache.
Abnormal Hematologic and Clinical Chemistry Findings: Hematologic and clinical chemistry parameters were not evaluated during clinical trials with STIEPROX.
Post-Market Adverse Drug Reactions: No adverse reactions to STIEPROX have been reported by health professionals or consumers.

DRUG INTERACTIONS: Overview: No drug interactions have been reported with ciclopirox olamine. The possibility of interaction with alcohol has not been evaluated.
Drug-Food Interactions: Interactions with food have not been established.
Drug-Herb Interactions: Interactions with herbal products have not been established.
Drug-Laboratory Test Interactions: Interactions with laboratory tests have not been established.

DOSAGE AND ADMINISTRATION: Dosing Considerations: Situations that may affect the dosing of STIEPROX have not been established.
Recommended Dose and Dosage Adjustment: Dandruff: Use 2 or 3 times a week or as often as necessary.
Seborrhoeic dermatitis: Use 3 times a week or as often as necessary.
Missed Dose: Any missed application of the shampoo should be done the next day.
Administration: The hair should be wet and sufficient STIEPROX (ciclopirox olamine 1.5%) shampoo should be applied to produce an abundant lather. The affected areas (scalp and/or its edges) should be vigorously massaged with the fingertips for two to three minutes. The hair should then be thoroughly rinsed and the procedure repeated.

OVERDOSAGE:
There have been no clinical reports of acute overdosage with STIEPROX (ciclopirox olamine 1.5%) shampoo.
Symptoms: Oral ingestion is usually followed by nausea and vomiting due to the detergent.
Treatment: If ingested, treatment should be symptomatic. In the event of accidental ingestion, only supportive measures should be carried out. In order to avoid aspiration, neither emesis nor gastric lavage should be performed.

For management of a suspected drug overdose, CPhA recommends that you contact your **regional Poison Control Centre**. See the *CPS* Directory section for a list of Poison Control Centres.

ACTION AND CLINICAL PHARMACOLOGY: Mechanism of Action: Ciclopirox olamine is a synthetic antifungal which is structurally unrelated to the common imidazoles or other antifungals. Unlike most antifungals, ciclopirox olamine does not affect sterol biosynthesis. It has been suggested that ciclopirox olamine interferes with the active uptake and accumulation of some essential substrates and/or polyvalent cations which results in cell death because of cellular depletion. Ciclopirox olamine may act through chelation of polyvalent cations such as Fe^{3+} or Al^{3+}.
Pharmacodynamics: Except for its specific fungicidal activity, ciclopirox olamine when formulated in a 1.5% shampoo is not expected to exert any other pharmacodynamic effect when applied topically. No pharmacodynamic studies were conducted in humans with STIEPROX (ciclopirox olamine 1.5%) shampoo.
Pharmacokinetics: No pharmacokinetic studies were conducted in humans with STIEPROX (ciclopirox olamine 1.5%) shampoo.
Special Populations and Conditions: STIEPROX was not tested in special populations.

STORAGE AND STABILITY: Store STIEPROX between 4 and 30°C.

SPECIAL HANDLING INSTRUCTIONS: None.

INFORMATION FOR THE PATIENT: Published in e-CPS, available by subscription at www.e-cps.ca.

DOSAGE FORMS, COMPOSITION AND PACKAGING: Each bottle of shampoo contains: 1.5% ciclopirox olamine USP in a mild aqueous shampoo base. Nonmedicinal ingredients: citric acid monohydrate, cocamidopropyl betaine, coconut diethanolamide, disodium hydrogen phosphate, fragrance, hexylene glycol, oleyl alcohol, polyquaternium 10, polysorbate 80, purified water, sodium hydroxide and sodium lauryl ether sulphate. Bottles of 150 mL. Sample sachets of 10 mL.

Stieva-A® ℞

tretinoin

Acne Therapy

Stiefel, a GSK company

SUPPLIED: Cream: Each g of cream contains: tretinoin USP 0.01%, 0.025% or 0.05% in an emollient cream base. Nonmedicinal ingredients: butylated hydroxyanisole, butylated hydroxytoluene, edetate disodium, isopropyl palmitate, methyl paraben, polyoxyl 40 stearate, propyl paraben, propylene glycol, purified water, stearic acid, stearyl alcohol and white petrolatum. Tubes of 25 g. Store between 15 to 30°C.
Forte Cream: Each g of cream contains: tretinoin USP 0.1%. Nonmedicinal ingredients: butylated hydroxyanisole, butylated hydroxytoluene, edetate disodium, isopropyl palmitate, methyl paraben, polyoxyl 40 stearate, propyl paraben, propylene glycol, purified water USP, stearic acid, stearyl alcohol, titanium dioxide and white petrolatum. Tubes of 25 g. Store between 15 to 30°C.
Gel: Each g of gel contains: tretinoin USP 0.025% or 0.05% in an alcohol base gel. Nonmedicinal ingredients: anhydrous alcohol, butylated hydroxytoluene and hydroxypropyl cellulose. Tubes of 25 g. Store between 15 to 30°C.
Solution: Each mL of solution contains: tretinoin USP 0.025%. Nonmedicinal ingredients: anhydrous alcohol, butylated hydroxytoluene, hydroxypropyl cellulose and purified water USP. Bottles of 50 mL with snap-on Dab-O-Matic applicator. Store between 15 to 30°C.

Stievamycin® Preparations ℞

erythromycin—tretinoin

Topical Acne Therapy

Stiefel, a GSK company

PHARMACOLOGY: Tretinoin: The precise mechanism of action of tretinoin on the skin is not fully understood. It is known that tretinoin is both pharmacologically and structurally related to vitamin A which regulates epithelial cell growth and differentiation. Tretinoin itself is known to have an irritant and keratolytic effect on the skin. These two actions which occur simultaneously have been shown histologically in both animal and man to be associated with an increased growth rate and with a decrease in the cohesiveness of the epidermal cells. The result is a slightly thickened epidermis with an accelerated turnover rate and shedding of keratinized cells as very fine barely perceptible scales.

In acne vulgaris, the induced fine scaling of the skin surface is accompanied by an increased production of less cohesive epidermal sebaceous cells which consequently flow out of the follicle at a more rapid rate. The thickened mass of sebaceous cellular debris, the comedones, appear to be initially extruded and then prevented from recurring by these actions. Histopathologically, acne is the impaction plus distention of the sebaceous follicles by tightly packed horny cells and disruption of the follicular epithelium. It has been postulated that tretinoin inhibits the synthesis or quality of the substance which binds the horny cells within the sebaceous follicle.
Erythromycin: Erythromycin exerts its antibacterial action by binding to the 50S ribosomal subunit of susceptible bacteria and suppressing protein synthesis. Erythromycin is usually bacteriostatic but may be bactericidal in high concentrations or against highly susceptible organisms.

The precise mechanism of action of erythromycin in the treatment of acne has not been established.

INDICATIONS: In the treatment of acne vulgaris, primarily where comedones, papules and pustules predominate. Not effective in most cases of severe pustular and deep cystic nodular varieties (acne conglobata). Not indicated in Stage IV acne.

CONTRAINDICATIONS: In patients with known hypersensitivity to retinoids and/or erythromycin or any of the components of the preparations.

WARNINGS: Topical gels are intended for external use only and should be kept away from eyes, nose, mouth, and other mucous membranes because of its irritant effect. Do not apply to eyelids or to the skin at the corners of the eyes and mouth. Avoid the angles of the nose and nasolabial fold (if treatment in these areas is necessary, apply very sparingly). Topical use may induce severe local erythema and peeling at the site of application. If the degree of local irritation warrants, patients should be directed to use the medication less frequently, discontinue use temporarily or discontinue use altogether. Tretinoin has been reported to cause severe irritation of eczematous skin and should only be used with utmost caution in patients with this condition.
Pregnancy: **Topical tretinoin should be used by women of childbearing years only after contraceptive counselling. It is recommended that topical tretinoin should not be used by pregnant women.**

There have been rare reports of birth defects among babies born to women exposed to **topical** tretinoin during pregnancy. However, there are no well controlled prospective studies of the use of topical tretinoin in pregnant women. A retrospective study of mothers exposed to topical tretinoin during the first trimester of pregnancy found no increase in the incidence of birth defects.

Topical retinoid teratology studies in rats and rabbits have been inconclusive. As with all retinoids, tretinoin administered **orally** at high doses is teratogenic.

The safety of erythromycin during pregnancy has not been established. Erythromycin crosses the placental barrier.
Lactation: **It is unknown whether tretinoin is excreted in human milk but erythromycin is so excreted. Nevertheless, a decision should be made whether to discontinue nursing or to discontinue the drug taking into account the importance of the drug to the mother.**

PRECAUTIONS: The use of preparations containing antibiotics may be associated with overgrowth of antibiotic resistant organisms, including those initially sensitive to the drug. Cross-resistance between erythromycin and macrolide antibiotics can occur. If this should occur, therapy should be discontinued and appropriate measures taken. A cross-resistance between erythromycin and clindamycin has rarely been reported.

Excessive exposure to sunlight or ultraviolet rays (sun lamps) should be avoided during treatment with Stievamycin topical gels because the additional irradiation may lead to a more intense action.

If a sunburn occurs, it is advisable to interrupt therapy until the severe erythema and peeling subside. Patients whose occupations require considerable exposure to the sun should exercise particular caution.
Drug Interactions: Concomitant topical medications should be used with caution during therapy with Stievamycin topical gels because of possible intensified reactions. Particular caution should be exercised when using preparations containing a peeling agent concomitantly (such as sulfur, resorcinol, benzoyl peroxide or salicylic acid) with Stievamycin. It may be advisable to "rest" a patient's skin until the effects of previously used peeling agents subside before initiating Stievamycin therapy. Concurrent use of abrasive or medicated soaps, or cosmetic products containing alcohol, such as astringents and after-shave lotions, may also result in a cumulative drying or irritant effect in patients using Stievamycin topical gels.

ADVERSE EFFECTS: The skin of certain sensitive individuals, particularly those with fair complexion, may become excessively red, edematous, blistered or crusted when exposed to Stievamycin topical gels. Pain, burning sensation, tenderness, irritation or pruritus have also been occasionally reported. If any of these effects occur, the medication should be discontinued until the integrity of the skin has been restored or the treatment schedule adjusted to the level the patient can tolerate. Temporary hyper- or hypopigmentation has been reported with repeated application of tretinoin. To date, all adverse clinical effects of tretinoin encountered have been reversible upon discontinuance of therapy. In many instances, reinstitution of therapy with tretinoin failed to produce the adverse effect previously experienced.

Topical erythromycin may cause desquamation and excessive dryness. Mild to moderate irritation has been observed in many patients, but severe irritation is generally less frequent. Urticaria, oiliness, coriaceousness and fissuring around the mouth may occur.

OVERDOSE:
Symptoms: Topical: If medication is applied excessively, marked redness, peeling or discomfort may occur.
Accidental Ingestion: In oral doses of over 2 g erythromycin per day, abdominal discomfort, nausea or diarrhea may occur. There is no specific treatment. Gastric lavage should be considered, otherwise, the treatment should be symptomatic.
Treatment: See Symptoms.

For management of a suspected drug overdose, CPhA recommends that you contact your **regional Poison Control Centre**. See the *CPS* Directory section for a list of Poison Control Centres.

DOSAGE: Stievamycin topical gels should be applied to the affected area once a day, preferably before retiring. The area under treatment (not just clinical lesions) should be thoroughly cleansed with a mild soap, and dried, followed by application of the gel in a gentle rubbing motion, using fingertips to apply medication. Application may be accompanied by a transitory feeling of warmth or a stinging sensation. Treatment should be discontinued if a severe local inflammatory response is experienced.

In cases where it may be necessary to discontinue therapy or reduce the frequency of applications, therapy may be resumed, when the adverse effects have ceased. In some patients, during the early weeks of therapy, an apparent exacerbation of the acne lesions may occur.

Therapeutic results may be noticed after 2 to 3 weeks of therapy; however, results may not be optimal until after 8 to 10 weeks of treatment. Once the acne lesions have responded satisfactorily, it may be possible to maintain the improved state with less frequent applications.

Patients being treated with Stievamycin topical gels may continue to use cosmetics; however, astringents may produce exacerbation when used concurrently with Stievamycin topical gels. The area of skin to be treated should be thoroughly cleansed and dried before Stievamycin topical gels are applied.

INFORMATION FOR THE PATIENT: Published in e-CPS, available by subscription at www.e-cps.ca.

SUPPLIED: Forte: Each g of gel contains: tretinoin USP 0.05% and erythromycin USP 4.0% in an alcohol gel base. Nonmedicinal ingredients: BHT, ethyl alcohol and hydroxypropyl cellulose. Tubes of 25 g. Store between 15 and 30°C.
Mild: Each g of gel contains: tretinoin USP 0.01% and erythromycin USP 4.0% in an alcohol gel base. Nonmedicinal ingredients: BHT, ethyl alcohol and hydroxypropyl cellulose. Tubes of 25 g. Store between 15 and 30°C.
Regular: Each g of gel contains: tretinoin USP 0.025% and erythromycin USP 4.0% in an alcohol gel base. Nonmedicinal ingredients: BHT, ethyl alcohol and hydroxypropyl cellulose. Tubes of 25 g. Store between 15 and 30°C.

Stilamin® Ⓟ

somatostatin

Treatment of Acute Variceal Bleeding

EMD Canada

Date of Preparation: December 2000

PHARMACOLOGY: Somatostatin is a synthetic cyclic 14 amino acid peptide (identical in structure and activity to naturally occurring somatostatin) which decreases splanchnic blood flow and portal venous pressure in man, possibly through a direct action on the unstriated muscle cells mediated by a calcium-dependent mechanism. In anesthetized healthy volunteers, somatostatin—dosed as a 250 µg i.v. bolus followed by a 250 µg/hour continuous infusion—also reduced blood flow in the common hepatic artery (56%), in the splenic artery (26%) and in the upper and lower mesenteric branches. In cirrhotic patients, wedged hepatic pressure and estimated liver blood flow were decreased with the administration of somatostatin.

Somatostatin is rapidly metabolized by the liver (plasma half-life of 1.1 to 3 minutes in healthy subjects) and cleared (50.3±7.0 mL/kg/min) from the body. Consequently, its pharmacological effects are transient, and a return to basal levels is generally seen shortly after the cessation of an i.v. infusion. In cirrhotic patients, the plasma half-life (1.2 to 4.8 minutes) approximates that of healthy volunteers while in patients with chronic renal failure, the plasma half-life is prolonged (2.6 to 4.9 minutes, see Precautions and Dosage). Somatostatin is excreted renally, with excretion 70% complete within 24 hours after dosing.

INDICATIONS: For the symptomatic treatment of acute bleeding from esophageal varices. Other treatment options for long-term management of the condition may be considered if necessary, once initial control has been established.

CONTRAINDICATIONS: Cases of known hypersensitivity to the product, its excipients, or recommended diluents.
Pregnancy: The use of somatostatin in known or suspected pregnancy and during the immediate post partum period is contraindicated.

During preclinical studies in the rabbit, somatostatin doses of 0.2 mg/kg/day and higher were found to interfere with the early stages of embryonal development (e.g., implantation). Studies performed in pregnant women during labor indicated that somatostatin (500 µg infused over 30 minutes) crossed the placental barrier, with effects on fetal levels of growth hormone and thyrotrophin.

In the absence of data concerning the effects of somatostatin on human pregnancy, its use is not recommended.
Lactation: There is no information from animal or human studies concerning the passage of somatostatin in breast milk. As somatostatin has a wide variety of potential pharmacological effects, its use during lactation is contraindicated until further information can be obtained.

WARNINGS: Somatostatin has an inhibitory effect on the secretion of insulin and glucagon. Therefore, at the outset of treatment, somatostatin can lead to a transient fall in blood glucose levels. Caution should therefore be used in administering the product to insulin-dependent diabetics in whom blood glucose should be measured every 3 to 4 hours. Simultaneous administration of insulin-requiring sugars should be avoided if possible. Insulin should be administered as necessary.
Children: There is no information concerning the use of somatostatin in children. Use in this patient population should only be considered if the potential benefits outweigh the possible risks.

PRECAUTIONS: General: As somatostatin has a short plasma half-life, it is essential that the infusion be maintained continuously once it has been initiated. In the event that any interruption in the infusion occurs, a repeat bolus dose may be given to the patient, followed by resumption of the continuous infusion (see Dosage).
Patients with Renal Disease: The plasma half-life of somatostatin is increased in patients with chronic renal disease, and its rate of clearance is reduced (see Pharmacology). Somatostatin should therefore be administered to such patients with caution.
Drug Interactions: Somatostatin has been demonstrated to prolong or enhance the effects of barbiturates such as hexobarbital and pentetrazole, in preclinical studies. Caution should be used in administering such agents concomitantly with somatostatin.

The glucoregulatory properties of somatostatin may cause it to interfere with the insulin requirements of insulin-dependent diabetics (see Warnings).
Laboratory Tests: Somatostatin has produced transient hyperglycemia and thrombocytopenia in some patients (see Adverse Effects).

ADVERSE EFFECTS: The adverse reactions which were reported by more than one patient during the clinical trials with the product in 278 patients included: nausea (4.0%), vomiting (2.1%), hyperglycemia (generally transient) (1.8%), pyrexia (1.8%), hypocalcemia (0.7%), headache (0.7%), thrombocytopenia (0.7%) and ventricular extrasystoles (0.7%).

OVERDOSE:
Symptoms: Transient bradycardia and hypotension were observed in some preclinical studies and may be a sign of overdosage in humans. Cramping and vomiting have been reported as the result of an accidental overdosage with somatostatin.
Treatment: The infusion should be stopped immediately if overdosage is suspected. Given the short half-life of somatostatin, symptoms should resolve rapidly with the cessation of the infusion. Other treatment would consist of standard supportive measures until the symptoms have been resolved.

> For management of a suspected drug overdose, CPhA recommends that you contact your **regional Poison Control Centre**. See the *CPS* Directory section for a list of Poison Control Centres.

DOSAGE: Stilamin (somatostatin) should be given as a slow 250 µg i.v. bolus injection over 3 to 5 minutes, followed by a continuous infusion at a rate of 250 µg/h until bleeding from the varices has stopped (usually within 12 to 24 hours). Once bleeding has been controlled, it is recommended that the infusion be continued for at least another 48 to 72 hours, or out to a maximum of 120 hours to prevent recurrent bleeding.

The short plasma half-life of somatostatin makes it essential that the infusion be maintained continuously. It has therefore been the practice in some clinical trials to establish the continuous infusion line prior to administering the bolus dose to ensure that the administration of the drug is uninterrupted. If the continuous infusion is interrupted for any reason, a second bolus dose may be given to rapidly re-establish circulating levels of the drug.

Patients with decreased renal function should be closely monitored since the plasma half-life is prolonged.

Immediately prior to administration, the 250 µg lyophilized product should be reconstituted with the sterile normal saline solution provided. Storage of the reconstituted product is not recommended.

The 3 mg lyophilized powder for continuous infusion should be reconstituted in either sterile normal (0.9%) saline or in 5% dextrose to provide sufficient solution for a 12-hour infusion of somatostatin at a rate of 250 µg/h (approximately 3.5 µg/kg/h). Once reconstituted it should be used within 24 hours and should be protected from light during this time.
Parenteral Products: Stilamin must be reconstituted before use.
Direct I.V. Injection: The 250 µg ampul of Stilamin is accompanied by a 1 mL ampul of sterile, normal (0.9%) saline for reconstitution. Immediately before use, the sodium chloride solution should be added to the lyophilized material under aseptic conditions (creating a 250 µg/mL solution) and swirled gently until all particles have been dissolved. Only clear solutions should be administered.
Continuous Infusion: The 3 mg ampul is not provided with diluent. It should be reconstituted with either sterile normal saline (0.9%) or in 5% dextrose prior to administration. The 3 mg ampul contains sufficient somatostatin to deliver a 12-hour continuous infusion at a rate of 250 µg/h. The volume of dilution will depend on the infusion system used and should be adjusted to ensure a continuous rate of infusion over 12 hours.

As with all parenteral drug products, i.v. admixtures should be inspected visually for clarity, particulate matter, precipitation, discoloration and leakage prior to administration whenever solution and container permit.
Stability and Storage Recommendations: The ampuls are stable for 3 years at 25°C or below in the original containers. The product should be protected from light.
Reconstituted Solutions: Stilamin, reconstituted with sterile, normal (0.9%) saline or 5% dextrose to a concentration of 250 µg/mL, is stable for 24 hours when refrigerated and protected from light.

SUPPLIED: 250 µg: Each ampul of white, lyophilized, sterile, pyrogen-free powder contains: somatostatin 250 µg (present as acetate hydrate) and mannitol 5 mg. Intended for reconstitution and administration as an i.v. bolus dose. Each ampul of Stilamin 250 µg is accompanied by its diluent, a 3 mL ampul which contains 1 mL of sterile normal (0.9%) Sodium Chloride Injection. Cartons of 1 ampul of diluent and 1 ampul of somatostatin. Cartons of 5 ampuls of diluent and 5 ampuls of somatostatin.
3 mg: Each ampul of white, lyophilized, sterile, pyrogen-free powder contains: somatostatin 3 mg (present as acetate hydrate) and mannitol 5 mg. Intended for reconstitution and administration as a 12-hour continuous infusion (delivery 250 µg/hour). Cartons of 1 ampul of somatostatin.

Strattera® Ⓟ

atomoxetine HCl

Selective Norepinephrine Reuptake Inhibitor for Attention-Deficit/Hyperactivity Disorder (ADHD)

Lilly

Date of Revision: September 24, 2009

SUMMARY PRODUCT INFORMATION:

Route of Administration	Dosage Form/Strength	Nonmedicinal Ingredients
Oral	10, 18, 25, 40, 60, 80 or 100 mg capsules	The capsules also contain pregelatinized starch and dimethicone. The capsule shells contain gelatin, sodium lauryl sulfate, and other inactive ingredients. The capsule shells also contain one or more of the following: FD&C Blue No. 2, synthetic yellow iron oxide, red iron oxide, titanium dioxide.

INDICATIONS AND CLINICAL USE: STRATTERA (atomoxetine hydrochloride) is indicated for the treatment of Attention-Deficit/Hyperactivity Disorder (ADHD) in children 6 years of age and over, adolescents, and adults.

A diagnosis of ADHD (DSM-IV) implies the presence of hyperactive-impulsive or inattentive symptoms that cause impairment and that were present before age 7 years. The symptoms must be persistent, must be more severe than is typically observed in individuals at a comparable level of development, must cause clinically significant impairment, e.g., in social, academic, or occupational functioning, and must be present in 2 or more settings, e.g., school (or work) and at home. The symptoms must not be better accounted for by another mental disorder. For the Inattentive Type, at least 6 of the following symptoms must have persisted for at least 6 months: lack of attention to details/careless mistakes, lack of sustained attention, poor listener, failure to follow through on tasks, poor organization, avoids tasks requiring sustained mental effort, loses things, easily distracted, forgetful. For the Hyperactive-Impulsive Type, at least 6 of the following symptoms must have persisted for at least 6 months: fidgeting/squirming, leaving seat, inappropriate running/climbing, difficulty with quiet activities, "on the go," excessive talking, blurting answers, can't wait turn, intrusive. For a Combined Type diagnosis, both inattentive and hyperactive-impulsive criteria must be met.
Special Diagnostic Considerations: The specific etiology of ADHD is unknown, and there is no single diagnostic test. Adequate diagnosis requires the use not only of medical but also of special psychological, educational, and social resources. Learning may or may not be impaired. The diagnosis must be based upon a complete history and evaluation of the patient and not solely on the presence of the required number of DSM-IV characteristics.
Need for Comprehensive Treatment Program: STRATTERA is indicated as an integral part of a total treatment program for ADHD that may include other measures (psychological, educational, and social) for patients with this syndrome. Drug treatment may not be indicated for all patients with this syndrome. Drug treatment is not intended for use in the patient who exhibits symptoms secondary to environmental factors and/or other primary psychiatric disorders, including psychosis. Appropriate educational placement is essential in children and adolescents with this diagnosis and psychosocial intervention is often helpful. When remedial measures alone are insufficient, the decision to prescribe drug treatment medication will depend upon the physician's assessment of the chronicity and severity of the patient's symptoms.
Pediatrics (<6 years of age): The safety and efficacy of STRATTERA in pediatric patients less than 6 years of age have not been established.

CONTRAINDICATIONS:

- **Hypersensitivity:** STRATTERA (atomoxetine hydrochloride) is contraindicated in patients known to be hypersensitive to atomoxetine or other constituents of the product (see Warnings and Precautions).
- **Monoamine Oxidase Inhibitors:** STRATTERA should not be taken with monoamine oxidase inhibitors (MAOI), or within 2 weeks after discontinuing MAOI. Treatment with MAOI should not be initiated within 2 weeks after discontinuing STRATTERA. With other drugs that affect brain monoamine concentrations, there have been reports of serious, sometimes fatal, reactions (including hyperthermia, rigidity, myoclonus, autonomic instability with possible rapid fluctuations of vital signs, and mental status changes that include extreme agitation progressing to delirium and coma) when taken in combination with MAOI. Some cases presented with features resembling neuroleptic malignant syndrome. Such reactions may occur when these drugs are given concurrently or in close proximity.
- **Narrow Angle Glaucoma:** In clinical trials, STRATTERA use was associated with an increased risk of mydriasis and therefore its use is not recommended in patients with narrow angle glaucoma.
- Symptomatic cardiovascular disease.
- Moderate to severe hypertension.
- Advanced arteriosclerosis.
- Uncontrolled hyperthyroidism.

WARNINGS AND PRECAUTIONS: Potential Association with the Occurrence of Behavioural and Emotional Changes, Including Self-Harm: Pediatric Placebo-Controlled Clinical Trial Data: An increased risk over placebo for suicide-related events in children and adolescents taking STRATTERA, was identified in a pooled analysis of placebo-controlled trials of 6-8 weeks duration. Of 1357 patients who received STRATTERA, 5 (0.37%) had reports of **suicidal ideation** compared to 0% of 851 patients who received placebo. In addition, one **suicide attempt** (overdose) was identified, which occurred in a STRATTERA patient. No completed suicides occurred during these trials. (See also Warnings and Precautions, Special Populations, Pediatrics (6-18 years of age)).
Post-Marketing Data: There have been very rare reports of suicidal ideation, suicidal attempts, suicidal depression and completed suicides in children, adolescents and adults (see Adverse Reactions, Post-Market Adverse Drug Reactions, Table 5 and Table 6).

ADHD and its related co-morbidities may be associated with increased risk of suicidal ideation and/or behaviour. Rigorous clinical monitoring for suicidal ideation or other indicators of potential for suicidal behaviour is advised in patients of all ages. This includes monitoring for agitation-type of emotional and behavioural changes, and clinical worsening.
Screening Patients for Bipolar Disorder: Particular care should be taken in treating ADHD in patients with comorbid bipolar disorder because of concern for possible induction of a mixed/manic episode in patients at risk for bipolar disorder. Prior to initiating treatment with STRATTERA, patients with comorbid depressive symptoms should be adequately screened to determine if they are at risk for bipolar disorder; such screening should include a detailed psychiatric history, including a family history of suicide, bipolar disorder, and depression.

Emergence of New Psychotic or Manic Symptoms: Treatment emergent psychotic or manic symptoms, e.g., hallucinations, delusional thinking, or mania in children and adolescents without a prior history of psychotic illness or mania can occur with atomoxetine use at usual doses. If such symptoms occur, consideration should be given to a possible causal role of atomoxetine, and discontinuation of treatment should be considered. In a pooled analysis of multiple short-term, placebo-controlled studies, such symptoms occurred in about 0.2% (4 patients with events out of 1939 exposed to atomoxetine for several weeks at usual doses) of atomoxetine-treated patients compared to 0 out of 1056 placebo-treated patients.

Pre-Existing Psychosis: Administration of medications for ADHD may also exacerbate symptoms of behaviour disturbance and thought disorder in patients with a pre-existing psychotic disorder.

Hepatic/Biliary/Pancreatic: Severe Liver Injury: Post-marketing reports indicate that STRATTERA (atomoxetine) can cause severe liver injury in rare cases. Although no evidence of liver injury was detected in clinical trials of about 6000 patients, there have been rare cases in postmarketing experience of clinically significant liver injury that were considered probably or possibly related to STRATTERA. In one patient, liver injury, manifested by elevated hepatic enzymes (up to 40×upper limit of normal [ULN]) and jaundice (bilirubin up to 12×ULN), recurred upon rechallenge and was followed by recovery upon drug discontinuation, providing evidence that STRATTERA likely caused the liver injury. Such reactions may occur several months after therapy is started, but laboratory abnormalities may continue to worsen for several weeks after drug is stopped. Because of probable under-reporting, it is impossible to provide an accurate estimate of the true incidence of these events. The patient described above recovered from his liver injury, and did not require a liver transplant. However, severe liver injury due to any drug may potentially progress to acute liver failure resulting in death or the need for a liver transplant.

STRATTERA should be discontinued in patients with jaundice or laboratory evidence of liver injury, and should not be restarted. Laboratory testing to determine liver enzyme levels should be done upon the first symptom or sign of liver dysfunction (e.g., pruritus, dark urine, jaundice, right upper quadrant tenderness, or unexplained "flu-like" symptoms). (See also Information for the Patient.)

Allergic Events: Although uncommon, allergic reactions, including rash, angioneurotic edema, and urticaria, have been reported in patients taking STRATTERA.

Effects on Growth: Chronic open-label treatment studies (up to 3 years) indicate minimal, if any, long-term effects of STRATTERA on weight and height compared with normal growth curves.

In general, the weight and height gain of pediatric patients treated with STRATTERA lags behind that predicted by normative population data for about the first 9-12 months of treatment. Subsequently, weight gain rebounds and at about 3 years of treatment, patients treated with STRATTERA have gained 17.9 kg on average, 0.5 kg more than predicted by their baseline data. After about 12 months, gain in height stabilizes, and at 3 years, patients treated with STRATTERA have gained 19.4 cm on average, 0.4 cm less than predicted by their baseline data.

This growth pattern was generally similar regardless of pubertal status at the time of treatment initiation. Patients who were pre-pubertal at the start of treatment (girls ≤8 years old, boys ≤9 years old) gained an average of 2.1 kg and 1.2 cm less than predicted after three years. Patients who were pubertal (girls >8 to ≤13 years old, boys >9 to ≤14 years old) or late pubertal (girls >13 years old, boys >14 years old) had average weight and height gains that were close to or exceeded those predicted after three years of treatment.

Growth followed a similar pattern in both extensive and poor metabolizers (EMs, PMs). PMs treated for at least 2 years gained an average of 2.4 kg and 1.1 cm less than predicted, while EMs gained an average of 0.2 kg and 0.4 cm less than predicted.

During acute treatment studies (up to 9 weeks), STRATTERA-treated patients lost an average of 0.4 kg, while placebo patients gained an average of 1.5 kg. In a controlled trial that randomized patients to placebo or 1 of 3 atomoxetine doses, 1.3%, 7.1%, 19.3%, and 29.1% of patients lost at least 3.5% of their body weight in the placebo, 0.5, 1.2, and 1.8 mg/kg/day STRATTERA dose groups, respectively. During acute treatment studies, STRATTERA-treated patients grew an average of 0.9 cm while placebo-treated patients grew an average of 1.1 cm. Whether final adult height or weight is affected by treatment with STRATTERA is unknown. Growth should be monitored during treatment with STRATTERA.

Cardiovascular: Pre-Existing Cardiovascular and Cerebral Vascular Conditions: STRATTERA should be used with caution in patients with hypertension, tachycardia, congenital long QT syndrome, or cardiovascular or cerebrovascular disease because it can increase blood pressure and heart rate. Patients should be screened for pre-existing or underlying cardiovascular or cerebrovascular conditions before initiation of treatment with STRATTERA and monitored for new conditions of the heart or brain during the course of treatment. Pulse and blood pressure should be measured at baseline, following STRATTERA dose increases, and periodically while on therapy.

In pediatric placebo-controlled trials, STRATTERA-treated subjects experienced a mean increase in heart rate of about 6 beats/minute compared with placebo subjects. At the final study visit before drug discontinuation, 3.1% (16/518) of STRATTERA-treated subjects had heart rate increases of at least 25 beats/minute and a heart rate of at least 110 beats/minute, compared with 0.3% (1/338) of placebo subjects. 1.9% (10/518) of STRATTERA-treated subjects and 0.3% (1/338) of placebo subjects had a heart rate increase of at least 25 beats/minute and a heart rate of at least 110 beats/minute on 2 or more occasions. Tachycardia was identified as an adverse event for 0.5% (3/657) of these pediatric subjects compared with 0.0% (0/408) of placebo subjects. The mean heart rate increase in extensive metabolizer (EM) patients was 5.8 beats/minute, and in poor metabolizer (PM) patients 9.7 beats/minute.

STRATTERA-treated pediatric subjects experienced mean increases of about 1.5 mm Hg in systolic and diastolic blood pressures compared with placebo. At the final study visit before drug discontinuation, 5.2% (26/496) of STRATTERA-treated pediatric subjects had high systolic blood pressure measurements compared with 2.4% (8/327) of placebo subjects. High systolic blood pressures were measured on 2 or more occasions in 6.0% (30/496) of STRATTERA-treated subjects and 2.4% (8/327) of placebo subjects. At the final study visit before drug discontinuation, 3.0% (15/506) of STRATTERA-treated pediatric subjects had high diastolic blood pressure measurements compared with 0.9% (3/330) of placebo subjects. High diastolic blood pressures were measured on 2 or more occasions in 4.2% (21/506) of STRATTERA-treated subjects and 0.9% (3/330) of placebo subjects. (High systolic and diastolic blood pressure measurements were defined as those exceeding the 95th percentile, stratified by age, gender, and height percentile—National High Blood Pressure Education Working Group on Hypertension Control in Children and Adolescents.)

In adult placebo-controlled trials, STRATTERA-treated subjects experienced a mean increase in heart rate of 5 beats/minute compared with placebo subjects. Tachycardia was identified as an adverse event for 3% (8/269) of these adult atomoxetine subjects compared with 0.8% (2/263) of placebo subjects.

STRATTERA-treated adult subjects experienced mean increases in systolic (about 3 mm Hg) and diastolic (about 1 mm Hg) blood pressures compared with placebo. At the final study visit before drug discontinuation, 1.9% (5/258) of STRATTERA-treated adult subjects had systolic blood pressure measurements ≥150 mm Hg compared with 1.2% (3/256) of placebo subjects. At the final study visit before drug discontinuation, 0.8% (2/257) of STRATTERA-treated adult subjects had diastolic blood pressure measurements ≥100 mm Hg compared with 0.4% (1/257) of placebo subjects. No adult subject had a high systolic or diastolic blood pressure detected on more than one occasion.

Orthostatic hypotension has been reported in subjects taking STRATTERA. In short-term child- and adolescent-controlled trials, 5.2% (34/657) of STRATTERA-treated subjects experienced symptoms of postural hypotension compared with 2.0% (8/408) of placebo-treated subjects. STRATTERA should be used with caution in any condition that may predispose patients to hypotension.

Sudden Death and Pre-Existing Structural Cardiac Abnormalities or Other Serious Heart Problems: Children and Adolescents: Sudden death has been reported in association with atomoxetine treatment at usual doses in children and adolescents with structural cardiac abnormalities or other serious heart problems. Although some serious heart problems alone carry an increased risk of sudden death, atomoxetine generally should not be used in children or adolescents with known serious structural cardiac abnormalities, cardiomyopathy, serious heart rhythm abnormalities, or other serious cardiac problems that may place them at increased vulnerability to the noradrenergic effects of atomoxetine.

Adults: Sudden deaths, stroke, and myocardial infarction have been reported in adults taking atomoxetine at usual doses for ADHD. Although the role of atomoxetine in these adult cases is also unknown, adults have a greater likelihood than children of having serious structural cardiac abnormalities, cardiomyopathy, serious heart rhythm abnormalities, coronary artery disease, or other serious cardiac problems. Consideration should be given to not treating adults with clinically significant cardiac abnormalities.

General: Children: Theoretically there exists a pharmacological potential for all ADHD drugs to increase the risk of sudden/cardiac death. Although confirmation of an incremental risk for adverse cardiac events arising from treatment with ADHD medications is lacking, prescribers should consider this potential risk.

All drugs with sympathomimetic effects prescribed in the management of ADHD should be used with caution in patients who: a) are involved in strenuous exercise or activities, b) use stimulants, or c) have a family history of sudden/cardiac death. Prior to the initiation of treatment with sympathomimetic medications, a personal and family history (including assessment for a family history of sudden death or ventricular arrhythmia) and physical exam should be obtained to assess for the presence of cardiac disease. In patients with relevant risk factors and based on the clinician's judgment, further cardiovascular evaluation may be considered (e.g., electrocardiogram and echocardiogram). Patients who develop symptoms such as exertional chest pain, unexplained syncope, or other symptoms suggestive of cardiac disease during ADHD treatment should undergo a prompt cardiac evaluation. Patients who are considered to need extended treatment with STRATTERA should undergo periodic evaluation of their cardiovascular status (see Dosage and Administration).

Genitourinary: Effects on Urine Outflow From the Bladder: In adult ADHD controlled trials, the rates of urinary retention and urinary hesitation were increased among atomoxetine subjects compared with placebo subjects. A complaint of urinary retention or urinary hesitancy should be considered potentially related to atomoxetine.

Carcinogenesis, Mutagenesis, Impairment of Fertility: Carcinogenesis: Atomoxetine HCl was not carcinogenic in rats and mice when given in the diet for 2 years at time-weighted average doses up to 47 and 458 mg/kg/day, respectively. The highest dose used in rats is approximately 8 and 5 times the maximum human dose in children and adults, respectively, on a mg/m^2 basis. Plasma levels (AUC) of atomoxetine at this dose in rats are estimated to be 1.8 times (extensive metabolizers) or 0.2 times (poor metabolizers) those in humans receiving the maximum human dose. The highest dose used in mice is approximately 39 and 26 times the maximum human dose in children and adults, respectively, on a mg/m^2 basis.

Mutagenesis: Atomoxetine HCl was negative in a battery of genotoxicity studies that included a reverse point mutation assay (Ames Test), an in vitro mouse lymphoma assay, a chromosomal aberration test in Chinese hamster ovary cells, an unscheduled DNA synthesis test in rat hepatocytes, and an in vivo micronucleus test in mice. However, there was a slight increase in the percentage of Chinese hamster ovary cells with diplochromosomes, suggesting endoreduplication (numerical aberration).

The metabolite N-desmethylatomoxetine HCl was negative in the Ames Test, mouse lymphoma assay, and unscheduled DNA synthesis test.

Impairment of Fertility: Atomoxetine HCl did not impair fertility in rats when given in the diet at doses of up to 57 mg/kg/day, which is approximately 6 times the maximum human dose on a mg/m^2 basis.

Teratogenicity: Pregnant rabbits were treated with up to 100 mg/kg/day of atomoxetine by gavage throughout the period of organogenesis. At this dose, in 1 of 3 studies, a decrease in live fetuses and an increase in early resorptions was observed. Slight increases in the incidences of atypical origin of carotid artery and absent subclavian artery were observed. These findings were observed at doses that caused slight maternal toxicity. The no-effect dose for these findings was 30 mg/kg/day. The 100-mg/kg dose is approximately 23 times the maximum human dose on a mg/m^2 basis; plasma levels (AUC) of atomoxetine at this dose in rabbits are estimated to be 3.3 times (extensive metabolizers) or 0.4 times (poor metabolizers) those in humans receiving the maximum human dose.

Rats were treated with up to approximately 50 mg/kg/day of atomoxetine (approximately 6 times the maximum human dose on a mg/m^2 basis) in the diet from 2 weeks (females) or 10 weeks (males) prior to mating through the periods of organogenesis and lactation. In 1 of 2 studies, decreases in pup weight and pup survival were observed. The decreased pup survival was also seen at 25 mg/kg (but not at 13 mg/kg). In a study in which rats were treated with atomoxetine in the diet from 2 weeks (females) or 10 weeks (males) prior to mating throughout the period of organogenesis, a decrease in fetal weight (female only) and an increase in the incidence of incomplete ossification of the vertebral arch in fetuses were observed at 40 mg/kg/day (approximately 5 times the maximum human dose on a mg/m^2 basis) but not at 20 mg/kg/day. No adverse fetal effects were seen when pregnant rats were treated with up to 150 mg/kg/day (approximately 17 times the maximum human dose on a mg/m^2 basis) by gavage throughout the period of organogenesis.

Special Populations: Pregnant Women: No adequate and well-controlled studies have been conducted in pregnant women. STRATTERA should not be used during pregnancy unless the potential benefit justifies the potential risk to the fetus. The effect of STRATTERA on labour and delivery in humans is unknown.

The extent of exposure in pregnancy during clinical trials was very limited.

Nursing Women: Atomoxetine and/or its metabolites were excreted in the milk of rats. It is not known if atomoxetine is excreted in human milk. Caution should be exercised if STRATTERA is administered to a nursing woman.

Pediatrics (<6 years of age): The safety and efficacy of STRATTERA in pediatric patients less than 6 years of age have not been established.

Pediatrics (6-18 years of age): Risk of suicide-related behaviours and ideation in children (see also Warnings and Precautions, Potential Association with the Occurrence of Behavioural and Emotional Changes, Including Self-Harm).

Pediatric Placebo-Controlled Clinical Trial Data: An increased risk over placebo, for suicide-related events in children and adolescents taking STRATTERA was identified in a combined analysis of 12 short-term (6-18 weeks) placebo-controlled trials (11 in ADHD and 1 in enuresis). Of 1357 patients who received STRATTERA, 5 (0.37%) had reports of **suicidal ideation** compared to 0% of 851 patients who received placebo. In addition, one **suicide attempt** (overdose) was identified which occurred in a STRATTERA patient. These 6 events occurred in STRATTERA patients 7 to 12 years of age who were male. There were no events in older adolescents, who comprised about 25 percent of the study population. Time to onset ranged from 9 to 32 days, and doses ranged from 0.48 to 1.40 mg/kg/day. A similar analysis in adult patients treated with STRATTERA for either ADHD or major depressive disorder (MDD) found no increased risk over placebo of suicidal ideation or behaviour with the use of STRATTERA.

Not included in these numerators were 6 cases (3 in the STRATTERA arms and 3 in the placebo arms) of non-fatal potentially self-injurious actions where the intent is unknown, including burns and taking more than one dose of medication at a time.

Post-Marketing Data: There have been very rare reports of suicidal ideation, suicidal attempts, suicidal depression and completed suicides in children and adolescents (see Adverse Reactions, Post-Market Adverse Drug Reactions, Table 5 and Table 6).

Rigorous clinical monitoring for suicidal ideation or other indicators of potential for suicidal behaviour is advised in patients of all ages. This includes monitoring for agitation-type of emotional and behavioural changes, and clinical worsening.

Irritability and Mood Swings: Clinical Trial Data: Clinical trial data in children and adolescents show higher rates than placebo for irritability, mood swings, aggression, crying and tearfulness (see Adverse Reactions, Table 1 and Table 2). The relationship, if any, between these events and suicide-related behaviours in children and adolescents with ADHD is unclear.

Aggressive Behaviour or Hostility: Aggressive behaviour or hostility has been observed in children and adolescents with ADHD, and has been reported with some medications indicated for the treatment of ADHD. Although there is no conclusive evidence that atomoxetine causes aggressive behaviour or hostility, this was observed more frequently in clinical trials among children and adolescents treated with atomoxetine compared to placebo (overall risk ratio of 1.33—not statistically significant). Patients beginning treatment for ADHD should be monitored for the appearance of, or worsening of, aggressive behaviour or hostility.

Caregivers/patients should be instructed to call their doctor as soon as possible should they notice an increase in aggression or hostility.

Animal Data: Growth and Neurobehavioural/Sexual Development: A study was conducted in young rats to evaluate the effects of atomoxetine on growth and neurobehavioral and sexual development. Rats were treated with 1, 10, or 50 mg/kg/day (approximately 0.2, 2, and 8 times, respectively, the maximum human dose on a mg/m^2 basis) of atomoxetine given by gavage from the early postnatal period (Day 10 of age) through adulthood. Slight delays in onset of vaginal patency (all doses) and preputial separation (10 and 50 mg/kg), slight decreases in epididymal weight and sperm number (10 and 50 mg/kg), and a slight decrease in corpora lutea (50 mg/kg) were seen, but there were no effects on fertility or reproductive performance. A slight delay in onset of incisor eruption was seen at 50 mg/kg. A slight increase in motor activity was seen on Day 15 (males at 10 and 50 mg/kg and females at 50 mg/kg) and on Day 30 (females at 50 mg/kg) but not on Day 60 of age. There were no effects on learning and memory tests. The significance of these findings to humans is unknown.

Geriatrics (>65 years of age): The safety and efficacy of STRATTERA in geriatric patients have not been established.

Monitoring and Laboratory Tests: Routine laboratory tests are not required.

CYP2D6 Metabolism: Poor metabolizers (PMs) of CYP2D6 have a 10-fold higher AUC and a 5-fold higher peak concentration to a given dose of STRATTERA compared with extensive metabolizers (EMs). Approximately 7% of a Caucasian population are PMs. Laboratory tests are available to identify CYP2D6 PMs. The blood levels in PMs are similar to those attained by taking strong inhibitors of CYP2D6. The higher blood levels in PMs lead to a higher rate of some adverse effects of STRATTERA (see Adverse Reactions).

ADVERSE REACTIONS: STRATTERA was administered to 3262 children or adolescent patients with ADHD and 471 adults with ADHD in clinical studies. During the ADHD clinical trials, 1409 patients (1236 pediatric and 173 adults) were treated for longer than 1 year and 1940 patients (1704 pediatric and 236 adults) were treated for over 6 months.

The data in the following tables and text cannot be used to predict the incidence of side effects in the course of usual medical practice where patient characteristics and other factors differ from those that prevailed in the clinical trials. Similarly, the cited frequencies cannot be compared with data obtained from other clinical investigations involving different treatments, uses, or investigators. The cited data provide the prescribing physician with some basis for estimating the relative contribution of drug and non-drug factors to the adverse event incidence in the population studied.

Child and Adolescent Clinical Trials: Reasons for Discontinuation of Treatment Due to Adverse Events in Child and Adolescent Clinical Trials: In acute child and adolescent placebo-controlled trials, 4.1% (27/661) of atomoxetine subjects and 1.2% (5/410) placebo subjects discontinued for adverse events. For all studies, (including open-label and long-term studies), 5.8% of extensive metabolizer (EM) patients and 8.9% of poor metabolizer (PM) patients discontinued because of an adverse event. Among STRATTERA-treated patients, somnolence (0.8%, N=5); aggression (0.5%, N=3); irritability (0.5%, N=3); vomiting (0.5%, N=3) and abdominal pain (0.3%, N=2) were the reasons for discontinuation reported by more than 1 patient.

Commonly Observed Adverse Events in Acute Child and Adolescent, Placebo-Controlled Trials: Commonly observed adverse events associated with the use of STRATTERA (incidence of 2% or greater) and not observed at an equivalent incidence among placebo-treated patients (STRATTERA incidence greater than placebo) are listed in Table 1 for all acute placebo-controlled trials. Results were similar in the BID trials and QD trials except as shown in Table 2, which shows both BID and QD results for selected adverse events. The most commonly observed adverse events in patients treated with STRATTERA (incidence of 5% or greater and at least twice the incidence in placebo patients, for either BID or QD dosing) were: appetite decreased, dizziness, dyspepsia, fatigue and/or lethargy, irritability, nausea, somnolence, and vomiting (see Table 2).

Table 1: STRATTERA

Common Treatment-Emergent Adverse Events Reported in STRATTERA Placebo-Controlled Clinical Trials in Children and Adolescents with ADHD[a]

Adverse Event	Percentage of Patients Reporting Events	
	STRATTERA (N=657)	Placebo (N=408)
Gastrointestinal Disorders		
Abdominal Pain Upper	18	13
Dyspepsia	5	1
Nausea	9	6
Vomiting	11	6
General Disorders		
Fatigue and/or Lethargy	8	4
Investigations		
Weight Decreased	2	0
Metabolism and Nutritional Disorders		
Anorexia	2	<1
Appetite Decreased	16	6
Nervous System Disorders		
Dizziness	5	2
Headache	21	20
Somnolence	10	4
Psychiatric Disorders		
Irritability	7	4
Mood Swings	2	<1
Respiratory Disorders		
Rhinorrhea	4	2
Skin and Subcutaneous Tissue Disorders		
Rash	3	1

[a] Events reported by at least 2% of patients treated with atomoxetine, and greater than placebo. The following events did not meet this criterion but were reported by more atomoxetine-treated patients than placebo-treated patients and are possibly related to atomoxetine treatment: aggression, blood pressure increased, early morning awakening, flushing, mydriasis, sinus tachycardia, crying, tearfulness, suicidal ideation. The following events were reported by at least 2% of patients treated with atomoxetine, and equal to or less than placebo: cough, diarrhea, insomnia, nasal congestion, nasopharyngitis, pharyngitis, pyrexia, upper respiratory tract infection.

Table 2: STRATTERA

Common Treatment-Emergent Adverse Events Associated with the Use of STRATTERA in Acute (up to 9 weeks) Child and Adolescent Trials[a]

Adverse Event	Percentage of Patients Reporting Events from BID Trials		Percentage of Patients Reporting Events from QD Trials	
	STRATTERA (N=340)	Placebo (N=207)	STRATTERA (N=317)	Placebo (N=201)
Gastrointestinal Disorders				
Abdominal Pain	1	<1	3	<1
Abdominal Pain Upper	21	16	15	8
Constipation	3	1	<1	0
Dyspepsia	4	2	6	<1
Nausea	7	8	10	4
Vomiting	12	9	11	2
General Disorders				
Fatigue and/or Lethargy	5	5	11	2
Pyrexia	5	7	6	4
Infections and Infestations				
Ear Infection	3	1	1	<1
Influenza	3	1	1	<1
Pharyngitis Streptococcal	2	<1	<1	<1
Investigations				
Weight Decreased	3	0	2	0
Metabolism and Nutritional Disorders				
Anorexia	2	<1	3	<1
Appetite Decreased	13	6	19	5
Nervous System Disorders				
Dizziness	6	3	4	<1
Headache	28	25	14	15
Sedation	1	1	3	1
Somnolence	7	5	14	3
Psychiatric Disorders				
Aggression	1	1	3	<1
Crying	2	1	1	0
Mood Swings	2	0	3	1
Irritability	8	5	6	3
Respiratory Disorders				
Cough	11	7	6	9
Rhinorrhoea	4	3	3	1
Skin and Subcutaneous Tissue Disorders				
Rash	4	1	2	1

(cont'd)

Table 2: STRATTERA *(cont'd)*

[a] Events reported by at least 2% of patients treated with atomoxetine, and greater than placebo in either BID or QD trials.

The following adverse events occurred in at least 2% of PM patients and were either twice as frequent or statistically significantly more frequent in PM patients compared with EM patients: appetite decreased (24% of PMs, 17% of EMs); insomnia and middle insomnia (14% of PMs, 8% of EMs); sedation (4% of PMs, 2% of EMs); depression and/or depressed mood (5% of PMs, 3% of EMs); abrasion (4% of PMs, 2% of EMs); tremor (5% of PMs, 1% of EMs); early morning awakening (2% of PMs, 1% of EMs); enuresis (3% of PMs, 1% of EMs); pruritus (3% of PMs, 1% of EMs); mydriasis (2% of PMs, 1% of EMs); conjunctivitis (3% of PMs, 1% of EMs); syncope (2% of PMs, 1% of EMs); animal bite (2% of PMs, 1% of EMs).

Adult Clinical Trials: Reasons for Discontinuation of Treatment Due to Adverse Events in Acute Adult Placebo-Controlled Trials: In the acute adult placebo-controlled trials, 8.5% (23/270) atomoxetine subjects and 3.4% (9/266) placebo subjects discontinued for adverse events. Among STRATTERA-treated patients, insomnia (1.1%, N=3); chest pain (0.7%, N=2); palpitations (0.7%, N=2); and urinary retention (0.7%, N=2) were the reasons for discontinuation reported by more than 1 patient.

Commonly Observed Adverse Events in Acute Adult Placebo-Controlled Trials: Commonly observed adverse events associated with the use of STRATTERA (incidence of 2% or greater) and not observed at an equivalent incidence among placebo-treated patients (STRATTERA incidence greater than placebo) are listed in Table 3.

The most commonly observed adverse events in patients treated with STRATTERA (incidence of 5% or greater and at least twice the incidence in placebo patients) were: constipation, dry mouth, nausea, appetite decreased, dizziness, insomnia, decreased libido, ejaculatory problems, erectile disturbance, urinary hesitation and/or urinary retention and/or difficulty in micturition, and dysmenorrhea (see Table 3).

Table 3: STRATTERA

Common Treatment-Emergent Adverse Events Associated with the Use of STRATTERA in Acute (up to 10 weeks) Adult Trials

Adverse Event[a]	Percentage of Patients Reporting Event	
	STRATTERA (N=269)	Placebo (N=263)
Cardiac Disorders		
Palpitations	4	1
Gastrointestinal Disorders		
Constipation	10	4
Dry Mouth	21	6
Dyspepsia	6	4
Flatulence	2	1
Nausea	12	5

(cont'd)

Table 3: STRATTERA *(cont'd)*

Common Treatment-Emergent Adverse Events Associated with the Use of STRATTERA in Acute (up to 10 weeks) Adult Trials

Adverse Event[a]	Percentage of Patients Reporting Event	
	STRATTERA (N=269)	Placebo (N=263)
General Disorders		
Fatigue and/or Lethargy	7	4
Pyrexia	3	2
Chills	3	1
Infections		
Sinusitis	6	4
Investigations		
Weight Decreased	2	1
Metabolism and Nutritional Disorders		
Appetite Decreased	10	3
Musculoskeletal Disorders		
Myalgia	3	2
Nervous System Disorders		
Dizziness	6	2
Headache	17	17
Insomnia and/or Middle Insomnia	17	8
Paraesthesia	4	2
Sinus Headache	3	1
Psychiatric Disorders		
Abnormal Dreams	4	3
Libido Decreased	6	2
Sleep Disorder	4	2
Renal and Urinary Disorders		
Urinary Hesitation and/or Urinary Retention and Dysuria	8	0
Reproductive System and Breast Disorders		
Dysmenorrhea[c]	7	3
Ejaculation Failure[b] and/or Ejaculation Disorder[b]	5	2
Erectile Dysfunction[b]	7	1
Impotence[b]	3	0
Menses Delayed[c]	2	1
Menstrual Disorder[c]	3	2
Menstruation Irregular[c]	2	0
Orgasm Abnormal	2	1
Prostatitis[b]	3	0
Skin and Subcutaneous Tissue Disorders		
Rash	2	1
Sweating Increased	4	1
Vascular Disorders		
Hot Flushes	3	1

[a] Events reported by at least 2% of patients treated with atomoxetine, and greater than placebo. The following events did not meet this criterion but were reported by more atomoxetine-treated patients than placebo-treated patients and are possibly related to atomoxetine treatment: early morning awakening, peripheral coldness, tachycardia. The following events were reported by at least 2% of patients treated with atomoxetine, and equal to or less than placebo: abdominal pain upper, arthralgia, back pain, cough, diarrhea, influenza, irritability, nasopharyngitis, sore throat, upper respiratory tract infection, vomiting.

[b] Based on total number of males (STRATTERA, N=174; placebo, N=172).

[c] Based on total number of females (STRATTERA, N=95; placebo, N=91).

Male and Female Sexual Dysfunction: Atomoxetine appears to impair sexual function in some patients. Changes in sexual desire, sexual performance, and sexual satisfaction are not well assessed in most clinical trials because they need special attention and because patients and physicians may be reluctant to discuss them. Accordingly, estimates of the incidence of untoward sexual experience and performance cited in product labelling are likely to underestimate the actual incidence. Table 4 displays the incidence of sexual side effects reported by at least 2% of adult patients taking STRATTERA in placebo-controlled trials.

Table 4: STRATTERA

Incidence of Sexual Side Effects

	STRATTERA	Placebo
Erectile Dysfunction[a]	7%	1%
Libido Decreased	6%	2%
Ejaculation Failure[a] and/or Ejaculation Disorder[a]	5%	2%
Impotence[a]	3%	0%
Orgasm Abnormal	2%	1%

[a] Males only.

There are no adequate and well-controlled studies examining sexual dysfunction with STRATTERA treatment. While it is difficult to know the precise risk of sexual dysfunction associated with the use of STRATTERA, physicians should routinely inquire about such possible side effects.

Post-Market Adverse Drug Reactions: During the first 5 years of post-market experience, it is estimated that over 5 million patients have been treated with STRATTERA, for 1 715 000 patient-years of therapy.

Table 5 and Table 6 are based on post-market spontaneous adverse event reports. The percentages shown are calculated by dividing the number of adverse events reported to the company by the estimated number of patients exposed to the drug during the same time period. The causal relationship between STRATTERA and the emergence of these events has not been established.

Table 5: STRATTERA

STRATTERA Post-Market Spontaneous Adverse Event Reports in Children and Adolescents with ADHD

Adverse Event	Frequency			
	≥1%	<1% and ≥0.1%	<0.1% and ≥0.01%	<0.01%
Cardiac Disorders				
Palpitations				X
Sinus Tachycardia			X	
Electrocardiogram QT Prolonged[a]				X
Eye Disorders				
Mydriasis			X	
Gastrointestinal Disorders				
Abdominal Pain			X	
Dyspepsia				X
Hepatobiliary Effects				X
Liver Function Tests Abnormal				X
Nausea			X	
Vomiting			X	
General Disorders				
Sudden Death				X
Injury				
Overdose				X
Investigations				
Weight Decreased			X	
Metabolism and Nutritional Disorders				
Anorexia			X	
Appetite Decreased			X	
Nervous System Disorders				
Dizziness			X	
Seizure[b]			X	
Somnolence		X		
Syncope[c]				X
Tics				X
Psychiatric Disorders				
Aggression/Hostility			X	
Anxiety			X	
Depression and Depressed Mood			X	
Early Morning Awakening				X

(cont'd)

Table 5: STRATTERA *(cont'd)*

STRATTERA Post-Market Spontaneous Adverse Event Reports in Children and Adolescents with ADHD

Adverse Event	Frequency ≥1%	<1% and ≥0.1%	<0.1% and ≥0.01%	<0.01%
Irritability			X	
Mood Swings			X	
Suicidality[d]				X
Skin and Subcutaneous Tissue Disorders				
Pruritus				X
Rash			X	
Urogenital Disorders				
Painful or Prolonged Penile Erection				X
Vascular Disorders				
Peripheral Vascular Instability, e.g., Raynaud's Phenomenon				X

[a] These spontaneously reported cases are not well documented, and the method of correction is unknown.
[b] Frequency of seizures reported=0.01%.
[c] Includes reports of "loss of consciousness".
[d] Includes reports of completed suicide, suicidal ideation, suicide attempt and suicidal depression.

Table 6: STRATTERA

STRATTERA Post-Market Spontaneous Adverse Event Reports in Adult Patients with ADHD

Adverse Event	Frequency ≥1%	<1% and ≥0.1%	<0.1% and ≥0.01%	<0.01%
Cardiac Disorders				
Palpitations				X
Tachycardia			X	
Electrocardiogram QT Prolonged[a]				X
Gastrointestinal Disorders				
Abdominal Pain			X	
Constipation			X	
Dry Mouth			X	
Dyspepsia				X
Flatulence				X
Hepatobiliary Effects				X
Liver Function Tests Abnormal				X
Nausea			X	
General Disorders				
Fatigue			X	
Lethargy				X
Chills			X	
Sudden Death				X
Injury				
Overdose				X
Investigations				
Weight Decreased			X	
Metabolism and Nutritional Disorders				
Appetite Decreased			X	
Nervous System Disorders				
Dizziness			X	

(cont'd)

Table 6: STRATTERA *(cont'd)*

STRATTERA Post-Market Spontaneous Adverse Event Reports in Adult Patients with ADHD

Adverse Event	Frequency ≥1%	<1% and ≥0.1%	<0.1% and ≥0.01%	<0.01%
Insomnia			X	
Middle Insomnia				X
Seizure[b]				X
Sinus Headache				X
Syncope[c]				X
Tics				X
Psychiatric Disorders				
Anxiety			X	
Depression and Depressed Mood			X	
Early Morning Awakening				X
Libido Decreased				X
Sleep Disorder				X
Suicidality[d]				X
Renal and Urinary Disorders				
Difficulty in Micturition			X	
Urinary Hesitation			X	
Urinary Retention			X	
Reproductive System and Breast Disorders				
Dysmenorrhea				X
Ejaculation Disorder			X	
Ejaculation Failure				X
Erectile Dysfunction			X	
Male Genital Pain				X
Menstruation Irregular				X
Orgasm Abnormal				X
Prostatitis				X
Skin and Subcutaneous Tissue Disorders				
Dermatitis				X
Sweating Increased			X	
Vascular Disorders				
Hot Flushes			X	
Peripheral Coldness				X
Peripheral Vascular Instability, e.g., Raynaud's Phenomenon				X

[a] These spontaneously reported cases are not well documented, and the method of correction is unknown.
[b] Frequency of seizures reported=0.0035%.
[c] Includes reports of "loss of consciousness".
[d] Includes reports of completed suicide, suicidal ideation, suicide attempt, and suicidal depression.

In post-market experience, serious skin reactions were reported at a spontaneous reporting rate less than 0.001%.

Drug Abuse and Dependence: STRATTERA is not a controlled substance.

STRATTERA is not a stimulant drug. In a randomized, double-blind, placebo-controlled, abuse-potential study in adults comparing effects of STRATTERA and placebo, STRATTERA was not associated with a pattern of response that suggested stimulant or euphoriant properties.

Clinical trials data in over 4000 children, adolescents, and adults with ADHD showed only isolated incidents of drug diversion or inappropriate self-administration associated with STRATTERA. There was no evidence of symptom rebound or adverse events suggesting a drug-discontinuation or withdrawal syndrome.

In preclinical studies, atomoxetine did not show a behavioural profile or stimulant properties associated with drugs that have abuse liability.

DRUG INTERACTIONS: Overview: STRATTERA (atomoxetine hydrochloride) is primarily metabolized by the CYP2D6 pathway to 4-hydroxyatomoxetine. In extensive metabolizers (EMs), inhibitors of CYP2D6 (e.g., paroxetine, fluoxetine, quinidine) increase atomoxetine steady-state plasma concentrations to exposures similar to those observed in poor metabolizers (PMs). Dosage adjustment of STRATTERA may be necessary when coadministered with CYP2D6 inhibitors, e.g., paroxetine, fluoxetine, and quinidine (see Dosage and Administration). In EM individuals treated with paroxetine or fluoxetine, the AUC of atomoxetine is approximately 6- to 8-fold and $C_{ss,max}$ is about 3- to 4-fold greater than atomoxetine alone.

In vitro studies suggest that coadministration of cytochrome P450 inhibitors to PMs will not further increase the plasma concentration of atomoxetine.

Atomoxetine did not cause clinically significant inhibition or induction of cytochrome P450 enzymes, including CYP1A2, CYP3A, CYP2D6, and CYP2C9.

Drugs that affect norepinephrine should be used cautiously when co-administered with STRATTERA because of the potential for additive or synergistic pharmacological effects.

Drug-Drug Interactions: See Table 7.

Table 7: STRATTERA

Established or Potential Drug-Drug Interactions with STRATTERA

Drug	Ref	Effect	Clinical Comment
MAO Inhibitors	T	There have been reports of serious, sometimes fatal, reactions when MAO Inhibitors are given concurrently or in close proximity to other drugs that affect brain monoamine concentrations.	See Contraindications.
Desipramine	CT	Coadministration of STRATTERA with desipramine, a model compound for CYP2D6 metabolized drugs, did not alter the pharmacokinetics of desipramine.	Because desipramine has noradrenergic effects, it should not be used in combination with STRATTERA.
Fluoxetine, Paroxetine	CT	Coadministration of selective inhibitors of CYP2D6 (e.g. fluoxetine, paroxetine) may increase atomoxetine steady-state plasma concentrations to exposures similar to those observed in CYP2D6 poor metabolizer patients.	Slower titration of STRATTERA may be necessary in those patients who are also taking fluoxetine, paroxetine or other CYP2D6 inhibitor drugs (see Dosage and Administration, Dosage Adjustment for Special Populations).
Salbutamol or Other β-adrenergic Receptor Agonists	CT	In adult volunteers, the effects on blood pressure and heart rate of a standard inhaled dose of salbutamol (200 µg) are not clinically significant compared to IV administration, and not increased by coadministration of atomoxetine (80 mg QD for 5 days). Heart rate after multiple inhalations of salbutamol (800 µg) was similar in the presence or absence of atomoxetine.	STRATTERA may be used in combination with inhaled β2 agonists, e.g., salbutamol, but should be used with caution in patients being treated with systemically administered (oral or intravenous) β2 agonists, including salbutamol.
Pressor Agents	T	Possible effects on blood pressure.	STRATTERA should be used with caution in patients being treated with pressor agents.
Methylphenidate	CT	Co-administration of methylphenidate with STRATTERA did not increase cardiovascular effects beyond those seen with methylphenidate administration alone.	
Midazolam	CT	Co-administration of STRATTERA with midazolam, a model compound for CYP3A4 metabolized drugs, resulted in small increases in midazolam plasma concentrations.	No dosage adjustment required.
Drugs Highly Bound to Plasma Protein	In vitro	Atomoxetine did not affect the binding of warfarin, acetylsalicylic acid, phenytoin, or diazepam to human albumin in-vitro. Similarly, these compounds did not affect the binding of atomoxetine to human albumin.	No dosage adjustment required.
Drugs Affecting Gastric pH	CT	Drugs that elevate gastric pH (magnesium hydroxide/aluminum hydroxide, omeprazole) had no effect on STRATTERA bioavailability.	No dosage adjustment required.

Legend: C=case study; CT=clinical trial; T=theoretical.

Drug-Food Interactions: STRATTERA may be taken with or without food.

Drug-Lifestyle Interactions: Alcohol: Consumption of ethanol with STRATTERA did not change the intoxicating effects of ethanol.

DOSAGE AND ADMINISTRATION: Dosing Considerations: STRATTERA should be administered starting at the lowest possible dose. Dosage should then be individually and slowly adjusted to the lowest effective dose, since individual patient response to STRATTERA varies widely.

STRATTERA should not be used in patients with symptomatic cardiovascular disease and should not generally be used in patients with known structural cardiac abnormalities (see Contraindications and Warnings and Precautions).

Children: Theoretically there exists a pharmacological potential for all ADHD drugs to increase the risk of sudden/cardiac death. Although confirmation of an incremental risk for adverse cardiac events arising from treatment with ADHD medications is lacking, prescribers should consider this potential risk.

All drugs with sympathomimetic effects prescribed in the management of ADHD should be used with caution in patients who: a) are involved in strenuous exercise or activities, b) use stimulants, or c) have a family history of sudden/cardiac death. Prior to the initiation of treatment with sympathomimetic medications, a personal and family history (including assessment for a family history of sudden death or ventricular arrhythmia) and physical exam should be obtained to assess for the presence of cardiac disease. In patients with relevant risk factors and based on the clinician's judgment, further cardiovascular evaluation may be considered (e.g., electrocardiogram and echocardiogram). Patients who develop symptoms such as exertional chest pain, unexplained syncope, or other symptoms suggestive of cardiac disease during ADHD treatment should undergo a prompt cardiac evaluation. Patients who are considered to need extended treatment with STRATTERA should undergo periodic evaluation of their cardiovascular status (see Warnings and Precautions).

Rigorous clinical monitoring for suicidal ideation or other indicators of potential for suicidal behaviour is advised in patients of all ages. This includes monitoring of agitation-type emotional and behavioural changes, and clinical worsening (see Warnings and Precautions, Potential Association with the Occurrence of Behavioural and Emotional Changes, Including Self-Harm).

STRATTERA (atomoxetine hydrochloride) is intended for oral administration and may be taken with or without food, either as a single daily dose in the morning or as divided doses in the morning and late afternoon/early evening.

Initial improvement of ADHD symptoms is generally observed within 1 to 4 weeks of initiating therapy.

STRATTERA did not worsen tics in pediatric patients, and may be used in patients with ADHD and comorbid motor tics or diagnosis of Tourette's Disorder. STRATTERA did not worsen anxiety in either pediatric or adult patients, and may be used in patients with ADHD and comorbid anxiety disorders. See Action and Clinical Pharmacology, Special Populations and Conditions, Patients with Concomitant Illness.

If patients miss a dose, they should take it as soon as possible; however, they should not take more than the prescribed total daily amount of STRATTERA in any 24-hour period.

STRATTERA may be discontinued without tapering the dose.

Recommended Dose and Dosage Adjustment: Children (6 years and over) and Adolescents up to 70 kg Body Weight: Do not exceed the recommended initial dose and subsequent dose escalations of STRATTERA. More rapid dose escalation may be associated with increased rates of somnolence and digestive system complaints. Do not exceed the recommended maximum total daily dose of 1.4 mg/kg or 100 mg, whichever is less. No additional benefit has been demonstrated at doses greater than 1.2 mg/kg/day. The safety of single doses over 1.8 mg/kg/day and total daily doses above 1.8 mg/kg have not been systematically evaluated, and therefore should not be administered because of potential side-effects (see Action and Clinical Pharmacology, Cardiovascular Safety and Overdosage).

STRATTERA should be initiated at a total daily dose of approximately 0.5 mg/kg (Step 1) for 7 to 14 days. Based on tolerability, the dose should be successively increased to approximately 0.8 mg/kg/day (Step 2) for 7 to 14 days, and then to approximately 1.2 mg/kg/day (Step 3). Table 8 provides, for each titration step, the corresponding daily STRATTERA dose according to body weight. After a minimum of 30 days, dose should be reassessed and adjusted according to clinical response and tolerability.

The total daily dose in children and adolescents up to 70 kg should not exceed 1.4 mg/kg or 100 mg, whichever is less.

As the lowest available capsule strength is 10 mg, the child should weigh at least 20 kg at the time of initiation of therapy. Only whole capsules should be administered.

Table 8: STRATTERA

Daily STRATTERA Dose for Each Titration Step as per Body Weight, in Children and Adolescents up to 70 kg Body Weight

Body Weight	Step 1 (approx. 0.5 mg/kg/day)	Step 2 (approx. 0.8 mg/kg/day)	Step 3 (approx. 1.2 mg/kg/day)	Maximum Dose
20–29 kg	10 mg/day	18 mg/day	25 mg/day	1.4 mg/kg/day or 100 mg/day (whichever is less)
30–44 kg	18 mg/day	25 mg/day	40 mg/day	
45–64 kg	25 mg/day	40 mg/day	60 mg/day	
65–70 kg	40 mg/day	60 mg/day	80 mg/day	

Children and Adolescents Over 70 kg Body Weight, and Adults: Do not exceed the recommended initial dose and subsequent dose escalations of STRATTERA. Do not exceed the recommended maximum total daily dose of 100 mg. The safety of single doses over 120 mg and total daily doses above 150 mg have not been systematically evaluated and therefore should not be administered because of potential side effects (see Action and Clinical Pharmacology, Cardiovascular Safety and Overdosage).

STRATTERA should be initiated at a total daily dose of 40 mg/day (Step 1) for 7 to 14 days. Based on tolerability, the dose should be successively increased to 60 mg/day (Step 2) for 7 to 14 days, and then to 80 mg/day (Step 3). After 2 to 4 additional weeks, the total daily dose may be increased to a maximum of 100 mg in patients who have not achieved an optimal response.

The maximum recommended total daily dose in children and adolescents over 70 kg and adults is 100 mg.

Dosage Adjustment for Special Populations: Hepatic Impaired: Atomoxetine clearance may be reduced in ADHD patients with hepatic impairment. For patients with moderate hepatic impairment (Child-Pugh Class B), initial and target doses should be reduced to 50% of the normal dose. For patients with severe hepatic impairment (Child-Pugh Class C), initial dose and target doses should be reduced to 25% of the normal dose.

Renal Impaired: Subjects with end stage renal disease had higher systemic exposure to atomoxetine than healthy subjects (about a 65% increase), but there was no difference when exposure was corrected for mg/kg dose. STRATTERA can therefore be administered to ADHD patients with end stage renal disease or lesser degrees of renal insufficiency using the usual dosing regimen. Atomoxetine may exacerbate hypertension in patients with end stage renal disease.

Dosing Adjustment for Use with a Strong CYP2D6 Inhibitor: In children (≥6 years old) and adolescents up to 70 kg body weight administered strong CYP2D6 inhibitors, e.g., paroxetine, fluoxetine, and quinidine, STRATTERA should be initiated at 0.5 mg/kg/day and only increased to the next dose level if symptoms fail to improve after 14 days and the previous dose is well tolerated.

In children (≥6 years old) and adolescents over 70 kg body weight and adults administered strong CYP2D6 inhibitors, e.g., paroxetine, fluoxetine, and quinidine, STRATTERA should be initiated at 40 mg/day and only increased to the next dose level if symptoms fail to improve after 14 days and the previous dose is well tolerated.

Maintenance/Extended Treatment: Pharmacological treatment of ADHD may be needed for extended periods. The efficacy of STRATTERA in maintaining symptom response during long-term treatment in children and adolescents was studied in an 18-month trial (3 months of acute open-label treatment followed by up to 15 months of placebo-controlled maintenance treatment). The results from this study suggest that atomoxetine may be beneficial in the long-term treatment of ADHD. Too few patients completed the study to permit an adequate assessment of the long-term safety profile of STRATTERA in this study. The long-term safety of STRATTERA has been demonstrated in double-blind and open-label clinical trials of at least 24 months. The physician who elects to use STRATTERA for extended periods should periodically reevaluate the long-term usefulness of the drug for the individual patient (see Indications and Clinical Use).

OVERDOSAGE:

There is limited clinical trial experience with STRATTERA overdose and no fatalities were observed in clinical studies.

During post-marketing, there have been reports of non-fatal, acute and chronic overdoses of STRATTERA. The most commonly reported symptoms accompanying acute and chronic overdoses were somnolence, agitation, hyperactivity, abnormal behaviour, and gastrointestinal symptoms. Signs and symptoms consistent with mild to moderate sympathetic nervous system activation (e.g., mydriasis, tachycardia, dry mouth) have also been observed. Seizures have been reported in several cases, including myoclonus of the extremities. Less commonly, there have been reports of QT prolongation and mental changes, including disorientation and hallucinations. All patients recovered from these events.

In the first 18 months of market availability in the US, among the mixed overdose reports involving STRATTERA where at least one other drug was taken in overdose amounts, there were 3 deaths reported, all in adults. The largest quantity of STRATTERA alone in a single overdose was 1400 mg, taken by a 17 year old patient. He experienced chest pain and drowsiness and was treated with activated charcoal about 2 hours after the ingestion and recovered fully after an overnight hospital stay for observation.

There were no deaths involving overdose of STRATTERA alone.

Management of Overdose: There is no established antidote for STRATTERA overdose. Treatment has been supportive, including establishing an airway when necessary, monitoring of cardiac and vital signs, along with appropriate symptomatic and supportive measures. Gastric lavage may be indicated if performed soon after ingestion. Activated charcoal may be useful in limiting absorption. Because atomoxetine is highly protein-bound, dialysis is not likely to be useful in the treatment of overdose.

For management of a suspected drug overdose, CPhA recommends that you contact your **regional Poison Control Centre**. See the *CPS* Directory section for a list of Poison Control Centres.

ACTION AND CLINICAL PHARMACOLOGY: Mechanism of Action: STRATTERA (atomoxetine hydrochloride) is a selective norepinephrine reuptake inhibitor. Its therapeutic effect in ADHD is thought to be related to its potent inhibition of the pre-synaptic norepinephrine transporter, with minimal affinity for other noradrenergic receptors or for other neurotransmitter transporters or receptors.

Pharmacodynamics: In ex vivo uptake and neurotransmitter depletion studies, atomoxetine was found to selectively inhibit the pre-synaptic norepinephrine transporter without directly affecting the serotonin or dopamine transporters. Atomoxetine has minimal affinity for other receptor systems. Atomoxetine is primarily oxidized to 4-hydroxyatomoxetine, which is also a potent inhibitor of the pre-synaptic norepinephrine transporter.

Cardiovascular Safety: The safety and tolerability of gradually increasing multiple-dose regimes of atomoxetine 60 to 150 mg/day was studied in 16 healthy adults (10 EM subjects and 6 PM subjects). None of the mean or individual $QT_{c(F)}$ intervals exceeded the upper limits of normal for each gender. The EM group had no statistically significant changes in mean $QT_{c(F)}$ interval compared to the placebo treatment. No statistically significant changes in $QT_{c(F)}$ were noted 1 hour post dose (during peak plasma concentrations) in the PM group. The PM group had a statistically significant increase in the mean $QT_{c(F)}$ interval measured at time 0 (during trough plasma concentrations) on the last day of the 60- and 75-mg atomoxetine twice-daily dosing regimens compared to the placebo. The greatest mean prolongation was about 17 msec at the 60-mg BID dose level, with the mean interval length of 417.2 msec. At the 75-mg BID atomoxetine dose level, the greatest mean prolongation was 15 msec, and the mean interval length was 414.9 msec. The 60 mg BID and 75 mg BID doses correspond to 1.4-2.24 mg/kg/day and 1.75-2.8 mg/kg/day, respectively. Baseline ECGs obtained during screening of pediatric patients for atomoxetine clinical trials were reviewed for cases of QTc prolongation. Using a correction method based on data from baseline ECGs, there were 32/3902 cases (0.8%) with $QT_{c(D)}$ >450 msec and 5/3902 cases (0.1%) with $QT_{c(D)}$>500 msec. In a meta-analysis of ECG data from patients who received atomoxetine in pediatric clinical trials, no relationship was observed between changes from baseline to final $QT_{c(D)}$ and prescribed atomoxetine dose, or between changes from baseline to $QT_{c(D)}$ at time of expected peak exposure and prescribed atomoxetine dose.

Overall, the data do not suggest a meaningful relationship between atomoxetine plasma concentrations and the length of the QT interval corrected for heart rate in the recommended dosage range. However, since there is no requirement for a priori screening of ADHD patients for CYP2D6 metabolizer status before initiating treatment with atomoxetine, it is important that the lowest effective dose be used, so as to minimize potential cardiac side effects.

Pharmacokinetics: Atomoxetine is well-absorbed after oral administration and is minimally affected by food. It is eliminated primarily by oxidative metabolism through the cytochrome P450 2D6 (CYP2D6) enzymatic pathway and subsequent glucuronidation. Atomoxetine has a half-life of about 5 hours. A fraction of the population (about 7% of Caucasians and 2% of African Americans) are poor metabolizers (PMs) of CYP2D6 metabolized drugs. These individuals have reduced activity in this pathway resulting in 10-fold higher AUCs, 5-fold higher peak plasma concentrations, and slower elimination (plasma half-life of 21.6 hours) of atomoxetine compared with people with normal activity [extensive metabolizers (EMs)]. Drugs that inhibit CYP2D6, such as fluoxetine, paroxetine, and quinidine, cause similar increases in exposure.

The pharmacokinetics of atomoxetine have been evaluated in more than 400 children and adolescents in selected clinical trials using a population approach. Single-dose and steady-state individual pharmacokinetic data were also obtained in children, adolescents, and adults. When doses were normalized to a mg/kg basis, similar half-life, C_{max}, and AUC values were observed in children, adolescents, and adults. Clearance and volume of distribution after adjustment for body weight were also similar.

Atomoxetine pharmacokinetics are dose proportional within the therapeutic range; hence, administration of STRATTERA once- or twice-daily is expected to result in the same systemic exposure (AUC) over a 24-hour period. Results of efficacy analysis show that once-daily (QD) dosing with STRATTERA is efficacious in the treatment of ADHD.

STRATTERA 80 mg capsules are bioequivalent to 2x40 mg capsules. STRATTERA 100 mg capsules are bioequivalent to a combination of one 40 mg and one 60 mg capsule.

Absorption: Atomoxetine is rapidly absorbed after oral administration, with absolute bioavailability of about 63% in extensive metabolizers (EMs) and 94% in poor metabolizers (PMs). Mean maximal plasma concentrations (C_{max}) are reached approximately 1 to 2 hours after dosing.

STRATTERA can be administered with or without food. In clinical trials with children and adolescents, administration of STRATTERA with food resulted in a 9% lower C_{max}. Administration of STRATTERA with a standard high-fat meal in adults did not affect the extent of oral absorption of atomoxetine (AUC), but did decrease the rate of absorption, resulting in a 37% lower C_{max} and delayed T_{max} by 3 hours.

Distribution: The steady-state volume of distribution after intravenous administration was approximately 0.85 L/kg indicating that atomoxetine distributes primarily into total body water. In children and adolescents, volume of distribution increased nearly proportionally to increases in body weight. Volume of distribution is similar across the patient weight range after normalizing for body weight.

At therapeutic concentrations, 98% of atomoxetine in plasma is bound to protein, primarily albumin.

Metabolism: Atomoxetine undergoes biotransformation primarily through the cytochrome P450 2D6 (CYP2D6) enzymatic pathway. People with reduced activity in the CYP2D6 pathway (PMs) have higher plasma concentrations of atomoxetine compared with people with normal activity (EMs). For PMs, AUC of atomoxetine at steady-state is approximately 10-fold higher and $C_{ss,max}$ is about 5-fold greater than for EMs.

Coadministration of STRATTERA with potent inhibitors of CYP2D6, such as fluoxetine, paroxetine, or quinidine, results in a substantial increase in atomoxetine plasma exposure, and dosing adjustment may be necessary (see Drug Interactions, Drug-Drug Interactions). In EM patients treated with potent CYP2D6 inhibitors such as fluoxetine, and paroxetine, the AUC of atomoxetine is approximately 6- to 8-fold and $C_{ss,max}$ is about 3- to 4-fold greater than with atomoxetine alone.

In vitro studies suggest that coadministration of cytochrome P450 inhibitors to PMs will not increase the plasma concentration of atomoxetine.

Atomoxetine did not inhibit or induce the CYP2D6 pathway.

The major oxidative metabolite formed regardless of CYP2D6 status is 4-hydroxyatomoxetine, which is rapidly glucuronidated. 4-Hydroxyatomoxetine is equipotent to atomoxetine as an inhibitor of the norepinephrine transporter, but circulates in plasma at much lower concentrations (1% of atomoxetine concentration in EMs and 0.1% of atomoxetine concentration in PMs). 4-Hydroxyatomoxetine is primarily formed by CYP2D6. In individuals that lack CYP2D6 activity (poor metabolizers), 4-hydroxyatomoxetine is formed by several other cytochrome P450 enzymes, but at a slower rate. N-Desmethylatomoxetine is formed by CYP2C19 and other cytochrome P450 enzymes, but has much less pharmacological activity than atomoxetine, and plasma concentrations are lower (5% of atomoxetine concentration in EMs and 45% of atomoxetine concentration in PMs).

Excretion: The mean elimination half-life of atomoxetine after oral administration is 5.2 hours and 21.6 hours in EM and PM subjects, respectively. The elimination half-life of 4 hydroxyatomoxetine is similar to that of N-desmethylatomoxetine (6 to 8 hours) in EM subjects, while the half-life of N-desmethylatomoxetine is much longer in PM subjects (34 to 40 hours).

Atomoxetine is excreted primarily as 4-hydroxyatomoxetine-O-glucuronide, mainly in the urine (greater than 80% of the dose) and to a lesser extent in the feces (less than 17% of the dose). Only a small fraction (less than 3%) of the STRATTERA dose is excreted as unchanged atomoxetine, indicating extensive biotransformation.

Special Populations and Conditions: Pediatrics: The pharmacokinetics of atomoxetine in children and adolescents are similar to those in adults. The pharmacokinetics of atomoxetine have not been evaluated in children under 6 years of age.

Geriatrics: The pharmacokinetics of atomoxetine have not been systematically evaluated in the geriatric population.

Gender: Gender did not influence atomoxetine disposition.

Race: Ethnic origin did not influence atomoxetine disposition.

Hepatic Insufficiency: Single doses of STRATTERA administered to EM subjects with moderate to severe hepatic insufficiency (Child-Pugh Class B and C) resulted in increased atomoxetine exposure, reduced atomoxetine clearance, and prolonged half-life of parent drug compared with healthy subjects. Dosage adjustment is recommended for patients with moderate or severe hepatic impairment (see Dosage and Administration).

Renal Insufficiency: Single doses of STRATTERA administered to EM subjects with end stage renal disease resulted in higher atomoxetine exposure (AUC) than in healthy subjects (about a 65% increase), but there was no difference when exposure was corrected for mg/kg dose. STRATTERA can therefore be administered to ADHD patients with end stage renal disease or lesser degrees of renal insufficiency using the normal dosing regimen.

Genetic Polymorphism: There are two major phenotypes associated with CYP2D6: extensive metabolizers that comprise >90% of the population, and poor metabolizers. Approximately 7% of the Caucasian population and 2% of Black population are poor metabolizers of CYP2D6.

Patients with Concomitant Illness: Pediatric Patients with ADHD and Comorbid Tics: Study LYAS enrolled patients meeting DSM-IV criteria for ADHD and comorbid Tourette's Disorder or chronic motor tics. STRATTERA met the primary study objective of non-inferiority to placebo with respect to worsening of tics and had a beneficial effect in reducing tic severity. STRATTERA was also markedly superior to placebo in reducing symptoms of ADHD as assessed by the ADHDRS-IV-Parent: Inv Total score (p=0.002).

Patients with ADHD and Comorbid Anxiety Disorder: Study LYBP: Pediatric patients (n=176, age 8-17), who met DSM-IV criteria for ADHD and at least one of the anxiety disorders of separation anxiety disorder, generalized anxiety disorder or social phobia were randomized 1:1 into a 12-week double-blind, placebo-controlled trial. The statistical analysis plan specified that patients responding (i.e., >25% reduction in Pediatric Anxiety Rating Scale (PARS) total scores) during a blinded placebo lead-in period be excluded from the primary efficacy analyses. However, all of the enrolled patients with a baseline and at least one post-baseline score were included in the remaining efficacy analyses. Initial STRATTERA dose was 0.8 mg/kg/day, with increase to a target dose of 1.2 mg/kg/day (median dose 1.3 mg/kg/day ± 0.3 mg/kg/day). STRATTERA was markedly superior to placebo in reducing symptoms of ADHD as assessed by the ADHDRS-IV-Parent: Inv Total score (p<0.001) and mean PARS total score improved significantly for STRATTERA relative to placebo (p=0.011). Worsening of anxiety was defined post-hoc as a 25% increase in PARS, or patient-reported anxiety as an adverse event. Based on these criteria, patients on STRATTERA did not have worsening of anxiety relative to the placebo group. Of the 158 patients who completed the double-blind placebo lead-in, 26 (16%) discontinued the study.

Study LYDQ: Adult patients (n=442, age 18-65) , who met DSM-IV criteria for adult ADHD and social anxiety disorder (23% of whom also had Generalized Anxiety Disorder) were randomized into a 16-week double-blind, placebo-controlled trial. The statistical analysis plan specified that patients responding (i.e., >25% decrease in social anxiety symptoms as measured by the Liebowitz Social Anxiety Scale) during a blinded placebo lead-in period be excluded from the primary efficacy analyses. However, all of the enrolled patients with a baseline and at least one post-baseline score were included in the remaining efficacy analyses. STRATTERA was initiated at 40 mg/day to a maximum dose of 100 mg/day (mean daily dose 83 mg/day ±19.5 mg/day). STRATTERA was markedly superior to placebo in reducing symptoms of ADHD as assessed by the Conners' Adult ADHD Rating Scale (p<0.001) and mean LSAS total score improved significantly for STRATTERA relative to placebo (p≤0.01). Worsening of anxiety was defined post-hoc as a 25% increase in LSAS, or patient-reported anxiety as an adverse event. Based on these criteria, patients on STRATTERA did not have worsening of anxiety relative to the placebo group. Of the 436 patients who completed the double-blind placebo lead-in, 172 (39%) discontinued the study.

STORAGE AND STABILITY: Store at controlled room temperature, 15 to 30°C.

STRATTERA capsules are not intended to be opened, they should be taken whole.

INFORMATION FOR THE PATIENT: Published in e-CPS, available by subscription at www.e-cps.ca.

DOSAGE FORMS, COMPOSITION AND PACKAGING: 10 mg: Each opaque white, opaque white capsule, identified with LILLY 3227, contains: atomoxetine hydrochloride equivalent to 10 mg of atomoxetine. Nonmedicinal ingredients: dimethicone and pregelatinized starch; capsule shell: gelatin, sodium lauryl sulfate, and other inactive ingredients. The capsule shells also contain one or more of the following: FD&C Blue No. 2, red iron oxide, synthetic yellow iron oxide and titanium dioxide. Blisters packages of 28.

18 mg: Each gold, opaque white capsule, identified with LILLY 3238, contains: atomoxetine hydrochloride equivalent to 18 mg of atomoxetine. Nonmedicinal ingredients: dimethicone and pregelatinized starch; capsule shell: gelatin, sodium lauryl sulfate, and other inactive ingredients. The capsule shells also contain one or more of the following: FD&C Blue No. 2, red iron oxide, synthetic yellow iron oxide and titanium dioxide. Blisters packages of 28.

25 mg: Each opaque blue, opaque white capsule, identified with LILLY 3228, contains: atomoxetine hydrochloride equivalent to 25 mg of atomoxetine. Nonmedicinal ingredients: dimethicone and pregelatinized starch; capsule shell: gelatin, sodium lauryl sulfate, and other inactive ingredients. The capsule shells also contain one or more of the following: FD&C Blue No. 2, red iron oxide, synthetic yellow iron oxide and titanium dioxide. Blisters packages of 28.

40 mg: Each opaque blue, opaque blue capsule, identified with LILLY 3229, contains: atomoxetine hydrochloride equivalent to 40 mg of atomoxetine. Nonmedicinal ingredients: dimethicone and pregelatinized starch; capsule shell: gelatin, sodium lauryl sulfate, and other inactive ingredients. The capsule shells also contain one or more of the following: FD&C Blue No. 2, red iron oxide, synthetic yellow iron oxide and titanium dioxide. Blisters packages of 28.

60 mg: Each opaque blue, gold capsule, identified with LILLY 3239, contains: atomoxetine hydrochloride equivalent to 60 mg of atomoxetine. Nonmedicinal ingredients: dimethicone and pregelatinized starch; capsule shell: gelatin, sodium lauryl sulfate, and other inactive ingredients. The capsule shells also contain one or more of the following: FD&C Blue No. 2, red iron oxide, synthetic yellow iron oxide and titanium dioxide. Blisters packages of 28.

80 mg: Each opaque brown, opaque white capsule, identified with LILLY 3250, contains: atomoxetine hydrochloride equivalent to 80 mg of atomoxetine. Nonmedicinal ingredients: dimethicone and pregelatinized starch; capsule shell: gelatin, sodium lauryl sulfate, and other inactive ingredients. The capsule shells also contain one or more of the following: FD&C Blue No. 2, red iron oxide, synthetic yellow iron oxide and titanium dioxide. Blisters packages of 28.

100 mg: Each opaque brown, opaque brown capsule, identified with LILLY 3251, contains: atomoxetine hydrochloride equivalent to 100 mg of atomoxetine. Nonmedicinal ingredients: dimethicone and pregelatinized starch; capsule shell: gelatin, sodium lauryl sulfate, and other inactive ingredients. The capsule shells also contain one or more of the following: FD&C Blue No. 2, red iron oxide, synthetic yellow iron oxide and titanium dioxide. Blisters packages of 28.

(Shown in Product Identification Section)

Streptase®

streptokinase

Fibrinolytic Agent

CSL Behring

Date of Revision: March 29, 2007

PHARMACOLOGY: STREPTASE (streptokinase injection) acts with plasminogen (or plasmin) to produce an "activator complex" that converts residual plasminogen into the proteolytic enzyme, plasmin. Plasmin is capable of hydrolyzing fibrin into polypeptides; it also hydrolyzes fibrinogen and other plasma proteins. Since plasminogen is present in the thrombus/embolus, activation by STREPTASE occurs within the thrombus/embolus as well as on its surface.

The activity of streptokinase is expressed in International Units (IU) and is a measure of its ability to cause lysis of a fibrin clot via the plasmin system in vitro. The effect on coagulation after intravenous administration may persist for 12 to 24 hours after discontinuation due to a decrease in plasma levels of fibrinogen and an increase in the amount of circulating fibrin(ogen) degradation products (FDP). Studies with radioactive streptokinase indicate 2 disappearance rates: a "fast" half-life of approximately 18 minutes due to the action of antibodies, and a "slow" half-life, operative in the absence of antibodies, of approximately 83 minutes. Effective blood level and disappearance rate are dependent upon availability of substrates and, thus, are only relative indices of the pharmacologic effects of the drug. The efficacy of STREPTASE in the lysis of venous thrombi and massive pulmonary emboli has been established in clinical studies by angiographic evaluations, before and after treatment.

Two large, randomized, multicentre, placebo-controlled studies involving almost 30 000 patients have demonstrated that a 60-minute intravenous infusion of 1 500 000 IU of STREPTASE significantly reduces mortality rates following a myocardial infarction. Concomitant oral administration of low-dose acetylsalicylic acid (ASA) (160 mg/day) over a period of one month was shown to significantly enhance this beneficial effect.

INDICATIONS: Acute Myocardial Infarction: STREPTASE (streptokinase injection) is indicated for use in the management of suspected acute myocardial infarction, for the lysis of acute thrombi obstructing coronary arteries associated with evolving transmural myocardial infarction, for the improvement of ventricular function, and for the reduction of infarct size and mortality associated with acute myocardial infarction, when administered by the intravenous or intracoronary route, as well as for the reduction of congestive heart failure associated with AMI when administered by the intravenous route. In the high risk group with anterior myocardial infarction, one year mortality was significantly reduced in those patients who reperfused in response to streptokinase.

Thrombolysis following intravenous streptokinase is usually achieved within less than one hour. Early administration is correlated with greater clinical benefit.

Pulmonary Embolism: STREPTASE is indicated in adults for the lysis of acute massive pulmonary emboli, defined as obstruction or significant filling defects involving two or more lobar pulmonary arteries or an equivalent amount of emboli in other vessels. It is also indicated for embolization accompanied by unstable hemodynamics, i.e., failure to maintain blood pressure without supportive measures. The diagnosis should be confirmed by objective means, preferably pulmonary arteriography via an upper extremity vein, or non-invasive procedures such as lung scanning.

Deep Vein Thrombosis: STREPTASE is indicated for lysis of acute, extensive thrombi of the deep veins in adults such as those involving the popliteal and more proximal vessels. Diagnosis should be confirmed by ascending venography or other equally objective methods.

Studies have demonstrated a better salvage of valvular function and prevention of postphlebitic syndrome by the combined usage of STREPTASE and heparin than by heparin alone.

Arterial Thrombosis and Embolism: STREPTASE is indicated for the lysis of acute arterial thrombi and for the lysis of arterial emboli. However, the use of STREPTASE in arterial emboli originating from the left side of the heart (e.g., in mitral stenosis accompanied by atrial fibrillation) should be avoided due to the danger of new embolic phenomena including those to cerebral vessels.

Arteriovenous Cannula Occlusion: STREPTASE is indicated for clearing of totally or partially occluded arteriovenous cannulae as an alternative to surgical intervention when acceptable flow cannot otherwise be achieved.

CONTRAINDICATIONS: Because thrombolytic therapy increases the risk of bleeding, STREPTASE (streptokinase injection) is contraindicated in the following conditions: Active or recent internal bleeding. Recent (within 2 months) cerebrovascular accident, intracranial or intraspinal surgery (see Warnings). Intracranial neoplasm. Uncontrollable hypertension with systolic values above 200 mm Hg and/or diastolic values above 100 mm Hg, or hypertensive retinal changes Grades III/IV. All forms of reduced blood coagulability in particular spontaneous fibrinolysis and extensive clotting disorders. Recent head trauma. Known neoplasm with risk of hemorrhage. Acute pancreatitis.

STREPTASE should not be administered to patients having experienced severe allergic reaction to the product.

WARNINGS: Bleeding: The aim of STREPTASE (streptokinase injection) therapy is the production of sufficient amounts of plasmin for the lysis of intravascular deposits of fibrin; however, fibrin deposits which provide hemostasis, for example at sites of needle punctures, are also lyzed and bleeding from such sites may occur.

Following intravenous high-dose brief-duration STREPTASE therapy (1 500 000 IU over 60 minutes), in acute myocardial infarction, severe bleeding complications requiring transfusion are extremely rare (0.3-0.5%), and combined therapy with low-dose ASA (160 mg/day over a period of one month) does not appear to increase the risk of major bleeding. The addition of ASA to STREPTASE may cause a slight increase in the risk of minor bleeding (3.1% without ASA vs 3.9% with ASA).

Intramuscular injections and nonessential handling of the patient must be avoided during treatment with STREPTASE. Venipunctures should be performed carefully and as infrequently as possible.

Should an arterial puncture be necessary, upper extremity vessels are preferable. Pressure should be applied for at least 30 minutes, a pressure dressing applied and the puncture site checked frequently for evidence of bleeding. When internal bleeding occurs it may be more difficult to manage than that which occurs with conventional anticoagulant therapy.

In the following conditions, the risks of therapy may be increased and should be weighed against the anticipated benefits: Recent (within 10 days) major surgery. Recent delivery, abortion. Recent organ biopsy, previous puncture of non-compressible vessels, intramuscular injections or intubation. Recent (within 10 days) serious gastrointestinal bleeding. Recent (within 10 days) trauma including cardiopulmonary resuscitation. High likelihood of left heart thrombus, e.g., mitral stenosis with atrial fibrillation. Subacute bacterial endocarditis or pericarditis; isolated cases of a pericarditis, misdiagnosed as acute myocardial infarction and treated with STREPTASE, have resulted in pericardial effusions including tamponade. Hemostatic defects including those secondary to severe hepatic or renal disease. Pregnancy. Cerebrovascular disease. Pulmonary diseases with cavitation (e.g., open tuberculosis) or severe bronchitis. Severe diabetes mellitus. Diabetic hemorrhagic retinopathy. Diseases of the urogenital tract with potential sources of bleeding. Septic thrombophlebitis or occluded AV cannula at seriously infected site. Suspicion of severe arthrosclerotic degeneration. Any other condition in which bleeding constitutes a significant hazard or would be particularly difficult to manage because of its location.

Should serious spontaneous bleeding (not controllable by local pressure) occur, the infusion of STREPTASE should be terminated immediately and treatment instituted as described under Adverse Effects.

Arrhythmias: Rapid lysis of coronary thrombi may cause reperfusion atrial or ventricular dysrhythmia requiring immediate treatment. Careful monitoring for arrhythmia should be maintained during and immediately following administration of STREPTASE.

Hypotension: Hypotension, sometimes severe, not secondary to bleeding or anaphylaxis has been observed during intravenous STREPTASE infusion in 1 to 10% of patients. Patients should be monitored closely and should symptomatic or alarming hypotension occur, appropriate treatment should be administered. This treatment may include a decrease in the intravenous STREPTASE infusion rate. Smaller hypotensive effects are common and have not required treatment.

PRECAUTIONS: General: STREPTASE (streptokinase injection) should be used in hospitals where the recommended diagnostic and monitoring techniques are available.

Non-cardiogenic pulmonary edema has been reported rarely in patients treated with streptokinase. The risk of this appears greatest in patients who have large myocardial infarctions and are undergoing thrombolytic therapy by the intracoronary route.

Rarely, polyneuropathy has been temporally related to the use of streptokinase.

Should pulmonary embolism or recurrent pulmonary embolism occur during streptokinase therapy, the originally planned course of treatment should be completed in an attempt to lyze these emboli. While pulmonary embolism may occasionally occur during STREPTASE treatment, the incidence is no greater than when patients are treated with heparin alone.

Repeated Administration: Because of the increased likelihood of resistance due to antistreptokinase antibodies, STREPTASE may not be effective if administered more than 5 days after prior to streptokinase administration or streptokinase-containing products, particularly between 5 days and 12 months.

It is not known whether persisting high in vitro neutralization titres affect the efficacy and safety of repeat administration of streptokinase or steptokinase-containing compounds.

Likewise, the effect may be reduced in patients with recent streptococcal infections such as streptococcal pharyngitis, acute rheumatic fever, acute glomerulonephritis secondary to a streptococcal infection.

Pregnancy: Experience in pregnant women has not shown that STREPTASE increases the risk of fetal abnormalities if administered during pregnancy. If this drug is used during pregnancy, the possibility of fetal harm appears remote. Because studies cannot rule out the possibility of harm, however, STREPTASE should be used during pregnancy only if clearly needed.

Thrombolytic therapy should be avoided within the first 18 weeks of the pregnancy because of the risk of placental separation.

Children: Safety and effectiveness of STREPTASE in children have not been established.

Lactation: It is not known whether streptokinase is excreted in the breast milk nor whether it has harmful effects on the newborn. In the absence of further information, it is recommended that breast-feeding be discontinued in a woman who is to receive STREPTASE.

Drug Interactions: The potential for an additive hypotensive effect should be borne in mind when STREPTASE therapy is combined with antihypertensive agents, such as β-blockers and glyceryl trinitrate.

Until information regarding the interaction between STREPTASE and tissue plasminogen activator (tPA) is available, special care should be taken if such a combination is considered.

There is an increased risk of hemorrhage in:

- Patients previously receiving heparin or coumarin derivatives. The effect of heparin can, however, be rapidly neutralized by administering protamine sulphate. In the case of prior treatment with coumarin derivatives, the Quick value must be more than 50% before the beginning of lysis.
- Patients receiving simultaneous treatment with platelet-aggregation inhibitors, e.g., ASA (see below also), phenylbutazone, dipyridamole and non-steroidal anti-inflammatory drugs (NSAIDs).
- Patients receiving simultaneous or previous treatment with dextrans.

Combination of STREPTASE with ASA for Treatment of Myocardial Infarction: In the treatment of acute myocardial infarction with intravenous STREPTASE (1 500 000 IU over 1 hour) combined with enteric-coated ASA (160 mg/day for one month), it was shown that the combined treatment results in a further reduction in mortality rate, as well as a decreased risk of reinfarction and stroke in comparison to treatment with each of the drugs alone. The addition of ASA to STREPTASE may cause a slight increase in the risk of minor bleeding, but does not appear to increase the incidence of major bleeding. Unless contraindicated, concomitant administration of ASA is recommended (see Dosage).

Anticoagulation Treatment Following STREPTASE: Anticoagulation Following Treatment for Myocardial Infarction: The use of anticoagulants following administration of STREPTASE treatment for acute myocardial infarction increases the risk of bleeding, and has not been shown to be of unequivocal clinical benefit. Therefore, their use should be decided upon at the discretion of the treating physician.

Anticoagulation Following Intravenous Treatment for Other Indications: To prevent rethrombosis following termination of STREPTASE infusion treatment for pulmonary embolism or deep vein thrombosis, continuous intravenous infusion of heparin without a loading dose is recommended (see Patient Monitoring).

Patient Monitoring: Intravenous or Intracoronary Artery Infusion for Myocardial Infarction: Intravenous administration of STREPTASE will cause marked decreases in plasminogen and fibrinogen levels and increases in thrombin time (TT), activated partial thromboplastin time (APTT), and prothrombin time (PT), which usually normalize within 12-24 hours. These changes may also occur in some patients with intracoronary administration of the drug.

Intravenous Infusion for Other Indications: Before commencing thrombolytic therapy, it is desirable to obtain a thrombin time (TT), activated partial thromboplastin time (APTT), prothrombin time (PT), and a hematocrit and platelet count to obtain hemostatic status of the patient.

If heparin has been given, it should be discontinued and the TT or APTT should be less than twice the normal control value before thrombolytic therapy is started.

During the infusion, decreases in the plasminogen and fibrinogen levels and an increase in the level of FDP (the latter two serving to prolong the clotting times of coagulation tests) will generally confirm the existence of a lytic state. Therefore, therapy can be monitored by performing the TT, or APTT, or PT, approximately 4 hours after initiation of therapy.

To prevent rethrombosis following STREPTASE infusion, continuous intravenous heparin infusion without a loading dose is recommended. The effect of STREPTASE on thrombin time (TT) and activated partial thromboplastin time (APTT) will usually diminish within 3 to 4 hours after STREPTASE therapy. A thrombin time value should be obtained during this period, and heparin therapy without a loading dose can be initiated when TT or APTT is less than twice the normal control value. (See manufacturer's prescribing information for proper use of heparin.) This should be followed by conventional oral anticoagulation therapy.

ADVERSE EFFECTS: The following adverse reactions have been frequently associated with intravenous therapy but may also occur with intracoronary artery infusion of STREPTASE (streptokinase injection).

Bleeding: The reported incidence of bleeding (major or minor) has varied widely depending on the indication, dose, route and duration of administration and concomitant therapy.

Minor bleeding occurs often with thrombolytic therapy mainly at invaded or disturbed sites. When lytic therapy is continued while local measures are used to control minor bleeding, do not reduce the dose as this will increase the conversion of plasminogen to plasmin which may increase bleeding.

Severe internal bleeding including gastrointestinal and liver hemorrhages, genitourinary, retroperitoneal or rare cases of intracerebral hemorrhages with their complications (also with fatal outcome), may occur, splenic rupture or retroperitoneal hemorrhages have been observed.

Intracerebral bleeding in connection with the treatment of myocardial infarction has been reported with an incidence of 0.1-0.3%. Several fatalities due to cerebral and other serious internal hemorrhage have occurred during thrombolytic therapy.

In the treatment of acute myocardial infarction with intravenous STREPTASE, the GISSI and ISIS-2 studies reported a rate of major bleeding (requiring transfusion) of 0.3-0.5%. In the TIMI study, which required both invasive techniques and administration of anticoagulants, a frequency of 15.6% for major bleeding (intracranial, or decrease in hemoglobin >5 g/dL, or decrease in hematocrit >15%) was reported.

During thrombolitic treatment of acute myocardial infarction, hemorrhages into the pericardium including myocardial rupture can occur in individual cases.

Should uncontrollable bleeding occur, STREPTASE infusion should be terminated immediately; slowing the rate of administration may increase the bleeding. If necessary, bleeding can be reversed and blood loss effectively managed with appropriate replacement therapy (see Overdose, Treatment).

Allergic Reactions: If a severe allergic reaction or anaphylactic shock occurs, the infusion should be discontinued immediately.

Immediate reactions: Reactions attributed to possible anaphylaxis have been observed rarely in patients treated with STREPTASE. These ranged in severity from minor breathing difficulty, dyspnoea to bronchospasm, periorbital swelling or angioneurotic edema. Other, milder allergic effects such as rash, urticaria, itching, flushing, nausea, headache and musculoskeletal pain have also been observed. Anaphylactoid shock is very rare, having been reported in 0-0.1% of patients.

An anaphylactic reaction has been reported in a patient following a second course of streptokinase within 1 month for clearance of an occluded arteriovenous shunt. Therefore, the possibility of systemic absorption of streptokinase following its use for this purpose must be considered.

Mild or moderate reactions may be managed with concomitant antihistamine and/or corticosteroid therapy. Severe allergic reactions require immediate discontinuation of STREPTASE with adrenergics, antihistamines, or corticosteroids administered intravenously as required.

Late reactions: In individual cases serum sickness, arthritis, vasculitis, nephritis and neuroallergic symptoms (polyneuropathy, e.g. Guillain-Barré syndrome) have been reported in temporal coincidence with streptokinase administration.

Embolisms: The risk of pulmonary embolism in patients with deep vein thrombosis is not higher during treatment with streptokinase than during treatment with heparine alone. If acute or recurrent pulmonary embolism occurs during STREPTASE treatment, the course of STREPTASE therapy should be continued as originally planned, so as to lyse the emboli.

During local lysis of peripheral arteries, distal embolization cannot be excluded.

A few cases of cholesterol embolism have been described in temporal coincidence with thrombolytic therapy, particularly in patients undergoing angiography.

Fever: Although STREPTASE is nonpyrogenic in standard animal tests, approximately one-third of patients treated with STREPTASE have shown increases in body temperature >0.83°C. Chills may also occur under therapy.

Symptomatic treatment is usually sufficient to alleviate discomfort.

Other: Transient elevations of serum transaminases as well as of bilirubin may occur.

At the beginning of the therapy, a fall in blood pressure, tachycardia or bradycardia (in individual cases reaching as far as shock) are observed occasionally.

In individual cases, under thrombolytic therapy of acute myocardial infarction, rhythm disturbances, persistent angina pectoris as well as cardiac failure reaching as far as cardiac and respiratory arrest may occur. It could be demonstrated, however, that myocardial infarction cardiac arrest due to ventricular fibrillation is more rare in STREPTASE treated patients than in patients treated conventionally.

In a few instances, after intracoronary thrombolytic therapy in patients with extensive myocardial infarction, non cardiogenic pulmonary edema has been observed.

Individual cases of cerebral convulsion were reported under thrombolytic therapy, and in temporal coincidence with cardiovascular hypoxia and cerebral hemorrhage.

Headache and muscle pain, gastrointestinal complaints, back pain as well as asthenia and malaise may occur under therapy.

Hemorrhagic myocardial infarction has been reported.

OVERDOSE:

Treatment: Minor bleeding complications with STREPTASE (streptokinase injection) are usually overcome by increasing the dosage. Should serious uncontrollable bleeding occur as a result of overdosage, the infusion of STREPTASE and any other concomitant anticoagulant should be discontinued immediately. If necessary, blood loss and reversal of the bleeding tendency can be effectively managed with whole blood (fresh blood preferable), packed red cells and cryoprecipitate or fresh frozen plasma. Although the use of aminocaproic acid (or aprotinin) in humans as an antidote for streptokinase has not been documented, it may be considered in an emergency situation.

> For management of a suspected drug overdose, CPhA recommends that you contact your **regional Poison Control Centre**. See the *CPS* Directory section for a list of Poison Control Centres.

DOSAGE:

STREPTASE (streptokinase injection) should be administered by volumetric infusion pump. Do not use drop-counting infusion methods since STREPTASE may alter droplet size.

For complete instructions on the reconstitution of the lyophilized product, see Supplied.

Acute Myocardial Infarction: STREPTASE treatment of coronary thrombosis should be instituted as soon as possible after the onset of symptoms of acute myocardial infarction. The greatest benefit in mortality reduction was observed when STREPTASE was administered within 4 hours. The clinical benefit in terms of reduction of mortality could not conclusively be proven in controlled clinical trials in patients being treated beyond 12 hours after the onset of symptoms (see Table 1).

Table 1: STREPTASE

Treatment for Acute Myocardial Infarction

Route	Dosage/Duration
Intravenous infusion (see Intravenous Administration)	1 500 000 IU within 60 min
Intracoronary infusion (see Intracoronary Administration)	20 000 IU by bolus followed by 2000–4000 IU/min for 30–90 min (average 60 min)

Intravenous Administration: With the above regimen, 1 500 000 IU within 60 minutes, no coagulation tests are necessary to monitor streptokinase therapy. Unless contraindicated, the concomitant use of ASA at a dose of 160 mg/day p.o., starting prior to STREPTASE infusion and continued for 1 month is recommended.

Intracoronary Administration: STREPTASE treatment of coronary thrombosis should be undertaken only in medical centres where coronary arteriography is an established routine and appropriate after-treatment available. STREPTASE is administered selectively into the thrombosed coronary artery via coronary catheter positioned by the Judkins or Sones technique.

Deep Vein Thrombosis, Pulmonary or Arterial Embolism or Arterial Thrombosis: STREPTASE treatment should be instituted as soon as possible after onset of thrombotic event, preferably within 7 days. Any delay in instituting lytic therapy to evaluate the effect of heparin therapy decreases the potential for optimal efficacy, although slight enhancement of clot lysis has been shown with initiation of thrombolytic therapy up to 14 days after the onset of symptoms of deep vein thrombosis.

Since human exposure to streptococci is common, antibodies to streptokinase are prevalent. Thus, a loading dose of streptokinase sufficient to neutralize these antibodies is required. A dose of 250 000 IU of STREPTASE infused into a peripheral vein over 30 minutes has been found appropriate in over 90% of patients. If the thrombin time or any other parameter of fibrinolysis

Table 3: STREPTASE

Suggested Dilution and Infusion Rates

Indication/Dosage Route	Total Dose to Be Administered (IU)	Total Vials of STREPTASE Required	Volume of Dilution per Vial or Bottle (mL)	Loading		Maintenance	
				Loading Dose (IU)	Infusion Rate (mL/hr)	Maintenance Dose (IU)	Infusion Rate (mL/hr)
I. Acute Myocardial Infarction							
a. Intracoronary artery administration	140 000 IU	1 vial 250 000 IU	125	20 000 IU	10 mL bolus injection	2 000 IU/min	60 mL/hr
b. Intravenous administration	1 500 000 IU	i) 1 vial 1 500 000 IU	50[a]	—	—	1 500 000 IU	i) 50 mL/hr
		ii) 1 bottle 1 500 000 IU	50[a]	—	—	1 500 000 IU	ii) 50 mL/hr
		iii) 2 vials 750 000 IU	50[a]	—	—	1 500 000 IU	iii) 100 mL/hr
II. Deep Vein Thrombosis, Pulmonary Embolism, Arterial Thrombosis							
a. Intravenous infusion	2 650 000 to 7 450 000 IU	i) 11 to 30 vials 250 000 IU	45[b]	250 000 IU	i) 90 mL/hr for 30 min	100 000 IU/hr for 24 to 72 hr	i) 18 mL/hr
		ii) 4 to 10 vials 750 000 IU	45[b]	250 000 IU	ii) 30 mL/hr for 30 min	100 000 IU/hr for 24 to 72 hr	ii) 6.0 mL/hr
		iii) 2 to 5 vials 1 500 000 IU	45[b]	250 000 IU	iii) 15 mL/hr for 30 min	100 000 IU/hr for 24 to 72 h	iii) 3.0 mL/hr
		iv) 2 to 5 bottles 1 500 000 IU	45[b]	250 000 IU	iv) 15 mL/hr for 30 min	100 000 IU/hr for 24 to 72 h	iv) 3.0 mL/hr

[a] Volumes of solution of 50 to 250 mL have been used.
[b] If necessary, total volume may be increased, in increments of approximately 45 mL, to a maximum of 500 mL with the infusion pump rate adjusted accordingly. The total volume of approximately 45 mL or multiple thereof is recommended to facilitate setting the infusion pump for hourly dosage.

after 4 hours of treatment is not significantly different from the normal control level, discontinue STREPTASE because excessive resistance to streptokinase is present. Furthermore, if the thrombin time after 16 hours is still prolonged to more than fourfold the control level, the streptokinase dosage should be doubled for several hours until the thrombin time recedes.

The following dosage schedule is recommended: see Table 2.

Table 2: STREPTASE

Dosage Schedule

Indication	Loading Dose	IV Infusion Dosage/Duration
Pulmonary Embolism	250 000 IU/30 min	100 000 IU/hr for 24 hrs (72 hrs if concurrent deep vein thrombosis suspected)
Deep Vein Thrombosis	250 000 IU/30 min	100 000 IU/hr for 72 hrs
Arterial Thrombosis or Embolism	250 000 IU/30 min	100 000 IU/hr for 24 hrs

A continuous intravenous infusion of heparin, without a loading dose, is recommended to prevent rethrombosis following termination of STREPTASE infusion (see Patient Monitoring).

Arteriovenous Cannula Occlusion:

1. **Before Treatment:** Before using STREPTASE, an attempt should be made to clear the cannula by careful syringe technique, using heparinized saline solution. If adequate flow is not re-established, STREPTASE may be employed. Allow the effect of any pretreatment anticoagulants to diminish.
2. **STREPTASE Administration:** Instill 250 000 IU STREPTASE in 2 mL intravenous solution into each occluded limb of the cannula slowly. Clamp off cannula limb(s) for 2 hours. Observe the patient closely for possible adverse effects.
3. **After Treatment:** Aspirate contents of infused cannula limb(s), flush with saline, reconnect cannula.

In patients with occlusions of the central retinal vessels a better success rate can be expected if the therapy is started within 6 to 8 hours of arterial occlusions, within 10 days of venous occlusions and within 6 weeks for chronic arterial occlusive diseases (embolic occlusions).

Reconstitution and Dilution: Intracoronary Artery and Intravenous Administration: The protein nature and lyophilized form of STREPTASE require careful reconstitution and dilution.

The following procedure is recommended:

1. Add 5 mL Sodium Chloride Injection USP or Dextrose 5% Injection USP **slowly** to the vacuum packed STREPTASE container, directing the vehicle at the side of the container rather than into the lyophilized STREPTASE powder.
2. Roll and tilt the container **gently** to reconstitute. **Avoid shaking.** (Shaking may cause foaming.)
3. Dilute the entire reconstituted contents of the container, with Sodium Chloride Injection USP or Dextrose 5% Injection USP, to a total volume of approximately 45 mL (see Table 1). Dilute slowly and carefully; avoid shaking and agitation. (If necessary, total volume may be increased to a maximum of 500 mL with the infusion pump setting in Table 1 increased accordingly.) To facilitate setting the infusion pump rate, a total volume of approximately 45 mL—or multiples thereof—is suggested.
4. Solutions of STREPTASE reconstituted and diluted to 500 mL or 50 mL with Sodium Chloride Injection, USP, in glass containers, irrespective of which potency is used (250 000 IU; 750 000 IU; 1 500 000 IU), can be drawn through in-line filters without a reduction in drug potency providing the filter is of 0.80 µm or greater pore size (if of cellulose construct) or of 0.22 µm or greater pore size (if of PVC—acrylic polymer construct). Flocculated product should be discarded if filters of the above mentioned construct and/or pore size are not available.
5. Parenteral drug products should be inspected visually for particulate matter and discoloration prior to administration whenever solution and container permit. (The Albumin (Human) may impart a slightly yellow color to the solution.)
6. Do not add other medication to the container of reconstituted STREPTASE.

For Use in Arteriovenous Cannulae: Slowly reconstitute the contents of 250 000 IU STREPTASE vial with 2 mL Sodium Chloride Injection USP or Dextrose 5% Injection USP.

The suggested dilutions and infusion rates provided in Table 3 represent a practical means of STREPTASE administration without compromise of safety and efficacy considerations. Depending on the type of available infusion pump/bags, the solution/volume/rates cited may be adjusted to correspond with the particular dosage rate to be administered.

Stability and Storage of Reconstituted and Diluted Solutions: Reconstituted Solutions: STREPTASE reconstituted with 5 mL of saline (Sodium Chloride Injection USP, 0.9%) or dextrose (Dextrose Injection USP, 5%) is stable for 24 hours at room temperature (15-30°C) and refrigeration (2-4°C). For the recommended total period of use of the product, from reconstitution and dilution to the end of patient administration, see Diluted Solutions.

Diluted Solutions: Stability studies have been carried out on the three potencies, reconstituted and diluted with saline (Sodium Chloride Injection USP, 0.9%) or dextrose (Dextrose Injection USP, 5%), to 50 or 500 mL, in glass or plastic containers. The total period of use of the product, from reconstitution and dilution to end of patient administration, should not exceed the specific stability time indicated in Table 4.

Table 4: STREPTASE

Stability of Reconstituted/Diluted Solutions

Dosage (IU)	Final Volume (mL)	Diluent	Container	Temperature	Stable (hours)
250 000	50	saline or dextrose	plastic	RT[a]	24
	500	dextrose	glass	RT	12
	500	dextrose	glass	5°C	24
	500	dextrose	plastic	RT	12
	500	dextrose	plastic	5°C	24
750 000	50	dextrose	glass or plastic	RT	24
	50	dextrose	glass or plastic	5°C	24
	50	saline	plastic	RT	24
1 500 000	50	saline or dextrose	glass or plastic	RT	24
	500	saline or dextrose	glass	RT	24

[a] Room Temperature.

SUPPLIED: Each vial of sterile, white, lyophilized powder, contains: 250 000 IU (green), 750 000 IU (blue) or 1 500 000 IU (red) of purified streptokinase, 25 mg of cross-linked gelatin polypeptides, 25 mg of sodium L-glutamate, sodium hydroxide to adjust pH, and 100 mg of albumin (human) as stabilizer. Vials of 6.5 mL. When stored at room temperature below 25°C, the dried STREPTASE product is stable up to the expiration date indicated on the package.

Streptokinase

Fibrinolytic Agent

CPhA Monograph

Date of Revision: June 2009

This monograph has been compiled by CPhA and reviewed by experts. It may contain information different from that found in Health Canada-approved Product Monographs. The reader is referred to the *CPS* Editorial Policy for more information.

SUMMARY PRODUCT INFORMATION:

Route of Administration	Dosage Form	Product Strength
Intravenous	Single use vial: 6.5 mL	250 000, 750 000 and 1 500 000 IU
	Infusion bottle: 68 mL	1 500 000 IU

PHARMACOLOGY: Streptokinase indirectly accelerates clot lysis by binding to plasminogen. The complex formed converts residual plasminogen into plasmin, a proteolytic enzyme capable of hydrolysing fibrin. This occurs both within a thrombus and on its surface. Plasmin also digests fibrinogen and other plasma proteins, including factors V and VIII. Endogenous circulating inhibitors of plasmin are depleted during streptokinase therapy.

Streptokinase is antigenic. Antibodies produced as a result of past administration of streptokinase or the related thrombolytic anistreplase may diminish the thrombolytic effect of treatment or cause allergic reactions. Variable amounts of antistreptokinase antibodies may also be present due to recent streptococcal infections. The recommended dosage schedule usually overcomes the neutralizing effect of these antibodies.

Pharmacokinetics: After iv administration, plasma fibrinogen levels remain depressed for 24-36 hours. The fibrinolytic effect of streptokinase disappears within a few hours of discontinuation, however the effect on coagulation may persist for up to 12-24 hours. Depending on the dosage and duration of infusion, the thrombin time normally decreases to less than 2 times the normal control value within 4 hours and returns to normal by 24 hours.

Streptokinase is cleared from circulation by circulating antibodies and the reticuloendothelial system. It has a biphasic half-life; the initial half-life is 18 minutes in the presence of antibodies, subsequently increasing to 83 minutes as antibodies are depleted.

INDICATIONS: Streptokinase is approved for use in acute evolving transmural myocardial infarction as evidenced by characteristic ST segment elevation or new left bundle branch block (intravenous or intracoronary routes); acute pulmonary embolism involving obstruction of blood flow to a lobe or multiple segments, with or without hemodynamic instability; acute, extensive deep vein thrombosis; acute arterial thromboemboli originating from sources other than the left side of the heart.

The use of streptokinase to restore patency in totally or partially occluded arteriovenous cannulae has largely been replaced by safer alternatives.

In clinical trials, streptokinase has been shown to reduce mortality from acute MI when administered within 12 hours of symptom onset. This effect is time-dependant, decreasing as the duration of symptoms prior to administration increases. Combining treatment with low-dose ASA significantly enhances this benefit. Streptokinase use can also reduce the incidence of heart failure, limit infarct size and improve ventricular function. Benefit of administration more than 12 hours after symptom onset is uncertain. If a patient is to be treated within 6 hours of symptom onset, The American College of Chest Physicians recommends thrombolytic agents other than streptokinase be used [*Chest* 2008;133(6 Suppl):708S-75S].

Although the intracoronary route is approved for treatment of acute MI, this route is rarely used.

Early use of fibrinolytics in treatment of deep vein thrombosis (DVT) can reduce pain, swelling and loss of venous valves. In some studies they have also decreased the incidence of the postphlebitic syndrome. Streptokinase may be considered in patients with extensive clot and a low risk of bleeding.

Use of fibrinolytics followed by heparin as treatment of pulmonary embolus (PE) leads to more rapid resolution of thrombus than heparin alone. Though not without risk, The American College of Chest Physicians recommends fibrinolytic therapy be given to patients with hemodynamically unstable PE who are at low risk of bleeding complications [*Chest* 2008;133(6 Suppl):454S-545S].

CONTRAINDICATIONS: Streptokinase is contraindicated in patients with: previous hemorrhagic stroke at any time; other strokes or cerebrovascular events within the previous year; known intracranial neoplasm; intracranial vascular disease (e.g., aneurysm, arteriovenous malformation); active internal bleeding (not including menses); and suspected aortic dissection.

Streptokinase should not be administered to anyone with a history of severe allergic reaction to the product. The manufacturer also considers recent (<2 months) intracranial or intraspinal surgery or trauma an absolute contraindication.

In the context of treatment of acute MI, diabetic hemorrhagic retinopathy is not considered a contraindication. However, if streptokinase is considered for use in other settings in a patient with diabetic hemorrhagic retinopathy, the risks of treatment should be weighed against the expected benefits.

Relative contraindications to fibrinolytic therapy include history of prior cerebrovascular accident or known intracerebral pathology not described in absolute contraindications; current use of anticoagulants in therapeutic doses (INR ≥2-3); known bleeding diathesis or other hemostatic defects, including those associated with renal or hepatic disease; recent (2-4 weeks) trauma, including head trauma; recent (<3 weeks) traumatic or prolonged CPR or major surgery; recent (≤10 days) noncompressable vascular punctures, obstetrical delivery or organ biopsy; recent (2-4 weeks) internal bleeding; pregnancy; active peptic ulcer; severe hypertension (systolic blood pressure >180 mmHg and /or diastolic pressure >110 mmHg).

Streptokinase should not be used to restore patency in occluded iv catheters. Life-threatening adverse reactions (e.g., hypotension, hypersensitivity reactions, apnea, bleeding) have occurred when it has been used in this setting. Other situations where the risks of therapy may be increased include subacute bacterial endocarditis; age >75 years; conditions with a high likelihood of left heart thrombus; septic thrombophlebitis or occluded arteriovenous cannula at a seriously infected site; any condition where bleeding is a significant hazard or would be particularly difficult to manage because of its location. In patients with the above conditions, the risks of treatment should be weighed against the expected benefit.

WARNINGS: The patient's history and overall clinical status should be carefully assessed before beginning therapy with streptokinase. Fatalities have occurred when streptokinase was used to treat suspected MI in patients who actually had pancreatitis.

Following standard streptokinase therapy for acute MI, severe bleeding complications are rare (incidence 0.3-0.5%). If serious spontaneous bleeding occurs and cannot be controlled by local pressure, the infusion of streptokinase should be stopped immediately. Simply decreasing the rate of infusion may actually aggravate bleeding by increasing the conversion of plasminogen to plasmin. Other treatment measures should be instituted as described under Adverse Effects.

Patients who have received streptokinase or the related thrombolytic anistreplase in the past may have developed antibodies to streptokinase. These antibodies may interfere with the thrombolytic effect of streptokinase and/or put the patient at risk of allergic reactions, which may be severe. Therefore, because alternative thrombolytics are available, many clinicians recommend that the use of streptokinase be avoided in patients with prior exposure to either streptokinase or anistreplase, especially if it occurred within the previous 5 days to 2 years.

Use of streptokinase to restore patency of occluded iv catheters (not an approved indication) has been associated with an increased incidence of adverse effects, including hypotension, hypersensitivity reactions, apnea and bleeding.

The commercially available form of streptokinase contains human albumin, a blood product. The manufacturer states that due to donor screening and product manufacturing processes, the risk of viral disease transmission is extremely remote. The manufacturer also considers the theoretical risk of transmission of Creutzfeld-Jacob disease extremely remote and states that no cases of transmission of viral diseases or Creutzfeld-Jacob disease have been identified for albumin.

PRECAUTIONS: To prevent bleeding, minimize venipunctures and unnecessary handling of the patient; avoid intramuscular injections. If an arterial puncture is necessary, it should be performed by an experienced clinician. An upper extremity vessel (e.g., brachial, radial artery) is preferred. Pressure should be applied for at least 30 minutes, a pressure dressing applied and the site frequently checked for bleeding.

If iv streptokinase is used to treat venous or arterial thromboembolism, the thrombin time (TT), APTT, PT, hematocrit and platelet count should be determined prior to beginning therapy. If the TT or any other parameter of lysis is not significantly prolonged (e.g., is less than about 1.5 times control) after 4 hours of therapy, excessive resistance should be assumed and therapy discontinued.

Monitor blood pressure carefully during treatment with streptokinase and institute appropriate therapy if symptomatic hypotension occurs. Patients receiving the drug for acute MI should also be closely monitored for reperfusion arrhythmias and therapy instituted as appropriate.

Drug Interactions: ASA: Combined therapy with low-dose ASA does not appear to increase the risk of major bleeding but may slightly increase the incidence of minor bleeding (from 3.1% to 3.9%). When used in combination with fibrinolytic therapy, low-dose ASA significantly decreases the mortality rate from acute MI. Therefore, unless otherwise contraindicated, low-dose ASA should be administered with streptokinase for the treatment of acute MI.

Heparin: Consider concomitant iv heparin in patients with acute MI. Though controversial, there may be an overall reduction in rates of reinfarction and death. Heparin should be infused at a rate to maintain the APTT between 50 and 70 s.

Subcutaneous heparin 7500 to 12 500 units twice daily may be considered in patients treated with streptokinase for acute MI who do not have contraindications to heparin. If used, it should be continued for 48 hours.

Continuous infusion of heparin has been recommended to prevent rethrombosis after termination of streptokinase infusion for the management of DVT or PE. Heparin, without a loading dose, may be started when the TT or APTT is less than twice the normal control value.

Antifibrinolytic Agents: The fibrinolytic effects of streptokinase are inhibited by agents such as aminocaproic acid.

Children: Safety and efficacy in children have not been established in controlled clinical trials. There are anecdotal reports of streptokinase use in children ranging in age from less than 1 month to 16 years. The majority of these reports describe use of streptokinase in the management of arterial occlusions. The nature of adverse effects appears similar to those occurring in adults. However, rates of bleeding complications have been variable and bleeding at catheter sites has been as high as 50% in some studies. Transfusions have occasionally been required to manage bleeding. As with other patient groups, careful monitoring of patient status is necessary.

Pregnancy: Animal reproduction studies have not been conducted with streptokinase. However, it does not appear to present a major risk to the fetus, either directly or indirectly. Fetal losses have occurred that may have been related to therapy but neither fetal hemorrhage nor teratogenic effects have been reported. Only small amounts of streptokinase cross the placenta and these do not induce a fibrinolytic state in the fetus. The effect of streptokinase on placental implantation early in pregnancy has not been resolved but there is no apparent increased risk of preterm rupture of the membranes, premature labor or placental hemorrhage. Antibodies to streptokinase do cross the placenta but would have clinical importance only if the neonate subsequently required streptokinase therapy.

Lactation: There is little experience with the use of streptokinase in lactating women due to its short duration of use and because its usual indications are unusual in this population.

ADVERSE EFFECTS: The most common adverse effects of streptokinase therapy are bleeding, hypersensitivity and fever.

Body as a Whole: Fever, with or without chills, often occurs in patients receiving streptokinase (1-4%). Symptomatic treatment is suggested; however, ASA should not be used. Acetaminophen is recommended instead.

Cardiovascular: Hypotension not related to bleeding or anaphylaxis has occurred in 1-10% of patients receiving iv streptokinase and may be severe. It usually is transient and may respond to a reduction in the infusion rate if necessary. Other appropriate therapy may include patient repositioning (i.e., to Trendelenburg's position), volume expansion and vasopressors. Small reductions in blood pressure are common and usually do not require specific treatment.

Hypotension may be associated with reperfusion of certain portions of the myocardium (e.g., inferoposterior wall of the left ventricle) and may be accompanied by bradycardia; if necessary this may be controlled by atropine.

Myocardial reperfusion may also be associated with atrial and/or ventricular arrhythmias. These are usually transient but immediate treatment is sometimes required. The arrhythmias most commonly seen include accelerated idioventricular rhythm, ventricular premature complexes and, less frequently, ventricular fibrillation; other arrhythmias, including bradyarrhythmias, have also been observed.

Cholesterol embolization has rarely been reported in patients receiving streptokinase or other fibrinolytics. Signs and symptoms may include purple toe syndrome; livedo reticularis; gangrenous digits; retinal artery occlusion; acute renal failure; bowel, spinal cord, cerebral or myocardial infarction; and pancreatitis.

Phlebitis near the site of iv streptokinase has occurred and may respond to further dilution of the infusion.

Gastrointestinal: Transient elevations in serum transaminases have been reported. The cause and significance of these increases is not fully understood.

Hematologic: Like other fibrinolytics, streptokinase is not specific for pathologic fibrin deposits, but also affects those providing hemostasis (e.g., at sites of needle punctures or cuts). When this occurs, bleeding may result.

Severe spontaneous bleeding, including cerebral, gastrointestinal, genitourinary and retroperitoneal bleeding, has occurred during streptokinase therapy and may be fatal. Severe bleeding complications requiring transfusions are generally rare, occurring at an incidence of 0.3 to 0.5% in one major trial of streptokinase therapy for acute MI. However, rates as high as 16% have been reported in trials requiring administration of anticoagulants and invasive procedures. Risk factors associated with bleeding in one large trial of streptokinase use in acute MI were advanced age, female sex and lower body weight.

Mild bleeding (e.g., oozing from a wound) should be treated with local pressure and supportive care. If bleeding is more severe, streptokinase should be discontinued immediately. Simply decreasing the infusion rate is not sufficient, as this may actually increase bleeding. If necessary, blood loss should be managed with appropriate replacement therapy, including cryoprecipitate +/− fresh frozen plasma. Although the use of aminocaproic acid as an antidote to streptokinase has not been documented, it may be considered in an emergency situation.

Immune: Allergic reactions may occur in patients receiving streptokinase. These range from mild reactions that do not require discontinuation of streptokinase (e.g., urticaria, pruritus, flushing, nausea, headache) to life-threatening anaphylaxis. Anaphylactic shock is rare, and has been reported in 0 to 0.1% of patients. Mild reactions may be managed with concomitant antihistamine and/or corticosteroid therapy. Severe reactions require immediate discontinuation of streptokinase and institution of appropriate therapy, which may include corticosteroids and vasopressors.

Delayed hypersensitivity reactions such as interstitial nephritis and vasculitis, and serum sickness-like illness have also occurred.

Musculoskeletal: Transient back pain has been reported during iv infusion of streptokinase. Back pain generally resolves when the infusion is discontinued.

Nervous System: Guillain-Barré syndrome has been reported in a few patients within 1-2 weeks of streptokinase administration. Although a causal relationship has not been established, it is biologically plausible that streptokinase could cause segmental demyelination via immunogenic mechanisms.

Respiratory: Noncardiogenic pulmonary edema has been rarely reported, as has respiratory depression.

OVERDOSE:

Reports of overdose with streptokinase could not be located. However, effects would be expected to be an extension of the drug's pharmacologic and adverse effects. If overdose does occur, manage any bleeding and institute supportive care as appropriate.

For management of a suspected drug overdose, CPhA recommends that you contact your **regional Poison Control Centre**. See the *CPS* Directory section for a list of Poison Control Centres.

DOSAGE: Streptokinase should be administered via a controlled-infusion device. Because solutions of streptokinase may alter drop size, the accuracy of drop-counting infusion devices may be adversely affected. Therefore, either volumetric controlled-infusion devices or syringe pumps are recommended for streptokinase administration.

Children: Approved dosage and administration recommendations for children are not available. However, in children with arterial occlusions, a loading dose of 1000 IU/kg followed by a maintenance infusion of 1000 IU/kg/hour for 12 hours or less has been frequently reported in the literature. Other children have received loading doses of 3000 IU/kg. Maintenance doses of up to 1500 IU/kg/hour have also been employed. In addition, infusions have sometimes been continued for 12-24 hours.

Adults: Acute evolving transmural myocardial infarction: Administer streptokinase as soon as possible after onset of symptoms. The usual adult dose is 1 500 000 IU by iv infusion over 60 minutes.

Streptokinase may also be administered by the intracoronary route. In this case the approved dose is a 20 000 IU bolus followed by an infusion of 2000 IU/minute for 60 minutes (total dose 140 000 IU). However, the intracoronary route is now rarely used.

Pulmonary Embolism or Deep Vein Thrombosis: A loading dose of 250 000 IU (administered as an iv infusion over 30 minutes) is required to neutralize antibodies to streptokinase. This is followed by an iv infusion of 100 000 IU/hour, continued for 24 hours in the case of pulmonary embolus or 72 hours in the case of deep vein thrombosis. If the TT or any other parameter of lysis is not significantly prolonged (e.g., is less than about 1.5 times control) after 4 hours of therapy, excessive resistance should be assumed and therapy discontinued (see Precautions).

Arterial Thromboembolism: The approved regimen for treatment of arterial thromboembolism is a loading dose of 250 000 IU (administered as an iv infusion over 30 minutes) followed by an iv infusion of 100 000 IU/hour for 24-72 hours. However, in practice the iv route of administration is rarely used in adults. If thrombolytics are used for this indication, they are more commonly administered directly into the affected artery proximal to the occlusion. Doses of intra-arterial streptokinase used in the treatment of lower limb artery occlusion have ranged from 5000 to 10 000 IU/hour.

Occluded Arteriovenous Cannulae: Note: The use of streptokinase for this indication has largely been replaced by the use of safer alternatives. See also Contraindications and Warnings.

Streptomycin ℞
Antibiotic

CPhA Monograph

Date of Revision: March 2008

This monograph has been compiled by CPhA and reviewed by experts. It may contain information different from that found in Health Canada-approved Product Monographs. The reader is referred to the *CPS* Editorial Policy for more information.

SUMMARY PRODUCT INFORMATION:

Route of Administration	Dosage Form	Product Strength
IM[a]	Powder	1 g/vial

[a] Available through Health Canada's Special Access Programme.

INDICATIONS AND CLINICAL USE: The use of streptomycin should be limited to the treatment of infections caused by bacteria that have been shown to be susceptible to streptomycin, when other less toxic agents are ineffective or contraindicated. Increased global prevalence of resistance limits the use of streptomycin.

Streptomycin is used in the following clinical settings to treat infections caused by susceptible organisms:

- Treatment of *M. tuberculosis*. Used as a second-line agent in the treatment of tuberculosis in combination with other antituberculosis agents, when the infecting organisms are susceptible [Canadian Tuberculosis Standards 6th ed. http://www.phac-aspc.gc.ca/tbpc-latb/pubs/pdf/tbstand07_e.pdf].
- Treatment of tularemia, plague, severe *M. avium* complex and brucellosis, when caused by susceptible organisms. Used in combination with other drugs. No longer consider first-line therapy for plague.

CONTRAINDICATIONS: Patients with a history of ototoxic reactions or hypersensitivity reactions to streptomycin or other aminoglycosides.

WARNINGS AND PRECAUTIONS: Warnings: Extreme caution is advised in people with pre-existing eighth cranial nerve impairment. The risk of severe neurotoxic reactions is sharply increased in patients with impaired kidney function or prerenal azotemia. These include disturbances of the auditory nerve, optic nerve, peripheral neuritis, arachnoiditis and encephalopathy. Renal function should be carefully determined and patients with renal impairment should have adjusted dosing intervals according to the degree of renal impairment.

Ototoxicity: Streptomycin-induced eighth cranial nerve damage may result in permanent loss of inner ear function. Aminoglycoside-induced ototoxicity is usually not reversible, although some adaptation may occur. Some individuals are predisposed to aminoglycoside-associated ototoxicity because of a maternally inherited mutation in mitochondrial DNA that makes the human mitochondrial ribosome more closely resemble the bacterial ribosome, which is the site of action for these drugs [*BMJ* 2007;335:784-5]. Ototoxicity may be manifested by vestibular and/or auditory dysfunction. Vestibular symptoms are more common and may include nausea, vomiting, vertigo, nystagmus and ataxia. Auditory symptoms include tinnitus, roaring noises, a sense of fullness in the ears and varying degrees of hearing impairment. Loss of high-frequency perception, which can be detected by audiometric testing, usually occurs before clinical hearing loss. Loss of hearing may be permanent if damage is extensive.

The incidence of ototoxicity is directly proportional to duration and amount of the drug administered. Advanced age, dehydration and renal impairment predispose patients to ototoxicity.

Periodic assessment of eighth cranial nerve function may avert ototoxicity. Tinnitus, roaring noises or a sense of fullness in the ears indicates the need for audiometric examination or termination of therapy or both. Instruct patients to immediately report any of the above signs and symptoms of toxicity.

Precautions: Although streptomycin is thought to be less nephrotoxic than other aminoglycosides, impairment of renal function may occur. Adverse effects on kidneys may include tubular necrosis, reduced glomerular filtration rate, decreased creatinine clearance, and rarely, electrolyte disturbances. Monitor patients for increased serum creatinine, proteinuria and the presence of casts or cells in the urine. Aminoglycoside-induced nephrotoxicity is usually reversible when the drug is discontinued.

When using streptomycin to treat tuberculosis, Health Canada recommends performing audiography before beginning treatment and monthly during treatment.

Since streptomycin may aggravate muscle weakness, use with caution in patients with neuromuscular disorders (e.g., myasthenia gravis).

Special care should be taken by individuals handling or preparing streptomycin for injection to avoid contact with or inhalation of this antibiotic. Hypersensitivity reactions have been reported.

Streptomycin should be administered by deep im injection. The iv route is not recommended but may be used if im injections are contraindicated.

As with other antibiotics, use of this drug may result in overgrowth of nonsusceptible organisms, including fungi. If suprainfection occurs, institute appropriate therapy.

Special Populations: Pregnant Women: Pregnancy Category D_M. Streptomycin readily crosses the placenta. Adverse fetal effects of eighth cranial nerve damage and deafness have been reported.

Nursing Women: Small amounts of streptomycin are excreted in breast milk. Since the oral absorption of this antibiotic is poor, it is unlikely that renal or ototoxicity would occur in the infant. Streptomycin is considered compatible with breastfeeding according to the American Academy of Pediatrics.

Geriatrics: Elderly patients may be at greater risk for renal and ototoxicity due to decreased kidney function. Use reduced doses and monitor serum streptomycin concentrations, renal status and eighth cranial nerve function.

ADVERSE REACTIONS: Commonly noted are: ototoxicity manifested by nausea, vomiting and vertigo; perioral or peripheral paresthesias; rash; fever; urticaria, angioneurotic edema; eosinophilia. Less frequent are deafness, exfoliative dermatitis, anaphylaxis, azotemia, oliguria, proteinuria, leukopenia, thrombocytopenia, pancytopenia, hemolytic anemia, muscular weakness and amblyopia.

DRUG INTERACTIONS: Since neurotoxic, ototoxic, or nephrotoxic effects may be additive, avoid concurrent or sequential administration of other drugs with similar toxicities.

General Anesthetics and Neuromuscular Blocking Agents (e.g., succinylcholine, tubocurarine): The neurotoxicity of streptomycin can result in respiratory paralysis from neuromuscular blockade, especially when the drug is given concurrently with or soon after anesthesia and muscle relaxants.

DOSAGE AND ADMINISTRATION: Streptomycin should be administered by deep im injection into a large muscle mass such as the gluteus maximus or the mid-lateral thigh. Injection site should be rotated to decrease irritation.

Treatment of Active Tuberculosis Disease: As part of a multidrug regimen for active pulmonary tuberculosis, the usual adult dose is 15 mg/kg (up to 1 g) once daily during the first 2-4 months of treatment, depending on the effectiveness of other antituberculosis drugs in the regimen. Can use 25 mg/kg (up to 1.5 g) 2-3 times weekly as soon as clinically possible after culture conversion. Therapy with streptomycin may be discontinued if symptoms of toxicity occur, toxicity is anticipated, organisms become resistant, or when full treatment has been achieved.

For elderly patients (>59 y) or those with auditory or renal function impairment, lower daily doses based on age, renal function and eighth cranial nerve function are recommended. A geriatric dose of 10 mg/kg daily, to a maximum of 750 mg, has been suggested.

The pediatric dose of streptomycin is 20 to 40 mg/kg, to a maximum of 1 g, daily or 20 mg/kg twice weekly.

Treatment of Severe *M. avium* Complex: 15 mg/kg three times weekly for the first 2-3 months in combination with a macrolide, rifamycin and ethambutol [*Am J Respir Crit Care Med* 2007; 175:367-416].

Treatment of Brucellosis: 1 g daily for 14 to 21 days in combination with doxycycline 100 mg po twice daily for 6 weeks.

Treatment of Tularemia: 10 to 15 mg/kg daily (maximum 2 g daily) in divided doses for 7 to 10 days or until the patient has been afebrile for 5 to 7 days.

Treatment of Plague: 30 mg/kg daily (maximum 2 g daily) in divided doses may be required and continued until the patient has been afebrile for at least 3 days.

Renal Impairment: In selected patients with renal impairment, serum concentrations should be determined. Peak concentrations should be 15 to 25 µg/mL and trough concentrations should be below 5 µg/mL. For dosing information in renal impairment, see Table 1.

Table 1: Streptomycin
Dose in Adult Patients with Renal Impairment

Creatinine Clearance	Interval Adjustment
>50 mL/min	Q24H
10–50 mL/min	Q24–72H
<10 mL/min	Q72–96H

OVERDOSAGE:

For management of a suspected drug overdose, CPhA recommends that you contact your **regional Poison Control Centre**. See the *CPS* Directory section for a list of Poison Control Centres.

ACTION AND CLINICAL PHARMACOLOGY: Streptomycin is an aminoglycoside antibiotic obtained from cultures of *Streptomyces griseus*, a soil actinomycete. Streptomycin binds to the 30S ribosomal subunit, thereby disrupting the ability of the mRNA to translate into a polypeptide. It is used in combination with other antituberculosis agents in the treatment of tuberculosis. Streptomycin is active against *M. tuberculosis*, *M. avium*, *M. intracellulare*, *Y. pestis* (plague), *F. tularensis* (tularemia), Brucella species, *S. viridans*, enterococci and some Enterobacteriaceae.

Pharmacokinetics: Streptomycin is not absorbed from the gastrointestinal tract and is administered im for systemic action.

Following im injection of 1 g of the drug, a peak serum concentration of 25 to 50 µg/mL is reached within 1 to 2 hours. The elimination half-life in adults with normal renal function is usually 2 to 3 hours. In newborns and premature infants the half-life may range from 4 to 10 hours. Adults with severe renal impairment may have half-lives of up to 110 hours. Appreciable concentrations are found in all organ tissues except the brain. Significant amounts have been found in pleural fluid and tuberculous cavities. The drug has a reported protein binding of up to 35%. Streptomycin passes through the placenta with serum concentrations in the cord blood similar to maternal levels. Small amounts are excreted in milk, saliva, and sweat. It is excreted rapidly in the urine by glomerular filtration. In patients with normal kidney function, between 29 and 89% of a single 600 mg dose is excreted within 24 hours. Any reduction of glomerular filtration results in decreased excretion of the drug and concurrent rise in serum and tissue concentrations.

Streptomycin Injection USP ℞
streptomycin
Aminoglycoside Antibiotic

SteriMax

SUPPLIED: Each vial of sterile lyophilized powder contains: streptomycin sulfate USP equivalent to 1 g streptomycin base. After reconstitution each mL contains 200 mg streptomycin activity. Sterile reconstituted solutions should be protected from light. Store dry powder under controlled room temperature (15-30°C).

Stresstabs® Regular
vitamin B complex—ascorbic acid—vitamin E
Vitamin Supplement

Pfizer Consumer Healthcare

Stresstabs® for Women
vitamin B complex—ascorbic acid—vitamin E—iron
Vitamin and Mineral Supplement

Pfizer Consumer Healthcare

Stresstabs® for Men
vitamin B complex—ascorbic acid—vitamin E—zinc—copper—selenium—lycopene
Vitamin and Mineral Supplement

Pfizer Consumer Healthcare

Stresstabs® Plus
vitamin B complex—ascorbic acid—vitamin E—selenium—lycopene
Vitamin and Mineral Supplement

Pfizer Consumer Healthcare

Stresstabs® Z-BEC®
vitamin B complex—ascorbic acid—vitamin E—zinc—copper
Vitamin and Mineral Supplement

Pfizer Consumer Healthcare

INDICATIONS: For use as a nutritional supplement.

CONTRAINDICATIONS: Stresstabs for Women: Hemochromatosis, hemosiderosis, hemolytic anemia.

PRECAUTIONS: Product contains iron, which can be harmful to children if taken in large doses.

Folic acid may obscure pernicious anemia in that the peripheral blood picture may return to normal while neurological manifestations remain progressive.

Stresstabs Regular/Women: Contact a healthcare practitioner prior to use if you are liver impaired or taking levodopa. Discontinue use if you experience prolonged flushing, burning, tingling or itching sensation on face arms or chest. Do not exceed recommended daily dose. As with any drug, if you are pregnant or nursing, contact a healthcare professional before taking.

Stresstabs for Women: Iron compounds taken orally can impair the absorption of tetracycline antibiotics. Antacids given concomitantly with iron compounds decrease iron absorption.

Stresstabs Z-BEC/Plus: Do not exceed recommended daily dose. As with any drug, if you are pregnant or nursing, contact a healthcare professional before taking.

Stresstabs for Men: Take a few hours before or after taking other medications. Do not exceed recommended daily dose.

ADVERSE EFFECTS: Stresstabs for Women: Iron-containing medications may occasionally cause gastrointestinal discomfort, nausea, constipation or diarrhea.

OVERDOSE:
In case of accidental overdose, contact a physician or poison control centre immediately, even if there are no symptoms.

For management of a suspected drug overdose, CPhA recommends that you contact your **regional Poison Control Centre**. See the *CPS* Directory section for a list of Poison Control Centres.

DOSAGE: Adults: 1 tablet daily with food. Take a few hours before or after other medications.

SUPPLIED: Stresstabs Regular: Each oval, orange, film-coated, scored tablet, engraved "S" and "S1", contains: folic acid (folate) 0.4 mg, vitamin B_1 (thiamine mononitrate) 15 mg, vitamin B_2 (riboflavin) 15 mg, niacinamide 20 mg, vitamin B_6 (pyridoxine HCl) 10 mg, vitamin B_{12} (cyanocobalamin) 25 µg, biotin 30 µg, pantothenic acid (calcium pantothenate) 20 mg, vitamin C (ascorbic acid) 500 mg, vitamin E (dl-α-tocopheryl acetate) 13.5 mg/30 IU. Nonmedicinal ingredients: calcium carbonate, citric acid, corn starch, dibasic calcium phosphate, FD&C Yellow No. 6, hypromellose, lactose monohydrate, magnesium stearate, maltodextrin, methylcellulose, microcrystalline cellulose, mineral oil light, modified food starch, silicon dioxide, sodium benzoate, sodium citrate, sodium lauryl sulfate, sorbic acid, stearic acid and titanium dioxide. Bottles of 100. Store at room temperature (15-30°C). Protect from moisture.

Stresstabs for Women: Each oval, red, film-coated, scored tablet, engraved "S" and "S2", contains: folic acid (folate) 0.4 mg, vitamin B_1 (thiamine mononitrate) 15 mg, vitamin B_2 (riboflavin) 15 mg, niacinamide 20 mg, vitamin B_6 (pyridoxine HCl) 10 mg, vitamin B_{12} (cyanocobalamin) 25 µg, biotin 30 µg, pantothenic acid (calcium pantothenate) 20 mg, vitamin C (ascorbic acid) 500 mg, vitamin E (dl-α-tocopheryl acetate) 13.5 mg/30 IU, iron (ferrous fumarate) 18 mg. Nonmedicinal ingredients: calcium carbonate, citric acid, corn starch, dibasic calcium phosphate, FD&C Red No. 40, FD&C Yellow No. 6, hypromellose, lactose monohydrate, magnesium stearate, maltodextrin, methylcellulose, microcrystalline cellulose, mineral oil light, modified food starch, silicon dioxide, sodium benzoate, sodium citrate, sodium lauryl sulfate, sorbic acid, stearic acid and titanium dioxide. Bottles of 100. Store at room temperature (15-30°C). Protect from moisture.

Stresstabs for Men: Each oval, orange, film-coated, scored tablet, engraved "S" and "S3", contains: folate (folic acid) 0.4 mg, vitamin B_1 (thiamine mononitrate) 15 mg, vitamin B2 (riboflavin) 15 mg, niacinamide 20 mg, vitamin B_6 (pyridoxine HCl) 10 mg, vitamin B_{12} (cyanocobalamin) 25 µg, biotin 30 µg, pantothenic acid (calcium d-pantothenate) 20 mg, vitamin C (ascorbic acid) 500 mg, vitamin E (dl-α-tocopheryl acetate) 13.5 mg/30 IU, copper (copper sulfate) 1 mg, zinc (zinc oxide) 7.5 mg, selenium (sodium selenate) 70 µg, lycopene 1 mg. Nonmedicinal ingredients: ascorbyl palmitate, calcium carbonate, citric acid, corn starch, dibasic calcium phosphate, FD&C Yellow No. 6, food starch modified, gelatin, hypromellose, lactose monohydrate, magnesium stearate, maltodextrin, methylcellulose, microcrystalline cellulose, mineral oil light, modified food starch, pregelatinized starch, silicon dioxide, sodium ascorbate, sodium benzoate, sodium citrate, sodium lauryl sulfate, sorbic acid, stearic acid and titanium dioxide. Bottles of 100. Store at room temperature (15-30°C). Protect from moisture.

Stresstabs Plus: Each oval, orange, film-coated, scored tablet, engraved "S" and "S4", contains: folic acid (folate) 0.8 mg, vitamin B_2 (riboflavin) 15 mg, vitamin B_6 (pyridoxine HCl) 25 mg, vitamin B_{12} (cyanocobalamin) 50 µg, vitamin C (ascorbic acid) 500 mg, vitamin E (dl-α tocopheryl-acetate) 90 mg/200 IU, selenium (sodium selenate) 70 µg, lycopene 2 mg. Nonmedicinal ingredients: ascorbyl palmitate, calcium carbonate/phosphate, citric acid, corn starch, crospovidone, FD&C Yellow No. 6, gelatin, hypromellose, lactose, magnesium stearate, methylcellulose, microcrystalline cellulose, mineral oil, polysorbate, silicon dioxide, sodium benzoate, sodium citrate, sodium lauryl sulfate, sorbic acid, stearic acid, sucrose, titanium dioxide and triethyl citrate. Bottles of 80. Store at room temperature (15-30°C). Protect from moisture.

Stresstabs Z-BEC: Each oval, green, film-coated tablet, engraved "Z-BEC" contains: folic acid (folate) 0.5 mg, vitamin B_1 (thiamine mononitrate) 30 mg, vitamin B_2 (riboflavin) 10 mg, niacin (niacinamide) 20 mg, vitamin B_6 (pyridoxine HCl) 10 mg, vitamin B_{12} (cyanocobalamin) 25 µg, pantothenic acid (calcium pantothenate) 25 mg, vitamin C (ascorbic acid) 600 mg, vitamin E (dl-α-tocopheryl acetate) 20.3 mg/45 IU, copper (cupric oxide) 3 mg, zinc (zinc sulfate) 23.9 mg. Nonmedicinal ingredients: calcium carbonate, citric acid, corn starch, FD&C Blue No. 1, flavour, hydroxypropyl cellulose, hypromellose, lactose monohydrate, magnesium stearate, methylcellulose, microcrystalline cellulose, polysorbate, propylene glycol, silicon dioxide, sodium benzoate, sodium citrate, sorbic acid, stearic acid and titanium dioxide. Bottles of 60. Store at room temperature (15-30°C). Protect from moisture.

Suboxone™ Ⓝ

buprenorphine HCl—naloxone HCl dihydrate

Partial Opiate Agonist—Opiate Antagonist

Schering-Plough

Date of Preparation: May 17, 2007

SUMMARY PRODUCT INFORMATION:

Route of Administration	Dosage Form/ Strength	Clinically Relevant Nonmedicinal Ingredients
Sublingual	Sublingual tablets 2 mg buprenorphine/0.5 mg naloxone 8 mg buprenorphine/2 mg naloxone	Lactose monohydrate For a complete listing see Dosage Forms, Composition and Packaging.

INDICATIONS AND CLINICAL USE: Adults: SUBOXONE (buprenorphine and naloxone) is indicated for:

- substitution treatment in opioid drug dependence in adults.

The intention of the naloxone component is to deter intravenous (IV) misuse.

Patients prescribed SUBOXONE should be carefully monitored within a framework of medical, social, and psychological support as part of a comprehensive opioid dependence treatment program.

SUBOXONE sublingual tablets should only be prescribed by physicians who meet the following requirements:

i. **experience in substitution treatment in opioid drug dependence, and**
ii. **completion of an accredited SUBOXONE Education Program.**

The SUBOXONE Education Program is a risk management program that is founded on the following four core components that provide for the safe and effective use of the drug within a framework of medical, social and psychological treatment:

- **training of the prescribing physicians in the use of SUBOXONE sublingual tablets;**
- **maintenance of a list of SUBOXONE Education Program trained physicians;**
- **daily dosing supervised by a healthcare professional for a minimum of two months;**
- **take-home doses should only be considered after a period of two months based upon assessment of clinical stability, length of time in treatment and ability to safely store SUBOXONE. Take-home doses should be assessed and reviewed on a regular basis.**

Physicians should not prescribe SUBOXONE sublingual tablets unless the condition of daily intake supervised by a healthcare professional can be ensured, except for week-ends and holidays, for a minimum of two months and until the patient is clinically stable and able to safely store SUBOXONE take-home doses (see Warnings and Precautions).

Physicians may obtain more information about the SUBOXONE Education Program by calling the following toll-free phone number: 1-800-463-5442.

Geriatrics (>65 years of age): The safety and efficacy of SUBOXONE have not been established in adults over 65 years of age, therefore SUBOXONE is not recommended in this patient population.

Pediatrics (<18 years of age): The safety and efficacy of SUBOXONE have not been established in children, therefore SUBOXONE is not recommended in patients under 18 years of age.

CONTRAINDICATIONS:

- SUBOXONE sublingual tablet is contraindicated in patients with known hypersensitivity to buprenorphine, naloxone, or any other components of the drug. For a complete listing, see Dosage Forms, Composition and Packaging.
- SUBOXONE should not be administered to women who are breast-feeding, or to patients who have severe respiratory insufficiency, severe hepatic insufficiency, acute alcoholism, or delirium tremens.

WARNINGS AND PRECAUTIONS:

Serious Warnings and Precautions

- **Abuse and diversion of buprenorphine have been reported.**
- **Appropriate security measures should be taken to safeguard stocks of SUBOXONE against diversion.**
- **SUBOXONE must be dispensed daily under the supervision of a healthcare professional, for a minimum of two months and until the patient is clinically stable and able to safely store SUBOXONE take-home doses. (See Dosage and Administration.)**

General: SUBOXONE sublingual tablets are recommended only for the treatment of opioid drug dependence and, as with other opioid substitution medications, should be used within the framework of medical, social and psychological support as part of a comprehensive opioid dependence treatment program. Naloxone is included to deter IV misuse of this product due to its ability to induce withdrawal in opiate-dependent subjects.

SUBOXONE should be administered with caution in the elderly or debilitated and those with severe impairment of hepatic, pulmonary, or renal function; myxedema or hypothyroidism; adrenal cortical insufficiency (e.g., Addison's disease); hypotension; CNS depression or coma; toxic psychoses; prostatic hypertrophy or urethral stricture; acute alcoholism; delirium tremens; or kyphoscoliosis.

The clinician should consider the risk of abuse and misuse (e.g., IV administration), particularly at the beginning of the treatment. Due to the risk of abuse and misuse, particularly at the beginning of treatment, daily supervised dosing is required for minimally the first two months of treatment. Take-home doses may be considered during this period if supervised dosing is not available on week-ends and holidays. This should be based upon assessment of clinical stability and ability to safely store SUBOXONE. Once the patient has reached their maintenance dose the physician may consider a less than daily dosing schedule during this period (see Dosage and Administration, Less Than Daily Dosing).

Use in Ambulatory Patients: SUBOXONE may impair the mental or physical abilities required for the performance of potentially dangerous tasks such as driving a car or operating machinery. Patients should be cautioned about operating hazardous machinery, including automobiles, until they are reasonably certain that SUBOXONE therapy does not adversely affect their ability to engage in such activities. Like other opioids, SUBOXONE may produce orthostatic hypotension in ambulatory patients.

Acute Abdominal Conditions: As with other mu-opioid receptor agonists, the administration of SUBOXONE may obscure the diagnosis or clinical course in patients with acute abdominal conditions.

Cardiovascular: SUBOXONE may cause orthostatic hypotension.

Dependence/Tolerance: SUBOXONE can produce drug dependence of the opiate type. Diversion of buprenorphine has been reported.

Hepatic/Biliary/Pancreatic: Because buprenorphine is extensively metabolized by the liver, the activity of SUBOXONE may be increased and/or extended in those individuals with impaired hepatic function or those receiving other agents known to decrease hepatic clearance.

Buprenorphine has been shown to increase intracholedochal pressure as do other opioids, and thus should be administered with caution to patients with dysfunction of the biliary tract.

Hepatitis, Hepatic Events: Cases of cytolytic hepatitis and hepatitis with jaundice have been observed in the addict population receiving buprenorphine. A biological and etiological evaluation is recommended when a hepatic event is suspected. Depending on the case, the drug should be carefully discontinued to prevent withdrawal symptoms and strict monitoring of the patients should be initiated.

Serious cases of acute hepatic injury have also been reported in a context of misuse, especially by IV route. These hepatic injuries have mainly been observed at the high doses and may be promoted by viral infections particularly chronic hepatitis C, alcohol abuse, anorexia, and the concurrent use of other potentially hepatotoxic drugs.

Immune: Allergic Reactions: Cases of acute and chronic hypersensitivity to buprenorphine have been reported both in clinical trials and in the post-marketing experience. The most common signs and symptoms include rashes, hives, and pruritus. Cases of bronchospasm, angioneurotic edema, and anaphylactic shock have been reported. A history of hypersensitivity to buprenorphine or naloxone or any component of the formulation is a contraindication to SUBOXONE use.

Neurologic: As buprenorphine is an opioid analgesic, pain as a symptom of disease may be attenuated.

Interaction with Other Central Nervous System Depressants: Patients receiving SUBOXONE in the presence of other narcotic analgesics, general anesthetics, antihistamines, benzodiazepines, phenothiazines, other antipsychotics, sedative/hypnotics, or other CNS depressants (including alcohol) may exhibit increased CNS depression. When such combined therapy is contemplated, it is particularly important that the dose of one or both agents be reduced if necessary.

Head Injury and Increased Intracranial Pressure: SUBOXONE, like other potent opioids, may by itself elevate cerebrospinal fluid pressure and should be used with caution in patients with head injury, intracranial lesions, and other circumstances where cerebrospinal pressure may be increased. SUBOXONE can produce miosis and changes in the level of consciousness, which may interfere with patient evaluation.

Opiate Withdrawal Effects: SUBOXONE can cause opioid withdrawal symptoms if administered to an addicted patient less than 4 hours after the last use of the addicting drug (see Dosage and Administration).

Buprenorphine is a partial agonist at the mu-opioid receptor and chronic administration produces dependence of the opiate type, characterized by withdrawal upon abrupt discontinuation or rapid taper. The withdrawal syndrome is milder than seen with full agonists, and may be delayed in onset.

Neonatal Withdrawal: In France, neonatal withdrawal has been reported in infants of women treated with buprenorphine during pregnancy. Time to onset of withdrawal symptoms ranged from Day 1 to Day 8 of life with most occurring on Day 1 (69%). The most commonly-reported manifestations include abnormal crying, agitation, hypertonia, tremor and convulsions. Respiratory depression has occurred in neonates whose mothers had taken high doses, even for a short duration of time in the third trimester.

Respiratory: Respiratory Depression: As with other potent opioids, clinically significant respiratory depression may occur in patients receiving SUBOXONE. Some cases of death due to respiratory depression have been reported, particularly when buprenorphine was used in combination with benzodiazepines, or with concomitant administration of buprenorphine with other depressants such as alcohol or other opioids. Patients should be warned of the potential danger of the self-administration of IV benzodiazepines or other depressants while under treatment with SUBOXONE, particularly when SUBOXONE is misused.

Naloxone may not be effective in reversing the respiratory depression produced by buprenorphine. Therefore, as with other potent opioids, the primary management of overdose should be the re-establishment of adequate ventilation with mechanical assistance of respiration if required.

SUBOXONE should be used with caution in patients with compromised respiratory function (e.g., chronic obstructive pulmonary disease, cor pulmonale, decreased respiratory reserve, hypoxia, hypercapnia or preexisting respiratory depression), in the elderly and in debilitated patients. Particular caution is advised if SUBOXONE is to be administered to patients taking or recently receiving drugs with CNS/respiratory depressant effects, such as in the immediate postoperative period.

In patients with respiratory depression, symptomatic treatment following standard intensive care measures should be instituted (see Overdosage).

Special Populations: Pregnant Women: There is very limited experience with buprenorphine/naloxone in pregnant women. In preclinical studies, all buprenorphine/naloxone doses tested produced embryolethality in rats. There are no adequate and well-controlled studies of SUBOXONE in pregnant women. SUBOXONE should only be used in pregnancy if the potential benefit justifies the potential risk to the fetus.

Nursing Women: Buprenorphine passes into the mother's milk, thus nursing mothers treated with SUBOXONE should not breast feed. There is no information available on naloxone in breast milk.

Pediatrics: Use in Children: SUBOXONE is not recommended for use in patients below the age of 18 years. The safety and efficacy of SUBOXONE in children have not been established.

Information for Physicians to Convey to Patients: Patients should be advised to inform their family members that, in the event of overdose, the treating physician or emergency room staff should be informed that the patient is physically dependent on narcotics and that the patient is being treated with SUBOXONE.

Patients should be warned that overdose resulting in serious harm or death may occur if benzodiazepines, sedatives, tranquilizers, antidepressants or alcohol are taken at the same time of SUBOXONE.

SUBOXONE can cause drowsiness which may be exacerbated by other centrally acting agents, such as: alcohol, tranquilizers, sedatives and hypnotics. Therefore, caution is advised when driving motor vehicles or operating machinery. (See Drug Interactions.)

Patients should consult their physician if other prescription medications are currently being used or are prescribed for future use.

Patients should be advised to keep SUBOXONE out of reach of children to prevent accidental ingestion.

Like other opioids, SUBOXONE may cause orthostatic hypotension.

Athletes should be aware that this medicine may cause a positive reaction to "anti-doping tests".

Studies in animals, as well as clinical experience, have demonstrated that buprenorphine may produce dependence.

ADVERSE REACTIONS: Adverse Drug Reaction Overview: The most common-treatment related adverse events reported during clinical trials with SUBOXONE were those related to withdrawal symptoms (e.g., abdominal pain, diarrhea, muscle aches, anxiety, sweating).

Clinical Trial Adverse Drug Reactions: Because clinical trials are conducted under very specific conditions the adverse reaction rates observed in the clinical trials may not reflect the rates observed in practice and should not be compared to the rates in the clinical trials of another drug. Adverse drug reaction information from clinical trials is useful for identifying drug-related adverse events and for approximating rates.

In the pivotal clinical study (CR96/013 [double-blind] + CR96/014 [open label extension]), of 472 patients treated with sublingual tablets containing buprenorphine in combination with naloxone, 334 patients were treated for 3 months, 261 patients were treated for greater than 6 months and 100 patients were treated up to one year. The most used dose was 16 mg/day. Treatment-emergent adverse events reported in the pivotal clinical study of SUBOXONE (≥1.0% of SUBOXONE-treated patients) are listed in Table 1.

Table 1: SUBOXONE

Treatment-emergent Adverse Events Reported in the Pivotal Clinical Study of SUBOXONE (≥1.0% of SUBOXONE-treated patients)

	SUBOXONE N=472
Body as a Whole	
Headache	202 (42.8%)
Pain	197 (41.7%)
Withdrawal Syndrome	194 (41.1%)
Infection	149 (31.6%)
Pain Back	132 (28.0%)
Flu Syndrome	89 (18.9%)
Pain Abdominal	77 (16.3%)
Injury Accidental	72 (15.3%)
Asthenia	48 (10.2%)
Chills	44 (9.3%)
Fever	36 (7.6%)
Pain Chest	23 (4.9%)
Abscess	17 (3.6%)
Pain Neck	12 (2.5%)
Malaise	9 (1.9%)
Allergic Reaction	8 (1.7%)
Edema Face	8 (1.7%)
Cyst	7 (1.5%)
Infection Viral	5 (1.1%)
Neck Rigid	5 (1.1%)
Cardiovascular System	
Vasodilation	29 (6.1%)
Hypertension	17 (3.6%)
Migraine	13 (2.8%)
Digestive System	
Constipation	115 (24.4%)
Nausea	76 (16.1%)
Vomiting	61 (12.9%)
Diarrhea	50 (10.6%)
Dyspepsia	45 (9.5%)
Tooth Disorder	37 (7.8%)
Liver Function Abnormal	18 (3.8%)
Anorexia	16 (3.4%)
Nausea/Vomiting	13 (2.8%)
Flatulence	11 (2.3%)
Abscess Periodontal	10 (2.1%)
Gastrointestinal Disorder	7 (1.5%)
Ulcer Mouth	6 (1.3%)
Stomatitis	5 (1.1%)
Hemic and Lymphatic System	
Anemia	7 (1.5%)
Ecchymosis	6 (1.3%)
Lymphadenopathy	5 (1.1%)

(cont'd)

Table 1: SUBOXONE *(cont'd)*

Treatment-emergent Adverse Events Reported in the Pivotal Clinical Study of SUBOXONE (≥1.0% of SUBOXONE-treated patients)

	SUBOXONE N=472
Metabolism and Nutritional Disorders	
Peripheral Edema	24 (5.1%)
Weight Decreased	15 (3.2%)
Hyperglycemia	5 (1.1%)
Musculoskeletal System	
Myalgia	31 (6.6%)
Arthralgia	20 (4.2%)
Leg Cramps	13 (2.8%)
Joint Disorder	9 (1.9%)
Arthritis	5 (1.1%)
Nervous System	
Insomnia	138 (29.2%)
Depression	70 (14.8%)
Anxiety	65 (13.8%)
Nervousness	42 (8.9%)
Somnolence	40 (8.5%)
Dizziness	33 (7.0%)
Paresthesia	28 (5.9%)
Agitation	10 (2.1%)
Dream Abnormal	9 (1.9%)
Drug Dependence	9 (1.9%)
Hypertonia	9 (1.9%)
Libido Decreased	9 (1.9%)
Tremor	7 (1.5%)
Thinking Abnormal	6 (1.3%)
Respiratory System	
Rhinitis	75 (15.9%)
Pharyngitis	64 (13.6%)
Cough Increased	36 (7.6%)
Asthma	21 (4.4%)
Pneumonia	12 (2.5%)
Lung Disorder	10 (2.1%)
Bronchitis	9 (1.9%)
Dyspnea	9 (1.9%)
Respiratory Disorder	7 (1.5%)
Sinusitis	7 (1.5%)
Yawning	6 (1.3%)
Sputum Increased	5 (1.1%)
Skin and Appendages	
Sweating	74 (15.7%)
Rash	23 (4.9%)
Pruritus	11 (2.3%)
Dry Skin	6 (1.3%)
Herpes Simplex	6 (1.3%)
Nodule Skin	6 (1.3%)
Urticaria	6 (1.3%)
Acne	5 (1.1%)

(cont'd)

Table 1: SUBOXONE *(cont'd)*

Treatment-emergent Adverse Events Reported in the Pivotal Clinical Study of SUBOXONE (≥1.0% of SUBOXONE-treated patients)

	SUBOXONE N=472
Contact Dermatitis	5 (1.1%)
Special Senses	
Conjunctivitis	14 (3.0%)
Lacrimation Disorder	14 (3.0%)
Eye Disorder	8 (1.7%)
Pain Ear	8 (1.7%)
Amblyopia	5 (1.1%)
Urogenital System	
Dysmenorrhea	19 (4.0%)
Urinary Tract Infection	19 (4.0%)
Urine Abnormal	12 (2.5%)
Impotence	11 (2.3%)
Vaginitis	11 (2.3%)
Dysuria	9 (1.9%)
Hematuria	8 (1.7%)

The most common adverse events observed in this study are consistent with opioid withdrawal or agonist effects. Although it is not possible to compare adverse events across trials because of differences in methodology and patient populations, the undesirable effects observed in other studies are qualitatively similar.

Less Common Clinical Trial Adverse Drug Reactions (<1%): Treatment-emergent adverse events reported as less common (<1%) in the pivotal SUBOXONE clinical study included:

Body as a Whole: carcinoma, cellulitis, chills/fever, hangover, heat stroke, hernia, human immunodeficiency virus (HIV) test positive, hostility, hypothermia, infection fungal, infection parasitic, neoplasia, overdose, pain chest (substernal), pain flank, pain pelvic, photosensitivity, pain rib and suicide attempt.

Cardiovascular System: angina pectoris, bradycardia, electrocardiogram abnormal, hypotension, myocardial infarction, palpitation, phlebitis, tachycardia, thrombosis, thrombophlebitis (deep), vascular disorder and varicose vein.

Digestive System: appetite increased, colitis, dry mouth, dysphagia, eructation, gastritis, gamma glutamyl transpeptidase increased, gingivitis, glossitis, gum hemorrhage, rectal hemorrhage, hematemesis, hepatitis C, rectal disorder, saliva increased, stomatitis/ulcer, tenesmus, tooth caries, ulcer peptic, stomach ulcer hemorrhage and tongue discolouration.

Endocrine System: sexual function abnormal.

Hemic and Lymphatic System: leucocytosis, leucopenia, methemoglobin, thrombocythemia, thrombocytopenia and white blood cells abnormal.

Metabolism and Nutritional Disorders: alanine aminotransferase increased, albuminuria, alkaline phosphatase increased, aspartate aminotransferase increased, blood urea nitrogen increased, creatinine increased, edema, electrolytes abnormal, hypercholesteremia, hyperlipidemia, hypoglycemia, hypokalemia, lactate dehydrogenase increased, weight increased.

Musculoskeletal System: bursitis, myasthenia, pain bone, spasm general, tendon disorder and tenosynovitis.

Nervous System: amnesia, apathy, convulsion, depersonalization, emotional lability, euphoric mood, hallucination, hyperkinesia, miosis, neuralgia, neuropathy, paralysis facial, speech disorder, stupor, twitch, urinary retention and vertigo.

Respiratory System: emphysema, epistaxis, hemoptysis, hiccup, laryngitis, pleural disorder and voice alteration.

Skin and Appendages: alopecia, exfoliative dermatitis, fungus dermatitis, hair disorder, lichen dermatitis, melanoma skin, neoplasia skin, psoriasis, rash maculopapular, rash vesiculobullous, skin disorder and ulcer skin.

Special Senses: corneal lesion, deafness, ear disorder, otitis media, pain eye, tinnitus.

Urogenital System: amenorrhea, ejaculation abnormal, fibrocystic breast, leukorrhea, mastitis, menorrhagia, menstrual disorder, metrorrhagia, neoplasia breast, nephrolithiasis, orchitis, pain breast, pain kidney, papanikolaou smear suspicious, unintended pregnancy, prostate disorder, salpingitis, testis disorder, urethritis, urination impaired, urinary frequency, and urinary urgency.

Buprenorphine Used Alone: Buprenorphine used alone for treatment of opioid dependency has been associated with the following symptoms (>1 %): constipation, headache, insomnia, asthenia, drowsiness, nausea and vomiting, fainting and dizziness, orthostatic hypotension, and sweating. Other side effects (<0.1 %) have been reported in association with buprenorphine alone. These are: respiratory depression (see Warnings and Precautions and Drug Interactions); hepatic necrosis and hepatitis (see Warnings and Precautions); and hallucinations.

Cases of bronchospasm, angioneurotic edema and anaphylactic shock have also been reported.

In cases of IV misuse, local reactions, sometimes septic, and potentially serious acute hepatitis have been reported (see Warnings and Precautions).

In patients presenting with marked drug dependence, initial administration of buprenorphine can produce a withdrawal effect similar to that associated with naloxone.

DRUG INTERACTIONS: Overview: Alcohol: SUBOXONE should not be taken together with alcoholic drinks or medications containing alcohol. Alcohol increases the sedative effect of buprenorphine.

Drug-Drug Interactions: SUBOXONE should be used cautiously together with:

- Benzodiazepines: This combination may result in death due to respiratory depression of central origin, therefore, dosage reduction of one or both medications must be considered. Unless the benzodiazepines are prescribed by a physician, this combination should be avoided due to the risk of misuse (see Warnings and Precautions).
- Patients should be warned of the potential danger of the self-administration of other CNS depressants; other opioid derivatives (analgesics and antitussives); certain antidepressants, sedative H_1-receptor antagonists, barbiturates, anxiolytics other than benzodiazepines, neuroleptics, clonidine and related substances: This combination increases central nervous system depression and can make driving vehicles and operating machinery hazardous.
- Monoamine oxidase inhibitors (MAOI): Caution should be exercised when SUBOXONE is used in combination with MAO inhibitors.
- Inhibitors of cytochrome P450 3A4: buprenorphine is metabolized by cytochrome P450 3A4. Caution is advised when buprenorphine is administered concomitantly with drugs known to inhibit the cytochrome P450 3A4 enzyme system (i.e., some drugs in the drug classes of azolo antimycotics, protease inhibitors, calcium channel blockers and macrolide antibiotics). Therefore, concomitant use of specific inhibitors of CYP 3A4 (e.g. ritonavir, indinavir, ketoconazole, itraconazole, erythromycin, diltiazem, fluoxetine) may significantly increase levels of buprenorphine.

Drug-Food Interactions: Interactions with food have not been established.

Drug-Herb Interactions: Interactions with herbal products have not been established.

Drug-Laboratory Test Interactions: Interactions with laboratory tests have not been established.

DOSAGE AND ADMINISTRATION: Adults:

Appropriate security measures should be taken to safeguard stocks of SUBOXONE against diversion.
SUBOXONE must be dispensed on a daily basis under the supervision of a healthcare professional for a minimum of two months and until the patient is clinically stable and able to safely store SUBOXONE take-home doses.

SUBOXONE is indicated for substitution treatment in opioid drug dependence in adults. The intention of the naloxone component is to deter IV misuse.

Patients prescribed SUBOXONE should be carefully monitored within a framework of medical, social, and psychological support as part of a comprehensive opioid dependence treatment program.

SUBOXONE sublingual tablets should only be prescribed by physicians who meet the following requirements:

i. **experience in substitution treatment in opioid drug dependence, and**
ii. **completion of an accredited SUBOXONE Education Program.**

The SUBOXONE Education Program is a risk management program that is founded on the following four core components that provide for the safe and effective use of the drug within a framework of medical, social and psychological treatment:

- **training of the prescribing physicians in the use of SUBOXONE sublingual tablets;**
- **maintenance of a list of SUBOXONE Education Program trained physicians;**
- **daily dosing supervised by a healthcare professional for a minimum of two months.**
- **take-home doses should only be considered after a period of two months based upon assessment of clinical stability, length of time in treatment and ability to safely store SUBOXONE. Take-home doses should be assessed and reviewed on a regular basis.**

Physicians should not prescribe SUBOXONE sublingual tablets unless the condition of daily intake supervised by a healthcare professional can be ensured, except for week-ends and holidays, for a minimum of two months and until the patient is clinically stable and able to safely store SUBOXONE take-home doses (see Warnings and Precautions).

Physicians may obtain more information about the SUBOXONE Education Program by calling the following toll-free phone number: 1-800-463-5442.

Dosing Considerations:

- Prior to induction, consideration should be given to the type of opiate dependence (i.e., long- or short-acting opiate), the time since last opiate use, and the degree or level of opiate dependence.
- **Patients taking street heroin (or other short-acting opiates):**
  When treatment starts, the dose of SUBOXONE should be taken at least 4 hours after the patient last used opiates or when early signs of opiate withdrawal appear.
- **Patients on methadone:**
  Before beginning SUBOXONE therapy, the dose of methadone must be reduced to a maximum of 30 mg/day. The first dose of SUBOXONE must be taken at least 24 hours after the patient last used methadone or preferably, when the early signs of withdrawal appear. SUBOXONE may precipitate symptoms of withdrawal in patients dependent upon methadone.

Recommended Dose and Dosage Adjustment: Induction: When initiating treatment with SUBOXONE, the physician should be aware of the partial agonist profile of buprenorphine to the mu-opioid receptors, which may precipitate a withdrawal syndrome in opioid-dependent patients.

The recommended starting dose is 4 mg SUBOXONE on Day 1. An additional 4 mg dose may be administered depending on the individual patient's requirement.

Maintenance: The dose of SUBOXONE should be increased progressively according to individual patient need and should not exceed a maximum single daily dose of 24 mg. The dosage is titrated according to reassessment of the clinical and psychological status of the patient.

During the initiation of treatment, daily dispensing of SUBOXONE is required for a minimum of two months. After clinical stabilisation has been achieved, a graduated schedule of take-home doses may be granted.

Less Than Daily Dosing: Following successful induction and after the patient is receiving a stable dose, the frequency of SUBOXONE dosing may be decreased to dosing every other day at twice the individually titrated daily dose. For example, a patient who receives a stable daily dose of 8 mg may be given 16 mg on alternate days, with no medication on the intervening days. However, the dose given on any one day should not exceed 24 mg.

In some patients, following successful induction and after the patient is receiving a stable dose, the frequency of SUBOXONE dosing may be decreased to 3 times a week (for example on Monday, Wednesday and Friday). The dose on Monday and Wednesday should be twice the individually titrated daily dose, and the dose on Friday should be three times the individually titrated daily dose, with no medication on the intervening days. However, the dose given on any one day should not exceed 24 mg. Patients requiring a titrated daily dose >8 mg/day may not find this regimen adequate.

Reducing Dosage and Terminating Treatment: The decision to discontinue therapy with SUBOXONE should be made as part of a comprehensive treatment plan. Both gradual and abrupt discontinuation have been used but controlled trials to determine the best method of dose taper have not been done. Gradual discontinuation is recommended with careful monitoring of the patient's progress. The risk of relapse following withdrawal of treatment should be considered.

Administration: SUBOXONE sublingual tablets should be placed under the tongue until dissolved. Dissolution usually occurs within 2 to 10 minutes. When necessary, tablets should be dosed simultaneously (i.e., two 8 mg tablets should be placed under the tongue to achieve a dose of 16 mg).

DRUG ABUSE AND DEPENDENCE: Buprenorphine is a partial agonist at the mu-opioid receptor and chronic administration produces dependence of the opiate type, characterized by withdrawal upon abrupt discontinuation or rapid taper. The withdrawal syndrome is milder than seen with full agonists, and may be delayed (see Warnings and Precautions).

Abuse and diversion of buprenorphine by opiate addicts has been reported (see Warnings and Precautions).

OVERDOSAGE:

Manifestations: Manifestations of acute overdose include pinpoint pupils, sedation, hypotension, respiratory depression and death.

Treatment: The respiratory and cardiac status of the patient should be monitored carefully. If the patient vomits, care must be taken to prevent aspiration of the vomitus. In the event of depression of respiratory or cardiac function, primary attention should be given to the re-establishment of adequate respiratory exchange through provision of a patent airway and institution of assisted or controlled ventilation. Oxygen, IV fluids, vasopressors, and other supportive measures should be employed as indicated.

In the case of overdose, the primary management should be the re-establishment of adequate ventilation with mechanical assistance of respiration, if required. Naloxone may not be effective in reversing any respiratory depression produced by buprenorphine.

High doses of naloxone hydrochloride, 10-35 mg/70 kg may be of limited value in the management of buprenorphine overdose.

In addition, the long duration of action of SUBOXONE should be taken into consideration when determining length of treatment needed to reverse the effects of an overdose.

For management of a suspected drug overdose, CPhA recommends that you contact your **regional Poison Control Centre**. See the *CPS* Directory section for a list of Poison Control Centres.

ACTION AND CLINICAL PHARMACOLOGY: Mechanism of Action: Buprenorphine is a partial agonist at the mu-opioid receptor and an antagonist at the kappa-opioid receptor.

Naloxone is an antagonist at mu-opioid receptors. Because of its almost complete first pass metabolism and low sublingual bioavailability, naloxone administered orally or sublingually has no detectable pharmacological activity. However, when administered intravenously to opiate dependent persons, the presence of naloxone in SUBOXONE produces marked opiate antagonist effects and opiate withdrawal, thereby deterring IV abuse.

Subjective Effects: Comparison of buprenorphine with full agonists such as methadone and hydromorphone suggest that sublingual buprenorphine produces typical opiate agonist effects, which are limited by a ceiling effect.

Buprenorphine 16 mg had opioid agonist effects similar to 4 mg intramuscular hydromorphone, and equivalent to about 30 mg intramuscular morphine.

Opioid agonist ceiling effects were also observed in a double-blind parallel group, dose ranging comparison of single doses of 1, 2, 4, 8, 16 or 32 mg buprenorphine sublingual solution (comparable approximately to 1.5 mg, 3 mg, 6 mg, 12 mg, 24 mg and 48 mg, respectively, of the tablet form), oral methadone (15, 30, 45 or 60 mg) and placebo. The treatments were given in ascending dose order at intervals of at least one week to 16 opioid experienced, non-dependent male subjects. Both drugs produced typical opioid agonist effects. For all measures for which drugs produced an effect, buprenorphine produced a dose-related response but, in each case, there was a dose which produced no further effects. In contrast, the highest dose of methadone (60 mg) always produced the greatest effects.

Physiologic Effects: Buprenorphine administered intravenously at doses of 2 mg, 4 mg, 8 mg, 12 mg and 16 mg or sublingually at a dose of 12 mg to non-opioid dependent individuals showed no statistically significant differences, compared to placebo, among any of the treatment conditions for blood pressure, heart rate, respiratory rate, O_2 saturation or skin temperature across time. Systolic blood pressure was higher for the 8 mg buprenorphine IV group than placebo. Minimum and maximum effects were similar across all treatments. Subjects remained responsive to low voice and responded to computer prompts. Some subjects showed irritability, but no other changes were observed.

Respiratory effects of sublingual buprenorphine solution (1, 2, 4, 8, 16 or 32 mg) were compared to those of oral methadone (15, 30, 45 or 60 mg) in non-dependent, opioid experienced healthy male volunteers. Hypoventilation not requiring mechanical intervention was reported more frequently after buprenorphine sublingual solution doses of 4 mg and greater (4 mg solution comparable approximately to a 6 mg tablet dose) than after methadone. Both drugs decreased O_2 saturation to the same degree.

Effect of Naloxone: Naloxone had no clinically significant effect when administered by the sublingual route; plasma concentrations are low and decline rapidly. SUBOXONE, when administered sublingually even to an opioid-dependent population, was recognized as an opioid agonist, whereas when administered intramuscularly, combinations of buprenorphine with naloxone produced opioid antagonist actions similar to naloxone. In the methadone-maintained patients and heroin-dependent subjects, IV administration of buprenorphine/naloxone combinations precipitated opioid withdrawal and was perceived as unpleasant and dysphoric. In morphine-stabilized subjects, intravenously administered combinations of buprenorphine with naloxone produced opioid antagonist and withdrawal effects that were ratio-dependent; the most intense withdrawal effects were produced by 2:1 and 4:1 ratio, less intense by an 8:1 ratio. SUBOXONE tablets contain buprenorphine with naloxone at a ratio of 4:1.

Pharmacokinetics: Buprenorphine: Absorption: When taken orally, buprenorphine undergoes first-pass hepatic metabolism with N-dealkylation and glucuroconjugation in the small intestine. The use of this medication by the oral route is therefore ineffective.

When taken sublingually, there was a wide inter-patient variability in the absorption of buprenorphine but within subject variability was low. Plasma levels of buprenorphine increased with dose in the range of 4 mg to 16 mg, although the increase was not directly dose proportional. Mean C_{max} for buprenorphine 4 mg was 2.00 ng/mL and increased to 2.65 ng/mL at 8 mg and 4.42 ng/mL at 16 mg. Mean $AUC_{0-\infty}$ for sublingual tablet doses of 4 mg, 8 mg and 16 mg were, respectively, 13.90, 27.83 and 44.16 (h·ng/mL).

Distribution: Buprenorphine is approximately 96% protein-bound, primarily to alpha and beta globulin.

Metabolism: Buprenorphine is metabolized by 14-N-dealkylation and glucuroconjugation of the parent molecule and the dealkylated metabolite. The N-dealkylation pathway is mediated by cytochrome P-450 3A4 isozyme. N-dealkylbuprenorphine (norbuprenorphine) is considered to be an inactive metabolite.

Excretion: Buprenorphine is essentially eliminated in the feces by biliary excretion of the glucuroconjugated metabolites (approximately 70%), the rest being eliminated in the urine. In feces, almost all of the buprenorphine and norbuprenorphine were free (buprenorphine, 33% free and 5% conjugated; norbuprenorphine, 21% free and 2% conjugated). In urine, most of buprenorphine and norbuprenorphine were conjugated (buprenorphine, 1% free and 9.4% conjugated; norbuprenorphine, 2.7% free and 11% conjugated).

The overall mean elimination half-life of buprenorphine in plasma is 37 hours, although the levels are very low 10 hours after dosing (majority of AUC of buprenorphine is captured within 10 hours), indicating that the effective half-life may be shorter.

Naloxone: Absorption and Distribution: Following IV administration, naloxone is rapidly distributed (distribution half-life ~4 minutes). Following oral administration, naloxone is barely detectable in plasma; following sublingual administration of SUBOXONE, plasma naloxone concentrations are low and decline rapidly.

Metabolism: The drug is metabolized in the liver, primarily by glucuronide conjugation.

Excretion: The drug is excreted in the urine. Naloxone has a mean elimination half-life from plasma of 1.3 hours.

Special Populations and Conditions: Hepatic Insufficiency: Hepatic elimination plays a relatively large role (~ 70%) in the overall clearance of SUBOXONE and the action of buprenorphine may be prolonged in subjects with impaired hepatic clearance. Lower initial SUBOXONE doses and cautious titration of dosage may be required in patients with mild to moderate hepatic dysfunction. SUBOXONE is contraindicated in patients with severe hepatic dysfunction.

Renal Insufficiency: Renal elimination plays a relatively small role (~30%) in the overall clearance of SUBOXONE. No dose modification based on renal function is required but caution is recommended when dosing subjects with severe renal impairment.

STORAGE AND STABILITY: Store at 15 to 30°C.

SPECIAL HANDLING INSTRUCTIONS: Protect from light. Protect from moisture.

INFORMATION FOR THE PATIENT: Published in e-CPS, available by subscription at www.e-cps.ca.

DOSAGE FORMS, COMPOSITION AND PACKAGING: 2 mg/0.5 mg : Each white to creamy white hexagonal tablet embossed with sword logo on one side and "N2" on the reverse, contains: 2 mg buprenorphine (as hydrochloride) and 0.5 mg naloxone (as hydrochloride dihydrate). Nonmedicinal ingredients: acesulfame potassium, citric acid anhydrous, lactose monohydrate, magnesium stearate, maize starch, mannitol, natural lemon and lime flavour, povidone K30 and sodium citrate. Blister packages of 7. **8 mg/2 mg :** Each white to creamy white hexagonal tablet embossed with sword logo on one side and "N8" on the reverse, contains: 8 mg buprenorphine (as hydrochloride) and 2 mg naloxone (as hydrochloride dihydrate). Nonmedicinal ingredients: acesulfame potassium, citric acid anhydrous, lactose monohydrate, magnesium stearate, maize starch, mannitol, natural lemon and lime flavour, povidone K30 and sodium citrate. Blister packages of 7.

(Shown in Product Identification Section)

Sudafed® Cold & Cough Extra Strength

pseudoephedrine HCl—dextromethorphan HBr—acetaminophen

Nasal Decongestant—Antitussive—Analgesic

McNeil Consumer Healthcare

Sudafed® Decongestant 12 Hour

pseudoephedrine HCl

Nasal Decongestant

McNeil Consumer Healthcare

Sudafed® Head Cold and Sinus Extra Strength

pseudoephedrine HCl—acetaminophen

Nasal Decongestant—Analgesic

McNeil Consumer Healthcare

Sudafed® PE Decongestant

phenylephrine HCl

Nasal Decongestant

McNeil Consumer Healthcare

Date of Revision: August 13, 2009

INDICATIONS: Cold & Cough Extra Strength: For relief of nasal congestion, dry cough, headache, body ache, fever and sore throat pain.

Decongestant: Relief of nasal congestion associated with allergic rhinitis, acute coryza, vasomotor rhinitis, acute and subacute sinusitis, acute otitis media, postnasal drip, acute eustachian salpingitis.

Head Cold and Sinus Extra Strength: For relief of nasal congestion, sinus pain, headache and body aches.

CONTRAINDICATIONS: Sensitivity to pseudoephedrine or any of the other components. Patients receiving or having received MAO inhibitors in the preceding 2 weeks; known hypersensitivity to pressor amines. Patients with severe hypertension or severe coronary artery disease.

Dextromethorphan: Pre-existing respiratory depression.

WARNINGS: Massive acetaminophen overdose can be toxic and potentially fatal. In adults, hepatotoxicity from acetaminophen is unlikely to occur with overdoses of less than 10 g ingested at one time and fatalities are unlikely to occur with overdoses of less than 15 g ingested at one time.

PRECAUTIONS: As pseudoephedrine is a sympathomimetic amine, it should be used with caution in hypertensive and diabetic patients; patients with latent or clinically recognized angle closure glaucoma, coronary artery disease, congestive heart failure, prostatic hypertrophy, hyperthyroidism, urinary retention.

Geriatrics: The elderly (65 years and older) are more likely to have adverse reactions to sympathomimetics. Overdosage of sympathomimetics in this age group may cause hallucinations, convulsions, CNS depression and death.

In severe hepatic or renal dysfunction, a single dose should be given and the patient's response used as a guide to the dosage requirement for further administration.

Hypertension and unconsciousness following the ingestion of one Sudafed tablet by a normotensive individual has been reported and should be regarded as an extremely rare example of pseudoephedrine intolerance.

Pregnancy: Use with caution. Pseudoephedrine has been reported to be excreted into breast milk of lactating women. Consult a physician before using these products.

Lactation: See Pregnancy.

Drug Interactions: Concomitant use of pseudoephedrine with other sympathomimetic agents, such as decongestants, appetite suppressants, and amphetamine-like psychostimulants or with MAO inhibitors, which interfere with the catabolism of sympathomimetic amines, may occasionally cause a rise in blood pressure.

The antibacterial agent, furazolidone, is known to cause a dose-related inhibition of MAO. Although there are no reports of a hypertensive crisis caused by the concurrent administration of pseudoephedrine and furazolidone, they should not be taken together.

The effect of antihypertensive drugs which interfere with sympathetic activity may be partially reversed by pseudoephedrine (e.g., bretylium, bethanidine, guanethidine, debrisoquine, methyldopa, beta and/or alpha- adrenergic-blocking agents).

ADVERSE EFFECTS: Pseudoephedrine: As with other sympathomimetic amines, headache, dizziness, insomnia, tremor, confusion, CNS stimulation, muscular weakness, dry mouth, nausea, vomiting, difficulty in micturition, palpitations, tightness in the chest and syncope may be encountered. Fixed drug eruption has been reported and rarely hallucinations.

Dextromethorphan: drowsiness, dizziness, constipation, nausea, vomiting and confusion.

Guaifenesin: Nausea, gastrointestinal upset and drowsiness occur infrequently.

OVERDOSE:

Symptoms: Pseudoephedrine: Increase in pulse and respiratory rate, CNS stimulation, disorientation, headache, dry mouth, nausea and vomiting. Nervousness, dizziness or sleeplessness may occur.

Dextromethorphan: In severe cases, there may be respiratory depression due to the dextromethorphan component.

Acetaminophen: Typical Toxidrome: Hepatic injury is the principal toxic effect of a substantial acetaminophen overdose. The physician should be mindful that there is no early presentation that is pathognomonic for the overdose. A high degree of clinical suspicion must always be maintained.

Untreated acetaminophen overdoses may produce hepatotoxicity. Acetaminophen hepatotoxicity occurs as a threshold effect and is characterized by a lack of toxicity at lower/therapeutic doses. Acetaminophen hepatotoxicity occurs after major depletion of glutathione, an endogenous detoxifying substance. Once the threshold is exceeded, increasing acetaminophen doses may produce increasing degrees of hepatotoxicity, unless N-acetylcysteine (NAC) is administered. Situations in which acetaminophen overdose and resultant hepatotoxicity may occur include acute intentional overdose and repeated supratherapeutic overdose in adults and acute accidental ingestion or overdose and repeated supratherapeutic overdose in children.

The clinical course of acetaminophen overdose generally occurs in a three-phase sequential pattern. The first phase begins shortly after ingestion and lasts for 12 to 24 hours. The patient may manifest signs of gastrointestinal irritability, nausea, vomiting, anorexia, diaphoresis, pallor and general malaise. If toxicity continues, there is a latent phase of up to 48 hours. During this second phase, initial symptoms abate and the patient may feel better. However, hepatic enzymes, bilirubin, and prothrombin time or INR values will progressively rise. Right upper quadrant pain may develop as the liver becomes enlarged and tender. Most patients do not progress beyond this phase, especially if given N-acetylcysteine (NAC) treatment early in the course. Signs and symptoms of the third phase depend on the severity of hepatic damage and usually occur from three to five days following overdose ingestion. Symptoms may be limited to anorexia, nausea, general malaise, and abdominal pain in less severe cases or may progress to confusion, stupor and sequelae of hepatic necrosis including jaundice, coagulation defects, hypoglycemia, and encephalopathy, as well as renal failure and cardiomyopathy. Death, if it occurs, is generally the result of complications associated with fulminant hepatic failure. Mortality rates in patients with toxic plasma levels who do not receive antidote therapy range from 3% to 4%.

Due to the wide availability of acetaminophen, it is commonly involved in single and mixed drug overdose situations and the practitioner should screen for its presence in a patient's serum. Acute toxicity after single dose overdoses of acetaminophen can be anticipated when the overdose exceeds 150 mg/kg. Chronic alcohol abusers, cachectic individuals, and persons taking pharmacologic inducers of the hepatic P450 microsomal enzyme system may be at risk with lower exposures.

Treatment: Pseudoephedrine: Gastric lavage, repeated, if necessary. Acidify the urine and institute general supportive measures. If CNS excitement is prominent, a short-acting barbiturate may be used. Catheterization of the bladder may be necessary. Alpha-adrenergic blockade may be required to treat hypertensive crises and beta-adrenergic blockade for the control of supraventricular dysrhythmias. Elimination may be accelerated by dialysis.

Dextromethorphan: In severe cases of acute poisoning, where the respiratory depressive effects of dextromethorphan may be apparent, the following may be indicated: naloxone; Adults: 400 µg s.c. Children: 5 to 10 µg/kg s.c. Depending on the patient's response, the dose can be repeated at 2 to 3 minute intervals.

Acetaminophen: Specific Antidote: Any individual presenting with a possible acetaminophen overdose should be treated with N-acetylcysteine (NAC), even if the amount of acetaminophen ingested is unknown or questionable. A blood sample for determination of the plasma acetaminophen concentration should be obtained as early as possible, but no sooner than four hours following ingestion. Do not await the results of assays for plasma acetaminophen levels before initiating treatment NAC. If the acetaminophen plasma level is found to plot above the treatment line on the acetaminophen overdose nomogram, NAC treatment should be continued for a full course of therapy. NAC is used clinically to treat acute acetaminophen overdose, and acts by interacting with the oxidative intermediate, NAPQI. NAC administered by either the i.v. or the oral route is known to be a highly effective antidote for acetaminophen poisoning. It is most effective when administered within 8 hours of a significant overdose but reports have indicated benefits to treatment initiated well beyond this time period. It is imperative to administer the antidote as early as possible in the time course of acute intoxication to reap the full benefits of the antidote's protective effects. For full prescribing information, consult the product monograph for NAC.

General Management: When the possibility of acetaminophen overdose exists, treatment should begin immediately and include appropriate decontamination of the gastrointestinal tract, proper supportive care, careful assessment of appropriately timed serum acetaminophen estimations evaluated against the Rumack-Matthew nomogram, timely administration of NAC as required and appropriate follow-up care. Liver function tests should be performed initially and repeated at 24-hour intervals.

For management of a suspected drug overdose, CPhA recommends that you contact your **regional Poison Control Centre**. See the *CPS* Directory section for a list of Poison Control Centres.

DOSAGE: Not recommended for children under 12 years of age.

Cold & Cough Extra Strength: Adults and children 12 years and over: 1 caplet every 4 to 6 hours. Do not exceed 4 doses in 24 hours. Persons over 65: use only as directed by a physician.

Decongestant 12 Hour: Adults and children 12 years and older: 1 caplet every 12 hours. Do not exceed 2 doses in 24 hours. Persons over 65: use only as directed by a physician.

Head Cold and Sinus Extra Strength: Adults and children 12 years of age and over: 1 caplet every 4 to 6 hours. Do not exceed 4 doses in 24 hours. Persons over 65: use as directed by a physician.

PE Decongestant: Adults and children 12 years and over: 1 tablet every 4 hours. Do not exceed 6 tablets in 24 hours.

SUPPLIED: Cold & Cough Extra Strength: Each white, biconvex caplet, coded "SU" on one side and "WL 61" on the other side, contains: pseudoephedrine HCl 60 mg, dextromethorphan HBr 30 mg and acetaminophen 500 mg. Nonmedicinal ingredients: cellulose, magnesium stearate, povidone and sodium starch glycolate. Blister packages of 12 and 24. Store at 15 to 25°C. Protect from light. Keep dry.

Decongestant 12 Hour: Each white, biconvex caplet, printed "SUDAFED 12 HOUR", contains: pseudoephedrine HCl 120 mg. Nonmedicinal ingredients: celluloses, edible blue ink, magnesium stearate, polyethylene glycol, povidone, titanium dioxide and wax. Blister packages of 20. Store at 15 to 25°C. Protect from light. Keep dry.

Head Cold and Sinus Extra Strength: Each white caplet coded "SU" on one side and "WL 62" on the other side, contains: acetaminophen 500 mg and pseudoephedrine HCl 60 mg. Nonmedicinal ingredients: cellulose, magnesium stearate, povidone and sodium starch glycolate (potato). Blister packages of 12 and 24. Store at 15 to 25°C. Protect from light. Keep dry.

PE Decongestant: Each round, biconvex, unscored, red tablet with code number "WL80" on one side and PE on the other side, contains: phenylephrine HCl 10 mg. Nonmedicinal ingredients: acesulfame K, celluloses, FD&C Red No. 40 aluminum lake, FD&C Yellow No. 6 aluminum lake, hypromellose, magnesium stearate, polydextrose, polyethylene glycol, povidone, silicone dioxide, starch, stearic acid, titanium dioxide, triacetin and wax. Blister packages of 12, 24 and 48. Store between 15 and 30°C. Protect from light. Keep dry.

Sudafed® Sinus Advance

pseudoephedrine HCl—ibuprofen

Decongestant—Analgesic—Antipyretic

McNeil Consumer Healthcare

Date of Revision: July 17, 2008

INDICATIONS: For the temporary relief of symptoms associated with the common cold, sinusitis or flu including nasal congestion, headache, fever, body aches and pains.

CONTRAINDICATIONS: Should not be used in patients who have previously exhibited hypersensitivity to it, or its components (ibuprofen, pseudoephedrine), or in individuals with the angioedema syndrome of nasal polyps, and bronchospastic reactivity to ASA or other NSAIDs (see Warnings). Sudafed Sinus Advance should not be used in patients with hypertension, coronary artery disease and in patients on MAOI therapy (see Precautions, Drug Interactions).

Sudafed Sinus Advance should not be used during pregnancy, in nursing mothers or in pediatric patients because its safety under these conditions has not been established.

Aseptic meningitis, fever, or rash has been reported in connection with ibuprofen therapy in patients with systemic lupus erythematosus. Sudafed Sinus Advance should not be used by patients with systemic lupus erythematosus except under a physician's supervision. Sudafed Sinus Advance should not be taken by patients with active peptic ulcer disease or gastrointestinal bleeding unless directed by a physician.

WARNINGS: Anaphylactoid reactions have occurred in patients with known ASA hypersensitivity (see Contraindications).

Peptic ulcerations and gastrointestinal bleeding, sometimes severe, have been reported in patients receiving prescription doses of ibuprofen. Peptic ulcerations, perforation, or severe gastrointestinal bleeding can have a fatal outcome, and although few such reports have been received with ibuprofen, a cause and effect relationship has not been established. Patients with a history of upper gastrointestinal tract disease should take Sudafed Sinus Advance under the supervision of a physician.

Like other nonsteroidal anti-inflammatory agents, ibuprofen can inhibit platelet aggregation. However, compared to ASA, the effect is quantitatively less, of shorter duration, and reversible upon discontinuation of ibuprofen. Bleeding time has also been prolonged by ibuprofen though within the normal range in normal subjects. Because this effect on bleeding time may be exaggerated in patients with underlying hemostatic defects, Sudafed Sinus Advance should be avoided by persons with intrinsic coagulation defects and those on anticoagulant therapy.

Patients with high blood pressure, heart disease, diabetes, narrow angle glaucoma, thyroid disease or difficulty in urination due to enlargement of the prostate gland should take Sudafed Sinus Advance only under the advice and supervision of a physician.

PRECAUTIONS: Conditions associated with dehydration appear to increase the risk of renal toxicity. Sudafed Sinus Advance should therefore be used with caution in patients with chronic renal failure, congestive heart failure or hypertension being treated chronically with diuretics.

Geriatrics: Caution should be observed in elderly patients, due to increased susceptibility to effects of sympathomimetic amines and increased risk of toxicity with ibuprofen, and patients with diminished renal function.

Patients on Sudafed Sinus Advance should be cautioned to report to their physician if any signs or symptoms of gastrointestinal ulceration or bleeding, blurred vision or other eye symptoms, skin rash, weight gain, edema, tinnitus, dizziness or respiratory difficulties.

If Sudafed Sinus Advance is taken in conjunction with prolonged corticosteroid therapy and it is decided to discontinue the latter therapy, as under other circumstances, the corticosteroid dosage should be tapered slowly to avoid exacerbation of disease or adrenal insufficiency.

Pregnancy: Pregnant women or nursing mothers should seek the advice of a health professional before using Sudafed Sinus Advance.

Lactation: See Pregnancy.

There is a possibility of insomnia, if this medicine is taken before bedtime.

If the symptoms do not improve, or are accompanied by a high fever, the patient should be advised to report to his physician.

Drug Interactions: Coumarin-type Anticoagulants: Several short-term controlled studies failed to show that ibuprofen significantly affected prothrombin time or a variety of other clotting factors when administered to individuals on coumarin-type anticoagulants. The physician should be cautious when administering Sudafed Sinus Advance to patients on anticoagulants.

ASA: Animal studies show that ASA given with nonsteroidal anti-inflammatory agents including ibuprofen yields a net decrease in anti-inflammatory activity with lowered blood levels of the non-ASA drug. Single dose bioavailability studies in normal volunteers have failed to show an effect of ASA on ibuprofen blood levels. Correlative clinical studies have not been conducted.

Other NSAIDs: The addition of Sudafed Sinus Advance to a pre-existent prescribed NSAID regimen in patients with a condition such as rheumatoid arthritis may result in increased risk of adverse effects.

Diuretics: Because of its fluid retention properties, high doses of ibuprofen can decrease the diuretic and antihypertensive effects of diuretics, and increased diuretic dosage may be required. Patients with impaired renal function who are taking potassium-sparing diuretics should not take Sudafed Sinus Advance.

Hypoglycemic Agents: Ibuprofen may increase hypoglycemic effects of oral antidiabetic agents and insulin.

Acetaminophen: Although interactions have not been reported, concurrent use with Sudafed Sinus Advance is not advisable, it may increase the risk of adverse renal effect.

Other Drugs: Although ibuprofen binds extensively to plasma proteins, interactions with other protein-bound drugs occur rarely. Nevertheless, caution should be observed when other drugs, also having a high affinity for protein binding sites, are used concurrently. Some observations have suggested a potential for ibuprofen to interact with furosemide, pindolol, digoxin, phenytoin and lithium salts. However, the mechanisms and clinical significance of these observations are presently not known. No interactions have been reported when ibuprofen has been used in conjunction with hypoglycemic agents, probenecid, digitalis, thyroxine, steroids, antibiotics or benzodiazepines. Sudafed Sinus Advance may enhance the effects of MAOIs.

ADVERSE EFFECTS: Ibuprofen: The following adverse reactions have been noted in patients treated with prescription regimens of ibuprofen: Note: Reactions listed below under Causal Relationship Unknown are those which occurred under circumstances where a causal relationship could not be established. However, in these rarely reported events, the possibility of a relationship to ibuprofen cannot be excluded.

Gastrointestinal: The adverse reactions most frequently seen with prescribed ibuprofen therapy involve the gastrointestinal system. Incidence 3 to 9%: nausea, epigastric pain, heartburn. Incidence 1 to 3%: diarrhea, abdominal distress, nausea and vomiting, indigestion, constipation, abdominal cramps or pain, fullness of the gastrointestinal tract (bloating or flatulence). Incidence less than 1%: gastric or duodenal ulcer with bleeding and/or perforation, gastrointestinal hemorrhage, melena, hepatitis, jaundice, abnormal liver function (AST, serum bilirubin and alkaline phosphatases).

CNS: Incidence 3 to 9%: dizziness. Incidence 1 to 3%: headache, nervousness. Incidence less than 1%: depression, insomnia. Causal relationship unknown: paresthesia, hallucinations, dream abnormalities. Aseptic meningitis and meningoencephalitis, in 1 case accompanied by eosinophilia in the cerebrospinal fluid, have been reported in patients who took ibuprofen intermittently and did not have any connective tissue disease.

Dermatologic: Incidence 3 to 9%: rash (including maculopapular type). Incidence 1 to 3%: pruritus. Incidence less than 1%: vesiculobullous eruptions, urticaria, erythema multiforme. Causal relationship unknown: alopecia, Stevens-Johnson syndrome.

Special Senses: Incidence 1 to 3%: tinnitus. Incidence less than 1%: amblyopia (blurred and/or diminished vision, scotomata and/or changes in color vision). Any patient with eye complaints during ibuprofen therapy should have an ophthalmological examination. Causal relationship unknown: conjunctivitis, diplopia, optic neuritis.

Metabolic: Incidence 1 to 3%: decreased appetite, edema, fluid retention. Fluid retention generally responds promptly to drug discontinuation (see Precautions).

Hematologic: Incidence less than 1%: leukopenia and decreases in hemoglobin and hematocrit. Causal relationship unknown: hemolytic anemia, thrombocytopenia, granulocytopenia, bleeding episodes (e.g., purpura, epistaxis, hematuria, menorrhagia).

Cardiovascular: Incidence less than 1%: congestive heart failure in patients with marginal cardiac function, elevated blood pressure. Causal relationship unknown: arrhythmias (sinus tachycardia, sinus bradycardia, palpitations).

Allergic: Incidence less than 1%: anaphylaxis (see Contraindications). Causal relationship unknown: fever, serum sickness, lupus erythematosus.

Endocrine: Causal relationship unknown: gynecomastia, hypoglycemic reaction. Menstrual delays of up to 2 weeks and dysfunctional uterine bleeding occurred in 9 patients taking ibuprofen, 400 mg t.i.d., for 3 days before menses.

Renal: Causal relationship unknown: decreased creatinine clearance, polyuria, azotemia. Like other NSAIDs, ibuprofen inhibits renal prostaglandin synthesis, which may decrease renal function and cause sodium retention. Renal blood flow and glomerular filtration rate decreased in patients with mild impairment of renal function who took 1200 mg/day of ibuprofen for 1 week. Renal papillary necrosis has been reported. A number of factors appear to increase the risk of renal toxicity (see Precautions). In comparative clinical trials analyzed by The Boots Company involving 7624 ibuprofen-treated, 2822 ASA-treated and 2843 placebo-treated patients, adverse reactions involving renal function were reported by 0.6% of the ibuprofen group, 0.3% of the ASA group and 0.1% of the placebo group. The analysis included data from trials which employed doses greater than 1200 mg, used for longer periods than OTC recommendations and by patients being treated for serious conditions.

Pseudoephedrine: Pseudoephedrine may cause mild CNS stimulation, especially in patients who are hypersensitive to the effects of sympathomimetic drugs. Nervousness, excitability, restlessness, dizziness, weakness, and insomnia may occur. Headache and drowsiness have also been reported. Large doses may cause lightheadedness, nausea, and/or vomiting. In addition, the possibility of other adverse effects associated with sympathomimetic drugs, including fear, anxiety, tenseness, tremor, hallucinations, seizures, pallor, respiratory difficulty, dysuria, and cardiovascular collapse should be considered. Although oral administration of usual doses of pseudoephedrine to normotensive patients usually produced negligible pressor effects, the drug should be used with caution in hypertensive patients. Pseudoephedrine may increase the irritability of heart muscle and may alter the rhythmic function of the ventricles, especially in large doses or when administered to patients who are hypersensitive to the myocardial effects of sympathomimetic drugs. Tachycardia or palpitation may occur. One patient who received 120 mg of pseudoephedrine every 4 hours developed multifocal premature ventricular contractions which disappeared a few days after the drug was discontinued. In addition, pseudoephedrine may have precipitated an attack of atrial fibrillation in an infant. It was postulated that the patient may have had previously unsuspected idiopathic atrial fibrillation, and therefore may have been especially sensitive to the myocardial effects of the drug.

OVERDOSE:

Treatment: Due to the rapid absorption of pseudoephedrine and ibuprofen from the gut, emetics and gastric lavage must be instituted within 4 hours of overdosage to be effective. Charcoal is useful only if given within 1 hour. Cardiac status should be monitored and the serum electrolytes measured. If there are signs of cardiac toxicity, propranolol may be administered i.v. A slow infusion of a dilute solution of potassium chloride should be initiated in the event of a drop in the serum potassium level. Despite hypokalemia, the patient is unlikely to be potassium-depleted; therefore, overload must be avoided. Monitoring of the serum potassium is advisable for several hours after administration of the salt. For delirium or convulsions, i.v. administration of diazepam is indicated.

> For management of a suspected drug overdose, CPhA recommends that you contact your **regional Poison Control Centre**. See the *CPS* Directory section for a list of Poison Control Centres.

DOSAGE: Adults and children over 12 years: Take 1 or 2 caplets every 4 hours as needed. Do not exceed 6 caplets in 24 hours, unless directed by a physician. Do not give to children under 12 years of age, except under the advice and supervision of a physician.

INFORMATION FOR THE PATIENT: Published in e-CPS, available by subscription at www.e-cps.ca.

SUPPLIED: Each white caplet, embossed with "SU" on one side and "WL 45" on the other side, contains: ibuprofen 200 mg and pseudoephedrine HCl 30 mg. Nonmedicinal ingredients: calcium stearate, candelilla wax, pregelatinized starch, croscarmellose sodium, hydroxypropyl methylcellulose, methylparaben, microcrystalline cellulose, povidone, propylene glycol, propylparaben, sodium lauryl sulfate, stearic acid and titanium dioxide. Aluminum-backed blisters, packages of 20 and 40. Store between 15 and 25°C. Protect from light. Keep dry.

Sufentanil Ⓝ

CPhA Monograph

see *Opioids*

Sufentanil Citrate Injection USP Ⓝ

sufentanil citrate

Opioid Analgesic—Adjunct to Anesthesia

Sandoz

SUPPLIED: Each mL of sterile, aqueous solution contains: sufentanil citrate equivalent to sufentanil base 50 µg. Nonmedicinal ingredients: citric acid and/or sodium hydroxide to adjust pH, sodium chloride for isotonicity and water for injection. Preservative-free. Amber ampoules of 1 mL, boxes of 10. Single use, amber vials of 5 mL, boxes of 5. Store between 15 and 30°C. Protect from light. Discard unused portion.

Sulcrate® Ⓟ

sucralfate

Gastroduodenal Cytoprotective Agent

Axcan Pharma

Sulcrate® Suspension Plus Ⓟ

sucralfate

Gastroduodenal Cytoprotective Agent

Axcan Pharma

PHARMACOLOGY: SULCRATE (sucralfate) exerts a generalized gastric cytoprotective effect by enhancing natural mucosal defense mechanisms. Studies conducted in animals and clinical trials in humans have demonstrated that sucralfate can protect the gastric mucosa against various irritants such as alcohol, ASA, hydrochloric acid, sodium hydroxide or sodium taurocholate.

In addition, sucralfate has been demonstrated to have a greater affinity for ulcerated gastric or duodenal mucosa than for nonulcerated mucosa.

Sucralfate produces an adherent and cytoprotective barrier at the ulcer site. This barrier protects the ulcer site from the potential ulcerogenic properties of acid, pepsin and bile. Furthermore, sucralfate blocks acid diffusion across the sucralfate protein barrier and also complexes directly with pepsin and bile.

Pharmacokinetics: The action of sucralfate is nonsystemic as the drug is only minimally absorbed from the gastrointestinal tract. The minute amounts of the sulfated disaccharide which are absorbed are primarily excreted in the urine.

Each g of sucralfate contains approximately 200 mg of aluminum. The aluminum moiety can dissociate at low pH and aluminum release in the stomach can be expected; however, aluminum is poorly absorbed from the intact gastrointestinal tract. Following administration of 1 g of sucralfate (tablets or suspension) 4 times a day to individuals with normal renal function, approximately

0.001% to 0.017% of sucralfate's aluminum content is absorbed and excreted in the urine. This results in an aluminum load of between 0.008 mg and 0.136 mg following a 4 g daily dose. Individuals with normal renal function excrete absorbed aluminum and can respond to an increased aluminum load by increasing urinary excretion.

These values were determined in individuals with intact gastrointestinal mucosa. Available evidence does not indicate that absorption of aluminum would be different in individuals with ulcerated gastrointestinal mucosa.

Experiments have shown that sucralfate is not an antacid.

INDICATIONS: Tablets: For the treatment of duodenal and non-malignant gastric ulcer.

Also indicated for the prophylaxis of duodenal ulcer recurrence.

Suspension: For the treatment of duodenal ulcer and for the prophylaxis of gastrointestinal hemorrhage due to stress ulceration in critically ill patients.

CONTRAINDICATIONS: There are no known contraindications to the use of SULCRATE. However, the physician should read the Warnings section when considering the use of this drug in pregnant or pediatric patients, or patients of childbearing potential.

WARNINGS: *Pregnancy:* There has been no experience to date with the use of SULCRATE in pregnant women. Therefore, sucralfate should not be used in pregnant women or women of childbearing potential unless, in the judgment of the physician, the anticipated benefits outweigh the potential risk.

Children: Clinical experience in children is limited. Therefore, sucralfate therapy cannot be recommended for children under 18 unless, in the judgment of the physician, anticipated benefits outweigh the potential risk.

PRECAUTIONS: General: The following should be taken into account before treating patients with SULCRATE:

Recurrence may be observed in patients after a successful course of treatment for gastric or duodenal ulcers. While treatment with sucralfate can result in complete healing of the ulcer, a successful course of treatment with sucralfate should not be expected to alter the underlying cause of ulcer disease.

Proper diagnosis is important since symptomatic response to sucralfate therapy does not rule out the presence of a gastric malignancy.

Isolated reports of sucralfate tablet aspiration with accompanying respiratory complications have been received. Therefore, sucralfate tablets should be used with caution by patients who have known conditions that may impair swallowing, such as recent or prolonged intubation, tracheostomy, prior history of aspiration, dysphagia, or any other conditions that may alter gag and cough reflexes, or diminish oropharyngeal coordination or motility.

Drug Interactions: Antacids should not be taken within half an hour before or after sucralfate intake because of the possibility of decreased binding of sucralfate with the gastroduodenal mucosa as a consequence of a change of intragastric pH.

Animal studies have shown that simultaneous administration of sucralfate with tetracycline, phenytoin or cimetidine results in a statistically significant reduction in the bioavailability of these agents. Cimetidine absorption was not reduced in humans.

In clinical trials, the concomitant administration of sucralfate reduced the bioavailability of digoxin. In case of simultaneous administration, the extent of absorption of phenytoin, warfarin and fluoroquinolone antibiotics (e.g. ciprofloxacin and norfloxacin) is also reduced. These interactions appear to be nonsystemic and to result from the binding of sucralfate to the concomitantly administered drug in the gastrointestinal tract. In all cases, complete bioavailability was restored by separating the administration of sucralfate from that of the other agent by 2 hours.

Sucralfate, administered respectively 30 and 60 minutes before ASA or ibuprofen did not alter the bioavailability of these agents. In a study comparing the prior administration of a single dose of sucralfate tablets on the bioavailability of naproxen, indomethacin or ketoprofen versus administration in the absence of sucralfate, it was shown that the total amount of these drugs absorbed was not altered; however, the peak concentration of each was reduced, and the time to reach peak concentration was delayed. A single dose of SULCRATE Suspension Plus administered one-half hour before naproxen had a similar effect on the bioavailability of naproxen.

The physician should consider the possible clinical implications of these interactions. It is recommended to separate the administration of any drug from that of sucralfate when the potential for altered bioavailability is felt to be critical to the effectiveness of that drug.

Unless specified, the above data are based on studies carried out with SULCRATE tablets.

Chronic Renal Failure: Dialyzed Patients: Sucralfate should be used with caution in patients with chronic renal failure. When sucralfate is administered orally, small amounts of aluminum are absorbed from the gastrointestinal tract (see Pharmacology). Existing evidence indicates that patients with normal renal function receiving the recommended doses of sucralfate adequately excrete aluminum in the urine; however, patients with chronic renal failure or those receiving dialysis have impaired excretion of absorbed aluminum, and in these individuals, aluminum is known to accumulate in serum and in tissues. In particular, dialysis patients are at greater risk as aluminum does not cross dialysis membranes of the dialysis machine since it is bound to plasma proteins, most notably albumin and transferrin.

In patients with chronic renal failure undergoing dialysis, aluminum-related toxicity (encephalopathy and aluminum-related bone disease), associated with the administration of sucralfate and/or other sources of aluminum has been reported. Consideration should therefore be given to the total daily load of aluminum before administering sucralfate in combination with other aluminum-containing medications, such as aluminum-containing antacids.

Nondialyzed Patients: In a study of 6 nondialyzed chronic renal failure patients with glomerular filtration rates ranging from approximately 10 to 40% of normal, sucralfate administered at a dose of 1 g QID for 3 weeks resulted in elevated serum aluminum concentrations which plateaued at approximately 23 µg/L after 1 week of treatment from a pretreatment level of 3 µg/L. Renal aluminum clearance increased in relation to the increase in serum levels and returned to baseline within 2 weeks following discontinuation of sucralfate as did serum aluminum concentrations. No adverse events were reported in these patients.

These data indicate that the use of sucralfate in nondialyzed chronic renal failure patients requires physician discretion since the excretion of absorbed aluminum may be impaired in these individuals.

ADVERSE EFFECTS: Tablets: Very few side effects have been reported with SULCRATE (sucralfate) tablets. They are mild in nature and have only exceptionally led to discontinuation of therapy.

The main complaint has been constipation ranging from 1.7% to 3.3% of patients.

Other side effects reported included diarrhea, nausea, gastric discomfort, indigestion, dry mouth, skin rash, pruritus, back pain, dizziness, sleepiness and vertigo.

Bezoars have been reported in patients treated with sucralfate (SULCRATE tablets). The majority of patients had underlying medical conditions that may predispose to bezoar formation (such as delayed gastric emptying) or were receiving concomitant enteral tube feedings.

Suspension Plus: In a placebo-controlled clinical trial involving 184 patients, the adverse event rates for SULCRATE SUSPENSION PLUS were similar to that seen in the placebo group (SULCRATE SUSPENSION PLUS 10.2% vs placebo 7.4%). The most common adverse event was headache (3.4%), followed by nausea (2.3%), abdominal pain (2.3%), constipation (1.1%), diarrhea (1.1%), and urticaria (1.1%). Only headache, abdominal pain and nausea had a higher incidence in the SULCRATE SUSPENSION PLUS group relative to placebo.

Bezoars have also been reported in patients treated with sucralfate (SULCRATE SUSPENSION PLUS). The majority of patients had underlying medical conditions that may predispose to bezoar formation (such as delayed gastric emptying) or were receiving concomitant enteral tube feedings.

See Precautions for information on the potential for aluminum toxicity in dialyzed chronic renal failure patients.

OVERDOSE:

Symptoms: Overdosage has never been observed with SULCRATE (sucralfate) and appears to be unlikely since, using maximal doses of up to 12 g/kg/body weight in a variety of animal species, a lethal dose could not be established.

Overdosage is likely to be associated with symptoms similar to those described in Adverse Effects, such as constipation. These should be treated symptomatically.

Treatment: See Symptoms.

For management of a suspected drug overdose, CPhA recommends that you contact your **regional Poison Control Centre**. See the *CPS* Directory section for a list of Poison Control Centres.

DOSAGE: Tablets: Duodenal and gastric ulcers: Adults: One tablet of 1 g 4 times daily, 1 hour before meals and at bedtime, on an empty stomach. For duodenal ulcer, SULCRATE may also be administered as two 1 g tablets twice daily, on waking and at bedtime on an empty stomach.

In duodenal ulcers, while healing with SULCRATE often occurs within 2 to 4 weeks, treatment should be continued for a maximum of 8 to 12 weeks unless healing has been demonstrated by x-ray and/or endoscopic examination.

In the case of gastric ulcers, an alternative treatment should be considered if no objective improvement is observed following 6 weeks of SULCRATE therapy. However, patients with a large gastric ulcer that has demonstrated a progressive healing tendency may require an additional 6 weeks of treatment.

For the prophylaxis of duodenal ulcer recurrence, the recommended dosage is 1 tablet of 1 g twice daily, on an empty stomach. Treatment may be continued for up to 1 year.

For relief of pain, antacids may be added to the treatment. However, antacids should not be taken within ½ hour before or after SULCRATE intake.

Suspension Plus (1 g/5 mL): Adults: (Acute) duodenal ulcer: 2 g (10 mL) twice a day on waking and at bedtime on an empty stomach.

Prophylaxis of gastrointestinal hemorrhage due to stress ulceration: 1 g (5 mL) orally or via nasogastric tube 4 to 6 times a day. To prevent clogging of the nasogastric tube flush with 10 mL of water following each administration.

The duration of treatment for prophylaxis of stress ulceration must be individually determined. Treatment should be continued for as long as one or more of the risk factors for stress ulceration is present but normally not for more than 14 days.

Duration of continuous treatment in patients with chronic renal failure receiving dialysis should be evaluated by periodic monitoring of serum aluminum levels, due to the possibility of aluminum accumulation in these patients (see Precautions). According to information widely available in the literature, patients with serum aluminum concentrations that approach 100 µg/L should be carefully monitored for symptoms of aluminum toxicity and treatment should be discontinued if such symptoms appear.

There is no evidence to indicate that patients with chronic renal failure, who do not require dialysis, are at risk of developing aluminum toxicity while receiving the recommended doses of sucralfate. Physician discretion should be exercised when considering the duration of treatment (see Precautions).

SUPPLIED: Tablets: Each white, capsule-shaped, biconvex tablet, embossed on one side with SULCRATE and debossed on the other side with HMR, contains: sucralfate 1 g. Nonmedicinal ingredients: calcium carboxymethylcellulose, hydrogenated vegetable oil, magnesium stearate and microcrystalline cellulose. Bottles of 100. Store and dispense in a well-closed container. **Suspension Plus:** Each 5 mL of off-white, creamy suspension with a caramel odor contains: sucralfate 1 g. Nonmedicinal ingredients: artificial caramel flavor, glycerin, sodium methylparaben, sodium phosphate monobasic, sodium propylparaben and xanthan gum. Bottles of 500 mL. Shake well before using. Store at room temperature. Avoid freezing.

(Shown in Product Identification Section)

Sulfacet-R® ℞

sulfacetamide sodium—sulfur

Acne Therapy

sanofi-aventis

Date of Revision: October 29, 2009

INDICATIONS: Severe acne vulgaris, seborrheic dermatitis, bacterial folliculitis and related conditions.

CONTRAINDICATIONS: Hypersensitivity to the sulfonamides as indicated by a previous toxic reaction to them (e.g. agranulocytosis, acute hemolytic anemia, purpura hemorrhagica, drug fever, jaundice, or contact dermatitis).

PRECAUTIONS: Sulfur may cause reddening and scaling of the epidermis, but if undue skin irritation develops or increases, discontinue use and consult a physician. Keep away from eyes.

OVERDOSE:

For management of a suspected drug overdose, CPhA recommends that you contact your **regional Poison Control Centre**. See the *CPS* Directory section for a list of Poison Control Centres.

DOSAGE: For external use only. Keep away from eyes. Shake lotion well. Apply a small quantity with fingertips 2 or 3 times daily.

SUPPLIED: Each mL of lotion contains: Sodium sulfacetamide 10% w/v, colloidal sulfur 5% w/v. Nonmedicinal ingredients: 2-bromo-2-nitropropane-1,3-diol (Bronopol), attapulgite, butylparaben, diethanolamine, hydroxyethyl cellulose, iron oxides, lauric myristic, methylparaben, naphthalene sulfonic acid, polyethylene glycol monolaurate, precipitated sulfur, propylene glycol, purified water, silicone emulsion, sodium chloride, sodium metabisulfite, talc, xanthan gum and zinc oxide. Bottles of 25 g.

Sulfamethoxazole–Trimethoprim ℞

Antibacterial

CPhA Monograph

Date of Preparation: November 2005

This monograph has been compiled by CPhA and reviewed by experts. It may contain information different from that found in Health Canada-approved Product Monographs. The reader is referred to the *CPS* Editorial Policy for more information.

SUMMARY PRODUCT INFORMATION:

Route of Administration	Dosage Form	Product Strength
Oral	Tablets	Regular strength: sulfamethoxazole 400 mg and trimethoprim 80 mg Double strength (DS): sulfamethoxazole 800 mg and trimethoprim 160 mg
	Suspension	Sulfamethoxazole 40 mg/mL and trimethoprim 8 mg/mL
Intravenous	Solution for injection	Sulfamethoxazole 80 mg/mL and trimethoprim 16 mg/mL

INDICATIONS AND CLINICAL USE: Sulfamethoxazole-trimethoprim is used in the treatment of urinary tract infections, upper and lower respiratory tract infections, gastrointestinal tract infections (including cholera and bacillary dysentery), and skin and soft tissue infections when caused by susceptible organisms. Sulfamethoxazole-trimethoprim is also indicated for treatment of brucellosis, mycetoma, nocardiosis and South American blastomycosis. Selected bacteria against which sulfamethoxazole-trimethoprim has been effective are listed in Table 1.

Sulfamethoxazole-trimethoprim is a drug of choice for the treatment of *Pneumocystis carinii* pneumonia (PCP). It is also used for both primary and secondary prophylaxis of PCP in immunocompromised individuals at increased risk (e.g., some HIV-positive patients). In addition, many clinicians consider it a first-line treatment for acute exacerbations of chronic bronchitis or chronic obstructive pulmonary disease in low risk patients (FEV_1 >50% predicted, fewer than 4 exacerbations per year and no significant cardiac disease) and for acute infective exacerbations of bronchiectasis that do not involve Pseudomonas species.

Sulfamethoxazole-trimethoprim is the drug of choice for treatment of infections caused by cyclospora (*C. cayetanensis*), *S. maltophilia* and *I. belli*. It is also effective against *L. pneumophila* and *L. monocytogenes*, though it is not the antibiotic of choice for infections due to either organism.

Some clinicians state that sulfamethoxazole-trimethoprim may be used as empiric treatment of community-acquired infectious diarrhea in children, pending results of fecal testing, if there is evidence of inflammation (fever, tenesmus, dysentery, fecal leukocytes or lactoferrin) and the diarrhea is not thought to be due to Shiga toxin-producing *E. coli*. The use of sulfamethoxazole-trimethoprim for the treatment of travellers' diarrhea and/or shigellosis is limited by high rates of resistance worldwide.

Sulfamethoxazole-trimethoprim, alone or with clindamycin, may be used to treat moderate to severe infection of bite wounds (cat, dog, wild animal, human) in patients who are allergic to beta-lactam antibiotics.

Sulfamethoxazole-trimethoprim may be used to treat acute sinusitis in adults and children. However, its usefulness is limited by increased resistance rates in *S. pneumoniae* and *H. influenzae*. For this reason, many clinicians consider it a second-line drug for this indication.

Sulfamethoxazole-trimethoprim (IV) is considered by some clinicians to be a second-line drug for the treatment of bacterial meningitis in adults over 50 years of age or with alcoholism and/or other debilitating illnesses. Sulfamethoxazole-trimethoprim has also been used to treat acute otitis media in children but its role has been limited by increased resistance rates in *S. pneumoniae* and *H. influenzae*. It is also considered by some clinicians to be a third-line drug for treatment of pertussis (whooping cough).

Sulfamethoxazole-trimethoprim was formerly a drug of choice for the treatment of typhoid fever. Fluoroquinolones are now considered the drugs of choice for typhoid, partly due to increasing resistance to sulfamethoxazole-trimethoprim in some parts of the world. Sulfamethoxazole-trimethoprim may still be used in areas where resistance is not a concern and where fluoroquinolones are either not available or not affordable. It can also be used to eradicate the causative organism (*S. typhii*) from the gastrointestinal tract.

Sulfamethoxazole-trimethoprim has been used as part of the treatment regimen for Whipple's disease and for the treatment of granuloma inguinale (donovanosis).

Table 1: Sulfamethoxazole–Trimethoprim

Selected organisms against which sulfamethoxazole-trimethoprim has been effective[a]

Gram-negative organisms	*E. aerogenes, E. coli, H. influenzae*, Klebsiella species, *N. gonorrhoeae, P. mirabilis, P. vulgaris, S. maltophilia*, Salmonella species, Shigella species[b], *V. cholerae*
Gram-positive organisms	*L. monocytogenes, S. aureus, S. albus, S. pneumoniae, S. pyogenes, S. viridans, T. whippelii*
Other organisms	*B. malitensis, C. cayetanensis, I. belli, L. pneumophila, N. asteroides, N. brasiliensis, P. brasiliensis, P. carinii, S. somaliensis, T. gondii*

[a] Resistance to sulfamethoxazole-trimethoprim has appeared or increased in some species, including *S. pneumoniae* and *H. influenzae*.
[b] Widespread resistance.

Though sulfamethoxazole-trimethoprim is approved for the treatment of uncomplicated gonococcal urethritis, it is no longer included in Canadian treatment recommendations for the treatment of gonorrhea.

Sulfamethoxazole-trimethoprim is not as effective as penicillin for the treatment of streptococcal pharyngitis and should not be used for this indication. It is also not effective for the treatment of viral infections, or infections caused by Pseudomonas or Mycoplasma species.

Pediatrics: Sulfamethoxazole-trimethoprim is indicated for the treatment of infants and children diagnosed with *P. carinii* pneumonitis, especially if they are immunosuppressed.

CONTRAINDICATIONS:

- Patients who are hypersensitive to sulfamethoxazole-trimethoprim or to any ingredient in the formulation or component of the container. However, cautious desensitization has been performed in selected patients in whom therapy with sulfamethoxazole-trimethoprim was deemed essential and in whom the benefit of continued therapy was thought to outweigh the risk of adverse effects.
- Documented megaloblastic anemia.
- Marked hepatic parenchymal damage.
- Blood dyscrasias.
- Porphyria, since sulfonamides may precipitate an acute attack.
- Severe renal function impairment when renal status cannot be monitored during therapy.
- Infants less than 2 months of age, since it may cause jaundice, hemolytic anemia and, theoretically, kernicterus. However, in exceptional circumstances, sulfamethoxazole-trimethoprim has been used in this age group.

WARNINGS AND PRECAUTIONS:

> **Serious Warnings and Precautions**
> - Rarely, death has occurred due to serious adverse effects of sulfamethoxazole-trimethoprim. These adverse effects have included Stevens-Johnson syndrome, toxic epidermal necrolysis, fulminant hepatic necrosis, agranulocytosis, aplastic anemia, other blood dyscrasias and hypersensitivity of the respiratory tract. Patients receiving sulfamethoxazole-trimethoprim should be monitored for signs and symptoms of such reactions (e.g., rash, sore throat, fever, pallor, arthralgia, cough, shortness of breath, purpura or jaundice) and the drug should be discontinued immediately if these occur.

General: Patients should be instructed to report any rash, fever, sore throat, pallor, cough, shortness of breath, arthralgia, jaundice or purpura, as these may be early signs and symptoms of serious adverse reactions.

Sulfamethoxazole-trimethoprim should be used with caution in patients with impaired renal or hepatic function, severe allergy or bronchial asthma or possible G-6-PD deficiency.

Sulfamethoxazole-trimethoprim should also be used with caution in those at higher risk of folate deficiency (e.g., geriatric patients, alcoholics, those taking anticonvulsants, the malnourished, those with malabsorption syndrome). The manufacturers recommend that complete blood counts be obtained regularly in these patients, as well as those on long-term therapy. Sulfamethoxazole-trimethoprim should be discontinued and leucovorin (folinic acid) administered if bone marrow suppression (e.g., megaloblastic anemia, neutropenia, thrombocytopenia) occurs. Suggested leucovorin doses range from 5 to15 mg/day; treatment should be continued until hematopoiesis returns to normal.

Patients with AIDS appear to have a particularly high risk of adverse effects due to sulfamethoxazole-trimethoprim (especially fever and hematologic and dermatologic reactions) and should be carefully monitored.

Patients should be instructed to maintain an adequate fluid intake to prevent crystalluria and stone formation. Some references suggest that urinalysis and renal function tests be performed weekly to detect any renal complications. This may be particularly important in patients with reduced renal function.

Local irritation and inflammation may result from extravascular infiltration of sulfamethoxazole-trimethoprim injection. If extravascular infiltration occurs, discontinue the infusion and restart at another site.

Endocrine and Metabolism: Hemolysis may occur if sulfamethoxazole-trimethoprim is administered to individuals who are G-6-PD deficient. This reaction is frequently dose-related.

Serum potassium should be monitored in patients at risk of hyperkalemia.

Gastrointestinal: Pseudomembranous colitis should be considered in the differential diagnosis of patients who develop diarrhea during treatment with sulfamethoxazole-trimethoprim.

Hematologic: Serious hematologic effects have occurred secondary to use of sulfamethoxazole-trimethoprim (see Warnings and Precautions, General).

Sulfonamides may precipitate an acute attack of porphyria in susceptible individuals.

Hepatic/Biliary/Pancreatic: Use sulfamethoxazole-trimethoprim with caution in patients with hepatic dysfunction. Dosage adjustment may be required.

Immune: Severe hypersensitivity reactions have occurred during treatment with sulfamethoxazole-trimethoprim, including Stevens-Johnson syndrome, toxic epidermal necrolysis, fulminant hepatic failure and blood dyscrasias. In some cases, these have resulted in death. See Warnings and Precautions, General for more information.

Use with caution in patients with a history of hypersensitivity to sulfonamide-derivatives such as acetazolamide, thiazide diuretics or tolbutamide.

Sulfamethoxazole-trimethoprim injectable may contain sodium metabisulfite as a preservative. This agent may provoke an allergic reaction in individuals who are hypersensitive to sulfites.

Renal: Dosage adjustment is recommended when sulfamethoxazole-trimethoprim is used in patients with reduced renal function in order to avoid accumulation of trimethoprim in the blood (see Table 6). Some references suggest avoiding sulfamethoxazole-trimethoprim if the creatinine clearance is estimated to be less than 10 mL/minute unless plasma concentrations of trimethoprim are monitored, while others do not.

Sexual Function/Reproduction: Combinations of trimethoprim and sulfonamides have been reported to decrease sperm counts by 7 to 88% after one month of continuous therapy. It has been postulated that trimethoprim deprives the spermatogeneic cells of folate by inhibiting dihydrofolate reductase.

Skin: Rash is a relatively common adverse effect of sulfamethoxazole-trimethoprim therapy. In many cases it is benign, but it may be an early sign of severe, potentially fatal, adverse reactions. See Warnings and Precautions, General for more information. Sulfamethoxazole-trimethoprim should be discontinued at the first sign of rash.

Photosensitivity reactions can occur. Advise patients to avoid sun exposure, use sunscreen and wear protective clothing.

Special Populations: Pregnant Women: Both trimethoprim and sulfamethoxazole cross the placenta. Trimethoprim levels are similar in maternal and fetal serum and in amniotic fluid. Sulfamethoxazole levels in fetal serum are 70 to 90% of maternal serum levels.

Sulfonamides as a group do not appear to pose a significant teratogenic risk. Trimethoprim use during the first trimester may be associated with structural defects. One study using data from a large, multicentre, case-control surveillance program for birth defects found an increased risk of cardiovascular defects if trimethoprim was taken in the second or third month of pregnancy (relative risk 4.2). Risk of neural tube defects was also increased. The use of multivitamins containing folate attenuated the increase in risk of both types of defect.

Significant levels of sulfamethoxazole may persist in neonatal circulation for several days after delivery if given near term. This may cause jaundice, hemolytic anemia and, theoretically, kernicterus in the neonate. Because of the potential toxicity to the newborn, sulfamethoxazole-trimethoprim should be avoided near term.

Nursing Women: Both trimethoprim and sulfamethoxazole are excreted into breast milk in low concentrations. Sulfonamide excretion into breast milk does not appear to pose a significant risk for the healthy, full-term neonate. However, sulfonamides should be avoided if the infant is ill, stressed or premature or has hyperbilirubinemia or G-6-PD deficiency. The American Academy of Pediatrics considers the combination of trimethoprim and sulfamethoxazole generally compatible with breast-feeding.

Pediatrics: Sulfamethoxazole-trimethoprim is generally contraindicated in infants under 2 months of age because of the risk of sulfamethoxazole-induced jaundice, hemolytic anemia or, theoretically, kernicterus. However, in exceptional circumstances its use may be justified.

The safety of repeated courses of sulfamethoxazole-trimethoprim in children under 2 years of age who do not have PCP has not been fully evaluated.

Folate depletion may worsen the psychomotor regression sometimes seen with fragile X chromosome associated with delayed mental development. Therefore, caution is advised when administering sulfamethoxazole-trimethoprim to children with this disorder.

Geriatrics: Elderly patients may have an increased risk of severe adverse reactions to sulfamethoxazole-trimethoprim. This may be especially true if complicating conditions exist (e.g., impaired renal or hepatic function, concomitant use of interacting drugs). The most frequently reported severe adverse reactions in this population are dermatologic reactions, generalized bone marrow suppression and thrombocytopenia.

Monitoring and Laboratory Tests: Renal function tests and urinalysis should be performed in patients with renal dysfunction. Some clinicians recommend these also be performed weekly in all patients. The complete blood count should be monitored in those at higher risk of folate deficiency (see Warnings and Precautions, General) or during long-term therapy. Serum potassium should be monitored in those at risk of hyperkalemia.

ADVERSE REACTIONS: Overview: Although sulfamethoxazole-trimethoprim is generally well-tolerated, rarely deaths have been associated with hypersensitivity reactions, fulminant hepatocellular necrosis, agranulocytosis, aplastic anemia or other blood dyscrasias.

More Common Adverse Drug Reactions (≥1%): See Table 2.

Table 2: Sulfamethoxazole–Trimethoprim

More Common Adverse Drug Reactions (≥1%)

Body System	Effect	Clinical Comment
Gastrointestinal (3–4%)	Nausea, vomiting, anorexia	Incidence and severity are generally dose related.
Dermatologic/immunologic (3–4%)	Sensitivity reactions (e.g., rash, urticaria)	

Less Common Adverse Drug Reactions (<1%): Body as a Whole: Chills and myalgia have occurred.

Cardiovascular: Hypotension and periarteritis nodosa have been reported.

Central Nervous System: Apathy, ataxia, fatigue, muscle weakness, headache, insomnia, vertigo, tinnitus, peripheral neuritis, mental depression, nervousness, aseptic meningitis, seizures and hallucinations have occurred during therapy with sulfamethoxazole-trimethoprim.

Dermatologic: See Adverse Effects, Immunologic.

Endocrine: Hypoglycemia has been reported.

Fluid and Electrolyte: Diuresis and hyperkalemia have been reported.

Gastrointestinal: Abdominal pain, diarrhea, glossitis, pancreatitis (sometimes fatal), pseudomembranous enterocolitis and stomatitis have occurred.

Hematologic: The following reactions have rarely been reported: aplastic anemia, agranulocytosis, eosinophilia, hypoprothrombinemia, leukopenia, neutropenia, methemoglobinemia, pancytopenia, thrombocytopenia, purpura, megaloblastic and/or hemolytic anemia. These reactions may occur more frequently in folate-depleted patients (i.e., those who are geriatric, malnourished, alcoholic, pregnant, debilitated); patients receiving folate antimetabolites (e.g., phenytoin) or diuretics; patients treated with hemodialysis or with impaired renal dysfunction; patients receiving high doses and/or prolonged courses (>6 months).

Immunologic: Immunologic adverse effects include anaphylaxis, drug fever, serum sickness, arthralgia, lupus erythematosus phenomenon, allergic myocarditis, periorbital edema, corneal ring infiltrates, conjunctival and scleral injection. Immune-mediated skin reactions include epidermal necrolysis, exfoliative dermatitis, Stevens-Johnson syndrome, erythema multiforme, Schönlein-Henoch purpura, pruritus, urticaria, photosensitivity.

When mild-moderate rashes occur, it is usually after 7 to 14 days of therapy. These are usually erythematous, maculopapular, morbilloform and/or pruritic. Generalized pustular dermatosis and fixed drug eruption have also been reported. Patients with AIDS are at increased risk of rash, which is usually diffuse, erythematous and maculopapular.

Musculoskeletal: Rhabdomyolysis has rarely been reported.

DRUG INTERACTIONS: Overview: If sulfamethoxazole-trimethoprim is administered concomitantly with drugs that form cations at normal physiologic pH and are also partly excreted by active renal secretion, plasma concentrations of one or both drugs may be increased.

Folic acid may be administered during therapy with sulfamethoxazole-trimethoprim without interfering with the latter's antibacterial effect.

Drug-Drug Interactions: See Table 3.

Table 3: Sulfamethoxazole–Trimethoprim

Drug-Drug Interactions

Interacting Drug	Effect	Clinical Comment
ACE inhibitors	Combined use may increase risk of hyperkalemia.	Monitor serum potassium and renal function, especially if there are other co-existing risk factors for hyperkalemia such as diabetes mellitus or pre-existing renal dysfunction.
Antidiabetic agents (oral)	Sulfamethoxazole-trimethoprim may increase serum concentrations of some oral antidiabetic agents (e.g., glyburide, glipizide, chlorpropamide, tolbutamide).	Monitor for hypoglycemia.
Cyclosporine	Sulfamethoxazole-trimethoprim may decrease the serum concentration of cyclosporine. Risk of nephrotoxicity may also be increased.	Avoid co-administration if possible. If not, monitor cyclosporine levels and serum creatinine closely.

(cont'd)

Table 3: Sulfamethoxazole–Trimethoprim *(cont'd)*

Drug-Drug Interactions

Interacting Drug	Effect	Clinical Comment
Dapsone	Serum concentrations of both drugs may increase, possibly leading to increased toxicity from either agent.	Monitor for signs and symptoms of toxicity.
Dofetilide	Serum concentrations of dofetilide may be increased during concomitant therapy with sulfamethoxazole-trimethoprim, increasing risk of ventricular arrhythmias, including torsades de pointes.	Avoid this combination.
Lamivudine	The AUC of lamivudine is increased by approximately 44% during concomitant therapy with sulfamethoxazole-trimethoprim.	Dosage alteration unneccessary, since increased lamivudine concentrations unlikely to have toxic effects.
Methotrexate	The risk of methotrexate-induced bone marrow suppression may be increased. Methotrexate may increase the risk of sulfamethoxazole-trimethoprim-induced megaloblastic anemia.	If concomitant treatment is necessary, monitor patients closely for signs of hematologic toxicity. Leucovorin may be helpful for treating any resulting neutropenia or megaloblastic anemia.
Metronidazole	Co-administration with injectable sulfamethoxazole-trimethoprim may result in a disulfarim-like reaction due to the ethanol content of the sulfamethoxazole-trimethoprim formulation.	Does not occur with oral sulfamethoxazole-trimethoprim.
Warfarin	At the beginning of combination therapy, the INR may increase due to decreased metabolism of warfarin. When sulfamethoxazole-trimethoprim is discontinued, the opposite effect will occur.	If possible, avoid combination by using another antibiotic or substituting heparin for warfarin. If the combination is used, monitor the patient's INR carefully at the beginning and end of sulfamethoxazole-trimethoprim therapy and adjust doses of warfarin as needed .

Drug-Laboratory Interactions: May result in overestimation (approximately 10% in the normal range) of serum creatinine when measured with the Jaffe alkaline picrate reaction assay. Also may interfere with measurement of serum methotrexate levels as determined by the competitive binding protein technique when bacterial dihydrofolate reductase is used as a binding protein. This does not occur when methotrexate is measured by radioimmunoassay.

DOSAGE AND ADMINISTRATION: Dosing Considerations: IV: Serious systemic infections, adults: The dose depends on the severity of infection. A dose of trimethoprim 160 to 240 mg and sulfamethoxazole 800 to 1200 mg may be given every 6, 8 or 12 hours. For doses for specific indications, see Table 4.

IV: Serious systemic infections, children: The recommended daily dose for children in general is trimethoprim 5 to 10 mg/kg/day and sulfamethoxazole 25 to 50 mg/kg/day. For doses for specific indications, see Table 5.

Recommended Dose and Dosage Adjustment: Adults: See Table 4.

Table 4: Sulfamethoxazole–Trimethoprim

Dose in Adult Patients

Indication	Usual Dose	Duration of Treatment	Clinical Comment
Acute UTI (female, >12 years old, uncomplicated) or asymptomatic bacteriuria associated with pregnancy[a]	Sulfamethoxazole 800 mg and trimethoprim 160 mg BID PO	3 days	
Recurrent cystitis (female, recurrence <1 month)	Sulfamethoxazole 800 mg + trimethoprim 160 mg BID PO	10–14 days	
Recurrent cystitis (female, frequent recurrence)	Sulfamethoxasole 400 mg + trimethoprim 80 mg PO QHS, daily or postcoitally	Reassess after 6 months of therapy	If less than 3 recurrences annually, an alternative is short-course self-treatment.
Acute cystitis, pregnant woman[a]	Sulfamethoxazole 800 mg + trimethoprim 160 mg BID PO	3 days	Second-line therapy. Follow-up cultures should be obtained.
Complicated UTI	Sulfamethoxazole 800 mg + trimethoprim 160 mg BID PO	10–14 days	Includes structural abnormalities or any UTI in men. Patients with indwelling catheters should not be treated unless there is evidence of systemic infection.
Pyelonephritis	Sulfamethoxazole 800 mg + trimethoprim 160 mg BID PO IV: 5–10 mg/kg (trimethoprim component) Q6–12H	10–14 days	
Acute prostatitis (mild to moderate)	Sulfamethoxazole 800 mg + trimethoprim 160 mg BID PO	2–4 weeks	

(cont'd)

Table 4: Sulfamethoxazole–Trimethoprim *(cont'd)*

Dose in Adult Patients

Indication	Usual Dose	Duration of Treatment	Clinical Comment
P. carinii pneumonia (treatment)	PO: 15–20 mg/kg/day (trimethoprim component) in 3 or 4 divided doses IV: 10–15 mg/kg/day	14–21 days	
P. carinii pneumonia (primary and secondary prophylaxis)	160 mg (trimethoprim component) PO once daily		
Chronic prostatitis	Sulfamethoxazole 800 mg + trimethoprim 160 mg BID PO	4–6 weeks	Second-line treatment
Meningitis (selected patients)	IV: 10–20 mg/kg/day (trimethoprim component) divided Q6–12H	Optimal duration of treatment uncertain. 7–28 days depending on causative pathogen	Second-line treatment for select group of patients. See Indications and Clinical Use for more information.
Sinusitis	Sulfamethoxazole 800 mg + trimethoprim 160 mg BID PO	10–14 days	Second-line treatment
Acute exacerbations of COPD	Sulfamethoxazole 800 mg + trimethoprim 160 mg BID PO	7–10 days	See Indications and Clinical Use for more information on selection of suitable patients.
Pertussis	Sulfamethoxazole 800 mg + trimethoprim 160 mg BID PO	10–14 days	Third line treatment. To be of benefit, treatment must be started within 3 weeks of symptom onset.
Soft-tissue infections	Sulfamethoxazole 800 mg + trimethoprim 160 mg BID PO	10–14 days	
Treatment of Nocardia infections	640 mg/day PO (trimethoprim component)	Months	Consult specialized references for more information.
Treatment of isosporiasis	160 mg (trimethoprim component) PO QID	10 days	
Treatment of Cyclospora infections	160 mg (trimethoprim component) PO BID	7–10 days	HIV-infected patients may require higher dosage and longer-term therapy.
Cholera (treatment)	Sulfamethoxazole 800 mg+ trimethoprim 160 mg BID PO	3 days	Resistance to sulfamethoxazole-trimethoprim present in some areas. Use in conjunction with fluid and electrolyte replacement.

[a] See Warnings and Precautions, Pregnant Women for more information on use of sulfamethoxazole-trimethoprim in pregnancy.

Pediatrics: See Table 5.

Table 5: Sulfamethoxazole–trimethoprim

Dose in Pediatric Patients

Indication	Usual Dose	Duration of Treatment	Clinical Comment
Acute UTI	5–10 mg/kg/day (trimethoprim component) divided q12h PO	7–10 days	
Acute otitis media	5–10 mg/kg/day (trimethoprim component) divided BID PO	If >2 years old and uncomplicated UTI: 5 days If <2 years old or complicated UTI: 10 days	Third-line treatment
Acute sinusitis	5–10 mg/kg/day (trimethoprim component) divided BID PO	10–14 days	Third-line treatment
P. carinii pneumonia (treatment)	PO: 15–20 mg/kg/day (trimethoprim component) in 3 or 4 divided doses	14–21 days	
P. carinii pneumonia (primary and secondary prophylaxis)	PO: 150 mg/m^2 daily in 2 divided doses for 3 consecutive days each week		Alternate regimens: 150 mg/m^2 daily for 3 consecutive days each week; in 2 divided doses daily, or in 2 divided daily doses 3 times a week on alternate days.
Treatment of isosporiasis	5 mg/kg (trimethoprim component) PO BID	10 days	

(cont'd)

Table 5: Sulfamethoxazole–trimethoprim *(cont'd)*

Dose in Pediatric Patients

Indication	Usual Dose	Duration of Treatment	Clinical Comment
Treatment of Cyclospora infections	5 mg/kg (trimethoprim component) PO BID	7–10 days	HIV-infected patients may require higher dosage and longer-term therapy.
Cholera (treatment)	4–5 mg/kg (trimethoprim component) PO BID	3 days	Resistance to sulfamethoxazole-trimethoprim present in some areas. Use in conjunction with fluid and electrolyte replacement.

Renal Impairment: See Table 6.

Table 6: Sulfamethoxazole-trimethoprim

Dose in Adult Patients with Renal Impairment

Route	Creatinine Clearance	Dose Adjustment	Comments
PO/IV	>25 mL/min	No change	
PO/IV	15–25 mL/min	Half normal dose	Adjust either dose or interval
PO/IV	<15 mL/min	Not routinely recommended.	

Administration:
- Oral dosage forms may be taken with or without food, though food may decrease the incidence of gastrointestinal side effects.
- Oral dosage forms should be taken with a glass of water.
- Oral suspension should be shaken before use.
- Sulfamethoxazole-trimethoprim injection must be diluted in one of the following: Ringer's solution; sodium chloride 0.9% solution; sodium chloride 0.18% + dextrose 4% solution; dextrose 5% solution; dextrose 10% solution; 10% Dextran 40 in sodium chloride 0.9% solution; 10% Dextran 40 in dextrose 5% solution; 6% dextran 70 in sodium chloride 0.9% solution; 6% Dextran 70 in dextrose 5% solution.

  Dilute each 400 mg sulfamethoxazole + 80 mg trimethoprim in 100 to 125 mL of diluent. In cases of fluid restriction, each 400 mg sulfamethoxazole + 80 mg trimethoprim may be diluted in 75 mL sodium chloride 0.9% solution or dextrose 5% solution.
- I.V. solutions of sulfamethoxazole-trimethoprim should be administered over 60 to 90 minutes.
- Avoid rapid or direct i.v. injection. Do not administer i.m.

OVERDOSAGE:

Symptoms: Acute: Signs and symptoms of acute overdose reported with sulfonamides and/or trimethoprim include anorexia, colic, nausea, vomiting, dizziness, headache, mental depression, confusion and bone marrow depression. Pyrexia, hematuria or crystalluria may also be noted. Blood dyscrasias and jaundice are potential late manifestations of acute overdose.

Chronic: Use of sulfamethoxazole-trimethoprim at high doses and/or for extended periods of time may cause bone marrow depression resulting in thrombocytopenia, leukopenia and/or megaloblastic anemia.

> For management of a suspected drug overdose, CPhA recommends that you contact your **regional Poison Control Centre**. See the *CPS* Directory section for a list of Poison Control Centres.

ACTION AND CLINICAL PHARMACOLOGY: Mechanism of Action: Sulfamethoxazole and trimethoprim act on sequential steps in the enzymatic pathway of bacterial synthesis of tetrahydrofolic acid. Sulfamethoxazole competitively inhibits the enzyme tetrahydropteroic acid synthetase, preventing the incorporation of para-aminobenzoic acid (PABA) into tetrahydropteroic acid, the immediate precursor of folic acid. Trimethoprim inhibits the enzyme dihydrofolate reductase, preventing the conversion of dihydrofolic acid into tetrahydrofolic acid. The combination has a synergistic effect. The net result is a decrease in bacterial ability to synthesize thymidine. Sulfamethoxazole alone is bacteriostatic and trimethoprim is bactericidal. The combination of the two is usually bactericidal.

Sulfamethoxazole-trimethoprim is selective for microorganisms for two reasons: (i) mammalian cells are unable to synthesize folic acid and must use dietary folate; (ii) though the reactions catalyzed by dihydrofolate reductase are also essential for mammals, trimethoprim is 50 000 to 100 000 fold more active against bacterial enzyme than against human enzyme.

Pharmacokinetics: Adults: Absorption: Both components of sulfamethoxazole-trimethoprim are rapidly and well absorbed after oral administration. After a single oral dose of sulfamethoxazole 800 mg + trimethoprim 160 mg, blood levels peak in 1 to 4 hours at approximately 40 to 60 µg/mL (sulfamethoxazole) and 1 to 2 µg/mL (trimethoprim) and are sustained for about 7 hours. After repeated intravenous administration of sulfamethoxazole 800 mg + trimethoprim 160 mg, every 8 hours, mean steady state peak concentrations of up to 105 µg/mL (sulfamethoxazole) and 9 µg/mL (trimethoprim) are attained. Steady state trough concentrations under the same conditions are approximately 70 µg/mL (sulfamethoxazole) and 6 µg/mL (trimethoprim).

Distribution: Trimethoprim is approximately 44% and sulfamethoxazole approximately 70% bound to plasma proteins. Trimethoprim is more widely distributed than is sulfamethoxazole with an apparent volume of distribution of 100 to 120 L compared to 12 to 18 L for sulfamethoxazole. Both drugs are distributed into the CNS, with trimethoprim and sulfamethoxazole concentrations of 50% and 40%, respectively, of concurrent serum concentrations. Both drugs are distributed into sputum, aqueous humor, middle ear fluid, prostatic fluid, vaginal fluid and bile. Trimethoprim is also distributed into bronchial secretions.

Sulfamethoxazole-trimethoprim crosses the placenta. Concentrations of trimethoprim and sulfamethoxazole in amniotic fluid are approximately 80 and 50%, respectively, of concurrent maternal serum concentrations. Sulfamethoxazole-trimethoprim is also excreted into breast milk in low concentrations. Concentrations of trimethoprim and sulfamethoxazole in human milk are approximately 125 and 10%, respectively, of concurrent maternal serum concentrations.

Metabolism: Both trimethoprim and sulfamethoxazole undergo hepatic metabolism. Trimethoprim may be metabolized into one of four oxide or hydroxyl derivatives. Sulfamethoxazole is primarily N-acetylated but may also be conjugated with glucuronic acid.

Excretion: The biological half-lives of trimethoprim and sulfamethoxazole are approximately 8 to 11 and 10 to 13 hours respectively. Approximately 40 to 50% of orally ingested trimethoprim is excreted unchanged in the urine within 24 hours. Some trimethoprim is excreted into the bile, but is almost completely reabsorbed so that less than 4% is excreted in the feces. Approximately 60% of orally administered sulfamethoxazole is excreted in the urine within 48 hours.

In adults with creatinine clearances of 10 to 30 mL/min, the serum half-life of trimethoprim may increase to 15 hours. It further increases to over 26 hours if the creatinine clearance is 0 to 10 mL/min. In adults with chronic renal failure, the serum half-life of sulfamethoxazole may triple.

Both trimethoprim and active sulfamethoxazole are moderately removed by hemodialysis.

Special Populations: Pediatrics: Trimethoprim may have a shorter half-life in children. Serum half-lives of about 7.7 and 5.5 hours have been reported in children less than 1 year old and between 1 and 10 years old respectively. Data for sulfamethoxazole are not available.

STORAGE AND STABILITY: Tablets: Store at 15 to 30°C. Protect from light and keep dry.

Suspension: Store at 15 to 25°C. Protect from light and freezing.

Injection: Store at 15 to 30°C. Protect from light.

Sulfapyridine

Antibacterial Sulfonamide

CPhA Monograph

Date of Revision: October 2009

> This monograph has been compiled by CPhA and reviewed by experts. It may contain information different from that found in Health Canada-approved Product Monographs. The reader is referred to the *CPS* Editorial Policy for more information.

SUMMARY PRODUCT INFORMATION:

Drug[a]	Route of Administration	Dosage Form	Strength
Sulfapyridine	Oral	Tablet	500 mg

[a] Sulfapyridine tablets are available through Health Canada's Special Access Programme (see Appendix 2).

PHARMACOLOGY: Sulfapyridine is a sulfonamide antibacterial agent. Sulfonamides are structural analogs of para-aminobenzoic acid and exert their bacteriostatic activity by interfering with folic acid metabolism and ultimately with DNA synthesis in susceptible bacteria. Because of its toxicity (see Warnings), sulfapyridine is used only for dermatitis herpetiformis and related skin disorders when alternate treatment cannot be used.

Pharmacokinetics: Sulfapyridine is slowly and incompletely absorbed from the gastrointestinal tract. It is metabolized in the liver and excreted renally with up to 80% being reabsorbed by the renal tubules. Sulfapyridine readily crosses the placenta and is distributed into CSF and breast milk. It reaches its peak concentration within 4 to 6 hours, has a half-life of 6 to 14 hours and is approximately 50% protein bound.

INDICATIONS: As a second-line agent in the treatment of dermatitis herpetiformis in patients who fail to respond to dapsone.

Sulfapyridine is also used as a second-line agent in the treatment of subcorneal pustular dermatosis, bullous pemphigoid and pyoderma gangrenosum.

CONTRAINDICATIONS: History of hypersensitivity to sulfonamides.

Sulfapyridine should not be used in: patients with G-6-PD deficiency as it may cause hemolytic anemia in this group; patients with porphyria as sulfapyridine may precipitate an acute attack; patients with blood dyscrasias.

WARNINGS: Fatalities have occurred due to severe reactions such as Stevens-Johnson syndrome, toxic epidermal necrolysis, fulminant hepatic necrosis, anaphylaxis and blood dyscrasias such as agranulocytosis and aplastic anemia. Therapy should be stopped at the first sign of skin rash, fever or any serious adverse effect.

Sulfapyridine is known to cause oligospermia and infertility in men.

PRECAUTIONS: Patients taking sulfapyridine should be advised to maintain adequate fluid intake to prevent crystalluria.

Periodic CBCs may be required for patients on long-term therapy, because of the risk of blood dyscrasias.

Sulfapyridine should be used with caution in patients with impaired renal or hepatic function.

Use with caution in patients with a history of hypersensitivity to sulfonamide derivatives such as furosemide, thiazide diuretics, sulfonylureas or carbonic anhydrase inhibitors.

Patients taking sulfapyridine should be monitored for early signs of serious reactions (e.g., sore throat, rash, arthralgia, purpura, shortness of breath).

<u>*Drug Interactions*</u>: Sulfapyridine may inhibit the metabolism of anticoagulants, anticonvulsants, methotrexate or sulfonylureas leading to increased or prolonged therapeutic and toxic effects. Dosage adjustments may be necessary.

Bone Marrow Suppressants or Hepatotoxic Drugs: Concurrent use with sulfapyridine may lead to increased toxic effects.

Pregnancy: Sulfapyridine readily crosses the placenta. The use of sulfapyridine during pregnancy has not been associated with a significant teratogenic risk; however, because it can cause kernicterus in neonates, its use is not recommended late in the 3rd trimester.

Lactation: Sulfapyridine is excreted in breast milk in significant amounts (30 to 60% of serum concentrations). Its use in nursing mothers does not pose a significant risk for most healthy full-term neonates. Exposure to sulfapyridine through breast-feeding should be avoided in premature infants, or infants with hyperbilirubinemia or G-6-PD deficiency.

Drug-Laboratory Test Interactions: Administration of sulfapyridine within 3 days prior to a bentiromide test (for pancreatic insufficiency) may invalidate the results as sulfapyridine is also metabolized to arylamines.

ADVERSE EFFECTS: Endocrine: goiter or thyroid function disturbance.

Gastrointestinal: diarrhea, anorexia, nausea and vomiting are common.

Hematologic: leukopenia, thrombocytopenia, agranulocytosis, aplastic anemia.

Hypersensitivity: skin rash, pruritus, fever and photosensitivity occur more frequently. Hypersensitivity reactions reported less frequently include urticaria, erythema nodosum, Stevens-Johnson syndrome, Lyell's syndrome, Behcet's syndrome, toxic epidermal necrolysis, serum sickness syndrome and hepatitis. Anaphylaxis has been reported rarely (see Warnings).

Renal: crystalluria, hematuria.

OVERDOSE:

Symptoms: Gastrointestinal symptoms such as nausea, vomiting and diarrhea are likely to occur. Other symptoms may include headache and dizziness. Crystalluria, possibly progressing to acute renal failure, can occur with sulfonamide overdose. Methemoglobinemia has occurred with acute overdose and chronic use. Hypersensitivity reactions may also occur (see Adverse Effects).

Treatment: If anaphylaxis occurs, management includes establishment of an open airway, administration of epinephrine and diphenhydramine, cardiac monitoring. Bronchodilators or inotropes may also be required.

Activated charcoal should be administered if a large amount has been ingested. Oxygen or methylene blue may be required if cyanosis and methemoglobinemia occur.

> For management of a suspected drug overdose, CPhA recommends that you contact your **regional Poison Control Centre**. See the *CPS* Directory section for a list of Poison Control Centres.

<u>**DOSAGE:**</u> Sulfapyridine is available through the Special Access Programme, Health Canada (see Appendix 2).

Dermatitis Herpetiformis: Adults: 250 to 1000 mg 4 times daily until improvement occurs. Reduce daily dose by 250 to 500 mg at 3-day intervals until a symptom-free maintenance dose is achieved.

Subcorneal Pustular Dermatosis: Adults: 500 mg twice daily to 750 mg 4 times daily.

Pemphigoid: Adults: 500 mg twice daily to 750 mg 4 times daily.

Pyoderma Gangrenosum: Adults: 1000 or 2000 mg 3 or 4 times daily.

Sulfonylureas

chlorpropamide
gliclazide
glimepiride
glyburide
tolbutamide

Oral Antihyperglycemics

CPhA Monograph

Date of Revision: November 2007

This monograph has been compiled by CPhA and reviewed by experts. It may contain information different from that found in Health Canada-approved Product Monographs. The reader is referred to the *CPS* Editorial Policy for more information.

SUMMARY PRODUCT INFORMATION:

Drug	Route of Administration	Dosage Form	Strength
Chlorpropamide	Oral	Tablet	100 mg, 250 mg
Gliclazide	Oral	Tablet	80 mg
			30 mg extended-release
Glimepiride	Oral	Tablet	1 mg, 2 mg, 4 mg
Glyburide	Oral	Tablet	2.5 mg, 5 mg
Tolbutamide	Oral	Tablet	500 mg

PHARMACOLOGY: Sulfonylurea antihyperglycemic agents stimulate insulin secretion from functioning beta cells of the pancreas. During long-term use, extrapancreatic effects of sulfonylureas (e.g., reduction of basal hepatic glucose production, enhanced peripheral tissue sensitivity to insulin) may contribute to glycemic control.
Pharmacokinetics: See Table 1. Sulfonylureas are readily absorbed from the gastrointestinal tract and are highly bound to plasma proteins (>90%). Sulfonylureas are metabolized in the liver and excreted in the urine and feces. Metabolites of the sulfonylureas do not appear to have clinically significant hypoglycemic effects. The metabolism and excretion of sulfonylureas may be slowed in patients with impaired renal or hepatic function.

Table 1: Sulfonylureas

Pharmacokinetics

Drug	Half-life (hours)	Time to Peak Concentration (hours)	Duration of Action (hours)
Chlorpropamide	36	2–4	24–72
Gliclazide	10	4–6	12–24
Glimepiride	5	2–3	24
Glyburide	10	2–4	18–24
Tolbutamide	4–7	3–4	6–12

INDICATIONS: Sulfonylureas are used alone or in combination with other oral agents or insulin as an adjunct to exercise and diet in the management of type 2 diabetes mellitus.

Sulfonylureas are not approved for the treatment of gestational diabetes mellitus, for which insulin is the treatment of choice [*Diabetes Care* 2007;30(11):2976-9]. Although not approved for this indication, glyburide could be considered to be an alternative to insulin for the treatment of gestational diabetes mellitus in patients who cannot or will not use insulin [*Diabetes Care* 2007;30(11):2980-82], and has been compared with insulin in a randomized trial [*N Engl J Med* 2000; 343:1134-8]. In this study of 404 women with gestational diabetes, there were no significant differences in mean blood glucose concentrations between individuals randomized to glyburide or insulin, and no significant differences in neonatal or maternal outcomes among those exposed to glyburide or insulin. Glyburide was undetectable in serum collected from the umbilical cord after birth. The use of glyburide for gestational diabetes is not a common practice in Canada.

Experience with sulfonylureas in children is limited and the drugs are not approved for use in this population. Glimepiride has been compared with metformin in children aged 8 to 17 years with type 2 diabetes mellitus. Improvement in glycosylated hemoglobin (HbA_{1c}) were similar in the two treatment groups: 42.4% of glimepiride recipients and 48.1% of metformin recipients had HbA_{1c} <7.0% after 24 weeks of treatment. Treatment was well tolerated [*Diabetes Care* 2007;30:790-4].

Glyburide has been used to treat diabetes mellitus in children aged >3 months with mutations (KCNJ11) in the Kir6.2 subunit of the ATP-sensitive potassium channel [*N Engl J Med* 2006;355:467-77].

CONTRAINDICATIONS: Known hypersensitivity or allergy to any of the sulfonylureas; type 1 diabetes mellitus; ketoacidosis; coma; during stress conditions such as severe infections, trauma or surgery; in the presence of severe liver, thyroid or renal impairment.

WARNINGS: Sulfonylureas should be used in conjunction with a proper diet and exercise regimen and not as a substitute for these important measures.

Over a period of time, patients may become progressively less responsive to therapy with oral antihyperglycemic agents. After 5 years of therapy with glyburide, 34% of patients experienced treatment failure in a randomized double-blind study of first-line therapy for patients with newly diagnosed type 2 diabetes mellitus. Treatment failure was defined as a fasting plasma glucose >9.9 mmol/L (>180 mg/dL) on consecutive tests while receiving the maximum dose prescribed by the protocol (7.5 mg twice daily) or tolerated by the patient [*N Engl J Med* 2006;355:2427-43]. Therefore, patients should be monitored with regular clinical and laboratory evaluations, including blood glucose and HbA_{1c} determinations, to determine the minimum effective dosage and to detect primary failure (inadequate lowering of blood glucose concentrations at the maximum recommended dosage) or secondary failure (progressive deterioration in blood sugar control following an initial period of effectiveness). Regular self-monitoring of blood glucose is an integral component of the therapeutic plan for most patients taking sulfonylureas.

The rate of primary failure will vary greatly depending upon patient selection and adherence to diet and exercise. The etiology of secondary failure is multifactorial and may involve progressive beta cell failure as well as exogenous diabetogenic factors such as obesity, illness or drugs, or tolerance to the sulfonylurea. If a loss of adequate blood glucose lowering response to a sulfonylurea is detected, the addition of a drug from a different class may be considered, although insulin is often required. Certain patients who demonstrate an inadequate response or true primary or secondary failure to one sulfonylurea may benefit from a switch to another sulfonylurea.

PRECAUTIONS: The importance of patient education, monitoring and follow-up cannot be overstated. Adequate control of blood sugar is crucial in preventing the microvascular and, perhaps, the macrovascular complications of diabetes.
Hypoglycemic Reactions: Severe hypoglycemia can be induced by all sulfonylureas (see Overdose). Particularly susceptible are the elderly, lean or underweight individuals and those with impaired hepatic or renal function. Also at risk are those who are debilitated or malnourished, and patients with primary or secondary adrenal insufficiency (Addison's disease). Hypoglycemia is more likely to occur when caloric intake is inadequate or after strenuous or prolonged exercise. The incidence of hypoglycemia in elderly patients is been reported to be higher during treatment with glyburide than with either gliclazide or glimepiride [*Can J Diabetes* 2003;27 (Suppl 2):S106-9]. If a patient becomes hypoglycemic during therapy with chlorpropamide, the drug should be withdrawn and the patient should be kept under close supervision for 5 to 6 days because of the long half-life of the drug. Subsequent reinstitution of the drug at a lower dose may be considered.
Drug Interactions: Sulfonylureas can potentially interact with numerous other drugs. Mechanisms include displacement from plasma proteins, increased or decreased metabolism or urinary excretion, and hyperglycemic or hypoglycemic effects of other drugs. Some sulfonylureas are known substrates or inhibitors of specific cytochrome P450 isoenzymes.

Enhanced glycemic monitoring should be instituted when therapy with other drugs is initiated, discontinued, or the dosages are changed.
Alcohol: Intolerance to alcohol (disulfiram-like reaction: flushing, sensation of warmth, giddiness, nausea and occasionally tachycardia) may occur in patients treated with sulfonylureas. This reaction occurs more frequently with chlorpropamide. Unpredictable fluctuations in serum glucose levels, most commonly hypoglycemia, may also occur following alcohol ingestion.
Anticoagulants, Oral: Coadministration of coumarin derivatives and sulfonylureas may initially result in increased plasma concentrations of both drugs. With continued therapy, decreased anticoagulant concentrations and increased hepatic metabolism of sulfonylureas may occur. Adjustment in dosage for both drugs may be required.
Hyperglycemia: Drugs that may cause hyperglycemia and have the potential to interfere with the action of sulfonylureas include: atypical antipsychotic agents, beta-adrenergic antagonists, corticosteroids, pentamidine, protease inhibitors and thiazide diuretics. Rifampin induces the metabolism of sulfonylureas. This results in a reduced elimination half-life and increased clearance of the sulfonylurea and may interfere with control of blood sugar levels. The dose of the sulfonylurea may need to be increased during and after concomitant therapy with any of these agents.
Hypoglycemia: Hypoglycemia may be potentiated when sulfonylureas are used concurrently with agents such as: ACE inhibitors, allopurinol, ethanol, fibrates, fluconazole, and sulfonamides.
Pregnancy: There are significant differences in the extent to which individual sulfonylureas cross the placenta. Higher amounts of first-generation agents (chlorpropamide, tolbutamide) cross the placenta than second-generation agents (glipizide, glyburide). In particular, glyburide does not cross the placenta to a great extent and does not appear to be teratogenic. Glyburide was not detected in cord blood collected after delivery from women with gestational diabetes mellitus who took the drug to control blood sugar in a randomized clinical trial.

Glyburide is preferentially transported by multidrug resistance-associated proteins (MRP) and the breast cancer resistance protein (BCRP), which is thought to limit the passage of the drug across the placental barrier [*Placenta* 2006;27:1096-102].
Lactation: Glyburide was not detected in the milk of women who received single (5 mg or 10 mg) or multiple doses (5 mg/day) during breast-feeding [*Diabetes Care* 2005;28:1851-5]. Moreover, the blood glucose profile of infants who were breast-fed by these women was not altered during treatment with glyburide. In contrast, chlorpropamide and tolbutamide enter breast milk in significant amounts and should not be administered during lactation. It is not known whether glimepiride or gliclazide enter human milk.
Children: There is limited experience with sulfonylureas in children with type 2 diabetes mellitus (see Indications and Dosage).

ADVERSE EFFECTS: The most common significant adverse effect of sulfonylureas is hypoglycemia (see Precautions). During a median of 3.3 years of treatment with glyburide, 38.7% of 1441 patients with newly diagnosed type 2 diabetes mellitus experienced hypoglycemia in a randomized clinical trial [*N Engl J Med* 2006;355:2427-2443]. Weight gain is not uncommon in patients taking sulfonylureas. Newly diagnosed patients with type 2 diabetes mellitus gained an average of 1.6 kg during the first year of treatment with glyburide in a randomized clinical trial [*N Engl J Med* 2006;355:2427-2443]. Other less commonly occurring adverse effects include:
Dermatologic: Allergic skin reactions such as pruritus, erythema, urticaria, morbiliform or maculopapular eruptions have been observed. These may subside on continued use of sulfonylureas but if they persist, the sulfonylurea should be discontinued. Porphyria cutanea tarda and photosensitivity reactions have been reported.
Gastrointestinal: Nausea, epigastric fullness and heartburn are the most common reactions. These tend to be dose-related and may disappear when dosage is reduced or the total daily dose is administered in divided doses.
Hematologic: Leukopenia, thrombocytopenia, agranulocytosis, hemolytic anemia and aplastic anemia have been reported.
Hepatic: Jaundice has been reported rarely. Discontinue therapy. Abnormalities in liver function tests have occasionally occurred.
Metabolic: The syndrome of inappropriate secretion of antidiuretic hormone (SIADH) has been associated with chlorpropamide. This is characterized by excessive water retention and hyponatremia, low serum osmolality and high urine osmolality. These adverse effects have occurred especially in the elderly and patients with congestive heart failure or hepatic cirrhosis or those taking diuretics.
Miscellaneous: Hepatic porphyria and disulfiram-like reactions have been reported.

OVERDOSE:

Symptoms: Sulfonylurea overdose manifests principally as hypoglycemia, which may be severe and can lead to death. The dosage that causes hypoglycemia varies widely, and may be within the daily dosage range in sensitive individuals. The onset of hypoglycemia after an ingestion may be delayed; hypoglycemic episodes may last for several days, especially in susceptible individuals (e.g., the elderly, malnourished individuals, those with renal or hepatic impairment); and hypoglycemia may recur after an apparent recovery.

The manifestations of hypoglycemia include agitation, confusion, diaphoresis and tachycardia. Severe hypoglycemia may result in seizures and coma. Hypokalemia, hypomagnesemia and their associated arrhythmias may occur. Hypothermia may occur. The symptoms of hypoglycemia may be mistaken for cerebrovascular insufficiency or alcohol intoxication.

Treatment: The goal of treatment for patients with sulfonylurea overdose is correction of hypoglycemia. Physicians should anticipate recurrence of hypoglycemia because of the long duration of action of sulfonylureas.

Confirm the presence of hypoglycemia by blood glucose testing, but do not delay treatment of symptomatic patients. Symptomatic patients should receive 0.5 to 1 g/kg of concentrated dextrose by iv infusion ($D_{50}W$ in adults, $D_{25}W$ in children and $D_{10}W$ in infants). Administer 5 to 10% dextrose solutions as needed to maintain a normal blood glucose. Fluid and electrolyte balance should be monitored and corrected if necessary. Monitor blood glucose concentrations and mental status frequently (for example every 1 or 2 hours initially) then decrease the frequency to every 4 to 6 hours. When appropriate the patient should be fed.

Octreotide inhibits glucose-stimulated release of insulin from pancreatic beta cells and is used in conjunction with dextrose in the management of refractory sulfonylurea-induced hypoglycemia. The recommended adult dose of octreotide is 50 to 100 µg sc or iv every 6 hours as needed. Children should receive 4 to 5 µg/kg/day sc or iv in divided doses every 6 hours to a maximum of 200 µg/day. Several days of therapy may be required depending on the duration of action of the hypoglycemic agent. Monitoring should continue for 24 hours after termination of octreotide therapy.

Diazoxide has been used in combination with iv dextrose to treat refractory hypoglycemia, but is probably less effective than octreotide.

Glucagon is generally not recommended as an antidote for sulfonylurea overdose.

Hemodialysis is not effective in removing sulfonylureas.

For management of a suspected drug overdose, CPhA recommends that you contact your **regional Poison Control Centre**. See the *CPS* Directory section for a list of Poison Control Centres.

DOSAGE: Adults: Sulfonylureas are generally administered with or before a meal (e.g., breakfast). For patients requiring higher doses, divided doses should be administered, usually before the morning and evening meals. This regimen may improve gastrointestinal tolerance and improve glycemic control in some patients. When initiating therapy, a night snack is recommended.

In patients with diabetes mellitus there is no fixed dosage regimen for management of blood glucose concentrations. Individual determination of the minimum dose that will lower the blood glucose adequately should be made (see Table 2). Since lean or elderly diabetic patients appear to be more sensitive to the effects of sulfonylureas, these patients should be started on lower initial doses with dosage adjustments being made cautiously. Patients with renal or hepatic impairment may require dosage reduction. Overweight patients or those with symptomatic hyperglycemia (polyuria and polydipsia) may be started on higher initial doses.

The response to a sulfonylurea will generally be evident within an initial trial period of 1 week; nevertheless, 4 weeks of therapy should be attempted before determining whether a patient is responding.

Blood glucose levels can sometimes be lowered further through combination therapy with other classes of antihyperglycemic agents. During the course of sulfonylurea therapy, a loss of effectiveness may occur (secondary failure). This can be detected by gradual deterioration in glycemic control, in which case the intensity of the regimen should be increased, either by increasing the dose, or by adding another oral medication or insulin.

Elderly: In elderly patients (i.e., those aged ≥60 years) the initial dose of a sulfonylurea should generally be 50% of that used in younger individuals and doses should be increased more slowly [*Can J Diabetes* 2003;27 (Suppl 2):S106-9]. Gliclazide and glimepiride are preferred over glyburide in this population because they are reported to have a lower propensity for hypoglycemia (Precautions).

Pediatric: Glimepiride has been studied as a treatment for type 2 diabetes mellitus in children aged 8 to 17 years. The initial dose of glimepiride was 1 mg once daily in the morning. If the target blood sugar level (<7.8 mmol/L) was not achieved, the dose was doubled at 4-week intervals. The maximum dose was 8 mg once daily [*Diabetes Care* 2007;30:790-4].

Glyburide has been used to treat diabetes mellitus in children aged >3 months with mutations (KCNJ11) in the ATP-sensitive potassium channel. Children were switched from ongoing insulin therapy to glyburide at an initial dose of 0.1 mg/kg/day (in 2 divided doses). The dose was increased in increments of 0.1 mg/kg/day at weekly intervals with concomitant reductions in the dose of insulin. The median equivalent dose required for insulin independence was 0.45 mg/kg/day (range 0.05 to 1.5 mg/kg/day) [*N Engl J Med* 2006;355:467-477].

Table 2: Sulfonylureas

Adult Dosage

Drug	Daily Dose (mg)	Usual Initial Dose (mg)	Equivalent Dose (mg)	Doses/Day
Chlorpropamide	100–500	250	250	1
Gliclazide	80–320[a,b]	160[a,b]	80	1–2[a,b]
Glimepiride	1–8	1	1	1
Glyburide	2.5–20	5	5	1–2
Tolbutamide	500–3000	1000	1000	1–3

a Daily doses of gliclazide immediate-release tablets ≥160 mg should be taken as two divided daily doses.
b The dose of gliclazide modified-release ranges from 30 to 120 mg once daily. The usual initial dose is 30 mg once daily.

The reader is referred to individual product monographs for more specific prescribing information.

Supeudol® Ⓝ

oxycodone HCl

Opioid Analgesic

Sandoz

PHARMACOLOGY: Oxycodone is a semi-synthetic opioid analgesic which exerts an agonist effect at specific, saturable opioid receptors in the CNS and other tissues. In man, oxycodone produces a variety of effects including analgesia, constipation from decreased gastrointestinal motility, suppression of the cough reflex, respiratory depression from reduced responsiveness of the respiratory center to CO_2, nausea and vomiting via stimulation of the chemoreceptor trigger zone, changes in mood including euphoria and dysphoria, sedation, mental clouding, and alterations of the endocrine and autonomic nervous systems.

Oxycodone retains at least one-half of its analgesic activity when administered orally and with acute dosing is approximately twice as potent as orally administered morphine.

Studies with oxycodone hydrochloride tablets in normal volunteers and patients demonstrate a consistent relationship between oxycodone dosage and plasma oxycodone concentrations as well as between concentrations and pharmacodynamic effects.

There is no intrinsic limit to the analgesic effect of oxycodone; like morphine, adequate doses will relieve even the most severe pain. Clinically, however, dosage limitations are imposed by the adverse effects, primarily respiratory depression, nausea and vomiting, which can result from high doses.

Pharmacokinetics: After oral administration, oxycodone is absorbed from the gastrointestinal tract and has a relatively high bioavailability of approximately 60-87%. Unlike morphine, oxycodone does not undergo high first pass metabolism, possibly due to the protective effect of a methoxy group in the 3-position which is a site of morphine glucuronidation. Oxycodone is metabolized in the liver by demethylation to noroxycodone and oxymorphone (via CYP2D6), and by conjugation, to a variety of glucuronide metabolites. Oxymorphone is known to possess analgesic activity but concentrations in the plasma are very low and not as closely correlated to opioid effects as oxycodone concentrations. Although the AUC ratio of noroxycodone to oxycodone is about 0.6 following oral dosing, noroxycodone is reported to be a considerably weaker analgesic than oxycodone and is unlikely to contribute significantly to the analgesic effect of oxycodone. The analgesic activity profile of other metabolites is not known. The terminal elimination half-life after immediate release tablets is approximately 4 hours. The majority of metabolites and unchanged drug (conjugated 2.2%, unconjugated 5.5%) are excreted in the urine.

One bioavailability study has been performed with the oral formulation using healthy human volunteers. The rate and extent of absorption after a single oral administration of OXY-IR (Purdue Pharma, Canada) and Supeudol 20 (oxycodone hydrochloride, Sandoz Canada Inc., Canada), were measured and compared. The results can be summarized as follows: see Table 1.

Table 1: SUPEUDOL

Table of the Comparative Bioavailability Data Oxycodone Hydrochloride (1×20 mg). From Measured Data. Geometric Mean. Arithmetic Mean (CV %)

Parameter	Test SUPEUDOL 20	Reference OXY·IR[a]	% Ratio of Geometric Means	90% Confidence Interval
AUC_T (ng·h/mL)	203.04 207.05 (19%)	220.45 227.70 (25%)	92%	87% to 97%
AUC_I (ng·h/mL)	206.12 210.19 (19%)	223.90 231.41 (26%)	92%	87% to 97%
C_{max} (ng/mL)	31.96 33.72 (33%)	39.98 43.02 (42%)	80%	72% to 88%
T_{max}[b] (h)	1.55 (84%)	1.31 (86%)		
$t_{½}$[b] (h)	3.78 (13%)	3.82 (13%)		

a Oxy·IR is manufactured by Purdue Pharma Inc. and was purchased in Canada.
b Expressed as arithmetic mean (CV%) only.

INDICATIONS: SUPEUDOL (oxycodone hydrochloride) is indicated for relief of moderate to severe pain.

CONTRAINDICATIONS: Oxycodone hydrochloride should not be given to patients with: hypersensitivity to opioid analgesics; acute asthma or other obstructive airway disease and acute respiratory depression; cor pulmonale; acute alcoholism; delirium tremens; severe CNS depression; convulsive disorders; increased cerebrospinal or intracranial pressure; head injury; suspected surgical abdomen; concomitant MAO inhibitors (or within 14 days of such therapy).

WARNINGS: Drug Dependence: As with other opioids, tolerance and physical dependence may develop upon repeated administration of oxycodone and there is a potential for development of psychological dependence. SUPEUDOL (oxycodone hydrochloride) should therefore be prescribed and handled with the degree of caution appropriate to the use of a drug with abuse potential. Drug abuse is not a problem in patients with pain in whom oxycodone is appropriately indicated. Withdrawal symptoms may occur following abrupt discontinuation of therapy or upon administration of an opioid antagonist. Therefore, patients on prolonged therapy should be withdrawn gradually from the drug if it is no longer required for pain control.

CNS Depression: Oxycodone should be used with caution and in reduced dosage during concomitant administration of other opioid analgesics, general anaesthetics, phenothiazines and other tranquilizers, sedative-hypnotics, tricyclic antidepressants and other CNS depressants, including alcohol. Respiratory depression, hypotension and profound sedation or coma may result.

Severe pain antagonizes the subjective and respiratory depressant actions of opioid analgesics. Should pain suddenly subside, these effects may rapidly become manifest. Patients who are scheduled for cordotomy or other interruption of pain transmission pathways should not receive SUPEUDOL within 24 hours of the procedure.

Pregnancy: While animal reproduction studies have revealed no evidence of harm to the fetus due to oxycodone, safe use in pregnancy has not been established. SUPEUDOL should be given to pregnant patients only when the anticipated benefits outweigh the potential risks to the fetus.

PRECAUTIONS: General: The respiratory depressant effects of oxycodone, and the capacity to elevate cerebrospinal fluid pressure, may be greatly increased in the presence of an already elevated intracranial pressure produced by trauma. Also, oxycodone may produce confusion, miosis, vomiting and other side effects which obscure the clinical course of patients with head injury. In such patients, oxycodone must be used with extreme caution and only if it is judged essential.

Oxycodone should be used with extreme caution in patients with substantially decreased respiratory reserve, pre-existing respiratory depression, hypoxia or hypercapnia. Such patients are often less sensitive to the stimulatory effects of carbon monoxide on the respiratory centre and the respiratory depressant effects of oxycodone may reduce respiratory drive to the point of apnea.

Oxycodone administration may result in severe hypotension in patients whose ability to maintain adequate blood pressure is compromised by reduced blood volume, or concurrent administration of such drugs as phenothiazines or certain anaesthetics.

Abdominal Conditions: Oxycodone and other morphine-type opioids have decreased bowel motility. Oxycodone may obscure the diagnosis or clinical course of patients with acute abdominal conditions.

Special Risk Groups: Oxycodone should be administered with caution and in reduced dosages, to debilitated patients, to patients with severely reduced hepatic or renal function, and in patients with Addison's disease, hypothyroidism, prostatic hypertrophy or urethral stricture.

Lactation: In view of the potential for opioids to cross the placental barrier and to be excreted in breast milk, oxycodone should be used with caution in nursing mothers.

Labor/Delivery: Physical dependence or respiratory depression may occur in the infant if opioids are administered during labor.

Occupational Hazards: Driving and Operating Dangerous Machinery: Oxycodone may impair the mental and/or physical abilities needed for certain potentially hazardous activities such as driving a car or operating machinery. Patients should be cautioned accordingly. Patients should also be cautioned about the combined effects of oxycodone with other CNS depressants, including other opioids, phenothiazines, sedative/hypnotics and alcohol.

Drug Interactions: CNS depressants, such as other opioids, anesthetics, sedatives, hypnotics, barbiturates, phenothiazines, chloral hydrate and glutethimide may enhance the depressant effects of oxycodone. Monoamine oxidase inhibitors, (including procarbazine hydrochloride), pyrazolidone antihistamines, beta-blockers and alcohol may also enhance the depressant effect of oxycodone.

Mixed agonist/antagonist opioid analgesics such as butorphanol, buprenorphine, nalbuphine and pentazocine need to be used cautiously in patients using pure opioid agonist analgesics such as oxycodone. Mixed agonist/antagonist analgesics might lessen the analgesic effect of oxycodone and/or may cause withdrawal symptoms in these patients.

ADVERSE EFFECTS: Adverse effects of SUPEUDOL (oxycodone hydrochloride) are similar to those of other opioid analgesics, and represent an extension of pharmacological effects of the drug class. The major hazards of opioids include respiratory and central nervous system depression and to a lesser degree, circulatory depression, respiratory arrest, shock and cardiac arrest.

The most frequently observed adverse effects of SUPEUDOL are constipation, nausea, somnolence, dizziness, vomiting, pruritus, headache, dry mouth, asthenia and sweating.

Sedation: Sedation is a common side effect of opioid analgesics, especially in opioid naive individuals. Sedation may also occur partly because patients often recuperate from prolonged fatigue after the relief of persistent pain. Most patients develop tolerance to the sedative effects of opioids within three to five days and, if the sedation is not severe, will not require any treatment except reassurance. If excessive sedation persists beyond a few days, the dose of the opioid should be reduced and alternate causes investigated. Some of these are: concurrent CNS depressant medication, hepatic or renal dysfunction, brain metastases, hypercalcemia and respiratory failure. If it is necessary to reduce the dose, it can be carefully increased again after three or four days if it is obvious that the pain is not being well controlled. Dizziness and unsteadiness may be caused by postural hypotension, particularly in elderly or debilitated patients, and may be alleviated if the patient lies down.

Nausea and Vomiting: Nausea is a common side effect on initiation of therapy with opioid analgesics and is thought to occur by activation of the chemoreceptor trigger zone, stimulation of the vestibular apparatus and through delayed gastric emptying. The prevalence of nausea declines following continued treatment with opioid analgesics. When instituting therapy with an opioid for chronic pain, the routine prescription of an antiemetic should be considered. In the cancer patient, investigation of nausea should include such causes as constipation, bowel obstruction, uremia, hypercalcemia, hepatomegaly, tumor invasion of celiac plexus and concurrent use of drugs with emetogenic properties. Persistent nausea which does not respond to dosage reduction may be caused by opioid-induced gastric stasis and may be accompanied by other symptoms including anorexia, early satiety, vomiting and abdominal fullness. These symptoms respond to chronic treatment with gastrointestinal prokinetic agents.

Constipation: Practically all patients become constipated while taking opioids on a persistent basis. In some patients, particularly the elderly or bedridden, fecal impaction may result. It is essential to caution the patients in this regard and to institute an appropriate regimen of bowel management at the start of prolonged opioid therapy. Stimulant laxatives, stool softeners, and other appropriate measures should be used as required.

The following adverse effects occur less frequently with opioid analgesics and include those reported in clinical trials of oxycodone, whether related or not to oxycodone.

General and CNS: dysphoria, euphoria, anxiety, depression, depersonalization, nervousness, agitation, hyperkinesia, hypotonia, muscular rigidity, twitching, tremor, seizure, speech disorder, vision abnormalities, hypesthesia, paresthesia, amnesia, thought abnormalities, abnormal dreams, hallucinations, confusion, delirium, abnormal gait, insomnia, vertigo, headache, miosis and tinnitus.

Cardiovascular: tachycardia, palpitation, faintness, syncope, vasodilation, postural hypotension, chest pain, ST depression, and migraine.

Respiratory: bronchospasm, pharyngitis, bronchitis, cough, pneumonia, dyspnea, sinusitis, and yawning.

Gastrointestinal: dysphagia, anorexia, taste alterations, abdominal pain, diarrhea, dyspepsia, eructation, flatulence, hiccups, gastritis, increased appetite, biliary spasm, ileus and stomatitis.

Genitourinary: urinary retention or hesitancy, dysuria, polyuria, hematuria, antidiuretic effects, and impotence.

Dermatologic: urticaria, exfoliative dermatitis, other skin rashes, and edema.

Other: allergic reaction, asthenia, lymphadenopathy, malaise, chills, fever, dehydration, hypoglycemia, weight loss, and thirst.

Withdrawal (Abstinence) Syndrome: Physical dependence with or without psychological dependence tend to occur on chronic administration. An abstinence syndrome may be precipitated when opioid administration is discontinued or opioid antagonists administered. The following withdrawal symptoms may be observed after opioids are discontinued: body aches, diarrhea, gooseflesh, loss of appetite, nervousness or restlessness, runny nose, sneezing, tremors or shivering, stomach cramps, nausea, trouble with sleeping, unusual increase in sweating and yawning, weakness, tachycardia and unexplained fever. In patients who are appropriately treated with opioid analgesics and who undergo gradual withdrawal from the drug, these symptoms are usually mild.

OVERDOSE:

Symptoms: Serious overdosage with oxycodone may be characterized by respiratory depression (a decrease in respiratory rate and/or tidal volume, Cheyne-Stokes respiration, cyanosis), extreme somnolence progressing to stupor or coma, skeletal muscle flaccidity, cold and clammy skin, and sometimes bradycardia and hypotension. Severe overdosage may result in apnea, circulatory collapse, cardiac arrest and death.

Treatment: Primary attention should be given to the establishment of adequate respiratory exchange through the provision of a patent airway and controlled or assisted ventilation. The opioid antagonist naloxone hydrochloride is a specific antidote against respiratory depression due to overdosage or as a result of unusual sensitivity to oxycodone. An appropriate dose of an opioid antagonist should therefore be administered, preferably by the intravenous route. The usual initial IV adult dose of naloxone is 0.4 mg or higher. Concomitant efforts at respiratory resuscitation should be carried out. Since the duration of action of oxycodone, particularly sustained release formulations, may exceed that of the antagonist, the patient should be under continued surveillance and doses of the antagonist should be repeated as needed to maintain adequate respiration.

An antagonist should not be administered in the absence of clinically significant respiratory or cardiovascular depression. Oxygen, intravenous fluids, vasopressors and other supportive measures should be used as indicated.

In individuals physically dependent on opioids, the administration of the usual dose of narcotic antagonist will precipitate an acute withdrawal syndrome. The severity of this syndrome will depend on the degree of physical dependence and the dose of antagonist administered. The use of narcotic antagonists in such individuals should be avoided if possible. If a narcotic antagonist must be used to treat serious respiratory depression in the physically dependent patient, the antagonist should be administered with extreme care by using dosage titration, commencing with 10 to 20% of the usual recommended initial dose.

Evacuation of gastric contents may be useful in removing unabsorbed drug.

For management of a suspected drug overdose, CPhA recommends that you contact your **regional Poison Control Centre**. See the *CPS* Directory section for a list of Poison Control Centres.

DOSAGE: Adults: Individual dosing requirements vary considerably based on each patient's age, weight, severity and cause of pain, and medical and analgesic history.

The usual initial adult dose of SUPEUDOL for patients who have not previously received opioid analgesics is 5 or 10 mg, every 6 hours.

For patients who are receiving an alternate opioid, the "oral oxycodone equivalent" of the analgesic presently being used should be determined. Having determined the total daily dosage of the present analgesic, Table 2 can be used to calculate the approximate daily oral oxycodone dosage that should provide equivalent analgesia. It is usually appropriate to treat a patient with only one opioid at a time.

If a non-opioid analgesic is being provided, it may be continued. If the non-opioid is discontinued, consideration should be given to increasing the opioid dose to compensate for the non-opioid analgesic. SUPEUDOL can be safely used concomitantly with usual doses of other non-opioid analgesics.

Dose Titration: Dose titration is the key to success with opioid analgesic therapy. Proper optimization of doses scaled to the relief of the individual's pain should aim at the regular administration of the lowest dose which will maintain the patient free of pain at all times. Dosage adjustments should be based on the patient's clinical response. If breakthrough pain repeatedly occurs at the end of the dosing interval it is generally an indication for a dosage increase rather than more frequent administration.

Adjustment or Reduction of Dosage: Following successful relief of pain, periodic attempts to re-assess the opioid analgesic requirements should be made. If treatment discontinuation is required, the dose of opioid may be decreased as follows: one-half of the previous daily dose given q6h (SUPEUDOL) for the first two days, followed thereafter by a 25% reduction every two days.

Opioid analgesics may only be partially effective in relieving dysesthetic pain, postherpetic neuralgia, stabbing pains, activity-related pain and some forms of headache. That is not to say that patients with these types of pain should not be given an adequate trial of opioid analgesics, but it may be necessary to refer such patients at an early time to other forms of pain therapy.

Table 2: SUPEUDOL

Opioid Analgesics: Approximate Analgesic Equivalences[a]

Drug	Equivalent Dose (mg)[b] (compared to morphine 10 mg IM)		Duration of Action (Hours)
	Parenteral	Oral	
Strong Opioid Agonists			
Morphine	10	60[c]	3–4
Oxycodone[d]	15	30	2–4
Hydromorphone	1.5	7.5	2–4
Anileridine	25	75	2–3
Levorphanol	2	4	4–8
Meperidine[f]	75	300	1–3
Oxymorphone	1.5	5 (rectal)	3–4
Methadone[e]	—	—	—
Heroin	5–8	10–15	3–4
Weak Opioid Agonists			
Codeine	120	200	3–4
Propoxyphene	50	100	2–4
Mixed Agonist-Antagonists[g]			
Pentazocine[f]	60	180	3–4
Nalbuphine	10	—	3–6
Butorphanol	2	—	3–4

[a] References:
Cancer Pain: A Monograph on the Management of Cancer Pain, Health and Welfare Canada, 1984.
Foley, K.M., New Engl. J. Med. 313: 84-95, 1985.
Aronoff, G.M. and Evans, W.O., In: Evaluation and Treatment of Chronic Pain, 2nd Ed., G.M. Aronoff (Ed.), Williams and Wilkins, Baltimore, pp. 359-368, 1992.
Cherny, N.I. and Portenoy,R.K., In: Textbook of Pain, 3rd Ed., P.D. Wall and R. Melzack (Eds.), Churchill Livingstone, London, pp. 1437-1467, 1994.

[b] Most of these data were derived from single-dose, acute pain studies and should be considered an approximation for selection of doses when treating chronic pain.

[c] For acute pain, the oral or rectal dose of morphine is six times the injectable dose. However, for chronic dosing, clinical experience indicates that this ratio is 2-3:1 (i.e., 20-30 mg of oral or rectal morphine is equivalent to 10 mg of parenteral morphine).

[d] Based on single entity oral oxycodone in acute pain.

[e] Extremely variable equianalgesic dose. Patients should undergo individualized titration starting at an equivalent to 1/10 of the morphine dose.

[f] Not recommended for the management of chronic pain.

[g] Mixed agonist-antagonists can precipitate withdrawal in patients on pure opioid agonists.

SUPPLIED: Suppositories: 10 mg: Each torpedo-shaped suppository, ivory in color, contains: oxycodone HCl 10 mg. Nonmedicinal ingredients: semi-synthetic glycerides. Boxes of 12. Store between 15 and 30°C.

20 mg: Each torpedo-shaped suppository, ivory in color, contains: oxycodone HCl 20 mg. Nonmedicinal ingredients: semi-synthetic glycerides. Boxes of 12. Store between 15 and 30°C.

Tablets: 5 mg: Each blue, round tablet, scored on one side and printed "5" in "V" on the other side, contains: oxycodone HCl 5 mg. Nonmedicinal ingredients: croscarmellose sodium, dibasic calcium phosphate, FD&C Blue #1, magnesium stearate and microcrystalline cellulose. Bottles of 100. Store between 15 and 30°C.

10 mg: Each white, round tablet, scored on one side and printed "10" in "V" on the other side, contains: oxycodone HCl 10 mg. Nonmedicinal ingredients: croscarmellose sodium, dibasic calcium phosphate, magnesium stearate and microcrystalline cellulose. Bottles of 100. Store between 15 and 30°C.

20 mg: Each white, oval tablet, scored on one side with a "S" printed on each side of the score and printed "20" in "V" on the other side, contains: oxycodone HCl 20 mg. Nonmedicinal ingredients: croscarmellose sodium, dibasic calcium phosphate, magnesium stearate and microcrystalline cellulose. Bottles of 50. Store between 15 and 30°C. Protect from light. Protect from moisture.

(Shown in Product Identification Section)

Supprane® Ⓟ

desflurane

Inhalation Anesthetic

Baxter

PHARMACOLOGY: Desflurane is a volatile inhalational anesthetic whose low solubility (blood/gas partition coefficient equals 0.42) permits rapid variation in anesthetic depth. If anesthesia is maintained with inflow rates of greater than 2 L/min, the alveolar concentration is usually within 10% of the inspired concentration. It is not necessary to deliver concentrations of desflurane far in excess of the desired end-tidal concentration ("overpressurization" technique) due to the low blood and tissue solubilities of desflurane and the resulting rapid equilibrium of alveolar concentration with inspired and delivered concentrations (see Warnings).

Since awakening is rapid, care should be taken that appropriate analgesia has been administered to the patient at the end of the procedure or early in the postanesthesia care unit.

MAC varies widely with age. In 45-year-old patients, MAC is 6% in 100% oxygen and 2.8% in 60% nitrous oxide (see Dosage, Table 2).

Desflurane is not useful for mask induction as it causes an unacceptably high incidence of laryngospasm, coughing, secretions, breath holding and apnea (see Adverse Effects).

Approximately 0.02% of absorbed desflurane is metabolized. In normal volunteers, there was no increase in serum or urine fluoride concentrations. Studies in patients with chronic renal insufficiency and patients undergoing renal transplantation showed no effects on renal function. Hepatic dysfunction has been reported after desflurane use. A causal relationship may or may not exist.

Desflurane is a profound respiratory depressant, producing a progressive decrease in tidal volume and increase in arterial carbon dioxide tension. Apnea is common at concentrations above 1.5 MAC (Minimum Alveolar Concentration). This depression may be partly reversed by surgical stimulation. Nitrous oxide diminishes the inspired concentration of desflurane required to reach a desired level of anesthesia (see Dosage, Table 2).

Desflurane potentiates the effect of depolarizing and nondepolarizing neuromuscular relaxants. When compared to nitrous oxide/opioid anesthesia, the requirements for depolarizing and nondepolarizing agents are reduced by 30% and 50%, respectively.

Desflurane, like other volatile anesthetics, induces malignant hyperthermia in genetically susceptible swine (see Precautions).

Hemodynamic Effects: Cardiovascular Effects: In healthy male volunteers, desflurane produced a progressive decrease in blood pressure (15% at 1.2 MAC), due mainly to vasodilation, and an increase in heart rate (15% at 1.2 MAC) when administered in oxygen or 60% nitrous oxide during controlled ventilation at normocapnia. The cardiac output was unchanged at 1.7 MAC in oxygen, but decreased 20% at 1.2 MAC in 60% nitrous oxide. Similar changes were seen during spontaneous ventilation.

Effect on Sympathetic Activity: Constant or slowly increasing concentrations of desflurane blunt or block sympathetic responses to noxious stimuli. The increased heart rate response to hypotension is reduced in this setting. However, rapid changes to concentrations above 6%, as well as rapid changes above 6% can result in tachycardia and hypertension. The physiology of this response is unknown. In unpremedicated volunteers, desflurane can unpredictably induce transient (approximately 4 minutes) increases in sympathetic activity, heart rate and blood pressure. The hemodynamic changes are more common at concentrations ≥6% and more severe with large (≥1%), sudden increments. A single clinical study of CABG patients showed similar effects (see Clinical Studies, Cardiovascular Surgery). This transient cardiovascular response can be blunted substantially by fentanyl (1.5 μg/kg), alfentanil (10 or 20 μg/kg), or clonidine 4 μg/kg as a premedication. Esmolol decreases the heart rate, but not blood pressure. The sympathetic stimulation is not obtunded by i.v. or endotracheal lidocaine or by i.v. propofol.

Desflurane does not alter the human myocardial arrhythmogenic threshold for epinephrine (approximately 7 μg/kg).

Clinical Studies: The safety and efficacy of desflurane have been established in large, multicentre clinical trials in adult outpatients (ASA I, II and III), in cardiovascular surgery (ASA II, III and IV) patients, in elderly (ASA II and III) patients and in pediatric (ASA I and II) patients.

Ambulatory Surgery: Desflurane was compared to isoflurane in multicentre studies (21 sites) of 792 ASA physical status I, II or III patients aged 18 to 76 years (median 32). Desflurane with or without nitrous oxide or other anesthetics was generally well tolerated. Patients receiving desflurane emerged significantly faster than those receiving isoflurane, and there were no differences in the incidence of nausea and vomiting.

Cardiovascular Surgery: Desflurane was compared to isoflurane, sufentanil or fentanyl for the anesthetic management of coronary artery bypass graft (CABG), abdominal aortic aneurysm, peripheral vascular and carotid endarterectomy surgery in 7 studies at 15 centres involving a total of 558 patients (ASA physical status II, III and IV).

Cardiac Studies: The effects of desflurane in patients undergoing CABG surgery were investigated in 3 studies.

Using echocardiography in addition to Holter monitoring to detect myocardial ischemia, 1 study compared desflurane with sufentanil in groups of 100 patients each. The opioid group received a small dose of thiopental, and sufentanil, 5 to 10 μg/kg followed by an infusion of 0.07 μg/kg/min, and no halogenated inhaled anesthetic. The desflurane group received no opioid for induction of anesthesia, and after i.v. thiopental had a rapid inhaled induction of anesthesia with desflurane concentrations exceeding 10% end-tidal. The desflurane group had increases in heart rate (HR) and mean arterial pressure (MAP) during induction of anesthesia and a 13% incidence of myocardial ischemia during induction of anesthesia which was greater than the zero incidence during induction in the sufentanil group. During the precardiopulmonary bypass period, more desflurane patients required cardiovascular adjuvants to control hemodynamics than the sufentanil patients. During maintenance of anesthesia, the sufentanil group had myocardial ischemia of greater duration and intensity than did the desflurane group. There were no differences in incidence of myocardial infarction or death between the 2 groups.

The second study compared desflurane with fentanyl in groups of 26 and 25 patients, respectively. The fentanyl group received 50 μg/kg and no halogenated inhaled anesthetic. The desflurane group received fentanyl 10 μg/kg and a maximum desflurane concentration of 6%. The groups did not differ in the incidence of ECG changes suggestive of ischemia, myocardial infarction, or death.

In the third study, investigators compared desflurane with isoflurane in groups of 57 and 58 patients, respectively. Both groups were given up to 10 μg/kg fentanyl during induction of anesthesia. The mean end-tidal anesthetic concentrations prior to coronary bypass were 6% desflurane or 0.9% isoflurane. Desflurane and isoflurane provided clinically acceptable anesthesia prior to and after coronary bypass. A subanalysis was performed for data collected at one of the study centres. At this centre desflurane was administered to 21 patients and 20 patients received isoflurane. Both groups were given fentanyl 10 μg/kg; during induction of anesthesia the maximum end-tidal anesthetic concentrations were 6% desflurane or 1.4% isoflurane. The groups had similar incidences of ischemia (as detected by Holter monitoring), myocardial infarction and death.

In the desflurane vs sufentanil study, investigators increased desflurane concentration rapidly to 10.2% end-tidal, without having administered any opioid, thereby increasing HR and MAP and observing a 13% incidence of myocardial ischemia in their patients with coronary artery disease. These rapid increases in desflurane concentration without pretreatment with an opioid, have been demonstrated to increase sympathetic activity, HR and MAP in volunteers. The other studies avoided these increases in HR and MAP by applying lower desflurane concentrations (less than 1 MAC), and by administering substantial doses of fentanyl (10 and 50 μg/kg) as part of the induction technique.

Peripheral Vascular Studies: Four randomized, open-label trials were conducted to assess the hemodynamic stability of patients administered desflurane vs isoflurane for maintenance anesthesia in peripheral vascular surgeries. These studies are summarized in Table 1.

Table 1: Suprane

Peripheral Vascular Studies

Type of Surgery	Desflurane/O_2		Isoflurane/O_2	
	# of patients	mean dose (%)	# of patients	mean dose (%)
Abdominal Aorta	25	5.2	29	0.74
Peripheral Vascular	24	2.9[a]	24	0.43[a]
Carotid	31	4.4	30	0.7

(cont'd)

Table 1: Suprane *(cont'd)*

Peripheral Vascular Studies

	Desflurane/O_2		Isoflurane/O_2	
Type of Surgery	**# of patients**	**mean dose (%)**	**# of patients**	**mean dose (%)**
Endarterectomy	15	6.1	15	0.65

[a] Desflurane and isoflurane administered with 60% N_2O.

In all patients, the volatile anesthetics were supplemented with fentanyl. Blood pressure and heart rate were controlled by changes in concentrations of the volatile anesthetics or opioids and cardiovascular drugs, if necessary. No differences were found in cardiovascular outcome (death, myocardial infarction, ventricular tachycardia or fibrillation, heart failure) for desflurane and isoflurane in these studies.

Desflurane should not be used as the sole anesthetic in patients with coronary artery disease or in patients where increases in the heart rate or blood pressure are undesirable (see Warnings).

Geriatric Surgery: Desflurane plus nitrous oxide was compared to isoflurane plus nitrous oxide in a multicentre study (6 sites) of 203 ASA physical status II or III elderly patients, aged 57 to 91 years (median 71). Heart rate and arterial blood pressure remained within 20% of preinduction baseline values during administration of desflurane 0.5 to 7.7% (average 3.6%) with 50 to 60% nitrous oxide. Maintenance and recovery cardiovascular measurements did not differ from those during isoflurane plus nitrous oxide administration, nor did the postoperative incidence of nausea and vomiting. The most common cardiovascular adverse event was hypotension for both isoflurane (6%) as well as desflurane (8%).

Neurosurgery: Desflurane was studied in 38 patients aged 26 to 76 years (median 48 years), ASA physical status II or III undergoing neurosurgical procedures for intracranial lesions. Due to the limited number of patients studied, the safety of desflurane has not been established and is not recommended for use in neurosurgical procedures.

Pediatric Surgery: Desflurane was compared to halothane, with or without nitrous oxide, in 235 patients aged 2 weeks to 12 years (median 2 years), ASA physical status I or II. The concentration of desflurane required for maintenance of anesthesia is age dependent (see Dosage, Table 2). Changes in blood pressure during maintenance of and recovery from anesthesia were similar between desflurane N_2O/O_2 and halothane/N_2O/O_2. Heart rate during maintenance of anesthesia was approximately 10 beats/min faster with desflurane than with halothane. There were no differences in the incidences of nausea and vomiting between desflurane and halothane.

INDICATIONS: As an inhalation agent for maintenance of general anesthesia.

Desflurane is not recommended for mask induction of anaesthesia because of a high incidence of moderate to severe upper airway adverse events (see Adverse Effects).

CONTRAINDICATIONS: When general anesthesia is contraindicated. Known sensitivity to desflurane or other halogenated anesthetics. Patients in whom liver dysfunction, jaundice or unexplained fever, leukocytosis, or eosinophilia has occurred after a previous halogenated anesthetic administration (see Warnings). Known or suspected genetic susceptibility to malignant hyperthermia or in patients with a history of malignant hyperthermia (see Precautions).

WARNINGS: Desflurane should be administered only by persons trained in the administration of general anesthesia, using a vaporizer specifically designed and designated for use with desflurane. Facilities for maintenance of a patent airway, artificial ventilation, oxygen enrichment and circulatory resuscitation must be immediately available. Hypotension and respiratory depression increase as anesthesia is deepened.

Respiration must be monitored closely and supported when necessary.

Desflurane is not recommended for mask induction as it causes a high incidence of laryngospasm, coughing, breath holding, apnea, increase in secretions and oxyhemoglobin desaturation (see Adverse Effects).

Since awakening is rapid, care should be taken that appropriate analgesia has been administered to the patient at the end of the procedure or early in the postanesthesia care unit. Rapid awakening with pain may be associated with agitation, particularly in pediatric patients.

As with other halogenated anesthetics, desflurane may cause sensitivity hepatitis in patients who have been sensitized by previous exposure to halogenated anesthetics (see Contraindications and Adverse Effects). In these patients, or in patients with pre-existing hepatic conditions, appropriate alternative therapy should be considered.

In healthy volunteers, in the absence of concomitant N_2O and/or opioid administration, sudden step increases in the end-tidal concentration of desflurane may cause transient increases in sympathetic activity with associated increases in heart rate and blood pressure. The hemodynamic changes are more common at concentrations ≥6% and more severe with large (≥1%), sudden increments. Without treatment, and without further increases in desflurane concentration, these increases in heart rate and blood pressure resolve in approximately 4 minutes. At the new, higher end-tidal desflurane concentration blood pressure is likely to be lower and heart rate higher than at the previous, lower steady-state desflurane concentration. The transient increases of heart rate and blood pressure are less if the end-tidal concentration of desflurane is increased in increments of 1% or less. However, if during the transiently increased heart rate and blood pressure the end-tidal concentration of desflurane is again rapidly increased, further increase of heart rate and blood pressure may result. Administration of sympatholytic drugs (fentanyl, alfentanil, esmolol, clonidine) prior to a sudden step increase of desflurane blunts or blocks the increase in heart rate and blood pressure. The sympathetic response is not obtunded by i.v. or endotracheal lidocaine or by i.v. propofol (see Pharmacology).

When desflurane is used in the clinical setting, the following should be considered:

Desflurane should not be used as the sole anesthetic in patients with coronary artery disease or in patients where increases in heart rate or blood pressure are undesirable. Rapid inhaled induction of anesthesia with desflurane alone, without concomitant administration of an opioid, in patients with coronary artery disease, has been associated with an increased incidence of myocardial ischemia. Desflurane, when given in conjunction with opioids for maintenance of anesthesia in patients with coronary artery disease, has not produced an incidence of ischemia different from that produced by other anesthetics. Thus, when desflurane is to be used in patients with coronary artery disease, it should always be used in combination with other medications, such as i.v. opioids or hypnotics and it should not be used for induction (see Pharmacology).

When changing the depth of anesthesia, rapid increases in the end-tidal concentration of desflurane should be avoided and the end-tidal concentration increased in small increments of 1% or less. It is not necessary to deliver concentrations of desflurane far in excess of the desired end-tidal concentration ("overpressurization" technique) due to the low blood and tissue solubilities of desflurane and the resulting rapid equilibrium of alveolar concentration with inspired and delivered concentrations; thus the transient and self-limiting increases in heart rate and blood pressure may be avoided.

During maintenance of anesthesia, increases in heart rate and blood pressure occurring after rapid incremental increases in end-tidal concentration of desflurane may not represent inadequate anesthesia. The changes due to sympathetic activation resolve in approximately 4 minutes. Increases in heart rate and blood pressure occurring before or in the absence of a rapid increase in desflurane concentration, may be interpreted as light anesthesia. Thus, in such patients, incremental increases of 0.5 to 1% end-tidal desflurane may attenuate these signs of light anesthesia, as may concomitant administration of analgesics. Should raised heart rate and blood pressure persist, then other causes should be sought.

There are no data regarding the cardiovascular effects of desflurane in hypovolemic and hypotensive patients.

PRECAUTIONS: General: As with any inhalation agent, the use of desflurane proportionately decreases the concentration of all other gases administered concurrently, including O_2. For example, the addition of 10% desflurane to 70% N_2O and 30% O_2 reduces the O_2 concentration to 27%.

Nitrous oxide diminishes the inspired concentration of desflurane required to reach a desired level of anesthesia (see Dosage, Table 2).

As with other rapidly acting anesthetic agents, rapid emergence with desflurane should be taken into account in cases where postanesthesia pain is anticipated. Care should be taken that appropriate analgesia has been administered to the patient at the end of the procedure or early in the postanesthesia care unit stay (see Warnings).

As with other halogenated anesthetic agents, there is some elevation of glucose intraoperatively. Glucose elevation should be considered in diabetic patients.

Desflurane can react with desiccated carbon dioxide (CO_2) absorbents to produce carbon monoxide which may result in elevated levels of carboxyhemoglobin in some patients. In clinical practice, cases of elevated carboxyhemoglobin have been reported in association with desflurane. Case reports suggest that barium hydroxide lime and sodalime become desiccated when fresh gases are passed through the CO_2 absorber cannister at high flow rates over many hours or days. When a clinician suspects that CO_2 absorbent may be desiccated, it should be replaced before the administration of desflurane.

Geriatrics: The MAC in geriatric patients is approximately 70% of the adult dose in 100% oxygen and 40% the adult dose in 60% nitrous oxide (see Dosage).

Pregnancy: There are no adequate and well-controlled studies in pregnant women. Desflurane should be used during pregnancy only if the potential benefit justifies the potential risk to the fetus.

Obstetrics: Due to the limited number of patients studied, safety of desflurane in obstetrics has not been established at this time.

Children: The MAC of desflurane in pediatric patients is higher than that in young adults (see Dosage). Several publications in the literature have reported frequent agitation upon emergence from desflurane anesthesia in children. It is unknown whether this is related to desflurane or to the rapid transition from anesthesia to consciousness.

Renal and Hepatic Impairment: No dosage adjustments are required in these patients. Hepatic dysfunction has been reported after desflurane use (see Adverse Effects, Laboratory Findings). A causal relationship may or may not exist.

Neurosurgery: Due to the limited number of patients studied, the safety of desflurane has not been established and is not recommended for use in neurosurgical procedures (see Pharmacology, Clinical Studies).

Drug Interactions: Benzodiazepines: Midazolam (25 to 50 μg/kg) decreases the MAC of desflurane by 16%.

Opioids: Immediately following the administration of fentanyl (3 to 6 μg/kg) the MAC of desflurane decreases by 50%.

Neuromuscular Relaxants: Desflurane potentiates the effect of depolarizing and nondepolarizing neuromuscular relaxants. When compared to nitrous oxide/opioid anesthesia, the requirements for depolarizing and nondepolarizing agents are reduced by 30% and 50%, respectively.

Other Drugs: The effects of desflurane on the disposition of other drugs has not been determined.

Pheochromocytoma/Neuroblastoma: There are insufficient data on the use of desflurane in patients with pheochromocytoma and neuroblastoma. Since desflurane can cause stimulation of the sympathetic nervous system, its use is not recommended in patients with these conditions (see Warnings).

Malignant Hyperthermia: In susceptible individuals, desflurane anesthesia may trigger a skeletal muscle hypermetabolic state leading to high oxygen demand and the clinical syndrome known as malignant hyperthermia. The clinical syndrome includes nonspecific features such as muscle rigidity, tachycardia, tachypnea, cyanosis, arrhythmias and unstable blood pressure. Some of these nonspecific signs may also appear during light anesthesia, acute hypoxia, hypercapnia and hypovolemia. An increase in overall metabolism may be reflected in an elevated temperature (which may rise rapidly early or late in the case, but usually is not the first sign of augmented metabolism) and an increased usage of the CO_2 absorption system (hot canister). PaO_2 and pH may decrease, and hyperkalemia and a base deficit may appear. Treatment includes discontinuation of desflurane, administration of i.v. dantrolene sodium, and application of supportive therapy. Such therapy includes vigorous efforts to restore body temperature to normal, respiratory and circulatory support as indicated, and management of electrolyte-fluid-acid-base derangements. (Consult prescribing information for dantrolene sodium i.v. for additional information on patient management.) Renal failure may appear later, and urine flow should be sustained if possible.

ADVERSE EFFECTS: Adverse event information is derived from controlled clinical trials. The studies were conducted using a variety of premedications, other anesthetics, and surgical procedures of varying length. Of the 1 843 patients exposed to desflurane in clinical trials, 1 209 were used in estimating the incidence of adverse reactions below. Of these, 370 adults and 152 children were induced with desflurane alone and 687 patients were maintained principally with desflurane. Frequencies reflect the percent of patients with the event and each patient was counted once for each type of adverse event. They are presented in alphabetical order within each body system.

Probably Causally Related: Incidence Greater than 1%. Induction (Use as a Mask Inhalation Agent): Adult Patients (n=370): coughing 34%, breath holding 27%, apnea 15%, increased secretions 9%, laryngospasm 8%, oxyhemoglobin desaturation (SpO_2 <90%) 8%, pharyngitis 4% (see Warnings). Pediatric patients (n=152): coughing 72%, breath holding 63%, laryngospasm 50%, oxyhemoglobin desaturation (SpO_2 <90%) 26%, increased secretions 21%, bronchospasm 3% (see Warnings).

Maintenance or Recovery: Adult and Pediatric Patients (n=687):

Body as a Whole: headache 1%.

Cardiovascular: bradycardia 1%, hypertension 1%, nodal arrhythmia 1%, tachycardia 1%.

Digestive: nausea 27%, vomiting 16%.

Nervous System: increased salivation 1%.

Respiratory: apnea 7%, breath holding 2%, cough increased 4%, laryngospasm 3%, pharyngitis 1%.

Special Senses: conjunctivitis (conjunctival hyperemia) 2%.

Probably Causally Related: Incidence Less than 1% and Reported in 3 or More Patients, Regardless of Severity (n=1 843):

Body as a Whole: fever.

Cardiovascular: arrhythmia, bigeminy, ECG abnormal, myocardial ischemia, vasodilation.

Nervous System: agitation, dizziness.

Respiratory: asthma, dyspnea, hypoxia.

Causal Relationship Unknown: Incidence Less than 1% and Reported in 3 or More Patients, Regardless of Severity (n=1 843):

Cardiovascular: hemorrhage, myocardial infarct.

Metabolic and Nutrition: creatinine phosphokinase increased.

Musculoskeletal System: myalgia.

Skin and Appendages: pruritus.

See Precautions for information regarding pediatric use and malignant hyperthermia.

Laboratory Findings: Transient elevations in glucose and white blood cell count may occur as with the use of other anesthetic agents. Abnormal liver function tests were observed in <1% of patients. Hepatitis has been reported very rarely.

OVERDOSE:

Symptoms: Marked hypotension, tachycardia and apnea.

Treatment: Stop drug administration. Support respiration and circulation as required.

For management of a suspected drug overdose, CPhA recommends that you contact your **regional Poison Control Centre**. See the *CPS* Directory section for a list of Poison Control Centres.

DOSAGE: General: Deliver from a vaporizer specifically designed and designated for use with desflurane.

Premedication should be selected according to the need of the individual patient. There is no evidence of interaction between desflurane and commonly used anticholinergic drugs. Desflurane is potentiated by benzodiazepines and opioids (see Precautions, Drug Interactions).

Desflurane is not recommended for mask induction as it causes a high incidence of laryngospasm, coughing, secretions, breath holding, apnea, and increase in secretions and oxyhemoglobin desaturation (see Adverse Effects).

Maintenance:

Adults: Surgical levels of anesthesia in adults may be maintained with concentrations of 2.5 to 8.5% desflurane with or without the concomitant use of nitrous oxide.

Children: Surgical anesthesia is maintained with concentrations of 5.2 to 10% desflurane in children with or without the concomitant use of nitrous oxide.

Geriatrics: Geriatric patients require approximately 70% the adult dose in 100% oxygen and approximately 40% the adult dose in 60% nitrous oxide.

Table 2 provides mean relative potency based on age in ASA physical status I and II patients.

Table 2: Suprane

Effect of Age on MAC of Suprane; Mean±SD (Percent Atmospheres)

Age	N	100% O_2	N	60% N_2O
2 weeks	6	9.2±0.0	—	—
10 weeks	5	9.4±0.4	—	—
9 months	4	10.0±0.7	5	7.5±0.8
2 years	3	9.1±0.6	—	—
3 years	—	—	5	6.4±0.4

(cont'd)

Table 2: Suprane *(cont'd)*

Effect of Age on MAC of Suprane; Mean±SD (Percent Atmospheres)

Age	N	100% O_2	N	60% N_2O
4 years	4	8.6±0.6	—	
7 years	5	8.1±0.6	—	
25 years	4	7.3±0.0	4	4.0±0.3
45 years	4	6.0±0.3	6	2.8±0.6
70 years	6	5.2±0.6	6	1.7±0.4

Legend:
N=Number of crossover pairs (using up-and-down method of quantal response).

Desflurane should not be used as the sole anesthetic in patients with coronary artery disease or in patients where increases in heart rate or blood pressure are undesirable. Rapid inhaled induction of anesthesia with desflurane alone, without concomitant administration of an opioid, in patients with coronary artery disease, has been associated with an increased incidence of myocardial ischemia. Desflurane, when given in conjunction with opioids for maintenance of anesthesia in patients with coronary artery disease, has not produced an incidence of ischemia different from that produced by other anesthetics. Thus, when desflurane is to be used in patients with coronary artery disease, it should always be used in combination with other medications, such as i.v. opioids or hypnotics and it should not be used for induction (see Pharmacology).

When changing the depth of anesthesia, rapid increases in the end-tidal concentration of desflurane should be avoided and the end-tidal concentration increased in small increments of 1% or less. It is not necessary to deliver concentrations far in excess of the desired end-tidal concentration ("overpressurization" technique) due to the low blood and tissue solubilities of desflurane and the resulting rapid equilibrium of alveolar concentration with inspired and delivered concentrations; thus the transient and self-limiting increases in heart rate and blood pressure may be avoided.

During maintenance of anesthesia, increases in heart rate and blood pressure occurring after rapid incremental increases in end-tidal concentration of desflurane may not represent inadequate anesthesia. The changes due to sympathetic activation resolve in approximately 4 minutes. Increases in heart rate and blood pressure occurring before or in the absence of a rapid increase in desflurane concentration may be interpreted as light anesthesia. Thus, in such patients, incremental increases of 0.5 to 1% end-tidal desflurane may attenuate these signs of light anesthesia, as may concomitant administration of analgesics. Should raised heart rate and blood pressure persist, then other causes should be sought.

SUPPLIED: Each bottle contains: desflurane 240 mL. Amber glass bottles of 250 mL. Store at or below 30°C.

Suprax® Ⓟ

cefixime

Antibiotic

sanofi-aventis

Date of Revision: October 27, 2009

PHARMACOLOGY: Cefixime exerts its bactericidal effect by attaching to penicillin-binding proteins and inhibiting peptidoglycan synthesis, thus causing damage to the bacterial cell wall.

Pharmacokinetics: Following oral dosing, cefixime attains peak serum levels in approximately 4 hours. The half-life is about 3 to 4 hours and is not dose dependent. Cefixime is excreted by renal and biliary mechanisms. About 50% of the absorbed dose is excreted unchanged in the urine within 24 hours. There is no evidence of metabolism of cefixime in vivo.

INDICATIONS: Treatment of the following infections caused by susceptible strains of the designated microorganisms:

Middle Ear: Otitis media caused by *S. pneumoniae*, *H. influenzae* (beta-lactamase positive and negative strains), *M. catarrhalis* (former *B. catarrhalis*) (beta-lactamase positive and negative strains) and *S. pyogenes*.

Paranasal Sinuses: Sinusitis caused by *S. pneumoniae*, *H. influenzae* (beta-lactamase positive and negative strains), and *M. catarrhalis* (former *B. catarrhalis*) (beta-lactamase positive and negative strains).

Urinary Tract: Acute uncomplicated cystitis and urethritis caused by *E. coli*, *P. mirabilis*, and Klebsiella species.

Upper Respiratory Tract: Pharyngitis and tonsillitis caused by *S. pyogenes*.

Lower Respiratory Tract: Acute bronchitis caused by *S. pneumoniae*, *M. catarrhalis* (former *B. catarrhalis*) (beta-lactamase positive and negative strains) and *H. influenzae* (beta-lactamase positive and negative strains).

Urinary Tract: Acute uncomplicated cystitis and urethritis caused by *E. coli*, *P. mirabilis*, and Klebsiella species.

Uncomplicated Gonorrhea: Uncomplicated gonorrhea (cervical/urethral and rectal) caused by *N. gonorrhoeae*, including penicillinase (beta-lactamase-positive) and nonpenicillinase (beta-lactamase-negative) producing strains.

Appropriate cultures should be taken for susceptibility testing before initiating treatment with cefixime. If warranted, therapy may be instituted before susceptibility results are known; however, once these are obtained, therapy may need to be adjusted.

CONTRAINDICATIONS: Patients with known allergies to the cephalosporin or penicillin antibiotics.

WARNINGS: In penicillin-sensitive patients, cefixime should be administered cautiously. Patients may be sensitive to penicillins and not to cephalosporins such as cefixime or be sensitive to both. Medical literature indicates that patients sensitive to cephalosporins are very likely to be penicillin sensitive.

Antibiotics, including cefixime, should be administered cautiously to any patient who has demonstrated some form of allergy, particularly to drugs.

C. difficile-associated disease (CDAD) has been reported with use of many antibacterial agents, including SUPRAX. CDAD may range in severity from mild diarrhea to fatal colitis. It is important to consider this diagnosis in patients who present with diarrhea, or symptoms of colitis, pseudomembranous colitis, toxic megacolon, or perforation of colon subsequent to the administration of any antibacterial agent. CDAD has been reported to occur over 2 months after the administration of antibacterial agents.

Treatment with antibacterial agents may alter the normal flora of the colon and may permit overgrowth of *C. difficile*. *C. difficile* produces toxins A and B, which contribute to the development of CDAD. CDAD may cause significant morbidity and mortality. CDAD can be refractory to antimicrobial therapy.

If the diagnosis of CDAD is suspected or confirmed, appropriate therapeutic measures should be initiated. Mild cases of CDAD usually respond to discontinuation of antibacterial agents not directed against *C. difficile*. In moderate to severe cases, consideration should be given to management with fluids and electrolytes, protein supplementation, and treatment with an antibacterial agent clinically effective against *C. difficile*. Surgical evaluation should be instituted as clinically indicated, as surgical intervention may be required in certain severe cases.

PRECAUTIONS: General: If an allergic reaction to cefixime occurs, the drug should be discontinued, and, if necessary, the patient should be treated with appropriate agents, e.g., pressor amines, antihistamines, or corticosteroids. The possibility of the emergence of resistant organisms which might result in overgrowth should be kept in mind, particularly during prolonged treatment. In such use, careful observation of the patient is essential. If superinfection occurs during therapy, appropriate measures should be taken.

Broad-spectrum antibiotics such as cefixime should be prescribed with caution in individuals with a history of gastrointestinal disease.

Once daily dosing only must be used for urinary tract infections, since twice daily dosing was shown to be not as effective in clinical studies.

Do not use cefixime to treat *S. aureus* as this strain of staphylococci is resistant to cefixime.

Renal Impairment: Cefixime may be administered in the presence of impaired renal function, but dose modification is recommended for patients with moderate or severe renal impairment (i.e., creatinine clearance of <40 mL/min) (see Dosage).

Bioavailability Differences Between Tablet and Suspension: The area under the time versus concentration curve is greater by approximately 26.4% and the C_{max} is greater by approximately 20.7% with the oral suspension when compared to the tablet after doses of 400 mg. This increased absorption should be taken into consideration if the oral suspension is to be substituted for the tablet. Because of the lack of bioequivalence, tablets should not be substituted for oral suspension particularly in the treatment of otitis media where clinical trial experience with the suspension only is available (see Dosage).

Drug/Laboratory Interactions: A false-positive reaction for ketones in the urine may occur with tests using nitroprusside but not with those using nitroferricyanide.

The administration of beta-lactams may result in a false-positive reaction for glucose in the urine using Clinitest, Benedict's solution, or Fehling's solution. It is recommended that glucose tests based on enzymatic glucose oxidase reactions (such as Clinistix) be used.

A false-positive direct Coombs test has been reported during treatment with cephalosporin antibiotics; therefore, it should be recognized that a positive Coombs test may be due to the drug.

Pregnancy: The safety of cefixime in the treatment of infection in pregnant women has not been established.

Reproduction studies have been performed in mice and rats at doses up to 400 times the human dose and have revealed no evidence of impaired fertility or harm to the fetus due to cefixime. Because animal reproduction studies are not always predictive of human response, this drug should be used during pregnancy only if the likely benefits of using cefixime outweighs the potential risk to the fetus and/or the mother.

Labor and Delivery: Cefixime has not been studied for use during labor and delivery.

Lactation: It is not known whether cefixime is excreted in human milk. Because many drugs are excreted in human milk, caution should be exercised when cefixime is administered to a nursing woman.

Children: Safety and effectiveness of cefixime in children less than 6 months old have not been established.

ADVERSE EFFECTS: Clinical Trials: Five percent of patients in the clinical trials discontinued therapy because of drug-related adverse reactions. Thirty-six percent of the pediatric patient population experienced at least one adverse reaction (mild 25%, moderate 9%, severe 2%). Forty-seven percent of the adult patients experienced at least one adverse reaction (mild 24%, moderate 19%, severe 4%). The most commonly seen adverse reactions in the clinical trials of the tablet formulation were gastrointestinal events, which were reported in 37% of all adult patients treated (mild 21%, moderate 13%, severe 3%). The predominant adverse events seen in adults in clinical trials with cefixime were diarrhea 15%, (mild 7.2%, moderate 6.2%, severe 1.5%), headache 11%, stool changes 12%, nausea 9%, abdominal pain 5%, and dyspepsia 3%. The rates of the most prevalent adverse reactions were similar in the once a day and twice a day dosing regimens with the exception of headache which appears slightly more frequently in adults dosed once a day (12.9%) versus twice a day (8%). Other than for generally mild rashes or emesis which were each observed in 5% of children treated, the incidence of adverse reactions in pediatric patients receiving the suspension was generally comparable to the incidence seen in adult patients receiving tablets.

These symptoms usually responded to symptomatic therapy or ceased when cefixime was discontinued.

Several patients developed severe diarrhea and/or documented pseudomembranous colitis, and a few required hospitalization.

When cefixime was used as single 400 mg dose therapy in clinical trials in the treatment of uncomplicated gonorrhea, adverse reactions which were considered to be related to cefixime therapy, were reported for 5.9% (21/358) of patients. Clinically mild gastrointestinal side effects occurred in 3.7% of all patients, moderate events occurred in 0.9% of all patients and no adverse reactions were reported as severe. Individual event rates included diarrhea 1% and loose or frequent stools 1%. Incidence rates for all other adverse reactions reported for adults in these trials were less than 1%.

Other Adverse Events including Post-Marketing Surveillance Data: The following adverse reactions have been reported following the use of cefixime. Incidence rates were less than 1 in 50 (less than 2%), except as otherwise noted.

Central Nervous System: headaches (11%) and dizziness (3%).

Gastrointestinal: diarrhea (15%), stool changes (12%), nausea (9%), abdominal pain (5%), dyspepsia (3%), flatulence (3%) and vomiting (2%).

Pseudomembranous colitis has been reported rarely.

Hepatic: transient elevations of AST, ALT and alkaline phosphatase.

Renal: transient elevations in Blood Urea Nitrogen (BUN) or creatinine.

Hemic and Lymphatic: transient thrombocytopenia, thrombocytosis, leukopenia, eosinophilia, neutropenia and agranulocytosis. Prolongation in prothrombin time was seen rarely.

Hypersensitivity: skin rashes, drug fever and pruritus. Anaphylactic reactions (urticaria and angioedema) have been reported rarely.

Other: Genital pruritus, vaginitis and candidiasis has been reported.

Skin: Bullous skin reactions (erythema multiforme and Stevens-Johnson syndrome) have been reported very rarely.

In addition to the adverse reactions listed above which have been observed in patients treated with cefixime, the following adverse reactions and altered laboratory tests have been reported for cephalosporin-class antibiotics. Allergic reactions were reported including anaphylaxis, Stevens-Johnson syndrome, erythema multiforme, toxic epidermal necrolysis, superinfection, renal dysfunction, toxic nephropathy, hepatic dysfunction including cholestasis, aplastic anemia, hemolytic anemia, and hemorrhage. Abnormal laboratory tests were reported including positive Coombs test, elevated bilirubin, elevated LDH, pancytopenia, neutropenia and agranulocytosis.

Several cephalosporins have been implicated in triggering seizures, particularly in patients with renal impairment when the dosage was not reduced (see Dosage and Overdose). If seizures associated with cefixime occur, the drug should be discontinued. Anticonvulsant therapy can be given if clinically indicated.

OVERDOSE:

Treatment: Gastric lavage may be indicated; otherwise, no specific antidote exists. Cefixime is not removed in significant quantities from the circulation by hemodialysis or peritoneal dialysis.

> For management of a suspected drug overdose, contact your **regional Poison Control Centre**. See the *CPS* Directory section for a list of Poison Control Centres.

DOSAGE: Adults: The recommended dose is 400 mg once daily. When necessary, a dose of 200 mg (one-half of a 400 mg tablet) given twice daily may be considered except for urinary tract infections where once daily dosing must be used.

For treatment of uncomplicated gonococcal infections, a single oral dose of 400 mg is recommended.

Children: The recommended dose is 8 mg/kg/day once daily (see Table 1). When necessary, a dose of 4 mg/kg given twice daily may be considered except for urinary tract infections where once daily dosing must be used.

Table 1: Suprax

Pediatric Dosage Chart

Weight (kg)	Dose/Day (mg)	Dose/Day (mL)
6	48	2.4
12.5	100	5.0
19	152	7.6
25	200	10.0
35	280	14.0

Children weighing more than 50 kg or older than 12 years should be treated with the recommended adult dose. Safety and effectiveness in infants aged less than 6 months have not been established.

Otitis media should be treated with the suspension. Clinical studies of otitis media were conducted with the suspension only and the suspension results in higher peak blood levels than the tablet when administered at the same dose. Therefore, the tablet should not be substituted for the suspension in the treatment of otitis media (see Precautions).

Duration of Therapy: Duration of dosage in clinical trials was 10 to 14 days. The duration of treatment should be guided by the patient's clinical and bacteriological response.

In the treatment of infections due to *S. pyogenes*, a therapeutic dose of cefixime should be administered for at least 10 days.

Renal Impairment: Cefixime may be administered in the presence of impaired renal function. Normal dose and schedule may be employed in patients with creatinine clearances of 40 mL/min or greater. Patients whose clearance is between 20 and 40 mL/min should be given 75% of the standard daily dosage. Patients whose creatinine clearance is less than 20 mL/min should be given 50% of the standard daily dosage.

Experience in children with renal impairment is very limited.

Note: Neither hemodialysis, nor peritoneal dialysis remove significant amounts of cefixime from the body.

Reconstitution Directions for Oral Suspensions: See Table 2.

Table 2: Suprax

Reconstitution Directions for Oral Suspensions

Size	Reconstitution Directions
50 mL	Suspend with 33 mL water
Method: Tap the bottle several times to loosen powder contents prior to reconstitution. Add 33 mL of water in **2 portions**. Mix well after each addition. Provides 20 mg/mL.	

After mixing, the suspension may be kept for 14 days at room temperature or under refrigeration without significant loss of potency. Keep container tightly closed. Shake well before using. Discard unused portion after 14 days.

SUPPLIED: Powder for Oral Suspension: Each 5 mL of reconstituted suspension contains: cefixime 100 mg. Nonmedicinal ingredients: artificial strawberry flavor, sodium benzoate, sucrose and xanthan gum. Gluten- and lactose-free. Bottles of 50 mL. Store at controlled room temperature 15 to 30°C.

Tablets: Each biconvex, oblong, white film-coated tablet, with rounded flattened corners, breaking scores on both sides and engraved EM 400 on one side, contains: cefixime 400 mg. The 400 mg tablet can be split into two equal parts of 200 mg. Nonmedicinal ingredients: calcium phosphate dibasic dihydrate, hydroxypropyl methylcellulose, light mineral oil, magnesium stearate, microcrystalline cellulose, pregelatinized starch, sodium lauryl sulfate and titanium dioxide. Gluten- and lactose-free. Blister packs of 7 and 10 tablets. Store at controlled room temperature 15 to 30°C.

(Shown in Product Identification Section)

Suprefact® Ⓟ

buserelin acetate

Luteinizing Hormone-Releasing Hormone (LHRH) Analog

sanofi-aventis

Date of Revision: August 10, 2010

SUMMARY PRODUCT INFORMATION:

Route of Administration	Dosage Form/ Strength	Clinically Relevant Nonmedicinal Ingredients
Subcutaneous Injection	Solution 1 mg/mL	For a complete listing see Dosage Forms, Composition and Packaging.
Intranasal	Solution 1 mg/mL	For a complete listing see Dosage Forms, Composition and Packaging.

INDICATIONS AND CLINICAL USE: SUPREFACT (buserelin acetate) is indicated for:

Subcutaneous Injection:

- The palliative treatment (initial and maintenance treatment) of patients with hormone-dependent advanced carcinoma of the prostate gland (Stage D).

Nasal Solution:

- The palliative treatment (maintenance treatment) of patients with hormone-dependent advanced carcinoma of the prostate gland (Stage D).
- The treatment of endometriosis in patients who do not require surgery as primary therapy. The duration of treatment is usually six months and should not exceed nine months.

SUPREFACT injection should be administered under the supervision of a health care professional.

Geriatrics: No data is available.

Pediatrics (<18 years of age): Experience with SUPREFACT for the management of endometriosis has been limited to women 18 years of age and older.

CONTRAINDICATIONS:

- SUPREFACT is contraindicated in patients who are hypersensitive to this drug, to any ingredient in the formulation or component of the container. Isolated cases of anaphylaxis have been reported. For a complete listing, see Dosage Forms, Composition and Packaging.

Patients with Prostatic Cancer:

- SUPREFACT is contraindicated in patients who do not present with hormone-dependent carcinoma and in patients who have undergone orchiectomy.

Patients with Endometriosis:

- SUPREFACT is contraindicated in women who are pregnant. As with other LHRH agonists, it is not known whether SUPREFACT causes fetal abnormalities in humans. Women of childbearing potential should be carefully examined before treatment to exclude pregnancy.
- The use of SUPREFACT in patients who are breast-feeding is not recommended.
- SUPREFACT should not be administered to females having undiagnosed abnormal vaginal bleeding.

WARNINGS AND PRECAUTIONS:

Serious Warnings and Precautions

SUPREFACT should be prescribed by a qualified physician experienced in the use of hormonal therapy in endometriosis and prostate cancer.

SUPREFACT Injection should be administered under the supervision of a healthcare professional (see Dosage and Administration).

The following are clinically significant adverse events:

- Clinical testosterone flare reaction in men with prostate cancer (see General and Adverse Reactions, Clinical Trial Adverse Drug Reactions)
- Osteoporosis (see Musculoskeletal)

General: Certain adverse effects (e.g. dizziness) may impair the patient's ability to concentrate and react, and therefore, constitute a risk in situations where these abilities are of special importance (e.g. operating a vehicle or machinery).

Initially, SUPREFACT transiently increases serum testosterone in males, serum estradiol in females and other gonadal hormones.

The administration of LHRH agonists is occasionally related with early, transient (less than 10 days duration usually) exacerbation of the signs and symptoms of metastatic prostatic cancer or endometriosis, which are sometimes, but not necessarily, associated with a transient rise in serum testosterone or estradiol.

Patients with Prostatic Cancer: SUPREFACT, like other LHRH agonists, causes a transient increase in serum concentration of testosterone during the first weeks of treatment. Patients may experience worsening of symptoms or onset of new symptoms, including bone pain, neuropathy, hematuria, or ureteral or bladder outlet obstruction. Cases of spinal cord compression, which may contribute to paralysis with or without complications, have been reported with LHRH agonists. If spinal cord compression or renal impairment due to ureteral obstruction develops, standard treatment of these complications should be instituted.

Patients with metastatic vertebral lesions and/or with urinary tract obstruction should begin buserelin therapy under close supervision.

It is strongly recommended that administration of an antiandrogen be started as adjunctive therapy before starting treatment with SUPREFACT.

This adjunctive therapy must be continued in parallel with SUPREFACT therapy for 4-5 weeks. After this time testosterone levels have usually fallen to the castrate level thus therapy with SUPREFACT as a single agent can be continued.

Co-administration of anti-androgens with SUPREFACT should be initiated to block testosterone flare.

The majority of clinical studies demonstrating the efficacy of SUPREFACT were completed without concomitant therapy with antiandrogens during the first weeks of treatment.

Patients with Endometriosis: Oral contraceptives must be discontinued before starting LHRH treatment; and non-hormonal methods of contraception (e.g. condoms) should be employed during therapy (see Warnings and Precautions, Special Populations, Pregnant Women).

Worsening of the clinical condition may occasionally require discontinuation of therapy and/or surgical intervention.

Cardiovascular: In treated hypertensive patients, hypertensive crisis may occur. It is recommended that blood pressure be monitored regularly in these patients.

Patients with Prostatic Cancer: There may be a relationship between androgen deprivation therapy and cardiovascular risk in men with prostate cancer on the basis of the demonstrated adverse impact of androgen deprivation on traditional cardiovascular risk factors, including serum lipoproteins, insulin sensitivity, and obesity.

Physicians should consider whether the benefits of androgen deprivation therapy outweigh the potential cardiovascular risk.

Androgen deprivation therapy has the potential to prolong QT/QTc interval on ECG. Physicians should also consider whether the benefits of androgen deprivation therapy outweigh the potential risk in patients with congenital long QT syndrome, electrolyte abnormalities, or congestive heart failure and in patients taking Class IA (e.g. quinidine, procainamide), Class III (e.g. amiodarone, sotalol, dofetilide, ibutilide), or Class IC (e.g. flecainide, propafenone) antiarrhythmic medications.

Assessment of cardiovascular risk and management according to local clinical practice and guidelines should be considered.

Endocrine and Metabolism: Isolated cases of loss of diabetic control (reduction in glucose tolerance) have been observed. Blood glucose levels should be checked regularly in diabetic patients.

Patients with Prostatic Cancer: While hypogonadism is a pharmacologic consequence of long-term LHRH agonist treatment, its reversibility has not been established in patients suffering with prostatic carcinoma.

Reduction in glucose tolerance: A reduction in glucose tolerance and an increase in diabetic risk have been observed in men treated with androgen deprivation therapy through orchiectomy or a LHRH agonist.

Therefore, diabetic patients and other patients at risk may require more frequent monitoring of blood glucose when receiving androgen deprivation therapy.

Hematologic: Patients with Prostatic Cancer: Anemia is a known physiologic consequence of testosterone suppression. Assessment of anemia risk and management according to local clinical practice and guidelines should be considered.

Hepatic/Biliary/Pancreatic: Studies have not been conducted in patients with hepatic impairment.

Immune: The hypersensitivity reactions may become manifest as, e.g. reddening of the skin, itching, skin rash (including urticaria) and allergic asthma with dyspnea as well as in isolated cases, anaphylactic/ anaphylactoid shock have been observed in patients treated with SUPREFACT, necessitating early treatment of such conditions.

Musculoskeletal: Decreased bone mineral density (BMD) can be anticipated with long term use of an LHRH agonist. Loss of BMD may lead to osteoporosis and an increased risk of skeletal bone fracture. The risk of fracture increases with the duration of therapy. Assessment of osteoporosis risk and management according to clinical practice and guidelines should be considered.

Patients with Endometriosis: Changes in Bone Density: Since bone loss can be anticipated as part of natural menopause, it may also be expected to occur during a medically induced hypoestrogenic state caused by SUPREFACT.

In patients with major risk factors for decreased bone mineral content such as chronic alcohol and/or tobacco use, presumed or strong family history of osteoporosis or chronic use of drugs that can reduce bone mass such as anticonvulsants or corticosteroids, SUPREFACT, like other LHRH analogues, may pose an additional risk. In these patients, the risks and benefits must be weighed carefully before therapy with SUPREFACT is instituted.

Use of SUPREFACT for longer than the recommended six months or in the presence of other known risk factors for decreased bone mineral content may cause additional bone loss.

Psychiatric: Patients with a history of depression or depressed moods should be observed closely for evidence of mood changes and treated accordingly.

Renal: Studies have not been conducted in patients with renal impairment.

Special Populations: Pregnant Women: Safe use of the drug in pregnancy has not been established; therefore, a non-hormonal method of contraception (e.g. condoms) should be used during treatment.

To exclude pre-existing pregnancy at the beginning of therapy, it is recommended that treatment be started on the first or second day of menstruation. If there is any doubt, a pregnancy test is recommended (see Contraindications).

Patients should be advised that if they miss or postpone a dose of SUPREFACT, ovulation may occur with the potential for conception.

If a patient becomes pregnant during treatment, she should discontinue treatment and consult her physician.

Nursing Women: SUPREFACT passes into breast milk in small amounts. Although negative effects on the infant have not been observed, it is recommended that breast-feeding be avoided during treatment with SUPREFACT in order to prevent the infant from ingesting small quantities of SUPREFACT with breast milk.

Pediatrics (<18 years of age): Experience with SUPREFACT for the management of endometriosis has been limited to women 18 years of age and older.

Geriatrics: No data is available.

Monitoring and Laboratory Tests: LHRH agonist treatment will affect selected hormonal and other serum/urine parameters in the first week of treatment: elevation of testosterone and dihydrotestosterone, as well as acid phosphatase and estradiol can be expected. With chronic drug administration, these elevated values of these variables will fall below baseline.

It is recommended that blood pressure be monitored regularly in patients with hypertension (See Warnings and Precautions, Cardiovascular).

Glycemic control tests such as blood glucose levels should be performed regularly in diabetic patients (See Warnings and Precautions, Endocrine and Metabolism).

Patients with Prostatic Cancer: Regular clinical assessment of patients and appropriate laboratory tests are recommended.

The response to treatment may be monitored by measuring serum testosterone, prostatic acid phosphatase (PAP) or acid phosphatase, and prostate-specific antigen (PSA). If cancer is responsive to SUPREFACT therapy, the prostate cancer tumor markers (PAP and PSA), if elevated prior to the commencement of treatment, are usually reduced by the end of the first month.

The status of bone lesions may be monitored by bone scans and that of the prostate lesions may be followed by ultrasonography and/or CT scan in addition to digital rectal examination.

Evaluation for obstructive uropathy may be undertaken by ultrasonography, intravenous pyelogram or CT scan in addition to clinical examination.

Evaluation of blood glucose levels may be undertaken at baseline and periodically thereafter for patients at risk.

Evaluation for QT prolongation may be undertaken for patients at risk by baseline ECG recording. Baseline measurements of serum potassium, calcium, and magnesium levels should be considered. Monitoring of serum electrolytes during treatment should be considered in those patients at risk for an electrolyte abnormality.

ADVERSE REACTIONS: Adverse Drug Reaction Overview: The adverse effects observed in patients treated with SUPREFACT are, principally, directly related to its anticipated pharmacologic action, i.e. suppression of pituitary (gonadotropin) and gonadal (testosterone or estradiol) hormone production with resulting clinical signs and symptoms of hypogonadism.

The most frequent adverse events reported in patients with prostatic cancer receiving SUPREFACT are hot flushes, loss of libido, impotence, nasal irritation (nasal solution) and headache (nasal solution).

The most frequent adverse events reported in patients with endometriosis receiving SUPREFACT are hot flushes, vaginal dryness, menorrhagia, headache and loss of libido.

Clinical Trial Adverse Drug Reactions: Patients with Prostatic Cancer: An early in treatment transient increase in serum testosterone levels usually occurs. Occasionally, this may be associated with transient worsening of clinical status with secondary reactions such as: occurrence or exacerbation of bone pain in patients with bone metastases, signs of neurological deficit due to spinal cord compression, impaired micturition, hydronephrosis, lymphostasis or thrombosis with pulmonary embolism. This transient initial rise in serum androgen will be followed by a progressive decrease to castration levels (see Warnings and Precautions, General). Serious clinical (flare) reactions were reported in approximately 1% of patients in SUPREFACT efficacy trials.

Such reactions can be largely avoided when an antiandrogen is given concomitantly in the initial phase of SUPREFACT treatment. However, even with concomitant anti-androgen therapy, a mild but transient increase in tumor pain as well as a deterioration in general well-being may develop in some patients.

In a large, North American multicentre study of SUPREFACT, the following reactions were encountered as listed in Table 1.

Table 1: SUPREFACT

Listing of Adverse Reactions, Arranged by Body System, Possibly or Probably Related to SUPREFACT That Occurred at an Incidence of 1% or Greater in Patients with Prostatic Cancer

	SUPREFACT	
Adverse Reactions	**Subcutaneous (%)**	**Intranasal (%)**
Gastrointestinal Disorders		
Gastrointestinal Disturbances	3.0	
Dry Mouth	—	1.8
General Disorders and Administration Site Conditions		
Transient Injection Site Reactions[a]	11.9	5.4
Pain	4.6	
Irritation	3.3	3.6
Swelling	3.3	
Urticaria	2.0	1.8
Other	4.6	
Clinical Flare Reaction	1.3	
Nervous System Disorders		
Headache[b]	—	28.5
Psychiatric Disorders		
Loss of Libido[c]	84.8	75.0
Reproductive System and Breast Disorders		
Impotence[c]	79.4	75.0
Gynecomastia	2.6	
Respiratory, Thoracic and Mediastinal Disorders		
Nasal Irritation[b]	—	12.5
Dry Nose		1.8
Skin and Subcutaneous Tissue Disorders		
Pruritus	1.3	—
Increased Sweating		1.8
Vascular Disorders		
Hot Flushes	71.6	66.1

[a] None of the transient injection site reactions were severe or required discontinuation of therapy.
[b] Not all of the cases were considered (by investigators) to be drug related.
[c] Over 50% of patients enrolled reported loss of libido.

Patients with Endometriosis: During the first two weeks of treatment with intranasal SUPREFACT, estradiol levels may increase but, thereafter decrease to basal or lower levels. This transient increase in estradiol may result in a temporary exacerbation of signs and symptoms (see Warnings and Precautions).

In two multicentre, open-label, randomized clinical trials, SUPREFACT was compared to danazol in the treatment of patients with mild to severe endometriosis. Reported adverse reactions, which were considered by the treating physician to have a possible or probable relationship to treatment and which occurred in 5% or more of patients are listed in Table 2.

Table 2: SUPREFACT

Possible or Probable Adverse Reactions in ≥5% of Patients Taking SUPREFACT in Two Trials in the Treatment of Mild to Severe Endometriosis

Adverse Reaction	**SUPREFACT (n=168) n (%)**	**Danazol (n=109) n (%)**
Hot Flushes[a]	121 (72.0)	42 (38.5)
Vaginal Dryness[a]	48 (28.6)	8 (7.3)
Menorrhagia	40 (23.8)	24 (22.0)
Headache[a]	34 (20.2)	18 (16.5)
Libido Decreased[a]	20 (11.9)	8 (7.3)
Dizziness	15 (8.9)	6 (5.5)
Application Site Reaction	13 (7.7)	0 (0.0)
Depression[a]	13 (7.7)	6 (5.5)
Emotional Lability[a]	12 (7.1)	15 (13.8)
Asthenia	12 (7.1)	24 (22.0)
Nausea	11 (6.5)	9 (8.3)
Acne[b]	9 (5.4)	35 (32.1)

(cont'd)

Table 2: SUPREFACT *(cont'd)*

[a] Physiological effects of decreased estrogen.
[b] Androgenic-like effects.

In addition, in these same studies, other adverse reactions possibly or probably related to SUPREFACT therapy that occurred between 1% and 5% of patients are listed in Table 3.

Table 3: SUPREFACT

Listing of Adverse Reactions, Arranged by Body System, Possibly or Probably Related to SUPREFACT That Occurred Between 1% and 5% in Patients with Endometriosis

Body System Adverse Reactions (Preferred Term)	**SUPREFACT (n=168) n (%)**
Cardiac Disorders	
Palpitation	2 (1.2)
Gastrointestinal Disorders	
Constipation	2 (1.2)
Gastrointestinal Fullness	5 (3.0)
Infections and Infestations	
Rhinitis	3 (1.8)
Upper Respiratory Infection	2 (1.2)
Vaginitis	3 (1.8)
Investigations	
Weight Gain	5 (3.0)
Weight Loss	4 (2.4)
Metabolism and Nutrition Disorders	
Edema	5 (3.0)
Musculoskeletal and Connective Tissue Disorders	
Arthralgia	8 (4.8)
Myalgia	3 (1.8)
Neck Rigidity	2 (1.2)
Pain in Extremity	3 (1.8)
Nervous System Disorders	
Migraine	5 (3.0)
Paresthesia	4 (2.4)
Taste Perversion	3 (1.8)
Psychiatric Disorders	
Anxiety	2 (1.2)
Hostility	2 (1.2)
Insomnia	8 (4.8)
Nervousness	4 (2.4)
Reproductive System and Breast Disorders	
Breast Pain	5 (3.0)
Dyspareunia	3 (1.8)
Menstrual Disorder	2 (1.2)
Skin and Subcutaneous Tissue Disorders	
Dry Skin	3 (1.8)
Hirsutism	2 (1.2)

(cont'd)

Table 3: SUPREFACT *(cont'd)*

Listing of Adverse Reactions, Arranged by Body System, Possibly or Probably Related to SUPREFACT That Occurred Between 1% and 5% in Patients with Endometriosis

Body System Adverse Reactions (Preferred Term)	SUPREFACT (n=168) n (%)
Purpura	2 (1.2)
Skin Disorder	3 (1.8)

In other clinical trials comprising a total of 968 patients with endometriosis treated with SUPREFACT, adverse events not listed above which occurred in 1% or more of patients are included in Table 4 (not all cases were assessed for causality to SUPREFACT).

Table 4: SUPREFACT

Listing of Adverse Reactions, Arranged by Body System, That Occurred in 1% or More of Patients with Endometriosis (Causality Not Assessed in All Cases)

Body System Adverse Reactions (Preferred Term)	SUPREFACT (n=968) 1200 µg/day (n=152) n (%)	900 µg/day (n=816)[a] n (%)
Gastrointestinal Disorders		
Diarrhea	12 (7.9)	8 (1.0)
Dry Mouth	4 (2.6)	9 (1.1)
Flatulence	23 (15.1)	4 (0.5)
Vomiting	6 (3.9)	9 (1.1)
General Disorders and Administration Site Conditions		
Ill-defined Symptoms	23 (15.1)	16 (2.0)
Malaise	12 (7.9)	4 (0.5)
Infections and Infestations		
Infection	11 (7.2)	—
Metabolism and Nutrition Disorders		
Generalized Edema	9 (5.9)	1 (0.1)
Peripheral Edema	3 (2.0)	12 (1.5)
Musculoskeletal and Connective Tissue Disorders		
Back Pain	42 (27.6)	30 (3.7)
Psychiatric Disorders		
Sleep Disorder	2 (1.3)	10 (1.2)
Reproductive System and Breast Disorders		
Leukorrhea	—	36 (4.4)
Pelvic Pain	1 (0.7)	17 (2.1)
Premenstrual Syndrome	—	12 (1.5)
Vaginal Discharge	—	14 (1.7)
Vaginal Discomfort	—	11 (1.3)
Respiratory, Thoracic and Mediastinal Disorders		
Sore Throat	8 (5.3)	4 (0.5)
Skin and Subcutaneous Tissue Disorders		
Pruritus	—	12 (1.5)

[a] 16 patients received 450-1800 µg/day.

Less Common Clinical Trial Adverse Drug Reactions (<1%): Patients with Prostatic Cancer: Other adverse reactions, arranged by body system possibly or probably related to the administration of SUPREFACT that occurred at an incidence below 1% included:
Body as a Whole: fever (subcutaneous), pain (subcutaneous).
Digestive System: (subcutaneous) diarrhea, nausea.
Endocrine System: feminization (subcutaneous).
Skin and Appendages: hirsutism (subcutaneous).
Urogenital System: urinary retention (subcutaneous).
Patients with Endometriosis: Other adverse reactions possibly or probably related to SUPREFACT therapy reported in less than 1% of patients included:
Body as a Whole: abdominal pain, allergic reaction, pain, photosensitivity.
Cardiovascular System: syncope, vasodilatation.
Digestive System: gastrointestinal disorder, gastrointestinal pain, increased appetite, mouth ulceration.
Nervous System: amnesia, somnolence, sweating increased, thinking abnormal, tremor, vertigo.
Respiratory System: epistaxis.
Skin and Appendages: breast atrophy, breast enlargement, rash.
Special Senses: abnormality of accommodation, dry eyes, ear disorder, ear pain, eye disorder, parosmia, tinnitus.
Urogenital System: vaginal hemorrhage.

Abnormal Hematologic and Clinical Chemistry Findings: LHRH agonist treatment will affect selected hormonal and other serum/urine parameters in the first week of treatment: elevation of testosterone and dihydrotestosterone, as well as acid phosphatase and estradiol can be expected. With chronic drug administration, these elevated values of these variables will fall below baseline.

In addition, changes in blood lipids, increase in bilirubin levels, increase in serum liver enzymes levels (e.g. transaminases), leucopenia, thrombopenia have been observed with the use of SUPREFACT.

Post-Market Adverse Drug Reactions: Very rare cases of pituitary adenomas were reported during treatment with LHRH agonists, including SUPREFACT.

Patients with Prostatic Cancer: In the international adverse effect database other adverse events have been observed in patients treated with buserelin with all reports probably or possibly related to the administration of SUPREFACT:
Endocrine disorder: atrophy of the testes.
Metabolic and Nutritional Disorders: mild edemas of the ankles and lower legs.
Nervous System: mood changes.
Respiratory System: rhinorrhea.
Special senses: eye dryness and irritation.
Skin and Appendages: articular pains, skin reaction (wheal) allergy.
Patients with Endometriosis: In the international database, other adverse events have been observed in patients treated with buserelin, as itemized below (not all events were considered to be related to buserelin therapy):
Digestive System: increased thirst.
Haemic and Lymphatic System: leucopenia, thrombopenia.
Nervous System: concentration and memory disturbances, drowsiness, tiredness.
Skin and Appendages: articular pains, application site pain, irritation of the mucosa in the nasopharynx due to nasal solution administration (which may lead to nosebleeds, hoarseness, disturbances of smell or taste), brittle finger nails, female lactation, decrease or increase in scalp hair, decrease in body hair.
Special Senses: feeling of pressure behind the eyes, impaired vision (e.g. blurred vision).
Urogenital System: ovarian cysts (during the initial phase of therapy).

DRUG INTERACTIONS: Drug-Drug Interactions: During treatment with SUPREFACT, the effect of antidiabetic agents may be attenuated.

Patients with Prostatic Cancer: Co-administration of androgen deprivation therapy with medicinal products known to prolong the QTc interval or to induce torsades de pointes should be carefully evaluated. Such medicinal products include but are not limited to the examples that follow: Class IA (e.g. quinidine, disopyramide), Class III (e.g. amiodarone, sotalol, dofetilide, ibutilide), or Class IC (e.g. flecainide, propafenone) antiarrhythmic medicinal products, antipsychotics (e.g. chlorpromazine), antidepressants (e.g. amitriptyline, nortriptyline), opioids (e.g. methadone), macrolide antibiotics and analogues (e.g. erythromycin, clarithromycin, azithromycin), quinolone antibiotics (e.g. moxifloxacin), pentamidine, antimalarials (e.g. quinine), azole antifungals, 5-hydroxytryptamine (5-HT3) receptor antagonists (e.g. ondansetron), and beta-2 adrenoceptor agonists (e.g. salbutamol).

Patients with Endometriosis: In concomitant treatment with sexual hormones ("add-back"), the dosage is to be selected so as to ensure that the overall therapeutic effect is not affected.

Drug-Herb Interactions: Interactions with herbal products have not been established.

Drug-Laboratory Test Interactions: Administration of SUPREFACT in therapeutic doses results in suppression of the pituitary-gonadal system. Normal function is usually restored after a few weeks of last dose of SUPREFACT. Diagnostic tests of pituitary-gonadal function conducted during the treatment and within a few weeks after discontinuation of SUPREFACT therapy may therefore be misleading.

DOSAGE AND ADMINISTRATION:

Dosing Considerations: SUPREFACT should be administered at approximately equal time intervals to ensure that the desired therapeutic effect is maintained.

Recommended Dose and Dosage Adjustment: Patients with Prostatic Cancer: Initial Treatment: For the first seven days of treatment give SUPREFACT 500 µg (0.5 mL) every 8 hours by subcutaneous injection. For patient comfort, vary the injection site.

Maintenance Treatment: Depending upon patient preference, or physician recommendation, maintenance treatment may be by daily subcutaneous injection or by intranasal administration three times daily.

During maintenance dosing by the subcutaneous injection route, the SUPREFACT dose is 200 µg (0.2 mL) daily. For patient comfort, vary the site of injection.

During maintenance dosing by the intranasal administration route, the SUPREFACT dose is 400 µg (200 µg into each nostril) three times daily using the metered-dose pump (nebulizer) provided. Each pump action delivers 100 µg buserelin (as buserelin acetate) or 0.1 mL solution.

Patients with Endometriosis: The dose of SUPREFACT in patients with endometriosis is 400 µg (200 µg into each nostril) three times daily using the metered-dose pump (nebulizer) provided. Each pump action delivers 100 µg buserelin (as buserelin acetate) or 0.1 mL solution. The treatment duration is usually six months and should not exceed nine months.

Missed Dose: Should the patient forget to take a dose, the dose should be administered as soon as they remember. However, if it is almost time for the next dose, the patients should skip the missed dose and go back to their regular dosing schedule. The patient should not double doses.

Administration: SUPREFACT Injection: The SUPREFACT vial is supplied with a plastic cap which can be removed by pressing upwards with the thumb. This cap serves to ensure that the vial has not been previously entered. After removal (the cap can be discarded) the rubber diaphragm of the vial is exposed. Proceed as follows:

1. Wash your hands, with soap and water, and dry on a clean towel.
2. Clean the rubber diaphragm of the SUPREFACT vial with a cotton swab previously dipped in alcohol. Leave to dry.
3. Select an appropriate sterile, disposable syringe and needle assembly and remove it from its sterile packaging.
4. Draw the syringe piston as far back as the volume (see syringe cylinder graduation) of solution you wish to withdraw from the vial.
5. Remove the needle sheath (protector).
6. Without touching the needle with your fingers, push the needle through the centre of the rubber diaphragm of the vial.
7. Push on the syringe plunger so that the selected air volume is expelled into the vial.
8. Keeping the needle in the vial, invert the vial into the vertical position adjusting the needle tip to a position below the surface of the solution in the vial.
9. Draw the required solution from the vial by withdrawing the syringe piston.
10. Carefully withdraw the needle and syringe assembly from the vial.
11. Choose the injection site (vary the site for each injection) and clean the skin with an alcohol impregnated swab
12. Pinch the site, if you wish, between index finger and thumb and, with the needle at an angle introduce the needle quickly under the skin as far as possible.
13. Withdraw the syringe piston a little and, if no blood is withdrawn into the syringe, then push on the piston steadily to inject the solution.
14. Upon completion of the injection, and resting the alcohol-impregnated swab over the needle entry site, remove the needle in a reverse fashion of the entry motion. Hold swab to injection site for a few seconds, then remove.
15. Discard needle and syringe assembly along with the swab in a safe manner. Return the SUPREFACT vial to its storage area.

There is no information available on possible incompatibilities between SUPREFACT solution or SUPREFACT injection and other agents.

OVERDOSAGE:

From acute studies of buserelin acetate in rodents, neither 0.5 mg/kg/IV (mouse) nor 1 mg/kg/IV (rat) produced evidence of toxic signs.

Two groups of 6 and 4 healthy volunteers, aged 26-40 years and 31-40 years respectively, were given 1 mg buserelin or 5 mg buserelin orally as a single dose. No luteinizing hormone (LH) or follicle stimulating hormone (FSH) release was observed. No clinical effects were observed.

Overdose may lead to signs and symptoms such as asthenia, headache, nervousness, hot flushes, dizziness, nausea, abdominal pain, edemas of the lower extremities, and mastodynia.

For the injectable formulation, local reactions at the injection site such as pain, haemorrhage and induration.

Therapy for overdose is directed to the symptoms.

For management of a suspected drug overdose, contact your regional Poison Control Centre. See the *CPS Directory* section for a list of Poison Control Centres.

ACTION AND CLINICAL PHARMACOLOGY: Mechanism of Action: Buserelin acetate is a synthetic peptide analog of the natural gonadotropin releasing hormone (GnRH/LHRH) with enhanced biological activity. After repeated administration of SUPREFACT, the secretion of gonadotrophin release and gonadal steroids is significantly inhibited. The pharmacological effect is attributable to the down-regulation of pituitary LHRH receptors.

In male individuals the elimination of gonadotrophin release results in a reduction in the synthesis and secretion of testosterone. In female individuals the elimination of pulsatile gonadotrophin release inhibits the secretion of estrogen.

Pharmacodynamics: The substitution of glycine in position 6 by D-serine, and that of glycinamide in position 10 by ethylamide, leads to a nonapeptide with a greatly enhanced LHRH effect. The effects of buserelin on FSH and LH release are 20 to 170 times greater than those of LHRH. Buserelin also has a longer duration of action than natural LHRH.

Investigations in healthy adult males and females have demonstrated that the increase in plasma LH and FSH levels persist for at least 7 hours and that a return to basal values requires about 24 hours.

Clinical inhibition of gonadotropin release, and subsequent reduction of serum testosterone or estradiol to castration level, was found when large pharmacologic doses (50-500 µg SC/day or 300-1200 µg IN/day) were administered for periods greater than 1 to 3 months. Chronic administration of such doses of buserelin results in sustained inhibition of gonadotropin production, suppression of ovarian and testicular steroidogenesis and, ultimately, reduced circulating levels of gonadotropin and gonadal steroids. These effects form the basis for buserelin use in patients with hormone-dependent metastatic carcinoma of the prostate gland as well as in patients with endometriosis.

Pharmacokinetics: Absorption: SUPREFACT is water-soluble; when administered by subcutaneous injection it is reliably absorbed. After subcutaneous injection of 200 µg, SUPREFACT is 70% bioavailable; in contrast, after oral administration, SUPREFACT is ineffective.

If administered correctly by the nasal route, it is absorbed via the nasal mucosa in such a way that sufficiently high plasma levels are guaranteed. The nasal absorption of SUPREFACT from SUPREFACT nasal solution is 1 to 3%.

Distribution: SUPREFACT circulates in serum predominantly in intact active form. SUPREFACT accumulates preferentially in the liver and kidneys as well as in the anterior pituitary lobe, the biological target organ. Protein binding is approximately 15%.

Metabolism: SUPREFACT is metabolized and subsequently inactivated by peptidase (pyroglutamyl peptidase and chymotrypsin-like endopeptidase) in the liver and kidneys as well as in the gastrointestinal tract. In the pituitary gland, receptor-bond SUPREFACT is inactivated by membrane-located enzymes.

Excretion: SUPREFACT and inactive SUPREFACT metabolites are excreted via the renal and biliary routes. In man approximately 50% of SUPREFACT excreted in urine is intact.

The elimination half-life is approximately 50 to 80 minutes following intravenous administration, 80 minutes after subcutaneous administration and approximately 1 to 2 hours after intranasal administration.

Special Populations and Conditions: Hepatic Insufficiency: The effect of hepatic impairment on the pharmacokinetics of SUPREFACT has not been studied.

Renal Insufficiency: The effect of renal impairment on the pharmacokinetics of SUPREFACT has not been studied.

STORAGE AND STABILITY: Solution for Subcutaneous Injection: Store at controlled room temperature 15-25°C in the original container, protect from heat and light, do not freeze.

Do not use beyond the expiration date printed on the container label.

The product can be kept up to 14 days after the first opening when stored at room temperature.

Keep in a safe place out of reach of children.

Solution for Intranasal Administration: Store at controlled room temperature 15-25°C in the original container, protect from heat and light, do not freeze.

Do not use beyond the expiration date printed on the container label.

The product can be kept up to 5 weeks after the first opening when stored at room temperature.

Keep in a safe place out of reach of children.

INFORMATION FOR THE PATIENT: Published in e-CPS, available by subscription at www.e-cps.ca.

DOSAGE FORMS, COMPOSITION AND PACKAGING: Injection: Each mL of sterile aqueous injection solution contains: buserelin acetate 1.05 mg (equivalent to 1 mg pure anhydrous buserelin free base). Nonmedicinal ingredients: benzyl alcohol, monobasic sodium phosphate, sodium chloride and sodium hydroxide. Clear glass, multidose vials of 10 mL containing 5.5 mL (net) ready for administration direct from the container. Cartons of 2, each containing 1 vial of 5.5 mL.

Nasal Solution: Each mL of aqueous intranasal solution contains: buserelin acetate 1.06 mg (equivalent to 1 mg pure anhydrous buserelin free base). Nonmedicinal ingredients: benzalkonium chloride, citric acid/sodium citrate and sodium chloride. Amber glass bottles of 10 mL (net) with metered-dose pump (nebulizer) ready for administration direct from the container. Cartons of 1 bottle and 1 metered-dose pump. The metered-dose pump (nebulizer) provided has a mechanical action and contains no propellants.

Suprefact® Depot ℞

buserelin acetate

Luteinizing Hormone-Releasing Hormone (LHRH) Analog

sanofi-aventis

Date of Revision: August 10, 2010

PHARMACOLOGY: Buserelin is a synthetic peptide analogue of the natural gonadotropin releasing hormone (GnRH/LH-RH). The substitution of glycine in position 6 by D-serine, and that of glycinamide in position 10 by ethylamide, leads to a nonapeptide with a greatly enhanced LH-RH effect. The effects of buserelin on follicle stimulating hormone (FSH) and luteinizing hormone (LH) release are 20 to 170 times greater than those of LH-RH. Buserelin also has a longer duration of action than natural LH-RH.

Investigations in healthy adult males and females have demonstrated that the increase in plasma LH and FSH levels persist for at least 7 hours and that a return to basal values requires about 24 hours.

Clinical inhibition of gonadotropin release, and subsequent reduction of serum testosterone or estradiol to castration level, was found when large pharmacologic doses (50 to 500 µg s.c./day or 300 to 1200 µg intranasal/day) were administered for periods greater than 1 to 3 months. Chronic administration of such doses of buserelin results in sustained inhibition of gonadotropin production, suppression of ovarian and testicular steroidogenesis and, ultimately, reduced circulating levels of gonadotropin and gonadal steroids. These effects form the basis for buserelin use in patients with hormone-dependent metastatic carcinoma of the prostate gland.

In the clinical pharmacology studies with the buserelin implant 2 months, the time-concentration curves of buserelin release from implants were reproducible and similar to those observed in preclinical studies. Maximum release on day 1 was followed by an extended plateau phase which lasted for 8 weeks. After this period, an accelerated biodegradation of the implant material was observed with a terminal half-life of release of 20 to 30 days. The single dose studies performed in healthy male subjects and in patients with benign prostatic hypertrophy showed a therapeutic release rate for 8 weeks (dosage interval); a minimum therapeutic release rate of 4.95 µg/day after 2 months was fully effective in maintaining testosterone levels in the surgical castration range by controlled release of buserelin. At the end of the dosage interval, the average fraction of the buserelin dose released from the implants based on urinary excretion data was 84% (in healthy subjects) and 92% (in patients with benign prostatic hypertrophy). Chronic administration of the implant every 2 months ensures continuous suppression of testosterone secretion with no cumulation of buserelin release after repeated dosing.

Similarly the release profile of the buserelin implant 3 months is biphasic; the initial release (T_{max} <1 day) is followed by a phase with slow, steady-release lasting more than the 3-month dosing interval. A second small increase in the serum buserelin concentration was detected between weeks 12 and 16. At 16 weeks, median serum levels of buserelin were far above the detection limit (0.05 ng/mL), indicating considerable release reserve, and testosterone levels were in the surgical castration range. Sixteen weeks after single-dose administration of buserelin implant 3 months, urinary excretion of buserelin is between 2 and 31 µg/g creatinine (estimated threshold for suppression of testosterone secretion is 1 µg/g creatinine). This indicates that the release characteristics of buserelin from the implant ensure therapeutically effective systemic concentrations for at least 3 weeks after the end of the proposed dosing interval (3 months).

INDICATIONS AND CLINICAL USE: SUPREFACT DEPOT 2 months and SUPREFACT DEPOT 3 months are indicated for the palliative treatment of patients with hormone-dependent advanced carcinoma of the prostate gland (Stage D).

CONTRAINDICATIONS: SUPREFACT DEPOT 2 months and SUPREFACT DEPOT 3 months are contraindicated in: patients with known hypersensitivity to buserelin or any other formulation component; patients who do not present with hormone-dependent carcinoma; and in patients who have undergone orchiectomy (in these patients, no further reduction of testosterone level is to be expected with buserelin therapy).

> **Serious Warnings and Precautions**
> SUPREFACT DEPOT 2 months and SUPREFACT DEPOT 3 months should be prescribed by a qualified physician experienced in the use of hormonal therapy in prostate cancer.
> SUPREFACT DEPOT 2 months and SUPREFACT DEPOT 3 months should be administered by a healthcare professional (see Dosage).
> The following are clinically significant adverse events:
> - Clinical testosterone flare reaction in men with prostate cancer (see Warnings, General; Precautions and Adverse Reactions)
> - Osteoporosis (see Precautions)

WARNINGS: General: Cases of early, transient exacerbation of disease signs and symptoms have been reported during treatment with LH-RH agonists (see Precautions). At the start of treatment, there is a temporary rise in male sex hormones. In a few patients, this rise may be associated with isolated cases of short-term worsening of signs and symptoms such as bone pain, urinary signs and symptoms (usually occurring in patients with a previous history of obstructive uropathy) or muscular weakness in the legs. Worsening of clinical conditions may occasionally require discontinuation of therapy and/or surgical intervention.

The majority of clinical studies demonstrating the efficacy of buserelin injection and nasal solution were completed without concomitant therapy with antiandrogens during the first weeks of treatment. For the clinical studies with buserelin implant 2 months and buserelin implant 3 months, however, an antiandrogen was administered as initial concurrent treatment for a duration of 5 weeks, starting 7 days before the start of buserelin implant therapy.

Patients with Vertebral Metastases: Due to the possibility of early, transient, lesion exacerbation, and consequent possible spinal cord compression, these patients should be closely monitored when LH-RH agonist treatment is initiated.

Patients with Genitourinary Tract Symptoms: Patients with genitourinary symptoms may experience a transient increase in such symptoms early in LH-RH agonist treatment. These patients should be particularly closely observed for events indicative of obstruction.

Reversibility of LH-RH Agonist-induced Hypogonadism: While hypogonadism is a pharmacologic consequence of long-term LH-RH agonist treatment, its reversibility has not been established in patients suffering with prostatic carcinoma.

PRECAUTIONS: General: Transient Exacerbation of Disease Signs and Symptoms: The administration of LH-RH agonists is occasionally related with early, transient (less than 10 days duration usually) exacerbation of the signs and symptoms of metastatic prostatic cancer which sometimes occurs in association with a transient rise in serum testosterone. Special precautions are recommended in the following patients since symptoms may progress to warrant, in rare cases, additional or alternate interventions:

- patients with metastatic vertebral lesions
- patients with history of obstructive uropathy (see Warnings).

From clinical trials with SUPREFACT DEPOT 2 months and SUPREFACT DEPOT 3 months, administration of an antiandrogen before and concurrently at the start of buserelin implant therapy may avoid the occurrence of such signs and symptoms of the disease (in clinical trials, the antiandrogen was primarily given for the first five weeks, beginning seven days prior to the first buserelin implant injection).

Cardiovascular: In treated hypertensive patients, hypertensive crisis may occur. It is recommended that blood pressure be monitored regularly in these patients.

There may be a relationship between androgen deprivation therapy and cardiovascular risk in men with prostate cancer on the basis of the demonstrated adverse impact of androgen deprivation on traditional cardiovascular risk factors, including serum lipoproteins, insulin sensitivity, and obesity.

Physicians should consider whether the benefits of androgen deprivation therapy outweigh the potential cardiovascular risk.

Androgen deprivation therapy has the potential to prolong QT/QTc interval on ECG. Physicians should also consider whether the benefits of androgen deprivation therapy outweigh the potential risk in patients with congenital long QT syndrome, electrolyte abnormalities, or congestive heart failure and in patients taking Class IA (e.g. quinidine, procainamide), Class III (e.g. amiodarone, sotalol, dofetilide, ibutilide), or Class IC (e.g. flecainide, propafenone) antiarrhythmic medications.

Assessment of cardiovascular risk and management according to local clinical practice and guidelines should be considered.

Endocrine and Metabolism: Isolated cases of loss of diabetic control have been observed. Blood glucose levels should be checked regularly in diabetic patients.

Reduction in glucose tolerance: A reduction in glucose tolerance and an increase in diabetic risk have been observed in men treated with androgen deprivation therapy through orchiectomy or a LHRH agonist.

Therefore, diabetic patients and other patients at risk may require more frequent monitoring of blood glucose when receiving androgen deprivation therapy.

Hematologic: Anemia is a known physiologic consequence of testosterone suppression. Assessment of anemia risk and management according to local clinical practice and guidelines should be considered.

Immune: Allergic Reactions: Allergic asthma with dyspnea as well as in isolated cases, anaphylactic/anaphylactoid shock have been observed in patients treated with buserelin, necessitating early treatment of such conditions. For patients experiencing anaphylactic/anaphylactoid reactions who were given buserelin implant 2 months or buserelin implant 3 months, it may be necessary to surgically remove the implant.

Muscoloskeletal: Changes in Bone Density: Bone loss can be expected as part of natural aging and can also be anticipated during medically induced hypoandrogenic status caused by long-term use of LH-RH agonists such as buserelin. In patients with significant risk factors for decreased bone mineral content and/or bone mass such as family history of osteoporosis, chronic use of corticosteroids or anticonvulsants or chronic abuse of alcohol or tobacco, LH-RH agonists may pose additional risk. In these patients, risk and benefits must be weighed carefully before initiation of LH-RH agonist therapy. Assessment of osteoporosis risk and management according to local clinical practice and guidelines should be considered during androgen deprivation therapy.

Psychiatric: Patients with a history of depression or depressed moods should be observed closely for evidence of mood changes and treated accordingly.

Monitoring of Patients: Regular clinical assessment of patients and appropriate laboratory tests are recommended.

The response to treatment may be monitored by measuring serum testosterone, prostatic acid phosphatase (PAP) or acid phosphatase, and prostate-specific antigen (PSA). If cancer is responsive to buserelin acetate therapy, the prostate cancer tumor markers (PAP and PSA), if elevated prior to the commencement of treatment, are usually reduced by the end of the first month.

The status of bone lesions may be monitored by bone scans and that of the prostate lesions may be followed by ultrasonography and/or CT scan in addition to digital rectal examination.

Evaluation for obstructive uropathy may be undertaken by ultrasonography, intravenous pyelogram or CT scan in addition to clinical examination.

It is recommended that blood pressure be monitored regularly in patients with hypertension (See Precautions, Cardiovascular).

Glycemic control tests such as blood glucose levels should be performed regularly in diabetic patients (See Precautions, Endocrine and Metabolism).

Evaluation of blood glucose levels may be undertaken at baseline and periodically thereafter for patients at risk.

Evaluation for QT prolongation may be undertaken for patients at risk by baseline ECG recording. Baseline measurements of serum potassium, calcium, and magnesium levels should be considered. Monitoring of serum electrolytes during treatment should be considered in those patients at risk for an electrolyte abnormality.

Effect on Clinical Laboratory Tests: LH-RH agonist treatment will affect selected hormonal and other serum/urine parameters in the first week of treatment: elevation of testosterone and dihydrotestosterone, as well as acid phosphatase can be expected. With chronic drug administration, these elevated values of these variables will fall below baseline.

Renal function tests, blood urea nitrogen and creatinine may rarely be elevated during the first few days of LH-RH agonist therapy in prostate cancer patients before returning to normal.

Drug Interactions: During treatment with buserelin, the effect of antidiabetic agents may be attenuated (see also Adverse Reactions).

Co-administration of androgen deprivation therapy with medicinal products known to prolong the QTc interval or to induce torsades de pointes should be carefully evaluated. Such medicinal products include but are not limited to the examples that follow: Class IA (e.g. quinidine, disopyramide), Class III (e.g. amiodarone, sotalol, dofetilide, ibutilide), or Class IC (e.g. flecainide, propafenone) antiarrhythmic medicinal products, antipsychotics (e.g. chlorpromazine), antidepressants (e.g. amitriptyline, nortriptyline), opioids (e.g. methadone), macrolide antibiotics and analogues (e.g. erythromycin, clarithromycin, azithromycin), quinolone antibiotics (e.g. moxifloxacin), pentamidine, antimalarials (e.g. quinine), azole antifungals, 5-hydroxytryptamine ($5\text{-}HT_3$) receptor antagonists (e.g. ondansetron), and beta-2 adrenoceptor agonists (e.g. salbutamol).

ADVERSE REACTIONS: The adverse effects observed in patients treated with SUPREFACT DEPOT 2 months or SUPREFACT DEPOT 3 months are, principally, directly related to its anticipated pharmacologic action, i.e. suppression of pituitary (gonadotropin) and gonadal (testosterone) hormone production with resulting clinical signs and symptoms of hypogonadism (hypoandrogenism).

An early in treatment transient increase in serum testosterone levels usually occurs. Occasionally, this may be associated with transient worsening of clinical status and secondary reactions such as: occurrence or exacerbation of bone pain in patients with bone metastases, signs of neurological deficit due to tumor compression, impaired micturition, hydronephrosis, lymphostasis or thrombosis with pulmonary embolism. This transient initial rise in serum androgen will be followed by a progressive decrease to castration levels (see Warnings and Precautions).

In patients treated with buserelin implant 2 months or buserelin implant 3 months, such reactions can be avoided when an antiandrogen is given concomitantly in the initial phase of buserelin treatment (see Precautions). Some of these patients may, nevertheless, develop a mild, transient increase in tumor pain and a deterioration in general well-being.

Very rare cases of pituitary adenomas were reported during treatment with LH-RH agonists including buserelin.

SUPREFACT DEPOT 2 months and SUPREFACT DEPOT 3 months

No serious clinical flare reactions were reported in patients (n=379) enrolled in clinical studies with SUPREFACT DEPOT 2 months and SUPREFACT DEPOT 3 months.

Table 1 provides a listing of adverse reactions, incidence ≥1%, considered to be at least possibly or probably related to buserelin acetate implant during a 5 year study with SUPREFACT DEPOT 2 months and a single dose, 16 week study with SUPREFACT DEPOT 3 months. Both studies were non-comparative, open label studies.

Table 1: Suprefact Depot

Listing Of Adverse Reactions (At Least Possibly Or Probably Related), Incidence ≥1%

	Suprefact Depot 2 months (buserelin acetate implant equivalent to 6.3 mg of buserelin base) Multidose 5-year study N=299		Suprefact Depot 3 months (buserelin acetate implant equivalent to 9.45 mg of buserelin base)[a] Single dose 16-week study N=22			
			Cyproterone acetate + Buserelin		Buserelin (>1 week after cyproterone acetate intake[b])	
Adverse Event	**n**	**%**	**n**	**%**	**n**	**%**
Hot Flashes	47	15.7	5	22.7	3	13.6
Libido Decrease	7	2.3	—	—	1	4.5
Hypertension	6	2.0	2	9.1	1	4.5
Depression	6	2.0	—	—	—	—
Pain	5	1.7	—	—	—	—
Impotence	5	1.7	5	22.7	2	9.1
Injection Site Reaction	4	1.3	1	4.5	—	—
Edema	3	1.0	—	—	—	—
Asthenia	—	<1.0%	3	13.6	3	13.6
Myalgia	—	—	1	4.5	1	4.5
Arthralgia	—	—	—	—	1	4.5
Increased Appetite	—	—	—	—	1	4.5
Insomnia	—	<1.0%	1	4.5	—	—
Nausea	—	—	1	4.5	—	—
Palpitation	—	—	1	4.5	—	—
Dizziness	—	—	1	4.5	—	—

a Cyproterone acetate given from 1 week before until 4 weeks after buserelin injection.

b >1 week after discontinuation of cyproterone acetate.

Legend: — Not detected as at least possibly or probably related.

Other adverse reactions, arranged by body system, and, at least possibly or probably related to the administration of buserelin implant 2 months or buserelin implant 3 months (individual signs/symptoms occurred at an incidence of less than 1%) were:

Body as a Whole: non-serious clinical flare reaction, asthenia and fever.

Cardiovascular: heart failure, tachycardia and thrombophlebitis.

Digestive: constipation, fecal incontinence and nausea.

Endocrine: exacerbation of pre-existing diabetes mellitus and hyperglycemia.

Musculoskeletal: muscle cramps and myopathy.

Metabolic and Nutritional: weight gain and weight loss.

Nervous System: hyperalgesia, nervousness, sleep disorder (insomnia), suicide attempt and sweating increased.

Respiratory: dyspnea and pharyngitis.

Skin and Appendages: gynecomastia, injection site hemorrhage, pruritus and rash.

Special Senses: blindness in one eye (temporary).

Urogenital: abnormal ejaculation, male genital pain and urogenital disorder.

Hemic and Lymphatic: myeloid metaplasia.

Arthritis, eye disorder, eczema, headaches, thrombosis and palpitations have been reported as remotely related to the administration of buserelin implant 2 months or buserelin implant 3 months.

Miscellaneous: In the literature and in our international database, other adverse events, including events which were observed only in females (excluding female gender-specific events) or for other unlabeled indications, have been observed in patients treated with buserelin, as itemized below (not all events were considered to be related to buserelin therapy):

Digestive: changes in appetite (e.g., anorexia), increased thirst and vomiting.

Endocrine Disorder: atrophy of the testes.

Hemic and Lymphatic: leukopenia and thrombopenia.

Laboratory Values: changes in blood lipids (e.g. hypercholesterolemia, hyperlipidemia), increase in bilirubin levels and increase serum liver enzymes levels (e.g., transaminases).

Musculoskeletal System: The use of LHRH-agonists may be associated with musculoskeletal discomfort and pain (including shoulder pain/stiffness in women). It may be associated with decreased bone density and may lead to osteoporosis and an increased risk of bone fracture. The risk of skeletal fracture increases with the duration of therapy.

Nervous System: concentration and memory disturbances, dizziness, drowsiness, emotional instability, feelings of anxiety, mood changes, nervousness and tiredness.

Skin and Appendages: articular pains, irritation of the mucosa in the nasopharynx due to nasal solution administration (which may lead to nosebleeds, hoarseness, disturbances of smell or taste), rhinorrhea and skin reaction (wheal) allergy, changes in scalp and body hair (increase or decrease).

Special Senses: eye dryness and irritation, feeling of pressure behind the eyes, impaired vision (e.g., blurred vision), hearing disorders and tinnitus.

OVERDOSE:

There have been no clinical reports of acute overdosage with buserelin implant 2 months or buserelin implant 3 months.

From acute studies of buserelin in rodents, neither 0.5 mg/kg/i.v. (mouse) nor 1 mg/kg/i.v. (rat) produced evidence of toxic signs.

Two groups of 6 and 4 healthy volunteers, aged 26 to 40 years and 31 to 40 years respectively, were given 1 mg buserelin or 5 mg buserelin **orally** as a single dose. No LH or FSH release was observed. No clinical effects were observed.

> For management of a suspected drug overdose, contact your regional Poison Control Centre. See the *CPS* Directory section for a list of Poison Control Centres.

DOSAGE: SUPREFACT DEPOT 2 months and SUPREFACT DEPOT 3 months is intended for the long-term treatment of prostatic carcinoma. SUPREFACT DEPOT 2 months and SUPREFACT DEPOT 3 months should be administered at approximately equal time intervals to ensure that the desired therapeutic effect is maintained.

The applicator containing the implant rods should be kept horizontal before injection (see Instructions for Using the Applicator). Before injection, a local anesthetic may be used if desired.

SUPREFACT DEPOT 2 months (buserelin acetate implant): The contents of 1 applicator, consisting of 2 implant rods, equivalent to a total of 6.3 mg buserelin base is injected s.c. every 2 months into the lateral abdominal wall. It is important to maintain a regular, 2-month rhythm for the dosage interval. In exceptional cases, the dosage interval may be shortened or extended by a few days.

SUPREFACT DEPOT 3 months (buserelin acetate implant): The contents of 1 applicator, consisting of 3 implant rods, equivalent to a total of 9.45 mg buserelin base is injected s.c. every 3 months into the lateral abdominal wall. It is important to maintain a regular, 3-month rhythm for the dosage interval. In exceptional cases, the dosage interval may be shortened or extended by a few days.

Initial Antiandrogen Comedication: About seven days before the first injection of SUPREFACT DEPOT 2 months or SUPREFACT DEPOT 3 months, an antiandrogen should be administered in accordance with the manufacturer's directions. This comedication is to be continued for four weeks after the first SUPREFACT DEPOT 2 months or SUPREFACT DEPOT 3 months injection, when testosterone levels can be expected to have entered the surgical castration range.

Instructions for Using the Applicator: (See package insert for illustrations.)

Please Note: To prevent the implant rods from falling out of the injection needle, hold the applicator in a vertical position until immediately prior to puncture, with the needle pointing upwards.

1. After removing the applicator from the foil wrapping, check that the implant rods are located in the window of the handle. If necessary, tap the protective cap of the needle lightly to reposition them in the window.
2. Disinfect the injection site of the lateral abdominal wall and administer a local anesthetic, if desired. After removing the protective case from the plunger, remove the cap from the injection needle.
3. Lift a fold of skin and insert the needle approximately 3 cm (somewhat more than 1 inch) into the subcutaneous tissue, with the tip of the needle pointed slightly upwards. Withdraw the applicator about 1 to 2 cm prior to injection of the implant rods.
4. While fully depressing the plunger, inject the implant rods into the subcutaneous tissue. Compress the puncture channel while withdrawing the needle so that the implant rods are retained in the tissue.
5. When the plunger is completely inserted to its final position (plunger knob is touching the body of applicator), the front end of the plunger protrudes the top of the cannula, protecting the needle and minimizing the risks of needle stick injuries.
6. To ensure that the implant rods have been injected, check the tip of the plunger to see if it is visible at the tip of the needle.

INFORMATION FOR THE PATIENT: Published in e-CPS, available by subscription at www.e-cps.ca.

SUPPLIED: Depot 2 Months: Each applicator contains 1 implant dose consisting of 2 identical cream-colored, biodegradable and biocompatible rods. Each implant dose contains a total of buserelin acetate 6.6 mg equivalent to buserelin base 6.3 mg. Nonmedicinal ingredients: poly-(D,L-lactide-co-glycolide). Sterile ready-to-use disposable applicator with an integrated safety engineered needle (internal needle diameter of 1.4 mm) for s.c. injection. Cartons supplied with 1 sterile foil bag containing 1 applicator prefilled with 1 implant dose. Consists of 2 identical rods. Store the intact package between 15 and 30°C. **Protect from excessive heat** and do not use beyond the expiration date printed on the container label.

Depot 3 Months: Each applicator contains 1 implant dose consisting of 3 identical cream-colored, biodegradable and biocompatible rods. Each implant dose contains a total of buserelin acetate 9.9 mg equivalent to buserelin base 9.45 mg. Nonmedicinal ingredients: poly-(D,L-lactide-co-glycolide). Sterile ready-to-use disposable applicator with an integrated safety engineered needle (internal needle diameter of 1.4 mm) for s.c. injection. Cartons supplied with 1 sterile foil bag containing 1 applicator prefilled with 1 implant dose. Consists of 3 identical rods. Store the intact package between 15 and 30°C. **Protect from excessive heat** and do not use beyond the expiration date printed on the container label.

Survanta® Ⓟ

beractant

Lung Surfactant (Bovine)

Abbott

Date of Preparation: January 29, 1993

Date of Revision: April 7, 2009

SUMMARY PRODUCT INFORMATION:

Route of Administration	Dosage Form/ Strength	Clinically Relevant Nonmedicinal Ingredients
Intratracheal	100 mg phospholipids/4 mL suspension 200 mg phospholipids/8 mL suspension	Sodium Chloride 0.9% For a complete listing see Dosage Forms, Composition and Packaging.

DESCRIPTION: SURVANTA (beractant, intratracheal suspension) is a sterile, non-pyrogenic pulmonary surfactant and natural bovine lung extract. It is supplemented with three synthetically derived lipids; colfosceril palmitate (dipalmitoylphosphatidylcholine), palmitic acid and tripalmitin. These latter lipids are added to standardize the composition and to mimic the surface-tension lowering properties of natural lung surfactant. The resulting composition provides an average concentration of 25 mg/mL phospholipids and less than 1.0 mg/mL protein. The formulation is an off-white to light brown opaque liquid.

INDICATIONS AND CLINICAL USE: SURVANTA (beractant, intratracheal suspension) is indicated for:

- Prevention (prophylaxis) and
- Treatment (rescue) of Respiratory Distress Syndrome (RDS/Hyaline Membrane Disease) in premature infants

Prevention: For **prophylactic** treatment of infants at risk of developing RDS or who have evidence of pulmonary immaturity.

In premature infants less than 1250 g birth weight or with evidence of surfactant deficiency, give SURVANTA as soon as possible after an airway has been established, preferably within 15 minutes of birth.

Rescue Treatment: For **rescue** treatment of infants who have developed RDS.

To treat infants with RDS confirmed by X-ray and who require mechanical ventilation, give SURVANTA as soon as possible after an airway has been established, preferably by eight hours of age.

SURVANTA significantly reduces the incidence of RDS, mortality due to RDS and air leak complications.

The use of SURVANTA (beractant, intratracheal suspension) in infants less than 600 g birth weight or greater than 1750 g birth weight has not been evaluated in controlled trials. There is no controlled experience with the use of SURVANTA in conjunction with experimental therapies for RDS (e.g., high frequency ventilation or extra-corporeal membrane oxygenation).

CONTRAINDICATIONS: There are no known contraindications to treatment with SURVANTA (beractant, intratracheal suspension).

WARNINGS AND PRECAUTIONS:

> **Serious Warnings and Precautions**
> - Administer in a highly supervised clinical setting
> - SURVANTA can rapidly affect oxygenation and lung compliance. Therefore, frequent and careful clinical observation and monitoring of systemic oxygenation are essential to avoid hyperoxia.
> - Transient episodes of bradycardia and decreased oxygen saturation may occur during dosing.

General: SURVANTA (beractant, intratracheal suspension) is intended for intratracheal use only (see Dosage and Administration).

No information is available on the effects of doses other than 100 mg phospholipids/kg, more than four doses, dosing more frequently than every 6 hours, or administration after 48 hours of age.

Usage of SURVANTA should be restricted to a highly supervised clinical setting with immediate availability of experienced neonatologists and other clinicians experienced with intubation, ventilator management, and general care of premature infants. Vigilant clinical attention should be given to all infants prior to, during, and after administration of SURVANTA. Infants receiving SURVANTA should be frequently monitored with arterial or transcutaneous measurement of systemic oxygen and carbon dioxide.

During the dosing procedure, transient episodes of bradycardia and decreased oxygen saturation have been reported (see Adverse Reactions). If these occur, stop the dosing procedure and initiate appropriate measures to alleviate the condition. After stabilization, resume the dosing procedure.

The use of SURVANTA in infants less than 600 g birth weight or greater than 1750 g birth weight has not been evaluated in controlled trials. There is no controlled experience with the use of SURVANTA in conjunction with experimental therapies for RDS (e.g., high frequency ventilation or extra-corporeal membrane oxygenation).

Intracranial Hemorrhage: In one of the single-dose rescue studies and one of the multi-dose prevention studies, the rate of intracranial hemorrhage was significantly higher in SURVANTA patients than in control patients (63.3% vs. 30.8%, p=0.001 and 48.8% vs. 34.2%, p=0.047, respectively). However, when all controlled studies were pooled, there was no difference between treatment groups in incidences of intracranial hemorrhage.

Carcinogenesis and Mutagenesis: Mutagenicity studies were negative. Carcinogenicity studies were not conducted with SURVANTA.

Immune: Increased probability of post-treatment nosocomial sepsis in SURVANTA-treated infants was observed in clinical trials (see Table 2). The increased risk for sepsis among SURVANTA-treated infants was not associated with increased mortality among these infants.

Respiratory: Endotracheal Tube Blockage Due to Mucous Plugs: Infants whose ventilation becomes markedly impaired during or shortly after dosing may have mucous plugging of the endotracheal tube, particularly if pulmonary secretions were prominent prior to drug administration. Suctioning of all infants prior to dosing may lessen the chance of mucous plugs obstructing the endotracheal tube. If endotracheal tube obstruction from such plugs is suspected, and suctioning is unsuccessful in removing the obstruction, the blocked endotracheal tube should be replaced immediately. In the multiple-dose studies performed with SURVANTA, there were 4 reports of endotracheal tube blockage out of 1691 doses (0.2%).

Oxygenation: SURVANTA can rapidly affect oxygenation and lung compliance. In some infants, hyperoxia may occur within minutes of administration of SURVANTA. If hyperoxia develops, and transcutaneous oxygen saturation is in excess of 95%, FiO_2 should be reduced until saturation is 90 to 95%. If the improvement in chest expansion seems excessive, peak ventilator inspiratory pressures should be immediately reduced. Failure to reduce inspiratory ventilatory pressures rapidly can result in lung overdistention and fatal pulmonary air leaks.

Hyperoxia, cyanosis and reflux through the endotracheal tube, additionally to bradycardia and decreased oxygen saturation, have been the most frequently reported complications in clinical trials. If reflux occurs, drug administration should be stopped and if necessary, peak inspiratory pressure on the ventilator should be increased by 4 to 5 cm H_2O until clearing of the endotracheal tube occurs.

Rales: Rales and moist breath sounds can occur transiently after administration. Endotracheal suctioning or other remedial action is necessary if clear-cut signs of airway obstruction are present.

Sexual Function/Reproduction: Beractant up to 500 mg phospholipids/kg/day, approximately one-third the premature infant dose based on mg/m²/day, was administered subcutaneously to newborn rats for five days. These rats reproduced normally and there were no observable adverse effects in their offspring.

Monitoring and Laboratory Tests: Vigilant clinical attention should be given to all infants prior to, during, and after administration of SURVANTA. Infants receiving SURVANTA should be frequently monitored with arterial or transcutaneous measurement of systemic oxygen and carbon dioxide.

ADVERSE REACTIONS: Adverse Drug Reaction Overview: The most commonly reported adverse experiences were associated with the dosing procedure.

In the multiple-dose controlled clinical trials, each dose of SURVANTA (beractant, intratracheal suspension) was divided into four quarter-doses. Each quarter dose was instilled through a catheter inserted into the endotracheal tube by briefly disconnecting the endotracheal tube from the ventilator.

Transient bradycardia occurred with 11.9% of doses. Oxygen desaturation occurred with 9.8% of doses. Other reactions during the dosing procedure occurred with fewer than 1% of doses and included endotracheal tube reflux, pallor, vasoconstriction, hypotension, endotracheal tube blockage, hypertension, hypocarbia, hypercarbia, and apnea. No deaths occurred during the dosing procedure, and all reactions resolved with symptomatic treatment.

Clinical Trial Adverse Drug Reactions: Because clinical trials are conducted under very specific conditions the adverse reaction rates observed in the clinical trials may not reflect the rates observed in practice and should not be compared to the rates in the clinical trials of another drug. Adverse drug reaction information from clinical trials is useful for identifying drug-related adverse events and for approximating rates.

Table 1 summarizes all adverse experiences reported during controlled clinical trials.

There were no statistically significant differences between treatments in the type or number of events reported.

Table 1: SURVANTA

Number of Infants with Adverse Events (All Controlled Studies) (Events with an Incidence ≥0.2% are Specified)

	SURVANTA		Sham Air	
Body System/Event	**n=840**	**(%)**	**n=851**	**(%)**
Respiratory				
Decreased oxygenation	9	1.1	3	0.4
Problems with ET tube	4	0.5	1	0.1
Blood from ET tube	3	0.4	0	0.0
Pulmonary hemorrhage N=225 for SURVANTA N=238 for Sham Air	2	0.9	1	0.1
Other respiratory adverse events	4	0.5	3	0.4
Cardiovascular				
Aortic thrombosis	3	0.4	0	0.0
Hypotension	3	0.4	0	0.0
Bradycardia	2	0.2	1	0.1
Other cardiovascular adverse events	7	0.8	9	1.0
Gastrointestinal				
Intestinal perforations	2	0.2	5	0.6
Volvulus	2	0.2	0	0.0
Other gastrointestinal adverse events	4	0.5	5	0.6
Renal				
Renal failure	2	0.2	2	0.2
Other renal adverse events	2	0.2	1	0.1
Hematologic				
Coagulopathy	2	0.2	0	0.0
Other hematologic adverse events	0	0	3	0.4
Central Nervous System				
Seizure	6	0.7	6	0.7
Other CNS adverse events	0	0.0	1	0.1
Systemic				
Sepsis	2	0.2	1	0.1
Other systemic adverse events	2	0.2	3	0.4
Other Adverse Events	3	0.4	3	0.4
At Least 1 Event	49	5.8	40	4.7

A clinical study compared the above quarter-dose administration regimen to the same procedure using two half-doses ar another two half-dose procedure with uninterrupted ventilation accomplished by passing the catheter through a neonatal suctic valve in the endotracheal tube. With the first dose there was significantly less endotracheal tube reflux observed in the group wi the quarter-dose regimen (p=0.007) than in the group with uninterrupted ventilation. With the first dose there was significant less oxygen desaturation in the group with uninterrupted ventilation (p=0.008) than in the other group receiving two half dose There were no differences in these events after later doses and no differences in heart rate after any doses (see Dosage ar Administration, Administration, Dosing Procedures).

The occurrence of concurrent illnesses common in premature infants was evaluated in the controlled trials. The rates in a controlled studies are in Table 2.

Table 2: SURVANTA

Percentage of Infants with Concurrent Events

	SURVANTA (%)	Control (%)
Patent ductus arteriosus	46.9	47.1
Intracranial hemorrhage	48.1	45.2
Severe intracranial hemorrhage	24.1	23.3
Pulmonary air leaks	10.9	24.7[a]
Pulmonary interstitial emphysema	20.2	38.4[a]
Necrotizing enterocolitis	6.1	5.3
Apnea	65.4	59.6
Severe apnea	46.1	42.5
Post-treatment sepsis	20.7	16.1[b]
Post-treatment infection	10.2	9.1
Pulmonary hemorrhage	7.2	5.3

[a] p <0.001.
[b] p <0.05.

In one of the single-dose rescue studies and one of the multi-dose prevention studies, the rate of intracranial hemorrhage wa significantly higher in SURVANTA patients than in control patients (63.3% vs. 30.8%, p=0.001 and 48.8% vs. 34.2%, p=0.04 respectively). However, when all controlled studies were pooled, there was no difference between treatment groups in incidence of intracranial hemorrhage.

Follow-up Evaluations: To date, no long-term complications or sequelae of SURVANTA therapy have been found.

Single-Dose Studies: Six-month adjusted-age follow-up evaluations of 232 infants (115 treated) demonstrated no clinical important differences between treatment groups in pulmonary and neurologic sequelae, incidence or severity of retinopathy prematurity, rehospitalizations, growth, or allergic manifestations.

Multiple-Dose Studies: Six-month adjusted-age follow-up evaluations have been completed in 631 (345 treated) of 916 survi ing infants. There was significantly less cerebral palsy and need for supplemental oxygen in SURVANTA infants than control Wheezing at the time of examination was more frequent among SURVANTA infants, although there was no difference in bro chodilator therapy.

Final twelve-month follow-up data from the multiple-dose studies are available from 521 (272 treated) of 909 surviving infant There was significantly less wheezing in SURVANTA infants than controls in contrast to the six-month results. There was r difference in the incidence of cerebral palsy at twelve months.

Twenty-four month adjusted-age evaluations were completed in 429 (226 treated) of 906 surviving infants. There were significantly fewer SURVANTA infants with rhonchi, wheezing, tachypnea or neurological findings, compared to infants treated with Sham Air, at the time of examination. No other differences were found.

Abnormal Hematologic and Clinical Chemistry Findings: In the controlled clinical trials, there was no effect of SURVANTA on results of common laboratory tests: white blood cell count, serum sodium, potassium, bilirubin, and creatinine. IgG or IgM antibodies to surfactant-associated proteins SP-B and SP-C were not detected.

Post-Market Adverse Drug Reactions: No new adverse reactions have been reported, nor has there been an increase in the incidence of known adverse reactions identified in the clinical trials completed to date.

DRUG INTERACTIONS: No formal drug-drug interaction studies were conducted.

DOSAGE AND ADMINISTRATION: Dosing Considerations: For Intratracheal Administration Only.

SURVANTA (beractant, intratracheal suspension) should be administered by or under the supervision of clinicians experienced in intubation, ventilator management, and general care of premature infants.

During the dosing procedure, transient episodes of bradycardia and decreased oxygen saturation have been reported (see Adverse Reactions). If these occur, stop the dosing procedure and initiate appropriate measures to alleviate the condition. After stabilization, resume the dosing procedure.

Marked improvements in oxygenation may occur within minutes of administration of SURVANTA. Therefore, **frequent** and careful clinical observation and monitoring of systemic oxygenation are essential to avoid hyperoxia.

Review of audiovisual instructional materials describing dosage and administration procedures is recommended before using SURVANTA. Materials are available upon request.

Recommended Dose and Dosage Adjustment: No information is available on the effects of doses other than 100 mg phospholipids/kg, more than four doses, dosing more frequently than every six hours, or administration after 48 hours of age.

Each dose of SURVANTA is 100 mg of phospholipids/kg birth weight (4 mL/kg). The SURVANTA Dosing Chart (Table 3) shows the total dosage for a range of birth weights.

Table 3: SURVANTA

SURVANTA Dosing Chart

Weight (g)	Total Dose (mL)	Weight (g)	Total Dose (mL)
600–650	2.6	1301–1350	5.4
651–700	2.8	1351–1400	5.6
701–750	3.0	1401–1450	5.8
751–800	3.2	1451–1500	6.0
801–850	3.4	1501–1550	6.2
851–900	3.6	1551–1600	6.4
901–950	3.8	1601–1650	6.6
951–1000	4.0	1651–1700	6.8
1001-1050	4.2	1701-1750	7.0
1051–1100	4.4	1751–1800	7.2[a]
1101–1150	4.6	1801–1850	7.4[a]
1151–1200	4.8	1851–1900	7.6[a]
1201–1250	5.0	1901–1950	7.8[a]
1251–1300	5.2	1951–2000	8.0[a]

[a] Suggested dosages based on limited clinical experience in uncontrolled trials.

Four doses of SURVANTA can be administered in the first 48 hours of life. Doses should be given no more frequently than every six hours.

Administration: Directions for Use: SURVANTA should be inspected visually for discolouration prior to administration. The colour of SURVANTA is off-white to light brown.

If settling occurs during storage, swirl the vial gently (do not shake) to redisperse. Some foaming at the surface may occur during handling and is inherent to the nature of the product. SURVANTA does not require sonication before use.

SURVANTA is stored refrigerated (2 to 8°C). Before administration, SURVANTA should be warmed by standing at room temperature for at least 20 minutes or warmed in the hand for at least eight minutes.

Artificial warming methods should not be used. If a prevention dose is to be given, preparation of SURVANTA should begin before the infant's birth.

Unopened, unused vials of SURVANTA that have been warmed to room temperature may be returned to the refrigerator within 24 hours of warming, and stored for future use. SURVANTA should not be warmed and returned to the refrigerator more than once. Each single-use vial of SURVANTA should be entered only once. Used vials with residual drug should be discarded.

Dosing Procedures: General: SURVANTA is administered intratracheally. It can be instilled through a 5 French end-hole catheter inserted into the infant's endotracheal tube by briefly disconnecting the endotracheal tube from the ventilator OR by inserting the catheter through a neonatal suction valve without disconnecting the endotracheal tube from the ventilator or by instillation through the secondary lumen of a double lumen endotracheal tube.

If the drug is instilled through an end-hole catheter, the length of the catheter should be shortened so that the tip of the catheter protrudes just beyond the endotracheal tube above the infant's carina. SURVANTA should not be instilled into a mainstem bronchus.

To ensure homogenous distribution of SURVANTA throughout the lungs, each dose is divided into fractional doses. Each dose can be administered in **two half-doses** or in **four quarter-doses**. Each fractional dose is administered with the infant in a different position.

To administer SURVANTA in two half-doses, the recommended positions are:

- Head and body turned approximately 45° to the right
- Head and body turned approximately 45° to the left

To administer SURVANTA in four quarter-doses, the recommended positions are:

- Head and body inclined 5 to 10° down, head and body turned to the right
- Head and body inclined 5 to 10° down, head and body turned to the left
- Head and body inclined 5 to 10° up, head and body turned to the right
- Head and body inclined 5 to 10° up, head and body turned to the left

The positions for four quarter-doses are illustrated in Figure 1.

The dosing procedure is facilitated if one person administers the dose while another person positions and monitors the baby.

The different methods of administering SURVANTA were evaluated in clinical trials. In the six single-dose and four multiple-dose controlled clinical trials that established safety and efficacy, SURVANTA was instilled through a catheter that was inserted into the infant's endotracheal tube by briefly disconnecting the endotracheal tube from the ventilator. Each dose was administered in four quarter-doses as described above.

This method of administering SURVANTA was compared to two other methods in a multi-centre, randomized clinical study involving 299 infants weighing 600 g or more with RDS requiring mechanical ventilation. The other methods evaluated were:

- Two half-doses administered by inserting the catheter through the endotracheal tube while the endotracheal tube was briefly disconnected from the ventilator. The half-doses were administered in the two positions described above.
- Two half-doses administered without disconnecting the endotracheal tube from the ventilator by inserting the catheter through a neonatal suction valve into the endotracheal tube. The half-doses were administered in the two positions described above.

There were no significant differences among the three groups in average FiO_2, a/APO_2, or MAP at 72 hours of age, or in the incidence of pulmonary air leaks, pulmonary interstitial emphysema, patent ductus arteriosus, or mortality at 72 hours of age.

Administration of SURVANTA using a double-lumen endotracheal tube is functionally equivalent to the use of the neonatal suction valve; i.e., delivery of SURVANTA at the distal end of the endotracheal tube without interrupting mechanical ventilation. If an infant is already intubated with a single-lumen endotracheal tube, the infant should not be reintubated with a double-lumen endotracheal tube solely for the purpose of administering SURVANTA.

Figure 1: SURVANTA

Positions for Four Quarter-Doses

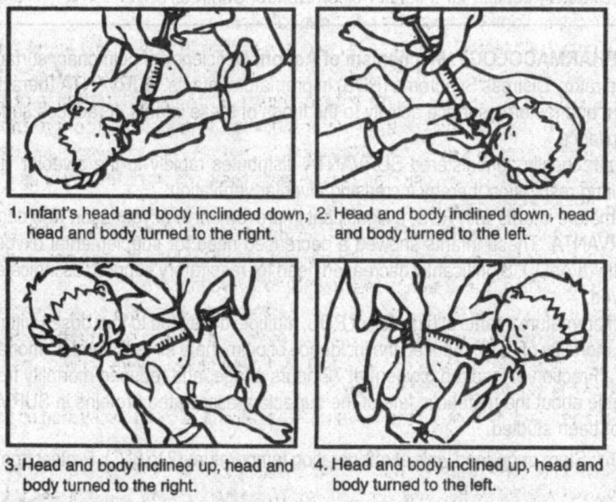

1. Infant's head and body inclined down, head and body turned to the right.
2. Head and body inclined down, head and body turned to the left.
3. Head and body inclined up, head and body turned to the right.
4. Head and body inclined up, head and body turned to the left.

First Dose: Instillation Through End-Hole Catheter: Determine the total dose of SURVANTA from the SURVANTA Dosing Chart (Table 3) based on the infant's birth weight. Slowly withdraw the entire contents of the vial into a plastic syringe through a large-gauge needle (e.g., at least 20 gauge). Do not filter SURVANTA and avoid shaking.

Attach the pre-measured 5 French end-hole catheter to the syringe. Fill the catheter with SURVANTA. Discard excess SURVANTA through the catheter so that only the total dose to be given remains in the syringe.

Before administering SURVANTA, assure proper placement and patency of the endotracheal tube. At the discretion of the clinician, the endotracheal tube may be suctioned before administering SURVANTA. The infant should be allowed to stabilize before proceeding with dosing.

First Fractional Dose—Prevention Strategy: In the prevention strategy, weigh, intubate and stabilize the infant. Administer the dose as soon as possible after birth, preferably within 15 minutes. Position the infant appropriately and gently inject the first fractional dose through the catheter over two to three seconds.

After administration of the first fractional dose, remove the catheter from the endotracheal tube.

Manually ventilate with a hand-bag with sufficient oxygen to prevent cyanosis, at a rate of 60 breaths/minute and sufficient positive pressure to provide adequate air exchange and chest wall excursion.

First Fractional Dose—Rescue Strategy: In the rescue strategy, the first dose should be given as soon as possible after the infant is placed on a ventilator for management of RDS. In the clinical trials, immediately before instilling the first fractional dose, the infant's ventilator settings were changed to rate 60/minute, inspiratory time 0.5 second, and FiO_2 1.0.

Position the infant appropriately and gently inject the first fractional dose through the catheter over two to three seconds. After administration of the first fractional dose, remove the catheter from the endotracheal tube. Return the infant to the mechanical ventilator.

Remaining Fractional Doses—Prevention and Rescue Strategies: In both strategies, ventilate the infant for at least 30 seconds or until stable. Reposition the infant for instillation of the next fractional dose.

Instill the remaining fractional doses using the same procedures. After instillation of each fractional dose, remove the catheter and ventilate for at least 30 seconds or until the infant is stabilized. After instillation of the final fractional dose, remove the catheter without flushing it.

Do not suction the infant for one hour after dosing unless signs of significant airway obstruction occur.

After completion of the dosing procedure, resume usual ventilator management and clinical care.

Instillation Through Secondary Lumen of a Double-Lumen Endotracheal Tube: Ensure that the infant is intubated with the appropriate size double-lumen endotracheal tube. Determine the total dose of SURVANTA from the SURVANTA Dosing Chart (Table 3) based on the infant's birth weight. Slowly withdraw the total dose from the vial into a plastic syringe through a large-gauge needle (e.g., at least 20 gauge). Do not filter SURVANTA and avoid shaking.

Before administering SURVANTA, assure proper placement and patency of the endotracheal tube. At the discretion of the clinician, the endotracheal tube may be suctioned before administering SURVANTA. The infant should be allowed to stabilize before proceeding with dosing.

First Fractional Dose—Prevention Strategy: In the prevention strategy, weigh, intubate and stabilize the infant. Administer the dose as soon as possible after birth, preferably within 15 minutes. Attach the syringe containing SURVANTA to the secondary lumen. Position the infant appropriately and gently inject the first fractional dose through the secondary lumen over two to three seconds without interrupting ventilation. If manually ventilated, ventilate with a hand-bag with sufficient oxygen to prevent cyanosis, at a rate of 60 breaths/minute, and sufficient positive pressure to provide adequate air exchange and chest wall excursion.

First Fractional Dose—Rescue Strategy: In the rescue strategy, the first dose should be given as soon as possible after the infant is placed on a ventilator for management of RDS. Immediately before instilling the first fractional dose, change the infant's ventilator settings to rate 60/minute, inspiratory time 0.5 second, and FiO_2 1.0.

Position the infant appropriately and gently inject the first fractional dose through the secondary lumen over two to three seconds without interrupting mechanical ventilation.

Remaining Fractional Doses—Prevention and Rescue Strategies: In both strategies, ventilate the infant for at least 30 seconds or until stable. Reposition the infant for instillation of the next fractional dose.

Instill the remaining fractional doses using the same procedures. After instillation of each fractional dose, ventilate for at least 30 seconds or until the infant is stabilized. After instillation of the final fractional dose, remove the syringe from the secondary lumen, inject 0.5 mL of air to flush the secondary lumen and cap it.

After completion of the dosing procedure, resume usual ventilator management and clinical care.

Repeat Doses: The need for additional doses of SURVANTA is determined by evidence of continuing respiratory distress.

- Dose no sooner than six hours after the preceding dose if the infant remains intubated and requires at least 30% inspired oxygen to maintain a PaO_2 less than or equal to 80 torr. In controlled clinical trials, 60% of patients (prevention) and 79% of patients (rescue) required more than one dose of SURVANTA. 34.8% of patients (prevention) and 52.2% of patients (rescue) required four doses.
- Radiographic confirmation of RDS should be obtained before administering additional doses to those who received a prevention dose.

The dosage of SURVANTA for each repeat doses is also 100 mg phospholipids/kg and is based on the infant's birth weight. The infant should not be reweighed for determination of the SURVANTA dosage. Use the SURVANTA Dosing Chart to determine the total dosage.

Prepare SURVANTA and position the infant for administration of each fractional dose as previously described. After instillation of each fractional dose, remove the dosing catheter from the endotracheal tube and ventilate the infant for at least 30 seconds or until stable.

In the clinical studies, ventilator settings used to administer repeat doses were different than those used for the first dose. For repeat doses, the FiO_2 was increased by 0.20 or an amount sufficient to prevent cyanosis. The ventilator delivered a rate of 30/minute with an inspiratory time less than 1.0 second. If the infant's pretreatment rate was 30 or greater, it was left unchanged during SURVANTA instillation.

Manual hand-bag ventilation should not be used to administer repeat doses. During the dosing procedure, ventilator settings may be adjusted at the discretion of the clinician to maintain appropriate oxygenation and ventilation.

After completion of the dosing procedure, resume usual ventilator management and clinical care.

Dosing Precautions: If an infant experiences bradycardia or oxygen desaturation during the dosing procedure, stop the dosing procedure and initiate appropriate measures to alleviate the condition. After the infant has stabilized, resume the dosing procedure.

Rales and moist breath sounds can occur transiently after administration of SURVANTA. Endotracheal suctioning or other remedial action is necessary if clear-cut signs of airway obstruction are present.

OVERDOSAGE:
Overdosage with SURVANTA (beractant, intratracheal suspension) has not been reported. Based on animal data, overdosage might result in acute airway obstruction. Treatment should be symptomatic and supportive.

For management of a suspected drug overdose, CPhA recommends that you contact your **regional Poison Control Centre**. See the *CPS* Directory section for a list of Poison Control Centres.

ACTION AND CLINICAL PHARMACOLOGY: Mechanism of Action: Deficiency of pulmonary surfactant is an important factor in the development of Respiratory Distress Syndrome (RDS) in premature infants. SURVANTA (beractant, intratracheal suspension) replenishes surfactant and restores surface activity to the lungs of these infants. It reduces surface tension and concomitantly increases lung compliance.

Pharmacodynamics: Intratracheally administered SURVANTA distributes rapidly to the alveolar surfaces and stabilizes the alveoli against collapse during respiration thereby increasing alveolar ventilation.

In clinical studies of premature infants with RDS, a significant improvement in oxygenation was demonstrated after treatment with a single dose of SURVANTA. These infants showed a decreased need for supplemental oxygen and an increase in the arterial/alveolar oxygen ratio (a/ApO_2). Significantly decreased need for respiratory support, as indicated by a lower mean airway pressure, was also observed.

In prophylactic studies of premature infants at high risk of RDS, multiple doses (up to four doses within 48 hours) of SURVANTA reduced the incidence and mortality of RDS, reduced the incidence of pulmonary air leaks and pulmonary interstitial emphysema, improved a/ApO_2 and FiO_2 (Fraction of inspired oxygen) at 72 hours of age, and reduced mortality from any cause.

No information is available about the metabolic fate of the surfactant-associated proteins in SURVANTA. The metabolic disposition in humans has not been studied.

STORAGE AND STABILITY: Store unopened vials at refrigeration temperature (2 to 8°C). Protect from light. Store vials in carton until ready for use.

Unopened, unused vials of SURVANTA that have been warmed to room temperature may be returned to the refrigerator within twenty-four hours of warming, and stored for future use. Drug should not be warmed and returned to the refrigerator more than once. Each single use vial of SURVANTA should be entered with a needle only once. Used vials with residual drug should be discarded.

INFORMATION FOR THE PATIENT: Published in e-CPS, available by subscription at www.e-cps.ca.

DOSAGE FORMS, COMPOSITION AND PACKAGING: Each mL of an off-white to light brown opaque liquid contains: phospholipids 25 mg (100 mg phospholipids/4 mL and 200 mg phospholipids/8 mL) (including 11.0 to 15.5 mg/mL disaturated phosphatidylcholine), 0.5 to 1.75 mg/mL triglycerides; 1.4 to 3.5 mg/mL free fatty acids, 0.1 to 0.4 mg/mL protein and 9.0 mg/mL sodium chloride. Fortification lipids are added to standardize the composition and to mimic surface-tension lowering properties of natural lung surfactant. SURVANTA is heat-sterilized and does not contain preservatives. Its protein content includes two hydrophobic surfactant-associated proteins of low molecular weight, commonly known as SP-B and SP-C. It does not contain the hydrophilic, large molecular weight surfactant-associated protein know as SP-A. Single-use glass vials of 4 and 8 mL.

Sustiva® Ⓟ

efavirenz

Antiretroviral Agent

Bristol-Myers Squibb

Date of Preparation: March 18, 1999
Date of Revision: April 7, 2010

SUMMARY PRODUCT INFORMATION:

Route of Administration	Dosage Form/ Strength	Clinically Relevant Nonmedicinal Ingredients
Oral	Capsules/50 and 200 mg	Lactose monohydrate For a complete listing, see Dosage Forms, Composition and Packaging.
	Tablets/600 mg	Lactose monohydrate For a complete listing, see Dosage Forms, Composition and Packaging.

INDICATIONS AND CLINICAL USE: SUSTIVA (efavirenz) is indicated for the treatment of HIV-1 infection in combination with other antiretroviral agents.

CONTRAINDICATIONS: SUSTIVA (efavirenz) is contraindicated in patients with clinically significant hypersensitivity to any of its components. For a complete listing, see Dosage Forms, Composition and Packaging.

SUSTIVA should not be administered concurrently with cisapride, midazolam, triazolam, pimozide or ergot derivatives because competition for CYP3A4 by efavirenz could result in inhibition of metabolism of these drugs and create the potential for serious and/or life-threatening adverse events (e.g., cardiac arrhythmias, prolonged sedation or respiratory depression). (See Table 1.)

Table 1: SUSTIVA

Drugs That Should Not Be Coadministered with SUSTIVA

Drug Class	Drugs Within Class Not to Be Coadministered with SUSTIVA	Clinical Comment
Benzodiazepines	midazolam, triazolam	**Contraindicated** due to potential for serious and/or life-threatening reactions such as prolonged or increased sedation or respiratory depression.
GI Motility Agents	cisapride	**Contraindicated** due to potential for serious and/or life-threatening reactions such as cardiac arrhythmias.
Anti-Migraine	ergot derivatives (dihydroergotamine, ergonovine, ergotamine)	**Contraindicated** due to potential for serious and/or life-threatening reactions such as acute ergot toxicity characterized by peripheral vasospasm and ischemia of the extremities and other tissues.
Neuroleptic	pimozide	**Contraindicated** due to potential for serious and/or life-threatening reactions such as cardiac arrhythmias.

WARNINGS AND PRECAUTIONS: SUSTIVA (efavirenz) must not be used as a single agent to treat HIV or added on as a sole agent to a failing regimen. As with all other non-nucleoside reverse transcriptase inhibitors, resistant virus emerges rapidly when efavirenz is administered as monotherapy. The choice of new antiretroviral agents to be used in combination with efavirenz should take into consideration the potential for viral cross-resistance. (Please refer to the most recent antiretroviral guidelines for further information.)

General: Coadministration of SUSTIVA with ATRIPLA, a fixed-dose combination tablet containing efavirenz, emtricitabine and tenofovir disoproxil fumarate, is not recommended.

Psychiatric Symptoms: Serious psychiatric adverse experiences have been reported in patients treated with SUSTIVA. In controlled trials of 1008 patients treated with regimens containing SUSTIVA for an average of 2.1 years and 635 patients treated with control regimens for an average of 1.5 years, the frequency of specific serious psychiatric events among patients who received efavirenz or control regimens respectively, were: severe depression (2.4%, 0.9%), suicidal ideation (0.7%, 0.3%), non-fatal suicide attempts (0.5%, 0%), aggressive behavior (0.4%, 0.5%), paranoid reactions (0.4%, 0.3%), and manic reactions (0.2%, 0.3%). When psychiatric symptoms similar to those noted above were combined and evaluated as a group in a multifactorial analysis of data from Study AI266-006, treatment with efavirenz was associated with an increase in the occurrence of these selected psychiatric symptoms. Other factors associated with an increase in the occurrence of these psychiatric symptoms were history of injection drug use, psychiatric history, and receipt of psychiatric medication at study entry; similar associations were observed in both the SUSTIVA and control treatment groups. In Study AI266-006, onset of new serious psychiatric symptoms occurred throughout the study for both SUSTIVA-treated and control-treated patients. One percent of SUSTIVA-treated patients discontinued or interrupted treatment because of one or more of these selected psychiatric symptoms. There have also been occasional post marketing reports of death by suicide, delusions, and psychosis—like behavior, although a causal relationship to the use of SUSTIVA cannot be determined from these reports. Patients with serious psychiatric adverse experiences should seek immediate medical evaluation to assess the probability that the symptoms may be related to the use of SUSTIVA, and if so, to determine whether the risks of continued therapy outweigh the benefits (see Adverse Reactions).

Nervous System Symptoms: Fifty-three percent of patients receiving SUSTIVA in controlled clinical trials reported central nervous system symptoms compared to 25% of patients receiving control regimens. These symptoms included, but were not limited to, dizziness (28.1%), insomnia (16.3%), impaired concentration (8.3%), somnolence (7.0%), abnormal dreams (6.2%), and hallucinations (1.2%). In controlled trials, these symptoms were severe in 2.0% of patients receiving SUSTIVA 600 mg daily and in 1.3% of patients receiving control regimens. In clinical trials, 2.1% of SUSTIVA-treated patients discontinued therapy because of nervous system symptoms. These symptoms usually begin during the first or second day of therapy and generally resolve after the first 2-4 weeks. After 4 weeks of therapy the prevalence of nervous system symptoms of at least moderate severity ranged from 5-9% in patients treated with regimens containing SUSTIVA and from 3-5% in patients treated with a control regimen. Patients should be informed that these common nervous system symptoms are likely to improve with continued therapy. Dosing at bedtime improves tolerability of these symptoms (see Adverse Reactions and Dosage and Administration).

Analysis of long-term data from Study AI266-006 (median follow-up 180 weeks, 102 weeks, and 76 weeks for patients treated with SUSTIVA + zidovudine + lamivudine, SUSTIVA + indinavir, and indinavir + zidovudine + lamivudine, respectively) showed that, beyond 24 weeks of therapy, the incidences of new-onset nervous system symptoms among SUSTIVA-treated patients were generally similar to those in the indinavir-containing control arm.

Patients receiving SUSTIVA should be alerted to the potential for additive central nervous system effects when SUSTIVA is used concomitantly with alcohol or psychoactive drugs.

Patients should be informed that SUSTIVA may cause dizziness, impaired concentration, and/or drowsiness. Patients should be instructed that if they experience these symptoms they should avoid potentially hazardous tasks such as driving or operating machinery (see Effects on Ability to Drive and to Use Machines).

St. John's Wort: Concomitant use of St. John's wort (Hypericum perforatum) or St. John's wort-containing products with efavirenz is not recommended. Coadministration of non-nucleoside reverse transcriptase inhibitors (NNRTIs), including SUSTIVA, with St. John's Wort is expected to substantially decrease NNRTI concentrations. Decreased concentrations may result in suboptimal levels of efavirenz and lead to loss of virologic response and possible resistance to efavirenz or to the class of NNRTIs (see Drug Interactions).

Reproductive Risk Potential: Efavirenz may cause fetal harm when administered during the first trimester to a pregnant woman.

Pregnancy should be avoided in women receiving SUSTIVA and for 12 weeks after discontinuation. Barrier contraception must always be used in combination with other methods of contraception (e.g., oral or other hormonal contraceptives) (see Pregnancy and Drug Interactions). Women of childbearing potential should undergo pregnancy testing prior to initiation of SUSTIVA (see Pregnancy and Antiretroviral Pregnancy Registry).

Efavirenz should be used during pregnancy only if the potential benefit justifies the risk to the fetus such as in pregnant women without other therapeutic options (see Pregnancy).

Fat Redistribution: Redistribution/accumulation of body fat including central obesity, dorsocervical fat enlargement (buffalo hump), peripheral wasting, facial wasting, breast enlargement, and "cushingoid appearance" have been observed in patients receiving antiretroviral therapy. The mechanism and long-term consequences of these events are currently unknown. A causal relationship has not been established.

Rash: In controlled clinical trials, 26% (266/1008) of patients treated with 600 mg SUSTIVA experienced new onset skin rash compared with 17% (111/635) of patients treated in control groups. Rash associated with blistering, moist desquamation or ulceration occurred in 0.9% (9/1008) of patients treated with SUSTIVA. The median time to onset of rash in adults was 11 days and the median duration, 16 days. The discontinuation rate for rash in clinical trials was 6.4% (17/266) among patients with rash and 1.7% (17/1008) overall.

In clinical trials, grade 4 rash (including Stevens-Johnson syndrome, erythema multiforme, toxic epidermal necrolysis and exfoliative dermatitis) was uncommon (<1%) in patients treated with SUSTIVA. SUSTIVA should be discontinued in patients developing severe rash associated with blistering, desquamation, mucosal involvement or fever.

Rash was reported in 26 of 57 pediatric patients (46%) treated with SUSTIVA capsules. One pediatric patient experienced Grade 3 rash (confluent rash with fever), and two patients had Grade 4 rash (erythema multiforme). The median time to onset of rash in children was eight days. Prophylaxis with appropriate antihistamines prior to initiating therapy with SUSTIVA in children may be considered (see Adverse Reactions).

Pancreatitis: In controlled clinical studies the rate of clinical pancreatitis was similar in patients receiving 1/1008 (0.1%) and not receiving efavirenz 2/635 (0.3%).

Asymptomatic increases in serum amylase levels were observed in a significantly higher number of patients treated with efavirenz 600 mg than in control patients (see Adverse Reactions, Laboratory Abnormalities).

Elevated triglycerides have been reported in patients receiving efavirenz, in some cases to levels which can predispose a patient to pancreatitis. Among patients with elevated triglycerides, there have been no cases of pancreatitis. Because these triglyceride levels were not obtained in a fasting state, the exact clinical relevance of these measurements is not known.

Seizures: Caution should be taken in any patient with a history of seizures. Convulsions have been observed infrequently in patients receiving efavirenz, generally in the presence of known medical history of seizures. Overall, the rate of seizure in controlled clinical trials has been 0.89% in SUSTIVA treated patients and 0.63% in the control patients. Patients who are receiving concomitant anticonvulsant medications primarily metabolized by the liver such as phenytoin, carbamazepine, and phenobarbital, may require periodic monitoring of plasma levels (see Drug Interactions).

Hypersensitivity Reactions: In clinical trials, hypersensitivity reactions were uncommon (<1%) in patients treated with SUSTIVA.

Immune: Immune Reconstitution: Immune reconstitution syndrome has been reported in patients treated with combination antiretroviral therapy, including SUSTIVA. During the initial phase of treatment, patients responding to antiretroviral therapy may develop an inflammatory response to indolent or residual opportunistic infections (such as MAC, CMV, PCP, and TB), which may necessitate further evaluation and treatment.

Special Populations: Geriatrics: Clinical studies of SUSTIVA did not include sufficient numbers of subjects aged 65 and over to determine whether they respond differently from younger subjects. In general, dose selection for an elderly patient should be cautious, reflecting the greater frequency of decreased hepatic, renal, or cardiac function and of concomitant disease or other therapy.

Pediatrics: ACTG 382 is an ongoing open-label uncontrolled 48-week study in 57 NRTI-experienced pediatric patients to characterize the safety, pharmacokinetics, and antiviral activity of SUSTIVA in combination with nelfinavir (20-30 mg/kg TID) and NRTIs. Mean age was 8 years (range 3-16). SUSTIVA has not been studied in pediatric patients below 3 years of age or who weigh less than 13 kg. At 48 weeks, the type and frequency of adverse experiences was generally similar to that of adult patients with the exception of a higher incidence of rash which was reported in 46% (26/57) of pediatric patients compared to 26% of adults, and a higher frequency of Grade 3 or 4 rash reported in 5% (3/57) of pediatric patients compared to 0.9% of adults (see Adverse Reactions).

The starting dose of SUSTIVA was 600 mg daily adjusted to body size, based on weight, targeting AUC levels in the range of 190-380 μM·h. The pharmacokinetics of efavirenz in pediatric patients were similar to adults. In 48 pediatric patients receiving the equivalent of a 600 mg dose of SUSTIVA, steady-state C_{max} was 14.2±5.8 μM (mean±SD), steady-state C_{min} was 5.6±4.1 μM, and AUC was 218±104 μM·h (see also Action and Clinical Pharmacology).

Carcinogenesis, Mutagenesis and Impairment of Fertility: Long-term carcinogenicity studies in mice and rats were carried out with efavirenz. Mice were dosed with 0, 25, 75, 150, or 300 mg/kg/day for 2 years. Incidences of hepatocellular adenomas and carcinomas and pulmonary alveolar/bronchiolar adenomas were increased above background in females. No increases in tumor incidence above background were seen in males. In studies in which rats were administered efavirenz at doses of 0, 25,

50, or 100 mg/kg/day for 2 years, no increases in tumor incidence above background were observed. The systemic exposure (based on AUCs) in mice was approximately 1.7-fold that in human receiving the 600 mg/day dose. The exposure in rats was lower than that in humans.

The mechanism of the carcinogenic potential is unknown. However, in genetic toxicology assays, efavirenz showed no evidence of mutagenic or clastogenic activity in a battery of in vitro and in vivo studies. These included bacterial mutation assays in *S. typhimurium* and *E. coli*, mammalian mutation assays in Chinese hamster ovary cells, chromosome aberration assays in human peripheral blood lymphocytes or Chinese hamster ovary cells, and an in vivo mouse bone marrow micronucleus assay. Given the lack of genotoxic activity of efavirenz, the relevance to humans of neoplasms in efavirenz-treated mice is not known.

Efavirenz did not impair mating or fertility of male or female rats, and did not affect sperm (i.e. sperm count, viability, and motility) of treated male rats. The reproductive performance of offspring born to female rats given efavirenz was not affected. As a result of the rapid clearance of efavirenz in rats, systemic drug exposures achieved in these studies were equivalent to or below those achieved in humans given therapeutic doses of efavirenz.

Pregnancy: Efavirenz may cause fetal harm when administered during the first trimester to a pregnant woman. Pregnancy should be avoided in women receiving SUSTIVA. Barrier contraception must always be used in combination with other methods of contraception (eg, oral or other hormonal contraceptives). Because of the long half-life of efavirenz, use of adequate contraceptive measures for 12 weeks after discontinuation of SUSTIVA is recommended. Women of childbearing potential should undergo pregnancy testing prior to initiation of SUSTIVA (see Reproductive Risk Potential).

There are no adequate and well-controlled studies in pregnant women. SUSTIVA should be used during pregnancy only if the potential benefit justifies the potential risk to the fetus, such as in pregnant women without other therapeutic options.

Antiretroviral Pregnancy Registry: To monitor fetal outcomes of pregnant women exposed to SUSTIVA, an Antiretroviral Pregnancy Registry has been established. Physicians are encouraged to register patients, http://www.apregistry.com. Telephone: (800) 258-4263. Fax: (800) 800-1052.

As of July 2009, the Antiretroviral Pregnancy Registry has received prospective reports of 661 pregnancies exposed to efavirenz-containing regimens, nearly all of which were first-trimester exposures (606 pregnancies). Birth defects occurred in 14 of 501 live births (first-trimester exposure) and 2 of 55) live births (second-/third-trimester exposure). One of these prospectively reported defects with first-trimester exposure was a neural tube defect. A single case of anophthalmia with first trimester exposure to efavirenz has also been prospectively reported; however, this case included severe oblique facial clefts and amniotic banding, a known association with anophthalmia. There have been six retrospective reports of findings consistent with neural tube defects, including meningomyelocele. All mothers were exposed to efavirenz containing regimens in the first trimester. A causal relationship of these events to the use of SUSTIVA cannot be established.

Malformations have been observed in 3 of 20 fetuses/infants from efavirenz-treated cynomolgus monkeys (versus 0 of 20 concomitant controls) in a developmental toxicity study. The pregnant monkeys were dosed throughout pregnancy (postcoital days 20-150) with efavirenz 60 mg/kg daily, a dose which resulted in plasma drug concentrations similar to those in humans given 600 mg/day of SUSTIVA. Anencephaly and unilateral anophthalmia were observed in one fetus, microophthalmia was observed in another fetus, and cleft palate was observed in a third fetus. Efavirenz crosses the placenta in cynomolgus monkeys and produces fetal blood concentrations similar to maternal blood concentrations. Efavirenz has been shown to cross the placenta in rats and rabbits and produces fetal blood concentrations of efavirenz similar to maternal concentrations. An increase in fetal resorptions was observed in rats at efavirenz doses that produced peak plasma concentrations and AUC values in female rats equivalent to or lower than those achieved in humans given 600 mg once daily of SUSTIVA. Efavirenz produced no reproductive toxicities when given to pregnant rabbits at dose that produced peak plasma concentrations similar to and AUC values approximately half of those achieved in humans given 600 mg once daily of SUSTIVA.

Nursing Mothers: It is currently recommended that HIV-infected women should not breast-feed to avoid postnatal transmission of HIV. Studies in rats have demonstrated that efavirenz is excreted in milk. **Mothers should be instructed not to breast-feed if they are receiving SUSTIVA.**

Hepatic Impairment: The pharmacokinetics of efavirenz have not been adequately studied in patients with hepatic impairment and its use is not recommended in patients with severe hepatic impairment (Child-Pugh Class C). Because of the extensive cytochrome P450-mediated metabolism of efavirenz and limited clinical experience in patients with mild or moderate hepatic impairment, caution should be exercised in administering SUSTIVA to these patients. Patients should be monitored carefully for adverse events, and laboratory tests to evaluate the liver disease should be performed at periodic intervals (see Monitoring and Laboratory Tests; Adverse Reactions, Laboratory Abnormalities and Dosage and Administration).

Renal Impairment: The pharmacokinetics of efavirenz have not been studied in patients with renal insufficiency. However, less than 1% of efavirenz is excreted unchanged in the urine; consequently, the impact of renal impairment on efavirenz elimination should be minimal. There is no experience in patients with severe renal failure and close safety monitoring is recommended in this population (see Dosage and Administration).

Effects on Ability to Drive and to Use Machines: SUSTIVA may cause dizziness, impaired concentration, and/or drowsiness. Patients should be instructed that, if they experience these symptoms, they should avoid potentially hazardous tasks such as driving or operating machinery (see Nervous System Symptoms).

Resistance: Clinical isolates with reduced susceptibility in cell culture to efavirenz have been obtained. The most frequently observed amino acid substitution in clinical studies with efavirenz is K103N (54%). One or more RT substitutions at amino acid positions 98, 100, 101, 103, 106, 108, 188, 190, 225, 227, and 230 were observed in patients failing treatment with efavirenz in combination with other antiretrovirals. Other resistance mutations observed to emerge commonly included L100I (7%), K101E/Q/R (14%), V108I (11%), G190S/T/A (7%), P225H (18%), and M230I/L (11%).

Cross-Resistance: Cross-resistance has been recognized among NNRTIs. Clinical isolates previously characterized as efavirenz-resistant were also phenotypically resistant in cell culture to delavirdine and nevirapine compared to baseline. Delavirdine- and/or nevirapine-resistant clinical viral isolates with NNRTI resistance-associated substitutions (A98G, L100I, K101E/P, K103N/S, V106A, Y181X, Y188X, G190X, P225H, F227L, or M230L) showed reduced susceptibility to efavirenz in cell culture.

Monitoring and Laboratory Tests: Lipids: Monitoring of cholesterol and triglycerides should be considered in patients treated with SUSTIVA. (See Adverse Reactions, Laboratory Abnormalities.)

Liver Enzymes: In patients with known or suspected history of Hepatitis B or C infection and in patients treated with other medications associated with liver toxicity, monitoring of liver enzymes is recommended. Postmarketing reports of hepatic failure have occurred including some cases in patients with no pre-existing hepatic disease or other identifiable risk factors (see Adverse Reactions, Post-Market Adverse Drug Reactions). Liver enzyme monitoring should also be considered for patients without pre-existing hepatic dysfunction or other risk factors. In patients with persistent elevations of serum transaminases to greater than five times the upper limit of the normal range, the benefit of continued therapy with SUSTIVA needs to be weighed against the potential risks of significant liver toxicity (see Adverse Reactions, Laboratory Abnormalities).

ADVERSE REACTIONS: Adverse Drug Reaction Overview: SUSTIVA (efavirenz) has been studied in 9200 patients. The most significant adverse events observed in patients treated with SUSTIVA are nervous system symptoms, psychiatric symptoms, and rash.

The long-term safety profile of SUSTIVA-containing regimens was evaluated in a controlled trial, in which patients received SUSTIVA + zidovudine + lamivudine (n=412, median duration 180 weeks), SUSTIVA + indinavir (n=415, median duration 102 weeks), or indinavir + zidovudine + lamivudine (n=401, median duration 76 weeks). Long-term use of SUSTIVA in this study was not associated with any new safety concerns.

Clinical Trial Adverse Drug Reactions: Because clinical trials are conducted under very specific conditions the adverse drug reaction rates observed in the clinical trials may not reflect the rates observed in practice and should not be compared to the rates in the clinical trials of another drug. Adverse drug reaction information from clinical trials is useful for identifying drug-related adverse events and for approximating rates.

Nervous System Symptoms: Fifty-three percent of patients receiving SUSTIVA reported central nervous system symptoms (see Warnings and Precautions, General). Table 2 lists the frequency of the symptoms of different degrees of severity, and gives the discontinuation rates in clinical trials for one or more of the following nervous system symptoms: dizziness, insomnia, impaired concentration, somnolence, abnormal dreaming, euphoria, confusion, agitation, amnesia, hallucinations, stupor, abnormal thinking, and depersonalization. The frequencies of specific central and peripheral nervous system symptoms are provided in Table 2.

Analysis of long-term data (median treatment duration 180 weeks, 102 weeks, and 76 weeks for patients treated with SUSTIVA + zidovudine + lamivudine, SUSTIVA + indinavir, and indinavir + zidovudine + lamivudine, respectively) showed that, beyond 24 weeks of therapy, the incidences of new-onset nervous system symptoms among SUSTIVA-treated patients were generally similar to those in the control arm.

Psychiatric Symptoms: Serious psychiatric adverse experiences have been reported in patients treated with SUSTIVA. In controlled trials the frequency of specific serious psychiatric symptoms among patients who received SUSTIVA or control regimens, respectively, were: severe depression (2.4%, 0.9%), suicidal ideation (0.7%, 0.3%), non-fatal suicide attempts (0.5%, 0%), aggressive behavior (0.4%, 0.5%), paranoid reactions (0.4%, 0.3%) and manic reactions (0.2%, 0.3%) (see Warnings and Precautions, Psychiatric Symptoms). Additional psychiatric symptoms observed at a frequency of >2% among patients treated with SUSTIVA or control regimens respectively, in controlled clinical trials were depression (19%, 16%), anxiety (13%, 9%) and nervousness (7%, 2%).

Table 2: SUSTIVA

Percent of Patients with One or More Selected Nervous System Symptoms[a,b]

Percent of Patients with	SUSTIVA 600 mg daily (N=1008) %	Control Groups (N=635) %
Mild Symptoms[c]	33.3	15.6
Moderate Symptoms[d]	17.4	7.7
Severe Symptoms[e]	2	1.3
Symptoms of Any Severity	52.7	24.6
Treatment discontinuation as a result of symptoms	2.1	1.1

a Includes events reported regardless of causality.
b Data from Studies 006, 020 and two Phase II studies.
c "Mild"=Symptoms which do not interfere with patient's daily activities.
d "Moderate"=Symptoms which may interfere with daily activities.
e "Severe"=Symptoms which interrupt patient's usual daily activities.

Skin Rash: Rashes are usually mild-to-moderate maculopapular skin eruptions that occur within the first two weeks of initiating therapy with SUSTIVA. In most patients rash resolves with continuing SUSTIVA therapy within one month. SUSTIVA can be reinitiated in patients interrupting therapy because of Grades 1 and 2 rash. SUSTIVA should be discontinued in patients developing severe rash associated with blistering, desquamation, mucosal involvement or fever. The frequency of rash by NCI grade and the discontinuation rates as a result of rash are provided in Table 3.

Table 3: SUSTIVA

Percent of Patients with Treatment-Emergent Rash[a,b]

Percent of Patients with	Description of Rash Grade[c]	SUSTIVA 600 mg once daily Adults (N=1008) %	SUSTIVA Pediatric Patients (N=57) %	Control Groups Adults (N=635) %
Grade 1 Rash	erythema, pruritus	10.7	8.8	9.8
Grade 2 Rash	diffuse maculopapular rash, dry desquamation	14.7	31.6	7.4
Grade 3 Rash	vesiculation, moist desquamation, ulceration	0.8	1.8	0.3
Grade 4 Rash	erythema multiforme, Stevens-Johnson syndrome, toxic epidermal necrolysis, necrosis requiring surgery, exfoliative dermatitis	0.1	3.5	0
Rash of Any Grade	—	26.3	45.6	17.5
Treatment discontinuation as a result of rash	—	1.7	8.8	0.3

a Includes events reported regardless of causality.
b Data from studies 006, 020, and two Phase II studies.
c NCI (National Cancer Institute) Grading System.

As seen in Table 3, rash is more common in children and more often of higher grade (i.e., more severe) (see Warnings and Precautions, General).

Experience with SUSTIVA in patients who discontinued other antiretroviral agents of the NNRTI class is limited. Nineteen patients who discontinued nevirapine because of rash have been treated with SUSTIVA. Nine of these patients developed mild-to-moderate rash while receiving therapy with SUSTIVA, and two of these patients discontinued because of rash.

Selected clinical adverse experiences of moderate or severe intensity observed in ≥2% of SUSTIVA-treated patients in three controlled clinical trials are presented in Table 4.

Lipodystrophy (any severity, regardless of relationship to study regimen) was reported in 3%, 4%, and 5% of patients treated with SUSTIVA + zidovudine + lamivudine, SUSTIVA + indinavir, and indinavir + zidovudine + lamivudine, respectively. The frequencies of other adverse event terms that may be associated with lipodystrophy (abdomen enlarged, breast enlargement, cachexia, gynecomastia, lipidosis, lipoma, and obesity) ranged from <1% to 3% and were similar among the treatment groups.

Clinical adverse experiences observed in ≥10% of 57 pediatric patients aged 3 to 16 years who received SUSTIVA capsules, nelfinavir, and one or more NRTIs were: rash (46%), diarrhea/loose stools (39%), fever (21%), cough (16%), dizziness/lightheaded/fainting (16%),ache/pain/discomfort (14%), nausea/vomiting (12%), and headache (11%). The incidence of nervous system symptoms was 18% (10/57). One patient experienced Grade 3 rash, two patients had Grade 4 rash, and five patients (9%) discontinued because of rash (see Warnings and Precautions, Pediatrics).

Adverse clinical experiences of moderate to severe intensity observed in less than 2% of patients receiving SUSTIVA in all Phase II/III studies, including the North American expanded access program as well as post-marketing spontaneous reports, and considered at least possibly related or of unknown relationship to treatment are listed below by body system:

Body as a Whole: alcohol intolerance, allergic reaction, asthenia, fever, hot flushes, influenza-like symptoms, malaise, pain, peripheral edema, syncope, dysregulated body temperature, flank pain, hypersensitivity reaction. Redistribution/accumulation of body fat (see Warnings and Precautions, Fat Redistribution).

Cardiovascular: arrhythmia, flushing, palpitations, tachycardia, thrombophlebitis, hypertension, congestive heart failure, chest pain.

Central and Peripheral Nervous Systems: ataxia, confusion, convulsions, impaired coordination, migraine headaches, neuralgia, paresthesia, hypoesthesia, peripheral neuropathy, speech disorder, stupor, tremor, neuromuscular paresis, paranoid reaction.

Gastrointestinal: dry mouth, pancreatitis, constipation, malabsorption.

Liver and Biliary System: hepatic enzymes increased (including ALT, AST and GGT), hepatitis, jaundice, hepatomegaly (see Post-Market Adverse Drug Reactions).

Metabolic and Nutritional: hypercholesterolemia, hypertriglyceridemia.

Miscellaneous: thrombocytopenia, proteinuria, anemia, pancytopenia, increased sweating.

Musculoskeletal: arthralgia, myalgia, myopathy, involuntary muscle contraction, muscle weakness, polyarthritis.

Psychiatric: aggressive reactions, abnormal thinking, aggravated depression, agitation, delusions, amnesia, anxiety, apathy, delirium, depersonalization, emotional lability, euphoria, hallucination, manic reaction, psychosis, neurosis, paranoia, suicide.

Respiratory: asthma, apnea, dyspnea.

Table 4: SUSTIVA
Selected Treatment-Emergent[a] Adverse Events of Moderate or Severe Intensity Reported in ≥2% of of SUSTIVA-Treated Patients in Studies DMP 266-006, ACTG 364 and DMP 266-020

	Study DMP 266-006 3TC, NNRTI and Protease Inhibitor-Naive Patients			Study ACTG 364 NRTI-experienced NNRTI and Protease Inhibitor-Naive Patients			Study DMP 266-020 NRTI-Experienced NNRTI and Protease Inhibitor-Naive Patients	
Adverse Events	SUSTIVA[b] + ZDV/3TC (N=412) 180 weeks[c] %	SUSTIVA[b] + Indinavir (N=415) 102 weeks[c] %	Indinavir + ZDV/3TC (N=401) 76 weeks[c] %	SUSTIVA[b] + Nelfinavir + NRTIs (N=64) %	SUSTIVA[b] + NRTIs (N=65) %	Nelfinavir + NRTIs (N=66) %	SUSTIVA[b] + Indinavir + NRTIs (N=154) %	Indinavir + NRTIs (N=168) %
Body as a Whole								
Fatigue	8	5	9	0	2	3	5	1
Pain	1	2	8	13	6	17	4	3
Central and Peripheral Nervous Systems								
Dizziness	9	9	2	2	6	6	7	1
Headache	8	5	3	5	2	3	5	4
Gastrointestinal								
Nausea	10	6	24	3	2	2	10	10
Vomiting	6	3	14	—	—	—	6	5
Diarrhea	3	5	6	14	3	9	11	3
Dyspepsia	4	4	6	0	0	2	3	1
Abdominal Pain	2	2	5	3	3	3	3	1
Psychiatric								
Concentration Impaired	5	3	<1	0	0	0	3	1
Insomnia	7	7	2	0	0	2	3	1
Anxiety	2	4	<1	—	—	—	2	1
Abnormal Dreams	3	1	0	—	—	—	2	1
Somnolence	2	2	<1	0	0	0	2	2
Depression	5	4	<1	3	0	5	2	0
Anorexia	1	<1	<1	0	2	2	5	1
Nervousness	2	2	0	2	0	2	1	0
Skin and Appendages								
Rash	11	16	5	9	5	9	10	6
Pruritus	<1	1	1	9	5	9	2	1

[a] Includes those adverse events at least possibly related to study drug or of unknown relationship for Studies 006 and 020. Includes all adverse events regardless of relationship to study drug for study ACTG 364.
[b] SUSTIVA provided as 600 mg daily.
[c] Median duration of treatment
Legend: — =Not specified; ZDV=zidovudine; 3TC=lamivudine.

Table 5: SUSTIVA
Selected Grade 3-4 Laboratory Abnormalities Reported in ≥2% of SUSTIVA-Treated Patients in Studies 006 and ACTG 364

		Study 006 3TC-, NNRTI-, and Protease Inhibitor-Naive Patients			Study ACTG 364 NRTI-Experienced, NNRTI- and Protease Inhibitor-Naive Patients		
Variable	**Limit**	SUSTIVA[a] + ZDV/3TC (n=412) 180 weeks[b]	SUSTIVA[a] + Indinavir (n=415) 102 weeks[b]	Indinavir + ZDV/3TC (n=401) 76 weeks[b]	SUSTIVA[a] + Nelfinavir + NRTIs (n=64) 71.1 weeks[b]	SUSTIVA[a] + NRTIs (n=65) 70.9 weeks[b]	Nelfinavir + NRTIs (n=66) 62.7 weeks[b]
Chemistry							
ALT	>5×ULN	5%	8%	5%	2%	6%	3%
AST	>5×ULN	5%	6%	5%	6%	8%	8%
GGT[c]	>5×ULN	8%	7%	3%	5%	0	5%
Amylase	>2×ULN	4%	4%	1%	0	6%	2%
Glucose	>250 mg/dL	3%	3%	3%	5%	2%	3%
Triglycerides[d]	≥751 mg/dL	9%	6%	6%	11%	8%	17%
Hematology							

(cont'd)

Table 5: SUSTIVA *(cont'd)*

Selected Grade 3-4 Laboratory Abnormalities Reported in ≥2% of SUSTIVA-Treated Patients in Studies 006 and ACTG 364

		Study 006 3TC-, NNRTI-, and Protease Inhibitor-Naive Patients			Study ACTG 364 NRTI-Experienced, NNRTI- and Protease Inhibitor-Naive Patients		
Variable	**Limit**	**SUSTIVA[a] + ZDV/3TC (n=412) 180 weeks[b]**	**SUSTIVA[a] + Indinavir (n=415) 102 weeks[b]**	**Indinavir + ZDV/3TC (n=401) 76 weeks[b]**	**SUSTIVA[a] + Nelfinavir + NRTIs (n=64) 71.1 weeks[b]**	**SUSTIVA[a] + NRTIs (n=65) 70.9 weeks[b]**	**Nelfinavir + NRTIs (n=66) 62.7 weeks[b]**
Neutrophils	<750/mm^3	10%	3%	5%	2%	3%	2%

[a] SUSTIVA provided as 600 mg once daily.
[b] Median duration of treatment.
[c] Isolated elevations of GGT in patients receiving SUSTIVA may reflect enzyme induction not associated with liver toxicity.
[d] Nonfasting.
Legend: ZDV=zidovudine; 3TC=lamivudine; ULN=Upper limit of normal; ALT=alanine aminotransferase; AST=aspartate aminotransferase; GGT=gamma-glutamyltransferase.

Skin and Appendages: acne, alopecia, eczema, folliculitis, skin exfoliation, urticaria, erythema nodosum, erythema multiforme, Stevens-Johnson syndrome, verruca, nail disorders, skin disorders, photosensitivity reaction.
Special Senses: abnormal vision, diplopia, glaucoma, iritis, parosmia, taste perversion, tinnitus
Urinary System: polyuria.
Laboratory Abnormalities: Table 5 summarizes clinically important laboratory abnormalities reported in Study 006 and ACTG 364.
Liver Enzymes: Liver function should be monitored in patients with a prior history of Hepatitis B and/or C (see Warnings and Precautions, Monitoring and Laboratory Tests).

In the long-term data set from Study 006, 137 patients treated with SUSTIVA-containing regimens (median duration of therapy, 68 weeks) and 84 treated with a control regimen (median duration, 56 weeks) were seropositive at screening for hepatitis B (surface antigen positive) and/or C (hepatitis C antibody positive). Among these co-infected patients, elevations in AST to greater than five times ULN developed in 13% of patients in the SUSTIVA arms and 7% of those in the control arm, and elevations in ALT to greater than five times ULN developed in 20% of patients in the SUSTIVA arms and 7% of patients in the control arm. Among co-infected patients, 3% of those treated with SUSTIVA-containing regimens and 2% in the control arm discontinued from the study because of liver or biliary system disorders.
Lipids: Increases in total cholesterol of 10-20% have been observed in some uninfected volunteers receiving SUSTIVA. In patients treated with SUSTIVA + ZDV + 3TC, increases in non-fasting total cholesterol and HDL of approximately 20% and 25%, respectively, were observed. In patients treated with SUSTIVA + IDV, increases in non-fasting cholesterol and HDL of approximately 40% and 35%, respectively, were observed. Nonfasting total cholesterol levels ≥6.2 mmol/L and ≥7.8 mmol/L were reported in 34% and 9%, respectively, of patients treated with SUSTIVA + ZDV + 3TC; 54% and 20%, respectively, of patients treated with SUSTIVA + indinavir; and 28% and 4%, respectively, of patients treated with indinavir + ZDV + 3TC. The effects of SUSTIVA on triglycerides and LDL were not well-characterized since samples were taken from non-fasting patients. The clinical significance of these findings is unknown (see Warnings and Precautions, General and Monitoring and Laboratory Tests).
Serum Amylase: Asymptomatic elevations in serum amylase greater than 1.5 times the upper limit of normal were seen in 10% of patients treated with SUSTIVA and in 6% of patients treated with control regimens. The clinical significance of asymptomatic increases in serum amylase is unknown (see Warnings and Precautions, General).
Cannabinoid Test Interaction: Efavirenz does not bind to cannabinoid receptors. False positive urine cannabinoid test results have been reported in uninfected volunteers receiving SUSTIVA when the CEDIA DAU Multi-Level THC assay (Microgenics) was used for screening. Negative results were obtained when more specific confirmatory testing was performed with gas chromatography/mass spectrometry. Of three assays analyzed only the CEDIA DAU Multi-Level THC assay showed false-positive results. The Cannabinoid Enzyme Immunoassay (Diagnostic Reagents, Inc) and AxSYM (Cannabinoid Assay (Abbott Laboratories) provided true negative results. The effects of SUSTIVA on cannabinoid screening tests other than these three are unknown.
Post-Market Adverse Drug Reactions: Additional undesirable effects reported in postmarketing surveillance include neurosis, gynecomastia, rhabdomyolysis, increased CPK, blurred vision, photoallergic dermatitis, immune reconstitution syndrome and cerebellar coordination and balance disturbances.

Hepatic failure has been reported postmarketing, including some cases in patients with no pre-existing hepatic disease or other identifiable risk factors and also some cases characterized by a fulminant course, sometimes progressing to transplantation or death.

Additional cases of pancreatitis have been reported in postmarketing surveillance. Please see Warnings and Precautions, Pancreatitis.

DRUG INTERACTIONS: Overview: Efavirenz has been shown in vivo to induce CYP3A4. Other compounds that are substrates of CYP3A4 may have decreased plasma concentrations when coadministered with SUSTIVA (efavirenz). In vitro studies have demonstrated that efavirenz inhibits 2C9, 2C19 and 3A4 isozymes in the range of observed efavirenz plasma concentrations. Coadministration of efavirenz with drugs primarily metabolized by these isozymes may result in altered plasma concentrations of the coadministered drug. Therefore, appropriate dose adjustments may be necessary for these drugs.
Drug-Drug Interactions: Drugs which induce CYP3A4 activity (e.g., phenobarbital, rifampin, rifabutin) would be expected to increase the clearance of efavirenz resulting in lowered plasma concentrations. Drug interactions with SUSTIVA are summarized in Table 1, Table 6 and Table 7. (See also Action and Clinical Pharmacology, Pharmacokinetics, Drug-Drug Interactions and Contraindications.)

The drugs listed in Table 1, Table 6 and Table 7 are based on either drug interaction case reports or studies, or potential interactions due to the expected magnitude and seriousness of the interaction.
Other Drugs: Based on the results of drug interaction studies, no dosage adjustment of either SUSTIVA or the following coadministered drugs is recommended: aluminum/magnesium hydroxide antacids, azithromycin, cetirizine, famotidine, fluconazole, lamivudine, nelfinavir, paroxetine, zidovudine and tenofovir disoproxil fumarate. (See Action and Clinical Pharmacology, Pharmacokinetics, Table 9 and Table 10.)

No dosage adjustment for lorazepam is recommended when coadministered with SUSTIVA.

Specific drug interaction studies have not been performed with SUSTIVA and NRTIs other than lamivudine and zidovudine. Clinically significant interactions would not be expected since the NRTIs are metabolized via a different route than efavirenz and would be unlikely to compete for the same metabolic enzymes and elimination pathways.

Table 6: SUSTIVA

Established Drug Interactions[a]

Concomitant Drug Class: Drug Name	Effect on Concentration	Clinical Comment
Antiretroviral Agents		
Protease Inhibitor: atazanavir	↓ atazanavir	SUSTIVA decreases atazanavir exposure (see Table 9). **For treatment-naive patients:** If atazanavir is combined with SUSTIVA, atazanavir 400 mg with ritonavir 100 mg should be administered once daily all as a single dose with food, and SUSTIVA should be administered on an empty stomach, preferably at bedtime. **For treatment-experienced patients:** Do not coadminister atazanavir with SUSTIVA in treatment-experienced patients due to decreased atazanavir exposure.
Protease Inhibitor: fosamprenavir calcium	↓ amprenavir	For coadministration with fosamprenavir and ritonavir, the complete prescribing information for fosamprenavir calcium should be consulted.

(cont'd)

Table 6: SUSTIVA *(cont'd)*

Established Drug Interactions[a]

Concomitant Drug Class: Drug Name	Effect on Concentration	Clinical Comment
Protease Inhibitor: indinavir	↓ indinavir	The optimal dose of indinavir, when given in combination with SUSTIVA, is not known. Increasing the indinavir dose to 1000 mg every 8 hours does not compensate for the increased indinavir metabolism due to SUSTIVA. When indinavir at an increased dose (1000 mg every 8 hours) was given with SUSTIVA (600 mg once daily), the indinavir AUC and C_{min} were decreased on average by 33%-46% and 39-57%, respectively, compared to when indinavir (800 mg every 8 hours) was given alone.
Protease Inhibitor: lopinavir/ritonavir	↓ lopinavir	For lopinavir/ritonavir capsules or oral solution, a dose increase to 533/133 mg (4 capsules or 6.5 mL) twice daily taken with food is recommended when used in combination with SUSTIVA in patients for whom reduced susceptibility to lopinavir is clinically suspected (by treatment history or laboratory evidence). **Lopinavir/ritonavir tablets should not be administered once-daily in combination with SUSTIVA.** In antiretroviral-naive patients, lopinavir/ritonavir tablets can be used twice daily in combination with SUSTIVA with no dose adjustment. A dose increase of lopinavir/ritonavir tablets to 600/150 mg (3 tablets) twice daily may be considered when used in combination with SUSTIVA in treatment-experienced patients where decreased susceptibility to lopinavir is clinically suspected (by treatment history or laboratory evidence).
CCR5 co-receptor antagonist: maraviroc	↓ maraviroc	Refer to the full prescribing information for maraviroc for guidance on coadministration with efavirenz.
Protease Inhibitor: ritonavir	↑ritonavir ↑efavirenz	When ritonavir 500 mg q12h was coadministered with SUSTIVA 600 mg once daily, the combination was associated with a higher frequency of adverse clinical experiences (e.g., dizziness, nausea, paresthesia) and laboratory abnormalities (elevated liver enzymes). Monitoring of liver enzymes is recommended when SUSTIVA is used in combination with ritonavir.
Protease Inhibitor: saquinavir	↓ saquinavir	Should not be used as sole protease inhibitor in combination with SUSTIVA.
Other Agents		
Anticonvulsants: carbamazepine	↓ carbamazepine[a] ↓ efavirenz[a]	Plasma concentrations of carbamazepine and SUSTIVA decreased. Periodic monitoring of carbamazepine plasma levels should be conducted. There are insufficient data to make a dose recommendation. Alternative anticonvulsant treatment should be considered.
Antidepressant: sertraline	↓ sertraline	Since SUSTIVA reduces sertraline levels, it may be necessary to retitrate the sertraline dose in order to achieve the desired clinical effect. In a drug interaction study in healthy subjects, an increased incidence of impaired concentration was seen in subjects receiving sertraline concomitantly with SUSTIVA.
Antifungal: itraconazole	↓ itraconazole[a] ↓ hydroxyitraconazole[a]	Since no dose recommendation for itraconazole can be made, alternative antifungal treatment should be considered.
Antifungal: posaconazole	↓ posaconazole	Avoid concomitant use of posaconazole and efavirenz unless the benefit to the patient outweighs the risk.
Antifungal: voriconazole	↓voriconazole ↑efavirenz	Standard doses of voriconazole and SUSTIVA should not be used concurrently. When voriconazole is coadministered with SUSTIVA, the voriconazole maintenance dose should be increased to 400 mg every 12 hours and SUSTIVA dose should be decreased to 300 mg once daily using the capsule formulation. SUSTIVA tablets should not be broken.
Anti-Infective: clarithromycin	↓ clarithromycin ↑14-OH metabolite	Plasma concentrations decreased by SUSTIVA; clinical significance unknown. In uninfected volunteers, 46% developed rash while receiving SUSTIVA and clarithromycin. No dose adjustment of SUSTIVA is recommended when given with clarithromycin. Alternatives to clarithromycin, such as azithromycin, should be considered (see Other Drugs, below Table 7). Not all macrolide antibiotics have been studied in combination with SUSTIVA.

(cont'd)

Table 6: SUSTIVA *(cont'd)*

Established Drug Interactions[a]

Concomitant Drug Class: Drug Name	Effect on Concentration	Clinical Comment
Antimycobacterial: rifabutin	↓ rifabutin	Consider an increase of the daily dose of rifabutin by 50%. Consider doubling the rifabutin dose in regimens where rifabutin is given 2 or 3 times a week.
Antimycobacterial: rifampin	↓ efavirenz	Rifampin has the potential to decrease serum concentration of SUSTIVA. Increase dose of efavirenz to 800 mg once daily.
Calcium Channel Blocker: diltiazem	↓ diltiazem[a] ↓ desacetyl diltiazem[a] ↓ N-monodesmethyl diltiazem[a]	Diltiazem levels are markedly decreased when coadministered with SUSTIVA. SUSTIVA levels increased to a lesser extent (see Table 9 and Table 10). Patients should be closely monitored for possible decreased diltiazem effects and increased adverse events and laboratory abnormalities associated with SUSTIVA. Refer to the prescribing information for diltiazem for guidance on dose adjustment).
HMG-CoA Reductase Inhibitors: atorvastatin pravastatin simvastatin	↓ atorvastatin[a] ↓ pravastatin[a] ↓ simvastatin[a]	Plasma concentrations of atorvastatin and pravastatin decreased. Consult the complete prescribing information for the HMG-CoA reductase inhibitor for guidance on individualizing the dose. A marked decrease in simvastatin plasma concentrations was seen when coadministered with SUSTIVA (see Table 9). Alternative statins should be considered.
Hormonal Contraceptive:		A reliable method of barrier contraception must be used in addition to hormonal contraceptives.
Oral: ethinyl estradiol/ norgestimate	↓ active metabolites of norgestimate	Efavirenz had no effect on ethinyl estradiol concentrations, but progestin levels (norelgestromin and levonorgestrel) were markedly decreased. The clinical significance of these effects is not known. No effect of ethinyl estradiol/norgestimate on efavirenz plasma concentrations was observed.
Implant: etonogestrel	↓ etonogestrel	The interaction between etonogestrel and efavirenz has not been studied. Decreased exposure of etonogestrel may be expected (CYP3A4 induction), and there have been occasional postmarketing reports of contraceptive failure with etonogestrel in efavirenz-exposed patients.
Narcotic Analgesic: methadone	↓ methadone	Coadministration in HIV-infected individuals with a history of injection drug use resulted in decreased plasma levels of methadone and signs of opiate withdrawal. Patients should be monitored for signs of withdrawal and their methadone dose increased as required to alleviate withdrawal symptoms.

[a] For magnitude of interactions, see Table 9 and Table 10.

Table 7: SUSTIVA

Other Potentially Clinically Significant Drug or Herbal Product Interactions with SUSTIVA[a]

Anticoagulants: warfarin	Plasma concentrations and effects potentially increased or decreased by SUSTIVA. It is recommended that INR be monitored.
Anticonvulsants: phenytoin phenobarbital	Potential for reduction in anticonvulsant and/or efavirenz plasma levels; periodic monitoring of anticonvulsant plasma levels should be conducted (see Warnings and Precautions).
Antifungals: ketoconazole	See Contraindications for other antifungals. Drug interaction studies with SUSTIVA and ketoconazole have not been conducted. SUSTIVA has the potential to decrease plasma concentrations of ketoconazole.
Anti-HIV Protease Inhibitors: saquinavir/ritonavir combination	No pharmacokinetic data are available. (See Table 6.)
Calcium Channel Blockers: felodipine, nifedipine, verapamil	No data are available on the potential interactions of efavirenz with calcium channel blockers that are substrates of the CYP3A4 enzyme, other than diltiazem (see Table 6). The potential exists for reduction in plasma concentrations of the calcium channel blocker. Dose adjustments should be guided by clinical response (refer to the prescribing information for the calcium channel blocker).
Immunosuppressants: cyclosporine, tacrolimus, sirolimus	When an immunosuppressant metabolized by CYP3A4 is administered with efavirenz, decreased exposure of the immunosuppressant may be expected due to CYP3A4 induction. Dose adjustments of the immunosuppressant may be required. Close monitoring of immunosuppressant concentrations for at least 2 weeks (until stable concentrations are reached) is recommended when starting or stopping treatment with SUSTIVA.
Non-nucleoside Reverse Transcriptase Inhibitors	No studies have been performed with other NNRTIs.
St. John's Wort (hypericum perforatum)	Expected to substantially decrease plasma levels of efavirenz; has not been studied in combination with SUSTIVA (see Warnings and Precautions).

[a] This table is not all inclusive.

DOSAGE AND ADMINISTRATION: Dosing Considerations: Adults: The recommended dosage of SUSTIVA (efavirenz) capsules and tablets in combination with other antiretroviral agents is 600 mg orally, once daily. SUSTIVA must be given in combination with other antiretroviral medications. It is recommended that SUSTIVA be taken on an empty stomach, preferably at bedtime. The increased efavirenz concentrations observed following administration of SUSTIVA with food may lead to an increase in frequency of adverse events (see Actions and Clinical Pharmacology, Effect of Food on Oral Absorption). Dosing at bedtime may improve the tolerability of nervous system symptoms (see Warnings and Precautions, General and Adverse Reactions).

Recommended Dose and Dosage Adjustment: Pediatric Patients and Adolescents: It is recommended that SUSTIVA be taken on an empty stomach, preferably at bedtime. The recommended dosage of SUSTIVA in combination with other antiretroviral agents for patients 3 to 17 years of age is described in Table 8. There are insufficient data to recommend a dose in pediatric patients below 3 years of age or who weigh less than 13 kg. SUSTIVA capsules must only be administered to children who are able to reliably swallow capsules. SUSTIVA tablets are not suitable for children weighing less than 40 kg. The recommended dosage of SUSTIVA for pediatric patients weighing greater than 40 kg is 600 mg, once daily.

Table 8: SUSTIVA

Pediatric Dose to Be Administered Once Daily

Body Weight (kg)	SUSTIVA Dose (mg)
13 to <15	200
15 to <20	250
20 to <25	300
25 to <32.5	350
32.5 to <40	400
≥40	600

Information is based on one study, ACTG 382. Patients were administered SUSTIVA in combination with nelfinavir and NRTIs. Further dose adjustments may be required if other products are used concomitantly. (See Action and Clinical Pharmacology, Pharmacokinetics, Drug-Drug Interactions and Drug Interactions.)

Renal Impairment: See Warnings and Precautions, Renal Impairment.

Hepatic Impairment: See Warnings and Precautions, Hepatic Impairment.

OVERDOSAGE:
Treatment of overdose with SUSTIVA (efavirenz) should consist of general supportive measures, including monitoring of vital signs and observation of the patient's clinical status. Administration of activated charcoal should be used to aid removal of unabsorbed drug, as recommended in American College of Emergency Physicians guidelines. There is no specific antidote for overdose with SUSTIVA. Since efavirenz is highly protein bound, dialysis is unlikely to significantly remove the drug from blood.

Some patients accidentally taking 600 mg twice daily have reported increased nervous system symptoms. One patient experienced involuntary muscle contractions and a second patient experienced vomiting after taking twice the recommended dose.

> For management of a suspected drug overdose, contact your regional Poison Control Centre. See the *CPS* Directory section for a list of Poison Control Centres.

ACTION AND CLINICAL PHARMACOLOGY: Mechanism of Action: Efavirenz is a selective non-nucleoside reverse transcriptase (RT) inhibitor of human immunodeficiency virus type 1 (HIV-1). Efavirenz is predominantly a non-competitive inhibitor of HIV-1 RT. HIV-2 RT and human cellular DNA polymerases α, β, γ and δ are not inhibited by concentrations of efavirenz well in excess of those achieved clinically.

Pharmacokinetics: Absorption: Peak efavirenz plasma concentrations were attained within 5 hours following single oral doses of 100 mg to 1600 mg administered to uninfected volunteers. Dose-related increases in C_{max} and AUC were seen for doses up to 1600 mg.

In HIV-infected patients at steady-state, mean C_{max}, mean C_{min}, and mean AUC were dose proportional.

Effect of Food on Oral Absorption: Capsules: Administration of a single 600 mg dose of efavirenz capsules with a high fat/high caloric meal (894 kcal, 54 g fat, 54% calories from fat) or a reduced fat/normal caloric meal (440 kcal, 2 g fat, 4% calories from fat) was associated with a mean increase of 22% and 17% in efavirenz AUC and a mean increase of 39% and 51% in efavirenz C_{max}, respectively, relative to the exposures achieved when given under fasted conditions. (See Dosage and Administration.)

Tablets: Administration of a single 600 mg dose of efavirenz tablet with a high fat/high caloric meal (approximately 1000 kcal, 500-600 kcal from fat) was associated with a 28% increase in mean AUC of efavirenz and a 79% increase in mean C_{max} of efavirenz relative to the exposures achieved under fasted conditions. (See Dosage and Administration.)

Distribution: Efavirenz is highly bound (approximately 99.5-99.75%) to human plasma proteins, predominantly albumin. In HIV-1 infected patients (N=9), efavirenz cerebrospinal fluid concentrations ranged from 0.26 to 1.19% (mean 0.69%) of the corresponding plasma concentration; approximately 3-fold higher than the non-protein-bound (free) fraction of efavirenz in plasma.

Metabolism: In vivo and in vitro studies demonstrated that efavirenz is principally metabolized by the cytochrome P450 system to hydroxylated metabolites with subsequent glucuronidation of these hydroxylated metabolites. These metabolites are essentially inactive against HIV-1.

Efavirenz has been shown to induce P450 enzymes, resulting in the induction of its own metabolism.

Elimination: Efavirenz has a long terminal half-life of 52-76 hours after single doses and 40-55 hours after multiple doses. Approximately 14-34% of the radiolabel was recovered in the urine and 16-61% was recovered in the feces. Nearly all of the urinary excretion of the radiolabelled drug was in the form of metabolites. Efavirenz accounted for the majority of the total radioactivity measured in feces.

Drug-Drug Interactions: Table 9 and Table 10 show drug-drug interactions of SUSTIVA with various coadministrated drugs and their pharmacokinetic profiles (see Drug Interactions).

Table 9: SUSTIVA

Effect of Efavirenz on Coadministered Drug Plasma C_{max}, AUC and C_{min}

Coadministered Drug Class: Drug Name	Dose	Efavirenz Dose	Coadministered Drug (Mean % change) C_{max}	AUC	C_{min}
Antiretroviral Agents					
Protease Inhibitor: atazanavir	400 mg daily×20 days	600 mg d 7–20	↓ 59%	↓ 74%	↓ 93%
atazanavir/ritonavir	400 mg daily d 1–6, then 300 mg daily d 7–20 with ritonavir 100 mg daily and a light meal	600 mg daily 2 h after atazanavir and ritonavir d 7–20	↑ 14%[a]	↑ 39%[a]	↑ 48%[a]
	300 mg qd/ritonavir 100 mg qd d 1–10 (pm), then 400 mg qd/ritonavir 100 mg qd d 11–24 (pm) (simultaneous with efavirenz)	600 mg d 11–24 (pm)	↑ 17%	↔	↓ 42%
Protease Inhibitor: indinavir	1000 mg q8h×10 days	600 mg×10 days			
	after morning dose		↔[b]	↓ 33%[b]	↓ 39%[b]
	after afternoon dose		↔[b]	↓ 37%[b]	↓ 52%[b]
	after evening dose		↓ 29%[b]	↓ 46%[b]	↓ 57%[b]

(cont'd)

Table 9: SUSTIVA *(cont'd)*

Effect of Efavirenz on Coadministered Drug Plasma C_{max}, AUC and C_{min}

Coadministered Drug Class: Drug Name	Dose	Efavirenz Dose	Coadministered Drug (Mean % change) C_{max}	AUC	C_{min}
Protease Inhibitor: indinavir/ritonavir	Indinavir 800 mg + ritonavir 100 mg q12h d 1–29	600 mg d 15–29	↓ 17%[e]	↓ 25%[e]	↓ 50%[e]
Protease Inhibitor: lopinavir/ritonavir	400/100 mg capsule q12h×9 days	600 mg×9 days	↔[c]	↓ 19%[c]	↓ 39%[c]
	600/150 mg tablet q12h×10 days with efavirenz compared to 400/100 mg q12h alone	600 mg×9 days	↑ 36%	↑ 36%	↑ 32%
CCR5 co-receptor antagonist: maraviroc	100 mg bid	600 mg	↓ 51%	↓ 45%	↓ 45%
Protease Inhibitor: nelfinavir	750 mg q8h×7 days	600 mg×7 days	↑ 21%	↑ 20%	↔
Metabolite AG-1402			↓ 40%	↓ 37%	↓ 43%
Protease Inhibitor: ritonavir	500 mg q12h×8 days	600 mg×10 days			
	after AM dose		↑ 24%	↑ 18%	↑ 42%
	after PM dose		↔	↔	↑ 24%
Protease Inhibitor: saquinavir (SGC)[g]	1200 mg q8h×10 days	600 mg×10 days	↓ 50%	↓ 62%	↓ 56%
Nucleoside Reverse Transcriptase Inhibitor: lamivudine	150 mg q12h×14 days	600 mg×14 days	↔	↔	↑ 265%
Nucleoside Reverse Transcriptase Inhibitor: zidovudine	300 mg q12h×14 days	600 mg×14 days	↔	↔	↑ 225%
Nucleoside Reverse Transcriptase Inhibitor: tenofovir disoproxil fumarate	300 mg daily	600 mg×14 days	↔	↔	↔
Other Agents					
Anticonvulsant: carbamazepine	200 mg daily×3 days, 200 mg bid×3 days, then 400 mg daily×29 days	600 mg×14 days	↓ 20%	↓ 27%	↓ 35%
epoxide metabolite			↔	↔	↓ 13%
Antidepressant: paroxetine	20 mg daily×14 days	600 mg×14 days	↔	↔	↔
Antidepressant: sertraline	50 mg daily×14 days	600 mg×14 days	↓ 29%	↓ 39%	↓ 46%
N desmethylsertraline			↓ 17%	↓ 20%	↓ 20%
Antifungal: fluconazole	200 mg×7 days	400 mg×7 days	↔	↔	↔
Antifungal: itraconazole	200 mg q12h×28 days	600 mg×14 days	↓ 37%	↓ 39%	↓ 44%
hydroxyitraconazole			↓ 35%	↓ 37%	↓ 43%
Antifungal: posaconazole	400 mg (oral suspension) bid×10 and 20 days	400 mg×10 and 20 days	↓ 45%	↓ 50%	NA
Antifungal: voriconazole	400 mg q12h d-1 200 mg q12h d 2-9	400 mg×9 days	↓ 61%	↓ 77%	NA
	300 mg po q12h d 2–7	300 mg×7 days	↓ 36%[f]	↓ 55%[f]	NA
	400 mg po q12h d 2–7	300 mg×7 days	↑ 23%[f]	↔[f]	NA
Anti-Infective: azithromycin	600 mg single dose	400 mg×7 days	↑ 22%	↔	NA
Anti-Infective: clarithromycin	500 mg q12h×7 days	400 mg×7 days	↓ 26%	↓ 39%	↓ 53%
14-OH metabolite			↑ 49%	↑ 34%	↑ 26%
Antimycobacterial: rifabutin	300 mg daily×14 days	600 mg×14 days	↓ 32%	↓ 38%	↓ 45%

(cont'd)

Table 9: SUSTIVA *(cont'd)*

Effect of Efavirenz on Coadministered Drug Plasma C_{max}, AUC and C_{min}

Coadministered Drug Class: Drug Name	Dose	Efavirenz Dose	Coadministered Drug (Mean % change) C_{max}	AUC	C_{min}
25-0-desacetylrifabutin			↓ 49%[d]	↓ 74%[d]	NA
Anxiolytic: lorazepam	2 mg single dose	600 mg×10 days	↑ 16%	↔	NA
Calcium Channel Blocker: diltiazem	240 mg×21 days	600 mg×14 days	↓ 60%	↓ 69%	↓ 63%
desacetyl diltiazem			↓ 64%	↓ 75%	↓ 62%
N-monodesmethyl diltiazem			↓ 28%	↓ 37%	↓ 37%
H_1 Receptor Antagonist: cetirizine	10 mg single dose	600 mg×10 days	↓ 24%	↔	NA
HMG-CoA Reductase Inhibitor: atorvastatin	10 mg qd daily×4 days	600 mg×15 days	↓ 14%	↓ 43%	↓ 69%
total active (including metabolites)			↓ 15%	↓ 32%	↓ 48%
HMG-CoA Reductase Inhibitor: pravastatin	40 mg daily×4 days	600 mg×15 days	↓ 32%	↓ 44%	↓ 19%
HMG-CoA Reductase Inhibitor: simvastatin	40 mg daily×4 days	600 mg×15 days	↓ 72%	↓ 68%	↓ 45%
total active (including metabolites)			↓ 68%	↓ 60%	NA
Narcotic Analgesic: methadone	Stable maintenance 35–100 mg daily	600 mg×14–21 days	↓ 45%	↓ 52%	NA
Oral Contraceptive:					
ethinyl estradiol/ norgestimate	0.035 mg/ 0.25 mg×14 days	600 mg×14 days			
ethinyl estradiol			↔	↔	↔
norelgestromin			↓ 46%	↓ 64%	↓ 82%
levonorgestrel			↓ 80%	↓ 83%	↓ 86%

a Compared with atazanavir 400 mg daily alone.
b Comparator dose of indinavir was 800 mg q8h×10 days.
c Values are for lopinavir. C_{min} of lopinavir was significantly decreased by 39%. C_{max} and AUC of lopinavir were decreased by 3% and 19% respectively (not significant). The pharmacokinetics of ritonavir 100 mg q12h are unaffected by concurrent efavirenz.
d Based on arithmetic mean values.
e Compared to indinavir 800 twice daily given with ritonavir 100 mg twice daily without efavirenz. The geometric Cmin for indinavir (0.33 mg/L) when given with ritonavir and efavirenz was higher than the mean historical Cmin (0.15 mg/L) when indinavir was given alone at 800 mg every 8 hours. When efavirenz 600 mg once daily was given with indinavir/ritonavir 800/100 mg twice daily in HIV-1-infected patients (n=6), the pharmacokinetics of indinavir and efavirenz were generally comparable to these data from uninfected volunteers.
f Relative to steady-state administration of voriconazole (400 mg for 1 day, then 200 mg po q12h for 2 days).
g SGC=Soft Gelatin Capsule.
Legend: ↑ Indicates increase; ↓ Indicates decrease; ↔ Indicates no change or a mean increase or decrease of <10%.

Table 10: SUSTIVA

Effect of Coadministered Drug on Efavirenz Plasma C_{max}, AUC and C_{min}

Coadministered Drug Class: Drug Name	Dose	Efavirenz Dose	Efavirenz (Mean % change) C_{max}	AUC	C_{min}
Antiretroviral Agents					
Protease Inhibitor: atazanavir	400 mg daily×20 days	600 mg d 7–20	↔	↔	NA
Protease Inhibitor: indinavir	800 mg q8h×14 days	200 mg×14 days	↔	↔	↔
Protease Inhibitor: lopinavir/ritonavir	400/100 mg q12h ×9 days	600 mg×9 days	↔	↓ 16%	↓ 16%
Protease Inhibitor: nelfinavir	750 mg q8h×7 days	600 mg×7 days	↓ 12%	↓ 12%	↓ 21%
Protease Inhibitor: ritonavir	500 mg q12h×8 days	600 mg×10 days	↑ 14%	↑ 21%	↑ 25%
Protease Inhibitor: saquinavir (SGC)[b]	1200 mg q8h×10 days	600 mg×10 days	↓ 13%	↓ 12%	↓ 14%

(cont'd)

Table 10: SUSTIVA *(cont'd)*

Effect of Coadministered Drug on Efavirenz Plasma C_{max}, AUC and C_{min}

Coadministered Drug Class: Drug Name	Dose	Efavirenz Dose	Efavirenz (Mean % change) C_{max}	AUC	C_{min}
Nucleotide Reverse Transcriptase Inhibitor: tenofovir disoproxil fumarate	300 mg daily	600 mg×14 days	↔	↔	↔
Other Agents					
Antacid: aluminum hydroxide 400 mg magnesium hydroxide 400 mg, + simethicone 30 mg	30 mL single dose	400 mg single dose	↔	↔	NA
Anticonvulsant: carbamazepine	200 mg daily×3 days, 200 mg bid×3 days, then 400 mg daily×15 days	600 mg×35 days	↓ 21%	↓ 36%	↓ 47%
Antidepressant: paroxetine	20 mg daily×14 days	600 mg×14 days	↔	↔	↔
Antidepressant: sertraline	50 mg daily×14 days	600 mg×14 days	↑ 11%	↔	↔
Antifungal: fluconazole	200 mg×7 days	400 mg×7 days	↔	↑ 16%	↑ 22%
Antifungal: itraconazole	200 mg q12h×14 days	600 mg×28 days	↔	↔	↔
Antifungal: voriconazole	400 mg q12h d-1 200 mg q12h d 2–9	400 mg×9 days	↑ 38%	↑ 44%	NA
	300 mg po q12h d 2–7	300 mg×7 days	↓ 14%[a]	↔[a]	NA
	400 mg po q12h d 2–7	300 mg×7 days	↔[a]	↑ 17%[a]	NA
Anti-infective: azithromycin	600 mg single dose	400 mg×7 days	↔	↔	↔
Anti-infective: clarithromycin	500 mg q12h×7 days	400 mg×7 days	↑ 11%	↔	↔
Antimycobacterial: rifabutin	300 mg daily×14 days	600 mg×14 days	↔	↔	↓ 12%
Antimycobacterial: rifampin	600 mg×7 days	600 mg×7 days	↓ 20%	↓ 26%	↓ 32%
Calcium Channel Blocker: diltiazem	240 mg×14 days	600 mg×28 days	↑ 16%	↑ 11%	↑ 13%
H_1 Receptor Antagonist: cetirizine	10 mg single dose	600 mg×10 days	↔	↔	↔
H_2 Receptor Antagonist: famotidine	40 mg single dose	400 mg single dose	↔	↔	NA
HMG-CoA Reductase Inhibitor: atorvastatin	10 mg daily×4 days	600 mg×15 days	↔	↔	↔
HMG-CoA Reductase Inhibitor: pravastatin	40 mg daily×4 days	600 mg×15 days	↔	↔	↔
HMG-CoA Reductase Inhibitor: simvastatin	40 mg daily×4 days	600 mg×15 days	↓ 12%	↔	↓ 12%

[a] Relative to steady-state administration of efavirenz (600 mg once daily for 9 days).
[b] SGC=Soft Gelatin Capsule
Legend: ↑ Indicates increase; ↓ Indicates decrease; ↔ Indicates no change or a mean increase or decrease of <10%.

STORAGE AND STABILITY: SUSTIVA (efavirenz) capsules or tablets should be stored at 25°C; excursions permitted to 15-30°C (see USP Controlled Room Temperature).

INFORMATION FOR THE PATIENT: Published in e-CPS, available by subscription at www.e-cps.ca.

DOSAGE FORMS, COMPOSITION AND PACKAGING: Capsules: 50 mg: Each gold and white capsule, printed with "SUSTIVA" on the gold cap and purple oval reverse printed with "50 mg" on the white body, contains: efavirenz 50 mg. Nonmedicinal ingredients: lactose monohydrate, magnesium stearate, sodium lauryl sulfate and sodium starch glycolate; capsule shell: gelatin, sodium lauryl sulfate, titanium dioxide and/or yellow iron oxide (may also contain silicon dioxide); ink: carmine, FD&C Blue No. 2 and titanium dioxide. Bottles of 30.

200 mg: Each gold capsule, reverse printed with "SUSTIVA" on the body and imprinted "200 mg" on the cap, contains: efavirenz 200 mg. Nonmedicinal ingredients: lactose monohydrate, magnesium stearate, sodium lauryl sulfate and sodium starch glycolate; capsule shell: gelatin, sodium lauryl sulfate, titanium dioxide and/or yellow iron oxide (may also contain silicon dioxide); ink: carmine, FD&C Blue No. 2 and titanium dioxide. Bottles of 90.

Tablets: Each yellow, capsular-shaped, film-coated tablet, printed with "SUSTIVA" on both sides, contains: efavirenz 600 mg. Nonmedicinal ingredients: croscarmellose sodium, hydroxypropyl cellulose, lactose monohydrate, magnesium stearate, microcrystalline cellulose and sodium lauryl sulfate; tablet shell: film-coated with Opadry Yellow and Opadry Clear. The tablets are polished with carnauba wax and printed with purple ink, Opacode WB. Bottles of 30.

(Shown in Product Identification Section)

Sutent® Ⓡ

sunitinib malata

Tyrosine Kinase Inhibitor—Antitumor Agent

Pfizer

Date of Revision: April 12, 2010

SUMMARY PRODUCT INFORMATION:

Route of Administration	Dosage Form/ Strength	Clinically Relevant Nonmedicinal Ingredients
Oral	Hard Gelatin Capsule 12.5 mg; 25 mg; 50 mg	Not applicable For a complete listing see Dosage Forms, Composition and Packaging.

INDICATIONS AND CLINICAL USE: SUTENT (sunitinib malate) is indicated for the treatment of gastrointestinal stromal tumour (GIST) after failure of imatinib mesylate treatment due to resistance or intolerance.

Approval of SUTENT is based on Time to Tumour Progression (TTP). Overall survival advantage could not be confirmed.

SUTENT is also indicated for the treatment of metastatic renal cell carcinoma (MRCC) of clear cell histology.

Approval for MRCC is based on statistically significant progression free survival in patients with good performance status (ECOG 0-1). There was a trend for overall survival advantage.

Geriatrics (>65 years of age): Of the 450 patients with solid tumours reported from clinical studies of SUTENT, 115 (25.6%) were 65 and over. No overall differences in safety or effectiveness were observed between younger and older patients.

Pediatrics: The safety and efficacy of SUTENT in pediatric patients have not been established (see Warnings and Precautions).

CONTRAINDICATIONS: Use of SUTENT (sunitinib malate) is contraindicated in patients with hypersensitivity to sunitinib malate or to any other component of SUTENT. For a complete listing, see Dosage Forms, Composition and Packaging.

SUTENT is contraindicated in pregnant women.

WARNINGS AND PRECAUTIONS:

Serious Warnings and Precautions

Patients receiving therapy with SUTENT (sunitinib malate) should be monitored by a qualified physician experienced in the use of anti-cancer agents.

- Tumour Hemorrhage (see Hemorrhage)
- Decreases in left ventricular ejection fraction (LVEF) (see Left Ventricular Dysfunction)
- Hypertension (see Hypertension)
- SUTENT has not been studied in patients with severe renal or severe hepatic impairment.
- Myopathy and/or rhabdomyolysis (see Adverse Reactions, Post-Marketing Experience)
- Cardiomyopathy, including fatal cases (see Adverse Reactions, Post-Marketing Experience)
- Pulmonary embolism, including fatal cases (see Adverse Reactions, Post-Marketing Experience)

Carcinogenesis and Mutagenesis: Carcinogenicity studies with sunitinib have not been completed.

Sunitinib has been tested for genotoxicity in a series of in vitro assays (bacterial mutation, human lymphocyte chromosome aberration) and an in vivo rat bone marrow micronucleus test and did not cause genetic damage.

Cardiovascular: Hypertension: Blood pressure was monitored on a routine basis in the clinical studies. In the treatment-naïve study, 3 patients were discontinued due to treatment-related hypertension, including one with malignant hypertension.

In the GIST trial (Study A), hypertension (all grades) was reported as an adverse event in 51/257 (19%) patients on SUTENT and 7/102 (7%) patients on placebo. Severe hypertension (>200 mmHg systolic or >110 mmHg diastolic) occurred in 9/237 (4%) patients on SUTENT and no patients on placebo. SUTENT dosing was neither delayed nor reduced due to hypertension in any of the GIST patients in the GIST pivotal trial.

Treatment-related hypertension was reported in approximately 30% of patients receiving SUTENT for treatment-naïve MRCC compared to 2% of patients receiving interferon-alfa (IFN-α). Severe hypertension (>200 mmHg systolic or >110 mmHg diastolic) occurred in 9% of treatment-naïve patients on SUTENT and 1% of patients on IFN-α.

In the cytokine-refractory metastatic RCC (MRCC) trials, hypertension (all grades) was reported as an adverse event in 47/169 (28%) patients on SUTENT. Hypertension (>150 mmHg systolic or >100 mmHg diastolic) occurred at least once during the study for 86/165 (52%) patients on SUTENT; severe hypertension (>200 mmHg systolic or >110 mmHg diastolic) occurred in 10/165 (6%) patients on SUTENT. SUTENT dosing was delayed or reduced due to hypertension in 8/165 (4%) cytokine-refractory MRCC patients.

Patients should be monitored for hypertension and treated as appropriate with standard antihypertensive therapy. Temporary suspension of SUTENT is recommended in patients with severe hypertension. Treatment may be resumed once hypertension is controlled.

Patients with hypertension that is not controlled by medications should not be treated with SUTENT.

Left Ventricular Dysfunction: Cardiovascular events, including heart failure, myocardial disorders and cardiomyopathy, some of which were fatal, have been reported through post-marketing experience. Decreases in left ventricular ejection fraction (LVEF) of ≥20% and below the lower limit of normal (LLN) occurred in approximately 2% of SUTENT-treated GIST patients, 4% of SUTENT-treated cytokine-refractory MRCC patients and 2% of placebo-treated patients.

In the double-blind treatment phase of GIST Study A, 22 patients (11%) on SUTENT and 3 patients (3%) on placebo had treatment-emergent LVEF values below LLN. Nine (9) of 22 GIST patients on SUTENT with LVEF changes recovered without intervention. Five (5) patients had documented LVEF recovery following intervention (dose reduction- 1 patient; addition of anti-hypertensive or diuretic medications- 4 patients). Six (6) patients went off study without documented recovery. Additionally, 3 patients (1%) on SUTENT had Grade 3 reductions in left ventricular systolic function to LVEF <40%; 2 of these patients died without receiving further study drug.

In the treatment-naïve MRCC study, 27% and 15% of patients on SUTENT and IFN-α, respectively, had an LVEF value below the LLN. Two (<1%) patients who received SUTENT were diagnosed with congestive heart failure (CHF). One of the two patients with CHF discontinued the study.

In cytokine-refractory MRCC Studies 1 and 2, a total of 24 patients (14%) had treatment-emergent LVEF values below the LLN. Five (5) of 24 patients on SUTENT with LVEF changes recovered without intervention. Five (5) patients had documented LVEF recovery following intervention (dose reduction- 3 patients; addition of antihypertensive or diuretic medications- 2 patients). Eight (8) patients went off study without documented recovery and 6 patients are ongoing on study without recovery.

Patients who presented with cardiac events within 12 months prior to SUTENT administration, such as myocardial infarction (including severe/unstable angina), coronary/peripheral artery bypass graft, symptomatic CHF, cerebrovascular accident or transient ischemic attack, or pulmonary embolism were excluded from SUTENT clinical studies. It is unknown whether patients with these concomitant conditions may be at a higher risk of developing drug-related left ventricular dysfunction. Physicians are advised to weigh this risk against the potential benefits of the drug. **These patients should be carefully monitored for clinical signs and symptoms of CHF while receiving SUTENT. Baseline and periodic evaluations of LVEF should also be considered while these patients are receiving SUTENT. In patients without cardiac risk factors, a baseline evaluation of ejection fraction should be considered.**

In the presence of clinical manifestations of CHF, discontinuation of SUTENT is recommended. The dose of SUTENT should be interrupted and/or reduced in patients without clinical evidence of CHF but with an ejection fraction <50% and >20% below baseline.

QT Interval Prolongation: There is clinical evidence that SUTENT prolongs QT interval, PR interval, and decreases the heart rate. Patients with QTc interval prolongation, atrioventricular (AV) block, and those taking concomitant drugs with dysrhythmic potential were excluded from the pivotal trials, therefore there is no information regarding safety of SUTENT therapy in this group. Because excessive prolongation of the PR interval can result in AV block, caution should be used if SUTENT is prescribed to patients in combination with other drugs that also cause PR interval prolongation, such as beta-blockers, calcium channel blockers, digitalis, or HIV protease inhibitors.

Pre-clinical data (in vitro and in vivo) demonstrate SUTENT causes QT interval prolongation.

Particular care should be exercised when administering SUTENT to patients who are at an increased risk of experiencing torsade de pointes during treatment with a QTc-prolonging drug, or who are taking concomitant drugs with potential to cause QTc interval prolongation (see Drug Interactions).

Bradycardia and AV block are recognized risk factors for torsade de pointes. For this reason, because SUTENT causes QTc prolongation in association with prolongation of the PR and RR intervals, this raises particular concern with respect to proarrhythmic potential. QT interval prolongation may lead to an increased risk of torsade de pointes. Torsade de pointes has been observed in <0.1% of SUTENT-exposed patients.

SUTENT therapy should be discontinued if symptoms suggestive of arrhythmia occur.

Venous Thromboembolic Events/Pulmonary Embolism: Seven (7) patients (3%) on SUTENT and none on placebo in the double-blind treatment phase of a Phase 3 GIST study experienced venous thromboembolic events; 5 of the 7 were Grade 3 deep vein thrombosis (DVT), and 2 were Grade 1 or 2. Four (4) of these 7 GIST patients discontinued treatment following first observation of DVT. Four (4) GIST patients receiving SUTENT experienced a Grade 3/4 pulmonary embolism. All 4 GIST patients had a dose interruption or delay, but were able to continue on SUTENT. Two (2) patients receiving placebo experienced pulmonary embolism. No fatalities related to pulmonary embolism were reported.

Thirteen (3%) patients receiving SUTENT for treatment-naïve MRCC and 4 (2%) patients on the 2 cytokine-refractory MRCC studies had treatment-emergent venous thromboembolic events reported. Seven (7) of the treatment-naïve MRCC patients had pulmonary embolism, 1 was Grade 2 and 6 were Grade 4. Six (6) of the treatment-naïve MRCC patients had DVT, including 3 Grade 3. Dose interruption occurred in 1 of these cases. In treatment-naïve MRCC patients receiving IFN-a , 6 (2%) venous thromboembolic events occurred; 1 patient (<1%) experienced a Grade 3 DVT and 5 patients (1%) had pulmonary embolism, all Grade 4.

Other Cardiovascular Warnings: There have been no cases of myocardial ischemia or myocardial infarction in patients with GIST exposed to either SUTENT or placebo. Two (2) patients with treatment-naïve MRCC experienced treatment-related myocardial infarction (Grade 4), while 2 patients had Grade 3 myocardial ischaemia. Two (2) patients with cytokine-refractory MRCC experienced Grade 3 myocardial ischemia, 1 had Grade 2 "cardiovascular toxicity" reported as an adverse event and 1 patient experienced a fatal myocardial infarction while on treatment.

Drug Interactions: Sunitinib is metabolized primarily by CYP3A4. Potential interactions may occur with drugs that are inhibitors or inducers of this enzyme system (see Drug Interactions).

Endocrine and Metabolism: Adrenal Function Effects: Adrenal toxicity was noted in pre-clinical repeat dose studies of 14 days to 9 months in rats and monkeys at plasma exposures as low as 1.1 times the AUC observed in clinical studies. Histological changes of the adrenal gland were characterized as hemorrhage, necrosis, congestion, hypertrophy and inflammation. In clinical studies, CT or MRI scanning performed on 336 patients treated with SUTENT demonstrated no evidence of adrenal gland hemorrhage or necrosis. ACTH stimulation testing was conducted in over 400 patients across multiple clinical trials of SUTENT. In the GIST studies, 13 patients with normal baseline testing had abnormalities at post-baseline testing consisting of: peak cortisol levels post-stimulation less than normal (497 nmol/L, or 18 µg/dL); failure of stimulation to increase cortisol level by a normal amount (193 nmol/L, or 7 µg/dL); or failure of ACTH Gel test to detect doubling of cortisol level post-stimulation. None of these patients were reported to have clinical evidence of adrenal insufficiency. In the cytokine-refractory MRCC studies, 28 patients with normal baseline testing had abnormalities at post-baseline testing and 3 patients had a treatment-emergent adverse event of adrenal insufficiency, which were not considered by the investigator to be related to SUTENT.

Patients treated with SUTENT should be monitored for adrenal insufficiency when they experience stress such as surgery, trauma, or severe infection.

Thyroid Dysfunction: Treatment-emergent acquired hypothyroidism was noted in 4% of GIST patients on SUTENT versus 1% on placebo. Although not prospectively studied in clinical trials, treatment-related hypothyroidism was reported as an adverse event in 15% of patients on SUTENT in the treatment-naïve MRCC study and two patients (0.6%) in the IFN-α arm, and in 4% of patients across the two cytokine-refractory MRCC studies. Additionally, TSH elevations were reported in 2% of cytokine-refractory MRCC patients.

All patients should be observed closely for signs and symptoms of thyroid dysfunction on sunitinib treatment. Patients with signs and/or symptoms suggestive of hypothyroidism thyroid dysfunction, such as fatigue, should have laboratory monitoring of thyroid function performed and be treated as per standard medical practice.

Rare cases of hyperthyroidism, some followed by hypothyroidism, have been reported in clinical trials and through post-marketing experience.

Gastrointestinal: Gastrointestinal Perforation: Serious, sometimes fatal gastrointestinal complications including gastrointestinal perforation, (likely linked to tumour necrosis) have occurred rarely in patients with intra-abdominal malignancies treated with SUTENT.

Hemorrhage: Hemorrhagic events reported through post-marketing experience, some of which were fatal, have included GI, respiratory, tumor, urinary tract and brain hemorrhages. In the double-blind treatment phase of GIST pivotal trial (Study A), bleeding events occurred in 20% of patients (41/202) receiving SUTENT, compared to 11% (11/102) receiving placebo. In GIST Study A, 14/202 patients (7%) receiving SUTENT and 9/102 patients (9%) on placebo had Grade 3 or 4 bleeding events. In addition, 1 patient in Study A taking placebo had a fatal gastrointestinal bleeding event during cycle 2.

In patients receiving SUTENT for treatment-naïve MRCC, 28% of patients had treatment-related bleeding events compared with 3% of patients receiving IFN-α. Eleven (2.1%) patients on SUTENT versus 1 (0.3%) of patients on IFN-α experienced Grade 3 or greater treatment-related bleeding events.

Bleeding events occurred in 50/169 (26%) patients receiving SUTENT for cytokine-refractory MRCC. Most events in cytokine-refractory MRCC patients were Grade 1 or 2; there was one Grade 3 event (bleeding foot wound). Two (2) cytokine-refractory MRCC study patients with pulmonary metastases experienced hemoptysis considered to be related to SUTENT administration.

Epistaxis was the most common hemorrhagic adverse event reported. Less common bleeding events in MRCC or GIST patients included rectal, gingival, upper GI, genital and wound bleeding.

Treatment-related tumour hemorrhage has been observed in patients receiving SUTENT. These events may occur suddenly, and in the case of pulmonary tumours, may present as severe and life-threatening hemoptysis or pulmonary hemorrhage. Fatal pulmonary hemorrhage occurred in 2 patients receiving SUTENT in a clinical trial of patients with metastatic non-small cell lung cancer (NSCLC). Both patients had squamous cell histology. SUTENT is not approved for use in patients with NSCLC. Treatment-related Grade 3 and 4 tumour hemorrhage occurred in 4/257 (approximately 2%) of GIST patients treated with SUTENT. One (1) patient with tumour hemorrhage had the SUTENT dose temporarily delayed. No patients discontinued treatment due to tumour hemorrhage.

Routine assessment of this event should include serial complete blood counts (CBCs) and physical examination.

Hematologic: Decreased absolute neutrophil counts of Grade 3 and 4 severity were reported in 13.1% and 0.9% patients, respectively. One (1) case of febrile neutropenia was reported in a patient receiving SUTENT on the GIST pivotal trial (Study A). Decreased platelet counts of grade 3 and 4 severity were reported in 4% and 0.5% of patients respectively. The above events were not cumulative, were typically reversible and generally did not result in treatment discontinuation. Complete blood counts should be performed at the beginning of each treatment cycle for patients receiving treatment with SUTENT. Supportive care for hematologic events may include colony stimulating factors.

Hepatic/Biliary/Pancreatic: Grade 3 and 4 increases in serum lipase have been observed in 20 SUTENT patients (10%) versus 7 placebo patients (7%) with GIST. Grade 3 and 4 increases in amylase have been observed in 10 SUTENT patients (5%) versus 3 placebo patients (3%) with GIST. In patients with treatment-naïve MRCC, Grade 3 or 4 increases in amylase and lipase have been observed in 6% and 18% of SUTENT-treated patients and in 3% and 7% of patients receiving IFN-α. In the cytokine-refractory MRCC studies, grade 3 or 4 increases in amylase and lipase have been observed in 4.8% and 16.9% of SUTENT-treated patients, respectively. Increases in lipase levels were transient and were generally not accompanied by signs or symptoms of pancreatitis in subjects receiving SUTENT for GIST or MRCC. Pancreatitis was observed in 2 solid tumour patients (0.4%). Hepatic failure was observed in <1% of solid tumour patients treated with SUTENT. If symptoms of pancreatitis or hepatic failure are present, patients should have SUTENT discontinued and be provided with appropriate medical care.

Neurologic: Seizures: SUTENT has not been studied in patients with known brain metastases. In clinical studies of SUTENT, seizures have been observed in <1% of subjects with radiological evidence of brain metastases.

In addition, there have been rare (<1%) reports of subjects presenting with seizures and radiological evidence of reversible posterior leukoencephalopathy syndrome (RPLS). None of these subjects had a fatal outcome to the event. Patients with seizures and signs/symptoms consistent with RPLS, such as hypertension, headache, decreased alertness, altered mental functioning and visual loss, including cortical blindness should be controlled with medical management including control of hypertension. Discontinuation of SUTENT is recommended; following resolution, treatment may be resumed at the discretion of the treating physician, although the evidence to support this recommendation (restarting treatment) is extremely limited.

Skin and Tissues: Skin discoloration, possibly due to the active substance color (yellow) is a common treatment-related adverse event occurring in approximately 30% of patients. Patients should be advised that depigmentation of the hair or skin may also occur during treatment with SUTENT. Other possible dermatologic effects may include dryness, thickness or cracking of the skin, blisters or occasional rash on the palms of the hands and soles of the feet.

The above events were not cumulative, were typically reversible, generally did not result in treatment discontinuation and may include topical therapies for symptomatic relief.

Special Populations: Pregnant Women: There are no adequate and well-controlled studies of SUTENT in pregnant women. Repeat-dose studies in animals have shown effects in reproductive organs. SUTENT should not be used during pregnancy or in any woman not employing adequate contraception. If the drug is used during pregnancy, or if the patient becomes pregnant while receiving this drug, the patient should be apprised of the potential hazard to the fetus. Women of childbearing potential should be advised to avoid becoming pregnant while receiving treatment with SUTENT.

Nursing Women: Sunitinib and/or its metabolites are excreted in rat milk. It is not known whether sunitinib or its primary active metabolite are excreted in human milk. Because drugs are commonly excreted in human milk and, because of the potential for serious adverse reactions in nursing infants, women should be advised against breastfeeding while taking SUTENT.

Male Contraception: Male patients should be surgically sterile or agree to use effective contraception during the period of therapy with SUTENT. SUTENT may cause embryonal and fetal developmental effects should the female partner of a male taking SUTENT become pregnant as the drug may be present in the semen.

Pediatrics: The safety and efficacy of SUTENT in pediatric patients have not been established (see Indications and Clinical Use). However, physeal dysplasia was observed in Cynomolgus monkeys with open growth plates treated for 3 months with sunitinib at doses that were approximately 0.4 times the recommended human dose (RHD) based on systemic exposure (AUC). The incidence and severity of physeal dysplasia were dose-related and were reversible upon cessation of treatment.

Hepatic: A single 50 mg dose of SUTENT was administered to patients with mild (Child-Pugh Class A) and moderate (Child-Pugh Class B) hepatic impairment, and to control group of patients with normal hepatic function. The pharmacokinetic parameters evaluated demonstrated that dose adjustments might not be necessary for patients with mild (Child-Pugh Class A) or moderate (Child-Pugh Class B) hepatic impairment. However, SUTENT was not studied in subjects with severe (Child-Pugh Class C) hepatic impairment. In addition, repeated administration of SUTENT was not studied in subjects with hepatic impairment.

Renal: SUTENT has not been studied in patients with renal impairment.

Monitoring and Laboratory Tests: CBCs and serum chemistries (including liver function tests, creatinine, electrolytes, magnesium, calcium, phosphate, amylase, and lipase) should be performed at the beginning of each treatment cycle for patients receiving treatment with SUTENT. In the event of an electrolyte abnormality, there should be prompt correction of the imbalance. Thyroid testing should be considered periodically.

Baseline ECG should be conducted prior to starting SUTENT, and ECGs should be performed periodically during therapy. SUTENT should generally not be prescribed to patients with abnormally long baseline QT/QTc intervals or AV block. If there are symptoms suggestive of arrhythmia or if the QT/QTc interval becomes markedly prolonged while the patient is on SUTENT, the drug should be discontinued.

ADVERSE REACTIONS: Adverse Drug Reaction Overview: Two thousand, two hundred and eight (2208) patients with solid tumours, including 853 (39%) patients with GIST and 927 (42%) patients with MRCC, have been treated with SUTENT (sunitinib malate) in 25 completed and ongoing clinical trials. Most of these patients received SUTENT (sunitinib malate) once daily as a 50 mg oral capsule, as a starting dose, on Schedule 4/2. One hundred two (102) patients received placebo in the randomized, double-blind, placebo-controlled clinical trial conducted in patients with GIST. Three hundred and sixty (360) patients received IFN-α in the randomized clinical trial in patients with treatment-naïve MRCC. Most adverse events are reversible and do not need to result in discontinuation. If necessary, these events can be managed through dose adjustments or interruptions.

The most common treatment-related adverse reactions (≥20%) in patients with GIST or MRCC are fatigue, asthenia, diarrhea, nausea, mucositis/stomatitis, vomiting, dyspepsia, hypertension, rash, hand-foot syndrome, skin discoloration, dry skin, hair color changes, altered taste, and anorexia. The potentially serious adverse reactions of left ventricular dysfunction, QT interval prolongation, hemorrhage, hypertension, thyroid dysfunction, and adrenal function are discussed in Warnings and Precautions. Other adverse reactions reported in studies of GIST and MRCC patients are described below

Because clinical trials are conducted under widely varying conditions, adverse reaction rates observed in the clinical trials of a drug cannot be directly compared to rates in the clinical trials of another drug and may not reflect the rates observed in clinical practice.

Adverse Events in GIST Placebo-Controlled Study (Study A): The median duration of blinded study treatment was 2 cycles for patients on the SUTENT arm (mean 3, range 0-9) and one cycle (mean 1.6, range 0-6) for patients on placebo at the time of the interim analysis. Dose reductions occurred in 23 patients (11%) on SUTENT and none on placebo. Dose interruptions occurred in 57 patients (28%) on SUTENT and 20 (20%) on placebo. The rate of permanent discontinuation due to treatment-related, non-fatal adverse events was 9% (19/202) vs. 8% (8/102), SUTENT vs. placebo.

Most treatment-related adverse events reported for both treatment arms were Grade 1 or 2 in severity. Grade 3 or 4 treatment-related adverse events were reported in 48% of SUTENT patients and 29% of placebo patients, respectively, in the double-blind treatment phase of the trial. Fatigue was the most common treatment-related adverse event of any maximum severity grade reported for 42% of SUTENT patients and 36% of placebo patients. Diarrhea, nausea, stomatitis, altered taste, skin abnormalities, hypertension and bleeding were all more common in patients receiving SUTENT than in those receiving placebo. Alopecia has been observed in 9 (4.5%) subjects exposed to sunitinib in Study A as compared to 1 (1%) subject exposed to placebo. All events were NCI CTC Grade 1 severity. Hair color changes have been observed in 14 (6.9%) subjects exposed to sunitinib in Study A as compared to 2 (2%) subjects exposed to placebo. Table 1 presents the treatment-emergent adverse events commonly reported (≥10% of patients) in Study A.

Table 1: SUTENT

Treatment-Emergent Adverse Events Reported in at Least 10% of GIST Patients Who Received SUTENT or Placebo in Study A in the Double-Blind Treatment Phase of Study A

	GIST			
	SUTENT (n=202)		Placebo (n=102)	
Adverse Event, n (%)	**All Grades**	**Grade 3/4**	**All Grades**	**Grade 3/4**
Any	**190 (94)**	**97 (48)**	**99 (97)**	**30 (29)**
Blood and Lymphatic System Disorders	60 (30)	34 (17)	9 (9)	3 (3)
Anaemia NOS	39 (19)	16 (8)	7 (7)	2 (2)
Gastrointestinal	171 (85)	40 (20)	75 (74)	19 (19)
Diarrhea NOS	82 (41)	9 (5)	21 (21)	0 (0)
Nausea	66 (33)	2 (1)	23 (23)	3 (3)
Abdominal pain NOS	61 (30)	12 (6)	28 (29)	10 (10)
Vomiting NOS	50 (25)	3 (2)	18 (18)	3 (3)
Constipation	43 (21)	0 (0)	16 (16)	2 (2)
Stomatitis	33 (16)	1 (1)	2 (2)	0 (0)
Dyspepsia	30 (15)	1 (1)	6 (6)	0 (0)
Abdominal pain upper	22 (11)	3 (2)	8 (8)	0 (0)
Metabolism and Nutritional Disorders	81 (40)	15 (8)	26 (26)	1 (1)
Anorexia	62 (31)	1 (1)	19 (19)	1 (1)

(cont'd)

Table 1: SUTENT *(cont'd)*

Treatment-Emergent Adverse Events Reported in at Least 10% of GIST Patients Who Received SUTENT or Placebo in Study A in the Double-Blind Treatment Phase of Study A

	GIST			
	SUTENT (n=202)		Placebo (n=102)	
Adverse Event, n (%)	**All Grades**	**Grade 3/4**	**All Grades**	**Grade 3/4**
Musculoskeletal and Connective Tissue Disorders	90 (45)	11 (5)	35 (34)	5 (5)
Arthralgia	24 (12)	2 (1)	10 (10)	0 (0)
Back pain	21 (10)	1 (1)	13 (13)	3 (3)
General Disorders and Administration Site Conditions	147 (73)	27 (13)	65 (64)	7 (7)
Fatigue	84 (42)	15 (7)	37 (36)	4 (4)
Asthenia	44 (22)	10 (5)	10 (10)	2 (2)
Pyrexia	32 (16)	2 (1)	9 (9)	1 (1)
Mucosal inflammation NOS	30 (15)	0 (0)	0 (0)	0 (0)
Nervous System Disorders	89 (44)	8 (4)	29 (28)	3 (3)
Dysgeusia	40 (20)	0 (0)	2 (2)	0 (0)
Headache	38 (19)	2 (1)	17 (17)	0 (0)
Psychiatric Disorders	36 (18)	1 (1)	15 (15)	1 (1)
Insomnia	24 (12)	0 (0)	10 (10)	1 (1)
Skin and Subcutaneous Tissue Disorders	125 (62)	12 (6)	31 (30)	0 (0)
Skin Discoloration	52 (26)	0 (0)	8 (8)	0 (0)
Rash NOS	30 (15)	2 (1)	6 (6)	0 (0)
PPE syndrome	28 (14)	9 (5)	2 (2)	0 (0)
Vascular Disorders	50 (25)	17 (8)	12 (12)	0 (0)
Hypertension NOS	28 (14)	8 (4)	7 (7)	0 (0)

Common Terminology Criteria for Adverse Events (CTCAE) Version 3.0.
Legend: PPE=palmar plantar erythrodyaesthesia syndrome; NOS=not otherwise specified.

Table 2 depicts common (≥10%) treatment-emergent laboratory abnormalities.

Table 2: SUTENT

Treatment-Emergent Laboratory Abnormalities in ≥10% of GIST Patients who Received SUTENT or Placebo in the Double-Blind Treatment Phase of Study A

	SUTENT (n=202)		Placebo (n=102)	
Adverse Event, n (%)	**All Grades**	**Grade 3/4[a]**	**All Grades**	**Grade 3/4[b]**
Any		68 (34)		22 (22)
Gastrointestinal				
AST/ALT	78 (39)	3 (2)	23 (23)	1 (1)
Alkaline phosphatase	48 (24)	7 (4)	21 (21)	4 (4)
Total Bilirubin	32 (16)	2 (1)	8 (8)	0 (0)
Indirect Bilirubin	20 (10)	0 (0)	4 (4)	0 (0)
Amylase	35 (17)	10 (5)	12 (12)	3 (3)
Lipase	50 (25)	20 (10)	17 (17)	7 (7)
Cardiac				
Decreased LVEF	22 (11)	2 (1)	3 (3)	0 (0)
Renal/Metabolic				
Creatinine	25 (12)	1 (1)	7 (7)	0 (0)
Hypokalemia	24 (12)	1 (1)	4 (4)	0 (0)
Hypernatremia	20 (10)	0 (0)	4 (4)	1 (1)
Uric acid	31 (15)	16 (8)	16 (16)	8 (8)
Hematology				
Neutropenia	107 (53)	20 (10)	4 (4)	0 (0)
Lymphopenia	76 (38)	0 (0)	16 (16)	0 (0)

(cont'd)

Table 2: SUTENT *(cont'd)*

Treatment-Emergent Laboratory Abnormalities in ≥10% of GIST Patients who Received SUTENT or Placebo in the Double-Blind Treatment Phase of Study A

	SUTENT (n=202)		Placebo (n=102)	
Adverse Event, n (%)	**All Grades**	**Grade 3/4[a]**	**All Grades**	**Grade 3/4[b]**
Anemia	52 (26)	6 (3)	22 (22)	2 (2)
Thrombocytopenia	76 (38)	10 (5)	4 (4)	0 (0)

[a] Grade 4 AEs in patients on SUTENT included alkaline phosphatase (1%), lipase (2%), creatinine (1%), hypokalemia (1%), neutropenia (2%), anemia (2%), and thrombocytopenia (1%).
[b] Grade 4 AEs in patients on placebo included amylase (1%), lipase (1%), anemia (2%), and thrombocytopenia (1%).
Common Terminology Criteria for Adverse Events (CTCAE) Version 3.0.

Grade 3 or 4 treatment-emergent laboratory abnormalities were seen in 68 SUTENT patients (34%) versus 22 placebo patients (22%). Elevated liver function tests, pancreatic enzymes and creatinine were all more common in SUTENT patients than placebo patients. Decreased LVEF, myelosuppression and electrolyte disturbances were all more common in SUTENT patients than placebo patients. Treatment-emergent acquired hypothyroidism was noted in 4% of GIST patients on SUTENT versus 1% on placebo.

After a positive interim analysis, the study was unblinded, and patients on the placebo arm were given the opportunity to receive open-label SUTENT treatment. For 241 patients randomized to the SUTENT arm, including 139 who received SUTENT in both the double-blind and open-label treatment phases, the median duration of SUTENT treatment was 6 cycles (mean 8.5, range 1-44). For the 255 patients who ultimately received open-label SUTENT treatment, median duration of study treatment was 6 cycles (mean 7.8, range 1-37) from the time of the unblinding. A total of 118 patients (46%) required dosing interruptions, and a total of 72 patients (28%) required dose reductions during the open-label treatment phase. The incidence of treatment-emergent adverse reactions resulting in permanent discontinuation was 20%. The most common Grade 3 or 4 treatment-related adverse reactions experienced by patients receiving SUTENT in the open-label treatment phase were neutropenia (11%), fatigue (10%), hypertension (8%), asthenia (5%), diarrhea (5%), hand-foot syndrome (5%), nausea (4%), abdominal pain (3%), anorexia (3%), mucositis (2%), vomiting (2%), and hypothyroidism (2%).

Adverse Reactions in MRCC Patient Population: Treatment-Naive: The as-treated patient population for the interim safety analysis of the Phase 3 MRCC study included 735 patients, 375 randomized to SUTENT and 360 randomized to IFN-α. The median duration of treatment was 11.1 months (range: 0.4-46.1) for SUTENT treatment and 4.1 months (range: 0.1-45.6) for IFN-α treatment. Dose interruptions occurred in 202 patients (54%) on SUTENT and 141 patients (39%) on IFN-α. Dose reductions occurred in 194 patients (52%) on SUTENT and 98 patients (27%) on IFN-α. Discontinuation rates due to adverse reactions were 20% for SUTENT and 23% for IFN-α. Most treatment-related adverse events in both study arms were Grade 1 or 2 in severity. Grade 3 or 4 treatment-related adverse events were reported in 69% and 38% of patients on SUTENT versus IFN-α, respectively. Common treatment-related adverse events of any grade for patients receiving SUTENT are fatigue, diarrhea, nausea, stomatitis, hypertension, hand-foot syndrome, ejection fraction decline. Table 3 compares the incidence of common (≥10%) treatment-related adverse events for patients receiving SUTENT versus those on IFN-α.

Table 3: SUTENT

Treatment-Related Adverse Events Reported in at Least 10% of Patients with Treatment-Naive MRCC Who Received SUTENT or IFN-α

	SUTENT (n=375)		IFN-α (n=360)	
Adverse Event, n (%)	**All Grades n (%)**	**Grade 3/4 n (%)**	**All Grades n (%)**	**Grade 3/4 n (%)**
Any adverse event	**358 (95.5%)**	**258 (68.8%)**	**331 (91.9%)**	**139 (38.6%)**
Blood and Lymphatic System Disorders				
Thrombocytopenia	69 (18.4%)	33 (8.8%)	11 (3.1%)	2 (0.6%)
Neutropenia	70 (18.7%)	40 (10.7%)	31 (8.6%)	12 (3.3%)
Anemia	51 (13.6%)	19 (5.1%)	31 (8.6%)	7 (1.9%)
Leukopenia	40 (10.7%)	12 (3.2%)	14 (3.9%)	3 (0.8%)
Metabolism and Nutrition Disorders				
Anorexia	129 (34.4%)	7 (1.9%)	101 (28.1%)	6 (1.7%)
Decreased appetite	37 (9.9%)	1 (0.3%)	38 (10.6%)	0 (0%)
Nervous System Disorders				
Dysgeusia	175 (46.7%)	1 (0.3%)	52 (13.9%)	0 (0%)
Headache	53 (14.1%)	2 (0.5%)	55 (15.3%)	0 (0%)
Vascular Disorders				
Hypertension	113 (30.1%)	46 (12.3%)	6 (1.7%)	1 (0. 3%)
Respiratory, Thoracic and Mediastinal Disorders				
Epistaxis	67 (17.9%)	3 (0.8%)	5 (1.4%)	0 (0%)
Gastrointestinal Disorders				
Diarrhea	229 (61.1%)	33 (8.8%)	49 (13.6%)	1 (0.3%)
Nausea	195 (52.0%)	17 (4.5%)	124 (34.4%)	4 (1.1%)
Dyspepsia	118 (31.5%)	7 (1.9%)	13 (3.6%)	0 (0%)
Stomatitis	110 (29.3%)	5 (1.3%)	10 (2.8%)	1 (0. 3%)
Vomiting	117 (31.2%)	14 (3.7%)	41 (11.4%)	2 (0.6%)
Abdominal pain[a]	70 (18.7%)	7 (1.9%)	15 (4.2%)	0 (0%)
Dry mouth	45 (12.0%)	0 (0%)	24 (6.7%)	1 (0. 3%)

(cont'd)

Table 3: SUTENT *(cont'd)*

Treatment-Related Adverse Events Reported in at Least 10% of Patients with Treatment-Naïve MRCC Who Received SUTENT or IFN-α

Adverse Event, n (%)	SUTENT (n=375)		IFN-α (n=360)	
	All Grades n (%)	Grade 3/4 n (%)	All Grades n (%)	Grade 3/4 n (%)
Constipation	44 (11.7%)	1 (0.3%)	14 (3.9%)	0 (0.0%)
Flatulence	43 (11.5%)	0 (0.0%)	6 (1.6%)	0 (0.0%)
Skin and Subcutaneous Tissue Disorders				
Rash[b]	115 (30.7%)	4 (1.1%)	33 (9.2%)	3 (0.8%)
Palmar-plantar erythrodysesthesia syndrome	108 (30.0%)	32 (8.5%)	2 (0.6%)	0 (0%)
Dry Skin	79 (21.1%)	1 (0.3%)	19 (5.3%)	0 (0%)
Skin discoloration	89 (23.7%)	1 (0.3%)	0 (0%)	0 (0%)
Hair color changes	75 (20.0%)	0 (0%)	1 (0.3%)	0 (0%)
Erythema	39 (10.4%)	2 (0.5%)	3 (0.8%)	0 (0.0%)
Musculoskeletal and Connective Tissue Disorders				
Pain in extremity	66 (17.6%)	5 (1.3%)	11 (3.1%)	0 (0%)
Arthralgia	43 (11.5%)	1 (0.3%)	49 (13.6%)	0 (0%)
Myalgia	32 (8.5%)	1 (0. 3%)	60 (16.7%)	2 (0. 6%)
General Disorders and Administration Site Conditions				
Fatigue	206 (54.9%)	43 (11.5%)	186 (51.7%)	48 (13.3%)
Mucosal inflammation	98 (26.1%)	7 (1.9%)	6 (1.7%)	1 (0. 3%)
Asthenia	76 (20.3%)	28 (7.5%)	67 (18.6%)	14 (3.9%)
Pyrexia	31 (8.3%)	3 (0.8%)	125 (34.7%)	1 (0.3%)
Chills	28 (7.5%)	2 (0.5%)	105 (29.2%)	0 (0%)
Investigations				
Ejection fraction decreased	51 (13.6%)	10 (2.7%)	11 (3.1%)	3 (0.8%)
Weight decreased	46 (12.3%)	1 (0.3%)	50 (13.9%)	1 (0.3%)

[a] The following terms have been combined: abdominal pain and abdominal pain upper.
[b] The following terms have been combined: rash, rash erythematous, exfoliative rash, rash follicular, rash macular, rash papular, rash pruritic, rash maculo-papular, rash psoriaform, and rash generalised.

In the treatment-naïve MRCC study, 75 (20%) versus 37 (10%) patients experienced treatment-emergent Grade 4 chemistry laboratory abnormalities on SUTENT versus IFN-α, respectively. The most common Grade 4 chemistry abnormalities were hyperuricemia (14% on SUTENT, 8% on IFN-α) and increased lipase (3% on SUTENT, 1% on IFN-α). The most common Grade 3 chemistry abnormalities observed on both arms were increased lipase (15% on SUTENT, 7% on IFN α) and hypophosphatemia (6% on SUTENT, 6% on IFN-α). Other common Grade 3 laboratory abnormalities on SUTENT were hyponatremia (8%) and increased amylase (5%), and on IFN-α was hyperglycemia (6%). Hematologic laboratory abnormalities in the treatment-naïve MRCC patient population are presented in Table 4.

Grade 4 hematology laboratory abnormalities in the Phase 3 MRCC study include neutropenia (2% on SUTENT, 1% on IFN-α) and anemia (2% on SUTENT, <1% on IFN-α). Grade 3 hematology laboratory abnormalities included neutropenia (15% on SUTENT, 8% on IFN-α), lymphopenia (16% on SUTENT, 24% on IFN-α), thrombocytopenia (8% on SUTENT, 1% on IFN-α), leukopenia (8% on SUTENT, 2% on IFN-α) and anemia (6% on SUTENT, 5% on IFN-α).

Table 4: SUTENT

Treatment-Emergent Laboratory Abnormalities Reported in at Least 10% of Treatment-Naïve MRCC Patients Who Received SUTENT or IFN-α

Laboratory Parameter, n (%)	Treatment-Naïve RCC			
	SUTENT (n=375)		IFN-a (n=360)	
	All Grades[a]	Grade 3/4[a,b]	All Grades[a,b]	Grade 3/4[a,c]
Gastrointestinal				
AST	211 (56)	6 (2)	136 (38)	8 (2)
ALT	192 (51)	10 (3)	144 (40)	9 (2)
Lipase	211 (56)	69 (18)	165 (46)	29 (8)
Alkaline phosphatase	171 (46)	7 (2)	132 (37)	6 (2)
Amylase	130 (35)	22 (6)	114 (32)	12 (3)
Total bilirubin	75 (20)	3 (1)	8 (2)	0 (0)
Indirect bilirubin	49 (13)	4 (1)	3 (1)	0 (0)
Renal/Metabolic				
Creatinine	262 (70)	2 (<1)	183 (51)	1 (<1)
Creatine kinase	183 (49)	9 (2)	40 (11)	4 (1)
Uric acid	173 (46)	54 (14)	119 (33)	29 (8)
Calcium decreased	156 (42)	4 (1)	145 (40)	4 (1)
Phosphorus	116 (31)	22 (6)	87 (24)	23 (6)
Albumin	106 (28)	4 (1)	72 (20)	0 (0)
Glucose increased	86 (23)	21 (6)	55 (15)	22 (6)
Sodium decreased	75 (20)	31 (8)	55 (15)	13 (4)
Glucose decreased	65 (17)	0 (0)	43 (12)	1 (<1)
Potassium increased	61 (16)	13 (3)	61 (17)	15 (4)
Calcium increased	50 (13)	2 (<1)	35 (10)	5 (1)
Potassium decreased	49 (13)	3 (1)	7 (2)	1 (<1)
Sodium increased	48 (13)	0 (0)	38 (10)	0 (0)
Hematology				
Neutrophils	289 (77)	65 (17)	178 (49)	31 (9)
Hemoglobin	298 (79)	29 (8)	250 (69)	18 (5)
Platelets	255 (68)	35 (9)	85 (24)	2 (1)
Lymphocytes	256 (68)	66 (18)	245 (68)	93 (26)
Leukocytes	293 (78)	29 (8)	202 (56)	8 (2)

[a] Common Terminology Criteria for Adverse Events (CTCAE), Version 3.0.
[b] Grade 4 laboratory abnormalities in patients on SUTENT included uric acid (14%), lipase (3%), neutrophils (2%), lymphocytes (2%), hemoglobin (2%), platelets (1%), amylase (1%), ALT (<1%), creatine kinase (<1%), creatinine (<1%), glucose increased (<1%), calcium decreased (<1%), phosphorous (<1%), potassium increased (<1%), and sodium decreased (<1%).
[c] Grade 4 laboratory abnormalities in patients on IFN-a included uric acid (8%), lymphocytes (2%), lipase (1%), neutrophils (1%), amylase (<1%), calcium increased (<1%), glucose decreased (<1%), potassium increased (<1%) and hemoglobin (<1%).

Cytokine-Refractory MRCC: The data described below reflect exposure to SUTENT in 169 patients with cytokine-refractory MRCC enrolled in Studies 1 and 2. The median duration of treatment was 5.5 months (range: 23 days to 11.2 months) for Study 1 and 7.9 months (range: 6 days to 1.3 years) for Study 2. Dose interruptions occurred in 48 patients (45%) on Study 1 and 45 patients (71%) on Study 2; one or more dose reductions occurred in 23 patients (22%) on Study 1 and 22 patients (35%) on Study 2. Permanent discontinuation from the study due to treatment-related adverse events occurred in 7 patients (8%) on Study 1 and 6 patients (10%) on Study 2. Treatment-related adverse events are presented by maximum severity grade for at least 10% of the MRCC patient population in Table 5. Treatment-related adverse events were experienced by nearly all of the patients with MRCC. Fatigue; gastrointestinal disorders, such as nausea, diarrhea, stomatitis, dyspepsia, vomiting and constipation; dysgeusia; skin discoloration; anorexia and rash were the most common treatment-related adverse events (experienced by at least 20% of the patients). The relative frequency of the most common all-causality adverse events was similar to that of these treatment-related adverse events.

Table 5: SUTENT

Treatment-Related Adverse Events Reported in at Least 10% of Patients Treated with SUTENT in the Two Cytokine-Refractory MRCC Studies

Adverse Event	All Grades n (%)	Grade 3/4 n (%)
Any Treatment-Related AE Experienced by ≥10% Patients	**166 (98.2)**	**91 (53.9)**
Blood and Lymphatic System Disorders	**57 (33.7)**	**30 (15.8)**
Anemia	21 (12.4)	6 (3.6)
Leukopenia	24 (14.2)	10 (5.9)
Neutropenia	24 (14.2)	14 (8.3)
Thrombocytopenia	23 (13.6)	11 (6.5)
Eye Disorders	**17 (10.1)**	**0 (0.0)**
Gastrointestinal Disorders	**156 (92.3)**	**15 (8.9)**
Constipation	34 (20.1)	0 (0.0)
Diarrhoea	83 (49.1)	5 (3.0)
Dyspepsia	69 (40.8)	1 (0.6)
Glossodynia	25 (14.8)	0 (0.0)
Nausea	84 (49.7)	2 (1.2)
Stomatitis	70 (41.4)	6 (3.6)

(cont'd)

Table 5: SUTENT *(cont'd)*

Treatment-Related Adverse Events Reported in at Least 10% of Patients Treated with SUTENT in the Two Cytokine-Refractory MRCC Studies

Adverse Event	All Grades n (%)	Grade 3/4 n (%)
Vomiting	52 (30.8)	2 (1.2)
General Disorders and Administration Site Conditions	**118 (69.8)**	**19 (11.2)**
Fatigue	102 (60.4)	18 (10.7)
Mucosal inflammation	30 (17.8)	1 (0.6)
Infections and infestations	21 (12.4)	4 (2.4)
Investigations[a]	**65 (38.5)**	**31 (20.1)**
Ejection fraction decreased	24 (14.2)	4 (2.4)
Lipase increased	17 (10.1)	15 (8.9)
Metabolism and Nutrition Disorders	**68 (40.2)**	**9 (5.3)**
Anorexia	47 (27.8)	1 (0.6)
Musculoskeletal and Connective Tissue Disorders	**45 (26.6)**	**3 (1.8)**
Pain in extremity	21 (12.4)	1 (0.6)
Nervous System Disorders	**101 (59.8)**	**6 (3.6)**
Dysgeusia	71 (42.0)	0 (0.0)
Headache	25 (14.8)	1 (0.6)
Psychiatric Disorders	**17 (10.1)**	**2 (1.2)**
Respiratory, Thoracic and Mediastinal Disorders	**40 (23.7)**	**3 (1.8)**
Skin and Subcutaneous Tissue Disorders	**122 (72.2)**	**12 (7.1)**
Dry skin	22 (13.0)	0 (0.0)
Erythema	20 (11.8)	0 (0.0)
Hair color changes	24 (14.2)	0 (0.0)
Palmar-plantar erythrodysesthesia syndrome	21 (12.4)	6 (3.6)
Rash	44 (26.0)	1 (0.6)
Skin discoloration	54 (32.0)	0 (0.0)
Vascular Disorders	**40 (23.7)**	**11 (6.5)**
Hypertension	28 (16.6)	7 (4.1)

[a] 1 patient (0.6%) was missing.
Severity grading was consistent with Common Terminology Criteria for Adverse Events (CTCAE) Version 3.0.
Abbreviations: n=number of subjects, MRCC=metastatic renal cell carcinoma.

Treatment-emergent laboratory abnormalities are presented by maximum severity grade for at least 10% of the MRCC patient population in Table 6. Hematologic laboratory abnormalities in the MRCC patient population were comparable to that observed in the overall solid tumour patient population.

Table 6: SUTENT

Abnormal Post-Baseline Laboratory Tests Occurring in at Least 10% of Cytokine-Refractory MRCC Patients (As-Treated Population)

Laboratory Test	Total 50 mg QD, Schedule 4/2 (N=169)	
	Grade 1-4 n (%)	Grade 3/4 n (%)
Any		105 (62.1%)
Gastrointestinal		
Albumin (Hypoalbuminemia)	47 (27.8)	0 (0.0)
Alkaline Phosphatase	93 (55.0)	3 (1.8)
Amylase	47 (27.8)	8 (4.7)
AST/ALT	97 (57.4)	6 (3.6)
Lipase	84 (49.7)	28 (16.6)
Total Bilirubin	20 (11.8)	1 (0.6)
Renal/Metabolic		
Calcium (Hypercalcemia)	19 (11.2)	1 (0.6)
Calcium (Hypocalcemia)	72 (42.6)	1 (0.6)
Creatine Kinase	65 (38.5)	2 (1.2)
Creatinine	100 (59.2)	2 (1.2)
Glucose (Hyperglycemia)	30 (17.8)	6 (3.6)
Glucose (Hypoglycemia)	34 (20.1)	0 (0.0)
Hypophosphatemia	37 (21.9)	15 (8.9)
Potassium (Hyperkalemia)	23 (13.6)	7 (4.1)
Sodium (Hypernatremia)	22 (13.0)	1 (0.6)
Sodium (Hyponatremia)	17 (10.1)	6 (3.6)
Uric Acid	83 (49.1)	25 (14.8)
Hematology		
Anemia	125 (74.0)	12 (7.1)
Neutropenia	116 (68.6)	22 (13.0)
Lymphopenia	99 (58.6)	33 (19.5)
Thrombocytopenia	99 (58.6)	5 (3.0)

Grading is based on Common Terminology Criteria for Adverse Events (CTCAE) Version 3.0 criteria; the grading criteria are not available for all lab tests performed on study; if applicable, a subject was summarized only once for each test under the maximum post-baseline grade.
Legend: n=number of subjects, MRCC=metastatic renal cell carcinoma.

Other Adverse Reactions: Musculoskeletal: Rhabdomyolysis has been reported in some cases from non-pivotal clinical trials (see Warnings and Precautions and Post-Marketing Experience).
Cardiovascular: See Warnings and Precautions.
Pulmonary Embolism: See Warnings and Precautions.
Pancreatic Function: See Warnings and Precautions.
Seizures: See Warnings and Precautions.
Post-Marketing Experience: The following adverse reactions have been identified during postapproval use of SUTENT. Because these reactions are reported voluntarily from a population of uncertain size, it is not always possible to reliably estimate their frequency or establish a causal relationship to drug exposure.
Blood and Lymphatic System Disorders: Rare cases of thrombotic microangiopathy have been reported. Temporary suspension of sunitinib is recommended; following resolution, treatment may be resumed at the discretion of the treating physician.
Cardiovascular: Left ventricular failure, cardiac failure, cardiovascular ischemia-related events and rhythm disorder events have been reported in patients with pre-existing disease and/or cardiovascular risk factors, but a causal association with sunitinib could not be ruled out.

Rare cases of cardiomyopathy, in some cases with fatal outcome attributed to SUTENT, have been reported.
Endocrine Disorders: Rare cases of hyperthyroidism, some followed by hypothyroidism, have been reported in clinical trials and through post-marketing experience (see Warnings and Precautions, Thyroid Dysfunction).
Hemorrhage: Epistaxis is one of the most common hemorrhagic adverse events reported with sunitinib (see Warnings and Precautions, Hemorrhage). Although most cases are mild and self-limited, serious cases have been reported through post-marketing experience.

Hemorrhagic events reported through post-marketing experience, some of which were fatal, have included GI, respiratory, tumor, urinary tract and brain hemorrhages. In addition, cases of fatal hemorrhage associated with thrombocytopenia have been reported.
Immune System Disorders: Hypersensitivity reactions, including angioedema, have been reported.
Infections and Infestations: Cases of serious infection (with or without neutropenia), in some cases with fatal outcome, have been reported.
Musculoskeletal and Connective Tissue Disorders: Rare cases of myopathy and/or rhabdomyolysis, some with acute renal failure, have been reported. Most of these patients had pre-existing risk factors and/or were receiving concomitant medications known to be associated with these adverse reactions. Patients with signs or symptoms of muscle toxicity should be managed as per standard medical practice. (See Warnings and Precautions.)
Nervous System Disorders: Taste disturbance, including ageusia, has been reported.
Renal and Urinary Disorders: Cases of renal impairment and/or failure, in some cases with fatal outcome, have been reported.

Cases of proteinuria and rare cases of nephrotic syndrome have been reported. Baseline urinalysis is recommended, and patients should be monitored for the development or worsening of proteinuria. The safety of continued sunitinib treatment in patients with moderate to severe proteinuria has not been systematically evaluated. Discontinue sunitinib in patients with nephrotic syndrome.
Respiratory Disorders: Rare cases of pulmonary embolism, in some cases with fatal outcome attributed to SUTENT, have been reported.
Other: Fistula formation: Cases of fistula formation, sometimes associated with tumour necrosis and/or regression, in some cases with fatal outcome, have been reported.
DRUG INTERACTIONS: Overview: Sunitinib is metabolized primarily by CYP3A4. Potential interactions may occur with drugs/foods/herbs that are inhibitors or inducers of this enzyme system.
Drug-Drug Interactions: CYP3A4 Inhibitors: Co-administration of SUTENT (sunitinib malate) with inhibitors of the CYP3A4 family may increase SUTENT concentrations (see Action and Clinical Pharmacology). Concomitant administration of SUTENT with CYP3A4 inhibitors should be avoided. These include, but are not limited to: non-dihydropyridine calcium channel blockers (e.g. diltiazem, verapamil); antifungals (e.g. ketoconazole, fluconazole, itraconazole, voriconazole); macrolide antibiotics (e.g. erythromycin, clarithromycin, telithromycin); fluoroquinolone antibiotics (e.g. ciprofloxacin, norfloxacin); and some HIV antivirals (e.g. ritonavir, indinavir).
CYP3A4 Inducers: Co-administration of SUTENT with inducers of the CYP3A4 family may decrease SUTENT concentrations (see Action and Clinical Pharmacology). Concomitant administration of SUTENT with CYP3A4 inducers should be avoided. CYP3A4 inducers include, but are not limited to: barbiturates (e.g. phenobarbital); anticonvulsants (e.g. carbamazepine, phenytoin); rifampin; glucocorticoids; pioglitazone; and some HIV antivirals (e.g. efavirenz, nevirapine).
Drugs Which Prolong the QT/QTc Interval: The concomitant use of SUTENT with another QT/QTc-prolonging drug is discouraged. However, if it is necessary, particular care should be used. Drugs that have been associated with QT/QTc interval prolongation and/or torsade de pointes include, but are not limited to, the examples in the following list. Chemical/pharmacological classes are listed if some, although not necessarily all, class members have been implicated in QT/QTc prolongation and/or torsade de pointes:

- Antiarrhythmics (Class IA, e.g., quinidine, procainamide, disopyramide; Class III, e.g. amiodarone, sotalol, ibutilide; Class IC, e.g. flecainide, propafenone)

- Antipsychotics (e.g. thioridazine, chlorpromazine, pimozide, haloperidol, droperidol)
- Antidepressants (e.g. amitriptyline, imipramine, maprotiline, fluoxetine, venlafaxine)
- Opioids (e.g. methadone)
- Macrolide antibiotics (e.g. erythromycin, clarithromycin, telithromycin)
- Quinolone antibiotics (e.g. moxifloxacin, gatifloxacin, ciprofloxacin)
- Antimalarials (e.g. quinine)
- Pentamidine
- Azole antifungals (e.g. ketoconazole, fluconazole, voriconazole)
- Gastrointestinal drugs (e.g. domperidone, 5HT3 antagonists, such as granisetron, ondansetron, dolasetron)
- Beta 2-adrenoreceptor agonists (e.g. salmeterol, formoterol)
- Tacrolimus

Drugs Which Prolong the PR Interval: Caution should be used if SUTENT is prescribed to patients in combination with other drugs that also cause PR interval prolongation, such as beta blockers, calcium channel blockers, digitalis, or HIV protease inhibitors (see Warnings and Precautions, Cardiovascular, QT Interval Prolongation).

The above list of potentially interacting drugs is not comprehensive. Current scientific literature should be consulted for more information.

Drug-Food Interactions: Grapefruit juice has CYP3A4 inhibitory activity. Therefore, ingestion of grapefruit juice while on SUTENT therapy may lead to decreased SUTENT metabolism and increased SUTENT plasma concentrations (see Drug-Drug Interactions). Concomitant administration of SUTENT with grapefruit juice should be avoided.

Drug-Herb Interactions: St. John's Wort is a potent CYP3A4 inducer. Co-administration with SUTENT may lead to increased SUTENT metabolism and decreased SUTENT plasma concentrations (see Drug-Drug Interactions). Patients receiving SUTENT should not take St. John's Wort concomitantly.

DOSAGE AND ADMINISTRATION: The recommended dose of SUTENT (sunitinib malate) is one 50 mg oral dose taken once daily, on a schedule of 4 weeks on treatment followed by 2 weeks off. SUTENT may be taken with or without food.

Recommended Dose and Dosage Adjustment: Daily doses should not exceed 50 mg nor be decreased below 25 mg. Dose modification of 12.5 mg is recommended based on individual safety and tolerability.

CYP3A4 Inhibitors: Concurrent administration of sunitinib malate with the CYP3A4 inhibitor, ketoconazole, resulted in 49% and 51% increases in combined (sunitinib + active metabolite) C_{max} and $AUC_{0-\infty}$ values, respectively, after a single dose of sunitinib malate in healthy volunteers. Doses of SUTENT may need to be reduced to a minimum of 25 mg daily, and clinical response and tolerability should be carefully monitored, in patients receiving a potent CYP3A4 inhibitor such as ketoconazole (see Drug Interactions and Action and Clinical Pharmacology). Selection of an alternate concomitant medication with no or minimal enzyme inhibition potential should be considered. **Note:** This recommendation is based on pharmacokinetic data from healthy volunteers. In clinical trials conducted to date, the safety and efficacy of SUTENT with concomitant use of CYP3A4 inhibitors has not been established. In the 2 cytokine-refractory MRCC studies, 14 of the 169 patients used a potent CYP 3A4 inhibitor concomitantly with SUTENT with no modification of the starting dose of SUTENT.

CYP3A4 Inducers: Concurrent administration of sunitinib malate with the potent CYP3A4 inducer, rifampin, resulted in a more than 23% and 46% reduction in combined (sunitinib + active metabolite) C_{max} and $AUC_{0-\infty}$ values, respectively, after a single dose of SUTENT in healthy volunteers. The dose of SUTENT may need to be increased (maximum 50 mg), and clinical response and tolerability should be carefully monitored, in patients receiving SUTENT with a potent CYP3A4 inducer, such as rifampin (see Drug Interactions and Action and Clinical Pharmacology). Selection of an alternate concomitant medication with no or minimal enzyme induction potential should be considered. **Note:** This recommendation is based on pharmacokinetic data from healthy volunteers. In clinical trials conducted to date, the safety and efficacy of SUTENT with concomitant use of CYP3A4 inducers has not been established. In the two cytokine-refractory MRCC studies, 33 of the 169 patients received a potent CYP3A4 inducer concomitantly with SUTENT with no modification of the starting dose of SUTENT.

Special Populations: No dose adjustment is required on the basis of patient age, body weight, creatine clearance, race, gender or ECOG score. (See Action And Clinical Pharmacology, Special Populations and Conditions.)

OVERDOSAGE:

Treatment of overdose with SUTENT should consist of general supportive measures. There is no specific antidote for overdosage with SUTENT. If indicated, elimination of unabsorbed drug should be achieved by emesis or gastric lavage. A few cases of accidental overdose have been reported; these cases were associated with adverse reactions consistent with the known safety profile of SUTENT, or without adverse reactions. A case of intentional overdose involving the ingestion of 1500 mg of SUTENT in an attempted suicide was reported without adverse reaction.

> For management of a suspected drug overdose, contact your regional Poison Control Centre. See the *CPS Directory* section for a list of Poison Control Centres.

ACTION AND CLINICAL PHARMACOLOGY: SUTENT (sunitinib malate) is a small molecule that inhibits multiple receptor tyrosine kinases (RTKs), some of which are implicated in tumour growth, pathologic angiogenesis, and metastatic progression of cancer. Sunitinib was evaluated for its inhibitory activity against a variety of kinases (>80 kinases) and was identified as a potent inhibitor of platelet-derived growth factor receptors (PDGFRα and PDGFRβ), vascular endothelial growth factor receptors (VEGFR1, VEGFR2 and VEGFR3), stem cell factor receptor (KIT), Fms-like tyrosine kinase-3 (FLT3), colony stimulating factor receptor (CSF-1R), and the glial cell-line derived neurotrophic factor receptor (RET). Inhibition of the activity of these RTKs by sunitinib has been demonstrated in biochemical and/or cellular assays, and inhibition of function has been demonstrated in cell proliferation or viability assays. The primary metabolite exhibits similar potency compared to sunitinib in biochemical and cellular assays.

Sunitinib inhibited the phosphorylation of multiple RTKs (PDGFRβ, VEGFR2, KIT) in tumour xenografts expressing RTK targets in vivo and demonstrated inhibition of tumour growth or tumour regression and/or inhibited metastases in some experimental models of cancer. Sunitinib demonstrated the ability to inhibit growth of tumour cells expressing dysregulated target RTKs (PDGFR, RET, or KIT) in vitro and to inhibit PDGFRβ- and VEGFR2-dependent tumour angiogenesis in vivo.

Pharmacodynamics: QT/QTc Interval Prolongation: In a phase I clinical QT study, patients with advanced solid tumours received SUTENT 150 mg on Days 3 and 9, and SUTENT 50 mg daily Days 4 to 8 (positive control given Day 1 and placebo given Day 2). Manual serial ECG readings were conducted in accordance with current guidelines. At approximately twice therapeutic concentrations, **SUTENT was associated with QTc prolongation. On both Day 3 and Day 9, SUTENT was associated with a progressive increase in the QTc interval that continued throughout the 24-hour observation period, without reaching any obvious peak, plateau, or offset.** Because of this, the peak effect could not be characterized with confidence. At the last observation (24 h), the maximum mean placebo-adjusted increase from baseline was 9.6 (90% CI 4.1, 15.1) msec for Day 3 and 15.4 (90% CI 8.4, 22.4) msec for Day 9 using a time-matched baseline and Fridericia's heart rate correction. The magnitude of these increases is considered to justify cause for concern. However, no subjects experienced an effect on the QTc interval greater than grade 2 (CTCAE version 3.0). No patient presented with a cardiac arrhythmia (see Warnings and Precautions).

T wave Morphology: At baseline, the incidence of patients with T wave abnormalities and the proportion of ECGs with abnormal T waves was high in this population of cancer patients. After 7 days of SUTENT therapy, however, these incidences had increased.

QTc prolongation in association with changes in T wave morphology has been suggested to merit intensified concern with respect to proarrhythmic potential.

PR Interval and Heart Rate: Mean placebo-adjusted changes in the PR interval were positive at all time points, with the maximum increase occurring 7 to 12 hours post-dosing, followed by a decline at 24 hours. Outlier analyses for the PR interval (>200 msec) were consistent with a shift toward a higher proportion of outliers in patients treated with SUTENT. Excessive PR interval prolongation can result in AV block. Progressive levels of AV block are associated with increasing morbidity and mortality.

On Days 3 and 9, heart rate decreased progressively over the 24 hours period following SUTENT dosing, but was not affected by the positive control. During the study, an event of bradycardia occurred that was considered treatment-related, and dizziness was experienced by 7 of 48 patients.

Bradycardia and AV block are recognized risk factors for torsade de pointes. For this reason, a drug that causes QTc prolongation in association with prolongation of the PR and RR intervals raises particular concerns with respect to proarrhythmic potential.

Pharmacokinetics: The pharmacokinetics of sunitinib and its primary active metabolite have been evaluated in 135 healthy volunteers and in 266 patients with solid tumours.

Absorption and Distribution: Maximum plasma concentrations (C_{max}) of sunitinib are generally observed from 6 to 12 hours (T_{max}) post-dose. Food has no effect on the bioavailability of sunitinib. Following administration of a single oral dose in healthy volunteers, the terminal half-lives of sunitinib and its primary active metabolite are approximately 40 to 60 hours and 80 to 110 hours, respectively. After repeated daily administration, in the dosing ranges of 25 to 100 mg, the area under the plasma concentration-time curve (AUC) and C_{max} for sunitinib and total drug increases proportionally with dose. With repeated daily administration, sunitinib accumulates 3- to 4-fold while the primary metabolite accumulates 7- to 10-fold. Steady-state concentrations of sunitinib and its primary active metabolite, are achieved within 10 to 14 days. By Day 14, combined trough plasma concentrations of sunitinib and its active metabolite are 62.9-101 ng/mL. No significant changes in the pharmacokinetics of sunitinib or the primary active metabolite are observed with repeated daily administration or with repeated cycles in the dosing regimens tested. The apparent volume of distribution (Vd/F) for sunitinib was 2230 L.

The pharmacokinetics were similar in healthy volunteers and in the solid tumour patient populations tested, including patients with GIST or MRCC.

Binding of sunitinib and its primary active metabolite to human plasma protein in vitro was 95% and 90%, respectively, with no apparent concentration dependence.

Metabolism and Excretion: Sunitinib is metabolized primarily by the cytochrome P450 enzyme, CYP3A4, to produce its primary active metabolite, which is further metabolized by CYP3A4. The primary active metabolite comprises 23 to 37% of the total exposure. Elimination is primarily via feces. In a human mass balance study of [^{14}C] sunitinib, 61% of the radioactive dose was eliminated in feces, with renal elimination of drug and metabolites accounting for 16% of the administered radioactive dose. Sunitinib and its primary active metabolite are the major drug-related compounds identified in plasma, urine and feces, representing 91.5%, 86.4% and 73.8% of radioactivity in pooled samples, respectively. Minor metabolites were identified in urine and feces, but were generally not found in plasma. Total oral clearance (CL/F) was 34-62 L/hr with an inter-patient variability of 40%.

Special Populations and Conditions: Population pharmacokinetic analyses of demographic data suggest that there are no clinically relevant effects of age, body weight, creatinine clearance, race, gender or ECOG score on the pharmacokinetics of sunitinib or the active metabolite.

There are no pharmacokinetic data available in pediatric patients.

Hepatic Insufficiency: A single 50 mg dose of SUTENT was administered to patients with mild (Child-Pugh Class A) and moderate (Child-Pugh Class B) hepatic impairment, and to control group of patients with normal hepatic function. The pharmacokinetic parameters evaluated demonstrated that dose adjustments might not be necessary for patients with mild (Child-Pugh Class A) or moderate (Child-Pugh Class B) hepatic impairment. However, SUTENT was not studied in subjects with severe (Child-Pugh Class C) hepatic impairment. In addition, repeated administration of SUTENT was not studied in subjects with hepatic impairment.

Renal Insufficiency: No clinical studies were conducted in patients with impaired renal function. Studies that were conducted excluded patients with serum creatinine >2.0×ULN. No relationship was observed between renal function (as measured by calculated creatinine clearance, range 42-347 mL/min) and sunitinib pharmacokinetics in a population pharmacokinetic analysis.

Drug-Drug Interactions: In vitro studies indicate that sunitinib does not induce or inhibit major CYP enzymes.

In vitro Studies of CYP Inhibition and Induction: The in vitro studies in human liver microsomes and hepatocytes of the activity of CYP isoforms CYP1A2, CYP2A6, CYP2B6, CYP2C8, CYP2C9, CYP2C19, CYP2D6, CYP2E1, CYP3A4/5, and CYP4A9/11 indicated that sunitinib and its primary active metabolite are unlikely to have any clinically relevant drug-drug interactions with drugs that may be metabolized by these enzymes.

CYP3A4 Inhibitors: Concurrent administration of SUTENT with the potent CYP3A4 inhibitor, ketoconazole, resulted in a 49% and 51% increase in the combined (sunitinib + active metabolite) C_{max} and $AUC_{0-\infty}$ values, respectively, after a single dose of SUTENT in healthy volunteers.

Administration of SUTENT with potent inhibitors of the CYP3A4 family may increase SUTENT concentrations. Concomitant administration of SUTENT with inhibitors should be avoided or the selection of an alternate concomitant medication with no, or minimal potential to inhibit CYP3A4 should be considered. If this is not possible, the dose of SUTENT may need to be reduced (see Dosage and Administration). **Note:** In clinical trials conducted to date, the safety and efficacy of SUTENT with concomitant use of CYP3A4 inhibitors has not been established.

CYP3A4 Inducers: Concurrent administration of SUTENT with the potent CYP3A4 inducer, rifampin, resulted in a 23% and 46% reduction in the combined (sunitinib + active metabolite) C_{max} and $AUC_{0-\infty}$ values, respectively, after a single dose of SUTENT in healthy volunteers.

Administration of SUTENT with potent inducers of CYP3A4 may decrease SUTENT concentrations. Concomitant administration of SUTENT should be avoided or selection of an alternate concomitant medication with no or minimal potential to induce CYP3A4 should be considered. If this is not possible, the dose of SUTENT may need to be increased (see Dosage and Administration). **Note:** In clinical trials conducted to date, the safety and efficacy of SUTENT with concomitant use of CYP3A4 inducers have not been established.

STORAGE AND STABILITY: Store between 15-30°C.

SPECIAL HANDLING INSTRUCTIONS: Not applicable.

INFORMATION FOR THE PATIENT: Published in e-CPS, available by subscription at www.e-cps.ca.

DOSAGE FORMS, COMPOSITION AND PACKAGING: 12.5 mg: Each hard gelatin capsule with orange cap and orange body, printed with white ink "Pfizer" on the cap, "STN 12.5 mg" on the body, contains: sunitinib malate equivalent to sunitinib 12.5 mg. Nonmedicinal ingredients: croscarmellose sodium, magnesium stearate, mannitol and povidone (K-25); orange capsule shell: gelatin, red iron oxide and titanium dioxide; imprinting ink: povidone, propylene glycol, shellac, sodium hydroxide and titanium dioxide. Bottles of 28.

25 mg: Each hard gelatin capsule with caramel cap and orange body, printed with white ink "Pfizer" on the cap, "STN 25 mg" on the body, contains: sunitinib malate equivalent to sunitinib 25 mg. Nonmedicinal ingredients: croscarmellose sodium, magnesium stearate, mannitol and povidone (K-25); orange capsule shell: gelatin, red iron oxide and titanium dioxide; caramel capsule shell also contain: black iron oxide and yellow iron oxide; imprinting ink: povidone, propylene glycol, shellac, sodium hydroxide and titanium dioxide. Bottles of 28.

50 mg: Each hard gelatin capsule with caramel cap and caramel body, printed with white ink "Pfizer" on the cap, "STN 50 mg" on the body, contains: sunitinib malate equivalent to sunitinib 50 mg. Nonmedicinal ingredients: croscarmellose sodium, magnesium stearate, mannitol and povidone (K-25); orange capsule shell: gelatin, red iron oxide and titanium dioxide; caramel capsule shell also contain: black iron oxide and yellow iron oxide; imprinting ink: povidone, propylene glycol, shellac, sodium hydroxide and titanium dioxide. Bottles of 28.

(Shown in Product Identification Section)

Symbicort® Turbuhaler® ℞

budesonide—formoterol fumarate dihydrate

Corticosteroid—Bronchodilator for Inhalation

AstraZeneca

Date of Preparation: February 5, 2002
Date of Revision: July 20, 2009

SUMMARY PRODUCT INFORMATION:

Route of Administration	Dosage Form/Strength	All Nonmedicinal Ingredients
Oral inhalation	Turbuhaler/ 100 µg budesonide/6 µg formoterol fumarate dihydrate 200 µg budesonide/6 µg formoterol fumarate dihydrate	Lactose

INDICATIONS AND CLINICAL USE: Asthma: SYMBICORT (budesonide and formoterol fumarate dihydrate) is indicated for regular treatment of asthma in patients 12 years and older with reversible obstructive airways disease, where the use of a combination product is appropriate. This may include:

- Patients on effective maintenance doses of long-acting beta$_2$-agonists and inhaled corticosteroids.
- Patients who are symptomatic on current inhaled corticosteroid therapy.

When treating asthma patients, SYMBICORT should be used only in patients whose conditions are not adequately controlled using low-to-medium dose inhaled corticosteroids or whose disease severity clearly warrants the initiation of treatment with two maintenance therapies (see Warnings and Precautions).

SYMBICORT should not be used in patients whose asthma can be managed by occasional use of short-acting, inhaled beta$_2$-agonists or for patients whose asthma can be successfully managed by inhaled corticosteroids along with occasional use of inhaled short-acting beta$_2$-agonists.

For SYMBICORT there are two treatment approaches:

A. **SYMBICORT Maintenance Therapy:** SYMBICORT is taken as regular maintenance treatment with a separate rapid-acting bronchodilator as rescue.

B. **SYMBICORT Maintenance and Reliever Therapy:** SYMBICORT is taken as regular maintenance treatment and as needed in response to symptoms.

See Dosage and Administration and Warnings and Precautions.

Chronic Obstructive Pulmonary Disease (COPD: SYMBICORT TURBUHALER is indicated for the maintenance treatment of moderate to severe COPD including chronic bronchitis and emphysema, in patients with persistent symptoms and a history of exacerbations, where the use of a combination product is considered appropriate.

SYMBICORT TURBUHALER is **not** indicated for the relief of acute bronchospasm in COPD patients.

See Dosage and Administration and Warnings and Precautions.

CONTRAINDICATIONS: SYMBICORT (budesonide/formoterol fumarate dihydrate) is contraindicated in patients with a known hypersensitivity to budesonide, formoterol or inhaled lactose.

WARNINGS AND PRECAUTIONS:

Warning for asthma patients:

- Data from a large placebo-controlled US study (Salmeterol Multi-center Asthma Research Trial) comparing the safety of the long-acting beta$_2$-adrenergic agonist salmeterol to that of a placebo added to the original asthma therapy showed an increase in asthma-related deaths in patients receiving salmeterol. Although the trial results were specific to salmeterol, one of the conclusions derived from this study is that long-acting beta$_2$-adrenergic agonists may increase the risk of asthma exacerbation and possibly asthma-related death. Post-hoc analysis of the trial data suggests that the risks may be lower in those patients who were using inhaled corticosteroids (ICS) at study entry. However, these post-hoc analysis results are not conclusive. The actual ICS dosage used by these patients was not assessed in the study.
- Available data for formoterol fumarate dihydrate do not suggest increased risk, however it can not be excluded that the findings with salmeterol may apply to all long-acting beta$_2$-adrenergic agonists including formoterol fumarate dihydrate, one of the active ingredients in SYMBICORT.
- SYMBICORT contains a combination of formoterol fumarate dihydrate and budesonide (an inhaled corticosteroid). Given that the actual ICS dosage used by patients in the salmeterol trial was not assessed, it is not known whether the potential risk associated with long-acting beta$_2$-adrenergic agonist would apply to SYMBICORT.
- When treating asthma patients, SYMBICORT should be used only in patients whose conditions are not adequately controlled using low-to-medium dose inhaled corticosteroids or whose disease severity clearly warrants the initiation of treatment with two maintenance therapies.

General: When beginning treatment with SYMBICORT (budesonide/formoterol fumarate dihydrate), patients who have been taking inhaled beta$_2$-agonist on a regular basis should be instructed to discontinue the regular use of these drugs.

It is crucial to inform patients with asthma to have medication for rescue use available at all times. Asthma patients should be clearly instructed to use medication for rescue (e.g., SYMBICORT, formoterol, terbutaline, or salbutamol) if they develop asthma symptoms while taking SYMBICORT.

The reliever inhalations of SYMBICORT should be taken in response to symptoms but is not intended for regular prophylactic use before exercise.

Do not exceed recommended dosage of SYMBICORT.

Use in Adolescents and Asthma Severity Reassessment: In adolescents the severity of asthma may vary with age and periodic reassessment should be considered to determine if continued therapy with SYMBICORT is still indicated.

Discontinuance: Treatment with inhaled corticosteroids should not be stopped abruptly, but tapered gradually under the supervision of a physician.

Cardiovascular: Cardiovascular Effects: Although clinically not significant, a small increase in QTc interval has been reported with therapeutic doses of formoterol. It is not known if this becomes clinically significant when concomitant medications causing similar effects are prescribed and/or in the presence of heart diseases, hypokalemia, or hypoxia.

No clinically significant effect on the cardiovascular system is usually seen after the administration of inhaled formoterol in recommended doses, but the cardiovascular and central nervous system effects seen with all sympathomimetic drugs (e.g., increased blood pressure, heart rate, excitement) can occur after use of formoterol. Formoterol, like all sympathomimetic amines, should be used with caution in patients with cardiovascular disorders, especially coronary insufficiency, cardiac arrhythmias, and hypertension; in patients with convulsive disorders or thyrotoxicosis; diabetes mellitus, and in patients who are unusually responsive to sympathomimetic amines.

With beta-adrenergic agonist bronchodilators, changes in systolic and/or diastolic blood pressure, pulse rate, and electrocardiograms have been noted. No clinically important differences have been observed with SYMBICORT within the recommended dosages.

Ear/Nose/Throat: Candidiasis: Therapeutic dosages of budesonide may cause the appearance of *C. albicans* (thrush) in the mouth and throat. The development of pharyngeal and laryngeal candidiasis is a cause for concern because the extent of its penetration into the respiratory tract is unknown. Symptomatic candidiasis can be treated with topical anti-fungal therapy while continuing to use SYMBICORT.

Endocrine and Metabolism: Metabolic Changes: In common with other beta-adrenergic agents, formoterol can induce reversible metabolic changes (hyperglycemia, hypokalemia).

Metabolic Effects: Due to reversible hyperglycemic effect of beta$_2$-agonists, additional blood glucose monitoring is recommended initially in diabetic patients.

Hypothyroidism: There is an enhanced effect of corticosteroids on patients with hypothyroidism.

Systemic Steroid Replacement by Inhaled Steroid: Particular care is needed in asthmatic patients who are transferred from systemically active corticosteroids to inhaled corticosteroids because deaths due to adrenal insufficiency have occurred during and after transfer. For the transfer of patients treated with oral corticosteroids, inhaled corticosteroids should first be added to the existing oral steroid therapy which is then gradually withdrawn.

Patients with adrenocortical suppression should be monitored regularly and the oral steroid reduced cautiously. Some depression of plasma cortisol may occur in a small number of patients on higher doses of inhaled budesonide (for example greater than 800 µg/day). However, in most but not all patients on inhaled budesonide therapy, adrenal function and adrenal reserve remain within normal range. Some patients transferred from other inhaled steroids or oral steroids remain at risk of impaired adrenal reserve for a considerable time after transferring to inhaled budesonide.

After withdrawal from long-term treatment with systemic corticosteroids, a number of months are required for recovery of hypothalamic-pituitary-adrenal (HPA) function. During this period of HPA suppression, patients may exhibit signs and symptoms of adrenal insufficiency when exposed to trauma, surgery or infections, particularly gastroenteritis. Although inhaled budesonide may provide control of asthmatic symptoms during these episodes, it does not provide the systemic steroid which is necessary for coping with these emergencies. The physician may consider supplying oral steroids for use in times of stress (e.g. asthma exacerbations, chest infections, surgery).

During periods of stress or a severe asthmatic attack, patients who have been withdrawn from systemic corticosteroids should be instructed to resume systemic steroids immediately and to contact their physician for further instruction. These patients should also be instructed to carry a warning card indicating that they may need supplementary systemic steroids during periods of stress or asthma exacerbation. To assess the risk of adrenal insufficiency in emergency situations, routine tests of adrenal cortical function, including measurement of early morning and evening cortisol levels, should be performed periodically in all patients. An early morning resting cortisol level may be accepted as normal only if it falls at or near the normal mean level.

Hepatic/Biliary/Pancreatic: Cirrhosis: There is an enhanced effect of corticosteroids on patients with cirrhosis. Reduced liver function may affect the elimination of corticosteroids. The intravenous pharmacokinetics of budesonide however, are similar in cirrhotic patients and in healthy subjects. The pharmacokinetics after oral ingestion of budesonide were affected by compromised liver function as evidenced by increased systemic availability. This is however, of little importance for budesonide, as after inhalation, the oral contribution to systemic availability is very small (see Dosage and Administration, Special Populations, Hepatic/Renal Impairment and Action and Clinical Pharmacology, Pharmacokinetics, Excretion).

Immune: Effect on Infection: Patients who are on drugs that suppress the immune system are more susceptible to infections than healthy individuals. Chickenpox and measles, for example, can have a more serious or even fatal course in susceptible children or adults on immunosuppressant corticosteroids. In such children or adults who have not had these diseases, particular care should be taken to avoid exposure. How the dose, route, and duration of corticosteroid administration affect the risk of developing a disseminated infection is not known. The contribution of the underlying disease and/or prior corticosteroid treatment to the risk is also not known. If exposed to chickenpox, prophylaxis with varicella zoster immune globulin (VZIG) may be indicated. If exposed to measles, prophylaxis with pooled intravenous immunoglobulin (IG) may be indicated. If chickenpox develops, treatment with antiviral agents may be considered.

Corticosteroids may mask some signs of infection and new infections may appear. A decreased resistance to localized infection has been observed during corticosteroid therapy.

Respiratory: Infection: Physicians should remain vigilant for the possible development of pneumonia in patients with COPD as the clinical features of pneumonia and exacerbations frequently overlap. Lower respiratory tract infections, including pneumonia, have been reported following the inhaled administration of corticosteroids.

The incidence of pneumonia and lung infections other than pneumonia have been assessed in two 12-month studies of 1834 patients with COPD. In these two studies, there was a slightly higher incidence of lung infections other than pneumonia (e.g., bronchitis, viral lower respiratory tract infections, etc.) in patients receiving SYMBICORT TURBUHALER 2×200/6 µg bid (13.0%) in comparison with those receiving formoterol 2×6 µg bid (11.4%), budesonide 2×200 µg bid (9.9%), or placebo (8.2%). Pneumonia occurred in 4.1% of patients treated with SYMBICORT TURBUHALER compared with 2.4% treated with formoterol, 3.1% treated with budesonide, and 2.8% treated with placebo (see Adverse Reactions).

Paradoxical Bronchospasm: As with other inhalation therapy, paradoxical bronchospasm may occur characterized by an immediate increase in wheezing after dosing. In this event, SYMBICORT should be discontinued immediately, the patient assessed, and if necessary, alternative therapy instituted.

Special Populations: Pregnant Women: In experimental animal studies, budesonide was found to cross the placental barrier. Like other glucocorticosteroids, budesonide is teratogenic to rodent species. High doses of budesonide administered subcutaneously produced fetal malformations, primarily skeletal defects, in rabbits, rats and mice. Results from world-wide post marketing experience indicate inhaled budesonide during pregnancy has no adverse effects on the health of the fetus/new born child. Review of published literature of orally inhaled budesonide, including results from a large case control study performed with cases identified from 3 Swedish health registers showed that there was no association between exposure to inhaled budesonide and overall congenital malformations. Results from a similar study performed with intranasal budesonide, using the same 3 Swedish health registers showed that the use of intranasal budesonide was associated with a subgroup "less severe cardiovascular defects"; however, there was no statistically significant association between the use of intranasal budesonide during pregnancy and overall congenital malformations, or overall frequency of cardiovascular defects in the offspring. The safety of formoterol during pregnancy has not yet been established. SYMBICORT should be used during pregnancy only if the potential benefit justifies the potential risk to the fetus.

Use in Labour and Delivery: There are no well-controlled human studies that have investigated effects of formoterol on preterm labour or labour at term. Because of the potential for beta-agonist interference with uterine contractility, use of SYMBICORT during labour should be restricted to those patients in whom the benefits clearly outweigh the risks.

Nursing Women: A clinical pharmacology study has shown that inhaled budesonide is excreted in breast milk. It is not known whether formoterol passes into human breast milk. In rats, small amounts of formoterol have been detected in maternal milk. Administration of SYMBICORT to women who are breast-feeding should only be considered if the expected benefit to the mother is greater than any possible risk to the child.

Pediatrics: SYMBICORT is not currently recommended in children younger than 12 years of age due to limited clinical data in this age group.

Geriatrics: There is no need to adjust the dose in elderly patients.

Monitoring and Laboratory Tests: Monitoring Control of Asthma or COPD: With asthma, a persistent increase in the use of medication for rescue (e.g. SYMBICORT, formoterol, terbutaline or salbutamol), indicates a deterioration of asthma control and the patient's condition should be re-evaluated (see Dosage and Administration).

Asthma or COPD may deteriorate acutely over a period of hours or chronically over several days or longer. If patients find the rescue medication less effective (e.g. increased or persistent use), or exceeds the highest recommended dose of SYMBICORT, medical attention must be sought as this could be indicative of disease deterioration.

Sudden and progressive deterioration in control of asthma or COPD (e.g. exacerbations) is potentially life threatening and the patient should undergo urgent medical assessment. It is recognized that exacerbations are the most frequent cause of medical visits, hospital admissions and mortality among patients with asthma or COPD. With asthma and COPD, consideration should be given to the need for increased therapy with corticosteroids, e.g. a course of oral corticosteroids. Antibiotic treatment should be considered if an infection is present. Treatment with SYMBICORT should not be initiated to treat a severe exacerbation.

As with any asthma or COPD therapy, before introducing SYMBICORT, adequate education on how to use the drug and what to do during periods of worsening disease should be provided to the patient.

ADVERSE REACTIONS: Adverse Drug Reaction Overview: Since SYMBICORT (budesonide/formoterol fumarate dihydrate) contains both budesonide and formoterol, the same type and intensity of undesirable effects as reported for these substances may occur. No increased incidence of adverse reactions has been seen following concurrent administration of the two compounds. The most common drug related adverse reactions are pharmacologically predictable side-effects of beta$_2$-agonist therapy, such as headaches, tremor, palpitations, and coughing. These tend to be mild and disappear within a few days of treatment.

Adverse reactions that have been associated with use of budesonide or formoterol, reported from either clinical trials for asthma or COPD, or SYMBICORT post-marketing use are noted in Table 1.

Table 1: SYMBICORT TURBUHALER

Adverse Reactions Associated with Use of Budesonide or Formoterol

Frequency	System Organ Class (SOC) Disorders	Reaction
Common 1% to 10% (>1/100, <1/10)	Cardiac Disorders	Palpitations
	Infections and Infestations	Candida infections in the oropharynx
	Nervous System Disorders	Headache, tremor
	Respiratory, Thoracic and Mediastinal Disorders	Mild irritation in the throat, coughing, hoarseness
Uncommon 0.1% to 1% (>1/1000, <1/100)	Cardiac Disorders	Tachycardia
	Gastrointestinal Disorders	Nausea
	Musculoskeletal and Connective Tissue Disorders	Muscle cramps
	Nervous System Disorders	Dizziness
	Psychiatric Disorders	Agitation, restlessness, nervousness, sleep disturbances
Rare 0.01 to 0.1% (>1/10 000, <1/1000)	Cardiac Disorders	Cardiac arrhythmias, e.g. atrial fibrillation, supraventricular tachycardia, extrasystoles
	Immune System Disorders	Immediate and delayed hypersensitivity reactions, e.g., dermatitis, exanthema, urticaria, pruritus, angioedema and anaphylactic reaction
	Respiratory, Thoracic and Mediastinal Disorders	Bronchospasm
	Skin and Subcutaneous Tissue Disorders	Skin bruising

(cont'd)

Table 1: SYMBICORT TURBUHALER *(cont'd)*

Adverse Reactions Associated with Use of Budesonide or Formoterol

Frequency	System Organ Class (SOC) Disorders	Reaction
Very Rare <0.01% (<1/10 000)	Cardiac Disorders	Angina pectoris
	Endocrine Disorders	Signs or symptoms of systemic glucocorticosteroid effects, e.g. hypofunction of the adrenal gland
	Metabolism and Nutrition Disorders	Hyperglycemia
	Psychiatric Disorders	Depression, behavioural disturbances

Clinical Trial Adverse Drug Reactions: Because clinical trials are conducted under very specific conditions the adverse reaction rates observed in the clinical trials may not reflect the rates observed in practice and should not be compared to the rates in the clinical trials of another drug. Adverse drug reaction information from clinical trials is useful for identifying drug related adverse events and for approximating rates.

COPD: Clinical trial adverse event data is provided from two 12-month, randomised, double-blind, placebo-control multicentre trials comparing SYMBICORT (2×200/6 µg) bid with placebo, budesonide 2×200 µg bid, and formoterol 2×6 µg bid. A total of 1834 COPD patients were enrolled in these studies. The most frequently reported adverse events are presented in Table 2. These adverse reactions were mostly mild to moderate in severity.

Table 2 includes all events (whether considered drug-related or non-drug related by the investigator) that occurred at a rate of 3% or greater in the SYMBICORT treatment group, and were more common than in the placebo group.

Table 2: SYMBICORT TURBUHALER

Overall Adverse Experiences with ≥3% and More Common Than Placebo in the SYMBICORT Group in Controlled Clinical Trials (0629 and 0670) with SYMBICORT in Patients with COPD

Adverse Event System Organ Class Preferred Term	Symbicort (n=462) %	Budesonide (n=455) %	Formoterol (n=456) %	Placebo (n=461) %
% of patients reporting at least one adverse event	63	64	67	61
Infections and Infestations				
Nasopharyngitis	9	7	7	6
Pneumonia	4	3	2	3
General Disorders and Administration Site Conditions				
Chest pain	3	2	2	2
Nervous System Disorders				
Headache	3	2	3	2
Musculoskeletal and Connective Tissue Disorders				
Muscle spasms	3	2	2	1

COPD Clinical Trial Adverse Drug Reactions (1-3%): Gastrointestinal Disorders: diarrhea, dyspepsia, constipation, abdominal pain, abdominal pain upper, vomiting.

General Disorders and Administration Site Conditions: pyrexia.

Infections and Infestations: influenza, respiratory tract infection, upper respiratory tract infection, rhinitis, pharyngitis, cystitis, oral candidiasis.

Musculoskeletal and Connective Tissue Disorders: myalgia, arthralgia, pain in extremity.

Nervous System Disorders: tremor.

Psychiatric Disorders: insomnia, anxiety.

Respiratory, Thoracic and Mediastinal Disorders: dysphonia, oropharyngeal pain, nasal congestion.

All cause mortality was assessed in COPD trials 0629 and 0670. Of the 1834 patients in the pooled data, there were 56 (3.1%) deaths: 20 (4.4%) in the formoterol group, 14 (3.0%) in the placebo group, 11 (2.4%) in the budesonide group, and 11 (2.4%) in the SYMBICORT group. The most common cause of death overall was COPD (formoterol=9, placebo=7, budesonide=3, and SYMBICORT=3 cases).

Post-Market Adverse Drug Reactions: The following adverse reactions have been reported during post-approval use of SYMBICORT. Because these reactions are reported voluntarily from a population of uncertain size, it is not always possible to reliably estimate their frequency or establish a causal relationship to drug exposure. Some of these adverse reactions may also have been observed in clinical studies with SYMBICORT.

Cardiac Disorders: angina pectoris, tachycardia, cardiac arrhythmias (e.g. atrial fibrillation, extrasystoles), palpitations.

Endocrine Disorders: hypercorticism, growth retardation.

Eye Disorders: cataract, glaucoma, increased intraocular pressure.

Gastrointestinal Disorders: oropharyngeal candidiasis, nausea.

Immune System Disorders: immediate and delayed hypersensitivity reactions, such as anaphylactic reaction, angioedema, brochospasm, urticaria, rash, dermatitis, pruritus.

Metabolic and Nutrition Disorders: hyperglycemia, hypokalemia.

Musculoskeletal, Connective Tissue, and Bone Disorders: muscle spasms.

Nervous System Disorders: tremor, dizziness, headache.

Psychiatric Disorders: behaviour disturbances, sleep disturbances, nervousness, agitation, depression, restlessness.

Respiratory, Thoracic, and Mediastinal Disorders: dysphonia, cough, throat irritation.

Skin and Subcutaneous Tissue Disorders: skin bruising.

Vascular Disorders: hypotension, hypertension.

DRUG INTERACTIONS: Overview: Pharmacokinetic Interactions: The metabolism of budesonide is primarily mediated by the enzyme CYP3A4. CYP3A4 inhibitors like ritonavir and azole antifungals (e.g., ketoconazole and itraconazole), increase the systemic exposure to budesonide. Therefore, concomitant use of budesonide and ritonavir or azole antifungals should be avoided unless the potential benefit outweighs the risk of systemic corticosteroid side-effects.

Pharmacodynamic Interactions: Beta-adrenergic blockers (including eye drops) can weaken or inhibit the effect of formoterol.

Budesonide and formoterol have not been observed to interact with any other drug used in the treatment of asthma.

DOSAGE AND ADMINISTRATION: SYMBICORT (budesonide/formoterol fumarate dihydrate) is for oral inhalation only. The medication from SYMBICORT is delivered to the lungs as the patient inhales, and, therefore, it is important to instruct the patient to breathe in forcefully and deeply through the mouthpiece. The patient may not taste or feel any medication when using SYMBICORT due to the small amount of drug dispensed.

Clinically equivalent doses of SYMBICORT and PULMICORT plus OXEZE TURBUHALER are defined as follows: see Table 3.

Table 3: SYMBICORT TURBUHALER

Clinically Equivalent Doses of SYMBICORT and PULMICORT plus OXEZE TURBUHALER

SYMBICORT TURBUHALER	PULMICORT TURBUHALER plus OXEZE TURBUHALER
SYMBICORT 100 TURBUHALER	PULMICORT TURBUHALER: (100 µg budesonide per metered dose) plus OXEZE TURBUHALER: (6 µg formoterol per metered dose)
SYMBICORT 200 TURBUHALER	PULMICORT TURBUHALER: (200 µg budesonide per metered dose) plus OXEZE TURBUHALER: (6 µg formoterol per metered dose)

Dosing Considerations for Asthma: When treating asthma patients, SYMBICORT should be used only in patients whose conditions are not adequately controlled using low-to-medium dose inhaled corticosteroids or whose disease severity clearly warrants the initiation of treatment with two maintenance therapies (see Warnings and Precautions).

SYMBICORT should not be used in patients whose asthma can be managed by occasional use of short-acting, inhaled beta$_2$-agonists or for patients whose asthma can be successfully managed by inhaled corticosteroids along with occasional use of inhaled short-acting beta$_2$-agonists.

It is crucial to inform patients to have a medication for rescue use (e.g., SYMBICORT, formoterol, terbutaline or salbutamol) available at all times to relieve acute asthmatic symptoms. If the patient's medication for rescue becomes less effective medical attention should be sought.

The patient should be made aware that for optimum benefit, SYMBICORT should be taken regularly, even when they are asymptomatic. Rescue inhalations only need to be taken to relieve acute asthma symptom (see Warnings and Precautions).

A reassessment of asthma therapy should be considered in patients using an increasing number of rescue inhalations for symptom relief without achieving improved asthma control.

SYMBICORT therapy should not be initiated to treat an asthma exacerbation.

Recommended Dose and Dosage Adjustment for Asthma: When starting a patient on SYMBICORT, the dose should first be selected so that effective symptom control is obtained. Subsequently, the dose should be adjusted to the lowest dose at which symptom control is maintained.

The dosage of SYMBICORT should be individualized according to disease severity. Patients should be regularly reassessed so that the dosage of SYMBICORT they are receiving remains optimal.

There are two strategies for the treatment of asthma with SYMBICORT:

A. SYMBICORT Maintenance Therapy (SMT): With SYMBICORT maintenance therapy, patients use SYMBICORT TURBUHALER as a daily maintenance dose and a separate fast-acting inhaled bronchodilator (e.g., formoterol, terbutaline or salbutamol) for symptom relief. Patients should be advised to have a fast-acting bronchodilator available at all times.

Adults and Adolescents (12 years and older): 1-2 inhalations SYMBICORT 100 TURBUHALER once or twice daily. The maximum recommended daily **maintenance** dose is 4 inhalations.

or

1-2 inhalations SYMBICORT 200 TURBUHALER once or twice daily. The maximum recommended daily **maintenance** dose is 4 inhalations.

In adults and adolescents the recommended starting dose is one or two inhalations of SYMBICORT 200 TURBUHALER twice daily.

During periods of worsening of asthma, the dose may temporarily be increased up to a maximum of 4 inhalations of SYMBICORT 100 TURBUHALER or SYMBICORT 200 TURBUHALER twice daily.

Missed Dose for Asthma: If a dose of SYMBICORT is missed, it should be taken as soon as possible; the patient should then resume their regular schedule. A double dose of SYMBICORT should not be taken to make up for doses that are missed.

B. SYMBICORT Maintenance and Reliever Therapy (SYMBICORT SMART): Patients use SYMBICORT TURBUHALER both as a daily maintenance dose plus additional inhalations as needed for rapid symptom relief and a timely increase in controller therapy for improved asthma control. Patients should be advised to always have SYMBICORT TURBUHALER available for rescue use. A persistent increase in the use of SYMBICORT as needed indicates a deterioration of asthma control, and the patient's condition should be re-evaluated.

Adults and Adolescents (12 years and older): 1-2 inhalations SYMBICORT 100 TURBUHALER twice daily or 2 inhalations once daily. Additional doses can be used as needed to provide rapid symptom relief and improved asthma control as follows. Patients should take 1 additional inhalation as needed in response to symptoms. If symptoms persist after a few minutes, an additional inhalation should be taken. Not more than 6 inhalations should be taken on any single occasion. The maximum recommended total daily dose is 8 inhalations.

or

1-2 inhalations SYMBICORT 200 TURBUHALER twice daily or 2 inhalations once daily. Additional doses can be used as needed to provide rapid symptom relief and improved asthma control as follows. Patients should take 1 additional inhalation as needed in response to symptoms. If symptoms persist after a few minutes, an additional inhalation should be taken. Not more than 6 inhalations should be taken on any single occasion. The maximum recommended total daily dose is 8 inhalations.

SYMBICORT Maintenance and Reliever Therapy and SYMBICORT Maintenance Therapy: SYMBICORT is not currently recommended for children younger than 12 years of age due to the limited clinical data in this age group.

Dosing Considerations for Chronic Obstructive Pulmonary Disease (COPD): SYMBICORT therapy should not be initiated to treat acute symptoms of COPD.

Recommended Dose and Dosage Adjustment for COPD: Maintenance for Adults (18 years and older): 2 inhalations SYMBICORT 200 TURBUHALER twice daily. The maximum recommended daily dose is 4 inhalations.

Special Populations: Geriatrics: There are no special dosage requirements for elderly patients.

Hepatic/Renal Impairment: There are no data available for the use of SYMBICORT in patients with hepatic or renal impairment. As budesonide and formoterol are primarily eliminated via hepatic metabolism an increased exposure can be expected in patients with severe liver disease (see Warnings and Precautions, Hepatic/Biliary/Pancreatic and Action and Clinical Pharmacology, Pharmacokinetics, Excretion).

OVERDOSAGE:

There are no data available from clinical trials on overdose with SYMBICORT (budesonide/formoterol fumarate dihydrate). An overdose of formoterol would likely lead to effects that are typical for beta$_2$-adrenergic agonists: tremor, headache, palpitations, and tachycardia. Hypotension, metabolic acidosis, hypokalemia and hyperglycemia may also occur. Supportive and symptomatic treatment may be indicated. A metered dose of 120 µg formoterol administered during three hours in patients with acute bronchial obstruction raised no safety concerns.

Acute overdosage with budesonide even in excessive doses, is not expected to be a clinical problem. When used chronically in excessive doses, systemic glucocorticosteroid effects, such as hypercorticism and adrenal suppression, may appear.

> For management of a suspected drug overdose, contact your regional Poison Control Centre. See the *CPS* Directory section for a list of Poison Control Centres.

ACTION AND CLINICAL PHARMACOLOGY: Mechanism of Action: SYMBICORT contains formoterol fumarate dihydrate and budesonide, which have different modes of action and show additive effects in terms of reduction of asthma and COPD exacerbations. In asthma, SYMBICORT can offer a more convenient regime for patients requiring concurrent long-acting beta$_2$-agonist and inhaled corticosteroid therapy—dosing with SYMBICORT may be adjusted to meet the condition of the patients' disease. SYMBICORT can be used both as a maintenance and reliever medication in asthma, due to the rapid bronchodilator effect of formoterol and the anti-inflammatory effects of budesonide.

Pharmacodynamics: The respective mechanisms of action of budesonide and formoterol are discussed below.

Budesonide: Budesonide is a potent synthetic glucocorticosteroid with strong topical and weak systemic effects. Budesonide has a high local anti-inflammatory potency and it is rapidly biotransformed in the liver. This favorable separation between topical anti-inflammatory activity and systemic effect is due to strong glucocorticosteroid receptor affinity and an effective first pass metabolism with a short half-life. The anti-anaphylactic and anti-inflammatory effects of budesonide manifest themselves as decreased bronchial obstruction in the early as well as the late phase allergic reactions. When administered by inhalation at therapeutic doses, it has a direct, potent anti-inflammatory action within the lungs, resulting in reduced symptoms and exacerbations of asthma, without the adverse effects observed when corticosteroids are administered systemically. Budesonide has also been shown to decrease airway reactivity to both direct and indirect challenge in hyperreactive patients. Therapy with inhaled budesonide has been effective when used for prevention of exercise-induced asthma.

Formoterol: Formoterol is a potent, selective, fast and long-acting $beta_2$-adrenergic stimulant used for the prevention and relief of asthma symptoms. Formoterol produces relaxation of bronchial smooth muscle in patients with reversible airways obstruction. The bronchodilating effect sets in as rapidly as short-acting bronchodilators (salbutamol, terbutaline), within 1-3 minutes after inhalation, and has a duration of 12 hours after a single dose. Formoterol offers more effective protection against carbachol, histamine- or methacholine-induced bronchoconstriction than other short (e.g., salbutamol) and long-acting (e.g., salmeterol) $beta_2$-agonists. Formoterol provides dose-related benefits in pulmonary function and in bronchoprotective effects against methacholine, histamine and AMP challenges, indicating a dose-related reduction in airways responsiveness to both direct and indirect stimuli and a greater protection against asthma triggers such as allergens and exercise.

SYMBICORT: In clinical trials in asthma and COPD, combination treatment with formoterol and budesonide improved symptoms and lung function, and reduced exacerbations.

In asthma, the effect on lung function of SYMBICORT was clinically equivalent to that of the free combination of budesonide and formoterol in separate inhalers in adults and exceeded that of budesonide alone in adults and adolescents. There was no sign of attenuation of the anti-asthmatic effect over time. SYMBICORT and the short-acting bronchodilator salbutamol have been shown to have similarly rapid onsets of effect. The combination of budesonide and formoterol does not mask the onset or severity of exacerbations.

Pharmacokinetics: Absorption: After the administration of budesonide, formoterol or the fixed combination, pharmacokinetic parameters, for the respective substances, were comparable. Specifically, for budesonide, AUC was slightly higher, rate of absorption more rapid and maximal plasma concentration higher after administration of the fixed combination. For formoterol, maximal plasma concentration was slightly lower after administration of the fixed combination.

SYMBICORT and the monoproducts (PULMICORT TURBUHALER and OXEZE TURBUHALER) were bioequivalent with regard to systemic bioavailability of budesonide and formoterol.

Inhaled budesonide is rapidly absorbed and the maximum plasma concentration is reached within 30 minutes after inhalation. In studies, mean lung deposition of budesonide after inhalation via TURBUHALER ranged from 32 to 44% of the delivered dose (25 to 30% of the metered dose). The systemic bioavailability is about 49% of the delivered dose and 38% of the metered dose.

Inhaled formoterol is rapidly absorbed and the maximum plasma concentration is reached within 10 minutes after inhalation. In studies the mean lung deposition of formoterol after inhalation via TURBUHALER ranged from 28-49% of the delivered dose (21-37% of the metered dose). Because of the low therapeutic dose, systemic levels of formoterol are low or undetectable after inhalation.

Distribution: Plasma protein binding is approximately 50% for formoterol and 90% for budesonide. Volume of distribution is about 4 L/kg for formoterol and 3 L/kg for budesonide.

Metabolism: Formoterol is inactivated via conjugation reactions (active O-demethylated and deformylated metabolites are formed, but they are seen mainly as inactivated conjugates).

Budesonide undergoes an extensive degree (≈90%) of biotransformation on first passage through the liver to metabolites of low glucocorticosteroid activity. The glucocorticosteroid activity of the major metabolites, 6β-hydroxy-budesonide and 16α-hydroxy-prednisolone, is less than 1% of that of budesonide. There are no indications of any metabolic interactions or any displacement reactions between formoterol and budesonide.

Excretion: The major part of a dose of formoterol is eliminated via hepatic metabolism followed by renal excretion. After inhalation 8-13% of the delivered dose of formoterol is excreted unmetabolised in the urine. Formoterol has a high systemic clearance (approximately 1.4 L/min) and the late elimination half-life averages 17 hours.

Budesonide is eliminated via metabolism mainly catalysed by the enzyme CYP3A4. The metabolites of budesonide are excreted in urine as such or in conjugated form. Only negligible amounts of unchanged budesonide have been detected in the urine. Budesonide has a high systemic clearance (approximately 1.2 L/min) and the plasma elimination half-life after i.v. dosing averages 4 hours.

Special Populations and Conditions: Pediatrics: Budesonide has a systemic clearance of approximately 0.5 L/min in 4-6 year old asthmatic children. Per kg body weight children have a clearance which is approximately 50% greater than in adults. The terminal half-life of budesonide after inhalation is approximately 2.3 hours in asthmatic children. The pharmacokinetics of formoterol in children has not been studied.

STORAGE AND STABILITY: SYMBICORT TURBUHALER (budesonide/formoterol fumarate dihydrate) should be stored at room temperature between 15 and 30°C with the cover tightened.

SPECIAL HANDLING INSTRUCTIONS: SYMBICORT TURBUHALER (budesonide/formoterol fumarate dihydrate) cannot be refilled and should be discarded when finished.

INFORMATION FOR THE PATIENT: Published in e-CPS, available by subscription at www.e-cps.ca.

DOSAGE FORMS, COMPOSITION AND PACKAGING: SYMBICORT 100 TURBUHALER: Each dry powder inhaler contains: budesonide 100 µg and formoterol fumarate dihydrate 6 µg per dose. Also contains lactose (may contain milk protein residue) which acts as a "carrier". The amount added does not normally cause problems in lactose-intolerant people. Pack sizes of 60 and 120 doses.

SYMBICORT 200 TURBUHALER: Each dry powder inhaler contains: budesonide 200 µg and formoterol fumarate dihydrate 6 µg per dose. Also contains lactose (may contain milk protein residue) which acts as a "carrier". The amount added does not normally cause problems in lactose-intolerant people. Pack sizes of 60 and 120 doses.

(Shown in Product Identification Section)

Synacthen® Depot ℞

cosyntropin—zinc hydroxide

Adrenocorticotropic Hormone

Novartis Pharmaceuticals

Date of Preparation: May 8, 1980
Date of Revision: August 16, 2005

PHARMACOLOGY: Natural adrenocorticotropin is a straight-chain polypeptide containing 39 amino acids which, by convention, are numbered from the N-terminal end of the molecule. The sequence of amino-acid occupying positions 25 to 33 varies among species and it is this part of the molecule which is most antigenic when ACTH of foreign origin is administered to man. In contrast, the N-terminal 24 amino-acid sequence is common to all species and is relatively non-antigenic, and it is only these amino-acids which are involved in its biological activities.

The most important physiological effects of ACTH involve the adrenal cortex and include the maintenance of adrenal weight and the control of adrenal corticosteroid synthesis and release. In its absence, adrenal blood flow is diminished, adrenal atrophy invariably ensues and cortisol secretion is markedly reduced. In addition to controlling corticosteroid secretion, ACTH also increases the synthesis and release of the other adrenal steroids, namely aldosterone and the adrenal androgens. It also has some degree of melanotropic activity and lipolytic effect.

SYNACTHEN DEPOT (cosyntropin zinc hydroxide suspension), a long-acting synthetic β1-24-corticotropin, exhibits the same activity as natural ACTH with regard to all its biological activities. The complex results in a product whose absorption in man is effected over a longer period of time as compared to corticotropin. Therefore, therapy may be maintained with less frequent administration.

The long-term administration of SYNACTHEN DEPOT produces the same effects as those produced by cortisone, cortisol and their synthetic analogues. In addition, there is also hypertrophy and hyperplasia of the adrenal cortex, in contrast to the effect of the exogenous corticoids.

INDICATIONS: Adrenal Function Test: The assessment of adrenocortical function based on its response to exogenous ACTH is well established. Nuki, G., et al. (1969) found that there was no significant difference in plasma 11-hydroxycorticosteroid response over 4 hours after a cosyntropin infusion or a single intramuscular injection of 1 mg of depot cosyntropin (SYNACTHEN DEPOT) in a group of patients with varying degrees of adrenocortical insufficiency secondary to corticosteroid therapy; suggesting its use to test for adrenocortical insufficiency without recourse of intravenous infusion, which is frequently unpleasant for both patient and clinician. Grant, J.K. (1969) found that the speed of response in the first 20-30 minutes is also virtually the same after cosyntropin intravenously as after cosyntropin depot intramuscularly; reasonably inferring that, except perhaps in states of extreme collapse, little advantage is to be gained in speed of response by giving cosyntropin (short acting) intravenously rather than cosyntropin depot intramuscularly.

Galvao-Teles, A., et al. (1971) proposed as a test of adrenal function that plasma-cortisol be estimated before and 4-6 hours after an intramuscular injection of 1 mg SYNACTHEN DEPOT, generally recommended to be given at about 10 a.m. The results may be interpreted as shown in Table 1.

Table 1: SYNACTHEN DEPOT

Interpretation of Plasma Cortisol Levels and Urinary Free Cortisol Excretion After Injection of 1 mg SYNACTHEN DEPOT

	Normal Subjects	Steroid-treated or Hypopituitary Patients with Abnormal Reserve		Addisonian Subjects
		Moderately Impaired	Severely Impaired	
Plasma-cortisol[a] 4–6 h after injection (µg/100 mL)	≥35	20–35	<20	<10
Urinary-free cortisol				
1st day (µg/day):	>700	—	<350	<150
2nd day (µg/day):	Less than 1st day	—	More than 1st day	<150

[a] By specific method; add one-third if plasma 11-OHCS is measured.

In hypoadrenal subjects, a further sample at 12-16 hours is indicated. Intermediate responses may then be clarified by measuring plasma-cortisol after three further injections of cosyntropin depot at 48-hour intervals during which period secondary hypoadrenalism may be expected to show recovery. The response to the first injection indicates the extent of adrenal atrophy or destruction, and that to the subsequent injections its recoverability.

SYNACTHEN DEPOT offers two advantages: first, the longer duration of action might help to provide stronger adrenal stimulation; second, the delay in response to corticotropin in cases of secondary adrenal atrophy which can be shown by prolonged corticotropin stimulation might be elicited by a single injection of SYNACTHEN DEPOT.

Performance of Adrenal Function Tests:

1. The 30-Minute SYNACTHEN DEPOT Screening Test: Preparation: The subject need not be fasted. The procedure should be started at about 10:00 a.m. and can be performed as an out-patient procedure.
   Procedure: i) A 5-7 mL blood sample is taken for determination of plasma cortisol levels at time 0. This will serve as a base against which to compare later values. ii) 1 mg of SYNACTHEN DEPOT is given by intramuscular injection immediately after the blood sample has been taken. iii) A further 5-7 mL blood sample is taken exactly 30 minutes after the injection.
   Note: Some clinicians take an additional sample 45-60 minutes after the injection (in case the 30-minute sample is lost or the assay is invalid for any reason).
   Interpretation of Results: In normal subjects the plasma cortisol level at 30 minutes reaches at least 20 µg/100 mL (0.55 µmol/L) with an increment which exceeds 7 µg/100 mL (0.19 µmol/L).
   Note: This simple procedure should be used only for screening purposes with any abnormal results requiring confirmation by more prolonged ACTH stimulation. However, a normal response does exclude primary adrenocortical insufficiency, and may also be of value in the serial assessment of adrenocortical function in patients who are, or were, receiving corticosteroid therapy.
2. The 5-Hour SYNACTHEN DEPOT Test: Preparation: The subject need not be fasted. The procedure should be started at about 10:00 a.m., at least 30 minutes after the insertion of an indwelling catheter.
   Procedure: i) A 5-7 mL blood sample is taken for determination of plasma cortisol levels at time 0. This will serve as a base against which to compare later values. ii) 1 mg of SYNACTHEN DEPOT is given by intramuscular injection immediately after the blood sample has been taken. iii) Further samples are taken after 0.5, 1, 2, 3, 4 and 5 hours for plasma cortisol assay. This assay of several samples avoids a single, possibly inaccurate result which might lead to an erroneous conclusion.
   Note: The amount of SYNACTHEN DEPOT used exceeds the amount required to induce a maximum adrenocortical response, ensuring an accurate assessment of the reserve capacity of the adrenal cortex.
   Interpretation of Results: In normal subjects, plasma cortisol levels more than double in the first hour, and then rise more slowly. After five hours normal values lie within the range of 37 to 66 µg/100 mL (1.02-1.82 µmol/L).
3. The 3-Day SYNACTHEN DEPOT Test Preparation: For Procedure A, hospitalization is not required, nor does the patient need to be fasted. Admission to hospital is usually required for Procedure B, however, the patient can eat a normal diet and remain ambulant during his in-patient stay.
   Procedure A: A 30-minute SYNACTHEN DEPOT test (see 30-Minute SYNACTHEN DEPOT Test) is performed at 9:00 a.m. on day 1. The patient then receives 1 mg of SYNACTHEN DEPOT injected intramuscularly on days 2 and 3. On day 4 a second 30-minute SYNACTHEN DEPOT test is performed at 10:00 a.m.
   Procedure B: Urinary cortisol levels are determined on complete 24-hour collections for 5 consecutive days. The first two days serve as a control period. Starting on day 3 the patient is given, once daily, intramuscular injections of 1 mg SYNACTHEN DEPOT. See Table 2.

Table 2: SYNACTHEN DEPOT

The 3-Day SYNACTHEN DEPOT Test: Procedure B

Day 1	Day 2	Day 3	Day 4	Day 5
Daily Urinary Cortisol Determinations				
		1 mg i.m. daily SYNACTHEN DEPOT at 9:30 a.m.		

Interpretation of Results: Note: Prolonged ACTH stimulation tests offer advantages over the shorter tests only in differentiating between primary and secondary adrenocortical insufficiency. No response is found in patients with the primary type (Addison's disease) whereas, with prolonged stimulation, in the great majority of patients there is a marked but delayed corticosteroid response in secondary adrenal atrophy.

Procedure A provides this information, i.e. a marked improvement in the second 30-minute SYNACTHEN DEPOT test is consistent with secondary adrenocortical insufficiency whereas no improvement is found in the primary type. As concerns procedure B, in normal subjects, urinary cortisol excretion at least doubles on the first day of SYNACTHEN DEPOT stimulation (i.e. day 3) and continues to increase during the remainder of the test.

Caution: The administration of ACTH for three consecutive days may rarely cause sodium and water retention with the risk of edema while the marked and prolonged increase in circulating corticosteroid levels that may occur in patients with bilateral adrenal hyperplasia, can cause a severe exacerbation of the symptoms of Cushing's syndrome. On extremely rare occasions, adrenal crisis has supervened during prolonged ACTH stimulation in patients with marked adrenal insufficiency. For this reason, some clinicians give 1 mg of dexamethasone daily through the 3 days on which SYNACTHEN DEPOT is given to provide steroid cover. This does not interfere with the test.

SYNACTHEN DEPOT has been used in the following:
Collagen Diseases: acute rheumatic fever; rheumatoid arthritis, lupus erythematosus; periarteritis nodosa, psoriatic arthritis; scleroderma; rheumatoid spondylitis; Still's disease.
Dermatologic Diseases: exfoliative dermatitis; dermatomyositis; pemphigus.
Endocrine Diseases: panhypopituitarism.
Eye Diseases: choroiditis; conjunctivitis; iritis; keratitis; optic neuritis; sympathetic ophthalmia; uveitis.
Hemolytic Diseases: acquired hemolytic jaundice.
Other Diseases: nephrotic syndrome; ulcerative colitis; Bell's palsy; acute exacerbations of multiple sclerosis, and as adjuvant treatment in cases of acute gout.

CONTRAINDICATIONS: Known or suspected hypersensitivity to cosyntropin and or ACTH of animal origin or to any of the excipients of SYNACTHEN (cosyntropin zinc hydroxide suspension); premature babies and neonates, due to the presence of benzylalcohol; pregnancy and lactation; untreated bacterial, fungal and viral infections, Cushing's syndrome; refractory congestive heart failure; active or latent peptic ulcer; acute psychosis; adrenocortical insufficiency; adrenogenital syndrome.

In view of the increased risk of anaphylactic reactions, SYNACTHEN DEPOT must not be employed to treat asthma or other allergic affections. Since SYNACTHEN DEPOT contains benzyl alcohol, it is contra-indicated in neonates (especially premature infants), in whom benzyl alcohol can cause severe poisoning.

WARNINGS: SYNACTHEN DEPOT (cosyntropin zinc hydroxide suspension), **must not be given intravenously**.

Due to the presence of benzylalcohol, SYNACTHEN DEPOT is not recommended in infants and children up to 3 years old, as it may cause toxic reactions and allergic reactions.

In rare cases, particularly in patients subject to asthma and/or other forms of allergy—severe anaphylactic reactions may occur. Such reactions set in usually within 30 minutes after administration of SYNACTHEN DEPOT.

If SYNACTHEN DEPOT is used in any of the following conditions, the risks should be weighed against the possible benefits: non-specific ulcerative colitis; diverticulitis; recent intestinal anastomosis; renal insufficiency; hypertension; thromboembolic tendencies; acute or chronic infections, especially varicella or vaccinia; exanthematous and fungal diseases; osteoporosis and myasthenia gravis.

PRECAUTIONS: Before employing SYNACTHEN DEPOT (cosyntropin zinc hydroxide suspension) the physician must ascertain whether the patient is suffering from an allergic disorder (especially asthma) or is susceptible in general to allergies (see Contraindications and Warnings). The physician should also enquire whether the patient has been treated with ACTH preparations in the past, and, if so, make sure that the treatment gave rise to no hypersensitivity reactions (see Contraindications).

Allergic reactions may occur in response to SYNACTHEN DEPOT, which tend to be more severe in patients susceptible to allergies (especially asthma) (see Contraindications). Because of the possibility of an allergic reaction occurring with SYNACTHEN DEPOT, the injection should be given under medical supervision and the patient kept under observation for about 1 hour. Self-injection by patients is not recommended. Should any prodomal signs occur, stop further treatment. Allergic reactions of this type include: marked redness and pain at the injection site, dizziness, nausea, vomiting, urticaria, pruritus, flushings, severe malaise, dyspnea or angioneurotic edema or Quincke's edema. If local or systemic hypersensitivity reactions occur during or after an injection, treatment with cosyntropin must be discontinued and all use of ACTH preparations avoided in the future.

Treatment of Anaphylactic Reactions: Severe anaphylactic reactions usually can be avoided by discontinuing the use of the drug at the earliest sign of local or systemic hypersensitivity. In the rare event of a serious incident occurring despite these precautions, initiate the following emergency measures as treatment for shock: Initial treatment or for less severe reactions: 0.3-0.5 mL S.C. or I.M. of a 1 mg/mL aqueous solution of epinephrine. For more severe or life threatening reactions, or if no response to S.C. or I.M. route: 1 to 5 mL I.V. **slowly** of a 1 mg/mL aqueous epinephrine solution diluted to 10 mL physiologic saline. As well, corticosteroid i.v., e.g., hydrocortisone or methylprednisolone, should be given immediately in large doses, repeated if necessary, in the event of a serious anaphylactic reaction.

Prolonged repeated cosyntropin administration may increase the risk of hypersensitivity reaction.

The blood pressure and weight should be carefully observed. Urinalysis should be done at intervals; if sugar is present the fasting blood glucose should be determined. Salt and water retention in response to SYNACTHEN DEPOT can often be avoided or eliminated by prescribing a low-sodium diet; diuretics may be employed when strict sodium restriction is impossible.

Potassium supplement should be administered in cases of prolonged use.

Psychological disturbances such as euphoria, depression, insomnia, psychosis, mood swings, personality changes may occur during therapy. Existing emotional disorders or psychoses may be aggravated.

Prolonged use of cosyntropin may be associated with development of posterior subcapsular cataracts and glaucoma.

Infections must be treated simultaneously with appropriate antibiotics; the signs and symptoms of inflammation may be masked by the anti-inflammatory effects of cortisol produced by the over-active adrenal glands.

Vaccination: Patients on therapy with cosyntropin should not be vaccinated against smallpox. If other immunization procedures are considered, these should be undertaken with caution because of decrease in antibody response and possible hazard of neurological complications.

Surgery: Patients who are subjected to the stress of surgical operations or trauma while being treated, or within one year after treatment has been terminated, should have their SYNACTHEN DEPOT therapy augmented or reinstated and continued for the duration of the stress period and immediately following it. In stressful conditions, additional use of rapidly acting corticosteroids may be required.

Although the action of cosyntropin is similar to that of exogenous adrenocortical steroids, the quantity of endogenous corticosteroids produced by the adrenal glands may be variable.

The lowest effective dose of cosyntropin should be used to control the condition under treatment. When reduction of the dosage is indicated, this should be gradual. Relative insufficiency of the pituitary-adrenal axis is induced by prolonged administration, therefore gradual reduction of cosyntropin dosage is essential. On discontinuation of therapy this type of insufficiency may persist for several months. During this period in cases of stressful conditions appropriate adrenocortical therapy should be considered.

It is advisable to verify the adrenal responsiveness before and during cosyntropin therapy.

Patients with Special Diseases and Conditions: Patients already receiving medication for diabetes mellitus or for moderate to severe hypertension must have the dosage of their medication readjusted if treatment with SYNACTHEN DEPOT is instituted.

An enhanced effect of corticotropin therapy has been observed in patients with hypothyroidism and in those with cirrhosis of the liver.

SYNACTHEN DEPOT should be used cautiously in patients with ocular herpes simplex owing to possible corneal perforation.

SYNACTHEN DEPOT may activate latent amoebiasis. It is therefore recommended that latent or active amoebiasis be ruled out before initiating therapy.

If SYNACTHEN DEPOT is indicated in patients with latent tuberculosis or tuberculin reactivity, close observation is necessary because the disease may be reactivated. During prolonged therapy, such patients should receive chemoprophylaxis.

Pediatric: Provided the dosage is carefully individualized SYNACTHEN DEPOT is unlikely to inhibit growth in children. Nevertheless, in children undergoing long-term treatment, growth should be monitored.

In infants and small children treated with SYNACTHEN DEPOT, echocardiographic recordings should be made regularly, because during long-term treatment with high doses reversible myocardial hypertrophy may occur.

SYNACTHEN DEPOT is contraindicated in neonates.

Drug Interactions: Since SYNACTHEN DEPOT increases the adrenocortical production of glucocorticoids and mineralocorticoids, drug interactions of the type seen with these corticosteroids may occur. Patients already receiving medication for diabetes mellitus or for moderate to severe hypertension must have their dosage adjusted if treatment with SYNACTHEN DEPOT is started.

SYNACTHEN DEPOT contains an active substance that may interfere with routine drug testing in athletes.

ADVERSE EFFECTS: Adverse reactions may be related to Cosyntropin Zinc Hydroxide, to the presence of benzylalcohol or the stimulation of glucocorticoids and mineralocorticoid secreation during the use of SYNACTHEN DEPOT.

Adverse reactions related to Cosyntropin Zinc Hydroxide: Cosyntropin Zinc Hydroxide can provoke hypersensitivity reactions (see Contraindications and Warnings), which tend to be more severe (anaphylactic shock) in patients susceptible to allergies (especially asthma). Hypersensitivity reactions may include skin reactions at the injection site, dizziness, nausea, vomiting, urticaria, pruritus, flushing, dyspnea, and angioneurotic edema or Quincke's edema.

Adrenal haemorrhage: Isolated cases have been reported with SYNACTHEN DEPOT.

Adverse reactions related to benzyl alcohol: In rare cases the benzyl alcohol contained SYNACTHEN DEPOT may also give rise to hypersensitivity reactions. The benzyl alcohol contained as an excipient in SYNACTHEN DEPOT may provoke toxic reactions and allergic reactions especially in children below 3 years old.

Adverse reactions related to glucocorticoid and mineralocorticoid effects: The adverse reactions related to glucocorticoid and mineralocorticoid effects are unlikely to be observed with short-term use of SYNACTHEN DEPOT as a diagnostic tool, but may be reported when SYNACTHEN DEPOT is used in therapeutic indications.

Fluid and Electrolyte Disturbances: sodium retention, fluid retention, potassium loss, hypokalemic alkalosis, calcium loss.

Musculoskeletal: muscle weakness, steroid myopathy, loss of muscle mass, osteoporosis, vertebral compression fractures, aseptic necrosis of femoral and humeral heads, pathologic fracture of long bones, tendon rupture.

Gastrointestinal: peptic ulcer with possible perforation and hemorrhage, pancreatitis, abdominal distention, ulcerative esophagitis.

Dermatologic: impaired wound healing, thin fragile skin, petechiae and ecchymoses, facial erythema, increased sweating, suppression of skin test reactions, acne, hyperpigmentation.

Cardiovascular: hypertension, necrotizing angiitis, congestive heart failure.

In infants and small children treated over a prolonged period with high dosages, reversible myocardial hypertrophy may occur in isolated instances.

Neurological: convulsions, increased intracranial pressure with papilledema (pseudo-tumor cerebri) usually after treatment; headache; vertigo; psychic changes.

Endocrine: menstrual irregularities; development of Cushingoid state; suppression of growth in children; secondary adrenocortical and pituitary unresponsiveness, particularly in times of stress, as in trauma, surgery or illness; decreased carbohydrate tolerance; hyperglycemia; manifestations of latent diabetes mellitus; increased requirements for insulin or oral hypoglycemic agents in diabetics; hirsutism.

Ophthalmic: posterior subcapsular cataracts, increased intraocular pressure, glaucoma, exophthalmos.

Metabolic: negative nitrogen balance due to protein catabolism.

Allergic Reactions: Especially in patients with allergic responses to proteins manifesting as dizziness, nausea and vomiting, anaphylactic shock, skin reactions.

Miscellaneous: increased susceptibility to infection; abscess; thromboembolism; weight gain; increased appetite; leucocytosis; prolonged ACTH may result in antibodies and loss of stimulatory effect.

OVERDOSE:

Symptoms: Edema, hypertension or signs of excessive adrenocortical activity (Cushings's syndrome) during therapy usually indicate overdosage. In such cases the dosage should be reduced, frequency of administration decreased (i.e. to 5-7 days), or the drug withdrawn according to the severity of the condition.

Treatment: There is no known antidote for corticotropin. Toxic effects should be treated symptomatically.

> For management of a suspected drug overdose, CPhA recommends that you contact your **regional Poison Control Centre**. See the *CPS* Directory section for a list of Poison Control Centres.

DOSAGE: Test of Adrenal Function: 1 mg SYNACTHEN DEPOT (cosyntropin zinc hydroxide suspension), injected intramuscularly at about 10 a.m. Plasma 11-hydroxycorticosteroids to be measured before and 4-6 hours after the injection. For interpretation of results, and further measurement and caution in certain cases, see Indications.

Dosage for Other Clinical Disorders: In general, the correct dose is the smallest one given at the longest possible interval necessary to produce control of the clinical disorder.

The average dose is 0.5-1 mg I.M. twice a week, tailoring the dose according to the individual requirements. In acute cases, or after prolonged steroid therapy, 1 mg I.M. daily for three days. However, the interval should be extended as soon as an adequate response is obtained.

Once the acute manifestations have subsided or for chronic conditions, the dose should be adjusted according to the patient's needs. Some may be best maintained on a dose of 0.5-1 mg every 2 or 3 days while others may respond better to 2 mg at weekly, or even longer intervals.

Children: Due to the presence of benzyl alcohol, SYNACTHEN DEPOT is contraindicated in premature babies and in neonates and is not recommended in children below 3 years of age (see Contraindications and Warnings).

Based on a number of clinical studies, the following dosage schedule in Table 3 is suggested for children.

Table 3: SYNACTHEN DEPOT

Dosage Schedule for Children

Age	Initial Dosage	Maintenance Dosage
3–6 years	0.25–0.5 mg/day	0.25–0.5 mg every 2–8 days
6–15 years	0.5–1 mg/day	0.25–1 mg every 2–8 days

Route of Administration: The preferred route of administration is by intramuscular injection, slowly and deeply into the gluteal region.

The ampoules and vials should be slightly shaken until the suspension shows a uniform appearance.

Transferring from Corticoids: Administer 1 mg SYNACTHEN DEPOT daily to elicit full adrenal response. At the same time withdraw the steroid gradually, reducing by a quarter the original dose on successive days. Once the steroid has been withdrawn, adjust SYNACTHEN DEPOT dosage to individual patient's requirements.

Transferring from ACTH of Animal Origin: 1 mg of Synacthen has approximately the same corticotropic activity as 100 international units of ACTH (as defined in the 3rd International Working Standard). This equivalence is not, however, valid for depot preparations since the effect of SYNACTHEN DEPOT lasts appreciably longer than ACTH gel and coniderably longer than ACTH in carboxymethyl cellulose. To transfer a patient receiving, for example, 40 units ACTH gel daily, give 0.5 mg SYNACTHEN DEPOT I.M. instead on alternate days. The response should then be assessed and the dosage adjusted, preferably by lengthening the interval between injections.

SUPPLIED: Each ampul of milky-white, sterile suspension for intramuscular injection contains: cosyntropin 1 mg as zinc hydroxide complex. Nonmedicinal ingredients: benzyl alcohol, sodium chloride, sodium hydroxide (to adjust pH), disodium phosphate dodecahydrate and sterile water for injection. Approximately 2.5 mg of Zn^{2+} is present per mL. Alcohol: 1 % w/v. Sodium: <1 mmol (1.13 mg)/mL. Bisulfite-, gluten-, lactose-, parabens- and tartrazine-free. Ampuls of 1 mL, cartons of 1. Store in a refrigerator (2-8°C); protect from light. Store in the original package or keep the ampoules in the outer carton. Must be kept out of reach of children.

Synagis® Ⓟ

palivizumab

Passive Immunizing Agent (Humanized Monoclonal Antibody)

Abbott

Date of Preparation: May 15, 2002

Date of Revision: December 16, 2009

SUMMARY PRODUCT INFORMATION:

Route of Administration	Dosage Form/ Strength	Clinically Relevant Nonmedicinal Ingredients
Intramuscular injection	Lyophilized powder/50 mg Lyophilized powder/100 mg	Glycine, histidine, and mannitol For a complete listing see Dosage Forms, Composition and Packaging.

DESCRIPTION: SYNAGIS (palivizumab) is a humanized monoclonal antibody (IgG1κ) produced by recombinant DNA technology, directed to an epitope in the A antigenic site of the F protein of respiratory syncytial virus (RSV). Palivizumab is a composite of (95%) human and (5%) murine amino acid sequences. The human heavy chain sequence was derived from the constant domains of human IgG1 and the variable framework regions of the V_H genes Cor and Cess. The human light chain sequence was derived from the constant domain of Cκ and the variable framework regions of the V_L gene K104 with Jκ-4. The murine sequences were derived from a murine monoclonal antibody, Mab 1129, in a process which involved the grafting of the murine complementarity determining regions into the human antibody frameworks. Palivizumab is composed of two heavy chains and two light chains and has a molecular weight of approximately 148 000 Daltons.

INDICATIONS AND CLINICAL USE: SYNAGIS (palivizumab) is indicated for:

- prevention of serious lower respiratory tract disease caused by respiratory syncytial virus (RSV) in pediatric patients at high risk of RSV disease. Safety and efficacy were established in infants with bronchopulmonary dysplasia (BPD), infants with a history of prematurity (≤35 weeks gestational age), and children with hemodynamically significant congenital heart disease (CHD).

Distribution restrictions: This product should be administered under the supervision of a qualified health professional.

Geriatrics (≥65 years of age): SYNAGIS is not indicated for adult usage.

Pediatrics (≤35 weeks gestational age): See Indications and Clinical Use.

CONTRAINDICATIONS:

- SYNAGIS (palivizumab) is contraindicated in patients with known hypersensitivity to palivizumab or to any of its excipients. It is also contraindicated in patients with known hypersensitivity to other humanized monoclonal antibodies. For a complete listing, see Dosage Forms, Composition and Packaging.

WARNINGS AND PRECAUTIONS:

> **Serious Warnings and Precautions**
> - If anaphylaxis or severe allergic reaction occurs, administer epinephrine in appropriate pediatric dosage, and provide supportive care as required.

General: No studies have been performed to assess the administration of more than seven SYNAGIS doses in an RSV season.
Carcinogenesis and Mutagenesis: Carcinogenesis and mutagenesis studies have not been performed with SYNAGIS.
Hematologic: SYNAGIS is **for intramuscular use only**. As with any intramuscular injection, SYNAGIS should be given with caution to patients with thrombocytopenia or any coagulation disorder.
Immune: In Study I, the incidence of anti-humanized antibody following the fourth injection was 1.1% in the placebo group and 0.7% in the SYNAGIS group. In pediatric patients receiving SYNAGIS for a second season, one of fifty-six patients had transient, low titer reactivity. This reactivity was not associated with adverse events or alteration in palivizumab serum concentrations. Immunogenicity was not assessed in Study II.

These data reflect the percentage of patients whose test results were considered positive for antibodies to palivizumab in an ELISA assay, and are highly dependent on the sensitivity and specificity of the assay. Additionally, the observed incidence of antibody positivity in an assay may be influenced by several factors including sample handling, concomitant medications, and underlying disease. For these reasons, comparison of the incidence of antibodies to SYNAGIS with the incidence of antibodies to other products may be misleading.

In the Extended Dose Study (Study IV), transient, low levels of antipalivizumab antibody (1:20) were observed in one child after the second dose of SYNAGIS that dropped to undetectable levels (<1:10) at the fifth and seventh dose.
Respiratory: A moderate to severe acute infection or febrile illness may warrant delaying the use of SYNAGIS, unless, in the opinion of the physician, withholding SYNAGIS entails a greater risk. A mild febrile illness, such as a mild upper respiratory infection, is not usually reason to defer administration of SYNAGIS.
Sensitivity/Resistance: Allergic reactions including very rare cases of anaphylaxis have been reported following SYNAGIS administration. (See Adverse Reactions, Post-Market Adverse Drug Reactions.)

Symptoms of immediate hypersensitivity and anaphylaxis were observed in two adult volunteers receiving 30 mg/kg in one of the pharmacodynamic studies.

Medications for the treatment of severe hypersensitivity reactions, including anaphylaxis, should be available for immediate use following administration of SYNAGIS. If a severe hypersensitivity reaction occurs, therapy with SYNAGIS should be permanently discontinued. As with other agents administered to this population, if milder hypersensitivity reactions occur, caution should be used on re-administration of SYNAGIS.
Sexual Function/Reproduction: Reproductive toxicity studies have not been performed with SYNAGIS.
Special Populations: Pregnant Women: SYNAGIS is not indicated for adult usage and animal reproduction studies have not been conducted. It is also not known whether palivizumab can cause fetal harm when administered to a pregnant woman or whether it could affect reproductive capacity.
Pediatrics (≤35 weeks gestational age): See Indications and Clinical Use.
Geriatrics (≥65 years of age): SYNAGIS is not indicated for adult usage.
Monitoring and Laboratory Tests: There is not known interference between SYNAGIS and laboratory tests.

ADVERSE REACTIONS: Adverse Drug Reaction Overview: In the combined pediatric prophylaxis studies of pediatric patients with BPD or prematurity involving 520 subjects receiving placebo and 1168 subjects receiving SYNAGIS (palivizumab), the proportions of subjects in the placebo and SYNAGIS groups who experienced any adverse event or any serious adverse event were similar.
Clinical Trial Adverse Drug Reactions : Because clinical trials are conducted under very specific conditions the adverse reaction rates observed in the clinical trials may not reflect the rates observed in practice and should not be compared to the rates in the clinical trials of another drug. Adverse drug reaction information from clinical trials is useful for identifying drug-related adverse events and for approximating rates.
Study I: Adverse events which occurred in more than 1% of patients receiving SYNAGIS in Study I for which the incidence in the SYNAGIS group was 1% greater than in the placebo group are presented in Table 1.

Table 1: SYNAGIS

Adverse Events Occurring in Study I at Greater Frequency in the SYNAGIS Group

	SYNAGIS n=1002 (%)	Placebo n=500 (%)
Body as a Whole	49.6	49.4
Upper respiratory infection	52.6	49.0
Otitis media	41.9	40.0
Rhinitis	28.7	23.4
Rash	25.6	22.4
Pain	8.5	6.8
Hernia	6.3	5.0
AST increased	4.9	3.8
Pharingitis	2.6	1.4

Other adverse events reported in more than 1% of the SYNAGIS group included:
Blood and Lymphatic System Disorders: anemia.
Ear and Labyrinth Disorders: ear disorder.
Gastrointestinal Disorders: constipation, diarrhea, flatulence, gastrointestinal disorder and vomiting.
General Disorders and Administration Site Conditions: fever and study drug injection site reaction.
Hepato-biliary Disorders: liver function abnormality.
Infections and Infestations: bronchitis, bronchiolitis, croup, conjunctivitis, flu syndrome, fungal dermatitis, gastroenteritis, oral moniliasis, pneumonia, RSV, sinusitis and viral infection.
Injury, Poisoning and Procedural Complications: accidental injury and miscellaneous procedure.
Investigations: ALT increase.
Metabolism and Nutrition Disorders: failure to thrive and feeding abnormalities.
Psychiatric Disorders: nervousness.
Respiratory, Thoracic and Mediastinal Disorders: asthma, apnea, cough, dyspnea, respiratory disorder and wheeze.
Skin and Subcutaneous Tissue Disorders: eczema and seborrhoea.

There were no statistically significant differences in the incidence of adverse events between the SYNAGIS and placebo groups.
Study II: In the randomized, double-blind, placebo-controlled trial of RSV disease prophylaxis among children with hemodynamically significant congenital heart disease, the proportion of subjects in the placebo and SYNAGIS groups who experienced any adverse event or any serious adverse events were similar. No significant differences in morbidity or mortality were observed.

Adverse events that occurred in more than 1% of patients receiving SYNAGIS and for which the incidence was 1% greater in the SYNAGIS group than in the placebo group are shown in Table 2.

Table 2: SYNAGIS

Adverse Events Occurring in Study II at Greater Frequency in the SYNAGIS Group

	SYNAGIS n=639 (%)	Placebo n=648 (%)
Upper respiratory infection	47.4	46.1
Fever	27.1	23.9
Conjunctivitis	11.3	9.3
Cyanosis	9.1	6.9
Infection	5.6	2.9
Study drug injection site reaction	3.4	2.2
Arrhythmia	3.1	1.7

Other adverse events reported in 1% or more of the SYNAGIS group included:
Blood and Lymphatic System Disorders: anemia, coagulation disorder and thrombocytopenia.
Cardiac Disorders: bradycardia, congestive heart failure, heart failure, cardiovascular disorder, pericardial effusion and tachycardia.
Ear and Labyrinth Disorders: ear disorder.
Gastrointestinal Disorders: constipation, diarrhea, flatulence, gastrointestinal disorder, pain (primarily teething) and vomiting.
General Disorders and Administration Site Conditions: asthenia and edema.
Infections and Infestations: bacterial infection, bronchitis, bronchiolitis, croup, flu syndrome, fungal infection, fungal dermatitis, gastroenteritis, otitis media, oral moniliasis, pneumonia, pharyngitis, RSV, rhinitis, urinary tract infection, sepsis, sinusitis and viral infection.
Injury, Poisoning and Procedural Complications: accidental injury.
Metabolism and Nutrition Disorders: failure to thrive, feeding abnormalities and hypokalemia.
Nervous System Disorders: hyperkinesia and somnolence.
Psychiatric Disorders: nervousness.
Respiratory, Thoracic and Mediastinal Disorders: apnea, atelectasis, cough, dyspnea, hypoxia, hyperventilation, lung edema, respiratory disorders, pleural effusion, pulmonary hypertension, pneumothorax, stridor and wheeze.
Skin and Subcutaneous Tissue Disorders: eczema and rash.
Vascular Disorders: hemorrhage.
Study IV: No reported adverse events were considered related to SYNAGIS and no deaths were reported in any of the 18 patients in this study.
Less Common Clinical Trial Adverse Drug Reactions (<1%): Both clinical and laboratory adverse drug reactions are displayed by system organ class.
Gastrointestinal Disorders: diarrhea and vomiting.
General Disorders and Administration Site Conditions: pain.
Infections and Infestations: upper respiratory infections, rhinitis and viral infection.
Investigations: aspartate aminotransferase (AST) increase, abnormal liver function test, and alanine aminotransferase (ALT) increase.
Respiratory, Thoracic and Mediastinal Disorders: cough and wheeze.
Skin and Subcutaneous Tissue Disorders: rash.
Abnormal Hematologic and Clinical Chemistry Findings: Mild or moderate elevations of AST occurred in 1.6% placebo and 3.7% SYNAGIS; for ALT, these percentages were 2.0% and 2.3% respectively. Reported adverse events related to the liver and deemed by the blinded investigator to be related to study drug were balanced between the two groups.
Post-Market Adverse Drug Reactions: The following adverse reactions have been very rarely (<1 in 10 000 reported cases) reported with SYNAGIS therapy.
Blood and Lymphatic System Disorders: thrombocytopenia.
Immune System Disorders: anaphylaxis.
Nervous System Disorders: convulsion.
Skin and Subcutaneous Tissue Disorders: urticaria.

SYNAGIS treatment schedule and adverse events were monitored in a group of nearly 20 000 infants tracked through a patient compliance registry, the REACH program. Of this group, 1250 enrolled infants received 6 injections, 183 infants received 7 injections, and 27 infants received either 8 or 9 injections each respectively. Fifteen (1%) adverse events were observed in patients following a sixth or greater dose. All 15 of the adverse events occurred following the administration of the sixth dose and not with subsequent doses (up to 9 doses). Adverse events from this registry as well as through routine post-marketing surveillance were similar in character and frequency to those after the initial 5 doses.

DRUG INTERACTIONS: Overview: No formal drug-drug interaction studies were conducted. In Study I, the proportions of patients in the placebo and SYNAGIS (palivizumab) groups who received routine childhood vaccines, influenza vaccine, bronchodilators or corticosteroids were similar and no incremental increase in adverse reactions was observed among patients receiving these agents, in either of the two groups. Since the monoclonal antibody is specific for RSV, SYNAGIS is not expected to interfere with the immune response to vaccines, including live viral vaccines.
Drug-Drug Interactions: No formal drug-drug interaction studies were conducted with SYNAGIS.
Drug-Food Interactions: Interactions with food have not been established with SYNAGIS.
Drug-Herb Interactions: Interactions with herbal products have not been established with SYNAGIS.
Drug-Laboratory Test Interactions: Interactions with laboratory tests have not been established with SYNAGIS.
Drug-Lifestyle Interactions: No data available.

DOSAGE AND ADMINISTRATION: Recommended Dose and Dosage Adjustment: The recommended dose of SYNAGIS (palivizumab) is 15 mg/kg of body weight, **intramuscular injection only**, given once a month during anticipated periods of RSV risk in the community. Where possible, the first dose should be administered prior to commencement of the RSV season, and subsequent doses should be administered monthly throughout the RSV season. To avoid risk of reinfection, it is recommended that children receiving SYNAGIS who become infected with RSV continue to receive monthly doses of SYNAGIS throughout the RSV season.

In temperate climates, the RSV season typically commences in the fall months and lasts through the spring; however, there have been reported cases during the summer. During this period, children normally receive 5 consecutive monthly intramuscular doses of palivizumab. (See Warnings and Precautions.)
Missed Dose: If your child misses an injection of SYNAGIS, you should contact your doctor as soon as possible. Each injection of SYNAGIS can only help protect your child for about one month before another injection is needed.
Administration: SYNAGIS should be administered in a once monthly dose of 15 mg/kg intramuscularly using aseptic technique, preferably in the anterolateral aspect of the thigh. The gluteal muscle should not be used routinely as an injection site because of the risk of damage to the sciatic nerve. The dose per month = [patient weight (kg)×15 mg/kg÷100 mg/mL of SYNAGIS]. Injection volumes over 1 mL should be given as a divided dose.

Reconstituted SYNAGIS is to be administered by **intramuscular injection only**.
Reconstitution: Parenteral Products:

Vial Size	Volume of Diluent to be Added to Vial	Approximate Available Volume	Nominal Concentration per mL
50 mg	0.6 mL	0.6 mL	50 mg/0.5 mL
100 mg	1.0 mL	1.0 mL	100 mg/mL

Note: Both the 50 mg and 100 mg vial contain an overfill to allow the withdrawal of 50 mg or 100 mg respectively when reconstituted if following the directions described below.

Reconstituted product is stable for up to 6 hours when left at room temperature. **However, since the single dose vial of SYNAGIS does not contain a preservative, unless it is reconstituted under controlled and validated aseptic conditions, the product should be administered within 3 hours of reconstitution.**

SYNAGIS should not be mixed with any medications or diluents other than sterile Water for Injection (WFI). WFI is provided in the SYNAGIS kit and it is to be used solely for reconstitution with SYNAGIS.

Reconstitution of the 50 mg Vial:

- Using aseptic technique, to reconstitute, remove the tab portion of the vial cap and clean the rubber stopper with 70% ethanol or equivalent.
- Carefully tap the top of the ampoule of sterile water for injection, provided in the kit, until all the droplets have fallen to the bottom of the ampoule. In one hand, hold the ampoule with the red dot facing you. With the other hand, hold a 2×2 gauze pad or equivalent at the top, near the red dot, and snap off the upper portion of the ampoule away from you. The glass will break off cleanly and easily.
- To minimize foaming, **slowly** add **0.6 mL** of sterile Water for Injection, provided in the kit, along the inner side of the **50 mg vial**. Ideally, the sterile water should be "dripped in" along the inner side of the vial. Rotate the sides of the vial after half the sterile water has been added to the SYNAGIS powder, and add the balance of the sterile water down the other side of the vial.
- After removing the syringe from the vial, gently turn the vial between your fingers for approximately 30 seconds. This allows you to visually ensure that all the SYNAGIS has **been saturated** by the sterile water. **Do not shake or vigorously agitate the vial.**
- **Do not invert the vial during the reconstitution process.**

Reconstitution of the 100 mg Vial:

- Using aseptic technique, to reconstitute, remove the tab portion of the vial cap and clean the rubber stopper with 70% ethanol or equivalent.
- Carefully tap the top of the ampoule of sterile water for injection, provided in the kit, until all the droplets have fallen to the bottom of the ampoule. In one hand, hold the ampoule with the red dot facing you. With the other hand, hold a 2×2 gauze pad or equivalent at the top, near the red dot, and snap off the upper portion of the ampoule away from you. The glass will break off cleanly and easily.
- To minimize foaming, **slowly** add **1.0 mL** of sterile Water for Injection, provided in the kit, along the inner side of the **100 mg vial**. Ideally, the sterile water should be "dripped in" along the inner side of the vial. Rotate the sides of the vial after half the sterile water has been added to the SYNAGIS powder and add the balance of the sterile water down the other side of the vial.
- After removing the syringe from the vial, gently turn the vial between your fingers for approximately 30 seconds. This allows you to visually ensure that all the SYNAGIS has **been saturated** by the sterile water. **Do not shake or vigorously agitate the vial.**
- **Do not invert the vial during the reconstitution process.**

Reconstituted SYNAGIS should stand undisturbed at room temperature for a minimum of 20 minutes until the solution clarifies. If excessive foaming has occurred and a full dose of either 1.0 mL or 0.5 mL is required, allow more time for the foam to dissipate (typically 1 hour or longer). The reconstituted solution should appear clear or slightly opalescent.

Before drawing up the solution, invert the vial for approximately 30 seconds. This allows the solution to collect at the bottom of the vial, and facilitates the withdrawal process.

It is most important to work slowly and not rush the reconstitution process.

Reconstituted product is stable for up to 6 hours when left at room temperature. **SYNAGIS is supplied as a single-dose vial and does not contain a preservative. It is recommended that unless it is reconstituted under controlled and validated aseptic conditions, the product should be administered within 3 hours of reconstitution.**

Discard any unused product.

To prevent the transmission of infectious diseases, sterile disposable syringes and needles should be used. Do not reuse syringes and needles.

OVERDOSAGE:

In clinical studies, three children received an overdose of more than 15 mg/kg. These doses were 20.25 mg/kg, 21.1 mg/kg and 22.27 mg/kg. No medical consequences were identified in these instances. From the post-marketing experience, overdoses as high as 60 mg/kg have been reported without any untoward medical events.

No clinical data are available from human subjects who have received more than 7 monthly SYNAGIS doses during a single RSV season.

For management of a suspected drug overdose, contact your regional Poison Control Centre. See the *CPS* Directory section for a list of Poison Control Centres.

ACTION AND CLINICAL PHARMACOLOGY: Mechanism of Action: SYNAGIS (palivizumab) exhibits neutralizing and fusion-inhibitory activity against RSV. These activities inhibit RSV replication in laboratory experiments. Although resistant RSV strains may be isolated in laboratory studies, a panel of clinical RSV isolates were all neutralized by SYNAGIS. Palivizumab serum concentrations of approximately 30 µg/mL have been shown to produce a mean 99% reduction in pulmonary RSV replication in the cotton rat model.

The in vivo neutralizing activity of the active ingredient in SYNAGIS was assessed in a randomized, placebo-controlled study of 35 pediatric patients tracheally intubated because of RSV disease. In these patients, SYNAGIS significantly reduced the quantity of RSV in the lower respiratory tract compared to control patients.

Pharmacokinetics: Absorption: Adult (intramuscular and intravenous): Palivizumab has a time to maximum serum concentration of 1.6 hours when administered intravenously, and 5 days when administered intramuscularly.

In adult volunteer studies, SYNAGIS administered either intravenously or intramuscularly had a pharmacokinetic profile similar to a human IgG1 antibody in regards to the volume of distribution (mean 57 mL/kg) and the half-life (mean 18 days).

Pediatric (intramuscular and intravenous): In pediatric patients less than 24 months of age, the mean half-life of palivizumab was 20 days (range 16.8 to 26.8 days), and monthly intramuscular doses of 15 mg/kg achieved mean±SD 30-day trough serum drug concentrations of 37±21 µg/mL after the first injection, 57±41 µg/mL after the second injection, 68±51 µg/mL after the third injection, and 72±50 µg/mL after the fourth injection. In pediatric patients given palivizumab for a second season, the mean±SD serum concentrations following the first and fourth injections were 61±17 µg/mL and 86±31 µg/mL, respectively.

Thirty days after the first intravenous infusion, the mean trough concentration in patients receiving 15 mg/kg was 60.6 µg/mL (range 21.4 to 149.8 µg/mL). Thirty days after the second infusion, the mean trough concentration in patients receiving 15 mg/kg was 70.7 µg/mL (range 20.2 to 112.6 µg/mL).

In pediatric patients ≤24 months of age with hemodynamically significant congenital heart disease (CHD) who received palivizumab and underwent cardio-pulmonary bypass for open-heart surgery, the mean serum palivizumab concentration was 98±52 µg/mL before bypass and declined to 41±33 µg/mL after bypass, a reduction of 58%.

The results of a prospective, phase 2, open-label trial designed to evaluate pharmacokinetics, safety and immunogenicity after administration of 7 doses of palivizumab within a single RSV season showed that adequate mean palivizumab target levels (30 µg/mL or greater) were achieved in all 18 children enrolled.

Special Populations and Conditions: Pediatrics: See [Action And Clinical Pharmacology, Pharmacokinetics, Absorption, Pediatric (intramuscular and intravenous)] for details.

Geriatrics: SYNAGIS pharmacokinetics has not been studied in geriatric population. SYNAGIS is not indicated for adult usage.

Gender: No gender related pharmacokinetic differences have been observed in adult patients.

Race: Pharmacokinetics differences due to race have not been identified.

Hepatic Insufficiency: No pharmacokinetic data are available in patients with hepatic impairment.

Renal Insufficiency: No pharmacokinetic data are available in patients with renal impairment.

Genetic Polymorphism: No data available on genetic polymorphism.

STORAGE AND STABILITY: Upon receipt and until reconstitution for use, SYNAGIS should be stored between 2 and 8°C in its original container. Do not freeze. Do not use beyond the expiration date.

SPECIAL HANDLING INSTRUCTIONS: After Reconstitution: Reconstituted SYNAGIS should stand at room temperature for a minimum of 20 minutes until the solution clarifies. The reconstituted solution should appear clear or slightly opalescent.

Reconstituted product is stable for up to 6 hours when left at room temperature. **However, since the single-dose vial of SYNAGIS does not contain a preservative, unless it is reconstituted under controlled and validated aseptic conditions, the product should be administered within 3 hours of reconstitution.**

Discard any unused product.

To prevent the transmission of infectious diseases, sterile disposable syringes and needles should be used. Do not reuse syringes and needles.

INFORMATION FOR THE PATIENT: Published in e-CPS, available by subscription at www.e-cps.ca.

DOSAGE FORMS, COMPOSITION AND PACKAGING: 50 mg: Each vial of lyophilized powder contains: palivizumab 50 mg. Nonmedicinal ingredients: glycine, histidine, mannitol and sterile Water for Injection. Kits contain a 50 mg single-dose 4 mL vial with a 1 mL ampoule of sterile Water for Injection. See Dosage and Administration, Administration, Reconstitution, Parenteral Products and Special Handling Instructions, After Reconstitution for more information on the reconstituted solution.

100 mg: Each vial of lyophilized powder contains: palivizumab 100 mg. Nonmedicinal ingredients: glycine, histidine, mannitol and sterile Water for Injection. Kits contain a 100 mg single-dose 10 mL vial with a 1 mL ampoule of sterile Water for Injection. See Dosage and Administration, Administration, Reconstitution, Parenteral Products and Special Handling Instructions, After Reconstitution for more information on the reconstituted solution.

Synarel® ℞

nafarelin acetate

Gonadotropin-releasing Hormone (GnRH) Analogue

Pfizer

PHARMACOLOGY: Nafarelin is an agonistic analogue of the gonadotropin releasing hormone (GnRH). Given as a single intranasal dose, nafarelin stimulates release of the pituitary gonadotropins, LH and FSH, with consequent increase of ovarian steroidogenesis. Repeated intranasal dosing abolishes the stimulatory effect on the pituitary gland. Twice daily administration of 200 µg, as a nasal spray, leads to decreased secretion of gonadal steroids by about 4 weeks. Consequently, tissues and functions that depend on gonadal steroids for their maintenance become quiescent.

Pharmacokinetics: Nafarelin is rapidly absorbed from the nasal mucosa into the systemic circulation after intranasal administration. The relative bioavailability of intranasally administered nafarelin averaged 2.8% (range 1.2 to 5.6%). This was determined by comparing nafarelin AUC values after a single 400 µg intranasal dose and a 25 µg i.v. dose and adjusting for the lower i.v. dose administered. The low relative bioavailability results from the drug not being well absorbed by the nasal mucosa. Maximum plasma concentrations are achieved 10 to 40 minutes after dosing. Following a single intranasal dose of 200 µg base, the observed average peak concentration of nafarelin is 0.6 ng/mL, whereas following a single dose of 400 µg base, the observed average peak concentration is 1.8 ng/mL (range 1.52 to 2.0 ng/mL). The average serum half-life of nafarelin following intranasal administration is 3 hours (range 2 to 4 hours).

The effect of rhinitis or a topical decongestant on intranasally administered Synarel has not yet been determined with the presently available formulation.

Clinical Use: In controlled clinical studies, nafarelin at doses of 400 and 800 µg/day for 6 months was shown to relieve the clinical symptoms of endometriosis (pelvic pain, dysmenorrhea, and dyspareunia) and to reduce the size of endometrial implants as determined by laparoscopy. The clinical significance of a decrease in endometriotic lesions is not known at this time. Laparoscopic staging of endometriosis did not necessarily correlate with severity of symptoms.

In 73 patients, Synarel 400 µg daily induced amenorrhea in approximately 65%, 80% and 90% of the patients after 60, 90 and 120 days, respectively. Most of the remaining patients reported episodes of only light bleeding or spotting. In the first, second and third post-treatment months normal menstrual cycles resumed in 4%, 82% and 100%, respectively, of those patients who did not become pregnant.

The distribution of patients, treated with 400 µg/day, by symptom severity at admission, end of treatment and 6 months after treatment is shown in Table 1.

Table 1: Synarel

Symptom Severity Score

	N	0 None	1–2 Mild	3–5 Moderate	6–9 Severe
At admission	73	6 (8%)	26 (36%)	28 (38%)	13 (18%)
End of treatment	73	44 (60%)	23 (32%)	5 (7%)	1 (1%)
6 months after treatment	73	37 (51%)	24 (33%)	12 (16%)	—

INDICATIONS: For hormonal management of endometriosis, including pain relief and reduction of endometriotic lesions. Experience with nafarelin for the management of endometriosis has been limited to women 18 years of age and older and treated for 6 months. There is no evidence that pregnancy rates are enhanced or adversely affected by its use.

CONTRAINDICATIONS: Should not be administered to patients who: are hypersensitive to GnRH, GnRH agonist analogues or any of the excipients in this product; have undiagnosed abnormal vaginal bleeding; are pregnant or who may become pregnant while receiving the drug (see Warnings). It is not known whether nafarelin causes fetal abnormalities in humans; are breast feeding (see Warnings).

WARNINGS: General: Isolated cases of short-term worsening of signs and symptoms or enlargement of ovarian cysts have been reported during initiation of nafarelin therapy: they are sometimes, but not necessarily, associated with a stimulation of the pituitary gland and an initial increase in the levels of circulating gonadal hormones. Many, but not all, of these events occurred in patients with polycystic ovarian disease. These cystic enlargements may resolve spontaneously, generally by about four to six weeks of therapy, but in some cases, worsening of the clinical condition may occasionally require discontinuation of therapy and/or surgical intervention.

Pregnancy: Safe use of nafarelin in pregnancy has not been established clinically. Before starting treatment, pregnancy must be excluded.

When used regularly at the recommended dose, nafarelin usually inhibits ovulation and stops menstruation. Contraception is not ensured, however, by taking nafarelin, particularly if patients miss successive drug doses. Therefore, **patients should use nonhormonal methods of contraception**. Patients should be advised to see their physician if they believe they may be pregnant. If a patient becomes pregnant during treatment, the drug must be discontinued, and the patient must be informed of the potential risk to fetal development. There is no experience with nafarelin in pregnant women.

Lactation: It is not known whether or to what extent nafarelin is excreted into human breast milk. The effects, if any, on the breast-fed child have not been determined and therefore, nafarelin should not be used in breast feeding women.

Children: The safety and effectiveness in children have not been established and therefore, nafarelin should not be used.

PRECAUTIONS: Information to Be Provided to the Patient: An information pamphlet for patients is included with the product and should be read carefully before initiating treatment with nafarelin. Patients should be made aware of the following information.

Menstruation: Since menstruation should stop with effective doses of nafarelin, the patient should notify her physician, if regular menstruation persists. Patients missing successive doses of the drug may experience break through vaginal bleeding.

Pregnancy: Patients should not use nafarelin if they are pregnant or suspected pregnant, are breast-feeding, have undiagnosed abnormal vaginal bleeding or are allergic to any of the ingredients in nafarelin. The patient must be informed of the potential risk to fetal development.

Lactation: See Pregnancy.

Use in Women of Childbearing Potential: Safe use of the drug in pregnancy has not been established clinically. Therefore, **a nonhormonal method of contraception should be used during treatment**. Patients should be advised that if they miss successive doses of nafarelin, ovulation may occur with the potential for conception. If a patient becomes pregnant during treatment, she should discontinue treatment and consult her physician. The patient must be informed of the potential risk to fetal development.

Adverse Events: Adverse events associated with the hypoestrogenic state induced by nafarelin, occurred in clinical studies. The most frequently reported adverse events were hot flashes (90%), decrease in libido (22%), headache (19%), vaginal dryness (19%), emotional lability (15%), acne (13%), myalgia (10%) and reduction in breast size (10%). Estrogen levels returned to normal after treatment was discontinued with resolution of the hypoestrogenic effects. Nasal irritation occurred in about 10% of all patients who used intranasal nafarelin.

Bone Density: The induced hypoestrogenic state caused by nafarelin results in a small loss in bone density over the course of treatment, some of which may not be reversible. During one 6-month treatment period, this bone loss should not be important. In patients with major risk factors for decreased bone mineral content such as chronic alcohol and/or tobacco use, strong family history of osteoporosis or chronic use of drugs that can reduce bone mass such as anticonvulsants or corticosteroids, nafarelin therapy may pose an additional risk. In these patients, the risks and benefits must be weighed carefully before therapy is instituted. Repeated courses of treatment with gonadotropin releasing hormone analogues are not advisable in patients with major risk factors for loss of bone mineral content.

Retreatment: The safety of retreatment as well as of treatment beyond 6 months with nafarelin has not yet been established, and therefore retreatment cannot be recommended.

Drug Interactions: No pharmacokinetic drug interaction studies have been conducted with nafarelin. However, because nafarelin is a peptide that is primarily degraded by peptidases and not by cytochrome P-450 enzymes, and because the drug is only about 80% bound to plasma proteins at 4°C, drug interactions would not be expected to occur.

Patients with intercurrent rhinitis should consult with their physician before the use of a topical nasal decongestant. If the use of a topical nasal decongestant is required during treatment with nafarelin, the decongestant must be used at least 30 minutes after dosing to decrease the possibility of reducing drug absorption. The effect of rhinitis or a topical decongestant on nafarelin absorption by the nasal mucosa has not yet been determined.

Sneezing during or immediately after dosing may impair absorption of nafarelin acetate. If sneezing occurs upon administration, repeating the dose may be advisable.

Diagnostic Interference: Administration of nafarelin in therapeutic doses results in suppression of the pituitary-gonadal system. Normal function is usually restored within 4 to 8 weeks after treatment is discontinued. Diagnostic tests of pituitary-gonadal function conducted during the treatment and within 8 weeks after discontinuation of nafarelin therapy may therefore be misleading.

Fertility Studies: Use of nafarelin in human pregnancy has not been studied. After 6 months of therapy, 56 patients, who were treated with 400 µg/day, desired and attempted pregnancy. By the end of 18 months post treatment, 17 (30%) patients became pregnant. In the 800 µg/day group, out of 48 patients attempting pregnancy, 25 of them (52%) became pregnant within 18 months post treatment. Full term delivery occurred in 82% and 68% of patients in the 400 and 800 µg/day groups respectively. All newborns were normal except for one male baby who had hydrocele. The mother of the baby was in the 400 µg/day group.

The serum concentration of gonadotropins and estradiol returned promptly to normal after cessation of therapy.

Mutagenicity and Carcinogenicity: As seen with other GnRH agonists, high parenteral doses (up to 100 µg/kg/day in mice for 18 months and 500 µg/kg/day in rats for 24 months) induced hyperplasia and/or neoplasia (without metastasis) of endocrine organs including the pituitary (adenoma/carcinoma). Rodents are particularly sensitive to hormonal stimulation when tested for tumorigenicity. No evidence of tumorigenicity has been reported in monkeys or man. No indication of a mutagenic potential for nafarelin has been reported.

ADVERSE EFFECTS: As would be expected with a drug which lowers serum estradiol levels, the most frequently reported adverse reactions were those related to hypoestrogenism.

Controlled studies included 203 evaluable women (mean age 32 years) treated on average for 170 days with nafarelin 400 µg/day. The adverse reactions most frequently reported and thought to be drug related are listed below (% incidence (n=203)).

Central Nervous System: headache 19%, emotional lability 15%, nervousness 9%, insomnia 8%, depression 2%, dizziness 1%, vertigo 1%, incoordination 0.5%, neurosis 0.5%, increased sweating 0.5%.

Skin and Appendages: acne 13%, breast atrophy 10%, seborrhea 8%, hirsutism 2%, dry skin 2%, alopecia 0.5%, chloasma 0.5%, gynecomastia 0.5%, herpes simplex 0.5%, maculopapular rash 0.5%.

Urogenital: vaginal dryness 19%, dyspareunia 1%, menstrual disorder 0.5%, cystitis 0.5%, dysuria 0.5%, urinary incontinence 0.5%, vaginal hemorrhage 0.5%.

Metabolic and Nutritional Disorders: weight gain 8%, edema 8%, weight loss 1%.

Musculoskeletal: myalgia 10%, arthralgia 1%, myasthenia 0.5%.

Digestive: nausea, gastrointestinal fullness 5%, increased appetite 1%, anorexia 1%, constipation 0.5%, diarrhea 0.5%, gastritis 0.5%, vomiting 0.5%.

Respiratory: rhinitis 10%, epistaxis 1%, dry nose 0.5%, sinusitis 0.5%, voice alteration 0.5%.

Special Senses: taste perversion 3%, conjunctivitis 1%, ear pain 0.5%, eye pain 0.5%.

Body as a Whole: asthenia 1%, mucous membrane disorder 0.5%.

Cardiovascular: hot flashes 90.0%, palpitation 0.5%.

Others: breast pain 3%, decreased libido 22%, increased libido 1%.

In approximately 2% of adult patients, symptoms suggestive of drug sensitivity, such as chest pain, pruritus, rash, shortness of breath and urticaria have occurred.

In other clinical trials and post-marketing experience, paresthesia and blood pressure changes were also reported. In very rare instances, uterine hemorrhage can occur.

Changes in Bone Density: After 6 months of treatment, vertebral trabecular bone density and total vertebral bone mass, measured by quantitative computed tomography (QCT), decreased by an average of 8.7% and 4.3%, respectively, compared to pretreatment levels. There was partial recovery of bone density, when assessed 6 months after end of treatment, the average trabecular bone density and total bone mass were 4.9% and 3.3% less than the pretreatment levels, respectively. Total vertebral bone mass, measured by dual photon absorptiometry (DPA), decreased by a mean of 5.9% at the end of treatment. Mean total vertebral mass, re-examined by DPA 6 months after completion of treatment, was 1.4% below pretreatment levels. There was little, if any, decrease in the mineral content in compact bone of the distal radius and second metacarpal. Use of nafarelin for longer than the recommended 6 months or in the presence of other known risk factors for decreased bone mineral content may cause additional bone loss.

Changes in Laboratory Values: Plasma Enzymes: After 6 months of therapy with 400 µg/day of nafarelin, elevations in AST outside the normal range were observed in 5 (3%) of 180 patients with normal baseline values. Post- treatment evaluations were available for 4 of these patients: the level of AST was within the normal range. For ALT, 2 (3 %) of 68 patients with normal baseline had increases outside the normal range. 1 patient, for which data are available, returned to normal during the post-treatment observation. For alkaline phosphatase, 10 (5%) out of 182 patients with normal baseline level had increases outside the normal range at the end of treatment. Post-treatment evaluations were available for 8 of these patients: 4 patients were within the normal range, the other 4 patients were above the normal range but this was not considered clinically significant.

Lipids: At enrollment, 9% of the patients receiving nafarelin 400 µg/day had total cholesterol values above 250 mg/dL. These patients also had cholesterol values above 250 mg/dL at the end of treatment.

Of those patients whose pretreatment cholesterol values were below 250 mg/dL, 6% in the nafarelin group, had post-treatment values above 250 mg/dL.

The mean (±SEM) pretreatment values for total cholesterol from all nafarelin patients were 191.8 (4.3) mg/dL. At the end of the treatment period, the mean values for total cholesterol from all patients in the nafarelin group were 204.5 (4.8) mg/dL. The increase from the pretreatment value was statistically significant ($p<0.05$).

Triglycerides were increased above the upper limit of 150 mg/dL in 12% of the patients who received nafarelin.

Following completion of treatment, no patients receiving nafarelin had abnormally low HDL cholesterol fractions (less than 30 mg/dL) and none of the patients receiving nafarelin had abnormally high LDL cholesterol fractions (greater than 190 mg/dL). There was no increase in the LDL/HDL ratio in patients receiving nafarelin.

Other Changes: In comparative studies, the following changes were seen in approximately 10% to 15% of patients. Nafarelin treatment was associated with elevations of plasma phosphorus and eosinophil counts, and decreases in serum calcium and WBC counts.

OVERDOSE:

Symptoms: In experimental animals a single s.c. administration of up to 60 times the recommended human dose (expressed on a µg/kg basis not adjusted for bioavailability) had no adverse effects. Orally administered nafarelin is subject to enzymatic degradation in the gastrointestinal tract and is therefore inactive. There is no clinical experience with overdosage of nafarelin acetate. At present, there is no clinical evidence of adverse effects following overdosage of GnRH analogues.

> For management of a suspected drug overdose, CPhA recommends that you contact your **regional Poison Control Centre**. See the *CPS* Directory section for a list of Poison Control Centres.

DOSAGE: For the management of endometriosis, the recommended daily dose is 400 µg. This is achieved by 1 spray (200 µg of nafarelin free base) into 1 nostril in the morning and 1 spray into the other nostril in the evening. Treatment should be started between days 2 and 4 of the menstrual cycle.

In an occasional patient, the 400 µg daily dose may not produce amenorrhea. For these patients with persistent regular menstruation after 2 months of treatment, the dose may be increased to 800 µg daily. The 800 µg dose is administered as 1 spray into each nostril in the morning (a total of 2 sprays) and again in the evening.

The recommended duration of administration is 6 months. The safety of retreatment as well as of treatment beyond 6 months with nafarelin has not yet been established. If the symptoms of endometriosis recur after a course of therapy, and further treatment is contemplated, it is recommended that bone density be assessed before retreatment begins to ensure that values are within normal limits.

If the use of a topical nasal decongestant is necessary during treatment with this product, the decongestant should not be used until at least 30 minutes after nafarelin dosing (see Precautions).

At 400 µg/day, a 8 mL bottle of nafarelin provides a 30-day (about 60 sprays) supply. If the daily dose is increased, increase the supply to the patient to ensure uninterrupted treatment for the recommended duration of therapy.

INFORMATION FOR THE PATIENT: Published in e-CPS, available by subscription at www.e-cps.ca.

SUPPLIED: Each mL of nasal solution contains: nafarelin acetate 2 mg (as nafarelin base). Nonmedicinal ingredients: benzalkonium chloride, glacial acetic acid, hydrochloric acid or sodium hydroxide, sorbitol and purified water. Bottles of 8 mL. Each bottle is supplied with a metered spray pump. A dust cover and a leaflet of patient instructions are also included.

After priming the pump unit, each actuation of the unit delivers approximately 100 µL of the metered droplet spray containing approximately 200 µg nafarelin base. The contents of one 8 mL spray bottle is intended to deliver at least 60 sprays. Store upright between 15 and 25°C. Protect from light and freezing.

(Shown in Product Identification Section)

Synergy Defense™

enzyme blend

To help break down fats, carbohydrates, proteins, and sugars, resulting in healthier digestion and improved nutrient absorption. Improves overall digestion and strengthens the body's natural defences

Awareness Corporation/dba AwarenessLife

SUPPLIED: Each capsule contains: amylase (aspergillus oryzae) 8000 FCC units, protease (aspergillus oryzae) 17 000 FCC units, cellulase (Aspergillus niger) 400 FCC units, lactase (aspergillus oryzae) 700 FCC units, diastase (Barley malt) 500 FCC units, invertase (Saccharomyces) 10 FCC units. Nonmedicinal ingredients: lactobacillus, Mediterranean Herbal Blend: green tea leaf extract, grape seed extract, tomato fruit concentrate (5000 ppm; 25 µg of lycopene), olive leaf extract, pomegranate fruit extract, rosemary leaf extract. Prebiotic & Digestive Blend: purified plant fiber, chicory root extract (90% inulin) (FOS), acacia gum, beet root fiber, blessed thistle (leaves and flowering tops), fennel seed, fenugreek seed, Jerusalem artichoke tuber. Ionic Plan Trace Mineral Blend (from ocean plant). No artificial colors, caffeine, flavors, preservatives, or salt. Boxes of 30. Store in cool, dry place. For occasional use only. Keep out of reach of children.

(Shown in Product Identification Section)

Synflorix™

pneumococcal conjugate vaccine (non-typeable H. influenzae (NTHi) protein D, diphtheria or tetanus toxoid conjugates) adsorbed

Active Immunizing Agent

GlaxoSmithKline

Date of Preparation: May 5, 2009

SUMMARY PRODUCT INFORMATION:

Route of Administration	Dosage Form/ Strength	Clinically Relevant Nonmedicinal Ingredients
Intramuscular	Suspension for injection 1 dose (0.5 mL) contains: Pneumococcal polysaccharide serotype 1[a] 1 µg Pneumococcal polysaccharide serotype 4[a] 3 µg Pneumococcal polysaccharide serotype 5[a] 1 µg Pneumococcal polysaccharide serotype 6B[a] 1 µg Pneumococcal polysaccharide serotype 7F[a] 1 µg Pneumococcal polysaccharide serotype 9V[a] 1 µg Pneumococcal polysaccharide serotype 14[a] 1 µg Pneumococcal polysaccharide serotype 18C[b] 3 µg Pneumococcal polysaccharide serotype 19F[c] 3 µg Pneumococcal polysaccharide serotype 23F[a] 1 µg	Aluminum phosphate, sodium chloride, water for injections For a complete listing see Dosage Forms, Composition and Packaging.

[a] Conjugated to protein D (derived from Non-Typeable *H. influenzae*) carrier protein.
[b] Conjugated to tetanus toxoid carrier protein.
[c] Conjugated to diphtheria toxoid carrier protein.

DESCRIPTION: SYNFLORIX [(pneumococcal conjugate vaccine (Non-Typeable *H. influenzae* (NTHi) protein D, diphtheria or tetanus toxoid conjugates) adsorbed] is a 10-valent pneumococcal polysaccharide conjugate vaccine using protein D derived from Non-Typeable *H. influenzae* as a carrier protein for 8 out of the 10 serotypes (1, 4, 5, 6B, 7F, 9V, 14 and 23F). Serotypes 18C and 19F are conjugated to tetanus toxoid and to diphtheria toxoid, respectively. All conjugates are adsorbed onto aluminum phosphate.

INDICATIONS AND CLINICAL USE: SYNFLORIX is indicated for active immunization of infants and children from 6 weeks up to 2 years of age against *S. pneumoniae* serotypes 1, 4, 5, 6B, 7F, 9V, 14, 18C, 19F and 23F and invasive disease caused by these serotypes (including sepsis, meningitis, bacteraemic pneumonia, pleural empyema and bacteraemia).

Geriatrics (>65 years of age): Studies have not been conducted in adults 65 years and older.

CONTRAINDICATIONS: SYNFLORIX should not be administered to subjects with known hypersensitivity to any component of the vaccine. For a complete listing, see Dosage Forms, Composition and Packaging.

WARNINGS AND PRECAUTIONS: General: It is good clinical practice to precede vaccination by a review of the medical history (especially with regard to previous vaccination and possible occurrence of undesirable events) and a clinical examination.

As with other vaccines, the administration of SYNFLORIX should be postponed in subjects suffering from acute severe febrile illness. However, the presence of a minor infection, such as a cold, should not result in the deferral of vaccination.

SYNFLORIX should under no circumstances be administered intravascularly or intradermally. No data are available on subcutaneous administration of SYNFLORIX.

SYNFLORIX will not protect against pneumococcal serogroups that are not included in the vaccine. The observed immune responses to the vaccine varied with each of the vaccine serotypes. Although antibody response to diphtheria toxoid, tetanus toxoid and protein D (protein D is highly conserved in all *H. influenzae* strains including NTHi) occurs, immunization with SYNFLORIX does not substitute routine immunization with diphtheria, tetanus or *H. influenzae* type b vaccines. Official recommendations for the immunizations against diphtheria, tetanus and *H. influenzae* type b should also be followed.

Safety and immunogenicity data in children with increased risk for pneumococcal infections (sickle cell disease, congenital and acquired splenic dysfunction, HIV-infected, malignancy, nephrotic syndrome) are not available.

Children with impaired immune responsiveness, whether due to the use of immunosuppressive therapy, a genetic defect, HIV infection, or other causes, may have reduced antibody response to vaccination.

Prophylactic administration of antipyretics before or immediately after vaccine administration can reduce the incidence and intensity of post-vaccination febrile reactions. Data however, suggest that the use of prophylactic acetaminophen might reduce the immune response to SYNFLORIX. The clinical relevance of this observation as well as the impact of antipyretics other than acetaminophen remains unknown.

The potential risk of apnoea and the need for respiratory monitoring for 48-72h should be considered when administering the primary immunization series to very premature infants (born ≤28 weeks of gestation) and particularly for those with a previous history of respiratory immaturity. As the benefit of vaccination is high in this group of infants, vaccination should not be withheld or delayed.

SYNFLORIX is indicated and intended for use in children up to 24 months of age. For appropriate usage of SYNFLORIX across age groups, children below 2 years of age should receive the appropriate-for-age SYNFLORIX vaccination series (see Indications and Clinical Use).

Hematologic: As for other vaccines administered intramuscularly, SYNFLORIX should be given with caution to individuals with thrombocytopenia or any coagulation disorder since bleeding may occur following an intramuscular administration to these subjects.

Immune: As with all injectable vaccines, appropriate medical treatment and supervision should always be readily available in case of a rare anaphylactic event following the administration of the vaccine.

Syringe components contain latex.

As with any vaccine, a protective immune response may not be elicited in all vaccinees.

Special Populations: Pregnant Women: As SYNFLORIX is not intended for use in adults, adequate human data on use during pregnancy and adequate animal reproduction studies are not available.

Nursing Women: As SYNFLORIX is not intended for use in adults, adequate human data on use during lactation and adequate animal reproduction studies are not available.

Geriatrics (>65 years of age): Studies have not been conducted in adults 65 years and older.

ADVERSE REACTIONS: Clinical Trial Adverse Drug Reactions: Because clinical trials are conducted under very specific conditions the adverse reaction rates observed in the clinical trials may not reflect the rates observed in practice and should not be compared to the rates in the clinical trials of another drug. Adverse drug reaction information from clinical trials is useful for identifying drug-related adverse events and for approximating rates.

Clinical trials involved the administration of 12 879 doses of SYNFLORIX to 4595 healthy children as primary vaccination. Three thousand, eight hundred and seventy infants received a booster dose of SYNFLORIX in the second year of life. In all trials, SYNFLORIX was administered concurrently with the recommended childhood vaccines.

No increase in the incidence or severity of the adverse reactions was seen with subsequent doses of the primary vaccination series.

An increase in reactogenicity was reported after booster vaccination compared to the doses of the primary course with SYNFLORIX.

The most common adverse reactions observed after primary vaccination were redness at the injection site and irritability which occurred after 38.3% and 52.3% of all doses respectively. Following booster vaccination, these adverse reactions occurred at 52.6% and 55.4% respectively. The majority of these reactions were of mild to moderate severity and were not long lasting.

Adverse reactions (following primary immunization or booster dose) considered as being at least possibly related to vaccination have been categorised by frequency (see Table 1).

Table 1: SYNFLORIX

Adverse Reactions Considered as Being at Least Possibly Related to Vaccination

Frequency	Adverse Reactions
Very common (≥1/10)	drowsiness, appetite loss, pain, redness, swelling at the injection site, fever (≥38°C rectally), irritability
Common (≥1/100 to <1/10)	injection site induration, fever (>39°C rectally)
Uncommon (≥1/1000 to <1/100)	diarrhoea, vomiting, injection site haematoma, haemorrhage and nodule, fever (>40°C rectally)[a], crying abnormal, apnoea in very premature infants (≤28 weeks of gestation)
Rare (≥1/10 000 to <1/1000)	febrile and non-febrile convulsions, rash, urticaria, allergic reactions (such as allergic dermatitis, atopic dermatitis, eczema)

[a] Reported following booster vaccination.

The incidence of solicited local and general adverse events reported within 4 days after each vaccination dose of SYNFLORIX was within the same range as after vaccination with PREVNAR (see Table 2).

Table 2: SYNFLORIX

Percentage of Subjects Reporting Local and General Adverse Events Within 4 Days (day 0-3) Following Each Dose in Primary Vaccination Course and After a Booster Dose of SYNFLORIX or PREVNAR in Primary Study 10PN-PD-DIT-001 and Subsequent Booster Study 10PN-PD-DIT-007

	Dose 1		Dose 2		Dose 3		Dose 4	
	SYN-FLORIX	PRE-VNAR	SYN-FLORIX	PRE-VNAR	SYN-FLORIX	PRE-VNAR	SYN-FLORIX	PRE-VNAR
Local Symptom	N=1230	N=415	N=1217	N=414	N=1216	N=411	N=735	N=91
Pain	35.5	27.2	27.8	26.8	22.8	23.4	56.6	49.5
Redness	37.3	38.3	37.6	39.1	37.8	36.3	51.7	57.1
Swelling	28.9	26	30.1	27.8	28.3	24.6	36.9	38.5
General Symptom								
Fever ≥38°C	36.7	30.1	35.3	39.6	25.6	31.4	33.3	36.3
Fever >39°C	2	1.4	2.2	2.4	1.8	2.4	3.3	7.7
Irritability	66.1	64.6	61.5	61.8	51.2	55.5	59.6	60.4
Drowsiness	58	54.7	47.5	45.2	33.1	35.3	41.2	52.7
Loss of appetite	29.8	28.4	23.7	23.4	16.9	21.9	31.3	34.1

Study 10PN-PD-DIT-001=3 doses of SYNFLORIX or PREVNAR+ DTPa-HBV-IPV/Hib at 2, 3 and 4 months of age.
Study 10PN-PD-DIT-007=1 dose of SYNFLORIX or PREVNAR + DTPa-HBV-IPV/Hib at 12 to 18 months of age

Swelling Reactions: In the clinical programme, the occurrence of large swelling reactions (i.e. swelling with a diameter >50 mm, noticeable diffuse swelling or noticeable increase of limb circumference) was solicited in subjects ≥11 months of age, following booster or catch-up vaccination. Seven (out of 2086) subjects reported large swelling reactions after a booster dose at the SYNFLORIX injection site and four (out of 300) subjects reported a large swelling reaction after catch-up immunization. All swellings were local and limited to the injection site, all occurred within three days of vaccination, and all resolved within three days.

Serious Adverse Events (SAE): Five out of 4145 subjects (0.1%) receiving primary vaccination with SYNFLORIX and two out of 1072 PREVNAR vaccinees (0.2%) experienced an SAE that was assessed by the investigator as causally related to vaccination. In booster studies four out of 3725 subjects (0.1%) receiving a booster dose of SYNFLORIX and none of the 449 PREVNAR vaccinees reported an SAE that was assessed by the investigator as causally related to vaccination.

Deaths: In primary vaccination studies, two (out of 4145) SYNFLORIX vaccinees (receiving 12 137 doses) experienced serious adverse events with a fatal outcome. These serious adverse events included one case of Sudden Infant Death Syndrome (SIDS) and one case of brain neoplasm. One out of 1072 PREVNAR vaccinees died due to muscle atrophy. None of the fatal cases were assessed by the investigator as causally related to vaccination. No fatal serious adverse events were reported in the completed booster and catch-up immunization studies.

DRUG INTERACTIONS: Drug-Drug Interactions: Use with Other Vaccines: SYNFLORIX can be given concomitantly with any of the following monovalent or combination vaccines [including DTPa-HBV-IPV/Hib]: diphtheria-tetanus-acellular pertussis vaccine (DTPa), hepatitis B vaccine (HBV), inactivated polio vaccine (IPV), *H. influenzae* type b vaccine (Hib), measles-mumps-rubella vaccine (MMR), varicella vaccine, meningococcal serogroup C conjugate vaccine (CRM_{197} and TT conjugates), and rotavirus vaccine. Different injectable vaccines should always be given at different injections sites.

Clinical studies demonstrated that the immune responses of the co-administered vaccines were unaffected, with the exception of the inactivated poliovirus type 2 response, for which inconsistent results were observed across studies (seroprotection ranging from 78% to 100%). The clinical relevance of this observation is not known. No negative interference was observed with meningococcal conjugate vaccines irrespective of the carrier protein (CRM_{197} and TT conjugates). Enhancement of antibody response to Hib-TT conjugate, diphtheria and tetanus antigens was observed.

The safety profiles of the co-administered vaccines appeared unaffected.

Use with Systemic Immunosuppressive Medications: As with other vaccines it may be expected that in patients receiving immunosuppressive treatment an adequate response may not be elicited.

Use with Propylatic Administration of Antipyretics: See Warnings and Precautions, General.

Drug-Food Interactions: Interactions with food have not been established.

Drug-Herb Interactions: Interactions with herbal products have not been established.

Drug-Laboratory Test Interactions: Interactions with laboratory tests have not been established.

DOSAGE AND ADMINISTRATION: Dosing Considerations: Official recommendations should be taken into account when immunizing with SYNFLORIX.

It is recommended that subjects who receive a first dose of SYNFLORIX complete the full vaccination course with SYNFLORIX.

Recommended Dose and Dosage Adjustment: Infants from 6 Weeks to 6 Months of Age: The primary vaccination schedule consists of three doses of 0.5 mL with an interval of at least 1 month between doses.

Results available to date suggest a 2-4-6 month schedule provides a better immune response as compared with 2-3-4 or 3-4-5 month schedules.

A booster dose is recommended at least 6 months after the last priming dose and preferably between 12 and 15 months of age.

Previously Unvaccinated Older Infants and Children: Infants Aged 7-11 Months: The vaccination schedule consists of two doses of 0.5 mL with an interval of at least 1 month between doses. A third dose is recommended in the second year of life with an interval of at least 2 months between doses.

Children Aged 12-23 Months: The vaccination schedule consists of two doses of 0.5 mL with an interval of at least 2 months between doses.

The immune response elicited after two doses of SYNFLORIX in children 12-23 months of age is comparable to the response elicited after three doses in infants. The immune response to a booster dose after two doses in children aged 12-23 months has not been evaluated, but a booster dose may be needed to ensure optimal protection. A 2-dose schedule in 12-23 month children with high risk of pneumococcal disease (such as children with sickle-cell disease, asplenia, HIV infection, chronic illness or who are immunocompromised) may not be sufficient to provide optimal protection.

Administration: Use of pre-filled syringes: see Special Handling Instructions.

SYNFLORIX should be given by intramuscular injection. The preferred sites are anterolateral aspect of the thigh in infants or the deltoid muscle of the upper arm in children.

A fine white deposit with a clear colourless supernatant may be observed upon storage of the syringe/vial. This does not constitute a sign of deterioration.

The content of the syringe/vial should be inspected visually both before and after shaking for any foreign particulate matter and/or abnormal physical appearance prior to administration. In the event of either being observed, discard the vaccine.

Shake well before use.

Any unused product or waste material should be disposed of in accordance with local requirements.

OVERDOSAGE:
Insufficient data are available.

For management of a suspected drug overdose, CPhA recommends that you contact your **regional Poison Control Centre**. See the *CPS* Directory section for a list of Poison Control Centres.

ACTION AND CLINICAL PHARMACOLOGY: Epidemiological Data: Invasive Pneumococcal Disease (IPD): IPD is a severe illness that occurs when bacteria invade normally sterile sites. *S. pneumoniae* is the primary cause of IPD, which manifests as bacteraemia, bacteraemic pneumonia and meningitis. IPD can result in serious morbidity and mortality, particularly in children, even in developed countries with high standards of healthcare. Routine use of PREVNAR has decreased the incidence of IPD considerably: a Calgary research team that collected population-based surveillance data from 1998 to 2004 found an 81.6% decrease in the overall incidence of IPD in children 23 months of age and younger (63.6 to 11.7 cases/100 000 population). However, there has been an emergence of cases in Canada and worldwide from serotypes not included in the vaccine. Rates of IPD due to serotypes 1, 7F and 19A have increased in children, while serotype 5 has led to IPD outbreaks in adults. The causes of this changing epidemiology are unknown.

Mechanism of Action: SYNFLORIX is a conjugate vaccine, adsorbed, composed of 10 active ingredients: the *S. pneumoniae* polysaccharide serotypes 1, 4, 5, 6B, 7F, 9V, 14, 18C, 19F and 23F, each conjugated to a carrier protein (protein D (PD), tetanus toxoid (TT) or diphtheria toxoid (DT)).

The carrier proteins (PD, TT and DT) provide T-cell help to B-cells to produce a boostable antibody response of high affinity to the polysaccharide antigens, thereby providing protection against bacterial tract infections caused by *S. pneumoniae*.

The amount of pneumococcal capsular polysaccharide antibodies elicited by the vaccine is measured by enzyme-linked immunosorbent assay (ELISA). These antibodies help to protect the host by facilitating opsonization of pneumococci and thus facilitating phagocytosis. The ability of a serum sample to facilitate opsonization of bacteria can be measured by in vitro opsonophagocytosis assays. It is generally agreed that opsonophagocytic activity (OPA) is the best functional correlate of protection against IPD.

STORAGE AND STABILITY: Store in a refrigerator (2-8°C). Do not freeze. Discard the vaccine if frozen.

Store in the original package in order to protect from light.

Do not use after the expiry date shown on the label.

SYNFLORIX should be administered as soon as possible after being removed from the refrigerator. However, stability data generated indicate that SYNFLORIX remains stable and can be administered in case the vaccine has been stored outside the refrigerator up to three days at temperatures between 8°C and 25°C or up to one day at temperatures between 25°C and 37°C. These data are not recommendations for storage. If exposed to temperatures >37°C, discard vaccine.

SPECIAL HANDLING INSTRUCTIONS: In the absence of compatibility studies, SYNFLORIX must not be mixed with other medicinal products.

Use of Pre-Filled Syringes: Do not remove the white back-stop from the syringe. Prior to administration, ensure that the plunger rod is firmly attached to the rubber stopper by turning the plunger clockwise until slight resistance is felt. **Do not** over tighten. Remove syringe LUER Tip-cap and needle cap. Attach needle by pressing and twisting in a clockwise rotation until secured to the syringe.

INFORMATION FOR THE PATIENT: Published in e-CPS, available by subscription at www.e-cps.ca.

DOSAGE FORMS, COMPOSITION AND PACKAGING: SYNFLORIX is available as a suspension for injection.

Table 3: SYNFLORIX

Composition: One dose (0.5 mL) contains

Pneumococcal polysaccharide serotype 1[a,b]	1 µg
Pneumococcal polysaccharide serotype 4[a,b]	3 µg
Pneumococcal polysaccharide serotype 5[a,b]	1 µg
Pneumococcal polysaccharide serotype 6B[a,b]	1 µg

(cont'd)

Table 3: SYNFLORIX *(cont'd)*

Composition: One dose (0.5 mL) contains

Pneumococcal polysaccharide serotype 7F[a,b]	1 µg
Pneumococcal polysaccharide serotype 9V[a,b]	1 µg
Pneumococcal polysaccharide serotype 14[a,b]	1 µg
Pneumococcal polysaccharide serotype 18C[a,c]	3 µg
Pneumococcal polysaccharide serotype 19F[a,d]	3 µg
Pneumococcal polysaccharide serotype 23F[a,b]	1 µg

[a] Adsorbed on aluminium phosphate: 0.5 mg Al^{3+}.
[b] Conjugated to protein D (derived from Non-Typeable *H. influenzae*) carrier protein: 9-16 µg.
[c] Conjugated to tetanus toxoid carrier protein: 5-10 µg.
[d] Conjugated to diphtheria toxoid carrier protein: 3-6 µg.

Additional Excipients: sodium chloride and water for injection.

Pre-filled Syringes: 0.5 mL of suspension in a pre-filled syringe (type I glass) for 1 dose with a plunger stopper (rubber butyl) with or without needles, pack sizes of 1 and 10. Syringe components contain latex.

Vials: 0.5 mL of suspension in a vial (type I glass) for 1 dose with a stopper (rubber butyl), pack sizes of 1, 10 and 100; 1 mL of suspension in a vial (type I glass) for 2 doses with a stopper (rubber butyl), pack size of 100.

Synphasic® ℞

norethindrone—ethinyl estradiol

Oral Contraceptive

Pfizer

PHARMACOLOGY: Estrogen-progestogen combinations act primarily through the mechanism of gonadotropin suppression due to the estrogenic and progestational activity of their components. Although the primary mechanism of action is inhibition of ovulation, alterations in the cervical mucus and the endometrium may also contribute to effectiveness.

INDICATIONS: Prevention of pregnancy.

CONTRAINDICATIONS: History of or actual thrombophlebitis or thromboembolic disorders; history of or actual cerebrovascular disorders; history of or actual myocardial infarction or coronary arterial disease; active liver disease or history of or actual benign or malignant liver tumors; history of or known or suspected carcinoma of the breast; history of or known or suspected estrogen-dependent neoplasia; undiagnosed abnormal vaginal bleeding; any ocular lesion arising from ophthalmic vascular disease, such as partial or complete loss of vision or defect in visual fields; when pregnancy is suspected or diagnosed.

WARNINGS: Predisposing Factors for Coronary Artery Disease: Cigarette smoking increases the risk of serious cardiovascular side effects and mortality. Birth control pills increase this risk, especially with increasing age. Convincing data are available to support an upper age limit of 35 years for oral contraceptive use in women who smoke.

Other women who are independently at high risk for cardiovascular disease include those with diabetes, hypertension, abnormal lipid profile, or a family history of these. Whether oral contraceptives accentuate this risk is unclear.

In low risk, nonsmoking women of any age, the benefits of oral contraceptive use outweigh the possible cardiovascular risks associated with low-dose formulations. Consequently, oral contraceptives may be prescribed for these women up to the age of menopause.

> Cigarette smoking increases the risk of serious adverse effects on the heart and blood vessels. This risk increases with age and becomes significant in oral contraceptive users over 35 years of age. Women should be counselled not to smoke.

Discontinue Medication at the Earliest Manifestation of the Following:

A. Thromboembolic and cardiovascular disorders such as: thrombophlebitis, pulmonary embolism, cerebrovascular disorders, myocardial ischemia, mesenteric thrombosis and retinal thrombosis.

B. Conditions that predispose to venous stasis and to vascular thrombosis, e.g., immobilization after accidents or confinement to bed during long-term illness. Other nonhormonal methods of contraception should be used until regular activities are resumed. For use of oral contraceptives when surgery is contemplated, see Precautions.

C. Visual defects, partial or complete.

D. Papilledema or ophthalmic vascular lesions.

E. Severe headache of unknown etiology or worsening of pre-existing migraine headache.

PRECAUTIONS: Physical Examination and Followup: Before oral contraceptives are used, a thorough history and physical examination should be performed, including a blood pressure determination. Breasts, liver, extremities and pelvic organs should be examined and a Papanicolaou smear should be taken if the patient has been sexually active.

The first followup visit should be done 3 months after oral contraceptives are prescribed. Thereafter, examinations should be performed at least once a year or more frequently if indicated. At each annual visit, examination should include those procedures that were done at the initial visit as outlined above or per recommendations of the Canadian Workshop on Screening for Cancer of the Cervix. Their suggestion was that, for women who had 2 consecutive negative Pap smears, screening could be continued every 3 years up to the age of 69.

Pregnancy: Fetal abnormalities have been reported to occur in the offspring of women who have taken estrogen-progestogen combinations in early pregnancy. Rule out pregnancy as soon as it is suspected.

Lactation: The use of oral contraceptives during the period a mother is breast-feeding her infant may not be advisable. The hormonal components are excreted in breast milk and may reduce its quantity and quality. The long-term effects on the developing child are not known.

Hepatic Function: Patients who have had jaundice including a history of cholestatic jaundice during pregnancy should be given oral contraceptives with great care and under close observation.

The development of severe generalized pruritus or icterus requires that the medication be withdrawn until the problem is resolved.

If a patient develops jaundice that proves to be cholestatic in type, the use of oral contraceptives should not be resumed. In patients taking oral contraceptives, changes in the composition of the bile may occur and an increased incidence of gallstones has been reported.

Hepatic nodules have been reported to be associated with use of oral contraceptives, particularly in long-term users of oral contraceptives. These nodules include benign hepatic adenomas, focal nodular hyperplasia and other hepatic lesions. In addition, hepatocellular carcinoma has been reported. Although these lesions are extremely rare, they have caused fatal intra-abdominal hemorrhage and should be considered in women presenting with an abdominal mass, acute abdominal pain, or evidence of intra-abdominal bleeding.

Hypertension: Patients with essential hypertension whose blood pressure is well-controlled may be given oral contraceptives but only under close supervision. If a significant elevation of blood pressure in previously normotensive or hypertensive subjects occurs at any time during the administration of the drug, cessation of medication is necessary.

Migraine and Headache: The onset or exacerbation of migraine or the development of headache of a new pattern which is recurrent, persistent or severe, requires discontinuation of oral contraceptives and evaluation of the cause.

Diabetes: Current low dose oral contraceptives exert minimal impact on glucose metabolism. Diabetic patients, or those with a family history of diabetes, should be observed closely to detect any worsening of carbohydrate metabolism. Patients predisposed to diabetes who can be kept under close supervision may be given oral contraceptives. Young diabetic patients whose disease is of recent origin, well-controlled, and not associated with hypertension or other signs of vascular disease such as ocular fundal changes should be monitored more frequently while using oral contraceptives.

Ocular Disorders: Patients who are pregnant or are taking oral contraceptives may experience corneal edema that may cause visual disturbances and changes in tolerance to contact lenses, especially of the rigid type. Soft contact lenses usually do not cause disturbances. If visual changes or alterations in tolerance to contact lenses occur, temporary or permanent cessation of wear may be advised.

Breasts: Increasing age and a strong family history are the most significant risk factors for the development of breast cancer. Other established risk factors include obesity, nulliparity and late age at first full-term pregnancy. The identified groups of women that may be at increased risk of developing breast cancer before menopause are long-term users of oral contraceptives (more than 8 years) and starters at early age. In a few women, the use of oral contraceptives may accelerate the growth of an existing but undiagnosed breast cancer. Since any potential increased risk related to oral contraceptive use is small, there is no reason to change prescribing habits at present.

Women receiving oral contraceptives should be instructed in self-examination of their breasts. Their physicians should be notified whenever any masses are detected. A yearly clinical breast examination is also recommended because, if a breast cancer should develop, drugs that contain estrogen may cause a rapid progression.

Vaginal Bleeding: Persistent irregular vaginal bleeding requires assessment to exclude underlying pathology.

Fibroids: Patients with fibroids (leiomyomata) should be carefully observed. Sudden enlargement, pain, or tenderness requires discontinuation of the use of oral contraceptives.

Emotional Disorders: Patients with a history of emotional disturbances, especially the depressive type, may be more prone to have a recurrence of depression while taking oral contraceptives. In cases of a serious recurrence, a trial of an alternate method of contraception should be made which may help to clarify the possible relationship. Women with premenstrual syndrome (PMS) may have a varied response to oral contraceptives, ranging from symptomatic improvement to worsening of the condition.

Metabolic and Endocrine Diseases: In metabolic or endocrine diseases and when metabolism of calcium and phosphorus is abnormal, careful clinical evaluation should precede medication and a regular followup is recommended.

Connective Tissue Disease: The use of oral contraceptives in some women has been associated with positive lupus erythematous cell tests and with clinical lupus erythematous. In some instances exacerbation of rheumatoid arthritis and synovitis have been observed.

Laboratory Tests: Results of laboratory tests should be interpreted in light of the fact that the patient is on oral contraceptives. The laboratory tests listed below are modified.

A. Liver function tests: Aspartate serum transaminase (AST): variously reported elevations. Alkaline phosphatase and gamma glutamine transaminase (GGT): slightly elevated.

B. Coagulation tests: Minimal elevation of test values reported for such parameters as Factors VII, VIII, IX and X. Increased platelet aggregation. Decreased antithrombin III.

C. Thyroid function tests: Protein binding of thyroxine is increased as indicated by increased total serum thyroxine concentrations and decreased T_3 resin uptake.

D. Lipoproteins: Small changes of unproven clinical significance may occur in lipoprotein cholesterol fractions.

E. Gonadotropins: LH and FSH levels are suppressed by the use of oral contraceptives. Wait 2 weeks after discontinuing the use of oral contraceptives before measurements are made.

Tissue Specimens: Pathologists should be advised of oral contraceptive therapy when specimens obtained from surgical procedures and Pap smears are submitted for examination.

Return to Fertility: After discontinuing oral contraceptive therapy, the patient should delay pregnancy until at least 1 normal spontaneous cycle has occurred in order to date the pregnancy. An alternative contraceptive method should be used during this time.

Amenorrhea: Women having a history of oligomenorrhea, secondary amenorrhea, or irregular cycles may remain anovulatory or become amenorrheic following discontinuation of estrogen-progestin combination therapy.

Amenorrhea, especially if associated with breast secretion, that continues for 6 months or more after withdrawal, warrants a careful assessment of hypothalamic-pituitary function.

Thromboembolic Complications—Postsurgery: There is an increased risk of postsurgery thromboembolic complications in oral contraceptive users, after major surgery. If feasible, oral contraceptives should be discontinued and an alternative method substituted at least 1 month prior to **major** elective surgery. Oral contraceptives should not be resumed until the first menstrual period after hospital discharge following surgery.

Drug Interactions: The concurrent administration of oral contraceptives with other drugs may result in an altered response to either agent. Reduced effectiveness of the oral contraceptive, should it occur, is more likely with the low dose formulations. It is important to ascertain all drugs that a patient is taking, both prescription and nonprescription, before oral contraceptives are prescribed.

Refer to the revised 1994 Report on Oral Contraceptives, Health Canada, for possible drug interactions with oral contraceptives.

Noncontraceptive Benefits of Oral Contraceptives: Several health advantages other than contraception have been reported.

Effects on menses: Increased menstrual cycle regularity; decreased menstrual blood loss; decreased incidence of iron deficiency anemia secondary to reduced menstrual blood loss; decreased incidence of dysmenorrhea.

Effects related to ovulation inhibition: Decreased incidence of functional ovarian cysts; decreased incidence of ectopic pregnancy.

Effects on other organs of the reproductive tract: Decreased incidence of acute salpingitis; decreased incidence of endometrial cancer (50%); decreased incidence of ovarian cancer (40%); potential beneficial effects on endometriosis; improvement of acne vulgaris, hirsutism, and other androgen-mediated disorders.

Effects on breasts: Decreased incidence of benign breast disease (fibroadenomas and fibrocystic breast disease); decreased incidence of breast biopsies.

The noncontraceptive benefits of oral contraceptives should be considered in addition to the efficacy of these preparations when counselling patients regarding contraceptive method selection.

> Oral contraceptives **do not protect** against sexually transmitted diseases (STDs) including HIV/AIDS. For protection against STDs, it is advisable to use latex condoms **in combination with** oral contraceptives.

ADVERSE EFFECTS: An increased risk of the following serious adverse reactions has been associated with the use of oral contraceptives: thrombophlebitis; pulmonary embolism; mesenteric thrombosis; neuro-ocular lesions, e.g., retinal thrombosis; myocardial infarction; cerebral thrombosis; cerebral hemorrhage; hypertension; benign hepatic tumors; gallbladder disease.

The following adverse reactions also have been reported in patients receiving oral contraceptives: Nausea and vomiting, usually the most common adverse reaction, occurs in approximately 10% or less of patients during the first cycle. Other reactions, as a general rule, are seen less frequently or only occasionally.

Other adverse reactions: gastrointestinal symptoms (such as abdominal cramps and bloating); breakthrough bleeding; spotting; change in menstrual flow; dysmenorrhea; amenorrhea during and after treatment; infertility after discontinuance of treatment; edema; chloasma or melasma which may persist; breast changes: tenderness, enlargement, and secretion; change in weight (increase or decrease); endocervical hyperplasias; possible diminution in lactation when given immediately post-partum; cholestatic jaundice; migraine; increase in size of uterine leiomyomata; rash (allergic); mental depression; reduced tolerance to carbohydrates; vaginal candidiasis; premenstrual-like syndrome; intolerance to contact lenses; change in corneal curvature (steepening); cataracts; optic neuritis; retinal thrombosis; changes in libido; chorea; changes in appetite; cystitis-like syndrome; rhinitis; headache; nervousness; dizziness; hirsutism; loss of scalp hair; erythema multiforme; erythema nodosum; hemorrhagic eruption; vaginitis; porphyria; impaired renal function; Raynaud's phenomenon; auditory disturbances; hemolytic uremic syndrome; pancreatitis; arterial thromboembolism.

OVERDOSE:

Symptoms: Numerous cases of the ingestion, by children, of estrogen-progestogen combinations have been reported. Although mild nausea may occur, there appears to be no other reaction.

Treatment: Treatment should be limited to a laxative such as citrate of magnesia with the aim of removing unabsorbed material as rapidly as possible.

> For management of a suspected drug overdose, CPhA recommends that you contact your **regional Poison Control Centre**. See the *CPS* Directory section for a list of Poison Control Centres.

DOSAGE: Information for the Patient on How to Take the Birth Control Pill:

1. **Read these directions:**
   - before you start taking your pills, and
   - any time you are not sure what to do.
2. **Look at your pill pack** to see if it has 21 or 28 pills:
   - 21-Pill Pack: 21 active pills (with hormones) taken daily for 3 weeks, and then take no pills for 1 week

or

- 28-Pill Pack: 21 active pills (with hormones) taken daily for 3 weeks, and then 7 "reminder" pills (no hormones) taken daily for 1 week.

 Also check the pill pack for instructions on (1) where to start and (2) directions to take pills (see package insert for illustrations).

3. It is recommended that you use a second method of birth control (e.g., latex condoms and spermicidal foam or gel) for the first 7 days of the first cycle of pill use. This will provide a back-up in case pills are forgotten while you are getting used to taking them.
4. **When receiving any medical treatment, be sure to tell your doctor that you are using birth control pills.**
5. **Many women have spotting or light bleeding or may feel sick to their stomach during the first 3 months on the pill.** If you do feel sick, do not stop taking the pill. The problem will usually go away. If it does not go away, check with your doctor or clinic.
6. **Missing pills also can cause some spotting or light bleeding**, even if you make up the missed pills. You also could feel a little sick to your stomach on the days you take 2 pills to make up for missed pills.
7. **If you miss pills at any time, you could get pregnant. The greatest risks for pregnancy are:**
   - when you start a pack late, or
   - when you miss pills at the beginning or at the very end of the pack.
8. **Always be sure you have ready:**
   - **another kind of birth control** (such as latex condoms and spermicidal foam or gel) to use as a backup in case you miss pills, and
   - **an extra, full pack of pills.**
9. **If you experience vomiting or diarrhea, or if you take certain medicines**, such as antibiotics, your pills may not work as well. Use a backup method, such as latex condoms and spermicidal foam or gel, until you can check with your doctor or clinic.
10. **If you forget more than 1 pill 2 months in a row**, talk to your doctor or clinic about how to make pill-taking easier or using another method of birth control.
11. **If your questions are not answered here, call your doctor or clinic.**

When to start the first pack of pills: Be sure to read these instructions:

- before you start taking your pills, and
- any time you are not sure what to do.

Decide with your doctor or clinic what is the best day for you to start taking your first pack of pills. Your pills may be either a 21-day or a 28-day type.

A. 21-Day Combination: With this type of birth control pill, you are on pills for 21 days and off pills for 7 days. You must not be off the pills for more than 7 days in a row.

1. **The first day of your menstrual period (bleeding) is Day 1 of your cycle.** Your doctor may advise you to start taking the pills on Day 1, on Day 5, or on the first Sunday after your period begins. If your period starts on Sunday, start that same day.
2. Take 1 pill at approximately the same time every day for 21 days; **then take no pills for 7 days**. Start a new pack on the 8th day. You will probably have a period during the 7 days off the pill. (This bleeding may be lighter and shorter than your usual period.)

B. 28-Day Combination: With this type of birth control pill, you take 21 pills which contain hormones and 7 pills which contain no hormones.

1. **The first day of your menstrual period (bleeding) is Day 1 of your cycle.** Your doctor may advise you to start taking the pills on Day 1, on Day 5, or on the first Sunday after your period begins. If your period starts on Sunday, start that same day.
2. Take 1 pill at approximately the same time every day for 28 days. Begin a new pack the next day, **not missing any days**. Your period should occur during the last 7 days of using that pill pack.

What to do during the month:

1. **Take a pill at approximately the same time every day until the pack is empty.**
   - Try to associate taking your pill with some regular activity like eating a meal or going to bed.
   - Do not skip pills even if you have bleeding between monthly periods or feel sick to your stomach (nausea).
   - Do not skip pills even if you do not have sex very often.
2. **When you finish a pack:**
   - **21 pills: Wait 7 days** to start the next pack. Your will have your period during that week.
   - **28 pills:** Start the next pack **on the next day**. Take 1 pill every day. Do not wait any days between packs.

What to do if you miss pills: Table 1 outlines the actions you should take if you miss 1 or more of your birth control pills. Match the number of pills missed with the appropriate starting time for your type of pill pack.

Table 1: Synphasic

What to Do if You Miss Pills

Sunday Start	**Other Than Sunday Start**
Miss 1 pill	**Miss 1 pill**
Take it as soon as you remember, and take the next pill at the usual time. This means that you might take 2 pills in one day.	Take it as soon as you remember, and take the next pill at the usual time. This means that you might take 2 pills in one day.
Miss 2 pills in a row	**Miss 2 pills in a row**
First 2 Weeks: 1. Take 2 pills the day you remember and 2 pills the next day. 2. Then take 1 pill a day until you finish the pack. 3. Use a backup method of birth control if you have sex in the 7 days after you miss the pills. **Third Week:** 1. Keep taking 1 pill a day until Sunday. 2. On Sunday, safely discard the rest of the pack and start a new pack that day. 3. Use a backup method of birth control if you have sex in the 7 days after you miss the pills. 4. You may not have a period this month. **If you miss 2 periods in a row, call your doctor or clinic.**	**First 2 Weeks:** 1. Take 2 pills the day you remember and 2 pills the next day. 2. Then take 1 pill a day until you finish the pack. 3. Use a backup method of birth control if you have sex in the 7 days after you miss the pills. **Third Week:** 1. Safely dispose of the rest of the pill pack and start a new pack that same day. 2. Use a backup method of birth control if you have sex in the 7 days after you miss the pills. 3. You may not have a period this month. **If you miss 2 periods in a row, call your doctor or clinic.**
Miss 3 or more pills in a row	**Miss 3 or more pills in a row**
Anytime in the Cycle: 1. Keep taking 1 pill a day until Sunday. 2. On Sunday, safely discard the rest of the pack and start a new pack that day. 3. Use a backup method of birth control if you have sex in the 7 days after you miss the pills. 4. You may not have a period this month. **If you miss 2 periods in a row, call your doctor or clinic.**	**Anytime in the Cycle:** 1. Safely dispose of the rest of the pill pack and start a new pack that same day. 2. Use a backup method of birth control if you have sex in the 7 days after you miss the pills. 3. You may not have a period this month. **If you miss 2 periods in a row, call your doctor or clinic.**

Note: 28-Day Pack: If you forget any of the 7 "reminder" pills (without hormones) in Week 4, just safely dispose of the pills you missed. Then keep taking 1 pill each day until the pack is empty. You do not need to use a backup method.

Always be sure you have on hand:

- a backup method of birth control (such as latex condoms and spermicidal foam or gel) in case you miss pills, and
- an extra, full pack of pills.

If you forget more than 1 pill 2 months in a row, talk to your doctor or clinic about ways to make pill-taking easier or about using another method of birth control.

Dosage: **A. 21-Day Pack:** With this type of birth control pill, the patient is 21 days on pills with 7 days off pills. The patient must not be off the pills for more than 7 days in a row.

1. **The first day of the patient's menstrual period (bleeding) is day 1 of a cycle.** The doctor may advise the patient to start taking the pills on Day 1, on Day 5, or on the first Sunday after a period begins. If a period starts on Sunday, the patient starts that same day.
2. The pack must be labelled correctly before starting. The pack is pre-printed with a Sunday starting day. If the patient is starting on a day other than a Sunday, she should use the Flexi-start sticker labels provided. The patient peels off the label with the chosen starting day and applies it over the pre-printed days on top of the card.
3. The patient takes 1 pill at approximately the same time every day for 21 days; **then she takes no pills for 7 days**. She starts a new pack on the 8th day. She will probably have a period during the 7 days off the pill. (This bleeding may be lighter and shorter than a usual period.)

B. 28-Day Pack: With this type of birth control pill, the patient takes 21 pills which contain hormones and 7 pills which contain no hormones.

1. **The first day of the patient's menstrual period (bleeding) is day 1 of a cycle.** The doctor may advise the patient to start taking the pills on Day 1, on Day 5, or on the first Sunday after a period begins. If a period starts on Sunday, the patient starts that same day.
2. The pack must be labelled correctly before starting. The pack is pre-printed with a Sunday starting day. If the patient is starting on a day other than a Sunday, she should use the Flexi-start sticker labels provided. The patient peels off the label with the chosen starting day and applies it over the pre-printed days on top of the card.
3. The patient takes 1 pill at approximately the same time every day for 28 days. She begins a new pack the next day, **not missing any days on the pills**. The patient's period should occur during the last 7 days of using that pill pack.

What to do during the month:

1. **The patient takes a pill at approximately the same time every day until the pack is empty.**
   - The patient should try to associate taking the pill with some regular activity like eating a meal or going to bed.
   - The patient must not skip pills even if she has bleeding between monthly periods or feels sick to her stomach (nausea).
   - The patient must not skip pills even if she does not have sex very often.
2. **When a pack is finished:**
   - **21 Pills: The patient must wait 7 days** to start the next pack. A period will begin during that week.
   - **28 Pills:** The patient starts the next pack **on the next day**. She takes 1 pill every day. She does not wait any days between packs.

INFORMATION FOR THE PATIENT: Published in e-CPS, available by subscription at www.e-cps.ca.

SUPPLIED: Each white circular tablet, impressed "SEARLE" on one side and "BX" on the other side, contains: norethindrone 1 mg and ethinyl estradiol 0.035 mg, and each blue circular tablet, impressed "SEARLE" on one side and "BX" on the other side, contains: norethindrone 0.5 mg and ethinyl estradiol 0.035 mg. Inert orange tablets are impressed "SEARLE" on one side and "P" on the other. Nonmedicinal ingredients: Active tablets: cornstarch, FD&C Blue No. 2, lactose hydrous, magnesium stearate and polyvidone. Placebo tablets: FD&C Yellow No. 6 Lake, lactose, lactose monohydrate, magnesium stearate and microcrystalline cellulose. Available in 21-day and 28-day dispensers. Store below 25°C.

(Shown in Product Identification Section)

Synthroid® P

levothyroxine sodium

Thyroid Hormone

Abbott

Date of Preparation: September 21, 2005

Date of Revision: May 25, 2010

SUMMARY PRODUCT INFORMATION:

Route of Administration	Dosage Form/ Strength	Clinically Relevant Nonmedicinal Ingredients
Oral	Tablet/25 μg, 50 μg, 75 μg, 88 μg, 100 μg, 112 μg, 125 μg, 137 μg, 150 μg, 175 μg, 200 μg and 300 μg	Acacia, confectioner's sugar, lactose, magnesium stearate, povidone, talc and colour additives For a complete listing see Dosage Forms, Composition and Packaging.

INDICATIONS AND CLINICAL USE: SYNTHROID (levothyroxine sodium, USP) is indicated for:

- replacement or supplemental therapy in patients of any age or state (including pregnancy) with hypothyroidism of any etiology except transient hypothyroidism during the recovery phase of subacute thyroiditis;

  Specific indication include: primary hypothyroidism resulting from thyroid dysfunction, primary atrophy, or partial or total absence of thyroid gland, or from the effects of surgery, radiation or drugs, with or without the presence of goiter, including subclinical hypothyroidism; secondary (pituitary) hypothyroidism; and tertiary (hypothalamic) hypothyroidism.
- a pituitary TSH suppressant in the treatment or prevention of various types of euthyroid goiters, including thyroid nodules, subacute or chronic lymphocytic thyroiditis (Hashimoto's), multinodular goiter, and in conjunction with surgery and radioactive iodine therapy in the management of thyrotropin-dependent well-differentiated papillary or follicular carcinoma of the thyroid.

CONTRAINDICATIONS: SYNTHROID (levothyroxine sodium, USP) is contraindicated in:

- Patients with an apparent hypersensitivity to thyroid hormones or any of the inactive product constituents. For a complete listing of nonmedicinal ingredients, see Dosage Forms, Composition and Packaging. (Note: The 50 μg tablet is formulated without colour additives for patients who are sensitive to dyes.) There is no well-documented evidence of true allergic or idiosyncratic reactions to thyroid hormone.
- Patients with untreated subclinical (suppressed serum thyroid-stimulating hormone [TSH] with normal L-triiodothyronine/liothyronine $[T_3]$ and L-thyroxine/levothyroxine $[T_4]$ levels) or overt thyrotoxicosis of any etiology.
- Patients with acute myocardial infarction.
- Patients with uncorrected adrenal insufficiency, as thyroid hormones increase tissue demands for adrenocortical hormones and may thereby precipitate acute adrenal crisis. (See Warnings and Precautions.)

WARNINGS AND PRECAUTIONS:

Serious Warnings and Precautions

Thyroid hormones, including SYNTHROID, either alone or with other therapeutic agents, should not be used for the treatment of obesity or for weight loss. In euthyroid patients, doses within the range of daily hormonal requirements are ineffective for weight reduction. Larger doses may produce serious or even life threatening manifestations of toxicity, particularly when given in association with sympathomimetic amines such as those used for their anorectic effects.

General: SYNTHROID (levothyroxine sodium, USP) has a narrow therapeutic index. Regardless of the indication for use, careful dosage titration is necessary to avoid the consequences of over- or under-treatment. These consequences include, among others, effects on growth and development, cardiovascular function, bone metabolism, reproductive function, cognitive function, emotional state, gastrointestinal function, and on glucose and lipid metabolism. Many drugs interact with SYNTHROID necessitating adjustments in dosing to maintain therapeutic response. (See Drug Interactions.)

The bioavailability of levothyroxine may differ to some extent among marketed brands. Once the patient is stabilized on a particular brand of levothyroxine sodium, caution should be exercised when a change in drug product brand is implemented.

It has been shown that differences in formulations of levothyroxine, despite an identical content of active ingredient, may be associated with differences in fractional gastrointestinal absorption. These differences may not be observed through measurement of total T_3 and T_4 serum levels. It is therefore, recommended that patients who are switched from one levothyroxine formulation to another be retitrated to the desired thyroid function. Accuracy in retitration can best be achieved by using sensitive thyrotropin assays.

Seizures have been reported rarely in association with the initiation of levothyroxine sodium therapy, and may be related to the effect of thyroid hormone on seizure threshold.

Lithium blocks the TSH-mediated release of T_4 and T_3. Thyroid function should therefore be carefully monitored during lithium initiation, stabilization, and maintenance. If hypothyroidism occurs during lithium treatment, a higher than usual SYNTHROID dose may be required.

Carcinogenesis and Mutagenesis: Although animal studies to determine the mutagenic or carcinogenic potential of thyroid hormones have not been performed, synthetic T_4 is identical to that produced by the human thyroid gland. A reported association between prolonged thyroid hormone therapy and breast cancer has not been confirmed and patients receiving SYNTHROID for established indications should not discontinue therapy.

Cardiovascular: SYNTHROID should be used with caution in patients with cardiovascular disorders, including angina, coronary artery disease, and hypertension, and in the elderly who have a greater likelihood of occult cardiac disease. In these patients, levothyroxine sodium therapy should be initiated at lower doses than those recommended in younger individuals or in patients without cardiac diseases. (See Warnings and Precautions, Special Populations, Geriatrics (>50 years of age) and Dosage and Administration.) If cardiac symptoms develop or worsen, the levothyroxine sodium dose should be reduced or withheld for one week and then cautiously restarted at a lower dose. Over-treatment with SYNTHROID may have adverse cardiovascular effects such as an increase in heart rate, cardiac wall thickness, and cardiac contractility and may precipitate angina or arrhythmias. Patients with coronary artery disease who are receiving levothyroxine sodium therapy should be monitored closely during surgical procedures, since the possibility of precipitating cardiac arrhythmias may be greater in those treated with levothyroxine. Concomitant administration of thyroid hormone and sympathomimetic agents to patients with coronary artery disease may increase the risk of coronary insufficiency.

Endocrine and Metabolism: Thyroid hormones, either alone or together with other therapeutic agents, should not be used for the treatment of obesity or for weight loss. In euthyroid patients, doses within the range of daily hormonal requirements are ineffective for weight reduction. Larger doses may produce serious or even life-threatening manifestations of toxicity, particularly when given in association with sympathomimetic amines such as those used for their anorectic effects.

Patients treated concomitantly with SYNTHROID and orlistat should be monitored for changes in thyroid function. (See Drug Interactions.) Hypothyroidism and/or reduced control of hypothyroidism may occur. The mechanism may involve a decreased absorption of iodine salts and/or levothyroxine.

Effects on Bone Mineral Density: In women, long-term levothyroxine therapy has been associated with increased bone resorption, thereby decreasing bone mineral density, especially in postmenopausal women on greater replacement doses or in women who are receiving suppressive doses of levothyroxine sodium. The increased bone resorption may be associated with increased serum levels and urinary excretion of calcium and phosphorous, elevations in bone alkaline phosphatase and suppressed serum parathyroid hormone levels. Therefore, it is recommended that patients receiving SYNTHROID be given the minimum dose necessary to achieve the desired clinical and biochemical response.

Patients with Nontoxic Diffuse Goiter or Nodular Thyroid Disease: In patients with non-toxic diffuse goiter or nodular thyroid disease, particularly the elderly or those with underlying cardiovascular disease, levothyroxine therapy is contraindicated if the serum TSH level is already suppressed due to the risk of precipitating overt thyrotoxicosis. (See Contraindications.) If the serum TSH level is not suppressed, SYNTHROID should be used with caution in conjunction with careful monitoring of thyroid function for evidence of hyperthyroidism and clinical monitoring for potential associated adverse cardiovascular signs and symptoms of hyperthyroidism.

Associated Endocrine Disorders: Hypothalamic/Pituitary Hormone Deficiencies: In patients with secondary or tertiary hypothyroidism, additional hypothalamic/pituitary hormone deficiencies should be considered, and, if diagnosed, treated for adrenal insufficiency.

Autoimmune Polyglandular Syndrome: Use of SYNTHROID in patients with concomitant diabetes mellitus, diabetes insipidus or adrenal cortical insufficiency may aggravate the intensity of their symptoms. Appropriate adjustments of the various therapeutic measures directed at these concomitant endocrine diseases may therefore be required. Treatment of myxedema coma may require simultaneous administration of glucocorticoids. (See Dosage and Administration.)

Hematologic: T_4 enhances the response to anticoagulant therapy. Prothrombin time should be closely monitored in patients taking both SYNTHROID and oral anticoagulants, and the dosage of anticoagulant adjusted accordingly.

Sexual Function/Reproduction: The use of SYNTHROID is also unjustified in the treatment of male or female infertility unless this condition is associated with hypothyroidism.

Special Populations: Pregnant Women: Studies in pregnant women have not shown that SYNTHROID increases the risk of fetal abnormalities if administered during pregnancy. If levothyroxine sodium is used during pregnancy, the possibility of fetal harm appears remote.

Thyroid hormones cross the placental barrier to some extent. T_4 levels in the cord blood of athyroid fetuses have been shown to be about one-third of maternal levels. Nevertheless, maternal-fetal transfer of T_4 may not prevent in utero hypothyroidism.

Hypothyroidism during pregnancy is associated with a higher rate of complications, including spontaneous abortion, preeclampsia, stillbirth and premature delivery. Maternal hypothyroidism may have an adverse effect on fetal and childhood growth and development. On the basis of current knowledge, SYNTHROID should therefore not be discontinued during pregnancy, and hypothyroidism diagnosed during pregnancy should be treated. Studies have shown that during pregnancy T_4 concentrations may decrease and TSH concentrations may increase to values outside normal ranges. Postpartum values are similar to preconception values. Elevations in TSH may occur as early as the fourth week of gestation.

Pregnant women who are maintained on SYNTHROID should have their TSH measured periodically. An elevated TSH should be corrected by an increase in levothyroxine sodium dose. After pregnancy, the dose can be decreased to the optimal preconception dose. A serum TSH level should be obtained six to eight weeks postpartum.

Nursing Women: Minimal amounts of thyroid hormones are excreted in human milk. Thyroid hormones are not associated with serious adverse reactions and do not have known tumorigenic potential. While caution should be exercised when SYNTHROID is administered to a nursing woman, adequate replacement doses of levothyroxine sodium are generally needed to maintain normal lactation.

Pediatrics (all ages including neonates): Congenital Hypothyroidism: Infants with congenital hypothyroidism appear to be at increased risk for other congenital anomalies, with cardiovascular anomalies (pulmonary stenosis, atrial septal defect, and ventricular septal defect) being the most common association.

Rapid restoration of normal serum T_4 concentrations is essential to prevent deleterious neonatal thyroid hormone deficiency effects on intelligence, overall growth, and development. Treatment should be initiated immediately upon diagnosis and generally maintained for life. The therapeutic goal is to maintain serum total T_4 or free T_4 (FT_4) in the upper half of the normal range and serum TSH in the normal range.

An initial starting dose of 10 to 15 μg/kg/day (ages 0 to 3 months) will generally increase serum T_4 concentrations to the upper half of the normal range in less than 3 weeks. Clinical assessment of growth, development, and thyroid status should be monitored frequently. In most cases, the SYNTHROID dose per body weight will decrease as the patient grows through infancy and childhood. (See Dosage and Administration, Recommended Dose and Dosage Adjustment, Pediatric Dosage, Table 2.) Prolonged use of large doses in infants may be associated with temperament problems, which appear to be transient.

Thyroid function tests (serum total T_4 or FT_4, and TSH) should be monitored closely and used to determine the adequacy of levothyroxine sodium therapy. Serum T_4 normalization is usually followed by a rapid decline in TSH. Nevertheless, TSH normalization may lag behind T_4 normalization by 2 to 3 months or longer. The relative serum TSH elevation is more marked in the early months, but can persist to some degree throughout life. In rare patients TSH remains relatively elevated despite clinical euthyroidism and age-specific normal total T_4 or FT_4 levels. Increasing the levothyroxine sodium dosage to suppress TSH into the normal range may produce overtreatment, with an elevated serum T_4 and clinical features of hyperthyroidism including: irritability, increased appetite with diarrhea, and sleeplessness. Another risk of prolonged overtreatment in infants is premature cranial synostosis.

Acquired Hypothyroidism: The initial SYNTHROID dose varies with age and body weight, and should be adjusted to maintain serum total T_4 or free T_4 levels in the upper half of the normal range. In general, unless there are overriding clinical concerns, children should be started on a full replacement dose. Children with underlying heart disease should be started at lower dosages, with careful upward titration. Children with severe, longstanding hypothyroidism may also be started on a lower initial dose followed by an upward titration, attempting to avoid premature epiphyseal closure. The recommended dose per body weight decreases with age. (See Dosage and Administration, Recommended Dose and Dosage Adjustment, Pediatric Dosage, Table 2.)

Treated children may resume growth at a greater than normal rate (period of transient catch-up growth). In some cases the catch-up may be adequate to normalize growth. However, severe and prolonged hypothyroidism may reduce adult height. Excessive thyroxine replacement may initiate accelerated bone maturation, producing disproportionate skeletal age advancement and shortened adult stature.

If transient hypothyroidism is suspected hypothyroidism permanence may be assessed after the child reaches 3 years of age. Levothyroxine therapy may be interrupted for 30 days and serum T_4 and TSH measured. Low T_4 and elevated TSH confirm permanent hypothyroidism; therapy should be re-instituted. If T_4 and TSH remain in the normal range, a presumptive diagnosis of transient hypothyroidism can be made. In this instance, continued clinical monitoring and periodic thyroid function test reevaluation may be warranted.

Since some more severely affected children may become clinically hypothyroid when treatment is discontinued for 30 days, an alternate approach is to reduce the replacement dose of SYNTHROID by half during the 30-day trial period. If, after 30 days, the serum TSH is elevated above 20 mU/L, the diagnosis of permanent hypothyroidism is confirmed, and full replacement therapy should be resumed. However, if the serum TSH has not risen to greater than 20 mU/L, SYNTHROID treatment should be discontinued for another 30-day trial period followed by repeat serum T_4 and TSH testing.

Geriatrics (>50 years of age): Because of the increased prevalence of cardiovascular disease among the elderly, levothyroxine therapy should not be initiated at the full replacement dose. (See Warnings and Precautions and Dosage and Administration.)

Monitoring and Laboratory Tests: Treatment of patients with SYNTHROID requires periodic assessment of thyroid status by appropriate laboratory tests and clinical evaluation. Selection of appropriate tests for the diagnosis and management of thyroid disorders depends on patient variables such as presenting signs and symptoms, pregnancy, and concomitant medications. A measurement of free T_4 and TSH levels, using a sensitive TSH assay, is recommended to confirm a diagnosis of thyroid disease. Normal ranges for these parameters are age-specific in newborns and younger children.

TSH alone or initially may be useful for thyroid disease screening and for monitoring therapy for primary hypothyroidism as a linear inverse correlation exists between serum TSH and free T_4. Measurement of total serum T_4 and T_3, resin T_3 uptake, and free T_3 concentrations may also be useful. Antithyroid microsomal antibodies are an indicator of autoimmune thyroid disease. Positive microsomal antibody presence in an euthyroid patient is a major risk factor for the development of hypothyroidism. An elevated serum TSH in the presence of a normal T_4 may indicate subclinical hypothyroidism. Intracellular resistance to thyroid hormone is quite rare, and is suggested by clinical signs and symptoms of hypothyroidism in the presence of high serum T_4 levels. Adequacy of levothyroxine sodium therapy for hypothyroidism of pituitary or hypothalamic origin should be assessed by measuring free T_4, which should be maintained in the upper half of the normal range. Measurement of TSH is not a reliable indicator of response to therapy for this condition. Adequacy of levothyroxine sodium therapy for congenital and acquired pediatric hypothyroidism should be assessed by measuring serum total T_4 or free T_4; these should be maintained in the upper half of the normal range. In congenital hypothyroidism, serum TSH normalization may lag behind serum T_4 normalization by 2 to 3 months or longer. In rare patients, serum TSH remains relatively elevated despite clinical euthyroidism and age-specific normal T_4 or free T_4 levels. (See Warnings and Precautions, Special Populations, Pediatrics (all ages including neonates).)

ADVERSE REACTIONS: Adverse Drug Reaction Overview: Adverse reactions other than those indicative of thyrotoxicosis as a result of therapeutic overdosage, either initially or during the maintenance periods, are rare. (See Overdosage.) Seizures have been reported rarely with the institution of levothyroxine sodium therapy. Pseudotumor cerebri and slipped capital femoral epiphysis have also been reported in children receiving levothyroxine therapy. Over treatment in children may result in craniosynostosis and premature closure of the epiphyses with resultant compromised adult height.

Inadequate doses of SYNTHROID (levothyroxine sodium, USP) may produce or fail to resolve symptoms of hypothyroidism. Hair loss may occur during the initial months of therapy, but is generally transient. The incidence of continued hair loss is unknown.

Post-Market Adverse Drug Reactions: Adverse reactions associated with SYNTHROID are primarily those of hyperthyroidism due to therapeutic overdosage. (See Warnings and Precautions and Overdosage.) They include the following:

Cardiovascular System: palpitations, tachycardia, arrhythmias, increased pulse and blood pressure, heart failure, angina, myocardial infarction and cardiac arrest.

Central Nervous System: headache, hyperactivity, nervousness, anxiety, irritability, emotional lability, and insomnia.

Dermatologic: hair loss, flushing.

Endocrine System: decreased bone mineral density.

Gastrointestinal System: diarrhea, vomiting, abdominal cramps, and elevations in liver function tests.

General: fatigue, increased appetite, weight loss, heat intolerance, fever, and excessive sweating.

Musculoskeletal System: tremors, muscle weakness.

Reproductive System: menstrual irregularities, impaired fertility.

Respiratory System: dyspnea.

Seizures have been reported rarely with the institution of levothyroxine sodium therapy.

Hypersensitivity reactions to inactive ingredients have occurred in patients treated with thyroid hormone products. These include urticaria, pruritus, skin rash, flushing, angioedema, various GI symptoms (abdominal pain, nausea, vomiting and diarrhea), fever, arthralgia, serum sickness and wheezing. Hypersensitivity to levothyroxine itself is not known to occur.

DRUG INTERACTIONS: Overview: The magnitude and relative clinical importance of the effects noted below are likely to be patient-specific and may vary by such factors as age, gender, race, intercurrent illnesses, dose of either agents, additional concomitant medications, and timing of drug administration. Any agent that alters thyroid hormone synthesis, secretion, distribution, effect on target tissues, metabolism, or elimination may alter the optimal therapeutic dose of SYNTHROID (levothyroxine sodium, USP).

Drug-Drug Interactions: Many drugs affect thyroid hormone pharmacokinetics and metabolism (e.g., absorption, synthesis, secretion, catabolism, protein binding, and target tissue response) and may alter the therapeutic response to SYNTHROID. In addition, thyroid hormones and thyroid status have varied effects on the pharmacokinetics and actions of other drugs. A listing of drug-thyroidal axis interactions is contained in Table 1.

The list of drug-thyroidal axis interactions in Table 1 may not be comprehensive due to the introduction of new drugs that interact with the thyroidal axis or the discovery of previously unknown interactions. The prescriber should be aware of this fact and should consult appropriate reference sources (e.g., package inserts of newly approved drugs, medical literature) for additional information if a drug-drug interaction with levothyroxine is suspected.

Anticoagulants: Levothyroxine levels increase the response to oral anticoagulant therapy. Therefore, a decrease in the dose of anticoagulant may be warranted with correction of the hypothyroid state or when the levothyroxine sodium dose is increased. Prothrombin time should be closely monitored to permit appropriate and timely dosage adjustments (see Table 1).

Digitalis Glycosides: The therapeutic effects of digitalis glycosides may be reduced by SYNTHROID. Serum digitalis glycoside levels may be decreased when a hypothyroid patient becomes euthyroid, necessitating an increase in the dose of digitalis glycosides (see Table 1).

Orlistat: Hypothyroidism and/or reduced control of hypothyroidism may occur. The mechanism, although not proven, may involve a decreased absorption of iodine salts and/or levothyroxine. Patients treated concomitantly with SYNTHROID and orlistat should be monitored for changes in thyroid function.

Table 1: SYNTHROID

Drug-Thyroidal Axis Interactions

Drug or Drug Class	Effect
Drugs that may reduce TSH secretion—the reduction is not sustained; therefore, hypothyroidism does not occur	
Dopamine/Dopamine Agonists Glucocorticoids Octreotide	Use of these agents may result in a transient reduction in TSH secretion when administered at the following doses: Dopamine (greater than or equal to 1 μg/kg/min); Glucocorticoids (hydrocortisone greater than or equal to 100 mg/day or equivalent); Octreotide (greater than 100 μg/day).
Drugs that alter thyroid hormone secretion	
Drugs that may decrease thyroid hormone secretion, which may result in hypothyroidism	

(cont'd)

Table 1: SYNTHROID *(cont'd)*

Drug-Thyroidal Axis Interactions

Drug or Drug Class	Effect
Aminoglutethimide Amiodarone Iodide (including iodine-containing radiographic contrast agents) Lithium Thioamides - Methimazole - Propylthiouracil (PTU) - Carbimazole Sulfonamides Tolbutamide	Long-term lithium therapy can result in goiter in up to 50% of patients, and either subclinical or overt hypothyroidism, each in up to 20% of patients. The fetus, neonate, elderly and euthyroid patients with underlying thyroid disease (e.g., Hashimotos's thyroiditis or with Grave's disease previously treated with radioiodine or surgery) are among those individuals who are particularly susceptible to iodine-induced hypothyroidism. Oral cholecystographic agents and amiodarone are slowly excreted, producing more prolonged hypothyroidism than parenterally administered iodinated contrast agents. Long-term aminoglutethimide therapy may minimally decrease T_4 and T_3 levels and increase TSH, although all values remain within normal limits in most patients.
Drugs that may increase thyroid hormone secretion, which may result in hyperthyroidism	
Amiodarone Iodide (including iodine-containing radiographic contrast agents)	Iodide and drugs that contain pharmacologic amounts of iodide may cause hyperthyroidism in euthyroid patients with Grave's disease previously treated with antithyroid drugs or in euthyroid patients with thyroid autonomy (e.g., multinodular goiter or hyperfunctioning thyroid adenoma). Hyperthyroidism may develop over several weeks and may persist for several months after therapy discontinuation. Amiodarone may induce hyperthyroidism by causing thyroiditis.
Drugs that may decrease T_4 absorption, which may result in hypothyroidism	
Antacids - Aluminum & Magnesium Hydroxides - Simethicone Bile Acid Sequestrants - Cholestyramine - Colestipol Calcium Carbonate Cation Exchange Resins - Kayexalate Ferrous Sulfate Orlistat Sucralfate	Concurrent use may reduce the efficacy of levothyroxine by binding and delaying or preventing absorption, potentially resulting in hypothyroidism. Calcium carbonate may form an insoluble chelate with levothyroxine, and ferrous sulfate likely forms a ferric-thyroxine complex. Administer levothyroxine at least four (4) hours apart from these agents. Patients treated concomitantly with orlistat and levothyroxine should be monitored for changes in thyroid function.
Drugs that may alter T_4 and T_3 serum transport—but FT_4 concentration remains normal; and therefore, the patient remains euthyroid	
Drugs that may increase serum TBG concentration	**Drugs that may decrease serum TBG concentration**
Clofibrate Estrogen-containing Oral Contraceptives Estrogens (oral) Heroin/Methadone 5-Fluorouracil Mitotane Tamoxifen	Androgens/Anabolic Steroids Asparaginase Glucocorticoids Slow-release Nicotinic Acid
Drugs that may cause protein-binding site replacement	
Furosemide (greater than 80 mg IV) Heparin Hydantoins Non Steroidal Anti-Inflammatory Drugs - Fenamates - Phenylbutazone Salicylates (greater than 2 g/day)	Administration of these agents with levothyroxine results in an initial transient increase in FT_4. Continued administration results in a decrease in Serum T_4 and normal FT_4 and TSH concentrations and, therefore, patients are clinically euthyroid. Salicylates inhibit binding of T_4 and T_3 to TBG and transthyretin. An initial increase in serum FT_4 is followed by return of FT_4 to normal levels with sustained therapeutic serum salicylate concentrations, although total T_4 levels may decrease by as much as 30%.
Drugs that may alter T_4 and T_3 metabolism	
Drugs that may increase hepatic metabolism, which may result in hypothyroidism	
Carbamazepine Hydantoins Phenobarbital Rifampin	Stimulation of hepatic microsomal drug-metabolizing enzyme activity may cause increased hepatic degradation of levothyroxine, resulting in increased levothyroxine requirements. Phenytoin and carbamazepine reduce serum protein binding of levothyroxine, and total and free T_4 may be reduced by 20 to 40%, but most patients have normal serum TSH levels and are clinically euthyroid.
Drugs that may decrease T_4 5'-deiodinase activity	
Amiodarone Beta-adrenergic Antagonists - (e.g., Propranolol greater than 160 mg/day) Glucocorticoids - (e.g., Dexamethasone greater than or equal to 4 mg/day) Propylthiouracil (PTU)	Administration of these enzyme inhibitors decreases the peripheral conversion of T_4 to T_3, leading to decreased T_3 levels. However, serum T_4 levels are usually normal but may occasionally be slightly increased. In patients treated with large doses of propranolol (greater than 160 mg/day), T_3 and T_4 levels change slightly, TSH levels remain normal, and patients are clinically euthyroid. It should be noted that actions of particular beta-adrenergic antagonists may be impaired when the hypothyroid patient is converted to the euthyroid state. Short-term administration of large doses of glucocorticoids may decrease serum T_3 concentrations by 30% with minimal change in serum T_4 levels. However, long-term glucocorticoid therapy may result in slightly decreased T_3 and T_4 levels due to decreased TBG production (see above).
Miscellaneous	

(cont'd)

Table 1: SYNTHROID *(cont'd)*

Drug-Thyroidal Axis Interactions

Drug or Drug Class	Effect
Anticoagulants (oral) - Coumarin Derivatives - Indandione Derivatives	Thyroid hormones appear to increase the catabolism of vitamin K-dependent clotting factors, thereby increasing the anticoagulant activity of oral anticoagulants. Concomitant use of these agents impairs the compensatory increases in clotting factor synthesis. Prothrombin time should be carefully monitored in patients taking levothyroxine and oral anticoagulants and the dose of anticoagulant therapy adjusted accordingly.
Antidepressants - Tricyclics (e.g., Amitriptyline) - Tetracyclics (e.g., Maprotiline) - Selective Serotonin Reuptake Inhibitors (SSRIs; e.g., Sertraline)	Concurrent use of tri/tetracyclic antidepressants and levothyroxine may increase the therapeutic and toxic effects of both drugs, possibly due to increased receptor sensitivity to catecholamines. Toxic effects may include increased risk of cardiac arrhythmias and CNS stimulation; onset of action of tricyclics may be accelerated. Administration of sertraline in patients stabilized on levothyroxine may result in increased levothyroxine requirements.
Antidiabetic Agents - Biguanides - Meglitinides - Sulfonylureas - Thiazolidinediones - Insulin	Addition of levothyroxine to antidiabetic or insulin therapy may result in increased antidiabetic agent or insulin requirements. Careful monitoring of diabetic control is recommended, especially when thyroid therapy is started, changed, or discontinued.
Cardiac Glycosides	Serum digitalis glycoside levels may be reduced in hyperthyroidism or when the hypothyroid patient is converted to the euthyroid state. Therapeutic effect of digitalis glycosides may be reduced.
Cytokines - Interferon-alpha - Interleukin-2	Therapy with interferon-alpha has been associated with the development of antithyroid microsomal antibodies in 20% of patients and some have transient hypothyroidism, hyperthyroidism, or both. Patients who have antithyroid antibodies before treatment are at higher risk for thyroid dysfunction during treatment. Interleukin-2 has been associated with transient painless thyroiditis in 20% of patients. Interferon-beta and-gamma have not been reported to cause thyroid dysfunction.
Growth Hormones - Somatrem - Somatropin	Excessive use of thyroid hormones with growth hormones may accelerate epiphyseal closure. However, untreated hypothyroidism may interfere with growth response to growth hormone.
Ketamine	Concurrent use may produce marked hypertension and tachycardia; cautious administration to patients receiving thyroid hormone therapy is recommended.
Methylxanthine Bronchodilators - (e.g., Theophylline)	Decreased theophylline clearance may occur in hypothyroid patients; clearance returns to normal when the euthyroid state is achieved.
Radiographic Agents	Thyroid hormones may reduce the uptake of ^{123}I, ^{131}I, and ^{99m}Tc.
Sympathomimetics	Concurrent use may increase the effects of sympathomimetics or thyroid hormone. Thyroid hormones may increase the risk of coronary insufficiency when sympathomimetic agents are administered to patients with coronary artery disease.
Chloral Hydrate Diazepam Ethionamide Lovastatin Metoclopramide 6-Mercaptopurine Nitroprusside Para-aminosalicylate Sodium Perphenazine Resorcinol (excessive topical use) Thiazide Diuretics	These agents have been associated with thyroid hormone and/or TSH level alterations by various mechanisms.

Legend: TBG=thyroxine-binding globulin.

Drug-Food Interactions: Consumption of certain foods may affect levothyroxine absorption thereby necessitating adjustments in dosing. Soybean flour (infant formula), cotton seed meal, walnuts, calcium and calcium-fortified orange juice, and dietary fibre may bind and decrease the absorption of levothyroxine sodium from the gastrointestinal tract.

Drug-Laboratory Test Interactions: A number of drugs or moieties are known to alter serum levels of TSH, T_4 and T_3 and may thereby influence the interpretation of laboratory tests of thyroid function. (See Drug Interactions.)

Drugs such as estrogens and estrogen-containing oral contraceptives increase serum thyroxine-binding globulin (TBG) concentrations. TBG concentrations may also be increased during pregnancy, in infectious hepatitis and acute intermittent porphyria. Decreases in TBG concentrations are observed in nephrosis, severe hypoproteinemia, severe liver disease, acromegaly, and after androgen or corticosteroid therapy. Familial hyper- or hypothyroxine-binding-globulinemias have been described. The incidence of TBG deficiency is approximately 1 in 9000. Certain drugs such as salicylates inhibit the protein binding of T_4. In such cases, the unbound (free) hormone should be measured and/or determination of the free T_4 index (FT_4I) should be done.

Persistent clinical and laboratory evidence of hypothyroidism despite an adequate replacement dose suggests either poor patient compliance, impaired absorption, drug interactions, or decreased potency of the preparation due to improper storage.

DOSAGE AND ADMINISTRATION:

Dosing Considerations: The dosage and rate of administration of SYNTHROID (levothyroxine sodium, USP) is determined by the indication, and must in every case be individualized according to patient response and laboratory findings.

Adult Dosage: Hypothyroidism: The goal of therapy for primary hypothyroidism is to achieve and maintain a clinical and biochemical euthyroid state with consequent resolution of hypothyroid signs and symptoms. The starting dose of SYNTHROID, the frequency of dose titration, and the optimal full replacement dose must be individualized for every patient, and will be influenced by such factors as age, weight, cardiovascular status, presence of other illness, and the severity and duration of hypothyroid symptoms.

In patients with hypothyroidism resulting from pituitary or hypothalamic disease, the possibility of secondary adrenal insufficiency should be considered, and if present, treated with glucocorticoids prior to initiation of SYNTHROID. The adequacy of levothyroxine sodium therapy should be assessed in these patients by measuring FT_4, which should be maintained in the upper half of the normal range, in addition to clinical assessment. Measurement of TSH is not a reliable indicator of response to therapy for this condition.

TSH Suppression in Thyroid Cancer and Thyroid Nodules: The rationale for TSH suppression therapy is that a reduction in TSH secretion may decrease the growth and function of abnormal thyroid tissue. Exogenous thyroid hormone may inhibit recurrence of tumour growth and may produce regression of metastases from well-differentiated (follicular and papillary) carcinoma of the thyroid. It is used as ancillary therapy of these conditions following surgery or radioactive iodine therapy. Medullary and anaplastic carcinoma of the thyroid is unresponsive to TSH suppression therapy. TSH suppression is also used in treating nontoxic solitary nodules and multinodular goiters.

No controlled studies have compared the various degrees of TSH suppression in the treatment of either benign or malignant thyroid nodular disease. Further, the effectiveness of TSH suppression for benign nodular disease is controversial. The dose of SYNTHROID used for TSH suppression should therefore be individualized by the nature of the disease, the patient being treated, and the desired clinical response, weighing the potential benefits of therapy against the risks of iatrogenic thyrotoxicosis. In general, SYNTHROID should be given in the smallest dose that will achieve the desired clinical response.

Pediatric Dosage: Congenital or Acquired Hypothyroidism: The SYNTHROID pediatric dosage varies with age and body weight. SYNTHROID should be given at a dose that maintains T_4 or free T_4 in the upper half of the normal range and serum TSH in the normal range. (See Warnings and Precautions, Special Populations, Pediatrics (all ages including neonates).) Normalization of TSH may lag significantly behind T_4 in some infants. In general, despite the smaller body size of children, the dosage (on a weight basis) required to sustain full development and general thriving is higher than in adults (see Table 2).

Recommended Dose and Dosage Adjustment: Adult Dosage: Hypothyroidism: The usual full replacement dose of SYNTHROID for younger, healthy adults is approximately 1.7 μg/kg/day administered once daily. In the elderly, the full replacement dose may be altered by decreases in T_4 metabolism and levothyroxine sodium absorption. Older patients may require less than 1 μg/kg/day. Children generally require higher doses. (See Pediatric Dosage.) Women who are maintained on SYNTHROID during pregnancy may require increased doses. (See Warnings and Precautions, Special Populations, Pregnant Women.)

Therapy is usually initiated in younger, healthy adults at the anticipated full replacement dose. Clinical and laboratory evaluations should be performed at 6 to 8 week intervals (2 to 3 weeks in severely hypothyroid patients), and the dosage adjusted by 12.5 to 25 μg increments until the serum TSH concentration is normalized and signs and symptoms resolve. For most patients older than 50 years and for patients under 50 years of age with a history of underlying cardiac disease, an initial starting dose of 25 to 50 μg/day of SYNTHROID is recommended, with gradual increments in dose at six to eight week intervals, as needed. The recommended starting dose of SYNTHROID in elderly patients with cardiac disease is 12.5 to 25 μg/day, with gradual dose increments at four to six week intervals. If cardiac symptoms develop or worsen, the cardiac disease should be evaluated and the dose of levothyroxine sodium reduced. Rarely, worsening angina or other signs of cardiac ischemia may prevent achieving a TSH in the normal range.

Treatment of subclinical hypothyroidism may require lower than usual replacement doses, e.g. 1.0 μg/kg/day. Patients for whom treatment is not initiated should be monitored yearly for changes in clinical status, TSH, and thyroid antibodies.

Few patients require doses greater than 200 μg/day. An inadequate response to daily doses of 300 to 400 μg/day is rare, and may suggest malabsorption, poor patient compliance, and/or drug interactions.

Once optimal replacement is achieved, clinical and laboratory evaluations should be conducted at least annually or whenever warranted by a change in patient status. Levothyroxine sodium products from different manufacturers should not be used interchangeably unless retesting of the patient and retitration of the dosage, as necessary, accompanies the product switch.

Myxedema Coma: Myxedema coma represents the extreme expression of severe hypothyroidism and is considered a medical emergency. It is characterized by hypothermia, hypotension, hypoventilation, hyponatremia, and bradycardia. In addition to restoration of normal thyroid hormone levels, therapy should be directed at the correction of electrolyte disturbances and possible infection. Because the mortality rate of patients with untreated myxedema coma is high, treatment must be started immediately, and should include appropriate supportive therapy and corticosteroids to prevent adrenal insufficiency. Possible precipitating factors should also be identified and treated.

Myxedema coma is a life-threatening emergency characterized by poor circulation and hypometabolism, and may result in unpredictable absorption of levothyroxine sodium from the gastrointestinal tract. Therefore, oral thyroid hormone drug products, such as SYNTHROID, are not recommended to treat this condition. Thyroid hormone products formulated for intravenous administration should be administered.

TSH Suppression in Thyroid Cancer and Thyroid Nodules: For well-differentiated thyroid cancer, TSH is generally suppressed to less than 0.1 mU/L. Doses of SYNTHROID greater than 2 μg/kg/day are usually required. The efficacy of TSH suppression in reducing the size of benign thyroid nodules and in preventing nodule regrowth after surgery is controversial. Nevertheless, when treatment with SYNTHROID is warranted, TSH is generally suppressed to a higher target range (e.g. 0.1 to 0.3 mU/L) than that employed for the treatment of thyroid cancer. SYNTHROID therapy may also be considered for patients with nontoxic multinodular goiter who have a TSH in the normal range, to moderately suppress TSH (e.g. 0.1 to 0.3 mU/L).

SYNTHROID should be administered with caution to patients in whom there is a suspicion of thyroid gland autonomy, in view of the fact that the effects of exogenous hormone administration will be additive to endogenous thyroid hormone production.

Pediatric Dosage: Congenital or Acquired Hypothyroidism: Therapy is usually initiated at the full replacement dose (see Table 2). Infants and neonates with very low (<5 μg/dL) or undetectable serum T_4 levels should be started at higher end of the dosage range (e.g. 50 μg daily). A lower dose (e.g. 25 μg daily) should be considered for neonates at risk of cardiac failure, increasing every few days until a full maintenance dose is reached. In children with severe, long-standing hypothyroidism, SYNTHROID should be initiated gradually, with an initial 25 μg dose for two weeks, then increasing by 25 μg every 2 to 4 weeks until the desired dose, based on serum T_4 and TSH levels, is achieved.

Table 2: SYNTHROID

Dosage Guidelines for Pediatric Hypothyroidism

Age	Daily dose (μg) per kg of body weight[a]
0– 3 months	10–15
3–6 months	8–10
6–12 months	6–8
1–5 years	5–6
6–12 years	4–5
>12 years but growth and puberty incomplete	2–3
Growth and puberty complete	1.6

[a] To be adjusted on the basis of clinical response and laboratory tests. (See Warnings and Precautions, Special Populations, Pediatrics (all ages including neonates).)

Serum T_4 and TSH measurements should be evaluated at the following intervals, with subsequent dosage adjustments to normalize serum total T_4 or FT_4 and TSH: 2 and 4 weeks after therapy initiation, every 1 to 2 months during the first year of life, every 2 to 3 months between 1 and 3 years of age, every 3 to 12 months thereafter until growth is completed

Evaluation at more frequent intervals is indicated when compliance is questioned or abnormal laboratory values are obtained. Patient evaluation is also advisable approximately 2 to 4 weeks after any change in SYNTHROID dose.

Missed Dose: A missed dose of one tablet can be taken with the next dose. If more than 2 tablets are missed, the patient should consult with their doctor.

Administration: Pediatrics: SYNTHROID Tablets may be given to infants and children who cannot swallow intact tablets by crushing the tablet and suspending the freshly crushed tablet in a small amount of water (5 to 10 mL), breast milk or non-soybean based formula. The suspension can be given by spoon or dropper. **Do not store the suspension for any period of time.** The crushed tablet may also be sprinkled over a small amount of food, such as apple sauce. Foods or formula containing large amounts of soybean, fibre, or iron should not be used for administering SYNTHROID.

Table 3 summarizes the Dosage and Administration of SYNTHROID.

Table 3: SYNTHROID

Dosing and Administration

Medical Condition(s)	Patient Population	Starting Dose	Dosing Increment	Interval for Monitoring/ Dosing Increment	Therapeutic Goal
Congenital Hypothyroidism	Neonate	10–15 μg/kg/day	12.5 μg/day	4–6 weeks	Free T_4 level in upper half of normal range
Congenital/ Acquired Hypothyroidism	Infants/ Children	See Table 2	25 μg/day	1–2 months (until 1 year), 2–3 months (until 3 years), 3–12 months thereafter	Free T_4 level in upper half of normal range, normal TSH
Congenital Hypothyroidism with Risk of Heart Failure	Neonate	25 μg/day	12.5 μg/day	4–6 weeks	Free T_4 level in upper half of normal range, normal TSH
Severe Congenital Hypothyroidism (T_4<5 μg/dL)	Neonate	50 μg/day	25 μg/day	2–4 weeks	Free T_4 level in upper half of normal range, normal TSH
Hypothyroidism with Completed Growth and Puberty	Children	1.6–1.7 μg/kg/day	25–50 μg/day	6–8 weeks	Normal TSH (age-specific reference range)
Hypothyroidism	Adults <50 years	1.7 μg/kg/day	25–50 μg/day	6–8 weeks	Normal TSH (between 0.5 and 2.0 mU/L)
	Adults >50 years	25–50 μg/day	12.5–25 μg/day	6–8 weeks	Normal TSH (between 0.5 and 2.0 mU/L)
Hypothyroidism with Cardiac Disease	Adults <50 years	25–50 μg/day	12.5–25 μg/day	6–8 weeks	Normal TSH (between 0.5 and 2.0 mU/L)
	Adults >50 years	12.5–25 μg/day	12.5–25 μg/day	4–6 weeks	Normal TSH (between 0.5 and 2.0 mU/L)
Severe Hypothyroidism	Adults <50 years	12.5–25 μg/day	25 μg/day	2–4 weeks	Normal TSH (between 0.5 and 2.0 mU/L)
	Infants/ Children	25 μg/day	25 μg/day	2–4 weeks	Normal TSH (age-specific reference range)
Hypothyroidism (short period) or Recently Treated with Hyperthyroidism	Adults >50 years	<1.7 μg/kg/day	25–50 μg/day	6–8 weeks	Normal TSH (between 0.5 and 2.0 mU/L)
Hypothyroidism with Pregnancy	Pregnant Women	1.7 μg/kg/day (Increased dose may be required)	25–50 μg/day	Each trimester and 6–8 weeks postpartum	Normal TSH and FT_4 in the upper third of normal range
Secondary Hypothyroidism	Not Specified	[a]	[a]	[a]	Free T_4 level in upper third of normal range
Tertiary Hypothyroidism	Not Specified	[a]	[a]	[a]	Free T_4 level in upper third of normal range
Subclinical Hypothyroidism	Not Specified	25–50 μg/day	Adjust as necessary	6–8 weeks	Normal TSH (between 0.5 and 2.0 mU/L)
Well-differentiated (Papillary or Follicular) Thyroid Cancers	Not Specified	>2 μg/kg/day	25–50 μg/day	6–8 weeks	TSH <0.1 mU/L TSH <0.01 mU/L for patients with high risk tumors
Benign Nodules and Nontoxic Multinodular Goiter	Not Specified	1.7–2 μg/kg/day (Suppression not <0.1 mU/L)	25–50 μg/day	6–8 weeks	TSH 0.1–0.3 mU/L for nodules and for multinodular goiter

[a] Depending on age, duration of hypothyroidism and cardiovascular risk factor.

OVERDOSAGE:

Signs and Symptoms: Excessive doses of SYNTHROID (levothyroxine sodium, USP) result in a hypermetabolic state indistinguishable from thyrotoxicosis of endogenous origin. Signs and symptoms of thyrotoxicosis include exophthalmic goiter, weight loss, increased appetite, palpitations, nervousness, diarrhea, abdominal cramps, sweating, tachycardia, increased pulse and blood pressure, cardiac arrhythmias, angina pectoris, tremors, insomnia, heat intolerance, fever, and menstrual irregularities. In addition, confusion and disorientation may occur. Cerebral embolism, shock, coma, and death have been reported. Seizures have occurred in a child ingesting 18 mg of levothyroxine. Symptoms are not always evident or may not appear until several days after ingestion of SYNTHROID.

Treatment of Overdosage: SYNTHROID should be reduced in dose or temporarily discontinued if signs and symptoms of overdosage appear.

In the treatment of acute massive SYNTHROID overdosage, symptomatic and supportive therapy should be instituted immediately. Treatment is aimed at reducing gastrointestinal absorption and counteracting central and peripheral effects, mainly those of increased sympathetic activity. The stomach should be emptied immediately by emesis or gastric lavage if not otherwise contraindicated (e.g. by coma, convulsions or loss of gag reflex). Cholestyramine and activated charcoal have also been used to decrease levothyroxine sodium absorption. Beta-receptor antagonists, particularly propranolol, are useful in counteracting many of the effects of increased central and peripheral sympathetic activity, especially when no contraindications exist for its use. Provide respiratory support as needed; control congestive heart failure and arrhythmia, control fever, hypoglycemia, and fluid loss as necessary. Large doses of antithyroid drugs (e.g. methimazole, carbimazole, or propylthiouracil) followed in one to two hours by large doses of iodine may be given to inhibit synthesis and release of thyroid hormones. Cardiac glycosides may be administered if congestive heart failure develops. Glucocorticoids may be administered to inhibit the conversion of T_4 to T_3. Plasmapheresis, charcoal hemoperfusion and exchange transfusion have been reserved for cases in which continued clinical deterioration occurs despite conventional therapy. Since T_4 is extensively protein bound, very little drug will be removed by dialysis.

> For management of a suspected drug overdose, contact your regional Poison Control Centre. See the *CPS* Directory section for a list of Poison Control Centres.

ACTION AND CLINICAL PHARMACOLOGY: Mechanism of Action: The synthesis and secretion of the major thyroid hormones, T_3 and T_4, from the normally functioning thyroid gland are regulated by complex feedback mechanisms of the hypothalamic-pituitary-thyroid axis. The thyroid gland is stimulated to secrete thyroid hormonesby the action of thyrotropin (thyroid stimulating hormone, TSH), which is produced in the anterior pituitary gland. TSH secretion is in turn controlled by thyrotropin-releasing hormone (TRH) produced in the hypothalamus, circulating thyroid hormones, and possibly other mechanisms. Thyroid hormones circulating in the blood act as feedback inhibitors of both TSH and TRH secretion. Thus, when serum concentrations of T_3 and T_4 are increased, secretion of TSH and TRH decreases. Conversely, when serum thyroid hormone concentrations are decreased, secretion of TSH and TRH is increased. Administration of exogenous thyroid hormones to euthyroid individuals results in suppression of endogenous thyroid hormone secretion.

The mechanisms by which thyroid hormones exert their physiologic actions have not been completely elucidated, but it is thought that their principal effects are exerted through control of DNA transcription and protein synthesis. T_3 and T_4 are transported into cells by passive and active mechanisms. T_3 in cell cytoplasm and T_3 generated from T_4 within the cell diffuse into the nucleus and bind to thyroid receptor proteins, which appear to be primarily attached to DNA. Receptor binding leads to activation or repression of DNA transcription, thereby altering the amounts of mRNA and resultant proteins. Changes in protein concentrations are responsible for the metabolic changes observed in organs and tissues.

Thyroid hormones enhance oxygen consumption of most body tissues and increase the basal metabolic rate and metabolism of carbohydrates, lipids, and proteins. Thus, they exert a profound influence on every organ system and are of particular importance in the development of the central nervous system. Thyroid hormones also appear to have direct effects on tissues, such as increased myocardial contractility and decreased systemic vascular resistance.

The physiologic effects of thyroid hormones are produced primarily by T_3, a large portion of which (approximately 80%) is derived from the deiodination of T_4 in peripheral tissues. About 70 to 90 percent of peripheral T_3 is produced by monodeiodination of T_4 at the 5 position (outer ring). Peripheral monodeiodination of T_4 at the 5 position (inner ring) results in the formation of reverse triiodothyronine (rT_3), which is calorigenically inactive.

Levothyroxine, at doses individualized according to patient response, is effective as replacement or supplemental therapy in hypothyroidism of any etiology, except transient hypothyroidism during the recovery phase of subacute thyroiditis.

Levothyroxine is also effective in the suppression of pituitary TSH secretion in the treatment or prevention of various types of euthyroid goiters, including thyroid nodules, Hashimoto's thyroiditis, multinodular goiter and, as adjunctive therapy in the management of thyrotropin-dependent well-differentiated thyroid cancer. (See Indications and Clinical Use, Warnings and Precautions and Dosage and Administration.)

Pharmacokinetics: Absorption: Few clinical studies have evaluated the kinetics of orally administered thyroid hormone. In animals, the most active sites of absorption appear to be the proximal and mid-jejunum. T_4 is not absorbed from the stomach and little, if any, drug is absorbed from the duodenum. There seems to be no absorption of T_4 from the distal colon in animals. A number of human studies have confirmed the importance of an intact jejunum and ileum for T_4 absorption and have shown some absorption from the duodenum. Studies involving radioiodinated T_4 fecal tracer excretion methods, equilibration, and AUC methods have shown that absorption varies from 48 to 80 percent of the administered dose. The extent of absorption is increased in the fasting state and decreased in malabsorption syndromes, such as sprue. Absorption may also decrease with age. The degree of T_4 absorption is dependent on the product formulation as well as on the character of the intestinal contents, the intestinal flora, including plasma protein and soluble dietary factors, which bind thyroid hormone, making it unavailable for diffusion. Decreased absorption may result from administration of infant soybean formula, ferrous sulfate, sodium polystyrene sulfonate, aluminum hydroxide, sucralfate, or bile acid sequestrants. T_4 absorption following intramuscular administration is variable. The relative bioavailability of SYNTHROID (levothyroxine sodium, USP) tablets, compared to an equal nominal dose of oral levothyroxine sodium solution, is approximately 93%.

Distribution: Distribution of thyroid hormones in human body tissues and fluids has not been fully elucidated. More than 99% of circulating hormones is bound to serum proteins, including thyroxine-binding globulin (TBG), thyroxine-binding prealbumin (TBPA), and albumin (TBA). T_4 is more extensively and firmly bound to serum proteins than is T_3. Only unbound thyroid hormone is metabolically active. The higher affinity of TBG and TBPA for T_4 partly explains the higher serum levels, slower metabolic clearance, and longer serum elimination half-life of this hormone.

Certain drugs and physiologic conditions can alter the binding of thyroid hormones to serum proteins and/or the concentrations of the serum proteins available for thyroid hormone binding. These effects must be considered when interpreting the results of thyroid function tests. (See Warnings and Precautions, Monitoring and Laboratory Tests and Drug Interactions.)

Metabolism: The liver is the major site of degradation for both hormones. T_3 and T_4 are conjugated with glucuronic and sulfuric acids and excreted in the bile. There is an enterohepatic circulation of thyroid hormones, as they are liberated by hydrolysis in the intestine and reabsorbed. A portion of the conjugated material reaches the colon unchanged, is hydrolyzed there, and is eliminated as free compounds in the feces. In man, approximately 20 to 40 percent of T_4 is eliminated in the stool. About 70 percent of the T_4 secreted daily is deiodinated to yield equal amounts of T_3 and rT_3. Subsequent deiodination of T_3 and rT_3 yields multiple forms of diiodothyronine. A number of other minor T_4metabolites have also been identified. Although some of these metabolites have biologic activity, their overall contribution to the therapeutic effect of T_4 is minimal.

Excretion: Thyroid hormones are primarily eliminated by the kidneys. T_4 is eliminated slowly from the body (see Table 4), with a half-life of 6 to 7 days. T_3 has a half-life of 1 to 2 days.

Table 4: SYNTHROID

Pharmacokinetic Parameters of Thyroid Hormones in Euthyroid Patients

Hormone	Ratio in Thyroglobulin	Biologic Potency	t½ (days)	Protein Binding (%)[b]
Levothyroxine, T_4	10 to 20	14	6 to 7[a]	99.96
Liothyronine, T_3	1	4	≤2	99.5

[a] Three to four days in hyperthyroidism, nine to ten days in hypothyroidism.
[b] Includes TBG, TBPA, and TBA.

STORAGE AND STABILITY: Store at controlled room temperature 15 to 25°C. SYNTHROID (levothyroxine sodium, USP) Tablets should be protected from light and moisture.

INFORMATION FOR THE PATIENT: Published in e-CPS, available by subscription at www.e-cps.ca.

DOSAGE FORMS, COMPOSITION AND PACKAGING: 25 µg: Each orange, round, color-coded, scored tablet, debossed with "SYNTHROID" on one side and potency on the other side contains: levothyroxine sodium, USP 25 µg. Nonmedicinal ingredients: acacia, confectioner's sugar, FD&C Yellow No. 6, lactose, magnesium stearate, povidone and talc. Bottles of 100 and 1000.

50 µg: Each white, round, color-coded, scored tablet, debossed with "SYNTHROID" on one side and potency on the other side contains: levothyroxine sodium, USP 50 µg. Nonmedicinal ingredients: acacia, confectioner's sugar, lactose, magnesium stearate, povidone and talc. Bottles of 100 and 1000.

75 µg: Each violet, round, color-coded, scored tablet, debossed with "SYNTHROID" on one side and potency on the other side contains: levothyroxine sodium, USP 75 µg. Nonmedicinal ingredients: acacia, confectioner's sugar, FD&C Blue No. 2, FD&C Red No. 40, lactose, magnesium stearate, povidone and talc. Bottles of 100 and 1000.

88 µg: Each olive, round, color-coded, scored tablet, debossed with "SYNTHROID" on one side and potency on the other side contains: levothyroxine sodium, USP 88 µg. Nonmedicinal ingredients: acacia, confectioner's sugar, D&C Yellow No. 10, FD&C Blue No. 1, FD&C Yellow No. 6, lactose, magnesium stearate, povidone and talc. Bottles of 100 and 1000.

100 µg: Each yellow, round, color-coded, scored tablet, debossed with "SYNTHROID" on one side and potency on the other side contains: levothyroxine sodium, USP 100 µg. Nonmedicinal ingredients: acacia, confectioner's sugar, D&C Yellow No. 10, FD&C Yellow No. 6, lactose, magnesium stearate, povidone and talc. Bottles of 100 and 1000.

112 µg: Each rose, round, color-coded, scored tablet, debossed with "SYNTHROID" on one side and potency on the other side contains: levothyroxine sodium, USP 112 µg. Nonmedicinal ingredients: acacia, confectioner's sugar, D&C Red No. 27 & 30, lactose, magnesium stearate, povidone and talc. Bottles of 100 and 1000.

125 µg: Each brown, round, color-coded, scored tablet, debossed with "SYNTHROID" on one side and potency on the other side contains: levothyroxine sodium, USP 125 µg. Nonmedicinal ingredients: acacia, confectioner's sugar, FD&C Blue No. 1, FD&C Red No. 40, FD&C Yellow No. 6, lactose, magnesium stearate, povidone and talc. Bottles of 100 and 1000.

137 µg: Each turquoise, round, color-coded, scored tablet, debossed with "SYNTHROID" on one side and potency on the other side contains: levothyroxine sodium, USP 137 µg. Nonmedicinal ingredients: acacia, confectioner's sugar, FD&C Blue No. 1, lactose, magnesium stearate, povidone and talc. Bottles of 100 and 1000.

150 µg: Each blue, round, color-coded, scored tablet, debossed with "SYNTHROID" on one side and potency on the other side contains: levothyroxine sodium, USP 150 µg. Nonmedicinal ingredients: acacia, confectioner's sugar, FD&C Blue No. 2, lactose, magnesium stearate, povidone and talc. Bottles of 100 and 1000.

175 µg: Each lilac, round, color-coded, scored tablet, debossed with "SYNTHROID" on one side and potency on the other side contains: levothyroxine sodium, USP 175 µg. Nonmedicinal ingredients: acacia, confectioner's sugar, D&C Red No. 27 & 30, FD&C Blue No. 1, lactose, magnesium stearate, povidone and talc. Bottles of 100 and 1000.

200 µg: Each pink, round, color-coded, scored tablet, debossed with "SYNTHROID" on one side and potency on the other side contains: levothyroxine sodium, USP 200 µg. Nonmedicinal ingredients: acacia, confectioner's sugar, FD&C Red No. 40, lactose, magnesium stearate, povidone and talc. Bottles of 100 and 1000.

300 µg: Each green, round, color-coded, scored tablet, debossed with "SYNTHROID" on one side and potency on the other side contains: levothyroxine sodium, USP 300 µg. Nonmedicinal ingredients: acacia, confectioner's sugar, D&C Yellow No. 10, FD&C Blue No. 1, FD&C Yellow No. 6, lactose, magnesium stearate, povidone and talc. Bottles of 100.

(Shown in Product Identification Section)

Synvisc®

hylan G-F 20

Viscosupplementation

Genzyme

Date of Revision: July 18, 2008

DESCRIPTION: Synvisc (hylan G-F 20) is a sterile, nonpyrogenic, elastoviscous fluid containing hylans. Hylans are derivatives of hyaluronan (sodium salt of hyaluronic acid) and consist of repeating disaccharide units of N-acetylglucosamine and sodium glucuronate. Hylan A has an average molecular weight of approximatley 6 000 000 and hylan B is a hydrated gel. Synvisc contains hylan A and hylan B (8.0 mg±2.0 mg/mL) in buffered physiological sodium chlroide solution (pH 7.2±3).

Synvisc is biologically similar to hyaluronan. Hyaluronan is a component of synovial fluid which is responsible for its viscoelasticity. The mechanical (elastoviscous) properties of Synvisc are, however, superior to those of synovial fluid and hyaluronan solutions of comparable concentration. Synvisc has an elasticity (storage modulus, G') at 2.5 Hz of 111±13 Pascals (Pa) and a viscosity (loss modulus, G") of 25±2 Pa. Elasticity and viscosity of knee joint synovial fluid of 18- to 27-year-old humans measured with comparable method at 2.5 Hz are G'=117±13 Pa and G"=45±8 Pa. Hylans are degraded in the body by the same pathway as hyaluronan, and breakdown products are nontoxic.

INDICATIONS: Synvisc is a temporary replacement and supplement for synovial fluid. Synvisc is beneficial for patients in all stages of joint pathology. Synvisc is most effective in patients who are actively and regularly using the affected joint. Synvisc is only intended for intra-articular use by a physician to treat pain associated with osteoarthritis of the knee, hip, ankle and shoulder.

Synvisc achieves its therapeutic effect through viscosupplementation, a process whereby the physiological and rheological states of the arthritic joint tissues are restored. Viscosupplementation with Synvisc is a treatment to decrease pain and discomfort, allowing more extensive movement of the joint. In vitro studies have shown that Synvisc protects cartilage cells against certain physical and chemical damage.

CONTRAINDICATIONS: If venous or lymphatic stasis is present in the relevant limb, Synvisc should not be injected into the joint.

Synvisc should not be used in infected or severely inflamed joints or in patients having skin diseases or infections in the area of the injection site.

WARNINGS: Do not inject intravascularly. Do not inject extra-articularly or into synovial tissues and capsule. Adverse events, generally in the area of injection, have occurred following extra-articular injection of Synvisc. Do not concomitantly use disinfectants containing quaternary ammonium salts for skin preparation because hyaluronan can precipitate in their presence.

PRECAUTIONS: Synvisc should not be used if there is a large intra-articular effusion prior to the injection.

As with any invasive joint procedure, it is recommended that the patient avoid any strenuous activities following the intra-articular injection, and resume full activities within a few days.

Synvisc has not been tested in pregnant women or children under 18 years of age.

Synvisc contains small amounts of avian protein and should not be used in patients with related hypersensitivities.

ADVERSE EFFECTS: Adverse events involving the injected joint: transient pain and/or swelling and/or effusion in the injected joint may occur after intra-articular injections of Synvisc. In some cases, the effusion may be large and can cause pronounced pain; it is important to remove and to analyze the fluid to rule out infection or crystalline arthropathies. These reactions generally abate within a few days. Clinical benefit from the treatment may still be apparent after such reactions. Intra-articular infections did not occur during any of the clinical trials and have been reported only rarely during clinical use of Synvisc.

The post marketing experience has identified the following systemic events to occur rarely with Synvisc administration: rash hives, itching, fever, nausea, headache, dizziness, chills, muscle cramps, paresthesia, peripheral oedema, malaise, respiratory difficulties, flushing and facial swelling. In the controlled clinical trials, there were no statistically significant differences in the number or types of systemic adverse events between the group of patients that received Synvisc and the group that received control treatments.

OVERDOSE:

> For management of a suspected drug overdose, CPhA recommends that you contact your **regional Poison Control Centre**. See the *CPS* Directory section for a list of Poison Control Centres.

DOSAGE: Remove synovial fluid or effusion before each Synvisc injection. Do not use Synvisc if package is opened or damaged. Inject at room temperature. To remove the syringe from the blister (or tray), take hold of it by the body, without touching the plunger rod. Administer using strict aseptic procedures, taking particular care when removing the tip cap. Twist the grey tip cap before pulling it off, as this will minimize product leakage. Use an appropriate size of needle (e.g. 18 to 22 gauge) and length of needle, depending on joint to be treated. To ensure a tight seal and prevent leakage during administration secure the needle tightly while firmly holding the Luer hub. Do not tighten or apply excessive leverage when attaching the needle or removing the needle guard, as this may break the tip of the syringe. Do not resterilize Synvisc. Inject into the synovial space only, using if necessary, appropriate guidance such as fluoroscopy especially in joints such as the hip and shoulder. The syringe contents are for single use only. When using fluoroscopic guidance, ionic or nonionic contrast agent may be utilized. No more than 1 mL of contrast agent should be used for 2 mL of Synvisc.

The dosage regimen for Synvisc is dependent on the joint being treated.

Osteoarthritis of the Knee: The recommended treatment regimen for Synvisc is three injections in the knee, one week apart. To achieve maximum effect, it is essential to administer all three injections. The maximum recommended dosage is six injections within six months, with a minimum of four weeks between treatment regimens.

Osteoarthritis of the Hip: The recommended initial treatment regimen is a single injection. If however, adequate symptomatic relief is not achieved after this injection, it is recommended to administer a second injection. Clinical data have demonstrated that patients benefit from this second injection when administered between 1 and 3 months after the first injection.
Osteoarthritis of the Ankle: The recommended initial treatment regimen is a single injection. If however, adequate symptomatic relief is not achieved after this injection, it is recommended to administer a second injection. Clinical data have demonstrated that patients benefit from this second injection when administered between 1 and 3 months after the first injection.
Osteoarthritis of the Shoulder: The recommended initial treatment regimen is a single injection. If however, adequate symptomatic relief is not achieved after this injection, it is recommended to administer a second injection. Clinical data have demonstrated that patients benefit from this second injection when administered between 1 and 3 months after the first injection.
Duration of Effect: Generally the duration of effect for those patients who respond to treatment has been reported up to twenty-six weeks, although shorter and longer periods have also been observed. However, prospective clinical data in knee OA patients have shown benefit of treatment up to 52 weeks, following a single course of three Synvisc injections.

Synvisc treatment affects only the injected joint; it does not produce a general systemic effect.

SUPPLIED: Each mL of sterile, nonpyrogenic, elastoviscous fluid contains: hylan 8 mg. Nonmedicinal ingredients: disodium hydrogen phosphate, sodium chloride, sodium dihydrogen phosphate hydrate and sterile water for injection. Glass syringes of 2.25 mL containing 2 mL Synvisc. Store between 2 and 30°C. Do not freeze.

Synvisc One®

hylan G-F 20

Viscosupplementation

Genzyme

Date of Revision: March 2, 2009

DESCRIPTION: Synvisc-One (hylan G-F 20) is a sterile, nonpyrogenic, elastoviscous fluid containing hylans. Hylans are derivatives of hyaluronan (sodium salt of hyaluronic acid) and consist of repeating disaccharide units of N-acetylglucosamine and sodium glucuronate. Hylan A has an average molecular weight of approximately 6 000 000 daltons and hylan B is a hydrated gel. Hylan G-F 20 contains hylan A and hylan B (8.0 mg±2.0 mg per mL) in buffered physiological sodium chloride solution (pH 7.2±0.3).
Characteristics: Synvisc-One is biologically similar to hyaluronan. Hyaluronan is a component of synovial fluid which is responsible for its elastoviscosity. The mechanical (elastoviscous) properties of hylan G-F 20 are, however, superior to those of synovial fluid and hyaluronan solutions of comparable concentration.

Synvisc-One has an elasticity (storage modulus G') at 2.5 Hz of 111±13 Pascals (Pa) and a viscosity (loss modulus G") of 25±2 Pa. Elasticity and viscosity of knee synovial fluid of 18- to 27-year-old humans measured with comparable method at 2.5 Hz are G'=117±13 Pa and G"= 45±8 Pa. Hylans are degraded in the body by the same pathway as hyaluronan, and breakdown products are nontoxic.

INDICATIONS: Synvisc-One is a temporary replacement and supplement for synovial fluid. Synvisc-One is beneficial for patients in all stages of knee pathology. Synvisc-One is most effective in patients who are actively and regularly using the affected knee. Synvisc-One achieves its therapeutic effect through viscosupplementation, a process whereby the physiological and rheological states of the arthritic knee tissues are restored.

Viscosupplementation with Synvisc-One is a treatment to decrease pain and discomfort, allowing more extensive movement of the knee. In vitro studies have shown that hylan G-F 20 protects cartilage cells against certain physical and chemical damage.

Synvisc-One is only intended for intra-articular use by a physician to treat pain associated with osteoarthritis of the knee.

CONTRAINDICATIONS: If venous or lymphatic stasis is present, Synvisc-One should not be injected into the knee.

Synvisc-One should not be used in infected or severely inflamed knees or in patients having skin diseases or infections in the area of the injection site.

WARNINGS: Do not inject intravascularly.

Do not inject extra-articularly or into the synovial tissues and capsule. Adverse events, generally in the area of the injection, have occurred following extra-articular injection of Synvisc*.

Do not concomitantly use disinfectants containing quaternary ammonium salts for skin preparation because hyaluronan can precipitate in their presence.

PRECAUTIONS: Synvisc-One should not be used if there is a large intra-articular effusion prior to the injection.

As with any invasive joint procedure, it is recommended that the patient avoid any strenuous activities following the intra-articular injection, and resume full activities within a few days.

Synvisc-One has not been tested in pregnant women or children under 18 years of age.

Synvisc-One contains small amounts of avian protein and should not be used in patients with related hypersensitivities.

ADVERSE EFFECTS: Adverse events involving the injected knee: transient pain and/or, swelling and/or effusion in the injected knee may occur after intra-articular injections of Synvisc-One. Post-marketing experience with Synvisc has shown that in some cases the effusion may be large and can cause pronounced pain; it is important to remove and to analyse the fluid to rule out infection or crystalline arthropathies. These reactions generally abate within a few days. Clinical benefit from the treatment may still be apparent after such reactions. Intra-articular infections did not occur in any of the clinical trials of Synvisc/Synvisc-One and have been reported only rarely during clinical use of Synvisc.

The post marketing experience has identified the following systemic events to occur rarely with Synvisc administration: rash, hives, itching, fever, nausea, headache, dizziness, chills, muscle cramps, paresthesia, peripheral oedema, malaise, respiratory difficulties, flushing and facial swelling.

In the controlled clinical trial with Synvisc-One, the frequency and types of adverse events were similar between the group of patients that received Synvisc-One and the group that received placebo.

OVERDOSE:

For management of a suspected drug overdose, CPhA recommends that you contact your **regional Poison Control Centre**. See the *CPS* Directory section for a list of Poison Control Centres.

DOSAGE: Remove synovial fluid or effusion before injecting Synvisc-One. Do not use Synvisc-One if package is opened or damaged. Inject at room temperature. To remove the syringe from the blister (or tray), take hold of it by the body, without touching the plunger rod. Administer using strict aseptic procedures, taking particular care when removing the tip cap. Twist the grey tip cap before pulling it off, as this will minimise product leakage. Use an 18-20 gauge needle. To ensure a tight seal and prevent leakage during administration secure the needle tightly while firmly holding the Luer hub. Do not over tighten or apply excessive leverage when attaching the needle or removing the needle guard, as this may break the tip of the syringe. Do not resterilise Synvisc-One. Inject into the synovial space only. The syringe contents are for single use only.
Dosage Guidelines: The recommended treatment regimen is one injection in the knee. The injection may be repeated 6 months after the first injection, if justified by the patient's symptoms.
Duration of Effect: Hylan G-F 20 treatment affects only the injected knee; it does not produce a general systemic effect. Prospective clinical data in knee osteoarthritis patients have shown benefit of treatment up to 26 weeks, following a single Synvisc-One injection.

SUPPLIED: Each mL of sterile, nonpyrogenic, elastoviscous fluid contains: hylan 8 mg. Nonmedicinal ingredients: disodium hydrogen phosphate, sodium chloride, sodium dihydrogen phosphate hydrate and water for injection. Glass syringes of 10 mL containing 6 mL hylan G-F 20. Store between 2 and 30°C. Do not freeze.

* Synvisc (hylan G-F 20) is a 3×2 mL treatment regimen supplied in a 2.25 mL syringe. Synvisc is administered by intra-articular injection once a week (one week apart) for a total of three injections.

COMBAT

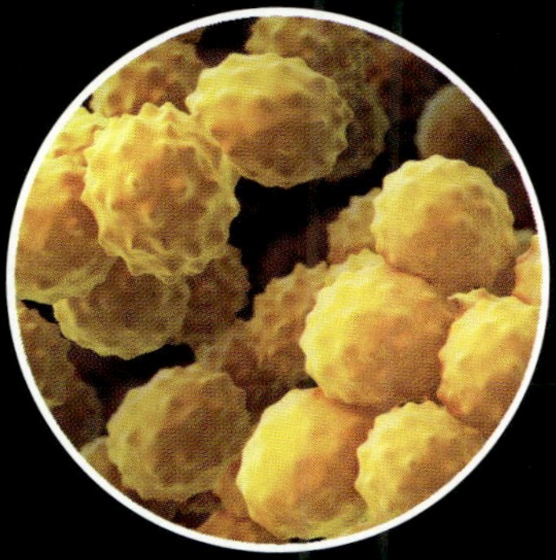

Our battle against infectious diseases starts here.

What will help the battle against infectious disease?
Research. Surveillance. Preparedness. Commitment to treatment.

Pfizer supports the battle against infectious disease – and the people behind it. From the frontline healthcare worker to the laboratory researcher, Pfizer is committed to helping all achieve their goals in the united fight against infectious disease.

T

Anti-fungals

Pr VFEND® (voriconazole)

Pr Eraxis™ (anidulafungin IV)

Anti-bacterials

Pr ZYVOXAM® IV/Oral (linezolid)

® Tygacil® tigecycline for injection

Infectious Diseases Pfizer
Joining forces against disease

T

There are many physiological symptoms of Overactive Bladder[1]

Choose PrDETROL LA® to treat ANY and ALL of the following:[2]

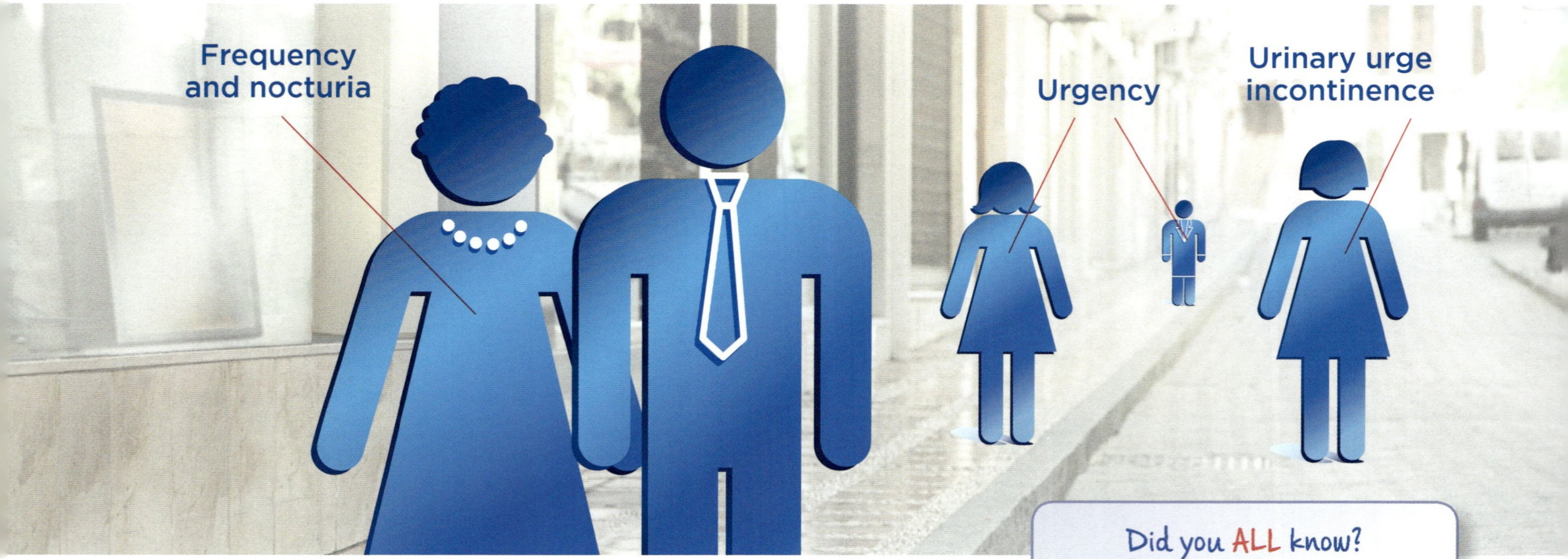

Did you ALL know?
DETROL LA is the #1 selling Overactive Bladder brand in Canada[6]

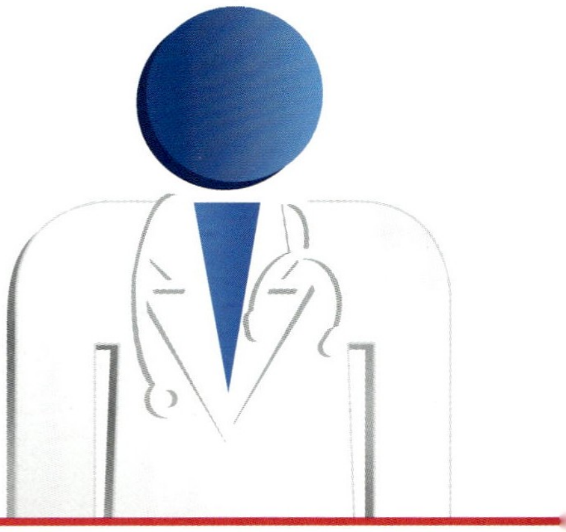

DETROL LA demonstrated significant improvement of

- **Frequency and nighttime micturitions**
  - p=0.0001 and p=0.0086 vs. placebo, respectively[3,4†‡]
- **Urgency**
  - p<0.001 vs. placebo[5§]
- **Urinary urge incontinence**
  - p=0.0001 vs. placebo[3‡]

DETROL LA – a once-daily formulation[2]

- **ALL the potential of DETROL LA in one dose each day**

And, to top it ALL off, DETROL LA has a favourable tolerability profile

- Most common adverse events ≥5%: dry mouth (23.4%), headache (6.3%), constipation (5.9%)[2]

DETROL LA (tolterodine L-tartrate capsules) is indicated for the symptomatic management of patients with an overactive bladder with symptoms of urinary frequency, urgency, or urge incontinence, or any combination of these symptoms (see WARNINGS AND PRECAUTIONS and DETAILED PHARMACOLOGY: Electrophysiology). The maximum recommended daily dose of 4 mg should not be exceeded.

Particular care should be exercised in patients who are at an increased risk of experiencing *torsade de pointes* during treatment with QT/QTc-prolonging drugs. This especially holds true in patients with abnormally long baseline QT/QTc intervals or when taking potent CYP3A4 inhibitors.

Discontinuation of the drug should be considered if symptoms suggestive of arrhythmia occur.

The most commonly reported adverse events with DETROL LA were dry mouth (23.4%), headache (6.3%), constipation (5.9%), abdominal pain (3.8%) and dyspepsia (3.0%).

DETROL LA is contraindicated in patients with urinary retention, gastric retention or uncontrolled narrow-angle glaucoma.

Patients with hepatic function impairment, patients with renal impairment or patients treated with potent CYP3A4 inhibitors should not receive doses greater than 2 mg od.

† Data from a 12-week, double-blind, randomized, placebo-controlled study. Patients taking DETROL LA demonstrated a reduction in frequency of -17% vs. -8% for those taking placebo (p=0.031) and a reduction in OAB-related nocturia episodes of -30% vs. -22% reduction with placebo (p=0.0086).

‡ Data based on a 12-week, double-blind, multicentre, randomized, placebo-controlled trial. Patients were randomized to either DETROL LA or placebo. After 12 weeks taking DETROL LA, patients experienced a mean reduction of -11.8 in UUI vs. -6.9 for those taking placebo (p=0.0001). DETROL LA significantly reduced micturitions/24 hrs vs. placebo by -3.5 (vs. -2.2 for placebo; p=0.0001).

§ Data based on a 12-week, double-blind, multicentre, randomized, placebo-controlled trial. Patients were randomized to receive either 4 mg DETROL LA OD or placebo for 12 weeks. Urgency was defined as the ability to finish a task before voiding. After 12 weeks taking DETROL LA, 33% of patients were able to perform tasks before voiding vs. 18% with placebo (p<0.001).

References: 1. Abrams P *et al.* The standardisation of terminology of lower urinary tract function: report from the Standardisation Sub-committee of the International Continence Society. *Neurourol Urodyn* 2002;21:167-178. 2. Pfizer Canada Inc. DETROL LA Product Monograph. February 2010. 3. Van Kerrebroeck P *et al.* Tolterodine once-daily: superior efficacy and tolerability in the treatment of the overactive bladder. *Urology* 2001;57:414-421. 4. Rackley R *et al.* Nighttime dosing with tolterodine reduces overactive bladder-related nocturnal micturitions in patients with overactive bladder and nocturia. *Urology* 2006;67:731-736. 5. Freeman R *et al.* Reduced perception of urgency in treatment of overactive bladder with extended-release tolterodine. *Obstet Gynecol* 2003;102:605-611. 6. IMS HEALTH. Canadian CompuScript National TRx for OAB market. February 2006 to January 2010.

Once-Daily Detrol LA
tolterodine L-tartrate extended-release capsules

Pfizer Working together for a healthier world™

Member R&D PAAB

T

Talwin® Injection Ⓝ

pentazocine lactate

Narcotic Analgesic

Hospira

PHARMACOLOGY: Pentazocine is a member of the benzazocine series of synthetic benzomorphans. It produces both analgesic (agonist) and narcotic antagonist effects. Following i.m. injection, a dose of 30 mg pentazocine is approximately equivalent to a 10 mg dose of morphine or a 75 to 100 mg dose of meperidine. Analgesia usually begins within 2 to 3 minutes after i.v. administration or 15 to 20 minutes after i.m. or s.c. injection and lasts about 3 hours. Opioid pharmacologic effects of pentazocine appear to be dose related and include miosis, respiratory depression, mild increase in biliary pressure, decreased intestinal motility and sedation.

Opiate antagonism: Pentazocine weakly antagonizes the analgesic effects of morphine, meperidine and phenazocine. In addition, it produces incomplete reversal of cardiovascular, respiratory and behavioral depression produced by morphine and meperidine. Pentazocine has about 1/50 the antagonistic activity of nalorphine. Pentazocine is well absorbed after i.m. or s.c. administration and is extensively metabolized in the liver. The metabolites are excreted by the kidney with only a small amount of unchanged drug excreted in the urine. Peak plasma concentrations occur 15 minutes to 1 hour after i.m. administration and the elimination half-life in plasma ranges between 2 and 5 hours.

INDICATIONS: For the relief of moderate to severe pain. Also for preoperative or preanesthetic medication, and as a supplement to surgical anesthesia.

CONTRAINDICATIONS: Pentazocine should not be administered to patients with known hypersensitivity to pentazocine or to any of the excipients contained in the formulation.

WARNINGS: Drug Abuse and Dependence: In chronic usage, care should be exercised to avoid any unnecessary increase in dosage since prolonged use of high doses of pentazocine may produce dependence. Patients with a history of drug abuse should be under close supervision when receiving pentazocine. Cases of myositis after long-term administration have been reported. As with all medication, the oral form of pentazocine is preferable for chronic administration.

When pentazocine is abruptly discontinued after extended use, withdrawal symptoms such as abdominal cramps, nausea, vomiting, elevated temperature, chills, rhinorrhea, restlessness, anxiety or lacrimation may occur. However, even when these symptoms have occurred, discontinuance has been accomplished with minimal difficulty. In the rare patient in whom more than minor difficulty has been encountered, reinstitution of pentazocine with gradual withdrawal has ameliorated the patient's symptoms.

Pregnancy: There have been rare reports of a withdrawal syndrome in newborns after prolonged use of pentazocine by the mother during pregnancy.

PRECAUTIONS: Head Injury and Increased Intracranial Pressure: The respiratory depressant effects of pentazocine and its potential for elevating cerebrospinal fluid pressure may be markedly exaggerated in the presence of head injury, other intracranial lesions or a pre-existing increase in intracranial pressure. Pentazocine can produce effects which may obscure the clinical course of patients with head injuries. Pentazocine must be used with caution in such patients, and only if its use is deemed essential.

Acute CNS Manifestations: There have been reported instances of the acute onset of hallucinations (usually visual), disorientation, and confusion in patients receiving therapeutic doses of pentazocine. These manifestations have cleared spontaneously within hours upon discontinuation of the drug. The mechanism responsible for this reaction is not known. Patients demonstrating this reaction should be closely observed and if therapy with pentazocine is to be restarted, administration should proceed cautiously since the acute CNS manifestations may recur.

Occupational Hazards: Ambulatory Patients: Since CNS effects have been noted with the use of pentazocine, ambulatory patients should be warned not to operate machinery, drive cars, or unnecessarily expose themselves to hazards.

Patients Dependent on Narcotics: Because pentazocine is a weak narcotic antagonist, patients who are addicted to narcotics may experience withdrawal symptoms and therefore it should be given with special caution to such persons. In nonaddicted patients receiving narcotics for a short period, symptoms believed to be related to antagonism may be observed. Intolerance or untoward reactions are usually not observed following administration of pentazocine to patients who have received single doses of or who have had limited exposure to narcotics.

Impaired Renal or Hepatic Function: Although laboratory tests have not indicated that pentazocine causes or increases renal or hepatic impairment, the drug should be administered with caution to patients with such impairment. Extensive liver disease appears to predispose to a higher incidence of side effects (e.g., marked apprehension, anxiety, dizziness, sleepiness) with the usual clinical dose, and may be the result of decreased metabolism of the drug by the liver.

Sphincter of Oddi: Until further experience is gained with the effects of pentazocine on the sphincter of Oddi, the drug should be used with caution in patients with acute cholecystitis or pancreatitis or in those about to undergo surgery of the biliary tract.

Obstructive Uropathy: Because urinary retention has been observed in a few patients receiving pentazocine, caution is advised in administration of the drug to patients with obstructive uropathy.

Respiratory Conditions: Because respiratory depression is a side effect of agonist opioid therapy, particular caution should be observed when administering pentazocine to patients with respiratory conditions such as bronchial asthma, established respiratory depression, limited respiratory reserve or obstructive respiratory conditions.

Patients with Cardiovascular Disease: Pentazocine can elevate blood pressure, possibly through the release of endogenous catecholamines. Particular caution should be observed in conditions where alterations in vascular resistance and blood pressure might be particularly undesirable such as in the acute phase of myocardial infarction.

Patients with Porphyria: Particular caution should be exercised in administering pentazocine to patients with porphyria, since it may provoke an acute attack in susceptible individuals.

Seizure-prone Patients: Caution should be observed in patients who are prone to convulsions; convulsions have occurred in a few such patients in association with the use of pentazocine, although no cause and effect relationship has been established.

Tissue Damage at Injection Site: Sclerosis of the skin, s.c. tissues, and underlying muscle have been reported at the injection sites of patients who have received multiple doses of pentazocine. If frequent daily injections are needed over long periods, the i.m. route is preferable to the s.c. route. To reduce risk of local tissue damage, injection sites should be systematically varied.

Use in Anesthesia: Concomitant use of CNS depressants with parenteral pentazocine may produce additive CNS depression. Adequate equipment and facilities should be available to identify and treat systemic emergencies should they occur.

Other: Caution should also be observed when administering pentazocine in patients with hypothyroidism, adrenocortical insufficiency, prostate hypertrophy, inflammatory or obstructive bowel disease, acute abdominal syndromes of unknown etiology, cholecystitis, pancreatitis, or acute alcohol intoxication and delirium tremens.

Drug Interactions: Concomitant use of MAOIs with pentazocine may cause CNS excitation and hypertension through their respective effects on catecholamines. Caution should, therefore, be observed in administering pentazocine to patients who are currently receiving MAOIs or who have received them within the preceding 14 days. Agents with CNS depressant properties including phenothiazine, tricyclic antidepressants, and ethyl alcohol can enhance the CNS depressant effects of pentazocine. Tobacco smoking could enhance the metabolic clearance rate of pentazocine reducing the clinical effectiveness of a standard dose of pentazocine. Pentazocine can antagonize the effects of opiate agonists such as diamorphine, morphine, and heroin and is itself antagonized by naloxone. Because pentazocine has narcotic antagonist activity, it may provoke withdrawal symptoms if given to narcotic addicts. It should be given with caution to patients recently being treated with large doses of narcotics.

Pregnancy: In animal reproduction studies (rodents), teratogenic effects were reported only at doses high enough to cause maternal toxicity. The safe use of pentazocine in pregnant women (other than during labor) has not been established. Pentazocine should be used during pregnancy only if the physician judges the potential benefit to outweigh the risk. Patients receiving pentazocine during labor have experienced no adverse effects other than those that occur with commonly used narcotic analgesics. Pentazocine can cross the placental barrier and can cause CNS depression in the newborn and, if used regularly throughout pregnancy, may lead to symptoms of withdrawal in the newborn. Pentazocine should be used with caution in women delivering premature infants.

Lactation: Pentazocine is excreted in human milk. Caution should be observed in administering pentazocine to breast-feeding mothers.

ADVERSE EFFECTS: The most frequently observed reactions after parenteral administration of pentazocine are nausea, vomiting, sedation, sweating, dizziness, euphoria and lightheadedness.

Dermatologic/Allergic: soft tissue induration, nodules, cutaneous depression at injection sites, ulceration (sloughing) and severe sclerosis of the skin and s.c. tissues (and, rarely, underlying muscle), sting on injection, diaphoresis, flushed skin including plethora, dermatitis including pruritus.

Infrequently occurring reactions are:

Respiratory: respiratory depression, dyspnea, transient apnea in a small number of newborn infants whose mothers received pentazocine during labor.

Cardiovascular: circulatory depression, shock, hypertension, hypotension, tachycardia.

Central and Peripheral Nervous Systems: hallucinations, visual blurring and focusing difficulty, headache, disorientation, dizziness, lightheadedness, sedation, disturbed dreams, insomnia, paresthesia, infrequent weakness, depression, syncope, euphoria, grand mal convulsions, increase in intracranial pressure, confusion, rarely tremor, irritability, excitement, tinnitus.

Gastrointestinal: constipation, dry mouth, biliary tract spasm, abdominal pain.

Other: urinary retention, headache, paresthesia, alterations in rate or strength of uterine contractions during labor, muscle tremor, chills.

Rarely reported reactions include:

Neuromuscular and Psychiatric: muscle tremor, insomnia, disorientation, hallucinations.

Gastrointestinal: taste alteration, diarrhea and cramps.

Ophthalmic: blurred vision, nystagmus, diplopia, miosis.

Hematologic: depression of white blood cell count with rare cases of agranulocytosis, which is usually reversible, moderate transient eosinophilia.

Other: tachycardia, weakness or faintness, chills, allergic reactions sometimes severe have been reported including edema of the face or anaphylactic shock, erythema multiforme and toxic epidermal necrolysis.

Compatibility with Other Drugs: Pentazocine has been compatible with other concurrently administered medication, such as diazepoxides, phenothiazines, meprobamate, barbiturates, chloral hydrate, digitalis, digitoxin, aminophylline, antibiotics and oncolytic drugs. Pentazocine did not alter insulin requirements in 5 diabetic patients. Pentazocine should not be mixed in the same syringe with soluble barbiturates, chlordiazepoxide or diazepam since precipitation will occur.

OVERDOSE:

Symptoms: The symptoms and clinical signs of pentazocine overdosage may resemble those of morphine or other opioids. They may include somnolence, respiratory depression, hypotension, hypertension, tachycardia, hallucinations or seizures. Circulatory failure and deepening coma may occur in more severe cases, particularly in patients who have also ingested other CNS depressants such as alcohol, sedative/hypnotics or antihistamines.

Treatment: Adequate measures to maintain ventilation and general circulatory support should be employed. For respiratory depression due to overdosage or unusual sensitivity to pentazocine, parenteral naloxone is a specific and effective antagonist. Initial doses of 0.4 to 2 mg of naloxone are recommended, repeated at 2- to 3-minute intervals if needed, up to a total of 10 mg. Anticonvulsant therapy may be necessary.

> For management of a suspected drug overdose, CPhA recommends that you contact your **regional Poison Control Centre**. See the *CPS* Directory section for a list of Poison Control Centres.

DOSAGE: Adults (Excluding Patients in Labor): Pentazocine injections may be administered s.c., i.m. or i.v. An initial single dose of 30 mg is recommended. Then the dosage may be adjusted according to patient response and pain severity. In selected situations, 45 to 60 mg administered s.c. or i.m. may be required. The injections may be repeated as necessary every 3 to 4 hours. A single dose should not normally exceed 1 mg/kg body weight s.c. or i.m., or 0.5 mg/kg i.v. The total daily dose should not exceed 360 mg.

Patients in Labor: Pentazocine may be administered as a single i.m. dose of 30 mg. In some patients, an i.v. dose of 20 mg, repeated 2 or 3 times as needed, at intervals of 2 to 3 hours has given adequate pain relief once contractions become regular.

Geriatrics: Elderly patients may require smaller and/or less frequent doses of pentazocine since renal or hepatic function impairment is often associated with aging.

Children: Since clinical experience in children under 12 years of age is limited, the use of pentazocine in this age group is not recommended.

SUPPLIED: Each mL contains: pentazocine 30 mg as pentazocine lactate. Also contains sodium chloride in water for injection. pH adjusted between 4.0 and 5.0 with lactic acid and sodium hydroxide. Alcohol-, bisulfite-, parabens- and tartrazine-free. Ampuls of 1 mL, boxes of 25.

Talwin® Tablets Ⓝ

pentazocine HCl

Narcotic Analgesic

sanofi-aventis

Date of Revision: September 29, 2009

PHARMACOLOGY: Talwin (pentazocine hydrochloride) is a member of the benzazocine series of synthetic benzomorphans. It produces both analgesic (agonist) and narcotic antagonist effects. The analgesic effect of 50 mg of pentazocine administered orally is approximately equivalent to 60 mg of codeine. An oral pentazocine dose of 90 to 100 mg is approximately equal in analgesic effect to 10 mg of i.m. morphine or 75 to 100 mg of i.m. meperidine (pethidine). Opioid pharmacologic effects of pentazocine appear to be dose related and include miosis, respiratory depression, mild increase in biliary pressure, decreased intestinal motility and sedation.

Opiate Antagonism: Pentazocine weakly antagonizes the analgesic effects of morphine, meperidine and phenazocine. In addition, it produces incomplete reversal of cardiovascular, respiratory and behavioral depression produced by morphine and meperidine. Pentazocine has about 1/50 the antagonistic activity of nalorphine.

Talwin is well absorbed from the gastrointestinal tract and is extensively metabolized in the liver. The metabolites are excreted by the kidney with only a small amount of unchanged drug excreted in the urine. Approximately 60% of an oral dose is eliminated in the urine in 24 hours. Oral bioavailability is low and somewhat variable between patients.

The onset of analgesia following oral administration of Talwin can occur within 15 to 30 minutes and the duration of effect is usually 3 hours or longer. The onset and duration of analgesia are, in part, related to the dose and severity of pretreatment pain. Peak serum levels of Talwin occur between 1 and 3 hours after oral administration and the elimination half-life in plasma ranges between 2 to 5 hours. There is considerable variability between individuals in terms of the rate of Talwin metabolism which may also account for the variability in analgesic response.

INDICATIONS: Talwin is indicated for the relief of chronic or acute pain of moderate to severe degree.

CONTRAINDICATIONS: Talwin should not be administered to patients with known hypersensitivity to pentazocine or any of its excipients.

WARNINGS: Drug Abuse and Dependence: In chronic usage, care should be exercised to avoid any unnecessary increase in dosage since prolonged use of high doses of Talwin may produce dependence. Patients with a history of drug abuse should be under close supervision when receiving Talwin.

When Talwin is abruptly discontinued after extended use, withdrawal symptoms such as abdominal cramps, nausea, vomiting, elevated temperature, chills, rhinorrhea, restlessness, anxiety or lacrimation may occur. However, even when these symptoms have occurred, discontinuance has been accomplished with minimal difficulty. In the rare patient in whom more than minor difficulty has been encountered, reinstitution of Talwin with gradual withdrawal has ameliorated the patient's symptoms.

There have been rare reports of a withdrawal syndrome in newborns after prolonged use of Talwin by the mother during pregnancy.

Head Injury and Increased Intracranial Pressure: The respiratory depressant effects of Talwin and its potential for elevating cerebrospinal fluid pressure may be markedly exaggerated in the presence of head injury, other intracranial lesions or a pre-existing increase in intracranial pressure. Talwin can produce effects which may obscure the clinical course of patients with head injuries. Talwin must be used with caution in such patients, and only if its use is deemed essential.

Acute CNS Manifestations: There have been reported instances of the acute onset of hallucinations (usually visual), disorientation, and confusion in patients receiving therapeutic doses of Talwin. These manifestations have cleared spontaneously within hours upon discontinuation of the drug. The mechanism responsible for this reaction is not known. Patients demonstrating this reaction should be closely observed, and if therapy with Talwin is to be restarted, administration should proceed cautiously since the acute CNS manifestations may recur.

Talwin tablets contain sodium metabisulfite, a sulfite that may cause allergic-type reactions including anaphylactic symptoms and life-threatening or less severe asthmatic episodes in certain susceptible people. The overall prevalence of sulfite sensitivity in the general population is unknown and probably low. Sulfite sensitivity is seen more frequently in asthmatic than in nonasthmatic people.

PRECAUTIONS: Occupational Hazards: Ambulatory Patients: Since CNS effects have been noted with the use of Talwin, ambulatory patients should be warned not to operate machinery, drive cars or unnecessarily expose themselves to hazards.

Patients Dependent on Narcotics: Because Talwin is a weak **narcotic antagonist**, patients who are addicted to narcotics may experience withdrawal symptoms, and therefore it should be given with special caution to such persons. In non-addicted patients receiving narcotics for a short period, symptoms believed to be related to antagonism may be observed. Intolerance or untoward reactions are usually not observed following administration of Talwin to patients who have received single doses of, or who have had limited exposure to narcotics.

Impaired Renal or Hepatic Function: Although laboratory tests have not indicated that Talwin causes or increases renal or hepatic impairment, the drug should be administered with caution to patients with such impairment. Extensive liver disease appears to predispose to a higher incidence of side effects (e.g., marked apprehension, anxiety, dizziness, sleepiness) with the usual clinical dose, and may be the result of decreased metabolism of the drug by the liver.

Sphincter of Oddi: Until further experience is gained with the effects of Talwin on the sphincter of Oddi, the drug should be used with caution in patients with acute cholecystitis or pancreatitis or in those about to undergo surgery of the biliary tract.

Obstructive Uropathy: Because urinary retention has been observed in a few patients receiving Talwin, caution is advised in administration of the drug to patients with obstructive uropathy.

Respiratory Conditions: Because respiratory depression is a side effect of agonist opioid therapy, particular caution should be observed when administering Talwin to patients with respiratory conditions such as bronchial asthma, established respiratory depression, limited respiratory reserve or obstructive respiratory conditions.

Patients with Cardiovascular Disease: Talwin can elevate blood pressure, possibly through the release of endogenous catecholamines. Particular caution should be observed in conditions where alterations in vascular resistance and blood pressure might be particularly undesirable such as in the acute phase of myocardial infarction.

Patients with Porphyria: Particular caution should be exercised in administering Talwin to patients with porphyria, since it may provoke an acute attack in susceptible individuals.

Seizure-prone Patients: Caution should be observed in patients who are prone to convulsions; convulsions have occurred in a few such patients in association with the use of Talwin, although no cause and effect relation has been established.

Other: Caution should also be observed when administering Talwin in patients with hypothyroidism, adrenocortical insufficiency, prostate hypertrophy, inflammatory or obstructive bowel disease, acute abdominal syndromes of unknown etiology, cholecystitis, pancreatitis, or acute alcohol intoxication and delirium tremens.

Drug Interactions: Concomitant use of MAOIs with Talwin may cause CNS excitation and hypertension through their respective effects on catecholamines. Caution should, therefore, be observed in administering Talwin to patients who are currently receiving MAOIs or who have received them within the preceding 14 days.

Agents with CNS depressant properties including phenothiazine, tricyclic antidepressants, and ethyl alcohol can enhance the CNS depressant effects of Talwin.

Tobacco smoking could enhance the metabolic clearance rate of Talwin reducing the clinical effectiveness of a standard dose of Talwin.

Talwin can antagonize the effects of opiate agonists such as diamorphine, morphine, and heroin and is itself antagonized by naloxone.

Pregnancy: In animal reproduction studies (rodents), teratogenic effects were reported only at doses high enough to cause maternal toxicity.

The safe use of Talwin in pregnant women (other than during labor) has not been established. Talwin should be used during pregnancy only if the physician judges the potential benefit to outweigh the risk.

Patients receiving Talwin during labor have experienced no adverse effects other than those that occur with commonly used narcotic analgesics. Pentazocine can cross the placental barrier and can cause CNS depression in the newborn and, if used regularly throughout pregnancy, may lead to symptoms of withdrawal in the newborn. Talwin should be used with caution in women delivering premature infants.

Lactation: Pentazocine is excreted in human milk. Caution should be observed in administering Talwin to breast-feeding mothers.

ADVERSE EFFECTS: The most frequently observed reactions after oral administration of Talwin are sedation or somnolence, vertigo, nausea, vomiting, dizziness, lightheadedness and sweating. Sedation may be more marked in the elderly.

Less frequent reactions have been:

Gastrointestinal: constipation, abdominal distress, anorexia, diarrhea, dry mouth, biliary tract spasm.

Central and Peripheral Nervous Systems: euphoria, lightheadedness, headache, dizziness, weakness, disturbed dreams, hallucinations, visual disturbances, insomnia, tinnitus, irritability, excitement, sweating, infrequently flushing or chills, disorientation, paresthesia, syncope, grand mal convulsions, increased intracranial pressure, confusion, tremor.

Cardiovascular: infrequently hypotension, tachycardia, hypertension, and circulatory depression.

Dermatologic/Allergic: allergic reactions, sometimes severe, have been reported including edema of the face or anaphylactic shock, flushed skin including plethora, dermatitis including pruritus. Erythema multiforme and toxic epidermal necrolysis have been reported.

Hematologic: depression of white blood cell count, with rare cases of agranulocytosis, which is usually reversible, moderate transient eosinophilia.

Ophthalmic: miosis.

Respiratory: respiratory depression.

Other: urinary retention, muscle tremor, chills, alterations in rate of strength of uterine contractions during labor, alterations in maturation. Scattered reports of abnormal liver function of questionable significance were noted during the clinical trials. Hallucinations were noted to occur more frequently when doses exceeding that recommended were employed.

OVERDOSE:

Symptoms: The symptoms and clinical signs of Talwin overdosage may resemble those of morphine or other opioids. They may include somnolence, respiratory depression, hypotension, hypertension, tachycardia, hallucinations or seizures. Circulatory failure and deepening coma may occur in more severe cases, particularly in patients who have also ingested other CNS depressants such as alcohol, sedative/hypnotics or antihistamines.

Treatment: Adequate measures to maintain ventilation and general circulatory support should be employed and consideration given to gastric lavage and gastric aspiration. For respiratory depression due to overdosage or unusual sensitivity to Talwin, parenteral naloxone is a specific and effective antagonist. Initial doses of 0.4 to 2 mg of naloxone are recommended, repeated at 2- to 3-minute intervals if needed, up to a total of 10 mg. Anticonvulsant therapy may be necessary.

For management of a suspected drug overdose, CPhA recommends that you contact your **regional Poison Control Centre**. See the *CPS* Directory section for a list of Poison Control Centres.

DOSAGE: The usual starting dose is 50 mg every 4 hours after meals. Dosage should be adjusted to individual requirements and tolerance within the range of 50 to 100 mg (1-2 tabs) every 3 to 4 hours.

In light of the tendency to marked sedation among the elderly, dosage should be kept low in this group of patients.

Concomitant Medication: When anti-inflammatory or antipyretic effects are desired in addition to analgesia, ASA can be administered concomitantly with Talwin.

Duration of Therapy: There have been rare reports of withdrawal symptoms upon abrupt discontinuance of Talwin therapy after prolonged administration of the product for chronic pain. Therefore, it would be prudent to reduce the dose gradually when the drug is no longer required.

SUPPLIED: Each round, flat, bevelled white tablet, engraved with "FtL" on one side and "50" on the other side contains: pentazocine HCl equivalent to 50 mg base. Nonmedicinal ingredients: calcium phosphate (dibasic), colloidal silicon dioxide, corn starch, magnesium stearate, microcrystalline cellulose, sodium lauryl sulfate and sodium metabisulfite. Gluten-, lactose- and tartrazine-free. Blisters of 100 and 500 tablets.

(Shown in Product Identification Section)

Tambocor™ Ⓟ

flecainide acetate

Antiarrhythmic

Graceway

PHARMACOLOGY: Flecainide belongs to the membrane stabilizing group of antiarrhythmic agents; it has electrophysiologic effects characteristic of the 1C class of the modified Vaughan-Williams classification. It also possesses local anesthetic properties.

In single cell preparations from canine cardiac tissue (Purkinje fibres) flecainide decreased the rate of rise (V_{max}, Phase O) of the action potential without greatly affecting its duration; the duration of the effective refractory period was lengthened and a small change was observed in the slope of Phase 4 depolarization. In ventricular muscle, some lengthening of the action potential duration has been observed.

Flecainide produces a dose-related decrease in intracardiac conduction in all parts of the heart with the greatest effect on the His-Purkinje system (H-V conduction). Effects upon atrioventricular (AV) nodal conduction time and intra-atrial conduction times, although present, are less pronounced than those on ventricular conduction velocity. Significant effects on refractory periods were observed only in the ventricle. Sinus node recovery times (corrected) following pacing and spontaneous cycle lengths are somewhat increased. This latter effect may become significant in patients with sinus node dysfunction (see Warnings).

Decreases in ejection fraction, consistent with a negative inotropic effect, have been observed after single administration of 200 to 250 mg flecainide; both increases and decreases in ejection fraction have been encountered during multidose therapy in patients at usual therapeutic doses (see Warnings).

During long-term clinical studies, some patients have developed congestive heart failure (CHF) while taking flecainide (see Warnings and Adverse Effects).

Flecainide does not usually alter heart rate, although bradycardia and tachycardia have been reported. In clinical studies, systolic and diastolic blood pressures increased slightly during therapy. A few patients have required changes in antihypertensive medication.

Following oral administration, flecainide is nearly completely absorbed with bioavailability of 90 to 95%. Peak plasma levels are attained at about 3 hours in most individuals (range, 1 to 6 hours). Food and antacids do not affect absorption. Flecainide does not undergo any consequential presystemic biotransformation.

The plasma half-life averages about 20 hours (range, 12 to 27 hours) after multiple oral doses in patients with premature ventricular complexes and normal renal function; this is similar to that in patients with CHF (mean, 19 hours), but it is moderately longer than for healthy subjects (mean, 14 hours). In patients with renal impairment the plasma half-life of flecainide is often prolonged and ranges from about 14 to 190 hours. Flecainide elimination from plasma is somewhat slower in healthy elderly subjects ($t½$=18 hours) than in young healthy subjects.

Steady-state plasma levels are reached within 3 to 5 days; once steady state is attained, no additional drug accumulation in plasma occurs. Therapeutic plasma concentrations of flecainide range from 0.2 to 1.0 µg/mL. The plasma levels are not directly proportional to dose. Within the usual therapeutic dose range, plasma levels deviate upwards from direct proportionality (average deviation about 10 to 15% per 100 mg).

The extent of flecainide binding to plasma proteins is about 40% and is independent of plasma drug level over the range of 0.015 to 3.4 µg/mL.

In healthy subjects, about 30% of a single oral dose (range, 10 to 50%) is excreted in urine as unchanged flecainide. The 2 major metabolites are meta-O-dealkylated flecainide (active, but about one fifth as potent) and the meta-O-dealkylated lactam of flecainide (nonactive metabolite). These 2 metabolites (primarily conjugated) account for most of the remaining portion of the dose in urine. Several minor metabolites (3% of the dose or less) are also found in urine; only 5% of an oral dose is excreted in feces. In patients, free (unconjugated) plasma levels of the 2 major metabolites are very low (less than 0.05 µg/mL).

With increasing renal impairment, the extent of unchanged drug excretion in urine is reduced. Since flecainide is also extensively metabolized, there is no simple relationship between creatinine clearance and the rate of flecainide elimination from plasma (see Dosage). When urine is very alkaline (pH 8 or higher), as may occur in rare conditions (e.g., renal tubular acidosis, strict vegetarian diet), flecainide elimination from plasma is much slower.

Hemodialysis removes only about 1% of an oral dose as unchanged flecainide.

INDICATIONS:

No antiarrhythmic drug has been shown to reduce the incidence of sudden death in patients with asymptomatic ventricular arrhythmias. Most antiarrhythmic drugs have the potential to cause dangerous arrhythmias; some have been shown to be associated with an increased incidence of sudden death. In light of the above, physicians should carefully consider the risks and benefits of antiarrhythmic therapy for all patients with ventricular arrhythmias.

In patients without structural heart disease and with disabling symptoms, flecainide is indicated for the prevention of: paroxysmal supraventricular tachycardias (PSVT), including AV nodal reentrant tachycardia, AV reentrant tachycardia and other supraventricular tachycardias of unspecified mechanism; paroxysmal atrial fibrillation/flutter (PAF).

Patients treated with flecainide for supraventricular arrhythmias having impaired left ventricular function (ejection fraction<40) and/or ischemic heart disease may be at increased risk for cardiac adverse reactions. Use of flecainide in chronic atrial fibrillation has not been adequately studied and is not recommended (see Warnings).

Flecainide is also indicated for the treatment of documented ventricular arrhythmias, such as sustained ventricular tachycardia (sustained VT), that in the judgment of the physician, are life-threatening.

Because of the proarrhythmic effects of flecainide, its use should be reserved for patients in whom, in the opinion of the physician, the benefits of treatment outweigh the risks. The use of flecainide is not recommended in patients with less severe ventricular arrhythmias, even if the patients are symptomatic (see Warnings). Use of flecainide for treatment of sustained ventricular tachycardia should be initiated in the hospital.

Tambocor should not be used in patients with recent myocardial infarction (see Warnings).

CONTRAINDICATIONS: In patients with: second- or third-degree AV block, unless a pacemaker is present to sustain rhythm; bifascicular or trifascicular bundle branch block unless a pacemaker is present to sustain rhythm; cardiogenic shock; and hypersensitivity to the drug.

WARNINGS:

Mortality: The results of the Cardiac Arrhythmia Suppression Trial (CAST) in postmyocardial infarction patients with asymptomatic ventricular arrhythmias showed a significant increase in mortality and in nonfatal cardiac arrest rate in patients treated with encainide or flecainide compared with a matched placebo-treated group. This rate was 19/323 (5.8%) for flecainide and 7/318 (2.2%) for its matched placebo. The average duration of treatment with flecainide was 10 months. CAST was continued using a revised protocol with the moricizine and placebo arms only. The trial was prematurely terminated because of a trend towards an increase in mortality in the moricizine treated group.

The applicability of these results to other populations or other antiarrhythmic agents is uncertain, but at present it is prudent to consider these results when using any antiarrhythmic agent.

Ventricular Proarrhythmic Effects in Patients with Atrial Fibrillation/Flutter: A review of the world literature revealed reports of 568 patients treated with flecainide for paroxysmal atrial fibrillation/flutter (PAF). Ventricular tachycardia was experienced in 0.4% (2/568) of these patients. Of 19 patients in the literature with chronic atrial fibrillation, 10.5% (2/19) experienced ventricular tachycardia or ventricular fibrillation. **Flecainide is not recommended for use in patients with chronic atrial fibrillation.** Case reports of ventricular proarrhythmic effects in patients treated with flecainide for atrial fibrillation/flutter have included increased premature ventricular contractions (PVCs), ventricular tachycardia (VT), ventricular fibrillation (VF), and death.

As with other class I agents, patients treated with flecainide atrial flutter have been reported with 1:1AV conduction due to slowing of the atrial rate. A paradoxical increase in the ventricular rate also may occur in patients with atrial fibrillation who receive flecainide. Concomitant negative chronotropic therapy such as digoxin or beta-blockers may lower the risk of this complication.

Proarrhythmic Effects: Flecainide, like other antiarrhythmic agents, can cause new or worsened arrhythmias. Such proarrhythmic effects range from an increase in frequency of PVCs to the development of more severe ventricular tachycardia, e.g., tachycardia that is more sustained or more resistant to conversion to sinus rhythm, with potentially fatal consequences. In studies of 225 patients with supraventricular arrhythmia (108 with paroxysmal supraventricular tachycardia and 117 with paroxysmal atrial fibrillation), there were nine (4%) proarrhythmic events, eight of them in patients with paroxysmal atrial fibrillation. Of the nine, seven (including the one in a PSVT patient) were exacerbations of supraventricular arrhythmias (longer duration, more rapid rate, harder to reverse). Two were ventricular arrhythmias, including one fatal case of VT/VF and one wide complex VT (the patient showed inducible VT, however, after withdrawal of flecainide), both in patients with paroxysmal atrial fibrillation and known coronary artery disease.

In studies of patients with ventricular arrhythmias, flecainide proarrhythmic effects were reported in 6.8% of patients. Three fourths of the proarrhythmic events were new or worsened ventricular tachyarrhythmias, the remainder being increased frequency of PVCs or new supraventricular arrhythmias.

In patients with complex ventricular arrhythmias, it is often difficult to distinguish a spontaneous variation in the patient's underlying rhythm disorder from drug-induced worsening, so that the following occurrence rates must be considered approximations. Their frequency appears to be related to dose and to the underlying cardiac disease. Among patients treated for sustained VT (who frequently also had heart failure, a low ejection fraction, a history of myocardial infarction and/or an episode of cardiac arrest), the incidence of proarrhythmic events was 13% when dosage was initiated at 200 mg/day with slow upward titration, and did not exceed 300 mg/day in most patients. In early studies in patients with sustained VT utilizing a higher initial dose (400 mg/day) the incidence of proarrhythmic events was 26%; moreover, in about 10% of the patients treated, proarrhythmic events resulted in death, despite prompt medical attention. With lower initial doses, the incidence of proarrhythmic events resulting in death decreased to 0.5% of these patients. Accordingly, it is extremely important to follow the recommended dosage schedule (see Dosage).

The relatively high frequency of proarrhythmic events in patients with sustained ventricular tachycardia and serious underlying heart disease, and the need for careful titration and monitoring, requires that flecainide therapy be started in the hospital (see Dosage).

Heart Failure: Because flecainide has a negative inotropic effect, it may cause or worsen congestive heart failure, particularly in patients with cardiomyopathy, pre-existing severe heart failure (NYHA functional class III or IV) or low ejection fractions (less than 40%). In patients with supraventricular arrhythmias new or worsened CHF developed in 0.4% (1/225) of patients. New or worsened CHF which might be attributed to flecainide treatment occurred in approximately 5% of patients studied in various trials. CHF developed rarely (1%) in patients who had no previous history of CHF. Flecainide should be used cautiously in patients who are known to have a history of CHF or myocardial dysfunction. The initial dose should be no more than 100 mg twice daily in such patients (see Dosage) and they should be carefully monitored. Careful attention must be given to maintenance of cardiac function, including optimization of digitalis, diuretic or other therapy. In the cases where CHF has occurred or worsened during flecainide therapy, the onset has ranged from a few hours to several months after starting therapy. Patients who develop evidence of reduced myocardial function while on flecainide should have their dose reduced or discontinued. It is recommended that plasma flecainide levels be monitored. Attempts should be made to keep trough plasma levels below 0.7 to 1 µg/mL.

Effects on Cardiac Conduction: In most patients flecainide slows cardiac conduction sufficiently to produce dose-related increases in the duration of the PR, QRS and QT intervals on the ECG.

PR interval increases on average about 25% (0.04 seconds) and as much as 118% in some patients. Approximately one-third of patients may develop new first degree AV heart block (PR interval 0.20 seconds). The QRS complex increases on average about 25% (0.2 seconds) and as much as 150% in some patients. Many patients develop QRS complexes with a duration of 0.12 seconds or more. In one study, 4% of patients developed new bundle branch block while on flecainide. The degree of lengthening of PR and QRS intervals does not predict either efficacy or the development of cardiac adverse effects. In clinical trials, it was unusual for PR intervals to increase to 0.30 seconds or more, or for QRS intervals to increase to 0.18 seconds or more. Thus, caution should be used when such intervals occur, and dose reductions may be considered. The QT interval widens about 8%, but most of this widening (about 60 to 90%) is due to widening of the QRS duration. The JT interval (QT minus QRS) only widens about 4% on the average. Significant JT prolongation occurs in less than 2% of patients. There have been a few cases of torsades de pointes-type arrhythmia associated with flecainide-induced QT prolongation and bradycardia.

Clinically significant conduction changes have been observed with these incidences: sinus node dysfunction such as sinus pause, sinus arrest and symptomatic bradycardia (1.2%); second-degree AV block (0.5%); and third-degree AV block (0.4%). An attempt should be made to manage the patient on the lowest effective dose in an effort to minimize these effects (see Dosage). If second- or third-degree AV block, or right bundle branch block associated with a left hemiblock occurs, therapy should be discontinued unless a temporary or implanted ventricular pacemaker is in place to ensure an adequate ventricular rate.

Sinus Node Dysfunction: In patients with sinus node dysfunction (e.g., sick sinus syndrome), flecainide should be used with extreme caution because it may cause sinus bradycardia, sinus pause or sinus arrest.

Digitalis Intoxication: Flecainide has not been evaluated in the treatment of arrhythmias secondary to digitalis intoxication, and it increases the plasma level of digoxin. Therefore, it is not recommended for such use.

Electrolyte Disturbances: The presence of potassium excess or deficit may alter the effects of antiarrhythmic drugs. Any pre-existing hypokalemia or hyperkalemia should be corrected before drug administration.

Effects of Pacemaker Thresholds: Flecainide is known to increase endocardial pacing thresholds and may suppress ventricular escape rhythms. These effects are reversible if flecainide is discontinued. It should be used with caution in patients with permanent pacemakers or temporary pacing electrodes and should not be administered to patients with existing poor thresholds or nonprogrammable pacemakers unless suitable pacing rescue is available.

The pacing threshold in patients with pacemakers should be determined prior to instituting therapy with flecainide, again after 1 week of administration and at regular intervals thereafter. Generally threshold changes are within the range of multiprogrammable pacemakers and, when these occur, a doubling of either voltage or pulse width is usually sufficient to regain capture.

Concomitant Antiarrhythmic Therapy: Due to limited experience, the concomitant use of flecainide and other antiarrhythmic agents is not recommended.

Both disopyramide and verapamil have negative inotropic properties and the effects of giving them with flecainide are unknown. Therefore, neither disopyramide or verapamil should be administered concurrently with flecainide unless, in the judgment of the physician, the possible benefit of this combination therapy clearly outweighs the risks.

When flecainide and amiodarone are coadministered, plasma flecainide levels may increase two-fold or more. If the combination therapy is required, the dose should be reduced (see Dosage).

Lidocaine has been used occasionally with flecainide while awaiting the therapeutic effect of flecainide. No adverse drug interactions were apparent. However, no studies have been performed to demonstrate the usefulness of this regimen.

Pregnancy: Flecainide has been shown to have teratogenic effects (club paws, sternebrae and vertebrae abnormalities, pale hearts with contracted ventricular septum) and an embryotoxic effect (increased resorptions) in one breed of rabbit (New Zealand White) but not in another breed of rabbit (Dutch Belted) when given in doses about 4 times (but not 3 times) the usual human dose (assuming a patient weight of 50 kg). No teratogenic effects were observed in rats and mice given doses up to 50 to 80 mg/kg/day, respectively; however, delayed sternebral and vertebral ossification was observed at the high dose in rats. There is no information about the effect on human fetuses. Flecainide should not be used during pregnancy unless as a drug of last resort in life-threatening arrhythmias.

Labor and Delivery: It is not known whether the use of flecainide during labor or delivery has immediate or delayed adverse effects on the mother or fetus, affects the duration of labor or delivery, or increases the possibility of forceps delivery or other obstetrical intervention.

PRECAUTIONS: Hepatic Impairment: Since flecainide elimination from plasma can be markedly slower in patients with significant hepatic impairment, it should not be used in such patients unless the potential benefits clearly outweigh the risks. If used, frequent and early plasma level monitoring is required to guide dosage (see Dosage); dosage increases should be made very cautiously when plasma levels have plateaued (after more than 4 days).

Abnormalities of liver function have rarely occurred in patients treated with flecainide (see Adverse Effects). In foreign post-marketing surveillance studies, there have been rare reports of hepatic dysfunction including reports of cholestasis and hepatic failure. Although no causal relationship has been established, periodic monitoring of liver function tests should be carried out during flecainide therapy. In patients who develop unexplained jaundice or signs of hepatic dysfunction, it is advisable to discontinue flecainide in order to eliminate the drug as the possible causative agent.

Renal Impairment: The elimination of flecainide from the body depends on renal function (i.e., 10 to 50% appears in urine as unchanged drug). With increasing renal impairment, the extent of unchanged drug excretion in urine is reduced and the plasma half-life of flecainide is prolonged. Different dosage regimens are recommended for patients with various degrees of renal insufficiency (see Pharmacology and Dosage).

Blood Dyscrasias: There have been extremely rare reports of blood dyscrasias (pancytopenia, anemia, thrombocytopenia, leukopenia, granulocytopenia). Although no causal relationship has been established, it is advisable to discontinue flecainide in patients who develop blood dyscrasia in order to eliminate it as the possible causative agent.

Occupational Hazards: Since flecainide can cause dizziness, light-headedness, faintness and visual disturbance, patients should be cautioned about engaging in activities requiring judgment and physical co-ordination (such as driving an automobile or operating dangerous machinery) when these effects occur.

Geriatrics: Flecainide elimination from plasma is somewhat slower in this age group (see Dosage).

Lactation: Flecainide is excreted in human milk. Because of the drug's potential for serious adverse reactions in nursing infants, a decision should be made whether to discontinue nursing or discontinue the drug, taking into account the importance of the drug to the mother.

Children: The safety and effectiveness in children below the age of 18 years have not been established.

Drug Interactions: Flecainide has been administered to patients receiving digitalis preparations or beta-adrenergic blocking agents without adverse effects. During multiple oral doses to healthy subjects stabilized on a maintenance dose of digoxin, a 13 to 19% increase in plasma digoxin levels occurred at 6 hours postdose.

In a study involving healthy subjects receiving flecainide and propranolol concurrently, plasma flecainide levels were increased about 20% and propranolol levels were increased about 30% compared with control values. In this study, flecainide and propranolol were each found to have negative inotropic effects; when the drugs were administered together, the effects were additive. The effects of concomitant administration on the PR interval were less than additive. In flecainide clinical trials, patients who were receiving beta-blockers concurrently did not experience an increased incidence of side effects. Nevertheless, the possibility of additive negative inotropic effects of beta-blockers and flecainide should be recognized.

Flecainide has been used in a large number of patients receiving diuretics without apparent interaction.

Interactions with antiarrhythmics, see Warnings.

Limited data in patients receiving known enzyme inducers (phenytoin, phenobarbital, carbamazepine) indicate a 30% increase in the rate of flecainide elimination.

In healthy subjects receiving cimetidine (1 g daily) for 1 week, plasma flecainide levels increased by about 30% and half-life increased by about 10%.

Flecainide is not extensively bound to plasma proteins. In vitro studies with several drugs which may be administered concomitantly showed that the extent of flecainide binding to human plasma proteins is either unchanged or only slightly less.

ADVERSE EFFECTS: In postmyocardial infarction patients, flecainide was found to be associated with a 5.8% rate of mortality and nonfatal cardiac arrest (see Warnings).

Flecainide has been evaluated in 225 patients with supraventricular arrhythmias. The most serious adverse reaction reported for flecainide patients with supraventricular arrhythmias were new or worsened supraventricular or ventricular arrhythmias which were reported in 4% of patients (see Warnings), conduction disturbance which occurred in 2% of patients, and new or worsened CHF occurred in 0.4% of patients.

The most commonly reported non-cardiac adverse reactions for supraventricular patients remain consistent with those known for patients treated with flecainide for ventricular arrhythmias: vision disturbance 38%, dizziness 37%, headache 18%, nausea 18%, dyspnea 13%, fatigue 13%, chest pain 12%, palpitations 11%. Although these incidences are higher than those reported in ventricular patients it is difficult to compare supraventricular and ventricular data bases because many of the supraventricular patients were dosed to tolerance in the clinical trials.

Flecainide has been evaluated in 1 224 patients which included both life threatening and non life threatening ventricular arrhythmias. The separate figures for these 2 groups of patients are not available at this time. The possibility exists that the incidences of adverse reactions in patients with life threatening ventricular arrhythmias for which this drug is indicated, might be different than that listed below. The most serious adverse reactions reported were new or exacerbated ventricular arrhythmias which occurred in 6.8% of patients, and new or worsened congestive heart failure which occurred in 3.9% of patients (or 5% of 717 patients in controlled clinical studies).

In some patients, treatment has been associated with episodes of unresuscitatable ventricular tachycardia or ventricular fibrillation. There have also been instances of second (0.5%) or third degree (0.4%) AV block. A total of 1.2% of patients developed sinus bradycardia, sinus pause, or sinus arrest (see Warnings). The frequency of most of these serious adverse reactions probably increases with higher trough plasma levels, especially when these trough levels exceed 0.7 mg/mL.

The most commonly reported noncardiac adverse reactions experienced by patients with ventricular arrhythmias participating in clinical trials were dizziness 26.6%, visual disturbance 25.9% (includes blurred vision, diplopia, visual field defects, photophobia), headache 10.4%, nausea 10.1%, and dyspnea 8.6%. Other adverse reactions occurring in over 3% of the patients in clinical trials:

Body as a Whole: fatigue 7.4%, asthenia 4.7%.
Cardiovascular: palpitations 6.0%, chest pain 6.0%.
Gastrointestinal: constipation 4.2%, abdominal pain 3.3%.
Nervous System: tremor 5.6%, nervousness 3.1%, paresthesia 3.1%.
Skin: rash 4.1%.

The following additional adverse reactions, possibly related to flecainide therapy and occurring in 1 to less than 3% of patients have been reported in clinical trials:

Body as a Whole: pain, increased sweating, flushing, dry mouth, arthralgia, fever, myalgia.
Cardiovascular: edema, syncope, tachycardia, angina pectoris, conduction disturbance.
Gastrointestinal: vomiting, diarrhea, anorexia.
Nervous System: hypoesthesia, somnolence, insomnia, ataxia.
Respiratory: coughing.
Skin: pruritus.
Special Senses: tinnitus.
Urinary System: micturition disorder (includes urinary retention, frequency, polyuria, dysuria).

The following additional adverse experiences, possibly related to flecainide, have been reported in less than 1% of patients:

Body as a Whole: impotence, decreased libido, gynecomastia, malaise.
Cardiovascular: bradycardia, ECG abnormality, hypertension, hypotension, heart disorder, myocardial infarction, peripheral ischemia, pulmonary edema.
Gastrointestinal: dyspepsia, flatulence, gastrointestinal hemorrhage.
Nervous System: anxiety, twitching, convulsions, nystagmus, stupor, dysphonia, speech disorder, coma, amnesia, confusion, depersonalization, hallucination, paranoid reaction, euphoria, apathy.
Respiratory: bronchospasm, laryngismus.
Skin: dermatitis, hypertrichosis, photosensitivity reaction, skin discoloration.
Special Senses: deafness, parosmia, loss of taste, taste perversion.
Urinary System: renal failure, hematuria.
Laboratory Abnormalities: hyperglycemia, increased nonprotein in nitrogen, increased serum alkaline phosphatase, increased serum ALT and AST. Patients with elevations of liver function tests have been asymptomatic and no cause and effect relationship with flecainide has been established.

Adverse reactions leading to discontinuation of therapy occurred in 18.5% of the patients. The two most common were noncardiac adverse reactions 9.0% and new or worsened arrhythmias 6.8%.

OVERDOSE:

Symptoms: Animal studies suggest the following events might occur with overdosage: lengthening of the PR interval; increase in the QRS duration, QT interval and amplitude of the T-wave; a reduction in myocardial rate and contractility; conduction disturbances; hypotension; and death from respiratory failure or asystole.

Treatment: No specific antidote has been identified for the treatment of flecainide overdosage. Treatment of overdosage should be supportive and may include the following: removal of unabsorbed drug from the gastrointestinal tract, administration of inotropic agents or cardiac stimulants such as dopamine, dobutamine or isoproterenol; mechanically assisted respiration; circulatory assists such as intra-aortic balloon pumping; and transvenous pacing in the event of conduction block. Because of the long plasma half-life of flecainide (range from 12 to 27 hours in patients), and the possibility of markedly nonlinear elimination kinetics at very high doses, these supportive treatments may need to be continued for extended periods of time.

Hemodialysis is not an effective means of removing flecainide from the body.

Since flecainide elimination is much slower when urine is very alkaline (pH 8 or higher), acidification of urine to promote drug excretion may, theoretically, be beneficial in overdose cases with very alkaline urine. There is no evidence that acidification from normal urinary pH increases excretion.

For management of a suspected drug overdose, CPhA recommends that you contact your **regional Poison Control Centre**. See the *CPS* Directory section for a list of Poison Control Centres.

DOSAGE: Supraventricular Arrhythmias: The recommended starting dose for patients with paroxysmal supraventricular tachycardias or patients with paroxysmal atrial fibrillation/flutter is 50 mg every 12 hrs. Flecainide may be increased in increments of 50 mg b.i.d. every 4 days until efficacy is achieved. The maximum recommended dose is 300 mg/day.

Ventricular Arrhythmias: For patients with sustained ventricular tachycardia, flecainide should be started in the hospital with rhythm monitoring. The recommended starting dose for patients with ventricular arrhythmias is 100 mg every 12 hours. Flecainide may be increased in increments of 50 mg b.i.d. every 4 days until efficacy is achieved. Most patients do not require more than 150 mg every 12 hours (300 mg/day). The maximum dose is 400 mg/day.

Use of higher initial doses and more rapid dosage adjustments has resulted in an increased incidence of proarrhythmic events and congestive heart failure, particularly during the first few days of dosing (see Warnings). Therefore, a loading dose is not recommended.

An occasional patient not adequately controlled by (or intolerant to) a dose given at 12-hour intervals may be given flecainide at 8-hour intervals.

Once adequate control of the arrhythmia has been achieved, it may be possible in some patients to reduce the dose as necessary to minimize side effects or effects on conduction. In such patients, efficacy at the lower dose should be evaluated.

In patients with a history of CHF or myocardial dysfunction, the initial dose should be no more than 100 mg every 12 hours. If needed to achieve efficacy, the dosage may be increased cautiously in increments of 50 mg twice a day every 4 days, and the maximum dosage should not exceed 200 mg every 12 hours (400 mg/day), because higher doses are associated with a greater incidence of worsened CHF (see Warnings).

In patients with severe renal impairment (creatinine clearance of 35 mL/min/1.73 m² or less), the initial dosage should be 50 mg to 100 mg once daily; when used in such patients, daily plasma level monitoring is required to guide dosage adjustments (see Plasma Level Monitoring). In patients with less severe renal disease, the initial dosage should be 100 mg every 12 hours; plasma level monitoring is also recommended in these patients during dosage adjustment. In both groups of patients, dosage increases should be made very cautiously when plasma levels have plateaued, observing the patient closely for signs of adverse cardiac effects or other toxicity. It should be borne in mind that in these patients it is likely to take longer than 4 days before a new steady state plasma level is reached following a dosage change. Therefore the interval between dose increases should be longer than the 4 days recommended for patients with normal renal function.

In elderly patients flecainide elimination from plasma is somewhat slower. The initial dosage need not be adjusted, however, daily trough plasma flecainide level monitoring is recommended during dosage adjustment.

Plasma Level Monitoring: Therapeutic trough plasma flecainide levels were found to range between 0.2 and 1.0 µg/mL. The probability of adverse experiences, especially cardiac, may increase with higher trough plasma levels, especially when these exceed 0.7 µg/mL. Periodic monitoring of trough plasma levels may be useful in patient management. Because elimination of flecainide from plasma may be markedly slower in patients with severe chronic renal failure or severe hepatic disease, plasma level monitoring is required in these patients. Plasma level monitoring is recommended in patients with congestive heart failure, moderate renal disease, and the elderly.

Based on theoretical considerations, rather than experimental data, the following suggestion is made: when transferring patients from another antiarrhythmic drug to flecainide or from flecainide to another antiarrhythmic, allow at least 2 to 4 plasma half-lives to elapse for the drug being discontinued before starting the alternative at the usual dosage. In patients where withdrawal of a previous antiarrhythmic agent is likely to produce life-threatening arrhythmias, the physician should consider hospitalizing the patient.

If flecainide is given in the presence of amiodarone (see Warnings) the usual dose of flecainide should be reduced by 50% and the patient should be monitored closely for adverse reactions. Plasma level monitoring is strongly recommended to guide dosage with such combination therapy.

SUPPLIED: 50 mg: Each white, round, unscored tablet, imprinted with 3M on one side and TR 50 on the other side, contains: flecainide acetate 50 mg. Nonmedicinal ingredients: croscarmellose sodium, hydrogenated vegetable oil, magnesium stearate, microcrystalline cellulose and starch. Tartrazine-free. Bottles of 100.

100 mg: Each white, round, scored tablet, embossed with 3M on one side and TR 100 on the other side, contains: flecainide acetate 100 mg. Nonmedicinal ingredients: croscarmellose sodium, hydrogenated vegetable oil, magnesium stearate, microcrystalline cellulose and starch. Tartrazine-free. Bottles of 100.

Store between 15 to 30°C. Protect from light.

Tamiflu® ℞

oseltamivir phosphate

Antiviral Agent

Roche

Date of Revision: November 9, 2009

SUMMARY PRODUCT INFORMATION:

Route of Administration	Dosage Form/ Strength	Clinically Relevant Nonmedicinal Ingredients
Oral	Capsule/30 mg, 45 mg and 75 mg oseltamivir	None For a complete listing see Dosage Forms, Composition and Packaging.
Oral	Powder for Oral Suspension/ 12 mg/mL oseltamivir when reconstituted	Sorbitol (see Warnings and Precautions) For a complete listing see Dosage Forms, Composition and Packaging.

INDICATIONS AND CLINICAL USE: Treatment of Influenza: TAMIFLU (oseltamivir phosphate) is indicated for:

- The treatment of uncomplicated acute illness due to influenza infection in adults and adolescents (>13 years) who have been symptomatic for no more than 2 days.

  The treatment indication is based on two Phase III clinical studies of naturally occurring influenza in adults in which the predominant infection was influenza A (95%) and a limited number with influenza B (3%) and influenza of unknown type (2%), reflecting the distribution of these strains in the community. The indication is also supported by influenza A and B challenge studies. No data are available to support the safety and efficacy of TAMIFLU in adult patients who commenced treatment after 40 hours of onset of symptoms.
- The treatment of uncomplicated acute illness due to influenza in pediatric patients 1 year and older who have been symptomatic for no more than 2 days.

The pediatric indication is based on one Phase III clinical study of naturally occurring influenza in pediatric patients aged 1 to 12 years in which 67% of influenza infected patients were infected with influenza A and 33% with influenza B.

TAMIFLU, when taken as recommended for the treatment of influenza, alleviates the symptoms and reduces their duration.

Prevention/Prophylaxis of Influenza: The decision to administer TAMIFLU for prophylaxis to close contacts should be based on the knowledge that influenza is circulating in the area and the index case demonstrates characteristic symptoms of influenza. TAMIFLU is not effective in providing prophylaxis for respiratory infections other than influenza therefore a proper diagnosis of the index case is important.

TAMIFLU is not a substitute for influenza vaccination. Vaccination is the preferred method of prophylactic prevention against influenza. The use of TAMIFLU should not affect the evaluation of individuals for annual influenza vaccination, in accordance to "Health Canada. An Advisory Committee Statement on Influenza Vaccination for the Current Year/Season."

The use of antivirals for the treatment and prevention of influenza should be determined on the basis of official recommendations taking into consideration variability of epidemiology and the impact of the disease in different geographical areas and patient populations.

TAMIFLU is indicated for:

- The prevention of influenza illness in adults and adolescents 13 years and older following close contact with an infected individual (the index case).

  The prevention indication is based on a phase III clinical study programme consisting of 4 Phase III clinical trials.
- The prevention of influenza illness in pediatric patients 1 year and older following close contact with an infected individual (the index case).

  This indication is based on a substudy of pediatric patients in a Phase III clinical trial.

CONTRAINDICATIONS:

- TAMIFLU (oseltamivir phosphate) is contraindicated in patients with known hypersensitivity to any of the components of the product. For a complete listing, see Dosage Forms, Composition and Packaging.

WARNINGS AND PRECAUTIONS: General: No increased efficacy was demonstrated in adult subjects receiving 150 mg TAMIFLU (oseltamivir phosphate) twice daily for 5 days compared to those receiving 75 mg twice daily for the treatment of influenza.

There is no evidence for efficacy of TAMIFLU in any illness caused by agents other than influenza viruses Types A and B. Data on treatment of influenza B are limited.

Efficacy of TAMIFLU in patients who begin treatment after 48 hours of symptoms has not been established.

Efficacy of TAMIFLU in the treatment of subjects with chronic cardiac disease and/or respiratory disease has not been established. No difference in the incidence of complications was observed between the treatment and placebo groups in this population. No information is available regarding treatment of influenza in patients with any medical condition sufficiently severe or unstable to be considered at imminent risk of requiring hospitalization.

Safety and efficacy of repeated treatment or prevention courses have not been studied.

Efficacy of TAMIFLU for treatment or prevention of influenza in immunocompromised patients has not been established.

Endocrine and Metabolism: A bottle of 30 g TAMIFLU powder for oral suspension contains 25.713 g of sorbitol. One dose of 45 mg oseltamivir administered twice daily delivers 2.6 g of sorbitol which is unsuitable for subjects with hereditary fructose intolerance.

Hepatic: There have been post-marketing reports of elevated liver enzymes and hepatotoxicity including fulminant hepatitis/hepatic failure, in some cases with fatal outcome, where a causal relationship with oseltamivir could not be excluded, especially in patients with pre-existing liver disease.

The safety, efficacy and pharmacokinetics of oseltamivir in patients with severe hepatic impairment have not been studied (see Dosage and Administration, Dosage Adjustment, Hepatic Impairment).

Neuropsychiatric: There have been post-marketing reports (mostly from Japan) of delirium and self-injury, in some cases resulting in fatal outcomes, in patients with influenza who were receiving TAMIFLU. Because these events were reported voluntarily during clinical practice, estimate of frequency cannot be made but they appear to be uncommon based on TAMIFLU usage data. These events were reported primarily among pediatric patients. The contribution of TAMIFLU to these events has not been established. Patients with influenza should be closely monitored for signs of abnormal behaviour. If neuropsychiatric symptoms occur, the risks and benefits of continuing treatment should be evaluated for each patient (see Adverse Reactions, Post-Market Adverse Drug Reactions, Neurologic, Psychiatric).

Influenza can be associated with a variety of neurologic and behavioural symptoms which can include events such as hallucinations, delirium, and abnormal behaviour, in some cases resulting in fatal outcomes. These events may occur in the setting of encephalitis or encephalopathy but can occur without obvious severe disease.

Renal: Renal Impairment: No dosing recommendation is available for patients undergoing routine hemodialysis and continuous peritoneal dialysis with end stage renal disease and for patients with creatinine clearance ≤10 mL/min (see Action and Clinical Pharmacology and Dosage and Administration, Dosage Adjustment).

Resistance: In clinical studies of naturally acquired infection, the cumulative incidence of oseltamivir-resistant virus by phenotyping alone or by phenotyping and genotyping was 0.32% (4/1245) or 0.4% (5/1245) respectively in adult/adolescent patients. In children with naturally acquired influenza virus infection, resistance was determined in 6 clinical studies WV15731 (0%; 0/5), WV15758 (8%; 15/183), WV15759/WV15871 (0%, 0/60), JV16284 (19%, 8/43), WV16193 (0%, 0/147), NV16871 (8%, 2/26). From the data obtained in these studies, the cumulative incidence of oseltamivir resistance in pediatric patients aged 1 to 12 years was 4.1% (19/464) based on phenotyping and 5.4% (25/464) based on phenotyping and genotyping (full genotyping was not performed on all patients). The patients cleared the virus normally and showed no clinical deterioration.

There has been no evidence for emergence of drug resistance associated with the use of TAMIFLU in clinical studies conducted to date in post-exposure (7 days), post-exposure within the household groups (10 days) and seasonal (42 days) prophylaxis of influenza.

Insufficient information is available to fully characterize the risk of emergence of resistance to TAMIFLU in clinical use.

Skin and Hypersensitivity Reactions: Severe skin and hypersensitivity reactions have been reported since marketing in patients treated with TAMIFLU (see Adverse Reactions, Post-Market Adverse Drug Reactions).

Special Populations: Pregnant Women: At present, insufficient data are available in pregnant women taking TAMIFLU to enable an evaluation of the potential for TAMIFLU to cause fetal malformations or fetal toxicity. TAMIFLU should therefore be used during pregnancy only if the potential benefit justifies the potential risk to the fetus.

Studies for effects on embryo-fetal development were conducted in rats (50, 250 and 1500 mg/kg/day) and rabbits (50, 150 and 500 mg/kg/day) by the oral route. Relative exposures at these doses were, respectively, 2, 13 and 100 times human exposure in the rat and 4, 8 and 50 times human exposure in the rabbit. Pharmacokinetic studies indicated that fetal exposure was seen in both species. In the rat study, minimal maternal toxicity was reported in the 1500 mg/kg/day group. In the rabbit study, slight and marked maternal toxicities were observed, respectively, in the 150 and 500 mg/kg/day groups. An increased incidence of abortion was seen in the 500 mg/kg/day group. There was a dose-dependent increase in the incidence rates of a variety of minor skeletal individual abnormalities and variants in the exposed offspring in these studies. However, the individual incidence rate of each skeletal abnormality or variant remained within the background rates of occurrence in the species studied. In view of the isolated nature of this finding it was considered to be of doubtful toxicological significance. For the results of administration of oseltamivir to juvenile rats see Warnings and Precautions, Nursing Women.

Nursing Women: It is not known whether oseltamivir or the active metabolite are excreted in human milk. In lactating rats, oseltamivir and the active metabolite are excreted in the milk. TAMIFLU should not be used by mothers who are nursing children under one year of age due to the potential risk to the nursing infant. Administration of oseltamivir to juvenile rats resulted in a high mortality rate.

Pediatrics (<1 year of age): TAMIFLU should not be used in children under 1 year of age. The safety and efficacy of TAMIFLU in infants younger than 1 year of age have not been established.

Geriatrics (≥65 years of age): Efficacy of TAMIFLU in the treatment of elderly patients has not been evaluated. Safety data in 372 elderly patients (≥65 years old) showed no overall difference between these subjects and younger adults. Based on drug exposure and tolerability, dosage adjustments are not anticipated for elderly patients (see Action and Clinical Pharmacology, Special Populations and Conditions, Geriatrics).

Safety has been demonstrated in elderly residents of nursing homes who took TAMIFLU for the prevention of influenza. Many of these individuals had cardiac and/or respiratory disease, and most had received vaccine that season.

ADVERSE REACTIONS: Adverse Drug Reaction Overview: In adult treatment studies with TAMIFLU (oseltamivir phosphate) the most frequently reported adverse events were nausea and vomiting. In the prevention studies adverse events were qualitatively very similar to those seen in the treatment studies. In the pediatric treatment and prophylaxis studies the most frequently reported adverse event was vomiting.

Clinical Trial Adverse Drug Reactions: Because clinical trials are conducted under very specific conditions the adverse reaction rates observed in the clinical trials may not reflect the rates observed in practice and should not be compared to the rates in the clinical trials of another drug. Adverse drug reaction information from clinical trials is useful for identifying drug-related adverse events and for approximating rates.

Adult Treatment Studies: In a total of 2107 patients, including patients on placebo and 75 mg b.i.d. TAMIFLU, in adult phase III studies in the treatment of influenza, the most frequently reported adverse events were nausea and vomiting. These events were transient and generally occurred with first dosing. These events did not lead to patient discontinuation of study drug in the vast majority of instances. At the recommended dose of 75 mg twice daily, three patients withdrew because of nausea and the same number withdrew because of vomiting.

In adult phase III treatment studies, some adverse events occurred more frequently in patients taking TAMIFLU compared to those taking placebos. The adverse events that occurred the most frequently at the recommended dose, either for treatment or prophylaxis, are shown in Table 1. This summary includes healthy young adults and "at risk" patients (patients at higher risk of developing complications associated with influenza e.g. elderly patients and patients with chronic cardiac or respiratory disease). Those events with an incidence of ≥1% and which were more frequently in patients taking TAMIFLU compared with placebo, irrespective of causality, were nausea, vomiting, abdominal pain and headache.

Table 1: TAMIFLU

Most Frequent Adverse Events in Studies in Naturally Acquired Influenza

Adverse Event System Organ Class (MedDRA)	Treatment[a]				Prevention			
	TAMIFLU 75 mg twice daily for 5 days N=1057		Placebo N=1050		TAMIFLU 75 mg once daily N=1480		Placebo N=1434	
Ear and Labyrinth Disorders								
Vertigo[b]	9	(0.9%)	6	(0.6%)	4	(0.3%)	3	(0.2%)
Gastrointestinal Disorders								
Nausea (without vomiting)	113	(10.7%)	71	(6.8%)	104	(7.0%)	56	(3.9%)
Vomiting	85	(8.0%)	32	(3.0%)	31	(2.1%)	15	(1.0%)
Diarrhea	58	(5.5%)	84	(8.0%)	48	(3.2%)	38	(2.6%)
Abdominal Pain	23	(2.2%)	21	(2.0%)	30	(2.0%)	23	(1.6%)
General Disorders and Administration Site Reactions								
Fatigue[b]	8	(0.8%)	7	(0.7%)	117	(7.9%)	107	(7.5%)
Infections and Infestations								
Bronchitis	39	(3.7%)	52	(5.0%)	11	(0.7%)	17	(1.2%)
Nervous System Disorders								
Dizziness	20	(1.9%)	31	(3.0%)	24	(1.6%)	21	(1.5%)
Headache	17	(1.6%)	16	(1.5%)	298	(20.1%)	251	(17.5%)
Insomnia	11	(1.0%)	10	(1.0%)	18	(1.2%)	14	(1.0%)
Respiratory, Thoracic and Mediastinal Disorders								
Cough[b]	10	(0.9%)	12	(1.1%)	83	(5.6%)	86	(6.0%)

a Adverse events included are all events reported the most frequently in the treatment studies in the oseltamivir 75 mg b.i.d. Group, and events are ordered by decreasing incidence in that group.
b These events no longer qualify as among the most-frequently recorded events for the treatment group but are included here for completeness as they were included in a previous version of this table which was based on a smaller dataset.

Additional adverse events occurring in <1% of patients receiving TAMIFLU for treatment included unstable angina, anemia, pseudomembranous colitis, humerus fracture, pneumonia, pyrexia, and peritonsillar abscess.

Adult Prevention Studies: A total of 3434 subjects (adolescents, healthy adults and elderly) participated in 3 phase III prevention studies, of whom 1480 received the recommended dose of 75 mg once daily. Adverse events were qualitatively very similar to those seen in the treatment studies (see Table 1). Additional adverse events ≥1% in the prevention studies included aches and pains, rhinorrhea, dyspepsia and upper respiratory tract infections. However, the difference in incidence between TAMIFLU and placebo for these events was less than 1%. There were no clinically relevant differences in the safety profile of the 942 elderly subjects who received TAMIFLU or placebo, compared with the younger population.

In a fourth study, an additional 399 subjects received 75 mg of TAMIFLU once daily for 10 days following the identification of a household index case. Similar to previous studies, nausea (8.3%), vomiting (4.5%), diarrhea (0.8%) and headache (7.8%) were among the most commonly reported adverse events.

Pediatric Treatment Studies: A total of 1032 pediatric patients aged 1 to 12 years (including 698 otherwise healthy pediatric patients aged 1 to 12 and 334 asthmatic pediatric patients aged 6 to 12) participated in Phase III studies of TAMIFLU given for the treatment of influenza. A total of 515 pediatric patients received treatment with TAMIFLU oral suspension.

Adverse events occurring in >1% of pediatric patients receiving TAMIFLU are listed in Table 2. The most frequently reported adverse event was vomiting. Other events reported more frequently by pediatric patients treated with TAMIFLU included abdominal pain, epistaxis, ear disorder and conjunctivitis. These events generally occurred once and resolved despite continued dosing. They did not cause discontinuation of drug in the vast majority of cases.

Although otitis media, pneumonia, sinusitis and bronchitis were all reported in >1% of pediatric patients receiving TAMIFLU, the incidence of these events in the group treated with TAMIFLU was lower than that in the placebo treated group.

The adverse event profile in adolescents is similar to that described for adult patients and pediatric patients aged 1 to 12 years.

Adverse events included are: all events reported in the treatment studies with frequency ≥1% in the oseltamivir 75 mg bid group.

Pediatric Prevention Studies: Pediatric patients aged 1 to 12 years participated in a post-exposure prophylaxis study in households, both as index cases (n=134) and as contacts (n=222). Gastrointestinal events were the most frequent, particularly vomiting. TAMIFLU was well tolerated in this study, the adverse events noted being consistent with those previously observed (see Table 2).

Post-Market Adverse Drug Reactions: The following adverse reactions have been identified during post-marketing use of TAMIFLU. Because these reactions are reported voluntarily from a population of uncertain size, it is not possible to reliably estimate their frequency or establish a causal relationship to TAMIFLU exposure.

Skin and Hypersensitivity Reactions: dermatitis, rash, eczema, urticaria, erythema multiforme, Stevens-Johnson syndrome, toxic epidermal necrolysis, anaphylactic/anaphylactoid reactions and face edema.

Liver and Biliary System elevated liver enzymes, hepatotoxicity including fulminant hepatitis/hepatic failure, in some cases with fatal outcome.

Gastrointestinal Disorders: gastrointestinal bleeding, hemorrhagic colitis.

Neurologic: seizure.

Psychiatric: delirium, including symptoms such as altered level of consciousness, confusion, abnormal behavior leading to self-injury, delusions, hallucinations, agitation, anxiety, nightmares (see Warnings and Precautions).

DRUG INTERACTIONS: Overview: Oseltamivir is extensively converted to oseltamivir carboxylate by esterases, located predominantly in the liver. Drug interactions involving competition for esterases have not been extensively reported in literature. Low protein binding of oseltamivir and oseltamivir carboxylate suggests that the probability of drug displacement interactions is low.

In vitro studies demonstrated that neither oseltamivir nor the active metabolite are good substrates for P450 mixed-function oxidases or for glucuronyl transferases.

Table 2: TAMIFLU

Most Frequent Adverse Events Occurring in Children Aged 1 to 12 Years in Studies in Naturally Acquired Influenza

Adverse Events System Organ Class (MedDRA)	Treatment[a]		Treatment[b]	Prophylaxis[b]
	TAMIFLU 2 mg/kg twice daily N=515	Placebo N=517	TAMIFLU Unit Dose[c] N=158	TAMIFLU Unit Dose[c] N=99
Blood and Lymphatic System Disorders				
Lymphadenopathy	5 (1.0%)	8 (1.5%)	1 (0.6%)	—
Ear and Labyrinth Disorders				
Ear Disorder	9 (1.7%)	6 (1.2%)	—	—
Tympanic Membrane Disorder	5 (1.0%)	6 (1.2%)	—	—
Eye Disorders				
Conjunctivitis	5 (1.0%)	2 (0.4%)	—	—
Gastrointestinal Disorders				
Vomiting	77 (15.0%)	48 (9.3%)	31 (19.6%)	10 (10.1%)
Diarrhea	49 (9.5%)	55 (10.6%)	5 (3.2%)	1 (1.0%)
Abdominal Pain	24 (4.7%)	20 (3.9%)	3 (1.9%)	3 (3.0%)
Nausea	17 (3.3%)	22 (4.3%)	10 (6.3%)	4 (4.0%)
Infections and Infestations				
Otitis Media	45 (8.7%)	58 (11.2%)	2 (1.3%)	2 (2.0%)
Pneumonia	10 (1.9%)	17 (3.3%)	—	—
Sinusitis	9 (1.7%)	13 (2.5%)	—	—
Bronchitis	8 (1.6%)	11 (2.1%)	3 (1.9%)	—
Respiratory, Thoracic and Mediastinal Disorders				
Asthma (including aggravated)	18 (3.5%)	19 (3.7%)	—	1 (1.0%)
Epistaxis	16 (3.1%)	13 (2.5%)	2 (1.3%)	1 (1.0%)
Skin and Subcutaneous Tissue Disorders				
Dermatitis	5 (1.0%)	10 (1.9%)	1 (0.6%)	—

a Pooled data from Phase III trials of TAMIFLU treatment of naturally acquired influenza.
b Uncontrolled study comparing treatment (twice-daily dosing for 5 days) with prophylaxis (once-daily dosing for 10 days).
c Unit dose=age-based dosing (see Dosage and Administration).

Drug-Drug Interactions: Cimetidine, a non-specific inhibitor of cytochrome P450 isoforms and competitor for renal tubular secretion of basic or cationic drugs, has no effect on plasma levels of oseltamivir or its active metabolite.

Clinically important drug interactions involving competition for renal tubular secretion are unlikely due to the known safety margin for most of these drugs, the elimination characteristics of the active metabolite (glomerular filtration and anionic tubular secretion) and the excretion capacity of these pathways. Co-administration of probenecid results in an approximate two-fold increase in exposure to the active metabolite due to a decrease in active anionic tubular secretion in the kidney. However, due to the wide safety margin of the active metabolite, no dose adjustments are required when co-administering with probenecid. Other drugs excreted via anionic tubular secretion have not been evaluated.

Co-administration with amoxicillin does not alter plasma levels of either compound, indicating that competition for the anionic secretion pathway is weak.

In six subjects, co-administration with acetaminophen did not alter plasma levels of oseltamivir, its active metabolite, or acetaminophen.

Co-administration with paracetamol does not alter plasma levels of oseltamivir, its active metabolite, or paracetamol.

No pharmacokinetic interactions between oseltamivir or its major metabolite have been observed when co-administering oseltamivir with paracetamol, acetyl-salicylic acid, cimetidine or with antacids (magnesium and aluminum hydroxides and calcium carbonates).

In phase III treatment and prophylaxis clinical studies, TAMIFLU (oseltamivir phosphate) has been administered with commonly used drugs such as ACE inhibitors (enalapril, captopril), thiazide diuretics (bendrofluazide), antibiotics (penicillin), H_2-receptor blockers (cimetidine), and analgesic agents (acetylsalicylic acid, ibuprofen and paracetamol). No change in adverse event profile or frequency has been observed as a result of co-administration of TAMIFLU with these compounds.

Drug-Food Interactions: Interactions with food have not been established.

Drug-Herb Interactions: Interactions with herbs have not been established.

Drug-Laboratory Test Interactions: Interactions with laboratory tests have not been established.

DOSAGE AND ADMINISTRATION: Dosing Considerations: Hepatic Impairment: The safety, efficacy and pharmacokinetics in patients with severe hepatic impairment have not been studied. No studies have been carried out in pediatric patients with hepatic impairment.

Infants: The safety and efficacy of TAMIFLU (oseltamivir phosphate) in infants younger than 1 year of age have not been established. TAMIFLU should not be used in children under 1 year of age. Administration of TAMIFLU to infants younger than 1 year of age is contraindicated (see Contraindications).

For information on renal impairment and elderly patients see Dosage Adjustment.

Recommended Dose—Treatment of Influenza: Treatment should begin no more than two days after the onset of symptoms of influenza.

Adults and Adolescents (≥13 years): The recommended oral dose of TAMIFLU capsules for the treatment of influenza in adults and adolescents 13 years and older is 75 mg twice daily, for 5 days.

Pediatrics (1 to 12 years): The recommended oral dose of TAMIFLU oral suspension for pediatric patients 1 year and older is shown in Table 3. TAMIFLU oral suspension may also be used by adult patients who cannot swallow a capsule. If TAMIFLU oral suspension is not available, TAMIFLU capsules may be opened and mixed with sweetened liquids such as regular or sugar-free chocolate syrup. For children old enough to safely swallow capsules, the 30 and 45 mg capsules can also be taken as outlined in Table 3.

An oral dosing dispenser with 30 mg, 45 mg, and 60 mg graduations is provided with the oral suspension; the 75 mg dose can be measured using a combination of 30 mg and 45 mg.

Table 3: TAMIFLU

Recommended Oral Dose of TAMIFLU Oral Suspension for Pediatric Patients 1 Year and Older or Adult Patients Who Cannot Swallow a Capsule

Body Weight in kg	Recommended Dose for 5 Days
≤15 kg	30 mg twice daily
>15 kg to 23 kg	45 mg twice daily
>23 kg to 40 kg	60 mg twice daily
>40 kg	75 mg twice daily

Recommended Dose—Prevention of Influenza: Therapy should begin within 2 days of exposure after the onset of symptoms in the index case and continue for at least ten days. Viral shedding may continue for up to 14 days in children and elderly after the onset of influenza illness. Therefore, if the index case is a child or an elderly person, therapy with TAMIFLU for prevention may continue for up to 14 days.

Patients should be instructed to complete the entire course of therapy.

Adults and Adolescents (≥13 years): The recommended oral dose of TAMIFLU for prevention of influenza following close contact with an infected individual (the index case) is 75 mg once daily.

Pediatrics (1 to 12 years): The recommended dose of TAMIFLU oral suspension for prevention in pediatric patients 1 year and older is shown in Table 4. TAMIFLU oral suspension may also be used by adult patients who cannot swallow a capsule. If TAMIFLU oral suspension is not available, TAMIFLU capsules may be opened and mixed with sweetened liquids such as regular or sugar-free chocolate syrup. For children old enough to safely swallow capsules, the 30 and 45 mg capsules can also be taken as outlined in Table 4.

Table 4: TAMIFLU

Recommended Dose of TAMIFLU Oral Suspension for Pediatric Patients 1 Year and Older

Body Weight in kg	Recommended Dose for at Least 10 Days
≤15 kg	30 mg once daily
>15 kg to 23 kg	45 mg once daily
>23 kg to 40 kg	60 mg once daily
>40 kg	75 mg once daily

An oral dosing dispenser with 30 mg, 45 mg, and 60 mg graduations is provided with the oral suspension; the 75 mg dose can be measured using a combination of 30 mg and 45 mg.

Dosage Adjustment: Hepatic Impairment: No dose adjustment is required in adult patients with mild or moderate hepatic impairment (see Actions and Clinical, Pharmacology, Special Populations and Conditions, Hepatic Impairment).

Renal Impairment: No dose adjustment is necessary for patients with creatinine clearance above 30 mL/min.

No dosing recommendation is available for patients undergoing routine hemodialysis and continuous peritoneal dialysis with end stage renal disease and for patients with creatinine clearance ≤10 mL/min (see Action and Clinical Pharmacology, Special Populations and Conditions, Renal Impairment).

Treatment of Influenza: In patients with a creatinine clearance of 10-30 mL/min, it is recommended that the dose be reduced to 75 mg of TAMIFLU once daily for 5 days.

Prevention of Influenza: In patients with a creatinine clearance of 10-30 mL/min, it is recommended that the dose be reduced to 75 mg of TAMIFLU every other day, or alternatively, one 30 mg capsule or 30 mg suspension once daily.

Elderly Patients: No dose adjustment is required for elderly patients (see Warnings and Precautions: Special Populations, Geriatrics (≥65 years of age)).

Missed Dose: The missed dose should be taken as soon as remembered, then the regular dosing schedule should be continued. Two doses of TAMIFLU should not be taken at the same time.

Administration: TAMIFLU may be taken with or without food (see Action and Clinical Pharmacology, Pharmacokinetics, Absorption). However, taking with food may enhance tolerability in some patients.

Reconstitution of Oral Suspension: It is recommended that TAMIFLU powder for oral suspension be reconstituted by the pharmacist prior to dispensing to the patient.

1. Tap the closed bottle several times to loosen the powder.
2. Measure 52 mL of water in a graduated cylinder.
3. Add the total amount of water for reconstitution to the bottle and shake the closed bottle well for 15 seconds.
4. Remove the child resistant cap and push bottle adapter into neck of bottle.
5. Close bottle with child resistant cap tightly. This will assure the proper seating of the bottle adapter in the bottle and child resistant status of the cap.

Dispense with patient information leaflet and oral dispenser. It is recommended to write the date of expiration of the reconstituted suspension on the bottle label. (The shelf life of the reconstituted suspension is 10 days if stored at room temperature (not above 25°C) or 17 days if stored in a refrigerator (2-8°C)).

A bottle of 30 g TAMIFLU powder for oral suspension contains 25.713 g of sorbitol. One dose of 45 mg oseltamivir administered twice daily delivers 2.6 g of sorbitol which is unsuitable for subjects with hereditary fructose intolerance (see Warnings and Precautions, Endocrine and Metabolism).

Note: Shake the TAMIFLU oral suspension well before each use.

Emergency Compounding of an Oral Suspension from TAMIFLU Capsules (Final Concentration 15 mg/mL): The following directions are provided for use only during emergency situations. These directions are not intended to be used if the Health Canada-approved, commercially manufactured TAMIFLU for Oral Suspension is readily available from wholesalers or the manufacturer.

Compounding an oral suspension with this procedure will provide one patient with enough medication for a 5-day course of treatment or a 10-day course of prophylaxis.

Commercially manufactured TAMIFLU for Oral Suspension (12 mg/mL) is the preferred product for pediatric and adult patients who have difficulty swallowing capsules or where lower doses are needed. In the event that TAMIFLU for Oral Suspension is not available, the pharmacist may compound a suspension (15 mg/mL) from TAMIFLU (oseltamivir phosphate) Capsules 75 mg using one of the following three vehicles: Cherry Syrup (Humco), Ora-Sweet SF (sugar-free) (Paddock Laboratories) **or** purified water containing 0.1% w/v sodium benzoate added as preservative. Other vehicles have not been studied. **This compounded suspension should not be used for convenience or when the Health Canada-approved TAMIFLU for Oral Suspension is commercially available.**

First, calculate the Total Volume of an oral suspension needed to be compounded and dispensed for each patient. The Total Volume required is determined by the weight of each patient. Refer to Table 5.

Second, determine the number of capsules and the amount of vehicle (Cherry Syrup (Humco), Ora-Sweet SF **or** purified water containing 0.1% w/v sodium benzoate added as preservative) that are needed to prepare the Total Volume (calculated from Table 5: 30 mL, 40 mL, 50 mL, or 60 mL) of compounded oral suspension (15 mg/mL). Refer to Table 6.

Third, follow the procedure below for compounding the oral suspension (15 mg/mL) from TAMIFLU Capsules 75 mg:

1. Carefully separate the capsule body and cap and transfer the contents of the required number of TAMIFLU 75 mg Capsules into a clean mortar.
2. Triturate the granules to a fine powder.
3. Add one-third (1/3) of the specified amount of vehicle and triturate the powder until a uniform suspension is achieved.
4. Transfer the suspension to an amber glass or amber polyethyleneterephthalate (PET) bottle. A funnel may be used to eliminate any spillage.
5. Add another one-third (1/3) of the vehicle to the mortar, rinse the pestle and mortar by a triturating motion and transfer the vehicle into the bottle.
6. Repeat the rinsing (Step 5) with the remainder of the vehicle.
7. Close the bottle using a child-resistant cap.
8. Shake well to completely dissolve the active drug and to ensure homogeneous distribution of the dissolved drug in the resulting suspension. (Note: The active drug, oseltamivir phosphate, readily dissolves in the specified vehicle. The suspension is caused by some of the inert ingredients of TAMIFLU Capsules which are insoluble in the vehicle.)
9. Put an ancillary label on the bottle indicating "Shake Gently Before Use". [This compounded suspension should be gently shaken prior to administration to minimize the tendency for air entrapment.]
10. Instruct the parent or guardian that any remaining material following completion of therapy must be discarded by either affixing an ancillary label to the bottle or adding a statement to the pharmacy label instructions.
11. Place an appropriate expiration date label according to storage condition (see below).

Table 5: TAMIFLU

Volume of an Oral Suspension (15 mg/mL) Needed to be Compounded Based Upon the Patient's Weight

Body Weight (kg)	Total Volume to Compound Per Patient (mL)
≤15 kg	30 mL
16 to 23 kg	40 mL
24 to 40 kg	50 mL
≥41 kg	60 mL

Table 6: TAMIFLU

Number of TAMIFLU 75 mg Capsules and Amount of Vehicle (Cherry Syrup (Humco), Ora-Sweet SF or purified water containing 0.1% w/v sodium benzoate added as preservative) Needed to Prepare the Total Volume of a Compounded Oral Suspension (15 mg/mL)

Total Volume of Compounded Oral Suspension Needed to be Prepared	30 mL	40 mL	50 mL	60 mL
Required Number of TAMIFLU 75 mg Capsules	6 capsules (450 mg oseltamivir)	8 capsules (600 mg oseltamivir)	10 capsules (750 mg oseltamivir)	12 capsules (900 mg oseltamivir)
Required Volume of Vehicle				
Cherry Syrup (Humco) or Ora-Sweet SF (Paddock Laboratories) or purified water containing 0.1% w/v sodium benzoate added as preservative	29 mL	38.5 mL	48 mL	57 mL

Storage of the Pharmacy-Compounded Suspension: Compounded with Ora-Sweet SF: Stable for 5 weeks (35 days) when stored at 25°C.

Compounded with Cherry Syrup (Humco): Stable for 5 weeks (35 days) when stored in a refrigerator at 2 to 8°C.

Compounded with purified water containing 0.1% w/v sodium benzoate added as preservative: Room temperature storage conditions: Stable for 3 weeks (21 days) when stored at room temperature. Do not store above 25°C.

Refrigerated storage conditions: Stable for 6 weeks when stored at 2-8°C.

Note: The storage conditions are based on stability studies of compounded oral suspensions, using the above mentioned vehicle, which were placed in amber glass and amber polyethyleneterephthalate (PET) bottles. Stability studies have not been conducted with other vehicles or bottle types.

Place a pharmacy label on the bottle that includes the patient's name, dosing instructions, and drug name and any other required information to be in compliance with all Provincial and Federal Pharmacy Regulations. **Refer to Table 7 for the proper dosing instructions.**

Note: This compounding procedure results in a 15 mg/mL suspension, which is different from the commercially available TAMIFLU for Oral Suspension, which has a concentration of 12 mg/mL.

Table 7: TAMIFLU

Dosing Chart for Pharmacy-Compounded Suspension from TAMIFLU Capsules 75 mg

Body Weight (kg)	Dose (mg)	Volume per Dose 15 mg/mL	Treatment Dose (for 5 days)	Prophylaxis Dose (for 10 days)
≤15 kg	30 mg	2 mL	2 mL two times a day	2 mL once daily
16 to 23 kg	45 mg	3 mL	3 mL two times a day	3 mL once daily
24 to 40 kg	60 mg	4 mL	4 mL two times a day	4 mL once daily
≥41 kg	75 mg	5 mL	5 mL two times a day	5 mL once daily

Note: 1 teaspoon=5 mL.

Consider dispensing the suspension with a graduated oral syringe for measuring small amounts of suspension. If possible, mark or highlight the graduation corresponding to the appropriate dose (2 mL, 3 mL, 4 mL, or 5 mL) on the oral syringe for each patient. The dosing device dispensed with the commercially available TAMIFLU for Oral Suspension should NOT be used with the compounded suspension since they have different concentrations.

For the suspension compounded with purified water containing 0.1% w/v sodium benzoate added as a preservative, the appropriate dose must be withdrawn from the dispensed bottle by the caregiver. Using a separate container, the withdrawn dose must be mixed with an equal amount of sweetened liquid, such as sugar water, chocolate syrup, cherry syrup, dessert toppings (like caramel or fudge sauce) to mask the bitter taste.

OVERDOSAGE:

Activated charcoal may be administered to aid in the removal of unabsorbed drug. General supportive measures are recommended.

At present there has been no experience with overdose. Single doses of up to 1000 mg of TAMIFLU (oseltamivir phosphate) have been associated with nausea and/or vomiting.

> For management of a suspected drug overdose, contact your **regional Poison Control Centre**. See the *CPS Directory* section for a list of Poison Control Centres.

ACTION AND CLINICAL PHARMACOLOGY: Mechanism of Action: TAMIFLU (oseltamivir phosphate) is an ethyl ester prodrug requiring ester hydrolysis for conversion to the active metabolite, oseltamivir carboxylate. The active metabolite is a selective inhibitor of influenza A and B virus neuraminidase enzymes which are glycoproteins found on the virion surface. Viral neuraminidase is important both for viral entry into uninfected cells and for the release of recently formed virus particles from infected cells and the further spread of infectious virus in the body. The proposed mechanism of action of oseltamivir is via inhibition of influenza virus neuraminidase with the possibility of alteration of virus particle aggregation and release.

Oseltamivir is readily absorbed after oral administration and converted by hepatic esterases to its active metabolite. The mean volume of distribution (V_{ss}) of the active metabolite is approximately 23 L. The active metabolite is not further metabolized and is eliminated in the urine. The half-life of elimination of this metabolite is 6 to 10 hours. Renal clearance (18.8 L/h) exceeds glomerular filtration rate (7.5 L/h), indicating that tubular secretion in addition to glomerular filtration occurs. The prodrug which reaches the systemic circulation (less than 5%) is eliminated by renal excretion also. The binding of oseltamivir to human plasma protein is 42% and that of the active metabolite is negligible, approximately 3%.

Exposure to the active metabolite is inversely proportional to declining renal function.

Pharmacokinetics: Absorption: Oseltamivir is readily absorbed from the gastrointestinal tract after oral administration of TAMIFLU and is extensively converted predominantly by hepatic esterases to the active metabolite. At least 75% of an oral dose reaches the systemic circulation as the active metabolite. Exposure to the prodrug is less than 5% relative to the active metabolite. Plasma concentrations of active metabolite are proportional to dose and are not significantly affected by co-administration with food (see Dosage and Administration).

Distribution: The mean volume of distribution (V_{ss}) of the active metabolite is approximately 23 L in humans.

The binding of oseltamivir to human plasma protein is 42% and that of the active metabolite is negligible, approximately 3%.

Metabolism: Oseltamivir is extensively converted to the active metabolite by esterases located predominantly in the liver. Neither oseltamivir nor the active metabolite are substrates for, or inhibitors of, cytochrome P450 isoforms.

Excretion: Absorbed oseltamivir is primarily (>90%) eliminated by conversion to the active metabolite. The active metabolite is not further metabolized and is eliminated in the urine. Peak plasma concentrations of the active metabolite decline with a half-life of 6 to 10 hours in most subjects. The active drug is eliminated entirely (>99%) by renal excretion. Renal clearance (18.8 L/h) exceeds glomerular filtration rate (7.5 L/h), indicating that tubular secretion in addition to glomerular filtration occurs. Less than 20% of an oral radiolabelled dose is eliminated in feces.

Special Populations and Conditions: Pediatrics: The pharmacokinetics of oseltamivir have been evaluated in single dose pharmacokinetic studies in pediatric patients aged 1 to 16 years. Multiple dose pharmacokinetics were studied in a small number of pediatric patients aged 3-12 years enrolled in a clinical trial. Younger pediatric patients cleared both the prodrug and the active metabolite faster than adults resulting in lower exposure for a given mg/kg dose. Doses of 2 mg/kg give oseltamivir carboxylate exposures comparable to those achieved in adults receiving a single 75 mg capsule dose (approximately 1 mg/kg). The pharmacokinetics of oseltamivir in pediatric patients over 12 years of age are similar to those in adults.

TAMIFLU should not be used in children under 1 year of age.

Geriatrics: Exposure to the active metabolite at steady-state was 25% to 35% higher in elderly patients (age range 65 to 78) compared to young adults given comparable doses of TAMIFLU. Half-lives observed in the elderly patients were similar to those seen in young adults. On the basis of drug exposure and tolerability, dosage adjustments are not required for elderly patients for either treatment or prevention (see Dosage and Administration, Dosage Adjustment).

Hepatic Impairment: The safety, efficacy and pharmacokinetics of TAMIFLU in patients with severe hepatic impairment have not been studied (see Warnings and Precautions, Hepatic). In a clinical study of adult patients with moderate hepatic impairment (N=11), compared with healthy volunteers (N=23), metabolic conversion of oseltamivir into the active metabolite oseltamivir carboxylate was not significantly altered (see Dosage and Administration, Dosage Adjustment, Hepatic Impairment). No studies have been carried out in pediatric patients with hepatic impairment.

Renal Impairment: Administration of 100 mg of TAMIFLU twice daily for five days to patients with various degrees of renal impairment showed that exposure to the active metabolite is inversely proportional to declining renal function.

No dosing recommendation is available for patients undergoing routine hemodialysis and continuous peritoneal dialysis with end stage renal disease and for patients with creatinine clearance ≤10 mL/min.

Treatment of Influenza: In patients with a creatinine clearance of 10-30 mL/min, it is recommended that the dose be reduced to 75 mg of TAMIFLU once daily for 5 days.

Prevention of Influenza: In patients with a creatinine clearance of 10-30 mL/min, it is recommended that the dose be reduced to 75 mg of TAMIFLU every other day, or alternatively, one 30 mg capsule or 30 mg suspension every day (see Dosage and Administration, Dosage Adjustment).

STORAGE AND STABILITY: TAMIFLU (oseltamivir phosphate) Capsules: Store at 15 to 25°C.

TAMIFLU Powder for Oral Suspension: Store dry powder at 15 to 25°C. Store reconstituted suspension: a) at room temperature (not above 25°C). Discard unused portion within **10 days** of reconstitution.

or

b) in a refrigerator (2-8°C). Discard unused portion within **17 days** of reconstitution. Do not freeze reconstituted suspension.

TAMIFLU Pharmacy-Compounded Suspension: Store reconstituted suspension:

(a) compounded with Ora-Sweet SF: Stable for 5 weeks (35 days) when stored at 25°C.

(b) compounded with Cherry Syrup (Humco): Stable for 5 weeks (35 days) when stored in a refrigerator at 2 to 8°C.

(c) compounded with purified water containing 0.1% w/v sodium benzoate added as a preservative:

Room temperature storage conditions: Stable for 3 weeks (21 days) when stored at room temperature. Do not store above 25°C.

Refrigerated storage conditions: Stable for 6 weeks when stored at 2-8°C.

INFORMATION FOR THE PATIENT: Published in e-CPS, available by subscription at www.e-cps.ca.

DOSAGE FORMS, COMPOSITION AND PACKAGING: Capsules: 30 mg: Each light yellow, hard gelatin capsule for oral use, with "ROCHE" printed in blue ink on the light yellow body and "30 mg" printed in blue ink on the light yellow cap, contains: oseltamivir 30 mg as oseltamivir phosphate. Nonmedicinal ingredients: corn starch, croscarmellose sodium, povidone K30, sodium stearyl fumarate and talc; shell: gelatin, red iron oxide, yellow iron oxide and titanium dioxide. Each capsule is printed with blue ink, which includes FD&C Blue No. 2 as a colorant. Blister packages of 10.

45 mg: Each grey, hard gelatin capsule for oral use, with "ROCHE" printed in blue ink on the grey body and "45 mg" printed in blue ink on the grey cap, contains: oseltamivir 45 mg as oseltamivir phosphate. Nonmedicinal ingredients: corn starch, croscarmellose sodium, povidone K30, sodium stearyl fumarate and talc; shell: gelatin, black iron oxide and titanium dioxide. Each capsule is printed with blue ink, which includes FD&C Blue No. 2 as a colorant. Blister packages of 10.

75 mg: Each grey/light yellow, hard gelatin capsule for oral use, with "ROCHE" printed in blue ink on the grey body and "75 mg" printed in blue ink on the light yellow cap, contains: oseltamivir 75 mg as oseltamivir phosphate. Nonmedicinal ingredients: corn starch, croscarmellose sodium, povidone K30, sodium stearyl fumarate and talc; shell: gelatin, black iron oxide, red iron oxide, yellow iron oxide and titanium dioxide. Each capsule is printed with blue ink, which includes FD&C Blue No. 2 as a colorant. Blister packages of 10.

Powder for Oral Suspension: Each bottle of white powder blend for reconstitution to a white tutti-frutti-flavored suspension, contains: oseltamivir 900 mg as oseltamivir phosphate, which when reconstituted contains 12 mg/mL oseltamivir. Net contents after reconstitution: 75 mL. Nonmedicinal ingredients: monosodium citrate, saccharin sodium, sodium benzoate, sorbitol, titanium dioxide, tutti-frutti flavoring and xanthan gum. Glass bottles of 100 mL with a bottle adapter and 1 oral dispenser.

(Shown in Product Identification Section)

Tamofen® Pr

tamoxifen citrate

Antineoplastic

sanofi-aventis

Date of Revision: May 22, 2007

> Tamoxifen therapy was associated with serious and life-threatening events including uterine malignancies, stroke, pulmonary embolism, and deep vein thrombosis in the National Surgical Adjuvant Breast and Bowel Project (NSABP) P-1 breast cancer prevention trial. The use of tamoxifen for breast cancer prevention is not an approved indication in Canada. The following risks associated with tamoxifen therapy have been estimated from the NSABP P-1 breast cancer prevention trial. The relative risk of tamoxifen compared to placebo was 3.1 for endometrial cancer, 4.0 for uterine sarcomas, 1.6 for stroke, 3.0 for pulmonary embolism, and 1.6 for deep vein thrombosis. These events were fatal in some patients. Health care providers should be aware of the possible risks associated with tamoxifen therapy and should discuss them with their patients.
>
> The benefits of tamoxifen therapy outweigh the risks in the majority of women being treated according to the approved Canadian indication for the treatment of breast cancer (see Warnings).

PHARMACOLOGY: Tamoxifen is a nonsteroidal agent which has demonstrated potent antiestrogenic properties in animal test systems. The antiestrogenic effects are related to is ability to compete with estrogen for binding sites in target tissues such as breast and uterus. Tamoxifen inhibits the induction of rat mammary carcinoma induced by dimethylbenzanthracene (DMBA) and causes the regression of already established DMBA-induced tumors. In this rat model tamoxifen appears to exert its antitumor effects by binding to estrogen receptors.

In cytosols derived from human endometrium and human breast and uterine adenocarcinomas tamoxifen competes with estradiol for estrogen receptor protein.

Reports of advanced breast cancer trials conducted world-wide, however, indicate that, using established criteria, there is an objective response rate (complete and partial remission) to tamoxifen of approximately 10% in patients with estrogen receptor negative tumors which may indicate other mechanisms of action. A further small percentage of patients show positive benefit in that they are reported to have disease stabilization. This may be explained by the shortcomings of the assay procedure or by actions of tamoxifen at loci other than the estrogen receptor.

Ranges as large as 0 to 300 fmoL/mg protein have been reported in histologically comparable portions of the same tumor. In addition, the collection, transport and storage of tumor specimens can affect the validity of current estrogen receptor assays.

The apparent discrepancy in correlation between estrogen receptor status and clinical response may also be explained by recent in vitro evidence indicating that not all of the growth inhibiting effects of tamoxifen are mediated through the estrogen receptor. Tamoxifen has been shown to have a low affinity for the androgen receptor and on a binding site distinct from the estrogen receptor. The possibility also exists that tamoxifen interferes with the action of hormonal steroids on cell growth, that it could modulate the action of peptide hormones at their receptors by effects on cell membranes, and that it inhibits prostaglandin synthetase thereby having the potential to limit tumor growth.

It is recognized that tamoxifen also displays estrogenic-like effects on several body systems including the endometrium, bone and blood lipids.

INDICATIONS: The adjuvant treatment of early breast cancer in women with estrogen receptor positive tumors. Tamoxifen is indicated for the treatment of women with hormone responsive locally advanced/metastatic breast cancer.

CONTRAINDICATIONS: When used in the prevention setting (an indication not approved in Canada), tamoxifen is contraindicated in patients with a history of stroke, deep venous thrombosis or pulmonary embolism, and in patients who are at an increased risk of developing endometrial cancer. Tamoxifen is not indicated for the prevention of breast cancer in Canada.

Pregnancy: Tamoxifen must not be given during pregnancy. There have been a small number of reports of spontaneous abortions, birth defects and fetal deaths after women have taken tamoxifen, although no causal relationship has been established.

Reproductive toxicology studies in rats, rabbits and monkeys have shown no teratogenic potential.

In rodent models of fetal reproductive tract development, tamoxifen was associated with changes similar to those caused by estradiol, ethynylestradiol, clomiphene and diethylstilboestrol (DES). Although the clinical relevance of these changes is unknown, some of them, especially vaginal adenosis, are similar to those seen in young women who were exposed to DES in utero and who have a 1 in 1 000 risk of developing clear-cell carcinoma of the vagina or cervix. Only a small number of pregnant women have been exposed to tamoxifen. Such exposure has not been reported to cause subsequent vaginal adenosis or clear-cell carcinoma of the vagina or cervix in young women exposed in utero to tamoxifen.

Women should be advised not to become pregnant while taking tamoxifen and should use barrier or other nonhormonal contraceptive methods if sexually active. Premenopausal patients must be carefully examined before treatment to exclude the possibility of pregnancy. Women should be appraised of the potential risks to the fetus, should they become pregnant while taking tamoxifen or within 2 months of cessation of therapy.

Tamoxifen is contraindicated in patients with hypersensitivity to tamoxifen or any of its components.

WARNINGS: An increased incidence of uterine malignancies has been reported in association with tamoxifen treatment. The underlying mechanism is unknown, but may be related to the estrogen-like effect of tamoxifen. Most uterine malignancies seen in association with tamoxifen are classified as adenocarcinoma of the endometrium. However, rare uterine sarcomas, including malignant mixed Mullerian tumours, have also been reported. Uterine sarcoma is generally associated with a higher FIGO stage (III/IV) at diagnosis, poorer prognosis, and shorter survival. Uterine sarcoma has been reported to occur more frequently among long-term users (≥2 years) of tamoxifen than non-users.

There is evidence of an increased incidence of thromboembolic events, including deep vein thrombosis and pulmonary embolism, during tamoxifen therapy. When tamoxifen is co-administered with chemotherapy, there may be a further increase in the incidence of thromboembolic effects. For treatment of breast cancer, the risks and benefits of tamoxifen should be carefully considered in women with a history of thromboembolic events.

An increased risk of stroke has been found to be associated with tamoxifen therapy in high-risk patients being treated for the prevention of breast cancer. The use of tamoxifen for the prevention of breast cancer is not an approved indication in Canada.

Incidence rates for the above events were estimated from a long-term clinical study called the National Surgical Adjuvant Breast and Bowel Project Breast Cancer Prevention (NSABP P-1) Trial. In this trial, high-risk patients were randomized to either tamoxifen therapy or placebo, for the prevention of breast cancer. Uterine malignancies were separated into cases of endometrial adenocarcinomas and uterine sarcomas. The relative risk of tamoxifen compared to placebo was 3.1 for endometrial cancer, 4.0 for uterine sarcomas 1.6 for stroke, 3.0 for pulmonary embolism, and 1.6 for deep vein thrombosis.

In rats, tamoxifen can induce preneoplastic and neoplastic changes of the liver including hepatocellular carcinomas when administered at high doses for prolonged periods. In that species tamoxifen behaves as a partial agonist whereas it is primarily an antiestrogen in humans. For this reason and considering the high dosage used in the rat studies (up to 100 times the normal human therapeutic dose), the relevance of these findings to human use is unknown.

Hepatocellular carcinomas have been reported in a 2 year oncogenicity study in rats receiving tamoxifen. In addition, gonadal tumors have been reported in mice receiving tamoxifen in long-term studies. The clinical relevance of these cancer findings has not been established.

Cataracts were also reported in the 2 year oncogenicity study in rats, and since then it has been established that treatment with tamoxifen has been associated with an increased incidence of cataracts.

A number of second primary tumors, occurring at sites other than the endometrium and the opposite breast, have been reported in clinical trials, following the treatment of breast cancer patients with tamoxifen. No causal link has been established and the clinical significance of these observations remains unclear.

Tamoxifen should be used only for the conditions listed under the Indications section.

PRECAUTIONS: Use tamoxifen cautiously in patients with existing thrombocytopenia or leukopenia. Transient decreases in platelet counts usually to 50 000 to 100 000/mm³ have been observed occasionally during treatment. However, no hemorrhagic tendency was reported and platelet counts returned to normal even though treatment was continued.

Transient decreases in leukocytes also have been observed occasionally during treatment. Although it was uncertain that these incidences of leukopenia and thrombocytopenia were due to tamoxifen therapy, complete blood counts, including platelet counts, should be obtained periodically.

As with other additive hormonal therapy (estrogens and androgens) hypercalcemia has been reported in some breast cancer patients with bone metastases within a few weeks of starting treatment with tamoxifen. Patient who have metastatic bone disease should have periodic serum calcium determinations during the first few weeks of tamoxifen therapy and any symptoms suggestive of hypercalcemia should be evaluated promptly. If hypercalcemia is present, appropriate measures should be taken, and, if severe, tamoxifen should be discontinued.

The first patient follow-up should be done within 1 month following initiation of treatment. Thereafter, examinations may be performed at 1- to 2-month intervals. If adverse reactions such as hot flushes, nausea or vomiting occur, and are severe, they may be controlled in some patients by a dosage reduction without loss of effect on the disease.

Bone pain, if it should occur, may require analgesics.

Any patients receiving tamoxifen or having previously received tamoxifen who report abnormal vaginal bleeding should be promptly investigated.

In clinical studies, the median duration of treatment before the onset of a definite objective response has been 2 months. However, approximately 25% of patients who eventually responded were treated for 4 or more months before a definite objective response was recorded.

The duration of tamoxifen treatment will depend on the patient's response. The drug should be continued as long as there is a favorable response.

With obvious disease progression, discontinue tamoxifen. However, because an occasional patient will have a local disease flare (see Adverse Effects) or an increase in bone pain shortly after starting tamoxifen, it is sometimes difficult during the first few weeks of treatment to determine whether the patient's disease is progressing, or whether it will stabilize or respond to continued treatment. There are data to suggest that, if possible, treatment should not be discontinued before a minimum of 3 to 4 weeks.

Drug Interactions: When tamoxifen is used in combination with cytotoxic agents, there is increased risk of thromboembolic events occurring.

ADVERSE EFFECTS: The most frequent adverse reactions to tamoxifen are hot flushes, nausea and vomiting. These may occur in up to 25% of patients and are rarely severe enough to require discontinuation of treatment.

Less frequently reported adverse reactions are vaginal bleeding and vaginal discharge. Any patients reporting these symptoms should be promptly investigated. An increased incidence of uterine cancer and uterine sarcomas has been reported in association with tamoxifen treatment (see Warnings).

Skin rashes, have also been reported. Usually these have not been severe enough to require dosage reduction or discontinuation of treatment.

Increased bone and tumor pain and also local disease flare have occurred. These are sometimes associated with good tumor response. Patients with soft tissue disease may have sudden increases in the size of pre-existing lesions, sometimes associated with marked erythema within and surrounding the lesions, and/or the development of new lesions. When they occur, the bone pain or disease flare are seen shortly after starting tamoxifen and generally subside rapidly.

Ocular changes have been reported in a few breast cancer patients who, as part of a clinical trial, were treated for periods longer than 1 year with doses of tamoxifen that were at least 4 times the highest recommended daily dose of 40 mg. In each instance, the total amount of drug exceeded 100 g. These changes were a retinopathy and, in a few patients, corneal changes and decreased visual acuity. There were multiple light refractile opacities in the paramacular area, and macular edema. The corneal lesions consist of whorl-like superficial opacities.

A number of cases of visual disturbances, including infrequent reports of corneal changes, and retinopathy have been described in patients receiving tamoxifen therapy. An increased incidence of cataracts has been reported in association with the administration of tamoxifen.

Leukopenia has been observed following the administration of tamoxifen, sometimes in association with anemia and/or thrombocytopenia. Neutropenia has been reported on rare occasions; this can sometimes be severe.

Elevations of ALT, AST and GGT levels have been reported on rare occasions in association with tamoxifen therapy. The incidence of overt cholestasis appears to be very low (<1%) but it should be kept in mind while administering tamoxifen over the long-term.

There have been infrequent reports of thromboembolic events occurring during tamoxifen therapy. As an increased incidence of these events is known to occur in patients with malignant disease, a causal relationship with tamoxifen has not been established.

Other adverse reactions noted infrequently are hypercalcemia, peripheral edema, benign symptomatic hepatic cysts, peliosis hepatitis, distaste for food, pruritus vulvae, depression, dizziness, lightheadedness and headache.

Uterine fibroids, endometriosis and other endometrial changes including hyperplasia and polyps have been reported. Ovarian cysts have been observed in a small number of pre-menopausal patients with advanced breast cancer who have been treated with tamoxifen.

Importantly, increased incidence of uterine malignancies, including endometrial adenocarcinomas and uterine sarcomas, have been reported in association with tamoxifen therapy (see Warnings).

In the prevention section, treatment with tamoxifen has been associated with an increased risk of stroke (see Warnings).

OVERDOSE:

Symptoms: Acute overdosage in humans has not been reported. Possible overdosage effects might include hot flushes, nausea, vomiting and vaginal bleeding.

Treatment: Symptomatic treatment. In the case of childhood accidental ingestion, gastric emptying is suggested.

> For management of a suspected drug overdose, CPhA recommends that you contact your **regional Poison Control Centre**. See the *CPS* Directory section for a list of Poison Control Centres.

DOSAGE: The usual dose is 20 to 40 mg/day in a single or 2 divided doses. Use the lowest effective dose.

In early disease, the recommended duration of therapy is 5 years. The optimal duration of therapy remains to be determined.

INFORMATION FOR THE PATIENT: Published in e-CPS, available by subscription at www.e-cps.ca.

SUPPLIED: 10 mg: Each white, round, scored, biconvex tablet, marked "T/10" on one side and scored on the other contains: tamoxifen citrate 15.2 mg equivalent to tamoxifen base 10 mg. Nonmedicinal ingredients: cornstarch, lactose monohydrate, magnesium stearate, povidone, purified water, silica colloidal anhydrous and talc. Plastic containers of 60. Boxes of 60 in aluminum film strips (unit dose packages).

20 mg: Each white, round, biconvex tablet, marked "T/20" on one side, contains: tamoxifen citrate 30.4 mg equivalent to tamoxifen base 20 mg. Nonmedicinal ingredients: cornstarch, lactose monohydrate, magnesium stearate, povidone, purified water, silica colloidal anhydrous and talc. Plastic containers of 60. Boxes of 30 and 60 in aluminum film strips (unit dose packages).

Store at room temperature (between 15 and 30°C) in a well closed container. Protect from light.

(Shown in Product Identification Section)

Tapazole® Ⓟ

methimazole

Antithyroid Agent

Paladin

Date of Revision: May 30, 2007

SUMMARY PRODUCT INFORMATION:

Route of Administration	Dosage Form/ Strength	Clinically Relevant Nonmedicinal Ingredients
Oral	Tablet 5, 10 mg	Lactose monohydrate For a complete listing see Dosage Forms, Composition and Packaging.

INDICATIONS AND CLINICAL USE:

- Tapazole (methimazole) is indicated in the medical treatment of hyperthyroidism. Long-term therapy may lead to remission of the disease.
- Tapazole may be used to ameliorate hyperthyroidism in preparation for subtotal thyroidectomy or radioactive iodine therapy.
- Tapazole is also used when thyroidectomy is contraindicated or not advisable.

CONTRAINDICATIONS:

- Patients who are hypersensitive to this drug or to any ingredient in the formulation or component of the container. For a complete listing, see Dosage Forms, Composition and Packaging.
- Nursing mothers, as the drug is excreted in breast milk.

WARNINGS AND PRECAUTIONS: General: Patients who receive methimazole should be under close surveillance. Physicians should encourage patients to immediately report any evidence of illness or unusual clinical symptoms, particularly sore throat, skin eruptions, fever, headache or general malaise. In such cases, white blood cell and differential counts should be made to determine whether agranulocytosis has developed. Particular care should be exercised with patients who are receiving additional drugs known to cause agranulocytosis.

The development of arthralgias should prompt drug discontinuation, since this symptom may indicate a severe transient migratory polyarthritis known as "the antithyroid arthritis syndrome".

Carcinogenesis and Mutagenesis: Rats treated for 2 years with methimazole demonstrated thyroid hyperplasia and thyroid adenoma and carcinoma formation. Such findings are seen with continuous suppression of thyroid function by sufficient doses of a variety of antithyroid agents. Pituitary adenomas have also been observed.

Hematologic: Agranulocytosis is potentially the most serious side effect of therapy with methimazole. Patients should be instructed to report to their physicians any symptoms of agranulocytosis, such as fever or sore throat. Leukopenia, thrombocytopenia, and aplastic anemia (pancytopenia) may also occur. The drug should be discontinued in the presence of agranulocytosis, aplastic anemia (pancytopenia), hepatitis, or exfoliative dermatitis. The patient's bone marrow function should be monitored.

Hepatic/Biliary/Pancreatic: Due to the similar hepatic toxicity profiles of methimazole and propylthiouracil, attention is drawn to the severe hepatic reactions, which have occurred with both drugs. There have been rare reports of fulminant hepatitis, hepatic necrosis, encephalopathy and death. Symptoms suggestive of hepatic dysfunction (anorexia, pruritis, right upper quadrant pain, etc.) should prompt evaluation of liver function. Drug treatment should be discontinued promptly in the event of clinically significant evidence of liver abnormality, including hepatic transaminase values exceeding 3 times the upper limit of normal.

Special Populations: Pregnant Women: Methimazole can cause fetal harm when administered to a pregnant woman. Methimazole readily crosses the placental membranes and can induce goiter and even cretinism in the developing fetus. In addition, rare instances of aplasia cutis, as manifested by scalp defects have occurred in infants born to mothers who received methimazole during pregnancy. If methimazole is used during pregnancy or if the patient becomes pregnant while taking this drug, the patient should be warned of the potential hazard to the fetus.

Since scalp defects have not been reported in offspring of patients treated with propylthiouracil, this agent may be preferable to methimazole in pregnant women requiring treatment with antithyroid drugs.

Methimazole used judiciously is an effective drug in the treatment of hyperthyroidism complicated by pregnancy. In many pregnant women, the thyroid dysfunction diminishes as the pregnancy proceeds; consequently, a reduction in dosage may be possible. In some instances, use of methimazole can be discontinued 2 or 3 weeks before delivery.

Nursing Women: Methimazole is excreted in human breast milk and its use is contraindicated in nursing mothers.

Pediatrics: No data is available.

Geriatrics: No data is available.

Monitoring and Laboratory Tests: Because methimazole may cause hypoprothrombinemia and bleeding, prothrombin time should be monitored during therapy with the drug, especially before surgical procedures.

Periodic monitoring of thyroid function is warranted. A laboratory result indicating elevated TSH warrants a decrease in the dosage of methimazole.

ADVERSE REACTIONS: Adverse Drug Reaction Overview: Adverse reactions occur in less than 1 percent of patients.

Serious adverse reactions (which occur less frequently than the minor less serious adverse reactions) include inhibition of myelopoiesis (agranulocytosis, granulocytopenia and thrombocytopenia), aplastic anemia, drug fever, a lupus-like syndrome, insulin autoimmune syndrome (which can result in hypoglycemic coma), hepatitis (jaundice may persist for several weeks after discontinuation of the drug), periarteritis and hypoprothrombinemia. Nephritis occurs very rarely.

Less serious adverse reactions include skin rash, urticaria, nausea, vomiting, epigastric distress, arthralgia, paresthesia, loss of taste, abnormal loss of hair, myalgia, headache, pruritus, drowsiness, neuritis, edema, vertigo, skin pigmentation, jaundice, sialadenopathy and lymphadenopathy.

Abnormal Hematologic and Clinical Chemistry Findings: It should be noted that about 10% of patients with untreated hyperthyroidism have leucopenia (white-blood-cell count of less than 4000/mm^3), often with relative granulopenia.

DRUG INTERACTIONS: Drug-Drug Interactions: The activity of anticoagulants may be potentiated by the anti-vitamin K activity attributed to methimazole.

Drug-Food Interactions: Interactions with foods have not been studied.

Drug-Herb Interactions: Interactions with herbal products have not been studied.

Drug-Laboratory Test Interactions: Interactions with laboratory tests have not been studied.

DOSAGE AND ADMINISTRATION: Dosing Considerations:

- Methimazole is administered orally.
- It is usually given in three equal doses a day at approximately eight-hour intervals.

Recommended Dose and Dosage Adjustment: Adult: The initial daily dose is 15 mg for mild hyperthyroidism, 30 to 40 mg for moderately severe hyperthyroidism and 60 mg for severe hyperthyroidism, divided into three doses at eight-hour intervals. The maintenance dosage is 5 to 15 mg daily.

Pediatric: Initially, the daily dosage is 0.4 mg/kg of body weight divided into three doses and given at eight-hour intervals. The maintenance dosage is approximately ½ of the initial dose.

Missed Dose: No data is available.

OVERDOSAGE:

Symptoms: Symptoms may include nausea, vomiting, epigastric distress, headache, fever, joint pain, pruritus and edema. Aplastic anemia (pancytopenia) or agranulocytosis may be manifested in hours to days. Less frequent events are hepatitis, nephrotic syndrome, exfoliative dermatitis, neuropathies and CNS stimulation or depression. Although not well studied, methimazole-induced agranulocytosis is generally associated with doses of 40 mg or more in patients older than 40 years of age.

No information is available on the median lethal dose of the drug or the concentration of methimazole in biologic fluids associated with toxicity and/or death.

Treatment: In managing overdosage, consider the possibility of multiple drug overdoses, interaction among drugs, and unusual drug kinetics in your patient.

Protect the patient's airway and support ventilation and perfusion. Meticulously monitor and maintain, within acceptable limits, the patient's vital signs, blood gases, serum electrolytes, etc. The patient's bone marrow function should be monitored. Absorption of drugs from the gastrointestinal tract may be decreased by giving activated charcoal, which, in many cases, is more effective than emesis or lavage; consider charcoal instead of or in addition to gastric emptying. Repeated doses of charcoal over time may hasten elimination of some drugs that have been absorbed. Safeguard the patient's airway when employing gastric emptying or charcoal.

Forced diuresis, peritoneal dialysis, hemodialysis or charcoal hemoperfusion have not been established as beneficial for an overdose of methimazole.

> For management of a suspected drug overdose, CPhA recommends that you contact your **regional Poison Control Centre**. See the *CPS* Directory section for a list of Poison Control Centres.

ACTION AND CLINICAL PHARMACOLOGY: Mechanism of Action: Methimazole inhibits the synthesis of thyroid hormones and thus is effective in the treatment of hyperthyroidism. The drug does not inactivate existing thyroxine and triiodo-thyroxine that are stored in the thyroid or circulating in the blood, nor does it interfere with the effectiveness of thyroid hormones given by mouth or by injection.

The actions and use of methimazole are similar to those of propylthiouracil. On a weight basis, the drug is at least ten times as potent as propylthiouracil, but methimazole may be less consistent in action.

Pharmacokinetics: Absorption: Methimazole is readily absorbed from the gastrointestinal tract.

Metabolism: It is metabolized rapidly and requires frequent administration.

Excretion: Methimazole is excreted in the urine.

STORAGE AND STABILITY: Store at room temperature (15 to 30°C). Protect from light. Keep tightly closed.

INFORMATION FOR THE PATIENT: Published in e-CPS, available by subscription at www.e-cps.ca.

DOSAGE FORMS, COMPOSITION AND PACKAGING: 5 mg : Each round, white, scored tablet, debossed with "J94" on one side and scored on the other side, contains: methimazole 5 mg. Nonmedicinal ingredients: corn starch, lactose monohydrate, magnesium stearate and talc. Bottles of 100.

10 mg : Each round, white tablet, debossed with "10" on one side and plain on the other side, contains: methimazole 10 mg. Nonmedicinal ingredients: corn starch, lactose monohydrate, magnesium stearate and talc. Bottles of 100.

(Shown in Product Identification Section)

Tarceva® Ⓟ

erlotinib HCl

Epidermal Growth Factor Receptor (EGFR) Tyrosine Kinase Inhibitor

Roche

Date of Preparation: June 28, 2005
Date of Revision: June 10, 2009

SUMMARY PRODUCT INFORMATION:

Route of Administration	Dosage Form/ Strength	Clinically Relevant Nonmedicinal Ingredients
Oral	Tablet 25 mg, 100 mg, 150 mg	Lactose monohydrate For a complete list of ingredients see Dosage Forms, Composition and Packaging.

INDICATIONS AND CLINICAL USE: TARCEVA (erlotinib) is indicated as monotherapy for the treatment of patients with locally advanced or metastatic non-small cell lung cancer (NSCLC) after failure of at least one prior chemotherapy regimen, and whose EGFR expression status is positive or unknown.

Geriatrics (>65 years of age): There have been no specific studies in elderly patients. Of the total number of patients participating in the phase III study, BR.21 (n=731), 62% were less than 65 years of age and 38% of patients were aged 65 years or older. The survival benefit was maintained across both age groups. No meaningful differences in safety or pharmacokinetics were observed between younger and older patients. Therefore, no dosage adjustments are recommended in elderly patients.

Pediatrics: The safety and efficacy of TARCEVA in the pediatric population has not been established.

CONTRAINDICATIONS: TARCEVA is contraindicated in patients with

- severe hypersensitivity to erlotinib or to any component of TARCEVA. For a complete listing, see Dosage Forms, Composition and Packaging.

WARNINGS AND PRECAUTIONS:

Serious Warnings and Precautions

TARCEVA should be administered under the supervision of a qualified health professional who is experienced in the treatment and management of patients with cancer.

- Fatal cases in patients with moderate hepatic impairment (see Warnings and Precautions, Special Populations, Patients with Hepatic Impairment)
- Fatal cases of gastrointestinal perforation (see Warnings and Precautions, Gastrointestinal, Gastrointestinal Perforation)

Drug Interactions: Erlotinib is metabolized in the liver by the hepatic cytochromes in humans, primarily CYP3A4 and to a lesser extent by CYP1A2 and the pulmonary isoform CYP1A1. Potential interactions may occur with drugs which are metabolized by, or are inhibitors or inducers of, these enzymes (see Drug Interactions).

Gastrointestinal: Diarrhea, Dehydration, Electrolyte Imbalance and Renal Failure: Diarrhea has occurred in patients on TARCEVA and moderate or severe diarrhea should be treated with loperamide. In some cases, dose reduction may be necessary. In the event of severe or persistent diarrhea, nausea, anorexia, or vomiting associated with dehydration, TARCEVA therapy should be interrupted and appropriate measures should be taken to treat the dehydration (see Dosage and Administration).

Gastrointestinal Hemorrhage: Gastrointestinal hemorrhage was seen in 2% of patients receiving TARCEVA therapy on study BR.21 in NSCLC. No cases were reported on the placebo arm. Confounding factors include concomitant NSAID use and history of ulcer disease. In patients who develop gastrointestinal hemorrhage while receiving TARCEVA, the drug should be discontinued (see Adverse Reactions, Clinical Trial Adverse Drug Reactions, Gastrointestinal Disorders).

Gastrointestinal Perforation: Patients receiving TARCEVA are at increased risk of developing gastrointestinal perforation, which was observed uncommonly. Patients receiving concomitant anti-angiogenic agents, corticosteroids, NSAIDs, and/or taxane based chemotherapy, or who have prior history of peptic ulceration or diverticular disease are at increased risk. However, in reported cases, not all patients had predisposing risk factors. One third of cases were fatal. TARCEVA should be permanently discontinued in patients who develop gastrointestinal perforation (see Adverse Reactions, Clinical Trial Adverse Drug Reactions, Gastrointestinal Disorders).

Hepatotoxicity: Hepatitis: Asymptomatic increases in liver transaminases have been observed in patients receiving TARCEVA. Therefore, periodic liver function testing (transaminases, bilirubin, and alkaline phosphatase) should be considered. Dose reduction or interruption of TARCEVA therapy should be considered if liver function changes are severe (see Adverse Reactions).

Hepatic Failure: Fatal cases of hepatic failure including hepatorenal syndrome have been reported during use of TARCEVA. Confounding factors in some patients have included pre-existing liver disease, impaired hepatic function and/or concomitant hepatotoxic medications. Close monitoring of liver function testing should be considered in these patients. TARCEVA dosing should be interrupted or discontinued if significant changes in liver function are observed. TARCEVA treatment is not recommended in patients with severe hepatic impairment including those with total bilirubin of >3×ULN and/or transaminases of >5×ULN. (See Warnings and Precautions, Special Populations, Patients with Hepatic Impairment and Adverse Reactions.)

Ocular: Very rare cases of corneal perforation or ulceration have been reported during use of TARCEVA. Permanent vision loss has been reported in one patient. Other ocular disorders including abnormal eyelash growth, keratoconjunctivitis sicca or keratitis have been observed with TARCEVA treatment which are also risk factors for corneal perforation/ulceration. Recent corneal surgery and contact lens wearing could be a risk factor for corneal ulceration/perforation for patients receiving TARCEVA. The optimum timing of TARCEVA therapy in relation to ophthalmic/corneal surgery is not known. TARCEVA therapy should be interrupted or discontinued if patients present with acute/worsening ocular disorders such as eye pain (see Adverse Reactions, Clinical Trial Adverse Drug Reactions).

Renal: There have been rare reports of hypokalaemia and renal failure (including fatalities) mainly in patients receiving concomitant chemotherapy but also in a few patients receiving TARCEVA as monotherapy. Some reports of renal failure were secondary to severe dehydration due to diarrhea, vomiting and/or anorexia while others were confounded by concomitant use of chemotherapy. In more severe or persistent cases of diarrhea, or cases leading to dehydration, particularly in groups of patients with aggravating risk factors (known renal disease, concurrent vomiting, concomitant medications, symptoms or diseases or other predisposing conditions including advanced age), TARCEVA therapy should be interrupted and appropriate measures taken to intensively rehydrate the patients intravenously. In addition, renal function and serum electrolytes including potassium should be monitored particularly in patients at high risk of dehydration (see Warnings and Precautions, Gastrointestinal).

Respiratory: Interstitial Lung Disease (ILD): Cases of ILD-like events, including fatalities, have been reported uncommonly in patients receiving TARCEVA for treatment of NSCLC or other advanced solid tumours. In the pivotal study BR.21 in NSCLC, the incidence of serious ILD-like events was 0.8% in both the TARCEVA and placebo arms. The overall incidence in TARCEVA treated patients from all studies (including uncontrolled studies and studies with concurrent chemotherapy) is approximately 0.6%. Some examples of reported diagnoses in patients suspected of having ILD-like events include pneumonitis, radiation pneumonitis, hypersensitivity pneumonitis, interstitial pneumonia, interstitial lung disease, obliterative bronchiolitis, pulmonary fibrosis, Acute Respiratory Distress Syndrome, lung infiltration and alveolitis. Symptoms started from 5 days to more than 9 months (median 47 days) after initiating TARCEVA. Most of the cases were associated with confounding or contributing factors such as concomitant or prior chemotherapy, prior radiotherapy, pre-existing parenchymal lung disease, metastatic lung disease, or pulmonary infections.

In patients who develop acute onset of new and/or progressive unexplained pulmonary symptoms, such as dyspnea, cough and fever, TARCEVA therapy should be interrupted pending diagnostic evaluation. If ILD is diagnosed, TARCEVA should be discontinued and appropriate treatment initiated as necessary (see Adverse Reactions and Dosage and Administration).

Skin: Bullous and Exfoliative Skin Disorders: Bullous, blistering and exfoliative skin conditions have been reported, including very rare cases suggestive of Stevens-Johnson syndrome/Toxic epidermal necrolysis, which in some cases were fatal (see Adverse Reactions, Clinical Trial Adverse Drug Reactions). TARCEVA treatment should be interrupted or discontinued if the patient develops severe bullous, blistering or exfoliating conditions.

Rash: In pivotal trial BR.21, over three quarters of patients developed a rash. Nine percent (9%) of patients had severe rash, and 6% required dose reduction. Median time to onset of rash was 8 days.

Special Populations: Patients with Brain Metastases: Pivotal trial BR.21 excluded patients with CNS metastases that were symptomatic, and those with asymptomatic metastases but not on a stable dose of corticosteroids for at least 4 weeks prior to randomization. Therefore, the safety of TARCEVA in this patient population is unknown.

Pregnant Women: There are no adequate or well-controlled studies in pregnant women using TARCEVA. Studies in animals have shown reproductive toxicity. The potential risk for humans is unknown. Women of childbearing potential must be advised to avoid pregnancy while on TARCEVA. Adequate contraceptive methods should be used during therapy, and for at least 2 weeks after completing therapy. Treatment should only be continued in pregnant women if the potential benefit to the mother outweighs the risk to the fetus. If TARCEVA is used during pregnancy, the patient must be informed of the potential hazard to the fetus or potential risk for loss of the pregnancy.

Nursing Women: It is not known whether erlotinib is excreted in human milk. Because of the potential harm to the infant, mothers should be advised against breast-feeding while receiving TARCEVA.

Patients with Hepatic Impairment: TARCEVA is eliminated by hepatic metabolism and biliary excretion. A pharmacokinetic study was conducted in patients with advanced solid tumours comparing patients with moderate hepatic impairment (Child-Pugh score 7-9) and patients with adequate hepatic function. Ten of the fifteen patients with moderate hepatic impairment died during TARCEVA treatment or within 30 days of the last dose. Five of the 10 patients died within the first month after initiating TARCEVA treatment. Six of the 10 patients who died had baseline total bilirubin >3×ULN suggesting severe hepatic impairment. Patients with hepatic impairment should be closely monitored during therapy with TARCEVA. TARCEVA dosing should be interrupted or discontinued if significant changes in liver function are observed. The use of TARCEVA in patients with severe hepatic impairment is not recommended (see Warnings and Precautions, Hepatotoxicity and Adverse Reactions).

In pivotal trial BR.21, adequate hepatic function was defined as total bilirubin <1.5×ULN and ALT/SGPT <2×ULN, unless clearly attributable to liver metastases, in which cases <5×ULN was allowed. Approximately 20% of patients on BR.21 had liver metastases. Asymptomatic increases in liver transaminases have been observed in TARCEVA treated patients; therefore, periodic liver function testing (transaminases, bilirubin, and alkaline phosphatase) should be considered. Dose reduction or interruption of TARCEVA should be considered if significant changes in liver function are observed (see Adverse Reactions, Abnormal Hematologic and Clinical Chemistry Findings).

Monitoring and Laboratory Tests: International Normalized Ratio (INR) elevations and bleeding events including gastrointestinal bleeding have been reported in clinical studies, some associated with concomitant warfarin administration (see Adverse Reactions). Patients taking warfarin or other coumarin derivative anticoagulants should be monitored regularly for any changes in prothrombin time or INR (see Drug Interactions). Close monitoring of liver function testing should be considered in patients with hepatic impairment (see Warnings and Precautions, Hepatotoxicity, Hepatic Failure). In addition, renal function and serum electrolytes including potassium should be monitored particularly in patients at high risk of dehydration (see Warnings and Precautions, Renal).

Other: TARCEVA tablets contain lactose and should not be administered to patients with rare hereditary problems of galactose intolerance, Lapp lactase deficiency or glucose-galactose malabsorption.

ADVERSE REACTIONS: Clinical Trial Adverse Drug Reactions: The ADRs listed in Table 1 are based on data from a randomized double-blind study (BR.21) conducted in 731 patients with locally advanced or metastatic NSCLC after failure of at least one prior chemotherapy regimen. Patients were randomized 2:1 to receive TARCEVA (erlotinib) 150 mg or placebo. Study drug was taken orally once daily until disease progression or unacceptable toxicity.

The most frequent ADRs were rash and diarrhea (any Grade 75% and 54%, respectively), most were Grade 1/2 in severity and manageable without intervention. Grade 3/4 rash and diarrhea occurred in 9% and 6%, respectively in TARCEVA-treated patients and each resulted in study discontinuation in 1% of patients. Dose reduction for rash and diarrhea was needed in 6% and 1% of patients, respectively. In study BR 21, the median time to onset of rash was 8 days, and the median time to onset of diarrhea was 12 days.

Table 1: TARCEVA

ADRs Occurring More Frequently (≥3%) in the TARCEVA Group Than in the Placebo Group and in ≥10% of Patients in the TARCEVA Group in Study BR.21

	Erlotinib N=485			Placebo N=242		
NCI-CTC Grade	**Any Grade**	**3**	**4**	**Any Grade**	**3**	**4**
MedDRA Preferred Term	**%**	**%**	**%**	**%**	**%**	**%**
Total patients with any AE	99	40	22	96	36	22
Eye Disorders						
Conjunctivitis	12	<1	0	2	<1	0
Keratoconjunctivitis sicca	12	0	0	3	0	0
Gastrointestinal Disorders						
Diarrhea	54	6	<1	18	<1	0
Nausea	33	3	0	24	2	0
Vomiting	23	2	<1	19	2	0
Stomatitis	17	<1	0	3	0	0
Abdominal Pain	11	2	<1	7	1	<1
General Disorders and Administration Site Conditions						
Fatigue	52	14	4	45	16	4
Infections and infestations[a]						
Infection	24	4	0	15	2	0
Metabolism and Nutrition Disorders						
Anorexia	52	8	1	38	5	<1
Respiratory, Thoracic and Mediastinal Disorders						
Dyspnea	41	17	11	35	15	11
Cough	33	4	0	29	2	0
Skin and Subcutaneous Tissue Disorders						
Rash	75	8	<1	17	0	0
Pruritus	13	<1	0	5	0	0
Dry skin	12	0	0	4	0	0

[a] Severe infections, with or without neutropenia, have included pneumonia, sepsis, and cellulitis.

In pivotal trial BR.21, serious gastrointestinal hemorrhage was seen in 8 patients treated with TARCEVA (2%) and there were no cases in placebo treated patients. The gastrointestinal hemorrhage was fatal in 2 patients treated with TARCEVA. Confounding factors include concomitant NSAID use and history of peptic ulcer disease. The incidence of serious interstitial lung disease in BR.21 was 0.8% in each treatment arm. There was 1 case of fatal pneumonitis (fatal outcome of ILD) in each treatment arm.

Other Observations: The primary safety population was defined as the 856 patients treated with at least one 150 mg dose of TARCEVA monotherapy during Phase II and Phase III studies in NSCLC (A248-1007, BR.21) and other Phase I through II studies in populations other than NSCLC. This population also takes into consideration the 242 patients who received placebo in study BR.21. The following common and uncommon adverse reactions have been observed in patients who received TARCEVA monotherapy in the primary safety population.

The following terms are used to rank the undesirable effects by frequency: very common (>1/10); common (>1/100, <1/10); uncommon (>1/1000, <1/100); rare (>1/10 000, <1/1000); very rare (<1/10 000) including isolated reports.

Gastrointestinal Disorders: Gastrointestinal perforations have been reported uncommonly (in less than 1% of patients) with TARCEVA treatment (see Warnings and Precautions, Gastrointestinal).

Cases of gastrointestinal bleeding have been commonly reported in clinical studies, some associated with concomitant warfarin administration (see also Drug Interactions) and some with concomitant NSAID administration.

Eye Disorders: Keratitis has been reported commonly in clinical trials of TARCEVA. Corneal ulcerations or perforations have been reported very rarely in patients receiving TARCEVA treatment (see Warnings and Precautions, Ocular).

Skin and Subcutaneous Tissue Disorders: Rash has been reported very commonly in patients receiving TARCEVA and in general, manifests as a mild or moderate erythematous and papulopustular rash, which may occur or worsen in sun exposed areas. For patients who are exposed to sun, protective clothing, and/or use of sun screen (e.g. mineral-containing) may be advisable. Other mild skin reactions such as hyperpigmentation have been observed uncommonly (in less than 1% of patients).

Bullous, blistering and exfoliative skin conditions have been reported, including very rare cases suggestive of Stevens-Johnson syndrome/Toxic epidermal necrolysis, which in some cases were fatal (see Warnings and Precautions, Skin).

Hair and nail changes, mostly non-serious, were reported in clinical trials, e.g. paronychia was reported commonly and hirsutism, and brittle and loose nails were reported uncommonly. Abnormal eyelash growth including; in-growing eyelashes, excessive growth and thickening of the eyelashes have been reported.

Abnormal Hematologic and Clinical Chemistry Findings: Hepato-Biliary Disorders: Liver function test abnormalities (including elevated alanine aminotransferase [ALT], aspartate aminotransferase [AST], bilirubin) have been observed commonly. These were mainly mild or moderate in severity, transient in nature or associated with liver metastases]. Grade 2 (>2.5-5.0×ULN) ALT elevations occurred in 4% and <1% of TARCEVA and placebo treated patients, respectively. Grade 3 (<5.0-20.0×ULN) elevations were not observed in TARCEVA treated patients. Fatal cases of hepatic failure including hepatorenal syndrome have been reported during use of TARCEVA. Confounding factors in some cases have included pre-existing liver disease, hepatic impairment and/or concomitant hepatotoxic medications (see Warnings and Precautions).

Less Common Clinical Trial Adverse Drug Reactions (<1%): Respiratory, Thoracic and Mediastinal Disorders: There have been uncommon reports of serious interstitial lung disease (ILD)-like events, including fatalities, in patients receiving TARCEVA for treatment of NSCLC and other advanced solid tumors (see Warnings and Precautions).

Post-Market Adverse Drug Reactions: Nervous System Disorders: headaches and dizziness.

Skin and Subcutaneous Tissue Disorders: hair and nail changes, dermatitis acneiform, erythema, hirsutism, eyelash/eyebrow changes, paronychia and brittle and loose nails, radiotherapy induced cutaneous phototoxicity.

DRUG INTERACTIONS: Overview: Erlotinib is metabolized in the liver by the hepatic cytochromes in humans, primarily CYP3A4 and to a lesser extent by CYP1A2, and the pulmonary isoform CYP1A1. Potential interactions may occur with drugs which are metabolized by, or are inhibitors or inducers of, these enzymes.

Drug-Drug Interactions: Comprehensive testing of drug-drug interactions with TARCEVA (erlotinib) has not been done.

Potent inhibitors of CYP3A4 activity decrease erlotinib metabolism and increase erlotinib plasma concentrations. Inhibition of CYP3A4 metabolism by ketoconazole (200 mg po BID for 5 days) resulted in increased exposure to erlotinib (86% in median erlotinib exposure [AUC]) and a 69% increase in C_{max} when compared to erlotinib alone. When TARCEVA was co-administered with ciprofloxacin, an inhibitor of both CYP3A4 and CYP1A2, the erlotinib exposure [AUC] and maximum concentration (C_{max}) increased by 39% and 17%, respectively. Therefore caution should be used when administering TARCEVA with potent CYP3A4 or combined CYP3A4/CYP1A2 inhibitors. These include, but are not limited to, calcium channel blockers (eg. diltiazem, verapamil); antifungals (eg. ketoconazole, fluconazole, itraconazole, voriconazole); macrolide antibiotics (eg. erythromycin, clarithromycin); fluoroquinalone antibiotics (eg. ciprofloxacin, norfloxacin); some HIV antivirals (eg. ritonavir, indinavir); and grapefruit juice. In these situations, the dose of TARCEVA should be reduced if toxicity is observed (see Dosage and Administration).

Potent inducers of CYP3A4 activity increase erlotinib metabolism and significantly decrease erlotinib plasma concentrations. Induction of CYP3A4 metabolism by rifampicin (600 mg po QD for 7 days) resulted in a 69% decrease in the median erlotinib AUC, following a 150 mg dose of TARCEVA, as compared to TARCEVA alone. In a separate study, pre-treatment and co-administration of rifampicin with a single 450 mg dose of TARCEVA reduced the mean erlotinib exposure [AUC] to 57.5% of what was observed at a single 150 mg TARCEVA dose in the absence of rifampicin treatment. On the other hand, systemic exposure of the active metabolites (OSI-413 and OSI-420) of TARCEVA was largely unaffected by rifampicin treatment. As a result, the active metabolites consist of 18% of the total erlotinib exposure following the concomitant administration compared to only 5% when TARCEVA was given alone. Alternative treatments lacking potent CYP3A4 inducing activity should be considered when possible.

Other CYP3A4 inducers include, but are not limited to, barbiturates (eg. phenobarbital); anticonvulsants (eg. carbamazepine, phenytoin); glucocorticoids; pioglitazone; St. John's wort, and some HIV antivirals (eg. efavirenz, nevirapine). Alternate treatments lacking potent CYP3A4 inducing activity should be considered when possible.

Pre-treatment or co-administration of TARCEVA did not alter the clearance of the prototypical CYP3A4 substrates midazolam and erythromycin. Significant interactions with the clearance of other CYP3A4 substrates are therefore unlikely. Oral availability of midazolam did appear to decrease by up to 24%, which was however not attributed to effects on CYP3A4 activity.

The solubility of erlotinib is pH dependent. Erlotinib solubility decreases as pH increases. Co-administration of TARCEVA with omeprazole, a proton pump inhibitor, decreased the erlotinib exposure [AUC] and [C_{max}] by 46% and 61%, respectively. There was no change to T_{max} or half-life. Increasing the dose of TARCEVA when co-administered with such agents is not likely to compensate for this loss of exposure.

International Normalized Ratio (INR) elevations and bleeding events including gastrointestinal bleeding (see Warnings and Precautions and Adverse Reactions) have been reported in clinical studies, some associated with concomitant warfarin administration. Patients taking warfarin or other coumarin derivative anticoagulants should be monitored regularly for any changes in prothrombin time or INR.

Drug-Food Interactions: Grapefruit juice has CYP3A4 inhibitory activity, therefore ingestion of grapefruit juice while on TARCEVA therapy may lead to decreased erlotinib metabolism and increased erlotinib plasma concentrations (see Drug-Drug Interactions).

Drug-Herb Interactions: St. John's wort is a potent CYP3A4 inducer. Co-administration with erlotinib can lead to increased erlotinib metabolism and decreased erlotinib plasma concentrations (see Drug-Drug Interactions).

Drug-Lifestyle Interactions: Smokers should be advised to stop smoking as cigarette smoking, which is known to induce CYP1A1 and CYP1A2, has been shown to reduce erlotinib exposure by 50-60% (see Dosage and Administration, Dosing Considerations).

DOSAGE AND ADMINISTRATION: The recommended daily dose of TARCEVA is 150 mg taken orally with a glass of plain water, at least one hour before or two hours after the ingestion of food.

Dosage Adjustment: When dose reduction is necessary, it is recommended to reduce in 50 mg steps.

Diarrhea can mostly be managed by loperamide. Patients with severe diarrhea that are unresponsive to loperamide or associated with dehydration may require a dose reduction or temporary interruption of therapy. Patients with severe skin reactions may also require a dose reduction or temporary interruption of therapy (see Warnings and Precautions).

In patients who develop acute onset of new and/or progressive unexplained pulmonary symptoms, such as dyspnea, cough and fever, TARCEVA therapy should be interrupted pending diagnostic evaluation. If ILD is diagnosed, TARCEVA should be discontinued and appropriate treatment initiated as necessary (see Warnings and Precautions).

In patients being concomitantly treated with a potent CYP3A4 inhibitor such as, but not limited to, ketoconazole, itraconazole, voriconazole, clarithromycin, telithromycin, troleandomycin, or atanazavir, a dose reduction should be considered in the presence of severe adverse events (see Drug Interactions).

Dosing Considerations: Hepatic impairment: Erlotinib is eliminated by hepatic metabolism and biliary excretion. Although erlotinib exposure following a single 150 mg was similar in patients with moderately impaired hepatic function (Child-Pugh score 7-9) compared with patients with adequate hepatic function, ten of the fifteen patients with hepatic impairment died during treatment or within 30 days of the last dose of TARCEVA. A reduced dose should be considered for patients with moderate hepatic impairment. Hepatic function should be closely monitored in patients with pre-existing liver disease, hepatic impairment and/or taking concomitant hepatotoxic medications. TARCEVA dosing should be interrupted or discontinued if significant changes in liver function tests are observed. The use of TARCEVA in patients with severe hepatic dysfunction including total bilirubin of >3×ULN and/or transaminases of >5×ULN is not recommended (see Warnings and Precautions, Special Populations, Patients with Hepatic Impairment).

Renal Impairment: The safety and efficacy of TARCEVA has not been studied in patients with renal impairment.

Geriatrics: No meaningful differences in safety or pharmacokinetics were observed between younger and older patients, therefore, no dosing adjustment is necessary (see Indications and Clinical Use).

Smokers: Cigarette smoking has been shown to reduce erlotinib exposure by 50-60%. The maximum tolerated dose of TARCEVA in NSCLC patients who concurrently smoked cigarettes was 300 mg. Efficacy and long term safety of a dose higher than the recommended 150 mg has not been established in patients who continue to smoke cigarettes (see Drug Interactions, Drug-Lifestyle Interactions).

Missed Dose: A double-dose should not be administered to make up for forgotten individual doses.

OVERDOSAGE:

Single oral doses of TARCEVA up to 1000 mg in healthy subjects, and up to 1600 mg given as a single dose once weekly in cancer patients have been tolerated. Repeated twice daily doses of 200 mg in healthy subjects were poorly tolerated after only a few days of dosing. Based on the data from these studies, severe adverse events such as diarrhea, rash and possibly liver transaminase elevation may occur above the recommended dose of 150 mg. In case of suspected overdose, TARCEVA should be withheld and symptomatic treatment initiated.

For management of a suspected drug overdose, contact your **regional Poison Control Centre**. See the *CPS* Directory section for a list of Poison Control Centres.

ACTION AND CLINICAL PHARMACOLOGY: TARCEVA is a Human Epidermal Growth Factor Receptor Type 1/Epidermal Growth Factor Receptor (HER1/EGFR) tyrosine kinase inhibitor.

Mechanism of Action: The mechanism of clinical antitumour action of erlotinib is not fully characterized. Erlotinib potently inhibits the intracellular phosphorylation of HER1/EGF receptor. HER1/EGF receptor is expressed on the cell surface of normal cells and cancer cells. Specificity of erlotinib inhibition on other tyrosine kinase receptors of the ErbB family has not been characterized.

Pharmacokinetics: Absorption: Oral erlotinib is well absorbed and has an extended absorption phase, with mean peak plasma levels occurring at 4 hours after oral dosing. A study in normal healthy volunteers provided an estimate of bioavailability of 59%. The exposure after an oral dose may be increased by food.

Following absorption, erlotinib is highly bound in blood, with approximately 95% bound to blood components, primarily to plasma proteins (i.e. albumin and alpha-1 acid glycoprotein [AAG]), with a free fraction of approximately 5%.

Distribution: Erlotinib has a mean apparent volume of distribution of 232 L and distributes into tumor tissue of humans. In a study of 4 patients (3 with non-small cell lung cancer [NSCLC], and 1 with laryngeal cancer) receiving 150 mg daily oral doses of TARCEVA, tumor samples from surgical excisions on Day 9 of treatment revealed tumor concentrations of erlotinib that averaged 1185 ng/g of tissue. This corresponded to an overall average of 63% of the steady state observed peak plasma concentrations. The primary active metabolites were present in tumors at concentrations averaging 160 ng/g tissue, which corresponded to an overall average of 113% of the observed steady state peak plasma concentrations. Tissue distribution studies using whole body autoradiography following oral administration with [^{14}C] labeled erlotinib in athymic nude mice with HN5 tumor xenografts have shown rapid and extensive tissue distribution with maximum concentrations of radiolabeled drug (approximately 73% of that in plasma) observed at 1 hour. Higher radioactivity exposure (4-8 fold as measured in other peripheral tissues) was observed in kidney and liver in these studies.

Metabolism: Erlotinib is metabolized in the liver by the hepatic cytochromes in humans, primarily CYP3A4 and to a lesser extent by CYP1A2, and the pulmonary isoform CYP1A1. In vitro studies indicate approximately 80-95% of erlotinib metabolism is by the CYP3A4 enzyme. There are three main metabolic pathways identified: 1) O-demethylation of either side chain or both, followed by oxidation to the carboxylic acids; 2) oxidation of the acetylene moiety followed by hydrolysis to the aryl carboxylic acid; and 3) aromatic hydroxylation of the phenyl-acetylene moiety. The primary metabolites of erlotinib produced by O-demethylation of either side chain are present in plasma at levels that are <10% of erlotinib and display similar pharmacokinetics as erlotinib. The metabolites and trace amounts of erlotinib are excreted predominantly via the feces (>90%), with renal elimination accounting for only a small amount of an oral dose.

Excretion: Clearance: A population pharmacokinetic analysis in 591 patients receiving single agent TARCEVA shows a mean apparent clearance of 4.47 L/hour with a median half-life of 36.2 hours. Therefore, the time to reach steady state plasma concentration would be expected to occur in approximately 7-8 days. No significant relationships between predicted apparent clearance and patient age, body weight, gender, and ethnicity were observed.

Serum total bilirubin, AAG concentrations and smoking are major confounding factors for erlotinib clearance. Increased serum concentration of total bilirubin or AAG was associated with reduced erlotinib clearance and an increase in systemic exposure. Smokers had a 24% higher rate of erlotinib clearance.

Exposure: Following a 150 mg oral dose of TARCEVA, at steady state, the median time to reach maximum plasma concentrations is approximately 4.0 hours with median maximum plasma concentrations achieved of 1995 ng/mL. Prior to the next dose at 24 hours, the median minimum plasma concentrations are 1238 ng/mL. Median AUC achieved during the dosing interval at steady state are 41 300 ng·h/mL.

Special Populations: Hepatic Impairment: Erlotinib is mainly cleared by the liver. A pharmacokinetic study was conducted in patients with advance solid tumors comparing patients with moderate hepatic impairment (Child-Pugh score 7-9) and those with adequate hepatic function. Erlotinib exposure following a single 150 mg dose was similar in patients with moderate hepatic impairment and those with adequate hepatic function whereas the steady-state pharmacokinetic parameters following TARCEVA daily dosing were not measured. Safety and pharmacokinetics of TARCEVA in patients with severe hepatic impairment is unknown (see Warnings and Precautions and Dosage and Administration, Dosing Considerations).

Renal Impairment: Erlotinib and its metabolites are not significantly excreted by the kidneys, as less than 9% of a single dose is excreted in the urine. No clinical studies have been conducted in patients with compromised renal function.

Smokers: A pharmacokinetic study in nonsmoking and currently cigarette smoking healthy subjects has shown that cigarette smoking leads to increased clearance of, and decreased exposure to, erlotinib. The $AUC_{0\text{-infinity}}$ in smokers was about 1/3 of that in never/former smokers (n=16 in each of smoker and never/former smoker arms). This reduced exposure in current smokers is presumably due to induction of CYP1A1 in lung and CYP1A2 in the liver.

In the pivotal Phase III NSCLC trial, current smokers achieved erlotinib steady state trough plasma concentration of 0.65 µg/mL (n=16) which was approximately 2-fold less than the former smokers or patients who had never smoked (1.28 µg/mL, n=108). This effect was accompanied by a 24% increase in apparent erlotinib plasma clearance.

In a phase I dose escalation study in NSCLC patients who were current smokers, pharmacokinetic analyses at steady-state indicated a dose proportional increase in erlotinib exposure when the TARCEVA dose was increased from 150 mg to 300 mg (see Drug Interactions, Drug-Lifestyle Interactions).

STORAGE AND STABILITY: Store TARCEVA between 15-30°C. Do not use after the expiry date stated on the carton.

SPECIAL HANDLING INSTRUCTIONS: Keep out of the reach of children.

INFORMATION FOR THE PATIENT: Published in e-CPS, available by subscription at www.e-cps.ca.

DOSAGE FORMS, COMPOSITION AND PACKAGING: 25 mg: Each white to yellowish, round, biconvex, film-coated tablet, with "Tarceva 25" and logo printed in brownish yellow on one side, contains: erlotinib hydrochloride corresponding to 25 mg of erlotinib. Nonmedicinal ingredients: tablet core: lactose monohydrate, magnesium stearate, microcrystalline cellulose, sodium lauryl sulfate and sodium starch glycolate; tablet coat: hydroxypropyl cellulose, hydroxypropyl methylcellulose, polyethylene glycol and titanium dioxide. PVC blisters sealed with aluminum foil of 10 tablets, cartons of 3.

100 mg: Each white to yellowish, round, biconvex, film-coated tablet with "Tarceva 100" and logo printed in grey on one side, contains: erlotinib hydrochloride corresponding to 100 mg of erlotinib. Nonmedicinal ingredients: tablet core: lactose monohydrate, magnesium stearate, microcrystalline cellulose, sodium lauryl sulfate and sodium starch glycolate; tablet coat: hydroxypropyl cellulose, hydroxypropyl methylcellulose, polyethylene glycol and titanium dioxide. PVC blisters sealed with aluminum foil of 10 tablets, cartons of 3.

150 mg: Each white to yellowish, round, biconvex, film-coated tablet with "Tarceva 150" and logo printed in brown on one side, contains: erlotinib hydrochloride corresponding to 150 mg of erlotinib. Nonmedicinal ingredients: tablet core: lactose monohydrate, magnesium stearate, microcrystalline cellulose, sodium lauryl sulfate and sodium starch glycolate; tablet coat: hydroxypropyl cellulose, hydroxypropyl methylcellulose, polyethylene glycol and titanium dioxide. PVC blisters sealed with aluminum foil of 10 tablets, cartons of 3.

(Shown in Product Identification Section)

Tardan®

coal tar—salicylic acid—triclosan

Antiseborrheic—Antipsoriasis

Odan

SUPPLIED: Each mL contains: coal tar solution 5%, salicylic acid 2% and triclosan 0.3%. Nonmedicinal ingredients: acrylates copolymer, cocamide diethanolamine, disodium cocoamphodipropionate, hydrolyzed wheat protein, perfume, sodium laureth sulfate, triethanolamine and water. Plastic bottles of 250 and 500 mL with dispensing caps.

Targel
coal tar
Antipsoriasis

Odan

Targel S.A.
coal tar—salicylic acid
Antipsoriasis

Odan

SUPPLIED: Targel: Each g contains: liquor carbonis detergens (coal tar solution) 10% in a water washable gel base. Nonmedicinal ingredients: carbomer, perfume, propylene glycol, purified water and triethanolamine. Plastic jars of 100 g.
Targel S.A.: Each g contains: liquor carbonis detergens (coal tar solution) 10% and salicylic acid 3% in a water washable gel base. Nonmedicinal ingredients: carbomer, perfume, purified water and triethanolamine. Plastic jars of 100 g.

Tarka® Ⓟ
trandolapril—verapamil HCl
Antihypertensive

Abbott

Date of Preparation: June 22, 2001
Date of Revision: May 20, 2008

SUMMARY PRODUCT INFORMATION:

Route of Administration	Dosage Form/ Strength	Clinically Relevant Nonmedicinal Ingredients
Oral	Film-coated tablets/ 2/240 mg 4/240 mg	Corn starch, dioctyl sodium sulfosuccinate, hydroxypropyl cellulose, hydroxypropyl methylcellulose, lactose monohydrate, magnesium stearate, microcrystalline cellulose, polyethylene glycol, povidone, purified water, silicon dioxide, sodium alginate, sodium stearyl fumarate, synthetic iron oxides, talc, titanium dioxide

INDICATIONS AND CLINICAL USE: TARKA (trandolapril/verapamil hydrochloride) is indicated for:
- treatment of mild to moderate essential hypertension in patients for whom combination therapy is appropriate.

Patients should be titrated with the individual drugs. If the fixed combination represents the dosage determined by this titration, the use of TARKA may be more convenient in the management of patients. If during maintenance therapy dosage adjustment is necessary, it is advisable to use individual drugs.

Both trandolapril and verapamil SR should normally be used in those patients in whom treatment with a diuretic or a beta-blocker were found to be ineffective or were associated with unacceptable adverse effects. They can be tried as initial agents in those patients in whom diuretics and/or beta-blockers are contraindicated or in patients with medical conditions in which these drugs frequently cause serious adverse effects.

TARKA is not indicated for initial therapy. Patients in whom trandolapril and verapamil SR are initiated simultaneously can develop symptomatic hypotension (see Warnings and Precautions, Hypotension).

In using trandolapril, consideration should be given to the risk of angioedema (see Warnings and Precautions).

Geriatrics (>65 years of age): In placebo-controlled studies, where 23% of patients receiving TARKA were 65 years and older, and 2.4% were 75 years and older, no overall differences on effectiveness or safety were observed between these patients and younger patients. However, greater sensitivity of some older individual patients cannot be ruled out.

Pediatrics (<18 years of age): TARKA has not been studied in children and therefore use in this age group is not recommended.

CONTRAINDICATIONS:
- Patients who are hypersensitive to one of these two drugs or to any ingredient in the formulation or component of the container. For a complete listing, see Dosage Forms, Composition and Packaging.
- Complicated myocardial infarction (patients who have ventricular failure manifested by pulmonary congestion).
- Severe left ventricular dysfunction (see Warnings and Precautions, Heart Failure).
- Hypotension (systolic pressure less than 90 mmHg) or cardiogenic shock.
- Second or third degree AV block (except in patients with a functioning artificial ventricular pacemaker).
- Sick sinus syndrome (except in patients with a functioning artificial ventricular pacemaker).
- Marked bradycardia.
- Patients with atrial flutter or atrial fibrillation and an accessory bypass tract (e.g. Wolff-Parkinson-White, Lown-Ganong-Levine syndromes) (see Warnings and Precautions, Accessory Bypass Tract (Wolff-Parkinson-White or Lown-Ganong-Levine)).
- A history of angioedema associated with prior angiotensin converting enzyme inhibitor (ACE) therapy.
- Pregnancy (see Warnings and Precautions, Special Populations, Pregnant Women).
- Nursing women (see Warnings and Precautions, Special Populations, Nursing Women).

WARNINGS AND PRECAUTIONS:

> **Serious Warnings and Precautions**
> When used in pregnancy, ACE inhibitors can cause injury to or even death of the developing fetus. When pregnancy is detected or if the patient is planning to become pregnant, TARKA should be discontinued as soon as possible (see Warnings and Precautions, Pregnant Women).

Cardiovascular: Hypotension: Concomitant therapy with ACE inhibitors and verapamil may result in hypotension. In controlled studies, hypotension was observed in 0.6% of uncomplicated hypertensive patients receiving TARKA (trandolapril/verapamil hydrochloride). Dizziness occurred more frequently than with placebo (see Adverse Reactions). In patients with angina or arrhythmias using antihypertensive drugs, the additional antihypertensive effect of TARKA should be taken into consideration.

Hypotensive symptoms of lethargy and weakness with faintness have been reported following single oral doses of verapamil and even after some months of treatment. In some patients it may be necessary to reduce the dose.

Symptomatic hypotension has occurred after administration of trandolapril, usually after the first or second dose, or when the dose was increased. It is more likely to occur in patients who are volume depleted as a result of diuretic therapy, dietary salt restriction, dialysis, diarrhea or vomiting. In patients with ischemic heart disease or cerebrovascular disease, an excessive fall in blood pressure could result in a myocardial infarction or cerebrovascular accident. Because of the potential fall in blood pressure in these patients, therapy with trandolapril should be started under close medical supervision. Such patients should be followed closely for the first weeks of treatment and whenever the dose of trandolapril is increased. In patients with severe congestive heart failure, with or without associated renal insufficiency, ACE inhibitor therapy may cause excessive hypotension and has been associated with oliguria, and/or progressive azotemia, and rarely, with acute renal failure and/or death.

If hypotension occurs, the patient should be placed in a supine position and, if necessary, receive an intravenous infusion of 0.9% sodium chloride. A transient hypotensive response is not a contraindication to further doses which can be given usually without difficulty once the blood pressure has increased after volume expansion. If symptoms persist, the dosage should be reduced or the drug discontinued.

Heart Failure: Because of the drug's negative inotropic effect, verapamil should not be used in patients with poorly compensated congestive heart failure, unless the failure is complicated by or caused by a dysrhythmia. If verapamil is used in such patients, they must be digitalized prior to treatment.

It has been reported that digoxin plasma levels may increase with chronic verapamil administration (see Drug Interactions, Drug-Drug Interactions: Digoxin). The use of verapamil in the treatment of hypertension is not recommended in patients with heart failure caused by systolic dysfunction.

Trandolapril, as an ACE inhibitor, may cause excessive hypotension in patients with congestive heart failure (see Warnings and Precautions, Hypotension).

Conduction Disturbance: Verapamil slows conduction across the A-V node and rarely may produce second or third degree A-V block, bradycardia and in extreme cases, asystole.

Because of the verapamil component, use TARKA with caution in patients with first degree AV block.

Verapamil causes dose-related suppression of the S-A node. In some patients, sinus bradycardia may occur, especially in patients with a sick sinus syndrome (S-A nodal disease), which is more common in older patients (see Contraindications).

Bradycardia: The total incidence of bradycardia with verapamil (ventricular rate less than 50 beats/min.) was 1.4% in controlled studies. Asystole in patients other than those with sick sinus syndrome is usually of short duration (few seconds or less), with spontaneous return to A-V nodal or normal sinus rhythm. If this does not occur promptly, appropriate treatment should be initiated immediately (see Overdosage).

Accessory Bypass Tract (Wolff-Parkinson-White or Lown-Ganong-Levine): Verapamil may result in significant acceleration of ventricular response during atrial fibrillation or atrial flutter in the Wolff-Parkinson-White (WPW) or Lown-Ganong-Levine syndromes after receiving intravenous verapamil. Although a risk of this occurring with oral verapamil has not been established, such patients receiving oral verapamil may be at risk and its use in these patients is contraindicated (see Contraindications).

Concomitant Use with Beta-blockers: Generally, oral verapamil should not be given to patients receiving beta blockers since the depressant effects on myocardial contractility, heart rate and A-V conduction may be additive. However, in exceptional cases when in the opinion of the physician concomitant use in angina and arrhythmia is considered essential, such use should be instituted gradually under careful supervision. If combined therapy is used, close surveillance of vital signs and clinical status should be carried out and the need for continued concomitant treatment periodically assessed.

Verapamil gives no protection against the dangers of abrupt beta-blocker withdrawal and such withdrawal should be done by the gradual reduction of the dose of beta blocker. Then verapamil may be started with the usual dose.

Patients with Hypertrophic Cardiomyopathy: In 120 patients with hypertrophic cardiomyopathy (most of them refractory or intolerant to propranolol) who received therapy with verapamil at doses up to 720 mg/day, a variety of serious adverse effects were seen. Three patients died in pulmonary edema; all had severe left ventricular outflow obstruction and a past history of left ventricular dysfunction. Eight other patients had pulmonary edema and/or severe hypotension; abnormally high (over 20 mmHg) capillary wedge pressure and a marked left ventricular outflow obstruction were present in most of these patients. Sinus bradycardia occurred in 11% of the patients, second-degree AV block in 4% and sinus arrest in 2%. It must be appreciated that this group of patients had a serious disease with a high mortality rate. Most adverse effects responded well to dose reduction, but in some cases verapamil use had to be discontinued.

Aortic Stenosis: TARKA should not be used in patients with aortic stenosis.

Immune: Angioedema: Angioedema has been reported in patients taking ACE inhibitors, including trandolapril. Angioedema associated with laryngeal involvement may be fatal. If laryngeal stridor or angioedema of the face, tongue, or glottis occurs, trandolapril should be discontinued immediately, the patient treated appropriately in accordance with accepted medical care, and carefully observed until the swelling disappears. In instances where swelling is confined to the face and lips, the condition generally resolves without treatment. Where there is involvement of tongue, glottis, or larynx, likely to cause airway obstruction, appropriate therapy (including, but not limited to 0.3 to 0.5 mL of subcutaneous epinephrine solution 1:1000) should be administered promptly (see Adverse Reactions).

Patients with a history of angioedema unrelated to ACE inhibitor therapy may be at increased risk of angioedema while receiving an ACE inhibitor (see Contraindications).

The incidence of angioedema during ACE inhibition therapy has been reported to be higher in black than in non-black patients.

Hematologic: Neutropenia/Agranulocytosis: Agranulocytosis and bone marrow depression have been caused by ACE inhibitors. Current experience with trandolapril shows the incidence to be rare. Periodic monitoring of white blood cell counts should be considered, especially in patients with collagen vascular disease and/or renal disease.

Hepatic/Biliary/Pancreatic: Hepatic Failure/Elevated Liver Enzymes: Elevations of transaminases, with and without concomitant elevations in alkaline phosphatase and bilirubin, have been reported. Several cases of hepatocellular injury related to verapamil have been proven by rechallenge. Clinical symptoms of malaise, fever, and/or right upper quadrant pain, in addition to elevations of AST, ALT, and alkaline phosphatase have been reported. Periodic monitoring of liver function in patients receiving TARKA is, therefore, prudent.

In rare instances, ACE inhibitors have been associated with a syndrome of cholestatic jaundice, fulminant hepatic necrosis and death. The mechanism of this syndrome is not understood.

Patients receiving TARKA who develop jaundice should discontinue therapy and receive appropriate medical follow-up.

Liver abnormalities (increased AST, increased ALT, increased liver enzyme and liver function abnormal) associated to TARKA were noted in only 1.2% of patients during TARKA clinical studies.

Use in Patients with Hepatic Impairment: In patients with impaired liver function, the elimination $t_{½}$ of verapamil is prolonged four-fold and the plasma concentrations of trandolapril and, to a lesser extent, of its principle active metabolite, trandolaprilat, are increased (see Action and Clinical Pharmacology, Pharmacokinetics). Accordingly, a decreased dosage of TARKA should be used in these patients (see Dosage and Administration).

In these patients, careful monitoring for abnormal prolongation of the PR interval or other signs of excessive pharmacologic effects should be carried out during TARKA therapy.

Renal: Use in Patients with Renal Impairment: About 70% of an administered dose of verapamil is excreted as metabolites in the urine. In one study in healthy volunteers, the total body clearance after intravenous administration of verapamil was 12.08 mL/min/kg, while in patients with advanced renal disease it was reduced to 5.33 mL/min/kg. This pharmacokinetic finding suggests that renal clearance of verapamil in patients with renal disease is decreased. In two studies with oral verapamil no difference in pharmacokinetics could be demonstrated. Therefore, until further data are available, verapamil should be used with caution in patients with impaired renal function. These patients should be carefully monitored for abnormal prolongation of the PR interval or other signs of excessive pharmacologic effect (see Dosage and Administration).

As a consequence of inhibiting the renin-angiotensin-aldosterone system, changes in renal function have been seen in susceptible individuals. In patients whose renal function may depend on the activity of the renin-angiotensin-aldosterone system, such as patients with bilateral renal artery stenosis, unilateral renal artery stenosis to a solitary kidney, or severe congestive heart failure, treatment with agents that inhibit this system has been associated with oliguria, progressive azotemia, and rarely, acute renal failure and/or death. In susceptible patients, concomitant diuretic use may further increase risk.

Use of trandolapril should include appropriate assessment of renal function.

Anaphylactoid Reactions During Membrane Exposure: Anaphylactoid reactions have been reported in patients dialyzed with high-flux membranes (e.g., polyacrylonitrile [PAN]) and treated concomitantly with an ACE inhibitor. Dialysis should be stopped immediately if symptoms such as nausea, abdominal cramps, burning, angioedema, shortness of breath and severe hypotension occur. Symptoms are not relieved by antihistamines. In these patients consideration should be given to using a different type of dialysis membrane or a different class of antihypertensive agents.

Ear/Nose/Throat: As with other ACE inhibitors, dry, persistent cough, which usually disappears only after withdrawal or lowering of the dose of trandolapril, has been reported. Such possibility should be considered as part of the differential diagnosis of cough.

Special Populations: Pregnant Women: ACE inhibitors can cause fetal and neonatal morbidity and mortality when administered to pregnant women. When pregnancy is detected or if the patient is planning to become pregnant, TARKA should be discontinued as soon as possible.

The use of ACE inhibitors during the second and third trimesters of pregnancy has been associated with fetal and neonatal injury including hypotension, neonatal skull hypoplasia, anuria, reversible or irreversible renal failure, and death. Oligohydramnios has also been reported, presumably resulting from decreased fetal renal function, associated with fetal limb contractures, craniofacial deformation, and hypoplastic lung development.

Prematurity, and patent ductus arteriosus and other structural cardiac malformations, as well as neurologic malformations, have also been reported following ACE inhibitor exposure in the first trimester of pregnancy.

Infants with a history of in utero exposure to ACE inhibitors should be closely observed for hypotension, oliguria, and hyperkalemia. If oliguria occurs, attention should be directed toward support of blood pressure and renal perfusion. Exchange transfusion or dialysis may be required as a means of reversing hypotension and/or substituting for impaired renal function; however, limited experience with those procedures has not been associated with significant clinical benefit.

Verapamil hydrochloride cannot be removed by hemodialysis. It is not known if trandolapril or trandolaprilat can be removed from the body by hemodialysis.

Nursing Women: The presence of concentrations of ACE inhibitor have been reported in human milk. Use of ACE inhibitors is not recommended during breast-feeding. If breast-feeding needs to be continued, alternative measures to control the patient's blood pressure need to be put in place.

TARKA is not recommended in these patients because of the potential for adverse reactions in nursing infants. The verapamil component of TARKA is secreted in human milk. Following administration of radio-labelled trandolapril to lactating rats, radioactivity has been detected in the milk.

Breast feeding should be discontinued during TARKA therapy.

Labor and Delivery: It is not known whether the use of verapamil during labour or delivery has immediate or delayed adverse effects on the fetus, or whether it prolongs the duration of labour or increases the need for forceps delivery or other obstetric intervention.

Pediatrics (<18 years of age): The safety and effectiveness of TARKA in children below the age of 18 have not been established. Therefore, use in this group is not recommended.

Geriatrics (>65 years of age): Although clinical experience has not identified differences in response between the elderly (≥65 years) and younger patients (<65 years), greater sensitivity of some older individuals to TARKA cannot be ruled out (see Action and Clinical Pharmacology, Pharmacokinetics).

Caution should be exercised when verapamil is administered to elderly patients (≥65 years) especially those prone to developing hypotension or those with a history of cerebrovascular insufficiency (see Dosage and Administration). The adverse reactions occurring more frequently include dizziness and constipation. Serious adverse events associated with heart block have occurred in the elderly.

Carcinogenesis and Mutagenesis: There was no evidence of a carcinogenic effect when verapamil hydrochloride was administered orally (diet) to male and female rats at doses up to 112.2 and 102.5 mg/kg/day, respectively, for 24 months, or when trandolapril was administered by gavage for 18 months to mice at doses up to 25 mg/kg/day and to rats at doses up to 8 mg/kg/day.

The mutagenic potential trandolapril/verapamil hydrochloride (1:60) was evaluated in four assays: the Salmonella/microsome (AMES) assay, the HPRT test on the V79 cell line, an in vitro chromosomal aberration test, and the chromosomal aberration test in the bone marrow of the Chinese hamster. The results obtained from these studies indicated that there were no gene mutations induced by the combination in any of the five salmonella typhimurium mutants or at the HPRT locus in V79 cells, and that the induction of structural chromosome aberrations and numerical aberrations by trandolapril and verapamil hydrochloride could be ruled out.

ADVERSE REACTIONS: Overview: The combination of trandolapril and verapamil SR has been evaluated in over 1957 subjects and patients. Of these, 541 patients (including 23% elderly patients) participated in North American placebo-controlled clinical trials, and 251 were studied in European placebo-controlled clinical trials. This combination has been evaluated for long-term safety in 272 patients treated for 1 year or more.

The most frequent adverse events in controlled clinical trials conducted in North America with trandolapril and verapamil SR were (n=541): first degree AV block (3.9%); cough (4.6%); constipation (3.3%) and dizziness (3.1%).

The most serious adverse reactions with TARKA (trandolapril/verapamil hydrochloride) are second degree AV block, angina, hypotension and angioedema.

Discontinuation of therapy because of adverse events in North American placebo-controlled hypertension studies was required in 2.6% and 1.9% of patients treated with (trandolapril/verapamil hydrochloride) and placebo, respectively.

Hypotension: In hypertensive patients in controlled and uncontrolled trials, hypotension occurred in 0.6% and near syncope occurred in 0.1% (possibly, probably or definitely related to combination treatment). Hypotension or syncope was a cause for discontinuation of therapy in 0.4% of hypertensive patients in North American controlled studies (see Warnings and Precautions, Hypotension).

Adverse experiences occurring more commonly with combination therapy than placebo in 1% or more of the 541 patients in North American placebo-controlled hypertension trials are shown in Table 1.

Clinical Trial Adverse Drug Reactions: Because clinical trials are conducted under very specific conditions the adverse reaction rates observed in the clinical trials may not reflect the rates observed in practice and should not be compared to the rates in the clinical trials of another drug. Adverse drug reaction information from clinical trials is useful for identifying drug-related adverse events and for approximating rates.

Most Common Drug Adverse Reactions (≥1%): Adverse experiences occurring more commonly with combination therapy than placebo in 1% or more of the 541 patients in North American placebo-controlled hypertension trials are shown in Table 1.

Table 1: TARKA

Adverse Drug Reactions in North American Placebo-Controlled Trials

	TARKA (N=541) % Incidence (% Discontinuance)	Placebo (N=206) % Incidence (% Discontinuance)
AV Block, First Degree	3.9 (0.2)	0.5 (0.0)
Bradycardia	1.8 (0.0)	0.0 (0.0)
Bronchitis	1.5 (0.0)	0.5 (0.0)
Chest Pain	2.2 (0.0)	1.0 (0.0)
Constipation	3.3 (0.0)	1.0 (0.0)
Cough	4.6 (0.0)	2.4 (0.0)
Diarrhea	1.5 (0.2)	1.0 (0.0)
Dizziness	3.1 (0.0)	1.9 (0.5)
Dyspnea	1.3 (0.4)	0.0 (0.0)
Edema	1.3 (0.0)	2.4 (0.0)
Fatigue	2.8 (0.4)	2.4 (0.0)
Increased Liver Enzymes[a]	2.8 (0.2)	1.0 (0.0)
Nausea	1.5 (0.2)	0.5 (0.0)
Pain Extremity(ies)	1.1 (0.2)	0.5 (0.0)
Pain Joint(s)	1.7 (0.0)	1.0 (0.0)

[a] Also includes increase in ALT, AST, alkaline phosphatase.

Less Common Clinical Trail Adverse Drug Reactions (≤1%): Other clinical adverse experiences possibly, probably, or definitely related to drug treatment, occurring in 0.3% or more of patients treated with (trandolapril/verapamil hydrochloride) in controlled, or uncontrolled trials (N=990) and less frequent, clinically significant events (in italics) include the following:

Cardiovascular: angina, second degree AV block, bundle branch block, edema, flushing, hypotension, myocardial infarction, palpitations, premature ventricular contractions, nonspecific ST-T changes, near syncope, tachycardia.

Central Nervous System: drowsiness, hypesthesia, insomnia, loss of balance, paresthesia, vertigo.

Dermatologic: pruritus, rash.

Emotional, Mental, Sexual States: anxiety, impotence, abnormal mentation.

Eye, Ear, Nose, Throat: epistaxis, tinnitus, upper respiratory tract infection, blurred vision.

Gastrointestinal: dyspepsia, dry mouth, nausea.

General Body Function: chest pain, malaise, weakness.

Genitourinary: endometriosis, hematuria, nocturia, polyuria, proteinuria.

Hemopoietic: decreased leukocytes, decreased neutrophils.

Metabolism and Endocrine Function: increased alkaline phosphatase, increased liver enzymes, increased potassium, increased AST.

Musculoskeletal System: arthralgia, myalgia, gout, increased uric acid.

Pulmonary: dyspnea.

Angioedema: Angioedema and/or facial edema has been reported in 3 (0.15%) patients receiving (trandolapril/verapamil hydrochloride) in North American and European studies (N=1957). Angioedema associated with laryngeal edema may be fatal. If angioedema of the face, extremities, lips, tongue, glottis, and/or larynx occurs, treatment with (trandolapril/verapamil hydrochloride) should be discontinued and appropriate therapy instituted immediately (see Warnings and Precautions, Angioedema).

In addition to those reported above, other adverse experiences have previously been reported with the individual components, verapamil hydrochloride and trandolapril:

Verapamil Component Adverse Reactions: Cardiovascular: CAF/pulmonary edema, third degree AV block, atrioventricular dissociation, claudication, syncope (see Warnings and Precautions, Hypotension).

Digestive System: nausea, gingival hyperplasia, reversible paralytic ileus.

Hemic and Lymphatic: ecchymosis or bruising.

Nervous System: cerebrovascular accident, confusion, psychotic symptoms, shakiness, somnolence.

Skin: exanthema, hair loss, hyperkeratosis, purpura (vasculitis), sweating, urticaria, Stevens-Johnson syndrome, erythema multiforme.

Urogenital: gynecomastia, galactorrhea/hyperprolactinemia, increased urination, spotty menstruation.

Trandolapril Component Adverse Reactions: Body as a Whole: asthenia, abnormal feeling, abdominal pain, pain in extremities.

Cardiovascular: hypertension, migraine, syncope.

Dermatology: urticaria, pemphigus, Stevens-Johnson Syndrome.

Gastrointestinal: gastrointestinal pain, gastrointestinal disorder, anorexia, abnormal liver function test, vomiting, pancreatitis.

Nervous System: depression, sleep disorder, decreased libido, hot flushes.

Respiratory System: bronchitis, pharyngitis.

Other: cramps, increased urinary frequency, edema, taste disorders, anaphylactoid reaction.

A symptom complex has been reported which may include fever, vasculitis, myalgia, arthralgia/arthritis, a positive ANA, elevated ESR, eosinophilia and leucocytosis. Rash, photosensitivity or other dermatologic manifestations may also occur.

Clinical Laboratory Testing Findings: Hematology: leucopenia, neutropenia, lymphopenia, thrombocytopenia (see Warnings and Precautions, Neutropenia/Agranulocytosis).

Serum Electrolytes: Hyperkalemia (see Drug Interactions, Hyperkalemia and Potassium—Sparing Diuretics), hyponatremia.

Renal Function Tests: Increases in creatinine and blood urea nitrogen levels occurred in 1.1 percent and 0.3 percent, respectively, of patients receiving (trandolapril/verapamil hydrochloride) with or without hydrochlorothiazide therapy. None of these increases required discontinuation of treatment. Increases in these laboratory values are more likely to occur in patients with renal insufficiency or those pretreated with a diuretic and, based on experience with other ACE inhibitors, would be expected to be especially likely in patients with renal artery stenosis. (See Warnings and Precautions, Use in Patients with Renal Impairment.)

Liver Function Tests: Elevations of liver enzymes (AST, ALT, LDH, and alkaline phosphatase) and/or serum bilirubin occurred. Discontinuation for elevated liver enzymes occurred in 0.9 percent of patients. (See Warnings and Precautions, Hepatic Failure/Elevated Liver Enzymes.)

DRUG INTERACTIONS: Overview: As with all drugs, care should be exercised when treating patients with multiple medications. Verapamil undergoes biotransformation by the CYP3A4, CYP1A2, CYP2C9 isoenzymes of the cytochrome P450 system. Verapamil has been shown to be an inhibitor of CYP3A4 enzymes. Coadministration of verapamil with other drugs which follow the same route of biotransformation or are inhibitors or inducers of these enzymes may result in altered bioavailability of verapamil or these drugs. Dosages of similarly metabolized drugs, particularly those of low therapeutic ratio, and especially in patients with renal and/or hepatic impairment, may require adjustment when starting or stopping concomitantly administered verapamil to maintain optimum therapeutic blood levels.

Drug-Drug Interactions: Vasodilators: Concomitant use with vasodilators may cause a potentiation of the hypotensive effect.

Interactions Due to Verapamil Hydrochloride Component: Table 2 summarizes potential drug interactions with TARKA due to the verapamil hydrochloride component.

Table 2: TARKA

Potential Drug Interactions Associated with Verapamil

Concomitant Drug Class: Drug Name	Effect on Concentration of Verapamil or Concomitant Drug	Clinical Comment
Alpha Blockers: Prazosin,	↑ prazosin C_{max} (~40%) with no effect on $t_{½}$	
Terazosin	↑ terazosin AUC (~24%) and C_{max} (~25%)	Clinically significant transient orthostatic hypotension may occur upon initiation of combined therapy.
Antiarrhythmics: Flecainide, Quinidine	Minimal effect on flecainide plasma clearance (<~10%); no effect on verapamil plasma clearance.	The concomitant administration of flecainide and verapamil may have additive effects on myocardial contractility, AV conduction, and repolarisation. May also have negative inotropic effect and prolongation of atrioventricular conduction.
	↓ oral quinidine clearance (~35%)	In a small number of patients with hypertrophic cardiomyopathy, concomitant use of verapamil and quinidine resulted in significant hypotension and may result in pulmonary edema. Until further data are obtained, combined therapy of TARKA and quinidine in patients with hypertrophic cardiomyopathy should be avoided. The electrophysiological effects of quinidine and verapamil on AV conduction were studied in 8 patients. Verapamil significantly counteracted the effects of quinidine on AV conduction. There has been a report of increased quinidine levels during verapamil therapy.
Antiasthmatics: Theophylline	↓ oral and systemic clearance of theophylline by ~20%. Reduction of clearance was lessened in smokers.	Caution should be exercised when co-administering theophylline and TARKA.
Anticonvulsants: Carbamazepine	↑ carbamazepine AUC (~46%) in refractory partial epilepsy patients	Concomitant oral use may potentiate the effects of carbamazepine neurotoxicity. Symptoms include nausea, diplopia, headache, ataxia or dizziness.
Antidepressants: Imipramine	↑ imipramine AUC (~15%). No effect on level of active metabolite desipramine	As with all antihypertensive agents, there is an elevated risk of orthostatic hypotension when combining TARKA with major tranquilizers or tricyclic antidepressants, such as imipramine.
Antidiabetics: Glibenclamide	↑ glibenclamide C_{max} (~28%), AUC (~26%)	

(cont'd)

Table 2: TARKA *(cont'd)*

Potential Drug Interactions Associated with Verapamil

Concomitant Drug Class: Drug Name	Effect on Concentration of Verapamil or Concomitant Drug	Clinical Comment
Anti-infectives: Rifampin, Erythromycin, Telithromycin	Rifampin: ↓ verapamil AUC (~97%), C_{max} (~94%) oral bioavailability (~92%) Possible ↑ in verapamil when used in combination with either erythromycin or telithromycin	Blood pressure lowering effect of verapamil may be reduced when used concomitantly with rifampin.
Antineoplastics: Doxorubicin	↑ doxorubicin AUC (89%) and C_{max} (61%) with oral verapamil administration in patients with small cell lung cancer. In patients with advanced neoplasm, intravenous verapamil did not change significantly doxorubicin PK.	Verapamil inhibits P-glycoprotein mediated transport of anti-neoplastic agents out of tumour cells, resulting in their decreased metabolic clearance. Dosage adjustments of anti-neoplastic agents should be considered when verapamil is administered concomitantly.
Barbiturates: Phenobarbital	↑ oral verapamil clearance (~5-fold)	
Benzodiazepines and Other Anxiolytics: Buspirone, Midazolam	↑ buspirone AUC, C_{max} by ~3.4-fold ↑ midazolam AUC (~3-fold) and, C_{max} (~2-fold)	
Beta Blockers: Atenolol, Metoprolol, Propranolol, Timolol	A variable increase in atenolol plasma concentration at steady state has been reported in patients with angina pectoris.	Concomitant therapy may result in additive negative effects on heart rate, atrioventricular conduction and/or cardiac contractility. (See Warnings and Precautions.)
	↑ metoprolol AUC (~32.5%) and C_{max} (~41%) in patients with angina pectoris ↑ propranolol AUC (~65%), C_{max} (~94%) in patients with angina pectoris	Asymptomatic bradycardia (<36 beats/min) with a wandering atrial pacemaker has been observed in a patient receiving concomitant timolol (a beta-adrenergic blocker) eye drops and oral verapamil.
Cardiac Glycosides: Digitoxin, Digoxin	↓ digitoxin total body CL (~27%) and extrarenal clearance (~29%) ↑ digoxin levels ~50–75% during the first week of therapy ↑ digoxin AUC (~32%), C_{max} (~98%) in hepatic cirrhosis patients Healthy subjects: ↑ digoxin C_{max} by ~45% to 53% ↑ digoxin C_{ss} by ~42% and ↑ AUC by ~52%	The increase in digoxin levels can result in digoxin toxicity. Maintenance digoxin doses should be reduced when verapamil is administered, and the patient should be carefully monitored to avoid over- or under-digitalization. Whenever overdigitalization is suspected, the daily dose of digoxin should be reduced or temporarily discontinued. Upon discontinuation of TARKA, the patient should be reassessed to avoid underdigitalization. (See Warnings and Precautions.)
H2 Receptor Antagonists: Cimetidine	In healthy subjects, ↑ AUC of R-(~25%) and S-(~40%) verapamil with corresponding ↓ in R- and S-verapamil clearance	
HIV Antiviral Agents		Due to the metabolic inhibitory potential of some of the HIV antiviral agents, such as ritonavir, plasma concentrations of verapamil may increase. Caution should be used or the dose of verapamil may be decreased.
Immunologics: Cyclosporine, Sirolimus, Tacrolimus	↑ cyclosporine AUC, C_{ss}, C_{max} by ~45% in renal transplant patients Possible ↑ sirolimus levels Possible ↑ tacrolimus levels	
Inhalation Anesthetics:		Animal experiments have shown that inhalation anesthetics depress cardiovascular activity by decreasing the inward movement of calcium ions. When used concomitantly, inhalation anesthetics and calcium antagonists, such as verapamil, should be titrated carefully to avoid excessive hemodynamic effects.
Lipid Metabolism Regulators: Atorvastatin, Lovastatin, Simvastatin	Possible ↑ atorvastatin levels Possible ↑ lovastatin levels ↑ simvastatin AUC (~4.6-fold), C_{max} (~2.6-fold) in healthy subjects	Treatment with HMG CoA reductase inhibitors (e.g., simvastatin/lovastatin) in a patient taking verapamil should be started at the lowest possible dose and titrated upwards. If verapamil treatment is to be added to patients already taking and HMG CoA reductase inhibitor (e.g., simvastatin/ lovastatin), consider a reduction in the statin dose and retitrate against serum cholesterol concentrations. There is no direct in vivo clinical evidence for an interaction between atorvastatin and verapamil, however, there is strong potential for verapamil to significantly affect atorvastatin pharmacokinetics in a similar manner to simvastatin and lovastatin. Consider using caution when atorvastatin and verapamil are concomitantly administered. Fluvastatin, pravastatin and rosuvastatin are not metabolized by CYP3A4 and are less likely to interact with verapamil.
Lithium		Increased sensitivity to the effects of lithium (neurotoxicity) has been reported during concomitant verapamil-lithium therapy with either no change or an increase in serum lithium levels. Lithium based drugs should be administered with caution, and frequent monitoring of serum lithium levels is recommended. If a diuretic is also used, the risk of lithium toxicity may be further increased.

(cont'd)

Table 2: TARKA *(cont'd)*

Potential Drug Interactions Associated with Verapamil

Concomitant Drug Class: Drug Name	Effect on Concentration of Verapamil or Concomitant Drug	Clinical Comment
Neuromuscular Blocking Agents		Clinical data and animal studies suggest that verapamil may potentiate the activity of neuromuscular blocking agents (curare-like and depolarizing). It may, therefore, be necessary to decrease the dose of verapamil and/or the dose of the neuromuscular blocking agent when the drugs are used concomitantly.
Non-steroidal Anti-inflammatory Agents: Acetylsalicylic acid		Potential adverse reactions in terms of bleeding due to synergistic antiplatelet effects of acetylsalicylic acid and verapamil should be taken into consideration in patients taking the two agents concomitantly.
Serotonin Receptor Agonists: Almotriptan	↑ almotriptan AUC (~20%) ↑ C_{max} (~24%)	
Uricosurics: Sulfinylpyrazone	↑ verapamil oral clearance (~3-fold). ↓ bioavailability (~60%)	The blood pressure lowering effect of verapamil may be reduced.

Disopyramide: Data on possible interactions between verapamil and disopyramide are not available. Therefore, disopyramide should not be administered within 48 hours before or 24 hours after TARKA administration.

Use in Patients with Attenuated (Decreased) Neuromuscular Transmission: It has been reported that verapamil decreases neuromuscular transmission in patients with Duchenne's muscular dystrophy, and that verapamil prolongs recovery from the neuromuscular blocking agent vecuronium. Accordingly, it may be necessary to decrease the dosage of verapamil when it is administered to patients with attenuated neuromuscular transmission. (See Drug interactions, Use in Surgery/Anaesthesia.)

Interactions Due to Trandolapril Component: Table 3 summarizes potential drug interactions with TARKA due to the trandolapril component.

Table 3: TARKA

Potential Drug Interactions Associated with Trandolapril and Trandolaprilat

Concomitant Drug Class: Drug Name	Effect on Concentration of Trandolapril/trandolaprilat or Concomitant Drug	Clinical Comment
Antacids	Antacids decrease the bioavailability of ACE inhibitors.	It is recommended to ingest these products separately.
Anticoagulants: Warfarin		In a multi-dose placebo-controlled pharmacodynamic study in healthy volunteers, the anticoagulant effect of warfarin was not significantly changed by trandolapril.
Beta Blockers: Propranolol	No effect on C_{max} and AUC of trandolaprilat. Trandolapril did not affect C_{max} and AUC of propranolol.	
Cardiac Glycosides: Digoxin	In one open-label study conducted in eight healthy male volunteers, in which multiple therapeutic doses of both trandolapril and digoxin were administered, no changes were found in serum levels of trandolapril, trandolaprilat and digoxin.	Pharmacodynamically, the combination had a synergistic effect on left ventricular functions, as evidenced by the improvement in systolic time-intervals.
Diuretics: Furosemide	No effect on C_{max} and AUC of trandolapril and trandolaprilat	Patients concomitantly taking antihypertensive therapy with diuretics, especially those on recently instituted diuretic therapy, may occasionally experience an excessive reduction of blood pressure after initiation of non-diuretic therapy. If it is not possible to discontinue the diuretic, the initial dose of antihypertensive therapy should be reduced and the patient observed closely for several hours following initiation of therapy (see Warnings and Precautions, Hypotension, and Dosage and Administration).
Non-steroidal Anti-inflammatory Agents		The antihypertensive effects of ACE inhibitors may be reduced with concomitant administration of non-steroidal anti-inflammatory agents. The combination of trandolapril with non-steroidal anti-inflammatory agents predisposes to a risk of hyperkalemia particularly in cases of renal failure. Blood pressure and cardiac functions monitoring should be increased when any non-steroidal anti-inflammatory agent is added or discontinued in a patient treated with trandolapril.
H2 Receptor Antagonists: Cimetidine	No effect of cimetidine on C_{max} and AUC of trandolapril and trandolaprilat	
Lithium	Increased serum lithium levels have been reported in patients receiving concurrently ACE inhibitors and lithium.	Symptoms of lithium toxicity have been reported in patients receiving concurrently ACE inhibitors and lithium.

Agents Causing Renin Release: The antihypertensive effect of trandolapril is augmented by antihypertensive agents that cause renin release (e.g. diuretics).

Agents Increasing Serum Potassium: Since trandolapril decreases aldosterone production, elevation of serum potassium may occur. Potassium sparing diuretics such as spironolactone, triamterene or amiloride, or potassium supplements should be given only for documented hypokalemia and with caution and frequent monitoring of serum potassium, since a significant increase in serum potassium could occur.

Salt substitutes which contain potassium should be used with caution.

Allopurinol, Cytostatic, Immunosuppressive Agents, Systemic Corticosteroids or Procainamide: Concomitant administration with ACE-inhibitors may lead to an increased risk of leucopenia.

Anaphylactoid Reactions During LDL Apheresis: Rarely, patients receiving ACE inhibitors during low density lipoprotein apheresis with dextran sulfate have experienced life-threatening anaphylactoid reactions. These reactions were avoided by temporarily withholding ACE inhibitor therapy prior to each apheresis.

Anaphylactoid Reactions During Desensitization: There have been isolated reports of patients experiencing sustained life threatening anaphylactoid reactions while receiving ACE inhibitors during desensitization treatment with hymenoptera (bees, wasps) venom. In the same patients, these reactions have been avoided when ACE inhibitors were temporarily withheld for at least 24 hours, but they have reappeared upon inadvertent rechallenge.

Use in Surgery/Anaesthesia: In patients undergoing major surgery or during anaesthesia with agents that produce hypotension, trandolapril will block angiotensin II formation secondary to compensatory renin release. If hypotension occurs and is considered to be due to this mechanism, it can be corrected by volume expansion (see Drug Interactions, Use in Patients with Attenuated (Decreased) Neuromuscular Transmission).

Hyperkalemia and Potassium—Sparing Diuretics: In clinical trials, hyperkalemia (serum potassium >6.00 mEq/L) occurred in approximately 0.4 % of hypertensive patients receiving trandolapril and in 0.8% of patients receiving trandolapril concurrently with verapamil SR. In most cases, elevated serum potassium levels were isolated values, which resolved despite continued therapy. None of these patients were discontinued from the trials because of hyperkalemia.

Risk factors for the development of hyperkalemia include renal insufficiency, diabetes mellitus, and the concomitant use of potassium-sparing diuretics, potassium supplements, and/or potassium-containing salt substitutes (see Drug Interactions, Agents Increasing Serum Potassium).

Drug-Food Interactions: Administration of TARKA with a high-fat meal does not alter the bioavailability of trandolapril, whereas verapamil peak concentrations and area under the curve (AUC) decrease 42% and 27%, respectively, relative to administration in the fasting state. Norverapamil values are also decreased 22% and 17%, respectively, in the fed state. Food thus decreases verapamil bioavailability, and results in a narrower peak to trough ratio.

In healthy volunteers, multiple high doses of grapefruit juice increased the AUC for S-verapamil and R-verapamil by up to 49% and 37%, respectively. The increase in C_{max} for S-verapamil and R-verapamil were up to 75% and 51%, respectively. Elimination half-life and renal clearance of both S- and R-verapamil were not affected.

Drug-Herb Interactions: In healthy volunteers, multiple doses of St John's wort decreased the AUC for R- and S- verapamil by 78% and 80%, respectively, with similar decreases in C_{max}.

Drug-Laboratory Interactions: Interactions with laboratory tests have not been evaluated.

Drug-Lifestyle Interactions: Verapamil may increase blood alcohol concentrations and prolong its effects. Alcohol enhances the bioavailability of ACE inhibitors.

Depending on individual susceptibility, the patients' ability to drive a vehicle or operate machinery may be impaired, especially in the initial stages of treatment. TARKA may increase the blood levels of alcohol and slow its elimination. The effects of alcohol may therefore be exaggerated.

DOSAGE AND ADMINISTRATION:

Dosing Considerations: Dosage must be individualized. The fixed combination is not for initial therapy. The dose of TARKA (trandolapril/verapamil hydrochloride) should be determined by titration of the individual components.

Once the patient has been successfully titrated with the individual components as described below, TARKA can be substituted if the titrated doses and dosing schedule can be achieved by the fixed combination (see Indications and Clinical Use, and Warnings and Precautions, Hypotension). TARKA is available at doses of 2/240 mg and 4/240 mg of trandolapril and verapamil SR, respectively.

For Verapamil Monotherapy: The dosage should be individualized by titration depending on patient tolerance and responsiveness to verapamil. Titration should be based on therapeutic efficacy and safety, evaluated weekly and approximately 24 hours after the previous dose.

The antihypertensive effects of verapamil SR are evident within the first week of therapy. Optimal doses are usually lower in patients also receiving diuretics since additive antihypertensive effects can be expected.

Patients with Hepatic and Renal Impairment: Verapamil SR should be administered cautiously to patients with liver or renal function impairment. The dosage should be carefully and gradually adjusted depending on patient tolerance and response. These patients should be monitored carefully for abnormal prolongation of the PR interval or other signs of overdosage. Verapamil SR should not be used in severe hepatic dysfunction (see Warnings and Precautions, Use in Patients with Hepatic Impairment).

Switching from Verapamil Tablets to Verapamil SR: When switching from verapamil tablets to verapamil SR, the total daily dose in milligrams may remain the same.

For Trandolapril Monotherapy: In some patients treated once daily, the antihypertensive effect may diminish toward the end of the dosing interval. This can be evaluated by measuring blood pressure just prior to dosing to determine whether satisfactory control is being maintained for 24 hours. If it is not, an increase in dose should be considered. If blood pressure is not controlled alone, a diuretic may be added.

Diuretic-treated Patients: Symptomatic hypotension occasionally may occur following the initial dose of trandolapril and is more likely in patients who are currently being treated with a diuretic. The diuretic should, if possible, be discontinued for two to three days before beginning therapy with trandolapril to reduce the likelihood of hypotension. If the diuretic cannot be discontinued, an initial dose of 0.5 mg trandolapril should be used with careful medical supervision for several hours and until blood pressure has stabilized. The dosage of trandolapril should subsequently be titrated to the optimal response.

Recommended Dose and Dosage Adjustment: For Verapamil Monotherapy: Adult: The usual initial adult dose is 180 to 240 mg/day. If required, the dose may be increased up to 240 mg twice a day. A maximum daily dose of 480 mg should not be exceeded.

Recommended dosing intervals for specific daily dosages are given below in Table 4.

Table 4: TARKA

Recommended Dosing Intervals for Specific Daily Dosages

Total Daily Verapamil SR Dose	Recommended Dosing Intervals
180 mg	Once each morning with food
240 mg	Once each morning with food
360 mg	180 mg each morning plus 180 mg each evening, with food; or 240 mg each morning plus 120 mg each evening, with food.
480 mg	240 mg each morning plus 240 mg each evening with food.

Elderly: Lower dosages of verapamil SR, i.e. 120 mg a day, may be warranted in elderly patients (i.e., 65 years and older). The dosage should be carefully and gradually adjusted depending on patient tolerability and response.

For Trandolapril Monotherapy: Adult: The recommended initial dosage for trandolapril is 1 mg once daily. Dosage should be adjusted according to blood pressure response at intervals of 2 to 4 weeks up to a maximum of 4 mg once daily. The usual maintenance dose is 1 to 2 mg once daily.

Elderly: In elderly patients with normal renal and hepatic function, no dosage adjustment is necessary.

However, as some elderly patients may be particularly susceptible to ACE inhibitors, administration of low initial doses and evaluation of the blood pressure response and of the renal function at the beginning of the treatment is recommended.

Dosage in Renal Impairment: For patients with a creatinine clearance below 30 mL/min/ 1.73 m², the recommended initial dose is 0.5 mg trandolapril once daily. Dosage may be titrated upward until blood pressure is controlled or to a maximum total daily dose of 1 mg.

In patients with severe renal impairment (creatinine clearance below 10 mL/min/1.73 m²) a daily dosage of 0.5 mg in a single dose should not be exceeded.

Use in Hepatic Impairment: The recommended initial dose is 0.5 mg trandolapril once daily.

Administration: TARKA tablets should not be divided, crushed or chewed. TARKA should be taken with food (see Drug Interactions, Drug-Food Interactions).

OVERDOSAGE:

During overdose with TARKA (trandolapril/verapamil hydrochloride), fatalities have occurred.

Verapamil Overdosage: Based on reports of intentional overdosage of verapamil hydrochloride, the following symptoms have been observed. Hypotension occurs, varying from transient to severe. Conduction disturbances seen included: prolongation of A-V conduction time, A-V dissociation, nodal rhythm, ventricular fibrillation and ventricular asystole.

Treatment of overdosage should be supportive. Gastric lavage should be undertaken, even later than 12 hours after ingestion, if no gastrointestinal motility is present. Beta-adrenergic stimulation or parenteral administration of calcium solutions may increase calcium ion influx across the slow channel.

These pharmacologic interventions have been effectively used in treatment of overdosage with verapamil. Clinically significant hypotensive reactions should be treated with vasopressor agents. A-V block is treated with atropine and cardiac pacing. Asystole should be handled by the usual Advanced Cardiac Life Support measures including the use of vasopressor agents, e.g. isoproterenol hydrochloride. Verapamil is not removed by hemodialysis.

In case of overdosage with large amounts of verapamil SR it should be noted that the release of the active drug and the absorption in the intestine may take more than 48 hours. Depending on the time of ingestion, incompletely dissolved tablets may be present along the entire length of the gastrointestinal tract which function as active drug depots. Extensive elimination measures are indicated, such as induced vomiting, removal of the contents of the stomach and the small intestine under endoscopy, intestinal lavage and high enemas.

Actual treatment and dosage should depend on the severity of the clinical situation and the judgment of the treating physician. Patients with hypertrophic cardiomyopathy treated with verapamil should not be administered positive inotropic agents. (Marked by letter a in Table 5.) See Table 5.

Table 5: TARKA

Overdosage Adverse Reactions and Recommended Treatments

Adverse Reaction	Proven Effective Treatment	Treatment with Good Theoretical Rationale	Supportive Treatment
Shock, cardiac failure, severe hypotension	Calcium salt e.g. calcium gluconate i.v.; i.v. metaraminol bitartrate[a]	i.v. dopamine HCl[a] i.v. dobutamine HCl[a]	i.v. fluids; Trendelenburg position
Bradycardia, A-V block, asystole	i.v. isoproterenol HCl[a]; i.v. atropine sulphate; cardiac pacing		i.v. fluids (slow drip)
Rapid ventricular rate (due to antegrade conduction in flutter/fibrillation with W-P-W or L-G-L syndrome)	D.C. cardioversion (high energy may be required); i.v. procainamide; i.v. lidocaine HCl		i.v. fluids (slow drip)

[a] Positive inotropic agent.

Trandolapril Overdosage: The most likely clinical manifestations of overdosage of trandolapril would be symptoms attributable to severe hypotension, which should normally be treated by intravenous volume expansion with normal saline. It is not known if trandolapril or trandolaprilat can be removed from the body by hemodialysis.

No data are available to suggest that physiological maneuvers (e.g. maneuvers to change pH of the urine) might accelerate elimination of trandolapril and its metabolites.

For management of a suspected drug overdose, CPhA recommends that you contact your **regional Poison Control Centre**. See the *CPS* Directory section for a list of Poison Control Centres.

ACTION AND CLINICAL PHARMACOLOGY: Mechanism of Action: TARKA (trandolapril/verapamil hydrochloride) is a formulation containing slow-release verapamil, a phenylalkylamine calcium channel blocker, along with immediate-release trandolapril, an angiotensin converting enzyme (ACE) inhibitor.

Verapamil is a calcium channel blocker that exerts its pharmacologic effects by modulating the influx of ionic calcium across the cell membrane of the arterial smooth muscle as well as in conductile and contractile myocardial cells. Verapamil exerts antihypertensive effects by decreasing systemic vascular resistance, usually without reflex tachycardia. During isometric or dynamic exercise, verapamil does not blunt hemodynamic response in patients with normal ventricular function. Verapamil does not alter total serum calcium levels.

Trandolapril is a pro-drug. Trandolaprilat, its major active metabolite, inhibits ACE in human subjects and in animals. ACE is a peptidyl dipeptidase that catalyzes the conversion of angiotensin I to the more pharmacologically active substance, angiotensin II. Angiotensin II has vasoconstrictor activity and also stimulates aldosterone secretion by the adrenal cortex.

Inhibition of ACE results in decreased plasma angiotensin II, which leads to decreased vasopressor activity. Removal of angiotensin II negative feedback on renin secretion leads to increased plasma renin activity.

ACE is identical to kininase II, an enzyme that degrades bradykinin. Whether increased levels of bradykinin, a potent vasodepressor, play a role in the therapeutic effect of TARKA remains to be elucidated.

Pharmacodynamics: Controlled clinical studies have shown that the effects of concurrent use of verapamil SR and trandolapril are additive with respect to lowering systolic and diastolic blood pressure.

The antihypertensive effect of angiotensin converting enzyme inhibitors is generally lower in black patients than in non-blacks.

Pharmacokinetics: Absorption: Following a single oral dose of TARKA in healthy subjects, peak plasma concentrations are reached within 0.5 to 2 hours for trandolapril and within 4 to 15 hours for verapamil. Peak plasma concentrations of the active desmethyl metabolite of verapamil, norverapamil, are reached within 5 to 15 hours. Trandolapril disappears very rapidly from plasma and its $t_{½}$ is less than one hour. Cleavage of the ester group by hydrolysis converts trandolapril to its active diacid metabolite, trandolaprilat, which reaches peak plasma concentrations within 2 to 12 hours.

Trandolaprilat has an effective elimination $t_{½}$ of approximately 10 hours while that of verapamil, as verapamil SR, is 6 to 11 hours. Steady-state plasma concentrations of the two components are achieved after about a week of once-daily dosing of TARKA. At steady-state, plasma concentrations of verapamil and trandolaprilat are up to twofold higher than those observed after a single oral dose of TARKA.

Verapamil SR is a racemic mixture consisting of equal portions of the R enantiomer and the S enantiomer. More than 90% of the orally administered dose of verapamil SR is absorbed. Upon oral administration, there is rapid stereo selective biotransformation during the first pass of verapamil through the portal circulation. The S enantiomer is pharmacologically more active than the R enantiomer. There is a nonlinear correlation between the verapamil dose administered and verapamil plasma levels.

Metabolism: In healthy men, orally administered verapamil undergoes extensive metabolism by the cytochrome P-450 system. The particular isoenzymes involved are CYP3A4, CYP1A2, and CYP2C family. Thirteen metabolites have been identified in urine. Norverapamil can reach steady-state plasma concentrations approximately equal to those of verapamil itself. The cardiovascular activity of norverapamil appears to be approximately 20% that of verapamil. R-verapamil is 94% bound to plasma albumin, while S-verapamil is 88% bound. In addition, R-verapamil is 92% and S-verapamil 86% bound to alpha-1 acid glycoprotein. The degree of biotransformation during the first pass of verapamil may vary according to the status of the liver in different patient populations. In patients with hepatic insufficiency, metabolism is delayed and elimination $t_{½}$ prolonged up to 14 to 16 hours (see Warnings and Precautions, Hepatic/Biliary/Pancreatic, and Dosage and Administration).

Approximately 40 to 60% of an administered oral dose of trandolapril is absorbed. Trandolapril undergoes extensive first-pass metabolism in the liver, and this is the reason that its bioavailability is low: 7.5% (ranging from 4% to 14%). Minor metabolic pathways lead to the formation of diketopiperazine derivatives of trandolapril and trandolaprilat. These molecules have no ACE inhibitory activity. Glucuronide conjugated derivatives of trandolapril and trandolaprilat are also produced.

Distribution: Verapamil crosses the placental barrier and can be detected in umbilical vein blood at delivery. Verapamil is excreted in human milk.

Excretion: Approximately 70% of an administered dose of verapamil is excreted as metabolites in the urine and 16% or more in the feces within 5 days. About 3% to 4% is excreted in the urine as unchanged drug.

Special Populations and Conditions: Geriatrics: The pharmacokinetics of verapamil and trandolaprilat are significantly different in the elderly (≥65 years), compared to younger subjects. AUCs are increased approximately 80% with verapamil and 35% with trandolaprilat. In the elderly, verapamil clearance is reduced resulting in increases in elimination $t_{½}$ (see Warnings and Precautions, Geriatrics (>65 years of age)).

Hepatic Insufficiency: In patients with hepatic insufficiency, verapamil clearance is reduced by 30% and the elimination $t_{½}$ is prolonged up to 14 to 16 hours (see Warnings and Precautions, Use in Patients with Hepatic Impairment, and Dosage and Administration).

In patients with moderate to severe impairment of liver function, plasma trandolapril levels were approximately ten times higher than in healthy subjects. The plasma concentrations of trandolaprilat and the quantities excreted in the urine were also increased, although to a lesser degree. The dose should therefore be reduced in these patients.

In one study, cirrhotic patients who received a single dose of trandolapril 2 mg exhibited a 9-fold increase in trandolapril C_{max} and AUC values. The C_{max} and AUC values of trandolaprilat were about doubled.

Renal Insufficiency: The results of an intravenous pharmacokinetic study suggest that renal clearance of verapamil may be decreased in patients with renal disease (see Dosage and Administration).

In patients with creatinine clearance ≤30 mL/min/1.73 m², the C_{max} and AUC of trandolaprilat were approximately doubled after repeated oral administration of trandolapril, as compared to those of normal subjects.

STORAGE AND STABILITY: Store at 15 to 25°C. Protect from light and moisture. Do not use beyond the expiry date indicated on the label.

INFORMATION FOR THE PATIENT Published in e-CPS, available by subscription at www.e-cps.ca.

DOSAGE FORMS, COMPOSITION AND PACKAGING: 2/240 mg: Each gold, oval, film-coated tablet, embossed with an arched triangle mark and "242", contains: trandolapril 2 mg in an immediate-release form and verapamil hydrochloride 240 mg in a sustained-release form. Nonmedicinal ingredients: cornstarch, dioctyl sodium sulfosuccinate, hydroxypropyl cellulose, hydroxypropyl methylcellulose, lactose, magnesium stearate, microcrystalline cellulose, polyethylene glycol, povidone, purified water, silicon dioxide, sodium alginate, sodium stearyl fumarate, synthetic iron oxides, talc and titanium dioxide. Bottles of 100. 10 strips by 10 tablets of PVC/aluminum blisters.

4/240 mg: Each reddish-brown, oval, film-coated tablet, embossed with an arched triangle mark and "244", contains: trandolapril 4 mg in an immediate-release form and verapamil hydrochloride 240 mg in a sustained-release form. Nonmedicinal ingredients: cornstarch, dioctyl sodium sulfosuccinate, hydroxypropyl cellulose, hydroxypropyl methylcellulose, lactose, magnesium stearate, microcrystalline cellulose, polyethylene glycol, povidone, purified water, silicon dioxide, sodium alginate, sodium stearyl fumarate, synthetic iron oxides, talc and titanium dioxide. Bottles of 100. 10 strips by 10 tablets of PVC/aluminum blisters.

The reader is invited to consult CPhA's monograph **Corticosteroids: Topical**.

Taro-Amcinonide Pr

amcinonide

Topical Corticosteroid

Taro

SUPPLIED: Each tube of cream contains: 1 mg/g amcinonide in a base of benzyl alcohol (as preservative), emulsifying wax, glycerin, isopropyl palmitate, lactic acid, purified water, and sorbitol solution 70%. Laminated tubes of 15, 30 and 60 g. Store at controlled room temperature 15-30°C. Avoid freezing.

Taro-Carbamazepine Pr

carbamazepine

Anticonvulsant—Symptomatic Relief of Trigeminal Neuralgia—Antimanic

Taro

SUPPLIED: 100 mg: Each white with pink speckles, round, flat chewable tablet, scored on one side, engraved "TARO" above the score and "16" under the score, contains: carbamazepine 100 mg. Nonmedicinal ingredients: croscarmellose sodium, diethyl phthalate, Eudragit RS 30D, FD&C Red No. 40 Lake, magnesium stearate, microcrystalline cellulose, natural cherry flavor, pregelatinized starch and sorbitol. Gluten- and tartrazine-free. Bottles of 100. Store at room temperature (15 to 30°C). Protect from light and humidity.

200 mg: Each white, with pink speckles, oval, flat chewable tablet, both sides scored, one side engraved "T" above the score and "27" under the score, contains: carbamazepine 200 mg. Nonmedicinal ingredients: croscarmellose sodium, diethyl phthalate, Eudragit RS 30D, FD&C Red No. 40 Lake, magnesium stearate, microcrystalline cellulose, natural cherry flavor, pregelatinized starch and sorbitol. Gluten- and tartrazine-free. Bottles of 100. Store at room temperature (15 to 30°C). Protect from light and humidity.

Taro-Clindamycin Pr

clindamycin phosphate

Antibiotic

Taro

SUPPLIED: Each mL of topical solution contains: clindamycin phosphate equivalent to clindamycin 10 mg (1%). Nonmedicinal ingredients: isopropyl alcohol 50% v/v, propylene glycol, purified water and, if necessary, sodium hydroxide to adjust pH. Bottles of 30 and 60 mL. A dab-o-matic applicator and cap is provided external to each bottle for placement into the bottle. To assist the patient, the pharmacist may assemble the bottle upon dispensing as follows: remove cap from bottle and discard, firmly press applicator into bottle, seal firmly by tightening domed-cap. Store at controlled room temperature (15-30°C).

The reader is invited to consult CPhA's monograph **Corticosteroids: Topical**.

Taro-Clobetasol Pr

clobetasol 17-propionate

Topical Corticosteroid

Taro

SUPPLIED: Cream: Each g contains: clobetasol 17-propionate 0.5 mg (0.05%). Nonmedicinal ingredients: cetyl alcohol, chlorocresol, citric acid, glyceryl monostearate, glyceryl stearate/PEG 100 stearate, propylene glycol, purified water, sodium citrate, stearyl alcohol and white wax. Tubes of 15 and 50 g. Jars of 454 g.

Ointment: Each g contains: clobetasol 17-propionate 0.5 mg (0.05%). Nonmedicinal ingredients: propylene glycol, sorbitan sesquioleate and white petrolatum. Tubes of 15 and 50 g.

Topical Solution: Each mL contains: clobetasol 17-propionate 0.5 mg (0.05%). Nonmedicinal ingredients: carbomer 934-P, isopropyl alcohol, purified water, sodium hydroxide for pH adjustment. Bottles of 60 mL.

Store at room temperature (15 to 30°C).

The reader is invited to consult CPhA's monograph **Corticosteroids: Topical**.

Taro-Mometasone Pr

mometasone furoate

Topical Corticosteroid

Taro

SUPPLIED: Lotion (Topical Solution) : Each g contains: mometasone furoate 1 mg (0.1%). Nonmedicinal ingredients: hydroxypropylcellulose, isopropyl alcohol, phosphoric acid, propylene glycol, purified water and sodium phosphate monobasic. Bottles of 30 and 75 mL. Store at room temperature (15-30°C).

Ointment : Each g contains: mometasone furoate 1 mg (0.1%). Nonmedicinal ingredients: hexylene glycol, propylene glycol stearate, white petrolatum and white wax. Tubes of 15 and 50 g. Store at room temperature between 15 and 30°C.

Taro-Mupirocin

mupirocin

Topical Antibiotic

Taro

SUPPLIED: Each g of ointment contains: mupirocin 20 mg (2%) in a bland water-soluble ointment base consisting of polyethylene glycol 400 and polyethylene glycol 3350. Tubes of 15 and 30 g. Store at 15-25°C.

Taro-Phenytoin Pr

phenytoin

Anticonvulsant

Taro

SUPPLIED: Each 5 mL of orange-vanilla flavoured, orange colored suspension contains: phenytoin (free acid form) 125 mg. Nonmedicinal ingredients: carboxymethylcellulose sodium, citric acid anhydrous, FD&C Yellow No. 6, magnesium aluminum silicate, orange flavour spray dry natural and artificial, polysorbate 60, sodium benzoate, sucrose and vanilla flavour powder, artificial. PET bottles of 237 mL. Store at controlled room temperature (15-30°C). Protect from freezing.

Taro-Sone Pr

betamethasone dipropionate

Topical Corticosteroid

Taro

SUPPLIED: Each g of cream contains: betamethasone dipropionate USP, 0.64 mg equivalent to 0.5 mg of betamethasone, USP (0.05%) in a water miscible base of white petrolatum, mineral oil, cetostearyl alcohol, cetomagrogol 1000, purified water, sodium phosphate monobasic, chlorocresol and propylene glycol with sodium hydroxide and phosphoric acid for pH correction. Tubes of 50 g. Store at room temperature (15-30°C).

Taro-Terconazole Pr

terconazole

Antifungal

Taro

SUPPLIED: Each g of white to off-white, water washable vaginal cream contains: terconazole 0.4%. Nonmedicinal ingredients: butylated hydroxyanisole, cetyl alcohol, isopropyl myristate, polysorbate 60, polysorbate 80, propylene glycol, purified water and stearyl alcohol. Tubes of 45 g with a vaginal applicator. Store at room temperature (15-30°C).

Taro-Warfarin Pr

warfarin sodium

Anticoagulant

Taro

SUPPLIED: 1 mg: Each pink, single scored tablet with WARFARIN/1 on one side and TARO on the other, contains: warfarin sodium 1 mg. Nonmedicinal ingredients: D&C Red No. 6 Lake, lactose anhydrous, magnesium stearate and pregelatinized cornstarch. Bottles of 100, 250 and 1000. Unit dose packages of 100 (for institutional use only).

2 mg: Each lavender, single scored tablet with WARFARIN/2 on one side and TARO on the other, contains: warfarin sodium 2 mg. Nonmedicinal ingredients: FD&C Blue No. 2 Lake, FD&C Red No. 40 Lake, lactose anhydrous, magnesium stearate and pregelatinized cornstarch. Bottles of 100, 250 and 1000. Unit dose packages of 100 (for institutional use only).

2.5 mg : Each green, single scored tablet with WARFARIN/2½ on one side and TARO on the other, contains warfarin sodium 2.5 mg. Nonmedicinal ingredients: D&C Yellow No. 10 Lake, FD&C Blue No. 2 Lake, lactose anhydrous, magnesium stearate and pregelatinized cornstarch. Bottles of 100, 250 and 1000. Unit dose packages of 100 (for institutional use only).

3 mg: Each tan, single scored tablet with WARFARIN/3 on one side and TARO on the other, contains warfarin sodium 3 mg. Nonmedicinal ingredients: D&C Yellow No. 10 Lake, FD&C Blue No. 2 Lake, FD&C Red No. 40 Lake, lactose anhydrous, magnesium stearate and pregelatinized cornstarch. Bottles of 100. Unit dose packages of 100 (for institutional use only).

4 mg: Each blue, single scored tablet with WARFARIN/4 on one side and TARO on the other, contains: warfarin sodium 4 mg. Nonmedicinal ingredients: FD&C Blue No. 1 Lake, lactose anhydrous, magnesium stearate and pregelatinized cornstarch. Bottles of 100 and 250. Unit dose packages of 100 (for institutional use only).

5 mg: Each peach, single scored tablet with WARFARIN/5 on one side and TARO on the other, contains: warfarin sodium 5 mg. Nonmedicinal ingredients: D&C Red No. 6 Lake, D&C Yellow No. 10 Lake, lactose anhydrous, magnesium stearate and pregelatinized cornstarch. Bottles of 100, 250 and 1000. Unit dose packages of 100 (for institutional use only).

6 mg: Each teal, single scored tablet with WARFARIN/6 on one side and TARO on the other, contains: warfarin sodium 6 mg. Nonmedicinal ingredients: D&C Yellow No. 10 Lake, FD&C Blue No. 2 Lake, lactose anhydrous, magnesium stearate and pregelatinized cornstarch. Bottles of 100.

7.5 mg: Each yellow, single scored tablet with WARFARIN/7½ on one side and TARO on the other, contains: warfarin sodium 7.5 mg. Nonmedicinal ingredients: D&C Yellow No. 10 Lake, lactose anhydrous, magnesium stearate and pregelatinized cornstarch. Bottles of 100.

10 mg: Each white, single scored tablet with WARFARIN 10 on one side and TARO on the other, contains: warfarin sodium 10 mg. Nonmedicinal ingredients: lactose anhydrous, magnesium stearate and pregelatinized cornstarch. Dye-free. Bottles of 100. Unit dose packages of 100 (for institutional use only).

Protect from light. Store at controlled room temperature (15 to 30°C). Dispense in a tight, light-resistant container as defined in the USP.

Tasigna® ℞

nilotinib HCl monohydrate

Protein-tyrosine Kinase Inhibitor

Novartis Pharmaceuticals

Date of Preparation: December 4, 2006
Date of Revision: July 20, 2010

TASIGNA (nilotinib capsules), indicated for, the treatment of chronic phase and accelerated phase Philadelphia chromosome positive chronic myeloid leukemia (CML) in adult patients resistant to or intolerant of at least one prior therapy including imatinib, has been issued marketing authorization with conditions, pending the results of studies to verify its clinical benefit. Patients should be advised of the conditional nature of the authorization.

Conditional approval of TASIGNA in CML-AP is based on the interim analysis of the confirmed hematologic and the unconfirmed major cytogenetic response rates. In CML-CP, it is based on the interim analysis of the unconfirmed major cytogenetic and hematologic response rates. Overall survival benefit has not been demonstrated.

TASIGNA should only be prescribed by a qualified healthcare professional who is experienced in the use of antineoplastic therapy and in the treatment of chronic myeloid leukemia.

SUMMARY PRODUCT INFORMATION:

Route of Administration	Dosage Form/ Strength	Clinically Relevant Nonmedicinal Ingredients
Oral	Capsule 200 mg	Capsule content: Lactose monohydrate For a complete listing see Dosage Forms, Composition and Packaging.

INDICATIONS AND CLINICAL USE:

- TASIGNA (nilotinib capsules) is indicated for the treatment of chronic phase and accelerated phase Philadelphia chromosome positive chronic myeloid leukemia (CML) in adult patients resistant to or intolerant of at least one prior therapy including imatinib.

Conditional approval of TASIGNA in CML-AP is based on the interim analysis of the confirmed hematologic and the unconfirmed major cytogenetic response rates. In CML-CP, it is based on the interim analysis of the unconfirmed major cytogenetic and hematologic response rates.

Overall survival benefit has not been demonstrated.

Geriatrics: Approximately 30% of subjects in clinical studies were 65 or over. No major differences were observed for safety and efficacy in patients ≥65 years of age as compared to adults 18 to 65 years of age.

Pediatrics: Clinical studies have not been conducted in children and adolescents.

CONTRAINDICATIONS: Do not use in patients with a known long QTc prolongation or with a persistent QTc of >480 msec (see Warnings and Precautions). Do not use in patients with uncorrectable hypokalemia or hypomagnesemia.

Do not use in patients with known hypersensitivity to nilotinib or to any of the excipients (for a complete listing, see Dosage Forms, Composition and Packaging).

WARNINGS AND PRECAUTIONS:

Serious Warnings and Precautions

- Sudden Cardiac Deaths (see Warnings and Precautions and Adverse Reactions)
- QT interval prolongation (see Warnings and Precautions, Drug Interactions, Drug-Food Interactions and Warnings and Precautions, Monitoring and Laboratory Tests)
- Should not be used in patients with uncorrectable hypokalemia or hypomagnesemia (see Warnings and Precautions)
- Hepatotoxicity/Hepatic failure (in some cases, fatal) (see Warnings and Precautions)
- Pancreatitis (see Warnings and Precautions)
- Myelosuppression (thrombocytopenia, neutropenia and anemia) (see Warnings and Precautions)

TASIGNA should only be prescribed by a qualified healthcare professional who is experienced in the use of antineoplastic therapy and in the treatment of chronic myeloid leukemia.

Sudden Cardiac Deaths: Fourteen cases of sudden cardiac deaths have been reported out of 5300 patients receiving TASIGNA (uncommon frequency of 0.26%). Of the 14, 12 documented cases had a past medical history of cardiac disease or significant cardiac risk factors for sudden cardiac death. In 2 of the 14 cases of sudden cardiac death, patients had no prior medical history of cardiac disease. Comorbidities in addition to the underlying malignancy were also frequently present as were concomitant medications. Ventricular repolarization abnormalities may have been contributory factors.

QT Prolongation: In vitro data indicate that nilotinib has the potential to prolong cardiac ventricular repolarization (QT interval). In the Phase II study in imatinib-resistant and intolerant CML patients in chronic and accelerated phase, the change from baseline in mean time-averaged QTcF interval at steady state was 6 and 8 msec, respectively. QTcF of >500 msec was observed in 3 (<1%) of these patients. QTcF >60 msec change from baseline was observed in 9 (2.1%) of patients.

In a healthy volunteer study, peak plasma concentrations were 26% lower than in the clinical study. The maximum mean placebo-adjusted QTcF increase from baseline was 18 msec (1-sided 95% Upper CI:26 msec). No clinically relevant arrhythmias were observed during the conduct of the trial. In particular, no episodes of Torsade de Pointes (transient or sustained) were observed.

Significant prolongation of the QT interval may occur when TASIGNA is inappropriately taken with food, and/or strong CYP3A4 inhibitors and/or medicinal products with a known potential to prolong QT. Therefore, co-administration with food must be avoided and concomitant use with strong CYP3A4 inhibitors and/or medicinal products with a known potential to prolong QT should be avoided (see Drug Interactions, Drug-Drug Interactions and Drug-Food Interactions). The presence of hypokalemia and hypomagnesemia may further enhance this effect (see Dosage and Administration).

TASIGNA should be avoided in patients who are at significant risk of developing prolongation of QTc interval, such as: patients taking anti-arrhythmic medicines or other drugs that may lead to QT prolongation, and cumulative high-dose anthracycline therapy. Hypokalemia or hypomagnesemia must be corrected prior to TASIGNA administration (see Drug Interactions, Drug-Drug Interactions and Dosage and Administration).

TASIGNA should be used with caution in patients with uncontrolled or significant cardiac disease including recent myocardial infarction, congestive heart failure, unstable angina or clinically significant bradycardia.

Cardiovascular: In clinical studies, patients with any of the following uncontrolled or significant cardiac disease were excluded (recent myocardial infarction, congestive heart failure (CHF), unstable angina, complete left bundle branch block and/or right bundle branch block plus left anterior hemiblock, bifascicular block, or clinically significant bradycardia). ECG and cardiac enzyme monitoring were conducted in some patients throughout the study. Left ventricular ejection fraction (LVEF) was assessed by echocardiography or MUGA scan at baseline (within 14 days prior to the initial dose of nilotinib in 49/438 patients in the core safety population). LVEF assessment was repeated in these patients as clinically indicated thereafter, and at the time of study completion. There was no clinically significant change in LVEF from baseline in the assessed patients.

The following cardiovascular adverse reactions have been observed in patients in the TASIGNA clinical studies at a frequency of less than 5% including congestive heart failure observed in <1% of patients in the core safety population (see Adverse Reactions).

Common: palpitations, electrocardiogram QT prolonged. Uncommon: myocardial infarction, cardiac failure, angina pectoris, atrial fibrillation, pericardial effusion, coronary artery disease, cardiomegaly, cardiac murmur, bradycardia. Unknown frequency: myocarditis, ventricular dysfunction, pericarditis, cardiac flutter, extrasystoles (see Adverse Reactions).

Hemorrhage: Gastrointestinal and CNS hemorrhage were reported in 1% and <1% of patients, respectively (see Adverse Reactions).

Hematologic: Myelosuppression: Treatment with TASIGNA is often associated with thrombocytopenia, neutropenia and anemia (NCI CTC Grade 3/4). Occurrence is more frequent in patients with Accelerated Phase CML (AP). Complete blood counts should be performed every two weeks for the first 2 months and then monthly thereafter, or as clinically indicated. Myelosuppression was generally reversible and usually managed by withholding TASIGNA temporarily or reducing the dose (see Dosage and Administration).

Hepatic/Biliary/Pancreatic: Hepatotoxicity/Hyperbilirubinemia: TASIGNA may result in elevation of bilirubin due to competitive inhibition of Uridine-Diphosphate-Glucuronyl Transferase (UGT1A1) and in elevation of AST, ALT and alkaline phosphatase (see Drug Interactions, Drug-Drug Interactions and Adverse Reactions). Patients taking TASIGNA who may be predisposed to or who may have Gilbert's syndrome may have a higher risk of unconjugated hyperbilirubinemia. This may also occur in patients who are taking drugs known to inhibit UGT1A1.

Hepatic Failure: Eight cases of hepatic failure were reported. Four of these were fatal including one case with no previous hepatic impairment. There were 17 cases of ascites and 3 cases of hepatic steatosis. Two cases of hepatic necrosis were reported in clinical trial patients (see Dosage and Administration).

Elevated Serum Lipase/Amylase: Grade 3/4 elevation in serum lipase and amylase have been observed. Few of these elevations were associated with abdominal pain or pancreatitis. There were 6 cases (1.36%) of pancreatitis reported in the core safety population (N=438). Caution is recommended in patients with previous history of pancreatitis (see Dosage and Administration).

Endocrine and Metabolism: New-onset diabetes (uncommon frequency) and 11% incidence of Grade 3/4 hyperglycemia has been reported (see Adverse Reactions).

Fluid Retention: Fluid retention including pericardial effusion (uncommon frequency), pleural effusion (uncommon frequency) and peripheral oedema (common frequency) have been reported (see Adverse Reactions).

Immune: Four cases of vasculitis (including 1 cerebral) have been reported (see Adverse Reactions).

Musculoskeletal: Five cases of rhabdomyolysis, some with concomitant elevations in serum creatinine, creatine kinase and hepatic transaminases, have been reported (see Adverse Reactions).

Sexual Function/Reproduction: Fertility: No effects on sperm count/motility, and on fertility were noted in male and female rats up to the highest tested dose of approximately 5-folder greater than the recommended dosage for humans.

Women of Childbearing Potential: Women of childbearing potential must be advised to use effective contraception during treatment with TASIGNA.

Carcinogenesis and Mutagenesis: Carcinogenicity studies have not been performed. TASIGNA is not mutagenic.

Special Populations: Renal Impairment: Clinical studies have not been performed in patients with impaired renal function. Clinical studies have excluded patients with serum creatinine concentration >1.5 times the upper limit of the normal range.

TASIGNA and its metabolites are not renally excreted (see Action and Clinical Pharmacology, Pharmacokinetics).

Hepatic Impairment: Hepatic impairment has an effect on the pharmacokinetics of TASIGNA. Single dose administration of TASIGNA 200 mg resulted in increases in AUC of 35%, 35% and 56% in subjects with mild, moderate and severe hepatic impairment, respectively, compared to a control group of subjects with normal hepatic function. The steady-state C_{max} of TASIGNA will likely to be increased by up to approximately 29% in subjects with hepatic impairment. Clinical studies have excluded patients with ALT and/or AST >2.5 (or >5, if related to disease) times the upper limit of the normal range and/ or total bilirubin >1.5 times the upper limit of the normal range. Metabolism of nilotinib is mainly hepatic. TASIGNA should be used with caution and careful clinical monitoring (including close monitoring of the QTc interval) in patients with hepatic impairment (see Dosage and Administration).

Gilbert's Syndrome: Due to a polymorphism in the enzyme UGT1A1 in patients who may be predisposed to Gilbert's syndrome, or in patients with Gilbert's syndrome, a higher risk unconjugated hyperbilirubinemia with nilotinib can occur, but is clinically benign and potentially persistent. No specific medical intervention is warranted (see Dosage and Administration).

Peri-Operative Considerations: Total Gastrectomy: The bioavailability of nilotinib was shown to be reduced in patients administered 400 mg bid TASIGNA with total gastrectomy versus non-gastrectomized patients (see Action and Clinical Pharmacology, Pharmacokinetics).

Sensitivity/Intolerance: Since the capsules contain lactose, TASIGNA is not recommended for patients with rare hereditary problems of galactose intolerance, severe lactase deficiency or of glucose-galactose malabsorption.

Pregnant Women: There are no data adequate on the use of TASIGNA in pregnant women. Studies in animals showed no teratogenicity, but embryo- and foetotoxicity was seen at doses which also showed maternal toxicity. TASIGNA should not be used during pregnancy unless necessary. If the drug is used during pregnancy, the patient must be informed of the potential risk to the foetus. One case of fatal congenital transposition of great vessels in a neonate whose mother was being treated with TASIGNA (see Adverse Reactions).

Nursing Women: It is not known whether nilotinib is excreted in human milk. Studies in animals demonstrate that it is excreted into breast milk. Women should not breast-feed while taking TASIGNA, as a risk to the infant cannot be excluded.

Pediatrics: Clinical studies have not been conducted in children and adolescents.

Geriatrics: Approximately 30% of subjects in clinical studies were 65 or over. No major differences were observed for safety and efficacy in patients ≥65 years of age as compared to adults 18 to 65 years of age.

Monitoring and Laboratory Tests: Complete blood counts should be performed every two weeks for the first 2 months and then monthly thereafter or as clinically indicated (see Warnings and Precautions). ECGs should be obtained before treatment, seven days after initiation and periodically thereafter, as well as following dose adjustments (see Warnings and Precautions and Dosage and Administration).

Liver function, (transaminases, total bilirubin and alkaline phosphatase) needs to be monitored before treatment, frequently during treatment, following dose adjustments or as clinically indicated (see Warnings and Precautions and Dosage and Administration).

Serum electrolytes as well as serum lipase/amylase, fasting glucose, creatine kinase (CPK) and creatinine levels need to be monitored before treatment and frequently during treatment with TASIGNA and as clinically indicated (see Warnings and Precautions and Dosage and Administration).

Patients should be weighed and monitored regularly for signs and symptoms of fluid retention (see Warnings and Precautions).

ADVERSE REACTIONS: Adverse Drug Reaction Overview: Sudden Cardiac Deaths: From all clinical trials, fourteen cases of sudden cardiac deaths have been reported out of 5300 patients receiving TASIGNA (uncommon frequency of 0.26%). Of the 14, 12 documented cases had a past medical history of cardiac disease or significant cardiac risk factors for sudden cardiac death. In 2 of the 14 cases of sudden cardiac death, patients had no prior medical history of cardiac disease. Comorbidities in addition to the underlying malignancy were also frequently present as were concomitant medications. Ventricular repolarization abnormalities may have been contributory factors.

Clinical Trial Adverse Drug Reactions: The data described below reflect exposure to TASIGNA in 438 patients (318 patients and 120 patients with Chronic Phase CML and Accelerated Phase CML respectively) in an open-label multicenter study. At cut-off, 46% of patients in CML-CP had durations of exposure of 6 to 12 months and 18% of patients had durations of exposure more than 12 months; 62% of patients in CML-AP had durations of exposure of 3 to 12 months and 10% of patients had durations of exposure more than 12 months. The patient population consisted of 51% males, 90% Caucasian, 8% black or Asian and 30% over the age of 65. The dose was 400 mg twice-daily. The median duration of exposure in days for these CML-CP and CML-AP patients were 245 (1-502 days) and 138 (2-503 days), respectively.

The most frequent non-hematologic drug-related adverse events were rash, pruritus, nausea, fatigue, headache, constipation and diarrhea. Most of these adverse events were mild to moderate in severity. Bone pain, arthralgia, muscle spasms, and peripheral oedema were observed less commonly and have been of mild to moderate severity. Discontinuation for adverse events regardless of causality was observed in 16 % of CP and 14 % of AP patients.

Treatment-emergent hematologic toxicities included thrombocytopenia (27%), neutropenia (15%), and anemia (13%). Pleural and pericardial effusions as well as complications of fluid retention occurred in <1% of patients receiving TASIGNA.

Congestive heart failure was observed in <1% of patients. QTcF exceeding 500 msec was observed in 3 (<1%) of these patients. No episodes of Torsade de Pointes (transient or sustained) were observed.

Gastrointestinal and CNS hemorrhage was reported in 1% and <1% of patients, respectively.

Non-hematologic adverse reactions (excluding laboratory abnormalities) that are reported in at least 5% of the patients in TASIGNA clinical studies are shown in Table 1. These are ranked under heading of frequency, the most frequent first, using the following convention: very common (≥1/10) or common (≥1/100, ≤1/10).

Less Common Clinical Trial Adverse Drug Reactions: Additional Data from Clinical Trials: The following adverse reactions were reported in patients in the TASIGNA clinical studies at a frequency of less than 5% (common is ≥1/100 and <1/10; uncommon is >1/1000 and <1/100; single events are captured as unknown in frequency). For laboratory abnormalities, very common events (≥1/10) not included in Table 1 are also reported. These adverse reactions are included based on clinical relevance and ranked in order of decreasing seriousness within each category.

Cardiac Disorders: Common: palpitations, electrocardiogram QT prolonged. Uncommon: myocardial infarction, cardiac failure, angina pectoris, atrial fibrillation, pericardial effusion, coronary artery disease, cardiomegaly, cardiac murmur, bradycardia. Unknown frequency: myocarditis, ventricular dysfunction, pericarditis, cardiac flutter, extrasystoles, congenital transposition of great vessels in neonate (fatal).

Table 1: TASIGNA
Adverse Reactions Reported in (≥5% of all Patients in Clinical Studies, N=438)

System Organ Class	Frequency	Adverse Reaction	Total N=438 All grades %	Total N=438 Grade 3/4 %	Chronic Phase N=318 Grade 3/4 %	Accelerated Phase N=120 Grade 3/4 %
Metabolism and Nutrition Disorders	Common	Anorexia	5	0	0	0
Nervous System Disorders	Very common	Headache	15	1	2	<1
Gastrointestinal Disorders	Very common	Nausea	19	<1	<1	<1
	Very common	Constipation	11	0	0	0
	Very common	Diarrhea	10	2	2	<1
	Common	Vomiting	9	<1	<1	0
	Common	Abdominal pain	5	<1	<1	<1
Skin and Subcutaneous Tissue Disorders	Very common	Rash	26	1	<1	0
	Very common	Pruritus	22	<1	<1	0
	Common	Alopecia	7	0	0	0
Musculoskeletal and Connective Tissue Disorders	Common	Myalgia	8	<1	<1	<1
	Common	Arthralgia	6	<1	<1	0
	Common	Muscle spasms	6	0	0	0
	Common	Bone pain	6	<1	<1	0
General Disorders and Administration Site Conditions	Very common	Fatigue	16	<1	<1	<1
	Common	Asthenia	6	0	0	0
	Common	Edema peripheral	5	0	0	0

Infections and Infestations: Uncommon: pneumonia, urinary tract infection, gastroenteritis, pharyngitis. Unknown frequency: sepsis, bronchitis, herpes simplex, candidiasis.
Blood and Lymphatic System Disorders: Common: febrile neutropenia, pancytopenia. Unknown frequency: thrombocythemia, leukocytosis.
Endocrine Disorders: Uncommon: hyperthyroidism. Unknown frequency: hypothyroidism, thyroiditis.
Metabolism and Nutrition Disorders: Common: hypomagnesemia, hyperkalemia, hyperglycemia. Uncommon: hypokalemia, hyponatremia, hypocalcemia, hypophosphatemia, dehydration, decreased appetite, increased appetite, new-onset diabetes. Unknown frequency: hypercalcemia, hyperphosphatemia.
Psychiatric Disorders: Common: insomnia. Uncommon: depression, anxiety. Unknown frequency: disorientation, confusional state.
Nervous System Disorders: Common: dizziness, paresthesia. Uncommon: intracranial hemorrhage, migraine, tremor, hypoaesthesia, hyperaesthesia. Unknown frequency: brain oedema, loss of consciousness, optic neuritis, peripheral neuropathy.
Eye Disorders: Uncommon: eye hemorrhage, visual acuity reduced, periorbital oedema, conjunctivitis, eye irritation, dry eye. Unknown frequency: papilloedema, diplopia, vision blurred, photophobia, eye swelling, blepharitis, eye pain.
Ear and Labyrinth Disorders: Common: vertigo. Unknown frequency: hearing impaired, ear pain.
Immune: Unknown frequency: vasculitis (cerebral, leukocytoclastic).
Vascular Disorders: Common: hypertension, flushing. Uncommon: hypertensive crisis, hematoma. Unknown frequency: shock hemorrhagic, hypotension, thrombosis.
Respiratory, Thoracic and Mediastinal Disorders: Common: dyspnea, dyspnea exertional, cough, dysphonia. Uncommon: pulmonary oedema, pleural effusion, interstitial lung disease, pleuritic pain, pleurisy, epistaxis, pharyngolaryngeal pain, throat irritation. Unknown frequency: pulmonary hypertension.
Gastrointestinal Disorders: Common: abdominal discomfort, dyspepsia, flatulence. Uncommon: pancreatitis, gastrointestinal hemorrhage, melaena, abdominal distension, mouth ulceration, gastroesophageal reflux, stomatitis, dry mouth. Unknown frequency: gastrointestinal ulcer perforation, retroperitoneal hemorrhage, hematemesis, gastric ulcer, esophagitis ulcerative, subileus.
Hepatobiliary Disorders: Uncommon: hepatic failure, hepatotoxicity, hepatitis, ascites. Unknown frequency: hepatic necrosis, hepatic steatosis, hepatomegaly, jaundice.
Skin and Subcutaneous Tissue Disorders: Common: night sweats, eczema, urticaria, erythema, hyperhidrosis, dry skin. Uncommon: exfoliative rash, ecchymosis, swelling face. Unknown frequency: erythema nodosum, skin ulcer, petechiae, photosensitivity.
Musculoskeletal and Connective Tissue Disorders: Common: musculoskeletal chest pain, musculoskeletal pain. Uncommon: muscular weakness. Unknown frequency: rhabdomyolysis, arthritis, joint swelling.
Renal and Urinary Disorders: Uncommon: dysuria, micturition urgency, nocturia, pollakiuria, acute renal failure. Unknown frequency: renal failure, hematuria, urinary incontinence.
Reproductive System and Breast Disorder: Uncommon: breast pain, gynecomastia, erectile dysfunction.
General Disorders and Administration Site Conditions: Common: pyrexia. Uncommon: chest pain, face edema, gravitational edema, influenza-like illness, chills, malaise.
Investigations: Very common: lipase increased. Common: blood total bilirubin increased, blood amylase increased, alanine aminotransferase increased, aspartate aminotransferase increased, blood alkaline phosphatase increased, gamma-glutamyltransferase increased, blood creatine phosphokinase increased, blood glucose increased, weight decreased, weight increased. Uncommon: blood lactate dehydrogenase increased, blood glucose decreased, blood creatinine increased, blood urea increased. Unknown frequency: troponin increased, blood potassium decreased, blood bilirubin unconjugated increased.
Abnormal Hematologic and Clinical Chemistry Findings: Clinically relevant or severe abnormalities of routine hematologic or biochemistry laboratory values are presented in Table 2.
Abnormal Electrocardiographic (ECG) Findings: QTcF exceeding 500 msec was observed in 3 (<1%) of these patients. QTcF >60 msec change from baseline was observed in 9 (2.1%) of patients. No episodes of Torsade de Pointes (transient or sustained) were observed (see Warnings and Precautions and Adverse Reactions).
Post-Market Adverse Drug Reactions: The following additional adverse reactions have been identified during post approval use of TASIGNA. Because these reactions are reported voluntarily from a population of uncertain size, it is not always possible to reliably estimate their frequency or establish a causal relationship to drug exposure.
Cardiovascular: anaphylaxis, cardiac tamponade.
Digestive: induced and therapeutic abortions due to fetal malformation (omphalocele).
Respiratory: bronchospasm.
Endocrine and Metabolism: diabetes mellitus exacerbation.

Table 2: TASIGNA
Adverse Reactions Grade 3/4 Lab Abnormalities

	CML-CP N=318 % Grade 3/4	CML-AP N=120 % Grade 3/4
Hematologic Parameters		
Myelosuppression		
Neutropenia	28	37
Thrombocytopenia	28	37
Anemia	8	23
Biochemistry Parameters		
Elevated creatinine	<1	0
Elevated lipase	15	17
Elevated AST	1	<1
Elevated ALT	4	2
Hypophosphatemia	10	10
Elevated bilirubin (total)	9	10
Hyperglycemia	11	4
Hyperkalemia	4	3
Hyponatremia	3	3
Hypokalemia	1	5
Hypocalcemia	1	4
Decreased albumin	1	1
Elevated alkaline phosphatase	1	3

Table 3: TASIGNA
Number (%) of Patients with Notable Values in QTcF Intervals-Studies 2101E2 and 2101E1

ECG Parameter	CML-CP (2101E2) N=318 n (%)	CML-AP (2101E1) N=120 n (%)	Total N=438 n (%)
Increase from baseline >30 msec	105 (33.0)	49 (40.8)	154 (35.2)
Increase from baseline >60 msec	6 (1.9)	3 (2.5)	9 (2.1)
Absolute value >450 msec	38 (11.9)	14 (11.7)	52 (11.9)
Absolute value >480 msec	5 (1.6)	0	5 (1.1)
Absolute value >500 msec	3 (0.9)	0	3 (0.7)

Legend: n=number of patients who meet the criterion for at least one post-baseline value.

DRUG INTERACTIONS:

Serious Drug Interactions and Drug-Food Interactions
- CYP3A4 inhibitors should be avoided as they can increase nilotinib serum concentrations.
- Concomitant use of drugs that prolong QT interval should be avoided.
- Co-administration with drugs with a narrow therapeutic index and that are eliminated by certain enzymes.
- TASIGNA absorption is increased if taken with food. TASIGNA must not be taken with food and should be taken 2 hours after a meal. No food should be consumed at least 1 hour after the drug is taken.

Overview: Drug-Drug Interactions: Drugs That May Increase Nilotinib Serum Concentrations: The administration of TASIGNA with agents that are strong CYP3A4 inhibitors should be avoided. Should treatment with any of these agents be required, it is recommended that therapy with TASIGNA be interrupted if possible. If transient interruption of treatment with TASIGNA is not possible, close monitoring of the individual for prolongation of the QT interval is indicated (see Dosage and Administration and Action and Clinical Pharmacology).

Nilotinib is mainly metabolized in the liver, and is also a substrate for the multi-drug efflux pump, P-glycoprotein (P-gp). Therefore, absorption and subsequent elimination of systemically absorbed nilotinib may be influenced by drugs that affect CYP3A4 and/or P-gp.

In a Phase I study of nilotinib given in combination with imatinib (a substrate and moderator of P-gP and CYP3A4), both drugs had individually an inhibitory effect on CYP3A4 and/or P-gP When the two drugs were administered concomitantly, the AUC of imatinib was increased by 18% to 39%, and the AUC of nilotinib was increased by 18% to 40%.

The bioavailability of nilotinib in healthy subjects was increased by 3-fold when co-administered with the strong CYP3A4 inhibitor **ketoconazole**. Concurrent treatment with strong CYP3A4 inhibitors should therefore be avoided (including but not limited to **ketoconazole, itraconazole, voriconazole, ritonavir, clarithromycin, and telithromycin**). For additional drugs, also refer to http://www.intermed-rx.ca (see Dosage and Administration and Warnings and Precautions regarding QT prolongation). Alternative concomitant medications with no or minimal CYP3A4 inhibition should be considered.
Drugs That May Decrease Nilotinib Serum Concentrations: Inducers of CYP3A4 activity could increase the metabolism of nilotinib and thereby decrease plasma concentrations of nilotinib. The concomitant administration of medications that induce CYP3A4 (e.g. **phenytoin, rifampin carbamazepine, phenobarbital, and St. John's Wort**) may reduce exposure to nilotinib to a

clinically relevant extent. In patients for whom CYP3A4 inducers are indicated, concomitant use of alternative therapeutic agents with less potential for CYP3A4 enzyme induction potential should be considered. In healthy subjects receiving the CYP3A4 inducer, **rifampicin**, at 600 mg daily for 12 days, systemic exposure (AUC) to TASIGNA was decreased approximately 80%. For additional drugs, also refer to http://www.intermed-rx.ca.

Nilotinib has pH-dependent solubility, with lower solubility at higher pH. In 22 healthy subjects receiving multiple doses of esomeprazole at 40 mg once daily for 5 days, gastric pH was markedly increased. Co-administration of a single 400 mg dose of nilotinib and 40 mg esomeprazole was associated with a modest decrease in nilotinib absorption (27% decrease in nilotinib C_{max} and 34% decrease in nilotinib $AUC_{0-\infty}$). TASIGNA may be used concurrently with esomeprazole or other proton pump inhibitors as needed.

Drugs That May Have Their Systemic Concentration Altered by Nilotinib: Nilotinib is identified as a competitive inhibitor of CYP3A4, CYP2C8, CYP2C9, and CYP2D6 and UGT1A1 in vitro, with Ki value being lowest for CYP2C9 (Ki=0.13 μM) (Substrates of UGT1A1: including but not limited to **buprenorphine, phenytoin**). A single-dose drug-drug interaction study with 25 mg warfarin, a sensitive CYP2C9 substrate, and 800 mg nilotinib was conducted in 24 healthy subjects. Nilotinib at clinically relevant concentrations was not found to alter the pharmacokinetics or pharmacodynamics of warfarin, a sensitive CYP2C9 substrate. TASIGNA can be used concurrently with warfarin without increasing the anticoagulant effect. Due to lack of steady-state data, control of warfarin pharmacodynamic markers (INR or PT) following initiation of nilotinib therapy (at least during the first 2 weeks) is recommended. In addition, single-dose administration of TASIGNA (600 mg) with midazolam (4 mg) to 18 healthy subjects increased **midazolam** exposure by 30%, however the metabolic ratio of 1-hydroxy-midazolam to midazolam was not altered. For additional drugs, also refer to http://www.intermed-rx.ca).

Nilotinib is a P-gP inhibitor in vitro. Therefore, concentration of drugs which are substrates of P-gP (including but not limited to **verapamil, digoxin, morphine, phenytoin, cefazolin, cyclosporine A, ondansetron**) may be increased. Alternative concomitant medications which are not P-gp substrates should be considered.

Anti-Arrhythmic Medicines and Other Drugs That May Prolong QT: Concomitant use of TASIGNA with **anti-arrhythmic medicines** (including, but not limited to **amiodarone, disopyramide, procainamide, quinidine and sotalol**) and other drugs that may prolong the QT interval (including, but not limited to **chloroquine, halofantrine, clarithromycin, and other macrolides, haloperidol, methadone, moxifloxacin, bepridil and pimozide**) should be avoided (see Warnings and Precautions).

Concomitant use of **anti-emetic medicines** (including but not limited to **metoclopramide, prochlorperazine, ondansetron and dolasetron**) should be avoided.

The concomitant use of TASIGNA with another QT/QTc-prolonging drug is discouraged. Drugs that have been associated with QT/QTc interval prolongation and/or torsade de pointes include, but are not limited to, the examples in the following list. Chemical/pharmacological classes are listed if some, although not necessarily all, class members have been implicated in QT/QTc prolongation and/or torsade de pointes:

- Class IA antiarrhythmics (e.g., quinidine, procainamide, disopyramide);
- Class III antiarrhythmics (e.g., amiodarone, sotalol, ibutilide);
- Class 1C antiarrhythmics (e.g., flecainide, propafenone);
- antipsychotics (e.g., chlorpromazine, pimozide, haloperidol, droperidol, ziprasidone);
- antidepressants (e.g., fluoxetine, citalopram, venlafaxine, tricyclic/tetracyclic antidepressants e.g., amitriptyline, imipramine, maprotiline);
- opioids (e.g., methadone);
- macrolide antibiotics and analogues (e.g., erythromycin, clarithromycin, telithromycin, tacrolimus);
- quinolone antibiotics (e.g., moxifloxacin, levofloxacin, ciprofloxacin);
- pentamidine;
- antimalarials (e.g., quinine, chloroquine);
- azole antifungals (e.g., ketoconazole, fluconazole, voriconazole);
- domperidone;
- 5-hydroxytryptamine (5-HT)3 receptor antagonists (e.g., dolasetron, ondansetron);
- tyrosine kinase inhibitors (e.g., sunitinib, lapatinib);
- histone deacetylase inhibitors (e.g., vorinostat);
- beta-2 adrenoceptor agonists (e.g., salmeterol, formoterol).

Drug-Food Interactions: Other Interactions That May Affect Serum Concentrations: Food Effect: The bioavailability of nilotinib is increased by food. TASIGNA must not be taken in conjunction with food (see Dosage and Administration; Warnings and Precautions and Action and Clinical Pharmacology) and should be taken 2 hours after a meal. No food should be consumed for at least one hour after the dose is taken. Products and juices containing grapefruit, star fruit, pomegranate, Seville oranges and other similar fruits that are known to inhibit CYP3A4 should be avoided at any time.

The absorption of TASIGNA is increased if it is taken with food, resulting in higher serum concentration (see Dosage and Administration; Warnings and Precautions and Action and Clinical Pharmacology).

Drug-Herb Interactions: St. John's Wort is a potent CYP3A4 inducer. Co-administration with TASIGNA may lead to increased TASIGNA metabolism, therefore decreased TASIGNA serum concentrations (see Drug Interactions, Drug-Drug Interactions).

Drug-Laboratory Test Interactions: Interactions with laboratory tests have not been established.

Drug-Lifestyle Interactions: Effects on Ability to Drive and Use Machines: No studies on the effects of nilotinib on the ability to drive and operate machines have been performed. Patients experiencing dizziness, visual impairment or other undesirable effects with a potential impact on the ability to safely drive or use machines should refrain from these activities as long as these undesirable effects persist (see Adverse Reactions).

DOSAGE AND ADMINISTRATION:

Dosing Considerations: Patients with Renal Impairment: Clinical studies have not been performed in patients with impaired renal function. Clinical studies have excluded patients with serum creatinine concentration >1.5 times the upper limit of the normal range.

TASIGNA and its metabolites are not renally excreted (see Action and Clinical Pharmacology, Pharmacokinetics).

Patients with Hepatic Impairment: Hepatic impairment has an effect on the pharmacokinetics of nilotinib. Dose adjustment is not considered necessary in hepatically impaired subjects, but patients with hepatic impairment should be treated with caution and careful clinical monitoring, including close monitoring of the QTc interval (see Warnings and Precautions).

Cardiac Disorders: In clinical studies, patients with any of the following uncontrolled or significant cardiac disease were excluded (recent myocardial infarction, congestive heart failure (CHF), unstable angina, complete left bundle branch block and/or right bundle branch block plus left anterior hemiblock, bifascicular block, or clinically significant bradycardia). Caution should be exercised in patients with relevant cardiac disorders (see Warnings and Precautions).

Recommended Dose and Dosage Adjustment: Therapy with TASIGNA (nilotinib capsules) should be initiated by a physician experienced in the treatment of patients with CML.

The recommended dose of TASIGNA is 400 mg twice daily (see Action and Clinical Pharmacology). Treatment should continue as long as the patient does not show evidence of progression or unacceptable toxicity.

TASIGNA should be taken twice daily, at approximately 12 hour intervals and must not be taken with food. The capsules should be swallowed whole with water. No food should be consumed for at least 2 hours before the dose is taken and no additional food should be consumed for at least one hour after the dose is taken (see Warnings and Precautions; Drug Interactions and Action and Clinical Pharmacology).

In the clinical study, TASIGNA was allowed to be given in combination with hematopoietic growth factors such as erythropoietin or G-CSF if clinically indicated. TASIGNA was also allowed to be given with hydroxyurea (permitted during the first 28 days of treatment, up to 5 g/day for a maximum of 7 days) or anagrelide (permitted during the first 28 days of treatment) if clinically indicated.

A baseline ECG is recommended prior to initiating therapy with TASIGNA and should be repeated after 7 days and as clinically indicated. Hypokalemia or hypomagnesemia must be corrected prior to TASIGNA administration and potassium and magnesium blood levels should be monitored periodically during therapy, particularly in patients at risk for these electrolyte abnormalities (see Warnings and Precautions).

Dose Adjustments or Modifications: TASIGNA may need to be temporarily withheld and/or dose reduced for hematological toxicities (neutropenia, thrombocytopenia) that are not related to underlying leukemia (see Table 4).

QT Interval Prolongation: See Table 5.

See Table 6 for dose adjustments for elevations of lipase, amylase, bilirubin, and/or hepatic transaminases (see Adverse Reactions).

If clinically significant moderate or severe non-hematologic toxicity develops, dosing should be interrupted, and may be resumed at 400 mg once daily once the toxicity has resolved. If clinically appropriate, re-escalation of the dose to 400 mg twice daily should be considered.

Serum lipase elevations were observed. Few of these elevations were associated with clinical symptoms such as abdominal pain or a diagnosis of pancreatitis. There were 6 cases (1.36%) of pancreatitis reported in the core safety population (N=438).

Missed Dose: If a dose is missed, the patient should not take an additional dose, but take the next scheduled usual prescribed dose.

Table 4: TASIGNA

Dose Adjustments for Neutropenia and Thrombocytopenia

Chronic Phase CML or Accelerated Phase CML at 400 mg b.i.d.	(ANC)[a] <1.0×10⁹/L and/or platelet counts <50×10⁹/L	1. Stop TASIGNA, and monitor blood counts. 2. Resume within 2 weeks at prior dose if ANC >1.0×10⁹/L and/or platelets >50×10⁹/L. 3. If blood counts remain low a dose reduction to 400 mg once daily may be required.

[a] ANC=absolute neutrophil count.

Table 5: TASIGNA

Dose Adjustments for QT Prolongation

ECGs with a QTc >480 msec	1. Withhold TASIGNA, and perform an analysis of serum potassium and magnesium, and if below lower limit of normal, correct with supplements to within normal limits. Concomitant medication usage must be reviewed. 2. Resume within 2 weeks at prior dose if QTcF returns to <450 msec and to within 20 msec of baseline. 3. If QTcF is between 450 msec and 480 msec after 2 weeks reduce the dose to 400 mg once daily. 4. If, following dose-reduction to 400 mg once daily, QTcF returns to >480 msec, TASIGNA should be discontinued. 5. An ECG should be repeated approximately 7 days after any dose adjustment.

Table 6: TASIGNA

Dose Adjustments for Selected Non-Hematologic Laboratory Abnormalities

Elevated serum lipase or amylase ≥ Grade 3	1. Withhold TASIGNA, and monitor serum lipase or amylase. 2. Resume treatment at 400 mg once daily if serum lipase or amylase return to ≤ Grade 1.[a]
Elevated Total bilirubin ≥ Grade 3	1. Withhold TASIGNA, and monitor total bilirubin. 2. Resume treatment at 400 mg once daily if total bilirubin return to ≤ Grade 1.[b] 3. Total bilirubin levels should be tested monthly or as clinically indicated.
Elevated hepatic transaminases ≥ Grade 3	1. Withhold TASIGNA, and monitor hepatic transaminases. 2. Resume treatment at 400 mg once daily if bilirubin return to ≤ Grade 1. 3. Hepatic transaminases levels should be tested monthly or as clinically indicated.

[a] Serum lipase levels should be tested frequently or as clinically indicated.
[b] Total bilirubin and hepatic transaminases levels should be tested frequently or as clinically indicated.

OVERDOSAGE:

Isolated reports of intentional overdose with nilotinib were reported, where an unspecified number of TASIGNA capsules were ingested in combination with alcohol and other drugs. Events included neutropenia, vomiting and drowsiness. No ECG changes or hepatotoxicity were reported. Outcomes were reported as recovered. One case of accidental overdose in a patient who took a second dose of TASIGNA 400mg shortly after having ingested a first dose of 400 mg. Approximately 8 hours after ingestion, the patient reported feeling weak, abdominal pain, tachycardia and epistaxis.

In the event of overdose, the patient should be observed and appropriate supportive treatment given.

For management of a suspected drug overdose, contact your regional Poison Control Centre. See the *CPS Directory* section for a list of Poison Control Centres.

ACTION AND CLINICAL PHARMACOLOGY: Mechanism of Action: Pharmacotherapeutic group: Antineoplastic agents—Protein-tyrosine kinase inhibitor ATC code: under assessment.

TASIGNA is a potent inhibitor of the Abl tyrosine kinase activity of the Bcr-Abl oncoprotein both in cell lines and in primary Philadelphia-chromosome positive leukemia cells. The drug binds strongly within the ATP-binding site in such a manner that it is a potent inhibitor of wild-type Bcr-Abl and maintains activity against 32/33 imatinib-resistant mutant forms of Bcr-Abl with the T315I mutant being the exception. As a consequence of this biochemical activity, nilotinib selectively inhibits the proliferation and induces apoptosis in cell lines and in primary Philadelphia-chromosome positive leukemia cells from CML patients. In murine models of CML, as a single agent nilotinib reduces tumour burden and prolongs survival following oral administration.

TASIGNA has also little or no effect against the majority of other protein kinases examined, except for PDGFRα, PDGFRβ, KIT, CSF-1R, DDR-1 and DDR-2 and Ephrin receptor kinases which it inhibits at concentrations within the range achieved following oral administration at therapeutic doses recommended for the treatment of CML (see Table 7).

Table 7: TASIGNA

Kinase Profile of Nilotinib (Phosphorylation IC_{50} nM)

Bcr-Abl	PDGFR	KIT
20	69	210

Pharmacodynamics: A dose response in the Phase IA component of Study 2101 was explored using the following initial dose cohorts based on daily exposure to nilotinib. The twice daily doses were associated with higher exposures as compared to the once daily doses (see Table 8).

Pharmacokinetics: See Table 9.

Absorption: Peak concentrations of nilotinib are reached 3 hours after oral administration. Nilotinib absorption following oral administration was approximately 30%. In healthy volunteers, C_{max} and area under the serum concentration-time curve (AUC) of nilotinib are increased by 112% and 82%, respectively compared to fasting conditions when TASIGNA is given with food. Administration of TASIGNA 30 minutes or 2 hours after food increased bioavailability of nilotinib by 29% or 15%, respectively (see Dosage and Administration and Drug Interactions). Nilotinib absorption (relative bioavailability) was reduced by approximately 48% and 22% in patients with total gastrectomy and partial gastrectomy, respectively. Mean steady state trough concentration of nilotinib in patients with total gastrectomy was 599 ng/mL vs. 1035 ng/mL in patients without prior GI resection.

Distribution: Blood-to-plasma ratio of nilotinib is 0.68. Plasma protein binding is approximately 98% on the basis of in vitro experiments.

Metabolism: Main metabolic pathways identified in healthy subjects are oxidation and hydroxylation. Nilotinib is the main circulating component in the serum. None of the metabolites contribute significantly to the pharmacological activity of nilotinib.

Excretion: After a single dose of radiolabelled nilotinib in healthy subjects, greater than 90% of the dose was eliminated within 7 days mainly in feces. Parent drug accounted for 69% of the dose.

Linearity/Non-Linearity: Steady-state nilotinib exposure was dose-dependent with less than dose-proportional increases in systemic exposure at dose levels higher than 400 mg given as once daily dosing. Daily serum exposure to nilotinib of 400 mg twice-daily dosing at steady state was 35% higher than with 800 mg once-daily dosing. There was no relevant increase in exposure to nilotinib when the dose was increased from 400 mg twice-daily to 600 mg twice-daily.

Characteristics in Patients: Steady-state conditions were essentially achieved by day 8. An increase in serum exposure to nilotinib between the first dose and steady state was approximately 2-fold for daily dosing and 3.8-fold for twice-daily dosing. The apparent elimination half-life estimated from the multiple dose PK with daily dosing was approximately 17 hours. Inter-patient variability in nilotinib PK was moderate to high.

Table 8: TASIGNA

Dose and Corresponding Exposure in all Patients or CML-AP Patients

Group	Nilotinib			Steady-state (day 15) $AUC_{0\text{-}24h}$ (ng·h/mL)	
	Initial Dose (mg)	Regimen	Exposure	All Patients[a]	CML-AP Patients[b]
1	50–200	o.d.	Low	6880 (4750)	6610 (2350–14 600)
2	400–1200	o.d.	Middle	26 000 (13 800)	24 900 (5770–65 900)
3	400	b.i.d.	High	36 000 (11 800)	35 200 (14 600–61 000)
4	600	b.i.d.	High	32 800 (13 800)	28 900 (16 000–61 500)

[a] Mean (SD) of dose group.
[b] Median (range) of dose group.

Table 9: TASIGNA

Summary of Nilotinib's Pharmacokinetic Parameters in Serum Plasma After a Single 400 mg Oral Dose in Healthy Male Volunteers (n=4)[a]

T_{max}	C_{max}	$t_{½}$ (h)	$AUC_{0-\infty}$	Clearance (CL/F)	Volume of Distribution (Vz/F)
3.5 hours	599 ng/mL	17 hours	20 700 ng·h/mL	29.1 L/hour	579 L

[a] Values are median for tmax and mean for all others.

Special Populations and Conditions: Effect of Age or Gender on PK: Age, body weight, or ethnic origin do not affect the pharmacokinetics of nilotinib, whereas there is an effect of gender, with exposure to nilotinib in female patients being approximately 20% greater than in male patients.

Pharmacogenomics: TASIGNA can lead to elevated bilirubin levels. A pharmacogenetic analysis of 101 patients was conducted to evaluate the polymorphisms of UGT1A1 and its potential association with hyperbilirubinemia during TASIGNA treatment. In this study, the (TA)7/(TA)7 genotype was associated with a statistically significant increase in the risk of hyperbilirubinemia relative to the (TA)6/(TA)6 and (TA)6/(TA)7 genotypes. The largest increases in bilirubin were observed in patients with the (TA)7/(TA)7 genotype. Caution is recommended in patients with (TA)7/(TA)7 genotype (see Warnings and Precautions and Dosage and Administration).

Patients with Hepatic Impairment: Hepatic impairment has an effect on the pharmacokinetics of TASIGNA. Single dose administration of TASIGNA 200 mg resulted in increases in AUC of 35%, 35% and 56% in subjects with mild, moderate and severe hepatic impairment respectively, compared to a control group of subjects with normal hepatic function. The steady-state C_{max} of TASIGNA will likely to be increased by up to approximately 29% in subjects with hepatic impairment (see Dosage and Administration).

STORAGE AND STABILITY: Store at room temperature (15-30°C).

Store in the original package.

TASIGNA must be kept out of reach and sight of children.

SPECIAL HANDLING INSTRUCTIONS: No special requirements.

INFORMATION FOR THE PATIENT: Published in e-CPS, available by subscription at www.e-cps.ca.

DOSAGE FORMS, COMPOSITION AND PACKAGING: Each light yellow opaque hard gelatin capsule, size 0, with red axial imprint "NVR/TKI", contains: nilotinib base 200 mg (as hydrochloride, monohydrate) as a white to slightly yellowish powder. Nonmedicinal ingredients: capsule: colloidal silicon anhydrous, crospovidone, lactose monohydrate, magnesium stearate and poloxamer 188; shell: gelatin, iron oxide yellow and titanium dioxide; printing ink: includes red iron oxide. Blister packs (2 strips of 14 blisters/card, 4 cards/carton).

(Shown in Product Identification Section)

Taxol™ Ⓟ

paclitaxel

Antineoplastic

Bristol-Myers Squibb

Date of Preparation: December 24, 1992
Date of Revision: February 22, 2010

TAXOL (paclitaxel) should be administered under the supervision of a physician experienced in the use of cancer chemotherapeutic agents.

Patients receiving TAXOL should be pretreated with corticosteroids, antihistamines, and H_2 antagonists (such as dexamethasone, diphenhydramine and cimetidine or ranitidine) to minimize hypersensitivity reactions (see Dosage). Severe hypersensitivity reactions characterized by dyspnea and hypotension requiring treatment, angioedema, and generalized urticaria have occurred in patients receiving TAXOL. These reactions are probably histamine mediated. Rare fatal reactions have occurred in patients despite pretreatment. Patients who experience severe hypersensitivity reactions to paclitaxel should not be rechallenged with the drug.

PHARMACOLOGY: TAXOL (paclitaxel) is a novel antimicrotubule agent that promotes the assembly of microtubules from tubulin dimers and stabilizes microtubules by preventing depolymerization.

In vitro, TAXOL exhibits cytotoxic activity against a wide variety of both human and rodent tumor cell lines including leukemia, non-small cell lung carcinoma, small cell lung carcinoma, colon carcinoma, CNS carcinoma, melanoma, renal carcinoma, ovarian carcinoma and breast carcinoma.

Pharmacokinetics: The pharmacokinetics of paclitaxel have been evaluated over a wide range of doses, up to 300 mg/m², and infusion schedules ranging from 3 to 24 hours. Following i.v. administration of TAXOL, the drug exhibited a biphasic decline in plasma concentrations. The initial rapid decline represents distribution to the peripheral compartment and elimination of the drug. The later phase is due, in part, to a relatively slow efflux of paclitaxel from the peripheral compartment. In patients treated with doses of 135 and 175 mg/m² given as 3 and 24 hour infusions, mean terminal half-life has ranged from 3.0 to 52.7 hours, and total body clearance has ranged from 11.6 to 24.0 L/h/m². Mean steady-state volume of distribution has ranged from 198 to 688 L/m², indicating extensive extravascular distribution and/or tissue binding.

Following 3 hour infusions of 175 mg/m², mean terminal half-life was estimated to be 9.9 hours; mean total body clearance was 12.4 L/h/m².

Variability in systemic paclitaxel exposure, as measured by $AUC_{0\rightarrow\infty}$ for successive treatment courses was minimal; there was no evidence of accumulation of paclitaxel with multiple treatment courses.

The pharmacokinetics of paclitaxel have been shown to be nonlinear. There is a disproportionately large increase in C_{max} and AUC with increasing dose, accompanied by an apparent dose-related decrease in total body clearance. These findings are most readily observed in patients in whom high plasma concentrations of paclitaxel are achieved. Saturable processes in distribution and elimination/metabolism may account for these findings.

In vitro studies of binding to human serum proteins, using paclitaxel concentrations ranging from 0.1 to 50 µg/mL, indicated that on average 89% of drug is bound; the presence of cimetidine, ranitidine, dexamethasone, or diphenhydramine did not affect protein binding of paclitaxel.

In vitro studies with human liver microsomes and tissue slices showed that paclitaxel was metabolized primarily to 6α-hydroxypaclitaxel by the cytochrome P450 isozyme CYP2C8; and to 2 minor metabolites, 3-p-hydroxypaclitaxel and 6α, 3'-p-dihydroxypaclitaxel by CYP3A4. In vitro, the metabolism of paclitaxel to 6α-hydroxypaclitaxel was inhibited by a number of agents (see Precautions, Drug Interactions). The effect of renal or hepatic dysfunction on the disposition of paclitaxel has not been investigated.

The disposition of paclitaxel has not been fully elucidated in humans. After i.v. administration of TAXOL, mean values for cumulative urinary recovery of unchanged drug ranged from 1.3 to 12.7% of the dose, indicating extensive nonrenal clearance. In 5 patients administered a 225 or 250 mg/m² dose of radiolabeled TAXOL as a 3-hour infusion, 14% of the radioactivity was recovered in the urine and 71% was excreted in the feces in 120 hours. Total recovery of radioactivity ranged from 56% to 101% of the dose. Paclitaxel represented a mean of 5% of the administered radioactivity recovered in the feces while metabolites, primarily 6α-hydroxypaclitaxel, accounted for the balance.

INDICATIONS: TAXOL (paclitaxel) is indicated, alone or in combination, for the treatment of carcinoma of the ovary, breast, lung or AIDS-related Kaposi's Sarcoma.

Ovarian Carcinoma: First-line treatment in combination with other chemotherapeutic agents. Second-line treatment of metastatic carcinoma of the ovary after failure of standard therapy.

Breast Carcinoma: Adjuvant treatment of node-positive breast cancer administered sequentially to standard combination therapy. In the clinical trial, there was an overall favorable effect on disease-free and overall survival in the total population of patients with receptor-positive and receptor-negative tumors, but the benefit has been specifically demonstrated by available data (median follow-up 30 months) only in the patients with estrogen and progesterone receptor-negative tumors. Second-line treatment of metastatic carcinoma of the breast after failure of standard therapy.

Lung Carcinoma: First-line treatment of advanced non-small cell lung cancer.

Kaposi's Sarcoma: Treatment of advanced, liposomal anthracycline-refractory AIDS-related Kaposi's Sarcoma.

CONTRAINDICATIONS: TAXOL (paclitaxel) is contraindicated in patients who have a history of severe hypersensitivity reactions to paclitaxel or other drugs formulated in Cremophor EL (polyethoxylated castor oil).

TAXOL should not be used in patients with severe baseline neutropenia (<1500 cells/mm³) nor in patients with AIDS-related Kaposi's Sarcoma with baseline or subsequent neutrophil counts of <1000 cells/mm³.

WARNINGS: TAXOL (paclitaxel) should be administered under the supervision of a physician experienced in the use of cancer chemotherapeutic agents.

TAXOL should be administered as a diluted infusion. Patients receiving TAXOL should be pretreated with corticosteroids, antihistamines, and H_2 antagonists (such as dexamethasone, diphenhydramine and cimetidine or ranitidine) to minimize hypersensitivity reactions (see Dosage). Anaphylaxis and severe hypersensitivity reactions characterized by dyspnea and hypotension requiring treatment, angioedema, or generalized urticaria have occurred in approximately 2% of patients receiving TAXOL. These reactions are probably histamine-mediated. Rare fatal reactions have occurred in patients despite pretreatment. In case of a severe hypersensitivity reaction, TAXOL infusion should be discontinued immediately and the patient should not be rechallenged with the drug (see Adverse Effects).

TAXOL should not be administered to patients with baseline neutrophil counts of less than 1500 cells/mm³ (<1000 cells/mm³ for patients with Kaposi's Sarcoma). Bone marrow suppression (primarily neutropenia) is dose and schedule dependent and is the dose-limiting toxicity within a regimen. Neutrophil nadirs occurred at a median of 11 days. Frequent monitoring of blood counts should be instituted during TAXOL treatment. Patients should not be retreated with subsequent cycles of TAXOL until neutrophils recover to a level >1500 cells/mm³ (>1000 cells/mm³ for patients with Kaposi's Sarcoma) and platelets recover to a level >100 000 cells/mm³ (see Dosage).

Severe cardiac conduction abnormalities have been reported in <1% of patients during TAXOL therapy. If patients develop significant conduction abnormalities during administration, appropriate therapy should be administered and continuous electrocardiographic monitoring should be performed during subsequent therapy with TAXOL (see Adverse Effects).

Pregnancy: TAXOL may cause fetal harm when administered to a pregnant woman. TAXOL has been shown to be embryotoxic and fetotoxic in rabbits and to decrease fertility in rats. There are no studies in pregnant women. Women of childbearing potential should be advised to avoid becoming pregnant during therapy with TAXOL. If TAXOL is used during pregnancy, or if the patient becomes pregnant while receiving this drug, the patient should be apprised of the potential hazard.

Lactation: It is not known whether TAXOL is excreted in human milk. Breast-feeding should be discontinued for the duration of TAXOL therapy.

Children: The safety and effectiveness of TAXOL in pediatric patients have not been established. There have been reports of CNS toxicity (rarely associated with death) in a clinical trial in pediatric patients in which TAXOL was infused i.v. over 3 hours at doses ranging from 350 to 420 mg/m². The toxicity is most likely attributable to the high dose of the ethanol component of the TAXOL vehicle given over a short infusion time. The use of concomitant antihistamines may intensify this effect. Although a direct effect of the paclitaxel itself cannot be discounted, the high doses used in this study (over twice the recommended adult dosage) must be considered in assessing the safety of TAXOL for use in this population.

PRECAUTIONS: Contact of the undiluted concentrate with plasticized polyvinyl chloride (PVC) equipment or devices used to prepare solutions for infusion is not recommended. In order to minimize patient exposure to the plasticizer DEHP [di-(2-ethylhexyl)phthalate], which may be leached from PVC infusion bags or sets, diluted paclitaxel solutions should preferably be stored in bottles (glass, polypropylene) or plastic bags (polypropylene, polyolefin) and administered through polyethylene-lined administration sets.

Drug Interactions: Cisplatin: In a Phase 1 trial in which TAXOL was administered as a 24-hour infusion and cisplatin was administered as a 1 mg/min infusion, myelosuppression was more profound when TAXOL was given after cisplatin than with the alternate sequence (i.e., TAXOL before cisplatin). When TAXOL is given before cisplatin, the safety profile of TAXOL is consistent with that reported for single-agent use. Pharmacokinetic data from these patients demonstrated a decrease in paclitaxel clearance of approximately 33% when TAXOL was administered following cisplatin. Therefore, TAXOL should be given before cisplatin when used in combination. Patients treated with TAXOL and cisplatin may have an increased risk of renal failure during the combination therapy of paclitaxel and cisplatin in gynecological cancers as compared to cisplatin alone.

Cimetidine: The effect of cimetidine premedication on the metabolism of paclitaxel has been investigated; the clearance of paclitaxel was not affected by cimetidine pretreatment.

Substrates, Inducers, Inhibitors of Cytochrome P450 2C8 and 3A4: The metabolism of TAXOL is catalyzed by cytochrome P450 isoenzymes CYP2C8 and CYP3A4. Caution should be exercised when administering TAXOL concomitantly with known substrates, inducers or inhibitors of the cytochrome P450 isoenzymes CYP2C8 and CYP3A4. In vitro, the metabolism of paclitaxel to 6α-hydroxypaclitaxel was inhibited by a number of agents (ketoconazole, verapamil, diazepam, quinidine, dexamethasone, cyclosporine, teniposide, etoposide, and vincristine), but the concentrations used exceeded those found in vivo following normal therapeutic doses. Testosterone, 17α-ethinyl estradiol, retinoic acid, montelukast and quercetin, a specific inhibitor of CYP2C8, also inhibited the formation of 6α-hydroxypaclitaxel in vitro. The pharmacokinetics of paclitaxel may also be altered in vivo as a result of interactions with compounds that are substrates, inducers, or inhibitors of CYP2C8 and/or CYP3A4.

Potential interactions between TAXOL, a substrate of CYP3A4, and protease inhibitors (ritonavir, saquinavir, indinavir, and nelfinavir), which are substrates and/or inhibitors of CYP3A4, have not been evaluated in clinical trials. Caution and close monitoring of liver function is required; further, no unapproved (e.g., investigational) protease inhibitor should be administered with TAXOL.

Doxorubicin: Sequence effects characterized by more profound neutropenic and stomatitis episodes, have been observed with combination use of TAXOL and doxorubicin when TAXOL was administered **before** doxorubicin and using longer than recommended infusion times (TAXOL administered over 24 hours; doxorubicin administered over 48 hours). Plasma levels of doxorubicin (and its active metabolite doxorubicinol) may be increased when TAXOL and doxorubicin are used in combination. However, data from a trial using bolus doxorubicin and 3-hour TAXOL infusion found no sequence effects on the pattern of toxicity.

Hematology: TAXOL should not be administered to patients with baseline neutrophil counts of less than 1500 cells/mm³ (see Warnings and Contraindications). In order to monitor the occurrence of myelotoxicity, it is recommended that frequent peripheral blood cell counts be performed on all patients receiving TAXOL. Patients should not be retreated with subsequent cycles of TAXOL until neutrophils recover to a level >1500 cells/mm³ and platelets recover to a level >100 000 cells/mm³. In the case of severe neutropenia (<500 cells/mm³) during a course of TAXOL therapy, a 20% reduction in dose for subsequent courses of therapy is recommended. For patients with advanced HIV disease and poor-risk AIDS-related Kaposi's Sarcoma, TAXOL, at the recommended dose for this disease, can be initiated and repeated if the neutrophil count is at least 1000 cells/mm³ (see Dosage).

Hypersensitivity Reactions: Patients with a history of severe hypersensitivity reactions to products containing Cremophor EL should not be treated with TAXOL (see Warnings and Contraindications). Minor symptoms such as flushing, skin reactions, dyspnea, hypotension or tachycardia do not require interruption of therapy. However, severe reactions, such as hypotension requiring treatment, dyspnea requiring bronchodilators, angioedema or generalized urticaria require immediate discontinuation of TAXOL and aggressive symptomatic therapy. Patients who have developed severe hypersensitivity reactions should not be rechallenged with TAXOL.

Cardiovascular: Hypotension, hypertension and bradycardia have been observed during TAXOL administration; patients are usually asymptomatic and generally do not require treatment. In severe cases, TAXOL infusions may need to be interrupted or discontinued at the discretion of the treating physician. Frequent monitoring of vital signs, particularly during the first hour of TAXOL infusion, is recommended. Continuous cardiac monitoring is not required except for patients who develop serious conduction abnormalities (see Warnings and Adverse Effects). When TAXOL is used in combination with doxorubicin for treatment of metastatic breast cancer, monitoring of cardiac function is recommended.

Nervous System: Although the occurrence of peripheral neuropathy is frequent, the development of severe symptomatology is unusual. A dose reduction of 20% is recommended for all subsequent courses of TAXOL for severe neuropathy (see Adverse Effects and Dosage).

TAXOL contains dehydrated ethanol, 396 mg/mL; consideration should be given to possible CNS and other effects of ethanol. Children may be more sensitive than the adults to the effects of ethanol (see Warnings, Children).

Hepatic: There is evidence that the toxicity of TAXOL is enhanced in patients with elevated liver enzymes. Patients with hepatic impairment may be at increased risk of toxicity, particularly grade III-IV myelosuppression. Caution should be exercised when administering TAXOL to patients with moderate to severe hepatic impairment. Patients should be monitored closely for the development of profound myelosuppression. (See Adverse Effects.)

Injection Site Reaction: Injection site reactions, including reactions secondary to extravasation, were usually mild and consisted of pain, erythema, tenderness, skin discoloration, or swelling at the injection site. These reactions have been observed more frequently with the 24-hour infusion than with the 3-hour infusion. Recurrence of skin reactions at a site of previous extravasation following administration of TAXOL at a different site, i.e., "recall", has been reported rarely.

Rare reports of more severe events such as phlebitis, cellulitis, induration, skin exfoliation, necrosis and fibrosis have been received as part of the continuing surveillance of TAXOL safety. In some cases the onset of the injection site reaction either occurred during a prolonged infusion or was delayed by a week to 10 days.

A specific treatment for extravasation reactions is unknown at this time. Given the possibility of extravasation, it is advisable to closely monitor the infusion site for possible infiltration during drug administration.

Occupational Hazards: Driving/Operating Machinery: Since TAXOL contains ethanol, consideration should be given to the possibility of CNS and other effects.

ADVERSE EFFECTS: The frequency and severity of adverse events are generally similar between patients receiving TAXOL for the treatment of ovarian, breast non-small cell lung carcinoma, or Kaposi's Sarcoma, but patients with AIDS-related Kaposi's Sarcoma may have more frequent and severe hematologic toxicity, infections, and febrile neutropenia. These patients require a lower dose intensity and supportive care.

The incidences of adverse reactions in Table 1 are derived from 10 clinical trials in carcinoma of the ovary and of the breast involving 812 patients treated with single-agent TAXOL at doses ranging from 135 to 300 mg/m²/day and schedules of 3 or 24 hours. Data from a subset of 181 patients treated at the recommended dose of 175 mg/m² and a 3-hour infusion schedule is also included in Table 1.

Table 1: TAXOL

Summary of Adverse Events

	135–300 mg/m² % of Patients N=812	175 mg/m² % of Patients N=181
Bone Marrow		
Neutropenia		
<2000/mm³	90	87
<500/mm³	52	27
Leukopenia		
<4000/mm³	90	86
<1000/mm³	17	4
Thrombocytopenia		
<100 000/mm³	20	6
<50 000/mm³	7	1
Anemia		
<11 g/dL	78	62
<8 g/dL	16	6
Infections	30	18
Bleeding	14	9
Red Cell Transfusions	25	13
Red Cell Transfusions (normal baseline)	12	6
Platelet Transfusions	2	0
Hypersensitivity Reaction		
All	41	40
Severe	2	1
Cardiovascular		
Bradycardia (first 3 hours of infusion)	3	3
Hypotension (first 3 hours of infusion)	12	11
Severe events	1	2
Abnormal ECG		

(cont'd)

Table 1: TAXOL *(cont'd)*

Summary of Adverse Events

	135–300 mg/m² % of Patients N=812	175 mg/m² % of Patients N=181
All Patients	23	13
Patients with normal baseline	14	8
Peripheral Neuropathy		
Any symptoms	60	64
Severe symptoms	3	4
Myalgia/Arthralgia		
Any symptoms	60	54
Severe symptoms	8	12
Gastrointestinal		
Nausea and vomiting	52	44
Diarrhea	38	25
Mucositis	31	20
Alopecia	87	93
Hepatic (Patients with normal baseline)		
Bilirubin elevations	7	4
Alkaline phosphatase elevations	22	18
AST elevations	19	18
Injection Site Reactions	13	4

Safety referring to a large randomized trial of TAXOL (135 mg/m² over 24 hours)/cisplatin (75 mg/m²) versus cyclophosphamide/cisplatin, including 410 patients (196 receiving TAXOL), has been evaluated. The combination of TAXOL with platinum agents has not resulted in any clinically relevant changes to the safety profile of the drug when used at the recommended dosage.

Safety data were collected for 3121 patients in the Phase III adjuvant breast carcinoma study. The adverse event profile for the patients who received TAXOL subsequent to cyclophosphamide and doxorubicin was consistent with that seen in the pooled analysis of data from 812 patients treated with single-agent TAXOL in 10 clinical studies.

Summary of 3-hour infusion data at a dose of 175 mg/m²: Unless otherwise stated, the following safety data relate to 62 patients with ovarian cancer and 119 patients with breast cancer treated at a dose of 175 mg/m² and a 3-hour infusion schedule, in phase III clinical trials. All patients were premedicated to minimize hypersensitivity reactions. Data from these clinical trials demonstrate that TAXOL given at this dose and schedule is well tolerated. Bone marrow suppression and peripheral neuropathy were the principal dose-related adverse effects associated with TAXOL. Compared to 24-hour infusion schedules, neutropenia was less common when TAXOL was given as a 3-hour infusion. Neutropenia was generally rapidly reversible and did not worsen with cumulative exposure. The frequency of neurologic symptoms increased with repeated exposure.

None of the observed toxicities were influenced by age.

AIDS-related Kaposi's Sarcoma: Table 2 shows the frequency of important adverse events in the 85 patients with KS treated with 2 different single-agent TAXOL regimens.

Table 2: TAXOL

Frequency[a] of Important[b] Adverse Events in the AIDS-related Kaposi's Sarcoma Studies

	Percent of Patients	
	Study CA139–174 135/3[c]/3 wk (n=29)	Study CA139–281 100/3[c]/2 wk (n=56)
Bone Marrow		
Neutropenia		
<2000/mm³	100	95
<500/mm³	76	35
Thrombocytopenia		
<100 000/mm³	52	27
<50 000/mm³	17	5
Anemia		
<11 g/dL	86	73
<8 g/dL	34	25
Febrile Neutropenia	55	9
Opportunistic Infections		
Any	76	54
Cytomegalovirus	45	27
Herpes Simplex	38	11

(cont'd)

Table 2: TAXOL *(cont'd)*

Frequency[a] of Important[b] Adverse Events in the AIDS-related Kaposi's Sarcoma Studies

	Percent of Patients	
	Study CA139–174 135/3[c]/3 wk (n=29)	Study CA139–281 100/3[c]/2 wk (n=56)
P. carinii	14	21
M. avium intracellulare	24	4
Candidiasis, esophageal	7	9
Cryptosporidiosis	7	7
Cryptococcal meningitis	3	2
Leukoencephalopathy	—	2
Hypersensitivity Reaction[d]		
All	14	9
Cardiovascular		
Hypotension	17	9
Bradycardia	3	—
Peripheral Neuropathy		
Any	79	46
Severe[e]	14	16
Myalgia/Arthralgia		
Any	93	48
Severe[e]	14	16
Gastrointestinal		
Nausea and vomiting	69	70
Diarrhea	90	73
Mucositis	45	20
Renal (Creatinine elevation)		
Any	34	18
Severe[e]	7	5
Discontinuation for Drug Toxicity	7	16

a Based on worst course analysis.
b Clinically relevant and/or possibly related.
c TAXOL dose in mg/m^2/infusion duration in hours.
d All patients received premedication.
e Severe events are defined as at least Grade III toxicity.

As demonstrated in Table 2, toxicity was more pronounced in the study utilizing TAXOL at a dose of 135 mg/m^2 every 3 weeks than in the study utilizing TAXOL at a dose of 100 mg/m^2 every 2 weeks. Notably, severe neutropenia (76% vs 35%), febrile neutropenia (55% vs 9%), and opportunistic infections (76% vs 54%) were more common with the former dose and schedule. The differences between the two studies with respect to dose escalation and use of hematopoietic growth factors, as described below, should be taken into account.

Adverse Experiences by Body System: Unless otherwise noted, the following discussion refers to the overall safety database of 812 patients with solid tumors treated with single-agent TAXOL in 10 clinical studies. Toxicities that occurred with greater severity or frequency in previously untreated patients with ovarian carcinoma or NSCLC who received TAXOL in combination with cisplatin or in patients with breast cancer who received TAXOL after doxorubicin/cyclophosphamide in the adjuvant setting, or in patients with AIDS-related Kaposi's Sarcoma, and that occurred with a difference that was clinically significant in these populations are also described. In addition, rare events have been reported from postmarketing experience or from other clinical studies.

The frequency and severity of adverse events have been generally similar for all patients receiving TAXOL. However, patients with AIDS-related Kaposi's Sarcoma may have more frequent and severe hematologic toxicity, infections, and febrile neutropenia. These patients require a lower dose intensity and supportive care. Toxicities that were observed only in or were noted to have occurred with greater severity in the population with Kaposi's Sarcoma and that occurred with a difference that was clinically significant in this population are described.

Hematologic: The most frequent significant undesirable effect of TAXOL was bone marrow suppression. Neutropenia was dose and schedule dependent and was generally rapidly reversible. Severe neutropenia (<500 cells/mm^3) occurred in 27% of patients treated at a dose of 175 mg/m^2, but was not associated with febrile episodes. Only 1% of patients experienced severe neutropenia for 7 days or more. Neutropenia was not more frequent or severe in patients who received prior radiation therapy, nor did it appear to be affected by treatment duration or cumulative exposure.

When TAXOL was administered to patients with ovarian carcinoma at a dose of 175 mg/m^2/3 hours in combination with cisplatin versus the control arm of cyclophosphamide plus cisplatin, the incidences of severe neutropenia and of febrile neutropenia were similar in the TAXOL plus cisplatin arm and in the control arm.

When TAXOL was administered in combination with cisplatin to patients with advanced NSCLC in the Eastern Cooperative Oncology Group (ECOG) study, the incidence of neutropenia (Grade IV) was 74% (TAXOL 135 mg/m^2/24 hours plus cisplatin) and 65% (TAXOL 250 mg/m^2/24 hours plus cisplatin and G-CSF) compared with 55% in patients who received cisplatin/etoposide. Considerably less Grade IV neutropenia was observed in the European Organization for Research and Treatment of Cancer (EORTC) (28%) and CA139-208 (45%) studies for TAXOL 175 mg/m^2/3 hours plus cisplatin (without G-CSF).

Fever was frequent (12% of all treatment courses). Infectious episodes occurred in 30% of all patients and 9% of all courses; these episodes were fatal in 1% of all patients, and included sepsis, pneumonia and peritonitis. In the Phase 3 second-line ovarian study, infectious episodes were reported in 20% of the patients given 135 mg/m^2 and 26% of the patients given 175 mg/m^2 by a 3-hour infusion. Urinary tract infections and upper respiratory tract infections were the most frequently reported infectious complications. In the immunosuppressed patient population with advanced HIV disease and poor-risk AIDS-related Kaposi's Sarcoma, 61% of the patients reported at least 1 opportunistic infection. The use of supportive therapy, including G-CSF, is recommended for patients who have experienced severe neutropenia (see Dosage).

Twenty percent of the patients experienced a drop in their platelet count below 100 000 cells/mm^3 at least once while on treatment; 7% had a platelet count <50 000 cells/mm^3 at the time of their worst nadir. Bleeding episodes were reported in 4% of all courses and by 14% of all patients, but most of the hemorrhagic episodes were localized and the frequency of these events was unrelated to the TAXOL dose and schedule. In the Phase III second-line ovarian cancer study, bleeding episodes were reported in 10% of the patients who received study medication; however, none of the patients treated with the 3-hour infusion received platelet transfusions. In the adjuvant breast carcinoma trial, the incidence of severe thrombocytopenia and platelet transfusions increased with higher doses of doxorubicin.

Anemia (Hb<11 g/dL) was observed in 78% of all patients and was severe (Hb<8 g/dL) in 16% of the cases. No consistent relationship between dose or schedule and the frequency of anemia was observed. Among all patients with normal baseline hemoglobin, 69% became anemic on study but only 7% had severe anemia. Red cell transfusions were required in 25% of all patients and in 12% of those with normal baseline hemoglobin levels.

Hypersensitivity Reactions (HSR): All patients received premedication prior to TAXOL (see Warnings). The frequency and severity of HSR were not affected by the dose or schedule of TAXOL administration. In the Phase III second-line ovarian study, the 3-hour infusion was not associated with a greater increase in HSR when compared to the 24-hour infusion. Hypersensitivity reactions were observed in 20% of all courses and in 41% of all patients. These reactions were severe in less than 2% of the patients and 1% of the courses. No severe reactions were observed after course 3 and severe symptoms occurred generally within the first hour of TAXOL infusion. The most frequent symptoms observed during these severe reactions were dyspnea, flushing, chest pain and tachycardia. Abdominal pain, pain in the extremities, diaphoresis, and hypertension are also noted.

The minor hypersensitivity reactions consisted mostly of flushing (28%), rash (12%), hypotension (4%), dyspnea (2%), tachycardia (2%) and hypertension (1%). The frequency of hypersensitivity reactions remained relatively stable during the entire treatment period.

Rare reports of chills and reports of back pain in association with hypersensitivity reactions have been received as part of the continuing surveillance of TAXOL safety.

Cardiovascular: Hypotension, during the first 3 hours of infusion, occurred in 12% of all patients and 3% of all courses administered. Bradycardia, during the first 3 hours of infusion, occurred in 3% of all patients and 1% of all courses. In the Phase III second-line ovarian study, neither dose nor schedule had an effect on the frequency of hypotension and bradycardia. These vital sign changes most often caused no symptoms and required neither specific therapy nor treatment discontinuation. The frequency of hypotension and bradycardia were not influenced by prior anthracycline therapy.

Significant cardiovascular events possibly related to single-agent TAXOL occurred in approximately 1% of all patients. These events included syncope, rhythm abnormalities, hypertension and venous thrombosis. One of the patients with syncope treated with TAXOL at 175 mg/m^2 over 24 hours had progressive hypotension and died. The arrhythmias included asymptomatic ventricular tachycardia, bigeminy and complete AV block requiring pacemaker placement. The incidence of Grade III or greater cardiovascular events was 13% (TAXOL 135 mg/m^2/24 hours plus cisplatin), 12% (TAXOL 250 mg/m^2/24 hours plus cisplatin and G-CSF), and 6% (TAXOL 175 mg/m^2/3 hours plus cisplatin) when TAXOL followed by cisplatin was administered to patients with advanced NSCLC; there was a similar incidence in the non-TAXOL control arms. The apparent increase in these cardiovascular events in patients with NSCLC compared to patients with breast or ovarian cancer is possibly related to the difference in cardiovascular risk factors among patients with lung cancer.

ECG abnormalities were common among patients at baseline. ECG abnormalities on study did not usually result in symptoms, were not dose-limiting, and required no intervention. ECG abnormalities were noted in 23% of all patients. Among patients with a normal ECG prior to study entry, 14% of all patients developed an abnormal tracing while on study. The most frequently reported ECG modifications were nonspecific repolarization abnormalities, sinus bradycardia, sinus tachycardia and premature beats. Among patients with normal ECG at baseline, prior therapy with anthracyclines did not influence the frequency of ECG abnormalities.

Cases of myocardial infarction have been reported rarely. Congestive heart failure (cardiac dysfunction and reduction of left ventricular ejection fraction or ventricular failure) has been reported typically in patients who have received other chemotherapy, notably anthracyclines (see Precautions, Drug Interactions).

Rare reports of atrial fibrillation and supraventricular tachycardia have been received as part of the continuing surveillance of TAXOL safety.

Respiratory: Rare reports of interstitial pneumonia, lung fibrosis and pulmonary embolism, have been received as part of the continuing surveillance of TAXOL safety. Rare reports of radiation pneumonitis have been received in patients receiving concurrent radiotherapy.

Neurologic: The frequency and severity of neurologic manifestations were influenced by prior and concomitant therapy with cisplatin. In general, the frequency and severity of neurologic manifestations were dose-dependent in patients receiving single-agent TAXOL. Paresthesia commonly occurs in the form of hyperesthesia. Peripheral neuropathy was observed in 60% of all patients (3% severe) and in 52% (2% severe) of the patients without pre-existing neuropathy.

The frequency of peripheral neuropathy increased with cumulative dose. Neurologic symptoms were observed in 27% of the patients after the first course of treatment and in 34 to 51% from course 2 to 10. Peripheral neuropathy was the cause of TAXOL discontinuation in 1% of all patients. Sensory symptoms have usually improved or resolved within several months of TAXOL discontinuation. The incidence of neurologic symptoms did not increase in the subset of patients previously treated with cisplatin. Pre-existing neuropathies resulting from prior therapies are not a contraindication for TAXOL therapy. In the Intergroup first-line ovarian carcinoma study, the regimen with TAXOL 175 mg/m^2 by 3-hour infusion followed by cisplatin 75 mg/m^2 resulted in greater incidence and severity of neurotoxicity (reported as neuromotor or neurosensory events) than the regimen containing cyclophosphamide 750 mg/m^2 followed by cisplatin 75 mg/m^2, 87% (21% severe) vs 52% (2% severe), respectively. In the GOG first-line ovarian carcinoma study, the regimen with TAXOL (135 mg/m^2 over 24 hours) followed by cisplatin (75 mg/m^2) resulted in an incidence of neurotoxicity (reported as peripheral neuropathy) that was similar to the regimen containing cyclophosphamide 750 mg/m^2 followed by cisplatin 75 mg/m^2, 25% (3% severe) vs 20% (0% severe), respectively. Cross-study comparison of neurotoxicity in Intergroup and GOG trials suggests that when TAXOL is given in combinations with cisplatin 75 mg/m^2, the incidence of severe neurotoxicity is more common at a TAXOL dose of 175 mg/m^2 given by 3-hour infusion (21%) than at a dose of 135 mg/m^2 given by 24-hour infusion (3%). In patients with NSCLC, administration of TAXOL followed by cisplatin resulted in greater incidence of severe neurotoxicity compared to the incidence in patients with ovarian or breast cancer treated with single-agent paclitaxel. Severe neurosensory symptoms were noted in 13% of NSCLC patients receiving TAXOL 135 mg/m^2 by 24-hour infusion followed by cisplatin 75 mg/m^2 and 8% of NSCLC patients receiving cisplatin/etoposide.

Other than peripheral neuropathy, serious neurologic events following TAXOL administration have been rare (<1%) and have included grand mal seizures, ataxia and encephalopathy.

Rare reports of autonomic neuropathy resulting in paralytic ileus and motor neuropathy with resultant minor distal weakness have been received as part of the continuing surveillance of TAXOL safety. Optic nerve and/or visual disturbances (scintillating scotoma) have also been reported, particularly in patients who have received higher doses than those recommended. These effects generally have been reversible. However, rare reports in the literature of abnormal visual evoked potentials in patients have suggested persistent optic nerve damage. Postmarketing reports of ototoxicity (hearing loss and tinnitus) have been received.

Arthralgia/myalgia: There was no consistent relationship between dose or schedule of TAXOL and the frequency or severity of arthralgia/myalgia. Sixty percent of all patients treated in single-agent trials experienced arthralgia/myalgia; 8% experienced severe symptoms. The symptoms were usually transient, occurred 2 or 3 days after TAXOL administration, and resolved within a few days. The frequency and severity of musculoskeletal symptoms remained unchanged throughout the treatment period.

Alopecia: Alopecia was observed in almost all patients.

Gastrointestinal: Nausea/vomiting, diarrhea and mucositis were reported by 52%, 38% and 31% of all patients, respectively. These manifestations were usually mild to moderate. Mucositis was schedule dependent and occurred more frequently with the 24-hour than with the 3-hour infusion.

In the first-line Phase III ovarian carcinoma study, the incidence of nausea and vomiting when TAXOL was administered in combination with cisplatin appeared to be greater compared with the database for single-agent TAXOL in ovarian and breast carcinoma. In the same study, diarrhea of any grade was reported more frequently (16%) compared to the control arm (8%) (p=0.008), but there was no difference for severe diarrhea.

Rare reports of intestinal obstruction, intestinal perforation, pancreatitis, ischemic colitis, and dehydration have been received as part of the continuing surveillance of TAXOL safety. Rare reports of neutropenic enterocolitis (typhlitis), despite the coadministration of G-CSF, were observed in patients treated with TAXOL alone and in combination with other chemotherapeutic agents.

In patients with poor-risk AIDS-related Kaposi's Sarcoma, nausea/vomiting, diarrhea, and mucositis were reported by 69%, 79% and 28% of patients, respectively. One third of patients with Kaposi's Sarcoma complained of diarrhea prior to study start.

Hepatic: No relationship was observed between liver function abnormalities and either dose or schedule of TAXOL administration. Among patients with normal baseline liver function 7%, 22% and 19% had elevations in bilirubin, alkaline phosphatase and AST, respectively. There is no evidence that TAXOL when given as a 3-hour infusion to patients with mildly abnormal liver function causes exacerbation of abnormal liver function. Prolonged exposure to TAXOL was not associated with cumulative hepatic toxicity.

Rare reports of hepatic necrosis and hepatic encephalopathy leading to death have been received as part of the continuing surveillance of TAXOL safety.

Renal: Among the patients treated for Kaposi's Sarcoma with TAXOL, 5 patients had renal toxicity of grade III or IV severity. One patient with suspected HIV nephropathy of grade IV severity had to discontinue therapy. The other 4 patients had renal insufficiency with reversible elevations of serum creatinine.

Injection Site Reactions: Injection site reactions, including reactions secondary to extravasation, were usually mild and consisted of pain, erythema, tenderness, skin discoloration, or swelling at the injection site. These reactions have been observed more frequently with the 24-hour infusion than with the 3-hour infusion. Recurrence of skin reactions at a site of previous extravasation following administration of TAXOL at a different site, i.e., "recall", has been reported rarely.

Rare reports of more severe events such as phlebitis, cellulitis, induration, skin exfoliation, necrosis and fibrosis have been received as part of the continuing surveillance of TAXOL safety. In some cases the onset of the injection site reaction either occurred during a prolonged infusion or was delayed by 1 week to 10 days.

A specific treatment for extravasation reactions is unknown at this time. Given the possibility of extravasation, it is advisable to closely monitor the infusion site for possible infiltration during drug administration.

Other: Transient skin changes due to TAXOL-related hypersensitivity reactions have been observed, but no other skin toxicities were significantly associated with TAXOL administration. Nail changes (changes in pigmentation or discoloration of nail bed) were uncommon (2%). Edema was reported in 21% of all patients (17% of those without baseline edema); only 1% had severe edema and none of these patients required treatment discontinuation. Edema was most commonly focal and disease-related. Edema was observed in 5% of all courses for patients with normal baseline and did not increase with time on study.

Rare reports of skin abnormalities related to radiation recall as well as reports of maculopapular rash, pruritus, Stevens-Johnson syndrome, and toxic epidermal necrolysis have been received as part of the continuing surveillance of TAXOL safety.

Reports of asthenia and malaise have been received as part of the continuing surveillance of TAXOL safety. In the Phase III trial of TAXOL 135 mg/m² over 24 hours in combination with cisplatin as first-line therapy of ovarian cancer, asthenia was reported in 17% of the patients, significantly greater than the 10% incidence observed in the control arm of cyclophosphamide/cisplatin.

Post-Market Adverse Drug Reactions : Unless otherwise indicated, Table 3 lists undesirable effects regardless of severity associated with the administration of single agent TAXOL (812 patients treated in clinical trials) or as reported in the postmarketing surveillance* of TAXOL.

The frequency of undesirable effects listed below is defined using the following convention: very common (≥1/10); common (≥1/100, <1/10); uncommon (≥1/1000, <1/100); rare (≥1/10 000, <1/1000); very rare (<1/10 000).

Table 3: TAXOL

Post-Marketing Adverse Drug Events

Infections and Infestations	Very common: infection Uncommon: septic shock Rare*: pneumonia, sepsis
Blood and the Lymphatic System Disorders	Very common: myelosuppression, neutropenia, anemia, thrombocytopenia, leukopenia, fever, bleeding Rare: febrile neutropenia Very rare*: acute myeloid leukemia, myelodysplastic syndrome
Immune System Disorders	Very common: minor hypersensitivity reactions (mainly flushing and rash) Uncommon: significant hypersensitivity reactions requiring therapy (eg, hypotension, angioneurotic edema, respiratory distress, generalised urticaria, edema, back pain, chills) Rare*: anaphylactic reactions (with fatal outcome) Very rare*: anaphylactic shock
Metabolism and Nutrition Disorders	Very rare*: anorexia
Psychiatric Disorders	Very rare*: confusional state
Nervous System Disorders	Very common: neurotoxicity (mainly: peripheral neuropathy) Rare*: motor neuropathy (with resultant minor distal weakness) Very rare*: autonomic neuropathy (resulting in paralytic ileus and orthostatic hypotension), grand mal seizures, convulsions, encephalopathy, dizziness, headache, ataxia
Eye Disorders	Very rare*: reversible optic nerve and/or visual disturbances (scintillating scotomata), particularly in patients who have received higher doses than recommended, photopsia, visual floaters
Ear and Labyrinth Disorders	Very rare*: hearing loss, tinnitus, vertigo, ototoxicity
Cardiac Disorders	Very common: abnormal ECG Common: bradycardia Uncommon: cardiomyopathy, asymptomatic ventricular tachycardia, tachycardia with bigeminy, AV block and syncope, myocardial infarction. Very rare*: atrial fibrillation, supraventricular tachycardia
Vascular Disorders	Very common: hypotension Uncommon: hypertension, thrombosis, thrombophlebitis Very rare*: shock
Respiratory, Thoracic and Mediastinal Disorders	Rare*: dyspnea, pleural effusion, respiratory failure, interstitial pneumonia, lung fibrosis, pulmonary embolism Very rare*: cough
Gastrointestinal Disorders	Very common: nausea, vomiting, diarrhea, mucosal inflammation Rare*: bowel obstruction, bowel perforation, ischemic colitis, pancreatitis Very rare*: mesenteric thrombosis, pseudomembranous colitis, esophagitis, constipation, ascites
Hepato-biliary Disorders	Very rare*: hepatic necrosis (with fatal outcome), hepatic encephalopathy (with fatal outcome)
Renal Disorders	Unknown*: renal failure
Skin and Subcutaneous Tissue Disorders	Very common: alopecia Common: transient and mild nail and skin changes Rare*: pruritus, rash, erythema, phlebitis, cellulitis, skin exfoliation, necrosis and fibrosis, radiation recall Very rare*: Stevens-Johnson syndrome, epidermal necrolysis, erythema multiforme, exfoliative dermatitis, urticaria, onycholysis (patients on therapy should wear sun protection on hands and feet), scleroderma-like changes preceded by chronic edema
Musculoskeletal, Connective Tissue and Bone Disorders	Very common: arthralgia, myalgia

(cont'd)

Table 3: TAXOL *(cont'd)*

Post-Marketing Adverse Drug Events

General Disorders and Administration Site Conditions	Common: injection site reactions (including localised edema, pain, erythema, induration, on occasion extravasation can result in cellulitis) Rare*: asthenia, malaise, pyrexia, dehydration, edema
Investigations	Common: severe elevation in AST, severe elevation in alkaline phosphatase Uncommon: severe elevation in bilirubin Rare*: Increase in blood creatinine

OVERDOSE:

Symptoms: The primary anticipated complications of overdosage would consist of bone marrow suppression, peripheral neurotoxicity and mucositis. Overdoses in pediatric patients may be associated with acute ethanol toxicity (see Warnings, Children).

Treatment: There is no known antidote for TAXOL overdosage.

For management of a suspected drug overdose, CPhA recommends that you contact your **regional Poison Control Centre**. See the *CPS* Directory section for a list of Poison Control Centres.

DOSAGE: Note: Undiluted concentrate should not come in contact with plasticized PVC equipment. In order to minimize patients exposure to the plasticizer DEHP [di-(2-ethylhexyl) phthalate], which may be leached from PVC infusion bags or sets, diluted TAXOL solutions should preferably be stored in bottles (glass, polypropylene) or plastic bags (polypropylene, polyolefin) and administered through polyethylene-lined administration sets.

TAXOL should be administered through an in-line filter with a microporous membrane not greater than 0.22 microns. Use of filter devices such as IVEX-2 filters which incorporate short inlet and outlet PVC-coated tubing has not resulted in significant leaching of DEHP.

All patients should be premedicated prior to TAXOL administration in order to reduce the risk of severe hypersensitivity reactions. Such premedication may consist of dexamethasone 20 mg orally (or its equivalent) approximately 12 and 6 hours before TAXOL, diphenhydramine 50 mg i.v. (or its equivalent) 30 to 60 minutes prior to TAXOL, and cimetidine (300 mg) or ranitidine (50 mg) i.v. 30 to 60 minutes before TAXOL.

Metastatic Carcinoma of the Ovary: The administration of TAXOL at a dose of 175 mg/m² over 3 hours in combination with cisplatin 75 mg/m² every 3 weeks is recommended for the primary treatment of patients with advanced carcinoma of the ovary. TAXOL should be given before cisplatin when used in combination.

In patients previously treated with chemotherapy, the recommended regimen is 175 mg/m² administered i.v. over 3 hours every 3 weeks.

Carcinoma of the Breast: For the adjuvant treatment of node-positive breast cancer, the recommended regimen is TAXOL, at a dose of 175 mg/m² i.v. over 3 hours every 3 weeks for 4 courses administered sequentially to standard combination therapy.

After failure of initial chemotherapy for metastatic disease or relapse within 6 months of adjuvant chemotherapy, TAXOL at a dose of 175 mg/m² administered i.v. over 3 hours every 3 weeks has been shown to be effective.

Non-small Cell Lung Carcinoma: The recommended regimen, given every 3 weeks, is TAXOL administered i.v. over 3 hours at a dose of 175 mg/m² followed by cisplatin.

Single courses of TAXOL should not be repeated until the neutrophil count is at least 1500 cells/mm³ and the platelet count is at least 100 000 cells/mm³. Patients who experience severe neutropenia (neutrophil <500 cells/mm³) or severe peripheral neuropathy during TAXOL therapy should have the dosage reduced by 20% for subsequent courses of TAXOL.

AIDS-related Kaposi's Sarcoma: TAXOL 135 mg/m² administered i.v. over 3 hours with a 3 week interval between courses or 100 mg/m² administered i.v. over 3 hours with a 2 week interval between courses (dose intensity 45 to 50 mg/m²/week). In the 2 clinical trials evaluating these schedules, the former schedule (135 mg/m² every 3 weeks) was more toxic than the latter. In addition, all patients with low performance status were treated with the latter schedule (100 mg/m² every 2 weeks).

Based upon the immunosuppression observed in patients with advanced HIV disease, the following modifications are recommended in these patients.

1) the dose of dexamethasone as 1 of the 3 premedication drugs should be reduced to 10 mg orally.
2) treatment with TAXOL should be initiated or repeated only if the neutrophil count is at least 1000 cells/mm³.
3) the dose of subsequent courses of TAXOL should be reduced by 20% for those patients who experience severe neutropenia (<500 cell/mm³ for a week or longer).
4) concomitant hematopoietic growth factor (G-CSF), should be initiated as clinically indicated.

Preparation and Administration Precautions: TAXOL is a cytotoxic anticancer drug and, as with other potentially toxic compounds, caution should be exercised in handling TAXOL. The use of gloves is recommended. Following topical exposure, tingling, burning, redness have been observed. If TAXOL solution contacts the skin, wash the skin immediately and thoroughly with soap and water.

If TAXOL contacts mucous membranes, the membranes should be flushed thoroughly with water. Upon inhalation, dyspnea, chest pain, burning eyes, sore throat and nausea have been reported. Given the possibility of extravasation, it is advisable to closely monitor the infusion site for possible infiltration during drug administration (see Precautions and Adverse Effects, Injection Site Reaction).

Preparation for I.V. Administration: TAXOL for Injection must be diluted prior to infusion. TAXOL should be diluted in 0.9% Sodium Chloride Injection, 5% Dextrose Injection, 5% Dextrose and 0.9% Sodium Chloride Injection, or 5% Dextrose in Ringer's Injection to a final concentration of 0.3 to 1.2 mg/mL. The solutions are physically and chemically stable for up to 27 hours at ambient temperature (15 to 30°C) and room lighting conditions; infusions should be completed within this time frame. There have been rare reports of precipitation with longer than the recommended 3-hour infusion schedules. Excessive agitation, vibration or shaking may induce precipitation and should be avoided. Infusion sets should be flushed thoroughly with a compatible diluent before use.

Upon preparation, solutions may show haziness, which is attributed to the formulation vehicle. No significant loss in potency has been noted following simulated delivery of the solution through i.v. tubing containing an in-line (0.22 micron) filter.

Data collected for the presence of the extractable plasticizer DEHP [di-(2-ethylhexyl)phthalate] show that levels increase with time and concentration when dilutions are prepared in PVC containers. Consequently, the use of plasticized PVC containers and administration sets is not recommended. TAXOL solutions should be prepared and stored in glass, polypropylene, or polyolefin containers. Non-PVC containing administration sets, such as those which are polyethylene-lined, should be used.

Devices with spikes should not be used with vials of TAXOL since they can cause the stopper to collapse resulting in loss of sterile integrity of TAXOL solution.

Contact of undiluted TAXOL with plasticized PVC equipment or devices used to prepare solutions for infusion is not recommended (see Dosage).

Prior to infusion, TAXOL should be diluted in 0.9% Sodium Chloride Injection, 5% Dextrose Injection, 5% Dextrose and 0.9% Sodium Chloride Injection or 5% Dextrose in Ringer's Injection to a final concentration of 0.3 to 1.2 mg/mL.

As with all parenteral drug products, i.v. admixtures should be inspected visually for clarity, particulate matter, precipitate, discoloration and leakage prior to administration, whenever solution and container permit.

TAXOL should be administered through an in-line filter with a microporous membrane not greater than 0.22 microns.

Special Instructions: 1) Preparation of TAXOL should be done in a vertical laminar flow hood (Biological Safety Cabinet—Class II).
2) Personnel preparing TAXOL should wear PVC gloves, safety glasses, disposable gowns and masks.
3) All needles, syringes, vials and other materials which have come in contact with TAXOL should be segregated and incinerated at 1000°C or more. Sealed containers may explode. Intact vials should be returned to the manufacturer for destruction. Proper precautions should be taken in packaging these materials for transport.
4) Personnel regularly involved in the preparation and handling of TAXOL should have biannual blood examinations.
5) Directions for Dispensing from Pharmacy Bulk Vial: The use of Pharmacy Bulk Vial is restricted to hospitals with a recognized i.v. admixture program. The Pharmacy Bulk Vial is intended for single puncture, multiple dispensing and for i.v. use only. Dispensing from the Pharmacy Bulk Vial should be completed within 24 hours after initial entry.

Stability and Storage Recommendations: TAXOL for Injection should be stored at room temperature (15-30°C). Retain in the original package and protect from light. Once punctured, the 5 and 16.7 mL vials of TAXOL are stable for 28 days at room temperature. The 50 mL pharmacy bulk vial should be used within 24 hours after initial entry.

Solutions for infusion prepared as recommended may be stored at room temperature (15 to 30°C) only if necessary. However, the infusion should be initiated within 24 hours of reconstitution.

If unopened vials are refrigerated, a precipitate may form which redissolves with little or no agitation upon reaching room temperature. Product quality is not affected. If the solution remains cloudy or if an insoluble precipitate is noted, the vial should be discarded.

SUPPLIED: Each mL contains: paclitaxel 6 mg. Nonmedicinal ingredients: dehydrated ethanol 49.7% v/v and purified Cremophor EL (polyoxyethylated castor oil 527 mg). Multidose vials of 5 and 16.7 mL and pharmacy bulk vials of 50 mL, containing respectively 30 mg, 100 mg, and 300 mg paclitaxel at a concentration of 6 mg/mL.

Taxotere® Ⓟ

docetaxel

Antineoplastic

sanofi-aventis

Date of Revision: January 4, 2010

TAXOTERE, in combination with doxorubicin and cyclophosphamide, indicated for adjuvant treatment of patients with operable node-positive breast cancer, has been issued marketing authorization with conditions. This conditional approval is based on the promising nature of the clinical evidence of TAXOTERE in these patients and the need for further follow-up to confirm the clinical results. Patients should be advised of the nature of the authorization.

TAXOTERE has received non-conditional approvals for the treatment of advanced breast cancer, non small cell lung cancer, ovarian cancer, prostate cancer, and squamous cell carcinoma of the head and neck.

TAXOTERE should be administered under the supervision of a qualified physician experienced in the use of anti-cancer agents.

SUMMARY PRODUCT INFORMATION:

Route of Administration	Dosage Form/ Strength	Clinically Relevant Nonmedicinal Ingredients
Intravenous Infusion	Concentrate for Injection 80 mg/2 mL and 20 mg/0.5 mL	Polysorbate 80
	Diluent	Ethanol 95% v/v/ water for injection (13/87 w/w)

INDICATIONS AND CLINICAL USE: Breast Cancer: TAXOTERE (docetaxel for injection) in combination with doxorubicin and cyclophosphamide is indicated for the adjuvant treatment of patients with operable node-positive breast cancer.

The effectiveness of TAXOTERE in combination with doxorubicin and cyclophosphamide is based on improved disease free survival and overall survival in comparison to the combination of fluorouracil, doxorubicin and cyclophosphamide at a median follow up of 55 months. However long-term data are not yet available.

TAXOTERE is indicated for the treatment of patients with locally advanced or metastatic breast cancer. TAXOTERE, in combination with doxorubicin as first line therapy, should be reserved for patients with potentially life threatening disease (such as visceral or lung metastatic disease).

TAXOTERE in combination with Xeloda (capecitabine) is indicated for the treatment of patients with advanced or metastatic breast cancer after failure of prior anthracycline containing chemotherapy.

Non-Small Cell Lung Cancer: TAXOTERE is indicated for the treatment of patients with locally advanced or metastatic non-small cell lung cancer in monotherapy or in combination with platinum derivatives.

Ovarian Cancer: TAXOTERE is indicated for the treatment of metastatic carcinoma of the ovary after failure of first-line or subsequent chemotherapy.

Prostate Cancer: TAXOTERE in combination with prednisone or prednisolone is indicated for the treatment of patients with androgen-independent (hormone-refractory) metastatic prostate cancer.

Squamous Cell Carcinoma of the Head and Neck: TAXOTERE is indicated as monotherapy in the treatment of patients with recurrent and/or metastatic squamous cell carcinoma of the head and neck after failure of a previous chemotherapy regimen.

TAXOTERE should be administered under the supervision of a physician experienced in the use of antineoplastic agents.

CONTRAINDICATIONS:

- TAXOTERE (docetaxel for injection) is contraindicated in:
  - patients who have a history of hypersensitivity reactions to TAXOTERE or to other drugs formulated with polysorbate 80
  - pregnant women, (see Warnings and Precautions, Special Populations, Pregnant Women)
  - women who are breast-feeding, (see Warnings and Precautions, Special Populations, Nursing Women) and
  - patients with severe liver impairment.
- TAXOTERE should not be used in patients with baseline neutrophil counts of <1500 cells/mm³.

Contraindications for other drugs also apply when combined with docetaxel:

- Contraindications for Xeloda (capecitabine) also apply to the capecitabine plus TAXOTERE combination (please refer to Xeloda Product Monograph).
- Contraindications to prednisone also apply to the combination with TAXOTERE (please refer to Product Monograph for prednisone).

WARNINGS AND PRECAUTIONS:

Serious Warnings and Precautions

TAXOTERE should be administered under the supervision of a physician experienced in the use of antineoplastic agents (see Indications and Clinical Use).

TAXOTERE therapy should not be given to patients with neutrophil counts of less than 1500 cells/mm³ (see Hematologic).

Severe hypersensitivity reactions requiring immediate discontinuation of TAXOTERE may occur (see Hypersensitivity Reactions).

Treatment related acute myeloid leukemia may occur. No studies have been conducted to assess the carcinogenic potential of TAXOTERE (see Acute Myeloid Leukemia/Myelodysplastic Syndrome and Carcinogenesis and Mutagenesis).

General: All patients should be premedicated with an oral corticosteroid such as dexamethasone 16 mg per day (e.g., 8 mg BID) for 3 days starting one day prior to TAXOTERE administration to reduce the incidence and severity of fluid retention as well as the severity of hypersensitivity reactions.

The pretreatment regimen for prostate cancer (given the concurrent use of prednisone or prednisolone) is oral dexamethasone 8 mg, 12 hours, 3 hours and 1 hour before the TAXOTERE infusion (see Dosage and Administration, Premedication).

Concomitant use of TAXOTERE and drugs that inhibit CYP3A4 may increase exposure to docetaxel and should be avoided. In patients receiving treatment with TAXOTERE, close monitoring for toxicity and a TAXOTERE dose reduction could be considered if systemic administration of a potent CYP3A4 inhibitor cannot be avoided (see Drug Interactions).

There are no clinical data with a dose adjustment in patients receiving strong CYP3A4 inhibitors. Based on extrapolation from a pharmacokinetic study with ketoconazole in 7 patients, consider a 50% docetaxel dose reduction if patients require coadministration of a strong CYP3A4 inhibitor.

Acute Myeloid Leukemia/Myelodysplastic Syndrome: Treatment related acute myeloid leukemia may occur. In the adjuvant breast cancer trial (TAX316) at a median follow-up of 83 months, 3 of 744 women who received TAXOTERE, doxorubicin and cyclophosphamide (TAC) were diagnosed with AML and one additional patient was diagnosed with suspected MDS. One of 736 women who received 5-fluorouracil, doxorubicin and cyclophosphamide (FAC) in the other arm of this study was diagnosed with AML.

In patients treated with TAXOTERE, doxorubicin and cyclophosphamide (TAC) as adjuvant therapy for breast cancer, the risk of delayed myelodysplasia or myeloid leukemia requires hematological follow-up (see Adverse Reactions).

Carcinogenesis and Mutagenesis: TAXOTERE has been shown to be mutagenic in the in vitro chromosome aberration test in CHO-K1 cells and in the in vivo micronucleus test in the mouse.

The carcinogenic potential of TAXOTERE has not been studied. However, given that TAXOTERE is unequivocally genotoxic, it should be presumed to be a human carcinogen.

Fluid Retention: Severe fluid retention has been reported following TAXOTERE therapy. Therefore, patients should be premedicated with oral corticosteroids prior to each TAXOTERE administration to reduce the incidence and severity of fluid retention (see Dosage and Administration). Patients with preexisting severe fluid retention such as pleural effusion, pericardial effusion and ascites should be closely monitored from the first dose for the possible exacerbation of the effusions.

Hematologic: Neutropenia is the most frequently reported adverse event. Neutrophil nadirs occurred at a median of 7 days but this interval may be shorter in heavily pretreated patients. TAXOTERE therapy should not be administered until the neutrophil count is over 1500 cells/mm³. In order to monitor the occurrence of myelotoxicity, it is recommended that frequent blood cell counts be performed on all patients receiving TAXOTERE. Patients should not be retreated with subsequent cycles of TAXOTERE until neutrophils recover to a level of >1500 cells/mm³. In cases of severe neutropenia (<500 cells/mm³) for seven days or more during a course of TAXOTERE therapy, a reduction in dose for subsequent courses of therapy or the use of appropriate systematic measures are recommended (see Dosage and Administration).

Hepatic: In patients treated with TAXOTERE at 100 mg/m² as a single agent who have transaminase (ALT and/or AST) greater than 1.5 times the upper limit of normal (ULN) concurrent with alkaline phosphatase greater than 2.5 times the ULN, there is a higher risk of developing severe adverse reactions such as toxic deaths including sepsis and gastrointestinal hemorrhage which can be fatal, febrile neutropenia, infections, thrombocytopenia, stomatitis and asthenia. If TAXOTERE is considered essential for a patient with above specified hepatic function impairment, the recommended dose of TAXOTERE in patients with elevated liver function test (LFTs) is 75 mg/m² and LFTs should be measured at baseline and before each cycle (see Dosage and Administration).

No data are available in patients with hepatic impairment treated by TAXOTERE in combination.

Hypersensitivity Reactions: Severe hypersensitivity reactions characterized by severe hypotension, bronchospasm, generalized rash/erythema or very rarely fatal anaphylaxis have been reported in patients who received premedication. These reactions resulted in immediate discontinuation in approximately 0.4% (5 of 1260) of patients. Severe symptoms resolve after discontinuation of the infusion and administration of appropriate therapy.

Patients should be observed closely for hypersensitivity reactions especially during the first and second infusions. Hypersensitivity reactions may occur within a few minutes following the initiation of the infusion of TAXOTERE, thus facilities for the treatment of hypotension and bronchospasm should be available. Severe reactions require immediate discontinuation of TAXOTERE and aggressive therapy. Patients who have developed severe hypersensitivity reactions should not be rechallenged with TAXOTERE. If minor reactions such as flushing or localized skin reactions occur, therapy with TAXOTERE does not have to be discontinued. All patients should be premedicated with an oral corticosteroid prior to the initiation of the infusion of TAXOTERE (see Dosage and Administration).

Neurologic: The development of severe peripheral neurotoxicity is infrequent and requires a reduction in dose (see Dosage and Administration). If symptoms persist, treatment should be discontinued.

Renal: A dose reduction of Xeloda (capecitabine) to 75% is recommended when used in combination with docetaxel in patients with moderate renal impairment (please refer to Xeloda Product Monograph).

Skin: Localized erythema of the extremities (palm of the hands and soles of the feet) with edema, followed by desquamation has been observed. In case of severe skin toxicity during a course of TAXOTERE therapy, a reduction in dose for subsequent courses of therapy is recommended (see Dosage and Administration).

Special Populations: Pregnant Women: TAXOTERE may cause fetal harm when administered to a pregnant woman. There is no information on the use of TAXOTERE during pregnancy. No evidence of teratogenic effect was found when TAXOTERE was administered at 1.8 or 1.2 mg/m²/day, in rats or rabbits, respectively. However, TAXOTERE has been shown to be both embryotoxic and fetotoxic in rabbits and rats—causing intrauterine mortality, reduced fetal weight and fetal ossification delays—and to reduce fertility in rats. These effects are consistent with maternal toxicity. As with other cytotoxic drugs, TAXOTERE may cause fetal harm when administered to pregnant women. Therefore, TAXOTERE must not be used during pregnancy. Women of childbearing age and receiving TAXOTERE should be advised to avoid becoming pregnant, and to inform the treating physician immediately should this occur. Should TAXOTERE be used during pregnancy, or if the patient becomes pregnant while receiving this drug, the patient should be apprised of the potential hazard to the fetus.

Nursing Women: It is not known whether TAXOTERE is excreted in human milk. Because many drugs are excreted in human milk, and because of the potential for serious adverse reactions in nursing infants from TAXOTERE, it is recommended that women be advised not to breast-feed during TAXOTERE therapy.

Pediatrics: The safety and effectiveness of TAXOTERE in children have not been established.

Geriatrics: Those with poor performance status, or otherwise non-life threatening indolent disease (such as relatively asymptomatic metastatic disease limited to the bone) should be considered as possible candidates for less toxic therapies prior to consideration of a TAXOTERE based therapy.

An analysis of safety data in patients equal or greater than 60 years of age showed an increase in the incidence of treatment-related grade 3 and 4 adverse events when treated with TAXOTERE in combination with Xeloda. Treatment-related serious adverse events and early withdrawals from treatment due to adverse events were lower in patients of less than 60 years of age.

Of the 332 patients treated with TAXOTERE every three weeks plus prednisone in the prostate cancer study (TAX327), 208 patients were 65 years of age or greater and 67 patients were older than 75 years. In patients treated with TAXOTERE every three weeks, the following TEAEs occurred at rates ≥10% higher in patients 65 years of age or greater compared to younger patients: anemia (71% vs 59%) infection (37% vs 24%), nail changes (34% vs 23%), anorexia (21% vs 10%), weight loss (15% vs 5%) respectively.

ADVERSE REACTIONS: Clinical Trial Experience: TAXOTERE (Docetaxel for Injection) as a Single Agent: Adverse Drug Reaction Overview: Two thousand one hundred and six (2106) patients received an initial dose of 100 mg/m² of TAXOTERE as a single agent over a one-hour infusion independently of the pre-medication for the treatment of various tumor types. The patients were enrolled in 40 clinical trials conducted in North America and Europe (breast carcinoma, n=991; non-small cell lung cancer, n=634). Table 1 lists adverse reaction data from 2045 patients with normal LFTs at baseline and 61 patients with elevated LFTs at baseline.

Additionally, 96 patients enrolled in 3 clinical trials received an initial dose of 100 mg/m² of TAXOTERE as a single agent over a one-hour infusion every 3 weeks for the treatment of recurrent and/or metastatic squamous cell carcinoma of the head and neck.

These reactions were considered possibly or probably related to TAXOTERE. The safety profile is generally similar in all patients whether they were treated for breast carcinoma or for other tumor types (e.g. ovarian cancer).

Clinical Trials Adverse Drug Reactions:

Table 1: TAXOTERE

Summary of Adverse Events in Patients Receiving TAXOTERE as a Single Agent

	TAXOTERE as Single Agent (100 mg/m²)		
	Various Tumor Types Including: Breast Carcinoma, Non-Small Cell Lung Cancer and Ovarian Cancer		Squamous Cell Carcinoma of the Head and Neck
	Normal LFTs[a] at Baseline N=2045 (%)	Elevated LFTs at Baseline N=61 (%)	Normal LFTs[a] at Baseline N=96 (%)
Alopecia	75.8	62.3	85.4
Arthralgia			
All Grades	9.2	6.6	5.5 [n=54]
Severe	0.6	0	0 [n=54]
Asthenia			

(cont'd)

Table 1: TAXOTERE *(cont'd)*

Summary of Adverse Events in Patients Receiving TAXOTERE as a Single Agent

	TAXOTERE as Single Agent (100 mg/m²)		
	Various Tumor Types Including: Breast Carcinoma, Non-Small Cell Lung Cancer and Ovarian Cancer		Squamous Cell Carcinoma of the Head and Neck
	Normal LFTs[a] at Baseline N=2045 (%)	Elevated LFTs at Baseline N=61 (%)	Normal LFTs[a] at Baseline N=96 (%)
All Grades	61.8	52.5	63.5
Severe	12.8	24.6	20.8
Cutaneous			
All Grades	47.6	57.4	39.6
Grades III-IV	4.8	9.8	3.1
Fever in Absence of Infection			
All Grades	32.1	41.0	29.2 [n=65]
Grades III-IV	2.1	8.2	1.5 [n=65]
Fluid Retention			
All Grades	47.0	54.1	28.1
Severe	6.9	9.8	4.2
Gastrointestinal			
Nausea (All)	38.9	37.7	19.8[c]
Severe (Grades III-IV)	3.9	4.9	—
Diarrhea (All)	39.0	32.8	15.6
Severe (Grades III-IV)	4.7	4.9	—
Vomiting (All)	22.3	23.0	15.6[c]
Severe (Grades III-IV)	2.7	4.9	—
Hypersensitivity Reactions			
All Grades	21.0	19.7	16.7
Severe	4.2	9.8	3.1
Infusion Site Reaction			
All Grades	4.4	3.3	—
Myalgia			
All Grades	18.9	16.4	16.7 [n=66]
Severe	1.5	1.6	0 [n=66]
Nail Changes			
All Grades	30.6	23.0	28.1
Severe	2.5	4.9	—
Neuromotor			
All Grades	13.8	6.6	7.1 [n=41]
Grades III-IV	3.6	1.6	1.0 [n=41]
Neurosensory			
All Grades	49.3	34.4	37.9 [n=66]
Grade III	4.3	0	3.1 [n=66][b]
Non-septic Death	0.3	6.6	NR
Septic Death	1.4	3.3	1.0
Stomatitis			
All Grades	41.7	49.2	29.2

(cont'd)

Table 1: TAXOTERE *(cont'd)*

Summary of Adverse Events in Patients Receiving TAXOTERE as a Single Agent

	TAXOTERE as Single Agent (100 mg/m²)		
	Various Tumor Types Including: Breast Carcinoma, Non-Small Cell Lung Cancer and Ovarian Cancer		Squamous Cell Carcinoma of the Head and Neck
	Normal LFTs[a] at Baseline N=2045 (%)	Elevated LFTs at Baseline N=61 (%)	Normal LFTs[a] at Baseline N=96 (%)
Grades III-IV	5.5	13.1	6.3

[a] Normal liver function tests (LFTs): transaminase ≤1.5 times upper limit of normal or alkaline phosphatase ≤2.5 times upper limit of normal or isolated elevations of transaminase or alkaline phosphatase up to 5 times upper limit of normal.
[b] Includes 2 patients who were counted as having peripheral neuropathy.
[c] Includes one patient with combined nausea/vomiting.
Legend: NR=not reported.

Table 2: TAXOTERE

Summary of Haematologic Adverse Events in Patients Receiving TAXOTERE as a Single Agent

	TAXOTERE as Single Agent (100 mg/m²)		
	Various Tumor Types Including: Breast Carcinoma, Non-Small Cell Lung Cancer and Ovarian Cancer		Squamous Cell Carcinoma of the Head and Neck
	Normal LFTs[a] at Baseline N=2045 (%)	Elevated LFTs at Baseline N=61 (%)	Normal LFTs[a] at Baseline N=96 (%)
Anemia <11 g/dL	90.4	91.8	90.8 [n=65]
Grades III IV <8 g/dL	8.8	31.2	0 [n=65]
Febrile Neutropenia	11.0	24.5	24.0[b]
Infection			
All Grades	21.6	32.8	—
Grades III-IV	6.1	16.4	—
Leukopenia <4000 cells/mm³	95.6	98.3	86.3 [n=95]
Grade IV <1000 cells/mm³	31.6	46.6	20.0 [n=95]
Neutropenia <2000 cells/mm³	95.5	96.4	95.4 [n=65]
Grade IV <500 cells/mm³	75.4	87.5	69.2 [n=65]
Thrombocytopenia <100 000 cells/mm³	8.0	24.6	3.1 [n=65]
Grade IV	0.5	4.9	—

[a] Normal liver function tests (LFTs): transaminase ≤1.5 times upper limit of normal or alkaline phosphatase ≤2.5 times upper limit of normal or isolated elevations of transaminase or alkaline phosphatase up to 5 times upper limit of normal.
[b] Includes 16 patients who were counted as having febrile leukopenia requiring hospitalization (defined as WBC count ≤1000/µL associated with fever ≥38°C requiring hospitalization).

Cardiovascular: Hypotension occurred in 3% of the patients and required therapy in 0.5% of the patients treated with TAXOTERE as a single agent for various tumor types. Dysrhythmia occurred in 2% of the patients and was severe in 0.4% of the patients. Clinically meaningful events occurred in less than 2% of patients. These events included: heart failure (0.3%), tachycardia (1.4%) and hypertension (1.6%).

Cutaneous: Cutaneous reactions have been observed in 48% of the patients treated with TAXOTERE as a single agent for various tumor types. These reactions were characterized by a rash, including localized eruptions mainly on feet and hands (including severe hand and foot syndrome), but also on arms, face or thorax. They were frequently associated with pruritus. Eruptions generally occurred within one week following the TAXOTERE infusion, resolved before the next infusion, and were not disabling.

Severe symptoms such as eruptions followed by desquamation occurred less frequently (5%). These reactions rarely led to interruption or discontinuation of TAXOTERE treatment.

Severe nail disorders occurred in 3% of the patients treated with TAXOTERE as a single agent. These reactions were characterized by hypo- or hyperpigmentation, and infrequently onycholysis and pain.

Alopecia was observed in 76% of patients treated with TAXOTERE as a single agent for various tumor types (0.5% severe), and in 85% of patients treated for recurrent and/or metastatic SCCHN.

Fluid Retention: Fluid retention which includes edema, and less frequently, pleural effusion, ascites, pericardial effusion, and weight gain, usually begins at the lower extremities and may become generalized with a weight gain of 3 kg or more. Fluid retention is cumulative in incidence and severity (see Warnings and Precautions).

The incidence of fluid retention in patients treated with TAXOTERE as a single agent and without premedication was 81.6%; of these 22.4% were severe. In patients treated for various tumor types and premedicated for 3 days with oral corticosteroids, the incidence of fluid retention was 64.1% (6.5% were severe). Fluid retention was reported in 24% for patients treated for recurrent and/or metastatic SCCHN. Table 3 is a table describing the effect on fluid retention with corticosteroid premedication (see Dosage and Administration for premedication regimen).

Table 3: TAXOTERE

Effects of Corticosteroid Premedication on the Incidence of Fluid Retention

	Incidence	Severe
Without Premedication	81.6%	22.4%
3-Day Premedication[a]	64.1%	6.5%

[a] Fluid retention adverse reactions have been obtained from 92 patients treated with TAXOTERE as single agent, 100 mg/m² from a retrospective analysis on the 3 day premedication regimen.

In patients treated by docetaxel as single agent, at 100 mg/m², the median cumulative dose to treatment discontinuation was more than 1000 mg/m² and the median time to fluid retention reversibility was 16.4 weeks (range 0 to 42 weeks). The onset of moderate and severe retention is delayed (median cumulative dose: 818.9 mg/m²) in patients with premedication compared with patients without premedication (median cumulative dose: 489.7 mg/m²); however, it has been reported in some patients during early courses of therapy. Fluid retention has not been accompanied by oliguria or hypotension, and was slowly reversible after TAXOTERE treatment was stopped.

Gastrointestinal: Nausea (39%), diarrhea (39%) and vomiting (22%), were observed in patients treated with TAXOTERE as a single agent for various tumor types. They were less frequent in patients treated for recurrent and/or metastatic SCCHN (20%, 16% and 16% respectively). These reactions were generally mild to moderate. Severe gastrointestinal reactions generally occurred in less than 5% of the cases reported. Stomatitis was reported by 42% and by 29% of patients treated for various tumor types and for recurrent and/or metastatic SCCHN, respectively. Other gastrointestinal events included anorexia, taste perversion, constipation, abdominal pain, gastrointestinal bleeding and esophagitis.

Hematologic: Bone marrow suppression and other hematologic adverse reactions to TAXOTERE include neutropenia, febrile neutropenia, thrombocytopenia and anemia, have been reported.

Neutropenia was the most frequent adverse reaction associated with TAXOTERE; it was reversible and not cumulative. The median time to nadir was 7 days, while the median duration of severe neutropenia (<500 cells/mm³) was 7 days. Severe neutropenia occurred in 75% of the patients treated with TAXOTERE as a single agent for various tumor types and 69% in patients with recurrent and/or metastatic SCCHN.

When treated with TAXOTERE as a single agent, fever was associated with neutropenia (<500 cells/mm³) in 11% of the patients with normal liver function (3% of the cycles) treated for various tumor types and in 24% of patients treated for recurrent and/or metastatic SCCHN. The incidence of severe infections associated with neutrophil counts <500 cells/mm³ was 6% of the patients (1.3% of the cycles). Infectious episodes which included sepsis and pneumonia occurred in 22% of the patients (6% of the cycles) and were fatal in approximately 1.7% of patients treated with TAXOTERE as a single agent for various tumor types. Septic death was reported less frequently (1%) in patients treated for recurrent and/or metastatic SCCHN.

Thrombocytopenia (<100 000 cells/mm³) has been reported in 8% of the patients treated with TAXOTERE as a single agent for various tumor types and 3.1% of patients treated for recurrent and/or metastatic SCCHN. Bleeding episodes were reported in 1% of the patients; this was associated with severe thrombocytopenia (<50 000 cells/mm³) in only two patients. A fatal gastrointestinal hemorrhage due to thrombocytopenia was reported in one patient.

Anemia (<11 g/dL) was observed in 90% of the patients treated with TAXOTERE as a single agent and was severe (<8 g/dL) in 9% of the cases. It was not reported in patients treated for recurrent and/or metastatic SCCHN.

Hepatic: Increases in alanine transferase (ALT), aspartate transferase (AST), bilirubin, and alkaline phosphatase which were greater than 2.5 times the upper limit of normal were observed in less than 5% of patients treated with TAXOTERE as a single agent for various tumor types.

Hypersensitivity Reactions: Hypersensitivity reactions occurred in 21% of the patients treated with TAXOTERE as a single agent for various tumor types and in 17% of patients treated for recurrent and/or metastatic SCCHN. The reactions occurred generally within a few minutes following the start of the infusion of TAXOTERE and were usually mild to moderate. The most frequent minor manifestations were flushing, rash with or without pruritus, chest tightness, back pain, dyspnea, drug fever or chills.

Severe reactions characterized by hypotension, bronchospasm, or generalized rash/erythema have occurred within a few minutes following the initiation of infusion of TAXOTERE as a single agent. Severe symptoms were observed in 4% of the patients treated for various tumor types; however, 1.2% (25 of 2045) had immediate discontinuation of treatment. All hypersensitivity reactions resolved after discontinuation of the infusion and appropriate therapy.

Infusion Site Reactions: Infusion site reactions occurred in 6% of the patients treated with TAXOTERE as a single agent for various tumor types and were generally mild. These reactions included skin sensitivities such as hyperpigmentation, inflammation, local erythema, redness or dryness of the skin, or swelling of the vein. Phlebitis or extravasation was observed less frequently.

Neurologic: Neurosensory symptoms characterized by paresthesia, dysesthesia or pain (including burning sensation) were reported in 49% of patients treated with TAXOTERE as a single agent for various tumor types and in 38% of patients treated for recurrent and/or metastatic SCCHN. Severe reactions were observed in less than 4% of the patients.

Neuromotor events (mainly characterized by weakness) were reported in 14% of patients treated with TAXOTERE as a single agent for various tumor types. These reactions were severe in 4% of patients.

When these symptoms occur, dosage must be adjusted. If symptoms persist, treatment should be discontinued (see Dosage and Administration, Dosing Adjustment).

Patients who experienced neurotoxicity in clinical trials and for whom follow-up information on the complete resolution of the event was available, had spontaneous reversal of symptoms with a median of 81 days from onset (range 0 to 741 days).

Other: Asthenia was reported by 62% of all patients and was considered severe in 13% of patients treated for various tumor types and in 21% of patients treated for recurrent and/or metastatic SCCHN. Arthralgias (5.5% to 9%) and myalgias (19%) were reported by patients but were generally considered to be mild to moderate.

Respiratory: Dyspnea has been reported.

TAXOTERE (Docetaxel for Injection) in Combination: Adverse Drug Reaction Overview: The percentage of events related to combination therapy might be different from those related to monotherapy with TAXOTERE. Please refer to Table 4, Table 5, Table 6, Table 7 for adverse drug reactions related to different combination therapies.

Clinical Trials Adverse Drug Reactions: Adjuvant Treatment of Breast Cancer—TAXOTERE in Combination with Doxorubicin and Cyclophosphamide: Table 4 presents the treatment emergent adverse events (TEAEs) possibly or probably related to treatment observed in the TAX316 study in which 744 patients, who were treated with 75 mg/m² of TAXOTERE every 3 weeks in combination with 50 mg/m² of doxorubicin and 500 mg/m² of cyclophosphamide (TAC) and 736 were treated with the combination of 500 mg/m² of 5-fluorouracil, 50 mg/m² of doxorubicin, and 500 mg/m² of cyclophosphamide every 3 weeks (FAC).

Table 4: TAXOTERE

Clinically Important Treatment Related Adverse Events in Patients in the TAX 316 Study

	TAXOTERE (75 mg/m²) in Combination with Doxorubicin (50 mg/m²) and Cyclophosphamide (500 mg/m²) [TAC regimen] N=744 (%)		5-fluorouracil (500 mg/m²) in Combination with Doxorubicin (50 mg/m²) and Cyclophosphamide (500 mg/m²) [FAC regimen] N=736 (%)	
Adverse Event	**Any**	**Grade 3/4**	**Any**	**Grade 3/4**
Body as a Whole				
Abdominal Pain	7.3	0.5	3.3	0.0
Asthenia	79.2	11.0	69.4	5.2
Fever in Absence of Infection	43.1	1.2	13.2	0.0
Cardiovascular System				
Cardiac Dysrhythmias	3.9	0.1	2.9	0.3
Hypotension	1.5	0.0	0.5	0.0
Phlebitis	0.7	0.0	0.4	0.0
Syncope	0.5	0.0	0.4	0.0
Vasodilatation	20.3	0.9	15.9	0.4
Digestive System				
Anorexia	19.9	2.2	16.4	1.2
Constipation	22.6	0.4	21.5	1.2
Diarrhea	30.9	3.2	23.5	1.0
Nausea	80.4	5.1	87.4	9.5
Stomatitis	69.1	7.1	52.6	2.0
Vomiting	42.6	4.3	58.2	7.3
Hematologic				
Anemia	91.5	4.3	71.7	1.6
Febrile Neutropenia[a]	24.7	N/A	2.5	N/A
Lymphedema	0.3	0.0	0.0	0.0
Neutropenia	71.4	65.5	82.0	49.3
Thrombocytopenia	39.4	2.0	27.7	1.2
Immune System				
Hypersensitivity Reactions	10.5	1.1	2.2	0.0
Infections and Infestations				
Infection	27.2	3.2	17.4	1.4
Neutropenic Infection[b]	12.1	N/A	6.3	N/A
Metabolic and Nutritional Disorders				
Peripheral Edema	26.7	0.4	7.2	0.0
Weight Gain or Loss	15.2	0.3	9.2	0.0
Musculoskeletal System				
Arthralgia	15.1	0.4	5.7	0.3
Myalgia	22.8	0.8	8.0	0.0
Nervous System				
Neuro-cerebellar	1.1	0.1	0.8	0.0
Neuro-cortical	2.8	0.3	3.9	0.3
Neuropathy Motor	2.8	0.0	1.5	0.0
Neuropathy Sensory	23.8	0.0	7.9	0.0
Respiratory System				
Cough	3.1	0.0	2.2	0.1
Skin and Appendages				
Alopecia	97.7	N/A	97.1	N/A
Nail Disorders	18.4	0.4	13.9	0.1
Skin Toxicity	18.4	0.7	10.9	0.3
Special Senses				
Conjunctivitis	4.6	0.3	6.0	0.1
Lacrimation Disorder	9.8	0.1	6.4	0.0
Taste Perversion	27.4	0.7	15.1	0.0
Urogenital System				
Amenorrhea	57.6	N/A	48.1	N/A

(cont'd)

[a] Febrile neutropenia was defined as grade ≥2 NCI term "fever in absence of infection" (oral temperature ≥38.1°C) concomitant (i.e., measured within 24 hours) with grade 4 neutropenia (ANC <0.5×10⁹/L), requiring IV antibiotics and/or hospitalization.

[b] Neutropenic infection was defined as grade ≥2 NCI term "infection" concomitant (i.e., measured within 24 hours) with grade ≥3 neutropenia (ANC <1.0×10⁹/L).

Of the 744 patients treated with TAC in the TAX316 study, 33.1% experienced severe TEAEs possibly or probably related to treatment compared to 22.1% of the 736 patients treated with FAC. Dose reductions due to hematologic toxicity occurred in 1% of cycles in the TAC arm compared to 0.1% of cycles in the FAC arm. Six percent of patients treated with TAC discontinued treatment due to adverse events, compared to 1.1% treated with FAC; fever in the absence of infection and allergy being the most common reasons for withdrawal among TAC-treated patients. Two TAC-treated patients died within 30 days of their last study treatment; 1 death was considered to be related to study drug. Two FAC-treated patients died within 30 days of their last study treatment; 1 death was considered to be related to study drug.

Fever and Infection: Treatment related fever in the absence of infection was seen in 43.1% (Gr 3/4: 1.2%) of TAC-treated patients and in 13.2% (Gr 3/4: 0.0%) of FAC-treated patients. Treatment related infection was seen in 27.2% (Gr 3/4: 3.2%) of TAC-treated patients and in 17.4% (Gr 3/4: 1.4%) of FAC-treated patients. There were no septic deaths in either treatment arm. G-CSF was used as treatment or secondary prophylaxis in 29.2% of TAC-treated patients compared to 5.6% of FAC-treated patients.

Gastrointestinal Events: In addition to gastrointestinal events reflected in Table 4, 4 patients in the TAC treatment arm and 1 patient in the FAC treatment arm were reported to have treatment related colitis/enteritis/large intestine perforation. Two of the 4 TAC-treated patients required treatment discontinuations; no deaths due to these events occurred.

Cardiovascular Events: More cardiovascular events were reported in the TAC arm than in the FAC arm: treatment related dysrhythmias, all grades (3.9% vs 2.9%), treatment related hypotension, all grades (1.5% vs 0.5%) and clinically significant treatment-emergent congestive heart failure (CHF), cardiac function grade 3-4 (1.6% vs 0.5%). One TAC-treated patient died due to heart failure. While left ventricular ejection fraction (LVEF) was measured at baseline as a study requirement in the TAX316 study, repeat measurements were not performed unless considered clinically relevant by the investigator. Of the patients with repeat LVEF assessment, 14/66 (21%) in the TAC treatment group and 4/48 (8.3%) in the FAC treatment group were reported to have LVEF declines to levels below the lower limit of normal.

Acute Myeloid Leukemia/Myelodysplastic Syndrome: At a median follow-up time of 83 months, 3 of 744 patients treated with TAC were diagnosed with acute myeloid leukemia (AML) and one additional patient was diagnosed with suspected myelodysplastic syndrome (MDS). In the other arm of the study, one of 736 patients treated with FAC was diagnosed with AML. In the MDS case, the chromosome abnormality t(11; 14)(q23;q24) was present. In two of the TAC-associated AML cases, abnormalities of chromosome 11 were present.

Other Persistent Reactions: The following events were observed to be ongoing at the median follow-up time of 55 months: alopecia (22/687), amenorrhea (133/233), neurosensory (9/73) and peripheral edema (18/112).

Locally-advanced and/or Metastatic Breast Cancer—TAXOTERE in Combination with Doxorubicin: Table 5 and Table 6 show data from a combination study with TAXOTERE and doxorubicin in patients with locally advanced and/or metastatic breast cancer. In this study, 258 patients received 75 mg/m² of TAXOTERE with 50 mg/m² of doxorubicin.

Table 5: TAXOTERE

Summary of Adverse Events Possibly or Probably Related to Study Treatment in Patients with Locally-advanced and/or Metastatic Breast Cancer Receiving TAXOTERE in Combination with Doxorubicin

	TAXOTERE in Combination (75 mg/m²) with Doxorubicin (50 mg/m²) N=258 (%)
Alopecia	94.6
Arthralgia	
All Grades	5.4
Severe	0.4
Asthenia	
All Grades	54.7
Severe	8.1
Cutaneous	
All Grades	13.6
Grades III-IV	0
Fever in Absence of Infection	
All Grades	50.4[a]
Grades III-IV	0.4[a]
Fluid Retention	
All Grades	35.7
Severe	1.2
Gastrointestinal	
Nausea (All)	64.0
Severe (Grades III-IV)	5.0
Diarrhea (All)	45.7
Severe (Grades III-IV)	6.2
Vomiting (All)	45.0
Severe (Grades III-IV)	5.0
Hypersensitivity Reactions	
All Grades	4.7
Severe	1.2
Infusion Site Reaction	
All Grades	3.5
Myalgia	
All Grades	8.5
Severe	0
Nail Changes	
All Grades	20.2

(cont'd)

Table 5: TAXOTERE *(cont'd)*

Summary of Adverse Events Possibly or Probably Related to Study Treatment in Patients with Locally-advanced and/or Metastatic Breast Cancer Receiving TAXOTERE in Combination with Doxorubicin

	TAXOTERE in Combination (75 mg/m²) with Doxorubicin (50 mg/m²) N=258 (%)
Severe	0.4
Neuromotor	
All Grades	2.3
Grades III-IV	0.4
Neurosensory	
All Grades	30.2
Grade III	0.4
Non-septic Death	2.3
Septic Death	0
Stomatitis	
All Grades	58.1
Grades III-IV	7.8

[a] In study TAX 306 (n=213), it included febrile neutropenia.

Table 6: TAXOTERE

Summary of Haematologic Adverse Events Possibly or Probably Related to Study Treatment in Patients with Locally-advanced and/or Metastatic Breast Cancer Receiving TAXOTERE in Combination with Doxorubicin

	TAXOTERE in Combination (75 mg/m²) with Doxorubicin (50 mg/m²) N=258 (%)
Anemia <11 g/dL	96.1
Grades III-IV <8 g/dL	9.4
Febrile Neutropenia	34.1
Infection	
All Grades	35.3
Grades III-IV	7.8
Leukopenia <4000 cells/mm³	99.6
Grade IV <1000 cells/mm³	53.5
Neutropenia <2000 cells/mm³	99.2
Grade IV <500 cells/mm³	91.7
Thrombocytopenia <100 000 cells/mm³	28.1
Grade IV	0.8

Locally-advanced and/or Metastatic Breast Cancer—TAXOTERE in Combination with Capecitabine: The following text and Table 7 provide data for the combination study with TAXOTERE and capecitabine in 506 patients with locally advanced and/or metastatic breast cancer. In the TAXOTERE-capecitabine combination arm (251 patients), the treatment was capecitabine administered orally 1250 mg/m² twice daily as intermittent therapy (2 weeks of treatment followed by one week without treatment) for at least 6 weeks and TAXOTERE administered as a 1 hour intravenous infusion at a dose of 75 mg/m² on the first day of each 3 week cycle for at least 6 weeks. In the monotherapy arm (255 patients), TAXOTERE was administered as a one-hour intravenous infusion at a dose of 100 mg/m² on the first day of each 3 week cycle for at least 6 weeks. The mean duration of treatment was 129 days in the combination arm and 98 days in the monotherapy arm. A total of 66 patients (26%) in the combination arm and 49 (19%) in the monotherapy arm withdrew from the study because of adverse events. The percentage of patients requiring dose reductions due to adverse events were 65% in the combination arm and 36% in the monotherapy arm. The hospitalization rate for treatment-related adverse events was 28.7% in the combination arm and 26.3% in the monotherapy arm.

Table 7: TAXOTERE

Adverse Events Considered Related to Treatment in ≥5% of Patients Participating in the Combination Study of TAXOTERE and Capecitabine in Patients with Locally-advanced and/or Metastatic Breast Cancer

Adverse Event	Capecitabine 1250 mg/m²/bid (Intermittent Regimen) with TAXOTERE 75 mg/m²/3 weeks (N=251)			TAXOTERE 100 mg/m²/3 weeks (N=255)		
	NCIC Grade					
Body System/Adverse Event	**Total %**	**Grade 3 %**	**Grade 4 %**	**Total %**	**Grade 3 %**	**Grade 4 %**
GI						
Stomatitis	67	17.1	0.4	43	4.7	—
Diarrhea	64	13.5	0.4	45	5.4	0.4

(cont'd)

Table 7: TAXOTERE *(cont'd)*

Adverse Events Considered Related to Treatment in ≥5% of Patients Participating in the Combination Study of TAXOTERE and Capecitabine in Patients with Locally-advanced and/or Metastatic Breast Cancer

Adverse Event	Capecitabine 1250 mg/m²/bid (Intermittent Regimen) with TAXOTERE 75 mg/m²/3 weeks (N=251)			TAXOTERE 100 mg/m²/3 weeks (N=255)		
	NCIC Grade					
Body System/Adverse Event	**Total %**	**Grade 3 %**	**Grade 4 %**	**Total %**	**Grade 3 %**	**Grade 4 %**
Nausea	43	6.4	—	35	2	—
Vomiting	33	3.6	0.8	22	0.8	—
Constipation	14	1.2	—	12	—	—
Abdominal Pain	14	2	—	9	0.8	—
Dyspepsia	12	—	—	5	0.4	—
Abdominal Pain Upper	9	—	—	6	—	—
Dry Mouth	5	0.4	—	4	—	—
Skin and Subcutaneous						
Hand-and-Foot Syndrome	63	24.3	—	8	12	—
Alopecia	41	6	—	42	6.7	—
Nail Disorder	14	2	—	15	—	—
Dermatitis	8	—	—	9	0.8	—
Rash Erythematous	8	0.4	—	4	—	—
Nail Discolouration	6	—	—	4	0.4	—
Onycholysis	5	1.2	—	5	0.8	—
Pruritus	2	—	—	5	—	—
General						
Pyrexia	21	0.8	—	29	0.4	—
Asthenia	23	3.2	0.4	22	5.5	—
Fatigue	21	4.4	—	25	5.1	—
Weakness	13	1.2	—	9	2	—
Pain in Limb	9	0.4	—	8	0.4	—
Lethargy	6	—	—	5	1.2	—
Pain	6	—	—	2	—	—
Neurological						
Taste Disturbance	15	0.4	—	14	0.4	—
Headache	7	0.4	—	8	—	—
Paraesthesia	11	0.4	—	15	0.8	—
Dizziness	9	—	—	6	0.4	—
Insomnia	4	—	—	5	0.4	—
Peripheral Neuropathy	5	—	—	10	0.8	—
Hypoaesthesia	4	—	—	7	0.4	—
Metabolism						
Anorexia	12	0.8	—	10	0.8	—
Appetite Decreased	10	—	—	4	—	—
Dehydration	8	2	—	5	0.4	0.4
Eyes						
Lacrimation Increased	12	—	—	5	—	—
Musculoskeletal						
Arthralgia	11	1.2	—	18	2.4	—
Myalgia	14	1.6	—	24	2	—
Back Pain	7	0.8	—	6	0.8	—
Cardiac						

(cont'd)

Table 7: TAXOTERE *(cont'd)*

Adverse Events Considered Related to Treatment in ≥5% of Patients Participating in the Combination Study of TAXOTERE and Capecitabine in Patients with Locally-advanced and/or Metastatic Breast Cancer

Adverse Event	Capecitabine 1250 mg/m²/bid (Intermittent Regimen) with TAXOTERE 75 mg/m²/3 weeks (N=251)			TAXOTERE 100 mg/m²/3 weeks (N=255)		
	NCIC Grade					
Body System/Adverse Event	**Total %**	**Grade 3 %**	**Grade 4 %**	**Total %**	**Grade 3 %**	**Grade 4 %**
Edema Lower Limb	14	0.8	—	12	1.2	—
Edema NOS	4	—	—	5	—	0.8
Edema Peripheral	4	—	—	5	0.4	—
Hematologic						
Neutropenia	17	4.8	10.8	16	2.7	11.8
Neutropenic Fever	16	2.8	13.1	21	4.7	16.1
Anaemia	13	2.8	0.8	11	3.9	—
Respiratory						
Dyspnea	7	0.8	—	9	0.4	—
Cough	6	0.4	—	9	—	—
Sore Throat	11	1.6	—	7	0.4	—
Epistaxis	5	0.4	—	5	—	—
Infections and Infestations						
Oral Candidiasis	6	0.4	—	7	0.4	—

Cutaneous: Hand-and-foot syndrome was more **common** in patients in the combination therapy arm than in the TAXOTERE monotherapy arm (63% vs 8%).

Hematology: In 251 patients who received TAXOTERE in combination with capecitabine, 68% had grade 3 or 4 neutropenia, 2.8% had grade 3 or 4 thrombocytopenia and 9.6% had grade 3 or 4 anemia.

Hyperbilirubinemia: In 251 patients who received a combination of capecitabine and TAXOTERE, grade 3 and 4 hyperbilirubinemia occurred in 6.8% (n=17) and 2% (n=5), respectively.

Table 8: TAXOTERE

Patients with Laboratory Abnormalities Participating in the Combination Study of TAXOTERE with Capecitabine in Patients with Locally-advanced and/or Metastatic Breast Cancer

Adverse Event	Capecitabine 1250 mg/m²/bid (Intermittent Regimen) with TAXOTERE 75 mg/m²/3 weeks (N=251)			TAXOTERE 100 mg/m²/3 weeks (N=255)		
Body System/Adverse Event	**Total %**	**Grade 3 %**	**Grade 4 %**	**Total %**	**Grade 3 %**	**Grade 4 %**
Hematologic						
Leukopenia	91	37	24	88	42	33
Neutropenia/Granulocytopenia	86	20	49	87	10	66
Thrombocytopenia	41	2	7	23	1	2
Anemia	80	7	3	83	5	<1
Lymphocytopenia	99	48	41	98	44	40
Hepatobiliary						
Hyperbilirubinemia	20	7	2	6	2	2

Shown below by body system are the adverse events in <5% of patients in the overall clinical trial safety database of 251 patients reported as related to the administration of capecitabine in combination with TAXOTERE and that were clinically at least remotely relevant. In parentheses is the incidence of grade 3 and 4 occurrences of each adverse event.

Cardiovascular: supraventricular tachycardia (0.39), hypotension (1.20), venous phlebitis and thrombophlebitis (0.39), blood pressure increase (0.39), postural hypotension (0.80).

Gastrointestinal: hemorrhoids (0.39), ileus (0.39), necrotizing enterocolitis (0.39), esophageal ulcer (0.39), hemorrhagic diarrhea (0.80).

General: rigors (0.39), injection site infection (0.39), neuralgia (0.39).

Hematologic: agranulocytosis (0.39), prothrombin decreased (0.39).

Hepatobiliary: jaundice (0.39), abnormal liver function tests (0.39), hepatic failure (0.39), hepatic coma (0.39), hepatotoxicity (0.39).

Immune System: hypersensitivity (1.20).

Infections: neutropenic sepsis (2.39), lower respiratory tract infection nos (0.39), pharyngitis (0.39), otitis media (0.39), sepsis (0.39), bronchopneumonia (0.39).

Neurological: ataxia (0.39), syncope (1.20), taste loss (0.80), polyneuropathy (0.39), migraine (0.39).

Renal: renal failure (0.39).

Prostate Cancer—TAXOTERE in Combination with Prednisone or Prednisolone: The following data are based on the experience of 332 patients, who were treated with TAXOTERE 75 mg/m² every 3 weeks in combination with prednisone or prednisolone 5 mg orally twice daily (see Table 9).

Table 9: TAXOTERE

Clinically Important Treatment-related Adverse Events in Patients with Prostate Cancer who Received TAXOTERE in Combination with Prednisone or Prednisolone (TAX 327)

Body System/Adverse Event	TAXOTERE 75 mg/m² Every 3 Weeks with Prednisone (or Prednisolone) 5 mg Twice Daily (N=332)	
	NCI Grade	
	Total %	Grade 3/4 %
Alopecia	65.1	—
Allergic Reactions	6.9	0.6
Anemia	66.5	4.9
Anorexia	12.7	0.6
Arthralgia	3.0	0.3
Cardiac Left Ventricular Function Decrease	3.9	0.3
Cough	1.2	0.0
Diarrhea	24.1	1.2
Dyspnea	4.5	0.6
Epistaxis	3.0	0.0
Fatigue	42.8	3.9
Febrile Neutropenia	2.7	—
Fluid Retention	24.4	0.6
Infection	12.0	3.3
Myalgia	6.9	0.3
Nail Changes	28.3	—
Nausea	35.5	2.4
Neuropathy Motor	3.9	0.0
Neuropathy Sensory	27.4	1.2
Neutropenia	40.9	32.0
Rash/Desquamation	3.3	0.3
Stomatitis/Pharyngitis	17.8	0.9
Taste Disturbance	17.5	—
Tearing	9.3	0.6
Thrombocytopenia	3.4	0.6
Vomiting	13.3	1.2

Of the 332 patients treated with TAXOTERE every three weeks in the prostate cancer study (TAX 327), 208 patients were 65 years of age or greater and 67 patients were older than 75 years. In patients treated with TAXOTERE every three weeks, the incidence of anemia, infection, nail changes, anorexia, weight loss, regardless of relationship to TAXOTERE, occurred at rates ≥10% higher in patients who were 65 years of age or greater compared to younger patients. Fatigue, all grades, was one of the most commonly reported TEAEs (regardless of relationship to TAXOTERE in patients treated with TAXOTERE every three weeks, but grade 3-4 were experienced in only 1.6% of subjects <65 years old, 6.3% in those ≥65 years, and 10.4% in those ≥75 years old. Similarly diarrhea, all grades, was also commonly reported, but the incidence of grade 3-4 diarrhea was much lower for each age category, 1.6%, 2.4% and 3.0% respectively. There was a similar pattern for the incidence of infection grade 3-4, in the three age categories the incidence was 4.0%, 6.7%, and 9.0%, respectively.

Post-Market Adverse Drug Reactions: Acute Myeloid Leukemia/Myelodysplastic Syndrome: Cases of acute myeloid leukemia (AML) and myelodysplastic syndrome (MDS) have been reported in association with TAXOTERE when used in combination with other chemotherapy agents and/or radiotherapy.

Cardiovascular: Cases of venous thromboembolic events and myocardial infarction have been reported.

Cutaneous: Cases of cutaneous lupus erythematosus and bullous eruptions such as erythema multiforme, Stevens-Johnson syndrome, toxic epidermal necrolysis, and scleroderma-like changes usually preceded by peripheral lymphedema have been reported with TAXOTERE. In some cases, multiple factors such as concomitant infections, concomitant medications and underlying disease may have contributed to the development of these effects.

Fluid Retention: Dehydration and pulmonary oedema have been reported.

Gastrointestinal: Cases of gastrointestinal perforation, dehydration as a consequence of gastrointestinal events, ischemic colitis, colitis and neutropenic enterocolitis have been reported.

Cases of ileus and intestinal obstruction have been reported.

Hematologic: Disseminated intravascular coagulation (DIC), often in association with sepsis, or multiorgan failure, has been reported.

Hepatic: Cases of hepatitis, sometimes fatal primarily in patients with pre-existing liver disorders, have been reported.

Hypersensitivity Reactions: Cases of severe hypersensitivity reactions/anaphylactic shock have been reported. Cases of anaphylactic shock with a fatal outcome have been reported in patients who received premedication.

Neurologic: Cases of convulsion or transient loss of consciousness have been observed with TAXOTERE administration. These reactions sometimes appear during the infusion of the drug.

Ophthalmologic: Cases of lacrimation with or without conjunctivitis have been reported and cases of lacrimal duct obstruction resulting in excessive tearing have been reported primarily in patients receiving other anti-tumor agents concomitantly. Cases of transient visual disturbances (flashes, flashing lights, scotomata) typically occurring during drug infusion and in association with hypersensitivity reactions have been reported. These were reversible upon discontinuation of the infusion.

Other: Generalised and localised pain including chest pain without any cardiac or respiratory involvement.

Ototoxicity and Hearing Disorders: Ear and labyrinth disorders include cases of ototoxicity, hearing disorders and/or hearing loss which have been reported, including cases associated with other ototoxic drugs.

Renal: Cases of renal insufficiency, including renal failure, have been reported in clinical trials with docetaxel, and they are typically associated with concomitant nephrotoxic drugs.

Respiratory: Acute respiratory distress syndrome, interstitial pneumonia, pulmonary fibrosis and radiation recall phenomena have been reported. Cases of radiation pneumonitis have been reported in patients receiving concomitant radiotherapy.

DRUG INTERACTIONS: There have been no formal clinical studies to evaluate the drug interactions of TAXOTERE with other medications. In vitro studies have shown that the metabolism of TAXOTERE may be modified by the concomitant administration of compounds, which induce, inhibit or are metabolised by (and thus may inhibit the enzyme competitively) cytochrome P450-3A such as cyclosporine, terfenadine, ketoconazole, erythromycin and troleandomycin. As a result, caution should be exercised when treating patients with these drugs as concomitant therapy since there is a potential for a significant interaction. There is no evidence of a pharmacokinetic interaction between TAXOTERE and doxorubicin.

TAXOTERE is highly protein bound (>95%). Although the possible in vivo interaction of TAXOTERE with concomitantly administered medication has not been investigated formally, in vitro interactions with tightly protein-bound drugs, such as erythromycin, diphenhydramine, propranolol, propafenone, phenytoin, salicylate, sulfamethoxazole and sodium valproate did not affect protein binding of TAXOTERE. TAXOTERE did not influence the binding of digoxin.

The effect of daily oral prednisone administration on the pharmacokinetics of TAXOTERE administered with dexamethasone premedication prior to infusion has been evaluated in 42 patients treated for prostate cancer. No effect of prednisone on the pharmacokinetics of TAXOTERE was observed.

The exposure of docetaxel increased 2.2-fold when it was coadministered with ketoconazole, a potent inhibitor of CYP3A4. Protease inhibitors, particularly ritonavir, may increase the exposure of docetaxel. Concomitant use of TAXOTERE and drugs that inhibit CYP3A4 may increase exposure to docetaxel and should be avoided. In patients receiving treatment with TAXOTERE, close monitoring for toxicity and a TAXOTERE dose reduction could be considered if systemic administration of a potent CYP3A4 inhibitor cannot be avoided.

The pharmacokinetics of docetaxel given in combination with doxorubicin and cyclophosphamide, have been studied in 30 patients treated for advanced breast cancer. There was no evidence of a pharmacokinetic interaction between the three drugs.

DOSAGE AND ADMINISTRATION: Recommended Dose: Metastatic Breast Cancer, Non-Small Cell Lung Cancer, Ovarian Cancer, and Squamous Cell Carcinoma of the Head and Neck: The recommended dosage of TAXOTERE (docetaxel for injection) is 100 mg/m² administered as a one-hour infusion every 3 weeks. When used in combination, TAXOTERE is administered at the recommended dosage of 75 mg/m².

Prostate Cancer: The recommended dosage of TAXOTERE is 75 mg/m² administered as a one-hour infusion every 3 weeks. Concomitant treatment with prednisone or prednisolone 5 mg orally twice daily is administered continuously.

Adjuvant Treatment of Operable Node-Positive Breast Cancer: The TAXOTERE (docetaxel for injection) dose is 75 mg/m² administered 1-hour after doxorubicin 50 mg/m² and cyclophosphamide 500 mg/m² every 3 weeks for 6 courses (see also Dosing Adjustment).

Premedication: Premedication Regimen (see below for prostate cancer): In order to reduce the incidence and severity of fluid retention, all patients should be pretreated with oral corticosteroids. The recommended premedication should consist only of oral corticosteroids, such as dexamethasone 16 mg per day (e.g. 8 mg BID), for 3 days starting one day prior to each TAXOTERE administration. Antihistamines have not been shown to be useful in controlling fluid retention.

Premedication Regimen for Prostate Cancer: For prostate cancer, given the concurrent use of prednisone or prednisolone, the recommended premedication regimen is oral dexamethasone 8 mg, 12 hours, 3 hours and 1 hour before the TAXOTERE infusion.

Other Dosing Considerations: Prophylactic Use of Antibiotics: In order to reduce the incidence of febrile neutropenia and infections, the prophylactic use of antibiotics is recommended to patients treated for head and neck cancer. The treatment should consist of oral fluroquinolone antibiotics, or equivalent oral or intravenous antibiotics, for 10 days starting on day 5 of each cycle of TAXOTERE administration.

Prophylactic Use of G-CSF: Prophylactic G-CSF may be used to mitigate the risk of hematological toxicities. See Dosing Adjustment. In addition to G-CSF, the prophylactic use of antibiotics may provide additional benefit.

Geriatrics: Based on the population pharmacokinetics, there are no special instructions for the use in the elderly (see Warnings and Precautions).

Dosing Adjustment: Patients with Neutropenia, Cutaneous Reactions or Peripheral Neuropathy: Like many other chemotherapeutic agents, careful monitoring of neutrophil counts are an essential part of TAXOTERE therapy. TAXOTERE should not be administered until the neutrophil count is at least 1500 cells/mm³. Patients who experience either febrile neutropenia, severe neutropenia (neutrophil <500 cells/mm³ for more than one week), severe or cumulative cutaneous reaction, or severe neurosensory signs and/or symptoms during TAXOTERE therapy should have the dosage of TAXOTERE reduced from 100 mg/m² to 75 mg/m². When TAXOTERE is given in combination, the dose of TAXOTERE should be reduced from 75 mg/m² to 60 mg/m². If the patient continues to experience these reactions at 60 mg/m², the treatment should be discontinued. Alternatively, prophylactic G-CSF may be used in patients with either prior febrile neutropenia or severe infection in order to maintain dose intensity (see Warnings and Precautions).

Patients who receive adjuvant therapy for breast cancer and who experience febrile neutropenia should receive G-CSF in all subsequent cycles. Patients who continue to experience this reaction should remain on G-CSF and have their TAXOTERE dose reduced to 60 mg/m². If G-CSF is not used, the TAXOTERE dose should be reduced from 75 to 60 mg/m².

Patients with Hepatic Impairment: Based on pharmacokinetic data obtained with TAXOTERE at 100 mg/m² as single agent, patients who have both elevations of transaminase values (ALT and/or AST) greater than 1.5 times the upper limit of normal (ULN) and alkaline phosphatase greater than 2.5 times the ULN, the recommended dose of TAXOTERE is 75 mg/m². For those patients with serum bilirubin greater than ULN and/or ALT and AST greater than 3.5 times ULN associated with alkaline phosphatase greater than 6 times ULN, TAXOTERE should not be used unless strictly indicated. There are no data available in patients with hepatic impairment treated with TAXOTERE combination (see Warnings and Precautions).

TAXOTERE in Combination with Capecitabine: See Table 10.

Table 10: TAXOTERE

Recommended Dose Modifications for Combination Therapy with Capecitabine

	Grade 2	Grade 3	Grade 4
1st appearance	Interrupt treatment until resolved to grade 0-1 then continue at same doses with prophylaxis where possible	Grade 3 at time TAXOTERE treatment due: interrupt treatment and delay for a maximum of two weeks until grade 0-1 then continue at 75% of original capecitabine dose and at 55 mg/m² of TAXOTERE with prophylaxis where possible. If no recovery to grade 0-1 within two weeks delay, patient will stop TAXOTERE therapy but may restart capecitabine at 75% of original capecitabine dose when grade 0-1. Grade 3 occurring between cycles with recovery to grade 0-1 by the time the next treatment due: continue at 75% of original capecitabine dose and at 55 mg/m² of TAXOTERE with prophylaxis where possible	Discontinue capecitabine and TAXOTERE treatment unless treating physician considers it to be in the best interest of the patient to continue with capecitabine monotherapy at 50% of original dose

(cont'd)

Table 10: TAXOTERE *(cont'd)*

Recommended Dose Modifications for Combination Therapy with Capecitabine

	Grade 2	Grade 3	Grade 4
2nd appearance of same toxicity	Interrupt treatment until resolved to grade 0-1, then continue at 75% of original capecitabine dose and at 55 mg/m² of TAXOTERE	Discontinue TAXOTERE treatment and interrupt capecitabine treatment until resolved to grade 0-1, then continue at 50% of original capecitabine dose	
3rd appearance of same toxicity	Interrupt treatment until resolved to grade 0-1, then continue at 50% of original capecitabine dose and discontinue TAXOTERE	Discontinue treatment	
4th appearance of same toxicity	Discontinue treatment		

Administration: Precautions: TAXOTERE must be administered intravenously. It is extremely important that the intravenous needle or catheter be properly positioned before any TAXOTERE is injected. Leakage into surrounding tissue during intravenous administration of TAXOTERE may cause considerable irritation, local tissue necrosis and/or thrombophlebitis. If extravasation occurs, the injection should be discontinued immediately, and any remaining portion of the dose should be introduced into another vein.

Please refer to the Special Handling Instructions as well.

Reconstitution of Solutions: Preparation and Administration Precautions: TAXOTERE concentrated solution requires dilution prior to administration. Please follow the preparation instructions provided below.

A) Preparation of the Premix Solution:

1. If the vials are stored under refrigeration, allow the required number of TAXOTERE concentrate and diluent vials to stand at room temperature for approximately 5 minutes.
2. Using a syringe fitted with a needle, aseptically withdraw the entire contents of the solvent for TAXOTERE by partially inverting the vial. Inject the entire contents of the syringe into the corresponding TAXOTERE concentrate vial.
3. Remove the syringe and needle and mix manually by repeated inversions for at least 45 seconds. Do not shake.
4. The TAXOTERE premix solution (10 mg docetaxel/mL) should be clear; however, there may be some foam on top of the solution due to the polysorbate 80. Allow the premix solution to stand for 5 minutes to allow any foam to dissipate. It is not required that all foam dissipate prior to continuing the preparation process.

After reconstitution, the TAXOTERE premix is stable for 8 hours at room temperature or between 2 and 8°C (see Storage and Stability).

B) Preparation of the Infusion Solution:

1. Aseptically withdraw the required amount of TAXOTERE premix solution (10 mg docetaxel/mL) with a calibrated syringe and inject the required volume of premix solution into a 250 mL infusion bag or bottle of either 0.9% Sodium Chloride solution or 5% Dextrose solution to produce a final concentration of 0.3 to 0.74 mg/mL. If a dose greater than 200 mg of TAXOTERE is required, use a larger volume of the infusion vehicle so that a concentration of 0.74 mg/mL TAXOTERE is not exceeded.
2. Thoroughly mix the infusion by manual rotation.
3. As with all parenteral products, TAXOTERE should be inspected visually for particulate matter or discoloration prior to administration whenever the solution and container permit. If the TAXOTERE for Injection premix solution or infusion solution is not clear or appears to have precipitation, the solution should be discarded.

TAXOTERE infusion solution should be aseptically administered intravenously as a 1-hour infusion under ambient room temperature and lighting conditions.

Contact of the undiluted concentrate with plasticized PVC equipment or devices used to prepare solution for infusion is not recommended. In order to minimize patient exposure to plasticizer DEHP (di-2-ethylhexyl phthalate), which may be leached from PVC infusion bags or sets, TAXOTERE infusion solution should be stored in bottles (glass, polypropylene) or plastic bags (polypropylene, polyolefin) and administered through polyethylene-lined administration sets.

OVERDOSAGE:

There is no known antidote for TAXOTERE (docetaxel for injection) overdosage. In case of overdosage, the patient should be kept in a specialized unit where vital functions can be closely monitored and supportive treatment administered as necessary. Anticipated complications of overdosage include: bone marrow suppression, peripheral neurotoxicity, and mucositis. Patients should receive therapeutic G-CSF as soon as possible after discovery of overdose. Other appropriate symptomatic measures should be taken, as needed.

There were a few reports of overdose. One patient received 150 mg/m² and the other received 200 mg/m² as one-hour infusion. Some patients experienced severe neutropenia, mild asthenia, cutaneous reactions, and mild paresthesia, and recovered without incident.

For management of a suspected drug overdose, CPhA recommends that you contact your **regional Poison Control Centre**. See the *CPS* Directory section for a list of Poison Control Centres.

ACTION AND CLINICAL PHARMACOLOGY: Mechanism of Action: TAXOTERE (docetaxel for injection) is an antineoplastic agent, which acts by disrupting the microtubular network in cells that is essential for vital mitotic and interphase cellular functions. TAXOTERE promotes the assembly of tubulin into stable microtubules while simultaneously inhibiting their disassembly. TAXOTERE binds to free tubulin thereby decreasing the critical intracellular concentration of tubulin. The promoted polymerization of microtubules leads to the production of microtubule bundles without normal function and to the stabilization of microtubules, resulting in the inhibition of mitosis in cells. The binding of TAXOTERE to microtubules does not alter the number of protofilaments in the bound microtubules; in that, it differs from other spindle poisons.

TAXOTERE was found to be cytotoxic in vitro against various murine and human tumor cell lines, and against freshly excised human tumor cells in clonogenic assays.

In addition, TAXOTERE was found to be active on a number of cell lines overexpressing the p-glycoprotein, which is encoded by the multidrug resistant gene.

Pharmacokinetics: At doses of 70-115 mg/m², the kinetic profile of TAXOTERE is dose independent and consistent with a three-compartment pharmacokinetic model, with half lives for the α, β and γ phases of 4 min, 36 min and 11.1 h, respectively. Mean values for total body clearance and steady state volume of distribution were 21 L/h/m² and 113 L, respectively.

A population pharmacokinetic analysis has been performed in patients receiving TAXOTERE. Pharmacokinetic parameters estimated by the model were very close to those estimated from Phase I studies. The pharmacokinetics of TAXOTERE were not altered by the age or sex of the patient. In a small number of patients with clinical chemistry data suggestive of mild to moderate liver function impairment (ALT, AST ≥1.5 times the upper limit of normal associated with alkaline phosphatase ≥2.5 times the upper limit of normal), total clearance was lowered by 27% on average (see Dosage and Administration).

The effect of daily oral prednisone administration on the pharmacokinetics of TAXOTERE administered with dexamethasone premedication prior to infusion has been evaluated in 42 patients treated for prostate cancer. No effect of prednisone on the pharmacokinetics of TAXOTERE was observed.

Based on in vitro studies, isoenzymes of the cytochrome P450-3A subfamily appear to be involved in TAXOTERE metabolism. TAXOTERE is more than 95% protein bound. Dexamethasone does not affect the protein binding of TAXOTERE.

STORAGE AND STABILITY: Stability: Unopened vials of TAXOTERE (docetaxel for injection) are stable until the expiration date indicated on the package when stored between 2 and 25°C and protected from light. Freezing does not adversely affect the product.

Storage: Store the unopened vials between 2-25°C. Retain in the original package to protect from bright light.

TAXOTERE premix solution (10 mg docetaxel/mL) should be used as soon as possible after preparation. However the chemical and physical stability of the premix solution has been demonstrated stable for 8 hours when stored either between 2 and 8°C or at room temperature.

TAXOTERE infusion solutions, if stored between 2 and 25°C is stable for 4 hours. Fully prepared TAXOTERE infusion solution (in either 0.9% sodium chloride solution or 5% dextrose solution) should be used within 4 hours (including the 1 hour i.v. administration).

SPECIAL HANDLING INSTRUCTIONS: TAXOTERE is a cytotoxic anticancer drug and, as with other potentially toxic compounds, caution should be exercised when handling and preparing TAXOTERE solutions. The use of gloves is recommended.

If TAXOTERE concentrate, premix solution or infusion solution should come into contact with the skin, immediately and thoroughly wash with soap and water. If TAXOTERE concentrate, premix solution, or infusion solution should come into contact with mucosa, immediately and thoroughly wash with water.

Procedures for proper handling and disposal of anticancer drugs should be considered. Several guidelines on this subject have been published. There is no general agreement that all of the procedures recommended in the guidelines are necessary or appropriate.

INFORMATION FOR THE PATIENT: Published in e-CPS, available by subscription at www.e-cps.ca.

DOSAGE FORMS, COMPOSITION AND PACKAGING: 20 mg/0.5 mL: Each single-dose vial of sterile, non-pyrogenic, nonaqueous, clear yellow to brownish-yellow viscous solution contains: docetaxel (anhydrous) 20 mg in 0.5 mL polysorbate 80 (Fill: docetaxel 24.4 mg in 0.61 mL polysorbate 80) with an accompanying sterile, non-pyrogenic diluent vial containing 1.98 mL of ethanol 13% in water for injection. This overfill ensures that there is a minimal extractable premix volume of 2 mL containing 10 mg/mL docetaxel which corresponds to the labelled amount of 20 mg/vial. Nonmedicinal ingredients: ethyl alcohol, polysorbate 80 and water for injection. Both items are in blister packs in 1 carton.

80 mg/2 mL: Each single-dose vial of sterile, non-pyrogenic, nonaqueous, clear yellow to brownish-yellow viscous solution contains: docetaxel (anhydrous) 80 mg in 2 mL polysorbate 80 (Fill: docetaxel 94.4 mg in 2.36 mL polysorbate 80) with an accompanying sterile, non-pyrogenic diluent vial containing 7.33 mL of ethanol 13% in water for injection. This overfill ensures that there is a minimal extractable premix volume of 8 mL containing 10 mg/mL docetaxel which corresponds to the labelled amount of 80 mg/vial. Nonmedicinal ingredients: ethyl alcohol, polysorbate 80 and water for injection. Both items are in blister packs in 1 carton.

TAXOTERE concentrated solution requires dilution prior to use. A sterile, non-pyrogenic, single-dose diluent is supplied for that purpose. The diluent for TAXOTERE contains ethanol 95% v/v/water for injection (13/87 w/w), and is supplied in 1.5 mL (to be used with 20 mg TAXOTERE) and 6 mL (to be used with 80 mg TAXOTERE) vials.

Tazocin® Ⓟ

piperacillin sodium—tazobactam sodium

Antibiotic—Beta-lactamase Inhibitor

Pfizer

Date of Revision: August 20, 2008

PHARMACOLOGY: TAZOCIN (sterile piperacillin sodium/tazobactam sodium) is an injectable antibacterial combination consisting of the semisynthetic antibiotic piperacillin sodium and the β-lactamase inhibitor tazobactam sodium for intravenous administration.

Piperacillin sodium exerts bactericidal activity by inhibiting septum formation and cell wall synthesis. In vitro, piperacillin is active against a variety of gram-positive and gram-negative aerobic and anaerobic bacteria. Tazobactam sodium is a β-lactamase inhibitor. Tazobactam, in combination with piperacillin enhances and extends the antibiotic spectrum of piperacillin to include ß-lactamase producing bacteria normally resistant to piperacillin.

Piperacillin is metabolized to a minor microbiologically active desethyl metabolite. Tazobactam is metabolized to a single metabolite which lacks pharmacological and antibacterial activities. Both tazobactam and piperacillin are eliminated by the kidney via glomerular filtration and tubular secretion. Tazobactam and its metabolite are eliminated primarily by renal excretion with 80% of the dose as unchanged drug and the remainder as the single metabolite. Piperacillin is excreted rapidly as unchanged drug, with 68% of the dose in the urine. Piperacillin, tazobactam and desethyl piperacillin are also secreted into the bile.

Tazobactam and piperacillin are widely distributed into tissues and body fluids including, but not limited to, intestinal mucosa, gallbladder, lung, female reproductive tissues (uterus, ovary and fallopian tube) interstitial fluid and bile. Mean tissue concentrations were generally 50-100% of those in plasma. Distribution of tazobactam and piperacillin into cerebrospinal fluid is low in subjects with non-inflamed meninges, as with other penicillins.

In subjects with renal impairment, the half-lives of tazobactam and piperacillin, after single doses, increase with decreasing creatinine clearance. At creatinine clearance below 20 mL/min., the increase in half-life is four-fold for tazobactam and two-fold for piperacillin compared to subjects with normal renal function. Dosage adjustments for TAZOCIN are recommended when creatinine clearance is below 40 mL/min in patients receiving the recommended daily dose of TAZOCIN (see Dosage).

Hemodialysis removes 30-40% of a TAZOCIN dose with an additional 5% of the tazobactam dose removed as the tazobactam metabolite. Peritoneal dialysis removes approximately 21% and 6% of the tazobactam and piperacillin doses, respectively, with up to 16% of the tazobactam dose removed as the tazobactam metabolite. For dosage recommendations for patients undergoing hemodialysis, see Dosage.

Tazobactam and piperacillin half-lives increase by approximately 18 % and 25% respectively, in patients with hepatic cirrhosis compared to healthy subjects. However, dosage adjustment of TAZOCIN due to hepatic cirrhosis is not necessary.

INDICATIONS: TAZOCIN (sterile piperacillin sodium/tazobactam sodium) is indicated for the treatment of patients with systemic and/or local bacterial infections, caused by piperacillin resistant, piperacillin/tazobactam susceptible, β-lactamase producing strains of the designated microorganisms in the specified conditions listed below.

Intra-abdominal Infections: Appendicitis (complicated by rupture or abscess) and peritonitis caused by piperacillin resistant, β-lactamase producing strains of *E. coli* or members of the *B. fragilis* group.

Skin and Skin Structure Infections: Uncomplicated and complicated skin and skin structure infections, including cellulitis, cutaneous abscess, acute ischemic diabetic foot infections caused by piperacillin resistant β-lactamase producing strains of *S. aureus* (not methicillin-resistant strains).

Gynecological Infections: Postpartum endometritis or pelvic inflammatory disease caused by piperacillin resistant, β-lactamase producing strains of *E. coli*.

Community-acquired Lower Respiratory Tract Infections: Community-acquired pneumonia (moderate severity only) caused by piperacillin resistant, β-lactamase producing strains of *H. influenzae*.

Nosocomial Pneumonia: Nosocomial pneumonia (moderate to severe) caused by piperacillin-resistant, β-lactamase producing strains of *S. aureus* and by piperacillin/tazobactam-susceptible Acinetobacter baumannii, *H. influenzae*, *K. pneumoniae*, and *P. aeruginosa* (Nosocomial pneumonia caused by *P. aeruginosa* should be treated in combination with an aminoglycoside) (see Dosage).

While TAZOCIN is indicated only for the conditions listed above, infections caused by piperacillin susceptible organisms are also amenable to TAZOCIN treatment due to its piperacillin content. The tazobactam component of this combination product does not decrease the activity of the piperacillin component against piperacillin susceptible organisms. Therefore, the treatment of polymicrobial infections caused by piperacillin susceptible organisms and β-lactamase producing organisms susceptible to TAZOCIN should not require the addition of another antibiotic.

TAZOCIN may be useful as presumptive therapy in the indicated conditions prior to identification of causative organisms because of its broad spectrum of bactericidal activity against gram-positive and gram-negative aerobic and anaerobic organisms.

Appropriate cultures should usually be performed before initiating antimicrobial treatment in order to isolate and identify the organisms causing infection and to determine their susceptibility to TAZOCIN. Antimicrobial therapy should be adjusted, if appropriate, once results of culture(s) and antimicrobial susceptibility testing are known.

CONTRAINDICATIONS: The use of TAZOCIN (sterile piperacillin sodium/tazobactam sodium) is contraindicated in patients with a history of allergic reactions to any of the penicillins and/or cephalosporins or β-lactamase inhibitors.

WARNINGS: Serious and occasionally fatal hypersensitivity (anaphylactic/anaphylactoid [including shock]) reactions have been reported in individuals receiving therapy with penicillins. These reactions are more apt to occur in individuals with a history of sensitivity to multiple allergens. There have been reports of individuals with a history of penicillin hypersensitivity who have experienced severe hypersensitivity reactions when treated with cephalosporins. Before initiating therapy with TAZOCIN (piperacillin sodium/tazobactam sodium), careful inquiry should be made concerning previous hypersensitivity reactions to penicillins, cephalosporins, or other allergens. If an allergic reaction occurs during therapy with TAZOCIN, the antibiotic should be discontinued and appropriate therapy instituted. Serious anaphylactoid reactions require immediate emergency treatment with epinephrine, oxygen and intravenous steroids and airway management, including intubation, should also be administered as indicated.

C. difficile-associated disease (CDAD) has been reported with use of many antibacterial agents, including TAZOCIN. CDAD may range in severity from mild diarrhea to fatal colitis. It is important to consider this diagnosis in patients who present with diarrhea, or symptoms of colitis, pseudomembranous colitis, toxic megacolon, or perforation of colon subsequent to the administration of any antibacterial agent. CDAD has been reported to occur over 2 months after the administration of antibacterial agents.

Treatment with antibacterial agents may alter the normal flora of the colon and may permit overgrowth of *C. difficile. C. difficile* produces toxins A and B, which contribute to the development of CDAD. CDAD may cause significant morbidity and mortality. CDAD can be refractory to antimicrobial therapy.

If the diagnosis of CDAD is suspected or confirmed, appropriate therapeutic measures should be initiated. Mild cases of CDAD usually respond to discontinuation of antibacterial agents not directed against *C. difficile*. In moderate to severe cases, consideration should be given to management with fluids and electrolytes, protein supplementation, and treatment with an antibacterial agent clinically effective against *C. difficile*. Surgical evaluation should be instituted as clinically indicated, as surgical intervention may be required in certain severe cases (see Adverse Effects).

PRECAUTIONS: General: Bleeding manifestations or significant leukopenia following prolonged administration have occurred in some patients receiving β-lactam antibiotics, including piperacillin. These reactions have sometimes been associated with abnormalities of coagulation tests such as clotting time, platelet aggregation and prothrombin time and are more likely to occur in patients with renal failure. If bleeding manifestations occur, the antibiotic should be discontinued and appropriate therapy instituted.

The possibility of the emergence of resistant organisms that might cause superinfections should be kept in mind. If this occurs, appropriate measures should be taken.

As with other penicillins, patients may experience neuromuscular excitability or convulsions if higher than recommended doses are given intravenously (particularly in the presence of renal failure).

TAZOCIN contains a total of 2.79 mEq (64 mg) of sodium (Na^+) per g of piperacillin in the combination product. This should be considered when treating patients requiring restricted salt intake. Periodic electrolyte determinations should be performed in patients with low potassium reserves, and the possibility of hypokalemia should be kept in mind with patients who have potentially low potassium reserves and who are receiving cytotoxic therapy or diuretics.

Leukopenia and neutropenia may occur, especially during prolonged therapy. Therefore, periodic assessment of hematopoietic function should be performed.

As with other semisynthetic penicillins, piperacillin therapy has been associated with an increased incidence of fever and rash in cystic fibrosis patients.

In patients with creatinine clearance <40 mL/min and dialysis patients [hemodialysis and chronic ambulatory peritoneal dialysis (CAPD)], the intravenous dose should be adjusted to the degree of renal function impairment (see Dosage).

Because of chemical instability, TAZOCIN should not be used for intravenous administration with solutions containing **only** sodium bicarbonate (see Dosage, Incompatibilities).

TAZOCIN should not be added to blood products or albumin hydrolysates.

Children: Safety and efficacy in children below the age of 12 have not been established.

Pregnancy: Obstetrics and Teratology: Reproduction studies have been performed in rats and have revealed no evidence of impaired fertility due to piperacillin/tazobactam administered up to a dose which is similar to the maximum recommended human daily dose based on body-surface area (mg/m²). Teratology studies have been performed in mice and rats and have revealed no evidence of harm to the fetus due to piperacillin/tazobactam at doses 1-2 and 2-3 times the human dose of piperacillin and tazobactam, respectively, based on body-surface area (mg/m²).

Piperacillin: Reproduction and teratology studies have been performed in mice and rats and have revealed no evidence of impaired fertility or harm to the fetus due to piperacillin administered up to a dose which is half (mice) or similar (rats) to the human dose based on body-surface area (mg/m²).

Tazobactam: Reproduction studies have been performed in rats and have revealed no evidence of impaired fertility due to tazobactam administered up to a dose 3 times the human dose based on body-surface area (mg/m²). Teratology studies have been performed in mice and rats and have revealed no evidence of harm to the fetus due to tazobactam up to a dose which is 6 (mice) and 14 (rats) times the human dose based on body-surface area (mg/m²). In rats, tazobactam crosses the placenta. Concentrations in the fetus are less than or equal to 10% of that found in maternal plasma.

There are no adequate and well-controlled studies with the piperacillin/tazobactam combination or with piperacillin or tazobactam alone in pregnant women. Piperacillin and tazobactam cross the placenta. Because animal reproduction studies are not always predictive of human response pregnant women should be treated with TAZOCIN only if the expected benefit outweighs the possible risks to the pregnant woman and fetus.

Lactation: Caution should be exercised when TAZOCIN is administered to nursing mothers. Piperacillin is excreted in low concentrations in human milk; tazobactam concentrations in milk have not been studied. Women who are breast-feeding should be treated only if the expected benefit outweighs the possible risks to the woman and child.

Geriatrics: Patients over 65 years of age are not at an increased risk of developing adverse effects solely because of age. However, dosage should be adjusted in the presence of renal insufficiency (see Dosage).

In general, dose selection for an elderly patient should be approached with caution, usually starting at the low end of the dosing range, reflecting the greater frequency of decreased hepatic, renal, or cardiac function, and of concomitant disease or other drug therapy.

Tazocin contains 64 mg (2.79 mEq) of sodium per gram of piperacillin in the combination product. At the usual recommended doses, patients would receive between 768 and 1024 mg/day (33.5 and 44.6 mEq) of sodium. The geriatric population may respond with a blunted natriuresis to salt loading. This may be clinically important with regard to diseases such as congestive heart failure.

This drug is known to be substantially excreted by the kidney, and the risk of toxic reactions to this drug may be greater in patients with impaired renal function. Elderly patients are more likely to have decreased renal function and therefore care should be taken in dose selection. It may be useful to monitor renal function.

Drug Interactions: Aminoglycosides: The mixing of beta-lactam antibiotics with aminoglycosides in vitro can result in substantial inactivation of the aminoglycoside. However, amikacin and gentamicin were determined to be compatible in vitro with reformulated TAZOCIN containing EDTA in certain diluents at specific concentrations for a simultaneous Y-site infusion (see Dosage).

The inactivation of aminoglycosides in the presence of penicillin-class drugs has been recognized. It has been postulated that penicillin-aminoglycoside complexes form; these complexes are microbiologically inactive and of unknown toxicity. Sequential administration of TAZOCIN with tobramycin to patients with normal renal function and mild to moderate renal impairment has been shown to modestly decrease serum concentrations of tobramycin but does not significantly affect tobramycin pharmacokinetics. When aminoglycosides are administered in combination with piperacillin to patients with end-stage renal disease requiring hemodialysis, the concentrations of the aminoglycosides (especially tobramycin) may be significantly altered and should be monitored. Since aminoglycosides are not equally susceptible to inactivation by piperacillin, consideration should be given to the choice of the aminoglycoside when administered in combination with piperacillin to these patients.

Probenecid: Concomitant administration of TAZOCIN and probenecid results in prolonged half-life of piperacillin (21%), and tazobactam (71%) and lower renal clearance for both piperacillin and tazobactam; however, peak plasma concentrations of either drug are unaffected.

Vancomycin: No pharmacokinetic interactions are found between TAZOCIN and vancomycin.

Heparin: Coagulation parameters should be tested more frequently and monitored regularly, during simultaneous administration of high doses of heparin, oral anticoagulants and other drugs that may affect the blood coagulation system and/or the thrombocyte function.

Vecuronium: Piperacillin used concomitantly with vecuronium has been implicated in the prolongation of the neuromuscular blockade of vecuronium. TAZOCIN (piperacillin/tazobactam) could produce the same phenonemon if given along with vecuronium. Due to their similar mechanism of action, it is expected that the neuromuscular blockade produced by any of the non-depolarizing muscle relaxants could be prolonged in the presence of piperacillin (see package information for vecuronium bromide).

Methotrexate: Piperacillin may reduce the excretion of methotrexate; therefore, serum levels of methotrexate should be monitored in patients to avoid drug toxicity.

Where TAZOCIN is administered concurrently with another antibiotic the drugs should **not** be mixed in the same solution but must be administered separately.

Drug/Laboratory Test Interactions: As with other penicillins, the administration of TAZOCIN may result in a false-positive reaction for glucose in the urine using a copper-reduction method (CLINITEST). It is recommended that glucose tests based on enzymatic glucose oxidase reactions (such as DIASTIX or TES-TAPE) be used.

There have been reports of positive test results using the Bio-Rad Laboratories Platelia Aspergillus EIA test in patients receiving piperacillin/tazobactam injection who were subsequently found to be free of Aspergillus infection. Cross-reactions with non-Aspergillus polysaccharides and polyfuranoses with Bio-Rad Laboratories Platelia Aspergillus EIA test have been reported. Therefore, positive test results in patients receiving piperacillin/tazobactam should be interpreted cautiously and confirmed by other diagnostic methods.

ADVERSE EFFECTS: Adverse Events from Clinical Trials: During the clinical investigations, 2621 patients worldwide were treated with TAZOCIN in phase 3 trials. In the key North American clinical trials (n=830 patients), 90% of the adverse events reported were mild to moderate in severity and transient in nature. However, in 3.2% of the patients treated worldwide, TAZOCIN was discontinued because of adverse events primarily involving the skin (1.3%), including rash and pruritus; the gastrointestinal system (0.9%), including diarrhea, nausea, and vomiting; and allergic reactions (0.5%).

Adverse local reactions that were reported, irrespective of relationship to therapy with TAZOCIN, were phlebitis (1.3%), injection site reaction (0.5%), pain (0.2%), inflammation (0.2%), thrombophlebitis (0.2%), and edema (0.1%).

Based on patients from the North American trials (n=1063), the events with the highest incidence in patients, irrespective of relationship to TAZOCIN therapy, were diarrhea (11.3%); headache (7.7%); constipation (7.7%); nausea (6.9%); insomnia (6.6%); rash (4.2%), including maculopapular, bullous, urticarial, and eczematoid; vomiting (3.3%); dyspepsia (3.3%); pruritus (3.1 %); stool changes (2.4%); fever (2.4%); agitation (2.1 %); pain (1.7%); moniliasis (1.6%); hypertension (1.6%); dizziness (1.4%); abdominal pain (1.3%); chest pain (1.3%); edema (1.2%); anxiety (1.2%); rhinitis (1.2%); and dyspnea (1.1%).

Additional adverse systemic clinical events reported in 1.0% or less of the patients are listed below within each body system:

Autonomic Nervous System: hypotension, ileus, syncope.

Body as a Whole: rigors, back pain, malaise, candidal superinfection.

Cardiovascular: tachycardia, including supraventricular and ventricular; bradycardia; arrhythmia, including atrial fibrillation, ventricular fibrillation, cardiac arrest, cardiac failure, circulatory failure, myocardial infarction.

CNS: tremor, convulsions, vertigo.

Gastrointestinal: melena, flatulence, hemorrhage, gastritis, hiccough, ulcerative stomatitis, jaundice.

Pseudomembranous colitis was reported in one patient during the clinical trials. The onset of pseudomembranous colitis symptoms may occur during or over 2 months after the administration of antibacterial treatment (see Warnings).

Hearing: tinnitus.

Hypersensitivity: anaphylaxis (including shock). Incidence of rash and fever is higher in patients with cystic fibrosis.

Metabolic and Nutritional: symptomatic hypoglycemia, thirst.

Musculoskeletal: myalgia, arthralgia.

Platelet, Bleeding, Clotting: mesenteric embolism, purpura, epistaxis, pulmonary embolism (see Precautions, General).

Psychiatric: confusion, hallucination, depression.

Reproduction, Female: leukorrhea, vaginitis.

Respiratory: pharyngitis, pulmonary edema, bronchospasm, coughing.

Skin and Appendages: genital pruritus, diaphoresis, toxic epidermal necrolysis.

Special Senses: taste perversion.

Urinary: retention, dysuria, oliguria, hematuria, incontinence.

Vision: photophobia.

Vascular (extracardiac): flushing.

Nosocomial Pneumonia Trials: In a completed study of nosocomial pneumonia, 222 patients were treated with TAZOCIN in a dosing regimen of **4.5 g every 6 hours in combination with an aminoglycoside and 215 patients were treated with a comparator in combination with an aminoglycoside**. In this trial, treatment-emergent adverse events were reported by 402 patients, 204 (91.9%) in the piperacillin/tazobactam group and 198 (92.1%) in the comparator group. Twenty-five (25, 11.0%) patients in the piperacillin/tazobactam group and 14 (6.5%) in the comparator group (p >0.05) discontinued treatment due to an adverse event.

In this study of TAZOCIN in combination with an aminoglycoside, adverse events that occurred in more than 1% of patients and were considered by the investigator to be drug-related were: diarrhea (17.6%), fever (2.7%), vomiting (2.7%), urinary tract infection (2.7%), rash (2.3%), abdominal pain (1.8%), generalized edema (1.8%), moniliasis (1.8%), nausea (1.8%), oral moniliasis (1.8%), BUN increased (1.8%), creatinine increased (1.8%), peripheral edema (1.8%), abdomen enlarged (1.4%), headache (1.4%), constipation (1.4%), liver function tests abnormal (1.4%), thrombocythemia (1.4%), excoriations (1.4%), and sweating (1.4%).

Drug-related adverse events reported in 1% or less of patients in the nosocomial pneumonia study of TAZOCIN with an aminoglycoside were: acidosis, acute kidney failure, agitation, alkaline phosphatase increased, anemia, asthenia, atrial fibrillation, chest pain, CNS depression, colitis, confusion, convulsion, cough increased, thrombocytopenia, dehydration, depression, diplopia, drug level decreased, dry mouth, dyspepsia, dysphagia, dyspnea, dysuria, eosinophilia, fungal dermatitis, gastritis, glossitis, grand mal convulsion, hematuria, hyperglycemia, hypernatremia, hypertension, hypertonia, hyperventilation, hypochromic anemia, hypoglycemia, hypokalemia, hyponatremia, hypophosphatemia, hypoxia, ileus, injection site edema, injection site pain, injection site reaction, kidney function abnormal, leukocytosis, leukopenia, local reaction to procedure, melena, pain, prothrombin decreased, pruritus, respiratory disorder, AST increased, ALT increased, sinus bradycardia, somnolence, stomatitis, stupor, tremor, tachycardia, ventricular extrasystoles, and ventricular tachycardia.

Post-Marketing Experience: Additional adverse events reported from worldwide marketing experience with TAZOCIN occuring under circumstances where causal relationship to TAZOCIN is uncertain:

Gastrointestinal: hepatitis, cholestatic jaundice.

Hematologic: hemolytic anemia, anemia, thrombocytosis, agranulocytosis, pancytopenia.

Immune: hypersensitivity reactions, anaphylactic/anaphylactoid reactions (including shock).

Infections: candidial superinfections.

Renal: interstitial nephritis, renal failure.

Skin and Appendages: erythema multiforme, Stevens-Johnson syndrome, toxic epidermal necrolysis.

Adverse Laboratory Events: Changes in laboratory parameters, without regard to drug relationship, were reported in all studies, including studies of nosocomial pneumonia in which a higher dose of TAZOCIN (piperacillin and tazobactam for injection) was used in combination with an aminoglycoside. The changes in laboratory parameters include:

Hematologic: agranulocytosis, pancytopenia, anemia, decreases in hemoglobin and hematocrit, thrombocytopenia, increases in platelet count, eosinophilia, leukopenia, neutropenia. The leukopenia/neutropenia associated with TAZOCIN administration appears to be reversible and most frequently associated with prolonged administration, i.e., ≥21 days of therapy. These patients were withdrawn from therapy; some had accompanying systemic symptoms (e.g., fever, rigors, chills).

Coagulation: positive direct Coombs test, prolonged prothrombin time, prolonged partial thromboplastin time, bleeding time prolonged.

Hepatic: transient elevations of AST , ALT, alkaline phosphatase, bilirubin, gamma-glutamyltransferase increased.

Renal: Increases in serum creatinine, blood urea nitrogen, renal failure.

Urinalysis: Proteinuria, hematuria, pyuria.

Additional laboratory events include abnormalities in electrolytes (i.e., increases and decreases in sodium, potassium, and calcium), hyperglycemia, decreases in total protein or albumin. In individuals with liver disease or those receiving cytotoxic therapy or diuretics, TAZOCIN has been reported rarely to produce a decrease in serum potassium levels at high doses of piperacillin.

The following adverse reactions have also been reported for PIPRACIL (sterile piperacillin sodium):

Skin and Appendages: erythema multiforme and Stevens-Johnson syndrome, rarely reported.

Gastrointestinal: cholestatic hepatitis.

Renal: rarely, interstitial nephritis.

Skeletal: prolonged muscle relaxation (see Precautions, Drug Interactions).

OVERDOSE:

Symptoms: There have been post-marketing reports of overdose with TAZOCIN. The majority of those events experienced including nausea, vomiting, and diarrhea have also been reported with the usual recommended dosages. Patients may experience neuromuscular excitability or convulsions if higher than recommended doses are given intravenously (particularly in the presence of renal failure).

Treatment: Treatment should be supportive and symptomatic according to the patient's clinical presentation.

Excessive serum levels of either tazobactam or piperacillin may be reduced by hemodialysis, although no specific antidote is known. As with other penicillins, neuromuscular excitability or convulsions have occurred following large intravenous doses, primarily in patients with impaired renal function.

In the case of motor excitability or convulsions, general supportive measures, including administration of anticonvulsive agents (eg. diazepam or barbiturates) may be considered.

For management of a suspected drug overdose, contact your **regional Poison Control Centre**. See the *CPS* Directory section for a list of Poison Control Centres.

DOSAGE: The usual total daily dose of TAZOCIN (sterile piperacillin sodium/tazobactam sodium) for adults is 12 g/1.5 g, given as 3 g/0.375 g every six hours.

Clinical trial data in the treatment of intra-abdominal infections support the efficacy of 4 g/0.5 g given every eight hours.

nitial presumptive treatment of patients with nosocomial pneumonia should start with TAZOCIN at a dosage of 4.5 g **every hours plus an aminoglycoside, totalling 18.0 g (16.0 g piperacillin sodium/2.0 g tazobactam sodium)**. Treatment with e aminoglycoside should be continued in patients from whom *P. aeruginosa* is isolated. If *P. aeruginosa* is not isolated, the minoglycoside may be discontinued at the discretion of the treating physician.

Due to the in vitro inactivation of the aminoglycoside by beta-lactam antibiotics, TAZOCIN and the aminoglycoside should be reconstituted and diluted separately when concomitant therapy with aminoglycosides is indicated (see Precautions, Drug Interactions).

When concomitant therapy with an aminoglycoside is indicated, TAZOCIN and the aminoglycoside should be administered separately.

In certain circumstances where co-administration is preferred, compatibility for simultaneous co-administration via Y-site infusion has been established for the TAZOCIN formulation containing EDTA supplied in vials with the following aminoglycosides under the following conditions:

The following compatibility information only applies to the reformulated TAZOCIN containing EDTA, and does not apply to other formulations of piperacillin/tazobactam including the previous TAZOCIN (piperacillin/tazobactam) brand formulation, see Table 1.

Table 1: TAZOCIN

Compatibility Information

Aminoglycoside	Piperacillin/ tazobactam (g) dose	Piperacillin/ tazobactam Diluent Volume (mL)	Aminoglycoside Concentration Range[a] (mg/mL)	Acceptable Diluents
Amikacin	2.25, 3.375, 4.5	50, 100, 150	1.75–7.5	0.9% sodium chloride or 5% dextrose
Gentamicin	2.25, 3.375, 4.5	100, 150	0.7–3.32	0.9% sodium chloride

[a] The dose of aminoglycoside should be based on patient weight, status of infection (serious or life threatening) and renal function (creatinine clearance).

TAZOCIN is not compatible with tobramycin for simultaneous coadministration via Y-site infusion. Compatibility of TAZOCIN with other aminoglycosides has not been established. Only the concentration and diluents of amikacin or gentamicin with the dosages of TAZOCIN listed in Table 1 have been established as compatible for co-administration via Y-site infusion. Simultaneous administration via Y-site infusion in any manner other than listed above may result in inactivation of the aminoglycoside by TAZOCIN.

Renal Insufficiency: In patients with renal insufficiency, the intravenous dose should be adjusted to the degree of actual renal function impairment. In patients with nosocomial pneumonia receiving concomitant aminoglycoside therapy, the aminoglycoside dosage should be adjusted according to the recommendations of the aminoglycoside used. The recommended daily doses of Tazocin for patients with renal insufficiency are in Table 2.

Table 2: TAZOCIN

Recommended Dosing of TAZOCIN in Patients with Normal Renal Function and Renal Insufficiency (As total g piperacillin/tazobactam)

Renal Function (Creatinine Clearance, mL/min)	All Indications (except Nosocomial Pneumonia)	Nosocomial Pneumonia
>40 mL/min	3.375 q6h	4.5 q6h
20–40 mL/min[a]	2.25 q6h	3.375 q6h
<20 mL/min[a]	2.25 q8h	2.25 q6h
Hemodialysis[b]	2.25 q12h	2.25 q8h
CAPD	2.25 q12h	2.25 q8h

[a] Creatinine clearance for patients not receiving hemodialysis.
[b] 0.75 g should be administered following each hemodialysis session on hemodialysis days.

For patients on hemodialysis, the maximum dose is 2.25 g piperacillin/tazobactam given every twelve hours for all indications other than nosocomial pneumonia and 2.25 g every eight hours for nosocomial pneumonia. In addition, because hemodialysis removes 30% to 40% of TAZOCIN dose in four hours, one additional dose of 0.75 g piperacillin/tazobactam should be administered following each dialysis period. For patients with renal failure, measurement of serum levels of TAZOCIN will provide additional guidance for adjusting dosage.

Dosage adjustment is based on pharmacokinetic data. Clinical studies with TAZOCIN have not been performed in patients with impaired renal function.

Duration of Therapy: The usual duration of TAZOCIN treatment is from seven to ten days. However, the recommended duration of TAZOCIN treatment of nosocomial pneumonia is 7 to 14 days. In all conditions, the duration should be guided by the severity of the infection and the patient's clinical and bacteriological progress.

Administration: TAZOCIN should be administered by intravenous infusion over 30 minutes (see Pharmacology).

Reconstituted Solutions: Reconstitute TAZOCIN with at least 5 mL of a suitable diluent per gram of piperacillin from the list of diluents provided below. Swirl until dissolved. It should be further diluted to the desired final volume with an acceptable diluent (see Table 3 and Table 4).

Table 3: TAZOCIN

Reconstitution

Vial Size (piperacillin/ tazobactam)	Volume of Diluent to be Added to Vial	Approximate Available Volume	Nominal Concentration per mL
2.25 g (2 g/0.25 g)	10 mL	11.60 mL	0.194 g/mL (0.172 g/mL/0.022 g/mL)
3.375 g (3 g/0.375 g)	15 mL	17.36 mL	0.194 g/mL (0.172 g/mL/0.022 g/mL)
4.5 g (4 g/0.5 g)	20 mL	23.15 mL	0.194 g/mL (0.172 g/mL/0.022 g/mL)

Lactated Ringer's Injection is only compatible with the reformulated TAZOCIN containing EDTA.

Intermittent Intravenous Infusion: Reconstitute as previously described, with 5 mL of an acceptable diluent per 1 g of piperacillin and then further dilute in the desired volume (at least 50 mL). This diluted solution must be used immediately. Administer by infusion over a period of at least 30 minutes. During the infusion it is desirable to discontinue the primary infusion solution.

Stability of TAZOCIN Following Reconstitution: TAZOCIN is stable in glass and plastic containers (plastic syringes, I.V. bags and tubing) when reconstituted with acceptable diluents.

Stability studies of TAZOCIN in glass vials have demonstrated chemical stability [potency, pH of reconstituted solution, appearance and description, and clarity of solution] for up to 24 hours at room temperature and up to 48 hours at refrigerated temperatures. Discard unused portions after storage for 24 hours at room temperature or 48 hours when refrigerated.

Due to microbial considerations, intravenous admixtures are usually recommended for use within a maximum of 24 hours at room temperature or 72 hours when refrigerated (2-8°C).

Stability studies of TAZOCIN in polyolefin I.V. bags have demonstrated chemical stability (potency, appearance and description and clarity of solution) for up to 24 hours at room temperature and up to 72 hours at refrigerated temperature. Stability and compatibility of Tazocin in PVC I.V. bags have not been established. TAZOCIN contains no preservatives. Appropriate consideration of aseptic technique should be used.

As with all parenteral drug products, intravenous admixtures should be inspected visually for clarity, particulate matter, precipitate, discoloration and leakage prior to administration, whenever solution and container permit. Solutions showing haziness, particulate matter, precipitate, discoloration or leakage should not be used. Discard unused portion.

Incompatibilities: Not to be added to blood products or albumin hydrolysates.

Because of chemical instability, TAZOCIN should not be used for intravenous administration with solutions containing sodium bicarbonate alone. It may be used with intravenous admixtures containing other ingredients as well as sodium bicarbonate for up to 24 hours at room temperature and 48 hours refrigerated.

Solutions containing TAZOCIN and protein hydrolysates or amino acids should be used within 12 hours if stored at room temperature and 24 hours if refrigerated.

TAZOCIN should not be mixed with other drugs in a syringe or infusion bottle since compatibility has not been established.

Table 4: TAZOCIN

Reconstitution

Reconstitute TAZOCIN per g of piperacillin with 5 mL of a **Compatible Reconstitution Diluent** (listed below).	**Further dilute** the reconstituted TAZOCIN with 50 mL to 150 mL of a **Compatible I.V. Solution** (listed below).
0.9% Sodium Chloride Injection Sterile Water for Injection 5% Dextrose Injection	0.9% Sodium Chloride Injection Sterile Water for Injection[a] 5% Dextrose Injection Lactated Ringer's Injection (Only compatible with reformulated TAZOCIN containing EDTA)[b]
Bacteriostatic Sodium Chloride Injection (with benzyl alcohol) Bacteriostatic Water for Injection (with benzyl alcohol) Bacteriostatic Water for Injection (with parabens)	0.9% Sodium Chloride Injection

[a] Maximum recommended volume per dose of Sterile Water for Injection is 50 mL.
[b] Compatibility was studied in 250 mL IV bags only.

SUPPLIED: Sensitivity Discs: Tazocin 110 µg sensitivity discs (piperacillin 100 µg + tazobactam 10 µg) are available and must be refrigerated upon receipt.

Vials: 2.25 g: Each vial contains: piperacillin sodium equivalent to piperacillin 2 g and tazobactam sodium equivalent to tazobactam 0.25 g. Also contains citric acid (monohydrate) and edetate disodium (dihydrate). Sodium: 5.58 mEq (128 mg). Glass vials of 2.25 g, boxes of 10.

3.375 g: Each vial contains: piperacillin sodium equivalent to piperacillin 3 g and tazobactam sodium equivalent to tazobactam 0.375 g. Also contains citric acid (monohydrate) and edetate disodium (dihydrate). Sodium: 8.38 mEq (192 mg). Glass vials of 3.375 g, boxes of 10.

4.5 g: Each vial contains: piperacillin sodium equivalent to piperacillin 4 g and tazobactam sodium equivalent to tazobactam 0.5 g. Also contains citric acid (monohydrate) and edetate disodium (dihydrate). Sodium: 11.17 mEq (256 mg). Glass vials of 4.5 g, boxes of 10.

Store at controlled room temperature 15 to 30°C. Single dose vials. Discard unused portions.

Tazorac® Cream ℞

tazarotene

Antipsoriasis—Antiacne—Agent for the Treatment of Photodamaged Skin

Allergan

PHARMACOLOGY: Tazarotene is a retinoid prodrug which is converted to its active form, M1 ("tazarotenic acid", or AGN 190299), by rapid deesterification in most biological systems. "Tazarotenic acid" binds to and regulates gene expression through all three members of the RAR family of retinoid nuclear receptors, RARα, RARβ, and RARγ, but shows selectivity for RARβ and RARγ.

Psoriasis: The exact mechanisms of tazarotene action in psoriasis are not completely defined. Among its specific pharmacological activities, demonstrated in cellular and in in vivo studies, topical tazarotene blocks induction of epidermal ornithine decarboxylase (ODC) activity, which is associated with cell proliferation and hyperplasia, suppresses expression of MRP8, an inflammatory marker present in psoriatic epidermis at high levels, and inhibits cornified envelope formation and build-up, which is an element of psoriatic scale. Improvement in psoriatic patients appears to occur in association with restoration of normal cutaneous morphology and reduction of the inflammatory markers ICAM-1 and HLA-DR. There is also a diminution of markers of epidermal hyperplasia and abnormal differentiation such as keratinocyte transglutaminase, involucrin and keratin 16.

Tazarotene also induces the expression to TIG3 (tazarotene induced gene 3), a tumor suppressor, which may inhibit epidermal hyperproliferation in treated plaques. Tazarotene, therefore, has multiple effects on keratinocyte differentiation and proliferation, as well as on inflammatory processes which contribute to the pathogenesis of psoriasis. The clinical significance of these findings is unknown.

In two 12-week vehicle-controlled clinical studies, tazarotene 0.05 and 0.1% creams were significantly more effective than vehicle in reducing the severity of plaque psoriasis. Tazarotene creams demonstrated effectiveness as early as 1 week after starting treatment, and initial treatment success (global response to treatment of moderate, marked, almost cleared or completely cleared) was reached significantly earlier than with vehicle. Treatment success rates with the 0.1% cream were generally superior (numerically) to those with the 0.05% cream.

During these studies, the number of patients with none, minimal or mild overall disease was significantly greater with tazarotene 0.05 and 0.1% vs vehicle at most follow-up visits.

In 1 of these studies, patients were evaluated for 12 weeks following cessation of therapy, and it was found that subjects treated with the 0.05 and 0.1% tazarotene creams continued to show a therapeutic effect during the 12-week post-treatment period.

Improvements in plaque elevation, scaling, and erythema were generally significantly greater with tazarotene cream 0.1 and 0.05% than with vehicle. Tazarotene cream 0.1% was generally more effective than the 0.05% concentration in reducing the severity of the individual signs of disease. However, tazarotene 0.1% was associated with a somewhat greater degree of local irritation than the 0.05% cream.

Acne: The mechanism of tazarotene action in acne is not defined. Acne is a multifactorial disease. The 4 main factors involved in its development are excessive follicular keratinization, hyperactivity of the sebaceous gland, proliferation of *P. acnes* and other microbes found in sebum-rich skin, and perifollicular inflammation. Acne vulgaris is the most common form of acne and is characterized by a mixture of inflammatory lesions (papules, pustules, and nodules) and non-inflammatory lesions (open comedones and closed comedones).

The basis of tazarotene's therapeutic effect in acne vulgaris appears to be due to its antihyperproliferative, normalizing-of-differentiation and anti-inflammatory effects. Its primary mechanisms of action in humans are believed to be the normalizing of keratinization and a decrease in the coherence of follicular keratinocytes as evidenced by animal and in vitro studies that show that tazarotene inhibits corneocyte accumulation in rhino mouse skin (in vivo) and cross-linked envelope formation in cultured human keratinocytes (in vitro). Both mechanisms contribute to a comedolytic effect against existing comedones and prevention of the development of new microcomedones. The anti-inflammatory effect is suggested by data from skin rafts, where it inhibits the expression of a presumed pro-inflammatory marker, migration inhibitory factor related protein type 8 (MRP8). Furthermore, tazarotene indirectly hinders the development of inflammatory acne by suppressing the microcomedo, the precursor acne lesion. In addition, by clearing obstructed follicles, tazarotene also allows aeration and release of accumulated sebum, making the follicles a less desirable environment for *P. acnes* and indirectly halting the progression of inflammatory acne.

In two 12-week vehicle-controlled clinical studies, tazarotene 0.1% cream was significantly more effective than vehicle in reducing the total number of lesions, the number of inflammatory lesions and the number of non-inflammatory lesions. Tazarotene cream 0.1% demonstrated effectiveness in reducing the total number of lesions as early as 4 weeks after starting treatment.

After 12 weeks, the number of patients whose overall acne assessment improved from baseline by 1 or more grades (clinical improvement rate) was significantly greater with tazarotene cream 0.1% than with vehicle.

Tazarotene cream 0.1% was also associated with a significantly higher treatment success rate, based upon numbers of patients with a moderate response to treatment or better, than vehicle cream.

Photodamage: The mechanism of tazarotene action in photodamage is unknown. Photodamaged or photoaged skin, resulting from over-exposure to the sun, is characterized by wrinkles, laxity, uneven pigmentation, brown spots, and a leathery appearance. In contrast, chronologically aged skin that has been protected from the sun is thin and has reduced elasticity, but is otherwise smooth and unblemished.

Improvement in the appearance of photodamaged patients appears to occur in association with increased epidermal thickness, decrease in percentage area of melanin, and compaction of the stratum corneum. A study of the histological safety of tazarotene cream 0.1% applied to photodamaged but otherwise normal skin for 24 weeks showed that tazarotene is not associated with the formation or worsening of keratinocytic atypia or melanocytic atypia. Tazarotene cream 0.1% was associated with significant improvements in the distribution/severity of melanocytic atypia when compared with vehicle. Furthermore, tazarotene cream 0.1% was shown to be associated with (i) significant increases in epidermal thickness and (ii) significantly greater proportions of patients who showed an increase from baseline in the number of granular cell layers. Tazarotene cream 0.1% was also associated with significantly greater proportions of patients who showed an increase from baseline in epidermal edema. The clinical significance of these changes is unknown.

In two 24-week vehicle-controlled clinical studies, tazarotene cream 0.1% was significantly more effective than vehicle in reducing the severity of fine wrinkling, mottled hyperpigmentation, elastosis, lentigines, pore size, and irregular depigmentation and in showing improvement in Overall Integrated Assessment (OIA) of Photodamage. (OIA is an assessment by the investigator of the overall severity of facial photodamage.)

The incidence rates of patients who improved by 1 grade or more from baseline were significantly higher for tazarotene cream 0.1% than vehicle as early as Week 2 for mottled hyperpigmentation and Week 8 for fine wrinkling. Improvement for lentigines was observed as early as Week 4, elastosis and pore size as early as Week 12, and irregular depigmentation as early as Week 16. Improvement in OIA was observed as early as Week 8. Tazarotene cream 0.1% was also associated with a significantly higher treatment success rate (based upon the numbers of patients with a moderate response to treatment or better, than vehicle cream).

The distribution of patients' overall self-assessment of photodamage scores in the tazarotene-treated group demonstrated significantly greater improvement from baseline compared with the vehicle-treated group. (Patients' Overall Assessment was a measure in which at each follow-up visit patients evaluated their overall response to treatment compared to their condition at baseline.) According to the Patients' Overall Assessment, in each study, more than 60% were either somewhat or much improved after Week 4, more than 70% were somewhat or much improved after Week 8, and more than 80% were somewhat or much improved after Weeks 12, 16, 20 and 24. In one study 93.1% were somewhat to much improved after Week 24.

Pharmacokinetics: Following application, the drug undergoes esterase hydrolysis to its primary active metabolite, "tazarotenic acid" (the only metabolite of tazarotene known to have retinoid activity), and oxidative metabolism to inactive sulfoxide and sulfone derivatives. Little parent compound can be detected in the plasma. "Tazarotenic acid" is highly bound to plasma proteins (>99%). The half-life of "tazarotenic acid" following topical application of tazarotene is similar in normal and psoriatic subjects, approximately 18 hours.

During clinical trials for the treatment of psoriasis with 0.05 and 0.1% tazarotene creams, plasma concentrations of tazarotene and "tazarotenic acid" were monitored. In 139 patients tested, quantifiable tazarotene was detected in only 3 patients, with the highest concentration at 0.09 ng/mL. The majority of plasma samples were quantitated at less than the limit of the assay for "tazarotenic acid" (<0.1 ng/mL). Only 6 patients had plasma "tazarotenic acid" concentrations greater than 1 ng/mL, the highest of which was 2.4 ng/mL.

In a Phase 3 clinical trial, tazarotene 0.1% cream was applied once daily to each patient with facial acne vulgaris for 12 weeks. The mean ±SD values of plasma tazarotenic acid at weeks 4 and 8 were 0.078±0.073 ng/mL (N=47) and 0.052±0.037 ng/mL (N=42), respectively. The highest observed individual plasma tazarotenic acid concentration was 0.41 ng/mL at week 4 from a female patient. The magnitude of plasma tazarotenic acid concentrations appears to be independent of gender, age, and body weight.

In a phase 3 study tazarotene cream 0.1% was applied once daily for 24 weeks under clinical conditions (double-blind period) to patients with photodamaged skin. The mean plasma tazarotenic acid concentrations following topical treatment with tazarotene cream 0.1% were 0.092±0.073 ng/mL (week 2; N=55), 0.108±0.081 ng/mL (week 12; N=54), and 0.108±0.098 ng/mL (week 24; N=50). The single highest observed tazarotenic acid concentration throughout the 24-week study was 0.423 ng/mL (observed at week 24). Systemic availability of tazarotenic acid was minimal and remained steady following once daily application of tazarotene cream 0.1% to the faces of patients with photodamaged facial skin for up to 24 weeks. The plasma tazarotenic concentrations observed are much lower than the endogenous concentrations of retinoids which are naturally present in plasma: all-trans retinoic acid has been reported to be present at concentrations of 1.32±0.46 ng/mL, 13-cis retinoic acid at 1.63±0.85 ng/mL, and 13-cis-4-oxo retinoic acid at 3.68±0.99 ng/mL.

Results from the well-controlled clinical pharmacokinetic and therapeutic drug monitoring studies using tazarotene cream in the treatment of plaque psoriasis, acne vulgaris, and photodamaged skin demonstrated limited systemic exposure after daily topical applications of tazarotene cream.

INDICATIONS: Tazarotene cream 0.05% and 0.1% are indicated for topical application in the treatment of plaque psoriasis.

Tazarotene cream 0.1% is indicated for the topical treatment of acne vulgaris.

Tazarotene cream 0.1% is indicated for the topical treatment of signs and symptoms (appearance and texture) of premature aging of the skin due to overexposure to the sun, including fine wrinkling, mottled hyperpigmentation, lentigines, elastosis, pore size, and irregular depigmentation.

CONTRAINDICATIONS: In individuals who have shown hypersensitivity to retinoid compounds, or to any of the product excipients (see Supplied). Topical retinoids should not be used in the presence of seborrheic dermatitis.

WARNINGS: General: Tazarotene cream 0.1% in the treatment of photodamaged (sun-damaged) skin should be used under medical supervision as part of a comprehensive skin protection programme, including use of sunscreen products and protective clothing.

Retinoids can cause severe irritation of eczematous skin and should therefore be used with the utmost caution in patients with this condition.

Excessive use of tazarotene cream 0.05 and 0.1% should be avoided. Keep away from the eyes, nose, mouth, and other mucous membranes. When using tazarotene for the treatment of photodamaged skin, care should be used when treating wrinkles around the eyes (Crow's feet) and mouth. In the event of contact with the eye, flush with cold water. Tazarotene should not be applied to severely inflamed skin or open lesions.

In some patients, temporary skin irritation may occur, especially during the early weeks of treatment. If excessive pruritus, burning, skin redness or peeling occur, the medication should either be discontinued until the integrity of the skin is restored, or the dosing should be adjusted to a level or interval the patient can tolerate. Efficacy at reduced frequency of application has not been established.

Pregnancy: **Topical tazarotene should be used by a female of childbearing age only after contraceptive counselling. It is recommended that topical tazarotene should not be used by pregnant women.**

There have been no adequate and well-controlled prospective studies on the use of tazarotene or other **topical** retinoids in pregnant women. There have been rare reports of birth defects among babies born to women exposed to topical retinoids during pregnancy, although a causal relationship has not been determined. A retrospective study of mothers exposed to topical tretinoin during the first trimester of pregnancy found no increase in the incidence of birth defects.

As with all retinoids **oral** tazarotene is teratogenic.

Tazarotene 0.05% gel, administered topically during gestation days 6 through 17 in rats and days 6 through 18 in rabbits, has been shown to be nonteratogenic and nonfetotoxic at maximum tolerated doses of 0.25 mg/kg/day. However, at these doses, slightly reduced fetal body weights and reduced skeletal ossification occurred in rats. These changes may be considered variants of normal development and were usually corrected after weaning. Multiple topical dosing to pregnant rats at 0.2 mg/kg daily resulted in undetectable radioactivity in the fetus. These findings indicate very little drug exposure to the rat fetus via placental transfer after topical treatment with tazarotene.

PRECAUTIONS: General: For external use only.

Because of heightened susceptibility to sunlight, excessive exposure to ultraviolet light, either natural source (sunlight) or artificial (ultraviolet lamps) should be minimized or avoided unless deemed medically necessary. Patients who have considerable sun exposure due to occupation and those inherently sensitive to the sun should exercise particular caution when using tazarotene. Sunscreen (minimum SPF of 15) and protective clothing should be used when using tazarotene and exposure to sunlight cannot be avoided.

Patients with sunburn should be advised not to use tazarotene until fully recovered.

Weather extremes such as wind or cold may be more irritating to patients using tazarotene.

The treatment area should not be covered with dressings or bandages.

Application to normal skin should be avoided in the treatment of psoriasis. In acne the whole of the skin prone to acne sho[uld] be treated. In the treatment of photodamaged skin, the entire face should be treated.

<u>*Drug Interactions:*</u> Concomitant dermatologic medications and cosmetics that have a strong drying effect or high amounts [of] alcohol, astringents, spices, lime peel, medicated soaps or shampoos, permanent wave solution, or other products that ma[y] irritate the skin should be avoided. It is also advisable to "rest" a patient's skin until the effects of such preparations subside before use of tazarotene cream 0.05 or 0.1% begins.

Tazarotene should be administered with caution if the patient is also taking drugs known to be photosensitizers (e.g., thiazides, tetracyclines, fluoroquinolones, phenothiazines, sulfonamides) because of the increased possibility of augmented photosensitivity.

Lactation: After single topical doses of ^{14}C-tazarotene gel to the skin of lactating rats, secretion of radioactivity at very low levels was detected in milk, suggesting that there would be limited transfer of drug-related material to the offspring via milk. It is not known whether this drug is excreted in human milk. Because many drugs are excreted in human milk, caution should be exercised when tazarotene is administered to a nursing woman.

Children: The safety and efficacy of tazarotene have not been established in pediatric patients under the age of 12 years.

ADVERSE EFFECTS: Psoriasis: The most frequent adverse reactions (≥5%) reported as being treatment related during Phase 3 clinical trials with tazarotene cream in the treatment of psoriasis (n=860) included pruritus (20.7%), erythema (14.3%), burning (12.7%), and irritation (8.3%). Reported less frequently (≥1% to <5%) were desquamation (2.9%), skin pain (2.4%), contact irritant dermatitis (2.3%), worsening of psoriasis (2.3%), stinging (2.1%), rash (2.1%), dermatitis (2%), eczema (1.5%), dry skin (1.1%), hypertriglyceridemia (1%). The incidence and severity of these adverse reactions appeared to be dose-related.

Acne: The most frequent adverse reactions (≥5%) reported as being treatment-related during Phase 3 clinical trials with tazarotene cream 0.1% in the treatment of acne (n=424) included desquamation (29.2%), dry skin (26.9%), erythema (20.5%), and burning sensation (13.9%). Reported less frequently (≥1-<5%) were pruritus (4.5%), irritation (4.0%), face pain (1.9%), and stinging (1.7%).

Photodamage: The most frequent treatment-related adverse reactions (≥5%) reported during the clinical trials with tazaortene in the treatment of signs and symptoms of premature aging of the skin due to overexposure to the sun (n=567) included desquamation (39.3%), erythema (33.2%), burning sensation (24.5%), dry skin (15.7%), skin irritation (9.3%), pruritus (8.8%), irritant contact dermatitis (7.2%). Reported less frequently (>1-<5%) were stinging (3.2%), acne (2.3%), and rash (1.9%).

In human topical safety studies, tazarotene 0.1 and 0.05% creams were moderately irritating under the exaggerated conditions of the studies, but did not induce allergic contact sensitization, phototoxicity or photoallergy.

OVERDOSE:

Symptoms: Excessive topical use of tazarotene creams 0.05 and 0.1% may lead to marked redness, peeling, or discomfort (see Warnings). Inadvertent oral ingestion of tazarotene may lead to the same adverse effects as those associated with excessive oral intake of vitamin A including teratogenesis in women of child-bearing age.

Treatment: If accidental oral ingestion occurs, the patient should be monitored, and appropriate supportive measures should be administered as necessary, including pregnancy testing in women of childbearing age.

For management of a suspected drug overdose, CPhA recommends that you contact your **regional Poison Control Centre**. See the *CPS* Directory section for a list of Poison Control Centres.

DOSAGE: General: **For dermatological (topical) use only.**

If affected areas are washed just prior to application, the skin should be dry prior to applying tazarotene. Application may cause a transitory feeling of burning or stinging. If irritation becomes problematic, therapy may be temporarily discontinued or the dosage may be altered by choosing the lower drug concentration or temporarily reducing the frequency of application. Therapy can be resumed or the frequency of application can be increased as the patient becomes able to tolerate the treatment. Frequency of application should be closely monitored by careful observation of the clinical therapeutic response and skin tolerance. Efficacy has not been established for less than once-daily dosing frequencies.

Excessive exposure to sun or ultraviolet light should be minimized or avoided. Sunscreen (minimum SPF of 15) and protective clothing should be used when exposed to sunlight.

For Psoriasis: Apply tazarotene cream 0.05% or 0.1% once a day, in the evening, to psoriatic lesions, using enough to cover only the lesion with a thin film. If emollients are used, they should be applied and allowed to absorb into the skin before application of tazarotene. Because unaffected skin may be more susceptible to irritation, application of tazarotene to these areas should be carefully avoided.

For Acne: Cleanse the skin gently. After the skin is dry, apply a thin film of tazarotene cream 0.1% once a day, to the entire face as delineated by the hairline, jawline and ears. Use enough to cover the entire affected area.

For Photodamage: For photodamage (premature aging of the skin due to overexposure to the sun), apply a pea-sized amount once a day to lightly cover the entire face, including the eyelids if desired. Facial moisturizers may be used as frequently as desired. Moisturizers may be applied either before or after tazarotene cream, but whichever is applied first should be allowed to absorb into the skin before the next one is applied. If any makeup is present it should be removed before applying tazarotene to the face.

INFORMATION FOR THE PATIENT: Published in e-CPS, available by subscription at www.e-cps.ca.

SUPPLIED: 0.05%: Each g of white to slightly off-white emollient cream contains: tazarotene 0.05% (w/w). Nonmedicinal ingredients: benzyl alcohol (as preservative), Carbomer 934P, Carbomer 1342, edetate disodium, medium chain triglycerides, mineral oil, purified water, sodium thiosulfate, sodium hydroxide (to adjust the pH) and sorbitan monooleate. Collapsible aluminum tubes of 30 g. Physician's sample sizes of 3.5 g.

0.1%: Each g of white to slightly off-white emollient cream contains: tazarotene 0.1% (w/w). Nonmedicinal ingredients: benzyl alcohol (as preservative), Carbomer 934P, Carbomer 1342, edetate disodium, medium chain triglycerides, mineral oil, purified water, sodium thiosulfate, sodium hydroxide (to adjust the pH) and sorbitan monooleate. Collapsible aluminum tubes of 30 g. Physician's sample sizes of 3.5 g.

Store at room temperature (15 to 25°C).

Tazorac™ Gel ℞

tazarotene

Antipsoriasis—Antiacne

Allergan

PHARMACOLOGY: Tazarotene is a retinoid prodrug which is converted to its active form, M1 ("tazarotenic acid", or AGN 190299), by rapid de-esterification in most biological systems. "Tazarotenic acid" binds to and regulates gene expression through all three members of the RAR family of retinoid nuclear receptors, RAR_{α}, RAR_{β}, and RAR_{γ}, but shows selectivity for RAR_{β} and RAR_{γ}.

Psoriasis: The exact mechanisms of tazarotene action in psoriasis are not completely defined. Among its specific pharmacological activities, demonstrated in cellular and in in vivo studies, topical tazarotene blocks induction of epidermal ornithine decarboxylase (ODC) activity, which is associated with cell proliferation and hyperplasia, suppresses expression of MRP8, an inflammatory marker present in psoriatic epidermis at high levels, and inhibits cornified envelope formation and build-up, which is an element of psoriatic scale. Improvement in psoriatic patients appears to occur in association with restoration of normal cutaneous morphology and reduction of the inflammatory markers ICAM-1 and HLA-DR. There is also a diminution of markers of epidermal hyperplasia and abnormal differentiation such as keratinocyte transglutaminase, involucrin and keratin 16.

In 2 large vehicle-controlled clinical studies, tazarotene 0.1 and 0.05% gels applied once daily were significantly more effective than vehicle in reducing the severity of the clinical signs of plaque psoriasis. Tazarotene gels demonstrated effectiveness as early as 1 week after starting treatment, with initial treatment success (good or excellent response or complete clearing) reached significantly earlier than with vehicle. The 0.1% gel was more effective than the 0.05% gel, but the 0.05% gel was associated with less local irritation than the 0.1% gel. In one of these studies, patients were also evaluated for 12 weeks following cessation of therapy, and it was found that subjects treated with the 0.1 and 0.05% tazarotene gels continued to show a therapeutic effect during the 12-week post-treatment period.

Acne: Tazarotene is thought to act against several of the factors that contribute to acne vulgaris. Animal and in vitro studies show that tazarotene inhibits corneocyte accumulation in rhino mouse skin (in vivo) and cross-linked envelope formation in cultured human keratinocytes (in vitro). The primary mechanisms of action in humans are believed to be the normalizing of keratinization and a decrease in the coherence of follicular keratinocytes. Both mechanisms contribute to a comedolytic effect against existing comedones and prevention of the development of new microcomedones. Tazarotene also exhibits activity against inflammatory acne.

In 2 large vehicle-controlled studies, tazarotene 0.1 and 0.05% gels applied once daily were significantly more effective than their vehicle in the treatment of acne vulgaris. The 0.1% gel was more effective than the 0.05% gel, but the 0.05% gel was associated with less local irritation than the 0.1% gel.

Pharmacokinetics: Controlled clinical pharmacokinetic studies with 0.1% ^{14}C-tazarotene gel indicate that less than 1% of the dose is systemically absorbed when applied topically (unoccluded) to psoriatic plaques, and approximately 5% of the dose is absorbed after application to normal skin under occlusion. After a 7-day topical dosing period with tazarotene 0.1% gel to normal skin over 20% of the body surface area (0.1 mg/kg/day), the mean maximum plasma concentration was 0.72±0.58 ng/mL at 9 hours, and the area under the plasma concentration time curve over a 24-hour time period was 10.1±7.2 ng·hr/mL. A clinical pharmacokinetic study conducted in 5 psoriatic patients where treatment conditions were maximized to ensure sufficiently high plasma concentrations, showed that tazarotene absorption through the skin increased over the 2-week course of the study. The maximal plasma concentration was 12.0±7.6 ng/mL at 6 hours, and the area under the plasma concentration time curve over a 24-hour time period was 105±55 ng·hr/mL. This increased absorption through the skin in psoriatic may be due not only to a reduction of thick scale prior to normalization of indurated plaques, but also in part to a possible thinning of the stratum corneum. Following topical dosing of tazarotene, the half-life of "tazarotenic acid", the primary active metabolite, was approximately 18 hours. The terminal half-lives of tazarotene and "tazarotenic acid" were 6 and 14 hours respectively, following i.v. dosing to normal volunteers.

Following application, the drug undergoes esterase hydrolysis to its primary active metabolite, tazarotenic acid (the only metabolite of tazarotene known to have retinoid activity), and oxidative metabolism to inactive sulfoxide and sulfone derivatives. Following topical dosing with ^{14}C-tazarotene under occlusion to healthy subjects, 2.6 and 2.7% of the dose were excreted in urine and feces, respectively, over a 7-day period. Following a topical unoccluded dose to psoriatic patients, 0.3% of the dose was excreted in the urine and 0.4% excreted in the feces. Greater than 75% of total drug excretion was completed within 72 hours after drug removal, with equal excretion of radioactivity in urine and feces. The drug's rapid systemic metabolism limits the propensity for tissue distribution and body exposure to tazarotene.

INDICATIONS: For topical application in the treatment of plaque psoriasis and acne vulgaris.

CONTRAINDICATIONS: Individuals who have shown hypersensitivity to retinoic compounds, or to any of the product excipients (see Supplied). Topical retinoids should not be used in the presence of seborrheic dermatitis.

WARNINGS: Topical retinoids should not be used on eczematous skin.

Keep away from the eyes, nose, mouth, and other mucous membranes. In the event of contact with the eye, flush with cold water.

In some patients, temporary skin irritation may occur, especially during the early weeks of treatment. If excessive pruritus, burning, skin redness or peeling occur, the medication should either be discontinued until the integrity of the skin is restored, or the dosing should be adjusted to a level or interval the patient can tolerate.

Pregnancy: **Topical tazarotene should be used by females of childbearing age only after contraceptive counselling. It is recommended that topical tazarotene should not be used by pregnant females.**

Tazarotene 0.05% gel, administered topically during gestation days 6 through 17 in rats and days 6 through 18 in rabbits, has been shown to be nonteratogenic and nonfetotoxic at maximum tolerated doses of 0.25 mg/kg/day. However, at these doses, slightly reduced fetal body weights and reduced skeletal ossification occurred in rats. These changes may be considered variants of normal development and were usually corrected after weaning. As with other retinoids, teratogenic effects were seen when tazarotene was given orally to rats and rabbits at doses of 0.25 and 0.2 mg/kg/day, respectively. Very low drug exposure to the fetus was observed after oral administration of ^{14}C-tazarotene to pregnant rats and rabbits. Multiple topical dosing to pregnant rats at 0.2 mg/kg daily resulted in undetectable radioactivity in the fetus. These finding indicate very little drug exposure to the rat fetus via placental transfer after topical treatment with tazarotene. There are no adequate and well-controlled studies in pregnant women.

PRECAUTIONS: General: For external use only. Excessive use should be avoided.

Excessive exposure to sun or ultraviolet light should be minimized or avoided. Sunscreen and protective clothing should be used when exposed to sunlight.

The safety of use over more than 20% of body surface area has not been established.

The treatment area should not be covered with dressings or bandages.

In patients with psoriasis, application to normal skin should be avoided.

Drug Interactions: Concomitant dermatologic medications and cosmetics that have a strong drying effect should be avoided. It is also advisable to "rest" a patient's skin until the effects of such preparations subside before use of tazarotene gels begins.

Carcinogenesis, Mutagenesis, Impairment of Fertility: Long-term studies of tazarotene following topical application in mice and oral administration to rats showed no indications of increased carcinogenic risks related to treatment. Marked skin irritation, possibly contributing to enhancement of photocarcinogenesis, was observed in hairless mice following chronic topical dosing with intercurrent exposure to ultraviolet radiation at tazarotene concentrations of 0.001, 0.005, and 0.01% for up to 40 weeks. Relevance of these studies to use in humans has not been established, but patients should minimize exposure to sun or ultraviolet light.

Tazarotene was found to be nonmutagenic and nonclastogenic in a standard battery of in vitro and in vivo tests.

No impairment of fertility occurred in rats when male animals were treated for 70 days prior to mating and female animals were treated for 14 days prior to mating and continuing through gestation and lactation with topical doses of tazarotene gel.

Reproductive capabilities of F1 animals, including F2 survival and development, were not affected by topical administration of tazarotene gel to female F0 parental rats from gestation day 16 through lactation day 20 at the maximum tolerated dose of 0.125 mg/kg/day.

Lactation: After single topical doses of ^{14}C-tazarotene to the skin of lactating rats, secretion of radioactivity at very low levels was detected in milk, suggesting that there would be limited transfer of drug-related material to the offspring via milk. It is not known whether this drug is excreted in human milk. Because many drugs are excreted in human milk, caution should be exercised when tazarotene is administered to a nursing woman.

Children: The safety and efficacy of tazarotene have not been established in pediatric patients under the age of 12 years.

ADVERSE EFFECTS: Psoriasis: The most frequent adverse reactions (≥5%) reported during clinical trials with tazarotene gel included pruritus, burning, erythema, skin irritation, skin pain, and worsening of psoriasis. Reported less frequently (1 to <5%) were desquamation, rash, contact irritant dermatitis, skin inflammation, stinging, and dry skin. Rarely reported reactions (<1%) included fissuring of the skin, bleeding, skin discharge, increased skin fragility, and localized edema. The incidence and severity of adverse reactions appeared to be dose related.

Acne: The most frequent adverse reactions (≥5%) reported during clinical trials with tazarotene gels in the treatment of acne included burning, desquamation, dry skin, erythema, and pruritus. Reported less frequently (1 to <5%) were skin irritation, and stinging. The following reactions were reported rarely (<1%) by study subjects: skin pain, skin tightness, fissuring of the skin, cheilitis, skin discoloration, worsening of acne, contact irritant dermatitis, and localized edema. The incidence and severity of adverse reactions appeared to be dose related.

In human topical safety studies, tazarotene 0.1% and 0.05% gels did not induce contact sensitization, phototoxicity or photoallergy.

OVERDOSE:

Symptoms: Excessive topical use of tazarotene may lead to marked redness, peeling, or discomfort (see Warnings). Inadvertent oral ingestion of tazarotene may lead to the same adverse effects as those associated with excessive oral intake of vitamin A including teratogenesis in women of childbearing age.

Treatment: If accidental oral ingestion occurs, the patient should be monitored, and appropriate supportive measures should be administered as necessary, including pregnancy testing in women of childbearing age.

For management of a suspected drug overdose, CPhA recommends that you contact your **regional Poison Control Centre**. See the *CPS* Directory section for a list of Poison Control Centres.

DOSAGE: General: Application may cause a transitory feeling of burning or stinging. If irritation becomes problematic, the dosage may be altered by choosing the lower drug concentration or temporarily reducing the frequency of application.

Excessive exposure to sun or ultraviolet light should be minimized or avoided. Sunscreen and protective clothing should be used when exposed to sunlight.

Psoriasis: Apply once a day, in the evening, to psoriatic lesions, using enough to cover only the lesion with a thin film. If a bath or shower is taken prior to application, the skin should be dry before applying the gel. If emollients are used, they should be applied and allowed to absorb into the skin before application. Because unaffected skin may be more susceptible to irritation, application to these areas should be carefully avoided.

Acne: Cleanse the skin gently. After the skin is dry, apply a thin film once a day, in the evening, to the skin where acne lesions appear. Use enough to cover the entire affected area.

INFORMATION FOR THE PATIENT: Published in e-CPS, available by subscription at www.e-cps.ca.

SUPPLIED: Each g of colorless to light yellow, translucent homogeneous gel contains: tazarotene 0.05% or 0.1% (w/w). Nonmedicinal ingredients: ascorbic acid, benzyl alcohol, butylated hydroxyanisole, butylated hydroxytoluene, carbomer 934P, edetate disodium, hexylene glycol, poloxamer 407, polyethylene glycol, polysorbate 40, purified water and tromethamine. Collapsible aluminum tubes of 30 g. Sample sizes of 3.5 g for physicians. Store at room temperature (15 to 25°C).

Td Adsorbed

tetanus and diphtheria toxoids adsorbed

Active Immunizing Agent

sanofi pasteur

Date of Revision: July 2010

SUMMARY PRODUCT INFORMATION:

Route of Administration	Dosage Form/ Strength	Clinically Relevant Nonmedicinal Ingredients
Intramuscular injection	Suspension for injection. Each 0.5 mL dose is formulated to contain: active ingredients tetanus toxoid, diphtheria toxoid	Excipients: Aluminum phosphate (adjuvant), 2-phenoxyethanol, isotonic solution of sodium chloride in water for injection. Manufacturing process residuals: formaldehyde is present in trace amounts. For a complete listing see Dosage Forms, Composition and Packaging.

DESCRIPTION: Td ADSORBED [Tetanus and Diphtheria Toxoids Adsorbed], is a sterile, cloudy, white, uniform suspension of tetanus and diphtheria toxoids adsorbed separately on aluminum phosphate and suspended in isotonic sodium chloride solution.

INDICATIONS AND CLINICAL USE: Td ADSORBED is indicated for active primary and booster immunization for the prevention of tetanus and diphtheria as a single dose in persons 7 years of age and older.

Persons who have had tetanus or diphtheria should still be immunized since these clinical infections do not always confer immunity.

Human Immunodeficiency Virus (HIV)-infected persons, both asymptomatic and symptomatic, should be immunized against tetanus and diphtheria according to standard schedules.

Td ADSORBED is not to be used for the treatment of disease caused by *C. diphtheriae* or *C. tetani* infections.

Pediatrics: Td ADSORBED is not indicated for immunization of children below the age of 7 years.

Geriatrics: Td ADSORBED is indicated for immunization of persons 7 years of age and older.

Tetanus Prophylaxis in Wound Management: The need for active immunization with a tetanus toxoid-containing preparation such as Td ADSORBED, with or without passive immunization with Tetanus Immune Globulin, depends on both the condition of the wound and the patient's vaccination history. (See Dosage and Administration.)

CONTRAINDICATIONS: Hypersensitivity: Known systemic hypersensitivity reaction to any component of Td ADSORBED or a life-threatening reaction after previous administration of the vaccine or a vaccine containing one or more of the same components are contraindications to vaccination. (See Summary Product Information.) Alternatively, such persons may be referred to an allergist for evaluation if further immunizations are considered.

WARNINGS AND PRECAUTIONS: General: Before administration of Td ADSORBED, health-care providers should inform the recipient, the parent or guardian of the recipient of the benefits and risks of immunization, inquire about the recent health status of the recipient, review the recipient's history concerning possible hypersensitivity to the vaccine or similar vaccine, previous immunization history, the presence of any contraindications to immunization and comply with any local requirements regarding information to be provided to the recipient/guardian before immunization.

It is extremely important that the recipient, parent or guardian be questioned concerning any signs or symptoms of an adverse reaction after a previous dose of vaccine (see Contraindications and Adverse Reactions).

The rates and severity of adverse events in recipients of tetanus toxoid are influenced by the number of prior doses and level of pre-existing antitoxins.

As with any vaccine Td ADSORBED may not protect 100% of vaccinated persons.

Administration Route Related Precautions: Do not administer Td ADSORBED by intravascular injection; ensure that the needle does not penetrate a blood vessel.

Intradermal or subcutaneous routes of administration are not to be utilized.

Td ADSORBED should not be administered into the buttocks.

Febrile and Acute Disease: Vaccination should be postponed in cases of an acute or febrile disease. However, a disease with low-grade fever should not usually be a reason to postpone vaccination.

Hematologic: Because any intramuscular injection can cause an injection site hematoma in persons with any bleeding disorders, such as hemophilia or thrombocytopenia, or in persons on anticoagulant therapy, intramuscular injections with Td ADSORBED should not be administered to such persons unless the potential benefits outweigh the risks of administration. If the decision is made to administer any product by intramuscular injection to such persons, it should be given with caution, with steps taken to avoid the risk of hematoma formation following injection.

Immune: The possibility of allergic reactions in persons sensitive to components of the vaccine should be evaluated. Hypersensitivity reactions may occur following the use of Td ADSORBED even in persons with no prior history of hypersensitivity to the product components. (See Dosage Forms, Composition and Packaging.)

As with all other products, epinephrine hydrochloride solution (1:1000) and other appropriate agents should be available for immediate use in case an anaphylactic or acute hypersensitivity reaction occurs. Health-care providers should be familiar with current recommendations for the initial management of anaphylaxis in non-hospital settings, including proper airway management. For instructions on recognition and treatment of anaphylactic reactions, see the current edition of the Canadian Immunization Guide or visit the Health Canada website.

Immunocompromised persons (whether from disease or treatment) may not achieve the expected immune response. If possible, consideration should be given to delaying vaccination until after the completion of any immunosuppressive treatment. Nevertheless, vaccination of persons with chronic immunodeficiency such as HIV infection is recommended even if the immune response might be limited.

Neurologic: A review by the US Institute of Medicine (IOM) found evidence for a causal relation between tetanus toxoid and both brachial neuritis and Guillain-Barré syndrome (GBS). If GBS occurred within 6 weeks of receipt of prior vaccine containing tetanus toxoid, the decision to give Td ADSORBED or any vaccine containing tetanus toxoid should be based on careful consideration of the potential benefits and possible risks.

A few cases of demyelinating diseases of the central nervous system, peripheral mononeuropathies and cranial mononeuropathies have been reported following vaccines containing tetanus and/or diphtheria toxoids, although the IOM concluded that the evidence is inadequate to accept or reject a causal relation between these conditions and vaccination.

Special Populations: Pregnant Women: Animal reproduction and fertility studies have not been conducted with Td ADSORBED. It is also not known whether Td ADSORBED can cause foetal harm when administered to a pregnant woman or can affect reproduction capacity. Td ADSORBED should be given to a pregnant woman only if clearly needed, as per national recommendations.

Nursing Women: It is not known whether the active substances included in Td ADSORBED are excreted in human milk. The effect of administration of Td ADSORBED during lactation has not been assessed. As Td ADSORBED is inactivated, any risk to the mother or the infant is improbable. However, the risks and benefits of vaccination should be assessed before making the decision to immunize a nursing woman.

ADVERSE REACTIONS: Clinical Trial Adverse Drug Reactions: Because clinical trials are conducted under widely varying conditions, adverse reaction rates observed in the clinical trials of a vaccine cannot be directly compared to rates in the clinical trials of another vaccine and may not reflect rates observed in practice. The adverse reaction information from clinical trials does, however, provide a basis for identifying the adverse events that appear to be related to vaccine use and for approximating rates of those events.

During clinical trials, the most common adverse reactions associated with the administration of Td ADSORBED were pain, swelling and redness at the injection site in all age groups and following both primary and booster immunization.

In a clinical study of primary immunization conducted in Canada, Td ADSORBED was administered as a three dose primary series to 18 subjects, 8 of whom were 6-9 years of age and 10 of whom were 17-56 years of age. In three booster immunization studies conducted in Canada, Td ADSORBED was administered to 773 subjects overall, ranging in age from 12-59 years.

In two of the booster immunization studies, one dose of Td ADSORBED was administered to subjects who were presumed to have previously received primary immunization against tetanus and diphtheria, and had not received tetanus or diphtheria toxoid within 5 years prior to enrollment. The results from these studies are presented in Table 1.

No serious adverse events were reported following vaccination with Td ADSORBED in these studies.

Table 1: Td ADSORBED

Frequencies of Selected Solicited Adverse Events within 72 Hours Following a Dose of Td ADSORBED in Presumably Previously Primed Subjects.

	TC9704		TD9707
Event	Adolescents[a] N=37 (%)	Adults N=263 (%)	Adults N=126 (%)
Injection Site Reactions			
Redness	5.4	8.4	21.4
Swelling	16.2	13.3	10.3
Pain	81.1	84.8	84.9
Systemic Reactions			
Fever (≥38.0°C)	2.7	4.2	0.8
Chills	8.1	4.6	5.6
Sore or Swollen Joints	8.1	5.3	5.6

[a] Ages 12–17 years.

Post-Market Adverse Drug Reactions: The following additional adverse events have been spontaneously reported during the post-marketing use of Td ADSORBED or a similar vaccine manufactured by Sanofi Pasteur, one of identical antigenic content but with thimerosal instead of 2-phenoxyethanol, one of identical tetanus antigen content but lower diphtheria antigen content and thimerosal instead of 2-phenoxyethanol. Because these events are reported voluntarily from a population of uncertain size, it is not always possible to reliably estimate their frequency or establish a causal relationship to vaccine exposure. Decisions to include these events in labelling were based on one or more of the following factors: 1) severity of the event, 2) frequency of reporting, or 3) strength of causal connection to Td ADSORBED.

Blood and Lymphatic System Disorders: lymphadenopathy.

Immune System Disorders: Allergic reactions (such as rash, urticaria, pruritus, rash erythematous, rash maculopapular), anaphylactoid reactions (bronchospasm and edema of the mouth) have also been reported.

Nervous System Disorders: paresthesia, dizziness, syncope.

Guillain-Barré syndrome (GBS) has been exceptionally reported.

Gastrointestinal Disorders: vomiting.

Musculoskeletal, Connective Tissue and Bone Disorders: myalgia, pain in extremities.

General Disorders and Administration Site Conditions: injection site reactions (including inflammation, mass, edema, induration, warmth, pruritus, cellulitis, discomfort).

fatigue, edema peripheral.

Physicians, nurses and pharmacists should report any adverse occurrences temporally related to the administration of the product in accordance with local requirements and to the Global Pharmacovigilance Department, Sanofi Pasteur Limited, 1755 Steeles Avenue West, Toronto, ON, M2R 3T4 Canada. 1-888-621-1146 (phone) or 416-667-2435 (fax).

DRUG INTERACTIONS: Vaccine-Drug Interactions: Immunosuppressive treatments may interfere with the development of the expected immune response. (See Warnings and Precautions.)

Concomitant Vaccine Administration: There are no data available on the concomitant administration of Td ADSORBED with other live or inactivated parenteral vaccines. Vaccine administered simultaneously should be given using separate syringes at separate sites, as appropriate for the recipient's age and previous vaccination status.

The vaccine must not be mixed with other medicinal products.

DOSAGE AND ADMINISTRATION: Recommended Dose and Dosage Adjustment: Primary Immunization: For primary immunization of persons 7 years of age and older, a series of three (0.5 mL) doses is required. The first two doses should be given 4 to 8 weeks apart and the third dose 6 to 12 months later.

Interruption of the recommended schedule with a delay between doses should not interfere with the final immunity achieved with Td ADSORBED. There is no need to start the series over, regardless of the time elapsed between doses.

Booster Immunization: For booster immunization of persons 7 years of age and older a single (0.5 mL) dose is required. There are currently no data upon which to base a recommendation for the optimal interval for administering subsequent booster doses with Td ADSORBED. For persons who have previously been immunized against tetanus and diphtheria, a dose of 0.5 mL should be administered as a reinforcing dose at approximately 10 year intervals.

Fractional doses (doses <0.5 mL) should not be given. The effect of fractional doses on safety and efficacy has not been determined.

Table 2: Td ADSORBED

NACI Recommended Use of Immunizing Agents in Wound Management

	Clean, Minor Wounds		All Other Wounds	
History of Tetanus Immunization	Td[a]	TIG[b] (Human)	Td	TIG (Human)
Uncertain or <3 doses of an immunization series[c]	Yes	No	Yes	Yes
≥3 doses received in an immunization series[c]	No[d]	No	Yes[e]	No[f]

[a] Adult-type tetanus and diphtheria toxoid.
[b] Tetanus immune globulin, given at a separate site from the Td.
[c] Primary immunization is at least 3 doses at age appropriate intervals.
[d] Yes, if >10 years since last booster.
[e] Yes, if >5 years since last booster.
[f] Yes, if persons are known to have a significant humoral immune deficiency state (eg, HIV, agammaglobulinemia) since immune response to tetanus toxoid may be suboptimal.

Health-care professionals should refer to the NACI guidelines for tetanus prophylaxis in routine wound management shown in Table 2.

A thorough attempt must be made to determine whether a patient has completed primary immunization. Persons who have completed primary immunization against tetanus and who sustain wounds that are minor and uncontaminated should receive a booster dose of a tetanus toxoid-containing preparation if they have not received tetanus toxoid within the preceding 10 years. For tetanus-prone wounds (eg, wounds contaminated with dirt, feces, soil and saliva, puncture wounds, avulsions and wounds resulting from missiles, crushing, burns or frostbite), a booster is appropriate if the patient has not received a tetanus toxoid-containing preparation within the preceding 5 years.

Administration: Inspect for extraneous particulate matter and/or discolouration before use. (See Description.) If these conditions exist, the product should not be administered.

Shake the vial well until a uniform, cloudy, suspension results. Cleanse the vial stopper with a suitable germicide prior to withdrawing the dose. Do not remove either the stopper or the metal seal holding it in place. Aseptic technique must be used. Use a separate sterile needle and syringe, or a sterile disposable unit for each individual recipient, to prevent disease transmission. Needles should not be recapped but should be disposed of according to biohazard waste guidelines. (See Warnings and Precautions.)

Before injection, the skin over the site to be injected should be cleansed with a suitable germicide. Administer the total volume of 0.5 mL **intramuscularly** (IM). The preferred site of injection is the deltoid muscle.

Give the patient a permanent personal immunization record. In addition, it is essential that the physician or nurse record the immunization history in the permanent medical record of each patient. This permanent office record should contain the name of the vaccine, date given, dose, manufacturer and lot number.

OVERDOSAGE:

For management of a suspected drug overdose, contact your regional Poison Control Centre. See the *CPS* Directory section for a list of Poison Control Centres.

ACTION AND CLINICAL PHARMACOLOGY: Tetanus and Diphtheria: Tetanus is an acute and often fatal disease caused by an extremely potent neurotoxin produced by *C. tetani*. The toxin causes neuromuscular dysfunction, with rigidity and spasms of skeletal muscles. Protection against disease attributable to *C. tetani* is due to the development of neutralizing antibodies to tetanus toxin. A serum tetanus antitoxin level of at least 0.01 IU/mL, measured by neutralization assay, is considered the minimum protective level. A tetanus antitoxin level of at least 0.1 IU/mL as measured by the ELISA used in clinical studies of Td ADSORBED is considered as protective for tetanus. Levels of 1.0 IU/mL have been associated with long-term protection.

Strains of *C. diphtheriae* that produce diphtheria toxin can cause severe or fatal illness characterized by membranous inflammation of the upper respiratory tract and toxin-induced damage to the myocardium and nervous system. Protection against disease attributable to *C. diphtheriae* is due to the development of neutralizing antibodies to diphtheria toxin. A serum diphtheria antitoxin level of 0.01 IU/mL is the lowest level giving some degree of protection. Antitoxin levels of at least 0.1 IU/mL are generally regarded as protective. Levels of 1.0 IU/mL have been associated with long-term protection.

STORAGE AND STABILITY: Store at 2° to 8°C. **Do not freeze.** Discard product if exposed to freezing.

Do not use after expiration date.

INFORMATION FOR THE PATIENT: Published in e-CPS, available by subscription at www.e-cps.ca.

DOSAGE FORMS, COMPOSITION AND PACKAGING: Td ADSORBED is supplied as a sterile, cloudy, white, uniform suspension in a vial.

Each single dose (0.5 mL) contains: tetanus toxoid (5 Lf), diphtheria toxoid (2 Lf). Other ingredients: aluminum phosphate (adjuvant) 1.5 mg, 2-phenoxyethanol 0.6% v/v and isotonic solution of Sodium Chloride in Water for Injection q.s. 0.5 mL. Manufacturing Process Residuals: Formaldehyde is present in trace amounts. Single-dose glass vials of 0.5 mL, packages of 5. The vials are made of Type 1 glass. The container closure system of Td ADSORBED is free of latex (natural rubber).

Td Polio Adsorbed

tetanus and diphtheria toxoids adsorbed and inactivated poliomyelitis vaccine

Active Immunizing Agent

sanofi pasteur

Date of Revision: April 10, 2006

SUMMARY PRODUCT INFORMATION:

Route of Administration	Dosage Form/Strength	Clinically Relevant Nonmedicinal Ingredients
Intramuscular injection	Suspension for injection Each dose (0.5 mL) is formulated to contain: 5 Lf tetanus toxoid, 2 Lf diphtheria toxoid Purified inactivated poliomyelitis vaccine: Type 1 (Mahoney) 40 D-antigen units, Type 2 (MEF1) 8 D-antigen units, Type 3 (Saukett) 32 D-antigen units	2-phenoxyethanol, aluminum phosphate, formaldehyde, polysorbate 80, bovine serum albumin, trace amounts of neomycin and polymyxin B For a complete listing see Dosage Forms, Composition and Packaging.

DESCRIPTION: Td POLIO ADSORBED [Tetanus and Diphtheria Toxoids Adsorbed and Inactivated Poliomyelitis Vaccine] produced by Sanofi Pasteur Limited, is a sterile, cloudy, white, uniform suspension of tetanus and diphtheria toxoids adsorbed on aluminum phosphate and suspended in phosphate buffered saline solution and combined with Inactivated Poliomyelitis Vaccine for intramuscular injection only.

INDICATIONS AND CLINICAL USE: Td POLIO ADSORBED [Tetanus and Diphtheria Toxoids Adsorbed and Inactivated Poliomyelitis Vaccine] is indicated for active immunization of persons 7 years of age and older for prevention of tetanus, diphtheria and poliomyelitis. Td POLIO ADSORBED may be used for primary immunization and for boosters.

Persons who have had tetanus or diphtheria should still be immunized since these clinical infections do not always confer immunity. Persons who have had poliomyelitis may receive IPV, as they may not be fully protected against all 3 poliovirus serotypes.

HIV-infected individuals, both asymptomatic and symptomatic, should be immunized against tetanus, diphtheria and poliomyelitis according to standard schedules.

Tetanus: Tetanus is an acute and often fatal disease caused by an extremely potent neurotoxin produced by *C. tetani*. The organism is ubiquitous and its occurrence in nature cannot be controlled. Immunization is highly effective, provides long-lasting protection and is recommended for the whole population. Only 1 to 7 cases of tetanus were reported annually in Canada during the 1990s.

Neonatal tetanus occurs among infants born under unhygienic conditions to inadequately vaccinated mothers. Vaccinated mothers confer protection to their infants through transplacental transfer of maternal antibody.

Diphtheria: Diphtheria is a serious communicable disease caused by toxigenic strains of *C. diphtheriae*. The organism may be harboured in the nasopharynx, skin or other sites of asymptomatic carriers, making eradication of the disease difficult. Routine immunization against diphtheria in infancy and childhood has been widely practiced in Canada since 1930. Fewer than 2 cases are now reported annually in Canada. The case-fatality rate remains at 5 to 10%, with the highest death rates in the very young and elderly. The disease occurs most frequently in unimmunized or partially immunized persons.

Poliomyelitis: Poliomyelitis is a disease that may cause irreversible paralysis in a certain proportion of infected individuals. It is a highly infectious disease caused by three types of the enterovirus poliovirus. It is primarily spread by the fecal-oral route of transmission but may also be spread by the pharyngeal route. Following introduction of poliovirus vaccines in Canada in 1955, the indigenous disease has been virtually eliminated. However, circulation of wild viruses does occur in rare circumstances, and it remains crucial that the highest possible level of vaccine-induced immunity be maintained in the population.

Pediatrics: Td POLIO ADSORBED is indicated for persons 7 years of age and older.

CONTRAINDICATIONS: Known systemic hypersensitivity to any component of Td POLIO ADSORBED [Tetanus and Diphtheria Toxoids Adsorbed and Inactivated Poliomyelitis Vaccine], after previous administration of the vaccine, or after a vaccine containing the same substances is a contraindication to vaccination. (See components listed in Dosage Forms, Composition and Packaging.)

Immunization with Td POLIO ADSORBED should be deferred in the presence of any acute illness, including febrile illness to avoid superimposing adverse effects from the vaccine on the underlying illness or mistakenly identifying a manifestation of the underlying illness as a complication of vaccine use. A minor illness such as mild upper respiratory infection is not a reason to defer immunization. The National Advisory Committee on Immunization (NACI) has published guidelines for vaccination of persons with recent acute illness.

WARNINGS AND PRECAUTIONS: General: Td POLIO ADSORBED [Tetanus and Diphtheria Toxoids Adsorbed and Inactivated Poliomyelitis Vaccine] should not be administered into the buttocks due to the varying amount of fatty tissue in this region, nor by the intradermal route, since these methods of administration may induce a weaker immune response.

As with any vaccine, immunization with Td POLIO ADSORBED may not protect 100% of susceptible individuals.

Do not inject into a blood vessel.

Aseptic technique must be used. Use a separate sterile needle and syringe, or a sterile disposable unit, for each individual dose to prevent disease transmission.

Before administration, take all appropriate precautions to prevent adverse reactions. This includes a review of the patient's history concerning possible hypersensitivity to the vaccine or similar vaccine, previous immunization history, the presence of any contraindications to immunization, and current health status.

Before administration of Td POLIO ADSORBED [Tetanus and Diphtheria Toxoids Adsorbed and Inactivated Poliomyelitis Vaccine], health-care providers should inform the patient, parent or guardian of the benefits and risks of immunization, inquire about the recent health status of the patient and comply with any local requirements regarding information to be provided to the patient before immunization and the importance of completing the immunization series.

It is extremely important that the patient, parent or guardian be questioned concerning any symptoms and/or signs of an adverse reaction after a previous dose of vaccine. (See Contraindications and Adverse Reactions.)

Hematologic: Because of the risk of bleeding and hematoma formation following an intramuscular injection, Td POLIO ADSORBED should be given with caution in persons with any bleeding disorder, such as hemophilia or thrombocytopenia, or to persons on anticoagulant therapy.

Immune: As with all other products, Epinephrine Hydrochloride Solution (1:1000) and other appropriate agents should be available for immediate use in case an anaphylactic or acute hypersensitivity reaction occurs. Health-care providers should be familiar with current recommendations for the initial management of anaphylaxis in nonhospital settings, including proper airway management. For instructions on recognition and treatment of anaphylactic reactions, see the current edition of the Canadian Immunization Guide or visit the Health Canada website.

The possibility of allergic reactions in persons sensitive to components of the vaccine should be evaluated.

Immunocompromised persons (whether from disease or treatment) may not obtain the expected immune response. If possible, consideration should be given to delaying routine vaccination until after the completion of any immunosuppressive treatment.

Neurologic: If Guillain-Barré Syndrome occurred within 6 weeks of immunization with a previous dose of vaccine containing tetanus toxoid, the decision to give subsequent doses of Td POLIO ADSORBED or any vaccine containing tetanus toxoid should be based on careful consideration of the potential benefits and possible risks.

Special Populations: Pregnant Women: There is no experience with Td POLIO ADSORBED in clinical trials in pregnant women. Animal reproduction studies have not been conducted with Td POLIO ADSORBED. It is also not known whether Td POLIO ADSORBED can cause fetal harm when administered to a pregnant woman or can affect reproduction capacity.

NACI states that there is no evidence that tetanus toxoid is teratogenic, but it is prudent to wait until the second trimester of pregnancy to administer a routinely required dose, to minimize concern about the theoretic possibility of a relationship with any observed birth defect. In the event of a tetanus-prone wound during pregnancy the recommendations in Table 2 should be followed.

Nursing Women: The effect of administration of Td POLIO ADSORBED during lactation has not been assessed.

NACI states that lactating mothers who have not received the recommended immunizations may safely be given vaccines.

ADVERSE REACTIONS: In a clinical trial involving 40 individuals previously immunized against tetanus, diphtheria and poliomyelitis who received a single (0.5 mL) injection of Td POLIO ADSORBED [Tetanus and Diphtheria Toxoids Adsorbed and Inactivated Poliomyelitis Vaccine], the vaccinees experienced only a low level of reactions associated with the injections. Discomfort at the injection site was usually of short duration. Systemic complaints included headache, malaise and dizziness. No fever was reported.

The percent of vaccinees reporting local and general reactions on the day of immunization (day 0) and for the following 3 days are shown in Table 1. Except for muscle aches at the injection site, all reactions were mild or moderate in severity.

Table 1: Td POLIO ADSORBED

Frequencies of Selected Solicited Adverse Events Within 72 Hours Following a Dose of Td POLIO ADSORBED in Presumably Previously Primed Subjects (N=40)

Reaction	Percent Reactivity Time Post Injection			
	Day 0	Day 1	Day 2	Day 3
Local				
Redness	3	3	3	3
Tenderness	38	43	0	0
Induration	3	5	3	0
Swelling	3	3	3	0
Pain	25	33	10	0
Itchiness	5	3	0	0
Muscle Ache, All (severe)	55 (3)	55 (3)	0	0
Systemic				
Headache	8	5	8	0
Dizziness	0	3	0	0
Malaise	3	3	0	0

Because clinical trials are conducted under widely varying conditions, adverse reaction rates observed in the clinical trials of a vaccine cannot be directly compared to rates in the clinical trials of another vaccine and may not reflect the rates observed in practice. The adverse reaction information from clinical trials does, however, provide a basis for identifying the adverse events that appear to be related to vaccine use and for approximating rates.

Post-Market Spontaneous Adverse Drug Reactions: The adverse events reported during the commercial use of Td POLIO ADSORBED are presented below. Because these are reported voluntarily from a population of uncertain size, it is not always possible to reliably estimate their frequency or establish a causal relationship to vaccine exposure.

The most commonly reported adverse drug reactions were injection site reactions and pyrexia, both described in 29% of the spontaneous adverse event reports.

Data are organized by MedDRA system organ class and within the system organ class, by decreasing frequency.

Immune System Disorders: allergic reactions (including urticaria, pruritus, rash).

Nervous System Disorders: dizziness, paraesthesia, headache. Guillain-Barré syndrome has been exceptionally reported.

Musculoskeletal, Connective Tissue and Bone Disorders: arthralgia, myalgia.

General Disorders and Administration Site Conditions: injection site reactions (including injection site inflammation, injection site mass, injection site pain, injection site pruritus); pyrexia; asthenic conditions: fatigue, asthenia, malaise.

Additional Adverse Drug Reactions: Additional adverse reactions have been reported following immunization with vaccines containing tetanus toxoid and/or diphtheria toxoid.

Arthus-type hypersensitivity reactions, characterized by severe local reactions (generally starting 2-8 hours after an injection), may follow immunization with tetanus toxoid. Such reactions may be associated with high levels of circulating antitoxin in persons who have had overly frequent injections of tetanus toxoid.

Persistent nodules at the site of injection have been reported following the use of adsorbed products.

Cases of allergic or anaphylactic reaction (i.e., hives, swelling of the mouth, difficulty breathing, hypotension, or shock) have been reported after receiving some preparations containing diphtheria and/or tetanus toxoid. Death following vaccine-caused anaphylaxis has been reported.

Certain neurological conditions have been reported in temporal association with some tetanus toxoid-containing vaccines or tetanus and diphtheria toxoid-containing vaccines. A review by the US Institute of Medicine (IOM) concluded that the evidence favours acceptance of a causal relation between tetanus toxoid and both brachial neuritis and Guillain-Barré syndrome. Other neurological conditions that have been reported include: demyelinating diseases of the central nervous system, peripheral mononeuropathies, cranial mononeuropathies, and EEG disturbances with encephalopathy (with or without permanent intellectual and/or motor function impairment). The IOM has concluded that the evidence is inadequate to accept or reject a causal relation between these conditions and vaccines containing tetanus and/or diphtheria toxoids. In the differential diagnosis of polyradiculoneuropathies following administration of a vaccine containing tetanus toxoid, tetanus toxoid should be considered as a possible etiology.

Physicians, nurses, and pharmacists should report any adverse occurrences temporally associated with the administration of the product in accordance with local requirements and to the Global Pharmacovigilance Department, Sanofi Pasteur Limited, 1755 Steeles Avenue West, Toronto, ON, M2R 3T4, Canada. 1-888-621-1146 (phone) or 416-667-2435 (fax).

DRUG INTERACTIONS: Immunosuppressive therapies, including irradiation, antimetabolites, alkylating agents, cytotoxic drugs and corticosteroids (used in greater than physiologic doses), may reduce the immune response to vaccines. (See Warnings and Precautions, Immune.)

Administering the most widely used live and inactivated vaccines during the same patient visit has produced seroconversion rates and rates of adverse reactions similar to those observed when the vaccines are administered separately. Simultaneous administration using separate syringes at separate sites is suggested, particularly when there is concern that an individual may not return for subsequent vaccination.

DOSAGE AND ADMINISTRATION:

Booster: For persons who have previously been immunized against tetanus, diphtheria and poliomyelitis, a dose of 0.5 mL should be administered as a reinforcing dose at approximately 10 year intervals.

For individuals planning to travel to developing countries where safe tetanus toxoid administration may not be available if required, it may be prudent to offer an early tetanus toxoid-containing booster prior to travel if more than 5 years have elapsed since the last dose.

Primary Immunization: For primary immunization of persons aged 7 years and older a series of three (0.5 mL) doses is required. The first two doses should be given 2 months apart and the third dose 6-12 months later. Thereafter booster doses are recommended at approximately 10 year intervals. NACI states that the first 2 doses should be given 4-8 weeks apart.

Interruption of the recommended schedule with a delay between doses should not interfere with the final immunity achieved with Td POLIO ADSORBED [Tetanus and Diphtheria Toxoids Adsorbed and Inactivated Poliomyelitis Vaccine]. There is no need to start the series over again, regardless of the time elapsed between doses.

Diphtheria Prophylaxis for Case Contacts: NACI has published recommendations on vaccination for diphtheria prophylaxis in persons who have had contact with a person with confirmed or suspected diphtheria.

Tetanus Prophylaxis in Wound Management: Table 2 summarizes the recommended use of immunizing agents in wound management. It is important to ascertain the number of doses of tetanus toxoid previously given and the interval since the last dose. If not clearly documented, a history of immunization should be regarded as "uncertain". When a tetanus booster is required the combined preparation formulated for adults containing 5 Lf of tetanus toxoid and 2 Lf of diphtheria toxoid per 0.5 mL dose is preferable (i.e., Td POLIO ADSORBED). Appropriate cleansing and debridement of the wound is imperative.

Some persons with humoral immune deficiency, including those with HIV infection, may not respond adequately to tetanus toxoid. Therefore, tetanus immune globulin (TIG) should be used in addition to tetanus toxoid if a wound occurs that is not clean, regardless of the time elapsed since the last booster.

Table 2: Td POLIO ADSORBED

Summary Guide to Tetanus Prophylaxis in Routine Wound Management for Persons 7 Years of Age or Older

History of Adsorbed Tetanus Toxoid (Doses)	Clean, Minor Wounds		All Other Wounds	
	Td[a]	TIG[b]	Td[a]	TIG
Uncertain or <3 doses of an immunization series[c]	Yes	No	Yes	Yes
≥3 doses received in an immunization series[c]	No[d]	No	No[e]	No[f]

[a] Adult type tetanus and diphtheria toxoids-containing vaccine (for 7 years and older) such as Td Polio Adsorbed. If the patient is <7 years old, an appropriate tetanus combination vaccine such as QUADRACEL or PENTACEL is given.

[b] Tetanus immune globulin, given at a separate site from Td POLIO with separate syringe.

[c] Primary immunization is at least 3 doses at age appropriate intervals.

[d] Yes, if >10 years since last booster.

[e] Yes, unless there is documentation of a booster within the last 5 years.

[f] Yes, if individuals are known to have a significant humoral immune deficiency state (e.g., HIV, agammaglobulinemia) since immune response to tetanus toxoid may be suboptimal.

Administration: Inspect for extraneous particulate matter and/or discolouration before use. If these conditions exist, the product should not be administered.

Shake the vial well to uniformly distribute the suspension before withdrawing each dose. When administering a dose from a stoppered vial, do not remove either the stopper or the metal seal holding it in place. Aseptic technique must be used. Use a separate sterile needle and syringe, or a sterile disposable unit, for each individual dose to prevent disease transmission. (See Warnings and Precautions.)

Administer the vaccine **intramuscularly**. The preferred site is into the deltoid muscle. Do not inject intravenously.

Needles should not be recapped and should be disposed of according to biohazard waste guidelines.

For information on vaccine administration see the current edition of the Canadian Immunization Guide or visit the Health Canada website.

Give the patient a permanent personal immunization record. In addition, it is essential that the physician or nurse record the immunization history in the permanent medical record of each patient. This permanent office record should contain the name of the vaccine, date given, dose, manufacturer and lot number.

OVERDOSAGE: Not applicable.

For management of a suspected drug overdose, contact your regional Poison Control Centre. See the *CPS* Directory section for a list of Poison Control Centres.

ACTION AND CLINICAL PHARMACOLOGY: Mechanism of Action: Protection against disease attributable to *C. tetani* is due to the development of neutralizing antibodies to tetanus toxin. A serum tetanus antitoxin level of at least 0.01 IU/mL, measured by neutralization assay, is considered the minimum protective level. Protection against disease attributable to *C. diphtheriae* is due to the development of neutralizing antibodies to diphtheria toxin. A serum diphtheria antitoxin level of 0.01 IU/mL is the lowest level giving some degree of protection. Antitoxin levels of at least 0.1 IU/mL are generally regarded as protective for both tetanus and diphtheria. Levels of 1.0 IU/mL have been associated with long-term protection.

Poliomyelitis is caused by poliovirus Types 1, 2 or 3. Inactivated poliomyelitis vaccine induces the production of detectable levels of neutralizing antibodies against each type of poliovirus. The detection of type-specific neutralizing antibodies has been correlated with protection. A primary series induces protective antibody levels in more than 99% of recipients.

Pharmacokinetics: Not applicable.
Duration of Effect: After completion of a primary series, circulating antibodies to tetanus and diphtheria toxoids gradually decline but are thought to persist at protective levels for up to 10 years. Tetanus and diphtheria boosters are recommended every 10 years.

STORAGE AND STABILITY: Store at 2 to 8°C. **Do not freeze.** Discard product if exposed to freezing. Do not use after expiration date.

INFORMATION FOR THE PATIENT: Published in e-CPS, available by subscription at www.e-cps.ca.

DOSAGE FORMS, COMPOSITION AND PACKAGING: Each dose of 0.5 mL contains: tetanus toxoid 5 Lf, diphtheria toxoid 2 Lf, purified inactivated poliomyelitis vaccine Type 1 (Mahoney) 40 D-antigen units, Type 2 (MEF1) 8 D-antigen units, Type 3 (Saukett) 32 D-antigen units. Other ingredients per dose include 0.5% v/v of 2-phenoxyethanol (not as a preservative), 1.5 mg of aluminum phosphate equivalent to 0.33 mg of aluminum as the adjuvant, and 27 ppm of formaldehyde. The vaccine also contains approximately 10 ppm polysorbate 80 and ≤50 ng of bovine serum albumin (by calculation). Trace amounts of neomycin and polymyxin B may be present from the cell growth medium. Single-dose vials of 0.5 mL, packages of 5. The stopper of the vial for this product does not contain dry natural latex rubber.

Tears Plus®

polyvinyl alcohol—povidone

Ocular Lubricant

Allergan

SUPPLIED: Each mL of an aqueous, sterile, nonbuffered isotonic solution contains: polyvinyl alcohol 1.4% and povidone with chlorobutanol (preservative). Plastic dropper bottles of 15 and 30 mL.

Tebrazid® Ⓟ

pyrazinamide

Antituberculosis Agent

Valeant

PHARMACOLOGY: Pyrazinamide may be bacteriostatic or bacteriocidal in action, depending on the concentration of the drug attained at the site of the infection and the susceptibility of the infecting organism. In vitro and in vivo, the drug is active only at a slightly acidic pH. The exact mechanism of action of pyrazinamide has not been fully elucidated. The antimycobacterial activity of pyrazinamide appears to partly depend on conversion of the drug to pyrazinoic acid (POA). Susceptible strains of *M. tuberculosis* produce pyrazinamidase, an enzyme that deaminates pyrazinamide to POA, and the in vitro susceptibility of a given strain of the organism appears to correspond to its pyrazinamidase activity. In vitro studies indicate that POA has specific antimycobacterial activity against *M. tuberculosis*. In addition, the fact that POA lowers the pH of the environment below that which is necessary for growth of *M. tuberculosis* appears to contribute to the drug's antimycobacterial activity in vitro.

Pyrazinamide is a highly specific agent and is active only against *M. tuberculosis*. Results of in vitro susceptibility testing with pyrazinamide are affected by the test media, inoculum size, and pH. In vitro, in media with a pH of 5.5, the minimum inhibitory concentration (MIC) of pyrazinamide for *M. tuberculosis* is generally less than 20 µg/mL. In one in vitro study in 7H12 liquid media, MICs of the drug reported for *M. tuberculosis* were 50 µg/mL at pH 5.5 and 400 µg/mL at pH 5.95.

Resistance: Natural and acquired resistance to pyrazinamide have been demonstrated in vitro and in vivo in strains of *M. tuberculosis*. Resistant strains of initially susceptible organisms develop rapidly if pyrazinamide is used alone in the treatment of clinical tuberculosis. When pyrazinamide is combined with other antituberculosis agents in the treatment of the disease, emergence of resistant strains may be delayed or prevented. Although the exact mechanism(s) of resistance to pyrazinamide has not been determined, some strains of pyrazinamide-resistant *M. tuberculosis* do not appear to produce pyrazinamidase and therefore cannot convert the parent drug to pyrazinoic acid (POA), its microbiologically active metabolite. There is no evidence of cross-resistance between pyrazinamide and other antituberculosis agents currently available on the market.

Pharmacokinetics: Absorption: Pyrazinamide is well absorbed from the gastrointestinal tract. Following a single 500 mg oral dose in healthy adults, peak plasma concentrations of pyrazinamide ranging from 9 to 12 µg/mL are attained within 2 hours; plasma concentrations of the drug average 7 µg/mL at 8 hours and 2 µg/mL at 24 hours. Plasma concentrations following doses of 20 to 25 mg/kg reportedly range from 30 to 50 µg/mL. Plasma concentrations of pyrazinoic acid, the major active metabolite of pyrazinamide, generally are greater than those of the parent drug and peak within 4 to 8 hours after an oral dose of the drug. In a single dose study in healthy fasting males, the extent of absorption (as measured by area under the plasma concentration-time curve) of isoniazid, rifampin, or pyrazinamide in dosages of 250, 600, or 1500 mg, respectively, was similar whether the drugs were administered individually as capsules (rifampin) and tablets (isoniazid and pyrazinamide) or as a fixed combination containing isoniazid 50 mg, rifampin 120 mg, and pyrazinamide 300 mg per tablet.

Distribution: Pyrazinamide is widely distributed into body tissues and fluids including the liver, lungs, kidneys, and CSF. In a limited number of adults with tuberculous meningitis, mean serum and CSF concentrations of pyrazinamide 2 hours after an oral dose of approximately 41 mg/kg were 52 and 39 µg/mL, respectively. Within 5 hours after an oral dose, CSF concentrations of pyrazinamide are reported to be approximately equal to concurrent plasma concentrations of the drug. Plasma protein binding of pyrazinamide (determined by ultrafiltration) in a limited number of healthy men averaged approximately 17% at a pyrazinamide concentration of 20 µg/mL. It is not known if pyrazinamide crosses the placenta or if it is distributed into milk.

Elimination: The plasma half-life of pyrazinamide is 9 to 10 hours in patients with normal renal and hepatic function. The plasma half-life of the drug may be prolonged in patients with impaired renal (approximately 26 hours) or hepatic function.

Pyrazinamide is hydrolyzed in the liver to pyrazinoic acid, the major active metabolite; some hydrolysis may also occur in the stomach and bladder. Pyrazoic acid is hyroxylated to 5-hydroxypyrazinoic acid, the major excretory product. Within 24 hours, approximately 70% of an oral dose of pyrazinamide is excreted as unchanged drug; the remainder is excreted as metabolites.

A single 3 to 4 hour hemodialysis session reduced serum pyrazinamide concentrations by approximately 55% and pyrazinoic acid concentrations by 50 to 60%.

INDICATIONS: In combination with other antituberculosis agents in the treatment of clinical tuberculosis.

CONTRAINDICATIONS: Pyrazinamide should be used only when close observation of the patient is possible. Serum AST, ALT, and uric acid concentrations should be determined prior to and every 2 to 4 weeks during pyrazinamide therapy. If signs of hepatic damage occur, pyrazinamide should be discontinued.

Pyrazinamide should be used with caution in patients with renal failure or a history of gout. The drug should also be used with caution in diabetics because the management of diabetes mellitus may become more difficult during pyrazinamide therapy. Pyrazinamide is contraindicated in patients with severe hepatic damage and in patients with known hypersensitivity to the drug. Patients hypersensitive to ethionamide, isoniazid, niacin (nicotinic acid), or other chemically related medications may be hypersensitive to this medication also.

Children: Safe use of pyrazinamide in children has not been definitely established. Because of the drug's potential toxicity, the manufacturer recommends that its use in children be avoided unless essential to therapy.

Geriatrics: Appropriate studies on the relationship of age to the effects of pyrazinamide have not been performed in the geriatric population. However, no geriatric-specific problems have been documented to date.

Carcinogenicity: Pyrazinamide was administered in the diet of rats and mice. The estimated daily dose was 2 g/kg, or 40 times the maximum human dose, for the mice, and 0.5 g/kg, or 10 times the maximum human dose, for the rat. Pyrazinamide was not carcinogenic in rats or male mice. No conclusion was possible for female mice due to insufficient numbers of surviving control mice.

Mutagenicity: Pyrazinamide was not mutagenic in the Ames bacterial test (Salmonella), but it did induce chromosomal aberrations in human lymphocyte cell cultures.

Pregnancy: Animal reproduction studies have not been conducted with pyrazinamide. Adequate and well-controlled studies in humans have not been done. The risk for teratogenicity has not been determined. If the organism is drug-susceptible, pregnant women can be safely treated with isoniazid, rifampin, and ethambutol for 9 months. If resistance to any of these medications is probable and susceptibility to pyrazinamide is likely, its use should be considered.

Lactation: See Pregnancy.

WARNINGS:

Reports from the Centers for Disease Control and Prevention of the USA showed high rates of hospitalization and death from liver injury following the combined use of Tebrazid (pyrazinamide) and rifampin for the treatment of **latent** tuberculosis because of a higher potential hepatotoxicity.

Hepatic Effects: The most frequent adverse effect of pyrazinamide is hepatotoxicity. Transient increases in serum aminotransaminase concentrations, jaundice, hepatitis, and a syndrome of fever, anorexia, malaise, liver tenderness, hepatomegaly, and splenomegaly have been reported in patients receiving pyrazinamide. Acute yellow atrophy of the liver and death have occurred. Hepatotoxicity appears to be dose related and may occur at any time during therapy. With a dosage of 3 g daily, hepatotoxicity occurs in approximately 15% of patients, and jaundice occurs in 2 to 3%. Recent studies in adults with tuberculosis indicate that the incidence of drug-induced adverse hepatic effects in patients who receive 25 to 35 mg/kg of pyrazinamide daily in the initial phase (i.e., first 2 months) of isoniazid and rifampin therapy is the same as that in patients who receive isoniazid and rifampin therapy without pyrazinamide.

Other Effects: Pyrazinamide inhibits renal excretion of urates, frequently resulting in hyperuricemia. This effect is usually asymptomatic, but acute gout has occurred in some patients. Nongouty polyarthralgia, which appears to be related to increased serum uric acid concentrations, reportedly occurs in up to 40% of patients receiving pyrazinamide. Uricosuric agents administered concurrently may reduce pyrazinamide-induced hyperuricemia; however, if hyperuricemia is severe or is accompanied by acute gouty arthritis, pyrazinamide should be discontinued.

Laboratory Value Alterations: Urine Ketone Determinations: Pyrazinamide may react with sodium nitroprusside tests; both pyrazinamide and pyrazinoic acid produce an interfering ping-brown color reaction with nitroprusside.

ALT and AST: Values may be increased.

Serum Uric Acid: Concentration may be increased.

Drug Interactions: Interactions between pyrazinamide and the following medications (or combinations containing the following medications) have been reported: allopurinol; colchicine; probenecid; sulfinpyrazone (pyrazinamide may increase serum uric acid concentrations and decrease the efficacy of gout therapy; dosage adjustments of these medications may be necessary to control hyperuricemia and gout when antigout medications are used concurrently with pyrazinamide). Cyclosporine (concurrent use with pyrazinamide may decrease the serum concentrations of cyclosporine, possibly leading to inadequate immunosuppression; cyclosporine serum concentrations should be monitored).

PRECAUTIONS: See Contraindications.

ADVERSE EFFECTS: More Frequent Incidence: arthralgia (pain and swelling of joints, especially big toe, ankle, and knee; tense, hot skin over affected joints); hepatotoxicity (loss of appetite, unusual tiredness or weakness, yellow eyes or skin), mostly related to large doses, i.e., 40 to 50 mg/kg of body weight/day for prolonged periods of time.

Rare Incidence: maculopapular rash, fever, acne, porphyria, dysuria, and photosensitivity with reddish-brown discoloration of exposed skin.

OVERDOSE:

No data supplied by the manufacturer.

For management of a suspected drug overdose, CPhA recommends that you contact your **regional Poison Control Centre**. See the *CPS* Directory section for a list of Poison Control Centres.

DOSAGE: Since bacterial resistance may develop rapidly when pyrazinamide is administered alone in the treatment of tuberculosis, it should only be administered concurrently with other antituberculosis agents.

Usual Adult and Adolescent Dose: Tuberculosis: In combination with other antitubercular drugs: oral, 15 to 30 mg/kg of body weight once a day; or 50 to 70 mg/kg of body weight 2 or 3 times a week, depending on the treatment regimen.

Note: The usual dose of pyrazinamide for persons infected with human immunodeficiency virus (HIV) is 20 to 30 mg/kg of body weight/day for the first 2 months of therapy.

Usual Adult Prescribing Limits: up to a maximum of 2 g when taken daily, 3 g per dose for the 3 times a week regimen, 4 g per dose for the 2 times a week regimen.

Pediatric Dose if Indicated: 30 mg/kg of body weight daily or less.

Note: The usual maximum dose in children is 2 g when taken daily, 3 g per dose for the 3 times a week regimen, 4 g per dose for the 2 times a week regimen.

SUPPLIED: Each white, round, compressed tablet, single-scored on one side and embossed ICN T11 on the other contains pyrazinamide, USP 500 mg. Nonmedicinal ingredients: cornstarch, silicone dioxide and talc. Bottles of 500. Store in well-closed containers at controlled room temperature (15 to 30°C).

Technetium Tc 99m Sestamibi Injection, Kit for the Preparation of

tetrakis (2-methoxy isobutyl isonitrile) copper (1) tetrafluoroborate

Radiodiagnostic Agent (Myocardial Imaging)—Kit for Intravenous and Diagnostic Use

tyco Healthcare

Date of Preparation: June 16, 2009

SUMMARY PRODUCT INFORMATION:

Route of Administration	Dosage Form/ Strength	Clinically Relevant Nonmedicinal Ingredients
Intravenous	1.0 mg/vial	None For a complete listing see Dosage Forms, Composition and Packaging.

DESCRIPTION: Physical Characteristics: Technetium Tc 99m decays by isomeric transition with a physical half-life of 6.02 hours. Photons that are useful for detection and imaging studies are listed in Table 1.

Table 1: Technetium Tc 99m Sestamibi Injection, Kit for the Preparation of

Principal Radiation Emission Data

Radiation	Mean %/Disintegration	Mean Energy (KeV)
Gamma-2	89.07	140.5

External Radiation: The specific gamma ray constant for Tc 99m is 5.4 microcoulombs/Kg-MBq-hr (0.78 R/mCi-hr) at 1 cm. The first half value layer is 0.017 cm of Pb. A range of values for the relative attenuation of the radiation emitted by this radionuclide that results from interpolition of various thicknesses of Pb is shown in Table 2. To facilitate control of the radiation exposure from Megabequerel (millicurie) amounts of this radionuclide, the use of a 0.25 cm thickness of Pb will attenuate the radiation emitted by a factor of 1000.

To correct for physical decay of this radionuclide, the fractions that remain at selected intervals after the time of calibration are shown in Table 3.

INDICATIONS AND CLINICAL USE: Kit for the Preparation of Technetium Tc-99m Sestamibi Injection is indicated for:

Myocardial Imaging: Technetium Tc 99m Sestamibi is useful in myocardial perfusion imaging for the diagnosis and localization of myocardial infarction; and for the diagnosis and localization of ischaemic heart disease and coronary artery disease.

Technetium Tc 99m Sestamibi is also useful in the assessment of global ventricular function by the first pass technique.

Table 2: Technetium Tc 99m Sestamibi Injection, Kit for the Preparation of Radiation Attenuation by Lead Shielding

Shield Thickness (Pb) cm	Coefficient of Attenuation
0.017	0.5
0.08	10^{-1}
0.16	10^{-2}
0.25	10^{-3}
0.33	10^{-4}

Table 3: Technetium Tc 99m Sestamibi Injection, Kit for the Preparation of Physical Decay Chart; Tc 99m Half-Life 6.02 Hours

Hours	Fraction Remaining	Hours	Fraction Remaining
0[a]	1.000	7	0.447
1	0.891	8	0.398
2	0.794	9	0.355
3	0.708	10	0.316
4	0.631	11	0.282
5	0.562	12	0.251
6	0.501		

a Calibration Time.

CONTRAINDICATIONS: None known. However, patients who are hypersensitive to this drug or to any ingredient in the formulation or component of the container should advise their physician.

WARNINGS AND PRECAUTIONS:

> **Serious Warnings and Precautions**
> Radiopharmaceuticals should be used only by those health professionals who are appropriately qualified in the use of radioactive prescribed substances in or on humans.

In studying patients in whom cardiac disease is known or suspected, care should be taken to assure continuous monitoring and treatment in accordance with safe, accepted clinical procedure.

Caution should be exercised and emergency equipment should be available when administering Technetium Tc 99m Sestamibi. Also, before administering Technetium Tc 99m Sestamibi, patients should be asked about the possibility of allergic reactions to the drug.

General: The contents of the vial are intended only for use in the preparation of Technetium Tc 99m Sestamibi and are not to be administered directly to the patient without first undergoing the preparative procedure.

Radioactive drugs must be handled with care and appropriate safety measures should be used to minimize radiation exposure to clinical personnel. Also, care should be taken to minimize radiation exposure to the patients consistent with proper patient management.

Contents of the kit before preparation are not radioactive. However, after the Sodium Pertechnetate Tc 99m Injection is added, adequate shielding of the final preparation must be maintained.

The components of the kit are sterile and non-pyrogenic. It is essential to follow directions carefully and to adhere to strict aseptic procedures during preparation.

Technetium Tc 99m labeling reactions depend on maintaining the stannous ion in the reduced state. Hence, Sodium Pertechnetate Tc 99m Injection containing oxidants should not be used.

Technetium Tc 99m Sestamibi should not be used more than six hours after preparation.

Radiopharmaceuticals should be used only by physicians who are qualified by training and experience in the safe use and handling of radionuclides and whose experience and training have been approved by the appropriate government agency authorized to license the use of radionuclides.

Stress testing should be performed only under the supervision of a qualified physician and in a laboratory equipped with appropriate resuscitation and support apparatus.

Carcinogenesis and Mutagenesis: No long-term animal studies have been performed to evaluate carcinogenic potential or whether Technetium Tc99m Sestamibi affects fertility in males or females. As with other radiopharmaceuticals which distribute intracellularly, there may be an increased risk of chromosomal damage from Auger electrons if nuclear uptake occurs.

In comparison with most other diagnostic technetium labeled radiopharmaceuticals, the radiation dose to the ovaries (1.5 rads/30 mCi at rest, 1.2 rads/30 mCi at exercise) is high. Minimal exposure (ALARA) is necessary in women of childbearing capability. (See Radiation Dosimetry.)

The active intermediate, $Cu(MIBI)_4BF_4$, was evaluated for genotoxic potential in a battery of five tests. No genotoxic activity was observed in the Ames, CHO/HPRT and sister chromatid exchange tests (all in vitro). At cytotoxic concentrations (≥20 µg/mL), an increase in cells with chromosome aberrations was observed in the in vitro human lymphocyte assay. $Cu(MIBI)_4BF_4$ did not show genotoxic effects in the in vivo mouse micronucleus test at a dose which caused systemic and bone marrow toxicity (9 mg/kg, >600×maximal human dose).

Contamination: The following measures should be taken for up to 12 hours after receiving the radiopharmaceutical product: Toilet should be used instead of urinal. Toilet should be flushed several times after use. If blood or urine gets onto clothing such clothing should be washed separately or stored for 1 to 2 weeks to allow for decay.

Special precautions such as bladder catherization should be taken following administration to incontinent patients to minimize the risk of radioactive contamination of clothing, bed linen and the patient's environment.

Special Populations: Pregnant Women: Animal reproduction and teratogenicity studies have not been conducted with Technetium Tc 99m Sestamibi. It is also not known whether Technetium Tc 99m Sestamibi can cause fetal harm when administered to a pregnant woman or can affect reproductive capacity. There have been no studies in pregnant women. Technetium Tc 99m Sestamibi should be given to a pregnant woman only if clearly needed. Ideally, examinations using radiopharmaceuticals, especially those elective in nature, of a woman of childbearing capability, should be performed during the first ten days following the onset of menses.

Nursing Women: Technetium Tc 99m Pertechnetate is excreted in human milk during lactation. It is not known whether Technetium Tc 99m Sestamibi is excreted in human milk. Therefore, formula feedings should be substituted for breast feedings.

Pediatrics (below 18 years of age): Safety and effectiveness in the pediatric population have not been established.

* The ethanol used in this procedure should be 95% or greater. Absolute ethanol (99%) should remain at ≥95% ethanol content for one week after opening if stored tightly capped, in a cool dry place.

Monitoring and Laboratory Tests: Blood pressure, laboratory or other tests are required to monitor response to therapy and possible adverse reactions. Please refer to Warnings and Precautions.

ADVERSE REACTIONS: Adverse Drug Reaction Overview: An overview of selected adverse events is reported in Table 4.

Clinical Trial Adverse Drug Reactions: Because clinical trials are conducted under very specific conditions the adverse reaction rates observed in the clinical trials may not reflect the rates observed in practice and should not be compared to the rates in the clinical trials of another drug. Adverse drug reaction information from clinical trials is useful for identifying drug-related adverse events and for approximating rates.

Adverse events were evaluated in 3741 adults who were evaluated in clinical studies. Of these patients, 3068 (77% men, 22% women, and 0.7% of the patients' genders were not recorded) were in cardiac clinical trials and 673 (100% women) in breast imaging trials. Cases of angina, chest pain, and death have occurred in cardiac imaging studies. Adverse events reported at a rate of 0.5% or greater after receiving Technetium Tc 99m Sestamibi administration are shown in Table 4:

Table 4: Technetium Tc 99m Sestamibi Injection, Kit for the Preparation of Selected Adverse Events Reported in >0.5% of Patients Who Received Technetium Tc 99m Sestamibi in Either Breast or Cardiac Clinical Studies[a]

Body System	Breast Studies	Cardiac Studies		
	Women n=673	Women n=685	Men n=2361	Total n=3046
Headache	11 (1.6%)	2 (0.3%)	4 (0.2%)	6 (0.2%)
Chest Pain/Angina	0 (0%)	18 (2.6%)	46 (1.9%)	64 (2.1%)
ST Segment Changes	0 (0%)	11 (1.6%)	29 (1.2%)	40 (1.3%)
Nausea	4 (0.6%)	1 (0.1%)	2 (0.1%)	3 (0.1%)
Taste Perversion	129 (19.2%)	60 (8.8%)	157 (6.6%)	217 (7.1%)
Parosmia	8 (1.2%)	6 (0.9%)	10 (0.4%)	16 (0.5%)

a Excludes the 22 patients whose genders were not recorded.

In the clinical studies for breast imaging, breast pain was reported in 12 (1.7%) of the patients. In 11 of these patients the pain appears to be associated with biopsy/surgical procedures.

The following adverse reactions have been reported in ≤0.5% of patients: signs and symptoms consistent with seizure occurring shortly after administration of the agent; transient arthritis; angioedema, arrhythmia, dizziness, syncope, abdominal pain, vomiting, and severe hypersensitivity characterized by dyspnea, hypotension, bradycardia, asthenia, and vomiting within two hours after a second injection of Technetium Tc 99m Sestamibi. A few cases of flushing, edema, injection site inflammation, dry mouth, fever, pruritus, rash, urticaria and fatigue have also been attributed to administration of the agent.

It should be noted that the above data on Adverse Events Reported in Breast Studies is provided for safety information purposes; the Mallinckrodt Sestamibi product is not indicated for breast imaging.

DOSAGE AND ADMINISTRATION: Dosage: The suggested dose range for I.V. administration to be employed in the average patient (70 kg) is: 370-1110 MBq (10-30 mCi).

Administration: The patient dose should be measured by a suitable radioactivity calibration system immediately prior to patient administration. Radiochemical purity should be checked prior to patient administration. Do not use if radiochemical purity is less than 90%.

Parenteral drug products should be inspected visually for particulate matter and discoloration prior to administration whenever solution and container permit.

Store at 15-25°C before and after reconstitution.

Instructions for Preparation and Use: Preparation of the Technetium Tc 99m Sestamibi from the Kit for the Preparation of Technetium Tc 99m Sestamibi Injection is done by the following aseptic procedure:

a. Prior to adding the Sodium Pertechnetate Tc 99m Injection to the vial, inspect the vial carefully for the presence of damage, particularly cracks, and do not use the vial if found. Tear off a radiation symbol and attach it to the neck of the vial.
b. Waterproof gloves should be worn during the preparation procedure. Remove the plastic disc from the vial and swab the top of the vial closure with alcohol to sanitize the surface.
c. Place the vial in a suitable radiation shield with a fitted radiation cap.
d. With a sterile shielded syringe, aseptically obtain additive-free, sterile, non-pyrogenic Sodium Pertechnetate Tc 99m Injection [925-5550 MBq, (25-150 mCi)] in approximately 1 to 3 mL.
e. Aseptically add the Sodium Pertechnetate Tc 99m Injection to the vial in the lead shield. Without withdrawing the needle, remove an equal volume of headspace to maintain atmospheric pressure within the vial.
f. Shake vigorously, about 5 to 10 quick upward-downward motions.
g. Remove the vial from the lead shield and place upright in an appropriately shielded and contained boiling water bath, such that the vial is suspended above the bottom of the bath, and boil for 10 minutes. Timing for 10 minutes is begun as soon as the water begins to boil again. Do not allow the boiling water to come in contact with the aluminum crimp.
h. Remove the vial from the water bath, place in the lead shield and allow to cool for fifteen minutes.
i. Using proper shielding, the vial contents should be visually inspected. Use only if the solution is clear and free of particulate matter and discoloration.
j. Assay the reaction vial using a suitable radioactivity calibration system. Record the Technetium Tc 99m concentration, total volume, assay time and date, expiration time and lot number on the radioassay information label and affix the label to the shield.
k. Store the reaction vial containing the Technetium Tc 99m Sestamibi at 15 to 25°C until use; at such time the product should be aseptically withdrawn. Technetium Tc 99m Sestamibi should be used within six hours of preparation. The vial contains no preservative.

Note: Adherence to the above product reconstitution instructions is recommended.

Mallinckrodt Inc.'s Kit for the Preparation of Technetium Tc 99m Sestamibi Injection is not to be used with the Recon-o-Stat thermal cycler due to the smaller vial size requirements of this heating device.

The potential for cracking and significant contamination exists whenever vials containing radioactive material are heated.

Product should be used within 6 hours after preparation.

Determination of Radiochemical Purity in Technetium Tc 99m Sestamibi: Final product with radiochemical purity of at least 90% was used in the clinical trials that established safety and effectiveness. The radiochemical purity was determined by the following method.

1. Obtain a Baker-Flex Aluminum Oxide coated, plastic TLC plate, #1 B-F, pre-cut to 2.5 cm×7.5 cm.
2. Dry the plate or plates at 100°C for 1 hour and store in a desiccator. Remove pre-dried plate from the desiccator just prior to use.
3. Apply 1 drop of ethanol* using a 1 mL syringe with a 22-26 gauge needle, 1.5 cm from the bottom of the plate. **The spot should not be allowed to dry.**
4. Add 2 drops of Technetium Tc 99m Sestamibi solution, side by side on top of the ethanol* spot. Return the plate to a desiccator and allow the sample spot to dry (typically 15 minutes).
5. The TLC tank is prepared by pouring ethanol* to a depth of 3-4 mm. Cover the tank and let it equilibrate for ~10 minutes.
6. Develop the plate in the covered TLC tank in ethanol* for a distance of 5 cm from the point of application.
7. Cut the TLC plate 4 cm from the bottom and measure the Tc 99m activity in each piece by appropriate radiation detector.
8. Calculate the % Tc 99m Sestamibi as:

$$\% \text{ Tc 99m Sestamibi} = \frac{\mu\text{Ci Top Piece}}{\mu\text{Ci Both Pieces}} \times 100$$

TLC Plate Diagram

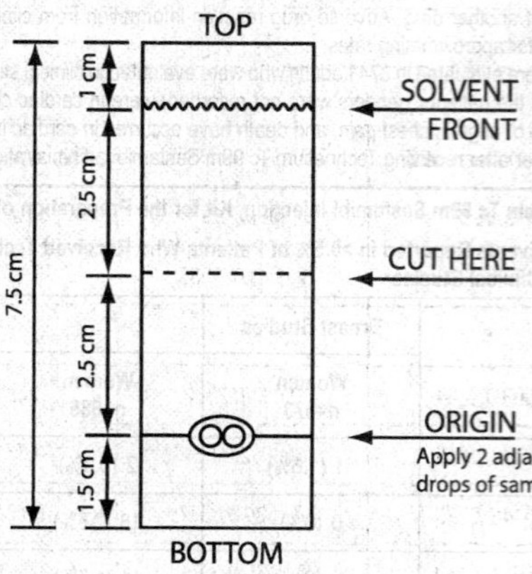

9. The dose should contain Tc 99m Sestamibi ≥90%. Do not use if radiochemical purity is less than 90%.

OVERDOSAGE:

Clinical consequences of overdosage with Kit for the Preparation of Technetium Tc-99m Sestamibi Injection have not been reported.

> For management of a suspected drug overdose, CPhA recommends that you contact your **regional Poison Control Centre**. See the *CPS* Directory section for a list of Poison Control Centres.

ACTION AND CLINICAL PHARMACOLOGY: Technetium Tc99m Sestamibi is a cationic Tc99m complex which has been found to accumulate in viable myocardial tissue in proportion to regional blood flow, in a manner analogous to that of Thallous Chloride Tl-201.

Animal cross-over experiments using Tl-201 and Tc99m Sestamibi have confirmed that the myocardial distribution of Tc99m Sestamibi correlates well with regional myocardial perfusion.

Scintigraphic images obtained in animals and humans after the intravenous administration of the drug have been comparable to those obtained with Thallous Chloride Tl-201 in normal and infarcted myocardial tissue.

The major metabolic pathway for clearance of Tc99 Sestamibi is the hepatobiliary system; Activity from the gallbladder appears in the intestines within one hour of injection. Twenty-seven percent of the injected dose is excreted in the urine, and approximately thirty-three percent of the injected dose is cleared through the feces in 48 hours. The agent is excreted without any evidence of metabolism.

Pulmonary activity is negligible even immediately after injection. Blood clearance studies indicate that the fast clearing component clears with a $t_{½}$ of 4.3 minutes at rest, and clears with a $t_{½}$ of 1.6 minutes under exercise conditions. At five minutes post injection about 8% of the injected dose remains in circulation. There is less than 1% protein binding of Technetium Tc 99m Sestamibi in plasma. The myocardial biological half-life is approximately seven hours after a rest or exercise injection. The biological half-life for the liver is approximately 35 minutes after a rest or exercise injection. The ideal imaging time reflects the best compromise between heart count rate and surrounding organ uptake. There is no evidence for change in myocardial distribution (redistribution), therefore imaging at delayed times is possible.

Myocardial uptake which is coronary flow dependent is 1.5% of the injected dose at exercise and 1.2% of the injected dose at rest. Animal studies have shown that uptake is not blocked when the sodium pump mechanism is inhibited.

Radiation Dosimetry: Estimates of radiation doses to organs and tissues of an average patient (70 Kg) per 1110 MBq (30 mCi) of Technetium Tc 99m Sestamibi injected intravenously are shown in Table 5.

Table 5: Technetium Tc 99m Sestamibi Injection, Kit for the Preparation of

Radiation Absorbed Doses from Tc 99m Sestamibi

	Estimated Radiation Absorbed Dose			
	Rest			
	2.0 Hour Void		4.8 Hour Void	
Organ	**rads/30 mCi**	**mGy/1110 MBq**	**rads/30 mCi**	**mGy/1110 MBq**
Breasts	0.2	2.0	0.2	1.9
Gallbladder Wall	2.0	20.0	2.0	20.0
Small Intestine	3.0	30.0	3.0	30.0
Upper Large Intestine Wall	5.4	55.5	5.4	55.5
Lower Large Intestine Wall	3.9	40.0	4.2	41.1
Stomach Wall	0.6	6.1	0.6	5.8
Heart Wall	0.5	5.1	0.5	4.9
Kidneys	2.0	20.0	2.0	20.0
Liver	0.6	5.8	0.6	5.7
Lungs	0.3	2.8	0.3	2.7
Bone Surfaces	0.7	6.8	0.7	6.4
Thyroid	0.7	7.0	0.7	2.4
Ovaries	1.5	15.5	1.6	15.5
Testes	0.3	3.4	0.4	3.9
Red Marrow	0.5	5.1	0.5	5.0
Urinary Bladder Wall	2.0	20.0	4.2	41.1
Total Body	0.5	4.8	0.5	4.8
	rem/30 mCi	mSv/1110 MBq	rem/30 mCi	mSv/1110 MBq
Effective Dose Equivalent	1.5	15.5	1.7	16.7
	Stress			
	2.0 Hour Void		4.8 Hour Void	
Organ	**rads/30 mCi**	**mGy/1110 MBq**	**rads/30 mCi**	**mGy/1110 MBq**
Breasts	0.2	2.0	0.2	1.8
Gallbladder Wall	2.8	28.9	2.8	27.8
Small Intestine	2.4	24.4	2.4	24.4
Upper Large Intestine Wall	4.5	44.4	4.5	44.4
Lower Large Intestine Wall	3.3	32.2	3.3	32.2
Stomach Wall	0.6	5.3	0.5	5.2
Heart Wall	0.5	5.6	0.5	5.3
Kidneys	1.7	16.7	1.7	16.7
Liver	0.4	4.2	0.4	4.1
Lungs	0.3	2.6	0.2	2.4
Bone Surfaces	0.6	6.2	0.6	6.0
Thyroid	0.3	2.7	0.2	2.4
Ovaries	1.2	12.2	1.3	13.3
Testes	0.3	3.1	0.3	3.4
Red Marrow	0.5	4.6	0.5	4.4
Urinary Bladder Wall	1.5	15.5	3.0	30.0
Total Body	0.4	4.2	0.4	4.2
	rem/30 mCi	mSv/1110 MBq	rem/30 mCi	mSv/1110 MBq
Effective Dose Equivalent	1.3	13.3	1.4	14.4

(cont'd)

Table 5: Technetium Tc 99m Sestamibi Injection, Kit for the Preparation of *(cont'd)*

Radiation Absorbed Doses from Tc 99m Sestamibi

Stabin, M., July, 1990, Oak Ridge Associated Universities, P.O. Box 117, Oak Ridge, TN 37831, (423) 576-3449.

Comparative Animal Biodistribution: The following study compared the biodistribution of a generic formulation of technetium 99m labelled sestamibi (MIBI) with the innovator formulation of technetium 99m labelled sestamibi, Cardiolite. In this study, rats (3 males and 3 females) were randomized to 1 of 8 treatment/time point groups. Each rat was injected with approximately 50 µCi of either generic MIBI or Cardiolite. Animals were euthanized at 0.5, 1, 6 or 24 hours after injection of radioactivity. After euthanasia, the following organs or tissues were collected and the amount of radioactivity present measured: liver, lungs, heart, spleen, kidneys, testes/ovaries, skeletal muscle, bone, urinary bladder, urine, stomach wall, small intestine, large intestine, cecum, feces, blood and site of injection. Data from this study demonstrate that the biodistribution of generic MIBI and Cardiolite are equivalent.

Dosing: Each animal was dosed at a volume of 0.2 mL which contained 66.7 µg, and 50 µCi/rat.

Methodology: A single intravenous bolus injection of either the generic formulation of MIBI or the innovator formulation of Cardiolite was administered via the lateral tail vein injection to six Sprague-Dawley rats. After injection, rats were placed in metabolism cages until the time of sacrifice. Animals were sacrificed at 30 minutes and 1, 6, and 24 hours after injection via cervical dislocation. Urine was collected from each rat at sacrifice. The organs, tissue/fluid specimens or excreta from multiple sites were collected and assayed for radioactivity.

Biodistribution Comparison: The biodistribution (percent injected dose per gram) data for both products are comparable in all organs at both time points tested as shown in following Table 6 and Table 7. At one hour post-administration (Table 6), compared to Cardiolite, there were statistically significant differences in the biodistribution of generic MIBI. The concentration of generic MIBI was slightly higher in the lung, bone, and urine ($P<0.05$). At six hours post administration, there were no statistically significant differences in the biodistribution of Cardiolite and Mallinckrodt Sestamibi (Table 7).

STORAGE AND STABILITY: Kit for the Preparation of Technetium Tc 99m Sestamibi Injection should be stored at 15 to 25°C before and after reconstitution. Protect from light prior to reconstitution. Expiration of the unreconstituted kit is 24 months from the date of manufacture. Expiration after reconstitution is 6 hours.

SPECIAL HANDLING INSTRUCTIONS: As with any other radioactive material, care should be taken to minimize radiation exposure to patients consistent with proper patient management, and to minimize radiation exposure to occupational workers.

Drug Handling: The patient dose should be measured by a suitable radioactivity calibration system immediately prior to patient administration. Radiochemical purity should be checked prior to patient administration.

Parenteral drug products should be inspected visually for particulate matter and discoloration prior to administration whenever solution and container permit.

INFORMATION FOR THE PATIENT: Published in e-CPS, available by subscription at www.e-cps.ca.

DOSAGE FORMS, COMPOSITION AND PACKAGING: Kit for the Preparation of Technetium Tc 99m Sestamibi Injection is supplied as a 10 mL vial in a kit of 5 or a carton of 30, sterile and non-pyrogenic.

Each 10 mL vial contains a sterile, non-pyrogenic, lyophilized mixture of: tetrakis (2-methoxy isobutyl isonitrile) copper (1) tetrafluoroborate 1 mg, sodium citrate dihydrate 2.6 mg, L-cysteine hydrochloride monohydrate 1 mg, mannitol 20 mg, stannous chloride, dihydrate, minimum ($SnCl_2{\cdot}2H_2O$) 0.025 mg, stannous chloride, dihydrate ($SnCl_2{\cdot}2H_2O$) 0.075 mg, tin chloride (stannous and stannic) dihydrate, maximum (as $SnCl_2{\cdot}2H_2O$) 0.086 mg.

Prior to lyophilization the pH is between 5.6-5.7. The contents of the vial are lyophilized and stored under nitrogen. Protect from light prior to reconstitution. Technetium Tc 99m Sestamibi contains no preservatives. Store at 15-25°C before and after reconstitution. Included in each 5 vial kit is 1 package insert and 5 radioassay information labels. Included in each 30 vial carton is 1 package insert and 30 radioassay information labels.

Table 6: Technetium Tc 99m Sestamibi Injection, Kit for the Preparation of 1 Hour Biodistribution Data

	Cardiolite vs. Generic MIBI 1 Hour Data, % ID/g							
	Both Sexes							
	Generic MIBI		Cardiolite		Males—Generic MIBI	Males—Cardiolite	Females—Generic MIBI	Females—Cardiolite
Organ/Tissue	Mean	SD	Mean	SD	Mean/SD	Mean/SD	Mean/SD	Mean/SD
Blood	0.0141	0.0021	0.0136	0.0037	0.0133/0.0003	0.0145/0.0055	0.0149/0.0030	0.0128/0.0012
Liver	0.4687	0.2036	0.3564	0.0396	0.4217/0.098	0.3642/0.0472	0.5157/0.2956	0.3487/0.0387
Kidney	1.7225	0.5356	1.2621	0.5410	1.3569/0.3284	0.907/0.2369	2.088/0.4564	1.6171/0.5454
Heart	3.1785	0.3801	3.0508	0.5683	2.9854/0.2325	2.6892/0.524	3.3716/0.4418	3.423/0.3753
Lung[a]	0.4827	0.0614	0.3517	0.0381	0.5014/0.0733	0.3524/0.0527	0.4641/0.0550	0.3510/0.0291
Spleen	0.4895	0.0836	0.3995	0.0755	0.4806/0.0460	0.3436/0.0275	0.4985/0.1229	0.4553/0.0642
Muscle	0.5565	0.1001	0.5562	0.1068	0.5037/0.1093	0.5401/0.0371	0.6093/0.0689	0.5722/0.1624
Bone[a]	0.2258	0.0306	0.1823	0.0331	0.2431/0.0322	0.1705/0.0356	0.2084/0.0201	0.1941/0.0325
Stomach	0.6436	0.0743	0.5734	0.1105	0.6489/0.1001	0.5187/0.0925	0.6384/0.0607	0.6281/0.1140
Sm. Int.	1.8429	0.1918	1.8442	0.7066	1.7475/0.1855	1.2200/0.1030	1.9384/0.1737	2.4685/0.2619
Lg. Int.	0.4657	0.0819	0.3763	0.1368	0.3992/0.0468	0.2812/0.1176	0.5322/0.0361	0.4715/0.0764
Cecum	0.5154	0.1265	0.416	0.1882	0.5773/0.0635	0.2559/0.0786	0.4536/0.1564	0.5762/0.0739
Gonads	0.3914	0.4318	0.2982	0.3122	0.0273/0.0091	0.0275/0.0020	0.7555/0.2615	0.5690/0.1542
Bladder	0.6957	0.5907	0.8487	0.8309	1.0156/0.7379	1.3114/1.0303	0.3758/0.1441	0.3860/0.1489
Inj. Site	0.4672	0.4286	0.1911	0.0554	0.5875/0.6331	0.2038/0.0689	0.3469/0.1229	0.1783/0.0493
Urine[a]	0.2383	0.0344	0.1245	0.0544	0.2659/0.0247	0.1085/0.0335	0.2107/0.0079	0.1404/0.0742

[a] Denotes significant differences ($P<0.05$) between the generic MIBI group and the Cardiolite group by student's t-test.

Table 7: Technetium Tc 99m Sestamibi Injection, Kit for the Preparation of 6 Hour Biodistribution Data

	Cardiolite vs. Generic MIBI 6 Hour Data, % ID/g							
	Both Sexes							
	Generic MIBI		Cardiolite		Males—Generic MIBI	Males—Cardiolite	Females—Generic MIBI	Females—Cardiolite
Organ/Tissue	Mean	SD	Mean	SD	Mean/SD	Mean/SD	Mean/SD	Mean/SD
Blood	0.0056	0.003	0.0056	0.0033	0.0062/0.0013	0.0074/0.0023	0.0051/0.0044	0.0038/0.0033
Liver	0.1002	0.0387	0.0748	0.0141	0.0807/0.0198	0.0645/0.0051	0.1198/0.0471	0.0850/0.0125
Kidney	0.5994	0.1407	0.535	0.0757	0.5351/0.0645	0.4744/0.0459	0.6637/0.1814	0.5957/0.0345
Heart	2.8825	0.4371	2.4945	0.2951	2.6170/0.4619	2.2286/0.0443	3.1481/0.2298	2.7604/0.0599
Lung	0.1153	0.023	0.1115	0.0143	0.1092/0.0101	0.1120/0.0138	0.1215/0.0334	0.1109/0.0180
Spleen	0.0971	0.0146	0.0976	0.0113	0.0973/0.0085	0.1018/0.0159	0.0968/0.0215	0.0934/0.0038
Muscle	0.6905	0.103	0.6071	0.1801	0.6994/0.0744	0.4955/0.1582	0.6815/0.1441	0.7207/0.1344
Bone	0.083	0.0172	0.0808	0.0150	0.0848/0.0217	0.0840/0.0123	0.0812/0.01601	0.0776/0.0195
Stomach	0.4245	0.0792	0.4032	0.0588	0.4113/0.0724	0.4109/0.0677	0.4376/0.0996	0.3955/0.0623
Sm. Int.	0.4280	0.1073	0.3446	0.1103	0.3820/0.0782	0.2703/0.0521	0.4739/0.1279	0.4190/0.1054
Lg. Int.	3.3495	1.0090	3.0252	1.0066	2.8055/0.5190	2.5158/0.8001	3.8935/1.1781	3.5345/1.0556
Cecum	5.7852	1.9189	4.8287	1.8961	4.1980/0.9791	3.1459/0.4327	7.3723/0.8304	6.5106/0.5614
Gonads	0.1580	0.1336	0.1940	0.1769	0.0372/0.0121	0.0336/0.0064	0.2788/0.0269	0.3544/0.0310
Bladder	0.2785	0.1586	0.3012	0.3379	0.3931/0.1478	0.3929/0.5035	0.1638/0.0400	0.2094/0.0822
Inj. Site	0.2172	0.0631	0.1526	0.0875	0.2124/0.0963	0.1313/0.0328	0.2219/0.0247	0.1739/0.1293
Urine	0.3907	0.1706	0.2965	0.1047	0.5221/0.0921	0.3363/0.1434	0.2594/0.1120	0.2568/0.0461

Tecta™ ℞

pantoprazole magnesium
H+, K+-ATPase Inhibitor

Nycomed

Date of Revision: December 1, 2008

SUMMARY PRODUCT INFORMATION:

Route of Administration	Dosage Form/ Strength	Clinically Relevant Nonmedicinal Ingredients
Oral	Enteric-Coated Tablet 40 mg pantoprazole	None For a complete listing see Dosage Forms, Composition and Packaging.

Note: As with all proton pump inhibitors, when TECTA (pantoprazole magnesium) is prescribed in combination with clarithromycin, amoxicillin or metronidazole for the eradication of an *H. pylori* infection, the Product Monograph for the antibiotics used should be consulted and followed.

INDICATIONS AND CLINICAL USE: TECTA (pantoprazole magnesium) is indicated for the treatment of conditions where a reduction of gastric acid secretion is required, such as the following:
- Duodenal ulcer
- Gastric ulcer
- Reflux esophagitis
- Symptomatic gastro-esophageal reflux disease (such as, acid regurgitation and heartburn).
- *H. pylori* associated duodenal ulcer
- Pantoprazole, in combination with clarithromycin and either amoxicillin or metronidazole, is indicated for the treatment of patients with an active duodenal ulcer who are *H. pylori* positive. Clinical trials using combinations of pantoprazole with appropriate antibiotics have indicated that such combinations are successful in eradicating *H. pylori*.

Geriatrics (>65 years of age): No dosage adjustment is recommended based on age. The daily dose used in elderly patients, as a rule, should not exceed the recommended dosage regimens. See Action and Clinical Pharmacology.

Pediatrics: The safety and effectiveness of pantoprazole in children have not yet been established.

CONTRAINDICATIONS: Patients who are hypersensitive to this drug or to any ingredient in the formulation or component of the container. For a complete listing, see Dosage Forms, Composition and Packaging.

Pantoprazole, like all PPIs, should not be concurrently administered with atazanavir. See Drug Interactions.

WARNINGS AND PRECAUTIONS: General: In the presence of any alarm symptom (e.g. significant unintentional weight loss, recurrent vomiting, dysphagia, haematemesis, anaemia, or melaena) and when gastric ulcer is suspected, the possibility of malignancy should be excluded before therapy with TECTA (pantoprazole magnesium) is instituted since treatment with pantoprazole magnesium may alleviate symptoms and delay diagnosis.

Further investigation should be considered if symptoms persist despite adequate treatment.

Carcinogenesis and Mutagenesis: Effects of long-term treatment include hypergastrinemia, possible enterochromaffin-like (ECL) cell hyperplasia and carcinoid formation in the stomach, adenomas and carcinomas in the liver and neoplastic changes in the thyroid.

In the rat, the mechanism leading to the formation of gastric carcinoids is considered to be due to the elevated gastrin level occurring during chronic treatment. Similar observations have also been made after administration of other acid secretion inhibitors.

Short-term and long-term treatment with pantoprazole sodium in a limited number of patients up to 6 years have not resulted in any significant pathological changes in gastric oxyntic exocrine cells.

Hepatic/Biliary/Pancreatic and Renal: Pantoprazole 40 mg daily is not recommended in patients with severe liver disease. For more details please see Action and Clinical Pharmacology, Special Populations and Conditions.

The daily dose used in renal insufficient patients, as a rule, should not exceed the recommended dosage regimens. See Action and Clinical Pharmacology, Special Populations and Conditions.

Pantoprazole should not be used in combination treatment for the eradication of *H. pylori* in patients with severe hepatic or renal dysfunction since currently no data are available on the efficacy and safety of pantoprazole in combination treatment of these patients.

Special Populations: Pregnant Women: There are no adequate or well-controlled studies in pregnant women. TECTA (pantoprazole magnesium) should not be administered to pregnant women unless the expected benefits outweigh the potential risks to the fetus.

Nursing Women: Limited data is available around pantoprazole use in nursing women. Pantoprazole excretion in human milk has been detected in a study of a single nursing mother after a single 40 mg oral dose. The clinical relevance of this finding is not known. Pantoprazole should not be given to nursing mothers unless its use is believed to outweigh the potential risks to the infant.

Pediatrics: The safety and effectiveness of pantoprazole in children have not yet been established.

Geriatrics (>65 years of age): No dose adjustment is recommended based on age. The daily dose used in elderly patients, as a rule, should not exceed the recommended dosage regimens. See Action and Clinical Pharmacology.

ADVERSE REACTIONS: In a short term study (40 mg pantoprazole magnesium tablet, once daily for 7 days) in patients with GERD, and in a 4 to 8-week clinical trial in 636 GERD patients, the adverse event profile seen with TECTA (pantoprazole magnesium) 40 mg tablet was similar to that seen with the pantoprazole sodium 40 mg tablet.

No differences in adverse reactions are expected between pantoprazole magnesium and pantoprazole sodium.

Adverse Drug Reaction Overview: Pantoprazole is well tolerated. Most adverse events have been mild and transient showing no consistent relationship with treatment. Adverse events have been recorded during controlled clinical investigations in 13 000 patients exposed to pantoprazole sodium as the single therapeutic agent for treatment of conditions requiring acid suppression.

The following adverse events (the most frequently reported) have been reported in individuals receiving pantoprazole sodium therapy (40 mg once daily) in controlled clinical trials of at least 6 months duration: headache (2.1%), diarrhea (1.6%), nausea (1.2%).

The following adverse reactions considered possibly, probably, or definitely related by the investigator have been reported in individuals receiving pantoprazole sodium therapy (20 mg or 40 mg once daily) in long-term clinical trials (duration of at least 6 months).

There were a limited number of *H. pylori* positive patients in these studies and therefore, definitive conclusions with regard to long-term consequences of *H. pylori* infection and acid suppressive treatment on gastric inflammation in this sub-group cannot be made.

Table 1: TECTA

Adverse Drug Reactions with a Frequency of ≥1% Related to 40 mg Pantoprazole Sodium, Assessed as Possibly, Probably or Definitely Related by the Investigator

Preferred Term	Number of Patients	Percentage of Patients
Headache	24	2.137
Diarrhoea	18	1.603
Nausea	13	1.158

Adverse Drug Reactions with a Frequency of 0.1 to 1% Related to 40 mg Pantoprazole Sodium: Cardiovascular System: blood pressure increased, hypertension, ECG abnormal.

Gastrointestinal Disorders: flatulence, abdominal distension, abdominal pain, abdominal pain upper, loose stools, oesophageal reflux aggravated, gastric polyps, abdominal discomfort, abdominal tenderness, constipation, eructation, vomiting, dyspepsia, gastroesophageal reflux, oesophagitis.

General Disorders: fatigue, peripheral oedema, pyrexia.

Hepatobiliary Disorders: alanine aminotransferase increased, aspartate aminotransferase increased, liver function tests abnormal, transaminases increased.

Laboratory Parameters: hypertriglyceridaemia.

Metabolic and Nutritional: appetite decreased, weight increase.

Nervous System Disorders: dysgeusia, dizziness, migraine, vertigo.

Respiratory System: cough.

Skin and Subcutaneous Tissue Disorders: pruritus, rash.

Special Senses: mouth dry, vision blurred.

Other: neoplasm.

The following adverse reactions considered possibly, probably, or definitely related by the investigator have been reported in individuals receiving pantoprazole therapy (20 mg or 40 mg pantoprazole sodium once daily) in short-term clinical trials (duration of up to 3 months).

Adverse Events with a Frequency of 0.1 to 1% Related to Pantoprazole Sodium 20 mg or 40 mg: Gastrointestinal Disorders: diarrhoea, flatulence, nausea, constipation, abdominal pain.

Nervous System Disorders: headache, dizziness.

Skin and Subcutaneous Tissue Disorders: pruritus.

In addition, the following adverse events considered unrelated, or unlikely related by the investigator have been reported in individuals receiving pantoprazole sodium therapy (20 mg or 40 mg once daily) in short-term and long-term clinical trials.

Adverse Events with a Frequency of >1%, 20 or 40 mg Pantoprazole Sodium: influenza like illness, headache, diarrhoea.

Adverse Events with a Frequency of 0.1 to 1%, 20 or 40 mg Pantoprazole Sodium: bronchitis, nausea, back pain, abdominal pain upper, upper respiratory tract infection, non-accidental injury, sinusitis, abdominal pain, dizziness, arthralgia, vomiting, pharyngitis, chest pain, gastroenteritis, dyspepsia, urinary tract infection, eructation, pyrexia, cough, depression, hypertension, pain in limb, constipation, fatigue, operation, neck pain, nasopharyngitis, alanine aminotransferase increased, haemorrhoids, pain, flatulence, viral infection, hypertriglyceridaemia, toothache, hypersensitivity, rash, abdominal pain lower, pneumonia, abdominal distension, dyspnoea, muscle cramp, rhinitis, peripheral oedema, tonsillitis, angina pectoris, cholelithiasis, sinus congestion, influenza, vertigo, insomnia, infection, osteoarthritis, hypercholesterolaemia, pruritus, eczema, sleep disorder, migraine, aspartate aminotransferase increased, hyperglycaemia, musculoskeletal discomfort, blood triglycerides increased, myocardial infarction, tendonitis, weight increased, rectal haemorrhage, cystitis, nasal congestion, arthritis, contusion, abdominal discomfort, enteritis.

The following Serious Adverse Events regardless of causality were reported with a frequency of <0.1% in either 20 mg or 40 mg: sepsis.

A total of 1217 patients were treated with triple combination therapy including pantoprazole sodium and two antibiotics. Adverse events noted at a frequency of greater than or equal to 1% when pantoprazole sodium was used in combination with antibiotics for the eradication of an *H. pylori* infection included the following:

In combination with clarithromycin and metronidazole (n=725):

Body as a Whole: headache (1.8%), tiredness (1.1%).

Central and Peripheral Nervous System: dizziness (1.4%).

Gastrointestinal: diarrhea (4.8%), nausea (3.7%), upper abdominal pain (1.9%), tongue pain (1.2%), loose stools (1.0%), buccal inflammation (1.0%).

Liver/Biliary: hepatic enzymes increased (1.2%).

Special Senses: bitter taste (4.0%), metallic taste (2.1%).

In combination with amoxicillin and clarithromycin (n=492):

Body as a Whole: headache (1.8%), pain (1.0%).

Skin and Appendages: exanthema (1.2%).

Gastrointestinal: diarrhea (10.0%), bitter taste (3.0%), upper abdominal pain (1.4%), nausea (1.2%).

Regardless of the combination regimen, the most frequently reported events were gastrointestinal system disorders, followed by autonomic nervous system disorders and "body as a whole", or generalized disorders.

Abnormal Hematologic and Clinical Chemistry Findings: Please refer to Adverse Reactions, Hepatobiliary Disorders and Laboratory Parameters, Action and Clinical Pharmacology, Special Populations and Conditions, and Warnings and Precautions, Hepatic/Biliary/Pancreatic and Renal.

Post-Market Adverse Drug Reactions: The following adverse events were reported in post-marketing use and causal relation to pantoprazole sodium treatment could not be ruled out:

Skin and Subcutaneous Tissue Disorders: allergic reactions such as skin rash. Very rare cases of angioedema, severe skin reactions such as Stevens-Johnson Syndrome, erythema multiforme, toxic epidermal necrolysis and photosensitivity. Isolated cases of alopecia, acne, maculopapular rash, urticaria, exfoliative dermatitis.

Nervous System Disorders: hypokinesia, disturbances in vision (blurred vision). Rare cases of somnolence, insomnia; in isolated cases vertigo, tremor, tinnitus, paresthesia, nervousness, photophobia.

Eye Disorders: anterior ischemic optic neuropathy.

Gastrointestinal Disorders: occasionally upper abdominal pain, flatulence; rare cases of increased appetite, dry mouth, nausea/vomiting, constipation, dyspeptic symptoms, acid eructation, pancreatitis, increased salivation.

Urogenital: isolated cases of hematuria and impotence. Interstitial nephritis.

Laboratory Parameters: in rare cases, increased liver enzymes (transaminases, γ-GT), elevated triglycerides.

Hematologic and Lymphatic System: pancytopenia, isolated cases of eosinophilia. Very rare cases of leukopenia, and thrombocytopenia.

General Disorders: speech disorder. Very rare cases of peripheral edema, increased body temperature.

Hepatobiliary Disorders: Very rare cases of severe hepatocellular damage leading to jaundice with or without hepatic failure.

Immune System Disorders: anaphylactic reactions including anaphylactic shock.

Musculoskeletal, Connective Tissue and Bone Disorders: elevated creatine phosphokinase, in rare cases, myalgia and arthralgia. In very rare cases rhabdomyolysis.

Psychiatric Disorders: confusion, rare cases of depression, hallucination, disorientation, confusion especially in pre-disposed patients, as well as the aggravation of these symptoms in the case of pre-existence.

Other: in isolated cases malaise.

DRUG INTERACTIONS: Overview: Pantoprazole undergoes extensive hepatic metabolism via cytochrome P450-mediated oxidation followed by sulphate conjugation via a Phase II reaction (non-saturable, non-cytochrome P450 dependent). Pharmacokinetic drug interaction studies in man did not demonstrate the inhibition of the oxidative metabolism of the drug. No induction of the CYP 450 system by pantoprazole was observed during chronic administration of pantoprazole sodium with antipyrine as a marker. Changes in absorption should be taken into account when drugs whose absorption is pH dependent, e.g., ketoconazole, are taken concomitantly.

It has been shown that co-administration of atazanavir 300 mg/ritonavir 100 mg with omeprazole (40 mg once daily) or atazanavir 400 mg with lansoprazole (60 mg single dose) to healthy volunteers resulted in a substantial reduction in the bioavailability of atazanavir. The absorption of atazanavir is pH dependent. Therefore all PPIs, including pantoprazole, should not be co-administered with atazanavir. See Contraindications.

Drug-Drug Interactions: The magnesium content of a 40 mg tablet is negligibly low, and thus far below the amount of magnesium taken with food or dietary supplements. No differences in drug-drug interactions are expected between pantoprazole magnesium and pantoprazole sodium.

Pantoprazole sodium does not interact with carbamazepine, caffeine, diclofenac, naproxen, piroxicam, ethanol, glibenclamide, metoprolol, antipyrine, diazepam, phenytoin, nifedipine, theophylline, digoxin, oral contraceptives, or cyclosporine. Concomitant use of antacids does not affect the pharmacokinetics of pantoprazole sodium.

Clinical studies have shown that there is no pharmacokinetic interaction between pantoprazole sodium and the following antibiotic combinations: metronidazole plus clarithromycin, metronidazole plus amoxicillin, amoxicillin plus clarithromycin.

In a preclinical study, pantoprazole sodium in combination therapy with various antibiotics (including tetracycline, clarithromycin, and amoxicillin) was shown to have a potentiating effect on the elimination rate of *H. pylori* infection.

Although no interaction during concomitant administration of warfarin has been observed in clinical pharmacokinetic studies, a few isolated cases of changes in INR have been reported during concomitant treatment in the post-marketing period. Therefore, in patients being treated with coumarin anticoagulants, monitoring of prothrombin time/INR is recommended after initiation, termination or during irregular use of pantoprazole.

Drug-Food Interactions: Consumption of food does not affect the pharmacokinetics (AUC and C_{max}) of pantoprazole sodium.

Drug-Laboratory Test Interactions: There have been reports of false-positive results in urine screening tests for tetrahydrocannabinol (THC) in patients receiving most proton pump inhibitors, including pantoprazole. To some extent, a cross-reactivity of proton pump inhibitors to the THC assay in the OnTrak TesTcard 9 has been seen, though this may not be limited to this screening test. In order to verify positive urine screening results, a confirmatory method should be considered.

Other: Generally, daily treatment with any acid-blocking medicines over a long time (e.g. longer than 3 years) may lead to malabsorption of cyanocobalamin caused by hypo- or achlorhydria. Rare cases of cyanocobalamin deficiency under acid-blocking therapy have been reported in the literature and should be considered if respective clinical symptoms are observed.

DOSAGE AND ADMINISTRATION: Recommended Dose and Dosage Adjustment: Duodenal Ulcer: The recommended adult dose of TECTA (pantoprazole magnesium) for the oral treatment of duodenal ulcer is 40 mg given once daily in the morning. Healing usually occurs within 2 weeks. For patients not healed after this initial course of therapy, an additional course of 2 weeks is recommended.

Gastric Ulcer: The recommended adult oral dose of TECTA (pantoprazole magnesium) for the oral treatment of gastric ulcer is 40 mg given once daily in the morning. Healing usually occurs within 4 weeks. For patients not healed after this initial course of therapy, an additional course of 4 weeks is recommended.

***H. pylori* Associated Duodenal Ulcer: Pantoprazole/Clarithromycin/Metronidazole Triple Combination Therapy:** The recommended dose for *H. pylori* eradication is treatment for seven days with TECTA (pantoprazole magnesium) 40 mg together with clarithromycin 500 mg and metronidazole 500 mg, all twice daily.

Pantoprazole/Clarithromycin/Amoxicillin Triple Combination Therapy: The recommended dose for *H. pylori* eradication is treatment for seven days with TECTA (pantoprazole magnesium) 40 mg together with clarithromycin 500 mg and amoxicillin 1000 mg, all twice daily.

Symptomatic Gastro-Esophageal Reflux Disease (GERD): The recommended adult oral dose for the treatment of symptoms of GERD, including heartburn and regurgitation, is TECTA (pantoprazole magnesium) 40 mg once daily for up to 4 weeks. If significant symptom relief is not obtained in 4 weeks, further investigation is required.

Reflux Esophagitis: The recommended adult oral dose of TECTA (pantoprazole magnesium) is 40 mg, given once daily in the morning. In most patients, healing usually occurs within 4 weeks. For patients not healed after this initial course of therapy, an additional 4 weeks of treatment is recommended.

Patients with healed gastroesophageal reflux disease, who require greater than usual maintenance doses of PPIs to avoid recurrence of reflux esophagitis, may consider 40 mg TECTA once daily in the morning.

Missed Dose: If a dose is forgotten, the missed dose should be taken as soon as possible unless it is close to the next scheduled dose. Two doses should never be taken at one time to make up for a missed dose; patients should just return to the regular schedule.

Administration: TECTA (pantoprazole magnesium) is formulated as an enteric-coated tablet. A whole tablet should not be chewed or crushed, and should be swallowed with fluid in the morning either before, during, or after breakfast.

Reconstitution: Not applicable.

OVERDOSAGE:

Some reports of overdosage with pantoprazole sodium have been received. No consistent symptom profile was observed after ingestion of high doses of pantoprazole sodium. Daily doses of up to 272 mg pantoprazole sodium i.v., and single doses of up to 240 mg i.v. administered over 2 minutes, have been administered and were well tolerated.

Treatment of overdosage should be supportive and symptomatic. Pantoprazole is not removed by hemodialysis.

For management of a suspected drug overdose, contact your **regional Poison Control Centre**. See the *CPS* Directory section for a list of Poison Control Centres.

ACTION AND CLINICAL PHARMACOLOGY: Mechanism of Action: TECTA (pantoprazole magnesium) is a specific inhibitor of the gastric H^+, K^+-ATPase enzyme (the proton pump) that is responsible for acid secretion by the parietal cells of the stomach.

Pantoprazole is a substituted benzimidazole that accumulates in the acidic environment of the parietal cells after absorption. Pantoprazole is then converted into the active form, a cyclic sulphenamide, which binds to the H^+, K^+-ATPase, thus inhibiting both the basal and stimulated gastric acid secretion. Pantoprazole exerts its effect in an acidic environment (pH <3), and it is mostly inactive at higher pH. Its pharmacological and therapeutic effect is achieved in the acid-secretory parietal cells.

Daily oral doses of pantoprazole magnesium 40 mg tablet showed a consistent and effective acid control. Information from a pharmacodynamic trial in patients with GERD indicates that TECTA (pantoprazole magnesium) 40 mg tablets demonstrate similar inhibition of acid secretion, and effect on intragastric pH, as pantoprazole sodium 40 mg tablets.

In clinical studies investigating intravenous (i.v.) and oral administration, pantoprazole sodium inhibited pentagastrin-stimulated gastric acid secretion. With a daily oral dose of 40 mg, inhibition was 51% on Day 1 and 85% on Day 7. Basal 24-hour acidity was reduced by 37% and 98% on Days 1 and 7, respectively.

Fasting gastrin values increased during pantoprazole sodium treatment, but in most cases the increase was only moderate. An extensive evaluation of clinical laboratory results has not revealed any clinically important changes during pantoprazole sodium treatment (except for gastrin which increased to 1.5- fold after 4 to 8 weeks).

Treatment with pantoprazole sodium alone has a limited effect on infections of *H. pylori*, a bacterium implicated as a major pathogen in peptic ulcer disease. Approximately 90-100% of patients with duodenal ulcers, and 80% of patients with gastric ulcers, are *H. pylori* positive. Preclinical evidence suggests that there is a synergistic effect between pantoprazole sodium and selected antibiotics in eradicating *H. pylori*. In infected patients, eradication of the infection with pantoprazole sodium and appropriate antibiotic therapy leads to ulcer healing, accompanied by symptom relief and a decreased rate of ulcer recurrence.

In single dose clinical pharmacology studies, pantoprazole sodium was administered concomitantly with combinations of amoxicillin, clarithromycin, and/or metronidazole. When a single dose of pantoprazole sodium was administered to healthy volunteers in combination with metronidazole plus amoxicillin, with clarithromycin plus metronidazole, or with clarithromycin plus amoxicillin, lack of interaction between any of the medications was shown.

Pharmacodynamics: Pantoprazole is a proton pump inhibitor. It inhibits H^+, K^+-ATPase, the enzyme responsible for gastric acid secretion in the parietal cells of the stomach, in a dose-dependent manner. The drug is a substituted benzimidazole that accumulates in the acid canaliculi of parietal cells after absorption. There, pantoprazole is converted into the active form, a cyclic sulfenamide that binds selectively to the proton translocating region of the H^+, K^+-ATPase. Pantoprazole's selectivity is due to the fact that it only exerts its maximal effect in a strongly acidic environment (pH <3). Pantoprazole remains mostly inactive at higher pH values. As pantoprazole action is distal to the receptor levels, it can inhibit gastric acid secretion irrespective of the nature of the stimulus (acetylcholine, histamine, gastrin).

Pharmacokinetics: Pantoprazole magnesium and pantoprazole sodium are not bioequivalent in terms of plasma AUC and C_{max}. In healthy, adult male volunteers, kinetic studies comparing the two salts show that the AUC of pantoprazole magnesium is almost 100% relative to that of pantoprazole sodium, under both fed and fasted conditions. C_{max} is lower for pantoprazole magnesium (approximately 65-73% of pantoprazole sodium values).

Absorption: Pantoprazole magnesium is absorbed rapidly following administration of a 40 mg enteric-coated tablet. Following an oral dose of 40 mg, mean maximum serum concentrations of approximately 1.3 µg/mL and 1.4 µg/mL are reached after about 2.5 and 6 hours under fasting and fed conditions respectively. The AUC is approximately 4 µg.h/mL.

Distribution: Pantoprazole is 98% bound to serum proteins. Elimination half-life, clearance and volume of distribution are independent of the dose.

Metabolism: Pantoprazole is almost completely metabolized in the liver. Studies with pantoprazole sodium in humans reveal no inhibition or activation of the cytochrome P450 (CYP 450) system of the liver.

Excretion: Renal elimination represents the major route of excretion (about 82%) for the metabolites of pantoprazole, the remaining metabolites are excreted in feces. The main metabolite in both the serum and urine is desmethylpantoprazole as a sulphate conjugate. The half-life of the main metabolite (about 1.5 hours) is not much longer than that of pantoprazole (approximately 1 hour).

Pantoprazole sodium shows linear pharmacokinetics, i.e., AUC and C_{max} increase in proportion with the dose within the dose-range of 10 to 80 mg after both i.v. and oral administration. Elimination half-life, clearance and volume of distribution are considered to be dose-independent. Following repeated i.v. or oral administration, the AUC of pantoprazole was similar to a single dose.

Special Populations and Conditions: Pediatrics: The safety and effectiveness of pantoprazole in children have not yet been established.

Geriatrics: An increase in AUC (35%) and C_{max} (22%) for pantoprazole occurs in elderly volunteers when compared to younger volunteers after 7 consecutive days oral dosing with pantoprazole sodium 40 mg. After a single oral dose of pantoprazole sodium 40 mg, an increase in AUC (43%) and C_{max} (26%) occurs in elderly volunteers when compared to younger volunteers. No dose adjustment is recommended based on age. The daily dose in elderly patients, as a rule, should not exceed the recommended dosage regimens.

Hepatic Insufficiency: The half-life increased to between 7 and 9 h, the AUC increased by a factor of 5 to 7, and the C_{max} increased by a factor of 1.5 in patients with liver cirrhosis compared with healthy subjects following administration of 40 mg pantoprazole sodium. Similarly, following administration of a 20 mg dose, the AUC increased by a factor of 5.5 and the C_{max} increased by a factor of 1.3 in patients with severe liver cirrhosis compared with healthy subjects. Considering the linear pharmacokinetics of pantoprazole sodium, there is an increase in AUC by a factor of 2.75 in patients with severe liver cirrhosis following administration of a 20 mg dose compared to healthy volunteers following administration of a 40 mg dose.

Renal Insufficiency: In patients with severe renal impairment, pharmacokinetic parameters for pantoprazole sodium were similar to those of healthy subjects. No dosage adjustment is necessary in patients with renal impairment or in patients undergoing hemodialysis, as the difference in AUCs between patients who are dialyzed and those who are not is 4%.

STORAGE AND STABILITY: Store at 15 to 30°C in the recommended packaging.

SPECIAL HANDLING INSTRUCTIONS: None.

INFORMATION FOR THE PATIENT: Published in e-CPS, available by subscription at www.e-cps.ca.

DOSAGE FORMS, COMPOSITION AND PACKAGING: Each enteric-coated, yellow, round, biconvex tablet for oral administration, marked 40 on one side, contains: pantoprazole 40 mg (pantoprazole magnesium). Nonmedicinal ingredients: anhydrous sodium carbonate, calcium stearate, crospovidone, ferric oxide, hypromellose, mannitol, povidone, poly (ethylacrylate, methacrylic acid), propylene glycol, titanium dioxide and triethyl citrate. Blisters of 30.

(Shown in Product Identification Section)

Tegretol® Ⓟ

carbamazepine

Anticonvulsant—Symptomatic Relief of Trigeminal Neuralgia—Antimanic

Novartis Pharmaceuticals

Date of Preparation: April 26, 1976
Date of Revision: June 16, 2010

PHARMACOLOGY: Carbamazepine has anticonvulsant properties which have been found useful in the treatment of partial seizures (simple or complex) with and without secondary generalization, and generalized tonic-clonic seizures. A mild psychotropic effect has been observed in some patients, which seems related to the effect of carbamazepine in localization-related epilepsies and syndromes.

Clinical Trials: Evidence supporting the efficacy of carbamazepine as an anticonvulsant was derived from active drug-controlled studies that enrolled patients with the following seizure types: partial seizures with simple or complex symptomatology; generalized tonic-clonic seizures; mixed seizure patterns which include the above, or other partial or generalized seizures.

Carbamazepine relieves or diminishes the pain associated with trigeminal neuralgia often within 24 to 48 hours.

Carbamazepine given as a monotherapy or in combination with lithium or neuroleptics has been found useful in the treatment of acute mania and the prophylactic treatment of bipolar (manic-depressive) disorders.

Like other tricyclic compounds, carbamazepine has a moderate anticholinergic action which is responsible for some of its side effects. A tolerance may develop to the action of carbamazepine after a few months of treatment and should be watched for. Carbamazepine may suppress ventricular automaticity due to its membrane-depressant effect, similar to that of quinidine and procainamide, associated with suppression of phase 4 depolarization of the heart muscle fibre.

A number of investigators have reported a deterioration of EEG abnormalities with regard to focal alterations and a higher incidence of records with nil β-activity during carbamazepine-combined treatment.

Pharmacokinetics: The absorption of carbamazepine in man is relatively slow. When taken in a single oral dose, the carbamazepine tablets and chewable tablets yield peak plasma concentrations of unchanged carbamazepine within 4 to 24 hours. With respect to the quantity of carbamazepine absorbed, there is no clinically relevant difference between the various dosage forms. However, carbamazepine suspension is absorbed somewhat faster than the tablet; peak plasma levels are reached within 2 hours. Following b.i.d. dosage regimens, higher peak levels and lower trough levels are obtained with the suspension than with the tablets. Steady-state plasma levels are comparable for carbamazepine suspension given t.i.d. and carbamazepine tablets given b.i.d., when administered at the same total daily dose.

Ingestion of food has no significant influence on the rate and extent of absorption regardless of the dosage form of carbamazepine.

When carbamazepine controlled-release tablets are administered repeatedly, they yield a lower average maximal concentration of carbamazepine in the plasma, without a reduction in the average minimal concentration. This tends to result in a lower incidence of intermittent concentration-dependent adverse drug reactions. It also ensures that the plasma concentrations remain largely stable throughout the day, thereby making it possible to manage with a twice-daily dosage.

Carbamazepine becomes bound to serum proteins to the extent of 70 to 80%. The concentration of unchanged substance in the saliva reflects the nonprotein-bound portion present in the serum (20 to 30%).

The elimination half-life of unchanged carbamazepine in the plasma averages approximately 36 hours following a single oral dose, whereas after repeated administration, which leads to autoinduction of hepatic enzymes, it averages only 16 to 24 hours, depending on the duration of the medication. In patients receiving concomitant treatment with other enzyme-inducing antiepileptic agents, half-life values averaging 9 to 10 hours have been found. One study in 39 children (aged 3 to 10 years) and 79 adults (aged 15 to 65 years) has indicated that carbamazepine elimination may be slightly enhanced in children. This data suggests that children may require higher doses of carbamazepine (in mg/kg) than adults.

Only 2 to 3% of the dose, whether given singly or repeatedly, is excreted in the urine in unchanged form. Approximately 30% of carbamazepine is renally eliminated via the epoxide pathway. The primary metabolite is the pharmacologically active 10, 11-epoxide. The mean elimination half-life of this active metabolite in the plasma is about 6 hours following single oral doses of the epoxide itself.

In man, the main urinary metabolite of carbamazepine is the trans-diol derivative originating from the 10,11-epoxide; a small portion of the epoxide is converted into 9-hydroxymethyl-10 carbamoyl-acridan. Other important biotransformation products are various monohydroxylated compounds, as well as the N-glucuronide of carbamazepine produced by UGT2B7.

In patients with epilepsy, the therapeutic range for the steady-state plasma concentration of carbamazepine generally lies between 4 to 10 µg/mL.

INDICATIONS: Epilepsy: For use as an anticonvulsant drug either alone or in combination with other anticonvulsant drugs.

Carbamazepine is not effective in controlling absence, myoclonic or atonic seizures, and does not prevent the generalization of epileptic discharge. Moreover, exacerbation of seizures may occasionally occur in patients with atypical absences.

Trigeminal Neuralgia: For the symptomatic relief of pain of trigeminal neuralgia only during periods of exacerbation of true or primary trigeminal neuralgia (tic douloureux). It should not be used preventively during periods of remission. In some patients, carbamazepine has relieved glossopharyngeal neuralgia. For patients who fail to respond to carbamazepine, or who are sensitive to the drug, recourse to other accepted measures must be considered.

Carbamazepine is not a simple analgesic and should not be used to relieve trivial facial pains or headaches.

Treatment of Acute Mania and Prophylaxis in Bipolar (Manic-Depressive) Disorders: Carbamazepine may be used as a monotherapy or as an adjunct to lithium in the treatment of acute mania or prophylaxis of bipolar (manic-depressive) disorders in patients who are resistant to or intolerant of conventional antimanic drugs. Carbamazepine may be a useful alternative to neuroleptics in such patients. Patients with severe mania, dysphoric mania or rapid cycling who are nonresponsive to lithium may show a positive response when treated with carbamazepine.

It is important to note that these recommendations are based on extensive clinical experience and some clinical trials versus active comparison agents.

CONTRAINDICATIONS: Carbamazepine should not be administered to patients with hepatic disease, a history of bone marrow depression, a history of hepatic porphyria (acute intermittent porphyria, variegate porphyria, porphyria cutanea tarda), or serious blood disorder.

Carbamazepine should not be administered immediately before, in conjunction with, or immediately after an MAO inhibitor (see Precautions, Drug Interactions).

Coadministration of carbamazepine and voriconazole is contraindicated, until data become available from drug interactions studies. CYP3A4 is one of the enzymes thought to be involved in the metabolism of voriconazole. Therefore, coadministration of carbamazepine, a potent inducer of CYP3A4, could diminish the therapeutic effect of voriconazole (see Precautions, Drug Interactions, Effects of Carbamazepine on Plasma Levels of Concomitant Agents).

Carbamazepine should not be administered to patients presenting AV heart block (see Pharmacology and Precautions).

Carbamazepine should not be administered to patients with known hypersensitivity to carbamazepine, to any of the components of the tablets or suspension, or to any of the tricyclic compounds, such as amitriptyline, trimipramine, imipramine, or their analogues or metabolites, because of the similarity in chemical structure.

WARNINGS:

Haematologic: Although reported infrequently, serious adverse effects have been observed during the use of carbamazepine. Agranulocytosis and aplastic anemia, with a fatal outcome, have occurred very rarely. Leukopenia, thrombocytopenia, hepatocellular and cholestatic jaundice, and hepatitis have also been reported. However, in the majority of cases, leukopenia and thrombocytopenia were transient and did not signal the onset of either aplastic anemia or agranulocytosis. It is important that carbamazepine should be used carefully and close clinical and frequent laboratory supervision should be maintained throughout treatment in order to detect as early as possible signs and symptoms of a possible blood dyscrasia. Carbamazepine should be discontinued if any evidence of significant bone marrow depression appears (see Precautions).

Dermatologic: Stevens-Johnson Syndrome and Toxic Epidermal Necrolysis: Serious and sometimes fatal dermatologic reactions, including Toxic Epidermal Necrolysis (TEN) and Stevens-Johnson Syndrome (SJS), have been reported with carbamazepine. In countries with mainly Caucasian populations, these reactions are estimated to occur in 1 to 6 per 10 000 new users, but in some Asian countries (e.g., Taiwan, Malaysia and the Philippines) the risk is estimated to be about 10 times higher.

HLA-B 1502: In studies that included small samples of patients of Han Chinese ancestry a strong association was found between the risk of developing SJS/TEN and the presence of HLA-B 1502, an inherited allelic variant of the HLA-B gene. The HLA-B 1502 allele is found almost exclusively in individuals with ancestry across broad areas of Asia*. Results of these studies suggest that the presence of the HLA-B 1502 allele may be one of the risk factors for carbamazepine-associated SJS/TEN in patients with Asian ancestry. Therefore, physicians should consider HLA-B 1502 genotyping as a screening tool in these patients. Until further information is available, the use of carbamazepine and other anti-epileptic drugs associated with SJS/TEN should also be avoided in patients who test positive for the HLA-B 1502 allele (see Warnings, Asian Ancestry and Allelic Variation in the HLA-B Gene and Important Limitations of HLA-B Genotyping).

Treatment Recommendations for Dermatological Reactions: Carbamazepine should be discontinued at the first sign of a rash, unless the rash is clearly not drug-related. If signs or symptoms suggest SJS/TEN, use of this drug should not be resumed and alternative therapy should be considered. The use of other anti-epileptic drugs associated with SJS/TEN should be avoided in patients who have shown severe dermatological reactions during carbamazepine treatment.

Carcinogenicity: Long-term toxicity studies in rats indicated a potential carcinogenic risk. Therefore, the possible risk of the drug must be weighed against the potential benefits before prescribing carbamazepine to individual patients.

Asian Ancestry and Allelic Variation in the HLA-B Gene: In studies that included small samples of patients of Han Chinese ancestry a strong association was found between the risk of developing SJS/TEN and the presence of HLA-B 1502, an inherited allelic variant of the HLA-B gene. The HLA-B 1502 allele is found almost exclusively in individuals with ancestry across broad areas of Asia. Results of these studies suggest that the presence of the HLA-B 1502 allele may be one of the risk factors for carbamazepine-associated SJS/TEN in patients with Asian ancestry. Therefore, physicians should consider HLA-B 1502 genotyping as a screening tool in these patients. Until further information is available, the use of carbamazepine and other anti-epileptic drugs associated with SJS/TEN should also be avoided in patients who test positive for the HLA-B 1502 allele.

Important Limitations of HLA-B Genotyping: HLA-B 1502 genotyping as a screening tool has important limitations and must never substitute for appropriate clinical vigilance and patient management. Many HLA-B 1502-positive Asian patients treated with carbamazepine will not develop SJS/TEN, and these reactions can still occur infrequently in HLA-B 1502-negative patients of any ethnicity. The role of other possible factors in the development of, and morbidity from, SJS/TEN, such as antiepileptic drug (AED) dose, compliance, concomitant medications, co-morbidities, and the level of dermatologic monitoring have not been studied.

In addition, it should be kept in mind that over 90% of carbamazepine treated patients who will experience SJS/TEN have this reaction within the first few months of treatment. This information may be taken into consideration when deciding whether to screen genetically at-risk patients currently on carbamazepine.

Should signs and symptoms suggest a severe skin reaction such as SJS or TEN, carbamazepine should be withdrawn at once.

Hypersensitivity: Carbamazepine may trigger hypersensitivity reactions, including multi-organ hypersensitivity reactions, which can affect the skin, liver (including intrahepatic bile ducts), hematopoietic organs and lymphatic system or other organs, either individually or together in the context of a systemic reaction (see Adverse Effects).

In general, if signs and symptoms suggestive of hypersensitivity reactions occur, carbamazepine should be withdrawn immediately, and alternative therapy should be considered.

Patients who have exhibited hypersensitivity reactions to carbamazepine should be informed that approximately 25 to 30 % of these patients may experience hypersensitivity reactions with oxcarbazepine (Trileptal).

Cross-hypersensitivity can occur between carbamazepine and phenytoin.

Pregnancy: **Women with epilepsy who are pregnant, or intend to become pregnant, should be treated with special care.**

In women of childbearing potential, carbamazepine should, whenever possible, be prescribed as monotherapy, because the incidence of congenital abnormalities in the offspring of women treated with more than one antiepileptic drug is greater than in those of women receiving a single antiepileptic.

Minimum effective doses should be given and the plasma levels monitored.

If pregnancy occurs in a woman receiving carbamazepine, or if the problem of initiating carbamazepine arises during pregnancy, the drug's potential benefits must be weighed against its hazards, particularly during the first 3 months of pregnancy. Carbamazepine should not be discontinued or withheld from patients if required to prevent major seizures because of the risks posed, to both mother and fetus, by status epilepticus with attendant hypoxia.

The possibility that carbamazepine, like all major antiepileptic drugs, increases the risk of malformations has been reported. Developmental disorders and malformations, including spina bifida, and also other congenital anomalies, e.g., craniofacial defects, cardiovascular malformations, hypospadias, and anomalies involving various body systems, have been reported in association with carbamazepine.

Conclusive evidence from controlled studies with carbamazepine monotherapy is lacking. Patients should be counselled regarding the possibility of an increased risk of malformations and given the opportunity of antenatal screening.

During pregnancy, an effective antiepileptic treatment should not be interrupted, since the aggravation of the illness is detrimental to both the mother and the fetus.

Folic acid deficiency is known to occur in pregnancy. Antiepileptic drugs have been reported to aggravate folic acid deficiency. This deficiency may contribute to the increased incidence of birth defects in the offspring of treated epileptic women. Folic acid supplementation has therefore been recommended before and during pregnancy.

To prevent neonatal bleeding disorders, Vitamin K_1 administration to the mother during the last weeks of pregnancy, as well as to the newborn, has been recommended.

A few cases of neonatal seizures and respiratory depression have been associated with maternal carbamazepine and other concomitant anticonvulsant drug use. A few cases of neonatal vomiting, diarrhea, and/or decreased feeding have also been associated with maternal carbamazepine use. These reactions may represent a neonatal withdrawal syndrome.

* The following rates provide a rough estimate of the prevalence of HLA-B 1502 in various populations. Greater than 15% of the population is reported positive in Hong Kong, Thailand, Malaysia, and parts of the Philippines, compared to about 10% in Taiwan and 4% in North China. South Asians, including Indians, appear to have intermediate prevalence of HLA-B 1502, averaging 2 to 4%, but this may be higher in some groups. HLA-B 1502 is present in <1% of the population in Japan and Korea. HLA-B 1502 is largely absent in individuals not of Asian origin (e.g., Caucasians, African-Americans, Hispanics, and Native Americans). The estimated prevalence rates have limitations due to the wide variability in rates that exist within ethnic groups, the difficulties in ascertaining ethnic ancestry and the likelihood of mixed ancestry.

† Increased levels of the active 10, 11-epoxide.

‡ Decreased levels of carbamazepine and increased levels of the 10, 11-epoxide.

Lactation: **Carbamazepine passes into breast milk in concentrations of about 25 to 60% of the plasma level. No reports are available on the long-term effect of breast-feeding. The benefits of breast-feeding should be weighed against the possible risks to the infant. Should the mother taking carbamazepine nurse her infant, the infant must be observed for possible adverse reactions, e.g., somnolence, allergic skin reaction.**

It should be noted that the reliability of oral contraceptives may be adversely affected by carbamazepine (see Precautions, Drug Interactions).

Fertility: There have been very rare reports of impaired male fertility and/or abnormal spermatogenesis.

PRECAUTIONS: Clinical Monitoring of Adverse Reactions: Carbamazepine should be prescribed only after a critical risk-benefit appraisal in patients with a history of cardiac, hepatic or renal damage, adverse hematological reactions to other drugs, or interrupted courses of therapy with carbamazepine. **Careful clinical and laboratory supervision should be maintained throughout treatment.** Should any signs or symptoms or abnormal laboratory findings be suggestive of blood dyscrasia or liver disorder, carbamazepine should be immediately discontinued until the case is carefully reassessed.

Bone Marrow Function: Complete blood counts, including platelets and possibly reticulocytes and serum iron, should be carried out before treatment is instituted, and periodically thereafter.

If definitely low or decreased white blood cell or platelet counts are observed during treatment, the patient and the complete blood count should be monitored closely. Nonprogressive fluctuating asymptomatic leukopenia, which is encountered, does not generally call for the withdrawal of carbamazepine. However, treatment with carbamazepine should be discontinued if the patient develops leukopenia which is progressive or accompanied by clinical manifestations, e.g., fever or sore throat, as this could indicate the onset of significant bone marrow depression.

Because the onset of potentially serious blood dyscrasias may be rapid, patients should be made aware of early toxic signs and symptoms of a potential hematological problem, as well as symptoms of dermatological or hepatic reactions. If reactions such as fever, sore throat, rash, ulcers in the mouth, easy bruising, petechial or purpuric hemorrhage appear, the patient should be advised to consult his/her physician immediately.

Hepatic Function: Baseline and periodic evaluations of hepatic function must be performed, particularly in elderly patients and patients with a history of liver disease. Carbamazepine should be withdrawn immediately in cases of aggravated liver dysfunction or active liver disease.

Kidney Function: Pretreatment and periodic complete urinalysis and BUN determinations should be performed.

Ophthalmic Examinations: Carbamazepine has been associated with pathological eye changes. Periodic eye examinations including slit-lamp funduscopy and tonometry are recommended.

Plasma Levels: Although correlations between dosage and plasma levels of carbamazepine, and between plasma levels and clinical efficacy or tolerability, are rather tenuous, monitoring plasma levels may be useful in the following situations: dramatic increase in seizure frequency/verification of patient compliance; during pregnancy; when treating children or adolescents; in suspected absorption disorders; in suspected toxicity, especially where more than one drug is being used (see Drug Interactions).

Increased Seizure Frequency: Carbamazepine should be used with caution in patients with mixed seizures which include absences, either typical or atypical. In all these conditions, carbamazepine may exacerbate seizures. In the event of exacerbation of seizures, carbamazepine should be discontinued.

Dermatologic: Mild skin reactions, e.g., isolated macular or maculopapular exanthema, usually disappear within a few days or weeks, either during a continued course of treatment or following a decrease in dosage. However, the patient should be kept under close surveillance because of the rare possibility of Stevens-Johnson Syndrome or Toxic Epidermal Necrolysis occurring (see Warnings, Dermatologic).

Urinary Retention and Increased Intraocular Pressure: Because of its anticholinergic action, carbamazepine should be given cautiously, if at all, to patients with increased intraocular pressure or urinary retention. Such patients should be followed closely while taking the drug.

Psychiatric: Because it is closely related to the other tricyclic drugs, there is some possibility that carbamazepine might activate a latent psychosis, or, in elderly patients, produce agitation or confusion, especially when combined with other drugs. Caution should also be exercised in alcoholics.

Suicidal Ideation and Behaviour: Suicidal ideation and behaviour have been reported in patients treated with antiepileptic agents in several indications.

All patients treated with antiepileptic drugs, irrespective of indication, should be monitored for signs of suicidal ideation and behaviour and appropriate treatment should be considered. Patients (and caregivers of patients) should be advised to seek medical advice should signs of suicidal ideation or behaviour emerge.

An FDA meta-analysis of randomized placebo controlled trials, in which antiepileptic drugs were used for various indications, has shown a small increased risk of suicidal ideation and behaviour in patients treated with these drugs. The reason for this risk is not known.

There were 43 892 patients treated in the placebo controlled clinical trials that were included in the meta-analysis. Approximately 75% of patients in these clinical trials were treated for indications other than epilepsy and, for the majority of non-epilepsy indications the treatment (antiepileptic drug or placebo) was administered as monotherapy. Patients with epilepsy represented approximately 25% of the total number of patients treated in the placebo controlled clinical trials and, for the majority of epilepsy patients, treatment (antiepileptic drug or placebo) was administered as adjunct to other antiepileptic agents (i.e., patients in both treatment arms were being treated with one or more antiepileptic drug). Therefore, the small increased risk of suicidal ideation and behaviour reported from the meta-analysis (0.43% for patients on antiepileptic drugs compared to 0.24% for patients on placebo) is based largely on patients that received monotherapy treatment (antiepileptic drug or placebo) for non-epilepsy indications. The study design does not allow for an estimation of the risk of suicidal ideation and behaviour for patients with epilepsy that are taking antiepileptic drugs, due both to this population being the minority in the study, and the drug-placebo comparison in this population being confounded by the presence of adjunct antiepileptic drug treatment in both arms.

Risk of Suicide in Patients with Bipolar Disorder: Patients with bipolar disorder may experience worsening of their depressive symptoms and/or the emergence of suicidal ideation and behaviors (suicidality) whether or not they are taking medications for bipolar disorder. Patients should be closely monitored for clinical worsening (including development of new symptoms) and suicidality, especially at the beginning of a course of treatment, or at the time of dose changes.

In addition, patients with a history of suicidal behavior or thoughts, those patients exhibiting a significant degree of suicidal ideation prior to commencement of treatment, and young adults, are at an increased risk of suicidal thoughts or suicide attempts, and should receive careful monitoring during treatment.

Patients (and caregivers of patients) should be alerted about the need to monitor for any worsening of their condition (including development of new symptoms) and /or the emergence of suicidal ideation/behavior or thoughts of harming themselves and to seek medical advice immediately if these symptoms present.

Prescriptions for all medications, including carbamazepine, should be written for the smallest quantity of tablets consistent with good patient management, in order to reduce the risk of overdose.

Patients with Cardiovascular Disorders: Carbamazepine should be used cautiously in patients with a history of coronary artery disease, organic heart disease or congestive heart failure. If a defective conductive system is suspected, an ECG should be performed before administering carbamazepine in order to exclude patients with AV block.

Occupational Hazards: Driving and Operating Hazardous Machinery: Because dizziness and drowsiness are possible side effects of carbamazepine, patients should be warned about the possible hazards of operating machinery or driving automobiles.

Others: Tegretol oral suspension contains parahydroxybenzoates which may cause allergic reactions (possibly delayed). It also contains sorbitol and, therefore, should not be administered to patients with rare hereditary problems of fructose intolerance.

Drug Interactions: Cytochrome P450 3A4 (CYP3A4) is the main enzyme responsible for metabolizing carbamazepine. Coadministration of CYP3A4 inhibitors may increase carbamazepine plasma concentrations and induce adverse reactions. Drugs that have been shown, or would be expected, to increase plasma carbamazepine levels include: cimetidine, danazol, diltiazem, macrolides, erythromycin, troleandomycin, clarithromycin, fluoxetine, fluvoxamine, nefazodone, loratadine, terfenadine, isoniazid, niacinamide, nicotinamide, propoxyphene, azoles (e.g., ketaconazole, itraconazole, fluconazole), acetazolamide, verapamil, grapefruit juice, protease inhibitors, valproate.†

Coadministration of CYP3A4 inducers may increase the rate of carbamazepine metabolism leading to potential decreases in the carbamazepine serum levels and therapeutic effect. Similarly, discontinuation of a CYP3A4 inducer may decrease the rate of metabolism of carbamazepine, leading to an increase in carbamazepine plasma levels. Drugs that have been shown, or that would be expected, to decrease plasma carbamazepine levels include: cisplatin, doxorubicin HCl, felbamate‡, rifampin, phenobarbital, phenytoin, primidone, methsuximide, theophylline.

Carbamazepine is a potent inducer of CYP3A4 and other phase I and phase II enzyme systems in the liver, and may therefore reduce plasma concentrations of comedications mainly metabolized by CYP3A4 by induction of their metabolism.

Human microsomal epoxide hydrolase has been identified as the enzyme responsible for the formation of the 10,11-transdiol derivative from carbamazepine-10,11 epoxide. Coadministration of inhibitors of human microsomal epoxide hydrolase may result in increased carbamazepine-10,11 epoxide plasma concentrations.

Effects of Carbamazepine on Plasma Levels of Concomitant Agents: Carbamazepine may lower the plasma level, or diminish or even abolish the activity of certain drugs. The dosage of the following drugs may have to be adjusted to clinical requirements when administered with carbamazepine:

Analgesics, anti-inflammatory agents: buprenorphine, methadone, paracetamol, phenazone (antipyrine), tramadol.
Antibiotics: doxycycline.
Anticoagulants: oral anticoagulants (warfarin, phenprocoumon, dicoumarol and acenocoumarol).
Antidepressants: bupropion, citalopram, mianserin, nefadozone, sertraline, trazodone, tricyclic antidepressants (e.g. imipramine, amitriptyline, nortryptyline, clomipramine). The use of carbamazepine is not recommended in combination with monoamine-oxidase inhibitors (MAOIs). Before administering carbamazepine, MAOIs should be discontinued for a minimum of 2 weeks, or longer if the clinical situation permits (see Contraindications).
Antiepileptics: oxcarbazepine, clobazam, clonazepam, ethosuximide, primidone, valproic acid, felbamate lamotrigine, zonisamide tiagabine, topiramate. Phenytoin plasma levels have been reported both to be raised and lowered by carbamazepine, and mephenytoin plasma levels have been reported in rare instances to increase.
Antifungals: caspofungin, itraconazole, voriconazole (see Contraindications).
Antihelmintics: praziquantel.
Antineoplastics: imatinib, irinotecan, gefitinib.
Antipsychotics: clozapine, haloperidol and bromperidol, olanzapine, quetiapine, risperidone, zisprasidone.
Antivirals: protease inhibitors for HIV treatment, e.g. indinavir, ritonavir, saquinavir.
Anxiolytics: alprazolam, midazolam.
Bronchodilatators or anti-asthma drugs: theophylline.
Contraceptives: hormonal contraceptives.
Cardiovascular drugs: calcium channel blockers (dihydropyridine group), e.g. felodipine, digoxin, disopyramide, quinidine, propranolol.
Corticosteroids: corticosteroids (e.g., prednisolone, dexamethasone).
Immunosuppressants: cyclosporin, everolimus, tacrolimus.
Thyroid agents: levothyroxine.
Other drug interactions: products containing estrogens and/or progesterones

Agents That May Raise Carbamazepine and/or Carbamazepine-10,11-epoxide Plasma Levels: Since an increase in carbamazepine and/or carbamazepine-10,11-epoxide plasma levels may result in adverse reactions (e.g., dizziness, drowsiness, ataxia, diplopia), the dosage of carbamazepine should be adjusted accordingly and the blood levels monitored when used concomitantly with the substances described below.

Analgesics, anti-inflammatory drugs: dextropropoxyphene, ibuprofen.
Androgens: danazol.
Antibiotics: macrolide antibiotics (e.g. erythromycin, troleandomycin, josamycin, clarithromycin, telithromycin).
Antidepressants: possibly desipramine fluoxetine, fluvoxamine, nefadozone, paroxetine, trazodone, viloxazine.
Antiepileptics: stiripentol, vigabatrin.
Antifungals: azoles (itraconazole, ketoconazole, fluconazole, voriconazole).
Antihistamines: terfenadine, loratadine.
Antipsychotics: loxapine, olanzapine, quetiapine.
Antituberculosis: isoniazid.
Antivirals: protease inhibitors for HIV treatment (e.g. ritonavir).
Carbonic anhydrase inhibitors: acetazolamide.
Cardiovascular drugs: verapamil, diltiazem.
Gastrointestinal drugs: cimetidine, omeprazole.
Muscle relaxants: oxybutynin, dantrolene.
Platelet aggregation inhibitors: ticlopidine.
Other interactions: grapefruit juice, nicotinamide (raises carbamazepine plasma levels in children, but only at high dosage in adults).

Loxapine, felbamate, quetiapine, primidone, valproic acid and valpromide were reported to increase concentration of the active metabolite carbamazepine-10,11-epoxide.

Agents That May Decrease Carbamazepine Plasma Levels: The dose of carbamazepine may consequently have to be adjusted when used concomitantly with the substances described below.

Antiepileptics: felbamate (might decrease the carbamazepine serum concentration associated with an increase in carbamazepine epoxide levels, and might decrease the serum felbamate levels), methsuximide, oxcarbazepine, phenobarbitone, phensuximide, phenytoin and fosphenytoin, primidone, progabide, and possibly by clonazepam, valproic acid or valpromide.
Antineoplastics: cisplatin or doxorubicin.
Antituberculosis: rifampicin.
Bronchodilatators or anti-asthma drugs: theophylline, aminophylline.
Dermatological drugs: isotretinoin.
Other interactions: herbal preparations containing St. John's wort (Hypericum perforatum).

Combination That Require Specific Consideration: Concomitant use of carbamazepine and levetiracetam has been reported to increase carbamazepine-induced toxicity (e.g., nystagmus, nausea, vomiting).

Combined use of carbamazepine with lithium, metoclopramide or haloperidol may increase the risk of neurotoxic side effects (even in the presence of "therapeutic plasma levels").

Concomitant use of carbamazepine and isoniazid has been reported to increase isoniazid-induced hepatotoxicity.

Carbamazepine, like other anticonvulsants, may adversely affect the reliability of hormonal contraceptives; breakthrough bleeding may occur. Patients should accordingly be advised to use some alternative, nonhormonal method of contraception while taking carbamazepine. Due to enzyme induction carbamazepine may cause failure of the therapeutic effect of estrogen and/or progesterone containing drugs (e.g., failure of contraception).

Concomitant medication with carbamazepine and some diuretics (hydrochlorothiazide, furosemide) may lead to symptomatic hyponatremia.

Carbamazepine may antagonize the effects of nondepolarizing muscle relaxants (e.g., pancuronium); their dosage may need to be raised and patients should be monitored closely for more rapid recovery from neuromuscular blockade than expected.

Isotretinoin has been reported to alter the bioavailability and/or clearance of carbamazepine and carbamazepine 10,11-epoxide; carbamazepine plasma levels should be monitored.

Carbamazepine, like other psychoactive drugs, may reduce the patient's alcohol tolerance; it is therefore advisable to abstain from alcohol consumption during treatment.

Carbamazepine should not be administered in conjunction with an MAO inhibitor (see Contraindications).

Information to Be Provided to the Patient: See Information for the Patient.

ADVERSE EFFECTS: The reactions which have been most commonly reported with carbamazepine are CNS disturbances (e.g., drowsiness, headache, unsteadiness on the feet, diplopia, dizziness), gastrointestinal disturbances (nausea, vomiting), and allergic skin reactions. These reactions usually occur only during the initial phase of therapy, if the initial dose is too high, or when treating elderly patients. They have rarely necessitated discontinuing carbamazepine therapy and can be minimized by initiating treatment at a low dosage.

The occurrence of CNS adverse reactions may be a manifestation of relative overdosage or significant fluctuation in plasma levels. In such cases it is advisable to monitor the plasma levels.

The more serious adverse reactions observed are the hematologic, hepatic, cardiovascular and dermatologic reactions, which require discontinuation of therapy.

Abrupt withdrawal of carbamazepine may precipitate seizures. In epileptic patients, the switch to the new antiepileptic compound should be made under cover of a suitable drug (e.g., diazepam i.v. or phenytoin i.v.).

The following adverse reactions have been reported (Frequency estimate: Very common: (≥1/10); common: (≥1/100, <1/10); uncommon: (≥1/1000, <1/100); rare (≥1/10 000 <1/1000); very rare: (<1/10 000):

Hematologic: Very common: leukopenia; Common: eosinophilia, thrombocytopenia; Rare: leukocytosis, lymphadenopathy, folic acid deficiency; Very rare: agranulocytosis, aplastic anemia, pancytopenia, pure red cell aplasia, anemia, macrocytic anemia, megaloblastic anemia, acute intermittent porphyria, variegate porphyria, prophyria cutanea tarda, reticulocytosis, thrombocytopenic purpura and possibly hemolytic anemia. In a few instances, deaths have occurred.

Hepatic: Very common: increased gamma-GT (due to hepatic enzyme induction), usually not clinically relevant; Common: increased blood alkaline phosphatase; Uncommon: increased transaminases; Rare: jaundice, hepatitis of a cholestatic, parenchymal (hepatocellular), or mixed type, vanishing bile duct syndrome; Very rare: granulomatous hepatitis, hepatic failure.

¶ In some Asian countries also reported as rare. See Warnings.

Dermatologic: Very common: dermatitis allergic and rashes, erythematous rashes, urticaria which may be severe; Uncommon: exfoliative dermatitis and erythroderma; Rare: systemic lupus erythematosus, pruritus; Very rare: Stevens-Johnson syndrome¶, toxic epidermal necrolysis (Lyell's syndrome), photosensitivity reaction, erythema multiforme and nodosum, skin pigmentation changes, purpura, acne, diaphoresis, alopecia, neurodermatitis, hirsutism.

Neurologic: Very common: dizziness, drowsiness, ataxia and fatigue; Common: an increase in motor seizures (see Indications), headache, diplopia, accommodation disorders (e.g., blurred vision); Uncommon: abnormal involuntary movements (e.g., tremor, asterixis, dystonia, tics), nystagmus; Rare: orofacial dyskinesia, paresis, eye movement disturbances, speech disorders (e.g., dysarthria, slurred speech), neuropathy peripheral, paraesthesia, muscle weakness, choreoathetosis; Very rare: neuroleptic malignant syndrome.

Cardiovascular: Rare: cardiac conduction disorders (including second and third degree atrioventricular heart block), hypertension or hypotension; Very rare: bradycardia, arrhythmias, Stokes-Adams in patients with atrioventricular block, circulatory collapse, congestive heart failure, aggravation of coronary artery disease, thrombophlebitis, thromboembolism (e.g. pulmonary embolism). Some of these cardiovascular complications have had fatal outcomes. Myocardial infarction and arrhythmia have been associated with other tricyclic compounds. Very rare cases of suicide attempt and completed suicide have been reported, however a causal relationship has not been established.

Psychiatric: Rare: hallucinations (visual or auditory), depression with agitation, talkativeness, agitation, anorexia, restlessness, aggression, confusional state; Very rare: activation of psychosis.

Genitourinary: Very rare: interstitial nephritis and renal failure, renal impairment (e.g., albuminuria, glycosuria, hematuria, oliguria sometimes associated with elevated blood pressure, and blood urea nitrogen increased/azotemia), urinary frequency, urinary retention and sexual dysfunction/impotence spermatogenesis abnormal (with decreased sperm count and/or motility).

Gastrointestinal: Very common: nausea, vomiting; Common: dry mouth and throat; Uncommon: diarrhea, constipation; Rare: abdominal pain; Very rare: glossitis, stomatitis, pancreatitis.

Sense Organs: Very rare: lenticular opacities, conjunctivitis, intraocular pressure increased, retinal changes, taste disturbances, hearing disorders (e.g., tinnitus, hyperacusis, hypoacusis), change in pitch perception.

Endocrine System and Metabolism: Common: edema, fluid retention, weight increase, hyponatremia and blood osmolarity decreased due to antidiuretic hormone (ADH)-like effect occurs, leading in rare cases to water intoxication accompanied by lethargy, vomiting, headache, confusional state, neurological disorders; Very rare: blood prolactin increased with or without clinical manifestations (e.g. galactorrhea), gynecomastia, abnormal thyroid function tests: decreased L-thyroxine (free thyroxine, thyroxine, tri-iodothyronine) and increased blood thyroid stimulating hormone, usually without clinical manifestations, bone metabolism disorders (decrease in plasma calcium and blood 25- hydroxy-calciferol), leading to osteomalacia/osteoporosis, increased blood cholesterol, including HDL cholesterol and triglycerides.

Musculoskeletal: Very rare: arthralgia, muscle pain, muscle spasms.

Respiratory: Very rare: pulmonary hypersensitivity characterized by fever, dyspnea, pneumonitis or pneumonia.

Hypersensitivity Reactions: Rare: delayed multiorgan hypersensitivity disorder with fever, rashes, vasculitis, lymphadenopathy, pseudo lymphoma, arthralgia, leukopenia, eosinophilia, hepatosplenomegaly, abnormal liver function tests and vanishing bile duct syndrome (destruction and disappearance of the intrahepatic bile ducts), occurring in various combinations. Other organs may also be affected (e.g., lungs, kidneys, pancreas, myocardium, colon); Very rare: aseptic meningitis with myoclonus and peripheral eosinophilia, anaphylactic reaction, angioneurotic edema.

Investigations: Very rare: hypogammaglobulinaemia.

OVERDOSE:

Lowest known lethal dose: estimated 3.2 g (24-year-old woman). Highest known doses survived: 80 g (34-year-old man); 34 g (13-year-old girl); 1.4 g (23-month-old girl).

Symptoms: The presenting signs and symptoms of overdosage usually involve the central nervous, cardiovascular and respiratory systems.

Central Nervous System: CNS depression, disorientation, tremor, restlessness, somnolence, agitation, hallucination, coma, blurred vision, nystagmus, mydriasis, slurred speech, dysarthria, ataxia, dyskinesia, abnormal reflexes (slowed/hyperactive), convulsions, psychomotor disturbances, myoclonus, opisthotonia, hypothermia/hyperthermia, flushed skin/cyanosis, EEG changes.

Respiratory: respiratory depression, pulmonary edema.

Cardiovascular: tachycardia, hypotension/hypertension, conduction disturbance with widening of QRS complex, syncope in association with cardiac arrest.

Gastrointestinal: nausea, vomiting, delayed gastric emptying, reduced bowel motility.

Renal Function: urinary retention, oliguria or anuria; fluid retention, and water intoxication.

Laboratory Findings: hyponatremia, hypokalemia, leukocytosis, reduced white cell count, metabolic acidosis, hyperglycemia, glycosuria, acetonuria, increased muscle creatine phosphokinase.

Treatment: There is no known specific antidote to carbamazepine.

Evacuate the stomach, with an emetic or by gastric lavage, then administer activated charcoal. Delay in evacuating the stomach may result in delayed absorption, leading to relapse during recovery from intoxication.

Vital signs should be watched and symptomatic treatment should be administered as required. Hyperirritability or convulsions may be controlled by the administration of parenteral diazepam or barbiturates but they may induce respiratory depression, particularly in children. Paraldehyde may be used to counteract muscular hypertonus without producing respiratory depression.

When barbiturates are employed, it is advisable to have equipment available for artificial ventilation and resuscitation. Barbiturates should not be used if drugs that inhibit monoamine oxidase have been taken by the patient, either in overdosage or in recent therapy (within 2 weeks).

Hyponatremia should be treated by restricting fluids and a slow and careful NaCl 0.9% infusion i.v. These measures may be useful in preventing brain damage.

Shock (circulatory collapse) should be treated with supportive measures, including i.v. fluids, oxygen and corticosteroids. For hypotension unresponsive to measures taken to increase plasma volume, dopamine or dobutamine i.v. may be administered.

It is recommended that the ECG be monitored, particularly in children, to detect any cardiac arrhythmias or conduction defects.

Charcoal hemoperfusion has been recommended. Forced diuresis, hemodialysis and peritoneal dialysis have been reported to be ineffective.

Relapse and aggravation of the symptomatology on the 2nd or 3rd day after overdose, due to delayed absorption, should be anticipated.

> For management of a suspected drug overdose, contact your regional Poison Control Centre. See the *CPS* Directory section for a list of Poison Control Centres.

DOSAGE: Epilepsy (see Indications): Carbamazepine may be used alone or with other anticonvulsants. A low initial daily dosage of carbamazepine with a gradual increase in dosage is advised. Dosage should be adjusted to the needs of the individual patient. Carbamazepine should be taken with meals whenever possible.

Tegretol tablets, Chewtabs and suspension should be taken in 2 to 4 divided doses daily.

Tegretol suspension should be well shaken before use since improper resuspension may lead to administering an incorrect dose. Since a given dose of Tegretol suspension produces higher peak carbamazepine levels than the same dose in tablet form, it is advisable to start with low doses and to increase slowly to avoid adverse reactions. When switching a patient from Tegretol tablets to Tegretol suspension, the same number of mg/day should be given in smaller, more frequent doses (i.e., b.i.d. tablets to t.i.d. suspension).

Tegretol Chewtabs and the suspension are particularly suitable for patients who have difficulty swallowing tablets or who need initial careful adjustment of dosage.

The controlled release characteristics of Tegretol CR reduce the daily fluctuations of plasma carbamazepine. Tegretol CR tablets (either whole or, if so prescribed, only half a tablet) should be swallowed unchewed with a little liquid during or after a meal. These controlled release tablets should be prescribed as a twice-daily dosage. If necessary, 3 divided doses may be prescribed. Some patients have been reported to require a dosage increase when switching from tablets to CR tablets. Dosage adjustments should be individualized based on clinical response and, if necessary, plasma carbamazepine levels.

Adults and Children Over 12 Years of Age: Initially: 100 to 200 mg once or twice a day depending on the severity of the case and previous therapeutic history. The initial dosage is progressively increased, in divided doses, until the best response is obtained. The usual optimal dosage is 800 to 1200 mg daily. In rare instances, some adult patients have received 1600 mg. As soon as disappearance of seizures has been obtained and maintained, dosage should be reduced very gradually until a minimum effective dose is reached.

Children 6 to 12 Years of Age: Initially: 100 mg in divided doses on the first day. Increase gradually by adding 100 mg/day until the best response is obtained. Dosage should generally not exceed 1000 mg daily. As soon as disappearance of seizures has been obtained and maintained, dosage should be reduced very gradually until a minimum effective dose is reached.

Combination Therapy: When added to existing anticonvulsant therapy, the drug should be added gradually while the other anticonvulsants are maintained or gradually decreased, except for phenytoin, which may be increased (See Precautions, Drug Interactions and Warnings, Pregnancy and Lactation).

Trigeminal Neuralgia: The initial daily dosage should be small; 200 mg taken in 2 doses of 100 mg each is recommended. Total daily dosage can be increased by 200 mg/day until relief of pain is obtained. This is usually achieved at dosage between 200 and 800 mg daily, but occasionally up to 1200 mg/day may be necessary. As soon as relief of pain has been obtained and maintained, progressive reduction in dosage should be attempted until a minimal effective dosage is reached. Because trigeminal neuralgia is characterized by periods of remission, attempts should be made to reduce or discontinue the use of carbamazepine at intervals of not more than 3 months, depending upon the individual clinical course.

Prophylactic use of the drug in trigeminal neuralgia is not recommended.

Mania and Bipolar (Manic-Depressive) Disorders: The initial daily dosage should be low, 200 to 400 mg/day, administered in divided doses, although higher starting doses of 400 to 600 mg/day may be used in acute mania. This dose may be gradually increased until patient symptomatology is controlled or a total daily dose of 1600 mg is achieved. Increments in dosage should be adjusted to ensure optimal patient tolerability. The usual dose range is 400 to 1200 mg/day administered in divided doses. Doses used to achieve optimal acute responses and tolerability should be continued during maintenance treatment. When given in combination with lithium and neuroleptics, the initial dosage should be low, 100 to 200 mg daily, and then increased gradually. A dose higher than 800 mg/day is rarely required when given in combination with neuroleptics and lithium, or with other psychotropic drugs such as benzodiazepines. Plasma levels are probably not helpful for guiding therapy in bipolar disorders.

INFORMATION FOR THE PATIENT: Published in e-CPS, available by subscription at www.e-cps.ca.

SUPPLIED: Tegretol: Chewtabs: 100 mg: Each white with red specks, round, flat-faced, beveled-edge tablet, engraved GEIGY on one side and M/R with bisect on the other, contains: carbamazepine 100 mg. Nonmedicinal ingredients: cherry-mint flavor, cornstarch, erythrosine, gelatin, glycerin, magnesium stearate, silicon dioxide, sodium starch glycolate, stearic acid and sugar. Energy: 4.5 kJ (1.08 kcal). Sodium: <1 mmol (0.12 mg). Bottles of 100. Store below 30°C. Protect from humidity and light.

200 mg: Each white with red specks, oval, biconvex tablet, engraved GEIGY on one side and P/U with bisect on the other, contains: carbamazepine 200 mg. Nonmedicinal ingredients: cherry-mint flavor, cornstarch, erythrosine, gelatin, glycerin, magnesium stearate, silicon dioxide, sodium starch glycolate, stearic acid and sugar. Energy: 8.9 kJ (2.12 kcal). Sodium: <1 mmol (0.12 mg). Bottles of 100. Store below 30°C. Protect from humidity and light.

Suspension: Each 5 mL of orange suspension contains: carbamazepine 100 mg. Nonmedicinal ingredients: citric acid, citrus-vanilla flavor, FD&C Yellow No. 6, pluronic polyol, potassium sorbate, propylene glycol, sucrose, sorbitol, water and xanthan gum. Energy: 37.63 kJ (8.96 kcal)/5 mL. Bottles of 450 mL. Store below 30°C. Protect from humidity and light.

Tablets: Each white, round, flat-faced and beveled-edge tablet, one side bearing the imprint CG, the other G/K and a score, contains: carbamazepine 200 mg. Nonmedicinal ingredients: cellulose compounds, magnesium stearate and silicon dioxide. Energy: nil. Sodium: <1 mmol (0.3 mg). Bottles of 100 and 500. Store below 30°C. Protect from humidity.

Tegretol CR: 200 mg: Each beige-orange, oval, slightly biconvex, controlled-release tablet, C/G engraved on one side and H/C engraved on the other, fully bisected on both sides, contains: carbamazepine 200 mg. Nonmedicinal ingredients: acrylic esters, castor oil derivative, cellulose compounds, iron oxides, magnesium stearate, silicon dioxide, talc and titanium dioxide. Energy: nil. Sodium: <1 mmol (2.1 mg). Bottles of 100. Store below 25°C. Protect from humidity.

400 mg: Each brown-orange, oval, slightly biconvex, controlled-release tablet, CG/CG engraved on one side and ENE/ENE engraved on the other, fully bisected on both sides, contains: carbamazepine 400 mg. Nonmedicinal ingredients: acrylic esters, castor oil derivative, cellulose compounds, iron oxides, magnesium stearate, silicon dioxide, talc and titanium dioxide. Energy: nil. Sodium: <1 mmol (4.3 mg). Bottles of 100. Store below 25°C. Protect from humidity.

All Tegretol products are alcohol-, bisulfite-, gluten-, lactose-, parabens- and tartrazine-free. Keep out of reach of children.

(Shown in Product Identification Section)

Telebrix® 38 Oral

meglumine ioxitalamate—sodium ioxitalamate

Radiopaque Contrast Medium

tyco Healthcare

Date of Revision: June 21, 2002

INDICATIONS: As a bowel opacifier during CT scanning of the abdomen and pelvis.

CONTRAINDICATIONS: Hypersensitivity to ioxitalamate acid salts. Severe oliguria or anuria.

WARNINGS: Although there have been no reports to date of adverse effects arising from the use of Telebrix 38 Oral, the possibility of an allergic reaction due to iodine sensitivity should be kept in mind.

Sensitivity to iodine per se, or to other contrast media is not an absolute contraindication to ioxitalamates, but extreme caution is called for.

PRECAUTIONS: General: Diagnostic procedures which involve the use of iodinated contrast agents should be carried out under the direction of radiologists skilled and experienced in the particular procedure to be performed.

The possibility of an idiosyncratic reaction occurring in patients who have previously received a contrast medium without ill effect should always be considered.

A positive history of bronchial asthma or allergy, a family history of allergy, or a previous reaction or hypersensitivity to a contrast agent implies a greater than usual risk. Such a history may be more accurate than pre-testing in predicting the potential for reaction, although not necessarily the severity or type of reaction in the individual case. A positive history of this type does not absolutely contraindicate the use of a contrast agent, when a diagnostic procedure is deemed essential, but does call for extreme caution. Premedication with antihistamines or corticosteroids as a means of avoiding or at least decreasing possible allergic reactions in such patients should be considered.

Pregnancy: Safety of the use of Telebrix 38 during pregnancy has not been established, therefore the product should be used during pregnancy only if the benefit to the mother clearly outweighs the risk to the fetus.

Lactation: It is not known whether Telebrix 38 is excreted in human milk. Because of possible adverse effects in the nursing infant, bottle feeding should be substituted for at least 24 hours following administration of Telebrix 38.

ADVERSE EFFECTS: There have been no reports of adverse reactions to date following the use of oral ioxitalamate.

OVERDOSE:

Treatment: Treatment of an overdose should be directed towards the support of all vital functions and prompt institution of specific therapy. As much as possible of the contrast medium should be removed from the stomach by gastric suction and lavage.

For management of a suspected drug overdose, CPhA recommends that you contact your **regional Poison Control Centre**. See the *CPS* Directory section for a list of Poison Control Centres.

DOSAGE: Telebrix 38 Oral has to be diluted to a 2% w/v salt solution before use. This can be accomplished, for example, by adding 12 mL of Telebrix 38 Oral to 450 mL of water (see Directions for Dilution).

The diluted solution is used orally for opacification of the bowel lumen in individual patients in the following doses, taken in small aliquots over a period of time.

Adults: For opacification of the colon: 450 mL of the diluted solution may be given several hours before the examination and 450 mL at least 1/2 hour before.

For small bowel opacification: 450 mL is given several hours before the examination followed by 450 mL at least 1/2 hour before and 150 mL immediately before the examination. The maximum total dose is 1050 mL.

Children: The oral dose of the diluted solution, for children 1 to 12 years of age, will be limited to 8 mL/kg or 400 mL total dose, whichever is less. For opacification of the colon, one half of the dose may be ingested several hours before the examination and the other half at least 1/2 hour before the examination.

Directions for Dilution: Telebrix 38 Oral may be diluted with tap water. Twelve mL of Telebrix 38 Oral is added to 450 mL of water. This will produce 462 mL of a 2% salt solution. This solution has been found to be stable for 2 weeks at room temperature (15 to 30°C). However, the solution should be kept at room temperature and discarded within 48 hours of preparation to avoid the risk of microbial growth.

SUPPLIED: Telebrix 38 Oral is an aqueous solution for oral use subsequent to dilution. Each mL contains: meglumine ioxitalamate 513 mg and sodium ioxitalamate 255 mg, equivalent to a combined content of 38% w/v organically bound iodine. Nonmedicinal ingredients: edetate calcium disodium and monobasic sodium phosphate. The pH is approximately 7.0. Bottles of 120 mL.

Store at 15 to 30°C. Do not freeze. If product is frozen or if crystallization of the salt has occurred, examine the container for physical damage. If no damage has occurred, the container should be brought to room temperature. Intermittent shaking may be necessary to completely redissolve the crystals. Before use, examine the product to ensure that all solids are redissolved. This preparation is sensitive to light and must be protected from strong daylight or direct exposure to the sun.

Telzir® Pr

fosamprenavir calcium

Antiretroviral Agent

ViiV Healthcare ULC

Date of Revision: May 17, 2010

SUMMARY PRODUCT INFORMATION:

Route of Administration	Dosage Form/ Strength	Clinically Relevant Nonmedicinal Ingredients
Oral	Tablet/ 700 mg fosamprenavir	None For a complete listing, see Dosage Forms, Composition and Packaging.
	Suspension/ 50 mg/mL fosamprenavir	Methyl parahydroxybenzoate, propyl parahydroxybenzoate. For a complete listing, see Dosage Forms, Composition and Packaging.

INDICATIONS AND CLINICAL USE: TELZIR (fosamprenavir calcium) in combination with low-dose ritonavir is indicated for:

- the treatment of HIV-1 infection in adults and pediatric patients ≥6 years old, in combination with other antiretroviral agents.

The following points should be considered when indicating therapy with TELZIR in combination with low-dose ritonavir in protease inhibitor-experienced adults and in pediatric patients ≥6 years old:

- The study in protease inhibitor-experienced patients was not large enough to reach a definitive conclusion that TELZIR/ritonavir combination is clinically equivalent to lopinavir/ritonavir combination used as a comparator in the study. No comparative studies were conducted in pediatric patients.
- Once-daily administration of TELZIR/ritonavir combination is not recommended in protease inhibitor-experienced patients or in pediatric patients.
- In protease inhibitor-experienced patients the choice of TELZIR should be based on individual viral resistance and treatment therapy.

CONTRAINDICATIONS:

- TELZIR (fosamprenavir calcium) must not be administered concurrently with medicinal products with a narrow therapeutic window that are substrates of cytochrome P450 3A4 (CYP 3A4). Coadministration may result in competitive inhibition of metabolism of these medicinal products and create the potential for serious and/or life-threatening adverse events such as cardiac arrhythmia (for example terfenadine, astemizole, cisapride, pimozide), prolonged sedation or respiratory depression (for example triazolam, midazolam, diazepam, flurazepam) or peripheral vasospasm or ischemia (for example ergot derivatives).
- Ritonavir also inhibits CYP2D6 in vitro and in vivo but to a lesser extent than CYP3A4. TELZIR in combination with ritonavir should not be coadministered with medicinal products that are highly dependent on CYP2D6 metabolism and for which elevated plasma concentrations are associated with serious and/or life-threatening results. These medicinal products include flecainide and propafenone (please refer to the full prescribing information for ritonavir for further details).
- TELZIR should not be given with rifampin. Rifampin reduces trough plasma concentrations of amprenavir by approximately 92% (see Drug Interactions).
- TELZIR is contraindicated in patients with previously demonstrated clinically significant hypersensitivity (e.g. Stevens-Johnson syndrome) to fosamprenavir calcium, amprenavir, ritonavir, or to any of the excipients of the products. For a complete listing, see Dosage Forms, Composition and Packaging.

Table 1: TELZIR

Drugs That Are Contraindicated with TELZIR

Drug Class	Drugs
Ergot Derivatives	Dihydroergotamine, ergonovine, ergotamine, methylergotamine
GI Motility Agents	Cisapride[a]
Antihistamine	Astemizole[a], terfenadine[a]
Antiarrhythmic	Flecainide, propafenone
Neuroleptic	Pimozide
Sedatives/Hypnotics	Midazolam, triazolam, diazepam, flurazepam

[a] Products no longer marketed in Canada.

WARNINGS AND PRECAUTIONS: General: Serious and/or life-threatening drug interactions could occur between TELZIR (fosamprenavir calcium) and amiodarone, lidocaine (systemic), halofantrine, tricyclic antidepressants, quinidine or warfarin (monitor International Normalized Ratio). Concentration monitoring of these agents is recommended if these agents are used concomitantly with TELZIR. Severe and life-threatening skin reactions, including Stevens-Johnson syndrome, were reported in less than 1% of subjects included in the clinical development programme. The TELZIR/ritonavir combination should be permanently discontinued in case of severe rash, or in case of rash of moderate intensity with systemic or mucosal symptoms (see Adverse Reactions).

Rifampin should not be used in combination with TELZIR since it reduces the C_{min} of amprenavir by 92% and AUC by 82% (see Contraindications and Drug Interactions).

Phenobarbital, phenytoin, carbamazepine and dexamethasone may decrease amprenavir concentrations (see Drug Interactions).

HMG-CoA reductase inhibitors (statins) may interact with protease inhibitors and increase the risk of myopathy including rhabdomyolysis. Concomitant use of protease inhibitors with lovastatin or simvastatin is not recommended. Other HMG-CoA reductase inhibitors (statins), may also interact with protease inhibitors.

Use the lowest possible dose of atorvastatin with careful monitoring or consider the use of pravastatin or fluvastatin as alternative HMG-CoA reductase inhibitors in combination with TELZIR (see Drug Interactions).

The concomitant use of TELZIR/ritonavir with lopinavir/ritonavir is not recommended because of significant pharmacokinetic interactions (see Drug Interactions).

Coadministration of protease inhibitors with PDE5 inhibitors is expected to substantially increase PDE5 inhibitor concentrations and may result in an increase in PDE5 inhibitor-associated adverse events, including hypotension, syncope, visual changes, and priapism (see Drug Interactions and the complete prescribing information for PDE5 inhibitors). Concomitant use of PDE5 inhibitors (e.g. tadalafil, vardenafil or sildenafil) in patients receiving TELZIR is not recommended (see Drug Interactions).

Concomitant use of St. John's Wort (Hypericum perforatum) or St. John's Wort- containing products and TELZIR is not recommended. Coadministration of St. John's Wort with protease inhibitors, including TELZIR, is expected to substantially decrease protease inhibitor concentrations and may result in suboptimal levels of amprenavir and lead to loss of virologic response and possible resistance to amprenavir or the class of protease inhibitors (see Drug Interactions).

Although the isozyme(s) responsible for bepridil metabolism has (have) not been elucidated, the metabolic pathways primarily responsible for bepridil metabolism are mediated by the CYP450 enzyme system. Because amprenavir and ritonavir are inhibitors of the CYP3A4 isozyme, the CYP450 isozyme most commonly responsible for drug metabolism, and because increased plasma bepridil exposure may increase the risk of life-threatening arrhythmia, caution is warranted when TELZIR and ritonavir are coadministered with bepridil (see Drug Interactions).

Coadministration of amprenavir with rifabutin results in a 200% increase in rifabutin plasma concentrations (AUC). When ritonavir is coadministered with TELZIR, a larger increase in rifabutin concentrations is expected. A reduction of rifabutin dosage of at least 75% of the recommended dose is recommended when administered with TELZIR and ritonavir and patients should be clinically monitored (see Drug Interactions).

The TELZIR oral suspension contains propyl and methyl parahydroxybenzoate. These products may cause an allergic reaction in some individuals. This reaction may be delayed.

Use of TELZIR with ritonavir at higher than approved dosages has resulted in elevated transaminase levels in some subjects and is not recommended for use (see Dosage and Administration).

Sulphonamide Allergies: TELZIR should be used with caution in patients with a known sulphonamide allergy. Fosamprenavir calcium contains a sulphonamide moiety. The potential for cross-sensitivity between drugs in the sulphonamide class and TELZIR is unknown. In the clinical studies where patients received TELZIR as the sole protease inhibitor or in combination with low-dose ritonavir, the incidence of rash was similar in patients with a history of sulphonamide allergy as compared to those who did not have a sulphonamide allergy.

Contraceptives: There may be an increased risk of clinically significant hepatic transaminase elevations and hormonal levels may be altered with coadministration of fosamprenavir, ritonavir and oral contraceptives. Therefore, concomitant use of fosamprenavir, ritonavir and oral contraceptives is not recommended and alternate methods of non-hormonal contraception are recommended for women of childbearing potential (see Drug Interactions).

Hormonal Replacement Therapies: No data are available on the coadministration of fosamprenavir and ritonavir with estrogens and/or progestogens when used as hormonal replacement therapies. The efficacy and safety of these therapies with fosamprenavir and ritonavir has not been established.

Carcinogenesis and Mutagenesis: Data from long-term carcinogenicity studies with amprenavir has revealed histopathological evidence for hepatocellular adenomas in males at the high dose of 500 mg/kg/day in mice or 750 mg/kg/day in rats, and altered hepatocellular foci were seen in male mice only at doses of 275 and 500 mg/kg/day. The clinical relevance of these findings is unknown.

Endocrine and Metabolism: New-onset diabetes mellitus, exacerbation of pre-existing diabetes mellitus and hyperglycemia have been reported during post-marketing surveillance in HIV-infected patients receiving protease inhibitor therapy. Some required either initiation or dose adjustments of insulin or oral hypoglycemic agents for treatment of these events. In some cases diabetic ketoacidosis has occurred. In those patients who discontinued protease inhibitor therapy, hyperglycemia persisted in some cases. Because these events have been reported voluntarily during clinical practice, estimates of frequency cannot be made and causal relationship between protease inhibitor therapy and these events has not been established (see Adverse Reactions).

Fat Redistribution: Redistribution/accumulation of body fat, including central obesity, dorsocervical fat enlargement ("buffalo hump"), peripheral wasting, breast enlargement, and "cushingoid appearance", have been observed in patients receiving antiretroviral therapies. The mechanism and long-term consequences of these events are currently unknown. A causal relationship has not been established (see Adverse Reactions).

Lipid Elevations: Treatment with TELZIR plus ritonavir has resulted in increases in the concentration of triglycerides and cholesterol (see Adverse Reactions). Triglycerides and cholesterol testing should be performed prior to initiating therapy with TELZIR and at periodic intervals during therapy. Lipid disorders should be managed as clinically appropriate (see Drug Interactions).

Hematologic: Acute hemolytic anemia has been reported in a patient treated with TELZIR.

Patients with Hemophilia: There have been reports of increased bleeding, including spontaneous skin hematomas and hemarthroses, in hemophiliac patients type A and B treated with protease inhibitors. In some patients additional factor VIII was given. In more than half of the reported cases, treatment with protease inhibitors was continued or reintroduced if treatment had been discontinued. A causal relationship has been evoked, although the mechanism of action has not been elucidated. Hemophiliac patients should therefore be made aware of the possibility of increased bleeding (see Adverse Reactions).

Hepatic/Biliary/Pancreatic: Amprenavir and ritonavir are principally metabolized by the liver. TELZIR with ritonavir at higher than recommended doses may result in transaminase elevations and should not be used. TELZIR with ritonavir should be used with caution and at reduced doses in adults with mild, moderate or severe hepatic impairment because amprenavir concentrations may be increased (see Dosage and Administration).

Patients with underlying hepatitis B or C or marked elevations in transaminases prior to treatment may be at increased risk of developing or worsening of transaminase elevations. Appropriate laboratory testing should be conducted prior to initiating therapy and at periodic intervals during treatment.

Immune: Immune Reconstitution: During the initial phase of treatment, patients responding to antiretroviral therapy may develop an inflammatory response to indolent or residual opportunistic infections (such as MAC, CMV, PCP and TB), which may necessitate further evaluation and treatment.

Renal: The safety and efficacy of TELZIR have not been studied in patients with renal impairment. Since the renal clearance of amprenavir and ritonavir is negligible, increased plasma concentrations are not expected in patients with renal impairment. Because amprenavir and ritonavir are highly protein bound, it is unlikely that hemodialysis or peritoneal dialysis will significantly remove them (see Action and Clinical Pharmacology).

Sensitivity/Resistance: Resistance/Cross-Resistance: Because the potential for HIV cross-resistance among protease inhibitors has not been fully explored, it is unknown what effect therapy with TELZIR will have on the activity of subsequently administered protease inhibitors. TELZIR has been studied in patients who have experienced treatment failure with protease inhibitors.

Skin: Severe and life-threatening skin reactions, including Stevens-Johnson syndrome, have occurred in patients treated with amprenavir (see Adverse Reactions).

Special Populations: Pregnant Women: There are no adequate and well-controlled studies in pregnant women. Animal reproduction studies are not always predictive of human response; therefore, administration of TELZIR in pregnancy should be considered only if the benefit to the mother outweighs the possible risk to the fetus.

Antiretroviral Pregnancy Registry: To monitor maternal-fetal outcomes of pregnant women exposed to TELZIR, an Antiretroviral Pregnancy Registry has been established. Physicians are encouraged to register patients by calling ViiV Healthcare ULC's Drug Safety Department (1-877-393-8448).

Nursing Women: Although it is not known if amprenavir is excreted in human milk, amprenavir is secreted into the milk of lactating rats. Because of both the potential for HIV transmission and possible adverse effects of amprenavir, mothers should be instructed not to breastfeed if they are receiving TELZIR.

Pediatrics: No pharmacokinetics, safety or efficacy data are available for pediatric patients <2 years old (see Dosage and Administration).

Geriatrics: The pharmacokinetics of TELZIR in combination with ritonavir has not been studied in patients over 65 years of age. When treating elderly patients consideration should be given to potential hepatic, renal or cardiac dysfunction, concomitant disease or other drug therapy (see Dosage and Administration and Action and Clinical Pharmacology).

ADVERSE REACTIONS: Adverse Drug Reaction Overview: New onset of diabetes mellitus, hyperglycemia or exacerbations of existing diabetes mellitus has been reported in patients receiving antiretroviral protease inhibitors (see Warnings and Precautions).

An increase in CPK, myalgia, myositis, and rarely, rhabdomyolysis, has been reported with protease inhibitors, more specifically in association with nucleoside analogues.

There have been reports of increased spontaneous bleeding in hemophiliac patients receiving antiretroviral protease inhibitors (see Warnings and Precautions).

Clinical Trial Adverse Drug Reactions: Because clinical trials are conducted under very specific conditions the adverse reaction rates observed in the clinical trials may not reflect the rates observed in practice and should not be compared to the rates in the clinical trials of another drug. Adverse drug reaction information from clinical trials is useful for identifying drug-related adverse events and for approximating rates.

Studies in Adults: The safety of TELZIR (fosamprenavir calcium) in combination with ritonavir has been studied in adults in controlled clinical trials, in combination with various other antiretroviral agents. The most frequently (>5% of adult subjects treated) reported undesirable effects were gastrointestinal events (nausea, diarrhea, abdominal pain and vomiting), headache and rash. Most undesirable effects associated with TELZIR/ritonavir combination therapies were mild to moderate in severity, early in onset and rarely treatment limiting. For many of these events, it is unclear whether they are related to the TELZIR/ritonavir combination, to concomitant treatment used in the management of HIV disease or to the disease process.

Adverse events are listed by MedDRA system, organ class and frequency category. Frequencies are defined as common (≥1% to <10%), uncommon (≥0.1% to <1%) and rare (≥0.01% to <0.1%).

Frequency categories for the events below have been based on clinical trials.

Most of the adverse events below come from two large clinical trials in adults. The most frequent clinical adverse events related to study drugs, of at least moderate intensity (Grade 2 or more) and occurring in at least 2% of subjects treated with the TELZIR/ritonavir combinations are included.

Table 2: TELZIR

Clinical Trial Adverse Drug Reactions

Frequency	Body System	Adverse Drug Reaction
Common	Gastrointestinal Disorders	abdominal pain, diarrhea, flatulence, nausea and vomiting
	General Disorders	fatigue
	Metabolic and Nutrition Disorders	hypertriglyceridemia
	Nervous System Disorders	headache, oral paraesthesia
	Skin and Subcutaneous Tissue Disorders	rash
Uncommon	Urogenital Disorders	nephrolithiasis
Rare	Skin and Subcutaneous Tissue Disorders	Stevens-Johnson syndrome, angioedema

The adverse event profile was similar across all the respective adult studies: antiretroviral-naïve (APV30002, n=322) and PI-experienced (once- or twice-daily dosing, APV30003 n=105 and n=107 respectively), with the exception of flatulence. This was only reported at a frequency of >2% in study APV30003 (PI-experienced subjects, TELZIR/ritonavir 700/100 mg twice daily).

In antiretroviral-naïve patients (APV30002) receiving TELZIR/ritonavir in combination with abacavir and lamivudine, drug hypersensitivity was commonly reported. All cases were reported as possibly related to abacavir. In cases of reported drug hypersensitivity, abacavir was discontinued and an alternative antiretroviral drug substituted. Few patients withdrew from the study due to these events.

Erythematous or maculopapular cutaneous eruptions, with or without pruritus, may occur during therapy. The rash generally will resolve spontaneously without the necessity of discontinuing of treatment with the TELZIR/ritonavir combination.

Severe or life threatening rash, including Stevens-Johnson syndrome, has been reported in less than 1% of subjects included in the clinical studies of TELZIR. Treatment with TELZIR should be discontinued for severe or life-threatening rashes and for moderate rashes accompanied by systemic symptoms or mucosal signs.

In some patients, fat redistribution, including a decrease in subcutaneous peripheral fat, an increase in intra-abdominal fat, breast hypertrophy and an accumulation of retrocervical fat ("buffalo hump") has been reported with antiretroviral regimen containing a protease inhibitor. Metabolic abnormalities including hypertriglyceridemia, hypercholesterolemia, resistance to insulin and hyperglycemia have also been reported with protease inhibitor-containing regimens.

Studies in Pediatric Patients: TELZIR with and without ritonavir was studied in 144 pediatric patients 2 to 18 years of age in 2 open-label studies. Safety information was obtained from 75 pediatric patients receiving TELZIR twice daily with or without ritonavir.

All adverse events, regardless of causality, all drug-related adverse events, and all laboratory events occurred with similar frequency in pediatrics as compared to adults, with the exception of vomiting. Vomiting, regardless of causality, occurred more frequently among pediatric patients receiving TELZIR twice daily with ritonavir (30% in patients between 2 and 18 years old) and without ritonavir (56%, in patients between 2 and 5 years old) as compared to adults receiving TELZIR twice daily with ritonavir (10%) and without ritonavir (16%). The median duration of drug-related vomiting episodes was 1 day (range 1 to 62 days). Vomiting required the permanent discontinuation of treatment in 1 pediatric patient and temporary discontinuation of treatment in 3 pediatric patients, all of whom were receiving TELZIR twice daily with ritonavir.

Abnormal Hematologic and Clinical Chemistry Findings: Clinical laboratory abnormalities (Grade 3 or 4) potentially related to treatment with TELZIR in combination with ritonavir and reported in greater than or equal to 2% of adult subjects are summarized in Table 3.

Table 3: TELZIR

Clinical Laboratory Abnormalities (Grade 3 or 4) Potentially Related to Treatment with TELZIR in Combination with Ritonavir and Reported in Greater Than or Equal to 2% of Adult Subjects

Clinical Abnormality (increased levels)	APV30002 (naïve patients)	APV30003 (experienced patients)
ALT	8%	5%
AST	6%	4%
Serum Lipase	6%	4%
Triglycerides	6%	6%

Grade 3 /4 neutropenia was documented in a higher proportion of pediatric subjects in Study APV20003 (20%) than in Study APV29005 (4%). The reason for the amount of neutropenia seen in APV20003 is unclear, and confounded by several factors (concomitant medications, compromised sample integrity, and changes in the toxicity grading scale). In APV29005, the rate of neutropenia was comparable to that seen in the adult population.

Post-Market Adverse Drug Reactions: Body as a Whole: redistribution/accumulation of body fat (see Warnings and Precautions, Fat Redistribution).

Cardiovascular: myocardial infarction.

Endocrine and Metabolism: New-onset diabetes mellitus, exacerbation of pre-existing diabetes mellitus, hyperglycemia and hypercholesterolemia have been reported during post-marketing surveillance in HIV-infected patients receiving protease inhibitor therapy (see Warnings and Precautions, Endocrine and Metabolism).

Urogenital: nephrolithiasis.

Skin and Subcutaneous Tissue Disorders: Stevens-Johnson syndrome and angioedema.

DRUG INTERACTIONS: Overview: When TELZIR (fosamprenavir calcium) and ritonavir are coadministered, the ritonavir metabolic drug interaction profile may predominate because ritonavir is a more potent CYP3A4 inhibitor. The full prescribing information for ritonavir must therefore be consulted prior to initiation of therapy with TELZIR and ritonavir.

Interaction studies have only been performed in adults.

Amprenavir, the active metabolite of TELZIR, is metabolized in the liver by the cytochrome P450 enzyme system. Amprenavir inhibits CYP3A4. Caution should be used when coadministering medications that are substrates, inhibitors, or inducers of CYP3A4. TELZIR should not be administered concurrently with medications with a narrow therapeutic window that are substrates of CYP3A4. Ritonavir also inhibits CYP2D6 and induces CYP3A4, CYP1A2, CYP2C9 and glucuronosyl transferase. Therefore, the combination of ritonavir with TELZIR may result in increased plasma concentrations of medicinal products that are primarily metabolized by CYP2D6. There are also other agents that may result in serious and/or life-threatening drug interactions (see Contraindications).

Drug-Drug Interactions: Drug interaction studies were performed with TELZIR tablets and amprenavir formulations. The effects of coadministration of amprenavir on the AUC, C_{max}, and C_{min} are summarized in Table 4. The effects of TELZIR on the pharmacokinetics of other drugs are summarized in Table 5.

Table 4: TELZIR

Drug Interactions: Pharmacokinetic Parameters for Amprenavir After Administration of TELZIR (fosamprenavir calcium) in the Presence of Coadministered Drug

Coadministered Drug(s) and Dose(s)	Dose of TELZIR[a]	n	% Change in Amprenavir Pharmacokinetic Parameters (90% CI)		
			C_{max}	AUC	C_{min}
Antacid (MAALOX TC) 30 mL single dose	1400 mg single dose	30	↓35 (↓24 to ↓42)	↓18 (↓9 to ↓26)	↑14 (↓7 to ↑39)
Atazanavir 300 mg q.d. for 10 days	700 mg b.i.d plus ritonavir 100 mg b.i.d. for 10 days	22	↔	↔	↔
Atorvastatin 10 mg q.d. for 4 days	1400 mg b.i.d. for 2 weeks	16	↓18 (↓34 to ↑1)	↓27 (↓41 to ↓12)	↓12 (↓27 to ↓6)
Atorvastatin 10 mg q.d. for 4 days	700 mg b.i.d. plus ritonavir 100 mg b.i.d. for 2 weeks	16	↔	↔	↔
Efavirenz 600 mg q.d. for 2 weeks	1400 mg q.d. plus ritonavir 200 mg q.d. for 2 weeks	16	↔	↓13 (↓30 to ↑7)	↓36 (↓8 to ↓56)
Efavirenz 600 mg q.d. plus Ritonavir 100 mg q.d for 2 weeks	1400 mg q.d. plus ritonavir 200 mg q.d. for 2 weeks	16	↑18 (↑1 to ↑38)	↑11 (0 to ↑24)	↔
Efavirenz 600 mg q.d. for 2 weeks	700 mg b.i.d. plus ritonavir 100 mg b.i.d. for 2 weeks	16	↔	↔	↓17 (↓4 to ↓29)
Ethinyl estradiol/norethisterone 0.035 mg/0.5 mg q.d. for 21 days	700 mg b.i.d. plus ritonavir 100 mg b.i.d. for 21 days	23	↔[b]	↔[b]	↔[b]
Lopinavir/ritonavir 533 mg/133 mg b.i.d.	1400 mg b.i.d. for 2 weeks	18	↓13	↓26	↓42
Lopinavir/ritonavir 400 mg/100 mg b.i.d. for 2 weeks	700 mg b.i.d. plus ritonavir 100 mg b.i.d. for 2 weeks	18	↓58 (↓42 to ↓ 70)	↓63 (↓51 to ↓72)	↓65 (↓54 to ↓73)
Methadone 70 to 120 mg q.d. for 2 weeks	700 mg b.i.d. plus ritonavir 100 mg b.i.d. for 2 weeks	19	↔[b]	↔[b]	↔[b]
Phenytoin 300 mg q.d. for 10 days	700 mg b.i.d. plus ritonavir 100 mg b.i.d. for 10 days	13	↔	↑20 (↑8 to ↑34)	↑19 (↑6 to ↑33)
Ranitidine 300 mg single dose	1400 mg single dose	30	↓51 (↓43 to ↓58)	↓30 (↓22 to ↓37)	↔ (↓19 to ↑21)
Nevirapine 200 mg b.i.d for 14 days[c]	700 mg b.i.d plus ritonavir 100 mg b.i.d for 14 days	17	↔	↓11 (↓23 to ↑3)	↓19 (↓32 to ↓4)

[a] Concomitant medication is also shown in this column where appropriate.
[b] Compared with historical control.
[c] Patients were receiving nevirapine for at least 12 weeks prior to study.
Legend: ↑=increase; ↓=decrease; ↔=no change (↑ or ↓<10%).

Table 5: TELZIR

Drug Interactions: Pharmacokinetic Parameters for Coadministered Drug in the Presence of Amprenavir After Administration of TELZIR (fosamprenavir calcium)

Coadministered Drug(s) and Dose(s)	Dose of TELZIR[a]	n	% Change in Pharmacokinetic Parameters of Coadministered Drug (90% CI)		
			C_{max}	AUC	C_{min}
Atazanavir 300 mg q.d. for 10 days	700 mg b.i.d plus ritonavir 100 mg b.i.d. for 10 days	21	↓24[b]	↓22[b]	↔[b]
Ritonavir 100 mg b.i.d. for 10 days	700 mg b.i.d plus atazanavir 300 mg q.d. for 10 days	22	↑96[f]	↑93[f]	↑37[f]
Atorvastatin 10 mg q.d. for 4 days	1400 mg b.i.d. for 2 weeks	16	↑304 (↑205 to ↑437)	↑130 (↑100 to ↑164)	↓10 (↓27 to ↑12)
Atorvastatin 10 mg q.d. for 4 days	700 mg b.i.d. plus ritonavir 100 mg b.i.d. for 2 weeks	16	↑184 (↑126 to ↑257)	↑153 (↑115 to ↑199)	↑73 (↑45 to ↑108)
Ethinyl estradiol[d] 0.035 mg q.d. for 21 days	700 mg b.i.d. plus ritonavir 100 mg b.i.d. for 21 days	25	↓28 (↓21 to ↓35)	↓37 (↓30 to ↓42)	ND
Lopinavir/ritonavir[c] 533 mg/133 mg b.i.d. for 2 weeks	1400 mg b.i.d. for 2 weeks	18	↔	↔	↔
Lopinavir/ritonavir[c] 400 mg/100 mg b.i.d. for 2 weeks	700 mg b.i.d. plus ritonavir 100 mg b.i.d. for 2 weeks	18	↑30 (↓15 to ↑ 47)	↑37 (↓20 to ↑55)	↑52 (↓28 to ↑82)

(cont'd)

Table 5: TELZIR *(cont'd)*

Drug Interactions: Pharmacokinetic Parameters for Coadministered Drug in the Presence of Amprenavir After Administration of TELZIR (fosamprenavir calcium)

Coadministered Drug(s) and Dose(s)	Dose of TELZIR[a]	n	% Change in Pharmacokinetic Parameters of Coadministered Drug (90% CI)		
			C_{max}	AUC	C_{min}
Methadone 70 to 120 mg q.d. for 2 weeks	700 mg b.i.d. plus ritonavir 100 mg b.i.d. for 2 weeks	19	R-Methadone (active)		
			↓21[e] (↓30 to ↓12)	↓18[e] (↓27 to ↓8)	↓11[e] (↓21 to ↑1)
			S-Methadone (inactive)		
			↓43[e] (↓49 to ↓37)	↓43[e] (↓50 to ↓36)	↓41[e] (↓49 to ↓31)
Norethisterone[d] 0.5 mg q.d. for 21 days	700 mg b.i.d. plus ritonavir 100 mg b.i.d. for 21 days	25	↓38 (↓32 to ↓44)	↓34 (↓30 to ↓37)	↓26 (↓20 to ↓32)
Phenytoin 300 mg q.d. for 10 days	700 mg b.i.d. plus ritonavir 100 mg b.i.d. for 10 days	14	↓20 (↓12 to ↓27)	↓22 (↓17 to ↓27)	↓29 (↓23 to ↓34)
Nevirapine 200 mg b.i.d for 2 weeks[g]	700 mg b.i.d. plus ritonavir 100 mg b.i.d. for 2 weeks	17	↑13 (↑3 to ↑24)	↑14 (↑5 to ↑24)	↑22 (↑9 to ↑35)

[a] Concomitant medication is also shown in this column where appropriate.
[b] Relative to values obtained from atazanavir (300 mg once daily) plus ritonavir (100 mg once daily).
[c] Data represent lopinavir concentrations.
[d] Administered as a combination oral contraceptive tablet: ethinyl estradiol 0.035 mg/norethisterone 0.5 mg.
[e] Dose normalized to 100 mg methadone. The unbound concentration of the active moiety, R-methadone, was unchanged.
[f] Compared to coadministration of fosamprenavir 700 mg twice daily plus 100 mg twice daily.
[g] Patients were receiving nevirapine for at least 12 weeks prior to study.
Legend: ↑=increase; ↓=decrease; ↔=no change (↑ or ↓<10%); ND=interaction cannot be determined as C_{min} was below the lower limit of quantification.

Although interactions with TELZIR to the following drugs have not been studied, since fosamprenavir calcium is metabolized to the active moiety, amprenavir, the information is included for reference in Table 6.

Table 6: TELZIR

Drug Interactions: Pharmacokinetic Parameters after Administration of Amprenavir

Pharmacokinetic Parameters for Amprenavir in the Presence of the Coadministered Drug			Coadministered Drug	Pharmacokinetic Parameters for Coadministered Drug in the Presence of Amprenavir		
C_{max}	AUC	C_{min}		C_{max}	AUC	C_{min}
↑47%	↑29%	↑27%	Abacavir	↔	↔	↔
↑15%	↑18%	↑39%	Clarithromycin	↓10%	↔	↔
↑18%	↑33%	↑25%	Indinavir	↓22%	↓38%	↓27%
↓16%	↑31%	NA	Ketoconazole (sd)	↑19%	↑44%	NA
↔	↔	NA	Lamivudine (sd)	↔	↔	NA
↓14%	↔	↑189%	Nelfinavir	↑12%	↑15%	↑14%
↔	↓15%	↓15%	Rifabutin	↑119%	↑193%	↑271%
↓70%	↓82%	↓92%	Rifampin	↔	↔	ND
↓37%	↓32%	↓14%	Saquinavir[a]	↑21%	↓19%	↓48%
↔	↑13%	NA	Zidovudine (sd)	↑40%	↑31%	NA
NA[b]	NA[b]	NA[b]	R-methadone (active)	↓25%	↓13%	↔
NA[b]	NA[b]	NA[b]	S-methadone (inactive)	↓48%	↓40%	↓23%
↔	↓22%	↓20%	Ethinyl estradiol	↔	↔	↑32%
			norethindrone	↔	↑18%	↑45%

[a] Soft gelatine capsules.
[b] See Other Possible Interactions, Methadone.
Legend: ↑=increase; ↓=decrease; ↔=no significant change; NA=not applicable; sd=single-dose study; ND=interaction cannot be determined as C_{min} was below lower limit of quantitation.

The following drug interaction data was obtained in adults (see Table 7).

Table 7: TELZIR

Established or Potential Drug-Drug Interactions

Concomitant Class Name: Drug Name	Effect on Concentration of Amprenavir or Concomitant Drug	Clinical Comment
Antiretroviral Agents		
HIV Protease Inhibitors (see Table 4 and Table 5)		

(cont'd)

Table 7: TELZIR *(cont'd)*

Established or Potential Drug-Drug Interactions

Concomitant Class Name: Drug Name	Effect on Concentration of Amprenavir or Concomitant Drug	Clinical Comment
Lopinavir/ritonavir	↓ Lopinavir ↓ Amprenavir	An increased rate of adverse events has been reported with coadministration of these medications: lopinavir and ritonavir. Appropriate doses of the combinations with respect to safety and efficacy have not been established.
Atazanavir/ritonavir	↓ Atazanavir	Coadministration of fosamprenavir (700 mg twice daily) plus ritonavir (100 mg twice daily) with atazanavir (300 mg once daily) for 10 days had no effect on steady state plasma amprenavir pharmacokinetics. Atazanavir plasma AUC(0-τ) decreased by 22%, C_{max} by 24% and Cτ remained unchanged relative to values obtained from atazanavir (300 mg once daily) plus ritonavir (100 mg once daily).
	↑ Ritonavir	Coadministration of fosamprenavir 700 mg twice daily plus ritonavir 100 mg twice daily with atazanavir 300 mg once daily increased plasma ritonavir AUC(0-τ) by 93%, C_{max} by 96%, and Cτ by 37%, compared to coadministration of fosamprenavir 700 mg twice daily plus ritonavir 100 mg twice daily.
Nucleoside Analogue Reverse Transcriptase Inhibitors (NRTIs)		
Abacavir	No effect	There were no clinically significant effects of amprenavir, administered as AGENERASE on abacavir in subjects receiving both agents based on historical data.
Tenofovir		In a phase III clinical trial (APV 30003), plasma amprenavir trough concentrations were similar for subjects receiving tenofovir disoproxil fumurate in combination with TELZIR and ritonavir as compared to subjects not receiving tenofovir.
Non-Nucleoside Reverse Transcriptase Inhibitors (NNRTIs)		
Efavirenz	↓ Amprenavir	An additional 100 mg/day (300 mg total) of ritonavir is recommended when efavirenz is administered with TELZIR plus ritonavir once daily. No change in the ritonavir dose is required when efavirenz is administered with TELZIR plus ritonavir twice daily.
Nevirapine	↓ Amprenavir	The AUC and C_{min} of amprenavir were decreased by 11% and 19% respectively, with C_{max} unchanged when fosamprenavir (700 mg twice daily) plus ritonavir (100 mg twice daily) was given concomitantly with nevirapine (200 mg twice daily). The AUC, C_{max} and C_{min} of nevirapine were increased by 14%, 13% and 22% respectively. Therefore, if nevirapine is given in combination with fosamprenavir (700 mg twice daily) plus ritonavir (100 mg twice daily), no dose adjustment is necessary. The fosamprenavir with ritonavir once daily regimen has not been studied.
Delavirdine	↓ Delavirdine	Appropriate doses of the combination of TELZIR plus ritonavir and delavirdine have not been established. Coadministration of fosamprenavir and delavirdine is not recommended because significant reductions in delavirdine concentrations are observed.
Antimalarial Agents		
Halofantrine	↑ Halofantrine	Coadministration of fosamprenavir with halofantrine is not recommended as halofantrine concentrations may be increased, potentially increasing the risk of serious adverse effects such as cardiac arrhythmia. Concomitant use is not recommended.
Antiarrhythmics		
Amiodarone Bepridil Lidocaine (systemic) Quinidine	↑ Antiarrhythmics	Use with caution. Increased exposure may be associated with life threatening reactions such as cardiac arrhythmias. Therapeutic concentration monitoring, if available, is recommended for antiarrhythmics.
Antibiotics/Antifungals		
Clarithromycin	↑ Clarithromycin	Ritonavir increases plasma concentrations of clarithromycin. A reduction in the clarithromycin dose should be considered when coadministered with fosamprenavir calcium and ritonavir in patients with renal impairment.
Dapsone Erythromycin	↑ Dapsone ↑ Erythromycin	The plasma concentrations of these medicinal products may be increased when coadministered with TELZIR. No pharmacokinetic study has been performed with fosamprenavir calcium in combination with erythromycin or dapsone; however, the plasma concentrations of these medicinal products may be increased when coadministered with TELZIR. Erythromycin may also increase amprenavir serum concentration.
Itraconazole Ketoconazole	↑ Itraconazole ↑ Ketoconazole	Coadministration may increase plasma concentrations of either drug. Amprenavir and ritonavir both increase plasma concentrations of ketoconazole and are expected to increase itraconazole concentrations. Itraconazole can increase amprenavir concentrations. High doses of ketoconazole and itraconazole (>200 mg/day) should not be used concomitantly with fosamprenavir calcium and ritonavir without assessing the risk/benefit ratio and increased monitoring for adverse events due to ketoconazole and itraconazole.
Rifampin	↓ Amprenavir	The pharmacokinetic parameters of amprenavir are affected when both drugs are administered in combination. Rifampin should not be used in combination with fosamprenavir calcium since it reduced C_{min} of amprenavir by 92% and the AUC by 82% (see Contraindications).

(cont'd)

Table 7: TELZIR *(cont'd)*

Established or Potential Drug-Drug Interactions

Concomitant Class Name: Drug Name	Effect on Concentration of Amprenavir or Concomitant Drug	Clinical Comment
Rifabutin	↓ Amprenavir ↑ Rifabutin	The pharmacokinetic parameters of both drugs are affected when administered in combination. Coadministration of amprenavir with rifabutin results in a 15% decrease in amprenavir plasma AUC and a 200% increase in rifabutin plasma AUC. A dosage reduction of rifabutin to at least 75% of the recommended dose is required when fosamprenavir calcium and ritonavir are coadministered with rifabutin. Further dose reduction may be necessary. A complete blood count should be performed weekly and as clinically indicated in order to monitor for neutropenia in patients receiving fosamprenavir calcium, ritonavir, and rifabutin.
Anticoagulants		
Warfarin		Concentrations of warfarin may be affected. It is recommended that INR (international normalized ratio) be monitored.
Anticonvulsants		
Carbamazepine Phenobarbital	↓ Amprenavir	Concomitant administration of anticonvulsant agents known to be enzymatic inducers (e.g., phenobarbital, carbamazepine) has not been studied but may lead to a decrease in the plasma concentrations of amprenavir.
Phenytoin	↓ Amprenavir	Coadministration of TELZIR and phenytoin may result in a decrease in the plasma concentrations of amprenavir.
	↑ Amprenavir ↓ Phenytoin	The AUC and C_{min} of amprenavir were increased by 20% and 19 % respectively, with C_{max} unchanged when TELZIR (700 mg twice daily) plus ritonavir (100 mg twice daily) was given concomitantly with phenytoin (300 mg once daily). The AUC, C_{max} and C_{min} of phenytoin were decreased by 22 %, 20 % and 29 % respectively. Plasma concentrations of phenytoin should be monitored and phenytoin dose increased as appropriate. No change to the TELZIR/ritonavir dosage regimen is required. The TELZIR/ritonavir once daily regimen has not been studied.
Antidepressants		
Paroxetine	↓ Paroxetine	Plasma concentrations of paroxetine may be significantly decreased when coadministered with TELZIR and ritonavir. Any paroxetine dose adjustment should be guided by clinical effect (tolerability and efficacy).
Trazodone	↑ Trazodone	Concomitant use of trazodone and TELZIR with or without ritonavir may increase plasma concentrations of trazodone. Adverse events of nausea, dizziness, hypotension and syncope have been observed following coadministration of trazodone and ritonavir. If trazodone is used with a CYP3A4 inhibitor such as TELZIR, the combination should be used with caution and a lower dose of trazodone should be considered.
Narcotic Analgesic		
Methadone	↓ Methadone	Coadministration of TELZIR 700 mg and ritonavir 100 mg twice daily with methadone once daily (≤200 mg) for 14 days decreased the active (R-) methadone enantiomer AUC(0-τ) and C_{max} by 18 % and 21 % respectively. The clinical significance of these alterations is unknown; however patients should be monitored for withdrawal syndrome. The impact of coadministration of a once daily regimen of TELZIR 1200 mg and ritonavir 200 mg on the pharmacokinetics of methadone has not been studied. On the basis of these data no dose adjustment is necessary when TELZIR/ritonavir is coadministered with methadone.
Oral Contraceptives		
Ethinylestradiol/norethisterone	↓ Ethinylestradiol ↓ Norethisterone	Coadministration of fosamprenavir with ritonavir and ethinylestradiol/norethisterone resulted in clinically significant hepatic transaminase elevations in some healthy subjects. Coadministration of fosamprenavir 700 mg twice daily + ritonavir 100 mg twice daily with ethinyl estradiol (EE) 0.035 mg/norethisterone (NE) 0.5 mg once daily decreased plasma EE AUC(0-τ) and C_{max} by 37% and 28%, respectively, and decreased plasma NE AUC(0-τ), C_{max}, and Cτ by 34%, 38%, and 26%, respectively. Steady state plasma amprenavir pharmacokinetic parameters were not significantly affected by coadministration with ethinylestradiol/norethisterone; however, ritonavir AUC(0-τ) and C_{max} were 45% and 63% higher, respectively, compared to historical data in female subjects dosed with fosamprenavir/ritonavir alone. Therefore alternative non-hormonal methods of contraception are recommended for women of childbearing potential (see Warnings and Precautions).
Antacids		
Aluminum hydroxide/Magnesium hydroxide	↓ Amprenavir	The pharmacokinetic parameters of amprenavir are affected when administered in combination. The AUC and C_{max} of amprenavir were decreased by 18% and 35% respectively, while the C_{min} (C12) was increased by 14%, when a single 1400 mg dose of fosamprenavir calcium was coadministered with a single 30 mL dose of antacid suspension (equivalent to 2.75 grams aluminum hydroxide and 1.8 grams magnesium hydroxide). No dose adjustment for any of the respective medicinal products is considered necessary when administered concomitantly.
Benzodiazepines		

(cont'd)

Table 7: TELZIR *(cont'd)*

Established or Potential Drug-Drug Interactions

Concomitant Class Name: Drug Name	Effect on Concentration of Amprenavir or Concomitant Drug	Clinical Comment
Alprazolam Clorazepate Diazepam Flurazepam Midazolam Triazolam	↑ Benzodiazepines	Possible increased benzodiazepine activity. Alprazolam, clorazepate, diazepam, flurazepam, midazolam and triazolam may have their serum concentrations increased by fosamprenavir calcium, which could increase their activity (see Contraindications).
Calcium Channel Blockers		
Diltiazem Amlodipine Nifedipine Felodipine Verapamil Nimodipine	↑ Calcium channel blockers	Possible increased calcium channel blocker activity. Diltiazem, amlodipine, nifedipine, felodipine, verapamil, and nimodipine may have their serum concentrations increased by fosamprenavir calcium, which could increase their activity.
Corticosteroids		
Dexamethasone	↓ Amprenavir	May induce CYP3A4 and decrease plasma concentrations of amprenavir.
PDE5 Inhibitors		
Sildenafil Vardenafil Tadalafil	↑ Sildenafil ↑ Vardenafil ↑ Tadalafil	Coadministration of TELZIR and ritonavir with erectile dysfunction agents is expected to substantially increase PDE5 inhibitor plasma concentrations and may result in PDE5 inhibitor associated adverse events, including hypotension, syncope, visual changes and priapism. Concomitant use of PDE5 inhibitors (e.g., sildenafil, vardenafil or tadalafil) in patients receiving TELZIR is not recommended.
Glucocorticoids		
Fluticasone propionate	↑ Fluticasone	Systemic corticosteroid effects including Cushing's syndrome and adrenal suppression have been reported in patients receiving ritonavir and inhaled or intranasally administered fluticasone propionate; this interaction is also expected with other corticosteroids metabolised via the P450 3A pathway. Concomitant use of fluticasone propionate and ritonavir should be avoided, unless the potential benefit to the patient outweighs the risk of systemic corticosteroid side effects.
Histamine H2 Receptor Antagonists		
Cimetidine Ranitidine Famotidine Nizatidine	↓ Amprenavir	The pharmacokinetic parameters of amprenavir are affected when administered in combination. Serum levels of amprenavir can be reduced by concomitant use of histamine H2 receptor antagonists (for example ranitidine and cimetidine). Concurrent administration of ranitidine (300 mg single dose) with fosamprenavir calcium (1400 mg single dose) decreased plasma amprenavir AUC by 30% and C_{max} by 51%. There was, however, no change observed in the amprenavir C_{min} (C12). No dose adjustment for any of the respective medicinal products is considered necessary when administered concomitantly.
HMG-CoA Reductase Inhibitors		
Atorvastatin Lovastatin Simvastatin	↑ Atorvastatin ↑ Lovastatin ↑ Simvastatin	HMG-CoA reductase inhibitors (statins) may interact with protease inhibitors and increase the risk of myopathy including rhabdomyolysis. Concomitant use of protease inhibitors with lovastatin or simvastatin is not recommended. Other HMG-CoA reductase inhibitors (statins), may also interact with protease inhibitors. Use the lowest possible dose of atorvastatin with careful monitoring or consider the use of pravastatin or fluvastatin as alternative HMG-CoA reductase inhibitors in combination with TELZIR (see Warnings and Precautions). The C_{max} and AUC of atorvastatin were increased by 304% and 130% respectively and C_{min} was decreased 10% when atorvastatin (10 mg once daily for 4 days) was given with fosamprenavir (1400 mg BID for two weeks). The C_{max}, AUC and C_{min} of amprenavir were decreased 18%, 27% and 12% respectively. When used with fosamprenavir, doses of atorvastatin no greater than 20 mg/dose should be administered with careful monitoring for atorvastatin toxicity. The same recommendation is also made with atorvastatin administered with fosamprenavir and ritonavir.
Immunosuppressants		
Cyclosporin Rapamycin Tacrolimus	↑ Immunosuppressants	Plasma concentrations of cyclosporin, rapamycin and tacrolimus may be increased when coadministered with fosamprenavir calcium and ritonavir. Therefore, frequent therapeutic concentration monitoring is recommended until levels have stabilized.
Proton Pump Inhibitors (PPIs)		
Esomeprazole Omeprazole Lansoprazole Pantoprazole Rabeprazole	No effect	Coadministration of esomeprazole with fosamprenavir did not alter plasma amprenavir AUC, C_{max}, or C_{min}; plasma esomeprazole AUC was increased 55% and t_{max} was delayed 1 hour; while C_{max} was unchanged. Coadministration with fosamprenavir in combination with ritonavir for 14 days did not alter plasma amprenavir AUC, C_{max}, or C_{min} and did not alter plasma esomeprazole AUC or C_{max}; esomeprazole t_{max} was delayed 1 hour. No dose adjustment is considered necessary when administered concomitantly.
Tricyclic Antidepressants		
Amitriptyline Imipramine	↑ Tricyclics	Therapeutic concentration monitoring is recommended for tricyclic antidepressants.

Drug-Food Interactions: Interactions with food have not been established.

Drug-Herb Interactions:

Table 8: TELZIR

Established or Potential Drug-Drug Interactions

Proper Name	Effect	Clinical Comment
St. John's wort	May result in reduced plasma concentrations of amprenavir.	Patients on TELZIR should not use products containing St. John's wort (Hypericum perforatum) since it may result in reduced plasma concentrations of amprenavir (see Warnings and Precautions).

Drug-Laboratory Interactions: Interactions with laboratory tests have not been established.

DOSAGE AND ADMINISTRATION: A physician experienced in the management of HIV infection should initiate therapy.

Higher than approved dose combinations of TELZIR (fosamprenavir calcium) with ritonavir is not recommended for use (see Warnings and Precautions) due to risk of transaminase elevations.

Recommended Dose and Dosage Adjustment: Once-daily administration of TELZIR/ritonavir combination is not recommended in protease inhibitor-experienced patients or any pediatric patients.

Adults (≥18 years of age): Low doses of ritonavir may be used to enhance the pharmacokinetic profile of amprenavir. Higher than approved dose combinations of fosamprenavir with ritonavir is not recommended for use. The recommended oral dose of fosamprenavir, in combination with ritonavir is outlined below.

Tablets: Therapy Naïve Patients: Once Daily: 1400 mg TELZIR and 200 mg ritonavir.

Twice Daily: 700 mg TELZIR and 100 mg ritonavir.

Protease Inhibitor-Experienced Patients: Twice Daily: 700 mg TELZIR and 100 mg ritonavir.

TELZIR tablets can be taken with or without food.

Oral Suspension: Therapy Naïve Patients: Once Daily: 1400 mg TELZIR and 200 mg ritonavir.

Twice Daily: 700 mg TELZIR and 100 mg ritonavir.

Protease Inhibitor-Experienced Patients: Twice Daily: 700 mg TELZIR and 100 mg ritonavir.

TELZIR oral suspension should be taken by adults without food and on an empty stomach. Shake the bottle vigorously before use.

Pediatric Patients (≥6 years old): The recommended dosage of TELZIR in patients ≥6 years of age should be calculated based on body weight (kg) and should not exceed the recommended adult dose. The data in pediatrics are insufficient to recommend: (1) once daily dosing or (2) any dosing in patients <6 years old.

TELZIR oral suspension is the recommended option for the most accurate dosing based on body weight. Pediatric patients should take oral suspension with food to aid palatability and assist adherence. The dose recommendations for this population are based on studies where the TELZIR oral suspension was administered with ritonavir and with food, and therefore take into account the observed food effect. Should vomiting occur within 30 minutes after dosing, the oral suspension should be re-dosed.

Oral Suspension: Therapy Naive and Protease Inhibitor Experienced: Twice daily: 18 mg/kg plus ritonavir 3 mg/kg administered twice daily not to exceed the adult dose of 700 mg plus ritonavir 100 mg.

Tablets: Therapy Naive and Protease Inhibitor Experienced: Twice daily: not to exceed 700 mg plus ritonavir 100 mg.

The adult tablet regimens of TELZIR/ritonavir may be used in patients who weigh at least 39 kg (ritonavir tablets may be used in patients who weight at least 33 kg) and can swallow the tablets whole (see Dosage and Administration, Adults (≥18 years of age)).

Pediatrics (<2 years of age): The safety and efficacy of TELZIR in combination with ritonavir have not yet been established in this patient population.

Geriatrics (≥65 years of age): The safety and efficacy of TELZIR in combination with ritonavir have not yet been established in this patient population.

Patients with Hepatic Impairment : TELZIR and ritonavir should be used with caution and at reduced doses in adults with mild, moderate or severe hepatic impairment (see Warnings and Precautions). There are no data on the use of TELZIR with ritonavir in pediatric patients with any degree of hepatic impairment; no dose recommendation can be made in this patient population.

Adults with Mild Hepatic Impairment (Child-Pugh score 5-6): TELZIR 700 mg twice daily plus ritonavir 100 mg once daily.

Adults with Moderate Hepatic Impairment (Child-Pugh score 7-9): TELZIR 450 mg twice daily plus ritonavir 100 mg once daily.

Adults with Severe Hepatic Impairment (Child-Pugh score: 10-15): TELZIR 300 mg twice daily plus ritonavir 100 mg once daily.

Even with these dose adjustments for adults with hepatic impairment, some subjects may have higher than anticipated amprenavir and ritonavir plasma concentrations due to inter-patient variability. Therefore, appropriate laboratory tests for liver function should be conducted prior to initiating therapy and at periodic intervals during treatment (see Warnings and Precautions).

Although it is not possible to achieve the 300 mg and 450 mg dose using the tablet formulation, they can be obtained with the TELZIR oral suspension.

Patients with Renal Impairment : No initial dose adjustment is considered necessary in patients with renal impairment.

OVERDOSAGE:

There is no known antidote for TELZIR (fosamprenavir calcium). It is not known whether amprenavir can be removed by peritoneal dialysis or hemodialysis. If overdosage occurs, the patient should be monitored for evidence of toxicity and standard supportive treatment applied as necessary. Although no data are available, administration of activated charcoal may be used to aid in removal of unabsorbed drug.

For management of a suspected drug overdose, contact your regional Poison Control Centre. See the *CPS Directory* section for a list of Poison Control Centres.

ACTION AND CLINICAL PHARMACOLOGY: Mechanism of Action: Fosamprenavir calcium is a pro-drug of amprenavir, a non-peptidic competitive inhibitor of HIV-1 protease. It blocks the ability of viral protease to process gag and gag-pol polyproteins necessary for viral replication.

Fosamprenavir calcium is rapidly hydrolyzed to amprenavir by enzymes in the gut epithelium as it is absorbed.

Pharmacokinetics: Absorption and Bioavailability: After multiple-dose oral administration of fosamprenavir calcium 1400 mg once daily and ritonavir 200 mg once daily, amprenavir was rapidly absorbed with a geometric mean (95% CI) steady-state peak plasma amprenavir concentration (C_{max}) of 7.24 (6.32-8.28) µg/mL occurring approximately 2 (0.8-5.0) hours after dosing (t_{max}). The geometric mean steady-state plasma amprenavir trough concentration (C_{min}) was 1.45 (1.16-1.81) µg/mL and $AUC_{24,ss}$ was 69.4 (59.7-80.8) h· µg/mL.

After multiple-dose oral administration of fosamprenavir calcium 700 mg twice daily and ritonavir 100 mg twice daily, amprenavir was rapidly absorbed with a geometric mean (95% CI) steady-state peak plasma amprenavir concentration (C_{max}) of 6.08 (5.38-6.86) µg/mL occurring approximately 1.5 (0.75-5.0) hours after dosing (t_{max}). The mean steady-state plasma amprenavir trough concentration (C_{min}) was 2.12 (1.77-2.54) µg/mL and $AUC_{24,ss}$ was 79.2 (69.0-90.6) h· µg/mL. The absolute oral bioavailability of amprenavir in humans has not been established.

Fosamprenavir calcium tablet and oral suspension formulations, both given fasted, delivered equivalent plasma amprenavir AUC_{∞} values and the TELZIR oral suspension formulation delivered a 14% higher plasma amprenavir C_{max} as compared to the oral tablet formulation.

Effects of Food on Oral Absorption: Tablets: The relative bioavailability of fosamprenavir calcium tablets was assessed in the fasted and fed states in healthy volunteers (standardized high-fat meal: 967 kcal, 67 grams fat, 33 grams protein, 58 grams carbohydrate). Administration of a single 1400 mg dose of TELZIR in the fed state compared to the fasted state was associated with no changes in C_{max}, T_{max} or $AUC_{0-\infty}$. TELZIR tablets may be taken with or without food.

Suspension: The administration of fosamprenavir calcium oral suspension formulation with a high-fat meal reduced plasma amprenavir AUC by approximately 28% and C_{max} by approximately 46% as compared to the administration of this formulation in the fasted state. The TELZIR oral suspension should be taken without food and on an empty stomach at the same dose as the tablets in the adult population; however, with food in the children and adolescent population (see Dosage and Administration).

Special Populations and Conditions: Pediatrics (≥6 years old): The pharmacokinetics parameters of amprenavir were evaluated in 47 pediatric patients (6 to 18 years old) following administration of TELZIR (oral suspension or tablets), with ritonavir and with food (see Table 9).

Geriatrics: The pharmacokinetics of fosamprenavir calcium have not been studied in patients over 65 years of age.

Gender: The pharmacokinetics of fosamprenavir calcium does not differ between males and females.

Table 10: TELZIR

Pharmacokinetics of Amprenavir (APV) Following the Administration of TELZIR and Ritonavir for 14 Days To HIV-1-Infected Adults with Hepatic Impairment vs. Adults with Normal Hepatic Function

	Normal Hepatic Function[a] (FPV 700 mg BID+RTV 100 mg BID) n=10	Mild Hepatic Impairment (Child Pugh 5–6) (FPV 700 mg BID+RTV 100 mg BID) n=9		Moderate Hepatic Impairment (Child Pugh 7–9) (FPV 300 mg BID+RTV 100 mg QD) n=10		Normal Hepatic Function[b] (FPV 700 mg BID+RTV 100 mg BID) n=7	Severe Hepatic Impairment (Child Pugh 10–15) (FPV 300 mg BID+RTV 100 mg QD) n=8	
APV Parameter	Parameter Estimate Geometric Mean [95% CI] (CVb%)	Parameter Estimate Geometric Mean [95% CI] (CVb%)	Mild vs Normal[a] GLS Mean Ratio [90% CI]	Parameter Estimate Geometric Mean [95% CI] (CVb%)	Moderate vs Normal[a] GLS Mean Ratio [90% CI]	Parameter Estimate Geometric Mean [95% CI] (CVb%)	Parameter Estimate Geometric Mean [95% CI] (CVb%)	Severe vs Normal[b] GLS Mean Ratio [90% CI]
AUC_{0-t} (µg· h/mL)	38.1 [31.6, 46.0] (27)	46.6 [39.0, 55.5] (25)	1.22 [0.94, 1.59]	27.8 [19.9, 38.7] (49)	0.73 [0.56, 0.95]	39.4 [34.5, 45.0] (14)	30.3 [22.6, 40.7] (36)	0.77 [0.60, 0.99]
C_{max} (µg/mL)	6.00 [4.97, 7.25] (27)	7.04 [5.72, 8.66] (30)	1.17 [0.90, 1.53]	4.38 [3.08, 6.22] (52)	0.73 [0.56, 0.95]	5.94 [5.05, 6.99] (18)	4.80 [3.52, 6.54] (38)	0.81 [0.62, 1.06]
Free Fraction (%) unbound at C_{max}	7.53[c] [6.10, 9.29] (28)	8.92 [7.68, 10.4] (21)	1.18 [0.94, 1.50]	10.1[c] [7.49, 13.5] (40)	1.33 [1.05, 1.69]	8.97[e] [5.14, 15.7] (57)	8.37[f] [6.57, 10.7] (27)	0.93 [0.62, 1.40]
C_t (µg/mL)	2.62 [2.14, 3.21] (29)	2.38 [1.80, 3.15] (40)	0.91 [0.63, 1.32]	1.13 [0.74, 1.71] (64)	0.43 [0.30, 0.62]	2.19 [1.82, 2.64] (20)	1.36 [0.85, 2.16] (60)	0.62 [0.42, 0.92]
Free Fraction (%) unbound at C_t	6.16[c] [4.52, 8.38] (42)	10.9[d] [8.88, 13.3] (25)	1.77 [1.37, 2.27]	12.5[c] [9.98, 15.5] (29)	2.02 [1.58, 2.58]	5.69[g] [3.72, 8.69] (35)	9.37 [6.24, 14.1] (52)	1.65 [1.05, 2.58]

a First normal hepatic function group matched for sex, age (+/−5 years), and BMI (+/−5kg) to subjects with moderate hepatic impairment and compared to subjects with mild and moderate hepatic impairment.
b Second normal hepatic function group matched for sex, age (+/−5 years), and BMI (+/−5kg) to subjects with severe hepatic impairment and compared to subjects with severe hepatic impairment.
c n=9.
d n=8.
e n=6.
f n=7.
g n=5.

Table 9: TELZIR

Geometric Mean (95% CI) Steady-State Plasma Amprenavir Pharmacokinetic Parameters in Pediatric Patients (≥6 years old) Receiving TELZIR Plus Ritonavir Twice Daily

	6 to 11 Years		12 to 18 Years	
Parameter	n	Fosamprenavir 18 mg/kg Plus Ritonavir 3 mg/kg b.i.d.	n	Fosamprenavir 700 mg Plus Ritonavir 100 mg b.i.d.
$AUC_{(0-24)}$ (µg· h/mL)	9	93.4 (67.8, 129)	8	58.8 (38.8, 89.0)
C_{max} (µg/mL)	9	6.07 (4.40, 8.38)	8	4.33 (2.82, 6.65)
C_{min} (µg/mL)	17	2.69 (2.15, 3.36)	24	1.61 (1.21, 2.15)

Hepatic Insufficiency: The pharmacokinetics of amprenavir were studied following the administration of TELZIR and ritonavir for 14 days to HIV-1-infected adults with hepatic impairment and to matched controls with normal hepatic function. Following 2 weeks of dosing with TELZIR plus ritonavir, the AUC of amprenavir was increased by approximately 22% in patients with mild hepatic impairment and by approximately 70% in patients with moderate hepatic impairment compared with HIV-1-infected patients with normal hepatic function. Protein binding of amprenavir was decreased in both mild and moderate hepatic impairment, with the unbound fraction at 2 hours (approximate C_{max}) increasing by 18% to 57% and the unbound fraction at the end of the dosing interval (C_{min}) increasing 50% to 102%. In patients with severe hepatic impairment (Child-Pugh score of 10-13), a reduced dose of TELZIR 300 mg twice daily with a reduced dosing frequency of ritonavir 100 mg once daily delivered 19% lower plasma amprenavir C_{max}, 23% lower AUC $_{(0-t)}$ and 38% lower C_t values, but similar unbound plasma amprenavir C_t values than achieved in patients with normal hepatic function receiving the standard TELZIR with ritonavir 700 mg/100 mg twice daily regimen. Despite reducing the dosing frequency of ritonavir, patients with severe hepatic impairment had 64% higher ritonavir C_{max}, 40% higher ritonavir C_{avg}, and 38% higher ritonavir C_t than achieved in patients with normal hepatic function receiving the standard TELZIR with ritonavir 700 mg/100 mg twice daily regimen. The pharmacokinetic parameters for amprenavir are summarized in Table 10.

Renal Insufficiency: Adults with Impaired Renal Function: The safety and efficacy of TELZIR have not been studied in patients with renal impairment. The renal elimination of unchanged amprenavir represents <1% of the administered dose. Renal elimination of ritonavir is also negligible; therefore, the impact of renal impairment on amprenavir elimination should be minimal.

STORAGE AND STABILITY: Tablets: TELZIR (fosamprenavir calcium) tablets should be stored between 15 and 30°C.
Suspension: TELZIR suspension should be stored between 2 and 30°C. **Do not freeze. The suspension should be discarded 28 days after first opening.**

SPECIAL HANDLING INSTRUCTIONS: Not applicable.

INFORMATION FOR THE PATIENT: Published in e-CPS, available by subscription at www.e-cps.ca.

DOSAGE FORMS, COMPOSITION AND PACKAGING: Suspension: Each mL of white to off-white oral suspension with grape bubblegum and peppermint flavoring contains: fosamprenavir 50 mg as calcium salt (equivalent to approximately 43 mg/mL amprenavir). Nonmedicinal ingredients: artificial grape bubblegum flavor, calcium chloride dihydrate, hypromellose, methyl parahydroxybenzoate, natural peppermint flavor, polysorbate 80, propylene glycol, propyl parahydroxybenzoate, purified water and sucralose. Bottles of 225 mL. A 10 mL dosing syringe is provided in the pack.
Tablets: Each pink, capsule-shaped tablet, with the letters "GX LL7" printed on one side contains: fosamprenavir 700 mg as fosamprenavir calcium (equivalent to approximately 600 mg of amprenavir). Nonmedicinal ingredients: colloidal silicon dioxide, croscarmellose sodium, magnesium stearate, microcrystalline cellulose and povidone K30; film-coating: hypromellose, iron oxide red, titanium dioxide, and triacetin. Bottles of 60 with child-resistant closures.

(Shown in Product Identification Section)

Temazepam

CPhA Monograph

see *Benzodiazepines*

Temodal®

temozolomide

Antineoplastic Agent

Schering-Plough

Date of Revision: January 5, 2009

SUMMARY PRODUCT INFORMATION:

Route of Administration	Dosage Form/ Strength	Clinically Relevant Nonmedicinal Ingredients
Oral	Capsule 5 mg, 20 mg, 100 mg, 140 mg, 180 mg and 250 mg	For a complete listing see Dosage Forms, Composition and Packaging.
Intravenous (IV) Injection	Powder for Solution for Injection 100 mg/vial	For a complete listing see Dosage Forms, Composition and Packaging.

INDICATIONS AND CLINICAL USE: TEMODAL (temozolomide) is indicated for:

- treatment of adult patients with newly diagnosed glioblastoma multiforme concomitantly with radiotherapy and then as maintenance treatment.
- treatment of adult patients with glioblastoma multiforme or anaplastic astrocytoma and documented evidence of recurrence or progression after standard therapy.

CONTRAINDICATIONS:

- TEMODAL is contraindicated in patients who have a history of hypersensitivity reaction to its components or to dacarbazine (DTIC).
- The use of TEMODAL is not recommended in patients with severe myelosuppression.

WARNINGS AND PRECAUTIONS:

Serious Warnings and Precautions

TEMODAL should be prescribed by a qualified healthcare professional who is experienced in the use of antineoplastic therapy.

The following are clinically significant adverse events:

- Myelosuppression including Neutropenia and Thrombocytopenia (see Warnings and Precautions, Hematologic, Myelosuppression).

TEMODAL may have to be discontinued or the dose may have to be adjusted (see Dosage and Administration).

General: The treating physician should use his discretion with respect to the use of TEMODAL in patients with poor performance status, severe debilitating diseases or infection when the risk of treatment outweighs the potential benefit to the patient.

Drug Interactions: Co-administration with valproic acid was associated with a small but statistically significant decrease in clearance of TEMODAL.

The combination of TEMODAL with other chemotherapeutic agents has not been fully evaluated. Combination with other alkylating agents is likely to result in increased myelosuppression.

Gastrointestinal: Antiemetic Therapy: Nausea and vomiting are very commonly associated with TEMODAL, and guidelines are provided:

Patients with newly diagnosed glioblastoma multiforme:

- anti-emetic prophylaxis is recommended prior to the initial dose of **concomitant** TEMODAL,
- anti-emetic prophylaxis is strongly recommended during the **maintenance phase.**

Patients with recurrent or progressive glioma: Patients who have experienced severe (Grade 3 or 4) vomiting in previous treatment cycles may require anti-emetic therapy.

Hematologic: Myelosuppression: TEMODAL is an alkylating antitumor drug. Severe myelosuppression can occur, and is a dose limiting side effect. TEMODAL is associated with Grade 3 and Grade 4 neutropenia and Grade 3 and Grade 4 thrombocytopenia. Prior to dosing and during treatment, proper hematologic monitoring must be performed. TEMODAL may have to be discontinued or the dose may have to be adjusted (see Adverse Reactions and Dosage and Administration, Administration).

Hepatic/Biliary/Pancreatic: In the absence of formal studies in patients suffering from severe hepatic dysfunction the treating physician should use his discretion in weighing the benefits of using TEMODAL in this patient population against the potential risks.

Renal: In the absence of formal studies in patients suffering from severe renal failure the treating physician should use his discretion in weighing the benefits of using TEMODAL in this patient population against the potential risks.

Respiratory: Patients who received concomitant TEMODAL and radiotherapy in a pilot trial for the prolonged 42 day schedule were shown to be at particular risk for developing *P. carinii* pneumonia. Thus prophylaxis against *P. carinii* pneumonia (PCP) is required for all patients receiving concomitant TEMODAL and radiotherapy for the 42 day regimen (with a maximum of 49 days). There may be a higher occurrence of PCP when TEMODAL is administered during a longer dosing regimen. However, all patients receiving TEMODAL, particularly patients receiving steroids should be observed closely for the development of PCP regardless of the regimen.

Cases of interstitial pneumonitis/pneumonitis have been reported in post-marketing experience. These events have the potential to be fatal.

Sexual Function/Reproduction: Male Patients: TEMODAL can have genotoxic effects. Effective contraception should also be used by male patients taking TEMODAL. Men being treated with TEMODAL are advised not to father a child during or up to 6 months after treatment and to seek advice on cryoconservation of sperm prior to treatment because of the possibility of irreversible infertility due to therapy with TEMODAL.

Skin: Serious dermatologic reactions including Stevens-Johnson syndrome (SJS) and toxic epidermal necrolysis (TEN) have been reported in post-marketing experience. These events have the potential to be fatal. When SJS/TEN is suspected, appropriate action should be taken, including close monitoring of the patient. Discontinuation of all concomitant medications suspected to contribute to SJS/TEN and TEMODAL should be evaluated.

Special Populations: Pregnant Women: There are no studies in pregnant women. In preclinical studies in rats and rabbits administered 150 mg/m², teratogenicity and/or fetal toxicity were demonstrated. Therefore, TEMODAL should not beadministered to pregnant women. If use during pregnancy must be considered, the patient should be apprised of the potential risks to the fetus. Women of childbearing potential should be advised to avoid pregnancy while they are receiving TEMODAL therapy and in the six months after discontinuation of treatment.

Nursing Women: It is not known whether TEMODAL is excreted in human milk. Lactating mothers should be advised to stop lactation while under treatment.

Pediatrics (<18 years and >3 years): The safety and effectiveness of TEMODAL in pediatric patients has not yet been fully established.

Geriatrics (>70 years of age): Elderly patients appear to be at increased risk of neutropenia and thrombocytopenia, compared with younger patients.

Monitoring and Laboratory Tests: Prior to dosing, on Day 1 of each cycle, the following values must be met: absolute neutrophil count (ANC) $\geq 1.5 \times 10^9$/L and platelets $\geq 100 \times 10^9$/L.

A complete blood count must also be obtained on Day 22 (21 days after the first dose) or within 48 hours of that day, and weekly until ANC is above 1.5×10^9/L and platelet count exceeds 100×10^9/L. If the ANC falls to $<1.0 \times 10^9$/L or the platelet count is $<50 \times 10^9$/L during any cycle, the next cycle should be reduced by one dose level, based upon the nadir blood count (see Dosage and Administration). Dose levels include 100 mg/m², 150 mg/m² and 200 mg/m². The lowest recommended dose is 100 mg/m².

ADVERSE REACTIONS: Clinical trial experience in patients treated with TEMODAL Capsules: Newly Diagnosed Patients with Glioblastoma Multiforme: Table 1 provides treatment emergent adverse events, in (causality not determined during clinical trials) patients with newly diagnosed glioblastoma multiforme during the concomitant and maintenance phases of treatment.

Table 1: TEMODAL

TEMODAL and Radiotherapy: Treatment-Emergent Events During Concomitant and Maintenance Treatment

Body System/Adverse Event	TEMODAL + Concomitant Radiotherapy n=288[a] n (%)	TEMODAL Maintenance Therapy n=224 n (%)	Total n=288 n (%)
Infections and Infestations			
Candidiasis oral	4 (1%)	5 (2%)	7 (2%)
Herpes simplex	4 (1%)	2 (1%)	6 (2%)
Herpes zoster	0 (0%)	3 (1%)	3 (1%)
Infection	4 (1%)	8 (4%)	12 (4%)
Influenza–like symptoms	0 (0%)	3 (1%)	3 (1%)
Pharyngitis	2 (1%)	1 (<1%)	3 (1%)
Wound infection	2 (1%)	0 (0%)	2 (1%)
Blood and the Lymphatic System Disorders			
Anemia	3 (1%)	4 (2%)	6 (2%)
Febrile neutropenia	2 (1%)	4 (2%)	6 (2%)
Leukopenia	6 (2%)	5 (2%)	10 (3%)
Lymphopenia	7 (2%)	2 (1%)	7 (2%)
Neutropenia	6 (2%)	7 (3%)	10 (3%)
Thrombocytopenia	11 (4%)	19 (8%)	29 (10%)
Petechiae	1 (<1%)	2 (1%)	3 (1%)
Endocrine Disorders			
Cushingoid	4 (1%)	2 (1%)	6 (2%)
Metabolism and Nutrition Disorders			
Anorexia	56 (19%)	61 (27%)	91 (32%)
Alkaline phosphatase increased	3 (1%)	1 (<1%)	4 (1%)
Hyperglycemia	7 (2%)	3 (1%)	9 (3%)
Hypokalemia	2 (1%)	1 (<1%)	3 (1%)
Weight decreased	5 (2%)	7 (3%)	11 (4%)
Weight increased	4 (1%)	3 (1%)	6 (2%)
Psychiatric Disorders			
Agitation	2 (1%)	1 (<1%)	3 (1%)

(cont'd)

Table 1: TEMODAL *(cont'd)*

TEMODAL and Radiotherapy: Treatment-Emergent Events During Concomitant and Maintenance Treatment

Body System/Adverse Event	TEMODAL + Concomitant Radiotherapy n=288[a] n (%)	TEMODAL Maintenance Therapy n=224 n (%)	Total n=288 n (%)
Amnesia	0 (0%)	2 (1%)	2 (1%)
Anxiety	5 (2%)	8 (4%)	10 (3%)
Apathy	2 (1%)	1 (<1%)	3 (1%)
Behavior disorder	2 (1%)	1 (<1%)	2 (1%)
Depression	3 (1%)	6 (3%)	8 (3%)
Emotional lability	5 (2%)	7 (3%)	10 (3%)
Hallucination	2 (1%)	2 (1%)	4 (1%)
Insomnia	14 (5%)	9 (4%)	18 (6%)
Nervous System Disorders			
Aphasia	9 (3%)	5 (2%)	11 (4%)
Ataxia	3 (1%)	3 (1%)	5 (2%)
Cerebral hemorrhage	2 (1%)	0 (0%)	2 (1%)
Balance impaired	5 (2%)	4 (2%)	9 (3%)
Cognition impaired	2 (1%)	0 (0%)	2 (1%)
Concentration impaired	6 (2%)	6 (3%)	10 (3%)
Confusion	11 (4%)	12 (5%)	22 (8%)
Consciousness decreased	5 (2%)	1 (<1%)	6 (2%)
Convulsions	17 (6%)	25 (11%)	36 (13%)
Coordination abnormal	0 (0%)	2 (1%)	2 (1%)
Dizziness	12 (4%)	12 (5%)	22 (8%)
Dysphasia	4 (1%)	9 (4%)	10 (3%)
Extrapyramidal disorder	2 (1%)	0 (0%)	2 (1%)
Gait abnormal	4 (1%)	3 (1%)	7 (2%)
Headache	56 (19%)	51 (23%)	87 (30%)
Hemiparesis	4 (1%)	8 (4%)	10 (3%)
Hemiplegia	0 (0%)	2 (1%)	2 (1%)
Hyperesthesia	2 (1%)	2 (1%)	3 (1%)
Hypoesthesia	2 (1%)	1 (<1%)	3 (1%)
Memory impairment	8 (3%)	16 (7%)	21 (7%)
Neurological disorder (NOS)	3 (1%)	6 (3%)	7 (2%)
Neuropathy	8 (3%)	6 (3%)	12 (4%)
Paresthesia	6 (2%)	4 (2%)	7 (2%)
Peripheral neuropathy	2 (1%)	4 (2%)	5 (2%)
Sensory disturbance	0 (0%)	2 (1%)	2 (1%)
Somnolence	5 (2%)	5 (2%)	10 (3%)
Speech disorder	6 (2%)	9 (4%)	14 (5%)
Status epilepticus	2 (1%)	0 (0%)	2 (1%)
Tremor	7 (2%)	9 (4%)	14 (5%)
Eye Disorders			
Diplopia	1 (<1%)	5 (2%)	6 (2%)
Eye pain	3 (1%)	2 (1%)	4 (1%)
Eyes dry	1 (<1%)	2 (1%)	2 (1%)
Hemianopia	2 (1%)	1 (<1%)	2 (1%)
Vision blurred	26 (9%)	17 (8%)	33 (11%)
Vision disorder	2 (1%)	2 (1%)	4 (1%)
Visual acuity reduced	2 (1%)	3 (1%)	4 (1%)

(cont'd)

Table 1: TEMODAL *(cont'd)*

TEMODAL and Radiotherapy: Treatment-Emergent Events During Concomitant and Maintenance Treatment

Body System/Adverse Event	TEMODAL + Concomitant Radiotherapy n=288[a] n (%)	TEMODAL Maintenance Therapy n=224 n (%)	Total n=288 n (%)
Visual field defect	4 (1%)	5 (2%)	7 (2%)
Ear and Labyrinth Disorders			
Deafness	1 (<1%)	2 (1%)	2 (1%)
Earache	3 (1%)	3 (1%)	5 (2%)
Hearing impairment	8 (3%)	10 (4%)	13 (5%)
Hyperacusis	2 (1%)	1 (<1%)	2 (1%)
Otitis media	2 (1%)	0 (0%)	2 (1%)
Tinnitus	4 (1%)	4 (2%)	6 (2%)
Vertigo	1 (<1%)	3 (1%)	3 (1%)
Cardiac Disorders			
Palpitation	2 (1%)	0 (0%)	2 (1%)
Vascular Disorders			
Deep venous thrombosis	5 (2%)	4 (2%)	8 (3%)
Edema	6 (2%)	2 (1%)	8 (3%)
Edema leg	6 (2%)	4 (2%)	9 (3%)
Edema peripheral	0 (0%)	3 (1%)	3 (1%)
Embolism pulmonary	0 (0%)	2 (1%)	2 (1%)
Hemorrhage	7 (2%)	7 (3%)	13 (5%)
Hypertension	2 (1%)	1 (<1%)	3 (1%)
Respiratory, Thoracic and Mediastinal Disorders			
Bronchitis	0 (0%)	2 (1%)	2 (1%)
Coughing	15 (5%)	19 (8%)	26 (9%)
Dyspnea	11 (4%)	12 (5%)	19 (7%)
Nasal congestion	2 (1%)	1 (<1%)	3 (1%)
Pneumonia	4 (1%)	2 (1%)	6 (2%)
Upper respiratory infection	4 (1%)	2 (1%)	6 (2%)
Sinusitis	1 (<1%)	2 (1%)	3 (1%)
Gastrointestinal Disorders			
Abdominal distension	1 (<1%)	2 (1%)	3 (1%)
Abdominal pain	7 (2%)	11 (5%)	15 (5%)
Constipation	53 (18%)	49 (22%)	87 (30%)
Diarrhea	18 (6%)	23 (10%)	36 (13%)
Dyspepsia	9 (3%)	4 (2%)	10 (3%)
Dysphagia	6 (2%)	6 (3%)	9 (3%)
Fecal incontinence	0 (0%)	2 (1%)	2 (1%)
Gastrointestinal disorder	1 (<1%)	2 (1%)	3 (1%)
Gastroenteritis	0 (0%)	2 (1%)	2 (1%)
Hemorrhoids	1 (<1%)	2 (1%)	3 (1%)
Mouth dry	1 (<1%)	5 (2%)	6 (2%)
Nausea	105 (36%)	110 (49%)	165 (57%)
Stomatitis	19 (7%)	20 (9%)	36 (13%)
Vomiting	57 (20%)	66 (29%)	106 (37%)
Skin and Subcutaneous Tissue Disorders			
Alopecia	199 (69%)	124 (55%)	208 (72%)
Dermatitis	8 (3%)	1 (<1%)	9 (3%)
Dry skin	7 (2%)	11 (5%)	17 (6%)

(cont'd)

Table 1: TEMODAL *(cont'd)*

TEMODAL and Radiotherapy: Treatment-Emergent Events During Concomitant and Maintenance Treatment

Body System/Adverse Event	TEMODAL + Concomitant Radiotherapy n=288[a] n (%)	TEMODAL Maintenance Therapy n=224 n (%)	Total n=288 n (%)
Erythema	14 (5%)	2 (1%)	16 (6%)
Exfoliation dermatitis	4 (1%)	0 (0%)	4 (1%)
Photosensitivity reaction	2 (1%)	0 (0%)	2 (1%)
Pigmentation abnormal	4 (1%)	1 (<1%)	5 (2%)
Pruritus	11 (4%)	11 (5%)	20 (7%)
Rash	56 (19%)	29 (13%)	74 (26%)
Sweating increased	1 (<1%)	2 (1%)	3 (1%)
Musculoskeletal and Connective Tissue Disorders			
Arthralgia	7 (2%)	14 (6%)	17 (6%)
Back pain	2 (1%)	3 (1%)	5 (2%)
Musculoskeletal pain	2 (1%)	4 (2%)	6 (2%)
Muscle weakness	8 (3%)	6 (3%)	11 (4%)
Myalgia	3 (1%)	7 (3%)	9 (3%)
Myopathy	3 (1%)	3 (1%)	5 (2%)
Renal and Urinary Disorders			
Dysuria	1 (<1%)	2 (1%)	2 (1%)
Micturition frequency	5 (2%)	1 (<1%)	6 (2%)
Urinary incontinence	6 (2%)	4 (2%)	10 (3%)
Reproductive System and Breast Disorders			
Amenorrhea	0 (0%)	1 (1%)	1 (1%)
Breast pain	0 (0%)	1 (1%)	1 (1%)
Impotence	1 (1%)	0 (0%)	1 (1%)
Menorrhagia	0 (0%)	1 (1%)	1 (1%)
Vaginal haemorrhage	0 (0%)	1 (1%)	1 (1%)
Vaginitis	0 (0%)	1 (1%)	1 (1%)
General Disorders and Administration Site Conditions			
Allergic reaction	13 (5%)	6 (3%)	17 (6%)
Asthenia	3 (1%)	2 (1%)	5 (2%)
Condition aggravated	2 (1%)	2 (1%)	4 (1%)
Face edema	8 (3%)	3 (1%)	9 (3%)
Fatigue	156 (54%)	137 (61%)	205 (71%)
Fever	12 (4%)	8 (4%)	18 (6%)
Flushing	2 (1%)	1 (<1%)	3 (1%)
Hot flushes	2 (1%)	1 (<1%)	2 (1%)
Pain	5 (2%)	5 (2%)	9 (3%)
Parosmia	2 (1%)	0 (0%)	2 (1%)
Radiation injury	20 (7%)	5 (2%)	22 (8%)
Rigors	2 (1%)	3 (1%)	4 (1%)
Taste perversion	18 (6%)	11 (5%)	22 (8%)
Thirst	3 (1%)	0 (0%)	3 (1%)
Tooth disorder	0 (0%)	2 (1%)	2 (1%)
Tongue discolouration	2 (1%)	0 (0%)	2 (1%)
Investigation			
Gamma GT increased	4 (1%)	0 (0%)	4 (1%)
Hepatic enzymes increased	3 (1%)	1 (<1%)	3 (1%)
AST increased	3 (1%)	0 (0%)	3 (1%)

(cont'd)

Table 1: TEMODAL *(cont'd)*

TEMODAL and Radiotherapy: Treatment-Emergent Events During Concomitant and Maintenance Treatment

Body System/Adverse Event	TEMODAL + Concomitant Radiotherapy n=288[a] n (%)	TEMODAL Maintenance Therapy n=224 n (%)	Total n=288 n (%)
ALT increased	12 (4%)	5 (2%)	13 (5%)

[a] A patient who was randomised to the RT arm only, received TEMODAL+ RT.

Laboratory Results: Myelosuppression, (neutropenia and thrombocytopenia), which are known dose limiting toxicities for most cytotoxic agents, including TEMODAL, were observed. When laboratory abnormalities and adverse events were combined across concomitant and maintenance treatment phases, Grade 3 or Grade 4 neutrophil abnormalities including neutropenic events were observed in 8% of the patients. Grade 3 or Grade 4 platelets abnormalities, including thrombocytopenic events were observed in 14% of the patients who received TEMODAL.

Table 2: TEMODAL

Grade 3 or Grade 4 Abnormalities Related to Neutrophils and Platelet. Protocol No. P00458

	TEMODAL
Neutrophils	8% (24/288)
Platelets	14% (39/288)

Includes patients with Grade 3 or 4 abnormalities based on either the lowest observed post-baseline laboratory values (Common Toxicity Criteria) for hematology assessments and/or adverse events related to hematological abnormalities.

Table 3: TEMODAL

TEMODAL + Radiotherapy: Grade 3/4 Abnormalities During Concomitant and Maintenance Phases Related to Neutrophils and Platelets

	Concomitant Phase (n=288)	Maintenance (n=224)
Neutrophil Abnormalities	**13 (5%)[a]**	**14 (6%)[a]**
Febrile neutropenia	2 (1%)	3 (1%)
Neutropenia	2 (1%)	5 (2%)
Lab only	9 (3%)[b]	6 (3%)
Platelet Abnormalities	**12 (4%)[c]**	**28 (13%)[c]**
Cerebral hemorrhage	2 (1%)	0
Hemorrhage[d]	4 (1%)	3 (1%)
Thrombocytopenia	8 (3%)[e]	8 (4%)
Lab only	2 (1%)	18 (8%)

[a] Three patients reported neutrophil abnormalitiesin both phases. A total of 24 patients (8%) reported Grade 3/4 neutropenia.
[b] Two of the 9 patients (182 & 194) reported event of neutropenia in Maintenance phase and Lab Only neutropenia in Concomitant Phase and are included in both categories.
[c] One patient reported platelet abnormality in both phases. A total of 39 patients (14%) reported Grade 3/4 platelet abnormalities.
[d] All reports of hemorrhage were associated with Grade 3/4 thrombocytopenia.
[e] One of 8 events of thrombocytopenia was Grade 5=fatal.

Malignant Gliomas Showing Recurrence or Progression After Standard Therapy: A total of 1030 patients with advanced malignancies, among which 400 glioma patients, were treated with TEMODAL in clinical trials. The most common treatment-related adverse events in the total population analyzed for safety were gastrointestinal disturbances, specifically nausea (43%) and vomiting (36%). These effects were usually Grade 1 or 2 mild to moderate in severity, (0-5 episodes of vomiting in 24 hours) and were either self-limiting or readily controlled with standard anti-emetic therapy. The incidence ofsevere nausea and vomiting was 4% each.

The grade 3 or 4 treatment-related hematologic adverse events (defined as those laboratory hematologic events leading to discontinuation, hospitalization, or transfusion) of thrombocytopenia, neutropenia, and anemia, occurred in 9%, 3%, and 3% of the total population analyzed for safety (1030 patients), respectively. In the glioma population (400 patients), these events occurred in 9%, 4%, and 1% of patients, respectively.

Myelosuppression was predictable (typically within the first 2-4 cycles with platelet and neutrophil nadirs between Days 21 to 28) and recovery was rapid, usually within 2 weeks. Myelosuppression was not cumulative. Pancytopenia and leukopenia have been reported. Lymphopenia has been commonly reported.

Table 4: TEMODAL

Treatment-Related Grade 3 and 4 Adverse Events[a] for All Cycles—Glioma Population

Body System/Adverse Event	Number (%) of Patients; N=400 Grade 3 Adverse Events Reported in At Least 2 Patients	Grade 4 Adverse Events Reported in All Patients
Number of Subjects With any Adverse Events	**87 (22%)**	**26 (7%)**
Body as a Whole, General	**25 (6%)**	**2 (<1%)**
Asthenia	6 (2%)	2 (<1%)
Fatigue	9 (2%)	0
Fever	2 (<1%)	0
Headache	6 (2%)	0
Central and Peripheral Nervous Systems	**11 (3%)**	**1 (<1%)**
Confusion	2 (<1%)	0

(cont'd)

Table 4: TEMODAL *(cont'd)*

Treatment-Related Grade 3 and 4 Adverse Events[a] for All Cycles—Glioma Population

Body System/Adverse Event	Number (%) of Patients; N=400 Grade 3 Adverse Events Reported in At Least 2 Patients	Grade 4 Adverse Events Reported in All Patients
Consciousness decreased	0	1 (<1%)
Convulsions	2 (<1%)	0
Hemiparesis	2 (<1%)	0
Paresis	2 (<1%)	0
Transient ischemic attack	0	1 (<1%)
Gastrointestinal System	**33 (8%)**	**1 (<1%)**
Abdominal pain	2 (<1%)	0
Constipation	2 (<1%)	0
Dehydration	2 (<1%)	0
Diarrhea	2 (<1%)	0
Nausea	18 (5%)	0
Vomiting	14 (4%)	1 (<1%)
Metabolic and Nutritional	**2 (<1%)**	**0**
Hyperglycemia	2 (<1%)	0
Platelet, Bleeding and Clotting	**17 (4%)**	**19 (5%)**
Thrombocytopenia	17 (4%)	19 (5%)
Psychiatric Disorders	**3 (1%)**	**0**
Somnolence	3 (1%)	0
Red Blood Cells	**3 (1%)**	**3 (1%)**
Anemia	2 (<1%)	2 (<1%)
Pancytopenia	1 (<1%)	1 (<1%)
Respiratory System	**3 (1%)**	**1 (<1%)**
Pneumonia	2 (<1%)	0
Pulmonary infection	1 (<1%)	1 (<1%)
Vascular (extracardiac)	**1 (<1%)**	**5 (1%)**
Embolism pulmonary	0	1 (<1%)
Hemorrhage intracranial	0	1 (<1%)
Hemorrhage, NOS	0	2 (<1%)
Purpura	1 (<1%)	0
Thrombophlebitis, deep	0	2 (<1%)
White Cell and RES	**14 (4%)**	**10 (3%)**
Leukopenia	10 (3%)	6 (2%)
Neutropenia	7 (2%)	7 (2%)

[a] Only lab abnormalities that led to discontinuation, hospitalization or transfusion were reported as adverse events and are included in this table. A patient is counted only once if >1 occurrence of a specific adverse event. Body system total numbers and percentages reflect all patients reporting any adverse events within that body system.

Among all patients treated with TEMODAL, changes in hematologic laboratory data from Grade 0-2 at Baseline to Grade 3-4 during treatment (thrombocytopenia, neutropenia, and anemia) occurred in 19%, 17% and 7% of the total population analyzed for safety, respectively and in 20%, 14%, and 5% of glioma patients respectively.

Table 5: TEMODAL

Changes in Hematologic Laboratory Data From Grade 0-2 at Baseline to Grade 3-4 During Treatment (Overall and Glioma Population)

	Overall Population (N=1030)[a]	Glioma Population (N=400)[a]
Platelets	19% (180/950)	20% (79/394)
Neutrophils	17% (154/907)	14% (52/366)
Hemoglobin	7% (63/969)	5% (20/397)

[a] Percents were based on the number of patients with data available at baseline and at least one subsequent visit for each parameter.

In a population pharmacokinetics analysis of clinical trial experience there were 101 female and 169 male subjects for whom nadir neutrophil counts were available and 110 female and 174 male subjects for whom nadir platelet counts were available. There were higher rates of Grade 4 neutropenia (ANC <500 cells/μL), 12% versus 5%, and thrombocytopenia (<20 000 cells/μL), 9% versus 3%, in women vs men in the first cycle of therapy. In a 400 subject recurrent glioma data set, Grade 4 neutropenia occurred in 8% of female versus 4% of male subjects and Grade 4 thrombocytopenia in 8% of female vs 3% of male subjects in the first cycle of therapy. In a study of 288 subjects with newly diagnosed glioblastoma multiforme, Grade 4 neutropenia occurred in 3% of female vs 0% of male subjects and Grade 4 thrombocytopenia in 1% of female vs 0% of male subjects in the first cycle of therapy.

Other adverse events reported frequently in the total population analyzed for safety included fatigue (22%), constipation (17%), and headache (14%). Anorexia (11%), diarrhea (8%), rash, fever, asthenia, and somnolence (6% each) were also reported. Less common adverse events (2% to 5%) and in descending order of frequency, were abdominal pain, pain, dizziness, weight decrease, malaise, dyspnea, alopecia, rigors, pruritus, dyspepsia, taste perversion, paresthesia and petechiae.

Table 6 shows the treatment-related adverse events reported in ≥2% of patients in clinical trials involving a total of 400 glioma patients treated with TEMODAL.

Table 6: TEMODAL

Treatment-Related Adverse Events[a] Reported in ≥2% of Glioma Patients

Body System/Adverse Event	Number (%) of Patients
Number of Subjects With any Adverse Event	**304 (76%)**
Body as a Whole, General	**154 (39%)**
Fatigue	90 (23%)
Headache	42 (11%)
Fever	15 (4%)
Asthenia	19 (5%)
Pain	10 (3%)
Malaise	7 (2%)
Rigors	2 (<1%)
Weight decrease	4 (1%)
Central and Peripheral Nervous Systems	**52 (13%)**
Convulsions	10 (3%)
Dizziness	9 (2%)
Paresthesia	6 (2%)
Gastrointestinal System	**230 (58%)**
Nausea	162 (41%)
Vomiting	137 (34%)
Constipation	60 (15%)
Anorexia	35 (9%)
Diarrhea	28 (7%)
Abdominal pain	13 (3%)
Dyspepsia	9 (2%)
Musculoskeletal System	**8 (2%)**
Myalgia	3 (1%)
Platelet, Bleeding and Clotting	**35 (9%)**
Thrombocytopenia	35 (9%)
Psychiatric Disorders	**37 (9%)**
Somnolence	18 (4%)
Depression	4 (1%)
Insomnia	6 (2%)
Red Blood Cells	**10 (2%)**
Anemia	8 (2%)
Pancytopenia	2 (<1%)
Resistance Mechanism	**31 (8%)**
Candidiasis oral	9 (2%)
Respiratory System	**27 (7%)**
Dyspnea	6 (2%)
Special Senses	**4 (1%)**
Taste perversion	4 (1%)
Skin and Appendages	**73 (18%)**
Rash	21 (5%)
Alopecia	15 (4%)
Pruritus	12 (3%)

(cont'd)

Table 6: TEMODAL *(cont'd)*

Treatment-Related Adverse Events[a] Reported in ≥2% of Glioma Patients

Body System/Adverse Event	Number (%) of Patients
Petechiae	14 (4%)
White Cell and Reticulo-Endothelial System	**21 (5%)**
Neutropenia	14 (4%)
Leukopenia	15 (4%)

[a] Only lab abnormalities that led to discontinuation, hospitalization or transfusion were reported as adverse events and are included in this table. A patient is counted only once if >1 occurrence of a specific adverse event. Body system total numbers and percentages reflect all patients reporting any adverse event within that body system.

In the phase II malignant glioma trials, serious adverse events were reported in 278 (70%) patients treated with TEMODAL. The majority of serious adverse events were hospitalizations due to disease progression or disease-related complications, and were unrelated to TEMODAL. Hematologic toxicity, usually grade 3 or 4 thrombocytopenia or neutropenia, was the most common serious adverse event. The majority of these reports were at the 200 mg/m²/day dose level, and most cases resolved with one dose level reduction. Non-hematologic serious adverse events were uncommon.

Within 30 days of the last dose of TEMODAL, forty glioma patients died, the majority due to disease progression or disease-related complications. Two deaths were judged as possibly related to the administration of TEMODAL (grade 4 intratumoral hemorrhage with grade 3 cerebral edema in one patient and grade 4 cerebral ischemia in one patient).

Patients treated with TEMODAL Powder for Solution for Injection: TEMODAL Powder for Solution for Injection delivers equivalent temozolomide dose and exposure to both temozolomide and monomethyl triazeno imidazole carboxamide (MTIC) as the corresponding TEMODAL Capsules. Adverse events probably related to treatment that were reported from the two studies with the IV formulation (n=35) and that were not reported in studies using the TEMODAL Capsules, were those at the infusion site: pain, irritation, pruritus, warmth, swelling, and erythema at infusion site; as well as hematoma.

Post-Market Adverse Drug Reactions: The following adverse events have been reported from post-marketing experience:

- Allergic reactions, including anaphylaxis
- Erythema multiforme, toxic epidermal necrolysis (TEN), Stevens-Johnson syndrome (SJS)
- Opportunistic infections including *P. carinii* pneumonia (PCP)
- Myelodysplastic syndrome (MDS) and secondary malignancies including myeloid leukemia
- Pancytopenia, which may result in aplastic anemia
- Interstitial pneumonitis/pneumonitis

DRUG INTERACTIONS: Drug Interactions with Oral TEMODAL: Antiemetic therapy may be administeredprior to or following administration of TEMODAL.

Administration of TEMODAL with ranitidine or with food did not result in clinically significant alterations in the extent of absorption of TEMODAL. Analyses of data obtained from population pharmacokinetics in the phase II studies demonstrated that co-administration of dexamethasone, prochlorperazine, phenytoin, carbamazepine, ondansetron, H_2-receptor antagonists, or phenobarbital did not alter the clearance of TEMODAL. Co-administration with valproic acid was associated with a small but statistically significant decrease in clearance of TEMODAL.

No studies have been conducted to determine the effect of TEMODAL on the metabolism or elimination of other medicinal products. However, since TEMODAL does not require hepatic metabolism, has a short half-life, and exhibits low protein binding, it is unlikely that it would affect the pharmacokinetics of other medicinal products.

The combination of TEMODAL with other chemotherapeutic agents has not been fully evaluated. Combination with other alkylating agents is likely to result in increased myelosuppression.

Drug-Food Interactions: TEMODAL interactions with food have not been established.

Drug-Herb Interactions: TEMODAL interactions with herbal products have not been established.

Drug-Laboratory Test Interactions: TEMODAL interactions with laboratory tests have not been established.

DOSAGE AND ADMINISTRATION: Recommended Dose and Dosage Adjustment: Adults Patients with Newly Diagnosed Glioblastoma Multiforme: Concomitant Phase: TEMODAL is administered at a dose of 75 mg/m² daily for 42 days concomitant with radiotherapy (60 Gy administered in 30 fractions) followed by maintenance TEMODAL for 6 cycles. No dose reductions are recommended; however, dose interruptions may occur based on patient tolerance. The TEMODAL dose can be continued throughout the 42 day concomitant period up to 49 days if all of the following conditions are met: absolute neutrophil count $\geq 1.5\times10^9$/L platelet count $\geq 100\times10^9$/L common toxicity criteria (CTC) non-hematological toxicity ≤Grade 1 (except for alopecia, nausea and vomiting). During treatment a complete blood count should be obtained weekly. TEMODAL dosing should be interrupted or discontinued during concomitant phase according to the hematological and non-hematological toxicity criteria as noted in Table 7.

Table 7: TEMODAL

TEMODAL Dosing Interruption or Discontinuation During Concomitant Radiotherapy and TEMODAL

Toxicity	TEMODAL Interruption[a]	TEMODAL Discontinuation
Absolute neutrophil count	≥ 0.5 and $<1.5\times10^9$/L	$<0.5\times10^9$/L
Platelet count	≥ 10 and $<100\times10^9$/L	$<10\times10^9$/L
CTC non-hematological toxicity (except for alopecia, nausea, vomiting)	CTC Grade 2	CTC Grade 3 or 4

[a] Treatment with concomitant TEMODAL could be continued when all of the following conditions were met: absolute neutrophil count $\geq 1.5\times10^9$/L; platelet count $\geq 100\times10^9$/L;CTC non-hematological toxicity ≤Grade 1 (except for alopecia, nausea, vomiting).

Legend: CTC=Common Toxicity Criteria.

Maintenance Phase: Four weeks after completing the TEMODAL+ RT (Radiotherapy) phase, TEMODAL is administered for an additional 6 cycles of maintenance treatment. Dosage in Cycle 1 (maintenance) is 150 mg/m² once daily for 5 days followed by 23 days without treatment. At the start of Cycle 2, the dose is escalated to 200 mg/m², if the CTC non-hematologic toxicity for Cycle 1 is Grade ≤2 (except for alopecia, nausea and vomiting), absolute neutrophil count (ANC) is $\geq 1.5\times10^9$/L, and the platelet count is $\geq 100\times10^9$/L. If the dose was not escalated at Cycle 2, escalation should not be done in subsequent cycles. The dose remains at 200 mg/m² per day for the first 5 days of each subsequent cycle except if toxicity occurs. Dose reductions during the maintenance phase should be applied according to Table 8 and Table 9.

During treatment a complete blood count should be obtained on day 22 (21 days after the first dose of TEMODAL). The TEMODAL dose should be reduced or discontinued according to Table 9.

Table 8: TEMODAL

TEMODAL Dose Levels for Maintenance Treatment

Dose Level	Dose (mg/m²/day)	Remarks
–1	100	Reduction for prior toxicity
0	150	Dose during Cycle 1
1	200	Dose during Cycles 2–6 in absence of toxicity

Table 9: TEMODAL

TEMODAL Dose Reduction or Discontinuation During Maintenance Treatment

Toxicity	Reduce TEMODAL by 1 Dose Level[a]	Discontinue TEMODAL
Absolute neutrophil count	$<1.0\times10^9$/L	See [b]
Platelet count	$<50\times10^9$/L	See [b]
CTC non-hematological toxicity (except for alopecia, nausea, vomiting)	CTC Grade 3	CTC Grade 4[b]

[a] TEMODAL dose levels are listed in Table 8.
[b] TEMODAL is to be discontinued if dose reduction to <100 mg/m² is required or if the same Grade3 non-hematological toxicity (except for alopecia, nausea, vomiting) recurs after dose reduction.
Legend: CTC=Common Toxicity Criteria.

Malignant Gliomas Showing Recurrence or Progression After Standard Therapy: Adult Patients: In patients previously untreated with chemotherapy, TEMODAL is administered at a dose of 200 mg/m² once daily for 5 days per 28-day cycle. For patients previously treated with chemotherapy, the initial dose is 150 mg/m² once daily for 5 days, to be increased in the second cycle to 200 mg/m² once daily for 5 days, providing there is no hematologic toxicity (see Warnings and Precautions).

In the reference controlled trial of GBM, the majority of patients treated with TEMODAL (90%) received more than one cycle and 22% of patients received 6 or more cycles. These patients received a total of 484 cycles of TEMODAL in total; 60% of cycles at 200 mg/m²/day and 36% at 150 mg/m²/day. In the single arm AA trial, 93% of patients received more than one cycle and 25% of patients continued on study for 12 months or greater. Eighty-eight percent of patients were receiving either their initial dose or a higher dose at the last cycle. However, limited experience is available on the prolonged use of TEMODAL in this patient population.

Administration: Prior to dosing and during treatment, proper hematologic monitoring must be performed (see Warnings and Precautions) to ensure that the following laboratory parameters are met: absolute neutrophil count (ANC) $\geq1.5\times10^9$/L and platelets $\geq100\times10^9$/L. If the ANC falls to $<1.0\times10^9$/L or the platelet countis $<50\times10^9$/L during any cycle, the next cycle should be reduced one dose level. Dose levels include 100 mg/m²,150 mg/m², and 200 mg/m². The lowest recommended dose is 100 mg/m². Dose modification for TEMODAL should be based on toxicities according to nadir ANC or platelet counts.

Since women taking TEMODAL were reported to have a higher incidence of grade 4 neutropenia and thrombocytopenia than men in the first cycle of therapy, they must be closely monitored for abnormal neutrophil and platelet counts.

TEMODAL therapy can be continued until disease progression.

TEMODAL Capsules: TEMODAL should be administered in the fasting state, at least one hour before a meal. Antiemetic therapy may be administered prior to or following administration of TEMODAL. If vomiting occurs after the dose is administered, a second dose should not be administered.

Store TEMODAL capsules between 15 and 30°C. Protect from moisture.

TEMODAL Powder for Solution for Injection: Reconstitution:

Vial Size	Volume of Diluent to be Added to Vial	Approximate Available Volume	Nominal Concentration per mL
100 mg as lyophilized powder	41 mL Sterile water for injection, USP	transfer into an empty 250 mL PVC infusion bag 40 mL from each vial to make up the total dose	2.5 mg

Preparation and Administration Instructions: TEMODAL Powder for Solution for Injection single use vial contains temozolomide lyophilized powder. When reconstituted with 41 mL Sterile Water for Injection, the resulting solution will contain 2.5 mg/mL temozolomide. The vial should be gently swirled and not shaken. The vials upon reconstitution and upon transfer into PVC bag should be inspected for discoloration, haziness, particulate matter and leakage prior to administration. Discard unused portion. Reconstituted product must be used within 14 hours, including infusion time.

Using aseptic technique, withdraw up to 40 mL from each vial to make up the total dose and transfer into an empty 250 mL PVC infusion bag. Compatibility studies with non-PVC bags have not been conducted. TEMODAL Powder for Solution for Injection should be infused intravenously using a pump over a period of 90 minutes. TEMODAL Powder for Solution for Injection should be administered only by IV infusion.

Because no data are available on the compatibility of TEMODAL Powder for Solution for Injection with other intravenous substances or additives, other medications should not be infused simultaneously through the same IV line.

As with other similar chemotherapeutic agents caution is recommended to avoid extravasation. Local injection site adverse reactions which were mostly mild and short lived were reported in patients receiving TEMODAL Powder for Solution for Injection. Preclinical studies did not show permanent tissue damage.

Store in a refrigerator (2-8°C). Do not freeze.

OVERDOSAGE:

Doses of 500, 750, 1000, and 1250 mg/m² (total dose per cycle over 5 days) have been evaluated clinically in patients. Dose-limiting toxicity was hematological and was reported at any dose but is expected to be more severe at higher doses. An overdose of 2000 mg per day for 5 days was taken by one patient and the adverse events reported were pancytopenia, pyrexia, multi-organ failure and death. There are reports of patients who have taken more than 5 consecutive days of treatment (up to 64 consecutive days) with adverse events reported including bone marrow suppression, with or without infection, in some cases severe and prolonged and resulting in death. In the event of an overdose, hematologic evaluation is needed. Supportive measures should be provided as necessary.

> For management of a suspecteddrug overdose, CPhA recommends that you contact your **regional Poison Control Centre**. See the *CPS* Directorysection for a list of Poison Control Centres.

ACTION AND CLINICAL PHARMACOLOGY: Mechanism of Action: Temozolomide is an imidazotetrazine alkylating agent with antitumor activity that can be used orally. It undergoes rapid chemical conversion in the systemic circulation at physiologic pH to the active compound, MTIC. The cytotoxicity of MTIC is thought to be due primarily to alkylation at the O^6 position of guanine with additional alkylation also occurring at the N^7 position. Cytotoxic lesions that develop subsequently are thought to involve aberrant repair of the methyl adduct.

After oral administration to adult patients, temozolomide is absorbed rapidly with peak plasma concentrations reached as early as 20 minutes post-dose (mean T_{max} range between 0.5 and 1.5 hours).

Plasma concentrations are dose-dependent, while plasma clearance, volume of distribution and half-life are independent of dose. Temozolomide demonstrates low protein binding (10% to 20%), and thus is not expected to interact with highly protein bound agents. After oral administration of ^{14}C labelled temozolomide, mean fecal elimination of ^{14}C over 7 days post-dose was 0.8% indicating complete absorption. Following oral administration, approximately 5% to 10% of the dose is recovered unchanged in the urine over 24 hours, and the remainder excreted as AIC (4-amino-5-imidazole-carboxamide hydrochloride) or unidentified polar metabolites.

Analysis of population based pharmacokinetics of temozolomide revealed that plasma temozolomide clearance was independent of age, renal function, hepatic function, or tobacco use.

Pediatric patients (<18 years old and >3 years old) had a higher area under the curve (AUC) than adult patients; however, the maximum tolerated dose (MTD) was 1000 mg/m² per cycle both in children and in adults.

STORAGE AND STABILITY: TEMODAL Capsules: Store between 15 and 30°C. Protect from moisture.

TEMODAL Powder for Solution for Injection: Store in a refrigerator (2-8°C). Do not freeze.

Upon reconstitution of TEMODAL Powder for Solution for Injection may be stored at room temperature for up to 14 hours, including infusion time. Single use vial. Partially used vials must be discarded.

SPECIAL HANDLING INSTRUCTIONS: TEMODAL Capsules: TEMODAL Capsules must not be opened or chewed, but are to be swallowed whole with a glass of water. If a capsule becomes damaged, avoid contact of the powder contents with skin or mucous membrane. In the case of accidental contact with skin or mucous membrane, flush with water.

Keep out of reach of children.

TEMODAL Powder for Solution for Injection: Caution must be exercised in handling TEMODAL Powder for Solution for Injection. The use of gloves is required. If TEMODAL comes into contact with skin or mucosa, wash immediately and thoroughly with soap and water. TEMODAL must be handled and disposed of in a manner consistent with that of other anticancer medicinal products in accordance with local requirements.

Keep out of reach of children.

INFORMATION FOR THE PATIENT: Published in e-CPS, available by subscription at www.e-cps.ca.

DOSAGE FORMS, COMPOSITION AND PACKAGING: Capsules: 5 mg: Each size No. 3 capsule, with opaque green cap and opaque white body, the cap imprinted in black ink with "TEMODAL", the body imprinted in black ink with 2 stripes, "5 mg", and the Schering Plough logo, contains: temozolomide 5 mg. Nonmedicinal ingredients: colloidal silicon dioxide, lactose anhydrous, sodium starch glycolate, stearic acid and tartaric acid; capsule shells: FD&C blue no. 2, gelatin, sodium lauryl sulfate, titanium dioxide and yellow iron oxide and are branded with black printing ink consisting of shellac, propylene glycol, ammonium hydroxide, black iron oxide and sometimes potassium hydroxide. Bottles of 5 and 20.

20 mg: Each size No. 2 capsule, with yellow cap and opaque white body, the cap imprinted in black ink with "TEMODAL", the body imprinted in black ink with 2 stripes, "20 mg", and Schering-Plough logo, contains: temozolomide 20 mg. Nonmedicinal ingredients: colloidal silicon dioxide, lactose anhydrous, sodium starch glycolate, stearic acid and tartaric acid; capsule shells: gelatin, sodium lauryl sulfate, titanium dioxide and yellow iron oxide and are branded with black printing ink consisting of shellac, propylene glycol, ammonium hydroxide, black iron oxide and sometimes potassium hydroxide. Bottles of 5 and 20.

100 mg: Each size No. 1 capsule, with opaque pink cap and opaque white body, the cap imprinted in black ink with "TEMODAL", the body imprinted in black ink with 2 stripes, "100 mg", and the Schering-Plough logo, contains: temozolomide 100 mg. Nonmedicinal ingredients: colloidal silicon dioxide, lactose anhydrous, sodium starch glycolate, stearic acid and tartaric acid; capsule shells: gelatin, sodium lauryl sulfate, red iron oxide and titanium dioxide and are branded with black printing ink consisting of shellac, propylene glycol, ammonium hydroxide, black iron oxide and sometimes potassium hydroxide. Bottles of 5 and 20.

140 mg: Each size No. 0 capsules with a blue cap and opaque white body, the cap imprinted in black ink with "TEMODAL", the body imprinted in black ink with 2 stripes, "140 mg", and the Schering-Plough logo, contains: temozolomide 140 mg. Nonmedicinal ingredients: colloidal silicon dioxide, lactose anhydrous, sodium starch glycolate, stearic acid and tartaric acid; capsule shells: FD&C blue no. 2, gelatin, sodium lauryl sulfate and titanium dioxide and are branded with black printing ink consisting of shellac, propylene glycol, ammonium hydroxide, black iron oxide and sometimes potassium hydroxide. Bottles of 5 and 20.

180 mg: Each size No. 0 capsules with an opaque orange cap and opaque white body, the cap imprinted in black ink with "TEMODAL", the body imprinted in black ink with 2 stripes, "180 mg", and the Schering-Plough logo, contains: temozolomide 180 mg. Nonmedicinal ingredients: colloidal silicon dioxide, lactose anhydrous, sodium starch glycolate, stearic acid and tartaric acid; capsule shells: gelatin, sodium lauryl sulfate, red iron oxide, titanium dioxide and yellow iron oxide and are branded with black printing ink consisting of shellac, propylene glycol, ammonium hydroxide, black iron oxide and sometimes potassium hydroxide. Bottles of 5 and 20.

250 mg: Each size No. 0 capsule, with opaque white cap and opaque white body, the cap imprinted in black ink with "TEMODAL", the body imprinted in black ink with 2 stripes, "250 mg" and the Schering-Plough logo, contains: temozolomide 250 mg. Nonmedicinal ingredients: colloidal silicon dioxide, lactose anhydrous, sodium starch glycolate, stearic acid and tartaric acid; capsule shells: gelatin, sodium lauryl sulfate and titanium dioxide and are branded with black printing ink consisting of shellac, propylene glycol, ammonium hydroxide, black iron oxide and sometimes potassium hydroxide. Bottles of 5.

Powder for Solution for Injection: Each glass vial contains: temozolomide lyophilized powder 100 mg. Nonmedicinal ingredients: hydrochloric acid, L-threonine, mannitol, polysorbate-80 and sodium citrate dihydrate. Upon reconstitution with 41 mL Sterile Water for Injection, the resulting solution will contain 2.5 mg/mL temozolomide. Single use 100 mL glass vials with rubber stopper, and aluminum seal.

(Shown in Product Identification Section)

Tempra®

acetaminophen

Antipyretic—Analgesic

Bristol-Myers Squibb

Date of Revision: April 30, 2010

INDICATIONS: For fast and effective relief of infant and children's fever or pain caused by immunization, teething, colds, or flu.

WARNINGS: Do not use with other drugs containing **acetaminophen.**

Do not take more than the recommended dose unless advised by a doctor. Taking more than the maximum daily dose may cause **severe or possibly fatal liver damage.**

Do not take if allergic to acetaminophen.

Consult a doctor if:

- you develop allergic reactions such as wheezing, rash or itching;
- your symptoms last for more than five days, or fever lasts more than 3 days.

OVERDOSE:

In the case of an overdose, even if there are no signs or symptoms, call your Poison Control Centre or physician immediately. Within the first 24 hours your infant or child may experience nausea or vomiting, increased sweating, diarrhea, loss of appetite and stomach pain. Medical attention is critical, even in the absence of symptoms.

> For management of a suspected drug overdose, contact your regional Poison Control Centre. See the *CPS* Directory section for a list of Poison Control Centres.

DOSAGE: Administer single dose orally, every 4-6 hours, according to the weights listed in Table 1 with a daily maximum of 5 doses/24 hours.

Table 1: TEMPRA

Dosage

Dosage[a]		Infant TEMPRA Drops 80 mg/1 mL 0–under 2 years Use supplied dropper only	Children's TEMPRA Syrup Regular Strength 80 mg/5 mL 2–6 years Use supplied dosage cup only	Double-Strength Children's TEMPRA Syrup 160 mg/5 mL 4–10 years Use supplied dosage cup only
lbs	kg			
6–11	2.0–5.4	Consult a physician	—	—
12–17	5.5–7.9	1.0 mL	—	—
18–23	8.0–10.9	1.5 mL	—	—
24–35	11.0–15.9	—	10 mL	5 mL
36–47	16.0–21.9	—	15 mL	7.5 mL
48–59	22.0–26.9	—	—	10 mL
60–71	27.0–31.9	—	—	12.5 mL

(cont'd)

Table 1: TEMPRA *(cont'd)*

Dosage

Dosage[a]		Infant TEMPRA Drops 80 mg/1 mL 0–under 2 years Use supplied dropper only	Children's TEMPRA Syrup Regular Strength 80 mg/5 mL 2–6 years Use supplied dosage cup only	Double-Strength Children's TEMPRA Syrup 160 mg/5 mL 4–10 years Use supplied dosage cup only
lbs	kg			
72–95	32.0–43.9	—	—	15 mL

[a] These doses are based on weight, not age, and offer more specific doses than in the general instructions on the label/carton.

- **Keep out of the reach of children.** Safety sealed bottle. Do not use if seal is broken.

SUPPLIED: Drops: 80 mg/1 mL: Each 1 mL of cherry- or banana-flavored liquid contains: acetaminophen 80 mg. Nonmedicinal ingredients: artificial flavoring, artificial coloring (in cherry flavored only), citric acid, glycerin, polyethylene glycol, propylene glycol, purified water, sodium citrate and sodium saccharin. Alcohol-, ASA- and sucrose-free. Banana flavored is dye free. Bottles of 15 mL (in cherry flavored only) and 24 mL with calibrated dropper.

Syrup: 80 mg/5 mL: Each 5 mL of cherry-flavored syrup contains: acetaminophen 80 mg. Nonmedicinal ingredients: artificial flavors and coloring, butylated hydroxyanisol, citric acid, polyethylene glycol, purified water, sodium benzoate, sodium chloride, sodium citrate and sucrose. Energy: 9 kcal/5 mL. Alcohol- and ASA-free. Bottles of 100 mL.

160 mg/5 mL: Each 5 mL of cherry- or banana-flavored syrup contains: acetaminophen 160 mg. Nonmedicinal ingredients: artificial flavors, artificial coloring (in cherry flavored only), butylated hydroxyanisol, citric acid, polyethylene glycol, purified water, sodium benzoate, sodium chloride, sodium citrate and sucrose. Energy: 9 kcal/5 mL. Alcohol- and ASA-free. Banana-flavored is dye free. Bottles of 100 mL.

Tenoretic® ℞

atenolol—chlorthalidone

Antihypertensive

AstraZeneca

Date of Preparation: September 23, 1993
Date of Revision: June 13, 2008

PHARMACOLOGY: TENORETIC (atenolol/chlorthalidone) combines the antihypertensive activity of two agents, a beta-adrenergic receptor blocking agent (atenolol) and a diuretic (chlorthalidone).

Atenolol is a beta$_1$-selective, beta adrenergic blocking agent, devoid of membrane stabilizing or intrinsic sympathomimetic (partial agonist) activities. It is a racemic mixture and the beta$_1$ properties reside in the S(-) enantiomer. Beta$_1$-selectivity decreases with increasing dose.

The mechanism of the antihypertensive effect of atenolol has not been established. Among the factors that may be involved are: a) competitive ability to antagonize catecholamine-induced tachycardia at the beta receptor sites in the heart, thus decreasing cardiac output. b) inhibition of renin release by the kidneys. c) inhibition of the vasomotor centres.

In man atenolol reduces both isoproterenol- and exercise-induced increases in heart rate over the dose range of 50 to 200 mg. At an oral dose of 100 mg the beta$_1$ blocking effects persist for at least 24 hours; the reduction in exercise-induced heart rate increase being about 32% and 13%, 2 and 24 hours after dosing, respectively. The logarithm of the plasma atenolol level correlates with the degree of beta$_1$ blockade but not with the antihypertensive effect.

Chlorthalidone, a monosulfonamyl diuretic, increases excretion of sodium and chloride. Natriuresis is accompanied by some loss of potassium. The mechanism by which chlorthalidone reduces blood pressure is not fully known but may be related to the excretion and redistribution of body sodium. Chlorthalidone usually does not decrease normal blood pressure.

The combination of atenolol with thiazide-like diuretics has been shown to be compatible and generally more effective than either drug used alone as an antihypertensive agent.

Pharmacokinetics: Approximately 40 to 50% of an oral dose of atenolol is absorbed from the gastrointestinal tract, the remainder being excreted unchanged in the feces. Peak plasma concentrations occur 2 to 4 hours after dosing and are subject to a 4-fold variability. The plasma levels are proportional to dose over the range 50 to 400 mg and 6 to 16% of atenolol is bound to plasma proteins. The plasma half-life is approximately 6 to 7 hours.

Approximately 60% of an oral dose of chlorthalidone is absorbed from the gastrointestinal tract and excreted unchanged in the urine. Following a single dose, the peak blood concentration of chlorthalidone occurs after approximately 12 hours and decreases thereafter according to first-order kinetics; the disposition half-life is approximately 50 hours. Approximately 75% of chlorthalidone is bound in plasma.

INDICATIONS: This fixed combination is not indicated for initial therapy of hypertension. Hypertension requires therapy titrated to the individual patient. It is always better to adjust the dosage of each antihypertensive drug separately, but when the fixed combination corresponds to the optimum drug and dose requirements of the patient, its use may be more convenient in patient management. For further adjustment of dosage, however, it is best to use the individual drugs again. The treatment of hypertension is not static, but must be re-evaluated as conditions in each patient warrant.

TENORETIC (atenolol/chlorthalidone) is indicated for the maintenance therapy of patients with hypertension who require atenolol and chlorthalidone in the dosage and ratios present in TENORETIC.

CONTRAINDICATIONS: TENORETIC (atenolol/chlorthalidone) should not be used in the presence of: sinus bradycardia, or bradycardia of other origin; second and third degree AV block; sick sinus syndrome; right ventricular failure secondary to pulmonary hypertension; uncontrolled heart failure; cardiogenic shock; hypotension; severe peripheral arterial disorders; anesthesia with agents that produce myocardial depression; pheochromocytoma, in the absence of alpha-blockade; metabolic acidosis; anuria; hypersensitivity to atenolol, chlorthalidone or to sulfonamide-derived drugs; pregnancy or lactation (see Pregnancy and Lactation).

WARNINGS: Cardiac Failure: Special caution should be exercised when administering TENORETIC to patients with a history of cardiac failure. Sympathetic stimulation is a vital component supporting circulatory function in congestive heart failure and inhibition with β-blockade always carries the potential hazard of further depressing myocardial contractility and precipitating cardiac failure.

In patients without a history of cardiac failure, continued depression of the myocardium with β-blocking agents over a period of time can, in some cases, lead to cardiac failure. Therefore, at the first sign or symptom of impending cardiac failure, patients should be fully digitalized and/or given additional diuretic and the response observed closely.

Atenolol acts selectively without blocking the inotropic action of digitalis on the heart muscle. However, the positive inotropic action of digitalis may be reduced by the negative inotropic effect of atenolol when the two drugs are used concomitantly. The effects of β-blockers and digitalis are additive in depressing AV conduction. If cardiac failure continues, despite adequate digitalization, TENORETIC therapy should be withdrawn immediately and diuretic therapy maintained (see below).

Abrupt Cessation of Therapy with TENORETIC: Patients with angina should be warned against abrupt discontinuation of TENORETIC. There have been reports of severe exacerbation of angina and of myocardial infarction or ventricular arrhythmias occurring in patients with angina pectoris, following abrupt discontinuation of β-blocker therapy. The last two complications may occur with or without preceding exacerbation of angina pectoris. Therefore, when discontinuation of TENORETIC is planned in patients with angina pectoris, the drug should be stopped and immediately replaced with atenolol and a diuretic given separately, so that the dose of atenolol may be gradually reduced over a period of about 2 weeks while the dose of diuretic is maintained. The same frequency of administration of both drugs should be maintained. The patients should be carefully observed.

In situations of greater urgency, TENORETIC should be discontinued stepwise over a shorter time and under closer observation. If angina markedly worsens or acute coronary insufficiency develops, it is recommended that treatment with TENORETIC be reinstituted promptly, at least temporarily.

Since ischemic heart disease may be unrecognized, the above advice should be followed in patients considered to be at risk of having asymptomatic ischemic heart disease.

Oculomucocutaneous Syndrome: Various skin rashes and conjunctival xerosis have been reported with β-blockers, including atenolol. A severe syndrome (oculomucocutaneous syndrome) whose signs include conjunctivitis sicca and psoriasiform rashes, otitis, and sclerosing serositis has occurred with the chronic use of one β-adrenergic blocking agent (practolol). This syndrome has not been observed with atenolol or any other such agent. However, physicians should be alert to the possibility of such reactions and should discontinue treatment with TENORETIC in the event that they occur.

Prinzmetal's Angina: Atenolol may increase the number and duration of angina attacks in patients with Prinzmetal's angina due to unopposed α-receptor mediated coronary artery vasoconstriction. TENORETIC, therefore, should only be used in these patients with the utmost care.

Sinus Bradycardia: Severe sinus bradycardia may occur with the use of atenolol from unopposed vagal activity remaining after blockade of β$_1$-adrenergic receptors; in such cases, the dose should be reduced.

Thyrotoxicosis: In patients with thyrotoxicosis, possible deleterious effects from long-term use of atenolol have not been adequately appraised. β-blockade may mask the clinical signs of continuing hyperthyroidism or its complications and give a false impression of improvement. Therefore, abrupt withdrawal of atenolol may be followed by an exacerbation of the symptoms of hyperthyroidism, including thyroid storm. Thiazides may decrease serum PBI levels without signs of thyroid disturbance.

Impaired Renal Function: TENORETIC should be used with caution since chlorthalidone may precipitate or increase azotemia. Cumulative effects may develop since both components of TENORETIC are excreted by the kidney. If progressive renal impairment becomes evident, TENORETIC should be discontinued.

When renal function is impaired, clearance of atenolol is closely related to the glomerular filtration rate. However, significant accumulation does not occur until the creatinine clearance falls below 35 mL/min/1.73 m^2.

Impaired Hepatic Function: In patients with impaired hepatic function or progressive liver disease, even minor alterations in fluid and electrolyte balance may precipitate hepatic coma. Hepatic encephalopathy, manifested by tremors, confusion and coma, has been reported in association with diuretic therapy, including chlorthalidone.

Hypersensitivity Reactions: In patients receiving chlorthalidone, sensitivity reactions may occur with or without a history of allergy or bronchial asthma.

Systemic Lupus Erythematosus: Possible exacerbation of systemic lupus erythematosus has been reported with thiazide-like diuretics.

Pregnancy: Use of TENORETIC is contraindicated during pregnancy.

Atenolol can cause fetal harm when administered to a pregnant woman. Atenolol crosses the placental barrier and appears in the cord blood.

No studies have been performed on the use of atenolol in the first trimester and the possibility of fetal injury cannot be excluded. Administration of atenolol, starting in the second trimester of pregnancy, has been associated with the birth of infants that are small for gestational age.

In a limited number of patients who were given atenolol during the last trimester of pregnancy, low birth weight, neonatal hypoglycemia, bradycardia in the fetus/newborn, and placental insufficiency were observed.

Neonates born to mothers who are receiving atenolol at parturition or breast-feeding may be at risk for hypoglycemia and bradycardia. (See Warnings, Lactation.)

Atenolol has been shown to produce a dose-related increase in embryo/fetal resorptions in rats at doses equal to or greater than 50 mg/kg/day or 25 or more times the maximum recommended human dose.

Thiazides cross the placental barrier and appear in cord blood. The use of chlorthalidone during pregnancy may cause fetal or neonatal jaundice, thrombocytopenia and, possibly, other adverse reactions, which have occurred in the adult.

Lactation: TENORETIC is contraindicated in lactating women.

There is a significant accumulation of atenolol in breast milk.

Neonates born to mothers who are receiving atenolol at parturition or breast-feeding may be at risk for hypoglycemia and bradycardia. (See Warnings, Pregnancy.)

PRECAUTIONS: Bronchospastic Disorders: Patients with bronchospastic diseases should, in general, not receive β-blockers. Due to the relative β$_1$-selectivity of atenolol, atenolol may be used with caution in patients with bronchospastic disease who do not respond to, or cannot tolerate, other antihypertensive treatment. Since β$_1$-selectivity is not absolute, a β$_2$-stimulating agent should be administered concomitantly and the lowest possible dose of atenolol should be used. Despite these precautions, the respiratory status of some patients may worsen, and, in such cases, TENORETIC should be withdrawn.

First Degree Heart Block: Due to atenolol's negative effect on A-V conduction time, TENORETIC should be used with caution in patients with first degree block.

Peripheral Arterial Circulatory Disorders: TENORETIC may aggravate less severe peripheral arterial circulatory disorders (see Contraindications).

Anaphylaxis—Epinephrine and β-blockers: There may be increased difficulty in treating an allergic type reaction in patients on β-blockers. In these patients, the reaction may be more severe due to pharmacological effects of β-blockers and problems with fluid changes. Epinephrine should be administered with caution since it may not have its usual effects in the treatment of anaphylaxis. On the one hand, larger doses of epinephrine may be needed to overcome the bronchospasm, while on the other, these doses can be associated with excessive α-adrenergic stimulation with consequent hypertension, reflex bradycardia and heart-block and possible potentiation of bronchospasm. Alternatives to the use of large doses of epinephrine include vigorous supportive care such as fluids and the use of β-agonists including parenteral salbutamol or isoproterenol to overcome bronchospasm and norepinephrine to overcome hypotension.

Diabetes and Patients Subject to Hypoglycemia: TENORETIC should be administered with caution to patients subject to spontaneous hypoglycemia, or to diabetic patients (especially those with labile diabetes) who are receiving insulin or oral hypoglycemic agents. β-adrenergic receptor blocking agents may mask the premonitory signs (e.g., tachycardia) and symptoms of acute hypoglycemia. Insulin requirements in diabetic patients may be increased, decreased, or unchanged by chlorthalidone. Diabetes mellitus which has been latent may become manifest during chlorthalidone administration.

Elective or Emergency Surgery: It is not advisable to withdraw β-adrenoceptor blocking drugs prior to surgery in the majority of patients. However, care should be taken when using TENORETIC with anesthetic agents such as those which may depress the myocardium. Vagal dominance, if it occurs, may be corrected with atropine (1 to 2 mg i.v.).

Some patients receiving β-adrenergic blocking agents have been subject to protracted severe hypotension during anesthesia. Difficulty in restarting and maintaining the heartbeat has also been reported.

In emergency surgery, since atenolol is a competitive inhibitor of β-adrenergic receptor agonists, its effects may be reversed, if necessary, by sufficient doses of such agonists as isoproterenol or norepinephrine.

Fluid or Electrolyte Imbalance: Patients receiving chlorthalidone should be carefully observed for clinical signs of fluid or electrolyte imbalance (hyponatremia, hypochloremic alkalosis and hypokalemia). Periodic determination of serum electrolytes should be performed at appropriate intervals. Serum and urine electrolyte determinations are particularly important when the patient is vomiting excessively or receiving parenteral fluids. Warning signs or symptoms of fluid and electrolyte imbalance include dryness of the mouth, thirst, weakness, lethargy, drowsiness, restlessness, muscle pains or cramps, muscular fatigue, hypotension, oliguria, tachycardia and gastrointestinal disturbances.

Hypokalemia may develop, especially with brisk diuresis, when severe cirrhosis is present, or during concomitant use of corticosteroids or ACTH. Interference with adequate oral electrolyte intake will also contribute to hypokalemia. Hypokalemia can sensitize or exaggerate the response of the heart to the toxic effects of digitalis (e.g., increased ventricular irritability). Hypokalemia may be avoided or treated by use of potassium supplements, potassium-sparing agents or foods with a high potassium content.

Any chloride deficit during chlorthalidone therapy is generally mild and usually does not require specific treatment except under extraordinary circumstances (as in liver disease or renal disease). Dilutional hyponatremia may occur in edematous patients in hot weather; appropriate therapy is water restriction rather than administration of salt except in rare instances when the hyponatremia is life threatening. In actual salt depletion, appropriate replacement is the therapy of choice.

Because calcium excretion is decreased by chlorthalidone, TENORETIC should be discontinued before carrying out tests for parathyroid function. Pathologic changes in the parathyroid glands, with hypercalcemia and hypophosphatemia, have been observed in a few patients on prolonged thiazide therapy; however, the common complications of hyperparathyroidism such as renal lithiasis, bone resorption and peptic ulceration have not been seen.

Post-sympathectomy Patients: The antihypertensive effects of thiazides may be enhanced in the post-sympathectomy patient.

Hyperuricemia: Hyperuricemia may occur or acute gout may be precipitated in certain patients receiving chlorthalidone.

Ethnic Populations: Atenolol appears to be effective and well-tolerated in most ethnic populations, although the response may be less in black patients than in Caucasians.

Children: The safety of use of atenolol in children has not been established; therefore, TENORETIC is not recommended in the pediatric age group.

Occupational Hazards: Activities Requiring Mental Alertness: Use of TENORETIC is unlikely to result in any impairment of the ability of patients to drive or operate machinery. However, it should be taken into account that dizziness or fatigue may occur.

Geriatrics: Clinical studies of TENORETIC did not include sufficient numbers of subjects aged 65 and over to determine whether they respond differently from younger subjects. Other reported clinical experience has not identified differences in responses between elderly and younger patients. In general, dose selection for an elderly patient should be cautious, usually starting at the low end of the dosing range, reflecting the greater frequency of decreased hepatic renal, or cardiac function, and concomitant diseases or other drug therapy.

Drug Interactions: Clonidine: β-blockers may exacerbate the rebound hypertension which can follow the withdrawal of clonidine. If the two drugs are coadministered, the β-blocker should be withdrawn several days before discontinuing clonidine. If replacing clonidine by β-blocker therapy, the introduction of β-blockers should be delayed for several days after clonidine administration has stopped. (Also see prescribing information for clonidine.)

Reserpine or Guanethidine: Patients receiving catecholamine-depleting drugs, such as reserpine or guanethidine, should be closely monitored because the added β-adrenergic blocking action of atenolol may produce an excessive reduction of sympathetic activity. TENORETIC should not be combined with other drugs containing β-blockers.

Antihypertensive Peripheral Vasodilator: The combination of TENORETIC with an antihypertensive peripheral vasodilator produces a greater fall in blood pressure than either drug alone. The same degree of blood pressure control can be achieved by lower than usual doses of each drug. Therefore, when using such concomitant therapy, careful monitoring of the doses is required until the patient is stabilized.

Norepinephrine: Thiazides may decrease arterial responsiveness to norepinephrine. This diminution is not sufficient to preclude the therapeutic effectiveness of the pressor agent in therapy.

Tubocurarine: Thiazide diuretics may increase the responsiveness to tubocurarine.

Lithium: Lithium generally should not be given with diuretics because they reduce its renal clearance and add a high risk of lithium toxicity. The Prescribing Information for lithium preparations should be read before use of such preparations with TENORETIC.

Alcohol, Barbiturates or Narcotics: Orthostatic hypotension may occur and may be potentiated by alcohol, barbiturates or narcotics.

Antiarrhythmic Agents: Class I antiarrhythmic drugs (e.g. disopyramide) and amiodarone may have potentiating effect on atrial-conduction time and induce negative inotropic effect.

Calcium Channel Blockers: Combined use of β-blockers and calcium channel blockers with negative inotropic effects can lead to prolongation of S-A and A-V conduction, particularly in patients with impaired ventricular function, conduction abnormalities, or diminished cardiac output. This may result in severe hypotension, bradycardia and cardiac failure. Concomitant therapy with dihydropyridines, e.g., nifedipine, may increase the risk of hypotension, and cardiac failure may occur in patients with latent cardiac insufficiency. On rare occasions the concomitant administration of i.v. beta-adrenergic blocking agents with i.v. verapamil has resulted in serious adverse effects, especially in patients with severe cardiomyopathy, congestive heart failure or recent myocardial infarction.

Digitalis Glycosides: Digitalis glycosides may potentiate the bradycardia of β-blockade.

Nonsteroidal Anti-inflammatory Agents: The concomitant use of nonsteroidal anti-inflammatory agents may blunt the antihypertensive effects of β-blockers.

Anesthetic Agents: Anesthetics can produce a hypotensive state with associated reflex tachycardia. Since β-blockade will inhibit reflex tachycardia, the hypotensive potential of anesthetic agents is increased with concomitant use of TENORETIC, thus the anesthetic used should be an agent with as little negative inotropic activity as possible (see Contraindications and Precautions, Elective or Emergency Surgery).

ADVERSE EFFECTS: Adverse reactions that have been reported with the individual components are listed below.

Atenolol: The most serious adverse reactions encountered are congestive heart failure, AV block and bronchospasm. Bronchospasm may occur in patients with bronchial asthma or a history of asthmatic complaints.

The most common adverse reactions reported in clinical trials with atenolol in 2500 patients are bradycardia (3%), dizziness (3%), vertigo (2%), fatigue (3%), diarrhea (2%) and nausea (3%).

Adverse reactions, occurring with an incidence of less than 1%, grouped by system, are as follows:

Cardiovascular: heart failure deterioration (see Warnings), heart block, palpitations, lengthening of PR interval, chest pain, lightheadedness, postural hypotension which may be associated with syncope, Raynaud's phenomenon, intermittent claudication, or worsening of pre-existing intermittent claudication, leg pain and cold extremities, edema.

Respiratory: dyspnea, wheeziness, cough, bronchospasm.

Central Nervous System: faintness, ataxia, tiredness, lethargy, nervousness, depression, drowsiness, vivid dreams, insomnia, paresthesia, headache, tinnitus, mood changes, visual disturbances, psychoses and hallucinations.

Gastrointestinal: abdominal discomfort, indigestion, constipation, anorexia.

Miscellaneous: skin rash, itchy and/or dry eyes, psoriasiform skin reactions, exacerbation of psoriasis, decreased exercise tolerance, alopecia, epistaxis, flushes, impotence, decreased libido, sweating, general body aches, thrombocytopenia and purpura.

Post-marketing Experience: During post-marketing experience with atenolol, cold extremities, gastrointestinal disturbances and fatigue were commonly reported. The following have been reported in temporal relationship to the use of the drug: elevated liver enzymes and/or bilirubin, headache, confusion, nightmares, impotence, Peyronie's disease, psoriasiform rash or exacerbation of psoriasis, purpura, reversible alopecia and thrombocytopenia. Rare cases of hepatic toxicity including intrahepatic cholestasis have been reported. Atenolol, like other beta blockers, has been associated with the development of antinuclear antibodies (ANA) and lupus syndrome.

In a long-term, well controlled trial of 1627 elderly patients with systolic hypertension, the incidence of dry mouth was significantly higher in patients taking atenolol (12.2%).

Potential Adverse Reactions: The following adverse reactions have occurred with other β-blockers but have not been reported with atenolol:

Cardiovascular: pulmonary edema, cardiac enlargement, hot flushes and sinus arrest.

Central Nervous System: aggressiveness, anxiety, short-term memory loss, and emotional lability with slightly clouded sensorium.

Allergic: laryngospasm, status asthmaticus and fever combined with aching and sore throat.

Dermatological: exfoliative dermatitis.

Ophthalmological: blurred vision, burning, and grittiness.

Hematological: agranulocytosis.

Gastrointestinal: mesenteric arterial thrombosis and ischemic colitis.

Chlorthalidone: The following adverse reactions have been reported:

Gastrointestinal: anorexia, gastric irritation, nausea, vomiting, cramping, diarrhea, constipation, jaundice (intrahepatic cholestatic jaundice), pancreatitis.

Central Nervous System: dizziness, vertigo, paresthesias, headache, xanthopsia.

Hematologic: leukopenia, agranulocytosis, thrombocytopenia, aplastic anemia.

Dermatologic-Hypersensitivity: purpura, photosensitivity, rash, urticaria, necrotizing angiitis (vasculitis) (cutaneous vasculitis), Lyell's syndrome (toxic epidermal necrolysis).

Cardiovascular: Orthostatic hypotension may occur and may be aggravated by alcohol, barbiturates or narcotics.

Other: hyperglycemia, glycosuria, hyperuricemia, hyponatremia, muscle spasm, weakness, restlessness, impotence and hypokalemia.

OVERDOSE:

Symptoms: No specific information is available with regard to overdosage of TENORETIC in humans.

Atenolol: Overdosage with atenolol has been reported with patients surviving acute doses as high as 5 g. One death was reported in a man who may have taken as much as 10 g acutely.

The predominant symptoms reported following atenolol overdosage are lethargy, disorder of respiratory drive, wheezing, sinus pause, and bradycardia. Additionally, common effects associated with overdosage of any β-adrenergic blocking agent are congestive heart failure, hypotension, bronchospasm and/or hypoglycemia.

Chlorthalidone: Symptoms of chlorthalidone overdose include nausea, weakness, dizziness and disturbances of electrolyte balance.

Treatment: Atenolol: Treatment should be symptomatic and supportive and directed to the removal of any unabsorbed drug by induced emesis, or administration of activated charcoal. Atenolol can be removed from the general circulation by hemodialysis. Further consideration should be given to dehydration, electrolyte imbalance and hypotension by established procedures.

Other treatment modalities should be employed at the physician's discretion and may include:

Bradycardia: Atropine 1 to 2 mg i.v. If there is no response to vagal blockade, give isoproterenol cautiously. In refractory cases, a transvenous cardiac pacemaker may be indicated. Glucagon in a 10 mg i.v. bolus has been reported to be useful. If required, this may be repeated or followed by an i.v. infusion of glucagon 1 to 10 mg/h depending on response. If no response to glucagon occurs or if glucagon is unavailable, a β-adrenoceptor stimulant such as dobutamine 2.5 to 10 µg/kg/min by i.v. infusion or isoproterenol 10 to 25 µg given as an infusion at a rate not exceeding 5 µg/min may be given, although larger doses may be required.

Heart Block (second or third degree): isoproterenol or transvenous pacemaker.

Congestive Heart Failure: Digitalize the patient and administer a diuretic. Glucagon has been reported to be useful.

Hypotension: vasopressors such as dopamine or norepinephrine. Monitor blood pressure continuously.

Bronchospasm: a β_2-stimulant such as isoproterenol or terbutaline, and/or i.v. aminophylline.

Hypoglycemia: i.v. glucose.

Electrolyte Disturbance: Monitor electrolyte levels and renal function. Institute measures to maintain hydration and electrolytes.

Based on the severity of symptoms, management may require intensive support care and facilities for applying cardiac and respiratory support.

For management of a suspected drug overdose, CPhA recommends that you contact your **regional Poison Control Centre**. See the *CPS* Directory section for a list of Poison Control Centres.

DOSAGE: Dosage must be determined for individual patients by titration of each component separately. Where the fixed combination in TENORETIC supplies the dosage so determined, the combination product may be used for maintenance therapy.

One TENORETIC tablet once daily can be used to administer up to 100 mg of atenolol and 25 mg of chlorthalidone.

If further lowering of the blood pressure is required, another antihypertensive agent may be added to the regimen.

In patients with renal impairment, the dose of the components should be carefully individualized. Recommendations for dosage adjustments for atenolol and chlorthalidone in renal disease are found in the TENORMIN and Hygroton prescribing information.

If dosage adjustment is necessary during maintenance therapy, it is advisable to use the individual drugs.

SUPPLIED: 50/25: Each white, round, biconvex tablet, scored and embossed 50/25 on one face and plain on the other, contains: atenolol 50 mg and chlorthalidone 25 mg. Nonmedicinal ingredients: magnesium stearate, microcrystalline cellulose, povidone and sodium starch glycolate. Calendar packs of 30. Protect from light and moisture. Store at room temperature.

100/25: Each white, round, biconvex tablet, scored and embossed with 100/25 on one face and plain on the other, contains: atenolol 100 mg and chlorthalidone 25 mg. Nonmedicinal ingredients: magnesium stearate, microcrystalline cellulose, povidone and sodium starch glycolate. Calendar packs of 30. Protect from light and moisture. Store at room temperature.

(Shown in Product Identification Section)

Tenormin® Ⓟ

atenolol

Beta-adrenergic Receptor Blocking Agent

AstraZeneca

Date of Preparation: June 18, 1993
Date of Revision: June 13, 2008

PHARMACOLOGY: Atenolol is a β_1-selective, β-adrenergic blocking agent, devoid of membrane stabilizing or intrinsic sympathomimetic (partial agonist) activities. It is a racemic mixture and the β_1-properties reside in the S(-) enantiomer. β_1-selectivity decreases with increasing dose.

The mechanism of the antihypertensive effect has not been established. Among the factors that may be involved are: competitive ability to antagonize catecholamine-induced tachycardia at the β-receptor sites in the heart, thus decreasing cardiac output; inhibition of renin release by the kidneys; inhibition of the vasomotor centres.

The mechanism of the antianginal effect is also uncertain. An important factor may be the reduction of myocardial oxygen requirements by blocking catecholamine-induced increases in heart rate, systolic blood pressure, and the velocity and extent of myocardial contraction.

In man atenolol reduces both isoproterenol- and exercise-induced increases in heart rate over the dose range of 50 to 200 mg. At an oral dose of 100 mg the β_1-blocking effects persist for at least 24 hours; the reduction in exercise-induced heart rate increase being about 32% and 13%, 2 and 24 hours after dosing, respectively. The logarithm of the plasma atenolol level correlates with the degree of β_1-blockade but not with the antihypertensive effect.

Pharmacokinetics: Approximately 40 to 50% of an oral dose of atenolol is absorbed from the gastrointestinal tract, the remainder being excreted unchanged in the feces. Peak plasma concentrations occur 2 to 4 hours after dosing and are subject to a 4-fold variability. The plasma levels are proportional to dose over the range 50 to 400 mg and 6 to 16% of atenolol is bound to plasma proteins. The mean peak plasma concentrations of atenolol were approximately 300 and 700 ng/mL following 50 and 100 mg, respectively. The plasma half-life is approximately 6 to 7 hours. Atenolol is extensively distributed to extravascular tissues, but only a small amount is found in the CNS.

There is no significant hepatic metabolism of atenolol in man and more than 90% of the absorbed dose reaches the systemic circulation unaltered. Small quantities of a hydroxy metabolite and a glucuronide are produced but neither has major pharmacological activity. As a consequence no accumulation occurs in patients with liver disease and no dosage adjustment is required. Approximately 47% and 53% of the oral dose is eliminated in the urine and feces, respectively. Recovery is complete after 72 hours.

Atenolol is primarily eliminated by the kidney, predominantly by glomerular filtration. The normal elimination half-life may increase in severe renal impairment but no significant accumulation occurs in patients who have creatinine clearance greater than 35 mL/min. The oral dose should be reduced in patients with a creatinine clearance less than 35 mL/min (see Dosage).

Following i.v. administration, peak plasma levels were reached within 5 minutes. Declines from peak plasma levels are rapid (5- to 10-fold) during the first 7 hours; thereafter, plasma levels decay with a half-life similar to that of orally administered drug. Over 85% of an i.v. dose is excreted in urine within 24 hours.

Atenolol is excreted in human breast milk and crosses the placental barrier—the maternal to cord blood ratio being about unity.

INDICATIONS: Hypertension: In patients with mild or moderate hypertension. It is usually used in combination with other drugs, particularly a thiazide diuretic. However, it may be tried alone as an initial agent in those patients in whom, in the judgement of the physician, treatment should be started with a β-blocker rather than a diuretic. Atenolol may be used in combination with diuretics and/or vasodilators to treat severe hypertension.

The combination of atenolol with a diuretic or peripheral vasodilator has been found to be compatible. Limited experience with other antihypertensive agents has not shown evidence of incompatibility with atenolol.

Atenolol is not recommended for the emergency treatment of hypertensive crises.

Angina Pectoris: In the long-term management of patients with angina pectoris due to ischemic heart disease.

CONTRAINDICATIONS: Sinus bradycardia, or bradycardia of other origin; second and third degree AV block; sick sinus syndrome; right ventricular failure secondary to pulmonary hypertension; uncontrolled heart failure; cardiogenic shock; hypotension; severe peripheral arterial disorders; anesthesia with agents that produce myocardial depression; pheochromocytoma, in the absence of α-blockade; metabolic acidosis; known hypersensitivity to the product.

WARNINGS: Cardiac Failure: Special caution should be exercised when administering atenolol to patients with a history of heart failure. Sympathetic stimulation is a vital component supporting circulatory function in congestive heart failure and inhibition with β-blockade always carries the potential hazard of further depressing myocardial contractility and precipitating cardiac failure. Atenolol acts selectively without abolishing the inotropic action of digitalis on the heart muscle. However, the positive inotropic action of digitalis may be reduced by the negative inotropic effect of atenolol when the two drugs are used concomitantly. The effects of β-blockers and digitalis are additive in depressing AV conduction. In patients without a history of cardiac failure, continued depression of the myocardium over a period of time can, in some cases, lead to cardiac failure. Therefore, at the first sign or symptom of impending cardiac failure, patients should be fully digitalized and/or given a diuretic and the response observed closely. If cardiac failure continues, despite adequate digitalization and diuretic therapy, atenolol therapy should be immediately withdrawn.

Abrupt Cessation of Therapy: Patients with angina should be warned against abrupt discontinuation of atenolol. There have been reports of severe exacerbation of angina and of myocardial infarction or ventricular arrhythmias occurring in patients with angina pectoris, following abrupt discontinuation of β-blocker therapy. The last two complications may occur with or without preceding exacerbation of angina pectoris. Therefore, when discontinuation of atenolol is planned in patients with angina pectoris, the dosage should be gradually reduced over a period of about 2 weeks and the patient should be carefully observed and advised to limit physical activity to a minimum. The same frequency of administration should be maintained. In situations of greater urgency, atenolol should be discontinued stepwise over a shorter time and under closer observation. If angina markedly worsens or acute coronary insufficiency develops, it is recommended that treatment with atenolol be reinstituted promptly, at least temporarily.

Oculomucocutaneous Syndrome: Various skin rashes and conjunctival xerosis have been reported with β-blockers, including atenolol. A severe syndrome (oculomucocutaneous syndrome) whose signs include conjunctivitis sicca and psoriasiform rashes, otitis, and sclerosing serositis has occurred with the chronic use of one β-adrenergic blocking agent (practolol). This syndrome has not been observed with atenolol or any other such agent. However, physicians should be alert to the possibility of such reactions and should discontinue treatment in the event that they occur.

Prinzmetal's Angina: Atenolol may increase the number and duration of angina attacks in patients with Prinzmetal's angina due to unopposed α-receptor mediated coronary artery vasoconstriction. Atenolol, therefore, should only be used in these patients with the utmost care.

Sinus Bradycardia: Severe sinus bradycardia may occur with the use of atenolol from unopposed vagal activity remaining after blockade of β_1-adrenergic receptors; in such cases, dosage should be reduced.

Thyrotoxicosis: In patients with thyrotoxicosis, possible deleterious effects from long-term use of atenolol have not been adequately appraised. β-blockade may mask the clinical signs of continuing hyperthyroidism or its complications and give a false impression of improvement. Therefore, abrupt withdrawal of atenolol may be followed by an exacerbation of the symptoms of hyperthyroidism, including thyroid storm.

Pregnancy: Atenolol can cause fetal harm when administered to a pregnant woman. Atenolol crosses the placental barrier and appears in the cord blood.

No studies have been performed on the use of atenolol in the first trimester and the possibility of fetal injury cannot be excluded. Administration of atenolol, starting in the second trimester of pregnancy, has been associated with the birth of infants that are small for gestational age.

Studies in humans have shown that transplacental passage of atenolol does occur in pregnant women, with fetal drug serum levels equal to those of the mother. In a limited number of patients who were given the drug during the last trimester of pregnancy, low birth weight, neonatal hypoglycemia, bradycardia in the fetus/newborn, and placental insufficiency were observed.

Neonates born to mothers who are receiving atenolol at parturition or breast-feeding may be at risk for hypoglycemia and bradycardia. Caution should be exercised when atenolol is administered during pregnancy or to a woman who is breast-feeding (see Precautions, Lactation).

Atenolol has been shown to produce a dose-related increase in embryo/fetal resorptions in rats at doses equal to or greater than 50 mg/kg/day or 25 or more times the maximum recommended human dose.

PRECAUTIONS: Bronchospastic Disorders: Patients with bronchospastic diseases should, in general, not receive β-blockers. Due to the relative β_1-selectivity of atenolol, atenolol may be used with caution in patients with bronchospastic disease who do not respond to, or cannot tolerate, other antihypertensive treatment. Since β_1-selectivity is not absolute, a β_2-stimulating agent should be administered concomitantly, and the lowest possible dose of atenolol should be used. Despite these precautions, the respiratory status of some patients may worsen, and, in such cases, atenolol should be withdrawn.

First Degree Heart Block: Due to its negative effect on A-V conduction time, atenolol should be used with caution in patients with first degree block.

Peripheral Arterial Circulatory Disorders: Atenolol may aggravate less severe peripheral arterial circulatory disorders (see Contraindications).

Anaphylaxis—Epinephrine and β-blockers: There may be increased difficulty in treating an allergic type reaction in patients on β-blockers. In these patients, the reaction may be more severe due to pharmacologic effects of β-blockers and problems with fluid changes. Epinephrine should be administered with caution since it may not have its usual effects in the treatment of anaphylaxis. On the one hand, larger doses of epinephrine may be needed to overcome the bronchospasm, while on the other, these doses can be associated with excessive α-adrenergic stimulation with consequent hypertension, reflex bradycardia and heart block and possible potentiation of bronchospasm. Alternatives to the use of large doses of epinephrine include vigorous supportive care such as fluids and the use of β_2-agonists including parenteral salbutamol or isoproterenol to overcome bronchospasm, and norepinephrine to overcome hypotension.

Diabetes and Patients Subject to Hypoglycemia: Atenolol should be administered with caution to patients subject to spontaneous hypoglycemia, or to diabetic patients (especially those with labile diabetes) who are receiving insulin or oral hypoglycemic agents. β-adrenergic blockers may mask the premonitory signs (e.g., tachycardia) and symptoms of acute hypoglycemia.

Impaired Renal Function: Atenolol should be used with caution in patients with impaired renal function (see Dosage).

When renal function is impaired, clearance of atenolol is closely related to the glomerular filtration rate; however, significant accumulation does not occur until the creatinine clearance falls below 35 mL/min/1.73 m².

Elective or Emergency Surgery: It is not advisable to withdraw β-adrenoceptor blocking drugs prior to surgery in the majority of patients. However, care should be taken when using atenolol with anesthetic agents such as those which may depress the myocardium. Vagal dominance, if it occurs, may be corrected with atropine (1 to 2 mg i.v.).

Some patients receiving β-adrenergic blocking agents have been subject to protracted severe hypotension during anesthesia. Difficulty in restarting and maintaining the heartbeat has also been reported.

In emergency surgery, since atenolol is a competitive inhibitor of β-adrenergic receptor agonists, its effects may be reversed, if necessary, by sufficient doses of such agonists as isoproterenol or norepinephrine.

Ethnic Populations: Atenolol appears to be effective and well-tolerated in most ethnic populations, although the responses may be less in black patients than in Caucasians.

Lactation: In humans, there is a significant accumulation of atenolol in the breast milk of lactating women. Neonates born to mothers who are breastfeeding may be at risk for hypoglycemia and bradycardia. If the use of atenolol is considered essential, then mothers should stop nursing.

Children: There is no experience with atenolol in the treatment of pediatric age groups.

Occupational Hazards: Activities Requiring Mental Alertness: Use of atenolol is unlikely to result in any impairment of the ability of patients to drive or operate machinery. However, it should be taken into account that dizziness or fatigue may occur.

Geriatrics: Clinical studies of atenolol did not include sufficient numbers of subjects aged 65 and over to determine whether they respond differently from younger subjects. Other reported clinical experience has not identified differences in responses between elderly and younger patients. In general, dose selection for an elderly patient should be cautious, usually starting at the low end of the dosing range, reflecting the greater frequency of decreased hepatic renal, or cardiac function, and concomitant diseases or other drug therapy.

Drug Interactions: Clonidine: β-blockers may exacerbate the rebound hypertension which can follow the withdrawal of clonidine. If the two drugs are coadministered, the β-blocker should be withdrawn several days before discontinuing clonidine. If replacing clonidine by β-blocker therapy, the introduction of β-blockers should be delayed for several days after clonidine administration has stopped (see also prescribing information for clonidine).

Reserpine or Guanethidine: Patients receiving catecholamine-depleting drugs, such as reserpine or guanethidine, should be closely monitored because the added β-adrenergic blocking action of atenolol may produce an excessive reduction of sympathetic activity. Atenolol should not be combined with other β-blockers.

Antiarrhythmic Agents: Class I antiarrhythmic drugs (e.g. disopyramide) and amiodarone may have potentiating effect on atrial-conduction time and induce negative inotropic effect.

Calcium Channel Blockers: Combined use of β-blockers and calcium channel blockers with negative inotropic effects can lead to prolongation of S-A and A-V conduction, particularly in patients with impaired ventricular function, conduction abnormalities, or diminished cardiac output. This may result in severe hypotension, bradycardia and cardiac failure. Concomitant therapy with dihydropyridines, e.g., nifedipine, may increase the risk of hypotension, and cardiac failure may occur in patients with latent cardiac insufficiency.

Digitalis Glycosides: Digitalis glycosides may potentiate the bradycardia of β_1-blockade.

Nonsteroidal Anti-inflammatory Agents: The concomitant use of nonsteroidal anti-inflammatory agents may blunt the antihypertensive effects of β-blockers.

Anesthetic Agents: Anesthetics can produce a hypotensive state with associated reflex tachycardia. Since β-blockade will inhibit reflex tachycardia, the hypotensive potential of anesthetic agents is increased with concomitant use of atenolol. The anesthetist should be informed and the choice of anesthetic should be an agent with as little negative inotropic activity as possible (Contraindications and Precautions, Elective or Emergency Surgery).

ADVERSE EFFECTS: The most serious adverse reactions encountered are congestive heart failure, AV block and bronchospasm. Bronchospasm may occur in patients with bronchial asthma or a history of asthmatic complaints.

The most common adverse reactions reported in clinical trials with oral Tenormin in 2500 patients are bradycardia (3%), dizziness (3%), vertigo (2%), fatigue (3%), diarrhea (2%) and nausea (3%).

Adverse reactions occurring with an incidence of less than 1%, grouped by system, are as follows:

Cardiovascular: heart failure deterioration (see Warnings), heart block, palpitations, lengthening of PR interval, chest pain, lightheadedness, postural hypotension which may be associated with syncope, Raynaud's phenomenon, intermittent claudication, or worsening of pre-existing intermittent claudication, leg pain and cold extremities, edema.

Respiratory: dyspnea, wheeziness, cough, bronchospasm.

Central Nervous System: faintness, ataxia, tiredness, lethargy, nervousness, depression, drowsiness, vivid dreams, insomnia, paresthesia, headache, tinnitus, mood changes, visual disturbances, psychoses and hallucinations.

Gastrointestinal: constipation, anorexia, abdominal discomfort, indigestion.

Miscellaneous: skin rash, itchy and/or dry eyes, psoriasiform skin reactions, exacerbation of psoriasis, decreased exercise tolerance, alopecia, epistaxis, flushes, impotence, decreased libido, sweating, general body aches, thrombocytopenia and purpura.

Postmarketing Experience: During the postmarketing experience with Tenormin, cold extremities, gastrointestinal disturbances and fatigue were commonly reported. The following have been reported in temporal relationship to the use of the drug: elevated liver enzymes and/or bilirubin, headache, confusion, nightmares, impotence, Peyronie's disease, psoriasiform rash or exacerbation of psoriasis, purpura, reversible alopecia and thrombocytopenia. Rare cases of hepatic toxicity including intrahepatic cholestasis have been reported. Tenormin, like other β-blockers, has been associated with the development of antinuclear antibodies (ANA) and lupus syndrome.

In a long-term, well-controlled trial of 1627 elderly patients with systolic hypertension, the incidence of dry mouth was significantly higher in patients taking atenolol (12.2%).

Potential Adverse Reactions: The following adverse reactions have occurred with other β-blockers but have not been reported with atenolol:

Cardiovascular: pulmonary edema, cardiac enlargement, hot flushes and sinus arrest.

Central Nervous System: aggressiveness, anxiety, short-term memory loss, and emotional lability with slightly clouded sensorium.

Allergic: laryngospasm, status asthmaticus and fever combined with aching and sore throat.

Dermatological: exfoliative dermatitis.

Ophthalmological: blurred vision, burning, and grittiness.

Hematological: agranulocytosis.

Gastrointestinal: mesenteric arterial thrombosis and ischemic colitis.

OVERDOSE:

Symptoms: Limited information is available with regard to overdosage with atenolol in humans. Overdosage with atenolol has been reported with patients surviving acute doses as high as 5 g. One death was reported in a man who may have taken as much as 10 g acutely.

The predominant symptoms reported following atenolol overdosage are lethargy, disorder of respiratory drive, wheezing, sinus pause and bradycardia. Additionally, common effects associated with overdosage of any β-adrenergic blocking agent are congestive heart failure, hypotension, bronchospasm and/or hypoglycemia.

Treatment: Treatment should be symptomatic and supportive and directed to the removal of any unabsorbed drug by induced emesis, or administration of activated charcoal. Atenolol can be removed from the general circulation by hemodialysis. Further consideration should be given to dehydration, electrolyte imbalance and hypotension by established procedures.

Other treatment modalities should be employed at the physician's discretion and may include:

Bradycardia: Atropine 1-2 mg intravenously. If there is no response to vagal blockade, give isoproterenol cautiously. In refractory cases, a transvenous cardiac pacemaker may be indicated. Glucagon in a 10 mg intravenous bolus has been reported to be useful. If required, this may be repeated or followed by an intravenous infusion of glucagon 1-10 mg/h depending on response. If no response to glucagon occurs or if glucagon is unavailable, a beta-adrenoceptor stimulant such as dobutamine 2.5 to 10 µg/kg/minute by intravenous infusion or isoproterenol 10 to 25 µg given as an infusion at a rate not exceeding 5 µg/minute may be given, although larger doses may be required.

Heart Block (second or third degree): Isoproterenol, or transvenous pacemaker.

Congestive Heart Failure: Digitalize the patient and administer a diuretic. Glucagon has been reported to be useful.

Hypotension: Vasopressors such as dopamine or norepinephrine. Monitor blood pressure continuously.

Bronchospasm: A β_2-stimulant such as isoproterenol or terbutaline and/or intravenous aminophylline.

Hypoglycemia: Intravenous glucose.

Based on the severity of symptoms, management may require intensive support care and facilities for applying cardiac and respiratory support.

For management of a suspected drug overdose, CPhA recommends that you contact your **regional Poison Control Centre**. See the *CPS* Directory section for a list of Poison Control Centres.

DOSAGE: Hypertension: Atenolol is usually used in conjunction with other antihypertensive agents, particularly a thiazide diuretic, but may be used alone (see Indications).

The dose of atenolol should be administered in accordance with individual patient's needs.

The following guidelines are recommended: Initial dose: 50 mg administered as 1 tablet a day either added to diuretic therapy or alone. The full effect of this dose will usually be seen within 1 to 2 weeks. If an adequate response is not achieved, the dose should be increased to atenolol 100 mg once daily. Increasing the dose beyond 100 mg a day is unlikely to produce any further benefit.

If further lowering of the blood pressure is required, another antihypertensive agent should be added to the regimen.

Angina Pectoris: Initial dose: 50 mg given as 1 tablet a day. The full effect of this dose will usually be seen within 1 to 2 weeks. If an optimal response is not achieved within 1 week, the dosage should be increased to 100 mg given as 1 tablet a day or 50 mg twice daily. Some patients may require a dosage of 200 mg a day for optimal effect.

Renal Impairment: Since atenolol is eliminated predominantly via the kidneys, dosage should be adjusted in patients with severe renal impairment. Significant accumulation of atenolol occurs when creatinine clearance falls below 35 mL/min/1.73 m² (normal range is 100 to 150 mL/min/1.73 m²).

The maximum dosages recommended for patients with renal impairment are found in Table 1.

Table 1: Tenormin

Dosage in Renal Impairment

Creatinine Clearance (mL/min/1.73 m²)	Atenolol Elimination Half-life (h)	Maximum Dosage
15–35	16–27	50 mg daily
<15	>27	50 mg every other day

Patients on hemodialysis should be given 50 mg after each dialysis; this should be done under hospital supervision as marked falls in blood pressure can occur.

Dosage requirements may be reduced in the elderly, especially in patients with impaired renal function.

SUPPLIED: 50 mg: Each scored, white to off-white, biconvex, film-coated tablet, embossed with TENORMIN 50 on one face and scored on the reverse, contains: atenolol 50 mg. Nonmedicinal ingredients: gelatin, glycerol, heavy magnesium carbonate, hydroxypropyl methylcellulose, magnesium stearate, maize starch, sodium lauryl sulfate and titanium dioxide. Calendar packs of 30.

100 mg: Each scored, white to off-white, biconvex, film-coated tablet, embossed with TENORMIN on one face and scored on the reverse, contains: atenolol 100 mg. Nonmedicinal ingredients: gelatin, glycerol, heavy magnesium carbonate, hydroxypropyl methylcellulose, magnesium stearate, maize starch, sodium lauryl sulfate and titanium dioxide. Calendar packs of 30.

Store between 15 and 25°C. Protect from light and moisture.

(Shown in Product Identification Section)

Terazol® Ⓟ

terconazole

Antifungal

Janssen-Ortho

PHARMACOLOGY: The exact pharmacologic mode of action of terconazole is uncertain; however, it may exert its antifungal activity by disruption of normal fungal cell membrane permeability. Terconazole exhibits fungicidal activity in vitro against the genus Candida. Both the yeast and mycelial forms of *C. albicans* are sensitive to terconazole.

Following intravaginal administration of terconazole in humans, absorption ranged from 5 to 8% in 3 hysterectomized patients and 12 to 16% in 2 nonhysterectomized subjects with tubal ligations. After single and multiple doses of terconazole 0.4% (20 mg) vaginal cream, the mean peak plasma concentration for both treatments was 0.004 μg, indicating no accumulation of terconazole following repeated intravaginal dosing.

INDICATIONS: For the local treatment of vulvovaginal candidiasis (moniliasis). The diagnosis of monilial infection should be confirmed by microscopic examination of a KOH smear and/or by culture.

The ovules and cream may be used in pregnant patients during the second and third trimesters if the physician considers it essential to the welfare of the patient (see Precautions, Pregnancy). The therapeutic effect of terconazole is not affected by oral contraceptive usage, menstruation or previous monilial infection.

CONTRAINDICATIONS: Patients known to be hypersensitive to terconazole or to any components of the ovule or cream.

WARNINGS: None.

PRECAUTIONS: General: Terconazole cream and ovules should be discontinued and patients should not be retreated if sensitization, vulvovaginal irritation, fever, chills or flu-like symptoms are reported during use.

Photosensitivity reactions were observed in some normal volunteers following repeated dermal application of terconazole 2.0% and 0.8% creams under conditions of filtered artificial ultraviolet light. Photosensitivity reactions have not been observed in clinical trials in patients who were treated vaginally with terconazole 0.4%, 0.8% or 1.6% vaginal cream.

The base contained in the ovule formulation may interact with certain natural rubber products, such as those used in vaginal contraceptive diaphragms or condoms. Concurrent use is not recommended. The cream may be considered for use under these conditions.

If there is a lack of response to terconazole therapy, appropriate microbiological studies (standard KOH smear and/or cultures) should be repeated to confirm the diagnosis and rule out other pathogens.

Intractable candidiasis may be the presenting symptom of unrecognized diabetes mellitus. In these cases, appropriate diagnostic tests for diabetes should be done.

Children: Safety and efficacy in children have not been established.

Pregnancy: Terconazole should not be used in the first trimester of pregnancy.

In studies, over 600 pregnant patients have used terconazole during the second and third trimesters with no apparent adverse effect on the course of pregnancy. These studies have not shown increased risk of abnormalities when administered during this period.

Pregnant patients should be advised to exercise caution in the use of the vaginal applicator.

Lactation: It is not known whether terconazole is excreted in human milk. Should the decision be made to use this drug, nursing should be discontinued during therapy.

ADVERSE EFFECTS: During controlled clinical studies conducted in the U.S., 284 patients with vulvovaginal candidiasis were treated with terconazole 80 mg vaginal ovules, 521 patients were treated with terconazole 0.4% vaginal cream and 297 patients were treated with terconazole 0.8% vaginal cream.

Terazol 3 Vaginal Ovules (terconazole 80 mg): Based on comparative analyses with placebo and a standard agent, the adverse experiences considered adverse reactions most likely related to terconazole 80 mg vaginal ovules are shown in Table 1.

Table 1: Terazol

Adverse Effects—Terazol 3 Vaginal Ovules

Event	Terazol	Placebo
Headache	30.3%	20.7%
Pain (female genitalia)	4.2%	0.7%
Burning	15.2%[a]	11.2%
Body Pain	3.9%[a]	1.7%
Fever	2.8%	1.4%
Chills	1.8%	0.75%

[a] Not statistically significantly different from placebo.

The adverse drug experience on terconazole 80 mg ovules most frequently causing discontinuation was burning (2.5% vs 1.4% with placebo) and pruritus (1.8% vs 1.4% with placebo). The terconazole therapy-related dropout rate was 3.5% and the placebo therapy-related dropout rate was 2.7%.

Terazol 7 Vaginal Cream (terconazole 0.4%): Based on comparative analyses with placebo and a standard agent, the adverse experiences considered to be most likely related to terconazole 0.4% vaginal cream are shown in Table 2.

Table 2: Terazol

Adverse Effects—Terazol 7 Vaginal Cream

Event	Terazol	Placebo
Headache	26.0%	17.0%
Body Pain	2.1%	0.0%
Fever	1.75%	0.5%
Chills	0.4%	0.0%

Vulvovaginal burning (5.2%), itching (2.3%) or irritation (3.1%) occurred less frequently with terconazole 0.4% vaginal cream than with the vehicle placebo. The adverse drug experience most frequently causing discontinuation of treatment with terconazole cream was vulvovaginal itching (0.6%) which was lower than the incidence for placebo (0.9%). The terconazole therapy and the placebo therapy-related dropout rate was 1.9%.

Terazol 3 Vaginal Cream (terconazole 0.8%): Based on comparative analyses with placebo and a standard agent, the only adverse experiences considered adverse reactions to terconazole 0.8% vaginal cream are shown in Table 3.

Table 3: Terazol

Adverse Effects—Terazol 3 Vaginal Cream

Event	Terazol	Placebo
Headache	21.0%	16.0%
Dysmenorrhea	6.0%	2.0%

Fever (1.0% vs. 0.3% with placebo) has been reported. The therapy-related dropout rate was 2.0%. The adverse drug experience on terconazole 0.8% most frequently causing discontinuation was vulvovaginal itching (0.7%), which was similar to the incidence for placebo (0.3%).

OVERDOSE:

Overdose of terconazole in humans has not been reported to date.

> For management of a suspected drug overdose, CPhA recommends that you contact your **regional Poison Control Centre**. See the *CPS* Directory section for a list of Poison Control Centres.

DOSAGE: **Terazol 3 Vaginal Ovules:** 1 ovule is administered intravaginally once daily at bedtime for 3 consecutive days.

Terazol 7 Vaginal Cream: One applicatorful (5 g) of vaginal cream (20 mg terconazole) is administered intravaginally once daily at bedtime for 7 consecutive days. In addition, a thin layer of vaginal cream (0.4% terconazole) is applied for 7 consecutive days directly to the vulva and massaged in gently.

Terazol 3 Vaginal Cream: One applicatorful (5 g) of vaginal cream (40 mg terconazole) is administered intravaginally once daily at bedtime for 3 consecutive days. In addition, a thin layer of vaginal cream (0.8% terconazole) is applied for 3 consecutive days directly to the vulva and massaged in gently.

Terazol 3 Dual-Pak Package: One vaginal ovule is administered intravaginally once daily at bedtime for 3 consecutive days. In addition, a thin layer of vaginal cream (0.8% terconazole) is applied for 3 consecutive days directly to the vulva and massaged in gently.

Before prescribing another course of therapy of terconazole, the diagnosis of monilial infection should be confirmed by microscopic examination of a KOH smear and/or by culture.

Intractable candidiasis may be the presenting symptom of unrecognized diabetes mellitus. In these cases appropriate diagnostic tests for diabetes should be done. The therapeutic effect of terconazole products is not affected by oral contraceptive usage or menstruation.

INFORMATION FOR THE PATIENT: Published in e-CPS, available by subscription at www.e-cps.ca.

SUPPLIED: Terazol 3 Vaginal Ovules: Each elliptically-shaped, white to off-white, 2.5 g ovule contains: terconazole 80 mg. Nonmedicinal ingredients: butylated hydroxyanisole and hydrogenated vegetable oils. Packages of 3 with an Ortho vaginal applicator.

Terazol 7 Vaginal Cream: Each g of white to off-white, water washable cream contains: terconazole 0.4%. Nonmedicinal ingredients: butylated hydroxyanisole, cetyl alcohol, isopropyl myristate, polysorbate 60, polysorbate 80, propylene glycol, purified water and stearyl alcohol. Tubes of 45 g with an Ortho vaginal applicator.

Terazol 3 Vaginal Cream: Each g of white to off-white, water washable cream contains: terconazole 0.8%. Nonmedicinal ingredients: butylated hydroxyanisole, cetyl alcohol, isopropyl myristate, polysorbate 60, polysorbate 80, propylene glycol, purified water and stearyl alcohol. Tubes of 20 g with an Ortho vaginal applicator.

Terazol 3 Dual-Pack Package: 3 Terazol 3 vaginal ovules, an Ortho vaginal applicator and a 9 g tube of Terazol 3 vaginal cream.

Store at controlled room temperature (15 to 30°C).

(Shown in Product Identification Section)

Tersaseptic®

triclosan

Antibacterial Cleanser

Stiefel, a GSK company

SUPPLIED: Each bottle contains: triclosan 0.5%. Nonmedicinal ingredients: citric acid, edetate disodium, fragrance #6218-1, glycol ether DE, lauramide DEA, PEG 600 distearate, purified water, sodium chloride and triethanolamine lauryl sulfate. Bottles of 200 and 450 mL.

Tersa-Tar®

tar distillate

Psoriasis—Seborrhea Therapy

Stiefel, a GSK company

SUPPLIED: Tersa-Tar: Each mL of shampoo contains: tar distillate "Doak" 3% in a soapless alkaline free solvent and emulsifying base. Nonmedicinal ingredients: D&C Yellow #8, edetate disodium, fragrance #6218-1, glycol ether DE, isopropyl alcohol, lauramide DEA, methylparaben, PEG 600 distearate, phosphoric acid 85%, propylparaben, purified water and triethanolamine lauryl sulfate. Bottles of 150 and 450 mL.

Tersa-Tar Mild: Each mL of shampoo contains: tar distillate "Doak" 1% in a soapless alkaline free solvent and emulsifying base with protein and an oil free conditioner. Nonmedicinal ingredients: citric acid, edetate disodium, fragrance A-833, glycol ether DE, hydrolysed collagen, isopropyl alcohol, lauramide DEA, methylparaben, PEG 600 distearate, polyquaternium-10, purified water, quaternium-15 and triethanolamine lauryl sulfate. Bottles of 150 and 450 mL.

Testim® 1%

testosterone

Androgens

Paladin

Date of Preparation: July 24, 2007
Date of Revision: October 1, 2009

SUMMARY PRODUCT INFORMATION:

Route of Administration	Dosage Form/ Strength	Clinically Relevant Nonmedicinal Ingredients
Topical	Gel 1%	Ethanol For a complete listing see Dosage Forms, Composition and Packaging.

INDICATIONS AND CLINICAL USE: Testim 1% (testosterone gel) is indicated for testosterone replacement therapy in adult males for conditions associated with a deficiency or absence of endogenous testosterone.

Testim 1% (testosterone gel) should not be used to treat non-specific symptoms suggestive of hypogonadism if testosterone deficiency has not been demonstrated and if other etiologies responsible for the symptoms have not been excluded. Testosterone deficiency should be clearly demonstrated by clinical features and confirmed by two separate validated biochemical assays (morning testosterone) before initiating therapy with any testosterone replacement, including Testim 1% treatment.

Geriatrics (>65 years of age): There are limited controlled clinical study data supporting the use of Testim 1% in the geriatric population (see Warnings and Precautions).

Pediatrics (<18 years of age): Testim 1% is not indicated for use in children <18 years of age since safety and efficacy have not been established in this patient population (see Warnings and Precautions, Special Populations).

CONTRAINDICATIONS:

- Testim 1% is not indicated for use in women.
- **Pregnant and nursing women should avoid skin contact with Testim 1% application sites on men. Testosterone may cause fetal harm. Testosterone exposure during pregnancy has been reported to be associated with fetal abnormalities (see Warnings and Precautions, Potential for Secondary Exposure to Testosterone and Special Populations).** In the event that unwashed or unclothed skin to which Testim 1% has been applied or clothing exposed to Testim 1% comes in direct contact with the skin of a pregnant or nursing woman, the general area of contact on the woman should be immediately washed with soap and water.
- Androgens are contraindicated in men with known or suspected carcinoma of the prostate or breast.
- Testim 1% should not be used in patients with known hypersensitivity to any of its ingredients, including testosterone that is chemically synthesized from soy. For a complete listing, see Dosage Forms, Composition and Packaging.

WARNINGS AND PRECAUTIONS:

Secondary Exposure to Testosterone
- Virilization has been reported in children who were secondarily exposed to testosterone gel, including Testim 1%.
- Children should avoid contact with unwashed or unclothed application sites in men using Testim 1%.
- Healthcare providers should advise patients to strictly adhere to recommended instructions for use.

(See Warnings and Precautions, Potential for Secondary Exposure to Testosterone. Strict adherence to the following precautions is advised in order to minimize the potential for secondary exposure to testosterone from skin treated with Testim 1%).

Potential for Secondary Exposure to Testosterone: Secondary exposure to testosterone in children and women can occur with testosterone gel use in men. Cases of secondary exposure resulting in virilization of children have been reported in postmarketing surveillance of testosterone-containing gel products. Signs and symptoms have included enlargement of the penis or clitoris, development of pubic hair, increased erections and libido, aggressive behavior, and advanced bone age. In most cases, these signs and symptoms regressed with removal of the exposure to testosterone. In a few cases, however, enlarged genitalia did not fully return to age-appropriate normal size, and bone age remained modestly greater than chronological age. The risk of transfer was increased in some of these cases by not adhering to precautions for the appropriate use of the testosterone gel product.

Inappropriate changes in genital size or development of pubic hair or libido in children, or changes in body hair distribution, significant increase in acne, or other signs of virilization in adult women should be brought to the attention of a physician, and the possibility of secondary exposure to testosterone gel should also be brought to the attention of a physician. Testosterone gel should be promptly discontinued until the cause of virilisation has been identified.

Strict adherence to the following precautions is advised in order to minimize the potential for secondary exposure to testosterone from Testim-treated skin:
- Children and women should avoid contact with Testim application sites on the skin of men using Testim.
- Testim should only be applied to the shoulders and/or upper (area of application should be limited to the area that will be covered by the patient's short sleeve t-shirt).
- Patients should wash their hands thoroughly and immediately with soap and water after application of Testim 1%. Topically applied testosterone can be removed from the skin surface by thorough washing with soap and water.
- Patients should cover the application site(s) with clothing (e.g., a shirt) after the gel has dried.
- Direct skin-to-skin contact should be avoided immediately following administration of a topical testosterone product. Prior to any situation in which skin-to-skin contact is anticipated, patients should wash the application site(s) thoroughly with soap and water to remove any testosterone residue.
- In the event that unwashed or unclothed skin to which Testim has been applied or the testosterone gel user's shirts and/or other fabrics (such as towels and sheets) comes in direct contact with the skin of another person, the general area of contact on the other person should be washed with soap and water as soon as possible. Studies show that residual testosterone is removed from the skin surface by washing with soap and water.

General: There is very limited data from clinical trials with Testim 1% in the geriatric male (>65 years of age) to support the efficacy and safety of prolonged use. Impacts to prostate and cardiovascular event rates and patient important outcomes are unknown.

If testosterone deficiency has not been established, testosterone replacement therapy should not be used to attempt to improve body composition, bone and muscle mass, increase lean body mass and decrease total fat mass. Efficacy and safety have not been established. Serious long term deleterious health issues may arise.

Testosterone replacement therapy has not been shown to be safe and effective for the enhancement of athletic performance. Because of the potential risk of serious adverse health effects, this drug should not be used for such purpose.

If testosterone deficiency has not been established, testosterone replacement therapy should not be used for the treatment of sexual dysfunction.

Testosterone replacement therapy is not a treatment for male infertility.

Gels are flammable. Following application of Testim 1% allow gel to dry completely before smoking or going near an open flame.

Special Populations: Pregnant Women: Pregnant and nursing women should avoid skin contact with Testim 1% application sites on men. Testosterone may cause fetal harm. Testosterone exposure during pregnancy has been reported to be associated with fetal abnormalities. In the event that unwashed or unclothed skin to which Testim 1% has been applied or clothing exposed to Testim 1% comes in direct contact with the skin of a pregnant or nursing woman, the general area of contact on the woman should be immediately washed with soap and water (see Contraindications).

Nursing Women: See Pregnant Women.

Pediatrics (<18 years old): Testim 1% is not indicated for use in children <18 years of age since the safety and efficacy has not been established in this patient population.

Androgen therapy should be used cautiously in males with hypogonadism causing delayed puberty. Androgens can accelerate bone maturation without producing compensatory gain in linear growth. This adverse effect may result in compromised adult stature. The younger the child is the greater risk of compromising final mature height. The effect of androgens on bone maturation should be monitored closely by assessing bone age of the wrist and hand on a regular basis.

Geriatrics (>65 years of age): There are very limited controlled clinical study data supporting the use of testosterone in the geriatric population and virtually no controlled clinical studies on subjects 75 years and over.

Geriatric patients treated with androgens may be at an increased risk for the development of prostatic hyperplasia and prostatic carcinoma.

Men with benign prostatic hyperplasia (BPH) treated with androgens are at an increased risk for worsening of BPH.

Geriatric patients and other patients with clinical or demographic characteristics that are recognized to be associated with an increased risk of prostate cancer should be evaluated for the presence of prostate cancer prior to initiation of testosterone replacement therapy. In men receiving testosterone replacement therapy, surveillance for prostate cancer should be consistent with current practices for eugonadal men (see Warnings and Precautions, Carcinogenesis).

Carcinogenesis: Prostatic: Geriatric patients treated with androgens may be at an increased risk for the development of prostatic hyperplasia and prostatic carcinoma (see Special Populations, Geriatrics (>65 years of age)).

Breast: Patients using long-term androgen therapy may be at an increased risk for the development of breast cancer.

Hepatic: Prolonged use of high doses of orally active 17-alpha-alkyl androgens (e.g., methyltestosterone) has been associated with serious hepatic adverse affects (peliosis hepatis, hepatic neoplasms, cholestatic hepatitis, and jaundice). Peliosis hepatis can be a life-threatening or fatal complication. Long-term therapy with testosterone enanthate, which elevates blood levels for prolonged periods, has produced multiple hepatic adenomas. Testim 1% is not known to produce these adverse effects.

Skeletal: Patients with skeletal metastases are at a risk of exacerbating hypercalcemia/hypercalciuria with concomitant androgen therapy.

Cardiovascular: Testosterone may increase blood pressure and should be used with caution in patients with hypertension.

Edema, with or without congestive heart failure, may be a serious complication in patients with pre-existing cardiac, renal, or hepatic disease. Diuretic therapy may be required, in addition to discontinuation of the drug.

Dependence/Tolerance: Testim 1% contains testosterone, a Schedule G controlled substance as defined by the Food and Drugs Act.

Endocrine and Metabolism: Androgens have been shown to alter glucose tolerance tests. Diabetics should be followed carefully and the insulin or oral hypoglycemic dosage adjusted accordingly (see Drug-Drug Interactions).

Hypercalciuria/hypercalcemia (caused by malignant tumors) may be exacerbated by androgen treatment. Androgens should be used with caution in cancer patients at risk of hypercalcemia (and associated hypercalciuria). Regular monitoring of serum calcium concentrations is recommended in patients at risk of hypercalciuria/hypercalcemia.

Hematologic: Hemoglobin and hematocrit levels should be checked periodically (to detect polycythemia) in patients on long-term androgen therapy (See Monitoring and Laboratory Tests).

Alkylated derivatives of testosterone such as methandrostenolone, have been reported to decrease the anticoagulant requirement of patients receiving oral anticoagulants (e.g. warfarin). Patients receiving oral anticoagulants therapy require close monitoring, especially when androgens are started or stopped (see Drug-Drug Interactions).

Respiratory: The treatment of hypogonadal men with testosterone may potentiate sleep apnea, particularly for those with risk factors such as obesity or chronic lung diseases.

Sexual Function/Reproduction: Gynecomastia may develop and occasionally persist in patients being treated for hypogonadism.

Priapism or excessive sexual stimulation may develop.

Oligospermia may occur after prolonged administration or excessive dosage.

Skin: Changes in body hair distribution, significant increase in acne, or other signs of virilization of the female partner or in any person (including children) exposed to skin-to-skin contact, should be brought to the attention of a physician.

Application site reactions associated with the use of transdermal testosterone may manifest as a skin irritation.

Monitoring and Laboratory Tests: The patient should be monitored (including serum testosterone levels) on a regular basis to ensure adequate response to treatment.

Currently there is no consensus about age specific testosterone levels. The normal serum testosterone level for young eugonadal men is generally accepted to be approximately 10.4-34.6 nmol/L (300-1000 ng/dL). However, it should be taken into account that physiologically testosterone levels (mean and range) decrease with increasing age.

The following laboratory tests, performed routinely, are recommended to ensure that adverse experience is detected and addressed: hemoglobin and hematocrit levels should be checked periodically (to detect polycythemia); liver function tests; to detect hepatoxicity associated with the use of 17-alpha-alkylated androgens (e.g. methyltestosterone); prostate specific antigen (PSA), Digital Rectal Examination (DRE), especially if the patient presents with progressive difficulty with urination or a change in voiding habits; lipid profile, total cholesterol, LDL, HDL, and triglycerides; diabetics should be followed carefully and the insulin or oral hypoglycemic dosage adjusted accordingly (see Drug-Drug Interactions).

ADVERSE REACTIONS: Adverse Drug Reaction Overview: See Table 1.

Table 1: Testim 1%

Incidence of Adverse Events Most Commonly Reported

Adverse Drug Event	% Incidence
Application Site Erythema	4.1%
Increased PSA	4.3%
Increased Hematocrit	3.9%
Increased Hemoglobin	3.7%

Clinical Trial Adverse Drug Reactions: Because clinical trials are conducted under very specific conditions the adverse reaction rates observed in the clinical trials may not reflect the rates observed in practice and should not be compared to the rates in the clinical trials of another drug. Adverse drug reaction information from clinical trials is useful for identifying drug-related adverse events and for approximating rates.

Safety Profile After Short Term Exposure to Testim 1% : Two randomized controlled clinical studies of 90 days duration were conducted. In one clinical trial, hypogonadal patients were treated with either Testim 1% 50 mg or 100 mg, testosterone patch or placebo gel. In the second clinical trial, hypogonadal patients were treated with either Testim 1% 50 mg or 100 mg or testosterone patch. Patients experiencing adverse events that were possibly related to the Testim 1% that occurred in ≥1% of the patients in the Testim 1% groups and with greater incidence than in the placebo group in both controlled clinical trials are presented in Table 2.

Table 2: Testim 1%

Double-Blind Phase III Studies: Summary of the Most Frequently Reported Adverse Events (≥1% of Subjects) Judged Possibly or Probably Related to Testim 1% by the Investigator

Body/Organ System MedDRA Preferred Term	Testim 1% 50 mg (n=171) %	Testim 1% 100 mg (n=221) %	Placebo (n=99) %
General Disorders/Administration Site Disorders			
Application Site Erythema	1.2	2.3	2.0
Application Site Irritation	1.2	0.5	0
ASR NOS	1.8	0.9	1.0
Nervous System Disorders			
Headache NOS	1.2	0.5	0
Insomnia	1.2	0	0

Legend: ASR=application site reaction; NOS=not otherwise specified.

Safety Profile After Long Term Exposure to Testim 1%: An extended use program was additionally conducted in order to provide additional safety and efficacy data. Two open label, longer-term studies involved patients who had completed the randomized, controlled 90 day Phase III studies and provide additional data for up to a further 12 months of treatment.

A summary of the most frequently reported (≥1% of total) adverse events judged possibly or probably related to Testim 1% by the investigator for all Testim 1% treated subjects for a period up to 15 months is provided in Table 3.

Table 3: Testim 1%

Summary of the Most Frequently Reported (≥1% of Total) Treatment Emergent Adverse Events Judged Possibly or Probably Related to Testim 1%

Body/Organ System MedDRA Preferred Term	Testim 1% 50 mg (n=443) %	Testim 1% 100 mg (n=395) %	Total (n=517) %
General Disorders/Administration Site Disorders			
Application Site Erythema	2.5	3.0	4.1
Application Site Rash	0.5	1.8	1.7
Application Site Reaction NOS	0.7	0.5	1.0
Investigations			
PSA Increased	2.0	3.5	4.3
Hematocrit Increased	0.7	4.3	3.9
Hemoglobin Increased	0.2	4.6	3.7
Red Blood Cell Count Increased	0.2	1.3	1.2
Reproductive System and Breast Disorders			

(cont'd)

Table 3: Testim 1% *(cont'd)*

Summary of the Most Frequently Reported (≥1% of Total) Treatment Emergent Adverse Events Judged Possibly or Probably Related to Testim 1%

Body/Organ System MedDRA Preferred Term	Testim 1% 50 mg (n=443) %	Testim 1% 100 mg (n=395) %	Total (n=517) %
Benign Prostatic Hyperplasia	0.2	1.3	1.2
Skin and Subcutaneous Tissue Disorders			
Acne NOS	0.5	1.5	1.4
Vascular Disorders			
Hypertension Aggravated	0.2	1.3	1.2

Legend: NOS=not otherwise specified; PSA=prostate specific antigen.

A total of 517 subjects participated in the Phase III clinical development program for Testim 1%. Some subjects received both Testim 1% 50 mg and Testim 1% 100 mg at different times during the duration of double-blind and/or open label extension trials. Consequently, 443 subjects received Testim 1% 50 mg at least once throughout the studies, 395 subjects received Testim 1% 100 mg at least once throughout the trials and 321 subjects received both Testim 1% 50 mg and Testim 1% 100 mg at some time during the clinical trials.

Although the safety analyses show that with longer term dosing, there is an increased number of adverse drug reactions reported at an incidence of ≥1% compared to the number reported in the 90 day double blind studies, this is as expected given the longer duration of exposure to Testim 1%.

Less Common Clinical Trial Adverse Drug Reactions (<1%): Adverse events possibly or probably related to Testim 1% administration occurring in less than 1% of patients are presented in Table 4.

Table 4: Testim 1%

Adverse Drug Reactions (<1%) Grouped by Body System

Body System	Preferred Term
Blood and lymphatic system disorders	polycythemia NOS
Cardiac disorders	angina pectoris
Eye disorders	lacrimation increase
Gastrointestinal disorders	dysgeusia
General disorders and administration site conditions	application site dryness
Investigations	activated partial thromboplastin time prolonged, blood creatinine increased, blood pressure diastolic decreased, blood pressure increased, blood pressure systolic increased, hematocrit increased, hemoglobin abnormal NOS, hemoglobin increased, international normalized ratio increased, prothrombin time prolonged, spontaneous penile erection, weight increased
Metabolism and nutrition disorders	appetite disorders,
Musculoskeletal and connective tissue disorders	arthralgia, soft tissue disorder NOS
Nervous system disorders	insomnia, migraine NOS, parosmia,
Psychiatric disorders	mood swings,
Reproductive system and breast disorders	nipple disorder, nipple pain, penile pain
Skin and subcutaneous tissue disorders	dermatitis acneiform, hair growth abnormal , skin disorder NOS
Vascular disorders	hot flushes NOS

The subset analysis on effect of age (subjects in age groups 18-45, 45-65, and >65 years) confirmed that age did not affect the overall adverse event profile for Testim 1%.

An analysis of the effect of race could not be determined due to the small number of non-Caucasian patients in the clinical trials.

Abnormal Hematologic and Clinical Chemistry Findings: Hematology: The known effects of testosterone on hematocrit, hemoglobin levels and red blood cell (RBC) counts were reported in the two controlled 90 day Phase III studies with small increases in hemoglobin and hematocrit observed in all active treatment groups. Increases in hemoglobin and hematocrit were greater in a dose-dependent manner from the placebo group, to the testosterone patch group, to the Testim 1% 50 and 100 mg groups. See Table 5.

Table 5: Testim 1%

Double-Blind Phase III Studies: Percent of Subjects Having a Clinically Important Hematology Parameter—All Treated Subjects

Hematology Parameter	Testim 1% 50 mg (n=171) %	Testim 1% 100 mg (n=221) %	Placebo (n=99) %
Eosinophils ≥10%	3.1	1.4	0
Hematocrit ≥58%	0.6	2.8	1.0
Hemoglobin ≥190 g/L	0.6	2.3	1.0
RBC ≥5.9×10[12] /L	4.9	7.4	1.0

Legend: RBC=red blood cell.

The long term safety data presented in Table 6 show that clinically important eosinophils values (≥10%) and hemoglobin values (≥190 g/L) were no more frequently reported in the long term data than in the short term double blind studies. Hematocrit values (≥58%) were most frequently reported during the >12 months exposure period (3.2%, seven subjects). A total of 8.1% of the subjects reported RBC values ≥5.9×10^{12}/L during the 3-6 months exposure period.

Table 6: Testim 1%

Long Term Studies with Testim 1%: Percent of Subjects Having a Clinically Important Hematology Parameter—All Treated Subjects

Hematology Parameter	Study Months				
	0–3 months (N=498) %	3–6 months (N=360) %	6–9 months (N=258) %	9–12 months (N=233) %	>12 months (N=220) %
Eosinophils ≥10%	2.2	1.7	0	1.3	0
Hematocrit ≥58%	1.2	1.1	1.2	0.9	3.2
Hemoglobin ≥190 g/L	1.2	1.4	1.2	0.9	0.5
RBC ≥5.9×10[12] /L	5.4	8.1	2.3	4.3	2.7

Legend: RBC=red blood cell.

Clinical Chemistry: In the two 90-day double blind Phase III studies, only three parameters (GGT, fasting serum glucose, and BUN) had an incidence of ≥1% of subjects with clinically important values for the Testim 1% groups. Additionally, mean total serum cholesterol and HDL-C were decreased for all treatment groups at the final evaluation in these studies. The changes were dose dependent for the Testim 1% 50 mg/day and 100 mg/day groups. For mean total serum cholesterol, the Testim 1% 100 mg group had a decrease of 0.34 mmol/L, while the Testim 1% 50 mg group had a decrease of 0.08 mmol/L. For HDL-C, the reduction for the Testim 1% 100 mg and 50 mg groups was 0.098 mmol/L and 0.135 mmol/L respectively. See Table 7.

Table 7: Testim 1%

Double-Blind Phase III Studies: Percent of Subjects Having a Clinically Important Chemistry Parameter—All Treated Subjects

Chemistry Parameter	Testim 1% 50 mg (n=171) %	Testim 1% 100 mg (n=221) %	Placebo (n=99) %
Gamma GT >3×ULN	0.6	1.4	0
BUN ≥10.7 mmol/L	3.6	2.8	5.1
BUN ≤2.86 mmol/L	1.8	4.2	1.0
Serum Glucose ≥16.7 mmol/L	0.6	1.9	1.0

Legend: ULN=Upper limit normal; BUN=blood urea nitrogen.

In long term studies, similar responses were seen with respect to clinically important values for GGT, serum glucose and BUN. In addition, in the 0-3 months exposure period to Testim 1%, a total of 2.6% of subjects had cholesterol levels greater than or equal to 7.77 mmol/L, 4.3% had LDL cholesterol levels greater than or equal to 5.05 mmol/L, 9.4% had triglycerides levels greater than or equal to 4.52 mmol/L, and 1.4% had HDL cholesterol levels less than or equal to 0.65 mmol/L. See Table 8.

Table 8: Testim 1%

Long Term Studies with Testim 1%: Percent of Subjects Having a Clinically Important Chemistry Parameter—All Treated Subjects

Hematology Parameter	Study Months				
	0–3 months (N=502) %	3–6 months (N=364) %	6–9 months (N=264) %	9–12 months (N=237) %	>12 months (N=225) %
Gamma GT >3×ULN	0.6	0.5	0.4	0.4	0.9
BUN ≥10.7 mmol/L	2.6	1.6	0.4	2.1	1.3
BUN ≤2.86 mmol/L	2.6	1.4	0.4	0.4	0
Serum Glucose ≥16.7 mmol/L	1.4	0.5	0	0.4	0
Cholesterol ≥7.77 mmol/L	2.6	0.5	0	0	0
LDL Cholesterol ≥5.05 mmol/L	4.3	1.4	0	0.4	0.9
HDL Cholesterol ≤0.65 mmol/L	1.4	1.6	0.4	0.4	0
Triglycerides ≥4.52 mmol/L	9.4	3.0	1.5	0.8	0.4

Post-Market Adverse Drug Reactions: Secondary Exposure to Testosterone in Children: Cases of secondary exposure to testosterone resulting in virilization of children have been reported in postmarketing surveillance of testosterone gel products. Signs and symptoms of these reported cases have included enlargement of the clitoris (with surgical intervention) or of the penis, premature development of pubic hair, increased erections and libido, aggressive behavior, and advanced bone age. In most cases with a reported outcome, these signs and symptoms were reported to have regressed with removal of the testosterone gel exposure. In a few cases, however, enlarged genitalia did not fully return to age-appropriate normal size, and bone age remained modestly greater than chronological age. In some of the cases, direct contact with the sites of application on the skin of men using testosterone gel was reported. In at least one reported case, the reporter considered the possibility of secondary exposure from items such as the testosterone gel user's shirts and/or other fabrics, such as towels and sheets (see Warnings and Precautions).

See Table 9.

Table 9: Testim 1%

Adverse Drug Reactions from Post-marketing Experience with Testim 1% and Known Adverse Drug Reactions of General Testosterone Treatment

MedDRA System Organ Class (SOC)	Adverse Drug Reaction
Blood and the lymphatic system disorders:	Polycythemia, erythropoiesis abnormal
Endocrine disorders:	Abnormal accelerated growth (growth accelerated)
Gastrointestinal disorders:	Nausea, vomiting, diarrhea, abdominal pain, gastrointestinal bleeding
General disorders and administration site conditions:	Edema, malaise, fatigue, application site burning, application site induration, application site rash, application site dermatitis, application site blister, application site erythema
Hepatobiliary disorders:	Hepatic neoplasms, peliosis hepatis
Immune system disorders:	Allergic reaction, hypersensitivity reaction
Investigations:	Weight increase, fluctuating testosterone levels, testosterone decreased, abnormal liver function tests (e.g. elevated GGTP), lipid abnormalities
Metabolism and nutrition disorders:	Increase appetite, electrolyte changes (nitrogen, potassium, phosphorus, sodium), urine calcium decrease, glucose tolerance impaired, elevated cholesterol
Musculoskeletal and connective tissue disorders:	Myalgia, arthralgia
Nervous system disorders:	Insomnia, headache, dizziness
Psychiatric disorders:	Personality disorder, confusion, anger, aggression, depression, anxiety, decreased libido, cognitive disturbance
Renal and urinary disorders:	Dysuria, hematuria, incontinence, bladder irritability
Reproductive system and breast disorders:	Prostate carcinoma, enlarged prostate (benign), free prostate-specific antigen increased, testicular atrophy, epididymitis, oligospermia, priapism, impotence, precocious puberty, gynecomastia, mastodynia
Respiratory, thoracic and mediastinal disorders:	Dyspnea, sleep apnea
Skin and subcutaneous tissue disorders:	Pruritus, rash, urticaria, vesiculo-bullous rash, seborrhea, acne, alopecia, male pattern baldness, hirsutism
Vascular disorders:	Hypertension

DRUG INTERACTIONS: Drug-Drug Interactions: Insulin: In diabetic patients, the metabolic effects of androgens may decrease blood glucose and, therefore, insulin requirements.

Propranolol: In a published pharmacokinetic study of an injectable testosterone product, administration of testosterone cypionate led to an increased clearance of propranolol in the majority of men tested. It is unknown if this would apply to Testim 1%.

Corticosteroids: The concurrent administration of testosterone with ACTH or corticosteroids may enhance edema formation; thus these drugs should be administered cautiously particularly in patients with cardiac, renal or hepatic disease.

Anticoagulants: Androgens may increase sensitivity to oral anticoagulants. Dosage of the anticoagulant may require reduction in order to maintain satisfactory therapeutic hypoprothrombinemia.

Drug-Food Interactions: Interactions with food have not been established.

Drug-Herb Interactions: It was found that some herbal products (e.g. St. John's wort) which are available as over-the-counter (OTC) products might interfere with steroid metabolism and therefore may decrease plasma testosterone levels.

Drug-Laboratory Test Interactions: Androgens may decrease levels of thyroxine-binding globulin, resulting in decreased total T_4 serum levels and increased resin uptake of T_3 and T_4. Free thyroid hormone levels remain unchanged, however, and there is no clinical evidence of thyroid dysfunction.

DOSAGE AND ADMINISTRATION: Dosing Considerations: Testim 1% is designed to provide consistent transdermal absorption of testosterone over 24 hours after a single dose.

Recommended Dose and Dosage Adjustment: The recommended starting dose of Testim 1% is 5 g of gel (one tube) containing 50 mg of testosterone applied once daily (preferably in the morning) to clean, dry intact skin of the shoulders and/or upper arms (area of application should be limited to the area that will be covered by the patient's short sleeve t-shirt).

Morning serum testosterone levels should be measured approximately 7-14 days after initiation of therapy to ensure proper serum testosterone levels are achieved. If the serum testosterone concentration is below the normal range, or if the desired clinical response is not achieved, the daily Testim 1% dose may be increased from 5 g (one tube) to 10 g (two tubes) as instructed by the physician. The duration of treatment and frequency of subsequent testosterone measurements should be determined by the physician. At any time during treatment, after initial titration, the dose may need to be reduced if serum testosterone levels are raised above the upper limit of the normal range. If serum testosterone levels are below the normal limit, the dose may be increased, not exceeding 100 mg per day.

Missed Dose: If a dose is missed, this dose should be taken only if the next scheduled dose is more than 12 hours away. The missed dose should not be taken if the next scheduled dose is less than 12 hours away. Resume a regular dosing schedule as soon as possible.

Administration: Upon opening the tube the entire contents should be squeezed into the palm of the hand and immediately applied to the shoulders and/or upper arms (area of application should be limited to the area that will be covered by the patient's short sleeve t-shirt). Application sites should be allowed to dry for a few minutes prior to dressing. Hands should be washed thoroughly with soap and water after Testim 1% has been applied.

Special Notes on Administration: The physician or health care professional should advise patients of the following:

- Testim 1% should not be applied to the scrotum.
- Testim 1% should be applied daily to clean dry skin.
- Avoid application of topical testosterone products to sunburned areas of the body.
- In order to maintain serum testosterone levels in the normal range, the sites of application should not be washed for at least two hours after application of Testim 1%.
- Men with known or suspected prostate or breast cancer should not use Testim.

Also advise patients of the risk of secondary exposure: Secondary exposure to testosterone in children and women can occur with the use of testosterone gel products in men. Cases of secondary exposure to testosterone have been reported in children with signs and symptoms including enlargement of the penis or clitoris, premature development of pubic hair, increased erections, and aggressive behavior.

Unexpected sexual development including inappropriate enlargement of the penis or clitoris, premature development of pubic hair, increased erections, and aggressive behavior in children, or changes in hair distribution, increase in acne, or other signs of testosterone effects in adult women should be brought to the attention of a physician and the possibility of secondary exposure to testosterone gel also should be brought to the attention of a physician. Testosterone gel should be promptly discontinued until the cause of virilization is identified.

Strict adherence to the following precautions is advised in order to minimize the potential for secondary exposure to testosterone from Testim-treated skin:

- Children and women should avoid contact with Testim application sites on the skin of men using Testim.
- Testim should only be applied to the shoulders and/or upper arms (area of application should be limited to the area that will be covered by the patient's short sleeve t-shirt).
- Patients should wash their hands thoroughly and immediately with soap and water after application of Testim.
- Patients should cover the application site(s) with clothing (e.g., a shirt) after the gel has dried.
- Prior to any situation in which skin-to-skin contact is anticipated, patients should wash the application site(s) thoroughly with soap and water to remove any testosterone residue.
- In the event that unwashed or unclothed skin to which testosterone gel has been applied or the testosterone gel user's shirts and/or other fabrics (such as towels and sheets) comes in direct contact with the skin of another person, the general area of contact on the other person should be washed with soap and water as soon as possible. Studies show that residual testosterone is removed from the skin surface by washing with soap and water.

Reconstitution: Not applicable.

OVERDOSAGE:

Symptoms of a testosterone overdose are not known. No specific antidote is available. Symptomatic and supportive treatment should be given.

> For management of a suspected drug overdose, CPhA recommends that you contact your **regional Poison Control Centre**. See the *CPS* Directory section for a list of Poison Control Centres.

ACTION AND CLINICAL PHARMACOLOGY: Mechanism of Action: Testim 1% delivers physiologic amounts of testosterone, producing circulating testosterone levels that approximate normal levels (e.g., 10.4-34.6 nmol/L [300-1000 ng/dL]) seen in healthy men.

Pharmacodynamics: Testosterone and Hypogonadism: Testosterone and dihydrotestosterone (DHT), endogenous androgens, are responsible for normal growth and development of the male sex organs and for maintenance of secondary sex characteristics. These effects include the growth and maturation of the prostate, seminal vesicles, penis, and scrotum; the development of male hair distribution, such as facial, pubic, chest, and axillary hair; laryngeal enlargement; vocal cord thickening; alterations in body musculature; and fat distribution.

Male hypogonadism results from insufficient secretion of testosterone and is characterized by low serum testosterone concentrations. Symptoms associated with male hypogonadism include decreased sexual desire with or without impotence, fatigue and loss of energy, mood depression, regression of secondary sexual characteristics, and osteoporosis. Hypogonadism is a risk factor for osteoporosis in men.

General Androgen Effects: Drugs in the androgen class also promote retention of nitrogen, sodium, potassium, phosphorus, and decreased urinary excretion of calcium.

Androgens have been reported to increase protein anabolism and decrease protein catabolism. Nitrogen balance is improved only when there is sufficient intake of calories and protein. Androgens have been reported to stimulate the production of red blood cells by enhancing erythropoietin production.

Androgens are responsible for the growth spurt of adolescence and for the eventual termination of linear growth brought about by fusion of the epiphyseal growth centers. In children, exogenous androgens accelerate linear growth rates but may cause a disproportionate advancement in bone maturation. Use over long periods may result in fusion of the epiphyseal growth centers and termination of the growth process.

During exogenous administration of androgens, endogenous testosterone release may be inhibited through feedback inhibition of pituitary luteinizing hormone (LH). At large doses of exogenous androgens, spermatogenesis may also be suppressed through feedback inhibition of pituitary follicle-stimulating hormone (FSH).

There is a lack of substantial evidence that androgens are effective in accelerating fracture healing or in shortening postsurgical convalescence.

Pharmacokinetics: The pharmacokinetics of Testim 1% have been evaluated using 50 mg and 100 mg doses of testosterone gel in adult hypogonadal males with morning testosterone levels ≤10.4 nmol/L (≤300 ng/dL).

Absorption: Testim 1% is a topical formulation that dries quickly when applied to the skin surface. The skin serves as a reservoir for the sustained release of testosterone into the systemic circulation. Approximately 10% of the testosterone applied on the skin surface is absorbed into the systemic circulation during a 24-hour period.

Single Dose: A single dose crossover study, Study 1, in 29 hypogonadal males was conducted to determine the bioavailability and pharmacokinetic profile of a single dose of 50 mg of Testim 1%.

Serum concentrations of testosterone increased rapidly and were within 10.4-34.6 nmol/L (300-1000 ng/dL) and lasted for at least 24 hours after application. See Figure 1.

Figure 1: Testim 1%

Testim 1% Serum Total Testosterone Concentration (single dose)

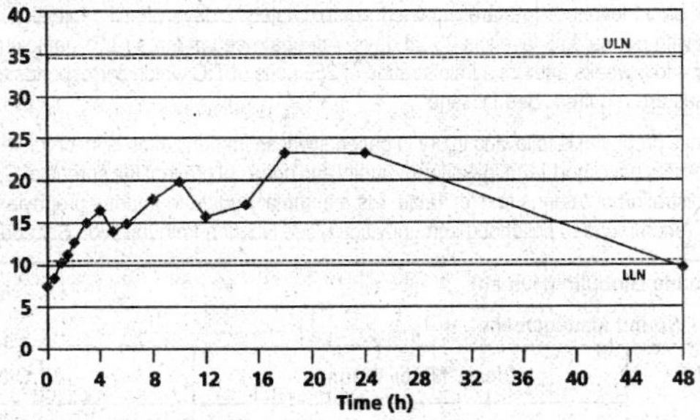

ULN: Upper Limit of Normal
LLN: Lower Limit of Normal

Multiple Dose: Pharmacokinetic data from two 90 day double blind phase III studies showed that treatment with Testim 1% resulted in increased levels of testosterone, DHT, and free testosterone when compared to baseline.

The average steady-state concentrations for testosterone showed a dose dependent response between the Testim 1% doses; 50 mg (12.7-14.2 nmol/L [365-409 ng/dL]) and 100 mg (17.9-21.3 nmol/L [515-612 ng/dL]) in both studies. The differences between the testosterone dose adjusted C_{avg} observed for Testim 1% 50 mg/d and 100 mg/d showed that these were slightly less than dose proportional.

With single daily applications of testosterone gel 50 mg and 100 mg, follow-up measurements at Days 30 and 90 after starting treatment confirmed that serum testosterone and DHT concentrations are generally maintained within the normal range.

Distribution: Circulating testosterone is chiefly bound in the serum to sex hormone-binding globulin (SHBG) and albumin. The albumin-bound fraction of testosterone easily dissociates from albumin and is presumed to be bioactive. The portion of testosterone bound to SHBG is not considered biologically active. Approximately 40% of testosterone in plasma is bound to SHBG, 2% remains unbound (free) and the rest is bound to albumin and other proteins. The amount of SHBG in the serum and the total testosterone level will determine the distribution of bioactive and non-bioactive androgen.

Metabolism: There is considerable variation in the half-life of testosterone as reported in the literature, ranging from ten to 100 minutes.

Testosterone is metabolized to two active metabolites. The major active metabolites of testosterone are estradiol and DHT. Testosterone is metabolized to DHT by steroid 5-α-reductase located in the skin, liver, and the urogenital tract of the male. Estradiol is formed by an aromatase enzyme complex in the brain, fat, and testes. DHT binds with greater affinity to SHBG than does testosterone. In many tissues, the activity of testosterone depends on its reduction to DHT, which binds to cytosol receptor proteins. The steroid-receptor complex is transported to the nucleus where it initiates transcription and cellular changes related to androgen action. In reproductive tissues, DHT is further metabolized to 3-α- and 3-β- androstanediol. Inactivation of testosterone occurs primarily in the liver.

DHT concentrations increased in parallel with testosterone concentrations during testosterone gel treatment. After 90 days of treatment, mean DHT concentrations remained generally within the normal range for testosterone gel-treated subjects.

Excretion: About 90% of a testosterone dose given intramuscularly is excreted in the urine as glucuronic and sulfuric acid conjugates of testosterone and metabolites; about 6% of a dose is excreted in the feces, mostly in the unconjugated form.
Special Populations and Conditions: In patients treated with testosterone gel there are no observed differences in the average daily serum testosterone concentration at steady-state based on age or cause of hypogonadism.
Pediatrics: Testim 1% is not indicated for use in the pediatrics aged <18 years.
Geriatrics: An evaluation of age on the clinical response to treatment with Testim 1% did not reveal any clinically significant findings.
Gender: Testim 1% is not indicated for females.
Race: In clinical studies, the small number of subjects who were non-Caucasian (6.5% overall) did not allow for a meaningful analysis of the response to treatment by subject race.
Hepatic/Renal Insufficiency: Since no formal studies were ever conducted involving patients with renal or hepatic insufficiencies, there are no dosing recommendations for the use of Testim 1% for these populations.
Genetic Polymorphism: No data is available.

STORAGE AND STABILITY: Store at room temperature (15-30°C).
Keep in a safe place out of reach of children.

SPECIAL HANDLING INSTRUCTIONS: Patients should wash their hands thoroughly and immediately with soap and water after application of Testim 1%.
Used Testim 1% tubes should be discarded in household trash in a manner that prevents accidental exposure of children or pets; contents flammable.

INFORMATION FOR THE PATIENT: Published in e-CPS, available by subscription at www.e-cps.ca.

DOSAGE FORMS, COMPOSITION AND PACKAGING: Each tube of clear to translucent hydroalcoholic topical gel contains: testosterone 1%. Nonmedicinal ingredients: carbomers, ethanol, glycerol, pentadecalactone, polyethylene glycol, propylene glycol, purified water and trometamol. Unit-dose aluminum tubes of 5 g with epoxy phenolic liners, cartons of 30.

Testosterone Cypionate Injection USP Ⓒ
testosterone cypionate
Androgens

Sandoz

SUPPLIED: Each mL of sterile solution contains: testosterone cypionate 100 mg. Nonmedicinal ingredients: benzyl alcohol, benzyl benzoate and cottonseed oil q.s. Multidose vials of 10 mL, boxes of 1. Store between 15 and 30°C. Protect from light.

Tetanus Immune Globulin (Human)
Tetanus Prophylaxis

CPhA Monograph

Date of Revision: September 2010

This monograph has been compiled by CPhA and reviewed by experts. It may contain information different from that found in Health Canada-approved Product Monographs. The reader is referred to the *CPS* Editorial Policy for more information.

SUMMARY PRODUCT INFORMATION:

Route of Administration	Dosage Form	Strength
Intramuscular	Solution	250 U single dose vial or prefilled syringe

PHARMACOLOGY: Tetanus immune globulin (human) (TIG) is a sterile solution of immunoglobulins (≥90% immunoglobulin G (IgG)), containing 15% to 18% protein and prepared from plasma of individuals immunized with tetanus toxoid. TIG provides passive immunity to those individuals who may have low or no immunity to tetanus. The tetanus antitoxin antibodies act to neutralize the exotoxin produced by the causative tetanus organism, *Clostridium tetani*, which is found in soil. Neutralization only occurs with unbound toxin; toxin already bound to neuroreceptors in the body are not neutralized. Passive immunization with TIG may be undertaken concomitantly with active immunization using tetanus toxoid.
Pharmacokinetics: Peak blood levels of IgG are obtained approximately 2 days after im injection. The half-life of IgG in the circulation of individuals with normal IgG levels is 23-28 days. Adequate serum titres (0.01 antitoxin units/mL) are expected to persist for approximately 4 to 6 weeks after im administration of 250 units of TIG which corresponds to an administration interval of 4 weeks if repeat doses are required. See Dosage.

INDICATIONS: For tetanus prophylaxis following injury in patients whose immunization is incomplete or uncertain (see Table 1). Administration of TIG provides only short-term, passive immunity and does not prevent the spread of *C. tetani*. Long-lasting, active immunity requires administration of tetanus toxoid. Table 1 is a summary guide to tetanus prophylaxis in wound management. For more information on recommended childhood immunizations, see Routine Immunization Schedules in the Clin-Info section.

Table 1: Tetanus Immune Globulin (Human)
Tetanus Prophylaxis in Wound Management

History of Tetanus Immunization	Clean, Minor Wounds		All Other Wounds	
	Td/Tdap[a]	TIG[b]	Td/Tdap[a]	TIG[b]
Uncertain or <3 doses of an immunization series	Yes	No	Yes	Yes
≥3 doses received in an immunization series	No[c]	No	No[d]	No[e]

[a] Adult type tetanus and diphtheria toxoid or a combined preparation of diphtheria, tetanus and acellular pertussis. If the patient is <7 years old DPT-Polio or DPT-Polio/Hib is given as part of the routine childhood immunization.
[b] Tetanus immune globulin. Give with a separate syringe at a separate site from Td/Tdap.
[c] Yes, if >10 years since last booster.
[d] Yes, if >5 years since the last booster. More frequent boosters are not required and can be associated with increased adverse events. The bivalent toxoid, Td, is not considered to be significantly more reactogenic than T alone and is recommended for use in this circumstance. For an adult that has not previously received a dose of pertussis vaccine substitute with Tdap. The patient should be informed that Td/Tdap has been given.
[e] Yes, if individuals are known to have a significant immune deficiency state (e.g., HIV, agammaglobulinemia) since immune response to tetanus toxoid may be suboptimal.

TIG is also used, although evidence of effectiveness is limited, in the treatment of active tetanus infection in conjunction with appropriate antibiotics (e.g., penicillin), muscle relaxants and sedatives.

CONTRAINDICATIONS: Patients who are hypersensitive to TIG or to any ingredient in the formulation or component of the container.
Immune serums should not be administered to persons with isolated immunoglobulin A (IgA) deficiency. These persons may develop antibodies to IgA and have anaphylactic reactions to subsequent administration of blood products containing IgA.

WARNINGS: Risk versus benefit should be weighed before im injections are administered to patients with thrombocytopenia or coagulation disorders.

Products derived from human plasma can contain infectious agents. During preparation of TIG, steps are taken to inactivate and remove infectious agents which greatly reduces the likelihood of transmitting viral diseases. Nevertheless, risk can never be fully eliminated and the patient should be informed of the risks and benefits of using the product.

PRECAUTIONS: TIG must not be given iv. Severe systemic reactions (e.g., severe fever, precipitous fall in blood pressure, fatal cardiovascular reactions, anaphylactoid reactions) have occurred following iv injection of immunoglobulin intended for im use. IM injections are preferably administered in the anterolateral aspects of the upper thigh and the deltoid muscle of the upper arm. The gluteal region is not recommended as a routine site of injection.
Skin tests should not be performed prior to the administration of TIG. The intradermal injection of concentrated IgG solutions often causes a localized area of inflammation due to tissue irritation, which can be misinterpreted as a positive allergic reaction. True allergic responses to human IgG are rare as this is a product of human origin; however, severe systemic reactions to immune serum globulin have occurred, and epinephrine should be available.
Drug Interactions: Antibodies in immunoglobulin preparations may interfere with the response to live virus vaccines such as measles, mumps, polio, rubella and varicella. Therefore, use of such vaccines should be deferred until 3 months after TIG administration.
TIG does not interfere with the immune response to tetanus toxoid, although the two should not be given in the same syringe nor injected at the same site, as neutralization of the toxoid may occur.
No interactions with other products are known.
Pregnant Women: Safety of TIG has not been studied in pregnancy, although no adverse effects on the fetus have been reported.
Nursing Women: It is not known if TIG antibodies are excreted in breast milk.
Pediatrics: Safety and efficacy has not been established.

ADVERSE EFFECTS: Reactions are usually of a mild nature. Soreness at the injection site is common. Some patients may react more strongly with localized tenderness, muscle stiffness and erythema, persisting for several hours. Low grade fever may occur. Hives, local inflammation and angioedema occur occasionally. Nephrotic syndrome and anaphylactic reactions are rare.
Sensitization to TIG, with severe local and systemic responses, has occurred after repeated injections of TIG, especially in individuals with previous history of allergy.

OVERDOSAGE:
Symptoms: Although few data are available, clinical experience with other immunoglobulin preparations suggests that the only manifestations would be pain and tenderness at the injection site.

For management of a suspected drug overdose, CPhA recommends that you contact your **regional Poison Control Centre**. See the *CPS* Directory section for a list of Poison Control Centres.

DOSAGE: The use of TIG is adjunctive to proper initial wound care. **TIG must be administered im.**
Adults and children ≥1 year of age should receive im injections into the deltoid muscle. IM injections in infants and children <1 year or children with small muscle mass should be made into the anterolateral aspect of the thigh. The plunger of the syringe should be drawn back before injection to ensure that the needle is not in a blood vessel.
Prophylaxis of Tetanus (see Indications): A dose of 250 units should be given by deep im injection. In cases of severe or grossly contaminated wounds, or when treatment is delayed >24 hours, a dose of 500 units may be required.
At the same time, but in a different extremity and with a separate syringe, tetanus toxoid should be administered (see Table 1). Further injections are required to complete the series for producing active immunity.
If the threat of tetanus infection persists, repeat doses of TIG can be given at 4-week intervals.
Children (<7 years of age): 4 units/kg im. Alternatively, 250 units may be used regardless of age or size since the amount of bacterial toxin produced is the same whether in an adult or child.
Immunocompromised Patients: Current recommendations on the use of TIG in patients with altered immunocompetence, including those with HIV infection, are the same as those for patients who are not immunocompromised.
Treatment of Tetanus: Standard therapy for the treatment of tetanus infection must be initiated promptly. The effectiveness of TIG at the recommended dosage has not been established. The currently accepted dosage is 3000 to 6000 units im, usually given in divided doses because of the large injection volume. For neonates a dosage of 500 units im has been suggested.
Storage and Stability: Store at 2°C to 8°C. Do not freeze. Discard if frozen.

Tetracyclines Ⓟ
doxycycline hyclate
minocycline HCl
tetracycline HCl

Antibiotic

CPhA Monograph

Date of Revision: November 2007

This monograph has been compiled by CPhA and reviewed by experts. It may contain information different from that found in Health Canada-approved Product Monographs. The reader is referred to the *CPS* Editorial Policy for more information.

SUMMARY PRODUCT INFORMATION:

Drug[a,b]	Route of Administration	Dosage Form	Strength
Doxycycline	Oral	Capsule	20 mg, 100 mg
		Tablet	100 mg
	Subgingival	Gel	44 mg/unit
Minocycline	Oral	Capsule	50 mg, 100 mg
Tetracycline	Oral	Capsule	250 mg
		Tablet	250 mg
	Ophthalmic	Ointment	1%

[a] For specific product information consult Health Canada's Drug Product Database http://www.hc-sc.gc.ca/dhp-mps/prodpharma/databasdon/index_e.html.
[b] Doxycycline injection and demeclocycline are available through Health Canada's Special Access Programme (see Appendix 2).

PHARMACOLOGY: The tetracyclines are semisynthetic derivatives obtained from Streptomyces cultures. They contain the tetracycline nucleus with various substitutions which impart different degrees of antibacterial activity, gastrointestinal absorption, affinity for divalent or trivalent cations and protein binding. Tetracyclines are mainly bacteriostatic agents which inhibit bacterial protein synthesis by binding to the 30S and to some extent the 50S ribosomal subunits. They may also alter the cytoplasmic membrane leading to leakage of intracellular components such as nucleotides from the cell.
Members of the tetracycline class have similar spectra of activity. They are active against a wide variety of organisms including Rickettsia, Chlamydia and Mycoplasma species, gram-positive bacteria such as *B. anthracis*, *C. perfringens*, *C. tetani*, *L. monocytogenes*, Nocardia, *P. acnes*, some strains of staphylococci and streptococci (although resistance is increasing) and gram-negative bacteria including *B. pertussis*, Brucella, Campylobacter, *H. ducreyi*, *H. influenzae*, *N. gonorrhoeae* (increasingly resistant), *N. meningitidis*, Shigella, *V. cholerae* and *Y. pestis*. Although susceptible in vitro, most strains of Acinetobacter, Bacteroides, *E. aerogenes*, *E. Coli* and Klebsiella are resistant to tetracyclines.

Spirochetes including Borrelia, Leptospira and Treponema species are generally inhibited in vivo by tetracyclines. *B. burgdorferi* (Lyme disease) has a higher minimum bactericidal concentration than other organisms.

Resistance to tetracyclines may be natural or acquired and usually results in decreased permeability of the organism's cell wall to tetracycline. Complete cross-resistance occurs among members of the tetracycline class, with the exception of minocycline which exhibits only partial cross-resistance.

Pharmacokinetics: (see Table 1): Tetracycline and demeclocycline are between 60 and 80% absorbed after oral administration. Minocycline and doxycycline are 90 to 100% absorbed. Absorption takes place mainly in the stomach and upper small intestine. The presence of food or milk can significantly decrease the extent of absorption of tetracycline and demeclocycline. Iron or antacids containing aluminum, calcium or magnesium can decrease the absorption of all tetracyclines. Tetracyclines are poorly and erratically absorbed after im injection.

Tetracyclines are distributed into most body tissues and fluids. They are distributed into the bile and undergo varying degrees of enterohepatic recirculation. The tetracyclines tend to localize in tumors, necrotic or ischemic tissue, liver and spleen, and to form tetracycline-calcium orthophosphate complexes at sites of new bone formation or tooth development.

Tetracyclines readily cross the placenta and are excreted in high amounts in breast milk.

For the most part, the tetracyclines are excreted unchanged in the urine and bile or secreted into the GI tract. Only minocycline is significantly metabolized in the liver.

Hemodialysis removes 20 to 30% of tetracycline but has little effect on doxycycline or minocycline. Peritoneal dialysis has no effect on any of the tetracyclines.

Table 1: Tetracyclines

Pharmacokinetics of Tetracyclines

Drug	Protein Binding (approx. %)	Normal Serum Half-life (hours)	Half-life in Anuric Patients (hours)	% Excreted Unchanged in Urine
Demeclocycline	36 to 91	10 to 17	40 to 60	39
Doxycycline	25 to 93	12 to 22	12 to 22	30 to 42
Minocycline	55 to 88	11 to 26	11 to 23	6 to 12
Tetracycline	20 to 67	6 to 12	57 to 108	60

INDICATIONS: Tetracyclines are indicated in the treatment of infections caused by susceptible strains of Rickettsiae (e.g., Rocky Mountain spotted fever, typhus fever, Q fever, rickettsialpox and Brill-Zinsser disease), Chlamydiae (psittacosis, lymphogranuloma venereum, uncomplicated sexually transmitted infections in adults or adolescents), *M. pneumoniae*, *B. burgdorferi* (Lyme disease), certain uncommon gram-negative infections such as brucellosis, bartonellosis, granuloma inguinale caused by *C. granulomatis*, cholera.

Although not the drugs of first choice, tetracyclines are sometimes used alternatively in the treatment of plague, tularemia, *Campylobacter fetus* infections, *Leptotrichia buccalis* (Vincent's) infection, chancroid, pertussis, anthrax and actinomycosis.

Oral doxycycline is indicated for the acute treatment of pelvic inflammatory disease following initial treatment with iv antibiotics. Doxycycline or tetracycline may be used to treat syphilis (except neurosyphilis) in penicillin-allergic patients.

Tetracycline is used in combination with bismuth subsalicylate, metronidazole and a proton pump inhibitor for treatment of *H. pylori* infection.

Doxycycline is used for chemoprophylaxis of malaria caused by chloroquine-resistant and/or mefloquine-resistant *P. falciparum*.

Low-dose doxycycline is used with adjunctive scaling and root planing for adult periodontitis.

Demeclocycline has been effective in the treatment of the syndrome of inappropriate antidiuretic hormone secretion (SIADH).

Minocycline and tetracycline have been used in some mycobacterial infections.

Tetracyclines have been used in the treatment of rosacea and inflammatory acne vulgaris. Tetracycline has been used in the treatment of bullous pemphigoid.

Due to an increasingly high level of resistance, tetracyclines should not be used empirically to treat the more common gram-negative or gram-positive bacterial infections such as Acinetobacter, Bacteroides species, *E. aerogenes*, *E. coli*, *H. influenzae*, Shigella, *K. pneumoniae*, streptococci or staphylococci. They should only be used to treat susceptible strains of these infections when other appropriate anti-infectives are ineffective or contraindicated.

Doxycycline has been used as a sclerosing agent in the treatment of malignant pleural effusions.

Minocycline has been used in the management of rheumatoid arthritis.

Ophthalmic tetracycline is indicated for treatment of superficial ocular infections caused by: *S. aureus*, *S. epidermicus* (*S. pyogenes*), *S. pneumoniae*, *N. gonorrhoeae* or *E. coli*, and for prophylaxis of ophthalmia neonatorum caused by *N. gonorrhoeae* or *C. trachomatis*.

CONTRAINDICATIONS: Hypersensitivity to any of the tetracyclines; severe renal or hepatic dysfunction; during pregnancy or lactation unless the potential benefit to the patient outweighs the risk to the fetus or child (see Precautions); therapy of common infections in children under 8 years.

Doxycycline is contraindicated in patients with myasthenia gravis because of a possible association with muscle weakness.

PRECAUTIONS: If renal impairment exists, tetracycline or demeclocycline dosage must be modified according to the degree of impairment. Usual doses of doxycycline or minocycline may be used in patients with impaired renal function.

The antianabolic action of the tetracyclines, with the exception of doxycycline, may cause an increase in BUN, which is not problematic in patients with normal renal function. However, in patients with significantly impaired renal function, higher serum levels of tetracycline may lead to azotemia, hyperphosphatemia and acidosis. Consequently, increasing levels of BUN may not accurately reflect changes in renal function; the serum creatinine will provide a more reliable index.

Commercial preparations of tetracyclines may contain sulfites which may cause hypersensitivity reactions including anaphylaxis, with a higher incidence among asthmatic individuals.

Photosensitivity manifested by an exaggerated sunburn reaction has been observed in some individuals taking tetracyclines. Patients should be warned to avoid exposure to direct sunlight or ultraviolet light while taking tetracycline drugs and treatment should be discontinued at the first sign of skin discomfort.

Tetracyclines form a stable calcium complex in any bone-forming tissue. A decrease in the fibula growth rate has been observed in premature infants receiving oral tetracycline in doses of 25 mg/kg every 6 hours. This reaction was reversible when the drug was discontinued.

Tetracycline administration may result in overgrowth of nonsusceptible organisms. Suprainfections due to staphylococci and other organisms may occur. If suprainfections are encountered, tetracyclines should be discontinued and appropriate therapy started. Although rare, suprainfection of the bowel involving staphylococci may be life-threatening.

In rare instances, oral tetracyclines have caused esophagitis and esophageal ulceration. Patients should be advised not to take tetracyclines at bedtime and to take each dose with a large glass of water, while standing or sitting upright.

During long-term therapy, periodic laboratory evaluation of organ systems, including hematopoietic, renal and hepatic studies should be performed.

Since sensitivity reactions are more likely to occur in persons with a history of allergy, asthma, hay fever, or urticaria, tetracyclines should be used with caution in such individuals.

Drug Interactions: Antacids: Antacids containing aluminum, calcium or magnesium and laxatives containing magnesium may impair the absorption of oral tetracyclines and should be given 2 hours before or after the tetracycline.

Anticoagulants: Tetracyclines may potentiate the effects of oral anticoagulants; INR or prothrombin times should be monitored more frequently in patients receiving concomitant anticoagulant therapy and dosage of the anticoagulant should be adjusted as required.

Contraceptives, Oral: Whether antibiotics such as tetracyclines decrease the effectiveness of oral contraceptives is controversial. Some clinicians recommend using an additional contraceptive method for the remainder of the cycle in which a tetracycline is taken.

Digoxin: Bioavailability of digoxin may be increased by tetracyclines in a small subset of patients (<10%) who metabolize significant amounts of digoxin in the gut, apparently by altering the GI flora. Increased serum digoxin may result and may occur up to several months after the discontinuation of tetracyclines. If these drugs are used together, monitor for potential increases in the response to digoxin; a lower dose of digoxin may be needed in certain patients.

Hepatotoxic Drugs: Other potentially hepatotoxic drugs should be avoided, if possible.

Insulin: Tetracyclines may reduce insulin requirements. Controlled studies are needed. Monitor blood glucose.

Iron: Iron salts may impair the gastrointestinal absorption of tetracyclines. It is also possible that tetracyclines may reduce iron absorption. If concurrent use cannot be avoided, give iron 3 hours before or 2 hours after the tetracycline.

Methoxyflurane: Concurrent use of methoxyflurane anesthesia and tetracyclines has been reported to seriously impair renal function, leading in some cases to death. Extreme caution is advised if the concurrent use of these drugs is contemplated.

Penicillin: Since bacteriostatic drugs may interfere with the bactericidal action of penicillin, it is advisable to avoid giving tetracycline in conjunction with penicillin.

Retinoids: Concurrent use of isotretinoin or acitretin with tetracyclines may increase the risk of pseudotumor cerebri. Avoid the combination if possible or monitor for signs and symptoms of pseudotumor cerebri such as headache, nausea, vomiting, visual disturbances and papilledema.

Other: Antidiarrheal agents containing kaolin and pectin or bismuth subsalicylate may impair absorption of oral tetracyclines and it is recommended to avoid concurrent use.

Barbiturates, carbamazepine and phenytoin may increase the rate of metabolism, and therefore, decrease the half-life of doxycycline. Adjustment of doxycycline dosage or substitution of another tetracycline may be necessary.

Drug-Food Interactions: Food and milk can decrease the absorption of tetracycline and demeclocycline due to chelate formation in the gut. These agents should be administered on an empty stomach, 1 hour before or 2 hours after food or milk ingestion. Doxycycline and minocycline may be administered with food or milk.

Pregnancy: Tetracyclines may cause adverse effects on fetal teeth and bone, maternal liver toxicity and congenital defects. They should be used with extreme caution, if at all, in pregnancy. Tetracyclines are contraindicated in the second and third trimesters of pregnancy.

Lactation: Tetracyclines are distributed into breast milk in low concentrations. Exposed infants have been reported to have undetectable serum concentrations. The short-term exposure of infants to tetracyclines through breast-feeding is not contraindicated (i.e., less than three weeks of treatment). Effects of exposure to even small amounts on a long-term basis are unknown but could result in dental staining.

Children: The use of tetracyclines during tooth development may cause permanent tooth discoloration (yellow/gray/brown). This reaction is more common during long-term use of the tetracyclines but has been observed following repeated short-term courses. Enamel hypoplasia has also been reported. Tetracyclines should be avoided in children younger than 8 years of age since the formation of dental enamel is incomplete, unless other drug therapy options are not likely to be effective, are contraindicated, or are more toxic. Doxycycline is usually the preferred agent if a tetracycline must be given to children <8 years old since it carries a lower risk of dental staining than other tetracyclines.

Geriatrics: Because of the greater prevalence of renal impairment in the elderly, renal function should be evaluated and dosage should be reduced or dosing intervals increased accordingly.

Occupational Hazards: Patients taking minocycline may experience headache, light-headedness, dizziness or vertigo and should be cautioned about the operation of hazardous machinery or motor vehicles.

ADVERSE EFFECTS: CNS: Lightheadedness, dizziness, vertigo, ataxia, drowsiness and fatigue may occur with minocycline and are often associated with nausea and vomiting. These reactions may occur in 30 to 90% of patients treated with minocycline. Tinnitus, hearing loss and visual disturbances have also been reported with tetracycline.

Increased intracranial pressure (pseudotumor cerebri) has been reported rarely in adults receiving tetracycline. Bulging fontanels have occurred in infants taking the drug. While both conditions tend to resolve when tetracycline is discontinued, the possibility of permanent sequelae exists.

Dermatologic: maculopapular and erythematous rashes. Exfoliative dermatitis has been reported but is uncommon. Onycholysis and discoloration of the nails have been reported rarely. Photosensitivity has occurred (see Precautions). Abnormal pigmentation of the skin has been reported with the use of minocycline.

Gastrointestinal: anorexia, epigastric distress, nausea, vomiting, diarrhea, bulky loose stools, stomatitis, sore throat, glossitis, black hairy tongue, dysphagia, hoarseness, enterocolitis and inflammatory lesions with candidal overgrowth in the anogenital region, including proctitis and pruritus ani. Rarely, pancreatitis, esophagitis and esophageal ulceration have occurred. See Precautions.

Hematologic: Anemia, hemolytic anemia, thrombocytopenia, thrombocytopenic purpura, neutropenia and eosinophilia have been reported.

Hepatic: Hepatic cholestasis has been reported rarely and is associated primarily with high serum levels of tetracycline. Hepatic toxicity, associated with pancreatitis in some cases, has been attributed to the long-term use of doses larger than those recommended in patients with renal insufficiency or to the concomitant administration of other potentially hepatotoxic drugs. This serious reaction has occurred most often in pregnant or in postpartum patients with pyelonephritis. Fatty infiltration of the liver has been associated primarily with iv tetracycline and appears to be particularly significant in pregnant women who were given large doses (≥2 g/day).

Hypersensitivity Reactions: urticaria, angioneurotic edema, anaphylaxis, anaphylactoid purpura, pericarditis, exacerbation of systemic lupus erythematosus, serum sickness-like reactions such as fever, rash and arthralgia. When given over prolonged periods, tetracyclines have been reported to produce brown-black microscopic discoloration of thyroid glands. No abnormalities of thyroid function are known to occur.

A Jarisch-Herxheimer reaction has occurred occasionally when tetracyclines were used to treat brucellosis or spirochetal infections. This reaction is characterized by fever, chills, myalgias, headache and increased heart and respiratory rates. It is presumably caused by pyrogen and/or endotoxin release from phagocytized organisms and occurs 12 to 24 hours after initiation of treatment.

Musculoskeletal: Rarely, minocycline has been associated with drug-induced lupus erythematosus, involving polyarthralgia, vasculitis, hepatitis and positive ANA.

Renal: Rise in BUN with or without increased serum creatinine concentrations has been reported and is apparently dose-related (see Precautions).

OVERDOSE:

Symptoms: Severe toxicity following acute overdose is unlikely. Symptoms may include nausea and vomiting, esophagitis or esophageal ulceration, hypersensitivity reactions including anaphylaxis.

Treatment: Dilute well with water or milk due to the possibility of esophageal ulceration. Antacids may relieve nausea and abdominal pain (e.g., calcium carbonate or lactate, milk of magnesia, aluminum hydroxide). Measures to reduce absorption may be beneficial in certain patients.

For management of a suspected drug overdose, CPhA recommends that you contact your **regional Poison Control Centre**. See the *CPS* Directory section for a list of Poison Control Centres.

DOSAGE: Antacids containing aluminum, calcium or magnesium and iron salts impair absorption of tetracyclines (see Precautions). Food and milk interfere with the absorption of tetracycline and demeclocycline. These drugs should be given 1 hour before or 2 hours after meals. Doxycycline and minocycline may be given orally with food and/or milk without a clinically important reduction in GI absorption. To reduce the risk of esophageal irritation and ulceration, tetracyclines should not be given at bedtime and should be taken with a full glass of water, while standing or sitting upright.

Demeclocycline: Oral: Children (>8 years): 8 to 12 mg/kg/day divided every 6 to 12 hours (see Precautions, Children).

Adults: SIADH: 3.25 to 3.75 mg/kg every 6 hours.

Renal Impairment: Avoid.

Doxycycline: Oral: Adults: 100 mg every 12 hours on the first day, then 100 mg daily. For severe infections, the dose can be increased to 200 mg daily in 1 or 2 doses.

Children (>8 years): 2 to 4 mg/kg/day divided every 12 to 24 hours, not to exceed 200 mg/day (see Precautions, Children).

Adults: Acne Vulgaris: 100 mg daily.

Rosacea: 100 mg daily for 12 weeks.

Malaria Prophylaxis: Adults: 100 mg once daily, beginning 1 or 2 days before travel to the malarious area and continuing for 4 weeks after leaving the area.

Children (>8 years): 2 mg/kg/day orally as a single daily dose to a maximum of 100 mg/day (see Precautions, Children). Start 1 to 2 days before travel to the malarious area and continue for 4 weeks after leaving the area with a maximum duration of prophylaxis of 4 months.

Periodontitis: 20 mg orally twice daily for up to 9 months.

Nongonococcal Urethritis and Uncomplicated Chlamydial Infections: 100 mg twice daily for at least 7 days.

Syphilis: Primary, secondary and early latent (duration of infection <1 year): 100 mg twice daily for 14 days. Late latent: 100 mg twice daily for 28 days.

Lyme Disease: 100 mg twice daily for 14 to 21 days.

Renal Impairment: No dosage adjustment required. Doxycycline is the tetracycline agent of choice for patients with renal failure.

Doxycycline injection is available through the Special Access Programme, Health Canada (see Appendix 2).
Minocycline: Adults: 200 mg initially, then 100 mg every 12 hours.
Children (>8 years): 4 mg/kg initially, then 2 mg/kg/dose every 12 hours (see Precautions, Children).
Acne Vulgaris: Adults: Initial dose is 100 mg daily, followed by a maintenance dose of 50 mg daily.
Rosacea: Adults: 50 to 100 mg daily for 6 to 8 weeks.
Tetracycline: Adults and adolescents: 250 mg 4 times daily. Higher dosages such as 500 mg 4 times daily may be required for pneumonia or other severe infections.
Acne Vulgaris: Initially, 500 mg twice daily; maintenance, 250 to 500 mg daily.
Rosacea: 500 mg twice daily for 2 weeks, then 500 mg daily until controlled, then 250 mg daily for 3 to 4 weeks.
Brucellosis: 500 mg every 6 hours for 3 weeks, with concurrent streptomycin.
Syphilis: Primary, secondary and early latent (duration of infection <1 year): 500 mg 4 times daily for 14 days. Late latent: 500 mg 4 times daily for 28 days.
Uncomplicated Nongonococcal Sexually Transmitted Diseases: 500 mg 4 times daily for at least 7 days.
Lyme Disease: 500 mg 4 times daily.
Renal Impairment: Patients with mild renal failure (ClCr >50 mL/min) should receive tetracycline every 8 to 12 hours; patients with ClCr between 10 and 50 mL/min should receive tetracycline every 12 to 24 hours; and patients with ClCr <10 mL/min should receive tetracycline every 24 hours.
Children (>8 years): 25 to 50 mg/kg/day up to a maximum of 3 g/day for severe infections, administered in 2 to 4 divided doses (see Precautions, Children).

Teva-5 ASA ℞
5-ASA
Lower Gastrointestinal Anti-inflammatory

Teva Canada

SUPPLIED: Each brown-red, capsule-shaped, enteric-coated tablet contains: 5-aminosalicylic acid 400 mg. Nonmedicinal ingredients: ethyl acrylate, hydroxypropyl methylcellulose, magnesium stearate, mannitol, methacrylic acid, polyethyl acrylate-co-methylmethacrylate, potassium sorbate, povidone, propylene glycol, sodium citrate, sodium starch glycolate, synthetic black iron oxide, synthetic red iron oxide, talc, titanium dioxide, triethyl citrate and xantham gum. Gluten- and tartrazine-free. Bottles of 100 and 500.

The reader is invited to consult CPhA's monograph **Bisphosphonates: Oral**.

Teva-Alendronate ℞
alendronate sodium
Bone Metabolism Regulator

Teva Canada

SUPPLIED: 5 mg: Each white to off-white, round, flat, beveled tablet, engraved with "N" on one side and "5" on the other side, contains: alendronic acid 5 mg as alendronate sodium monohydrate. Nonmedicinal ingredients: colloidal silicon dioxide, hydroxypropylcellulose, low-substituted hydroxypropylcellulose and sodium stearyl fumarate. Blister packages of 30. White high density polyethylene bottles of 100. Store between 15 and 30°C.
10 mg: Each white to off-white, oval tablet, engraved with "N" on one side and "10" on the other side, contains: alendronic acid 10 mg as alendronate sodium monohydrate. Nonmedicinal ingredients: colloidal silicon dioxide, hydroxypropylcellulose, low-substituted hydroxypropylcellulose and sodium stearyl fumarate. Blister packages of 30. White high density polyethylene bottles of 100. Store between 15 and 30°C.
70 mg: Each white to off-white, convex oval tablet, debossed with "N" on one side and "70" on the other side, contains: alendronic acid 70 mg as alendronate sodium monohydrate. Nonmedicinal ingredients: croscarmellose sodium, magnesium stearate and microcrystalline cellulose. Blister packages of 4. White high density polyethylene bottles of 50. Store between 15 and 30°C.

The reader is invited to consult CPhA's monograph **Calcium Channel Blockers**.

Teva-Amlodipine ℞
amlodipine besylate
Antihypertensive— Antianginal

Teva Canada

SUPPLIED: 5 mg: Each white octagonal tablet, engraved with 2 "N"s and a vertical scoreline on one side and "5" on the other side contains: amlodipine besylate 5 mg. Nonmedicinal ingredients: calcium phosphate (dibasic) anhydrous, magnesium stearate, microcrystalline cellulose and sodium starch glycolate. Bottles of 100, 250 and 500. Gluten-free. Store at 15-30°C. Protect from light.
10 mg: Each white octagonal tablet, engraved with "N" on one side and "10" on the other side contains: amlodipine besylate 10 mg. Nonmedicinal ingredients: calcium phosphate (dibasic) anhydrous, magnesium stearate, microcrystalline cellulose and sodium starch glycolate . Bottles of 100 and 250. Gluten-free. Store at 15-30°C. Protect from light.

Teva-Amoxicillin ℞
amoxicillin trihydrate
Antibiotic

Teva Canada

SUPPLIED: Capsules: 250 mg: Each hard gelatin capsule with opaque scarlet cap and yellow body, size #2, printed white NOVO and 250 on opposing cap and body portions of the capsule, contains: amoxicillin USP (as the trihydrate) 250 mg. Nonmedicinal ingredients: colloidal silicon dioxide, D&C Yellow #10, dry-flo starch, FD&C Blue #1, FD&C Red #3, FD&C Red #40, FD&C Yellow #6, gelatin, magnesium stearate, sodium lauryl sulfate, talc and titanium dioxide. Gluten- and tartrazine-free. Bottles of 100 and 1000. Unit dose strips of 100. Store between 15 and 30°C. Unit dose strips should be stored between 15 and 25°C and protected from high humidity.
500 mg: Each hard gelatin capsule with opaque scarlet cap and yellow body, size #0, printed white NOVO and 500 on opposing cap and body portions of the capsule, contains: amoxicillin USP (as the trihydrate) 500 mg. Nonmedicinal ingredients: colloidal silicon dioxide, D&C Yellow #10, dry-flo starch, FD&C Blue #1, FD&C Red #3, FD&C Red #40, FD&C Yellow #6, gelatin, magnesium stearate, sodium lauryl sulfate, talc and titanium dioxide. Gluten- and tartrazine-free. Bottles of 100 and 500. Unit dose strips of 100. Store between 15 and 30°C. Unit dose strips should be stored between 15 and 25°C and protected from high humidity.
Chewable Tablets: 125 mg: Each chewable, rose colored, mottled, oval-shaped, biconvex compressed tablet with cherry aroma, engraved no|vo on one side and 125 on the reverse, contains: amoxicillin 125 mg as the trihydrate. Nonmedicinal ingredients: artificial cherry flavor, aspartame, colloidal silicon dioxide, D&C Red #30 Lake, dipac white, FD&C Red #40 Lake, magnesium stearate, mannitol and microcrystalline cellulose. Gluten- and tartrazine-free. Bottles of 100. Store between 15 and 30°C.
250 mg: Each chewable, rose colored, mottled, oval-shaped, biconvex compressed tablet with cherry aroma, engraved no|vo on one side and 250 on the reverse, contains: amoxicillin 250 mg as the trihydrate. Nonmedicinal ingredients: artificial cherry flavor, aspartame, colloidal silicon dioxide, D&C Red #30 Lake, dipac white, FD&C Red #40 Lake, magnesium stearate, mannitol and microcrystalline cellulose. Gluten- and tartrazine-free. Bottles of 100. Store between 15 and 30°C.
Suspension: 125 mg: Following reconstitution, each 5 mL of finely granulated, off-white to pinkish powder cherry raspberry flavored contains: amoxicillin trihydrate equivalent to amoxicillin 125 mg. Nonmedicinal ingredients: artificial flavors, benzyl alcohol, cornstarch, FD&C Red #40, maltodextrin, propylene glycol, silicon dioxide, sodium benzoate, sodium citrate, sucrose and xanthan gum. Gluten- and tartrazine-free. Bottles of 75, 100 and 150 mL. Store granules for oral suspension at room temperature (between 15 and 30°C). Keep bottle tightly closed. The reconstituted formulation is stable for 14 days under refrigeration (between 2 and 8°C) or 7 days at room temperature (between 15 and 30°C).
250 mg: Following reconstitution, each 5 mL of finely granulated, off-white to pinkish powder cherry raspberry flavored contains: amoxicillin trihydrate equivalent to amoxicillin 250 mg. Nonmedicinal ingredients: artificial flavors, benzyl alcohol, cornstarch, FD&C Red #40, maltodextrin, propylene glycol, silicon dioxide, sodium benzoate, sodium citrate, sucrose and xanthan gum. Gluten- and tartrazine-free. Bottles of 75, 100 and 150 mL. Store granules for oral suspension at room temperature (between 15 and 30°C). Keep bottle tightly closed. The reconstituted formulation is stable for 14 days under refrigeration (between 2 and 8°C) or 7 days at room temperature (between 15 and 30°C).
Sugar-Reduced Suspension: 125 mg: Following reconstitution, each 5 mL of off-white to pale pink colored strawberry-flavored granular powder mix contains: amoxicillin trihydrate equivalent to amoxicillin 125 mg. Nonmedicinal ingredients: artificial flavors, carboxymethylcellulose, colloidal silicon dioxide, corn starch, FD&C Red #40, maltodextrin, mannitol, natural and artificial strawberry flavor, nipagin-M sodium, nipasol-M sodium, sodium citrate (dihydrate), sucrose and xanthan gum. Gluten- and tartrazine-free. Bottles of 75, 100 and 150 mL. Store granules for oral suspension at room temperature (between 15 and 30°C). Keep bottle tightly closed. The reconstituted formulation is stable for 14 days under refrigeration (between 2 and 8°C) or 7 days at room temperature (between 15 and 30°C).
250 mg: Following reconstitution, each 5 mL of off-white to pale yellow colored banana-flavored granular powder mix contains: amoxicillin trihydrate equivalent to amoxicillin 250 mg. Nonmedicinal ingredients: artificial and natural banana flavor, colloidal silicon dioxide, BHA, cornstarch, D&C Yellow #10, maltodextrin, mannitol, nipagin-M sodium, nipasol-M sodium, sodium ascorbate, sodium citrate (dihydrate), sodium pyrophosphate, sucrose, tricalcium phosphate, triglycerides and xanthan gum. Gluten- and tartrazine-free. Bottles of 75, 100 and 150 mL. Store granules for oral suspension at room temperature (between 15 and 30°C). Keep bottle tightly closed. The reconstituted formulation is stable for 14 days under refrigeration (between 2 and 8°C) or 7 days at room temperature (between 15 and 30°C).

Teva-Ampicillin ℞
ampicillin trihydrate
Antibiotic

Teva Canada

SUPPLIED: 250 mg: Each black cap and opaque scarlet body capsule, size #2, imprinted NOVO and 250 on opposing cap and body portions of the capsule in white contains: ampicillin 250 mg. Nonmedicinal ingredients: acid red 27, D&C Yellow #10, FD&C Blue #1, FD&C Red #3, FD&C Yellow #6, gelatin, lactose monohydrate, magnesium stearate, sodium lauryl sulfate, talc and titanium dioxide. Bottles of 100.
500 mg: Each black cap and opaque scarlet body capsule, size #0, imprinted NOVO and 500 on opposing cap and body portions of the capsule in white contains: ampicillin 500 mg. Nonmedicinal ingredients: acid red 27, colloidal silicon dioxide, D&C Yellow #10, FD&C Blue #1, FD&C Red #3, FD&C Yellow #6, gelatin, lactose monohydrate, magnesium stearate, sodium lauryl sulfate, talc and titanium dioxide. Bottles of 100.

Teva-Atenolol ℞
atenolol
Beta-Adrenergic Receptor Blocking Agent

Teva Canada

SUPPLIED: 25 mg: Each white, round, scored uncoated tablet engraved N|N on the scored side and 25 on the other side contains: atenolol 25 mg. Nonmedicinal ingredients: colloidal silicon dioxide, magnesium stearate, microcrystalline cellulose, sodium lauryl sulfate, sodium starch glycolate and starch 1500 (pregelatinized maize starch). Gluten-free. Bottles of 100. Store at room temperature protected from light and moisture. Store between 15-30°C.
50 mg: Each white tablet, engraved with novo 50 on one side, contains: atenolol 50 mg. Nonmedicinal ingredients: colloidal silicon dioxide, magnesium stearate, microcrystalline cellulose, sodium lauryl sulfate, sodium starch glycolate and starch 1500 (pregelatinized maize starch). Gluten-free. Bottles of 100 and 500. Patient packs of 30. Unit dose strips of 100. Store at room temperature protected from light and moisture. Store between 15-30°C.
100 mg: Each white tablet, engraved with no|vo on one side and 100 on the other side, contains: atenolol 100 mg. Nonmedicinal ingredients: colloidal silicon dioxide, magnesium stearate, microcrystalline cellulose, sodium lauryl sulfate, sodium starch glycolate and starch 1500 (pregelatinized maize starch). Gluten-free. Bottles of 100 and 500. Patient packs of 30. Unit dose strips of 100. Store at room temperature protected from light and moisture. Store between 15-30°C.

Teva-Betahistine ℞
betahistine dihydrochloride
Antivertigo Agent

Teva Canada

SUPPLIED: 16 mg: Each white to almost white, round, biconvex, bevelled-edge scored tablet, engraved "N" on one side and "16" on the scored side, contains: betahistine dihydrochloride 16 mg. Nonmedicinal ingredients: mannitol, microcrystalline cellulose and sodium stearyl fumarate. Blisters of 100. Bottles of 100 and 500. Store at controlled room temperature (15-30°C) and protect from exposure to heat and moisture.
24 mg: Each white to almost white, round, biconvex, bevelled-edge scored tablet, engraved "N" on one side and "24" on the scored side, contains: betahistine dihydrochloride 24 mg. Nonmedicinal ingredients: mannitol, microcrystalline cellulose and sodium stearyl fumarate. Blisters of 100. Bottles of 100 and 500. Store at controlled room temperature (15-30°C) and protect from exposure to heat and moisture.

Teva-Cephalexin ℞
cephalexin
Antibiotic

Teva Canada

SUPPLIED: Capsules: 250 mg: Each hard gelatin orange capsule, imprinted NOVO and 250 on opposing body and cap portions of the capsule, contains: cephalexin monohydrate 250 mg. Gluten- and tartrazine-free. Nonmedicinal ingredients: colloidal silicon dioxide, D&C Red #28, FD&C Red #40, FD&C Yellow #6, gelatin, magnesium stearate, pregelatinized starch, sodium lauryl sulfate, starch and titanium dioxide. Bottles of 100.
500 mg: Each hard gelatin, opaque orange body and opaque grey cap, imprinted NOVO and 500 on opposing body and cap portions of the capsule, contains: cephalexin 500 mg. Gluten- and tartrazine-free. Nonmedicinal ingredients: black iron oxide, colloidal silicon dioxide, D&C Red #28, FD&C Red #40, FD&C Yellow #6, gelatin, magnesium stearate, pregelatinized starch, sodium lauryl sulfate, starch and titanium dioxide. Bottles of 100 and 500.

Suspension: 125 mg/5 mL: Each 5 mL of reconstituted suspension contains: cephalexin equivalent to 125 mg off-white to yellowish colored granular powder. On constitution it forms an orange colored orange-banana-flavored suspension. Nonmedicinal ingredients: citric acid, edetate disodium, FD&C Yellow #6, flavour natural and artificial orange and banana, sodium benzoate, sodium citrate, sodium lauryl sulfate and sucrose. Gluten- and tartrazine-free. Bottles of 100 and 150 mL. The reconstituted formulation is stable for 14 days under refrigeration (2-8°C).
250 mg/5 mL: Each 5 mL of reconstituted suspension contains: cephalexin equivalent to 250 mg off-white to pinkish colored granular powder. On constitution it forms a pink colored wild cherry-flavored suspension. Nonmedicinal ingredients: citric acid, edetate disodium, FD&C Red #3, flavour natural and artificial wild cherry, sodium benzoate, sodium citrate, sodium lauryl sulfate and sucrose. Gluten- and tartrazine-free. Bottles of 100 and 150 mL. The reconstituted formulation is stable for 14 days under refrigeration (2-8°C).
Tablets: 250 mg: Each orange, paramette-shaped, biconvex, film-coated tablet, engraved N 250 with partial bisect on one side and plain on the reverse, contains: cephalexin 250 mg. Nonmedicinal ingredients: artificial vanilla flavor, colloidal silicon dioxide, D&C Yellow #10 Lake, dibutyl sebacata, ethylcellulose, FD&C Red #40, FD&C Yellow #6, hydroxypropyl methylcellulose, magnesium stearate, microcrystalline cellulose, polyethylene glycol, polysorbate 80, sodium lauryl sulfate, sodium starch glycolate, starch and titanium dioxide. Gluten- and tartrazine-free. Bottles of 100 and 1000.
500 mg: Each orange, paramette-shaped, biconvex, film-coated tablet, engraved N 500 with partial bisect on one side and plain on the reverse, contains: cephalexin 500 mg. Nonmedicinal ingredients: artificial vanilla flavor, colloidal silicon dioxide, D&C Yellow #10 Lake, dibutyl sebacata, ethylcellulose, FD&C Red #40, FD&C Yellow #6, hydroxypropyl methylcellulose, magnesium stearate, microcrystalline cellulose, polyethylene glycol, polysorbate 80, sodium lauryl sulfate, sodium starch glycolate, starch and titanium dioxide. Gluten- and tartrazine-free. Bottles of 100 and 500.

Teva-Chloroquine ℞
chloroquine diphosphate
Antimalarial

Teva Canada

SUPPLIED: Each white, round, biconvex compressed tablet, bisected on one side and plain on the reverse, contains: chloroquine diphosphate 250 mg equivalent to chloroquine 150 mg base. Nonmedicinal ingredients: dibasic calcium phosphate, lactose monohydrate, magnesium stearate, microcrystalline cellulose, povidone and pregelatinized starch. Bottles of 100. Store between 15 and 30°C.

Teva-Chlorpromazine ℞
chlorpromazine HCl
Antipsychotic

Teva Canada

SUPPLIED: 25 mg: Each white, round, biconvex, film-coated tablet, engraved "2|5" on one side and modified "N" on the reverse, contains: chlorpromazine 25 mg (as hydrochloride). Nonmedicinal ingredients: colloidal silicon dioxide, hydroxypropyl methylcellulose, hypromellose, isopropyl alcohol, magnesium stearate, maltodextrin, microcrystalline cellulose, polyethylene glycol, polydextrose, pregelatinized starch, sodium lauryl sulfate, titanium dioxide and triacetin. Bottles of 100 and 500. Protect from light.
50 mg: Each white, round, biconvex, film-coated tablet, engraved "N|N" on one side and "C50" on the other side, contains: chlorpromazine 50 mg (as hydrochloride). Nonmedicinal ingredients: colloidal silicon dioxide, hydroxypropyl methylcellulose, hypromellose, isopropyl alcohol, magnesium stearate, maltodextrin, microcrystalline cellulose, polyethylene glycol, polydextrose, pregelatinized starch, sodium lauryl sulfate, titanium dioxide and triacetin. Bottles of 100 and 500. Protect from light.
100 mg: Each white, round, biconvex, film-coated tablet, engraved 100 overscore line on one side and modified "N" on the reverse, contains: chlorpromazine 100 mg (as hydrochloride). Nonmedicinal ingredients: colloidal silicon dioxide, hydroxypropyl methylcellulose, hypromellose, isopropyl alcohol, magnesium stearate, maltodextrin, microcrystalline cellulose, polyethylene glycol, polydextrose, pregelatinized starch, sodium lauryl sulfate, titanium dioxide and triacetin. Bottles of 100 and 500. Protect from light.

The reader is invited to consult CPhA's monograph **Selective Serotonin Reuptake Inhibitors**.

Teva-Citalopram ℞
citalopram HBr
Antidepressant

Teva Canada

SUPPLIED: 10 mg: Each white, round, biconvex film-coated tablet, engraved C11 on one side and plain on the other side contains: citalopram hydrobromide corresponding to citalopram 10 mg. Nonmedicinal ingredients: copovidone, croscarmellose sodium, glycerine, hydroxypropylmethylcellulose, lactose monohydrate, magnesium stearate, maize starch, microcrystalline cellulose, polyoxyethylene stearate and titanium dioxide. Gluten-free. Bottles of 100. Store in a dry place at room temperature between 15-30°C.
20 mg: Each white, oval, biconvex film-coated tablet, scored on one side contains: citalopram hydrobromide corresponding to citalopram 20 mg. Nonmedicinal ingredients: copovidone, croscarmellose sodium, glycerine, hydroxypropylmethylcellulose, lactose monohydrate, magnesium stearate, maize starch, microcrystalline cellulose, polyoxyethylene stearate and titanium dioxide. Gluten-free. Bottles of 100 and 500. Blister packages of 30. Store in a dry place at room temperature between 15-30°C.
40 mg: Each white, oval, biconvex film-coated tablet, scored on one side contains: citalopram hydrobromide corresponding to citalopram 40 mg. Nonmedicinal ingredients: copovidone, croscarmellose sodium, glycerine, hydroxypropylmethylcellulose, lactose monohydrate, magnesium stearate, maize starch, microcrystalline cellulose, polyoxyethylene stearate and titanium dioxide. Gluten-free. Bottles of 100. Blister packages of 30. Store in a dry place at room temperature between 15-30°C.

The reader is invited to consult CPhA's monograph **Calcium Channel Blockers**.

Teva-Diltiazem ℞
diltiazem HCl
Antianginal

Teva Canada

Teva-Diltiazem CD ℞
diltiazem HCl
Antihypertensive—Antianginal

Teva Canada

SUPPLIED: Teva-Diltiazem: 30 mg: Each green, round, biconvex, film-coated tablet, engraved novo on one side and 30 on the reverse, contains: diltiazem hydrochloride 30 mg. Nonmedicinal ingredients: colloidal silicon dioxide, D&C Yellow #10 Lake, FD&C Blue #1 Lake, hydroxypropyl methylcellulose, hypromellose, lactose monohydrate, magnesium stearate, methocel and polyethylene glycol. Gluten-free. Bottles of 100. Unit dose strips of 100. Store between 15 and 25°C. Protect from high humidity.
60 mg: Each light yellow, round, biconvex, film-coated tablet, engraved novo over scoreline, 60 under it, plain on the reverse, contains: diltiazem hydrochloride 60 mg. Nonmedicinal ingredients: colloidal silicon dioxide, D&C Yellow #10 Lake, FD&C Yellow #6 Lake, hydroxypropyl methylcellulose, hypromellose, lactose monohydrate, magnesium stearate, methocel and polyethylene glycol. Gluten-free. Bottles of 100. Unit dose strips of 100. Store between 15 and 25°C. Protect from high humidity.
Teva-Diltiazem CD: 120 mg: Each light turquoise blue, controlled delivery capsule, imprinted with "N" and "120" on the body and cap, axial print in black ink, contains: diltiazem hydrochloride 120 mg. Nonmedicinal ingredients: black iron oxide, FD&C Blue #1, gelatin, hydroxypropylmethylcellulose, magnesium stearate, microcrystalline cellulose, polyacrylate dispersion (30%), polysorbate 80, povidone K30, silicon dioxide, simethicone C emulsion, sodium lauryl sulphate, sucrose stearate, talc and titanium dioxide. Gluten-free. Bottles of 100 (38 mm plastic closure) and 500 (53 mm metal closure). Store between 15 and 30°C. Protect from light.
180 mg: Each light blue/light turquoise blue, controlled delivery capsule, imprinted with "N" and "180" on the body and cap, axial print in white ink, contains: diltiazem hydrochloride 180 mg. Nonmedicinal ingredients: black iron oxide, FD&C Blue #1, gelatin, hydroxypropylmethylcellulose, magnesium stearate, microcrystalline cellulose, polyacrylate dispersion (30%), polysorbate 80, povidone K30, silicon dioxide, simethicone C, sodium lauryl sulphate, sucrose stearate, talc and titanium dioxide. Bottles of 100 (38 mm plastic closure) and 500 (53 mm metal closure). Gluten-free. Store between 15 and 30°C. Protect from light.
240 mg: Each light blue/light blue, controlled delivery capsule, imprinted with "N" and "240" on the body and cap, axial print in white ink, contains: diltiazem hydrochloride 240 mg. Nonmedicinal ingredients: black iron oxide, FD&C Blue #1, gelatin, hydroxypropylmethylcellulose, magnesium stearate, microcrystalline cellulose, polyacrylate dispersion (30%), polysorbate 80, povidone K30, silicon dioxide, simethicone C, sodium lauryl sulphate, sucrose stearate, talc and titanium dioxide. Gluten-free. Bottles of 100 (38 mm plastic closure) and 500 (53 mm metal closure). Store between 15 and 30°C. Protect from light.
300 mg: Each light blue/light gray, controlled delivery capsule, imprinted with "N" and "300" on the body and cap, axial print in white ink, contains: diltiazem hydrochloride 300 mg. Nonmedicinal ingredients: black iron oxide, FD&C Blue #1, gelatin, hydroxypropylmethylcellulose, magnesium stearate, microcrystalline cellulose, polyacrylate dispersion (30%), polysorbate 80, povidone K30, silicon dioxide, simethicone C, sodium lauryl sulphate, sucrose stearate, talc and titanium dioxide. Gluten-free. Bottles of 100 (38 mm plastic closure) and 500 (53 mm metal closure). Store between 15 and 30°C. Protect from light.

The reader is invited to consult CPhA's monograph **ACE Inhibitors**.

Teva-Enalapril ℞
enalapril maleate
Angiotensin Converting Enzyme Inhibitor

Teva Canada

SUPPLIED: 2.5 mg: Each white to off-white, oval-shaped, scored, biconvex compressed tablet, engraved N|N on one the scored side and 2.5 on the other side contains: enalapril maleate 2.5 mg that appears as enalapril sodium 2 mg. Nonmedicinal ingredients: colloidal silicon dioxide, corn starch, lactose monohydrate, magnesium stearate, povidone, pregelatinized starch, sodium bicarbonate and talc. Bottles of 100. Unit dose of 30. Store at controlled room temperature (15-30°C). Keep container tightly closed. Protect from light, moisture and high humidity. **Note: 100 tablet bottle: Discard remaining tablets six months after opening bottle.**
5 mg: Each white to off-white, barrel-shaped, biconvex, scored, compressed tablet, engraved N|N on the scored side and 5 on the other side contains enalapril maleate 5 mg that appears as enalapril sodium 4 mg. Nonmedicinal ingredients: colloidal silicon dioxide, corn starch, lactose monohydrate, magnesium stearate, povidone, pregelatinized starch, sodium bicarbonate and talc. Bottles of 100 and 500. Unit dose of 30. Store at controlled room temperature (15-30°C). Keep container tightly closed. Protect from light, moisture and high humidity. **Note: 100 and 500 tablet bottle: Discard remaining tablets six months after opening bottle.**
10 mg: Each rust-red, barrel-shaped, biconvex, scored, compressed tablet, engraved 1|0 on the scored side and N on the other side contains: enalapril maleate 10 mg that appears as enalapril sodium 8 mg. Nonmedicinal ingredients: colloidal silicon dioxide, corn starch, D&C Red #30 Aluminum Lake, FD&C Blue #1 Aluminum Lake HT, FD&C Yellow #6 Aluminum Lake HT, lactose monohydrate, magnesium stearate, povidone, pregelatinized starch, sodium bicarbonate and talc. Bottles of 100 and 500. Unit dose of 30. Store at controlled room temperature (15-30°C). Keep container tightly closed. Protect from light, moisture and high humidity. **Note: 100 and 500 tablet bottle: discard remaining tablets six months after opening bottle.**
20 mg: Each peach coloured, barrel-shaped, biconvex, scored, compressed tablet, engraved 2|0 on the scored side and N on the other side contains: enalapril maleate 20 mg that appears as enalapril sodium 16 mg. Nonmedicinal ingredients: colloidal silicon dioxide, corn starch, D&C Red #30 Aluminum Lake, FD&C Blue #1 Aluminum Lake HT, FD&C Yellow #6 Aluminum Lake HT, lactose monohydrate, magnesium stearate, povidone, pregelatinized starch, sodium bicarbonate and talc. Bottles of 100 and 500. Unit dose of 30. Store at controlled room temperature (15-30°C). Keep container tightly closed. Protect from light, moisture and high humidity. **Note: 100 and 500 tablet bottle: discard remaining tablets six months after opening bottle.**
40 mg: Each peach, rounded triangle-shaped, scored, compressed tablet, engraved N|N on one side and 40 on the other side contains: enalapril maleate 40 mg that appears as enalapril sodium 32 mg. Nonmedicinal ingredients: colloidal silicon dioxide, corn starch, D&C Red #30 Aluminum Lake, FD&C Blue #1 Aluminum Lake HT, FD&C Yellow #6 Aluminum Lake HT, lactose monohydrate, magnesium stearate, povidone, pregelatinized starch, sodium bicarbonate and talc. Unit dose of 30. Store at controlled room temperature (15-30°C). Keep container tightly closed. Protect from light, moisture and high humidity.

The reader is invited to consult CPhA's monograph **ACE Inhibitors** and **Thiazide Diuretics**.

Teva-Enalapril/HCTZ ℞
enalapril—hydrochlorothiazide
Angiotensin Converting Enzyme Inhibitor—Diuretic

Teva Canada

SUPPLIED: 5/12.5 mg: Each green, squared capsule-shaped, compressed tablet, engraved with N on one side and 5 on the other contains: enalapril maleate 5 mg that appears as enalapril sodium 4 mg and hydrochlorothiazide 12.5 mg. Nonmedicinal ingredients: corn starch, FD&C Blue # 2 aluminum lake, lactose, magnesium stearate, pregelatinized starch, sodium bicarbonate powder and yellow ferric oxide. Blister packages of 30. Store at controlled room temperature (15-30°C). Protect from moisture.
10/25 mg: Each rust, oval-shaped, scored tablet, engraved with N on one side and 10 scoreline 25 (10|25) on the scored side contains: enalapril maleate 10 mg that appears as enalapril sodium 8 mg and hydrochlorothiazide 25 mg. Nonmedicinal ingredients: corn starch, lactose, magnesium stearate, pregelatinized starch, red ferric oxide and sodium bicarbonate powder. Bottles of 100. Blister packages of 30. Store at controlled room temperature (15-30°C). Protect from moisture.

Teva-Erythromycin Estolate Pr
erythromycin estolate
Antibiotic

Teva Canada

Teva-Erythromycin Ethylsuccinate Pr
erythromycin ethylsuccinate
Antibiotic

Teva Canada

SUPPLIED: Teva-Erythromycin Estolate: 125 mg/5 mL: Each 5 mL of light orange suspension with an orange aroma, contains: erythromycin 125 mg as estolate. Nonmedicinal ingredients: antifoaming emulsion, benzoic acid, citric acid, disodium EDTA, FD&C Yellow #6, orange extract flavour, polysorbate, sucrose, sodium citrate, sodium chloride, sodium lauryl sulfate and tragacanth. Bottles of 100 and 500 mL. Shake well before using.
250 mg/5 mL: Each 5 mL of light pink suspension with a cherry aroma, contains: erythromycin 250 mg as estolate. Nonmedicinal ingredients: antifoaming emulsion, artificial cherry flavour, benzoic acid, citric acid, disodium EDTA, FD&C Red #2, polysorbate, sucrose, sodium citrate, sodium chloride, sodium lauryl sulfate and tragacanth. Bottles of 100 and 500 mL. Shake well before using.
Teva-Erythromycin Ethylsuccinate: 200 mg/5 mL: Each 5 mL of light-buff coloured powder mix with banana aroma on constitution yields a tan coloured, viscous suspension, contains: erythromycin 200 mg as ethylsuccinate USP. Nonmedicinal ingredients: artificial banana flavour, aspartame, caramel colour, sodium citrate, sorbitan monolaurate, sucrose and xanthan gum. Bottles of 100 and 150 mL. Store below 25°C. Discard any unused medication after 35 days.
400 mg/5 mL: Each 5 mL of light-buff coloured powder mix with banana aroma on constitution yields a tan coloured, viscous suspension, contains: erythromycin 400 mg as ethylsuccinate USP. Nonmedicinal ingredients: artificial banana flavour, aspartame, caramel colour, sodium citrate, sorbitan monolaurate, sucrose and xanthan gum. Bottles of 100 and 150 mL. Store below 25°C. Discard any unused medication after 35 days.

Teva-Fentanyl Pr
fentanyl transdermal system
Opioid Analgesic

Teva Canada

SUPPLIED: 25 µg/h: Each rectangular unit with round corners consisting of an opaque tan backing imprinted overall with "Fentanyl 25 mcg/hr" in pink contains: fentanyl 2.76 mg. Cartons containing 5 individually packaged systems. Stored in sealed pouch between 15 and 25°C. Do not refrigerate or freeze. Keep out of the reach of children before and after use.
50 µg/h: Each rectangular unit is imprinted overall with "Fentanyl 50 mcg/hr" in green and contains: fentanyl 5.52 mg. Cartons containing 5 individually packaged systems. Stored in sealed pouch between 15 and 25°C. Do not refrigerate or freeze. Keep out of the reach of children before and after use.
75 µg/h: Each rectangular unit is imprinted overall with "Fentanyl 75 mcg/hr" in teal and contains: fentanyl 8.28 mg. Cartons containing 5 individually packaged systems. Stored in sealed pouch between 15 and 25°C. Do not refrigerate or freeze. Keep out of the reach of children before and after use.
100 µg/h: Each rectangular unit is imprinted overall with "Fentanyl 100 mcg/hr" in gray and contains: fentanyl 11.04 mg. Cartons containing 5 individually packaged systems. Stored in sealed pouch between 15 and 25°C. Do not refrigerate or freeze. Keep out of the reach of children before and after use.

TEVA-FENTANYL is comprised of a release liner, a functional layer and a backing. Proceeding from the outer surface towards the surface adhering to the skin, these layers are 1) a backing layer of polyester film, 2) an adhesive matrix containing isopropyl myristate, octyldodecanol, polybutene and polyisobutene and the active ingredient, fentanyl and 3) a protective release liner made of polyester. The peelable release liner must be removed before the system can be applied.

The reader is invited to consult CPhA's monograph **Selective Serotonin Reuptake Inhibitors**.

Teva-Fluoxetine Pr
fluoxetine HCl
Antidepressant—Antiobsessional—Antibulimic

Teva Canada

SUPPLIED: 10 mg: Each hard gelatin capsule, size #3, with opaque green cap and opaque grey body, imprinted with black ink novo on cap and 10 on opposing cap and body portions of the capsule, contains: fluoxetine hydrochloride equivalent to fluoxetine 10 mg. Nonmedicinal ingredients: black iron oxide, colloidal silicon dioxide, D&C Yellow #10, FD&C Blue #1, FD&C Yellow #6, gelatin, magnesium stearate, pregelatinized starch, sodium starch glycolate, talc and titanium dioxide. Gluten-free. Bottles of 100. Store between 15 to 30°C. Protect from high humidity and light.
20 mg: Each hard gelatin capsule, size #3, with opaque light green cap and opaque ivory body, imprinted with black ink novo and 20 on opposing cap and body portions of the capsule, contains: fluoxetine hydrochloride equivalent to fluoxetine 20 mg. Nonmedicinal ingredients: colloidal silicon dioxide, D&C Yellow #10, FD&C Blue #1, FD&C Yellow #6, gelatin, magnesium stearate, pregelatinized starch, sodium starch glycolate, talc and titanium dioxide. Gluten-free. Bottles of 100 and 500. Boxes of 100 as unit dose strips. Store bottles between 15 to 30°C. Protect from light. Unit dose boxes should be kept between 15 to 25°C. Protect from light.

Teva-Gabapentin Pr
gabapentin
Antiepileptic

Teva Canada

SUPPLIED: Capsules: 100 mg: Each white, opaque cap and body, hard gelatin capsule, size #3, with "N" and "100" printed in blue ink on opposing caps and body portions of the capsule, contains: gabapentin 100 mg. Nonmedicinal ingredients: colloidal silicon dioxide, FD&C Blue #2, gelatin, lactose monohydrate, pregelatinized starch, sodium lauryl sulfate, talc and titanium dioxide. Gluten-free. White HDPE bottles of 100 and 500. Store at room temperature between 15-30°C.
300 mg: Each yellow, opaque cap and body, hard gelatin capsule, size #1, with "N" and "300" printed in blue ink on opposing cap and body portions of the capsule, contains: gabapentin 300 mg. Nonmedicinal ingredients: colloidal silicon dioxide, FD&C Blue #2, gelatin, lactose monohydrate, pregelatinized starch, sodium lauryl sulfate, yellow iron oxide, talc, titanium dioxide and yellow iron oxide. Gluten-free. White HDPE bottles of 100 and 500. Store at room temperature between 15-30°C.
400 mg: Each orange, opaque cap and body, hard gelatin capsule, size #0, with "N" and "400" printed in blue ink on opposing cap and body portions of the capsule, contains: gabapentin 400 mg. Nonmedicinal ingredients: colloidal silicon dioxide, FD&C Blue #2, gelatin, lactose monohydrate, pregelatinized starch, red iron oxide, talc and titanium dioxide. Gluten-free. White HDPE bottles of 100 and 500. Store at room temperature between 15-30°C.
Tablets: 600 mg: Each white, elliptical film coated tablet, engraved "N" on one side and "600" on the other, contains: gabapentin 600 mg. Nonmedicinal ingredients: black iron oxide, crospovidone, hydrogenated vegetable oil, macrogol, microcrystalline cellulose, polyethylene glycol, polyvinyl alcohol, povidone, talc and titanium dioxide. White HDPE bottles of 100. Store at room temperature between 15-30°C.
800 mg: Each white, elliptical film coated tablet, embossed "N" on one side and "800" on the other, contains: gabapentin 800 mg. Nonmedicinal ingredients: black iron oxide, crospovidone, hydrogenated vegetable oil, hydroxypropyl methylcellulose, microcrystalline cellulose, polyethylene glycol, povidone, talc and titanium dioxide. White HDPE bottles of 100. Store at room temperature between 15-30°C.

Teva-Ketotifen Pr
ketotifen fumarate
Pediatric Asthma Prophylactic—Antiallergic

Teva Canada

SUPPLIED: Syrup: Each 5 mL of ketotifen syrup contains: ketotifen 1 mg. Nonmedicinal ingredients: alcohol USP 95%, artificial strawberry flavour, citric acid (anhydrous), dibasic sodium phosphate (anhydrous), methylparaben, propylparaben, sorbitol solution USP/BP 70% and sucrose. Gluten-free. Bottles of 250 mL, to be administered orally. Store at temperatures not exceeding 25°C.
Tablets: Each white, round, flat-faced compressed tablet, engraved "N|N" on one side and "1" on the reverse contains: ketotifen fumarate 1.38 mg equivalent to ketotifen 1 mg. Nonmedicinal ingredients: corn starch, lactose monohydrate and magnesium stearate. Bottles of 100. Store between 15-25°C and protect from high humidity.

Teva-Lansoprazole Pr
lansoprazole
H+, K+-ATPase Inhibitor

Teva Canada

SUPPLIED: 15 mg: Each pink and green coloured, opaque, delayed-release capsule, printed with "N" on one portion and "15" on the other, filled with off white to beige delayed release pellets contains: lansoprazole 15 mg. Nonmedicinal ingredients: capsule fill: hypromellose, magnesium carbonate, methacrylic acid ethylacrylate copolymer, sugar spheres, talc, titanium dioxide and triethyl citrate; capsule shell: erythrosin (FD&C Red 3), brilliant blue (FD&C Blue 1), gelatin, quinoline yellow, sunset yellow (FD&C Yellow 6) and titanium dioxide; printing ink: povidone, propylene glycol, shellac, sodium hydroxide and titanium dioxide. Gluten-free. Bottles of 30 and 100. Store in a tight container protected from light and moisture. Store between 15-25°C.
30 mg: Each pink and black coloured, opaque, delayed-release capsule, printed with "N" on one portion and "30" on the other, filled with off white to beige delayed release pellets contains: lansoprazole 30 mg. Nonmedicinal ingredients: capsule fill: hypromellose, magnesium carbonate, methacrylic acid ethylacrylate copolymer, sugar spheres, talc, titanium dioxide and triethyl citrate; capsule shell: erythrosin (FD&C Red 3), brilliant blue (FD&C Blue 1), gelatin, quinoline yellow, sunset yellow (FD&C Yellow 6) and titanium dioxide; printing ink: povidone, propylene glycol, shellac, sodium hydroxide and titanium dioxide. Gluten-free. Bottles of 30, 100 and 500. Store in a tight container protected from light and moisture. Store between 15-25°C.

Teva-Maprotiline Pr
maprotiline HCl
Antidepressant

Teva Canada

SUPPLIED: 25 mg: Each round, orange-colored, beveled-edged, biconvex, film-coated tablet, engraved N/25 on one side, plain on the reverse, contains: maprotiline HCl 25 mg. Nonmedicinal ingredients: dibasic calcium phosphate, FD&C Yellow #6, hydroxypropyl methylcellulose, lactose monohydrate, magnesium stearate, polyethylene glycol, pregelatinized starch, stearic acid, talc, titanium dioxide, triacetin and triethyl citrate. Gluten- and tartrazine-free. Bottles of 100. Store between 15-30°C in well-closed containers.
50 mg: Each round, orange-colored, beveled-edged, biconvex, film-coated tablet, engraved N/50 on one side, plain on the reverse, contains: maprotiline HCl 50 mg. Nonmedicinal ingredients: dibasic calcium phosphate, erythrosine Aluminum Lake, FD&C Yellow #6, hydroxypropyl methylcellulose, lactose monohydrate, magnesium stearate, polyethylene glycol, polysorbate 80, pregelatinized starch, stearic acid, talc, titanium dioxide and triethyl citrate. Gluten- and tartrazine-free. Bottles of 100. Store between 15-30°C in well-closed containers.
75 mg: Each round, orange-red-colored, shallow, biconvex, film-coated tablet, engraved N/75 on one side, plain on the reverse, contains: maprotiline HCl 75 mg. Nonmedicinal ingredients: D&C Yellow #10, dibasic calcium phosphate, erythrosine Aluminum Lake, hydroxypropyl methylcellulose, lactose monohydrate, magnesium stearate, polyethylene glycol, pregelatinized starch, stearic acid, talc, titanium dioxide, triacetin and triethyl citrate. Gluten- and tartrazine-free. Bottles of 100. Store between 15-30°C in well-closed containers.

Teva-Metoprolol Pr
metoprolol tartrate
Antihypertensive—Antianginal

Teva Canada

SUPPLIED: 50 mg: Film-coated: Each pink, capsule-shaped, biconvex, film-coated tablet, engraved N|50 on one side, plain on the reverse, contains: metoprolol tartrate 50 mg. Nonmedicinal ingredients: cornstarch, D&C Red #30 Lake, FD&C Yellow #6, hydroxypropyl methylcellulose, lactose monohydrate, magnesium stearate, microcrystalline cellulose, polyethylene glycol, silicon dioxide, sodium starch glycolate and titanium dioxide. Gluten- and tartrazine-free. Bottles of 100 and 500. Unit dose strips of 100. Store bottles between 15 to 30°C and unit dose boxes between 15 to 25°C. Protect from heat, light and humidity.
Uncoated: Each white, round, biconvex tablet, engraved N over 50 on one side, plain on the reverse, contains: metoprolol tartrate 50 mg. Nonmedicinal ingredients: cornstarch, lactose monohydrate, magnesium stearate, microcrystalline cellulose, silicon dioxide and sodium starch glycolate. Gluten- and tartrazine-free. Bottles of 100 and 500. Store bottles between 15 to 30°C. Protect from heat, light and humidity.
100 mg: Film-coated: Each light blue, capsule-shaped, biconvex, film-coated tablet, engraved N|100 on one side, plain on the reverse, contains: metoprolol tartrate 100 mg. Nonmedicinal ingredients: cornstarch, FD&C Blue #2, hydroxypropyl methylcellulose, lactose, magnesium stearate, microcrystalline cellulose, polyethylene glycol, silicon dioxide, sodium starch glycolate and titanium dioxide. Gluten- and tartrazine-free. Bottles of 100 and 500. Unit dose strips of 100. Store bottles between 15 to 30°C and unit dose boxes between 15 to 25°C. Protect from heat, light and humidity.
Uncoated: Each white, round, biconvex tablet, engraved N over 100 on one side, plain on the reverse, contains: metoprolol tartrate 100 mg. Nonmedicinal ingredients: cornstarch, lactose monohydrate, magnesium stearate, microcrystalline cellulose, silicon dioxide and sodium starch glycolate. Gluten- and tartrazine-free. Bottles of 100 and 500. Store bottles between 15 to 30°C. Protect from heat, light and humidity.

Teva-Mexiletine ℞
mexiletine HCl
Antiarrhythmic

Teva Canada

SUPPLIED: 100 mg: Each opaque scarlet cap and opaque orange body, hard gelatin capsule, with N and 100 imprinted on opposing cap and body portions of the capsule, contains: mexiletine HCl 100 mg. Nonmedicinal ingredients: colloidal silicon dioxide, D&C Red No. 33, FD&C Blue No. 1, FD&C Red No. 3, FD&C Red No. 40, FD&C Yellow No. 6, gelatin, magnesium stearate, parabens, pregelatinized starch, silicon dioxide, sodium lauryl sulfate, talc and titanium dioxide. Gluten- and tartrazine-free. Bottles of 100. Store between 15-30°C.
200 mg: Each scarlet, hard gelatin capsule, with N and 200 imprinted on opposing cap and body portions of the capsule, contains: mexiletine HCl 200 mg. Nonmedicinal ingredients: colloidal silicon dioxide, D&C Red No. 33, FD&C Blue No. 1, FD&C Red No. 40, gelatin, magnesium stearate, parabens, pregelatinized starch, silicon dioxide, sodium lauryl sulfate, talc and titanium dioxide. Gluten- and tartrazine-free. Bottles of 100. Store between 15-30°C.

Teva-Naproxen ℞
naproxen
Nonsteroidal Anti-Inflammatory

Teva Canada

Teva-Naproxen-EC ℞
naproxen
Nonsteroidal Anti-Inflammatory

Teva Canada

Teva-Naproxen Sodium ℞
naproxen sodium
Nonsteroidal Anti-Inflammatory

Teva Canada

Teva-Naproxen Sodium DS ℞
naproxen sodium
Nonsteroidal Anti-Inflammatory

Teva Canada

SUPPLIED: Teva-Naproxen: 250 mg: Each yellow, oval, compressed tablet engraved with NOVO on one side and 250 on the other side, contains: naproxen USP 250 mg. Nonmedicinal ingredients: colloidal silicon dioxide, D&C Yellow #10 Lake, FD&C Yellow #6 Lake, magnesium stearate, microcrystalline cellulose, povidone, sodium lauryl sulfate and sodium starch glycolate. Gluten- and tartrazine-free. Bottles of 100 and 500. Unit dose strips of 100.
375 mg: Each peach, capsule-shaped, compressed tablet engraved with no|vo on one side and 375 on the reverse, contains: naproxen USP 375 mg. Nonmedicinal ingredients: colloidal silicon dioxide, FD&C Yellow #6 Lake, magnesium stearate, microcrystalline cellulose, povidone, sodium lauryl sulfate and sodium starch glycolate. Gluten- and tartrazine-free. Bottles of 100 and 500.
500 mg: Each yellow, capsule-shaped, compressed tablet with N|500 engraved on one side, plain on the reverse, contains: naproxen USP 500 mg. Nonmedicinal ingredients: colloidal silicon dioxide, D&C Yellow #10 Lake, FD&C Yellow #6 Lake, magnesium stearate, microcrystalline cellulose, povidone, sodium lauryl sulfate and sodium starch glycolate. Gluten- and tartrazine-free. Bottles of 100 and 500.
Teva-Naproxen-EC: 250 mg: Each white to off-white, round biconvex, enteric-coated tablet, printed in black on one side with N and 250 on the other side, contains: naproxen 250 mg USP. Nonmedicinal ingredients: colloidal silicon dioxide, croscarmellose sodium, hydroxypropyl methylcellulose, magnesium stearate, methylacrylic acid, polyethylene glycol, polysorbate 80, povidone, sodium citrate, sodium lauryl sulfate, talc, titanium dioxide and triethyl citrate. Gluten- and tartrazine-free. Bottles of 100.
375 mg: Each white to off-white, capsule-shaped enteric-coated tablet, printed in black on one side with N and 375 on the other side, contains: naproxen 375 mg USP. Nonmedicinal ingredients: colloidal silicon dioxide, croscarmellose sodium, hydroxypropyl methylcellulose, magnesium stearate, methylacrylic acid, polyethylene glycol, polysorbate 80, povidone, sodium citrate, sodium lauryl sulfate, talc, titanium dioxide and triethyl citrate. Gluten- and tartrazine-free. Bottles of 100.
500 mg: Each white to off-white, capsule-shaped enteric-coated tablet, printed in black on one side with N and 500 on the other side, contains: naproxen 500 mg USP. Nonmedicinal ingredients: colloidal silicon dioxide, croscarmellose sodium, hydroxypropyl methylcellulose, magnesium stearate, methylacrylic acid, polyethylene glycol, polysorbate 80, povidone, sodium citrate, sodium lauryl sulfate, talc, titanium dioxide and triethyl citrate. Gluten- and tartrazine-free. Bottles of 100.
Teva-Naproxen Sodium: Each blue, oval shaped, biconvex, film-coated tablet, engraved NOVO on one side and 275 on the other, contains: naproxen sodium 275 mg. Nonmedicinal ingredients: colloidal silicon dioxide, FD&C Blue No. 2, hydroxypropyl methylcellulose, magnesium stearate, microcrystalline cellulose, polyethylene glycol, polysorbate 80, povidone, sodium lauryl sulfate, sodium starch glycolate and titanium dioxide. Gluten-and tartrazine-free. Bottles of 100 and 500.
Teva-Naproxen Sodium DS: Each blue, oval shaped, biconvex, bevelled-edged, film-coated tablet, engraved novo on one side and 550 on the other, contains: naproxen sodium 550 mg. Nonmedicinal ingredients: colloidal silicon dioxide, FD&C Blue No. 2, hydroxypropyl methylcellulose, magnesium stearate, microcrystalline cellulose, polyethylene glycol, polysorbate 80, povidone, sodium lauryl sulfate, sodium starch glycolate and titanium dioxide. Gluten- and tartrazine-free. Bottles of 100 and 500.

Teva-Olanzapine ℞
olanzapine
Antipsychotic—Antimanic Agent

Teva Canada

SUPPLIED: 2.5 mg: Each white, round, film coated tablet, engraved with "2.5" on one side and "N" on the other side, contains: olanzapine 2.5 mg. Nonmedicinal ingredients: crospovidone, glycerol triacetate, hypromellose, hydroxypropyl cellulose, lactose monohydrate, macrogol, magnesium stearate, polydextrose, silicified microcrystalline cellulose and titanium dioxide. Gluten-free. White HDPE bottles of 100. Store at 15-30°C. Protect from light and moisture.
5 mg: Each white, round, film coated tablet, engraved with "5" on one side and "N" on the other side, contains: olanzapine 5 mg. Nonmedicinal ingredients: crospovidone, glycerol triacetate, hypromellose, hydroxypropyl cellulose, lactose monohydrate, macrogol, magnesium stearate, polydextrose, silicified microcrystalline cellulose and titanium dioxide. Gluten-free. White HDPE bottles of 100. Store at 15-30°C. Protect from light and moisture.
7.5 mg: Each white, round, film coated tablet, engraved with "7.5" on one side and "N" on the other side, contains: olanzapine 7.5 mg. Nonmedicinal ingredients: crospovidone, glycerol triacetate, hypromellose, hydroxypropyl cellulose, lactose monohydrate, macrogol, magnesium stearate, polydextrose, silicified microcrystalline cellulose and titanium dioxide. Gluten-free. White HDPE bottles of 100. Store at 15-30°C. Protect from light and moisture.
10 mg: Each white, round, film coated tablet, engraved with "10" on one side and "N" on the other side, contains: olanzapine 10 mg. Nonmedicinal ingredients: crospovidone, glycerol triacetate, hypromellose, hydroxypropyl cellulose, lactose monohydrate, macrogol, magnesium stearate, polydextrose, silicified microcrystalline cellulose and titanium dioxide. Gluten-free. White HDPE bottles of 100 and 500. Store at 15-30°C. Protect from light and moisture.
15 mg: Each light blue, elliptical, film coated tablet, engraved with "15" on one side and "N" on the other side, contains: olanzapine 15 mg. Nonmedicinal ingredients: crospovidone, FD&C Blue # 2 indigo carmine aluminium lake, hypromellose, hydroxypropyl cellulose, lactose monohydrate, macrogol, magnesium stearate, polydextrose, silicified microcrystalline cellulose and titanium dioxide. Gluten-free. White HDPE bottles of 100. Store at 15-30°C. Protect from light and moisture.

Teva-Pantoprazole ℞
pantoprazole sodium
H+, K+-ATPase Inhibitor

Teva Canada

SUPPLIED: 20 mg: Each yellow, oval shaped tablet, imprinted with black ink on the one side "93/11", plain on the other side, contains: pantoprazole sodium sesquihydrate 20 mg. Nonmedicinal ingredients: black iron oxide, calcium carbonate, calcium stearate, D&C Yellow #10 Aluminium Lake, FD&C Yellow #6 Aluminium Lake, hypromellose, iron oxide yellow, lactose monohydrate, low-substituted hydroxypropyl cellulose, methacrylic acid copolymer, microcrystalline cellulose, polyethylene glycol, propylene glycol, shellac glaze, sodium carbonate anhydrous, stearic acid, talc, titanium dioxide and triethyl citrate. Bottles of 100 tablets. Store at room temperature (15-30°C). Protect from light.
40 mg: Each yellow, oval shaped tablet, imprinted with black ink on the one side "93/12", plain on the other side, contains: pantoprazole sodium sesquihydrate 40 mg. Nonmedicinal ingredients: black iron oxide, calcium carbonate, calcium stearate, D&C Yellow #10 Aluminium Lake, FD&C Yellow #6 Aluminium Lake, hypromellose, iron oxide yellow, lactose monohydrate, low-substituted hydroxypropyl cellulose, methacrylic acid copolymer, microcrystalline cellulose, polyethylene glycol, propylene glycol, shellac glaze, sodium carbonate anhydrous, stearic acid, talc, titanium dioxide and triethyl citrate. Bottles of 100 tablets. Store at room temperature (15-30°C). Protect from light.

The reader is invited to consult CPhA's monograph **Fluoroquinolones**.

Teva-Paroxetine ℞
paroxetine HCl
Antidepressant—Antiobsessional—Antipanic—Anxiolytic—Social Phobia (Social Anxiety Disorder)—Post-traumatic Stress Disorder Therapy

Teva Canada

SUPPLIED: 10 mg: Each yellow, oval, biconvex, film-coated tablet, engraved with N on one side and 10 on the other side, contains: paroxetine HCl 10 mg. Nonmedicinal ingredients: D&C Yellow No. 10 aluminum lake, FD&C Yellow No. 6 aluminum lake, hydroxypropyl methylcellulose, isomalt D.C., magnesium hydroxide, magnesium stearate, microcrystalline cellulose, polyethylene glycol 3350, povidone, sodium stearyl fumarate, talc and titanium dioxide. Bottles of 30 and 100 packaged in white, high density polyethylene bottles. Patient packs of 30. Store between 15-30°C.
20 mg: Each pink, oval, bisected, biconvex, film-coated tablet, engraved with N on one side and 2 vertical bisect 0 on the other side, contains: paroxetine HCl 20 mg. Nonmedicinal ingredients: D&C Red No. 30 aluminum lake, hydroxypropyl methylcellulose, isomalt D.C., magnesium hydroxide, magnesium stearate, microcrystalline cellulose, polyethylene glycol 3350, povidone, sodium stearyl fumarate, talc and titanium dioxide. Bottles of 100 and 500 packaged in white, high density polyethylene bottles. Patient packs of 30. Store between 15-30°C.
30 mg: Each blue, oval, biconvex, film-coated tablet, engraved with N on one side and 30 on the other side, contains: paroxetine HCl 30 mg. Nonmedicinal ingredients: FD&C Blue No. 2 aluminum lake, hydroxypropyl methylcellulose, isomalt D.C., magnesium hydroxide, magnesium stearate, microcrystalline cellulose, polyethylene glycol 3350, povidone, sodium stearyl fumarate, talc and titanium dioxide. Bottles of 30 and 100 packaged in white, high density polyethylene bottles. Patient packs of 30. Store between 15-30°C.

The reader is invited to consult CPhA's monograph **HMG-CoA Reductase Inhibitors**.

Teva-Pravastatin ℞
pravastatin sodium
Lipid Metabolism Regulator

Teva Canada

SUPPLIED: 10 mg: Each pink to peach, rounded, rectangular-shaped, biconvex compressed tablet, engraved N on one side and 10 on the other side, contains: pravastatin sodium 10 mg. Nonmedicinal ingredients: calcium phosphate dibasic anhydrous, croscarmellose sodium, crospovidone, ferric oxide red, lactose anhydrous, microcrystalline cellulose, povidone and sodium stearyl fumarate. Bottles of 100. Patient packs of 30. Store at room temperature (15 to 30°C). Protect from moisture and light.
20 mg: Each yellow, rounded, rectangular-shaped, biconvex compressed tablet, engraved N on one side and 20 on the other side, contains: pravastatin sodium 20 mg. Nonmedicinal ingredients: calcium phosphate dibasic anhydrous, croscarmellose sodium, crospovidone, ferric oxide yellow, lactose anhydrous, microcrystalline cellulose, povidone and sodium stearyl fumarate. Bottles of 100. Patient packs of 30. Store at room temperature (15 to 30°C). Protect from moisture and light.
40 mg: Each green, rounded, rectangular-shaped, biconvex compressed tablet, engraved N on one side and 40 on the other side, contains: pravastatin sodium 40 mg. Nonmedicinal ingredients: calcium phosphate dibasic anhydrous, D&C Yellow No.10 Aluminum Lake 18-24%, FD&C Blue No.1 Aluminum Lake 11-13%, croscarmellose sodium, crospovidone, lactose anhydrous, microcrystalline cellulose, povidone and sodium stearyl fumarate. Bottles of 100. Patient packs of 30. Store at room temperature (15 to 30°C). Protect from moisture and light.

Teva-Quetiapine ℞
quetiapine fumarate
Antipsychotic

Teva Canada

SUPPLIED: 25 mg: Each peach, round, biconvex, film-coated tablet, engraved with "N" on one side and "25" on the other side, contains: quetiapine fumarate 25 mg. Nonmedicinal ingredients: colloidal silicon dioxide, dibasic calcium phosphate, hydroxypropyl methylcellulose, iron oxide red, iron oxide yellow, lactose monohydrate, magnesium stearate, microcrystalline cellulose, polydextrose, polyethylene glycol, polysorbate 80, povidone, sodium starch glycolate, titanium dioxide and triacetin. Gluten-free. Blister packages of 30. High-density polyethylene (HDPE) bottles of 100 and 500. Store at room temperature (15-30°C).
100 mg: Each yellow, round, biconvex, film-coated tablet, engraved with "N" on one side and "100" on the other side, contains: quetiapine fumarate 100 mg. Nonmedicinal ingredients: colloidal silicon dioxide, dibasic calcium phosphate, FD&C Yellow #6/sunset yellow FCF aluminum lake, hydroxypropyl methylcellulose, iron oxide yellow, lactose monohydrate, magnesium

stearate, microcrystalline cellulose, polydextrose, polyethylene glycol, polysorbate 80, povidone, sodium starch glycolate, titanium dioxide and triacetin. Gluten-free. Blister packages of 30. High-density polyethylene (HDPE) bottles of 100 and 500. Store at room temperature (15-30°C).
150 mg: Each pale yellow, round, biconvex, film-coated tablet, engraved with "N" on one side and "150" on the other side, contains: quetiapine fumarate 150 mg. Nonmedicinal ingredients: colloidal silicon dioxide, dibasic calcium phosphate, hydroxypropyl methylcellulose, iron oxide yellow, lactose monohydrate, magnesium stearate, microcrystalline cellulose, polydextrose, polyethylene glycol, polysorbate 80, povidone, sodium starch glycolate, titanium dioxide and triacetin. Gluten-free. High-density polyethylene (HDPE) bottles of 100. Store at room temperature (15-30°C).
200 mg: Each white, round, biconvex, film-coated tablet, engraved with "N" on one side and "200" on the other side, contains: quetiapine fumarate 200 mg. Nonmedicinal ingredients: colloidal silicon dioxide, dibasic calcium phosphate, hydroxypropyl methylcellulose, lactose monohydrate, magnesium stearate, microcrystalline cellulose, povidone, polydextrose, polyethylene glycol, polysorbate 80, sodium starch glycolate, titanium dioxide and triacetin. Gluten-free. Blister packages of 30. High-density polyethylene (HDPE) bottles of 100. Store at room temperature (15-30°C).
300 mg: Each white, capsule-shaped, biconvex, film-coated tablet, engraved with "N" on one side and "300" on the other side, contains: quetiapine fumarate 300 mg. Nonmedicinal ingredients: colloidal silicon dioxide, dibasic calcium phosphate, hydroxypropyl methylcellulose, lactose monohydrate, magnesium stearate, microcrystalline cellulose, povidone, polydextrose, polyethylene glycol, polysorbate 80, sodium starch glycolate, titanium dioxide and triacetin. Gluten-free. Blister packages of 30. High-density polyethylene (HDPE) bottles of 100. Store at room temperature (15-30°C).

Teva-Rabeprazole EC Ⓟ
rabeprazole sodium
H+, K+-ATPase Inhibitor

Teva Canada

SUPPLIED: 10 mg: Each pink, round tablet, imprinted in black ink with "N10" on one side and plain on the other side, contains: rabeprazole sodium 10 mg. Nonmedicinal ingredients: anatase titanium dioxide, hydroxypropyl cellulose, hydroxypropyl methylcellulose, hypromellose, hypromellose phthalate, industrial methylated spirit, iron oxide black, isopropyl alcohol, iron oxide red, iron oxide yellow, lactose monohydrate, low-substituted hydroxypropyl cellulose, magnesium oxide, magnesium stearate, mannitol, microcrystalline cellulose, n-butyl alcohol, polyethylene glycol, propylene glycol, shellac glaze, stearic acid, titanium dioxide and triethyl citrate. Gluten-free. Bottles of 100. Store at room temperature (15 to 30°C) protected from moisture.
20 mg: Each yellow, round tablet, imprinted in black ink with "93" over "64" on one side, contains: rabeprazole sodium 20 mg. Nonmedicinal ingredients: anatase titanium dioxide, antifoam, FD&C Yellow #6 aluminum lake, hydroxypropyl cellulose, hydroxypropyl methylcellulose, hypromellose, hypromellose phthalate, industrial methylated spirit, iron oxide black, isopropyl alcohol, lactose monohydrate, low-substituted hydroxypropyl cellulose, magnesium oxide, magnesium stearate, mannitol, microcrystalline cellulose, n-butyl alcohol, polyethylene glycol, propylene glycol, shellac glaze, stearic acid, titanium dioxide and triethyl citrate. Gluten-free. Bottles of 100. Unit dose blister packages of 30. Store at room temperature (15 to 30°C) protected from moisture.

The reader is invited to consult CPhA's monograph **ACE Inhibitors**.

Teva-Ramipril Ⓟ
ramipril
Angiotensin Converting Enzyme Inhibitor

Teva Canada

SUPPLIED: 2.5 mg: Each opaque orange cap and opaque white body, size no. 4 hard gelatin capsule, printed in black ink N and 2.5 on opposing cap and body portions of the capsule, contains: ramipril 2.5 mg. Nonmedicinal ingredients: calcium phosphate (dibasic), colloidal silicon dioxide, magnesium hydroxide, magnesium stearate, pregelatinized starch and talc; empty gelatin capsules: D&C Yellow No. 10, FD&C Red No. 40, gelatin and titanium dioxide. Gluten-free. Bottles of 100 and 500. Unit dose cartons of 30 capsules. Store bottles between 15-30°C. Store blister packs between 15-25°C.
5 mg: Each opaque red cap and opaque white body, size no. 4 hard gelatin capsule, printed in black ink N and 5 on opposing cap and body portions of the capsule, contains: ramipril 5 mg. Nonmedicinal ingredients: calcium phosphate (dibasic), colloidal silicon dioxide, magnesium hydroxide, magnesium stearate, pregelatinized starch and talc; empty gelatin capsules: D&C Red No. 33, FD&C Blue No. 1, FD&C Red No. 40, gelatin and titanium dioxide. Gluten-free. Bottles of 100 and 500. Unit dose cartons of 30 capsules. Store bottles between 15-30°C. Store blister packs between 15-25°C.
10 mg: Each opaque blue cap and opaque white body, size no. 4 hard gelatin capsule, printed in black ink N and 10 on opposing cap and body portions of the capsule, contains: ramipril 10 mg. Nonmedicinal ingredients: calcium phosphate (dibasic), colloidal silicon dioxide, magnesium hydroxide, magnesium stearate, pregelatinized starch and talc; empty gelatin capsules: D&C Red No. 28, FD&C Blue No. 1, FDA/E172 Black Iron Oxide, gelatin and titanium dioxide. Gluten-free. Bottles of 100 and 500. Unit dose cartons of 30 capsules. Store bottles between 15-30°C. Store blister packs between 15-25°C.

The reader is invited to consult CPhA's monograph **Selective Serotonin Reuptake Inhibitors**.

Teva-Sertraline Ⓟ
sertraline HCl
Antidepressant—Antipanic—Antiobsessional

Teva Canada

SUPPLIED: 25 mg: Each yellow body and yellow cap, hard gelatin capsule, printed N and 25 in black ink on opposing cap and body portions of the capsule, contains: sertraline HCl equivalent to sertraline 25 mg. Nonmedicinal ingredients: colloidal silicon dioxide, D&C Yellow #10, FD&C Yellow #6, gelatin, lactose monohydrate, magnesium stearate, pregelatinized starch, sodium lauryl sulfate, talc and titanium dioxide. Gluten- and tartrazine-free. White, opaque HDPE bottles of 100. Store at controlled room temperature between 15 and 30°C.
50 mg: Each white body and yellow cap, hard gelatin capsule, printed N and 50 in black ink on opposing cap and body portions of the capsule, contains: sertraline HCl equivalent to sertraline 50 mg. Nonmedicinal ingredients: colloidal silicon dioxide, D&C Yellow #10, FD&C Yellow #6, gelatin, lactose monohydrate, magnesium stearate, pregelatinized starch, sodium lauryl sulfate, talc and titanium dioxide. Gluten- and tartrazine-free. White opaque HDPE bottles of 100 and 250. Store at controlled room temperature between 15 and 30°C.
100 mg: Each orange body and orange cap, hard gelatin capsule, printed N and 100 in black ink on opposing cap and body portions of the capsule, contains: sertraline HCl equivalent to sertraline 100 mg. Nonmedicinal ingredients: colloidal silicon dioxide, D&C Yellow #10, FD&C Red #40, gelatin, lactose monohydrate, magnesium stearate, pregelatinized starch, sodium lauryl sulfate, talc and titanium dioxide. Gluten- and tartrazine-free. White, opaque HDPE bottles of 100. Store at controlled room temperature between 15 and 30°C.

New CPhA monographs in 2011 include bisoprolol, dantrolene and propafenone. Consult the CPhA Monographs Index in the front pages of the *CPS* to obtain a complete list.

The reader is invited to consult CPhA's monograph **HMG-CoA Reductase Inhibitors**.

Teva-Simvastatin Ⓟ
simvastatin
Lipid Metabolism Regulator

Teva Canada

SUPPLIED: 5 mg: Each buff colored, shield-shaped, film-coated tablet, engraved with N on one side and 5 on the other side, contains: simvastatin 5 mg. Nonmedicinal ingredients: ascorbic acid, butylated hydroxyanisole, citric acid monohydrate, glycerol triacetate, hypromellose, iron oxide yellow, lactose monohydrate, magnesium stearate, microcrystalline cellulose, polydextrose, polyethylene glycol, polysorbate 80, pregelatinized starch, titanium dioxide and triacetin. White high density polyethylene bottles of 100. Blister packages of 30. Store at room temperature (15-30°C).
10 mg: Each peach colored, shield-shaped, film-coated tablet, engraved with N on one side and 10 on the other side, contains: simvastatin 10 mg. Nonmedicinal ingredients: ascorbic acid, butylated hydroxyanisole, citric acid monohydrate, glycerol triacetate, hypromellose, iron oxide red, lactose monohydrate, magnesium stearate, microcrystalline cellulose, polydextrose, polyethylene glycol, polysorbate 80, pregelatinized starch, titanium dioxide and triacetin. White high density polyethylene bottles of 100 and 500. Blister packages of 30. Store at room temperature (15-30°C).
20 mg: Each tan colored, shield-shaped, film-coated tablet, engraved with N on one side and 20 on the other side, contains: simvastatin 20 mg. Nonmedicinal ingredients: ascorbic acid, butylated hydroxyanisole, citric acid monohydrate, glycerol triacetate, hypromellose, iron oxide red, iron oxide yellow, lactose monohydrate, magnesium stearate, microcrystalline cellulose, polydextrose, polyethylene glycol, polysorbate 80, pregelatinized starch, titanium dioxide and triacetin. White high density polyethylene bottles of 100. Blister packages of 30. Store at room temperature (15-30°C).
40 mg: Each brick red colored, shield-shaped, film-coated tablet, engraved with N on one side and 40 on the other side, contains: simvastatin 40 mg. Nonmedicinal ingredients: ascorbic acid, butylated hydroxyanisole, citric acid monohydrate, FD&C Blue #2, FD&C Red # 40, FD&C Yellow # 6, glycerol triacetate, hypromellose, lactose monohydrate, magnesium stearate, microcrystalline cellulose, polydextrose, polyethylene glycol, polysorbate 80, pregelatinized starch, titanium dioxide and triacetin. White high density polyethylene bottles of 100. Blister packages of 30. Store at room temperature (15-30°C).
80 mg: Each brick red colored, capsule-shaped, film-coated tablet, engraved with N on one side and 80 on the other side, contains: simvastatin 80 mg. Nonmedicinal ingredients: ascorbic acid, butylated hydroxyanisole, citric acid monohydrate, FD&C Blue #2, FD&C Red # 40, FD&C Yellow # 6, glycerol triacetate, hypromellose, lactose monohydrate, magnesium stearate, microcrystalline cellulose, polydextrose, polyethylene glycol, polysorbate 80, pregelatinized starch, titanium dioxide and triacetin. White high density polyethylene bottles of 100. Blister packages of 30. Store at room temperature (15-30°C).

Teva-Spironolactone Ⓟ
spironolactone
Aldosterone Antagonist

Teva Canada

SUPPLIED: 25 mg: Each cream-colored, round, biconvex, compressed tablet, and with a peppermint aroma, engraved N on one side and 2|5 on the reverse, contains: spironolactone 25 mg. Nonmedicinal ingredients: D&C Yellow #10 Lake, FD&C Yellow #6 Lake, lactose monohydrate, magnesium stearate, natural peppermint flavor, sodium lauryl sulfate and sodium starch glycolate. Gluten- and tartrazine-free. Bottles of 500. Unit dose strips of 100.
100 mg: Each cream-colored, round, biconvex tablet, and with a peppermint aroma, engraved N|N on one side and 100 on the reverse, contains: spironolactone 100 mg. Nonmedicinal ingredients: D&C Yellow #10 Lake, FD&C Yellow #6 Lake, lactose monohydrate, magnesium stearate, natural peppermint flavor, sodium lauryl sulfate and sodium starch glycolate. Gluten- and tartrazine-free. Bottles of 100. Unit dose strips of 100.

Teva-Spironolactone HCTZ Ⓟ
hydrochlorothiazide—spironolactone
Diuretic—Aldosterone Antagonist

Teva Canada

SUPPLIED: 25 mg: Each round, biconvex, compressed, ivory tablet, with a peppermint aroma, engraved 25 over 25 on one side and novo on the other side, contains: spironolactone 25 mg and hydrochlorothiazide 25 mg. Nonmedicinal ingredients: colloidal silicon dioxide, D&C Yellow #10 Lake, FD&C Yellow #6 Lake, lactose monohydrate, magnesium stearate, natural peppermint flavor, sodium lauryl sulfate and sodium starch glycolate. Gluten- and tartrazine-free. Bottles of 100. Store between 15-30°C.
50 mg: Each round, biconvex, compressed, white tablet, with a peppermint aroma, engraved 50 over 50 on one side and novo on the other side, contains: spironolactone 50 mg and hydrochlorothiazide 50 mg. Nonmedicinal ingredients: colloidal silicon dioxide, lactose monohydrate, magnesium stearate, natural peppermint flavor, sodium lauryl sulfate and sodium starch glycolate. Gluten- and tartrazine-free. Bottles of 100. Store between 15-30°C.

Teva-Sulfamethoxazole Trimethoprim Ⓟ
sulfamethoxazole—trimethoprim
Antibacterial

Teva Canada

Teva-Sulfamethoxazole Trimethoprim DS Ⓟ
sulfamethoxazole—trimethoprim
Antibacterial

Teva Canada

SUPPLIED: Teva-Sulfamethoxazole Trimethoprim: Oral Suspension: Each 5 mL of light pink, cherry flavored suspension contains: trimethoprim 40 mg and sulfamethoxazole 200 mg. Nonmedicinal ingredients: cherry flavor, citric acid, FD&C Red #40, sorbitol, sodium chloride, sodium cyclamate, sodium methyl hydroxybenzoate, sodium propyl hydroxybenzoate, polysorbate 80 and tragacanth. Gluten- and tartrazine-free. Bottles of 100 and 400 mL.
Tablets: Each white, round, biconvex, compressed tablet, engraved N over scoreline 80 under scoreline on one side and plain on the reverse, contains: trimethoprim 80 mg and sulfamethoxazole 400 mg. Nonmedicinal ingredients: gelatin, glycerin, magnesium stearate, sodium lauryl sulfate and sodium starch glycolate. Gluten- and tartrazine-free. Bottles of 100, 500 and 1000. Unit dose strips of 100.
Teva-Sulfamethoxazole Trimethoprim DS: Each white, oval-shaped, biconvex, compressed tablet, N, scoreline and 160 engraved on one side, plain on the reverse, contains: trimethoprim 160 mg and sulfamethoxazole 800 mg. Nonmedicinal ingredients: gelatin, glycerin, magnesium stearate, sodium lauryl sulfate and sodium starch glycolate. Gluten- and tartrazine-free. Bottles of 100 and 500. Unit dose strips of 100.

Teva-Sumatriptan ℞
sumatriptan succinate
5-HT1 Receptor Agonist—Migraine Therapy

Teva Canada

Teva-Sumatriptan DF ℞
sumatriptan succinate
5-HT1 Receptor Agonist—Migraine Therapy

Teva Canada

SUPPLIED: Teva-Sumatriptan: Each pink, triangular, film-coated tablet, engraved with N on one side and 100 on the other side, contains: sumatriptan (base) 100 mg as the succinate salt. Nonmedicinal ingredients: colloidal silicon dioxide, lactose, magnesium stearate, microcrystalline cellulose and sodium starch glycolate; film-coating: hydroxypropyl methylcellulose, polydextrose, polyethylene glycol, synthetic red iron oxide, titanium dioxide and triacetin. Blister pack boxes of 6. Store between 15 and 30°C.
Teva-Sumatriptan DF: 25 mg: Each white, triangular, film-coated tablet, engraved with N on one side and 25 on the other side, contains: sumatriptan (base) 25 mg as the succinate salt. Nonmedicinal ingredients: colloidal silicon dioxide, crospovidone, lactose, magnesium stearate and microcrystalline cellulose; film-coating: hydroxypropyl methylcellulose, polydextrose, polyethylene glycol, titanium dioxide and triacetin. Blister pack boxes of 6 (1 sheet of 6 unit dose tablets). Store between 15 and 30°C.
50 mg: Each white, triangular, film-coated tablet, engraved with N on one side and 50 on the other side, contains: sumatriptan (base) 50 mg as the succinate salt. Nonmedicinal ingredients: colloidal silicon dioxide, crospovidone, lactose, magnesium stearate and microcrystalline cellulose; film-coating: hydroxypropyl methylcellulose, polydextrose, polyethylene glycol, titanium dioxide and triacetin. Blister pack boxes of 6 (1 sheet of 6 unit dose tablets). Store between 15 and 30°C.
100 mg: Each pink, triangular, film-coated tablet, engraved with N N on one side and 100 on the other side, contains: sumatriptan (base) 100 mg as the succinate salt. Nonmedicinal ingredients: colloidal silicon dioxide, crospovidone, lactose, magnesium stearate and microcrystalline cellulose; film-coating: hydroxypropyl methylcellulose, polydextrose, polyethylene glycol, synthetic red iron oxide, titanium dioxide and triacetin. Bottles of 50. Blister pack boxes of 6 (1 sheet of 6 unit dose tablets). Store between 15 and 30°C.

Teva-Topiramate ℞
topiramate
Antiepileptic—Migraine Prophylaxis

Teva Canada

SUPPLIED: 25 mg: Each white to off-white, round, film-coated tablet, engraved "N" on one side and "25" on the other side contains: topiramate 25 mg. Nonmedicinal ingredients: colloidal silicon dioxide, HPMC 2910/Hypromellose 3cP, HPMC 2910/Hypromellose 6cP, HPMC 2910/Hypromellose 50cP, lactose monohydrate, Macrogol/PEG 8000, magnesium stearate, microcrystalline cellulose, polydextrose, sodium starch glycolate, starch 1500, triacetin and titanium dioxide. Gluten-free. Pack sizes of 100. Store at 15-30°C. Protect from moisture.
100 mg: Each yellow, round, film-coated tablet, engraved "N" on one side and "100" on the other side contains: topiramate 100 mg. Nonmedicinal ingredients: colloidal silicon dioxide, hypromellose, lactose monohydrate, magnesium stearate, microcrystalline cellulose, polyethylene glycol, polysorbate 80, sodium starch glycolate, starch 1500, titanium dioxide and yellow iron oxide. Gluten-free. Pack sizes of 60. Store at 15-30°C. Protect from moisture.
200 mg: Each salmon-coloured, round, film-coated tablet, engraved "N" on one side and "200" on the other side contains: topiramate 200 mg. Nonmedicinal ingredients: colloidal silicon dioxide, hypromellose, iron oxide red, lactose monohydrate, magnesium stearate, microcrystalline cellulose, polyethylene glycol, sodium starch glycolate, starch 1500 and titanium dioxide. Gluten-free. Pack sizes of 60. Store at 15-30°C. Protect from moisture.

Teva-Venlafaxine XR ℞
venlafaxine HCl
Antidepressant—Anxiolytic

Teva Canada

SUPPLIED: 37.5 mg: Each extended-release, hard gelatin capsule, with a grey cap and peach body, filled with white to off-white pellets, imprinting on Body: 37.5 Cap: N, contains: venlafaxine HCl 37.5 mg. Nonmedicinal ingredients: black iron oxide, D&C Yellow #10, dibutyl sebacate, ethylcellulose, FD&C Yellow #6, gelatin, isopropyl alcohol, polyethylene glycol, povidone, propylene glycol, shellac, starch, sucrose, talc and titanium dioxide. Gluten-free. White HDPE bottles of 100. Store at room temperature (15-30°C), in a dry place.
75 mg: Each extended-release, hard gelatin capsule, with peach cap and peach body, filled with white to off-white pellets, imprinting on Body: 75 Cap: N, contains: venlafaxine HCl 75 mg. Nonmedicinal ingredients: black iron oxide, n-butyl alcohol, D&C Yellow #10, dibutyl sebacate, ethylcellulose, FD&C Yellow #6, gelatin, isopropyl alcohol, polyethylene glycol, povidone, propylene glycol, shellac, starch, sucrose, talc and titanium dioxide. Gluten-free. White HDPE bottles of 100 and 500. Store at room temperature (15-30°C), in a dry place.
150 mg: Each extended-release, hard gelatin capsule, with a dark orange cap and dark orange body, filled with white to off-white pellets, imprinting on Body: 150 Cap: N, contains: venlafaxine HCl 150 mg. Nonmedicinal ingredients: black iron oxide, dibutyl sebacate, ethylcellulose, FD&C Yellow #6, gelatin, isopropyl alcohol, polyethylene glycol, povidone, propylene glycol, shellac, starch, sucrose, talc and titanium dioxide. Gluten-free. White HDPE bottles of 100 and 500. Store at room temperature (15-30°C), in a dry place.

Teveten® ℞
eprosartan mesylate
Angiotensin II Receptor (AT1) Antagonist

Abbott Products

Date of Preparation: August 20, 1999
Date of Revision: June 2, 2010

SUMMARY PRODUCT INFORMATION:

Route of Administration	Dosage Form/ Strength	Clinically Relevant Nonmedicinal Ingredients
Oral	Tablet/400 mg and 600 mg	Lactose monohydrate For a complete listing see Dosage Forms, Composition and Packaging.

INDICATIONS AND CLINICAL USE: TEVETEN (eprosartan mesylate) is indicated for the treatment of mild to moderate essential hypertension.

TEVETEN may be used alone or concomitantly with thiazide diuretics.

The safety and efficacy of concurrent treatment with TEVETEN and angiotensin converting enzyme inhibitors have not been established.

Geriatrics: In elderly patients with essential hypertension eprosartan taken once daily for 12 weeks in doses of 600-800 mg is a well-tolerated and effective treatment. At study endpoint there were clinically significant and useful reductions in sitting SBP and DBP compared to baseline in both treatments. However, appropriate caution should nevertheless be used when prescribing to the elderly, as increased vulnerability to drug effect is possible in this patient population (see Action and Clinical Pharmacology, Special Populations and Conditions, Geriatrics, and Dosage and Administration).
Pediatrics: The safety and effectiveness in pediatric patients have not been established.

CONTRAINDICATIONS: Patients who are hypersensitive to TEVETEN (eprosartan mesylate) or to any ingredient in the formulation or component of the container (see Dosage Forms, Composition and Packaging).

TEVETEN is contraindicated in pregnancy and in nursing women (see Warnings and Precautions).

TEVETEN is also contraindicated in patients with hemodynamically significant bilateral renovascular disease or severe stenosis of a solitary functioning kidney (see Warnings and Precautions).

WARNINGS AND PRECAUTIONS:

> **Serious Warnings and Precautions**
> **When used in pregnancy, angiotensin receptor (AT_1) blockers (ARBs) can cause injury or even death of the developing fetus. When pregnancy is detected, TEVETEN should be discontinued as soon as possible (see Contraindications and Warnings and Precautions, Special Populations).**

General: Patients with rare hereditary problems of galactose intolerance, the Lapp lactase deficiency or glucose-galactose malabsorption should not take this medication.
Cardiovascular: There is concern on theoretical grounds that patients with aortic stenosis might be at particular risk of decreased coronary perfusion when treated with vasodilators because they do not develop as much afterload reduction.
Hypotension: Occasionally, symptomatic hypotension has occurred after administration of eprosartan, in some cases after the first dose. It is more likely to occur in patients who are volume-depleted by diuretic therapy, dietary salt restriction, dialysis, diarrhea, or vomiting. In those patients, because of the potential fall in blood pressure, these conditions should be corrected prior to starting therapy and under close medical supervision. Similar considerations apply to patients with ischemic heart or cerebrovascular disease, in whom an excessive fall in blood pressure could result in myocardial infarction or cerebrovascular accident.
Hepatic/Biliary/Pancreatic: Based on pharmacokinetic data which demonstrate increased plasma concentrations of eprosartan in hepatically impaired patients after administration of TEVETEN (eprosartan mesylate), a lower initial dose should be considered for patients with hepatic impairment or a history of hepatic impairment (see Dosage and Administration).
Renal: As a consequence of inhibiting the renin-angiotensin-aldosterone system, changes in renal function have been seen in susceptible individuals. In patients whose renal function may depend on the activity of the renin-angiotensin-aldosterone system, such as patients with bilateral renal artery stenosis, unilateral renal artery stenosis to a solitary kidney, or severe congestive heart failure, treatment with agents that inhibit this system has been associated with oliguria, progressive azotemia, and rarely, acute renal failure and/or death. In susceptible patients, concomitant diuretic use may further increase risk.

Use of eprosartan should include appropriate assessment of renal function (see Dosage and Administration).
Special Populations: Pregnant Women: Drugs that act directly on the renin-angiotensin-aldosterone system (RAAS) can cause fetal and neonatal morbidity and death when administered to pregnant women. When pregnancy is detected, TEVETEN should be discontinued as soon as possible (see Contraindications).

The use of ARBs is not recommended during pregnancy. Epidemiological evidence regarding the risk of teratogenicity following exposure to angiotensin converting enzyme inhibitors (another class of therapeutic products interfering with the RAAS) during the first trimester of pregnancy has not been conclusive; however a small increase in risk cannot be excluded. Given the current evidence available on the risk with ARBs, similar risk may exist for this class of drugs. Patients planning pregnancy should be changed to alternative antihypertensive treatments which have an established safety profile for use in pregnancy. When pregnancy is diagnosed, treatment with angiotensin II antagonists should be stopped immediately, and, if appropriate, alternative therapy should be started.

The use of ARBs during the second and third trimesters is known to induce human fetotoxicity (decreased renal function, oligohydramnios, skull ossification retardation) and neonatal toxicity (renal failure, hypotension, hyperkalaemia).

Infants with a history of in utero exposure to ARBs should be closely observed for hypotension, oliguria, and hyperkalemia. If oliguria occurs, attention should be directed toward support of blood pressure and renal perfusion. Exchange transfusion or dialysis may be required as a means of reversing hypotension and/or substituting for impaired renal function; however, limited experience with those procedures has not been associated with significant clinical benefit.

Eprosartan is not removed from plasma by dialysis.
Animal Data: Eprosartan mesylate has been shown to produce maternal and fetal toxicities (maternal and fetal mortality, low maternal body weight and food consumption, resorptions, abortions and litter loss) in pregnant rabbits given oral doses as low as 10 mg eprosartan/kg/day. No maternal or fetal adverse effects were observed at 3 mg/kg/day; this oral dose yielded a systemic exposure (AUC) to unbound eprosartan 0.8 times that achieved in humans given 400 mg b.i.d. No adverse effects on in utero or postnatal development and maturation of offspring were observed when eprosartan mesylate was administered to pregnant rats at oral doses up to 1000 mg eprosartan/kg/day (the 1000 mg eprosartan/kg/day dose in non-pregnant rats yielded systemic exposure to unbound eprosartan approximately 0.6 times the exposure achieved in humans given 400 mg b.i.d.).
Nursing Women: It is not known whether eprosartan is excreted in human milk but significant levels have been found in the milk of lactating rats. Because many drugs are excreted in human milk and because of their potential for affecting the nursing infant adversely, if the initiation of treatment with eprosartan is regarded necessary, nursing should be discontinued first. Nursing women should not be treated with TEVETEN (see Contraindications).
Pediatrics: The safety and effectiveness in pediatric patients have not been established.
Geriatrics: In elderly patients with essential hypertension eprosartan taken once daily for 12 weeks in doses of 600-800 mg is a well-tolerated and effective treatment. At study endpoint there were clinically significant and useful reductions in sitting SBP and DBP compared to baseline in both treatments. However, appropriate caution should nevertheless be used when prescribing to the elderly, as increased vulnerability to drug effect is possible in this patient population (see Action and Clinical Pharmacology, Special Populations and Conditions, Geriatrics, and Dosage and Administration, Recommended Dose and Dosage Adjustment, Use in the Elderly).

ADVERSE REACTIONS: Adverse Drug Reaction Overview: TEVETEN (eprosartan mesylate) has been evaluated for safety in more than 3300 healthy volunteers and patients, including more than 1460 patients treated for more than 6 months, and more than 980 patients treated for 1 year or longer.

Adverse experiences were similar in patients regardless of age, gender, or race.
Clinical Trial Adverse Drug Reactions: Because clinical trials are conducted under very specific conditions the adverse reaction rates observed in the clinical trials may not reflect the rates observed in practice and should not be compared to the rates in the clinical trials of another drug. Adverse drug reaction information from clinical trials is useful for identifying drug-related adverse events and for approximating rates.

In placebo-controlled clinical trials, about 4% of 1202 patients treated with TEVETEN discontinued therapy due to clinical adverse experiences, compared to 6.5% of 352 patients given placebo.
Adverse Events Occurring at an Incidence of 1% or More Among Eprosartan-treated Patients: Table 1 lists adverse events that occurred at an incidence of 1% or more among eprosartan-treated patients who participated in placebo-controlled trials of 8 to 13 weeks duration, using od and bid dosing. The overall incidence of adverse events reported with TEVETEN (54.4%) was similar to placebo (52.8%). The following potentially serious adverse reactions have been reported rarely with eprosartan: syncope, hypotension.

In addition, asthenia has been seen commonly in clinical trials.
Less Common Clinical Trial Adverse Drug Events (<1%): In addition to the adverse events above, potentially important events that occurred in at least two patients/subjects exposed to eprosartan or other adverse events that occurred in <1% of patients in clinical studies regardless of drug relationship are listed below.
Body as a Whole: alcohol intolerance, allergic reaction, allergy, substernal chest pain, leg edema, peripheral edema, fever, hot flushes, influenza-like symptoms, malaise, rigors.
Cardiovascular: angina pectoris, bradycardia, nonspecific ST-T changes, T-wave inversion, extrasystoles, atrial fibrillation, hypotension, tachycardia, peripheral ischemia.
Gastrointestinal: anorexia, constipation, dry mouth, esophagitis, flatulence, gastritis, gastroenteritis, gingivitis, nausea, periodontitis, toothache, vomiting.
Hematologic: anemia, purpura.
Metabolic and Nutritional: increased creatine phosphokinase, diabetes mellitus, glycosuria, gout, hypercholesterolemia, hyperglycemia, hyperkalemia, hypokalemia, hyponatremia.

Table 1: TEVETEN

Most Common[a] On-therapy Adverse Experiences for Patients in Placebo-controlled, Hypertension Studies

	Number of Patients with Adverse Experiences			
	Eprosartan (n=1202)		Placebo (n=352)	
	N	%	N	%
Central and Peripheral Nervous Systems				
Headache	121	10.1	38	10.8
Dizziness	35	2.9	13	3.7
Musculoskeletal System				
Myalgia	48	4	14	4
Arthralgia	22	1.8	4	1.1
Back Pain	16	1.3	4	1.1
Respiratory System				
Upper Respiratory Tract Infection	95	7.9	19	5.4
Rhinitis	48	4	10	2.8
Pharyngitis	44	3.7	9	2.6
Coughing	42	3.5	9	2.6
Sinusitis	38	3.2	12	3.4
Dyspnea	15	1.2	2	0.6
Bronchitis	13	1.1	8	2.3
Gastrointestinal System				
Diarrhea	30	2.5	9	2.6
Abdominal Pain	18	1.5	3	0.9
Dyspepsia	16	1.3	6	1.7
Body as a Whole, General				
Viral Infection	29	2.4	5	1.4
Injury	29	2.4	4	1.1
Chest Pain	25	2.1	7	2
Fatigue	18	1.5	4	1.1
Pain	14	1.2	4	1.1
Dependent Edema	13	1.1	8	2.3
Urinary System				
Urinary Tract Infection	16	1.3	1	0.3
Metabolic and Nutritional				
Hypertriglyceridemia	15	1.2	0	0
Heart Rate and Rhythm				
Palpitation	14	1.2	3	0.9
Psychiatric				
Depression	12	1	0	0
Total[b]	654	54.4	186	52.8

[a] Includes adverse experiences reported for ≥1% of patients who received oral eprosartan monotherapy.
[b] Total patients with at least 1 adverse experience. Patients with multiple adverse experiences are counted only once.

Musculoskeletal: arthritis, aggravated arthritis, arthrosis, leg cramps, skeletal pain, tendonitis.
Nervous System/Psychiatric: anxiety, ataxia, insomnia, migraine, neuritis, nervousness, paresthesia, somnolence, tremor, vertigo.
Resistance Mechanism: herpes simplex, otitis externa, otitis media, upper respiratory tract infection.
Respiratory: asthma, epistaxis.
Skin and Appendages: eczema, furunculosis, pruritus, rash, maculopapular rash, increased sweating.
Special Senses: conjunctivitis, abnormal vision, xerophthalmia, tinnitus.
Urinary: albuminuria, cystitis, hematuria, micturition frequency, polyuria, renal calculus, urinary incontinence.
Abnormal Hematologic and Clinical Chemistry Findings: In placebo-controlled studies, clinically important changes in standard laboratory parameters were rarely associated with administration of TEVETEN.
Creatinine, Blood Urea Nitrogen: Minor elevations in creatinine and in BUN occurred in 0.6% and 1.3%, respectively, of patients taking TEVETEN and 0.9% and 0.3%, respectively, of patients given placebo in controlled clinical trials. Two patients were withdrawn from clinical trials for elevations in serum creatinine and BUN, and three additional patients were withdrawn for increases in serum creatinine.
Liver Function Tests: Minor elevations of ALAT, ASAT, and alkaline phosphatase occurred for comparable percentages of patients taking TEVETEN (eprosartan mesylate) or placebo in controlled clinical trials. An elevated ALAT of >3.5×ULN occurred in 0.1% of patients taking TEVETEN (one patient) and in no patient given placebo in controlled clinical trials. Four patients were withdrawn from clinical trials for an elevation in liver function tests.
Hemoglobin: A greater than 20% decrease in hemoglobin was observed in 0.1% of patients taking TEVETEN (one patient) and in no patient given placebo in controlled clinical trials. Two patients were withdrawn from clinical trials for anemia.
Leukopenia: A WBC count of $\leq 3.0 \times 10^3/mm^3$ occurred in 0.3% of patients taking TEVETEN and in 0.3% of patients given placebo in controlled clinical trials. One patient was withdrawn from clinical trials for leukopenia.
Neutropenia: A neutrophil count of $\leq 1.5 \times 10^3/mm^3$ occurred in 1.3% of patients taking TEVETEN and in 1.4% of patients given placebo in controlled clinical trials. No patient was withdrawn from any clinical trials for neutropenia.
Thrombocytopenia: A platelet count of $\leq 100 \times 10^9$/L occurred in 0.3% of patients taking TEVETEN (one patient) and in no patient given placebo in controlled clinical trials. Four patients receiving TEVETEN in clinical trials were withdrawn for thrombocytopenia. In one case, thrombocytopenia was present prior to dosing with TEVETEN.
Serum Potassium: A potassium value of ≥5.6 mmol/L occurred in 0.9% of patients taking TEVETEN and 0.3% of patients given placebo in controlled clinical trials. One patient was withdrawn from clinical trials for hyperkalemia and three for hypokalemia.
Post-Market Adverse Drug Reactions: The following adverse reactions have been identified during post-marketing use of TEVETEN:

- Headaches, dizziness, and asthenia have been rarely reported.
- Hypotension, including postural hypotension, has been very rarely reported.
- Skin reactions (rash, pruritus, urticaria) have been very rarely reported.
- Angioedema (involving swelling of the face, lips and/or tongue) has been very rarely reported.

Cases of muscle pain, muscle weakness, myositis and rhabdomyolysis have been reported in patients receiving angiotensin II receptor blockers.

Since there is currently inadequate therapeutic experience in patients with severe cardiac insufficiency or renal artery stenosis, it cannot be ruled out that renal function may be impaired (including renal failure in patients at risk e.g. renal artery stenosis) with eprosartan due to inhibition of the renin-angiotensin-aldosterone system.

DRUG INTERACTIONS: Drug-Drug Interactions: See Table 2.

Table 2: TEVETEN

Established or Potential Drug-Drug Interactions

Proper Name	Ref.	Effect	Clinical Comment
Diuretics	T	Patients on diuretics, and especially those in whom diuretic therapy was recently instituted, may occasionally experience an excessive reduction in blood pressure after initiation of therapy with TEVETEN (eprosartan mesylate).	No drug interaction of clinical significance has been identified with thiazide diuretics. The possibility of symptomatic hypotension with the use of TEVETEN can be minimized by discontinuing the diuretic prior to initiation of treatment (see Warnings and Precautions, Cardiovascular, Hypotension and Dosage and Administration).
Agents Increasing Serum Potassium	T	Eprosartan decreases the production of aldosterone.	Potassium-sparing diuretics or potassium supplements should be given only for documented hypokalemia and with frequent monitoring of serum potassium. Potassium-containing salt substitutes should also be used with caution.
Lithium Salts	T	As with other drugs which eliminate sodium, lithium clearance may be reduced.	Serum lithium levels should be monitored carefully if lithium salts are to be administered.
Digoxin	CT	No effect on single oral-dose digoxin pharmacokinetics.	Concomitant administration of eprosartan and digoxin had no effect on single oral-dose digoxin pharmacokinetics.
Warfarin	CT	No effect on steady-state prothrombin time ratios (INR) in healthy volunteers.	Concomitant administration of eprosartan and warfarin had no effect on steady-state prothrombin time ratios (INR) in healthy volunteers.
Ranitidine	CT	No effect on eprosartan pharmacokinetics.	Concomitant administration of ranitidine has no effect on eprosartan pharmacokinetics.
Antifungals (ketoconazole and fluconazole)	CT	No effect on steady state pharmacokinetics of eprosartan.	Concomitant administration of ketoconazole or fluconazole had no effect on steady state pharmacokinetics of eprosartan.
Glyburide	CT	Does not affect 24-hour mean plasma glucose concentrations in diabetic patients.	Concomitant administration of eprosartan and glyburide in diabetic patients did not affect 24-hour mean plasma glucose concentrations.

Legend: C=Case Study; CT=Clinical Trial; T=Theoretical.

Eprosartan has been shown not to inhibit human cytochrome P450 enzymes CYP1A, 2A6, 2C9/8, 2C19, 2D6, 2E, and 3A in vitro.

DOSAGE AND ADMINISTRATION: Dosing Considerations: The dosage of TEVETEN (eprosartan mesylate) must be individualized.

Initiation of therapy requires consideration of recent antihypertensive drug treatment, the extent of blood pressure elevation, salt restriction, and other pertinent clinical factors (see Warnings and Precautions, Cardiovascular, Hypotension). The dosage of antihypertensive agents used with TEVETEN may need to be adjusted.

TEVETEN may be taken with or without food, but it should be taken consistently with respect to food intake and at the same time every day.

Recommended Dose and Dosage Adjustment: Monotherapy: The recommended initial dose of TEVETEN is 600 mg once daily.

Achievement of maximum blood pressure reduction in most patients may take 2-3 weeks after initiation of therapy.

In patients whose blood pressure is not adequately controlled, the dose may be increased to 800 mg once daily. In some patients treated once daily, the antihypertensive effect may diminish toward the end of the dosing interval. If satisfactory control is not being maintained for 24 hours, twice daily administration with the same total daily dosage should be considered. If blood pressure is not adequately controlled with TEVETEN alone, a thiazide diuretic may be administered concomitantly.

Concomitant Diuretic Therapy: In patients receiving diuretics, TEVETEN therapy should be initiated with caution, since these patients may be volume-depleted and thus more likely to experience hypotension following initiation of additional antihypertensive therapy. Whenever possible, all diuretics should be discontinued two to three days prior to the administration of TEVETEN to reduce the likelihood of hypotension (see Warnings and Precautions, Cardiovascular, Hypotension and Drug Interactions, Drug-Drug Interactions). If this is not possible because of the patient's condition, TEVETEN should be administered with caution and the blood pressure monitored closely. Thereafter, the dosage should be adjusted according to the individual response of the patient.

Use in the Elderly: A lower starting dose of 400 mg once daily should be considered (see Action and Clinical Pharmacology, Special Populations and Conditions, Geriatrics and Warnings and Precautions, Special Populations, Geriatrics).

Use in Patients with Impaired Renal Function: A lower starting dose of 400 mg once daily should be considered in patients with severe renal impairment. Patients with moderate to severe renal impairment (creatinine clearance <60 mL/min) requiring 600 mg once daily to control their blood pressure should be monitored carefully and 600 mg once daily should be the maximum dose in these patients (see Action and Clinical Pharmacology, Special Populations and Conditions, Renal Insufficiency and Warnings and Precautions, Renal).

Use in Patients with Impaired Hepatic Function: The starting dose of 400 mg once daily should be considered for patients with impaired hepatic function.
Use in Children: The safety and efficacy of TEVETEN have not been established in children.
Missed Dose: If a dose is forgotten, the missed dose should be taken as soon as possible. The next dose should be taken at the normal time. Two doses should not be taken within six hours of each other.
Administration: TEVETEN is formulated as an aqueous film-coated tablet. It may be taken with or without food, but it should be taken consistently with respect to food intake and at the same time every day.

OVERDOSAGE:
Limited data are available in regard to overdosage with TEVETEN (eprosartan mesylate). The most likely manifestations of overdosage would be hypotension and/or tachycardia. If symptomatic hypotension should occur, supportive treatment should be instituted. Eprosartan was poorly removed by hemodialysis (CL_{HD}<1 L/h).

For management of a suspected drug overdose, CPhA recommends that you contact your **regional Poison Control Centre**. See the *CPS* Directory section for a list of Poison Control Centres.

ACTION AND CLINICAL PHARMACOLOGY: Mechanism of Action: TEVETEN (eprosartan mesylate) antagonizes angiotensin II by blocking the angiotensin type 1 (AT_1) receptor. Angiotensin II is a potent vasoconstrictor, the primary vasoactive hormone of the renin-angiotensin system and an important component in the pathophysiology of hypertension. It also stimulates aldosterone secretion by the adrenal cortex. Eprosartan blocks the vasoconstrictor and aldosterone-secreting effects of angiotensin II by selectively blocking the binding of angiotensin II to the AT_1 receptor found in many tissues (e.g., vascular smooth muscle, adrenal gland). There is also an AT_2 receptor found in many tissues but it is not known to be associated with cardiovascular homeostasis. Eprosartan does not exhibit any partial agonist activity at the AT_1 receptor. Its affinity for the AT_1 receptor is 1000 times greater than for the AT_2 receptor. In vitro binding studies indicate that eprosartan is a reversible, competitive inhibitor of the AT_1 receptor.

TEVETEN does not inhibit angiotensin converting enzyme (ACE), also known as kininase II, the enzyme that converts angiotensin I to angiotensin II and degrades bradykinin, nor does it bind to or block other hormone receptors or ion channels known to be important in cardiovascular regulation.
Pharmacodynamics: Eprosartan inhibits the pharmacologic effects of angiotensin II infusions in healthy adult men. Single oral doses of eprosartan from 10 mg to 400 mg have been shown to inhibit the vasopressor, renal vasoconstrictive and aldosterone secretory effects of infused angiotensin II with complete inhibition evident at doses of 350 mg and above. Eprosartan inhibits the pressor effects of angiotensin II infusions. A single oral dose of 350 mg of eprosartan inhibits pressor effects by approximately 100% at peak, with approximately 30% inhibition persisting for 24 hours. In hypertensive patients treated chronically with eprosartan, there was a twofold rise in angiotensin II plasma concentration and a twofold rise in plasma renin activity, while plasma aldosterone levels remained unchanged. Serum potassium levels also remained unchanged in these patients.

Achievement of maximal blood pressure response to a given dose in most patients may take 2 to 3 weeks of treatment. Onset of blood pressure reduction is seen within 1 to 2 hours of dosing with few instances of orthostatic hypotension. Blood pressure control can be maintained with once- or twice-daily dosing over a 24-hour period. Attenuation of the effect towards the end of the 24 hour dosing period may occur in some patients with once daily dosing. Discontinuing treatment with eprosartan does not lead to a rebound increase in blood pressure.

There was no change in mean heart rate in patients treated with eprosartan in controlled clinical trials.

The antihypertensive effect of TEVETEN was similar in men and women, but was somewhat smaller in patients over 65.

Although data available to date indicate a similar pharmacodynamic effect of eprosartan in black and white hypertensive patients, this should be viewed with caution since antihypertensive drugs that affect the renin-angiotensin system, such as ACE inhibitors and angiotensin II AT_1 receptor blockers, have generally been found to be less effective in low-renin hypertensives (frequently blacks).
Pharmacokinetics: See Table 3.

Table 3: TEVETEN

Summary of Pharmacokinetic Parameter Estimates (arithmetic mean±S.D.) for Eprosartan after Single Doses of Eprosartan in Healthy Male Volunteers (n=17)

Dose Mean	C_{max} (ng/mL)	$t_{1/2}$ (h)	$AUC_{(0-t)}$ (ng·h/mL)	Cl (mL/min)	Vdss (L)
Eprosartan 300 mg oral (fasted)	1612±720	4.52±3.05	5657±2694	ND	ND
Eprosartan 300 mg oral (fed)	1205±484	7.25±4.61	4807±1907	ND	ND
Eprosartan 20 mg i.v.	2246±255	2.07±0.63	2631±576	131.8±36.2	12.6±2.6

Legend: C_{max}=peak plasma concentration; $t_{1/2}$=elimination half-life; $AUC_{(0-t)}$=area under plasma concentration time curve; Cl=clearance; Vdss=volume of distribution; ND=not determined.

Eprosartan pharmacokinetics was not influenced by weight, race, gender or severity of hypertension at baseline.
Absorption: Eprosartan plasma concentrations peak at 1 to 2 hours after an oral dose in the fasted state. Absolute bioavailability following a single 300 mg oral dose of eprosartan is approximately 13%. Administering eprosartan with food delays absorption, and causes variable changes (25%) in C_{max} and AUC values, which do not appear clinically important. Plasma concentrations of eprosartan increase in a slightly less than dose-proportional manner over the 100 to 800 mg dose-range. Eprosartan does not significantly accumulate with chronic use.
Distribution: Plasma protein binding of eprosartan is high (approximately 98%) and constant over the concentration range achieved with therapeutic doses. After intravenous dosing, the eprosartan volume of distribution is about 13 L and total plasma clearance is about 8 L/h. The mean steady-state volume of distribution (Vss/F) was 308 liters in patients of all ages.
Metabolism: Eprosartan is not metabolized by the cytochrome P450 system. No active metabolites were detected following oral and intravenous dosing with eprosartan in human subjects.
Excretion: Eprosartan is eliminated by biliary and renal excretion, primarily as unchanged compound. Less than 2% of an oral dose is excreted in the urine as a glucuronide. Eprosartan was the only drug-related compound found in the plasma and feces. Following administration of intravenous eprosartan, about 61% of the material is recovered in the feces and about 37% in the urine. Following an oral dose of eprosartan, about 90% is recovered in the feces and about 7% in the urine. Approximately 20% of the radioactivity excreted in the urine was an acyl glucuronide of eprosartan with the remaining 80% being unchanged eprosartan. The terminal elimination half-life of eprosartan following oral administration is 5 to 9 hours. Eprosartan exhibited a population mean oral clearance (CL/F) for an average 60-year-old patient of 48.5 L/h. Oral clearance was shown to be a linear function of age with CL/F decreasing 0.62 L/h for every year increase.
Special Populations and Conditions: Pediatrics: The safety and effectiveness in pediatric patients have not been established.
Geriatrics: Following single oral dose administration of eprosartan to healthy elderly men (aged 68 to 78 years), both AUC and C_{max} eprosartan values increased, on average by approximately 2-fold, compared to healthy young men (aged 20 to 39 years) who received the same dose. The extent of plasma protein binding was not influenced by age.
Gender: There were no differences in the pharmacokinetics and plasma protein binding between men and women following administration of a single oral dose of eprosartan.
Race: A pooled population pharmacokinetic analysis of 442 Caucasian and 29 non-Caucasian hypertensive patients showed that oral clearance and steady-state volume of distribution were not influenced by race.
Hepatic Insufficiency: Geometric mean eprosartan AUC values increased approximately 40% in a study of mild to moderate hepatically impaired men vs. healthy men who each received a single 100 mg oral dose of eprosartan. The extent of eprosartan plasma protein binding was not influenced by hepatic dysfunction (see Dosage and Administration).
Renal Insufficiency: Following administration of eprosartan 200 mg b.i.d. for 7 days, patients with mild renal impairment (CLcr 60 to 80 mL/min) showed mean eprosartan C_{max} and AUC values similar to subjects with normal renal function. Following treatment once daily of 600 mg for seven days, the AUC (0-24 hours) values were two-fold increased in patients with moderate (Clcr 30 to 59 mL/min) or severe renal impairment (Clcr 5 to 29 mL/min) from that in the patients with normal renal function. The C_{max} values were also 30-50% higher in patients with moderate or severe renal impairment than in patients with normal renal function. The unbound eprosartan fraction was not influenced by mild to moderate renal impairment but increased approximately 2-fold in a few patients with severe renal impairment. Eprosartan was poorly removed by hemodialysis (CL_{HD}<1 L/h) (see Dosage and Administration).
STORAGE AND STABILITY: TEVETEN (eprosartan mesylate) tablets should be stored at controlled room temperature, between 15 to 25°C. Protect from moisture.
SPECIAL HANDLING INSTRUCTIONS: None.
INFORMATION FOR THE PATIENT: Published in e-CPS, available by subscription at www.e-cps.ca.
DOSAGE FORMS, COMPOSITION AND PACKAGING: 400 mg: Each pink, oval, aqueous film-coated tablet, debossed with "SOLVAY" on one side and "5044" on the other side, contains: eprosartan mesylate equivalent to eprosartan 400 mg. Nonmedicinal ingredients: croscarmellose sodium, hypromellose, lactose monohydrate, magnesium stearate, microcrystalline cellulose, polyethylene glycol, pregelatinized starch and titanium dioxide. May also contain: iron oxide red, iron oxide yellow and polysorbate 80. Blister packs of 28.
600 mg: Each white, capsule-shaped, aqueous film-coated tablet, debossed with "SOLVAY" on one side and "5046" on the other side, contains: eprosartan mesylate equivalent to eprosartan 600 mg. Nonmedicinal ingredients: crospovidone, hypromellose, lactose monohydrate, magnesium stearate, microcrystalline cellulose, polyethylene glycol, pregelatinized starch and titanium dioxide. May also contain: iron oxide red, iron oxide yellow and polysorbate 80. Blister packs of 28.

(Shown in Product Identification Section)

Teveten® Plus 🄿

eprosartan mesylate—hydrochlorothiazide
Angiotensin II Receptor (AT1) Antagonist—Diuretic

Abbott Products

Date of Preparation: May 25, 2004
Date of Revision: May 31, 2010

PHARMACOLOGY: TEVETEN PLUS (eprosartan mesylate and hydrochlorothiazide) combines the actions of eprosartan mesylate, an angiotensin II (AT_1) receptor antagonist, and that of a thiazide diuretic, hydrochlorothiazide.
Eprosartan: Eprosartan antagonizes angiotensin II by blocking the angiotensin type 1 (AT_1) receptor. Angiotensin II is a potent vasoconstrictor, the primary vasoactive hormone of the renin-angiotensin system and an important component in the pathophysiology of hypertension. It also stimulates aldosterone secretion by the adrenal cortex. Eprosartan blocks the vasoconstrictor and aldosterone-secreting effects of angiotensin II by selectively blocking the binding of angiotensin II to the AT_1 receptor found in many tissues (e.g., vascular smooth muscle, adrenal gland). There is also an AT_2 receptor found in many tissues but it is not known to be associated with cardiovascular homeostasis. Eprosartan does not exhibit any partial agonist activity at the AT_1 receptor. Its affinity for the AT_1 receptor is 1000 times greater than for the AT_2 receptor. In vitro binding studies indicate that eprosartan is a reversible, competitive inhibitor of the AT_1 receptor.

Eprosartan does not inhibit angiotensin converting enzyme (ACE), also known as kininase II, the enzyme that converts angiotensin I to angiotensin II and degrades bradykinin, nor does it bind to or block other hormone receptors or ion channels known to be important in cardiovascular regulation.
Hydrochlorothiazide: Hydrochlorothiazide is a diuretic and antihypertensive which interferes with the renal tubular mechanisms of electrolyte reabsorption. It increases excretion of sodium and chloride in approximately equivalent amounts. Natriuresis may be accompanied by some loss of potassium and bicarbonate. While this compound is predominantly a saluretic agent, in vitro studies have shown that it has a carbonic anhydrase inhibitory action which seems to be relatively specific for the renal tubular mechanism. It does not appear to be concentrated in erthrocytes or the brain in sufficient amounts to influence the activity of carbonic anhydrase in those tissues.

Hydrochlorothiazide is useful in the treatment of hypertension. It may be used alone or as an adjunct to other antihypertensive drugs. Hydrochlorothiazide does not affect normal blood pressure.
Pharmacokinetics: Eprosartan: Absolute bioavailability following a single 300 mg oral dose of eprosartan is approximately 13%. Eprosartan plasma concentrations peak at 1 to 2 hours after an oral dose in the fasted state. Plasma concentrations of eprosartan increase in a slightly less than dose-proportional manner over the 100 to 800 mg dose-range. The terminal elimination half-life of eprosartan following oral administration is 5 to 9 hours. Eprosartan does not significantly accumulate with chronic use.

Plasma protein binding of eprosartan is high (approximately 98%) and constant over the concentration range achieved with therapeutic doses. After intravenous dosing, the eprosartan volume of distribution is about 13 liters and total plasma clearance is about 8 L/h.

Eprosartan exhibited a population mean oral clearance (CL/F) for an average 60-year-old patient of 48.5 L/h. The mean steady-state volume of distribution (Vss/F) was 308 liters in patients of all ages. Eprosartan pharmacokinetics were not influenced by weight, race, gender or severity of hypertension at baseline. Oral clearance was shown to be a linear function of age with CL/F decreasing 0.62 L/h for every year increase.

Eprosartan is not metabolized by the cytochrome P450 system. Eprosartan is eliminated by biliary and renal excretion, primarily as unchanged compound. Less than 2% of an oral dose is excreted in the urine as a glucuronide. No active metabolites were detected following oral and intravenous dosing with eprosartan in human subjects. Eprosartan was the only drug-related compound found in the plasma and feces. Following administration of i.v. eprosartan, about 61% of the material is recovered in the feces and about 37% in the urine. Following an oral dose of eprosartan, about 90% is recovered in the feces and about 7% in the urine. Approximately 20% of the radioactivity excreted in the urine was an acyl glucuronide of eprosartan with the remaining 80% being unchanged eprosartan.
Renal Insufficiency: Following administration of eprosartan 200 mg b.i.d. for 7 days, patients with mild renal impairment (creatinine clearance 60 to 80 mL/min) showed mean eprosartan C_{max} and AUC values similar to subjects with normal renal function. Compared to patients with normal renal function, mean AUC and C_{max} values were approximately 30% higher in patients with moderate renal impairment (creatinine clearance 30 to 59 mL/min) and 50% higher in patients with severe renal impairment (creatinine clearance 5 to 29 mL/min). The unbound eprosartan fraction was not influenced by mild to moderate renal impairment but increased approximately 2-fold in a few patients with severe renal impairment (see Dosage, Eprosartan Monotherapy). Hemodialysis resulted in very limited effects on clearance (CL_{HD}<1L/h) and was essentially not dialyzed.
Hepatic Insufficiency: Geometric mean eprosartan AUC values increased approximately 40% in a study of mild to moderate hepatically impaired men vs. healthy men who each received a single 100 mg oral dose of eprosartan. The extent of eprosartan plasma protein binding was not influenced by hepatic dysfunction (see Dosage).
Geriatrics: Following single oral dose administration of eprosartan to healthy elderly men (aged 68 to 78 years), both AUC and C_{max} eprosartan values increased, on average by approximately two-fold, compared to healthy young men (aged 20 to 39 years) who received the same dose. The extent of plasma protein binding was not influenced by age.
Gender: There were no differences in the pharmacokinetics and plasma protein binding between men and women following administration of a single oral dose of eprosartan.
Race: A pooled population pharmacokinetic analysis of 442 Caucasian and 29 non-Caucasian hypertensive patients showed that oral clearance and steady-state volume of distribution for eprosartan were not influenced by race.
Hydrochlorothiazide: Hydrochlorothiazide is not metabolized but is eliminated rapidly by the kidney. The plasma half-life is 5.6-14.8 hours when the plasma levels can be followed for at least 24 hours. At least 61% of the oral dose is eliminated unchanged within 24 hours. Hydrochlorothiazide crosses the placental but not the blood-brain barrier and is excreted in breast milk.
Eprosartan and Hydrochlorothiazide: Concomitant administration of eprosartan and hydrochlorothiazide has no clinically significant effect on the pharmacokinetics of either drug.
Pharmacodynamics: Eprosartan: Eprosartan inhibits the pharmacologic effects of angiotensin II infusions in healthy adult men. Single oral doses of eprosartan from 10 mg to 400 mg have been shown to inhibit the vasopressor, renal vasoconstrictive and aldosterone secretory effects of infused angiotensin II with complete inhibition evident at doses of 350 mg and above. Eprosartan inhibits the pressor effects of angiotensin II infusions. A single oral dose of 350 mg inhibits pressor effects by approximately 100% at peak, with approximately 30% inhibition persisting for 24 hours. In hypertensive patients treated chronically with eprosartan, there was a twofold rise in angiotensin II plasma concentration and a twofold rise in plasma renin activity, while plasma aldosterone levels remained unchanged. Serum potassium levels also remained unchanged in these patients.

Achievement of maximal blood pressure response to a given dose in most patients may take 2 to 3 weeks of treatment. Onset of blood pressure reduction is seen within 1 to 2 hours of dosing with few instances of orthostatic hypotension. Blood pressure control can be maintained with once- or twice-daily dosing over a 24-hour period. Attenuation of the effect towards the end of the 24 hour dosing period may occur in some patients with once daily dosing. Discontinuing treatment with eprosartan does not lead to a rebound increase in blood pressure.

There was no change in mean heart rate in patients treated with eprosartan in controlled clinical trials.

The antihypertensive effect of eprosartan was similar in men and women, but was somewhat smaller in patients over 65 years.

Although data available to date indicate a similar pharmacodynamic effect of eprosartan in black and white hypertensive patients, this should be viewed with caution since antihypertensive drugs that affect the renin-angiotensin system, such as ACE inhibitors and angiotensin II AT_1 receptor blockers, have generally been found to be less effective in low-renin hypertensives (frequently blacks).

Hydrochlorothiazide: Onset of diuretic action following oral administration occurs in 2 hours and the peak action in about 4 hours. Diuretic activity lasts about 6 to 12 hours.

Eprosartan and Hydrochlorothiazide: The components of TEVETEN PLUS have been shown to have an additive effect on blood pressure reduction, reducing blood pressure to a greater degree than either component alone.

The antihypertensive effect of TEVETEN PLUS is sustained over a 24 hour period. In clinical studies of one year's duration, the antihypertensive effect was maintained with continued therapy. Despite the significant decrease in blood pressure, administration of TEVETEN PLUS had no clinically significant effect on heart rate.

INDICATIONS: TEVETEN PLUS (eprosartan mesylate and hydrochlorothiazide) is indicated for the treatment of mild to moderate essential hypertension in patients for whom combination therapy is appropriate.

TEVETEN PLUS is not indicated for initial therapy (see Dosage).

CONTRAINDICATIONS: TEVETEN PLUS (eprosartan mesylate and hydrochlorothiazide) is contraindicated in patients who are hypersensitive to any component of this product. It is also contraindicated in pregnancy and in nursing women (see Warnings). Because of the hydrochlorothiazide component, it is also contraindicated in patients with anuria, or severe renal impairment, and in patients who are hypersensitive to thiazides or other sulfonamide-derived drugs.

WARNINGS:

Serious Warnings and Precautions
When used in pregnancy, angiotensin receptor (AT_1) blockers (ARBs) can cause injury or even death of the developing fetus. When pregnancy is detected, TEVETEN PLUS should be discontinued as soon as possible (see Contraindications and Warnings, Pregnancy).

Pregnancy: Drugs that act directly on the renin-angiotensin-aldosterone-system (RAAS) can cause fetal and neonatal morbidity and death when administered to pregnant women. When pregnancy is detected, TEVETEN PLUS (eprosartan mesylate and hydrochlorothiazide) should be discontinued as soon as possible (see Contraindications).

The use of ARBs is not recommended during pregnancy. Epidemiological evidence regarding the risk of teratogenicity following exposure to angiotensin converting enzyme inhibitors (another class of therapeutic products interfering with the RAAS) during the first trimester of pregnancy has not been conclusive; however a small increase in risk cannot be excluded. Given the current evidence available on the risk with ARBs, similar risks may exist for this class of drugs. Patients planning pregnancy should be changed to alternative antihypertensive treatments which have an established safety profile for use in pregnancy. When pregnancy is diagnosed, treatment with angiotensin II antagonists should be stopped immediately, and, if appropriate, alternative therapy should be started.

The use of ARBs during the second and third trimesters is known to induce human fetotoxicity (decreased renal function, oligohydramnios, skull ossification retardation) and neonatal toxicity (renal failure, hypotension, hyperkalaemia).

Infants with a history of in utero exposure to ARBs should be closely observed for hypotension, oliguria, and hyperkalemia. If oliguria occurs, attention should be directed toward support of blood pressure and renal perfusion. Exchange transfusion or dialysis may be required as a means of reversing hypotension and/or substituting for impaired renal function; however, limited experience with those procedures has not been associated with significant clinical benefit.

Eprosartan is not removed from plasma by dialysis.

Thiazides cross the placental barrier and appear in cord blood. The routine use of diuretics in otherwise healthy pregnant women is not recommended and exposes mother and fetus to unnecessary hazard including fetal or neonatal jaundice, thrombocytopenia and possibly other adverse experiences which have occurred in the adult. Diuretics do not prevent development of toxemia of pregnancy and there is no satisfactory evidence that they are useful in the treatment of toxemia.

Animal Data: Eprosartan has been shown to produce maternal and fetal toxicities (maternal and fetal mortality, low maternal body weight and food consumption, resorptions, abortions and litter loss) in pregnant rabbits given oral doses as low as 10 mg eprosartan/kg/day. No maternal or fetal adverse effects were observed at 3 mg/kg/day; this oral dose yielded a systemic exposure (AUC) to unbound eprosartan 0.8 times that achieved in humans given 400 mg twice daily. No adverse effects on in utero or postnatal development and maturation of offspring were observed when eprosartan mesylate was administered to pregnant rats at oral doses up to 1000 mg eprosartan/kg/day (the 1000 mg eprosartan/kg/day dose in nonpregnant rats yielded systemic exposure to unbound eprosartan approximately 0.6 times the exposure achieved in humans given 400 mg twice daily).

Lactation: It is not known whether eprosartan is excreted in human milk but significant levels have been found in the milk of lactating rats. Thiazides appear in human milk. Because many drugs are excreted in human milk and because of their potential for affecting the nursing infant adversely, if the initiation of treatment with eprosartan and hydrochlorothiazide is regarded necessary, nursing should be discontinued first. Nursing women should not be treated with TEVETEN PLUS (see Contraindications).

Hypotension: Occasionally, symptomatic hypotension has occurred after administration of eprosartan, in some cases after the first dose. It is more likely to occur in patients who are volume-depleted by diuretic therapy, dietary salt restriction, dialysis, diarrhea, or vomiting. In those patients, because of the potential fall in blood pressure, therapy should be started under close medical supervision. Similar considerations apply to patients with ischemic heart or cerebrovascular disease, in whom an excessive fall in blood pressure could result in myocardial infarction or cerebrovascular accident.

Azotemia: Azotemia may be precipitated or increased by hydrochlorothiazide. Cumulative effects of the drug may develop in patients with impaired renal function. If increasing azotemia and oliguria occur during treatment of severe progressive renal disease the diuretic should be discontinued.

Hypersensitivity Reactions: Hypersensitivity reactions to hydrochlorothiazide may occur in patients with or without a history of allergy or bronchial asthma.

Thiazide diuretics have been reported to cause exacerbation or activation of systemic lupus erythematosus.

PRECAUTIONS: Patients with Renal Impairment: As a consequence of inhibiting the renin-angiotensin-aldosterone system, changes in renal function have been seen in susceptible individuals. In patients whose renal function may depend on the activity of the renin-angiotensin-aldosterone system, such as patients with bilateral renal artery stenosis, unilateral renal artery stenosis to a solitary kidney, or severe congestive heart failure, treatment with agents that inhibit this system has been associated with oliguria, progressive azotemia, and rarely, acute renal failure and/or death. In susceptible patients, concomitant diuretic use may further increase risk.

Use of eprosartan should include appropriate assessment of renal function (see Dosage).

Thiazides should be used with caution in patients with renal disease. Because of the hydrochlorothiazide component, TEVETEN PLUS (eprosartan mesylate and hydrochlorothiazide) is not recommended in patients with severe renal impairment (creatinine clearance <30 mL/min) (see Dosage).

Patients with Liver Impairment: Based on pharmacokinetic data which demonstrate increased plasma concentrations of eprosartan in hepatically impaired patients after administration of eprosartan, a lower initial dose should be considered for patients with hepatic impairment or a history of hepatic impairment (see Dosage).

Thiazides should be used with caution in patients with impaired hepatic function or progressive liver disease, since minor alterations of fluid and electrolyte balance may precipitate hepatic coma (see Dosage).

Metabolism: Periodic determination of serum electrolytes to detect possible electrolyte imbalance should be performed at appropriate intervals.

All patients receiving thiazide therapy should be observed for clinical signs of fluid or electrolyte imbalance: hyokalemia, hyponatremia and hypochloremic alkalosis. Serum and urine electrolyte determinations are particularly important when the patient is vomiting excessively or receiving parenteral fluids. Warning signs or symptoms of fluid and electrolyte imbalance, irrespective of cause, include dryness of mouth, thirst, weakness, lethargy, drowsiness, restlessness, confusion, seizures, muscle pains or cramps, muscular fatigue, hypotension, oliguria, tachycardia, arrhythmias, and gastrointestinal disturbances such as nausea and vomiting.

Hypokalemia may develop, especially with brisk diuresis, when severe cirrhosis is present, or after prolonged therapy.

Interference with adequate oral electrolyte intake will also contribute to hypokalemia. Hypokalemia may cause cardiac arrhythmia and may also sensitize or exaggerate the response of the heart to the toxic effects of digitalis (e.g., increased ventricular irritability).

Although any chloride deficit is generally mild and usually does not require specific treatment except under extraordinary circumstances (as in liver disease or renal disease), chloride replacement may be required in the treatment of metabolic alkalosis. Dilutional hyponatremia may occur in edematous patients in hot weather; appropriate therapy is water restriction, rather than administration of salt except in rare instances when the hyponatremia is life-threatening. In actual salt depletion, appropriate replacement is the therapy of choice.

Hyperuricemia may occur or frank gout may be precipitated in certain patients receiving thiazide therapy. Thiazides may decrease serum protein-bound iodine levels without signs of thyroid disturbance.

Thiazides have been shown to increase the urinary excretion of magnesium; this may result in hypomagnesemia.

Thiazides may decrease urinary calcium excretion. Thiazides may cause intermittent and slight elevation of serum calcium in the absence of known disorders of calcium metabolism. Marked hypercalcemia may be evidence of hidden hyperparathyroidism. Thiazides should be discontinued before carrying out tests for parathyroid function.

The antihypertensive effects of hydrochlorothiazide may be enhanced in postsympathectomy patients.

Valvular Stenosis: There is concern on theoretical grounds that patients with aortic stenosis might be at particular risk of decreased coronary perfusion when treated with vasodilators because they do not develop as much afterload reduction.

Children: The safety and efficacy in children have not been established. Treatment of children is not recommended.

Geriatrics: No overall differences in safety were observed between elderly patients and younger patients, but appropriate caution should nevertheless be used when prescribing to the elderly, as increased vulnerability to drug effect is possible in this patient population.

Diabetes: In diabetic patients, dosage adjustment of insulin or oral hypoglycemic agents may be required. Hyperglycemia may occur with thiazide diuretics. Thus, latent diabetes mellitus may manifest during thiazide therapy.

Drug Interactions: Diuretics: Patients on diuretics, and especially those in whom diuretic therapy was recently instituted, may occasionally experience an excessive reduction in blood pressure after initiation of therapy with eprosartan. The possibility of symptomatic hypotension with the use of eprosartan can be minimized by discontinuing the diuretic prior to initiation of treatment (see Warnings, Hypotension, and Dosage). No pharmacokinetic drug interaction of clinical significance has been identified with eprosartan and thiazide diuretics.

Agents Affecting Serum Potassium: Since eprosartan decreases the production of aldosterone, potassium-sparing diuretics (e.g., spironolactone, triamterene, amiloride), or potassium supplements should be given only for documented hypokalemia and with frequent monitoring of serum potassium. Potassium-containing salt substitutes should also be used with caution.

Concomitant thiazide diuretic use may attenuate any effect that eprosartan may have on serum potassium. Concomitant use of laxatives may increase the risk of hypokalemia.

Lithium Salts: Lithium generally should not be given with diuretics. As with other drugs which eliminate sodium, lithium clearance may be reduced leading to lithium toxicity. Therefore, serum lithium levels should be monitored carefully if lithium salts are to be administered.

Digoxin and Antiarrhythmic Drugs: By lowering serum potassium levels, hydrochlorothiazide can increase effects and side-effects of digoxin and antiarrhythmic drugs. Hypokalemia resulting from thiazide therapy may increase the risk of quinidine-induced ventricular arrhythmias.

Alcohol, Barbiturates, or Narcotics: Potentiation of orthostatic hypotension may occur with diuretic therapy.

Antidiabetic Drugs (Oral Agents and Insulin): Insulin requirements in diabetic patients treated with diuretics may be increased, decreased or unchanged.

Nonsteroidal Anti-inflammatory Drugs: In some patients, the administration of a nonsteroidal anti-inflammatory agent can reduce the diuretic, natriuretic, and antihypertensive effects of loop, potassium sparing and thiazide diuretics. Therefore, when TEVETEN PLUS and nonsteroidal anti-inflammatory agents are used concomitantly, the patient should be observed closely to determine if the desired antihypertensive effect of the diuretic is obtained.

Cholestyramine and Colestipol Resins: Absorption of hydrochlorothiazide is impaired in the presence of anionic exchange resins. Single doses of either cholestyramine or colestipol resins bind hydrochlorothiazide and reduce its absorption from the gastrointestinal tract by up to 85% and 43%, respectively.

Pressor Amines (e.g. norepinephrine): In the presence of diuretics, possible decreased response to pressor amines may be seen but not sufficient to preclude their use.

Skeletal Muscle Relaxants, Non-Depolarizing (e.g. Tubocurarine-type): Thiazide diuretics may increase the effects of non-depolarizing (tubocurarine-type) skeletal muscle relaxants.

Corticosteroids, ACTH: Intensified electrolyte depletion, particularly hypokalemia, may occur when given concomitantly with diuretics.

Warfarin: Concomitant administration of eprosartan and warfarin had no effect on steady-state prothrombin time ratios (INR) in healthy volunteers.

Ranitidine: Eprosartan pharmacokinetics were not affected by concomitant administration of ranitidine.

Antifungals: Concomitant administration of ketoconazole or fluconazole (potent inhibitors of CYP 3A4 and 2C9, respectively) had no effect on steady state pharmacokinetics of eprosartan.

ADVERSE EFFECTS: The combination of eprosartan mesylate and hydrochlorothiazide contained in TEVETEN PLUS (eprosartan mesylate and hydrochlorothiazide) has been evaluated for safety in 1518 patients treated for hypertension. In open studies, 890 patients were treated from 6 months to 2 years. Of these, 528 patients were treated for at least 6 months and 449 patients were treated for 1 year or longer at various doses of eprosartan and at least 12.5 mg hydrochlorothiazide daily.

In controlled clinical trials, 268 patients were treated with eprosartan 600 mg plus hydrochlorothiazide 12.5 mg and about 3% of these patients discontinued therapy due to clinical adverse experiences.

The following potentially serious adverse reactions have been reported rarely in controlled clinical trials: syncope, hypotension.

Table 1 is based on double-blind controlled trials in patients treated at doses of 600 mg eprosartan and 12.5 mg hydrochlorothiazide. In double-blind controlled clinical trials, the following adverse events occurred amongst patients treated with combination therapy at an incidence of 1% or greater. Of the 268 patients who received such combination therapy during the double-blind treatment period in the controlled trials, 110 patients were reported to have adverse events.

Table 1: TEVETEN PLUS

Frequency of Adverse Events ≥1% During the Double-blind Treatment Period by Preferred Term and Treatment Group Regardless of Causality: Controlled Studies

	Eprosartan 600 mg/ Hydrochlorothiazide 12.5 mg (N=268) (%)	Eprosartan 600 mg (N=275) (%)	Hydrochlorothiazide 12.5 mg (N=117) (%)	Placebo (N=122) (%)
General				
Asthenia	1.1	1.1	0.9	0.8
Fatigue	1.9	1.8	0.9	0.8
Central and peripheral nervous				
Dizziness	4.1	1.8	1.7	1.6
Headache	3.4	3.6	3.4	9.0
Neuralgia	1.1	1.1	0.0	1.6
Paresthesia	1.1	0.7	0.0	0.8
Vertigo	1.5	0.0	0.0	1.6

(cont'd)

Table 1: TEVETEN PLUS *(cont'd)*

Frequency of Adverse Events ≥1% During the Double-blind Treatment Period by Preferred Term and Treatment Group Regardless of Causality: Controlled Studies

	Eprosartan 600 mg/ Hydrochlorothiazide 12.5 mg (N=268) (%)	Eprosartan 600 mg (N=275) (%)	Hydrochlorothiazide 12.5 mg (N=117) (%)	Placebo (N=122) (%)
Gastrointestinal				
Abdominal pain	1.5	0.4	0.9	0.8
Liver and biliary				
ALT increase	1.1	0	0.9	0
Metabolic and nutritional				
Hyperglycemia	1.5	0.7	2.6	0.8
Musculoskeletal				
Arthrosis	1.9	0.4	0.0	0.8
Back Pain	2.6	2.5	1.7	3.3
Psychiatric				
Insomnia	1.9	0.7	1.7	0.0
Depression	1.1	0.4	0.0	0.0
Respiratory				
Bronchitis	1.5	0.7	1.7	0
Urinary				
Albuminuria	1.9	0.7	1.7	1.6
Cystitis	1.1	0.0	0.9	0.8
Hematuria	1.1	0.7	1.7	0.8
Pyuria	1.5	1.1	1.7	0.8
Urinary tract infection	1.1	0.4	1.7	0.8
White cell and reticuloendothelial				
Leucocytosis	1.5	0.7	0.9	0.8

The most commonly reported adverse events in the eprosartan 600 mg and hydrochlorothiazide 12.5 mg group were dizziness (4.1%) and headache (3.4%).

In addition to the above, the following adverse reactions have been reported rarely in post-marketing experience: hypotension, including postural hypotension, skin reactions (rash, pruritus, urticaria), anemia, thrombocytopenia, myalgia and taste disorders.

Angioedema (involving swelling of the face, lips and/or tongue) has been very rarely reported.

Laboratory testing has demonstrated occasional elevation of liver enzymes.

Cases of muscle pain, muscle weakness, myositis and rhabdomyolysis have been reported in patients receiving angiotensin II receptor blockers.

For adverse reactions pertinent to the individual components of TEVETEN PLUS, please consult the Product Monographs for eprosartan mesylate and hydrochlorothiazide.

OVERDOSE: No specific information is available on the treatment overdosage with TEVETEN PLUS (eprosartan mesylate and hydrochlorothiazide). Treatment is symptomatic and supportive.

Symptoms: Eprosartan: Limited data are available in regard to overdosage with eprosartan. The most likely manifestations of overdosage would be hypotension and/or tachycardia. If symptomatic hypotension should occur, supportive treatment should be instituted. Eprosartan is not removed by hemodialysis.

Hydrochlorothiazide: The most common signs and symptoms observed are those caused by electrolyte depletion (hypokalemia, hypochloremia, hyponatremia) and dehydration resulting from excessive diuresis and may present as nausea and somnolence. If digitalis has also been administered, hypokalemia may accentuate cardiac arrhythmias. The degree to which hydrochlorothiazide is removed by hemodialysis has not been established.

Treatment: See Symptoms.

> For management of a suspected drug overdose, CPhA recommends that you contact your **regional Poison Control Centre**. See the *CPS* Directory section for a list of Poison Control Centres.

DOSAGE: Dosage must be individualized. The fixed combination is not for initial therapy. The dose of TEVETEN PLUS (eprosartan mesylate and hydrochlorothiazide) should be determined by the titration of the individual components.

Once the patient has been stabilized on the individual components as described below, one tablet of TEVETEN PLUS given once daily may be substituted if the doses on which the patient were stabilized are the same as those in the fixed combination (see Indications).

TEVETEN PLUS may be taken with or without food, but it should be taken consistently with respect to food intake and at the same time every day.

Eprosartan Monotherapy: The recommended initial dose of eprosartan monotherapy is 600 mg once daily. Achievement of maximum blood pressure reduction in most patients may take 2-3 weeks after initiation of therapy. In patients whose blood pressure is not adequately controlled, the dose may be increased to 800 mg once daily. In some patients treated once daily, the antihypertensive effect may diminish toward the end of the dosing interval. If satisfactory control is not being maintained for 24 hours, twice daily administration with the same total daily dosage should be considered. If blood pressure is not adequately controlled with eprosartan alone, a thiazide diuretic may be administered concomitantly.

Dosage Adjustment in Elderly and in Patients with Severe Renal Impairment: A lower initial starting dose of 400 mg eprosartan monotherapy once daily should be considered. The usual regimen of therapy with TEVETEN PLUS may generally be followed for patients with creatinine >30 mL/min. Because of the hydrochlorothiazide component, TEVETEN PLUS is not recommended in patients with severe renal impairment (creatinine clearance <30 mL/min) (see Precautions, Patients with Renal Impairment).

Patients with Hepatic Impairment: Since dosage adjustment of eprosartan is required in patients with liver impairment, and thiazide diuretics may precipitate hepatic coma, a fixed combination product such as TEVETEN PLUS is not advisable (see Precautions, Patients with Liver Impairment).

Patients Treated with Diuretics: In patients receiving diuretics, eprosartan therapy should be initiated with caution, since these patients may be volume-depleted and thus more likely to experience hypotension following initiation of additional antihypertensive therapy. Whenever possible, all diuretics should be discontinued two to three days prior to the administration of TEVETEN to reduce the likelihood of hypotension (see Warnings, Hypotension, and Precautions, Drug Interactions). If this is not possible because of the patient's condition, TEVETEN should be administered with caution and the blood pressure monitored closely. Thereafter, the dosage should be adjusted according to the individual response of the patient.

INFORMATION FOR THE PATIENT: Published in e-CPS, available by subscription at www.e-cps.ca.

SUPPLIED: Each film-coated, capsule-shaped, butterscotch-colored tablet, debossed with "SOLVAY" on one side and "5147" on the other side contains: eprosartan 600 mg as eprosartan mesylate and hydrochlorothiazide 12.5 mg. Nonmedicinal ingredients: crospovidone, iron oxide black, iron oxide yellow, lactose monohydrate, macrogol 3350, magnesium stearate, microcrystalline cellulose, polyvinyl alcohol, pregelatinized starch, talc and titanium dioxide. Blister packs of 28. Store between 15 and 25°C. Protect from moisture.

(Shown in Product Identification Section)

Thelin® Ⓟ

sitaxsentan sodium

Endothelin Receptor Antagonist

Pfizer

Date of Revision: April 26, 2010

SUMMARY PRODUCT INFORMATION:

Route of Administration	Dosage Form/ Strength	Clinically Relevant Nonmedicinal Ingredients
Oral	Tablet 100 mg	Lactose monohydrate

INDICATIONS AND CLINICAL USE: THELIN (sitaxsentan sodium) is indicated for treatment of primary pulmonary arterial hypertension or pulmonary hypertension secondary to connective tissue disease, in patients with WHO functional class III who have not responded to conventional therapy. THELIN is also indicated in patients with WHO functional class II who did not respond to conventional therapy and for whom no appropriate alternative can be identified.

Pediatrics: Safety and efficacy in pediatric patients have not been established.

CONTRAINDICATIONS:

- Pregnancy

  Endothelin-1 receptor antagonists, as a class, have consistently produced teratogenic effects in animals. Results from reproductive toxicology studies performed with sitaxsentan indicate that dosing during pregnancy in the rat results in several fetal malformations. Although the effects of THELIN on human development are unknown, THELIN is likely to produce major birth defects if used by pregnant women. Therefore, pregnancy must be excluded before the start of treatment with THELIN and prevented thereafter by the use of a reliable method of contraception. Monthly pregnancy tests during treatment with THELIN are recommended.

  The patient must be advised that if there is any delay in onset of menses or any other reason to suspect pregnancy, she must notify the physician immediately for pregnancy testing. If the pregnancy test is positive, the physician and patient must discuss the risk to the fetus.
- The co-administration of THELIN with cyclosporine is contraindicated, as cyclosporine induces a 6-fold increase in the pre-dose plasma concentrations of sitaxsentan.
- Hypersensitivity to sitaxsentan sodium or any component of the drug product (for a complete listing, see Dosage Forms, Composition and Packaging)
- Nursing women
- Prior liver impairment (mild to severe, Child-Pugh Class A-C)
- Elevated liver aminotransferases prior to initiation of treatment (aspartate aminotransferase (AST) and/or alanine aminotransferase (ALT) >3 × ULN).
- Elevated direct bilirubin (conjugated) of >2 × ULN prior to initiation of treatment.

WARNINGS AND PRECAUTIONS:

> **Serious Warnings and Precautions**
> - **Liver toxicity (see Hepatic/Biliary/Pancreatic)**
>
>   **THELIN has been associated with a reversible, dose-related increase in aspartate aminotransferase (AST) and alanine aminotransferase (ALT), accompanied in some cases by elevated bilirubin. THELIN has been associated with 4 cases of mild to severe hepatitis, with one case resulting in hepatic failure and death. These patients were taking doses ≥300 mg daily and had multiple co-morbidities and drug therapies; however, the contribution of THELIN in these cases could not be excluded. Doses of THELIN above 100 mg once daily are not recommended.**

General: THELIN is to be taken orally. The adult dose is 100 mg once daily. THELIN may be taken with or without food and without regard to the time of day.

Higher doses did not confer additional benefit sufficient to offset the increased risk of side effects, particularly liver injury (see Warnings and Precautions). A dose of 50 mg once daily did not demonstrate sufficient efficacy to support its use.

Safety and efficacy in pediatric patients have not been established.

Cardiovascular: THELIN should be initiated with caution if the patient has a systemic systolic blood pressure lower than 85 mm Hg.

Hematologic: Treatment with THELIN has been associated with a dose-related decrease in hemoglobin and hematocrit. The overall mean decrease in hemoglobin concentration in 149 THELIN-treated patients during placebo-controlled trials was 0.5 g/dL (change from baseline to end of treatment).

Most of the decrease in hemoglobin concentration was detected during the first few weeks of THELIN treatment and hemoglobin levels normally stabilized by week 4 of THELIN treatment. In the placebo-controlled studies, marked decreases in hemoglobin (>15% decrease from baseline with values below the lower limit of normal) were observed in 7% of patients treated with THELIN (10/149) and in 3% of placebo-treated patients (5/155).

A decrease in hemoglobin concentration by at least 1 g/dL was observed in 60% of patients treated with THELIN (83/149) as compared to 32% of placebo-treated patients (48/155). The origin of the change in hemoglobin is not known, but it does not appear to be due to hemorrhage or hemolysis.

It is recommended that hemoglobin concentrations be monitored 1 and 3 months following the initiation of THELIN and every 3 months thereafter. If a marked decrease in hemoglobin concentration occurs, a further evaluation should be undertaken to determine the cause and need for specific treatment.

Hepatic/Biliary/Pancreatic: THELIN has been associated with a reversible, dose-related increase in aspartate aminotransferase (AST) and alanine aminotransferase (ALT), accompanied in some cases by elevated bilirubin. THELIN has been associated with 4 cases of mild to severe hepatitis, with one case resulting in hepatic failure and death. These patients were taking doses ≥300 mg daily and had multiple co-morbidities and drug therapies; however, the contribution of THELIN in these cases could not be excluded. Doses of THELIN above 100 mg once daily are not recommended.

Liver aminotransaminase levels must be measured prior to initiation of treatment and subsequently at monthly intervals.

Pre-Existing Liver Impairment: Use in patients with baseline values of liver aminotransaminases, i.e., aspartate aminotransferase (AST) and/or alanine aminotransferase (ALT), greater than 3 times the upper limit of normal (ULN), particularly when the total bilirubin is increased to greater than 2 times the ULN, is contraindicated (see Contraindications).

Elevations of AST and/or ALT may be markers for liver injury, therefore liver aminotransferase levels must be measured prior to initiation of treatment and subsequently at regular monthly intervals. If AST and/or ALT are >3 x ULN prior to initiation of therapy, or direct bilirubin is >2 x ULN, use of sitaxsentan is contraindicated.

Management of Patients with Increased Liver Transaminases: ALT/AST levels and treatment/monitoring recommendations are as follows:

>3 and ≤8 × ULN—Confirm by another liver function test; if confirmed, stop treatment and monitor aminotransferase levels at least every 2 weeks. Once the aminotransferase levels return to pretreatment values consider reintroducing THELIN (see Reintroduction of Treatment).

>8 × ULN—Treatment must be stopped and reintroduction of THELIN is not to be considered.

If liver aminotransferase elevations are accompanied by clinical symptoms of liver injury (such as nausea, vomiting, anorexia, fever, abdominal pain, jaundice, or unusual lethargy or fatigue) or increases in total bilirubin above 2 × ULN, treatment should be stopped and reintroduction of THELIN is not to be considered.

Reintroduction of Treatment: Reintroduction of treatment with THELIN should only be considered if the potential benefits of treatment with THELIN outweigh the potential risks and when aminotransferase levels are within pretreatment values. The advice of a hepatologist is recommended. Aminotransferase levels must then be checked within 3 days after reintroduction, then again after further 2 weeks, and thereafter according to the recommendations above.

Special Populations: Pregnant Women: THELIN is contraindicated in pregnant women or in women intending to become pregnant (see Contraindications).

Nursing Women: Sitaxsentan was detected in the plasma of nursing pups from female rats treated with sitaxsentan, indicating that sitaxsentan was present in the breast milk. It is unknown whether sitaxsentan is excreted in human milk, but breastfeeding while taking THELIN is contraindicated (see Contraindications).

Pediatrics: Safety and efficacy of THELIN in pediatric patients have not been established.

Geriatrics: Of the 1487 patients treated with THELIN in clinical studies, 169 (11%) were aged 65 and over. The overall frequency of events and types of adverse events were similar in patients above and below 65 years of age.

In the 512 patients studied in the placebo-controlled PAH trials, the efficacy of THELIN in the geriatric population (≥65 years of age) was comparable to the efficacy observed in the non-elderly. Therefore, THELIN may be used in the patients aged 65 years and over as long as haematology and liver function assessments are performed regularly (see Warnings and Precautions).

ADVERSE REACTIONS: Adverse Drug Reaction Overview: The most commonly reported adverse events with THELIN treatment were headache, peripheral oedema, nasal congestion, nausea, constipation, epistaxis, insomnia; prothrombin time prolonged and increased INR (refer to Table 1).

Overall treatment discontinuations were less frequent in THELIN-treated patients (3%; 4/149 patients) than in placebo-treated patients (8%; 12/155 patients). In the STRIDE-2 study, 2/61 (3%) patients taking THELIN discontinued treatment due to adverse events, as compared to 6/62 (10%) placebo-treated. During continued treatment in the extension study following completion of STRIDE-2, 13/145 (9%) patients treated with THELIN were discontinued due to adverse events.

Serious Adverse Drug Reactions Related to the Administration of THELIN: hepatobiliary disorders (hepatitis), hepatic failure, investigations (elevated liver function test abnormal/hepatic enzymes increased [ALT/AST]).

Discontinuations Related to THELIN: Of the 774 subjects treated in the sitaxsentan >50 to ≤100 mg group, 34 (4%) discontinued study drug due to a drug-related, treatment-emergent AE. The only drug-related, treatment-emergent AE associated with discontinuation of study drug in at least 2% of subject in the >50 to ≤100 mg sitaxsentan group was LFT abnormal (13 subjects, 2%). None of the specific drug-related, treatment-emergent AEs associated with discontinuation of study drug were experienced in at least 2% of placebo subjects.

Clinical Trial Adverse Drug Reactions: Because clinical trials are conducted under very specific conditions the adverse drug reaction rates observed in the clinical trials may not reflect the rates observed in practice and should not be compared to the rates in the clinical trials of another drug. Adverse reaction information from clinical trials is useful for identifying drug-related adverse events and for approximate rates.

Safety data were obtained from 29 clinical studies, which comprised a total of 1487 subjects, including healthy volunteers and patients. Doses ranged from 50 mg to more than 1000 mg per day, and duration of treatment ranged from 1 day to 2.8 years (N=148 for 1 year or more). In PAH studies, safety data were obtained from 899 patients receiving THELIN.

Table 1 presents the adverse drug reactions that occurred during placebo-controlled PAH trials in >1% of THELIN patients, at a rate greater than placebo, and that were considered to be at least possibly related to THELIN treatment.

Table 1: THELIN

Adverse Drug Reactions Occurring in >1% of Patients Treated with THELIN, More Frequently Than Placebo, and Related to THELIN Treatment

System Organ Class Preferred Term	THELIN 100 mg N=149 (%)	Placebo N=155 (%)
Gastrointestinal Disorders		
Nausea	10 (6.7%)	6 (3.9%)
Constipation	5 (3.4%)	0
Upper Abdominal Pain	3 (2.0%)	2 (1.3%)
Vomiting	4 (2.7%)	2 (1.3%)
Dyspepsia	3 (2.0%)	1 (0.6%)
General Disorders and Administration Site Conditions		
Fatigue	4 (2.7%)	3 (1.9%)
Investigations		
INR Increased	9 (6.0%)	4 (2.6%)
PT Prolonged	7 (4.7%)	0
Metabolism and Nutrition		
Peripheral Oedema	13 (8.7%)	5 (3.2%)
Musculoskeletal, Connective Tissue and Bone		
Muscle Cramp	3 (2.0%)	1 (0.6%)
Nervous System Disorders		
Headache	23 (15.4%)	21 (13.5%)
Insomnia	3 (2.0%)	0
Respiratory, Thoracic, and Mediastinal Disorders		
Nasal Congestion	13 (8.7%)	7 (4.5%)
Epistaxis	5 (3.4%)	0
Skin and Subcutaneous Tissue		
Flushing	6 (4.0%)	1 (0.6%)

Less Common Clinical Trial Adverse Drug Reactions (<1%): Blood and Lymphatic System Disorders: eosinophilia, leukopenia, myeloproliferative disorder, thrombocytopenia, lymphoma, pancytopenia.

Cardiac Disorders: bradycardia, chest discomfort, right ventricular failure, angina pectoris, atrial flutter, atrioventricular block first degree, myocardial infarction, pericardial effusion, sinus bradycardia, supraventricular tachycardia, tachycardia, ventricular bigeminy, ventricular extrasystoles, ventricular tachycardia, cardiac disorder, cardiac failure, cardiac failure congestive, cardiac flutter, dilatation atrial, supraventricular extrasystoles.

Ear and Labyrinth Disorders: tinnitus, cerumen impaction, deafness, ear congestion, ear pain, sensation of block in ear, otitis media.

Endocrine Disorders: goiter.

Eye Disorders: conjunctival haemorrhage, lacrimation increased, photophobia, conjunctival hyperaemia, conjunctivitis, eye infection, eye oedema, visual disturbance, eye inflammation, eye irritation, eye pruritus, keratoconjunctivitis sicca, retinal tear, vitreous floaters.

Gastrointestinal Disorders: dry mouth, gastroenteritis viral, gingivitis, haematochezia, gastrointestinal discomfort, gingival pain, abdominal strangulated hernia, anal skin tags, appendicitis, colitis, colonic polyp, diverticulum, eructation, faecal incontinence, food poisoning, gastroenteritis bacterial, gastrointestinal fungal infection, gastrointestinal haemorrhage, gastrointestinal infection, glossodynia, haemorrhoids, mouth haemorrhage, oesophageal spasm, peptic ulcer, proctalgia, pruritus ani, retching, tongue blistering, tongue discolouration, tongue disorder, tongue ulceration, tooth abscess, abdominal hernia, abdominal tenderness, abscess, aptyalism, ascites, enteritis, frequent bowel movements, gastritis viral, gastroenteritis, gastrointestinal disorder, hiccups, oral pruritus, pancreatic pseudocyst, pancreatitis acute, stomatitis.

General Disorders and Administration Site Conditions: malaise, feeling hot, puncture site haemorrhage, feeling cold, inflammation localized, injection site dermatitis, venipuncture site inflammation, application site bruising, hyperthermia, multi-organ failure, pain, sensation of foreign body.

Hepatobiliary Disorders: gallbladder disorder, hepatomegaly, jaundice, cholecystitis chronic, cholelithiasis, cholestasis, hyperbilirubinaemia.

Immune System Disorders: hypersensitivity, conjunctivitis allergic, drug hypersensitivity, systemic lupus erythematosus.

Infections and Infestations: viral infection, candidiasis, fungal infection, oral candidiasis.

Injury, Poisoning and Procedural Complications: arthropod bite, joint injury, laceration, arthropod sting, drug toxicity, fall, head injury, sunburn, animal bite, ligament injury, post procedural haemorrhage, skin laceration, soft tissue injury, thermal burn.

Investigations: activated partial thromboplastin time prolonged, blood bicarbonate decreased, haemoglobin decreased, weight decreased, blood bilirubin increased, blood creatinine increased, blood glucose increased, blood pressure decreased, cardiac murmur, eosinophil count increased, haematocrit decreased, white blood cell count decreased, aspartate aminotransferase increased, blood creatine phosphokinase increased, blood lactate dehydrogenase increased, blood phosphorus increased, blood potassium decreased, blood potassium increased, blood pressure increased, body temperature increased, electrocardiogram QT prolonged, heart rate increased, heart rate irregular, oxygen saturation decreased, pregnancy test positive, red blood cell count decreased, venous pressure jugular increased, alanine aminotransferase increased, blood creatine phosphokinase-mb increased, blood uric acid increased, coagulation time prolonged, crystal urine, haematocrit increased, haemoglobin increased.

Metabolism and Nutrition Disorders: decreased appetite, anorexia, fluid retention, oedema, gout, hyperglycaemia, hyperkalaemia, hypocalcaemia, hypoglycaemia, increased appetite, lactic acidosis, localised oedema, weight fluctuation, dehydration, hypercholesterolaemia, hypernatraemia, polydipsia.

Musculoskeletal and Connective Tissue Disorders: flank pain, chest wall pain, facial pain, localised infection, osteochondrosis, arthritis, arthritis bacterial, arthritis infective, limb discomfort, muscle fatigue, muscle haemorrhage, muscle twitching, muscular weakness, musculoskeletal pain, musculoskeletal stiffness, osteoarthritis, pain in jaw, polyarthritis, rib fracture, tendonitis, connective tissue inflammation, fibromyalgia, groin pain, joint sprain, joint stiffness, muscle atrophy, musculoskeletal chest pain.

Neoplasms Benign, Malignant and Unspecified (Incl. Cysts and Polyps): ovarian cyst, skin papilloma, uterine leiomyoma, basal cell carcinoma.

Nervous System Disorders: sinus headache, somnolence, tremor, dizziness postural, ataxia, disturbance in attention, dysphonia, memory impairment, partial seizures, vertigo, confusional state, dysaesthesia, facial palsy, head discomfort, ischaemic stroke, paraesthesia oral, restless legs syndrome, restlessness, sciatica.

Pregnancy, Puerperium and Perinatal Conditions: abortion spontaneous.

Psychiatric Disorders: nervousness, agitation, sleep disorder, thinking abnormal.

Renal and Urinary Disorders: haematuria, pollakiuria, bladder disorder, dysuria, nephritis interstitial, renal impairment, renal insufficiency, proteinuria, urosepsis.

Reproductive System and Breast Disorders: menorrhagia, metrorrhagia, vaginal haemorrhage, amenorrhoea, nipple pain, breast tenderness, genital pruritus female, menopausal symptoms, testicular pain, vaginal mycosis, breast microcalcification, breast pain, vaginal infection, vaginal prolapse.

Respiratory, Thoracic and Mediastinal Disorders: sinusitis, hypoxia, sinus congestion, hoarseness, orthopnoea, pleurisy, rhinitis, acute sinusitis, alveolitis allergic, asthma, lower respiratory tract infection, nasal sinus drainage, nocturnal dyspnea, pleural effusion, pleuritic pain, pneumonia aspiration, pneumothorax, respiratory tract infection, sneezing, sputum purulent, wheezing, bronchitis acute, dry throat, dyspnoea exertional, dyspnoea paroxysmal nocturnal, lobar pneumonia, lung infection, nasal discomfort, paranasal sinus hypersecretion, pulmonary embolism, respiratory failure, sinus pain, sputum discoloured, tachypnoea, throat irritation.

Skin and Subcutaneous Tissue Disorders: contusion, alopecia, herpes simplex, herpes zoster, onychomycosis, urticaria, cellulitis, dermatitis allergic, dry skin, night sweats, petechiae, pruritus generalised, rash papular, rosacea, skin disorder, skin hyperpigmentation, skin necrosis, skin ulcer, subcutaneous abscess, dermatitis contact, furuncle, gouty tophus, intertrigo, nail hypertrophy, pallor, palmar erythema, paronychia, psoriasis, rash macular, rash pustular, skin desquamation, skin irritation, skin lesion.

Surgical and Medical Procedures: tooth extraction, endodontic procedure, medical device implantation, nasal polypectomy, radiofrequency ablation, stent placement, aneurysmectomy, atrial septal defect repair, detached retina repair.

Vascular Disorders: hypertension, haematoma, arteriovenous fistula-acquired, haemorrhage, migraine, orthostatic hypotension, phlebothrombosis, post thrombotic syndrome, thrombophlebitis superficial, catheter site haemorrhage, peripheral artery aneurysm.

Abnormal Hematologic and Clinical Chemistry Findings: Chemistry: During all PAH placebo-controlled trials, elevations in ALT or AST by more than 3 × ULN were observed in 2% of THELIN-treated PAH patients at the 100 mg dose (N=149) compared to 5% of placebo-treated patients (N=155). A higher dose of THELIN (300 mg), evaluated in STRIDE-1, demonstrated an increased frequency and severity of liver abnormalities (see Warnings and Precautions). In STRIDE-2, elevated LFTs >3 × ULN were observed in 2 patients (3%) treated with THELIN 100 mg per day versus 4 patients in the placebo group (6%).

Elevations in AST and/or ALT occurred both early and late in treatment with THELIN and usually progressed slowly. These changes were typically asymptomatic and were reversible when monitoring and discontinuation guidelines were followed. Liver aminotransferase elevations have reversed spontaneously while continuing treatment with THELIN (see Dosage and Administration, Management of Patients with Increased Liver Aminotransaminases; Hepatic/Biliary/Pancreatic; Warnings and Precautions and Dosage and Administration).

Table 2: THELIN

Treatment-Emergent Bleeding AEs Experienced by ≥1.0% of Subjects in THELIN 100 mg/day Combined Group (Phase 3, Long-Term, Oral Studies in Subjects with PAH Exposed ≥6 Months)

Preferred Term	Subjects (N=438)
Subjects with ≥1 Bleeding AE	74 (17%)
Epistaxis	35 (8%)
Haemoptysis	9 (2%)
Menorrhagia	6 (1%)
Haematoma	3 (1%)
Gingival Bleeding	6 (1%)

(cont'd)

Table 2: THELIN *(cont'd)*

Treatment-Emergent Bleeding AEs Experienced by ≥1.0% of Subjects in THELIN 100 mg/day Combined Group (Phase 3, Long-Term, Oral Studies in Subjects with PAH Exposed ≥6 Months)

Preferred Term	Subjects (N=438)
Haematuria	4 (1%)
Vaginal Haemorrhage	3 (1%)

Hematology: (See Warnings and Precautions.)

Post-Market Adverse Drug Reactions : Adverse events reported during the post-marketing period to date have been generally similar to those reported in clinical trials.

Cases of prolonged concurrent elevations of transaminases (ALT and/or AST) >8 × ULN and total bilirubin >2 × ULN have been reported following administration of sitaxsentan sodium. As with other endothelin receptor antagonists, this combination of factors may lead to hepatic failure which highlights the need for regular monitoring of transaminases and bilirubin.

DRUG INTERACTIONS:

Serious Drug Interactions
- **Cyclosporin: Contraindicated** due to a significant increase in the exposure of sitaxsentan (see Drug-Drug Interactions and Contraindications).
- **Warfarin: Reduced dosage** of warfarin is recommended due to enhanced effect on PT and INR (see Drug-Drug Interactions and Dosage and Administration).

Overview: In vitro data indicate that sitaxsentan is metabolized by CYP2C9 and CYP3A4/5.

Sitaxsentan is also a moderate inhibitor of CYP2C9 (K_i=0.46 μM) and, to a lesser extent, of CYP2C19 (K_i=1-4 μM) and CYP3A4/5 (K_i=20 μM). Plasma concentrations of drugs principally metabolized by these isoforms, particularly CYP2C9 (such as warfarin, phenytoin), may be increased during THELIN co-administration.

Drug-Drug Interactions: Cyclosporine: THELIN 100 mg once daily co-administered with cyclosporine 3.5 mg/kg twice daily did not alter the pharmacokinetic disposition of cyclosporine, which is extensively metabolized by CYP3A4/5. However, this co-administration resulted in a 6-fold increase in the pre-dose concentrations of sitaxsentan. The mechanism for this interaction is not known. Because of this increase in sitaxsentan exposure, the use of THELIN in patients receiving cyclosporine is contraindicated (see Contraindications).

Digoxin: Concomitant administration of digoxin 0.25 mg once daily and THELIN 100 mg did not alter the pharmacokinetics of digoxin, indicating no effect on the p-glycoprotein transporter.

Fluconazole: Concomitant administration of THELIN 100 mg once daily with fluconazole 400 mg once daily resulted, on average, in moderate increases in the C_{max} (17%) and AUC_{0-24} (9%) of sitaxsentan. These effects, however, varied on an individual basis, unrelated to genotype; although 52% of the subjects exhibited an increase in C_{max} and 38% exhibited an increase in AUC_{0-24}, the remaining subjects had either no change or a decrease in these parameters. Sitaxsentan is metabolized by CYP2C9 and CYP3A4/5, both of which are inhibited by fluconazole. While it is possible the predominant isoform may vary among individuals, this redundancy in metabolic pathways may minimize the effect of inhibition of either isoform on the overall clearance of sitaxsentan. There was no clinically significant effect on AEs. The results of this study, as well as an earlier study, indicate that it is not likely that a significant drug interaction would result when sitaxsentan and fluconazole are co-administered.

Ketoconazole: Ketoconazole is metabolized by CYP3A4/5. Co-administration of THELIN 100 mg once daily with ketoconazole 400 mg once daily resulted in reduced clearance of ketoconazole. The increases in mean C_{max} and AUC_{0-24} were approximately 18% and 20%, respectively. These changes were not considered clinically significant.

Ketoconazole is also a CYP3A4/5 inhibitor. During concomitant administration, sitaxsentan C_{max} was unchanged, but AUC_{0-24} was increased by approximately 20%, consistent with ketoconazole inhibiting CYP3A4/5 in vivo. This change was not considered clinically significant.

Nelfinavir: Nelfinavir is metabolized by both CYP2C19 and CYP3A4/5. Concomitant administration of THELIN 100 mg once daily and nelfinavir 1250 mg twice daily reduced the clearance of nelfinavir, resulting in a 14% increase in mean C_{max} and a 15% increase in mean AUC_{0-12}. In the one subject classified as a CYP2C19 poor metabolizer, mean C_{max} and mean AUC_{0-12} increased by 18% and 36%, respectively. These changes were not considered clinically significant.

Nelfinavir is also a CYP3A4/5 inhibitor. The sitaxsentan mean C_{max} decreased by 7% and mean AUC_{0-24} decreased by 17%. These changes were not considered clinically significant.

Nifedipine: THELIN 100 mg co-administered with nifedipine 10 mg every 8 hours increased C_{max} of nifedipine by 12% and mean AUC_{0-8} by 21%, while clearance was reduced. These changes were not considered clinically significant.

Omeprazole: THELIN 100 mg once daily co-administered with omeprazole 41.2 mg once daily increased the mean AUC_{0-24} by 27%; C_{max} was unchanged. The change in AUC was not considered clinically significant.

Oral Contraceptives: Concomitant administration of THELIN 100 mg once daily and Ortho-Novum 1/35 for a 28-day cycle resulted in increases in the mean exposure to ethinyl estradiol (59%) and norethindrone (47%). THELIN had no effect on the anti-ovulatory activity of the oral contraceptive as assessed by plasma concentrations of FSH, LH, and progesterone.

Sildenafil: A single dose of sildenafil 100 mg co-administered with THELIN 100 mg increased the mean C_{max} and AUC_{∞} of sildenafil by 18% and 28%, respectively. There was no change in mean C_{max} or AUC_{∞} for the active metabolite, n-desmethylsildenafil. These changes in sildenafil plasma concentrations were not considered clinically significant.

Warfarin: Sitaxsentan is an inhibitor of CYP2C9 and increases the AUC and C_{max} of drugs metabolized by CYP2C9. The AUC_{∞} of S-warfarin was increased by approximately 96%, and clearance was decreased by approximately 63% when a single 25 mg dose was co-administered with THELIN 100 mg once daily. An enhanced effect on PT and INR was observed, consistent with the increase in exposure to S-warfarin (see Dosage and Administration).

In clinical trials, it was recommended that the warfarin dose be decreased by 80% when starting THELIN and then increased in increments of no greater than 0.5 mg/day while titrating to the desired INR. The mean dose of warfarin at study endpoint in STRIDE 2 (18 weeks of dosing) was 2.2 mg/day for patients receiving THELIN, compared to 3.6 mg/day for patients treated with placebo. In STRIDE 2, the need to change the warfarin dose due to changes in INR was similar among the THELIN-treated and, placebo-treated patients.

Drug-Food Interactions: Food had no clinically significant interaction on THELIN 100 mg orally.

Drug-Herb Interactions: Interactions with herbal products have not been studied.

Drug-Laboratory Test Interactions: Interactions with laboratory tests have not been studied.

DOSAGE AND ADMINISTRATION: General: THELIN is to be taken orally. The adult dose is 100 mg once daily. THELIN may be taken with or without food and without regard to the time of day.

Higher doses did not confer additional benefit sufficient to offset the increased risk of side effects, particularly liver injury (see Warnings and Precautions). A dose of 50 mg once daily did not demonstrate sufficient efficacy to support its use.

Safety and efficacy in pediatric patients have not been established.

Dosage Adjustment and Monitoring in Patients Receiving Warfarin: Subjects receiving warfarin achieve therapeutic anti-coagulation (International Normalised Ratio (INR) target) with lower doses of the anticoagulant in the presence of THELIN. The mean dose of warfarin at study endpoint in STRIDE-2 (18 weeks of dosing) was 3.6 mg/day for patients treated with placebo, compared to 2.2 mg/day for patients receiving THELIN (approximately 40% lower). When initiating warfarin therapy in a patient taking THELIN, it is recommended to start at the lowest available dose of warfarin. In patients already taking warfarin, it is recommended that the warfarin dose be reduced when starting THELIN. In all cases, INR should be monitored on a regular schedule. Increases in the warfarin dose should be done in small increments to reach an appropriate target INR (see Drug Interactions).

Monitoring and Discontinuing THELIN in Patients Developing Liver Aminotransferase Abnormalities: Hepatic/Biliary/Pancreatic: THELIN has been associated with a reversible, dose-related increase in aspartate aminotransferase (AST) and alanine aminotransferase (ALT), accompanied in some cases by elevated bilirubin. THELIN has been associated with 4 cases of mild to severe hepatitis, with one case resulting in hepatic failure and death. These patients were taking doses ≥300 mg daily and had multiple co-morbidities and drug therapies; however, the contribution of THELIN in these cases could not be excluded. Doses of THELIN above 100 mg once daily are not recommended.

Liver transaminase levels must be measured prior to initiation of treatment and subsequently at monthly intervals.

Pre-Existing Liver Impairment: Use in patients with baseline values of liver aminotransaminases, i.e., aspartate aminotransferase (AST) and/or alanine aminotransferase (ALT), greater than 3 times the upper limit of normal (ULN), particularly when the total bilirubin is increased to greater than 2 times the ULN, is contraindicated (see Contraindications).

Management of Patients with Increased Liver Aminotransaminases: ALT/AST levels and treatment/monitoring recommendations are as follows:

>3 and ≤8 × ULN—Confirm by another liver function test; if confirmed, stop treatment and monitor aminotransferase levels at least every 2 weeks. Once the aminotransferase levels return to pretreatment values consider reintroducing THELIN (see Reintroduction of Treatment).

>8 × ULN—Treatment must be stopped and reintroduction of THELIN is not to be considered.

If liver aminotransferase elevations are accompanied by clinical symptoms of liver injury (such as nausea, vomiting, anorexia, fever, abdominal pain, jaundice, or unusual lethargy or fatigue) or increases in total bilirubin above 2 × ULN, treatment should be stopped and re-introduction of THELIN is not to be considered.

Reintroduction of Treatment: Reintroduction of treatment with THELIN should only be considered if the potential benefits of treatment with THELIN outweigh the potential risks and when aminotransferase levels are within pretreatment values. The advice of a hepatologist is recommended. Aminotransferase levels must then be checked within 3 days after reintroduction, then again after further 2 weeks, and thereafter according to the recommendations above.

Use in Women of Child-Bearing Potential: In women of child-bearing potential, THELIN treatment must only be initiated following a negative pregnancy test and only in those who practice adequate contraception. Monthly pregnancy tests during treatment with THELIN are recommended.

Dosage Adjustment in Hepatically Impaired Patients: Studies in patients with pre-existing liver impairment have not been conducted. THELIN is contraindicated with elevated liver aminotransferases prior to initiation of treatment (>3 × ULN) (see Contraindications).

Use in Patients Discontinuing Endothelin Receptor Antagonists (ERA) Due to Liver Function Abnormalities: STRIDE-6 was a 48 patient, 12-week study of sitaxsentan in patients who discontinued treatment with bosentan. In the 12 patients who had discontinued bosentan for elevated hepatic transaminases, sitaxsentan was initiated after hepatic enzymes returned to pre-bosentan baseline levels. Of these 12 patients, 1 experienced an increase (<5 × ULN) in hepatic transaminases during the 12-week study period.

Sixty-two patients discontinuing bosentan due to liver function abnormalities (of whom 32 failed attempts at dose reduction and/or interruption and re-challenge with bosentan) were treated using THELIN in clinical trials. Of these patients, 19% (12/62) experienced a recurrence of abnormalities during treatment with THELIN following a mean exposure of 28 weeks. Appropriate care should be exercised when initiating THELIN in this patient population.

OVERDOSAGE:

There is no specific experience with the management of THELIN overdose. In the event of an overdose, symptomatic and supportive measures should be employed.

At doses greater than or equal to 300 mg daily THELIN has been associated with 4 cases of mild to severe hepatitis, with one case resulting in hepatic failure and death. These patients had multiple co-morbidities and drug therapies; however, the contribution of THELIN in these cases could not be excluded.

For management of a suspected drug overdose, CPhA recommends that you contact your **regional Poison Control Centre**. See the *CPS* Directory section for a list of Poison Control Centres.

ACTION AND CLINICAL PHARMACOLOGY: Mechanism of Action: Endothelin-1 (ET-1) is a potent vasoconstricting paracrine and autocrine peptide found in the lungs. ET-1 concentrations are elevated in plasma and lung tissue of patients with pulmonary arterial hypertension (PAH). Additionally, PAH also is characterized by reduced nitric oxide activity. ET-1 actions are mediated through endothelin A receptors (ET_A), present on smooth muscle cells, and endothelin B receptors (ET_B), present on endothelial cells. Predominant actions of ET-1 binding to ET_A are vasoconstriction and vascular remodeling, while binding to ET_B results in ET-1 clearance, and vasodilatory/antiproliferative effects, due in part to nitric oxide and prostacyclin release.

Sitaxsentan is a potent (Ki 0.43 nM) and highly selective ET_A antagonist (approximately 6500-fold more selective for ET_A as compared to ET_B).

Pharmacokinetics: Absorption: THELIN is rapidly absorbed following oral administration. In PAH patients, peak plasma concentrations are generally achieved within 1-4 h. The absolute bioavailability of THELIN is between 70 and 100%.

When administered with a high fat meal, the rate of absorption of THELIN was decreased as evidenced by a 43% decrease in C_{max} and a delay in T_{max} (2-fold increase) compared to fasted conditions, but the extent of absorption (AUC) was the same.

Distribution: THELIN is widely distributed in tissues and more than 99% protein bound to plasma proteins, predominantly albumin. The degree of binding is independent of concentration in the clinically relevant range.

Sitaxsentan sodium does not penetrate into erythrocytes and does not appear to cross the blood-brain barrier.

Metabolism and Excretion: Following oral administration to healthy volunteers, sitaxsentan is highly metabolized. The 2 most common circulating metabolites (1, 3 keto and 1-keto-2-hydroxy derivatives) account for approximately 3 and 8.5%, respectively, of the parent compound activity. They are at least 20 and 30 times, respectively, less potent than sitaxsentan on ETA receptors and inactive on ETB receptors. In vitro, sitaxsentan is metabolized via CYP2C9 and CYP3A4. However, administration of sitaxsentan with inhibitors of these isoforms is not expected to result in clinically significant changes in sitaxsentan plasma concentrations.

Approximately 50-60% of an oral dose is excreted in the urine with the remainder eliminated in the feces. Approximately 1% of the dose is excreted as unchanged drug. The terminal elimination half-life (t½) is 10 hours. Steady state in PAH subjects is expected to be reached within 4-6 days. Apparent clearance increases with body weight in PAH subjects; however, no adjustment in dose is warranted.

No unexpected accumulation in the plasma was observed after multiple dosing at the recommended dose of 100 mg once daily. At doses of 300 mg or above non-linear pharmacokinetics resulted in disproportionately higher plasma concentrations of sitaxsentan, which may results in an increased incidence of liver injury (see Warnings and Precautions).

Special Populations and Conditions: Based on results of the population pharmacokinetic analysis and pooled pharmacokinetic data over several studies, it was found that sex, race, and age do not significantly affect the pharmacokinetics of sitaxsentan sodium.

Hepatic Insufficiency: The influence of liver impairment on the pharmacokinetics of sitaxsentan sodium has not been evaluated. THELIN is contraindicated with elevated liver aminotransferases prior to initiation of treatment (>3 × ULN) (see Contraindications).

Renal Insufficiency: No dose adjustment is required in patients with renal impairment.

STORAGE AND STABILITY: Temperature: Store at room temperature (15°C to 25°C). Protect from heat and moisture.

Others: Keep in a safe place out of the reach of children.

INFORMATION FOR THE PATIENT: Published in e-CPS, available by subscription at www.e-cps.ca.

DOSAGE FORMS, COMPOSITION AND PACKAGING: Each capsule-shaped, yellow-to-orange, film-coated oral tablet, debossed with T-100 on one side, contains: sitaxsentan sodium 100 mg. Nonmedicinal ingredients: ascorbyl palmitate, dibasic sodium phosphate, edetate disodium dehydrate, hydroxypropyl methylcellulose, lactose monohydrate, magnesium stearate, microcrystalline cellulose, monobasic sodium phosphate and sodium starch glycolate; film coating: anatose titanium dioxide, hydroxypropyl methylcellulose, microcrystalline cellulose, pharmaceutical talc, stearic acid and yellow iron oxide dehydrate. Bottles of 28.

(Shown in Product Identification Section)

Theolair™ Pr

theophylline

Bronchodilator

Graceway

SUPPLIED: Each 15 mL of alcohol-free, citrus berry flavored liquid contains: theophylline (anhydrous) 80 mg. Nonmedicinal ingredients: flavor, methyl- and propylparabens, purified water, sorbitol and sucrose. Tartrazine-free. Bottles of 500 mL.

Theophyllines

aminophylline
oxtriphylline
theophylline

Bronchodilator

CPhA Monograph

Date of Revision: September 2009

> This monograph has been compiled by CPhA and reviewed by experts. It may contain information different from that found in Health Canada-approved Product Monographs. The reader is referred to the *CPS* Editorial Policy for more information.

PHARMACOLOGY: Like caffeine, theophylline is a derivative of xanthine. Aminophylline is a complex of theophylline with ethylenediamine; oxtriphylline is the choline salt of theophylline. Both aminophylline and oxtriphylline dissociate in biological fluids to yield theophylline.

Theophylline's pharmacologic actions include stimulation of the central nervous system (CNS) specifically the medullary respiratory centre, stimulation of cardiac muscle, relaxation of bronchial smooth muscle and diuresis. Theophylline also increases diaphragm contractility. The mechanism of action of theophylline is unknown; however, the three basic cellular effects of theophylline are translocation of intracellular calcium, adenosine receptor blockade and accumulation of cyclic adenosine monophosphate (cAMP) through inhibition of phosphodiesterases. The accumulation of cAMP increases the release of endogenous epinephrine resulting in increased β-adrenergic stimulation.

Pharmacokinetics: Theophylline is well absorbed orally. Maximal plasma concentrations occur approximately 1 to 2 hours after ingestion of oral liquids and immediate-release tablets. Maximal plasma concentrations occur within 3 to 7 hours after ingestion of most sustained-release preparations; however, this varies with the individual preparation. Food delays but does not reduce absorption of uncoated tablets and liquids; however, it may affect absorption of extended-release preparations. The product manufacturers' guidelines on administration should be consulted.

The absorption of theophylline administered im is usually slow and incomplete. The im route is extremely painful and is not recommended. Absorption of theophylline from rectal suppositories is not dependable; a retention enema may be more reliable, but a preparation is not available in Canada. Theophylline iv produces the highest and most rapidly achieved theophylline serum concentrations, reaching peak serum levels within 30 minutes.

Theophylline is distributed throughout extracellular fluids and body tissues. It does not distribute into adipose tissue. Theophylline readily crosses the placenta and is secreted into breast milk in concentrations approaching 70% of those in maternal serum. The average volume of distribution is reported to be 0.45 L/kg for children and adults. At therapeutic concentrations plasma protein binding is approximately 60% in adults compared to 35% in neonates and in patients with hepatic cirrhosis.

Theophylline is metabolized by the cytochrome P450 isoenzymes, CYP1A2 and CYP3A4, to 1,3-dimethyluric acid, 1-methyluric acid and 3-methylxanthine. Theophylline and its metabolites are excreted mainly by the kidneys. Metabolites account for approximately 85% while renal elimination of unchanged drug is less than 15% of the overall plasma clearance of theophylline.

Table 1: Theophyllines

Average Plasma Half-Life of Theophylline

Adults (healthy, nonsmokers)	7–9 hours
Adults (smokers)	4–5 hours
Elderly (nonsmokers)	10 hours
Children	3–5 hours
Neonates (premature)	20–30 hours

Theophylline clearance is markedly reduced in neonates. Neonates excrete a larger proportion of unchanged theophylline in the urine and dosage must be adjusted in the presence of renal failure in this group. Theophylline half-life is much longer in neonates which allows for dosing intervals of 12 hours (see Table 1). Theophylline clearance increases during the first year of life and remains relatively constant during the first 9 years, thereafter decreasing to adult values by age 16. Clearance is decreased in hepatic cirrhosis, acute hepatitis, cholestasis, heart failure, cor pulmonale, febrile respiratory tract infections and in the elderly. Cigarette or marijuana smokers have a more rapid clearance. Diets low in carbohydrates and high in protein or charcoal broiled meats may contribute to an increased ability to clear theophylline.

There is significant interpatient variability in theophylline pharmacokinetics. Steady state is usually achieved within 48 hours with a consistent dosage schedule. Serum concentrations should be monitored more closely, regardless of steady state, in patients with acute respiratory illness, in neonates or in patients at risk of decreased theophylline clearance. Although the accepted therapeutic plasma concentration range has traditionally been 55 to 110 µmol/L in children and adults, side effects can be significantly reduced without compromising clinical benefit by aiming for serum concentrations of 28 to 55 µmol/L according to the Canadian Asthma Consensus Report, 1999 [*CMAJ* 1999;161(11 Suppl 2):S1-12].

Clinically, peak concentrations should be monitored. The peak level yields information about efficacy and potential for toxicity of the dosage regimen. Sampling time for peak concentration will vary depending on the route of administration and dosage form. If the patient becomes symptomatic at the end of the dosing interval, a trough concentration may be taken to determine whether or not the patient's dosing interval is appropriate. If toxicity or occult ingestion is suspected consider immediate and potentially delayed sampling. Saliva concentrations are not a reliable indicator of serum concentrations.

Concurrent administration of other drugs and xanthine-containing beverages can affect some assay results measured by spectrophotometric methods. These substances do not interfere with results when measured by high-pressure liquid chromatography or EMIT (enzyme multiplied immunoassay technique).

INDICATIONS: The symptomatic treatment of reversible bronchoconstriction associated with chronic obstructive pulmonary disease, asthma, chronic bronchitis and related bronchospastic disorders.

Theophylline is not a first-line agent in the management of chronic asthma. Long-acting formulations of oral theophylline may be useful as add-on therapy in adults who do not respond adequately to inhaled corticosteroids alone, or in children >5 years of age, who require high-dose inhaled corticosteroids despite optimal compliance and technique. In these clinical settings, theophylline has been shown to control day and night symptoms, and reduce the dose of the inhaled corticosteroid [Global Initiative for Asthma. *Global strategy for asthma management and prevention.* Updated 2007. Available from: http://www.ginasthma.com].

In patients with COPD, long-acting formulations of oral theophylline may be useful in those with severe symptoms despite the use of tiotropium plus a long-acting beta agonist/inhaled corticosteroid combination [*Can Respir J* 2007;14(Suppl B):5B-32B].

CONTRAINDICATIONS: Hypersensitivity to xanthines; active or symptomatic coronary artery disease. Aminophylline is contraindicated in patients allergic to ethylenediamine.

WARNINGS: Children: Children are very sensitive to xanthines, especially their CNS stimulant effects. Parents or other caregivers should be cautioned against overdosing children. The margin of safety above therapeutic doses is small. It is important to ensure that children receiving oral theophylline are not also receiving the drug by the rectal route.

Sustained-release dosage forms are not recommended in children ≤12 years of age as safety and efficacy have not been established.

PRECAUTIONS: There is marked interpatient variation in serum levels achieved following a given dose of theophylline. Dosage should be individualized to avoid excessive serum levels and serious adverse effects. Ideally, all individuals should have theophylline serum concentrations measured. Toxicity can occur when theophylline clearance is decreased in situations such as: premature or neonatal infants; age >60 years; high carbohydrate intake; concurrent methylxanthine intake; drug interactions (see Table 2); concurrent disease such as hepatic cirrhosis, congestive heart failure, acute pulmonary edema, chronic obstructive pulmonary disease, pneumonia, severe pulmonary obstruction, acute febrile episodes.

IV injections must be given slowly and cautiously, especially in patients with pronounced myocardial injury. Rapid iv injection may cause sudden and severe hypotension or cardiac arrest.

Theophylline should be used with caution in patients with confirmed or suspected peptic ulcer disease or esophagogastroduodenitis.

Extended-release preparations should be taken with adequate liquids to prevent esophageal erosion and ulceration.

For once-a-day dosage forms, dosage has not been established for children younger than 12 years.

Drug Interactions: As a substrate of CYP1A2 (major) and CYP3A4 (minor), theophylline's metabolism is susceptible to alteration when it is taken concurrently with inducers or inhibitors of these isoenzymes. Dose adjustments for drugs such as zafirlukast may be needed as concomitant administration with theophylline results in decreased zafirlukast levels.

In patients with hyperthyroidism, theophylline clearance increases. Monitor theophylline serum levels when initiating, discontinuing or changing dose of propylthiouracil and methimazole. In patients with hypothyroidism, theophylline clearance decreases. Monitor theophylline serum levels when initiating, discontinuing or changing dose of levothyroxine.

The drug interactions in Table 2 represent reported clinically significant interactions. Monitor theophylline serum concentrations and/or dosage adjustments when concurrent use of these medications with theophylline is initiated or discontinued.

There have been no documented interactions with newer macrolides.

Table 2: Theophyllines

Drug Interactions

Interacting Drug	Change in Theophylline Serum Concentration	Comments
Adenosine	—	Decreased cardiac effects of adenosine.
Allopurinol (≥600 mg/day)	↑	
Amiodarone	↑	
Barbiturates[a]	↓	
Benzodiazepines	—	Decreased sedative effects of benzodiazepines.
β-Blockers (nonselective)	↑	
Calcium Channel Blockers[b]	↑	
Carbamazepine	↓	
Cimetidine	↑	
Contraceptives, Oral	↑	
Fluvoxamine	↑	
Halothane	—	Arrhythmias.
Influenza Virus Vaccine	↑	Reports of seizures, headache, nausea and vomiting. Monitor theophylline toxicity in patients for 24 hours after influenza vaccine administration.
Interferon α, recombinant	↑	
Lithium	—	Decreased lithium serum concentrations.
Macrolides	↑	Mainly erythromycin, possibly clarithromycin. Has not occurred with azithromycin.
Methotrexate	↑	Reported with weekly methotrexate im injections.
Mexiletine	↑	
Muscle Relaxants, nondepolarizing	—	Decreased neuromuscular blockade.
Phenytoin[c]	↓	
Propafenone	↑	
Quinolones	↑	Ciprofloxacin, ofloxacin and norfloxacin only. No reports with newer fluoroquinolones.
Rifampin	↓	
Thiabendazole	↑	
Ticlopidine	↑	
Tobacco	↓	

[a] Includes primidone and its major metabolite, phenobarbital.
[b] Diltiazem and verapamil.
[c] Decreased phenytoin levels may also occur.

Pregnancy: Theophylline readily crosses the placenta. Transient tachycardia, irritability and vomiting have been reported in newborns exposed to theophylline in utero. Theophylline has not been associated with an increased risk of fetal malformations. If theophylline is used during pregnancy, careful titration of theophylline dose and regular monitoring of theophylline levels is recommended [*J Allergy Clin Immunol* 2005;115(1):34-46].

Nursing Women: Theophylline is excreted in breast milk and may occasionally cause irritability or other signs of toxicity in nursing infants. According to the American Academy of Pediatrics, theophylline is compatible with breast-feeding.

Children: See Warnings.

ADVERSE EFFECTS: Side effects most frequently experienced include: anorexia, nausea, vomiting, headache, abdominal discomfort, nervousness, insomnia, irritability and tremor. Tolerance to these effects may develop with continued dosing, or a reduction in dosage may alleviate the symptoms (see Pharmacology, Pharmacokinetics). About 5 to 15% of patients do not tolerate oral theophylline even if serum concentrations are less than 83 µmol/L.

Theophylline toxicity is frequently associated with large doses and high plasma concentrations of theophylline; severe effects are rare at concentrations below 110 µmol/L. Atrial and ventricular arrhythmias may occur with theophylline serum concentrations greater than 110 µmol/L, or at therapeutic concentrations in patients with heart disease. Focal or generalized seizures may occur at high serum concentrations, or at therapeutic serum concentrations in predisposed individuals. Toxicity of theophylline and its derivatives may present as follows:

Gastrointestinal: nausea, vomiting, diarrhea, abdominal cramps, epigastric pain, anorexia, reactivation of peptic ulcer, intestinal bleeding.

Central Nervous System: headache, nervousness, insomnia, dizziness, lightheadedness, excitement, irritability, restlessness, fever, convulsions.
Cardiovascular: palpitations, sinus tachycardia, atrial or ventricular arrhythmias, increased pulse rate, peripheral vascular constriction and/or collapse.
Urinary Tract: albuminuria.
Skin: rarely urticaria, generalized pruritus, angioedema, contact dermatitis.

OVERDOSE:

Symptoms: Patients, especially children, who are chronically overmedicated may develop severe toxicity with serum levels lower than those seen in an acute intoxication.

Seizures and death have occurred following large overdoses without prior symptoms of toxicity. The most common reactions observed with toxic overdoses of theophylline are:
Gastrointestinal: nausea, vomiting, epigastric pain, hematemesis, diarrhea.
Central Nervous System: hyperreflexia, fasciculations and tonic-clonic convulsions, hallucinations.
Cardiovascular: fatal arrhythmia or shock; marked hypotension and circulatory failure.
Respiratory: tachypnea and respiratory arrest.
Renal: albuminuria and microhematuria, increased excretion of renal tubular cells.
General Systemic Events: syncope, collapse, fever and dehydration.

Treatment: Induced vomiting is contraindicated because of the risk of sudden onset of seizures. Activated charcoal should be administered within 1 hour of ingestion ensuring that the airway remains protected. Multiple dose activated charcoal not only minimizes absorption but also enhances elimination of theophylline. Sorbitol may be given with the first dose of charcoal but should not be repeated. Theophylline serum concentrations should be monitored frequently until below the toxic range.

Seizures can be difficult to control and should be treated initially with an iv benzodiazepine. There may be a need to progress to barbiturates or propofol. Avoid phenytoin. Treatment also involves support of cardiac and respiratory functions, maintenance of fluid and electrolyte balance and ECG monitoring. A beta-adrenergic blocker may be used to control cardiac arrhythmias. Charcoal hemoperfusion and hemodialysis are effective in removing theophylline. Hemoperfusion is more effective than hemodialysis in removing theophylline, but carries a greater risk of complications.

For management of a suspected drug overdose, CPhA recommends that you contact your **regional Poison Control Centre**. See the *CPS* Directory section for a list of Poison Control Centres.

DOSAGE: Theophylline has a narrow therapeutic index; therefore, cautious dosage determination is essential. Individuals metabolize theophylline at different rates; appropriate dosages must be determined for each patient by carefully monitoring patient response and tolerance, pulmonary function and theophylline serum concentrations. Dosage adjustments are based on clinical response with careful monitoring for manifestations of toxicity. Symptoms of toxicity may even occur when serum concentrations are within the upper end of the therapeutic range (85 to 110 μmol/L), particularly during initiation of therapy (see Pharmacology, Pharmacokinetics). Although the accepted therapeutic plasma concentration range has traditionally been 55 to 110 μmol/L in children and adults, side effects can be significantly reduced without compromising clinical benefit by aiming for serum concentrations of 28 to 55 μmol/L, according to the Canadian Asthma Consensus Report, 1999.

Doses should be calculated based on ideal body weight.

Regardless of the preparation used, dosage should be based on theophylline content (see Table 3). Because of the significant differences among sustained-release theophylline formulations with respect to release characteristics, rate and/or extent of absorption, they are generally not considered interchangeable.

Table 3: Theophyllines

Theophylline Content

Xanthine	% Theophylline
Aminophylline	85
Oxtriphylline	65

Parenteral: Acute: The loading dose does not generally require adjustment in the presence of various disease states. The following loading doses are designed to achieve theophylline serum concentrations at the lower end of the therapeutic range (55 to 65 μmol/L).

If it has been established that the patient has not taken any theophylline preparation within the preceding 24 hours, the following loading dose is appropriate: Theophylline 5 mg/kg iv over 20 to 30 minutes (aminophylline 6 mg/kg iv over 20 to 30 minutes).

Ideally, if there is a strong suspicion that the patient has ingested some form of theophylline within the last 24 hours, the loading dose should be deferred until a theophylline serum determination is made. Since this is usually not possible, the use of other nonxanthine bronchodilators should be considered. If there is sufficient respiratory distress to warrant a small risk, a partial loading dose may be administered.

Partial Loading Dose: Theophylline 2.5 mg/kg iv over 20 to 30 minutes (aminophylline 3 mg/kg iv over 20 to 30 minutes).

This dose should produce an increase in serum theophylline concentration of approximately 25 to 30 μmol/L.

Alternatively, an increase in dosage of 1 mg/kg for every desired 10 μmol/L increase in theophylline serum concentration may be used at the discretion of the clinician.

Maintenance: These recommendations are not designed to replace theophylline serum concentrations as a guide for dosage adjustment, and should be used only until serum concentrations are available (see Table 4).

Table 4: Theophyllines

Parenteral Maintenance Dosage[a]

Group	Aminophylline IV (mg/kg/h)[a]	Theophylline IV (mg/kg/h)[b]
Neonates	0.2	0.17
6 weeks to 6 months	0.5	0.43
6 months to 1 year	0.6–0.7	0.5–0.6
1 to 9 years	1–1.2	0.85–1
9 to 12 years; young adult smokers	0.9	0.77
>12 years, nonsmoking	0.7	0.6
Older adults; patients with cor pulmonale, CHF or liver failure	0.25	0.21

[a] To be used only until serum level determinations are available to guide further dosage adjustment.
[b] Doses are designed to achieve a serum concentration of 55 μmol/L in most patients (see Pharmacology, Pharmacokinetics). Ideal body weight should be used to calculate dose.

Oral: Chronic Therapy: Children (over 1 year to 16 years): Starting dose (immediate-release formulations): 16 mg/kg/day to a maximum of 400 mg/day, administered in 3 to 4 divided doses at 6- to 8-hour intervals. Adults (>16 years): start with 400 mg/day.

The above dose may be increased, if tolerated, in approximately 25% increments at 2- to 3-day intervals, up to the maximum doses indicated in Table 5. When the recommended maximum dosage is exceeded, dosage adjustment should be based on measurement of peak theophylline serum concentration.

Dosage adjustments may be based on peak theophylline serum concentrations, clinical response and tolerance.

When adjusting the dose based on serum concentration, it is important that dosage in the previous 48 hours be reasonably typical of the prescribed regimen and that the patient has not missed a dose or taken an extra dose in this period. It is important that serum levels are obtained at steady state. If laboratory results appear questionable, serum levels should be repeated.

Table 5: Theophyllines

Maximum Recommended Oral Dosage

Age (years)	Dose of Theophylline[a]
1 to 9	16–22 mg/kg/day
9 to 12	16–20 mg/kg/day or 800 mg/day (whichever is less)
12 to 16	16–18 mg/kg/day or 900 mg/day (whichever is less)
Adults >16, nonsmoking	900 mg/day

[a] Use ideal body weight.

Infants: Elimination of the drug in children younger than 1 year, especially in neonates, generally appears to be reduced. Due to potential for toxicity, use of the drug in children younger than 1 year should be carefully considered and, if used, the initial and maintenance dosages (particularly the latter) should be conservative. The maintenance dose and dosing interval should be guided by monitoring of theophylline serum concentrations.

Caution is recommended in younger children who are not yet able to report minor side effects.

Extended-release Preparations: The actual dosing frequency for a given patient and preparation depends on the patient's individual pharmacokinetic parameters. Different extended-release formulations are generally not considered interchangeable.

Treatment of Asthma and COPD in Adults: Aminophylline: 225 to 350 mg po Q12H; theophylline 400 to 600 mg po with food given once daily, usually in the evening. Monitor and adjust dose based on serum levels.

Extended-release preparations are not indicated for the relief of acute conditions.

When extended-release preparations are to be administered, some clinicians recommend that the daily dosage requirement first be established by monitoring theophylline serum concentrations while the patient is receiving a rapidly absorbed dosage form. Therapy with an extended-release preparation may be started by administering one-half of the total daily dose every 12 hours. Follow the manufacturer's specific dosage and administration directions when initiating or transferring a patient to once daily extended-release preparations.

Extended-release preparations should not be chewed or crushed; the contents of extended-release capsules may be mixed with soft food and taken without chewing in patients who have difficulty swallowing solid dosage forms. For administration information with respect to meals, see Pharmacology, Pharmacokinetics.

Thiamine

CPhA Monograph

see *Vitamin B1*

Thiazide Diuretics

chlorthalidone
hydrochlorothiazide
indapamide
metolazone

Diuretic—Antihypertensive

CPhA Monograph

Date of Revision: October 2006

This monograph has been compiled by CPhA and reviewed by experts. It may contain information different from that found in Health Canada-approved Product Monographs. The reader is referred to the *CPS* Editorial Policy for more information.

SUMMARY PRODUCT INFORMATION:

Thiazide Diuretics	Dosage Form	Product Strength
Chlorthalidone	Tablets	50 mg, 100 mg
Hydrochlorothiazide	Tablets	25 mg, 50 mg, 100 mg
Indapamide	Tablets	1.25 mg, 2.5 mg
Metolazone	Tablets	2.5 mg, 5 mg

INDICATIONS: In this monograph the term "thiazides" refers to all drugs that inhibit the Na^+-Cl^--co-transporter. The information in this monograph therefore applies to both thiazides (e.g., hydrochlorothiazide) and thiazide-like (e.g., chlorthalidone, indapamide, metolazone) diuretics available in Canada.

Table 1: Thiazide Diuretics

Health Canada—Approved Indications for Thiazides Available in Canada

Thiazide Diuretic	Edema of Heart Failure	Hepatic Cirrhosis with Ascites	Drug-induced Edema[a]	Edema of Renal Origin[b]	Hypertension[c]
Chlorthalidone	Y	Y	Y	Y	Y
Hydrochlorthiazide	Y	Y	Y	Y	Y
Indapamide	N	N	N	N	Y
Metolazone	Y	N	N	Y	Y

[a] Approved in the treatment of corticosteroid and estrogen therapy-induced edema.
[b] Approved in the treatment of edema due to nephritic syndrome, acute glomerulonephritis, chronic renal disease.
[c] Approved for treatment of hypertension alone or in combination with other antihypertensive agents.
Legend: Y=yes, N=no.

Comparative Efficacy and Toxicity: There do not appear to be any significant differences in the clinical effect and toxicity of comparable doses of the various thiazide diuretics. Although evidence is weak, metolazone may be more effective in patients with renal impairment. Indapamide may have less potential to cause abnormalities in serum glucose and serum lipid levels; however, long-term studies are lacking. Low doses of thiazide diuretics for the treatment of hypertension appear to have negligible effects on serum glucose and lipid levels.

Hypertension: In the treatment of hypertension, thiazides may be used either alone or in combination with antihypertensive medications from other classes. They can be used as the initial agent or as add-on therapy in multiple drug regimens. When used in multiple drug regimens, antihypertensive effects of thiazide diuretics and other antihypertensive agents are additive or synergistic.

Edema: See Table 1. Thiazides are also effective as add-on therapy in patients whose response to loop diuretics has diminished over time (see Action and Clinical Pharmacology, Co-administration with Loop Diuretics).

Diabetes Insipidus: Thiazide diuretics have been used in the treatment of diabetes insipidus of both nephrogenic and neurohypophyseal origin.

Prophylaxis of Renal Calculus Formation: The thiazide-induced decrease in urinary excretion of calcium may be useful for prophylaxis of renal calculus formation associated with hypercalcemia. Regular, long-term administration of hydrochlorothiazide may have beneficial effects on bone mineral density. This effect may be a result of decreased calcium excretion during long-term thiazide therapy.

Geriatrics: Thiazide diuretics are safe and effective in elderly patients. However, the elderly may be at greater risk for developing electrolyte abnormalities due to age-related changes in renal function. In addition, the elderly may be more sensitive to the hypotensive effects of antihypertensive therapy, particularly upon initiation of therapy (see Warnings and Precautions, Geriatrics). Dosage adjustments are required in elderly patients, especially upon initiation of therapy (see Dosage and Administration, Geriatrics).

Pediatrics: Hydrochlorothiazide is the only thiazide diuretic approved for use in children (see Dosage and Administration, Pediatrics). Chlorthalidone, metolazone and indapamide are not approved for pediatric use; however, in practice chlorthalidone is used in this population. In addition, some hospitals use metolazone in infants and older children. Metolazone has also been used to induce diuresis in neonates unresponsive to furosemide.

CONTRAINDICATIONS: Anuria (discontinue if increasing azotemia and oliguria occur during treatment of severe progressive renal disease); hepatic coma or pre-coma (see Warnings and Precautions, Hepatic/Biliary/Pancreatic); known sensitivity to thiazides or related drugs; known sensitivity to other sulfonamide-derived drugs; known sensitivity to any ingredient in the formulation or component of the container (note: some commercially available hydrochlorothiazide products contain sulfites).

WARNINGS AND PRECAUTIONS: Cardiovascular: Orthostatic hypotension may occur. Alcohol, barbiturates, narcotics and concurrent therapy with other antihypertensives may potentiate this effect (see Drug Interactions, Alcohol, Barbiturates and Narcotics). When thiazide diuretics are used with antihypertensive agents from other classes, the hypotensive effects are additive or synergistic. Although combinations are often used to therapeutic advantage, the initial doses should be low and the doses of either agent should be increased slowly to reduce the risk of excessive hypotension. It may be prudent under certain circumstances to reduce the dose of the other antihypertensive before starting therapy with the thiazide diuretic (see Drug Interactions).

Endocrine and Metabolism: Electrolyte abnormalities (general): Electrolyte disturbances are more likely to occur in patients predisposed to electrolyte disorders (i.e., heart failure, renal diseases, hepatic cirrhosis and ascites) and when salt intake is severely restricted. Rarely, the rapid onset of severe hyponatremia and/or hypokalemia has been reported after the initial doses of thiazide diuretics. When symptoms consistent with a severe electrolyte imbalance (see Monitoring and Laboratory Tests) appear rapidly, the drug should be discontinued and supportive measures initiated immediately. The appropriateness of therapy with a thiazide diuretic should then be re-evaluated.

Unusually large or prolonged losses of fluid and electrolytes may result when metolazone or other thiazides are administered with loop diuretics (see Drug Interactions, Loop Diuretics). However, combination therapy with a thiazide and a loop diuretic may be advantageous under certain circumstances (see Action and Clinical Pharmacology, Co-administration with Loop Diuretics).

Hypokalemia: Hypokalemia, defined as serum potassium less than 3.5 mmol/L, is common with thiazide diuretics. Mild hypokalemia (serum potassium 3.0 to 3.5 mmol/L) may be associated with symptoms of generalized weakness, lassitude and constipation; however, often no symptoms are apparent. Severe hypokalemia (serum potassium <2.5 mmol/L) may be associated with muscle cramping due to muscle necrosis in addition to the above symptoms. Once serum potassium falls below 2.0 mmol/L, flaccid paralysis and respiratory collapse can occur.

In patients with pre-existing cardiac arrhythmias, cardiac ischemia, heart failure, left ventricular hypertrophy or in those receiving concomitant therapy with cardiac glycosides, hypokalemia, even of mild to moderate severity, significantly increases the probability of developing cardiac arrhythmias. Heart conduction abnormalities and arrhythmias are unusual in patients without underlying heart disease, even when the serum potassium is <3.0 mmol/L.

Hypokalemia is more common under the following circumstances: concomitant steroid or ACTH therapy; inadequate oral intake of potassium; excess extra-renal potassium losses such as with vomiting or diarrhea; rapid diuresis; severe liver disease; use of higher doses of thiazide and related diuretics (although hypokalemia can occur at any dose); and/or combination therapy with thiazide and loop diuretics.

Hypokalemia may be prevented or treated with mild salt restriction, consumption of potassium-rich foods (e.g., bananas, dried figs, dates and prunes, nuts, bran cereals, lima beans) or potassium supplements, or with the addition of a potassium-sparing diuretic.

Hyponatremia: Severe hyponatremia is defined as a serum sodium level <120 mmol/L. Hyponatremia may occur at any time during therapy. Dilutional hyponatremia occurs most commonly during hot weather in patients with heart failure or hepatic disease. Chronic thiazide therapy may aggravate dilutional hyponatremia. Patients with edematous conditions are at greater risk of dilutional hyponatremia.

Treatment of thiazide-induced hyponatremia includes withdrawal of the diuretic, fluid restriction and potassium and/or magnesium supplementation. Administration of sodium chloride is usually not required except in rare instances when hyponatremia may be life-threatening. Thiazide-induced hyponatremia has been associated with death and neurologic damage in elderly patients. CNS manifestations include seizures, coma and extensor-plantar response. Although improved outcomes are associated with correcting hyponatremia in the first 1 to 2 days, correcting serum sodium too quickly can cause rapid osmolar changes that are associated with development of central pontine myelinolysis. It has been suggested that a maximum correction of 20 mmol/L be achieved in the first 24 hours.

Hypochloremia: Hypochloremic alkalosis with thiazides may be more likely to occur in patients with renal or hepatic disease and may be accompanied by hypokalemia. Hypochloremia is generally mild and usually does not require specific treatment.

Hypomagnesemia: Hypomagnesemia is defined as a serum magnesium level less than 0.7 mmol/L (normal range 0.7 to 0.85 mmol/L). Hypomagnesemia may occur during thiazide therapy due to increased excretion of magnesium. Correction of thiazide-induced hypokalemia is impaired in the presence of hypomagnesemia (particularly when serum magnesium concentrations are less than 0.5 mmol/L) because hypomagnesemia induces hypokalemia independently of thiazide diuretic therapy. Magnesium improves co-existing hypokalemia. Serum magnesium levels should be monitored and maintained within the normal range during thiazide therapy. Particular care should be taken to maintain normal magnesium concentrations in patients at risk of cardiac conduction abnormalities in the presence of hypokalemia.

Hypercalcemia: Thiazides and related diuretics decrease urinary excretion of calcium and may cause intermittent and slight elevation of serum calcium in the absence of known disorders of calcium metabolism. Hyperparathyroidism should be suspected if marked hypercalcemia occurs. The use of thiazide and related diuretics has on rare instances been associated with physiologic and/or pathologic changes in the parathyroid glands; however, the common complications of hyperparathyroidism such as renal lithiasis, bone resorption and peptic ulcer have not been seen.

Hyperuricemia: Hyperuricemia may occur during thiazide therapy. Gout may be precipitated in predisposed patients. Use diuretics with caution in patients with a history of gout or hyperuricemia (see Drug Interactions). Uric acid levels should be monitored in these patients (see Monitoring and Laboratory Tests).

Hyperglycemia: Thiazide therapy may induce hyperglycemia and result in decreased glucose tolerance in a dose-related manner. Doses of insulin and/or other antidiabetic medications may require adjustment (see Drug Interactions, Antidiabetic Medications). Use of low doses of thiazide diuretics for the treatment of hypertension produce negligible effects on serum glucose and lipid levels in most patients. In the ALLHAT study (JAMA 2002;288(23):2981-97) thiazide-associated increases in fasting glucose levels did not offset the cardiovascular benefits of chlorthalidone.

Hyperlipidemia: Concentrations of total serum cholesterol, total triglycerides and LDL (but not HDL) may be slightly and transiently elevated in some patients in a dose-dependent manner. The currently recommended low doses of thiazide diuretics for the treatment of hypertension appear to have negligible effects on lipid levels. In addition, the results of ALLHAT indicate that modest thiazide-induced elevations in lipoproteins do not offset the cardiovascular benefit of these agents.

Hepatic/Biliary/Pancreatic: Patients with impaired hepatic function or progressive hepatic disease should be carefully monitored during thiazide therapy for electrolyte abnormalities. Patients with these conditions are at particular risk of hepatic encephalopathy due to thiazide-induced potassium depletion and resulting metabolic alkalosis.

Immune: Cross-sensitivity with sulfonamides may occur.

Some thiazide products contain tartrazine (FD&C yellow #5), which may precipitate allergic-type reactions (including bronchial asthma) in susceptible individuals. Although the incidence of sensitivity is low, it is frequently seen in patients who also have ASA hypersensitivity. For specific products containing tartrazine see specific product monographs.

Some thiazide products contain sulfites, which may cause allergic-type reactions in susceptible individuals. For specific products containing sulfites, see individual product monographs.

Neurologic: The antihypertensive effect of thiazides may be enhanced in the patient post sympathectomy.

Peri-operative Considerations: Hypokalemia may enhance the neuromuscular blocking action of curariform drugs leading to respiratory depression or apnea.

Renal: Thiazides and related diuretics may decrease GFR and precipitate or increase azotemia. Treatment should be discontinued or withheld in the presence of increasing azotemia and oliguria and in severe progressive renal disease.

Thiazide diuretics, with the possible exception of metolazone, are ineffective when the creatinine clearance is less than 30 mL/min (see Recommended Dose and Dosage Adjustment, Renal Impairment). Under these circumstances, if diuretic therapy is appropriate, treatment with a loop diuretic should be considered.

Skin: Photosensitivity: Photosensitization may occur during therapy with thiazides and related diuretics; therefore, caution patients to take protective measures (i.e., sunscreens, protective clothing) against exposure to ultraviolet light and/or sunlight until tolerance is determined.

Special Populations: Pregnant Women: Pregnancy Category B (chlorthalidone, hydrochlorothiazide, indapamide, metolazone).

Thiazides cross the placenta. Possible fetal risks include jaundice, thrombocytopenia and other adverse reactions that have occurred in adults. Increased concentrations of uric acid and creatinine have been found in the amniotic fluid of pregnant women near term who are taking thiazides. There is a theoretical risk to the fetus associated with plasma volume reduction induced by thiazide diuretics.

Thiazides do not prevent pre-eclampsia or eclampsia, nor are they useful in its treatment. Routine use of thiazide diuretics in otherwise healthy pregnant women with or without edema is not appropriate. Edema in pregnancy, resulting from restriction of venous return by the expanded uterus is treated by elevation of the lower extremities and use of support hose. A short course of diuretics may be appropriate in patients with severe hypervolemia that is not relieved by rest or other measures (i.e., reducing sodium intake and placement in a recumbent position). Therapy with a thiazide diuretic may be indicated in pathological cardiac, nephritic or hepatic edema if the benefits outweigh the risk to the fetus.

Nursing Women: Thiazides (including hydrochlorothiazide, chlorthalidone and metolazone) are excreted into the milk of nursing women, although apparently not in significant amounts. The distribution of indapamide into breast milk is unknown. The American Academy of Pediatrics considers chlorthalidone and hydrochlorothiazide to be compatible with breastfeeding. It should be noted that thiazides may partially suppress lactation and idiosyncratic or allergic reactions may occur in the infant.

Pediatrics (birth to 16 years old): Hydrochlorthiazide is safe and effective in children. The safety and efficacy of chlorthalidone, indapamide and metolazone have not been established in children. However chlorthalidone and metolazone have been used safely in children.

Geriatrics: Elderly patients may be at greater risk for development of electrolyte abnormalities due to age-related changes in renal function. In these patients, therapy should be initiated at half the usual starting dose and the minimum effective dose should be used. Serum electrolytes (particularly potassium) should be regularly monitored and interventions to maintain serum electrolytes within the desired range should be carried out as required (see Warnings and Precautions, Endocrine and Metabolism, Electrolyte Abnormalities).

Monitoring and Laboratory Tests: Baseline serum electrolyte (sodium, potassium, magnesium, chloride, calcium, phosphate) concentrations and baseline levels of blood glucose, lipids, uric acid, serum creatinine and blood urea nitrogen (BUN) should be determined before starting therapy with a diuretic. Weekly electrolyte assessments may be appropriate early during the course of therapy. Once the patient is stabilized, electrolyte assessments may be repeated at 3-month intervals and after increasing the dosage. More frequent monitoring of serum electrolytes is warranted in patients with risk factors for hypokalemia (see Warnings and Precautions, Endocrine and Metabolism, Hypokalemia) or hypokalemia-induced cardiac arrhythmias (patients with cardiac arrhythmias, cardiac ischemia, heart failure, left ventricular hypertrophy or those who are receiving concomitant therapy with cardiac glycosides). Potassium replacement strategies should be instituted promptly if hypokalemia develops. During therapy with thiazide diuretics, all patients should be monitored for signs of electrolyte abnormalities such as dry mouth, thirst, weakness, lethargy, drowsiness, restlessness, muscle pains or cramps, muscular fatigue, hypotension, oliguria, tachycardia, nausea, vomiting, seizures or confusion.

The serum creatinine and BUN should be monitored more frequently in patients with renal insufficiency. If azotemia and oliguria occur or worsen during treatment, the diuretic should be discontinued (see Warnings and Precautions, Renal).

Blood pressure should be monitored every 1 to 2 months after initiation of therapy and the dose of the thiazide diuretic should be adjusted according to response to achieve target blood pressure levels. The maximum antihypertensive effect of thiazides may not be apparent for several months.

Once target blood pressure levels are achieved and antihypertensive therapy is stabilized, blood pressure should be monitored at 3- to 6-month intervals. Consideration should be given to monitoring blood pressure in both seated and standing positions in geriatric patients and in those with orthostatic hypotension.

Occupational Hazards: Thiazides may cause dizziness and hypotension, especially upon initiation of therapy and after dose increases. Patients receiving a thiazide should be cautioned against engaging in hazardous occupations that require complete mental alertness such as operating machinery or driving a motor vehicle until they know how the drug will affect them.

DRUG INTERACTIONS: Overview: See Table 2.

Table 2: Thiazide Diuretics

Drug-Drug Interactions

Interacting Drug	Effect	Clinical Comment
ACTH	Additive hypokalemia. Reversal of antihypertensive efficacy may result from sodium and water retention induced by ACTH.	Monitor serum potassium levels and institute replacement therapy if necessary. Monitor blood pressure and adjust therapy as required.
Alcohol, barbiturates, narcotics	Orthostatic hypotension may occur. Alcohol, barbiturates and narcotics may potentiate the antihypertensive effects of thiazides.	Avoid alcohol, especially with initiation of therapy. Monitor and adjust therapy as required.
Allopurinol	An increased incidence of hypersensitivity reactions to allopurinol have been reported in patients receiving diuretics. Symptoms include fever, chills, eosinophilia, pruritus, maculopapular rash, hepatic and renal toxicity. Mechanism unknown.	No change in therapy is indicated. Monitor for hypersensitivity during combined therapy.

(cont'd)

Table 2: Thiazide Diuretics *(cont'd)*

Drug-Drug Interactions

Interacting Drug	Effect	Clinical Comment
Amphotericin B	Additive hypokalemia	Monitor serum potassium levels and institute replacement therapy if necessary.
Anesthetics	Anesthesia may be potentiated by thiazide diuretics.	Monitor and correct fluid and electrolyte abnormalities prior to surgery if possible. Dose adjustment of anesthetics may be required.
Anticholinergics	Increased therapeutic effect of the thiazide. Anticholinergics increase absorption of thiazides by decreasing gastrointestinal motility and delaying stomach emptying. In particular the rate at which thiazides pass through the optimal absorbing region in the small intestine is increased.	No clinical intervention is required. In patients on chronic anticholinergic therapy it may be possible to lower the thiazide dose.
Anticoagulants	Anticoagulant effects may be slightly diminished. Volume contraction induced by thiazide diuretics may effectively increase the concentration of clotting factors in the circulation and/or increase synthesis of clotting factors in the liver by reducing hepatic congestion and facilitating hepatic function.	The effect is not usually clinically significant; however increases in anticoagulant dose may sometimes be required. Monitor for decreased effect and adjust anticoagulant dose if required.
Antihyperglycemic medications: (alpha glucosidase inhibitors, biguanides, meglitinides, sulfonylureas, thiazolidinediones, insulin)	Thiazide-induced hyperglycemia may compromise blood glucose control. Thiazide-induced hypokalemia may inhibit insulin secretion or decrease tissue sensitivity to insulin. The effect is dose-related.	The clinical significance is minimal to moderate. Hyperglycemia may occur within days to months after initiating thiazide therapy. Monitor glycemic control, supplement potassium to ensure adequate levels, and/or adjust the dose of antihyperglycemic medications.
Antigout medications	Reemergence of previously controlled symptoms of gout. Thiazide-induced hyperuricemia may compromise control of gout symptoms.	In predisposed patients, monitor for symptoms of gout and adjust dose of antigout medications as required.
Antihypertensive medications	Excessive hypotension. Increased risk of hypotension with thiazide-ACE inhibitor combination due to synergistic effects on blood pressure. This interaction is often used to therapeutic advantage.	When starting combined therapy, use the lowest dose and titrate upwards carefully to avoid excessive hypotension. Under certain circumstances, it may be prudent to decrease the dose of the established antihypertensive prior to adding the second.
Beta-adrenergic antagonists	Additive increase in blood glucose, LDL and triglyceride levels. Patients with diabetes are most at risk. Propranolol is most likely to cause effect. Cardioselective agents may have lower potential to induce these effects. Agents with ISA or alpha-antagonist properties do not alter lipid levels.	Monitor blood glucose and lipid levels. Treat or adjust therapy as required. Counsel patients regarding diet. Choose cardioselective agents and avoid propranolol if possible.
Calcium salts and vitamin D (calcitriol, cholecalciferol, dihydrotachysterol, ergocalciferol)	Increased risk of hypercalcemia and associated calcium toxicity. Thiazides decrease renal excretion of calcium and increase calcium release from bone. Hypercalcemia may occur with chronic high doses of exogenous calcium. Hyperparathyroidism and concurrent administration of vitamin D further increase risk of calcium toxicity since thiazides may enhance the effect of parathyroid hormone and vitamin D on release of calcium from bone.	Monitor serum calcium. Signs and symptoms of hypercalcemia include anorexia, nausea, vomiting, constipation, polyuria, polydipsia, nocturia. Dose reduction or withdrawal of calcium and vitamin D supplements may be necessary.
Cholestyramine and colestipol resins (bile acid sequestrants)	Bile acid sequestrants bind thiazide diuretics in the gut and impair gastrointestinal absorption by 43–85%. Administration of thiazide 4 h after a bile acid sequestrant reduced absorption of hydrochlorothiazide by 30–35%.	Give the thiazide 2 h before or 6 h after the bile acid sequestrant. Maintain a consistent sequence of administration. Monitor blood pressure if a bile acid sequestrant is started, stopped or the dose is changed. Increase the thiazide dose if necessary.
Corticosteroids	Additive hypokalemia. Possible reversal of thiazide antihypertensive response via corticosteroid-induced salt and water retention.	Monitor serum potassium levels and replace potassium if required. Monitor blood pressure and adjust medications as required.
Digoxin	Thiazide-induced electrolyte disturbances (hypokalemia and hypomagnesemia) increase the risk of digoxin toxicity, the most serious manifestation of which is arrhythmia. Other signs and symptoms of digoxin toxicity include nausea, vomiting, anorexia, blurred or yellowed vision, confusion, bradycardia. Correction of thiazide-induced hypokalemia is impaired by hypomagnesemia (particularly when serum magnesium concentrations are <0.5 mmol/L; see Warnings, Electrolyte Abnormalities, Hypomagnesemia).	Clinical significance is high. Monitor serum electrolytes, particularly potassium and magnesium levels. Administer potassium and/or magnesium supplements as required. Consider adding a potassium-sparing diuretic. (Triamterene may be a better choice than spironolactone or amiloride, which can cause small increases in serum digoxin levels.)
Lithium	Thiazides increase serum lithium levels and can precipitate lithium toxicity within several days of initiating therapy. In a sodium depleted state, lithium is reabsorbed with or in place of sodium in the renal tubule. Signs and symptoms of lithium toxicity include nausea, vomiting, diarrhea, anorexia, coarse tremor, slurred speech, vertigo, confusion, lethargy. Symptoms can progress to severe seizures, stupor, coma and cardiovascular collapse.	If these drugs must be used together, decrease the lithium dose by 50% with close monitoring of lithium concentration, serum electrolytes and fluid intake. Observe for signs and symptoms of lithium toxicity. Thiazides and lithium can be co-administered safely with close lithium level monitoring.
Loop diuretics (e.g., furosemide)	Synergistic effects on sodium and water excretion and electrolyte disturbances. This combination has been used successfully in patients who become resistant to diuresis with loop diuretics (see Action and Clinical Pharmacology, Co-administration with Loop Diuretics). Unusually large or prolonged losses of fluids and electrolytes may result even when used for therapeutic effect.	When using for therapeutic effect, careful titration and small or intermittent doses should be used. Monitor for dehydration and electrolyte abnormalities.
Methenamine	Methenamine requires acidic urine for effect (pH <5.5). The urinary alkalizing effect of thiazides may decrease the efficacy of methenamine.	Consider monitoring urine pH in patients on this combination.
NSAIDs	NSAID-induced inhibition of renal prostaglandin synthesis and induction of sodium and water retention antagonizes the diuretic and antihypertensive effects of thiazides. Renal failure may be more likely due to the combination of NSAID-induced inhibition of renal prostaglandins, which decreases renal blood flow, and thiazide-induced decreases in GFR. Heart failure patients may be at particular risk. Changes are less apparent with sulindac, aspirin, and ibuprofen and more apparent with indomethacin, naproxen and piroxicam. Sulindac may enhance the diuretic effect of thiazides due to decreased renal clearance of HCTZ.	Avoid the combination if possible. Close monitoring of BUN, serum creatinine, potassium and the patient's weight is recommended if using this combination. Monitor blood pressure and diuretic effect and increase the dose if necessary or discontinue the NSAID.
Quinidine	Hypokalemia increases the risk of quinidine-induced ventricular arrhythmias. Urinary excretion of quinidine may be decreased in alkaline urine.	The effect is not usually clinically significant. Monitor for signs and symptoms of quinidine toxicity.
Skeletal muscle relaxants (nondepolarizing); curariform drugs	Thiazides may enhance the effects of nondepolarizing skeletal muscle relaxants. Thiazide-induced hypokalemia increases resistance to depolarization by hyperpolarizing the end plate resulting in enhanced myoneural blockade.	Monitor and correct thiazide-induced hypokalemia. Consider decreasing dose of nondepolarizing skeletal muscle relaxant if hypokalemia cannot be corrected before administration of a muscle relaxant. Discontinue metolazone 2–3 days before elective surgery. Clinical significance is unknown.
Sympathomimetics	May decrease the antihypertensive effect of the thiazide. May decrease arterial responsiveness to norepinephrine but this does not preclude use of pressor agents for therapeutic purposes.	Clinical significance is unknown.
Tetracyclines	Tetracyclines and thiazides can increase BUN levels. Patients with pre-existing renal disease are at increased risk.	Monitor BUN especially in patients with renal dysfunction.

Legend: ACTH=adrenocorticotropic hormone, LDL=low density lipoprotein, GFR=glomerular filtration rate, HCTZ=hydrochlorothiazide, ISA=intrinsic sympathomimetic activity.

Drug-Herb Interactions: The following herbal preparations may decrease the efficacy of thiazides and increase blood pressure; Coltsfoot; Eleuthero (Siberian ginseng); Ginkgo; Licorice; Ma huang; Puncture vine; Stinging nettle; Yarrow.

Table 3: Thiazide Diuretics

Drug-Laboratory Test Interactions

Interacting Laboratory Test	Effect	Clinical Comment
Estriol assay (spectrophotometric assay)	Hydrochlorothiazide interferes with the degradation of estriol resulting in falsely decreased values.	Apparently does not occur with chlorothiazide.
Parathyroid function tests	Thiazides may cause hypercalcemia in the absence of known disorders of calcium metabolism.	Discontinue thiazides before performing parathyroid function tests.
PSP excretion	Thiazides compete with phenolsulfonphthalein for secretion by proximal renal tubules.	Clinical significance is unknown.
Protein-bound iodine values	Test may show falsely decreased values in patients taking hydrochlorothiazide due to interference with formation of the Kober chromogen.	
Triiodothyronine resin uptake	Uptake may be decreased slightly but 24 h I^{131} uptake is not affected.	Thyroid function is not affected by thiazides.
Tyramine, phentolamine and possibly histamine tests for pheochromocytoma	False negative results may occur in patients taking thiazides.	
Urinary corticosteroid values	Thiazides may decrease urinary corticosteroid values. They may also decrease urinary excretion of cortisol.	Clinical significance unclear.

Legend: PSP=phenolsulfonphthalein.

ACTION AND CLINICAL PHARMACOLOGY: The main mechanism of action of thiazide diuretics involves inhibition of the Na+-Cl− co-transporter in the proximal part of the distal convoluted tubule of the kidney. This decreases tubular reabsorption of sodium and chloride, and increases urinary excretion of sodium and water.

Thiazide diuretics have moderate natriuretic and diuretic effects. These agents are able to excrete a maximum of 5% of the filtered sodium load since 90% is reabsorbed at more proximal sites before reaching the distal convoluted tubule. Inhibition of sodium and water reabsorption in the distal convoluted tubule results in increased delivery of sodium and solute to sites of sodium-potassium exchange in the late distal tubule and collecting duct. The result is a substantial increase in excretion of potassium. Increased urinary excretion of bicarbonate, chloride, magnesium, phosphate, bromide and iodide may also occur during therapy with thiazide diuretics.

The mechanism by which thiazide diuretics induce antihypertensive effects is not completely understood; although sodium depletion is thought to be of primary importance. Upon initiation of therapy, thiazide-induced natriuresis and diuresis reduces extracellular volume and decreases blood pressure. Volume contraction causes reflex activation of the renin-angiotensin system and the sympathetic nervous system, causing compensatory increases in proximal tubular sodium and water reabsorption and return of extracellular volume to near normal levels. In spite of the near normalization of plasma volume, peripheral vascular resistance is persistently lowered with continued thiazide therapy. Because of this, a direct action of these agents on vascular smooth muscle has been hypothesized. This effect may involve direct effects on vascular smooth muscle carbonic acid anhydrase and activation of calcium activated potassium channels in vascular smooth muscle cells. The equivalency of the different thiazide diuretics with respect to their direct actions on vascular smooth muscle cells is also unclear.

Diabetes Insipidus: The use of thiazide diuretics for diabetes insipidus is paradoxical. Diuretics usually increase urine volume; however, in patients with diabetes insipidus, these agents reduce urine volume. With chronic thiazide therapy, compensatory increases in proximal tubular sodium and water reabsorption decrease urine volume. Inhibition of the Na+-Cl− co-transporter in the distal convoluted tubule impairs maximal dilution of urine, helping to decrease urine volume.

Prophylaxis of Renal Calculus Formation: Thiazides increase both proximal and distal tubular reabsorption of calcium in the renal tubule, thus decreasing calcium concentrations in the urine.

Co-administration with Loop Diuretics: Thiazide diuretics are often used as add-on therapy in patients whose diuretic response to loop diuretics has diminished. During therapy with loop diuretics, inhibition of sodium reabsorption at sites in the ascending loop of Henle results in increased delivery of sodium and solute to the distal tubule. Increased delivery of solute to these tubule segments results in hypertrophy, which increases reabsorption of sodium and water at these locations. This decreases the efficacy of loop diuretics and produces "tolerance" to diuresis. Co-administration of a thiazide diuretic counteracts "tolerance" by blocking compensatory sodium reabsorption in the distal tubule.

Pharmacokinetics: The onset of antihypertensive action of thiazide diuretics requires several days and administration for 2 to 4 weeks is necessary for optimal therapeutic effect. The duration of antihypertensive effect of all thiazides is sufficiently long to adequately control blood pressure with a single daily dose. There is no relationship between plasma levels and diuretic effect.

At maximal therapeutic dosages all thiazides are approximately equal in diuretic efficacy.

Table 4: Thiazide Diuretics

Pharmacokinetics

Drug	Chlorthalidone	Hydrochlorothiazide	Indapamide	Metolazone
Usual $t_{1/2}$ (h)	40–80	2.5–14.8	4–22	4–20
Renal $t_{1/2}$ (h)	Unknown	12–20	No change	No data
Bioavailability	60–70%	65–75%	93%	65% (40% in patients with cardiac disease)
Clearance	Renal: 30–65 Other: 10–25%	Renal: >95%	Renal: 7% as unchanged drug Hepatic: extensive	Renal: 70–90% Hepatic: 10% Other: 10%
Volume of Distribution (L/kg)	3.9	3.0	0.3–1.3	1.6
Onset (h)	2–3	2	1–2	1
Peak (h)	2–6	4–6	2	2
Duration (h)	24–72	6–12	Up to 36	12–24
Relative potency	1	1	20	10
Equivalent dose (mg)	50	50	2.5	5
C_{max}			230–260 ng/mL	
Plasma protein binding	76–90%	40%	76–79%	90–95%

Absorption: See Table 4. The bioavailability of thiazide diuretics may be decreased in patients with heart failure.

Metabolism: Indapamide undergoes extensive hepatic metabolism; however, interactions with specific CYP450 isozymes have not been described. Chlorthalidone, hydrochlorothiazide and metolazone undergo negligible hepatic metabolism and do not induce or inhibit CYP450 isozymes.

Excretion: See Table 4. The clearance of hydrochlorothiazide may be decreased in patients with heart failure.

Special Populations and Conditions: Geriatrics: The clearance of hydrochlorothiazide may be decreased in the elderly.

Hepatic Insufficiency: Clearance of indapamide may be reduced in patients with advanced hepatic disease since indapamide undergoes extensive hepatic metabolism. Hepatic metabolism does not play a significant role in the elimination of hydrochlorothiazide, chlorthalidone or metolazone.

Thiazide diuretics are contraindicated in patients with hepatic coma or pre-coma. These agents should be used cautiously in patients with progressive hepatic disease.

Renal Insufficiency: The clearance of hydrochlorothiazide and chlorthalidone is decreased in patients with renal dysfunction. Since renal excretion of metolazone is high, clearance of this agent is also likely to be decreased. The clearance of indapamide may also be reduced since the metabolites are eliminated largely by the renal route.

Thiazide diuretics must be present at the site of action in the renal tubule in sufficient concentration in order to achieve their therapeutic effects. Thiazides reach their site of action almost exclusively by secretion into the tubular fluid via the organic acid cotransporter. In mild renal insufficiency, higher doses are required to achieve sufficient concentrations of drug at the site of action due to decreased renal tubular secretion. Most thiazide diuretics become ineffective once creatinine clearance drops below 30 to 50 mL/min. However, higher doses of metolazone are effective in patients with creatinine clearance less than 20 mL/min.

ADVERSE REACTIONS: Adverse Drug Reaction Overview: There do not appear to be any significant differences in toxicity of comparable doses of the various thiazide diuretics. The main adverse drug reactions associated with thiazide diuretics are electrolyte abnormalities.

Table 5: Thiazide Diuretics

Adverse Drug Reactions

Body System	Chlorthalidone (%)	Hydrochlorothiazide (%)	Indapamide (%)	Metolazone (%)
Cardiovascular				
Arrhythmia			2	
Chest pain (precordial)				3
Chest pain/discomfort			2	Y
Elevated cholesterol, triglycerides and LDL (see Warnings and Precautions)	Y	Y (transient hyperlipidemia)	Y (may have less effect on blood lipids than other thiazides but long term data are limited)	Y
Cold extremities, edema				<2
ECG abnormalities (non-specific ST)			<1 to 7 (non-specific ST changes)	
Edema			2	
Excessive volume depletion				Y
Hemoconcentration				Y
Hypotension		Y	<1	
Hypotension (orthostatic)		Y	<5	<2
Myocarditis (allergic)		Y		
Palpitations			<5	<2
Premature ventricular contractions, irregular heartbeat			<5	
Sinus bradycardia			3	
Stroke			PM	
Syncope			<1 (fainting)	Y
Tachycardia			<2	
Torsades de pointes			PM	
Vasculitis			PM	
Venous thrombosis				Y
Ventricular arrhythmia			PM	
CNS				
Asthenia			1.7 to 4	
Depression			<5	<2 (psychotic depression)
Dizziness/ light-headedness	Y	Y	1.9 to 7	10
Drowsiness			<5	Y
Fatigue/lethargy/ malaise/lassitude				4

(cont'd)

Table 5: Thiazide Diuretics *(cont'd)*

Adverse Drug Reactions

Body System	Chlorthalidone (%)	Hydrochlorothiazide (%)	Indapamide (%)	Metolazone (%)
Headache	Y	Y	3.4 to 17	9
Nervousness/Anxiety			1	<2
Neuropathy				Y
Paresthesias	Y	Y	<1	Y
Restlessness/ Insomnia	Y	Y	<5	Y
Tingling of extremities			<5	
Vertigo	Y	Y	<1	Y
Weakness	Y		<2 (and fatigue)	
Weird feeling/ neuropathy				<2
Xanthopsia	Y	Y		
Dermatologic				
Alopecia		Y		
Dry skin			<2	
Erythema multiforme, Stevens-Johnson syndrome		Y (hypersensitivity)		
Hives			<5	
Pruritus			<5	
Endocrine and Metabolism				
Acute gouty attacks			<1	Y
Dehydration			PM	
Glucosuria	Y	Y	<5	Y
Hyperglycemia	Y	Y	6	Y
Hyperosmolar coma			PM	
Hypochloremia			9.4	Y
Hypokalemia (total)			3–20	
Hypokalemia (requiring supplementation)			6.0	
Hypokalemia (symptomatic)			1.2 to 7	
Hyponatremia		Y	3.1	Y
Metabolic alkalosis			PM	
Uric acid (blood) elevated	Y	Y	<9	Y
Gastrointestinal				
Abdominal pain/ cramping/bloating	Y	Y	<5	<2
Anorexia	Y	Y	<5	Y
Constipation	Y	Y	<5	<2
Diarrhea	Y	Y	<5	<2
Dry mouth			<5	
Dyspepsia			4	
Gastric irritation/ epigastric distress	Y	Y	<5	Y
Hepatitis			PM	Y
Jaundice (intra-hepatic/cholestatic)	Y	Y		Y
Nausea	Y	Y	<5	<2
Pancreatitis	Y	Y	PM	Y
Sialadenitis		Y		
Vomiting	Y	Y	<5	<2

(cont'd)

Table 5: Thiazide Diuretics *(cont'd)*

Adverse Drug Reactions

Body System	Chlorthalidone (%)	Hydrochlorothiazide (%)	Indapamide (%)	Metolazone (%)
Genitourinary				
Elevated BUN			5.7	Y
Elevated serum creatinine				Y
Frequent urination, polyuria			<5	
Impotence/reduced libido	Y	Y	<5	<2 (impotence)
Interstitial nephritis		Y	PM (hypersensitivity reaction)	
Nocturia			<5	
Renal failure/ dysfunction		Y	PM (hypersensitivity reaction)	
Hematologic				
Agranulocytosis	Y	Y	PM	Y
Anemia			PM	
Aplastic/hypoplastic anemia	Y	Y		Y
Hemolytic anemia		Y		
Leukopenia	Y	Y		Y
Thrombocytopenia	Y	Y		
Immune				
Anaphylaxis		Y		
Angioedema			PM	
Bullous eruption			PM	
Erythema multiforme			PM	
Erythroderma			PM	
Exfoliative dermatitis/toxic epidermal necrolysis	Y	Y	PM	
Fever		Y	<1	
Necrotizing angiitis, (vasculitis, cutaneous vasculitis)	Y	Y	<5	Y
Photosensitivity with bullae			PM	
Photosensitivity/ photosensitivity dermatitis	Y	Y		Y
Purpura	Y	Y	PM	Y
Rash	Y	Y	<5	<2
Respiratory distress (including pneumonitis/ pulmonary edema)		Y		
Stevens Johnson Syndrome			PM	
Urticaria	Y	Y		Y
Musculoskeletal				
Back pain			5	
Hypertonia			3	
Joint disorders/ swelling of joints			<1	Y
Joint pain			<8	Y
Muscle cramps		Y	1.2	6
Muscle spasm		Y		
Rhabdomyolysis			PM	
Respiratory				
Cough			2	

(cont'd)

Table 5: Thiazide Diuretics *(cont'd)*

Adverse Drug Reactions

Body System	Chlorthalidone (%)	Hydrochlorothiazide (%)	Indapamide (%)	Metolazone (%)
Pharyngitis			2	
Rhinitis			5	
Rhinorrhea			<5	
Sinusitis			3	
Ophthalmologic				
Acute myopia			PM	
Blurred vision (may be transient), visual disturbance		Y	<1 to <5	Y
Cataract			PM	
Optic neuritis			PM	
Miscellaneous				
Chills				Y
Flu syndrome			3	
Flushing and weight loss			<5	
Infection			12	
Lithium toxicity			PM	

Legend: Y=yes (has been reported but frequency unknown), PM=post-marketing adverse drug reaction.

Adverse Drug Reactions for indapamide (<1%): Cardiovascular: angina pectoris, atrial fibrillation, atrial flutter, bundle branch block, supraventricular tachycardia, vasodilation, ventricular asystole.
CNS: amnesia, ataxia, coordination abnormality, dream abnormality, hyperesthesia, twitching.
Dermatologic: acne, bullous eruption, nail disorder, skin nodule.
Endocrine and Metabolism: thyroid disorder.
Gastrointestinal: duodenitis, dysphagia, esophagitis, flatulence, gastralgia, gastritis, gastroenteritis, gastrointestinal carcinoma, increased appetite, oral moniliasis, proctitis, rectal disorders, rectal hemorrhoids, stomatitis, tooth disorders.
Genitourinary: dysmenorrhea, dysuria, oliguria, prostate disorders, renal pain or calculus, urinary frequency or urgency, urinary tract infection, vaginitis.
Musculoskeletal: arthralgia, arthritis, bone disorders, bone fracture, bone pain, leg weakness, myalgia, myasthenia, myopathy.
Respiratory: bronchitis, dyspnea, increased sputum, laryngitis, lung disorders.
Miscellaneous: conjunctivitis, ear disorders, ear pain, eye itching, otitis, photophobia, taste perversion, tinnitus, vision abnormality, allergic reaction, ecchymosis, hernia, monilia, sweating.

DOSAGE AND ADMINISTRATION: Dosing Considerations: General: Therapy should be individualized according to patient response. The smallest effective dose to achieve the desired effect should be used to minimize the likelihood of adverse effects.
Edema: To reduce the chance of thiazide-induced electrolyte abnormalities, intermittent administration (every other day, or three days per week) may be advantageous.
Hypertension: When thiazide diuretics are used with antihypertensive agents from different classes, the hypotensive effects are additive or synergistic. Therapy should be initiated at low doses and titrated cautiously to reduce the risk of excessive hypotension. It may be prudent under certain circumstances to reduce the dose of the other antihypertensive before starting therapy with the thiazide diuretic (see Drug Interactions).
Concomitant administration: Due to their synergistic effects on diuresis, concurrent administration of thiazide diuretics (usually metolazone but others are also appropriate) and loop diuretics have been used in the management of patients refractory to monotherapy with loop diuretics (see Action and Clinical Pharmacology, Co-administration with Loop Diuretics). The thiazide diuretic should be introduced at a low dose and then progressively increased. Close monitoring for azotemia, electrolyte imbalance and volume depletion is required. Patients requiring 240 mg/day or more of furosemide are likely to benefit more from the addition of a thiazide diuretic such as metolazone than from further increases in the dose of furosemide. Thiazide diuretics can be given at the same time as a loop diuretic when they are both given orally. However, when a thiazide diuretic is given orally and a loop diuretic is given intravenously, the thiazide should be given 30 to 60 minutes in advance of furosemide.

Most thiazide diuretics are ineffective once creatinine clearance falls below 30 mL/min. Switching to a loop diuretic once creatinine clearance falls below 50 mL/min is recommended. Metolazone is the only thiazide-like diuretic that may produce diuresis in patients with creatinine clearances less than 20 mL/min. Indapamide may also be effective in patients with renal impairment but efficacy declines in proportion to renal function.

The use of diuretics in critically ill patients with acute renal failure has been associated with an increased risk of death and/or non-recovery of renal function. This may be a result of a direct toxic effect of diuretics on the kidney or indirect diuretic effects that may or may not be related to the kidney. Alternatively, use of diuretics in this population may delay initiation of dialysis, contributing to poorer outcomes. Prolonged use of diuretics in critically ill patients with acute renal failure is discouraged.
Dosage In Dialysis: Removal of thiazide diuretics by dialysis is negligible; however, the daily dose should be administered after dialysis.
Geriatrics: See Table 8 and Table 9.
Pediatrics: See Table 10.
Renal Impairment: See Table 11.
Hepatic Impairment: Indapamide is eliminated mainly by the liver and may therefore require dosage adjustment in hepatic impairment. The other thiazide diuretics do not undergo significant hepatic excretion. Dosage adjustment in hepatic impairment is unlikely to be necessary with these agents. However, in the presence of significant hepatic disease, use of thiazide diuretics is contraindicated due to the potential for precipitation of hepatic encephalopathy with even slight electrolyte disturbances (see Contraindications and Warnings and Precautions, Hepatic/Biliary/Pancreatic).
Administration: Oral: Time of day for optimal drug effect: Thiazides may be taken at any time of day. However, for the first week of therapy, morning administration of once daily doses may help decrease nocturnal urination. In multiple dose regimens, the last dose of the day should be taken 6 hours before bedtime. Effects on urination decrease with continued therapy and usually subside after 1-2 weeks of continuous therapy.

Timing of administration with respect to food: All thiazides may be taken with or without food. However, taking these drugs with food or milk decreases gastrointestinal side effects.

Table 6: Thiazide Diuretics

Dose of Thiazides Used in Adult Patients for Edema

Drug	Initial Dose	Titrate	Usual Dose	Maximum Dose	Detailed Information
Chlorthalidone	25–100 mg daily in 1–3 divided doses		25–100 mg daily in 1–3 divided doses	200 mg daily in 1–3 divided doses. Maximum maintenance dose: 50 mg/day	Large initial doses are given until the edema fluid is removed. After achievement of normal weight, a lower maintenance dose should be used. Administration on alternate days or 3–5 days weekly may help avoid excessive diuresis and side effects. Doses greater than 200 mg increase the severity of side effects but do not increase efficacy.
Hydrochlorothiazide	25–100 mg daily in 1–3 divided doses		25–100 mg daily in 1–3 divided doses	200 mg daily in 1–3 divided doses	In the treatment of edema, large initial doses are given until the edema fluid is removed. After several days of therapy and achievement of normal weight, a lower maintenance dose should be used. Administration on alternate days or 3–5 days weekly may help avoid excessive response and side effects in some patients. Doses greater than 200 mg increase the severity of side effects but do not increase efficacy.
Indapamide	2.5 mg once daily	Increase to 5 mg once daily after 1 wk if therapeutic effect is inadequate	2.5–5 mg daily as a single dose	5 mg daily as a single dose	Although an unapproved indication, indapamide is used for the management of edema associated with heart failure.
Metolazone			Cardiac: 5–10 mg once daily as a single dose Renal: 5–20 mg once daily as a single dose	20 mg daily as a single dose	Large initial doses are given until the edema fluid is removed. After achievement of normal weight, a lower maintenance dose should be used. Administration on alternate days or 3–5 days weekly may help avoid excessive diuresis and side effects.

Table 7: Thiazide Diuretics

Doses Used in Adults for Hypertension

Drug	Initial Dose	Titrate	Usual Dose	Maximum Dose	Detailed Information
Chlorthalidone	12.5 mg daily as a single dose	Increase by 12.5–25 mg increments every 1–2 mo according to blood pressure response.	Monotherapy: 12.5–50 mg once daily Multiple drug regimens: 12.5–25 mg once daily.	50 mg daily as a single dose. Some sources recommend 25 mg as the maximum daily dose.	Use the minimum required dose. Doses greater than 25–50 mg/day increase the severity of adverse effects without increasing therapeutic efficacy. Doses as high as 100 mg daily may rarely be useful in diuretic-resistant patients (consider risk:benefit ratio). If an adequate blood pressure response is not achieved with 25–50 mg of chlorthalidone, another antihypertensive agent from a different class should be added (see Dosing Considerations, Hypertension).
Hydrochlorothiazide	12.5 mg daily	Increase by 12.5–25 mg increments every 1–2 mo according to blood pressure response.	Monotherapy: 12.5–50 mg once daily. Multiple drug regimens: 12.5–25 mg once daily.	50 mg daily as a single dose. Some sources recommend 25 mg as the maximum daily dose.	Use the minimum required dose. Doses greater than 25–50 mg/day increase the severity of adverse effects with only a limited increase in therapeutic efficacy. Doses as high as 100 mg daily may rarely be useful in diuretic resistant patients (consider risk:benefit ratio). If an adequate blood pressure response is not achieved with 25–50 mg/day, add an antihypertensive agent from a different class (see Dosing Considerations, Hypertension).
Indapamide	1.25 mg daily as a single dose	Increase by 1.25 mg increments every 1–2 mo according to blood pressure response.	Monotherapy: 2.5 mg once daily. Multiple drug regimens: 1.25–2.5 mg once daily.	5 mg daily as a single dose. The manufacturer recommends 2.5 mg as the maximum daily dose.	Use the minimum required dose. Some sources recommend 2.5 mg as the maximum daily dose since the severity of electrolyte abnormalities is increased with higher doses. If an adequate blood pressure response is not achieved with 2.5–5 mg/day, add an antihypertensive agent from a different class (see Dosing Considerations, Hypertension).
Metolazone	2.5 mg daily as a single daily dose	Increase by 1.25–2.5 mg increments every 1–2 mo according to blood pressure response.	Monotherapy: 2.5–5 mg once daily. Multiple drug regimens: 1.25–5 mg once daily.	10 mg daily as a single dose.	Use the minimum required dose. If an adequate blood pressure response is not achieved with 5–10 mg/day, add an antihypertensive agent from a different class (see Dosing Considerations, Hypertension).

Table 8: Thiazide Diuretics

Thiazide Doses Used in Geriatric Patients for Edema

Drug	Initial Dose	Usual Dose	Maximum Dose	Detailed Information
Chlorthalidone	12.5–50 mg daily in 1–3 divided doses	25–100 mg daily in 1–3 divided doses	200 mg daily in 1–3 divided doses. Maximum maintenance dose: 50 mg/day	Large initial doses are given until the edema fluid is removed. After achievement of normal weight, a lower maintenance dose should be used. Administration on alternate days or 3–5 days weekly may help avoid excessive response and side effects. Doses greater than 200 mg/day increase the severity of side effects without increasing efficacy.
Hydrochlorothiazide	12.5–50 mg daily in 1–3 divided doses	25–100 mg daily in 1–3 divided doses	200 mg daily in 1–3 divided doses.	Large initial doses are given until the edema fluid is removed. After achievement of normal weight, a lower maintenance dose should be used. Administration on alternate days or 3–5 days weekly may help avoid excessive response and side effects. Doses greater than 200 mg/day increase the severity of side effects without increasing efficacy.
Indapamide	1.25–2.5 mg daily	2.5–5 mg daily	5 mg as a single daily dose. Some sources recommend 2.5 mg as the maximum daily dose.	Although an unapproved indication, indapamide is used for the management of edema associated with heart failure.
Metolazone	Cardiac: 2.5–5 mg once daily as a single dose. Renal: 2.5–10 mg once daily as a single dose	Cardiac: 5–10 mg once daily as a single dose. Renal: 5–20 mg once daily as a single dose	20 mg daily as a single dose.	Large initial doses are given until the edema fluid is removed. After achievement of normal weight, a lower maintenance dose should be used. Administration on alternate days or 3–5 days weekly may help avoid excessive response and side effects.

Table 9: Thiazide Diuretics

Doses Used in Geriatric Patients for Hypertension

Drug	Initial Dose	Titrate	Usual Dose	Maximum Dose	Detailed Information
Chlorthalidone	6.25–12.5 mg daily as a single dose	Increase by 6.25–12.5 mg increments every 1–2 mo according to blood pressure response.	Monotherapy: 12.5–50 mg daily as a single dose. Multiple drug regimens: 12.5–25 mg daily as a single dose	50 mg as a single daily dose. Some sources recommend 25 mg as the maximum daily dose in elderly patients.	Use the minimum required dose. Doses greater than 25–50 mg/day increase the severity of adverse effects with only a limited increase in efficacy. Doses as high as 100 mg/day daily may be useful in diuretic resistant patients (consider risk:benefit ratio). If an adequate blood pressure response is not achieved with 25–50 mg/day, add an antihypertensive agent from a different class (see Dosing Considerations, Hypertension).
Hydrochlorothiazide	6.25–12.5 mg daily as a single dose	Increase by 6.25–12.5 mg increments every 1–2 mo according to blood pressure response.	Monotherapy: 12.5–50 mg daily as a single dose. Multiple drug regimens: 12.5–25 mg once daily	50 mg once daily. Some sources recommend 25 mg as the maximum daily dose in elderly patients.	Use the minimum required dose. Doses greater than 25–50 mg/day significantly increases the severity of adverse effects with only a limited increase in efficacy. Doses as high as 100 mg/day may be useful in diuretic resistant patients (consider risk:benefit ratio). If an adequate blood pressure response is not achieved with 25–50 mg/day, add an antihypertensive agent from a different class (see Dosing Considerations, Hypertension).
Indapamide	0.625 mg once daily	Increase by 0.625–1.25 mg increments every 1–2 mo according to blood pressure response.	Monotherapy: 0.625–2.5 mg daily as a single dose. Multiple drug regimens: 0.625–2.5 mg daily as a single dose	5 mg once daily. Some sources recommend 2.5 mg daily as the maximum dose.	Use the minimum required dose. Some sources recommend 2.5 mg/day as the maximum dose due to the increased severity of electrolyte abnormalities at higher doses. As elderly patients may be more likely to experience electrolyte abnormalities related to thiazide therapy, doses greater than 2.5 mg/day should be avoided. If an adequate blood pressure response is not achieved with 2.5–5 mg/day, add an antihypertensive agent from a different class (see Dosing Considerations, Hypertension).
Metolazone	1.25 mg once daily	Increase by 1.25 mg increments every 1–2 mo according to blood pressure response.	Monotherapy: 1.25–5 mg daily as a single dose. Multiple drug regimens: 1.25–5 mg once daily	10 mg once daily.	Use the minimum required dose. If an adequate blood pressure response is not achieved with 5–10 mg/day, add an antihypertensive agent from a different class (see Dosing Considerations, Hypertension).

Table 10: Thiazide Diuretics

Dose in Pediatric Patients

Drug	Age/Weight	Usual Dose	Maximum Dose	Detailed Information
Chlorthalidone	Children	1–2 mg/kg daily as a single dose. 2 mg/kg administered as a single daily dose on 3 days each wk		Not approved for use in children.
Hydrochlorothiazide	Neonates and infants <6 mo of age	Approved dose: 2.5–3.5 mg/kg/day in 2 divided doses. Usual dose: 2–4 mg/kg/day in 2 divided doses	37.5 mg once daily	Some commercial hydrochlorothiazide solutions contain sodium benzoate, which displaces bilirubin from protein binding sites. Avoid use of these solutions in neonates.
Hydrochlorothiazide	Infants older than 6 mo of age and children under 12 y of age	Approved dose: 2.5 mg/kg/day divided into 2 doses. Usual dose: 2 mg/kg/day divided into 2 doses	Up to 2 y: 37.5 mg daily. 2–12 y: 100 mg daily.	Some commercial hydrochlorothiazide solutions contain sodium benzoate, which displaces bilirubin from protein binding sites. Avoid use of these solutions in neonates.
Metolazone	Children	0.2–0.4 mg/kg/day in 1–2 divided doses		Not approved for use in children.

Table 11: Thiazide Diuretics

Dose in Adult Patients with Renal Impairment

Drug/Indication	Creatinine Clearance	Dose Adjustment	Comment
Hydrochlorothiazide: Edema	20–50 mL/min	50–100 mg daily in 1–2 divided doses in combination with a loop diuretic	In patients with renal insufficiency, thiazides alone are ineffective. Loop diuretics should be given instead and a thiazide added if the patient does not have an adequate response to maximal doses of the loop diuretic (e.g., furosemide 240 mg). Because thiazides must reach the lumen of the nephron to be effective, higher doses are required in patients with renal insufficiency than in other patients.
Hydrochlorothiazide: Edema	10–20 mL/min	100–200 mg daily in 1–2 divided doses in combination with a loop diuretic	In patients with renal insufficiency, thiazides alone are ineffective. Loop diuretics should be given instead and a thiazide added if the patient does not have an adequate response to maximal doses of the loop diuretic (e.g., furosemide 240 mg), Because thiazides must reach the lumen of the nephron to be effective, higher doses are required in patients with renal insufficiency than in other patients.
Hydrochlorothiazide: Hypertension		Daily; titrate dose to response.	
Chlorthalidone: Hypertension	Mild–moderately impaired	Daily; titrate dose to response	
Indapamide			Indapamide is mainly metabolized by the hepatic route. However, significant renal excretion of hepatic metabolites is believed to occur. It appears that no dosage adjustment is required in renal failure but comprehensive data are lacking. Use caution when administering indapamide to patients with renal failure.
Metolazone: Hypertension		Daily; titrate dose to response	
Metolazone: Edema		If a loop diuretic is ineffective, some clinicians recommend adding metolazone 2.5–10 mg/day. The dose of metolazone is doubled every 24 h until the desired response is achieved (maximum 20 mg/day).	If synergistic diuresis occurs with the first dose of metolazone, the dose of the loop diuretic may be decreased. Hydrochlorothiazide (50 mg) may also be used and may be safer because of its shorter duration of action.

OVERDOSE:

Signs and Symptoms: Toxicity due to thiazide diuretics can occur after acute ingestion of large doses or with chronic abuse (e.g., patients with anorexia or bulimia).

Thiazide toxicity associated with acute ingestion of large doses is mainly related to fluid and electrolyte status. Symptoms usually appear approximately 2 hours after ingestion and often include a brisk diuresis, possible hypovolemia and electrolyte abnormalities. Other symptoms may include lethargy, confusion, dizziness, drowsiness, depressed respiration and coma. Muscle weakness, cramps, hypertonia and convulsions may also be evident. Hemodynamic changes secondary to plasma volume depletion may result in hypotension and syncope. Rarely, arrhythmias and noncardiogenic pulmonary edema have occurred. Hypercalcemia, hyperglycemia and temporary increases in BUN (especially in patients with renal failure) have been reported. Hemoconcentration due to fluid losses may aggravate these effects. Gastrointestinal irritation and hypermotility, usually of short duration, may occur due to osmotic effects in the gut.

It is important to note that lethargy of varying degrees can progress to coma within just a few hours even in the absence of other symptoms such as depression of respiration, depression of cardiovascular function, dehydration or serum electrolyte changes.

Recommended Management: Monitor the patient's vital signs, mental status, serum glucose, and fluid and electrolyte status. Correct any fluid or electrolyte abnormalities and provide symptomatic and supportive care. Avoid cathartics such as sorbitol, which might aggravate diuretic-induced electrolyte abnormalities.

For management of a suspected drug overdose, CPhA recommends that you contact your **regional Poison Control Centre**. See the *CPS* Directory section for a list of Poison Control Centres.

Thiopental ©

CPhA Monograph

see *Barbiturates*

Thymoglobulin® ℞

anti-thymocyte globulin (rabbit)

Immunosuppressant

Genzyme

Date of Revision: January 22, 2008

SUMMARY PRODUCT INFORMATION:

Route of Administration	Dosage Form/ Strength	Clinically Relevant Nonmedicinal Ingredients
Intravenous infusion	Lyophilized powder Thymoglobulin formulation 25 mg	Glycine, sodium chloride, D-mannitol For a complete listing see Dosage Forms, Composition and Packaging.

DESCRIPTION: Thymoglobulin (Anti-thymocyte Globulin [Rabbit]) is a purified, pasteurized, gamma immune globulin obtained by immunization of rabbits with human thymocytes. Gamma immune globulin or immunoglobulins are heavy plasma proteins, often with added sugar chains on N-terminal.

INDICATIONS AND CLINICAL USE: Thymoglobulin (Anti-thymocyte Globulin [Rabbit]) is indicated for the treatment of renal transplant acute rejection in conjunction with concomitant immunosuppression and for induction in adult renal transplant recipients.

CONTRAINDICATIONS: Thymoglobulin (Anti-thymocyte Globulin [Rabbit]) is contraindicated in patients with:
- Hypersensitivity to rabbit proteins or to any product excipients
- Active acute or chronic infections, which would contraindicate any additional immunosuppression

WARNINGS AND PRECAUTIONS:

Serious Warnings and Precautions
- Thymoglobulin (Anti-thymocyte Globulin [Rabbit]) should only be used by physicians experienced in immunosuppressive therapy for the treatment of renal transplant patients.
- In rare instances, serious immune-mediated reactions have been reported with the use of Thymoglobulin and consist of anaphylaxis or severe cytokine release syndrome (CRS) (see Immune).

Medical surveillance is required during Thymoglobulin infusion.

General: Appropriate dosing for Thymoglobulin is different from dosing for other anti-thymocyte globulin (ATG) products, as protein composition and concentrations vary depending on the source of ATG used. Physicians should therefore exercise care to ensure that the dose prescribed is appropriate for the ATG product being administered.

Thymoglobulin should be used under strict medical supervision in a hospital setting, and patients should be carefully monitored during the infusions. Close compliance with the recommended dosage and infusion time may reduce the incidence and severity of IARs. Additionally, reducing the infusion rate may minimize many of these acute infusion-associated reactions (IARs). Premedication with antipyretics, corticosteroids, and/or antihistamines may decrease both the incidence and severity of these adverse reactions.

Rapid infusion rates have been associated with case reports consistent with CRS. In rare instances, severe CRS can be fatal (see Immune).

Immune: In rare instances, serious immune-mediated reactions have been reported with the use of Thymoglobulin and consist of anaphylaxis or severe cytokine release syndrome (CRS).

Very rarely, fatal anaphylaxis has been reported (see Adverse Reactions, Post-Market Adverse Drug Reactions). If an anaphylactic reaction occurs, the infusion should be terminated immediately. Medical personnel should be available to treat patients who experience anaphylaxis. Emergency treatment such as 0.3 mL to 0.5 mL aqueous epinephrine (1:1000 dilution) subcutaneously and other resuscitative measures including oxygen, intravenous fluids, antihistamines, corticosteroids, pressor amines, and airway management, as clinically indicated, should be provided. Thymoglobulin or other rabbit immunoglobulins should not be administered again for such patients.

Severe, acute infusion-associated reactions (IARs) are consistent with CRS attributed to the release of cytokines by activated monocytes and lymphocytes. In rare instances, these reported reactions are associated with serious cardiorespiratory events and/or death (see Warnings and Precautions and Adverse Reactions, Post-Market Adverse Drug Reactions).

Thymoglobulin contains a mixture primarily of antibodies to T cell antigens, but it is largely unknown which specificities mediate the alteration in immunoregulation. Thymoglobulin may potentially contain or promote undesired or harmful antibody specificities, but which may be difficult to predict, identify or to exclude.

Live vaccines should not be administered to patients about to receive, receiving, or after treatment with Thymoglobulin. Concomitant administration of Thymoglobulin with live virus vaccines carries a potential of uncontrolled viral replication in the immunosuppressed patient. There is insufficient information to fully define the extent of the risk, or the period of time during which the risk exists. If administered, live viruses may interfere with Thymoglobulin treatment.

Skin testing is not advised prior to Thymoglobulin administration.

Infection: Thymoglobulin is routinely used in combination with other immunosuppressive agents. Infections (bacterial, fungal, viral, and protozoal), reactivation of infection (particularly cytomegalovirus [CMV]), and sepsis have been reported after Thymoglobulin administration in combination with multiple immunosuppressive agents. In rare cases, these infections have been fatal. Careful patient monitoring and appropriate anti-infective prophylaxis are recommended.

Malignancy: Use of immunosuppressive agents, including Thymoglobulin, may increase the incidence of malignancies, including lymphoma or post-transplant lymphoproliferative disease (PTLD) (see Adverse Reactions, Post-Market Adverse Drug Reactions). Appropriate antiviral, antibacterial, antiprotozoal, and/or antifungal prophylaxis is recommended.

Carcinogenesis and Mutagenesis: The carcinogenic and mutagenic potential of Thymoglobulin and its potential to impair fertility have not been studied.

Special Considerations for Thymoglobulin Infusion: As with any infusion, reactions at the infusion site can occur and may include pain, swelling, and erythema.

The recommended route of administration for Thymoglobulin is intravenous infusion using a high flow vein; however, it may be administered through a peripheral vein. When Thymoglobulin is administered through a peripheral vein, concomitant use of heparin and hydrocortisone in an infusion solution of 0.9% sodium chloride may minimize the potential for superficial thrombophlebitis and deep vein thrombosis. The combination of Thymoglobulin, heparin, and hydrocortisone in a dextrose infusion solution has been noted to precipitate and is not recommended.

Hematologic: Thrombocytopenia and/or leukopenia (including lymphopenia and neutropenia) have been identified and are reversible following dose adjustments. When thrombocytopenia and/or leukopenia are not part of the underlying disease or associated with the condition for which Thymoglobulin is being administered, the following dose reductions are suggested:
- A reduction in dosage must be considered if the platelet count is between 50 000 and 75 000 cells/mm^3 or if the white blood cell count is between 2000 and 3000 cells/mm^3;
- Stopping Thymoglobulin treatment should be considered if persistent and severe thrombocytopenia (<50 000 cells/mm^3) occurs or leukopenia (<2000 cells/mm^3) develops.

White blood cell and platelet counts should be monitored during and after Thymoglobulin therapy.

Occupational Hazards: Effects on Ability to Drive and Handle Heavy Machinery: Given the possible adverse events that can occur during the period of Thymoglobulin infusion, in particular CRS, it is recommended that patients should not drive or operate machinery during the course of Thymoglobulin therapy.

Special Populations: Pregnant Women: Females of childbearing age should be informed of the lack of information on the risks associated with the administration of Thymoglobulin during pregnancy and that adequate/appropriate contraception is recommended, during, and for a period after treatment. Therefore, Thymoglobulin should only be given to a pregnant woman if the benefits clearly outweigh the risks.

Animal reproduction studies have not been conducted with Thymoglobulin. It is also not known whether Thymoglobulin can cause fetal harm or can affect reproduction capacity.

Nursing Women: Thymoglobulin has not been studied in nursing women. It is not known whether this drug is excreted in human milk. Because other immunoglobulins are excreted in human milk, breast-feeding should be discontinued during Thymoglobulin therapy.

Pediatrics: The safety and effectiveness of Thymoglobulin in pediatric patients has not been established in controlled trials. However, the dose, efficacy, and adverse event profile are not thought to be different from adults based on limited studies undertaken in Europe and data collected in the United States.

Monitoring and Laboratory Tests: In some clinical studies, changes in lymphocyte subsets, including reversal of the CD4/CD8 ratio, have been observed for periods of up to 1 year after treatment with Thymoglobulin (the longest duration of observation in these trials). Appropriate monitoring of lymphocyte subsets is recommended.

During Thymoglobulin therapy, monitoring the lymphocyte count (i.e., total lymphocyte and/or T-cell subset) may help assess the degree of T-cell depletion (see Action and Clinical Pharmacology, Pharmacokinetics). For safety, WBC and platelet counts should also be monitored (see Dosage and Administration). Thymoglobulin contains a mixture primarily of antibodies to T cell antigens, but it is largely unknown which specificities mediate the alteration in immunoregulation.

ADVERSE REACTIONS: Adverse Drug Reaction Overview: Medical surveillance is required during Thymoglobulin infusion. See Contraindications and Warnings and Precautions sections for serious adverse drug reactions.

Thymoglobulin adverse events are generally manageable or reversible. The most frequent reported adverse events (more than 25% of patients) include: fever, chills, leukopenia, pain, headache, abdominal pain, diarrhea, hypertension, nausea, thrombocytopenia, peripheral edema, dyspnea, asthenia, hyperkalemia, tachycardia, and infection.

Serious immune-mediated reactions have been reported with the use of Thymoglobulin and consist of anaphylaxis or severe cytokine release syndrome (CRS). Fatal anaphylaxis has been reported. Severe, acute infusion-associated reactions (IARs) are consistent with CRS and can cause serious cardiorespiratory events and/or death. IARs may occur as soon as the first or second infusion during a single course of Thymoglobulin treatment. During post-marketing surveillance, fever, rash, arthralgia and/or myalgia have been reported to occur 5 to 15 days after onset of Thymoglobulin therapy, indicating possible serum sickness. These symptoms are manageable with corticosteroid treatment. Infections, reactivation of infection, sepsis, malignancies including post-transplant lymphoproliferative disorder (PTLD) and other lymphomas as well as solid tumors have been reported after Thymoglobulin administration in combination with multiple immunosuppressive agents.

Prolonged use or overdose of Thymoglobulin in association with other immunosuppressive agents may cause over-immunosuppression. During Thymoglobulin therapy, monitoring the lymphocyte count may help assess the degree of T-cell depletion. WBC and platelet counts should also be monitored (refer to Warnings and Precautions, Monitoring and Laboratory Tests).

Clinical Trial Adverse Drug Reactions: Adverse Reactions in US Phase III Study on Acute Renal Graft Rejection: Thymoglobulin (Anti-thymocyte Globulin [Rabbit]) adverse events are generally manageable or reversible. In the US Phase III controlled clinical trial (n=163) comparing the efficacy and safety of Thymoglobulin and Atgam in acute renal graft rejection, there were no significant differences in clinically significant adverse events between the two treatment groups (Table 1). Malignancies were reported in three patients who received Thymoglobulin and in three patients who received Atgam during the one-year follow-up period. These included two PTLDs in the Thymoglobulin group and two PTLDs in the Atgam group. In the Thymoglobulin group one additional patient was diagnosed with leukemia (LGL).

Table 1: Thymoglobulin

Frequently Reported and Significant Adverse Events in Patients Receiving Thymoglobulin or Atgam for Treatment of Acute Rejection[a]

Preferred Term	Thymoglobulin n=82 No. of Patients (%)	Atgam n=81 No. of Patients (%)	p-value[b]
Frequently Reported Events			
Fever	52 (63.4)	51 (63.0)	1.0
Chills	47 (57.3)	35 (43.2)	0.086
Leukopenia	47 (57.3)	24 (29.6)	<0.001
Pain	38 (46.3)	35 (43.2)	0.753
Headache	33 (40.2)	28 (34.6)	0.518
Abdominal Pain	31 (37.8)	22 (27.2)	0.181
Diarrhea	30 (36.6)	26 (32.1)	0.622
Hypertension	30 (36.6)	23 (28.4)	0.316
Nausea	30 (36.6)	23 (28.4)	0.316
Thrombocytopenia	30 (36.6)	36 (44.4)	0.341
Peripheral Edema	28 (34.1)	28 (34.6)	1.0
Dyspnea	23 (28.0)	16 (19.8)	0.271

(cont'd)

Table 1: Thymoglobulin *(cont'd)*

Frequently Reported and Significant Adverse Events in Patients Receiving Thymoglobulin or Atgam for Treatment of Acute Rejection[a]

	Thymoglobulin n=82	Atgam n=81	
Preferred Term	**No. of Patients (%)**	**No. of Patients (%)**	**p-value**[b]
Asthenia	22 (26.8)	26 (32.1)	0.495
Hyperkalemia	22 (26.8)	15 (18.5)	0.262
Tachycardia	22 (26.8)	19 (23.5)	0.719
Significant Events[c]			
Leukopenia	47 (57.3)	24 (29.6)	<0.001
Malaise	11 (13.4)	3 (3.7)	0.047
Dizziness	7 (8.5)	20 (24.7)	0.006

[a] Frequently reported adverse events are those reported by more than 25% of patients in a treatment group regardless of causality; significant adverse events are those where the incidence rate differed between treatment groups by a significance level of ≤0.05.
[b] p-value comparing treatment groups using Fisher's exact test.
[c] Statistically significant differences in adverse event incidence between treatment groups.

Infections occurring in both treatment groups during the 3-month follow-up are summarized in Table 2. No significant differences were seen between the Thymoglobulin and Atgam groups for all types of infections, and the incidence of CMV infection was equivalent in both groups. (Viral prophylaxis was by the center's discretion during antibody treatment, but all centers used gancyclovir infusion during treatment).

Table 2: Thymoglobulin

Infections in Patients Receiving Thymoglobulin or Atgam for Treatment of Acute Rejection

	Thymoglobulin n=82			Atgam n=81			
Body System Preferred Term	**No. of Patients**	**(%)**	**Total Reports**	**No. of Patients**	**(%)**	**Total Reports**	**p-value**[a]
Body as a Whole	30	(36.6)	36	22	(27.2)	29	0.240
Infection	25	(30.5)	26	19	(23.5)	21	0.378
Other	14	(17.1)	15	11	(13.6)	12	0.665
CMV	11	(13.4)	11	9	(11.1)	9	0.812
Sepsis	10	(12.2)	10	7	(9.6)	7	0.610
Moniliasis	0	(0.0)	0	1	(1.2)	1	0.497
Digestive	5	(6.1)	5	3	(3.7)	3	0.720
Gastrointestinal Moniliasis	4	(4.9)	4	1	(1.2)	1	0.367
Oral Moniliasis	3	(3.7)	0	2	(2.5)	1	0.497
Gastritis	1	(1.2)	1	0	(0.0)	0	1.000
Respiratory	0	(0.0)	0	1	(1.2)	1	0.497
Pneumonia	0	(0.0)	0	1	(1.2)	1	0.497
Skin	4	(4.9)	4	0	(0.0)	0	0.120
Herpes Simplex	4	(4.9)	4	0	(0.0)	0	0.120
Urogenital	15	(18.3)	15	22	(29.2)	22	0.195
Urinary Tract Infection	15	(18.3)	15	21	(25.9)	21	0.262
Vaginitis	0	(0.0)	0	1	(1.2)	1	0.497
Not Specified	0	(0.0)	0	2	(2.5)	2	0.245

[a] p-value comparing treatment groups using Fisher's exact test.

Adverse Reactions in US Phase II Prophylaxis Trial: In the phase II study for the prophylaxis of acute organ rejection, leukopenia (white blood cells <3000/mm³) occurred almost exclusively during the induction period and more commonly among the Thymoglobulin-treated patients (56.3%) than among the Atgam-treated patients (4.2%) (p<0.0001). Lymphopenia persisted for more than 180 days in the Thymoglobulin patients but resolved by day 14 in Atgam patients (p=0.012). Thrombocytopenia was equal between groups. An additional subset analysis of 17 Thymoglobulin-treated patients and 13 Atgam-treated patients, at 22 months, showed that the long-term CD4 counts were lower for Thymoglobulin (237/mm³ versus 466/mm³; p=0.007). The CD4/CD8 ratio showed a tendency to be lower in the Thymoglobulin group (1.6 versus 2.4; p=0.103).

Table 3: Thymoglobulin

Selected Adverse Events of Special Interest in Transplant Patients Receiving Immunosuppressive Therapy: Incidence During 1 year of Follow-up

Variable	Thymoglobulin	Atgam	p-value	Overall
Delayed Graft Function, n (%)	1 (2.1)	0	1.0	1 (1.4)
CMV Disease, n (%)	6 (12.6)	8 (33.3)	0.0560	14 (19.4)
Malignancy, n (%)	1 (2.1)	0	1.00	1 (1.4)
Leukopenia, n (%)	27 (56.3)	1 (4.2)	<0.0001	28 (38.9)
Thrombocytopenia, n (%)	5 (10.4)	2 (8.3)	1.0	7 (9.7)
Infection, n (%)	27 (56.3)	18 (75.0)	0.196	45 (62.5)
Infections per Patient				
mean±SD median (range)	1.2±1.9 1 (0–7)	1.8±1.9 1.0 (0–7)	0.149 0.162[a]	1.4±1.7 1 (0–7)
Serious Adverse Events per Patient				
mean±SD median (range)	1.2±2.3 0 (0–11)	1.8±1.5 1.0 (0–5)	0.258 0.013[a]	1.3±2.0 1 (0–11)

[a] Wilcoxon rank sums test.

Despite this, there was no difference between groups in the incidence of infections. Among recipients of Thymoglobulin, 56.3% developed infection at any time during the study, compared with 75% of Atgam recipients. The mean number of infections was 1.2±1.9 versus 1.8±1.9 for Thymoglobulin and Atgam-treated patients, respectively (p=NS). The incidence of CMV disease at 6 months was lower among Thymoglobulin-treated patients (5 of 48, 10.4%) than among those treated with Atgam (8 of 24, 33.3%) (p=0.025). Over 1 year, CMV disease tended to be less common among Thymoglobulin-treated patients than among Atgam-treated patients: 6 of 48 (12.5%) versus 8 of 24 (33.3%) (p=0.056). Calculation of the relative risk of development of CMV disease for the Thymoglobulin group compared with the Atgam group yielded a RR of 0.28 (95% CI, 0.10-0.81). This represented a 72% reduction in the incidence of CMV over the course of 1 year in recipients of Thymoglobulin. Pertinently, all CMV disease reported in this study developed after discontinuation of prophylactic oral ganciclovir.

Post-Market Adverse Drug Reactions: Infusion-Associated Reactions and Immune System Disorders: IARs may occur following the administration of Thymoglobulin and may occur as soon as the first or second infusion during a single course of Thymoglobulin treatment. Clinical manifestations of IARs have included some of the following signs and symptoms: fever, chills/rigors, dyspnea, nausea/vomiting, diarrhea, hypotension or hypertension, malaise, rash, and/or headache. IARs with Thymoglobulin are usually mild and transient and are managed with reduction in infusion rates and/or with medications (see Warnings and Precautions). Serious, and in very rare instances, fatal anaphylactic reactions have been reported (see Warnings and Precautions). The fatalities occurred in patients who did not receive epinephrine during the event.

IARs consistent with CRS have been reported (see Warnings and Precautions). Severe and potentially life threatening CRS is rarely reported. Post-marketing reports of severe CRS have been associated with cardiorespiratory dysfunction (including hypotension, acute respiratory distress syndrome [ARDS], pulmonary edema, myocardial infarction, tachycardia, and/or death).

During post-marketing surveillance, reactions such as fever, rash, arthralgia, and/or myalgia, indicating possible serum sickness, have been reported. Serum sickness tends to occur 5 to 15 days after onset of Thymoglobulin therapy. Symptoms are usually self-limited or resolve rapidly with corticosteroid treatment.

Adverse Events Due to Immunosuppression: Infections, reactivation of infection, and sepsis have been reported after Thymoglobulin administration in combination with multiple immunosuppressive agents (see Warnings and Precautions). In rare instances, malignancies including, but not limited to PTLD and other lymphomas as well as solid tumors have been reported (see Warnings and Precautions). These adverse events were always associated with a combination of multiple immunosuppressive agents.

DRUG INTERACTIONS: Overview: Because Thymoglobulin (Anti-thymocyte Globulin [Rabbit]) is administered to patients receiving a standard immunosuppressive regimen, this may predispose patients to over-immunosuppression. Many transplant centers decrease maintenance immunosuppression therapy during the period of antibody therapy.

Thymoglobulin can stimulate the production of antibodies which cross react with rabbit immune globulins (see Action and Clinical Pharmacology, Pharmacokinetics).

Pharmaceutical Incompatibilities: Based on a single compatibility study, the combination of Thymoglobulin, heparin, and hydrocortisone in a dextrose infusion solution has been noted to precipitate and is not recommended. In the absence of additional pharmaceutical incompatibility data, Thymoglobulin should not be mixed with other medicinal products in the same infusion.

Drug-Drug Interactions: No drug interaction studies have been performed.

Drug-Food Interactions: Interactions with food and drink are unlikely.

Drug-Laboratory Test Interactions: Thymoglobulin has not been shown to interfere with any routine clinical laboratory tests which do not use immunoglobulins. Thymoglobulin may interfere with rabbit antibody-based immunoassays and with cross-match or PRA cytotoxicity assays, in particular.

DOSAGE AND ADMINISTRATION: Dosing Considerations: Appropriate dosing for Thymoglobulin (Anti-thymocyte Globulin [Rabbit]) is different from dosing for other anti-thymocyte globulin (ATG) products, as protein composition and concentrations vary depending on the source of ATG used. Physicians should therefore exercise care to ensure that the dose prescribed is appropriate for the ATG product being administered.

Recommended Dose and Dosage Adjustment: The recommended dosage of Thymoglobulin for treatment of acute renal graft rejection is 1.5 mg/kg of body weight administered daily for 7 to 14 days. For prophylaxis in adult renal transplant recipients the recommended dose is 1.5 mg/kg/day intravenously for at least seven days beginning intraoperatively, through a high-flow vein. Thymoglobulin should be infused over a minimum of 6 hours for the first infusion and over at least 4 hours on subsequent days of therapy. For vial reconstitution, dilution in infusion solution and infusion procedure (see Preparation for Administration). Investigations indicate that Thymoglobulin is well tolerated and less likely to produce side effects when administered at the recommended rate. Additionally, reducing the infusion rate may minimize IARs (see Warnings and Precautions, General).

The Thymoglobulin dose should be reduced by one-half if the WBC count is between 2000 and 3000 cells/mm³ or if the platelet count is between 50 000 and 75 000 cells/mm³. Stopping Thymoglobulin treatment should be considered if the WBC counts falls below 2000 cells/mm³ or platelets below 50 000 cells/mm³.

Administration: The recommended route of administration is intravenous infusion using a high-flow vein; however, it may be administered through a peripheral vein. When Thymoglobulin is administered through a peripheral vein, concomitant use of heparin and hydrocortisone in an infusion solution of 0.9% sodium chloride may minimize the potential for superficial thrombophlebitis and deep vein thrombosis. The combination of Thymoglobulin, heparin, and hydrocortisone in a dextrose infusion solution has been noted to precipitate and is not recommended (see Drug Interactions, Pharmaceutical Incompatibilities).

Thymoglobulin should be administered through an in-line 0.22 µm filter.

Administration of antiviral prophylactic therapy is recommended. Premedication with corticosteroids, acetaminophen, and/or antihistamine one hour prior to the infusion is recommended and may reduce the incidence and intensity of side effects during the infusion (see Warnings and Precautions, General). Medical personnel should monitor patients for adverse events during and after infusion. Monitoring T-cell counts (absolute and/or subsets) to assess the level of T-cell depletion is recommended. Total white blood cell and platelet counts should be monitored.

Reconstitution: Parenteral Products:

Vial Size	Volume to be Added to Vial	Approximate Available Volume	Nominal Concentration per mL
10 mL	5 mL SWFI	5 mL	5 mg/mL (25 mg/5 mL)

Reconstituted Solutions: Reconstitution: After calculating the number of vials needed, using aseptic technique, reconstitute each vial of Thymoglobulin with 5 mL Sterile Water for Injections (SWFI), immediately before use. As Thymoglobulin contains no preservatives, reconstituted product should be used as soon as possible. Infusion solutions of Thymoglobulin must be used as soon as possible.

1. Allow Thymoglobulin vials to reach room temperature before reconstituting the lyophilized product.
2. Aseptically remove caps to expose rubber stoppers.
3. Clean stoppers with germicidal or alcohol swab.
4. Aseptically reconstitute each vial of Thymoglobulin lyophilized powder with the 5 mL of SWFI.

5. Rotate vial gently until powder is completely dissolved. Each reconstituted vial contains 25 mg or 5 mg/mL of Thymoglobulin.
6. Inspect solution for particulate matter after reconstitution. Should some particulate matter remain, continue to gently rotate the vial until no particulate matter is visible. If particulate matter persists, discard this vial.

Dilution:

1. Transfer the contents of the calculated number of Thymoglobulin vials into the bag of infusion solution (saline or dextrose). Recommended volume: per one vial of Thymoglobulin use 50 mL of infusion solution (total volume usually between 50 to 500 mL).
2. Mix the solution by inverting the bag gently only once or twice.
3. Do not mix Thymoglobulin with other solutions.

Infusion:

1. Follow the manufacturer's instructions for the infusion administration set. Infuse using a central line through a 0.22 µm filter into a high-flow vein.
2. Set the flow rate to deliver the dose over a minimum of 6 hours for the first dose and over at least 4 hours for subsequent doses.

OVERDOSAGE:

Inadvertent overdosage of Thymoglobulin may induce leukopenia (including lymphopenia and neutropenia) and thrombocytopenia, which can be managed with dose reduction (see Dosage and Administration).

> For management of a suspected drug overdose, CPhA recommends that you contact your **regional Poison Control Centre**. See the *CPS* Directory section for a list of Poison Control Centres.

ACTION AND CLINICAL PHARMACOLOGY: Mechanism of Action: The in vitro mechanism of action by which polyclonal antilymphocyte preparations suppress immune responses is not fully understood. Thymoglobulin (Anti-thymocyte Globulin [Rabbit]) includes antibodies against T cell markers such as CD2, CD3, CD4, CD8, CD11a, CD18, CD 44, CD45, HLA-DR, HLA Class I heavy chains, and β2 microglobulin. In vitro Thymoglobulin (concentrations >0.1 mg/mL) mediates T cell suppressive effects via inhibition of proliferative responses to several mitogens. In patients, T cell depletion is usually observed within a day from initiating Thymoglobulin therapy. Thymoglobulin has not been shown to be effective for treating antibody (humoral) mediated rejections.

The in vivo mechanism of action of Thymoglobulin, is also not fully understood. The possible mechanisms by which Thymoglobulin may induce immunosuppression in vivo include the following:

i. T cell clearance from the circulation.
ii. Modulation of T cell activation, homing and cytotoxic activities.

Following clinical administration of Thymoglobulin, T cell depletion is promptly observed. This may result from the complement-dependent lysis in the intravascular space or the opsonization and subsequent phagocytosis by macrophages. When Thymoglobulin is given with other immunosuppressive therapies, such as corticosteroids, azathioprine, cyclosporine, etc., there is a decrease in the patient's own antibody formation. Monitoring Thymoglobulin therapy reveals that T cell depletion in peripheral blood persists for several days to several weeks following cessation of Thymoglobulin therapy.

Thymoglobulin is a potent immunosuppressive agent that demonstrates a rapid and profound pharmacodynamic effect resulting in lower white blood cell, T cell and T cell subset counts. The magnitude and duration of lymphopenia is consistent; reductions of 83% to 92% from pre-treatment values were seen after a single dose of Thymoglobulin and were sustained throughout the daily dosing period in four clinical pharmacology studies. Recovery from treatment-induced lymphocyte depletion was gradual, beginning two months after initiation of therapy, with most recovery by three months, but was not seen in all cases even at six months. T cell subsets determined by flow cytometry also demonstrate similar dramatic decreases.

Pharmacodynamics: The pharmacodynamic effects of Thymoglobulin were assessed in the measurements of total lymphocytes and of lymphocyte subpopulations. Total lymphocyte values were used to assess the degree, time to induction, and duration of lymphopenia. Also assessed was the degree of lymphopenia in absolute values and percentages of lymphocyte subsets with phenotypes CD2 (T cells, sheep erythrocyte receptor), CD3 (T lymphocytes), CD4 (T cells, helper-inducer subset), CD8 (T cells, cytotoxic/suppressor subset), CD14 (monocytes), CD19 (B lymphocytes), CD25 (activated T and B lymphocytes and activated macrophages), CD56 (NK cells), and CD57 (NK cells). The pharmacodynamic effect of Thymoglobulin was demonstrated by a marked decrease in lymphocyte counts as well as nearly all subsets.

Pharmacokinetics: After an intravenous dose of 1.25 to 1.5 mg/kg/day, (over 4 hours for 7-11 days) 4-8 hours post-infusion. Thymoglobulin (Anti-thymocyte Globulin [Rabbit]) levels were on average 21.5 µg/mL (10-40 µg/mL) with a half-life of 2-3 days after the first dose, and 87 µg/mL (23-170 µg/mL) after the last dose. Rare allergic reactions such as serum sickness (fever, pruritus, rash associated with arthralgia, myalgia) may occur seven to fifteen days after onset of treatment. Immediate serious allergic reactions are rare. The most frequent, as well as the most severe adverse reactions, occur following the first infusion. The mechanism of some of these adverse reactions is more likely related to a cytokine release. Premedication with corticosteroids and antihistamines decreases both incidence and severity of these adverse reactions. Reducing the infusion rate may lead to a reduction of some of these adverse reactions.

During the Thymoglobulin Phase III randomized trial, of the 108 of 163 patients evaluated, no difference was seen in sensitization level to horse IgG after Atgam (lymphocyte immune globulin anti-thymocyte [equine] sterile solution) treatment (78.5%) or to rabbit IgG after Thymoglobulin treatment (69%) (p=0.4).

In a Phase II randomized trial for the prophylaxis of rejection, the assays used indicated that 6 of 48 (12%) of those receiving Thymoglobulin versus 1 of 25 (4%) of those receiving Atgam had detectable antibody to rabbit or horse immunoglobulin, respectively, prior to initiation of the study (p=0.412). The incidence of new onset sensitization was lower with Thymoglobulin than with Atgam when presensitized patients were excluded from the analysis (43% versus 78%; p=0.22). Including presensitized patients, fewer Thymoglobulin patients than Atgam patients had evidence of sensitization (51% versus 81%; p=0.031). In neither group did the presence of preformed antibody correlate with serious adverse events or effectiveness of therapy. No controlled studies have been conducted to study the effect of anti-rabbit antibodies on repeat use of Thymoglobulin. However, monitoring the lymphocyte count to ensure that T-cell depletion is achieved upon re-treatment with Thymoglobulin is recommended.

STORAGE AND STABILITY:

- Store in refrigerator between +2 and +8°C. A higher temperature of ≤37°C during transport for a total excursion time of ≤10 days will do the product no harm.
- Protect from light.
- Do not freeze.
- Do not use after the expiration dated indicated on the label.
- Any unused drug remaining after infusion must be discarded.

INFORMATION FOR THE PATIENT: Published in e-CPS, available by subscription at www.e-cps.ca.

DOSAGE FORMS, COMPOSITION AND PACKAGING: Each vial of sterile, lyophilized powder to be reconstituted with Sterile Water for Injections, EP, contains: anti-thymocyte globulin (rabbit) 25 mg. Nonmedicinal ingredients: glycine, D-mannitol and sodium chloride. Each package contains one 10 mL vial.

The reconstituted preparation contains approximately 5 mg/mL of Thymoglobulin of which >95% is rabbit gamma immune globulin (IgG). The reconstituted solution has a pH of 7.0±0.4. Human red blood cells are used in the manufacturing process to deplete cross-reactive antibodies to non T-cell antigens. The manufacturing process is validated to remove or inactivate potential exogenous viruses. All human red blood cells are from US registered or FDA licensed blood banks. A viral inactivation step (pasteurization, i.e., heat treatment of active ingredient at 60°C/10 hours) is performed for each lot.

This immunosuppressive product contains cytotoxic antibodies directed against antigens expressed on human T lymphocytes. Thymoglobulin is a sterile freeze-dried product for intravenous administration after reconstitution with Sterile Water for Injections, EP (SWFI).

Thyrogen® Ⓟ

thyrotropin alfa

Human Thyroid Stimulating Hormone

Genzyme

Date of Preparation: September 8, 2004
Date of Revision: August 28, 2009

SUMMARY PRODUCT INFORMATION:

Route of Administration	Dosage Form/ Strength	Clinically Relevant Nonmedicinal Ingredients
Intramuscular injection in the gluteal muscle	Lyophilized powder/0.9 mg/mL[a]	There are no clinically relevant nonmedicinal ingredients. Nonmedicinal ingredients: mannitol, sodium phosphate monobasic monohydrate, sodium phosphate dibasic heptahydrate, sodium chloride, nitrogen, sterile water for injection

[a] THYROGEN is supplied as a sterile lyophilized powder for reconstitution in a clear 5.0 mL Type I flint tubing vial; gray 20 mm siliconized butyl stopper; 20 mm aluminum 6 bridge seal with a plastic flip off cap dimethicone siliconizing agent.

INDICATIONS AND CLINICAL USE: THYROGEN (thyrotropin alfa for injection) is indicated for:

- use as an adjunctive treatment as pre-therapeutic stimulation for radioiodine ablation of thyroid tissue remnants in patients maintained on thyroid hormone suppression therapy who have undergone a near-total or total thyroidectomy for well-differentiated thyroid cancer without evidence of distant metastatic thyroid cancer.
- use as an adjunctive diagnostic tool for serum thyroglobulin (Tg) testing, with or without radioiodine imaging, in the follow-up of patients with well-differentiated thyroid cancer.

Potential Clinical Uses:

1. THYROGEN treatment may be used in combination with radioiodine (^{131}I) to ablate thyroid remnants following near-total or total thyroidectomy in patients without evidence of distant metastatic thyroid cancer.
2. THYROGEN Tg testing may be used in patients with an undetectable Tg on thyroid hormone suppressive therapy, to exclude the diagnosis of residual or recurrent thyroid cancer.
3. THYROGEN testing may be used in patients requiring serum Tg testing and radioiodine imaging, who are unwilling to undergo thyroid hormone withdrawal testing.
4. THYROGEN treatment and testing may be used in patients who are either unable to mount an adequate endogenous TSH response to thyroid hormone withdrawal or in whom withdrawal is medically contraindicated.

Considerations in the Use of THYROGEN:

1. Clinicians employ a wide range of ^{131}I activities to achieve remnant ablation. Published studies of the use of THYROGEN to achieve remnant ablation have used ^{131}I activities of 30 mCi to 110 mCi and the Genzyme study employed 100 mCi±10% in all patients. Multiple factors contribute to the decision about the activity of ^{131}I that should be administered for a given patient, such as the size of the remnant tissue (a function of aggressiveness of the surgical resection), and the perceived risk of the patient for thyroid cancer recurrence (a function of patient age, primary tumour type and size, extent of disease). Activities of ^{131}I in the 100 mCi range or above achieve remnant ablation more frequently than do lower activities, but may be associated more often with complications of ^{131}I treatment, such as salivary gland pain and swelling, persistent dry mouth, dry eyes or altered taste. Data are inadequate to determine if a lower dose of radioiodine would be effective when THYROGEN is used as an adjunct to radioiodine in postsurgical thyroid remnant ablation. There is evidence from the literature of lower efficacy of THYROGEN administration compared with withdrawal of THST when using 30 mCi. Therefore, efficacy of THYROGEN with doses of ^{131}I outside the range of 100 mCi±10% has not been established for ablation.
2. **Even when THYROGEN-stimulated Tg testing is performed in combination with radioiodine imaging, there remains a risk of missing a diagnosis of thyroid cancer or of underestimating the extent of disease. Therefore, thyroid hormone withdrawal Tg testing with radioiodine imaging continues to be the standard diagnostic modality to assess the presence, location and extent of thyroid cancer.**
3. Although THYROGEN appeared noninferior to thyroid hormone withholding, based on <0.1% uptake of radioactive tracer within the thyroid bed at 24 hours in a study of postsurgical thyroid remnant ablation, long-term clinical outcome data are limited. Due to the relatively small clinical experience with THYROGEN in remnant ablation, it is not possible to conclude whether long-term thyroid cancer outcomes would be equivalent after use of THYROGEN or use of thyroid hormone withholding for TSH elevation prior to remnant ablation.
4. THYROGEN Tg levels are generally lower than Tg levels after thyroid hormone withdrawal. The extent to which THYROGEN Tg levels correlate with Tg levels after thyroid hormone withdrawal has not been adequately studied.
5. A newly detectable Tg level or a Tg level rising over time after THYROGEN, or a high index of suspicion of metastatic disease, even in the setting of a negative or low-stage THYROGEN radioiodine scan, should prompt further evaluation such as thyroid hormone withdrawal to definitively establish the location and extent of thyroid cancer. On the other hand, none of the 31 patients studied with undetectable THYROGEN Tg levels (<2.5 ng/mL) had metastatic disease. Therefore, an undetectable THYROGEN Tg level suggests the absence of clinically significant disease.
6. The decisions whether to perform a THYROGEN radioiodine scan in conjunction with a THYROGEN serum Tg test and whether and when to withdraw a patient from thyroid hormone are complex. Pertinent factors in these decisions include the sensitivity of the Tg assay used, the THYROGEN Tg level obtained, and the index of suspicion of recurrent or persistent local or metastatic disease. In the clinical trials combination Tg and scan testing did enhance the diagnostic accuracy of THYROGEN in some cases.
7. The signs and symptoms of hypothyroidism which accompany thyroid hormone withdrawal are avoided with THYROGEN.

CONTRAINDICATIONS: Patients who are hypersensitive to THYROGEN (thyrotropin alfa for injection) or to any ingredient in the formulation or component of the container (see Warnings and Precautions, General). For a complete listing of ingredients in the formulation and components of the container, refer to the table in Summary Product Information.

WARNINGS AND PRECAUTIONS:

> **Serious Warnings and Precautions**
> - THYROGEN (thyrotropin alfa for injection) should be administered intramuscularly only. It should not be administered intravenously (see Warnings and Precautions, General).

General: Intravenous use has caused rapid onset of: severe nausea, vomiting, diaphoresis, hypotension and tachycardia. This occurred in one patient enrolled in a clinical trial who received 0.3 mg of THYROGEN as a single IV bolus, experienced severe nausea, vomiting, diaphoresis, hypotension (BP decreased from 115/66 mmHg to 81/44 mmHg) and tachycardia (pulse increased from 75 to 117 bpm) 15 minutes after injection.

THYROGEN injections should be supervised by a healthcare professional knowledgeable in the management of thyroid cancer. THYROGEN should only be administered intramuscularly in the gluteal muscle. It should not be administered intravenously.

Caution should be exercised when THYROGEN is administered to patients who have been previously treated with bovine thyroid stimulating hormone. In particular, patients who have experienced hypersensitivity reactions to bovine or human TSH may be at a greater risk for developing hypersensitivity reactions to THYROGEN, and appropriate precautions should be undertaken.

The combination of WBS (Whole Body Scan) and Tg testing after THYROGEN administration improves sensitivity for detection of thyroid remnants of cancer over either alone.

Due to elevation of TSH levels after THYROGEN administration (0.9 mg×2), thyroid cancer patients with metastatic disease, particularly in confined spaces (for example, brain, spinal cord, orbit or soft tissues of the neck) may be subject to local edema or focal hemorrhage at the site of these metastases. Enlargement of residual thyroid tissue or metastases can also occur, which may lead to acute symptoms depending on the anatomical location of the tissue. It is recommended that pre-treatment with glucocorticoids be considered for patients in whom local tumour expansion may compromise vital anatomic structures (such as trachea, central nervous system, or extensive macroscopic lung metastases) prior to the administration of THYROGEN (see Adverse Reactions).

THYROGEN adjunctive treatment for radioiodine ablation of thyroid tissue remnants after near-total or total thyroidectomy should not be used in patients with distant metastatic thyroid cancer.

Careful evaluation of benefit risk relationships should be assessed for high risk elderly patients with functioning thyroid tumours undergoing THYROGEN administration. This may result in palpitations or cardiac rhythm disorder (see Adverse Reactions).

Elimination of THYROGEN is significantly slower in dialysis-dependent end-stage renal disease (ESRD) patients, resulting in prolonged elevation of TSH levels (see Adverse Reactions).

In post-marketing experience, there have been rare reports of events leading to death that occurred within 24 hours of administration of THYROGEN in patients with multiple serious medical problems. For patients for whom THYROGEN-induced hyperthyroidism could have serious consequences, hospitalization for administration of THYROGEN and post-administration observation should be considered. Such patients might include those with known heart disease, extensive metastatic disease, or other known serious underlying illness.

Interpretation of Results: As with other diagnostic modalities, false negative results may occur with THYROGEN. If a high index of suspicion for metastatic disease persists, confirmatory WBS and Tg testing should be considered following thyroid hormone withdrawal.

Thyroglobulin (Tg) antibodies may confound the Tg assay and render Tg levels uninterpretable. Therefore, in such cases, even with a negative or low-stage THYROGEN radioiodine scan, consideration should be given to evaluating patients further with, for example, a confirmatory thyroid hormone withdrawal scan to determine the location and extent of thyroid cancer.

TSH antibodies have not been reported in patients treated to date. However, exposure has been limited to 27 patients who received THYROGEN in the clinical trials on more than one occasion and remained antibody negative. There have been several reports of hypersensitivity consisting of urticaria, rash, pruritus, flushing and respiratory signs and symptoms (see Adverse Reactions).

Carcinogenesis and Mutagenesis: Long-term toxicity studies in animals have not been performed with THYROGEN to evaluate the carcinogenic potential of the drug. THYROGEN was not mutagenic in the bacterial reverse mutation assay.

Cardiovascular: Three patients enrolled in clinical trials and/or the Compassionate Use Program developed thromboembolism. Amongst 152 patients in the diagnostic study TSH92-0601, one patient with extensive metastases had a fatal Pulmonary Embolism 8 days after receiving THYROGEN. Amongst 115 advanced cancer patients treated in the Compassionate Use Program, 2 had Deep Vein Thrombosis (DVT) AEs.

There are several reports in the post-marketing database of DVT and/or Pulmonary Embolism in patients who received THYROGEN. One patient was on concomitant oral contraceptive therapy, and the other patients had prolonged hospitalization and/or extensive metastatic disease prior to the thromboembolic event.

Caution should be exercised when administering THYROGEN to patients with a known history of heart disease and with significant residual thyroid tissue. THYROGEN is known to stimulate residual thyroid tissue to produce a transient but significant rise in serum thyroid hormone concentration when given to patients who have substantial thyroid tissue still in situ. Elevations in thyroid hormone levels may exacerbate underlying heart disease. When appropriate, physicians should undertake precautionary measures to prevent or mitigate hyperthyroidism, monitor patients for evidence of worsening heart disease, and treat signs and symptoms of hyperthyroidism and worsening heart disease.

Careful evaluation of benefit-risk with THYROGEN treatment should be assessed for high-risk elderly patients with heart disease (e.g., valvular heart disease, cardiomyopathy, coronary artery disease, and prior or current tachyarrhythmia).

See also: Overdosage.

Dependence/Tolerance: No studies have been conducted.

Ear/Nose/Throat: Not applicable.

Endocrine and Metabolism: Careful evaluation of benefit-risk relationships should be assessed for THYROGEN administration in high-risk elderly patients who have not yet undergone thyroidectomy.

Gastrointestinal: Not applicable.

Genitourinary: Not applicable.

Hematologic: Three patients enrolled in clinical trials and/or the Compassionate Use Program developed thromboembolism. Amongst 152 patients in the diagnostic study TSH92-0601, one patient with extensive metastases had a fatal Pulmonary Embolism 8 days after receiving THYROGEN. Amongst 115 advanced cancer patients treated in the Compassionate Use Program, 2 had Deep Vein Thrombosis (DVT) AEs.

There are several reports in the post-marketing database of DVT and/or Pulmonary Embolism in patients who received THYROGEN. One patient was on concomitant oral contraceptive therapy, and the other patients had prolonged hospitalization and/or extensive metastatic disease prior to the thromboembolic event.

Hepatic/Biliary/Pancreatic: The organ(s) of rhTSH clearance in humans have not been identified, but preclinical studies suggest the involvement of the liver and kidneys.

Immune: TSH antibodies have not been reported in patients treated with THYROGEN in the clinical trials, although only 27 patients who received THYROGEN treatment more than once underwent testing for the development of TSH antibodies. The occurrence of antibodies which could interfere with endogenous TSH assays cannot be excluded.

Neurologic: 4/55 patients [7.3%] with CNS metastases experienced acute hemiplegia, hemiparesis, pain or loss of vision within 72 hours of THYROGEN administration.

Ophthalmologic: See Neurologic.

Peri-Operative Considerations: Not applicable.

Psychiatric: Not applicable.

Renal: The organ(s) of rhTSH clearance in humans have not been identified, but preclinical studies suggest the involvement of the liver and kidneys.

Elimination of THYROGEN is significantly slower in dialysis-dependent end-stage renal disease (ESRD) patients, resulting in prolonged elevation of TSH levels (see Adverse Reactions).

Respiratory: Laryngeal oedema, pain at the site of metastases and respiratory distress requiring tracheotomy have occurred. Sudden rapid and painful enlargement of locally recurring papillary carcinoma has been reported 12-48 hours after THYROGEN administration. The enlargement was accompanied by dyspnoea, stridor or dysphonia. Rapid clinical improvement occurred following glucocorticoid therapy.

Sensitivity/Resistance: There have been several reports of hypersensitivity reactions (including urticaria, rash, pruritus, flushing and respiratory symptoms) requiring urgent treatment.

Sexual Function/Reproduction: Studies have not been conducted.

See also: Pregnant Women and Nursing Women.

Skin: See Sensitivity/Resistance.

Effects on Ability to Drive and Handle Heavy Machinery: Studies have not been conducted.

Special Populations: Effect on Tumour Growth: In patients with thyroid cancer, several cases of stimulated tumour growth have been reported during withdrawal of thyroid hormones for diagnostic procedures due to the subsequent prolonged elevation of thyroid stimulating hormone (TSH) levels.

There is a theoretical possibility that THYROGEN, like thyroid hormone withdrawal, may lead to stimulated tumour growth. In clinical trials with thyrotropin alfa, which produces a short-term increase in TSH levels, no case of tumour growth has been reported.

However, due to elevation of TSH levels after THYROGEN administration, thyroid cancer patients with metastatic disease, particularly in confined spaces (for example, brain, spinal cord, orbit or soft tissues of the neck) may be subject to local edema or focal hemorrhage at the site of these metastases. It is recommended that pre-treatment with corticosteroids be considered in these patients in whom local tumour expansion may compromise vital anatomic structures prior to the administration of THYROGEN.

Pregnant Women: No experience. Animal reproductive studies and studies to evaluate the effects on fertility have not been conducted with THYROGEN. It is also not known whether THYROGEN can cause fetal harm when administered to a pregnant woman or can affect reproductive capacity. THYROGEN should be used in pregnancy only if the benefit outweighs the risks. THYROGEN in combination with diagnostic radioiodine whole body scintigraphy is contraindicated in pregnancy, because of the consequent exposure of the foetus to a high dose of radioactive material.

Nursing Women: It is not known whether the drug is excreted in human milk. Because many drugs are excreted in human milk, caution should be exercised when THYROGEN is administered to a nursing woman. Patients should not breast-feed.

Pediatrics (<18 years of age): Safety and effectiveness in patients below the age of 18 years have not been established.

Geriatrics (>65 years of age): Results from controlled trials indicate no difference in the safety and efficacy of THYROGEN between adult patients less than 65 years and those greater than 65 years of age.

Careful evaluation of benefit risk relationships should be assessed for high risk elderly patients with functioning thyroid tumours and/or patients with heart disease (i.e. valvular heart disease, cardiomyopathy, coronary artery disease, and prior or current tachyarrhythmia) undergoing THYROGEN administration.

Monitoring and Laboratory Tests: Measurement of serum TSH 72 hours following the second dose of THYROGEN may show levels below the 25 mU/L normally observed in hypothyroid patients. In pharmacokinetic studies, peak serum TSH levels of 116±38 mU/L were reached between 3 and 24 hours following a single dose of THYROGEN (see Action and Clinical Pharmacology, Pharmacokinetics). THYROGEN has an elimination half-life of 25±10 hours, therefore, several days after the second dose of THYROGEN, the serum TSH levels can fall to levels below those normally observed in hypothyroid cancer patients.

In clinical trials, the reference standard for determining whether patients had thyroid remnant or cancer present was a hypothyroid Tg ≥2 ng/mL and/or a hypothyroid scan (either diagnostic or post-therapy). This analysis evaluated whether Tg testing after THYROGEN administration improved the diagnostic sensitivity of a Tg test in patients with a negative Tg on THST using a cut-off of 2 ng/mL. It should be noted that THYROGEN Tg levels are generally lower than hypothyroid Tg levels and thus physicians may need to use a lower Tg cut-off level when using THYROGEN than would be used with a hypothyroid Tg.

ADVERSE REACTIONS: Adverse Drug Reaction Overview: Adverse reaction data were derived from post-marketing surveillance and clinical trials. Table 1 represents adverse reactions experienced by 62 thyroid cancer patients who participated in the clinical trials for THYROGEN supporting the ablation indication (THYR-008-00 and THYR01605). Table 2 represents adverse reactions experienced by 381 thyroid cancer patients who participated in the clinical trials for THYROGEN supporting the diagnostic indication (TSH92-0601 and TSH95-0101).

Clinical Trial Adverse Drug Reactions: Because clinical trials are conducted under very specific conditions the adverse reaction rates observed in the clinical trials may not reflect the rates observed in practice and should not be compared to the rates in the clinical trials of another drug. Adverse drug reaction information from clinical trials is useful for identifying drug-related adverse events and for approximating rates.

Remnant Ablation Indication: Adverse reaction data for the remnant ablation indication are derived from 62 patients who received THYROGEN as adjunctive treatment for radioiodine ablation of thyroid tissue remnants in THYR-008-00 and follow-up study THYR01605.

In the THYR-008-00 study, patients were randomized to either the hypothyroid or euthyroid group after thyroidectomy. Patients randomised to the Euthyroid group received 0.9 mg THYROGEN IM once a day for 2 days prior to an ablative activity of ^{131}I (100 mCi±10%; 3.7 GBq) administered on the following day. Patients randomised to the Hypothyroid Group did not receive THYROGEN prior to ablation. An ablative activity of ^{131}I (100 mCi±10%; 3.7 GBq) was administered. Eight (±1) months later, patients in both groups were administered THYROGEN 0.9 mg IM once a day × 2 days for diagnostic purposes. Adverse events were collected in the Euthyroid group for the entire 8 month period including 5 days after the diagnostic dose of THYROGEN. The THYR01605 study was a follow-up study performed on a subset of patients from the THYR-008-00 study, with a median follow-up of 3.7 years (range 3.4-4.4 years) following radioiodine ablation. Therefore, the study has limited long-term safety data.

Very common adverse events (≥10%) reported in the THYR-008-00 clinical trial were insomnia (15.2%), nausea (12.1%), fatigue (12.1%), nasopharyngitis (12.1%) and anxiety (12.1%). All adverse events reported in the THYR01605 trial occurred in only one patient. The frequency of these adverse events was 3.7%. Events reported in patients in the trials are summarized in Table 1.

Table 1: THYROGEN

Summary of Treatment-Emergent Adverse Events by Euthyroid Group and Hypothyroid Group Occurring in Patients During the THYR-008-00 and THYR01605 Studies

	THYR-008-00						THYR01605					
	Euthyroid Group 33 Patients			Hypothyroid Group 29 Patients[a]			Former Euthyroid Group 27 Patients			Former Hypothyroid Group 21 Patients		
	AEs	Pts	(%)	AEs	Pts	(%)	AEs	Pts	(%)	AEs	Pts	(%)
Total AEs/ Patients with AEs	130	26	(78.8)	17	11	(37.9)	12	6	(22.2)	4	2	(9.5)
Blood and Lymphatic System Disorders	1	1	(3.0)	0	0	0	0	0	0	0	0	0
Lymphadenopathy	1	1	(3.0)	0	0	0	0	0	0	0	0	0
Cardiac Disorders	2	2	(6.1)	0	0	0	0	0	0	0	0	0
Palpitations	2	2	(6.1)	0	0	0	0	0	0	0	0	0
Ear and Labyrinth Disorders	1	1	(3.0)	0	0	0	0	0	0	0	0	0
Tinnitus	1	1	(3.0)	0	0	0	0	0	0	0	0	0
Gastrointestinal Disorders	18	11	(33.3)	2	2	(6.9)	2	2	(7.4)	2	1	(4.8)
Nausea	7	4	(12.1)	1	1	(3.4)	1	1	(3.7)	1	1	(4.8)
Diarrhoea	2	2	(6.1)	0	0	0	0	0	0	1	1	(4.8)
Dry mouth	2	2	(6.1)	0	0	0	0	0	0	0	0	0
Vomiting	0	0	0	0	0	0	1	1	(3.7)	0	0	0
Chapped lips	0	0	0	1	1	(3.4)	0	0	0	0	0	0
Constipation	1	1	(3.0)	0	0	0	0	0	0	0	0	0
Dysphagia	1	1	(3.0)	0	0	0	0	0	0	0	0	0
Haemorrhoids	1	1	(3.0)	0	0	0	0	0	0	0	0	0
Pancreatitis	1	1	(3.0)	0	0	0	0	0	0	0	0	0
Peptic ulcer	1	1	(3.0)	0	0	0	0	0	0	0	0	0
Salivary gland disorder	1	1	(3.0)	0	0	0	0	0	0	0	0	0
Salivary gland enlargement	1	1	(3.0)	0	0	0	0	0	0	0	0	0
General Disorders and Administration Site Conditions	17	8	(24.2)	3	3	(10.3)	0	0	0	1	1	(4.8)
Fatigue	4	4	(12.1)	1	1	(3.4)	0	0	0	0	0	0
Malaise	3	3	(9.1)	0	0	0	0	0	0	0	0	0
Asthenia	3	2	(6.1)	0	0	0	0	0	0	1	1	(4.8)
Temperature intolerance	1	1	(3.0)	1	1	(3.4)	0	0	0	0	0	0
Swelling	0	0	0	1	1	(3.4)	0	0	0	0	0	0
Peripheral coldness	2	1	(3.0)	0	0	0	0	0	0	0	0	0
Feeling cold	1	1	(3.0)	0	0	0	0	0	0	0	0	0

(cont'd)

Table 1: THYROGEN *(cont'd)*

Summary of Treatment-Emergent Adverse Events by Euthyroid Group and Hypothyroid Group Occurring in Patients During the THYR-008-00 and THYR01605 Studies

	THYR-008-00						THYR01605					
	Euthyroid Group 33 Patients			Hypothyroid Group 29 Patients[a]			Former Euthyroid Group 27 Patients			Former Hypothyroid Group 21 Patients		
	AEs	Pts	(%)	AEs	Pts	(%)	AEs	Pts	(%)	AEs	Pts	(%)
Feeling hot	1	1	(3.0)	0	0	0	0	0	0	0	0	0
Injection site warmth	1	1	(3.0)	0	0	0	0	0	0	0	0	0
Irritability	1	1	(3.0)	00	0	0	0	0	0	0	0	0
Hepatobiliary Disorders	1	1	(3.0)	0	0	0	0	0	0	0	0	0
Cholelithiasis	1	1	(3.0)	0	0	0	0	0	0	0	0	0
Immune System Disorders	1	1	(3.0)	0	0	0	0	0	0	0	0	0
Multiple allergies	1	1	(3.0)	0	0	0	0	0	0	0	0	0
Infections and Infestations	12	11	(33.3)	0	0	0	0	0	0	0	0	0
Nasopharyngitis	4	4	(12.1)	0	0	0	0	0	0	0	0	0
Urinary tract infection	3	3	(9.1)	0	0	0	0	0	0	0	0	0
Cellulitis	1	1	(3.0)	0	0	0	0	0	0	0	0	0
Ear infection	1	1	(3.0)	0	0	0	0	0	0	0	0	0
Lower respiratory tract infection	1	1	(3.0)	0	0	0	0	0	0	0	0	0
Pharyngitis	1	1	(3.0)	0	0	0	0	0	0	0	0	0
Sinusitis	1	1	(3.0)	0	0	0	0	0	0	0	0	0
Injury, Poisoning and Procedural Complications	1	1	(3.0)	0	0	0	0	0	0	0	0	0
Procedural pain	1	1	(3.0)	0	0	0	0	0	0	0	0	0
Investigations	2	2	(6.1)	5	5	(17.2)	0	0	0	0	0	0
Thyroglobulin present	2	2	(6.1)	3	3	(10.3)	0	0	0	0	0	0
Hepatic enzyme increased	0	0	0	1	1	(3.4)	0	0	0	0	0	0
Thyroglobulin increased	0	0	0	1	1	(3.4)	0	0	0	0	0	0
Metabolism and Nutrition Disorders	1	1	(3.0)	0	0	0	0	0	0	0	0	0
Appetite disorder	1	1	(3.0)	0	0	0	0	0	0	0	0	0
Musculoskeletal and Connective Tissue Disorders	20	13	(39.4)	4	3	(10.3)	1	1	(3.7)	0	0	0
Back pain	3	3	(9.1)	0	0	0	0	0	0	0	0	0
Shoulder pain	3	3	(9.1)	0	0	0	0	0	0	0	0	0
Arthralgia	3	2	(6.1)	1	1	(3.4)	0	0	0	0	0	0
Neck pain	2	2	(6.1)	1	1	(3.4)	0	0	0	0	0	0
Musculoskeletal stiffness	2	2	(6.1)	0	0	0	0	0	0	0	0	0
Pain in extremity	4	2	(6.1)	0	0	0	0	0	0	0	0	0
Muscle spasms	1	1	(3.0)	1	1	(3.4)	1	1	(3.7)	0	0	0
Bone pain	0	0	0	1	1	(3.4)	0	0	0	0	0	0
Muscle tightness	1	1	(3.0)	0	0	0	0	0	0	0	0	0
Sensation of heaviness	1	1	(3.0)	0	0	0	0	0	0	0	0	0
Nervous System Disorders	15	8	(24.2)	3	1	(3.4)	4	3	(11.1)	1	1	(4.8)
Headache	3	3	(9.1)	0	0	0	1	1	(3.7)	0	0	0
Paraesthesia	5	3	(9.1)	1	1	(3.4)	0	0	0	0	0	0
Ageusia	3	2	(6.1)	0	0	0	0	0	0	0	0	0
Hypoaesthesia	2	2	(6.1)	0	0	0	0	0	0	0	0	0

(cont'd)

Table 1: THYROGEN *(cont'd)*

Summary of Treatment-Emergent Adverse Events by Euthyroid Group and Hypothyroid Group Occurring in Patients During the THYR-008-00 and THYR01605 Studies

	THYR-008-00						THYR01605					
	Euthyroid Group 33 Patients			Hypothyroid Group 29 Patients[a]			Former Euthyroid Group 27 Patients			Former Hypothyroid Group 21 Patients		
	AEs	Pts	(%)	AEs	Pts	(%)	AEs	Pts	(%)	AEs	Pts	(%)
Dizziness	0	0	0	0	0	0	1	1	(3.7)	1	1	(4.8)
Disturbance in attention	0	0	0	0	0	0	1	1	(3.7)	0	0	0
Syncope	0	0	0	0	0	0	1	1	(3.7)	0	0	0
Tremor	1	1	(3.0)	1	1	(3.4)	0	0	0	0	0	0
Memory impairment	0	0	0	1	1	(3.4)	0	0	0	0	0	0
Migraine	1	1	(3.0)	0	0	0	0	0	0	0	0	0
Psychiatric Disorders	12	11	(33.3)	0	0	0	1	1	(3.7)	0	0	0
Insomnia	5	5	(15.2)	0	0	0	1	1	(3.7)	0	0	0
Anxiety	4	4	(12.1)	0	0	0	0	0	0	0	0	0
Acrophobia	1	1	(3.0)	0	0	0	0	0	0	0	0	0
Depression	1	1	(3.0)	0	0	0	0	0	0	0	0	0
Restlessness	1	1	(3.0)	0	0	0	0	0	0	0	0	0
Renal and Urinary Disorders	2	2	(6.1)	0	0	0	0	0	0	0	0	0
Glycosuria	1	1	(3.0)	0	0	0	0	0	0	0	0	0
Renal cyst	1	1	(3.0)	0	0	0	0	0	0	0	0	0
Reproductive System and Breast Disorders	2	2	(6.1)	0	0	0	1	1	(3.7)	0	0	0
Testicular swelling	0	0	0	0	0	0	1	1	(3.7)	0	0	0
Pelvic pain	1	1	(3.0)	0	0	0	0	0	0	0	0	0
Testicular pain	1	1	(3.0)	0	0	0	0	0	0	0	0	0
Respiratory, Thoracic and Mediastinal Disorders	11	9	(27.3)	0	0	0	1	1	(3.7)	0	0	0
Pharyngolaryngeal pain	3	3	(9.1)	0	0	0	0	0	0	0	0	0
Productive cough	2	2	(6.1)	0	0	0	0	0	0	0	0	0
Sinus congestion	1	1	(3.0)	0	0	0	1	1	(3.7)	0	0	0
Cough	1	1	(3.0)	0	0	0	0	0	0	0	0	0
Dysphonia	1	1	(3.0)	0	0	0	0	0	0	0	0	0
Dyspnoea	1	1	(3.0)	0	0	0	0	0	0	0	0	0
Rhinorrhoea	1	1	(3.0)	0	0	0	0	0	0	0	0	0
Throat tightness	1	1	(3.0)	0	0	0	0	0	0	0	0	0
Skin and Subcutaneous Tissue Disorders	10	8	(24.2)	0	0	0	2	2	(7.4)	0	0	0
Hyperhidrosis	3	3	(9.1)	0	0	0	0	0	0	0	0	0
Dry skin	2	2	(6.1)	0	0	0	0	0	0	0	0	0
Urticaria	2	2	(6.1)	0	0	0	0	0	0	0	0	0
Blister	0	0	0	0	0	0	1	1	(3.7)	0	0	0
Increased tendency to bruise	0	0	0	0	0	0	1	1	(3.7)	0	0	0
Alopecia	1	1	(3.0)	0	0	0	0	0	0	0	0	0
Rash	1	1	(3.0)	0	0	0	0	0	0	0	0	0
Skin discolouration	1	1	(3.0)	0	0	0	0	0	0	0	0	0
Surgical and Medical Procedures	1	1	(3.0)	0	0	0	0	0	0	0	0	0
Nasal polypectomy	1	1	(3.0)	0	0	0	0	0	0	0	0	0

[a] There were a total of 30 patients in the Hypothyroid group. One patient in the Hypothyroid group withdrew from study participation prior to the Month 8 primary efficacy assessment due to an adverse event and is excluded from this analysis.

Diagnostic Indication : Adverse reaction data are derived from the two clinical trials, in which 381 patients were treated with THYROGEN (thyrotropin alfa for injection).

Very common adverse events (≥10%) reported in the TSH92-0601 clinical trial was nausea (17.1%). Events reported in patients in the clinical trials supporting the diagnostic indication are summarized in Table 2.

Table 2: THYROGEN

Summary of Treatment-Emergent Adverse Events Occurring in Patients During the TSH92-0601 and TSH95-0101 Studies

	TSH92-0601			TSH95-0101		
	AEs	Pts	(%)	AEs	Pts	(%)
Total Number of Patients Treated with THYROGEN		152			229	
Total AEs/Patients with AEs	65	42	(27.6)	143	79	(34.5)
Blood and Lymphatic System Disorders	0	0	0	2	2	(0.9)
Anaemia	0	0	0	1	1	(0.4)
Lymphadenopathy	0	0	0	1	1	(0.4)
Cardiac Disorders	0	0	0	3	3	(1.3)
Palpitations	0	0	0	2	2	(0.9)
Tachycardia	0	0	0	1	1	(0.4)
Ear and Labyrinth Disorders	0	0	0	1	1	(0.4)
Ear discomfort	0	0	0	1	1	(0.4)
Endocrine Disorders	0	0	0	1	1	(0.4)
Thyroid pain	0	0	0	1	1	(0.4)
Eye Disorders	0	0	0	2	2	(0.9)
Eye inflammation	0	0	0	1	1	(0.4)
Eye pain	0	0	0	1	1	(0.4)
Gastrointestinal Disorders	33	31	(20.4)	37	26	(11.4)
Nausea	27	26	(17.1)	18	16	(7.0)
Vomiting	3	3	(2.0)	10	8	(3.5)
Abdominal pain	1	1	(0.7)	3	2	(0.9)
Diarrhoea	1	1	(0.7)	1	1	(0.4)
Abdominal discomfort	1	1	(0.7)	0	0	0
Abdominal pain upper	0	0	0	1	1	(0.4)
Constipation	0	0	0	1	1	(0.4)
Gastritis	0	0	0	1	1	(0.4)
Paraesthesia oral	0	0	0	1	1	(0.4)
Stomach discomfort	0	0	0	1	1	(0.4)
General Disorders and Administration Site Conditions	10	6	(3.9)	24	20	(8.7)
Fatigue	5	5	(3.3)	6	5	(2.2)
Pyrexia	0	0	0	4	4	(1.7
Asthenia	0	0	0	3	3	(1.3)
Chills	1	1	(0.7)	4	2	(0.9)
Feeling hot	1	1	(0.7)	1	1	(0.4)
Feeling cold	1	1	(0.7)	0	0	0
Pain	1	1	(0.7)	0	0	0
Thirst	1	1	(0.7)	0	0	0
Chest pain	0	0	0	1	1	(0.4)
Inflammation	0	0	0	1	1	(0.4)
Injection site discomfort	0	0	0	1	1	(0.4)
Injection site pruritus	0	0	0	1	1	(0.4)
Local swelling	0	0	0	1	1	(0.4)
Ulcer	0	0	0	1	1	(0.4)
Infections and Infestations	1	1	(0.7)	9	9	(3.9)
Influenza	0	0	0	4	4	(1.7)
Candidiasis	1	1	(0.7)	0	0	0
Nasopharyngitis	0	0	0	1	1	(0.4)
Oesophageal candidiasis	0	0	0	1	1	(0.4)
Parotitis	0	0	0	1	1	(0.4)
Pneumonia	0	0	0	1	1	(0.4)
Upper respiratory tract infection	0	0	0	1	1	(0.4)
Injury, Poisoning and Procedural Complications	0	0	0	2	2	(0.9)
Post procedural discomfort	0	0	0	1	1	(0.4)
Road traffic accident	0	0	0	1	1	(0.4)
Investigations	0	0	0	3	3	(1.3)
Blood cholesterol abnormal	0	0	0	1	1	(0.4)
Blood creatinine increased	0	0	0	1	1	(0.4)
White blood cell count decreased	0	0	0	1	1	(0.4)
Metabolism and Nutrition Disorders	0	0	0	4	3	(1.3)
Anorexia	0	0	0	1	1	(0.4)
Decreased appetite	0	0	0	1	1	(0.4)
Dehydration	0	0	0	1	1	(0.4)
Hypercholesterolemia	0	0	0	1	1	(0.4)
Musculoskeletal and Connective Tissue Disorders	1	1	(0.7)	5	5	(2.2)
Neck pain	1	1	(0.7)	0	0	0
Arthralgia	0	0	0	1	1	(0.4)
Back pain	0	0	0	1	1	(0.4)
Musculoskeletal pain	0	0	0	1	1	(0.4)
Myalgia	0	0	0	1	1	(0.4)
Shoulder pain	0	0	0	1	1	(0.4)
Neoplasms Benign, Malignant and Unspecified (incl cysts and polyps)	0	0	0	1	1	(0.4)
Neoplasm swelling	0	0	0	1	1	(0.4)
Nervous System Disorders	11	10	(6.6)	39	27	(11.8)
Headache	7	7	(4.6)	29	20	(8.7)
Dizziness	4	3	(2.0)	3	3	(1.3)
Paraesthesia	0	0	0	4	4	(1.7)
Dysgeusia	0	0	0	2	1	(0.4)
Tremor	0	0	0	1	1	(0.4)
Psychiatric Disorders	3	2	(1.3)	4	4	(1.7)
Disorientation	1	1	(0.7)	0	0	0
Insomnia	1	1	(0.7)	0	0	0
Nervousness	1	1	(0.7)	0	0	0
Agitation	0	0	0	1	1	(0.4)
Claustrophobia	0	0	0	1	1	(0.4)
Mood swings	0	0	0	1	1	(0.4)
Sleep disorder	0	0	0	1	1	(0.4)
Reproductive System and Breast Disorders	0	0	0	1	1	(0.4)
Metrorrhagia	0	0	0	1	1	(0.4)
Respiratory, Thoracic and Mediastinal Disorders	2	2	(1.3)	3	3	(1.3)
Dyspnoea	1	1	(0.7)	0	0	0

(cont'd)

Table 2: THYROGEN *(cont'd)*

Summary of Treatment-Emergent Adverse Events Occurring in Patients During the TSH92-0601 and TSH95-0101 Studies

	TSH92-0601			TSH95-0101		
	AEs	Pts	(%)	AEs	Pts	(%)
Pulmonary embolism	1	1	(0.7)	0	0	0
Epistaxis	0	0	0	1	1	(0.4)
Pharyngolaryngeal pain	0	0	0	1	1	(0.4)
Sinus congestion	0	0	0	1	1	(0.4)
Skin and Subcutaneous Tissue Disorders	3	3	(2.0)	2	2	(0.9)
Rash	2	2	(1.3)	0	0	0
Urticaria	0	0	0	2	2	(0.9)
Rash maculo-papular	1	1	(0.7)	0	0	0
Vascular disorders	1	1	(0.7)	0	0	0
Hypotension	1	1	(0.7)	0	0	0

TSH antibodies have not been reported in patients treated with THYROGEN in the clinical trials, although only 27 patients who received THYROGEN treatment more than once underwent testing for the development of TSH antibodies. The occurrence of antibodies which could interfere with endogenous TSH assays cannot be excluded.

Less Common Clinical Trial Adverse Drug Reactions (<1%): Very rare manifestations of hypersensitivity to THYROGEN reported in clinical trials, post-marketing settings and in special treatment programs involving patients with advanced disease classified by System Organ Class include:

Skin and Subcutaneous Tissue Disorder: urticaria, rash, pruritus, flushing.

Respiratory, Thoracic and Mediastinal Disorder: respiratory signs and symptoms including laryngeal oedema, pain at the site of metastases and respiratory distress requiring tracheotomy. Sudden rapid and painful enlargement of locally recurring papillary carcinoma has been reported 12-48 hours after THYROGEN administration. The enlargement was accompanied by dyspnoea, stridor or dysphonia. Rapid clinical improvement occurred following glucocorticoid therapy.

Post-Market Adverse Drug Reactions: Post-marketing surveillance indicates that the types of events most frequently reported are similar to those seen in the clinical trials (headache, nausea, vomiting and dizziness). Sudden rapid and painful enlargement of locally recurring papillary carcinoma has been reported 12-48 hours after THYROGEN administration. The enlargement was accompanied by dyspnea, stridor or dysphonia. Rapid clinical improvement occurred following glucocorticoid therapy. There have also been several reports of hypersensitivity reactions (including urticaria, rash, pruritus, flushing and respiratory difficulties requiring treatment) reported in the Post-Marketing setting.

Post-marketing experience indicates that THYROGEN administration may cause transient (<48 hours) influenza-like symptoms [also called flu-like symptoms (FLS)], which may include fever (>38°C), chills/shivering, myalgia/arthralgia, fatigue/asthenia/malaise, headache (non-focal), and chills.

A 77 year-old non-thyroidectomized patient with a history of heart disease and spinal metastases who received four THYROGEN injections over 6 days in a special treatment protocol experienced a fatal MI 24 hours after he received the last THYROGEN injection. The event was likely related to THYROGEN-induced hyperthyroidism (see Warnings and Precautions, Interpretation of Results).

Information from post-marketing surveillance, as well as from the literature, suggests that elimination of THYROGEN is significantly slower in dialysis-dependent end-stage renal disease (ESRD) patients, resulting in prolonged elevation of TSH levels. ESRD patients who receive THYROGEN may have markedly elevated TSH levels for several days after treatment, which may lead to increased risk of headache and nausea.

Post-marketing data include cases of atrial arrhythmias in elderly patients with pre-existing cardiac disease who received THYROGEN, and suggest that use of THYROGEN in this group should be considered carefully.

There are several reports in the post-marketing database of DVT and/or Pulmonary Embolism in patients who received THYROGEN. One patient was on concomitant oral contraceptive therapy, and the other patients had prolonged hospitalization and/or extensive metastatic disease prior to the thromboembolic event.

DRUG INTERACTIONS: Drug-Drug Interactions: Formal interaction studies between THYROGEN (thyrotropin alfa for injection) and other medicinal products have not been performed. In clinical trials, no interactions were observed between THYROGEN and the thyroid hormones triiodothyronine (T_3) and thyroxine (T_4) when administered concurrently.

The use of THYROGEN allows for radioiodine imaging while patients are euthyroid on T_3 and/or T_4. Data on radioiodine kinetics indicate that the clearance of radioiodine is approximately 50% greater while euthyroid than during the hypothyroid state when renal function is decreased, thus resulting in less radioiodine retention in the body at the time of imaging. This factor should be considered when selecting the activity of radioiodine for use in radioiodine imaging.

Drug-Food Interactions: Interactions with food have not been established.

Drug-Herb Interactions: Interactions with herbal products have not been established.

Drug-Laboratory Test Interactions: In clinical trials, the reference standard for determining whether patients had thyroid remnant or cancer present was a hypothyroid Tg ≥2 ng/mL and/or a hypothyroid scan (either diagnostic or post-therapy). This analysis evaluated whether Tg testing after THYROGEN administration improved the diagnostic sensitivity of a Tg test in patients with a negative Tg on thyroid hormone suppression therapy (THST) using a cut-off of 2 ng/mL. It should be noted that THYROGEN-Tg levels are generally lower than hypothyroid-Tg levels and thus physicians may need to use a lower Tg cut-off level when using THYROGEN than would be used with a hypothyroid-Tg.

DOSAGE AND ADMINISTRATION: Dosing Considerations:

- THYROGEN (thyrotropin alfa for injection) injections should be supervised by a healthcare professional knowledgeable in the management of thyroid cancer.
- THYROGEN should be administered intramuscularly only. It should not be administered intravenously.

Recommended Dose and Dosage Adjustment: A two-injection regimen is recommended for THYROGEN administration.

The two-injection regimen is THYROGEN 0.9 mg intramuscularly (IM), followed by a second 0.9 mg IM injection 24 hours later.

After reconstitution with 1.2 mL Sterile Water for injection, USP, 1 mL solution (containing 0.9 mg thyrotropin alfa), THYROGEN is administered by **intramuscular injection** in the gluteal muscle.

Parenteral Products:

Vial Size	Volume of Diluent to be Added to Vial	Approximate Available Volume	Nominal Concentration per mL
5 cc	1.2 mL	~1.2 mL	0.9 mg/mL

The following parameters were utilized in the second Phase 3 study and these parameters are recommended for radioimaging scanning:

- For radioiodine imaging or treatment, radioiodine administration should be given 24 hours following the final THYROGEN injection. Diagnostic scanning should be performed 48 hours after radioiodine administration whereas post-therapy scanning may be delayed additional days to allow background activity to decline.
- A diagnostic activity of 4 mCi (148 MBq) ^{131}I should be used.
- Whole body images should be acquired for a minimum of 30 minutes and/or should contain a minimum of 140 000 counts.
- Scanning times for single (spot) images of body regions should be 10-15 minutes or less if the minimum number of counts is reached sooner (i.e. 60 000 for a large field of view camera, 35 000 counts for a small field of view).

For radioiodine ablation of thyroid tissue remnants, the activity of ^{131}I is carefully selected at the discretion of the nuclear medicine physician. Studies with THYROGEN were conducted using 100 mCi±10% of ^{131}I.

For serum Tg testing, the serum sample should be obtained 72 hours after the final injection of THYROGEN.

Overdosage: In case of overdose, assessment of fluid balance and administration of fluids and/or an antiemetic may be considered.

Administration: THYROGEN has to be reconstituted with Sterile Water for Injection. Only one vial of THYROGEN is required per injection.

Instructions for Use (with Aseptic Technique): Reconstitution: Add 1.2 mL of Sterile Water for Injection, USP, to the THYROGEN powder in the vial. Swirl the contents of the vial gently until all material is dissolved. Do not shake the solution. When reconstituted as directed, the resulting solution has a concentration of 0.9 mg thyrotropin alfa per mL.

Reconstituted THYROGEN solution should be a clear, colourless solution. Do not use vials exhibiting foreign particles, cloudiness or discoloration. The pH of the reconstituted solution is 6.5-7.5.

Withdraw 1 mL of the THYROGEN solution from the product vial. This equals 0.9 mg thyrotropin alfa to be injected.

THYROGEN does not contain preservatives.

The THYROGEN solution should be injected within three hours, however the THYROGEN solution will stay chemically stable for up to 24 hours, if kept in a refrigerator (between 2-8°C). It is important to note that the microbiological safety depends on the aseptic conditions during the preparation of the solution.

Each vial of THYROGEN and each vial of diluent is intended for single use. Discard unused materials.

THYROGEN injection material should not be mixed with other substances.

OVERDOSAGE:

Data on exposure above the recommended dose is limited to clinical studies and a special treatment program. Three patients in clinical trials, and one patient in the special treatment program experienced symptoms after receiving THYROGEN (thyrotropin alfa for injection) doses higher than those recommended. Two patients had nausea after a 2.7 mg IM dose, and in one of these patients, the event was accompanied by weakness, dizziness and headache. The third patient experienced nausea, vomiting and hot flashes after 3.6 mg IM dose. In the special treatment program, a 77 year-old non-thyroidectomized patient received 4 doses of THYROGEN 0.9 mg over 6 days, developed atrial fibrillation, cardiac decompensation and terminal myocardial infarction 2 days later.

One additional patient enrolled in a clinical trial who received 0.3 mg THYROGEN as a single IV bolus, experienced severe nausea, vomiting, diaphoresis, hypotension (BP decreased from 115/66 mm Hg to 81/44 mm Hg) and tachycardia (pulse increased from 75 to 117 bpm) 15 minutes after injection.

When necessary, symptomatic treatment should be considered for potential cardiac symptoms.

For management of a suspected drug overdose, CPhA recommends that you contact your **regional Poison Control Centre**. See the *CPS* Directory section for a list of Poison Control Centres.

ACTION AND CLINICAL PHARMACOLOGY: Mechanism of Action: THYROGEN (thyrotropin alfa for injection) is a heterodimeric glycoprotein produced by recombinant DNA technology. It has comparable biochemical properties to human pituitary thyroid stimulating hormone (TSH). Binding of thyrotropin alfa to TSH receptors on normal thyroid epithelial cells or on well-differentiated thyroid cancer tissue stimulates iodine uptake and organification, and synthesis and secretion of thyroglobulin (Tg), triiodothyronine (T_3) and thyroxine (T_4).

THYROGEN is an alternative to thyroid hormone withdrawal for the radioablative treatment and follow-up of patients with a history of well-differentiated thyroid cancer while the patient remains euthyroid on THST (thyroid hormone suppressive therapy).

Pharmacodynamics: THYROGEN has comparable biochemical properties to human pituitary TSH. Binding of thyrotropin alfa to TSH receptors on normal thyroid epithelial cells or on well-differentiated thyroid cancer tissue stimulates iodine uptake and organification, and synthesis and secretion of Tg, T_3 and T_4.

In patients with well-differentiated thyroid cancer, a near total or total thyroidectomy is performed usually followed by radioiodine treatment to remove residual remnant tissue and microscopic residues of malignant tissue. Patients are placed on synthetic thyroid hormone supplements to replace endogenous hormone and to suppress serum levels of TSH in order to avoid TSH-stimulated tumour growth. Thereafter, patients are followed up for the presence of thyroid remnants or residual or recurrent cancer by Tg testing with or without radioiodine imaging. This follow-up testing is most effective when conducted under TSH stimulation, either while they remain on THST and are euthyroid using THYROGEN, or by Tg testing and radioiodine imaging following thyroid hormone withdrawal.

Pharmacokinetics: The pharmacokinetics of THYROGEN were studied in 16 patients with well-differentiated thyroid cancer given a single 0.9 mg IM dose. After injection, mean peak concentrations of 116±38 mU/L were reached between 3 and 24 hours after administration (median 10 hours). The mean apparent elimination half-life was found to be 25±10 hours. TSH clearance in man has not been fully elucidated, but studies with pituitary-derived TSH suggest that the liver and kidney are involved.

Absorption: Following a single intramuscular injection of 0.9 mg of thyrotropin alfa (0.9 mg/mL formulation), the mean±SD peak plasma level (C_{max}) was 116±38 mU/L which occurred approximately at 22±8.5 hours (T_{max}). The $AUC_{0\rightarrow\infty}$ was 5088±1728 mU·hr/L.

Distribution: As with endogenous TSH, rTSH binds to the TSH receptors on thyroid epithelial cells. The volume of distribution (Vd) is 68.7±32.05 L.

Metabolism: Since THYROGEN is a highly purified, recombinant form of the naturally occurring endogenous TSH, it is reasonable to assume that the metabolic pathway of rhTSH will be common to that of the endogenous TSH (i.e. broken down in the body to its component amino acids).

Excretion: The major elimination route of TSH is believed to be renal and to a lesser extent hepatic. In contrast, pre-clinical data on endogenous human pituitary derived TSH (phTSH) show that the kidney and liver appear to be the major organs of clearance for phTSH (Szkudlinski et al., 1995). The carbohydrate composition of rhTSH differs from phTSH in both the presence of terminal sialic acid residues and the absence of sulphated GalNAc. These differences may both contribute to the reduced clearance of rhTSH by the liver and enhanced clearance by the kidney (Szkudlinski et al., 1995). Based on these data, the kidney appears to be the major organ of clearance of rhTSH from the plasma, with a smaller additional clearance contributed by the liver. Serum clearance rate in humans was calculated as 36.3±11.6 mL/min.

STORAGE AND STABILITY: THYROGEN (thyrotropin alfa for injection) should be stored at 2-8°C. Each vial, after reconstitution with 1.2 mL Sterile Water for Injection, USP, should be inspected visually for particulate matter or discoloration before use. Any vials exhibiting particulate matter or discoloration should not be used.

Do not use THYROGEN after the expiration date on the vial. Protect from light.

The reconstituted solution should be injected within three hours, however it will stay chemically stable for up to 24 hours, if kept in a refrigerator (between 2-8°C). It is important to know that microbiological safety depends on the aseptic conditions during the preparation of the solution.

INFORMATION FOR THE PATIENT: Published in e-CPS, available by subscription at www.e-cps.ca.

DOSAGE FORMS, COMPOSITION AND PACKAGING: Each vial of sterile, nonpyrogenic lyophilized product, contains: thyrotropin alfa 1.1 mg. Nonmedicinal ingredients: mannitol, nitrogen, sodium chloride, sodium phosphate dibasic heptahydrate and sodium phosphate monobasic monohydrate. Preservative-free. Kits of two 1.1 mg (7-26 IU/mg) vials.

Tiamol® Ⓟ

fluocinonide

Topical Corticosteroid

TaroPharma

SUPPLIED: Each g of cream contains: fluocinonide 0.05% in an emollient base. Nonmedicinal ingredients: cetyl alcohol, citric acid, mineral oil, polysorbate-60, propylene glycol, sorbitan monostearate, stearyl alcohol and white petrolatum. Jars of 100 g. Tubes of 25 g. Store at room temperature (15-30°C).

The reader is invited to consult CPhA's monograph **Calcium Channel Blockers**.

Tiazac® Pr

diltiazem HCl

Antihypertensive—Antianginal

Biovail Pharmaceuticals

PHARMACOLOGY: Diltiazem is a calcium ion cellular influx inhibitor (calcium entry blocker or calcium ion antagonist).

Mechanism of Action: The therapeutic effect of this group of drugs is believed to be related to their specific cellular action of selectively inhibiting transmembrane influx of calcium ions into cardiac muscle and vascular smooth muscle. The contractile processes of these tissues are dependent upon the movement of extracellular calcium into the cells through specific ion channels. Diltiazem blocks transmembrane influx of calcium through the slow channel without affecting, to any significant degree, the transmembrane influx of sodium through the fast channel. This results in a reduction of free calcium ions available within cells of the above tissues. Diltiazem does not alter total serum calcium.

Hypertension: The antihypertensive effect of diltiazem is believed to be brought about largely by its vasodilatory action on peripheral blood vessels with resultant decrease in peripheral vascular resistance.

Angina: The precise mechanism by which diltiazem relieves angina has not been fully determined, but it is believed to be brought about largely by its vasodilatory action.

In angina of effort it appears that the action of diltiazem is related to the reduction of myocardial oxygen demand. This is probably caused by a decrease in blood pressure brought about by the reduction of peripheral resistance and of heart rate.

Hemodynamic and Electrophysiologic Effects: Diltiazem produces antihypertensive effects both in the supine and standing positions. Resting heart rate is usually slightly reduced. During dynamic exercise, increases in diastolic pressure are inhibited while maximum achievable systolic pressure is usually unaffected. Heart rate at maximum exercise is reduced. Studies to date, primarily in patients with normal ventricular function, have shown that cardiac output, ejection fraction and left ventricular end-diastolic pressure have not been affected.

Chronic therapy with diltiazem produces no change, or a decrease, in circulating plasma catecholamines. However, no increased activity of the renin-angiotensin-aldosterone axis has been observed. Diltiazem inhibits the renal and peripheral effects of angiotensin II.

In man, i.v. diltiazem in doses of 20 mg prolongs AH conduction time and AV node functional and effective refractory periods by approximately 20%. Chronic oral administration of diltiazem in doses up to 540 mg/day has resulted in small increases in PR interval. Second-degree and third-degree AV block have been observed (see Warnings). In patients with sick sinus syndrome, diltiazem significantly prolongs sinus cycle length (up to 50% in some cases).

Pharmacokinetics: Diltiazem is well absorbed from the gastrointestinal tract and is subject to an extensive first-pass effect giving absolute bioavailability (compared to i.v. dosing) of about 40%. Therapeutic blood levels appear to be in the range of 50 to 200 ng/mL range and the plasma elimination half-life (beta-phase) following single or multiple drug administration is approximately 3.5 to 6 hours. In-vitro human serum binding studies revealed that 70 to 80% of diltiazem is bound to plasma proteins. Following extensive hepatic metabolism, only 2 to 4% of the drug appears unchanged in the urine and 6 to 7% appears as metabolites.

The metabolic pathways of diltiazem include N-and O-demethylation (via cytochrome P450), deacetylation (via plasma and tissue esterases), in addition to conjugation (via sulfation and glucuridonation). In vitro studies have demonstrated that CYP 3A4 is the principal CYP isoenzyme involved in N-demethylation. The major metabolite, desacetyl diltiazem, is present in the plasma at levels 10 to 20% of the parent drug and is 25 to 50% as potent as diltiazem in terms of coronary vasodilation.

TIAZAC Capsules: When compared to a regimen of immediate-release tablets at steady-state, approximately 93% of drug is absorbed from the TIAZAC formulation. When TIAZAC was coadministered with a high fat content breakfast, the extent of diltiazem absorption was not affected; T_{max}, however, occurred slightly earlier. Dose-dumping does not occur. The apparent elimination half-life after single or multiple dosing is 4 to 9.5 hours (mean 6.5 hours).

TIAZAC demonstrates nonlinear pharmacokinetics. As the dose of TIAZAC is increased from a daily dose of 120 to 240 mg, there is an increase in the AUC of 2.4 times. When the dose is increased from 240 mg to 360 mg there is an increase in AUC of 1.5 times.

In a study with 14 healthy subjects, the steady-state pharmacokinetics of TIAZAC were compared with Cardizem CD at a dose of 240 mg/day. The bioavailability of TIAZAC relative to Cardizem CD based on mean diltiazem AUC was 124% (90% CI=111 to 139%). The relative mean C_{max} was 121%.

Pharmacodynamics: Hypertension: In a parallel-group, double-blind placebo-controlled study of 198 patients with mild to moderate essential hypertension, TIAZAC was given for 4 weeks. The changes in diastolic blood pressure measured at trough (24 hours after the dose) for placebo, 90 mg, 180 mg and 360 mg were −5.4, −6.3, −6.2, −8.2 mmHg, respectively.

Another double-blind placebo-controlled clinical trial in 56 patients with mild to moderate essential hypertension treated for 8 weeks, followed a dose-escalation design. Supine diastolic blood pressure measured at trough following 2-week intervals of treatment with TIAZAC was reduced by −3.7 mmHg with 120 mg/day vs −2.0 mmHg with placebo, by −7.6 mmHg after escalation to 240 mg/day vs −2.3 mmHg with placebo, by −8.1 mmHg after escalation to 360 mg/day versus −0.9 mmHg with placebo.

In a double-blind, multicentre study, 181 patients with mild to moderate essential hypertension controlled with Cardizem CD monotherapy, were randomized to the same dose of either Cardizem CD or TIAZAC. The least squares mean for the difference in diastolic blood pressure at trough between TIAZAC and Cardizem CD groups pooled was 0.19 mmHg (90% CI=1.2 to 1.6 mmHg). Data based on same dose comparisons were supportive of this result.

Angina: In a double-blind, parallel group placebo-controlled trial, 158 patients with chronic stable angina were, after titration, treated for 2 weeks on their target maintenance dose of TIAZAC.

TIAZAC increased exercise tolerance times in a Bruce exercise protocol, at trough, 24 hours after dosing. Exercise tolerance times increased by 14, 26, 41 and 33 seconds for placebo, 120 mg, 240 mg, and 360 mg/day treated patient groups respectively. At peak, 8 hours after dosing, exercise tolerance times were increased by 13, 38, 64 and 53 seconds for placebo, 120 mg, 240 mg and 360 mg/day treated groups, respectively.

INDICATIONS: Essential Hypertension: For the treatment of mild to moderate essential hypertension. TIAZAC should normally be used in those patients in whom treatment with diuretics or beta-blockers has been ineffective, or has been associated with unacceptable adverse effects.

TIAZAC can be tried as an initial agent in those patients in whom the use of diuretics and/or beta-blockers is contraindicated, or in patients with medical conditions in which these drugs frequently cause serious adverse effects.

Safety of concurrent use of TIAZAC with other antihypertensive agents has not been established.

Chronic Stable Angina: For the management of chronic stable angina (effort-associated angina) without evidence of vasospasm in patients who remain symptomatic despite adequate doses of beta-blockers and/or organic nitrates or who cannot tolerate these agents.

TIAZAC may be tried in combination with beta-blockers in chronic stable angina patients with normal ventricular function. When such concomitant therapy is introduced, patients must be monitored closely (see Warnings, Use with Beta-blockers).

Since the safety and efficacy of TIAZAC in the management of unstable or vasospastic angina has not been substantiated, its use for these indications is not recommended.

CONTRAINDICATIONS: Patients with sick sinus syndrome except in the presence of an implanted pacemaker; patients with second- or third-degree AV block except in the presence of an implanted pacemaker; patients with known hypersensitivity to diltiazem; patients with severe hypotension (less than 90 mmHg systolic); myocardial infarction patients, who have left ventricular failure manifested by congestion.

Pregnancy: In pregnancy and in women of childbearing potential. Fetal malformations and adverse effects on pregnancy have been reported in animals. In repeated dose studies a high incidence of vertebral column malformations were present in the offspring of mice receiving more than 50 mg/kg of diltiazem orally.

In the offspring of mice receiving a single oral dose of 50 or 100 mg/kg on day 12 of gestation, the incidence of cleft palate and malformed extremities was significantly higher. Vertebral malformations were most prevalent when they received the drug on day 9. In rats, a significantly higher fetal death rate was present when 200 and 400 mg/kg were given orally on days 9 to 14 of gestation. Single oral dose studies in rats resulted in a significant incidence of skeletal malformations in the offspring of the group receiving 400 mg/kg on day 11. In rabbits, all pregnant dams receiving 70 mg/kg orally from day 6 to 18 of gestation aborted; at 35 mg/kg, a significant increase in skeletal malformations was recorded in the offspring.

WARNINGS: Cardiac Conduction: Diltiazem prolongs AV node refractory periods without significantly prolonging sinus node recovery time, except in patients with sick sinus syndrome. This effect may rarely result in abnormally slow heart rates (particularly in patients with sick sinus syndrome) or second-or third-degree AV block (13 of 3 007 patients or 0.43%). Concomitant use of diltiazem with beta-blockers or digitalis may result in additive effects on cardiac conduction.

Congestive Heart Failure: Because diltiazem has a negative inotropic effect in vitro and it affects cardiac conduction, the drug should only be used with caution and under careful medical supervision in patients with congestive cardiac failure (see also Contraindications).

Use With Beta-blockers: The combination of diltiazem and beta-blockers warrants caution since in some patients additive effects on heart rate, cardiac conduction, blood pressure or left ventricular function have been observed. Close medical supervision is recommended.

Generally diltiazem should not be given to patients with impaired left ventricular function while they receive beta-blockers. However in exceptional cases, when in the opinion of the physician, concomitant use is considered essential, such use should be instituted gradually in a hospital setting.

Diltiazem gives no protection against the dangers of abrupt beta-blocker withdrawal and such withdrawal should be done by the gradual reduction of the dose of beta-blocker.

Hypotension: Decreases in blood pressure associated with diltiazem therapy may occasionally result in symptomatic hypotension.

Patients With Myocardial Infarction: Use of immediate release diltiazem at 240 mg/day started 3 to 15 days after a myocardial infarction was associated with an increase in cardiac events in patients with pulmonary congestion with no overall effect on mortality. Although there has not been a study of sustained release formulations of diltiazem in acute myocardial infarction, their use may have effects similar to those of immediate release diltiazem in acute myocardial infarction.

Acute Hepatic Injury: In rare instances, significant elevations in alkaline phosphatase, CPK, LDH, AST, ALT and symptoms consistent with acute hepatic injury have been observed. These reactions have been reversible upon discontinuation of drug therapy. Although a causal relationship to diltiazem has not been established in all cases, a drug induced hypersensitivity reaction is suspected (see Adverse Effects). As with any drug given over prolonged periods, laboratory parameters should be monitored at regular intervals.

PRECAUTIONS: Impaired Hepatic or Renal Function: Because diltiazem is extensively metabolized by the liver and excreted by the kidney and in bile, monitoring of laboratory parameters and cautious dosage titration are recommended in patients with impaired hepatic or renal function (see Adverse Effects).

Pediatrics: Safety and effectiveness in children have not been established.

Lactation: Diltiazem is excreted in human milk. One report suggests that concentrations in breast milk may approximate serum levels. If use of diltiazem is deemed essential, an alternative method of infant feeding should be instituted.

Geriatrics: Administration of diltiazem to elderly patients (over or equal to 65 years of age) requires caution. The incidence of adverse reactions is approximately 13% higher in this group. Those adverse reactions which occur more frequently include: peripheral edema, bradycardia, palpitation, dizziness, rash and polyuria. Therefore particular care in titration is advisable.

Drug Interactions: As with all drugs, care should be exercised when treating patients with multiple medications. Calcium channel blockers undergo biotransformation by the cytochrome P450 system. Coadministration of diltiazem with other drugs which follow the same route of biotransformation may result in altered bioavailability. Dosages of similarly metabolized drugs, particularly those of low therapeutic ratio, and especially in patients with renal and/or hepatic impairment, may require adjustment when starting or stopping concomitantly administered diltiazem to maintain optimum therapeutic blood levels.

Drugs known to be inhibitors of the cytochrome P450 system include: azole antifungals, cimetidine, cyclosporine, erythromycin, quinidine, warfarin.

Drugs known to be inducers of the cytochrome P450 system include: phenobarbital, phenytoin, rifampin.

Drugs known to be biotransformed via P450 include: benzodiazepines, flecainide, imipramine, propafenone, terfenadine, theophylline.

Anesthetics: The depression of cardiac contractility, conductivity, and automaticity as well as the vascular dilation associated with anesthetics may be potentiated by calcium channel blockers. When used concomitantly, anesthetics and calcium blockers should be titrated carefully.

Benzodiazepines: Diltiazem significantly increases peak plasma levels and the elimination half-life of triazolam and midazolam.

Beta-blockers: The concomitant administration of diltiazem with beta adrenergic blocking drugs warrants caution and careful monitoring. Such an association may have an additive effect on heart rate, on AV conduction or on blood pressure (see Warnings). Appropriate dosage adjustments may be necessary. A study in 5 normal subjects showed that diltiazem increased propranolol bioavailability by approximately 50%.

Carbamazepine: Concomitant administration of diltiazem with carbamazepine has been reported to result in elevated serum levels of carbamazepine (40 to 72% increase), resulting in toxicity in some cases. Patients receiving these drugs concurrently should be monitored for a potential drug interaction.

Cimetidine: A study in 6 healthy volunteers has shown a significant increase in peak diltiazem plasma levels (58%) and AUC (53%) after a 1-week course of cimetidine 1200 mg/day and a single dose of diltiazem 60 mg. Ranitidine produced smaller, nonsignificant increases. The effect may be mediated by cimetidine's known inhibition of hepatic cytochrome P450, the enzyme system responsible for the first-pass metabolism of diltiazem. Patients currently receiving diltiazem therapy should be carefully monitored for a change in pharmacological effect when initiating and discontinuing therapy with cimetidine. An adjustment in the diltiazem dose may be warranted.

Cyclosporine: A pharmacokinetic interaction between diltiazem and cyclosporine has been observed during studies involving renal and cardiac transplant patients. In renal and cardiac transplant recipients, a reduction of cyclosporine dose ranging from 15 to 48% was necessary to maintain cyclosporine trough concentrations similar to those seen prior to the addition of diltiazem. If these agents are to be administered concurrently, cyclosporine concentrations should be monitored, especially when diltiazem therapy is initiated, adjusted, or discontinued. The effect of cyclosporine on diltiazem plasma concentrations has not been evaluated.

Digitalis: Diltiazem and digitalis glycosides may have an additive effect in prolonging AV conduction. In clinical trials, concurrent administration of diltiazem and digoxin have resulted in increases in serum digoxin levels with prolongation of AV conduction. This increase may result from a decrease in renal clearance of digoxin. Patients on concomitant therapy, especially those with renal impairment, should be carefully monitored. The dose of digoxin may need downward adjustment.

Rifampin: Administration of diltiazem with rifampin markedly reduced plasma diltiazem concentrations and the therapeutic effect of diltiazem.

Short- and Long-Acting Nitrates: Diltiazem may be safely coadministered with nitrates.

Other Calcium Antagonists: Limited clinical experience suggests that in certain severe conditions not responding adequately to verapamil or to nifedipine, using diltiazem in conjunction with either of these drugs may be beneficial.

ADVERSE EFFECTS: Overall Diltiazem Safety Profile: In clinical trials with diltiazem involving over 3 300 patients, the most common adverse reactions were headache (4.6%), edema (4.6%), dizziness (3.5%), asthenia (2.7%), first degree AV block (2.4%), bradycardia (1.7%), flushing (1.5%), nausea (1.4%), rash (1.2%) and dyspepsia (1.0%).

In addition, the following events were reported with a frequency of less than 1%:

Cardiovascular: angina, arrhythmia, AV block (second- or third-degree), bundle branch block, congestive heart failure, ECG abnormalities, hypotension, palpitations, syncope, tachycardia, ventricular extrasystoles.

Nervous System: abnormal dreams, amnesia, depression, gait abnormality, hallucinations, insomnia, nervousness, paresthesia, personality change, somnolence, tinnitus, tremor.

Gastrointestinal: anorexia, constipation, diarrhea, dry mouth, dysgeusia, mild elevations of AST, ALT, LDH, and alkaline phosphatase (see Warnings), thirst, vomiting, weight increase.

Dermatological: petechiae, photosensitivity, pruritus.

Other: amblyopia, CPK increase, dyspnea, epistaxis, eye irritation, hyperglycemia, hyperuricemia, impotence, nasal congestion, nocturia, osteoarticular pain, polyuria, sexual difficulties, dry mouth.

The following postmarketing events have been reported infrequently in patients receiving diltiazem: alopecia, erythema multiforme, exfoliative dermatitis, Stevens-Johnson syndrome, angioedema, toxic epidermal necrolysis, extrapyramidal symptoms, gingival hyperplasia, hemolytic anemia, increased bleeding time, leukopenia, purpura, retinopathy, and thrombocytopenia. In addition, events such as myocardial infarction have been observed which are not readily distinguishable from the natural history of the disease in these patients. A number of well-documented cases of generalized rash, characterized as leukocytoclastic vasculitis, have been reported. However, a definitive cause and effect relationship between these events and diltiazem therapy is yet to be established.

TIAZAC (diltiazem hydrochloride): Hypertension: A safety evaluation was carried out in placebo-controlled studies in which 345 hypertensive patients (TIAZAC n=243; placebo n=102) were treated with TIAZAC at doses up to 360 mg/day. The most common adverse effects were: headache (13%); edema (5%); gastrointestinal disease (5%); pain (4%); vasodilation (3%); asthenia (3%); dizziness (3%) and palpitations (2%).

The following percentage of adverse effects, divided by system, were reported:

Cardiovascular: edema, including peripheral edema (5%), vasodilation, including hypotension, syncope and flushing (3%), palpitations (2%) and tachycardia (1%).
Central Nervous System: headache (13%), asthenia (3%), dizziness (3%), neck rigidity (1%), nervousness (1%), paresthesia (1%).
Gastrointestinal: gastrointestinal disease, including dyspepsia, nausea (5%), constipation (1%), anorexia (1%), dry mouth (1%).
Other: pain (4%), pharyngitis (2%), rhinitis (1%), dyspnea (1%), allergic reaction (1%), polyuria (1%), rash (1%).

The most common adverse effects for placebo treated patients in the above mentioned trials were: headache (17%), edema (3%), gastrointestinal disease (2%), pain (5%), vasodilation (1%), asthenia (6%), dizziness (4%), palpitations (2%), pharyngitis (2%), rhinitis (2%), dyspnea (1%), nervousness (2%), paresthesia (2%), tachycardia (2%).

Angina: The safety of TIAZAC was evaluated in 158 patients with chronic stable angina pectoris treated with TIAZAC at doses from 120 to 360 mg/day and in 50 patients treated with placebo. Thirty three percent of the TIAZAC treated patients had one or more adverse event compared to 18% in the placebo group. Discontinuation due to adverse events was required in 3 patients who were on TIAZAC 240 mg/day. The most common adverse events were: headache (8%), pain (4%), dizziness (3%) and peripheral edema (2%).

The following percentage of adverse effects, divided by system, were reported:
Cardiovascular: edema, peripheral (1.8%), palpitations (1.2%), arrhythmia (1.2%).
Central Nervous System: headache (8.2%), asthenia (0.6%), dizziness (3.1%).
Gastrointestinal: constipation (1.2%), dyspepsia (1.2%).
Other: pain (3.7%), pharyngitis (1.8%), cough increase (1.2%), gout (1.2%), rash (1.2%), hyperglycemia (1.2%), albuminuria (1.2%), crystalluria (1.2%), dyspnea (0.6%), infection (0.6%).

OVERDOSE:

Symptoms: There have been reports of diltiazem overdose in doses ranging from less than 1 to 18 g. In cases with fatal outcome, the majority involved multiple drug ingestion.

Events observed following diltiazem overdose included bradycardia, hypotension, heart block and cardiac failure.

Treatment: Most reports of overdose described some supportive medical measure and/or drug treatment. Bradycardia frequently responded favorably to atropine as did heart block, although cardiac pacing was also frequently utilized to treat heart block. Fluids and vasopressors were used to maintain blood pressure, and in cases of cardiac failure, inotropic agents were administered. In addition, some patients received treatment with ventilatory support, gastric lavage, activated charcoal, and i.v. calcium.

The effectiveness of i.v. calcium administration to reverse the pharmacological effects of diltiazem overdose has been inconsistent. In a few reported cases, overdose with calcium channel blockers associated with hypotension and bradycardia that was initially refractory to atropine became more responsive to atropine after the patients received i.v. calcium. In some cases i.v. calcium has been administered (1 g calcium chloride or 3 g calcium gluconate) over 5 minutes, and repeated every 10 to 20 minutes as necessary. Calcium gluconate has also been administered as a continuous infusion at a rate of 2 g/hour for 10 hours. Infusions of calcium for 24 hours or more may be required. Patients should be monitored for signs of hypercalcemia.

In the event of overdosage or exaggerated response, appropriate supportive measures should be employed in addition to gastric lavage. The following measures may be considered:
Bradycardia: Administer atropine. If there is no response to vagal blockage, administer isoproterenol cautiously.
High-degree AV Block: Treat as for bradycardia above. Fixed high-degree AV block should be treated with cardiac pacing.
Cardiac Failure: Administer inotropic agents (isoproterenol, dopamine or dobutamine) and diuretics.
Hypotension: Vasopressors (e.g., dopamine or norepinephrine bitartrate). Actual treatment and dosage should depend on the severity of the clinical situation and the judgment and experience of the treating physician.

For management of a suspected drug overdose, CPhA recommends that you contact your **regional Poison Control Centre**. See the *CPS* Directory section for a list of Poison Control Centres.

DOSAGE: TIAZAC should not be chewed or crushed. TIAZAC has not been shown to be bioequivalent to other diltiazem formulations (see Pharmacology, Pharmacokinetics).

Hypertension: When used as monotherapy, usual starting doses are 180 to 240 mg once daily, although some patients may respond to 120 mg once daily. Maximum antihypertensive effect is usually observed after approximately 2 to 4 weeks of therapy; therefore, dosage adjustments should be scheduled accordingly.

A maximum daily dose of 360 mg should not be exceeded.

The dosage of TIAZAC or concomitant antihypertensive agents may need to be adjusted when adding one to the other. See Warnings and Precautions regarding use with beta-blockers.

Angina: Dosages for the treatment of angina should be adjusted to each patient's needs, starting with a dose of 120 mg to 180 mg once daily. Individual patients may respond to higher doses of up to 360 mg once daily. When necessary, titration should be carried out over a 7- to 14-day period.

There is limited experience with doses above 360 mg. However, the incidence of adverse events increases as the dose increases with first-degree AV block, dizziness, and sinus bradycardia bearing the strongest realtionship to dose. Therefore, doses greater than 360 mg are not recommended.

INFORMATION FOR THE PATIENT: Published in e-CPS, available by subscription at www.e-cps.ca.

SUPPLIED: 120 mg: Each lavender/lavender extended-release capsule imprinted, in white ink, with a maple leaf on one end and "BVF 120" on the other, contains: diltiazem HCl 120 mg. Nonmedicinal ingredients: black iron oxide, D&C Red #28, eudragit, FD&C Blue #1, FD&C Red #40, gelatin, hydroxypropylmethylcellulose, magnesium stearate, microcrystalline cellulose, polysorbate, povidone, simethicone, sucrose stearate, talc and titanium dioxide. Bottles of 100.

180 mg: Each bluish green/white extended-release capsule imprinted, in black ink, with a maple leaf on one end and "BVF 180" on the other, contains: diltiazem HCl 180 mg. Nonmedicinal ingredients: black iron oxide, D&C Red #28, eudragit, FD&C Green #3, gelatin, hydroxypropylmethylcellulose, magnesium stearate, microcrystalline cellulose, polysorbate, povidone, simethicone, sucrose stearate, talc and titanium dioxide. Bottles of 100.

240 mg: Each lavender/bluish green extended-release capsule imprinted, in white ink, with a maple leaf on one end and "BVF 240" on the other, contains: diltiazem HCl 240 mg. Nonmedicinal ingredients: black iron oxide, D&C Red #28, eudragit, FD&C Blue #1, FD&C Green #3, FD&C Red #40, gelatin, hydroxypropylmethylcellulose, magnesium stearate, microcrystalline cellulose, polysorbate, povidone, simethicone, sucrose stearate, talc and titanium dioxide. Bottles of 100.

300 mg: Each lavender/white extended-release capsule imprinted, in black ink, with a maple leaf on one end and "BVF 300" on the other, contains: diltiazem HCl 300 mg. Nonmedicinal ingredients: black iron oxide, D&C Red #28, eudragit, FD&C Blue #1, FD&C Red #40, gelatin, hydroxypropylmethylcellulose, magnesium stearate, microcrystalline cellulose, polysorbate, povidone, simethicone, sucrose stearate, talc and titanium dioxide. Bottles of 100.

360 mg: Each bluish green/bluish green extended-release capsule imprinted, in white ink, with a maple leaf on one end and "BVF 360" on the other, contains: diltiazem HCl 360 mg. Nonmedicinal ingredients: black iron oxide, eudragit, FD&C Green #3, gelatin, hydroxypropylmethylcellulose, magnesium stearate, microcrystalline cellulose, polysorbate, povidone, simethicone, sucrose stearate, talc and titanium dioxide. Bottles of 100.

Store between 15 to 30°C. Avoid excessive humidity.

(Shown in Product Identification Section)

The reader is invited to consult CPhA's monograph **Calcium Channel Blockers**.

Tiazac® XC

diltiazem HCl

Antihypertensive—Antianginal

Biovail Pharmaceuticals

Date of Preparation: August 5, 2004
Date of Revision: July 13, 2007

SUMMARY PRODUCT INFORMATION:

Route of Administration	Dosage Form/ Strength	Clinically Relevant Nonmedicinal Ingredients[a]
Oral	Tablets: 120 mg, 180 mg, 240 mg, 300 mg, 360 mg	Microcrystalline cellulose, eudragit, povidone, sucrose stearate, magnesium stearate, talc, titanium dioxide, hydroxypropylmethylcellulose, polysorbate, simethicone, microcrystalline wax, pregelatinized starch, sodium starch glycolate, croscarmellose sodium, colloidal silicone dioxide, hydrogenated vegetable oil, polydextrose, polyethylene glycol, carnauba wax

[a] For Complete Information, see Dosage Forms, Composition and Packaging.

INDICATIONS AND CLINICAL USE: Essential Hypertension: For the treatment of mild to moderate essential hypertension. It is to be administered once daily at bedtime.

TIAZAC XC should normally be used in those patients in whom treatment with diuretics or beta-blockers has been ineffective, or has been associated with unacceptable adverse effects.

The safety of concurrent use of TIAZAC XC with other antihypertensive agents has not been established.

No morbidity and mortality studies have been carried out to support the use of TIAZAC XC (see Action and Clinical Pharmacology, Pharmacodynamics).

Chronic Stable Angina: For the management of chronic stable angina (effort-associated angina) without evidence of vasospasm in patients who remain symptomatic despite adequate doses of beta-blockers and/or organic nitrates or who cannot tolerate those agents.

TIAZAC XC may be tried in combination with beta-blockers in chronic stable angina in patients with normal ventricular function. When such concomitant therapy is introduced, these patients must be monitored closely (see Warnings and Precautions).

Since the safety and efficacy of TIAZAC XC in the management of unstable or vasospastic angina has not been substantiated, its use for these conditions is not recommended.

Geriatrics: Administration of diltiazem to elderly patients (over or equal to 65 years of age) requires caution. The incidence of adverse reactions is approximately 13% higher in this group.

Pediatrics: Safety and efficacy in children has not been studied.

CONTRAINDICATIONS: TIAZAC XC is contraindicated:
- In patients with sick sinus syndrome, except in the presence of an implanted pacemaker;
- In patients with second or third-degree AV block, except in the presence of an implanted pacemaker;
- In patients with known hypersensitivity to diltiazem;
- In patients with severe hypotension (less than 90 mm Hg systolic);
- In myocardial infarction patients, who have left ventricular failure manifested by pulmonary congestion;
- In pregnancy and in women of child-bearing potential. Fetal malformations and adverse effects on pregnancy have been reported in animals.

WARNINGS AND PRECAUTIONS: Cardiac Conduction: TIAZAC XC (diltiazem hydrochloride) prolongs AV node refractory periods without significantly prolonging sinus node recovery time, except in patients with sick sinus syndrome. This effect may rarely result in abnormally slow heart rates (particularly in patients with sick sinus syndrome) or second- or third-degree AV block (13 of 3007 patients or 0.43%). Concomitant use of diltiazem with beta-blockers or digitalis may result in additive effects on cardiac conduction.

Heart Failure: Because diltiazem has a negative inotropic effect in vitro and it affects cardiac conduction, the drug should only be used with caution and under careful medical supervision in patients with cardiac failure (see also Contraindications).

Postinfarction patients with reduced ejection fraction are at particular risk for subsequent heart failure when treated with diltiazem. Accordingly, diltiazem should be avoided in patients with substantially reduced ejection fraction.

Hypotension: Decreases in blood pressure associated with diltiazem hydrochloride therapy may occasionally result in symptomatic hypotension.

Patients with Myocardial Infarction: Use of immediate release diltiazem at 240 mg per day started 3 to 15 days after a myocardial infarction was associated with an increase in cardiac events in patients with pulmonary congestion with no overall effect on mortality. Although there has not been a study of a sustained-release formulation of diltiazem in acute myocardial infarction, their use may have effects similar to those of immediate-release diltiazem in acute myocardial infarction.

Acute Hepatic Injury: In rare instances, significant elevations in alkaline phosphatase, CPK, LDH, AST, ALT and symptoms consistent with hepatic injury have been observed. These reactions have been reversible upon discontinuation of drug therapy. Although a causal relationship to diltiazem has not been established in all cases, a drug induced hypersensitivity reaction is suspected (see Adverse Reactions). As with any drug given over prolonged periods, laboratory parameters should be monitored at regular intervals.

Use with Beta-Blockers: Generally, diltiazem should not be given to patients with impaired left ventricular function if they are already receiving beta-blockers. In exceptional cases, when in the opinion of the physician, concomitant use is considered essential, such use should be instituted gradually in a hospital setting under close medical supervision.

The combination of diltiazem and beta-blockers warrants caution since in some patients additive effects on heart rate, cardiac conduction, blood pressure or left ventricular function have been observed.

Diltiazem gives no protection against the dangers of abrupt beta-blocker withdrawal and such withdrawal should be done by the gradual reduction of the dose of beta-blocker.

Special Populations: Impaired Hepatic or Renal Function: Because TIAZAC XC (diltiazem hydrochloride) is extensively metabolized by the liver and excreted by the kidney and in bile, monitoring of laboratory parameters and cautious dosage titration are recommended in patients with severe hepatic or renal function (see Adverse Reactions).

Pediatrics: Safety and effectiveness in children has not been studied.

Nursing Women: Diltiazem is excreted in human milk. One report suggests that concentrations in breast milk may approximate serum levels. If use of TIAZAC XC is deemed essential, an alternative method of infant feeding should be instituted.

Geriatrics: Administration of diltiazem to elderly patients (over or equal to 65 years of age) requires caution. The incidence of adverse reactions is approximately 13% higher in this group. Those adverse reactions which occur more frequently include: peripheral edema, bradycardia, palpitation, dizziness, rash and polyuria. Therefore particular care in titration is advisable.

ADVERSE REACTIONS: Adverse Drug Reaction Overview: In clinical trials with diltiazem, involving over 3300 patients the most common adverse reactions were headache (4.6%), edema (4.6%), dizziness (3.5%), asthenia (2.7%), first degree AV block (2.4%), bradycardia (1.7%), flushing (1.5%), nausea (1.4%), rash (1.2%), and dyspepsia (1.0%).

Clinical Trial Adverse Drug Reactions: Because clinical trials are conducted under very specific conditions the adverse reaction rates observed in the clinical trials may not reflect the rates observed in practice and should not be compared to the rates in the clinical trials of another drug. Adverse drug reaction information from clinical trials is useful for identifying drug-related adverse events and for approximating rates.

Table 1: TIAZAC XC
Adverse Events >1%: Diltiazem HCl Extended-Release Formulation. Once-a-day PM Administration. Placebo-Controlled Hypertension Trials

Adverse Reactions	Placebo n=69 # pts (%)	Diltiazem HCl Extended-release 120–360 mg n=238 # pts (%)
Headache	10 (15)	29 (12)
Oedema Lower Limb	4 (6)	9 (4)
Upper Respiratory Tract Infection	2 (3)	12 (5)
Nasopharyngitis	1 (1)	7 (3)
Sinusitis	2 (3)	7 (3)

Hypertension: Table 1 presents the most common adverse reactions reported in the placebo-controlled hypertension trials in patients receiving a diltiazem hydrochloride extended-release formulation (once-a-day dosing) up to 360 mg.

Angina: In the angina clinical study, the adverse event profile of TIAZAC XC was consistent with that previously described for TIAZAC XC and other formulations of diltiazem HCl. The most frequent adverse effects experienced by TIAZAC XC patients are presented in Table 2.

Table 2: TIAZAC XC

Adverse Events >1%: Diltiazem Hydrochloride Extended-Release Formulation. Once-a-day Administration. Placebo-Controlled Angina Trial

Adverse Reactions	Placebo n=61 # pts (%)	Diltiazem HCl Extended-release 180, 360 & 420 mg n=250 # pts (%)
Oedema Lower Limb	2 (3.3)	17 (6.8)
Dizziness	0 (0)	16 (6.4)
Fatigue	3 (4.9)	12 (4.8)
Bradycardia	0 (0)	9 (3.6)
Atrioventricular Block First Degree	0 (0)	8 (3.2)
Cough	0 (0)	5 (2.0)

Uncommon Clinical Trial Adverse Drug Reactions (<1%): The following data is divided into two sections. The first represents ADRs <1% in TIAZAC XC Clinical trials. The second reflects ADRs <1% in other diltiazem products.

The following treatment related adverse drug reactions were reported with <1% incidence in the TIAZAC XC clinical trial:

Cardiac Disorders: atrioventricular block first degree, palpitations.

Eye Disorders: vitreous floaters, diplopia.

Gastrointestinal Disorders: dyspepsia, nausea.

General Disorders and Administration Site Conditions: feeling jittery, joint swelling, lethargy, neck swelling, oedema NOS, peripheral swelling, swelling NOS.

Investigations: aspartate aminotransferase increased.

Nervous System Disorders: dizziness (exc vertigo), sinus headache.

Renal and Urinary Disorders: urinary frequency.

Respiratory, Thoracic and Mediastinal Disorders: dyspnoea NOS.

Skin and Subcutaneous Disorders: dermatitis NOS, erythema NEC, face oedema, pruritus NOS, rash generalized.

Vascular Disorders: flushing.

In addition, the following events were reported with a frequency of less than 1% in other diltiazem products:

Cardiovascular: angina, arrhythmia, AV block (second- or third-degree), bundle branch block, congestive heart failure (left ventricular dysfunction), ECG abnormalities, hypotension, palpitations, syncope, tachycardia, ventricular extrasystoles.

Nervous System: abnormal dreams, amnesia, depression, gait abnormality, hallucinations, insomnia, nervousness, paresthesia, personality change, somnolence, tinnitus, tremor.

Gastrointestinal: anorexia, constipation, diarrhea, dry mouth, dysgeusia, mild elevations of AST, ALT, LDH, and alkaline phosphatase (see Warnings and Precautions, Acute Hepatic Injury), thirst, vomiting, weight increase.

Dermatological: petechiae, photosensitivity, pruritus.

Other: amblyopia, CPK increase, dyspnea, epistaxis, eye irritation, hyperglycemia, hyperuricemia, impotence, nasal congestion, nocturia, osteoarticular pain, polyuria, sexual difficulties, dry mouth.

The following postmarketing events have been reported infrequently in patients receiving diltiazem: alopecia, erythema multiforme, exfoliative dermatitis, Stevens-Johnson syndrome, angioedema, toxic epidermal necrolysis, extrapyramidal symptoms, gingival hyperplasia, hemolytic anemia, increased bleeding time, leukopenia, purpura, retinopathy, and thrombocytopenia. In addition, adverse reactions such as myocardial infarction have been observed which are not readily distinguishable from the natural history of the disease in these patients. A number of well-documented cases of generalized rash, characterized as leukocytoclastic vasculitis, have been reported. However, a definitive cause and effect relationship between these events and diltiazem therapy is yet to be established.

DRUG INTERACTIONS: Overview: As with all drugs, care should be exercised when treating patients with multiple medications. Calcium channel blockers undergo biotransformation by the cytochrome P450 system. Coadministration of diltiazem with other drugs which follow the same route of biotransformation may result in altered bioavailability. Dosages of similarly metabolized drugs, particularly those of low therapeutic ratio, and especially in patients with renal and/or hepatic impairment, may require adjustment when starting or stopping concomitantly administered diltiazem to maintain optimum therapeutic blood levels.

Drugs known to be inhibitors of the cytochrome P450 system include: azole antifungals, cimetidine, cyclosporine, erythromycin, quinidine, and warfarin. Drugs known to be inducers of the cytochrome P450 system include: phenobarbital, phenytoin, and rifampin.

Drugs known to be biotransformed via P450 include: benzodiazepines, flecainide, imipramine, propafenone, terfenadine, and theophylline.

Amoxicillin: There was no increased risk of sudden cardiac death among users of amoxicillin.

Anaesthetics: The depression of cardiac contractility, conductivity, and automaticity as well as the vascular dilation associated with anesthetics may be potentiated by calcium channel blockers. When used concomitantly, anesthetics and calcium blockers should be titrated carefully.

Benzodiazepines: Diltiazem significantly increases peak plasma levels and the elimination half-life of triazolam and midazolam.

Beta-Blockers: The concomitant administration of diltiazem with beta-adrenergic blocking drugs warrants caution, and requires close medical supervision. Such an association may have an additive effect on heart rate, on AV conduction or on blood pressure (see Warnings and Precautions). Appropriate dosage adjustments may be necessary. A study in five normal subjects showed that diltiazem increased propranolol bioavailability by 50%.

Carbamazepine: Concomitant administration of diltiazem with carbamazepine has been reported to result in elevated serum levels of carbamazepine (40% to 72% increase), resulting in toxicity in some cases. Patients receiving these drugs concurrently should be monitored for a potential drug interaction.

Cimetidine: A study in six healthy volunteers has shown a significant increase in peak diltiazem plasma levels (58%) and area-under-the-curve (53%) after a 1-week course of cimetidine 1200 mg per day and a single dose of diltiazem 60 mg. Ranitidine produced smaller, nonsignificant increases. The effect may be mediated by cimetidine's known inhibition of hepatic cytochrome P450, the enzyme system responsible for the first-pass metabolism of diltiazem. Patients currently receiving diltiazem therapy should be carefully monitored for a change in pharmacological effect when initiating and discontinuing therapy with cimetidine. An adjustment in the diltiazem dose may be warranted.

Cyclosporine: A pharmacokinetic interaction between diltiazem and cyclosporine has been observed during studies involving renal and cardiac transplant patients. In renal and cardiac transplant recipients, a reduction of cyclosporine dose ranging from 15% to 48% was necessary to maintain cyclosporine trough concentrations similar to those seen prior to the addition of diltiazem. If these agents are to be administered concurrently, cyclosporine concentrations should be monitored, especially when diltiazem therapy is initiated, adjusted, or discontinued. The effect of cyclosporine on diltiazem plasma concentrations has not been evaluated.

Digitalis: Diltiazem and digitalis glycosides may have an additive effect in prolonging AV conduction. In clinical trials, concurrent administration of diltiazem and digoxin have resulted in increases in serum digoxin levels with prolongation of AV conduction. This increase may result from a decrease in renal clearance of digoxin. Patients on concomitant therapy, especially those with renal impairment, should be carefully monitored. The dose of digoxin may need downward adjustment.

Erythromycin: The use of erythromycin should be avoided in patients treated with CYP3A inhibitors, including diltiazem. An analysis reported in the literature indicates that the risk of sudden death is increased in current users of erythromycin (incidence-rate ratio=2.01; 95% CI=1.08 to 3.75), and this risk is further elevated in concurrent users of CYP3A inhibitors (5.35; 95% CI=1.72 to 16.64), including diltiazem. Cohort analysis revealed one death in 106 person—years in diltiazem-treated patients.

Rifampin: Administration of diltiazem with rifampin markedly reduced plasma diltiazem concentrations and the therapeutic effect of diltiazem.

Short- and Long acting Nitrates: Diltiazem may be safely co-administered with nitrates.

Statins: The concomitant administration of diltiazem with statin drugs warrants caution, and requires close medical supervision. Rhabdomyolysis and hepatitis have been reported in patients treated with atorvastatin or simvastatin in combination with diltiazem, and in the case of simvastatin-treated patients, deaths have occurred. If diltiazem is prescribed to a patient already taking a statin, consideration should be given to decreasing the dose of the statin.

In a published study of 10 healthy volunteers treated with simvastatin 20 mg, after 2 weeks of treatment with diltiazem 240 mg, the mean C_{max} (3.6-fold) and AUC (5-fold) of simvastatin were increased significantly.

Alcohol: There is no known diltiazem reaction with alcohol.

DOSAGE AND ADMINISTRATION: Dosing Considerations: TIAZAC XC has an extended-release delivery system designed to deliver maximum effect in the morning when administered at night-time. Accordingly, TIAZAC XC should be administered once daily at bedtime. TIAZAC XC should not be chewed or crushed. TIAZAC XC may be taken with or without food, but should be so taken consistently.

Recommended Dose and Dose Adjustment: Hypertension: When used as monotherapy, usual starting doses for hypertension are 180 to 240 mg once daily. Maximum antihypertensive effect is usually observed after approximately 2 to 4 weeks of therapy; therefore, dosage adjustments should be scheduled accordingly.

A maximum daily dose of 360 mg should not be exceeded. The dosage of TIAZAC XC or concomitant antihypertensive agents may need to be adjusted when adding one to the other. See Warnings and Precautions regarding use with beta-blockers.

Angina: Dosage should be based on individual patient response. Treatment should start with 180 mg once daily; this may be increased at intervals of 7 to 14 days if adequate response is not obtained. Higher doses may not result in greater anti-anginal effect. The maximum dose is 360 mg once daily.

TIAZAC XC may be safely co-administered with short- and long-acting nitrates. Sublingual nitroglycerin may be taken as required to support acute anginal attacks during TIAZAC XC therapy.

OVERDOSAGE:

Significant diltiazem overdose causes cardiovascular and systemic toxicity and may be fatal. The onset of toxicity may be delayed in patients who have ingested a sustained release preparation such as TIAZAC XC. Symptomatic patients will have hypotension from peripheral vasodilation and impaired contractility. They will also have impaired conduction ranging from sinus bradycardia, atrioventricular blocks of varying degree, to asystole. Mental status will often be preserved although patients with hypotension may be drowsy or comatose. Hypoxia may be due to non-cardiogenic lung injury caused by precapillary vasodilation. Impaired gut motility may result in ileus. Patients are often hyperglycemic due to impaired insulin release. Fatalities may occur with large overdoses and in patients with coexisiting cardiac disease or with cardiotoxic coingestants.

Anyone who has ingested a significant overdose of diltiazem should be sent to hospital and expert advice from the local poison control center should be sought.

Severely symptomatic patients poisoned with diltiazem should receive supplemental oxygen and be stabilized in the usual fashion with attention to maintaining the airway and restoring circulation. An electrocardiogram and routine blood analysis including electrolytes, glucose, and the usual search for coingestants should be performed.

Induced emesis is contraindicated. Patients who present within an hour of a significant overdose of diltiazem should have gastric lavage followed by activated charcoal. Lavage is not indicated for patients with delayed presentations. Whole bowel irrigation may be considered in patients with significant ingestions of sustained-release diltiazem.

In the event of overdose or exaggerated response, appropriate supportive measures should be employed in addition to gastric lavage. The following measures may be considered:

Bradycardia: Atropine and intravenous fluids may suffice in patients with mild poisoning.

Hypotension: Calcium salts given intravenously (should be avoided in patients who may have coingested digoxin). Catecholamine pressors may be used to improve cardiac contractility (epinephrine, dopamine, dobutamine, isoproterenol) or vascular tone (norepinephrine, epinephrine, dopamine). High dose insulin together with glucose or glucagon may be effective in patients not responding to catecholamines.

Sustained release calcium channel blockers may cause delayed onset of toxicity and once established, toxicity may last for several days. Patients who have symptoms following a TIAZAC XC ingestion should be treated and monitored until all signs and symptoms of toxicity have resolved. Patients who remain asymptomatic with normal vital signs during a 24 hour period of observation in a monitored setting may be discharged.

For management of a suspected drug overdose, CPhA recommends that you contact your **regional Poison Control Centre**. See the *CPS* Directory section for a list of Poison Control Centres.

ACTION AND CLINICAL PHARMACOLOGY: TIAZAC XC (diltiazem hydrochloride) is a calcium ion cellular influx inhibitor (calcium channel blocker or calcium channel antagonist) of the benzothiazepine (non-dihydropyridine) class.

Mechanism of Action: The therapeutic effect of this group of drugs is believed to be related to their specific cellular action of selectively inhibiting transmembrane influx of calcium ions into cardiac muscle and vascular smooth muscle. The contractile processes of these tissues are dependent upon the movement of extracellular calcium into the cells through specific ion channels. Diltiazem blocks transmembrane influx of calcium through the slow channel without affecting, to any significant degree the transmembrane influx of sodium through the fast channel. This results in a reduction of free calcium ions available within cells of the above tissues. Diltiazem does not alter total serum calcium.

Hypertension: The antihypertensive effect of diltiazem is believed to be brought about largely by its vasodilatory action on peripheral blood vessels with resultant decrease in peripheral vascular resistance.

Angina: The precise mechanism by which diltiazem relieves angina has not been fully determined but it is believed to be brought about largely by its vasodilator action.

In angina due to coronary spasm, diltiazem increases myocardial oxygen delivery by dilating both large and small coronary arteries and by inhibiting coronary spasm at drug levels which cause little negative inotropic effect. The resultant increases in coronary blood flow are accompanied by dose-dependent decreases in systemic blood pressure and decreases in peripheral resistance.

In angina of effort it appears that the action of diltiazem is related to the reduction of myocardial oxygen demand. This is probably caused by a decrease in blood pressure brought about by the reduction of peripheral resistance and of heart rate.

Pharmacodynamics: Hypertension: In a double-blind clinical study, a diltiazem hydrochloride extended-release clinical trial formulation with the same bead coating as TIAZAC XC, administered daily at night for 7 weeks at doses of 120 mg, 240 mg, 360 mg and 540 mg was compared to administration of 360 mg in the morning. The 540 mg dose is not approved for use in Canada.

Group mean reductions in diastolic blood pressure between 6 AM and 12 NOON, as measured by ambulatory blood pressure monitoring (ABPM) for 120 mg, 240 mg, 360 mg and 540 mg taken at night were 4.7, 8.9, 10.2 and 14.8 mmHg, respectively, placebo-corrected. These reductions in diastolic blood pressure for all doses were significantly different from placebo and dose-related. Within this time period of 6 AM to 12 NOON, the 360 mg PM dose produced a statistically significant 3.3 mmHg greater reduction in diastolic blood pressure than the 360 mg AM dose.

When changes in mean seated office diastolic blood pressure from baseline were evaluated at 8 AM, the following decreases were noted: placebo 6.6 mmHg; 120 mg PM 10.5 mmHg; 240 mg PM 13.1 mmHg; 360 mg PM 15.5 mmHg; 540 mg PM 20.3 mmHg, with p<0.0001 for all comparisons with corresponding baseline measurements. For 360 mg AM, a mean decrease from baseline of 10.8 mmHg was seen, p<0.0001. When measured at 6 PM, the following decreases were noted: placebo 5.5 mmHg; 120 mg PM 5.2 mmHg; 240 mg PM 8.7 mmHg; 360 mg PM 10.3 mmHg; 540 mg PM 14.1 mmHg, with p<0.0001 for all comparisons with corresponding baseline measurements. For 360 mg AM, a mean decrease from baseline of 13.1 mmHg was seen, p<0.0001.

Angina: In a double-blind study involving 311 patients with chronic stable angina, evening doses of 180, 360 and 420 mg clinical trial formulation of TIAZAC XC were compared to placebo and to 360 mg administered in the morning. The 420 mg dose is not approved for use in Canada. All doses administered at night increased exercise tolerance when compared with placebo after 21 hours, during the diltiazem trough period. The median effect, placebo-subtracted, was 20 to 28 seconds for all three doses; no dose-response was demonstrated, ie. use of the higher doses tested did not consistently result in increased exercise tolerance. The 360 mg dose given in the morning also improved exercise tolerance when measured 25 hours later. As expected, the effect was smaller than the effects measured only 21 hours following nighttime administration. TIAZAC XC had a larger effect in increasing exercise tolerance at peak serum concentrations than at trough.

Hemodynamic and Electrophysiologic Effects: Diltiazem produces antihypertensive effects both in the supine and standing positions. Resting heart rate is usually slightly reduced. During dynamic exercise, increases in diastolic pressure are inhibited while maximum achievable systolic pressure is usually unaffected. Heart rate at maximum exercise is reduced. Studies to date, primarily in patients with normal ventricular function, have shown that cardiac output, ejection fraction and left ventricular end-diastolic pressure have not been affected.

Chronic therapy with diltiazem produces no change, or a decrease, in circulating plasma catecholamines. However, no increased activity of the renin-angiotensin-aldosterone axis has been observed.

Diltiazem inhibits the renal and peripheral effects of angiotensin II.

In man, intravenous diltiazem in doses of 20 mg prolongs atrio-His conduction time and atrioventricular node functional and effective refractory periods by approximately 20%. Chronic oral administration of diltiazem in doses up to 540 mg per day has resulted in small increases in PR interval. Second degree and third degree AV block have been observed (see Warnings and Precautions). In patients with sick sinus syndrome, diltiazem significantly prolongs sinus cycle length (up to 50% in some cases).

Pharmacokinetics: Absorption: Diltiazem is well absorbed from the gastrointestinal tract and is subject to an extensive first-pass effect giving absolute bioavailability (compared to intravenous dosing) of about 40%.

Distribution: Therapeutic blood levels appear to be in the range of 50-200 ng/mL. In vitro human serum binding studies revealed that 70 to 80% of diltiazem is bound to plasma proteins. The pharmacokinetics of diltiazem are non-linear.

Metabolism: The metabolic pathways of diltiazem include N- and O-demethylation (via cytochrome P450), deacetylation (via plasma and tissue esterases), in addition to conjugation (via sulfation and glucuridonation). In vitro studies have demonstrated that CYP 3A4 is the principal CYP isoenzyme involved in N-demethylation. The active metabolite, desacetyl diltiazem, is present in the plasma at levels 10-20% of the parent drug and is 25-50% as potent as diltiazem in terms of coronary vasodilation.

Excretion: Following extensive hepatic metabolism, only 2-4% of the drug appears unchanged in the urine and 6-7% appears as metabolites

TIAZAC XC Tablets: TIAZAC XC has an extended-release delivery system designed for night-time administration, resulting in maximum diltiazem plasma levels in the morning.

Administration of TIAZAC XC tablets in the fasted state at bedtime, in a single study, resulted in detectable dilitazem plasma levels after 3 to 4 hours, and peak plasma levels between 11 and 18 hours post dose. After single dosing, diltiazem bioavailability ranged from 2.5% to 16% over the first six hours. The apparent elimination half-life for TIAZAC XC after single or multiple dosing is 6 to 9 hours.

When a single dose of 360 mg TIAZAC XC tablets, administered at night, was compared to the same dose given in the morning, an 18% greater systemic exposure and 11% higher peak exposure were observed at night relative to morning. Under steady-state conditions, night-time administration resulted in 22% and 16% greater systemic and peak exposure, respectively, relative to morning administration.

When single doses of 360 mg TIAZAC XC tablets were given in the morning to assess potential food interaction, the observed ratios of means were AUC_{tau} 112.4% (90% C.I. 101.2-124.9) and C_{max} 104.0% (90% C.I. 92.9-116.5) for the fed/fasted comparison (see Dosage and Administration).

While both TIAZAC XC tablets and TIAZAC capsules possess the same immediate release diltiazem-containing bead cores, the release-controlling polymer bead coatings are different, resulting in different bioavailability profiles. Further, the TIAZAC beads are encapsulated in gelatin capsules to produce the TIAZAC formulation, while TIAZAC XC tablet beads are blended with inert wax beads and excipients, then compressed into tablets.

Diltiazem time course kinetics, as noted across studies in healthy volunteers that evaluated TIAZAC XC tablets and TIAZAC capsules respectively, are presented below in Figure 1.

Figure 1: TIAZAC XC

24-hour Diltiazem Plasma Concentration Time Course at Steady-state[a]

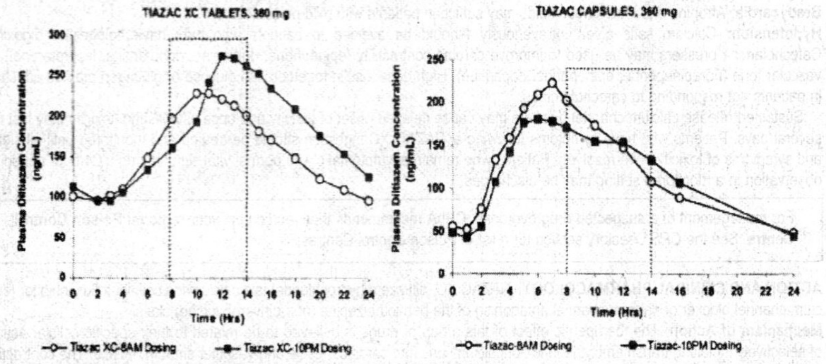

[a] Data for each graph were obtained from separate studies.

No studies are available that compare the relative bioavailability of TIAZAC XC tablets to TIAZAC capsules directly.

Special Populations and Conditions: Pediatrics: Pharmacokinetic studies with TIAZAC XC in children have not been conducted.

Geriatrics: Pharmacokinetic studies with TIAZAC XC in geriatrics have not been conducted. However it is known that administration of diltiazem to elderly patients (over or equal to 65 years of age) requires caution. The incidence of adverse reactions is approximately 13% higher in this group.

Sex: In pharmacokinetic studies in healthy volunteers, there were no statistically significant differences between male and female subjects with respect to the AUC (p=0.099) and C_{max} (p=0.295).

Race: The effect of race in pharmacokinetic studies has not been evaluated.

Hepatic Insufficiency: No pharmacokinetic studies have been conducted with TIAZAC XC in patients with hepatic insufficiency.

Renal Insufficiency: No pharmacokinetic studies have been conducted with TIAZAC XC in patients with renal insufficiency.

STORAGE AND STABILITY: Store at room temperature (15-30 °C). Avoid excessive humidity, and temperatures above 30 °C.

INFORMATION FOR THE PATIENT: Published in e-CPS, available by subscription at www.e-cps.ca.

DOSAGE FORMS, COMPOSITION AND PACKAGING: 120 mg: Each white, film-coated, extended-release tablet, debossed with "B" on one side, and the strength on the other, contains: diltiazem HCl 120 mg. Nonmedicinal ingredients: carnauba wax, colloidal silicone dioxide, croscarmellose sodium, eudragit, hydrogenated vegetable oil, hydroxypropylmethylcellulose, magnesium stearate, microcrystalline cellulose, microcrystalline wax, polydextrose, polyethylene glycol, polysorbate, povidone, pregelatinized starch, simethicone, sodium starch glycolate, sucrose stearate, talc and titanium dioxide. Bottles of 90.

180 mg: Each white, film-coated, extended-release tablet, debossed with "B" on one side, and the strength on the other, contains: diltiazem HCl 180 mg. Nonmedicinal ingredients: carnauba wax, colloidal silicone dioxide, croscarmellose sodium, eudragit, hydrogenated vegetable oil, hydroxypropylmethylcellulose, magnesium stearate, microcrystalline cellulose, microcrystalline wax, polydextrose, polyethylene glycol, polysorbate, povidone, pregelatinized starch, simethicone, sodium starch glycolate, sucrose stearate, talc and titanium dioxide. Bottles of 90.

240 mg: Each white, film-coated, extended-release tablet, debossed with "B" on one side, and the strength on the other, contains: diltiazem HCl 240 mg. Nonmedicinal ingredients: carnauba wax, colloidal silicone dioxide, croscarmellose sodium, eudragit, hydrogenated vegetable oil, hydroxypropylmethylcellulose, magnesium stearate, microcrystalline cellulose, microcrystalline wax, polydextrose, polyethylene glycol, polysorbate, povidone, pregelatinized starch, simethicone, sodium starch glycolate, sucrose stearate, talc and titanium dioxide. Bottles of 90.

300 mg: Each white, film-coated, extended-release tablet, debossed with "B" on one side, and the strength on the other, contains: diltiazem HCl 300 mg. Nonmedicinal ingredients: carnauba wax, colloidal silicone dioxide, croscarmellose sodium, eudragit, hydrogenated vegetable oil, hydroxypropylmethylcellulose, magnesium stearate, microcrystalline cellulose, microcrystalline wax, polydextrose, polyethylene glycol, polysorbate, povidone, pregelatinized starch, simethicone, sodium starch glycolate, sucrose stearate, talc and titanium dioxide. Bottles of 90.

360 mg: Each white, film-coated, extended-release tablet, debossed with "B" on one side, and the strength on the other, contains: diltiazem HCl 360 mg. Nonmedicinal ingredients: carnauba wax, colloidal silicone dioxide, croscarmellose sodium, eudragit, hydrogenated vegetable oil, hydroxypropylmethylcellulose, magnesium stearate, microcrystalline cellulose, microcrystalline wax, polydextrose, polyethylene glycol, polysorbate, povidone, pregelatinized starch, simethicone, sodium starch glycolate, sucrose stearate, talc and titanium dioxide. Bottles of 90.

(Shown in Product Identification Section)

Ticlopidine ℞

Platelet-aggregation Inhibitor

CPhA Monograph

Date of Preparation: October 2007

This monograph has been compiled by CPhA and reviewed by experts. It may contain information different from that found in Health Canada-approved Product Monographs. The reader is referred to the *CPS* Editorial Policy for more information.

SUMMARY PRODUCT INFORMATION:

Route of Administration	Dosage Form	Strength
Oral	Tablet	250 mg

INDICATIONS AND CLINICAL USE: Ticlopidine is indicated for reduction of risk of a first or recurrent stroke in patients who have had a previous thromboembolic stroke, minor stroke, reversible ischemic neurologic deficit or transient ischemic attack including transient monocular blindness.

Although approved for secondary prevention of thromboembolic stroke, ticlopidine is not the preferred antithrombotic therapy for this indication. Ticlopine has been compared with placebo and ASA for the secondary prevention of ischemic stroke. At a dose of 500 mg/day, ticlopidine was significantly more effective than placebo in preventing stroke, myocardial infarction or vascular death in the Canadian American Ticlopidine Study (CATS) [*Lancet* 1989;1(8649):1215-20]. The results of the randomized, double-blind Ticlopidine Aspirin Stroke Study (TASS) suggested that ticlopidine 500 mg/day was more effective than ASA 1300 mg/day in reducing the incidence of nonfatal stroke or all cause mortality (3 year event rate 17% for ticlopidine vs. 19% for ASA, p=0.48) [*N Engl J Med* 1989;321(8):501-7]. However, there was no statistically significant difference in the rate of the composite endpoint of recurrent stroke, myocardial infarction or vascular death in patients randomized to ticlopidine 500 mg/day (15%) or ASA 650 mg/day (12%) in a subsequent double-blind study [*JAMA* 2003;289(22):2947-57]. It should be noted that the dose of ASA used in these trials is higher than that currently recommended for prevention of ischemic stroke (50 to 325 mg/day). ASA and other antithrombotic agents are effective in the secondary prevention of ischemic stroke, but are associated with a lower incidence of blood dyscrasias than ticlopidine; thus, use of ticlopidine is not recommended in treatment guidelines for the secondary prevention of ischemic stroke [*Stroke* 2006;37(2):577-617].

In recipients of intracoronary stents, the combination of ticlopidine plus ASA is significantly more effective than ASA alone or ASA plus warfarin in preventing the composite endpoint of death, revascularization of the target lesion, thrombosis as evidenced by angiography or myocardial infarction within 30 days [*N Engl J Med* 1998; 339(23):1665-1671]. However, the 30-day incidence of major cardiac adverse events is lower in patients treated with the combination of clopidogrel plus ASA than with the combination of ticlopidine plus ASA, according to a meta-analysis of data from 13,955 patients [*J Am Coll Cardiol* 2002;39(1):9-14]. Because of the greater efficacy and better tolerability of clopidogrel over ticlopidine, the combination of clopidogrel plus ASA is the preferred antiplatelet regimen for prevention of thrombosis after placement of intracoronary stents [*Circulation* 2006; 113(1):156-175].

In patients with unstable angina or non-ST segment elevation myocardial infarction who are allergic to clopidogrel, ticlopidine is recommended for use in combination with ASA. This recommendation applies to patients treated with medical therapy without stents, and to those receiving bare-metal or drug-eluting stents [*Circulation* 2007;116(7):148-304]. Clopidogrel is preferred over ticlopidine in this setting because of its more rapid onset of action, especially after a loading dose, and its better tolerability profile.

Ticlopidine (or clopidogrel) may be substituted for ASA in patients presenting with ST segment elevation myocardial infarction who have a true allergy to ASA as indicated by a history of hives, nasal polyps, bronchospasm, or anaphylaxis [*Circulation* 2004;110(9):82-292].

CONTRAINDICATIONS:

- Hypersensitivity to ticlopidine
- Active bleeding (e.g., intracranial hemorrhage, peptic ulcer)
- Hematopoietic disorders (e.g., neutropenia, thrombocytopenia)
- Thrombotic thrombocytopenic purpura (TTP)
- Hemostatic disorders
- Severe liver dysfunction

WARNINGS AND PRECAUTIONS:

Serious Warnings and Precautions
- Severe, sometimes fatal hematologic and hemorrhagic adverse effects can occur.
- GI bleeding

Endocrine and Metabolism: Total serum cholesterol and triglyceride concentrations increased by up to 8% to 10% during the first month of treatment with ticlopidine in clinical trials. Further increases in serum lipids did not generally occur in these studies.

Hematologic: The most serious hematologic adverse effects of ticlopidine include neutropenia, TTP, agranulocytosis, and aplastic anemia.

TTP is a rare but potentially fatal adverse event that manifests as a multisystem disorder characterized by thrombocytopenia, microangiopathic hemolytic anemia, renal dysfunction, neurologic abnormalities, and fever. Prompt institution of therapeutic plasma exchange enhances the likelihood of survival, especially if the onset of TTP occurs more than 2 weeks after initiation of therapy [*J Am Coll Cardiol* 2007;50(12):1138-43].

Severe neutropenia (absolute neutrophil count <0.45×10^9 cells/L) may have a sudden onset, generally occurs during the first 3 to 12 weeks of treatment, and was reported in 0.8% of patients enrolled in clinical trials. Ticlopidine-associated neutropenia is generally reversible upon discontinuation of the drug, with recovery occurring within 1 to 3 weeks; however, the condition can be life threatening and deaths have occurred.

Thrombocytopenia, alone or in combination with neutropenia, has occurred during treatment with ticlopidine. The onset is generally within the first 3 to 12 weeks of treatment with the drug. Recovery of platelet counts generally occurs upon discontinuation of ticlopidine.

Hemorrhagic Complications: A wide range of hemorrhagic complications (post-traumatic bleeding, perioperative bleeding, ecchymosis, epistaxis, hematuria, conjunctival hemorrhage, petechiae, GI hemorrhage, hematemesis, gingival bleeding, melena, hemothorax, menorrhagia, and intracerebral hemorrhage) have been reported during treatment with ticlopidine.

Hepatic Considerations: Ticlopidine is a prodrug that is converted to its active form via hepatic metabolism. Use of the drug in patients with severe hepatic dysfunction is contraindicated.

Abnormal hepatic function tests were reported in 1% of patients enrolled in clinical trials of the drug; thus serum transaminase (ALT, AST) and alkaline phosphatase levels should be monitored during the first 4 months of therapy if liver dysfunction is suspected.

Peri-Operative Considerations: Ticlopidine should be discontinued 14 days prior to elective surgery or dental extraction. For urgent surgery, the effects of ticlopidine may be reversed by transfusion of platelets, but not by administration of fresh frozen plasma.

Renal: Ticlopidine is not eliminated by renal excretion, and routine dosage adjustments are not required in patients with renal impairment. Supplementary doses are not required after hemodialysis or peritoneal dialysis.

Special Populations: Pregnant Women: Category B. Ticlopidine was not teratogenic when administered to mice, rats and rabbits. It is not known whether the drug crosses the placenta and there is very limited experience with ticlopidine in human pregnancy; thus, it is not possible to make definitive statements regarding the safety of the drug in this setting.

Nursing Women: Ticlopidine is excreted in the breast milk of lactating rats; no human data are available. Given the potential hematologic complications associated with the drug it is best avoided during breastfeeding.
Pediatrics: The safety and efficacy of ticlopidine in children have not been established.
Monitoring and Laboratory Tests: All patients should be monitored for signs and symptoms of bleeding during treatment with ticlopidine. Monitor complete blood count with differential prior to ticlopidine therapy, every 2 weeks during the first three months of therapy and periodically thereafter. Monitor alkaline phosphatase and serum transaminase levels at baseline and during the first four months of therapy if liver dysfunction is suspected.
ADVERSE REACTIONS: Adverse Drug Reactions Overview: See Table 1.

Table 1: Ticlopidine
More Common Adverse Drug Reactions (≥1%) Reported in Placebo-controlled Trials

Body System	Effect	Ticlopidine (% of patients)	Placebo (% of patients)	Clinical Comment
Gastrointestinal	Diarrhea	13	5	Advise patients to take ticlopidine tablets with meals to minimize gastrointestinal adverse events
	Dyspepsia	7	1	
	Nausea	7	2	
	Gastrointestinal pain	4	1	
	Vomiting	2	1	
	Flatulence	2	0	
	Anorexia	1	0	
Dermatologic	Rash	5	1	Counsel patients to report rash if it occurs
	Purpura	2	0	
	Pruritus	1	0	
Hematologic	Neutropenia	2	1	Monitor CBC and differential in all patients
CNS	Dizziness	1	0	

Less Common Adverse Drug Reactions (<1%): Central Nervous System: headache, pain.
Allergic/Dermatologic: urticaria, rash, Stevens-Johnson syndrome, erythema multiforme, erythema nodosum, exfoliative dermatitis.
Hematologic: thrombocytopenia, TTP, agranulocytosis, aplastic anemia, eosinophilia, pancytopenia, thrombocytosis, bone marrow suppression, hemorrhage
Hepatic/Biliary/Pancreatic: elevated liver enzymes, cholestatic jaundice, hepatocellular jaundice, hepatitis.
Immunologic: anaphylaxis, angioedema, serum sickness, systemic lupus erythematosus (antinuclear antibody formation).
Musculoskeletal: arthropathy, myositis.
Neurologic: peripheral neuropathy, asthenia.
Pulmonary: bronchiolitis obliterans-organizing pneumonia.
Renal: renal failure, nephrotic syndrome.
Abnormal Hematologic and Clinical Chemistry Findings: See Table 2.

Table 2: Ticlopidine
Abnormal Hematologic and Clinical Chemistry Findings

Test	Effect	Clinical Comment
Complete blood count	Clinically significant blood dyscrasias (e.g., neutropenia in approximately 2% of patients, thrombocytopenia, TTP in <1% of patients)	Usually occurs between 3 and 12 weeks after starting therapy. Monitor CBC with differential at baseline and then every two weeks during the first 12 weeks of therapy and then periodically thereafter.
Hepatic	Alkaline phosphatase increase (>2×ULN)	Usually occurs within 1–4 months of starting therapy. Monitor alkaline phosphatase
Cholesterol	HDL-C, LDL-C, VLDL-C, triglycerides increased 8–10% after 1–4 months of therapy.	Consider monitoring serum lipid levels

DRUG INTERACTIONS:

Serious Drug Interactions
- Potential for bleeding is increased with concomitant use of heparin, oral anticoagulants and other antiplatelet agents. Close clinical and laboratory monitoring is required with concomitant use.

Drug-Drug Interactions: See Table 3.

Table 3: Ticlopidine
Drug-Drug Interactions

Interacting Drug	Effect	Clinical Comment
Antacids	Decreased ticlopidine levels	Separate administration by 1 to 2 hours
Anticoagulants (heparin, warfarin)	Increased bleeding potential	Monitor INR and aPTT
ASA	Increased bleeding potential	Monitor for signs of bleeding
Cimetidine	Increased ticlopidine levels	Avoid
Cyclosporine	Decreased cyclosporine levels	Monitor cyclosporine levels when starting or stopping ticlopidine

(cont'd)

Table 3: Ticlopidine *(cont'd)*
Drug-Drug Interactions

Interacting Drug	Effect	Clinical Comment
Nonsteroidal anti-inflammatory drugs other than ASA	Increased bleeding potential	Avoid if possible. Monitor for signs of bleeding if used concomitantly
Phenytoin	Increased phenytoin levels and toxicity	Monitor for signs of phenytoin toxicity. Monitor phenytoin levels and adjust dose, if necessary, when starting or stopping ticlopidine
Theophylline	Increased theophylline levels	Monitor for signs of theophylline toxicity. Monitor theophylline levels and adjust dose, if necessary, when starting or stopping ticlopidine
Thrombolytics (e.g., alteplase, streptokinase)	Increased bleeding potential	Monitor for signs of bleeding
Digoxin	Decreased digoxin levels	Monitor patients and adjust dose of digoxin, if necessary, when starting or stopping ticlopidine

Drug-Food Interactions: The oral bioavailability of ticlopidine is increased by 20% when taken after a meal. Administer with food to minimize GI intolerance.

DOSAGE AND ADMINISTRATION: Recommended Dose and Dosage Adjustment: Adults: See Table 4.

Table 4: Ticlopidine
Dose in Adult Patients

Indication	Route	Loading Dose	Usual Dose	Maximum Dose	Clinical Comment
As an antithrombotic agent	Oral	None	250 mg BID	250 mg BID	Take with meals to minimize GI intolerance. If diarrhea occurs, a temporary dose reduction (e.g., 125 mg BID) may be tried.
Unstable angina/non-ST segment elevation myocardial infarction (patients allergic to clopidogrel)	Oral	500 mg once	250 mg BID	250 mg BID	Administer in combination with ASA for at least 1 month and ideally for up to 1 year in patients receiving medical therapy only and in those receiving bare metal stents, or for at least 1 year in patients receiving drug-eluting stents.

Renal Impairment: Ticlopidine is not eliminated by renal excretion; thus, dosage adjustments are generally not required in patients with renal impairment. Supplemental doses are not required in patients receiving hemodialysis or peritoneal dialysis.
Hepatic Impairment: The average plasma concentration in patients with advanced cirrhosis was slightly higher than that seen in older subjects. Ticlopidine is converted to an active metabolite by hepatic metabolism; thus, use in patients with severe hepatic dysfunction is contraindicated.

OVERDOSAGE:

For management of a suspected drug overdose, CPhA recommends that you contact your **regional Poison Control Centre**. See the *CPS* Directory section for a list of Poison Control Centres.

ACTION AND CLINICAL PHARMACOLOGY: Mechanism of Action: Ticlopidine is an irreversible platelet aggregation inhibitor. The drug antagonizes the effects of ADP at P2Y12 receptors located on the platelet membrane, thereby inhibiting ADP-mediated platelet aggregation. The effect on platelet function is irreversible and persists for the life of the platelet, which is approximately 7 to 10 days.

The onset of platelet inhibition occurs within 24 to 48 hours, although maximal inhibition requires 5 to 7 days of administration.
Pharmacokinetics: Adults: Absorption: Ticlopidine is rapidly absorbed from the gastrointestinal tract (> 80%) after oral administration.
Distribution: Peak plasma levels occur approximately 2 hours after oral administration.
Metabolism: Ticlopidine is a prodrug that is converted to an active metabolite by hepatic cytochrome P450 (CYP)-mediated metabolism. CYP2C19 is thought to be responsible for generation of the active metabolite. Ticlopidine is extensively metabolized in the liver and only trace amounts of intact drug are detected in the urine. The initial half-life is about 7 hours; with chronic dosing, the half-life increases to approximately 4 days.
Excretion: Approximately 60% of a dose is excreted in urine, almost completely as metabolites. Clearance decreases with age. Steady-state trough values in elderly patients (mean age 70 years) are about twice those in younger populations.

Timentin® Ⓟ

ticarcillin disodium—potassium clavulanate
Antibiotic—β-Lactamase Inhibitor

GlaxoSmithKline

Date of Revision: March 16, 2009

PHARMACOLOGY: Ticarcillin exerts a bactericidal action against sensitive organisms during the stage of active multiplication, through the inhibition of the biosynthesis of bacterial cell wall mucopeptides. Clavulanic acid inhibits specific β-lactamases of some microorganisms and allows ticarcillin to inhibit ticarcillin resistant organisms which produce clavulanic acid sensitive β-lactamases.

INDICATIONS: Treatment: For the treatment of the following infections when caused by Timentin-susceptible strains of the designated bacteria: Bacterial septicemia when caused by β-lactamase (excluding Type I) producing strains of *E. coli*, *S. aureus*, and Klebsiella species.

Lower respiratory infections when caused by β-lactamase (excluding Type I) producing strains of *S. aureus*, *H. influenzae* and Klebsiella species.

Bone infections when caused by β-lactamase producing strains of *S. aureus*.

Skin structure infections when caused by β-lactamase (excluding Type I) producing strains of *S. aureus*, *E. coli* and Klebsiella species.

Urinary tract infections when caused by β-lactamase (excluding Type I) producing strains of *E. coli* and Klebsiella species.

Gynecologic infections when caused by β-lactamase (excluding Type I) producing strains of Bacteroides species, *E. coli*, *S. aureus*, *S. epidermidis* and Klebsiella species.

Intra-abdominal infections including peritonitis and intra-abdominal abscess, when caused by β-lactamase (excluding Type 1) producing strains of *E. coli*, *K. pneumoniae*, *B. fragilis*, and *P. aeruginosa*. The efficacy and safety of Timentin for the treatment of intra-abdominal infections in infants and children under the age of 12 have not been established.

Appropriate culture and susceptibility tests should be performed before treatment, in order to isolate and identify organisms causing infection and to determine their susceptibilities to Timentin. Therapy may, however, be initiated before results of such tests are known when there is reason to believe the infection may involve any of the β-lactamase (excluding Type I) producing organisms listed above. Modification of the treatment may be required once these results become available or if there is no clinical response.

The treatment of mixed infections caused by ticarcillin susceptible organisms and β-lactamase (excluding Type 1) producing organisms susceptible to Timentin should not require the addition of another antibiotic, due to the ticarcillin content of Timentin.

Prophylaxis: The administration of Timentin perioperatively (preoperatively, intraoperatively and postoperatively) may reduce the incidence of certain infections in patients undergoing elective surgical procedures (i.e., colorectal surgery and abdominal hysterectomy) that may be classified as contaminated or potentially contaminated.

In patients undergoing cesarean section, who are considered to be at increased risk of infection, intraoperative (after clamping the umbilical cord) and postoperative use of Timentin may reduce the incidence of surgery related postoperative infections.

The data from all the surgical prophylaxis trials were combined to obtain a sufficient number of patients to suggest that Timentin may be of value in reducing infection following colorectal surgery, abdominal hysterectomy or high-risk cesarean section.

If signs of postsurgical infection should appear, specimens for culture should be obtained for identification of the causative organism(s) so that appropriate therapy may be instituted.

CONTRAINDICATIONS: Patients with a history of hypersensitivity to beta-lactam antibiotics (e.g., penicillins, clavams, and cephalosporins).

WARNINGS: Serious and occasionally fatal hypersensitivity (anaphylactoid) reactions have been reported in patients on penicillin therapy. These reactions are more apt to occur in individuals with a history of penicillin hypersensitivity and/or a history of sensitivity to multiple allergens. There have been reports of individuals with a history of cephalosporin hypersensitivity who have experienced severe reactions when treated with penicillins. Before initiating therapy with Timentin, careful inquiry should be made concerning previous hypersensitivity reactions to beta-lactams (e.g., penicillins, cephalosporins, and clavams) or other allergens. If an allergic reaction occurs, the administration of Timentin should be discontinued and appropriate therapy should be instituted. Serious anaphylactoid reactions require immediate emergency treatment with epinephrine. Oxygen, i.v. steroids and airway management, including intubation, should also be used as indicated.

Patients with renal impairment or underlying hemostatic problems should be observed for bleeding manifestations. Such patients should be dosed strictly according to recommendations (see Dosage). If bleeding occurs, the administration of Timentin should be discontinued and appropriate therapy instituted.

Patients receiving Timentin may develop hemorrhagic manifestations associated with coagulation abnormalities, such as changes in bleeding time and platelet function, particularly if coadministered with drugs such as ASA or anticoagulants. If these occur, the administration of Timentin should be discontinued and appropriate therapy instituted. On withdrawal of the drug, the bleeding time and coagulation abnormalities should revert to normal after approximately 7 days. Other causes of abnormal bleeding should also be considered.

Gastrointestinal: *C. difficile*-associated Disease: *C. difficile*-associated disease (CDAD) has been reported with use of many antibacterial agents, including Timentin. CDAD may range in severity from mild diarrhea to fatal colitis. It is important to consider this diagnosis in patients who present with diarrhea, or symptoms of colitis, pseudomembranous colitis, toxic megacolon, or perforation of colon subsequent to the administration of any antibacterial agent. CDAD has been reported to occur over 2 months after the administration of antibacterial agents.

Treatment with antibacterial agents may alter the normal flora of the colon and may permit overgrowth of *C. difficile*. *C. difficile* produces toxins A and B, which contribute to the development of CDAD. CDAD may cause significant morbidity and mortality. CDAD can be refractory to antimicrobial therapy.

If the diagnosis of CDAD is suspected or confirmed, appropriate therapeutic measures should be initiated. Mild cases of CDAD usually respond to discontinuation of antibacterial agents not directed against *C. difficile*. In moderate to severe cases, consideration should be given to management with fluids and electrolytes, protein supplementation, and treatment with an antibacterial agent clinically effective against *C. difficile*. Surgical evaluation should be instituted as clinically indicated, as surgical intervention may be required in certain severe cases (see Adverse Effects).

PRECAUTIONS: General: The total daily dosage should be reduced when Timentin is administered to patients with transient or persistent reduction of urinary output due to renal insufficiency (see Dosage) because high and prolonged serum antibiotic concentrations can occur from usual doses.

Periodic assessment of organ system functions, including renal, hepatic and hematopoietic function should be made during prolonged therapy with Timentin.

Bleeding manifestations have occurred in some patients receiving beta-lactam antibiotics. These reactions have been associated with abnormalities of coagulation tests such as clotting time, platelet aggregation and prothrombin time and are more likely to occur in patients with renal impairment. If bleeding manifestations appear, Timentin treatment should be discontinued and appropriate therapy instituted.

The passage of any penicillin from blood into brain is facilitated by inflamed meninges and during cardiopulmonary bypass. In the presence of these conditions and particularly when accompanied by renal failure, sufficiently high serum ticarcillin concentration can be attained to produce CNS adverse effects: these include myoclonia, convulsive seizures and depressed consciousness.

Timentin has been reported to cause hypokalemia; therefore, the possibility of this occurring should be kept in mind particularly when treating patients with fluid and electrolyte imbalance. Periodic monitoring of serum potassium is advisable and, when necessary, corrective therapy should be implemented.

The theoretical sodium content is 4.75 mEq (109 mg)/g of Timentin. This should be included in the daily allowance of patients on sodium-restricted diets. Electrolyte levels and cardiac status should be monitored carefully during treatment, particularly in patients with hypertension or congestive heart failure.

The possibility of overgrowth by non-susceptible organisms and species originally sensitive to Timentin should be kept in mind, particularly during prolonged treatment. If superinfection occurs during therapy, appropriate measures should be taken.

In patients with renal impairment, dosage should be adjusted according to the degree of impairment (see Dosage).

Children: The safety and efficacy for the treatment of infections in infants from birth to 1 month of age have not been established.

Pregnancy: The safety of Timentin in the treatment of infections during human pregnancy is unknown. Timentin should only be used during pregnancy if the anticipated benefit to the mother justifies the potential risk to the fetus.

Lactation: Trace quantities of Timentin are excreted in breast milk. Timentin may be administered during the period of lactation. With the exception of the risk of sensitization, there are no detrimental effects for the breast-fed infant.

Drug Interactions: Timentin should not be mixed with an aminoglycoside in the same container. Penicillins can cause substantial inactivation of aminoglycosides.

Probenecid decreases the renal tubular secretion of ticarcillin, thereby increasing serum concentrations and prolonging serum half-life of the antibiotic. Concurrent administration of probenecid delays ticarcillin renal excretion but does not delay the excretion of clavulanic acid.

In common with other antibiotics, ticarcillin may affect the gut flora, leading to lower estrogen reabsorption and reduced efficacy of combined oral contraceptives.

Laboratory Test Interactions: High urine concentrations of ticarcillin (>1500 mg/L 2 hours after an i.v. injection of 3.1 g Timentin) may produce false positive protein reactions (pseudoproteinuria) with the following methods: sulfosalicylic acid and boiling test, acetic acid test, biuret reaction, and nitric acid test. The bromphenol blue (Multi-stix) reagent strip test has been reported to be reliable.

The presence of clavulanic acid in Timentin may cause a non-specific binding of IgG and albumin by red cell membranes, leading to a false positive Coombs' test.

ADVERSE EFFECTS: The following adverse reactions may occur during Timentin therapy:

Hypersensitivity: skin rash, pruritus, urticaria, arthralgia, myalgia, drug fever, chills, chest discomfort, bronchospasm, wheezing, and anaphylactic reactions.

Bullous reactions (including erythema multiforme, Stevens-Johnson syndrome and toxic epidermal necrolysis) have been reported very rarely.

CNS: headache, giddiness, or neuromuscular hyperirritability. Convulsions, particularly in patients with impaired renal function or in those receiving high doses.

Gastrointestinal: disturbances of taste and smell, stomatitis, flatulence, nausea, vomiting and diarrhea, epigastric pain. Pseudomembranous colitis has been reported (see Warnings, Gastrointestinal, *C. difficile*-associated Disease).

Hemic and Lymphatic: thrombocytopenia, leukopenia, neutropenia, eosinophilia and reduction of hemoglobin or hematocrit. Prolongation of prothrombin time and bleeding time. Bleeding manifestations have occurred.

Hepatic Effects: a moderate rise in ALT and/or AST. Elevation of serum alkaline phosphatase, serum LDH, and serum bilirubin. Hepatitis and cholestatic jaundice have been reported very rarely.

Local Reactions: pain, burning, erythema, swelling and induration at the injection site and phlebitis and thrombophlebitis with i.v. administration.

Other: Increased muscle weakness in patients with myasthenia gravis has been reported.

Renal and Urinary Effects: elevation of serum creatinine and/or BUN, hypernatremia. Reduction in serum potassium and uric acid. Hypokalaemia has been reported rarely. Hemorrhagic cystitis has been reported very rarely.

OVERDOSE:

Symptoms: Gastrointestinal effects such as nausea, vomiting and diarrhea may be evident and should be treated symptomatically.

Disturbances of the fluid and electrolyte balance may be evident and may be treated symptomatically.

Timentin overdosage has the potential to cause neuromuscular hyperirritability or convulsive seizures.

Treatment: Ticarcillin and clavulanic acid may be removed from circulation by hemodialysis.

> For management of a suspected drug overdose, contact your **regional Poison Control Centre**. Further management should be as clinically indicated. See the *CPS* Directory section for a list of Poison Control Centres.

DOSAGE: Timentin should be administered only by i.v. infusion over 30 minutes.

Adults: Treatment: Dosage for any individual patient must take into consideration the site and severity of infection, the susceptibility of the organisms causing infection, and the status of the patient's host defense mechanisms.

The recommended dosage for adults (60 kg or greater) is 3.1 g every 4 to 6 hours.

For patients weighing less than 60 kg, the recommended dosage is 200-300 mg/kg/day, based on ticarcillin content, given in divided doses every 4 to 6 hours.

The duration of therapy depends upon the severity of infection. Generally, Timentin should be continued for at least 2 days after signs and symptoms of infection have disappeared. The usual duration is 10 to 14 days; however, in difficult and complicated infections, more prolonged therapy may be required. In certain infections, involving abscess formation, appropriate surgical drainage should be performed in conjunction with antimicrobial therapy.

Adults with Impaired Renal Function: The serum half-life of Timentin in patients with renal insufficiency is prolonged, consequently, the dosage regimen must be adjusted. Clinical efficacy data are insufficient at present to establish an appropriate dosage regimen for Timentin in patients with renal dysfunction.

However, on the basis of theoretical pharmacokinetic considerations (namely absence of any change in the pharmacokinetics of ticarcillin due to clavulanic acid and the apparent greater tissue clearance of clavulanic acid as compared to ticarcillin), it is suggested that for infections complicated by renal dysfunction, the dosage regimen as used currently for ticarcillin alone may generally be adopted (see Table 1).

An initial loading dose of 3.1 g Timentin followed by doses indicated in Table 1.

Table 1: Timentin

Dosage in Adults with Impaired Renal Function

Creatinine Clearance mL/min	Dosage (based on ticarcillin content)
Over 60	3 g every 4 hours
30–60	2 g every 4 hour
10–30	2 g every 8 hours
Less than 10	2 g every 12 hours
Less than 10 with hepatic dysfunction	2 g every 24 hours
Patients on peritoneal dialysis	3 g every 12 hours
Patients on hemodialysis	2 g every 12 hours supplemented with 3 g after each dialysis

The half-lives of ticarcillin and clavulanic acid in patients with renal dysfunction (creatinine clearance <10 mL/min) are 8.5 and 2.9 hours, respectively.

To calculate creatinine clearance from a serum creatinine value, use the following formula:

$$C_{cr} = \frac{(140-\text{age})\ (\text{wt in kg})}{72 \times S_{cr}\ (\text{mg/dL})}$$

This is the calculated creatinine clearance for adult males, for females it is 15% less. To convert calculated creatinine clearance to SI units (mL/second), multiply result by 0.0167.

Prophylaxis: For surgical prophylaxis, administration should not exceed the recommended dosage regimen, since the continued administration of any antibiotic increases the risk of adverse reactions while, in the majority of surgical procedures, does not reduce the incidence of subsequent infection.

A 3-dosage regimen is recommended as follows: Patients Undergoing Cesarean Section: Administer the first dose of 3.1 g Timentin as soon as the umbilical cord is clamped. The second and third dosage of 3.1 g should be administered at 4 hour intervals after the initial dose, for a total of 3 doses.

Patients Undergoing Abdominal Hysterectomy or Colorectal Surgery: Administer the first dose of 3.1 g Timentin one-half to 1 hour prior to the initial incision. The second and third dosage of 3.1 g should be administered at 4-hour intervals after the initial dose for a total of 3 doses.

Infants and Children (under 40 kg, 1 month to 12 years of age): Clinical and pharmacokinetic data are limited in these age groups. However, the dosages in Table 2, based on the ticarcillin content have been used. The daily dosages should not exceed the adult dose.

Neonates: The safety and efficacy for the treatment of infections in neonates (birth to 1 month of age) have not been established.

Administration: Timentin must not be administered by bolus i.v. injection or by i.m. injection.

The further diluted intravenous solution of Timentin should be administered over a period of 30 minutes by direct infusion or through a Y-type intravenous infusion set which may already be in place. If this method or the "piggyback" method of administration is used, it is advisable to discontinue temporarily the administration of any other solutions during the infusion of Timentin.

Timentin should not be physically mixed or administered at the same site with any other antimicrobial agent such as an aminoglycoside.

Reconstituted Solutions: For I.V. Infusion: **3.1 g vial:** Reconstitute each vial with 13 mL Sterile Water for Injection USP; when dissolved, the concentration of ticarcillin will be approximately 200 mg/mL with a corresponding concentration of 6.7 mg/mL for clavulanic acid (stock solution). Conversely, each 5.0 mL of the 3.1 g dose reconstituted with approximately 13 mL of diluent will contain approximately 1 g of ticarcillin and 33 mg of clavulanic acid.

31 g vial: Reconstitute each vial with 76 mL Sterile Water for Injection USP; when dissolved, concentration of ticarcillin will be approximately 300 mg/mL with a corresponding concentration of 10 mg/mL for clavulanic acid (stock solution). Conversely, each 5.0 mL of the 31 g dose reconstituted with approximately 76 mL of diluent will contain approximately 1.5 g of ticarcillin and 50 mg of clavulanic acid.

The dissolved drug should be further diluted to the desired volume using a suitable solution listed below. The further diluted solution of reconstituted drug may then be administered over a period of 30 minutes by direct infusion or through a Y-type intravenous infusion set which may already be in place. If this method or the "piggyback" method of administration is used, it is advisable to discontinue temporarily the administration of any other solutions during the infusion of Timentin.

Solutions for I.V. Infusion: Sodium Chloride Injection USP, Dextrose Injection 5% USP, sterile water for injection USP and Lactated Ringer's solution USP.

Note: When Timentin is given in combination with another antimicrobial such as an aminoglycoside, each drug should be given separately in accordance with the recommended dosage and routes of administration for each drug.

After reconstitution and further dilution and prior to administration, Timentin, as with other parenteral drugs, should be inspected visually for particulate matter and discoloration.

The reconstitution solution is clear, colorless or pale yellow, with a pH of 5.5 to 7.5.

For a 3.1 g dose of Timentin (using either the 3.1 g or 31 g vial), the theoretical sodium content is 4.75 mEq (109 mg)/g of Timentin and the theoretical potassium content is 0.15 mEq (6 mg)/g of Timentin.

Stability and Storage Recommendations: Timentin stock solution at 200 mg/mL or 300 mg/mL (ticarcillin) is stable for up to 6 hours at room temperature (21 to 24°C) or up to 72 hours under refrigeration (4°C).

Further diluted solutions of 200 mg/mL Timentin stock solution should be used within the stated time periods as shown in Table 3.

Table 2: Timentin

Dosage in Infants and Children

Infections		Dosage Schedule (mg/kg)[a]	Total Daily Dosage (mg/kg/day)
Non U.T.I.	severe	50 mg/kg every 4 hours	300
	mild-moderate	50 mg/kg every 6 hours	200
U.T.I.	complicated	50 mg/kg every 4 hours	300
	uncomplicated	50 mg/kg every 6 hours	200

[a] Based on ticarcillin content.

Table 3: Timentin

Stability Period

I.V. Solution	Room Temp. (21–24°C)	Refrigeration (4°C)
Sodium Chloride Injection USP	16 hours	48 hours
Dextrose Injection 5% USP	8 hours	24 hours
Lactated Ringer's Injection USP	16 hours	48 hours

Further diluted solutions of 300 mg/mL Timentin stock solution should be used within the stated time periods as shown in Table 4.

Table 4: Timentin

Stability Period

I.V. Solution	Room Temp. (21–24°C)	Refrigeration (4°C)
Sodium Chloride Injection USP	24 hours	3 days
Dextrose Injection 5% USP	24 hours	3 days
Lactated Ringer's Injection USP	24 hours	3 days
Sterile Water for Injection USP	24 hours	3 days

SUPPLIED: 3.1 g: Each vial contains: sterile ticarcillin disodium equivalent to ticarcillin 3 g and sterile potassium clavulanate equivalent to clavulanic acid 0.1 g.

31 g: Each vial contains: sterile ticarcillin disodium equivalent to ticarcillin 30 g and sterile potassium clavulanate equivalent to clavulanic acid 1 g.

Store at or below 24°C.

Timoptic® Ⓟ

timolol maleate

Elevated Intraocular Pressure Therapy

Merck Frosst

Date of Preparation: October 5, 1978
Date of Revision: May 4, 2007

SUMMARY PRODUCT INFORMATION:

Route of Administration	Dosage Form/ Strength	Clinically Relevant Nonmedicinal Ingredients
Ophthalmic	Solution, 0.5% timolol	For a complete listing see Dosage Forms, Composition and Packaging.

INDICATIONS AND CLINICAL USE: TIMOPTIC (timolol maleate ophthalmic solution, USP) is indicated for the reduction of elevated intraocular pressure.

In clinical trials TIMOPTIC has been shown to reduce intraocular pressure in:

- Patients with chronic open-angle glaucoma
- Patients with ocular hypertension
- Aphakic patients having glaucoma, including those wearing contact lenses
- Patients with narrow angles and a history of spontaneous or iatrogenically-induced narrow-angle closure in the opposite eye in whom reduction of intraocular pressure is necessary (see Warnings and Precautions).

CONTRAINDICATIONS:

- Hypersensitivity to any component of this product. For a complete listing of components see the Dosage Forms, Composition and Packaging.
- Bronchospasm, including bronchial asthma or a history of bronchial asthma or chronic obstructive pulmonary disease.
- Sinus bradycardia; second-and third-degree atrioventricular block; overt cardiac failure; cardiogenic shock.

WARNINGS AND PRECAUTIONS: General: As with other topically applied ophthalmic drugs, this drug may be absorbed systemically. The same adverse reactions reported with systemic beta-adrenergic blocking agents may occur with topical administration.

TIMOPTIC should be used with caution in patients subject to spontaneous hypoglycemia or in diabetic patients (especially those with labile diabetes) who are receiving insulin or oral hypoglycemic agents. Beta-adrenergic blocking agents may mask the signs and symptoms of acute hypoglycemia.

In patients with angle-closure glaucoma, the immediate objective of treatment is to reopen the angle. This requires constricting the pupil with a miotic. Timolol maleate has little or no effect on the pupil. When TIMOPTIC is used to reduce elevated intraocular pressure in angle-closure glaucoma they should be used with a miotic and not alone.

Cardiac failure should be adequately controlled before beginning therapy with TIMOPTIC. In patients with a history of severe cardiac disease, signs of cardiac failure should be watched for and pulse rates should be checked.

Respiratory reactions and cardiac reactions, including death due to bronchospasm in patients with asthma and rarely death in association with cardiac failure, have been reported following administration of timolol maleate ophthalmic solutions.

Because of the potential effects of beta-adrenergic blocking agents on blood pressure and pulse, these agents should be used with caution in patient with cerebrovascular insufficiency. If signs or symptoms suggesting reduced cerebral blood flow develop following initiation of therapy with TIMOPTIC, alternative therapy should be considered.

Endocrine and Metabolism: Thyrotoxicosis: β-adrenergic blocking agents may mask certain clinical signs of hyperthyroidism (e.g., tachycardia). Patients suspected of developing thyrotoxicosis should be managed carefully to avoid abrupt withdrawal of β-adrenergic blocking agents which might precipitate a thyroid storm.

Immune: Risk from Anaphylactic Reaction: While taking beta blockers, patients with a history of atopy or a history of severe anaphylactic reaction to a variety of allergens may be more reactive to repeated challenge with such allergens, either accidental, diagnostic, or therapeutic. These patients may be more resistant to treatment of anaphylactic reactions with the usual doses of epinephrine since timolol may blunt the beta agonist effect of epinephrine. In such cases, alternatives to epinephrine should be considered.

Ophthalmologic: Choroidal Detachment: Choroidal detachment has been reported with administration of aqueous suppressant therapy (e.g., timolol, acetazolamide or combination) after filtration procedures. Management of eyes with chronic or recurrent choroidal detachment should include stopping all forms of aqueous suppressant therapy and treating endogenous inflammation vigorously.

As with the use of other antiglaucoma drugs, diminished responsiveness to TIMOPTIC after prolonged therapy has been reported in some patients. However, in clinical studies in which 164 patients have been followed for at least 3 years, no significant difference in mean intra ocular pressure has been observed after initial stabilization.

Contact Lenses: The preservative in TIMOPTIC is benzalkonium chloride. This preservative is a quaternary ammonium compound that may be absorbed by soft contact lenses. Therefore, TIMOPTIC should not be administered while wearing soft contact lenses. The contact lenses should be removed before application of the drops and not be reinserted earlier than 15 minutes after use.

Neurologic: Muscle Weakness: β-adrenergic blockade has been reported to increase muscle weakness consistent with certain myasthenic symptoms (e.g., diplopia, ptosis, and generalized weakness). Timolol has been reported rarely to increase muscle weakness in some patients with myasthenic symptoms.

Peri-Operative Considerations: Major Surgery: The necessity or desirability of withdrawal of β-adrenergic blocking agents prior to major surgery is controversial. Beta-adrenergic receptor blockade impairs the ability of the heart to respond to beta-adrenergically mediated reflex stimuli. This may augment the risk of general anesthesia in surgical procedures. Some patients receiving beta-adrenergic blocking agents have experienced protracted severe hypotension during anesthesia. Difficulty in restarting and maintaining the heartbeat has also been reported. For these reasons, in patients undergoing elective surgery, some authorities recommend gradual withdrawal of beta-adrenergic blocking agents. If necessary during surgery, the effects of β-adrenergic blocking agents may be reversed by sufficient doses of such agonists as isoproterenol, dopamine, dobutamine or levarterenol.

Special Populations: Pregnant Women: TIMOPTIC has not been studied in human pregnancy. The use of TIMOPTIC requires that the anticipated benefit be weighed against possible hazards.

Nursing Women: Timolol is detectable in human milk. Because of the potential for serious adverse reactions from timolol in nursing infants, a decision should be made whether to discontinue nursing or to discontinue the drug, taking into account the importance of the drug to the mother.

Pediatrics: Safety and effectiveness in children have not been established.

ADVERSE REACTIONS: Clinical Trial Adverse Drug Reactions: Because clinical trials are conducted under very specific conditions the adverse reaction rates observed in the clinical trials may not reflect the rates observed in practice and should not be compared to the rates in the clinical trials of another drug. Adverse drug reaction information from clinical trials is useful for identifying drug-related adverse events and for approximating rates.

TIMOPTIC is usually well tolerated.

The following adverse reactions have been reported with ocular administration of this or other timolol maleate formulations, either in clinical trials or since the drug has been marketed.

Body as a Whole: headache, asthenia, fatigue, chest pain.

Cardiovascular: Aggravation or precipitation of certain cardiovascular pulmonary and other disorders presumably related to effects of systemic beta blockade has been reported (see Contraindications and Warnings and Precautions). These include bradycardia, arrhythmia, hypotension, syncope, heart block, cerebrovascular accident, cerebral ischemia, palpitation, cardiac arrest, congestive heart failure, edema, claudication, Raynaud's phenomenon, cold hands and feet and in insulin-dependent diabetics masked symptoms of hypoglycemia have been reported rarely.

Digestive: nausea, diarrhea, dyspepsia, dry mouth.

Hypersensitivity: signs and symptoms of allergic reactions including anaphylaxis, angioedema, urticaria, localized and generalized rash.

Immunologic: systemic lupus erythematosus.

Integumentary: alopecia, psoriasiform rash or exacerbation of psoriasis.

Nervous System/Psychiatric: dizziness, depression, insomnia, nightmares, memory loss, increase in signs and symptoms of myasthenia gravis, paresthesia.

Respiratory: bronchospasm (predominantly in patients with pre-existing bronchospastic disease), respiratory failure, dyspnea, cough.

Special Senses: Signs and symptoms of ocular irritation: including burning and stinging, conjunctivitis, blepharitis, keratitis, decreased corneal sensitivity, and dry eyes.

Visual disturbances: including refractive changes (due to withdrawal of miotic therapy in some cases), diplopia, ptosis, and choroidal detachment following filtration surgery (see Warnings and Precautions).

Tinnitus.

Urogenital: decreased libido, Peyronie's disease.

Causal Relationship Unknown: The following adverse reactions have been reported but a causal relationship to therapy with TIMOPTIC has not been established: aphakic cystoid macular edema, nasal congestion, anorexia, CNS effects (e.g., behavioral changes including confusion, hallucinations, anxiety, disorientation, nervousness, somnolence, and other psychic disturbances), hypertension, retroperitoneal fibrosis and pseudopemphigoid.

Potential Adverse Reactions: Adverse reactions reported in clinical experience with systemic timolol maleate may be considered potential side effects of ophthalmic timolol maleate.

DRUG INTERACTIONS: Drug-Drug Interactions: Beta-adrenergic Blockers: Patients who are already receiving a beta blocker systemically and who are given TIMOPTIC should be observed for a potential additive effect on the intraocular pressure or on the known systemic effects of beta blockers (hypotension and/or bradycardia). The concomitant use of two topical beta-adrenergic blocking agents is not recommended.

Calcium Channel Blockers or Catecholamine-depleting Drugs: The potential exists for additive effects and production of hypotension and/or marked bradycardia when TIMOPTIC is administered together with an oral calcium channel blocker or catecholamine-depleting drugs such as reserpine.

Clonidine: Oral β-adrenergic blocking agents may exacerbate the rebound hypertension which can follow the withdrawal of clonidine. If the two drugs are coadministered, the β-adrenergic blocking agent should be withdrawn several days before the gradual withdrawal of clonidine. If replacing clonidine by β-blocker therapy, the introduction of β-adrenergic blocking agents should be delayed for several days after clonidine administration has stopped.

Epinephrine: Although TIMOPTIC used alone has little or no effect on pupil size, mydriasis resulting from concomitant therapy with timolol maleate ophthalmic solutions and epinephrine has been reported occasionally.

Quinidine: Potentiated systemic beta blockade (e.g., decreased heart rate, depression) has been reported during combined treatment with CYP2D6 inhibitors (e.g. quinidine, SSRIs) and timolol.

Drug-Herb Interactions: Interactions with herbal products have not been established.

Drug-Laboratory Test Interactions: Clinically important changes in standard laboratory parameters were rarely associated with the administration of systemic timolol maleate. Slight increases in blood urea nitrogen, serum potassium, serum uric acid and triglycerides and slight decreases in hemoglobin, hematocrit, and HDL-cholesterol occurred, but were not progressive or associated with clinical manifestations.

DOSAGE AND ADMINISTRATION: Recommended Dose and Dosage Adjustment: The dosage is one drop of TIMOPTIC in the affected eye twice a day.

If needed, concomitant therapy with other agent(s) for lowering intraocular pressure may be given with TIMOPTIC. The use of two topical beta-adrenergic blocking agents is not recommended (see Warnings and Precautions).

Since in some patients the pressure-lowering response to TIMOPTIC may require a few weeks to stabilize, evaluation should include a determination of intraocular pressure after approximately 4 weeks of treatment with TIMOPTIC.

If the intraocular pressure is maintained at satisfactory levels, many patients can be placed on once-a-day therapy. Because of naturally occurring diurnal variations in intraocular pressure, satisfactory response is best determined by measuring the intraocular pressure at different times during the day.

How to Transfer Patients from Other Therapy: When a patient is transferred from another topical ophthalmic beta-adrenergic blocking agent, that agent should be discontinued after proper dosing on one day and treatment with TIMOPTIC started on the following day with one drop of TIMOPTIC in the affected eye(s) twice a day.

When a patient is transferred from a single antiglaucoma agent, other than a topical ophthalmic beta-adrenergic blocking agent, continue the agent already being used and add one drop of TIMOPTIC in each affected eye twice a day. On the following day, discontinue the previously used antiglaucoma agent completely and continue with TIMOPTIC.

When a patient is transferred from several concomitantly administered antiglaucoma agents, individualization is required. The physician may be able to discontinue some or all of the other antiglaucoma agents. Adjustments should involve one agent at a time.

Clinical trials have shown the addition of TIMOPTIC to be useful in patients who respond inadequately to the maximum tolerable antiglaucoma drug therapy.

Missed Dose: If a dose is missed, it should be applied as soon as possible. However, if it is almost time for the next dose, the missed dose should be skipped and the next dose should be taken as usual.

OVERDOSAGE:
There have been reports of inadvertent overdosage with TIMOPTIC resulting in systemic effects similar to those seen with systemic beta-adrenergic blocking agents such as dizziness, headache, shortness of breath, bradycardia, bronchospasm, and cardiac arrest (see also Adverse Reactions).

The following additional therapeutic measures should be considered:

Gastric lavage: If ingested. Studies have shown that timolol does not dialyze readily.

Symptomatic bradycardia: Use atropine sulfate intravenously in a dosage of 0.25 to 2 mg to induce vagal blockade. If bradycardia persists, intravenous isoproterenol hydrochloride should be administered cautiously. In refractory cases the use of a transvenous cardiac pacemaker may be considered.

Hypotension: Use sympathomimetic pressor drug therapy, such as dopamine, dobutamine or levarterenol. In refractory cases the use of glucagon hydrochloride has been reported to be useful.

Bronchospasm: Use isoproterenol hydrochloride. Additional therapy with aminophylline may be considered.

Acute cardiac failure: Conventional therapy with digitalis, diuretics and oxygen should be instituted immediately. In refractory cases the use of intravenous aminophylline is suggested. This may be followed if necessary by glucagon hydrochloride which has been reported to be useful.

Heart block (second-or third-degree: Use isoproterenol hydrochloride or a transvenous cardiac pacemaker.

For management of a suspected drug overdose, CPhA recommends that you contact your **regional Poison Control Centre**. See the *CPS* Directory section for a list of Poison Control Centres.

ACTION AND CLINICAL PHARMACOLOGY: Mechanism of Action: Timolol maleate is a general beta-adrenergic receptor blocking agent that does not have significant intrinsic sympathomimetic, direct myocardial depressant, or local anesthetic (membrane-stabilizing) activity. Timolol maleate combines reversibly with a part of the cell membrane, the beta-adrenergic receptor, and thus inhibits the usual biologic response that would occur with stimulation of that receptor. This specific competitive antagonism blocks stimulation of the beta-adrenergic receptors by catecholamines having beta-adrenergic stimulating (agonist) activity, whether these originate from an endogenous or exogenous source. Reversal of this blockade can be accomplished by increasing the concentration of the agonist, which will restore the usual biologic response.

Pharmacokinetics: Timolol maleate (S(-) enantiomer) is significantly metabolized after oral and ophthalmic administration. The drug and the metabolites (hydroxyethylamino, hydroxyethylglycolamino derivatives and a third minor metabolite that results from the hydroxylation of a terminal methyl group on the tertiary butylamino moiety) are excreted primarily via the kidney. Based on correlation with debrisoquine metabolism, timolol metabolism is mediated primarily by cytochrome P-450 2D6. Timolol is moderately (<60%) bound to plasma proteins.

In a study of plasma drug concentration in six subjects, the systemic exposure to timolol was determined following twice-daily topical administration of timolol maleate ophthalmic solution 0.5% for 8 days. The mean peak plasma concentration following morning dosing was 0.46 ng/mL and following afternoon dosing was 0.35 ng/mL.

By comparison to plasma concentrations (10 to 20 ng/mL) following oral 5 mg dose, it was estimated that timolol was approximately 50% bio-available systemically following intraocular administration.

STORAGE AND STABILITY: Store at room temperature (15-25°C). Protect from light.

INFORMATION FOR THE PATIENT: Published in e-CPS, available by subscription at www.e-cps.ca.

DOSAGE FORMS, COMPOSITION AND PACKAGING: Each mL of clear, colorless to light yellow, sterile, isotonic, buffered, aqueous ophthalmic solution contains: timolol maleate 6.8 mg equivalent to timolol 5 mg (0.5%). Nonmedicinal ingredients: benzalkonium chloride 0.01% (as a preservative), monobasic and dibasic sodium phosphate, sodium hydroxide (to adjust pH) and water for injection. Translucent, high-density polyethylene OCUMETER PLUS ophthalmic dispenser of 10 mL, with a sealed dropper tip, a flexible fluted side area which is depressed to dispense the drops and a 2-piece cap assembly, color-coded with a dark pink label on the cap. The opaque, white, 2-piece cap mechanism punctures the dropper tip seal upon initial use, then locks to provide a single cap during the usage period. Tamper evidence is provided by a safety strip on the container label.

Timoptic-XE® Ⓟ
timolol maleate
Elevated Intraocular Pressure Therapy

Merck Frosst

Date of Preparation: October 5, 1978
Date of Revision: March 16, 2007

SUMMARY PRODUCT INFORMATION:

Route of Administration	Dosage Form/ Strength	Clinically Relevant Nonmedicinal Ingredients
Ophthalmic	Solution, 0.25% and 0.5% timolol	For a complete listing see Dosage Forms, Composition and Packaging.

INDICATIONS AND CLINICAL USE: TIMOPTIC-XE (timolol maleate ophthalmic gellan solution) is indicated for the reduction of elevated intraocular pressure.

In clinical trials TIMOPTIC-XE has been shown to reduce intraocular pressure in:

- Patients with chronic open-angle glaucoma
- Patients with ocular hypertension
- Aphakic patients having glaucoma, including those wearing contact lenses
- Patients with narrow angles and a history of spontaneous or iatrogenically-induced narrow-angle closure in the opposite eye in whom reduction of intraocular pressure is necessary (see Warnings and Precautions).

CONTRAINDICATIONS:

- Bronchospasm, including bronchial asthma or a history of bronchial asthma or chronic obstructive pulmonary disease.
- Sinus bradycardia; second-and third-degree atrioventricular block; overt cardiac failure; cardiogenic shock.
- Hypersensitivity to any component of this product. For a complete listing of components see Dosage Forms, Composition and Packaging.

WARNINGS AND PRECAUTIONS: General: As with other topically applied ophthalmic drugs, this drug may be absorbed systemically. The same adverse reactions reported with systemic beta-adrenergic blocking agents may occur with topical administration.

TIMOPTIC-XE should be used with caution in patients subject to spontaneous hypoglycemia or in diabetic patients (especially those with labile diabetes) who are receiving insulin or oral hypoglycemic agents. Beta-adrenergic blocking agents may mask the signs and symptoms of acute hypoglycemia.

In patients with angle-closure glaucoma, the immediate objective of treatment is to reopen the angle. This requires constricting the pupil with a miotic. Timolol maleate has little or no effect on the pupil. When TIMOPTIC-XE is used to reduce elevated intraocular pressure in angle-closure glaucoma they should be used with a miotic and not alone.

Cardiac failure should be adequately controlled before beginning therapy with TIMOPTIC-XE. In patients with a history of severe cardiac disease, signs of cardiac failure should be watched for and pulse rates should be checked.

Respiratory reactions and cardiac reactions, including death due to bronchospasm in patients with asthma and rarely death in association with cardiac failure, have been reported following administration of TIMOPTIC (timolol maleate ophthalmic solution, USP). These are also potential complications of therapy with TIMOPTIC-XE.

Because of the potential effects of beta-adrenergic blocking agents on blood pressure and pulse, these agents should be used with caution in patient with cerebrovascular insufficiency. If signs or symptoms suggesting reduced cerebral blood flow develop following initiation of therapy with TIMOPTIC-XE, alternative therapy should be considered.

Endocrine and Metabolism: Thyrotoxicosis: β-adrenergic blocking agents may mask certain clinical signs of hyperthyroidism (e.g., tachycardia). Patients suspected of developing thyrotoxicosis should be managed carefully to avoid abrupt withdrawal of β-adrenergic blocking agents which might precipitate a thyroid storm.

Immune: Risk from Anaphylactic Reaction: While taking beta blockers, patients with a history of atopy or a history of severe anaphylactic reaction to a variety of allergens may be more reactive to repeated challenge with such allergens, either accidental, diagnostic, or therapeutic. These patients may be more resistant to treatment of anaphylactic reactions with the usual doses of epinephrine since timolol may blunt the beta agonist effect of epinephrine. In such cases, alternatives to epinephrine should be considered.

Ophthalmologic: Choroidal Detachment : Choroidal detachment has been reported with administration of aqueous suppressant therapy (e.g., timolol, acetazolamide or combination) after filtration procedures. Management of eyes with chronic or recurrent choroidal detachment should include stopping all forms of aqueous suppressant therapy and treating endogenous inflammation vigorously.

As with the use of other antiglaucoma drugs, diminished responsiveness to TIMOPTIC (timolol maleate ophthalmic solution, USP) after prolonged therapy has been reported in some patients. However, in clinical studies in which 164 patients have been followed for at least 3 years, no significant difference in mean intra ocular pressure has been observed after initial stabilization.

Contact Lenses: The preservative in TIMOPTIC-XE is benzododecinium bromide. This preservative is a quaternary ammonium compound that may be absorbed by soft contact lenses. For TIMOPTIC-XE, studies have not been done in patients wearing contact lenses. However, in a clinical study, the time required to eliminate 50% of the gellan solution from the eye was up to 30 minutes.

Neurologic: Muscle Weakness: β-adrenergic blockade has been reported to increase muscle weakness consistent with certain myasthenic symptoms (e.g., diplopia, ptosis, and generalized weakness). Timolol has been reported rarely to increase muscle weakness in some patients with myasthenic symptoms.

Peri-Operative Considerations: Major Surgery : The necessity or desirability of withdrawal of β-adrenergic blocking agents prior to major surgery is controversial. Beta-adrenergic receptor blockade impairs the ability of the heart to respond to beta-adrenergically mediated reflex stimuli. This may augment the risk of general anesthesia in surgical procedures. Some patients receiving beta-adrenergic blocking agents have experienced protracted severe hypotension during anesthesia. Difficulty in restarting and maintaining the heartbeat has also been reported. For these reasons, in patients undergoing elective surgery, some authorities recommend gradual withdrawal of beta-adrenergic blocking agents. If necessary during surgery, the effects of β-adrenergic blocking agents may be reversed by sufficient doses of such agonists as isoproterenol, dopamine, dobutamine or levarterenol.

Special Populations: Pregnant Women: TIMOPTIC-XE has not been studied in human pregnancy. The use of TIMOPTIC-XE requires that the anticipated benefit be weighed against possible hazards.

Nursing Women: Timolol is detectable in human milk. Because of the potential for serious adverse reactions from timolol in nursing infants, a decision should be made whether to discontinue nursing or to discontinue the drug, taking into account the importance of the drug to the mother.

Pediatrics: Safety and effectiveness in children have not been established.

ADVERSE REACTIONS: Clinical Trial Adverse Drug Reactions: Because clinical trials are conducted under very specific conditions the adverse reaction rates observed in the clinical trials may not reflect the rates observed in practice and should not be compared to the rates in the clinical trials of another drug. Adverse drug reaction information from clinical trials is useful for identifying drug-related adverse events and for approximating rates.

TIMOPTIC-XE is usually well tolerated. The most frequent (6.0%) drug related complaint in the original clinical trials for TIMOPTIC-XE was transient blurred vision, lasting from 30 seconds to 5 minutes, following instillation.

The following possibly, probably, or definitely drug related adverse reactions occurred with frequency of at least 1% in active treatment controlled clinical trials:

Ocular: burning and stinging, discharge, foreign body sensation, itching.

The adverse reactions reported for TIMOPTIC (timolol maleate ophthalmic solution, USP) are potential adverse reactions for TIMOPTIC-XE. Please refer to the list below.

Body as a Whole: headache, asthenia, fatigue, chest pain.

Cardiovascular: Aggravation or precipitation of certain cardiovascular pulmonary and other disorders presumably related to effects of systemic beta blockade has been reported (see Contraindications and Warnings and Precautions). These include bradycardia, arrhythmia, hypotension, syncope, heart block, cerebrovascular accident, cerebral ischemia, palpitation, cardiac arrest, congestive heart failure, edema, claudication, Raynaud's phenomenon, cold hands and feet and in insulin dependent diabetics masked symptoms of hypoglycemia have been reported rarely.

Digestive: nausea, diarrhea, dyspepsia, dry mouth.

Hypersensitivity: signs and symptoms of allergic reactions including anaphylaxis, angioedema, urticaria, localized and generalized rash.

Immunologic: systemic lupus erythematosus.

Integumentary: alopecia, psoriasiform rash or exacerbation of psoriasis.

Nervous System/Psychiatric: dizziness, depression, insomnia, nightmares, memory loss, increase in signs and symptoms of myasthenia gravis, paresthesia.

Respiratory: bronchospasm (predominantly in patients with pre existing bronchospastic disease), respiratory failure, dyspnea, cough.

Special Senses: signs and symptoms of ocular irritation: including burning and stinging, conjunctivitis, blepharitis, keratitis, decreased corneal sensitivity, and dry eyes.

Visual disturbances: including refractive changes (due to withdrawal of miotic therapy in some cases), diplopia, ptosis, and choroidal detachment following filtration surgery. (See Warnings and Precautions.)

Tinnitus.

Urogenital: decreased libido, Peyronie's disease.

Causal Relationship Unknown: The following adverse reactions have been reported but a causal relationship to therapy with TIMOPTIC has not been established: aphakic cystoid macular edema, nasal congestion, anorexia, CNS effects (e.g., behavioral changes including confusion, hallucinations, anxiety, disorientation, nervousness, somnolence, and other psychic disturbances), hypertension, retroperitoneal fibrosis and pseudopemphigoid.

Adverse reactions reported in clinical experience with systemic timolol maleate may be considered potential side effects of ophthalmic timolol maleate.

DRUG INTERACTIONS: Drug-Drug Interactions: Beta-adrenergic Blockers: Patients who are already receiving a beta blocker systemically and who are given TIMOPTIC-XE should be observed for a potential additive effect on the intraocular pressure or on the known systemic effects of beta blockers (hypotension and/or bradycardia). The concomitant use of two topical beta-adrenergic blocking agents is not recommended.

Calcium Channel Blockers or Catecholamine-depleting Drugs: The potential exists for additive effects and production of hypotension and/or marked bradycardia when TIMOPTIC-XE is administered together with an oral calcium channel blocker or catecholamine-depleting drugs such as reserpine.

Clonidine: Oral β-adrenergic blocking agents may exacerbate the rebound hypertension which can follow the withdrawal of clonidine. If the two drugs are coadministered, the β-adrenergic blocking agent should be withdrawn several days before the gradual withdrawal of clonidine. If replacing clonidine by β-blocker therapy, the introduction of β-adrenergic blocking agents should be delayed for several days after clonidine administration has stopped.

Epinephrine: Although timolol maleate used alone has little or no effect on pupil size, mydriasis resulting from concomitant therapy with epinephrine has been reported occasionally.

The potential for mydriasis also exists from concomitant therapy with TIMOPTIC-XE and epinephrine.

Quinidine: Potentiated systemic beta blockade (e.g., decreased heart rate, depression) has been reported during combined treatment with CYP2D6 inhibitors (e.g., quinidine, SSRIs) and timolol.

Drug-Herb Interactions: Interactions with herbal products have not been established.

Drug-Laboratory Test Interactions: Clinical Laboratory Test: Clinically important changes in standard laboratory parameters were rarely associated with the administration of systemic timolol maleate. Slight increases in blood urea nitrogen, serum potassium, serum uric acid and triglycerides and slight decreases in hemoglobin, hematocrit, and HDL-cholesterol occurred, but were not progressive or associated with clinical manifestations.

DOSAGE AND ADMINISTRATION: Recommended Dose and Dosage Adjustment: The usual starting dosage is one drop of 0.25% TIMOPTIC-XE in the affected eye(s) once a day. If the clinical response is not adequate, the dosage may be changed to one drop of 0.5% TIMOPTIC-XE in the affected eye(s) once a day.

Invert the closed container and shake once before each use. It is not necessary to shake the container more than once.

If needed, concomitant therapy with miotics, epinephrine and systemically administered carbonic anhydrase inhibitors may be given with TIMOPTIC-XE. Other topically applied medications should be administered no less than 10 minutes before TIMOPTIC-XE.

How to Transfer Patients from Other Therapy: When a patient is transferred from TIMOPTIC (timolol maleate ophthalmic solution, USP) to TIMOPTIC-XE, TIMOPTIC should be discontinued after proper dosing on one day, and treatment with the same concentration of TIMOPTIC-XE started on the following day.

When a patient is transferred from another topical ophthalmic beta adrenergic blocking agent, that agent should be discontinued after proper dosing on one day and treatment with TIMOPTIC-XE started on the following day with one drop of 0.25% TIMOPTIC-XE in the affected eye(s) once a day. The dose may be increased to one drop of 0.5% TIMOPTIC-XE once a day if the clinical response is not adequate.

When a patient is transferred from a single antiglaucoma agent, other than a topical ophthalmic beta adrenergic blocking agent, continue the agent and add one drop of 0.25% TIMOPTIC-XE to each affected eye once a day. On the following day, discontinue the previously used antiglaucoma agent and continue TIMOPTIC-XE. If a greater response is required, substitute one drop of 0.5% TIMOPTIC-XE for the 0.25% dosage.

Missed Dose: If a dose is missed, it should be applied as soon as possible. However, if it is almost time for the next dose, the missed dose should be skipped and the next dose should be taken as usual.

OVERDOSAGE:

There have been reports of inadvertent overdosage with TIMOPTIC (timolol maleate ophthalmic solution, USP) resulting in systemic effects similar to those seen with systemic beta-adrenergic blocking agents such as dizziness, headache, shortness of breath, bradycardia, bronchospasm, and cardiac arrest (see Adverse Reactions).

The following additional therapeutic measures should be considered:

Gastric Lavage: If ingested. Studies have shown that timolol does not dialyze readily.

Symptomatic Bradycardia: Use atropine sulfate intravenously in a dosage of 0.25 to 2 mg to induce vagal blockade. If bradycardia persists, intravenous isoproterenol hydrochloride should be administered cautiously. In refractory cases the use of a transvenous cardiac pacemaker may be considered.

Hypotension: Use sympathomimetic pressor drug therapy, such as dopamine, dobutamine or levarterenol. In refractory cases the use of glucagon hydrochloride has been reported to be useful.

Bronchospasm: Use isoproterenol hydrochloride. Additional therapy with aminophylline may be considered.

Acute Cardiac Failure: Conventional therapy with digitalis, diuretics and oxygen should be instituted immediately. In refractory cases the use of intravenous aminophylline is suggested. This may be followed if necessary by glucagon hydrochloride which has been reported to be useful.

Heart Block (Second-or Third-Degree): Use isoproterenol hydrochloride or a transvenous cardiac pacemaker.

For management of a suspected drug overdose, CPhA recommends that you contact your **regional Poison Control Centre**. See the *CPS* Directory section for a list of Poison Control Centres.

ACTION AND CLINICAL PHARMACOLOGY: Mechanism of Action: Timolol maleate is a general beta-adrenergic receptor blocking agent that does not have significant intrinsic sympathomimetic, direct myocardial depressant, or local anesthetic (membrane-stabilizing) activity. Timolol maleate combines reversibly with a part of the cell membrane, the beta-adrenergic receptor, and thus inhibits the usual biologic response that would occur with stimulation of that receptor. This specific competitive antagonism blocks stimulation of the beta-adrenergic receptors by catecholamines having beta-adrenergic stimulating (agonist) activity, whether these originate from an endogenous or exogenous source. Reversal of this blockade can be accomplished by increasing the concentration of the agonist, which will restore the usual biologic response.

Pharmacokinetics: Timolol maleate (S(-) enantiomer) is significantly metabolized after oral and ophthalmic administration. The drug and the metabolites (hydroxyethylamino, hydroxyethylglycolamino derivatives and a third minor metabolite that results from the hydroxylation of a terminal methyl group on the tertiary butylamino moiety) are excreted primarily via the kidney. Based on correlation with debrisoquine metabolism, timolol metabolism is mediated primarily by cytochrome P-450 2D6. Timolol is moderately (<60%) bound to plasma proteins.

In a study of plasma drug concentration in six subjects, the systemic exposure to timolol was determined following twice-daily topical administration of timolol maleate ophthalmic solution 0.5% for 8 days. The mean peak plasma concentration following morning dosing was 0.46 ng/mL and following afternoon dosing was 0.35 ng/mL.

By comparison to plasma concentrations (10 to 20 ng/mL) following oral 5 mg dose, it was estimated that timolol was approximately 50% bio-available systemically following intraocular administration.

STORAGE AND STABILITY: Store at room temperature (15-25°C). Protect from light and freezing.

The contents of TIMOPTIC-XE should not be used for more than one month after the date on which the container is first opened.

INFORMATION FOR THE PATIENT: Published in e-CPS, available by subscription at www.e-cps.ca.

DOSAGE FORMS, COMPOSITION AND PACKAGING: 0.25%: Each mL of sterile, colorless to nearly colorless, slightly opalescent, slightly viscous, aqueous ophthalmic solution contains: timolol maleate 3.4 mg equivalent to timolol 2.5 mg (0.25%). Nonmedicinal ingredients: benzododecinium bromide 0.012% (as a preservative), gellan gum, mannitol, tromethamine and water for injection. Gellan gum used in this formulation contains a highly purified anionic heteropolysaccharide. Aqueous solutions of gellan gum form a clear transparent gel at low polymer concentrations in the presence of cations. The concentration of sodium cation in tears is ideally suited to cause gelation of the material when topically instilled in the conjunctival sac. When TIMOPTIC-XE contacts the pre corneal tear film, it becomes a gel. The vehicle of TIMOPTIC-XE, gellan gum, increases the contact time of the drug with the eye. Translucent, high-density polyethylene OCUMETER PLUS, 5 mL ophthalmic dispensers, with a sealed dropper tip, a flexible fluted side area which is depressed to dispense the drops and a 2-piece cap assembly, color-coded with a light blue label on the cap. The opaque, white, 2-piece cap mechanism punctures the dropper tip seal upon initial use, then locks to provide a single cap during the usage period. Tamper evidence is provided by a safety strip on the container label.
0.5%: Each mL of sterile, colorless to nearly colorless, slightly opalescent, slightly viscous, aqueous ophthalmic solution contains: timolol maleate 6.8 mg equivalent to timolol 5 mg (0.5%). Nonmedicinal ingredients: benzododecinium bromide 0.012% (as a preservative), gellan gum, mannitol, tromethamine and water for injection. Gellan gum used in this formulation contains a highly purified anionic heteropolysaccharide. Aqueous solutions of gellan gum form a clear transparent gel at low polymer concentrations in the presence of cations. The concentration of sodium cation in tears is ideally suited to cause gelation of the material when topically instilled in the conjunctival sac. When TIMOPTIC-XE contacts the pre corneal tear film, it becomes a gel. The vehicle of TIMOPTIC-XE, gellan gum, increases the contact time of the drug with the eye. Translucent, high-density polyethylene OCUMETER PLUS, 5 mL ophthalmic dispensers, with a sealed dropper tip, a flexible fluted side area which is depressed to dispense the drops and a 2-piece cap assembly, color-coded with a dark blue label on the cap. The opaque, white, 2-piece cap mechanism punctures the dropper tip seal upon initial use, then locks to provide a single cap during the usage period. Tamper evidence is provided by a safety strip on the container label.

Tinzaparin ℞

CPhA Monograph

see *Heparins: Low Molecular Weight*

The database, reporting form and monitoring procedures for adverse events related to vaccines are separate from those related to other drug products. See the APPENDICES for a description of the program and a copy of the reporting form.

Tisseel® Kit VH

fibrin sealant

Hemostatic Agent

Baxter

Date of Preparation: October 26, 2004
Date of Revision: October 2004

PHARMACOLOGY: TISSEEL KIT VH, Two-Component Fibrin Sealant (Human), Vapor Heated, is a tissue glue with sealing, hemostyptic and gluing properties, which does not interfere with but may enhance wound healing.

Numerous clinical studies investigating the safety and efficacy of the product as a hemostyptic and biodegradable tissue glue in various fields of surgery have been performed. A number of these were controlled studies in fields including orthopedic surgery, abdominal surgery, urology, and cardiovascular surgery. The recently concluded cardiovascular safety study using the heat treated product has shown that TISSEEL transmits neither hepatitis viruses nor HIV. Pre-clinical studies have shown that the vapor treated product is at least as effective as the heat treated product.

Use of the Sealant has invariably shown superior results in the groups treated as against the untreated controls who underwent the same types of surgery. These results were attributable to an improved hemostasis and, therefore, reduced blood loss, a tighter sealing of sutures preventing leakages or a fast and uncomplicated healing of the surgical wound.

In none of the studies have systemic side-effects been seen nor has any product related transmission of viral hepatitis or HIV occurred in any of the patients treated.

INDICATIONS: TISSEEL KIT VH, Two-Component Fibrin Sealant (Human), Vapor Heated, is used, in addition to standard measures, to achieve hemostasis, to seal or glue tissue, and to support wound healing.

Indications include: abdominal surgery; cardiovascular surgery; orthopedic surgery; thoracic surgery; urology.

CONTRAINDICATIONS: TISSEEL KIT VH, Two-Component Fibrin Sealant (Human), Vapor Heated, alone is not indicated for the treatment of massive and brisk arterial or venous bleeding.

Known hypersensitivity to bovine protein.

WARNINGS: This product is manufactured using components of human blood which may contain the causative agent of hepatitis and other viral diseases. Prescribed manufacturing procedures utilized in blood collection centres and the plasma testing laboratories are designed to reduce the risk of transmitting viral infection. However, the risk of viral infectivity from this product cannot be totally excluded.

TISSEEL KIT VH, Two-Component Fibrin Sealant (Human), Vapor Heated, should not be applied intravascularly, since this may lead to anaphylactic reactions and/or thromboembolic complications, which both may be life-threatening. Especially in coronary bypass surgery, TISSEEL KIT VH should be applied with caution to minimize any risk of intravascular application.

However, if in well-founded cases the injection of Tisseel and/or Thrombin Solution/s into a tissue or vessel is indicated, careful risk/benefit analysis of the individual case is to be carried out.

In the submucous injection of fibrin sealant into hollow organs (stomach, duodenum), the following points are to be considered:

1. Insertion of the needle into the organ wall may result in accidental perforation, which in rare cases may injure adjoining organs or vessels.
2. No case of thromboembolic events following accidental vessel puncture and intravascular injection of fibrin sealant has so far been observed in the treatment of ventricular or duodenal ulcers, but cannot be excluded with certainty.
3. Injection into the submucous membrane may cause a mechanical dissection between the tunica mucosa and the tunica muscularis propria, which in rare cases may lead to vessel injury or the formation of an intramural hematoma.

Injection into the nasal mucosa must be avoided, as severe allergic-anaphylactoid reactions have been seen and thromboembolic events may occur.

PRECAUTIONS: Neither of the two components, separately or combined, should be administered by the intravascular route, or thromboembolic complications will occur.

As Tisseel Sealer Protein Concentrate and Thrombin Solutions can be denatured by contact with alcohol, iodine or other antiseptics, any such substances should be removed before application.

This product must not be used in animals.

Fibrin Sealant can also be sprayed using pressurized gas. Any application of pressurized gas may be associated with a potential risk of gas emphysema, tissue rupture, or air embolism, which may be life-threatening. Be sure to take appropriate measures to exclude these risks.

Fibrin Sealant may be sprayed only by means of the Tissomat to application sites that are visible, the minimum required spraying distance being 10 cm. Thus, the Duploject system with the Spray Set must not be used in enclosed body areas.

The user is cautioned against the spray application of TISSEEL KIT VH, Sealer Protein Concentrate (Human), Vapor Heated, with devices produced by other manufacturers. The Tissomat control device and the Spray Set may be obtained from Baxter.

To prevent TISSEEL from adhering to gloves and instruments, wet these with saline before contact with sealant.

In order to avoid excess formation of granulation tissue and slow absorption of TISSEEL, only apply thin layers of the two components.

Drug Interactions: Are not known. The Sealant can even be applied in fully heparinised patients (e.g. extracorporeal circulation).

ADVERSE EFFECTS: TISSEEL KIT VH, Two-Component Fibrin Sealant (Human), Vapor Heated, should not be applied intravascularly, since this may lead to anaphylactic reactions and/or thromboembolic complications, which both may be life-threatening. Especially in coronary bypass surgery, TISSEEL KIT VH should be applied with caution to minimize any risk of intravascular application. However, if in well-founded cases the injection of Tisseel and/or Thrombin Solution/s into a tissue or vessel is indicated, careful risk/benefit analysis of the individual case is to be carried out.

In very rare cases allergic and/or anaphylactic reactions may occur in patients with a history of hypersensitivity against bovine protein and/or in the event of repeated administration. If symptoms require treatment to be initiated, this should be effected in the usual manner, as for instance with antihistamines, corticoids or adrenalin.

OVERDOSE:

No data supplied by the manufacturer.

For management of a suspected drug overdose, CPhA recommends that you contact your **regional Poison Control Centre**. See the *CPS* Directory section for a list of Poison Control Centres.

DOSAGE: The required dose of Tisseel Thrombin Solution depends on the size of the surface to be sealed or coated or on the size of the defect to be packed. As a rule, TISSEEL KIT VH 1.0, Two-Component Fibrin Sealant (Human), Vapor Heated, will provide for sealing of approximately 10 cm^2 when using the Application Needle, and 25 cm^2–100 cm^2 when using the Spray Set.

It is desirable for Tisseel to be absorbed slowly during the wound healing process. For that reason, Aprotinin Solution is used for reconstitution of the freeze-dried Tisseel Sealer Protein Concentrate. The concentration of the Aprotinin Solution supplied with the Kit may be varied to control the rate at which TISSEEL will be absorbed. If the Aprotinin Solution is diluted with Sterile Water for Injection, TISSEEL will be absorbed faster. This may also be desirable if a recipient surface is known to have a low fibrinolytic activity of its own.

The setting rate of the Tisseel Thrombin Solution, on the other hand, depends on the concentration of the Thrombin Solution used. While the Tisseel Thrombin Solution may take up to one minute to set with a thrombin concentration of 4 IU/mL, this setting process will be complete within seconds if the higher Thrombin concentration of 500 IU/mL is used. The higher thrombin concentration may be advantageous to achieve hemostasis, while the lower thrombin concentration is better apt to seal tissue because it allows time for approximation of the wound areas.

Various methods can be used to apply the two components of TISSEEL:

Simultaneous application: a) using Duploject and application needle; b) using Duploject and spray head; c) using Duploject and application catheters; d) by premixing.

Consecutive application.

Note: Simultaneous application by premixing requires a low thrombin concentration of 4 IU/mL. Either concentration is suitable for applications using Duploject and for the consecutive application.

1. **How to Prepare Tisseel Solution:** Freeze-dried Tisseel Sealer Protein Concentrate is reconstituted in the Aprotinin Solution of 3000 KIU/mL. To obtain lower concentrations, dilute the Aprotinin Solution with Sterile Water for Injection.

For example, to obtain a concentration of 100 KIU/mL dilute 0.1 mL (0.2 mL if TISSEEL KIT VH 5.0 is used) with 3 mL (5 mL) of Sterile Water for Injection using the blue-scaled syringe.

Reconstitution of Freeze-Dried Tisseel Sealer Protein Concentrate Using Fibrinotherm: For ease of handling, a combined heating and stirring device, Fibrinotherm, has been developed to meet the specific requirements of reconstituting freeze-dried Tisseel Sealer Protein Concentrate. Fibrinotherm is a thermoblock with a magnetic stirrer (the vials for freeze-dried Tisseel Sealer Protein Concentrate contain a magnetic spin propeller to stir the contents). Heating and stirring can be operated independently. In a first step, Fibrinotherm heats up to 37°C and then maintains that temperature constantly with minimum variation. Fibrinotherm has been designed to hold the various vial sizes of freeze-dried Tisseel Sealer Protein Concentrate and Aprotinin Solution.

Place vials containing freeze-dried Tisseel Sealer Protein Concentrate and Aprotinin Solution into the appropriate openings of the Fibrinotherm and operate flip switch. Wait until signal lamp goes out. Fibrinotherm has now reached 37°C. Preheat vials for ten minutes.

Transfer Aprotinin Solution into vial containing freeze-dried Tisseel Sealer Protein Concentrate using blue-scaled syringe of corresponding size (or syringe that has been used for dilution of Aprotinin Solution).

Note: Only combine **preheated** Aprotinin Solution with **preheated** Tisseel Sealer Protein Concentrate.

Place vial into largest opening of Fibrinotherm (if necessary, use adaptors). Turn on stirrer with flip switch and stir contents for 8 to 10 minutes.

Reconstitution of freeze-dried Tisseel Sealer Protein Concentrate is complete as soon as no undissolved particles are detectable in transparent light. Otherwise, replace into Fibrinotherm and agitate for another few minutes until the solution appears homogeneous.

Note: If not used immediately, keep Tisseel Solution at 37°C without stirring. To ensure homogeneity switch on stirrer of Fibrinotherm shortly before drawing up the solution.

Reconstitution of Freeze-Dried Tisseel Sealer Protein Concentrate Using a Water-Bath:

Preheat the vial with freeze-dried Tisseel Sealer Protein Concentrate and the vial with the Aprotinin Solution to about 37°C (but not beyond 40°C).

Transfer Aprotinin Solution into vial containing freeze-dried Tisseel Sealer Protein Concentrate using blue-scaled syringe of corresponding size (or syringe that has been used for dilution of Aprotinin Solution).

Allow vial to stand at 37°C for one minute.

Swirl briefly and vigorously with a circular motion (avoid excessive frothing) and replace vial into water-bath for another 10-15 minutes.

Reconstitution of freeze-dried Tisseel Sealer Protein Concentrate is complete as soon as no undissolved particles are detectable in transparent light. Otherwise, swirl again briefly and keep vial at 37°C for a few more minutes.

Draw up reconstituted Tisseel Solution into a sterile blue-scaled syringe using aseptic precautions (insert a needle through the rubber stopper at its center to allow access of air).

Note: If not used immediately, keep Tisseel Solution at 37°C. To ensure homogeneity, swirl with a circular motion (avoiding frothing) before drawing up the solution.

2. **How to Prepare Thrombin Solution:** Depending on the desired thrombin concentration, either transfer the contents of the vial with Calcium Chloride Solution into the vial containing freeze-dried Thrombin 500 (quick solidification) or Thrombin 4 (slow solidification).

Use one of the sterile black-scaled syringes for preparing Thrombin Solution.

Swirl briefly. Keep Thrombin Solution at 37°C until used. Draw up an amount of Thrombin Solution equal to the amount of Tisseel Solution that will be used into a sterile black-scaled syringe using aseptic precautions.

Note: Do not use the syringes and needles previously used for reconstitution of freeze-dried Tisseel Sealer Protein Concentrate to prevent premature setting.

3. **Application:** Simultaneous Application Using DUPLOJECT-System: The Duploject allows simultaneous application of the two components and ensures that they are quickly and thoroughly mixed, which is essential for TISSEEL to gain the optimum strength. Either Thrombin concentration can be used.

a) Simultaneous Application Using Duploject and Application Needle: The sterile Duploject consists of a clip for two identical disposable syringes and a common plunger which ensures that equal volumes of the two components are fed over a common joining piece before being mixed in the Application Needle and ejected.

Operating Instructions: Place syringes filled with Tisseel and Thrombin Solutions into the clip. Both syringes should be filled with equal amounts and should not contain any air bubbles.

Connect the nozzles of the two syringes with the Joining Piece. Ensure firm hold. Secure the Joining Piece by fastening the strap to the clip.

Fit Application Needle onto the Joining Piece. Do not remove remaining air from inside the Joining Piece or Application Needle. Otherwise the apertures of the needle may clog before application of the Tisseel Thrombin Solution.

Apply the Tisseel Thrombin Solution onto the recipient surface or surfaces if two parts of tissue need to be glued together.

Note: Only the syringes contained in the Kit for reconstitution and application are designed to perfectly fit into the Duploject clip. Any other syringe may cause problems since exact and firm adaptation to the Joining Piece cannot be granted for. If the procedure of applying the two components with Duploject is interrupted, replace the Application Needle by a new one when sealing is resumed (three spare needles come with the Kit). Only replace Application Needle immediately prior to resuming sealing. Otherwise, the apertures of the Joining Piece will clog, which requires it to be also replaced (one spare Joining Piece comes with the Kit).

b) Simultaneous Application Using Duploject, Spray Set and Tissomat: The spray set is particularly suitable for spraying of larger areas, e.g. to control oozing of parenchymatous organs. Duploject is used for this method of application except that a Spray Head is used instead of the Joining Piece. The two components are sprayed simultaneously using sterile propellent gas via Tissomat, and the volume of the Solutions ejected is controlled with the Duploject plunger. Spray at a distance of at least 10-20 cm. The user is cautioned against the spray application of TISSEEL with devices produced by other manufacturers.

Note: A detailed description of this application method is included in the leaflet of the Spray Set.

c) Simultaneous Application Using Duploject and Application Catheter: In operation sites where access is difficult or when using an endoscope or trocar, TISSEEL can be applied using Duploject with Application Catheter.

Note: A detailed description of this application method is included in the leaflet of the respective Application Catheter.

d) Simultaneous Application by Premixing: Mix equal volumes of the two components and immediately apply them to the recipient surface or surfaces. When the low thrombin concentration of 4 IU/mL is used, approximately one minute is allowed for mixing the components, applying them, and approximating the wound areas. If desired, the Tisseel Thrombin Solution can be mixed with spongiosa to pack bone defects. Hold in place for three minutes. Once turbid, TISSEEL can no longer be manipulated.

Consecutive Application: Apply the two components in two layers. Apply Tisseel Solution to the recipient surface or surfaces first, then apply an equal amount of Thrombin Solution on top of the Tisseel Solution using a separate syringe. Approximate surfaces and hold in place for three minutes. If a collagen fleece is used, soak the fleece with an appropriate amount of Tisseel Solution, cover the recipient area with Tisseel Solution and apply appropriate amounts of Thrombin Solution on top of both. Press the fleece onto the recipient area for about three minutes to allow TISSEEL to gain strength. Alternatively, when two parts are to be glued, apply one component to one surface, the other component to the opposite surface.

4. **Gluing of Tissue:** After the two components have been applied, approximate the wound areas. Fix or hold the glued parts in the desired position for three to five minutes to ensure that the setting Sealant adheres firmly to the surrounding tissue. Solidified Sealant reaches its ultimate strength after about two hours (70% after about ten minutes).

SUPPLIED: TISSEEL KIT VH, Two-Component Fibrin Sealant (Human), Vapor Heated, contains the following substances in five separate vials: 1. Tisseel Sealer Protein Concentrate (Human)*, sterile, freeze-dried, vapor-heated, reconstituted contains: Total protein, 100-130 mg/mL; including fibrinogen, 70-110 mg/mL; Plasma fibronectin (cold insoluble globulin), 2-9 mg/mL; Factor XIII, 10-50 U/mL†; plasminogen, 40-120 μg/mL. 2. Aprotinin Solution, sterile, bovine 3000 KIU/mL‡. 3. Thrombin 4, sterile, freeze-dried, vapor-heated, human reconstituted contains: 4 IU/mL§. 4. Thrombin 500, sterile, freeze-dried, vapor-heated, human reconstituted contains: 500 IU/mL§. 5. Calcium Chloride Solution, sterile 40 μmol/mL.

The Kit also contains an application set consisting of a Duploject-applicator, disposable syringes, two Joining Pieces and four Application Needles. In addition to the Kit, a Spray Set and Application Catheters are available.

* Each vial contains a magnetic spin propeller to facilitate reconstitution when placed in the FIBRINOTHERM warming and stirring device.

† One unit corresponds to the amount of Factor XIII contained in 1 mL of fresh normal plasma.

‡ 30 Kallidinogenase Inactivator Units (KIU) correspond to 1 FIP-Unit.

§ One International Unit (IU) of Thrombin is defined as the activity contained in 0.0853 mg of the First International Standard of Human Thrombin.

¶ HIQ-PCR=Hyland Immuno Quality Assured Polymerase Chain Reaction. With this method 500 genome equivalents/mL of the above viruses can be determined reliably, with the actual sensitivity of HIQ-PCR being below that. Therefore all pools which have been tested and evaluated as being positive lead to exclusion from further processing. No correlation has been demonstrated between infectivity and removal of pools containing these levels of genomic equivalents from further manufacturing.

Tisseel Sealer Protein Concentrate and Thrombin are made from human plasma. During manufacture they are subjected to a product-specific vapor heat treatment. Preclinical data show that this treatment produces a decrease in HIV-1 titer of 10^6 or more infectious units per mL.

Individual donations of human plasma are combined to form plasma pools. Prior to being used for manufacture of TISSEEL, each plasma pool is tested for the presence of genome sequences of the human immunodeficiency virus type 1 (HIV-1), hepatitis B virus (HBV) and hepatitis C virus (HCV) using the HIQ-PCR.¶

The action of TISSEEL simulates key features of the physiological process of wound closure. A highly concentrated fibrinogen aprotinin solution, which among other ingredients contains Factor XIII, and a solution of thrombin and calcium chloride are applied to the wound area, where the mixture coagulates. The presence of Factor XIII causes the fibrin to crosslink, which gives the coagulum additional resilience.

The substances in the Kit are used to prepare two components: Tisseel Solution and Thrombin Solution. Tisseel Solution is produced by dissolving Tisseel Sealer Protein Concentrate in Aprotinin Solution. Freeze-dried Thrombin, dissolved in Calcium Chloride Solution, yields the Thrombin Solution.

The two components are mixed either immediately before application to the recipient surface or in situ using one of the methods described under Application. Tisseel Thrombin Solution is a viscous solution adhering to wound surfaces and quickly sets to form a white, rubberlike mass, which continues to gain in strength within two hours following application. This process is made use of to achieve hemostasis, and to seal or glue tissue.

In this manner, the need for sutures may be reduced, although not totally eliminated. The time until Sealant sets can be used to approximate wound edges, to provide optimum conditions for healing. In the course of wound healing, Sealant is completely absorbed.

To prevent the transmission of infective agents by the administration of TISSEEL, prescribed procedures are used for the collection and testing of the source plasma and during the manufacture of the product. They include measures taken for donor and plasma selection**, as well as virus removal and inactivation steps during manufacturing.

The efficiency of these manufacturing steps employed during the production of TISSEEL has been demonstrated in validation studies using human immunodeficiency virus (HIV), hepatitis A virus, and model viruses for hepatitis B and hepatitis C viruses (HBV, HCV) as well as for non-enveloped viruses.

In an international multicenter safety study, coagulation factor concentrates that were virus-inactivated by steam treatment showed no evidence of transmission of hepatitis viruses or HIV.

Pharmaco-epidemiological surveillance of TISSEEL has shown no product-related transmission of infective agents.

Stability and Storage Recommendations: When stored between 2°C and 8°C, TISSEEL KIT VH, Two-Component Fibrin Sealant (Human), Vapor Heated, is stable until the expiry date indicated on the label.

Reconstituted Solutions: Reconstituted Tisseel and Thrombin Solutions must be used within four hours.

TISSEEL KIT VH, Two-Component Fibrin Sealant (Human), Vapor Heated, is supplied in the following three pack sizes:

TISSEEL KIT VH, 1.0 for 1.0 mL of reconstituted Tisseel Solution and 1.0 mL Thrombin Solution.

TISSEEL KIT VH, 2.0 for 2.0 mL of reconstituted Tisseel Solution and 2.0 mL Thrombin Solution.

TISSEEL KIT VH, 5.0 for 5.0 mL of reconstituted Tisseel Solution and 5.0 mL Thrombin Solution.

Accessories: The following accessories can be obtained from a Baxter representative:

FIBRINOTHERM: Combined heating and stirring device for the reconstitution of freeze-dried Tisseel Sealer Protein Concentrate.

Accessories for the use of DUPLOJECT with Spray Set:

TISSOMAT: Propellent gas control unit including foot switch, manometer, reducing valve, and pressure tube.

SPRAY-SET (sterile, disposable): Disposable set consisting of sterile filter with connection tube and a spray head.

Accessories for the use of DUPLOJECT with Application Catheter:

DUPLOCATH 25 Application Catheter: Length: approximately 25 cm (10"); Diameter: approximately 5 french (approx. 0.17 cm); Radiopaque.

DUPLOCATH 35 M.I.S.: Catheter: Length: approximately 35 cm (14"); Diameter: approximately 5 french (approx. 0.17 cm); Adapter: Length: approximately 30 cm (12"); Diameter: 15 french (0.5 cm); For insertion through a 5-6 mm trocar in minimally invasive surgery (M.I.S.); Radiopaque. Sterile. Disposable.

DUPLOCATH 180 Application Catheter: Length: approximately 180 cm (70"); Diameter: approximately 5 french (approx. 0.17 cm); For use with an endoscope. Radiopaque. The Application Catheter 180 can be shortened to any length necessary.

TNKase® Ⓟ

tenecteplase

Fibrinolytic Agent

Roche

Date of Preparation: October 17, 2001

Date of Revision: May 27, 2008

SUMMARY PRODUCT INFORMATION:

Route of Administration	Dosage Form/Strength	Clinically Relevant Nonmedicinal
IV bolus	Powder for solution sterile, lyophilized 50 mg/vial	None For a complete listing see Dosage Forms, Composition and Packaging.

INDICATIONS AND CLINICAL USE: TNKase (tenecteplase) is indicated for intravenous use in adults for the lysis of suspected occlusive coronary artery thrombi associated with evolving transmural myocardial infarction to reduce the mortality associated with acute myocardial infarction (AMI). Treatment should be initiated as soon as possible after the onset of AMI symptoms.

The ASSENT-2 clinical trial compared single bolus weight adjusted TNKase with accelerated ACTIVASE (rt-PA) (alteplase) in patients presenting within 6 hours of onset of AMI symptoms.

Geriatrics: For clinical use in geriatric patients please refer to Warnings and Precautions, Special Populations, Geriatrics.

CONTRAINDICATIONS: Therapy with TNKase (tenecteplase) in patients with acute myocardial infarction is contraindicated in the following situations because of an increased risk of bleeding (see Warnings and Precautions):

- Active internal bleeding
- History of cerebrovascular accident
- Intracranial or intraspinal surgery or trauma within 2 months
- Intracranial neoplasm, arteriovenous malformation, or aneurysm
- Known bleeding diathesis
- Severe uncontrolled hypertension

Patients who are hypersensitive to this drug or to any ingredient in the formulation or component of the container. For a complete listing, see Dosage Forms, Composition and Packaging.

WARNINGS AND PRECAUTIONS: General: Each patient being considered for therapy with TNKase (tenecteplase) should be carefully evaluated and anticipated benefits weighed against potential risks associated with therapy. In the following conditions, the risk of therapy with TNKase may be increased and should be weighed against the anticipated benefits: Recent major surgery, e.g., coronary artery bypass graft, obstetrical delivery, organ biopsy, previous puncture of noncompressible vessels. Cerebrovascular disease. Recent gastrointestinal or genitourinary bleeding. Recent trauma. Hypertension: systolic BP ≥180 mm Hg and/or diastolic BP ≥110 mm Hg. High likelihood of left heart thrombus, e.g., mitral stenosis with atrial fibrillation. Acute pericarditis. Subacute bacterial endocarditis. Hemostatic defects, including those secondary to severe hepatic or renal disease. Severe hepatic dysfunction. Pregnancy. Diabetic hemorrhagic retinopathy or other hemorrhagic ophthalmic conditions. Septic thrombophlebitis or occluded AV cannula at seriously infected site. Advanced age (see Warnings and Precautions, Geriatrics). Patients currently receiving oral anticoagulants, e.g., warfarin sodium. Recent administration of GP IIb/IIIa inhibitors. Any other condition in which bleeding constitutes a significant hazard or would be particularly difficult to manage because of its location.

** All plasma units used for manufacture are ALT tested and non-reactive in tests for Hbs-antigen and antibodies to HCV, HIV-1 and HIV-2. Before further processing all individual plasma donations are subjected to an inventory hold for a possible look-back of plasma donations suspected of infection.

Standard management of myocardial infarction should be implemented concomitantly with TNKase treatment. Arterial and venous punctures should be minimized. Noncompressible arterial puncture must be avoided and internal jugular and subclavian venous punctures should be avoided to minimize bleeding from the noncompressible sites. In the event of serious bleeding, heparin and antiplatelet agents should be discontinued immediately. Heparin effects can be reversed by protamine.

All plasminogen activators, including TNKase, should be used in conjunction with anticoagulants. There are some patients that may require further intervention to achieve reperfusion. Adherence to the ACC/AHA anticoagulation guidelines is recommended.

Bleeding: The most common complication encountered during therapy with TNKase is bleeding. The type of bleeding associated with thrombolytic therapy can be divided into two broad categories:

- Internal bleeding, involving intracranial and retroperitoneal sites, or the gastrointestinal, genitourinary, or respiratory tracts.
- Superficial or surface bleeding, observed mainly at vascular puncture and access sites (e.g., venous cutdowns, arterial punctures) or sites of recent surgical intervention.

Should serious bleeding (not controlled by local pressure) occur, any concomitant heparin and antiplatelet agents should be discontinued immediately.

In clinical studies of TNKase, patients were treated with both ASA and heparin. Heparin may contribute to the bleeding risks associated with TNKase. The safety of the use of TNKase with other antiplatelet agents has not been adequately studied (see Drug Interactions). Intramuscular injections and nonessential handling of the patient should be avoided for the first few hours following treatment with TNKase. Venipunctures should be performed and monitored carefully.

Should an arterial puncture be necessary during the first few hours following therapy with TNKase, it is preferable to use an upper extremity vessel that is accessible to manual compression. Pressure should be applied for at least 30 minutes, a pressure dressing applied, and the puncture site checked frequently for evidence of bleeding.

Carcinogenesis and Mutagenesis: Studies in animals have not been performed to evaluate the carcinogenic potential, mutagenicity, or the effect on fertility.

Cardiovascular: Arrhythmias: Coronary thrombolysis may result in arrhythmias associated with reperfusion. These arrhythmias (such as sinus bradycardia, accelerated idioventricular rhythm, ventricular premature depolarizations, ventricular tachycardia) are not different from those often seen in the ordinary course of acute myocardial infarction and may be managed with standard anti-arrhythmic measures. It is recommended that anti-arrhythmic therapy for bradycardia and/or ventricular irritability be available when TNKase is administered.

Use with Percutaneous Coronary Intervention (PCI): In patients with large ST segment elevation myocardial infarction, physicians should choose either thrombolysis or PCI as the primary treatment strategy for reperfusion. Rescue PCI or subsequent elective PCI may be performed after administration of thrombolytic therapies if medically appropriate; however, the optimal use of adjunctive antithrombotic and antiplatelet therapies in this setting is unknown.

Endocrine and Metabolism: Cholesterol Embolization: Cholesterol embolism has been reported rarely in patients treated with all types of thrombolytic agents; the true incidence is unknown. This serious condition, which can be lethal, is also associated with invasive vascular procedures (e.g., cardiac catheterization, angiography, vascular surgery) and/or anticoagulant therapy. Clinical features of cholesterol embolism may include livedo reticularis "purple toe" syndrome, acute renal failure, gangrenous digits, hypertension, pancreatitis, myocardial infarction, cerebral infarction, spinal cord infarction, retinal artery occlusion, bowel infarction, and rhabdomyolysis.

Sensitivity/Resistance: Readministration: Readministration of plasminogen activators, including TNKase, to patients who have received prior plasminogen activator therapy has not been systematically studied. Three of 487 patients tested for antibody formation to TNKase had a positive antibody titer at 30 days. The data reflect the percentage of patients whose test results were considered positive for antibodies to TNKase in a radioimmunoprecipitation assay, and are highly dependent on the sensitivity and specificity of the assay. Additionally, the observed incidence of antibody positivity in an assay may be influenced by several factors including sample handling, concomitant medications, and underlying disease. For these reasons, comparison of the incidence of antibodies to TNKase with the incidence of antibodies to other products may be misleading. Although sustained antibody formation in patients receiving one dose of TNKase has not been documented, readministration should be undertaken with caution. If an anaphylactic reaction occurs, appropriate therapy should be administered.

Special Populations: Pregnant Women: There are no adequate and well controlled studies in pregnant women. TNKase should be given to pregnant women only if the potential benefits justify the potential risk to the fetus.

Nursing Women: It is not known if TNKase is excreted in human milk. Because many drugs are excreted in human milk, caution should be exercised when TNKase is administered to a nursing woman.

Pediatrics: Safety and effectiveness of TNKase in pediatric patients have not been established.

Geriatrics: In elderly patients, the benefits of TNKase on mortality should be carefully weighed against the risk of increased adverse events, including bleeding (see Table 1).

Table 1: TNKase

ASSENT-2: Elderly Patients Who Received TNKase

	Age		
Event Rate	**<65 years n=4958 (59%)**	**65–74 years n=2256 (27%)**	**≥75 years n=1244 (15%)**
30-Day Mortality	2.5%	8.5%	16.2%
Intracranial Hemorrhage (ICH)	0.4%	1.6%	1.7%
Any Stroke	1.0%	2.9%	3.0%
Major Bleeding[a]	3.1%	6.4%	7.7%

[a] Defined as bleeding requiring blood transfusion or leading to hemodynamic compromise.

Monitoring and Laboratory Tests: During therapy with TNKase, results of coagulation tests and/or measures of fibrinolytic activity may be unreliable unless specific precautions are taken to prevent in vitro artifacts. Tenecteplase is an enzyme that when present in blood in pharmacologic concentrations remains active under in vitro conditions. This can lead to degradation of fibrinogen in blood samples removed for analysis.

ADVERSE REACTIONS: Adverse Drug Reaction Overview: Bleeding: The most frequent adverse reaction associated with TNKase (tenecteplase) is bleeding (see Warnings and Precautions).

Should serious bleeding occur, concomitant heparin and antiplatelet therapy should be discontinued. Death or permanent disability can occur in patients who experience stroke or serious bleeding episodes.

Clinical Trial Adverse Drug Reactions: Because clinical trials are conducted under very specific conditions the adverse reaction rates observed in the clinical trials may not reflect the rates observed in practice and should not be compared to the rates in the clinical trials of another drug. Adverse drug reaction information from clinical trials is useful for identifying drug-related adverse events and for approximating rates.

For TNKase treated patients in ASSENT-2, the incidence of intracranial haemorrhage was 0.9% and any stroke was 1.8%. The incidence of all strokes, including intracranial bleeding, increases with increasing age (see Warnings and Precautions, Geriatrics).

In the ASSENT-2 study, the following bleeding events were reported (see Table 2).

Table 2: TNKase

ASSENT-2: Non-ICH Bleeding Events

	TNKase (n=8461)	**Accelerated ACTIVASE (n=8488)**	**Relative Risk for TNKase/ACTIVASE (95% CI)**	**p-value**
Major Bleeding[a]	4.7%	5.9%	0.78 (0.69, 0.89)	0.0002
Minor Bleeding	21.8%	23.0%	0.94 (0.89, 1.00)	0.0553
Units of Transfused Blood				
Any	4.3%	5.5%	0.77 (0.67, 0.89)	0.0013
1-2	2.6%	3.2%		
>2	1.7%	2.2%		

[a] Defined as bleeding requiring blood transfusion or leading to hemodynamic compromise.

The incidence of non-intracranial major bleeding and the need for blood transfusions were statistically lower in patients treated with TNKase compared to an accelerated infusion of ACTIVASE.

Types of major bleeding reported in 1% or more of the patients were hematoma (1.7%) and gastrointestinal tract (1%). Types of major bleeding reported in less than 1% of the patients were urinary tract, puncture site (including cardiac catheterization site), retroperitoneal, respiratory tract, and unspecified. Types of minor bleeding reported in 1% or more of the patients were hematoma (12.3%), urinary tract (3.7%), puncture site (including cardiac catheterization site) (3.6%), pharyngeal (3.1%), gastrointestinal tract (1.9%), epistaxis (1.5%), and unspecified (1.3%).

Allergic Reactions: Allergic-type reactions (e.g., anaphylaxis, angioedema, laryngeal edema, rash, and urticaria) have rarely (<1%) been reported in patients treated with TNKase. Anaphylaxis was reported in <0.1% of patients treated with TNKase; however, causality was not established. When such reactions occur, they usually respond to conventional therapy.

Other Adverse Reactions: The following serious adverse reactions have been reported among patients receiving TNKase in the ASSENT-2 clinical trial. These reactions are frequent sequelae of the underlying disease, and the effect of TNKase on the incidence of these events is unknown. These events can be life-threatening and may lead to death (see Table 3).

Table 3: TNKase

Serious Non-Bleeding Events Reported in ≥1% of Patients in the ASSENT-2 Trial[a]

	TNKase (n=8258)	**AcceleratedACTIVASE (n=8299)**
Cardiovascular		
Cardiogenic Shock	3%	3%
Hypotension	3%	3%
Electromechanical Dissociation	2%	2%
Myocardial Reinfarction	2%	2%
Recurrent Myocardial Ischemia	2%	2%
Atrioventricular Block	1%	1%
Respiratory		
Pulmonary Edema	2%	3%

[a] Reported adverse events are without attribution.

Serious non-bleeding events reported in the ASSENT-2 trial at a frequency of <1% include arrhythmias, heart failure, cardiac arrest, myocardial rupture, cardiac tamponade, pericarditis, pericardial effusion, mitral regurgitation, thrombosis, embolism, nausea and/or vomiting, and fever.

Post-Market Adverse Drug Reactions: Adverse events that have been reported during the post-marketing period are consistent with those seen in clinical trials with TNKase.

DRUG INTERACTIONS: Drug-Drug Interactions: Formal interaction studies of TNKase (tenecteplase) with other drugs have not been performed. Patients studied in clinical trials of TNKase were routinely treated with heparin and ASA. Anticoagulants (such as heparin and vitamin K antagonists) and drugs that alter platelet function (such as acetylsalicylic acid, dipyridamole, and GP IIb/IIIa inhibitors) may increase the risk of bleeding if administered prior to, during, or after therapy with TNKase.

DOSAGE AND ADMINISTRATION: Recommended Dose and Dosage Adjustment: TNKase (tenecteplase) is for intravenous administration only. The recommended total dose should not exceed 50 mg and is based upon patient weight (see Table 4).

A single bolus dose should be administered over 5 seconds based on patient weight. Treatment should be initiated as soon as possible after the onset of AMI symptoms.

Table 4: TNKase

Dose Information Table

Patient Weight (kg)	**TNKase (mg)**	**Volume TNKase[a] to be administered (mL)**
<60	30	6
≥60 to <70	35	7
≥70 to <80	40	8
≥80 to <90	45	9
≥90	50	10

[a] From 1 vial of tenecteplase reconstituted with 10 mL SWFI.

The safety and efficacy of TNKase have only been investigated with concomitant administration of heparin and ASA.

Reconstitution: Note: Read all instructions completely before beginning reconstitution and administration

1. Remove the shield assembly from the supplied B-D 10 cc Syringe with TwinPak Dual Cannula Device and aseptically withdraw 10 mL of Sterile Water for Injection (SWFI), USP from the supplied diluent vial using the red hub cannula syringe filling device. Do not use Bacteriostatic Water for Injection, USP.
   Note: Do not discard the shield assembly.
2. Inject the entire contents of the syringe (10 mL) into the TNKase vial directing the diluent stream into the powder. Slight foaming upon reconstitution is not unusual; any large bubbles will dissipate if the product is allowed to stand undisturbed for several minutes.
3. Gently swirl until contents are completely dissolved. **Do not shake.** The reconstituted preparation results in a colourless to pale yellow transparent solution containing TNKase at 5 mg/mL at a pH of approximately 7.3. The osmolality of this solution is approximately 290 mOsm/kg.

4. Determine the appropriate dose of TNKase (see Table 4) and withdraw this volume (in mL) from the reconstituted vial with the syringe. Any unused solution should be discarded.
5. Once the appropriate dose of TNKase is drawn into the syringe, stand the shield vertically on a flat surface (with green side down) and passively recap the red hub cannula.
6. Remove the entire shield assembly, including the red hub cannula, by twisting counter-clockwise. Note: The shield assembly also contains the clear-ended blunt plastic cannula; retain for split septum IV access.

Administration:

1. The product should be visually inspected prior to administration for particulate matter and discoloration. TNKase may be administered as reconstituted at 5 mg/mL.
2. Precipitation may occur when TNKase is administered in an IV line containing dextrose. Dextrose containing lines should be flushed with a saline containing solution prior to and following single bolus administration of TNKase.
3. Reconstituted TNKase should be administered as a single IV bolus over 5 seconds.
4. Because TNKase contains no antibacterial preservatives, it should be reconstituted immediately before use. If the reconstituted TNKase is not used immediately, refrigerate the TNKase vial at 2-8°C and use within 8 hours.
5. Although the supplied syringe is compatible with a conventional needle, this syringe is designed to be used with needleless IV systems. From the information below, follow the instructions applicable to the IV system in use.

Table 5: TNKase

Administration

Split Septum I.V. System:	• Remove the green cap. • Attach the clear-ended blunt plastic cannula to the syringe. • Remove the shield and use the blunt plastic cannula to access the split septum injection port. • Because the blunt plastic cannula has two side ports, air or fluid expelled through the cannula will exit in two sideways directions; direct away from face or mucous membranes.
Luer-Lok System:	• Connect syringe directly to i.v. port.
Conventional Needle (not supplied in this kit):	• Attach a large bore needle, e.g., 18 gauge, to the syringe's universal Luer-Lok.

6. Dispose of the syringe, cannula and shield per established procedures.

OVERDOSAGE:
Single doses greater than 50 mg (10 000 units) have not been tested. The total dose should be based on patient weight, not to exceed 50 mg (see Dosage and Administration).

Any patients receiving greater than the recommended dosage should be carefully monitored. Bleeding complications, notably Intracranial Hemorrhage (ICH), are the most important adverse events associated with TNKase (tenecteplase), as with other thrombolytics. If bleeding occurs, standard medical management should be implemented.

For management of a suspected drug overdose, CPhA recommends that you contact your **regional Poison Control Centre**. See the *CPS* Directory section for a list of Poison Control Centres.

ACTION AND CLINICAL PHARMACOLOGY: Mechanism of Action: TNKase (tenecteplase) is a modified form of human tissue plasminogen activator (tPA) that binds to fibrin and converts plasminogen to plasmin. In the presence of fibrin, in vitro studies demonstrate that tenecteplase conversion of plasminogen to plasmin is increased relative to its conversion in the absence of fibrin. This fibrin specificity decreases systemic activation of plasminogen and the resulting degradation of circulating fibrinogen as compared to a molecule lacking this property. Following administration of 30, 40, or 50 mg of TNKase, there are decreases in circulating fibrinogen (4%-15%) and plasminogen (11%-24%). The clinical significance of fibrin specificity on safety (e.g., bleeding) or efficacy has not been established. Biological potency is determined by an in vitro clot lysis assay and is expressed in tenecteplase-specific units. The specific activity of TNKase has been defined as 200 units/mg.
Pharmacokinetics: In patients with acute myocardial infarction (AMI), administration of TNKase as a single bolus exhibits a biphasic disposition from the plasma. TNKase was cleared from the plasma with an initial half-life of 20 to 24 minutes. The terminal phase half-life of TNKase was 90 to 130 minutes. In 99 of 104 patients treated with TNKase, mean plasma clearance ranged from 99 to 119 mL/min.
Distribution: The initial volume of distribution is weight related and approximates plasma volume.
Metabolism: The major route of clearance of TNKase is liver metabolism.

STORAGE AND STABILITY: Store lyophilized TNKase at controlled room temperature not to exceed 30°C or under refrigeration (2-8°C). Do not use beyond the expiration date stamped on the vial.

Unused reconstituted TNKase (in the vial) may be stored at 2-8°C and used within 8 hours. After that time, any unused portion of the reconstituted material should be discarded.

INFORMATION FOR THE PATIENT: Published in e-CPS, available by subscription at www.e-cps.ca.

DOSAGE FORMS, COMPOSITION AND PACKAGING: Each vial of sterile, white to off-white, lyophilized powder for single i.v. bolus administration after reconstitution with Sterile Water for Injection, USP, contains: tenecteplase 52.5 mg*. Nonmedicinal ingredients: L-arginine, phosphoric acid and polysorbate 20. Each 50 mg (10 000 units) glass vial (20 mL) under partial vacuum is packaged with one 10 mL vial of Sterile Water for Injection, USP, for reconstitution, one B-D 10 mL Syringe with TwinPak Dual Cannula Device, and 3 alcohol prep pads.

* This includes a 5% overfill so that each vial will deliver 50 mg of tenecteplase.

TOBI® Tobramycin Inhalation Solution, USP ℞

tobramycin sulfate

Respiratory Antibiotic

Novartis Pharmaceuticals

PHARMACOLOGY: TOBI is a formulation of tobramycin designed specifically for administration by inhalation. When tobramycin solution for inhalation is inhaled, tobramycin can be detected at high concentration in the sputum of cystic fibrosis patients.

The drug substance, tobramycin, is an aminoglycoside antibiotic derived from *S. tenebrarius*. Tobramycin, a cationic polar molecule that does not readily cross epithelial membranes, is chemically and pharmacologically related to the aminoglycoside class of antibiotics. The primary mode of action is bactericidal resulting from disruption of protein synthesis in susceptible bacteria.
Pharmacokinetics: Concentrations of tobramycin in the sputum vary widely. This variation may be explained by individual differences in nebulizer performance and airway pathology. Following administration of tobramycin solution for inhalation, the drug remains concentrated primarily in sputum in the airways.
Sputum Concentrations: Ten minutes after inhalation of the first 300 mg dose of tobramycin solution for inhalation by cystic fibrosis patients, the mean (median) concentration of tobramycin in the sputum was 1 237 µg/g (959 µg/g) with the range from 35 to 7 417 µg/g. Tobramycin does not accumulate in sputum; after 20 weeks of therapy with the tobramycin solution for inhalation regimen, the mean (median) concentration of tobramycin at 10 minutes after inhalation was 1 154 µg/g (818 µg/g), ranging from below quantifiable limits to 8 085 µg/g. High intra- and inter-subject variability of tobramycin concentrations in the sputum was observed. Two hours after inhalation, sputum tobramycin concentrations declined to approximately 14% of sputum tobramycin concentrations at 10 minutes after inhalation.
Serum Concentrations: The mean (median) serum concentration of tobramycin 1 hour after inhalation of a single 300 mg dose of tobramycin solution for inhalation by cystic fibrosis patients was 0.95 µg/mL (0.91 µg/mL), ranging from below quantifiable limits to 3.62 µg/mL. After 20 weeks of therapy on the tobramycin solution for inhalation regimen, the mean (median) serum tobramycin concentration 1 hour after dosing was 1.05 µg/mL (0.94 µg/mL), ranging from below quantifiable limits to 3.41 µg/mL.
Elimination: The elimination half-life of tobramycin from serum is approximately 2 hours after i.v. administration. Assuming tobramycin absorbed following inhalation behaves similarly to tobramycin following i.v. administration, systemically absorbed tobramycin is eliminated principally by glomerular filtration. Unabsorbed tobramycin, following tobramycin solution for inhalation administration, may be eliminated in expectorated sputum or via the gastrointestinal tract.
Clinical Studies: Two identically designed, double-blind, randomized, placebo-controlled, parallel group, 24-week clinical studies (Study 1 and Study 2) at a total of 69 cystic fibrosis centers in the US were conducted in cystic fibrosis patients with *P. aeruginosa*. Subjects who were less than 6 years of age, had a baseline creatinine of >2 mg/dL, or had *B. cepacia* isolated from sputum were excluded. All subjects had baseline FEV_1% predicted between 25 and 75%. In these clinical studies, 258 patients received tobramycin solution for inhalation therapy on an outpatient basis (see Table 1) using a hand-held Pari LC Plus reusable nebulizer with a DeVilbiss Pulmo-Aide compressor.

Table 1: TOBI

Dosing Regimens in Clinical Studies

	Cycle 1		Cycle 2		Cycle 3	
	28 Days	28 Days	28 Days	28 Days	28 Days	28 Days
TOBI regimen n=258	TOBI 300 mg b.i.d.	no drug	TOBI 300 mg b.i.d.	no drug	TOBI 300 mg b.i.d.	no drug
Placebo regimen n=262	placebo b.i.d.	no drug	placebo b.i.d.	no drug	placebo b.i.d.	no drug

All patients received either tobramycin solution for inhalation or placebo (saline with 1.25 mg quinine for flavoring) in addition to standard treatment recommended for cystic fibrosis patients, which included oral and parenteral antipseudomonal therapy, β_2-agonists, cromolyn, inhaled steroids, and airway clearance techniques. In addition, approximately 77% of patients were concurrently treated with dornase alfa (Pulmozyme).

In each study, tobramycin solution for inhalation-treated patients experienced significant improvement in pulmonary function. Improvement was demonstrated in the tobramycin solution for inhalation group in Study 1 by an average increase in FEV_1 % predicted of about 11% relative to baseline (Week 0) during 24 weeks compared to no average change in placebo patients. In Study 2, tobramycin solution for inhalation-treated patients had an average increase of about 7% compared to an average decrease of about 1% in placebo patients. Figure 1 shows the average relative change in FEV_1 % predicted over 24 weeks for both studies.

In each study, tobramycin solution for inhalation therapy resulted in a significant reduction of approximately 1 log in the number of *P. aeruginosa* colony forming units (CFUs) in sputum during the on-drug periods. Sputum bacterial density returned to baseline during the off-drug periods. Reductions in sputum bacterial density were smaller in each successive cycle (see Figure 2).

Figure 1: TOBI

Mean Relative Change From Baseline in FEV_1 % Predicted

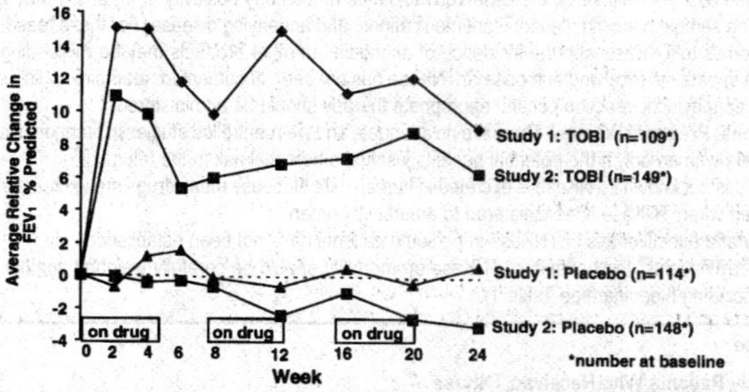

Figure 2: TOBI

Mean Absolute Change From Baseline in Log_{10} CFUs

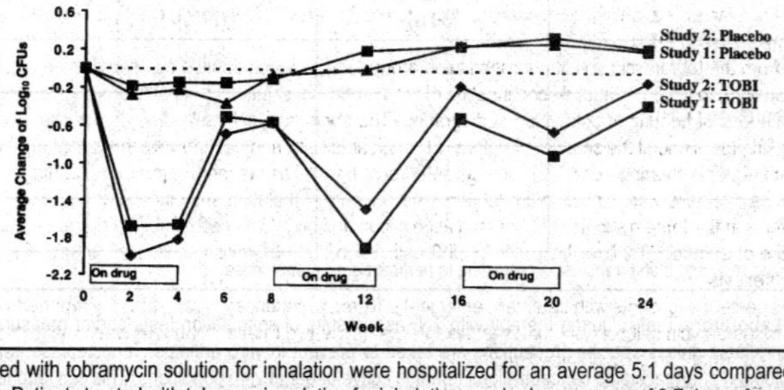

Patients treated with tobramycin solution for inhalation were hospitalized for an average 5.1 days compared to 8.1 days for placebo patients. Patients treated with tobramycin solution for inhalation required an average of 9.7 days of parenteral antipseudomonal antibiotic treatment compared to 14.1 days for placebo patients. During the 6 months of treatment, 40% of tobramycin solution for inhalation patients and 53% of placebo patients were treated with parenteral antipseudomonal antibiotics.

Treatment with tobramycin solution for inhalation for 3 cycles was associated with a decline in the in vitro susceptibility of *P. aeruginosa* isolates to tobramycin compared to placebo. The percentage of patients with *P. aeruginosa* isolates with tobramycin MICs ≥16 µg/mL was 13% at the beginning, and 23% at the end of 6 months of the tobramycin solution for inhalation regimen, compared to 10 and 8% in the placebo group.

The relationship between in vitro susceptibility test results and clinical outcome with tobramycin solution for inhalation therapy is not clear. However, 4 tobramycin solution for inhalation patients who began the clinical study with *P. aeruginosa* isolates having MIC values ≥128 µg/mL did not experience an improvement in FEV_1 or a decrease in sputum bacterial density.

Over 3 cycles of therapy with tobramycin solution for inhalation, the prevalence of *S. aureus* in sputum tended to decline while that of Aspergillis sp. and *C. albicans* increased.

INDICATIONS: For the management of cystic fibrosis patients with chronic pulmonary *P. aeruginosa* infections.

Demonstration of safety and efficacy of tobramycin solution for inhalation is limited to clinical trial data obtained over 3 cycles (6 months) of therapy for efficacy and up to 6 cycles (12 months) of therapy for safety.

Safety and efficacy have not been demonstrated in patients under the age of 6 years, patients with FEV_1 < 25% or >75% predicted, or patients colonized with *B. cepacia*.

Culture and sensitivity testing performed periodically will provide information on changing microbial flora and the possible emergence of bacterial resistance (see Pharmacology, Clinical Studies).

CONTRAINDICATIONS: In patients with a known hypersensitivity to any aminoglycoside.

WARNINGS: Caution should be exercised when prescribing tobramycin solution for inhalation to patients with known or suspected renal, auditory, vestibular, or neuromuscular dysfunction. Patients receiving concomitant parenteral aminoglycoside therapy should be monitored as clinically appropriate.
Pregnancy: Aminoglycosides can cause fetal harm when administered to a pregnant woman. Aminoglycosides cross the placenta, and streptomycin has been associated with several reports of total, irreversible, bilateral congenital deafness in pediatric patients exposed in utero. Patients who use tobramycin solution for inhalation during pregnancy, or become pregnant while taking tobramycin solution for inhalation should be apprised of the potential hazard to the fetus.

Ototoxicity: Ototoxicity, manifested as both auditory and vestibular toxicity, has been reported with aminoglycosides. Vestibular toxicity may be manifested by vertigo, ataxia or dizziness. Tinnitus is a sentinel symptom of ototoxicity, and therefore the onset of this symptom warrants caution.

In clinical studies, transient tinnitus occurred in 8 tobramycin solution for inhalation-treated patients vs no placebo patients.

In postmarketing experience, severe hearing loss has been reported in some patients who received tobramycin solution for inhalation therapy in association with either previous or concomitant parenteral aminoglycoside use (see Precautions and Adverse Effects).

Nephrotoxicity: Nephrotoxicity was not seen during 4 to 6 cycles of tobramycin solution for inhalation therapy in clinical studies but has been associated with aminoglycosides as a class. If nephrotoxicity occurs in a patient receiving tobramycin solution for inhalation, tobramycin therapy should be discontinued until serum concentrations fall below 2 µg/mL.

Muscular Disorders: Tobramycin solution for inhalation should be used cautiously in patients with muscular disorders, such as myasthenia gravis or Parkinson's disease, since aminoglycosides may aggravate muscle weakness because of a potential curare-like effect on neuromuscular function.

Bronchospasm: Bronchospasm can occur with inhalation of tobramycin solution for inhalation. In clinical studies of 3 cycles of tobramycin for inhalation therapy, acute changes in FEV_1% predicted, measured 30 minutes after the inhaled dose, documented decreases of ≥20% FEV_1% predicted in 12 tobramycin solution for inhalation patients (4.7%) and 2 placebo patients (0.8%). Bronchospasm should be treated as medically appropriate.

PRECAUTIONS: Laboratory Tests: Audiograms: Physicians should consider an audiogram for patients with known or suspected auditory dysfunction, or who are at increased risk for auditory dysfunction. Tinnitus may be a sentinel symptom of ototoxicity and therefore the onset of this symptom warrants caution.

Clinical studies of 4 to 6 cycles duration of tobramycin solution for inhalation therapy did not identify hearing loss using audiometric tests which used as criteria a bilateral, high frequency decrease of ≥15 dB at 2 consecutive frequencies, evaluating frequencies up to 8 000 Hz. However, tinnitus was documented in a small number of tobramycin solution for inhalation patients, and there have been occasional reports of severe hearing loss in postmarketing experience where patients received tobramycin solution for inhalation in association with previous or concomitant parenteral aminoclycoside use (see Warnings and Adverse Effects).

Serum Concentrations: In patients with normal renal function treated with tobramycin solution for inhalation, serum tobramycin concentrations are approximately 1 µg/mL 1 hour after dose administration and do not require routine monitoring. Serum concentrations of tobramycin in patients with renal dysfunction or patients treated with concomitant parenteral tobramycin should be monitored at the discretion of the treating physician.

Renal Function: The clinical studies of tobramycin solution for inhalation did not reveal any imbalance in the percentage of patients in the tobramycin solution for inhalation and placebo groups who experienced at least a 50% rise in serum creatinine from baseline through 3 cycles of therapy (see Adverse Effects). Laboratory tests of urine and renal function should be conducted at the discretion of the treating physician.

Drug Interactions: In clinical studies of tobramycin solution for inhalation, patients taking tobramycin solution for inhalation concomitantly with dornase alfa (Pulmozyme), β-agonists, inhaled corticosteroids, other antipseudomonal antibiotics, or parenteral aminoglycosides demonstrated adverse experience profiles similar to the study population as a whole. In postmarketing experience, some patients receiving tobramycin solution for inhalation with previous or concomitant parenteral aminoglycosides have reported severe hearing loss.

Concurrent and/or sequential use of tobramycin solution for inhalation with other drugs with neurotoxic or ototoxic potential should be avoided. Some diuretics can enhance aminoglycoside toxicity by altering antibiotic concentrations in serum and tissue. Tobramycin solution for inhalation should not be administered concomitantly with ethacrynic acid, furosemide, urea, or mannitol.

Pregnancy: No reproduction toxicology studies have been conducted with tobramycin solution for inhalation. However, s.c. administration of tobramycin at doses of 100 or 20 mg/kg/day during organogenesis was not teratogenic in rats or rabbits, respectively. Doses of tobramycin ≥40 mg/kg/day were severely maternally toxic to rabbits and precluded the evaluation of teratogenicity. Aminoglycosides can cause fetal harm (e.g., congenital deafness) when administered to a pregnant woman. Ototoxicity was not evaluated in offspring during nonclinical reproduction toxicity studies with tobramycin. If tobramycin solution for inhalation is used during pregnancy, or if the patient becomes pregnant while taking tobramycin solution for inhalation, the patient should be apprised of the potential hazard to the fetus.

Lactation: It is not known if tobramycin solution for inhalation will reach sufficient concentrations after administration by inhalation to be excreted in human breast milk. Because of the potential for ototoxicity and nephrotoxicity in infants, a decision should be made whether to terminate nursing or discontinue tobramycin solution for inhalation.

Children: The safety and efficacy of tobramycin solution for inhalation have not been studied in pediatric patients under 6 years of age.

ADVERSE EFFECTS: Tobramycin solution for inhalation was generally well tolerated during 2 clinical studies in 258 cystic fibrosis patients ranging in age from 6 to 48 years. Patients received tobramycin solution for inhalation in alternating periods of 28 days on and 28 days off drug in addition to their standard cystic fibrosis therapy for a total of 24 weeks.

Voice alteration and tinnitus were the only adverse experiences reported by significantly more tobramycin solution for inhalation-treated patients. Thirty-three patients (13%) treated with tobramycin solution for inhalation complained of voice alteration compared to 17 (7%) placebo patients. Voice alteration was more common in the on-drug periods. Episodes were transient and resolved during the off-drug period.

Eight patients from the tobramycin solution for inhalation group (3%) reported tinnitus compared to no placebo patients. All episodes were transient, resolved without discontinuation of the tobramycin solution for inhalation treatment regimen, and were not associated with loss of hearing in scheduled audiograms. (The audiogram schedule did not necessarily coincide with the tinnitus episode.) Tinnitus is one of the sentinel symptoms of cochlear toxicity, and patients with this symptom should be carefully monitored for high frequency hearing loss (see Warnings and Precautions). The numbers of patients reporting vestibular adverse experiences such as dizziness were similar in the tobramycin solution for inhalation and placebo groups.

Nine (3%) patients in the tobramycin solution for inhalation group and nine (3%) patients in the placebo group had increases in serum creatinine of at least 50% over baseline. In all 9 patients in the tobramycin solution for inhalation group, creatinine decreased at the next visit.

Table 2 lists the percent of patients with treatment-emergent adverse experiences (spontaneously reported and solicited) that occurred in >5% of tobramycin solution for inhalation patients during the two Phase III studies, where patients received up to 3 cycles of therapy (see Pharmacology, Clinical Studies).

Table 2: TOBI

Percent of Patients With Treatment Emergent Adverse Experiences Occurring in >5% of TOBI Patients During Phase III Studies (Up to 6 Months of Therapy)

Adverse Event	TOBI (n=258) %	Placebo (n=262) %
Body as a Whole		
Asthenia	35.7	39.3
Fever[a]	32.9	43.5
Headache	26.7	32.1
Chest Pain	26.0	29.8
Abdominal Pain	12.8	23.7
Pain	8.1	12.6
Back Pain	7.0	8.0
Malaise	6.2	5.3
Digestive		
Anorexia	18.6	27.9
Vomiting	14.0	22.1
Nausea	11.2	16.0
Diarrhea	6.2	10.3
Metabolic and Nutritional Disorders		
Weight Loss	10.1	15.3
Nervous System		
Dizziness	5.8	7.6
Respiratory		
Cough Increased	46.1	47.3
Pharyngitis	38.0	39.3
Sputum Increased	37.6	39.7
Rhinitis	34.5	33.6
Dyspnea	33.7	38.5
Lung Disorder	31.4	31.3
Sputum Discoloration	21.3	19.8
Hemoptysis	19.4	23.7
Lung Function Decreased[b]	16.3	15.3
Asthma	15.9	20.2
Voice Alteration	12.8	6.5
Sinusitis	8.1	9.2
Epistaxis	7.0	6.5
Lower Respiratory Tract Infection	5.8	8.0
Hyperventilation	5.4	9.9
Special Senses		
Ear Pain	7.4	8.8
Taste Perversion	6.6	6.9
Skin and Appendages		
Rash	5.4	6.1

[a] Includes subjective complaints of fever.
[b] Includes reported decreases in pulmonary function tests or decreased lung volume on chest radiograph associated with intercurrent illness or study drug administration.

In a follow-on study of tobramycin solution for inhalation, the following adverse experiences were observed at a higher frequency in patients who received 4 to 6 cycles (over 6 to 12 months) of tobramycin solution for inhalation therapy than that seen in patients who received ≤3 cycles (up to 6 months) (see Table 3). The role of chronic progression of disease on the increasing frequency of adverse experiences should be considered in the interpretation of these data.

Table 3: TOBI

Treatment Emergent Adverse Experiences[a] Occurring at Higher Frequency During 6 to 12 Months of TOBI Therapy

Adverse Event	4-6 Cycles (n=192) %	≤3 Cycles (n=204) %
Body as a Whole		
Asthenia	44.3	38.2
Chest Pain	36.5	35.3
Back Pain	10.4	5.9
Lymphadenopathy	8.3	6.9
Chills	6.8	5.9
Sweating	5.7	4.9
Digestive		
Anorexia	29.2	27.5
Diarrhea	16.7	12.7
Oral Monoliasis	6.3	2.5

(cont'd)

Table 3: TOBI *(cont'd)*

Treatment Emergent Adverse Experiences[a] Occurring at Higher Frequency During 6 to 12 Months of TOBI Therapy

Adverse Event	4-6 Cycles (n=192) %	≤3 Cycles (n=204) %
Dyspepsia	5.2	4.9
Musculoskeletal		
Myalgia	5.7	5.4
Respiratory		
Cough Increased	49.5	48.0
Pharyngitis	47.9	43.6
Sputum Increased	43.8	38.2
Dyspnea	41.7	33.8
Rhinitis	37.5	33.3
Hemoptysis	31.3	27.0
Lung Function Decreased	28.6	23.0
Asthma	28.1	23.5
Sputum Discoloration	24.5	19.1
Upper Respiratory Infection	13.5	9.8
Voice Alteration	12.0	6.4
Hyperventilation	8.9	5.4
Laryngitis	5.2	3.4
Special Senses		
Otitis Media	5.2	2.0

[a] Includes Adverse Experiences that were observed in >5% of patients in the 4 to 6 Cycles group and at a higher frequency than in the ≤3 Cycles group. (The ≤3 Cycles group received placebo during Phase III studies).

In open label follow-on clinical trials and postmarketing surveillance, the following additional adverse events have been reported infrequently in patients receiving tobramycin solution for inhalation concurrently with other medications: Allergic reactions, fungal infection, hearing loss, hypoxia, mouth ulcerations and photosensitivity reaction.

OVERDOSE:

Symptoms: Signs and symptoms of acute toxicity from overdosage of i.v. tobramycin might include dizziness, tinnitus, vertigo, loss of high-tone hearing acuity, respiratory failure, and neuromuscular blockade. Administration by inhalation results in low systemic bioavailability of tobramycin. Tobramycin is not significantly absorbed following oral administration. Tobramycin serum concentrations may be helpful in monitoring overdose.

Treatment: In all cases of suspected overdosage, physicians should contact the Regional Poison Control Centre for information about effective treatment. In the case of any overdosage, the possibility of drug interactions with alterations in drug disposition should be considered.

> For management of a suspected drug overdose, CPhA recommends that you contact your **regional Poison Control Centre**. See the *CPS* Directory section for a list of Poison Control Centres.

DOSAGE: The recommended dosage for both adults and pediatric patients 6 years of age and older is 1 single-use ampul (300 mg) administered twice a day (b.i.d.) for 28 days. The doses should be taken as close to 12 hours apart as possible; they should not be taken less than 6 hours apart.

Tobramycin solution for inhalation is administered b.i.d. in alternating periods of 28 days. After 28 days of therapy, patients should stop tobramycin solution for inhalation therapy for the next 28 days, and then resume therapy for the next 28 day on / 28 day off cycle.

Dosage is not adjusted by weight. All patients should be administered 300 mg b.i.d.

Administration: Tobramycin solution for inhalation is supplied as a single-use ampul and is administered by inhalation. Tobramycin solution for inhalation is not for s.c., i.v. or intrathecal administration.

Tobramycin solution for inhalation is administered using a hand-held Pari LC Plus reusable nebulizer with a DeVilbiss Pulmo-Aide compressor over a 15-minute period on average. Tobramycin solution for inhalation is inhaled while the patient is sitting or standing upright and breathing normally through the mouthpiece of the nebulizer. Nose clips may help the patient breathe through the mouth.

Tobramycin solution for inhalation should not be diluted or mixed with dornase alfa (Pulmozyme) in the nebulizer.

During clinical studies, patients on multiple therapies were instructed to take them first, followed by tobramycin solution for inhalation.

INFORMATION FOR THE PATIENT: Published in e-CPS, available by subscription at www.e-cps.ca.

SUPPLIED: TOBI is a tobramycin solution for inhalation. Each ampul of sterile, clear, slightly yellow, nonpyrogenic, aqueous solution, with a pH (6.0) and salinity specifically adjusted for administration by a compressed air driven reusable nebulizer, contains: tobramycin solution 300 mg (as sulfate). Nonmedicinal ingredients: nitrogen, sodium chloride, sodium hydroxide, sterile water for injection and sulfuric acid. Preservative-free. Low-density polyethylene plastic ampuls of 5 mL. Boxes of 56 (14 flexible, laminated foil over-pouches, each containing 4 ampuls).

Store under refrigeration at 2 to 8°C. Upon removal from the refrigerator, or if refrigeration is unavailable, the pouches (opened or unopened) may be stored at room temperature (up to 25°C). Do not use beyond the expiration date stamped on the ampul when stored under refrigeration (2 to 8°C) or beyond 28 days when stored at room temperature (25°C). Ampuls should not be exposed to intense light. The solution in the ampul is slightly yellow, but may darken with age if not stored in the refrigerator; however, the color change does not indicate any change in the quality of the product as long as it is stored within the recommended storage conditions.

(Shown in Product Identification Section)

Tobradex® Pr
tobramycin—dexamethasone
Antibiotic—Corticosteroid

Alcon

SUPPLIED: Ointment: Each g of sterile ophthalmic ointment contains: tobramycin 3 mg and dexamethasone 0.1% with chlorobutanol 0.5% as a preservative in a mineral oil and petrolatum base. Tubes of 3.5 g.

Suspension: Each mL of sterile, isotonic, aqueous suspension contains: tobramycin 3 mg and dexamethasone 0.1% with benzalkonium chloride 0.01% as a preservative. Nonmedicinal ingredients: edetate disodium, hydroxyethyl cellulose, purified water, sodium chloride, sodium hydroxide and/or sulfuric acid (to adjust pH), sodium sulfate and tyloxapol. Drop-Tainer dispensers of 5 mL. Shake well before use. Store in an upright position. Store at room temperature.

Tobramycin Pr
Antibacterial

CPhA Monograph

Date of Preparation: November 2007

> This monograph has been compiled by CPhA and reviewed by experts. It may contain information different from that found in Health Canada-approved Product Monographs. The reader is referred to the *CPS* Editorial Policy for more information.

SUMMARY PRODUCT INFORMATION:

Drug	Route of Administration	Dosage Form	Strength
Tobramycin	Injectable (IV, IM)	Solution	10 mg/mL (2 mL); 40 mg/mL (3 mL)
	Injectable (IV, IM)	Powder for solution	1.2 g/vial
	Ophthalmic	Solution	0.3% (5 mL); 3 mg/mL (5 mL)
	Inhalation	Solution	60 mg/mL [300 mg/5 mL]
Tobramycin/ dexamethasone	Ophthalmic	Ointment	Tobramycin (0.3%) 3 mg/g plus dexamethasone (0.1%) 1 mg/g (3.5 g)
	Ophthalmic	Suspension	Tobramycin 0.3% plus dexamethasone 0.1% (5 mL)

INDICATIONS AND CLINICAL USE: Tobramycin is an aminoglycoside antibacterial agent. The spectrum of activity of tobramycin includes primarily aerobic gram-negative bacteria including nosocomial pathogens.

Tobramycin is indicated for:

- treatment of nosocomial infections due to susceptible aerobic gram-negative bacteria
- treatment of serious or complicated infections including bone and joint infections, genitourinary tract infections, and intra-abdominal infections when used in combination with other antibacterial agents
- use in synergistic antibacterial combination regimens for empiric treatment of hospital-acquired pneumonia, ventilator-associated pneumonia in patients with late-onset disease or risk factors for multidrug-resistant pathogens
- empiric treatment of infections in febrile neutropenic patients in combination with another agent
- treatment of pulmonary infections in patients with cystic fibrosis
- prevention of exacerbations and maintenance of stable clinical status in patients with cystic fibrosis when administered as an inhalation aerosol
- topical therapy of superficial eye infections

Aminoglycosides are generally active against *P. aeruginosa*; however, tobramycin is considered to have 2 to 4 times more activity against this pathogen than gentamicin (on the basis of minimum inhibitory concentrations). In contrast, tobramycin has less activity than gentamicin in the setting of enterococcal infections. Among aerobic gram-negative bacteria, *S. maltophilia* and *B. cepacia* are unusual in that they are not considered to be susceptible to aminoglycosides. Tobramycin is the most active aminoglycoside antibiotic against *M. chelonae*, a species of rapidly growing mycobacteria that can cause skin, bone and soft tissue infections. Anaerobic bacteria are not susceptible to aminoglycosides.

Acquired resistance to aminoglycosides is mediated via numerous aminoglycoside-modifying enzymes produced by bacteria that alter specific amino or hydroxyl functions on the drug. Acquired resistance to one aminoglycoside does not necessarily confer resistance to other agents in the class.

Tobramycin is eliminated almost exclusively by renal excretion and is associated with nephrotoxicity. For this reason the drug must be used with caution and the dose must be individualized in patients with renal impairment. Monitoring of renal function (i.e., BUN and serum creatinine) is recommended during treatment.

Tobramycin is also associated with ototoxicity, which is usually not reversible. Some individuals are predisposed to aminoglycoside-associated ototoxicity because of a maternally inherited mutation in mitochondrial DNA that makes the human mitochondrial ribosome more closely resemble the bacterial ribosome, which is the site of action for these drugs [*BMJ* 2007;335:784-5].

Geriatrics: Elderly patients may be more susceptible to aminoglycoside-associated nephrotoxicity due to the age-related decline in renal function. The dosage regimen of tobramycin must be tailored to renal function.

Pediatrics: Aminoglycoside antibiotics have been used extensively in pediatric patients including neonates. Changes in renal function during the neonatal period (see Warnings and Precautions, Special Populations, Pediatrics) must be considered when selecting a dosing regimen for tobramycin or another aminoglycoside antibiotic.

CONTRAINDICATIONS:

- Patients who are hypersensitive to tobramycin, or other aminoglycoside antibiotics, or to any ingredient in the formulation.

WARNINGS AND PRECAUTIONS:

> **Serious Warnings and Precautions**
> - Nephrotoxicity and ototoxicity are serious adverse effects associated with tobramycin and other aminoglycosides. These effects may be seen in any patient treated with these drugs, but are more likely to occur in the following settings: pre-existing renal, vestibular or auditory impairment, older individuals, dehydration, concomitant therapy with other nephrotoxic or ototoxic agents, or prolonged therapy.
> - Neuromuscular blockade has been associated with aminoglycoside antibiotics.

Neurologic: Aminoglycosides are associated with eighth cranial nerve toxicity, which may affect the vestibular and the auditory senses and is generally not reversible. Symptoms of vestibular toxicity include nausea, vomiting, dizziness, nystagmus, vertigo and ataxia. Symptoms of cochlear (auditory) toxicity include tinnitus, roaring in the ears and hearing impairment. Loss of high frequency auditory perception, which may be detected by audiometric testing, usually precedes clinically detectable hearing loss. Some individuals have a genetic predisposition to aminoglycoside-induced ototoxicity. Ototoxicity has occurred within the recommended target serum concentration range. Patients receiving high cumulative doses of tobramycin or therapy for protracted periods are at increased risk of developing ototoxicity. In patients receiving protracted therapy, consideration should be given to performing regular audiograms (e.g., weekly) to detect signs of ototoxicity before it becomes clinically significant.

Neuromuscular blockade associated with aminoglycosides is dose-related and generally self-limiting, but may rarely lead to respiratory muscle paralysis. Clinical manifestations include flaccid paralysis, dilated pupils and weakness of the respiratory musculature. Neuromuscular effects occur more commonly after application to serosal surfaces (e.g., after intrapleural injection or peritoneal instillation), after administration to patients with neuromuscular disease (e.g., myasthenia gravis), hypocalcemia or hypomagnesemia, or after concomitant administration with neuromuscular blocking agents. Rapid injection of aminoglycoside antibiotics is a risk factor for neuromuscular blockade; therefore, these drugs should be infused over at least 30 minutes.

Perioperative Considerations: Aminoglycosides may produce neuromuscular blockade when used in combination with neuromuscular blocking agents (e.g., succinylcholine, tubocurarine).

Renal: Aminoglycosides are associated with renal tubular necrosis, which decreases the glomerular filtration rate and is reflected in increased concentrations of BUN and serum creatinine. Aminoglycoside-associated nephrotoxicity is most often evident as nonoliguric azotemia; oliguria is rare. Changes in renal function are usually reversible when the drug is discontinued.

Patient-related factors associated with an increased risk of aminoglycoside-associated nephrotoxicity include older age, pre-existing renal disease, volume depletion, hypotension, hepatic dysfunction and recent treatment with an aminoglycoside antibiotic. Concomitant administration of nephrotoxic drugs may increase the clinical risk of aminoglycoside-associated nephrotoxicity.

Factors that decrease the risk of aminoglycoside-associated nephrotoxicity include younger age, normal renal and hepatic function, use of smaller cumulative doses and treatment for less than 3 days, and use of extended interval ("once daily") dosing regimens (see Dosage and Administration).

Nephrotoxicity has occurred within the recommended target serum concentration range. Peak serum aminoglycoside levels are not a clinical risk factor for aminoglycoside-associated nephrotoxicity. In contrast, nephrotoxicity is associated with persistently elevated trough serum concentrations.

Special Populations: Pregnant Women: Tobramycin crosses the placenta and is distributed into the fetal circulation and amniotic fluid; it is not considered to be teratogenic and has been used to treat serious infections in pregnancy.

Nursing Women: Tobramycin is excreted in breast milk, but is considered to be compatible with breast-feeding because it is minimally absorbed from the gastrointestinal tract.

Pediatrics: Tobramycin is used in the pediatric setting including treatment of suspected or confirmed infections in neonates. The pharmacokinetics of tobramycin differs in neonates compared with older children in that renal clearance of the drug is prolonged in infants. Specific dosage guidelines for neonates and children should be consulted.

Geriatrics: Elimination of tobramycin is prolonged in elderly patients because of the age-related decline in glomerular filtration rate. Renal function should be determined at baseline and monitored during therapy with tobramycin. Specific dosage guidelines for patients with renal dysfunction should be consulted and the dosage regimen should be adjusted accordingly.

Monitoring and Laboratory Tests: Renal function (BUN and serum creatinine) should be monitored before and during therapy with tobramycin.

When extended interval dosing (Table 6) of tobramycin is employed it is not necessary to monitor peak serum drug levels. Some extended interval dosing protocols require measurement of the serum concentration.

It is necessary to measure serum drug concentrations and individualize the dose of tobramycin if achievement of specific peak and trough serum concentrations is desired. Some authors have argued that dose individualization is preferred to the use of dosing nomograms because of the wide interindividual variation in aminoglycoside pharmacokinetics [see *Clin Pharmacokinet* 1999;36(2):89-98 and *Pharmacotherapy* 2002;22(9):1077-1083].

If tobramycin is dosed in the conventional manner (Table 7), monitoring of peak and trough tobramycin levels is recommended in patients receiving prolonged courses of therapy, and in those with renal dysfunction or serious infections. Calculation of pharmacokinetic parameters is done with steady state versions of one-compartment equations. Serum concentrations should be measured at steady state, which is achieved after 3 to 5 half-lives have elapsed. If no loading dose is administered, steady state will usually be achieved after the third or fourth dose (this is also the case after each dose adjustment). Peak concentrations should be measured after the distribution phase is complete; ideally 30 to 60 minutes after the end of the infusion. Trough concentrations may be measured 30 minutes before infusion of the next dose. Specific target peak and trough concentrations are provided in Table 7. If a higher peak concentration is desired, the dose of tobramycin should be increased. If a lower trough concentration is desired, prolonging the dosing interval is preferred. Determination of peak and trough levels should be repeated after dosage adjustments to ensure the desired results have been obtained.

ADVERSE REACTIONS: More Common Adverse Drug Reactions (≥1%): See Table 1.

Table 1: Tobramycin

More Common Adverse Drug Reactions (≥1%)

Body System	Effect	Clinical Comment
Renal	Nephrotoxicity. Damage to proximal tubule marked by elevated BUN, elevated serum creatinine and decreased urine specific gravity. May involve proteinuria, nonoliguric azotemia, aminoaciduria and metabolic acidosis, electrolyte wasting and renal failure.	Monitor renal function at baseline and during treatment. Individualize dose based on renal function and adjust the dose based on changes in renal function and or serum drug levels. Consider alternative antibiotics in patients at risk.

Less Common Adverse Drug Reactions (<1%): Overview: Cardiovascular: tachycardia, hypotension, hypertension.

Central Nervous System: headache, dizziness, nystagmus, vertigo, ataxia, tinnitus, roaring in the ears, hearing impairment, loss of high frequency hearing perception.

Allergic/Dermatologic: local irritation, phlebitis, rash, urticaria, stomatitis, pruritus, fever, toxic epidermal necrolysis, erythema multiforme, Stevens-Johnson syndrome. Hypersensitivity reactions are rare with aminoglycosides. Cross-allergenicity with aminoglycosides has been reported.

Gastrointestinal: anorexia, weight loss, nausea and vomiting.

Hematologic: anemia, leukopenia, granulocytopenia, thrombocytopenia.

Hepatic/Biliary/Pancreatic: hepatic necrosis, hepatomegaly, splenomegaly, transient increase in serum transaminase, alkaline phosphatase and bilirubin levels.

Neurologic: peripheral neuropathy, numbness, tingling, muscle twitching, seizures, myasthenia gravis-like syndrome, tremor.

Abnormal Hematologic and Clinical Chemistry Findings: See Table 2.

Table 2: Tobramycin

Abnormal Hematologic and Clinical Chemistry Findings

Test	Effect	Clinical Comment
BUN	Increased	An increase in BUN and serum creatinine over baseline is an indication of nephrotoxicity.
Serum creatinine	Increased	In patients with a serum creatinine in the normal range before therapy, an increase to >133 µmol/L or an absolute increase of 35 µmol/L may indicate nephrotoxicity. In patients with a baseline serum creatinine concentration >133 µmol/L, an increase of >44 µmol/L is indicative of nephrotoxicity; in those with a baseline serum creatinine concentration >265 µmol/L, an increase of >88 µmol/L is indicative of nephrotoxicity. If nephrotoxicity occurs during treatment with tobramycin, the preferred strategy is discontinuation of the drug and substitution with an alternative non-nephrotoxic agent. If discontinuation is not possible, then the dosage should be adjusted accordingly and renal function monitored.

DRUG INTERACTIONS:

Serious Drug Interactions

- Concomitant administration of nephrotoxic drugs may increase the clinical risk of aminoglycoside-associated nephrotoxicity.
- Concomitant administration of tobramycin with neuromuscular blocking agents may result in an increased risk of neuromuscular blockade.

Overview: Because potential drug interactions involving tobramycin generally involve combinations that result in additive nephrotoxicity or ototoxicity, it is best to avoid combined use of tobramycin with any agent that is known to be nephrotoxic or ototoxic. If combined use cannot be avoided, monitoring of renal function and serum tobramycin levels and adjustment of the dosage of tobramycin are recommended. Tobramycin does not alter the pharmacokinetics of other drugs.

Drug-Drug Interactions: See Table 3.

DOSAGE AND ADMINISTRATION: Dosing Considerations: Tobramycin may be administered by iv or im injection. In addition, commercial preparations are available for ophthalmic application and for administration by inhalation.

In contemporary clinical practice there are two broad strategies used to dose tobramycin. Extended interval ("once daily") administration involves administration of single large iv doses of tobramycin at prolonged intervals (i.e., 24 hours or longer). The alternative (conventional) approach involves administering lower doses of the drug at more frequent intervals (e.g., Q8H) with monitoring of peak and trough serum concentrations.

Table 3: Tobramycin

Drug-Drug Interactions

Interacting Drug	Effect	Clinical Comment
Amphotericin B	Additive nephrotoxicity	Monitor renal function and adjust the dose of tobramycin if BUN or SCr increases.
Cisplatin	Additive nephrotoxicity	Monitor renal function and adjust the dose of tobramycin if BUN or SCr increases.
Cyclosporine	Additive nephrotoxicity	Monitor renal function and adjust the dose of tobramycin if BUN or SCr increases.
Vancomycin	Additive nephrotoxicity	Monitor renal function and adjust the dose of tobramycin if BUN or SCr increases.
Ethacrynic acid	Additive ototoxicity	Avoid combination use. Monitor for signs and symptoms of ototoxicity.
Furosemide or bumetanide	Increased risk of nephrotoxicity or ototoxicity	Monitor renal function and adjust the dose of tobramycin if BUN or SCr increases. Monitor for signs of ototoxicity.
Indomethacin	Increased tobramycin serum levels in infants	Monitor renal function and serum levels of tobramycin and adjust the dose of tobramycin accordingly.
Neuromuscular blocking agents	Additive neuromuscular blockade	Monitor respiratory function. Provide supportive care if an interaction occurs. May respond to neostigmine.
Botulinum toxin	Additive neuromuscular blockade	Avoid concurrent use. If given together, monitor respiratory function.

Whichever strategy is used, the dose of tobramycin should be individualized according to patient weight and renal function. Specialized references for pediatric patients should be consulted when prescribing tobramycin for neonates or children.

Several lines of evidence suggest that extended interval administration of aminoglycosides may be less toxic than conventional three-times-daily administration. The principles underlying extended interval administration include concentration-dependent killing of susceptible bacteria, the post-antibiotic effect, and time-dependent nephrotoxicity and ototoxicity. High peak serum concentrations of aminoglycoside antibiotics are not associated with an increased incidence of adverse events. Thus, extended interval administration of aminoglycosides may be preferred to administration of multiple daily doses for some but not all indications.

Situations in which extended interval dosing of aminoglycosides should not be considered are presented in Table 5.

Table 4: Tobramycin

Indications and Recommended Regimens

Indication	Route	Recommended Regimen (see also Table 5, Table 6, Table 7, Table 8, Table 9, Table 10)	Duration of Treatment	Clinical Comment
Treatment of infections in adults	IV/IM	Extended interval ("once daily") iv dosing. Alternative: conventional divided daily dosing.	Dependent upon susceptibility of organisms and response to therapy.	Usually used in combination with other agents. Switch to a suitable oral antibiotic as soon as feasible.
Empiric treatment of febrile neutropenic adults	IV/IM	Extended interval ("once daily") iv dosing. Alternative: conventional divided daily dosing.	Dependent upon susceptibility of organisms and response to therapy.	Administer in combination with a broad spectrum antipseudomonal agent (i.e., cephalosporin, antipseudomonal penicillin, carbapenem). Monitor renal function and adjust dosage (as per Table 8 recommendations).
Treatment of infections in neonates or children	IV	Conventional divided daily dosing. (Table 9, Table 10)	Dependent upon susceptibility of organisms and response to therapy.	Administer in combination with other antibacterial agents. Monitor renal function and adjust dose as appropriate.
Cystic fibrosis (patients aged >6 years)	Inhalation	80 mg TID Or High dose regimen: 300 mg via nebulizer Q12H × 28 days then stop × 28 days, then repeat		In patients who have moderate to severe lung disease and with *P. aeruginosa* persistently present in cultures of airways, chronic use of inhaled tobramycin improves lung function, prevents exacerbations and is strongly recommended [*Am J Crit Care Med* 2007;176:957–69]. In patients with mild disease and those who are asymptomatic with *P. aeruginosa* persistently present in cultures of airways, the drug prevents exacerbations and is recommended [*Am J Crit Care Med* 2007;176:957–69]. Administer over 15 minutes by nebulizer. A formulation for inhalation is available commercially.

There are several protocols for extended interval dosing of aminoglycosides. One approach is presented in Table 6. The Hartford method is an alternative in which the dose of tobramycin is 7 mg/kg. The serum concentration is determined 6 to 14 hours after the start of an infusion and the measured serum level is plotted on the nomogram to determine the dosage interval [*Antimicrob Agent Chemother* 1995;39:650-55]. The Hartford nomogram and more information on the use of this method is available online at www.bugsanddrugs.ca.

Ophthalmic: For the treatment of superficial ophthalmologic infections caused by susceptible bacteria, 1 or 2 drops in the affected eye(s) 4 times daily for 5 days. In severe infections instil 2 drops per hour initially and then decrease the frequency of administration to less frequent intervals as the infection resolves.

Alternatively, a strip of ointment may be placed in the affected eye(s) 2 or 3 times daily.

Recommended Dose and Dosage Adjustment: See Table 4, Table 5, Table 6, Table 7, Table 8, Table 9 and Table 10.

Dosage in Continuous Ambulatory Peritoneal Dialysis: In adult patients receiving continuous ambulatory peritoneal dialysis it is estimated that 3 to 4 mg of tobramycin will be lost per litre of dialysate each day. Thus in a patient receiving 8 L of dialysate per day a total of 24 to 32 mg will be lost daily and may be replaced intravenously.

Tobramycin may be added directly to peritoneal dialysis fluid for the treatment of peritonitis. In patients receiving continuous ambulatory peritoneal dialysis the recommended dose of tobramycin is 0.6 mg/kg in one exchange per day. In patients receiving automated peritoneal dialysis a loading dose of 1.5 mg/kg on day 1 is followed by 0.5 mg/kg once daily added to the first or second ambulatory dwell. The duration of treatment is determined by the clinical response. Systemic toxicity can occur when tobramycin is given by the intraperitoneal route. Thus patients should be closely monitored.

Table 5: Tobramycin

Situations in which Extended Interval ("Once Daily") Dosing of Tobramycin is Not Recommended in Adults

Extensive burns (>20% body surface area)
Ascites (altered volume of distribution)
Pregnancy/postpartum (altered volume of distribution)
Patients with gram-positive infections for which gentamicin is used for synergy (exception: endocarditis due to viridans group streptococci)
Surgical prophylaxis

Table 6: Tobramycin

Extended Interval ("Once Daily") Administration in Adults[a]

Estimated ClCr[b] (mL/min)	Dosage Interval (h)	Dose (mg/kg IBW[c])
100	24	5
90	24	5
80	24	5
70	24	4
60	24	4
50	24	3.5
40	24	2.5
30	24	2.5
20	48	4
10	48	3
Hemodialysis	48 (give after dialysis)	2

[a] Measure the trough level prior to the third dose. The desired trough level is <1 µg/mL.
[b] ClCr = creatinine clearance (estimate using the Cockcroft-Gault equation).

$$\text{ClCr (mL/min)} = \frac{1.2\ (140-\text{age})\ (\text{wt in kg})}{\text{serum creatinine (µmol/L)}}$$

For females, multiply the result by 0.85
[c] IBW = ideal body weight.
IBW (kg; males) = 50 + (2.3 × height in inches over 5 feet).
IBW (kg; females) = 45.5 + (2.3 × height in inches over 5 feet).
Adjusted body weight (ABW) has been recommended for dosing aminoglycosides in obese individuals (i.e., if total body weight is >25% above the IBW [see *Br J Clin Pharmacol* 2004;58(2):119-33 and *Antimicrob Agents Chemother* 1995;39(2):545-8].
ABW = IBW + 0.4 × (total body weight − IBW).

Table 7: Tobramycin

Conventional Dosing in Adults with ClCr >90 mL/min (as an alternative to extended interval dosing)

Route	Loading Dose	Maintenance Dose	Desired Serum Concentration	
			Peak	Trough
IV/IM	2 mg/kg (IBW[a])	1.7 mg/kg (IBW[a]) Q8H	5–10 µg/mL	0.5–2 µg/mL
Peak concentration is measured 30 to 60 minutes after infusion to allow for distribution. Trough concentration is measured 30 minutes prior to infusion of the next dose.				

[a] IBW = ideal body weight.
IBW (kg; males) = 50 + (2.3 × height in inches over 5 feet).
IBW (kg; females) = 45.5 + (2.3 × height in inches over 5 feet).
Adjusted body weight (ABW) has been recommended for dosing aminoglycosides in obese individuals (i.e., if total body weight is >25% above the IBW [see *Br J Clin Pharmacol* 2004;58(2):119-33 and *Antimicrob Agents Chemother* 1995;39(2):545-8].
ABW = IBW + 0.4 × (total body weight − IBW).

Table 8: Tobramycin

Conventional Dose in Adults with Renal Dysfunction (as an alternative to extended interval dosing)

Route	ClCr[a] (mL/min)	Dose	Clinical Comment
IV/IM	>50–90	60–90% of recommended dose Q8–12H (see Table 7)	Monitor serum concentration and adjust dosage regimen to achieve desired peak (4–10 µg/mL) and trough (1–2 µg/mL) serum levels.
IV/IM	10–50	30–70% of recommended dose Q12H (see Table 7)	
IV/IM	<10	20–30% of recommended dose Q24–48H (see Table 7)	
IV/IM	Hemodialysis	Dose as for ClCr <10 mL/min; give supplemental ½ dose after dialysis	

[a] ClCr = creatinine clearance (estimate using the Cockcroft-Gault equation).

$$\text{ClCr (mL/min)} = \frac{1.2\ (140-\text{age})\ (\text{wt in kg})}{\text{serum creatinine (µmol/L)}}$$

For females, multiply the result by 0.85

Dosage in Hemodialysis: See Table 6 and Table 8.

Hepatic Impairment: Tobramycin is not eliminated by hepatic metabolism; hence no dosage adjustments are required in patients with hepatic dysfunction. However, patients with severe hepatic dysfunction are at increased risk of nephrotoxicity, so careful monitoring of renal function is advised in these individuals.

Pediatrics: Regimens recommended in the SickKids Drug Handbook and Formulary 2007–2008 are presented in Table 9 for neonates and in Table 10 for older infants and children.

There have been numerous studies of extended interval dosing of aminoglycosides in children. A meta-analysis of 24 studies concluded that this approach simplifies administration and provides similar or better efficacy and safety compared with conventional multiple daily dose regimens [*Pediatrics* 2004;114(1):111-8]. Tobramycin was administered at dosages ranging from 8 to 15 mg/kg once daily in the studies that were considered in the analysis.

Table 9: Tobramycin

Dose in Neonates

Route	Age and Weight	Dose
IV	Neonates ≤7 days (PCA <34 weeks)[a]	3 mg/kg/dose Q24H
IV	Neonates ≤7 days (PCA ≥34 weeks)[a]	3 mg/kg/dose Q18H
IV	Neonates >7 days and ≤1 kg[a]	3.5 mg/kg/dose Q24H
IV	Neonates >7 days (PCA <37 weeks) and >1 kg[a]	2.5 mg/kg/dose Q12H
IV	Neonates >7 days (PCA ≥37 weeks) and >1 kg[a]	2.5 mg/kg/dose Q8H
The peak concentration is measured 30 to 60 minutes after infusion to allow for distribution. The desired peak is 5–9 µg/mL. The trough concentration is measured 30 minutes prior to infusion of the next dose. The desired trough level is 0.5–2 µg/mL.		

[a] Applies to neonates until a postconceptional age of >38 weeks and a postnatal age of 28 days is achieved [*SickKids Drug Handbook and Formulary* 2007-2008].
Abbreviations: PCA=postconceptional age.

Table 10: Tobramycin

Dose in Pediatric Patients

Route	Age and Weight	Dose
IM/IV	Infants >28 days and children	7.5 mg/kg/day divided Q8H (maximum 120 mg/dose prior to measuring serum levels)
IV	Females ≥14 years with cystic fibrosis[a]	7 mg/kg/day Q24H (no dose limit)
IV	All other patients with cystic fibrosis[a]	9 mg/kg/day Q24H (no dose limit)
If given Q8H the peak concentration is measured 30 to 60 minutes after infusion to allow for distribution. The desired peak is 5–9 µg/mL. If given Q8H the trough concentration is measured 30 minutes prior to infusion of the next dose. The desired trough level is 0.5–2 µg/mL.		

[a] See *J Antimicrob Chemother* 2007;59(6):1135-40 and *SickKids Drug Handbook and Formulary* 2007-2008.

Pulmonary Administration in Children: The recommended dose of tobramycin is 80 mg TID via nebulizer [*SickKids Drug Handbook and Formulary* 2007-2008]. There is a specific product that is indicated for inhalation.

Administration: Tobramycin may be administered by iv or im injection. It is impractical to administer large injection volumes, such as those required in extended interval regimens, by im injection. When large doses are given by iv infusion the drug should be infused over at least 30 minutes to minimize the possibility of neuromuscular blockade.

OVERDOSAGE:

For management of a suspected drug overdose, CPhA recommends that you contact your **regional Poison Control Centre**. See the *CPS* Directory section for a list of Poison Control Centres.

ACTION AND CLINICAL PHARMACOLOGY: Mechanism of Action: Tobramycin is highly water soluble, a property that limits its ability to cross lipid-rich cellular membranes. The drug is also positively charged, such that activity is enhanced at alkaline pH and decreased at acidic pH. Transport of aminoglycosides across bacterial cytoplasmic membranes is an energy-dependent process. Tobramycin binds to the 30S subunit of prokaryotic ribosomes. This results in a conformational change in the structure of the ribosomal subunit and impairs messenger RNA translation and translocation. The drug also binds electrostatically to the lipopolysaccharide layer of gram-negative bacteria, an effect that ultimately disrupts the permeability of the bacterial cell wall.

Aminoglycosides are bactericidal antibiotics that are characterized by concentration-dependent killing of susceptible bacteria. As the rate of killing increases in proportion to the serum concentration, achievement of higher serum concentrations may enhance efficacy. This phenomenon forms part of the rationale for extended interval dosing regimens.

Aminoglycosides are associated with a significant post-antibiotic effect. This phenomenon results in persistent suppression of bacterial growth after exposure to the antibiotic. The duration of the post-antibiotic effect is prolonged after exposure to high drug concentrations and persists after the concentration falls below the minimal inhibitory concentration of the organism. The post-antibiotic effect forms part of the rationale for extended interval dosing of aminoglycosides.

The uptake of aminoglycosides by gram-positive cocci is enhanced by concomitant exposure to cell-wall active agents, a phenomenon which forms the basis for the clinical use of aminoglycosides and penicillins as a synergistic combination against certain pathogens.

The antibacterial efficacy of aminoglycosides is not affected by the size of the inoculum.

Pharmacokinetics: Adults: Absorption: Aminoglycosides are minimally absorbed from the gastrointestinal tract and thus must be administered intravenously or intramuscularly in order to treat systemic infections. When administered as a 1 mg/kg im dose to patients with normal renal function, tobramycin peak serum concentrations of 4 to 6 µg/mL occur within 30 to 90 minutes and trough serum concentrations of ≤1 µg/mL occur 6 to 8 hours after injection. Absorption may be delayed in patients with hypotension or poor tissue perfusion.

Tobramycin is minimally absorbed into the systemic circulation after inhalation. Serum concentrations of 0.95 µg/mL were obtained 1 hour after inhalation of a single 300 mg dose in patients with cystic fibrosis. The mean sputum concentration was 1237 µg/g after inhalation of a 300 mg dose over 10 minutes via nebulizer.

Distribution: Aminoglycoside antibiotics are minimally bound to plasma proteins (~10%) and, given their high water solubility, are distributed in the vascular space and interstices of most tissues. Drug concentrations in interstitial fluids at steady state approximate those of plasma. The volume of distribution is typically on the order of 0.2 to 0.3 L/kg. However, the volume of distribution increases in certain clinical situations including extensive burns, ascites, pregnancy and the postpartum state.

Aminoglycosides accumulate in the cells of the proximal convoluted tubule to concentrations that exceed those in plasma. Nephrotoxicity is probably due to time-dependent accumulation of drug within cells of the proximal convoluted tubule. Thus, minimizing exposure to the drug, as with extended interval administration, may minimize the risk of nephrotoxicity. This reasoning supports the concept of extended interval administration of aminoglycosides.

Concentrations of aminoglycosides in vitreous humour are approximately 40% of serum levels. Aminoglycosides have poor penetration across the blood-brain barrier and into bronchial secretions, the biliary tract and abscesses.

Tobramycin crosses the placenta and is distributed into fetal circulation and amniotic fluid. Tobramycin is excreted in breast milk, but the drug is poorly absorbed orally so is unlikely to result in significant plasma levels in infants.

Excretion: Tobramycin is not metabolized, but rather is eliminated almost exclusively by glomerular filtration. In adults over the age of 6 months with normal renal function, the elimination half-life of tobramycin typically ranges from 2 to 3 hours. In adults with normal renal function, >90% of an administered dose is recoverable in urine within 24 hours. Peak urine concentrations range from 75 to 100 µg/mL (i.e., approximately 10-fold greater than serum levels of the drug).

The elimination half-life may be shortened in patients with febrile conditions and is prolonged in elderly patients and in those with renal dysfunction in proportion to the extent of the impairment in glomerular filtration rate.

Special Populations: Pediatrics The elimination half-life of aminoglycoside antibiotics is prolonged in neonates. In full term infants the mean elimination half-life is reported to be 4.6 hours in those weighing >2.5 kg and 8.7 hours in those weighing <1.5 kg. Specific dosing guidelines should be consulted when prescribing tobramycin for newborns.
Geriatrics: Due to the age-related decline in glomerular filtration rate, the terminal elimination half-life of tobramycin is prolonged in elderly patients. The dose must be individualized according to renal function.
Patients with Cystic Fibrosis: There is an approximate 20% increase in the total body clearance of tobramycin in patients with cystic fibrosis.

Tobramycin for Injection USP ℞
tobramycin sulfate
Antibiotic

SteriMax

SUPPLIED: Each vial of lyophilized powder contains: tobramycin 1.2 g (as sulfate). Preservative-free. Sterile reconstituted solutions should be dispensed and diluted within 8 hours. Unused reconstituted solution should be discarded after 8 hours. If the solution becomes discoloured, do not use. Pharmacy bulk vials of 50 mL, cartons of 6. Store dry powder under controlled room temperature 15-30°C, protect from light.

Tobramycin Injection USP ℞
tobramycin
Antibiotic

Sandoz

SUPPLIED: 10 mg/mL: Each mL contains: tobramycin 10 mg. Nonmedicinal ingredients: disodium edetate, sodium bisulfite, sulfuric acid and/or sodium hydroxide to adjust pH, and water for injection. Preservative-free. Single use vials of 2 mL, boxes of 10. Discard unused portion. Store between 15 and 30°C. Protect from light.
40 mg/mL: Each mL contains: tobramycin 40 mg. Nonmedicinal ingredients: disodium edetate, sodium bisulfite, sulfuric acid and/or sodium hydroxide to adjust pH, and water for injection. Preservative-free. Single use vials of 2 mL, boxes of 10. Discard unused portion. Store between 15 and 30°C. Protect from light.
Multidose: 40 mg/mL: Each mL contains: tobramycin 40 mg. Nonmedicinal ingredients: disodium edetate, phenol (as preservative), sodium bisulfite, sulfuric acid and/or sodium hydroxide to adjust pH, and water for injection. Multidose vials of 30 mL, boxes of 1. Multidose vials of 2 mL, boxes of 10. Discard unused portion 28 days after initial use. Store between 15 and 30°C. Protect from light.

Tobrex® ℞
tobramycin
Topical Antibiotic

Alcon

SUPPLIED: Ointment: Each g of sterile, ophthalmic ointment contains: tobramycin 3 mg and chlorobutanol 0.5% as preservative, in a mineral oil and petrolatum base. Tubes of 3.5 g. Keep tightly closed.
Solution: Each mL of sterile solution contains: tobramycin 0.3% (3 mg) and benzalkonium chloride 0.01% as preservative. Nonmedicinal ingredients: boric acid, purified water, sodium chloride, sodium hydroxide and/or sulfuric acid (to adjust pH), sodium sulfate and tyloxapol. Drop-Tainer dispensers of 5 mL. Keep tightly closed.

Tofranil® ℞
imipramine HCl
Antidepressant

Novartis Pharmaceuticals

Date of Preparation: February 18, 1985
Date of Revision: June 16, 2010

PHARMACOLOGY: TOFRANIL (imipramine hydrochloride) is a tricyclic antidepressant with general pharmacological properties similar to those of structurally related tricyclic antidepressant drugs such as amitriptyline and doxepin.

TOFRANIL possesses anticholinergic properties which are responsible for certain of its side effects. The mechanism of action of imipramine and other tricyclic antidepressants is not well established, but it is thought that it might be related to their action on the transmitter-uptake mechanism of monoaminergic neurons. The mechanism of action in childhood nocturnal enuresis is not fully known.

TOFRANIL is rapidly and almost completely absorbed from the gastrointestinal tract. Peak plasma levels are reached in 2 to 5 hours, and plasma half-life ranges from 9 to 20 hours. After oral administration of 50 mg 3 times daily for 10 days, the mean steady-state plasma concentration was 33 to 85 ng/mL for imipramine and 43 to 109 ng/mL for desmethylimipramine, an active metabolite. Approximately 86% of imipramine is bound to plasma proteins. It is excreted primarily as inactive metabolites, up to 80% in the urine and up to 20% in the feces.

Owing to the lower clearance of imipramine in plasma, elderly patients require lower doses of TOFRANIL than patients in younger age groups.

INDICATIONS: For the relief of symptoms of depression.

CONTRAINDICATIONS: In patients who have known or suspected hypersensitivity to the drug or its excipients, or have known or suspected hypersensitivity to tricyclic antidepressants belonging to the dibenzazepine group.

TOFRANIL should not be given in conjunction with, or within 14 days before or after treatment with a MAO inhibitor (see Precautions, Drug Interactions). The concomitant treatment with selective reversible MAO-A inhibitors, such as moclobemide, is also contraindicated. Symptoms such as hypertensive crises, hyperactivity, hyperpyrexia, spasticity, severe convulsions, and those consistent with serotonin syndrome, e.g. myoclonus, agitation, seizures, delirium or coma, and death have been reported in patients receiving such combinations.

TOFRANIL is contraindicated for use during the acute recovery phase following a myocardial infarction and in the presence of acute congestive heart failure.

TOFRANIL is contraindicated in patients with existing liver or kidney damage and should not be administered to patients with a history of blood dyscrasias.

TOFRANIL is contraindicated in patients with glaucoma, as the condition may be aggravated due to the atropine-like effects of the drug.

WARNINGS: Seizures: Tricyclic agents are known to lower the convulsive threshold and TOFRANIL (imipramine hydrochloride) should, therefore, be used with extreme caution in patients with a history of convulsive disorders and other predisposing factors, e.g., brain damage of varying etiology, concomitant use of neuroleptics, alcoholism and withdrawal from alcohol, and concomitant use with other drugs that lower the seizure threshold. It appears that the occurrence of seizures is dose dependent. Therefore, the recommended total daily doses should not be exceeded (see Dosage).

Concurrent administration of electroconvulsive therapy and TOFRANIL may be hazardous and such treatment should be limited to patients for whom it is essential. Physicians should discuss with patients the risk of taking TOFRANIL while engaging in activities in which a sudden loss of consciousness could result in serious injury to the patient or others e.g., the operation of complex machinery, driving, swimming, or climbing.

Cardiovascular: Tricyclic antidepressants, particularly in high doses, have been reported to produce sinus tachycardia, changes in conduction time and arrhythmias. A few instances of unexpected death have been reported in patients with cardiovascular disorders. Myocardial infarction and stroke have also been reported with drugs of this class. Therefore, TOFRANIL should be administered with extreme caution to patients with a history of cardiovascular disorders, especially those with cardiovascular insufficiency, conduction disorders (e.g., atrioventricular block grades I to III) or other arrhythmias, those with circulatory lability and elderly patients.

Isolated cases of QTc prolongation and very rare cases of ventricular tachycardia and sudden unexplained death have occurred at supra-therapeutic doses of TOFRANIL which have primarily occurred in conjunction with overdose, but also in a few reports of co-medication that itself can lead to a prolonged QTc interval (e.g. thioridazine). Isolated cases have also been reported in the absence of co-medication.

TOFRANIL also has a hypotensive action which may be detrimental in these circumstances. In such cases, treatment should be initiated at low doses with progressive increases only if required and tolerated, and the patients should be under close surveillance at all dosage levels. Monitoring of cardiac function and the ECG is indicated in such patients as well as in the elderly.
Serotonin Syndrome: Due to the risk of serotonergic toxicity, it is advisable to adhere to recommended doses and any increase in dose should be made with caution if other serotonergic agents are coadministered. Serotonin syndrome, with symptoms such as hyperpyrexia, myoclonus, agitation, seizures, delirium and coma, can possibly occur when imipramine is administered with serotonergic co-medications such as selective serotonin reuptake inhibitors (SSRIs), serotonin and noradrenaline reuptake inhibitors (SNRIs), tricyclic antidepressants or lithium (see Drug Interactions).
Potential Association with the Occurrence of Behavioural and Emotional Changes, Including Self-Harm: It is unknown whether increased risk of suicidal ideation and behaviour is associated with the use of older antidepressants (eg TOFRANIL) in pediatric patients and/or adults. However, recent analyses of placebo-controlled clinical trial safety databases from SSRIs and other newer antidepressants suggest that use of these drugs in patients under the age of 25 may be associated with behavioural and emotional changes, including an increased risk of suicidal ideation and behaviour over that of placebo. Thus, rigorous clinical monitoring for suicidal ideation or other indicators of potential for suicidal behaviour is advised in **patients of all ages** given any antidepressant drug. This includes monitoring for emotional and behavioural changes.
Use in Concomitant Illness: Caution should be observed when prescribing TOFRANIL for hyperthyroid patients or for patients receiving thyroid medication. Transient cardiac arrhythmias have occurred in rare instances in patients who have been receiving other tricyclic compounds concomitantly with thyroid medication.

Because of its anticholinergic properties, TOFRANIL should be used with caution in patients with increased intraocular pressure, narrow angle glaucoma or urinary retention, particularly in the presence of prostatic hypertrophy.

Tricyclic antidepressants may give rise to paralytic ileus, particularly in the elderly and in hospitalized patients. Therefore, appropriate measures should be taken if constipation occurs.

Caution is called for when employing TOFRANIL in patients with tumors of the adrenal medulla (e.g., pheochromocytoma, neuroblastoma), in whom the drug may provoke hypertensive crisis.
Pregnancy: The safety of use in pregnant women has not been established. Therefore, TOFRANIL should not be administered to women of childbearing potential, or during pregnancy, unless, in the opinion of the physician, the expected benefit to the patient outweighs the potential risk to the fetus. Withdrawal symptoms including: tremors, dyspnea, lethargy, colic, irritability, hypotonia/hypertonia, convulsions and respiratory depression have been reported in neonates whose mothers received tricyclic antidepressants during the third trimester of pregnancy. To avoid such symptoms, TOFRANIL should, if possible, be gradually withdrawn at least 7 weeks before the calculated date of confinement.
Lactation: Since imipramine passes into breast milk, TOFRANIL should be gradually withdrawn or the infant weaned if the patient is breast-feeding.

PRECAUTIONS: The possibility of a suicide attempt is inherent in depression. These patients should be carefully supervised during treatment with imipramine and hospitalization or concomitant electroconvulsive therapy may be required. Prescriptions for TOFRANIL should be written for the smallest possible quantity of tablets consistent with good patient management, in order to reduce the risk of overdose.
Psychosis, Mania-Hypomania and Other Neuropsychiatric Phenomena: In patients treated with tricyclic antidepressants, activation of latent schizophrenia or aggravation of existing psychotic manifestations in schizophrenic patients may occur. Patients with manic-depressive tendencies may experience hypomanic or manic shifts. Hyperactive or agitated patients may become over-stimulated. A reduction in dose or discontinuation of TOFRANIL should be considered under these circumstances.

In predisposed and elderly patients, tricyclic antidepressants may, particularly at night, provoke pharmacogenic (delirious) psychoses that disappear within a few days of withdrawing the drug.

Since TOFRANIL may produce sedation, particularly during the initial phase of therapy, patients should be cautioned about the danger of engaging in activities requiring mental alertness, judgment and physical coordination.
Cardiovascular: Before initiating treatment, it is advisable to check the patient's blood pressure, because individuals with hypotension or a labile circulation may react to the drug with a fall in blood pressure. Regular measurements of blood pressure should be performed in susceptible patients. Postural hypotension may be controlled by reducing the dosage or administering circulatory stimulants.

ECG abnormalities have been observed in patients treated with imipramine. The most common ECG changes were premature ventricular contractions (PVCs), ST-T wave changes, and abnormalities in intraventricular conduction. These changes were rarely associated with significant clinical symptoms. Nevertheless, caution is necessary when treating patients with heart disease, as well as elderly subjects. In these patients cardiac function should be monitored and ECG examinations performed during long-term therapy. Gradual dose titration is also recommended.
Hepatic Changes: Isolated cases of obstructive jaundice have been reported. Caution is indicated in treating patients with known liver disease and periodic monitoring of hepatic function is recommended in such patients.
Hematological Changes: Isolated cases of bone marrow depression with agranulocytosis have been reported. Leukocyte and differential blood cell counts are recommended in patients receiving treatment with TOFRANIL over prolonged periods, and should be performed for patients who develop fever, an influenzal infection or sore throat. In the event of an allergic skin reaction, TOFRANIL should be withdrawn.
Withdrawal Symptoms: A variety of withdrawal symptoms have been reported in association with abrupt discontinuation of TOFRANIL, including dizziness, nausea, vomiting, headache, malaise, sleep disturbance, hyperthermia and irritability. In addition, such patients may experience a worsening of psychiatric status. While the withdrawal effects of TOFRANIL have not been systematically evaluated in controlled trials, they are well known with closely related tricyclic antidepressants. If the decision has been made to discontinue treatment, medication should be tapered as rapidly as feasible, but with recognition that abrupt discontinuation can be associated with certain symptoms (see Adverse Effects).
Metabolic Effects: Tricyclic antidepressants have been associated with porphyrinogenicity in susceptible patients.
Renal Function: It is advisable to monitor renal function during long-term therapy with tricyclic antidepressants.
Dental Effects: Lengthy treatment with tricyclic antidepressants can lead to an increased incidence of dental caries.
Lacrimation: Decreased lacrimation and accumulation of mucoid secretions due to the anticholinergic properties of tricyclic antidepressants may cause damage to the corneal epithelium in patients with contact lenses.
Lactose and Sucrose: TOFRANIL coated tablets contain lactose and sucrose. Patients with rare hereditary problems of galactose intolerance, fructose intolerance, severe lactase deficiency, sucrase-isomaltase insufficiency or glucose-galactose malabsorption should not take TOFRANIL coated tablets.
Drug Interactions: Patients should be warned that, while taking TOFRANIL, their responses to alcoholic beverages, other CNS depressants (e.g., barbiturates, benzodiazepines or general anesthetics) or anticholinergic agents (e.g., atropine, antihistamines, biperiden, levodopa) may be exaggerated.

When tricyclic antidepressants are given in combination with anticholinergics or neuroleptics with an anticholinergic action, hyperexcitation states or delirium may occur, as well as attacks of glaucoma.

Tricyclic antidepressants should not be employed in combination with antiarrhythmic agents of the quinidine type (see Warnings, Cardiovascular).

Since TOFRANIL may diminish or abolish the antihypertensive effects of guanethidine, bethanidine, clonidine, reserpine, or alpha-methyldopa, patients requiring concomitant treatment for hypertension should be given antihypertensives of a different type (e.g., diuretics, vasodilators, beta-blockers).

TOFRANIL may potentiate the cardiovascular effects of norepinephrine or epinephrine, amphetamine, as well as nasal drops and local anesthetics containing sympathomimetics (e.g., isoprenaline, ephedrine, phenylephrine).

SSRIs such as fluoxetine, paroxetine, sertraline or citalopram are inhibitors of CYP2D6. Fluvoxamine is a potent inhibitor of CYP1A2 and a moderate inhibitor of CYP2D6. Thus, coadministration of SSRIs and TOFRANIL may result in increased exposure and accumulation of imipramine and desipramine. Dose adjustments of TOFRANIL may therefore be necessary.

Co-medication of other serotonergic agents may lead to additive effects on the serotonergic system. Serotonin syndrome can possibly occur when imipramine is administered with serotonergic co-medications such as SSRIs, SNRIs, tricyclic antidepressants or lithium (see Warnings).

Caution should be exercised if TOFRANIL is administered together with cimetidine or methylphenidate since these drugs have been shown to inhibit the metabolism of several tricyclic antidepressants. Clinically significant increases in plasma levels of TOFRANIL may occur, necessitating a dosage reduction.

Substances which activate the hepatic mono-oxygenase enzyme system (e.g., barbiturates, carbamazepine, phenytoin, nicotine and oral contraceptives) may lower plasma concentrations of tricyclic antidepressants and so reduce their antidepressive effects. In addition, TOFRANIL may increase plasma levels of phenytoin and carbamazepine, therefore, it may be necessary to adjust the dosage of these drugs.

TOFRANIL should not be administered for a period of at least 14 days after the discontinuation of treatment with MAO-inhibitors due to the potential for severe interactions (see Contraindications). The same caution should also be observed when administering a MAO-inhibitor after previous treatment with TOFRANIL.

TOFRANIL should be discontinued prior to elective surgery for as long as clinically feasible, since little is known about the interaction with general anesthetics.

Concomitant treatment with neuroleptic agents (e.g., phenothiazines and butyrophenones) may result in increased plasma concentrations of TOFRANIL, a lowered convulsion threshold and seizures. Combination with thioridazine may produce severe cardiac arrhythmias. No such effects are known to occur in combination with diazepam, but it might be necessary to lower the dosage of imipramine if administered concomitantly with alprazolam or disulfiram.

Tricyclic antidepressants may potentiate the anticoagulant effect of coumarin drugs by inhibiting hepatic metabolism of these drugs. Careful monitoring of plasma prothrombin is therefore advised.

If administered concomitantly with estrogens, the dose of imipramine should be reduced since steroid hormones inhibit the metabolism of imipramine.

Oral antifungal, terbinafine: Coadministration of TOFRANIL with terbinafine, a strong inhibitor of CYP2D6, may result in increased exposure and accumulation of imipramine and desipramine. Therefore, dose adjustments of TOFRANIL may be necessary when coadministered with terbinafine.

ADVERSE EFFECTS: If severe neurological or psychiatric reactions occur, TOFRANIL (imipramine hydrochloride) should be withdrawn.

Elderly patients are particularly susceptible to anticholinergic, psychiatric, neurological and cardiovascular effects.

The following adverse reactions have been reported with imipramine or other tricyclic antidepressants. Adverse reactions are ranked under heading of frequency, the most frequent first, using the following convention: very common (≥1/10); common (≥1/100, <1/10); uncommon (≥1/1000, <1/100); rare (≥1/10 000, <1/1000) very rare (<1/10 000), including isolated reports.

Infection and Infestations: Very rare: dental caries.

Neurological: Very common: tremors. Common: dizziness, headache, paresthesia (numbness, tingling sensation, symptoms suggestive of peripheral neuropathy), delirium. Rare: convulsions. Very rare: tinnitus, incoordination, ataxia, electroencephalogram abnormal, extrapyramidal disorder, myoclonus, speech disorders, asthenia.

Behavioral: Common: somnolence, fatigue, insomnia, confusional states with hallucinations (particularly in geriatric patients and patients suffering from Parkinson's disease), anxiety, agitation, restlessness, nightmares, hypomania, mania, decrease in memory, feeling of unreality, disorientation. Rare: psychotic disorders. Very rare: aggression.

Anticholinergic: Very common: dry mouth and rarely associated sublingual adenitis, blurred vision, disturbances of visual accommodation, lacrimation decreased, constipation, hyperhidrosis, hot flushes. Common: micturition disorders, dilation of the urinary tract. Very rare: mydriasis, glaucoma, paralytic ileus, urinary retention.

Cardiovascular: Very common: hypotension, particularly orthostatic hypotension with associated vertigo, sinus tachycardia, electrocardiogram abnormalities (including flattening or inversion of T wave, depressed S-T segments). Common: arrhythmia, disturbances in cardiac conduction (e.g., widening of QRS complex, PQ changes, bundle-branch block), palpitation, syncope. Very rare: hypertension, congestive heart failure, myocardial infarction, heart block, asystole, stroke, vasospasms, QT interval prolongation, ventricular arrhythmia, ventricular tachycardia, ventricular fibrillation, torsades de pointes.

Hematologic: Very rare: agranulocytosis, eosinophilia, leukopenia, purpura and thrombocytopenia may occur as an idiosyncratic response.

Gastrointestinal: Common: nausea, vomiting, anorexia, abdominal cramps, liver function test abnormal. Rare: diarrhea. Very rare: bitter taste, stomatitis, epigastric distress, black tongue, dysphagia, increased salivation, hepatitis with or without jaundice, abnormal disorders, tongue ulceration.

Respiratory: Very rare: bronchospasm.

Endocrine: Very common: weight gain. Common: increased or decreased libido, impotence. Very rare: gynecomastia in the male, hypertrophy breast and galactorrhea in the female, testicular swelling, elevation or depression of blood sugar levels, weight loss, inappropriate antidiuretic hormone (SIADH) secretion syndrome.

Allergic or Toxic: Common: dermatitis allergic, rash, urticaria. Very rare: petechiae, itching, photosensitization (avoid excessive exposure to sunlight), edema (general or of face and tongue), pyrexia, obstructive jaundice, nasal congestion, alopecia, cross-sensitivity with desipramine, allergic alveolitis (pneumonia) with or without eosinophilia, systemic anaphylactic/anaphylactoid reactions including hypotension, skin hyperpigmentation.

General: Very rare: sudden death.

Withdrawal Symptoms: Abrupt cessation of treatment with tricyclic antidepressants after prolonged administration may occasionally produce nausea, vomiting, abdominal pain, diarrhea, insomnia, nervousness, anxiety, headache and malaise. These symptoms are not indicative of addiction.

OVERDOSE:

Symptoms: These may vary in severity depending upon factors such as the amount of drug absorbed, the interval between drug ingestion and the start of treatment and the age of the patient. Accidental ingestion in children should be regarded as serious and potentially fatal.

Symptoms generally appear within 4 hours of ingestion and reach maximum severity after 24 hours. Owing to delayed absorption (increased anticholinergic effect due to overdose), long half-life and enterohepatic recycling of the drug, the patient may be at risk for up to 4 to 6 days.

Symptoms may include drowsiness, stupor, ataxia, vomiting, cyanosis, restlessness, agitation, delirium, severe perspiration, hyperactive reflexes, muscle rigidity, athetoid and choreiform movements and/or convulsions, serotonin syndrome. Hyperpyrexia, mydriasis, bowel and bladder paralysis, oliguria or anuria and respiratory depression may occur.

Hypotension and initial hypertension may occur. However, the usual finding is increasing hypotension which may eventually lead to shock. Serious cardiovascular disturbances are frequently present, including tachycardia, cardiac arrhythmias (flutter, atriofibrillation, premature ventricular beats and ventricular tachycardia), as well as impaired myocardial conduction, atrioventricular and intraventricular block, ECG abnormalities (such as widened QRS complexes and marked S-T shifts), signs of congestive heart failure and cardiac arrest. Coma may ensue. Isolated cases of QT prolongation, torsades de pointes and death have been reported in overdose.

Treatment: Patients in whom overdosage is suspected should be admitted to hospital without delay. No specific antidote is available and treatment is essentially symptomatic and supportive.

Gastric lavage or aspiration should be performed promptly and is recommended up to 12 hours or even more after the overdose, since the anticholinergic effect of the drug may delay gastric emptying. Administration of activated charcoal may help reduce absorption of the drug. As TOFRANIL is largely protein bound, forced diuresis, peritoneal dialysis and hemodialysis are unlikely to be of value.

Treatment should be designed to insure maintenance of the vital functions. An open airway should be maintained in comatose patients and assisted ventilation instituted, if necessary, but respiratory stimulants should not be used. Hyperpyrexia should be controlled by external measures, such as ice packs and cooling sponge baths. Acidosis may be treated by cautious administration of sodium bicarbonate. Adequate renal function should be maintained.

ECG monitoring in an intensive care unit is recommended in all patients, particularly in the presence of ECG abnormalities, and should be maintained for several days after the cardiac rhythm has returned to normal. Unexpected deaths attributed to cardiac arrhythmias have been reported several days following an apparent recovery from tricyclic antidepressant overdose. Correction of hypoxia and acidosis, if present, may be beneficial. Correction of metabolic acidosis and low potassium concentrations by means of bicarbonate i.v. and potassium substitution may also be effective for treatment of arrhythmias. If bradyarrhythmia or AV-block occur, consider temporary insertion of a cardiac pacemaker. Because of its effect on cardiac conduction, digitalis should be used only, with caution. If rapid digitalization is required for the treatment of congestive heart failure, special care should be exercised in using the drug.

External stimulation should be minimized to reduce the tendency to convulsions. If convulsions occur, anticonvulsants (preferably i.v. diazepam) should be administered. Barbiturates may intensify respiratory depression, and aggravate hypotension and coma. Prompt control of convulsions is essential since they aggravate hypoxia and acidosis and may thereby precipitate cardiac arrhythmias and arrest.

Shock should be treated with supportive measures such as i.v. fluids, plasma expanders, and oxygen. The use of corticosteroids in shock is controversial and may be contraindicated in tricyclic antidepressant overdose. Hypotension usually responds to elevation of the foot of the bed. Pressor agents, (but **not** epinephrine) should be given cautiously, if indicated. In the event of a reduced myocardial function, consider recourse to treatment with dopamine or dobutamine by i.v. drip.

Since it has been reported that physostigmine may cause severe bradycardia, asystole and seizures, its use is not recommended in cases of overdosage with TOFRANIL.

Deaths by deliberate or accidental overdosage have occurred with this class of drugs. Since the propensity for suicide is high in depressed patients, a suicide attempt by other means may occur during the recovery phase. The possibility of simultaneous ingestion of other drugs should also be considered.

> For management of a suspected drug overdose, CPhA recommends that you contact your **regional Poison Control Centre**. See the *CPS* Directory section for a list of Poison Control Centres.

DOSAGE: Depression: The dosage should be individualized according to the requirements of each patient. Treatment should be initiated at the lowest recommended dose and increased gradually noting carefully the clinical response and any evidence of intolerance, particularly when treating elderly and adolescent patients. It should be kept in mind that a lag in therapeutic response usually occurs at the onset of therapy, lasting from several days to a few weeks. Increasing the dosage does not normally shorten this latent period and may increase the incidence of side effects.

Initial Dosage: Adults: 25 mg 3 times daily. This should be increased gradually as required and tolerated, up to 150 mg/day. Dosages over 200 mg/day are not recommended. In severely ill, hospitalized patients, initially 100 mg/day in divided doses, gradually increasing to 200 mg/day, if required. If no significant response is observed after 3 weeks, dosage may be increased up to 250 to 300 mg/day.

Maintenance Dosage: Dosage during maintenance therapy should be kept at the lowest effective level. Medication should be continued for the expected duration of the depressive episode in order to minimize the possibility of relapse following clinical improvement.

When a maintenance dosage has been established as described above, TOFRANIL may be administered in a single daily dose at bedtime, provided such a dosage regimen is well tolerated.

INFORMATION FOR THE PATIENT: Published in e-CPS, available by subscription at www.e-cps.ca.

SUPPLIED: 25 mg: Each reddish brown, round, biconvex, sugar-coated tablet, contains: imipramine HCl 25 mg. Nonmedicinal ingredients: cellulose compounds, colloidal silicon dioxide, cornstarch, glycerin, iron oxides, lactose, magnesium stearate, polyethylene glycol, povidone, stearic acid, sucrose, talc and titanium dioxide. Energy: 1 kJ (0.25 kcal). Alcohol-, bisulfite-, gluten-, parabens-, sodium- and tartrazine-free. Bottles of 100. Protect from heat (store between 2 and 30°C) and humidity. Keep out of reach of children.

50 mg: Each reddish brown, round, biconvex, sugar-coated tablet, branded GEIGY on one side and LB on the other side in white, contains: imipramine HCl 50 mg. Nonmedicinal ingredients: cellulose compounds, colloidal silicon dioxide, cornstarch, glycerin, iron oxides, lactose, magnesium stearate, polyethylene glycol, povidone, stearic acid, sucrose, talc and titanium dioxide. Energy: 3.77 kJ (0.90 kcal). Alcohol-, bisulfite-, gluten-, parabens-, sodium- and tartrazine-free. Bottles of 100. Protect from heat (store between 2 and 30°C) and humidity. Keep out of reach of children.

75 mg: Each reddish brown, round, biconvex, sugar-coated tablet, branded GEIGY on one side and ATA on the other side in white, contains: imipramine HCl 75 mg. Nonmedicinal ingredients: cellulose compounds, colloidal silicon dioxide, cornstarch, glycerin, iron oxides, lactose, magnesium stearate, polyethylene glycol, povidone, stearic acid, sucrose, talc and titanium dioxide. Energy: 3.3 kJ (0.8 kcal). Alcohol-, bisulfite-, gluten-, parabens-, sodium- and tartrazine-free. Bottles of 30. Protect from heat (store between 2 and 30°C) and humidity. Keep out of reach of children.

(Shown in Product Identification Section)

Tolbutamide ℞

CPhA Monograph

see *Sulfonylureas*

Toloxin™ ℞

digoxin

Cardiotonic Glycoside

MM Therapeutics

Date of Preparation: November 25, 2009

SUMMARY PRODUCT INFORMATION:

Route of Administration	Dosage Form/ Strength	All Nonmedicinal Ingredients
Oral	Tablets: 0.0625 mg, 0.125 mg and 0.25 mg	Tablets: **0.0625 mg:** FD&C Yellow No. 6, lactose, magnesium stearate, and starch (corn). **0.125 mg:** D&C Yellow No. 10, lactose, magnesium stearate, starch (corn), and yellow ferric oxide. **0.25 mg:** lactose, magnesium stearate, and starch (corn).

INDICATIONS AND CLINICAL USE: TOLOXIN (Digoxin Tablets, C.S.D.) is indicated for:

Congestive Heart Failure: TOLOXIN is indicated for the treatment of mild to moderate heart failure. TOLOXIN increases left ventricular ejection fraction and improves heart failure symptoms as evidenced by exercise capacity and heart failure-related hospitalizations and emergency care, while having no effect on mortality. Where possible, TOLOXIN should be used with a diuretic and angiotensin-converting enzyme inhibitor, but an optimal order for starting these three drugs cannot be specified.

Digoxin is usually continued after failure is controlled unless some known precipitating factor is corrected. Studies have shown that withdrawal of digoxin may worsen functional status, exercise capacity, and the left ventricular ejection fraction in patients with heart failure. In patients in whom digoxin may be difficult to regulate, or in whom the risk of toxicity may be great (e.g., patients with unstable renal function or whose potassium levels tend to fluctuate) a cautious withdrawal of digoxin may be considered. If digoxin is discontinued, the patient should be regularly monitored for clinical evidence of recurrent heart failure.

Atrial Fibrillation: TOLOXIN is indicated for the control of ventricular response rate in patients with chronic atrial fibrillation.

Geriatrics (>70 years of age): Although appropriate studies on the relationship of age to the effects of digitalis glycosides have not been performed in the geriatric population, the majority of experience with digoxin is in this population. This drug is known to be substantially excreted by the kidneys, and the risk of toxic reactions to this drug may be greater in patients with impaired renal function. Because elderly patients may be more likely to have age-related renal function impairment, which may significantly increase the elimination half-life of digoxin, care should be taken in dose selection, which should be based on renal function, and it may be useful to monitor renal function (see Dosage and Administration).

Pediatrics (<10 years of age): Newborn infants display considerable variability in their tolerance to digoxin. Premature and immature infants are particularly sensitive to the effect of digoxin, and the dosage of the drug must not only be reduced but must be individualized according to their degree of maturity. Digitalization in infants and children must be individualized (see Dosage and Administration).

CONTRAINDICATIONS: Digitalis glycosides are contraindicated in ventricular fibrillation.

In a given patient, an untoward effect requiring permanent discontinuation of other digitalis preparations usually constitutes a contraindication to TOLOXIN (Digoxin Tablets, C.S.D.). Hypersensitivity to TOLOXIN itself is a contraindication to its use. Allergy to digoxin, though rare, does occur. It may not extend to all such preparations, and another digitalis glycoside may be tried with caution.

WARNINGS AND PRECAUTIONS:

Serious Warnings and Precautions
- **Do not take other prescription, non-prescription and herbal medications without advice from your doctor.**

General: Digitalis alone or with other drugs has been used in the treatment of obesity. This use of digoxin or other digitalis glycosides is unwarranted. Moreover, since they may cause potentially fatal arrhythmias or other adverse effects, the use of these drugs solely for the treatment of obesity is dangerous.

Anorexia, nausea, vomiting and arrhythmias may accompany heart failure or may be indications of digitalis intoxication. Clinical evaluation of the cause of the symptoms should be attempted before further digitalis administration. In such circumstances determination of the serum digoxin concentration may be an aid in deciding whether or not digitalis toxicity is likely to be present. If the possibility of digitalis intoxication cannot be excluded, cardiac glycosides should be temporarily withheld, if permitted by the clinical situation.

Patients with renal insufficiency require smaller than usual maintenance doses of TOLOXIN (Digoxin Tablets, C.S.D.) (see Dosage and Administration).

Heart failure accompanying acute glomerulonephritis requires extreme care in digitalization. Relatively low loading and maintenance doses and concomitant use of antihypertensive drugs may be necessary and careful monitoring is essential. TOLOXIN (Digoxin Tablets, C.S.D.) should be discontinued as soon as possible, especially if a therapeutic trial does not result in improvement. Patients with severe carditis, such as carditis associated with rheumatic fever or viral myocarditis, are especially sensitive to digoxin-induced disturbances of rhythm.

Newborn infants display considerable variability in their tolerance to digoxin. Premature and immature infants are particularly sensitive and dosage must not only be reduced but must be individualized according to their degree of maturity. Impaired renal function must also be carefully taken into consideration.

Dosage of digoxin must be carefully titrated and differences in the bioavailability of parenteral preparations, oral solution and tablets taken into account when changing patients from one preparation to another.

Carcinogenesis and Mutagenesis: There have been no long-term studies performed in animals to evaluate carcinogenic potential, nor have studies been conducted to assess the mutagenic potential of digoxin or its potential to affect fertility.

Cardiovascular: Use During Electrical Cardioversion: Reduction of digoxin dosage may be desirable prior to electrical cardioversion to avoid induction of ventricular arrhythmias, but the physician must consider the consequences of rapid increase in ventricular response to atrial fibrillation if digoxin is withheld 1 to 2 days prior to cardioversion. If there is a suspicion that digitalis toxicity exists, elective cardioversion should be delayed. If it is not prudent to delay cardioversion, the energy level selected should be minimal at first and carefully increased in an attempt to avoid precipitating ventricular arrhythmias.

Sinus Node Disease and AV Block: Incomplete AV block, especially in patients with Stokes-Adams attacks, may progress to advanced or complete heart block if digoxin is given. Heart failure in these patients can usually be controlled by other measures and by increasing the heart rate. If digitalization is essential, electrical pacing of the ventricles may be indicated. In some patients with sinus node disease (i.e., Sick Sinus Syndrome), digoxin may worsen sinus bradycardia or sinoatrial block. Digoxin is not indicated for the treatment of sinus tachycardia unless it is associated with heart failure.

Accessory AV Pathway (Wolff-Parkinson-White Syndrome): In patients with Wolff-Parkinson-White Syndrome and atrial fibrillation, digoxin can enhance transmission of impulses through the accessory pathway. This effect may result in extremely rapid ventricular rates and even ventricular fibrillation.

Use in Patients with preserved Left Ventricular Systolic Function: Digoxin may worsen the outflow obstruction in patients with idiopathic hypertrophic subaortic stenosis (IHSS). Unless cardiac failure is severe, it is doubtful whether digoxin should be employed. Patients with chronic constrictive pericarditis may fail to respond to digoxin. In addition, slowing of the heart rate by digoxin in some patients may further decrease cardiac output. Patients with heart failure from amyloid heart disease or constrictive cardiomyopathies respond poorly to treatment with digoxin. Patients with severe carditis, such as carditis associated with rheumatic fever or viral myocarditis, are especially sensitive to digoxin-induced disturbances of rhythm.

Use in Patients with Acute Myocardial Infarction: Digoxin should be used with caution in patients with acute myocardial infarction. The use of inotropic drugs in some patients in this setting may result in undesirable increases in myocardial oxygen demand and ischemia.

Dependence/Tolerance: No drug dependence has been reported with the use of digoxin.

Endocrine and Metabolism: In Patients with Electrolyte Disorders: In patients with hypokalemia, toxicity may occur despite serum digoxin concentrations within the normal range, because potassium depletion sensitizes the myocardium to digoxin. Therefore, it is desirable to maintain normal serum potassium levels in patients being treated with digoxin. Hypokalemia may result from diuretic, amphotericin B or corticosteroid therapy, and from peritoneal or hemodialysis or mechanical suction of gastrointestinal secretions. It may also accompany malnutrition, diarrhea, prolonged vomiting, old age, long-standing heart failure, long-standing wasting diseases and treatment with ion-exchange resins or carbenoxolone. In general, rapid changes in serum potassium or other electrolytes should be avoided, and i.v. treatment with potassium should be reserved for special circumstances as described below (see Overdosage).

Calcium, particularly when administered rapidly by the intravenous route, may produce serious arrhythmias in digitalized patients. Hypercalcemia from any cause predisposes the patient to digitalis toxicity. On the other hand, hypocalcemia can nullify the effects of digoxin in man; thus digoxin may be ineffective until serum calcium is restored to normal. These interactions are elated to the fact that calcium affects contractility and excitability of the heart in a manner similar to digoxin.

Hypomagnesemia may predispose to digitalis toxicity. If low magnesium levels are detected in a patient on digoxin, replacement therapy should be instituted.

Use in Thyroid Disorders and Hypermetabolic States: In hypothyroidism the digoxin requirements are reduced. Digoxin responses in patients with compensated thyroid disease are normal. Heart failure and/or atrial arrhythmias resulting from hypermetabolic or hyperdynamic states (e.g., hyperthyroidism, hypoxia, or arteriovenous shunt) are best treated by addressing the underlying condition. Atrial arrhythmias associated with hypermetabolic states are particularly resistant to digoxin treatment. Care must be taken to avoid toxicity if digoxin is used.

Renal: In Patients with Renal Disease: Patients with renal insufficiency require smaller than usual maintenance doses of digoxin (see Dosage and Administration).

If the patient has been given digoxin during the previous week or any other less rapidly excreted drug of the digitalis group during the previous 2 weeks, the dose of digoxin must be reduced accordingly. Digoxin toxicity develops more frequently and lasts longer in patients with renal impairment because of the decreased excretion of digoxin. Therefore, it should be anticipated that dosage requirements will be decreased in patients with moderate to severe renal disease (see Dosage and Administration). Because of impaired renal function and excretion in elderly patients, they frequently require lower than recommended doses. Because of the prolonged half-life, a longer period of time is required to achieve an initial or new steady-state concentration in patients with renal impairment than in patients with normal renal function.

Special Populations: Pregnant Women: Teratogenic Effects: Animal reproduction studies have not been conducted with digoxin. It is also not known whether digoxin can cause fetal harm when administered to a pregnant woman or can affect reproduction capacity, although there have been no reports of teratogenic effects following the use of digoxin in pregnancy since its availability in 1929. Digoxin should be given to pregnant women only if clearly needed.

Nursing Women: Studies have shown that digoxin concentrations in the mother's serum and milk are similar. However, the estimated daily dose to a nursing infant will be far below the usual infant maintenance dose. Therefore, this amount should have no pharmacologic effect upon the infant. Nevertheless, caution should be exercised when digoxin is administered to a nursing woman.

Pediatrics (<10 years of age): Digitalis glycosides are a major cause of poisoning in children. The tolerance of newborn infants to digitalis glycosides is variable, since their renal clearance of the medication is reduced. Premature and immature infants are especially sensitive. Dosage of digoxin should be reduced and individualized according to the infant's degree of maturity, since renal clearance increases as the infant matures. Children older than 1 month of age generally require proportionally larger doses than adults on the basis of body weight or body surface area.

Geriatrics (>70 years of age): Although appropriate studies on the relationship of age to the effects of digitalis glycosides have not been performed in the geriatric population, the majority of experience with digoxin is in this population. Elderly patients may be more likely to have age-related renal function impairment, which may significantly increase the elimination half-life of digoxin. Additionally, elderly patients may have a decreased volume of distribution of digitalis due to decreased muscle mass. These factors may contribute to digitalis toxicity in elderly patients.

Monitoring and Laboratory Tests: Patients receiving TOLOXIN (Digoxin Tablets, C.S.D.) should have their serum electrolytes and renal function (BUN and/or serum creatinine) assessed periodically; the frequency of assessments will depend on the clinical setting. For discussion of serum digoxin concentrations, see Dosage and Administration.

The use of therapeutic doses of digoxin may cause prolongation of the PR interval and depression of the ST segment on the electrocardiogram. Digoxin may produce false positive ST-T changes on the electrocardiogram during exercise testing. These electrophysiologic effects reflect an expected effect of the drug and are not indicative of toxicity.

ADVERSE REACTIONS: Adverse Drug Reaction Overview: In general, the adverse reactions of digoxin are dose-dependent and occur at doses higher than those needed to achieve a therapeutic effect. Hence, adverse reactions are less common when digoxin is used within the recommended dose range or therapeutic serum concentration range and when there is careful attention to concurrent medications and conditions.

Because some patients may be particularly susceptible to side effects with digoxin, the dosage of the drug should always be selected carefully and adjusted as the clinical condition of the patient warrants. In the past, when high doses of digoxin were used and little attention was paid to clinical status or concurrent medications, adverse reactions to digoxin were more frequent and severe. Cardiac adverse reactions accounted for about one-half, gastrointestinal disturbances for about one-fourth, and CNS and other toxicity for about one-fourth of these adverse reactions. However, available evidence suggests that the incidence and severity of digoxin toxicity has decreased substantially in recent years. In recent controlled clinical trials, in patients with predominantly mild to moderate heart failure, the incidence of adverse experiences was comparable in patients taking digoxin and in those taking placebo. In a large mortality trial, the incidence of hospitalization for suspected digoxin toxicity was 2% in patients taking TOLOXIN compared to 0.9% in patients taking placebo. In this trial, the most common manifestations of digoxin toxicity included gastrointestinal and cardiac disturbances; CNS manifestations were less common.

Clinical Trial Adverse Drug Reactions: Adults: Cardiac: Unifocal or multiform ventricular premature contractions, especially in bigeminal or trigeminal patterns, are the most common arrhythmias associated with digoxin toxicity in adults with heart disease. Persistent bigeminy at rest but not on exercise when the sinus rate increases has traditionally been acceptable in the management of some arrhythmias. Ventricular tachycardia and ventricular fibrillation may result from digitalis toxicity. Atrioventricular (AV) dissociation, accelerated junctional (nodal) rhythm and atrial tachycardia with block are also common arrhythmias caused by digoxin overdosage. Excessive slowing of the pulse is a clinical sign of digoxin overdosage. AV block (Wenckebach) of increasing degree may proceed to complete heart block (including asystole).

Note: The electrocardiogram is fundamental in determining the presence and nature of these cardiac disturbances.

Digoxin may also induce other changes in the ECG (e.g., PR prolongation, ST depression), which represent digoxin effect and may or may not be associated with digitalis toxicity. Cardiac toxicity can also occur at therapeutic doses in patients who have conditions which may alter their sensitivity to digoxin (see Warnings and Precautions).

Gastrointestinal: Anorexia, nausea, vomiting, and less commonly, diarrhea are common early symptoms of overdosage. However, uncontrolled heart failure may also produce such symptoms. Rarely, the use of digoxin has been associated with abdominal pain.

It is inadvisable to rely on nausea as an early warning of excessive digoxin as arrhythmias may occur first.

Central Nervous System: Visual disturbances (blurred or yellow vision), headache, weakness, apathy, psychosis, and mental disturbances (such as anxiety, depression, delirium, and hallucination) can occur.

Other: Gynecomastia is occasionally observed following prolonged use of digoxin. Thrombocytopenia and maculopapular rash and other skin reactions have been rarely observed.

Table 1 summarizes the incidence of those adverse experiences listed above for patients treated with TOLOXIN tablets or placebo from two randomized, double-blind, placebo-controlled withdrawal trials. Patients in these trials were also receiving diuretics with or without angiotensin-converting enzyme inhibitors. These patients had been stable on digoxin, and were randomized to digoxin or placebo. The results shown in Table 1 reflect the experience in patients following dosage titration with the use of serum digoxin concentrations and careful follow-up. These adverse experiences are consistent with results from a large, placebo-controlled mortality trial (DIG trial) wherein over half the patients were not receiving digoxin prior to enrollment.

Table 1: TOLOXIN

Adverse Experiences in Two Parallel, Double-Blind, Placebo-Controlled Withdrawal Trials with TOLOXIN Tablets (Number of Patients Reporting)

Adverse Experience	TOLOXIN Patients (n=123) (%)	Placebo Patients (n=125) (%)
Cardiac		
Palpitation	1 (0.8)	4 (3.2)
Ventricular extrasystole	1 (0.8)	1 (0.8)
Tachycardia	2 (1.6)	1 (0.8)
Heart arrest	1 (0.8)	1 (0.8)
Gastrointestinal		
Anorexia	1 (0.8)	4 (3.2)
Nausea	4 (3.3)	2 (1.6)
Vomiting	2 (1.6)	1 (0.8)
Diarrhea	4 (3.3)	1 (0.8)
Abdominal pain	0	6 (4.8)
CNS		
Headache	4 (3.3)	4 (3.2)
Dizziness	6 (4.9)	5 (4.0)
Mental disturbances	5 (4.1)	1 (0.8)
Other		
Rash	2 (1.6)	1 (0.8)
Death	4 (3.3)	3 (2.4)

Less Common Clinical Trial Adverse Drug Reactions (<1%): Gastrointestinal: Rarely, the use of digoxin has been associated with abdominal pain, intestinal ischemia, and hemorrhagic necrosis of the intestines.

Other: Thrombocytopenia and maculopapular rash and other skin reactions have been rarely observed.

Infants and Children: Toxicity differs from the adult in a number of respects. Anorexia, nausea, vomiting, diarrhea and CNS disturbances may be present but are rare as initial symptoms in infants. Cardiac arrhythmias are more reliable signs of toxicity. Digoxin in children may produce any arrhythmia. The most commonly encountered are conduction disturbances or supraventricular tachyarrhythmias, such as atrial tachycardia with or without block and junctional (nodal) tachycardia. Ventricular arrhythmias are less common. Sinus bradycardia may also be a sign of impending digoxin intoxication, especially in infants, even in the absence of first-degree heart block. Any arrhythmia or alteration in cardiac conduction that develops in a child taking digoxin should initially be assumed to be a consequence of digoxin intoxication, until further evaluation proves otherwise.

Post-Market Adverse Drug Reactions: Adverse reactions to digoxin are usually dose dependent and occur at dosages higher than those needed to achieve a therapeutic effect.

DRUG INTERACTIONS: Overview: Digitalis glycosides have a narrow therapeutic range and changes in digoxin pharmacokinetics and/or pharmacodynamics caused by a digoxin-drug interaction can result in toxicity or underdigitalization. The presence of or a change in an underlying disease state also can cause changes in digoxin pharmacokinetics and/or pharmacodynamics and may complicate or contribute to a digoxin-drug interaction. Because a risk of digoxin toxicity exists, and the clinical significance of an interaction may be variable and not necessarily predictable, it is important that the addition or withdrawal of a drug to or from a therapeutic regimen that includes digoxin be carefully evaluated in the context of the patient and the clinical situation.

Potassium-depleting corticosteroids and diuretics may be major contributing factors to digitalis toxicity. Calcium, particularly if administered rapidly by the intravenous route, may produce serious arrhythmias in digitalized patients. Quinidine, verapamil, amiodarone, propafenone, indomethacin, itraconazole, alprazolam, and spironolactone raise the serum digoxin concentration due to a reduction in clearance and/or in volume of distribution of the drug, cause a rise in serum digoxin concentration, with the implication that digitalis intoxication may result. This rise appears to be proportional to the dose.

Certain antibiotics [erythromycin, clarithromycin (and possibly other macrolide antibiotics) and tetracycline] may increase digoxin absorption in patients who inactivate digoxin by bacterial metabolism in the lower intestine, so that digitalis intoxication may result. Recent studies have shown that specific colonic bacteria in the lower gastrointestinal tract convert digoxin to cardioinactive reduction products, thereby reducing its bioavailability. Although inactivation of these bacteria by antibiotics is rapid, the serum digoxin concentration will rise at a rate consistent with the elimination half-life of digoxin. The magnitude of rise in serum digoxin concentration relates to the extent of bacterial inactivation, and may be as much as 2 fold in some cases.

Propantheline and diphenoxylate, by decreasing gut motility, may increase digoxin absorption. Antacids, kaolin-pectin, sulfasalazine, neomycin, cholestyramine, phenytoin, St. John's wort (Hypericum perforatum) and certain anticancer drugs may interfere with intestinal digoxin absorption, resulting in unexpectedly low serum concentrations. Thyroid administration to a digitalized hypothyroid patient may increase the dose requirement of digoxin. Concomitant use of digoxin and sympathomimetics increases the risk of cardiac arrhythmias because both enhance ectopic pacemaker activity. Succinylcholine may cause a sudden extrusion of potassium from muscle cells and may thereby cause arrhythmias in digitalized patients. Although α-adrenergic blockers or calcium channel blockers and digoxin may be useful in combination to control atrial fibrillation, their additive effects on AV node conduction can result in complete heart block.

Due to the considerable variability of these interactions, digoxin dosage should be carefully individualized when patients receive coadministered medications. Furthermore, caution should be exercised when combining digoxin with any drug that may cause a significant deterioration in renal function, since a decline in glomerular filtration or tubular secretion may impair the excretion of digoxin.

Drug-Drug Interactions: See Table 2.

Drug-Herb Interactions: St. John's wort (Hypericum perforatum) may interfere with intestinal digoxin absorption, resulting in unexpectedly low serum concentrations. Patients are advised to consult with their doctors before taking herbal products.

Drug-Laboratory Test Interactions: The use of therapeutic doses of digoxin may cause prolongation of the PR interval and depression of the ST segment on the electrocardiogram. Digoxin may produce false positive ST-T changes on the electrocardiogram during exercise testing. These electrophysiologic effects reflect an expected effect of the drug and are not indicative of toxicity.

Drug-Lifestyle Interactions: Serum digoxin concentration may decrease acutely during periods of exercise without any associated change in clinical efficacy due to increased binding of digoxin to skeletal muscle.

Table 2: TOLOXIN

Established or Potential Drug-Drug Interactions with Digoxin

Interacting Drugs	Ref	Effect	Clinical Comment
Albuterol	USP DI 2004	Concurrent use may decrease serum digoxin concentrations, possibly by redistributing digoxin to other tissues. Albuterol may also decrease serum potassium concentrations, which may increase the risk of digoxin toxicity.	
Alprazolam	USP DI 2004	Concurrent use may increase serum digoxin concentrations, possibly by decreasing the renal clearance of digoxin; although one small study performed in healthy volunteers concluded that alprazolam had no significant effect on digoxin clearance, contradictory evidence has been reported in patients [primarily elderly patients] receiving long-term digoxin therapy.	
Amiodarone	USP DI 2004	Increases in serum digoxin concentrations by as much as 100% have been reported with concurrent use. Although it is thought that amiodarone decreases renal and/or nonrenal clearance and/or the volume of distribution of digoxin, other contributing factors, such as amiodarone-induced displacement of digoxin from tissue binding sites, also may be involved. Amiodarone has a long elimination half-life [15 to 65 days or longer] and digoxin toxicity may not appear until several weeks after the addition of amiodarone or may persist long after discontinuation of amiodarone.	
Antacids or Antidiarrheal adsorbents (e.g., kaolin and pectin) or Sulfasalazine	USP DI 2004	Concurrent use may decrease digoxin bioavailability by decreasing digoxin absorption.	In the case of antidiarrheal adsorbents and sulfasalazine, the digoxin dose may be administered 8 hours before the interacting medication.
Antibiotics, oral, especially Macrolide antibiotics, such as: Clarithromycin or Erythromycin or Tetracycline	USP DI 2004	Concurrent use of some oral antibiotics may increase serum digoxin concentrations in patients who inactivate digoxin in the lower intestine by bacterial metabolism; in these individuals, altering the bowel flora with certain antibiotics may diminish digoxin conversion to inactive metabolites, resulting in increased serum digoxin concentration; the increase in serum digoxin concentration has been as much as twofold in some cases and correlates with the extent of bacterial inactivation. Although there are limited data, this interaction has been reported with oral use of clarithromycin, erythromycin, and tetracycline.	
Anticancer medications (such as bleomycin, cyclophosphamide, cytarabine, doxorubicin, procarbazine, and vincristine) or Radiation therapy	USP DI 2004	Concurrent use may decrease digoxin bioavailability by decreasing digoxin absorption; the reduced absorption that occurs during concurrent use with anticancer medications or radiation therapy may be due to temporary damage to the gastrointestinal mucosa and may continue for several days after treatment. However, digitoxin absorption does not appear to be affected by anticancer agents.	In the case of concurrent use of anticancer medications, a dosage form with greater bioavailability, such as the capsule or solution, may help to minimize decreased bioavailability.
Atorvastatin	USP DI 2004	Concurrent use may increase digoxin serum concentrations; steady-state serum concentration increases of approximately 20% have been reported.	
Beta-adrenergic blocking agents including Atenolol, Carvedilol, Metoprolol and Propranolol	USP DI 2004	Concurrent use with these agents may have additive effects on slowing atrioventricular [AV] nodal conduction; concurrent use with carvedilol in patients with hypertension increased the steady-state area under the plasma concentration—time curve [AUC] and trough concentrations of digoxin by 14% and 16%, respectively.	Plasma digoxin concentrations should be monitored when digoxin is coadministered with beta-adrenergic blocking agents.
Bran fiber, dietary	USP DI 2004	It is uncertain whether concurrent administration of dietary bran fiber decreases digoxin bioavailability. In one small study, there was presumed to be a decrease in digoxin absorption when concurrent administration of digoxin with 5 grams of fiber resulted in a decrease in urinary excretion of digoxin. Another small study found no change in steady-state serum digoxin concentrations when digoxin was administered 15 to 30 minutes before administration of 11 grams of bran [as a bran muffin], with a second bran muffin administered several hours later.	
Calcium channel blocking agents, especially Bepridil or Diltiazem or Nifedipine or Verapamil	USP DI 2004	Concurrent use with calcium channel blocking agents may have additive effects on AV nodal conduction, which could result in complete heart block; concurrent use also may increase serum digoxin concentrations by reducing digoxin renal clearance, possibly as a result of inhibition of active tubular secretion of digoxin; verapamil may increase serum digoxin concentrations by 30 to 200%; bepridil may increase serum digoxin concentrations by approximately 34%; some studies have reported no interaction with diltiazem while others have reported increases in serum digoxin concentrations of 20 to 60%; contradictory evidence of an interaction also exists for nifedipine, although serum digoxin increases of 15 to 50% have been reported; increases in serum digitoxin concentrations also have been reported with concurrent use of diltiazem and verapamil, although increases were less pronounced than with digoxin use and may be due to a reduction in extrarenal digitoxin clearance.	Serum digitalis concentrations and electrocardiogram [ECG] should be monitored and dosages should be adjusted accordingly.
Cholestyramine or Colestipol	USP DI 2004	Colestipol and cholestyramine may delay and reduce the absorption of digoxin.	Digoxin dose may be administered 8 hours before the interacting medication to minimize the interference with digoxin absorption.
Cyclosporine	USP DI 2004	Concurrent use has resulted in increases in serum digoxin concentrations, possibly as a result of decreased apparent volume of distribution and/or plasma clearance of digoxin.	
Diphenoxylate or Propantheline	USP DI 2004	Concurrent use may increase digoxin bioavailability; diphenoxylate and propantheline increase digoxin absorption by decreasing intestinal motility.	
Diuretics, potassium-depleting (such as bumetanide, ethacrynic acid, furosemide, indapamide, mannitol, or thiazides) or Hypokalemia-causing medications	USP DI 2004	Decreases in serum potassium concentrations that can occur with these medications may increase the risk of digitalis toxicity.	Frequent serum potassium concentration determinations are recommended when these medications are concurrently administered with digoxin.
Flecainide	USP DI 2004	Concurrent use has increased serum digoxin concentrations, on average, by 24%; it also has been speculated that concurrent use may cause a slight additive increase in the PR interval.	
Hepatic enzyme inducers, such as: Barbiturates or Phenytoin or Rifampin	USP DI 2004	Concurrent use may increase the metabolism of digitoxin; serum digitoxin concentrations have been reported to decrease by 50% in patients who received 180 mg of phenobarbital per day for 12 weeks; decreases in serum digoxin concentrations also have been reported with concurrent use of rifampin, although the mechanism for this interaction is not completely understood.	Serum digitalis concentrations should be monitored and dosages adjusted accordingly.
Indomethacin	USP DI 2004	Concurrent use may increase digoxin serum concentrations, possibly by inhibiting the renal elimination of digoxin; two small studies that evaluated the interaction in healthy adult patients did not find a clinically significant interaction. Another small study found a significant increase [about 40% on average] in serum digoxin concentrations in adult heart failure patients treated with digoxin on a long-term basis. A small study in premature infants treated conventionally with indomethacin for patent ductus arteriosus [PDA] found an increase in serum digoxin concentrations of approximately 50% with concurrent use.	

(cont'd)

Table 2: TOLOXIN *(cont'd)*

Established or Potential Drug-Drug Interactions with Digoxin

Interacting Drugs	Ref	Effect	Clinical Comment
Itraconazole	USP DI 2004	Concurrent use may increase serum digoxin concentrations, possibly by decreasing renal elimination of digoxin; serum digoxin concentration increases of approximately 50% have been reported.	
Metoclopramide	USP DI 2004	Concurrent use of metoclopramide may decrease digoxin absorption by increasing gastrointestinal motility; serum digoxin concentrations as determined by AUC have been reported to decrease by about 24%.	
Neomycin, oral	USP DI 2004	Concurrent use decreases the rate and extent of absorption of digoxin. In a study in healthy volunteers, the extent of absorption of digoxin was decreased by as much as 51% after single doses of digoxin and neomycin. The absorption of digoxin also was decreased when the antibiotic was given 3 or 6 hours before the digoxin dose. The mechanism of this interaction has not been established.	It is recommended that digoxin be administered at least 8 hours before neomycin.
Omeprazole	USP DI 2004	Concurrent use with digoxin may increase digoxin absorption, possibly by altering gastric acidity; on average, C_{max} and AUC values have been reported to be about 10% higher with concurrent use.	
Propafenone	USP DI 2004	Concurrent use of propafenone with digoxin results in an increase in serum digoxin concentrations ranging from 35 to 85%, which appears to be unrelated to digoxin renal clearance but may be related to a decrease in the volume of distribution and nonrenal clearance of digoxin.	Careful monitoring of digoxin concentrations and dosage reduction of digoxin are recommended when propafenone is initiated.
Quinidine or Quinine	USP DI 2004	Concurrent use with quinidine has resulted in increased digoxin plasma concentrations, possibly due to an initial displacement of digoxin from quinidine binding sites, and a reduction in the renal and nonrenal clearance and volume of distribution of digoxin; the extent of the interaction is proportional to plasma quinidine concentrations and, on average, concurrent use results in 100% increases in serum digoxin concentrations, although increases of over 300% have been reported; concurrent use of quinidine with digitoxin has resulted in increases in serum digitoxin concentrations of 30 to 67%, the smaller increases possibly resulting from impairment of extrarenal clearance of digitoxin by quinidine; increases in serum digoxin concentrations also have been reported with concurrent use of quinine.	Serum digitalis concentrations should be monitored and dosage adjusted as indicated.
Spironolactone	USP DI 2004	Concurrent use with digoxin may increase serum digoxin concentrations, possibly by decreasing digoxin renal and nonrenal clearance and/or digoxin volume of distribution; it has been estimated that digoxin plasma concentrations may increase by one third with concurrent use.	
Succinylcholine	USP DI 2004	Concurrent use may cause a sudden release of potassium from muscle cells, increasing the risk of arrhythmias in digitalized patients.	
Sucralfate	USP DI 2004	Sucralfate was reported to reduce digoxin plasma concentrations by about 19%, presumably by reducing the bioavailability of digoxin.	Sucralfate should not be taken within 2 hours of digoxin.
Sympathomimetics	USP DI 2004	Concurrent use may increase the risk of cardiac arrhythmias.	
Thyroid hormones	USP DI 2004	Patients with thyroid disease may have an altered sensitivity to digitalis: hyperthyroid patients may have a reduced response to digitalis and hypothyroid patients may have an increased risk of digitalis toxicity.	Increase in digitalis dose may be required with the use of thyroid hormones in a hypothyroid patient.

DOSAGE AND ADMINISTRATION:

General: Recommended dosages of digoxin may require considerable modification because of individual sensitivity of the patient to the drug, the presence of associated conditions, or the use of concurrent medications.

In selecting the dose of digoxin, several factors must be considered:

1. The body weight of the patient. Doses should be calculated based upon (i.e., ideal) body weight.
2. The patient's renal function, preferably evaluated on the basis of estimated creatinine clearance.
3. The patient's age. Infants and children require different doses of digoxin than adults. Also, advanced age may be indicative of diminished renal function even in patients with normal serum creatinine concentration (i.e., below 1.5 mg/dL).
4. Concomitant disease states, concurrent medication or other factors likely to alter the pharmacokinetic or pharmacodynamic profile of digoxin (see Warnings and Precautions).
5. To minimize toxic side effects, the lowest effective dose should be used as the maintenance dose.

Serum Digoxin Concentrations: In general, the dose of digoxin used should be determined on clinical grounds. However, measurement of serum digoxin concentrations can be helpful to the clinician in determining the adequacy of digoxin therapy and in assigning certain probabilities to the likelihood of digoxin intoxication. About two-thirds of adults considered adequately digitalized (without evidence of toxicity) have serum digoxin concentrations ranging from 0.8 to 2.0 ng/mL. However, digoxin may produce clinical benefits even at serum concentrations below this range. About two-thirds of adult patients with clinical toxicity have serum digoxin concentrations greater than 2.0 ng/mL. However, since one-third of patients with clinical toxicity have concentrations less than 2.0 ng/mL, values below 2.0 ng/mL do not rule out the possibility that a certain sign or symptom is related to digoxin therapy. Rarely, there are patients who are unable to tolerate digoxin at serum concentrations below 0.8 ng/mL. Consequently, the serum concentration of digoxin should always be interpreted in the overall clinical context, and an isolated measurement should not be used alone as the basis for increasing or decreasing the dose of the drug.

To allow adequate time for equilibration of digoxin between serum and tissue, sampling of serum concentrations should be done just before the next scheduled dose of the drug. If this is not possible, sampling should be done at least 6 to 8 hours after the last dose, regardless of the route of administration or the formulation used. On a once-daily dosing schedule, the concentration of digoxin will be 10% to 25% lower when sampled at 24 versus 8 hours, depending upon the patient's renal function. On a twice-daily dosing schedule, there will be only minor differences in serum digoxin concentrations whether sampling is done at 8 or 12 hours after a dose.

If a discrepancy exists between the reported serum concentration and the observed clinical response, the clinician should consider the following possibilities:

1. Analytical problems in the assay procedure.
2. Inappropriate serum sampling time.
3. Administration of a digitalis glycoside other than digoxin.
4. Conditions (described in Warnings and Precautions) causing an alteration in the sensitivity of the patient to digoxin.
5. Serum digoxin concentration may decrease acutely during periods of exercise without any associated change in clinical efficacy due to increased binding of digoxin to skeletal muscle.

Heart Failure: Adults: Digitalization may be accomplished by either of two general approaches that vary in dosage and frequency of administration, but reach the same endpoint in terms of total amount of digoxin accumulated in the body.

1. Rapid digitalization may be achieved by administering a loading dose based upon projected peak body digoxin stores, then calculating the maintenance dose as a percentage of the loading dose.
2. More gradual digitalization may be obtained by beginning an appropriate maintenance dose, thus allowing digoxin body stores to accumulate slowly. Steady-state serum digoxin concentrations will be achieved in approximately 5 half-lives of the drug for the individual patient. Depending upon the patient's renal function, this will take between 1 and 3 weeks.

Rapid Digitalization with a Loading Dose: Peak body digoxin stores of 8 to 12 µg/kg should provide therapeutic effect with minimum risk of toxicity in most patients with heart failure and normal sinus rhythm. Because of altered digoxin distribution and elimination, projected peak body stores for patients with renal insufficiency should be conservative (i.e., 6 to 10 µg/kg) [see Warnings and Precautions].

The loading dose should be administered in several portions, with roughly half the total given as the first dose. Additional fractions of this planned total dose may be given at 6- to 8-hour intervals, **with careful assessment of clinical response before each additional dose.**

If the patient's clinical response necessitates a change from the calculated dose of digoxin, then calculation of the maintenance dose should be based upon the amount actually given.

A single initial dose of 500 to 750 µg (0.5 to 0.75 mg) of TOLOXIN Tablets usually produces a detectable effect in 0.5 to 2 hours that becomes maximal in 2 to 6 hours. Additional doses of 125 to 375 µg (0.125 to 0.375 mg) may be given cautiously at 6- to 8-hour intervals until clinical evidence of an adequate effect is noted. The usual amount of TOLOXIN Tablets that a 70-kg patient requires to achieve 8 to 12 µg/kg peak body stores is 750 to 1250 µg (0.75 to 1.25 mg).

Digoxin injection is frequently used to achieve rapid digitalization, with conversion to TOLOXIN Tablets for maintenance therapy. If patients are switched from intravenous to oral digoxin formulations, allowances must be made for differences in bioavailability when calculating maintenance dosages (see Table 5).

Table 3: TOLOXIN

Usual Daily Maintenance Dose Requirements of TOLOXIN (µg) for Estimated Peak Body Stores of 10 µg/kg

		Lean Body Weight						
Corrected Ccr	kg	50	60	70	80	90	100	Number of Days Before Steady State Achieved[b]
(mL/min per 70 kg)[a]	lb	110	132	154	176	198	220	
0		62.5[c]	125	125	125	187.5	187.5	22
10		125	125	125	187.5	187.5	187.5	19
20		125	125	187.5	187.5	187.5	250	16
30		125	187.5	187.5	187.5	250	250	14
40		125	187.5	187.5	250	250	250	13
50		187.5	187.5	250	250	250	250	12
60		187.5	187.5	250	250	250	375	11
70		187.5	250	250	250	250	375	10
80		187.5	250	250	250	375	375	9
90		187.5	250	250	250	375	500	8
100		250	250	250	375	375	500	7

[a] Ccr is creatinine clearance, corrected to 70 kg body weight or 1.73 m^2 body surface area. For adults, if only serum creatinine concentrations (Scr) are available, a Ccr (corrected to 70 kg body weight) may be estimated in men as (140−Age)/Scr. For women, this result should be multiplied by 0.85. Note: This equation cannot be used for estimating creatinine clearance in infants or children.

[b] If no loading dose administered.

[c] 62.5 µg=0.0625 mg.

Example: Based on Table 3, a patient in heart failure with an estimated lean body weight of 70 kg and a Ccr of 60 mL/min, should be given 250 µg (0.25 mg) daily of TOLOXIN Tablet, usually taken after the morning meal. If no loading dose is administered, steady-state serum concentration in this patient should be anticipated at approximately 11 days.

Infants and Children: In general, divided daily dosing is recommended for infants and young children (under age 10). In the newborn period, renal clearance of digoxin is diminished and suitable dosage adjustments must be observed. This is especially pronounced in the premature infant. Beyond the immediate newborn period, children generally require proportionally larger doses than adults on the basis of body weight or body surface area. Children over 10 years of age require adult dosages in proportion to their body weight. Some researchers have suggested that infants and young children tolerate slightly higher serum concentrations than do adults.

Daily maintenance doses for each age group are given in Table 4 and should provide therapeutic effect with minimum risk of toxicity in most patients with heart failure and normal sinus rhythm. These recommendations assume the presence of normal renal function.

Table 4: TOLOXIN

Daily Maintenance Doses of TOLOXIN Tablets in Children with Normal Renal Function

Age	Daily Maintenance Dose (µg/kg)
2 to 5 years	10 to 15
5 to 10 years	7 to 10
Over 10 years	3 to 5

Additional Information for Digoxin Oral Solution: Rapid Digitalization with a Loading Dose: A pediatric digoxin injection can be used to achieve rapid digitalization, with conversion to an oral formulation of TOLOXIN for maintenance therapy. If patients are switched from intravenous to oral digoxin formulations, allowances must be made for differences in bioavailability when calculating maintenance dosages (see also dosing Table 5). Peak digoxin stores of 8 to 12 µg/kg should provide therapeutic effect with minimum risk of toxicity in most patients with heart failure and normal sinus rhythm. Because of altered digoxin distribution and elimination, projected peak body stores for patients with renal insufficiency should be conservative (i.e., 6 to 10 µg/kg) [see Warnings and Precautions].

Digitalizing and daily maintenance doses for each age are given in Table 5 and should provide therapeutic effect with minimum risk of toxicity in most patients with heart failure and normal sinus rhythm. These recommendations assume the presence of normal renal function.

The loading dose should be administered in several portions, with roughly half the total given as the first dose. Additional fractions of this planned total dose may be given at 6- to 8-hour intervals, **with careful assessment of clinical response before each additional dose**. If the patients' clinical response necessitates a change from the calculated loading dose of digoxin, then calculation of the maintenance dose should be based upon the amount actually given.

Table 5: TOLOXIN

Usual Digitalizing and Maintenance Dosages for Digoxin Oral Solution in Children with Normal Renal Function Based on Lean Body Weight

Age	Oral Digitalizing[a] Dose (µg/kg)	IV Digitalizing Dose (µg/kg)	Daily Maintenance Dose[b] (µg/kg)
Premature	20 to 30	15 to 25	20% to 30% of **oral** [or IV] digitalizing dose[c]
Full-term	25 to 35	20 to 30	25% to 35% of **oral** [or IV] digitalizing dose[c]
1 to 24 Months	35 to 60	30 to 50	
2 to 5 Years	30 to 40	25 to 35	
2 to 10 Years	20 to 35	15 to 30	
Over 10 Years	10 to 15	8 to 12	

[a] IV digitalizing doses are 80% of oral digitalizing doses.
[b] Divided daily dosing is recommended for children under 10 years of age.
[c] Projected or actual digitalizing dose providing clinical response.

In children with renal disease, digoxin must be carefully titrated based upon clinical response.

Gradual Digitalization with a Maintenance Dose: More gradual digitalization can also be accomplished by beginning an appropriate maintenance dose. The range of percentages provided in Table 4 can be used in calculating this dose for patients with normal renal function.

It cannot be overemphasized that both the adult and pediatric dosage guidelines provided are based upon average patient response and substantial individual variation can be expected. Accordingly, ultimate dosage selection must be based upon clinical assessment of the patient.

Missed Dose: If a dose is missed patients are advised to take the dose as soon as remembered if within 12 hours of scheduled dose and not taking if remembered later. Patients are advised not to double doses and to consult their doctor if a dose is missed for 2 days or more.

Administration: Digoxin is usually administered orally as a single daily dose. Divided daily dosing is recommended in infants and young children.

OVERDOSAGE:

Adults: Digoxin should be temporarily discontinued until the adverse reaction resolves.

Every effort should also be made to correct factors that may contribute to the adverse reaction (such as electrolyte disturbances or concurrent medications). Once the adverse reaction has resolved, therapy with digoxin may be reinstituted, following a careful reassessment of dose.

Withdrawal of digoxin may be all that is required to treat the adverse reaction. However, when the primary manifestation of digoxin overdosage is a cardiac arrhythmia, additional therapy may be needed.

If the rhythm disturbance is a symptomatic bradyarrhythmia or heart block, consideration should be given to the reversal of toxicity with DIGIBIND [Digoxin Immune Fab (Ovine)] (see Massive Digitalis Overdosage), the use of atropine, or the insertion of a temporary cardiac pacemaker. However, asymptomatic bradycardia or heart block related to digoxin may require only temporary withdrawal of the drug and cardiac monitoring of the patient.

If the rhythm disturbance is a ventricular arrhythmia, consideration should be given to the correction of electrolyte disorders, particularly if hypokalemia (see Administration of Potassium) or hypomagnesemia is present. DIGIBIND is a specific antidote for digoxin and may be used to reverse potentially life-threatening ventricular arrhythmias due to digoxin overdosage.

Administration of Potassium: Every effort should be made to maintain the serum potassium concentration between 4.0 and 5.5 mmol/L. Potassium is usually administered orally, but when correction of the arrhythmia is urgent and the serum potassium concentration is low, potassium may be administered cautiously by the intravenous route. The electrocardiogram should be monitored for any evidence of potassium toxicity (e.g., peaking of T waves) and to observe the effect on the arrhythmia. Potassium salts may be dangerous in patients who manifest bradycardia or heart block due to digoxin (unless primarily related to supraventricular tachycardia) and in the setting of massive digitalis overdosage (see Massive Digitalis Overdosage).

Massive Digitalis Overdosage: Manifestations of life-threatening toxicity include severe ventricular tachycardia or ventricular fibrillation, or progressive bradyarrhythmias or heart block. The administration of more than 10 mg of digoxin in a previously healthy adult, or more than 4 mg in a previously healthy child or a steady-state serum concentration greater than 10 ng/mL, often results in cardiac arrest.

DIGIBIND should be used to reverse the toxic effect of a massive overdose. The decision to administer DIGIBIND to a patient who has ingested a massive dose of digoxin but who has not yet manifested life-threatening toxicity should depend on the likelihood that the life-threatening toxicity will occur (see above).

Patients with massive digitalis ingestion should receive large doses of activated charcoal to prevent absorption and bind digoxin in the gut during enteroenteric recirculation. Emesis or gastric lavage may be indicated especially if ingestion has occurred within 30 minutes of the patient's presentation at the hospital. Emesis should not be induced in patients who are obtunded. If a patient presents more than 2 hours after ingestion or already has toxic manifestations, it may be unsafe to induce vomiting or attempt passage of a gastric tube, because such manoeuvers may induce an acute vagal episode that can worsen digitalis-related arrhythmias.

Severe digitalis intoxication can cause a massive shift of potassium from inside to outside the cell, leading to life-threatening hyperkalemia. The administration of potassium supplements in the setting of massive intoxication may be hazardous and should be avoided. Hyperkalemia caused by massive digitalis toxicity is best treated with DIGIBIND; initial treatment with glucose and insulin may also be required if hyperkalemia itself is acutely life-threatening.

For management of a suspected drug overdose, contact your regional Poison Control Centre. See the *CPS Directory* section for a list of Poison Control Centres.

ACTION AND CLINICAL PHARMACOLOGY: Mechanism of Action: The influence of digitalis glycosides on the myocardium is dose related, and involves both direct action on cardiac muscle and the specialized conduction system, and indirect actions on cardiovascular system mediated by the autonomic nervous system. The indirect actions mediated by the autonomic nervous system involve a vagomimetic action, which is responsible for the effects of digitalis on the sinoatrial (SA) and atrioventricular (AV) nodes; and also a baroreceptor sensitization which results in increased carotid sinus nerve activity and enhanced sympathetic withdrawal for any given increment in mean arterial pressure. The pharmacologic consequences of these direct and indirect effects are: an increase in the force and velocity of myocardial systolic contraction (positive inotropic action); a slowing of heart rate (negative chronotropic effect); and decreased conduction velocity through the AV node. In higher doses, digitalis increases sympathetic outflow from the CNS to both cardiac and peripheral sympathetic nerves. This increase in sympathetic activity may be an important factor in digitalis cardiac toxicity. Most of the extracardiac manifestations of digitalis toxicity are also mediated by the CNS.

Pharmacodynamics: Digoxin produces hemodynamic improvement in patients with heart failure. Short- and long-term therapy with the drug increases cardiac output and lowers pulmonary artery pressure, pulmonary capillary wedge pressure, and systemic vascular resistance. These hemodynamic effects are accompanied by an increase in the left ventricular ejection fraction and a decrease in end-systolic and end-diastolic dimensions.

The times to onset of pharmacologic effect and to peak effect of preparations of TOLOXIN are shown in Table 6.

Table 6: TOLOXIN

Time to Onset of Effect and Peak Effect for TOLOXIN and Digoxin Oral Solution Products

Product	Time to Onset of Effect[a]	Time to Peak Effect[a]
TOLOXIN (Digoxin Tablets, C.S.D.)	0.5 to 2 hours	2 to 6 hours
Digoxin Oral Solution, C.S.D.	0.5 to 2 hours	2 to 6 hours

[a] Documented for ventricular response rate in atrial fibrillation, inotropic effect and electrocardiograph changes.

Congestive Heart Failure: Two 12-week, double-blind, placebo-controlled studies enrolled 178 (RADIANCE trial) and 88 (PROVED trial) patients with NYHA class II or III heart failure previously treated with digoxin, a diuretic, and an ACE inhibitor (RADIANCE only) and randomized them to placebo or treatment with digoxin. Both trials demonstrated better preservation of exercise capacity in patients randomized to digoxin. Continued treatment with digoxin reduced the risk of developing worsening heart failure, as evidenced by heart failure-related hospitalizations and emergency care and the need for concomitant heart failure therapy. The larger study also showed treatment-related benefits in NYHA class and patients' global assessment. In the smaller trial, these trended in favour of a treatment benefit.

The Digitalis Investigation Group (DIG) main trial was a multicenter, randomized, double-blind, placebo-controlled mortality study of 6801 patients with heart failure and left ventricular ejection fraction ≤0.45. At randomization, 67% were NYHA class I or II, 71% had heart failure of ischemic etiology, 44% had been receiving digoxin, and most were receiving concomitant ACE inhibitor (94%) and diuretic (82%). Patients were randomized to placebo or digoxin, the dose of which was adjusted for the patient's age, sex, lean body weight, and serum creatinine (see Dosage and Administration), and followed for up to 58 months (median 37 months). The median daily dose prescribed was 0.25 mg. Overall all-cause mortality was 35% with no difference between groups (95% confidence limits for relative risk of 0.91 to 1.07). Digoxin was associated with a 25% reduction in the number of hospitalizations for heart failure, a 28% reduction in the risk of a patient having at least one hospitalization for heart failure, and a 6.5% reduction in total hospitalizations (for any cause).

Use of digoxin was associated with a trend to increase time to all-cause death or hospitalization. The trend was evident in subgroups of patients with mild heart failure as well as more severe disease, as shown in Table 7. Although the effect on all-cause death or hospitalization was not statistically significant, much of the apparent benefit derived from effects on mortality and hospitalization attributed to heart failure. In situations where there is no statistically significant benefit of treatment evident from a trial's primary end point, results pertaining to secondary endpoint should be interpreted cautiously.

Table 7: TOLOXIN

Subgroup Analyses of Mortality and Hospitalization During the First Two Years Following Randomization in the DIG Trial with TOLOXIN

		Risk of All-Cause Mortality or All-Cause Hospitalization[a]			Risk of HF-Related Mortality or HF-Related Hospitalization[a]		
	n	Placebo	Digoxin	Relative Risk[b]	Placebo	Digoxin	Relative Risk[b]
All patients (EF ≤0.45)	6801	604	593	0.94 (0.88–1.00)	294	217	0.69 (0.63–0.76)
NYHA I/II	4571	549	541	0.96 (0.89–1.04)	242	178	0.70 (0.62–0.80)
EF 0.25–0.45	4543	568	571	0.99 (0.91–1.07)	244	190	0.74 (0.66–0.84)
CTR ≤0.55	4455	561	563	0.98 (0.91–1.06)	239	180	0.71 (0.63–0.81)
NYHA III/IV	2224	719	696	0.88 (0.80–0.97)	402	295	0.65 (0.57–0.75)
EF <0.25	2258	677	637	0.84 (0.76–0.93)	394	270	0.61 (0.53–0.71)
CTR >0.55	2346	687	650	0.85 (0.77–0.94)	398	287	0.65 (0.57–0.75)
EF >0.45[c]	987	571	585	1.04 (0.88–1.23)	179	136	0.72 (0.53–0.99)

[a] Number of patients with an event during the first 2 years per 1000 randomized patients.
[b] Relative risk (95% confidence interval).
[c] DIG Ancillary Study.

Chronic Atrial Fibrillation: In patients with chronic atrial fibrillation, digoxin slows rapid ventricular response rate in a linear dose-response fashion from 0.25 to 0.75 mg/day. Digoxin should not be used for the treatment of multifocal atrial tachycardia.

Pharmacokinetics: Absorption: Gastrointestinal absorption of digoxin is a passive process. Absorption of digoxin from tablets is 60 to 80%. Absorption of Digoxin Oral Solution formulation has been demonstrated to be 70% to 85% complete compared to an identical intravenous dose of digoxin (absolute bioavailability). When digoxin oral solution/tablets are taken after meals, the rate of absorption is slowed, but the total amount of digoxin absorbed is usually unchanged. When taken with meals high in bran fibre; however, the amount absorbed from an oral dose may be reduced.

In some patients, orally administered digoxin is converted to cardioinactive reduction products (e.g., dihydrodigoxin) by colonic bacteria in the gut. Data suggest that 1 in 10 patients treated with digoxin tablets will degrade 40% or more of the ingested dose. As a result, certain antibiotics may increase the absorption of digoxin in such patients. Although inactivation of these bacteria by antibiotics is rapid, the serum digoxin concentration will rise at a rate constant with the extent of bacterial interaction and may be as much as two-fold in some cases.

Distribution: Following drug administration, a 6- to 8-hour distribution phase is observed. This is followed by a much more gradual serum concentration decline, which is dependent on digoxin elimination from the body. The peak height and slope of the early portion (absorption/distribution phases) of the serum concentration-time curve are dependent upon the route of administration and the absorption characteristics of the formulation. Clinical evidence indicates that the early high serum concentrations do not reflect the concentration of digoxin at its site of action, but that with chronic use, the steady-state postdistribution serum levels are in equilibrium with tissue levels and correlate with pharmacologic effects. In individual patients, these postdistribution serum concentrations are linearly related to maintenance dosage and may be useful in evaluating therapeutic and toxic effects.

Digoxin is concentrated in tissues and therefore has a large apparent volume of distribution. Digoxin crosses both the blood-brain barrier and the placenta. At delivery, serum digoxin concentration in the newborn is similar to the serum level in the mother. Approximately 20 to 25% of plasma digoxin is bound to protein. Serum digoxin concentrations are not significantly altered by large changes in fat tissue weight, so that its distribution space correlates best with lean (ideal) body weight, not total body weight.

Metabolism: Metabolism occurs partially in the stomach, but also may occur in the liver and, although only about 16% of a dose of digoxin is metabolized, several metabolites of digoxin and their metabolic pathways have been identified. The bis-digitoxoside and mono-digitoxoside metabolites are considered to be cardioactive. Other metabolites, such as digoxigenin, are considered to be less cardioactive than digoxin. In some patients (estimated to be approximately 10% of patients taking digoxin), other cardioinactive metabolites, such as dihydrodigoxin and dihydrodigoxigenin, may result from the metabolism of digoxin by intestinal bacteria. In these individuals, as much as 40% or more of the oral dose of digoxin may be converted to these inactive reduction products. The metabolism of digoxin is not dependent upon the cytochrome P-450 system.

Excretion: Elimination of digoxin follows first-order kinetics (that is, the quantity of digoxin eliminated at any time is proportional to the total body content). Following i.v. administration to normal subjects, 50 to 70% of a digoxin dose is excreted unchanged in the urine. Renal excretion of digoxin is proportional to glomerular filtration rate and is largely independent of urine flow. In subjects with normal renal function, digoxin has a half-life of 1.5 to 2 days.

Special Populations and Conditions: Pediatrics: The tolerance of newborn infants to digitalis glycosides is variable, since their renal clearance of the medication is reduced. Premature and immature infants are especially sensitive. Dosage should be reduced and individualized according to the infant's degree of maturity, since renal clearance increases as the infant matures. Children older than 1 month of age generally require proportionally larger doses than adults on the basis of body weight or body surface area (see Dosage and Administration).

Geriatrics: Elderly patients may be more likely to have age-related renal function impairment, which may significantly increase the elimination half-life of digoxin. Additionally, elderly patients may have a decreased volume of distribution of digitalis due to decreased muscle mass. These factors may contribute to digitalis toxicity in elderly patients.

Gender: Digoxin is primarily removed from the body by renal elimination. Although the digoxin clearance in women is about 10-15% lower than in men, the effect of gender on the pharmacokinetics of digoxin is not expected to be clinically significant when initiating and monitoring digoxin therapy in patients.

Race: Race differences in digoxin pharmacokinetics have not been formally studied. Because digoxin is primarily eliminated as unchanged drug via the kidney and because there are no important differences in creatinine clearance among races, pharmacokinetic differences due to race are not expected.

Hepatic Insufficiency: Plasma digoxin concentration profiles in patients with acute hepatitis generally fell within the range of profiles in a group of healthy subjects.

Renal Insufficiency: The clearance of digoxin can be primarily correlated with renal function as indicated by creatinine clearance. In children with renal disease, digoxin must be carefully titrated based on clinical response.

The half-life of digoxin in anuric patients is prolonged to 4 to 6 days. Digoxin is not effectively removed from the body by dialysis, exchange transfusion or during cardiopulmonary bypass because most of the drug is in the tissue rather than circulating in the blood.

Genetic Polymorphism: The effect of genetic polymorphism on the pharmacokinetics of TOLOXIN was not studied.

STORAGE AND STABILITY: Store between 15 to 30°C in a dry place and protect from light. Avoid exposure to excessive heat.

INFORMATION FOR THE PATIENT: Published in e-CPS, available by subscription at www.e-cps.ca.

DOSAGE FORMS, COMPOSITION AND PACKAGING: 0.0625 mg: Each round, peach, flat-faced, bevelled edge tablet, debossed "TOLOXIN" over a score line and "06" under it on one side and plain on the other side, contains: digoxin 0.0625 mg (62.5 µg). Nonmedicinal ingredients: FD&C Yellow No. 6, lactose, magnesium stearate and starch (corn). Tartrazine-free. Bottles of 100 and 250.

0.125 mg: Each round, yellow, flat-faced, bevelled edge tablet, debossed "TOLOXIN" over a score line and "12" under it on one side and plain on the other side, contains: digoxin 0.125 mg (125 µg). Nonmedicinal ingredients: D&C Yellow No. 10, lactose, magnesium stearate, starch (corn), and yellow ferric oxide. Tartrazine-free. Bottles of 100, 250, 500 and 1000.

0.25 mg: Each round, white, biconvex tablet, debossed "TOLOXIN" over a score line and "25" under it on one side and plain on the other side, contains: digoxin 0.25 mg (250 µg). Nonmedicinal ingredients: lactose, magnesium stearate, and starch (corn). Dye- and tartrazine-free. Bottles of 100, 250, 500 and 1000.

Tomudex® Ⓟ

raltitrexed disodium

Antineoplastic

Hospira

Date of Preparation: May 1, 2008

Caution: Raltitrexed should be administered only by, or under the supervision of, a physician who is experienced in cancer chemotherapy and in the management of related toxicities. This includes myelosuppression, hepatic and renal impairment. Raltitrexed should not be administered to patients with severe hepatic impairment.

PHARMACOLOGY: Raltitrexed is a quinazoline folate analogue that selectively inhibits thymidylate synthase (TS). Thymidylate synthase is a key enzyme in the de novo synthesis of thymidine triphosphate (TTP), a nucleotide required exclusively for deoxyribonucleic acid (DNA) synthesis. Inhibition of thymidylate synthase leads to DNA fragmentation and cell death.

Raltitrexed is transported into cells via a reduced folate carrier (RFC) and is then extensively polyglutamated by the enzyme folyl polyglutamate synthetase (FPGS) to polyglutamate forms that are retained in cells and are even more potent inhibitors of thymidylate synthase. Raltitrexed polyglutamation enhances thymidylate synthase inhibitory potency and increases the duration of thymidylate synthase inhibition in cells which may improve anti-tumoral activity. Polyglutamation could also contribute to increased toxicity due to drug retention in normal tissues.

Raltitrexed is 93% protein bound in humans.

Pharmacokinetics: Following i.v. administration at 3 mg/m², the concentration-time profile in patients is triphasic. Peak concentrations, at the end of infusion, are followed by a rapid initial decline in concentration. This is followed by a slow elimination phase. The key pharmacokinetic parameters are presented in Table 1.

Table 1: Tomudex

Key Pharmacokinetic Parameters of Raltitrexed

C_{max} (ng/mL)	$AUC_{0-\infty}$ (ng·h/mL)	CL (mL/min)	CL_r (mL/min)	V_{ss} (L)	$t_{1/2}\beta$ (h)	$t_{1/2}\gamma$ (h)
656	1856	51.6	25.1	548	1.79	198

Legend: C_{max}: peak plasma concentration; CL: clearance; CL_r: renal clearance; $t_{1/2}\beta$: half-life of the second phase; $t_{1/2}\gamma$: terminal half-life; AUC: area under plasma concentration-time curve; V_{ss}: volume of distribution at steady state.

The maximum concentrations of raltitrexed increased linearly with dose over the clinical dose range tested.

There is no clinically significant plasma accumulation of raltitrexed in patients with normal renal function during repeat administration at 3-week intervals. Apart from the expected intracellular polyglutamation, raltitrexed was mainly (approximately 50%) excreted unchanged in the urine. It is also excreted in the feces with approximately 15% of the dose being eliminated over a 10-day period. In the study following [^{14}C] labelled raltitrexed, approximately half of the radiolabel was not recovered during the study period suggesting that a proportion (50%) of the raltitrexed dose is retained within tissues, perhaps as raltitrexed polyglutamates, beyond the end of the measurement period. Trace levels of radiolabel were detected in red blood cells on Day 29.

Raltitrexed pharmacokinetics are independent of age and gender. Pharmacokinetics have not been evaluated in children.

Mild (WHO grade 2) to moderate (WHO grade 3) hepatic impairment led to a reduction in plasma clearance of less than 25%.

Mild to moderate renal impairment (creatinine clearance of 25 to 65 mL/min) led to a significant reduction (approximately 50%) in raltitrexed plasma clearance.

Clinical Experience: In clinical trials raltitrexed, administered as a single 3 mg/m² i.v. dose every 3 weeks, demonstrated clinical antitumor activity with an acceptable toxicity profile in patients with advanced colorectal cancer.

Four large clinical trials have been conducted with raltitrexed in advanced colorectal cancer. Of the 3 comparative trials, 2 showed no statistical difference between raltitrexed and the combination of 5-fluorouracil plus leucovorin for survival, while 1 trial showed a statistically significant difference in favor of the combination of 5-fluorouracil plus leucovorin. Raltitrexed as a single agent was as effective as the combination of 5-fluorouracil and leucovorin in terms of objective response rate in all trials.

INDICATIONS: In the treatment of advanced colorectal cancer.

CONTRAINDICATIONS: In patients with hypersensitivity to the drug or any of its components.

Pregnancy: Raltitrexed is contraindicated in pregnant women, in women who may become pregnant during treatment or women who are breastfeeding. Teratology studies in the rat indicate that raltitrexed caused embryolethality and fetal abnormalities in pregnant rats. Pregnancy should be excluded before treatment with raltitrexed is commenced and should be avoided during treatment and for at least 6 months after cessation of treatment if either partner is receiving raltitrexed.

Lactation: See Pregnancy.

Children: Raltitrexed is not recommended for use in children as safety and efficacy have not been established in this group of patients.

Raltitrexed is contraindicated in patients with severe renal and/or hepatic impairment.

WARNINGS: It is recommended that raltitrexed is only given by or under the supervision of a physician who is experienced in cancer chemotherapy, and in the management of chemotherapy-related toxicity. Patients undergoing therapy should be subject to appropriate supervision so that signs of possible toxic effects or adverse reactions (particularly diarrhea) may be detected and treated promptly (see Dosage).

As with other cytotoxic agents of this type, caution is necessary in patients with depressed bone marrow function, poor general condition, or prior radiotherapy.

A proportion of raltitrexed is excreted via the fecal route (see Pharmacology) therefore, patients with mild (WHO grade 2) to moderate (WHO grade 3) hepatic impairment should be treated with caution.

PRECAUTIONS: Raltitrexed is a cytotoxic agent and should be handled according to normal procedures adopted for such agents (see Dosage, Special Instructions).

Occupational Hazards: Raltitrexed may cause malaise or asthenia following infusion and the ability to drive or use machinery could be impaired while symptoms continue.

Geriatrics: Elderly patients are more vulnerable to the toxic effects of raltitrexed. Extreme care should be taken to ensure adequate monitoring of adverse reactions, especially signs of gastrointestinal toxicity (diarrhea or mucositis).

Drug Interactions: No specific clinical drug-drug interaction studies have been conducted.

Leucovorin (folinic acid), folic acid or vitamin preparations containing these agents must not be given immediately prior to or during administration of raltitrexed, since they may interfere with its action.

There is no experience to date in relation to the combined use of raltitrexed with other cytotoxic agents.

Raltitrexed is 93% protein bound and while it has the potential to interact with other highly protein bound drugs, no interactions due to displacement between raltitrexed and warfarin has been observed in vitro. Active tubular secretion may contribute to the renal excretion of raltitrexed, indicating a potential interaction with other actively secreted drugs such as NSAIDs. However, a review of the clinical trial safety database does not reveal evidence of clinically significant interaction in patients treated with raltitrexed who also received concomitant NSAIDs, warfarin and other commonly prescribed drugs.

ADVERSE EFFECTS: As with other cytotoxic drugs, the administration of raltitrexed is associated with certain adverse reactions; these mainly include reversible effects on the gastrointestinal tract, hematopoietic system and liver enzymes.

Gastrointestinal System: The most frequent effects were nausea (58%), vomiting (37%), diarrhea (38%) and anorexia (28%). Other less frequent effects were mucositis, stomatitis (including mouth ulceration), dyspepsia and constipation. Gastrointestinal bleeding which may be associated with mucositis and/or thrombocytopenia has been reported.

Diarrhea is usually mild or moderate (WHO grade 1 and 2) and can occur at any time following the administration of raltitrexed. However, severe diarrhea (WHO grade 3 and 4) can occur, and may be associated with concurrent hematological suppression, especially leukopenia (neutropenia in particular). Subsequent treatment may need to be discontinued or the dose reduced depending on the grade of toxicity (see Dosage).

Nausea and vomiting are usually mild (WHO grade 1 and 2), occur usually for the first week following the administration of raltitrexed, and are responsive to antiemetics.

Hematopoietic System: Leukopenia (neutropenia in particular), anemia and thrombocytopenia, alone and in combination, have been reported as possible adverse drug reactions in clinical trials (22%, 18% and 5% of patients, respectively). They are usually mild to moderate (WHO grade 1 and 2) and occur in the first or second week after treatment and recovering by the third week. Severe (WHO grade 3 and 4) leukopenia (neutropenia in particular) and thrombocytopenia of WHO grade 4 can occur and may be life-threatening or fatal, especially if associated with signs of gastrointestinal toxicity.

Hepatic: Reversible increases in AST and ALT have been commonly reported as adverse drug reactions in clinical trials (16% and 14% of patients, respectively). Such changes have usually been asymptomatic and self-limiting when not associated with progression of the underlying malignancy. Other less frequent effects were weight loss, dehydration, peripheral edema, hyperbilirubinemia and increases in alkaline phosphatase.

Cardiovascular System: A number of cardiac rhythm or cardiac function abnormalities have been reported in clinical trials in advanced colorectal cancer. These ranged from sinus tachycardia and supraventricular tachycardia to atrial fibrillation and congestive heart failure. The incidence of disorders of rhythm and function in patients treated with raltitrexed was 2.8% and 1.8% respectively compared to 1.9% and 1.4% for patients on the comparator treatment. A causal relationship could not be established since many of the abnormalities were concurrent with the underlying conditions such as sepsis and dehydration and more than one third of the patients reported cardiovascular abnormalities prior to treatment.

Musculoskeletal and Nervous System: Arthralgia and hypertonia (usually muscular cramps) have each been reported as possible adverse drug reactions in less than 2% of patients who received raltitrexed in clinical trials.

Skin, Appendages and Special Senses: Rash was commonly reported in clinical trials (14% of patients), sometimes associated with pruritus. Other less frequent effects were desquamation, alopecia, sweating, taste perversion and conjunctivitis.

Whole Body: The most frequent effects in clinical trials were asthenia (49% of patients) and fever (22% of patients) which were usually mild to moderate following the first week of administration of raltitrexed, and reversible. Severe asthenia can occur and may be associated with malaise and a flu-like syndrome. Other less frequent effects were abdominal pain, pain, headache, cellulitis and sepsis.

The following effects (see Table 2) were reported as possible adverse drug reactions occurring with an incidence of 2% or more in patients with colorectal cancer treated with raltitrexed in clinical trials.

Table 2: Tomudex

Drug-related Adverse Events Reported for at Least 2% of Patients Treated with Tomudex 3 mg/m² in Core Colorectal Cancer Trials

Body System and COSTART Term	Number and Percentage of Patients					
	Four Colorectal Cancer Trials		Controlled Colorectal Cancer Trials			
	Tomudex 3 mg/m² (N=861)		Tomudex 3 mg/m² (N=684)		5-FU-LV (N=656)	
Whole Body						
Asthenia	418	48.5%	315	46.1%	243	37%
Fever	192	2.3%	158	23.1%	108	16.5%
Mucous Membrane Disorder	103	12.0%	85	12.4%	269	41.0%
Flu Syndrome	70	8.1%	38	5.6%	17	2.6%
Abdominal Pain	146	17.0%	126	18.4%	115	17.5%
Headache	51	5.9%	44	6.4%	25	3.8%
Infection	25	2.9%	21	3.1%	15	2.3%
Cellulitis	27	3.1%	18	2.6%	0	0%
Pain	36	4.2%	30	4.4%	35	5.3%
Malaise	33	3.8%	27	3.9%	15	2.3%
Chills	31	3.6%	30	4.4%	15	2.3%
Sepsis	20	2.3%	18	2.6%	12	1.8%
Digestive						
Nausea	502	58.3%	390	57.0%	327	49.8%

(cont'd)

Table 2: Tomudex *(cont'd)*

Drug-related Adverse Events Reported for at Least 2% of Patients Treated with Tomudex 3 mg/m² in Core Colorectal Cancer Trials

Body System and COSTART Term	Number and Percentage of Patients					
	Four Colorectal Cancer Trials		Controlled Colorectal Cancer Trials			
	Tomudex 3 mg/m² (N=861)		Tomudex 3 mg/m² (N=684)		5-FU-LV (N=656)	
Diarrhea	324	37.6%	256	37.4%	382	58.2%
Vomiting	320	37.2%	257	37.6%	197	30.0%
Anorexia	238	27.6%	180	26.3%	98	14.9%
Stomatitis	94	10.9%	77	11.2%	229	34.9%
Constipation	115	13.4%	104	15.2%	77	11.7%
Dyspepsia	55	6.4%	38	5.6%	31	4.7%
Flatulence	20	2.3%	18	2.6%	14	2.1%
Dry Mouth	21	2.4%	18	2.6%	17	2.6%
Hemic and Lymphatic						
Leukopenia	188	21.8%	139	20.3%	231	35.2%
Anemia	152	17.7%	103	15.1%	50	7.6%
Thrombocytopenia	45	5.2%	39	5.7%	16	2.4%
Metabolic and Nutritional						
AST Increased	137	15.9%	121	17.7%	14	2.1%
ALT Increased	118	13.7%	104	15.2%	17	2.6%
Peripheral Edema	82	9.5%	69	10.1%	31	4.7%
Weight Loss	51	5.9%	39	5.7%	19	2.9%
Dehydration	49	5.7%	45	6.6%	35	5.3%
Alkaline Phosphatase Increased	20	2.3%	17	2.5%	4	0.6%
Creatinine Increased	20	2.3%	20	2.9%	1	0.2%
Bilirubinemia	19	2.2%	18	2.6%	9	1.4%
Hypokalemia	17	2.0%	15	2.2%	12	1.8%
Musculoskeletal						
Arthralgia[a]	8[a]	2%[a]	4	2%[a]	0	0%[a]
Myalgia	22	2.6%	17	2.5%	11	1.7%
Nervous System						
Insomnia	29	3.4%	28	4.1%	19	2.9%
Depression	22	2.6%	21	3.1%	11	1.7%
Dizziness	35	4.1%	33	4.8%	22	3.4%
Paresthesia	21	2.4%	18	2.6%	18	2.7%
Hypertonia[a]	9	2%[a]	5	2%[a]	0	0%[a]
Respiratory						
Cough Increased	41	4.8%	36	5.3%	26	4.0%
Dyspnea	37	4.3%	34	5.0%	25	3.8%
Pharyngitis	37	4.3%	36	5.3%	41	6.3%
Skin and Appendages						
Rash	123	14.3%	98	14.3%	127	19.4%
Alopecia	52	6.0%	42	6.1%	127	19.4%
Pruritus	28	3.3%	23	3.4%	18	2.7%
Sweating	27	3.1%	25	3.7%	19	2.9%
Special Senses						
Taste Perversion	48	5.6%	40	5.8%	31	4.7%
Conjunctivitis	21	2.4%	17	2.5%	34	5.2%
Urogenital						

(cont'd)

Table 2: Tomudex *(cont'd)*

Drug-related Adverse Events Reported for at Least 2% of Patients Treated with Tomudex 3 mg/m² in Core Colorectal Cancer Trials

Body System and COSTART Term	Number and Percentage of Patients					
	Four Colorectal Cancer Trials		Controlled Colorectal Cancer Trials			
	Tomudex 3 mg/m² (N=861)		Tomudex 3 mg/m² (N=684)		5-FU-LV (N=656)	
Urinary Tract Infection	22	2.6%	21	3.1%	17	2.6%

[a] These values are the results of only 2 clinical trials (study IL/002 and study IL/003). The incidence of these events when calculated for all 4 trials was less than 2%.
Legend: 5-FU-LV = 5-fluorouracil and leucovorin.

Table 3 lists the incidence of WHO Grade 3/4 adverse events reported for at least 2% of patients.

Table 3: Tomudex

Adverse Events of WHO Grade 3/4 (incidences 2% or more)

Adverse Event	Four Colorectal Trials 3.0 mg/m² n[a]=861		Controlled Colorectal Cancer Trials			
			Tomudex 3.0 mg/m² n[a]=684		5FU+LV (LD+HD) n[a]=656	
Nausea and Vomiting	100	11.6%	80	11.7%	58	8.8%
Diarrhea	96	11.1%	78	11.4%	100	15.2%
Constipation	17	2.0%	16	2.3%	11	1.7%
Oral Effects	18	2.1%	16	2.3%	105	16.0%
Pain	63	7.3%	54	7.9%	54	8.2%
Asthenia	–[b]	–[b]	64	9.4%	28	4.3%
Infection	43	5.0%	33	4.8%	32	4.9%
Hemoglobin Decreased	56	6.5%	53	7.7%	17	2.6%
Platelets	30	3.5%	28	4.1%	7	1.1%
Leukocytes	111	12.9%	85	12.4%	176	26.8%
Transaminase Increases	87	10.1%	69	10.1%	2	0.3%
Bilirubin	19	2.2%	11	1.6%	12	1.8%

[a] n=total number of patients.
[b] COSTART term not reported.

The number of serious adverse events reported in the 4 colorectal trials, including those where hospitalization was the criterion for seriousness, are presented in Table 4. In total, 37% of patients participating in these trials experienced a serious adverse event that included hospitalization.

Table 4: Tomudex

Number of SAEs Where Hospitalization Was a Criterion for Seriousness in Trials 1694IL/0002C, 1694IL/0003, 1694IL/0010 and 1694IL/0012

	1694IL/0002C 3 mg/m² n[a]=177		1694IL/0003 3 mg/m² n[a]=222		1694IL/0010 3 mg/m² n[a]=217		1694IL/0012 3 mg/m² n[a]=245		Total Four Colorectal Cancer Trials n[a]=861	
	N	%	N	%	N	%	N	%	N	%
Total number of SAEs	234	21	319	29	309	28	245	22	1107	—
Total number of SAEs where hospitalization was a criterion of seriousness	181	19	280	29	274	29	216	23	951	—
Total number of patients with an SAE	81	46	116	52	91	42	87	35	375	44
Total number of patients with an SAE where hospitalization was a criterion of seriousness	66	37	99	45	75	35	76	31	316	37

[a] n is the total number of patients in trial.
Legend: SAE=Serious Adverse Event.

OVERDOSE:

Symptoms: The expected manifestations of overdose are likely to be an exaggerated form of the adverse drug reactions anticipated with the administration of the drug. Patients should, therefore, be monitored carefully for signs of gastrointestinal and hematological toxicity. Symptomatic treatment and standard supportive care measures for the management of this toxicity should be applied.

Treatment: See Symptoms.

There is no clinically proven antidote available. In the case of inadvertent or accidental administration of an overdose, consideration should be given to the administration of leucovorin. From clinical experience with other antifolates, leucovorin may be given at a dose of 25 mg/m² i.v. every 6 hours. As the time interval between raltitrexed administration and leucovorin rescue increases, its effectiveness in counteracting toxicity may decrease. Data in animals show that delayed administration of leucovorin after raltitrexed produced earlier recovery from weight loss and some improvement to intestinal damage and neutrophil and platelet numbers.

For management of a suspected drug overdose, CPhA recommends that you contact your **regional Poison Control Centre**. See the *CPS* Directory section for a list of Poison Control Centres.

DOSAGE: The dose of raltitrexed is calculated on the basis of body surface area. The recommended dose is 3 mg/m² given i.v., as a single short, i.v. infusion in 50 to 250 mL diluted in 0.9% sodium chloride or 5% dextrose (glucose) solution. It is recommended that the infusion be given over a 15-minute period. In the absence of toxicity, treatment may be repeated every 3 weeks.

Other drugs should not be mixed with raltitrexed in the same infusion container.

Dose escalation above 3 mg/m² is not recommended, since higher doses have been associated with an increased incidence of life-threatening or fatal toxicity.

Prior to the initiation of treatment and before each subsequent treatment, a full blood count (including a differential count and platelets), liver transaminases, serum bilirubin and serum creatinine measurements should be performed. The total white cell count should be greater than 4000/mm³, the neutrophil count greater than 2000/mm³ and the platelet count greater than 100 000/mm³ prior to treatment.

In the event of toxicity the next scheduled dose should be withheld until signs of toxic effects regress. In particular, signs of gastrointestinal toxicity (diarrhea or mucositis) and hematological toxicity (neutropenia or thrombocytopenia) should have resolved completely before subsequent treatment is allowed. Patients who develop signs of gastrointestinal toxicity should have their full blood counts monitored at least weekly for signs of hematological toxicity. Treatment in patients with suspected drug-related rises in liver enzymes should be deferred until they show evidence of reversibility to at least WHO grade 2.

Based on the worst grade of gastrointestinal and hematological toxicity observed on the previous treatment and provided that such toxicity has resolved completely, the following dose reductions are recommended for subsequent treatment:

25% Dose Reduction: In patients with WHO grade 3 hematological toxicity (neutropenia or thrombocytopenia) or WHO grade 2 gastrointestinal toxicity (diarrhea or mucositis).

50% Dose Reduction: In patients with WHO grade 4 hematological toxicity (neutropenia or thrombocytopenia) or WHO grade 3 gastrointestinal toxicity (diarrhea or mucositis). Once a dose reduction has been made, all subsequent doses should be given at the reduced dose level.

Treatment should be discontinued in the event of any WHO grade 4 gastrointestinal toxicity (diarrhea or mucositis) or in the event of a WHO grade 3 gastrointestinal toxicity associated with WHO grade 4 hematological toxicity. Patients with such toxicity should be managed promptly with standard supportive care measures including i.v. hydration and bone marrow support to help neutrophil and platelet recovery thus reducing the likelihood of fatal sepsis or hemorrhage. Based on data in animals where delayed administration of leucovorin after raltitrexed produced earlier recovery from weight loss and some improvement to intestinal damage and recovery of neutrophil and platelet numbers, consideration should be given to the administration of leucovorin (folinic acid). From clinical experience with other antifolates leucovorin may be given at a dose of 25 mg/m² i.v. every 6 hours until the resolution of symptoms. Further use of raltitrexed in such patients is not recommended.

It is essential that the dose reduction scheme be adhered to since the potential for life threatening and fatal toxicity increases if the dose is not reduced or treatment not stopped as appropriate.

Geriatrics: Dosage and administration as for adults. However, as with other cytotoxics, raltitrexed should be used with caution in elderly patients (see Precautions).

Renal Impairment: For patients with abnormal serum creatinine, before the first or any subsequent treatment, a creatinine clearance should be performed or calculated. For patients with a normal serum creatinine when the serum creatinine may not correlate well with the creatinine clearance due to factors such as age or weight loss, the same procedure should be followed. If creatinine clearance is ≤65 mL/min, the following dose modifications are recommended (see Table 5).

Table 5: Tomudex

Dose Modifications Recommended in Renal Impairment

Creatinine Clearance	Dose as % of 3 mg/m²	Dosing Interval
>65 mL/min	Full dose	3-weekly
55-65 mL/min	75%	4-weekly
25-54 mL/min	% equivalent to mL/min[a]	4-weekly
<25 mL/min	No therapy	Not applicable

[a] For example, if the creatinine clearance=30 mL/min, 30% of the full dose should be given.

Patients with renal impairment may have an increased propensity for side effects and should be monitored appropriately.

Hepatic Impairment: No dosage adjustment is necessary for patients with mild (WHO grade 2) to moderate (WHO grade 3) hepatic impairment. However, given that a proportion of the drug is excreted via the fecal route (see Pharmacology) and that these patients usually form a poor prognosis group, patients with mild (WHO grade 2) to moderate (WHO grade 3) hepatic impairment need to be treated with caution. Treatment in patients with suspected drug-related rises in liver enzymes should be deferred until they show evidence of reversibility to at least WHO grade 2. Raltitrexed has not been studied in patients with severe hepatic impairment, clinical jaundice or decompensated liver disease and its use in such patients is not recommended.

Special Instructions: Raltitrexed is a cytotoxic agent and should be handled according to the normal procedures adopted for such agents in each institution. At minimum the following are recommended: Any unused injection or reconstituted solution should be discarded in a suitable manner for cytotoxics.

Raltitrexed should be reconstituted for injection by trained personnel in a designated area for the reconstitution of cytotoxic agents. Cytotoxic preparations such as raltitrexed should not be handled by pregnant women.

Reconstitution should normally be carried out in a partial containment facility with extraction capabilities, e.g., a laminar air-flow cabinet, and work surfaces should be covered with disposable plastic-backed absorbent paper.

Appropriate protective clothing, including surgical gloves and goggles, should be worn. In case of contact with skin, wash immediately with water. For splashes in the eyes irrigate with clean water, holding the eyelids apart, for at least 10 minutes. Seek medical attention.

Any spillage should be cleared up using standard procedures consistent with the handling of chemotherapeutic agents.

Waste material should be disposed of by incineration in a manner consistent with the handling of cytotoxic agents.

Stability and Storage Recommendations: Store at 2 to 25°C protected from light. Once reconstituted, raltitrexed is chemically stable for 24 hours at 25°C exposed to ambient light, however, it is recommended that raltitrexed should be refrigerated to avoid bacterial contamination (for further information see Reconstituted Solutions).

Reconstituted Solutions: Each vial, containing 2 mg of raltitrexed, should be reconstituted with 4 mL of sterile water for injection to produce a 0.5 mg/mL solution. The appropriate dose of solution, calculated on the basis of body surface area, is diluted in 50 to 250 mL of either 0.9% sodium chloride or 5% glucose (dextrose) injection and administered by a short i.v. infusion over a period of 15 minutes.

There is no preservative or bacteriostatic agent present in raltitrexed or the materials specified for reconstitution or dilution. Raltitrexed must therefore be reconstituted and diluted under aseptic conditions (see Special Instructions) and it is recommended that solutions of raltitrexed should be used as soon as possible. Reconstituted raltitrexed solution may be stored refrigerated (2 to 8°C) for up to 24 hours. The admixed solution must be completely used or discarded within 24 hours of reconstitution of raltitrexed i.v. injection.

Reconstituted and diluted solutions do not need to be protected from light.

Do not store partially used vials or admixed solutions for future patient use.

Parenteral Products: Continuous i.v. infusion (see Table 6).

Table 6: Tomudex

Reconstitution

Vial Size	Volume of Diluent to be Added to Vial	Approximate Available Volume	Nominal Concentration /mL
2 mg raltitrexed/vial[a]	4 mL sterile water for injection	4 mL	0.5 mg/mL

[a] As the disodium salt.

There is no information on incompatibilities at present and therefore raltitrexed should not be mixed with any other drug.

As with all parenteral drug products, i.v. admixtures should be inspected visually for clarity, particulate matter, precipitate, discoloration and leakage prior to administration whenever solutions and containers permit.

SUPPLIED: Each vial of sterile, lyophilized powder without preservative or bacteriostatic agent contains: raltitrexed 2 mg (as the disodium salt). Nonmedicinal ingredients: dibasic sodium phosphate, mannitol, nitrogen and sodium hydroxide. Single dose vials of 2 mg.

Topamax® Ⓟ

topiramate

Antiepileptic—Migraine Prophylaxis

Janssen-Ortho

Date of Preparation: March 6, 1997
Date of Revision: April 8, 2010

SUMMARY PRODUCT INFORMATION:

Route of Administration	Dosage Form/ Strength	All Nonmedicinal Ingredients
Oral	Tablet 25 mg, 100 mg, 200 mg	Carnauba wax, hypromellose, lactose monohydrate, magnesium stearate, pregelatinized starch, microcrystalline cellulose, polyethylene glycol, polysorbate 80, purified water, sodium starch glycolate, titanium dioxide, and may contain synthetic iron oxide
Oral	Sprinkle capsule 15 mg, 25 mg	black pharmaceutical ink, cellulose acetate, gelatin, povidone, sorbitan monolaurate, sodium lauryl sulfate, sugar spheres (sucrose and starch), and titanium dioxide

INDICATIONS AND CLINICAL USE: Epilepsy: TOPAMAX (topiramate) is indicated as monotherapy for the management of patients (adults and children six years and older) with newly diagnosed epilepsy.

TOPAMAX (topiramate) is also indicated as adjunctive therapy for the management of patients (adults and children two years and older) with epilepsy who are not satisfactorily controlled with conventional therapy.

Migraine: TOPAMAX (topiramate) is indicated in adults for the prophylaxis of migraine headache. Prophylactic treatment of migraine may be considered in situations such as: adults experiencing four or more migraine attacks per month who fail to respond adequately to acute abortive therapy; recurring attacks that significantly interfere with the patient's daily routine; a pattern of increasing migraine attacks over time, with the risk of developing rebound headache from acute abortive therapies; or failure of, or contraindication to, or troublesome side effects from acute abortive medications. Continuing therapy should be reviewed every six months. TOPAMAX should not be used in the acute treatment of migraine attacks. Safety and efficacy of topiramate in the management or prevention of cluster headache, hemiplegic, basilar, ophthalmoplegic, or transformed migraine headaches have not been established.

Geriatrics (>65 years of age): There is limited information in patients over 65 years of age (see Warnings and Precautions, Special Populations, Geriatrics (>65 years of age)).

CONTRAINDICATIONS: Patients who are hypersensitive to this drug or to any nonmedicinal ingredient in the formulation or component of the container. For a complete listing, see Dosage Forms, Composition and Packaging.

TOPAMAX for the indication prophylaxis of migraine is contraindicated in pregnancy and in women of childbearing potential who are not using an effective method of contraception (see Warnings and Precautions, Special Populations, Pregnant Women, Migraine, Adverse Reactions, Post-Market Adverse Drug Reactions, Pregnancy Registries to Date (August 2009) and Dosage and Administration, Dosing Considerations).

WARNINGS AND PRECAUTIONS: General: Antiepileptic drugs, including TOPAMAX (topiramate), should be withdrawn gradually to minimize the potential for seizures or increased seizure frequency. In clinical trials in adult patients with epilepsy, dosages were decreased by 50-100 mg/day at weekly intervals. In clinical trials of children, TOPAMAX was gradually withdrawn over a 2-8 week period (see Dosage and Administration, General and Epilepsy).

In patients without a history of seizures or epilepsy, TOPAMAX (topiramate) should be gradually withdrawn to minimize the potential for seizures or increased seizure frequency. In clinical trials in adult patients receiving TOPAMAX for migraine prophylaxis dosages were decreased by 25-50 mg/day at weekly intervals (see Dosage and Administration, General and Migraine).

In situations where rapid withdrawal of TOPAMAX is medically required, appropriate monitoring is recommended (see Dosage and Administration, General).

Hyperammonemia and Encephalopathy: There have been rare reports of patients, with or without previous history, experiencing hyperammonemia with or without encephalopathy while receiving topiramate alone or in combination with other antiepileptic medications. The majority of these cases indicate that concomitant administration of topiramate and valproic acid is associated with hyperammonemia with or without encephalopathy in patients who have tolerated either drug alone. In most cases, symptoms and signs abated with discontinuation of either drug. This adverse event is not due to a pharmacokinetic interaction. Patients with inborn errors of metabolism or reduced hepatic mitochondrial activity may be at an increased risk for hyperammonemia with or without encephalopathy. Although not studied, an interaction of topiramate and valproic acid may exacerbate existing defects or unmask deficiencies in susceptible persons (see Adverse Reactions, Post-Market Adverse Drug Reactions and Drug Interactions, Drug-Drug Interactions).

In patients who develop unexplained vomiting, lethargy, confusion or other changes in mental status, hyperammonemic encephalopathy should be considered and serum ammonia levels should be measured.

Endocrine and Metabolism: Oligohidrosis and Hyperthermia: Oligohidrosis (decreased sweating) and hyperthermia, infrequently resulting in hospitalization, including fatalities, have been reported in patients treated with topiramate. Oligohidrosis and hyperthermia may have potentially serious sequelae and may be preventable by prompt recognition of symptoms and appropriate treatment. Decreased sweating and elevation of body temperature above normal characterized the cases reported in patients treated with topiramate. Some of the cases were reported after exposure to elevated environmental temperatures.

These reports have primarily involved children. Patients treated with TOPAMAX, especially pediatric patients, should be monitored closely for evidence of decreased sweating and increased body temperature, particularly in hot weather. Proper hydration before and during activities such as exercise or exposure to warm temperatures is recommended.

Caution should be used when TOPAMAX is prescribed with other drugs that predispose patients to heat-related disorders; these drugs include, but are not limited to, other carbonic anhydrase inhibitors and drugs with anticholinergic activity (see Adverse Reactions, Post-Market Adverse Drug Reactions).

Metabolic Acidosis: Hyperchloremic, non-anion gap, metabolic acidosis (i.e. decreased serum bicarbonate below the normal reference range in the absence of respiratory alkalosis) is associated with topiramate treatment. This decrease in serum bicarbonate is due to the inhibitory effect of topiramate on renal carbonic anhydrase. Generally, the decrease in bicarbonate occurs early in treatment although it can occur at any time during treatment. These decreases are usually mild to moderate (average decrease of 4 mmol/L at doses of 100 mg/day or above in adults and at approximately 6 mg/kg/day in pediatric patients). Rarely, patients have experienced decreases to values below 10 mmol/L. Conditions or therapies that predispose to acidosis (such as renal disease, severe respiratory disorders, status epilepticus, diarrhea, surgery, ketogenic diet, or certain drugs) may be additive to the bicarbonate-lowering effects of topiramate.

In adults, the incidence of persistent treatment-emergent decreases in serum bicarbonate (levels of <20 mmol/L at two consecutive visits or at the final visit) in controlled clinical trials for adjunctive treatment of epilepsy was 32% for 400 mg/day, and 1% for placebo. Metabolic acidosis has been observed at doses as low as 50 mg/day. The incidence of a markedly abnormally low serum bicarbonate (i.e. absolute value <17 mmol/L and >5 mmol/L decrease from pre-treatment) in these trials was 3% for 400 mg/day, and 0% for placebo. Serum bicarbonate levels have not been systematically evaluated at daily doses greater than 400 mg/day.

In pediatric patients (<16 years of age), the incidence of persistent treatment-emergent decreases in serum bicarbonate in placebo-controlled trials for adjunctive treatment of Lennox-Gastaut Syndrome or refractory partial onset seizures was 67% for TOPAMAX (at approximately 6 mg/kg/day), and 10% for placebo. The incidence of a markedly abnormally low serum bicarbonate (i.e. absolute value <17 mmol/L and >5 mmol/L decrease from pre-treatment) in these trials was 11% for TOPAMAX and 0% for placebo. Cases of moderately severe metabolic acidosis have been reported in patients as young as 5 months old, especially at daily doses above 5 mg/kg/day.

The incidence of persistent treatment-emergent decreases in serum bicarbonate in placebo-controlled trials for adults for prophylaxis of migraine was 44% for 200 mg/day, 39% for 100 mg/day, 23% for 50 mg/day, and 7% for placebo. The incidence of a markedly abnormally low serum bicarbonate (i.e. absolute value <17 mmol/L and >5 mmol/L decrease from pre-treatment) in these trials was 11% for 200 mg/day, 9% for 100 mg/day, 2% for 50 mg/day, and <1% for placebo.

Safety and effectiveness in patients below the age of 2 years have not been established. Topiramate is associated with metabolic acidosis. Chronic untreated metabolic acidosis in pediatric patients may cause osteomalacia (rickets) and may reduce growth rates. A reduction in growth rate may eventually decrease the maximal height achieved. The effect of topiramate on growth and bone-related sequelae has not been systematically investigated.

Measurement of baseline and periodic serum bicarbonate during topiramate treatment is recommended. If metabolic acidosis develops and persists, consideration should be given to reducing the dose or discontinuing topiramate (using dose tapering). If the decision is made to continue patients on topiramate in the face of persistent acidosis, alkali treatment should be considered.

Decreases in Serum Potassium with Concomitant Treatment with Hydrochlorothiazide (HCTZ): In a drug interaction study, a greater decrease from baseline in serum potassium values was seen with concomitant treatment than for either drug alone. At the end of each treatment period, 27% (3/11) of subjects on topiramate treatment alone and 25% (3/12) of subjects on HCTZ treatment alone showed a serum potassium value of <3.6 mEq/L, compared to 61% (14/23) of subjects on concomitant drug treatment. One of the subjects who had hypokalemia with concomitant treatment also had an abnormal ECG (non-specific ST-T wave changes), which may have been related to the decrease in plasma potassium levels. Caution should be used when treating patients who are receiving TOPAMAX and hydrochlorothiazide concomitantly (see Drug Interactions).

Nutritional Supplementation: A dietary supplement or increased food intake may be considered if the patient is losing weight while on this medication.

Hepatic/Biliary/Pancreatic: Decreased Hepatic Function: In hepatically impaired patients, TOPAMAX should be administered with caution as the clearance of topiramate was decreased compared with normal subjects.

Neurologic: Central Nervous System Effects: Adverse events most often associated with the use of TOPAMAX were central nervous system related and were observed in both the epilepsy and migraine populations. In adults, the most significant of these can be classified into three general categories: 1) psychomotor slowing, difficulty with concentration and speech or language problems, in particular, word-finding difficulties, 2) somnolence or fatigue and 3) mood disturbances including irritability and depression.

In the controlled epilepsy adjunctive therapy trials, these events were generally mild to moderate and generally occurred early in therapy. While the incidence of psychomotor slowing does not appear to be dose related, both language problems and difficulty with concentration or attention increased in frequency with increasing dosage in the six double-blind trials, suggesting that these events are dose related (see Adverse Reactions, Post-Market Adverse Drug Reactions).

Central nervous system and psychiatric-related events were also more frequently reported in topiramate-treated subjects in the migraine prophylaxis trials. These included: anorexia, dizziness, difficulty with memory, somnolence, language problems, and difficulty with concentration and attention. Most of the events were mild or moderate in severity, some of which led to withdrawal from treatment (see Adverse Reactions, Migraine).

Additional non-specific CNS effects occasionally observed with TOPAMAX as add-on epilepsy therapy include dizziness or imbalance, confusion and memory problems. Although the duration of the epilepsy monotherapy studies was considerably longer than the epilepsy adjunctive therapy studies, these adverse events were reported at lower incidences in the monotherapy trials.

Paresthesia: Paresthesia, an effect associated with the use of other carbonic anhydrase inhibitors, appears to be a common effect of TOPAMAX. Paresthesia was more frequently reported in the migraine prophylaxis and epilepsy monotherapy trials versus the adjunctive therapy trials in epilepsy. The higher incidence in the epilepsy monotherapy studies may have been related to the higher topiramate plasma concentrations achieved in the monotherapy studies. In the majority of instances, paresthesia did not lead to treatment discontinuation.

Ophthalmologic: Acute Myopia and Secondary Angle Closure Glaucoma: A syndrome consisting of acute myopia associated with secondary angle closure glaucoma has been reported in patients receiving TOPAMAX. Symptoms include acute onset of decreased visual acuity and/or ocular pain. Ophthalmologic findings can include myopia, anterior chamber shallowing, ocular hyperemia (redness) and increased intraocular pressure. Mydriasis may or may not be present. This syndrome may be associated with supraciliary effusion resulting in anterior displacement of the lens and iris, with secondary angle closure glaucoma. Symptoms typically occur within a few days to 1 month of initiating TOPAMAX therapy. In contrast to primary narrow angle glaucoma, which is rare under 40 years of age, secondary angle closure glaucoma associated with TOPAMAX has been reported in pediatric patients as well as adults. The primary treatment to reverse symptoms is discontinuation of TOPAMAX as rapidly as possible, according to the judgment of the treating physician. Other measures, in conjunction with discontinuation of TOPAMAX, may be helpful (see Adverse Reactions, Post-Market Adverse Drug Reactions).

In all cases of acute visual blurring and/or painful/red eye(s), immediate consultation with an ophthalmologist/emergency room is recommended.

Elevated intraocular pressure of any etiology, if left untreated, can lead to serious sequelae including permanent vision loss.

Maculopathy, including visual field defect, has been observed very rarely in post-marketing reports (see Adverse Reactions, Post-Market Adverse Drug Reactions).

Psychiatric: Suicidal Ideation and Behaviour: Suicidal ideation and behaviour have been reported in patients treated with antiepileptic agents in several indications.

All patients treated with antiepileptic drugs, irrespective of indication, should be monitored for signs of suicidal ideation and behaviour and appropriate treatment should be considered. Patients (and caregivers of patients) should be advised to seek medical advice should signs of suicidal ideation or behaviour emerge.

An FDA meta-analysis of randomized placebo controlled trials, in which antiepileptic drugs were used for various indications, has shown a small increased risk of suicidal ideation and behaviour in patients treated with these drugs. The mechanism of this risk is not known.

There were 43 892 patients treated in the placebo controlled clinical trials that were included in the meta-analysis. Approximately 75% of patients in these clinical trials were treated for indications other than epilepsy and, for the majority of non-epilepsy indications the treatment (antiepileptic drug or placebo) was administered as monotherapy. Patients with epilepsy represented approximately 25% of the total number of patients treated in the placebo controlled clinical trials and, for the majority of epilepsy patients, treatment (antiepileptic drug or placebo) was administered as adjunct to other antiepileptic agents (i.e., patients in both treatment arms were being treated with one or more antiepileptic drug). Therefore, the small increased risk of suicidal ideation and behaviour reported from the meta-analysis (0.43% for patients on antiepileptic drugs compared to 0.24% for patients on placebo) is based largely on patients that received monotherapy treatment (antiepileptic drug or placebo) for non-epilepsy indications. The study design does not allow an estimation of the risk of suicidal ideation and behaviour for patients with epilepsy that are taking antiepileptic drugs, due both to this population being the minority in the study, and the drug-placebo comparison in this population being confounded by the presence of adjunct antiepileptic drug treatment in both arms.

Renal: Kidney Stones: A total of 32/1715 (1.9%) of patients exposed to TOPAMAX during its epilepsy adjunctive therapy development reported the occurrence of kidney stones, an incidence about 10 times that expected in a similar, untreated population (M/F ratio: 27/1092 male; 5/623 female). In double-blind epilepsy monotherapy studies, a total of 8/886 (0.9%) of adults reported the occurrence of kidney stones. In the general population, risk factors for kidney stone formation include gender (male), ages between 20-50 years, prior stone formation, family history of nephrolithiasis, and hypercalciuria. Based on logistic regression analysis of the clinical trial data, no correlation between mean TOPAMAX dosage, duration of TOPAMAX therapy, or age and the occurrence of kidney stones was established; of the risk factors evaluated, only gender (male) showed a correlation with the occurrence of kidney stones. In the pediatric patients studied, there were no kidney stones observed.

Carbonic anhydrase inhibitors, e.g. acetazolamide, promote stone formation by reducing urinary citrate excretion and by increasing urinary pH. Concomitant use of TOPAMAX, a weak carbonic anhydrase inhibitor, with other carbonic anhydrase inhibitors may create a physiological environment that increases the risk of kidney stone formation, and should therefore be avoided (see Drug Interactions, Drug-Drug Interactions).

Patients, especially those with a predisposition to nephrolithiasis, may have an increased risk of renal stone formation and associated signs and symptoms such as renal colic, renal pain or flank pain. Increased fluid intake increases the urinary output, lowering the concentration of substances involved in stone formation. Therefore, adequate hydration is recommended to reduce this risk. None of the risk factors for nephrolithiasis can reliably predict stone formation during TOPAMAX treatment.

Adjustment of Dose in Renal Failure: The major route of elimination of unchanged topiramate and its metabolites is via the kidney. Renal elimination is dependent on renal function and is independent of age. Patients with impaired renal function (CL_{CR} <70 mL/min/1.73 m^2) or with end-stage renal disease receiving hemodialysis treatments may take 10 to 15 days to reach steady-state plasma concentrations as compared to 4 to 8 days in patients with normal renal function. As with all patients, the titration schedule should be guided by clinical outcome (i.e. seizure control, avoidance of side effects) with the knowledge that patients with known renal impairment may require a longer time to reach steady state at each dose (see Dosage and Administration, Dosing Considerations).

Information to Be Provided to the Patient: Pregnant Women: Epilepsy: Patients should be reminded to inform their doctor if they are pregnant or intend to become pregnant while on TOPAMAX therapy. **TOPAMAX should be used during pregnancy only if potential benefit justifies the potential risk to the fetus.**

Patients should be encouraged to enroll in the North American Antiepileptic Drug (NAAED) Pregnancy Registry if they become pregnant. This registry is collecting information about the safety of antiepileptic drugs during pregnancy. To enroll, patients can call the toll free number, 1-888-233-2334. Information on the registry can also be found at the website http://www.aedpregnancyregistry.org/.

Migraine: Prophylactic treatment of migraine: Taking TOPAMAX to prevent migraine attacks does not outweigh the risk of malformations to the fetus. Consequently, TOPAMAX is contraindicated in pregnancy and in women of childbearing potential who are not using an effective method of contraception (see Contraindications, Warnings and Precautions, Special Populations, Pregnant Women, Migraine and Dosage and Administration, Dosing Considerations).

Adequate Hydration: Patients, especially those with predisposing factors, should be instructed to maintain an adequate fluid intake in order to minimize the risk of renal stone formation. Patients also should be instructed to increase and maintain fluid intake prior to and during activities such as exercise and exposure to warm temperatures to help prevent complications from decreased sweating.

Effects on Ability to Drive and Use Machines: Patients should be warned about the potential for somnolence, dizziness, confusion, and difficulty concentrating, and advised not to drive or operate machinery until they have gained sufficient experience on TOPAMAX to gauge whether it adversely affects their mental and/or motor performance.

Acute Myopia and Secondary Angle Closure Glaucoma: Patients taking TOPAMAX should be told to immediately contact their doctor and/or go to the Emergency Room if they/their child experience(s) sudden worsening of vision, blurred vision or painful/red eye(s).

Special Populations: Pregnant Women: Epilepsy: Like many other drugs, topiramate was teratogenic in mice, rats, and rabbits. In rats, topiramate crosses the placental barrier.

There are no studies using TOPAMAX in pregnant women. TOPAMAX therapy should be used during pregnancy only if the potential benefit outweighs the potential risk to the fetus.

In post-marketing experience, cases of hypospadias have been reported in male infants exposed in utero to TOPAMAX, with or without other anticonvulsants; however, a causal relationship with TOPAMAX has not been established.

Pregnancy registry data suggest that there may be an association between the use of TOPAMAX during pregnancy and congenital malformations (e.g., craniofacial defects, such as cleft lip/palate, hypospadias, and anomalies involving various body systems). This has been reported with topiramate monotherapy and topiramate as part of a polytherapy regimen (see Adverse Reactions, Post-Market Adverse Drug Reactions, Pregnancy Registries to Date (August 2009)).

In addition, data from these registries and other studies suggest that, compared with monotherapy, there may be an increased risk of teratogenic effects associated with the use of anti-epileptic drugs in combination therapy.

TOPAMAX should be used during pregnancy only if potential benefit justifies the potential risk to the fetus. In treating and counselling women of childbearing potential, the prescribing physician should weigh the benefits of therapy against the risks. If this drug is used during pregnancy or if the patient becomes pregnant while taking this drug, the patient should be apprised of the potential hazard to the fetus.

To provide information regarding the effects of in utero exposure to TOPAMAX, physicians are advised to recommend that pregnant patients taking TOPAMAX enroll in the North American Antiepileptic Drug (NAAED) Pregnancy Registry. This can be done by calling the toll free number, 1-888-233-2334, and must be done by patients themselves. Information on the registry can also be found at the website http://www.aedpregnancyregistry.org/.

The effect of TOPAMAX on labor and delivery in humans is unknown.

Migraine: Prophylactic treatment of migraine: In pregnancy, the occurrence of seizures presents a significant risk for the mother and child. Prescribing TOPAMAX to prevent seizures therefore outweighs the risk of malformations to the fetus. However, taking TOPAMAX to prevent migraine attacks does not outweigh this risk. Consequently, TOPAMAX is contraindicated in pregnancy and in women of child bearing potential who are not using an effective method of contraception (see Contraindications and Dosage and Administration, Dosing Considerations).

Nursing Women: Topiramate is excreted in the milk of lactating rats. The excretion of topiramate in human milk has not been evaluated in controlled studies. Limited observations in patients suggest an extensive excretion of topiramate into breast milk. Since the potential for serious adverse reactions in nursing infants exposed to TOPAMAX exists, the prescriber should decide whether to discontinue nursing or discontinue the drug, taking into account the importance of the drug to the mother and the risks to the infant.

Pediatrics (<2 years of age): Safety and effectiveness in children under 2 years of age have not been established.

Weight Loss in Pediatrics (>2 years of age): TOPAMAX administration is associated with weight loss in some children that generally occurs early in therapy. Of those pediatric subjects treated in clinical trials for at least a year who experienced weight loss, 96% showed a resumption of weight gain within the period tested. In 2-4-year-olds, the mean change in weight from baseline at 12 months (n=25) was +0.7 kg (range −1.1 to 3.2); at 24 months (n=14), the mean change was +2.2 kg (range −1.1 to 6.1). In 5-10-year-olds, the mean change in weight from baseline at 12 months (n=88) was +0.7 kg (range −6.7 to 11.8); at 24 months (n=67), the mean change was +3.3 kg (range −8.6 to 20.0). Weight decreases, usually associated with anorexia or appetite changes, were reported as adverse events for 9% of patients treated with TOPAMAX. The long-term effects of reduced weight gain in pediatric patients are not known.

Geriatrics (>65 years of age): There is limited information in patients over 65 years of age. The possibility of age-associated renal function abnormalities should be considered when using TOPAMAX (see Action and Clinical Pharmacology, Special Populations and Conditions).

Monitoring and Laboratory Tests: It has been observed in clinical trials that topiramate-treated subjects experienced an average decrease in serum bicarbonate level of 4 mmol/L and an average increase in serum chloride level of 4 mmol/L (see Warnings and Precautions, Endocrine and Metabolism).

Hypokalemia Observed During Concomitant Treatment with Hydrochlorothiazide: In a drug interaction study with the diuretic hydrochlorothiazide (HCTZ), the percentage of patients with a serum potassium measurement of <3.6 mEq/L was greater at the end of concomitant treatment than at the end of treatment for either drug alone: 27% (3/11) of subjects on topiramate treatment alone and 25% (3/12) of subjects on HCTZ alone versus 61% (14/22) of subjects on concomitant drug treatment (see Warnings and Precautions, Endocrine and Metabolism and Drug Interactions).

ADVERSE REACTIONS: The majority of the most common adverse events in clinical trials were mild-moderate in severity and dose-related. These dose-related adverse events typically began in the titration phase and often persisted into the maintenance phase, but infrequently began in the maintenance phase. Rapid titration rate and higher initial dose were associated with higher incidences of adverse events leading to discontinuation.

Epilepsy: Adverse Drug Reaction Overview for Monotherapy: Adults: The most commonly observed adverse events associated with the use of topiramate at dosages of 100 to 400 mg/day in controlled trials in adults with newly diagnosed epilepsy were: paresthesia, fatigue, headache, somnolence, dizziness, upper respiratory tract infection, anorexia, weight decrease, depression, and nausea (see Table 1).

Approximately 19% of the 886 adult patients who received topiramate as monotherapy in controlled clinical trials for patients with newly diagnosed epilepsy discontinued therapy due to adverse events. Adverse events associated with discontinuing therapy included paresthesia (2.6%), somnolence (2.5%), fatigue (2.3%), nausea (2.0%), and psychomotor slowing (1.6%).

Pediatrics: The most commonly observed adverse events associated with the use of topiramate at dosages of 100 to 400 mg/day in controlled trials in children with newly diagnosed epilepsy were: upper respiratory tract infection, headache, anorexia, difficulty with concentration/attention, weight decrease, somnolence, paresthesia, fever, and fatigue (see Table 2).

Approximately 10% of the 245 pediatric patients who received topiramate as monotherapy in controlled clinical trials for patients with newly diagnosed epilepsy discontinued therapy due to adverse events. Adverse events associated with discontinuing therapy included difficulty with concentration/attention (2.0%). No pediatric patients withdrew due to psychomotor slowing.

Clinical Trial Adverse Drug Reactions: Because clinical trials are conducted under very specific conditions the adverse reaction rates observed in the clinical trials may not reflect the rates observed in practice and should not be compared to the rates in the clinical trials of another drug. Adverse drug reaction information from clinical trials is useful for identifying drug-related adverse events and for approximating rates.

Table 1: TOPAMAX

Incidence of Treatment-emergent Adverse Events in Monotherapy Trials in Adults[a] Where Rate was ≥2% in Any Topiramate Group

Body System/Adverse Event	TOPAMAX Dosage (mg/day) 50–100 (n=444)	200–400 (n=329)	500 (n=113)
Body as a Whole—General Disorders			
Fatigue	18	18	19
Injury	9	8	4
Asthenia	4	5	4
Back Pain	3	2	5
Pain	3	2	5
Chest Pain	2	2	3
Fever	1	2	3
Syncope	2	1	1
Leg Pain	2	2	1
Peripheral Edema	1	<1	2
Central and Peripheral Nervous Systems Disorders			
Paresthesia	23	39	38
Headache	23	16	19
Dizziness	16	13	13
Hypoesthesia	5	5	12
Language Problems	4	5	6
Ataxia	3	5	4
Speech Disorders/Related Speech Problems	2	3	3
Vertigo	2	3	4
Tremor	3	2	3
Hypertonia	1	2	2
Involuntary Muscle Contractions	1	2	4
Sensory Disturbances	1	1	4
Migraine	2	1	1
Abnormal Co-ordination	1	1	3
Convulsions Aggravated	1	0	2
Convulsions Grand Mal	<1	1	2
Gait Abnormal	<1	<1	3
Dyskinesia	0	0	2
Gastrointestinal System Disorders			
Nausea	11	12	12
Diarrhea	6	8	12
Abdominal Pain	6	8	7
Dyspepsia	5	5	4
Vomiting	4	3	2
Constipation	2	3	1
Dry Mouth	1	2	6
Gastroenteritis	2	1	2
Gastritis	1	2	2
Toothache	1	1	2
Gastrointestinal Disorder NOS	<1	<1	2
Hemorrhoids	<1	<1	2
Stomatitis Ulcerative	<1	0	2
Hearing and Vestibular Disorders			
Tinnitus	1	2	2

(cont'd)

Table 1: TOPAMAX *(cont'd)*

Incidence of Treatment-emergent Adverse Events in Monotherapy Trials in Adults[a] Where Rate was ≥2% in Any Topiramate Group

Body System/Adverse Event	TOPAMAX Dosage (mg/day) 50–100 (n=444)	200–400 (n=329)	500 (n=113)
Heart Rate and Rhythm Disorders			
Palpitation	1	1	4
Tachycardia	1	0	2
Metabolic and Nutritional Disorders			
Weight Decrease	9	14	18
Musculoskeletal System Disorders			
Arthralgia	3	4	4
Myalgia	2	1	2
Muscle Weakness	1	1	2
Platelet, Bleeding & Clotting Disorders			
Epistaxis	1	2	1
Hematoma	0	0	2
Psychiatric Disorders			
Somnolence	11	15	19
Anorexia	8	14	11
Insomnia	9	8	9
Difficulty with Memory NOS	6	10	9
Depression	7	10	4
Difficulty with Concentration/Attention	6	9	8
Nervousness	6	7	8
Mood Problems	5	6	4
Anxiety	4	6	5
Confusion	4	5	7
Psychomotor Slowing	2	5	8
Cognitive Problems NOS	2	3	3
Agitation	2	2	3
Emotional Lability	1	3	2
Aggressive Reaction	2	1	2
Libido Decreased	1	2	1
Depression Aggravated	<1	2	3
Impotence	1	1	2
Reproductive Disorders, Female			
Menstrual Disorder	3	1	8
Dysmenorrhea	2	2	0
Intermenstrual Bleeding	2	1	0
Menorrhagia	1	1	2
Pregnancy Unintended	1	1	2
Mastitis	0	0	2
Reproductive Disorders, Male			
Premature Ejaculation	0	0	2
Resistance Mechanism Disorders			
Infection Viral	5	9	6
Otitis Media	2	1	2
Respiratory System Disorders			
Upper Respiratory Tract Infection	15	13	10
Pharyngitis	5	5	2

(cont'd)

Table 1: TOPAMAX *(cont'd)*

Incidence of Treatment-emergent Adverse Events in Monotherapy Trials in Adults[a] Where Rate was ≥2% in Any Topiramate Group

	TOPAMAX Dosage (mg/day)		
Body System/Adverse Event	**50–100 (n=444)**	**200–400 (n=329)**	**500 (n=113)**
Sinusitis	3	4	6
Rhinitis	3	3	5
Bronchitis	2	2	1
Coughing	2	2	2
Dyspnea	1	2	1
Pneumonia	1	<1	3
Skin and Appendages Disorders			
Rash	3	4	3
Alopecia	3	3	1
Acne	1	3	2
Pruritus	1	3	1
Increased Sweating	1	<1	2
Maculopapular Rash	1	0	2
Special Senses Other, Disorders			
Taste Perversion	3	5	6
Urinary System Disorders			
Urinary Tract Infection	2	2	5
Micturition Frequency	1	2	4
Dysuria	<1	2	1
Cystitis	<1	2	1
Renal Calculus	<1	2	2
Vision Disorders			
Vision Abnormal	3	4	4
Diplopia	1	1	2

[a] Values represent the percentage of patients reporting a given adverse event. Patients may have reported more than one adverse event during the study and can be included in more than one adverse event category.

Adverse Drug Reaction Overview for Adjunctive Therapy: Adults: The most commonly observed adverse events associated with the adjunctive use of TOPAMAX (topiramate) at dosages of 200 to 400 mg/day in controlled trials in adults that were seen at greater frequency in patients treated with TOPAMAX and did not appear to be dose related within this dosage range were: somnolence, dizziness, ataxia, speech disorders and related speech problems, psychomotor slowing, nystagmus, and paresthesia (see Table 3).

The most common dose-related adverse events at dosages of 200 to 1000 mg/day were: nervousness, difficulty with concentration or attention, confusion, depression, anorexia, language problems, and mood problems (see Table 4).

Pediatrics: Adverse events associated with the use of TOPAMAX at dosages of 5 to 9 mg/kg/day in worldwide pediatric clinical trials that were seen at greater frequency in patients treated with TOPAMAX were: fatigue, somnolence, anorexia, nervousness, difficulty with concentration/attention, difficulty with memory, aggressive reaction, and weight decrease (see Table 5).

Clinical Trial Adverse Drug Reactions: Because clinical trials are conducted under very specific conditions the adverse reaction rates observed in the clinical trials may not reflect the rates observed in practice and should not be compared to the rates in the clinical trials of another drug. Adverse drug reaction information from clinical trials is useful for identifying drug-related adverse events and for approximating rates.

Table 2: TOPAMAX

Incidence of Treatment-emergent Adverse Events in Monotherapy Trials in Children Ages 6 up to 16 Years[a] Where Rate was ≥2% in Any Topiramate Group

	TOPAMAX Dosage (mg/day)		
Body System/Adverse Event	**50–100 (n=125)**	**200–400 (n=106)**	**500[b] (n=14)**
Body as a Whole—General Disorders			
Fatigue	7	10	14
Fever	2	11	7
Injury	4	2	14
Asthenia	0	3	7
Back Pain	2	2	0
Allergic Reaction	1	1	7
Allergy	0	1	7
Influenza-like Symptoms	0	0	7

(cont'd)

Table 2: TOPAMAX *(cont'd)*

Incidence of Treatment-emergent Adverse Events in Monotherapy Trials in Children Ages 6 up to 16 Years[a] Where Rate was ≥2% in Any Topiramate Group

	TOPAMAX Dosage (mg/day)		
Body System/Adverse Event	**50–100 (n=125)**	**200–400 (n=106)**	**500[b] (n=14)**
Central and Peripheral Nervous Systems Disorders			
Headache	27	17	29
Dizziness	9	8	0
Paresthesia	4	11	7
Language Problems	0	3	7
Convulsions Grand Mal	2	0	7
Hypertonia	0	0	7
Hyperkinesia	2	0	21
Migraine	2	1	0
Muscle Contractions Involuntary	1	2	0
Tremor	2	0	0
Vertigo	0	3	0
Cramps Legs	2	0	0
Gait Abnormal	2	0	0
Collagen Disorders			
Auto-antibody Response	0	0	7
Gastrointestinal System Disorders			
Diarrhea	9	7	7
Vomiting	8	6	14
Abdominal Pain	6	4	14
Nausea	4	5	14
Gastroenteritis	6	0	7
Constipation	1	0	7
Gastrointestinal Disorder NOS	0	0	7
Dyspepsia	2	1	0
Toothache	1	1	7
Hearing and Vestibular Disorders			
Earache	2	0	0
Metabolic and Nutritional Disorders			
Weight Decrease	5	14	0
Acidosis	0	0	7
Musculoskeletal System Disorders			
Arthralgia	1	2	7
Platelet, Bleeding and Clotting Disorders			
Epistaxis	2	4	14
Psychiatric Disorders			
Anorexia	13	13	14
Somnolence	14	9	0
Difficulty with Concentration/Attention	6	13	7
Insomnia	5	4	14
Nervousness	5	6	0
Mood Problems	2	8	0
Difficulty with Memory NOS	4	2	14
Cognitive Problems NOS	1	6	0
Psychomotor Slowing	3	3	0
Aggressive Reaction	2	3	7

(cont'd)

Table 2: TOPAMAX *(cont'd)*

Incidence of Treatment-emergent Adverse Events in Monotherapy Trials in Children Ages 6 up to 16 Years[a] Where Rate was ≥2% in Any Topiramate Group

	TOPAMAX Dosage (mg/day)		
Body System/Adverse Event	**50–100 (n=125)**	**200–400 (n=106)**	**500[b] (n=14)**
Depression	0	5	0
Sleep Disorder	2	2	0
Personality Disorder (Behaviour Problems)	2	2	0
Anxiety	2	1	0
Confusion	0	3	0
Emotional Lability	2	1	0
Red Blood Cell Disorders			
Anemia	1	2	0
Reproductive Disorders, Female			
Vaginitis	0	0	13
Dysmenorrhea	2	2	0
Intermenstrual Bleeding	0	2	0
Reproductive Disorders, Male			
Testis Disorder	2	0	0
Resistance Mechanism Disorders			
Infection Viral	4	7	7
Infection	2	6	0
Otitis Media	2	1	7
Respiratory System Disorders			
Upper Respiratory Tract Infection	26	25	21
Pharyngitis	9	5	21
Rhinitis	5	6	21
Sinusitis	3	6	14
Bronchitis	2	4	0
Asthma	2	1	0
Coughing	2	1	0
Skin and Appendages Disorders			
Rash	3	4	21
Dermatitis	1	0	7
Alopecia	1	3	0
Acne	2	0	0
Nail Disorder	2	0	0
Pruritus	0	2	0
Rash Erythematous	2	0	0
Urinary System Disorders			
Urinary Incontinence	2	2	7
Renal Calculus	0	0	7
Micturition Frequency	0	2	0
Urinary Tract Infection	2	0	0
Vascular Disorders			
Flushing	1	4	7
Vision Disorders			
Conjunctivitis	2	2	0

a Values represent the percentage of patients reporting a given adverse event. Patients may have reported more than one adverse event during the study and can be included in more than one adverse event category.

b Due to n=14 in the 500 mg topiramate group, an incidence of 7% represents one patient.

Table 3: TOPAMAX

Incidence of Treatment-emergent Adverse Events in Placebo-controlled, Add-on Epilepsy Trials in Adults[a,b] (Events that occurred in ≥2% of patients treated with TOPAMAX and occurred more frequently in patients treated with TOPAMAX than placebo-treated patients)

		TOPAMAX Dosage (mg/day)	
Body System/Adverse Event	**Placebo (n=216)**	**200–400 (n=113)**	**600–1000 (n=414)**
Body as a Whole			
Asthenia	1.4	8.0	3.1
Back Pain	4.2	6.2	2.9
Chest Pain	2.8	4.4	2.4
Influenza-like Symptoms	3.2	3.5	3.6
Leg Pain	2.3	3.5	3.6
Hot Flushes	1.9	2.7	0.7
Nervous System			
Dizziness	15.3	28.3	32.1
Ataxia	6.9	21.2	14.5
Speech Disorders/Related Speech Problems	2.3	16.8	11.4
Nystagmus	9.3	15.0	11.1
Paresthesia	4.6	15.0	19.1
Tremor	6.0	10.6	8.9
Language Problems	0.5	6.2	10.4
Co-ordination Abnormal	1.9	5.3	3.6
Hypoesthesia	0.9	2.7	1.2
Abnormal Gait	1.4	1.8	2.2
Gastrointestinal System			
Nausea	7.4	11.5	12.1
Dyspepsia	6.5	8.0	6.3
Abdominal Pain	3.7	5.3	7.0
Constipation	2.3	5.3	3.4
Dry Mouth	0.9	2.7	3.9
Metabolic and Nutritional			
Weight Decrease	2.8	7.1	12.8
Neuropsychiatric			
Somnolence	9.7	30.1	27.8
Psychomotor Slowing	2.3	16.8	20.8
Nervousness	7.4	15.9	19.3
Difficulty with Memory	3.2	12.4	14.5
Confusion	4.2	9.7	13.8
Depression	5.6	8.0	13.0
Difficulty with Concentration/Attention	1.4	8.0	14.5
Anorexia	3.7	5.3	12.3
Agitation	1.4	4.4	3.4
Mood Problems	1.9	3.5	9.2
Aggressive Reaction	0.5	2.7	2.9
Apathy	0	1.8	3.1
Depersonalization	0.9	1.8	2.2
Emotional Lability	0.9	1.8	2.7
Reproductive Disorders, Female	(n=59)	(n=24)	(n=128)
Breast Pain, Female	1.7	8.3	0
Dysmenorrhea	6.8	8.3	3.1
Menstrual Disorder	0	4.2	0.8

(cont'd)

Table 3: TOPAMAX *(cont'd)*

Incidence of Treatment-emergent Adverse Events in Placebo-controlled, Add-on Epilepsy Trials in Adults[a,b] (Events that occurred in ≥2% of patients treated with TOPAMAX and occurred more frequently in patients treated with TOPAMAX than placebo-treated patients)

Body System/Adverse Event	Placebo (n=216)	TOPAMAX Dosage (mg/day) 200–400 (n=113)	600–1000 (n=414)
Reproductive Disorders, Male	(n=157)	(n=89)	(n=286)
Prostatic Disorder	0.6	2.2	0
Respiratory System			
Pharyngitis	2.3	7.1	3.1
Rhinitis	6.9	7.1	6.3
Sinusitis	4.2	4.4	5.6
Dyspnea	0.9	1.8	2.4
Skin and Appendages			
Pruritus	1.4	1.8	3.1
Vision			
Diplopia	5.6	14.2	10.4
Vision Abnormal	2.8	14.2	10.1
White Cell and RES			
Leukopenia	0.5	2.7	1.2

a Patients in these add-on trials were receiving 1 to 2 concomitant antiepileptic drugs in addition to TOPAMAX or placebo.
b Values represent the percentage of patients reporting a given adverse event. Patients may have reported more than one adverse event during the study and can be included in more than one adverse event category.

Table 4: TOPAMAX

Incidence (%) of Dose-related Adverse Events From Placebo-controlled, Add-on Epilepsy Trials in Adults

Adverse Event	Placebo (n=216)	TOPAMAX Dosage (mg/day) 200 (n=45)	400 (n=68)	600–1000 (n=414)
Fatigue	13.4	11.1	11.8	29.7
Nervousness	7.4	13.3	17.6	19.3
Difficulty with Concentration/Attention	1.4	6.7	8.8	14.5
Confusion	4.2	8.9	10.3	13.8
Depression	5.6	8.9	7.4	13.0
Anorexia	3.7	4.4	5.9	12.3
Language Problems	0.5	2.2	8.8	10.1
Anxiety	6.0	2.2	2.9	10.4
Mood Problems	1.9	0	5.9	9.2

In six double-blind clinical trials, 10.6% of subjects (n=113) assigned to a TOPAMAX dosage of 200 to 400 mg/day in addition to their standard AED therapy discontinued due to adverse events, compared to 5.8% of subjects (n=69) receiving placebo. The percentage of subjects discontinuing due to adverse events appeared to increase at dosages above 400 mg/day. Overall, approximately 17% of all subjects (n=527) who received TOPAMAX in the double-blind trials discontinued due to adverse events, compared to 4% of the subjects (n=216) receiving placebo.

Table 5 lists treatment-emergent adverse events that occurred in at least 2% of children treated with 5 to 9 mg/kg/day TOPAMAX in controlled trials that were numerically more common than in patients treated with placebo.

Table 5: TOPAMAX

Incidence (%) of Treatment-emergent Adverse Events in Worldwide Pediatric Add-on Epilepsy Clinical Trials Experience (2-16 Years of Age)[a,b] (Events that occurred in ≥2% of patients treated with TOPAMAX and occurred more frequently in patients treated with TOPAMAX than placebo-treated patients)

Body System/Adverse Event	Placebo (n=101)	Topiramate (n=98)
Body as a Whole—General Disorders		
Fatigue	5	16.3
Injury	12.9	14.3
Allergic Reaction	1	2
Central and Peripheral Nervous Systems Disorders		
Gait Abnormal	5	8.2
Ataxia	2	6.1
Hyperkinesia	4	5.1
Dizziness	2	4.1
Speech Disorders/Related Speech Problems	2	4.1
Convulsions Aggravated	3	3.1
Hyporeflexia	0	2
Gastrointestinal System Disorders		
Nausea	5	6.1
Saliva Increased	4	6.1
Constipation	4	5.1
Gastroenteritis	2	3.1
Metabolic and Nutritional Disorders		
Weight Decrease	1	9.2
Thirst	1	2
Platelet, Bleeding and Clotting Disorders		
Purpura	4	8.2
Epistaxis	1	4.1
Nervous Disorders		
Somnolence	15.8	25.5
Anorexia	14.9	24.5
Nervousness	6.9	14.3
Personality Disorder (Behaviour Problems)	8.9	11.2
Difficulty with Concentration/Attention	2	10.2
Aggressive Reaction	4	9.2
Insomnia	6.9	8.2
Mood Problems	6.9	7.1
Difficulty with Memory NOS[c]	0	5.1
Emotional Lability	5	5.1
Confusion	3	4.1
Psychomotor Slowing	2	3.1
Reproductive Disorders, Female		
Leukorrhea	0	2.3
Resistance Mechanism Disorders		
Infection Viral	3	7.1
Infection	3	3.1
Respiratory System Disorders		
Upper Respiratory Tract Infection	36.6	36.7
Pneumonia	1	5.1
Skin and Appendages Disorders		
Skin Disorder	2	3.1
Alopecia	1	2
Dermatitis	0	2
Hypertrichosis	1	2
Rash Erythematous	0	2
Urinary System Disorders		
Urinary Incontinence	2	4.1
Vision Disorders		
Eye Abnormality	1	2

(cont'd)

Table 5: TOPAMAX *(cont'd)*

Incidence (%) of Treatment-emergent Adverse Events in Worldwide Pediatric Add-on Epilepsy Clinical Trials Experience (2-16 Years of Age)[a,b] (Events that occurred in ≥2% of patients treated with TOPAMAX and occurred more frequently in patients treated with TOPAMAX than placebo-treated patients)

Body System/Adverse Event	Placebo (n=101)	Topiramate (n=98)
Vision Abnormal	1	2
White Cell and RES Disorders		
Leukopenia	0	2

[a] Patients in these add-on trials were receiving 1 to 2 concomitant antiepileptic drugs in addition to TOPAMAX or placebo.
[b] Values represent the percentage of patients reporting a given adverse event. Patients may have reported more than one adverse event during the study and can be included in more than one adverse event category.
[c] Not otherwise specified.

None of the pediatric patients who received TOPAMAX adjunctive therapy at 5 to 9 mg/kg/day in controlled clinical trials discontinued due to adverse events. In open extensions of the controlled clinical trials, approximately 9% of the 303 pediatric patients who received TOPAMAX at dosages up to 30 mg/kg/day discontinued due to adverse events. Adverse events associated with discontinuing therapy included aggravated convulsions (2.3%), language problems (1.3%), and difficulty with concentration/attention (1.3%).

When the safety experience of patients receiving TOPAMAX as adjunctive therapy in both double-blind and open-label trials (1446 adults and 303 children) was analyzed, a similar pattern of adverse events emerged.

Less Common Clinical Trial Adverse Drug Reactions (<2%): Adverse events that occurred less frequently but were considered potentially medically relevant included: taste perversion, cognitive problems (not otherwise specified) and psychosis/psychotic symptoms.

In adult and pediatric patients, nephrolithiasis was reported rarely. Isolated cases of thromboembolic events have also been reported; a causal association with the drug has not been established.

In clinical trials with topiramate, the occurrence rate for all potential cases of oligohidrosis (decreased sweating) was 0.25%.

In clinical trials for topiramate in epilepsy, migraine prophylaxis and other investigational indications (obesity, bipolar disorder and diabetic peripheral neuropathy), suicide-related adverse events* occurred at a rate of 0.8% (84 reports/10 846 patients) in topiramate versus 0.2% (5 reports/3150 patients) in placebo groups. Although the average exposure time for patients on topiramate (approximately 10 months) was longer than for those on placebo (approximately 5 months), these adverse events were reported randomly over the exposure period. Suicide attempts occurred in 0.3% (33 reports/10 846 patients) of the topiramate-treated patients compared to 0% in placebo groups. Of these 33 attempts, one completed suicide was reported in a double-blind bipolar disorder trial and 3 in the open-label phase of the bipolar disorder trials (see Warnings and Precautions, Neurologic, Central Nervous System Effects).

Migraine: Adverse Drug Reaction Overview: Table 6 includes those adverse events reported for patients in four multicentre, randomized, double-blind, placebo-controlled, parallel-group migraine prophylaxis clinical trials where the incidence rate in any topiramate treatment group was at least 2% and was greater than that for placebo patients. Most of the adverse events were mild or moderate in severity and most occurred more frequently during the titration period than during the maintenance period.

Clinical Trial Adverse Drug Reactions: Because clinical trials are conducted under very specific conditions the adverse reaction rates observed in the clinical trials may not reflect the rates observed in practice and should not be compared to the rates in the clinical trials of another drug. Adverse drug reaction information from clinical trials is useful for identifying drug-related adverse events and for approximating rates.

Of the 1135 patients exposed to topiramate in the placebo-controlled studies, 25% discontinued due to adverse events, compared to 10% of the 445 placebo patients. The most common adverse events associated with discontinuing therapy in the topiramate-treated patients included paresthesia (6.7%), fatigue (4.3%), nausea (4.0%), difficulty with concentration/attention (2.9%), insomnia (2.7%), anorexia (2.1%), and dizziness (2.0%).

In the 6-month migraine prophylaxis controlled trials, the proportion of patients who experienced one or more cognitive-related events was 19% for TOPAMAX 50 mg/day, 22% for 100 mg/day, 28% for 200 mg/day and 10% for placebo. These dose-related adverse reactions typically began in the titration phase and often persisted into the maintenance phase, but infrequently began in the maintenance phase.

Table 7 shows adverse events that were dose-dependent.

Other Adverse Events Observed During Migraine Clinical Trials: For the prophylactic treatment of migraine headache, topiramate has been administered to 1367 patients in all clinical studies (includes double-blind and open-label extension). During these studies, all adverse events were recorded by the clinical investigators using terminology of their own choosing. To provide a meaningful estimate of the proportion of individuals having adverse events, similar types of events were grouped into a smaller number of standardized categories using modified WHOART dictionary terminology.

The following additional adverse events that were not described earlier were reported by greater than 1% of the 1367 topiramate-treated patients in the controlled clinical trials:

Body as a Whole: pain, chest pain, allergic reaction.
Central and Peripheral Nervous Systems Disorders: headache, vertigo, tremor, sensory disturbance, migraine aggravated.
Gastrointestinal System Disorders: constipation, gastroesophageal reflux, tooth disorder.
Musculoskeletal System Disorders: myalgia.
Platelet, Bleeding and Clotting Disorders: epistaxis.
Reproductive Disorders, Female: intermenstrual bleeding.
Resistance Mechanism Disorders: infection, genital moniliasis.
Respiratory System Disorders: pneumonia, asthma.
Skin and Appendages Disorders: rash, alopecia.
Vision Disorders: abnormal accommodation, eye pain.

Post-Market Adverse Drug Reactions: In addition to the adverse events reported during clinical trial testing of TOPAMAX, the following adverse drug reactions have been reported in patients receiving marketed TOPAMAX from worldwide use since approval. Adverse drug reactions from spontaneous reports during the worldwide post-marketing experience with TOPAMAX are included in Table 8. The adverse drug reactions are ranked by frequency, using the following convention (all calculated per patient-years of estimated exposure): very common ≥1/10; common ≥1/100 and <1/10; uncommon ≥1/1000 and <1/100; rare ≥1/10 000 and <1/1000; very rare <1/10 000.

The frequencies provided below reflect reporting rates for adverse drug reactions from spontaneous reports, and do not represent more precise estimates that might be obtained in clinical or experimental studies.

Oligohidrosis (decreased sweating) has been rarely reported with the use of TOPAMAX. The majority of spontaneous post-marketing reports have been in children. Adverse events that may be related to potential cases of oligohidrosis include dehydration, hyperthermia, and heat intolerance. Adequate hydration prior to activities such as exercise or exposure to warm temperatures is recommended (see Warnings and Precautions, Endocrine and Metabolism).

To date, there have been rare spontaneous, post-marketing reports of metabolic acidosis. In some cases, acidosis resolved after dosage reduction or upon discontinuation of topiramate (see Warnings and Precautions, Endocrine and Metabolism).

Rare reports of encephalopathy with or without hyperammonemia have been received for patients treated with TOPAMAX while also taking valproate or other antiepileptic medications (see Warnings and Precautions, General and Drug Interactions, Drug-Drug Interactions).

There have been rare spontaneous post-marketing reports of suicide attempts and suicide-related adverse events, including fatalities, in patients treated with topiramate alone or in combination with other medications (see Warnings and Precautions, Neurologic, Central Nervous System Effects).

The following adverse experiences have not been listed above and data are insufficient to support an estimate of their incidence or to establish causation.

Reports of increases in liver function tests in patients taking TOPAMAX with and without other medications have been received. Isolated reports have been received of hepatitis and hepatic failure occurring in patients taking multiple medications while being treated with TOPAMAX.

* Suicide-related adverse events include suicidal ideation, suicide attempt, suicide and any evidence of self-harm.

Isolated reports have also been received for bullous skin and mucosal reactions (including Stevens-Johnson syndrome, toxic epidermal necrolysis, erythema multiforme and pemphigus). The majority of these reports have occurred in patients taking other medications that can be associated with bullous skin and mucosal reactions.

Pregnancy Registries to Date (August 2009): Post-marketing data from two prospective pregnancy registries have documented outcomes in approximately 648 women (445 from NA pregnancy registry and 203 from UK pregnancy registry) exposed to topiramate during the first trimester of pregnancy. Both registries reported an increase in the risk of malformations (see examples below) with exposure to topiramate monotherapy or in combination with other anti-epileptic drugs (AED's) over and above the reference population and background rates from the literature. Further information will be added as it becomes available (see Warnings and Precautions, Special Populations, Pregnant Women).

North American Registry: Of the 265 women exposed to topiramate monotherapy, 12 pregnancies resulted in major malformations (e.g., craniofacial defects, such as cleft lip/palate, hypospadias, and anomalies involving various body systems). The rate of all malformations for topiramate was 4.5% (45.3/1000, n=265) vs 2.2% (21.6/1000, n=3427) for the reference population and 1.8% (17.6/1000, n=340) for the background rates.

UK Registry: Of the 203 pregnancies that involved topiramate use (mono- and polytherapy), 16 pregnancies resulted in major malformations (e.g., cleft lip and palate, pyloric stenosis, anal atresia, hypospadias). The overall rate of major malformations among topiramate monotherapy exposures was 4.3% (43/1000; n=70).

When used for the treatment of epilepsy, TOPAMAX should be used during pregnancy only if potential benefit justifies the potential risk to the fetus.

When used for the prophylactic treatment of migraines, TOPAMAX is not to be used in pregnancy and in women of child bearing potential who are not using an effective method of contraception (see Contraindications, Warnings and Precautions, Special Populations, Pregnant Women, Migraine and Dosage and Administration, Dosing Considerations).

Table 6: TOPAMAX

Incidence % of Treatment-emergent Adverse Events in Placebo-controlled Migraine Trials Where Rate Was at Least 2% in Any Topiramate Group and Greater Than the Rate in Placebo-treated Patients[a]

Body System/Adverse Event	Placebo (n=445)	TOPAMAX Dosage (mg/day) 50 (n=235)	100 (n=386)	200 (n=514)
Body as a Whole—General Disorders				
Fatigue	11	14	15	19
Injury	7	9	6	6
Asthenia	1	<1	2	2
Fever	1	1	1	2
Influenza-like Symptoms	<1	<1	<1	2
Allergy	<1	2	<1	<1
Central and Peripheral Nervous Systems Disorders				
Paresthesia	6	35	51	49
Dizziness	10	8	9	12
Hypoesthesia	2	6	7	8
Language Problems	2	7	6	7
Involuntary Muscle Contractions	1	2	2	4
Ataxia	<1	1	2	1
Speech Disorders/Related Speech Problems	<1	1	<1	2
Gastrointestinal System Disorders				
Nausea	8	9	13	14
Diarrhea	4	9	11	11
Abdominal Pain	5	6	6	7
Dyspepsia	3	4	5	3
Dry Mouth	2	2	3	5
Vomiting	2	1	2	3
Gastroenteritis	1	3	3	2
Hearing and Vestibular Disorders				
Tinnitus	1	<1	1	2
Metabolic and Nutritional Disorders				
Weight Decrease	1	6	9	11
Thirst	<1	2	2	1
Musculoskeletal System Disorders				
Arthralgia	2	7	3	1
Neoplasms				
Neoplasm NOS	<1	2	<1	<1
Psychiatric Disorders				

(cont'd)

Table 6: TOPAMAX (cont'd)

Incidence % of Treatment-emergent Adverse Events in Placebo-controlled Migraine Trials Where Rate Was at Least 2% in Any Topiramate Group and Greater Than the Rate in Placebo-treated Patients[a]

Body System/Adverse Event	Placebo (n=445)	TOPAMAX Dosage (mg/day) 50 (n=235)	100 (n=386)	200 (n=514)
Anorexia	6	9	15	14
Somnolence	5	8	7	10
Difficulty with Memory NOS	2	7	7	11
Difficulty with Concentration/Attention	2	3	6	10
Insomnia	5	6	7	6
Anxiety	3	4	5	6
Mood Problems	2	3	6	5
Depression	4	3	4	6
Nervousness	2	4	4	4
Confusion	2	2	3	4
Psychomotor Slowing	1	3	2	4
Libido Decreased	1	1	1	2
Aggravated Depression	1	1	2	2
Agitation	1	2	2	1
Cognitive Problems NOS	1	<1	2	2
Reproductive Disorders, Female				
Menstrual Disorder	2	3	2	2
Reproductive Disorders, Male				
Ejaculation Premature	0	3	0	0
Resistance Mechanism Disorders				
Viral Infection	3	4	4	3
Otitis Media	<1	2	1	1
Respiratory System Disorders				
Upper Respiratory Tract Infection	12	13	14	12
Sinusitis	6	10	6	8
Pharyngitis	4	5	6	2
Coughing	2	2	4	3
Bronchitis	2	3	3	3
Dyspnea	2	1	3	2
Rhinitis	1	1	2	2
Skin and Appendages Disorders				
Pruritus	2	4	2	2
Special Sense Other, Disorders				
Taste Perversion	1	15	8	12
Taste Loss	<1	1	1	2
Urinary System Disorders				
Urinary Tract Infection	2	4	2	4
Renal Calculus	0	0	1	2
Vision Disorders				
Vision Abnormal	<1	1	2	3
Blurred Vision[b]	2	4	2	4
Conjunctivitis	1	1	2	1

[a] Values represent the percentage of patients reporting a given adverse event. Patients may have reported more than one adverse event during the study and can be included in more than one adverse event category.
[b] Blurred vision was the most common term considered as vision abnormal. Blurred vision was an included term that accounted for >50% of events coded as vision abnormal, a preferred term.

Table 7: TOPAMAX

Incidence (%) of Dose-related Adverse Events From Placebo-controlled Migraine Trials[a]

Adverse Event	Placebo (n=445)	TOPAMAX Dosage (mg/day) 50 (n=235)	100 (n=386)	200 (n=514)
Paresthesia	6	35	51	49
Fatigue	11	14	15	19
Nausea	8	9	13	14
Anorexia	6	9	15	14
Dizziness	10	8	9	12
Weight Decrease	1	6	9	11
Difficulty with Memory NOS	2	7	7	11
Diarrhea	4	9	11	11
Difficulty with Concentration/Attention	2	3	6	10
Somnolence	5	8	7	10
Hypoesthesia	2	6	7	8
Anxiety	3	4	5	6
Depression	4	3	4	6
Mood Problems	2	3	6	5
Dry Mouth	2	2	3	5
Confusion	2	2	3	4
Involuntary Muscle Contractions	1	2	2	4
Abnormal Vision	<1	1	2	3
Renal Calculus	0	0	1	2

[a] The incidence rate of the adverse event in the 200 mg/day group was ≥2% than the rate in both the placebo group and the 50 mg/day group.

Table 8: TOPAMAX

Post-marketing Reports of Adverse Drug Reactions

Adverse Event	Reporting Rate: Common	Uncommon	Rare	Very Rare
Blood and Lymphatic System Disorders				
Leucopenia and Neutropenia				X
Thrombocytopenia				X
Metabolism and Nutrition Disorders				
Anorexia			X	
Metabolic Acidosis[a]				X
Hyperammonemia[b]				X
Hypokalemia				X
Musculoskeletal and Connective Tissue Disorders				
Musculoskeletal Pain				X
Myalgia				X
Arthralgia				X
Psychiatric Disorders				
Depression[c]			X	
Agitation[c]			X	
Somnolence[c]			X	
Insomnia[c]				X
Mood Altered[c]				X
Confusional State[c]				X
Psychotic Disorder[c]				X

(cont'd)

Table 8: TOPAMAX *(cont'd)*

Post-marketing Reports of Adverse Drug Reactions

	Reporting Rate			
Adverse Event	**Common**	**Uncommon**	**Rare**	**Very Rare**
Aggression[c]				X
Hallucination[c]				X
Suicidal Ideation[c]				X
Suicidal Attempts[c]				X
Suicide[c]				X
Expressive Language Disorder				X
Delusion				X
Concentration Impaired				X
Nervous System Disorders				
Paresthesia[c]			X	
Convulsion			X	
Headache			X	
Dizziness			X	
Speech Disorder				X
Dysgeusia				X
Amnesia				X
Memory Impairment				X
Drug Withdrawal Convulsion				X
Ataxia				X
Hyperkinesia				X
Eye Disorders				
Visual Disturbance			X	
Vision Blurred			X	
Myopia[d]				X
Angle Closure Glaucoma[d]				X
Eye Pain				X
Maculopathy (including field vision defect)				X
Gastrointestinal Disorders				
Nausea			X	
Diarrhea				X
Abdominal Pain				X
Vomiting				X
Skin and Subcutaneous Tissue Disorders				
Alopecia			X	
Rash				X
Renal and Urinary Disorders				
Nephrolithiasis[e]			X	
General Disorders and Administration Site Conditions				
Fatigue[a]			X	
Oligohidrosis[a,f]			X	
Pyrexia				X
Feeling Abnormal				X
Asthenia				X
Dehydration				X

(cont'd)

Table 8: TOPAMAX *(cont'd)*

Post-marketing Reports of Adverse Drug Reactions

	Reporting Rate			
Adverse Event	**Common**	**Uncommon**	**Rare**	**Very Rare**
Flushing				X
Hot Flushes				X
Investigations				
Weight Decreased			X	
Hepatic Enzymes Increased				X

[a] See Warnings and Precautions, Endocrine and Metabolism.
[b] See Warnings and Precautions, Hyperammonemia and Encephalopathy and Drug Interactions, Drug-Drug Interactions.
[c] See Warnings and Precautions, Neurologic.
[d] See Warnings and Precautions, Ophthalmologic.
[e] See Warnings and Precautions, Renal and Drug Interactions, Drug-Drug Interactions.
[f] The majority of these reports have been in children.

DRUG INTERACTIONS: Drug-Drug Interactions: In all of the studies below, except where noted, the maximum TOPAMAX dose administered was 200 mg/day.

Antiepileptic Drugs: Potential interactions between TOPAMAX and standard AEDs were measured in controlled clinical pharmacokinetic studies in patients with epilepsy. The effects of these interactions on plasma concentrations are summarized in Table 9.

Table 9: TOPAMAX

Drug Interactions with TOPAMAX Therapy

AED Co-administered	AED Concentration	Topiramate Concentration
Phenytoin	↔[b]	↓59%
Carbamazepine (CBZ)	↔	↓40%
CBZ Epoxide[a]	↔	NS
Valproic Acid	↓11%	↓14%
Phenobarbital	↔	NS
Primidone	↔	NS
Lamotrigine	↔ at TOPAMAX doses up to 400 mg/day	13% decrease

[a] Is not administered but is an active metabolite of carbamazepine.
[b] Plasma concentrations increased 25% in some patients, generally those on a b.i.d. dosing regimen of phenytoin.
Legend: ↔=no effect on plasma concentration (≤15% change); ↓=plasma concentrations decrease in individual patients; NS=not studied; AED=antiepileptic drug.

Effects of TOPAMAX on Other Antiepileptic Drugs: The addition of TOPAMAX to other antiepileptic drugs (phenytoin, carbamazepine, valproic acid, phenobarbital, primidone) has no effect on their steady-state plasma concentrations, except in the occasional patient, where the addition of TOPAMAX to phenytoin may result in an increase of plasma concentrations of phenytoin.

The effect of TOPAMAX on the steady-state pharmacokinetics of phenytoin may be related to the frequency of phenytoin dosing. A slight increase in steady-state phenytoin plasma concentrations was observed, primarily in patients receiving phenytoin in two divided doses. The slight increase may be due to the saturable nature of phenytoin pharmacokinetics and inhibition of phenytoin metabolism CYP2C19.

The addition of TOPAMAX therapy to phenytoin should be guided by clinical outcome. In general, as evidenced in clinical trials, patients do not require dose adjustments. However, any patient on phenytoin showing clinical signs or symptoms of toxicity should have phenytoin levels monitored. The effects of these interactions on plasma concentrations are summarized in Table 9.

Effects of Other Antiepileptic Drugs on TOPAMAX: Phenytoin and Carbamazepine: Phenytoin and carbamazepine decrease the plasma concentration of topiramate. The addition or withdrawal of phenytoin and/or carbamazepine during adjunctive therapy with TOPAMAX may require adjustment of the dose of TOPAMAX. This should be done by titrating to clinical effect.

Valproic Acid: The addition or withdrawal of valproic acid does not produce clinically significant changes in plasma concentrations of topiramate, and therefore, does not warrant dosage adjustment of TOPAMAX. The effects of these interactions on plasma concentrations are summarized in Table 9.

Rare post-marketing reports of encephalopathy with or without hyperammonemia have been received for patients treated with TOPAMAX alone or in combination with valproic acid or other antiepileptic medications. The majority of the cases reported concomitant administration of topiramate and valproic acid. Thus, caution is advised when polytherapy is necessary (see Adverse Reactions, Post-Market Adverse Drug Reactions and Warnings and Precautions, General).

Other Drug Interactions: Digoxin: In a single-dose study, serum digoxin AUC decreased 12% due to concomitant TOPAMAX administration (200 mg/day). Multiple-dose studies have not been performed. When TOPAMAX is added or withdrawn in patients on digoxin therapy, careful attention should be given to the routine monitoring of serum digoxin.

CNS Depressants: Concomitant administration of TOPAMAX and alcohol or other CNS depressant drugs has not been evaluated in clinical studies. It is recommended that TOPAMAX not be used concomitantly with alcohol or other CNS depressant drugs.

Oral Contraceptives: TOPAMAX (50-200 mg/day) in Healthy Volunteers: In a pharmacokinetic interaction study in healthy volunteers, subjects were stratified into obese versus non-obese (n=12 versus n=12) with both groups concomitantly administered a combination oral contraceptive product containing 1 mg norethindrone plus 35 μg ethinyl estradiol and TOPAMAX (50 to 200 mg/day) given in the absence of other medications. For the ethinyl estradiol component, both obese and non-obese volunteers showed a decrease in mean AUC and C_{max} at 200 mg/day (−10.7% and −9.4% versus −15.2% and −11.3%, respectively) that were not statistically significant. Changes in individual subjects ranged from decreases of approximately 35% to 90% in 5 individuals to increases of approximately 35% to 60% in 3 individuals. At the 50 and 100 mg/day TOPAMAX doses, similar changes in mean C_{max} and AUC were observed for non-obese volunteers. The clinical significance of these changes is unknown. For the norethindrone component, only the non-obese group showed a decrease (−11.8%). In view of the dose-dependent decreases seen in the ethinyl estradiol component in epileptic patients receiving TOPAMAX as adjunctive therapy (below), and the fact that the recommended dose is up to 400 mg/day, there may be greater decreases seen at doses above 200 mg/day as monotherapy.

TOPAMAX as Adjunctive Therapy with Valproic Acid in Epileptic Patients: In a pharmacokinetic interaction study, epileptic patients received TOPAMAX as adjunctive therapy with valproic acid and a combination oral contraceptive product containing norethindrone (1 mg) plus ethinyl estradiol (35 μg). In this study, TOPAMAX did not significantly affect the oral clearance of norethindrone. The serum levels of the estrogenic component decreased by 18%, 21% and 30% at daily doses of 200, 400 and 800 mg of topiramate, respectively. There are minimal clinical data regarding interaction of valproic acid and oral contraceptives.

In view of both of the above study findings, the efficacy of low-dose (e.g. 20 μg) oral contraceptives may be reduced in both the monotherapy and adjunctive therapy situation with topiramate. For topiramate doses up to 200 mg/day, which includes the recommended dose for migraine prophylaxis of 100 mg/day, the mean reduction in norethindrone and ethinyl estradiol exposure from topiramate treatment is not significant, although marked changes in individual patients are possible. In the treatment of epilepsy at doses greater than 200 mg/day, significant dose-dependent decreases in ethinyl estradiol exposure are expected. Patients on topiramate doses greater than 200 mg/day who are taking oral contraceptives should receive a preparation containing not less than 30 μg of estrogen. Patients taking oral contraceptives should be asked to report any change in their bleeding patterns. Contraceptive efficacy can be decreased even in the absence of breakthrough bleeding.

Hydrochlorothiazide (HCTZ): A parallel-arm drug-drug interaction study conducted in healthy volunteers (12 males, 11 females) evaluated the steady-state pharmacokinetics of the diuretic HCTZ (25 mg q24h) and topiramate (96 mg q12h) when administered alone and concomitantly. The results of this study indicate that mean topiramate C_{max} increased by 27% and mean AUC increased by 29% when HCTZ was added to topiramate. The clinical significance of this statistically significant change is unknown. Thus, the concomitant use of topiramate and HCTZ may require a downward adjustment of the topiramate dose. The steady-state pharmacokinetics of HCTZ were not significantly influenced by the concomitant administration of topiramate. In addition, greater decreases in serum potassium were seen with concomitant treatment than with either drug alone, both in terms of percentage of patients with a serum potassium measurement of <3.6 mEq/L at the end of each treatment period [61% (14/23) with concomitant treatment versus 27% (3/11) with topiramate alone versus 25% (3/12) with HCTZ alone] and in mean change from baseline (approximately −0.60 mEq/L for concomitant treatment versus −0.25 mEq/L for topiramate alone versus −0.12 mEq/L for HCTZ alone). One of the subjects who had hypokalemia with concomitant treatment also had an abnormal ECG (non-specific ST-T wave changes), which may have been related to the decrease in plasma potassium levels. See also Warnings and Precautions, Endocrine and Metabolism.

Metformin: A drug-drug interaction study conducted in 18 healthy volunteers, ages 18-37, evaluated the steady-state pharmacokinetics of metformin and topiramate in plasma when metformin (500 mg b.i.d.) was given alone and when metformin and topiramate (50, 75 and 100 mg) were given simultaneously for 6 consecutive days. The results of this study indicated that metformin mean C_{max} and mean AUC_{0-12h} increased by 18% and 25%, respectively, while mean CL/F decreased 20% when metformin was co-administered with TOPAMAX (up-titrated to 100 mg b.i.d.). TOPAMAX did not affect metformin t_{max}. The effects of higher doses of topiramate (>100 mg b.i.d.) on metformin are unknown. The clinical significance of the effect of topiramate on metformin pharmacokinetics is unclear. Oral plasma clearance of topiramate appears to be reduced when administered with metformin. The extent of change in the clearance is unknown. The clinical significance of the effect of metformin on topiramate pharmacokinetics is unclear. When TOPAMAX is added or withdrawn in patients on metformin therapy, careful attention should be given to the routine monitoring for adequate control of their diabetic disease state.

Glyburide: A drug-drug interaction study conducted in 28 patients with type 2 diabetes, ages 38-68 years and BMIs 25-40 kg/m², evaluated the steady-state pharmacokinetics of glyburide and topiramate in plasma when glyburide (5 mg/day) was given alone and when glyburide and topiramate (150 mg/day) were given concomitantly for 48 consecutive days. Glyburide systemic exposure was statistically significantly reduced when combined with topiramate such that mean C_{max} and mean AUC_{24} decreased by 22% and 25%, respectively, while mean CL/F increased by 21%. Systemic exposure of the active metabolites, 4-trans-hydroxyglyburide and 3-cis-hydroxyglyburide, was also statistically significantly reduced by 13% and 15%, respectively. The steady-state pharmacokinetics of topiramate were unaffected by concomitant administration of glyburide. The clinical significance of the effect of glyburide on topiramate pharmacokinetics is unclear. Mild to moderate declines in serum bicarbonate without metabolic acidosis were associated with the addition of topiramate (see Warnings and Precautions, Endocrine and Metabolism, Metabolic Acidosis). The effects of higher doses of topiramate (>150 mg/day) on glyburide are unknown. When topiramate is added to glyburide therapy or glyburide is added to topiramate therapy, careful attention should be given to the routine monitoring of patients for adequate control of their diabetic disease state.

Pioglitazone: A drug-drug interaction study conducted in healthy volunteers (26 males, 26 females) evaluated the steady-state pharmacokinetics of topiramate and the antidiabetic agent, pioglitazone, when administered alone and concomitantly. The pharmacokinetic parameters of topiramate were not affected; mean pioglitazone AUC decreased by 15%, and mean C_{max} increased non-significantly by 10%, but with individual subjects showing large increases and 3 of the 4 highest values recorded by males. In addition, each of the active hydroxy-metabolite and the active keto-metabolite showed mean decreases in C_{max} and AUC (approximately 15% for the hydroxy-metabolite and 60% for the keto-metabolite). The clinical significance of these findings is not known. When TOPAMAX is added to pioglitazone therapy or pioglitazone is added to TOPAMAX therapy, careful attention should be given to the routine monitoring of patients for adequate control of their diabetic disease state.

Lithium: Healthy Volunteers: A drug-drug interaction study conducted in twelve healthy volunteers, ages 20-40 years, evaluated the steady-state pharmacokinetics of lithium in plasma when lithium (300 mg q8h) was administered for 14 days and topiramate (up-titrated to 100 mg q12h) was given concomitantly for the last 6 days. Based on the data analysis of twelve subjects, systemic exposure of lithium was statistically significantly reduced in the presence of topiramate such that C_{max} and AUC_{0-8h} decreased by 20% and 18%, respectively, while mean CL/F and CL_R increased by 36% and 12%, respectively. One subject did not have measurable trough lithium concentrations on Day 14, potentially indicating missed dose administration. By excluding this subject from the analyses, systemic exposure of lithium was slightly reduced in the presence of topiramate (12% for C_{max}, 10% for AUC_{0-8}) while mean CL/F and CL_R increased by 11% and 16%, respectively. The clinical significance of the effect of topiramate on lithium pharmacokinetics is unclear. The effects of higher doses of topiramate (>200 mg/day) on the pharmacokinetics of lithium are unknown.

Patients with Bipolar Disorder: A drug-drug interaction study conducted in 31 patients with various types of bipolar disorder, ages 20-60 years, evaluated the steady-state pharmacokinetics of lithium and topiramate when administered concomitantly. Subjects were randomized to receive either low doses of topiramate of up to 200 mg/day or high doses of topiramate of up to 600 mg/day. Pharmacokinetic profiles for lithium were obtained following 1 week and 3 weeks of continuous lithium dosing. The pharmacokinetics of lithium were unaffected during treatment with topiramate at doses of up to 200 mg/day, and were unaffected by short-term treatment with topiramate (1 week) at doses up to 600 mg/day. Following treatment with topiramate at doses of up to 600 mg/day for 3 weeks, there was an observed statistically significant increase in systemic exposure of lithium (about 27% for both C_{max} and AUC). Topiramate exposure for both the low and high dose groups was similar following 1 week and 3 weeks of continuous treatment in the presence of lithium. The effects of higher doses of topiramate (>600 mg/day) on lithium have not been studied and are unknown. Lithium levels should be monitored when co-administered with topiramate and dose adjustments for lithium should be based on both lithium levels and clinical outcome for the patient.

Risperidone: Healthy Volunteers: A drug-drug interaction study was conducted in 12 healthy volunteers (6 males, 6 females), ages 28-40 years, with single-dose administration of risperidone (2 mg) and multiple doses of topiramate (titrated up to 200 mg/day). In the presence of topiramate, systemic exposure of the total active moiety (risperidone + 9-hydroxyrisperidone) was reduced such that mean $AUC_{0-\infty}$ was 11% lower and mean C_{max} was statistically significantly (18%) lower. In the presence of topiramate, systemic exposure of risperidone was statistically significantly reduced such that mean C_{max} and $AUC_{0-\infty}$ were 29% and 23% lower, respectively. The pharmacokinetics of 9-hydroxyrisperidone were unaffected. The effects of a single dose (2 mg/day) of risperidone on the pharmacokinetics of multiple doses of topiramate have not been studied. Therefore, patients receiving risperidone in combination with topiramate should be closely monitored for clinical response to risperidone.

Patients with Bipolar Disorder: A drug-drug interaction study conducted in 52 patients with various types of bipolar disorder (24 males, 28 females), ages 19-56 years, evaluated the steady-state pharmacokinetics of risperidone and topiramate when administered concomitantly. Eligible subjects were stabilized on a risperidone dose of 1-6 mg/day for 2 to 3 weeks. Topiramate was then titrated up to escalating doses of 100, 250 and 400 mg/day along with risperidone for up to 6 weeks. Risperidone was then tapered and discontinued over 4 weeks while maintaining topiramate (up to 400 mg/day). There was a statistically significant reduction in risperidone systemic exposure (16% and 33% for AUC_{12} and 13% and 34% for C_{max} at the 250 and 400 mg/day doses, respectively). Minimal alterations were observed in the pharmacokinetics of the total active moiety (risperidone plus 9-hydroxyrisperidone) and 9-hydroxyrisperidone. Topiramate systemic exposure was slightly reduced (12.5% for mean C_{max} and 11% for mean AUC_{12}) in the presence of risperidone, which achieved statistical significance. There were no clinically significant changes in the systemic exposure of the risperidone total active moiety or of topiramate. The effects of higher doses of topiramate (>400 mg/day) are unknown. Patients with bipolar disorder receiving risperidone in combination with topiramate should be closely monitored for clinical response to risperidone.

Haloperidol: The pharmacokinetics of a single dose of the antipsychotic haloperidol (5 mg) were not affected following multiple dosing of topiramate (200 mg/day) in 13 healthy adults (6 males, 7 females).

Venlafaxine: A drug-drug interaction study was conducted in 26 healthy volunteers (16 males/10 females, ages 18-40 years, BMI ranging from 25 to 30 kg/m²) to evaluate the interaction between venlafaxine and topiramate. Subjects received single 150-mg doses of extended release venlafaxine and multiple doses of topiramate titrated up to 150 mg/day. The single-dose pharmacokinetics of venlafaxine were unaffected by treatment with topiramate. While the C_{max}, AUC_{∞} and CL/F of the active metabolite, O-desmethylvenlafaxine were unaffected, the renal clearance of the active metabolite was increased by 53% during treatment with topiramate. These observed increases in urinary excretion of O-desmethylvenlafaxine during treatment with topiramate did not affect systemic exposure. The steady-state pharmacokinetics of topiramate were unaffected by repeated daily-dose administration of venlafaxine for 5 days. The effects of higher doses of topiramate (>150 mg/day) on the pharmacokinetics of venlafaxine and higher doses of venlafaxine up to the maximum dose of 375 mg/day on the pharmacokinetics of topiramate are unknown.

Amitriptyline: There was a 12% increase in both AUC and C_{max} for the tricyclic antidepressant amitriptyline (25 mg/day) in 18 normal subjects (9 males, 9 females) receiving 200 mg/day of topiramate. Individual subjects experienced large changes in amitriptyline concentration, either up or down, in the presence of topiramate; any adjustments in amitriptyline dose should be made according to patients' clinical response and not on the basis of plasma levels.

Pizotifen: Multiple dosing of topiramate (200 mg/day) in 19 healthy volunteers (12 males, 7 females) had little effect on the pharmacokinetics of the antihistamine pizotifen following daily 1.5 mg doses. There was a mean 12% and 15% decrease respectively in topiramate C_{max} and AUC in the volunteers (12 males and 7 females) receiving 200 mg/day topiramate and 1.5 mg/day pizotifen. This is not considered to be clinically significant.

Dihydroergotamine: Multiple dosing of topiramate (200 mg/day) in 24 healthy volunteers (12 males, 12 females) had little effect on the pharmacokinetics of a 1 mg subcutaneous dose of dihydroergotamine and a 1 mg subcutaneous dose of dihydroergotamine similarly had little effect on the pharmacokinetics of a 200 mg/day dose of topiramate.

Sumatriptan: Multiple dosing of topiramate (200 mg/day) in 24 healthy volunteers (14 males, 10 females) had little effect on the pharmacokinetics of single doses of the anti-migraine medication sumatriptan, either orally (100 mg) or subcutaneously (6 mg).

Propranolol: Multiple dosing of topiramate (100, then 200, mg/day) in 34 healthy volunteers (17 males, 17 females) had little effect on the pharmacokinetics of propranolol following daily 160 mg doses. There was a 17% increase in C_{max} of the metabolite 4-OH propranolol at 100 mg/day topiramate. Propranolol doses of 80, then 160, mg/day in 39 volunteers (27 males, 12 females) had a dose-dependent effect on exposure to topiramate (200 mg/day), reaching approximately a 9% and 16% increase for C_{max} and a 9% and 17% increase for AUC at 80 and 160 mg/day propranolol respectively.

Diltiazem: A drug-drug interaction study was conducted in 28 healthy volunteers (13 males/15 females, ages 18-45 years and BMIs 25-35 kg/m²) to evaluate the interaction between topiramate and diltiazem. Eligible subjects received single 240-mg doses of extended-release diltiazem and multiple doses of topiramate titrated to 150 mg/day. Systemic exposure of diltiazem was statistically significantly reduced during topiramate treatment, where C_{max} and AUC_{∞} were 10% and 25% lower, respectively, following single-dose administration. There was an increase in diltiazem CL/F by approximately 30%. Systemic exposure of the active metabolite, desacetyl diltiazem, was statistically significantly reduced during treatment with topiramate where C_{max} and AUC_{36} were 27% and 18% lower, respectively. The single-dose pharmacokinetics of the active metabolite, N-demethyl-diltiazem, were unaffected by topiramate. Following repeated daily-dose administration of diltiazem for 5 days, steady-state systemic exposure of topiramate was greater during treatment with diltiazem, where C_{max} and AUC_{12} were approximately 17% and 20% higher, respectively, and CL/F was 16% lower. The effects of higher doses of topiramate (>150 mg/day) on the pharmacokinetics of diltiazem or its metabolites have not been studied. Overall, the clinical significance of these observations is unclear.

Flunarizine: Patients with Migraine: Effects of topiramate on the pharmacokinetics of flunarizine: The dose of flunarizine used in this study is one-half of the recommended daily dose. A drug-drug interaction study was conducted in forty seven patients with a history migraine (13 males, 34 females), ages 20-53 years, evaluated the steady-state pharmacokinetics of flunarizine when topiramate was administered concomitantly. Subjects were taking flunarizine for at least 4 weeks before study start. One subgroup was administered only flunarizine (5 mg q24h) for 81 days, and, a second subgroup received flunarizine (5 mg q24h) for 81 days and topiramate (up-titrated to 50 mg/day and then to 100 mg/day) from Day 4 to a.m. dose on Day 82 concomitantly.

Mean C_{max} of flunarizine decreased by 22% with concomitant administration of topiramate at 50 mg/day. During concomitant treatment with topiramate at 100 mg/day, C_{max} estimates returned to those observed during treatment with flunarizine alone. Mean AUC_{0-24} for flunarizine was similar with concomitant administration of topiramate at 50 mg/day and 16% higher with topiramate at 100 mg/day compared to treatment with flunarizine alone. Mean CL/F of flunarizine was unaffected by treatment with topiramate. Systemic exposure of topiramate (C_{max} and AUC_{0-12}) doubled with increasing topiramate dose from 50 mg/day to 100 mg/day. Mean CL/F was similar during both dose periods and was consistent with previously observed estimates in healthy volunteers. These alterations are unlikely to be of clinical significance. However, there are no data on the effects of higher doses of topiramate on flunarizine levels. There is also no information on the interaction of topiramate and flunarizine in patients with history of seizure or epilepsy.

Agents Predisposing to Nephrolithiasis: TOPAMAX, when used concomitantly with other agents predisposing to nephrolithiasis, such as carbonic anhydrase inhibitors, e.g. acetazolamide, may increase the risk of nephrolithiasis. While using TOPAMAX, agents like these should be avoided since they may create a physiological environment that increases the risk of renal stone formation (see Warnings and Precautions, Renal).

Drug-Food Interactions: There was no clinically significant effect of food on the bioavailability of topiramate.

Drug-Herb Interactions: Interactions with herbal products have not been established.

Drug-Laboratory Test Interactions: There are no known interactions of TOPAMAX with commonly used laboratory tests.

DOSAGE AND ADMINISTRATION:

General: In patients with or without a history of seizures or epilepsy, TOPAMAX (topiramate) should be gradually withdrawn to minimize the potential for seizures or increased seizure frequency (see Warnings and Precautions, General).

In clinical trials in adult patients with epilepsy, dosages were decreased by 50-100 mg/day at weekly intervals. In clinical trials of children, TOPAMAX was gradually withdrawn over a 2-8 week period.

In clinical trials in adult patients receiving TOPAMAX for migraine prophylaxis dosages were decreased by 25-50 mg/day at weekly intervals (see Warnings and Precautions, General).

In situations where rapid withdrawal of TOPAMAX is medically required, appropriate monitoring is recommended (see Warnings and Precautions, General).

Dosing Considerations:

- Patients with renal impairment
- Patients undergoing hemodialysis
- Patients with hepatic disease
- Prophylactic treatment of migraine: In pregnancy, the occurrence of seizures presents a significant risk for the mother and child. Prescribing TOPAMAX to prevent seizures therefore outweighs the risk of malformations to the fetus. However, taking TOPAMAX to prevent migraine attacks does not outweigh this risk. Consequently, TOPAMAX is contraindicated in pregnancy and in women of child bearing potential who are not using an effective method of contraception (see Contraindications).

Recommended Dose and Dosage Adjustment: TOPAMAX (topiramate) Tablets or Sprinkle Capsules can be taken without regard to meals.

Epilepsy: Monotherapy: Adults and Children (Age 6 years and older): The recommended initial target dose for topiramate monotherapy in adults and children 6 years of age and older is 100 mg/day and the maximum recommended dose is 400 mg/day, administered in two divided doses, as needed and tolerated.

The recommended titration rate for topiramate monotherapy to 100 mg/day is:

	Week 1	Weeks 2–3	Weeks 3–4
Morning Dose	None	25 mg	50 mg
Evening Dose	25 mg	25 mg	50 mg

If doses above 100 mg/day are required, the dose may be increased at weekly intervals in increments of 50 mg/day to a maximum of 400 mg/day. Dose and titration rate should be guided by clinical outcome. Some patients may benefit from a slower titration schedule. Daily doses above 400 mg have not been adequately studied. Only 14 pediatric patients have received 500 mg/day topiramate in controlled clinical trials (see Adverse Reactions, Epilepsy, Clinical Trial Adverse Drug Reactions, Table 2).

Adjunctive Therapy: Adults (Age 17 years and older): It is recommended that TOPAMAX as adjunctive therapy be initiated at 50 mg/day, followed by titration as needed and tolerated to an effective dose. At weekly intervals, the dose may be increased by 50 mg/day and taken in two divided doses. Some patients may benefit from lower initial doses, e.g. 25 mg and/or a slower titration schedule. Some patients may achieve efficacy with once-a-day dosing.

The recommended total daily maintenance dose is 200-400 mg/day in two divided doses. Doses above 400 mg/day have not been shown to improve responses and have been associated with a greater incidence of adverse events. The maximum recommended dose is 800 mg/day. Daily doses above 1600 mg have not been studied.

Children (Ages 2-16 years): It is recommended that TOPAMAX as adjunctive therapy be initiated at 25 mg (or less, based on a range of 1 to 3 mg/kg/day) nightly for the first week followed by titration as needed and tolerated to an effective dose. The dosage should then be increased at 1- or 2-week intervals by increments of 1 to 3 mg/kg/day (administered in two divided doses). Some patients may benefit from lower initial doses and/or a slower titration schedule.

The recommended total daily maintenance dose is approximately 5 to 9 mg/kg/day in two divided doses.

Drug Discontinuation: In patients with a history of seizures or epilepsy, TOPAMAX should be gradually withdrawn to minimize the potential for seizures or increased seizure frequency. In clinical trials, daily dosages were decreased in weekly intervals by 50-100 mg in adults with epilepsy.

In clinical trials of children, TOPAMAX was gradually withdrawn over a 2-8 week period.

In situations where rapid withdrawal of TOPAMAX is medically required, appropriate monitoring is recommended.

Migraine: Adults: The usual total daily dose of TOPAMAX as treatment for prophylaxis of migraine headache is 100 mg/day administered in two divided doses. Dose and titration rate should be guided by clinical outcome. If required, longer intervals between dose adjustments can be used. No extra benefit has been demonstrated from the administration of doses higher than 100 mg/day and the incidence of some adverse events increases with increasing dose (see Adverse Reactions, Migraine, Table 7).

The recommended titration rate for topiramate for migraine prophylaxis to 100 mg/day is:

	Morning Dose	Evening Dose
Week 1	None	25 mg
Week 2	25 mg	25 mg
Week 3	25 mg	50 mg
Week 4	50 mg	50 mg

Drug Discontinuation: In patients without a history of seizures or epilepsy, TOPAMAX should be gradually withdrawn to minimize the potential for seizures or increased seizure frequency. In clinical trials, daily dosages were decreased in weekly intervals by 25-50 mg in adults receiving TOPAMAX at doses up to 100 mg/day for migraine prophylaxis.

In situations where rapid withdrawal of TOPAMAX is medically required, appropriate monitoring is recommended.

Pediatrics: The safety and efficacy of topiramate in the management or prevention of migraine in pediatrics have not been established.

Patients with Renal Impairment: In renally impaired subjects (creatinine clearance less than 70 mL/min/1.73 m^2), one-half of the usual adult dose is recommended. Such patients will require a longer time to reach steady-state at each dose.

Patients Undergoing Hemodialysis: Topiramate is cleared by hemodialysis at a rate that is 4 to 6 times greater than a normal individual. Accordingly, a prolonged period of dialysis may cause topiramate concentration to fall below that required to maintain an antiseizure effect. To avoid rapid drops in topiramate plasma concentration during hemodialysis, a supplemental dose of TOPAMAX may be required. The actual adjustment should take into account 1) the duration of dialysis, 2) the clearance rate of the dialysis system being used, and 3) the effective renal clearance of topiramate in the patient being dialyzed.

Patients with Hepatic Disease: In hepatically impaired patients, topiramate plasma concentrations are increased approximately 30%. This moderate increase is not considered to warrant adjustment of the TOPAMAX dosing regimen. Initiate topiramate therapy with the same dose and regimen as for patients with normal hepatic function. The dose titration in these patients should be guided by clinical outcome, i.e. seizure control, and avoidance of adverse effects. Such patients will require a longer time to reach steady-state at each dose.

Geriatrics: See Warnings and Precautions.

Missed Dose: The missed dose should be taken as soon as possible. If it is almost time for the next dose, the missed dose should not be taken. Instead, the next scheduled dose should be taken. Doses should not be doubled.

Administration: Tablets should not be broken. TOPAMAX Sprinkle Capsules may be swallowed whole or may be administered by carefully opening the capsule and sprinkling the entire contents on a small amount (teaspoon) of soft food. This drug/food mixture should be swallowed immediately and not chewed. It should not be stored for future use. The sprinkle formulation is provided for those patients who cannot swallow tablets, e.g. pediatric and the elderly.

OVERDOSAGE:

Overdoses of topiramate have been reported. Signs and symptoms included convulsions, drowsiness, speech disturbances, blurred vision, diplopia, mentation impaired, lethargy, abnormal co-ordination, stupor, hypotension, abdominal pain, agitation, dizziness and depression. The clinical consequences were not severe in most cases but deaths have been reported after polydrug overdoses involving topiramate.

Topiramate overdose can result in severe metabolic acidosis (see Warnings and Precautions, Endocrine and Metabolism, Metabolic Acidosis).

The highest topiramate overdose reported was calculated to be between 96 and 110 g and resulted in coma lasting 20 to 24 hours followed by full recovery after 3 to 4 days.

In acute topiramate overdose, if the ingestion is recent, the stomach should be emptied immediately by lavage or by induction of emesis. Activated charcoal has been shown to adsorb topiramate in vitro. Treatment should be appropriately supportive. Hemodialysis has been shown to be an effective means of removing topiramate from the body. The patient should be well hydrated.

> For management of a suspected drug overdose, contact your regional Poison Control Centre. See the *CPS* Directory section for a list of Poison Control Centres.

ACTION AND CLINICAL PHARMACOLOGY: Pharmacodynamics: TOPAMAX (topiramate) is a novel agent classified as a sulfamate substituted monosaccharide. Three pharmacological properties of topiramate are believed to contribute to its anticonvulsant activity. First, topiramate reduces the frequency at which action potentials are generated when neurons are subjected to a sustained depolarization indicative of a state-dependent blockade of voltage-sensitive sodium channels. Second, topiramate markedly enhances the activity of GABA at some types of GABA receptors. Because the antiepileptic profile of topiramate differs markedly from that of the benzodiazepines, it may modulate a benzodiazepine-insensitive subtype of GABA$_A$ receptor. Third, topiramate antagonizes the ability of kainate to activate the kainate/AMPA subtype of excitatory amino acid (glutamate) receptors but has no apparent effect on the activity of N-methyl-D-aspartate (NMDA) at the NMDA receptor subtype.

In addition, topiramate inhibits some isoenzymes of carbonic anhydrase. This pharmacologic effect is much weaker than that of acetazolamide, a known carbonic anhydrase inhibitor, and is not thought to be a major component of topiramate's antiepileptic activity.

Pharmacokinetics: Topiramate exhibits low intersubject variability in plasma concentrations and therefore has predictable pharmacokinetics. The pharmacokinetics of topiramate are linear with plasma clearance remaining constant and area under the plasma concentration curve increasing in a dose-proportional manner over a 100 to 400 mg single oral dose range in healthy subjects. Patients with normal renal function may take 4 to 8 days to reach steady-state plasma concentrations. The mean C_{max} following multiple twice-a-day oral doses of 100 mg to healthy subjects was 6.76 µg/mL. The mean plasma elimination half-lives from multiple 50 mg and 100 mg q12h doses of topiramate were approximately 21 hours. The elimination half-life did not significantly change when switching from single dose to multiple dose.

In well-controlled add-on trials, no correlation has been demonstrated between trough plasma concentrations and its clinical efficacy. It is not necessary to monitor topiramate plasma concentrations to optimize therapy with TOPAMAX.

No evidence of tolerance requiring increased dosage has been demonstrated in patients during 5 years of use.

Concomitant multiple-dose administration of TOPAMAX, 100 to 400 mg q12h, with phenytoin or carbamazepine shows dose-proportional increases in plasma concentrations of topiramate.

Absorption: Topiramate is rapidly and well absorbed. Following oral administration of 100 mg topiramate to healthy subjects, a mean peak plasma concentration (C_{max}) of 1.5 µg/mL was achieved within 2 to 3 hours (T_{max}). The mean extent of absorption from a 100 mg oral dose of ^{14}C-topiramate was at least 81% based on the recovery of radioactivity from the urine.

There was no clinically significant effect of food on the bioavailability of topiramate.

Distribution: Approximately 13% to 17% of topiramate is bound to plasma proteins. A low capacity binding site for topiramate in/on erythrocytes that is saturable above plasma concentrations of 4 µg/mL has been observed.

The volume of distribution varied inversely with the dose. The mean apparent volume of distribution was 0.80 to 0.55 L/kg for a single-dose range of 100 to 1200 mg.

Metabolism: Topiramate is not extensively metabolized (≈20%) in healthy volunteers. It is metabolized up to 50% in patients receiving concomitant antiepileptic therapy with known inducers of drug-metabolizing enzymes. Six metabolites formed through hydroxylation, hydrolysis and glucuronidation have been isolated, characterized and identified from plasma, urine and feces of humans. Each metabolite represents less than 3% of the total radioactivity excreted following administration of ^{14}C-topiramate.

Two metabolites which retained most of the structure of topiramate were tested and found to have little or no pharmacological activity.

Excretion: In humans, the major route of elimination of unchanged topiramate and its metabolites is via the kidney (at least 81% of the dose). Approximately 66% of a dose of ^{14}C-topiramate was excreted unchanged in the urine within 4 days. The mean renal clearance for 50 mg and 100 mg of topiramate, following q12h dosing, was approximately 18 mL/min and 17 mL/min, respectively. Evidence exists for renal tubular reabsorption of topiramate. This is supported by studies in rats where topiramate was co-administered with probenecid, and a significant increase in renal clearance of topiramate was observed. This interaction has not been evaluated in humans. Overall, plasma clearance (CL/F) is approximately 20 to 30 mL/min in humans following oral administration.

Special Populations and Conditions: Pediatrics: Pharmacokinetics of topiramate were evaluated in patients aged 4 to 17 years receiving one or two other antiepileptic drugs. Pharmacokinetic profiles were obtained after one week at doses of 1, 3, and 9 mg/kg/day. As in adults, topiramate pharmacokinetics were linear with clearance independent of dose and steady-state plasma concentrations increasing in proportion to dose. Compared with adult epileptic patients, mean topiramate clearance is approximately 50% higher in pediatric patients. Steady-state plasma topiramate concentrations for the same mg/kg dose are expected to be approximately 33% lower in children compared to adults. As with adults, hepatic enzyme-inducing antiepileptic drugs (AEDs) decrease the plasma concentration of topiramate.

Geriatrics: Plasma clearance of topiramate is unchanged in elderly subjects in the absence of underlying renal disease.

Race, Gender and Age: Although direct comparison studies of pharmacokinetics have not been conducted, analysis of plasma concentration data from clinical efficacy trials has shown that race, gender and age appear to have no effect on the plasma clearance of topiramate. In addition, based on pooled analyses, race and gender appear to have no effect on the efficacy of TOPAMAX.

Hepatic Insufficiency: The plasma clearance of topiramate is decreased in patients with moderate to severe hepatic impairment.

Renal Insufficiency: The plasma and renal clearance of topiramate are decreased in patients with impaired renal function (CL_{CR} <70 mL/min/1.73 m^2), and the plasma clearance is decreased in patients with end-stage renal disease. As a result, higher steady-state topiramate plasma concentrations are expected for a given dose in renally impaired patients as compared to those with normal renal function.

Hemodialysis: Topiramate is effectively removed from plasma by hemodialysis (see Dosage and Administration).

STORAGE AND STABILITY: TOPAMAX Tablets or Sprinkle Capsules should be stored in tightly closed containers at controlled room temperature (15 to 30°C). Protect from moisture.

INFORMATION FOR THE PATIENT: Published in e-CPS, available by subscription at www.e-cps.ca.

DOSAGE FORMS, COMPOSITION AND PACKAGING: Tablets: 25 mg: Each white, embossed, round, coated tablet, marked "TOP" on one side, "25" on the other, contains: topiramate 25 mg. Nonmedicinal ingredients: carnauba wax, hypromellose, lactose monohydrate, magnesium stearate, pregelatinized starch, microcrystalline cellulose, polyethylene glycol, polysorbate 80, purified water, sodium starch glycolate, titanium dioxide, and may contain synthetic iron oxide. Bottles of 100 with desiccant.

100 mg: Each yellow, embossed, round, coated tablet, marked "TOP" on one side, "100" on the other, contains: topiramate 100 mg. Nonmedicinal ingredients: carnauba wax, hypromellose, lactose monohydrate, magnesium stearate, pregelatinized starch, microcrystalline cellulose, polyethylene glycol, polysorbate 80, purified water, sodium starch glycolate, titanium dioxide, and may contain synthetic iron oxide. Bottles of 60 with desiccant.

200 mg: Each salmon, embossed, round, coated tablet, marked "TOP" on one side, "200" on the other, contains: topiramate 200 mg. Nonmedicinal ingredients: carnauba wax, hypromellose, lactose monohydrate, magnesium stearate, pregelatinized starch, microcrystalline cellulose, polyethylene glycol, polysorbate 80, purified water, sodium starch glycolate, titanium dioxide, and may contain synthetic iron oxide. Bottles of 60 with desiccant.

Sprinkle Capsules: 15 mg: Each white and clear gelatin capsule, containing small white to off-white spheres, marked "TOP" and "15 mg" on the side, contains: topiramate-coated beads 15 mg. Nonmedicinal ingredients: black pharmaceutical ink, cellulose acetate, gelatin, povidone, sorbitan monolaurate, sodium lauryl sulfate, sugar spheres (sucrose and starch) and titanium dioxide. Bottles of 60 without desiccant.

25 mg: Each white and clear gelatin capsule, containing small white to off-white spheres, marked "TOP" and "25 mg" on the side, contains: topiramate-coated beads 25 mg. Nonmedicinal ingredients: black pharmaceutical ink, cellulose acetate, gelatin, povidone, sorbitan monolaurate, sodium lauryl sulfate, sugar spheres (sucrose and starch) and titanium dioxide. Bottles of 60 without desiccant.

(Shown in Product Identification Section)

> The reader is invited to consult CPhA's monograph **Corticosteroids: Topical.**

Topicort® Preparations

desoximetasone

Topical Corticosteroid

sanofi-aventis

Date of Revision: May 30, 2006

PHARMACOLOGY: Topicort preparations are primarily effective because of their anti-inflammatory, antipruritic and vasoconstrictive actions.

INDICATIONS: For the relief of acute or chronic corticosteroid-responsive dermatoses.

CONTRAINDICATIONS: Topical corticosteroids are contraindicated in untreated bacterial, tubercular, fungal and most viral lesions of the skin (including herpes simplex, vaccinia and varicella) and in those patients with a history of hypersensitivity to any of the components of the preparation.

Topicort preparations are not for ophthalmic use.

WARNINGS: Systemic side effects may occur with topical corticosteroid preparations, particularly when these preparations are used over large areas or for an extended period of time or with occlusive dressings. A patient who has been on prolonged therapy, especially occlusive therapy may develop adrenal suppression due to sufficient absorption of the steroid.

Pregnancy: The safety of topical corticosteroid preparations during pregnancy and lactation has not been established. The potential benefit should be weighed in these conditions against possible hazard to the fetus or the nursing infant. When indicated, they should not be used extensively, in large amounts or for prolonged periods of time in pregnant patients or nursing mothers.

Lactation: See Pregnancy.

PRECAUTIONS: General: Children may absorb proportionally larger amounts of topical corticosteroids and thus be more susceptible to systemic toxicity (see Children).

If local infection exists, suitable concomitant antimicrobial or antifungal therapy should be administered as primary therapy. If it is considered necessary, the topical corticosteroid may be used as an adjunct to control inflammation, erythema and itching. If a favorable response does not occur promptly, application of the corticosteroid should be discontinued until the infection is adequately controlled.

If local irritation or sensitization develops, desoximetasone creams, gel and ointment should be discontinued and appropriate therapy instituted.

The use of occlusive dressings increases the percutaneous absorption of corticosteroids; their extensive use increases the possibility of systemic effects and is therefore not advisable. For patients with extensive lesions it may be preferable to use a sequential approach, treating one portion of the body at a time. The patient should be kept under close observation if treated with large amounts of topical corticosteroid or with the occlusive technique over a prolonged period of time.

Occlusive dressings should not be applied if there is an elevation of body temperature.

Patients should be advised to inform subsequent physicians of the prior use of corticosteroids.

Topical corticosteroids should be used with caution on lesions close to the eyes.

Prolonged use of topical corticosteroid products may produce atrophy of skin and s.c. tissues, particularly on flexor surfaces and on the face. If this is noted, discontinue the use of this product.

The product should be used with caution in patients with stasis dermatitis and other skin diseases associated with impaired circulation.

Children: **Pediatric patients may demonstrate greater susceptibility to topical corticosteroid induced HPA axis suppression and Cushing's syndrome than mature patients because of a larger skin surface area to body weight ratio.**

Hypothalamic-pituitary-adrenal [HPA] axis suppression, Cushing's syndrome and intracranial hypertension have been reported in children receiving topical corticosteroids. Manifestations of adrenal suppression in children include linear growth retardation, delayed weight gain, low plasma cortisol levels and absence of response to ACTH stimulation. Manifestations of intracranial hypertension include bulging fontanelles, headaches and bilateral papilledema.

Administration of topical corticosteroids to children should be limited to the least amount compatible with an effective therapeutic regimen. Chronic corticosteroid therapy may interfere with the growth and development of children.

ADVERSE EFFECTS: Topicort preparations are well tolerated. Side effects have been rare. Similar to other topical corticosteroid preparations, they may cause: burning sensation, dryness, itching, erythema, change in skin pigmentation, folliculitis, pyoderma, striae, telangiectasia and skin atrophy. The following reactions are reported when corticosteroid preparations are used extensively on intertriginous areas or under occlusive dressings: maceration of the skin, secondary infection, striae, miliaria, hypertrichosis and localized skin atrophy.

Adrenal suppression has been shown to occur with prolonged use of large doses of topical corticosteroids, particularly under occlusion, due to increased percutaneous absorption.

Posterior subcapsular cataracts have been reported following systemic use of corticosteroids.

OVERDOSE:

Symptoms: Toxic effects due to prolonged percutaneous absorption of large amounts of corticosteroids may include: reversible suppression of adrenal function, skin striae, ecchymoses, discoloration or atrophy, acneiform eruptions, hirsutism, infection. Prolonged systemic corticosteroid action may cause hypertension, peptic ulceration, hypokalemia, muscle weakness and wastage and subcapsular cataracts.

Treatment: Treatment should include symptomatic therapy and discontinuation of corticosteroid administration. In chronically affected patients, a gradual discontinuation may prevent the development of steroid withdrawal symptoms.

> For management of a suspected drug overdose, CPhA recommends that you contact your **regional Poison Control Centre**. See the *CPS* Directory section for a list of Poison Control Centres.

DOSAGE: Apply a thin film to the affected skin areas twice daily. Rub in gently.

SUPPLIED: Topicort Cream: Each tube contains: desoximetasone, 0.25%. Nonmedicinal ingredients: isopropyl myristate, methylparaben, propylparaben, wool alcohols and wool alcohols ointment. Tubes of 20 and 60 g.

Topicort Mild Cream: Each tube contains: desoximetasone, 0.05%. Nonmedicinal ingredients: edetate disodium, isopropyl myristate, lactic acid, methylparaben, propylparaben, wool alcohols and wool alcohols ointment. Tubes of 20 and 60 g.

Topicort Gel: Each tube contains: desoximetasone, 0.05%. Nonmedicinal ingredients: alcohol, carbopol 940 (carboxypolymethylene), docusate sodium, edetate disodium, isopropyl myristate, trolamine and water. Extended-tip tubes of 20 and 60 g.

Topicort Ointment: Each tube contains: desoximetasone, 0.25%. Nonmedicinal ingredients: aluminum stearate, beeswax, butylated hydroxyanisole, citric acid, fatty acid pentaerythritol ester, fatty alcohol citrate, propylene glycol, sorbitan sesquioleate and white petrolatum. Tubes of 20 and 60 g.

Store at room temperature, below 25°C.

Topotecan for Injection ℞

topotecan HCl

Antineoplastic

Sandoz

SUPPLIED: Each vial of sterile lyophilized powder contains: topotecan 4 mg (topotecan hydrochloride 4.48 mg), mannitol and tartaric acid. Hydrochloric acid and/or sodium hydroxide may be added to adjust the pH. Single use vials of 4 mg (free base), boxes of 1. Store between 15 and 30°C, protected from light. Reconstituted vials diluted for infusion are stable for up to 24 hours at room temperature with ambient lighting conditions. If not used immediately, the diluted solution should be stored in a refrigerator between 2 and 8°C, up to 24 hours.

Torisel™ ℞

temsirolimus

mTOR Kinase Inhibitor—Antineoplastic Agent

Pfizer

Date of Revision: July 12, 2010

SUMMARY PRODUCT INFORMATION:

Route of Administration	Dosage Form/ Strength	Clinically Relevant Nonmedicinal Ingredients
Intravenous Infusion	Concentrate for Injection 25 mg/mL	Dehydrated alcohol
	Diluent	Dehydrated alcohol For a complete listing see Dosage Forms, Composition and Packaging.

INDICATIONS AND CLINICAL USE: TORISEL (temsirolimus concentrate for injection) is indicated for the treatment of metastatic renal cell carcinoma.

Geriatrics (≥65 years of age): No specific overall differences in safety were observed between patients younger than 65 or older than 65.

Overall survival in a subset of patients 65 years of age or older (N=64) treated with TORISEL was shorter than that observed with patients under 65 years of age. The clinical relevance of this subgroup analysis is unclear.

No specific dose adjustment is recommended for elderly patients.

Pediatrics: The safety and effectiveness of TORISEL in pediatric patients have not been established. No data are available on the use of TORISEL in pediatric patients.

CONTRAINDICATIONS: TORISEL (temsirolimus concentrate for injection) is contraindicated in patients who have a history of anaphylaxis after exposure to temsirolimus, sirolimus or any other component of TORISEL (see Dosage Forms, Composition and Packaging).

WARNINGS AND PRECAUTIONS:

> **Serious Warnings and Precautions**
> TORISEL should be prescribed by a qualified healthcare professional who is experienced in the management of metastatic renal cell carcinoma. TORISEL should be administered in an appropriate setting, under the supervision of a qualified healthcare professional. Appropriate management of therapy and complications is only possible when adequate diagnostic and treatment facilities are readily available.
> The following are clinically significant adverse events:
> - Hypersensitivity/Infusion reactions (see Sensitivity/Resistance)
> - Hyperglycemia/Glucose Intolerance (see Endocrine and Metabolism)
> - Infections (see Infections)
> - Interstitial Lung Disease (see Respiratory)
> - Renal Failure (see Renal and Hepatic Dysfunction)

Bleeding: Patients with central nervous system tumors (primary CNS tumors or metastases) and/or receiving anticoagulation therapy may be at an increased risk of developing intracerebral bleeding (including fatal outcomes) while receiving therapy with temsirolimus.

Bleeding events were noted in 103 (25%) of patients receiving temsirolimus. Epistaxis was the commonest bleeding event with 3-times the incidence in the temsirolimus arm than in the IFN arm (12.0% in the temsirolimus arm and 3.5% in the IFN arm). Most bleeding events were grade 1 or 2, with only 13 (3%) grade 3 and 4.

Carcinogenesis and Mutagenesis: Carcinogenicity studies have not been conducted with temsirolimus. However, sirolimus, the major metabolite of temsirolimus in humans, induced malignant lymphoma, hepatocellular adenoma and carcinoma, and testicular adenoma in mice and/or rats. Patients receiving immunosuppression regimens involving combinations of drugs, including sirolimus, are at increased risk of developing lymphomas and other malignancies, particularly of the skin.

Cardiovascular: TORISEL is associated with small (<10 msec) but statistically significant QT/QTc interval prolongation (see Action and Clinical Pharmacology, Cardiac Electrophysiology).

Hypertension has been reported in 14 patients (7%) receiving TORISEL compared with 8 patients (4%) receiving Interferon in the Renal Cell Carcinoma Study (3066K1-304-WW). In Study 3066K1-155-US, diastolic and systolic blood pressures of subjects continued to steadily increase up to 48 hours after administration of temsirolimus (see Adverse Reactions).

Drug-Drug Interactions: Agents Inducing CYP3A Metabolism: Agents such as carbamazepine, phenytoin, barbiturates, rifabutin, rifampicin, and St John's Wort are strong inducers of CYP3A4/5 and may decrease composite exposures of the active moieties, temsirolimus and its metabolite, sirolimus. Therefore, concomitant treatment with agents that have CYP3A4/5 induction potential should be avoided. The safety profile of temsirolimus at doses greater than 25 mg in the presence of a CYP3A4/5 inducer has not been evaluated in the context of compensation for the reduced sirolimus exposure (see Overdosage).

Agents Inhibiting CYP3A Metabolism: Agents such as protease inhibitors, anti-fungals, macrolide antibiotics, nefazodone, and selective serotonin inhibitors are strong CYP3A4 inhibitors and may increase blood concentrations of the active moieties, temsirolimus and its metabolite, sirolimus. Therefore, concomitant treatment with agents that have CYP3A4 inhibition potential should be avoided. Alternative treatments with agents that do not have CYP3A4 inhibition potential should be considered (see Drug Interactions).

Pharmacodynamic Drug Interactions: TORISEL in combination with sunitinib, gemcitabine or 5-fluorouracil has been associated with serious adverse drug reactions. Fatal events have been seen when TORISEL was combined with 5-fluorouracil.

Angioneurotic edema-type reactions (including delayed reactions occurring two months following initiation of therapy) have been observed in some patients who received TORISEL and angiotension-converting enzyme (ACE) inhibitors concomitantly.

Endocrine and Metabolism: Hyperglycemia/Glucose Intolerance: The use of TORISEL in renal cell carcinoma (RCC) patients was frequently associated with increases in serum glucose. In Study 1, hyperglycemia was present on at least one occasion in over 82% of patients receiving temsirolimus and was an adverse event (greater than 13.9 mmol/L) in 15.9% of patients. This may result in the need for an increase in the dose of, or initiation of, insulin and/or oral hypoglycemic agent therapy. Patients should be advised to report excessive thirst or any increase in the volume or frequency of urination.

Hyperlipidemia: The use of TORISEL in RCC patients was frequently associated with increases in serum triglycerides and cholesterol. In Study 1, hypercholesterolemia was present on at least one occasion in 80% of patients receiving temsirolimus, and hypertriglyceridemia was present in over 83% of patients. One or both dyslipidemias was an adverse event (cholesterol greater than 10.34 mmol/L, triglycerides greater than 5× upper limit of normal) in 45.2% of patients. This may require initiation, or increase in the dose of lipid lowering agents. Serum cholesterol and triglycerides should be tested before and during treatment with TORISEL.

Gastrointestinal: Cases of bowel perforation (including fatal outcomes) have occurred in patients who received TORISEL (see Adverse Reactions).

Stomatitis and mucositis were significantly more common in the temsirolimus arm, with combined incidences of 19 (10%) and 86 (41%) in the IFN and temsirolimus arms, respectively. Grade 3 or 4 stomatitis and mucositis was reported in 0 and 6 (3%) in each arm, respectively.

Hematologic: Anemia was very common across the treatment arms, with over 90% of patients reporting at least one low hemoglobin level. Grade 3 and 4 anemia was reported in 43 (21.5%) and 41 (19.7%) in the IFN and temsirolimus arms, respectively. Transfusion of at least one unit of blood was given to 51 (25.5%) and 63 (30.3%) patients in each arm respectively.

Leukopenia, neutropenia, lymphopenia and thrombocytopenia including grade 3 and 4 events were commonly reported in all treatment arms (see Table 2).

Immune: Infections: Infection related events were reported in patients receiving temsirolimus more than twice as frequently than in those receiving IFN only (31% vs. 15%). Temsirolimus may be immunosuppressive. Patients should be carefully observed for the occurrence of infections, including opportunistic infections (see Adverse Reactions).

Vaccinations: The use of live vaccines and close contact with people who have received live vaccines should be avoided during treatment with temsirolimus. Examples of live vaccines are: measles, mumps, rubella, oral polio, BCG, yellow fever, varicella, and TY21a typhoid vaccines.

Musculoskeletal and Connective Tissue Disorders: Myalgia, arthralgia, and increased serum creatine phosphokinase have been observed in subjects treated with TORISEL.

Peri-Operative Considerations: Wound Healing Complications: The use of TORISEL has been associated with abnormal wound healing. Therefore, caution should be exercised with the use of TORISEL in the peri-surgical period.

Renal and Hepatic Dysfunction: Renal insufficiency was a common treatment emergent adverse event. In study 1, elevated creatinine was present on at least one occasion in 57.2% of patients receiving temsirolimus and in 48.5% of patients receiving IFN. Increased creatinine was an adverse event (greater than 3× upper limit of normal) in 3.4% of patients receiving temsirolimus and 1% of patients receiving IFN.

Cases of rapidly progressive and sometimes fatal acute renal failure not clearly related to disease progression occurred in patients who received TORISEL.

Effect of renal impairment on TORISEL pharmacokinetics has not been studied.

Dose de-escalation and multiple dose interruption were observed in patients with mild hepatic impairment primarily due to thrombocytopenia. Study of TORISEL pharmacokinetics in patients with moderate to severe hepatic impairment has not been conducted.

Respiratory: Interstitial Lung Disease: Cases of interstitial lung disease, including some fatalities, have occurred in patients who received TORISEL. Some patients were asymptomatic with infiltrates detected on CT scan or chest X-ray. Others presented with symptoms such as dyspnea, cough, hypoxia, and fever. In a series of patients receiving intravenous temsirolimus 25 mg weekly for advanced neuroendocrine tumours or advanced endometrial carcinoma, 8 out of 22 patients developed pulmonary abnormalities compatible with drug-induced pneumonitis. Half were asymptomatic. Some patients required discontinuation of TORISEL or treatment with corticosteroids and/or antibiotics, while some patients continued treatment without additional intervention.

It is recommended that patients undergo baseline radiographic assessment by lung computed tomography scan or chest radiograph prior to the initiation of temsirolimus therapy. Follow such assessments periodically, even in the absence of clinical respiratory symptoms.

It is recommended that patients be followed closely for occurrence of clinical respiratory symptoms. If clinically significant respiratory symptoms develop, consider withholding temsirolimus administration until after recovery of symptoms and improvement of radiographic findings related to pneumonitis. Empiric treatment with corticosteroids and/or antibodies may be considered.

Sensitivity/Resistance: Hypersensitivity/Infusion Reactions: Hypersensitivity/infusion reactions (including some life-threatening and rare fatal reactions), including but not limited to flushing, chest pain, dyspnea, hypotension, apnea, loss of consciousness, hypersensitivity and anaphylaxis, have been associated with the administration of TORISEL. These reactions can occur very early in the first infusion, but may also occur with subsequent infusions. Patients should be monitored early during the infusion and appropriate supportive care should be available. TORISEL infusion should be interrupted in all patients with severe infusion reactions and appropriate medical therapy administered. A benefit-risk assessment should be done prior to the continuation of TORISEL therapy in patients with severe or life-threatening reactions.

Sirolimus is the major metabolite of temsirolimus, therefore, temsirolimus should be administered with caution in patients with a known hypersensitivity to sirolimus.

Because it is recommended that an H_1 antihistamine be administered to patients before the start of the intravenous temsirolimus infusion, TORISEL should be used with caution in patients with known hypersensitivity to an antihistamine, or patients who cannot receive an antihistamine for other medical reasons.

If a patient develops a hypersensitivity reaction during the TORISEL infusion despite the premedication, the infusion should be stopped and the patient should be observed for at least 30 to 60 minutes (depending on the severity of the reaction). At the discretion of the physician, treatment may be resumed with the administration of an H_1-receptor antagonist (such as diphenhydramine), if not previously administered (Dosage and Administration), and/or an H_2-receptor antagonist (such as intravenous famotidine 20 mg or intravenous ranitidine 50 mg) approximately 30 minutes before restarting the TORISEL infusion. The infusion may then be resumed at a slower rate (up to 60 minutes). Diluted TORISEL should be administered within 6 hours of mixing (see Dosage and Administration).

Skin: Rash NOS (all grades) was reported in 11 (5.5%) and 77 (37.0%) in the IFN and temsirolimus arms, respectively. Acne was common in the temsirolimus group with 21 (10.1%) reports, compared with 2 (1.0%) in the IFN arm.

Special Populations: Pregnant Women: There are no adequate and well-controlled studies in pregnant women using TORISEL. In animal toxicity studies with rats and rabbits, there was increased embryo/fetal mortality and decreased fetal growth.

Women of childbearing age should use medically acceptable contraception during (and up to 3 months after) treatment.

Temsirolimus should not be used during pregnancy.

In addition, men should be adequately counseled prior to starting treatment with TORISEL and need to understand the possible danger of taking a medicinal product whose effects on the fetus and sperm are unknown. Men with partners of childbearing potential should use medically acceptable contraception throughout treatment and are recommended to continue this for 12 weeks after the last dose of TORISEL.

Nursing Women: It is not known whether TORISEL is excreted into human milk. Because many drugs are excreted into human milk, and because the effects of temsirolimus excretion in human milk have not been studied, women should be advised against breast-feeding while receiving temsirolimus.

Pediatrics: The safety and effectiveness of TORISEL in pediatric patients have not been established. No data are available on the use of TORISEL in pediatric patients.

Geriatrics (≥65 years of age): No specific overall differences in safety were observed between patients younger than 65 or older than 65.

Overall survival in a subset of patients 65 years of age or older (N=64) treated with TORISEL was shorter than that observed with patients under 65 years of age. The clinical relevance of this subgroup analysis is unclear.

No specific dose adjustment is recommended for elderly patients.

Monitoring and Laboratory Tests: In the randomized phase 3 trial, complete blood counts were checked weekly, and chemistry panels were checked every two weeks. In addition, it is recommended to measure fasting glucose and lipids prior to starting treatment, with regular follow up tests during the treatment period. Laboratory monitoring for patients receiving TORISEL must be individualized at the discretion of the treating physician.

ADVERSE REACTIONS: Adverse Drug Reaction Overview: The following serious adverse reactions have been associated with TORISEL (temsirolimus concentrate for injection) in clinical trials and are discussed in greater detail in other sections of the label (see Warnings and Precautions): hypersensitivity reactions; hyperglycemia/glucose intolerance; infections; interstitial lung disease; renal failure.

The most common (≥30%) adverse reactions observed with TORISEL are rash, asthenia, mucositis, nausea, edema, and anorexia. The most common (≥30%) laboratory abnormalities observed with TORISEL are anemia, hyperglycemia, hyperlipidemia, hypertriglyceridemia, lymphopenia, elevated alkaline phosphatase, elevated serum creatinine, hypophosphatemia, thrombocytopenia, elevated AST, and leukopenia.

Clinical Trial Adverse Drug Reactions: Renal Cell Carcinoma Study 1 (3066K1-304-WW): Study 1 is a phase 3, three-arm, randomized, open-label study of Interferon alfa (IFN-α) alone, TORISEL alone, and TORISEL and IFN-α. A total of 616 patients were treated. Two hundred patients received IFN-α weekly, 208 received TORISEL 25 mg weekly, and 208 patients received a combination of IFN-α and TORISEL weekly.

Treatment with the combination of TORISEL 15 mg and IFN-α resulted in a statistically significant increase in the incidence of certain grade 3-4 adverse events (weight loss, hyperlipemia, anemia, neutropenia, thrombocytopenia and mucosal inflammation) when compared with the adverse events observed in the IFN-α or TORISEL 25 mg-alone arms. The combination did not result in a significant increase in overall survival when compared with IFN-α alone (8.4 vs 7.3 months, hazard ratio=0.96, p=0.6965).

Of the 208 patients treated in the temsirolimus alone arm, 88 (42.3%) patients had adverse events of nausea or vomiting or both. Of these 88 patients, 59 (67.0%) received at least one anti-emetic during their study participation. Temsirolimus was dose-reduced and discontinued in one patient due to vomiting. Of the 8 patients who reported grade 3 or 4 nausea or vomiting or both, 2 patients had a past medical history of nausea or vomiting at the time of screening, and 2 patients did not receive any anti-emetics to control their nausea or vomiting while on study.

Table 1 shows the percentage of patients experiencing treatment emergent adverse reactions reported in Study 1. Reactions reported in at least 10% of patients who received TORISEL 25 mg alone are listed. Data for the same adverse reactions in the IFN-α alone arm are shown for comparison.

Table 1: TORISEL

Adverse Reactions Reported in at Least 10% of Patients Who Received 25 mg IV TORISEL in Study 1

Adverse Reaction	TORISEL 25 mg n=208 All Grades[a] n (%)	TORISEL 25 mg n=208 Grades 3 & 4[a] n (%)	IFN-α n=200 All Grades[a] n (%)	IFN-α n=200 Grades 3 & 4[a] n (%)
Any	208 (100)	139 (67)	199 (100)	155 (78)
Blood and Lymphatic System Disorders				
Anemia	94 (45)	41 (20)	83 (42)	43 (22)
Thrombocytopenia	28 (14)	3 (1)	16 (8)	0 (0)
Gastrointestinal Disorders				
Nausea	77 (37)	5 (2)	82 (41)	9 (4)
Diarrhea	56 (27)	3 (1)	40 (20)	4 (2)
Abdominal Pain	44 (21)	9 (4)	34 (17)	3 (2)
Stomatitis[b]	86 (41)	6 (3)	19 (10)	0 (0)
Vomiting	40 (19)	4 (2)	57 (29)	5 (3)
General Disorders and Administrative Site Conditions				
Asthenia	106 (51)	23 (11)	127 (64)	52 (26)
Edema[c]	88 (42)	7 (3)	25 (13)	1 (1)
Pain	59 (28)	10 (5)	31 (16)	4 (2)
Pyrexia	50 (24)	1 (1)	99 (50)	7 (4)
Chest Pain	34 (16)	2 (1)	18 (9)	2 (1)
Infections and Infestations				
Infections[d]	52 (25)	6 (3)	19 (10)	4 (2)
Urinary Tract Infection[e]	39 (19)	3 (1)	30 (15)	4 (2)
Pharyngitis	25 (12)	0 (0)	3 (2)	0 (0)
Rhinitis	25 (10)	0 (0)	4 (2)	0 (0)
Investigations				
Blood Creatinine Increased	30 (14)	6 (3)	21 (10)	1 (1)
Metabolism and Nutrition Disorders				
Anorexia	66 (32)	5 (2)	87 (44)	8 (4)
Hyperlipidemia	57 (27)	6 (3)	28 (14)	2 (1)
Hyperglycemia	53 (26)	22 (11)	22 (11)	3 (2)
Hypercholesteremia	51 (25)	1 (1)	9 (4)	0 (0)
Weight Loss	39 (19)	3 (1)	50 (25)	4 (2)
Musculoskeletal and Connective Tissue Disorders				
Back Pain	41 (20)	6 (3)	28 (14)	3 (2)
Arthralgia	37 (18)	2 (1)	29 (15)	2 (1)
Nervous System Disorders				
Dysgeusia[f]	41 (20)	0 (0)	17 (9)	0 (0)
Insomnia	24 (12)	1 (1)	30 (15)	0 (0)
Respiratory, Thoracic and Mediastinal Disorders				
Dyspnea	58 (30)	18 (9)	48 (24)	11 (6)
Cough	53 (26)	2 (1)	29 (15)	0 (0)
Epistaxis	25 (12)	0 (0)	7 (4)	0 (0)
Skin and Subcutaneous Tissue Disorders				
Rash[g]	97 (47)	11 (5)	12 (6)	0 (0)
Pruritus	40 (19)	1 (1)	16 (8)	0 (0)
Nail Disorder	28 (14)	0 (0)	1 (1)	0 (0)
Dry Skin	22 (11)	1 (1)	14 (7)	0 (0)
Acne	21 (10)	0 (0)	2 (1)	0 (0)

(cont'd)

Table 1: TORISEL *(cont'd)*

a Common Toxicity Criteria for Adverse Events (CTCAE), Version 3.0.
b Includes aphthous stomatitis, glossitis, mouth ulceration, mucositis, and stomatitis.
c Includes facial edema and peripheral edema.
d Includes general infections and a variety of infections that occurred infrequently as distinct entities: cellulitis, herpes zoster, herpes simplex, bronchitis, and abscess.
e Includes dysuria, hematuria, urinary frequency, and cystitis.
f Includes taste loss and taste perversion.
g Includes pruritic rash, maculopapular rash, and pustular rash.

The following adverse reactions were commonly reported (≥1% and ≤10%) and may be associated with the use of TORISEL:

Eye Disorders: Conjunctivitis (including lacrimation disorder) occurred in 15 patients (7%).

Gastrointestinal Disorders : Abdominal distension occurred in 9 patients (4%). Gingivitis occurred in 5 patients (2%). Oral pain occurred in 5 patients (2%). Fatal bowel perforation occurred in 1 patient (1%).

General Disorders and Administrative Site Conditions: Impaired healing occurred in 3 patients (1%).

Immune System: Allergic/hypersensitivity reactions occurred in 18 patients (9%).

Infections and Infestations: Pneumonia occurred in 15 patients (7%). Upper respiratory tract infection occurred in 14 patients (7%). Folliculitis occurred in 4 patients (2%).

Investigations: Aspartate aminotransferase increase occurred in 17 patients (8%). Alanine aminotransferase increase occurred in 12 patients (6%).

Renal and Urinary Disorders: Renal Failure (see Warnings and Precautions) occurred in 7 patients (3%).

Respiratory, Thoracic and Mediastinal Disorders: Interstitial pneumonitis, including fatal episodes, has been reported in patients taking temsirolimus. Pleural effusion occurred in 10 patients (5%).

Skin and Subcutaneous Tissue Disorders: Exfoliative dermatitis occurred in 16 patients (8%).

Vascular: Hypertension occurred in 14 patients (7%) (see Warnings and Precautions); Venous thromboembolism (including deep vein thrombosis and pulmonary embolus [including fatal outcomes]) occurred in 5 patients (2%). Thrombophlebitis occurred in 2 patients (1%).

The following adverse reactions were uncommonly reported (≥0.1% and <1%) and may be associated with the use of TORISEL:

Cardiac Disorders: Pericardial effusion (including hemodynamically significant pericardial effusions requiring intervention) occurred in 2 patients (1%).

Nervous System Disorders: Convulsion occurred in 1 patient (0.5%).

Renal Cell Carcinoma Study 2 (3066K1-200-WW): Study 2 was a phase 2, randomized, double-blind, multi-center, outpatient trial to evaluate the efficacy, safety, and pharmacokinetics of three dose levels of TORISEL when administered to previously treated patients with advanced RCC. One hundred eleven (111) patients were randomly assigned in a 1:1:1 ratio to receive 25 mg, 75 mg, or 250 mg TORISEL IV weekly. The incidence and type of adverse events reported for the temsirolimus 25 mg arm were generally similar to those reported in the pivotal phase 3 study (Study 1).

Abnormal Hematologic and Clinical Chemistry Findings: See Table 2.

Post-Marketing Adverse Drug Reactions: The following adverse reactions have been identified during the post-approval use of temsirolimus. Frequency determination of adverse events reported from the post marketing environment is not possible since the size of the population receiving the drug is largely undetermined.

Hypersensitivity/Infusion Reactions: Hypersensitivity/infusion reactions (including some life-threatening and rare fatal reactions), have been associated with the administration of temsirolimus (see Warnings and Precautions).

Other adverse reactions observed in the post marketing environment include delayed angioneurotic edema-type reactions (occurring two months following initiation of therapy) observed in some patients who received concomitant therapy with temsirolimus and angiotensin-converting enzyme (ACE) inhibitors (see Warnings and Precautions), pleural effusion, pericardial effusion (including hemodynamically significant pericardial effusions requiring intervention), and convulsion.

There have been reports of Stevens-Johnson Syndrome, pulmonary embolus (including fatal outcomes) and hand-foot syndrome in patients who received TORISEL.

Table 2: TORISEL

Incidence of Clinically Important Laboratory Abnormalities Reported in at Least 10% of Patients Who Received 25 mg IV TORISEL in Study 1

	TORISEL 25 mg n=208		IFN-α n=200	
Laboratory Abnormality	**All Grades[a] n (%)**	**Grades 3 & 4[a] n (%)**	**All Grades[a] n (%)**	**Grades 3 & 4[a] n (%)**
Any	208 (100)	139 (67)	199 (100)	155 (78)
Hematology				
Hemoglobin Decreased	195 (94)	41 (20)	180 (90)	43 (22)
Lymphocytes Decreased[b]	110 (53)	33 (16)	106 (53)	48 (24)
Neutrophils Decreased[b]	39 (19)	10 (5)	58 (29)	19 (10)
Platelets Decreased	84 (40)	3 (1)	51 (26)	0 (0)
Leukocytes Decreased	67 (32)	1 (1)	93 (47)	11 (6)
Chemistry				
Alkaline Phosphatase Increased	141 (68)	7 (3)	111 (56)	13 (7)
AST Increased	79 (38)	5 (2)	103 (52)	14 (7)
Creatinine Increased	119 (57)	7 (3)	97 (49)	2 (1)
Glucose Increased	186 (89)	33 (16)	128 (64)	6 (3)
Phosphorus Decreased	102 (49)	38 (18)	61 (31)	17 (9)
Total Bilirubin Increased	16 (8)	2 (1)	25 (13)	4 (2)
Total Cholesterol Increased	181 (87)	5 (2)	95 (48)	2 (1)
Triglycerides Increased	173 (83)	92 (44)	144 (72)	69 (35)
Potassium Decreased	43 (21)	11 (5)	15 (8)	0 (0)
Potassium Increased	46 (22)	10 (5)	68 (34)	9 (5)
Calcium Increased	46 (22)	8 (4)	46 (23)	12 (6)
Calcium Decreased	82 (39)	9 (4)	83 (42)	9 (5)
Albumin Decreased	108 (52)	3 (1)	121 (61)	12 (6)

[a] NCI CTC version 3.0.
[b] Grade 1 toxicity may be under-reported for lymphocytes and neutrophils.

DRUG INTERACTIONS: Overview: TORISEL in combination with sunitinib, gemcitabine or 5-fluorouracil has been associated with serious adverse drug reactions. Fatal cases of bowel perforation have been observed when TORISEL was combined with 5-fluorouracil.

CYP3A4 is the major CYP isozyme responsible for the metabolism of temsirolimus and sirolimus. Potential interactions may occur with drugs/foods/herbs that are inhibitors or inducers of this enzyme system.

Drug-Drug Interactions: Agents Inducing CYP3A Metabolism: Co-administration of TORISEL with rifampicin (600 mg), a potent CYP3A4/5 inducer, had no significant effect on temsirolimus C_{max} (maximum concentration) and AUC, after intravenous administration, but decreased sirolimus C_{max} by 65% and AUC by 56%, and AUC_{sum} (composite of temsirolimus AUC plus sirolimus AUC) by 41% compared to temsirolimus treatment alone. Therefore, concomitant treatment with agents that have CYP3A4/5 induction potential should be avoided. The safety profile of temsirolimus at doses greater than 25 mg in the presence of a CYP3A4/5 inducer has not been evaluated in the context of compensation for the reduced sirolimus exposure (see Overdosage).

Agents Inhibiting CYP3A Metabolism: Co-administration of TORISEL (5 mg, 1/5th of the clinically recommended dose) with ketoconazole (400 mg), a potent CYP3A4 inhibitor to healthy subjects, had no significant effect on temsirolimus C_{max} or AUC; however, AUC of sirolimus increased 3.1-fold, and AUC_{sum} increased 2.3-fold compared to temsirolimus alone. A 51% increase in sirolimus half-life and 69% decrease in clearance were also observed.

Concomitant treatment of TORISEL with agents that have strong CYP3A4 inhibition potential should be avoided (see Warnings and Precautions).

Interactions with Drugs Metabolized by CYP3A4/5: Temsirolimus may inhibit the metabolic clearance of substrates of CYP3A4/5 including statins. Caution should be exercised if a statin is required for hyperlipidemia, since the risk of developing rhabdomyolysis may be increased. Patients on treatment with TORISEL who are co-prescribed a statin should be advised to report symptoms including muscle pain or weakness.

Interactions with Drugs Metabolized by CYP2D6: In a study with 23 healthy subjects, the concentration of desipramine (50 mg), a CYP2D6 substrate, was unaffected when 25 mg of TORISEL was co-administered. However, there was over 8 hour gap between the peak concentration of the two drugs when they were administered concurrently. The magnitude of the interaction may have been reduced. Caution should be taken when temsirolimus is co-administered with agents that are metabolized by CYP2D6.

Interactions with Drugs that are P-glycoprotein Substrates: In an in vitro study, temsirolimus inhibited the transport of digoxin, a P-gp substrate, with an IC50 value of 2 μM. Clinical implications related to concomitant administration of P-gp substrates are not known.

Anti-emetic Agents: The safety of concomitant use of temsirolimus with anti-emetic agents, including but not limited to: prochlorperazine, diphenhydramine, metoclopramide, ondansetron, or domperidone, has not been formally studied.

Interactions with QT/QTc-prolonging Drugs: The concomitant use of TORISEL with another QT/QTc-prolonging drug should be avoided to the extent possible.

Drug-Food Interactions: The effect of food on exposure following an intravenous dose of temsirolimus was not examined.

Drug-Herb Interactions: Interactions with herbal products have not been established. St John's Wort is a strong inducer of CYP3A4 and may decrease blood concentrations of temsirolimus metabolites (see Warnings and Precautions and Drug Interactions).

Drug-Laboratory Test Interactions: Interactions with laboratory tests have not been established.

DOSAGE AND ADMINISTRATION: Dosing Considerations:

- No special dosage modification is required for any of the populations that have been studied (e.g. gender, elderly).
- The safety and effectiveness of TORISEL in pediatric patients have not been established.
- Studies in patients with varying renal impairment or in patients undergoing hemodialysis have not been conducted (see Action and Clinical Pharmacology).
- Temsirolimus should be used with caution in patients with hepatic impairment.

Recommended Dose and Dosage Adjustment: The recommended dose of TORISEL for advanced renal cell carcinoma is 25 mg, infused over a 30-60 minute period once a week.

Treatment should continue until the patient is no longer clinically benefiting from therapy or until unacceptable toxicity occurs. No special dosage modification is required for any of the populations that have been studied (e.g. gender, elderly).

In Study 1, 19.2% of patients receiving temsirolimus alone reported vomiting as an adverse event. The emetogenic potential of temsirolimus is low.

Dose Modification: Management of suspected drug reactions may require temporary interruption and/or dose reduction of TORISEL therapy. If a suspected reaction is not manageable with dose delays, then TORISEL may be reduced by 5 mg/week decrements.

Hepatic Impairment: For patients with severe hepatic impairment (Child-Pugh class C or NCI-Organ Dysfunction Working Group [ODWG] group D) and who have baseline platelets ≥100×10^9/L, the recommended dose is 10 mg IV infused over a 30-60 minute period, once a week.

Administration: Instructions for Intravenous Administration: TORISEL must be stored under refrigeration at 2-8°C and protected from light. During handling and preparation of admixtures, TORISEL should be protected from excessive room light and sunlight. TORISEL should be inspected visually for particulate matter and discoloration prior to administration, whenever solution and container permit. Bags/containers that come in contact with TORISEL must be made of glass, polyolefin, or polyethylene.

Premedication: Patients should receive prophylactic medication of intravenous diphenhydramine 25 to 50 mg (or equivalent) approximately 30 minutes before the start of each dose of TORISEL. If a hypersensitivity reaction develops during the temsirolimus infusion, the infusion should be stopped. Upon adequate resolution, and at the discretion of the physician, treatment may be resumed with the administration of an H_1-receptor antagonist (or equivalent), if not previously administered, and/or an H_2-receptor antagonist (such as intravenous famotidine 20 mg or intravenous ranitidine 50 mg) approximately 30 minutes before restarting the temsirolimus infusion. The infusion may then be resumed at a slower rate (up to 60 minutes) (see Warnings and Precautions).

Dilution: In preparing the TORISEL administration solution, follow this two-step dilution process in an aseptic manner.

Step 1: Inject 1.8 mL of diluent for TORISEL concentrate into the vial containing TORISEL for injection. The vial containing TORISEL contains 30 mg of drug in 1.2 mL vehicle. The drug concentration after mixing will be 10 mg/mL. Allow sufficient time for air bubbles to subside. The solution is clear to slightly turbid, colorless to light yellow, essentially free from visual particulates. A 1.2 mL volume of drug concentrate contains a total of 30 mg of drug product. When 1.2 mL of drug concentrate is combined with 1.8 mL of diluent, a total volume of 3.0 mL is obtained. Thirty milligrams (30 mg) of drug product per 3.0 mL=10 mg of drug product/mL. The drug concentrate-diluent mixture is stable for up to 24 hours at room temperature 20 to 25°C and protected from light. Any unused diluted mixture should be discarded after 24 hours.

Vial Size	Volume of Diluent to be Added to Vial	Approximate Available Volume	Nominal Concentration per mL
25 mg/mL (1.2 mL of drug concentrate)	1.8 mL of diluent	3.0 mL	10 mg/mL

Step 2: Withdraw the required amount (2.5 mL) of TORISEL concentrate/diluent mixture from step 1 (10 mg/mL) and inject rapidly into 250 mL of 0.9% sodium chloride injection to ensure adequate mixing. Mix the admixture by inversion of the bag or bottle. Avoid excessive shaking as this may cause foaming.

Administration:

- Administration of the final diluted infusion solution should be completed within six hours from the time that the concentrate-diluent mixture is added to the sodium chloride injection.
- TORISEL is administered as an IV solution over a 30-60 minute period once a week. The use of an infusion pump is the preferred method of administration to ensure accurate delivery of the drug.
- Appropriate administration materials should be composed of glass, polyolefin, or polyethylene to avoid excessive loss of drug and to decrease the rate of di-(2-ethylhexyl) phthalate (DEHP) extraction. The administration materials should consist of non-DEHP non-polyvinyl chloride (PVC) tubing with the recommended filter. It is important that the recommendations in Dosage and Administration be followed closely.
  An in-line polyethersulfone filter with a pore size of not greater than 5 microns is recommended for administration.
- TORISEL concentrate, when constituted, contains polysorbate 80, which is known to increase the rate of di-(2-ethylhexyl)phthalate (DEHP) extraction from PVC. This should be considered during the preparation and administration of TORISEL, including storage time elapsed in a PVC container following constitution. It is important that the recommendations in Dosage and Administration be followed closely.

Compatibilities, Incompatibilities: TORISEL concentrate for injection should not be added directly to aqueous infusion solutions. Direct addition of TORISEL concentrate for injection to aqueous solutions will result in precipitation of drug. Always combine TORISEL concentrate for injection with diluent for TORISEL concentrate for injection before adding to infusion solutions. It is recommended that temsirolimus be administered in 0.9% sodium chloride injection after combining with diluent.

The stability of temsirolimus in other infusion solutions has not been evaluated. Addition of other drugs or nutritional agents to admixtures of temsirolimus in sodium chloride injection has not been evaluated and should be avoided. Temsirolimus is degraded by both acids and bases, and thus combinations of temsirolimus with agents capable of modifying solution pH should be avoided.

OVERDOSAGE:

There is no specific treatment for TORISEL intravenous overdose. TORISEL has been administered to patients with cancer with repeated intravenous doses as high as 220 mg/m^2 (396 mg). However, the risk of serious adverse events including thrombosis, CNS hemorrhage, melena, bowel perforation, interstitial lung disease (ILD), seizure, and psychosis, is increased with doses of TORISEL greater than 25 mg.

> For management of a suspected drug overdose, contact your regional Poison Control Centre. See the *CPS* Directory section for a list of Poison Control Centres.

ACTION AND CLINICAL PHARMACOLOGY: Mechanism of Action: Temsirolimus is a selective inhibitor of mTOR (mammalian target of rapamycin). mTOR inhibition is implicated in preventing the proliferation of a number of tumour cell types and angiogenesis. Temsirolimus binds to an intracellular protein (FKBP12), and the protein-drug complex binds and inhibits the activity of mTOR that controls cell division. Inhibition of mTOR activity results in a G1 growth arrest in treated tumor cells resulting from selective disruption of translation of cell cycle regulatory proteins, such as D-type cyclins, c-myc, and ornithine decarboxylase. Temsirolimus exerts its effect by binding in a complex with FKBP-12 and mTOR. When mTOR is bound in this complex, its ability to phosphorylate, and thereby control the activity of protein translation factors (4E-BP1 and S6K, both downstream of mTOR in the P13 kinase/AKT pathway) that control cell division, is blocked. In addition to regulating cell cycle proteins, mTOR can regulate translation of the hypoxia-inducible factors, HIF-1 and HIF-2 alpha. These transcription factors regulate the ability of tumors to adapt to hypoxic microenvironments and to produce the angiogenic factor vascular endothelial growth factor (VEGF). The anti-tumor effect of temsirolimus, therefore, may also in part stem from its ability to depress levels of HIF and VEGF in the tumor or tumor microenvironment, thereby impairing vessel development.

Pharmacodynamics: The effect of TORISEL on the inhibition of phosphorylation of S6-ribosomal protein in circulating lymphocytes was examined in 30 healthy male subjects. Data indicate that inhibition of protein phosphorylation was rapid and dose-dependent. Following a single 25 mg dose of TORISEL, 50% of maximal inhibition of S6-ribosomal protein in CD3+ cells was shown for at least 3 days.

Cardiac Electrophysiology: The cardiac electrophysiology of a single 25 mg intravenous dose of temsirolimus was studied in 58 healthy male volunteers (18-50 years) in a fixed sequence, three period crossover design trial. In periods 1 and 2, the subjects were randomized to receive single-blind placebo IV infusion either alone or with open label oral moxifloxacin 400 mg. In period 3, all subjects were administered single-blind temsirolimus 25 mg IV.

Temsirolimus resulted in a statistically significant increase in the QTc interval from 1 to 48 hours post-dosing. The 48 hour ECG collection period in this study was not sufficiently long to characterize the offset of the effect. The maximum increase was 8.05 ms (90% CI 5.77, 10.34 ms) at 36 hours post-dosing.

In a different trial in patients with a hematologic malignancy, 103 patients receiving TORISEL doses up to 175 mg were studied for QTc effects. One subject with normal QTcF at baseline exhibited a QTcF increase >60 ms by week 12 of treatment.

Many drugs that cause clinically significant QT/QTc prolongation are suspected to increase the risk of torsades de pointes. Temsirolimus should be administered with caution in patients who have or may develop prolongation of QTc interval. These include patients with hypokalemia or hypomagnesemia, patients with congenital long QT syndrome, patients taking anti-arrhythmic medicines or other medicinal products that lead to QTc prolongation, and cumulative high-dose anthracycline therapy.

Pharmacokinetics: Following a single 25 mg intravenous dose in patients with cancer, sirolimus AUC was 2.7-fold that of temsirolimus AUC, due principally to the longer half-life of sirolimus (see Table 3). Following varying IV temsirolimus doses, the AUC_{sum} in whole blood increased in a dose-related, but non-proportional manner.

Table 3: TORISEL

Mean (SD) Pharmacokinetic Parameters[a] of Temsirolimus and Sirolimus in Whole Blood of Patients Following a Single 25-mg Intravenous Dose of Temsirolimus

	C_{max} (ng/mL)	AUC (ng·h/mL)	AUC_{sum}[b] (ng Eq's·h/mL)	T_{max} (h)	T½ (h)
Temsirolimus	585.4±83.1	1627±425	—	1.0±0	17.3±5.9
Sirolimus	55.4±31.8	4151±1600	5778±1722	2.0±0	54.6±1.5

[a] N=13. For C_{max}, N=5; for T½, N=2.
[b] AUC_{sum} expressed relative to temsirolimus equivalents.

Distribution: Temsirolimus exhibits a polyexponential decline in whole blood concentrations and distribution and is attributable to preferential binding to FKBP-12 in blood cells. The mean (standard deviation, SD) dissociation constant (K_d) of binding was 5.1 (3.0) ng/mL, denoting the concentration at which 50% of binding sites in blood cells were occupied. Temsirolimus distribution is dose-dependent with mean (10th, 90th percentiles) maximal specific binding in blood cells of 1.4 mg (0.47 to 2.5 mg). Following a single 25 mg intravenous dose, mean steady-state volume of distribution in whole blood of patients with cancer was 172 liters. In vitro temsirolimus binding to plasma proteins was approximately 87% at the concentration of 100 ng/mL.

Metabolism: Temsirolimus is metabolized primarily by CYP3A4 in human liver. It is also a substrate and potential inhibitor of P-glycoprotein. Sirolimus, an equally potent metabolite to temsirolimus was observed as the principal metabolite in humans following intravenous administration. Additional metabolic pathways were hydroxylation, reduction and demethylation in in vitro temsirolimus metabolism studies.

Temsirolimus inhibited CYP3A4/5 and CYP2D6 in human liver microsome studies with C_{max}/K_i ratio values of 0.19 and 0.38, respectively. Following a single 25 mg intravenous dose in patients with cancer, sirolimus AUC was 2.7-fold that of temsirolimus AUC, due principally to the longer half-life of sirolimus.

Excretion: Following administration of a single dose of [^{14}C]-labeled temsirolimus, excretion was predominantly via the feces (78%), with renal elimination of drug and metabolites accounting for 4.6% of the administered radioactivity. Approximate 17% of the total radioactivity was not recovered from either route following 14-day sample collection. Mean (CV) systemic clearance was 16.2 (22%) L/h. Mean half-lives of temsirolimus and sirolimus were 17.3 hr and 54.6 hr, respectively.

Special Populations and Conditions: Pediatrics: There are no data available for pediatric patients.

Geriatrics: In population pharmacokinetic-based data analyses, age did not have a significant effect on the disposition of temsirolimus or sirolimus metabolite.

Gender: In population pharmacokinetic-based data analyses, gender did not have a significant effect on the disposition of temsirolimus or sirolimus metabolite.

Race: In a study of ten Japanese patients (mean [range] body surface area of 1.6 m² [1.4 to 1.8 m²]), seven patients received an intravenous administration of 15 mg/m² dose of temsirolimus (24 mg [21 to 28 mg]). In these patients, the whole blood mean (SD) C_{max} was 1014 (316) ng/mL, AUC_{sum} was 11 041 (1935) ng Eq's·h/mL, and clearance was 8.48 (1.73) L/h. The total exposure level and C_{max} of temsirolimus in Japanese patients were significantly higher than those of non-Japanese patients following a 25 mg dose (see Table 3 for comparison).

Renal Cell Carcinoma: In an integrated population pharmacokinetic-based data analysis, patients with RCC exhibited an increase in apparent clearance of sirolimus of 24.8% compared to healthy subjects and patients without RCC. Temsirolimus exposure was not affected by presence or absence of RCC.

Hematocrit: In a phase II study of RCC patients treated with temsirolimus, increased hematocrit was associated with increased trough drug concentrations in the blood [for hematocrit increase from 25% to 55%, end-of-week [temsirolimus+sirolimus] whole blood trough concentrations were 2.7 to 6.0 ng/mL; peak concentrations were unaffected (691 to 678 ng/mL)].

Hepatic Insufficiency: Temsirolimus is cleared predominantly by the liver. Temsirolimus should be used with caution in patients with hepatic impairment. Dose de-escalation and multiple dose interruption were observed in patients with mild hepatic impairment primarily due to thrombocytopenia. No data are currently available regarding the influence of moderate and severe hepatic dysfunction and/or hepatic metastases on temsirolimus disposition.

For 7 patients with severe (Organ Dysfunction Working Group D) hepatic impairment receiving the 10 mg dose, temsirolimus mean AUC was ~1.7-fold higher compared to 7 patients with mild hepatic function (ODWG group B). For patients with severe hepatic impairment, a reduction of the temsirolimus dose to 10 mg is recommended to provide a degree of temsirolimus and sirolimus exposures in blood (AUC_{sum} 6580 ng·h/mL), which approximates those following the 25 mg dose (AUC_{sum} 7225 ng·h/mL) in patients with normal liver function.

Renal Insufficiency: Studies in patients with varying renal impairment have not been conducted. Caution should be taken when TORISEL is administered to patients with renal impairment.

TORISEL concentrate for injection has not been studied in patients undergoing hemodialysis.

STORAGE AND STABILITY: TORISEL (temsirolimus concentrate for injection) must be stored refrigerated (2-8°C) and protected from light.

TORISEL (temsirolimus concentrate for injection) and Diluent for TORISEL are co-packaged in a single carton, and must be stored refrigerated (2-8°C). Protect from light.

TORISEL or Diluent for TORISEL should not be used after the expiry date stated on the label.

The drug concentrate-diluent mixture is stable for up to 24 hours at controlled room temperature 20-25°C and protected from light. Any unused diluted mixture should be discarded after 24 hours.

Admixtures containing temsirolimus with 0.9% sodium chloride for injection should be used within 6 hours of preparation and should be stored at room temperature and protected from excessive light and sunlight. Any unused admixture should be discarded after 6 hours.

SPECIAL HANDLING INSTRUCTIONS: TORISEL (temsirolimus concentrate for injection) should be protected from excessive room light and sunlight during handling and preparation of admixtures. TORISEL should be inspected visually for particulate matter and discoloration following reconstitution and prior to administration. Bags/containers that come in contact with TORISEL must be made of glass, polyolefin, or polyethylene.

Once the concentrate is combined with the provided diluent, inject the mixture rapidly into 0.9% sodium chloride for injection. Administration of the final diluted infusion solution should be completed within six hours from the time that the concentrate is first diluted with the diluent.

Intravenous admixtures should be inspected visually for clarity, particulate matter, precipitate, discoloration, and leakage prior to administration. Solutions showing haziness, particulate matter, precipitate, discoloration or leakage should not be used. Discard unused portion.

INFORMATION FOR THE PATIENT: Published in e-CPS, available by subscription at www.e-cps.ca.

DOSAGE FORMS, COMPOSITION AND PACKAGING: Each mL of concentrate for injection contains: temsirolimus 25 mg. Nonmedicinal ingredients: anhydrous citric acid, dehydrated alcohol, d,l-alpha-tocopherol and propylene glycol. Vials of 1.2 mL (30 mg). DILUENT for TORISEL (temsirolimus) concentrate for injection, 1.8 mL per vial. Nonmedicinal ingredients: dehydrated alcohol (anhydrous ethanol), polyethylene glycol 400 macrogol and polysorbate 80. These two vials are co-packaged in a single carton, and must be stored at 2-8°C. Protect from light. TORISEL concentrate for injection and diluent are filled in clear glass vials with butyl rubber stoppers. A color-coded seal will be used with TORISEL concentrate for injection and with the diluent.

Tracleer® Ⓟ

bosentan monohydrate

Endothelin Receptor Antagonist

Actelion

Date of Revision: January 4, 2010

SUMMARY PRODUCT INFORMATION:

Route of Administration	Dosage Form/ Strength	Clinically Relevant Nonmedicinal Ingredients
Oral	Tablet, 62.5 mg and 125 mg bosentan (from bosentan monohydrate)	Tablet contents: cornstarch, glyceryl behenate, magnesium stearate, povidone, pregelatinized starch and sodium starch glycolate Film coating: ethylcellulose, hydroxypropylmethylcellulose, iron oxide red, iron oxide yellow, talc, titanium dioxide and triacetin This is a complete listing.

INDICATIONS AND CLINICAL USE: TRACLEER (bosentan) is indicated for the treatment of pulmonary arterial hypertension in patients with WHO functional class III or IV primary pulmonary hypertension, or pulmonary hypertension secondary to scleroderma or congenital heart disease or human immunodeficiency virus in patients who did not respond adequately to conventional therapy. As well, a prolongation of time to clinical worsening was shown in patients with WHO functional class II.

CONTRAINDICATIONS: TRACLEER is contraindicated in patients:

- who are hypersensitive to bosentan or to any excipient in the formulation. For a complete listing, see Dosage Forms, Composition and Packaging.
- who are pregnant, or of childbearing potential unless adequate contraceptive measures are taken. Fetal malformations were reported in animals (see Warnings and Precautions, Special Populations, Pregnant Women);
- with moderate or severe liver impairment and/or with baseline values of liver transaminases, i.e., aspartate aminotransferase (AST) and/or alanine aminotransferase (ALT), greater than 3 times the upper limit of normal (ULN), particularly when the total bilirubin is increased to greater than 2 times the ULN (see Warnings and Precautions, Hepatic/Biliary/Pancreatic);
- concomitant use of cyclosporine A;
- concomitant use of glyburide.

WARNINGS AND PRECAUTIONS: Hepatic/Biliary/Pancreatic: TRACLEER has been associated with a reversible, dose-related increase in aspartate aminotransferase (AST) and alanine aminotransferase (ALT), accompanied in some cases by elevated bilirubin. Increases in liver enzymes usually occurred within the first 26 weeks following initiation of treatment and returned to pretreatment levels without sequelae within a few days to 9 weeks, either spontaneously or after dose reduction or discontinuation. These increases may also occur late in treatment.

In the post-marketing period, rare cases of unexplained hepatic cirrhosis were reported after prolonged (>12 months) therapy with TRACLEER in patients with multiple co-morbidities and drug therapies. There have also been rare reports of liver failure. The contribution of TRACLEER in these cases could not be excluded.

In at least one case the initial presentation (after >20 months of treatment) included pronounced elevations in aminotransferases and bilirubin levels accompanied by non-specific symptoms, all of which resolved slowly over time after discontinuation of TRACLEER. This case reinforces the importance of strict adherence to the monthly monitoring schedule for the duration of treatment and the treatment algorithm, which includes stopping TRACLEER with a rise of aminotransferases accompanied by signs or symptoms of liver dysfunction.

Liver transaminase levels must be measured prior to initiation of treatment and subsequently at monthly intervals.

Pre-existing Liver Impairment: Use in patients with baseline values of liver transaminases, i.e., aspartate aminotransferase (AST) and/or alanine aminotransferase (ALT), greater than 3 times the upper limit of normal (ULN), particularly when the total bilirubin is increased to greater than 2 times the ULN, is contraindicated (see Contraindications).

Management of Patients with Increased Liver Transaminases:

ALT/AST Levels	Treatment and monitoring recommendations are as follows:
>3 and ≤5×ULN	**Confirm by another liver function test; if confirmed, reduce the daily dose or stop treatment, monitor aminotransferase levels at least every 2 weeks. If the aminotransferase levels return to pretreatment values consider continuing or reintroducing TRACLEER as appropriate (see Reintroduction of Treatment).**
>5 and ≤8×ULN	**Confirm by another liver function test; if confirmed, stop treatment and monitor aminotransferase levels at least every 2 weeks. Once the aminotransferase levels return to pretreatment values consider reintroducing TRACLEER (see Reintroduction of Treatment).**
>8×ULN	**Treatment must be stopped and reintroduction of TRACLEER is not to be considered.**

In the case of elevations of aminotransferases accompanied by clinical symptoms of liver injury (such as nausea, vomiting, fever, abdominal pain, jaundice or unusual lethargy or fatigue) or of increases in bilirubin ≥2×ULN, treatment must be stopped and reintroduction of TRACLEER is not to be considered.

Reintroduction of Treatment: Reintroduction of treatment with TRACLEER should only be considered if the potential benefits of treatment with TRACLEER outweigh the potential risks and when aminotransferase levels are within pretreatment values. TRACLEER is to be reintroduced at the starting dose and aminotransferase levels must then be checked within 3 days after reintroduction, then again after further 2 weeks, and thereafter according to the recommendations above.

General: Treatment with TRACLEER in patients with severe chronic heart failure was associated with an increased incidence of hospitalization due to worsening of chronic heart failure during the first 4 to 8 weeks of treatment with TRACLEER, which could have been the result of fluid retention. It is recommended that patients be monitored for signs of fluid retention (e.g., leg edema, weight gain). Should this occur, starting treatment with diuretics or increasing the existing dose of diuretics is recommended. Treatment with diuretics is recommended in patients with evidence of fluid retention before the start of treatment with TRACLEER.

Hematologic: Treatment with TRACLEER has been associated with dose-related decreases in hemoglobin concentration (0.9 g/dL overall average), which is likely due to hemodilution. In placebo-controlled studies TRACLEER-related decreases in hemoglobin concentration were not progressive, and stabilized after the first 4-12 weeks of treatment. It is recommended that hemoglobin concentrations be checked prior to the initiation of treatment, after 1 month and after 3 months, and quarterly thereafter. If a marked decrease in hemoglobin concentration occurs, further evaluation should be undertaken to determine the cause and the need for specific treatment. In the post-marketing period, cases of anemia requiring red blood cell transfusion have been reported (see Adverse Reactions, Post-Market Adverse Drug Reactions).

Cardiovascular: TRACLEER should be initiated with caution if the patient has a systemic systolic blood pressure lower than 85 mm Hg.

Special Populations: Pregnant Women: TRACLEER should be considered a potential human teratogen. TRACLEER has been shown to be teratogenic in rats when given at doses ≥60 mg/kg/day (twice the human oral therapeutic dose of 125 mg b.i.d., on a mg/m² basis). In an embryo-fetal toxicity study in rats, TRACLEER showed dose-dependent teratogenic effects including malformations of the head and face and of the major vessels. No birth defects were observed in rabbits at doses of up to 1500 mg/kg/day; however, the plasma concentrations were lower than those reached in rats. The similarity of malformations induced by TRACLEER and those observed in endothelin-1 knockout mice and in animals treated by other endothelin receptor antagonists indicates that teratogenicity is a class effect of these drugs. There are no studies in pregnant women.

TRACLEER treatment must not be initiated in women of childbearing potential unless they practice reliable contraception and the result of the pretreatment pregnancy test is negative.

Before the initiation of TRACLEER treatment in women of childbearing potential, the absence of pregnancy should be checked, appropriate advice on reliable method of contraception provided, and reliable contraception initiated. Patients and prescribers must be aware that, due to potential pharmacokinetic interactions, TRACLEER may render hormonal contraceptives ineffective (see Drug Interactions, Drug-Drug Interactions, Hormonal Contraceptives). Therefore, women of childbearing potential must not use hormonal contraceptives (including oral, injectable, transdermal, and implantable forms) as the sole method of contraception but should use an additional or an alternative reliable method of contraception. If there is any doubt on what contraceptive advice should be given to the individual patient, consultation with a gynecologist is recommended.

Because of possible hormonal contraception failure during TRACLEER treatment and also bearing in mind the risk that pulmonary hypertension severely deteriorates with pregnancy, monthly pregnancy tests during treatment with TRACLEER are recommended to allow early detection of pregnancy.

Nursing Women: It is not known whether TRACLEER is excreted in human milk. Because many drugs are excreted in human milk, nursing women taking TRACLEER should be advised to discontinue breast-feeding.

Pediatrics (3-18 years of age): The safety and efficacy of TRACLEER in children was studied in a group of 19 patients ages 3-15 years with PAH either primary or secondary to various congenital heart defects, in WHO functional class II or III. Of the 19 patients, 10 were receiving concomitant Flolan (epoprostenol). After 12 weeks of treatment with TRACLEER, efficacy could not be demonstrated based on increased exercise capacity. However, statistically significant improvements in certain hemodynamic indices were noted (mean pulmonary artery pressure, mean systemic artery pressure, pulmonary vascular resistance and pulmonary vascular resistance index, systemic vascular resistance and systemic vascular resistance index, cardiac output and stroke index). No statistically significant improvement in respiratory parameters (oxygen and CO_2) or cardiac index was present. By treatment end, five patients had improved by one functional class and one deteriorated. No new safety concerns arose during the study, though one patient was withdrawn from treatment due to increased liver transaminases.

The dosing regimen used in the study was based on body-weight:

Body Weight (kg)	Initiation Dose	Maintenance Dose
10≤×≤20	31.25 mg q.d.	31.25 mg b.i.d.
20≤×≤40	31.25 mg b.i.d.	62.5 mg b.i.d.
>40 kg	62.5 mg b.i.d.	125 mg b.i.d.

Geriatrics (>65 years of age): Limited clinical experience with TRACLEER in patients aged 65 years or older has not identified any difference in response between elderly and younger patients, but the possibility of decreased hepatic function in the elderly should be considered (see Dosage and Administration).

Monitoring and Laboratory Tests: Liver Abnormalities Management: Liver transaminase levels must be measured prior to initiation of treatment and subsequently at monthly intervals. For liver abnormalities management (see Warnings and Precautions, Hepatic/Biliary/Pancreatic).

Hemoglobin Concentrations Management: Hemoglobin concentrations should be checked prior to the initiation of treatment, after 1 month and after 3 months, and quarterly thereafter. If a marked decrease in hemoglobin concentration occurs, further evaluation should be undertaken to determine the cause and the need for specific treatment. (See Warnings and Precautions, Hematologic.)

ADVERSE REACTIONS: Clinical Trial Adverse Drug Reactions: Because clinical trials are conducted under very specific conditions the adverse reaction rates observed in the clinical trials may not reflect the rates observed in practice and should not be compared to the rates in the clinical trials of another drug. Adverse drug reaction information from clinical trials is useful for identifying drug-related adverse events and for approximating rates.

In placebo-controlled studies 258 were patients with pulmonary arterial hypertension. They received TRACLEER at doses of 250 mg (n=188) or 500 mg (n=70) per day. Safety data on TRACLEER were obtained from placebo-controlled and open-label studies in 677 patients with pulmonary arterial hypertension or other conditions. Doses up to 8 times the currently recommended maintenance dose for pulmonary arterial hypertension were administered. The duration of treatment ranged from 1 day to 4.1 years. At the recommended maintenance dose of 125 mg b.i.d., adverse events that occurred at an incidence greater than 1% in TRACLEER-treated patients with pulmonary arterial hypertension are given in Table 1.

In placebo-controlled studies of TRACLEER in the treatment of pulmonary arterial hypertension and other diseases, a total of 677 patients were treated with TRACLEER and 288 patients were treated with placebo, with doses ranging from 100 mg to 2000 mg per day. The duration of treatment ranged from four weeks to six months. Adverse events that occurred at an incidence greater than 1% in TRACLEER-treated patients are given in Table 2.

Table 1: TRACLEER

Incidence of Adverse Events, Regardless of Drug Causality, Occurring in >1% of Patients Treated with TRACLEER (125 mg b.i.d.) in Placebo-Controlled Studies in Pulmonary Arterial Hypertension

	TRACLEER n=188		Placebo n=172	
System Organ Class/Adverse Events (AEs)	**n**	**(%)**	**N**	**(%)**
All System Organ Classes				
Total patients with at least one AE	155	(82)	135	(79)
Total number of AEs	504		548	
Infections and Infestations				
Nasopharyngitis	16	(9)	14	(8)
Upper respiratory tract infection	15	(8)	11	(6)
Sinusitis	7	(4)	4	(2)
Bronchitis	6	(3)	12	(7)
Urinary tract infection	5	(3)	6	(4)
Respiratory tract infection	5	(3)	5	(3)
Influenza	4	(2)	8	(5)
Lower respiratory tract infection	3	(2)	4	(2)
Pharyngitis	3	(2)	1	(1)
Ear infection	3	(2)		
Gastrointestinal Disorders				
Nausea	15	(8)	19	(11)
Diarrhea	8	(4)	13	(8)
Abdominal pain	5	(3)	7	(4)
Vomiting	4	(2)	10	(6)
Dyspepsia	4	(2)	4	(2)
Abdominal distension	4	(2)	3	(2)
Rectal hemorrhage	4	(2)		
Constipation	3	(2)	4	(2)
Dry mouth	3	(2)	2	(1)

(cont'd)

Table 1: TRACLEER *(cont'd)*

Incidence of Adverse Events, Regardless of Drug Causality, Occurring in >1% of Patients Treated with TRACLEER (125 mg b.i.d.) in Placebo-Controlled Studies in Pulmonary Arterial Hypertension

	TRACLEER n=188		Placebo n=172	
System Organ Class/Adverse Events (AEs)	**n**	**(%)**	**N**	**(%)**
Mouth ulceration	3	(2)		
Nervous System Disorders				
Headache	24	(13)	25	(15)
Dizziness	18	(10)	23	(13)
Syncope	8	(4)	7	(4)
General Disorders and Administration Site Conditions				
Edema peripheral	15	(8)	13	(8)
Chest pain	10	(5)	8	(5)
Edema	5	(3)	4	(2)
Influenza like illness	4	(2)	2	(1)
Respiratory, Thoracic and Mediastinal Disorders				
Cough	9	(5)	14	(8)
Pulmonary hypertension	8	(4)	23	(13)
Dyspnea	6	(3)	7	(4)
Epistaxis	6	(3)	7	(4)
Hemoptysis	4	(2)	4	(2)
Dyspnea exacerbated	3	(2)	6	(4)
Dyspnea exertional	3	(2)	1	(1)
Musculoskeletal and Connective Tissue Disorders				
Back pain	7	(4)	6	(4)
Arthralgia	6	(3)	3	(2)
Muscle spasms	5	(3)	6	(4)
Shoulder pain	4	(2)	4	(2)
Investigations				
Liver function test abnormal	8	(4)	3	(2)
Hepatic enzyme increased	3	(2)		
Vascular Disorders				
Flushing	8	(4)	5	(3)
Hypotension	6	(3)	3	(2)
Cardiac Disorders				
Palpitations	6	(3)	3	(2)
Eye Disorders				
Vision blurred	3	(2)	2	(1)
Blood and Lymphatic System Disorders				
Anemia	6	(3)		
Injury, Poisoning and Procedural Complications				
Contusion	4	(2)	1	(1)

Table 2: TRACLEER

Incidence of Adverse Events, Regardless of Drug Causality, Occurring in >1% of Patients Treated with TRACLEER in Placebo-Controlled Studies

	TRACLEER n=677		Placebo n=288	
System Organ Class/Adverse Events (AEs)	**n**	**(%)**	**n**	**(%)**
All System Organ Classes				
Total patients with at least one AE	529	(78)	220	(76)
Total number of AEs	1591		840	
Blood and Lymphatic System Disorders				

(cont'd)

Table 2: TRACLEER *(cont'd)*

Incidence of Adverse Events, Regardless of Drug Causality, Occurring in >1% of Patients Treated with TRACLEER in Placebo-Controlled Studies

	TRACLEER n=677		Placebo n=288	
System Organ Class/Adverse Events (AEs)	**n**	**(%)**	**n**	**(%)**
Anemia (NOS)	23	(3)	3	(1)
Cardiac Disorders				
Angina pectoris	15	(2)	3	(1)
Cardiac failure	120	(18)	64	(22)
Edema (NOS)	16	(2)	3	(1)
Edema—legs (edema lower limb)	32	(5)	4	(1)
Palpitations	18	(3)	5	(2)
Gastrointestinal Disorders				
Abdominal pain (NOS)	13	(2)	11	(4)
Constipation	15	(2)	7	(2)
Diarrhea (NOS)	30	(4)	18	(6)
Dyspepsia	11	(2)	3	(1)
Nausea	31	(5)	30	(10)
Vomiting	16	(2)	12	(4)
General Disorders				
Chest pain (NEC)	27	(4)	20	(7)
Fatigue	14	(2)	12	(4)
Pyrexia	13	(2)	5	(2)
Hepato-biliary Disorders				
Hepatic function abnormal	40	(6)	6	(2)
Infections and Infestations				
Influenza	20	(3)	14	(5)
Metabolic and Nutritional Disorders				
Gout	12	(2)	7	(2)
Musculoskeletal, Connective Tissue and Bone Disorders				
Arthralgia	14	(2)	10	(3)
Back pain	17	(3)	8	(3)
Pain in limb	12	(2)	7	(2)
Nervous System Disorders				
Dizziness (exc. vertigo)	80	(12)	39	(14)
Headache NOS	107	(16)	37	(13)
Vision blurred	20	(3)	7	(2)
Syncope	20	(3)	12	(4)
Respiratory, Thoracic and Mediastinal Disorders				
Bronchitis	19	(3)	10	(3)
Coughing	26	(4)	13	(5)
Dyspnea (NOS)	26	(4)	14	(5)
Nasopharyngitis	23	(3)	10	(3)
Pneumonia	11	(2)	2	(1)
Sinusitis	12	(2)	5	(2)
Lower respiratory tract infection	12	(2)	5	(2)
Upper respiratory tract infection	32	(5)	18	(6)
Renal and Urinary Disorders				
Urinary tract infection	18	(3)	12	(4)
Skin and Subcutaneous Tissue Disorders				
Pruritus (NOS)	12	(2)		

(cont'd)

Table 2: TRACLEER *(cont'd)*

Incidence of Adverse Events, Regardless of Drug Causality, Occurring in >1% of Patients Treated with TRACLEER in Placebo-Controlled Studies

	TRACLEER n=677		Placebo n=288	
System Organ Class/Adverse Events (AEs)	**n**	**(%)**	**n**	**(%)**
Vascular Disorders				
Epistaxis	12	(2)	5	(2)
Flushing	45	(7)	5	(2)
Hypotension (NOS)	46	(7)	22	(8)
Postural hypotension	13	(2)	14	(5)

Legend: NOS=not otherwise specified. NEC=not elsewhere classified.

Note: The population studied included patients with pulmonary arterial hypertension as well as patients with other conditions. The doses used in some placebo-controlled studies were higher than those recommended for pulmonary arterial hypertension.

Adverse events that occurred more frequently in patients treated with TRACLEER than those treated with placebo were headache, flushing, abnormal hepatic function, anemia, and leg edema.

Less Common Clinical Trial Adverse Drug Reactions (<1%): Blood and Lymphatic System Disorders: ecchymosis, thrombocytopenia.

Cardiac Disorders: complete atrioventricular block, cardiac arrest, myocardial infarction, tachycardia, ventricular arrhythmia, ventricular tachycardia.

Eye Disorders: conjunctivitis, eye inflammation, photophobia, xerophthalmia.

Gastrointestinal Disorders: anorexia, ascites, duodenal ulcer, flatulence, gastroenteritis, mouth ulceration, intestinal obstruction, loose stools.

General Disorders: chest pain (non cardiac), feeling hot, lethargy, pain, shivering, thirst, weakness.

Immune System Disorders: anaphylactic shock, urticaria.

Infections and Infestations: infection.

Investigations: blood alkaline phosphatase increased, blood lactate dehydrogenase increased, decreased weight, hyperglycemia, hypoglycemia, increased blood urea, increased eosinophil count, prolonged coagulation time, shortened coagulation time.

Metabolism and Nutrition Disorders: dehydration, hypokalemia, hyponatremia, impaired glucose tolerance.

Musculoskeletal Disorders: gout, muscle cramps, muscle twitching, musculoskeletal pain, sensation of heaviness.

Nervous System Disorders: central nervous system depression, cerebrovascular accident, hemiparesis, hydrocephalus, hypoesthesia, insomnia, paresthesia, somnolence, tinnitus, tremor, vasovagal attack, vertigo.

Psychiatric Disorders: anxiety, disturbance in attention, irritability, increased libido, mood swings, nightmares, panic attack.

Respiratory, Thoracic and Mediastinal Disorders: aspiration, asthma, bronchospasm, hemoptysis, nasal congestion, pneumonia, respiratory depression, respiratory failure, increased sputum.

Skin and Subcutaneous Tissue Disorders: dermatitis, dry skin, eczema, erythema multiforme, erythema, skin discoloration, Stevens-Johnson syndrome, increased sweating.

Renal Disorders: cystitis, dysuria, hematuria, renal failure, renal impairment, urinary frequency, urine discoloration.

Vascular Disorders: epistaxis, hypertension, peripheral ischemia, subarachnoid hemorrhage, restless leg syndrome.

Abnormal Hematologic and Clinical Chemistry Findings: In placebo-controlled studies, increases in alanine aminotransferase (ALT) and aspartate aminotransferase (AST) to more than three times the upper limit of normal (ULN) were observed in 11% of TRACLEER-treated patients (n=658) as compared to 2% of placebo-treated patients (n=280). Increase in aminotransferases equal or greater than 3 times of ULN was seen in 12.4% of 188 patients with pulmonary arterial hypertension treated with 125 mg b.i.d. and 14% of 70 patients with pulmonary arterial hypertension treated with 250 mg b.i.d. Increase in aminotransferases equal or greater than 8 times of ULN was seen in 3.8% of patients with pulmonary arterial hypertension on 125 mg b.i.d. and 7% of patients with pulmonary arterial hypertension on 250 mg b.i.d. Increases in bilirubin to more than three times the upper limit of normal were associated with aminotransferase increases in 2 of 658 (0.3%) of patients treated with TRACLEER.

Elevations in alanine aminotransferase (ALT) and aspartate aminotransferase (AST) associated with TRACLEER are dose-dependent, occur most often early but occasionally late in treatment, usually progress slowly, are typically asymptomatic, and to date have been reversible after treatment interruption or cessation. These aminotransferase elevations may reverse spontaneously while continuing treatment with TRACLEER. In the post-marketing period, rare cases of liver cirrhosis and liver failure have been reported (see Warnings and Precautions).

In the placebo-controlled trials of all uses of TRACLEER, marked decreases in hemoglobin (>15% decrease from baseline and <11 g/dL) were observed in 6.2% of TRACLEER-treated patients as compared to 2.9% of placebo-treated patients. In patients with pulmonary arterial hypertension treated with doses of 125 mg and 250 mg b.i.d., marked decreases in hemoglobin occurred in 4.3% of patients, compared to 1.2% in placebo-treated patients.

A decrease in hemoglobin concentration by at least 1 g/dL was observed in 57% of TRACLEER-treated patients as compared to 29% of placebo-treated patients. In 80% of those patients whose hemoglobin decreased by at least 1 g/dL, the decrease occurred during the first 6 weeks of TRACLEER treatment.

During the course of treatment, the hemoglobin concentration remained within normal limits in 68% of TRACLEER-treated patients compared to 76% of placebo patients. The explanation for the change in hemoglobin is not known, but it does not appear to be hemorrhage, hemolysis or bone marrow toxicity.

In the post-marketing period, cases of anemia requiring red blood cell transfusion have been reported (see Adverse Reactions, Post-Market Adverse Drug Reactions).

It is recommended that hemoglobin concentrations be checked after 1 month and after 3 months of treatment and every 3 months thereafter.

Pulmonary Veno-Occlusive Disease: Cases of pulmonary edema have been reported with vasodilators (mainly prostacyclins) when used in patients with pulmonary veno-occlusive disease. Consequently, should signs of pulmonary edema occur when TRACLEER is administered in patients with PAH, the possibility of associated veno-occlusive disease should be considered. In the post-marketing period there have been rare reports of pulmonary edema in patients treated with TRACLEER who had a suspected diagnosis of pulmonary veno-occlusive disease.

Fluid Retention: In a placebo-controlled study, 1611 patients with severe chronic heart failure were treated with TRACLEER for a mean duration of 1.5 years. In this study there was one new safety finding that was not previously observed in the pulmonary arterial hypertension studies. This was an early increased incidence of hospitalization due to worsening of chronic heart failure with no difference in mortality between TRACLEER and placebo-treated patients. At the end of the study, there was no difference in overall hospitalizations for heart failure or in mortality between TRACLEER and placebo-treated patients. This effect was observed during the first 4-8 weeks of treatment with TRACLEER and could have been the result of fluid retention. In this trial, fluid retention was reflected by early weight gain, decreased hemoglobin concentration, and increased incidence of leg edema.

In the placebo-controlled trials with pulmonary arterial hypertension patients, peripheral edema and decreased hemoglobin concentrations were reported with no evidence for increased incidence of early hospitalization due to clinical worsening.

It is recommended that patients be monitored for signs of fluid retention (e.g., leg edema, weight gain). Should this occur, starting treatment with diuretics or increasing the existing dose of diuretics is recommended. Treatment with diuretics is recommended in patients with evidence of fluid retention before the start of treatment with TRACLEER.

Pediatric Patients: In a study in children and adolescents 17 of the 19 patients (89.5%) reported at least one adverse event. The most frequent adverse events were flushing (four patients), headache, and abnormal hepatic function (three patients each). Dizziness, fluid retention, aggravated PAH, pyrexia, and a variety of infections occurred in two patients each.

Flushing was noted only in patients also on epoprostenol. Mild fluid retention was reported for two patients and moderate edema for one, but unlike most cases in previous studies did not occur early in treatment, but rather after at least 79 days of treatment. The incidences of these and other adverse events did not appear to have any relationship to weight group.

Combination with Epoprostenol: In study AC-052-355 (BREATHE-2) in adult patients, the most frequent adverse event experienced with the combination was jaw pain (59.1% on TRACLEER+epoprostenol and 90.9% on placebo+epoprostenol), a known side effect of epoprostenol therapy. Among the events associated with TRACLEER therapy, only leg edema was more frequent on TRACLEER plus epoprostenol than placebo plus epoprostenol (27.3% vs 9.1%). Few patients in either group experienced a serious adverse event or had treatment discontinued because of an adverse event. Two patients on combination therapy died during the study from progression of disease, and another died 36 days after having been withdrawn from the study because of a worsening condition. None of the deaths were considered by the investigator to be related to treatment but rather a reflection of the natural progression of the disease.

Incidences of elevated liver aminotransferases to clinically relevant values were higher on placebo plus epoprostenol (18.2%) than on TRACLEER plus epoprostenol therapy (9.5%). Similarly, the incidences of clinically relevant decreases in hemoglobin were higher on placebo plus epoprostenol (10.0%) than on TRACLEER plus epoprostenol therapy (0%). The clinical pattern of laboratory abnormalities in the TRACLEER plus epoprostenol group was consistent with previous findings. No meaningful changes in ECG parameters were seen in either group, and no change in pulse rate was observed with TRACLEER plus epoprostenol. Decreases in blood pressures were observed in both groups, but the decrease in systolic blood pressure was smaller in the group on combination therapy than on placebo plus epoprostenol. No cases of hypotension or postural hypotension were reported on the combination therapy.

Post-Market Adverse Drug Reactions: Based on an exposure of about 49 000 patients to TRACLEER in the post-marketing period, the majority of adverse events have been similar to those reported in clinical trials.

Undesirable effects are ranked under headings of frequency using the following convention: very common (≥1/10); common (>1/100, <1/10); uncommon (>1/1000, ≤1/100); rare (>1/10 000, ≤1/1000); very rare(≤1/10 000).

Gastrointestinal Disorders: Common: nausea. Uncommon: vomiting, abdominal pain, diarrhea.

Hepato-biliary Disorders: Uncommon: aminotransferase elevations associated with hepatitis and/or jaundice. Rare: hepatic cirrhosis and liver failure (see Warnings and Precautions).

Skin and Subcutaneous Tissue Disorders: Uncommon: hypersensitivity reaction including dermatitis pruritus and rash.

Immune System: Rare: anaphylaxis and/or angioedema.

Blood and Lymphatic System Disorders: Common: anemia or hemoglobin decreases, sometimes requiring red blood cell transfusion (see Warnings and Precautions). Uncommon: thrombocytopenia. Rare: neutropenia, leucopenia.

DRUG INTERACTIONS: Overview: Cytochrome P450 System: Bosentan had no relevant inhibitory effect on cytochrome P450 isoenzymes CYP1A2, CYP2A6, CYP2B6, CYP2C8, CYP2C9, CYP2C19, CYP2D6, CYP2E1, and CYP3A4. Consequently, TRACLEER is not expected to increase plasma concentrations of drugs metabolized by these enzymes.

Bosentan is an inducer of CYP3A4 and CYP2C9. Consequently, plasma concentrations of drugs metabolized by these two isoenzymes may be decreased when TRACLEER is coadministered. Concomitant administration of both a CYP2C9 inhibitor (such as fluconazole or voriconazole) and a CYP3A4 inhibitor (such as ketoconazole, itraconazole or ritonavir) with bosentan may theoretically lead to large increases in plasma concentrations of bosentan. Coadministration of such combinations of a potent CYP2C9 inhibitor plus a CYP3A4 inhibitor with TRACLEER is not recommended.

Drug-Drug Interactions: Warfarin: Coadministration of TRACLEER 500 mg twice daily decreased plasma concentrations of both S-warfarin and R-warfarin by approximately 30%. In patients with pulmonary arterial hypertension, TRACLEER 125 mg b.i.d. had no clinically significant effect on prothrombin time/INR when administered to patients receiving chronic warfarin therapy. No additional dose adjustment should be needed for warfarin, but routine INR monitoring is recommended.

Simvastatin and Other Statins: Coadministration of TRACLEER decreased the plasma concentrations of simvastatin, and of its active β-hydroxy acid metabolite, by approximately 50%. The plasma concentrations of TRACLEER were not affected. TRACLEER is also expected to reduce plasma concentrations of other statins that have significant metabolism by CYP3A4. The possibility of reduced efficacy should be considered for these statins.

Glyburide: An increased risk of elevated transaminases was observed in patients receiving concomitant therapy with glyburide. Therefore, the concomitant administration of TRACLEER and glyburide is contraindicated, and alternative hypoglycemic agents should be considered (see Contraindications).

Coadministration of TRACLEER decreased the plasma concentrations of glyburide by approximately 40%. The plasma concentrations of TRACLEER were also decreased by approximately 30%. TRACLEER is also expected to reduce plasma concentrations of other oral hypoglycemic agents that are predominantly metabolized by CYP2C9 or CYP3A4. The possibility of worsened glucose control in patients using these agents should be considered.

Ketoconazole: Coadministration of TRACLEER and ketoconazole increased the plasma concentrations of TRACLEER by approximately 2-fold. No dose adjustment is necessary. However, increased effects of TRACLEER should be considered.

Nimodipine, Digoxin, and Losartan: TRACLEER has been shown to have no pharmacokinetic interactions with digoxin and nimodipine. Losartan has no effect on plasma levels of TRACLEER.

Cyclosporine A: Coadministration of TRACLEER decreased the blood concentrations of cyclosporine A by approximately 50%. This is most likely due to induction of CYP3A4 by TRACLEER. Initial trough concentrations of TRACLEER were approximately 30-fold higher than those measured after TRACLEER alone. However, at steady state, TRACLEER plasma concentrations were only 3- to 4-fold higher. The mechanism of this interaction is most likely inhibition of transport protein-mediated uptake of bosentan into hepatocytes by cyclosporine. The concomitant administration of TRACLEER and cyclosporine A is contraindicated (see Contraindications).

Tacrolimus and Sirolimus: No drug-interaction study was performed with tacrolimus or sirolimus but a similar interaction with cyclosporine A can be expected. It is recommended to exclude concomitant administration of TRACLEER and tacrolimus or sirolimus.

Hormonal Contraceptives: Coadministration of bosentan decreased the plasma concentrations of ethinyl estradiol and norethindrone by 31 and 14% respectively. However, decreases in exposure were as much as 56% and 66%, respectively, in individual subjects. Bosentan is also expected to reduce plasma concentrations of other contraceptive steroids that have significant metabolism by CYP3A4. Therefore, hormone-based contraceptives alone, regardless of the route of administration (i.e. oral, injectable, transdermal, and implantable forms), are not considered as reliable methods of contraception (see Warnings and Precautions, Special Populations, Pregnant Women).

Sildenafil: In healthy volunteers coadministration of TRACLEER 125 mg twice daily (steady state) with sildenafil 80 mg three times a day (steady state) resulted in a 63% decrease of the sildenafil AUC and a 50% increase of the bosentan AUC. The combination was well tolerated. A dose adjustment of neither drug is considered necessary.

Rifampicin: Coadministration of TRACLEER 125 mg twice daily for 7 days and rifampicin, a potent inducer of CYP2C9 and CYP3A4, decreased the plasma concentrations of bosentan by 58%, and this decrease could achieve almost 90% in an individual case. Therefore a significantly reduced effect of bosentan is expected when it is coadministered with rifampicin. Data on other CYP3A4 inducers, e.g. carbamazepine, phenobarbital, phenytoin and St. John's wort are lacking, but their concomitant administration is expected to lead to reduced systemic exposure to bosentan. A clinically significant reduction of efficacy cannot be excluded.

Epoprostenol: Data obtained in a study in pediatric PAH patients show that after both single- and multiple-dose administration, the C_{max} and AUC values of bosentan were similar in patients with or without continuous infusion of epoprostenol.

Antiretroviral Agents: Lopinavir+Ritonavir (and other boosted protease inhibitors): Coadministration of TRACLEER 125 mg twice daily and lopinavir+ritonavir 400+100 mg twice daily during 9.5 days in healthy volunteers, resulted in initial trough plasma concentrations, on Day 3-4 of bosentan that were approximately 48-fold higher than those measured after TRACLEER administered alone. On day 9, plasma concentrations of bosentan declined to approximately 5-fold higher than with TRACLEER administered alone. Inhibition by ritonavir of transport protein mediated uptake into hepatocytes and of CYP3A4, thereby reducing the clearance of bosentan, most likely causes this interaction. When started in patients on concomitant lopinavir+ritonavir or other ritonavir-boosted protease inhibitors, TRACLEER should be initiated at a dose of 62.5 mg once daily and the patient's tolerability of TRACLEER should be closely monitored with special attention, at the beginning of the initiation phase and 17 during titration to the maintenance dose of 125 mg twice daily, to the risk of hypotension and to liver function tests.

After coadministration of TRACLEER for 9.5 days, the plasma exposures to lopinavir and ritonavir decreased to a clinically non significant extent (by approximately 14% and 17%, respectively). However, full induction by bosentan might not have been reached and further decrease of protease inhibitors cannot be excluded. Appropriate monitoring of the HIV therapy is recommended. Similar effects would be expected with other ritonavir-boosted protease inhibitors.

Other Antiretroviral Agents: No specific recommendation can be made with regard to other available antiretroviral agents due to the lack of data. It is emphasized that due to a marked hepatotoxicity of nevirapine that could cumulate with bosentan potential impact on the liver, this combination is not recommended.

Drug-Food Interactions: Coadministration of TRACLEER with food results in small clinically irrelevant increases in C_{max} (22%) and AUC (10%). Bosentan can be given with or without food.

Drug-Herb Interactions: Interactions with herbal products have not been established.

Drug-Laboratory Test Interactions: Interactions with laboratory tests have not been established. (See Adverse Reactions, Abnormal Hematologic and Clinical Chemistry Findings.)

DOSAGE AND ADMINISTRATION: Dosing Considerations:

- Dosage in Patients with Hepatic Impairment: No dose adjustment of TRACLEER is needed in patients with mild hepatic impairment (i.e., Child-Pugh class A). Use of TRACLEER in patients with moderate or severe liver impairment is contraindicated (see Action and Clinical Pharmacology, Contraindications and Warnings and Precautions).

Recommended Dose and Dosage Adjustment: TRACLEER should be initiated at a dose of 62.5 mg twice daily for 4 weeks and then increased to the recommended maintenance dose of 125 mg twice daily. Doses above 125 mg twice daily do not confer additional benefit sufficient to offset the increased risk of liver injury.

TRACLEER should be taken morning and evening, consistently, with or without food.

- Dosage in Pediatric Patients: There is only limited experience with TRACLEER in patients under the age of 18 years (see Warnings and Precautions, Pediatrics (3-18 years of age)).
- Dosage in the Elderly: Clinical studies of TRACLEER did not include a sufficient number of patients aged 65 and over to determine if they respond differently than younger patients with pulmonary arterial hypertension. In general, dose selection for an elderly patient should be made cautiously, reflecting a possible decrease in renal and/or cardiac function, concomitant disease, other drug therapy, and, particularly, decrease in hepatic function.
- Dosage in Patients with Renal Impairment: The effect of renal impairment on the pharmacokinetics of TRACLEER is small. No dosing adjustment is required including patients undergoing dialysis.

Missed Dose: If a scheduled dose of TRACLEER is missed, a double dose should not be taken to make up for the forgotten individual dose. The patient should take the next tablet at the usual scheduled time.

Discontinuation of Treatment : There is no experience with abrupt discontinuation of TRACLEER at the recommended doses in pulmonary arterial hypertension patients. However, to avoid the possible occurrence of sudden clinical deterioration as has been seen with the discontinuation of other medications for this disease, patients should be monitored closely and reducing the dose by half for 3 to 7 days prior to discontinuation should be considered.

OVERDOSAGE:

TRACLEER has been given as a single dose of up to 2400 mg in normal volunteers, or up to 2000 mg/day for two months in patients, without any major clinical consequences. The most common side effect was headaches of mild-to-moderate intensity. In the cyclosporine A interaction study, where doses of 500 and 1000 mg of TRACLEER were given concomitantly with cyclosporine A, initial trough plasma concentrations of TRACLEER increased 30-fold resulting in severe headaches, nausea, and vomiting, but no serious adverse events occurred. Mild decreases in blood pressure and increases in heart rate were observed.

Massive overdosage may result in pronounced hypotension requiring active cardiovascular support. In the post-marketing period there was one reported overdose of 10 000 mg of TRACLEER taken by an adolescent male patient. He had symptoms of nausea, vomiting, hypotension, dizziness, sweating, blurred vision. He recovered completely within 24 hours with blood pressure support. Note: bosentan is not removed through dialysis.

> For management of a suspected drug overdose, contact your **regional Poison Control Centre**. See the *CPS Directory* section for a list of Poison Control Centres.

ACTION AND CLINICAL PHARMACOLOGY: Mechanism of Action: Bosentan is a dual endothelin receptor antagonist with affinity for both ETA and ETB receptors. Bosentan decreases both pulmonary and systemic vascular resistance, resulting in increased cardiac output without increasing heart rate.

Pharmacodynamics: The neurohormone endothelin is a potent vasoconstrictor with the ability to promote fibrosis, cell proliferation, and tissue remodeling. Endothelin concentrations in plasma and tissues are increased in a number of cardiovascular disorders, including pulmonary hypertension, suggesting a pathological role for endothelin in these diseases. In pulmonary arterial hypertension, endothelin plasma concentrations strongly correlate with poor prognosis.

Bosentan is specific for endothelin receptors. Bosentan competes with the binding of endothelin for both ETA and ETB receptors with a slightly higher affinity for ETA receptors. In animal models of pulmonary hypertension, chronic oral administration of bosentan reduced pulmonary vascular resistance and reversed pulmonary vascular and right ventricular hypertrophy. In an animal model of pulmonary fibrosis, bosentan reduced collagen deposition.

Pharmacokinetics:

Table 3: TRACLEER

Summary of Bosentan's Pharmacokinetic Parameters in Patients with Pulmonary Arterial Hypertension

	C_{max}	$t_{½}$	$AUC_{0-\infty}$
14 days (125 mg twice a day)	2286 ng/mL (1234, 3337)	2.3 h (1.0–6.0)	8912 ng·h/mL (6296, 11531)

Data are expressed as arithmetic mean (and 95% confidence limits) or, for t_{max}, as median (and range). Data were obtained from PAH patients treated for at least two weeks with the maintenance dose of 125 mg b.i.d.

Absorption: The absolute bioavailability of bosentan is approximately 50% and is unaffected by food. Maximum plasma concentrations are attained within 3-5 hours after oral administration. Pharmacokinetic data following both oral and intravenous administration in adult patients with pulmonary arterial hypertension have been obtained. The data show that the exposure to bosentan in adult pulmonary arterial hypertension patients is about 2-fold greater than in healthy adult subjects.

Distribution: The volume of distribution is about 18 L and the clearance is about 8 L/h. Bosentan is highly bound (>98%) to plasma proteins, mainly albumin. Bosentan does not penetrate into erythrocytes.

Metabolism: Bosentan is metabolized in the liver by the cytochrome P450 isoenzymes, CYP3A4 and CYP2C9. Three metabolites of bosentan were identified in human plasma. Only one metabolite, Ro 48-5033, is pharmacologically active. In adult patients, the exposure to this active metabolite is greater than in healthy subjects and it may contribute up to 25% to the effect of bosentan. In patients with evidence of the presence of cholestasis, the exposure to the active metabolite may be increased.

Excretion: Bosentan is eliminated by biliary excretion. The apparent elimination half-life ($t_{1/2}$) is 5.4 hours.

Special Populations and Conditions: Pediatrics: The pharmacokinetics of single and multiple oral doses of bosentan have been studied (see Warnings and Precautions, Special Populations, Pediatrics (3-18 years of age)) in pediatric patients with pulmonary arterial hypertension. The exposure to bosentan decreased with time in a manner consistent with the known autoinduction properties of bosentan. The mean AUC (CV%) values of bosentan in pediatric patients treated with 31.25, 62.5 or 125 mg b.i.d. were 3496 (49), 5428 (79), and 6124 (27) ng·h/mL, respectively, and were lower than the value of 8149 (47) ng·h/mL observed in adult patients receiving 125 mg b.i.d.

Geriatrics: The pharmacokinetics of bosentan have not been evaluated in patients over the age of 65 years.

Gender: No significant relationship or trend was noted between bosentan pharmacokinetic parameters and gender.

Race: The pharmacokinetics of bosentan were compared between Caucasian and Japanese subjects both after single- and multiple-dose administration. The bosentan pharmacokinetics were similar and dose-proportional in Caucasian and Japanese subjects. Other ethnic differences in bosentan pharmacokinetics have not been evaluated.

Hepatic Insufficiency: In patients with mildly impaired liver function (Child-Pugh class A) no relevant changes in the pharmacokinetics have been observed and no dose adjustment is required in these patients. The steady-state AUC of bosentan was 9% greater and the AUC of the major metabolite, Ro 48-5033, was 33% greater in patients with mild hepatic impairment than in healthy volunteers. The pharmacokinetics of bosentan have not been studied in patients with Child-Pugh class B or C hepatic impairment and bosentan is contraindicated in this patient population. (See Contraindications and Warnings and Precautions.)

Renal Insufficiency: In patients with severe renal impairment (creatinine clearance 15-30 mL/min), plasma concentrations of bosentan decreased by approximately 10%, and plasma concentrations of the three metabolites increased about 2-fold as compared to volunteers with normal renal function. No dose adjustment is required in patients with renal impairment, as less than 3% of an administered dose is excreted in urine. The degree to which bosentan is removed by hemodialysis has not been established.

STORAGE AND STABILITY: TRACLEER should be stored at room temperature between 15 and 30°C.

SPECIAL HANDLING INSTRUCTIONS: There are no special handling requirements for TRACLEER.

INFORMATION FOR THE PATIENT: Published in e-CPS, available by subscription at www.e-cps.ca.

DOSAGE FORMS, COMPOSITION AND PACKAGING: 62.5 mg: Each film-coated, round, biconvex, orange-white tablet embossed with "62,5" on one side, contains: bosentan 62.5 mg (from bosentan monohydrate). Nonmedicinal ingredients: cornstarch, glyceryl behenate, magnesium stearate, povidone, pregelatinized starch and sodium starch glycolate; film-coating: ethylcellulose, hydroxypropylmethylcellulose, iron oxide red, iron oxide yellow, talc, titanium dioxide and triacetin. Blisters of 14 tablets, carton boxes of 4 blisters.

125 mg: Each film-coated, oval, biconvex, orange-white tablet embossed with "125" on one side, contains: bosentan 125 mg (from bosentan monohydrate). Nonmedicinal ingredients: cornstarch, glyceryl behenate, magnesium stearate, povidone, pregelatinized starch and sodium starch glycolate; film-coating: ethylcellulose, hydroxypropylmethylcellulose, iron oxide red, iron oxide yellow, talc, titanium dioxide and triacetin. Blisters of 14 tablets, carton boxes of 4 blisters.

(Shown in Product Identification Section)

Tramacet™ ℞

tramadol HCl—acetaminophen

Centrally Acting Analgesic

Janssen-Ortho

Date of Preparation: July 14, 2005
Date of Revision: March 28, 2008

SUMMARY PRODUCT INFORMATION:

Route of Administration	Dosage Form/ Strength	Clinically Relevant Nonmedicinal Ingredients
Oral	37.5 mg tramadol HCl/ 325 mg acetaminophen tablets	None For a complete listing of nonmedicinal ingredients see Dosage Forms, Composition and Packaging.

INDICATIONS AND CLINICAL USE: Adults: TRAMACET (tramadol hydrochloride/acetaminophen) is indicated for the management of moderate to moderately severe pain in adults.

TRAMACET has not been systematically evaluated beyond 12 weeks in controlled clinical trials. Therefore, the physician who elects to use TRAMACET for extended periods should periodically re-evaluate the long-term usefulness of the drug for the individual patient.

TRAMACET (tramadol hydrochloride/acetaminophen) is not recommended for minor pain that may be treated adequately through lesser means.

Geriatrics (>65 years of age): No overall differences with regard to safety or pharmacokinetics were noted between subjects ≥65 years of age and younger subjects. However, dose selection for an elderly patient should be cautious, reflecting the greater frequency of decreased hepatic, renal or cardiac function, of concomitant disease and multiple drug therapy.

Pediatrics (<18 years of age): The safety and effectiveness of TRAMACET has not been studied in the pediatric population. Therefore, use of TRAMACET tablets is not recommended in patients under 18 years of age.

CONTRAINDICATIONS:

- TRAMACET (tramadol hydrochloride/acetaminophen) tablets should not be administered to patients who have previously demonstrated hypersensitivity to tramadol, acetaminophen, opioids or any other component of this product. For a complete listing of nonmedicinal ingredients, see Dosage Forms, Composition and Packaging.
- TRAMACET is contraindicated in any situation where opioids are contraindicated, including acute intoxication with any of the following: alcohol, hypnotics, narcotics, centrally acting analgesics, opioids or psychotropic drugs. TRAMACET may worsen central nervous system and respiratory depression in these patients.
- The concomitant use of TRAMACET and MAO inhibitors (or within 14 days following discontinuation of such therapy) is contraindicated.

WARNINGS AND PRECAUTIONS Seizure Risk: Seizures have been reported in patients receiving tramadol within the recommended dosage range. Spontaneous post-marketing reports indicate that seizure risk is increased with doses of tramadol above the recommended range. Concomitant use of tramadol increases the seizure risk in patients taking:

- selective serotonin reuptake inhibitors (SSRI antidepressants or anorectics) (see Use with Serotonin Reuptake Inhibitors);
- tricyclic antidepressants (TCAs) and other tricyclic compounds (e.g. cyclobenzaprine, promethazine, etc.); or
- opioids.

Administration of tramadol may enhance the seizure risk in patients taking:

- MAO inhibitors (see Contraindications);
- neuroleptics; or
- other drugs that reduce the seizure threshold.

Risk of convulsions may also increase in patients with epilepsy, those with a history of seizures or in patients with a recognized risk for seizure (such as head trauma, metabolic disorders, alcohol and drug withdrawal, CNS infections). In tramadol overdose, naloxone administration may increase the risk of seizure.

Anaphylactoid Reactions: Serious and, rarely, fatal anaphylactoid reactions have been reported in patients receiving therapy with tramadol. When these rare reactions do occur, it is often following the first dose. Other reported allergic reactions include pruritus, hives, bronchospasm, angioedema, toxic epidermal necrolysis and Stevens-Johnson syndrome. Patients with a history of anaphylactoid reactions to codeine and other opioids may be at increased risk and therefore should not receive TRAMACET tablets (see Contraindications).

Drug Abuse and Dependence: Tramadol has a potential to cause psychic and physical dependence of the morphine-type (μ-opioid). The drug has been associated with craving, drug-seeking behaviour and tolerance development. Cases of abuse and dependence on tramadol have been reported. TRAMACET tablets should not be used in opioid-dependent patients. Tramadol can re-initiate physical dependence in patients who have been previously dependent or chronically using other opioids. In patients with a tendency to abuse drugs or a history of drug dependence, and in patients who are chronically using opioids, treatment with TRAMACET is not recommended.

A Risk Management strategy to support the safe and effective use of TRAMACET under Schedule F has been established. The following are considered to be the essential components of the Risk Management strategy:

a. Commitment to not emphasize or highlight the scheduling status of TRAMACET (i.e. Schedule F of the Food and Drug Regulations; not listed under a schedule to the CDSA) in its advertising or promotional activities.
b. Inclusion of an approved fair balance statement in all TRAMACET advertising and promotional materials.
c. Provision of progress reports to TPD, MHPD and HECSB from the ongoing drug abuse surveillance program, including data from four key informant Canadian sites in the program.
d. Reassessment of the success of the risk management strategy 2 years post product launch.

Withdrawal Symptoms: Withdrawal symptoms may occur if tramadol is discontinued abruptly. These symptoms may include: anxiety, sweating, insomnia, rigors, pain, nausea, tremors, diarrhea, upper respiratory symptoms, piloerection, and rarely, hallucinations. Other symptoms that have been seen less frequently with TRAMACET discontinuation include: panic attacks, severe anxiety, and paresthesias. Clinical experience suggests that withdrawal symptoms may be relieved by reinstitution of opioid therapy followed by a gradual, tapered dose reduction of the medication combined with symptomatic support.

Intracranial Pressure or Head Trauma: TRAMACET should be used with caution in patients with increased intracranial pressure or head injury. The respiratory depressant effects of opioids include carbon dioxide retention and secondary elevation of cerebrospinal fluid pressure and may be markedly exaggerated in these patients. Additionally, pupillary changes (miosis) from tramadol may obscure the existence, extent, or course of intracranial pathology. Clinicians should also maintain a high index of suspicion for adverse drug reaction when evaluating altered mental status in these patients if they are receiving TRAMACET (see Respiratory, Respiratory Depression).

Interaction with Central Nervous System (CNS) Depressants: TRAMACET tablets should be used with caution and in reduced dosages when administered to patients receiving CNS depressants such as alcohol, opioids, anaesthetic agents, narcotics, phenothiazines, tranquilizers or sedative hypnotics. Tramadol increases the risk of CNS and respiratory depression in these patients.

Use with Alcohol: TRAMACET should not be used concomitantly with alcohol consumption. The use of TRAMACET in patients with liver disease is not recommended.

Use with MAO Inhibitors: Concomitant use of TRAMACET with MAO inhibitors is contraindicated (see Contraindications).

Animal studies have shown increased deaths with combined administration of MAO inhibitors and tramadol. Concomitant use of tramadol with MAO inhibitors increases the risk of adverse events, including seizure (see Seizure Risk and Drug Interactions) and serotonin syndrome.

Use with Serotonin Reuptake Inhibitors: Concomitant use of tramadol with SRIs increases the risk of adverse events, including seizure (see Seizure Risk) and serotonin syndrome. When coadministration of tramadol and SRIs is indicated, monitor the patient for seizures and possible early signs and symptoms of serotonin syndrome. Early symptoms of serotonin syndrome may include myoclonus, tremors, hyper-reflexia, diaphoresis, fever, tachycardia, tachypnonea, and altered mental status (agitation, excitement).

Gastrointestinal: Acute Abdominal Conditions: The administration of TRAMACET may complicate the clinical assessment of patients with acute abdominal conditions.

Hepatic/Biliary/Pancreatic: Acetaminophen may cause hepatotoxicity in situations of overdose, including intentional, unintentional, accidental, and simultaneous use of multiple acetaminophen-containing preparations, or in very rare cases, after recommended doses, although causality has not been determined. The hepatotoxic reaction can be severe and life threatening (see Overdosage).

Use in Hepatic Disease: TRAMACET has not been studied in patients with impaired hepatic function. The use of TRAMACET tablets in patients with severe hepatic impairment is not recommended.

Theoretical risk factors for acetaminophen hepatotoxicity in patients with chronic liver disease include slower metabolism of acetaminophen, increased activity of the cytochrome P450 enzyme system, or depleted glutathione stores.

Use with Other Acetaminophen-containing Products: Due to the potential for acetaminophen hepatotoxicity at doses higher than the recommended dose, TRAMACET should not be used concomitantly with other acetaminophen-containing products.

Renal: Use in Renal Disease: TRAMACET has not been studied in patients with impaired renal function. Experience with tramadol suggests that impaired renal function results in a decreased rate and extent of excretion of tramadol and its active metabolite, M1. In patients with creatinine clearances of less than 30 mL/min, it is recommended that the dosing interval of TRAMACET be increased to not exceed 2 tablets every 12 hours (see Dosage and Administration).

Respiratory: Respiratory Depression: Administer TRAMACET cautiously in patients at risk for respiratory depression. In these patients, alternative non-opioid analgesics should be considered. When large doses of tramadol are administered with anaesthetic medications or alcohol, respiratory depression may result. Respiratory depression should be treated as an overdose. If naloxone is to be administered, use cautiously because it may precipitate seizures (see Seizure Risk and Overdosage).

Carcinogenesis, Mutagenesis, Impairment of Fertility: There are no animal or laboratory studies on the combination product (tramadol and acetaminophen) to evaluate carcinogenesis, mutagenesis, or impairment of fertility.

A slight but statistically significant increase in two common murine tumours, pulmonary and hepatic, was observed in a mouse carcinogenicity study, particularly in aged mice. Mice were dosed orally up to 30 mg/kg (90 mg/m^2 or 0.5 times the maximum daily human tramadol dosage of 185 mg/m^2) for approximately two years, although the study was not done with the Maximum Tolerated Dose. This finding is not believed to suggest risk in humans. No such finding occurred in rat carcinogenicity study (dosing orally up to 30 mg/kg, 180 mg/m^2, or 1 time the maximum daily human tramadol dosage).

Tramadol was not mutagenic in the following assays: Ames Salmonella microsomal activation test, CHO/HPRT mammalian cell assay, mouse lymphoma assay (in the absence of metabolic activation), dominant lethal mutation tests in mice, chromosome aberration test in Chinese hamsters, and bone marrow micronucleus tests in mice and Chinese hamsters. Weakly mutagenic results occurred in the presence of metabolic activation in the mouse lymphoma assay and micronucleus test in rats. Overall, the weight of evidence from these tests indicates that tramadol does not pose a genotoxic risk to humans.

No effects on fertility were observed for tramadol at oral dose levels up to 50 mg/kg (350 mg/m^2) in male rats and 75 mg/kg (450 mg/m^2) in female rats. These dosages are 1.6 and 2.4 times the maximum daily human tramadol dosage of 185 mg/m^2.

No drug-related teratogenic effects were observed in the progeny of rats treated orally with tramadol and acetaminophen. The tramadol/acetaminophen combination product was shown to be embryotoxic and fetotoxic in rats at a maternally toxic dose, 50/434 mg/kg tramadol/acetaminophen (300/2604 mg/m^2 or 1.6 times the maximum daily human tramadol/acetaminophen dosage of 185/1591 mg/m^2), but was not teratogenic at this dose level. Embryo and fetal toxicity consisted of decreased fetal weights and increased supernumerary ribs.

Tramadol alone was evaluated in peri- and post-natal studies in rats. Progeny of dams receiving oral (gavage) dose levels of 50 mg/kg (300 mg/m^2 or 1.6 times the maximum daily human tramadol dosage) or greater had decreased weights, and pup survival was decreased early in lactation at 80 mg/kg (480 mg/m^2 or 2.6 times the maximum daily human tramadol dosage).

Use in Ambulatory Patients: TRAMACET may impair mental or physical abilities required for the performance of potentially hazardous tasks such as driving a car or operating machinery.

Special Populations: Pregnant Women: There are no adequate and well-controlled studies in pregnant women. TRAMACET should be used during pregnancy only if the potential benefit justifies the potential risk to the fetus. Neonatal seizures, neonatal withdrawal syndrome, fetal death and stillbirth have been reported with tramadol hydrochloride during post-marketing.

TRAMACET should not be used in pregnant women prior to or during labor unless the potential benefits outweigh the risks. Safe use in pregnancy has not been established. Chronic use during pregnancy may lead to physical dependence and post-partum withdrawal symptoms in the newborn (see Drug Abuse and Dependence). Tramadol has been shown to cross the placenta. The mean ratio of serum tramadol in the umbilical veins compared to maternal veins was 0.83 for 40 women given tramadol during labor.

The effect of TRAMACET, if any, on the later growth, development, and functional maturation of the child is unknown.

Nursing Women: TRAMACET is not recommended for obstetrical pre-operative medication or for post-delivery analgesia in nursing mothers because its safety in infants and newborns has not been studied.

Following a single 100 mg i.v. dose of tramadol, the cumulative excretion in breast milk within 16 hours post-dose was 100 μg of tramadol (0.1% of the maternal dose) and 27 μg of M1.

Pediatrics (<18 years of age): The safety and effectiveness of TRAMACET has not been studied in the pediatric population. Therefore, use of TRAMACET tablets is not recommended in patients under 18 years of age.

Geriatrics (>65 years of age): In general, dose selection for an elderly patient should be cautious, reflecting the greater frequency of decreased hepatic, renal or cardiac function; of concomitant disease and multiple drug therapy.

ADVERSE REACTIONS: Clinical Trial Adverse Drug Reactions: Because clinical trials are conducted under very specific conditions the adverse reaction rates observed in the clinical trials may not reflect the rates observed in practice and should not be compared to the rates in the clinical trials of another drug. Adverse drug reaction information from clinical trials is useful for identifying drug-related adverse events and for approximating rates.

TRAMACET (tramadol hydrochloride/acetaminophen) tablets were administered to 1597 patients during the double-blind or open-label extension periods in studies of chronic non-malignant pain. Of these patients, 539 were 65 years old or older. The most frequently reported events were in the central nervous and gastrointestinal systems. These are common effects associated with other drugs with opioid agonist activity. See Table 1.

Table 1: TRAMACET

Treatment-emergent Adverse Events Reported in at Least 2% of TRAMACET Patients with Chronic Pain[a] and an Incidence Greater Than with Placebo

Body System Adverse Events	TRAMACET (N=481) %	Placebo (N=479) %
Body As a Whole		
Fatigue	7	2
Hot Flushes	2	0
Influenza-Like Symptoms	3	2
Cardiovascular Disorders		
Hypertension	3	1
Central and Peripheral Nervous System Disorders		
Headache	15	10
Dizziness	11	4
Hypoaesthesia	2	0
Gastro-Intestinal System Disorders		
Nausea	18	5

(cont'd)

Table 1: TRAMACET *(cont'd)*

Treatment-emergent Adverse Events Reported in at Least 2% of TRAMACET Patients with Chronic Pain[a] and an Incidence Greater Than with Placebo

Body System Adverse Events	TRAMACET (N=481) %	Placebo (N=479) %
Constipation	16	5
Mouth Dry	8	1
Vomiting	5	1
Abdominal Pain	5	4
Diarrhoea	5	3
Psychiatric Disorders		
Somnolence	14	2
Insomnia	5	1
Anorexia	4	1
Nervousness	2	0
Skin and Appendages Disorders		
Pruritus	6	1
Sweating Increased	4	0
Rash	3	1

[a] In placebo controlled trials of three months in duration.

Incidence at Least 1%—Causal Relationship at Least Possible or Greater: The following lists treatment-emergent adverse reactions that occurred with an incidence of at least 1% in clinical trials with a population of 2836 tramadol/acetaminophen-exposed subjects in the 18 acute and chronic pain studies combined.
Body as a Whole: asthenia, fatigue, hot flushes.
Central and Peripheral Nervous System: dizziness, headache, tremor.
Gastrointestinal System: abdominal pain, constipation, diarrhea, dyspepsia, flatulence, dry mouth, nausea, vomiting.
Psychiatric Disorders: anorexia, anxiety, confusion, euphoria, insomnia, nervousness, somnolence.
Skin and Appendages: pruritus, rash, increased sweating.

Among these, the most common (≥5% of subjects) treatment-emergent adverse events were nausea (14%), dizziness (10%), somnolence (9%), constipation (8%), vomiting (5%), and headache (5%). These data are consistent with data presented in Table 1.

Clinically Relevant Treatment-Emergent Adverse Events Occurring at Less than 1%: The following lists clinically relevant treatment-emergent adverse reactions that occurred with an incidence of less than 1% in tramadol/acetaminophen clinical trials.
Body as a Whole: chest pain, rigors, syncope, withdrawal syndrome, allergic reaction.
Cardiovascular Disorders: hypertension, aggravated hypertension, hypotension, dependent edema.
Central and Peripheral Nervous System: ataxia, convulsions, hypertonia, migraine, aggravated migraine, involuntary muscle contractions, paresthesia, stupor, vertigo.
Gastrointestinal System: dysphagia, melena, tongue edema.
Hearing and Vestibular Disorders: tinnitus.
Heart Rate and Rhythm Disorders: arrhythmia, palpitation, tachycardia.
Liver and Biliary System: abnormal hepatic function, ALT increased, AST increased.
Metabolic and Nutritional Disorders: weight decrease, hypoglycemia, increased alkaline phosphatase, weight increase.
Musculoskeletal System Disorders: arthralgia.
Platelets, Bleeding and Clotting Disorders: increased coagulation time, purpura.
Psychiatric Disorders: amnesia, depersonalisation, depression, drug abuse, emotional lability, hallucination, impotence, bad dreams, abnormal thinking.
Red Blood Cell Disorders: anemia.
Respiratory System: dyspnea, bronchospasm.
Skin and Appendages Disorders: dermatitis, erythematous rash.
Urinary System: albuminuria, micturition disorder, oliguria, urinary retention.
Vision Disorders: abnormal vision.
White Cell and RES Disorders: granulocytopenia and leukocytosis.

Other Clinically Significant Adverse Experiences Previously Reported in Clinical Trials or Post-marketing Reports with Tramadol Hydrochloride: Other events which have been reported with the use of tramadol products and for which a causal association has not been determined include: vasodilation, orthostatic hypotension, myocardial ischemia, pulmonary edema, allergic reactions (including anaphylaxis and urticaria, Stevens-Johnson syndrome/TENS), cognitive dysfunction, difficulty concentrating, depression, suicidal tendency, hepatitis liver failure and gastrointestinal bleeding. Reported laboratory abnormalities included elevated creatinine and liver function tests. Serotonin syndrome (whose symptoms may include mental status change, hyperreflexia, fever, shivering, tremor, agitation, diaphoresis, seizures and coma) has been reported with tramadol when used concomitantly with other serotonergic agents such as SSRIs and MAOIs.

Other Clinically Significant Adverse Experiences Previously Reported in Clinical Trials or Post-marketing Reports with Acetaminophen: Allergic reactions (primarily skin rash) or reports of hypersensitivity secondary to acetaminophen are rare and generally controlled by discontinuation of the drug and, when necessary, symptomatic treatment. There have been several reports that suggest that acetaminophen may produce hypoprothrombinemia when administered with warfarin-like compounds. In other studies, prothrombin time did not change.

Drug Abuse and Dependence: Tramadol may induce psychic and physical dependence of the morphine-type (μ-opioid) (see Warnings and Precautions, Drug Abuse and Dependence). Dependence and abuse, including drug-seeking behaviour and taking illicit actions to obtain the drug are not limited to those patients with a prior history of opioid dependence. The risk in patients with substance abuse has been observed to be higher. Tramadol is associated with craving and tolerance development.

A Risk Management strategy to support the safe and effective use of TRAMACET under Schedule F has been established. The following are considered to be the essential components of the Risk Management strategy:

a. Commitment to not emphasize or highlight the scheduling status of TRAMACET (i.e. Schedule F of the Food and Drug Regulations; not listed under a schedule to the CDSA) in its advertising or promotional activities.
b. Inclusion of an approved fair balance statement in all TRAMACET advertising and promotional materials.
c. Provision of progress reports to TPD, MHPD and HECSB from the ongoing drug abuse surveillance program, including data from four key informant Canadian sites in the program.
d. Reassessment of the success of the risk management strategy 2 years post product launch.

Withdrawal Symptoms: Withdrawal symptoms may occur if tramadol is discontinued abruptly. These symptoms may include: anxiety, sweating, insomnia, rigors, pain, nausea, tremors, diarrhea, upper respiratory symptoms, piloerection, and rarely, hallucinations. Other symptoms that have been seen less frequently with TRAMACET discontinuation include: panic attacks, severe anxiety, and paresthesias. Clinical experience suggests that withdrawal symptoms may be relieved by reinstitution of opioid therapy followed by a gradual, tapered dose reduction of the medication combined with symptomatic support.

DRUG INTERACTIONS: Overview: In vitro studies indicate that tramadol is unlikely to inhibit the CYP3A4-mediated metabolism of other drugs when tramadol is administered concomitantly at therapeutic doses. Tramadol does not appear to induce its own metabolism in humans, since observed maximal plasma concentrations after multiple oral doses are higher than expected based on single dose data. Tramadol is a mild inducer of selected drug metabolism pathways measured in animals.
Drug-Drug Interactions: Use with Carbamazepine: Patients taking carbamazepine may have a significantly reduced analgesic effect of tramadol. Because carbamazepine increases tramadol metabolism and because of the seizure risk associated with tramadol, concomitant administration of TRAMACET and carbamazepine is not recommended.
Use with Quinidine: Tramadol is metabolized to M1 by the CYP2D6 P450 isoenzyme. Quinidine is a selective inhibitor of that isoenzyme, so that concomitant administration of quinidine and tramadol results in increased concentrations of tramadol and reduced concentrations of M1. The clinical consequences of these findings are unknown. In vitro drug interaction studies in human liver microsomes indicate that tramadol has no effect on quinidine metabolism.
Use with Inhibitors of CYP2D6: In vitro drug interaction studies in human liver microsomes indicate that concomitant administration with inhibitors of CYP2D6 such as fluoxetine, paroxetine and amitriptyline could result in some inhibition of the metabolism of tramadol.
Use with Cimetidine: Concomitant administration of TRAMACET and cimetidine has not been studied. Concomitant administration of tramadol and cimetidine does not result in clinically significant changes in tramadol pharmacokinetics. Therefore, no alteration of the TRAMACET dosage regimen is recommended.
Use with MAO Inhibitors: TRAMACET is contraindicated in patients receiving MAO inhibitors or who have used them within the previous 14 days (see Contraindications, Warnings and Precautions).
Use with Digoxin: Postmarketing surveillance of tramadol has revealed rare reports of digoxin toxicity.
Use with Warfarin-like Compounds: Post-marketing surveillance of both tramadol and acetaminophen individual products have revealed rare alterations of warfarin effect, including elevation of prothrombin times.

While such changes have been generally of limited clinical significance for the individual products, periodic evaluation of prothrombin time should be performed when TRAMACET tablets and warfarin-like compounds are administered concurrently.
Drug-Food Interactions: When TRAMACET was administered with food, the time to peak plasma concentration was delayed for approximately 35 minutes for tramadol and almost one hour for acetaminophen. However, peak plasma concentration and the extent of absorption of either tramadol or acetaminophen were not affected. The clinical significance of this difference is unknown.

DOSAGE AND ADMINISTRATION: Dosing Considerations: TRAMACET (tramadol hydrochloride/acetaminophen) is not recommended for minor pain that may be treated adequately through lesser means where benefit does not outweigh the possible opioid-related side effects.

Do not co-administer TRAMACET tablets with other acetaminophen- or tramadol-containing products.

TRAMACET can be administered without regard to food.

The recommended dose of TRAMACET (tramadol hydrochloride/acetaminophen) should not be exceeded.
Recommended Dose and Dosage Adjustment: Adults: For the management of pain, the recommended dose of TRAMACET is 1 or 2 tablets every 4 to 6 hours as needed for pain relief up to a maximum of 8 tablets per day.

A titration period of several days with gradual dose increases at the initiation of TRAMACET therapy may be beneficial for some patients. Clinical studies with tramadol in patients with moderate to moderately severe chronic pain indicate that tolerability of tramadol can be improved by starting tramadol at a low dose with gradual upward dose titration to reach doses that provide sufficient pain relief.
Use in Renal Impairment: In patients with creatinine clearances of less than 30 mL/min, it is recommended that the dosing interval of TRAMACET be increased to not exceed 2 tablets every 12 hours.
Use in the Elderly: No overall differences with regard to safety or pharmacokinetics were noted between subjects ≥65 years of age and younger subjects. However, dose selection for an elderly patient should be cautious, in view of the greater frequency of decreased hepatic, renal or cardiac function, concomitant disease or drug therapy, and the potential for greater sensitivity to adverse events.
Pediatric Use: The safety and effectiveness of TRAMACET has not been studied in the pediatric population. Therefore, use of TRAMACET is not recommended in patients under 18 years of age.
Discontinuation: Withdrawal symptoms may occur if TRAMACET is discontinued abruptly. These symptoms may include: anxiety, sweating, insomnia, rigors, pain, nausea, tremors, diarrhea, upper respiratory symptoms, piloerection, and rarely, hallucinations. Other symptoms that have been seen less frequently with TRAMACET discontinuation include: panic attacks, severe anxiety, and paresthesias. Clinical experience suggests that withdrawal symptoms may be avoided by tapering TRAMACET at the time of discontinuation (see Drug Abuse and Dependence, Withdrawal Symptoms).

OVERDOSAGE:
TRAMACET is a combination product. The clinical presentation of overdose may include the signs and symptoms of tramadol toxicity, acetaminophen toxicity or both.
Tramadol: Serious potential consequences of overdosage are respiratory depression, lethargy, coma, seizure, cardiac arrest and death. Fatalities have been reported in post-marketing in association with both intentional and unintentional overdose with tramadol. The initial symptoms of tramadol overdosage may include respiratory depression and/or seizures. In treating an overdose, primary attention should be given to maintaining adequate ventilation along with general supportive treatment.
Acetaminophen: Serious potential consequences of overdosage with acetaminophen are hepatic centrilobular necrosis, leading to hepatic failure and death. Renal tubular necrosis, hypoglycemia and coagulation defects also may occur. The initial symptoms seen within the first 24 hours following an acetaminophen overdose are: anorexia, nausea, vomiting, malaise, pallor and diaphoresis. Clinical and laboratory evidence of hepatic toxicity may not be apparent until 48 to 72 hours post-ingestion. Emergency help should be sought immediately and treatment initiated immediately if overdose is suspected, even if symptoms are not apparent.
Treatment of Overdose: A single or multiple overdose with TRAMACET may be a potentially lethal polydrug overdose, and consultation with a regional poison control centre is recommended. In treating an overdose of TRAMACET, primary attention should be given to maintaining adequate ventilation along with general supportive treatment. While naloxone will reverse some, but not all, symptoms caused by overdosage with tramadol, the risk of seizures is also increased with naloxone administration. In animals, convulsions following the administration of toxic doses of tramadol could be suppressed with barbiturates or benzodiazepines but were increased with naloxone. Naloxone administration did not change the lethality of an overdose in mice. Based on experience with tramadol, hemodialysis is not expected to be helpful in an overdose because it removes less than 7% of the administered dose in a 4-hour dialysis period.

Standard recommendations should be followed for the treatment of acetaminophen overdose.

For management of a suspected drug overdose, CPhA recommends that you contact your **regional Poison Control Centre**. See the *CPS* Directory section for a list of Poison Control Centres.

ACTION AND CLINICAL PHARMACOLOGY: Mechanism of Action: Tramadol: Tramadol is a centrally acting synthetic opioid analgesic. Although its mode of action is not completely understood, from animal tests, at least two complementary mechanisms appear applicable: binding of parent and M1 metabolite to μ-opioid receptors and weak inhibition of reuptake of norepinephrine and serotonin.

Opioid activity is due to both low affinity binding of the parent compound and higher affinity binding of the O-demethylated metabolite M1 to μ-opioid receptors. In animal models, M1 is up to 6 times more potent than tramadol in producing analgesia and 200 times more potent in μ-opioid binding. Tramadol-induced analgesia is only partially antagonized by the opiate antagonist naloxone in several animal tests. The relative contribution of both tramadol and M1 to human analgesia is dependent upon the plasma concentrations of each compound (see Pharmacokinetics).

Tramadol has been shown to inhibit reuptake of norepinephrine and serotonin in vitro, as have some other opioid analgesics. These mechanisms may contribute independently to the overall analgesic profile of tramadol.

Apart from analgesia, tramadol administration may produce a constellation of symptoms (including dizziness, somnolence, nausea, constipation, sweating and pruritus) similar to that of opioids. In contrast to morphine, tramadol has not been shown to cause histamine release. At therapeutic doses, tramadol has no effect on heart rate, left-ventricular function or cardiac index. Orthostatic hypotension has been observed.
Acetaminophen: Acetaminophen is a non-opiate, non-salicylate analgesic.
Tramadol/Acetaminophen Combination: When evaluated in a standard animal model, the combination of tramadol and acetaminophen exhibited a synergistic effect. That is, when tramadol and acetaminophen were administered together, significantly less of each drug was needed to produce a given analgesic effect than would be expected if their effects were

merely additive. Tramadol reaches peak activity in 2 to 3 hours with a prolonged analgesic effect, so that its combination with acetaminophen, a rapid-onset, short-acting analgesic agent, provides substantial benefit to patients over either component alone.

Pharmacokinetics: Tramadol is administered as a racemate and both the (−) and (+) forms of both tramadol and M1 are detected in the circulation. The pharmacokinetics of plasma tramadol and acetaminophen following oral administration of one tablet are shown in Table 2. Tramadol has a slower absorption and longer half-life when compared to acetaminophen.

Table 2: TRAMACET

Summary of Mean (±SD) Pharmacokinetic Parameters of the (+) and (−) Enantiomers of Tramadol and M1, and Acetaminophen Following a Single Oral Dose of One Tramadol/Acetaminophen Combination Tablet (37.5 mg/325 mg) in Volunteers

Parameter[a]	(+)-Tramadol	(−)-Tramadol	(+)-M1	(−)-M1	Acetaminophen
C_{max} (ng/mL)	64.3 (9.3)	55.5 (8.1)	10.9 (5.7)	12.8 (4.2)	4.2 (0.8)
t_{max} (h)	1.8 (0.6)	1.8 (0.7)	2.1 (0.7)	2.2 (0.7)	0.9 (0.7)
CL/F (mL/min)	588 (226)	736 (244)	—	—	365 (84)
$t_{½}$ (h)	5.1 (1.4)	4.7 (1.2)	7.8 (3.0)	6.2 (1.6)	2.5 (0.6)

[a] For acetaminophen, C_{max} was measured as μg/mL.

A single dose pharmacokinetic study of TRAMACET in volunteers showed no drug interactions between tramadol and acetaminophen. Upon multiple oral dosing to steady state, however, the bioavailability of tramadol and metabolite M1 was lower for the combination tablets compared to tramadol administered alone. The decrease in AUC was 14% for (+)-tramadol, 10.4% for (−)-tramadol, 11.9% for (+)-M1 and 24.2% for (−)-M1. The cause of this reduced bioavailability is not clear. Following single or multiple dose administration of TRAMACET, no significant change in acetaminophen pharmacokinetics was observed when compared to acetaminophen given alone.

Absorption: The absolute bioavailability of tramadol from TRAMACET tablets has not been determined. Tramadol hydrochloride has a mean absolute bioavailability of approximately 75% following administration of a single 100 mg oral dose of tramadol HCl tablets. The mean peak plasma concentration of racemic tramadol and M1 after administration of two TRAMACET tablets occurs at approximately two and three hours, respectively, post-dose.

Peak plasma concentrations of acetaminophen occur within one hour and are not affected by coadministration with tramadol. Oral absorption of acetaminophen following administration of TRAMACET occurs primarily in the small intestine.

Food Effects: When TRAMACET was administered with food, the time to peak plasma concentration was delayed for approximately 35 minutes for tramadol and almost one hour for acetaminophen. However, peak plasma concentration and the extent of absorption of either tramadol or acetaminophen were not affected. The clinical significance of this difference is unknown.

Distribution: The volume of distribution of tramadol was 2.6 and 2.9 L/kg in male and female subjects, respectively, following a 100 mg intravenous dose. The binding of tramadol to human plasma proteins is approximately 20%, and binding also appears to be independent of concentration up to 10 μg/mL. Saturation of plasma protein binding occurs only at concentrations outside the clinically relevant range.

Acetaminophen appears to be widely distributed throughout most body tissues except fat. Its apparent volume of distribution is about 0.9 L/kg. A relatively small portion (~20%) of acetaminophen is bound to plasma protein.

Metabolism: Following oral administration, tramadol is extensively metabolized by a number of pathways, including CYP2D6 and CYP3A4, as well as by conjugation of parent and metabolites. Approximately 30% of the dose is excreted in the urine as unchanged drug, whereas 60% of the dose is excreted as metabolites. The major metabolic pathways appear to be N- and O-demethylation and glucuronidation or sulfation in the liver. Metabolite M1 (O-desmethyltramadol) is pharmacologically active in animal models. Formation of M1 is dependent on CYP2D6 and as such is subject to inhibition, which may affect the therapeutic response (see Drug Interactions).

Approximately 7% of the population has reduced activity of the CYP2D6 isoenzyme of cytochrome P450. These individuals are "poor metabolizers" of debrisoquine, dextromethorphan, and tricyclic antidepressants, among other drugs. Based on a population PK analysis of Phase I studies in healthy subjects, concentrations of tramadol were approximately 20% higher in "poor metabolizers" versus "extensive metabolizers", while M1 concentrations were 40% lower. In vitro drug interaction studies in human liver microsomes indicate that inhibitors of CYP2D6 such as fluoxetine and its metabolite norfluoxetine, amitriptyline and quinidine inhibit the metabolism of tramadol to various degrees. The full pharmacological impact of these alterations in terms of either efficacy or safety is unknown. Concomitant use of serotonin reuptake inhibitors and MAO inhibitors may enhance the risk of adverse events, including seizure (see Warnings and Precautions) and serotonin syndrome.

Acetaminophen is primarily metabolized in the liver by first-order kinetics and involves three principal separate pathways:

a. conjugation with glucuronide;
b. conjugation with sulfate; and
c. oxidation via the cytochrome, P450-dependent, mixed-function oxidase enzyme pathway to form a reactive intermediate metabolite, which conjugates with glutathione and is then further metabolized to form cysteine and mercapturic acid conjugates. The principal cytochrome P450 isoenzyme involved appears to be CYP2E1, with CYP1A2 and CYP3A4 additional pathways.

In adults, the majority of acetaminophen is conjugated with glucuronic acid and, to a lesser extent, with sulfate. These glucuronide-, sulfate- and glutathione-derived metabolites lack biologic activity. In premature infants, newborns and young infants, the sulfate conjugate predominates.

Elimination: Tramadol is eliminated primarily through metabolism by the liver and the metabolites are eliminated primarily by the kidneys. The plasma elimination half-lives of racemic tramadol and M1 are approximately 5-6 and 7 hours, respectively, after administration of TRAMACET. The apparent plasma elimination half-life of racemic tramadol increased to 7-9 hours upon multiple dosing of TRAMACET.

The half-life of acetaminophen is about 2 to 3 hours in adults. It is somewhat shorter in children and somewhat longer in neonates and in cirrhotic patients. Acetaminophen is eliminated from the body primarily by formation of glucuronide and sulfate conjugates in a dose-dependent manner. Less than 9% of acetaminophen is excreted unchanged in the urine.

Special Populations and Conditions: Renal Insufficiency: The pharmacokinetics of TRAMACET in patients with renal impairment have not been studied. Based on studies using tramadol alone, excretion of tramadol and metabolite M1 is reduced in patients with creatinine clearance of less than 30 mL/min, adjustment of dosing regimen in this patient population is recommended. The total amount of tramadol and M1 removed during a 4-hour dialysis period is less than 7% of the administered dose based on studies using tramadol alone (see Warnings and Precautions and Dosage and Administration).

Hepatic Insufficiency: The pharmacokinetics and tolerability of TRAMACET in patients with impaired hepatic function has not been studied. Since tramadol and acetaminophen are both extensively metabolized by the liver, the use of TRAMACET tablets in patients with hepatic impairment is not recommended (see Warnings and Precautions and Dosage and Administration).

Geriatrics: A population pharmacokinetic analysis of data obtained from a clinical trial in patients with chronic pain treated with TRAMACET which included 55 patients between 65 and 75 years of age and 19 patients over 75 years of age, showed no significant changes in pharmacokinetics of tramadol and acetaminophen in elderly patients with normal renal and hepatic function.

Gender: Tramadol clearance was 20% higher in female subjects compared to males on four Phase I studies of TRAMACET in 50 male and 34 female healthy subjects. The clinical significance of this difference is unknown.

Pediatrics: Pharmacokinetics of TRAMACET tablets have not been studied in pediatric patients below 18 years of age.

STORAGE AND STABILITY: Dispense in a tight container. Store at 15-30°C.

INFORMATION FOR THE PATIENT: Published in e-CPS, available by subscription at www.e-cps.ca.

DOSAGE FORMS, COMPOSITION AND PACKAGING: Each light yellow, film-coated, capsule-shaped tablet, engraved "J-C" on one side and "T/P" on the other side, contains: tramadol HCl 37.5 mg and acetaminophen 325 mg. Nonmedicinal ingredients: carnauba wax, hypromellose, magnesium stearate, polyethylene glycol, polysorbate 80, powdered cellulose, pregelatinized starch, sodium starch glycolate, starch, titanium dioxide and yellow iron oxide. PVC or PP blisters of 10.

(Shown in Product Identification Section)

Tramadol

CPhA Monograph

see *Opioids*

Trandate®

labetalol HCl

Antihypertensive

Paladin

Date of Revision: August 12, 2009

PHARMACOLOGY: Labetalol is an adrenergic receptor blocking agent possessing both $alpha_1$-(post-synaptic) and beta-receptor blocking activity. Its action on beta-receptors is 4 times stronger than that on alpha-receptors. It antagonizes $beta_1$- and $beta_2$-receptors equally.

The mechanism of the antihypertensive action of labetalol has not been fully established. It is considered that labetalol lowers blood pressure by partially blocking the alpha-adrenoreceptors in the peripheral arterioles, thus causing vasodilation and a resulting reduction of peripheral resistance. At the same time, blockade of the beta-adrenoreceptors in the myocardium prevents reflex tachycardia and subsequent elevation of cardiac output. Peripheral vasodilation is achieved with incomplete blockade of alpha-adrenoreceptors in the arterioles and the barostatic reflexes remain sufficiently active to reduce the incidence of postural hypotension.

At rest labetalol slightly reduces the heart rate, increases the stroke volume but does not significantly affect cardiac output. It reduces exercise-induced increases in systolic pressure and heart rate, again without significantly influencing cardiac output.

Following oral administration to hypertensive patients, labetalol decreases plasma renin activity and aldosterone levels, both at rest and during exercise, particularly when these were elevated prior to treatment. It is significantly more efficacious in hypertensive patients with high baseline plasma noradrenaline levels.

Labetalol is well absorbed from the gastrointestinal tract with peak blood levels occurring 1 to 2 hours after oral dosing. A single oral dose of 200 mg produced average peak plasma levels of 360 μg/100 mL. The drug undergoes extensive first pass metabolism following oral administration. The bioavailability of oral compared to i.v. labetalol is approximately 25%. When taken with food, the bioavailability of unchanged drug is increased although peak plasma levels remain the same. The drug is metabolized mostly by conjugation with glucuronic acid; the resulting metabolite is inactive. Rapid and extensive distribution within tissue compartments occurs after i.v. administration. The drug is approximately 50% bound to plasma proteins. Labetalol and its metabolites are rapidly excreted in urine, and via bile into the feces. The plasma half-life of labetalol is approximately 6 to 8 hours following oral administration.

Labetalol produces a significant fall in blood pressure in 1 to 4 hours after the first oral dose. The maximum blood pressure lowering effect at any particular dose level is usually achieved within 24 to 72 hours.

In a clinical pharmacologic study in severe hypertensives, an initial 0.25 mg/kg injection of labetalol administered to patients in the supine position decreased blood pressure by an average of 11/7 mm Hg. Additional injections of 0.5 mg/kg at 15-minute intervals up to a total cumulative dose of 1.75 mg/kg of labetalol caused further dose-related decreases in blood pressure. Some patients required cumulative doses of up to 3.25 mg/kg. The maximal effect of each dose level occurred within 5 minutes. Following discontinuation of i.v. treatment with labetalol, the blood pressure rose gradually and progressively, approaching pretreatment baseline values within an average of 16 to 18 hours in the majority of patients.

Similar results were obtained in the treatment of patients with severe hypertension requiring urgent blood pressure reduction with an initial dose of 20 mg (which corresponds to 0.25 mg/kg for an 80 kg patient) followed by additional doses of either 40 mg or 80 mg at 10-minute intervals to achieve the desired effect or up to a cumulative dose of 300 mg.

INDICATIONS: For treatment of hypertension. Labetalol is usually used in combination with other drugs, particularly a thiazide diuretic. However, it may be tried alone as an initial agent in those patients in whom, in the judgement of the physician, treatment should be started with an alpha-beta-blocker rather than with a diuretic. Labetalol may be used in combination with diuretics and/or other antihypertensive agents to treat severe hypertension.

The combination of labetalol with a diuretic has been found to be compatible. Limited experience with other antihypertensive agents has not shown evidence of incompatibility with labetalol.

CONTRAINDICATIONS: Uncontrolled congestive heart failure (see Warnings); asthma or a history of obstructive lung disease; greater than first degree AV block; cardiogenic shock and states of hypoperfusion; sinus bradycardia; known sensitivity to labetalol.

WARNINGS: Cardiac failure should be controlled with digitalis and diuretics before labetalol treatment is initiated. Labetalol should not be given to patients with digitalis-resistant heart failure. Sympathetic stimulation is a vital component supporting circulatory function in congestive heart failure and inhibition with beta-blockade always carries the potential hazard of further depressing myocardial contractibility and precipitating cardiac failure. A few patients developed heart failure while on labetalol. Therefore, administration of labetalol to patients with controlled failure or those likely to develop such failure, must be carried out under careful supervision. The drug does not abolish the inotropic action of digitalis on heart muscle.

Patients with angina should be warned against abrupt discontinuation of beta-adrenergic blocking agents. There have been reports of severe exacerbation of angina, and of myocardial infarction or ventricular arrhythmias occurring in patients with angina pectoris, following abrupt discontinuation of therapy. The last two complications may occur with or without preceeding exacerbation of angina pectoris. Therefore, when discontinuation of labetalol is planned in patients with angina pectoris, the dosage should be gradually reduced over a period of about 2 weeks and the patient should be carefully observed. The same frequency of administration should be maintained. In situations of greater urgency, labetalol therapy should be discontinued stepwise and under conditions of closer observation. If angina markedly worsens or acute coronary insufficiency develops, it is recommended that treatment with the drug be re-instituted promptly, at least temporarily.

Various skin rashes and conjunctival xerosis have been reported with beta-blockers. A severe syndrome (oculomucocutaneous syndrome) whose signs include conjunctivitis sicca and psoriasiform rashes, otitis, and sclerosing serositis has occurred with the chronic use of one beta-adrenergic blocking agent (practolol). This syndrome has not been observed in association with labetalol or any other such agent. However, physicians should be alert to the possibility of such reactions and should discontinue treatment in the event that they occur.

Animal studies have shown that labetalol binds to the melanin of the uveal tract. The significance of this in humans is not known but periodic ophthalmic examinations are advisable while the patient is taking labetalol.

There have been rare reports of severe hepatocellular injury with labetalol therapy. Injury has occurred after both short-term and long-term treatment and may be slowly progressive despite minimal symptomatology. The hepatic injury is usually reversible but rare cases of hepatic necrosis and death have been reported. Appropriate laboratory testing should be performed at regular intervals during labetalol therapy. Tests should also be done at the first sign or symptom of liver dysfunction (e.g., pruritus, dark urine, persistent anorexia, jaundice, right upper quadrant tenderness or unexplained flu-like symptoms). If there is laboratory evidence of liver injury or the patient is jaundiced, labetalol should be stopped and not restarted.

Severe sinus bradycardia may occur with the use of labetalol from unopposed vagal activity remaining after blockade of $beta_1$-adrenergic receptors; in such cases, dosage should be reduced.

In patients with thyrotoxicosis, possible deleterious effects from long-term use of labetalol have not been adequately appraised. Beta-blockade may mask the clinical signs of continuing hyperthyroidism or complications, and give a false impression of improvement. Therefore, abrupt withdrawal of labetalol may be followed by an exacerbation of the symptoms of hyperthyroidism, including thyroid storm.

While labetalol has been shown to be effective in lowering the blood pressure and relieving symptoms in patients with pheochromocytoma, paradoxical hypertensive responses have been reported in a few patients with this tumor. Use caution when administering labetalol to patients with pheochromocytoma.

PRECAUTIONS: Postural hypotension and syncope may occur in patients treated with labetalol, particularly if the initial dose is too high or if dose titration is too rapid (see Dosage). Treatment should start with small doses without additional alpha- or beta-adrenergic blocking drugs.

Beta-receptor blocking drugs may enhance hypoglycemia in patients prone to this condition. Also, diabetics on insulin or oral hypoglycemic medication may have an increased tendency towards hypoglycemia when treated with these drugs.

Care should be taken if labetalol is used concomitantly with either Class I antiarrhythmic agents or calcium antagonists of the verapamil class since these drugs may potentiate the cardiac depressant activities of labetalol.

In patients with chronic liver disease the oral bioavailability of labetalol is enhanced due to reduced first pass metabolism. Lower doses of labetalol are likely to be required in these patients.

There may be increased difficulty in treating an allergic-type reaction in patients on beta-blockers. In these patients, the reaction may be more severe due to pharmacological effects of beta blockers and problems with fluid changes. Epinephrine should be administered with caution since it may not have its usual effects in the treatment of anaphylaxis. On the one hand, larger doses of epinephrine may be needed to overcome the bronchospasm, while on the other, these doses can be associated with excessive alpha adrenergic stimulation with consequent hypertension, reflex bradycardia and heart block and possible potentiation of bronchospasm. Alternatives to the use of large doses of epinephrine include vigorous supportive care such as fluids and the use of beta agonists including parenteral salbutamol or isoproterenol to overcome bronchospasm and norepinephrine to overcome hypotension.

Geriatrics: The bioavailability and half-life of labetalol are increased in the elderly. In addition, the hypotensive response is greater in this age group following administration. Therefore, lower doses of labetalol are likely to be required in elderly patients.

Pregnancy: Although no teratogenic effects were seen in animal testing, the safety of the use of labetalol during pregnancy has not been established. Labetalol crosses the placental barrier in women and has been found to bind to the eyes of fetal animals. Labetalol should be used in pregnant women only if the expected benefit to the mother justifies the potential risk to the fetus.

Lactation: Labetalol has been found in the breast milk of lactating women. If the use of labetalol is considered essential, then mothers should stop nursing.

Children: Safety and effectiveness in children have not been established.

Drug Interactions: When used with diuretics and/or other antihypertensive agents the dose of labetalol must be appropriately adjusted (see Dosage).

Labetalol and halothane have additive hypotensive effects. High doses of halothane (3%) with labetalol predispose the patient to the myocardial depressant effects of halothane and an undesirable reduction in myocardial performance. The anesthesiologist should be informed when a patient is receiving labetalol.

Labetalol blunts the reflex tachycardia produced by nitroglycerin without preventing its hypotensive effect. When labetalol is used with nitroglycerin in patients with angina pectoris, additional antihypertensive effects may occur.

Cimetidine has been shown to increase the oral bioavailability of labetalol. As cimetidine might be given to patients with hypertension also receiving labetalol, special care should be used in establishing the dose required for blood pressure control in such patients.

In one survey, 2.3% of patients taking labetalol in combination with tricyclic antidepressants experienced tremor as compared to 0.7% reported to occur with labetalol alone. The contribution of each of the treatments to this adverse reaction is unknown, but the possibility of a drug interaction cannot be excluded.

Drug/Laboratory Test Interactions: The presence of a metabolite of labetalol in the urine may result in falsely elevated levels of urinary catecholamines when measured by a nonspecific trihydroxyindole (THI) reaction. In screening patients suspected of having a pheochromocytoma and being treated with labetalol, specific radioenzymatic or high performance liquid chromatographic assay techniques should be used to determine levels of catecholamines or their metabolites.

ADVERSE EFFECTS: The most serious reported adverse effects of labetalol are severe postural hypotension, jaundice and bronchospasm.

In well-controlled clinical trials, the most common transient adverse reactions reported at routinely administered therapeutic doses, were postural hypotension and/or dizziness (16.9%), fatigue/malaise (13.1%), and headache (8.0%). Other transient effects include acute retention of urine and difficulty in micturition. The following summarizes the adverse effects reported.

Cardiovascular: postural hypotension/dizziness (16.9%), angina pectoris (3.2%), Raynaud's phenomenon (3.2%), pedal edema (1.9%), palpitations (1.3%), bradycardia (<1.0%).

Gastrointestinal: nausea/vomiting (6.1%), dyspepsia (1.9%), constipation (1.6%), dry mouth/sore throat (1.6%).

Respiratory: dyspnea (3.8%), nasal congestion (1.3%).

Dermatological: drug rash (3.2%), paresthesia (especially "scalp tingling") (3.8%), pruritus (0.6%) and angioedema.

Urogenital: impotence (2.2%), failure of ejaculation (0.6%), dysuria (0.6%).

Musculoskeletal: aches/pains (3.5%), muscle cramps (1.3%).

Central Nervous System: fatigue/malaise (13.1%), headache (8.0%), depression (2.6%), loss of libido (1.3%), dreaming (1.3%).

Miscellaneous: visual blurring (4.2%), epistaxis (1.6%).

In addition, in the more extensive trials, bronchospasm and severe bradycardia, were reported with the incidence less than 1%. There are rare reports of raised liver function tests, jaundice (both hepatic and cholestatic), and hepatic necrosis (see Warnings).

Other published or unpublished reports describe other rare, isolated adverse events in patients who were taking labetalol (oral or injectable), as follows: bronchospasm and reduction in PEFR, difficulty in micturition including acute urinary retention, ejaculatory failure, Peyronie's disease, toxic myopathy, tremor, taste distortion, hypersensitivity, hypoesthesia, rashes of various types, such as generalized maculopapular, lichenoid, urticarial, bullous lichen planus, psoriasiform, facial erythema and reversible alopecia and very rarely drug fever. A skin lesion resembling disseminated lupus erythematosus occurred in one patient receiving a high dose of labetalol. There are rare reports of patients who developed lupus-like syndromes while on labetalol which cleared upon discontinuation of treatment. Positive antinuclear factor and antimitochondrial antibodies have been reported in patients receiving the drug, but the significance of these findings is not clear. There is a report of hemiparesis following a rapid fall in blood pressure in a patient who was given a single dose of labetalol i.v.

Clinical Laboratory Tests: Occasional elevations of serum transaminases and blood urea have been reported following administration.

OVERDOSE:

Symptoms: Excessive hypotension which is posture-sensitive, and sometimes, excessive bradycardia.

Treatment: Patients should be laid supine and their legs raised, if necessary.

Gastric lavage or pharmacologically-induced emesis (using syrup of ipecac) is useful for removal of the drug shortly after ingestion. Hemodialysis removes less than 1% of circulating labetalol, and is therefore not recommended.

The following additional measures should be employed if necessary:

Excessive Bradycardia: Administer atropine to induce vagal blockade. If bradycardia persists, isoproterenol may be administered cautiously. In refractory cases, the use of a cardiac pacemaker may be considered.

Congestive Heart Failure: Conventional therapy with cardiac glycosides and diuretics.

Hypotension: Administer vasopressors, e.g. norepinephrine.

Bronchospasm: Administer a $beta_2$-stimulating agent and/or a theophylline preparation.

Oliguric renal failure has been reported after massive overdosage of labetalol orally. In one case, the use of dopamine to increase blood pressure may have aggravated the renal failure.

> For management of a suspected drug overdose, CPhA recommends that you contact your **regional Poison Control Centre**. See the *CPS* Directory section for a list of Poison Control Centres.

DOSAGE: Labetalol should be taken preferably after food. The dosage must always be adjusted in accordance with the individual requirements of the patient. The recommended initial dose is 100 mg twice daily whether used alone or with a diuretic. Thereafter, the dose should be adjusted semi- weekly or weekly according to the response.

The usual maintenance dose is 200 to 400 mg twice daily. Patients may require up to 1200 mg/day, in 2 divided doses.

Optimal doses are usually lower in patients also receiving a diuretic since an additive antihypertensive effect can be expected.

Geriatrics: Lower doses of labetalol are likely to be required in elderly patients (see Precautions).

Children: Safe and effective use of labetalol in children have not presently been elucidated.

Patients with liver function impairment will likely require lower doses since metabolism of the drug will be diminished.

SUPPLIED: 100 mg: Each orange, capsule-shaped tablet, scored and engraved LAB 100 on one side, PLB on the other side, contains: labetalol HCl 100 mg. Bottles of 100.

200 mg: Each white, capsule-shaped tablet, scored and engraved LAB 200 on one side, PLB on the other side, contains: labetalol HCl 200 mg. Bottles of 100.

(Shown in Product Identification Section)

Trandolapril ℞

CPhA Monograph

see *ACE Inhibitors*

Transderm-Nitro®

nitroglycerin

Transdermal Antianginal

Novartis Pharmaceuticals

Date of Preparation: November 12, 1993
Date of Revision: July 13, 2005

PHARMACOLOGY: The principal pharmacological action of nitroglycerin is relaxation of vascular smooth muscle, producing a vasodilator effect on both peripheral arteries and veins, with more prominent effects on the latter. Dilation of the post-capillary vessels, including large veins, promotes peripheral pooling of blood and decreases venous return to the heart, thereby reducing left ventricular end-diastolic pressure (preload). Arteriolar relaxation reduces systemic vascular resistance and arterial pressure (afterload). Dilation of the coronary arteries also occurs. The relative importance of preload reduction, afterload reduction, and coronary dilation remains undefined.

When TRANSDERM-NITRO is applied to the skin, nitroglycerin is absorbed directly into the systemic circulation. Thus, the active drug reaches target organs before inactivation by the liver. The transdermal absorption of nitroglycerin occurs in a continuous and well-controlled manner. Nitroglycerin is rapidly metabolized, principally by a liver reductase, to form glycerol nitrate metabolites and inorganic nitrate. Two active major metabolites, the 1,2- and 1,3-dinitroglycerols, the products of hydrolysis, appear to be less potent than nitroglycerin as vasodilators but have longer plasma half-lives. The dinitrates are further metabolized to mononitrates (biologically inactive with respect to cardiovascular effects) and ultimately to glycerol and carbon dioxide. There is extensive first-pass deactivation by the liver following gastrointestinal absorption.

Single-blind, placebo-controlled studies in healthy volunteers revealed that uniform steady state plasma concentrations were reached within two hours after application of the patch and remained at the same level until removal of the patch at 24 hours. Between 2 and 24 hours, the mean concentration was 0.16±0.03 ng/mL (1×10 cm^2 patch), 0.25±0.04 ng/mL (2×10 cm^2 patch), and 0.57±0.11 ng/mL (4×10 cm^2 patch), the area under the curve showing a linear correlation between drug-release area and plasma concentration. Within one hour of removal of the patch, the plasma concentration declines to about 50% of steady state concentration and to undetectable concentrations by two hours.

Although dosing regimens for most chronically used drugs are designed to provide plasma concentrations that are continuously greater than a minimally effective concentration, such a strategy is probably inappropriate for organic nitrates. Some controlled clinical trials using exercise tolerance testing have shown maintenance of effectiveness when patches are worn continuously. The large majority of such controlled trials, however, have shown the development of tolerance (i.e. complete loss of effect as measured by exercise testing) within the first day. Tolerance has appeared even when doses greater than 4 mg/hour were delivered continuously. This dose is far in excess of the effective dose 0.2 to 0.8 mg/hour applied intermittently.

Efficacy of organic nitrates is restored after a period of absence of nitrates from the body. Drug-free intervals of 10 to 12 hours are known to be sufficient to restore response. Several studies have demonstrated that when nitroglycerin is administered according to an intermittent regimen, doses of TRANSDERM-NITRO 0.4-0.8 mg/h (20-40 cm^2) have increased exercise capacity for up to 8 hours, with a trend of increased exercise capacity to 12 hours. One controlled clinical trial suggested that the intermittent use of nitrates may be associated with a decreased, in comparison to placebo, exercise tolerance during the last part of the nitrate-free interval; the clinical relevance of this observation is unknown. In another clinical trial there was an increase in nocturnal angina attacks during the drug-free period in some patients treated with nitroglycerin as compared to placebo. Therefore, the possibility of increased frequency or severity of angina during the nitrate-free interval should be considered.

INDICATIONS: TRANSDERM-NITRO (nitroglycerin) used intermittently (see Pharmacology) is indicated for the prevention of anginal attacks in patients with stable angina pectoris associated with coronary artery disease. It can be used in conjunction with other antianginal agents such as β-blockers and/or calcium channel blockers.

TRANSDERM-NITRO is not intended for the immediate relief of acute attacks of angina pectoris. Sublingual nitroglycerin preparations should be used for this purpose.

CONTRAINDICATIONS: Known hypersensitivity to nitroglycerin and related organic nitrate compounds, known or suspected hypersensitivity to components of the patch, acute circulatory failure associated with marked hypotension (shock and states of collapse), postural hypotension, left ventricular dysfunction due to obstruction as in aortic or mitral stenosis or constrictive pericarditis, increased intracranial pressure, increased intraocular pressure, severe anemia.

Concomitant use of TRANSDERM-NITRO (nitroglycerin) either regularly and/or intermittently, with phosphodiesterase type 5 (PDE5) inhibitors such as VIAGRA (sildenafil), CIALIS (tadalafil) and LEVITRA (vardenafil) is absolutely contraindicated, because PDE5 inhibitors amplify the vasodilatory effects of TRANSDERM-NITRO which can lead to severe hypotension.

WARNINGS: TRANSDERM-NITRO (nitroglycerin) patches contain an aluminum layer. Therefore, the TRANSDERM-NITRO patch must be removed before applying a magnetic field to the body during procedures such as an MRI (magnetic resonance imaging) or an electrical field such as in a cardioversion or DC defibrillation, as well as before applying diathermy treatment, since it may be associated with damage to the paddles and burns to the patient.

The benefits and safety of transdermal nitroglycerin in angina patients with acute myocardial infarction or congestive heart failure have not been established. If one elects to use TRANSDERM-NITRO in these conditions, careful clinical or hemodynamic monitoring must be used to avoid the potentially deleterious effects of induced hypotension and tachycardia.

PRECAUTIONS: Headaches or symptoms of hypotension, such as weakness or dizziness, particularly when arising suddenly from a recumbent position, may occur. A reduction in dose or discontinuation of treatment may be necessary.

Caution should be exercised when using nitroglycerin in patients prone to, or who might be affected by hypotension. The drug therefore should be used with caution in patients who may have volume depletion from diuretic therapy or in patients who have low systolic blood pressure (e.g. below 90 mmHg). Paradoxical bradycardia and increased angina pectoris may accompany nitroglycerin-induced hypotension.

Nitrate therapy may aggravate the angina caused by hypertrophic cardiomyopathy.

In industrial workers who have had long-term exposure to unknown (presumably high) doses of nitroglycerin, tolerance clearly occurs. There is moreover, physical dependence since chest pain, acute myocardial infarction, and even sudden death have occurred during temporary withdrawal of nitroglycerin from these workers. In clinical trials of angina patients, there are reports of anginal attacks being more easily provoked and of rebound in the hemodynamic effects soon after nitrate withdrawal. The importance of these observations to the routine clinical use of nitroglycerin has not been fully elucidated, but patients should be monitored closely for increased anginal symptoms during drug-free periods.

Caution should be exercised in patients with arterial hypoxemia due to anemia (see Contraindications), because in such patients the biotransformation of nitroglycerin is reduced. Similarly, caution is called for in patients with hypoxemia and ventilation/perfusion imbalance due to lung disease or ischemic heart failure. Patients with angina pectoris, myocardial infarction, or cerebral ischemia frequently suffer from abnormalities of the small airways (especially alveolar hypoxia). Under these circumstances vasoconstriction occurs within the lung to shift perfusion from areas of alveolar hypoxia to better ventilated regions of the lung. As a potent vasodilator, nitroglycerin could reverse this protective vasoconstriction and thus result in increased perfusion to poorly ventilated areas, worsening of the ventilation/perfusion imbalance, and a further decrease in the arterial partial pressure of oxygen.

Tolerance to nitroglycerin with cross tolerance to other nitrates or nitrites may occur (see Pharmacology). Co-administration of other long-acting nitrates could jeopardize the integrity of the nitrate-free interval and therefore must be avoided. As tolerance to nitroglycerin patches develops, the effect of sublingual nitroglycerin on exercise tolerance, although still observable, is somewhat blunted.

Occupations Hazards: As patients may experience faintness and/or dizziness, reaction time when driving or operating machinery may be impaired, especially at the start of treatment.

Pregnancy: It is not known whether nitroglycerin can cause fetal harm when administered to a pregnant woman. Therefore use TRANSDERM-NITRO (nitroglycerin) only if the potential benefit justifies the risk to the fetus.

Lactation: It is not known whether nitroglycerin is excreted into breast milk. Benefits to the mother must be weighed against the risks to the child.

Pediatric: Safety and effectiveness have not been established in children.

Drug Interactions: Concomitant treatment with other vasodilators such as PDE5 inhibitors (see Contraindications), calcium channel blockers, ACE inhibitors, β-blockers, diuretics, antihypertensives, tricyclic antidepressants, and major tranquilizers may be expected to potentiate the blood pressure lowering effect of TRANSDERM-NITRO. Dose adjustment may be necessary.

Marked symptomatic orthostatic hypotension has been reported when calcium channel blockers and organic nitrates were used in combination. Dosage adjustments of either class of agents may be necessary.

Alcohol may enhance sensitivity to the hypotensive effects of nitrates.

Concurrent administration of TRANSDERM-NITRO with dihydroergotamine may increase the bioavailability of dihydroergotamine. This warrants special attention in patients with coronary artery disease, because dihydroergotamine antagonizes the effect of nitroglycerin and may lead to coronary vasoconstriction.

The possibility that the ingestion of acetylsalicylic acid and non-steroidal anti inflammatory drugs might diminish the therapeutic response to nitrates and nitroglycerin cannot be excluded.

Concomitant use of TRANSDERM-NITRO (nitroglycerin) and PDE5 inhibitors such as VIAGRA (sildenafil), CIALIS (tadalafil) and LEVITRA (vardenafil) potentiate the hypotensive effect of TRANSDERM-NITRO. This could result in life-threatening hypotension with syncope or myocardial infarction and death. Therefore, PDE5 inhibitors are absolutely contraindicated in patients receiving TRANSDERM-NITRO therapy in any manner (see Contraindications).

Information to Be Provided to the Patient: Daily headaches sometimes accompany treatment with nitroglycerin. In patients who get these headaches, the headaches may be a marker of the activity of the drug. Patients should resist the temptation to avoid headaches by altering the schedule of their treatment with nitroglycerin, since loss of headache may be associated with simultaneous loss of antianginal efficacy.

Treatment with nitroglycerin may be associated with lightheadedness on standing, especially just after rising from a recumbent or seated position. This effect may be more frequent in patients who have also consumed alcohol.

After normal use, there is enough residual nitroglycerin in discarded patches that they are a potential hazard to children and pets.

A patient leaflet is supplied with the patches (see Information for the Patient).

ADVERSE EFFECTS: Headache, which may be severe, is the most commonly reported side effect. Headache may be recurrent with each daily dose, especially at higher doses of nitroglycerin. Headaches may be treated with concomitant administration of mild analgesics. If such headaches are unresponsive to treatment, the nitroglycerin dosage should be reduced or the product discontinued. Transient episodes of lightheadedness, occasionally related to blood pressure changes, may also occur. Hypotension occurs infrequently, but in some patients it may be severe enough to warrant discontinuation of therapy.

Reddening of the skin (erythema), with or without a mild local itching (pruritus) or burning sensation, as well as allergic contact dermatitis may occasionally occur. Upon removal of the patch, any slight reddening of the skin will usually disappear within a few hours. The application site should be changed regularly to prevent local irritation.

Less frequently reported adverse reactions include dizziness, faintness, facial flushing, postural hypotension which may be associated with reflex tachycardia. Syncope, crescendo angina, and rebound hypertension have been reported but are uncommon. Rarely nausea, and vomiting.

OVERDOSE:

Symptoms: Nitroglycerin overdose may result in severe hypotension, persistent throbbing headache, vertigo, palpitations, visual disturbances, flushing and perspiring skin (later becoming cold and cyanotic), anorexia, nausea and vomiting (possibly with colic and even bloody diarrhea), syncope (especially in the upright posture), methemoglobinemia with cyanosis, hyperpnea, dyspnea and slow breathing, slow pulse (dicrotic and intermittent), heart block and bradycardia, increased intracranial pressure with cerebral symptoms of fever, confusion, and coma possibly followed by paralysis, clonic convulsions and death due to circulatory collapse.

Treatment: Keep the patient recumbent in a shock position and comfortably warm. Remove the TRANSDERM-NITRO patch.

Passive movement of the extremities may aid venous return. Administer oxygen and artificial ventilation if necessary.

Intravenous infusion of normal saline or similar fluid may also be required to produce sufficient central volume expansion. However, in patients with renal disease or congestive heart failure, therapy resulting in central volume expansion is not without hazard. Treatment of nitroglycerin overdose in these patients may be subtle and difficult, and invasive monitoring may be required.

Epinephrine is ineffective in reversing the severe hypotensive events associated with overdose; it and related compounds are contraindicated in this situation.

Methemoglobinemia:

Case reports of clinically significant methemoglobinemia are rare at conventional doses of nitroglycerin. The formation of methemoglobin is dose-related, and in the case of genetic abnormalities of hemoglobin that favour methemoglobin formation, even conventional doses of organic nitrates can produce harmful concentrations of methemoglobin. Methemoglobin levels are available from most clinical laboratories. The diagnosis should be suspected in patients who exhibit signs of impaired oxygen delivery despite adequate cardiac output and adequate arterial pO_2. Classically, methemoglobinemic blood is described as chocolate brown, without color change on exposure to air. If methemoglobinemia is present, administration of methylene blue (1% solution), 1 to 2 mg/kg intravenously, may be required.

For management of a suspected drug overdose, CPhA recommends that you contact your **regional Poison Control Centre**. See the *CPS* Directory section for a list of Poison Control Centres.

DOSAGE: Daily Dosage Schedule: The daily dosage schedule is based on intermittent therapy to prevent the development of tolerance to nitroglycerin. The optimal dose should be selected based upon the clinical response, side effects, and the effects of therapy on blood pressure.

Starting dose is one TRANSDERM-NITRO 0.2 patch (10 cm^2), usually applied in the morning. If 0.2 mg/hour (10 cm^2) is well tolerated, the dose can be increased to 0.4 mg/hour (20 cm^2) if required. A maximum of 0.8 mg/hour (40 cm^2) may be used.

Prevention of Tolerance: Although some controlled clinical trials using exercise tolerance testing have shown maintenance of effectiveness when patches are worn continuously, the large majority of such controlled trials have shown the development of tolerance (i.e. complete loss of effect) within the first 24 hours after therapy was initiated. Dose adjustments even to levels much higher than generally used did not prevent the development of tolerance.

Tolerance can be prevented or attenuated by use of an intermittent dosage schedule. Although the minimum nitrate-free interval has not been defined, clinical trials have demonstrated that an appropriate dosing schedule for nitroglycerin patches would provide for a daily patch-on period of 12-14 hours and a daily patch-off period of 10-12 hours. The patch-free time should coincide with the period in which angina pectoris is least likely to occur (usually at night). Patients should be watched carefully for an increase of angina pectoris during the patch-free period. Adjustment of background medication may be required.

The dose of TRANSDERM-NITRO should be periodically reviewed in relation to continuing antianginal control.

Site of Patch Application: TRANSDERM-NITRO can be applied to any area of skin **except** the distal extremities. Many patients prefer the chest. Each successive application should be to a different site to minimize local irritation.

The area should be clean, dry, and preferably hairless. If hair is likely to interfere with patch adhesion or removal, clipping may be necessary prior to application. Take care to avoid areas with cuts or irritations.

Table 1: TRANSDERM-NITRO

Rate of Nitroglycerin Release

	TRANSDERM-NITRO 0.2	TRANSDERM-NITRO 0.4	TRANSDERM-NITRO 0.6
Rated Release of Nitroglycerin in vivo	0.2 mg/hour	0.4 mg/hour	0.6 mg/hour
Nitroglycerin Content	25 mg	50 mg	75 mg
Drug Releasing Area	10 cm^2	20 cm^2	30 cm^2
Printed Code	TRANSDERM-NITRO 0.2 mg/hour CG DOD	TRANSDERM-NITRO 0.4 mg/hour CG DPD	TRANSDERM-NITRO 0.6 mg/hour CG EJE
Color of Protective Liner (peel off and discard)	off-white	off-white	off-white

INFORMATION FOR THE PATIENT: Published in e-CPS, available by subscription at www.e-cps.ca.

SUPPLIED: TRANSDERM-NITRO (nitroglycerin) transdermal therapeutic system, is a flat multilayer unit designed to release nitroglycerin continuously through a semipermeable membrane following its application to intact skin. In cases where permeability of the skin is excessive, drug release is limited by this release membrane.

The rate of nitroglycerin release is linearly dependent upon the drug releasing area of the applied patch (see Table 1). The nominal rate of nitroglycerin release in vivo is approximately 0.02 mg/cm^2/hour. Nitroglycerin remaining in the patch serves as a thermodynamic energy source to keep the pattern of drug delivery constant.

The patch comprises five layers: a tan-coloured backing layer (aluminized plastic) impermeable to nitroglycerin; a drug reservoir containing nitroglycerin adsorbed on lactose, colloidal silicon dioxide and silicone medical fluid; an ethylene/vinyl acetate copolymer membrane that is permeable to nitroglycerin; a layer of hypoallergenic silicone adhesive; a protective liner (peel strip) which is removed prior to use to expose the adhesive surface.

Store patches below 25°C. Do not freeze. Each patch is individually sealed in a separate pouch. Do not store out of the pouch. Keep TRANSDERM-NITRO out of reach of children and pets both before use and when disposing of used patches.

(Shown in Product Identification Section)

Transderm-V®

scopolamine

Antimotion Sickness Agent

Novartis Pharmaceuticals

PHARMACOLOGY: Scopolamine is a naturally occurring belladonna alkaloid. As a parasympatholytic agent it competitively antagonizes acetylcholine (or other direct parasympathomimetics) at the muscarinic receptor. This means that its effect can be abolished by high doses of a parasympathomimetic agent. The effect of scopolamine depends on the sensitivity of the target organs and on the size of the dose employed.

The principal actions of scopolamine are related to anticholinergic effects which include depressed motor function, decreased salivation and sweating, mydriasis, inhibition of visual accommodation, and tachycardia. Drowsiness may also occur at therapeutic doses.

The mechanism of action of scopolamine in the CNS is not well known but may include anticholinergic effects. The ability of scopolamine to prevent motion-induced nausea is believed to be associated with inhibition of vestibular input to the CNS, which results in inhibition of the vomiting reflex. In addition, scopolamine may have a direct action on the vomiting centre within the reticular formation of the brain stem.

After transdermal administration of scopolamine, the time necessary to reach maximum blood levels (estimated by urinary excretion of scopolamine) is approximately 12 hours. The disc is designed for continuous release of scopolamine over the 3 day functional lifetime. Scopolamine excretion continues for up to 12 hours after removal of the system. Approximately 5 to 8% of the administered drug is excreted unchanged.

INDICATIONS: For prevention of symptoms of motion sickness such as nausea and vomiting.

CONTRAINDICATIONS: Known hypersensitivity to scopolamine or any components of the system.

Glaucoma or a predisposition to angle-closure glaucoma (see Warnings).

WARNINGS: Occupational Hazards: Since drowsiness, disorientation and confusion may occasionally occur with the use of scopolamine, patients should be cautioned about engaging in activities that require mental alertness, such as driving a motor vehicle or operating dangerous machinery.

Potentially alarming idiosyncratic reactions may occur with ordinary therapeutic doses of scopolamine.

In patients with a history of possible raised intraocular pressure (pressure pain, blurred vision, glaucomatous halo), scopolamine should be employed only after ophthalmological examination excludes glaucoma (see Contraindications).

Scopolamine should be discontinued if it causes blurring of vision with pressure pain within the eye (see Contraindications).

PRECAUTIONS: Scopolamine should be used with caution in patients with dysuria, e.g., due to urinary bladder neck obstruction. Caution should be exercised when administering an antiemetic or antimuscarinic drug to patients suspected of having intestinal obstruction, e.g., pyloric stenosis.

Scopolamine should be used with caution in the elderly or in individuals with impaired metabolic, liver or kidney functions.

In certain cases, especially in the elderly, confusional states and/or visual hallucinations may occur. Should this occur, scopolamine should be removed at once. If severe symptoms persist, appropriate countermeasures should be taken (see Overdose: Symptoms and Treatment).

In epileptic patients, isolated cases of increased seizure frequency have been reported.

Children: Children are particularly susceptible to the side effects of belladonna alkaloids. Transderm-V should not be used in children because it is not known whether the amount of scopolamine released could produce serious adverse effects in children.

Pregnancy: Scopolamine should be used during pregnancy only if the anticipated benefit justifies the potential risk to the mother and fetus.

Lactation: Scopolamine should not be administered to nursing mothers since it is excreted into breast milk.

Drug Interactions: Scopolamine should be employed with caution in patients taking drugs which act on the CNS. This applies particularly to patients under treatment with drugs displaying anticholinergic properties, for example, belladonna alkaloids, antihistamines, antidepressants (tricyclics and MAO inhibitors), phenothiazines, amantadine and quinidine.

Any parasympatholytic or sympathomimetic agent or barbiturate should be administered with caution to persons wearing scopolamine.

Patients should refrain from consuming alcohol while using scopolamine. Alcohol may interfere with the metabolism of the drug and could thus cause plasma levels to become elevated, which could intensify the side effects.

Information to Be Provided to the Patient: Since scopolamine can cause temporary dilation of the pupils and blurred vision if it comes in contact with the eyes, patients should be strongly advised to wash their hands thoroughly with soap and water immediately after handling the disc and to avoid touching the disc while in place behind the ear.

Patients should be advised to remove the disc and contact a physician promptly in the unlikely event that they experience symptoms of angle-closure glaucoma (pain in and reddening of the eyes accompanied by dilated pupils).

Patients should be instructed to remove the disc if they develop difficulty urinating.

Patients should be advised to refrain from consuming alcohol while using scopolamine.

Patients should be warned against driving a motor vehicle or operating dangerous machinery.

A patient leaflet is supplied with the discs (see Information for the Patient).

ADVERSE EFFECTS: Gastrointestinal: Frequent: transient dryness of the mouth.

Ophthalmic: Frequent: transient impairment of eye accommodation (cycloplegia), including blurred (near) vision and dilatation of the pupils (sometimes in one eye only), especially if traces of active substance on the hands enter the eyes. Occasional: irritation of the eyelids. Isolated cases: dilatation of the pupils may provoke acute glaucoma, especially angle-closure glaucoma.

Central Nervous System: Occasional: drowsiness. Rare: impairment of memory and concentration, restlessness, giddiness, dizziness, disorientation, confusion and hallucinations.

Dermatological: Occasional: local irritation of the skin. Isolated cases: generalized skin rash.

Genitourinary: Rare: disturbances of micturition (retention of urine).

Cardiovascular: Isolated cases: slight variations in blood pressure.

Adverse Effects after Withdrawal of Scopolamine: In certain instances, there have been complaints of transient dizziness, nausea, vomiting, headache and disturbances of balance following discontinuation of scopolamine, usually after several days of use.

OVERDOSE:

Symptoms: The central actions of scopolamine in high doses are similar to those of atropine. They begin with restlessness, excitation states, disorientation and confusion. In response to higher doses, delirium, hallucinations and convulsions set in. At very high doses coma and respiratory paralysis occur.

Treatment: Remove the disc immediately.

Treatment of acute antimuscarinic overdose consists mainly of symptomatic and supportive treatments. Patients should be hospitalized and closely monitored, including continuous ECG monitoring.

The most effective antidote is physostigmine, which, depending on the severity of the poisoning, should be injected slowly i.v. in doses of 1 to 4 mg (0.5 mg in children). Since physostigmine is rapidly metabolized, the patients may lapse into coma again within 1 to 2 hours, thus necessitating renewed injections. It should, however, be noted that physostigmine has the potential for producing severe adverse effects (for instance, seizures, asystole). **The use of physostigmine should, therefore, be reserved for life-threatening situations only.**

Fairly small doses of diazepam may prove useful in the presence of excitation states and convulsions. Larger doses should be avoided in view of the possibility of additional respiratory depression. In severe cases artificial respiration may be necessary.

In the event of hyperthermia, urgent action should be taken to dissipate heat (e.g., cold baths).

For management of a suspected drug overdose, CPhA recommends that you contact your **regional Poison Control Centre**. See the *CPS* Directory section for a list of Poison Control Centres.

DOSAGE: Adults: To obtain optimum effect, Transderm-V should be applied to a dry, hairless area of post-auricular skin approximately 12 hours before the antiemetic effect is required. Only 1 disc should be worn at any time. Should the disc become displaced, it should be discarded and a fresh one placed on a different skin site.

Scopolamine provides protection over a 3 day period. If the disc is only needed for a shorter time, it should be removed at the end of the journey.

If therapy is required for longer periods, the first disc should be removed after 72 hours and a second disc applied behind the other ear.

Children: Scopolamine should not be used in children (see Precautions).

Transderm-V is designed to deliver in vitro 1 mg scopolamine at a constant rate over the 3 day functional lifetime. An initial priming dose of scopolamine, released from the adhesive layer of the system, saturates the skin binding sites for the drug and brings the plasma concentration to the required steady state level. Subsequently, there is continuous controlled release of scopolamine, from the drug reservoir through the rate-controlling membrane.

Handling: After the disc is applied on dry skin behind the ear, the hands should be washed thoroughly with soap and water, then dried. Once the disc has been affixed, it should not be touched again while it is being worn. Upon removal, the disc should be carefully discarded, and the hands and application site washed thoroughly with soap and water to prevent traces of scopolamine from coming in direct contact with the eyes. If scopolamine were to contact the eyes it could cause slight temporary blurring of vision and dilation of the pupils (sometimes in one eye only).

INFORMATION FOR THE PATIENT: Published in e-CPS, available by subscription at www.e-cps.ca.

SUPPLIED: Each flat, circular, multilayer, tan-colored, adhesive disc (contact surface 2.5 cm²), attached to a clear, oversized, hexagonal, protective liner (peel strip), contains: scopolamine 1.5 mg and is programmed to release in vitro 1 mg scopolamine over 3 days. Cartons of 2.

Transderm-V is a 0.2 mm-thick film with 5 layers. Proceeding from the visible surface towards the surface attached to the skin, these layers are: (1) a **backing layer** of tan-colored, aluminized polyester film; (2) a drug **reservoir** of scopolamine, mineral oil and polyisobutylene; (3) a microporous polypropylene **membrane** that controls the rate of delivery of scopolamine from the system to the skin surface; (4) an **adhesive** formulation of mineral oil, polyisobutylene and a priming dose of scopolamine; (5) a clear hexagonal **protective liner** (peel strip) of siliconized polyester, which is removed before applying the disc.

Store below 25°C. Do not freeze. Each disc is individually sealed in a separate pouch. Do not store out of the pouch. Apply immediately upon removal from the protective pouch. Keep out of the reach of children and pets both before use and when disposing of used discs.

Trasylol® Ⓟ

aprotinin

Hemostatic Agent

Bayer

Date of Revision: February 14, 2007

SUMMARY PRODUCT INFORMATION:

Route of Administration	Dosage Form/ Strength	Clinically Relevant Nonmedicinal Ingredients
Intravenous	Isotonic Solution, 10 000 KIU/mL	Sodium Chloride (BP), Water for Injection (BP) For a complete listing see Dosage Forms, Composition and Packaging.

DESCRIPTION: TRASYLOL (aprotinin) is a highly purified natural polypeptide proteinase inhibitor obtained from bovine lung.

INDICATIONS AND CLINICAL USE: TRASYLOL (aprotinin) is indicated for prophylactic use to reduce perioperative blood loss and the need for blood transfusion in those patients undergoing cardiopulmonary bypass in the course of coronary artery bypass graft (CABG) surgery who are at increased risk for blood loss and blood transfusion requirement.

CONTRAINDICATIONS:

- Patients who are hypersensitive to this drug or to any ingredient in the formulation or component of the container. For a complete listing, see Dosage Forms, Composition and Packaging.
- Administration of TRASYLOL to patients with a known or suspected previous aprotinin exposure during the last 12 months is contraindicated. For patients with known or suspected history of exposure to aprotinin greater than 12 months previously, see Warnings and Precautions. Aprotinin may also be a component of some fibrin sealant products and the use of these products should be included in the patient history.

WARNINGS AND PRECAUTIONS:

Serious Warnings and Precautions

- TRASYLOL administration may cause fatal anaphylactic or anaphylactoid reactions. Fatal reactions have occurred with an initial (test) dose as well as with any of the components of the dose regimen. Fatal reactions have also occurred in situations where the initial (test) dose was tolerated. The risk for anaphylactic or anaphylactoid reactions is increased among patients with prior aprotinin exposure and a history of any prior aprotinin exposure must be sought prior to TRASYLOL administration. The risk for a fatal reaction appears to be greater upon re-exposure within 12 months of the most recent prior aprotinin exposure. TRASYLOL should be administered only in operative settings where cardiopulmonary bypass can be rapidly initiated. The benefit of TRASYLOL to patients undergoing primary CABG surgery should be weighed against the risk of anaphylaxis associated with any subsequent exposure to aprotinin. (See Contraindications and Warnings and Precautions.)

General: Anaphylactic or anaphylactoid reactions have occurred with TRASYLOL administration, including fatal reactions in association with the initial (test) dose. The initial (test) dose does not fully predict a patient's risk for a hypersensitivity reaction, including a fatal reaction. Fatal hypersensitivity reactions have occurred among patients who tolerated an initial (test) dose.

Hypersensitivity reactions often manifest as anaphylactic/anaphylactoid reactions with hypotension the most frequently reported sign of the hypersensitivity reaction. Other symptoms of a hypersensitivity reaction include pruritis, rash, asthma, and nausea. The hypersensitivity reaction can progress to anaphylactic shock with circulatory failure. If a hypersensitivity reaction occurs during injection or infusion of TRASYLOL, administration should be stopped immediately and emergency treatment should be initiated. Even when a second exposure to TRASYLOL has been tolerated without symptoms, a subsequent administration may result in severe hypersensitivity/anaphylactic reactions.

TRASYLOL should be administered only in operative settings where cardiopulmonary bypass can be rapidly initiated. Before initiating treatment with TRASYLOL, the recommendations below should be followed to manage a potential hypersensitivity or anaphylactic reaction:

1. Have standard emergency treatments for hypersensitivity or anaphylactic reactions readily available in the operating room (e.g., epinephrine, corticosteroids).
2. Administration of the initial (test) dose and loading dose should be done only when the patient is intubated and when conditions for rapid cannulation and initiation of cardiopulmonary bypass are present.
3. Delay the addition of TRASYLOL into the pump prime solution until after the loading dose has been safely administered.

Re-exposure to Aprotinin: Administration of TRASYLOL, especially to patients who have received aprotinin in the past, requires a careful risk/benefit assessment because an allergic reaction may occur (see Contraindications and Adverse Reactions). Although the majority of cases of anaphylaxis occur upon re-exposure within the first 12 months, there are also case reports of anaphylaxis occurring upon re-exposure after more than 12 months.

In a retrospective review of 387 European patient records with documented re-exposure to TRASYLOL, the incidence of hypersensitivity/anaphylactic reactions was 2.7%. Two patients who experienced hypersensitivity/anaphylactic reactions subsequently died, 24 hours and 5 days after surgery, respectively. The relationship of these 2 deaths to TRASYLOL is unclear. This retrospective review also showed that the incidence of a hypersensitivity or anaphylactic reaction following re-exposure is increased when the re-exposure occurs within 6 months of the initial administration (5.0% for re-exposure within 6 months and 0.9% for re-exposure greater than 6 months). Other smaller studies have shown that in cases of re-exposure, the incidence of hypersensitivity/anaphylactic reactions may reach the five percent level.

An analysis of all spontaneous reports from the Bayer Global database covering a period from 1985 to March 2006 revealed that of 291 possibly associated spontaneous cases of hypersensitivity (fatal: n=52 and non-fatal: n=239), 47% (138/291) of hypersensitivity cases had documented previous exposure to TRASYLOL. Of the 138 cases with documented previous exposure, 110 had information on the time of the previous exposure. Ninety-nine of the 110 cases had previous exposure within the prior 12 months.

Initial (Test) Dose: All patients treated with TRASYLOL should first receive an initial (test) dose to minimize the extent of aprotinin exposure and to help assess the potential for allergic reactions (see Dosage and Administration). Initiation of this initial (test) dose should occur only in operative settings where cardiopulmonary bypass can be rapidly initiated. The initial (test) dose of 1 mL TRASYLOL should be administered intravenously at least 10 minutes prior to the loading dose and the patient should be observed for manifestations of possible hypersensitivity reaction.

However, even after the uneventful administration of the 1 mL initial (test) dose, any subsequent dose may cause an anaphylactic reaction. If this happens, the infusion of aprotinin should immediately be stopped, and the standard emergency treatment for anaphylaxis be applied.

It should be noted that serious, even fatal, hypersensitivity/anaphylactic reactions can occur with administration of the initial (test) dose.

Loading Dose: The loading dose of TRASYLOL should be given intravenously to patients in the supine position over a 20-30 minute period. Rapid intravenous administration of TRASYLOL can cause a transient fall in blood pressure (see Dosage and Administration).

Immune: Patients with a history of allergic reactions to drugs and other agents may be at a greater risk of developing hypersensitivity or anaphylactic reactions to TRASYLOL (see Warnings and Precautions, General).

Renal: TRASYLOL administration increases the risk for renal dysfunction and may increase the need for dialysis in the perioperative period. This risk may be especially increased for patients with pre-existing renal impairment or those who receive aminoglycoside antibiotics or drugs that alter renal function.

An analysis of Bayer's global pool of placebo-controlled studies in patients undergoing coronary artery bypass graft (CABG) surgery has found elevations of serum creatinine values >44.2 µmol/L (0.5 mg/dL) above baseline in patients with TRASYLOL therapy (see Adverse Reactions, Abnormal Hematologic and Clinical Chemistry Findings, Renal Function Tests). Careful consideration of the balance of risks and benefits is therefore advised before administering TRASYLOL to patients with pre-existing impaired renal function (creatinine clearance <60 mL/min), or to those with other risk factors for renal dysfunction (such as perioperative administration of aminoglycosides or products that alter renal function). Serum creatinine should be monitored regularly.

An increase in renal failure and mortality compared to age matched historical controls has been reported for TRASYLOL-treated patients undergoing cardiopulmonary bypass with deep hypothermic circulatory arrest during operation of the thoracic aorta. Caution should be exercised and a careful risk/benefit assessment made before TRASYLOL is used in this setting. Specifically, adequate anticoagulation with heparin must be assured (see Drug Interactions, Drug-Laboratory Test Interactions, Laboratory Monitoring of Anticoagulation during Cardiopulmonary Bypass).

Special Populations: Pregnant Women: No evidence of teratogenic or embryotoxic effects has been seen in animals. There are no adequate and well-controlled studies in pregnant women. TRASYLOL may be used in pregnancy only if the potential benefit justifies the potential risk. In case of severe adverse drug reactions (like anaphylactic reaction, heart arrest, etc.) and their consecutive therapeutic measures, damage to the fetus has to be taken into account for a risk/benefit evaluation.

Nursing Women: It is not known whether TRASYLOL is excreted in human milk. However, since TRASYLOL is not bioavailable after oral administration, any drug contained in the milk would have no effect on the baby.

Geriatrics (≥65 years of age): Of the total of 3083 subjects in clinical studies of TRASYLOL, 1100 (35.7%) were 65 years of age and over, while 297 (9.6%) were 75 and over. No overall differences in safety or effectiveness were observed between these subjects and younger subjects, and other reported clinical experience has not identified differences in responses between the elderly and younger patients.

Pediatrics (<18 years of age): Infants, toddlers, children and adolescents: efficacy and safety have not been established in this patient population.

ADVERSE REACTIONS: Adverse Drug Reaction Overview: Adverse drug reactions (ADRs) based on all placebo-controlled clinical studies with aprotinin sorted by CIOMS III categories of frequency (aprotinin n=3817 and placebo n=2682, status: April 2005) are listed below:

ADRs derived from post marketing reports (n=584 reports, status: April 2005) are printed in bold italic.

As with all venipunctures, local thrombophlebitic reactions (thrombophlebitis injection site) may occur after TRASYLOL injections or infusions.

Clinical Trial Adverse Drug Reactions: Because clinical trials are conducted under very specific conditions the adverse reaction rates observed in the clinical trials may not reflect the rates observed in practice and should not be compared to the rates in the clinical trials of another drug. Adverse drug reaction information from clinical trials is useful for identifying drug-related adverse events and for approximating rates. See Table 1.

Table 1: TRASYLOL

ADRs Based on all Placebo-Controlled Clinical Studies with Aprotinin

Clinical Description	Common ≥1% to <10%	Uncommon ≥0.1% to <1%	Rare ≥0.01% to <0.1%	Very Rare <0.01%
General Disorders or Administration Site Conditions				
Infusion Site Reactions				Injection and infusion site reactions Infusion site (thrombo-) phlebitis
Cardiac Disorders				
Myocardial Disorders		Myocardial ischemia Coronary occlusion/ thrombosis Myocardial infarction Thrombosis		
Pericardial Effusion		Pericardial effusion		
Vascular Disorders				
Embolism and Thrombosis		Thrombosis	Arterial thrombosis (and its organ-specific manifestations that might occur in vital organs such as kidney, lung or brain)	***Pulmonary embolism***

(cont'd)

Table 1: TRASYLOL *(cont'd)*

ADRs Based on all Placebo-Controlled Clinical Studies with Aprotinin

Clinical Description	Common ≥1% to <10%	Uncommon ≥0.1% to <1%	Rare ≥0.01% to <0.1%	Very Rare <0.01%
Blood and Lymphatic System Disorders				
Changes in Coagulation				***Disseminated intravascular coagulation Coagulopathy***
Immune System Disorders				
Acute Hypersensitivity Reactions			Allergic reaction Anaphylactic/ anaphylactoid reaction	***Anaphylactic shock (potentially life threatening)***
Renal and Urinary Disorders				
Renal Impairment		Oliguria, acute renal failure, renal tubular necrosis		

Myocardial Infarction: In the pooled analysis of placebo-controlled clinical studies with patients undergoing CABG surgery, the incidence of investigator-reported myocardial infarction (MI) in aprotinin treated patients was 5.8% compared to 4.8% placebo treated patients with a difference of 0.96% between the groups (aprotinin n=3817 and placebo n=2682, status: April 2005).

A numerically greater incidence of MI in association with aprotinin was observed in some studies, while other studies showed a lower incidence compared to placebo. The described studies were not designed to detect the difference of incidence of MI and might not have the statistical power to exclude a clinically significant adverse event.

Because no uniform criteria for the diagnosis of myocardial infraction were utilized by investigators, this issue was addressed prospectively in three studies. These data were analyzed by a blinded consultant employing an algorithm for possible, probable or definite MI. Data from these three studies are summarized in Table 2.

Table 2: TRASYLOL

Incidence of Myocardial Infarctions by Treatment Group Population: All CABG Patients Valid for Safety Analysis (Studies 466, 471, 472)

Treatment	Definite MI (%)	Definite or Probable MI (%)	Definite, Probable, or Possible MI (%)
TRASYLOL (n=646)	4.6	10.7	14.1
Placebo (n=661)	4.7	11.3	13.4

Mortality: There were 43 (2.65%) deaths in the group of patients who received placebo compared to 48 (2.85%) deaths in patients treated with aprotinin. From these data there seems to be no major difference regarding mortality between placebo and full dose aprotinin.

Graft Closure: In some studies, a numerical increase of graft closure, although not statistically significant, was observed in association with aprotinin. In a multi-centre study in patients undergoing primary coronary artery bypass graft surgery there was a statistically significant increased risk of graft closure (coronary occlusion) for TRASYLOL-treated patients compared to patients who received placebo. The graft closure rates observed in this study are shown in Table 3. This result was mainly negatively influenced by two centres. Subanalyses clearly demonstrated that for one centre inadequate heparinisation was the primary issue while the other centre used a non-standard graft conservation technique. In addition to the note on heparinisation, (see Drug Interactions, Drug-Laboratory Test Interactions) the practice of using blood from the aprotinin central infusion line is strongly discouraged (for determining ACT and other blood tests). No differences between the treatment groups were observed for the incidence of myocardial infarctions or of deaths in this study.

Table 3: TRASYLOL

Overall Graft Closure Rates[a]

	Aprotinin	Placebo	CI for the difference (%) (Aprotinin–Placebo)
All centers (n=703)	15.4%	10.9%	1.3% to 9.6%
North America centers (n=381)	9.4%	9.5%	−3.8% to 5.9%

[a] Population: All patients with assessable saphenous vein grafts.

A follow-up study was done on patients who survived the original study. Of the 870 patients in the study, 857 were alive at the end of the clinical trial and 645 (75%) responded to the follow-up survey. Final analysis showed that aprotinin administered intra-operatively to primary CABG patients did not affect mortality and cardiac-related morbidity after the conclusion of the trial.

Abnormal Hematologic and Clinical Chemistry Findings: Renal Function Tests: Data from Bayer's global pool of placebo-controlled studies in patients undergoing coronary artery bypass graft (CABG) surgery showed that the incidence of serum creatinine elevations >44.2 μmol/L (0.5 mg/dL) above pretreatment levels was statistically higher at 9.0% (185/2047) in the aprotinin group compared with 6.6% (129/1957) in the placebo group, with an odds ratio of 1.41 (1.12-1.79). In the majority of instances, postoperative renal dysfunction was not severe and was reversible. However, renal dysfunction may progress to renal failure and the incidence of serum creatinine elevations >176.8 μmol/L (2.0 mg/dL) above baseline was slightly higher in the aprotinin group (1.1% vs 0.8%) (see Warnings and Precautions).

As shown in Table 1, oliguria, acute renal failure, and renal tubular necrosis are uncommon (≥0.1% to <1%).

Serum Transaminases: Data pooled from all patients undergoing CABG surgery in placebo-controlled trials showed no evidence of an increase in the incidence of postoperative hepatic dysfunction in patients treated with TRASYLOL. The mean changes of ALT and AST from baseline to 24 hours postoperatively were not different between patients treated with TRASYLOL compared to patients treated with placebo.

Other Laboratory Findings: The incidence of treatment-emergent events in plasma glucose, AST (formerly SGOT), LDH, alkaline phosphatase, and CPK-MB was not notably different between TRASYLOL and placebo-treated patients undergoing CABG surgery. Significant elevations in the partial thromboplastin time (PTT) and celite Activated Clotting Time (Celite ACT) are expected in TRASYLOL-treated patients in the hours after surgery due to circulating concentrations of TRASYLOL, which are known to inhibit activation of the intrinsic clotting system by contact with a foreign material (e.g., celite), a method used in these tests (see Drug Interactions, Drug-Laboratory Test Interactions).

Post-Market Adverse Drug Reactions: Allergic/anaphylactic reactions are rare in patients with no prior exposure to aprotinin. In case of re-exposure the incidence of allergic/anaphylactic reactions may reach the five percent level. A retrospective review showed that the incidence of an allergic/anaphylactic reaction following re-exposure is increased when the re-exposure occurs within 6 months of the initial administration (5.0% for re-exposure within 6 months and 0.9% for re-exposures greater than 6 months). A retrospective review suggests that the incidence of severe anaphylactic reactions to aprotinin may further increase when patients are re-exposed more than twice within 6 months. Even when a second exposure to aprotinin has been tolerated without symptoms, a subsequent administration may result in severe allergic reactions or anaphylactic shock with, in rare cases, fatal outcome.

The symptoms of allergic/anaphylactic reactions may include:

Respiratory System: asthma (bronchospasm).

Skin and Appendages: pruritus, rash, urticaria.

Some of the following adverse drug reactions could be part of an allergic/anaphylactic reaction:

Cardiovascular System: bradycardia, heart arrest, heart failure, hypotension, tachycardia, thrombosis, vasodilation, ventricular fibrillation.

Digestive System: nausea.

If allergic reactions occur during injection or infusion, administration should be stopped immediately. Standard emergency treatment may be required, ie, adrenalin/epinephrine, volume substitution and corticosteroids.

During post marketing surveillance, single cases of reversible kidney failure have been reported.

DRUG INTERACTIONS: Drug-Drug Interactions: TRASYLOL has a dose-dependent inhibitory effect on the action of thrombolytic agents (ie streptokinase, tPA and urokinase).

In a study of nine patients with untreated hypertension, TRASYLOL, infused intravenously in a dose of 2 million KIU over two hours, blocked the acute hypotensive effect of 100 mg of captopril.

Drug-Laboratory Test Interactions: Laboratory Monitoring of Anticoagulation during Cardiopulmonary Bypass: TRASYLOL prolongs whole blood clotting times by a different mechanism than heparin. In the presence of aprotinin, prolongation is dependent on the type of whole blood clotting test employed. If an activated clotting time (ACT) is used to determine the effectiveness of heparin anticoagulation, the prolongation of the ACT by aprotinin may lead to an overestimation of the degree of anticoagulation, thereby leading to inadequate anticoagulation which may be associated with an increased risk of graft closure. During extended extracorporeal circulation, patients may require additional heparin, even in the presence of ACT levels that appear adequate.

In patients undergoing cardiopulmonary bypass with TRASYLOL therapy, one of the following methods is recommended to maintain adequate anticoagulation:

1. Activated Clotting Time (ACT)—An ACT is not a standardized coagulation test, and different formulations of the assay are affected differently by the presence of aprotinin. The test is further influenced by variable dilution effects and the temperature experienced during cardiopulmonary bypass. It has been observed that kaolin-based ACTs are not increased to the same degree by aprotinin as are diatomaceous earth-based (celite) ACTs.

   While protocols vary, a minimal celite-ACT of 750 seconds or kaolin-ACT of 480 seconds, independant of the effects of haemodilution and hypothermia, is recommended in the presence of aprotinin. The manufacturer of the ACT test should be consulted regarding interpretation of the assay in the presence of TRASYLOL.
2. Fixed Heparin Dosing—A standard loading dose of heparin, administered prior to cannulation of the heart, plus the quantity of heparin added to the prime volume of the cardiopulmonary bypass circuit, should total at least 350 IU/kg. Additional heparin should be administered in a fixed dose regimen based on patient weight and duration of cardiopulmonary bypass.
3. Heparin Titration—Protamine titration, a method that is not affected by aprotinin, can be used to measure heparin levels. A heparin dose response, assessed by protamine titration, should be performed prior to administration of aprotinin to determine the heparin loading dose. Additional heparin should be administered on the basis of heparin levels measured by protamine titration. Heparin levels during bypass should not be allowed to drop below 2.7 IU/mL (2.0 mg/kg) or below the level indicated by heparin dose-response testing performed prior to administration of aprotinin.

In TRASYLOL treated patients the neutralisation of heparin by protamine after discontinuation of cardiopulmonary bypass should either be based on a fixed ratio to the amount of heparin administered or be guided by a protamine titration method.

TRASYLOL is not a heparin-sparing agent.

DOSAGE AND ADMINISTRATION: Recommended Dose and Dosage Adjustment: TRASYLOL, given prophylactically to patients undergoing CABG surgery, significantly reduced the donor blood transfusion requirement relative to placebo treatment. TRASYLOL is supplied as a solution containing 10 000 KIU/mL, which is equal to 1.4 mg/mL. All intravenous doses of TRASYLOL should be administered through a central line. **Do not administer any other drug using the same line.** The dosing regimen includes a 1 mL test dose, a loading dose, a dose to be added while **recirculating** the priming fluid of the cardiopulmonary bypass circuit ("pump prime" dose), and a constant infusion dose. To avoid physical incompatibility of TRASYLOL and heparin when adding to the pump prime solution, each agent must be added **during recirculation** of the pump prime to assure adequate dilution prior to admixture with the other component. The dosing regimen (incorporating a 1 mL test dose) is described in Table 4.

Table 4: TRASYLOL

Dosing Regimen for CABG Surgery

	Initial (Test) Dose	Loading Dose	"Pump Prime" Dose	Constant Infusion Dose
TRASYLOL	1 mL (1.4 mg, or 10 000 KIU)	200 mL (280 mg, or 2.0 million KIU)	200 mL (280 mg, or 2.0 million KIU)	50 mL/h (70 mg/h, or 500 000 KIU/h)

Administration: Initial (Test) Dose: Owing to the risk of allergic/anaphylactic reactions, a 1 mL initial (test) dose should be administered intravenously at least 10 minutes before the loading dose. After the uneventful administration of the 1 mL test-dose, the loading dose may be given. An H_1-antagonist and an H_2-antagonist may be administered 15 minutes prior to the initial (test) dose of TRASYLOL. In any case, standard emergency treatments for anaphylactic and allergic reactions should be readily available. Initiation of this initial (test) dose should occur only in operative settings where cardiopulmonary bypass can be rapidly initiated.

Loading Dose: With the patient in a supine position, the loading dose is given slowly over 20-30 minutes, after induction of anesthesia but prior to sternotomy. In patients with known previous exposure to TRASYLOL, the loading dose should be given just prior to cannulation. When the loading dose is complete, it is followed by the constant infusion dose, which is continued until surgery is complete. The "pump prime" dose is added to the **recirculating** priming fluid of the cardiopulmonary bypass circuit, by replacement of an aliquot of the priming fluid, prior to the institution of cardiopulmonary bypass. Total doses of more than 7 million KIU have not been studied in controlled trials.

Parenteral drug products should be inspected visually for particulate matter and discoloration prior to administration whenever solution and container permit. Discard any unused portion.

Reconstitution: Parenteral Products: TRASYLOL is compatible with glucose 20% solution, hydroxyethyl starch solution and Ringers lactate solution.

TRASYLOL (aprotinin) has been shown to be physically incompatible with corticosteroids, heparin, nutrient solutions containing amino acids or fat emulsions, and tetracyclines.

Administration of TRASYLOL in mixed infusions (particularly with beta-lactam antibiotics) should be avoided.

OVERDOSAGE:

Although TRASYLOL (aprotinin) has been used extensively in clinical medicine, no symptoms of overdosing have come to our knowledge. There is no specific antidote.

> For management of a suspected drug overdose, CPhA recommends that you contact your **regional Poison Control Centre**. See the *CPS* Directory section for a list of Poison Control Centres.

ACTION AND CLINICAL PHARMACOLOGY: Mechanism of Action: Aprotinin is a broad spectrum protease inhibitor which has antifibrinolytic properties. By forming reversible stoichiometric enzyme-inhibitor complexes, aprotinin acts as an inhibitor of human trypsin, plasmin, plasma kallikrein and tissue kallikrein, thus inhibiting fibrinolysis.

It also inhibits the contact phase activation of coagulation which both initiates coagulation and promotes fibrinolysis. In the special situation of cardiopulmonary bypass and foreign-surface mediated contact activation, additional inhibition of plasma kallikrein appears to contribute to the desired effect, which in general can be described as minimizing derangements in the coagulation and fibrinolysis system.

Aprotinin modulates the systemic inflammatory response (SIR) associated with cardiopulmonary bypass (CPB) surgery. SIR results in the interrelated activation of the hemostatic, fibrinolytic, cellular and humoral inflammatory systems. Aprotinin, through its inhibition of multiple mediators (e.g., kallikrein, plasmin) results in the attenuation of inflammatory responses, fibrinolysis, and thrombin generation. Aprotinin has a dose-dependent inhibitory effect on the action of thrombolytic agents (ie, streptokinase, tPA and urokinase).

Aprotinin inhibits pro-inflammatory cytokine release and maintains glycoprotein homeostasis. In platelets, aprotinin reduces glycoprotein loss (e.g., GpIb, GpIIb/IIIa), while in granulocytes it prevents the expression of pro-inflammatory adhesive glycoproteins (e.g., CD11b).

Pharmacodynamics: The effects of aprotinin use in CPB involves a reduction in inflammatory response which translates into a decreased need for allogeneic blood transfusions, reduced bleeding, and decreased mediastinal re-exploration for bleeding.

Pharmacokinetics: The studies comparing the pharmacokinetics of aprotinin in healthy volunteers, cardiac patients undergoing surgery with cardiopulmonary bypass, and women undergoing hysterectomy suggest linear pharmacokinetics over the dose range of 500 000 KIU to 2 million KIU.

Absorption: After intravenous (I.V.) injection, rapid distribution of aprotinin occurs into the total extracellular space, leading to a rapid initial decrease in plasma aprotinin concentration.

Distribution: Average steady state intraoperative plasma concentrations were 137 KIU/mL (n=10) after administration of the following dosage regimen: 1 million KIU I.V. loading dose, 1 million KIU into the pump prime volume, 250 000 KIU per hour of operation as continuous intravenous infusion.

Average steady state intraoperative plasma concentrations were 175-281 KIU/mL in patients treated with aprotinin during cardiac surgery (2 million KIU I.V. loading dose, 2 million KIU into the pump prime volume 500 000 KIU per hour of operation as continuous intravenous infusion).

Animal studies have shown that aprotinin is accumulated primarily in the kidney. Aprotinin, after being filtered by the glomeruli, is actively reabsorbed by the proximal tubules in which it is stored in phagolysosomes.

Metabolism: Aprotinin is slowly degraded by lysosomal enzymes. The physiological renal handling of aprotinin is similar to that of other small proteins, e.g., insulin.

Excretion: TRASYLOL is rapidly excreted from the body. In humans, a biphasic elimination pattern with an initial half-life of 0.3-0.7 hours and a terminal half-life of 5-10 hours is observed.

Following a single I.V. dose of radiolabelled aprotinin, approximately 25-40% of the radioactivity is excreted in the urine over 48 hours. After a 30 minute infusion of 1 million KIU, about 2% is excreted as unchanged drug. After a larger dose of 2 million KIU infused over 30 minutes, urinary excretion of unchanged aprotinin accounts for approximately 9% of the dose.

Special Populations and Conditions: Renal Insufficiency: No pharmacokinetic studies are available in patients with terminal renal insufficiency. Studies in patients with renal impairment revealed no clinically significant pharmacokinetic alterations or obvious side effects. A special dose adjustment is not warranted.

Duration of Effect: TRASYLOL is administered as a continuous intravenous infusion throughout the duration of the surgery and acts as a hemostatic agent. Since TRASYLOL inhibits multiple mediators (e.g., kallikrein, plasmin), there is an attenuation of inflammatory responses, fibrinolysis and thrombin generation post-surgery.

STORAGE AND STABILITY: TRASYLOL (aprotinin) is stable when stored in sealed vials at room temperature. Do not store above 25°C. Avoid freezing. If a precipitate or particulate matter is present, or if the contents are cloudy, the drug should not be used. Once a vial has been opened, it should be used immediately.

SPECIAL HANDLING INSTRUCTIONS: Not applicable.

INFORMATION FOR THE PATIENT: Published in e-CPS, available by subscription at www.e-cps.ca.

DOSAGE FORMS, COMPOSITION AND PACKAGING: Each mL of clear almost colorless aqueous, isotonic solution contains: aprotinin 10 000 KIU (Kallikrein Inhibitory Units). Nonmedicinal ingredients: sodium chloride and water for injection. pH of the concentrate is adjusted to 5 to 7 during manufacture. Preservative-free. Single dose vials of 50 and 200 mL. TRASYLOL is administered intravenously. Do not make repeated withdrawals from the vial. It should be used only as a single dose vial.

Travatan® Z Ⓟ

travoprost

Elevated Intraocular Pressure Therapy—Prostaglandin F2α Analogue

Alcon

Date of Revision: June 1, 2010

PHARMACOLOGY: Mechanism of Action: Travoprost, an isopropyl ester prodrug, is rapidly hydrolyzed by esterases in the cornea to the biologically active free acid. Travoprost free acid is a highly selective, potent agonist for the FP prostanoid receptor. FP receptor agonists are thought to reduce intraocular pressure (IOP) by increasing the outflow of aqueous humor, primarily by increased uveoscleral outflow.

Pharmacokinetics/Pharmacodynamics: TRAVATAN Z (travoprost) Ophthalmic Solution, when applied topically to the eye, reduces elevated as well as normal intraocular pressure, whether or not accompanied by glaucoma. Elevated intraocular pressure is a major risk factor in the pathogenesis of glaucomatous visual field loss. The higher the level of intraocular pressure, the greater the likelihood of glaucomatous visual field loss and optic nerve damage. The Advanced Glaucoma Intervention Study (AGIS) established elevated intraocular pressure as a positive risk factor for glaucomatous visual field loss. Eyes with intraocular pressures below 18 mmHg at all visits were found to have little to no visual field loss during the six-year monitoring period.

Absorption: Travoprost is absorbed through the cornea. Studies in rabbits have shown peak concentrations in aqueous humor were reached one to two hours following topical administration. In humans, peak plasma concentrations of travoprost free acid were low (25 pg/mL or less) and occurred within 30 minutes following topical ocular administration of one drop of 0.004% travoprost ophthalmic solution.

Distribution: Travoprost free acid is moderately distributed into body tissues with a volume of distribution of 2.6 L/kg in rats. Radioactivity levels in rat tissues following a single s.c. dose of ^{14}C-travoprost dropped rapidly during the first 3 hours and by 24 hours were below or near detection limits (<0.2-6 ng equiv./g). Binding of travoprost free acid to plasma proteins is moderate at 80% and linear over a 10 000-fold concentration range (0.10-100 ng/mL).

Metabolism: Metabolism was studied in rats, dogs and monkeys. Systemically, travoprost free acid is rapidly and extensively metabolized in the kidney, liver and lung to inactive metabolites. Biotransformations include beta-oxidation of the α(carboxylic acid) chain to give the 1,2-dinor and 1,2,3,4-tetranor analogs, oxidation of the 15-hydroxyl moiety, as well as reduction of the 13,14 double bond.

Excretion: In rats, 95% of a subcutaneous radiolabeled dose was eliminated within 24 hours. The major route of elimination was via the bile (61%) with the remainder excreted by the kidneys. In humans, elimination from plasma was rapid resulting in concentrations below the limit of quantitation (<10 pg/mL) by one hour.

Clinical Studies: TRAVATAN Z (travoprost) Ophthalmic Solution is a benzalkonium chloride-free formulation of TRAVATAN (travoprost) Opthalmic Solution. In three controlled clinical studies, with durations from 6 to 12 months, patients with open angle glaucoma or ocular hypertension were treated once daily in the evening with TRAVATAN Solution, 0.004%. TRAVATAN Solution reduced IOP 6.7 to 9.0 mmHg. Stable diurnal IOP reductions were achieved as early as 2 weeks after initiation of therapy and were maintained over the 6 to 12 month treatment period.

In a multi-center, randomized, controlled trial, patients with mean baseline intraocular pressure of 24 to 26 mmHg on TIMOPTIC 0.5% BID, who were treated with TRAVATAN Solution 0.004% dosed QD adjunctively to TIMOPTIC 0.5% dosed BID, demonstrated 6-7 mmHg additional reductions in intraocular pressure.

There are no plasma interactions with the concomitant administration of travoprost and timolol.

A 9-month pivotal clinical study with a 5-year extension phase was conducted to evaluate the long-term safety of once-daily evening dosing of TRAVATAN Solution. Overall, 196 patients were enrolled into the 5-year extension clinical trial, 67 of which were exposed to TRAVATAN Solution, 0.004%. TRAVATAN Solution maintained clinically relevant long-term IOP control in all patients for nearly 6 years. The overall incidence of iris discoloration in patients treated with TRAVATAN Solution was 11.9%. The adverse events of iris discoloration were mild and did not interrupt patient continuation in the study. The observation of increased iris discoloration did not affect the incidence, nature or severity of adverse events recorded in the study. IOP reduction was similar regardless of the development of increased iris discoloration.

In a 3 month clinical study, TRAVATAN Z Solution dosed QD in the evening produced equivalent IOP lowering efficacy compared to TRAVATAN Solution QD. The maximum mean IOP reductions for TRAVATAN Z Solution (8.5 mmHg) and TRAVATAN Solution (8.4 mmHg) correspond to approximate 31% IOP reductions in each group. All mean reductions were clinically relevant and statistically significant (p<0.0001).

Table 1: TRAVATAN

Summary of Patient Demographics for Clinical Trials in Specific Indication

Study #	Trial Design	Dosage, Route of Administration and Duration	Study Subjects	Mean Age (Range)	Gender
1 - C-97-71	Randomised, triple masked, multicentre, parallel group, active control in patients with open-angle glaucoma or ocular hypertension.	1 drop QD of placebo (8 AM) + 1 drop QD (8 PM) travoprost 0.004% or 0.0015%; 1 drop QD of placebo (8 AM) + 1 drop QD (8 PM) latanoprost 0.005%; or 1 drop BID of TIMOPTIC 0.5% (8 AM and 8 PM). 12 months.	787	64.2 years (22–94)	392 M 395 F
2 - C-97-72	Randomised, triple masked, multicentre, parallel group, active control in patients with open-angle glaucoma or ocular hypertension.	1 drop QD of placebo (8 AM) + 1 drop QD (8 PM) travoprost 0.004% or 0.0015%; or 1 drop of TIMOPTIC 0.5% (8 AM and 8 PM). 6 months.	594	63.7 years (21–91)	293 M 301 F
3 - C-97-73	Randomised, multicentre, triple-masked, vehicle-controlled, parallel group study in patients with open-angle glaucoma or ocular hypertension who were uncontrolled after a 3-week run-in on TIMOPTIC 0.5% dosed BID.	1 drop QD (8 PM) of travoprost 0.004% or 0.0015% plus 1 drop BID of open-label TIMOPTIC 0.5% (8 AM and 8 PM); or 1 drop QD (8 PM) of placebo plus 1 drop BID of open-label TIMOPTIC 0.5% (8 AM and 8 PM). 6 months.	410	63.7 years (11–89)	180 M 230 F
4 - C-97-79	Randomised, multicenter, triple-masked, active controlled, parallel group study in patients with open-angle glaucoma or ocular hypertension.	1 drop QD of placebo (9 AM) + 1 drop QD (9 PM) travoprost 0.004% or 0.0015%; or 1 drop BID of TIMOPTIC 0.5% (9 AM and 9 PM). 9 months.	572	63.3 years (31–88)	284 M 288 F
5 - C-01-74	Randomized, double-masked, multicenter, parallel group, active-controlled in patients with open-angle glaucoma or ocular hypertension.	1 drop QD of placebo (9 AM) + 1 drop QD (9 PM) travoprost 0.004%; or 1 drop QD of latanoprost/timolol 0.5% (9 AM) + 1 drop QD of placebo (9 PM). 6 weeks	106	68.0 years (34–86)	46 M 60 F

Table 2: TRAVATAN

Mean Baseline IOP and Mean Change from Baseline IOP Measurements

Study (Duration)	Baseline Mean IOP (mmHg)			Mean IOP Change from Baseline (mmHg)		
	8 AM	10 AM	4 PM	8 AM	10 AM	4 PM
C-97–71						
TRAVATAN	26.8	25.2	24.6	−7.6	−7.4	−6.9
Timolol	26.9	25.3	24.6	−6.7[c]	−6.1[c]	−5.3[c]
Latanoprost	26.9	25.2	24.9	−7.7	−6.9	−6.3[c]
C-97–72						
TRAVATAN	27.3	25.7	25.1	−7.6	−7.2	−7.0
Timolol	27.4	25.8	25.4	−6.8[c]	−6.0[c]	−5.1[c]
C-97–73						
TRAVATAN/timolol	26.0	24.5	24.6	−6.8	−6.4	−6.0
Timolol	26.4	24.8	24.4	−2.6[c]	−1.8[c]	−1.6[c]
C-97–79[a]						
TRAVATAN	27.4	26.5	25.6	−8.8	−8.7	−8.2
Timolol	27.0	26.2	25.1	−7.7[c]	−7.5[c]	−6.6[c]
C-01–74[b]						
TRAVATAN	25.3	—	24.3	−6.9	—	−6.8
latanoprost/timolol	24.6	—	23.9	−6.4	—	−6.1

[a] The C-97-79 IOP measurements were taken at 9 AM, 11 AM and 4 PM.
[b] The C-01-74 IOP measurements were taken at 9 AM and 5 PM.
[c] P<0.05 for between group comparisons versus TRAVATAN.

INDICATIONS: TRAVATAN Z (travoprost) Ophthalmic Solution is indicated for the reduction of intraocular pressure in patients with open-angle glaucoma or ocular hypertension.

CONTRAINDICATIONS: Known hypersensitivity to any of the ingredients in this product (see Supplied). TRAVATAN Z (travoprost) Ophthalmic Solution may interfere with the maintenance of pregnancy and should not be used by women during pregnancy or by women attempting to become pregnant.

WARNINGS: Ocular Effects: TRAVATAN Z (travoprost) Ophthalmic Solution may gradually change eye color, increasing the amount of brown pigmentation in the iris by increasing the number of melanosomes (pigment granules) in melanocytes. The long term effects on the melanocytes and any consequences of potential injury to the melanocytes and/or deposition of pigment granules to other areas of the eye are currently unknown. Typically, the brown pigmentation around the pupil spreads concentrically towards the periphery in affected eyes, but the entire iris or parts of it may become more brownish. The change in iris color occurs slowly and may not be noticeable for months to years. In clinical trials, iris pigmentation was detected as early as 3 months. This change in eye color has predominantly been seen in patients with mixed colored irides, i.e., blue-brown, grey-brown, yellow-brown and green-brown; however, it has also been observed in patients with brown eyes. These changes may be permanent. Patients should be informed of the possibility of iris color change. There are no clinical data on treatment with TRAVATAN solution beyond five years.

Periorbital and/or eyelid skin darkening has been reported in association with the use of TRAVATAN Z (travoprost) Ophthalmic Solution.

TRAVATAN Z (travoprost) Ophthalmic Solution may gradually change eyelashes in the treated eye; these changes include: increased length, thickness, pigmentation, and/or number of lashes. During long-term clinical trials, eyelash photographs taken periodically during the studies, revealed an overall incidence of eyelash changes of 61%. The overall incidence of patient complaints regarding these changes was 0.8%. Changes in eyelashes may be noticed as early as one and a half months after initiation of treatment. The mechanism of eyelash changes and their long term consequence are currently unknown.

Patients who receive treatment in only one eye may experience increased brown pigmentation of the iris, periorbital and/or eyelid tissue, and eyelashes in the treated eye. They may also experience disparity between the eyes in length, thickness, and/or number of eyelashes. These changes in pigmentation and lash growth may be permanent.

There is no experience of TRAVATAN Z (travoprost) Ophthalmic Solution in inflammatory ocular conditions; nor in neovascular or angle-closure glaucoma.

Systemic Effects: *Pregnancy:* No adequate and well-controlled studies have been performed in pregnant women. Travoprost, like all FP agonists, may interfere with the maintenance of pregnancy and should not be used by women during pregnancy or by women attempting to become pregnant.

Teratogenic Effects: Travoprost was teratogenic in rats. Travoprost administered i.v. to pregnant rats from gestation Days 6-17 at a dose of 10 μg/kg/day, induced a slight increase in the incidence of skeletal malformations such as fused sternebrae, domed head and hydrocephaly. No effect was observed at 3 μg/kg/day (75 times the maximum recommended human dose of 0.04 μg/kg/day). The no effect level for fetal external, visceral or skeletal malformation was observed after 1.0 μg/kg/day s.c. administration during gestation days 6 to 16 to pregnant mice, though postimplantation loss was increased at that dose, but not at 0.3 μg/kg/day.

PRECAUTIONS: There have been reports of bacterial keratitis associated with the use of multiple-dose containers of topical ophthalmic products. These containers had been inadvertently contaminated by patients who, in most cases, had a concurrent corneal disease or a disruption of the epithelial surface (see Information to Be Provided to the Patient).

Patients may slowly develop increased brown pigmentation of the iris. This change may not be noticeable for months to years (see Warnings).

TRAVATAN Z (travoprost) Ophthalmic Solution should be used with caution in patients with active intraocular inflammation (iritis/uveitis).

Macular edema, including cystoid macular edema, has been reported during treatment with prostaglandin $F_{2\alpha}$ analogues. These reports have mainly occurred in aphakic patients, pseudophakic patients with a torn posterior lens capsule, or in patients with known risk factors for macular edema. TRAVATAN Z Solution should be used with caution in these patients.

TRAVATAN Z (travoprost) Ophthalmic Solution is a benzalkonium chloride-free formulation of TRAVATAN (travoprost) Ophthalmic Solution. In phase III clinical trials, TRAVATAN Solution was studied adjunctively with TIMOPTIC. No additional adjunctive studies have been done.

TRAVATAN solution has been studied in patients with mild to severe hepatic impairment (Childs-Pugh Classification A-C) and also in patients with mild to severe renal impairment (creatinine clearance from as low as 14 mL/min/1.73 m^2 to 77 mL/min/1.73 m^2). No clinically relevant changes in hematology, blood chemistry, urinalysis laboratory data or plasma concentrations of free acid were observed in patients with impaired (mild, moderate, or severe) hepatic or renal function. No dosage adjustment is necessary in patients with hepatic or renal impairment.

Patients should remove contact lenses prior to administration of the solution. Lenses may be reinserted 15 minutes following administration of TRAVATAN Z Solution.

Since prostaglandins are biologically active and may be absorbed through the skin, women who are pregnant or attempting to become pregnant should exercise appropriate precautions to avoid direct exposure to the contents of the bottle. In case of accidental contact with the contents of the bottle, thoroughly cleanse the exposed area with soap and water immediately.

Lactation: A study in lactating rats demonstrated that radiolabeled travoprost and/or its metabolites were excreted in milk. It is not known whether this drug or its metabolites are excreted in human milk. Because many drugs are excreted in human milk, caution should be exercised when TRAVATAN Z Solution is administered to a nursing woman.

Children: Safety and effectiveness in pediatric patients have not been established.

Information to Be Provided to the Patient: Patients should be advised concerning all the information contained in the Warnings and Precautions sections.

Patients should also be instructed to avoid allowing the tip of the dispensing container to contact the eye or surrounding structures because this could cause the tip to become contaminated by common bacteria known to cause ocular infections. Serious damage to the eye and subsequent loss of vision may result from using contaminated solutions.

Patients also should be advised that if they develop an intercurrent ocular condition (e.g., trauma, or infection) or have ocular surgery, they should immediately seek their physician's advice concerning the continued use of the multi-dose container.

Patients should be advised that if they develop symptoms of hypersensitivity, particularly conjunctivitis and lid reactions, they should immediately seek their physician's advice.

Contact lenses should be removed prior to administration of TRAVATAN Z solution. Lenses may be reinserted 15 minutes following administration.

If more than one topical ophthalmic drug is being used, the drugs should be administered at least five (5) minutes apart.

ADVERSE EFFECTS: TRAVATAN Z (travoprost) Ophthalmic Solution is a benzalkonium chloride-free formulation of TRAVATAN (travoprost) Ophthalmic Solution. Ocular hyperemia was reported in 40% of all patients receiving TRAVATAN (travoprost) Ophthalmic Solution and TRAVATAN Z (travoprost) Ophthalmic Solution. Approximately 80 to 90% of the ocular hyperemia was mild in intensity and subsided over time without treatment. Up to 3% of the patients discontinued therapy due to conjunctival hyperemia. Table 3 summarizes adverse reactions reported with TRAVATAN Solution.

During clinical studies, there were extremely rare reports of the following: choroidal nevus, retinal detachment, retinal hemorrhage, retinal pigmentation, and vitreous detachment.

Table 3: TRAVATAN

Overall (Related and Unrelated) Frequency and Incidence of Adverse Events Occurring at an Incidence ≥1.0%

	TRAVATAN 0.004% N=656		TRAVATAN 0.004% + Timolol 0.5% N=145	
	N	%	N	%
Ocular				
Hyperemia Eye	259	39.5	52	35.9
Discomfort Eye	35	5.3	7	4.8
Pruritus Eye	48	7.3	5	3.4
Visual Acuity Decrease	29	4.4	6	4.1
Iris Discoloration[a]	15	2.3	0	
Dry Eye	20	3.0	8	5.5
Foreign Body Sensation	24	3.7	4	2.8
Pain Eye	33	5.0	6	4.1
Keratitis	17	2.6	3	2.1
Vision Blurred	13	2.0	3	2.1
Cataract NOS	13	2.0	1	0.7
Blepharitis	11	1.7	2	1.4
Cells	7	1.1	6	4.1
Hemorrhage Subconjunctival	7	1.1	0	
Conjunctivitis	10	1.5	2	1.4
Flare	7	1.1	2	1.4
Photophobia	8	1.2	4	2.8
Tearing	7	1.1	3	2.1
Lid Disorder	1[b]	0.2	3[c]	2.1
Eye Fatigue	2	0.3	2	1.4
Sticky Sensation	1	0.2	2	1.4
Nonocular				
Body as a Whole				
Surgical/Medical Procedure	31	4.7	4	2.8
Infection	24	3.7	3	2.1
Headache	20	3.0	2	1.4
Pain	14	2.1	0	
Injury Accidental	17	2.6	1	0.7
Cold Syndrome	10	1.5	3	2.1
Flu Syndrome	17	2.6	2	1.4
Allergy	3	0.5	2	1.4
Cardiovascular System				
Hypertension	27	4.1	2	1.4
Digestive System				
GI Disorder	10	1.5	1	0.7
Metabolic and Nutritional				
Hypercholesteremia	11	1.7	0	
Nervous				
Depression	9	1.4	2	1.4
Respiratory System				
Sinusitis	11	1.7	3	2.1
Bronchitis	7	1.1	1	0.7
Rhinitis	7	1.1	1	0.7
Urogenital System				
Infection Urinary Tract	7	1.1	3	2.1
Prostate Disorder	6	0.9	2	1.4

(cont'd)

[a] Increase in brown pigmentation of the iris.
[b] Lid pigment (1).
[c] Prominent vessel (1), sore soot (1), lid lesion (1).

A similar safety profile was observed in a clinical trial of 3 months duration, comparing therapy with TRAVATAN Z Solution (399 patients dosed QD in the evening) to TRAVATAN Solution (400 patients dosed QD in the evening).

The following serious, unexpected reactions reported during the post-market use of TRAVATAN Solution in clinical practice and in the literature have been included based on the frequency of reporting, possible causal connection to TRAVATAN Solution, or a combination of these factors:

Ocular Disorders: corneal edema and macular edema.

Nonocular Disorders: Cardiac disorders: bradycardia and tachycardia. General disorders and administration site conditions: chest discomfort. Respiratory, thoracic and mediastinal disorders: asthma and dyspnea.

A few case reports of iritis/uveitis associated with the use of travoprost have been published. These cases occurred a few days after travoprost use in patients without a history of iritis/uveitis. All of these cases resolved after stopping travoprost with or without corticosteroid treatment.

OVERDOSE:

Symptoms: A single-dose intravenous study in rats was conducted to elucidate maximal acute hazard. The dose employed was 250 000- times the proposed daily clinical exposure and over 5000-times the possible exposure from the entire contents of 1 product container. No treatment related pharmacotoxic signs were present in the animals receiving travoprost.

Treatment: If overdosage with TRAVATAN Z (travoprost) Ophthalmic Solution occurs, treatment should be symptomatic.

For management of a suspected drug overdose, including oral ingestion, contact your regional Poison Control Centre. See the *CPS* Directory section for a list of Poison Control Centres.

DOSAGE: The recommended dosage is one drop in the affected eye(s) once-daily. Optimal effect is observed with evening dosing. The dosage of TRAVATAN Z (travoprost) Ophthalmic Solution should not exceed once-daily since it has been shown that more frequent administration may decrease the intraocular pressure lowering effect.

Reduction of intraocular pressure starts approximately 2 hours after administration and the maximum effect is reached after 12 hours.

TRAVATAN Z Solution may be used concomitantly with topical ophthalmic beta-blockers to lower intraocular pressure. If more than 1 topical ophthalmic drug is being used, the drugs should be administered at least five (5) minutes apart.

INFORMATION FOR THE PATIENT: Published in e-CPS, available by subscription at www.e-cps.ca.

SUPPLIED: Each mL of sterile, isotonic, buffered, preserved aqueous solution contains: travoprost 40 µg. Nonmedicinal ingredients: polyoxyl 40 hydrogenated castor oil, purified water, sofZia preservative system (boric acid, propylene glycol, sorbitol, zinc chloride), and sodium hydroxide and/or hydrochloric acid (to adjust pH). Preserved in the bottle with an ionic buffered system, sofZia. pH: approx. 5.7. Osmolality: approx. 290 mOsm/kg. Alcon oval DROP-TAINER dispenser bottle. This plastic, oval-shaped dispenser bottle, containing 2.5 mL or 5 mL, includes a tamper evident neck-band which shrinks to conform around the closure and neck area of the package. Store between 2 to 25°C.

Trelstar™ 3.75 mg (1 month slow-release) Ⓟ

triptorelin pamoate

Luteinizing Hormone-Releasing Hormone (LHRH) Analog

Paladin

Trelstar™ 11.25 mg (3 month slow-release) Ⓟ

triptorelin pamoate

Luteinizing Hormone-Releasing Hormone (LHRH) Analog

Paladin

Date of Preparation: June 18, 2010

SUMMARY PRODUCT INFORMATION:

Route of Administration	Dosage Form/ Strength	Clinically Relevant Nonmedicinal Ingredients
Intramuscular	Powder (microgranules) for slow release suspension 3.75 mg of triptorelin peptide base units/vial; 11.25 mg of triptorelin peptide base units/vial	For a complete listing see Dosage Forms, Composition and Packaging.

INDICATIONS AND CLINICAL USE: TRELSTAR (triptorelin pamoate for injectable suspension) is indicated for:

- the palliative treatment of hormone dependent advanced carcinoma of the prostate gland (stage D2).

Geriatrics (>65 years of age): The majority of the patients studied in the clinical trials for TRELSTAR were 65 years and older.

Pediatrics (<18 years of age): The safety and effectiveness of TRELSTAR in pediatric patients have not been established (see Warnings and Precautions).

TRELSTAR must be administered under the supervision of a physician.

CONTRAINDICATIONS:

- TRELSTAR is contraindicated in patients with hypersensitivity to gonadotropin releasing hormone or luteinizing hormone-releasing hormone (GnRH or LHRH), GnRH agonist analogs or any ingredient in the formulation or component of the container. Anaphylactic reactions to synthetic GnRH or GnRH agonist analogs have been reported (see Warnings and Precautions). For a complete listing, see Dosage Forms, Composition and Packaging.
- TRELSTAR is contraindicated in women who are or may become pregnant while receiving the drug. TRELSTAR may cause fetal harm when administered to a pregnant woman. If this drug is used during pregnancy or if the patient becomes pregnant while taking this drug, she should be apprised of the potential hazard to the fetus (see Warnings and Precautions).
- TRELSTAR is contraindicated in nursing women (see Warnings and Precautions).

WARNINGS AND PRECAUTIONS: General: TRELSTAR (triptorelin pamoate for injection), like other LH-RH agonists, cause a transient increase in serum concentration of testosterone during the first weeks of treatment. Patients may experience worsening of symptoms or onset of new symptoms, including bone pain, neuropathy, hematuria, or ureteral or bladder outlet obstruction. Cases of spinal cord compression, which may contribute to paralysis with or without fatal complications, have been reported with LH-RH agonists. If spinal cord compression or renal impairment due to ureteral obstruction develops, standard treatment of these complications should be instituted. Patients with metastatic vertebral lesions and/or with urinary tract obstruction should begin triptorelin therapy under close supervision.

Hypersensitivity and anaphylactic reactions have been reported with triptorelin as with other LHRH agonists (see Adverse Reactions, Post-Market Adverse Drug Reactions).

Carcinogenesis and Mutagenesis: Carcinogenicity and mutagenicity studies have been performed in animals.

Endocrine and Metabolism: Changes in Bone Density: Bone loss can be expected as part of natural aging and can also be anticipated during the hypoandrogenic state caused by long-term use of triptorelin. In patients with significant risk factors for decreased bone mineral content and/or bone mass such as family history of osteoporosis, chronic use of corticosteroids or anticonvulsants or chronic abuse of alcohol or tobacco, triptorelin may pose additional risk. In these patients, risk versus benefit must be weighed carefully before initiation of triptorelin therapy.

Long-term administration of triptorelin will cause suppression of pituitary gonadotropins and gonadal hormone production with clinical symptoms of hypogonadism. These changes have been observed to reverse on discontinuation of therapy. However, whether the clinical symptoms of induced hypogonadism will reverse in all patients has not yet been established.

In prostate cancer patients, an assessment of bone lesions may require the use of bone scans. Prostatic lesions may be monitored by ultrasonography/or CT scan in addition to digital rectal examination. The status of obstructive uropathy may be assessed and/or diagnosed using intravenous pyelography, ultrasonography or CT scan.

Renal and Hepatic: Triptorelin exposure was higher in patients with renal or hepatic insufficiency than in healthy volunteers. Clinical consequences of the increase and potential need for dose adjustment are unknown.

Special Populations: Pregnant Women: The safe use of triptorelin during pregnancy has not been established clinically. If a woman becomes pregnant while receiving TRELSTAR, therapy should be discontinued and the patient advised of the potential risk to the fetus. The possibility exists that spontaneous abortion may occur if the drug is administered during pregnancy (see Contraindications).

Nursing Women: It is not known to what extent triptorelin is excreted into human milk and caution should be exercised when TRELSTAR is administered to nursing women (see Contraindications).

Pediatrics (<18 years of age): The safety and effectiveness of TRELSTAR in pediatric patients have not been established.

Geriatrics (>65 years of age): The majority of the patients studied in the clinical trials for TRELSTAR were 65 years and older.

Race: The effects of race on triptorelin pharmacokinetics, safety, and efficacy have not been systematically studied. In the three controlled clinical studies conducted to compare a controlled release formulation of triptorelin acetate with orchiectomy, no race data were collected. The study that compared TRELSTAR (1-month, 3.75 mg triptorelin pamoate formulation) and TRELSTAR (3-month, 11.25 mg triptorelin pamoate formulation), included 47.7% Caucasian, 37.6% Black, and 14.7% Colored patients.

Monitoring and Laboratory Tests: During therapy with TRELSTAR, patients should be routinely monitored by physical examinations and appropriate laboratory tests. Response to TRELSTAR may be monitored by periodically measuring serum concentrations of testosterone and prostate specific antigen. Results of testosterone determinations are dependant on assay methodology. It is advisable to be aware of the type and precision of the assay methodology to make appropriate clinical and therapeutic decisions.

ADVERSE REACTIONS: Adverse Drug Reaction Overview: Triptorelin pamoate has been found to be generally well tolerated in clinical trials. Adverse reactions reported in these trials were rarely severe enough to result in patient withdrawal from triptorelin treatment. Three postmarketing reports of anaphylactic shock and seven postmarketing reports of angioedema related to triptorelin administration have been reported since 1986 (see Warnings and Precautions). In clinical trials, no serious adverse events that were considered to be related to study drug administration were reported.

As seen with other LHRH agonist therapies, the most commonly observed adverse events during triptorelin treatment were due to the expected physiological effects related to decreased testosterone levels. These effects included hot flushes, impotence, and decreased libido. TRELSTAR, like other LH-RH analogs, caused a transient increase in serum testosterone concentrations during the first weeks of treatment. Therefore, potential exacerbations of signs and symptoms of the disease during the first few weeks of treatment are of concern in patients with vertebral metastases and/or urinary obstruction or hematuria. If these conditions are aggravated, it may lead to neurological problems such as weakness and/or paresthesia of the lower limbs or worsening of urinary symptoms (see Warnings and Precautions).

Clinical Trial Adverse Drug Reactions: Because clinical trials are conducted under very specific conditions the adverse reaction rates observed in the clinical trials may not reflect the rates observed in practice and should not be compared to the rates in the clinical trials of another drug. Adverse drug reaction information from clinical trials is useful for identifying drug-related adverse events and for approximating rates.

Clinical Studies with Triptorelin Acetate: Three controlled clinical studies were conducted on 265 patients to compare a controlled release formulation of triptorelin acetate (N=160) with orchiectomy (N=105).

In the first study, all patients received an i.m. injection of 3.75 mg triptorelin and every month thereafter for 24 months, with the exception of 3 patients who received 100 µg triptorelin s.c. for the first month. In the second study, all patients received 100 µg triptorelin s.c. for the first 7 days, and 3.75 mg i.m. on Days 8, 28, and every month thereafter for up to 18 months. In the third study, all patients received an i.m. injection of 3.75 mg triptorelin on Days 0 and 28, and every month thereafter for 24 months.

In these studies, the most commonly observed adverse events reported in 5% or more of patients were: impotence (50.0% in the triptorelin group and 41.2% in the orchiectomy group), decreased libido (44.9% of patients in the triptorelin group and 39.2% in the orchiectomy group), hot flushes (44.9% in the triptorelin group and 43.3% in the orchiectomy group) and reduced size of genitalia (12.2% in the triptorelin group). These events are known to be related to biochemical or surgical castration.

Clinical Study with Triptorelin Pamoate: The safety of triptorelin was also evaluated in a study that compared TRELSTAR (1-month, 3.75 mg triptorelin pamoate formulation) and TRELSTAR (3-month, 11.25 mg triptorelin pamoate formulation). The patients in this study were randomized to receive either three injections of triptorelin pamoate 3-month formulation (11.25 mg), administered i.m. every 84 days for 9 months, or nine injections of triptorelin pamoate 1-month formulation (3.75 mg), administered i.m. every 28 days for 9 months.

The following possibly or probably related systemic adverse events were reported by 1% or more of patients in this study: see Table 1.

Table 1: TRELSTAR 3.75 mg (1 month slow-release)/TRELSTAR 11.25 mg (3 month slow-release)

Incidence (%) of Possibly or Probably Related Systemic Adverse Events Reported by 1% or More of Patients in Either Treatment Group Treated with TRELSTAR 3.75 mg (1 injection every 28 days for 9 months) and TRELSTAR 11.25 mg (1 injection every 84 days for 9 months)

	TRELSTAR (3.75 mg) N=172 n (%)	TRELSTAR (11.25 mg) N=174 n (%)
Application Site Disorders		
Injection site pain	2 (1.2)	7 (4.0)
Body as a Whole		
Hot flushes[a]	114 (66.3)	127 (73.0)
Back pain	6 (3.5)	5 (2.9)
Pain	10 (5.8)	6 (3.4)
Leg pain	5 (2.9)	9 (5.2)
Fatigue	5 (2.9)	4 (2.3)
Chest pain	0 (0.0)	3 (1.7)
Asthenia	2 (1.2)	2 (1.1)
Oedema peripheral	3 (1.7)	2 (1.1)
Allergic reaction	2 (1.2)	0 (0.0)
Cardiovascular Disorders		
Hypertension	8 (4.7)	7 (4.0)
Oedema dependant	0 (0.0)	4 (2.3)
Central and Peripheral Nervous Systems Disorders		
Headache	7 (4.1)	12 (6.9)
Dizziness	5 (2.9)	5 (2.9)
Cramps legs	1 (0.6)	3 (1.7)
Endocrine Disorders		
Breast pain male	5 (2.9)	4 (2.3)
Gynecomastia	0 (0.0)	3 (1.7)
Gastrointestinal System Disorders		
Constipation	4 (2.3)	3 (1.7)

(cont'd)

Table 1: TRELSTAR 3.75 mg (1 month slow-release)/TRELSTAR 11.25 mg (3 month slow-release) *(cont'd)*

Incidence (%) of Possibly or Probably Related Systemic Adverse Events Reported by 1% or More of Patients in Either Treatment Group Treated with TRELSTAR 3.75 mg (1 injection every 28 days for 9 months) and TRELSTAR 11.25 mg (1 injection every 84 days for 9 months)

	TRELSTAR (3.75 mg) N=172 n (%)	TRELSTAR (11.25 mg) N=174 n (%)
Nausea	7 (4.1)	5 (2.9)
Diarrhoea	4 (2.3)	2 (1.1)
Abdominal pain	1 (0.6)	2 (1.1)
Dyspepsia	2 (1.2)	3 (1.7)
Heart Rate and Rhythm Disorders		
Palpitation	3 (1.7)	0 (0.0)
Liver and Biliary System Disorders		
Hepatic function abnormal	0 (0.0)	2 (1.1)
Metabolic and Nutritional Disorders		
Oedema legs	14 (8.1)	11 (6.3)
Diabetes mellitus	2 (1.2)	1 (0.6)
Musculo-skeletal Disorders		
Skeletal pain	20 (11.6)	23 (13.2)
Arthralgia	4 (2.3)	4 (2.3)
Myalgia	1 (0.6)	2 (1.1)
Psychiatric Disorders		
Insomnia	2 (1.2)	3 (1.7)
Depression[a]	3 (1.7)	1 (0.6)
Impotence[a]	7 (4.1)	4 (2.3)
Anorexia	1 (0.6)	3 (1.7)
Libido decreased[a]	1 (0.6)	4 (2.3)
Respiratory System Disorders		
Coughing	1 (0.6)	3 (1.7)
Dyspnoea	3 (1.7)	2 (1.1)
Pharyngitis	0 (0.0)	2 (1.1)
Skin and Appendages Disorders		
Rash	1 (0.6)	3 (1.7)
Pruritus	2 (1.2)	0 (0.0)
Urinary System Disorders		
Urinary tract infection	3 (1.7)	0 (0.0)
Dysuria	3 (1.7)	8 (4.6)
Urinary retention	0 (0.0)	2 (1.1)
Vision Disorders		
Eye pain	1 (0.6)	2 (1.1)
Conjunctivitis	0 (0.0)	2 (1.1)

[a] Expected pharmacological consequence of testosterone suppression.

Less Common Clinical Trial Adverse Drug Reactions (<1%): Adverse drug reactions that were reported by 1% or less of subjects in both the TRELSTAR 3.75 mg and TRELSTAR 11.25 mg treatment groups, and were considered to be possibly or probably related to study drug, included the following: injection site reaction, malaise, muscle weakness, rhinitis, skin disorder, and hematuria.

Abnormal Hematologic and Clinical Chemistry Findings: The incidence rate greater than 15% for low abnormal laboratory values (hemoglobin and erythrocyte count) and high abnormal laboratory values (fasting glucose, BUN, and alkaline phosphatase) were comparable for both TRELSTAR 3.75 mg and TRELSTAR 11.25 mg.

Post-Market Adverse Drug Reactions: During post-marketing surveillance, three cases of anaphylactic shock and two cases of angioedema have been reported that were related to triptorelin.

DRUG INTERACTIONS: Overview: No formal drug interaction studies have been conducted with TRELSTAR and no data are available on the interaction with alcohol. In the absence of relevant data and as a precaution, hyperprolactinemic drugs should not be prescribed concomitantly with triptorelin pamoate since hyperprolactinemia reduces the number of pituitary GnRH receptors.

Drug-Drug Interactions: Interactions with other drugs have not been established.

Drug-Food Interactions: Interactions with food have not been established.

Drug-Herb Interactions: Interactions with herbal products have not been established.

Drug-Laboratory Test Interactions: Administration of LHRH analogs, including triptorelin, in therapeutic doses results in suppression of the pituitary-gonadal system. Normal function is usually restored within 4 to 12 weeks after treatment is discontinued. Diagnostic tests of pituitary-gonadal function conducted during treatment and within 4 to 12 weeks after discontinuation of therapy with a LHRH agonist may therefore be misleading.

DOSAGE AND ADMINISTRATION:

Recommended Dose and Dosage Adjustment: Triptorelin pamoate is intended for long-term administration unless clinically inappropriate.

TRELSTAR (1 month slow release) 3.75 mg triptorelin/vial: The recommended dose of TRELSTAR 3.75 mg (triptorelin for injectable suspension) is 3.75 mg (as peptide base) incorporated in a depot formulation, monthly. The lyophilized microgranules are to be reconstituted either with 2 mL of sterile water for injection utilizing a 21-gauge needle or using one of the single dose delivery systems (MIXJECT). Administer monthly as a single intramuscular injection, in accordance with the Instructions for use (see below).

TRELSTAR (3 month slow release) 11.25 mg triptorelin/vial: The recommended dose of TRELSTAR 11.25 mg (triptorelin for injectable suspension) is 11.25 mg (as peptide base), incorporated in a depot formulation, every 3 months. The lyophilized microgranules are to be reconstituted either with 2 mL of sterile water for injection utilizing a 21-gauge needle or using one of the single dose delivery systems (MIXJECT). Administer every 3 months as a single intramuscular injection, in accordance with the Instructions for use (see below).

Missed Dose: Maintaining testosterone suppression is important in treating the symptoms of hormone-dependent prostate cancer. Missing an appointment by a few days should not disrupt the benefits of treatment, but keeping a consistent schedule of TRELSTAR injections is an important part of treatment.

Administration: TRELSTAR is administered as a single intramuscular injection.

Reconstitution: TRELSTAR is supplied in single-dose vials containing lyophilized microgranules. These microgranules are to be reconstituted with 2 mL of sterile water for injection. Instructions are provided (see below) for reconstitution using the TRELSTAR dose delivery system (with Sterile Water for Injection), MIXJECT and the TRELSTAR vial (without Sterile Water for Injection).

When 2 mL of Sterile Water for Injection is added to the lyophilized triptorelin pamoate microgranules and mixed, a suspension is formed. For TRELSTAR 3.75 mg (1 month slow release) this is equivalent to 3.75 mg of triptorelin peptide base units intended as a single monthly intramuscular injection. For TRELSTAR 11.25 mg (3 month slow release) this is equivalent to 11.25 mg of triptorelin peptide base units intended as a single 3 month intramuscular injection.

The suspension should be discarded if not used immediately after reconstitution. As with other drugs administered by intramuscular injection, the injection site should be varied periodically.

As with all parenteral admixtures, the reconstituted product should be examined for the presence of foreign particulate matter, agglomeration or discoloration. Any defective units should be discarded.

Single use only. Inject immediately after reconstitution and discard unused portion.

Instructions for Use—TRELSTAR Vial (with Sterile Water for Injection), MIXJECT: Please read the instructions completely before you begin.

MIXJECT Preparation: Wash your hands with soap and hot water and put on gloves immediately prior to preparing the injection. Place the sealed tray on a clean, flat surface that is covered with a sterile pad or cloth. Peel the cover away from the tray and remove the MIXJECT components and the TRELSTAR vial. Remove the Flip-Off button from the top of the vial, revealing the rubber stopper. Place the vial in a standing upright position on the prepared surface. Disinfect the rubber stopper with the alcohol wipe. Discard the alcohol wipe and allow the stopper to dry. Proceed to MIXJECT Activation.

MIXJECT Activation:

1. Peel the cover away from the blister pack containing the vial adapter. **Do not remove the vial adapter from the blister pack.** Place the blister pack containing the vial adapter firmly on the vial top, piercing the vial. Push down gently until you feel it snap in place. Remove the blister pack from the vial adapter.
2. (a) Screw the plunger rod into the barrel end of the syringe. Remove the cap from the syringe barrel.
(b) Connect the syringe to the vial adapter by screwing it clockwise into the opening on the side of the vial adapter. Be sure to gently twist the syringe until it stops turning to ensure a tight connection.
3. While holding the vial, place your thumb on the plunger rod and push the plunger rod in all the way to transfer the diluent from the pre-filled syringe into the vial. Do not release the plunger rod.
4. Keeping the plunger rod depressed, gently swirl the vial so that the diluent rinses the sides of the vial. This will ensure complete mixing of TRELSTAR and the sterile water diluent. The suspension will now have a milky appearance. In order to avoid separation of the suspension, proceed to the next steps without delay.
5. (a) Invert the MIXJECT system so that the vial is at the top. Grasp the MIXJECT system firmly by the syringe and pull back the plunger rod slowly to draw the reconstituted TRELSTAR into the syringe.
(b) Return the vial to its upright position, and disconnect the vial adapter and vial from the MIXJECT syringe assembly by turning the plastic cap of the vial adapter clockwise. **Grasp only the plastic cap when removing.**
6. Lift up the safety cover and remove the clear plastic needle shield by pulling it from the assembly. The safety cover should be perpendicular to the needle, with the needle facing away from you. The syringe containing the TRELSTAR suspension is now ready for administration. **The suspension should be administered immediately after reconstitution.**

MIXJECT Disposal:

1. After administering the injection, immediately activate the safety mechanism by centering your thumb or forefinger on the textured finger pad area of the safety cover and pushing it forward over the needle until you hear or feel it lock. Use the one-handed technique and activate the mechanism away from yourself and others. Activation of the safety cover causes virtually no splatter.
2. Immediately discard the syringe assembly after a single use into a suitable sharps container.

Instructions for Use—TRELSTAR Vial (without Sterile Water for Injection): The lyophilized microgranules are to be reconstituted **in sterile water. No other diluent should be used.** It is necessary for an aseptic technique to be maintained throughout preparation.

Preparation:

1. Using a syringe fitted with a sterile 21-gauge needle, withdraw 2 mL **sterile water** for injection, USP, and after removing the flip-off seal from the vial, inject into the vial.
2. Shake well to thoroughly disperse particles to obtain a uniform suspension. The suspension will appear milky.
3. Withdraw the entire content of the reconstituted suspension into the syringe and inject it immediately.

Disposal: Dispose of the syringe and vial into a suitable sharps container.

OVERDOSAGE:

The pharmacologic properties of triptorelin pamoate and its mode of administration make accidental or intentional overdosage unlikely. There is no experience of overdosage from clinical trials. Acute animal toxicity of the drug is low and high multiples of clinical dose did not cause any adverse effects. If overdosage occurs, it should be managed symptomatically.

> For management of a suspected drug overdose, CPhA recommends that you contact your **regional Poison Control Centre**. See the *CPS* Directory section for a list of Poison Control Centres.

ACTION AND CLINICAL PHARMACOLOGY: Triptorelin is a synthetic decapeptide agonist analog of naturally occurring luteinizing hormone-releasing hormone (LHRH), also called gonadotropin releasing hormone (GnRH). This analog possesses greater potency than the natural hormone.

Triptorelin, a LHRH agonist, acts as a potent inhibitor of gonadotropin secretion when given continuously in therapeutic doses. On administration of triptorelin there is an initial and transient increase in circulating levels of luteinizing hormone (LH), follicle stimulating hormone (FSH), and testosterone. However, chronic and continuous administration of triptorelin results in decreased LH and FSH secretion and suppression of testicular steroidogenesis. A reduction of serum testosterone levels into the range normally seen in surgically castrated men occurs approximately 2 to 4 weeks after initiation of therapy. This results in accessory sexual organ atrophy which is generally reversible upon discontinuation of drug therapy.

Following a single intramuscular injection of TRELSTAR 3.75 mg (triptorelin pamoate for injectable suspension) as a 1 month sustained release formulation to healthy male volunteers, serum testosterone levels first increased, peaking on day 4, and thereafter declined to low levels by 4 weeks. By week 8, following this single injection, low levels of testosterone were no longer maintained. A similar serum testosterone profile was observed in patients with advanced prostate cancer after intramuscular injection.

Following intramuscular injection of TRELSTAR 11.25 mg (triptorelin pamoate for injectable suspension) in patients with advanced prostate cancer, serum testosterone levels first increased, peaking around day 2, and thereafter declined to low levels by 4 weeks. This suppression of testosterone, similar to castrate levels (<50 ng/dL), was maintained for 3 months after the first injection and on repeat administration. Intramuscular injection of TRELSTAR every 3 months ensures that exposure to triptorelin is maintained with no clinically significant accumulation.

Pharmacokinetics: Absorption: Triptorelin is not active when given orally. The pharmacokinetic parameters following single intramuscular injections of triptorelin 3.75 mg and 11.25 mg sustained release formulations are listed in Table 2. The plasma concentrations for the 3.75 mg formulation declined to 0.084 ng/mL at 4 weeks.

Table 2: TRELSTAR 3.75 mg (1 month slow-release)/TRELSTAR 11.25 mg (3 month slow-release)

Pharmacokinetic Parameters of Triptorelin (Mean±SD or Median (Range) for T_{max})

Triptorelin Pharmacokinetics				
Dose No. of Subjects	C_{max} (ng/mL)	T_{max} (h)	AUC (h·ng/mL)	F (%)[a] (No. of days)
3.75 mg 20 healthy male volunteers	28.43±7.31	1.0 (1.0– 3.0)	223.15±46.96[b]	83 (28 d)
11.25 mg 13 prostate cancer patients	38.5±10.5	2.0 (2.0– 4.0)	2268.0±444.63[c]	103 (85 d)

[a] Computed as the mean AUC of the study divided by the mean AUC of healthy volunteers corrected for dose (AUC=36.1 h·ng/mL; 500 µg IV bolus of triptorelin).
[b] AUC (0-28 d).
[c] AUC (0-85 d).

Distribution: The volume of distribution of triptorelin following IV administration of 0.5 mg triptorelin was approximately 30 L in healthy male volunteers. Since there is no evidence that triptorelin at clinically relevant concentrations binds to plasma proteins, drug interactions involving binding-site displacement are unlikely (see Drug Interactions).
Metabolism: Metabolites of triptorelin have not been determined in humans. However, human pharmacokinetic data suggest that C-terminal fragments produced by degradation are either completely degraded within tissues or are rapidly further degraded in plasma, or cleared by the kidneys.
Excretion: Triptorelin is eliminated by both the liver and the kidneys. Following IV administration of 0.5 mg triptorelin peptide to 6 healthy male volunteers with a creatinine clearance of 149.9 mL/min, 41.7% of the dose was excreted in urine as intact peptide with a total triptorelin clearance of 211.9 mL/min. This percentage increased to 62.3% in patients with liver disease who have a lower creatinine clearance (89.9 mL/min). It has also been observed that the non-renal clearance of triptorelin (patient anuric, Cl_{creat}=0) was 76.2 mL/min, thus indicating that the nonrenal elimination of triptorelin is mainly dependant on the liver (see Special Populations and Conditions).
Special Populations and Conditions: Renal and Hepatic Impairment: After an IV injection of 0.5 mg triptorelin peptide, the two distribution half-lives were unaffected by renal and hepatic impairment, but renal insufficiency led to a decrease in total triptorelin clearance proportional to the decrease in creatinine clearance as well as an increase in volume of distribution and consequently an increase in elimination half-life (see Table 3). The decrease in triptorelin clearance was more pronounced in subjects with liver insufficiency, but the half-life was prolonged similarly in subjects with renal insufficiency, since the volume of distribution was only minimally increased.
Age and Race: The effects of age and race on triptorelin pharmacokinetics have not been systematically studied. However, pharmacokinetic data obtained in young healthy male volunteers aged 20 to 22 years with an elevated creatinine clearance (approximately 250 mL/min) indicates that triptorelin was eliminated twice as fast in this young population (see Special Populations and Conditions, Renal and Hepatic Impairment) as compared to patients with moderate renal insufficiency. This is related to the fact that triptorelin clearance is partly correlated to total creatinine clearance, which is well known to decrease with age.

Table 3: TRELSTAR 3.75 mg (1 month slow-release)/TRELSTAR 11.25 mg (3 month slow-release)

Pharmacokinetic Parameters (Mean±SD) in Healthy Volunteers and Special Populations

Group	C_{max} (ng/mL)	AUC_{inf} (h·ng/mL)	Cl_p (mL/min)	Cl_{renal} (mL/min)	$T_{1/2}$ (h)	Cl_{creat} (mL/min)
6 healthy male volunteers	48.2 ±11.8	36.1 ±5.8	211.9 ±31.6	90.6 ±35.3	2.81 ±1.21	149.9 ±7.3
6 males with moderate renal impairment	45.6 ±20.5	69.9 ±24.6	120.0 ±45.0	23.3 ±17.6	6.56 ±1.25	39.7 ±22.5
6 males with severe renal impairment	46.5 ±14.0	88.0 ±18.4	88.6 ±19.7	4.3 ±2.9	7.65 ±1.25	8.9 ±6.0
6 males with liver disease	54.1 ±5.3	131.9 ±18.1	57.8 ±8.0	35.9 ±5.0	7.58 ±1.17	89.9 ±15.1

STORAGE AND STABILITY: Store TRELSTAR 3.75 mg and TRELSTAR 11.25 mg vial supplied with MIXJECT Dose Delivery System (with Sterile Water for Injection) at 20-25°C; excursions permitted: 15-30°C.
Store TRELSTAR 3.75 mg and TRELSTAR 11.25 mg vial (without Sterile Water for Injection) at 4-25°C.
No refrigeration necessary. Protect from freezing. Protect from light.
Unused portion of reconstituted TRELSTAR should be discarded immediately.

INFORMATION FOR THE PATIENT: Published in e-CPS, available by subscription at www.e-cps.ca.

DOSAGE FORMS, COMPOSITION AND PACKAGING: TRELSTAR (1 month slow release) 3.75 mg triptorelin/vial: Each vial of sterile lyophilized microgranules contains: triptorelin pamoate which are equivalent to triptorelin peptide base 3.75 mg, poly-d,l-lactide-co-glycolide (170 mg), mannitol, USP (85 mg), carboxymethylcellulose sodium, USP (30 mg), and polysorbate 80, USP (2 mg). When 2 mL Sterile Water for Injection is added to the microgranules and mixed, a suspension is formed, which is intended as a single, monthly intramuscular injection.
TRELSTAR (3 month slow release) 11.25 mg triptorelin/vial: Each vial of sterile lyophilized microgranules contains: triptorelin pamoate which are equivalent to triptorelin peptide base 11.25 mg, poly-d,l-lactide-co-glycolide (145 mg), mannitol, USP (85 mg), carboxymethylcellulose sodium, USP (30 mg), and polysorbate 80, USP (2 mg). When 2 mL Sterile Water for Injection is added to the microgranules and mixed, a suspension is formed, which is intended as a single, 3 month intramuscular injection.
TRELSTAR is available in two presentations:
TRELSTAR dose delivery system (with Sterile Water for Injection), MIXJECT: The accompanying pre-filled syringe contains 2 mL Sterile Water for Injection.
TRELSTAR vial (without Sterile Water for Injection).

Trelstar™ (Endometriosis) ℞

triptorelin pamoate

Luteinizing Hormone-Releasing Hormone (LHRH) Analog

Paladin

Date of Preparation: March 1, 2006
Date of Revision: June 18, 2010

SUMMARY PRODUCT INFORMATION:

Route of Administration	Dosage Form/ Strength	Clinically Relevant Nonmedicinal Ingredients
Intramuscular	Powder (microgranules) for slow release suspension 3.75 mg of triptorelin peptide base units/vial	For a complete listing see Dosage Forms, Composition and Packaging.

INDICATIONS AND CLINICAL USE: TRELSTAR (triptorelin pamoate for injectable suspension) is indicated for:
- The management and relief of chronic pain associated with endometriosis.

TRELSTAR must be administered under the supervision of a physician.
Experience in women has been limited to women 18 years of age or older treated for 6 months.
Geriatrics (>65 years of age): No data are available.
Pediatrics (<18 years of age): Safety and effectiveness of TRELSTAR in women with endometriosis under the age of 18 years have not been established.

CONTRAINDICATIONS:
- TRELSTAR is contraindicated in patients with hypersensitivity to gonadotropin releasing hormone or luteinizing hormone-releasing hormone (GnRH or LHRH), GnRH agonist analogs or any ingredient in the formulation or component of the container. Anaphylactic reactions to synthetic GnRH or GnRH agonist analogs have been reported (see Warnings and Precautions). For a complete listing, see Dosage Forms, Composition and Packaging.
- TRELSTAR is contraindicated in women who are or may become pregnant while receiving the drug. TRELSTAR may cause fetal harm when administered to a pregnant woman. If this drug is used during pregnancy or if the patient becomes pregnant while taking this drug, she should be apprised of the potential hazard to the fetus (see Warnings and Precautions).
- TRELSTAR is contraindicated in nursing women (see Warnings and Precautions).
- TRELSTAR is contraindicated in women with undiagnosed abnormal vaginal bleeding.

WARNINGS AND PRECAUTIONS: General: During the early phase of therapy, sex hormones usually rise above baseline levels because of the physiologic effect of the drug. An increase in clinical signs and symptoms of endometriosis is often observed during the initial days of therapy. These will subside with continued treatment.
Worsening of the clinical condition may occasionally require discontinuation of therapy.
Hypersensitivity and anaphylactic reactions have been reported with triptorelin as with other LHRH agonists. TRELSTAR should not be administered to individuals who are hypersensitive to triptorelin, other LHRH agonists, or LHRH (see Adverse Reactions, Post-Market Adverse Drug Reactions). In the event of a hypersensitivity reaction, TRELSTAR therapy should be discontinued immediately and the appropriate supportive and symptomatic care should be administered.
Before initiating treatment with TRELSTAR, pregnancy must be ruled out (see Special Populations, Pregnant Women).
Retreatment cannot be recommended since safety data beyond 6 months are not available.
Carcinogenesis and Mutagenesis: Carcinogenicity and mutagenicity studies have been performed in animals.
Endocrine and Metabolism: Changes in Bone Mineral Density: Bone loss can be expected as part of natural aging and can also be anticipated during the hypoestrogenic state caused by long-term use of triptorelin. Some of the bone density loss over the course of triptorelin therapy may not be reversible. For a period up to 6 months, this bone loss should not be important.
In patients with significant risk factors for decreased bone mineral content and/or bone mass such as family history of osteoporosis, chronic use of corticosteroids or anticonvulsants or chronic use of alcohol or tobacco, triptorelin may pose additional risk. In these patients, risk versus benefit must be weighted carefully before initiation of triptorelin therapy. Repeated courses of therapy with gonadotropin-releasing hormone analogs beyond 6 months are not advisable for patients with major risk factors for loss of bone mineral content.
Long-term administration of triptorelin will cause suppression of pituitary gonadotropins and gonadal hormone production with clinical symptoms of hypogonadism. These changes have been observed to reverse on discontinuation therapy. However, whether the clinical symptoms of induced hypogonadism will reverse in all patients has not yet been established.
Genitourinary: Vaginal Bleeding: Since menstruation should stop with effective doses of TRELSTAR, the patient should notify her physician if regular menstruation persists. Patients missing successive doses of TRELSTAR may experience breakthrough bleeding.
Renal and Hepatic: Triptorelin exposure was higher in patients with renal or hepatic insufficiency than in healthy volunteers. Clinical consequences of the increase and potential need for dose adjustment are unknown.
Sexual Function/Reproduction: Ovarian Cysts: As with other drugs that stimulate the release of gonadotropin or that induce ovulation, ovarian cysts have been reported to occur, usually within the first 2 months of treatment. In most cases, these enlargements resolve spontaneously in 4 to 6 weeks. However, in some cases they may require discontinuation of drug and/or surgical intervention.
Special Populations: Pregnant Women: The safe use of triptorelin during pregnancy has not been established clinically (see Adverse Reactions). Before starting therapy with TRELSTAR, pregnancy must be excluded. When used regularly and at therapeutic doses, TRELSTAR inhibits ovulation and subsequently menstruation. However, contraception cannot be insured. Women should use nonhormonal methods of contraception while on therapy and should be advised to see their physician if they think they may be pregnant. If a woman becomes pregnant while receiving TRELSTAR, therapy should be discontinued and the patient advised of the potential risk to the fetus. The possibility exists that spontaneous abortion may occur if the drug is administered during pregnancy.
Nursing Women: It is not known to what extent TRELSTAR is excreted into human milk. Because there are no well-controlled studies on the effect of TRELSTAR in nursing women and because many drugs are excreted into human milk, caution should be exercised when TRELSTAR is administered to nursing women (see Contraindications).
Pediatrics (<18 years of age): Safety and effectiveness of TRELSTAR in women with endometriosis under the age of 18 years have not been established.
Race: The effects of race on triptorelin pharmacokinetics, safety, and efficacy have not been systematically studied. The controlled study comparing triptorelin [3.75 mg] and leuprolide [3.75 mg] administered monthly for 6 months to endometriosis patients included 97.1% Caucasian, 2.2% Asian, and 0.7% Afro-Caribbean patients.
Monitoring and Laboratory Tests: Before starting therapy with TRELSTAR, pregnancy must be excluded.

ADVERSE REACTIONS: Adverse Drug Reaction Overview: Triptorelin has been found to be generally well tolerated in clinical trials. Adverse reactions reported in these trials were rarely severe enough to result in patient withdrawal from triptorelin treatment. Three postmarketing reports of anaphylactic shock and seven postmarketing reports of angioedema related to triptorelin administration have been reported since 1986 (see Warnings and Precautions). In a controlled study comparing triptorelin [3.75 mg] and leuprolide [3.75 mg] administered monthly for 6 months to endometriosis patients, one case of severe acute abdominal pain was judged probably related to therapy.
As seen with other LHRH agonist therapies, the most commonly observed adverse events during triptorelin treatment were due to the expected physiological effects related to hypoestrogenism. These effects included hot flushes, vaginal dryness, and amenorrhea. During the first 1-2 weeks following the initial injection, estradiol levels increase and then decline to menopausal levels. The transient increase in estradiol levels may be associated with temporary worsening of signs and symptoms of endometriosis (see Warnings and Precautions).
Triptorelin 3.75 mg was found to be generally safe and well tolerated in women with endometriosis treated for up to 6 months with the drug. Most adverse reactions did not result in discontinuation and most resolved spontaneously without further medical intervention. The most frequently reported adverse reactions were those related to hypoestrogenism.
A small number of women have been inadvertently exposed to triptorelin during pregnancy. Of 28 pregnant women in France exposed to triptorelin in fertility trials, one case of trisomy 13 was reported in a women who received triptorelin 15 days after conception. One case of trisomy 18 has been reported in Italy. In both cases, a causal relationship could not be established. In another study, very long fetal exposure to triptorelin in a woman who became pregnant during a clinically-induced pseudomenopause resulted in the term delivery of a healthy newborn.
Clinical Trial Adverse Drug Reactions: Because clinical trials are conducted under very specific conditions the adverse reaction rates observed in the clinical trials may not reflect the rates observed in practice and should not be compared to the rates in the clinical trials of another drug. Adverse drug reaction information from clinical trials is useful for identifying drug-related adverse events and for approximating rates.
In a controlled study comparing triptorelin [3.75 mg] and leuprolide [3.75 mg] administered monthly for 6 months to endometriosis patients, the following adverse events were reported by 1% or more of patients in the triptorelin study group regardless of relationship or association to treatment: see Table 1.

Table 1: TRELSTAR (Endometriosis)

Adverse Events Reported by 1% or More of Patients During Treatment With Triptorelin

Adverse Event	Triptorelin (n=67) % of patients
Body as a Whole	
Ankle Edema (edema dependent)	23.9

(cont'd)

Table 1: TRELSTAR (Endometriosis) *(cont'd)*

Adverse Events Reported by 1% or More of Patients During Treatment With Triptorelin

Adverse Event	**Triptorelin (n=67) % of patients**
Pain, nos[a]	11.9
Back Pain	9.0
Accidental Injury	7.5
Bruising	6.0
Fatigue	3.0
Central and Peripheral Nervous Systems Disorders	
Headache	59.7
Dizziness	6.0
Endocrine Disorders	
Breast Disorder	31.3
Gastrointestinal Disorders	
Nausea	13.4
Abdominal Pain	10.4
Vomiting	3.0
Musculoskeletal Disorders	
Arthralgia	7.5
Psychiatric	
Insomnia	68.7
Depression	56.7
Decreased Libido	53.7
Irritability	44.8
Reproductive Disorders	
Vaginal Dryness	49.3
Pelvic Pain	3.0
Resistance Mechanism Disorders	
Viral Infection	13.4
Skin and Appendages Disorders	
Increased Sweating	85.1
Seborrhea	43.3
Acne	29.9
Urinary System	
Urinary Tract Infection	6.0
Vascular (extracardiac) Disorders	
Hot Flushes	91.0

[a] nos=not otherwise specified.
Dose of drug administered was 3.75 mg IM every four weeks for six months (6 injections).

Frequently reported adverse events for both the triptorelin and leuprolide groups included hot flushes, depression, irritability, headache, breast disorder, arthralgia, insomnia, decreased libido, acne, seborrhea, increased sweating, and vaginal dryness.

Infrequent (<5% of women) adverse events included, but were not limited to, injection site reaction, chest pain, rash, peripheral edema, leg cramps, diarrhea, irritable bowel, arthritis, arthrosis, myalgia, amnesia, apathy, leukorrhea, and vaginal hemorrhage.

Changes in Bone Mineral Density: After 6 months of treatment with triptorelin in 32 women, the average decrease in bone mineral density, as measured by dual energy x-ray absorptiometry, was 5.3% and 2.3% in lumbar spine and hip, respectively, compared to pretreatment values. Lumbar spine and hip bone mineral density were still slightly decreased by 12 months follow-up (1.7% and 1.3%, respectively).

Abnormal Hematologic and Clinical Chemistry Findings: For the most part, hematology test results were within normal limits throughout the study for patients in each treatment group with available data. Minor fluctuations in values were observed at various time points in each of the treatment groups, none of which were considered clinically meaningful. With the exception of serum and urine creatinines, which were relatively low throughout the study, chemistry results were generally within normal limits for most patients throughout the study.

Post-Market Adverse Drug Reactions: Three postmarketing reports of anaphylactic shock and seven postmarketing reports of angioedema related to triptorelin administration have been reported since 1986 (see Warnings and Precautions).

DRUG INTERACTIONS: Overview: No formal drug interaction studies have been conducted with TRELSTAR and no data are available on the interaction with alcohol. In the absence of relevant data and as a precaution, hyperprolactinemic drugs would not be prescribed concomitantly with triptorelin since hyperprolactinemia reduces the number of pituitary GnRH receptors.

Drug-Drug Interactions: Interactions with other drugs have not been established.

Drug-Food Interactions: Interactions with food have not been established.

Drug-Herb Interactions: Interactions with herbal products have not been established.

Drug-Laboratory Test Interactions: Administration of LHRH analogs, including triptorelin, in therapeutic doses results in suppression of the pituitary-gonadal system. Normal function is usually restored within 4 to 12 weeks after treatment is discontinued. Diagnostic tests of pituitary-gonadal function conducted during treatment and within 4 to 12 weeks after discontinuation of therapy with a LHRH agonist may therefore be misleading.

In clinical trials, there were no clinically meaningful changes in laboratory values during or following triptorelin therapy. Triptorelin therapy had no significant effect on liver enzymes (ALT/AST), alkaline phosphatase, LDH, total bilirubin, urea or inorganic phosphorous during the study. Likewise, there was no significant treatment effect on hematology parameters (WBC, RBC, hemoglobin, hematocrit, platelet count, or WBC differential).

DOSAGE AND ADMINISTRATION: Recommended Dose and Dosage Adjustment: The recommended dose of TRELSTAR (triptorelin pamoate for injectable suspension) for the management and relief of chronic pain associated with endometriosis is a monthly intramuscular injection of 3.75 mg (as peptide base) incorporated in a depot formulation every 28 days for no longer than 6 months.

Missed Dose: Maintaining estradiol suppression is important in the management and relief of chronic pain associated with endometriosis. Missing an appointment by a few days should not disrupt the benefits of treatment, but keeping a consistent schedule of TRELSTAR injections is an important part of treatment.

Administration: TRELSTAR is administered monthly as a single intramuscular injection.

Reconstitution: TRELSTAR is supplied in a single-dose vial containing lyophilized microgranules. These microgranules are to be reconstituted with 2 mL of sterile water for injection. Instructions are provided (see below) for reconstitution using the TRELSTAR dose delivery system (with Sterile Water for Injection), MIXJECT and the TRELSTAR vial (without Sterile Water for Injection).

When 2 mL of Sterile Water for Injection is added to the lyophilized triptorelin pamoate microgranules and mixed, a suspension is formed. This is equivalent to 3.75 mg of triptorelin peptide base units intended as a single monthly intramuscular injection.

The suspension should be discarded if not used immediately after reconstitution. As with other drugs administered by intramuscular injection, the injection site should be varied periodically.

As with all parenteral admixtures, the reconstituted product should be examined for the presence of foreign particulate matter, agglomeration or discoloration. Any defective units should be discarded.

Single use only. Inject immediately after reconstitution and discard unused portion.

Instructions for Use—TRELSTAR Vial (with Sterile Water for Injection), MIXJECT: Please read the instructions completely before you begin.

MIXJECT Preparation: Wash your hands with soap and hot water and put on gloves immediately prior to preparing the injection. Place the sealed tray on a clean, flat surface that is covered with a sterile pad or cloth. Peel the cover away from the tray and remove the MIXJECT components and the TRELSTAR vial. Remove the Flip-Off button from the top of the vial, revealing the rubber stopper. Place the vial in a standing upright position on the prepared surface. Disinfect the rubber stopper with the alcohol wipe. Discard the alcohol wipe and allow the stopper to dry. Proceed to MIXJECT Activation.

MIXJECT Activation:

1. Peel the cover away from the blister pack containing the vial adapter. **Do not remove the vial adapter from the blister pack.** Place the blister pack containing the vial adapter firmly on the vial top, piercing the vial. Push down gently until you feel it snap in place. Remove the blister pack from the vial adapter.
2. (a) Screw the plunger rod into the barrel end of the syringe. Remove the cap from the syringe barrel.
   (b) Connect the syringe to the vial adapter by screwing it clockwise into the opening on the side of the vial adapter. Be sure to gently twist the syringe until it stops turning to ensure a tight connection.
3. While holding the vial, place your thumb on the plunger rod and push the plunger rod in all the way to transfer the diluent from the pre-filled syringe into the vial. Do not release the plunger rod.
4. Keeping the plunger rod depressed, gently swirl the vial so that the diluent rinses the sides of the vial. This will ensure complete mixing of TRELSTAR and the sterile water diluent. The suspension will now have a milky appearance. In order to avoid separation of the suspension, proceed to the next steps without delay.
5. (a) Invert the MIXJECT system so that the vial is at the top. Grasp the MIXJECT system firmly by the syringe and pull back the plunger rod slowly to draw the reconstituted TRELSTAR into the syringe.
   (b) Return the vial to its upright position, and disconnect the vial adapter and vial from the MIXJECT syringe assembly by turning the plastic cap of the vial adapter clockwise. **Grasp only the plastic cap when removing.**
6. Lift up the safety cover and remove the clear plastic needle shield by pulling it from the assembly. The safety cover should be perpendicular to the needle, with the needle facing away from you. The syringe containing the TRELSTAR suspension is now ready for administration. **The suspension should be administered immediately after reconstitution.**

MIXJECT Disposal:

1. After administering the injection, immediately activate the safety mechanism by centering your thumb or forefinger on the textured finger pad area of the safety cover and pushing it forward over the needle until you hear or feel it lock. Use the one-handed technique and activate the mechanism away from yourself and others. Activation of the safety cover causes virtually no splatter.
2. Immediately discard the syringe assembly after a single use into a suitable sharps container.

Instructions for Use—TRELSTAR Vial (without Sterile Water for Injection): The lyophilized microgranules are to be reconstituted **in sterile water. No other diluent should be used.** It is necessary for an aseptic technique to be maintained throughout preparation.

Preparation:

1. Using a syringe fitted with a sterile 21-gauge needle, withdraw 2 mL **sterile water** for injection, USP, and after removing the flip-off seal from the vial, inject into the vial.
2. Shake well to thoroughly disperse particles to obtain a uniform suspension. The suspension will appear milky.
3. Withdraw the entire content of the reconstituted suspension into the syringe and inject it immediately.

Disposal: Dispose of the syringe and vial into a suitable sharps container.

OVERDOSAGE:

The pharmacologic properties of TRELSTAR (triptorelin pamoate for injectable suspension) and its mode of administration make accidental or intentional overdosage unlikely. There is no experience of overdosage from clinical trials. Acute animal toxicity of the drug is low and high multiples of clinical dose did not cause any adverse effects. If overdosage occurs, it should be managed symptomatically.

For management of a suspected drug overdose, CPhA recommends that you contact your **regional Poison Control Centre**. See the *CPS* Directory section for a list of Poison Control Centres.

ACTION AND CLINICAL PHARMACOLOGY: TRELSTAR (triptorelin for injectable suspension) is a synthetic decapeptide agonist analog of naturally occurring luteinizing hormone-releasing hormone (LHRH), also called gonadotropin releasing hormone (GnRH). This analog possesses greater potency than the natural hormone.

Triptorelin acts as a potent inhibitor of gonadotropin secretion when given continuously in therapeutic doses. On administration of triptorelin there is an initial and transient increase in circulating levels of luteinizing hormone (LH), follicle-stimulating hormone (FSH), and estradiol. However, chronic and continuous administration of triptorelin results in decreased LH and FSH secretion and suppression of ovarian steroidogenesis. In premenopausal women, circulating estrogen is decreased to postmenopausal levels (see Table 2). This results in accessory sexual organ atrophy which is generally reversible upon discontinuation of drug therapy.

Table 2: TRELSTAR (Endometriosis)

Estradiol Level (pmol/L) Profile Over 24 Weeks of Treatment with Triptorelin (n=66)

	Week 0 Pretreatment	Week 4	Week 8	Week 12	Week 16	Week 20	Week 24
Mean	124	48	48	52	51	52	46
SD	77	42	36	37	35	36	25

A single intramuscular (IM) dose of 1.9, 3.75, or 7.5 mg to women with endometriosis, uterine myoma or dysfunctional bleeding resulted in transient dose-dependent increase in LH and estradiol following injection. By day 14, serum LH and estradiol concentrations decreased to levels typically seen in postmenopausal women. On day 28 and up to day 42 after injection, estradiol levels were still suppressed (<184 pmol/L) in the mid- and high-dose groups. Following LHRH challenge (100 mg) on day 28, 7/10 patients in the 1.9 mg group, 3/10 patients in the 3.75 mg group, and 0/10 patients in the 7.5 mg group responded to stimulation with increased LH levels. By day 56, estradiol concentrations returned to pretreatment levels in the mid-dose group but were still suppressed in the high dose group (7/8 patients).

Pharmacokinetics: Results of pharmacokinetic investigations conducted in both women and men indicate that after IV bolus administration, triptorelin is distributed and eliminated according to a 3-compartment model with elimination from the central compartment and corresponding distribution half-lives of approximately 3 minutes, 47 minutes, and 5 hours in women and 6 minutes, 45 minutes, and 3 hours in men.

Absorption: Triptorelin is not active when given orally. Following a single intramuscular injection of the sustained release formulation in healthy male volunteers, mean peak triptorelin serum concentration was 28.4 ng/mL at 1-3 hours and 0.084 ng/mL at 4 weeks (see Table 3). In this study, absolute bioavailability of intramuscular triptorelin relative to intravenous triptorelin (F based on AUC) was approximately 83%.

Table 3: TRELSTAR (Endometriosis)

Pharmacokinetic Parameters of Triptorelin Following an Intramuscular Administration of TRELSTAR in Healthy Male Volunteers (mean±SD or median (range) for T_{max})

	Triptorelin Pharmacokinetics			
No. of Subjects	C_{max} (ng/mL)	T_{max} (h)	AUC (h·ng/mL)	F (%)[a] (No. of days)
20	28.43±7.31	1.0 (1.0–3.0)	223.15±46.96	83 (28 d)

[a] Computed as the mean AUC of the study divided by the mean AUC of healthy volunteers corrected for dose (AUC=36.1 h·ng/mL; 500 µg IV bolus of triptorelin).

Distribution: The volume of distribution of triptorelin following IV administration of 0.5 mg triptorelin was approximately 30-33 L in healthy male volunteers and women with endometriosis.

Metabolism: Metabolites of triptorelin have not been determined in humans. However, human pharmacokinetic data suggest that C-terminal fragments produced by degradation are either completely degraded within tissues or are rapidly further degraded in plasma, or cleared by the kidneys.

Excretion: Triptorelin is eliminated by both the liver and the kidneys. Following IV administration of 0.5 mg triptorelin peptide to 6 healthy male volunteers with a creatinine clearance of 149.9 mL/min, 41.7% of the dose was excreted in urine as intact peptide with a total triptorelin clearance of 211.9 mL/min. This percentage increased to 62.3% in patients with liver disease who have a lower creatinine clearance (89.9 mL/min). It has also been observed that the non-renal clearance of triptorelin (patient anuric, Cl_{creat}=0) was 76.2 mL/min, thus indicating that the nonrenal elimination of triptorelin is mainly dependant on the liver (see Special Populations and Conditions).

Following a 0.5 mg IV bolus dose to 19 women, the total clearance was estimated to be 110 mL/min. Twenty percent of the dose was eliminated in the urine (see Table 4).

Table 4: TRELSTAR (Endometriosis)

Pharmacokinetic Parameters Following IV Administration of Triptorelin to Women with Endometriosis or Uterine Myoma

Dose (No. of subjects)	C_{max} (ng/mL)[a]	T_{max} (h)[b]	AUC (h·ng/mL)[a]	$t_{½}$[c] (h)[a]	Cl_p (mL/min)[a]	V_{ss} (L)[a]	% elimin. Urine[a]
0.5 mg IVB (n=19)	115,8 ±59,0	0,03 (0,03–0,17)	81,9 ±32,9	5,37 ±2,29	110 ±40	32,9 ± 16,8	20 ±10

[a] Mean±SD.
[b] Median (range).
[c] Elimination half-life.

Special Populations and Conditions: Renal and Hepatic Impairment: After an IV injection of 0.5 mg triptorelin peptide, the two distribution half-lives were unaffected by renal and hepatic impairment, but renal insufficiency led to a decrease in total triptorelin clearance proportional to the decrease in creatinine clearance as well as an increase in volume of distribution and consequently an increase in elimination half-life (see Table 5). The decrease in triptorelin clearance was more pronounced in subjects with liver insufficiency, but the half-life was prolonged similarly in subjects with renal insufficiency, since the volume of distribution was only minimally increased.

Table 5: TRELSTAR (Endometriosis)

Pharmacokinetic Parameters (mean ±SD) in Healthy Volunteers and Special Populations

Group	C_{max} (ng/mL)	AUC_{inf} (h·ng/mL)	Cl_p (mL/min)	Cl_{renal} (mL/min)	$t_{½}$ (h)	Cl_{creat} (mL/min)
6 healthy male volunteers	48.2 ±11.8	36.1 ±5.8	211.9 ±31.6	90.6 ±35.3	2.81 ±1.21	149.9 ±7.3
6 males with moderate renal impairment	45.6 ±20.5	69.9 ±24.6	120.0 ±45.0	23.3 ±17.6	6.56 ±1.25	39.7 ±22.5
6 males with severe renal impairment	46.5 ±14.0	88.0 ±18.4	88.6 ±19.7	4.3 ±2.9	7.65 ±1.25	8.9 ±6.0
6 males with liver disease	54.1 ±5.3	131.9 ±18.1	57.8 ±8.0	35.9 ±5.0	7.58 ±1.17	89.9 ±15.1

Age and Race: The effects of age and race on triptorelin pharmacokinetics have not been systematically studied. However, pharmacokinetic data obtained in young healthy male volunteers aged 20 to 22 years with an elevated creatinine clearance (approximately 250 mL/min) indicates that triptorelin was eliminated twice as fast in this young population (see Special Populations and Conditions, Renal and Hepatic Impairment) as compared to patients with moderate renal insufficiency. This is related to the fact that triptorelin clearance is partly correlated to total creatinine clearance, which is well known to decrease with age

STORAGE AND STABILITY: Store TRELSTAR vial supplied with MIXJECT Dose Delivery System (with Sterile Water for Injection) at 20-25°C; excursions permitted: 15-30°C.

Store TRELSTAR vial (without Sterile Water for Injection) at 4-25°C.

No refrigeration necessary. Protect from freezing. Protect from light.

Unused portion of reconstituted TRELSTAR should be discarded immediately.

INFORMATION FOR THE PATIENT: Published in e-CPS, available by subscription at www.e-cps.ca.

DOSAGE FORMS, COMPOSITION AND PACKAGING: TRELSTAR is supplied in a vial containing sterile lyophilized triptorelin pamoate microgranules which are equivalent to 3.75 mg triptorelin peptide base, incorporated in a biodegradable copolymer of lactic and glycolic acids. When 2 mL Sterile Water for Injection is added to the microgranules and mixed, a suspension is formed, which is intended as a single, monthly intramuscular injection.

TRELSTAR Dose Delivery System (with Sterile Water for Injection), MIXJECT: Each vial contains: triptorelin pamoate (equivalent to triptorelin 3.75 mg), poly-d,l-lactide-co-glycolide (170 mg), mannitol, USP (85 mg), carboxymethylcellulose sodium, USP (30 mg), and polysorbate 80, USP (2 mg). The accompanying pre-filled syringe contains 2 mL Sterile Water for Injection.

TRELSTAR Vial (without Sterile Water for Injection): Each vial contains: triptorelin pamoate (equivalent to triptorelin 3.75 mg), poly-d,l-lactide-co-glycolide (170 mg), mannitol, USP (85 mg), carboxymethylcellulose sodium, USP (30 mg), and polysorbate 80, USP (2 mg).

Trental® Ⓟ

pentoxifylline

Vasoactive Agent

sanofi-aventis

Date of Revision: February 17, 2009

SUMMARY PRODUCT INFORMATION:

Route of Administration	Dosage Form/ Strength	Clinically Relevant Nonmedicinal Ingredients
Oral	Sustained release tablet 400 mg	For a complete listing see Dosage Forms, Composition and Packaging.

INDICATIONS AND CLINICAL USE: Trental (pentoxifylline) is indicated for the symptomatic treatment of:

- patients with chronic occlusive peripheral vascular disorders of the extremities.

In such patients Trental may give relief of signs and symptoms of impaired blood flow, such as intermittent claudication or trophic ulcers.

CONTRAINDICATIONS: The use of Trental (pentoxifylline) is contraindicated in:

- Patients who are hypersensitive to pentoxifylline or other xanthines such as caffeine, theophylline and theobromine or to any ingredient in the formulation or component of the container (see Dosage Forms, Composition and Packaging).
- Patients with acute myocardial infraction;
- Patients with severe coronary artery disease when, in the physician's judgement, myocardial stimulation might prove harmful;
- Patients with hemorrhage (e.g. extensive retinal bleeding) or at risk of increased bleeding;
- Patients with peptic ulcers or recent history thereof.

WARNINGS AND PRECAUTIONS: General: Patients with hepatic impairment should be closely monitored during Trental therapy and may require lower doses. Since Trental (pentoxifylline) is extensively metabolized in the liver, the use of this drug is not recommended in patients with severe hepatic impairment of liver function (Child-Pugh class C, score >9).

Patients with renal impairment (creatinine clearance below 80 mL/min) should be closely monitored during Trental therapy and may require lower doses. Since Trental (pentoxifylline) is eliminated through the kidneys, the use of this drug is not recommended in patients with severe renal impairment (creatinine clearance below 30 mL/min).

Cardiovascular: Low, Labile Blood Pressure: Caution should be exercised when administering Trental (pentoxifylline) to patients with low or labile blood pressure. In such patients any dose increase should be done gradually.

Hematologic: The administration of Trental has been associated with bleeding and/or prolonged prothrombin time (see Drug Interactions). The risk of bleeding may be increased by combined treatment with anticoagulant agents or use in coagulation disorders. Therefore, in patients with coagulation disorders or being treated with anticoagulant therapy, Trental should be used with caution and only when, in the physician's judgement, the potential benefit outweighs the risk.

Special Populations: Pregnant Women: Reproduction studies have been performed in rats, mice and rabbits at doses up to 23,2 and 11 times the maximum recommended daily human dose and have revealed no evidence of impaired fertility or harm to the fetus due to pentoxifylline. The drug has been shown to cross the blood-placenta barrier in mice. There is no adequate experience in pregnant women. Therefore, Trental is not recommended for women who are, or may become, pregnant unless the expected benefits for the mothers outweigh the potential risk to the fetus.

Nursing Women: Pentoxifylline and its major metabolites are excreted in human milk, following a 400 mg single oral dose of Trental. The patient should be advised to discontinue nursing or to discontinue taking the drug depending on the importance of the drug to the mother.

Pediatrics: The use of Trental in patients below the age of 18 years is not recommended as safety and effectiveness have not been established in this age group.

Geriatrics: Trental should be used with caution in elderly patients as peak plasma levels of pentoxifylline and its metabolites are moderately higher in this age group. Elderly patients had a slight increase in the incidence of some adverse effects. Careful dose adjustment is therefore recommended.

ADVERSE REACTIONS: Clinical Trial Adverse Drug Reactions: Because clinical trials are conducted under very specific conditions the adverse reaction rates observed in the clinical trials may not reflect the rates observed in practice and should not be compared to the rates in the clinical trials of another drug. Adverse drug reaction information from clinical trials is useful for identifying drug-related adverse events and for approximating rates.

The most frequent adverse event reported with Trental (pentoxifylline) is nausea (14%). Individual signs/symptoms listed in Table 1 occurred at an incidence between 1 and 3%, except when stated otherwise.

Table 1: Trental

Individual Signs/Symptoms Occurred at an Incidence Between 1 and 3%, Except When Stated Otherwise

	Symptoms
Body as a Whole	Malaise
Cardiovascular System	Flushing
Central Nervous System	Dizziness/light-headedness (9.4%), headache (4.9 %)
Gastrointestinal System	Nausea (14%), vomiting (3.4%), abdominal discomfort, bloating, diarrhea, dyspepsia

Less Common Clinical Trial Adverse Drug Reactions (<1%): Body as a Whole: muscle aches/spasm, weight change, backache, bad taste in mouth, leg cramps, fever, weakness, sweating.

Cardiovascular: chest pain, arrhythmia, hypertension, dyspnea, edema, hypotension, angina, tachycardia.

Central Nervous System: drowsiness/sleepiness, tremor, agitation anxiety, confusion, insomnia, restlessness.

Gastrointestinal: abdominal burning, abdominal pain, anorexia flatus, constipation, haemorrhage, heartburn, salivation, dry mouth/throat, hepatitis, jaundice, increased liver enzymes.

Hemic and Lymphatic: decreased serum fibrinogen, pancytopenia, purpura, thrombocytopenia, leucopenia, anemia, aplastic anemia.

Hypersensitivity Reactions: pruritus, rash, urticaria, angioedema.

Organs of Special Sense: blurred vision, scotoma, lacrimation, epistaxis.

Post-Market Adverse Drug Reactions: Hepatobiliary Disorders: intrahepatic cholestasis.

Immune System Disorders: severe anaphylactic/anaphylactoid reaction with, for example, angioneurotic edema, bronchospasms, sometimes shock.

Infections and Infestations: aseptic meningitis.

Investigations: transaminase elevation.

Psychiatric: sleep disturbances.

Skin and Subcutaneous Tissue Disorders: reddening of skin.

DRUG INTERACTIONS: Drug-Drug Interactions: Antacids: In patients with digestive side effects, antacids may be administered with Trental. In comparative bioavailability study, no interference with absorption of Trental by antacids was observed.

Antihypertensive Agents: Trental (pentoxifylline) may potentiate the action of antihypertensive agents. Patients receiving these agents require blood pressure monitoring and possibly a dose reduction of the antihypertensive agents.

Anticoagulants: There have been reports of bleeding and/or prolonged prothrombin time in patients treated with Trental with and without anticoagulants or platelet aggregation inhibitors. Patients on warfarin should have more frequent monitoring of prothrombin time, while patients with other risk factors complicated by hemorrhage (e.g. recent surgery) should have periodic examinations for signs of bleeding, including hematocrit and haemoglobin.

Cimetidine: During concurrent use of cimetidine and pentoxifylline, cimetidine has been shown to significantly increase the steady-state plasma concentration of pentoxifylline, which may enhance the possibility of adverse effects.

Erythromycin: No data are available on the possible interaction of Trental and erythromycin. However concurrent administration of erythromycin and theomycin has resulted in significant elevation of serum theophylline levels with toxic reactions.

Hypoglycemic Agents: The blood-sugar lowering effect of insulin or oral antidiabetic agents may be potentiated. In patients treated with hypoglycemic agents, a moderate adjustment in the dose of these agents may be required when Trental is prescribed.

Sympathomimetics: Combined use with other xanthines or with sympathomimetics may cause excessive CNS stimulation.

Theophylline: Although causality has not been established, concurrent use of pentoxifylline with theophylline has resulted in elevated theophylline plasma levels, which may enhance the possibility of adverse effects.

Drug-Food Interactions: Interactions with food have not been established.

Drug-Herb Interactions: Interactions with herbal product have not been established.

Drug-Laboratory Test Interactions: Interactions with laboratory tests have not been established.

Drug-Lifestyle Interactions: Interactions with lifestyles have not been established.

DOSAGE AND ADMINISTRATION: Recommended Dose and Dosage Adjustment: The recommended starting dosage of Trental (pentoxifylline) is 400 mg twice daily after meals. The usual dose is 400 mg twice or three times daily. A maximum of 400 mg three times daily should not be exceeded.

It may take up to two months to obtain full results.

Trental 400 mg sustained release tablets must be swallowed whole.

OVERDOSAGE:

Overdosage with Trental (pentoxifylline) has been reported in children and adults. Symptoms appear to be dose related and usually occurred 4-5 hours after ingestion and lasted about 12 hours. Initial manifestations of acute overdose with pentoxifylline may be nausea, dizziness, tachycardia, fever, gastrointestinal bleeding—coffee-ground vomiting and areflexia. The highest amount ingested was 80 mg/kg with which flushing, hypotension, convulsions, somnolence, loss of consciousness, fever, and agitation have been observed. All patients recovered.

No specific antidote is known. In addition to symptomatic treatment and gastric lavage, special attention must be given to supporting respiration, maintaining systemic blood pressure, and controlling convulsions with intravenous diazepam. Activated charcoal has been used to absorb pentoxifylline in patients who have overdosed.

> For management of a suspected drug overdose, CPhA recommends that you contact your **regional Poison Control Centre**. See the *CPS* Directory section for a list of Poison Control Centres.

ACTION AND CLINICAL PHARMACOLOGY: Mechanism of Action: Trental (pentoxifylline) is a xanthine derivative. It belongs to a group of vasoactive drugs which improve peripheral blood flow and thus enhance peripheral tissue oxygenation. The mechanism by which Trental achieves this effect has not been determined, but it is likely that the following factors are involved:

- Trental, as with other xanthine derivatives, relaxes certain smooth muscles including those of the peripheral vessels, thus causing vasodilatation or preventing spasm. This action, however, may have a limited role in patients with chronic obstructive arterial disease when peripheral vessels are already maximally dilated.
- Trental improves flexibility of red blood cells. This increase in the flexibility of red blood cells probably contributes to the improvement of the ability of blood to flow through peripheral vessels (haemorheologic action). This property was seen during in vitro and in vivo experiments with Trental but the correlation between it and the clinical improvement of patients with peripheral vascular diseases has not been determined.
- Trental promotes platelet deaggregation.

Improvement of red blood cell flexibility and platelet deaggregation contribute to the decrease in blood viscosity.

Pharmacokinetics: Pentoxifylline is almost completely absorbed after oral administration. The Trental 400 mg sustained release tablet showed an initial peak plasma pentoxifylline concentration 2 to 3 hours post-administration. The drug is extensively metabolized. Biotransformation products are almost exclusively eliminated by the kidneys.

Food intake before the administration of Trental delayed the absorption but did not decrease it.

STORAGE AND STABILITY: Store at room temperature (15 to 30°C). Protect from light. Protect from moisture and excessive heat.

INFORMATION FOR THE PATIENT: Published in e-CPS, available by subscription at www.e-cps.ca.

DOSAGE FORMS, COMPOSITION AND PACKAGING: Each pink, oblong, film-coated, sustained release tablet, one face embossed with "Trental", the other face plain, contains: pentoxifylline 400 mg. Nonmedicinal ingredients: benzyl alcohol, FD&C Red No. 3, hydroxyethyl cellulose, hydroxypropyl methylcellulose, magnesium stearate, polyethylene glycol 8000, povidone, talc and titanium dioxide. Unit pack cartons of 6×10 clear PVC film and aluminium foil blister-packed tablets.

(Shown in Product Identification Section)

> The reader is invited to consult CPhA's monograph **Corticosteroids: Topical**.

Triaderm Pr

triamcinolone acetonide

Topical Corticosteroid

Taro

SUPPLIED: Each g contains: triamcinolone acetonide USP 0.1% in an aqueous vanishing cream base containing cetyl alcohol, cetyl esters wax, glyceryl monostearate, isopropyl palmitate, polysorbates, propylene glycol and purified water. Paraben-free. Jars of 500 g. Store at room temperature (15-30°C).

Triamcinolone Pr

CPhA Monograph

see *Corticosteroids: Eye Ear Nose*

see *Corticosteroids: Systemic*

see *Corticosteroids: Topical*

Triamcinolone Acetonide Injectable Suspension USP Pr

triamcinolone acetonide

Corticosteroid—Anti-inflammatory

Sandoz

SUPPLIED: 10 mg/mL: Each mL of sterile, aqueous suspension contains: triamcinolone acetonide 10 mg. Nonmedicinal ingredients: benzyl alcohol 0.9% v/v (as preservative), polysorbate 80, sodium carboxymethylcellulose, sodium chloride for isotonicity, sodium hydroxide and/or hydrochloric acid to adjust pH and water for injection. Multidose vials of 5 mL, boxes of 1. Shake well before use. Protect from light. Do not freeze. Store between 15 and 30°C. Store in outer carton until last dose has been dispensed.

40 mg/mL: Each mL of sterile, aqueous suspension contains: triamcinolone acetonide 40 mg. Nonmedicinal ingredients: benzyl alcohol 0.9% v/v (as preservative), polysorbate 80, sodium carboxymethylcellulose, sodium chloride to adjust isotonicity, sodium hydroxide and/or hydrochloric acid to adjust pH and water for injection. Multidose vials of 1 and 5 mL, boxes of 1. Shake well before use. Protect from light. Do not freeze. Store between 15 and 30°C. Store in outer carton until last dose has been dispensed.

Trianal Ⓒ

ASA—caffeine—butalbital

Analgesic—Sedative

Trianon

Trianal C¼, C½ Ⓝ

ASA—caffeine—codeine phosphate—butalbital

Analgesic—Sedative

Trianon

SUPPLIED: Trianal: Capsules: Each hard gelatin, oblong capsule, blue opaque cap printed "TRIANAL" and purple insert part printed "△", contains: butalbital USP 50 mg, caffeine USP 40 mg and ASA USP 330 mg. Nonmedicinal ingredients: cellulose and stearic acid. Alcohol-, gluten-, lactose-, sulfite- and tartrazine-free. Bottles of 100 and 500.

Tablets: Each white compressed tablet embossed "TRIANAL" on one side and "△" on the other, contains: butalbital USP 50 mg, caffeine USP 40 mg and ASA USP 330 mg. Nonmedicinal ingredients: cellulose, croscarmellose sodium, sodium lauryl sulfate and stearic acid. Alcohol-, gluten-, lactose-, sulfite- and tartrazine-free. Bottles of 100 and 500.

Trianal C¼: Each hard gelatin, oblong capsule, blue opaque cap printed "TRIANAL C¼" and white insert part printed "△", contains: butalbital USP 50 mg, caffeine USP 40 mg, ASA USP 330 mg and codeine phosphate USP 15 mg. Nonmedicinal ingredients: cellulose, croscarmellose sodium and stearic acid. Alcohol-, gluten-, lactose-, sulfite- and tartrazine-free. Bottles of 100 and 500.

Trianal C½: Each hard gelatin, oblong capsule, blue opaque cap printed "TRIANAL C½" and pale blue insert part printed "△", contains: butalbital USP 50 mg, caffeine USP 40 mg, ASA USP 330 mg and codeine phosphate USP 30 mg. Nonmedicinal ingredients: cellulose, starch and stearic acid. Alcohol-, gluten-, lactose-, sulfite- and tartrazine-free. Bottles of 100 and 500.

Triatec-8 Ⓝ

acetaminophen—codeine phosphate—caffeine citrate

Analgesic—Antipyretic—Antitussive

Trianon

Triatec-8 Strong Ⓝ

acetaminophen—codeine phosphate—caffeine citrate

Analgesic—Antipyretic—Antitussive

Trianon

Triatec-30 Ⓝ

acetaminophen—codeine phosphate

Analgesic—Antipyretic—Antitussive

Trianon

SUPPLIED: Triatec-8: Each oblong-shaped, white tablet contains: acetaminophen 325 mg, codeine phosphate 8 mg and caffeine citrate 30 mg. Nonmedicinal ingredients: cellulose, citric acid, croscarmellose sodium, magnesium stearate and stearic acid. Alcohol-, gluten-, lactose-, sulfite- and tartrazine-free. Bottles of 30, 100 and 200.

Triatec-8 Strong: Each oblong-shaped, white tablet contains: acetaminophen 500 mg, codeine phosphate 8 mg and caffeine citrate 30 mg. Nonmedicinal ingredients: cellulose, citric acid, croscarmellose sodium, magnesium stearate and stearic acid. Alcohol-, gluten-, lactose-, sulfite- and tartrazine-free. Bottles of 50.

Triatec-30: Each round, scored, salmon-colored, flat-faced tablet, engraved TRIATEC-30, contains: acetaminophen 300 mg and codeine phosphate 30 mg. Nonmedicinal ingredients: cellulose, colloidal silicon dioxide FD&C yellow #6 aluminum lake, lactose, sodium starch glycolate, stearic acid and talc. Alcohol-, gluten-, sulfite- and tartrazine-free. Bottles of 100 and 500.

Triazolam

CPhA Monograph

see *Benzodiazepines*

Tri-Cyclen® Pr

norgestimate—ethinyl estradiol

Oral Contraceptive

Janssen-Ortho

Date of Preparation: May 4, 1993

Date of Revision: January 13, 2010

PHARMACOLOGY: The primary mechanism of action of Tri-Cyclen is an inhibition of ovulation. Additionally, other effects caused by the treatment (for example, alteration of the endometrium and the thickening of the cervical mucus) appear to interfere with implantation and conception.

INDICATIONS: Treatment of moderate acne vulgaris in females who have no known contraindications to oral contraceptive therapy. Conception control.

CONTRAINDICATIONS: History of/or actual thrombophlebitis or thromboembolic disorders. Known thrombophilic conditions. History of/or actual cerebrovascular disorders. History of/or actual myocardial infarction or coronary arterial disease. Active liver disease or history of/or actual benign or malignant liver tumors. Known or suspected carcinoma of the breast. Known or suspected estrogen-dependent neoplasia. Undiagnosed abnormal vaginal bleeding. Any ocular lesion arising from ophthalmic vascular disease, such as partial or complete loss of vision or defect in visual fields. When pregnancy is suspected or diagnosed. Valvular heart disease with complications. Persistent blood pressure values ≥160 mm Hg systolic or ≥100 mm Hg diastolic. Diabetes with vascular involvement. Cholestatic jaundice or history of jaundice of pregnancy. Migraine with focal aura. Hypersensitivity to any component of this product.

WARNINGS: Predisposing Factors for Coronary Artery Disease: Cigarette smoking increases the risk of serious cardiovascular side effects and mortality. Birth control pills increase this risk, especially with increasing age. Convincing data are available to support an upper age limit of 35 years for oral contraceptive use by women who smoke.

Other women who are independently at high risk for cardiovascular disease include those with diabetes, hypertension (persistent blood pressure values ≥140 mm Hg systolic or ≥90 mm Hg diastolic), abnormal lipid profile, or a family history of these. Whether oral contraceptives accentuate this risk is unclear.

In low-risk, nonsmoking women of any age, the benefits of oral contraceptive use outweigh the possible cardiovascular risks associated with low-dose formulations. Consequently, oral contraceptives may be prescribed for these women up to the age of menopause.

> Cigarette smoking increases the risk of serious adverse effects on the heart and blood vessels. This risk increases with age and becomes significant in oral contraceptive users older than 35 years of age. Women should be counselled not to smoke.

Venous and Arterial Thrombosis and Thromboembolism: Venous thrombosis and thromboembolism: Epidemiological studies have shown that the incidence of venous thromboembolism (VTE) in users of oral contraceptives with low estrogen content (<50 µg ethinyl estradiol) ranges from about 20 to 40 cases per 100 000 women-years, but this risk estimate varies according to the progestogen. This compares with 5 to 10 cases per 100 000 women-years for non-users.

The use of any combined oral contraceptive carries an increased risk of VTE compared with no use. The excess risk of VTE is highest during the first year a woman ever uses a combined oral contraceptive. The increased risk is less than the risk of VTE associated with pregnancy, which is estimated as 60 cases per 100 000 pregnancies. VTE is fatal in 1-2% of cases.

Other generalized risk factors for venous thromboembolism include but are not limited to a personal history, a family history (the occurrence of VTE in a direct relative at a relatively early age may indicate genetic predisposition), severe obesity (body mass index >30 kg/m^2) and systemic lupus erythematosus. The risk of VTE also increases with age and smoking. The risk of VTE may be temporarily increased with prolonged immobilization, major surgery, or trauma. Also, patients with varicose veins and leg cast should be closely supervised.

If a hereditary or acquired predisposition for venous thromboembolism is suspected, the woman should be referred to a specialist for advice before deciding on any combination oral contraceptives (COC) use.

Arterial thrombosis and thromboembolism: The use of COCs increases the risk of arterial thrombotic and thromboembolic events. Reported events include myocardial infarction and cerebrovascular events (ischemic and hemorrhagic stroke, transient ischemic attack).

The risk of arterial thrombotic and thromboembolic events is further increased in women with underlying risk factors. Caution must be exercised when prescribing COCs for women with risk factors for arterial thrombotic and thromboembolic events.

Discontinue medication at the earliest manifestation of the following:

A. Thromboembolic and cardiovascular disorders such as: thrombophlebitis, pulmonary embolism, cerebrovascular disorders, myocardial ischemia, mesenteric thrombosis and retinal thrombosis.
B. Conditions that predispose to venous stasis and to vascular thrombosis, (e.g., immobilization after accidents or confinement to bed during long-term illness). Other non-hormonal methods of contraception should be used until regular activities are resumed. For use of oral contraceptives when surgery is contemplated, see Precautions.
C. Visual defects—partial or complete.
D. Papilledema, or ophthalmic vascular lesions.
E. Severe headache of unknown etiology or worsening of pre-existing migraine headache.

PRECAUTIONS: Physical Examination and Follow-up: Before oral contraceptives are used, a thorough history and physical examination should be performed, including a blood pressure determination. Breasts, liver, extremities and pelvic organs should be examined. A Papanicolaou smear should be taken if the patient has been sexually active.

The first follow-up visit should be 3 months after oral contraceptives are prescribed. Thereafter, examinations should be performed at least once a year, or more frequently if indicated. At each annual visit, examination should include those procedures that were done at the initial visit as outlined above or per recommendations of the Canadian Workshop on Screening for Cancer of the Cervix. Their suggestion was that, for women who had 2 consecutive negative Pap smears, screening could be continued every 3 years up to the age of 69.

Pregnancy: Oral contraceptives should not be taken by pregnant women. However, if conception accidentally occurs while taking the pill, there is no conclusive evidence that the estrogen and progestin contained in the oral contraceptive will damage the developing child.

Lactation: In breast-feeding women, the use of oral contraceptives results in the hormonal components being excreted in breast milk and may reduce its quantity and quality. If the use of oral contraceptives is initiated after the establishment of lactation, there does not appear to be any effect on the quantity and quality of the milk. There is no evidence that low-dose oral contraceptives are harmful to the nursing infant.

Hepatic Function: Patients who have had jaundice, including a history of cholestatic jaundice during pregnancy, should be given oral contraceptives with great care and under close observation.

The development of severe generalized pruritus or icterus requires that the medication be withdrawn until the problem is resolved.

If the patient develops jaundice that proves to be cholestatic in type, the use of oral contraceptives should not be resumed. In patients taking oral contraceptives, changes in the composition of the bile may occur and an increased incidence of gallstones has been reported.

Hepatic nodules (adenoma and focal nodular hyperplasia) have been reported, particularly in long-term users of oral contraceptives. Although these lesions are extremely rare, they have caused fatal intra-abdominal hemorrhage and should be considered in women with an abdominal mass, acute abdominal pain, or evidence of intra-abdominal bleeding.

Hypertension: Patients with essential hypertension whose blood pressure (BP) is well controlled may be given oral contraceptives but only under close supervision. If a significant persistent elevation of blood pressure in previously normotensive or hypertensive subjects occurs at any time during the administration of the drug, cessation of medication is necessary and an alternate method of contraception should be prescribed (see Contraindications).

Migraine and Headache: The onset or exacerbation of migraine or the development of headache of a new pattern that is recurrent, persistent or severe requires discontinuation of oral contraceptives and evaluation of the cause.

Diabetes: Current low-dose oral contraceptives exert minimal impact on glucose metabolism. Diabetic patients, or those with a family history of diabetes, should be observed closely to detect any worsening of carbohydrate metabolism. Patients predisposed to diabetes who can be kept under close supervision may be given oral contraceptives. Young diabetic patients whose disease is of recent origin, well-controlled, and not associated with hypertension or other signs of vascular disease such as ocular fundal changes, should be monitored more frequently while using oral contraceptives.

Ocular Disease: Patients who are pregnant or are taking oral contraceptives may experience corneal edema that may cause visual disturbances and changes in tolerance to contact lenses, especially of the rigid type. Soft contact lenses usually do not cause disturbances. If visual changes or alterations in tolerance to contact lenses occur, temporary or permanent cessation of wear may be advised.

Breasts: Increasing age and a strong family history are the most significant risk factors for the development of breast cancer. Other established risk factors include obesity, nulliparity and late age for first full-term pregnancy. The identified groups of women that may be at increased risk of developing breast cancer before menopause are long-term users of oral contraceptives (more than 8 years) and starters at an early age. In a few women, the use of oral contraceptives may accelerate the growth of an existing but undiagnosed breast cancer. Since any potential increased risk related to oral contraceptive use is small, there is no reason to change prescribing habits at present.

Women receiving oral contraceptives should be instructed in self-examination of their breasts. Their physicians should be notified whenever any masses are detected. A yearly clinical breast examination is also recommended because, if a breast cancer should develop, drugs that contain estrogen may cause a rapid progression.

Vaginal Bleeding: Persistent irregular vaginal bleeding requires assessment to exclude underlying pathology.

Fibroids: Patients with fibroids (leiomyomata) should be carefully observed. Sudden enlargement, pain, or tenderness requires discontinuation of the use of oral contraceptives.

Emotional Disorders: Patients with a history of emotional disturbances, especially the depressive type, may be more prone to have a recurrence of depression while taking oral contraceptives. In cases of a serious recurrence, a trial of an alternative method of contraception should be made which may help to clarify the possible relationship. Women with premenstrual syndrome (PMS) may have a varied response to oral contraceptives, ranging from symptomatic improvement to worsening of the condition.

Laboratory Tests: Results of laboratory tests should be interpreted in light of the fact that the patient is on oral contraceptives. The following laboratory tests are modified.

A. Liver Function Tests: Bromsulphthalein Retention Test (BSP), moderate increase; AST and GGT, minor increase; alkaline phosphatase, variable increase; serum bilirubin, increased, particularly in conditions predisposing to or associated with hyperbilirubinemia.
B. Coagulation Tests: Factors II, VII, IX, X, XII and XIII, increased; Factor VIII, mild increase; platelet aggregation and adhesiveness, mild increase in response to common aggregating agents; fibrinogen, increased; plasminogen, mild increase; antithrombin III, mild decrease; prothrombin time, increased.
C. Thyroid Function Tests: Protein-bound Iodine (PBI), increased; Total Serum Thyroxine (T_4), increased; Thyroid Stimulating Hormone (TSH), unchanged; T_3 resin-uptake, decreased.
D. Adrenocortical Function Tests: plasma cortisol, increased.
E. Miscellaneous Tests: serum folate, occasionally decreased; glucose tolerance test, variable increase with return to normal after 6 to 12 months; insulin response, mild to moderate increase; c-peptide response, mild to moderate increase.

Tissue Specimens: Pathologists should be advised of oral contraceptive therapy when specimens obtained from surgical procedures and Pap smears are submitted for examination.

Return to Fertility: After discontinuing oral contraceptive therapy, the patient should delay pregnancy until at least 1 normal spontaneous cycle has occurred in order to date the pregnancy. An alternative contraceptive method should be used during this time.

Amenorrhea: Women having a history of oligomenorrhea, secondary amenorrhea, or irregular cycles may remain anovulatory or become amenorrheic following discontinuation of estrogen-progestin combination therapy.

Amenorrhea, especially if associated with breast secretion, that continues for 6 months or more after withdrawal, warrants a careful assessment of hypothalamic-pituitary function.

Thromboembolic Complications—Post-surgery: There is an increased risk of thromboembolic complications in oral contraceptive users after major surgery. If feasible, oral contraceptives should be discontinued and an alternative method substituted at least 1 month prior to **major** elective surgery. Oral contraceptives should not be resumed until the first menstrual period after hospital discharge following surgery.

Drug Interactions: The concurrent administration of oral contraceptives with other drugs may result in an altered response to either agent (see Table 1 and Table 2). Reduced effectiveness of the oral contraceptive, should it occur, is more likely with the low-dose formulations.

It is important to ascertain all drugs that a patient is taking, both prescription and non-prescription, including herbal preparations/remedies, before oral contraceptives are prescribed.

Table 1: Tri-Cyclen

Drugs That May Decrease the Efficacy of Oral Contraceptives

Class of Compound	Drug	Proposed Mechanism	Suggested Management
Anticonvulsants	Carbamazepine Ethosuximide Phenobarbital Phenytoin Primidone	Induction of hepatic microsomal enzymes: Rapid metabolism of estrogen and increased binding of progestin and ethinyl estradiol to SHBG.	Use higher dose OCs (50 µg ethinyl estradiol), another drug or another method.
Antibiotics	Ampicillin Cotrimoxazole Penicillin	Enterohepatic circulation disturbance, intestinal hurry.	For short course, use additional method or use another drug. For long course, use another method.
	Rifampin	Increased metabolism of progestins. Suspected acceleration of estrogen metabolism.	Use another method.
	Chloramphenicol Metronidazole Neomycin Nitrofurantoin Sulfonamides Tetracyclines	Induction of hepatic microsomal enzymes. Also disturbance of enterohepatic circulation.	For short course, use additional method or use another drug. For long course, use another method.
	Troleandomycin	May retard metabolism of OCs, increasing the risk of cholestatic jaundice.	
Antifungals	Griseofulvin	Stimulation of hepatic metabolism of contraceptive steroids may occur.	Use another method.
Cholesterol Lowering Agent	Cholestyramine	May result in hastened elimination and impaired effectiveness.	
Sedatives and Hypnotics	Benzodiazepines Barbiturates Chloral hydrate Glutethimide Meprobamate	Induction of hepatic microsomal enzymes.	For short course, use additional method or another drug. For long course, use another method or higher dose OCs.
Antacids		Decreased intestinal absorption of progestins.	Dose 2 hours apart.
Other Drugs	Phenylbutazone Antihistamines Analgesics Antimigraine preparations Vitamin E	Reduced OC efficacy has been reported. Remains to be confirmed.	
	Bosentan	Induction of hepatic microsomal enzymes.	Consider switching to a non-hormonal contraceptive method or adding a barrier method to oral contraceptive therapy.

Changes in Contraceptive Effectiveness Associated With Co-Administration of Other Drugs: If a woman on hormonal contraceptives takes a drug or herbal product that induces enzymes, including CYP3A4, that metabolize contraceptive hormones, she should be counselled to use additional contraception or a different method of contraception. Drugs or herbal products that induce such enzymes may decrease the plasma concentrations of contraceptive hormones, and may decrease the effectiveness of hormonal contraceptives or increase breakthrough bleeding. Some drugs or herbal products that may decrease the effectiveness of hormonal contraceptives include:*

- modafinil
- oxcarbazepine
- St. John's wort
- topiramate

HIV protease inhibitors and non-nucleoside reverse transcriptase inhibitors: Significant changes (increase or decrease) in the plasma levels of the estrogen and progestin have been noted in some cases of co-administration of HIV protease inhibitors and non-nucleoside reverse transcriptase inhibitors.

Antibiotics: There have been reports of pregnancy while taking hormonal contraceptives and antibiotics, but clinical pharmacokinetic studies have not shown consistent effects of antibiotics on plasma concentrations of synthetic steroids.

Table 2: Tri-Cyclen

Modification of Other Drug Action by Oral Contraceptives

Class of Compound	Drug	Modification of Other Drug Action	Suggested Management
Alcohol		Possible increased levels of ethanol or acetaldehyde.	Use with caution.
Alpha-II Adrenoreceptor Agents	Clonidine	Sedation effect increased.	Use with caution.
Anticoagulants	All	OCs increase clotting factors, decrease efficacy. However, OCs may potentiate action in some patients.	Use another method.
Anticonvulsants	All	Fluid retention may increase risk of seizures.	Use another method.
	Lamotrigine	Significantly decreased lamotrigine levels (due to induction of lamotrigine glucuronidation) may lead to breakthrough seizures.	Adjust dose of drug if necessary.
Antidiabetic Drugs	Oral hypoglycemics and insulin	OCs may impair glucose tolerance and increase blood glucose.	Use low-dose estrogen and progestin OC or another method. Monitor blood glucose.
Antihypertensive Agents	Guanethidine and methyldopa	Estrogen component causes sodium retention, progestin has no effect.	Use low-dose estrogen OC or use another method.
	Beta-blockers	Increased drug effect (decreased metabolism).	Adjust dose of drug if necessary. Monitor cardiovascular status.
Antipyretics	Acetaminophen	Increased metabolism and renal clearance.	Dose of drug may have to be increased.
	Antipyrine	Impaired metabolism.	Decrease dose of drug.
	ASA	Effects of ASA may be decreased by the short-term use of OCs.	Patients on chronic ASA therapy may require an increase in ASA dosage.
Aminocaproic Acid		Theoretically, a hypercoagulable state may occur because OCs augment clotting factors.	Avoid concomitant use.
Betamimetic Agents	Isoproterenol	Estrogen causes decreased response to these drugs.	Adjust dose of drug as necessary. Discontinuing OCs can result in excessive drug activity.
Caffeine		The actions of caffeine may be enhanced as OCs may impair the hepatic metabolism of caffeine.	Use with caution.
Corticosteroids	Prednisone Prednisolone	Markedly increased serum levels.	Possible need for decrease in dose.
Cyclosporine		May lead to an increase in cyclosporine levels and hepatotoxicity.	Monitor hepatic function. The cyclosporine dose may have to be decreased.
Folic Acid		OCs have been reported to impair folate metabolism.	May need to increase dietary intake, or supplement.
Meperidine		Possible increased analgesia and CNS depression due to decreased metabolism of meperidine.	Use combination with caution.
Phenothiazine Tranquilizers	All phenothiazines, reserpine and similar drugs	Estrogen potentiates the hyperprolactinemia effect of these drugs.	Use other drugs or lower dose OCs. If galactorrhea or hyperprolactinemia occurs, use other method.
Sedatives and Hypnotics	Chlordiazepoxide Lorazepam Oxazepam Diazepam	Increased effect (increased metabolism).	Use with caution.
Theophylline	All	Decreased oxidation, leading to possible toxicity.	Use with caution. Monitor theophylline levels.
Tricyclic Antidepressants	Clomipramine (possibly others)	Increased side effects, i.e., depression.	Use with caution.
Vitamin B_{12}		OCs have been reported to reduce serum levels of Vitamin B_{12}.	May need to increase dietary intake, or supplement.

* Additional drugs are listed in Table I.
† Additional drugs are listed in Table II.

Increase in Plasma Hormone Levels Associated With Co-Administered Drugs: Some drugs and grapefruit juice may increase the plasma levels of ethinyl estradiol if co-administered. Examples include:

- acetaminophen
- ascorbic acid
- CYP3A4 inhibitors (including itraconazole, ketoconazole, voriconazole and fluconazole)
- grapefruit juice
- HMG-CoA reductase inhibitors (including atorvastatin and rosuvastatin)

Changes in Plasma Levels of Co-Administered Drugs: Combination hormonal contraceptives may also affect the pharmacokinetics of some other drugs if used concomitantly. Examples of drugs whose plasma levels may be increased (due to CYP inhibition) include:†

- omeprazole
- voriconazole

Examples of drugs whose plasma levels may be decreased (due to induction of glucuronidation) include:†

- morphine
- salicylic acid
- temazepam

Physicians are advised to consult the labelling of concurrently used drugs to obtain further information about interactions with hormonal contraceptives or the potential for enzyme alterations.

Refer to Oral Contraceptives 1994 (Chapter 8), Health Canada, for other possible drug interactions with OCs.

Non-contraceptive Benefits of Oral Contraceptives: Several health advantages other than contraception have been reported.

1. Combination oral contraceptives reduce the incidence of cancer of the endometrium and ovaries.
2. Oral contraceptives reduce the likelihood of developing benign breast disease and, as a result, decrease the incidence of breast biopsies.
3. Oral contraceptives reduce the likelihood of development of functional ovarian cysts.
4. Pill users have less menstrual blood loss and have more regular cycles, thereby reducing the chance of developing iron-deficiency anemia.
5. The use of oral contraceptives may decrease the severity of dysmenorrhea and premenstrual syndrome, and may improve acne vulgaris, hirsutism and other androgen-mediated disorders. Tri-Cyclen tablets are also used to treat moderate acne in females who are able to take oral contraceptives.
6. Oral contraceptives decrease the incidence of acute pelvic inflammatory disease and, thereby, reduce as well the incidence of ectopic pregnancy.
7. Oral contraceptives have potential beneficial effects on endometriosis.

Oral contraceptives **do not protect** against sexually transmitted diseases (STDs) including HIV/AIDS. For protection against STDs, it is advisable to use latex condoms **in combination with** oral contraceptives.

ADVERSE EFFECTS: An increased risk of the following serious adverse reactions has been associated with the use of oral contraceptives: thrombophlebitis and venous thrombosis with or without embolism, arterial thromboembolism, pulmonary embolism, mesenteric thrombosis, neuro-ocular lesions (e.g., retinal thrombosis), myocardial infarction, cerebral thrombosis, cerebral hemorrhage, hypertension, benign hepatic tumors, gallbladder disease.

The following adverse reactions also have been reported in patients receiving oral contraceptives: nausea and vomiting, usually the most common adverse reaction, occurs in approximately 10% or less of patients during the first cycle. Other reactions, as a general rule, are seen less frequently or only occasionally, as follows:

Cardiovascular System: edema, slight rise of blood pressure.

Genital Tract: breakthrough bleeding, spotting, change in menstrual flow, dysmenorrhea, amenorrhea during and after treatment, vaginal candidiasis, premenstrual-like syndrome, temporary infertility after discontinuance of treatment, vaginitis, endocervical hyperplasias, increase in cervical erosion and secretion.

Neoplasms: malignant hepatic tumors, cervical cancer, increase in size of uterine leiomyomata, breast cancer.

Breast: pain, tenderness, enlargement, and secretion, possible diminution in lactation when given immediately, postpartum.

Skin and Subcutaneous Tissue: chloasma or melasma which may persist, rash (allergic), hirsutism, loss of scalp hair, erythema multiforme, erythema nodosum, Raynaud's phenomenon, hemorrhagic eruption, porphyria, acne, seborrhea, pemphigoid (herpes gestationis), urticaria, angioedema.

CNS: migraine, depression, headache, nervousness, dizziness, changes in libido, chorea.

Metabolic: reduced tolerance to carbohydrates, change in weight (increase or decrease), changes in appetite.

Gastro-intestinal Tract: gastrointestinal symptoms (such as abdominal cramps and bloating), colitis, pancreatitis.

Hepatobiliary: cholestatic jaundice, Budd-Chiari syndrome.

Eyes: intolerance to contact lenses, change in corneal curvature (steepening), cataracts, optic neuritis, retinal thrombosis.

Urinary: impaired renal function, hemolytic uremic syndrome, cystitis-like syndrome.

Others: rhinitis, auditory disturbances.

OVERDOSE:

Treatment: In case of overdose or accidental ingestion by children, the physician should observe the patient closely, although generally no treatment is required. Gastric lavage may be utilized if considered necessary. Overdosage may cause nausea and vomiting and withdrawal bleeding may occur in females. There are no antidotes and treatment should be symptomatic.

For management of a suspected drug overdose, contact your regional Poison Control Centre. See the *CPS* Directory section for a list of Poison Control Centres.

DOSAGE: Information for the Patient on How to Take the Birth Control Pill:

1. **Read these directions:**
   - before you start taking your pills, and
   - any time you are not sure what to do.
2. **Look at your pill pack** to see if it has 21 or 28 pills:
   - **21-Pill Pack:** 21 active pills (with hormones) taken daily for 3 weeks, and then take no pills for 1 week or
   - **28-Pill Pack:** 21 active pills (with hormones) taken daily for 3 weeks, and then 7 "reminder" pills (no hormones) taken daily for 1 week.

   Also check the pill pack for instructions on (1) where to start and (2) directions to take pills (see package insert for illustrations).
3. You may wish to use a second method of birth control (e.g. latex condoms and spermicidal foam or gel) for the first 7 days of the first cycle of pill use. This will provide a back-up in case pills are forgotten while you are getting used to taking them.
4. **When receiving any medical treatment, be sure to tell your doctor that you are using birth control pills.**
5. **Many women have spotting or light bleeding, or may feel sick to their stomach during the first 3 months on the pill.** If you do feel sick, do not stop taking the pill. The problem will usually go away. If it does not go away, check with your doctor or clinic.
6. **Missing pills also can cause some spotting or light bleeding**, even if you make up the missed pills. You also could feel a little sick to your stomach on the days you take 2 pills to make up for missed pills.
7. **If you miss pills at any time, you could get pregnant. The greatest risks for pregnancy are:**
   - when you start a pack late, and
   - when you miss pills at the beginning or at the very end of the pack.
8. **Always be sure you have ready:**
   - **another kind of birth control** (such as latex condoms and spermicidal foam or gel) to use as a back-up in case you miss pills, and
   - **an extra, full pack of pills.**
9. **If you experience vomiting or diarrhea, or if you take certain medicines**, such as antibiotics, your pills may not work as well. Use a back-up method, such as latex condoms and spermicidal foam or gel, until you can check with your doctor or clinic.
10. **If you forget more than 1 pill 2 months in a row,** talk to your doctor or clinic about how to make pill-taking easier or about using another method of birth control.
11. **If your questions are not answered here, call your doctor or clinic.**

When to Start the First Pack of Pills: Be sure to read these instructions:

- before you start taking your pills, and

- any time you are not sure what to do.

Decide with your doctor or clinic what is the best day for you to start taking your first pack of pills. Your pills may be either a 21-day or a 28-day type.

Directions for 21-Day and 28-Day Pill Packs:

1. **The first day of your menstrual period (bleeding) is Day 1 of your cycle.** The pills may be started up to Day 6 of your cycle. Your starting day will be chosen in discussion with your doctor. You will **always** begin taking your pill on this day of the week. Your doctor may advise you to start taking the pills on Day 1, on Day 5, or on the first Sunday after your period begins. If your period starts on Sunday, start that same day.
2. **If you are using a:**
   21-Day Pill Pack: With this type of birth control pill, you are on pills for 21 days and off pills for 7 days. You must not be off the pills for more than 7 days in a row.
   Take 1 pill at approximately the same time every day for 21 days. **Then do not take a pill for 7 days.** Start a new pack on the 8th day. You will probably have a period during the 7 days off the pill. (This bleeding may be lighter and shorter than your usual period.)
   28-Day Pill Pack: With this type of birth control pill, you take 21 pills that contain hormones and seven pills that contain no hormones.
   Take 1 pill at approximately the same time every day for 28 days. Begin a new pack the next day, **not missing any days on the pills.** Your period should occur during the last 7 days of using that pill pack.

Instructions for Using Your Discreet Package for Both 21-Day and 28-Day Packs: Follow these instructions carefully:

1. **For Day 1 start:** Label the Discreet package by selecting the day label that starts with Day 1 of your menstrual period (the first day of menstruation is Day 1). For example, if your first day of menstruation is Tuesday, attach the day label that begins with **TUE** in the space provided.
   or
   For Day 5 start: Label the Discreet package by selecting the day label that starts with the day that is 5 days after your period begins. (Count 5 days **including** the first day of menstruation.) For example, if your first day of menstruation is Saturday, place the day label that starts with **WED** in the space provided.
   or
   For Sunday start: No day label is required. The Discreet package is printed for a Sunday start. (The first Sunday **after** your period begins, or, if your period starts on Sunday, start that **same day.**)
2. Place the day label in the space where you see the words "Place day label here". Having the DISCREET Package labelled with the days of the week will help remind you to take your pill every day.
3. To begin taking your pills, start with the pill inside the red circle (where you see the word **START**). This pill should correspond to the day of the week that you are taking your first pill. To remove the pill, push through the back of the Discreet Package.
4. On the following day, take the next pill in the same row, always proceeding from left to right (→). Each row will always begin on the same day of the week.

What to do during the month:

1. **Take a pill at approximately the same time every day until the pack is empty.**
   - Try to associate taking your pill with some regular activity like eating a meal or going to bed.
   - Do not skip pills even if you have bleeding between monthly periods or feel sick to your stomach (nausea).
   - Do not skip pills even if you do not have sex very often.
2. **When you finish a pack:**
   - **21 pills: Wait 7 days** to start the next pack. You will have your period during that week.
   - **28 pills:** Start the next pack **on the next day.** Take 1 pill every day. Do not wait any days between packs.

What to do if you miss pills: Table 3 outlines the actions you should take if you miss 1 or more of your birth control pills. Match the number of pills missed with the appropriate starting time for your type of pill pack.

Note: 28-Day Pack: If you forget any of the 7 "reminder" pills (without hormones) in Week 4, just safely dispose of the pills you missed. Then keep taking 1 pill each day until the pack is empty. You do not need to use a back-up method.

Always be sure you have on hand:

- a back-up method of birth control (such as latex condoms and spermicidal foam or gel) in case you miss pills, and
- an extra full pack of pills.

If you forget more than 1 pill 2 months in a row, talk to your doctor or clinic about ways to make pill-taking easier or about using another method of birth control.

Table 3: Tri-Cyclen

What To Do if you Miss Pills

Sunday Start	Other Than Sunday Start
Miss 1 pill	**Miss 1 pill**
Take it as soon as you remember and take the next pill at the usual time. This means that you might take 2 pills in one day.	Take it as soon as you remember, and take the next pill at the usual time. This means that you might take 2 pills in one day.
Miss 2 pills in a row	**Miss 2 pills in a row**
First 2 Weeks: 1. Take 2 pills the day you remember and 2 pills the next day. 2. Then take 1 pill a day until you finish the pack. 3. Use a back-up method of birth control if you have sex in the 7 days after you miss the pills. **Third Week:** 1. Keep taking 1 pill a day until Sunday. 2. On Sunday, safely discard the rest of the pack and start a new pack that day. 3. Use a back-up method of birth control if you have sex in the 7 days after you miss the pills. 4. You may not have a period this month. **If you miss 2 periods in a row, call your doctor or clinic.**	**First 2 Weeks:** 1. Take 2 pills the day you remember and 2 pills the next day. 2. Then take 1 pill a day until you finish the pack. 3. Use a back-up method of birth control if you have sex in the 7 days after you miss the pills. **Third Week:** 1. Safely dispose of the rest of the pill pack and start a new pack that same day. 2. Use a back-up method of birth control if you have sex in the 7 days after you miss the pills. 3. You may not have a period this month. **If you miss 2 periods in a row, call your doctor or clinic.**
Miss 3 or more pills in a row	**Miss 3 or more pills in a row**
Anytime in the Cycle: 1. Keep taking 1 pill a day until Sunday. 2. On Sunday, safely discard the rest of the pack and start a new pack that day. 3. Use a back-up method of birth control if you have sex in the 7 days after you miss the pills. 4. You may not have a period this month. **If you miss 2 periods in a row, call your doctor or clinic.**	**Anytime in the Cycle:** 1. Safely dispose of the rest of the pill pack and start a new pack that same day. 2. Use a back-up method of birth control if you have sex in the 7 days after you miss the pills. 3. You may not have a period this month. **If you miss 2 periods in a row, call your doctor or clinic.**

INFORMATION FOR THE PATIENT: Published in e-CPS, available by subscription at www.e-cps.ca.

SUPPLIED: Each white tablet contains: norgestimate 0.18 mg and ethinyl estradiol 0.035 mg. Each light blue tablet contains: norgestimate 0.215 mg and ethinyl estradiol 0.035 mg. Each blue tablet contains: norgestimate 0.25 mg and ethinyl estradiol 0.035 mg. Nonmedicinal ingredients: white, light blue, and blue tablets: lactose, magnesium stearate and starch. Light blue and blue tablets also contain FD&C Blue #2 Aluminum Lake. In the 28 day regimen the green tablets contain inert ingredients, namely: D&C Yellow #10 Aluminum Lake, FD&C Blue #2 Aluminum Lake, lactose, magnesium stearate, microcrystalline cellulose and starch. Available in 21-day (7 white tablets, 7 light blue tablets and 7 blue tablets) or 28-day (7 white tablets, 7 light blue tablets, 7 blue tablets and 7 green tablets) Discreet Packages. Store between 15 and 25°C. Leave contents in protective packaging until time of use.

(Shown in Product Identification Section)

Tri-Cyclen® LO ℞

norgestimate—ethinyl estradiol

Oral Contraceptive

Janssen-Ortho

Date of Preparation: June 27, 2003
Date of Revision: April 28, 2006

PHARMACOLOGY: Oral Contraception: Combination oral contraceptives act by suppression of gonadotropins. Although the primary mechanism of this action is inhibition of ovulation, other alterations include changes in the cervical mucus (which increase the difficulty of sperm entry into the uterus) and the endometrium (which reduce the likelihood of implantation).

Receptor binding studies, as well as studies in animals and humans, have shown that norgestimate and 17-deacetyl norgestimate (norelgestromin), the major serum metabolite, combine high progestational activity with minimal intrinsic androgenicity. Norgestimate, in combination with ethinyl estradiol, does not counteract the estrogen-induced increases in sex hormone binding globulin (SHBG), resulting in lower serum testosterone.

INDICATIONS: TRI-CYCLEN LO Tablets are indicated for conception control.

In an active controlled clinical trial including 1673 subjects completing 11 003 cycles of TRI-CYCLEN LO use, a total of 20 pregnancies were reported among TRI-CYCLEN LO users. This represents an overall use-efficacy (typical user efficacy) pregnancy rate of 2.36 per 100 women-years of use. This figure for Pearl Index is slightly higher than other Pearl Indices for similar products marketed in Canada and may be attributed to differences in clinical trial design.

Table 1: TRI-CYCLEN LO

Percentage of Women Experiencing an Unintended Pregnancy During the First Year of Typical Use and the First Year of Perfect Use of Contraception and the Percentage Continuing Use at the End of the First Year

	% of Women Experiencing an Unintended Pregnancy Within the First Year of Use		
Method	**Typical Use**[a]	**Perfect Use**[b]	**% of Women Continuing Use at One Year**[c]
Chance[d]	85	85	
Spermicides[e]	26	6	40
Periodic Abstinence	25		
Calendar		9	
Ovulation Method		3	
Sympto-thermal[f]		2	
Post-ovulation		1	
Withdrawal	19	4	
Cap[g]			
Parous Women	40	26	42
Nulliparous Women	20	9	56
Sponge			
Parous Women	40	20	42
Nulliparous Women	20	9	56
Diaphragm[g]	20	6	56
Condom[h]			
Female (Reality)	21	5	56
Male	14	3	61
Pill	5		
Progestin Only		0.5	
Combined		0.1	
IUD			
Progesterone T	2.0	1.5	81
CopperT380A	0.8	0.6	78
LNg 20	0.1	0.1	81
Depo-Provera	0.3	0.3	70
Female Sterilization	0.5	0.5	100

(cont'd)

Table 1: TRI-CYCLEN LO *(cont'd)*

Percentage of Women Experiencing an Unintended Pregnancy During the First Year of Typical Use and the First Year of Perfect Use of Contraception and the Percentage Continuing Use at the End of the First Year

Method	% of Women Experiencing an Unintended Pregnancy Within the First Year of Use		% of Women Continuing Use at One Year[c]
	Typical Use[a]	Perfect Use[b]	
Male Sterilization	0.15	0.10	100

[a] Among typical couples who initiate use of a method (not necessarily for the first time), the percentage who experience an accidental pregnancy during the first year if they do not stop for any other reason.
[b] Among couples who initiate use of a method (not necessarily for the first time) and who use it perfectly (both consistently and correctly), the percentage who experience an accidental pregnancy during the first year if they do not stop use for any other reason.
[c] Among couples attempting to avoid pregnancy, the percentage who continue to use a method for one year.
[d] The percents becoming pregnant in columns (2) and (3) are based on data from populations where contraception is not used and from women who cease using contraception in order to become pregnant. Among such populations, about 89% become pregnant within one year. This estimate was lowered slightly (to 85%) to represent the percent who would become pregnant within one year among women now relying on reversible methods of contraception if they abandoned contraception altogether.
[e] Foams, creams, gels, vaginal suppositories, and vaginal films.
[f] Cervical mucus (ovulation) method supplemented by calendar in the pre-ovulatory and basal body temperature in the post-ovulatory phases.
[g] With spermicidal cream or jelly.
[h] Without spermicides.
Source:
Trussell J. Contraceptive efficacy. In Hatcher RA, Trussell J, Stewart F, Cates W, Stewart GK, Kowel D, Guest F, Contraceptive Technology: Seventeenth Revised Edition. New York NY: Irvington Publishers, 1998.

CONTRAINDICATIONS: Oral contraceptives should not be used in women who currently have the following conditions:
1. History of or actual thrombophlebitis or thromboembolic disorders.
2. History of or actual cerebrovascular disorders.
3. History of or actual myocardial infarction or coronary arterial disease.
4. Active liver disease or history of or actual benign or malignant liver tumors.
5. Known or suspected carcinoma of the breast.
6. Known or suspected estrogen-dependent neoplasia.
7. Undiagnosed abnormal vaginal bleeding.
8. Any ocular lesion arising from ophthalmic vascular disease, such as partial or complete loss of vision or defect in visual fields.
9. When pregnancy is suspected or diagnosed.
10. Valvular heart disease with complications.
11. Severe hypertension (persistent systolic values of ≥160 or persistent diastolic values of ≥100 mmHg).
12. Diabetes with vascular involvement.
13. Cholestatic jaundice or history of jaundice of pregnancy.
14. Migraine with focal aura.
15. Hypersensitivity to any of the components of this product.

WARNINGS: The following information is provided from studies for combination oral contraceptives. The use of combination hormonal contraceptives is associated with increased risks of several serious conditions including myocardial infarction, thromboembolism, stroke, hepatic neoplasia and gallbladder disease, although the risk of serious morbidity and mortality is small in healthy women without underlying risk factors. The risk of morbidity and mortality increases significantly if associated with the presence of other risk factors such as hypertension, hyperlipidemias, obesity and diabetes.

The information contained in this section is principally on studies carried out in women who used combination oral contraceptives with higher formulations of estrogens and progestins than those in common use today. The effect of long-term use of combination hormonal contraceptives with lower doses of both estrogen and progestin administered orally remains to be determined.

Predisposing Factors for Coronary Artery Disease: Cigarette smoking increases the risk of serious cardiovascular side effects and mortality. Birth control pills increase this risk, especially with increasing age. Convincing data are available to support an upper age limit of 35 years for oral contraceptive use by women who smoke.

Other women who are independently at high risk for cardiovascular disease include those with diabetes, hypertension, abnormal lipid profile, or a family history of these. Whether oral contraceptives accentuate this risk is unclear.

In low-risk, non-smoking women of any age, the benefits of oral contraceptive use outweigh the possible cardiovascular risks associated with low-dose formulations. Consequently, oral contraceptives may be prescribed for these women up to the age of menopause.

> Cigarette smoking increases the risk of serious adverse effects on the heart and blood vessels. This risk increases with age and becomes significant in oral contraceptive users older than 35 years of age. Women should be counselled not to smoke.

Discontinue Medication at the Earliest Manifestation of the Following:
A. Thromboembolic and cardiovascular disorders such as thrombophlebitis, pulmonary embolism, cerebrovascular disorders, myocardial ischemia, mesenteric thrombosis, and retinal thrombosis.
B. Conditions that predispose to venous stasis and to vascular thrombosis (e.g. immobilization after accidents or confinement to bed during long-term illness). Other non-hormonal methods of contraception should be used until regular activities are resumed. For use of oral contraceptives when surgery is contemplated, see Precautions.
C. Visual defects—partial or complete.
D. Papilledema or ophthalmic vascular lesions.
E. Severe headache of unknown etiology or worsening of pre-existing migraine headache.

PRECAUTIONS: Physical Examination and Follow-up: Before oral contraceptives are used, a thorough history and physical examination should be performed, including a blood pressure determination. Breasts, liver, extremities, and pelvic organs should also be examined. A Papanicolaou smear should be taken if the patient has been sexually active.

The first follow-up visit should be three months after oral contraceptives are prescribed. Thereafter, examinations should be performed at least once a year, or more frequently if indicated. At each annual visit, examination should include those procedures that were done at the initial visit as outlined above or per recommendations of the Canadian Workshop on Screening for Cancer of the Cervix. Their suggestion was that, for women who had two consecutive negative Pap smears, screening could be continued every three years up to the age of 69.

Pregnancy: Oral contraceptives should not be taken by pregnant women. However, if conception accidentally occurs while taking the pill, there is no conclusive evidence that the estrogen and progestin contained in the oral contraceptive will damage the developing child.

Lactation: In breast-feeding women, the use of oral contraceptives results in the hormonal components being excreted in breast milk and may reduce its quantity and quality. If the use of oral contraceptives is initiated after the establishment of lactation, there does not appear to be any effect on the quantity and quality of the milk. There is no evidence that low-dose oral contraceptives are harmful to the nursing infant.

Hepatic Function: Patients who have had jaundice, including a history of cholestatic jaundice during pregnancy, should be given oral contraceptives with great care and under close observation.

The development of severe generalized pruritus or icterus requires that the medication be withdrawn until the problem is resolved.

If a patient develops jaundice that proves to be cholestatic in type, the use of oral contraceptives should not be resumed. In patients taking oral contraceptives, changes in the composition of the bile may occur and an increased incidence of gallstones has been reported.

Hepatic nodules (adenoma and focal nodular hyperplasia) have been reported, particularly in long-term users of oral contraceptives. Although these lesions are extremely rare, they have caused fatal intra-abdominal hemorrhage and should be considered in women with an abdominal mass, acute abdominal pain, or evidence of intra-abdominal bleeding.

Hypertension: Patients with essential hypertension whose blood pressure is well controlled may be given oral contraceptives but only under close supervision. If a significant elevation of blood pressure in previously normotensive or hypertensive subjects occurs at any time during the administration of the drug, cessation of medication is necessary.

Migraine and Headache: The onset or exacerbation of migraine or the development of headache of a new pattern that is recurrent, persistent or severe, requires discontinuation of oral contraceptives and evaluation of the cause.

Diabetes: Current low-dose oral contraceptives exert minimal impact on glucose metabolism. Diabetic patients, or those with a family history of diabetes, should be observed closely to detect any worsening of carbohydrate metabolism. Patients predisposed to diabetes who can be kept under close supervision may be given oral contraceptives. Young diabetic patients whose disease is of recent origin, well-controlled, and not associated with hypertension or other signs of vascular disease such as ocular fundal changes, should be monitored more frequently while using oral contraceptives.

Ocular Disease: Patients who are pregnant or are taking oral contraceptives, may experience corneal edema that may cause visual disturbances and changes in tolerance to contact lenses, especially of the rigid type. Soft contact lenses usually do not cause disturbances. If visual changes or alterations in tolerance to contact lenses occur, temporary or permanent cessation of wear may be advised.

Breasts: Increasing age and a strong family history are the most significant risk factors for the development of breast cancer. Other established risk factors include obesity, nulliparity and late age for first full-term pregnancy. The identified groups of women that may be at increased risk of developing breast cancer before menopause are long-term users of oral contraceptives (more than eight years) and starters at early age. In a few women, the use of oral contraceptives may accelerate the growth of an existing but undiagnosed breast cancer. Since any potential increased risk related to oral contraceptive use is small, there is no reason to change prescribing habits at present.

Women receiving oral contraceptives should be instructed in self-examination of their breasts. Their physicians should be notified whenever any masses are detected. A yearly clinical breast examination is also recommended because, if a breast cancer should develop, drugs that contain estrogen may cause a rapid progression.

Vaginal Bleeding: Persistent irregular vaginal bleeding requires assessment to exclude underlying pathology.

Fibroids: Patients with fibroids (leiomyomata) should be carefully observed. Sudden enlargement, pain, or tenderness require discontinuation of the use of oral contraceptives.

Emotional Disorders: Patients with a history of emotional disturbances, especially the depressive type, may be more prone to have a recurrence of depression while taking oral contraceptives. In cases of a serious recurrence, a trial of an alternative method of contraception should be made which may help to clarify the possible relationship. Women with premenstrual syndrome (PMS) may have a varied response to oral contraceptives, ranging from symptomatic improvement to worsening of the condition.

Laboratory Tests: Results of laboratory tests should be interpreted in light of the fact that the patient is on oral contraceptives. The following laboratory tests are modified.

Liver Function Tests: Bromsulphthalein Retention Test (BSP), moderate increase; AST and GGT, minor increase; alkaline phosphatase, variable increase; serum bilirubin, increased, particularly in conditions predisposing to or associated with hyperbilirubinemia.

Coagulation Tests: Factors II, VII, IX, X, XII and XIII, increased; Factor VIII, mild increase; platelet aggregation and adhesiveness, mild increase in response to common aggregating agents; fibrinogen, increased; plasminogen, mild increase; antithrombin III, mild decrease; prothrombin time, increased.

Thyroid Function Tests: Protein-bound Iodine (PBI), increased; Total Serum Thyroxine (T_4), increased; Thyroid Stimulating Hormone (TSH), unchanged; T_3 resin-uptake, decreased.

Adrenocortical Function Tests: plasma cortisol, increased.

Miscellaneous Tests: serum folate, occasionally decreased; glucose tolerance test, variable increase with return to normal after 6 to 12 months; insulin response, mild to moderate increase; c-peptide response, mild to moderate increase.

Tissue Specimens: Pathologists should be advised of oral contraceptive therapy when specimens obtained from surgical procedures and Pap smears are submitted for examination.

Return to Fertility: After discontinuing oral contraceptive therapy, the patient should delay pregnancy until at least one normal spontaneous cycle has occurred in order to date the pregnancy. An alternative contraceptive method should be used during this time.

Amenorrhea: Women having a history of oligomenorrhea, secondary amenorrhea, or irregular cycles may remain anovulatory or become amenorrheic following discontinuation of estrogen-progestin combination therapy.

Amenorrhea, especially if associated with breast secretion, that continues for six months or more after withdrawal, warrants a careful assessment of hypothalamic-pituitary function.

Thromboembolic Complications—Post-surgery: There is an increased risk of thromboembolic complications in oral contraceptive users after major surgery. If feasible, oral contraceptives should be discontinued and an alternative method substituted at least one month prior to **major** elective surgery. Oral contraceptive use should not be resumed until the first menstrual period after hospital discharge following surgery.

Drug Interactions: The concurrent administration of oral contraceptives with other drugs may result in an altered response to either agent (Table 2 and Table 3). Reduced effectiveness of the oral contraceptive, should it occur, is more likely with the low-dose formulations. It is important to ascertain all drugs that a patient is taking, both prescription and non-prescription, including herbal preparations/remedies, before oral contraceptives are prescribed.

The metabolism of oral contraceptives may be influenced by various drugs and herbal preparations including St. John's wort. Of potential clinical importance are drugs and herbal supplements that are known to affect the induction of enzymes that are responsible for the degradation of contraceptive steroid hormones (e.g. St. John's wort). Decreased effectiveness of the estrogenic component of oral contraceptives may result in spotting, breakthrough bleeding and possible pill failure. It is possible that induction of these enzymes may lead to reductions in the circulating levels of the progestational component of TRI-CYCLEN LO Tablets. In actual practice, reduced efficacy has been associated with concomitant use of St. John's wort.

Some drugs, such as cholestyramine, may impair the enterohepatic circulation of estrogens, and may result in hastened elimination and impaired effectiveness.

Some data has indicated a decrease in the serum levels of the estrogenic component of oral contraceptives in conjunction with topiramate. Therefore, the efficacy of low-dose oral contraceptives may be reduced with concomitant use. Patients should be encouraged to report any change in bleeding patterns.

Some protease inhibitors and some anti-retroviral agents have been found to either increase (e.g. indinavir) or decrease (e.g. ritonavir) circulating levels of combination hormonal contraceptives.

Refer to Oral Contraceptives 1994 (Chapter 8), Health Canada, for other possible drug interactions with OCs.

Table 2: TRI-CYCLEN LO

Drugs That May Decrease the Efficacy of Oral Contraceptives

Class of Compound	Drug	Proposed Mechanism	Suggested Management
Anticonvulsants	Carbamazepine Ethosuximide Phenobarbital Phenytoin Primidone	Induction of hepatic microsomal enzymes. Rapid metabolism of estrogen and increased binding of progestin and ethinyl estradiol to SHBG.	Use higher dose OCs (50 µg ethinyl estradiol), another drug or another method.
Antibiotics	Ampicillin Cotrimoxazole Penicillin	Enterohepatic circulation disturbance, intestinal hurry.	For short course, use additional method or use another drug. For long course, use another method.
	Rifampin	Increased metabolism of progestins. Suspected acceleration of estrogen metabolism.	Use another method.

(cont'd)

Table 2: TRI-CYCLEN LO *(cont'd)*
Drugs That May Decrease the Efficacy of Oral Contraceptives

Class of Compound	Drug	Proposed Mechanism	Suggested Management
	Chloramphenicol Metronidazole Neomycin Nitrofurantoin Sulfonamides Tetracyclines	Induction of hepatic microsomal enzymes. Also disturbance of enterohepatic circulation.	For short course, use additional method or use another drug. For long course, use another method.
	Troleandomycin	May retard metabolism of OCs, increasing the risk of cholestatic jaundice.	
Antifungals	Griseofulvin	Stimulation of hepatic metabolism of contraceptive steroids may occur.	Use another method.
Cholesterol Lowering Agents	Clofibrate	Reduces elevated serum triglycerides and cholesterol; this reduces OC efficacy.	Use another method.
Sedatives and Hypnotics	Benzodiazepines Barbiturates Chloral Hydrate Glutethimide Meprobamate	Induction of hepatic microsomal enzymes.	For short course, use additional method or another drug. For long course, use another method or higher dose OCs.
Antacids		Decreased intestinal absorption of progestins.	Dose two hours apart.
Other Drugs	Phenylbutazone Antihistamines Analgesics Antimigraine preparations Vitamin E	Reduced OC efficacy has been reported. Remains to be confirmed.	

Table 3: TRI-CYCLEN LO
Modification of Other Drug Action by Oral Contraceptives

Class of Compound	Drug	Modification of Drug Action	Suggested Management
Alcohol		Possible increased levels of ethanol or acetaldehyde.	Use with caution.
Alpha-II Adrenoreceptor Agents	Clonidine	Sedation effect increased.	Use with caution.
Anticoagulants	All	OCs increase clotting factors, decrease efficacy. However, OCs may potentiate action in some patients.	Use another method.
Anticonvulsants	All	Fluid retention may increase risk of seizures.	Use another method.
Antidiabetic Drugs	Oral Hypoglycemics and Insulin	OCs may impair glucose tolerance and increase blood glucose.	Use low-dose estrogen and progestin OC or another method. Monitor blood glucose.
Antihypertensive Agents	Guanethidine and Methyldopa	Estrogen component causes sodium retention, progestin has no effect.	Use low-dose estrogen OC or use another method.
	Beta-Blockers	Increased drug effect (decreased metabolism).	Adjust dose of drug if necessary. Monitor cardiovascular status.
Antipyretics	Acetaminophen	Increased metabolism and renal clearance.	Dose of drug may have to be increased.
	Antipyrine	Impaired metabolism.	Decrease dose of drug.
	ASA	Effects of ASA may be decreased by the short-term use of OCs.	Patients on chronic ASA therapy may require an increase in ASA dosage.
Aminocaproic Acid		Theoretically, a hypercoagulable state may occur because OCs augment clotting factors.	Avoid concomitant use.
Betamimetic Agents	Isoproterenol	Estrogen causes decreased response to these drugs.	Adjust dose of drug as necessary. Discontinuing OCs can result in excessive drug activity.
Caffeine		The actions of caffeine may be enhanced as OCs may impair the hepatic metabolism of caffeine.	Use with caution.
Cholesterol Lowering Agents	Clofibrate	Their action may be antagonized by OCs. OCs may also increase metabolism of clofibrate.	May need to increase dose of clofibrate.
Corticosteroids	Prednisone	Markedly increased serum levels.	Possible need for decrease in dose.
Cyclosporine		May lead to an increase in cyclosporine levels and hepatotoxicity.	Monitor hepatic function. The cyclosporine dose may have to be decreased.
Folic Acid		OCs have been reported to impair folate metabolism.	May need to increase dietary intake, or supplement.
Meperidine		Possible increased analgesia and CNS depression due to decreased metabolism of meperidine.	Use combination with caution.
Phenothiazine Tranquilizers	All Phenothiazines, Reserpine and similar drugs	Estrogen potentiates the hyperprolactinemia effect of these drugs.	Use other drugs or lower dose OCs. If galactorrhea or hyperprolactinemia occurs, use other method.
Sedatives and Hypnotics	Chlordiazepoxide Lorazepam Oxazepam Diazepam	Increased effect (increased metabolism).	Use with caution.
Theophylline	All	Decreased oxidation, leading to possible toxicity.	Use with caution. Monitor theophylline levels.
Tricyclic Antidepressants	Clomipramine (possibly others)	Increased side effects; i.e. depression.	Use with caution.
Vitamin B_{12}		OCs have been reported to reduce serum levels of Vitamin B_{12}.	May need to increase dietary intake, or supplement.

Non-contraceptive Benefits of Oral Contraceptives: Several health advantages other than contraception have been reported.

1. Combination oral contraceptives reduce the incidence of cancer of the endometrium and ovaries.
2. Oral contraceptives reduce the likelihood of developing benign breast disease and, as a result, decrease the incidence of breast biopsies.
3. Oral contraceptives reduce the likelihood of development of functional ovarian cysts.
4. Pill users have less menstrual blood loss and have more regular cycles, thereby reducing the chance of developing iron-deficiency anemia.
5. The use of oral contraceptives may decrease the severity of dysmenorrhea and premenstrual syndrome, and may improve acne vulgaris, hirsutism, and other androgen-mediated disorders. TRI-CYCLEN LO Tablets are also used to treat moderate acne in females who are able to take oral contraceptives.
6. Oral contraceptives decrease the incidence of acute pelvic inflammatory disease and, thereby, reduce as well the incidence of ectopic pregnancy.
7. Oral contraceptives have potential beneficial effects on endometriosis.

> Oral contraceptives **do not protect** against sexually transmitted diseases including HIV/AIDS. For protection against STDs, it is advisable to use latex condoms **in combination with** oral contraceptives.

ADVERSE EFFECTS: An increased risk of the following serious adverse reactions has been associated with the use of oral contraceptives: thrombophlebitis, pulmonary embolism, mesenteric thrombosis, neuro-ocular lesions (e.g. retinal thrombosis), myocardial infarction, cerebral thrombosis, cerebral hemorrhage, hypertension, benign hepatic tumours, gallbladder disease.

The following adverse reactions also have been reported in patients receiving oral contraceptives: Nausea and vomiting, usually the most common adverse reaction, occurs in approximately 10 per cent or less patients during the first cycle. Other reactions, as a general rule, are seen less frequently or only occasionally, as follows: gastrointestinal symptoms (such as abdominal cramps and bloating), breakthrough bleeding, spotting, change in menstrual flow, dysmenorrhea, amenorrhea during and after treatment, temporary infertility after discontinuance of treatment, edema, chloasma or melasma which may persist, breast changes: tenderness, enlargement, and secretion, change in weight (increase or decrease), endocervical hyperplasias, possible diminution in lactation when given immediately postpartum, cholestatic jaundice, migraine, increase in size of uterine leiomyomata, rash (allergic), depression, reduced tolerance to carbohydrates, vaginal candidiasis, premenstrual-like syndrome, intolerance to contact lenses, change in corneal curvature (steepening), cataracts, optic neuritis, retinal thrombosis, changes in libido, chorea, changes in appetite, cystitis-like syndrome, rhinitis, headache, nervousness, dizziness, hirsutism, loss of scalp hair, erythema multiforme, erythema nodosum, hemorrhagic eruption, vaginitis, porphyria, impaired renal function, raynaud's phenomenon, auditory disturbances, hemolytic uremic syndrome, pancreatitis.

OVERDOSE:

Treatment: In case of overdose or accidental ingestion by children, the physician should observe the patient closely although generally no treatment is required. Gastric lavage may be utilized if considered necessary.

> For management of a suspected drug overdose, CPhA recommends that you contact your **regional Poison Control Centre**. See the *CPS* Directory section for a list of Poison Control Centres.

DOSAGE: Information to Patient on How to Take the Birth Control Pill:

1. **Read these directions:**
   - before you start taking your pills, and
   - any time you are not sure what to do.
2. **Look at your pill pack** to see if it has 21 or 28 pills:
   - 21-Pill Pack: 21 active pills (with hormones) taken daily for 3 weeks, and then no pills taken for 1 week or
   - 28-Pill Pack: 21 active pills (with hormones) taken daily for 3 weeks, and then 7 "reminder" pills (no hormones) taken daily for 1 week.

   Also check the pill pack for instructions on 1) where to start and 2) direction to take pills.
3. You may wish to use a second method of birth control (e.g. latex condoms and spermicidal foam or gel) for the first seven days of the first cycle of pill use. This will provide a back-up in case pills are forgotten while you are getting used to taking them.
4. **When receiving any medical treatment, be sure to tell your doctor that you are using birth control pills.**
5. **Many women have spotting or light bleeding, or may feel sick to their stomach during the first three months on the pill.** If you do feel sick, do not stop taking the pill. The problem will usually go away. If it does not go away, check with your doctor or clinic.
6. **Missing pills also can cause some spotting or light bleeding**, even if you make up the missed pills. You also could feel a little sick to your stomach on the days you take 2 pills to make up for missed pills.
7. **If you miss pills at any time, you could get pregnant. The greatest risks for pregnancy are:**
   - when you start a pack late, or
   - when you miss pills at the beginning or at the very end of the pack.
8. **Always be sure you have ready:**
   - **another kind of birth control** (such as latex condoms and spermicidal foam or gel) to use as a back-up in case you miss pills, and
   - **an extra, full pack of pills.**
9. **If you experience vomiting or diarrhea, or if you take certain medicines**, such as antibiotics, your pills may not work as well. Use a back-up method, such as latex condoms and spermicidal foam or gel, until you can check with your doctor or clinic.

(cont'd)

10. **If you forget more than 1 pill 2 months in a row**, talk to your doctor or clinic about how to make pill-taking easier or about using another method of birth control.
11. **If your questions are not answered here, call your doctor or clinic.**

When to start the first pack of pills: Be sure to read these instructions:

- before you start taking your pills, and
- any time you are not sure what to do.

Decide with your doctor or clinic what is the best day for you to start taking your first pack of pills. Your pills may be either a 21-day or a 28-day type.

Directions for 21-day and 28-day pill packs:

1. **The first day of your menstrual period (bleeding) is day 1 of your cycle.** The pills may be started up to Day 6 of your cycle. Your starting day will be chosen in discussion with your doctor. You will **always** begin taking your pill on this day of the week. Your doctor may advise you to start taking the pills on Day 1, on Day 5, or on the first Sunday after your period begins. If your period starts on Sunday, start that same day.
2. **If you are using a: 21-Day Pill Pack:** With this type of birth control pill, you are on pills for 21 days and off pills for 7 days. You must not be off the pills for more than 7 days in a row.

   Take 1 pill at approximately the same time every day for 21 days. **Then do not take a pill for seven days.** Start a new pack on the eighth day. You will probably have a period during the 7 days off the pill. (This bleeding may be lighter and shorter than your usual period.)

28-Day Pill Pack: With this type of birth control pill, you take 21 pills that contain hormones and seven pills that contain no hormones.

Take 1 pill at approximately the same time every day for 28 days. Begin a new pack the next day, **not missing any days on the pills**. Your period should occur during the last 7 days of using that pill pack.

Instructions For Using Your DISCREET Package for Both 21-Day and 28-Day Packs: Follow These Instructions Carefully:

1. **For Day 1 start:** Label the DISCREET Package by selecting the day label that starts with Day 1 of your menstrual period (the first day of menstruation is Day 1). For example, if your first day of menstruation is Tuesday, attach the day label that begins with **TUE** in the space provided.

   or

   For Day 5 start: Label the DISCREET Package by selecting the day label that starts with the day that is 5 days after your period begins. (Count 5 days **including** the first day of menstruation.) For example, if your first day of menstruation is Saturday, place the day label that starts with **WED** in the space provided.

   or

   For Sunday start: No day label is required. The DISCREET Package is printed for a Sunday start. (The first Sunday **after** your period begins, or, if your period starts on Sunday, start that **same day**.)
2. Place the day label in the space where you see the words "Place day label here". Having the DISCREET Package labelled with the days of the week will help remind you to take your pill every day.
3. To begin taking your pills, start with the pill inside the coloured circle (where you see the word **START**). This pill should correspond to the day of the week that you are taking your first pill. To remove the pill, push through the back of the DISCREET Package.
4. On the following day, take the next pill in the same row, always proceeding from left to right (→). Each row will always begin on the same day of the week.

What to Do During The Month:

1. **Take a pill at approximately the same time every day until the pack is empty.**
   - Try to associate taking your pill with some regular activity such as eating a meal or going to bed.
   - Do not skip pills even if you have bleeding between monthly periods or feel sick to your stomach (nausea).
   - Do not skip pills even if you do not have sex very often.
2. **When you finish a pack:**
   - **21 pills: Wait 7 days** to start the next pack. You will have your period during that week.
   - **28 pills:** Start the next pack **on the next day**. Take 1 pill every day. Do not wait any days between packs.

What to Do if You Miss Pills: Table 4 outlines the actions you should take if you miss one or more of your birth control pills. Match the number of pills missed with the appropriate starting time for your type of pill pack.

Table 4: TRI-CYCLEN LO

What to Do if You Miss Pills

Sunday Start	Other Than Sunday Start
Miss 1 pill	**Miss 1 pill**
Take it as soon as you remember and take the next pill at the usual time. This means that you might take 2 pills in 1 day.	Take it as soon as you remember and take the next pill at the usual time. This means that you might take 2 pills in 1 day.
Miss 2 pills in a row	**Miss 2 pills in a row**
First 2 Weeks: 1. Take 2 pills the day you remember and 2 pills the next day. 2. Then take 1 pill a day until you finish the pack. 3. Use a back-up method of birth control if you have sex in the seven days after you miss the pills. **Third Week:** 1. Keep taking 1 pill a day until Sunday. 2. On Sunday, safely discard the rest of the pack and start a new pack that day. 3. Use a back-up method of birth control if you have sex in the seven days after you miss the pills. 4. You may not have a period this month. **If you miss 2 periods in a row, call your doctor or clinic.**	**First 2 Weeks:** 1. Take 2 pills the day you remember and 2 pills the next day. 2. Then take 1 pill a day until you finish the pack. 3. Use a back-up method of birth control if you have sex in the seven days after you miss the pills. **Third Week:** 1. Safely dispose of the rest of the pill pack and start a new pack that same day. 2. Use a back-up method of birth control if you have sex in the seven days after you miss the pills. 3. You may not have a period this month. **If you miss 2 periods in a row, call your doctor or clinic.**
Miss 3 or more pills in a row	**Miss 3 or more pills in a row**
Any Time in the Cycle: 1. Keep taking 1 pill a day until Sunday. 2. On Sunday, safely discard the rest of the pack and start a new pack that day. 3. Use a back-up method of birth control if you have sex in the seven days after you miss the pills. 4. You may not have a period this month. **If you miss 2 periods in a row, call your doctor or clinic.**	**Any Time in the Cycle:** 1. Safely dispose of the rest of the pill pack and start a new pack that same day. 2. Use a back-up method of birth control if you have sex in the 7 days after you miss the pills. 3. You may not have a period this month. **If you miss 2 periods in a row, call your doctor or clinic.**

Note: 28-Day Pack—If you forget any of the 7 "reminder" pills (without hormones) in Week 4, just safely dispose of the pills you missed. Then keep taking 1 pill each day until the pack is empty. You do not need to use a back-up method.

Always be sure you have on hand:

- a back-up method of birth control (such as latex condoms and spermicidal foam or gel) in case you miss pills, and
- an extra, full pack of pills.

If you forget more than 1 pill 2 months in a row, talk to your doctor or clinic about ways to make pill-taking easier or about using another method of birth control.

INFORMATION FOR THE PATIENT: Published in e-CPS, available by subscription at www.e-cps.ca.

SUPPLIED: Each white tablet contains: norgestimate 0.180 mg and ethinyl estradiol 0.025 mg. Each light blue tablet contains: norgestimate 0.215 mg and ethinyl estradiol 0.025 mg. Each dark blue tablet contains: norgestimate 0.250 mg and ethinyl estradiol 0.025 mg. Nonmedicinal ingredients: white, light blue and dark blue tablets: carnauba wax, croscarmellose sodium, hydroxypropylmethylcellulose, lactose, magnesium stearate, microcrystalline cellulose, polyethylene glycol and titanium dioxide. Light blue tablet also contains: FD&C Blue # 2 aluminum lake, Dark blue tablet also contains: FD&C Blue #2 aluminum lake and polysorbate 80. In the 28 day regimen, the green tablet contains inert ingredients. Nonmedicinal ingredients: FD&C Blue #2 aluminum lake, lactose, magnesium stearate, polyethylene glycol, polyvinyl alcohol, starch, talc, titanium dioxide and yellow iron oxide. Store between 15-30°C. Leave contents in protective packaging until time of use.

(Shown in Product Identification Section)

Tridural® Ⓟ

tramadol HCl

Opioid Analgesic

Labopharm

Date of Revision: July 27, 2010

SUMMARY PRODUCT INFORMATION:

Route of Administration	Dosage Form/ Strength	Clinically Relevant Nonmedicinal Ingredients
Oral	Extended-release tablets 100 mg, 200 mg, 300 mg	None For a complete listing see Dosage Forms, Composition and Packaging.

INDICATIONS AND CLINICAL USE: Adults: TRIDURAL (tramadol hydrochloride extended-release tablets) is indicated for the management of moderate to moderately severe pain in adults who require treatment for several days or more.

Geriatrics (>65 years of age): Healthy elderly subjects aged 65 to 75 years, administered an immediate release formulation of tramadol, have plasma concentrations and elimination half-lives comparable to those observed in healthy subjects less than 65 years of age. TRIDURAL should be administered with greater caution in patients older than 75 years due to the greater potential for adverse events in this population (see Warnings and Precautions and Dosage and Administration).

Pediatrics (<18 years of age): The safety and effectiveness of TRIDURAL has not been studied in the pediatric population. Therefore, use of TRIDURAL tablets is not recommended in patients under 18 years of age.

CONTRAINDICATIONS:

- TRIDURAL should not be administered to patients who have previously demonstrated hypersensitivity to tramadol, opioids or any other component of this product. For a complete listing, see Dosage Forms, Composition and Packaging.
- TRIDURAL is contraindicated in any situation where opioids are contraindicated, including acute intoxication with any of the following: alcohol, hypnotics, centrally acting analgesics, opioids or psychotropic drugs. TRIDURAL may worsen central nervous system and respiratory depression in these patients.
- TRIDURAL is contraindicated with concomitant MAO inhibitors (or within 14 days of such therapy).
- TRIDURAL is contraindicated in severe renal or hepatic impairment (creatinine clearance of less than 30 mL/min and/or Child-Pugh Class C).

WARNINGS AND PRECAUTIONS: General: TRIDURAL (tramadol hydrochloride extended-release tablets) must be swallowed whole and should not be broken, chewed or crushed, since this can lead to the rapid release of tramadol and absorption of a potentially fatal dose of tramadol.

Seizure Risk: Seizures have been reported in patients receiving tramadol hydrochloride within the recommended dosage range. Spontaneous postmarketing reports indicate that seizure risk is increased with doses above the recommended range. Concomitant use of tramadol hydrochloride increases the seizure risk in patients taking:

- Selective serotonin reuptake inhibitors (SSRI antidepressants or anorectics),
- Tricyclic antidepressants (TCAs), and other tricyclic compounds (e.g., cyclobenzaprine, promethazine, etc.), or
- Other opioids.

Administration of tramadol may enhance the seizure risk in patients taking:

- MAO inhibitors (see Contraindications),
- Neuroleptics, or
- Other drugs that reduce the seizure threshold.

Risk of convulsions may also increase in patients with epilepsy, those with a history of seizures, or in patients with a recognized risk for seizure (such as head trauma, metabolic disorders, alcohol and drug withdrawal, CNS infections). In tramadol overdose, naloxone administration may increase the risk of seizures.

Anaphylactoid Reactions: Serious and rarely fatal anaphylactoid reactions have been reported in patients receiving therapy with tramadol. When these events do occur, it is often following the first dose. Other reported allergic reactions include pruritus, hives, bronchospasm, angioedema, toxic epidermal necrolysis and Stevens-Johnson syndrome. Patients with a history of anaphylactoid reactions to codeine and other opioids may be at increased risk and therefore should not receive TRIDURAL (see Contraindications).

Drug Abuse, Addiction and Dependence: Tramadol has the potential to cause psychic and physical dependence of the morphine-type (μ-opioid). The drug has been associated with craving, drug-seeking behaviour and tolerance development. Cases of abuse and dependence on tramadol have been reported. TRIDURAL should not be used in opioid-dependent patients. Tramadol has been shown to reinitiate physical dependence in some patients that have been previously dependent on other opioids. Dependence and abuse, including drug-seeking behaviour and taking illicit actions to obtain the drug, are not limited to those patients with prior history of opioid dependence. In patients with a tendency to abuse drugs or a history of drug dependence, and in patients who are chronically abusing opioids, treatment with TRIDURAL is not recommended.

Proper assessment of the patient, proper prescribing practices, periodic re-evaluation of therapy, and proper dispensing and storage are appropriate measures that help to limit abuse of opioid drugs.

A Risk Management program to support the safe and effective use of TRIDURAL has been established. The following are considered to be the essential components of the Risk Management program: a) Commitment to not emphasize or highlight the scheduling status of TRIDURAL (i.e., not listed under a schedule to the CDSA) in its advertising or promotional activities; b) Inclusion of a PAAB-approved fair balance statement in all TRIDURAL advertising and promotional materials; c) Provision of progress reports to TPD, MHPD and HECSB from a drug abuse surveillance program for TRIDURAL; d) Assurance that health-care education activities on pain management with TRIDURAL include balanced, evidence-based and current information. Commitment to take reasonable actions to inform health-care professionals that there is Health Canada-approved patient information on benefits and risks, and to ensure that this information can be readily accessed through electronic and/or hard copy sources; e) Reassessment of the risk management program 2 years post product launch.

TRIDURAL is intended for oral use only. Extended-release tablets may be abused by breaking, crushing, chewing, snorting, or injecting the dissolved product. These practices will result in the uncontrolled delivery of the opioid and pose a significant risk to the abuser that could result in overdose and death. This risk is increased with concurrent abuse of alcohol and other substances. With parenteral abuse, the tablet excipients can be expected to result in local tissue necrosis, infection, pulmonary granulomas, and increased risk of endocarditis and valvular heart injury.

TRIDURAL should not be used to treat the symptoms of opioid withdrawal in opioid-dependent patients since it cannot suppress morphine withdrawal symptoms, even though it is an opioid agonist.

Abuse and addiction are separate and distinct from physical dependence and tolerance. In addition, abuse of opioids can occur in the absence of true addiction and is characterized by misuse for non-medical purposes, often in combination with other psychoactive substances. Tolerance as well as both physical and psychological dependence may develop upon repeated administration of opioids, and are not by themselves evidence of an addictive disorder or abuse.

Concerns about abuse, addiction, and diversion should not prevent the proper management of pain. The development of addiction to opioid analgesics in properly managed patients with pain has been reported to be rare. However, data are not available to establish the true incidence of addiction in chronic pain patients.

Careful record-keeping of prescribing information, including quantity, frequency, and renewal requests is strongly advised.

Withdrawal Symptoms: Withdrawal symptoms may occur if TRIDURAL is discontinued abruptly. These symptoms may include: anxiety, sweating, insomnia, rigors, pain, nausea, tremors, diarrhea, upper respiratory symptoms, piloerection, and rarely hallucinations. Other symptoms that have been seen less frequently with tramadol discontinuation include: panic attacks, severe anxiety and paresthesias.

Clinical experience suggests that signs and symptoms of withdrawal may be avoided by tapering medication when discontinuing tramadol therapy. Patients on prolonged therapy should be withdrawn gradually from the drug if it is no longer required for pain control. Clinical experience suggests that withdrawal symptoms may be relieved by reinstitution of tramadol therapy followed by a gradual, tapered dose reduction of the medication combined with symptomatic support.

Risk of Overdosage: Serious potential consequences of overdosage with TRIDURAL are central nervous system depression, respiratory depression and death. In treating an overdose, primary attention should be given to maintaining adequate ventilation along with general supportive treatment (see Overdosage).

Do not prescribe TRIDURAL for patients who are suicidal or addiction-prone.

TRIDURAL should not be taken in doses higher than those recommended by the physician. The judicious prescribing of tramadol is essential to the safe use of this drug. With patients who are depressed or suicidal, consideration should be given to the use of non-narcotic analgesics. Patients should be cautioned about the concomitant use of tramadol products and alcohol because of potentially serious CNS-additive effects of these agents. Because of its added depressant effects, tramadol should be prescribed with caution for those patients whose medical condition requires the concomitant administration of sedatives, tranquilizers, muscle relaxants, antidepressants, or other CNS-depressant drugs. Patients should be advised of the additive depressant effects of these combinations.

Intracranial Pressure or Head Trauma: TRIDURAL should be used with caution in patients with increased intracranial pressure or head injury. The respiratory depressant effects of opioids include carbon dioxide retention and secondary elevation of cerebrospinal fluid pressure, and may be markedly exaggerated in these patients. Additionally, pupillary changes (miosis) from tramadol may obscure the existence, extent, or course of intracranial pathology. Clinicians should also maintain a high index of suspicion for adverse drug reaction when evaluating altered mental status in these patients if they are receiving TRIDURAL (see Warnings and Precautions, Respiratory Depression).

Respiratory Depression: Administer TRIDURAL cautiously in patients at risk for respiratory depression, such as patients with significant chronic obstructive pulmonary disease or corpulmonale, and in patients having a substantially decreased respiratory reserve, hypoxia, or hypercapnia. In these patients alternative non-opioid analgesics should be considered and opioids should be employed only under careful medical supervision at the lowest effective dose. When large doses of tramadol are administered with anesthetic medications or alcohol, respiratory depression may result. Respiratory depression should be treated as an overdose. If naloxone is to be administered, use cautiously because it may precipitate seizures (see Warnings and Precautions, Seizure Risk and Overdosage).

Interaction with Central Nervous System (CNS) Depressants: TRIDURAL should be used with caution and in reduced dosages when administered to patients receiving CNS depressants such as alcohol, opioids, anesthetic agents, narcotics, phenothiazines, tranquilizers or sedative hypnotics. Tramadol increases the risk of CNS and respiratory depression in these patients.

TRIDURAL may be expected to have additive effects when used in conjunction with alcohol, other opioids, or illicit drugs that cause central nervous system depression.

In Vitro Dissolution Studies of Interaction with Alcohol: Increasing concentrations of ethanol resulted in a decrease in the rate of release of TRIDURAL tablets.

Use with Alcohol: TRIDURAL should not be used concomitantly with alcohol consumption. The use of TRIDURAL in patients with liver disease is not recommended.

Use in Ambulatory Patients: TRIDURAL may impair the mental and or physical abilities required for the performance of potentially hazardous tasks such as driving a car or operating machinery. The patient using this drug should be cautioned accordingly.

Use with Serotonin Reuptake Inhibitors: Concomitant use of tramadol products with SSRIs increases the risk of adverse events, including seizure and serotonin syndrome (see Warnings and Precautions, Seizure Risk and Drug Interactions).

Acute Abdominal Conditions: The administration of TRIDURAL may complicate the clinical assessment of patients with acute abdominal conditions.

Use in Drug and Alcohol Addiction: TRIDURAL is an opioid with no approved use in the management of addictive disorders.

Special Populations: Hepatic/Biliary/Pancreatic Impairment: Metabolism of tramadol and M1 is reduced in patients with advanced cirrhosis of the liver, resulting in both a larger area under the concentration time curve for tramadol and longer tramadol and M1 elimination half-lives (13 hours for tramadol and 19 hours for M1). TRIDURAL is contraindicated in patients with severe hepatic impairment (see Dosage and Administration).

Renal Impairment: Impaired renal function results in a decreased rate and extent of excretion of tramadol and its active metabolite, M1. TRIDURAL is contraindicated in severe renal impairment. The total amount of tramadol and M1 removed during a 4-hour dialysis period is less than 7% of the administered dose (see Dosage and Administration).

Pregnant Women: There are no adequate and well-controlled studies in pregnant women. Therefore, TRIDURAL should not be used during pregnancy and labour, unless in the opinion of the physician, the expected benefit to the patient outweighs the possible risk to the fetus.

Chronic use during pregnancy may lead to physical dependence and post-partum withdrawal symptoms in the newborn (see Drug Abuse, Addiction and Dependence). Tramadol has been shown to cross the placenta. The mean ratio of serum tramadol in the umbilical veins compared to maternal veins was 0.83 for 40 women given tramadol during labour. Neonatal seizures, neonatal withdrawal syndrome, fetal death and stillbirth have been reported with tramadol during post-marketing.

The effect of tramadol, if any, on the later growth, development and functional maturation of the child is unknown.

Nursing Women: TRIDURAL is not recommended for obstetrical preoperative medication or for post-delivery analgesia in nursing mothers because its safety in infants and newborns has not been studied.

Following a single IV 100 mg dose of tramadol, the cumulative excretion in breast milk within 16 hours postdose was 100 µg of tramadol (0.1% of the maternal dose) and 27 µg of M1.

Pediatrics (<18 years of age): The safety and use of TRIDURAL in patients under 18 years of age has not been established. The use of TRIDURAL in the pediatric population is not recommended.

Geriatrics (>65 years of age): In general, caution should be used when selecting the dose for an elderly patient. The elimination half-life of tramadol may be prolonged in patients over 75 years, thereby increasing the potential for adverse events. Usually, dose administration should start at the low end of the dosing range, reflecting the greater frequency of decreased hepatic, renal or cardiac function and of concomitant disease or other drug therapy (see Action and Clinical Pharmacology and Dosage and Administration).

In clinical trials, TRIDURAL was administered to 1013 patients aged 65 years and older. Of those, 89 patients were 75 years of age and older. Comparable incidence rates of patients experiencing adverse events were observed for patients older than 65 years of age compared with younger patients (<65 years of age), except constipation for which the incidence was higher in older patients. TRIDURAL should be used with caution in patients older than 75 years of age (see Action and Clinical Pharmacology and Dosage and Administration).

ADVERSE REACTIONS: Clinical Trial Adverse Drug Reactions: Because clinical trials are conducted under very specific conditions the adverse reaction rates observed in the clinical trials may not reflect the rates observed in practice and should not be compared to the rates in the clinical trials of another drug. Adverse drug reaction information from clinical trials is useful for identifying drug-related adverse events and for approximating rates.

TRIDURAL was administered to a total of 2707 subjects (2406 patients and 301 healthy volunteers) during clinical studies, including four randomized double-blind studies (treatment ≥12 weeks) and two open-label long-term studies (treatment up to 12 months) in patients with moderate to severe pain due to osteoarthritis of the knee. A total of 1901 patients were exposed to TRIDURAL during 12-week studies, 493 for a 6-month period and 243 for a 12-month period. A total of 1013 patients were 65 years and older, including 89 patients 75 years of age and older. A summary of adverse events occurring at an incidence of 1% or more is given in Table 1, which includes all events, whether considered by the clinical investigator to be related to the study drug or not.

The majority of patients who experienced the most common adverse events (≥1%) reported mild to moderate symptoms. Less than 3% of adverse events were rated as severe. Overall, onset of these adverse events usually occurred within the first two weeks of treatment.

Adverse Events with an Incidence of <1.0% (whether considered by the clinical investigator to be related to the study drug or not): Blood and Lymphatic System Disorders: anaemia, lymphadenopathy, thrombocytopenia.

Cardiac Disorders: acute myocardial infarction, angina pectoris, angina unstable, atrial fibrillation, bradycardia, cardiovascular disorder, palpitations, sinus tachycardia, tachycardia.

Ear and Labyrinth Disorders: cerumen impaction, ear congestion, ear discomfort, ear pain, labyrinthitis, tinnitus.

Table 1: TRIDURAL

Percentage of Patients with Incidence of Adverse Events ≥1% from Three 12-Week Placebo-Controlled Studies (MDT3-002, MDT3-003 and MDT3-005)[a]

	TRIDURAL				
Adverse Events	**100 mg N=216**	**200 mg N=311**	**300 mg N=530**	**Total N=1095**	**Placebo N=668**
Any TEAE	125 (57.9%)	184 (59.2%)	302 (57.0%)	690 (63.0%)	338 (50.6%)
Ear and Labyrinth Disorders					
Vertigo	3 (1.4%)	3 (1.0%)	8 (1.5%)	27 (2.5%)	3 (0.4%)
Gastrointestinal Disorders					
Abdominal pain	2 (0.9%)	5 (1.6%)	8 (1.5%)	17 (1.6%)	7 (1.0%)
Abdominal pain upper	3 (1.4%)	4 (1.3%)	9 (1.7%)	18 (1.6%)	4 (0.6%)
Constipation	21 (9.7%)	38 (12.2%)	53 (10.0%)	143 (13.1%)	27 (4.0%)
Diarrhea	6 (2.8%)	1 (0.3%)	10 (1.9%)	21 (1.9%)	20 (3.0%)
Dry mouth	7 (3.2%)	17 (5.5%)	7 (1.3%)	38 (3.5%)	8 (1.2%)
Dyspepsia	3 (1.4%)	6 (1.9%)	4 (0.8%)	13 (1.2%)	7 (1.0%)
Nausea	29 (13.4%)	50 (16.1%)	88 (16.6%)	202 (18.4%)	39 (5.8%)
Vomiting	8 (3.7%)	19 (6.1%)	36 (6.8%)	71 (6.5%)	6 (0.9%)
General Disorders and Administration Site Conditions					
Fatigue	6 (2.8%)	10 (3.2%)	9 (1.7%)	29 (2.6%)	6 (0.9%)
Pain exacerbated	6 (2.8%)	3 (1.0%)	6 (1.1%)	18 (1.6%)	16 (2.4%)
Weakness	3 (1.4%)	5 (1.6%)	4 (0.8%)	12 (1.1%)	1 (0.1%)
Infections and Infestations					
Influenza	2 (0.9%)	1 (0.3%)	8 (1.5%)	11 (1.0%)	3 (0.4%)
Nasopharyngitis	4 (1.9%)	7 (2.3%)	7 (1.3%)	20 (1.8%)	18 (2.7%)
Upper respiratory tract infection	3 (1.4%)	5 (1.6%)	6 (1.1%)	16 (1.5%)	17 (2.5%)
Urinary tract infection	2 (0.9%)	3 (1.0%)	6 (1.1%)	12 (1.1%)	10 (1.5%)
Investigations					
Weight decreased	1 (0.5%)	5 (1.6%)	11 (2.1%)	20 (1.8%)	1 (0.1%)
Metabolism and Nutrition Disorders					
Anorexia	5 (2.3%)	4 (1.3%)	11 (2.1%)	27 (2.5%)	2 (0.3%)
Musculoskeletal and Connective Tissue Disorders					
Arthralgia	2 (0.9%)	3 (1.0%)	8 (1.5%)	15 (1.4%)	14 (2.1%)
Nervous System Disorders					
Dizziness	18 (8.3%)	31 (10.0%)	59 (11.1%)	119 (10.9%)	21 (3.1%)
Headache	13 (6.0%)	18 (5.8%)	26 (4.9%)	64 (5.8%)	43 (6.4%)
Somnolence	12 (5.6%)	23 (7.4%)	26 (4.9%)	82 (7.5%)	13 (1.9%)
Tremor	1 (0.5%)	3 (1.0%)	6 (1.1%)	11 (1.0%)	1 (0.1%)
Psychiatric Disorders					
Anxiety NEC	1 (0.5%)	6 (1.9%)	4 (0.8%)	11 (1.0%)	1 (0.1%)
Insomnia	3 (1.4%)	9 (2.9%)	11 (2.1%)	25 (2.3%)	8 (1.2%)
Skin and Subcutaneous Tissue Disorders					
Pruritus	11 (5.1%)	16 (5.1%)	23 (4.3%)	60 (5.5%)	7 (1.0%)
Sweating increased	1 (0.5%)	10 (3.2%)	16 (3.0%)	38 (3.5%)	6 (0.9%)
Vascular Disorders					
Hot flushes	1 (0.5%)	3 (1.0%)	7 (1.3%)	12 (1.1%)	1 (0.1%)

[a] Due to the difference in study design of MDT3-005, only the results of the double-blind phase of the study are presented and the dose specific results include maintenance period data only.

Endocrine Disorders: hypothyroidism.

Eye Disorders: cataract, dry eyes, eye pain, eyelid disorder, lacrimation increased, photopsia, scleral haemorrhage, blurred vision, visual disturbance.

Gastrointestinal Disorders: abdominal discomfort, abdominal distension, lower abdominal pain, abdominal tenderness, change in bowel habit, constipation aggravated, diverticulitis, dyspepsia aggravated, dysphagia, faecal impaction, feces discoloured, flatulence, food poisoning, gastric irritation, gastritis, gastrointestinal haemorrhage, gastrointestinal irritation, gastro-oesophageal reflux disease, hiccups, lip blister, loose stools, pancreatitis aggravated, rectal haemorrhage, rectal prolapse, retching, small intestinal obstruction, toothache.

General Disorders and Administration Site Conditions: asthenia, chest pain, chest tightness, fall, feeling abnormal, feeling cold, inflammation localised, inflammation, influenza like illness, lethargy, malaise, mass, oedema peripheral, pain, rigors, thirst.

Hepatobiliary Disorders: biliary tract disorder, cholelithiasis.
Immune System Disorders: hypersensitivity, seasonal allergy.
Infections and Infestations: abscess limb, bladder infection, bronchitis, ear infection, erysipelas, foot infection fungal, fungal infection, gastroenteritis, gastroenteritis viral, gastrointestinal infection, helicobacter infection, herpes simplex, herpes zoster, laryngitis acute, nail fungal infection, otitis externa, otitis media, otitis media serous, pharyngitis, respiratory tract infection viral, sinusitis, stye, tooth abscess, tooth infection, tracheitis, vaginosis fungal, viral infection, wound infection.
Injury, Poisoning and Procedural Complications: abrasion, arthropod bite, back injury, blister, concussion, eye injury, face injury, hand fracture, head injury, joint sprain, laceration, ligament injury, limb injury, muscle injury, muscle strain, neck injury, postoperative wound complication, soft tissue injury, tendon injury, wrist fracture.
Investigations: alanine aminotransferase decreased, alanine aminotransferase increased, aspartate aminotransferase decreased, aspartate aminotransferase increased, blood amylase increased, blood calcium increased, blood cholesterol increased, blood creatinine increased, blood glucose abnormal, blood glucose increased, blood in stool, blood potassium abnormal, blood pressure increased, blood urea increased, body temperature increased, cardiac murmur, c-reactive protein increased, gamma-glutamyltransferase increased, haematocrit decreased, haematocrit increased, haemoglobin decreased, haemoglobin increased, low density lipoprotein increased, lymphocyte count increased, mammogram abnormal, mean platelet volume decreased, neutrophil count decreased, protein total decreased, red blood cell count decreased, red blood cell count increased, red blood cell sedimentation rate increased, red cell distribution with increased, white blood cell count increased.
Metabolism and Nutrition Disorders: decreased appetite, dehydration, diabetes mellitus, gout, hypercholesterolemia, hyperglycaemia, hyperlipidemia, hypertriglyceridaemia, hyperuricaemia, hypocalcaemia, hypokalaemia.
Musculoskeletal and Connective Tissue Disorders: back disorder, back pain, bone pain, bone spur, bursitis, ganglion, groin pain, joint crepitation, joint disorder, joint stiffness, joint swelling, muscle cramps, muscle spasms, musculoskeletal discomfort, musculoskeletal stiffness, myalgia, neck pain, neck stiffness, osteoarthritis aggravated, osteopenia, osteoporosis, pain in limb, plantar fasciitis, polyarthralgia, rheumatoid arthritis, temporomandibular joint arthralgia, tendonitis.
Neoplasms Benign, Malignant and Unspecified (including cysts and polyps): benign breast neoplasm, breast cancer invasive, breast cancer, thyroid neoplasm, uterine fibroids.
Nervous System Disorders: ataxia, burning sensation, disturbance in attention, dysarthria, dysgeusia, gait abnormal, headache aggravated, hypoaesthesia, mental impairment, migraine, neuralgia, paraesthesia, sedation, sinus headache, sleep apnoea syndrome, syncope.
Psychiatric Disorders: abnormal behaviour, agitation, bipolar disorder, confusion, depression, emotional disturbance, euphoric mood, indifference, irritability, libido decreased, nervousness, sleep disorder.
Renal and Urinary Disorders: calculus renal, difficulty in micturition, dysuria, haematuria, micturition urgency, nocturia, renal impairment, renal pain, urinary frequency, urinary hesitation, urinary incontinence, urinary retention.
Reproductive System and Breast Disorders: dysmenorrhoea, erectile dysfunction, genital pruritus female, menometrorrhagia, prostatitis, sexual dysfunction, vaginal cyst, vaginal discharge.
Respiratory, Thoracic and Mediastinal Disorders: asthma aggravated, asthma, chest wall pain, cough, crackles lung, dry throat, dyspnoea, epistaxis, nasal congestion, nasal oedema, pharyngolaryngeal pain, productive cough, rhinitis allergic, rhinitis, rhinorrhea, rhonchi, sinus congestion, sinus pain, throat irritation.
Skin and Subcutaneous Tissue Disorders: acne, cold sweat, contusion, dermatitis allergic, dermatitis contact, dermatitis, dermatitis aggravated, dermatosis, dry skin, eczema exacerbated, eczema, erythema, hyperkeratosis, ingrowing nail, night sweat, pallor, piloerection, prurigo, pruritus generalised, rash, rash pruritic, rosacea, skin ulcer, urticaria.
Surgical and Medical Procedures: cardiac pacemaker replacement, colon polypectomy, endodontic procedure, foot operation, hernia repair, lesion excision, tumour excision.
Vascular Disorders: aortic aneurysm, deep venous thrombosis, flushing, haematoma, hot flushes aggravated, hypertension aggravated, hypertension, hypotension, orthostatic hypotension, poor peripheral circulation, vascular insufficiency, wound haemorrhage.
Abnormal Hematologic and Clinical Chemistry Findings: In clinical trials where clinical abnormalities were recorded (n=106), the following abnormalities were reported: Sedimentation rate increased (0.7%), glucose abnormalities (0.5%), GGT increased (0.4%).

The following abnormalities occurred in 0.2% of patients: cholesterol abnormalities, LDH increased, uric acid increased, hemoglobin decreased, red cell count decreased.

The following abnormalities occurred in <0.1% of patients: hematocrit decreased, alanine aminotransferase increased, aspartate aminotransferase increased, urea increased, liver function tests abnormal.

The following abnormalities were single occurrences: alanine aminotransferase decreased, aspartate aminotransferase decreased, amylase increased, bilirubin increased, calcium increased, creatinine increased, potassium abnormal, C-Reactive Protein increased, hematocrit increased, hemoglobin increased, low density lipoprotein increased, lymphocyte count decreased, mean platelet volume decreased, neutrophil count decreased, platelet count decreased, protein total decreased, red cell count increased, red cell distribution width increased, white cell count increased.

Other Adverse Experiences Previously Reported in Clinical Trials or Post-Marketing Reports with Tramadol Hydrochloride: Adverse events which have been reported with the use of tramadol products include: allergic reactions (including anaphylaxis, angioneurotic edema and urticaria), bradycardia, convulsions, drug dependence, drug withdrawal (including agitation, anxiety, gastrointestinal symptoms, hyperkinesia, insomnia, nervousness, tremors), hyperactivity, hypoactivity, hypotension and respiratory depression. Other adverse events which have been reported with the use of tramadol products and for which a causal association has not been determined include: difficulty concentrating, hepatitis, liver failure, pulmonary edema, Stevens-Johnson syndrome and suicidal tendency.

Serotonin syndrome (whose symptoms may include mental status change, hyperreflexia, fever, shivering, tremor, agitation, diaphoresis, seizures and coma) has been reported with tramadol when used concomitantly with other serotonergic agents such as SSRIs and MAOIs.

Drug Abuse, Addiction and Dependence: Tramadol may induce psychic and physical dependence of the morphine-type (μ-opioid) (see Warnings and Precautions, Drug Abuse, Addiction and Dependence). Dependence and abuse, including drug-seeking behavior and taking illicit actions to obtain the drug are not limited to those patients with prior history of opioid dependence. The risk in patients with substance abuse has been observed to be higher. Tramadol is associated with craving and tolerance development.

A Risk Management program to support the safe and effective use of TRIDURAL has been established. The following are considered to be the essential components of the Risk Management program: a) commitment to not emphasize or highlight the scheduling status of TRIDURAL (i.e., not listed under a schedule to the CDSA) in its advertising or promotional activities; b) inclusion of a PAAB-approved fair balance statement in all TRIDURAL advertising and promotional materials; c) provision of progress reports to TPD, MHPD and HECSB from a drug abuse surveillance program for TRIDURAL; d) assurance that health-care education activities on pain management with TRIDURAL include balanced, evidence-based and current information. Commitment to take reasonable actions to inform health-care professionals that there is Health Canada approved patient information on benefits and risks, and to ensure that this information can be readily accessed through electronic and/or hard copy sources; e) reassessment of the risk management program 2 years post product launch.

Withdrawal Symptoms: Withdrawal symptoms may occur if tramadol is discontinued abruptly. These symptoms may include: anxiety, sweating, insomnia, rigors, pain, nausea, tremors, diarrhea, upper respiratory symptoms, piloerection, and rarely hallucinations. Other symptoms that have been seen less frequently with tramadol hydrochloride discontinuation include: panic attacks, severe anxiety, and paresthesias.

Withdrawal symptoms have been studied in 325 patients, 3 and 7 days after discontinuation of treatment with TRIDURAL. The majority of symptoms were mild to moderate in nature. Onset of the post-treatment adverse events occurred more frequently within the first 3 days after treatment was stopped. Less than 1% of patients taking TRIDURAL met the DSM-IV criteria for a diagnosis of opioid withdrawal.

Clinical experience suggests that signs and symptoms of withdrawal may be avoided by tapering medication when discontinuing tramadol therapy.

DRUG INTERACTIONS: Overview: In vitro studies indicate that tramadol is unlikely to inhibit the CYP3A4-mediated metabolism of other drugs when it is administered concomitantly at therapeutic doses. Tramadol does not appear to induce its own metabolism in humans, since observed maximal plasma concentrations after multiple oral doses are higher than expected based on single dose data. Tramadol is a mild inducer of selected drug metabolism pathways measured in animals.

Administration of CYP3A4 inhibitors, such as ketoconazole and erythromycin, or inducers, such as rifampin and St. John's Wort, with TRIDURAL may affect the metabolism of tramadol leading to altered tramadol exposure.

Drug-Drug Interactions: MAO Inhibitors: Tramadol is contraindicated in patients receiving MAO inhibitors or who have used them within the previous 14 days (see Contraindications, Warnings and Precautions).

Drugs that Lower Seizure Threshold: Tramadol can increase the potential for selective serotonin reuptake inhibitors (SSRIs), tricyclic anti-depressants (TCAs), anti-psychotics and other seizure threshold lowering drugs to cause convulsions (see Warnings and Precautions).

CNS Depressants: Concurrent administration of tramadol with other centrally acting drugs, including alcohol, centrally acting analgesics, opioids and psychotropic drugs may potentiate CNS depressant effects.

Use with Carbamazepine: Patients taking carbamazepine, a CYP3A4 inducer, may have a significantly reduced analgesic effect. Because carbamazepine increases tramadol metabolism and because of the seizure risk associated with tramadol, concomitant administration of TRIDURAL and carbamazepine is not recommended.

Use with Quinidine: Tramadol is metabolized to M1 by CYP2D6. Quinidine is a selective inhibitor of that isoenzyme, so that concomitant administration of quinidine and tramadol products results in increased concentrations of tramadol and reduced concentrations of M1. The clinical consequences of these findings are unknown. In vitro drug interaction studies in human liver microsomes indicate that tramadol has no effect on quinidine metabolism.

Use with Inhibitors of CYP2D6: In vitro drug interaction studies in human liver microsomes indicate that concomitant administration with inhibitors of CYP2D6 such as fluoxetine, paroxetine, and amitriptyline could result in some inhibition of the metabolism of tramadol.

Inhibitors or Inducers of CYP3A4: Administration of CYP3A4 inhibitors, such as ketoconazole and erythromycin, or inducers, such as rifampin and St. John's Wort may affect the metabolism of tramadol, leading to altered tramadol exposure.

Use with Cimetidine: Concomitant administration of tramadol immediate-release tablets with cimetidine does not result in clinically significant changes in tramadol pharmacokinetics. No alteration of the TRIDURAL dosage regimen with cimetidine is recommended.

Protease Inhibitors, e.g., Ritonavir: Co-administered ritonavir may increase the serum concentration of tramadol, resulting in tramadol toxicity.

Use with Digoxin: Post-marketing surveillance of tramadol has revealed rare reports of digoxin toxicity.

Use with Warfarin-Like Compounds: Post-marketing surveillance of tramadol has revealed rare reports of alteration of warfarin effect, including elevation of prothrombin times.

While such changes have been generally of limited clinical significance for tramadol, periodic evaluation of prothrombin time should be performed when TRIDURAL tablets and warfarin-like compounds are administered concurrently.

Drug-Food Interactions: Co-administration with food did not significantly change the overall exposure to tramadol; however, peak plasma concentrations increased. In the presence of food, the availability and controlled-release properties of TRIDURAL tablets were maintained with no evidence of dose dumping. TRIDURAL was administered either with breakfast or before breakfast in all clinical trials.

DOSAGE AND ADMINISTRATION: Dosing Considerations: TRIDURAL (tramadol hydrochloride) is not recommended for minor pain that may be treated adequately through lesser means where benefit does not outweigh the possible opioid-related side effects.

TRIDURAL tablets must be swallowed whole and should not be broken, chewed or crushed, since this can lead to the rapid release of tramadol and absorption of a potentially fatal dose of tramadol.

Due to possible differences in pharmacokinetic properties, TRIDURAL tablets are not interchangeable with other tramadol-containing products.

The maximum recommended daily dose of TRIDURAL should not be exceeded.

TRIDURAL is contraindicated in patients with severe hepatic or renal impairment.

Do not co-administer TRIDURAL tablets with other tramadol containing products.

Good pain management practice dictates that analgesic dose be individualized according to patient need using the lowest beneficial dose. Studies with tramadol products in adults have shown that starting at the lowest possible dose and titrating upward will result in fewer discontinuations and increased tolerability.

TRIDURAL extended-release tablets should be taken once a day at breakfast. The tablets should be swallowed whole with liquid and not split, chewed, dissolved or crushed.

TRIDURAL tablets have a continuous release of active ingredient over 24 hours: a repeat dosage within 24 hours is not recommended.

Recommended Dose and Dosage Adjustment: Adults: Treatment with TRIDURAL should be initiated at a dose of 100 mg/day. Daily doses should be titrated by 100 mg/day increments every 2 days (i.e., start 200 mg/day on day 3 of therapy) to achieve a balance between adequate pain control and tolerability for the individual patient. For patients requiring the 300 mg daily dose, titration should take at least 4 days (i.e., 300 mg/day on day 5). The daily dose and titration should be individualized for each patient. Therapy should be continued with the lowest effective dose. TRIDURAL should not be administered at a dose exceeding 300 mg per day.

The correct dosage for any individual patient is that which controls the pain for a full 24 hours with no or tolerable side effects.

Patients Not Receiving Opioids at the Time of Initiation of Tramadol Treatment: The usual initial dose of TRIDURAL for patients who have not previously received opioid analgesics is 100 mg q24h.

Patients Currently Receiving Other Tramadol Formulations: Patients currently receiving other oral immediate-release tramadol preparations may be transferred to TRIDURAL tablets at the same or lowest nearest total daily tramadol dosage.

Geriatric Patients (65 years of age and older): In general, dose selection for patients over 65 years of age, who may have decreased hepatic or renal function, or other concomitant diseases, should be initiated cautiously, usually starting at the low end of the dosing range. TRIDURAL should be administered with greater caution at the lowest effective dose in patients over 75 years, due to the potential for greater frequency of adverse events in this population.

Pediatric Use: The safety and effectiveness of TRIDURAL has not been studied in the pediatric population. Therefore, the use of TRIDURAL is not recommended in patients under 18 years of age.

Renal and Hepatic Disease: TRIDURAL is contraindicated in patients with:

- creatinine clearance less than 30 mL/min,
- severe hepatic impairment.

The elimination half-life of tramadol and its active metabolite may be prolonged in mild to moderate renal and/or hepatic disease. A starting dose of 100 mg daily is recommended, and upward dosage titration should be done with careful monitoring.

Management of Patients Requiring Rescue Medication: If rescue medications are warranted for episodes of pain in the course of appropriate adjustments of TRIDURAL dose, acetaminophen or ibuprofen may be given. If immediate release tramadol is used as rescue medication, the total daily dose of tramadol should not exceed 300 mg. Selection of rescue medication should be based on individual patient conditions. Fentanyl products should not be used as rescue medication in patients taking TRIDURAL.

Missed Dose: If a patient forgets to take one or more doses, they should take their next dose at the normal time and in the normal amount.

Discontinuation: Withdrawal symptoms may occur if TRIDURAL is discontinued abruptly. These symptoms may include: anxiety, sweating, insomnia, rigors, pain, nausea, tremors, diarrhea, upper respiratory symptoms, piloerection, and rarely, hallucinations. Other symptoms that have been seen less frequently with tramadol discontinuation include: panic attacks, severe anxiety, and paresthesias. Clinical experience suggests that signs and symptoms of withdrawal may be avoided by tapering medication when discontinuing tramadol therapy (see Adverse Reactions, Drug Abuse, Addiction and Dependence, Withdrawal Symptoms).

OVERDOSAGE:
Deaths due to overdose have been reported with abuse and misuse of tramadol, by ingesting, inhaling, or injecting the crushed tablets. Review of case reports has indicated that the risk of fatal overdose is further increased when tramadol is abused concurrently with alcohol or other CNS depressants, including other opioids.

Symptoms: Acute overdosage with tramadol can be manifested by respiratory depression, somnolence progressing to stupor or coma, skeletal muscle flaccidity, cold and clammy skin, constricted pupils, bradycardia, hypotension, and death.

Treatment: A single or multiple overdose with TRIDURAL may be a potentially lethal drug overdose, and consultation with a regional poison control centre is recommended.

In treating an overdose, primary attention should be given to maintaining adequate ventilation along with general supportive treatment. Supportive measures (including oxygen and vasopressors) should be employed in the management of circulatory shock and pulmonary edema accompanying overdose as indicated. Cardiac arrest or arrhythmias may require cardiac massage or defibrillation.

While naloxone will reverse some, but not all, symptoms caused by overdosage with tramadol, the risk of seizures is also increased with naloxone administration. In animals, convulsions following the administration of toxic doses of tramadol could be suppressed with barbiturates or benzodiazepines but were increased with naloxone. Naloxone administration did not change the lethality of an overdose in mice.

Hemodialysis is not expected to be helpful in an overdose because it removes less than 7% of the administered dose in a 4-hour dialysis period.

Emptying of the gastric contents may be useful to remove any unabsorbed drug.

For management of a suspected drug overdose, CPhA recommends that you contact your **regional Poison Control Centre**. See the *CPS* Directory section for a list of Poison Control Centres.

ACTION AND CLINICAL PHARMACOLOGY: Mechanism of Action: Tramadol is a centrally acting synthetic opioid analgesic. Although its mode of action is not completely understood, from animal tests, at least two complementary mechanisms appear applicable: binding of parent and M1 metabolite to μ-opioid receptors and weak inhibition of reuptake of norepinephrine and serotonin. Opioid activity is due to both low affinity binding of the parent compound and higher affinity binding of the O-demethylated metabolite M1 to μ-opioid receptors. In animal models, M1 is up to 6 times more potent than tramadol in producing analgesia and 200 times more potent in μ-opioid binding. Tramadol-induced analgesia is only partially antagonized by the opiate antagonist naloxone in several animal tests. The relative contribution of both tramadol and M1 to human analgesia is dependent upon the plasma concentrations of each compound (see Pharmacokinetics).

Tramadol has been shown to inhibit reuptake of norepinephrine and serotonin in vitro, as have some other opioid analgesics. These mechanisms may contribute independently to the overall analgesic profile of TRIDURAL.

Apart from analgesia, tramadol administration may produce a constellation of symptoms (including dizziness, somnolence, nausea, constipation, sweating and pruritus) similar to that of opioids. In contrast to morphine, tramadol has not been shown to cause histamine release. At therapeutic doses, tramadol has no effect on heart rate, left-ventricular function or cardiac index. Orthostatic hypotension has been observed.

Pharmacokinetics: The analgesic activity of tramadol hydrochloride is due to both parent drug and the M1 metabolite (see Clinical Pharmacology, Mechanism of Action).

In a single-dose study, the dose adjusted bioavailability of the 100 mg, 200 mg and 300 mg tablets were equivalent confirming a linear pharmacokinetic response (in relation to both tramadol and O-desmethyltramadol) over this range of strengths. Dose proportionality of the 100 mg, 200 mg and 300 mg tablets has been demonstrated.

Absorption: Following oral administration of a single dose, tramadol is almost completely absorbed and the absolute bioavailability is approximately 70%. There is no lag time in drug absorption following administration of TRIDURAL. TRIDURAL exhibits a plasma/time concentration profile with a sharp initial slope similar to immediate-release tramadol tablets followed by a sustained release phase. This behavior is due to the two phases of drug release which work together to provide a smooth plasma concentration/time profile (Figure 1).

The mean peak steady-state plasma concentrations of tramadol and M1 after multiple dose administration of TRIDURAL 200 mg tablets to healthy subjects are attained at about 4.3 h and 7.4 h, respectively (Table 2).

Steady-state levels with TRIDURAL were reached within 48 hours (Figure 2). This is clinically meaningful in that it forms the basis for the titration schedule in all clinical studies and the dosing recommendations related to titration (see Dosage and Administration).

Food Effect: Co-administration with food did not significantly change the overall exposure to tramadol; however, peak plasma concentrations increased. TRIDURAL was administered either with breakfast or before breakfast in all efficacy and safety clinical trials.

In Vitro Dissolution Studies of Interaction with Alcohol: Increasing concentrations of ethanol resulted in a decrease in the rate of release of TRIDURAL tablets.

Distribution: The volume of distribution of tramadol is 2.6 and 2.9 L/kg in males and females, respectively, following a 100 mg intravenous dose. The binding of tramadol to human plasma proteins is approximately 20%. Protein binding also appears to be independent of concentration up to 10 μg/mL. Saturation of plasma protein binding occurs only at concentrations outside the clinically relevant range.

Figure 1: TRIDURAL

Mean Tramadol and M1 Plasma Concentrations over the 24-Hour Dosing Interval Following a Single Oral Dose of TRIDURAL 200 mg

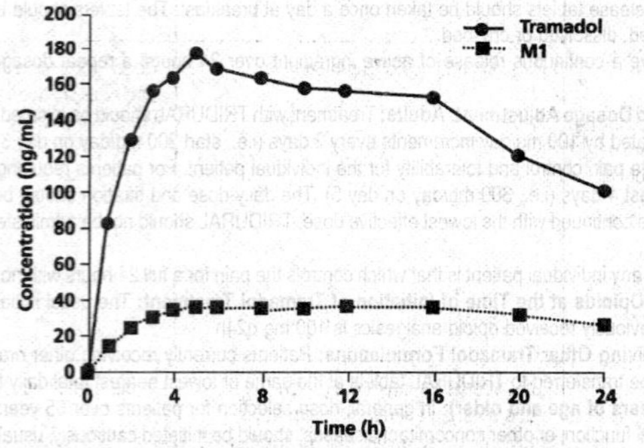

Table 2: TRIDURAL

Mean (%CV) Steady-State Pharmacokinetic Parameter Values (n=26)

Pharmacokinetic Parameter	Tramadol TRIDURAL 200 mg Tablet Once-Daily	M1 Metabolite TRIDURAL 200 mg Tablet Once-Daily
$AUC_{0\text{-}24}$ (ng·h/mL)	5991 (22)	1361 (27)
C_{max} (ng/mL)	345 (21)	71 (27)
C_{min} (ng/mL)	157 (31)	41 (30)
T_{max} (hr)[a]	4.0 (3.0–9.0)	5.0 (3.0–20.0)
Fluctuation (%)	77 (26)	53 (29)

[a] T_{max} is presented as Median (Range).

Figure 2: TRIDURAL

Mean Tramadol Plasma Concentrations at Steady-State Following Oral Administration of TRIDURAL 200 mg Once Daily

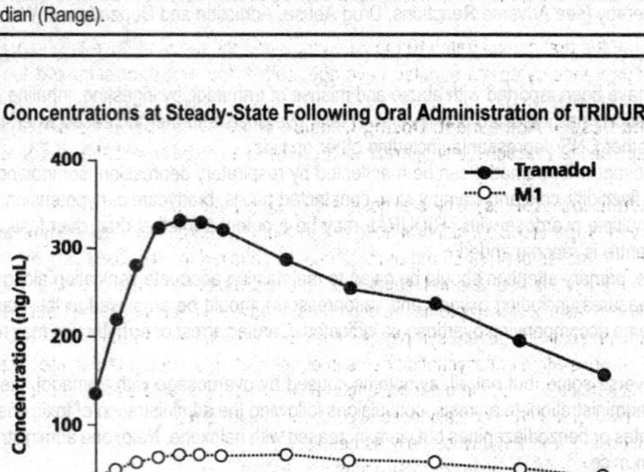

Metabolism: Tramadol is extensively metabolized after oral administration. The major metabolic pathways appear to be N- and O-demethylation and glucuronidation or sulfation in the liver. One metabolite (O-desmethyltramadol, denoted M1) is pharmacologically active in animal models. Formation of M1 is dependent on CYP2D6 and as such is subject to inhibition, which may affect the therapeutic response (see Drug Interactions).

Excretion: Tramadol is eliminated primarily through metabolism by the liver and the metabolites are eliminated primarily by the kidneys. Approximately 30% of the dose is excreted in the urine as unchanged drug, whereas 60% of the dose is excreted as metabolites. The remainder is excreted either as unidentified or as unextractable metabolites. After single administration of TRIDURAL, the mean terminal plasma elimination half-lives of racemic tramadol and racemic M1 are 6.5±1.5 and 7.5±1.4 hours, respectively.

Special Populations and Conditions: Renal Insufficiency: Impaired renal function results in a decreased rate and extent of excretion of tramadol and its active metabolite, M1. TRIDURAL has not been studied in patients with severe renal impairment (creatinine clearances of less than 30 mL/min), and therefore should not be used in these patients (see Contraindications, Warnings and Precautions, Renal Impairment and Dosage and Administration). The total amount of tramadol and M1 removed during a 4-hour dialysis period is less than 7% of the administered dose.

Hepatic Insufficiency: TRIDURAL is contraindicated in patients with severe hepatic impairment. The elimination half-life of tramadol and its active metabolite may be prolonged in patients with hepatic impairment. TRIDURAL has not been studied in patients with severe hepatic impairment and, therefore should not be used (see Contraindications, Warnings and Precautions, Hepatic/Biliary/Pancreatic Impairment and Dosage and Administration).

Geriatrics: Healthy elderly subjects aged 65 to 75 years, administered an immediate-release formulation of tramadol, have plasma concentrations and elimination half-lives comparable to those observed in healthy subjects less than 65 years of age. The elimination half-life of tramadol may be prolonged in patients over 75 years, thereby increasing the potential for adverse events. Adjustment of the daily dose is recommended for patients older than 75 years (see Dosage and Administration).

Gender: Following a 100 mg IV dose of tramadol, plasma clearance was 6.4 mL/min/kg in males and 5.7 mL/min/kg in females. This difference is not likely to be clinically significant; therefore, dosage adjustment based on gender is not recommended.

Pediatrics: Pharmacokinetics of TRIDURAL tablets have not been studied in pediatric patients below 18 years of age.

STORAGE AND STABILITY: Store at room temperature (15-30°C).

INFORMATION FOR THE PATIENT: Published in e-CPS, available by subscription at www.e-cps.ca.

DOSAGE FORMS, COMPOSITION AND PACKAGING: 100 mg: Each white, beveled edge, round biconvex extended-release tablet, plain on one side and printed "LP 100" in black ink on the other side, contains: tramadol hydrochloride 100 mg. Nonmedicinal ingredients: ammonium hydroxide, colloidal silicon dioxide, Contramid (modified starch), hydrogenated vegetable oil, iron oxide black, isopropyl alcohol, magnesium stearate, n-butyl alcohol, polyvinyl acetate, povidone, propylene glycol, shellac glaze, sodium lauryl sulfate and xanthan gum. Bottles of 30, 90, 100 and 500. Blister packs of 20, 2 cards of 10 single-dose units. Tablets are comprised of a dual-matrix delivery system with an outer compression coat (containing tramadol hydrochloride) providing immediate release characteristics and a controlled-release core containing tramadol hydrochloride and Contramid, which provides the controlled-release characteristics.

200 mg: Each white, beveled edge, round biconvex extended-release tablet, plain on one side and printed "LP 200" in black ink on the other side, contains: tramadol hydrochloride 200 mg. Nonmedicinal ingredients: ammonium hydroxide, colloidal silicon dioxide, Contramid (modified starch), hydrogenated vegetable oil, iron oxide black, isopropyl alcohol, magnesium stearate, n-butyl alcohol, polyvinyl acetate, povidone, propylene glycol, shellac glaze, sodium lauryl sulfate and xanthan gum. Bottles of 30, 90, 100 and 500. Blister packs of 20, 2 cards of 10 single-dose units. Tablets are comprised of a dual-matrix delivery system with an outer compression coat (containing tramadol hydrochloride) providing immediate release characteristics and a controlled-release core containing tramadol hydrochloride and Contramid, which provides the controlled-release characteristics.

300 mg: Each white, beveled edge, round biconvex extended-release tablet, plain on one side and printed "LP 300" in black ink on the other side, contains: tramadol hydrochloride 300 mg. Nonmedicinal ingredients: ammonium hydroxide, colloidal silicon dioxide, Contramid (modified starch), hydrogenated vegetable oil, iron oxide black, isopropyl alcohol, magnesium stearate, n-butyl alcohol, polyvinyl acetate, povidone, propylene glycol, shellac glaze, sodium lauryl sulfate and xanthan gum. Bottles of 30, 90, 100 and 500. Blister packs of 20, 2 cards of 10 single-dose units. Tablets are comprised of a dual-matrix delivery system with an outer compression coat (containing tramadol hydrochloride) providing immediate release characteristics and a controlled-release core containing tramadol hydrochloride and Contramid, which provides the controlled-release characteristics.

(Shown in Product Identification Section)

Trifluoperazine

Antipsychotic

CPhA Monograph

Date of Revision: October 2010

This monograph has been compiled by CPhA and reviewed by experts. It may contain information different from that found in Health Canada-approved Product Monographs. The reader is referred to the *CPS* Editorial Policy for more information.

SUMMARY PRODUCT INFORMATION:

Route of Administration	Dosage Form	Strength
Oral	Tablet	1 mg, 2 mg, 5 mg, 10 mg, 20 mg
Oral	Syrup	1 mg/mL, 10 mg/mL

INDICATIONS AND CLINICAL USE: Health Canada-approved indications for trifluoperazine include:

- management of psychotic disorders including schizophrenia
- prevention or treatment of nausea and vomiting (not currently recommended for this indication)
- management of anxiety (not currently recommended for this indication)

CONTRAINDICATIONS:

- Patients who are hypersensitive to trifluoperazine or to any ingredient in the formulation or component of the container.
- Patients with:
  - severe CNS depression or coma
  - bone marrow suppression
  - blood dyscrasias
  - severe hepatic disease

WARNINGS AND PRECAUTIONS:

Serious Warnings and Precautions

- The use of phenothiazines such as trifluoperazine has been associated with acute and chronic extrapyramidal reactions including dystonias, akathisia, parkinsonian symptoms, neuroleptic malignant syndrome (NMS) and tardive dyskinesia (TD). NMS can be life-threatening, especially when not recognized and addressed early, and TD may not resolve after drug discontinuation. See Adverse Effects. These reactions may be more common and more severe with the use of high-potency phenothiazines such as trifluoperazine.
- The use of antipsychotic agents in elderly patients has been associated with a dose-related increase in all-cause mortality, with an inverse relationship to duration of use. The risk may be higher with first-generation or "conventional" antipsychotics compared to second-generation or "atypical" agents [*N Engl J Med* 2005;353(22):2335-41; *CMAJ* 2007;176(5):627-32. doi:10.1503/cmaj.061250]. The use of antipsychotics in older patients should be carefully considered, and first-generation agents should be avoided whenever possible.

Cardiovascular: Hypotension and tachycardia may occur in patients taking phenothiazines, though more commonly with low-potency agents. Trifluoperazine should be used with caution in patients with cardiovascular disease.

CNS: See also Serious Warnings and Precautions and Adverse Effects. Because phenothiazines can lower the seizure threshold, trifluoperazine should be used with caution in patients with a history of seizures or additional risk factors such as hyponatremia or alcohol withdrawal.

Phenothiazines, particularly high potency agents such as trifluoperazine, can cause extrapyramidal reactions (see Adverse Effects).

Because phenothiazines can affect the hypothalamic regulation of body temperature, they should be used with caution in patients exposed to extreme heat or cold.

Due to their pharmacologic antagonism of dopamine D_2 receptors in the nigrostriatal region, phenothiazines can cause or exacerbate movement disorders and should be used with caution in patients with Parkinson's disease.

Because of their anticholinergic properties, phenothiazines should be used with caution in patients with angle closure glaucoma, benign prostatic hyperplasia, or other conditions that could be aggravated by anticholinergic effects.

Endocrine and Metabolism: Patients with hypocalcemia may be more susceptible to dystonic reactions (see Adverse Effects). May cause hyperprolactinemia and resultant sexual dysfunction, galactorrhea, amenorrhea and gynecomastia. Weight gain and lipid/glucose abnormalities are also possible.

Immune: The oral syrup contains sodium bisulfite. Caution is advised in patients with sulfite allergy.

Special Populations: Pregnant Women: Phenothiazines readily cross the placenta but have not been associated with an increased risk of congenital abnormalities and are considered relatively safe during pregnancy when used in low doses. They should be used in the lowest effective dose for the shortest possible time and avoided near term if possible, to prevent adverse effects in the fetus.

Nursing Women: Phenothiazines are distributed into breast milk but are likely safe due to a low milk:plasma concentration ratio. If the decision is made to use trifluoperazine while breastfeeding, use with caution at the lowest effective dose for the shortest possible time to minimize infant exposure, and monitor for signs of adverse effects in the infant such as drowsiness, lethargy or extrapyramidal symptoms.

Pediatrics: Children may be more susceptible to extrapyramidal reactions than adults, particularly if they have acute infectious illnesses or are dehydrated. Use lower doses in children and monitor therapy closely.

Geriatrics: See Serious Warnings and Precautions.

Older individuals may be more susceptible than younger adults to the CNS, anticholinergic and cardiovascular side effects of phenothiazines. Hypotension and sedation may increase the risk of falls and associated hip fractures. Lower doses should be used in older patients and therapy should be closely monitored.

Occupational Hazards: Because trifluoperazine can cause drowsiness and dizziness, especially at the beginning of the therapy, it is important to avoid driving a car, operating machinery or participating in activities that require mental alertness until this effect has subsided.

ADVERSE EFFECTS: Overview: Two of the most serious potential adverse effects of trifluoperazine therapy are neuroleptic malignant syndrome and tardive dyskinesia.

Tardive Dyskinesia (TD): The use of antipsychotic agents such as trifluoperazine has been associated with the chronic, potentially irreversible movement disorder, tardive dyskinesia. Duration of use, daily dose and possibly total cumulative dose are important risk factors for the development of tardive dyskinesia, although it has occurred following as little as 6 months of continuous therapy. Other proposed risk factors include age, history of acute extrapyramidal side effects, poor antipsychotic response to the drug and female gender. There is no standard treatment for tardive dyskinesia, although discontinuing the antipsychotic, when possible, may lead to remission of symptoms. Fine vermicular movements of the tongue may be an early sign of tardive dyskinesia; discontinuing the drug when this occurs may prevent full onset of the syndrome.

Neuroleptic Malignant Syndrome (NMS): This potentially fatal syndrome characterized by muscle rigidity, fever/hyperthermia, labile blood pressure and fluctuating levels of consciousness, can occur in patients taking trifluoperazine or other antipsychotics. NMS appears to occur more commonly in young males. Dehydration is an additional risk factor. Patients need to be aware of the importance of adequate hydration, particularly in situations involving environmental exposure to extreme heat.

More Common Adverse Drug Reactions: See Table 1.

Table 1: Trifluoperazine

More Common Adverse Drug Reactions (≥1%)

Body System	Effect	Clinical Comment
Anticholinergic Effects	Dry mouth, dry eyes, constipation, urinary retention, blurred vision, cognitive impairment	May remit over time or respond to dosage reduction. Some side effects may be ameliorated by symptomatic measures such as fibre and fluids for constipation or artificial tears for dry eyes.
Cardiovascular	Hypotension, orthostatic hypotension, peripheral edema (1-3%), QTc interval prolongation	Monitor blood pressure during first few hours following initiation of therapy. Use caution in patients where a sudden drop in blood pressure may be particularly hazardous (e.g., older individuals or patients with cardiovascular disease). Avoid concurrent administration of other drugs known or suspected to cause QTc interval prolongation (see Table 2).
Central Nervous System	Extrapyramidal symptoms such as pseudoparkinsonism (tremor, rigidity, bradykinesia), akathisia, dystonias, tardive dyskinesia (less common with doses ≤6 mg and common with doses of 10-40 mg); dizziness, headache, sedation	Initial management includes dosage reduction; if not effective consider switching to a 2nd generation antipsychotic. Acute dystonia can be treated with im benztropine or diphenhydramine. To prevent tardive dyskinesia, use the lowest effective doses. If symptoms of tardive dyskinesia appear, discontinue trifluoperazine and, if necessary, switch to an antipsychotic with lower propensity to cause EPS. Bedtime administration may prevent daytime sedation.
Endocrine and Metabolic	Hyperprolactinemia (amenorrhea, mastalgia, gynecomastia, galactorrhea, sexual dysfunction), weight gain, dysglycemia	Hyperprolactinemic symptoms may respond to dosage reduction or consider switching to an alternate antipsychotic agent. Encourage healthy diet and lifestyle to minimize cardiovascular risk factors.
Gastrointestinal	Constipation, stomach pain, xerostomia	
Genitourinary	Difficult urination, ejaculatory dysfunction	
Hepatic	Hepatotoxicity, abnormal liver function tests (dose-related)	
Ocular	Pigmentary retinopathy, cornea and lens changes	

Less Common Adverse Drug Reactions (<1%): Cardiovascular: QT prolongation, torsades de pointes.

Central Nervous System: neuroleptic malignant syndrome (see Adverse Effects, Overview), impairment of temperature regulation (heat stroke or hypothermia), seizures.

Gastrointestinal: obstipation (severe constipation), paralytic ileus.

Genitourinary: priapism, sexual dysfunction.

Hematologic: blood dyscrasias, agranulocytosis (very rare and usually occurs in the first 2 months of therapy), leukocytopenia, thrombocytopenia.

Hepatic/Biliary/Pancreatic: cholestatic jaundice (usually occurs in first 2 to 4 weeks of therapy).

Immune: systemic lupus erythematosus-like syndrome.

Ocular: Lenticular pigmentation with long-term use; presents as glare or halo around lights or hazy vision.

DRUG INTERACTIONS: Overview: Trifluoperazine is a major substrate of the CYP1A2. Inhibitors of CYP1A2 may increase the levels of trifluoperazine, enhancing its effects; CYP1A2 inducers produce the opposite effect.

Drug-Drug Interactions: See Table 2.

Table 2: Trifluoperazine

Drug-Drug Interactions

Interacting Drug	Effect	Clinical Comment
Anticholinergics (e.g., benztropine, trihexyphenidyl, orphenadrine, procyclidine)	May delay gastric emptying, decrease absorption and increase gut wall metabolism of trifluoperazine. Additive anticholinergic side effects (e.g., constipation, urinary retention, blurred vision, dry eyes, dry mouth, cognitive impairment).	Reserve for situations where extrapyramidal symptoms occur and lowering of the antipsychotic dose is not possible. Re-evaluate anticholinergic use regularly (e.g., every 3 months).
Antihypertensives	Potential additive hypotension.	Monitor blood pressure as appropriate.
Chloroquine	May increase trifluoperazine levels.	Mechanism unknown; monitor for enhanced pharmacologic and adverse effects of trifluoperazine.
CNS depressants (e.g., opioid analgesics, ethanol, barbiturates, cyclic antidepressants, antihistamines, sedative-hypnotics)	May produce additive CNS depression.	Advise patients to monitor for additive effects and to modify activities accordingly (e.g., driving).
CYP1A2 inducers (e.g., carbamazepine, cigarette smoking, phenobarbital, rifampin)	May result in decreased trifluoperazine plasma concentrations.	Monitor for decreased therapeutic effects of trifluoperazine and adjust dose as indicated.
CYP1A2 inhibitors (e.g., amiodarone, ciprofloxacin, fluvoxamine, ketoconazole, ofloxacin, propranolol)	May result in increased trifluoperazine plasma concentrations.	Monitor for increased pharmacologic and adverse effects of trifluoperazine and adjust dose as indicated.
Drugs that prolong the QTc interval (e.g., amiodarone, chlorpromazine, clarithromycin, disopyramide, domperidone, droperidol, erythromycin, indapamide, lithium, moxifloxacin, pimozide, procainamide, quetiapine, quinidine, quinine, tricyclic antidepressants, ziprasidone)	Potential additive QTc prolongation.	Coadministration of phenothiazines with other medications that might also prolong the QTc interval is not recommended.
Dopaminergic agents (e.g., bromocriptine, cabergoline, levodopa, pramipexole, ropinirole)	Trifluoperazine may antagonize the dopaminergic effects of these drugs resulting in decreased efficacy/worsening of parkinsonian symptoms.	Avoid combination.
Lithium	Rarely, concurrent use of lithium with phenothiazines has resulted in acute encephalopathic syndrome, even with normal lithium levels.	Caution and close monitoring for neurologic symptoms are advised.

Drug-Herb Interactions: Avoid concurrent use of phenothiazines with kava kava, gotu kola, valerian and St. John's wort because these herbs may increase CNS depression. Kava kava may also provide additive dopamine antagonism. Avoid dong quai because of a possible increased risk of photosensitization. Case reports indicate seizures have occurred in patients taking evening primrose oil with phenothiazines.

Drug-Laboratory Interactions: Trifluoperazine use may cause a false positive reading for phenylketonuria.

DOSAGE AND ADMINISTRATION: Dosing Considerations:

- Individualization of the dose is important when using trifluoperazine. Once the maximum response is achieved, the dose may need to be reduced gradually to a maintenance level. The lowest effective dose should be used. To prevent withdrawal syndromes, reduce gradually over 1-2 weeks.
- In older adults, it is advisable to start low and titrate up gradually to minimize the risk of hypotension and neuromuscular reactions.
- To enhance palatability of the oral concentrate (10 mg/mL syrup), add the required dose to at least 60 mL of tomato or fruit juice, milk, simple syrup, orange syrup, carbonated beverage, coffee, tea, water, or semisolid food (soup, puddings), and administer immediately after preparing.

Recommended Dose and Dosage Adjustment: Dosing Considerations: To minimize the risk of dose-related or long-term side effects, such as extrapyramidal reactions, trifluoperazine should be used at the lowest effective dose for the shortest possible duration.

Psychotic Disorders: Adults (outpatients): The oral dose is 1 to 2 mg twice daily.

Adults (hospitalized or well supervised): Initial oral dose is 2 to 5 mg twice daily with optimum response usually seen in the 15 to 20 mg/day range. Higher doses of 40 to 80 mg or more may be required in rare cases.

Children (6 to 12 years): If hospitalized or are well supervised, the recommended initial oral dose is 1 mg once or twice daily. The dose is then gradually increased until symptoms are controlled or adverse effects become troublesome. Older children may require higher doses if they present with severe symptoms. Maximum daily dose is 15 mg.

Geriatrics: Avoid using first-generation antipsychotic agents in elderly patients when possible (see Warnings and Precautions, Serious Warnings and Precautions). If used in older patients, initial oral dose should start at the low end of the dosage range and should be increased more gradually. The daily dose should not exceed 6 mg.

Antiemetic: Adults: Oral dose is 1 to 2 mg twice daily as needed.

Administration: Administer with food to minimize gastrointestinal distress.

OVERDOSAGE:

Signs and Symptoms: Symptoms of trifluoperazine overdose are an extension of its pharmacologic actions. The primary symptoms observed are sedation and hypotension. Mild or early intoxication may appear as restlessness and confusion, which may progress to coma. Altered temperature regulation can occur; both hypothermia and hyperthermia have been reported. Neuroleptic malignant syndrome can occur in overdose, though it most often occurs with therapeutic doses (see also Adverse Effects). Other symptoms may include anticholinergic manifestations (mydriasis, dry mouth, agitation, urinary retention, decreased bowel sounds), tachycardia, cardiac arrhythmias, seizures and respiratory and/or vasomotor collapse.

Recommended Management: Patients who have ingested trifluoperazine in overdose may require respiratory and hemodynamic support. This may include intubation, ventilation, boluses of isotonic iv fluids and inotropic support. Once the patient's airway is adequately protected, 1 dose of activated charcoal (1 g/kg body weight) can be administered up to 120 minutes after oral overdose to minimize absorption of trifluoperazine. The utility of this intervention decreases with time, and it may not influence clinical outcome. Patients with seizures should be treated with benzodiazepines, or if necessary, barbiturates. Ventricular arrhythmias are uncommon, and should be treated with boluses of sodium bicarbonate as well as conventional antiarrhythmics such as lidocaine. In the rare patient with torsades de pointes, iv magnesium sulfate and/or an overdrive pacemaker should be used. Acute dystonic reactions may be treated with iv benztropine or diphenhydramine.

> For management of a suspected drug overdose, CPhA recommends that you contact your **regional Poison Control Centre**. See the *CPS* Directory section for a list of Poison Control Centres.

ACTION AND CLINICAL PHARMACOLOGY: Mechanism of Action: Trifluoperazine is a high potency piperazine phenothiazine antipsychotic. The pharmacologic effect of phenothiazines on positive symptoms of psychotic disorders (hallucinations, delusions) is believed to be mediated by antagonism of postsynaptic dopamine D_2 receptors in the mesolimbic pathway. Antagonism of D_2 receptors in the nigrostriatal and tuberoinfundibular regions may result in extrapyramidal side effects (EPS) and hyperprolactinemia, respectively. Trifluoperazine also antagonizes histamine H_1 receptors (associated with sedation and weight gain), alpha$_1$ adrenergic receptors (orthostatic hypotension and reflex tachycardia) and muscarinic M_1 receptors (anticholinergic effects such as dry mouth, dry eyes, blurred vision, constipation and urinary retention). Because trifluoperazine has a higher affinity for D_2 receptors than for H_1, M_1 or alpha$_1$ adrenergic receptors, it has a higher propensity to cause EPS than side effects associated with the other receptors.

Trifluoperazine inhibits indirect stimulation of the vomiting centre, consequently preventing or treating nausea and vomiting. It is not effective in preventing vertigo or motion sickness.

Pharmacokinetics: Adults: Absorption: Trifluoperazine is readily absorbed. Absorption from tablets is sometimes erratic; however, it may be less so with the liquid formulation. When taken orally, trifluoperazine reaches its peak concentration within 2 to 4 hours. The onset of action of trifluoperazine is 0.5 to 1 hour following tablet administration. Slightly faster onset is achieved with the oral suspension since no disintegration time is involved.

Distribution: Trifluoperazine is >90% plasma protein bound. Because of its highly lipophilic nature, CNS trifluoperazine concentrations exceed those in plasma. The volume of distribution is 10 to 35 L/kg.

Metabolism: Trifluoperazine is metabolized in the liver, primarily by CYP1A2. The half-life of trifluoperazine ranges from 7 to 18 hours.

Excretion: The inactive metabolites are excreted primarily in the urine. Trifluoperazine is not dialyzable.

SPECIAL HANDLING INSTRUCTIONS: Avoid skin contact with oral suspension as contact dermatitis has been reported.

Trihexyphenidyl Ⓟ
Antiparkinsonian Agent

CPhA Monograph

Date of Revision: November 2005

> This monograph has been compiled by CPhA and reviewed by experts. It may contain information different from that found in Health Canada-approved Product Monographs. The reader is referred to the *CPS* Editorial Policy for more information.

PHARMACOLOGY: Trihexyphenidyl is a synthetic tertiary amine with antimuscarinic and antiparkinsonian effects. Its mechanism of action is not well understood, but it appears that by reducing cholinergic activity it helps to restore the functional balance between acetylcholine and dopamine in the basal ganglia of patients with Parkinsonian symptoms. The proposed ability of trihexyphenidyl to inhibit reuptake and storage of dopamine, thereby prolonging the action of dopamine, may also contribute to an effect on the equilibrium between acetylcholine and dopamine.

Trihexyphenidyl also exhibits a direct antispasmodic effect on smooth muscle. In small doses, trihexyphenidyl causes CNS depression while in larger doses it may cause CNS stimulation.

Pharmacokinetics: Following oral administration, trihexyphenidyl is rapidly absorbed from the gastrointestinal tract. Onset of action is within 1 hour of administration. Peak effects of the drug last for 2 to 3 hours and the duration of action is 6 to 12 hours. Trihexyphenidyl is excreted in the urine, probably as unchanged drug.

INDICATIONS: Adjunctive therapy in the symptomatic treatment of Parkinsonism and drug-induced parkinsonian symptoms.

CONTRAINDICATIONS: Trihexyphenidyl is contraindicated in patients with a known hypersensitivity to trihexyphenidyl or any of its excipients, and in patients with angle-closure glaucoma or severe ulcerative colitis.

WARNINGS: See Precautions.

PRECAUTIONS: Because of its anticholinergic properties, trihexyphenidyl should be used with caution in patients with cardiac arrhythmias, hypertension or hypotension, prostatic hypertrophy, liver or kidney disease or obstructive disease of the gastrointestinal or genitourinary tract.

Trihexyphenidyl, alone or in combination with antipsychotics or other anticholinergics, may cause anhidrosis and/or hyperthermia, which may be fatal. Patients should avoid overheating from prolonged exposure to high environmental temperatures or from sustained heavy exercise. The elderly, the chronically ill, alcoholics and those with CNS disease may be particularly vulnerable. If there is evidence of anhidrosis, dosage should be decreased so that the ability to maintain body temperature equilibrium through perspiration is not impaired. Trihexyphenidyl should also be used with caution in patients with fever.

Some experts recommend gonioscopic examination and monitoring of intraocular pressure (IOP) at regular intervals during prolonged therapy with trihexyphenidyl. The drug may precipitate the onset of incipient angle-closure glaucoma and should not be used in predisposed patients (see Contraindications). Patients with primary open-angle glaucoma controlled with medication are at minimal risk of induction of an increase in IOP and many clinicians do not consider this condition a contraindication to therapy with trihexyphenidyl.

Tardive dyskinesia may appear in some patients on long-term treatment with antipsychotics and related agents, or may occur after these drugs have been discontinued. Antiparkinsonian agents usually do not alleviate the symptoms of tardive dyskinesia and in some instances may aggravate or unmask such symptoms. Trihexyphenidyl is not recommended in tardive dyskinesia.

When trihexyphenidyl is used to treat parkinsonian symptoms caused by antipsychotic therapy, there may be an intensification of the psychiatric illness being treated. Although trihexyphenidyl need not be discontinued when this occurs, its psychotogenic potential should be considered when planning the management of patients with psychiatric illness. When using trihexyphenidyl in these patients, they should be carefully observed, especially at the beginning of treatment or if dosage is increased.

Use trihexyphenidyl with extreme caution in patients with mild to moderate ulcerative colitis since antimuscarinic agents may suppress intestinal motility and produce paralytic ileus with resultant precipitation or aggravation of toxic megacolon. Trihexyphenidyl is contraindicated in patients with severe ulcerative colitis (see Contraindications). Use trihexyphenidyl cautiously in those patients with known or suspected gastrointestinal infections since it may decrease gut motility and prolong symptomatology by causing retention of the causative organism or toxin.

Antimuscarinics in general may delay gastric emptying with possible antral stasis in patients with gastric ulcer; therefore trihexyphenidyl should be used cautiously in these patients. Antimuscarinics may also relax the lower esophageal sphincter. This, combined with their effects on gastric emptying, may result in increased esophageal reflux in patients with gastroesophageal reflux disease or hiatus hernia associated with reflux esophagitis.

Due to its drying effects on bronchial secretions, trihexyphenidyl should be used with caution in patients with chronic obstructive pulmonary disease. It should also be used with extreme caution in patients with autonomic neuropathy.

Drug Interactions: Amantadine: Trihexyphenidyl and other anticholinergic drugs may potentiate the CNS side effects of amantadine. Monitor patients for this effect and reduce the dose of one or both drugs as necessary.

Anticholinergics: Trihexyphenidyl may enhance the anticholinergic effects of drugs including atropine, MAO inhibitors, tricyclic antidepressants and phenothiazines. Paralytic ileus (sometimes fatal), hyperthermia and heat stroke may occur. Advise patients to report gastrointestinal problems, fever or heat intolerance promptly.

CNS depressants: Trihexyphenidyl in small doses, may enhance the CNS depressant effects of drugs including alcohol, anticonvulsants, barbiturates, MAO inhibitors, opioid analgesics, phenothiazines and tricyclic antidepressants.

Cholinesterase Inhibitors: Theoretically, trihexyphenidyl and other anticholinergic drugs that readily penetrate the blood-brain barrier may interfere with the action of centrally acting cholinesterase inhibitors (e.g., donepezil, galantamine, rivastigmine).In addition, cholinesterase inhibitors have the potential to interfere with the activity of anticholinergic medications.

Levodopa: When trihexyphenidyl is used in combination with levodopa, the dosage of each drug may have to be reduced.

Occupational Hazards: Trihexyphenidyl may impair mental and/or physical abilities required for performance of hazardous tasks such as operating machinery or driving a motor vehicle.

Pregnancy: Safe use in children, or pregnant or lactating women has not been established.

Lactation: See Pregnancy.

Children: See Pregnancy.

Geriatrics: Geriatric patients are frequently more sensitive to the adverse effects of anticholinergic medications, including trihexyphenidyl. These patients may require lower doses, especially at the onset of therapy, and slower dose titration than younger adults.

ADVERSE EFFECTS: The adverse effects of trihexyphenidyl are usually an extension of its pharmacologic action. They are usually dose-related and may be reduced by lowering the dose. Dry mouth, blurred vision, dizziness, mild nausea or anxiety will be experienced by 30 to 50% of patients.

Older patients, particularly those with underlying cognitive impairment, are especially prone to reactions such as mental confusion, agitation, disturbed behavior, or nausea and vomiting. Such patients should receive lower initial doses, with gradual increases until an effective level is reached. If a severe reaction should occur, the drug should be discontinued for a few days and then resumed at a lower dosage.

Withdrawal symptoms may occur in patients who were receiving large doses.

Cardiovascular: Tachycardia, postural hypotension, palpitations.

Central Nervous System: Dizziness, drowsiness, anxiety, headache. Less frequent reactions include confusion, disturbed behavior, restlessness, delirium, euphoria, delusions and hallucinations (patients with pre-existing dementia may be more susceptible).

Endocrine: Hyperthermia, anhidrosis, heat stroke.

Gastrointestinal: Dry mouth, constipation, nausea, vomiting. Isolated cases of dilatation of the colon, paralytic ileus and suppurative parotitis secondary to excessive dryness of the mouth have been reported. Dry mouth may be relieved by the use of saliva substitute or sugarless gum.

Genitourinary: Urinary hesitancy or retention.

Hypersensitivity: Skin rash may occur occasionally.

Musculoskeletal: Weakness.

Ophthalmic: Blurred vision, mydriasis, increased intraocular pressure, cycloplegia, photophobia, xerophthalmia.

OVERDOSE:

Symptoms: Symptoms of trihexyphenidyl overdose are primarily extensions of its anticholinergic actions. Tachycardia; flushed, hot, dry skin; dry mucous membranes; mydriasis and blurred vision are common. Drowsiness, nervousness and lightheadedness may progress to, or alternate with, agitation, confusion, delirium and hallucinations, especially in children or the elderly. Urinary retention, hypertension, hyperthermia, photophobia, thirst and decreased gastrointestinal motility are also seen. Pupils may be fixed. Susceptible patients may experience angle-closure glaucoma. In severely poisoned patients coma or seizures may occur. Psychosis, rash, dystonic reactions, respiratory depression, cardiac arrhythmia and rhabdomyolysis have been reported.

Treatment: Treatment is symptomatic and supportive. If ingestion occurred within 4 hours prior to presentation for medical care, administer activated charcoal with or without a cathartic. Cathartics should not be given to patients with an ileus or impaired renal function. Monitor vital signs, urine output and bowel sounds; monitor ECG in severely poisoned patients. Maintain respiration, fluid and electrolyte balance. Mydriasis and cycloplegia may be treated with a local miotic such as pilocarpine. Hyperthermia can be managed with physical measures and control of agitation. Treat agitation and seizures with i.v. benzodiazepines. Avoid antipsychotics and other anticholinergic drugs. If rhabdomyolysis does occur, alkalinize urine and maintain good urine output. Peritoneal dialysis and hemodialysis are of no value in the management of trihexyphenidyl overdose.

> For management of a suspected drug overdose, CPhA recommends that you contact your **regional Poison Control Centre**. See the *CPS* Directory section for a list of Poison Control Centres.

DOSAGE: Trihexiphenidyl dosage should be individualized. The initial dosage should be low and then increased gradually, especially in patients over 60 years of age.

Parkinsonism: 1 mg orally the first day; increase by 2 mg daily at intervals of 3 to 5 days, up to 6 to 10 mg daily. In patients with post-encephalitic parkinsonism, dosages as high as 12 to 15 mg daily may be necessary. The total daily dose is best tolerated if divided into 3 doses and taken at mealtimes.

Drug-induced Parkinsonian Symptoms: The size and frequency of doses of trihexyphenidyl needed to control drug-induced parkinsonian symptoms, attributable especially to antipsychotics, must be determined empirically. The total daily dosage usually ranges between 5 and 15 mg; however, in some cases, these reactions have been satisfactorily controlled with as little as 1 mg daily. It may be advisable to commence therapy with a single 1 mg dose. If the extrapyramidal manifestations are not controlled in a few hours, the subsequent doses may be progressively increased until satisfactory control is achieved. Control may sometimes be more rapidly achieved by temporarily reducing the dosage of the antipsychotic or instituting trihexyphenidyl therapy and then adjusting the dosage of both drugs until the desired antipsychotic effect is retained without the reappearance of parkinsonian symptoms.

It is sometimes possible to maintain the patient on a reduced trihexyphenidyl dosage after the reactions have remained under control for several days. In the majority of patients, the use of anticholinergic agents is not required after 3 months of antipsychotic therapy.

Trileptal® Ⓟ
oxcarbazepine
Antiepileptic

Novartis Pharmaceuticals

Date of Preparation: April 6, 2000
Date of Revision: September 11, 2009

SUMMARY PRODUCT INFORMATION:

Route of Administration	Dosage Form/ Strength	Clinically Relevant Nonmedicinal Ingredients
Oral	Tablets, 150 mg, 300 mg and 600 mg	Not applicable For a complete listing see Dosage Forms, Composition and Packaging.
Oral	Oral Suspension, 60 mg/mL	Ethanol (less than 100 mg per dose) For a complete listing see Dosage Forms, Composition and Packaging.

INDICATIONS AND CLINICAL USE: Adults: TRILEPTAL (oxcarbazepine) is indicated for use as monotherapy or adjunctive therapy in the treatment of partial seizures.

Geriatrics (>65 years of age): Evidence from clinical studies indicates that there are differences in the pharmacokinetic profile of oxcarbazepine in the geriatric population relative to younger adults, which may be associated with differences in safety or effectiveness. A brief discussion can be found in the appropriate sections (see Warnings and Precautions, Special Populations, Geriatrics (>65 years of age); Action and Clinical Pharmacology; Dosage and Administration, Dosing Considerations).

Pediatrics (6 to 16 years of age): TRILEPTAL (oxcarbazepine) is indicated for use as monotherapy or adjunctive therapy in the treatment of partial seizures.

CONTRAINDICATIONS:

- Patients with a known hypersensitivity to oxcarbazepine or to any of the components of TRILEPTAL. For a complete listing, see Dosage Forms, Composition and Packaging.

WARNINGS AND PRECAUTIONS: Serious Dermatological Reactions: Serious dermatological reactions, including Stevens-Johnson syndrome (SJS) and toxic epidermal necrolysis (TEN), have been reported in both children and adults in association with TRILEPTAL use. The median time of onset for reported cases was 19 days. Such serious skin reactions may be life-threatening, and some patients have required hospitalization with very rare reports of fatal outcome. Recurrence of the serious skin reactions following re-challenge with TRILEPTAL has also been reported.

The reporting rate of TEN and SJS associated with TRILEPTAL use, which is generally accepted to be an underestimate due to underreporting, exceeds the background incidence rate estimates by a factor of 3- to 10-fold. Estimates of the background incidence rate for these serious skin reactions in the general population range between 0.5 to 6 cases per million-person years. Therefore, if a patient develops a skin reaction while taking TRILEPTAL, consideration should be given to discontinuing TRILEPTAL use and prescribing another antiepileptic medication.

Hypersensitivity: Class I (immediate) hypersensitivity reactions including rash, pruritus, urticaria, angioedema and reports of anaphylaxis have been received in the post-marketing period. Cases of anaphylaxis and angioedema involving the larynx, glottis, lips and eyelids have been reported in patients after taking the first or subsequent doses of TRILEPTAL. The reporting rate of anaphylaxis and angioedema associated with TRILEPTAL use, which is generally accepted to be an underestimate due to underreporting, does not exceed the background incidence rate estimates. Estimates of the background incidence rate for severe anaphylaxis in the general population ranges between 50 and 300 cases per million-person years and the estimated lifetime prevalence of anaphylaxis ranges between 0.05% and 2.0% and that of angioedema ranges between 0.05% and 1%. If a patient develops these reactions after treatment with TRILEPTAL, the drug should be discontinued and an alternative treatment started.

Patients with a Past History of Hypersensitivity Reaction to Carbamazepine: Patients who have had hypersensitivity reactions to carbamazepine should be informed that approximately 25%-30% of them will experience hypersensitivity reactions with TRILEPTAL. For this reason patients should be specifically questioned about any prior experience with carbamazepine, and patients with a history of hypersensitivity reactions to carbamazepine should ordinarily be treated with TRILEPTAL only if the potential benefit justifies the potential risk. Hypersensitivity reactions may also occur in patients without a history of hypersensitivity to carbamazepine. In general, if signs or symptoms of hypersensitivity develop, TRILEPTAL should be discontinued immediately.

Multi-Organ Hypersensitivity: Multi-organ hypersensitivity reactions have occurred in close temporal association (median time to detection 13 days: range 4-60) to the initiation of TRILEPTAL therapy in adult and pediatric patients. Although there have been a limited number of reports, many of these cases resulted in hospitalization and some were considered life threatening. Signs and symptoms of this disorder were diverse; however, patients typically, although not exclusively, presented with fever and rash associated with other organ system involvement. Other associated manifestations included hemic and lymphatic system disorders (e.g., eosinophilia, thrombocytopenia, lymphadenopathy, leucopenia, neutropenia, splenomegaly), hepatobiliary disorders (e.g. hepatitis, liver function test abnormalities), renal disorders (e.g. proteinura, nephritis, oliguria, renal failure), muscles and joints disorders (e.g. joint swelling, myalgia, arthralgia, asthenia), nervous system disorders (hepatic encephalopathy), respiratory disorders (e.g. dyspnea, pulmonary oedema, asthma, bronchospasms, interstitial lung disease), hepatorenal syndrome, pruritus, and angioedema. Because the disorder is variable in its expression, other organ system symptoms and signs, not noted here, may occur. If this reaction is suspected, TRILEPTAL should be discontinued and an alternative treatment started. Although there are no case reports to indicate cross sensitivity with other drugs that produce this syndrome, the experience amongst drugs associated with multi-organ hypersensitivity would indicate this to be a possibility.

Oral Suspension: TRILEPTAL oral suspension contains parabenes which may cause allergic reactions (possibly delayed) (see Contraindications).

Carcinogenesis and Mutagenesis: In 2-year carcinogenicity studies, oxcarbazepine was administered orally at doses up to 100 mg/kg/day in mice and up to 250 mg/kg in rats, and the pharmacologically active 10-hydroxy metabolite (MHD) was administered orally at doses up to 600 mg/kg/day in rats. The following dose-related increases in the incidences of liver tumors were noted: hepatocellular carcinomas in the female rats (oxcarbazepine 25 mg/kg/day), hepatocellular adenomas in mice (oxcarbazepine 70 mg/kg/day) and hepatocellular adenomas and/or carcinomas in males at 600 mg/kg/day and in females at >250 mg/kg/day with MHD. There was a marginal increase in the incidence of benign testicular interstitial cell tumors in rats at 250 mg MHD/kg/day and an increase in the incidence of granular cell aggregates or tumors in the cervix and vagina in rats at 75 mg MHD/kg/day.

The occurrence of liver tumors was attributed to the induction of hepatic microsomal enzymes, an effect which is weak or absent in patients treated with TRILEPTAL. Interstitial cell tumors are common spontaneous tumors in aged rats and are considered to be without risk for man. The significance of granular cell tumors to therapy with TRILEPTAL is unknown, however as the tumors were microscopic in size and bland in appearance, they are considered to be of little importance in human safety assessment.

In a series of in vitro and in vivo mutagenicity studies there was no evidence of a mutagenic potential for oxcarbazepine or MHD.

Cardiovascular: In clinical trials with TRILEPTAL, patients with significant cardiovascular disease or electrocardiographic abnormalities were systematically excluded. Thus, TRILEPTAL should be used with caution in patients with cardiac conduction abnormalities and in patients taking concomitant medications which depress AV conduction. It is recommended that TRILEPTAL should not be used in patients with AV block. For patients with cardiac insufficiency and secondary heart failure for whom treatment with TRILEPTAL is considered clinically indicated, body weight should be monitored to determine the occurrence of fluid retention. In case of fluid retention or worsening of the cardiac condition, serum sodium should be checked. If hyponatremia is observed, water restriction is an important counter-measurement.

Dependence/Tolerance: Withdrawal of AEDs: As with all antiepileptic drugs, TRILEPTAL should be withdrawn gradually to minimize the potential of increased seizure frequency.

Abuse and Dependence Liability: The abuse potential of TRILEPTAL has not been evaluated in human studies.

Intragastric injections of oxcarbazepine to four cynomolgus monkeys demonstrated no signs of physical dependence as measured by the desire to self administer oxcarbazepine by lever pressing activity.

Endocrine and Metabolism: Hyponatremia : Clinically significant hyponatremia (sodium <125 mmol/L) can develop during TRILEPTAL (oxcarbazepine) use. In the 14 controlled epilepsy studies 2.5% of TRILEPTAL treated patients (38/1524) had a sodium of less than 125 mmol/L at some point during treatment, compared to no such patients assigned placebo or active control (carbamazepine and phenobarbital for adjunctive and monotherapy substitution studies, and phenytoin and valproate for the monotherapy initiation studies). Clinically significant hyponatremia generally occurred during the first 3 months of treatment with TRILEPTAL, although there were patients who first developed a serum sodium <125 mmol/L more than 1 year after initiation of therapy. Most patients who developed hyponatremia were asymptomatic but patients in the clinical trials were frequently monitored and some had their TRILEPTAL dose reduced, discontinued, or had their fluid intake restricted for hyponatremia. Whether or not these maneuvers prevented the occurrence of more severe events is unknown. Cases of symptomatic hyponatremia have been reported during post-marketing use. In clinical trials, patients whose treatment with TRILEPTAL was discontinued due to hyponatremia generally experienced normalization of serum sodium within a few days without additional treatment.

In patients with pre-existing renal conditions associated with low sodium or in patients treated concomitantly with sodium–lowering drugs (e.g. diuretics, drugs associated with inappropriate ADH secretion), serum sodium levels should be measured prior to initiating therapy. Thereafter, serum sodium levels should be measured after approximately two weeks and then at monthly intervals for the first three months during clinical therapy, or according to clinical need. These risk factors may apply especially to elderly patients. For patients on TRILEPTAL therapy when starting on sodium-lowering drugs, the same approach for sodium checks should be followed. In general, if clinical symptoms suggestive of hyponatremia (e.g., nausea, malaise, headache, lethargy, confusion, or obtundation) occur on TRILEPTAL therapy, serum sodium measurement may be considered. Other patients may have serum sodium assessed as part of their routine laboratory studies.

Patients with Fructose Intolerance: TRILEPTAL oral suspension contains sorbitol and, therefore, should not be administered to patients with rare hereditary problems of fructose intolerance.

Thyroid Hormone: Decreases in TT_4 and/or FT_4 (total and/or free thyroxine, respectively), usually without changes in T_3 or TSH, have been reported in pediatric and adult patients during short-term and long-term treatment with oxcarbazepine (see Warnings and Precautions, Monitoring and Laboratory Tests; Adverse Reactions, Post-Market Adverse Drug Reactions). Although patients with oxcarbazepine-induced reductions in T_4 may remain clinically euthyroid, some patients present with symptoms of hypothyroidism. Discontinuation of oxcarbazepine treatment has been shown to be associated with a return to normal levels of T_4.

Evaluation of thyroid hormone status should be considered for patients treated with oxcarbazepine, particularly for pediatric patients, due to the potential risk of sub-clinical or clinical hypothyroidism and long-term adverse effects on development that can occur in relation to undetected changes in thyroid hormone status.

Hematologic: Very rare reports of agranulocytosis, aplastic anemia and pancytopenia have been seen in patients treated with TRILEPTAL during post-marketing experience (see Adverse Reactions, Post-Market Adverse Drug Reactions). However, due to the very low incidence of these conditions and confounding factors (e.g. underlying disease, concomitant medication), causality cannot be established.

Discontinuation of the drug should be considered if any evidence of significant bone marrow depression develops.

Hepatic/Biliary/Pancreatic: Very rare cases of hepatitis and hepatic failure have been reported. Symptoms suggestive of hepatic dysfunction (nausea/vomiting, anorexia, pruritis, right upper quadrant pain, etc.) should prompt evaluation of liver function. In the event of a clinically significant liver abnormality, treatment with TRILEPTAL should be promptly discontinued.

Neurologic: Use of TRILEPTAL (oxcarbazepine) has been associated with central nervous system related adverse events. The most significant of these can be classified into three general categories: 1) cognitive symptoms including psychomotor slowing, difficulty with concentration, and speech or language problems, 2) somnolence or fatigue, and 3) coordination abnormalities, including ataxia and gait disturbances.

Adult Patients: In one, large, fixed dose study, TRILEPTAL was added to existing AED therapy (up to three concomitant AEDs). By protocol, the dosage of the concomitant AEDs could not be reduced as TRILEPTAL was added, reduction in TRILEPTAL dosage was not allowed if intolerance developed, and patients were discontinued if unable to tolerate their highest target maintenance doses. In this trial, 65% of patients were discontinued because they could not tolerate the 2400 mg/day dose of TRILEPTAL on top of existing AEDs. The adverse events seen in this study were primarily CNS related and the risk for discontinuation was dose related.

In this trial, 7.1% of oxcarbazepine treated patients and 4% of placebo treated patients experienced a cognitive adverse event. The risk of discontinuation for these events was about 6.5 times greater on oxcarbazepine than on placebo. In addition, 26% of oxcarbazepine-treated patients and 12% of placebo-treated patients experienced somnolence. The risk of discontinuation for somnolence was about 10 times greater on oxcarbazepine than on placebo. Finally, 28.7% of oxcarbazepine-treated patients and 6.4% of placebo-treated patients experienced ataxia or gait disturbances. The risk for discontinuation for these events was about 7 times greater on oxcarbazepine than on placebo.

In a single placebo-controlled monotherapy trial evaluating 2400 mg/day of TRILEPTAL, no patients in either treatment group discontinued double-blind treatment because of cognitive adverse events, somnolence, ataxia, or gait disturbance.

In the two dose-controlled conversion to monotherapy trials comparing 2400 mg/day and 300 mg/day TRILEPTAL, 1.1% of patients in the 2400 mg/day group discontinued double blind treatment because of somnolence or cognitive adverse events compared to 0% in the 300 mg/day group. In these trials, no patients discontinued because of ataxia or gait disturbances in either treatment group.

Pediatric Patients: A study was conducted in pediatric patients with inadequately controlled partial seizures in which TRILEPTAL was added to existing AED therapy (up to two concomitant AEDs). By protocol, the dosage of concomitant AEDs could not be reduced as TRILEPTAL was added. TRILEPTAL was titrated to reach a target dose ranging from 30 mg/kg to 46 mg/kg (based on a patient's body weight with fixed doses for predefined weight ranges).

Cognitive adverse events occurred in 5.8% of oxcarbazepine-treated patients (the single most common event being concentration impairment, 4 of 138 patients) and in 3.1% of patients treated with placebo. In addition, 34.8% of oxcarbazepine-treated patients and 14.0% of placebo-treated patients experienced somnolence. (No patient discontinued due to a cognitive adverse event or somnolence.) Finally, 23.2% of oxcarbazepine-treated patients and 7.0% of placebo-treated patients experienced ataxia or gait disturbances. Two (1.4%) oxcarbazepine-treated patients and 1 (0.8%) placebo-treated patient discontinued due to ataxia or gait disturbances.

The use of TRILEPTAL has been associated with dizziness and somnolence. Therefore, patients should be advised that physical and/or mental abilities required for operating machinery, including automobiles, may be impaired.

Psychiatric: Suicidal Ideation and Behaviour: Suicidal ideation and behaviour have been reported in patients treated with antiepileptic agents in several indications.

All patients treated with antiepileptic drugs, irrespective of indication, should be monitored for signs of suicidal ideation and behaviour and appropriate treatment should be considered. Patients (and caregivers of patients) should be advised to seek medical advice should signs of suicidal ideation or behaviour emerge.

An FDA meta-analysis of randomized placebo controlled trials, in which antiepileptic drugs were used for various indications, has shown a small increased risk of suicidal ideation and behaviour in patients treated with these drugs. The mechanism of this risk is not known.

There were 43 892 patients treated in the placebo controlled clinical trials that were included in the meta-analysis. Approximately 75% of patients in these clinical trials were treated for indications other than epilepsy and, for the majority of non-epilepsy indications the treatment (antiepileptic drug or placebo) was administered as monotherapy. Patients with epilepsy represented approximately 25% of the total number of patients treated in the placebo controlled clinical trials and, for the majority of epilepsy patients, treatment (antiepileptic drug or placebo) was administered as adjunct to other antiepileptic agents (i.e., patients in both treatment arms were being treated with one or more antiepileptic drug). Therefore, the small increased risk of suicidal ideation and behaviour reported from the meta-analysis (0.43% for patients on antiepileptic drugs compared to 0.24% for patients on placebo) is based largely on patients that received monotherapy treatment (antiepileptic drug or placebo) for non-epilepsy indications. The study design does not allow an estimation of the risk of suicidal ideation and behaviour for patients with epilepsy that are taking antiepileptic drugs, due both to this population being the minority in the study, and the drug-placebo comparison in this population being confounded by the presence of adjunct antiepileptic drug treatment in both arms.

Renal: In renally-impaired patients (creatinine clearance <30 mL/min), the elimination half-life of MHD is prolonged with a corresponding two fold increase in AUC (see Action and Clinical Pharmacology, Special Populations and Conditions). TRILEPTAL therapy should be initiated at one-half the usual starting dose and increased, if necessary, at a slower than usual rate until the desired clinical response is achieved.

Special Populations: Pregnant Women: Data on a limited number of pregnancies indicate that oxcarbazepine may cause serious birth defects (e.g. cleft palate and other malformations) when administered during pregnancy. In animal studies, increased incidences of fetal structural abnormalities and other manifestations of developmental toxicity (embryolethality, growth retardation) were observed in the offspring of animals treated with either oxcarbazepine or its active 10-hydroxy metabolite (MHD) during pregnancy at doses similar to the maximum recommended human dose.

Taking this data into consideration:

- If women receiving TRILEPTAL become pregnant, plan to become pregnant, or if the need to initiate treatment with TRILEPTAL arises during pregnancy, the drug's potential benefits must carefully be weighed against its hazards, particularly during the first 3 months of pregnancy.
- As is usual clinical practice, women of childbearing potential should, whenever possible, be prescribed antiepileptic drugs as monotherapy because the incidence of congenital abnormalities in the offspring of women treated with more than one antiepileptic drug is greater than in those women receiving a single antiepileptic.
- Minimum effective doses should be given and plasma levels monitored.
- Patients should be counselled regarding the possibility of an increased risk of malformations and given the opportunity of antenatal screening.
- During pregnancy, effective antiepileptic treatment should not be interrupted, since the aggravation of the illness is detrimental to both the mother and the foetus.

Like many antiepileptic drugs, TRILEPTAL may contribute to folic acid deficiency, a possible contributory cause of foetal abnormality. Folic acid supplementation is recommended before and during pregnancy.

Due to physiological changes during pregnancy, plasma levels of the active metabolite of oxcarbazepine, the 10-monohydroxy derivative (MHD), may gradually decrease throughout pregnancy. It is recommended that clinical response should be monitored carefully in women receiving TRILEPTAL treatment during pregnancy and determination of changes in MHD plasma concentrations should be considered to ensure that adequate seizure control is maintained throughout pregnancy. Postpartum MHD plasma levels may also be considered for monitoring, especially in the event that medication was increased during pregnancy, to minimize the risk of concentration dependent adverse events.

Bleeding disorders in the newborn caused by antiepileptic agents have been reported. As a precaution, vitamin K_1 should be administered as a preventive measure in the last few weeks of the woman's pregnancy and to the newborn.

Nursing Women: Oxcarbazepine and its active metabolite (MHD) are excreted in human breast milk. A milk-to-plasma concentration ratio of 0.5 was found for both. The effects on the infant exposed to TRILEPTAL by this route are unknown. Therefore, TRILEPTAL should not be used during breast-feeding.

Pediatrics (6-16 years of age): TRILEPTAL is indicated for use as monotherapy or as adjunctive therapy for partial seizures in patients aged 6-16 years old. TRILEPTAL has been given to about 623 patients between the ages of 3-17 in controlled clinical trials (185 treated as monotherapy) and about 615 patients between the ages of 3-17 in other trials. (See Adverse Reactions, Adjunctive Therapy in Pediatric Patients Previously Treated with Other AEDs, for a description of the adverse events associated with TRILEPTAL use in this population.)

Geriatrics (>65 years of age): There were 52 patients over age 65 in controlled trials and 565 patients over the age of 65 in other trials. Following administration of single (300 mg) and multiple (600 mg/day) doses of TRILEPTAL in elderly volunteers (60-82 years of age), the maximum plasma concentration and AUC values of MHD were 30%-60% higher than in younger volunteers (18-32 years of age). Comparisons of creatinine clearance in young and elderly volunteers indicate that the difference was due to age-related reductions in creatinine clearance (see Dosage and Administration, Dosing Considerations).

Monitoring and Laboratory Tests: Serum sodium levels below 125 mmol/L have been observed in patients treated with TRILEPTAL (see Warnings and Precautions). Experience from clinical trials indicates that serum sodium levels return toward normal when the TRILEPTAL dosage is reduced or discontinued, or when the patient was treated conservatively (e.g., fluid restriction).

Laboratory data from clinical trials suggest that TRILEPTAL use was associated with decreases in T_4, without changes in T_3 or TSH. Evaluation of thyroid hormone status should be considered for patients treated with oxcarbazepine, particularly for pediatric patients, due to potential risk of sub-clinical or clinical hypothyroidism and adverse effects on development that can occur in relation to undetected changes in thyroid hormone status (see Warnings and Precautions, Endocrine and Metabolism).

ADVERSE REACTIONS: Clinical Trial Adverse Drug Reactions: Because clinical trials are conducted under very specific conditions the adverse reaction rates observed in the clinical trials may not reflect the rates observed in practice and should not be compared to the rates in the clinical trials of another drug. Adverse drug reaction information from clinical trials is useful for identifying drug-related adverse events and for approximating rates.

Most Common Adverse Events in All Clinical Studies: Adjunctive Therapy/Monotherapy in Adults Previously Treated with Other AEDs: The most commonly observed (≥5%) adverse experiences seen in association with TRILEPTAL (oxcarbazepine) and substantially more frequent than in placebo-treated patients were: Dizziness, somnolence, diplopia, fatigue, nausea, vomiting, ataxia, abnormal vision, abdominal pain, tremor, dyspepsia, abnormal gait.

Approximately 23% of these 1537 adult patients discontinued treatment because of an adverse experience. The adverse experience most commonly associated with discontinuation were: dizziness (6.4%), diplopia (5.9%), ataxia (5.2%), vomiting (5.1%), nausea (4.9%), somnolence (3.8%), headache (2.9%), fatigue (2.1%), abnormal vision (2.1%), tremor (1.6%), abnormal gait (1.7%), rash (1.4%), hyponatremia (1.0%).

Monotherapy in Adults not Previously Treated with other AEDs: The most commonly observed (≥5%) adverse experiences seen in association with TRILEPTAL in these patients were similar to those in previously treated patients.

Approximately 9% of these 295 adult patients discontinued treatment because of an adverse experience. The adverse experiences most commonly associated with discontinuation were: dizziness (1.7%), nausea (1.7%), rash (1.7%), headache (1.4%).

Adjunctive Therapy in Pediatric Patients Previously Treated with Other AEDs: The most commonly observed (≥5%) adverse experiences seen in association with TRILEPTAL in these patients were similar to those seen in adults.

Approximately 11% of these 456 pediatric patients discontinued treatment because of an adverse experience. The adverse experiences most commonly associated with discontinuation were: somnolence (2.4%), vomiting (2.0%), ataxia (1.8%), diplopia (1.3%), dizziness (1.3%), fatigue (1.1%), nystagmus (1.1%).

Monotherapy in Pediatric Patients not Previously Treated with Other AEDs: The most commonly observed (≥5%) adverse experiences seen in association with TRILEPTAL in these patients were similar to those in adults.

Approximately 9.2% of 152 pediatric patients discontinued treatment because of an adverse experience. The adverse experiences most commonly associated (≥1%) with discontinuation were rash (5.3%) and maculopapular rash (1.3%).

Incidence in Controlled Clinical Studies: The prescriber should be aware that the figures in Table 1, Table 2, Table 3, Table 4 and Table 5 cannot be used to predict the frequency of adverse experiences in the course of usual medical practice where patient characteristics and other factors may differ from those prevailing during clinical studies. Similarly, the cited frequencies cannot be directly compared with figures obtained from other clinical investigations involving different treatments, uses or investigators. An inspection of these frequencies, however, does provide the prescriber with one basis to estimate the relative contribution of drug and nondrug factors to the adverse event incidences in the population studies.

Controlled Clinical Studies of Adjunctive Therapy/Monotherapy in Adults Previously Treated with Other AEDs: Table 1 lists treatment-emergent signs and symptoms that occurred in at least 2% of adult patients with epilepsy treated with TRILEPTAL or placebo as adjunctive treatment and were numerically more common in the patients treated with any dose of TRILEPTAL. Table 2 lists treatment-emergent signs and symptoms in patients converted from other AEDs to either high dose TRILEPTAL or low dose (300 mg) TRILEPTAL. Note that in some of these monotherapy studies patients who dropped out during a preliminary tolerability phase are not included in the tables.

Table 1: TRILEPTAL

Treatment-Emergent Adverse Event Incidence in a Controlled Clinical Study of Adjunctive Therapy in Adults (events in at least 2% of patients treated with 2400 mg/day of TRILEPTAL and numerically more frequent than in the placebo group)

Body System/ Adverse Event	Oxcarbazepine Dosage (mg/day)			
	OXC 600 N=163 %	OXC 1200 N=171 %	OXC 2400 N=126 %	Placebo N=166 %
Body as a Whole				
Fatigue	15	12	15	7
Asthenia	6	3	6	5
Edema Legs	2	1	2	1
Weight Increase	1	2	2	1
Feeling Abnormal	0	1	2	0
Cardiovascular System				
Hypotension	0	1	2	0
Digestive System				
Nausea	15	25	29	10
Vomiting	13	25	36	5
Pain Abdominal	10	13	11	5
Diarrhea	5	6	7	6
Dyspepsia	5	5	6	2
Constipation	2	2	6	4
Gastritis	2	1	2	1
Metabolic and Nutritional Disorders				
Hyponatremia	3	1	2	1
Musculoskeletal System				
Muscle Weakness	1	2	2	0
Sprains and Strains	0	2	2	1
Nervous System				
Headache	32	28	26	23
Dizziness	26	32	49	13
Somnolence	20	28	36	12
Ataxia	9	17	31	5
Nystagmus	7	20	26	5
Gait Abnormal	5	10	17	1
Insomnia	4	2	3	1
Tremor	3	8	16	5
Nervousness	2	4	2	1
Agitation	1	1	2	1
Coordination Abnormal	1	3	2	1
EEG Abnormal	0	0	2	0
Speech Disorder	1	1	3	0
Confusion	1	1	2	1
Cranial Injury	1	0	2	1
Dysmetria	1	2	3	0
Thinking Abnormal	0	2	4	0
Respiratory System				
Rhinitis	2	4	5	4
Skin and Appendages				
Acne	1	2	2	0
Special Senses				
Diplopia	14	30	40	5
Vertigo	6	12	15	2
Vision Abnormal	6	14	13	4
Accommodation Abnormal	0	0	2	0

Table 2: TRILEPTAL

Treatment-Emergent Adverse Event Incidence in Controlled Clinical Studies of Monotherapy in Adults Previously Treated with Other AEDs (events in at least 2% of patients treated with 2400 mg/day of TRILEPTAL and numerically more frequent than in the low dose control group)

Body System/ Adverse Event	Oxcarbazepine Dosage (mg/day)	
	2400 N=86 %	300 N=86 %
Body as a Whole		
Fatigue	21	5
Fever	3	0
Allergy	2	0
Edema Generalized	2	1
Pain Chest	2	0
Digestive System		
Nausea	22	7
Vomiting	15	5
Diarrhea	7	5
Dyspepsia	6	1
Anorexia	5	3
Pain Abdominal	5	3

(cont'd)

Table 2: TRILEPTAL *(cont'd)*

Treatment-Emergent Adverse Event Incidence in Controlled Clinical Studies of Monotherapy in Adults Previously Treated with Other AEDs (events in at least 2% of patients treated with 2400 mg/day of TRILEPTAL and numerically more frequent than in the low dose control group)

Body System/ Adverse Event	Oxcarbazepine Dosage (mg/day) 2400 N=86 %	300 N=86 %
Mouth Dry	3	0
Hemorrhage Rectum	2	0
Toothache	2	1
Hemic and Lymphatic System		
Lymphadenopathy	2	0
Infections and Infestations		
Infection Viral	7	5
Infection	2	0
Metabolic and Nutritional Disorders		
Hyponatremia	5	0
Thirst	2	0
Nervous System		
Headache	31	15
Dizziness	28	8
Somnolence	19	5
Anxiety	7	5
Ataxia	7	1
Confusion	7	0
Nervousness	7	0
Insomnia	6	3
Tremor	6	3
Amnesia	5	1
Convulsions Aggravated	5	2
Emotional Lability	3	2
Hypoesthesia	3	1
Coordination Abnormal	2	1
Nystagmus	2	0
Speech Disorder	2	0
Respiratory System		
Upper Respiratory Tract Infection	10	5
Coughing	5	0
Bronchitis	3	0
Pharyngitis	3	0
Skin and Appendages		
Hot Flushes	2	1
Purpura	2	0
Special Senses		
Vision Abnormal	14	2
Diplopia	12	1
Taste Perversion	5	0
Vertigo	3	0
Ear Ache	2	1
Ear Infection	2	0

(cont'd)

Table 2: TRILEPTAL *(cont'd)*

Treatment-Emergent Adverse Event Incidence in Controlled Clinical Studies of Monotherapy in Adults Previously Treated with Other AEDs (events in at least 2% of patients treated with 2400 mg/day of TRILEPTAL and numerically more frequent than in the low dose control group)

Body System/ Adverse Event	Oxcarbazepine Dosage (mg/day) 2400 N=86 %	300 N=86 %
Urogenital and Reproductive System		
Urinary Tract Infection	5	1
Micturition Frequency	2	1
Vaginitis	2	0

Controlled Clinical Study of Monotherapy in Adults Not Previously Treated with Other AEDs: Table 3 lists treatment-emergent signs and symptoms in a controlled clinical study of monotherapy in adults not previously treated with other AEDs that occurred in at least 2% of adult patients with epilepsy treated with TRILEPTAL or placebo and were numerically more common in the patients treated with TRILEPTAL.

Table 3: TRILEPTAL

Treatment-Emergent Adverse Event Incidence in a Controlled Clinical Study of Monotherapy in Adults not Previously Treated with Other AEDs (events in at least 2% of patients treated with TRILEPTAL and numerically more frequent than in the placebo group)

Body System/ Adverse Event	Oxcarbazepine N=55 %	Placebo N=49 %
Body as a Whole		
Falling Down	4	0
Digestive System		
Nausea	16	12
Diarrhea	7	2
Vomiting	7	6
Constipation	5	0
Dyspepsia	5	4
Musculoskeletal System		
Back Pain	4	2
Nervous System		
Dizziness	22	6
Headache	13	10
Ataxia	5	0
Nervousness	5	2
Amnesia	4	2
Coordination Abnormal	4	2
Tremor	4	0
Respiratory System		
Upper Respiratory Tract Infection	7	0
Epistaxis	4	0
Infection Chest	4	0
Sinusitis	4	2
Skin and Appendages		
Rash	4	2
Special Senses		
Vision Abnormal	4	0

Controlled Clinical Studies of Adjunctive Therapy/Monotherapy in Pediatric Patients Previously Treated with Other AEDs: Table 4 lists treatment-emergent signs and symptoms that occurred in at least 2% of pediatric patients with epilepsy treated with TRILEPTAL or placebo as adjunctive treatment and were numerically more common in the patients treated with TRILEPTAL.

Controlled Clinical Studies of Monotherapy in Pediatric Patients Not Previously Treated with Other AEDs: Table 5 lists treatment-emergent signs and symptoms regardless of relationship to study drug, in controlled clinical studies of monotherapy in pediatric patients not previously treated with other AEDs. The signs and symptoms listed are the ones that occurred in at least 2% of pediatric patients with epilepsy treated with TRILEPTAL or placebo and were numerically more frequent in the patients treated with TRILEPTAL.

Table 4: TRILEPTAL

Treatment-Emergent Adverse Event Incidence in a Controlled Clinical Study of Adjunctive Therapy in Pediatric Patients Previously Treated with Other AEDs (Events in at least 2% of patients treated with TRILEPTAL and numerically more frequent than in the placebo group)

Body System/ Adverse Event	Oxcarbazepine N=171 %	Placebo N=139 %
Body as a Whole		
Fatigue	13	9
Allergy	2	0
Asthenia	2	1
Digestive System		
Vomiting	33	14
Nausea	19	5
Constipation	4	1
Dyspepsia	2	0
Nervous System		
Headache	31	19
Somnolence	31	13
Dizziness	28	8
Ataxia	13	4
Nystagmus	9	1
Emotional Lability	8	4
Gait Abnormal	8	3
Tremor	6	4
Speech Disorder	3	1
Concentration Impaired	2	1
Convulsions	2	1
Muscle Contractions Involuntary	2	1
Respiratory System		
Rhinitis	10	9
Pneumonia	2	1
Skin and Appendages		
Bruising	4	2
Sweating Increased	3	0
Special Senses		
Diplopia	17	1
Vision Abnormal	13	1
Vertigo	2	0

Table 5: TRILEPTAL

Treatment-Emergent Adverse Event Incidence Regardless of Relationship to Study Drug, in Controlled Clinical Studies of Monotherapy in Pediatric Patients Not Previously Treated with Other AEDs (events in at least 2% of patients treated with TRILEPTAL and numerically more frequent than in the placebo group).

Body System/ Adverse Event	Oxcarbazepine N=129 %	Placebo N=17 %
Body as a Whole		
Fever	14.7	5.9
Chest Pain	3.9	0
Cardiovascular System		
Syncope	3.9	0
Digestive System		
Abdominal Pain	7.8	5.9
Vomiting	7.8	5.9
Anorexia	6.2	5.9
Diarrhea	4.7	0
Gum Hyperplasia	2.3	0
Infections and Infestations		
Viral Infection	18.6	17.6
Parasitic Infection	6.2	0
Musculoskeletal System		
Arthralgia	3.1	0
Leg Pain	3.1	0
Nervous System		
Headache	45.0	17.6
Somnolence	25.6	0
Dizziness	15.5	0
Apathy	9.3	0
Learning Difficulties NOS	3.9	0
Aggressive Reaction	3.1	0
Respiratory System		
Upper Respiratory Tract Infection	7.8	5.9
Epistaxis	3.9	0
Rhinitis	2.3	0
Skin and Appendages		
Acne	6.2	0
Pruritus	4.7	0
Impetigo	2.3	0
Urogenital and Reproductive System		
Dysmenorrhea	2.3	0

Other Events Observed in Association with the Administration of TRILEPTAL: In the paragraphs that follow, the adverse events other than those in the preceding tables or text, that occurred in a total of 565 children and 1574 adults exposed to TRILEPTAL and that are reasonably likely to be related to drug use are presented. Events common in the population, events reflecting chronic illness and events likely to reflect concomitant illness are omitted particularly if minor. They are listed in order of decreasing frequency. Because the reports cite events observed in open label and uncontrolled trials, the role of TRILEPTAL in their causation cannot be reliably determined.

Body as a Whole: fever, malaise, pain chest precordial, rigors, weight decrease.

Cardiovascular System: bradycardia, cardiac failure, cerebral hemorrhage, hypertension, hypotension postural, palpitation, syncope, tachycardia.

Digestive System: appetite increased, blood in stool, cholelithiasis, colitis, duodenal ulcer, dysphagia, enteritis, eructation, esophagitis, flatulence, gastric ulcer, gingival bleeding, gum hyperplasia, hematemesis, hemorrhage rectum, hemorrhoids, hiccup, mouth dry, pain biliary, pain right hypochondrium, retching, sialoadenitis, stomatitis, stomatitis ulcerative.

Hemic and Lymphatic System: leucopenia, thrombocytopenia.

Laboratory Abnormality: gamma-GT increased, hyperglycemia, hypocalcemia, hypoglycemia, hypokalemia, liver enzymes elevated, serum transaminase increased.

Musculoskeletal System: hypertonia muscle.

Nervous System: aggressive reaction, amnesia, anguish, anxiety, apathy, aphasia, aura, convulsions aggravated, delirium, delusion, depressed level of consciousness, dysphonia, dystonia, emotional lability, euphoria, extra pyramidal disorder, feeling drunk, hemiplegia, hyperkinesia, hyperreflexia, hypoesthesia, hypokinesia, hyporeflexia, hypotonia, hysteria, libido decreased, libido increased, manic reaction, migraine, muscle contractions involuntary, nervousness, neuralgia, oculogyric crisis, panic disorder, paralysis, paroniria, personality disorder, psychoses, ptosis, stupor, tetany.

Respiratory System: asthma, dyspnea, epistaxis, laryngismus, pleurisy.

Skin and Appendages: acne, alopecia, angioedema, bruising, dermatitis contact, eczema, facial rash, flushing, folliculitis, heat rash, hot flushes, photosensitivity reaction, pruritis genital, psoriasis, purpura, rash erythematous, rash maculopapular, vitiligo.

Special Senses: accommodation abnormal, cataract, conjunctival hemorrhage, edema eye, hemianopia, mydriasis, otitis externa, photophobia, scotoma, taste perversion, tinnitus, xerophthalmia.

Surgical and Medical Procedures: procedure dental oral, procedure female reproductive, procedure musculoskeletal, procedure skin.

Urogenital and Reproductive System: dysuria, hematuria, intermenstrual bleeding, leukorrhea, menorrhagia, micturition frequency, pain renal, pain urinary tract, polyuria, priapism, renal calculus.

Other: system lupus erythematosus.

Post-Market Adverse Drug Reactions: The following adverse events not seen in controlled clinical trials have been observed in named patient programs or post-marketing experience:

Body as a Whole: multi-organ hypersensitivity disorders characterized by features such as rash, fever, lymphadenopathy, abnormal liver function tests, eosinophilia and arthralgia (see Warning and Precautions, Multi-Organ Hypersensitivity), anaphylactic reactions (see Warning and Precautions, Hypersensitivity).

Digestive System: pancreatitis and/or lipase and/or amylase increase.

Hemic and Lymphatic System: bone marrow depression, agranulocytosis, aplastic anemia, pancytopenia, neutropenia (see Warning and Precautions, Hematologic).

Metabolism and Nutrition Disorders: folic acid deficiency, abnormal thyroid function tests (decreased total T_4 and/or free T_4), hypothyroidism (see Warnings and Precautions, Endocrine and Metabolism).

Skin and Appendages: erythema multiforme, Stevens-Johnson syndrome, toxic epidermal necrolysis (see Warning and Precautions, Serious Dermatological Reactions).

DRUG INTERACTIONS: Overview: Enzyme Inhibition: Oxcarbazepine was evaluated in human liver microsomes to determine its capacity to inhibit the major cytochrome P450 enzymes responsible for the metabolism of other drugs. The results demonstrate that oxcarbazepine and its pharmacologically active metabolite (the monohydroxy derivative, MHD) inhibit the CYP2C19. Therefore, interactions could arise when co-administering high doses (e.g. 2400 mg/day) of TRILEPTAL with drugs that are metabolised by CYP2C19 (e.g. phenobarbital, phenytoin, see below). In some patients treated with TRILEPTAL and drugs metabolized via CYP2C19 a reduction of the co-administered drugs might be necessary. In human liver microsomes, oxcarbazepine and MHD have little or no capacity to function as inhibitors for the following enzymes: CYP1A2, CYP2A6, CYP2C9, CYP2D6, CYP2E1, CYP4A9 and CYP4A11.

Enzyme Induction: Oxcarbazepine and MHD induce in vitro and in vivo, the cytochromes CYP3A4 and CYP3A5 responsible for the metabolism of dihydropyridine calcium antagonists, oral contraceptives, and AEDs (e.g. carbamazepine) resulting in a lower plasma concentration of these medicinal products (see below). Such level of decrease in plasma concentrations may also be observed in other drugs mainly metabolized by CYP3A4 and CYP3A5, for example immunosuppressants (e.g. cyclosporine).

In vitro, oxcarbazepine and MHD are weak inducers of UDP–glucuronyl transferase and, therefore, in vivo they are unlikely to have an effect on drugs which are mainly eliminated by conjugation through the UDP-glucuronyl transferases (e.g. valproic acid, lamotrigine). Even in view of the weak induction potential of oxcarbazepine and MHD, a higher dose of concomitantly used drugs which are metabolized via CYP3A4 or via conjugation (UDPGT) may be necessary. In the case of discontinuation of TRILEPTAL therapy, a dose reduction of the concomitant medication may be necessary. Induction studies conducted with human hepatocytes confirmed oxcarbazepine and MHD as weak inducers of isoenzymes of the 2B and 3A4 CYP sub-family. The induction potential of oxcarbazepine/MHD on other CYP isoenzymes is not known.

Drug-Drug Interactions: Antiepileptic Drugs: Potential interactions between TRILEPTAL and other AEDs were assessed in clinical studies. The effect of these interactions on mean AUCs and C_{min} are summarized in Table 6.

In vivo, the plasma levels of phenytoin increased by up to 40% when TRILEPTAL was given at doses above 1200 mg/day. Therefore, when using doses of TRILEPTAL greater than 1200 mg/day during adjunctive therapy, a decrease in the dose of phenytoin may be required (see Dosage and Administration). The increase of phenobarbital level, however, is small (15%) when given with TRILEPTAL.

Strong inducers of cytochrome P450 enzymes (i.e., carbamazepine, phenytoin and phenobarbital) have been shown to decrease the plasma levels of MHD (29%-40%).

No autoinduction has been observed with TRILEPTAL.

Table 6: TRILEPTAL

Summary of AED Interactions with TRILEPTAL

AED Coadministered	Dose of AED (mg/day)	TRILEPTAL Dose (mg/day)	Influence of TRILEPTAL on AED Concentration (Mean Change, 90% Confidence Interval)	Influence of AED on MHD Concentration (Mean Change, 90% Confidence Interval)
Carbamazepine	400–1200	900	nc[a]	40% decrease [CI: 17% decrease, 57% decrease]
Phenobarbital	100–150	600–1800	14% increase [CI: 2% increase, 24% increase]	25% decrease [CI: 12% decrease, 51% decrease]
Phenytoin	250–500	600–1800 >1200–2400	nc[a,b] up to 40% increase[c] [CI: 12% increase, 60% increase]	30% decrease [CI: 3% decrease, 48% decrease]
Valproic acid	400–2800	600–1800	nc[a]	18% decrease [CI: 13% decrease, 40% decrease]

a nc denotes a mean change of less than 10%.
b Pediatrics.
c Mean increase in adults at high TRILEPTAL doses.

Hormonal Contraceptives: Co-administration of TRILEPTAL with an oral contraceptive has been shown to influence the plasma concentrations of the two hormonal components, ethinylestradiol (EE) and levonorgestrel (LNG). The mean AUC values of EE were decreased by 48% [90% CI: 22-65] in one study and 52% [90% CI: 38-52] in another study. The mean AUC values of LNG were decreased by 32% [90% CI: 20-45] in one study and 52% [90% CI: 42-52] in another study. Therefore, concurrent use of TRILEPTAL with hormonal contraceptives may render these contraceptives ineffective. Studies with other oral or implant contraceptives have not been conducted.

Calcium Antagonists: After repeated co-administration of TRILEPTAL, the AUC of felodipine was lowered by 28% [90% CI: 20-33]. Verapamil produced a decrease of 20% [90% CI: 18-27] of the plasma levels of MHD.

Other Drug Interactions: Cimetidine, erythromycin and dextropropoxyphene had no effect on the pharmacokinetics of MHD. Results with warfarin show no evidence of interaction with either single or repeated doses of TRILEPTAL.

Drug-Laboratory Test Interactions: There are no known interactions of TRILEPTAL with commonly used laboratory tests.

DOSAGE AND ADMINISTRATION: Dosing Considerations:

- Patients with Hepatic Impairment: In general, dose adjustments are not required in patients with mild to moderate hepatic impairment (see Action and Clinical Pharmacology,Special Populations and Conditions).
- Patients with Renal Impairment: In patients with impaired renal function (creatinine clearance <30 mL/min) TRILEPTAL therapy should be initiated at one-half the usual starting dose (300 mg/day) and increased slowly to achieve the desired clinical response (see Action and Clinical Pharmacology, Special Populations and Conditions).
- Geriatrics: There were 52 patients over age 65 in controlled trials and 565 patients over the age of 65 in other trials. Following administration of single (300 mg) and multiple (600 mg/day) doses of TRILEPTAL to elderly volunteers (60-82 years of age), the maximum plasma concentrations and AUC values of MHD were 30%-60% higher than in younger volunteers (18-32 years of age). Comparisons of creatinine clearance in young and elderly volunteers indicate that the difference was due to age-related reductions in creatinine clearance. Dosage should be carefully titrated in the elderly.

Recommended Dose and Dosage Adjustment: TRILEPTAL (oxcarbazepine) is indicated for use as monotherapy or adjunctive therapy in the treatment of partial seizures in adults and children ages 6-16. All dosing should be given in a twice a day (BID) regimen.

Adults: Adjunctive Therapy: Treatment with TRILEPTAL should be initiated with a dose of 600 mg/day, given in a BID regimen. If clinically indicated, the dose may be increased by a maximum of 600 mg/day at approximately weekly intervals; the recommended daily dose is 1200 mg/day. Daily doses above 1200 mg/day show somewhat greater effectiveness in controlled trials, but most patients were not able to tolerate the 2400 mg/day dose, primarily because of CNS effects. It is recommended that the patient be observed closely and plasma levels of the concomitant AEDs be monitored during the period of TRILEPTAL titration, as these plasma levels may be altered, especially at TRILEPTAL doses greater than 1200 mg/day (see Drug Interactions).

Conversion to Monotherapy: Patients receiving concomitant AEDs may be converted to monotherapy by initiating treatment with TRILEPTAL at 600 mg/day (given in a BID regimen) while simultaneously initiating the reduction of the dose of the concomitant AEDs. The concomitant AEDs should be completely withdrawn over 3-6 weeks, while the maximum dose of TRILEPTAL should be reached in about 2-4 weeks.TRILEPTAL may be increased as clinically indicated by a maximum increment of 600 mg/day at approximately weekly intervals to achieve the daily dose of 2400 mg/day. A daily dose of 1200 mg/day has been shown in one study to be effective in patients in whom monotherapy has been initiated with TRILEPTAL. Patients should be observed closely during this transition phase.

Initiation of Monotherapy: Patients not currently being treated with AEDs may have monotherapy initiated with TRILEPTAL. In these patients, TRILEPTAL should be initiated at a dose of 600 mg/day (given in a BID regimen); the dose should be increased by 300 mg/day every third day to a dose of 1200 mg/day. Controlled trials in these patients examined the effectiveness of a 1200 mg/day dose; a dose of 2400 mg/day has been shown to be effective in patients converted from other AEDs to TRILEPTAL monotherapy (see above).

Pediatric Patients Ages 6-16: Adjunctive Therapy: Treatment should be initiated at a daily dose of 8-10 mg/kg generally not to exceed 600 mg/day, given in a BID regimen. The target maintenance dose of TRILEPTAL should be achieved over 2 weeks, and is dependent upon patient weight, according to the following chart:

20–29 kg	900 mg/day
29.1–39 kg:	1200 mg/day
>39 kg:	1800 mg/day

In the clinical trial, in which the intention was to reach these target doses, the median daily dose was 31 mg/kg with a range of 6-51 mg/kg.

The pharmacokinetics of TRILEPTAL are similar in older children (age >8 yrs) and adults. However, younger children (age <8 yrs) have an increased clearance (by about 30-40%) compared with older children and adults. In the controlled trial, pediatric patients 8 years old and below received the highest maintenance doses.

Conversion to Monotherapy: Patients receiving concomitant antiepileptic drugs may be converted to monotherapy by initiating treatment with TRILEPTAL at approximately 8-10 mg/kg/day given in a BID regimen, while simultaneously initiating the reduction of the dose of the concomitant antiepileptic drugs. The concomitant antiepileptic drugs can be completely withdrawn over 3-6 weeks while TRILEPTAL may be increased as clinically indicated by a maximum increment of 10 mg/kg/day at approximately weekly intervals to achieve the recommended daily dose. Patients should be observed closely during this transition phase.

The recommended total daily dose of TRILEPTAL is shown in Table 7.

Initiation of Monotherapy: Patients not currently being treated with antiepileptic drugs may have monotherapy initiated with TRILEPTAL. In these patients, TRILEPTAL should be initiated at a dose of 8-10 mg/kg/day given in a BID regimen. The dose should be increased by 5 mg/kg/day every third day to the recommended daily dose shown in Table 7.

Table 7: TRILEPTAL

Range of Maintenance Doses of TRILEPTAL for Children by Weight During Monotherapy

Weight in kg	From Dose (mg/day)	To Dose (mg/day)
20	600	900
25	900	1200
30	900	1200
35	900	1500
40	900	1500
45	1200	1500
50	1200	1800
55	1200	1800
60	1200	2100
65	1200	2100
70	1500	2100

Children below 2 years of age have not been studied in controlled clinical trials.

Administration: Before using TRILEPTAL oral suspension, shake the bottle well and prepare the dose immediately afterwards.The prescribed amount of oral suspension should be withdrawn from the bottle using the oral dosing syringe supplied. TRILEPTAL oral suspension can be mixed in a small glass of water just prior to administration or, alternatively, may be swallowed directly from the syringe. After use, rinse the syringe with water and shake out as much residual liquid as possible and leave out to dry.

TRILEPTAL can be taken with or without food.

OVERDOSAGE:

Human Overdose Experience: Isolated cases of overdose with TRILEPTAL (oxcarbazepine) have been reported. The maximum dose taken was approximately 24 000 mg. All patients recovered with symptomatic treatment. Symptoms of overdose include somnolence, dizziness, nausea, vomiting, hyperkinesia, hyponatremia, ataxia, and nystagmus.

Treatment and Management: There is no specific antidote. Symptomatic and supportive treatment should be administered as appropriate. Removal of the drug by gastric lavage and/or inactivation by administering activated charcoal should be considered.

> For management of a suspected drug overdose, contact your regional Poison Control Centre. See the *CPS* Directory section for a list of Poison Control Centres.

ACTION AND CLINICAL PHARMACOLOGY: Mechanism of Action: The pharmacological activity of TRILEPTAL (oxcarbazepine) is primarily exerted through the 10-monohydroxy metabolite (MHD) of oxcarbazepine (see Metabolism and Excretion). The precise mechanism by which oxcarbazepine and MHD exert their antiseizure effect is unknown; however, in vitro electrophysiological studies indicate that they produce blockade of voltage-sensitive sodium channels, resulting in stabilization of hyperexcited neural membranes, inhibition of repetitive neuronal firing, and diminution of propagation of synaptic impulses. These actions are thought to be important in the prevention of seizure spread in the intact brain. In addition, increased potassium conductance and modulation of high-voltage activated calcium channels may contribute to the anticonvulsant effects of the drug. No significant interactions of oxcarbazepine or MHD with brain neurotransmitter or modulator receptor sites have been demonstrated.

Pharmacodynamics: Oxcarbazepine and its active metabolite (MHD) exhibit anticonvulsant properties in animal seizure models. They protected rodents against electrically induced tonic extension seizures and, to a lesser degree, chemically induced clonic seizures, and abolished or reduced the frequency of chronically recurring focal seizures in Rhesus monkeys with aluminum implants. No development of tolerance (i.e., attenuation of anticonvulsive activity) was observed in the maximal electroshock test when mice and rats were treated daily for 5 days and 4 weeks, respectively, with oxcarbazepine or MHD.

Pharmacokinetics: Absorption: Following oral administration of TRILEPTAL, oxcarbazepine is completely absorbed and extensively metabolized to its pharmacologically active 10-monohydroxy metabolite (MHD). The half life of the parent is about 2 hours, while the half-life of MHD is about 9 hours, so that MHD is responsible for most antiepileptic activity.

After single dose administration of TRILEPTAL tablets to healthy male volunteers under fasted conditions, the median t_{max} was 4.5 (range 3 to 13 hours).

After single dose administration of 600 mg TRILEPTAL oral suspension to healthy male volunteers under fasted conditions, the mean C_{max} value of MHD was 24.9 µmol/L, with a corresponding median t_{max} of 6 hours.

The TRILEPTAL tablet and suspension dosage forms were found to be bioequivalent in an open-label, randomized, balanced, three-period cross-over study conducted in 20 healthy volunteers and comparing the 600 mg tablet formulation to 10 mL of the 60 mg/mL oral suspension. At steady-state under fasted conditions, the median T_{max} values were identical (4.0 h) and the mean C_{max} values were nearly identical (89.4 µmol/L versus 91.1 µmol/L, respectively for the tablet and suspension). The AUC $_{(0-12\ h)}$ was 900 h·µmol/L for the tablet and 916 h·µmol/L for the suspension.

In a mass balance study in people, only 2% of total radioactivity in plasma was due to unchanged oxcarbazepine, with approximately 70% present as MHD, and the remainder attributable to minor metabolites. Food has no effect on the rate and extent of absorption of oxcarbazepine.

Steady-state plasma concentrations of MHD are reached within 2-3 days in patients when TRILEPTAL is given twice a day. At steady-state the pharmacokinetics of MHD are linear and show dose proportionality over the dose range of 300 to 2400 mg/day.

Distribution: The apparent volume of distribution of MHD is 49 L.

Approximately 40% of MHD is bound to serum proteins, predominantly to albumin. Binding is independent of the serum concentration within the therapeutically relevant range. Oxcarbazepine and MHD do not bind to alpha-1-acid glycoprotein.

Metabolism: Oxcarbazepine is rapidly reduced by cytosolic enzymes in the liver to its 10-monohydroxy metabolite, MHD, which is primarily responsible for the pharmacological effect of TRILEPTAL. MHD is metabolized further by conjugation with glucuronic acid. Minor amounts (4% of the dose) are oxidized to the pharmacologically inactive 10,11 dihydroxy metabolite (DHD).

Excretion: Oxcarbazepine is cleared from the body mostly in the form of metabolites which are predominantly excreted by the kidneys. More than 95% of the dose appears in the urine, with less than 1% as unchanged oxcarbazepine. Fecal excretion accounts for less than 4% of the administered dose. Approximately 80% of the dose is excreted in the urine either as glucuronides of MHD (49%) or as unchanged MHD (27%); the inactive DHD accounts for approximately 3% and conjugates of MHD and oxcarbazepine account for 13% of the dose.

Special Populations and Conditions: Pediatrics: After a single-dose administration of 5 or 15 mg/kg of TRILEPTAL, the dose adjusted AUC values of MHD were 30%-40% lower in children below the age of 8 years than in children above 8 years of age. The clearance in children greater than 8 years old approaches that of adults.

Pregnancy: Due to physiological changes during pregnancy, MHD plasma levels may gradually decrease throughout pregnancy (see Warnings and Precautions, Special Populations, Pregnant Women).

Geriatrics: Following administration of single (300 mg) and multiple (600 mg/day) doses of TRILEPTAL to elderly volunteers (60-82 years of age), the maximum plasma concentrations and AUC values of MHD were 30%-60% higher than in younger volunteers (18-32 years of age). Comparisons of creatinine clearance in young and elderly volunteers indicate that the difference was due to age-related reductions in creatinine clearance.

Gender: No gender related pharmacokinetic differences have been observed in children, adults, or the elderly.

Race: No specific studies have been conducted to assess what effect, if any, race may have on the disposition of oxcarbazepine.

Hepatic Insufficiency: The pharmacokinetics and metabolism of oxcarbazepine and MHD were evaluated in healthy volunteers and hepatically-impaired subjects after a single 900 mg oral dose. Mild-to-moderate hepatic impairment did not affect the pharmacokinetics of oxcarbazepine and MHD. No dose adjustment for TRILEPTAL is recommended in patients with mild-to-moderate hepatic impairment. The pharmacokinetics of oxcarbazepine and MHD have not been evaluated in severe hepatic impairment.

Renal Insufficiency: There is a linear correlation between creatinine clearance and the renal clearance of MHD. When TRILEPTAL is administered as a single 300 mg dose in renally impaired patients (creatinine clearance <30 mL/min), the elimination half-life of MHD is prolonged to 19 hours, with a two fold increase in AUC. Dose adjustment for TRILEPTAL is recommended in these patients (see Warnings and Precautions and Dosage and Administration).

STORAGE AND STABILITY: Tablets: Store at 15-30°C.

Suspension: Store TRILEPTAL oral suspension at 15-30°C in the original package. Use within 7 weeks after first opening the bottle.

The suspension is off-white to slightly brown or slightly red.

TRILEPTAL must be kept out of the reach and sight of children.

INFORMATION FOR THE PATIENT: Published in e-CPS, available by subscription at www.e-cps.ca.

DOSAGE FORMS, COMPOSITION AND PACKAGING: Suspension: Each mL of off-white to slightly brown or slightly red oral suspension contains: oxcarbazepine 60 mg. Nonmedicinal ingredients: ascorbic acid, carboxymethylcellulose sodium, ethanol, microcrystalline cellulose, methylparaben, polyethylene glycol-400 stearate, propylene glycol, propylparaben, purified water, sodium saccharin, sorbic acid, sorbitol and yellow plum-lemon aroma. Brown (amber) glass bottles of 250 mL with safety closure (child-resistant cap), one 10 mL dosing syringe and one press-in bottle adaptor.

Tablets: 150 mg: Each film-coated, pale grey green, ovaloid, slightly biconvex tablet, scored on both sides, and imprinted with T/D on one side and C/G on the other side, contains: oxcarbazepine 150 mg. Nonmedicinal ingredients: colloidal silicon dioxide, crospovidone, hydroxypropyl methylcellulose, magnesium stearate, microcrystalline cellulose, polyethylene glycol, talc, titanium dioxide and yellow and/or black and/or red iron oxides. Blister packs of 50 (5 strips of 10).

300 mg: Each film-coated, yellow, ovaloid, slightly biconvex tablet, scored on both sides and imprinted with TE/TE on one side and CG/CG on the other side, contains: oxcarbazepine 300 mg. Nonmedicinal ingredients: colloidal silicon dioxide, crospovidone, hydroxypropyl methylcellulose, magnesium stearate, microcrystalline cellulose, polyethylene glycol, talc, titanium dioxide and yellow and/or black and/or red iron oxides. Blister packs of 50 (5 strips of 10).

600 mg: Each light pink, ovaloid, slightly biconvex tablet, scored on both sides and imprinted with TF/TF on one side and CG/CG on the other side, contains: oxcarbazepine 600 mg. Nonmedicinal ingredients: colloidal silicon dioxide, crospovidone, hydroxypropyl methylcellulose, magnesium stearate, microcrystalline cellulose, polyethylene glycol, talc, titanium dioxide and yellow and/or black and/or red iron oxides. Blister packs of 50 (5 strips of 10).

(Shown in Product Identification Section)

Trimethoprim
Antibacterial

CPhA Monograph

Date of Preparation: October 2007

This monograph has been compiled by CPhA and reviewed by experts. It may contain information different from that found in Health Canada-approved Product Monographs. The reader is referred to the *CPS* Editorial Policy for more information.

SUMMARY PRODUCT INFORMATION:

Route of Administration	Dosage Form	Strength
Oral	Tablet	100 mg, 200 mg

INDICATIONS AND CLINICAL USE: Trimethoprim is indicated for:

- treatment of acute, uncomplicated urinary tract infections (UTIs) due to susceptible strains of *E. coli*, *K. pneumoniae*, *P. mirabilis*, Enterobacter species and *S. saprophyticus*.

Trimethoprim is recommended empirically as a first-line agent for the treatment of acute, uncomplicated UTIs in women > 12 years; as a first-line prophylactic agent in patients with chronic recurrent cystitis in women; as a first-line in the treatment of uncomplicated, non-obstructive, mild pyelonephritis; and as first-line treatment of acute, mild to moderate prostatitis. Alternative therapy should be considered, however, in areas in which prevalence of *E. coli* resistance is > 20%.

Trimethoprim is recommended as a first-line prophylactic agent in asymptomatic bacteriuria in pregnant women and in those undergoing pre-operative genitourinary procedures. Trimethoprim is recommended as a second-line treatment in acute cystitis in pregnant women (see Warnings and Precautions, Special Populations, Pregnant Women). Alternative agents should be considered in areas in which prevalence to *E. coli* resistance is > 20%.

The combination of trimethoprim with dapsone is used as an alternative treatment for *P. jirovecii* pneumonia.

The spectrum of activity of trimethoprim includes gram-negative organisms including *E. coli*, Klebsiella spp, Enterobacter spp, *M. morganii*, *P. mirabilis* and *P. vulgaris*. Trimethoprim is active against certain nonbacterial pathogens such as *P. jirovecii*.

Pediatrics: Trimethoprim is used as a second-line agent in the treatment of acute urinary tract infection in children. It may be used as prophylaxis in children with vesicoureteral reflux. Trimethoprim is recommended as a second-line agent in children > 9 years for the treatment of nongonococcal urethritis.

CONTRAINDICATIONS:

- Patients who are hypersensitive to trimethoprim or to any ingredient in the formulation or component of the container.
- Patients with documented megaloblastic anemia due to folate deficiency.

WARNINGS AND PRECAUTIONS:

Serious Warnings and Precautions

- Death has occurred due to serious adverse effects of trimethoprim such as toxic epidermal necrolysis.
- Administer trimethoprim with caution to those with possible folate deficiency.
- Trimethoprim has been associated with cholestatic jaundice, megaloblastic anemia, thrombocytopenia, leukopenia and bone marrow toxicity.

Special Populations: Pregnant Women: Category C. Trimethoprim crosses the placenta. The drug levels are similar in maternal and fetal serum and in amniotic fluid. Trimethoprim use during the first trimester may limit the availability of folic acid to the fetus and therefore be associated with structural defects in the newborn. (See Indications and Clinical Use.) The risk of neural tube defects is increased by treatment with trimethoprim. An increased risk of cardiovascular defects was found in newborns when trimethoprim was taken in the second or third month of pregnancy.

Nursing Women: Because trimethoprim is excreted into breast milk in low concentrations, the levels may be negligible to the infant. According to the American Academy of Pediatrics, the combination of sulfamethoxazole and trimethoprim is compatible with breastfeeding.

Geriatrics: Elderly patients may have an increased risk of severe adverse reactions to trimethoprim, especially in those with impaired renal function or in those receiving drugs with the potential to interact with trimethoprim.

Monitoring and Laboratory Tests: Monitor renal function (serum creatinine, urea) and perform urinalysis in patients with renal impairment. Monitor complete blood count in those at higher risk of folate deficiency or during long-term therapy. Monitor serum potassium in patients at risk of hyperkalemia.

ADVERSE REACTIONS: Adverse Drug Reactions Overview: Although trimethoprim is generally well tolerated, deaths have rarely been associated with hypersensitivity reactions, fulminant hepatocellular necrosis, agranulocytosis, aplastic anemia or other blood dyscrasias.

More Common Adverse Drug Reactions: See Table 1.

Table 1: Trimethoprim

More Common Adverse Drug Reactions (≥1%)

Body System	Effect	Clinical Comment
Dermatologic	Pruritus, rash	Frequency of maculopapular rash increases with higher doses of trimethoprim.
Gastrointestinal	Nausea, vomiting	Incidence and severity may be dose-related.
Renal	↑ creatinine	May ↑ creatinine without affecting glomerular filtration rate due to inhibition of tubular secretion of creatinine.

Less Common Adverse Drug Reactions (< 1%): Central Nervous System: aseptic meningitis, encephalitis.

Allergic/Dermatologic: erythema multiforme, exfoliative dermatitis, Stevens-Johnson syndrome, toxic epidermal necrolysis, erythematous skin eruptions, fixed drug eruption.

Endocrine and Metabolism: hyperkalemia (dose dependent), hyponatremia, arthritis.

Gastrointestinal: glossitis.

Hematologic: leukopenia, megaloblastic anemia, neutropenia, thrombocytopenia.

Hepatic/Biliary/Pancreatic: elevated serum transaminases, cholestatic jaundice.

Immune: anaphylaxis, vasculitis.

Ophthalmologic: uveitis.

DRUG INTERACTIONS: Overview: Folic acid may be administered during therapy with trimethoprim without interfering with its antibacterial effect.

Drug-Drug Interactions: See Table 2.

Table 2: Trimethoprim

Drug-Drug Interactions

Interacting Drug	Effect	Clinical Comment
Angiotensin Converting Enzyme Inhibitors	↑ potassium levels	Monitor serum potassium and renal function, especially if other co-existing factors for hyperkalemia are present such as diabetes mellitus, pre-existing renal dysfunction and age-related decline in glomerular filtration rate.
Cyclosporine	↓ serum concentration of cyclosporine. Risk of nephrotoxicity may ↑ with combination.	If administered concomitantly, monitor renal function and cyclosporine levels. Adjust cyclosporine dose during trimethoprim treatment and upon discontinuation.
Dapsone	Serum levels of both drugs may ↑ due to interference with clearance. May lead to ↑ toxicity from either agent.	Monitor for signs and symptoms of toxicity (e.g., methemoglobinemia, leukopenia, rash, fever, vomiting). Combination of trimethoprim and dapsone may result in megaloblastic anemia in patients with underlying vitamin B_{12} deficiency, especially in AIDS patients.
Lamivudine	May ↑ plasma lamivudine levels through inhibiting renal secretion.	Not clinically significant. Consider adjusting lamivudine dose in renal impairment.
Methotrexate	May ↑ the risk of methotrexate-induced hematologic toxicity (e.g., bone marrow suppression, megaloblastic anemia, pancytopenia).	If concomitant treatment is necessary, monitor patients (e.g., elderly) closely for signs of hematologic toxicity. Monitor CBC with differential.
Phenytoin	Inhibition of hepatic metabolism of phenytoin. May ↑ serum phenytoin concentrations.	Monitor for ↑ pharmacologic and adverse effects of phenytoin. Monitor phenytoin levels during trimethoprim treatment and after discontinuation.

(cont'd)

Table 2: Trimethoprim *(cont'd)*

Drug-Drug Interactions

Interacting Drug	Effect	Clinical Comment
Procainamide	Reduces renal clearance through ↓ net tubular cationic secretion. May ↑ plasma concentrations of procainamide and its active metabolite, N-acetylprocainamide (NAPA).	Monitor procainamide and NAPA levels and adjust dose accordingly upon addition and discontinuation of trimethoprim.
Repaglinide	May ↑ repaglinide plasma concentration by inhibiting its CYP2C8 metabolism.	Monitor blood glucose levels during trimethoprim treatment and after discontinuation. Adjust repaglinide dose if necessary.
Rosiglitazone	May ↑ rosiglitazone plasma concentration by inhibiting its CYP2C8 metabolism.	Monitor blood glucose levels during trimethoprim treatment and after discontinuation. Adjust rosiglitazone dose if necessary.
Theophylline	May ↑ the risk of developing hyponatremia.	Monitor for symptoms of hyponatremia, e.g., fatigue, weakness, nausea, vomiting, dizziness.
Zidovudine	May ↑ plasma concentration of zidovudine by ↓ renal clearance	Monitor for increased pharmacologic and adverse effects (gastrointestinal disturbances, headache, fatigue) of zidovudine. Consider adjusting zidovudine dose in renal impairment.

Drug-Food Interactions: May be taken with food or milk to minimize gastrointestinal upset.
Drug-Laboratory Interactions: Trimethoprim does not interfere with the radioimmunoassay method for determining serum methotrexate levels; however, trimethoprim interferes with methotrexate assays that use a competitive binding protein technique with bacterial dihydrofolate reductase as the binding protein.

Falsely elevated creatinine values (overestimation of 10%) may result from trimethoprim therapy using creatinine assays using the Jaffe alkaline picrate reactions.

Serum alkaline phosphatase levels may be elevated by trimethoprim.

Serum potassium levels may be elevated by trimethoprim.

DOSAGE AND ADMINISTRATION: Recommended Dose and Dosage Adjustment: Adults: See Table 3.
Pediatrics: See Table 4.
Renal Impairment: See Table 5.
Dialysis: Trimethoprim is dialyzable. A maintenance dose is recommended after dialysis.

Table 3: Trimethoprim

Dose in Adult Patients

Indication	Usual Dose	Duration of Therapy	Clinical Comment
Bacteriuria, asymptomatic	100 mg po q12h or 200 mg po q24h	3 days	Avoid in first trimester of pregnancy due to concerns of limiting availability of folic acid to the fetus thereby increasing the risk of neural tube defects. Follow-up culture after completion of therapy and monthly culture is recommended in pregnancy. Screening for asymptomatic bacteriuria is recommended in patients undergoing pre-operative genitourinary procedures and in pregnancy.
Cystitis, recurrent (< 1 month)	100 mg po BID or 200 mg po daily	10–14 days	
Cystitis, recurrent (≥ 3 episodes/ year)	Prophylaxis: 100 mg po QHS or post-coital	≥ 3 UTIs/year: 12 months	With suppressive therapy, bacterial growth is suppressed. Active infection is not eliminated. If < 3 UTIs/year: consider short course self-treatment.
Urinary tract infection, acute uncomplicated	100 mg po q12h or 200 mg po q24h	7–10 days	First-line agent. May be used as an alternative in patients with a sulfa allergy. Monotherapy as effective as sulfamethoxazole-trimethoprim with comparatively fewer side effects. Avoid in first trimester of pregnancy. Recommended if prevalence of resistant *E. coli* is < 20%. Consider resistance in patients who have failed empiric therapy or who have had recent TMP therapy.
	100–200 mg po BID	3 days	First-line agent. Monotherapy as effective as sulfamethoxazole-trimethoprim with fewer side effects. Avoid in first trimester of pregnancy. Recommended if prevalence of resistant *E. coli* is < 20%. Consider resistance in patients who have failed empiric therapy or who have had recent TMP therapy.
Urinary tract infections, prophylaxis	100 mg po once daily	< 3 UTIs/year: 6 months ≥ 3 UTIs/year: 12 months	With suppressive therapy, bacterial growth is suppressed. Active infection is not eliminated.
Pneumonia, *P. jirovecii*	15–20 mg/kg po daily divided q6–8h	21 days	Alternative agent for mild to moderate disease. Administered in conjunction with dapsone 100 mg po daily × 21 days.
Prostatitis, acute	200 mg po q12h	4–12 weeks	For mild to moderate acute prostatitis. Only prescribed once culture and sensitivity results are available. Used in situations where prevalence of resistant *E. coli* is < 20%. Used in sulfa-allergic patients.
Prostatitis, chronic	200 mg po BID	4–6 weeks	Second-line agent.
Pyelonephritis, uncomplicated, non-obstruction, mild	100 mg po BID or 200 mg po daily	10–14 days	

Table 4: Trimethoprim

Dose in Pediatric Patients

Indication	Usual Dose	Duration of Therapy	Clinical Comment
Urethritis, nongonococcal	< 9 y: 4 mg/kg daily po divided q12h	10 days	Second- line agent.
Urinary tract infection, uncomplicated	< 12 y: 4 mg/kg daily po divided q12h, max 200 mg/day	10 days	Second- line agent.
Urinary tract infection, prophylaxis	2 mg/kg daily po divided BID or given as a single dose		
Vesicoureteral Reflux	¼ to ⅓ of the dose necessary to treat an acute infection given once daily	Continue until the child remains free of infection	Continue prophylaxis with trimethoprim until resolution of reflux or until the risk of reflux is considered low by the physician. Perform a urine culture and sensitivity test if there are signs and symptoms of a urinary tract infection.

Table 5: Trimethoprim

Dose in Adult Patients with Renal Impairment

Creatinine Clearance	Interval Adjustment
> 30 mL/min	q12h
10–30 mL/min	q18h
< 10 mL/min	q24h

OVERDOSAGE:

For management of a suspected drug overdose, CPhA recommends that you contact your **regional Poison Control Centre**. See the *CPS* Directory section for a list of Poison Control Centres.

ACTION AND CLINICAL PHARMACOLOGY: Mechanism of Action: Trimethoprim reversibly inhibits dihydrofolate reductase in susceptible bacteria preventing the conversion of dihydrofolic acid to tetrahydrofolic acid. Tetrahydrofolic acid is a precursor required for de novo synthesis of purines. By blocking the enzyme, trimethoprim inhibits bacterial DNA replication and transcription.

Trimethoprim is 50 000 to 100 000 times more active against bacterial dihydrofolate reductase than human dihydrofolate reductase. For this reason, human purine synthesis is not significantly affected.
Pharmacokinetics: Adults: See Table 6.

Table 6: Trimethoprim

Summary of the Pharmacokinetic Properties of Trimethoprim After Oral Administration

Oral bioavailability	80-90%	
Serum half-life	Normal renal function: 9–13 h End-stage renal disease: 20–49 h	
Peak serum concentration following single-dose oral administration (within 1–4 hours after administration)	100 mg	1 μg/L
	200 mg	2 μg/L
Range of urine concentration following single-dose oral administration of 100 mg	30–60 μg/mL	
Plasma protein binding (%)	30–70	
Volume of distribution (L/kg)	1.0–2.2	
Total clearance	0.12 L/hour/kg	
Primary route of elimination	60-80% renally excreted unchanged	

Trinipatch™

nitroglycerin

Antianginal

Paladin

Date of Preparation: January 13, 2009

SUMMARY PRODUCT INFORMATION:

Route of Administration	Dosage Form/ Strength	Clinically Relevant Nonmedicinal Ingredients
Dermal	Transdermal delivery system Patch 0.2 mg/h, 7 cm² Patch 0.4 mg/h, 14 cm² Patch 0.6 mg/h, 21 cm²	None

DESCRIPTION: The TRINIPATCH (nitroglycerin) transdermal system is a flat unit designed to provide continuous controlled release of nitroglycerin through intact skin. The rate of release of nitroglycerin is linearly dependent upon the area of the applied system; each cm² of applied system delivers approximately 0.03 mg of nitroglycerin per hour. Thus, the 7, 14 and 21 cm² systems deliver approximately 0.2, 0.4 and 0.6 mg of nitroglycerin per hour, respectively.

The remainder of the nitroglycerin in each system serves as a reservoir and is not delivered in normal use. After 12 hours, for example, each system has delivered approximately 10% of its original content of nitroglycerin.
The TRINIPATCH system comprises three layers:

1. a thin, occlusive, low density polyethylene (LDPE) backing film layer,
2. an acrylic adhesive matrix/drug reservoir layer,

3. a layer of siliconized polyester release liner comprised of overlapped liner strips that form an easy-opening tab.
Prior to use, a protective peel strip is removed from the adhesive surface.

INDICATIONS AND CLINICAL USE: TRINIPATCH (nitroglycerin) used intermittently (see Action and Clinical Pharmacology) is indicated for the prevention of anginal attacks in patients with stable angina pectoris associated with coronary artery disease. It can be used in conjunction with other antianginal agents such as beta-blockers and/or calcium antagonists.

TRINIPATCH is not intended for the immediate relief of acute attacks of angina pectoris. Sublingual nitroglycerin preparations should be used for this purpose.

CONTRAINDICATIONS:

1. Known hypersensitivity to nitroglycerin and related organic nitrate compounds.
2. Known or suspected hypersensitivity to components of the patch.
3. Acute circulatory failure associated with marked hypotension (shock and states of collapse).
4. Postural hypotension.
5. Left ventricular dysfunction due to obstruction as in aortic or mitral stenosis or of constrictive pericarditis.
6. Increased intracranial pressure.
7. Increased intraocular pressure.
8. Severe anemia.
9. Concomitant use of TRINIPATCH (nitroglycerin) either regularly and/or intermittently, with phosphodiesterase type 5 (PDE5) inhibitors such as VIAGRA (sildenafil), CIALIS (tadalafil) and LEVITRA (vardenafil) is absolutely contraindicated, because PDE5 inhibitors amplify the vasodilatory effects of TRINIPATCH which can lead to severe hypotension.

WARNINGS AND PRECAUTIONS: General: Daily headaches sometimes accompany treatment with nitroglycerin. In patients who get these headaches, the headaches may be a marker of the activity of the drug. Patients should resist the temptation to avoid headaches by altering the schedule of their treatment with nitroglycerin, since loss of headache may be associated with simultaneous loss of antianginal efficacy.

After normal use, there is enough residual nitroglycerin in discarded patches that they are a potential hazard to children and pets.

Cardiovascular: TRINIPATCH must be removed before cardioversion or DC defibrillation is attempted, as well as before applying diathermy treatment.

The benefits and safety of transdermal nitroglycerin in angina patients with acute myocardial infarction or congestive heart failure have not been established. If one elects to use TRINIPATCH in these conditions, careful clinical or hemodynamic monitoring must be used to avoid the potentially deleterious effects of induced hypotension and tachycardia.

Headaches or symptoms of hypotension, such as weakness or dizziness, particularly when arising suddenly from a recumbent position, may occur. A reduction in dose or discontinuation of treatment may be necessary.

Caution should be exercised when using nitroglycerin in patients prone to, or who might be affected by hypotension. The drug therefore should be used with caution in patients who may have volume depletion from diuretic therapy or in patients who have low systolic blood pressure (e.g. below 90 mmHg). Paradoxical bradycardia and increased angina pectoris may accompany nitroglycerin-induced hypotension.

Nitrate therapy may aggravate the angina caused by hypertrophic cardiomyopathy.

Dependence/Tolerance: In industrial workers who have had long-term exposure to unknown (presumably high) doses of nitroglycerin, tolerance clearly occurs. There is moreover, physical dependence since chest pain, acute myocardial infarction, and even sudden death have occurred during temporary withdrawal of nitroglycerin from these workers. In clinical trials of angina patients, there are reports of anginal attacks being more easily provoked and of rebound in the hemodynamic effects soon after nitrate withdrawal. The importance of these observations to the routine clinical use of nitroglycerin has not been fully elucidated, but patients should be monitored closely for increased anginal symptoms during drug-free periods.

Tolerance to nitroglycerin with cross tolerance to other nitrates or nitrites may occur (see Dosage and Administration). Co-administration of other long-acting nitrates could jeopardize the integrity of the nitrate-free interval and therefore must be avoided. As tolerance to nitroglycerin patches develops, the effect of sublingual nitroglycerin on exercise tolerance, although still observable, is somewhat blunted.

Respiratory: Caution should be exercised in patients with arterial hypoxemia due to anemia (see Contraindications), because in such patients the biotransformation of nitroglycerin is reduced. Similarly, caution is called for in patients with hypoxemia and ventilation/perfusion imbalance due to lung disease or ischemic heart failure. Patients with angina pectoris, myocardial infarction, or cerebral ischemia frequently suffer from abnormalities of the small airways (especially alveolar hypoxia). Under these circumstances vasoconstriction occurs within the lung to shift perfusion from areas of alveolar hypoxia to better ventilated regions of the lung. As a potent vasodilator, nitroglycerin could reverse this protective vasoconstriction and thus result in increased perfusion to poorly ventilated areas, worsening of the ventilation/perfusion imbalance, and a further decrease in the arterial partial pressure of oxygen.

Neurologic: Treatment with nitroglycerin may be associated with lightheadedness on standing, especially just after rising from a recumbent or seated position. This effect may be more frequent in patients who have also consumed alcohol.

As patients may experience faintness and/or dizziness, reaction time when driving or operating machinery may be impaired, especially at the start of treatment.

Hematologic: Case reports of clinically significant methemoglobinemia are rare at conventional doses of nitroglycerin. The formation of methemoglobin is dose-related, and in the case of genetic abnormalities of hemoglobin that favour methemoglobin formation, even conventional doses of organic nitrates can produce harmful concentrations of methemoglobin. Methemoglobin levels are available from most clinical laboratories. The diagnosis should be suspected in patients who exhibit signs of impaired oxygen delivery despite adequate cardiac output and adequate arterial pO_2. Classically, methemoglobinemic blood is described as chocolate brown, without color change on exposure to air. If methemoglobinemia is present, administration of methylene blue (1% solution), 1 to 2 mg/kg intravenously, may be required.

Special Populations: Pregnant Women: Animal reproduction studies have not been conducted with nitroglycerin. It is not known whether nitroglycerin can cause fetal harm when administered to a pregnant woman. Therefore use TRINIPATCH only if the potential benefit justifies the risk to the fetus.

Nursing Women: It is not known whether nitroglycerin is excreted into breast milk. Benefits to the mother must be weighed against the risks to the child.

Pediatrics: Safety and effectiveness have not been established in children.

ADVERSE REACTIONS: Adverse Drug Reaction Overview: Headache, which may be severe, is the most commonly reported side effect. Headache may be recurrent with each daily dose, especially at higher doses of nitroglycerin. Headaches may be treated with concomitant administration of mild analgesics. If such headaches are unresponsive to treatment, the nitroglycerin dosage should be reduced or the product discontinued. Transient episodes of lightheadedness, occasionally related to blood pressure changes, may also occur. Hypotension occurs infrequently, but in some patients it may be severe enough to warrant discontinuation of therapy.

Reddening of the skin (erythema), with or without a mild local itching (pruritus) or burning sensation, as well as allergic contact dermatitis may occasionally occur. Upon removal of the patch, any slight reddening of the skin will usually disappear within a few hours. The application site should be changed regularly to prevent local irritation.

Less frequently reported adverse reactions include dizziness, faintness, facial flushing, postural hypotension which may be associated with reflex tachycardia. Syncope, crescendo angina, and rebound hypertension have been reported but are uncommon. Rarely nausea, and vomiting.

Post-Market Adverse Drug Reactions: The most common adverse drug reaction reported post-market is localized skin reaction (local erythema, pruritus, rash). Other adverse reactions reported rarely in post-marketing use include:

Ophthalmic: blurred vision.

Renal: acute renal failure.

Skin: application site pruritus, eczema, rash.

Cardiovascular: hypotension, orthostatic hypotension.

DRUG INTERACTIONS:

Serious Drug Interactions

Concomitant use of TRINIPATCH (nitroglycerin) either regularly and/or intermittently, with phosphodiesterase type 5 (PDE5) inhibitors such as VIAGRA (sildenafil), CIALIS (tadalafil) and LEVITRA (vardenafil) is absolutely contraindicated, because PDE5 inhibitors amplify the vasodilatory effects of TRINIPATCH which can lead to severe hypotension.

Drug-Drug Interactions: See Table 1.

Table 1: TRINIPATCH

Established or Potential Drug-Drug Interactions

Nitroglycerin TTS	Ref	Effect	Clinical Comment
Phosphodiesterase 5 (PDE 5) inhibitors	T	↑ hypotensive effect	This could result in life-threatening hypotension with syncope or myocardial infarction and death.
Calcium channel blockers	T	↑ hypotensive effect	Marked symptomatic orthostatic hypotension has been reported when calcium channel blockers and organic nitrates were used in combination. Dosage adjustments of either class of agents may be necessary.
Angiotensin converting enzyme (ACE) inhibitors	T	↑ hypotensive effect	Reinforce the influence of nitroglycerin on the lowering arterial blood pressure. Dosage adjustment may be necessary.
Beta-Blockers	T	↑ hypotensive effect	Reinforce the influence of nitroglycerin on the lowering arterial blood pressure. Dosage adjustment may be necessary.
Diuretics	T	↑ hypotensive effect	Reinforce the influence of nitroglycerin on the lowering arterial blood pressure. Dosage adjustment may be necessary.
Tricyclic antidepressants	T	↑ hypotensive effect	Reinforce the influence of nitroglycerin on the lowering arterial blood pressure. Dosage adjustment may be necessary.
Major tranquilizers	T	↑ hypotensive effect	Reinforce the influence of nitroglycerin on the lowering arterial blood pressure. Dosage adjustment may be necessary.
Dihydroergotamine	T	↑ bioavailability of dihydroergotamine	Warrants special attention in patients with coronary artery disease, because dihydroergotamine antagonizes the action of nitroglycerin and this can lead to a coronary vasoconstriction.
Acetylsalicylic acid (ASA) and non-steroidal anti-inflammatory drugs (NSAIDs)	T	↓ therapeutic response	Ingestion of acetylsalicylic acid and non-steroidal anti-inflammatory drugs might diminish the therapeutic response to nitrates and nitroglycerin. Nitroglycerin's vasodilatory and hemodynamic effects may be altered by concomitant administration of acetylsalicylic acid and NSAIDs.
Heparin	T	↓ effectiveness of heparin	Use of nitroglycerin may decrease the effect of heparin. The effect of heparin should be frequently monitored when these two agents are used together. The dose of both agents may need to be adjusted.

Legend: T=Theoretical.

Drug-Food Interactions: Alcohol may enhance sensitivity to the hypotensive effects of nitrates.

Drug-Herb Interactions: Interaction with herbal products has not been established.

Drug-Laboratory Test Interactions: Interaction with laboratory tests has not been established.

Drug-Lifestyle Interactions: Driving and Using Machines: Dizziness, fatigue and postural hypotension may affect the patient's speed of reaction and impair the individual's ability to operate machinery and motor vehicles.

DOSAGE AND ADMINISTRATION: Dosing Considerations: Prevention of tolerance: Although some controlled clinical trials using exercise tolerance testing have shown maintenance of effectiveness when patches are worn continuously, the large majority of such controlled trials have shown the development of tolerance (i.e. complete loss of effect) within the first 24 hours after therapy was initiated. Dose adjustments even to levels much higher than generally used did not prevent the development of tolerance. Tolerance has appeared even when doses greater than 4 mg/hour were delivered continuously, a dose far in excess of the effective dose 0.2 to 0.8 mg/hour applied intermittently.

Efficacy of organic nitrates is restored after a period of absence of nitrates from the body. Thus, tolerance can be prevented or attenuated by use of an intermittent dosage schedule. Although the minimum nitrate-free interval has not been defined, clinical trials have demonstrated that an appropriate dosing schedule for nitroglycerin patches would provide for a daily patch-on period of 12-14 hours and a daily patch-off period of 10-12 hours. The patch-free time should coincide with the period in which angina pectoris is least likely to occur (usually at night). Patients should be watched carefully for an increase of angina pectoris during the patch-free period. Adjustment of background medication may be required.

Several studies have demonstrated that when nitroglycerin is administered according to an intermittent regimen, doses of 0.4-0.8 mg/hr have increased exercise capacity for up to 8 hours, with a trend of increased exercise capacity to 12 hours. One controlled clinical trial suggested that the intermittent use of nitrates may be associated with a decreased exercise tolerance, in comparison to placebo, during the last part of the nitrate-free interval; the clinical relevance of this observation is unknown, but the possibility of increased frequency or severity of angina during the nitrate-free interval should be considered.

The dose of TRINIPATCH should be periodically reviewed in relation to continuing antianginal control.

Recommended Dose and Dosage Adjustment: The daily dosage schedule is based on intermittent therapy to prevent the development of tolerance to nitroglycerin. The optimal dose should be selected based upon the clinical response, side effects, and the effects of therapy on blood pressure.

Starting dose is one TRINIPATCH 0.2 patch (7 cm^2), usually applied in the morning. If 0.2 mg/hour (7 cm^2) is well tolerated, the dose can be increased to 0.4 mg/hour (14 cm^2) if required. A maximum of 0.8 mg/hour may be used.

Administration: TRINIPATCH can be applied to any area of skin **except** the distal extremities. Many patients prefer the chest. Each successive application should be to a different site.

The area should be clean, dry, and preferably hairless. If hair is likely to interfere with patch adhesion or removal, clipping may be necessary prior to application. Take care to avoid areas with cuts or irritations.

OVERDOSAGE:

Symptoms: Nitroglycerin overdose may result in severe hypotension, persistent throbbing headache, vertigo, palpitations, visual disturbances, flushing and perspiring skin (later becoming cold and cyanotic), anorexia, nausea and vomiting (possibly with colic and even bloody diarrhea), syncope (especially in the upright posture), methemoglobinemia with cyanosis, hyperpnea, dyspnea and slow breathing, slow pulse (dicrotic and intermittent), heart block and bradycardia, increased intracranial pressure with cerebral symptoms of fever, confusion, and coma possibly followed by paralysis, clonic convulsions and death due to circulatory collapse.

Treatment: Keep the patient recumbent in a shock position and comfortably warm. Remove the TRINIPATCH.

Passive movement of the extremities may aid venous return. Administer oxygen and artificial ventilation if necessary.

Intravenous infusion of normal saline or similar fluid may also be required to produce sufficient central volume expansion. However, in patients with renal disease or congestive heart failure, therapy resulting in central volume expansion is not without hazard. Treatment of nitroglycerin overdose in these patients may be subtle and difficult, and invasive monitoring may be required.

Epinephrine is ineffective in reversing the severe hypotensive events associated with overdose; it and related compounds are contraindicated in this situation.

> For management of a suspected drug overdose, CPhA recommends that you contact your **regional Poison Control Centre**. See the *CPS* Directory section for a list of Poison Control Centres.

ACTION AND CLINICAL PHARMACOLOGY: Mechanism of Action: The principal pharmacological action of nitroglycerin is relaxation of vascular smooth muscle, producing a vasodilator effect on both peripheral arteries and veins, with more prominent effects on the latter. Dilation of the post-capillary vessels, including large veins, promotes peripheral pooling of blood and decreases venous return to the heart, thereby reducing left ventricular end-diastolic pressure (preload). Arteriolar relaxation reduces system vascular resistance and arterial pressure (afterload). Dilation of the coronary arteries also occurs. The relative importance of preload reduction, afterload reduction, and coronary dilation remains undefined.

Pharmacodynamics: TRINIPATCH transdermal system seems to cause redistribution of coronary blood flow in the endocardium. Nitroglycerin allows the improvement of balance between oxygen supply and demand, while dissipating spontaneously and completely the symptoms of angina pectoris attacks.

The response to nitrate products may differ from patient to patient, while absorption of nitroglycerin resulting from the system may vary between subjects.

Following the application of TRINIPATCH transdermal system onto the skin, constant, continued and prolonged absorption of the active ingredient (nitroglycerin) is initiated, resulting in prolonged venous diastolic action. Onset of action is achieved 30-60 minutes after the application of TRINIPATCH. The duration of action is approximately 24 hours.

Pharmacokinetics: Absorption: When TRINIPATCH is applied to the skin, nitroglycerin is absorbed directly into the systemic circulation. Thus, the active drug reaches target organs before inactivation by the liver. The transdermal absorption of nitroglycerin occurs in a continuous and well-controlled manner. Bioavailability studies in healthy volunteers have shown that the released amount of nitroglycerin (5 mg or 10 mg/24 hours) represents the mean release rate of nitroglycerin resulting from the system and represents the amount available for absorption.

Distribution: The volume of distribution of nitroglycerin is about 3 L/kg, and nitroglycerin is cleared from this volume at extremely rapid rates, with a resulting serum half-life of about 3 minutes. The serum therapeutic level remains undefined. With 50-500 ng/mL plasma concentrations, nitroglycerin is bound to plasma proteins at a rate of approximately 60%, while 1,2 and 1,3-dinitroglycerides are approximately 60% and 30% bound respectively.

The observed clearance rates (close to 1 L/kg/min.) greatly exceed hepatic blood flow, known sites of extrahepatic metabolism include red blood cells and vascular walls.

In healthy volunteers, after the application of the system in different dosages (2×7 cm^2 patch, 1×14 cm^2 patch and 1×21 cm^2 patch), the concentrations of nitroglycerin reached in the plasma were uniform and dose-related, i.e. dependent on drug-release area. They remained constant as long as the system is in contact with the skin (observations have been limited to 24 hours). Upon removal of the patch, the plasma concentrations were maintained for about 30 min. Since the rate of release of nitroglycerin is linearly dependent upon the area of the applied system, two patches of 0.4 mg (or one patch of 0.2 mg and one patch of 0.6 mg) can be used for a dose of 0.8 mg.

Metabolism: Nitroglycerin is rapidly metabolized, principally by a liver reductase, to form glycerol nitrate metabolites and inorganic nitrate. Two active major metabolites, the 1,2- and 1,3-dinitroglycerols, the products of hydrolysis, appear to be less potent than nitroglycerin as vasodilators but have longer plasma half-lives. The dinitrates are further metabolized to mononitrates (biologically inactive with respect to cardiovascular effects) and ultimately to glycerol and carbon dioxide. There is extensive first-pass deactivation by the liver following gastrointestinal absorption.

Excretion: Metabolic derivatives of nitroglycerin are excreted in the urine.

Special Populations and Conditions: Pediatrics: Safety and effectiveness have not been established in children.

Geriatrics: No special information is available on the use of TRINIPATCH in elderly people. However, there is no evidence suggesting that dosage should be adapted in these patients.

STORAGE AND STABILITY: Storage: under controlled room temperature (between 15-30°C).

Each patch is individually sealed in a separate pouch. Do not store out of the pouch. Keep TRINIPATCH out of reach of children and pets before use and when disposing of used patches.

Do not use beyond the expiry date indicated on the label. Do not refrigerate.

INFORMATION FOR THE PATIENT: Published in e-CPS, available by subscription at www.e-cps.ca.

DOSAGE FORMS, COMPOSITION AND PACKAGING: The TRINIPATCH transdermal system is a flat unit designed to provide continuous controlled release of nitroglycerin through intact skin. The rate of release of nitroglycerin is linearly dependent upon the area of the applied system; each cm^2 of applied system delivers approximately 0.03 mg of nitroglycerin per hour. Nitroglycerin remaining in the patch serves as a thermodynamic energy source to keep the pattern of delivery constant.

The drug product is a matrix transdermal patch design consisting of three laminated film layers: a) a thin, occlusive, low density polyethylene (LDPE) backing film layer; b) an acrylic adhesive matrix/drug reservoir layer, and c) siliconized polyester release liner layer comprised of overlapped liner that form an easy-opening tab.

TRINIPATCH 0.2 : Each TRINIPATCH 0.2 (7 cm^2) contains: 22.4 mg of nitroglycerin and delivers approximately 0.2 mg of active substance per hour. Nonmedicinal ingredients: DuroTak 80-1196 and sorbitan mono-oleate. Boxes of 30 and 100 systems. Each system is individually sealed in a separate pouch.

TRINIPATCH 0.4 : Each TRINIPATCH 0.4 (14 cm^2) contains: 44.8 mg of nitroglycerin and delivers approximately 0.4 mg of active substance per hour. Nonmedicinal ingredients: DuroTak 80-1196 and sorbitan mono-oleate. Boxes of 30 and 100 systems. Each system is individually sealed in a separate pouch.

TRINIPATCH 0.6 : Each TRINIPATCH 0.6 (21 cm^2) contains: 67.2 mg of nitroglycerin and delivers approximately 0.6 mg of active substance per hour. Nonmedicinal ingredients: DuroTak 80-1196 and sorbitan mono-oleate. Boxes of 30 and 100 systems. Each system is individually sealed in a separate pouch.

(Shown in Product Identification Section)

Triple Antibiotic Ointment

bacitracin zinc—polymyxin B sulfate—gramicidin

Antibiotic

Taro

SUPPLIED: Each g of ointment contains: polymyxin B sulfate 10 000 units, bacitracin zinc 500 units and gramicidin 0.25 mg. Nonmedicinal ingredients: vitamin E (dl-alpha tocopheryl acetate) and white petrolatum. Tubes of 15 and 30 g. Store at room temperature (15 to 30 °C).

Triquilar® 21 Ⓟ

levonorgestrel—ethinyl estradiol

Oral Contraceptive

Bayer

Triquilar® 28 Ⓟ

levonorgestrel—ethinyl estradiol

Oral Contraceptive

Bayer

Date of Revision: June 7, 2010

SUMMARY PRODUCT INFORMATION:

Route of Administration	Dosage Form/ Strength	Clinically Relevant Nonmedicinal Ingredients
Oral	0.05 mg levonorgestrel and 0.03 mg ethinyl estradiol tablets 0.075 mg levonorgestrel and 0.04 mg ethinyl estradiol tablets 0.125 mg levonorgestrel and 0.03 mg ethinyl estradiol tablets	Lactose monohydrate For a complete listing see Dosage Forms, Composition and Packaging.

INDICATIONS AND CLINICAL USE: TRIQUILAR (levonorgestrel and ethinyl estradiol) is indicated for:

- Conception control (prevention of pregnancy)

CONTRAINDICATIONS: TRIQUILAR should not be used in women with:

- a history of or actual thrombophlebitis or thromboembolic disorders;
- a history of or actual cerebrovascular disorders;
- a history of or actual myocardial infarction or coronary artery disease;
- a history of or actual prodromi of a thrombosis (eg, transient ischemic attack, angina pectoris)
- presence of severe or multiple risk factor(s) for arterial or venous thrombosis:
  - severe hypertension (persistent values of ≥160/100 mmHg)
  - hereditary or acquired predisposition for venous or arterial thrombosis, such as Factor V Leiden mutation and activated protein C (APC-) resistance, antithrombin-III-deficiency, protein C deficiency, protein S deficiency, hyperhomocysteinemia (eg, due to MTHFR C677T, A1298 mutations), prothrombin mutation G20210A, and antiphospholipid-antibodies (anticardiolipin antibodies, lupus anticoagulant)
  - severe dyslipoproteinemia
  - heavy smoking (>15 cigarettes per day) and over age 35
  - diabetes mellitus with vascular involvement
  - major surgery associated with an increased risk of postoperative thromboembolism
  - prolonged immobilization
- valvular heart disease with complications;
- active liver disease, or history of or actual benign or malignant liver tumours;
- known or suspected carcinoma of the breast;
- carcinoma of the endometrium or other known or suspected estrogen-dependent neoplasia;
- undiagnosed abnormal vaginal bleeding;
- steroid-dependent jaundice, cholestatic jaundice, history of jaundice of pregnancy;
- any ocular lesion arising from ophthalmic vascular disease, such as partial or complete loss of vision, or defect in visual fields;
- known or suspected pregnancy;
- current or history of migraine with focal aura;
- history of or actual pancreatitis if associated with severe hypertriglyceridemia;
- hypersensitivity to this drug or to any ingredient in the formulation or component of the container. For a complete listing, see Dosage Forms, Composition and Packaging.

WARNINGS AND PRECAUTIONS:

> **Serious Warnings and Precautions**
>
> Cigarette smoking increases the risk of serious adverse effects on the heart and blood vessels. The risk increases with age and becomes significant in oral contraceptive users older than 35 years of age. Women should be counselled not to smoke (see Cardiovascular).
>
> Patients should be counseled that birth control pills **do not protect** against sexually transmitted diseases including HIV/AIDS. For protection against STDs, patients should be counseled to use latex condoms **in combination with** birth control pills.

General: Discontinue Medication at the Earliest Manifestation of:

A. **Thromboembolic and cardiovascular disorders** such as, thrombophlebitis pulmonary embolism, cerebrovascular disorders, myocardial ischemia, mesenteric thrombosis, retinal thrombosis.
B. **Conditions which predispose to venous stasis and to vascular thrombosis** (eg, immobilization after accidents or confinement to bed during long-term illness). Other non-hormonal methods of contraception should be used until regular activities are resumed. For use of oral contraceptives when surgery is contemplated, see Peri-Operative Considerations.
C. **Visual defects, partial or complete.**
D. **Papilledema, or ophthalmic vascular lesions.**
E. **Severe headache of unknown etiology or worsening of pre-existing migraine headache.**
F. **Increase in epileptic seizures.**

The following information is provided from studies of combination oral contraceptives (COCs).

The use of combination hormonal contraceptives is associated with increased risks of several serious conditions including myocardial infarction, thromboembolism, stroke, hepatic neoplasia and gallbladder disease, although the risk of serious morbidity and mortality is small in healthy women without underlying risk factors. The risk of morbidity and mortality increases significantly if associated with the presence of other risk factors such as hypertension, hyperlipidemias, obesity and diabetes. Other medical conditions which have been associated with adverse circulatory events include, systemic lupus erythematosus, hemolytic uremic syndrome, chronic inflammatory bowel disease (Crohn's disease or ulcerative colitis), sickle cell disease, valvular heart disease and atrial fibrillation.

The following conditions have been reported to occur or deteriorate with both pregnancy and COC use, although a direct association with COC's has not been firmly established: porphyria, systemic lupus erythematosus, hemolytic uremic syndrome, Sydenham's chorea, herpes gestationis, and otosclerosis-related hearing loss.

The information contained in this section is principally from studies carried out in women who used COCs with higher formulations of estrogens and progestogens than those in common use today. The effect of long-term use of combination hormonal contraceptives with lower doses of both estrogen and progestogen administered orally remains to be determined.

Carcinogenesis and Mutagenesis: Breast Cancer: Increasing age and a strong family history are the most significant risk factors for the development of breast cancer. Other established risk factors include obesity, nulliparity and late age at first full-term pregnancy. The identified groups of women that may be at increased risk of developing breast cancer before menopause are long-term users of oral contraceptives (more than 8 years) and starters at early age. In a few women, the use of oral contraceptives may accelerate the growth of an existing but undiagnosed breast cancer. Since any potential increased risk related to oral contraceptives use is small, there is no reason to change prescribing habits at present.

Women receiving oral contraceptives should be instructed in self-examination of their breasts. Their physicians should be notified whenever any masses are detected. A yearly clinical breast examination is also recommended because, if a breast cancer should develop, drugs that contain estrogen may cause a rapid progression.

Cervical Cancer: The most important risk factor for cervical cancer is persistent human papillomavirus infection. Some epidemiological studies have indicated that long-term use of COCs may further contribute to this increased risk but there continues to be controversy about the extent to which this finding is attributable to confounding effects, eg, cervical screening and sexual behaviour including use of barrier contraceptives.

Hepatocellular Carcinoma: Hepatocellular carcinoma may be associated with oral contraceptives. The risk appears to increase with duration of hormonal contraceptive use. However, the attributable risk (the excess incidence) of liver cancers in oral contraceptive users is extremely small. A liver tumor should be considered in the differential diagnosis when severe upper abdominal pain, liver enlargement, or signs of intra-abdominal hemorrhage occur in women taking COCs.

Cardiovascular: Predisposing Factors for Coronary Artery Disease: Cigarette smoking increases the risk of serious cardiovascular side effects and mortality. Birth control pills increase this risk, especially with increasing age. Convincing data are available to support an upper age limit of 35 years for oral contraceptive use by women who smoke.

Other women who are independently at high risk for cardiovascular disease include those with diabetes, hypertension, abnormal lipid profile or a family history of these. Whether oral contraceptives accentuate this risk is unclear.

In low-risk, non-smoking women of any age, the benefits of oral contraceptive use outweigh the possible cardiovascular risks associated with low-dose formulations. Consequently, oral contraceptives may be prescribed for these women up to the age of menopause.

Hypertension: Patients with essential hypertension whose blood pressure is well-controlled may be given hormonal contraceptives but only under close supervision. If a significant elevation of blood pressure in previously normotensive or hypertensive subjects occurs at any time during the administration of the drug, cessation of medication is necessary.

Endocrine and Metabolism: Diabetes: Current low-dose oral contraceptives exert minimal impact on glucose metabolism. Diabetic patients, or those with a family history of diabetes, should be observed closely to detect any worsening of carbohydrate metabolism. Patients predisposed to diabetes who can be kept under close supervision may be given oral contraceptives. Young diabetic patients whose disease is of recent origin, well-controlled, and not associated with hypertension or other signs of vascular disease such as ocular fundal changes, should be monitored more frequently while using oral contraceptives.

Lipid and Other Metabolic Effects: A small proportion of women will have adverse lipid changes while on oral contraceptives. Alternative contraception should be used in women with uncontrolled dyslipidemias. (See also Contraindications.) Elevations of plasma triglycerides may lead to pancreatitis and other complications.

Gastrointestinal: Published epidemiological studies indicate a possible association of COC use and the development of Crohn's disease and ulcerative colitis, although this has not been firmly established.

Genitourinary: Vaginal Bleeding: Persistent, irregular vaginal bleeding requires assessment to exclude underlying pathology.

Fibroids: Patients with fibroids (leiomyomata) should be carefully observed. Sudden enlargement, pain or tenderness requires discontinuation of the use of oral contraceptives.

Hematologic: Epidemiological studies have suggested an association between the use of COCs and an increased risk of arterial and venous thrombotic and thromboembolic diseases such as myocardial infarction, deep venous thrombosis, pulmonary embolism, and of cerebrovascular accidents. These events occur rarely.

The use of any combined oral contraceptive carries an increased risk of VTE compared with no use. The excess risk of VTE is highest during the first year a woman ever uses a combined oral contraceptive or restarts (following a 4-week or greater pill-free interval) the same or a different COC. Data from a large, prospective 3-armed cohort study suggest that this increased risk is mainly present during the first 3 months. VTE is fatal in 1-2% of cases.

A large, prospective 3-armed cohort study has shown that the frequency of VTE diagnosis ranges from about 8 to 10 per 10 000 woman-years in users of oral contraceptives with low estrogen content (<50 µg ethinyl estradiol). The most recent data suggest that the frequency of VTE diagnosis is approximately 4.4 per 10 000 woman-years in nonpregnant, non-COC users and ranges from 20 to 30 per 10 000 pregnant women or postpartum.

Overall the risk for venous thromboembolism (VTE) in users of oral contraceptives with low estrogen content (<50 µg ethinyl estradiol) is two- to three-fold higher than for nonusers of COCs who are not pregnant and remains lower than the risk associated with pregnancy and delivery.

Venous thromboembolism (VTE), manifesting as deep venous thrombosis and/or pulmonary embolism may occur during the use of all COCs.

Extremely rarely, thrombosis has been reported to occur in other blood vessels (eg, hepatic, mesenteric, renal, cerebral or retinal veins and arteries) in COC users. There is no consensus as to whether the occurrence of these events is associated with the use of COCs.

Symptoms of deep vein thrombosis (DVT) can include: unilateral swelling of the leg or along a vein in the leg; pain or tenderness in the leg which may be felt only when standing or walking, increased warmth in the affected leg; red or discolored skin on the leg.

Symptoms of pulmonary embolism (PE) can include: sudden onset of unexplained shortness of breath or rapid breathing; sudden coughing which may bring up blood; sharp chest pain which may increase with deep breathing; sense of anxiety; severe light headedness or dizziness; rapid or irregular heartbeat. Some of these symptoms (eg, "shortness of breath", "coughing") are nonspecific and might be misinterpreted as more common or less severe events (eg, respiratory tract infections).

The risk for arterial thromboembolism (ATE) in users of oral contraceptives with low estrogen content (<50 µg ethinyl estradiol) ranges from about 1 to 3 cases per 10 000 woman-years. An arterial thromboembolic event can include cerebrovascular accident, vascular occlusion or myocardial infarction (MI). Symptoms of a cerebrovascular accident can include: sudden numbness or weakness of the face, arm, or leg, especially on one side of the body; sudden confusion, trouble speaking or understanding; sudden trouble seeing in one or both eyes; sudden trouble walking, dizziness, loss of balance or coordination; sudden, severe or prolonged headache with no known cause; loss of consciousness or fainting with or without seizure. Other signs of vascular occlusion can include: sudden pain, swelling and slight blue discoloration of an extremity; acute abdomen.

Symptoms of MI can include: pain, discomfort, pressure, heaviness, sensation of squeezing or fullness in the chest, arm, or below the breastbone; discomfort radiating to the back, jaw, throat, arm, stomach; fullness, indigestion or choking feeling; sweating, nausea, vomiting or dizziness; extreme weakness, anxiety, or shortness of breath; rapid or irregular heartbeats.

Arterial thromboembolic events may be fatal.

Other Risk Factors for Venous or Arterial Thromboembolism or of a Cerebrovascular Accident: Other generalized risk factors for venous or arterial thromboembolism include but are not limited to age, severe obesity (body mass index >30 kg/m^2), a personal history, a positive family history (the occurrence of VTE/ATE in a direct relative at a relatively early age may indicate genetic predisposition) and systemic lupus erythematosus.

If a hereditary or acquired predisposition of venous or arterial thromboembolism is suspected, the woman should be referred to a specialist for advice before deciding on any COC use. The risk of VTE/ATE may be temporarily increased with prolonged immobilization, major surgery, or trauma. In these situations it is advisable to discontinue COC use (in the case of elective surgery at least four weeks in advance) and not to resume COC use until two weeks after complete remobilization. Also, patients with varicose veins and leg cast should be closely supervised. Other risk factors may include smoking (with heavier smoking and increasing age, the risk further increases, especially in women over 35 years of age), dyslipoproteinemia, hypertension, migraine, valvular heart disease, and atrial fibrillation.

Biochemical factors that may be indicative of hereditary or acquired predisposition for venous or arterial thrombosis include Activated Protein C (APC) resistance, hyperhomocysteinemia, antithrombin-III deficiency, protein C deficiency, protein S deficiency, antiphospholipid antibodies (anticardiolipin antibodies, lupus anticoagulant).

When considering risk/benefit, the physician should take into account that adequate treatment of a condition may reduce the associated risk of thrombosis and that the risk associated with pregnancy is higher than that associated with low-dose COCs (<0.05 mg ethinyl estradiol).

Hepatic/Biliary/Pancreatic: Acute or chronic disturbances of liver function may necessitate the discontinuation of COC use until markers of liver function return to normal.

Jaundice: Patients who have had jaundice should be given oral contraceptives only with great care and under close observation. Oral contraceptive-related cholestasis has been described in women with a history of pregnancy-related cholestasis. Women with a history of cholestasis may have the condition recur with subsequent hormonal contraceptive use.

The development of severe generalized pruritus or icterus requires that the medication be withdrawn until the problem is resolved.

If a patient develops jaundice that proves to be cholestatic in type, the use of oral contraceptives should not be resumed. In patients taking hormonal contraceptives, changes in the composition of the bile may occur and an increased incidence of gallstones has been reported.

Gallbladder Disease: Patients taking oral contraceptives have a greater risk of developing gallbladder disease requiring surgery within the first year of use. The risk may double after four or five years.

Hepatic Nodules: Hepatic nodules (adenoma and focal nodular hyperplasia) have been reported, particularly in long-term users of oral contraceptives. Although these lesions are extremely rare, they have caused fatal intra-abdominal hemorrhage and should be considered in women with an abdominal mass, acute abdominal pain, or evidence of intra-abdominal bleeding.

Immune: Angioedema: Exogenous estrogens may induce or exacerbate symptoms of angioedema, in particular in women with hereditary angioedema.

Neurologic: Migraine and Headache : The onset or exacerbation of migraine or the development of headaches with a new pattern that is recurrent, persistent, or severe, requires discontinuation of hormonal contraceptives and evaluation of the cause. Women with migraine headaches who take oral contraceptives may be at increased risk of stroke (see Contraindications).

Ophthalmologic: Patients who are pregnant or are taking oral contraceptives may experience corneal edema that may cause visual disturbances and changes in tolerance to contact lenses, especially of the rigid type. Soft contact lenses usually do not cause disturbances. If visual changes or alterations in tolerance to contact lenses occur, temporary or permanent cessation of wear may be advised.

Peri-Operative Considerations: There is an increased risk of thromboembolic complications in oral contraceptive users, after major surgery. If feasible, oral contraceptives should be discontinued and an alternative method substituted at least one month prior to **major** elective surgery. Oral contraceptive use should not be resumed until the first menstrual period after hospital discharge following surgery.

Psychiatric: Patients with a history of emotional disturbances, especially the depressive type, may be more prone to have a recurrence of depression while taking oral contraceptives. In cases of a serious recurrence, a trial of an alternate method of contraception should be made, which may help to clarify the possible relationship. Women with premenstrual syndrome (PMS) may have a varied response to oral contraceptives, ranging from symptomatic improvement to worsening of the condition.

Renal: Fluid Retention: Hormonal contraceptives may cause some degree of fluid retention. They should be prescribed with caution, and only with careful monitoring, in patients with conditions which might be aggravated by fluid retention.

Sexual Function/Reproduction: Return to Fertility: After discontinuing oral contraceptive therapy, the patient should delay pregnancy until at least one normal spontaneous menstrual cycle has occurred in order to date the pregnancy. An alternate contraceptive method should be used during this time.

Amenorrhea: In some women, withdrawal bleeding may not occur during the tablet-free interval. If the COC has been taken according to directions, it is unlikely that the woman is pregnant. However, if the COC has not been taken according to directions prior to the first missed withdrawal bleed, or if two withdrawal bleeds are missed, pregnancy must be ruled out before COC use is continued.

Women having a history of oligomenorrhea, secondary amenorrhea, or irregular cycles may remain anovulatory or become amenorrheic following discontinuation of estrogen-progestin combination therapy.

Amenorrhea, especially if associated with breast secretion, that continues for six months or more after withdrawal, warrants a careful assessment of hypothalamic-pituitary function.

Reduced Efficacy: The efficacy of COCs may be reduced in the event of missed pills, gastrointestinal disturbances or concomitant medication (see Drug Interactions).

Skin: Chloasma may occasionally occur with use of COCs, especially in women with a history of chloasma gravidarum. Women with a tendency to chloasma should avoid exposure to the sun or ultraviolet radiation while taking COCs.

Special Populations: Pregnant Women: Oral contraceptives should not be taken by pregnant women. If pregnancy occurs during treatment with TRIQUILAR, further intake must be stopped. However, if conception accidentally occurs while taking the pill, there is no conclusive evidence that the estrogen and progestin contained in the oral contraceptive will damage the developing child.

Nursing Women: In breastfeeding women, the use of oral contraceptives results in the hormonal components being excreted in breast milk and may reduce its quantity and quality. Published studies have indicated that during lactation, 0.1% of the daily maternal dose of levonorgestrel and 0.02% of the daily maternal dose of ethinyl estradiol could be transferred to the newborn via milk. Adverse effects on the child have been reported, including jaundice and breast enlargement. The nursing mother should be advised not to use oral contraceptives but to use other forms of contraception until she has completely weaned her child. There have been no formal studies of TRIQUILAR in nursing women.

Pediatrics: Safety and efficacy of TRIQUILAR has not been established in women under the age of 16 years. Use of this product before menarche is not indicated.

Geriatrics: TRIQUILAR is not indicated for use in postmenopausal women. Oral contraceptives may mask the onset of the climacteric.

Monitoring and Laboratory Tests: Physical Examination and Followup: Before oral contraceptives are used, a thorough history and physical examination should be performed, including a blood pressure determination and the family case history carefully noted. In addition, disturbances of the clotting system must be ruled out if any members of the family have suffered from thromboembolic diseases (eg, deep vein thrombosis, stroke, myocardial infarction) at a young age. Breasts, liver, extremities and pelvic organs should be examined. A Papanicolaou (Pap) smear should be taken if the patient has been sexually active.

The first follow-up visit should be done three months after oral contraceptives are prescribed. Thereafter, examinations should be performed at least once a year, or more frequently if indicated. At each annual visit, examination should include those procedures that were done at the initial visit as outlined above or per recommendations of the Canadian Task Force on the Periodic Health Examination.

ADVERSE REACTIONS: Adverse Drug Reaction Overview: An increased risk of the following serious adverse reactions has been associated with the use of oral contraceptives: thrombophlebitis, pulmonary embolism, mesenteric thrombosis, neuro-ocular lesions (eg, retinal thrombosis), myocardial infarction, cerebral thrombosis, cerebral hemorrhage, hypertension, benign hepatic tumours, gallbladder disease, congenital anomalies.

The following other adverse reactions have also been reported in patients receiving oral contraceptives: Nausea and vomiting, usually the most common adverse reaction, occurs in approximately 10% or fewer of patients during the first cycle. The following other reactions, as a general rule, are seen less frequently or only occasionally: gastrointestinal symptoms (such as abdominal cramps and bloating); breakthrough bleeding; spotting;, change in menstrual flow; dysmenorrhea; amenorrhea during and after treatment; temporary infertility after discontinuation of treatment; edema; chloasma or melasma which may persist; breast changes (tenderness, enlargement, and secretion); change in weight (increase or decrease); endocervical hyperplasia; possible diminution in lactation when given immediately postpartum; cholestatic jaundice; migraine; increase in size of uterine leiomyomata; rash (allergic); mental depression; reduced tolerance to carbohydrates; vaginal candidiasis; premenstrual-like syndrome; intolerance to contact lenses; change in corneal curvature (steepening); cataracts; optic neuritis; retinal thrombosis; changes in libido; chorea; changes in appetite; cystitis-like syndrome; rhinitis; headache; nervousness; dizziness; hirsutism; loss of scalp hair; erythema multiforme; erythema nodosum; hemorrhagic eruption; vaginitis; porphyria; impaired renal function; Raynaud's phenomenon; auditory disturbances; hemolytic uremic syndrome; pancreatitis; abdominal pain; diarrhea; hypersensitivity; vaginal discharge; rash; urticaria

Clinical Trial Adverse Drug Reactions: Because clinical trials are conducted under very specific conditions, the adverse reaction rates observed in the clinical trials may not reflect the rates observed in practice and should not be compared to the rates in the clinical trials of another drug. Adverse drug reaction information from clinical trials is useful for identifying drug-related adverse events and for approximating rates.

The most frequently reported adverse events in the 8748 patients (50 793 cycles) monitored during clinical trials have been tabulated in Table 1. The reported frequencies are the numbers of patients exhibiting a certain symptom per total number of cycles monitored.

Table 1: TRIQUILAR

Clinical Trial Adverse Drug Reactions with a Reported Frequency of >1%

Adverse Events	Frequency of Observations per Cycle (%)
Gastrointestinal Disorders	
Nausea and/or vomiting	4.2
Nervous System Disorders	
Headache	5.6
Migraine	2.0
Psychiatric Disorders	
Libido, increase-decrease	2.0
Depression	2.0
Reproductive System and Breast Disorders	
Dysmenorrhea	6.5
Spotting	5.8
Breast tension or pain	4.2
Breakthrough bleeding	1.8
Skin and Subcutaneous Tissue Disorders	
Acne	2.3

(cont'd)

Table 1: TRIQUILAR *(cont'd)*

Clinical Trial Adverse Drug Reactions with a Reported Frequency of >1%

Adverse Events	Frequency of Observations per Cycle (%)
Chloasma	1.8
Vascular Disorders	
Varicose veins	3.5

In all studies, there was a decline in the incidence of symptoms with time. Most side effects were observed in the first three months of therapy, particularly such symptoms as nausea, dizziness, breast tension, headache and changes in libido occurred more frequently during Cycles 1 to 3 than during the pretreatment phase. However, from Cycles 4 to 24, the frequencies of all symptoms were lower than the pretreatment values.

Less Common Clinical Trial Adverse Drug Reactions (<1%): General Disorders and Administration Site Condition: edema.
Investigations: weight increased.
Metabolism and Nutrition Disorders: increased appetite.
Reproductive System and Breast Disorders: amenorrhea.
Vascular Disorders: thrombophlebitis.
Intermenstrual Bleeding: The incidence of intercyclic bleeding irregularities (defined as either spotting or breakthrough bleeding) was higher during the first cycle. The frequency of intercyclic bleeding episodes decreased with time, so that after the 12th cycle with TRIQUILAR bleeding irregularities were rarely encountered.

In the patient population studied, bleeding irregularities occurred during 8.5% of all cycles monitored. However, bleeding irregularities for those cycles associated with admitted pill errors were generally much higher (25.6%) (see Table 2). Overall the incidence of spotting was greater than that of breakthrough bleeding in most cycles.

Table 2: TRIQUILAR

Intermenstrual Bleeding

	Spotting		Breakthrough Bleeding		Spotting and Breakthrough Bleeding	
Pill error—1211 cycles	187	(14.60%)	107	(9.00%)	27	(2.20%)
All cycles—50 793 cycles	2946	(5.80%)	901	(1.80%)	455	(0.90%)

DRUG INTERACTIONS: Overview: The concurrent administration of oral contraceptives with other drugs may lead to breakthrough bleeding and/or may result in an altered response to either agent (Table 3 and Table 4). Reduced effectiveness of the oral contraceptive, should it occur, is more likely with the low-dose formulations. It is important to ascertain all drugs that a patient is taking, both prescription and non-prescription, before oral contraceptives are prescribed.
Drug-Drug Interactions:

Table 3: TRIQUILAR

Drugs Which May Decrease the Efficacy of Oral Contraceptives

Class of Compound	Drug	Proposed Mechanism	Suggested Management
Antacids		Decreased intestinal absorption of progestins.	Dose two hours apart.
Antibiotics	Ampicillin Cotrimoxazole Penicillin	Enterohepatic circulation disturbance, intestinal hurry.	For short course, use additional method or use another drug. For long course, use another method.
	Rifampin Rifabutin	Increased metabolism of progestins. Suspected acceleration of estrogen metabolism.	Use another method.
	Chloramphenicol Metronidazole Neomycin Nitrofurantoin Sulfonamides Tetracyclines	Induction of hepatic microsomal enzymes. Also disturbance of enterohepatic circulation.	For short course, use additional method or use another drug. For long course, use another method.
	Troleandomycin	May retard metabolism of oral contraceptives, increasing the risk of cholestatic jaundice.	
Anticonvulsants	Carbamazepine Ethosuximide Oxcarbazepine Phenobarbital Phenytoin Primidone Topiramate Lamotrigine Felbamate	Induction of hepatic microsomal enzymes. Rapid metabolism of estrogen and increased binding of progestin and ethinyl estradiol to SHBG.	Use higher dose oral contraceptives (50 µg ethinyl estradiol), another drug or another method.
Antifungals	Griseofulvin	Stimulation of hepatic metabolism of contraceptive steroids may occur.	Use another method.
Cholesterol Lowering Agents	Clofibrate	Reduces elevated serum triglycerides and cholesterol; this reduces oral contraceptive efficacy.	Use another method.
HIV Protease Inhibitors	Ritonavir	Induction of hepatic microsomal enzymes.	Use another drug or another method.
Non-nucleoside Reverse Transcriptase Inhibitors	Nevirapine	Induction of hepatic microsomal enzymes.	Use another drug or another method.

(cont'd)

Table 3: TRIQUILAR *(cont'd)*

Drugs Which May Decrease the Efficacy of Oral Contraceptives

Class of Compound	Drug	Proposed Mechanism	Suggested Management
Sedatives and Hypnotics	Benzodiazepines Barbiturates Chloral hydrate Glutethimide Meprobamate	Induction of hepatic microsomal enzymes.	For short course, use additional method or another drug. For long course, use another method or higher dose oral contraceptives.
Other Drugs	Phenylbutazone Antihistamines Analgesics Antimigraine preparations Vitamin E	Reduced oral contraceptive efficacy has been reported. Remains to be confirmed.	

Oral contraceptives may interfere with the metabolism of other drugs. Accordingly, plasma and tissue concentrations may either increase (eg, cyclosporine) or decrease (eg, lamotrigine).

Table 4: TRIQUILAR

Modification of Other Drug Action by Oral Contraceptives

Class of Compound	Drug	Modification of Drug Action	Suggested Management
Alcohol		Possible increased levels of ethanol or acetaldehyde.	Use with caution.
Alpha-II Adrenoreceptor Agents	Clonidine	Sedation effect increased.	Use with caution.
Anticoagulants	All	Oral contraceptives increase clotting factors, decrease efficacy. However, oral contraceptives may potentiate action in some patients.	Use another method.
Anticonvulsants	All	Estrogens may increase risk of seizures.	Use another method.
	Lamotrigine	Decreased lamotrigine levels may lead to breakthrough seizures.	Use another method.
Antidiabetic Drugs	Oral hypoglycemics and insulin	Oral contraceptives may impair glucose tolerance and increase blood glucose.	Use low-dose estrogen and progestin oral contraceptive or another method. Monitor blood glucose.
Antihypertensive Agents	Guanethidine and methyldopa	Estrogen component causes sodium retention, progestin has no effect.	Use low-dose estrogen oral contraceptive or use another method.
	Beta blockers	Increased drug effect (decreased metabolism).	Adjust dose of drug if necessary. Monitor cardiovascular status.
Antipyretics	Acetaminophen	Increased metabolism and renal clearance.	Dose of drug may have to be increased.
	Antipyrine	Impaired metabolism.	Decrease dose of drug.
	ASA	Effects of ASA may be decreased by the short-term use of oral contraceptives.	Patients on chronic ASA therapy may require an increase in ASA dosage.
Aminocaproic Acid		Theoretically, a hypercoagulable state may occur because oral contraceptives augment clotting factors.	Avoid concomitant use.
Betamimetic Agents	Isoproterenol	Estrogen causes decreased response to these drugs.	Adjust dose of drug as necessary. Discontinuing oral contraceptives can result in excessive drug activity.
Caffeine		The actions of caffeine may be enhanced as oral contraceptives may impair the hepatic metabolism of caffeine.	Use with caution.
Cholesterol Lowering Agents	Clofibrate	Their action may be antagonized by oral contraceptives. Oral contraceptives may also increase metabolism of clofibrate.	May need to increase dose of clofibrate.
Corticosteroids	Prednisone	Markedly increased serum levels.	Possible need for decrease in dose.
Cyclosporine		May lead to an increase in cyclosporine levels and hepatotoxicity.	Monitor hepatic function. The cyclosporine dose may have to be decreased.
Folic Acid		Oral contraceptives have been reported to impair folate metabolism.	May need to increase dietary intake, or supplement.

(cont'd)

Table 4: **TRIQUILAR** *(cont'd)*

Modification of Other Drug Action by Oral Contraceptives

Class of Compound	Drug	Modification of Drug Action	Suggested Management
Meperidine		Possible increased analgesia and CNS depression due to decreased metabolism of meperidine.	Use combination with caution.
Phenothiazine Tranquilizers	All phenothiazines, reserpine and similar drugs	Estrogen potentiates the hyperprolactinemia effect of these drugs.	Use other drugs or lower dose oral contraceptives. If galactorrhea or hyperprolactinemia occurs, use other method.
Sedatives and Hypnotics	Chlordiazepoxide Lorazepam Oxazepam Diazepam	Increased effect (increased metabolism).	Use with caution.
Theophylline	All	Decreased oxidation, leading to possible toxicity.	Use with caution. Monitor theophylline levels.
Tricyclic Antidepressants	Clomipramine (possibly others)	Increased side effects: ie, depression.	Use with caution.
Vitamin B_{12}		Oral contraceptives have been reported to reduce serum levels of Vitamin B_{12}.	May need to increase dietary intake, or supplement.

Several of the anti-HIV protease inhibitors (eg, ritonavir) and non-nucleoside reverse transcriptase inhibitors (eg, nevirapine) have been studied with coadministration of oral combination hormonal contraceptives; significant changes (increase and decrease) in the mean AUC of the estrogen and progestogen and the potential to affect hepatic metabolism have been noted in some cases. The efficacy and safety of oral contraceptive products may be affected. Health care professionals should refer to the label of the individual anti-HIV protease inhibitor for further drug-drug interaction information.

No formal drug-drug interaction studies have been conducted with TRIQUILAR.

Drug-Food Interactions: Interactions with food have not been established.

Drug-Herb Interactions: Herbal products containing St. John's wort (Hypericum perforatum) may induce hepatic enzymes (cytochrome P450) and p-glycoprotein transporter and may reduce the effectiveness of contraceptive steroids. This may also result in breakthrough bleeding.

Drug-Laboratory Test Interactions: Results of laboratory tests should be interpreted with the knowledge that the patient is on oral contraceptives. The following laboratory tests are modified:

Liver Function Tests: Aspartate serum transaminase (AST)—variously reported elevations Alkaline phosphatase and gamma glutamine transaminase (GGT)—slightly elevated.

Coagulation Tests: Minimal elevation of test values reported for such parameters as prothrombin and Factors VII, VIII, IX and X.

Thyroid Function Tests: Protein binding of thyroxine is increased as indicated by increased total serum thyroxine concentrations and decreased T_3 resin uptake.

Lipoproteins: Small changes of unproven clinical significance may occur in lipoprotein cholesterol fractions.

Gonadotropins: LH and FSH levels are suppressed by the use of oral contraceptives. Wait two weeks after discontinuing the use of oral contraceptives before measurements are made.

Glucose Tolerance: Glucose tolerance may be decreased.

Tissue Specimens: Pathologists should be advised of oral contraceptive therapy when specimens obtained from surgical procedures and Pap smears are submitted for examination.

Drug-Lifestyle Interactions: No studies on the effects of TRIQUILAR on the ability to drive or use machines have been performed.

Non-Contraceptive Benefits of Oral Contraceptives: Several health advantages other than contraception have been reported.

1. Combination oral contraceptives reduce the incidence of cancer of the endometrium and ovaries.
2. Oral contraceptives reduce the likelihood of developing benign breast disease, and as a result decrease the incidence of breast biopsies.
3. Oral contraceptives reduce the likelihood of development of functional ovarian cysts.
4. Pill-users have less menstrual blood loss and have more regular cycles, thereby reducing the chance of developing iron-deficiency anemia.
5. The use of oral contraceptives may decrease the severity of dysmenorrhea and premenstrual syndrome, and may improve acne vulgaris, hirsutism, and other androgen-mediated disorders.
6. Oral contraceptives decrease the incidence of acute pelvic inflammatory disease and thereby reduce as well the incidence of ectopic pregnancy.
7. Oral contraceptives have potential beneficial effects on endometriosis.

DOSAGE AND ADMINISTRATION: Pills must be taken in the order directed on the package every day at about the same time with some liquid as needed. The patient may begin using TRIQUILAR (levonorgestrel and ethinyl estradiol) on Day 1 of her menstrual cycle (ie, the first day of menstrual flow), on Day 5, or on the first Sunday after her period begins. If the patient's period begins on Sunday, she should start that same day. An additional (barrier) method of birth control is recommended for the first seven days of use.

TRIQUILAR 21 (21-day Regimen): One pill is to be taken daily for 21 consecutive days. Pills are then discontinued for 7 consecutive days. Withdrawal bleeding usually occurs within 2 to 3 days following discontinuation.

The patient begins each subsequent course of TRIQUILAR 21 pills on the same day of the week that she began her first course. She begins taking her next course on the 8th day after discontinuation, regardless of whether or not withdrawal bleeding is still in progress.

TRIQUILAR 28 (28-day Regimen): Pill taking is continuous. One pill is to be taken daily for 28 consecutive days. Withdrawal bleeding usually occurs within 2 to 3 days of starting the placebo pills (ie, while the patient is taking the last row of the slightly larger, hormone-free white pills).

The patient begins each subsequent course of TRIQUILAR 28 pills on the same day of the week that she began her first course. She begins taking her next course immediately after completion of the last course, regardless of whether or not withdrawal bleeding is still in progress. There is no need for the patient to count days between cycles because there are no "off pill days".

Management of Missed Pills: The patient should be instructed to use the following chart if she misses one or more of her birth control pills (see Table 5). She should be told to match the number of pills missed with the appropriate starting time for her dosing regimen.

Table 5: **TRIQUILAR**

Management of Missed Pills

Sunday Start	Other than Sunday Start
Miss One Pill at Any Time	**Miss One Pill at Any Time**
Take it as soon as you remember, and take the next pill at the usual time. This means that you might take two pills in one day.	Take it as soon as you remember, and take the next pill at the usual time. This means that you might take two pills in one day.
Miss Two Pills in a Row	**Miss Two Pills in a Row**
First Two Weeks 1. Take two pills the day you remember and two pills the next day. 2. Then take one pill a day until you finish the pack. 3. Use a back-up (barrier) method of birth control if you have sex in the seven days after you miss the pills. **Third Week** 1. Keep taking one pill a day until Sunday. 2. On Sunday, safely discard the rest of the pack and start a new pack that day. 3. Use a back-up (barrier) method of birth control if you have sex in the seven days after you miss the pills. 4. You may not have a period this month. **If you miss two periods in a row, call your doctor or clinic.**	**First Two Weeks** 1. Take two pills the day you remember and two pills the next day. 2. Then take one pill a day until you finish the pack. 3. Use a back-up (barrier) method of birth control if you have sex in the seven days after you miss the pills. **Third Week** 1. Safely dispose of the rest of the pill pack and start a new pack that same day. 2. Use a back-up (barrier) method of birth control if you have sex in the seven days after you miss the pills. 3. You may not have a period this month. **If you miss two periods in a row, call your doctor or clinic.**
Miss Three or More Pills in a Row	**Miss Three or More Pills in a Row**
Anytime in the Cycle 1. Keep taking one pill a day until Sunday. 2. On Sunday, safely discard the rest of the pack and start a new pack that day. 3. Use a back-up (barrier) method of birth control if you have sex in the seven days after you miss the pills. 4. You may not have a period this month. **If you miss two periods in a row, call your doctor or clinic.**	**Anytime in the Cycle** 1. Safely dispose of the rest of the pill pack and start a new pack that same day. 2. Use a back-up (barrier) method of birth control if you have sex in the seven days after you miss the pills. 3. You may not have a period this month. **If you miss two periods in a row, call your doctor or clinic.**

Patients Taking TRIQUILAR 28: If the patient forgets any of the seven slightly larger, hormone-free white pills in Week 4, she should be advised to safely dispose of the pills she missed, and then to keep taking one pill each day until the pack is empty. A backup method of birth control is not required.

Special Notes on Administration: Switching from Another Combined Hormonal Contraceptive (Combined Oral Contraceptive (COC), Vaginal Ring or Transdermal Patch): The patient should start TRIQUILAR on the day she would normally start her next pack of combination oral contraceptives. In case a vaginal ring or transdermal patch has been used, the woman should start using TRIQUILAR preferably on the day of removal, but at the latest when the next application would have been due.

Switching from a Progestogen-only Method (Mini-Pill, Injection) or from a Progestogen-releasing Intrauterine System (IUS): The patient may switch from the mini-pill to TRIQUILAR on any day of her cycle. Patients using a progestogen injection should start TRIQUILAR on the day the next injection is due. Patients using an IUS should start TRIQUILAR on the day the IUS is removed. In all cases, the patient should be advised to use an additional (barrier) method for the first 7 days of TRIQUILAR use.

Following First Trimester Abortion: The patient may start using TRIQUILAR immediately. When doing so, she need not take additional contraceptive measures.

Following Delivery or Second Trimester Abortion: Patients should be advised to start TRIQUILAR on day 21 to 28 after delivery or second trimester abortion, after consulting with their physician. When starting later, the patient should be advised to use an additional (barrier) method for the first seven days of TRIQUILAR use. However, if intercourse has already occurred, pregnancy should be excluded before the actual start of use, or the woman should be advised to wait for her next menstrual period prior to starting TRIQUILAR. When the pills are administered in the postpartum period, the increased risk of thromboembolic disease associated with the postpartum period must be considered.

Withdrawal/Breakthrough Bleeding: Withdrawal bleeding usually occurs within 3 days following the last hormone-containing pill. If spotting or breakthrough bleeding occurs while taking TRIQUILAR, the patient should be instructed to continue taking TRIQUILAR as instructed and by the regimen described above. She should be instructed that this type of bleeding is usually transient and without significance; however, if the bleeding is persistent or prolonged, the patient should be advised to consult her physician.

Although the occurrence of pregnancy is unlikely if TRIQUILAR is taken according to directions, if withdrawal bleeding does not occur, the possibility of pregnancy must be considered. If the patient has not adhered to the prescribed dosing schedule (missed one or more hormone-containing pills or started taking them on a day later than she should have), the probability of pregnancy should be considered at the time of the first missed period and appropriate diagnostic measures taken before the medication is resumed. If the patient has adhered to the regimen and misses two consecutive periods, pregnancy should be ruled out before continuing the contraceptive regimen.

Advice in Case of Vomiting: If vomiting occurs within 3 to 4 hours after a pill is taken, absorption may not be complete. In such an event, the advice concerning management of missed pills is applicable.

OVERDOSAGE:

Symptoms: With levonorgestrel and ethinyl estradiol, acute doses in excess of clinical levels, when administered to experimental animals, have been shown to have a minimal deleterious effect. In humans, however, the extent of ill effects to be expected following accidental ingestion of a large dose of any oral contraceptive has not been firmly established.

Overdosage may cause nausea and vomiting. Depending upon the amount ingested, liver toxicity, temporary interference with the function of the seminiferous tubules, or in the case of females, possible withdrawal bleeding within a few days of consumption, are theoretically possible. However, case histories of both male and female children, some of whom ingested more than half a month's supply of oral contraceptive pills, indicate that the effects are asymptomatic and without immediate consequence. Despite the frequency of nausea and vomiting in adult females during the first few cycles of use, none of these children presented such symptoms.

Treatment: There is no known antidote to overdosage. Treatment should be symptomatic, based on the knowledge of the pharmacological action of the constituents. Liver function tests should be conducted, particularly transaminase levels, 2 to 3 weeks after consumption.

> For management of a suspected drug overdose, contact your regional Poison Control Centre. See the *CPS* Directory section for a list of Poison Control Centres.

ACTION AND CLINICAL PHARMACOLOGY: Mechanism of Action: TRIQUILAR, a triphasic oral contraceptive, contains as active ingredients levonorgestrel and ethinyl estradiol. It acts primarily through the mechanism of gonadotrophin suppression by the estrogenic and progestational activity of the active ingredients. Although the primary activity is inhibition of ovulation, alterations in the genital tract, including changes in the cervical mucus (which make sperm penetration more difficult), and the endometrium (which reduce the likelihood of implantation) may also contribute to contraceptive effectiveness.

Levonorgestrel has been evaluated extensively in women to assess its progestational activity.

In women, the endometrium is transformed by the oral administration of 2.5 mg levonorgestrel given over a period of 10 days (total dose after pretreatment with estrogen). The endometrial transformation dose is 250 µg/day, corresponding to 5 µg/kg.

Levonorgestrel at a dose of 125 μg/day was also shown to be twice as potent as norethindrone in the delay of menstruation test by "Swyer and Greenblatt".

Pharmacodynamics: Effects on central and peripheral function before, during and after the use of TRIQUILAR were evaluated in 5 women.

The first and third cycles under TRIQUILAR differed considerably from the control cycle. Serum LH values remained at the level of the early follicular phase as a sign of central inhibitory effect, furthermore there was no increase at mid-cycle.

The 17 β-estradiol also failed to peak and serum progesterone reflected the absence of ovulation. As a result, cervical function was limited, the spinnbarkeit and degree of crystallization of the secretion were greatly reduced. The Caryopyknotic index ran in waves to achieve 25%. Finally, the basal body temperature increased as a result of the thermogenic effect of the progesterone, although this occurred later and more slowly than with preparations which contain a higher dose of progesterone in the first half of the cycle.

Upon discontinuation of TRIQUILAR after the third cycle of use, the serum values of LH, 17 β-estradiol and progesterone again displayed all signs of a normal ovulatory cycle pattern.

Overall the study results confirm that ovulation is inhibited and a distinct antifertile effect is exerted in the peripheral cycle function during therapy with TRIQUILAR.

Pharmacokinetics: Levonorgestrel: Absorption: Orally administered levonorgestrel is rapidly and completely absorbed. Following single ingestion of 0.125 mg levonorgestrel together with 0.03 mg ethinyl estradiol (which represents the combination with the highest levonorgestrel content of the triphasic formulation), peak serum concentrations of 4.3 ng/mL are reached at about one hour after single ingestion. Levonorgestrel is almost completely bioavailable after oral administration.

Distribution: Levonorgestrel is bound to serum albumin and to sex hormone binding globulin (SHBG). Only 1.4% of the total serum drug concentrations are present as free steroid, 55% are specifically bound to SHBG and about 44% are non-specifically bound to albumin. The ethinyl estradiol induced increase in SHBG influences the proportion of levonorgestrel bound to the serum proteins, causing an increase of the SHBG-bound fraction and a decrease of the albumin-bound fraction. The volume of distribution of levonorgestrel (V_z) is about 128 L after single oral administration of the highest levonorgestrel dose of TRIQUILAR.

Metabolism: Levonorgestrel is completely metabolized by the known pathways of steroid metabolism. The clearance rate from serum is approximately 1.0 mL/min/kg after single oral administration of the highest levonorgestrel dose of TRIQUILAR. The majority of an oral dose of levonorgestrel is eliminated as glucuronides, significantly smaller portions as free, very polar metabolites and as sulphates. The principal metabolite is d-3α-5β-tetrahydronorgestrel.

Excretion: Levonorgestrel serum levels decrease in two phases. The terminal disposition phase is characterized by a half-life of approximately 22 hours. Levonorgestrel is not excreted in unchanged form. Its metabolites are excreted at a urinary to biliary ratio of about 1:1. The half life of metabolite excretion is about 1 day.

Steady-state Conditions: Levonorgestrel pharmacokinetics are influenced by SHBG levels, which are increased about twofold during the 21-day treatment period with TRIQUILAR. Following daily ingestion drug serum levels increase about fourfold as compared to single oral administration of the highest levonorgestrel dose of TRIQUILAR, reaching steady-state conditions during the second half of a treatment cycle. At steady-state, the volume of distribution and the clearance rate are reduced to 52 L and 0.5 mL/min/kg, respectively, as compared to single oral administration of the highest levonorgestrel dose of TRIQUILAR.

Ethinyl Estradiol: Absorption: Orally administered ethinyl estradiol is rapidly and completely absorbed. Peak serum concentrations of about 116 pg/mL are reached within 1.3 hours after single oral ingestion of 0.03 mg ethinyl estradiol in combination with 0.125 mg levonorgestrel. During absorption and first liver passage, ethinyl estradiol is metabolized extensively, resulting in a mean oral bioavailability of about 45% with a large inter-individual variation of about 20-65%.

Distribution: Ethinyl estradiol is highly but non-specifically bound to serum albumin (approximately 95-98%), and induces an increase in the serum concentrations of SHBG. An apparent volume of distribution of about 2.8-8.6 L/kg was reported after intravenous administration.

Metabolism: Ethinyl estradiol is subject to presystemic conjugation in both small bowel mucosa and the liver. Ethinyl estradiol is primarily metabolized by aromatic hydroxylation but a wide variety of hydroxylated and methylated metabolites are formed, and these are present as free metabolites and as conjugates with glucuronides and sulfate. The clearance rate was reported to be 2.3-7 mL/min/kg after intravenous administration.

Excretion: Ethinyl estradiol serum levels decrease in two disposition phases characterized by half-lives of about 1 hour and 10-20 hours, respectively. Unchanged drug is not excreted. Ethinyl estradiol metabolites are excreted at a urinary to biliary ratio of 4:6 with a half-life of about 1 day.

Steady-state Conditions: According to the variable half-life of the terminal disposition phase from serum, and the daily ingestion, steady-state serum levels of ethinyl estradiol will be reached after about one week. After three cycles, the maximum ethinyl estradiol concentration of about 132 pg/mL is reached after about 1.3 h.

Special Populations and Conditions: Pediatrics: Safety and efficacy of TRIQUILAR has not been established in women under the age of 16 years. Use of this product before menarche is not indicated.

Geriatrics: TRIQUILAR is not indicated for use in postmenopausal women. Oral contraceptives may mask the onset of the climacteric.

Hepatic Insufficiency: TRIQUILAR is contraindicated in women with active liver diseases (see Contraindications).

Renal Insufficiency: TRIQUILAR has not been specifically studied in renally impaired patients. Available data do not suggest a change in treatment in this patient population.

STORAGE AND STABILITY: Store in original packaging between 15 and 30°C. Keep out of reach of children and pets.

Medicines should not be disposed of via wastewater or household waste. Ask your pharmacist how to dispose of medicines no longer required. These measures will help to protect the environment.

SPECIAL HANDLING INSTRUCTIONS: There are no special handling instructions.

INFORMATION FOR THE PATIENT: Published in e-CPS, available by subscription at www.e-cps.ca.

DOSAGE FORMS, COMPOSITION AND PACKAGING: TRIQUILAR 21: Days 1-6: Each hormone-containing light brown tablet contains: levonorgestrel 0.05 mg and ethinyl estradiol 0.03 mg. Days 7-11: Each hormone-containing white tablet contains: levonorgestrel 0.075 mg and ethinyl estradiol 0.04 mg. Days 12-21: Each hormone-containing ochreous tablet contains: levonorgestrel 0.125 mg and ethinyl estradiol 0.03 mg. Nonmedicinal ingredients: calcium carbonate, cornstarch, glycerin, lactose, magnesium stearate, montanglycol wax, polyethylene glycol, polyvinylpyrrolidone, red ferric oxide, sucrose, talc, titanium dioxide and yellow ferric oxide. Gluten- and tartrazine-free.

TRIQUILAR 28: Package contains the same tablets as TRIQUILAR 21 plus seven slightly larger inert hormone-free white tablets. Nonmedicinal ingredients: calcium carbonate, cornstarch, glycerin, lactose, magnesium stearate, montanglycol wax, polyethylene glycol, polyvinylpyrrolidone, red ferric oxide, sucrose, talc, titanium dioxide and yellow ferric oxide. Gluten- and tartrazine-free.

(Shown in Product Identification Section)

Trizivir® ℞

abacavir sulfate—lamivudine—zidovudine

Antiretroviral Agent

ViiV Healthcare ULC

Date of Revision: April 23, 2010

SUMMARY PRODUCT INFORMATION:

Route of Administration	Dosage Form/ Strength	Clinically Relevant Nonmedicinal Ingredients
Oral	Tablet/300 mg abacavir, 150 mg lamivudine and 300 mg zidovudine	None For a complete listing see Dosage Forms, Composition and Packaging.

INDICATIONS AND CLINICAL USE: TRIZIVIR (abacavir sulfate/lamivudine/zidovudine) is indicated for:

- the treatment of Human Immunodeficiency Virus (HIV) infection in adult patients. This fixed-dose combination is a simplified dosing alternative to the three components used separately in similar dosages.

This indication is supported by the results obtained in controlled clinical trials with the separate components (abacavir sulfate, lamivudine and zidovudine). The demonstration of benefit of this combination is mainly based on results of studies of antiretroviral naïve patients. In patients with high viral load (>100 000 copies/mL) choice of therapy needs special consideration.

TRIZIVIR was approved on pharmacokinetic and safety data only.

CONTRAINDICATIONS:

- TRIZIVIR (abacavir sulfate/lamivudine/zidovudine) is contraindicated in patients with previously demonstrated clinically significant hypersensitivity to any of the components of the product (see Dosage Forms, Composition and Packaging).
- TRIZIVIR is contraindicated in patients with end stage renal disease.
- Due to the active ingredient abacavir, TRIZIVIR is contraindicated in patients with hepatic impairment.
- Due to the active ingredient zidovudine, TRIZIVIR is contraindicated in patients with abnormally low neutrophil counts ($<0.75\times10^9$/L) or abnormally low hemoglobin levels (<7.5 g/dL or 4.65 mmol/L).

WARNINGS AND PRECAUTIONS:

Serious Warnings and Precautions

- **Fatal Hypersensitivity Reactions:** Fatal hypersensitivity reactions have been associated with therapy with abacavir sulfate and other abacavir containing products. Therapy with TRIZIVIR (abacavir sulfate/lamivudine/zidovudine) should be discontinued in patients developing signs or symptoms of hypersensitivity in 2 or more of the following groups: 1) fever, 2) rash, 3) gastrointestinal (including nausea, vomiting, diarrhea or abdominal pain), 4) constitutional (including generalized malaise, fatigue or achiness), 5) respiratory (including pharyngitis, dyspnea, cough and abnormal chest x-ray findings, predominantly infiltrates, which can be localized) (see Warnings and Precautions, Hypersensitivity Reactions to Abacavir). To minimize the risk of a life-threatening hypersensitivity reaction, TRIZIVIR should be permanently discontinued if hypersensitivity cannot be ruled out, even when other diagnoses are possible (acute onset of respiratory diseases, gastroenteritis or reactions to other medications).

  The symptoms of a hypersensitivity reaction can occur at any time during treatment with abacavir, but usually occur within the first six weeks of therapy. **TRIZIVIR or any other medicinal product containing abacavir (e.g. ZIAGEN, KIVEXA) must never be restarted following a hypersensitivity reaction, as more severe symptoms will recur within hours and may include life-threatening hypotension and death.** Severe or fatal hypersensitivity reactions can occur within hours after TRIZIVIR re-introduction in patients who have no identified history or undiagnosed symptoms of hypersensitivity during their initial period of use of TRIZIVIR.

  Patients who carry the HLA-B*5701 allele are at a significant increased risk for experiencing a hypersensitivity reaction to abacavir. Prior to initiating therapy with abacavir, it is recommended that screening for HLA-B*5701 status be undertaken. Screening is also recommended prior to re-initiation of abacavir in patients of unknown HLA-B*5701 status who have previously tolerated abacavir. Use of abacavir in patients known to carry the HLA-B*5701 allele is not recommended.

  Cases of abacavir hypersensitivity have occurred in patients who are HLA-B*5701 negative. The clinical diagnosis of suspected hypersensitivity to abacavir remains the basis for clinical decision making in all patients. Therefore, it is important to permanently discontinue abacavir and not rechallenge with abacavir if hypersensitivity cannot be ruled out, regardless of the presence or absence of the HLA-B*5701 allele due to the potential for a severe or even fatal reaction (see Warnings and Precautions, Hypersensitivity Reaction, Risk Factors: HLA-B*5701 Allele).
- **Lactic Acidosis and Severe Hepatomegaly with Steatosis:** Lactic acidosis and severe hepatomegaly with steatosis, including fatal cases, have been reported with the use of nucleoside analogues alone or in combination, including TRIZIVIR and other antiretrovirals. A majority of these cases have been in women. Obesity and prolonged nucleoside exposure may be risk factors. However, cases have also been reported in patients with no known risk factors. Treatment with TRIZIVIR should be suspended in any patient who develops clinical or laboratory findings suggestive of lactic acidosis or pronounced hepatotoxicity (which may include hepatomegaly and steatosis even in the absence of marked transaminase elevations) (see Warnings and Precautions, Hepatic/Biliary/Pancreatic).
- **Post-Treatment Exacerbation of Hepatitis:** It is recommended that all patients with HIV be tested for the presence of chronic hepatitis B virus (HBV) before initiating antiretroviral therapy. TRIZIVIR is not indicated for the treatment of chronic HBV infection and the safety and efficacy of TRIZIVIR have not been established in patients coinfected with HBV and HIV. Exacerbations of hepatitis B have been reported in patients after the discontinuation of antiretroviral therapy. Patients coinfected with HIV and HBV should be closely monitored with both clinical and laboratory follow-up for at least several months after stopping treatment with TRIZIVIR (see Adverse Reactions, Post-Market Adverse Drug Reactions).
- **Pancreatitis:** Pancreatitis has been observed in some patients receiving abacavir and lamivudine. However it is not clear whether these cases were due to drug treatment or to the underlying HIV disease. Pancreatitis must be considered whenever a patient develops abdominal pain, nausea, vomiting or elevated biochemical markers. Discontinue use of TRIZIVIR until diagnosis of pancreatitis is excluded (see Adverse Reactions, Post-Market Adverse Drug Reactions).
- **Pancreatitis in Pediatric Patients:** In pediatric patients with a history of prior antiretroviral nucleoside exposure, a history of pancreatitis, or other significant risk factors for the development of pancreatitis, lamivudine containing products should be used with caution. Treatment with lamivudine containing products should be stopped immediately if clinical signs, symptoms, or laboratory abnormalities suggestive of pancreatitis occur (see Adverse Reactions, Post-Market Adverse Drug Reactions).

General: TRIZIVIR is a fixed dose combination of abacavir sulfate, lamivudine and zidovudine. TRIZIVIR should not be administered concomitantly with either abacavir, lamivudine or zidovudine. The complete prescribing information for all agents being considered for use with TRIZIVIR should be consulted before combination therapy with TRIZIVIR is initiated.

The incidence of adverse reactions appears to increase with disease progression and patients should be monitored carefully, especially as disease progression occurs.

Hypersensitivity Reactions: Serious and sometimes fatal hypersensitivity reactions have been associated with therapy with abacavir sulfate, one of the three active ingredients of TRIZIVIR. Patients who carry the HLA-B*5701 allele are at a significantly increased risk for experiencing a hypersensitivity reaction to abacavir. Other less common signs or symptoms of hypersensitivity include fever, skin rash, fatigue, myolysis, edema, paresthesia, anaphylaxis, liver failure, renal failure, hypotension, adult respiratory distress syndrome, respiratory failure, and death have occurred in association with hypersensitivity reactions, gastrointestinal symptoms, such as nausea, vomiting, diarrhea or abdominal pain, and respiratory signs and symptoms such as pharngitis, dyspnea, cough and abnormal chest x-ray findings predominantly infiltrates, which can be localized.

Physical findings associated with hypersensitivity to abacavir in some patients include lymphadenopathy, mucous membrane lesions (conjunctivitis and mouth ulcerations), and rash. The rash usually appears maculopapular or urticarial, but may be variable in appearance. There have been reports of erythema multiforme. Hypersensitivity reactions have occurred without rash.

Laboratory abnormalities associated with hypersensitivity to abacavir in some patients include elevated liver function tests, elevated creatine phosphokinase, elevated creatinine, and lymphopenia.

The diagnosis of a hypersensitivity reaction should be carefully considered for patients presenting with symptoms of acute onset respiratory diseases, even if alternative respiratory diagnoses (pneumonia, bronchitis, pharyngitis or flu-like illness) are possible. **TRIZIVIR or any other medicinal product containing abacavir must never be restarted following a hypersensitivity reaction, as more severe symptoms will recur within hours and may include life-threatening hypotension and death.**

To avoid a delay in diagnosis and minimize the risk of a life-threatening hypersensitivity reaction, TRIZIVIR should be permanently discontinued if hypersensitivity cannot be ruled out, even when other diagnoses are possible (respiratory diseases, flu-like illness, gastroenteritis or reactions to other medications). TRIZIVIR or any other medicinal product containing abacavir should not be re-started, even if a recurrence of symptoms occurs following rechallenge with alternative medication(s).

Severe or fatal hypersensitivity reactions can occur within hours after TRIZIVIR re-introduction in patients who have no identified history or unrecognized symptoms of hypersensitivity during their initial period of use of TRIZIVIR.

Regardless of a patient's HLA-B*5701 status, if therapy with TRIZIVIR or any other medicinal product containing abacavir has been discontinued and restarting therapy is under consideration, the reason for discontinuation should be evaluated to ensure that the patient did not have symptoms of a hypersensitivity reaction. **If a hypersensitivity reaction cannot be ruled out, TRIZIVIR, or any other medicinal product containing abacavir (e.g. ZIAGEN, KIVEXA) should not be restarted.**

If symptoms consistent with hypersensitivity are not identified, reintroduction can be undertaken with continued monitoring for symptoms of a hypersensitivity reaction. Make patients aware that a hypersensitivity reaction can occur with reintroduction of TRIZIVIR or any other abacavir containing product and that reintroduction of TRIZIVIR or introduction of any other abacavir containing product needs to be undertaken only if medical care can be readily accessed by the patient or others.

Overall, in clinical trials conducted before the introduction of screening for the HLA-B*5701 allele, hypersensitivity to abacavir was reported in approximately 8% of 2670 patients (n=206) in 9 clinical trials (range: 2% to 9%) with enrolment from November 1999 to February 2002. Data on time to onset and symptoms of suspected hypersensitivity were collected on a detailed data collection module. This reaction is characterised by the appearance of symptoms indicating multi-organ/body-system involvement. Symptoms can occur at any time during therapy, however they usually appear within the first 6 weeks (median time to onset 11 days) of initiation of treatment with TRIZIVIR (see Adverse Reactions). See Figure 1.

Figure 1: TRIZIVIR

Hypersensitivity Related Symptoms Reported with ≥10% Frequency in Clinical Trials (n=206 Patients)

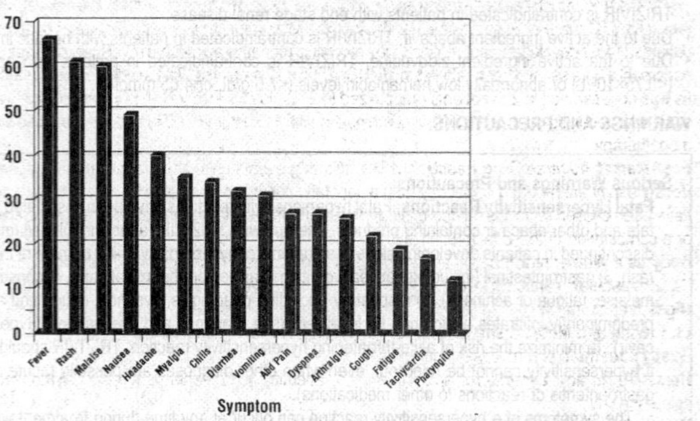

A warning card with information for the patient about this hypersensitivity reaction is included in the TRIZIVIR pack (see Information for the Patient, Warning Card).

Risk Factors: HLA-B*5701 Allele: Studies have shown that carriage of the HLA-B*5701 allele is associated with a significantly increased risk of a hypersensitivity reaction to abacavir. CNA106030 (PREDICT-1), a randomized, double blind study, evaluated the clinical utility of prospective HLA-B*5701 screening on the incidence of abacavir hypersensitivity reaction in abacavir-naive HIV-1 infected adults (n=1650). In this study, use of pre-therapy screening for the HLA-B*5701 allele and exclusion of subjects with this allele reduced the incidence of clinically suspected abacavir hypersensitivity reactions from 7.8% (66/847) to 3.4% (27/803) (p<0.0001). Based on this study, it is estimated that 61% of patients with the HLA-B*5701 allele will develop a clinically suspected hypersensitivity reaction during the course of abacavir treatment compared with 4% of patients who do not have the HLA-B*5701 allele.

Screening for carriage of the HLA-B*5701 allele is recommended prior to initiating treatment with abacavir. Screening is also recommended prior to re-initiating abacavir in patients of unknown HLA-B*5701 status who have previously tolerated abacavir. For HLA-B*5701-positive patients, initiating or re-initiating treatment with an abacavir containing regimen is not recommended and should be considered only with close medical supervision and under exceptional circumstances where potential benefit outweighs the risk.

Skin patch testing is used as a research tool and should not be used to aid in the clinical diagnosis of abacavir hypersensitivity.

In any patient treated with abacavir, the clinical diagnosis of a hypersensitivity reaction must remain the basis of clinical decision making. Even in the absence of the HLA- B*5701 allele, it is important to permanently discontinue abacavir and not rechallenge with abacavir if a hypersensitivity reaction cannot be ruled out on clinical grounds, due to the potential for a severe or even fatal reaction.

Carcinogenesis and Mutagenesis: Abacavir induced chromosomal aberrations both in the presence and absence of metabolic activation in an in vitro cytogenetic study in human lymphocytes. Abacavir was mutagenic in the absence of metabolic activation, although it was not mutagenic in the presence of metabolic activation in an L5178Y mouse lymphoma assay.

At systemic exposures approximately nine times higher than that in humans at the therapeutic dose, abacavir was clastogenic in males and not clastogenic in females in an in vivo mouse bone marrow micronucleus assay.

Abacavir was not mutagenic in bacterial mutagenicity assays in the presence and absence of metabolic activation.

Carcinogenicity studies with orally administered abacavir in mice and rats showed an increase in the incidence of malignant and non-malignant tumors. Malignant tumors occurred in the preputial gland of males and the clitoral gland of females of both species, and in the liver, urinary bladder, lymph nodes and subcutis of female rats. The majority of these tumors occurred at the highest abacavir dose in mice and rats, which correspond to 24-32 times the expected systemic exposure in humans.

Cardiovascular: The results of a prospective, observational, epidemiological study designed to investigate the rate of myocardial infarction in patients on combination antiretroviral therapy (N=33 347) suggest that current or recent use (within the past 6 months) of abacavir may be associated with a potential increased risk of myocardial infarction. This elevated risk does not appear to increase further over time, and no excess risk was present in patients who had stopped taking abacavir more than 6 months previously. The relative risk of myocardial infarction was estimated to be 1.9 (95% CI 1.47-2.45). The absolute myocardial infarction rate was 6.1/1000 patient years of exposure for those recently exposed to abacavir compared to an absolute myocardial infarction rate of 2.6/1000 patient years of exposure for those not recently exposed. In addition, the absolute myocardial infarction rate ranged from 3.4 to 3.7/1000 patient years of exposure for patients recently exposed to other NRTIs (i.e. zidovudine, stavudine and lamivudine).

In a pooled analysis of GSK sponsored clinical trials (N=9639), no increased risk of myocardial infarction was observed with abacavir use. At this time, though the available data do not allow a definitive conclusion regarding the association between the use of abacavir and an increased risk of myocardial infarction, it is recommended that physicians discuss the potential benefits and risks of abacavir with their patients.

As a precaution, the underlying risk of coronary heart disease should be considered when prescribing antiretroviral therapies, including abacavir, and action taken to minimize all modifiable risk factors (e.g. hypertension, hyperlipidemia, diabetes mellitus and smoking).

Endocrine and Metabolism: Fat Redistribution: Redistribution/accumulation of body fat including central obesity, dorsocervical fat enlargement ("buffalo hump"), peripheral wasting, facial wasting, breast enlargement, and "cushingoid appearance" have been observed in patients receiving antiretroviral therapy. The mechanism and long-term consequences of these events are currently unknown. A causal relationship has not been established.

Hematologic: Bone Marrow Suppression: Since TRIZIVIR contains zidovudine, TRIZIVIR should be used with extreme caution in patients who have bone marrow compromise evidenced by granulocyte count <1000 cells/mm^3 or hemoglobin <9.5 g/dL. In all of the placebo-controlled studies, but most frequently in patients with advanced symptomatic disease, anemia and granulocytopenia was the most significant adverse events observed (see Adverse Reactions). There have been reports of pancytopenia associated with the use of zidovudine, which was reversible in most instances after discontinuation of the drug.

Very rare occurrences of pure red cell aplasia have been reported with lamivudine or zidovudine use. Discontinuation of lamivudine and/or zidovudine has resulted in normalization of hematologic parameters in patients with suspected lamivudine or zidovudine induced pure red cell aplasia.

Anemia, neutropenia and leucopenia (usually secondary to neutropenia) can be expected to occur in patients receiving zidovudine. These occurred more frequently at higher zidovudine dosages (1200 to 1500 mg/day) and in patients with poor bone marrow reserve prior to treatment, particularly with advanced HIV disease. Hematological parameters should therefore be carefully monitored in patients receiving TRIZIVIR (see Contraindications).

These hematological effects are not usually observed before four to six weeks therapy. For patients with advanced symptomatic HIV disease, it is generally recommended that blood tests are performed at least every two weeks for the first three months of therapy and at least monthly thereafter. In patients with early HIV disease hematological adverse reactions are infrequent. Depending on the overall condition of the patient, blood tests may be performed less often, for example every one to three months.

Additionally dosage adjustment of zidovudine may be required if severe anemia or myelosuppression occurs during treatment with TRIZIVIR, or in patients with pre-existing bone marrow compromise e.g. haemoglobin less than 9 g/dL (5.59 mmol/L) or neutrophil count less than 1.0×10^9/L (see Dosage and Administration). As dosage adjustment of TRIZIVIR is not possible separate preparations of zidovudine, abacavir and lamivudine should be used.

Hepatic/Biliary/Pancreatic: Lactic Acidosis/Severe Hepatomegaly with Steatosis: Lactic acidosis and severe hepatomegaly with steatosis, including fatal cases, have been reported with the use of antiretroviral nucleoside analogues either alone or in combination, including abacavir, lamivudine and zidovudine. A majority of these cases have been in women.

Clinical features which may be indicative of the development of lactic acidosis include generalized weakness, anorexia, and sudden unexplained weight loss, gastrointestinal symptoms and respiratory symptoms (dyspnea and tachypnea).

Obesity and prolonged nucleoside exposure may be risk factors. Particular caution should be exercised when administering TRIZIVIR to any patient with known risk factors for liver disease; however, cases have also been reported in patients with no known risk factors. Treatment with TRIZIVIR should be suspended in any patient who develops clinical or laboratory findings suggestive of lactic acidosis or hepatotoxicity (which may include hepatomegaly and steatosis even in the absence of marked transaminase elevations).

Use with Interferon- and Ribavirin Based Regimens: In vitro studies have shown ribavirin can reduce the phosphorylation of pyrimidine nucleoside analogues such as lamivudine, a component of TRIZIVIR. Although no evidence of a pharmacokinetic or pharmacodynamic interaction (e.g., loss of HIV/HCV virologic suppression) was seen when ribavirin was coadministered with lamivudine in HIV/HCV co infected patients (see Drug Interactions), hepatic decompensation (some fatal) has occurred in HIV/HCV co infected patients receiving combination antiretroviral therapy for HIV and interferon alfa with or without ribavirin. Patients receiving interferon alfa with or without ribavirin and TRIZIVIR should be closely monitored for treatment associated toxicities, especially hepatic decompensation. Discontinuation of TRIZIVIR should be considered as medically appropriate. Dose reduction or discontinuation of interferon alfa, ribavirin, or both should also be considered if worsening clinical toxicities are observed, including hepatic decompensation.

Patients with Impaired Hepatic Function: TRIZIVIR is contraindicated for use in hepatically impaired patients (see Contraindications). There are no data available on the use of TRIZIVIR in hepatically impaired patients. Abacavir is contraindicated in patients with moderate to severe hepatic impairment and dose reduction is required in some patients with mild hepatic impairment. Because TRIZIVIR is a fixed dose combination and cannot be dose adjusted, TRIZIVIR is contraindicated for patients with hepatic impairment.

Abacavir is metabolized primarily by the liver. The pharmacokinetics of abacavir have been studied in patients with mild hepatic impairment (Child-Pugh score 5-6) who had confirmed cirrhosis.

The results showed that there was a mean increase of 1.89 fold in the abacavir AUC, and 1.58 fold in the half-life of abacavir. The AUCs of the metabolites were not modified by the liver disease. However, the rates of formation and elimination of these were decreased. Dosage reduction of abacavir is therefore required in patients with mild hepatic impairment. The pharmacokinetics of abacavir have not been studied in patients with moderate or severe hepatic impairment.

Limited data in patients with cirrhosis suggest that accumulation of zidovudine may occur, because of decreased glucuronidation. Data obtained in patients with moderate to severe hepatic impairment show that lamivudine pharmacokinetics are not significantly affected by hepatic dysfunction.

Patients co-infected with Hepatitis B Virus: Clinical trial and marketed use of lamivudine, have shown that some patients with chronic hepatitis B virus (HBV) disease may experience clinical or laboratory evidence of recurrent hepatitis upon discontinuation of lamivudine, which may have more severe consequences in patients with decompensated liver disease. If TRIZIVIR is discontinued in a patient with HIV and HBV co-infection, periodic monitoring of both liver function tests and markers of HBV replication should be considered.

Patients co-infected with Hepatitis C Virus: Exacerbation of anemia due to ribavirin has been reported when zidovudine is part of the regimen used to treat HIV although the exact mechanism remains to be elucidated. Therefore, the co-administration of ribavirin and zidovudine is not advised and consideration should be given to replacing zidovudine in a combination ART regimen if this is already established. This is particularly important in patients with a known history of zidovudine induced anemia.

Immune: Patients receiving TRIZIVIR or any other antiretroviral therapy may continue to develop opportunistic infections and other complications of HIV infection. Therefore, patients should remain under close observation by physicians experienced in the treatment of patients with HIV associated diseases.

Immune Reconstitution: During the initial phase of treatment, patients responding to antiretroviral therapy may develop an inflammatory response to indolent or residual opportunistic infections (such as MAC, CMV, PCP, and TB) which may necessitate further evaluation and treatment.

Therapy Experienced Patients: In clinical trials, patients with prolonged prior nucleoside reverse transcriptase inhibitor (NRTI) exposure or who had HIV-1 isolates that contained multiple mutations conferring resistance to NRTIs had limited response to abacavir. The potential for cross-resistance between abacavir and other NRTIs should be considered when choosing new therapeutic regimens in therapy experienced patients.

In heavily pre-treated NRTI patients, the reduction in viral load with abacavir sulfate was very low. The degree of viral load reduction as part of a new combination regimen will depend on the nature and duration of prior therapy which may have selected for HIV-1 variants with cross-resistance to abacavir.

Ophthalmologic: Myopathy: Myopathy and myositis with pathological changes similar to that produced by HIV disease have been associated with prolonged use of zidovudine and therefore may occur with TRIZIVIR therapy.

Renal: Patients with impaired renal function may be at a greater risk of toxicity from TRIZIVIR due to decreased renal clearance of lamivudine and zidovudine. Therefore a dosage adjustment of lamivudine and zidovudine may be necessary. The pharmacokinetic properties of abacavir have not been determined in patients with impaired renal function. Other drugs that are eliminated by acyl glucuronide formation are known to accumulate in patients with renal impairment, therefore it is possible the 5'glucuronide and 5'-carboxylic acid metabolites of abacavir might accumulate in patients with impaired renal function.

It is recommended that TRIZIVIR not be used in patients with reduced renal function (creatinine clearance ≤50 mL/min). For these patients, it is recommended that abacavir, lamivudine and zidovudine be administered. The individual Product Monographs for abacavir, lamivudine and zidovudine should be consulted for appropriate dosage adjustments.

TRIZIVIR is contraindicated in patients with end-stage renal disease (see Contraindications).

Respiratory: Severe respiratory symptoms, some indicative of adult respiratory distress syndrome (ARDS), occur in a small proportion of hypersensitivity reaction cases. ARDS or respiratory failure appear more likely to occur in a re-challenge situation.

Special Populations: Pregnant Women: The safety of TRIZIVIR in human pregnancy has not been established.

Lamivudine, abacavir and zidovudine have been associated with findings in animal reproductive studies. Therefore, administration of TRIZIVIR in pregnancy should be considered only if the benefit to the mother outweighs the possible risk to the fetus.

There have been reports of mild, transient elevations in serum lactate levels, which may be due to mitochondrial dysfunction, in neonates and infants exposed in utero or peri-partum to nucleoside reverse transcriptase inhibitors (NRTIs). The clinical relevance of transient elevations in serum lactate is unknown. There have also been very rare reports of developmental delay, seizures and other neurological disease.

However, a causal relationship between these events and NRTI exposure in utero or peri-partum has not been established. These findings do not affect current recommendations to use antiretroviral therapy in pregnant women to prevent vertical transmission of HIV.

To monitor maternal-fetal outcomes of pregnant women exposed to TRIZIVIR, an Antiretroviral Pregnancy Registry has been established. Physicians are encouraged to register patients by calling ViiV Healthcare ULC's Drug Safety Department (1-877-393-8448).

Nursing Women: It is recommend that HIV-infected women do not breast-feed their infants under any circumstances in order to avoid transmission of HIV. It is therefore recommended that mothers do not breast-feed their babies while receiving treatment with TRIZIVIR.

Both lamivudine and zidovudine are excreted in human milk at similar concentrations to those found in serum. It is expected that abacavir will also be secreted into human milk, although this has not been confirmed.

Pediatrics: TRIZIVIR is not recommended in children. There are no data on the use of TRIZIVIR in pediatric patients.

Geriatrics: Clinical studies of TRIZIVIR did not include sufficient numbers of subjects aged 65 and over to determine whether they respond differently from younger subjects. Other reported clinical experience has not identified differences in responses between the elderly and younger patients. In general, dose selection for an elderly patient should be cautious, reflecting the greater frequency of decreased hepatic, renal or cardiac function, and of concomitant disease or other drug therapy.

ADVERSE REACTIONS: Adverse Drug Reaction Overview: TRIZIVIR (abacavir sulphate/lamivudine/zidovudine) contains abacavir, lamivudine and zidovudine. The adverse events associated with these compounds listed in Table 1 may therefore be expected following treatment with TRIZIVIR. For many of these adverse events, it is unclear whether they are related to the active substance, the wide range of other medicinal products used in the management of HIV disease, or whether they are a result of the underlying disease process. The assessment of the safety profile of TRIZIVIR in clinical studies is not yet available.

Hypersensitivity Reactions: Fatal hypersensitivity reactions have been associated with therapy with abacavir sulfate. Therapy with TRIZIVIR or any medicinal product containing abacavir, **must not** be restarted following a hypersensitivity reaction because more severe symptoms will recur within hours and may include life-threatening hypotension and death. Patients developing signs or symptoms of hypersensitivity should discontinue treatment as soon as a hypersensitivity reaction is first suspected, and must seek medical evaluation immediately. To avoid a delay in diagnosis and minimize the risk of a life-threatening hypersensitivity reaction, TRIZIVIR should be permanently discontinued if hypersensitivity cannot be ruled out, even when other diagnoses are possible (respiratory diseases, flu-like illness, gastroenteritis or reactions to other medications). TRIZIVIR, or any other medicinal product containing abacavir should not be restarted even if a recurrence of symptoms occurs following rechallenge with alternative medication(s).

Severe or fatal hypersensitivity reactions can occur within hours after TRIZIVIR re-introduction in patients who have no identified history or unrecognized symptoms of hypersensitivity during their initial period of use of TRIZIVIR (see Warnings and Precautions).

Regardless of a patient's HLA-B*5701 status, if therapy with TRIZIVIR or any other medicinal product containing abacavir has been discontinued and restarting therapy is under consideration, the reason for discontinuation should be evaluated to ensure that the patient did not have symptoms of a hypersensitivity reaction. If a hypersensitivity reaction can not be ruled out TRIZIVIR or any other medicinal product containing abacavir (e.g. ZIAGEN, KIVEXA) should not be restarted.

Clinical Trial Adverse Drug Reactions: Because clinical trials are conducted under very specific conditions the adverse reaction rates observed in the clinical trials may not reflect the rates observed in practice and should not be compared to the rates in the clinical trials of another drug. Adverse drug reaction information from clinical trials is useful for identifying drug-related adverse events and for approximating rates.

Hypersensitivity Reactions: Overall, in clinical trials conducted before the introduction of screening for the HLA-B*5701 allele, hypersensitivity to abacavir was reported in approximately 8% of patients in 9 clinical trials (range: 2% to 9%). This reaction is characterized by the appearance of symptoms indicating multi-organ/body-system involvement. Symptoms can occur at any time during therapy however they usually appear within the first six weeks (median time to onset 11 days) of initiation of treatment with abacavir.

Almost all patients developing hypersensitivity reactions will have fever and/or rash (usually maculopapular or urticarial) as part of the syndrome, however reactions have occurred without rash or fever.

The signs and symptoms of this hypersensitivity reaction are listed below. Those reported **in at least 10% of patients** with a hypersensitivity reaction are in bold text:

Gastrointestinal Tract	**Abdominal pain**, **diarrhea**, mouth ulceration, **nausea**, **vomiting**
Hematological	Lymphopenia
Liver/Pancreas	**Elevated liver function tests**, hepatic failure
Miscellaneous	Anaphylaxis, conjunctivitis, edema, **fatigue**, **fever**, hypotension, lymphadenopathy, **malaise**
Musculoskeletal	Arthralgia, elevated creatine, **myalgia**, phosphokinase, rarely myolysis
Neurological/Psychiatry	**Headache**, paresthesia
Respiratory Tract	Adult respiratory distress syndrome, **cough**, **dyspnea**, respiratory failure, sore throat
Skin	**Rash** (usually maculopapular or urticarial)
Urology	Elevated creatinine, renal failure

Some patients who experienced a hypersensitivity reaction were initially thought to have acute onset or worsening respiratory disease. The diagnosis of hypersensitivity reaction should be carefully considered for patients presenting with symptoms of acute onset respiratory diseases, even if alternative respiratory diagnoses (pneumonia, bronchitis, pharyngitis) or flu-like illness, gastroenteritis or reactions to other medications are possible.

Symptoms worsen with continued therapy, and usually resolve upon discontinuation of TRIZIVIR (abacavir sulphate/lamivudine/zidovudine).

Restarting TRIZIVIR or any other medicinal product containing abacavir following a hypersensitivity reaction results in a prompt return of symptoms within hours.

This recurrence of the hypersensitivity reaction maybe more severe than on initial presentation, and may include life-threatening hypotension and death.

Regardless of their HLA-B*5701 status, patients who develop this hypersensitivity reaction must discontinue TRIZIVIR and must never be rechallenged with TRIZIVIR or any other medicinal product containing abacavir (e.g. ZIAGEN, KIVEXA).

Many of the adverse events listed above for abacavir (nausea, vomiting, diarrhea, fever, fatigue, rash) occur commonly as part of abacavir hypersensitivity. Therefore, patients with any of these symptoms should be carefully evaluated for the presence of this hypersensitivity reaction.

Hematological Adverse Events with Zidovudine: Anemia (which may require transfusions), neutropenia, leucopenia and aplastic anemia occurred more frequently at higher dosages (1200-1500 mg/day) and in patients with advanced HIV disease (especially when there is poor bone marrow reserve prior to treatment) and particularly in patients with CD_4 cell counts less than 100/mm³. Dosage reduction or cessation of therapy may become necessary (see Warnings and Precautions).

Table 1: TRIZIVIR

Adverse Events Reported with the Individual Components of TRIZIVIR (Adverse events occurring in at least 5% of patients are in bold)

	Abacavir	Lamivudine	Zidovudine
Cardiovascular			Cough, dyspnea
Gastrointestinal Tract	**Nausea, vomiting, diarrhea**	**Nausea, vomiting, diarrhea, upper abdominal pain**	**Nausea, vomiting, anorexia**, diarrhea, abdominal pain, oral mucosa pigmentation, dyspepsia and flatulence
Hematological		Anemia, pure red cell aplasia, neutropenia, thrombocytopenia	Anemia, neutropenia, leucopenia and aplastic anemia (see text below for further details), thrombocytopenia, pancytopenia (with marrow hypoplasia) and pure red cell aplasia
Liver/Pancreas	Pancreatitis	Transient rises in liver enzymes (AST, ALT), rises in serum amylase, pancreatitis	Liver disorders such as severe hepatomegaly with steatosis, rises in blood levels of liver enzymes and bilirubin, pancreatitis
Metabolic/ Endocrine	Lactic acidosis, hyperlactatemia Redistribution/ accumulation of body fat	Lactic acidosis, hyperlactatemia Redistribution/ accumulation of body fat	Lactic acidosis, hyperlactatemia Redistribution/ accumulation of body fat
Musculoskeletal		**Muscle disorders**, rarely rhabdomyolysis, arthralgia	**Myalgia**, myopathy
Neurological/ Psychiatry	**Headache**	**Headache**, peripheral neuropathy, paresthesia	**Headache, insomnia**, paresthesia, dizziness, somnolence, loss of mental acuity, convulsions, anxiety, depression
Respiratory Tract			Cough, dyspnea
Skin	Rash without systemic symptoms. Very rarely erythema multiforme, Stevens-Johnson Syndrome and toxic epidermal necrolysis	**Rash, alopecia**	Rash, nail and skin pigmentation, urticaria, pruritus, sweating
Miscellaneous	**Fever, lethargy, fatigue,** anorexia	**Fever, malaise, fatigue**	**Malaise**, fever, urinary frequency, taste perversion, generalized pain, chills, chest pain, influenza-like syndrome, gynecomastia, asthenia

The incidence of neutropenia was also increased in those patients whose neutrophil counts, hemoglobin levels and serum vitamin B_{12} levels were low at the start of zidovudine therapy.

Pancreatitis, which has been fatal in some cases, has been observed in antiretroviral nucleoside-experienced pediatric patients receiving 3TC alone or in combination with other antiretroviral agents. In an open-label dose-escalation study (NUCA2002), 14 patients (14%) developed pancreatitis while receiving monotherapy with 3TC. Three of these patients died of complications of pancreatitis. In a second open-label study (NUCA2005), 12 patients (18%) developed pancreatitis. In study ACTG300, pancreatitis was not observed in 236 patients randomized to 3TC plus RETROVIR (AZT). Pancreatitis was observed in one patient in this study who received open-label 3TC in combination with RETROVIR (AZT) and ritonavir following discontinuation of didanosine monotherapy.

Post-Market Adverse Drug Reactions: The following events have been identified during use of TRIZIVIR in clinical practice. Because they are reported voluntarily from a population of unknown size, estimates of frequency cannot be made. These events have been chosen for inclusion due to either their seriousness, frequency of reporting, potential causal connection to TRIZIVIR, or a combination of these factors.

Body as a Whole: redistribution/accumulation of body fat (see Warnings and Precautions, Endocrine and Metabolism).
Cardiovascular: cardiomyopathy.
Digestive: stomatitis.
Endocrine and Metabolism: lactic acidosis, hyperglycemia, hyperlactemia.
Gastrointestinal: oral mucosal pigmentation.
Hematologic and Lymphatic: aplastic anemia, anemia, neutropenia, leucopenia, lymphadenopathy, pure red cell aplasia, splenomegaly.
Hepatic/Biliary/Pancreatic: severe hepatomegaly with steatosis, cytolytic hepatitis, pancreatitis, posttreatment exacerbation of hepatitis B.
Hypersensitivity: sensitization reactions (including anaphylaxis), urticaria.
Musculoskeletal: myalgia, arthralgia, CPK elevation, rhabdomyolysis.
Miscellaneous: gynecomastia, asthenia.
Nervous: paresthesia, peripheral neuropathy, seizures.
Respiratory: abnormal breath sounds/wheezing, respiratory failure.
Skin: alopecia, erythema multiforme, Stevens-Johnson Syndrome, toxic epidermal necrolysis.

Serious Adverse Reactions: Abacavir: A patient with a diagnosis of AIDS dementia and a history of seizure disorder experienced a seizure 3 days after stopping abacavir therapy. In the absence of an autopsy, a definitive diagnosis could not be adequately made, and a possible relationship to abacavir therefore could not be ruled out.

Lamivudine: Several serious adverse events have been reported with use of lamivudine in clinical practice. Reports of anaphylaxis, rhabdomyolysis and peripheral neuropathy have been rare (<1 in 1000).

Zidovudine: Several serious adverse events have been reported with use of zidovudine in clinical practice. Reports of pancreatitis, sensitization reactions (including anaphylaxis in one patient), vasculitis and seizures have been rare. These adverse events, except for sensitization, have also been associated with HIV disease. Changes in skin and nail pigmentation have been associated with the use of zidovudine.

Coadministration of zidovudine with other drugs metabolized by glucuronidation should be avoided because the toxicity of either drug may be potentiated (see Drug Interactions).

DRUG INTERACTIONS: Overview: Dosage Adjustments: Separate preparations of abacavir, lamivudine and zidovudine should be administered where dosage adjustment is necessary. In these cases the physician should refer to the individual Product Monographs.

No clinically significant changes to pharmacokinetic parameters were observed for abacavir, lamivudine or zidovudine when administered together. As TRIZIVIR (abacavir sulphate/lamivudine/zidovudine) contains abacavir, lamivudine and zidovudine, any interactions that have been identified with these agents individually may occur with TRIZIVIR. The interactions listed below should not be considered exhaustive but are representative of the classes of medicinal products where caution should be exercised.

Drug-Drug Interactions: Interactions Relevant to Abacavir: Based on the results of in vitro experiments and the known major metabolic pathways of abacavir sulfate, the potential for drug interactions involving abacavir sulfate is low. Abacavir sulfate shows low potential to inhibit metabolism mediated by the cytochrome P450 3A4 enzyme. It has also been shown in vitro not to interact with drugs that are metabolized by CYP3A4, CYP2C9 or CYP2D6 enzymes. Induction of hepatic metabolism has not been observed in clinical studies. Therefore, there is little potential for drug interactions with antiretroviral protease inhibitors and other drugs metabolized by major P450 enzymes. Clinical studies have shown that there are no clinically significant interactions between abacavir sulfate, zidovudine and lamivudine. See Table 2.

Table 2: TRIZIVIR

Established or Potential Drug-Drug Interactions Relevant to Abacavir

Proper Name	Effect	Clinical Comment
Ethanol	In men, the metabolism of abacavir sulfate is altered.	In men, the metabolism of abacavir sulfate is altered by concomitant ethanol resulting in an increase in AUC of abacavir of about 41%. The clinical significance of this is unknown. In men, abacavir sulfate has no effect on the metabolism of ethanol. This interaction has not been studied in women.
Methadone	Changes in abacavir pharmacokinetics.	In a pharmacokinetic study, coadministration of 600 mg abacavir twice daily and methadone showed a 35% reduction in abacavir C_{max} and a 1 hour delay in t_{max}, but AUC was unchanged. The changes in abacavir pharmacokinetics are not considered clinically relevant. In this study abacavir increased methadone systemic clearance by 22%. This change is not considered clinically relevant for the majority of patients, however occasionally methadone re-titration may be required.
Retinoids	Interaction with elimination is possible.	Retinoid compounds such as isotretinoin, are eliminated via alcohol dehydrogenase. Interaction with abacavir is possible but has not been studied.

Interactions Relevant to Lamivudine: Zidovudine plasma levels are not significantly altered when coadministered with lamivudine. Zidovudine has no effect on the pharmacokinetics of lamivudine. See Table 3.

Table 3: TRIZIVIR

Established or Potential Drug-Drug Interactions Relevant to Lamivudine

Proper Name	Effect	Clinical Comment
Trimethoprim	Administration of trimethoprim, a constituent of co-trimoxazole, causes a 40% increase in lamivudine plasma levels.	However, unless the patient has renal impairment, no dosage adjustment of lamivudine is necessary. Lamivudine has no effect on the pharmacokinetics of co-trimoxazole. Administration of co-trimoxazole with the lamivudine/zidovudine combination in patients with renal impairment should be carefully assessed.
Zalcitabine	Lamivudine may inhibit the intracellular phosphorylation of zalcitabine when the two medicinal products are used concurrently.	Lamivudine is not recommended to be used in combination with zalcitabine.

The possibility of interactions with other drugs administered concurrently should be considered, particularly when the main route of elimination is renal.

Interactions Relevant to Zidovudine: Other medicinal products, including but not limited to, acetylsalicylic acid, codeine, morphine, indomethacin, ketoprofen, naproxen, oxazepam, lorazepam, cimetidine, clofibrate and isoprinosine, may alter the metabolism of zidovudine by competitively inhibiting glucuronidation or directly inhibiting hepatic microsomal metabolism. Careful thought should be given to the possibilities of interactions before using such medicinal products particularly for chronic therapy, in combination with TRIZIVIR.

Concomitant treatment, especially acute therapy, with potentially nephrotoxic or myelosuppressive medicinal products (such as systemic pentamidine, pyrimethamine, co-trimoxazole, amphotericin, ganciclovir and interferon) may also increase the risk of adverse reactions to zidovudine.

If concomitant therapy with TRIZIVIR and any of these medicinal products is necessary then extra care should be taken in monitoring renal function and hematological parameters and, if required, the dosage of one or more agents should be reduced.

Some patients receiving TRIZIVIR may continue to experience opportunistic infections, concomitant use of prophylactic antimicrobial therapy may have to be considered. Such prophylaxis has included co-trimoxazole, aerosolized pentamidine, pyrimethamine and acyclovir. Limited data from clinical trials do not indicate a significantly increased risk of adverse reactions to zidovudine with these medicinal products.

See Table 4.

Table 4: TRIZIVIR

Established or Potential Drug-Drug Interactions Relevant to Zidovudine

Proper Name	Effect	Clinical Comment
Atovaquone	Zidovudine does not appear to affect the pharmacokinetics of atovaquone.	Pharmacokinetic data have shown that atovaquone appears to decrease the rate of metabolism of zidovudine to its glucuronide metabolite (steady state AUC of zidovudine was increased by 33% and peak plasma concentration of the glucuronide was decreased by 19%). At zidovudine dosages of 500 or 600 mg/day it would seem unlikely that a three week, concomitant course of atovaquone for the treatment of acute PCP would result in an increased incidence of adverse reactions attributable to higher plasma concentrations of zidovudine. Extra care should be taken in monitoring patients receiving prolonged atovaquone therapy.
Bone Marrow Suppressive Agents/Cytotoxic Agents	Coadministration may increase risk of hematologic toxicity.	Coadministration of zidovudine with drugs that are cytotoxic or which interfere with RBC/WBC number or function (e.g. dapsone, flucytosine, vincristine, or adriamycin) may increase the risk of hematologic toxicity.
Clarithromycin	Clarithromycin tablets reduce the absorption of zidovudine.	This can be avoided by separating the administration of zidovudine and clarithromycin by at least two hours.
Fluconazole	Fluconazole interferes with the oral clearance and metabolism of zidovudine.	Preliminary data suggests that fluconazole interferes with the oral clearance and metabolism of zidovudine. In a pharmacokinetic interaction study in which 12 HIV-positive men received zidovudine alone and in combination with fluconazole, increases in the mean peak serum concentration (79%), AUC (70%) and half-life (38%) were observed at steady state. The clinical significance of this interaction is unknown.
Interferon-alpha	Hematologic toxicities have been seen when RETROVIR (AZT) is used concomitantly with interferon-alpha.	As with the concomitant use of RETROVIR (AZT) and ganciclovir, dose reduction or interruption of one or both agents may be necessary, and hematologic parameters should be monitored frequently.
Lamivudine	Coadministration resulted in a 13% increase in C_{max} of zidovudine and a 28% increase in peak plasma levels.	Zidovudine and lamivudine were coadministered to 12 asymptomatic HIV-positive patients in a single-center, open-label, randomized, crossover study. No significant differences were observed in AUC_{∞} or total clearance for lamivudine or zidovudine when the two drugs were administered together. Coadministration of zidovudine with lamivudine resulted in an increase of 39%±62% (mean±SD) in C_{max} of zidovudine. This increase is not considered significant to patient safety and therefore no dosage adjustments are necessary.
Methadone	Plasma levels of zidovudine can be elevated in some patients while remaining unchanged in others.	In a pharmacokinetic study of 9 HIV-positive patients receiving methadone-maintenance (30 to 90 mg daily) concurrent with 200 mg of zidovudine every 4 hours, no changes were observed in the pharmacokinetics of methadone upon initiation of therapy with zidovudine and after 14 days of treatment with zidovudine. No adjustments in methadone-maintenance requirements were reported. However, plasma levels of zidovudine were elevated in some patients while remaining unchanged in others. The exact mechanism and clinical significance of these data are unknown.
Phenytoin	A decrease in oral zidovudine clearance.	Phenytoin plasma levels have been reported to be low in some patients receiving zidovudine, while in one case a high level was documented. However, in a pharmacokinetic interaction study in which 12 HIV-positive volunteers received a single 300 mg phenytoin dose alone and during steady-state zidovudine conditions (200 mg every 4 hours), no change in phenytoin kinetics was observed. Although not designed to optimally assess the effect of phenytoin on zidovudine kinetics, a 30% decrease in oral zidovudine clearance was observed with phenytoin.
Probenecid	May increase zidovudine levels.	Limited data suggest that probenecid may increase zidovudine levels by inhibiting glucuronidation and/or reducing renal excretion of zidovudine. Some patients who have used zidovudine concomitantly with probenecid have developed flu-like symptoms consisting of myalgia, malaise, and/or fever and maculopapular rash.
Ribavarin	Coadministration of ribavirin and zidovudine may lead to increased ribavirin levels and increased risk of anemia.	Preliminary data suggest that the use of ribavirin and zidovudine lead to increased ribavirin levels and increased risk of anemia. The use of ribavirin concomitantly with zidovudine in the treatment of HIV/Hep C co-infected patients is not advised. Consideration should be given to replacing zidovudine in a combination ART regimen if this is already established.
Stavudine	Zidovudine may inhibit intracellular phosphorylation of stavudine	Zidovudine may inhibit the intracellular phosphorylation of stavudine when the two medicinal products are used concurrently. Stavudine is therefore not recommended to be used in combination with zidovudine.

(cont'd)

Table 4: TRIZIVIR *(cont'd)*

Established or Potential Drug-Drug Interactions Relevant to Zidovudine

Proper Name	Effect	Clinical Comment
Valproic Acid	Increase in zidovudine AUC and a decrease in the plasma GZDV AUC.	The concomitant administration of valproic acid 250 mg (n=5) or 500 mg (n=1) every 8 hours and zidovudine 100 mg orally every 8 hours for 4 days to 6 HIV-infected, asymptomatic male volunteers resulted in a 79%±61% (mean±SD) increase in the plasma zidovudine AUC and a 22%±10% decrease in the plasma GZDV AUC as compared to the administration of zidovudine in the absence of valproic acid. The GZDV/zidovudine urinary excretion ratio decreased 58%±12%. Because no change in the zidovudine plasma half-life occurred, these results suggest that valproic acid may increase the oral bioavailability of zidovudine through inhibition of first-pass metabolism. Although the clinical signification of this interaction is unknown, patients should be monitored more closely for a possible increase in zidovudine-related adverse effects. The effect of zidovudine on the pharmacokinetics of valproic acid was not evaluated.
Other Agents		Some drugs such as trimethoprim-sulfamethoxazole, pyrimethamine, and acyclovir may be necessary for the management or prevention of opportunistic infections. In the placebo-controlled trial in patients with advanced HIV disease, increased toxicity was not detected with limited exposure to these drugs. However, there is one published report of neurotoxicity (profound lethargy) associated with concomitant use of zidovudine and acyclovir. Preliminary data from a drug interaction study (n=10) suggest that coadministration of 200 mg zidovudine and 600 mg rifampin decreases the area under the zidovudine plasma concentration curve by an average of 48%±34%. However, the effect of once daily dosing of rifampin on multiple daily doses of zidovudine is unknown.
Miscellaneous		Other medicinal products, including but not limited to, acetylsalicyclic acid, codeine, morphine, methadone, indomethacin, ketoprofen, naproxen, oxazepam, lorazepam, cimetidine, clofibrate, dapsone and isoprinosine, may alter the metabolism of zidovudine by competitively inhibiting glucuronidation or directly inhibiting hepatic microsomal metabolism. Careful thought should be given to the possibilities of interactions before using such medicinal products particularly for chronic therapy, in combination with TRIZIVIR. Concomitant treatment, especially acute therapy, with potentially nephrotoxic or myelosuppressive medicinal products (such as systemic pentamidine, dapsone, pyrimethamine, co-trimoxazole, amphotericin, flucytosine, ganciclovir, interferon, vincristine, vinblastine and doxorubicin) may also increase the risk of adverse reactions to zidovudine. If concomitant therapy with TRIZIVIR and any of these medicinal products is necessary then extra care should be taken in monitoring renal function and hematological parameters and, if required, the dosage of one or more agents should be reduced.

DOSAGE AND ADMINISTRATION

Recommended Dose and Dosage Adjustment: The recommended oral dose of TRIZIVIR (abacavir sulfate/lamivudine/zidovudine) is one tablet twice daily.

TRIZIVIR can be taken with or without food.

Dose Adjustment: It is recommended that separate doses of abacavir, lamivudine and zidovudine be administered to patients with reduced renal function (see Warnings and Precautions), patients who weigh less than 50 kg or patients requiring dosing adjustments due to adverse events. See complete prescribing information for abacavir, lamivudine and zidovudine for dosage adjustments.

Missed Dose: If you forget to take your medicine, take it as soon as you remember. Then continue as before. Do not take a double dose to make up for forgotten individual doses.

OVERDOSAGE:

There is no known antidote for TRIZIVIR (abacavir sulfate/lamivudine/zidovudine).

If overdosage occurs, the patient should be monitored, and standard supportive treatment applied as required. Although no data is available, administration of activated charcoal may be used to aid in the removal of unabsorbed drug. It is not known whether abacavir can be removed by peritoneal dialysis or hemodialysis. Because a negligible amount of lamivudine was removed via (4-hour) hemodialysis, continuous ambulatory peritoneal dialysis, and automated peritoneal dialysis, it is not known if continuous hemodialysis would provide clinical benefit in a lamivudine overdose event. Hemodialysis and peritoneal dialysis appear to have a negligible effect on the removal of zidovudine, while elimination of its primary metabolite, GZDV is enhanced.

Limited data are available on the consequences of ingestion of acute overdoses in humans. No fatalities occurred, and the patients recovered.

Single doses up to 1200 mg and daily doses up to 1800 mg of abacavir sulfate have been administered to patients in clinical studies. No unexpected adverse reactions were reported. The effects of higher doses are not known. No specific signs or symptoms have been identified following such overdose.

One case of acute overdose in an adult ingesting 6 g of 3TC was reported; there were no clinical signs or symptoms noted and hematologic tests remained normal. One other adult patient in error ingested lamivudine 1200 mg per day plus zidovudine 1200 mg per day for approximately 2 weeks; he had a Grade 3 decrease in absolute neutrophil count that resolved upon reduction of doses of lamivudine and zidovudine. Two cases of pediatric overdose were reported in ACTG300. One case was a single dose of 7 mg/kg of 3TC; the second case involved the use of 5 mg/kg of 3TC twice daily for 30 days. There were no clinical signs or symptoms noted in either case.

In Phase I studies, lamivudine was administered at doses up to 20 mg/kg per day (i.e. approximately five times the usual recommended dose in adults) without serious consequences.

Cases of acute overdose of zidovudine in both children and adults have been reported with doses up to 50 g. The only consistent finding in these cases of overdosage was spontaneous or induced nausea and vomiting. Hematologic changes were transient and not severe. Some patients experienced non specific CNS symptoms such as headache, dizziness, drowsiness, lethargy, and confusion. One report of a grand mal seizure possible attributable to zidovudine occurred in a 35-year old male, 3 hours after ingesting 36 g of zidovudine. No other causes could be identified. All patients recovered without permanent sequelae.

> For management of a suspected drug overdose, contact your regional Poison Control Centre. See the *CPS* Directory section for a list of Poison Control Centres.

ACTION AND CLINICAL PHARMACOLOGY: Mechanism of Action: Abacavir sulfate, lamivudine and zidovudine are inhibitors of HIV-1 and HIV-2 replication in vitro. Abacavir is a synthetic carbocyclic nucleoside analogue. Lamivudine is the (-) enantiomer of a dideoxy analogue of cytidine. Zidovudine is a thymidine analogue in which the 3'-hydroxy (-OH) group is replaced by an azido (-N3) group. Intracellularly, abacavir, lamivudine and zidovudine are phosphorylated to their active 5'-triphosphate metabolites, carbovir-triphosphate, lamivudine triphosphate and zidovudine triphosphate. The principal mode of action of carbovir, lamivudine and zidovudine triphosphate is inhibition of HIV reverse transcription (RT) via viral DNA chain termination. Carbovir, lamivudine and zidovudine triphosphate show significantly less affinity for host cell DNA polymerases.

Pharmacokinetics: Abacavir sulfate is rapidly and well absorbed following oral administration. The absolute bioavailability of oral abacavir sulfate in adults is about 83%. Following oral administration, the mean time (t_{max}) to maximal serum concentrations of abacavir is about 1.5 hours for the tablet formulation and about 1.0 hour for the solution formulation. There are no differences observed between the AUC for the tablet or solution. At therapeutic dosages (300 mg twice daily), the steady state C_{max} of abacavir sulfate tablets is approximately 3 µg/mL, and the AUC over a dosing interval of 12 hours is approximately 6 µg·h/mL. The C_{max} value for the oral solution is slightly higher than the tablet. Food delayed absorption and decreased C_{max} but did not affect overall plasma concentrations (AUC). Therefore abacavir can be taken with or without food. The pharmacokinetic properties of lamivudine have been studied in asymptomatic, HIV-infected adult patients after administration of single oral, multiple oral and intravenous (IV) doses ranging from 0.25 to 10 mg/kg. After oral administration lamivudine is well absorbed from the gut. The bioavailability of lamivudine in adults is normally between 80 and 85% and the mean time (t_{max}) to maximal serum concentrations (C_{max}) is about an hour. After oral administration of 2 mg/kg, the peak plasma lamivudine concentration (C_{max}) was 1.5±0.5 µg/mL (mean±S.D.) and half-life was 2.6±0.5 hours. There were no significant differences in half-life across the range of single doses (0.25 to 8 mg/kg). The area under the plasma concentration versus time curve (AUC) and C_{max} increased in proportion to dose over the range from 0.25 to 10 mg/kg.

Pharmacokinetic studies of zidovudine following intravenous dosing in adults indicate dose-independent kinetics over the range of 1 to 5 mg/kg with a mean zidovudine half-life of 1.1 hours. Zidovudine is rapidly metabolized in the liver to 3'-azido-3'-deoxy-5'-O-β-D-glucopyranuronosylthymidine (GZDV, formerly called GAZT), and both are rapidly eliminated by the kidney. A second metabolite, 3'-amino-3'-deoxythymidine (AMT) has been identified in the plasma following single dose intravenous administration of zidovudine. After oral dosing in adults, zidovudine is rapidly absorbed from the gastrointestinal tract with peak serum concentrations occurring within 0.5 to 1.5 hours, with an average oral bioavailability of 65%.

STORAGE AND STABILITY: Store TRIZIVIR (abacavir sulfate/lamivudine/zidovudine) tablets between 15 and 30°C.

SPECIAL HANDLING INSTRUCTIONS: Not applicable.

INFORMATION FOR THE PATIENT: Published in e-CPS, available by subscription at www.e-cps.ca.

DOSAGE FORMS, COMPOSITION AND PACKAGING: Each blue/green, capsule-shaped, film-coated tablet, imprinted with GX LL1 on one face contains: abacavir 300 mg as abacavir sulfate, lamivudine 150 mg and zidovudine 300 mg. Nonmedicinal ingredients: hydroxypropyl methylcellulose, indigotine aluminium lake, iron oxide yellow, magnesium stearate, microcrystalline cellulose, polyethylene glycol, sodium starch glycolate and titanium dioxide. HDPE bottles of 60.

(Shown in Product Identification Section)

Trosec® Ⓟ
trospium chloride
Antispasmodic

Sepracor

Date of Preparation: November 9, 2009

SUMMARY PRODUCT INFORMATION:

Route of Administration	Dosage Form/ Strength	Clinically Relevant Nonmedicinal Ingredients
Oral	Coated tablet/20 mg	Lactose monohydrate For a complete listing of all nonmedicinal ingredients see Dosage Forms, Composition and Packaging.

INDICATIONS AND CLINICAL USE: TROSEC (trospium chloride) is indicated for:
- the treatment of overactive bladder with symptoms of urge or mixed urinary incontinence, urgency, and urinary frequency.

CONTRAINDICATIONS: TROSEC is contraindicated in patients:
- with urinary retention, gastric retention, or uncontrolled narrow-angle glaucoma and in patients who are at risk for these conditions,
- who have demonstrated hypersensitivity to the drug, its ingredients, or any component of the container. For a complete listing, see Dosage Forms, Composition and Packaging.

WARNINGS AND PRECAUTIONS: General: Patients should be informed that anticholinergic agents, such as TROSEC, may produce clinically significant adverse effects related to anticholinergic pharmacological activity. For example, heat prostration (fever and heat stroke due to decreased sweating) can occur when anticholinergics such as TROSEC are used in a hot environment. Because anticholinergics such as TROSEC may also produce dizziness or blurred vision, patients should be advised to exercise caution. Patients should be informed that alcohol may enhance the drowsiness caused by anticholinergic agents.
Carcinogenesis and Mutagenesis: Carcinogenicity studies with trospium chloride were conducted in mice and rats. A 78-week carcinogenicity study in mice and a 104-week carcinogenicity study in rats were conducted at doses of 2, 20, and 200 mg/kg/day. No evidence of a carcinogenic effect was found in either mice or rats. The 200 mg/kg/day dose in the mouse and rat represents approximately 25 and 60 times, respectively, the human dose based on body surface area. At 200 mg/kg/day in the mouse and rat after 4 weeks the AUC was 34 and 753 ng·h/mL, respectively. The exposure in the rat is 8.6-fold higher than the AUC following 40 mg daily exposure in healthy young or elderly subjects (88 ng·h/mL).

Trospium chloride was not mutagenic in tests for detection of gene mutations in bacteria (Ames test) and mammalian cells (L5178Y mouse lymphoma and Chinese Hamster Ovary [CHO] cells) or in vivo in the rat micronucleus test.
Cardiovascular: The effect of 20 mg twice daily (bid) and up to 100 mg bid TROSEC on QT interval was evaluated in a single-blind, randomized, placebo and active (moxifloxacin 400 mg qd) controlled 5 day parallel trial in 170 male and female healthy volunteer subjects aged 18 to 45 years. The QT interval was measured over a 24 hour period at steady state. The 100 mg bid dose of TROSEC was chosen because this dose achieves the C_{max} expected in severe renal impairment. TROSEC was not associated with an increase in individual corrected (QTcI) or Fridericia corrected (QTcF) QT interval at any time during steady state measurement, while moxifloxacin was associated with a 6.4 msec increase in QTcF.

In this study, asymptomatic, non-specific T wave inversions were observed more often in subjects receiving TROSEC than in subjects receiving moxifloxacin or placebo following five days of treatment. This finding was not observed during routine safety monitoring in two other U.S. placebo-controlled clinical trials in 591 TROSEC-treated overactive bladder patients. The clinical significance of T wave inversion in this study is unknown.

TROSEC is associated with an increase in heart rate that correlates with increasing plasma concentrations. In the study described above, TROSEC demonstrated a mean increase in heart rate compared to placebo of 9.1 bpm for the 20 mg dose and of 18.0 bpm for the 100 mg dose. In the two U.S. placebo-controlled trials in patients with overactive bladder, the mean increase in heart rate compared to placebo in Study 1 was observed to be 3.0 bpm and in Study 2 was 4.0 bpm.

TROSEC has not been formally evaluated in patients with conditions such as congestive heart failure, hypokalemia, myocardial infarction, etc., which potentiate proarrhythmic risk.
Gastrointestinal: TROSEC should be administered with caution to patients with gastrointestinal obstructive disorders because of the risk of gastric retention (see Contraindications). TROSEC, like other anticholinergic drugs, may decrease gastrointestinal motility and should be used with caution in patients with conditions such as ulcerative colitis, intestinal atony and myasthenia gravis.
Hepatic/Biliary/Pancreatic: Caution should be used when administering TROSEC in patients with moderate hepatic dysfunction (see Action and Clinical Pharmacology, Special Populations and Conditions). There is no experience in patients with severe hepatic dysfunction.
Ophthalmologic: In patients being treated for narrow-angle glaucoma, TROSEC should only be used if the potential benefits outweigh the risks and in that circumstance only with careful monitoring.
Renal: TROSEC should be administered with caution to patients with clinically significant bladder outflow obstruction because of the risk of urinary retention.

Dose modification is recommended in patients with severe renal insufficiency [Clcr 0.25-0.5 mL/sec (15-30 mL/min)]. In such patients, TROSEC should be administered as 20 mg once a day at bedtime (see Dosage and Administration). The use of TROSEC in patients with renal function <0.25 mL/sec (15 mL/min) has not been studied.
Sexual Function/Reproduction: No evidence of impaired fertility was observed in rats administered doses up to 200 mg/kg/day (about 10 multiples of the expected clinical exposure via AUC). The effect of TROSEC on sexual function/reproduction in humans has not been studied.
Special Populations: Pregnant Women: Trospium chloride has been shown to cause maternal toxicity in rats and a decrease in fetal survival in rats administered approximately 10 times the expected clinical exposure (AUC). The no effect levels for maternal and fetal toxicity were approximately equivalent to the expected clinical exposure in rats, and about 5-6 times the expected clinical exposure in rabbits. No malformations or developmental delays were observed. There are no adequate and well controlled studies in pregnant women. TROSEC should be used during pregnancy only if the potential benefit justifies the potential risk to the fetus.
Nursing Women: Trospium chloride (2 mg/kg po and 50 µg/kg iv) was excreted, to a limited extent (<1%), into the milk of lactating rats. The activity observed in the milk was primarily from the parent compound. It is not known whether this drug is excreted in human milk. Because many drugs are excreted in human milk, caution should be exercised when TROSEC is administered to a nursing woman. TROSEC should be used during lactation only if the potential benefit justifies the potential risk to the newborn.
Pediatrics: The safety and effectiveness of TROSEC in pediatric patients have not been established.
Geriatrics (≥75 years of age): Of the 262 patients with overactive bladder who received treatment with TROSEC in the US 12-week clinical study, 120 patients (45.8%) were 65 years of age and older. Forty-two TROSEC-treated patients (16%) were ≥75 years of age.

Age did not, independently, affect trospium pharmacokinetics. However, the population older than 75 years has greater heterogeneity with respect to hepatic and renal function and has been shown to have an increased incidence of anticholinergic side effects.

In this study, the incidence of commonly reported anticholinergic adverse events in patients treated with TROSEC (including dry mouth, constipation, dyspepsia, urinary tract infection (UTI), and urinary retention) was higher in patients 75 years of age and older as compared to younger patients. Therefore, based upon tolerability, the dose frequency of TROSEC may be reduced to 20 mg once daily in patients 75 years of age and older.

ADVERSE REACTIONS: Adverse Drug Reaction Overview: Trospium chloride antagonizes the effect of acetylcholine on cholinergically innervated organs and exhibits parasympatholytic action by reducing smooth muscle tone, such as in the urogenital and gastrointestinal tracts. Adverse events characteristically associated with the use of anticholinergic agents are dry mouth, constipation, urinary retention, dry eyes, blurred vision, tachycardia, increased heart rate, and palpitation. These adverse effects have been investigated for trospium chloride in animal pharmacology studies and were monitored in human clinical trials.
Clinical Trial Adverse Drug Reactions: Because clinical trials are conducted under very specific conditions the adverse reaction rates observed in the clinical trials may not reflect the rates observed in practice and should not be compared to the rates in the clinical trials of another drug. Adverse drug reaction information from clinical trials is useful for identifying drug-related adverse events and for approximating rates.

The safety of TROSEC was evaluated in Phase 2 and 3 controlled clinical trials in a total of 2975 patients, who were treated with TROSEC (N=1673), placebo (N=1056) or active control medications (N=246). Of this total, 1181 patients participated in two, twelve-week, Phase 3, US efficacy and safety studies and a 9-month open-label extension. Of this total, 591 patients received TROSEC 20 mg twice daily. In all controlled trials combined, 232 and 208 patients received treatment with TROSEC for at least 24 and 52 weeks, respectively.

In all placebo-controlled trials combined, the incidence of serious adverse events was 2.9% among patients receiving TROSEC 20 mg bid and 1.5% among patients receiving placebo. Of these, 0.2% and 0.3% were judged to be at least possibly related to treatment with TROSEC or placebo, respectively, by the investigator.

Table 1 lists treatment emergent adverse events from the combined 12-week US safety and efficacy trials that were judged to be at least possibly related to treatment with TROSEC by the investigator, were reported by at least 1% of patients, and were reported more frequently in the TROSEC group than in the placebo group.

The two most common adverse events reported by patients receiving TROSEC 20 mg bid were dry mouth and constipation. The single most frequently reported adverse event for TROSEC, dry mouth, occurred in 20.1% of TROSEC treated patients and 5.8% of patients receiving placebo. In the two Phase 3 US studies, dry mouth led to discontinuation in 1.9% of patients treated with TROSEC 20 mg bid. For the patients who reported dry mouth, most had their first occurrence of the event within the first month of treatment.

Other adverse events from the Phase 3, US placebo-controlled trials judged possibly related to treatment with TROSEC by the investigator, occurring in ≥0.5% of TROSEC-treated patients, and more common with TROSEC than placebo are: tachycardia NOS, vision blurred, abdominal distension, vomiting NOS, dysgeusia, dry throat, and dry skin.

During controlled clinical studies, one event of angioneurotic edema was reported.

Though not an adverse effect, heart rate was noted to increase by an average of 4 beats per minute in those subjects on active treatment.
Less Common Clinical Trial Adverse Drug Reactions (<1%): Blood and Lymphatic System Disorders: lymphadenopathy.
Cardiac Disorders: angina pectoris, coronary artery disease, palpitations, supraventricular extrasystoles, tachycardia.
Ear and Labyrinth Disorders: ear pain.
Endocrine Disorders: endocrine disorder.
Eye Disorders: accommodation disorder, dry eye, eye pain, vision blurred.
Gastrointestinal Disorders: abdominal discomfort, abdominal distension, abdominal pain upper, constipation aggravated, gastrointestinal disorder, mouth ulceration, vomiting.
General Disorders and Administration Site Conditions: chest pain, influenza like illness, oedema, oedema peripheral, thirst.
Infections and Infestations: urinary tract infection.
Investigations: electrocardiogram abnormal, heart rate increased, QRS axis abnormal, residual urine volume, weight increased.
Metabolism and Nutrition Disorders: appetite decreased, fluid retention, hyperuricaemia.
Musculoskeletal and Connective Tissue Disorders: back pain, muscle cramps, pain in jaw, peripheral swelling.
Nervous System Disorders: dysgeusia, migraine.
Renal and Urinary Disorders: bladder pain, dysuria, haematuria, micturition disorder, micturition urgency, renal pain, urinary hesitation, urine abnormal, urine odour abnormal.
Reproductive System and Breast Disorders: vaginal pain.
Respiratory, Thoracic and Mediastinal Disorders: dry throat, hoarseness, nasal dryness, respiratory tract congestion, rhinitis.
Skin and Subcutaneous Tissue Disorders: dermatitis contact, dry skin, eczema, hair growth abnormal, photosensitivity reaction, pruritus, rash erythematous, rash, sweating increased, urticaria.
Vascular Disorders: flushing, hot flushes, orthostatic hypotension.

Table 1: TROSEC

Incidence (%) of Adverse Events Judged at Least Possibly Related to Treatment with TROSEC, Reported in ≥1% of all Patients Treated with TROSEC and More Frequent with TROSEC (20 mg bid) Than Placebo in Studies 1 and 2 Combined

Adverse Event	Placebo (N=590)	TROSEC 20 mg bid (N=591)
Gastrointestinal Disorders		
Dry mouth	34 (5.8)	119 (20.1)
Constipation	27 (4.6)	57 (9.6)
Abdominal pain upper	7 (1.2)	9 (1.5)
Constipation aggravated	5 (0.8)	8 (1.4)
Dyspepsia	2 (0.3)	7 (1.2)
Flatulence	5 (0.8)	7 (1.2)
Nervous System Disorders		
Headache	12 (2.0)	25 (4.2)
General Disorders		
Fatigue	8 (1.4)	11 (1.9)
Renal and Urinary Disorders		

(cont'd)

Table 1: TROSEC *(cont'd)*

Incidence (%) of Adverse Events Judged at Least Possibly Related to Treatment with TROSEC, Reported in ≥1% of all Patients Treated with TROSEC and More Frequent with TROSEC (20 mg bid) Than Placebo in Studies 1 and 2 Combined

Adverse Event	Placebo (N=590)	TROSEC 20 mg bid (N=591)
Urinary retention	2 (0.3)	7 (1.2)
Eye Disorders		
Dry eyes NOS	2 (0.3)	7 (1.2)

Legend: bid=twice daily; NOS=not otherwise specified.

Abnormal Hematologic and Clinical Chemistry Findings: Analysis of laboratory data from 1 clinical pharmacology study and 2 controlled studies did not identify any trends to suggest that trospium chloride is associated with any relevant laboratory abnormalities in hematology, clinical chemistry, or urinalysis parameters.

Post-Market Adverse Drug Reactions: Additional spontaneous adverse events, regardless of relationship to drug, reported from marketing experience with trospium chloride include: gastritis, palpitations, supraventricular tachycardia, chest pain, Stevens-Johnson syndrome, anaphylactic reaction, syncope, rhabdomyolysis, vision abnormal, hallucinations and delirium, and "hypertensive crisis".

DRUG INTERACTIONS: Overview: Possible drug interactions, based on the anticholinergic properties of trospium chloride, could include potentiation of the anticholinergic action of agents possessing these properties. Also, trospium chloride could theoretically alter the absorption of some concomitantly administered drugs due to anticholinergic effects on gastrointestinal motility.

The major route of excretion of trospium chloride is the kidney. Consequently, concomitant drug therapy that significantly interferes with renal excretion of trospium chloride may cause drug-drug interactions (see Drug-Drug Interactions).

Drug-Drug Interactions: The concomitant use of TROSEC with other anticholinergic agents that produce dry mouth, constipation, and other anticholinergic pharmacological effects may increase the frequency and/or severity of such effects. Anticholinergic agents may potentially alter the absorption of some concomitantly administered drugs due to anticholinergic effects on gastrointestinal motility.

No in vivo drug-drug interaction studies have been performed to assess the effect of concomitant medications on the pharmacokinetics of TROSEC or to assess the effect of TROSEC on the pharmacokinetics of other drugs. TROSEC is metabolized by esterases and excreted by the kidneys by a combination of tubular secretion and glomerular filtration. Based on in vitro data, no clinically relevant interactions with the metabolism of trospium chloride are expected. However, drugs which are actively secreted (e.g. digoxin, procainamide, pancuronium, morphine, vancomycin, metformin and tenofovir) may interact with trospium chloride by competing for renal tubular secretion. Coadministration of TROSEC with drugs that are eliminated by active renal tubular secretion may increase the serum concentration of TROSEC and/or the coadministered drug due to competition for this elimination pathway. Careful patient monitoring is recommended in patients receiving such drugs (see Action and Clinical Pharmacology, Excretion).

Drug-Food Interactions: Coadministration of TROSEC with food has been shown to reduce drug absorption (see Action and Clinical Pharmacology, Pharmacokinetics, Effect of Food). TROSEC should therefore be taken at least one hour prior to meals or on an empty stomach (see Dosage and Administration).

Drug-Herb Interactions: Interactions with herbal products have not been established.

Drug-Laboratory Test Interactions: Interactions between TROSEC and laboratory tests have not been studied.

DOSAGE AND ADMINISTRATION: Dosing Considerations:

- Patients with severe renal impairment [CLcr 0.25-0.5 mL/sec (15-30 mL/min)] (see Warnings and Precautions, Renal).
- Geriatric patients ≥75 years of age (see Warnings and Precautions, Special Populations).

Recommended Dose and Dosage Adjustment: The recommended dose is 20 mg twice daily.

Dosage modification is recommended in the following patient populations:

For patients with severe renal impairment [CLcr 0.25-0.5 mL/sec (15-30 mL/min)], the recommended dose is 20 mg once daily at bedtime. The use of TROSEC in patients with renal function <0.25 mL/sec (15 mL/min) has not been studied.

In geriatric patients ≥75 years of age, dose may be titrated down to 20 mg once daily based upon tolerability (see Warnings and Precautions, Special Populations).

Caution should be used when administering TROSEC to patients with moderate or severe hepatic impairment.

Missed Dose: If a dose is skipped, patients are advised to take their next dose on an empty stomach 1 hour prior to their next meal.

Administration: TROSEC should be dosed at least one hour before meals or given on an empty stomach.

OVERDOSAGE:

Overdosage with TROSEC may result in severe anticholinergic effects. Treatment should be supportive and provided according to symptoms. In the event of overdosage, electrocardiographic (ECG) monitoring is strongly recommended.

A 7-month-old baby experienced tachycardia and mydriasis after administration of a single dose of trospium chloride 10 mg given by a sibling. The baby's weight was reported as 5 kg. Following admission into the hospital and about 1 hour after ingestion of the trospium chloride, medicinal charcoal was administered for detoxification. While hospitalized, the baby experienced mydriasis and tachycardia up to 230 beats/minute. Therapeutic intervention was not deemed necessary. The baby was discharged as completely recovered the following day.

> For management of a suspected drug overdose, CPhA recommends that you contact your **regional Poison Control Centre**. See the *CPS* Directory section for a list of Poison Control Centres.

ACTION AND CLINICAL PHARMACOLOGY: Mechanism of Action: TROSEC is an antispasmodic, antimuscarinic agent.

Trospium chloride antagonizes the effect of acetylcholine on muscarinic receptors in cholinergically innervated organs. Its parasympatholytic action reduces the tonus of smooth muscle in the bladder. Receptor assays showed that trospium chloride has negligible affinity for nicotinic receptors as compared to muscarinic receptors at concentrations obtained from therapeutic doses.

Pharmacodynamics: Placebo-controlled studies employing urodynamic variables were conducted in patients with conditions characterized by involuntary detrusor contractions. The results demonstrate that TROSEC increases maximum cystometric bladder capacity and volume at first detrusor contraction.

Pharmacokinetics: A summary of mean (±standard deviation) pharmacokinetic parameters for a single 20 mg dose of TROSEC is provided in Table 2.

Table 2: TROSEC

Mean (±SD) Pharmacokinetic Parameter Estimates for a Single 20 mg TROSEC Dose in Healthy Volunteers

C_{max} (ng/mL)	$AUC_{0-\infty}$ (ng/mL·h)	T_{max} (h)	$t_{½}$ (h)
3.5±4.0	36.4±21.8	5.3±1.2	18.3±3.2

The mean plasma concentration-time (±SD) profile for TROSEC is shown in Figure 1.

Absorption: After oral administration, less than 10% of the dose is absorbed. Mean absolute bioavailability of a 20 mg dose is 9.6% (range: 4.0-16.1%). Peak plasma concentrations (C_{max}) occur between 5 to 6 hours post-dose. Mean C_{max} increases greater than dose-proportionally; a 3-fold and 4-fold increase in C_{max} was observed for dose increases from 20 mg to 40 mg and from 20 mg to 60 mg, respectively. AUC exhibits dose linearity for single doses up to 60 mg. TROSEC exhibits diurnal variability in exposure with a decrease in C_{max} and AUC of up to 59% and 33%, respectively, for evening relative to morning doses.

Effect of Food: Administration with a high fat meal resulted in reduced absorption, with AUC and C_{max} values 70-80% lower than those obtained when TROSEC was administered while fasting. Therefore, it is recommended that TROSEC should be taken at least one hour prior to meals or on an empty stomach (see Dosage and Administration).

Figure 1: TROSEC

Mean (±SD) Concentration-Time Profile for a Single 20 mg Oral Dose of TROSEC in Healthy Volunteers

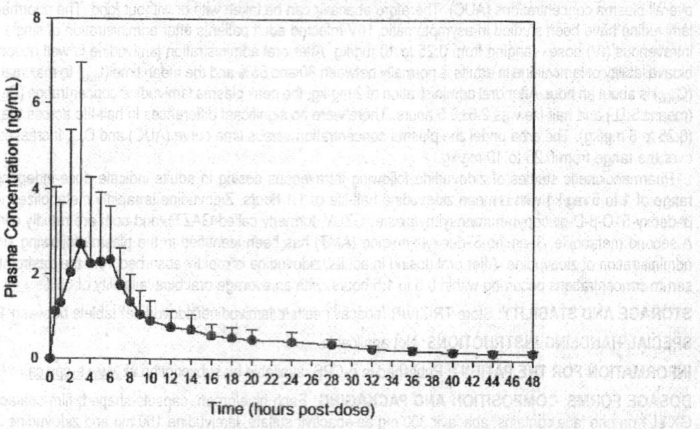

Distribution: Protein binding ranged from 50 to 85% when therapeutic concentration levels (0.5-50 ng/mL) were incubated with human serum in vitro.

The ^{3}H-trospium chloride ratio of plasma to whole blood was 1.6:1. This ratio indicates that the majority of ^{3}H-trospium chloride is distributed in plasma. The apparent volume of distribution for a 20 mg oral dose is 395 (±140) L.

Metabolism: The metabolic pathway of trospium chloride in humans has not been fully defined. Of the 10% of the dose absorbed, metabolites account for approximately 40% of the excreted dose following oral administration. The major metabolic pathway is hypothesized as ester hydrolysis with subsequent conjugation of benzylic acid to form azoniaspironortropanol with glucuronic acid. Cytochrome P450 is not expected to contribute significantly to the elimination of trospium chloride. In vitro data from human liver microsomes investigating the inhibitory effect of trospium chloride on seven cytochrome P450 isoenzyme substrates (CYP1A2, 2A6, 2C9, 2C19, 2D6, 2E1, and 3A4) suggest a lack of inhibition at clinically relevant concentrations of trospium chloride.

Excretion: The plasma half-life for TROSEC following oral administration is approximately 20 hours. After administration of oral ^{14}C-trospium chloride, the majority of the dose (85.2%) was recovered in feces and a smaller amount (5.8% of the dose) was recovered in urine; 60% of the radioactivity excreted in urine was unchanged trospium chloride.

The mean renal clearance for trospium chloride 8 mL/sec (29.07 L/h) is 4-fold higher than average glomerular filtration rate, indicating that active tubular secretion is a major route of elimination for trospium chloride. There may be competition for elimination with other compounds that are also renally eliminated (see Drug Interactions).

Special Populations and Conditions: Pediatrics: The pharmacokinetics of TROSEC were not evaluated in pediatric patients.

Geriatrics: Age did not appear to significantly affect the pharmacokinetics of TROSEC however, increased anticholinergic side effects unrelated to drug exposure were observed in patients ≥75 years of age (see Warnings and Precautions, Special Populations and Dosage and Administration).

Gender: Studies comparing the pharmacokinetics in different genders had conflicting results. When a single 40 mg TROSEC dose was administered to 16 elderly subjects, exposure was 45% lower in elderly females compared to elderly males. When 20 mg TROSEC was dosed bid for 4 days to 6 elderly males and 6 elderly females (60 to 75 years), AUC and C_{max} were 26% and 68% higher, respectively, in females without hormone replacement therapy than in males.

Race: Pharmacokinetic differences due to race have not been studied.

Hepatic Insufficiency: There is no information regarding the effect of severe hepatic impairment on exposure to TROSEC. Maximum trospium chloride concentration (C_{max}) increased 12% and 63% in subjects with mild and moderate hepatic impairment, respectively, compared to healthy subjects. Mean area under the plasma concentration-time curve (AUC) was similar. Caution should be used when administering TROSEC to patients with moderate and severe hepatic dysfunction (see Warnings and Precautions, Hepatic/Biliary/Pancreatic).

Renal Insufficiency: Severe renal impairment significantly altered the disposition of TROSEC. A 4.5-fold and 2-fold increase in mean $AUC_{0-\infty}$ and C_{max}, respectively, and the appearance of an additional elimination phase with a long half-life (~33 h) was detected in patients with severe renal insufficiency [Clcr 0.25-0.5 mL/sec (15-30 mL/min)] compared with healthy, nearly age-matched subjects. The different pharmacokinetic behavior of TROSEC in patients with severe renal insufficiency necessitates adjustment of dosage frequency. The pharmacokinetics of TROSEC have not been studied in people with moderate or mild renal impairment [CLcr ranging from 0.5-1.3 mL/sec (30-80 mL/min)] (see Warnings and Precautions, Renal, and Dosage and Administration). The use of TROSEC in patients with renal function <0.25 mL/sec (15 mL/min) has not been studied.

STORAGE AND STABILITY: Store at controlled room temperature 15 to 30°C.

Keep in a safe place out of reach of children.

SPECIAL HANDLING INSTRUCTIONS: None.

INFORMATION FOR THE PATIENT: Published in e-CPS, available by subscription at www.e-cps.ca.

DOSAGE FORMS, COMPOSITION AND PACKAGING: Each brownish yellow, biconvex, glossy coated tablet, imprinted with a "T", contains: trospium chloride 20 mg. Nonmedicinal ingredients: calcium carbonate, carboxymethylcellulose sodium, carnauba wax, colloidal silicon dioxide, croscarmellose sodium, ferric oxide, lactose monohydrate, microcrystalline cellulose, polyethylene glycol 8000, povidone, stearic acid, sucrose, talc, titanium dioxide, wheat starch and white wax. Blister packs of 10.

Trusopt® ℞

dorzolamide HCl

Elevated Intraocular Pressure Therapy—Topical Carbonic Anhydrase Inhibitor

Merck Frosst

Date of Revision: April 21, 2010

SUMMARY PRODUCT INFORMATION:

Route of Administration	Dosage Form/ Strength	Clinically Relevant Nonmedicinal Ingredients
Ophthalmic	Solution, each mL contains 20 mg dorzolamide (22.3 mg of dorzolamide hydrochloride)	For a complete listing see Dosage Forms, Composition and Packaging.

INDICATIONS AND CLINICAL USE: TRUSOPT (dorzolamide hydrochloride) ophthalmic solution 2% and TRUSOPT preservative-free formulation are indicated in the treatment of elevated intraocular pressure in patients with:

- ocular hypertension
- open-angle glaucoma

TRUSOPT preservative-free formulation is indicated in patients who may be sensitive to a preservative, or for whom the use of a preservative-free formulation is otherwise advisable.

A comparative crossover clinical trial consisting of two 6-week periods has been performed with TRUSOPT preservative-free formulation and TRUSOPT (with preservative) in 152 adult patients. The results have indicated that the efficacy and safety profile of these two formulations appear to be equivalent. No studies were conducted with TRUSOPT preservative-free formulation in special populations (pediatric, kidney or liver diseases, etc.). For details, please also refer to Dosage and Administration.

CONTRAINDICATIONS: TRUSOPT (dorzolamide hydrochloride) is contraindicated in patients who are hypersensitive to any component of this product. For a complete listing, see Dosage Forms, Composition and Packaging.

TRUSOPT has not been studied in patients with severe renal impairment (CrCl <0.5 mL/s). Because TRUSOPT and its metabolite are excreted predominantly by the kidney, TRUSOPT is not recommended in such patients.

There is a potential for an additive effect with the known systemic effects of carbonic anhydrase inhibition in patients receiving oral carbonic anhydrase inhibitor and TRUSOPT. The concomitant administration of TRUSOPT and oral carbonic anhydrase inhibitors has not been studied and is not recommended.

WARNINGS AND PRECAUTIONS: General: TRUSOPT (dorzolamide hydrochloride) is a sulfonamide and although administered topically, is absorbed systemically. Therefore the same types of adverse reactions that are attributable to sulfonamides may occur with topical administration, including severe reactions such as Stevens-Johnson syndrome and toxic epidermal necrolysis. If signs of serious reactions or hypersensitivity occur, discontinue the use of this preparation.

The management of patients with acute angle-closure glaucoma requires therapeutic interventions in addition to ocular hypotensive agents. TRUSOPT has not been studied in patients with acute angle-closure glaucoma.

Immune: Immunology and Hypersensitivity: In clinical studies, local ocular adverse effects, primarily conjunctivitis and eyelid reactions, were reported with chronic administration of TRUSOPT. Some of these reactions had the clinical appearance and course of an allergic-type reaction that resolved upon discontinuation of drug therapy. If such reactions are observed, discontinuation of treatment with TRUSOPT should be considered.

Ophthalmologic: Corneal Edema: There is an increased risk of developing irreversible corneal edema in a subset of glaucoma patients with endothelial abnormalities including cellular density and/or morphology. In this group of patients evaluation of the cornea with particular attention to the corneal endothelium is recommended prior and during treatment with TRUSOPT.

Corneal Edema and Irreversible Corneal Decompensation: Corneal edema and irreversible corneal decompensation has been reported in patients with pre-existing chronic corneal defects and/or a history of intraocular surgery while using dorzolamide. TRUSOPT should be used with caution in such patients.

Choroidal Detachment: Choroidal detachment has been reported with administration of aqueous suppressant therapy (e.g., dorzolamide) after filtration procedures.

Management of eyes with chronic or recurrent choroidal detachment should include stopping all forms of aqueous suppressant therapy and treating endogenous inflammation vigorously.

Contact Lenses: TRUSOPT has not been studied in patients wearing contact lenses. The preservative in TRUSOPT Ophthalmic Solution, benzalkonium chloride, may be absorbed by soft contact lenses. Patients should be instructed to remove their lenses before application of the drops and not to re-insert the lenses earlier than 15 minutes after use. TRUSOPT preservative-free formulation does not contain the preservative benzalkonium chloride.

Hepatic: Hepatic Impairment: TRUSOPT has not been studied in patients with hepatic impairment and should therefore be used with caution in such patients.

Special Populations: Pregnant Women: There are no adequate and well-controlled studies in pregnant women. TRUSOPT should be used during pregnancy only if the potential benefit justifies the potential risk to the fetus.

Nursing Women: It is not known whether dorzolamide is excreted in human milk. Because many drugs are excreted in human milk and because of the potential for serious adverse reactions from TRUSOPT in nursing infants, a decision should be made whether to discontinue nursing or to discontinue the drug, taking into account the importance of the drug to the mother.

In a study of dorzolamide hydrochloride in lactating rats, decreases in body weight gain of 5 to 7% in offspring at an oral dose of 7.5 mg/kg/day (94 times the maximum recommended human ophthalmic dose) were seen during lactation. A slight delay in postnatal development (incisor eruption, vaginal canalization and eye openings), secondary to lower fetal body weight, was noted at 7.5 mg/kg/day (94 times the maximum recommended human ophthalmic dose).

Pediatrics: Safety and effectiveness in children have not been established.

Geriatrics (>65 years of age): Of the total number of patients in clinical studies of TRUSOPT, 44% were 65 years of age and over, while 10% were 75 years of age and over. No overall differences in effectiveness or safety were observed between these patients and younger patients, but greater sensitivity of some older individuals to the product cannot be ruled out.

In a clinical study comparing TRUSOPT preservative-free formulation and TRUSOPT, 48% of all patients were over the age of 65, while 12% were over 75 years of age. No statistical analysis was performed based upon age.

Monitoring and Laboratory Tests: TRUSOPT was not associated with clinically meaningful electrolyte disturbances.

ADVERSE REACTIONS: Adverse Drug Reaction Overview: In long-term studies of 1108 patients treated with TRUSOPT (dorzolamide hydrochloride) as monotherapy or as adjunctive therapy with an ophthalmic beta-blocker, the most frequent cause of discontinuation (approximately 3%) from treatment with TRUSOPT was drug-related ocular adverse effects, primarily conjunctivitis and eyelid reactions (see Warnings and Precautions).

In clinical studies, the most common ocular complaints were burning and stinging, blurred vision, itching and tearing. Bitter taste was also frequently reported. If these local symptoms were considered clinically important by investigators they also appear as adverse experiences in the listing below.

In an active treatment, controlled, crossover clinical study of 12 weeks duration, 152 patients received TRUSOPT preservative-free formulation for 6 weeks and TRUSOPT for 6 weeks. Approximately 1.3% of patients receiving TRUSOPT preservative-free formulation discontinued therapy due to adverse experiences. Approximately 0.7% of all patients receiving TRUSOPT preservative-free formulation discontinued therapy because of adverse reactions suggestive of allergy and/or hypersensitivity.

The most frequently reported ocular drug related adverse effects for TRUSOPT preservative-free formulation were burning and stinging 41%, taste perversion 13%, corneal erosion 5%, follicular conjunctivitis 3%, conjunctival injection 3%, and blurred vision 1%. For TRUSOPT ophthalmic solution the most frequently reported ocular drug related adverse events were burning and stinging 38%, taste perversion 13%, conjunctival injection 5%, corneal erosion 4%, follicular conjunctivitis 3%, and blurred vision 3%.

Clinical Trial Adverse Drug Reactions: Adverse experiences that were reported during clinical studies as drug-related (possibly, probably, or definitely) in 1-5% of patients on TRUSOPT were in decreasing order of frequency:

Ocular: burning and stinging, conjunctivitis, eyelid inflammation, eye itching, eyelid irritation.

Systemic: headache, bitter taste, nausea, asthenia/fatigue.

Iridocyclitis and rash were each reported rarely. There was one report of urolithiasis.

Post-Market Adverse Drug Reactions: The following adverse reactions have been reported in post-marketing experience:

Hypersensitivity: Signs and symptoms of local reactions including palpebral reactions and systemic allergic reactions including angioedema, bronchospasm, urticaria and pruritus.

Nervous System: dizziness, paresthesia.

Ocular: pain, redness, superficial punctate keratitis, transient myopia (which resolved upon discontinuation of therapy), eyelid crusting, choroidal detachment following filtration surgery, corneal edema in glaucoma patients with endothelial abnormalities including cellular density and/or morphology.

Skin/Mucous Membranes: contact dermatitis, epistaxis, throat irritation, dry mouth, Stevens-Johnson syndrome, toxic epidermal necrolysis.

Urogenital: urolithiasis.

DRUG INTERACTIONS: Overview: Specific drug interaction studies have not been performed with TRUSOPT Ophthalmic Solution. In clinical studies, TRUSOPT was used concomitantly with the following medications without evidence of adverse interactions: timolol ophthalmic solution, betaxolol ophthalmic solution and systemic medications, including ACE-inhibitors, calcium channel blockers, diuretics, non-steroidal anti-inflammatory drugs including ASA, and hormones (e.g. estrogen, insulin, thyroxine).

Drug-Drug Interactions: The following drug interaction has been associated with the dorzolamide component of TRUSOPT or with other sulfonamides:

Acid-base Disturbances: TRUSOPT is a carbonic anhydrase inhibitor and although administered topically, is absorbed systemically. In clinical studies, TRUSOPT was not associated with acid-base disturbances. However, these disturbances have been reported with oral carbonic anhydrase inhibitors and have, in some instances, resulted in drug interactions (e.g. toxicity associated with high-dose salicylate therapy). Therefore, the potential for such drug interactions should be considered in patients receiving TRUSOPT.

Drug-Lifestyle Interactions: Effects on Ability to Drive and Use Machines: Possible side effects such as visual disturbances may affect the ability to drive and use machines (see Drug Interactions and Adverse Reactions).

DOSAGE AND ADMINISTRATION: Recommended Dose and Dosage Adjustment: When used as monotherapy, the dose is one drop of TRUSOPT (dorzolamide hydrochloride) or TRUSOPT preservative-free formulation ophthalmic solution 2% in the affected eye(s) three times daily.

When used as adjunctive therapy with an ophthalmic beta-blocker, the dose is one drop of TRUSOPT or TRUSOPT preservative-free formulation in the affected eye(s) two times daily.

A comparative crossover clinical trial of 12 weeks duration (two 6-week periods) has been performed with TRUSOPT preservative-free formulation and TRUSOPT with preservative in adult patients. The total duration of exposure to TRUSOPT preservative-free formulation was for 6 weeks. The results have indicated that the efficacy and safety profile of these two formulations appear to be equivalent. No studies were conducted with TRUSOPT preservative-free formulation in special populations (pediatric, kidney or liver diseases, etc.).

When substituting TRUSOPT or TRUSOPT preservative-free formulation for another ophthalmic antiglaucoma agent, discontinue the other agent after proper dosing on one day, and start TRUSOPT or TRUSOPT preservative-free formulation on the next day.

If more than one topical ophthalmic drug is being used, the drugs should be administered at least ten minutes apart.

Missed Dose: If a dose is missed, it should be applied as soon as possible. However, if it is almost time for the next dose, the missed dose should be skipped and the next dose should be taken as usual.

OVERDOSAGE:

No data are available in humans in regard to overdosage by accidental or deliberate ingestion. The most common signs and symptoms to be expected with overdosage of dorzolamide are electrolyte imbalance, development of an acidotic state, and possibly central nervous system effects (see Adverse Reactions).

Treatment should be symptomatic and supportive. Serum electrolyte levels (particularly potassium) and blood pH levels should be monitored.

Significant lethality was observed in female rats and mice after single oral doses of dorzolamide hydrochloride of 11 369 mg/m^2 or 1927 mg/kg (24 000 times the maximum recommended human ophthalmic dose) and 3960 mg/m^2 or 1320 mg/kg (16 000 times the maximum recommended human ophthalmic dose), respectively.

> For management of a suspected drug overdose, contact your regional Poison Control Centre. See the *CPS* Directory section for a list of Poison Control Centres.

ACTION AND CLINICAL PHARMACOLOGY: Mechanism of Action: TRUSOPT (dorzolamide hydrochloride) is a carbonic anhydrase inhibitor formulated for topical ophthalmic use.

Inhibition of carbonic anhydrase in the ciliary processes of the eye decreases aqueous humor secretion, presumably by slowing the formation of bicarbonate ions with subsequent reduction in sodium and fluid transport. The result is a reduction in intraocular pressure (IOP).

Pharmacokinetics: Unlike oral carbonic anhydrase inhibitors, topically-applied TRUSOPT exerts its effects at substantially low doses and therefore with less systemic exposure.

When applied topically, dorzolamide reaches the systemic circulation. To assess the potential for systemic carbonic anhydrase inhibition following topical administration, drug and metabolite concentrations in RBCs and plasma and carbonic anhydrase inhibition in RBCs were measured. Dorzolamide accumulates in RBCs during chronic dosing as a result of selective binding to CA-II while extremely low concentrations of free drug in plasma are maintained. The parent drug forms a single N-desethyl metabolite that inhibits CA-II less potently than the parent drug but also inhibits a less active isoenzyme (CA-I). The metabolite also accumulates in RBCs where it binds primarily to CA-I. Dorzolamide binds moderately to plasma proteins (approximately 33%). Dorzolamide is excreted unchanged in the urine; the metabolite is also excreted in urine. After dosing ends, dorzolamide washes out of RBCs in a non-linear manner, resulting in a rapid decline of drug concentration initially, followed by a slower elimination phase with a half-life of about four months.

To simulate the maximum systemic exposure after long term topical ocular administration, dorzolamide was given orally to eight healthy subjects for up to 20 weeks. The oral dose of 4 mg/day closely approximates the maximum amount of dorzolamide delivered by topical ocular administration of TRUSOPT 2% t.i.d. Dorzolamide and metabolite reached steady state by 4 and 13 weeks, respectively, and the following observations were noted:

- In plasma, concentrations of dorzolamide and metabolite were generally below the assay limit of quantitation (15 nM) indicating almost no free drug or metabolite;
- In RBCs, dorzolamide concentrations approached the binding capacity of CA-II (20-25 μM) and metabolite concentrations approached 12-15 μM, well below the binding capacity of CA-I (125-155 μM);
- In RBCs, inhibition of CA-II activity and total carbonic anhydrase activity was below the degree of inhibition anticipated to be necessary for a pharmacological effect on renal function and respiration.

STORAGE AND STABILITY: TRUSOPT Ophthalmic Solution: Store at 15-25°C. Protect from light.

TRUSOPT Preservative-free Formulation Ophthalmic Solution: Store at 15-25°C. Protect from light. Store in protective foil pouch.

INFORMATION FOR THE PATIENT: Published in e-CPS, available by subscription at www.e-cps.ca.

DOSAGE FORMS, COMPOSITION AND PACKAGING: TRUSOPT Ophthalmic Solution: Each mL of sterile, clear, colorless to nearly colorless, isotonic, buffered, slightly viscous, aqueous ophthalmic solution contains: dorzolamide 20 mg (equivalent to dorzolamide HCl 22.3 mg). Nonmedicinal ingredients: benzalkonium chloride (as preservative), hydroxyethyl cellulose, mannitol, sodium citrate dihydrate, sodium hydroxide and water for injection. Translucent, high-density polyethylene Ocumeter Plus ophthalmic dispensers of 5 mL, with a sealed dropper tip, a flexible fluted side area which is depressed to dispense the drops, and a 2-piece cap assembly. The opaque, white, 2-piece cap mechanism punctures the dropper tip seal upon initial use, then locks to provide a single cap during the usage period. Tamper evidence is provided by a safety strip on the container label.

TRUSOPT Preservative-Free Ophthalmic Solution: Each mL of sterile, clear, colorless to nearly colorless, isotonic, buffered, slightly viscous, aqueous ophthalmic solution contains: dorzolamide 20 mg (equivalent to dorzolamide HCl 22.3 mg). Nonmedicinal ingredients: hydroxyethyl cellulose, mannitol, sodium citrate dihydrate, sodium hydroxide and water for injection. Packages of 15 individual fill volume unit dose pipettes of 0.2 mL, pouches of 4.

Truvada® Pr

emtricitabine—tenofovir disoproxil fumarate

Antiretroviral Agent

Gilead Sciences

Date of Revision: May 25, 2009

SUMMARY PRODUCT INFORMATION:

Route of Administration	Dosage Form/ Strength	Clinically Relevant Nonmedicinal Ingredients
Oral	Tablet Emtricitabine 200 mg/Tenofovir Disoproxil Fumarate 300 mg	Lactose monohydrate, pregelatinized starch (gluten free). For a complete listing see Dosage Forms, Composition and Packaging.

TRUVADA Tablets are a fixed-dose combination containing emtricitabine (also known as EMTRIVA) and tenofovir disoproxil fumarate (also known as VIREAD).

INDICATIONS AND CLINICAL USE: TRUVADA is indicated in combination with other antiretroviral agents (such as non-nucleoside reverse transcriptase inhibitors or protease inhibitors) for the treatment of HIV-1 infection in adults.

Additional important information regarding the use of TRUVADA for the treatment of HIV-1 infection:

- It is not recommended that TRUVADA be used as a component of a triple nucleoside regimen.
- TRUVADA should not be administered with EMTRIVA, VIREAD, ATRIPLA or lamivudine-containing products (see Warnings and Precautions).
- In treatment-experienced patients, the use of TRUVADA should be guided by laboratory testing and treatment history.

Geriatrics (>65 years of age): Clinical studies of EMTRIVA or VIREAD did not include sufficient numbers of subjects aged 65 and over to determine whether they respond differently from younger subjects.

Pediatrics (<18 years of age): Safety and effectiveness in pediatric patients have not been established.

CONTRAINDICATIONS: TRUVADA is contraindicated in patients with previously demonstrated hypersensitivity to any of the components of the product. For a complete listing, see Dosage Forms, Composition and Packaging.

WARNINGS AND PRECAUTIONS:

Serious Warnings and Precautions

- **Lactic Acidosis and Severe Hepatomegaly with Steatosis:** Lactic acidosis and severe hepatomegaly with steatosis, including fatal cases, have been reported with the use of nucleoside analogs, including VIREAD, a component of TRUVADA, alone or in combination with other antiretrovirals (see Warnings and Precautions).
- **Post-Treatment Exacerbation of Hepatitis:** TRUVADA is not approved for the treatment of chronic hepatitis B virus (HBV) infection and the safety and efficacy of TRUVADA have not been established in patients co-infected with HBV and HIV. Severe acute exacerbations of hepatitis B have been reported in patients who are co-infected with HBV and HIV and have discontinued TRUVADA. Hepatic function should be monitored closely with both clinical and laboratory follow-up for at least several months in patients who are co-infected with HIV and HBV and discontinue TRUVADA. If appropriate, initiation of anti-hepatitis B therapy may be warranted (see Warnings and Precautions).
- **Nephrotoxicity:** Renal impairment, including cases of acute renal failure and Fanconi syndrome (renal tubular injury with severe hypophosphatemia) has been reported with the use of VIREAD during clinical practice (see Warnings and Precautions).

General: TRUVADA is a fixed-dose combination of emtricitabine and tenofovir disoproxil fumarate. TRUVADA should not be coadministered with EMTRIVA, VIREAD or ATRIPLA. Due to similarities between emtricitabine and lamivudine, TRUVADA should not be coadministered with other drugs containing lamivudine such as COMBIVIR, 3TC, HEPTOVIR, KIVEXA or TRIZIVIR.

TRUVADA should not be administered with HEPSERA (adefovir dipivoxil).

Clinical studies in HIV-infected patients have demonstrated that certain regimens that only contain three nucleoside reverse transcriptase inhibitors (NRTI) are generally less effective than triple drug regimens containing two NRTIs in combination with either a non-nucleoside reverse transcriptase inhibitor or a HIV-1 protease inhibitor. In particular, early virological failure and high rates of resistance mutations have been reported. Triple nucleoside regimens should therefore be used with caution. Patients on a therapy utilizing a triple nucleoside-only regimen should be carefully monitored and considered for treatment modification.

Bone Effects: In Study 903 through 144 weeks, decreases from baseline in bone mineral density (BMD) were seen at the lumbar spine and hip in both VIREAD and stavudine treatment arms of the study and significantly greater decreases were seen in the lumbar spine measurement in the VIREAD group relative to the stavudine group. Clinically relevant fractures were reported in both treatment groups. Increases in biochemical markers of bone metabolism (serum bone-specific alkaline phosphatase, serum osteocalcin, serum C-telopeptide, and urinary N-telopeptide) were observed, suggesting increased bone turnover. Except for bone specific alkaline phosphatase, these changes resulted in values that remained within the normal range. The effects of VIREAD-associated changes in BMD and biochemical markers on long-term bone health and future fracture risk are unknown.

Cases of osteomalacia (associated with proximal renal tubulopathy and infrequently contributing to fractures) have been reported in association with the use of VIREAD (see Adverse Reactions, Post-Market Adverse Drug Reactions).

Bone monitoring should be considered for HIV infected patients who have a history of pathologic bone fracture or are at risk for osteopenia. Although the effect of supplementation with calcium and vitamin D was not studied, such supplementation may be beneficial for all patients. If bone abnormalities are suspected then appropriate consultation should be obtained.

Carcinogenesis, Mutagenesis, Impairment of Fertility: Emtricitabine: In long-term oral carcinogenicity studies of emtricitabine, no drug-related increase in tumor incidence was found in mice at doses up to 750 mg/kg/day (26 times the human systemic exposure at the therapeutic dose of 200 mg/day) or in rats at doses up to 600 mg/kg/day (31 times the human systemic exposure at the therapeutic dose).

Emtricitabine was not genotoxic in the reverse mutation bacterial test (Ames test), mouse lymphoma or mouse micronucleus assays.

Emtricitabine did not affect fertility in male rats at approximately 140-fold or in male and female mice at approximately 60-fold higher exposures (AUC) than in humans given the recommended 200 mg daily dose. Fertility was normal in the offspring of mice exposed daily from before birth (in utero) through sexual maturity at daily exposures (AUC) of approximately 60-fold higher than human exposures at the recommended 200 mg daily dose.

Tenofovir disoproxil fumarate: Tenofovir DF did not show any carcinogenic potential in a long-term oral carcinogenicity study in rats. A long-term oral carcinogenicity study in mice showed a low incidence of duodenal tumors, considered likely related to high local concentrations in the gastrointestinal tract at the high dose of 600 mg/kg/day. The mechanism of tumor formation in mice and potential relevance for humans are uncertain.

Tenofovir disoproxil fumarate was mutagenic in the in vitro mouse lymphoma assay and negative in an in vitro bacterial mutagenicity test (Ames test). In an in vivo mouse micronucleus assay, tenofovir disoproxil fumarate was negative at doses up to 2000 mg/kg when administered orally to male mice.

There were no effects on fertility, mating performance or early embryonic development when tenofovir disoproxil fumarate was administered at 600 mg/kg/day to male rats for 28 days prior to mating and to female rats for 15 days prior to mating through day seven of gestation. There was, however, an alteration of the estrous cycle in female rats. A dose of 600 mg/kg/day is equivalent to 19 times the human dose based on body surface area comparisons.

Endocrine and Metabolism: Fat Redistribution: Redistribution/accumulation of body fat (lipodystrophy) including central obesity, dorsocervical fat enlargement (buffalo hump), peripheral wasting, facial wasting, breast enlargement, and "cushingoid appearance" have been observed in patients receiving antiretroviral therapy. The mechanism and long-term consequences of these events are currently unknown. A causal relationship has not been established.

Hepatic/Biliary/Pancreatic: Lactic Acidosis/Severe Hepatomegaly with Steatosis: Lactic acidosis and severe hepatomegaly with steatosis, including fatal cases, have been reported with the use of antiretroviral nucleoside analogs, including tenofovir disoproxil fumarate, a component of TRUVADA, alone or in combination with other antiretrovirals in the treatment of HIV infection. A majority of these cases have been in women. Obesity and prolonged nucleoside exposure may be risk factors. Particular caution should be exercised when administering nucleoside analogs to any patient with known risk factors for liver disease; however, cases have also been reported in patients with no known risk factors. Treatment with TRUVADA should be suspended in any patient who develops clinical or laboratory findings suggestive of lactic acidosis or pronounced hepatotoxicity (which may include hepatomegaly and steatosis even in the absence of marked transaminase elevations).

Hepatic Impairment: Tenofovir and tenofovir disoproxil are not metabolized by liver enzymes. Clinically relevant pharmacokinetic changes in patients with hepatic impairment are not observed. Therefore, no dose adjustment is required in patients with hepatic impairment. Emtricitabine has not been evaluated in patients with hepatic impairment; however, emtricitabine has not been shown to be metabolized by liver enzymes, so the impact of liver impairment is likely to be limited. The safety and efficacy of TRUVADA has not been established or specifically studied in patients with underlying liver disorders. Patients with chronic hepatitis B or C and treated with antiretroviral therapy are at increased risk for severe and potentially fatal hepatic adverse events. In case of concomitant antiviral therapy for hepatitis B or C, please refer also to the relevant product information for these medicinal products.

Pancreatitis: Pancreatitis has occurred during therapy with combination regimens that included tenofovir disoproxil fumarate (VIREAD). Caution should be used when administering nucleoside analogues (including TRUVADA) to patients with a history of pancreatitis or risk factors for the development of pancreatitis. Therapy should be suspended in patients with suspected pancreatitis.

Immune: Immune Reconstitution: During the initial phase of treatment, patients responding to antiretroviral therapy may develop an inflammatory response to indolent or residual opportunistic infections (such as MAC, CMV, PCP and TB), which may necessitate further evaluation and treatment.

Renal: Nephrotoxicity: Emtricitabine and tenofovir are principally eliminated by the kidney. Renal impairment, including cases of acute renal failure and Fanconi syndrome (renal tubular injury with severe hypophosphatemia) has been reported in association with the use of VIREAD in clinical practice (see Adverse Reactions, Post-Market Adverse Drug Reactions and Drug Interactions). The majority of these cases occurred in patients with underlying systemic or renal disease, or in patients taking nephrotoxic agents, however, some cases occurred in patients without identified risk factors.

It is recommended that creatinine clearance be calculated in all patients prior to initiating therapy and as clinically appropriate during therapy with TRUVADA. Routine monitoring of calculated creatinine clearance and serum phosphorus should be performed in patients at risk for renal impairment, including patients who have previously experienced renal events while receiving HEPSERA.

Particular caution should be exercised when administering TRUVADA to patients with known risk factors for renal disease and a history of renal dysfunction; however, cases of renal failure have also been reported in patients with no known risk factors. TRUVADA should be avoided with concurrent or recent use of a nephrotoxic agent.

Dosing interval adjustment of TRUVADA and close monitoring of renal function are recommended in all patients with creatinine clearance 30-49 mL/min, (see Dosage and Administration). No safety and efficacy data are available in patients with renal dysfunction who received TRUVADA using these guidelines, and so the potential benefit of TRUVADA should be assessed against the potential risk of renal toxicity. TRUVADA should not be administered to patients with creatinine clearance <30 mL/min or patients requiring hemodialysis.

Special Populations: Patients with HIV and Hepatitis B Virus Coinfection: It is recommended that all patients with HIV be tested for the presence of hepatitis B virus (HBV) before initiating antiretroviral therapy. TRUVADA is not approved for the treatment of chronic HBV infection and the safety and efficacy of TRUVADA have not been established in patients co-infected with HBV and HIV. Severe acute exacerbations of hepatitis B have been reported in patients who are coinfected with HBV and HIV after the discontinuation of TRUVADA. In some patients infected with HBV and treated with EMTRIVA, the exacerbations of hepatitis B were associated with liver decompensation and liver failure. Hepatic function should be closely monitored with both clinical and laboratory follow up for at least several months in patients who are co-infected with HIV and HBV and discontinue TRUVADA. If appropriate, initiation of anti-hepatitis B therapy may be warranted. In patients with advanced liver disease or cirrhosis, post-treatment exacerbation of hepatitis may lead to hepatic decompensation. Therefore, in these patients, discontinuation of treatment without initiation of alternative anti-hepatitis B therapy is not recommended.

Pregnant Women: There are no adequate and well-controlled studies in pregnant women. Because animal reproduction studies are not always predictive of human response, TRUVADA should be used in pregnant women only if the potential benefits outweigh the potential risks to the fetus.

Emtricitabine: The incidence of fetal variations and malformations was not increased in embryo-fetal toxicity studies performed with emtricitabine in mice at exposures (AUC) approximately 60-fold higher and in rabbits at approximately 120-fold higher than human exposures at the recommended daily dose.

Tenofovir disoproxil fumarate: Reproduction studies have been performed in rats and rabbits at doses up to 14 and 19 times the human dose based on body surface area comparisons and revealed no evidence of impaired fertility or harm to the fetus due to tenofovir. Reduced pup body weights, survival and delay in sexual maturation was observed in a peri- and postnatal toxicity study in rats at the maternally toxic doses of 450 and 600 mg/kg (approximately 14 and 19 times the human dose based on body surface area comparisons).

Antiretroviral Pregnancy Registry: To monitor fetal outcomes of pregnant women exposed to ART (antiretroviral therapy) including TRUVADA, an Antiretroviral Pregnancy Registry has been established. Healthcare providers are encouraged to register patients by calling 800-258-4263.

Nursing Women: HIV-infected mothers should not breast-feed their infants to avoid risking postnatal transmission of HIV. Studies in rats and rhesus monkeys have demonstrated that tenofovir is secreted in milk. It is not known whether emtricitabine or tenofovir is excreted in human milk. Because of both the potential for HIV transmission and the potential for serious adverse reactions in nursing infants, **mothers should be instructed not to breast-feed if they are receiving TRUVADA.**

Pediatrics (<18 years of age): Safety and effectiveness in pediatric patients have not been established.

Geriatrics (>65 years of age): Clinical studies of EMTRIVA or VIREAD did not include sufficient numbers of subjects aged 65 and over to determine whether they respond differently than younger subjects. In general, dose selection for the elderly patient should be cautious, keeping in mind the greater frequency of decreased hepatic, renal, or cardiac function, and of concomitant disease or other drug therapy.

ADVERSE REACTIONS: Clinical Trial Adverse Drug Reactions: Because clinical trials are conducted under very specific conditions the adverse reaction rates observed in the clinical trials may not reflect the rates observed in practice and should not be compared to the rates in the clinical trials of another drug. Adverse drug reaction information from clinical trials is useful for identifying drug-related adverse events and for approximating rates.

TRUVADA: Four hundred and forty-seven HIV-1 infected patients have received combination therapy with EMTRIVA or VIREAD with either a non-nucleoside reverse transcriptase inhibitor or protease inhibitor for 48 weeks in ongoing clinical studies.

Table 1: TRUVADA

Selected Treatment-emergent Adverse Events (Grades 2-4) Reported in ≥3% in Any Treatment Group in Study 934 (0-48 Weeks)

	EMTRIVA + VIREAD + EFV N=257	**AZT/3TC + EFV N=254**
Blood and Lymphatic System Disorders		
Anemia	<1%	5%
Gastrointestinal Disorder		
Diarrhea	7%	4%
Nausea	8%	6%
Vomiting	1%	4%
General Disorders and Administration Site Condition		
Fatigue	7%	6%
Infections and Infestations		
Sinusitis	4%	2%
Upper respiratory tract infections	3%	3%
Nasopharyngitis	3%	1%
Nervous System Disorders		
Somnolence	3%	2%
Headache	5%	4%
Dizziness	8%	7%
Psychiatric Disorders		
Depression	4%	7%
Insomnia	4%	5%
Abnormal Dreams	4%	3%
Skin and Subcutaneous Tissue Disorders		
Rash	5%	4%

Study 934—Treatment Emergent Adverse Events: Assessment of adverse reactions is based on data from Study 934 in which 511 antiretroviral-naïve patients received either EMTRIVA + VIREAD administered in combination with efavirenz (N=257) or Combivir (lamivudine/zidovudine) administered in combination with efavirenz (N=254). Adverse events observed in this study were generally consistent with those seen in other studies in treatment experienced or treatment-naïve patients (see Table 1).

Patients who received treatment up to 144 weeks in Study 934 reported adverse events similar in nature and severity to those reported in the first 48 weeks.

Through 48 weeks, 7 patients in the EMTRIVA + VIREAD group and 5 patients in the lamivudine/zidovudine group experienced a new CDC Class C event (10 and 6 patients, respectively, through 144 weeks). Renal safety assessed by laboratory abnormalities was similar in the two groups and no patient discontinued study drug due to renal events. At Weeks 48 and 144, total limb fat (as measured by dual-energy x-ray absorptiometry) was significantly less in a subgroup of patients in the lamivudine/zidovudine group compared to the tenofovir/emtricitabine subgroup (see Table 2).

Table 2: TRUVADA

Study 934 Total Limb Fat at Week 48 and 144 (Dual-Energy X-Ray Absorptiometry)

	EMTRIVA + VIREAD + EFV	AZT/3TC + EFV
Week 48[a]	**N=51**	**N=49**
Total Limb Fat (kg) (Mean±S.D.)	8.9±5.4	6.9±3.9
Week 144[b]	**N=145**	**N=124**
Total Limb Fat (kg) (Mean±S.D.)	9.2±5.4	6.5±4.3

a P=0.03 for the comparison between arms.
b P<0.001 for the comparison between arms.

Laboratory Abnormalities: Laboratory Abnormalities observed in this study were generally consistent with those seen in other studies (see Table 3).

Table 3: TRUVADA

Grade 3/4 Laboratory Abnormalities Reported in ≥1% in Any Treatment Group in Study 934 (0-48 Weeks)

	EMTRIVA + VIREAD + EFV N=257	AZT/3TC + EFV N=254
Any ≥ Grade 3 Laboratory Abnormality	25%	22%
Fasting Cholesterol (>240 mg/dL)	15%	17%
Creatine Kinase (M: >990 U/L) (F: >845 U/L)	7%	6%
Serum Amylase (>175 U/L)	7%	3%
Alkaline Phosphatase (>550 U/L)	1%	0%
AST (M: >180 U/L) (F: >170 U/L)	3%	2%
ALT (M: >215 U/L) (F: >170 U/L)	2%	2%
Hemoglobin (<8.0 mg/dL)	0%	3%
Hyperglycemia (>250 mg/dL)	1%	1%
Hematuria (>75 RBC/HPF)	2%	2%
Neutrophil (>750/mm³)	3%	4%
Fasting Triglycerides (>750 mg/dL)	4%	2%

Laboratory abnormalities in patients who received treatment up to 144 weeks in Study 934 were consistent with those observed in the first 48 weeks of treatment.

In addition to the events described above for Study 934, other adverse events that occurred in at least 3-5% of patients receiving EMTRIVA or VIREAD with other antiretroviral agents in clinical trials include: anorexia, anxiety, arthralgia, asthenia, increased cough, depressive disorders dyspepsia, fever, flatulence, myalgia, pain, abdominal pain, back pain, chest pain, paresthesia, peripheral neuropathy (including peripheral neuritis and neuropathy), pneumonia, rhinitis and rash event (including rash, pruritus, maculopapular rash, urticaria vesiculobullous rash, pustular rash and allergic reaction), sweating and weight loss.

Skin discoloration has been reported with higher frequency among EMTRIVA treated patients. Skin discoloration, mainly manifested by hyperpigmentation on the palms and/or soles was generally mild and asymptomatic and of little clinical significance. The mechanism is unknown.

In addition to the laboratory abnormalities described above for Study 934, Grade 3/4 elevations of bilirubin (>2.5×ULN), pancreatic amylase (>2.0×ULN), serum glucose (<40 or >250 mg/dL), serum lipase (>2.0×ULN), and urine glucose (≥3+) occurred in up to 3% of patients treated with EMTRIVA or VIREAD with other antiretroviral agents in clinical trials.

For more information, please consult the EMTRIVA and VIREAD Product Monographs.

In Study 903 through 144 weeks, decreases from baseline in bone mineral density (BMD) were seen at the lumbar spine and hip in both arms of the study. At Week 144, there was a significantly greater mean percentage decrease from baseline in BMD at the lumbar spine in patients in the VIREAD group compared with patients in the stavudine group (see Table 4). In both groups, the majority of the reduction in BMD occurred in the first 24-48 weeks of the study and this reduction was sustained through Week 144. Twenty-eight percent of VIREAD-treated patients vs. 21% of the stavudine-treated patients lost at least 5% of BMD at the spine or 7% of BMD at the hip. Clinically relevant fractures (excluding fingers and toes) were reported in 4 patients in the VIREAD group and 6 patients in the stavudine group. In addition, there were significant increases in biochemical markers of bone metabolism (serum bone-specific alkaline phosphatase, serum osteocalcin, serum C-telopeptide, and urinary N-telopeptide) in the VIREAD group relative to the stavudine group, suggesting increased bone turnover. Serum parathyroid hormone levels and 1,25 Vitamin D levels were also higher in the VIREAD group. Except for bone specific alkaline phosphatase, these changes resulted in values that remained within the normal range. The effects of VIREAD-associated changes in BMD and biochemical markers on long-term bone health and future fracture risk are unknown.

Post-Market Adverse Drug Reactions: EMTRIVA: The following adverse experiences have been reported in post-marketing experience without regard to causality. Because these events are voluntarily reported from a population of unknown size, estimates of frequency cannot be made.

Blood and Lymphatic System Disorders: thrombocytopenia.
Gastrointestinal Disorders: pancreatitis.
General Disorders and Administrative Site Conditions: pyrexia.
Metabolism and Nutrition Disorders: lactic acidosis.
Immune System Disorders: allergic reaction (including angioedema).
Metabolism and Nutrition Disorders: lactic acidosis, hypokalemia, hypophosphatemia.
Respiratory, Thoracic and Mediastinal Disorders: dyspnea.
Gastrointestinal Disorders: pancreatitis, increased amylase, abdominal pain.
Blood and Lymphatic System Disorders: thrombocytopenia.
Hepatobiliary Disorders: hepatic steatosis, hepatitis, increased liver enzymes (most commonly AST, ALT, GGT).
Skin and Subcutaneous Tissue Disorders: rash.
Musculoskeletal and Connective Tissue Disorders: rhabdomyolysis, osteomalacia (manifested as bone pain and infrequently contributing to fractures), muscular weakness, myopathy.
Renal and Urinary Disorders: acute renal failure, renal failure, acute tubular necrosis, Fanconi syndrome, proximal renal tubulopathy, interstitial nephritis (including acute cases), nephrogenic diabetes insipidus, renal insufficiency, increased creatinine, proteinuria, polyuria.
General Disorders and Administration Site Conditions: asthenia.

Table 4: TRUVADA

Changes in Bone Mineral Density Study 903

	Mean Percent Change (±SD) to Week 144 in BMD	
	VIREAD + 3TC+ EFV	d4T + 3TC +EFV
Lumbar Spine	−2.2%±3.9	−1.0%±4.6
Hip	−2.8%±3.5	−2.4%±4.5

The following adverse reactions, listed under the body system headings above sometimes appeared to be concurrent with proximal renal tubulopathy: rhabdomyolysis, osteomalacia (manifested as bone pain and infrequently contributing to fractures), hypokalemia, muscular weakness, myopathy, hypophosphatemia.

There have been three post marketing reports of acute renal failure in patients on concomitant NSAIDS therapy where a relationship to VIREAD could not be excluded. These events mostly occurred in medically complex patients, where underlying disease processes confound interpretation.

VIREAD and EMTRIVA: In HIV-infected patients with severe immune deficiency at the time of initiation of antiretroviral therapy an inflammatory reaction to infectious pathogens (active or inactive) may arise (see Warnings and Precautions).

In HIV infected patients coinfected with HBV, clinical and laboratory evidence of exacerbations of hepatitis have occurred after discontinuation of treatment (see Warnings and Precautions).

DRUG INTERACTIONS: Drug-Drug Interactions:

Serious Drug Interactions
- **Atazanavir and lopinavir/ritonavir increase tenofovir disoproxil fumarate concentrations which may lead to tenofovir-associated adverse events (see Warnings and Precautions)**
- **Tenofovir disoproxil fumarate decreases atazanavir concentrations—administer atazanavir with ritonavir (see below)**
- **Tenofovir disoproxil fumarate increases didanosine (ddI) concentrations—the dose of ddI may be reduced but use with caution and monitor for ddI-related adverse events and clinical response (see below)**

TRUVADA: No drug interaction studies have been conducted using TRUVADA Tablets.

Emtricitabine and Tenofovir Disoproxil Fumarate: The steady state pharmacokinetics of emtricitabine and tenofovir were unaffected when emtricitabine and tenofovir disoproxil fumarate were administered together versus each agent dosed alone.

In vitro and clinical pharmacokinetic drug-drug interaction studies have shown that the potential for CYP450 mediated interactions involving emtricitabine and tenofovir with other medicinal products is low.

Emtricitabine and tenofovir are primarily excreted by the kidneys by a combination of glomerular filtration and active tubular secretion. No drug-drug interactions due to competition for renal excretion have been observed. Since emtricitabine and tenofovir are primarily eliminated by the kidneys, coadministration of TRUVADA with drugs that reduce renal function or compete for active tubular secretion may increase serum concentrations of emtricitabine, tenofovir, and/or other renally eliminated drugs. Some examples include, but are not limited to cidofovir, acyclovir, valacyclovir, ganciclovir, and valganciclovir.

TRUVADA should not be administered with HEPSERA (adefovir dipivoxil).

No clinically significant drug interactions have been observed between emtricitabine and famciclovir, indinavir, zidovudine, stavudine, and tenofovir disoproxil fumarate (see Table 5 and Table 6). Similarly, no clinically significant drug interactions have been observed between tenofovir disoproxil fumarate and abacavir, efavirenz, emtricitabine, entecavir, indinavir, lamivudine, methadone, nelfinavir, oral contraceptives, ribavirin, saquinavir/ritonavir and tacrolimus in studies conducted in healthy volunteers (see Table 7 and Table 8).

Atazanavir and Lopinavir/Ritonavir: Atazanavir and lopinavir/ritonavir have been shown to increase tenofovir concentrations (see Table 7). The mechanism of this interaction is unknown. Higher tenofovir concentrations could potentiate tenofovir-associated adverse events, including renal disorders. Patients receiving atazanavir, lopinavir/ritonavir, and TRUVADA should be monitored for TRUVADA-associated adverse events.

Tenofovir decreases atazanavir concentrations (see Table 8). Although safety and efficacy data are limited, it is recommended that atazanavir, without ritonavir should not be coadministered with TRUVADA. The recommended regimen is atazanavir 300 mg given with ritonavir 100 mg when used in combination with TRUVADA (all as a single daily dose with food).

Table 5: TRUVADA

Drug Interactions: Changes in Pharmacokinetic Parameters for Emtricitabine in the Presence of the Coadministered Drug[a]

Coadministered Drug	Dose of Coadministered Drug (mg)	Emtricitabine Dose (mg)	N	% Change of Emtricitabine Pharmacokinetic Parameters[b] (90% CI)		
				C_{max}	AUC	C_{min}
Tenofovir DF	300 once daily×7 days	200 once daily×7 days	17	↔	↔	↑ 20 (↑ 12 to ↑ 29)
Zidovudine	300 twice daily×7 days	200 once daily×7 days	27	↔	↔	↔
Indinavir	800×1	200×1	12	↔	↔	NA
Famciclovir	500×1	200×1	12	↔	↔	NA
Stavudine	40×1	200×1	6	↔	↔	NA

a All interaction studies conducted in healthy volunteers.
b ↑=increase; ↓=decrease; ↔=no effect; NA=not applicable.

Didanosine: Pharmacokinetic studies have shown that coadministration of didanosine and tenofovir disoproxil fumarate results in 40-60% increase in C_{max} and AUC of didanosine (see Table 9). The mechanism of this interaction is unknown. **Increases in didanosine concentrations of this magnitude could potentiate didanosine-associated adverse events, including pancreatitis, lactic acidosis, and neuropathy.** In addition, suppression of CD4 counts has been observed in patients receiving tenofovir disoproxil fumarate with didanosine at a dose of 400 mg daily.

A reduced dose of Videx EC (ddI-EC) is recommended when coadministered with TRUVADA. When coadministered with TRUVADA, the Videx EC Product Monograph recommends a reduced dose of 250 mg ddI-EC for HIV infected adults with body weight ≥60 kg and creatinine clearance ≥60 mL/min. For patients with body weight <60 kg, and creatinine clearance ≥60 mL/min, the recommended dose of ddI-EC is 200 mg. Data are not available to recommend a dose adjustment for patients with creatinine clearance <60mL/min or for the buffered tablet formulation of didanosine (Videx).

Caution should be used when coadministering reduced-dose didanosine, tenofovir, and an NNRTI in treatment-naïve patients with high viral loads at baseline since such use has been associated with reports of a high rate of virologic failure and emergence of resistance at an early stage. All patients receiving tenofovir disoproxil fumarate and didanosine concomitantly should be closely monitored for didanosine-related adverse events and clinical response.

Table 6: TRUVADA

Drug Interactions: Changes in Pharmacokinetic Parameters for Coadministered Drug in the Presence of Emtricitabine[a]

Coadministered Drug	Dose of Coadministered Drug (mg)	Emtricitabine Dose (mg)	N	% Change of Coadministered Drug Pharmacokinetic Parameters[b] (90% CI) C_{max}	AUC	C_{min}
Tenofovir DF	300 once daily×7 days	200 once daily×7 days	17	↔	↔	↔
Zidovudine	300 twice daily×7 days	200 once daily×7 days	27	↑ 17 (↑ 0 to ↑ 38)	↑ 13 (↑ 5 to ↑ 20)	↔
Indinavir	800×1	200×1	12	↔	↔	NA
Famciclovir	500×1	200×1	12	↔	↔	NA
Stavudine	40×1	200×1	6	↔	↔	NA

[a] All interaction studies conducted in healthy volunteers.
[b] ↑=increase; ↓=decrease; ↔=no effect; NA=not applicable.

Table 7: TRUVADA

Drug Interactions: Changes in Pharmacokinetic Parameters for Tenofovir[a] in the Presence of the Coadministered Drug

Coadministered Drug	Dose of Coadministered Drug (mg)	N	% Change of Tenofovir Pharmacokinetic Parameters[b] (90% CI) C_{max}	AUC	C_{min}
Abacavir	300 once	8	↔	↔	NC
Atazanavir[c]	400 once daily×14 days	33	↑ 14 (↑ 8 to ↑ 20)	↑ 24 (↑ 21 to ↑ 28)	↑ 22 (↑ 15 to ↑ 30)
Didanosine (enteric-coated)	400 once	25	↔	↔	↔
Didanosine (buffered)	250 or 400 once daily×7 days	14	↔	↔	↔
Efavirenz	600 once daily×14 days	29	↔	↔	↔
Emtricitabine	200 once daily×7 days	17	↔	↔	↔
Entecavir	1 mg once daily×10 days	28	↔	↔	↔
Indinavir	800 three times daily×7 days	13	↑ 14 (↓ 3 to ↑ 33)	↔	↔
Lamivudine	150 twice daily×7 days	15	↔	↔	↔
Lopinavir/Ritonavir	400/100 twice daily ×14 days	24	↔	↑ 32 (↑ 26 to ↑ 38)	↑ 51 (↑ 32 to ↑ 66)
Nelfinavir	1250 twice daily×14 days	29	↔	↔	↔
Saquinavir/Ritonavir	1000/100 twice daily×14 days	35	↔	↔	↑23 (↑ 16 to ↑ 30)
Tacrolimus	0.05 mg/kg twice daily×7 days	21	↑ 13 (↑ 1 to ↑ 27)	↔	↔

[a] Patients received VIREAD 300 mg once daily.
[b] ↑=increase; ↓=decrease; ↔=no effect; NC=not calculated.
[c] REYATAZ Prescribing Information (Bristol-Myers Squibb).

Table 8: TRUVADA

Drug Interactions: Changes in Pharmacokinetic Parameters for Coadministered Drug in the Presence of Tenofovir

Coadministered Drug	Dose of Coadministered Drug (mg)	N	% Change of Coadministered Drug Pharmacokinetic Parameters[a] (90% CI) C_{max}	AUC	C_{min}
Abacavir	300 once	8	↑ 12 (↓ 1 to ↑ 26)	↔	NA
Atazanavir[b]	400 once daily×14 days	34	↓ 21 (↓ 27 to ↓ 14)	↓ 25 (↓ 30 to ↓ 19)	↓ 40 (↓ 48 to ↓ 32)
Atazanavir[b]	Atazanavir/Ritonavir 300/100 once daily×42 days	10	↓ 28 (↓ 50 to ↑ 5)	↓ 25[c] (↓ 42 to ↓ 3)	↓ 23[c] (↓ 46 to ↑ 10)
Efavirenz	600 once daily×14 days	30	↔	↔	↔
Emtricitabine	200 once daily×7 days	17	↔	↔	↔
Entecavir	1 mg once daily×10 days	28	↔	↑ 13 (↑ 11 to ↑ 15)	↔
Indinavir	800 three times daily×7 days	12	↓ 11 (↓ 30 to ↑ 12)	↔	↔
Lamivudine	150 twice daily×7 days	15	↓ 24 (↓ 34 to ↓ 12)	↔	↔
Lopinavir Ritonavir	Lopinavir/Ritonavir 400/100 twice daily×14 days	24	↔	↔	↔
Methadone[d]	40–110 once daily×14 days[e]	13	↔	↔	↔
Nelfinavir M8 metabolite	1250 twice daily×14 days	29	↔ ↔	↔ ↔	↔ ↔
Oral Contraceptives[f]	Ethinyl Estradiol/ Norgestimate (Ortho-Tricyclen) Once daily×7 days	20	↔	↔	↔
Ribavirin	600 once	22	↔	↔	NA
Saquinavir	1000/100 twice daily×14 days	32	↑ 22 (↑ 6 to ↑ 41)	↑ 29[g] (↑12 to ↑48)	↑ 47[g] (↑ 23 to ↑ 76)
Ritonavir			↔	↔	↑ 23 (↑ 3 to ↑ 46)
Tacrolimus	0.05 mg/kg twice daily×7 days	21	↔	↔	↔

(cont'd)

[a] ↑=increase; ↓=decrease; ↔=no effect; NA=not applicable.
[b] REYATAZ Prescribing Information (Bristol-Myers Squibb).
[c] In HIV-infected patients, addition of tenofovir DF to atazanavir 300 mg plus ritonavir 100 mg, resulted in AUC and C_{min} values of atazanavir that were 2.3 and 4-fold higher than the respective values observed for atazanavir 400 mg when given alone.
[d] R-(active), S-and total methadone exposures were equivalent when dosed alone or with VIREAD.
[e] Individual subjects were maintained on their stable methadone dose. No pharmacodynamic alterations (opiate toxicity or withdrawal signs or symptoms) were reported.
[f] Ethinyl estradiol and 17-deacetyl norgestimate (pharmacologically active metabolite) exposures were equivalent when dosed alone or with VIREAD.
[g] Increases in AUC and C_{min} are not expected to be clinically relevant; hence no dose adjustments are required when tenofovir DF and ritonavir-boosted saquinavir are coadministered.

Table 9: TRUVADA

Drug Interactions: Pharmacokinetic Parameters for Didanosine in the Presence of Tenofovir

Didanosine[a] Dose (mg)/Method of Administration[b]	Tenofovir Method of Administration[b]	N	% Difference (90% CI) vs. Didanosine 400 mg Alone, Fasted[c] C_{max}	AUC
Buffered tablets				
400 once daily[d] ×7 days	Fasted 1 hour after didanosine	14	↑ 28 (↑ 11 to ↑ 48)	↑ 44 (↑ 31 to ↑ 59)
Enteric coated capsules				
400 once, fasted	With food, 2 h after didanosine	26	↑ 48 (↑ 25 to ↑ 76)	↑ 48 (↑ 31 to ↑ 67)
400 once, with food	Simultaneously with didanosine	26	↑ 64 (↑ 41 to ↑ 89)	↑ 60 (↑ 44 to ↑ 79)
250 once, fasted	With food, 2 h after didanosine	28	↓ 10 (↓ 22 to ↑ 3)	↔
250 once, fasted	Simultaneously with didanosine	28	↔	↑ 14 (0 to ↑ 31)
250 once, with food	Simultaneously with didanosine	28	↓ 29 (↓ 39 to ↓ 18)	↓ 11 (↓ 23 to ↑ 2)

[a] See Warnings and Precautions regarding use of didanosine with VIREAD.
[b] Administration with food was with a light meal (~373 kcal, 20% fat).
[c] ↑=increase; ↓=decrease; ↔=no difference.
[d] Includes 4 subjects weighing <60 kg receiving ddI 250 mg.

Drug-Food Interactions: Interactions of TRUVADA with food have not been established (see Actions and Clinical Pharmacology, Effects of Food on Oral Absorption).
Drug-Herb Interactions: Interactions of TRUVADA with herbs have not been established.
Drug-Laboratory Test Interactions: Interactions of TRUVADA with laboratory tests have not been established.

DOSAGE AND ADMINISTRATION:

The dose of TRUVADA is one tablet (containing 200 mg of emtricitabine and 300 mg of tenofovir disoproxil fumarate) once daily taken orally with or without food.

Dose Adjustment for Renal Impairment: Significantly increased drug exposures occurred when EMTRIVA or VIREAD were administered to patients with moderate to severe renal impairment (see Action and Clinical Pharmacology, Special Populations and Conditions, Renal Insufficiency). Therefore, the dosing interval of TRUVADA should be adjusted in patients with baseline creatinine clearance 30-49 mL/min using the recommendations in Table 10. These dosing interval recommendations are based on modeling of single-dose pharmacokinetic data in non-HIV infected subjects with varying degrees of renal impairment, including end-stage renal disease requiring hemodialysis. The safety and effectiveness of these dosing interval adjustment recommendations have not been clinically evaluated in moderate to severe renal impairment, therefore, clinical response to treatment and renal function should be closely monitored in these patients. Routine monitoring of creatinine clearance and serum phosphorus should be performed for patients with mild renal impairment (creatinine clearance 50-80 mL/min). (See Warnings and Precautions.)

Table 10: TRUVADA

Dosage Adjustment for Patients with Altered Creatinine Clearance

	Creatinine Clearance (mL/min)[a] ≥50	30–49	<30 (Including Patients Requiring Hemodialysis)
Recommended Dosing Interval	Every 24 hours	Every 48 hours	TRUVADA should not be administered.

[a] Calculated using ideal (lean) body weight.

Missed Dose: If a patient misses a dose at the regularly scheduled time, but then remembers it that same day, the patient should take the missed dose immediately. The patient should not take more than 1 dose of TRUVADA in a day, or 2 doses of TRUVADA at the same time to make up for missing a dose.

OVERDOSAGE:
If overdose occurs the patient must be monitored for evidence of toxicity, and standard supportive treatment applied as necessary.
Emtricitabine: Limited clinical experience is available at doses higher than the therapeutic dose of EMTRIVA. In one clinical pharmacology study single doses of emtricitabine 1200 mg were administered to 11 patients. No severe adverse reactions were reported. The effects of higher doses are not known.

Hemodialysis treatment removes approximately 30% of the emtricitabine dose over a 3 hour dialysis period starting within 1.5 hours of emtricitabine dosing (blood flow rate of 400 mL/min and a dialysate flow rate of 600 mL/min), however, a single treatment does not significantly affect emtricitabine C_{max} or AUC. It is not known whether emtricitabine can be removed by peritoneal dialysis.
Tenofovir disoproxil fumarate: Limited clinical experience at doses higher than the therapeutic dose of VIREAD 300 mg is available. In one study, 600 mg tenofovir disoproxil fumarate was administered to 8 patients orally for 28 days. No severe adverse reactions were reported. The effects of higher doses are not known.

Tenofovir is efficiently removed by hemodialysis with an extraction coefficient of approximately 54%. Following a single 300 mg dose of VIREAD, a four-hour hemodialysis session removed approximately 10% of the administered tenofovir dose.

For management of a suspected drug overdose, contact your **regional Poison Control Centre**. See the *CPS* Directory section for a list of Poison Control Centres.

ACTION AND CLINICAL PHARMACOLOGY: Mechanism of Action: Emtricitabine: Emtricitabine, a synthetic nucleoside analog of cytidine, is phosphorylated by cellular enzymes to form emtricitabine 5'-triphosphate. Emtricitabine 5'-triphosphate inhibits the activity of the HIV-1 reverse transcriptase (RT) by competing with the natural substrate deoxycytidine 5'-triphosphate and by being incorporated into nascent viral DNA which results in chain termination. Emtricitabine 5'-triphosphate is a weak inhibitor of mammalian DNA polymerases α, β, ε, and mitochondrial DNA polymerase γ.
Tenofovir disoproxil fumarate: Tenofovir disoproxil fumarate is an acyclic nucleoside phosphonate diester analog of adenosine monophosphate. Tenofovir disoproxil fumarate requires initial diester hydrolysis for conversion to tenofovir and subsequent phosphorylations by cellular enzymes to form tenofovir diphosphate. Tenofovir diphosphate inhibits the activity of HIV-1 RT by competing with the natural substrate deoxyadenosine 5'-triphosphate and, after incorporation into DNA, by DNA chain termination. Tenofovir diphosphate is a weak inhibitor of mammalian DNA polymerases α, β, and mitochondrial DNA polymerase γ.
Pharmacodynamics: Antiviral Activity In Vitro: Emtricitabine and tenofovir disoproxil fumarate: In combination studies evaluating the in vitro antiviral activity of emtricitabine and tenofovir together, synergistic antiviral effects were observed.
Emtricitabine: The in vitro antiviral activity of emtricitabine against laboratory and clinical isolates of HIV was assessed in lymphoblastoid cell lines, the MAGI-CCR5 cell line, and peripheral blood mononuclear cells. The IC_{50} (50% inhibitory concentration) values for emtricitabine were in the range of 0.0013-0.64 µM (0.0003-0.158 µg/mL). In drug combination studies of emtricitabine with nucleoside reverse transcriptase inhibitors (abacavir, lamivudine, stavudine, zalcitabine, and zidovudine), non-nucleoside reverse transcriptase inhibitors (delavirdine, efavirenz, and nevirapine), and protease inhibitors (amprenavir, nelfinavir, ritonavir, and saquinavir), additive to synergistic effects were observed. Most of these drug combinations have not been studied in humans. Emtricitabine displayed antiviral activity in vitro against HIV-1 clades A, B, C, D, E, F, and G (IC_{50} values ranged from 0.007-0.075 µM) and showed strain specific activity against HIV-2 (IC_{50} values ranged from 0.007-1.5 µM).
Tenofovir disoproxil fumarate: The in vitro antiviral activity of tenofovir against laboratory and clinical isolates of HIV-1 was assessed in lymphoblastoid cell lines, primary monocyte/macrophage cells and peripheral blood lymphocytes. The IC_{50} values for tenofovir were in the range of 0.04-8.5 µM. In drug combination studies of tenofovir with nucleoside reverse transcriptase inhibitors (abacavir, didanosine, lamivudine, stavudine, zalcitabine, and zidovudine), non-nucleoside reverse transcriptase inhibitors (delavirdine, efavirenz, and nevirapine), and protease inhibitors (amprenavir, indinavir, nelfinavir, ritonavir, and saquinavir), additive to synergistic effects were observed. Most of these drug combinations have not been studied in humans. Tenofovir displayed antiviral activity in vitro against HIV-1 clades A, B, C, D, E, F, G, and O (IC_{50} values ranged from 0.5-2.2 µM).
Antiviral Activity In Vivo: The antiviral effects of emtricitabine and tenofovir disoproxil fumarate in terms of reducing HIV-1 viral load and the relationship with dose were assessed in clinical phase 1 studies in treatment-naive and treatment-experienced HIV-infected patients.
Emtricitabine: The in vivo activity of emtricitabine was evaluated in two clinical trials in which 101 patients were administered 25 to 400 mg a day of EMTRIVA as monotherapy for 10 to 14 days. A dose-related antiviral effect was observed, with a median decrease from baseline in plasma HIV-1 RNA of 1.3 log_{10} at a dose of 25 mg QD and 1.7 log_{10} to 1.9 log_{10} at a dose of 200 mg QD or BID.
Tenofovir disoproxil fumarate: The antiviral effects of tenofovir disoproxil fumarate monotherapy in reducing HIV-1 viral load and the relationship with dose were assessed in clinical phase 1 studies in treatment-naive and treatment-experienced HIV infected patients. Doses of tenofovir disoproxil fumarate ranging from 75 mg to 600 mg once daily resulted in statistically significant decreases in plasma HIV-1 RNA levels compared with placebo. In a mixed population of treatment-naive and treatment-experienced patients who received 28 days of repeat daily dosing with tenofovir disoproxil fumarate 300 mg QD (Study GS-97-901) the median decrease in plasma log_{10} HIV-1 RNA level was 1.22 log_{10} copies/mL.
Pharmacokinetics: TRUVADA: One TRUVADA Tablet was bioequivalent to one EMTRIVA Capsule (200 mg) plus one VIREAD Tablet (300 mg) following single-dose administration to fasting healthy subjects (N=39).
Emtricitabine: The pharmacokinetic properties of emtricitabine are summarized in Table 11. Following oral administration of EMTRIVA, emtricitabine is rapidly absorbed with peak plasma concentrations occurring at 1-2 hours post-dose. In vitro binding of emtricitabine to human plasma proteins is <4% and is independent of concentration over the range of 0.02-200 µg/mL. Following administration of radiolabelled emtricitabine, approximately 86% is recovered in the urine and 13% is recovered as metabolites. The metabolites of emtricitabine include 3'-sulfoxide diastereomers and their glucuronic acid conjugate. Emtricitabine is eliminated by a combination of glomerular filtration and active tubular secretion. Following a single oral dose of EMTRIVA, the plasma emtricitabine half-life is approximately 10 hours.
Tenofovir disoproxil fumarate: The pharmacokinetic properties of tenofovir disoproxil fumarate are summarized in Table 11. Following oral administration of VIREAD, maximum tenofovir serum concentrations are achieved in 1.0±0.4 hour. In vitro binding of tenofovir to human plasma proteins is <0.7% and is independent of concentration over the range of 0.01-25 µg/mL. Approximately 70-80% of the intravenous dose of tenofovir is recovered as unchanged drug in the urine. Tenofovir is eliminated by a combination of glomerular filtration and active tubular secretion. Following a single oral dose of VIREAD, the terminal elimination half-life of tenofovir is approximately 17 hours.

Table 11: TRUVADA

Single Dose Pharmacokinetic Parameters for Emtricitabine and Tenofovir in Adults

	Emtricitabine	Tenofovir
Fasted Oral Bioavailability[b] (%)	92 (83.1–106.4)	25 (NC–45.0)[a]
Plasma Terminal Elimination Half-Life[b] (h)	10 (7.4–18.0)	17 (12.0–25.7)
C_{max}[c] (µg/mL)	1.8±0.72[d]	0.30±0.09
AUC[c] (µg·h/mL)	10.0±3.12[d]	2.29±0.69
CL/F[c] (mL/min)	302±94	1043±115
CL_{renal}[c] (mL/min)	213±89	243±33

[a] NC=not calculated.
[b] Median (range).
[c] Mean±SD.
[d] Data presented as steady state values.

Effects of Food on Oral Absorption: TRUVADA may be administered with or without food. Administration of TRUVADA following a high fat meal (784 kcal; 49 grams of fat) or a light meal (373 kcal; 8 grams of fat) delayed the time of tenofovir C_{max} by approximately 0.75 hour. The mean increases in tenofovir AUC and C_{max} were approximately 35% and 15%, respectively, when administered with a high fat or light meal, compared to administration in the fasted state. In previous safety and efficacy studies, VIREAD (tenofovir) was taken under fed conditions. Emtricitabine systemic exposures (AUC and C_{max}) were unaffected when TRUVADA was administered with either a high fat or a light meal.

Special Populations and Conditions: Pediatrics and Geriatrics: Pharmacokinetics of emtricitabine and tenofovir have not been fully evaluated in children (<18 years) or in the elderly (>65 years).
Race: Emtricitabine: No pharmacokinetic differences due to race have been identified following the administration of EMTRIVA.
Tenofovir disoproxil fumarate: There were insufficient numbers from racial and ethnic groups other than Caucasian to adequately determine potential pharmacokinetic differences among these populations.
Gender: Emtricitabine and tenofovir disoproxil fumarate: Emtricitabine and tenofovir pharmacokinetics are similar in male and female patients.
Hepatic Insufficiency: The pharmacokinetics of tenofovir following a 300 mg single dose of VIREAD have been studied in non-HIV infected subjects with moderate to severe hepatic impairment. There were no substantial alterations in tenofovir pharmacokinetics in subjects with hepatic impairment compared with unimpaired subjects. The pharmacokinetics of TRUVADA or emtricitabine have not been studied in patients with hepatic impairment; however, emtricitabine has not been shown to be significantly metabolized by liver enzymes, so the impact of liver impairment is likely to be limited.
Renal Insufficiency: The pharmacokinetics of emtricitabine and tenofovir are altered in patients with renal insufficiency (see Warnings and Precautions, Nephrotoxicity). In patients with creatinine clearance <50 mL/min, C_{max} and $AUC_{0-\infty}$ of emtricitabine and tenofovir were increased. It is recommended that the dosing interval for TRUVADA be modified in patients with creatinine clearance 30-49 mL/min. TRUVADA should not be used in patients with creatinine clearance <30 mL/min and in patients with end-stage renal disease requiring dialysis (see Dosage and Administration).
STORAGE AND STABILITY: Store at 15-30°C.
Keep container tightly closed.
Dispense only in original container.
Do not use if seal over bottle opening is broken or missing.
SPECIAL HANDLING INSTRUCTIONS: There are no special handling instructions.
INFORMATION FOR THE PATIENT: Published in e-CPS, available by subscription at www.e-cps.ca.
DOSAGE FORMS, COMPOSITION AND PACKAGING: Each blue, capsule-shaped, film-coated tablet, debossed with "GILEAD" on one side and with "701" on the other side, contains: emtricitabine 200 mg and tenofovir disoproxil fumarate 300 mg (which is equivalent to 245 mg of tenofovir disoproxil). Nonmedicinal ingredients: croscarmellose sodium, lactose monohydrate, magnesium stearate, microcrystalline cellulose and pregelatinized starch (gluten free); coating: Opadry II Blue Y-30-10701, which contains FD&C Blue #2 aluminum lake, hydropropylmethylcellulose 2910, lactose monohydrate, titanium dioxide and triacetin. Bottles of 30 and a desiccant (silica gel canister or sachet) with a child-resistant closure.

Tryptan® Ⓟ

L-tryptophan

Adjunct in the Management of Affective Disorders

Valeant

PHARMACOLOGY: The rationale for the use of L-tryptophan in affective disorders is based on clinical findings more than 20 years ago, that L-tryptophan increases 5-HT (serotonin) synthesis in the CNS of humans. It has been demonstrated in clinical trials that oral ingestion of L-tryptophan in humans caused a significant increase in the level of the serotonin metabolite, 5-hydroxyindoleacetic acid (5-HIAA), in the lumbar cerebrospinal fluid, indicating an increased turnover of serotonin in the CNS.

L-tryptophan is 1 of the 8 essential amino acids. The minimum daily requirements are said to be 0.25 g for males and 0.15 g for females. It is present in the hydrolysates of most proteins, the average western diet containing between 1 and 3 g/day. There are 2 major metabolic pathways for L-tryptophan, the first to serotonin, the second to nicotinic acid. Approximately 98% of dietary L-tryptophan is metabolized into nicotinic acid and only a very small amount is being metabolized to serotonin via the intermediary stage of 5-hydroxy-tryptophan (5-HTP). Tryptophan hydroxylase, the enzyme responsible for this step, is the rate-limiting enzyme for serotonin production and is normally only about half- saturated. CNS serotonin is metabolized by monoamine oxidase to 5-HIAA.
INDICATIONS: As a valuable adjunct to antidepressant drug treatment in the management of patients suffering from depressive disorders (bipolar affective disorders). An adjunctive effect has been observed in some cases when L-tryptophan is given in combination with lithium in bipolar patients with mania or depression for whom lithium alone or in combination with neuroleptics or tricyclics has shown little or no effect. Clinical observations suggest the possibility that the combination of lithium and L-tryptophan may reduce the need for the higher, more toxic doses of lithium necessary in control acute mania.
CONTRAINDICATIONS: In patients with known sensitivity to L-tryptophan or any other compound in the formulation.
WARNINGS: L-tryptophan should not be given to patients suffering from the following conditions or should be prescribed only under close supervision.
Bladder Cancer: To minimize the risk of bladder cancer, it may be recommended to give vitamin B_6 supplements if the L-tryptophan doses are many times in excess of those consumed normally in dietary protein. An increased incidence rate of bladder cancer has been observed in experimental animals after implantation of pellets containing any of the 7 tryptophan metabolites formed by tryptophan pyrrolase. Active metabolites included kynurenine, 3-hydroxykynurenine, 3-hydroxyanthranillic acid, and xanthurenic acid, but not tryptophan itself. Vitamin B_6 has been reported to correct the metabolism of L-tryptophan and to reduce the metabolites to normal levels. A large study carried out by the National Cancer Institute did not find L-tryptophan to produce cancer in either rats or mice. Elevated levels of L-tryptophan metabolites in the urine have been reported both in bladder cancer patients relative to controls, in patients who had a recurrence of cancer relative to those who did not, and in patients taking oral contraceptives or hormones.
Diabetes Mellitus: Xanthurenic acid, which is increased on L-tryptophan loading, has a diabetogenic action in animals, possibly due to its ability to bind insulin, suggesting caution in the use of tryptophan in patients with a family history of diabetes.
Achlorhydria/Malabsorption: In ruminants, oral L-tryptophan caused pulmonary edema and emphysema, mediated by bacterial conversion of L-tryptophan to skatole (3-methylindole). This is not normally of concern in humans except where bacteria exist high in the gastrointestinal tract due to conditions such as achlorhydria, or where L-tryptophan reaches the bacterial populations lower in the gastrointestinal tract due to malabsorption.
Cataract Formation: Animal data suggest that photooxidation of L-tryptophan and some of its metabolites, such as kynurenine, may be involved in cataract formation. Although there is no evidence that this occurs in humans, L-tryptophan administration is likely to raise lenticular tryptophan and kynurenine concentrations, and this might make subjects more susceptible to cataract formation, particularly if exposed to ultraviolet light.
PRECAUTIONS: *Drug Interactions:* Drug interactions between tryptophan and other CNS affecting drugs have been reported. A higher occurrence of side effects was reported when tryptophan was given in combination with MAO inhibitors. The most common side effects caused by this drug combination were dizziness, nausea and headache. At a dosage of 20 to 50 mg/kg tryptophan in addition to MAO inhibitors, the following side effects have been reported: ethanol-like intoxication, drowsiness, hyperreflexia and clonus. Single case reports of adverse reactions to the drug combination include hypomanic behavior, ocular oscillation, ataxia, and myoclonus. Some of these reactions resemble the "serotonin syndrome" seen in experimental animals, which consists of tremor, hypertonus, myoclonus, and hyperreactivity. These symptoms disappear soon after cessation of tryptophan, and no detrimental long-term effects have been reported.

When tryptophan was given in combination with fluoxetine, the following side effects have been reported, but disappeared as soon as the medication was discontinued. Neither drug alone caused similar side effects: agitation, restlessness, poor concentration, nausea, diarrhea, and worsening of obsessive-compulsive disorder.

Patients taking high doses of L-tryptophan should not be protein deprived since an amino acid imbalance can ensue.
ADVERSE EFFECTS: L-tryptophan, in doses below 5 g/day may cause dry mouth and drowsiness. In higher doses (9 to 12 g/day) nausea, anorexia, dizziness and headache have been reported.

Side effects disappear when medication is continued and in most cases only a light dizziness may persist.

Sexual disinhibition has been reported in some patients with emotional disorders.

L-tryptophan, when given with lithium, might increase some side effects associated with lithium therapy by potentiating the lithium effect (nausea, vomiting, dermatological eruptions, psoriasis, alopecia).
OVERDOSE:
Symptoms: According to the toxicity described, symptoms of overdosage would include vomiting and might include serotonin syndrome symptoms.
Treatment: Treatment of overdosage would be symptomatic with close monitoring and support of vital systems as necessary.

For management of a suspected drug overdose, CPhA recommends that you contact your **regional Poison Control Centre**. See the *CPS* Directory section for a list of Poison Control Centres.

DOSAGE: Clinical reports on the use of L-tryptophan as an adjunct in the management of affective disorders have indicated the dose of 8 to 12 g/day to be the most effective one. Lower doses have been reported to be effective in combination with other antidepressants. Some patients may not tolerate 12 g/day but might still benefit from doses reduced to 8 g/day.

The treatment might be initiated with 12 g/day of L-tryptophan, given in 3 to 4 equally divided doses. Administration with meals or snacks is recommended to reduce the incidence of nausea. The dose and frequency of administration may have to be adjusted to the patient's need and tolerance.

A small number of bipolar patients are particularly sensitive to L-tryptophan and will not tolerate higher doses than 1 or 2 g/day. Patients on concomitant medication should be monitored for possible reduction of the concomitant medication since L-tryptophan may enhance their efficacy.

If L-tryptophan is used in the acute treatment of mania in conjunction with lithium it will potentiate some of the side effects associated with lithium such as nausea and vomiting. Thus, often it will be necessary to decrease the lithium dosage especially when it is given in doses above 900 to 1 200 mg/day. In manic-depressive illness chronically treated with lithium, the lithium dose may need to be decreased when L-tryptophan is added because of increased side effects. In these patients L-tryptophan tends to produce an increase in lithium concentrations, thus it is important to monitor the lithium concentration closely for at least 2 weeks after the addition of L-tryptophan.

With some of the more sedative neuroleptics and antidepressants, if L-tryptophan is added, an increased incidence of sedation may occur.

Information to Be Provided to the Patient: For better results, L-tryptophan should be taken with a protein-low, carbohydrate-rich snack or meal.

SUPPLIED: Capsules: Each opaque white capsule, size No. 00, imprinted with ICN T17, contains: L-tryptophan, USP 500 mg. Nonmedicinal ingredients: magnesium stearate and talc. Bottles of 100 and 250.

Tablets: 250 mg: Each white, oval, film-coated tablet, embossed "TRYPTAN" on one side and "250 mg" on the other side, contains: L-tryptophan, USP 250 mg. Nonmedicinal ingredients: calcium phosphate, croscarmellose sodium, film coating base solution (includes: acetylated monoglyceride, hydroxypropylmethyl cellulose, povidone, titanium dioxide), magnesium stearate, methylcellulose, opaspray white and wax solution. Bottles of 100.

500 mg: Each white, oval, biconvex, film-coated tablet, embossed "TRYPTAN" on one side and "500 mg" on the other side, contains: L-tryptophan, USP 500 mg. Nonmedicinal ingredients: calcium phosphate, croscarmellose sodium, film coating base solution (includes: acetylated monoglyceride, hydroxypropylmethyl cellulose, povidone, titanium dioxide), magnesium stearate, methylcellulose, opaspray white and wax solution. Bottles of 100 and 250.

750 mg: Each white, oval, biconvex, film-coated tablet, embossed "TRYPTAN" on one side and "750 mg" on the other side, contains: L-tryptophan, USP 750 mg. Nonmedicinal ingredients: calcium phosphate, croscarmellose sodium, film coating base solution (includes: acetylated monoglyceride, hydroxypropylmethyl cellulose, povidone, titanium dioxide), magnesium stearate, methylcellulose, opaspray white and wax solution. Bottles of 100.

1 g: Each white, oval, film-coated tablet, embossed "TRYPTAN" 1 g on one side, contains: L-tryptophan, USP 1 g. Nonmedicinal ingredients: calcium phosphate, croscarmellose sodium, film coating base solution (includes: acetylated monoglyceride, hydroxypropylmethyl cellulose, povidone, titanium dioxide), magnesium stearate, methylcellulose, opaspray white and wax solution. Bottles of 100 and 250.

Store at controlled room temperature (15 to 30°C). Protect from heat and light.

Tubersol®

tuberculin purified protein derivative (Mantoux)

Diagnostic Antigen

sanofi pasteur

Date of Revision: October 2005

PHARMACOLOGY: Intracutaneous tuberculin testing is an accepted aid in the diagnosis of tuberculosis infection.

The reaction to intracutaneously injected tuberculin is a delayed (cellular) hypersensitivity reaction. The reaction which characteristically shows a delayed course, reaching its peak more than 24 hours after administration, consists of induration due to cell infiltration and occasionally vesiculation and necrosis. Clinically, a delayed hypersensitivity reaction to tuberculin is a manifestation of previous infection with *M. tuberculosis* or a variety of non-tuberculosis bacteria. In most cases sensitization is induced by natural mycobacterial infection or by vaccination with BCG Vaccine.

The sensitization following infection with mycobacteria occurs primarily in the regional lymph nodes. Small lymphocytes (T lymphocytes) proliferate in response to the antigenic stimulus to give rise to specifically sensitized lymphocytes. After several weeks, these lymphocytes enter the blood stream and circulate for long periods of time. Subsequent restimulation of these sensitized lymphocytes with the same or a similar antigen, such as the intradermal injection of tuberculin, evokes a local reaction mediated by these cells.

The tuberculin reaction is characterized by the early predominance of mononuclear cells (small and medium sized lymphocytes and monocytes). Only a small proportion of these cells appear to be lymphocytes sensitized to tuberculin. Most cells are brought into the reaction through the release of biologically active substances by sensitized lymphocytes. An increase in vascular permeability leading to erythema and edema also occurs in tuberculin reactions.

Characteristically, delayed hypersensitivity reactions to tuberculin begin at 5 to 6 hours, are maximal at 48 to 72 hours and subside over a period of days. In those who are elderly or those who are being tested for the first time reactions may develop slowly and may not peak until after 72 hours. Immediate hypersensitivity reactions to tuberculin may occur.

INDICATIONS: TUBERSOL [Tuberculin Purified Protein Derivative (Mantoux)] is indicated to aid diagnosis of tuberculosis infection (TB) in persons at increased risk of developing active disease. There are two general situations where risk of disease is increased:

- Recent infection—most commonly contacts of a recently diagnosed patient with active contagious pulmonary TB, or immigrants within five years of their arrival in Canada from countries where TB is still common,
- Increased risk of reactivation due to impaired immunity. This includes HIV infection, diabetes, renal failure, corticosteroids or other immunosuppressant medication and pulmonary silicosis.

All health-care workers (HCWs) (pre-placement and presently employed) should have their TB infection status documented. Ongoing surveillance for TB in HCWs includes both regular ongoing screening and post-exposure screening.

Travellers at high risk of exposure to TB due to travel in a high-endemic environment, who have a medical condition increasing the risk of TB, have "high-risk" lengths of travel (>1 month), or participate in high-risk activities leading to probable exposure should have a pre-exposure Tuberculin Skin Test (TST). Post-exposure TST, or testing at least every 2 years, should be done for all tuberculin-negative reactors.

HIV-infected persons should be given a TST as soon as possible after HIV infection is diagnosed and as recommended.

Staff members in all correctional facilities should have tuberculin skin test screening (at hiring and routinely thereafter). Inmates in long-term correctional facilities should have tuberculin skin test screening on admission and routinely thereafter.

The tuberculin skin test is useful in epidemiologic surveys to define the prevalence of infection in population groups or to estimate prevalence or risk of infection in certain population groups.

Five (5) tuberculin units (TU) per test dose of 0.1 mL is the standard strength used for intradermal (Mantoux) testing.

Previous BCG vaccination is not a contraindication to tuberculin testing. TUBERSOL may be used as an aid in the diagnosis of tuberculosis infection in persons with a history of BCG vaccination.

The repeated testing of uninfected persons does not sensitize them to tuberculin.

CONTRAINDICATIONS: Allergy to any component of TUBERSOL [Tuberculin Purified Protein Derivative (Mantoux)] or its container, or an anaphylactic or other allergic reaction to a previous test of tuberculin PPD is a contraindication to the use of TUBERSOL (see Supplied).

TUBERSOL should not be administered to:

- known tuberculin positive reactors because of the severity of reactions (e.g., vesiculation, ulceration or necrosis) that may occur at the test site in highly sensitive persons,
- persons with severe blistering tuberculin reactions in the past,
- persons with documented active tuberculosis or a clear history of treatment for TB infection or disease,
- persons with extensive burns or eczema.

Deferral: Tuberculin skin testing should be deferred for patients with major viral infections or live-virus vaccination in the past month, for example vaccination against mumps or measles. Persons with the common cold may be tuberculin tested.

WARNINGS: Do not inject intravenously or intramuscularly.

Do not inject subcutaneously. If this occurs, the test cannot be interpreted.

Not all infected persons will have a delayed hypersensitivity reaction to a tuberculin test. A large number of factors have been reported to cause a decreased ability to respond to the tuberculin test in the presence of tuberculous infection (TB) including viral infections (measles, mumps, chickenpox and HIV), live virus vaccinations (measles, mumps, rubella, oral polio and yellow fever), overwhelming tuberculosis, other bacterial infections, drugs (corticosteroids and many other immunosuppressive agents), and malignancy.

PRECAUTIONS: As with all other products, Epinephrine Hydrochloride Solution (1:1,000) and other appropriate agents should be available for immediate use in case an anaphylactic or acute hypersensitivity reaction occurs. Health-care providers should be familiar with current recommendations for the initial management of anaphylaxis in non-hospital settings, including proper airway management.

The possibility of allergic reactions in persons sensitive to components of TUBERSOL [Tuberculin Purified Protein Derivative (Mantoux)] should be evaluated. Allergic reactions may occur following the use of TUBERSOL even in persons with no prior history of hypersensitivity to the product components.

For instructions on recognition and treatment of anaphylactic reactions, see the current edition of the Canadian Immunization Guide or visit the Health Canada website.

Proper use of the tuberculin skin test requires a knowledge of the antigen used (tuberculin), the immunological basis for the reaction to this antigen, the technique(s) of administering and reading the test, and the results of epidemiologic and clinical experience with the test. In any population, the likelihood that a positive test represents a true infection is influenced by the prevalence of infection with *M. tuberculosis*. False positive tuberculin reaction tests occur in individuals who have been infected with other mycobacteria, including vaccination with BCG. Some antigens in the tuberculin skin test are shared with other mycobacteria and thus can elicit a skin test response.

Anything that impairs or attenuates cell mediated immunity (CMI) potentially can cause a false negative tuberculin reaction (e.g., viral infections, live virus vaccines, leukemia, sarcoidosis, use of glucocorticosteroids and other immunosuppressive agents, bacterial infections, fungal infections, metabolic derangements, low protein states, diseases affecting lymphoid organs, age (newborns, elderly) or stress).

HIV-infected persons may have a compromised ability to react to tuberculin skin tests because of cutaneous anergy associated with progressive HIV immunosuppression.

Before administration, take all appropriate precautions to prevent adverse reactions. This includes a review of the patient's history concerning possible hypersensitivity to the product or similar products, previous testing history with TUBERSOL, the presence of any contraindications to the use of TUBERSOL, and the patient's current health status.

Use a separate, sterile needle and syringe, or a sterile disposable unit, for each individual dose to prevent disease transmission. There have been case reports of transmission of HIV and hepatitis by failure to scrupulously observe sterile technique. In particular, the same needle and/or syringe must never be used to re-enter a multi-dose vial to withdraw product even when it is to be used for testing of the same patient. This may lead to contamination of the vial contents and infection of patients who subsequently receive product from the vial.

Laboratory Tests: Tuberculin reactivity may indicate latent infection, prior infection and/or disease with *M. tuberculosis* and does not necessarily indicate the presence of active tuberculous disease. Persons showing tuberculin reactions considered positive by current public health guidelines should be evaluated by other diagnostic procedures, such as x-ray examination of the chest and microbiological examination of the sputum.

Drug Interactions: Reactivity to the test may be depressed or suppressed in persons who are receiving corticosteroids or immunosuppressive agents.

Vaccination with live-attenuated virus can cause suppression of the tuberculin test response in patients known to be infected with *M. tuberculosis*. Reactivity to PPD may be temporarily depressed by certain live virus vaccines (measles, mumps, rubella, oral polio, yellow fever, and varicella). When tuberculin screening is required at the same time as a measles-containing vaccine or other parenteral live attenuated virus vaccine, simultaneous administration of TUBERSOL and the vaccine at separate sites is the preferred option. If a parenteral live attenuated virus vaccine has been administered recently, tuberculin testing should be delayed for >1 month after vaccination.

Pregnancy: Animal reproduction studies have not been conducted with TUBERSOL. However, the Canadian Tuberculosis Standard states "persons can be skin tested if they are pregnant". No teratogenic effects of testing during pregnancy have been documented.

The risk of unrecognized tuberculosis and the close postpartum contact between a mother with active disease and an infant leaves the infant in grave danger of tuberculosis and complications such as tuberculous meningitis. Therefore, the prescribing physician should consider if the potential benefits outweigh the possible risks for performing the tuberculin test on a pregnant woman or a woman of childbearing age, particularly in certain "high risk populations".

Pediatric: There is no age contraindication to tuberculin skin testing of infants. Because their immune systems are immature, many infants <6 weeks of age who are infected with *M. tuberculosis* do not react to tuberculin tests. Older infants and children develop tuberculin sensitivity 3-6 weeks or more after initial infection.

ADVERSE EFFECTS: Local: Pain, pruritus and discomfort at the test site may occur.

Immediate erythematous or other reactions may occur at the injection site. The reason(s) for these occurrences are presently unknown.

Two to three percent of tested persons will have localized redness or rash (without induration) occurring within 12 hours of testing. These reactions do not indicate TB infection.

Injection site bleeding after the needle is withdrawn and hematoma and bruising up to three days after the administration of the test have been seen.

Very rare: Vesiculation, ulceration or necrosis may appear at the test site in highly sensitive persons.

Strongly positive reactions may result in scarring at the test site.

Systemic: There have been rare severe systemic hypersensitivity reactions (anaphylactic/anaphylactoid reactions) following TUBERSOL administration that were manifested by angioedema, upper respiratory stridor, dyspnea, skin rash, generalized rash and/or urticaria reported within 24 hours. These were treated with epinephrine, diphenhydramine and/or steroids. Some of these events were reported in patients who had no prior exposure to TUBERSOL. No cause and effect was able to be established with a specific component of the skin test.

Reporting of Adverse Events: Health-care providers should report any adverse occurrences temporally related to the administration of the product in accordance with local requirements and to the Global Pharmacovigilance Department, Sanofi Pasteur Limited, 1755 Steeles Avenue West, Toronto, ON, M2R 3T4 Canada. 1-888-621-1146 (phone) or 416-667-2435 (fax).

DOSAGE: TUBERSOL [Tuberculin Purified Protein Derivative (Mantoux)] is a clear, colorless liquid. Inspect for extraneous particulate matter and/or discoloration before use. If these conditions exist, the product should not be administered.

The Test: Five (5) Tuberculin units (TU) per test dose of 0.1 mL is the standard strength tuberculin test used for intradermal (Mantoux) testing.

The Mantoux test is performed by injecting intradermally, with a syringe and needle, 0.1 mL of TUBERSOL. For the intradermal (Mantoux) tuberculin test, the dose is 5 TU per test dose of 0.1 mL.

Method of Administration:

1. The preferred site of the test is the volar aspect of the forearm. Avoid areas on the skin that are red or swollen. Avoid visible veins.
2. The skin site is first cleansed with a suitable germicide and should be dry prior to injection of the antigen.
3. The test dose (0.1 mL) of TUBERSOL is administered with a 1 mL syringe calibrated in tenths and fitted with a short, one quarter to one half inch, 26 or 27 gauge needle.
4. The stopper of the vial should be wiped with a suitable germicide and should be dry before needle insertion. The needle is then inserted gently through the stopper and 0.1 mL of TUBERSOL is drawn into the syringe. Care should be taken to avoid injection of excess air with removal of each dose so as not to overpressurize the vial thus causing possible seepage at the puncture site.
5. The point of the needle is inserted into the most superficial layers of the skin with the needle bevel pointing upward. If the intradermal injection is performed properly, a definite pale bleb will rise at the needle point, about 10 mm (3/8") in diameter. This bleb will disperse within minutes. No dressing is required.
6. You may see a drop of blood when you withdraw the needle. This is normal. Offer the patient a gauze pad to remove the blood. Advise the patient not to press the gauze pad over the injection site but just to dab gently to remove the blood. This will avoid squeezing out the tuberculin thereby disrupting the test.

Needles should not be recapped and should be disposed of properly.

In the event of an improperly performed injection (i.e., no bleb formed), the test should be repeated immediately at another site, at least 2 inches from the first site and the second injection site circled as an indication that this is the site to be read.

Inform the patient of the need to return for the reading of the test by a trained health professional. Self-reading is inaccurate and is strongly discouraged.

Interpretation of the Test: The skin test should be read by a trained health professional 48 to 72 hours after administration of TUBERSOL. Sensitivity is indicated by induration only; redness should not be measured.

The diameter of induration should be measured transversely to the long axis of the forearm and recorded in millimetres (including 0). The tip of a ballpoint pen pushed at a 45° angle toward the site of injection will stop at the edge of induration. Presence and size of necrosis and edema (if present) should also be recorded, although it is not used in the interpretation of the test.

The significance of induration measurements in diagnosing latent TB infection must be considered in terms of the patient's history and his or her risk of developing active TB disease as indicated below: See Table 1.

Table 1: TUBERSOL
Interpretation of Tuberculin Test

Tuberculin Reaction Size, mm Induration	Setting in which Reaction Considered Significant (Meaning Probable TB Infection)
0–4	HIV infection and expected risk of tuberculosis infection is high (e.g., patient is an immigrant from a country where TB is endemic, is a household contact, or has an abnormal X-ray). This reaction size is not normally considered significant, but in the presence of immune suppression may be important.
5–9	HIV infection Contact of active contagious case Abnormal chest X-ray with fibronodular disease
≥10	All others

The possibility should be considered that skin test sensitivity may also be due to previous contact with atypical mycobacteria or previous BCG vaccination.

BCG vaccination may produce a PPD reaction that cannot be distinguished reliably from a reaction caused by infection with *M. tuberculosis*. However, a diagnosis of *M. tuberculosis* infection and the use of preventive therapy should be considered for any BCG-vaccinated person who has a tuberculin skin-test reaction of ≥10 mm of induration, especially if any of the following circumstances are present: a) the vaccinated person is a contact of another person who has infectious TB, particularly if the infectious person has transmitted *M. tuberculosis* to others; b) the vaccinated person was born or has resided in a country in which the prevalence of TB is high; or c) the vaccinated person is exposed continually to populations in which the prevalence of TB is high.

The Booster Effect and Two-step Testing: Infection of a person with tubercle bacilli or other mycobacteria results in a delayed hypersensitivity response to tuberculin which is demonstrated by the skin test. The delayed hypersensitivity response may gradually wane over a period of years. If a person receives a tuberculin test at this time (several years after infection) the response may be a reaction that is not significant. However, the stimulus of the test may boost or increase the size of the reaction to a second test, sometimes causing an apparent conversion or development of sensitivity.

To eliminate this potential confusion, two-step testing should be performed as a baseline, if tuberculin testing will subsequently be conducted at regular intervals, for instance among health-care or prison workers. If the first test shows either no reaction or a small reaction, the second test should be performed one to four weeks later. Both tests should be read and recorded at 48 to 72 hours. Patients with a second tuberculin test (booster) response of 10 mm or more should be considered to have experienced past or old infection.

Persons who do not boost when given repeat tests at one week, but whose tuberculin reactions change to positive after one year, should be considered to have newly-acquired tuberculosis infection and managed accordingly.

Since tuberculin reactivity may not necessarily indicate the presence of active tuberculous disease, persons showing a tuberculin reaction should be further evaluated with other diagnostic procedures.

Give the patient a permanent personal record. In addition, it is essential that the health professional record the testing history in the permanent medical record of each patient. This permanent office record should contain the name of the product, date given, dose, manufacturer and lot number, as well as the test result in millimetres of induration (including 0, if appropriate). Reporting results only as negative or positive is not satisfactory.

SUPPLIED: TUBERSOL [Tuberculin Purified Protein Derivative (Mantoux)] for intradermal tuberculin testing is prepared from a large Master Batch Connaught Tuberculin (CT68) and is a cell-free purified protein fraction obtained from a human strain of *M. tuberculosis* grown on a protein-free synthetic medium and inactivated. The use of a standard preparation derived from a single batch (CT68) has been adopted in order to eliminate batch to batch variation by the same manufacturer. TUBERSOL is a clear colourless liquid.

TUBERSOL contains: purified protein derivative of *M. tuberculosis* 5 TU per 0.1 mL, polysorbate 80 0.0006%, phenol 0.22% to 0.35% w/v in sterile isotonic phosphate buffered saline. Vials of 1 mL (5 TU per 0.1 mL test dose). Vials of 5 mL (5 TU per 0.1 mL test dose). The stopper of the vial for this product does not contain dry natural latex rubber.

Independent studies conducted by the U.S. Public Health Service in humans have determined the amount of CT68 in stabilized solution necessary to produce bio-equivalency with Tuberculin PPD-S (in phosphate buffer without polysorbate 80) using 5 US units (TU) Tuberculin PPD-S as the standard.

Before release, each successive lot is tested for potency in comparison with a Standard.

Store at 2 to 8°C. **Do not freeze.** Discard product if exposed to freezing. Tuberculin PPD solutions can be adversely affected by exposure to light. The product should be stored in the dark except when doses are actually being withdrawn from the vial. **A vial of TUBERSOL [Tuberculin Purified Protein Derivative (Mantoux)] which has been entered and in use for 30 days should be discarded because oxidation and degradation may have reduced the potency.** Failure to store and handle TUBERSOL as recommended will result in a loss of potency and inaccurate test results. Do not use after expiration date.

Tums® Tablets
calcium carbonate
Antacid—Calcium Supplement

GlaxoSmithKline Consumer Healthcare

INDICATIONS: Antacid: For relief of acid indigestion, heartburn and sour stomach caused by excess stomach acidity. Calcium Supplement: An excellent source of calcium. Calcium is a factor in the normal development and maintenance of bones and teeth, as well as in the maintenance of good health.

CONTRAINDICATIONS: No data supplied by the manufacturer.

WARNINGS: No data supplied by the manufacturer.

PRECAUTIONS: Do not take within 2 hours of another medicine because the effectiveness of the medicine may be altered. Keep out of reach of children.

ADVERSE EFFECTS: No data supplied by the manufacturer.

OVERDOSE:
No data supplied by the manufacturer.

> For management of a suspected drug overdose, CPhA recommends that you contact your **regional Poison Control Centre**. See the *CPS* Directory section for a list of Poison Control Centres.

DOSAGE: Regular Strength: Antacid: Adults and pregnant women: Chew 2 to 4 tablets as needed. Consult a physician if symptoms persist beyond 2 weeks or recur. Maximum: Adults: 16 tablets/day. Pregnant women: 7 tablets/day. Calcium supplement: Adults and pregnant women: Chew 2 tablets after meals or as directed by a physician. Maximum: 7 tablets/day.

Extra Strength: Antacid: Adults and pregnant women: Chew 2 to 3 tablets as needed. Consult a physician if symptoms persist beyond 2 weeks or recur. Maximum: Adults: 10 tablets/day. Pregnant women: 5 tablets/day. Calcium supplement: Adults and pregnant women: Chew 2 tablets after meals or as directed by a physician. Maximum: 5 tablets/day.

Ultra Strength: Antacid: Adults and pregnant women: Chew 1 to 2 tablets as needed. Consult a physician if symptoms persist beyond 2 weeks or recur. Maximum: Adults: 8 tablets/day. Pregnant women: 3 tablets/day. Calcium supplement: Adults and pregnant women: Chew 1 to 2 tablets after meals or as directed by a physician. Maximum: 3 tablets/day.

SUPPLIED: Regular Strength: Each peppermint or assorted fruit-flavoured tablet contains: calcium carbonate 500 mg equivalent to elemental calcium 200 mg. Security-sealed bottles of 75 and 150. Rolls of 12 and 36.
Extra Strength: Each peppermint, assorted fruit, assorted tropical fruit, assorted mint, banana-berry, cocoa and crème smoothies, tropical fruit smoothies, berry fusion, and assorted berries-flavoured tablet contains: calcium carbonate 750 mg equivalent to elemental calcium 300 mg. Security-sealed bottles of 50, 60, 100 and 350. Rolls of 8 and 24.
Ultra Strength: Each peppermint, assorted fruit, assorted tropical fruit, assorted berries-flavoured tablet contains: calcium carbonate 1000 mg equivalent to elemental calcium 400 mg. Security-sealed bottles of 72, 160 and 250.

Tussionex® Ⓝ
hydrocodone bitartrate—phenyltoloxamine
Antitussive—Antihistamine

sanofi-aventis

SUPPLIED: Suspension: Each 5 mL of neutral tasting, gold-colored, thixotropic suspension, contains: hydrocodone resin complex equivalent to hydrocodone bitartrate 5 mg and phenyltoloxamine resin complex equivalent to phenyltoloxamine citrate 10 mg. Nonmedicinal ingredients: ethanol, FD&C Yellow No. 6, FD&C Yellow No. 10, glycerin, methylparaben, peach flavor, pineapple flavor, propylene glycol, propylparaben, sorbitol, water and xanthan gum. Bottles of 500 mL. Store at room temperature.
Tablets: Each light brown tablet, scored on one side and marked 0894 on the other, contains: hydrocodone resin complex equivalent to hydrocodone bitartrate 5 mg and phenyltoloxamine resin complex equivalent to phenyltoloxamine citrate 10 mg. Nonmedicinal ingredients: calcium phosphate dibasic, colloidal silicon dioxide, lactose monohydrate, magnesium stearate, starch, sugar and water. Bottles of 100. Store at room temperature.

(Shown in Product Identification Section)

TuZen
lactobacillus plantarum 299v
Natural Health Product—Probiotic

Ferring

INDICATIONS: Helps to reduce flatulence and abdominal pain associated with flatulence in individuals with Irritable Bowel Syndrome (IBS).

CONTRAINDICATIONS: Do not use if you are experiencing nausea, fever, vomiting, bloody diarrhea or unusually severe abdominal pain. Discontinue use and consult a health care practitioner if symptoms of digestive upset (e.g. diarrhea) occur, worsen or persist beyond 3 days.

WARNINGS AND PRECAUTIONS: Not recommended for use in children. Do not take if pregnant, breastfeeding or if immune system is compromised. Has been in contact with soy.

OVERDOSE:

> For management of a suspected drug overdose, CPhA recommends that you contact your **regional Poison Control Centre**. See the *CPS* Directory section for a list of Poison Control Centres.

DOSAGE: Adults: Take 1 or 2 capsules daily with food.

SUPPLIED: Each capsule contains: lactobacillus plantarum 10 billion cfu. Nonmedicinal ingredients: ascorbic acid, hypromellose, lecithin, magnesium stearate, monopotassium phosphate, potassium phosphate dibasic, potato starch and saccharose. Store at room temperature (15-25 °C). May be stored in refrigerator to ensure temperature does not exceed 15°C.

Twinject™ 0.3 mg Auto-Injector
epinephrine
Allergy Therapy Auto-Injector

Paladin

Twinject™ 0.15 mg Auto-Injector
epinephrine
Allergy Therapy Auto-Injector

Paladin

Date of Preparation: May 17, 2005
Date of Revision: March 12, 2010

SUMMARY PRODUCT INFORMATION:

Route of Administration	Product	Dosage Form/ Strength	Clinically Relevant Nonmedicinal Ingredients
Injection	Twinject 0.3 mg Auto-Injector	Syringe, 1:1000 2 doses 0.3 mg each	For a complete listing see Dosage Forms, Composition and Packaging.
	Twinject 0.15 mg Auto-Injector	Syringe, 1:1000 2 doses 0.15 mg each	

INDICATIONS AND CLINICAL USE: Epinephrine is the drug of choice for the emergency treatment of severe allergic reactions (Type I) to allergens, such as those present in certain insect venoms, foods, latex, or drugs.

Twinject 0.3 mg Auto-Injector (0.3 mL Epinephrine Injection, USP, 1:1000) and Twinject 0.15 mg Auto-Injector (0.15 mL Epinephrine Injection, USP, 1:1000) are indicated for the emergency treatment of severe allergic reactions (Type 1) including anaphylaxis to:

- stinging insects (e.g. order Hymenoptera, which includes bees, wasps, hornets, yellow jackets and fire ants), and biting insects (e.g. triatoma, mosquitoes),
- allergen immunotherapy,
- foods (peanuts, tree nuts, such as walnuts, hazelnuts, almonds, cashews, pecans, pistachios, shellfish, fish, milk, eggs and wheat),
- latex,
- other allergens,
- drugs.

Epinephrine can also be used in the treatment of anaphylaxis of unknown cause (idiopathic anaphylaxis), exercise-induced anaphylaxis (anaphylaxis occurring when exercise takes place within 2 to 4 hours of ingesting a specific food such as celery, shellfish, or wheat]), or anaphylactoid reactions (these reactions are clinically indistinguishable from anaphylaxis, but are not IgE mediated and are seen in response to opiates, NSAIDs and radiocontrast agents).

The Canadian Pediatric Surveillance Program defines anaphylaxis as "a severe allergic reaction to any stimulus, having sudden onset and generally lasting less than 24 hours, involving one or more body systems and producing one or more symptoms such as hives, flushing, itching, angioedema, stridor, wheezing, shortness of breath, vomiting, diarrhea, or shock." Because anaphylaxis is a generalized reaction, a wide variety of clinical signs and symptoms may be observed.

In the general population, 1 to 2% is estimated to be at risk for anaphylaxis from food allergies and insect stings, with a lower reported prevalence for drugs and latex. Asthmatic subjects are at particular risk.

Clinical Signs and Symptoms of Anaphylaxis: (Sampson HA. Anaphylaxis and emergency treatment. *Pediatrics.* 2003 Jun: 111(6 Pt3): 1601-8)

Oral: pruritus of lips, tongue, and palate and edema of lips and tongue; metallic taste in the mouth.

Cutaneous: flushing, pruritus, urticaria, angioedema, morbilliform rash, and pilor erecti.

Gastrointestinal: nausea, abdominal pain (colic), vomiting (large amounts of "stringy" mucus), and diarrhea.

Respiratory (major shock organ): laryngeal: pruritus and "tightness" in the throat, dysphagia, dysphonia and hoarseness, dry "staccato" cough, and sensation of itching in the external auditory canals, "deep" cough, and wheezing; nose pruritus, congestion, rhinorrhea, and sneezing.

Cardiovascular: feeling of faintness, syncope, chest pain, dysrhythmia, hypotension.

Other: periorbital pruritus, erythema and edema, conjunctival erythema, and tearing; lower back pain and uterine contractions in women; aura of "doom".

Hypotension is a **late** sign of anaphylaxis. Patients should be treated in the early stages of anaphylaxis in order to **prevent** hypotension from developing.

The severity of previous anaphylactic reactions does not determine the severity of future reactions, and subsequent reactions could be the same, better, or worse. The unpredictability depends on the degree of allergy and the dose of allergen.

Epinephrine should be administered as early as possible after the onset of symptoms of severe allergic response. Patients requiring epinephrine will not always have predictable reactions. Adequate warning signs are not always present before serious reactions occur.

It is recommended that epinephrine be given at the start of any reaction occurring in conjunction with a known or suspected allergy contact. In patients with a history of a severe cardiovascular collapse to an allergen the physician may advocate that epinephrine be administered immediately after an insect sting or ingestion of the offending food and before any reaction has begun.

Epinephrine, when used as directed immediately following exposure to an allergen, may prove life-saving.

More than 2 sequential doses of epinephrine should only be administered under direct medical supervision.

Under physician supervised care, epinephrine can be re-injected every 5 to15 minutes until there is resolution of the anaphylaxis or signs of hyperadrenalism occur (including palpitations, tremor, uncomfortable apprehension and anxiety).

Epinephrine in the majority of cases will be effective after one injection. However, **all** patients receiving emergency epinephrine must immediately be transported to an emergency medical facility. Further treatments may be required and therefore observation in an emergency medical setting is necessary. It is strongly recommended that patients (including individuals with milder reactions) should be observed for 4 hours after initial symptoms of anaphylaxis subside.

Anaphylactic reactions typically follow a uniphasic course; however, 20% will be biphasic in nature. The second phase usually occurs after an asymptomatic period of 1 to 8 hours, but may occur up to 38 hours (mean 10 hours) after the initial reaction. About one-third of the second-phase reactions are more severe, one-third are as severe and one-third are less severe. The second-phase reactions can occur even following administration of corticosteroids. It is recommended that following successful treatment of anaphylaxis, the patient should stay where he or she can call 911 with timely delivery to hospital for the next 48 hours.

Protracted anaphylaxis, which is frequently associated with profound hypotension and sometimes lasts longer than 24 hours, is minimally responsive to aggressive therapy, and has a poor prognosis.

Epinephrine injections are designed as emergency supportive therapy only and are not a replacement or substitute for immediate medical care.

CONTRAINDICATIONS: There are no known contraindications to the use of epinephrine in a life-threatening allergic reaction.

WARNINGS AND PRECAUTIONS: General: Patients with a history of anaphylaxis are at risk for subsequent episodes and death. All patients who have had one or more episodes of anaphylaxis should have injectable epinephrine with them or with their parent or caregiver at all times, and should wear some form of medical identification bracelet or necklace.

Epinephrine Injection, USP (1:1000) is not intended as a substitute for medical attention or hospital care. In conjunction with the administration of epinephrine, the patient should seek appropriate medical care.

The alternatives to using epinephrine in a life-threatening situation may not be satisfactory.

Twinject 0.3 mg Auto-Injector and Twinject 0.15 mg Auto-Injector should only be injected into the anterolateral aspect of the thigh (mid outer thigh). Accidental injection into the hands or feet may result in loss of blood flow to the affected area and should be avoided.

Avoid possible inadvertent intravascular administration.

Do not inject intravenously. The marked pressor effects may be counteracted by use of rapidly acting vasodilators.

Larger doses or accidental intravenous administration may induce severe hypertension, or cerebrovascular hemorrhage due to a sharp rise in blood pressure.

It should be determined whether the patient is at risk for future anaphylaxis, since there are some concerns in specific patients with epinephrine administration. Despite these concerns, epinephrine is essential for the treatment of anaphylaxis.

The presence of these conditions is not a contraindication to epinephrine administration in an acute, life-threatening situation. Therefore, patients with these conditions, or any other person who might be in a position to administer epinephrine to a patient with these conditions experiencing anaphylaxis, should be instructed about the circumstances under which epinephrine should be used.

Carcinogenesis and Mutagenesis: There are no data from either animal or human studies regarding the carcinogenicity or mutagenicity of epinephrine.

Cardiovascular: Epinephrine use should be avoided in patients with cardiogenic, traumatic, or hemorrhagic shock; cardiac dilation; and/or cerebral arteriosclerosis.

Epinephrine should be used with caution in patients with cardiac arrhythmias, coronary artery or organic heart disease, hypertension, or in patients who are on medications that may sensitize the heart to arrhythmias, e.g., digitalis, diuretics, or antiarrhythmics. In such patients, epinephrine may precipitate or aggravate angina pectoris as well as produce ventricular arrhythmias.

In patients with coronary insufficiency or ischemic heart disease, epinephrine may precipitate or aggravate angina pectoris as well as produce potentially fatal ventricular arrhythmias.

Patients with hypertension or hyperthyroidism are prone to more severe or persistent effects, as are patients with coronary artery disease, who may experience angina.

Endocrine and Metabolism: Patients with diabetes may develop increased blood glucose levels following epinephrine administration.

Neurologic: Epinephrine use should be avoided in patients with organic brain damage.

Patients with Parkinson's disease may notice a temporary worsening of symptoms after treatment with epinephrine.

Ophthalmologic: Epinephrine use should be avoided in patients with narrow-angle glaucoma.

Respiratory: Studies have shown a significant increased risk of near fatal and fatal reactions in patients with coexistent asthma. Fatalities may also occur from pulmonary edema resulting from peripheral constriction and cardiac stimulation.

Sensitivity: Epinephrine is the preferred treatment for serious allergic or other emergency situations even though this product contains sodium bisulfite, a sulfite that may in other products cause allergic-type reactions including anaphylactic symptoms or life-threatening or less severe asthmatic episodes in certain susceptible persons.

The presence of sulfite(s) in this product should not deter administration of the drug for treatment of serious allergic or other emergency situations, even if the patient is sulfite-sensitive.

Reproduction: No studies have been conducted to determine epinephrine's potential for the impairment of fertility.

Special Populations: Geriatrics (>65 years of age): Elderly patients with hypertension, arteriopathies or known ischaemic heart disease are particularly at risk for epinephrine overdose. Careful monitoring and avoidance of epinephrine overdose is necessary in these patients.

Pediatrics (patients 15-30 kg): There are no data to suggest a difference in safety or effectiveness of epinephrine between adults and children.

See Dosage and Administration for dosage requirements based on weight.

Pregnancy: Teratogenic Effects. Pregnancy Category C: Epinephrine has been shown to have developmental effects in rabbits at a subcutaneous dose of 1.2 mg/kg (approximately 30 times the maximum recommended daily subcutaneous or intramuscular dose on a mg/m^2 basis), in mice at a subcutaneous dose of 1 mg/kg (approximately 7 times the maximum recommended daily subcutaneous or intramuscular dose on a mg/m^2 basis), and in hamsters at a subcutaneous dose of 0.5 mg/kg (approximately 5 times the maximum recommended daily subcutaneous or intramuscular dose on a mg/m^2 basis).

These effects were not seen in mice at a subcutaneous dose of 0.5 mg/kg (approximately 3 times the maximum recommended daily subcutaneous or intramuscular dose on a mg/m^2 basis).

Although there are no adequate and well-controlled studies in pregnant women, epinephrine crosses the placenta and could lead to fetal anoxia, spontaneous abortion or both.

Epinephrine Injection, USP (1:1000) should be used in pregnancy only if the potential benefit justifies the potential risk to the fetus.

ADVERSE REACTIONS: Adverse Drug Reaction Overview: Adverse reactions include transient, moderate anxiety; feelings of over stimulation; apprehensiveness; restlessness; tremor; weakness; shakiness; dizziness; sweating; an increase in pulse rate; the sensation of a more forceful heartbeat; palpitations; pallor; nausea and vomiting; headache, and/or respiratory difficulties.

While these symptoms occur in some patients treated with epinephrine, they are more likely to be pronounced in patients with hypertension or hypothyroidism.

These signs and symptoms usually subside rapidly, especially with rest, quiet, and recumbency.

Some patients may be at greater risk of developing adverse reactions after epinephrine administration. These include elderly individuals, pregnant women, and patients with diabetes.

Patients with coronary artery disease are prone to more severe or persistent effects, and may experience angina.

Excessive doses cause acute hypertension. Rapid rises in blood pressure have produced cerebral hemorrhage, particularly in elderly patients with cardiovascular disease.

Arrhythmias, including fatal ventricular fibrillation, have been reported, particularly in patients with underlying cardiac disease or those receiving certain drugs (see Drug Interactions).

The potential for epinephrine to produce these types of adverse reactions does not contraindicate its use in an acute life-threatening allergic reaction.

DRUG INTERACTIONS: Overview: There are no known contraindications to the use of epinephrine in a life-threatening allergic reaction.

Drug-Drug Interactions: Epinephrine should be used with caution in patients who are on medications that may sensitize the heart to arrhythmias, e.g., digitalis, diuretics, or anti-arrhythmias. In such patients, epinephrine may precipitate or aggravate angina pectoris as well as produce ventricular arrhythmias.

Caution is indicated in patients receiving cardiac glycosides or mercurial diuretics, since these agents may sensitize the myocardium to beta-adrenergic stimulation and make cardiac arrhythmias more likely.

The effects of epinephrine may be potentiated by tricyclic antidepressants, monoamine oxidase inhibitors, sodium levothyroxine, and certain antihistamines, notably chlorpheniramine, tripelennamine, and diphenhydramine.

The cardiostimulating and bronchodilating effects of epinephrine are antagonized by beta-adrenergic blocking drugs, such as propranolol. Anaphylaxis may be made worse by beta blockers, and these drugs decrease the effectiveness of epinephrine.

The vasoconstricting and hypertensive effects are antagonized by alpha-adrenergic blocking drugs, such as phentolamine.

Ergot alkaloids and phenothiazines may also reverse the pressor effects of epinephrine.

Deaths have been reported in asthmatics treated with epinephrine following the use of isoproterenol or orciprenaline.

Drug-Food Interactions: Interactions with food have not been established.

Drug-Herb Interactions: Interactions with herbal products have not been established.

Drug-Laboratory Interactions: Interactions with laboratory tests have not been established.

Drug-Lifestyle Interactions: Cocaine sensitizes the heart to catecholamines (as does uncontrolled hyperthyroidism), and epinephrine use in these patients should be administered cautiously.

DOSAGE AND ADMINISTRATION: Dosing Considerations: The prescribing physician should carefully assess each patient to determine the most appropriate dose of epinephrine, recognizing the life-threatening nature of the reactions for which this drug is being prescribed.

Since the dose of epinephrine delivered from Twinject 0.15 mg is fixed at 0.15 mg, the physician should consider other forms of injectable epinephrine if doses lower than 0.15 mg are felt to be necessary (e.g. for children weighing less than 15 kg).

The second dose should be injected in approximately 10 minutes if symptoms worsen or if there is no clinical improvement, and if the patient has not yet reached an emergency medical facility for treatment.

More than 2 sequential doses of epinephrine should only be administered under direct medical supervision.

Recommended Dose and Dosage Adjustment: Twinject 0.3 mg Auto-Injector: This product is intended for use by adults and children who weigh 30 kg or more only.

Twinject 0.3 mg is capable of delivering two doses of 0.3 mg (0.3 mL of 1:1000 dilution of epinephrine) each.

The first dose is available for auto-injection by the patient. With persistent symptoms of anaphylaxis, a second dose is available for manual injection by the patient following a partial disassembly of the Twinject 0.3 mg Auto-Injector.

Twinject 0.15 mg Auto-Injector: This product is intended for use by adults and children who weigh 15 to 30 kg. A dosage of 0.01 mg/kg body weight is usually recommended for pediatric patients.

Since the dose of epinephrine delivered from Twinject 0.15 mg is fixed at 0.15 mg, the physician should consider other forms of injectable epinephrine if doses lower than 0.15 mg are felt to be necessary (e.g. for children weighing less than 15 kg).

Twinject 0.15 mg is capable of delivering two doses of 0.15 mg (0.15 mL of 1:1000 dilution of epinephrine) each.

The first dose is available for auto-injection by the patient or caregiver. With persistent symptoms of anaphylaxis, a second dose is available for manual injection by the patient or caregiver following a partial disassembly of the Twinject 0.15 mg Auto-Injector.

Administration: Patients with a history of severe allergic reactions should be instructed about the circumstances under which epinephrine should be used (see Indications and Clinical Use).

The patient's physician or pharmacist should review the package insert in detail with the patient or caregiver to insure that he/she understands the indications and use of Twinject 0.3 mg or Twinject 0.15 mg Auto-Injector.

Actual demonstration of the injection technique by a physician or a pharmacist is recommended. A demonstrator unit which does not contain a needle or epinephrine is available for this purpose.

Product is intended for subcutaneous or intramuscular use. Do not inject into buttock.

The first dose is delivered automatically after the patient prepares the Twinject 0.3 mg Auto-Injector or Twinject 0.15 mg Auto-Injector for firing as directed.

Inject the delivered dose of the Twinject 0.3 mg Auto-Injector (0.3 mL epinephrine injection, USP, 1:1000) or the Twinject 0.15 mg Auto-Injector (0.15 mL epinephrine 1:1000) subcutaneously or intramuscularly into the anteriolateral (mid outer thigh) aspect of the thigh, through clothing if necessary.

A second, manually administered dose is available following a partial disassembly of the Twinject 0.3 mg or Twinject 0.15 mg Auto-Injector.

If the second dose is not needed, discard Twinject (including unused epinephrine) as directed at the end of this package insert or in the instructions inside each Twinject 0.3 mg and Twinject 0.15 mg package.

OVERDOSAGE:

Epinephrine is rapidly inactivated in the body, and treatment following overdose with epinephrine is primarily supportive. If necessary, pressor effects may be counteracted by rapidly acting vasodilators or alpha-adrenergic blocking drugs.

If prolonged hypotension follows such measures, it may be necessary to administer another pressor drug.

Overdosage of epinephrine may produce extremely elevated arterial pressure, which may result in cerebrovascular hemorrhage, particularly in elderly patients. If an epinephrine overdose induces pulmonary edema that interferes with respiration, treatment consists of a rapidly acting alpha-adrenergic blocking drug and/or intermittent positive-pressure respiration.

Epinephrine overdosage can also cause transient bradycardia followed by tachycardia, and these may be accompanied by potentially fatal cardiac arrhythmias. Treatment of arrhythmias consists of administration of a beta-adrenergic blocking drug such as propranolol.

Premature ventricular contractions may appear within one minute after injection and may be followed by multifocal ventricular tachycardia (prefibrillation rhythm).

Subsidence of the ventricular effects may be followed by atrial tachycardia and occasionally by atrioventricular block.

Overdosage sometimes also results in extreme pallor and coldness of the skin, metabolic acidosis and kidney failure. Suitable corrective measures must be taken in such situations.

> For management of a suspected drug overdose, CPhA recommends that you contact your **regional Poison Control Centre**. See the *CPS* Directory section for a list of Poison Control Centres.

STORAGE AND STABILITY: Patients should be instructed to periodically check the expiration date and visually inspect the epinephrine solution for particulate matter and discolouration.

Epinephrine deteriorates rapidly on exposure to air or light, turning pink from oxidation to adrenochrome and brown from the formation of melanin.

If the solution contains particulate matter or develops a pinkish color or becomes darker than slightly yellow, the patient should immediately contact their physician or pharmacist for a replacement, since these changes indicate that the effectiveness of the drug product may be decreased. Epinephrine solutions that show evidence of discoloration should be discarded.

Because epinephrine is light sensitive, the Twinject 0.3 mg Auto-Injector or Twinject 0.15 mg Auto-Injector should be stored in the case provided. Protect from light. Store at 20-25° C (with excursions permitted to 15-30° C). Protect from freezing. Do not refrigerate.

Keep out of reach of children.

INFORMATION FOR THE PATIENT: Published in e-CPS, available by subscription at www.e-cps.ca.

DOSAGE FORMS, COMPOSITION AND PACKAGING: The Twinject 0.3 mg or Twinject 0.15 mg Auto-Injector unit is designed to be compact and easy to carry, and to provide emergency treatment when medical care is not immediately available. Highly sensitive individuals should have the Twinject 0.3 mg and Twinject 0.15 mg auto-injectors readily available at all times.

Twinject 0.3 mg Auto-Injector: Each patient-actuated single-use auto-injection device contains: epinephrine 1.1 mL injection, USP (1:1000) in a sterile syringe designed to deliver 2 doses of 0.3 mL each. Once fired, the Twinject 0.3 mg will administer one 0.3 mL (0.3 mg) dose. A second 0.3 mL dose of epinephrine is available by manual administration. There is residual epinephrine left in the syringe following delivery of the second dose. Each 0.3 mL dose contains 0.3 mg l-epinephrine, 2.6 mg sodium chloride, 1.5 mg chlorobutanol, 0.45 mg sodium bisulfite and water for injection. Sealed under nitrogen. Single unit carton. It is also available in a Twinpack format, containing two Twinject auto-injectors and one demonstrator.

Twinject 0.15 mg Auto-Injector: A patient-actuated single-use auto-injection device that contains 1.1 mL Epinephrine Injection, USP (1:1000) in a sterile syringe designed to deliver 2 doses of 0.15 mL each. Once fired, the Twinject 0.15 mg will administer one 0.15 mL (0.15 mg) dose. A second 0.15 mL dose of epinephrine is available by manual administration. There is residual epinephrine left in the syringe following delivery of the second dose. Each 0.15 mL dose contains 0.15 mg l-epinephrine, 1.3 mg sodium chloride, 0.75 mg chlorobutanol, 0.225 mg sodium bisulfite, and water for injection. Sealed under nitrogen. Single unit carton. It is also available in a Twinpack format, containing two Twinject auto-injectors and one demonstrator.

Twinrix®

combined hepatitis A and hepatitis B vaccine

Active Immunizing Agent Against Infection by Hepatitis A and Hepatitis B Virus

GlaxoSmithKline

Date of Revision: September 16, 2008

SUMMARY PRODUCT INFORMATION:

Route of Administration	Dosage Form/ Strength	Clinically Relevant Nonmedicinal Ingredients
Intramuscular injection	Suspension for injection/ **TWINRIX:** 720 ELISA units HAV/20 μg HBV per 1 mL dose **TWINRIX Junior:** 360 ELISA units HAV/10 μg HBV per 0.5 mL dose	**Excipients:** aluminum hydroxide, aluminum phosphate, sodium chloride and water for injection **Residues:** amino acids for injection, formaldehyde, neomycin sulphate and polysorbate 20

DESCRIPTION: TWINRIX (combined hepatitis A and hepatitis B vaccine) confers immunity against hepatitis A virus (HAV) and hepatitis B virus (HBV) infection by inducing specific anti-HAV and anti-HBs antibodies.

INDICATIONS AND CLINICAL USE: TWINRIX (combined hepatitis A and hepatitis B vaccine) is indicated for:

- active immunization against hepatitis A and hepatitis B virus infection in adults, adolescents, children and infants.

The vaccine will not protect against infection caused by other agents such as hepatitis C, hepatitis E and other pathogens known to infect the liver. It can be expected that hepatitis D will also be prevented by immunization with TWINRIX as hepatitis D (caused by the delta agent) does not occur in the absence of hepatitis B infection.

CONTRAINDICATIONS: TWINRIX (combined hepatitis A and hepatitis B vaccine) should not be administered:

- to subjects with known hypersensitivity to any constituent of the vaccine, or to subjects having shown signs of hypersensitivity after previous administration of TWINRIX or the monovalent hepatitis A or hepatitis B vaccine. For a complete listing, see Dosage Forms, Composition and Packaging.

As with other vaccines, the administration of TWINRIX should be postponed in subjects suffering from acute severe febrile illness. The presence of a minor infection, however, is not a contraindication for vaccination.

WARNINGS AND PRECAUTIONS: General: As with all injectable vaccines, appropriate medication (e.g. adrenaline) should always be readily available in case of anaphylaxis or anaphylactoid reactions following administration of the vaccine. For this reason, the vaccinee should remain under medical supervision for 30 minutes after immunization.

Since there is a possibility that the vaccine may contain trace amounts of neomycin, the possibility of an allergic reaction in individuals sensitive to this substance should be kept in mind when considering the use of this vaccine (see Dosage Forms, Composition and Packaging).

It is possible that subjects may be in the incubation period of a hepatitis A or hepatitis B infection at the time of vaccination. It is not known whether TWINRIX (combined hepatitis A and hepatitis B vaccine) will prevent hepatitis A and hepatitis B in such cases.

Hematologic: TWINRIX should be administered subcutaneously to subjects with thrombocytopenia or bleeding disorders since bleeding may occur following an intramuscular administration to these subjects. Subcutaneous injection may result in a less than optimal antibody response.

Immune: As with other vaccines, persons with an impaired immune system, adequate anti-HAV and anti-HBs antibody titres may not be obtained after the primary immunization course and such patients may therefore require administration of additional doses of vaccine. However, no specific dosing recommendations can be made at this time.

Renal: As with other vaccines, hemodialysis patients may not obtain adequate anti-HAV and anti-HBs antibody titres after the primary immunization course and such patients may therefore require administration of additional doses of vaccine. However, no specific dosing recommendations can be made at this time.

Special Populations: Pregnant Women: TWINRIX should be used during pregnancy only when clearly needed, and when the possible advantages outweigh the possible risks for the fetus.

The effect of TWINRIX on embryo-fetal, peri-natal and post-natal survival and development has not been prospectively evaluated in clinical trials.

The effect of TWINRIX on embryo-fetal, peri-natal and post-natal survival and development has been assessed in rats. Such animal studies do not indicate direct or indirect harmful effects with respect to fertility, pregnancy, embryonal/fetal development, parturition or post-natal development.

Nursing Women: Adequate human data on use during lactation and adequate animal reproduction studies are not available. TWINRIX should therefore be used with caution in breastfeeding mothers.

ADVERSE REACTIONS: Clinical Trial Adverse Drug Reactions: Because clinical trials are conducted under very specific conditions the adverse reaction rates observed in the clinical trials may not reflect the rates observed in practice and should not be compared to the rates in the clinical trials of another drug. Adverse drug reaction information from clinical trials is useful for identifying drug-related adverse events and for approximating rates.

Adults: The safety profile presented in Table 1 is based on data from more than 6000 subjects who received either the standard 0, 1, 6 month schedule or the accelerated 0, 7, 21 days schedule.

In a comparative study it was noted that the frequency of the solicited adverse events following the administration of TWINRIX is not different from the frequency of the solicited adverse events following the administration of the monovalent vaccines.

In a clinical trial where TWINRIX was administered at 0, 7, 21 days, solicited general symptoms were reported with the same categories of frequency as defined above. After a fourth dose given at month 12, the incidence of systemic adverse reactions was comparable to that seen after vaccination at 0, 7, 21 days.

Pediatric: The safety profile presented in Table 2 is based on data from approximately 800 subjects.

Post-Market Adverse Drug Reactions: The following adverse reactions have been reported with either TWINRIX or with GlaxoSmithKline monovalent hepatitis A or B vaccines. See Table 3.

Table 1: TWINRIX

Adverse Reactions Considered by the Investigator as Being at Least Possibly Related to TWINRIX Vaccination in Adults

Frequency	Adverse Event	System/Organ Class
Very Common ≥10%	headache	Nervous system disorders
	pain and redness at the injection site, fatigue	General disorders and administration site conditions
Common ≥1% and <10%	gastrointestinal symptoms (such as diarrhea, nausea, vomiting)	Gastrointestinal disorders
	swelling at the injection site, injection site reaction, malaise	General disorders and administration site conditions
Uncommon ≥0.1% and <1%	upper respiratory tract infection	Infection and infestations
	dizziness	Nervous system disorders
	myalgia	Musculoskeletal and connective tissue disorders
	fever (≥37.5°C)	General disorders and administration site conditions
Rare ≥0.01% and <0.1%	lymphadenopathy	Blood and lymphatic system disorders
	decreased appetite	Metabolism and nutrition disorders
	hypoaesthesia, paraesthesia	Nervous system disorders
	hypotension	Vascular disorders
	rash, pruritus	Skin and subcutaneous tissue disorders
	arthralgia	Musculoskeletal and connective tissue disorders
	influenza like illness, chills	General disorders and administration site conditions
Very Rare <0.01%	urticaria	Skin and subcutaneous tissue disorders

Table 2: TWINRIX

Adverse Reactions Considered by the Investigator as Being at Least Possibly Related to TWINRIX Vaccination in Children

Frequency	Adverse Event	System/Organ Class
Very Common ≥10%	pain and redness at the injection site	General disorders and administration site conditions
Common ≥1% and <10%	appetite lost	Metabolism and nutrition disorders
	irritability	Psychiatric disorders
	drowsiness, headache	Nervous system disorders
	gastrointestinal symptoms (such as nausea, diarrhea, vomiting)	Gastrointestinal disorders
	swelling at the injection site, injection site reaction, fatigue, malaise, fever (≥37.5°C)	General disorders and administration site conditions
Uncommon ≥0.1% and <1%	rash	Skin and subcutaneous tissue disorders
Rare ≥0.01% and <0.1%	lymphadenopathy	Blood and lymphatic system disorders
	dizziness	Nervous system disorders
	urticaria	Skin and subcutaneous tissue disorders
Very Rare <0.01%	paraesthesia, hypoaesthesia	Nervous system disorders
	hypotension	Vascular disorders
	pruritus	Skin and subcutaneous tissue disorders
	myalgia, arthralgia	Musculoskeletal and connective tissue disorders
	influenza like illness, chills	General disorders and administration site conditions

Table 3: TWINRIX

Post-Market Adverse Reactions

Infections and Infestations	Meningitis
Blood and Lymphatic System Disorder	Thrombocytopenia, thrombocytopenic purpura
Immune System Disorders	Anaphylaxis, allergic reactions including anaphylactoid reactions and mimicking serum sickness
Nervous System Disorders	Encephalopathy, encephalitis, neuritis, neuropathy, paralysis, convulsions, multiple sclerosis[a], Guillain-Barre syndrome[a], optic neuritis, myelitis, facial palsy

(cont'd)

Table 3: TWINRIX (cont'd)

Post-Market Adverse Reactions

Vascular Disorders	Vasculitis
Skin and Subcutaneous Tissue Disorders	Angioneurotic oedema, lichen planus, erythema multiforme
Musculoskeletal and Connective Tissue Disorders	Arthritis, muscular weakness
Gastrointestinal Disorders	Abdominal pain
Hepatic System Disorders	Abnormal liver function tests

[a] "A number of studies have demonstrated no link between hepatitis B vaccine and multiple sclerosis, Guillain-Barre syndrome (GBS), ..." (Canadian Immunization Guide 7th Edition 2006).

DRUG INTERACTIONS: Overview: Clinical studies have demonstrated that TWINRIX (combined hepatitis A and hepatitis B vaccine) used in an alternate 2 dose schedule can be administered concomitantly with either diphtheria, tetanus, acellular pertussis, inactivated poliomyelitis *H. influenzae* type b (DTPa-IPV/Hib) or Measles-Mumps-Rubella (MMR) vaccines in the second year of life. In these trials, the injectable vaccines were given at different injection sites.

Although the concomitant administration of TWINRIX and other vaccines has not specifically been studied, it is anticipated that, if different syringes and other injection sites are used, no interaction will be observed.

As with other vaccines, it may be expected that in patients receiving immunosuppressive treatment or patients with immunodeficiency, an adequate response may not be achieved.

Drug-Drug Interactions: No data on concomitant administration of TWINRIX with specific hepatitis A immunoglobulin or hepatitis B immunoglobulin have been generated. However, when the monovalent hepatitis A and hepatitis B vaccines were administered concomitantly with specific immunoglobulins, no influence on seroconversion was observed although it may result in lower antibody titres.

Drug-Food Interactions: Interactions with food have not been established.

Drug-Herb Interactions: Interactions with herbal products have not been established.

Drug-Laboratory Test Interactions: Interactions with laboratory tests have not been established.

Drug-Lifestyle Interactions: Effects on the Ability to Drive and Use Machines: TWINRIX has no or negligible influence on the ability to drive and use machines.

DOSAGE AND ADMINISTRATION: Recommended Dose and Dosage Adjustment: See Table 4.

Table 4: TWINRIX

Dosage and Administration

Vaccination Schedule	Age	Vaccine	Dose/volume HAV ELU/ HBV µg	Dosing Schedule (months) 0	1	6	12
Standard (3 dose)	Adults over 19 years of age	Twinrix	(720/20)/1 mL	X	X	X	
Standard (3 dose)	1–18 years	Twinrix Junior	(360/10)/0.5 mL	X	X	X	
Rapid (4 dose)	Adults over 19 years of age	Twinrix	(720/20)/1 mL	0,7 d, 21 d XXX d=days			X
Alternate (2 dose)	1–15 years	Twinrix	(720/20)/1 mL	X		X or X	

Primary Course: Standard Schedule: The standard primary course of vaccination with TWINRIX (combined hepatitis A and hepatitis B vaccine) consists of three doses, the first administered at the elected date, the second one month later and the third six months after the first dose.

Rapid Schedule: In exceptional circumstances in adults, when travel is anticipated within one month or more after initiating the vaccination course, but where insufficient time is available to allow the standard 0, 1, 6 month schedule to be completed, a schedule of three intramuscular injections given at 0, 7 and 21 days may be used. When this schedule is applied, a fourth dose is recommended 12 months after the first dose.

Alternate Schedule: The alternate schedule, **for children and adolescents only**, consists of two doses of TWINRIX (720 ELU HAV/20 µg HBV), the first administered at the elected date and the second between six and twelve months after the first dose. The alternate schedule should be used where completion of the 2 dose vaccination course can be assured, such as school based vaccination programs.

Once initiated, the 2 dose course of vaccination should be completed with the same vaccine.

In situations where rapid protection is required in children and adolescents (1 to 15 years old), the standard 3 dose schedule is recommended. The alternate 2 dose schedule demonstrated similar antibody titres after completion of the vaccination course.

Booster Dose: Long-term antibody persistence data following vaccination with TWINRIX are available up to 60 months after vaccination in adults and up to 48 months in infants, children and adolescents. The anti-HBs and anti-HAV antibody titres observed following a primary vaccination course with the combined vaccine are in the range of what is seen following vaccination with the monovalent vaccines. The kinetics of antibody decline are shown to be similar.

General guidelines for booster vaccination can therefore be drawn from experience with the monovalent vaccines.

The anti-HBs and anti-HAV antibody titres observed following a 2 dose vaccination course with TWINRIX are in the same range of what is seen following vaccination with the standard 3 dose schedule.

For the Hepatitis B Component: Routine booster vaccinations in immunocompetent persons are not recommended since protection has been shown to last for at least 15 years. Studies of long-term protective efficacy, however, will determine whether booster doses of the vaccine are needed. It is important to recognise that the absence of detectable anti-HBs in a person who has been previously demonstrated to have anti-HBs, does not mean lack of protection, because immune memory persists. Booster doses in this situation are not indicated.

Immunocompromized persons often respond sub-optimally to the vaccine. Subsequent HBV exposures in these individuals can result in disease or the carrier state. Therefore, boosters may be necessary in this population. The optimal timing of booster doses for immunocompromized individuals who are at continued risk of HBV exposure is not known and should be based on the severity of the compromised state and annual monitoring for the presence of anti-HBs.

For the Hepatitis A Component: It is not yet fully established whether immunocompetent individuals who have responded to hepatitis A vaccination will require booster doses as protection in the absence of detectable antibodies. Guidelines for boosting are based on the extrapolation from the data available required for protection; anti-HAV antibodies have been predicted to persist for at least 20 years (based on mathematical calculations).

In situations where a booster dose of both hepatitis A and hepatitis B are desired, TWINRIX can be given. Alternatively, subjects primed with TWINRIX may be administered a booster dose of either of the monovalent vaccines.

Administration: TWINRIX is for **intramuscular** injection, preferably in the deltoid region, or in the anterolateral thigh in infants. The vaccine **should not** be administered intramuscularly in the gluteal region or subcutaneously/intradermally since administration by these routes may result in a less than optimal anti-HAV antibody response.

As with all parenterals, vaccine products should be inspected visually for any foreign particulate matter or discolouration prior to administration. Before use of TWINRIX, the vaccine should be well shaken to obtain a slightly opaque, white suspension. Discard if the contents of the vial or syringe appear otherwise.

Syringe Instructions: Do not remove the white back-stop from the syringe. Prior to administration, ensure that the plunger rod is firmly attached to the rubber stopper by turning the plunger clockwise until slight resistance is felt. **Do not** over tighten. Remove syringe LUER Tip-cap and needle cap. Attach needle by pressing and twisting in a clockwise rotation until secured to the syringe.

TWINRIX should never be administered intravenously.

OVERDOSAGE:

Cases of overdose have been reported during post-marketing surveillance. Adverse events reported following overdosage were similar to those reported with normal vaccine administration.

> For management of a suspected drug overdose, CPhA recommends that you contact your **regional Poison Control Centre**. See the *CPS* Directory section for a list of Poison Control Centres.

ACTION AND CLINICAL PHARMACOLOGY: Data has been obtained from clinical studies involving over 980 adults, adolescents, children and infants using the standard 3 dose vaccination schedule with TWINRIX (combined hepatitis A and hepatitis B vaccine) and TWINRIX Junior respectively, and a total of 819 children and adolescents aged 1-15 years of age using the alternate 2 dose vaccination schedule with TWINRIX.

TWINRIX in Adults: Standard Vaccination Schedule (3 doses at 0, 1, 6 months): 720 ELISA units HAV/ 20 µg HBV per 1 mL dose.

Anti-HAV Response: In a clinical study involving subjects 18-75 years of age, anti-HAV seropositivity rates were 91.1% one month after the first dose of vaccine, 97.6% one month after the second dose of vaccine and 99.5% one month after the third dose of vaccine.

Anti-HBV Response: The seroconversion rate one month after the second dose of vaccine was more than 96.5% in adult subjects. At month 7, one month after dose 3, seroprotection was close to 100%.

Anti-HAV Response and Anti-HBV Response: In a study conducted in subjects over 40 years old it was shown that the anti-HAV seropositivity and anti-HBs seroprotection rates were 97.2 and 91.7% at month 7 and 96.4 and 87.5% at month 12 respectively.

Rapid Dosing Schedule (4 doses at 0, 7, and 21 days and booster at 12 months): 720 ELISA units HAV/ 20 µg HBV per 1 mL dose.

Anti-HAV Response: In a clinical trial comparing TWINRIX at the 0, 7, 21 day primary schedule to the monovalent vaccines administered concomitantly (currently marketed ENGERIX-B and HAVRIX 1440), seropositivity rates for anti-HAV antibodies were 100 and 99.5% at 1 and 5 weeks respectively after the third dose, and reached 100% one month after the fourth dose.

Anti-HBV Response: TWINRIX given according to the 0, 7, 21 day primary schedule, resulted in 82 and 85% of vaccinees having seroprotective levels of anti-HBV antibodies at 1 and 5 weeks respectively following the third dose in adults. One month after the fourth dose, all vaccinees demonstrated seroprotective levels of anti-HBs antibodies.

Anti-HAV Response and Anti-HBV Response: After the fourth dose of the rapid schedule, the immune response to both antigen components was comparable to that seen after completion of the currently marketed schedule of TWINRIX (0, 1, 6 months).

No statistically significant differences in anti-HAV seropositivity or anti-HBs seroprotection rates were observed at any time point between the two cohorts receiving either TWINRIX or the monovalent vaccines.

TWINRIX Junior in Pediatrics: Standard Vaccination Schedule (3 doses at 0, 1, 6 months): 360 ELISA units HAV/ 10 µg HBV per 0.5 mL dose.

Anti-HAV Response: In clinical studies involving subjects 1-18 years of age, specific humoral antibodies against HAV were detected in more than 93% of the vaccinees at day 15, and 100% of vaccinees one month following vaccination with the 3 dose schedule.

Anti-HBV Response: The seroconversion rate one month after the second dose was >98.0% in subjects aged 1-18 years of age. Immunogenicity of the vaccine was analyzed one month after the third vaccine dose. The seroprotection rate (>10 IU/L) for hepatitis B was 100%. An anti-HBs antibody titre above 10 IU/L correlates with protection to HBV infection.

TWINRIX in Subjects Aged 1-15 Years: Alternate Vaccination Schedule (2 doses at 0, and 6 to 12 months): 720 ELISA units HAV/20 µg HBV per 1 mL dose.

Anti-HAV Response: In clinical trials using the alternate vaccination schedule subjects aged 1 to 15 years demonstrated seropositivity rates for anti-HAV antibodies to be 99.1% one month after the first dose and 100% one month after the second dose (i.e. month 7) when given at month 6. When the second dose was administered at month 12, seropositivity rates for anti-HAV were 99.0% one month later (i.e. month 13).

Anti-HAV antibodies have been shown to persist for at least 24 months following the initiation of a 0, 6 month schedule of TWINRIX (2 dose schedule). Seropositivity rates were 100% for anti-HAV antibodies at month 24.

Anti-HBV Response: For children and adolescents (1 to 15 years of age), using the alternate schedule, seropositivity rates for anti-HBs antibodies were shown to be 74.2% one month after the first dose and 100% one month after the second dose (i.e. month 7) when given at month 6. The anti-HBs seroprotection rates (titres ≥10 IU/L) at these time points were 37.4 and 98.2% respectively.

When the second dose was administered at month 12 with serology testing one month later (i.e. month 13), seropositivity rate for anti-HBs were 99.0%, with seroprotection rates of 97.0%.

Anti-HBs antibodies have been shown to persist for at least 24 months following the initiation of a 0, 6 month schedule. Seropositivity rates were 94.2% for anti-HBs antibodies at month 24. The seroprotection rate for anti-HBs at this time point was 93.3%.

In this 2 dose study, the immune response to both antigen components was comparable to that seen after a 3 dose regimen of the combined vaccine containing 360 ELISA units of hepatitis A virus and 10 µg of the hepatitis B surface antigen in a 0.5 mL dose.

The persistence of anti-HAV and anti-HBs antibodies at month 24 was shown to be similar following a 0, 6 month or a 0, 12 month schedule.

Duration of Effect: Adults: Protection against hepatitis A and hepatitis B develops within 2 to 4 weeks. In clinical studies, specific humoral antibodies against hepatitis A were observed in approximately 94% of the adults one month after the first dose and in 100% one month after the third dose (i.e. month 7). Specific humoral antibodies against hepatitis B were observed in 70% of the adults after the first dose and approximately 99% after the third dose.

Two clinical studies conducted in adults demonstrated the persistence of anti-HAV and anti-HBs antibodies up to 60 months following the initiation of a primary vaccination course of TWINRIX in the majority of vaccinees.

The seropositivity rates for anti-HAV and anti-HBs observed were 100% and 97.7% respectively at month 60, with a seroprotection rate of 93.2% for anti-HBs in one study.

All subjects were seropositive in the other study for both anti-HAV and anti-HBs antibodies at month 60, while 95.7% of vaccinees were seroprotected against hepatitis B.

Pediatrics: In clinical studies of the pediatric population, specific humoral antibodies against hepatitis A were observed in approximately 89% of the subjects one month after the first dose, and in 100% after the third dose (i.e. month 7). Specific humoral antibodies against hepatitis B were observed in approximately 67% of the subjects after the first dose and 100% after the third dose.

In a long-term clinical trial conducted in the pediatric population, persistence of anti-HAV and anti-HBs antibodies has been demonstrated up to 48 months following the course of vaccination in the majority of vaccinees.

From month 36 to month 48, the percentage of decrease in anti-HAV titres was generally similar in all studies when compared to the adult population titres. At month 48, the anti-HAV GMTs obtained in the pediatric study were in the range of those seen in the adult vaccinated population.

The anti-HBs GMTs obtained at either month 36 or 48 in the pediatric group, revealed similar or even higher titres than those reported in the adult vaccinated population.

STORAGE AND STABILITY: The expiry date of the vaccine is indicated on the label and packaging. TWINRIX (combined hepatitis A and hepatitis B vaccine) should be stored at +2 to +8°C.

Do not freeze; discard if the vaccine has been frozen.

INFORMATION FOR THE PATIENT: Published in e-CPS, available by subscription at www.e-cps.ca.

DOSAGE FORMS, COMPOSITION AND PACKAGING: TWINRIX Adult: Each 1 mL dose contains: hepatitis A 720 ELISA units and hepatitis B 20 µg. Single dose vials and syringes, packages of 1, 10 and 25 (adult presentation).

TWINRIX Junior: Each 0.5 mL dose contains: hepatitis A 360 ELISA units and hepatitis B 10 µg. Single dose vials, packages of 1, 3 and 10 and syringes, packages of 1 and 10 (pediatric/adolescent presentation).

The liquid suspension is made isotonic with sodium chloride in water for injection. Excipients: aluminum hydroxide, aluminum phosphate, sodium chloride and water for injection. Residues: amino acids for injection, formaldehyde, neomycin sulphate and polysorbate 20. TWINRIX meets the World Health Organization requirements for the manufacture of biological substances.

Tygacil® ℞
tigecycline
Tetracycline Antibiotic

Pfizer

Date of Revision: June 16, 2009

SUMMARY PRODUCT INFORMATION:

Route of Administration	Dosage Form/ Strength	Clinically Relevant Nonmedicinal Ingredients
Intravenous infusion	Sterile, lyophilized powder 50 mg tigecycline per vial	Lactose See Dosage Forms, Composition and Packaging.

INDICATIONS AND CLINICAL USE: TYGACIL (tigecycline) is indicated for the treatment of the following infections when caused by susceptible strains of the designated microorganisms in patients 18 years of age and older:

- Complicated skin and skin structure infections caused by *E. coli*, *E. faecalis* (vancomycin-susceptible strains only), *S. aureus* (methicillin-susceptible and -resistant strains), *S. agalactiae*, *S. anginosus*, *S. pyogenes*, *E. cloacae*, *K. pneumoniae*, and *B. fragilis*.

  Patients with severe underlying disease, such as those who were immunocompromised, patients with decubitus ulcer infections, or patients who had infections requiring longer than 14 days of treatment (for example, necrotizing fasciitis), were not enrolled in clinical trials.
- Complicated intra-abdominal infections caused by *C. freundii*, *E. cloacae*, *E. coli*, *K. oxytoca*, *K. pneumoniae*, *E. faecalis* (vancomycin-susceptible strains only), *S. aureus* (methicillin-susceptible only), *S. anginosus* grp. (includes *S. anginosus*, *S. intermedius*, and *S. constellatus*), *B. fragilis*, *B. thetaiotaomicron*, *B. uniformis*, *B. vulgatus*, *C. perfringens*, and *P. micros*.
- Community acquired pneumonia (mild to moderate infections only) caused by *H. influenzae*, *S. pneumoniae* (penicillin-susceptible isolates only), *M. pneumoniae*, and *C. pneumoniae*.

Appropriate specimens for bacteriological examination should be obtained in order to isolate and identify the causative organisms and to determine their susceptibility to tigecycline. Once these results are available, antimicrobial therapy should be adjusted if necessary. TYGACIL may be initiated as empiric therapy before results of these tests are known. Tigecycline has decreased in vitro activity against Proteus spp., Providencia spp., and Morganella spp. *P. aeruginosa* is inherently resistant to TYGACIL.

Geriatrics (≥65 years of age): Evidence from clinical studies suggests that use in the geriatric population is not associated with differences in safety or effectiveness. A brief discussion can be found in Warnings and Precautions, Special Populations, Geriatrics (≥65 years of age).

Pediatrics (<18 years of age): No data is available. (See Warnings and Precautions, Special Populations, Pediatrics (<18 years of age).)

CONTRAINDICATIONS: TYGACIL (tigecycline) is contraindicated for use in patients who have known hypersensitivity to tigecycline or tetracycline class of antibiotics.

WARNINGS AND PRECAUTIONS: General: Anaphylaxis/anaphylactoid reactions have been reported with TYGACIL, and may be life-threatening.

Glycylcycline class antibiotics are structurally similar to tetracycline class antibiotics and may have similar adverse events. Such effects may include photosensitivity, pseudotumor cerebri, and anti-anabolic action (which has led to increased BUN, azotemia, acidosis, and hyperphosphatemia). As with tetracyclines, pancreatitis has been reported with the use of tigecycline.

Tigecycline may be associated with permanent tooth discoloration in humans during tooth development (last half of pregnancy, infancy, and childhood to the age of 8 years). Results of studies in rats with tigecycline have shown bone discoloration.

During antibiotic therapy, colonization or superinfection with Candida, Proteus or Pseudomonas spp may occur in the GI, genitourinary, and respiratory tracts. Patients should be carefully monitored during therapy. If superinfection occurs, appropriate measures should be taken.

TYGACIL is **not** indicated for the treatment of severe community acquired pneumonia. Safety and efficacy of TYGACIL in severe community acquired pneumonia have not been studied. TYGACIL has not been evaluated in clinical trials for use against suspected or documented multiple drug resistant pathogens in pneumonia.

TYGACIL is **not** indicated for treatment of hospital acquired pneumonia. The safety and efficacy of TYGACIL in patients with hospital acquired pneumonia have not been established. In a study of hospital acquired pneumonia patients, the sub-group of patients with ventilator-associated pneumonia who received TYGACIL had lower cure rates (47.9% versus 70.1% for the clinically evaluable population) and greater mortality (25/131 [19.1%] versus 14/122 [11.5%]) than the comparator.

Caution should be exercised when considering TYGACIL monotherapy in patients with complicated intra-abdominal infections (cIAI) secondary to clinically apparent intestinal perforation. (See Adverse Reactions.) In Phase 3 cIAI studies (n=1642), 6 patients treated with TYGACIL and 2 patients treated with imipenem/cilastatin presented with intestinal perforations and developed sepsis/septic shock. The 6 patients treated with TYGACIL had higher APACHE II scores (median=13) vs the 2 patients treated with imipenem/cilastatin (APACHE II scores=4 and 6). Due to differences in baseline APACHE II scores between treatment groups and small overall numbers, the relationship of this outcome to treatment cannot be established.

Cardiovascular: An effect on cardiac repolarization following tigecycline administration cannot be definitively excluded from the clinical data (see Action and Clinical Pharmacology, Special Populations and Conditions, Cardiovascular).

There is limited clinical experience using tigecycline in patients with known prolongation of the QTc interval, patients with hypokalemia, patients receiving Class IA (e.g. quinidine, procainamide) or Class III (e.g., amiodarone, sotalol) antiarrhythmic agents, or in other pro-arrhythmic conditions.

Pharmacokinetic studies between tigecycline and drugs that prolong the QTc interval such as cisapride, erythromycin, antipsychotics, and tricyclic antidepressants have not been performed. The effect of tigecycline has also not been studied in patients with congenital prolongation of the QT interval. It is expected that these individuals may be more susceptible to drug-induced QT prolongation.

The magnitude of QTc prolongation may increase with increasing concentrations of drugs; therefore, the recommended dose and the recommended infusion rate for TYGACIL should not be exceeded (see Dosage and Administration).

Patients should be instructed to contact their physician if they experience palpitations or fainting spells while taking TYGACIL.

Gastrointestinal: *C. difficile*-associated disease: *C. difficile*-associated disease (CDAD) has been reported with use of many antibacterial agents, including TYGACIL. CDAD may range in severity from mild diarrhea to fatal colitis. It is important to consider this diagnosis in patients who present with diarrhea, or symptoms of colitis, pseudomembranous colitis, toxic megacolon, or perforation of colon subsequent to the administration of any antibacterial agent. CDAD has been reported to occur over 2 months after the administration of antibacterial agents.

Treatment with antibacterial agents may alter the normal flora of the colon and may permit overgrowth of *C. difficile*. *C. difficile* produces toxins A and B, which contribute to the development of CDAD. CDAD may cause significant morbidity and mortality. CDAD can be refractory to antimicrobial therapy.

If the diagnosis of CDAD is suspected or confirmed, appropriate therapeutic measures should be initiated. Mild cases of CDAD usually respond to discontinuation of antibacterial agents not directed against *C. difficile*. In moderate to severe cases, consideration should be given to management with fluids and electrolytes, protein supplementation, and treatment with an antibacterial agent clinically effective against *C. difficile*. Surgical evaluation should be instituted as clinically indicated, as surgical intervention may be required in certain severe cases (see Adverse Reactions).

Hepatic/Biliary/Pancreatic: Increases in total bilirubin concentration, prothrombin time and transaminases have been seen in patients treated with tigecycline. Isolated cases of significant hepatic dysfunction and hepatic failure have been reported in patients treated with tigecycline. Patients who develop abnormal liver function tests during tigecycline therapy should be monitored for evidence of worsening hepatic function and evaluated for risk/benefit of continuing tigecycline therapy. Adverse events may occur after the drug has been discontinued.

Cases of pancreatitis have been reported.

Special Populations: Pregnant Women: There are no adequate and well-controlled studies of TYGACIL in pregnant women. TYGACIL should not be used unless the potential benefit to the mother outweighs any possible risk to the fetus.

TYGACIL may cause fetal harm when administered to a pregnant woman. Results of animal studies indicate that tigecycline crosses the placenta and is found in fetal tissues. Tigecycline was not teratogenic in the rat or rabbit. Decreased fetal weights and increased incidence of minor skeletal anomalies in rats and rabbits (with associated delays in ossification) and fetal loss in rabbits have been observed with tigecycline.

TYGACIL has not been studied for use during labor and delivery.

Nursing Women: It is not known whether this drug is excreted in human milk. Because many drugs are excreted in human milk, and there is the potential risk of permanent discoloration of the teeth/bones (yellow gray-brown) of the child, TYGACIL should not be administered to a nursing woman unless the potential benefit to the mother outweighs any possible risk to the child. (See Warnings and Precautions, General.)

Results from animal studies using ^{14}C-labeled tigecycline indicate that tigecycline is excreted readily via milk of lactating rats. Consistent with the limited oral bioavailability of tigecycline there was little or no systemic exposure to tigecycline in nursing pups as a result of exposure via maternal milk.

Pediatrics (<18 years of age): TYGACIL should not be used in children under 8 years of age because of the risk of teeth discoloration. Safety and effectiveness in pediatric patients below the age of 18 have not been established. Therefore, use in patients under 18 years of age is not recommended.

Geriatrics (≥65 years of age): Of the total number of subjects who received TYGACIL in Phase 3 clinical studies (n=2514), 664 were 65 years of age and over, while 238 were 75 years of age and over. No overall differences in safety or effectiveness were observed between these subjects and younger subjects, but greater sensitivity to adverse events in some older individuals cannot be ruled out.

Monitoring and Laboratory Tests: Prothrombin time or other suitable anticoagulation test should be monitored if tigecycline is administered with warfarin.

Occupational Hazards: Driving a Vehicle or Operating Machinery: Tigecycline can cause dizziness which may impair the ability to drive and/or operate machinery.

ADVERSE REACTIONS: Adverse Drug Reaction Overview: The overall incidence of drug-related adverse reactions was 41.0%. The most common adverse drug reactions, as judged by investigators, in patients treated with TYGACIL (tigecycline) were nausea at 18.9% (11.6% mild; 6.4% moderate; 0.9% severe) and vomiting 12.4% (7.4% mild; 4.3% moderate; 0.6% severe). In general, nausea and vomiting occurred early in treatment (days 1-2) and on average over 2 to 4 days.

Tigecycline was discontinued due to an adverse event in 6.7% of subjects. Discontinuation from tigecycline was most frequently associated with nausea (1.1%) and vomiting (1.1%).

Clinical Trial Adverse Drug Reactions: Because clinical studies are conducted under varying conditions, adverse reaction rates observed in the clinical studies of a drug cannot be directly compared to rates in the clinical studies of another drug and may not reflect the rates observed in practice. The adverse reaction information from clinical studies does, however, provide a basis for identifying the adverse events that appear to be related to drug use and for approximating rates.

In Phase 3 clinical studies, 2514 patients were treated with TYGACIL. These patients received at least 1 dose of TYGACIL. In the active controlled studies that employed a 1:1 randomization, 2274 patients with complicated intra-abdominal infections, complicated skin and skin structure infections, community acquired pneumonia, and hospital acquired pneumonia were treated with TYGACIL for up to 14 days. In resistant pathogen clinical studies which were uncontrolled or employed a randomization of 3:1, 184 patients were treated for up to 14 days and 56 patients up to 28 days.

Table 1 shows the incidence (%) of treatment-emergent adverse drug reactions (as judged by the investigators) reported in ≥1% of patients treated with TYGACIL in Phase 3 clinical studies.

Table 1: TYGACIL

Incidence (%) of Adverse Drug Reactions Reported in ≥1% of Patients Treated with TYGACIL in Phase 3 Clinical Studies

Adverse Events	TYGACIL[a] (N=2514)	Comparator (N=2307)
Any adverse event	41.0	32.4
Body as a Whole	6.2	6.1
Abdominal pain	1.2	0.6
Headache	1.2	1.7
Cardiovascular System	3.7	5.0
Phlebitis	1.5	2.3
Digestive System	27.2	14.9
Nausea	18.9	7.8
Vomiting	12.4	4.2
Diarrhea	6.2	4.9
Anorexia	1.1	0.2
Liver function tests abnormal	1.0	0.8
Hemic and Lymphatic System	6.0	5.0
Thrombocythemia	2.1	1.8
Activated partial thromboplastin time prolonged	1.0	0.4
Metabolic and Nutritional	8.7	7.5
Lactic dehydrogenase increased	1.4	1.0
Alkaline phosphatase increased	1.9	1.5
ALT increased[b]	2.5	3.4
AST increased[b]	2.2	3.3
Amylase increased	1.4	1.0
Bilirubinemia	1.3	0.2
Skin and Appendages	2.7	3.8
Rash	1.2	1.7
Urogenital System	1.4	0.8
Vaginal moniliasis	1.0	0.6

[a] 100 mg initially, followed by 50 mg every 12 hours.

[b] Liver function test abnormalities in TYGACIL-treated patients were reported more frequently in the post-therapy period than those in comparator-treated patients, which occurred more often on therapy.

Legend: ALT=alanine transferase; AST=aspartate transferase.

Less Common Clinical Trial Adverse Drug Reactions (<1%): The following adverse drug reactions as judged by the investigators were reported infrequently (<1% and ≥0.1%) in patients receiving TYGACIL in Phase 3 clinical studies:

Body as a Whole: infection, fever, asthenia, septic shock, injection site inflammation, injection site pain, injection site reaction, chills, injection site edema, injection site phlebitis, pain, moniliasis, chest pain, chills and fever, malaise, peritonitis, allergic reaction.

Cardiovascular System: thrombophlebitis, hypertension, hypotension, bradycardia, vasodilatation, tachycardia, atrial fibrillation, AV block first degree, congestive heart failure, electrocardiogram abnormal, palpitation, QT interval prolonged, sinus bradycardia, syncope, tachycardia sinus, ventricular extrasystoles.

Digestive System: oral moniliasis, constipation, dry mouth, jaundice, stools abnormal, abdominal distension, fecal incontinence, flatulence, gastroesophageal reflux disease, glossitis, hepatic failure, liver damage, mucositis, pancreatitis, pseudomembranous colitis.

Hemic and Lymphatic System: eosinophilia, prothrombin time prolonged, anemia, leukocytosis, leukopenia, international normalized ratio increased, thrombocytopenia, coagulation disorder, ecchymosis, hemolysis, neutropenia, prothrombin decreased, prothrombin time shortened.

Metabolic and Nutritional: BUN increased, hypoproteinemia, creatinine increased, hypocalcemia, hyperkalemia, hyponatremia, peripheral edema, hypoglycemia, hypokalemia, creatine phosphokinase increased, healing abnormal, hyperglycemia, hyperphosphatemia, hypophosphatemia.

Musculoskeletal System: myalgia.

Nervous System: dizziness, somnolence, insomnia, nervousness, tremor, twitching, vertigo.

Respiratory System: cough increased, dyspnea, hiccup, pleural effusion, pneumonia, pulmonary physical finding, pharyngitis, sputum increased.

Skin and Appendages: pruritus, sweating, urticaria, fungal dermatitis, herpes simplex, maculopapular rash, pruritic rash, skin discoloration.

Special Senses: taste perversion, abnormal vision.

Urogenital System: vaginitis, kidney function abnormal, urinary tract infection, creatinine clearance decreased, leukorrhea, polyuria, scrotal edema, vulvovaginal disorder, vulvovaginitis.

Adverse Events Associated with Miscellaneous Factors: local reaction to procedure, device malfunction.

In addition to those noted above, the following adverse reactions judged as related as determined by the investigator were noted in Phase 2 studies in complicated skin and skin structure infections and complicated intra-abdominal infections: hypomagnesemia, confusion.

Adverse reactions for the Phase 1 clinical pharmacology studies are similar to those reported in Phase 3 and Phase 2 clinical trials. The most common adverse reactions in these trials were nausea, vomiting, headache, dizziness, and diarrhea.

Abnormal Hematologic and Clinical Chemistry Findings: See Table 1.

Adverse Events with Outcome of Death: In Phase 3 studies, which included controlled and uncontrolled studies, death occurred in 5.4% (137/2514) of patients receiving TYGACIL and 3.8% (87/2307) of patients receiving comparator drugs. In Phase 3 double blind controlled studies that included a comparator and employed a 1:1 randomization, death occurred in 4.7% (107/2274) of patients receiving TYGACIL and 3.8% (85/2264) of patients receiving comparator drugs. In a pooled analysis of these studies, the risk difference of all cause mortality was 1.0% (95% CI −0.3, 2.2) between tigecycline and comparator treated patients. Risk differences in the treatments by infection type are provided in Table 2. Generally, deaths represented complications of the underlying disease or progression of disease. A causal relationship to TYGACIL has not been established.

Infection-related Serious Adverse Events: In Phase 3 clinical studies, infection-related serious adverse events were more frequently reported for subjects treated with TYGACIL (6.7%) vs comparators (5.5%). Serious adverse events of sepsis/septic shock were more frequently reported for subjects treated with TYGACIL (1.8%) vs comparators (1.2%). Due to baseline differences between treatment groups in this subset of patients, the relationship of this outcome to treatment cannot be established (see Warnings and Precautions). Other events included abscess (1.4% vs 1.2%), infections, including wound infections (1.2% vs 0.9%) and pneumonia (1.1% vs 1.2%) for TYGACIL vs comparators, respectively.

Post-Market Adverse Drug Reactions: The following adverse reactions have been identified during postapproval use of tigecycline: acute pancreatitis, anaphylaxis/anaphylactoid reactions, and hepatic cholestasis.

There has been one case of ventricular arrhythmia (with positive dechallenge and rechallenge) associated with TYGACIL administration.

Table 2: TYGACIL

Patients with Adverse Events with Outcome of Death by Infection Type

	Tigecycline		Comparator		Risk Difference[a]
Infection Type	n/N	%	n/N	%	% (95% CI)
cSSSI	6/566	1.1	1/550	0.2	0.9 (−0.3, 2.2)
cIAI	24/817	2.9	17/825	2.1	0.9 (−0.8, 2.6)
CAP	12/424	2.8	11/422	2.6	0.2 (−2.3, 2.7)
HAP	65/467	13.9	56/467	12	1.9 (−2.6, 6.4)
Non-VAP[b]	40/336	11.9	42/345	12.2	-0.3 (−5.4, 4.9)
VAP[b]	25/131	19.1	14/122	11.5	7.6 (−0.2, 16.9)

[a] The difference between the percentage of patients who died in TYGACIL and comparator treatment groups.

[b] These are subgroups of the HAP population.

Legend: CAP=Community-acquired pneumonia; cIAI=Complicated intra-abdominal infections; cSSSI=Complicated skin and skin structure infections; HAP=Hospital-acquired pneumonia; VAP=Ventilator-associated pneumonia.

Note: The Phase 3 double blind controlled studies include 300 and 305 (cSSSI), 301and 306 (cIAI), 308 and 313 (CAP), 311 (HAP).

DRUG INTERACTIONS: Overview: In vitro studies in human liver microsomes indicate that tigecycline does not inhibit metabolism mediated by any of the following 6 cytochrome (CYP) P450 isoforms: 1A2, 2C8, 2C9, 2C19, 2D6, and 3A4. There has been no specific study conducted to examine the effects of tigecycline on microsomal enzyme induction. The exposure and safety data did not show any evidence of increased liver weight during multiple dosing which typically is associated with enzyme induction. Therefore, tigecycline is not expected to alter the metabolism of drugs metabolized by these enzymes. In addition, because tigecycline is not extensively metabolized, clearance of tigecycline is not expected to be affected by drugs that inhibit or induce the activity of these CYP450 isoforms.

Drug-Drug Interactions: Concurrent use of antibiotics with oral contraceptives may render oral contraceptives less effective.

Tigecycline (100 mg followed by 50 mg every 12 hours) and digoxin (0.5 mg followed by 0.25 mg every 24 hours) were coadministered to healthy subjects in a drug interaction study. Tigecycline slightly decreased the C_{max} of digoxin by 13%, but did not affect the AUC or clearance of digoxin. This small change in C_{max} did not affect the steady-state pharmacodynamic effects of digoxin as measured by changes in ECG intervals. In addition, digoxin did not affect the pharmacokinetic profile of tigecycline. Therefore, no dosage adjustment is necessary when tigecycline is administered with digoxin.

Concomitant administration of tigecycline (100 mg followed by 50 mg every 12 hours) and warfarin (25 mg single-dose) to healthy subjects resulted in a decrease in clearance of R-warfarin and S-warfarin by 40% and 23%, and an increase in AUC by 68% and 29%, respectively. Tigecycline did not significantly alter the effects of warfarin on INR. In addition, warfarin did not affect the pharmacokinetic profile of tigecycline. However prothrombin time or other suitable anticoagulation test should be monitored if tigecycline is administered with warfarin.

Drug-Food Interactions: Interactions with food have not been established.

Drug-Herb Interactions: Interactions with herbal products have not been established.

Drug-Laboratory Test Interactions: There are no reported drug-laboratory test interactions.

DOSAGE AND ADMINISTRATION: Dosing Considerations: Based on pharmacokinetic data in patients with severe hepatic impairment (Child-Pugh C), the dose of TYGACIL (tigecycline) should be altered (see Recommended Dose and Dosage Adjustment).

Recommended Dose and Dosage Adjustment: The recommended dosage regimen of TYGACIL is an initial dose of 100 mg, followed by 50 mg every 12 hours. Intravenous (IV) infusions of TYGACIL should be administered over approximately 30 to 60 minutes every 12 hours.

The recommended duration of treatment with TYGACIL for complicated skin and skin structure infections or for complicated intra-abdominal infections is 5 to 14 days.

The recommended duration of treatment with TYGACIL for community acquired pneumonia (mild to moderate infections only) is 7 to 14 days.

The duration of therapy should be guided by the severity and site of the infection and the patient's clinical and bacteriological progress.

Patients with Hepatic Insufficiency: No dosage adjustment of TYGACIL is warranted in patients with mild to moderate hepatic impairment (Child-Pugh A and Child-Pugh B). (See Action and Clinical Pharmacology, Special Populations and Conditions, Hepatic Insufficiency.)

Patients with Severe Hepatic Impairment: Based on the pharmacokinetic profile of tigecycline in patients with severe hepatic impairment (Child-Pugh C), the dose of TYGACIL should be altered to 100 mg followed by 25 mg every 12 hours. Patients with severe hepatic impairment (Child-Pugh C) should be treated with caution and monitored for treatment response. (See Action and Clinical Pharmacology, Special Populations and Conditions, Hepatic Insufficiency.)

Patients with Renal Insufficiency: Based on the pharmacokinetic data, no dosage adjustment of TYGACIL is necessary in patients with renal impairment or in patients undergoing hemodialysis. (See Action and Clinical Pharmacology, Special Populations and Conditions, Renal Insufficiency.)

Other: No dosage adjustment of TYGACIL is necessary based on age, gender or race. (See Action and Clinical Pharmacology, Special Populations and Conditions.)

Administration: Intravenous (IV) infusions of TYGACIL should be administered over approximately 30 to 60 minutes every 12 hours.

TYGACIL may be administered intravenously through a dedicated line or through a Y-site. If the same intravenous line is used for sequential infusion of several drugs, the line should be flushed before and after infusion of TYGACIL with either 0.9% Sodium Chloride Injection, USP, or 5% Dextrose Injection, USP. Injection should be made with an infusion solution compatible with TYGACIL and with any other drug(s) administered via this common line.

Reconstitution: Parenteral Products:

Vial Size	Volume of Diluent to be Added to Vial	Approximate Available Volume	Nominal Concentration per mL
5 mL	5.3 mL	5 mL	10 mg/mL[a]

[a] The pH of the reconstituted solution is 4.5-5.5.

Each Vial of TYGACIL should be reconstituted with 5.3 mL of 0.9% Sodium Chloride Injection, USP, or 5% Dextrose Injection, USP, or, Lactated Ringer's Injection, USP to achieve a concentration of 10 mg/mL of tigecycline. (Note: Each vial contains a 6% overage. Thus, 5 mL of reconstituted solution is equivalent to 50 mg of the drug.) The vial should be gently swirled until the drug dissolves.

Dilution: Withdraw 5 mL of the reconstituted solution from the vial and add to a 100 mL IV bag for infusion (for a 100 mg dose, reconstitute two vials; for a 50 mg dose, reconstitute one vial). The maximum concentration in the IV bag should be 1 mg/mL. **The reconstituted solution should be yellow to orange in color; if not, the solution should be discarded.** Parenteral drug products should be inspected visually for particulate matter and discoloration (e.g., green or black) prior to administration, whenever solution and container permit.

Compatible intravenous solutions include 0.9% Sodium Chloride Injection, USP, 5% Dextrose Injection USP, and Lactated Ringer's Injection, USP.

Once reconstituted, TYGACIL may be stored at room temperature for up to 24 hours (up to 6 hours in the vial and the remaining time in the IV bag). Alternatively, TYGACIL mixed with 0.9% Sodium Chloride Injection, USP, or 5% Dextrose Injection USP may be stored refrigerated at 2 to 8°C for up to 48 hours following immediate transfer of the reconstituted solution into the IV bag. (See Storage and Stability.)

The concentration of the admixture solution is 1 mg/mL (100 mg loading dose/100 mL) or 0.5 mg/mL (50 mg dose in 100 mL).

When administered through a Y-site, TYGACIL, is compatible with the following drugs or diluents when used with either 0.9% Sodium Chloride Injection, USP, or 5% Dextrose Injection USP:

- Dopamine HCl Injection, USP (1.6 mg/mL in 0.9% Sodium Chloride Injection)
- Lidocaine HCl Injection, USP (2.0 mg/mL in 0.9% Sodium Chloride Injection)
- Lactated Ringer's Injection, USP (250 mL bag)
- Potassium Chloride Injection concentrate, USP (0.04 mEq/mL in 0.9% Sodium Chloride Injection)
- Ranitidine Injection, USP (0.6 mg/mL in 0.9% Sodium Chloride Injection)
- Theophylline (1.6 mg/mL in 5% Dextrose Injection)
- Dobutamine Injection, USP (1.0 mg/mL in 0.9% Sodium Chloride Injection)
- Amikacin sulphate Injection, USP (2.5 and 5.0 mg/mL in 0.9% Sodium Chloride Injection)
- Gentamicin Injection, USP (1.4 mg/mL in 0.9% Sodium Chloride Injection)
- Tobramycin Injection, USP (1.4 mg/mL in 0.9% Sodium Chloride Injection)
- Haloperidol Injection, USP (0.2 mg/mL in 0.9% Sodium Chloride Injection)
- Metoclopramide Injection, USP (3 mg/mL in 0.9% Sodium Chloride Injection)
- Morphine sulphate Injection, USP (0.5 mg/mL in 0.9% Sodium Chloride Injection)
- Norepinephrine bitartrate Injection, USP (4 μg/mL in 5% Dextrose Injection)
- Propofol Injectable Emulsion 1% (10 mg/mL in 0.9% Sodium Chloride Injection)
- Piperacillin sodium/tazobactam sodium (EDTA formulation) powder for Injection (Piperacillin 40 mg/tazobactam 5 mg/mL in 0.9% Sodium Chloride Injection)

The following drugs should not be administered simultaneously through the same Y-site as TYGACIL: amphotericin B, amphotericin B lipid complex, diazepam, esomeprazole and omeprazole.

A generic schematic diagram for the Y-site coadministration is provided below: (see Figure 1).

Figure 1: TYGACIL

Generic Schematic Diagram for the Y-site Coadministration

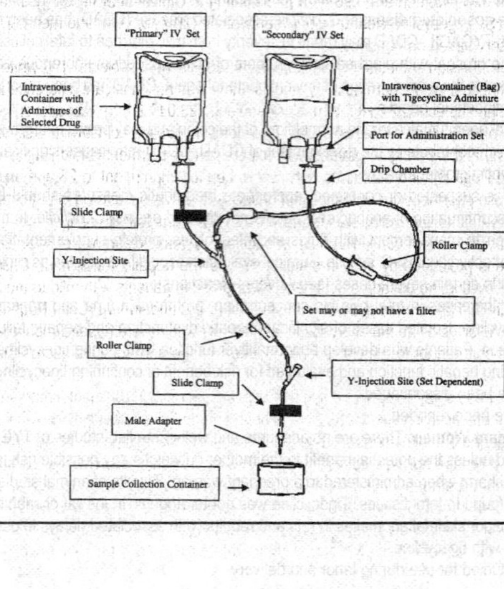

OVERDOSAGE:
No specific information is available on the treatment of overdosage with TYGACIL (tigecycline). Intravenous administration of tigecycline at a single dose of 300 mg over 60 minutes in healthy volunteers resulted in an increased incidence of nausea and vomiting. In single-dose IV toxicity studies conducted with tigecycline in mice, the estimated median lethal dose (LD_{50}) was 124 mg/kg in males and 98 mg/kg in females. In rats, the estimated LD_{50} was 106 mg/kg for both sexes. Tigecycline is not removed in significant quantities by hemodialysis.

For management of a suspected drug overdose, contact your **regional Poison Control Centre**. See the *CPS* Directory section for a list of Poison Control Centres.

ACTION AND CLINICAL PHARMACOLOGY: Mechanism of Action: Tigecycline, a glycylcycline, acts by inhibiting protein synthesis at the level of the bacterial ribosome by blocking the binding of amino-acyl tRNA to the A site of the ribosome. Tigecycline has in vivo and in vitro antibacterial activity against a broad-spectrum of pathogens. Tigecycline is active against bacterial strains that carry classical tetracycline resistant genes encoding either ribosomal protection or a tetracycline efflux pump. Several efflux-related resistance mechanisms have been identified that provide decreased activity (Proteus spp., Providencia spp., and Morganella spp.) or no activity (*P. aeruginosa* spp.).
Pharmacokinetics: The mean pharmacokinetic parameters of tigecycline after single and multiple intravenous doses are summarized in Table 3. Intravenous infusions of tigecycline were administered over approximately 30 to 60 minutes.

Table 3: TYGACIL
Mean (CV%) Pharmacokinetic Parameters of Tigecycline

	Single Doses 100 mg	Multiple Doses[a] 50 mg q12h
C_{max} (µg/mL)[b]	1.45 (22%)	0.87 (27%)
C_{max} (µg/mL)[c]	0.90 (30%)	0.63 (15%)
AUC (µg· h/mL)	5.19 (36%)	—
AUC_{0-24h} (µg· h/mL)	—	4.70 (36%)
C_{min} (µg/mL)	—	0.13 (59%)
$t_{½}$ (h)	27.1 (53%)	42.4 (83%)
CL (L/h)	21.8 (40%)	23.8 (33%)
CL_r (mL/min)	38.0 (82%)	51.0 (58%)
V_{ss} (L)	568 (43%)	639 (48%)

a 100 mg initially, followed by 50 mg every 12 hours.
b 30-minute infusion.
c 60-minute infusion.

Absorption: Tigecycline is administered intravenously and therefore has 100% bioavailability.
Distribution: The in vitro plasma protein binding of tigecycline ranges from approximately 71% to 89% at concentrations observed in clinical studies (0.1 to 1.0 µg/mL). Animal and human pharmacokinetic studies have demonstrated that tigecycline readily distributes to tissues. In rats receiving single or multiple doses of ^{14}C-tigecycline, radioactivity was well distributed to most tissues, with the highest overall exposure observed in bone, bone marrow, thyroid gland, kidney, spleen and salivary gland. In humans, the steady-state volume of distribution of tigecycline averaged 500 to 700 L (7 to 9 L/kg); indicating tigecycline is extensively distributed beyond the plasma volume and into the tissues of humans.

Two studies examined the steady-state pharmacokinetic profile of tigecycline in specific tissues or fluids of healthy subjects receiving tigecycline 100 mg followed by 50 mg every 12 hours. In a bronchoalveolar lavage study, the tigecycline AUC_{0-12h} (134 µg· h/mL) in alveolar cells was approximately 77.5-fold higher than the AUC_{0-12h} in the serum of these subjects, and the AUC_{0-12h} (2.28 µg· h/mL) in epithelial lining fluid was approximately 32% higher than the AUC_{0-12h} in serum. In a skin blister study, the AUC_{0-12h} (1.61 µg· h/mL) of tigecycline in skin blister fluid was approximately 26% lower than the AUC_{0-12h} in the serum of these subjects. In a single-dose study, tigecycline 100 mg was administered to subjects prior to undergoing elective surgery or medical procedure for tissue extraction. Tissue concentrations at 4 hours after tigecycline administration were measured in the following tissue and fluid samples: gallbladder, lung, colon, synovial fluid and bone. Tigecycline attained higher concentrations in tissues versus serum in gallbladder (38-fold, n=6), lung (8.6-fold, n=1), and colon (2.1-fold, n=5). The concentration of tigecycline in these tissues after multiple doses has not been studied.
Metabolism: Tigecycline is not extensively metabolized. In vitro studies with tigecycline using human liver microsomes, liver slices, and hepatocytes led to the formation of only trace amounts of metabolites. In healthy male volunteers, receiving ^{14}C-tigecycline, tigecycline was the primary ^{14}C-labeled material recovered in urine and feces, but a glucuronide, an N-acetyl metabolite and a tigecycline epimer (each at no more than 10% of the administered dose) were also present.
Excretion: The recovery of total radioactivity in feces and urine following administration of ^{14}C-tigecycline indicates that 59% of the dose is eliminated by biliary/fecal excretion, and 33% is excreted in urine. Overall, the primary route of elimination for tigecycline is biliary excretion of unchanged tigecycline. Glucuronidation and renal excretion of unchanged tigecycline are secondary routes.
Special Populations and Conditions: Pediatrics: The pharmacokinetics of tigecycline in patients less than 18 years of age have not been established. (See Warnings and Precautions, Special Populations, Pediatrics (<18 years of age).)
Geriatrics: No overall differences in pharmacokinetics were observed between healthy elderly subjects (n=15, age 65-75; n=13, age >75) and younger subjects (n=18) receiving a single 100-mg dose of tigecycline. Therefore, no dosage adjustment is necessary based on age. (See Warnings and Precautions, Special Populations, Geriatrics (≥65 years of age).)
Gender: In a pooled analysis of 38 women and 298 men participating in clinical pharmacology studies, there was no significant difference in the mean (±SD) tigecycline clearance between women (20.7±6.5 L/h) and men (22.8±8.7 L/h). Therefore, no dosage adjustment is necessary based on gender.
Race: In a pooled analysis of 73 Asian subjects, 53 black subjects, 15 Hispanic subjects, 190 white subjects, and 3 subjects classified as "other" participating in clinical pharmacology studies, there was no significant difference in the mean (±SD) tigecycline clearance among the Asian subjects (22.8±8.8 L/h), black subjects (23.0±7.8 L/h), Hispanic subjects (24.3±6.5 L/h), white subjects (22.1±8.9 L/h), and "other" subjects (25.0±4.8 L/h). Therefore, no dosage adjustment is necessary based on race.
Hepatic Insufficiency: In a study comparing 10 patients with mild hepatic impairment (Child-Pugh A), 10 patients with moderate hepatic impairment (Child-Pugh B), and 5 patients with severe hepatic impairment to 23 age and weight matched healthy control subjects, the single-dose pharmacokinetic disposition of tigecycline was not altered in patients with mild hepatic impairment. However, systemic clearance of tigecycline was reduced by 25% and the half-life of tigecycline was prolonged by 23% in patients with moderate hepatic impairment (Child-Pugh B). In addition, systemic clearance of tigecycline was reduced by 55%, and the half-life of tigecycline is prolonged by 43% in patients with severe hepatic impairment (Child-Pugh C). Based on the pharmacokinetic profile of tigecycline, no dosage adjustment is warranted in patients with mild to moderate hepatic impairment (Child-Pugh A and Child-Pugh B). However, in patients with severe hepatic impairment (Child-Pugh C), the dose of tigecycline should be reduced to 100 mg followed by 25 mg every 12 hours. Patients with severe hepatic impairment (Child-Pugh C) should be treated with caution and monitored for treatment response. (See Dosage and Administration, Patients with Severe Hepatic Impairment.)
Renal Insufficiency: A single dose study compared 6 subjects with severe renal impairment (creatinine clearance ≤30 mL/min), 4 end stage renal disease patients receiving tigecycline 2 hours before hemodialysis, 4 end stage renal disease patients receiving tigecycline after hemodialysis, and 6 healthy control subjects. The pharmacokinetic profile of tigecycline was not altered in any of the renally impaired patient groups nor was tigecycline removed by hemodialysis. No dosage adjustment of tigecycline is necessary in patients with renal impairment or in patients undergoing hemodialysis. (See Dosage and Administration.)
Cardiovascular: In a phase 2 study, ECG results are available from 88 subjects treated with tigecycline. Median change from baseline for QT corrected using the Fridericia formula (QTc(F)) and using a log-linear method (QTc(L)) were 8.5 msec and −4.9 msec, respectively. The upper bounds of a 2-sided 95% confidence interval (CI) were 14.0 and 0.6 msec, respectively. No apparent clinically important effects on cardiac repolarization were seen in subjects treated with tigecycline in this trial. Categorical analyses of QTc(F) and QTc(L) changes ≥60 msec from baseline occurred in 6.8% and 1.1% of the subjects, respectively. However, interpretation of these results is limited because of the relatively small sample size and lack of a control group in this trial.

The results from phase 3 studies involving ECGs from 773 subjects showed that the median changes from baseline for QTc(F) and QTc(L) were 6.0 and 3.3 msec, respectively, with an upper bound of a 2-sided 95% CI of 7 and 5 msec, respectively. Comparable median change values from subjects treated with comparator agents (n=788) were 3.0 and 1.2 msec, with upper bounds of the 95% CI of 5 and 3 msec, respectively. Categorical analyses of QTc(F) and QTc(L) changes ≥60 msec from baseline occurred, respectively, in 1.8% and 1.3% of tigecycline-treated subjects and in 0.8% and 0.6% of comparator subjects. The differences between the tigecycline and comparator groups were statistically significant for the QTc(F) analysis. QTc(F) and QTc(L) absolute values >500 msec occurred in 0.4% of tigecycline-treated subjects and in none of the comparator subjects. These differences between the tigecycline and comparator groups were not statistically significant. Although an effect on cardiac repolarization following administration of tigecycline cannot be absolutely excluded, the overall median changes from baseline in the phase 3 studies were generally small, with the upper bounds of the 95% CI ≤10 msec, without associated drug-related adverse cardiac events being reported in concert with any significant changes in QTc.

STORAGE AND STABILITY: Prior to reconstitution, TYGACIL (tigecycline) lyophilized powder should be stored at a controlled room temperature 20-25°C, excursions permitted to 15-30°C for up to the expiration date specified on the label. Once reconstituted, TYGACIL may be stored at room temperature for up to 24 hours (up to 6 hours in the vial and the remaining time in the IV bag). Alternatively, TYGACIL mixed with 0.9% Sodium Chloride Injection, USP, 5% Dextrose Injection USP may be stored refrigerated at 2 to 8°C for up to 48 hours following immediate transfer of the reconstituted solution into the IV bag.

The reconstituted solution should be yellow to orange in color; if not, the solution should be discarded. Parenteral drug products should be inspected visually for particulate matter and discoloration (e.g., green or black) prior to administration.

INFORMATION FOR THE PATIENT: Published in e-CPS, available by subscription at www.e-cps.ca.

DOSAGE FORMS, COMPOSITION AND PACKAGING: Each vial of orange lyophilized powder or cake for intravenous infusion contains: tigecycline 50 mg and lactose monohydrate 100 mg. The pH is adjusted with hydrochloric acid, and if necessary sodium hydroxide. Preservative-free. Single-dose Type I glass vials of 5 mL, boxes of 10.

Tykerb™ Ⓟ

lapatinib ditosylate
Antineoplastic

GlaxoSmithKline

Date of Revision: June 14, 2010

SUMMARY PRODUCT INFORMATION:

Route of Administration	Dosage Form/ Strength	Clinically Relevant Nonmedicinal Ingredients
Oral	Tablet/250 mg lapatinib as lapatinib ditosylate monohydrate	Hypromellose, iron oxide red, iron oxide yellow, macrogol/PEG 400, magnesium stearate, microcrystalline cellulose, polysorbate 80, povidone, sodium starch glycolate and titanium dioxide

INDICATIONS AND CLINICAL USE: TYKERB (lapatinib ditosylate) is indicated in combination with capecitabine for the treatment of patients with advanced or metastatic breast cancer whose tumours overexpress ErbB2 (HER2). Patients should have progressed on taxanes, anthracycline and trastuzumab before starting this therapy.

Approval is based on the surrogate endpoint, time to progression, without demonstration of an overall survival advantage or palliation due to therapy.

CONTRAINDICATIONS: TYKERB (lapatinib ditosylate) is contraindicated in patients who are hypersensitive to this drug or to any ingredient in the formulation or component of the container. For a complete listing, see Dosage Forms, Composition and Packaging.

Please refer to the capecitabine product monograph for relevant contraindications and safety information when administering TYKERB in combination with capecitabine.

WARNINGS AND PRECAUTIONS:

Serious Warnings and Precautions
TYKERB (lapatinib ditosylate) should only be administered by physicians experienced with antineoplastic drugs (see Indications and Clinical Use).
- Hepatotoxicity (see Hepatic/Biliary/Pancreatic)
- Decreases in left ventricular ejection fraction (LVEF) (see Cardiovascular)
- QT/QTc prolongation (see Cardiovascular)
- Diarrhea (see Gastrointestinal)

Cardiovascular: LVEF and Heart Failure: TYKERB has been reported to decrease left ventricular ejection fraction [LVEF] (see Adverse Reactions). In a randomized clinical trial, the majority (>60%) of LVEF decreases occurred within the first 9 weeks of treatment, but data on long-term exposure are limited. LVEF should be evaluated in all patients prior to initiation of treatment with TYKERB to ensure that the patient has a baseline LVEF that is within the institutions normal limits. LVEF should continue to be evaluated during treatment with TYKERB to ensure that LVEF does not decline to an unacceptable level. Caution should be taken if TYKERB is to be administered to patients with conditions that could impair left ventricular function (see Dosage and Administration, Recommended Dose and Dosage Adjustment, Cardiac Events).
QTc Prolongation: TYKERB is associated with QT/QTc interval prolongation (see Drug Interactions, Drug-Drug Interactions and Action and Clinical Pharmacology). Many drugs that cause QT/QTc prolongation are suspected to increase the risk of torsade de pointes. If sustained, torsade de pointes can progress to ventricular fibrillation and sudden cardiac death. Events of ventricular fibrillation, cardiac arrest, and sudden death have been reported with TYKERB in clinical trials.

Particular care should be exercised when administering TYKERB to patients who are suspected to be at an increased risk of experiencing torsade de pointes during treatment with a QT/QTc-prolonging drug. Risk factors for torsade de pointes in the general population include, but are not limited to, the following: female gender; age 65 years or older; baseline prolongation of the QT/QTc interval; presence of genetic variants affecting cardiac ion channels or regulatory proteins, especially congenital long QT syndromes; family history of sudden cardiac death at <50 years; cardiac disease (e.g., myocardial ischemia or infarction, congestive heart failure, left ventricular hypertrophy, cardiomyopathy, conduction system disease); history of arrhythmias (especially ventricular arrhythmias, atrial fibrillation, or recent conversion from atrial fibrillation); electrolyte disturbances (e.g., hypokalemia, hypomagnesemia, hypocalcemia); bradycardia (<50 beats per minute); acute neurological events (e.g., intracranial or subarachnoid haemorrhage, stroke, intracranial trauma); nutritional deficits (e.g., eating disorders, extreme diets); diabetes mellitus; autonomic neuropathy; hepatic dysfunction.

Physicians who prescribe drugs that prolong the QT/QTc interval should counsel their patients concerning the nature and implications of the ECG changes, underlying diseases and disorders that are considered to represent risk factors, demonstrated and predicted drug-drug interactions, symptoms suggestive of arrhythmia, risk management strategies, and other information relevant to the use of the drug.
Drug Interactions: Concomitant treatment with inhibitors or inducers of CYP3A4, including grapefruit juice, should be avoided due to risk of increased or decreased exposure to TYKERB, respectively (see Drug Interactions).

Co-administration of TYKERB with medications with narrow therapeutic windows that are substrates of CYP3A4 or CYP2C8 should be avoided (see Drug Interactions).

Concomitant treatment with other QT-prolonging drugs should be avoided to the extent possible (see Drug Interactions).

Gastrointestinal: Diarrhea, including severe diarrhea, has been reported with TYKERB treatment (see Adverse Reactions). Proactive management of diarrhea with anti-diarrhea agents is important and severe cases of diarrhea may require administration of oral or intravenous electrolytes and fluids, and interruption or discontinuation of TYKERB therapy (see Dosage and Administration, Recommended Dose and Dosage Adjustment, Other Toxicities). Please refer to the capecitabine product monograph for relevant safety information.

Hepatic/Biliary/Pancreatic: Hepatotoxicity (ALT or AST >3 times the upper limit of normal and total bilirubin >1.5 times the upper limit of normal) has been observed in clinical trials (<1% of patients) and post-marketing experience (see Adverse Reactions). The hepatotoxicity may be severe and deaths have been reported, although the relationship to TYKERB is uncertain. The hepatotoxicity may occur days to several months after initiation of treatment. Liver function tests (transaminases, bilirubin, and alkaline phosphatase) should be monitored before initiation of treatment, every 4 to 6 weeks during treatment, and as clinically indicated. If changes in liver function are severe, therapy with TYKERB should be discontinued and patients should not be retreated with lapatinib.

There is no clinical experience with TYKERB in patients with severe pre-existing hepatic impairment. If TYKERB is to be administered to patients with severe pre-existing hepatic impairment, a dose reduction is recommended based on pharmacokinetic modeling. In patients who develop severe hepatotoxicity while on therapy, lapatinib should be discontinued and patients should not be retreated with TYKERB (see Dosage and Administration, Recommended Dose and Dosage Adjustment, Hepatic Impairment).

Respiratory: TYKERB has been associated with reports of interstitial lung disease and pneumonitis (see Adverse Reactions). Patients should be monitored for pulmonary symptoms indicative of interstitial lung disease/pneumonitis. TYKERB should be discontinued in patients who experience pulmonary symptoms indicative of interstitial lung disease/pneumonitis which are ≥Grade 3 (see Dosage and Administration).

Special Populations: Pregnant Women: TYKERB can cause fetal harm when administered to a pregnant woman. There are no adequate and well-controlled studies of TYKERB in pregnant women. Women of childbearing potential should be advised to use adequate contraception and avoid becoming pregnant while receiving treatment with TYKERB. If this drug is used during pregnancy, or if the patient becomes pregnant while taking this drug, the patient should be apprised of the potential hazard to the fetus.

TYKERB was not teratogenic when studied in pregnant rats and rabbits but caused minor abnormalities at doses which were maternally toxic.

Nursing Women: It is not known whether TYKERB is excreted in human milk. Because many drugs are excreted in human milk and because of the potential for adverse reactions in breastfeeding infants from TYKERB, it is recommended that breastfeeding be discontinued in women who are receiving therapy with TYKERB.

Pediatrics: The safety and efficacy of TYKERB in pediatric patients have not been established.

Geriatrics (>65 years of age): There are limited data of the use of TYKERB in patients aged 65 years and older. Of the total number of metastatic breast cancer patients in clinical studies of TYKERB in combination with capecitabine (N=198) 16% were 65 and over and 1% were 75 and over. No overall differences in safety were observed between these subjects and younger subjects. Other reported clinical experience has not identified differences in responses between the elderly and younger patients, but greater sensitivity of some older individuals cannot be ruled out.

Monitoring and Laboratory Tests: Hypokalemia, hypomagnesemia, or hypocalcemia should be corrected prior to administration of TYKERB. The prescriber should consider baseline and on-treatment electrolyte measurements and electrocardiograms with QT measurement.

Prior to the initiation of treatment, left ventricular ejection fraction (LVEF) must be evaluated to ensure that baseline LVEF is within the institutional limits of normal (see Warnings and Precautions). LVEF must continue to be monitored during treatment with TYKERB to ensure that LVEF does not decline below the institutional lower limit of normal. LVEF was monitored at approximately 8 week intervals during treatment with TYKERB in clinical trials (see Dosage and Administration, Recommended Dose and Dosage Adjustment).

Liver function (transaminases, bilirubin and alkaline phosphatase) should be monitored before initiation of treatment, every 4 to 6 weeks during treatment and as clinically indicated. Lapatinib dosing should be discontinued if changes in liver function are severe and patients should not be retreated.

Ability to Perform Tasks That Require Judgement, Motor or Cognitive Skills: There have been no studies to investigate the effect of TYKERB on driving performance or the ability to operate machinery. A detrimental effect on such activities cannot be predicted from the pharmacology of lapatinib. The clinical status of the patient and the adverse event profile of TYKERB should be borne in mind when considering the patient's ability to perform tasks that require judgement, motor or cognitive skills.

ADVERSE REACTIONS: Clinical Trial Adverse Drug Reactions: TYKERB has been evaluated for safety as a single agent and in combination with other chemotherapies in more than 11 000 patients with various cancers.

The safety of TYKERB in combination with capecitabine in advanced and metastatic breast cancer was evaluated in 198 patients in a randomized, phase III trial. Adverse events (regardless of causality) which occurred in at least 5% of patients in either treatment arm are shown in Table 1.

Table 1: TYKERB

Adverse Events from Clinical Trial EGF100151 (Without Regard to Causality) Occurring in ≥5% of Patients

	TYKERB + Capecitabine (N=198)			Capecitabine (N=191)		
Event	**All Grades[a] %**	**Grade 3 %**	**Grade 4 %**	**All Grades[a] %**	**Grade 3 %**	**Grade 4 %**
Gastrointestinal Disorders						
Diarrhea	65	13	1	40	10	0
Nausea	44	2	0	43	2	0
Vomiting	26	2	0	21	2	0
Abdominal pain	13	1	0	16	1	0
Stomatitis	14	0	0	11	<1	0
Constipation	10	0	0	12	1	0
Abdominal pain upper	9	0	0	6	0	0
Dyspepsia	11	<1	0	3	0	0
General Disorders and Administrative Site Conditions						
Fatigue	23	3	0	25	3	<1
Mucosal inflammation	15	0	0	12	2	0
Asthenia	10	1	<1	13	2	0
Pyrexia	8	0	0	6	0	0
Oedema peripheral	6	<1	0	4	<1	0
Infections and Infestations						
Nasopharyngitis	4	0	0	7	0	0
Metabolism and Nutrition Disorders						
Anorexia	14	<1	0	19	<1	0
Musculoskeletal and Connective Tissue Disorders						
Pain in extremity	12	1	0	7	<1	0
Back pain	11	1	0	6	<1	0
Arthralgia	7	<1	0	4	0	0
Bone pain	7	<1	0	4	<1	0
Nervous System Disorders						
Headache	10	0	0	14	<1	<1
Dizziness	4	0	0	8	<1	<1
Psychiatric Disorders						
Insomnia	10	<1	0	6	0	0
Respiratory, Thoracic, and Mediastinal Disorders						
Dyspnea	12	3	0	8	2	0
Cough	7	0	0	8	0	0
Epistaxis	8	0	0	2	0	0
Skin and Subcutaneous Tissue Disorders						
Palmar-plantar erythrodysaesthesia	53	12	0	51	14	0
Rash[b]	28	2	0	14	1	0
Dry skin	10	0	0	6	0	0

[a] National Cancer Institute Common Toxicity Criteria for Adverse Events, version 3.

[b] Grade 3 dermatitis acneiform was reported in <1% of patients in TYKERB plus capecitabine group.

None of the listed Adverse Events met the criteria for Grade 5.

The most common adverse reactions during therapy with TYKERB plus capecitabine were gastrointestinal (diarrhea, nausea, and vomiting), dermatologic (palmar-plantar erythrodysaesthesia and rash), and fatigue. Diarrhea was the most common adverse reaction (60% all grades) resulting in discontinuation of study medication (5% of patients). The most common Grade 3 and 4 adverse reactions (NCI CTC v3) were diarrhea and palmar-plantar erythrodysaesthesia.

Selected laboratory abnormalities are shown in Table 2. The majority of adverse events and laboratory abnormalities were Grades 1 or 2.

Abnormal Hematologic and Clinical Chemistry Findings:

Table 2: TYKERB

Selected Laboratory Abnormalities

	TYKERB + Capecitabine			Capecitabine		
Event	**All Grades[a] %**	**Grade 3 %**	**Grade 4 %**	**All Grades[a] %**	**Grade 3 %**	**Grade 4 %**
Hematologic						
Hemoglobin	56	<1	0	53	1	0
Neutrophils	22	3	<1	31	2	1
Platelets	18	<1	0	17	<1	<1
Hepatic						
AST	49	2	<1	43	2	0
Total Bilirubin[b]	45	4	0	30	3	0
ALT	37	2	0	33	1	0

[a] National Cancer Institute Common Terminology Criteria for Adverse Events, version 3.

[b] Elevated bilirubin may be due to lapatinib inhibition by OATP1B1, Pgp or BCRP (see Drug Interactions).

Other Clinical Trial Adverse Drug Reactions: Cardiotoxicity: Rare but serious events of congestive heart failure, cardiac arrest and sudden death have been reported with TYKERB. Due to potential cardiac toxicity with HER2 (ErbB2) inhibitors, LVEF was monitored in clinical trials at approximately 8-week intervals. Decreases in LVEF were considered a Serious Adverse Event (SAE) if signs or symptoms of deterioration in LVEF were ≥Grade 3 (NCI CTCAE), or in cases of a ≥20% decrease in LVEF relative to baseline value and below the institution's lower limit of normal. In study EGF100151, among 177 patients who received lapatinib plus capecitabine and had screening, plus at least one on-treatment LVEF measurement, 10 patients (6%) experienced a ≥20% decrease in LVEF, including 4 patients (2%) that met the SAE criteria above. Amongst 150 patients who received capecitabine monotherapy and had screening, plus at least one on treatment LVEF measurement, 9 patients (6%) experienced a ≥20% decrease in LVEF, including 4 patients (3%) that met the SAE criteria.

In 3 supportive monotherapy studies, among 338 patients who had screening, plus at least one on treatment LVEF measurement, 17 patients (5%) experienced a ≥20% decrease in LVEF, including 7 patients (2.1%) that met the SAE criteria (see Warnings and Precautions, Cardiovascular).

Hepatotoxicity: TYKERB has been associated with hepatotoxicity. In clinical trials, it has been observed in <1% of patients, but may be severe and deaths have been reported. The causality of the deaths is uncertain. See Warnings and Precautions, Hepatic/Biliary/Pancreatic.

Respiratory, Thoracic and Mediastinal Disorders: TYKERB has been associated with interstitial lung disease and pneumonitis in monotherapy or in combination with other chemotherapies. See Warnings and Precautions, Respiratory.

Immune System Disorders: TYKERB has been associated with hypersensitivity reactions including anaphylaxis. See Contraindications.

Skin and Subcutaneous Tissue Disorders: Nail disorders including paronychia have been reported.

Post-Market Adverse Drug Reactions: No post marketing data are currently available.

DRUG INTERACTIONS: Drug-Drug Interactions: Lapatinib undergoes extensive metabolism by CYP3A4, and concomitant administration of strong inhibitors or inducers of CYP3A4 alter lapatinib concentrations (see Action and Clinical Pharmacology, Pharmacokinetics and Warnings and Precautions).

In healthy subjects receiving ketoconazole, a CYP3A4 inhibitor, at 200 mg twice daily for 7 days, systemic exposure (AUC) to lapatinib was increased approximately 3.6 fold of control and half-life increase to 1.7 fold of control. The concomitant use of strong CYP3A4 inhibitors should be avoided (e.g., ketoconazole, itraconazole, clarithromycin, atazanivir, indinavir, nefazodone, nelfinavir, ritonavir, saquinavir, telithromycin, voriconazole). Grapefruit may also increase plasma concentrations of lapatinib and should be avoided. If patients must be co-administered a strong CYP3A4 inhibitor, a dose reduction should be considered (see Dosage and Administration, Recommended Dose and Dosage Adjustment). Co-administration of lapatinib with moderate inhibitors of CYP3A4 should proceed with caution and clinical adverse reactions should be carefully monitored.

In healthy subjects receiving the CYP3A4 inducer, carbamazepine, at 100 mg twice daily for 3 days and 200 mg twice daily for 17 days, systemic exposure (AUC) to lapatinib was decreased approximately 72%. The concomitant use of strong CYP3A4 inducers should be avoided (e.g., dexamethasone, phenytoin, carbamazepine, rifampin, rifabutin, rifapentin, phenobarbital, St. John's Wort). If patients must be co-administered a strong CYP3A4 inducer, the dose of lapatinib should be adjusted (see Dosage and Administration, Recommended Dose and Dosage Adjustment).

The concomitant use of TYKERB with another QT/QTc-prolonging drug should be avoided to the extent possible. Drugs that have been associated with QT/QTc interval prolongation and/or torsade de pointes include, but are not limited to, the examples in the following list. Chemical/pharmacological classes are listed if some, although not necessarily all, class members have been implicated in QT/QTc prolongation and/or torsade de pointes:

Class IA antiarrhythmics (e.g., quinidine, procainamide, disopyramide), Class III antiarrhythmics (e.g., amiodarone, sotalol, ibutilide), Class 1C antiarrhythmics (e.g., flecainide, propafenone), anthracyclines, including a history of prior treatment (e.g., doxorubicin, epirubicin), tyrosine kinase inhibitors (e.g., sunitinib), antipsychotics (e.g., chlorpromazine, pimozide, haloperidol, droperidol, ziprasidone), antidepressants (e.g., fluoxetine, venlafaxine, tricyclic/tetracyclic antidepressants e.g., amitriptyline, imipramine, maprotiline), opioids (e.g., methadone), macrolide antibiotics and analogues (e.g., erythromycin, clarithromycin, telithromycin), quinolone antibiotics (e.g., moxifloxacin, levofloxacin), pentamidine, antimalarials (e.g., quinine, chloroquine), azole antifungals (e.g., ketoconazole, fluconazole, voriconazole), domperidone, 5-HT_3 receptor antagonists (e.g., dolasetron, ondansetron), tacrolimus, beta-2 adrenoceptor agonists (e.g., salmeterol, formoterol).

TYKERB is a substrate for CYP3A4. Plasma levels of lapatinib can be increased by inhibitors of CYP3A4. Prolongation of the QT/QTc interval by TYKERB is anticipated to be increased in the presence of CYP3A4 inhibitors. Drugs that inhibit CYP3A4 include ketoconazole, itraconazole, voriconazole, clarithromycin, erythromycin, telithromycin, atazanavir, indinavir, nelfinavir, ritonavir, saquinavir, and amiodarone. The concomitant use of these drugs with TYKERB is discouraged.

TYKERB is, itself, an inhibitor of CYP3A4. TYKERB is anticipated to decrease the metabolism/increase the bioavailability of the following drugs that also prolong the QT/QTc interval: clarithromycin, erythromycin, telithromycin, quinidine, quinine, ondansetron, haloperidol, pimozide, ziprasidone, salmeterol, methadone, and domperidone. The concomitant use of these drugs with TYKERB is discouraged.

The use of TYKERB is discouraged with drugs that can disrupt electrolyte levels, including, but not limited to, the following: loop, thiazide, and related diuretics; laxatives and enemas; amphotericin B; high dose corticosteroids.

The above lists of potentially interacting drugs are not comprehensive. Current information sources should be consulted for newly approved drugs that prolong the QT/QTc interval, inhibit CYP3A4, or cause electrolyte disturbances, as well as for older drugs for which these effects have recently been established.

TYKERB inhibits CYP3A4 and CYP2C8 in vitro at clinically relevant concentrations. Caution should be exercised and dose reduction of the concomitant substrate drug should be considered when dosing TYKERB concurrently with medications with narrow therapeutic windows that are substrates of CYP3A4 or CYP2C8 (see Warnings and Precautions and Action and Clinical Pharmacology, Pharmacokinetics).

TYKERB is a substrate for the transport proteins P-glycoprotein and BCRP. Inhibitors (e.g. quinidine and cyclosporine A) and inducers (e.g. rifampicin and dexamethasone) of these proteins may alter the exposure and/or distribution of lapatinib, and caution should be exercised (see Action and Clinical Pharmacology, Pharmacokinetics). The QT/QTc prolongation caused by TYKERB is expected to be increased in the presence of inhibitors of these transport proteins.

TYKERB inhibits the transport proteins P-glycoprotein, BCRP and OATP1B1 in vitro. The clinical relevance of this effect has not been evaluated, although it may cause elevated bilirubin due to lapatinib inhibition of hepatic uptake by OATP1B1 or inhibition of excretion into bile by Pgp or BCRP. If TYKERB is administered with drugs that are substrates of Pgp (e.g. digoxin), BCRP (e.g. topotecan) or OATP1B1 (e.g. rosuvastatin), increased concentrations of the substrate drug are likely, and caution should be exercised (see Action and Clinical Pharmacology, Pharmacokinetics).

Concomitant administration of TYKERB with capecitabine did not meaningfully alter the pharmacokinetics of either agent (or the metabolites of capecitabine).

Drug-Food Interactions: The bioavailability of TYKERB is increased by food. TYKERB should only be taken at least 1 hour before or at least 1 hour after a low-fat meal (see Dosage and Administration and Action and Clinical Pharmacology, Pharmacokinetics).

Grapefruit juice may inhibit CYP3A4 in the gut wall and increase the bioavailability of lapatinib and should therefore be avoided during treatment with lapatinib.

DOSAGE AND ADMINISTRATION: TYKERB (lapatinib ditosylate) should only be administered by physicians experienced with antineoplastic drugs (see Indications and Clinical Use).

Dosing Considerations: The bioavailability of lapatinib is increased by food. TYKERB should only be taken at least 1 hour before or at least 1 hour after a low-fat meal.

Recommended Dose and Dosage Adjustment: TYKERB is taken in combination with capecitabine.

The recommended dose of TYKERB is 1250 mg (i.e. five tablets) once daily every day. TYKERB should be taken at least one hour before, or at least one hour after a low fat meal (see Action and Clinical Pharmacology, Pharmacokinetics).

The recommended dose of capecitabine is 2000 mg/m²/day divided into two equal doses, each dose taken 12 hours apart on days 1-14 in a 21 day cycle. Capecitabine should be taken with food or within 30 minutes after food.

The prescribing information for capecitabine must be consulted for guidance on dose delay and dose reduction recommendations for capecitabine.

Cardiac Events: (See Warnings and Precautions.)

TYKERB should be discontinued in patients with symptoms associated with decreased LVEF that are National Cancer Institute Common Terminology Criteria for Adverse Events (NCI CTCAE) grade 3 or greater or if their LVEF drops below the institutions lower limit of normal. Consideration may be given to restarting TYKERB after a minimum of 2 weeks and only if the LVEF recovers to normal and the patient is asymptomatic. If TYKERB is restarted under these circumstances, a reduced dose (1000 mg/day) is recommended. Based on current data, the majority of LVEF decreases occur within the first 9 weeks of treatment, but there is limited data on long term exposure.

Interstitial Lung Disease/Pneumonitis: (See Warnings and Precautions and Adverse Reactions.) TYKERB should be discontinued in patients who experience pulmonary symptoms indicative of interstitial lung disease/pneumonitis which are NCI CTCAE grade 3 or greater.

Renal Impairment: There is no experience of TYKERB in patients with severe renal impairment; however, patients with renal impairment are unlikely to require dose modification of TYKERB given that less than 2% of an administered dose (TYKERB and metabolites) is eliminated by the kidneys (see Actions and Clinical Pharmacology, Pharmacokinetics, Special Populations and Conditions).

Hepatic Impairment: TYKERB is metabolised in the liver. Moderate and severe hepatic impairment have been associated respectively, with 56% and 85% increases in systemic exposure. Administration of TYKERB to patients with hepatic impairment should be undertaken with caution due to increased exposure to the drug. TYKERB dosing should be discontinued if changes in liver function are severe and patients should not be retreated (see Warnings and Precautions and Actions and Clinical Pharmacology, Pharmacokinetics, Special Populations and Conditions).

There is no safety data from clinical trials on the use of TYKERB in patients with severe hepatic impairment (Child-Pugh Class C). Based on pharmacokinetic modelling, a dose reduction to 750 mg/day in patients with severe hepatic impairment is predicted to adjust the area under the curve (AUC) to the normal range. However, the safety and efficacy of this dose has not been demonstrated (see Warnings and Precautions and Actions and Clinical Pharmacology, Pharmacokinetics, Special Populations and Conditions).

Concomitant Strong CYP3A4 Inhibitors: The concomitant use of strong CYP3A4 inhibitors should be avoided (see Warnings and Precautions and Drug Interactions). There are no clinical data recommending an appropriate dose adjustment in patients receiving strong CYP3A4 inhibitors. However, if patients must be co-administered a strong CYP3A4 inhibitor, based on pharmacokinetic studies, a dose reduction to 500 mg/day of TYKERB is predicted to adjust the lapatinib AUC to the range observed without inhibitors and should be considered. If the strong inhibitor is discontinued, a washout period of approximately 1 week should be allowed before the lapatinib dose is adjusted upward to the indicated dose.

Concomitant Strong CYP3A4 Inducers: The concomitant use of strong CYP3A4 inducers should be avoided (see Warnings and Precautions and Drug Interactions). There are no clinical data recommending an appropriate dose adjustment in patients receiving strong CYP3A4 inducers. If patients must be co-administered a strong CYP3A4 inducer, based on pharmacokinetic studies, the dose of TYKERB should be titrated gradually form 1250 mg/day up to 4500 mg/day based on tolerability. This dose of TYKERB is predicted to adjust the lapatinib AUC to the range observed without inducers and should be considered. If the strong inducer is discontinued the TYKERB dose should be reduced over approximately 2 weeks to the indicated dose.

Other Toxicities: Discontinuation or interruption of dosing with TYKERB may be considered when a patient develops toxicity greater than or equal to grade 2 on the NCI CTCAE. Dosing can be restarted at 1250 mg/day when the toxicity improves to grade 1 or less. If the toxicity recurs, then TYKERB should be restarted at a lower dose (1000 mg/day).

Missed Dose: Missed doses of TYKERB should not be replaced and the dosing should resume with the next scheduled daily dose (see Overdosage).

Administration: TYKERB tablets are to be taken orally.

OVERDOSAGE:

There is no specific antidote for the inhibition of ErbB1 (EGFR) and/or ErbB2 (HER2) tyrosine phosphorylation. The maximum oral dose of TYKERB (lapatinib ditosylate) that has been administered in clinical trials is 1800 mg once daily.

More frequent ingestion of TYKERB could result in serum concentrations exceeding those observed in clinical trials, therefore missed doses should not be replaced and dosing should resume with the next scheduled daily dose (see Dosage and Administration). Continuous ECG monitoring may be appropriate in cases of overdose.

Symptoms and Signs: Asymptomatic and symptomatic cases of overdose have been reported in patients being treated with TYKERB. Symptoms observed include known TYKERB associated adverse events (see Adverse Reactions), and in some cases sore scalp, sinus tachycardia (with an otherwise normal ECG), and/or mucosal inflammation.

Treatment: TYKERB is not significantly renally excreted and is highly bound to plasma proteins, therefore hemodialysis would not be expected to be an effective method to enhance the elimination of TYKERB.

For management of a suspected drug overdose, contact your regional Poison Control Centre. See the *CPS* Directory section for a list of Poison Control Centres.

ACTION AND CLINICAL PHARMACOLOGY: Mechanism of Action: Lapatinib ditosylate is a novel small molecule, dual 4-anilinoquinazoline kinase inhibitor with a unique mechanism of action, since it is a potent, reversible and selective inhibitor of the intracellular tyrosine kinase domains of both ErbB1 (EGFR) and of ErbB2 (HER2) receptors (estimated Ki^{app} values of 3nM and 13nM, respectively). Like other small-molecule tyrosine kinase inhibitors, lapatinib mimics adenosine triphosphate (ATP) and binds to the ATP binding site at the tyrosine kinase domain. As a result, lapatinib blocks ATP from binding to the tyrosine kinase domain and inhibits tyrosine kinase from using ATP as a cofactor for phosphorylation of tyrosine residues. Unlike other small molecule tyrosine kinase inhibitors which only inhibit one type of intracellular tyrosine kinase domain, lapatinib inhibits two members of the human epidermal growth family, i.e. both ErbB1 and ErbB2 tyrosine kinase.

Lapatinib has a slow off-rate from these receptors (half-life greater than or equal to 300 minutes). This dissociation rate was found to be slower than other 4-anilinoquinazoline kinase inhibitors studied. Lapatinib inhibits ErbB-driven tumour cell growth in vitro and in various animal models.

In addition to its activity as a single agent, an additive effect was demonstrated in an in vitro study when lapatinib and 5-Fluorouracil (the active metabolite of capecitabine) were used in combination in the four tumour cell lines tested. The clinical significance of these in vitro data is unknown.

The growth inhibitory effects of lapatinib were evaluated in trastuzumab-conditioned cell lines. Lapatinib retained significant activity against breast cancer cell lines selected for long-term growth in trastuzumab-containing medium in vitro. These findings suggest non-cross-resistance between these two ErbB2 (HER2) directed agents.

Cardiac Electrophysiology: In an uncontrolled, open-label, dose escalation study in patients with solid tumours receiving TYKERB at doses of 175 mg/kg to 1800 mg/kg for 14 days, concentration-dependent prolongation of the QTc interval was observed. The magnitude of QTc prolongation at maximal plasma concentrations based on pharmacokinetic-pharmacodynamic modelling was predicted to be as follows: see Table 3.

Table 3: TYKERB

Predicted Change from Baseline in QTc (ms) N=38

Condition[a]	Lapatinib Concentration (ng/mL)	Machine Read ECG		Manually Read ECG	
		Mean Slope	95th Percentile Slope	Mean Slope	95th Percentile Slope
Geometric mean C_{max} in EGF10005	3203	12	20	7	13
Maximum observed C_{max} in EGF10005	7487	27	47	16	29
Moderate[b] hepatic impairment (×1.15)	3683	13	23	8	14
Ketoconazole inhibition (×2.14)	6854	24	43	15	27
High-fat breakfast (×3.15)	10 089	36	63	22	39

[a] Geom. mean C_{max} value multiplied by geom. mean ratio of effect noted in parentheses for each condition.
[b] C_{max} was decreased in severe hepatic impairment so change due to moderate impairment is provided.
Legend: $QTc=QT/RR^{0.33}$.

Pharmacokinetics: Absorption: Absorption following oral administration of TYKERB is incomplete and variable (approximately 50 to 100% coefficient of variation in AUC). Serum concentrations appear after a median lag time of 0.25 hours (range 0 to 1.5 hour). Peak plasma concentrations (C_{max}) of TYKERB are achieved approximately 4 hours after administration. Daily dosing of 1250 mg produces steady state geometric mean (95% confidence interval) C_{max} values of 2.43 (1.57 to 3.77) µg/mL and AUC values of 36.2 (23.4 to 56) µg·hr/mL.

Systemic exposure to TYKERB is increased when administered with food (see Dosage and Administration and Drug Interactions). TYKERB AUC values were approximately 3- and 4-fold higher (C_{max} approximately 2.5 and 3-fold higher) when administered with a low fat (5% fat [500 calories]) or with a high fat (50% fat [1000 calories]) meal, respectively.

Distribution: TYKERB is highly bound (greater than 99%) to albumin and alpha-1 acid glycoprotein. In vitro studies indicate that TYKERB is a substrate for the transporters BCRP (ABCG1) and p-glycoprotein (ABCB1). TYKERB has also been shown in vitro to inhibit these efflux transporters, as well as the hepatic uptake transporter OATP 1B1, at clinically relevant concentrations (IC_{50} values were equal to 2.3 μg/mL). The clinical significance of these effects on the pharmacokinetics of other drugs or the pharmacological activity of other anti-cancer agents is not known.

Metabolism: TYKERB undergoes extensive metabolism, primarily by CYP3A4/5, with minor contributions from CYP2C19 and CYP2C8 to a variety of oxidated metabolites, none of which account for more than 14% of the dose recovered in the feces or 10% of TYKERB concentration in plasma.

TYKERB inhibits CYP3A4 (Ki 0.6 to 2.3 μg/mL) and CYP2C8 (0.3 μg/mL) in vitro at clinically relevant concentrations. TYKERB did not significantly inhibit the following enzymes in human liver microsomes: CYP1A2, CYP2C9, CYP2C19, and CYP2D6 or UGT enzymes (in vitro IC_{50} values were greater than or equal to 6.9 μg/mL).

In healthy volunteers receiving ketoconazole, a CYP3A4 inhibitor, at 200 mg twice daily for 7 days, systemic exposure to TYKERB was increased approximately 3.6-fold, and half-life increased 1.7-fold (see Drug Interactions, Drug-Drug Interactions).

In healthy volunteers receiving carbamazepine, a CYP3A4 inducer, at 100 mg twice daily for 3 days and 200 mg twice daily for 17 days, systemic exposure to TYKERB was decreased approximately 72% (see Drug Interactions, Drug-Drug Interactions).

Excretion: The half-life of TYKERB measured after single doses increases with increasing dose. However, daily dosing of TYKERB results in achievement of steady state within 6 to 7 days, indicating an effective half-life of 24 hours. TYKERB is predominantly eliminated through metabolism by CYP3A4/5. The primary route of elimination for TYKERB and its metabolites is in feces (median recovery 27% (range 3 to 67%)). Less than 2% is excreted in urine.

Special Populations and Conditions: Hepatic Insufficiency: The pharmacokinetics of TYKERB were examined in subjects with moderate (n=8) or severe (n=4) hepatic impairment and in 8 healthy control subjects. Systemic exposure (AUC) to TYKERB after a single oral 100 mg dose increased approximately 56% and 85% in subjects with moderate and severe hepatic impairment, respectively. Administration of TYKERB in patients with hepatic impairment should be undertaken with caution due to increased exposure to the drug. There is no safety data from clinical trials on the use of TYKERB in patients with severe hepatic impairment, however based on pharmacokinetic modeling, a dose reduction is recommended although the safety and efficacy of this dose has not been demonstrated (see Dosage and Administration, Recommended Dose and Dosage Adjustment). In patients who develop severe hepatotoxicity while on therapy, TYKERB should be discontinued and patients should not be retreated with lapatinib (see Dosage and Administration and Warnings and Precautions).

Renal Insufficiency: TYKERB pharmacokinetics have not been specifically studied in patients with renal impairment or in patients undergoing hemodialysis. However, renal impairment is unlikely to affect the pharmacokinetics of TYKERB given that less than 2% of an administered dose (as unchanged lapatinib and metabolites) is eliminated by the kidneys.

STORAGE AND STABILITY: Do not store TYKERB tablets above 30°C.

INFORMATION FOR THE PATIENT: Published in e-CPS, available by subscription at www.e-cps.ca.

DOSAGE FORMS, COMPOSITION AND PACKAGING: Each yellow, oval, biconvex, film-coated tablet, with one side plain and the opposite side debossed with GS XJG, contains: lapatinib ditosylate 250 mg. Nonmedicinal ingredients: tablet core: magnesium stearate, microcrystalline cellulose, povidone and sodium starch glycolate; coating: hypromellose, iron oxide red, iron oxide yellow, macrogol/PEG 400, polysorbate 80 and titanium dioxide.

Each pack of TYKERB contains 70 tablets in foil blisters of 10 tablets each. Each foil has a perforation down the middle to allow the blisters to be separated into two sections, each containing a daily dose of 5 tablets.

(Shown in Product Identification Section)

Tylenol® Allergy Extra Strength (Multi-Symptom Relief)

acetaminophen—phenylephrine HCl—chlorpheniramine maleate

Analgesic—Decongestant—Antihistamine

McNeil Consumer Healthcare

Tylenol® Sinus Extra Strength Daytime

acetaminophen—phenylephrine HCl

Analgesic—Decongestant

McNeil Consumer Healthcare

Tylenol® Sinus Extra Strength Nighttime

acetaminophen—phenylephrine HCl—chlorpheniramine maleate

Analgesic—Decongestant—Antihistamine

McNeil Consumer Healthcare

Tylenol® Sinus Regular Strength Daytime

acetaminophen—phenylephrine HCl

Analgesic—Decongestant

McNeil Consumer Healthcare

Date of Revision: July 17, 2008

SUMMARY PRODUCT INFORMATION:

Route of Administration	Dosage Form/ Strength	Clinically Relevant Nonmedicinal Ingredients
Oral	Extra Strength Allergy Tablet/ 500 mg acetaminophen, 5 mg phenylephrine HCl and 2 mg chlorpheniramine maleate	Alcohol-, gluten-, lactose- and sulfite-free For a complete listing of nonmedicinal ingredients, see Dosage Forms, Composition and Packaging.
	Extra Strength Sinus Daytime Tablet/ 500 mg acetaminophen and 5 mg phenylephrine HCl	Alcohol-, gluten-, lactose- sulfite- and tartrazine-free For a complete listing of nonmedicinal ingredients, see Dosage Forms, Composition and Packaging.
	Extra Strength Sinus Nighttime Tablet/ 500 mg acetaminophen, 5 mg phenylephrine HCl and 2 mg chlorpheniramine maleate	Alcohol-, gluten-, lactose-, sulfite- and tartrazine-free For a complete listing of nonmedicinal ingredients, see Dosage Forms, Composition and Packaging.
	Regular Strength Sinus Daytime Caplet/ 325 mg acetaminophen and 5 mg phenylephrine HCl	Alcohol-, gluten-, lactose-, sulfite- and tartrazine-free For a complete listing of nonmedicinal ingredients, see Dosage Forms, Composition and Packaging.

INDICATIONS AND CLINICAL USE: Extra Strength TYLENOL Allergy (Multi-Symptom Relief): For the effective relief of runny nose, sneezing, itchy watery eyes, sinus pain and pressure, sinus congestion and sinus headache due to hay fever or similar allergies.

Extra Strength and Regular Strength TYLENOL Sinus Daytime: A non-drowsy formulation for the effective relief of sinus pain and headache and sinus congestion and pressure caused by sinusitis and common colds.

Extra Strength TYLENOL Sinus Nighttime: For the effective relief of sinus pain and headache, sinus congestion and pressure, runny nose and sneezing caused by sinusitis and common colds.

CONTRAINDICATIONS: Hypersensitivity to acetaminophen, pressor amines or to the ingredients of this formulation (see Dosage Forms, Composition and Packaging). Allergic reactions (primarily skin rash) or reports of hypersensitivity secondary to acetaminophen are rare and generally are controlled by discontinuation of the drug and, when necessary, symptomatic treatment.

In patients receiving or having received MAO inhibitors in the preceding 2 weeks. Although phenylephrine is virtually without pressor effect in normotensive patients, it should be used with caution in hypertensives.

WARNINGS AND PRECAUTIONS: General: Consumers should not exceed 4 g/day of acetaminophen or use two or more acetaminophen-containing products together. This includes combination products that contain acetaminophen. Do not use with other products containing salicylates or any other pain or fever medicine.

Acetaminophen-containing products should be kept out of the reach of children.

Physicians should be cognizant of and supervise the use of acetaminophen in patients with chronic alcoholism, serious kidney or serious liver disease. Physicians should alert their patients who regularly consume large amounts of alcohol not to exceed the recommended doses of acetaminophen. Chronic heavy alcohol abusers may be at increased risk of liver toxicity from excessive doses of acetaminophen.

Patients should be counseled to consult a physician if redness or swelling is present in an area of pain, if symptoms do not improve or if they worsen, or if new symptoms such as high fever, rash, itching or persistent headache occur, as these may be signs of a condition which requires medical attention.

Acetaminophen should not be taken for pain for more than 5 days or if new symptoms appear, without consulting a physician.

In patients with high blood pressure, heart disease, diabetes, thyroid disease, difficulty in urination due to enlargement of the prostate gland or who are taking a prescription drug for high blood pressure or depression, phenylephrine HCl should be used with caution and only under close medical supervision.

Patients with asthma, glaucoma, emphysema, chronic pulmonary disease or shortness of breath should not use this medication unless directed by a physician.

Occupational Hazards: Preparations containing chlorpheniramine maleate may cause drowsiness. Alcoholic beverages, sedatives and tranquilizers may increase this effect and should be avoided. Advise caution when driving a motor vehicle or operating machinery or engaging in any activity requiring alertness. Patients taking tranquilizers or sedatives should not take this medication before consulting a physician.

Hepatic/Biliary/Pancreatic: Slower metabolism of acetaminophen, increased activity of the cytochrome P450 enzyme system, or depleted glutathione stores are cited as theoretical risk factors for acetaminophen hepatotoxicity in patients with chronic liver disease. However, acetaminophen has been studied in both adults and children with a wide variety of liver diseases including various types of cirrhosis, hepatitis (including hepatitis C), nodular transformation, congenital hepatic fibrosis, and α1-antitrypsin deficiency. In none of these conditions is there evidence of an increased risk for hepatotoxicity at currently recommended acetaminophen doses but the studies were insufficiently powered to definitely establish the extent of risk.

Forrest compared acetaminophen metabolism following a single 1500 mg dose in normal subjects, patients with mild liver disease, and patients with severe liver disease. There were no significant differences in overall 24-hour urinary excretion of acetaminophen and glucuronide, sulfate, cysteine, and mercapturic acid conjugates, evidence that acetaminophen metabolism was similar to that in normal subjects. However, the elimination half-life was significantly prolonged in patients with severe liver disease.

Acetaminophen has also been studied in pediatric patients with liver disease. Following a single (10 mg/kg) dose of acetaminophen, the pharmacokinetic profiles in pediatric patients with mild, moderate, or severe liver disease were not significantly different. Although the plasma half-life of acetaminophen was prolonged in patients with severe liver disease, there were no significant differences in the 36-hour (children) urinary excretion of acetaminophen or its conjugates.

Acetaminophen may cause hepatotoxicity in situations of intentional overdose (e.g. attempted suicide), unintentional overdose (e.g. overdosing when pain relief is not satisfactory), simultaneous use of multiple acetaminophen-containing preparations, accidental overdose or in very rare cases, after recommended doses, although causality has not been determined. The hepatotoxic reaction can be severe and life-threatening. Early symptoms following a hepatotoxic overdose may include nausea, vomiting, diaphoresis, lethargy, and general malaise. If appropriate treatment is not instituted, these may progress to upper quadrant pain, confusion, stupor, and sequelae of hepatic necrosis, such as jaundice, coagulation defects, hypoglycemia, and encephalopathy. Renal failure and cardiomyopathy may also occur. In the event of known or suspected overdosage, treatment with N-acetyl cysteine should be instituted immediately (see Overdosage), even when there are no obvious symptoms. Failure to promptly treat acetaminophen hepatotoxicity with N-acetyl cysteine can result in liver failure, leading to liver transplantation and/or death.

Chronic Alcohol Use: Excessive alcohol use may increase risk of liver toxicity from acetaminophen overdose (acute or chronic).

In prospective, placebo controlled studies, researchers evaluated an actively drinking group of alcoholics with a high prevalence of malnourishment. The study participants abruptly stopped their daily alcohol intake and took acetaminophen the next day. This should theoretically make them vulnerable to acetaminophen injury because their CYP2E1 would be maximally induced from the alcohol and there would be no alcohol present to compete with acetaminophen for metabolism by CYP2E1. There was no statistically significant difference in mean values for AST, ALT, or INR for alcoholics given four grams per day of acetaminophen compared to placebo. Additionally, the researchers performed an analysis of the malnourished patients that showed there was no increase in AST or ALT levels in these patients. Study limitations include a limited duration of 2 days and exclusion of patients with preexisting AST or ALT elevations greater than 120 U/L. Study results do not preclude the possibility of an idiosyncratic hepatic reaction.

Renal: Martin found that patients with chronic renal failure had higher plasma concentrations of acetaminophen and the inactive glucuronide and sulfate metabolites than healthy subjects during repeated dosing up to ten days. Several single-dose studies demonstrate accumulation of acetaminophen metabolites in patients with moderate chronic renal failure and in anephric patients for whom hemodialysis appeared to be the major route of elimination.

The habitual consumption of acetaminophen should be discouraged. If indicated medically, the long-term use of acetaminophen should be supervised by a physician.

A National Kidney Foundation position paper notes that physicians preferentially recommend acetaminophen to patients with renal failure because of the bleeding complications associated with ASA in these individuals.

Special Populations: Geriatrics: In a comprehensive metabolic study by Miners, the formation and clearance of glucuronide and glutathione conjugates were the same in young and elderly adults, although clearance of the sulphate conjugate and unchanged acetaminophen were reduced. This finding provides prospective scientific data that the amount of acetaminophen metabolized via the oxidative pathway, from which the highly reactive intermediate, NAPQI, is generated, does not increase with age. Recently, Bannwarth evaluated the multiple-dose pharmacokinetics of acetaminophen in elderly patients. After seven days of repeat dosing, acetaminophen did not accumulate in the plasma, and the elimination half-life was the same as that reported for young adults.

Elderly patients who require therapy for longer than 5 days should consult their physician for condition monitoring.

Glucose-6-Phosphate Dehydrogenase (G6PD) Deficiency: In therapeutic doses, acetaminophen does not shorten the lifespan of red blood cells and does not produce any clinically perceptible destruction of circulating red blood cells.

Obese Adults: O'Shea studied the pharmacokinetics of chlorzoxazone (a putative probe for CYP2E1 activity) to evaluate the effect of obesity on CYP2E1 activity. The authors concluded that CYP2E1 is induced in obese adults and that this could impact the metabolic pathway of a number of drugs metabolized by CYP2E1, including acetaminophen. However, acetaminophen pharmacokinetic data have been investigated in obese adults. In this prospective study, 650 mg acetaminophen was administered intravenously to obese men (297 lb), obese women (193 lb), control men (155 lb) and control women (121 lb). Acetaminophen distribution volume per total body weight was slightly lower in the obese adults but, more importantly, the half-life and metabolic clearance per total body weight did not differ among groups.

ADVERSE REACTIONS: Central Nervous System Effects: Acetaminophen at recommended doses has no obvious effects on central nervous system function. In an overdose situation, central nervous system effects are uncommon.

Chlorpheniramine maleate may cause excitability, especially in children.

Gastrointestinal Effects: Acetaminophen at recommended doses does not cause gastric irritation, gastric erosions, occult or overt gastrointestinal blood loss or ulcers.

Blot and McLaughlin conducted an independent analysis of case-control data from a study conducted by the American College of Gastroenterology. The risk of gastrointestinal bleeding increased two to three-fold among recent users of ASA, ibuprofen and other NSAIDs at OTC doses, and the risk was also dose-related. In contrast, the use of acetaminophen was not associated with an increased risk of gastrointestinal bleeding.

Hematologic Effects: Acetaminophen does not have any immediate or delayed effects on small vessel hemostasis, as measured by bleeding time. In normal volunteers receiving a single dose of acetaminophen (975 or 1950 mg) or multiple doses of acetaminophen (1950 mg daily for 6 weeks), no change in bleeding time or platelet aggregation was observed. In another study, a single 1000 mg dose of acetaminophen was given to normal volunteers and did not affect bleeding time or platelet aggregation. Patients with hemophilia receiving multiple doses of acetaminophen showed no significant changes in bleeding time.

Haematological reactions including thrombocytopenia, leucopenia, pancytopenia, neutropenia, and agranulocytosis have been reported, although these are rare and causality has not been established.

Hepatic Effects: As an illustration of the margin of safety of acetaminophen at supratherapeutic doses, a comparison of serum concentrations of acetaminophen over time for a standard 15 mg/kg dose and for a dose exceeding the standard by a multiple of 5 (75 mg/kg) are shown in Figure 1. The serum concentrations are drawn relative to the risk line for hepatotoxicity and treatment line of the Rumack-Matthew nomogram used to manage acute overdoses. The mean plasma concentrations for this supratherapeutic dose are well below the risk and treatment lines of the nomogram at all times. However, to minimize the risk for adverse effects, the maximum recommended dose should not be exceeded.

Figure 1: TYLENOL Allergy/Sinus

Mean Data for a Standard (1 g, 15 mg/kg) and Higher (5.6 g, 75 mg/kg) Dose Relative to Risk and Treatment Lines of the Acetaminophen Nomogram

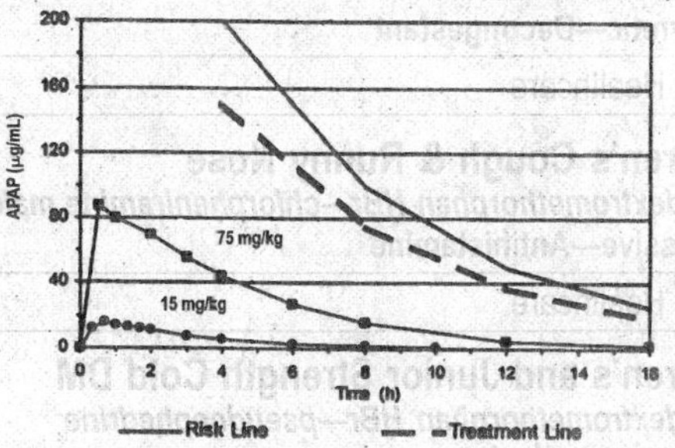

Acetaminophen in overdosage may cause hepatotoxicity. In adults and adolescents, hepatotoxicity may occur following ingestion of greater than 150 mg/kg over a period of 8 hours or less. Fatalities are infrequent (less than 3% to 4% of untreated cases in which blood levels exceed the treatment line) and have rarely been reported with overdoses less than 7.5 g. In children, amounts less than 150 mg/kg are unlikely to produce hepatotoxicity. In both adults and children, toxicity associated with acetaminophen is usually caused by ingestion of quantities of the drug that are significantly above the recommended dosage range. Hepatotoxicity, ranging from transient sharp transaminase elevations to fatal, fulminant hepatic failure, is the most common result of clinically significant overdosage.

In a double-blind, placebo-controlled clinical study, healthy adults were given 4, 6 and 8 g/d of acetaminophen over 3 days. Plasma concentrations did not accumulate with repeat doses. Clinically all doses were well tolerated by the subjects and aminotransferase values stayed within normal limits throughout the study. These data provide information related to the margin of safety but are not intended to support dosing beyond the maximum recommended dose of 4 g/day.

A report has suggested that hepatotoxicity following greater than the recommended dose of acetaminophen may be enhanced by both prolonged fasting and/or chronic alcohol abuse.

Acute Alcohol Use: Acute alcohol ingestion refers to the occasional or intermittent use of alcohol. When taken together, alcohol competes with acetaminophen for CYP2E1. CYP2E1 accepts alcohol more readily than acetaminophen; therefore, less NAPQI is produced. In the presence of alcohol, acetaminophen may be diverted to the glucuronidation and sulfation pathways. The overall result is that a smaller percentage of acetaminophen may be expected to be metabolized to the toxic intermediate, NAPQI, than would otherwise be the case. NAPQI production is increased above baseline for the period up to 18-24 hours post ethanol clearance from the body. In healthy adults, at normal labeled doses of acetaminophen, the temporary increase in NAPQI production is more than accommodated by normal glutathione stores in the liver.

Hypersensitivity: Sensitivity reactions are rare and may manifest as rash, urticaria, dyspnea, hypotension, laryngeal edema, angioedema, bronchospasm, or anaphylaxis. Cross-reactivity in ASA-sensitive persons has been rarely reported. If sensitivity is suspected, discontinue use of the drug.

Renal Effects: Acute nephrotoxicity has been reported following massive overdose either as a sequela of hepatic failure or, occasionally, in the absence of hepatic failure.

Clinical data have established that acetaminophen in recommended doses is not nephrotoxic.

Some studies suggest an association between the chronic long-term use of acetaminophen and renal effects. Results, however, are conflicting, limited by recall bias and confounded by the inability to determine whether analgesic use preceded or followed the onset of renal disease.

Case control studies have suggested a weak association between habitual acetaminophen use and prevalence of chronic renal failure and end stage renal disease. This National Kidney Foundation position paper concludes that acetaminophen has been preferentially recommended by physicians to patients with renal failure and that there is no evidence that occasional use of acetaminophen caused renal injury.

Special Populations: Pregnant Women and Nursing Women: As with any drug, patients who are pregnant or nursing a baby should consult a physician before taking this product.

Pregnant Women: Issues of risks in pregnancy are multifactorial. The information provided cannot be substituted for direct patient consultation. Acetaminophen is believed to be non-teratogenic in humans. However, existing studies have not assessed the effect of very high doses. The Motherrisk Collaborative Perinatal project monitored 50 282 mother-child pairs, of which 226 had first trimester exposure to acetaminophen and 781 had used acetaminophen at any time during their pregnancy. No evidence was found to suggest a relationship between acetaminophen use and major or minor malformations. In a surveillance study of Michigan Medicaid recipients conducted between 1985 and 1992 involving 229 101 completed pregnancies, 9146 newborns had been exposed to acetaminophen during the first trimester. This data do not support an association between acetaminophen use and the occurrence of birth defects. Another cohort study, using prescription monitoring, found no excess risk for malformation, and no evidence that acetaminophen influenced fetal growth. Finally, as part of a larger study, 697 women used acetaminophen with or without codeine in their first trimester. No teratogenic risk was found.

A prospective study investigated the outcome of pregnancy in 300 women who had self-administered an overdose of acetaminophen, either alone, or as part of a combined preparation. Exposure to overdose occurred in all trimesters. The majority of the pregnancies had normal outcomes. The malformation rate was within the expected range. There was no obvious relationship between the time of exposure and the time of delivery. The overall conclusion was that acetaminophen overdose is not an indication for termination of pregnancy.

In a long-term developmental follow-up study, acetaminophen did not adversely affect IQ or behavior measures at four years of age. Height, weight and head circumference were also not affected by exposure to acetaminophen in-utero.

Unlike ASA, which has been shown to profoundly effect platelet function, there does not seem to be a risk of hemorrhage associated with acetaminophen use at term.

Currently there is no evidence to suggest that acetaminophen is teratogenic when used as recommended. However, data for continuous high daily doses are not sufficient, and safety during pregnancy has not yet been established.

Nursing Women: Following a typical therapeutic dose, acetaminophen is excreted in breast milk in very low concentrations. Based on a number of published reports, infant exposure levels are at most 4.5% of a weight adjusted pediatric therapeutic dose. In addition, acetaminophen is considered compatible with breast-feeding by the American Academy of Pediatrics.

DRUG INTERACTIONS: Alcohol: Studies evaluating the metabolism of doses up to 20 mg/kg of acetaminophen in chronic alcohol abusers and a study evaluating the effects of 2 days of acetaminophen dosing at 4000 mg/d in chronic alcoholics undergoing detoxification, have yielded inconsistent results with regard to effects on acetaminophen pharmacokinetics and demonstrate no evidence of adverse effect on liver function tests.

Anticoagulants-Oral: Patients who concomitantly medicate with warfarin-type anticoagulants and regular doses of acetaminophen have occasionally been reported to have unforeseen elevations in their INR. Physicians should be cognizant of this potential interaction and monitor the INR in such patients closely while therapy is established. Many factors, including diet, medications, and environmental and physical states, may affect how a patient responds to anticoagulant therapy. There have been several reports that suggest that acetaminophen may produce hypoprothrombinemia (elevated international normalized ratio [INR] or prothrombin time) when administered with coumarin derivatives. In other studies, prothrombin time did not change. Reported changes have been generally of limited clinical significance, however, periodic evaluation of prothrombin time should be performed when these agents are administered concurrently.

In the period immediately following discharge from the hospital or whenever other medications are initiated, discontinued, or taken regularly, it is important to monitor patient response to anticoagulation therapy with additional prothrombin time or INR determinations. Despite the potential for interaction, acetaminophen is the least likely OTC analgesic to interfere with anticoagulant therapy.

Anticonvulsants: Some reports have suggested that patients taking long-term anticonvulsants, who overdose on acetaminophen, may be at increased risk of hepatotoxicity because of accelerated metabolism of acetaminophen. Available data are conflicting. A 7-year retrospective study of acetaminophen overdose admissions indicates that the overall mortality rate was not significantly different for patients taking concomitant anticonvulsant medications.

Hydantoins: Pharmacokinetic studies indicate that phenytoin primarily induces the glucuronidation pathway, whereas glutathione-derived metabolites are not increased in patients on chronic phenytoin therapy. Additionally, recent data demonstrate that phenytoin is metabolized primarily by CYP2C9 and CYP2C19, whereas acetaminophen is primarily metabolized by CYP2E1.

Carbamazepine: Carbamazepine is primarily metabolized by CYP3A4, whereas acetaminophen is metabolized primarily via CYP2E1. It is not known whether there is increased risk from an acetaminophen overdose in patients on chronic carbamazepine therapy.

Diflunisal: Professional literature from the manufacturer of diflunisal cautions that concomitant administration with acetaminophen produces an approximate 50% increase in plasma levels of acetaminophen in normal volunteers. Acetaminophen had no effect on diflunisal plasma levels. The clinical significance of these findings has not been established. However, caution should be used with concomitant administration of diflunisal and acetaminophen and patients should be monitored carefully.

Isoniazid: Some reports suggest that patients on chronic isoniazid therapy may be at risk for developing hepatotoxicity from an acetaminophen overdose. Since patients on isoniazid therapy may develop hepatic effects from isoniazid alone, data from individual case reports are unclear as to whether chronic administration of isoniazid may increase the risk of acetaminophen toxicity. Isoniazid is primarily metabolized by CYP2E1 and induces CYP2E1. Studies in healthy subjects demonstrate that isoniazid blocks the formation of the toxic metabolite NAPQI when administered concomitantly with acetaminophen, but increase NAPQI formation when acetaminophen is administered one day after discontinuation of isoniazid. Thus, concomitant use of isoniazid is unlikely to potentiate the risk of acetaminophen-induced hepatotoxicity at recommended doses. The isoniazid induction of CYP2E1 is short-lived, lasting only 12 to 48 hours after the discontinuation of isoniazid, it is during this period the toxicity of an acetaminophen overdose may be potentiated.

DOSAGE AND ADMINISTRATION:

Extra Strength TYLENOL Allergy: Adults (12 years of age and older): 1 to 2 tablets every 4 hours as needed. It is hazardous to exceed 8 tablets per day unless advised by a doctor. Reduce dose if nervousness or sleeplessness occurs.

Extra Strength TYLENOL Sinus (Daytime and Nighttime): Adults (12 years of age and older): 1 to 2 tablets every 4 hours as needed. It is hazardous to exceed a combined total of 8 tablets per day unless advised by a doctor. Reduce dosage if nervousness or sleeplessness occurs.

Regular Strength TYLENOL Sinus Daytime: Adults (12 years of age and older): 1 to 2 caplets every 4 hours as needed. It is hazardous to exceed 12 caplets per day unless advised by a doctor. Reduce dosage if nervousness or sleeplessness occurs.

OVERDOSAGE:

Symptoms and Treatment: Acetaminophen: Typical Toxidrome: Hepatic injury is the principal toxic effect of a substantial acetaminophen overdose. The physician should be mindful that there is no early presentation that is pathognomic for the overdose. A high degree of clinical suspicion must always be maintained.

Untreated acetaminophen overdoses may produce hepatotoxicity. Acetaminophen hepatotoxicity occurs as a threshold effect and is characterized by a lack of toxicity at lower/therapeutic doses. Acetaminophen hepatotoxicity occurs after major depletion of glutathione, an endogenous detoxifying substance. Once the threshold is exceeded, increasing acetaminophen doses may produce increasing degrees of hepatotoxicity, unless N-acetylcysteine (NAC) is administered. Situations in which acetaminophen overdose and resultant hepatotoxicity may occur include acute intentional overdose and repeated supratherapeutic overdose in adults and acute accidental ingestion or overdose and repeated supratherapeutic overdose in children.

The clinical course of acetaminophen overdose generally occurs in a three-phase sequential pattern. The first phase begins shortly after ingestion and lasts for 12 to 24 hours. The patient may manifest signs of gastrointestinal irritability, nausea, vomiting, anorexia, diaphoresis, pallor and general malaise. If toxicity continues, there is a latent phase of up to 48 hours. During this second phase, initial symptoms abate and the patient may feel better. However, hepatic enzymes, bilirubin, and prothrombin time or INR values will progressively rise. Right upper quadrant pain may develop as the liver becomes enlarged and tender. Most patients do not progress beyond this phase, especially if given N-acetylcysteine (NAC) treatment early in the course. Signs and symptoms of the third phase depend on the severity of hepatic damage and usually occur from three to five days following overdose ingestion. Symptoms may be limited to anorexia, nausea, general malaise, and abdominal pain in less severe cases or may progress to confusion, stupor and sequelae of hepatic necrosis including jaundice, coagulation defects, hypoglycemia, and encephalopathy, as well as renal failure and cardiomyopathy. Death, if it occurs, is generally the result of complications associated with fulminant hepatic failure. Mortality rates in patients with toxic plasma levels who do not receive antidote therapy range from 3% to 4%.

Due to the wide availability of acetaminophen, it is commonly involved in single and mixed drug overdose situations and the practitioner should screen for its presence in a patient's serum. Acute toxicity after single dose overdoses of acetaminophen can be anticipated when the overdose exceeds 150 mg/kg. Chronic alcohol abusers, cachectic individuals, and persons taking pharmacologic inducers of the hepatic P450 microsomal enzyme system may be at risk with lower exposures.

Specific Antidote: Any individual presenting with a possible acetaminophen overdose should be treated with N-acetylcysteine (NAC), even if the amount of acetaminophen ingested is unknown or questionable. A blood sample for determination of the plasma acetaminophen concentration should be obtained as early as possible, but no sooner than four hours following ingestion. Do not await the results of assays for plasma acetaminophen levels before initiating treatment NAC. If the acetaminophen plasma level is found to plot above the treatment line on the acetaminophen overdose nomogram, NAC treatment should be continued for a full course of therapy. NAC is used clinically to treat acute acetaminophen overdose, and acts by interacting with the oxidative intermediate, NAPQI. NAC administered by either the i.v. or the oral route is known to be a highly effective antidote for acetaminophen poisoning. It is most effective when administered within 8 hours of a significant overdose but reports have indicated benefits to treatment initiated well beyond this time period. It is imperative to administer the antidote as early as possible in the time course of acute intoxication to reap the full benefits of the antidote's protective effects. For full prescribing information, consult the product monograph for NAC.

General Management: When the possibility of acetaminophen overdose exists, treatment should begin immediately and include appropriate decontamination of the gastrointestinal tract, proper supportive care, careful assessment of appropriately timed serum acetaminophen estimations evaluated against the Rumack-Matthew nomogram, timely administration of NAC as required and appropriate follow-up care. Liver function tests should be performed initially and repeated at 24-hour intervals.

Phenylephrine HCl: Typical Toxidrome: sympathomimetic/stimulant.

Specific Antidote: None.

General Management: Stabilize the patient (A, B, Cs), undertake appropriate gastrointestinal tract decontamination procedures, initiate supportive care, consult with a Regional Poison Control Centre regarding ongoing management, and arrange for appropriate follow-up care.

Chlorpheniramine maleate: Typical Toxidrome: anticholinergic, CNS depressant (adult), CNS stimulant (child).

Specific Antidote: None.

General Management: Stabilize the patient (A, B, Cs), undertake appropriate gastrointestinal tract decontamination procedures, initiate supportive care, consult with a Regional Poison Control Centre regarding ongoing management, and arrange for appropriate follow-up care.

Overdose During Pregnancy: Acetaminophen is one of the most common overdoses in pregnancy. Hepatic toxicity of acetaminophen follows the formation of the highly reactive metabolite N-acetyl-p-benzoquinoneimine produced by acetaminophen metabolism through the cytochrome P450 mixed-function oxidase system. Hepatic failure can be prevented by timely administration of NAC either orally for 72 hours, or intravenously (IV) for 20 hours.

Acetaminophen crosses the human placenta though the fetus is theoretically at risk when maternal overdose of acetaminophen occurs. Acetaminophen can be transformed to its toxic metabolite since the oxidative capacity of fetal microsomes is present in the fetus by 14 weeks gestation.

Studies on placental transfer of NAC in rats and sheep yielded conflicting results. Placental transfer of N-acetylcysteine in humans was demonstrated in 4 women treated with NAC for acetaminophen overdose during labour. NAC blood levels in the fetuses were within the range associated with therapeutic doses of NAC administered to adults with acetaminophen poisoning.

Fetal toxicity and stillbirth after a large (e.g. 30 g) acetaminophen overdose has been reported, but others observed a normal outcome for the offspring after acetaminophen overdose in pregnancy. A large case series investigated the pregnancy outcome in 300 women who had overdosed with acetaminophen. In this group, 118 cases occurred in the first trimester, 103 in the second trimester and 79 in the third trimester. Forty-nine of these mothers were treated with specific antidotes (33 with NAC and

16 with methionine). There were 219 live-born infants, 11 having malformations (including minor); none had been exposed to acetaminophen during the first trimester. Nine women were treated with NAC during the first trimester; there were two elective terminations; two spontaneous abortions, and five healthy babies in this group.

In summary, acetaminophen overdose during pregnancy should be treated according to regular protocols in order to prevent maternal and potentially fetal toxicity. Unless severe maternal toxicity develops, an acetaminophen overdose does not increase the risk for birth defects or adverse pregnancy outcomes.

Physicians unfamiliar with the current management of acetaminophen overdose should consult with a Poison Control Centre immediately. Telephone numbers for local Poison Control Centres are available in the local phone directory. Delays in initiation of appropriate therapy may jeopardize the patient's chances for full recovery.

For management of a suspected drug overdose, CPhA recommends that you contact your **regional Poison Control Centre**. See the *CPS* Directory section for a list of Poison Control Centres.

ACTION AND CLINICAL PHARMACOLOGY: Mechanism of Action: Acetaminophen is a centrally acting analgesic and antipyretic drug. Although the precise mechanism of action is not totally understood, work by Boutaud suggests acetaminophen is an inhibitor of the peroxidase portion of cyclooxygenase (prostaglandin H synthase inhibitor). Depending on the redox state and substrate concentrations surrounding the enzymes, acetaminophen may or may not have a significant inhibitory effect. This accounts for its selective activity on pain and fever with little anti-inflammatory effect.

It is postulated that the analgesic effect is produced by elevation of the pain threshold and the antipyretic effect is produced through action on the hypothalamic heat-regulating centre.

The optimal effective analgesic dose of acetaminophen was demonstrated in dental pain studies and is 1000 mg every four to six hours, up to 4000 mg daily. At least 500 published and unpublished controlled clinical trials in adults and children have evaluated acetaminophen for the relief of pain or fever. These studies include single and multiple dose treatments. Most studies were less than 14 days in duration, although the longest study duration was two years. No significant safety issues were reported in any of these studies.

Moreover, at recommended doses, acetaminophen has not been shown to increase the risk of developing renal diseases or upper gastrointestinal ulceration/bleeding. This observation is consistent with its minimal inhibitory effect on peripheral prostaglandin synthesis and on gastric prostaglandin synthesis.

Acetaminophen is considered equipotent to ASA and ibuprofen, within the recommended OTC dosing ranges, in its analgesic and antipyretic effects. Acetaminophen at recommended doses does not cause the type of gastrointestinal complications associated with NSAID-containing products, such as gastric irritation, gastric erosions, occult or overt gastrointestinal blood loss, or ulcers. Unlike these drugs, however, it has no anti-inflammatory effect at clinically relevant doses in humans.

Pharmacokinetics: Absorption: Oral acetaminophen is rapidly and almost completely absorbed from the gastrointestinal tract primarily in the small intestine. This absorption process occurs by passive transport. Peak plasma concentrations occur within 0.4 to 1 hour depending on the product formulation. Although high-fat foods delay the time to peak concentration for up to an hour, the dose is completely absorbed.

Distribution: Acetaminophen is uniformly distributed throughout most body fluids, but not in fatty tissue. As a result, the volume of distribution in adults ranges between 0.8 and 1.0 L/kg. Since acetaminophen has low protein binding in plasma of only 10% to 25%, it does not compete with drugs that are highly protein bound.

Metabolism: Acetaminophen is primarily metabolized by the liver via three principal separate pathways: conjugation with glucuronide; conjugation with sulfate; oxidation via the cytochrome P450 mixed function oxidase system.

Both the glucuronic and oxidative pathways adhere to a first-order rate process, which means the concentration of acetaminophen metabolized increases as the concentration in the liver increases. The sulfate pathway adheres to Michaelis-Menten kinetics, which means the concentration of acetaminophen metabolized remains constant once the concentration in the liver increases above a saturation level. A schematic of acetaminophen metabolism is shown in Figure 2.

The major metabolic pathway is glucuronidation, where 47% to 62% of the acetaminophen dose conjugates with glucuronide. These glucuronide conjugates are inactive and nontoxic, and are secreted in bile and eliminated in the urine.

The second major pathway is sulfation, where 25% to 36% of the dose conjugates with sulfate. These sulfate ester conjugates are also inactive and nontoxic and are excreted in the urine.

The third pathway is oxidation, where 5% to 8% of the dose is metabolized via the cytochrome P450 enzyme system. The cytochrome P450 isoenzyme that is primarily responsible is CYP2E1. When acetaminophen is metabolized by CYP2E1, it forms a highly reactive intermediate, N-acetyl-p-benzoquinoneimine (NAPQI). Since NAPQI is highly reactive, it cannot be measured outside the liver nor can it accumulate. This intermediate is rapidly inactivated by hepatocellular stores of glutathione to form cysteine and mercapturate conjugates, which are both inactive and nontoxic. These conjugates are excreted in the urine.

Excretion: Acetaminophen undergoes first-order elimination from the body, and has a short plasma half-life that ranges from 2 to 3 hours in healthy young and elderly adults and from 1.5 to 2.9 hours in children. Since acetaminophen clears rapidly from the body, repeated doses do not lead to accumulation of acetaminophen plasma concentrations.

STORAGE AND STABILITY: Store at room temperature (15 to 30°C). Protect from moisture.

DOSAGE FORMS, COMPOSITION AND PACKAGING: Extra Strength TYLENOL Allergy tablets: Each round, light yellow coated tablet, with "TYLENOL" over "Allergy" printed in black ink on one side, blank on the other side and with a characteristic mint odour, contains: acetaminophen 500 mg, phenylephrine HCl 5 mg and chlorpheniramine maleate 2 mg. Nonmedicinal ingredients: carnauba wax, cellulose, corn starch, FD&C Red No. 40, FD&C Yellow No. 5, flavour, hypromellose, iron oxide black, magnesium stearate, polydextrose, polyethylene glycol, sodium starch glycolate, sucralose, titanium dioxide and triacetin. Energy: 1.3 kJ (0.3 kcal). Sodium: 0.4 mg. Alcohol-, gluten-, lactose- and sulfite-free. Plastic bottles of 20* and 40*.

Figure 2: TYLENOL Allergy/Sinus

Acetaminophen Metabolism

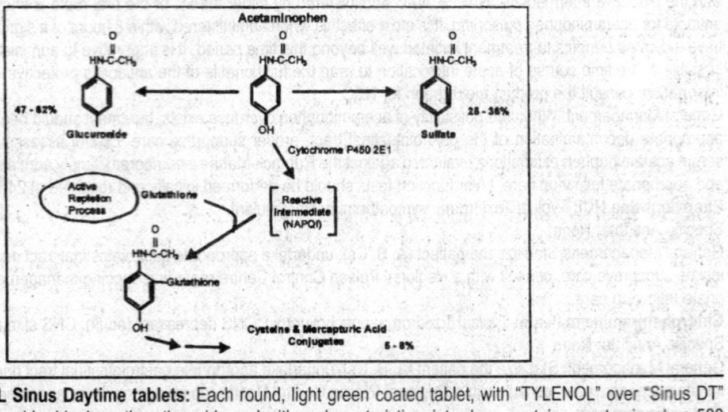

Extra Strength TYLENOL Sinus Daytime tablets: Each round, light green coated tablet, with "TYLENOL" over "Sinus DT" printed in black ink on one side, blank on the other side and with a characteristic mint odour, contains: acetaminophen 500 mg and phenylephrine HCl 5 mg. Nonmedicinal ingredients: carnauba wax, cellulose, corn starch, D&C Yellow No. 10, FD&C Blue No. 1, FD&C Blue No. 2, FD&C Red No. 40, flavour, hypromellose, iron oxide black, magnesium stearate, polydextrose, polyethylene glycol, sodium starch glycolate, sucralose, titanium dioxide and triacetin. Energy: 1.3 kJ (0.3 kcal). Sodium: 0.4 mg. Alcohol-, gluten-, lactose-, sulfite- and tartrazine-free. Plastic bottles 20* and 40*. Blister packs of 6 in combination with blister packs of 4 Extra Strength TYLENOL Sinus Nighttime tablets. Blister packs of 12 in combination with blister packs of 8 Extra Strength TYLENOL Sinus Nighttime tablets.

Extra Strength TYLENOL Sinus Nighttime tablets: Each round, dark green coated tablet, with "TYLENOL" over "Sinus NT" printed in black ink on one side, blank on the other side and with a characteristic mint odour, contains: acetaminophen 500 mg, phenylephrine HCl 5 mg and chlorpheniramine maleate 2 mg. Nonmedicinal ingredients: carnauba wax, cellulose, corn starch, D&C Yellow No. 10, FD&C Blue No. 1, FD&C Yellow No. 6, flavour, hypromellose, iron oxide black, magnesium stearate, polydextrose, polyethylene glycol, sodium starch glycolate, sucralose, titanium dioxide and triacetin. Energy: 1.3 kJ (0.3 kcal). Sodium: 0.4 mg. Alcohol-, gluten-, lactose-, sulfite- and tartrazine-free. Plastic bottles 20*. Blister packs of 4 in combination with blister packs of 6 Extra Strength TYLENOL Sinus Daytime tablets. Blister packs of 8 in combination with blister packs of 12 Extra Strength TYLENOL Sinus Daytime tablets.

Regular Strength TYLENOL Sinus Daytime caplets: Each light green, caplet-shaped tablet, with "TY C1080" printed in black ink on one side, contains: acetaminophen 325 mg and phenylephrine HCl 5 mg. Nonmedicinal ingredients: carnauba wax, cellulose, colloidal silicon dioxide, corn starch, D&C Yellow No. 10, FD&C Blue No. 1, FD&C Red No. 40, flavour, hypromellose, iron oxide black, magnesium stearate, polyethylene glycol, polysorbate 80, potassium sorbate, shellac glaze, sodium benzoate, sodium starch glycolate, stearic acid, sucralose and titanium dioxide. Energy: 1.3 kJ (0.3 kcal). Sodium: 0.4 mg. Alcohol-, gluten-, lactose-, sulfite- and tartrazine-free. Plastic bottles of 20*.

All packages are safety sealed.

* Container provided with a child-resistant closure.

Tylenol® Children's Decongestant
acetaminophen—pseudoephedrine HCl
Analgesic—Antipyretic—Decongestant

McNeil Consumer Healthcare

Tylenol® Children's Cough & Runny Nose
acetaminophen—dextromethorphan HBr—chlorpheniramine maleate
Analgesic—Antitussive—Antihistamine

McNeil Consumer Healthcare

Tylenol® Children's and Junior Strength Cold DM
acetaminophen—dextromethorphan HBr—pseudoephedrine HCl—chlorpheniramine maleate
Analgesic—Antipyretic—Antitussive—Decongestant—Antihistamine

McNeil Consumer Healthcare

Tylenol® Children's Cold & Cough Nighttime
acetaminophen—diphenhydramine HCl—dextromethorphan HBr
Analgesic—Antihistamine—Antitussive

McNeil Consumer Healthcare

Date of Revision: June 5, 2008

SUMMARY PRODUCT INFORMATION:

Route of Administration	Dosage Form/ Strength	Clinically Relevant Nonmedicinal Ingredients
Oral	Children's Decongestant Suspension/Per 5 mL: 160 mg acetaminophen and 15 mg pseudoephedrine HCl	Alcohol-, gluten-, lactose-, sucrose-, sulfite- and tartrazine-free For a complete listing of nonmedicinal ingredients, see Dosage Forms, Composition and Packaging.
	Children's Cold Suspension/Per 5 mL: 160 mg acetaminophen, 15 mg pseudoephedrine HCl and 1 mg chlorpheniramine maleate	Alcohol-, gluten-, lactose-, sucrose- and tartrazine-free For a complete listing of nonmedicinal ingredients, see Dosage Forms, Composition and Packaging.
	Children's Cough & Runny Nose Suspension/Per 5 mL: 160 mg acetaminophen, 5 mg dextromethorphan HBr, and 1 mg chlorpheniramine maleate	Alcohol-, gluten-, lactose-, sucrose-, sulfite- and tartrazine-free For a complete listing of nonmedicinal ingredients, see Dosage Forms, Composition and Packaging.
	Children's Cold & Cough Nighttime Suspension/Per 5 mL: 160 mg acetaminophen, 6.25 mg diphenhydramine HCl and 5 mg dextromethorphan HBr	Alcohol-, gluten-, lactose-, sucrose-, sulfite- and tartrazine-free For a complete listing of nonmedicinal ingredients, see Dosage Forms, Composition and Packaging.
	Children's Cold DM Suspension/Per 5 mL: 160 mg acetaminophen, 7.5 mg dextromethorphan HBr, 15 mg pseudoephedrine HCl and 1 mg chlorpheniramine maleate	Alcohol-, gluten-, lactose-, sucrose-and tartrazine-free For a complete listing of nonmedicinal ingredients, see Dosage Forms, Composition and Packaging.
	Children's Cold DM Tablets/80 mg acetaminophen, 3.75 mg dextromethorphan HBr, 7.5 mg pseudoephedrine HCl, 0.5 mg chlorpheniramine maleate	Gluten-, lactose-, sodium- and tartrazine-free For a complete listing of nonmedicinal ingredients, see Dosage Forms, Composition and Packaging.
	Junior Strength Cold DM Tablets/160 mg acetaminophen, 7.5 mg dextromethorphan HBr, 15 mg pseudoephedrine HCl and 1 mg chlorpheniramine maleate	Gluten-, lactose-, sodium- and tartrazine-free For a complete listing of nonmedicinal ingredients, see Dosage Forms, Composition and Packaging.

INDICATIONS AND CLINICAL USE: Children's TYLENOL Decongestant: For the temporary relief of earache pain, fever, other aches and pains and stuffy nose associated with colds and flu.

Children's TYLENOL Cough & Runny Nose: For the temporary relief of dry cough, sneezing, runny nose, fever, headache and sore throat pain due to common colds.

Children's TYLENOL Cold & Cough Nighttime: For the temporary relief of dry cough, sneezing, runny nose, fever, aches and pain, and sore throat pain due to common colds.

Children's and Junior Strength TYLENOL Cold DM: For the temporary relief of cough, stuffy nose, runny nose, sneezing, fever, headaches, aches and pain due to common colds, hayfever or other allergies.

CONTRAINDICATIONS: Hypersensitivity to acetaminophen, pressor amines or to the ingredients of this formulation (see Dosage Forms, Composition and Packaging). Allergic reactions (primarily skin rash) or reports of hypersensitivity secondary to acetaminophen are rare and generally are controlled by discontinuation of the drug and, when necessary, symptomatic treatment.

In patients receiving or having received MAO inhibitors in the preceding 2 weeks. Although pseudoephedrine is virtually without pressor effect in normotensive patients, it should be used with caution in hypertensives.

WARNINGS AND PRECAUTIONS: General: Children should not exceed 75 mg/kg of acetaminophen in 24 hours, never to exceed the maximum adult daily dose of 4000 mg, or use two or more acetaminophen-containing products together. This includes combination products that contain acetaminophen. Do not use with other products containing salicylates or any other pain or fever medicine.

Acetaminophen-containing products should be kept out of the reach of children.

Physicians should be cognizant of and supervise the use of acetaminophen in patients with chronic alcoholism, serious kidney or serious liver disease. Physicians should alert their patients who regularly consume large amounts of alcohol not to exceed the recommended doses of acetaminophen. Chronic heavy alcohol abusers may be at increased risk of liver toxicity from excessive doses of acetaminophen.

Patients should be counseled to consult a physician if redness or swelling is present in an area of pain, if symptoms do not improve or if they worsen, or if new symptoms such as high fever, rash, itching, excessive mucus, persistent or recurring cough or persistent headache occur, as these may be signs of a condition which requires medical attention.

Acetaminophen should not be taken for pain for more than 5 days, for fever for more than 3 days or if new symptoms appear, without consulting a physician.

In patients with high blood pressure, heart disease, diabetes, thyroid disease or who are taking a prescription drug for high blood pressure or depression, pseudoephedrine HCl should be used with caution and only under close medical supervision.

Patients with asthma, glaucoma, chronic pulmonary disease or shortness of breath should not use this medication unless directed by a physician. This product should not be used for persistent or chronic cough such as occurs with asthma unless directed by a physician.

Occupational Hazards: Preparations containing chlorpheniramine maleate or diphenhydramine HCl may cause drowsiness. Sedatives and tranquilizers may increase this effect and should be avoided. Advise caution when engaging in any activity requiring alertness. Patients taking tranquilizers or sedatives should not take this medication before consulting a physician.

Preparations may, in some cases, cause excitability or dizziness.

Hepatic/Biliary/Pancreatic: Slower metabolism of acetaminophen, increased activity of the cytochrome P450 enzyme system, or depleted glutathione stores are cited as theoretical risk factors for acetaminophen hepatotoxicity in patients with chronic liver disease. However, acetaminophen has been studied in both adults and children with a wide variety of liver diseases including various types of cirrhosis, hepatitis (including hepatitis C), nodular transformation, congenital hepatic fibrosis, and α1-antitrypsin deficiency. In none of these conditions is there evidence of an increased risk for hepatotoxicity at currently recommended acetaminophen doses but the studies were insufficiently powered to definitely establish the extent of risk.

Forrest compared acetaminophen metabolism following a single 1500 mg dose in normal subjects, patients with mild liver disease, and patients with severe liver disease. There were no significant differences in overall 24-hour urinary excretion of acetaminophen and glucuronide, sulfate, cysteine and mercapturic acid conjugates, evidence that acetaminophen metabolism was similar to that in normal subjects. However, the elimination half-life was significantly prolonged in patients with severe liver disease.

Acetaminophen has also been studied in pediatric patients with liver disease. Following a single (10 mg/kg) dose of acetaminophen, the pharmacokinetic profiles in pediatric patients with mild, moderate, or severe liver disease were not significantly different. Although the plasma half-life of acetaminophen was prolonged in patients with severe liver disease, there were no significant differences in the 36-hour (children) urinary excretion of acetaminophen or its conjugates.

Acetaminophen may cause hepatotoxicity in situations of intentional overdose (e.g. attempted suicide), unintentional overdose (e.g. overdosing when pain relief is not satisfactory), simultaneous use of multiple acetaminophen-containing preparations, accidental overdose or in very rare cases, after recommended doses, although causality has not been determined. The hepatotoxic reaction can be severe and life-threatening. Early symptoms following a hepatotoxic overdose may include nausea, vomiting, diaphoresis, lethargy, and general malaise. If appropriate treatment is not instituted, these may progress to upper quadrant pain, confusion, stupor, and sequelae of hepatic necrosis, such as jaundice, coagulation defects, hypoglycemia, and encephalopathy. Renal failure and cardiomyopathy may also occur. In the event of known or suspected overdosage, treatment with N-acetyl cysteine should be instituted immediately (see Overdosage), even when there are no obvious symptoms. Failure to promptly treat acetaminophen hepatotoxicity with N-acetyl cysteine can result in liver failure, leading to liver transplantation and/or death.

Chronic Alcohol Use: Excessive alcohol use may increase risk of liver toxicity from acetaminophen overdose (acute or chronic).

In prospective, placebo controlled studies, researchers evaluated an actively drinking group of alcoholics with a high prevalence of malnourishment. The study participants abruptly stopped their daily alcohol intake and took acetaminophen the next day. This should theoretically make them vulnerable to acetaminophen injury because their CYP2E1 would be maximally induced from the alcohol and there would be no alcohol present to compete with acetaminophen for metabolism by CYP2E1. There was no statistically significant difference in mean values for AST, ALT, or INR for alcoholics given four grams per day of acetaminophen compared to placebo. Additionally, the researchers performed an analysis of the malnourished patients that showed there was no increase in AST or ALT levels in these patients. Study limitations include a limited duration of 2 days and exclusion of patients with preexisting AST or ALT elevations greater than 120 U/L. Study results do not preclude the possibility of an idiosyncratic hepatic reaction.

Renal: Martin found that patients with chronic renal failure had higher plasma concentrations of acetaminophen and the inactive glucuronide and sulfate metabolites than healthy subjects during repeated dosing up to ten days.

Several single-dose studies demonstrate accumulation of acetaminophen metabolites in patients with moderate chronic renal failure and in anephric patients for whom hemodialysis appeared to be the major route of elimination.

The habitual consumption of acetaminophen should be discouraged. If indicated medically, the long-term use of acetaminophen should be supervised by a physician.

A National Kidney Foundation position paper notes that physicians preferentially recommend acetaminophen to patients with renal failure because of the bleeding complications associated with ASA in these individuals.

Special Populations: Glucose-6-Phosphate Dehydrogenase (G6PD) Deficiency: In therapeutic doses, acetaminophen does not shorten the lifespan of red blood cells and does not produce any clinically perceptible destruction of circulating red blood cells.

Obese Adults: O'Shea studied the pharmacokinetics of chlorzoxazone (a putative probe for CYP2E1 activity) to evaluate the effect of obesity on CYP2E1 activity. The authors concluded that CYP2E1 is induced in obese adults and that this could impact the metabolic pathway of a number of drugs metabolized by CYP2E1, including acetaminophen. However, acetaminophen pharmacokinetic data have been investigated in obese adults. In this prospective study, 650 mg acetaminophen was administered intravenously to obese men (297 lb), obese women (193 lb), control men (155 lb) and control women (121 lb). Acetaminophen distribution volume per total body weight was slightly lower in the obese adults but, more importantly, the half-life and metabolic clearance per total body weight did not differ among groups.

ADVERSE REACTIONS: Central Nervous System Effects: Acetaminophen at recommended doses has no obvious effects on central nervous system function. In an overdose situation, central nervous system effects are uncommon.

Chlorpheniramine maleate or diphenhydramine HCl may cause excitability, especially in infants and children.

Gastrointestinal Effects: Acetaminophen at recommended doses does not cause gastric irritation, gastric erosions, occult or overt gastrointestinal blood loss or ulcers.

Blot and McLaughlin conducted an independent analysis of case-control data from a study conducted by the American College of Gastroenterology. The risk of gastrointestinal bleeding increased two to three-fold among recent users of ASA, ibuprofen and other NSAIDs at OTC doses, and the risk was also dose-related. In contrast, the use of acetaminophen was not associated with an increased risk of gastrointestinal bleeding.

Hematologic Effects: Acetaminophen does not have any immediate or delayed effects on small vessel hemostasis, as measured by bleeding time. In normal volunteers receiving a single dose of acetaminophen (975 or 1950 mg) or multiple doses of acetaminophen (1950 mg daily for 6 weeks), no change in bleeding time or platelet aggregation was observed. In another study, a single 1000 mg dose of acetaminophen was given to normal volunteers and did not affect bleeding time or platelet aggregation. Patients with hemophilia receiving multiple doses of acetaminophen showed no significant changes in bleeding time.

Hematological reactions including thrombocytopenia, leucopenia, pancytopenia, neutropenia, and agranulocytosis have been reported, although these are rare and causality has not been established.

Hepatic Effects: As an illustration of the margin of safety of acetaminophen at supratherapeutic doses, a comparison of serum concentrations of acetaminophen over time for a standard 15 mg/kg dose and for a dose exceeding the standard by a multiple of 5 (75 mg/kg) are shown in Figure 1. The serum concentrations are drawn relative to the risk line for hepatotoxicity and treatment line of the Rumack-Matthew nomogram used to manage acute overdoses. The mean plasma concentrations for this supratherapeutic dose are well below the risk and treatment lines of the nomogram at all times. However, to minimize the risk for adverse effects, the maximum recommended dose should not be exceeded.

Acetaminophen in overdosage may cause hepatotoxicity. In adults and adolescents, hepatotoxicity may occur following ingestion of greater than 150 mg/kg over a period of 8 hours or less. Fatalities are infrequent (less than 3% to 4% of untreated cases in which blood levels exceed the treatment line) and have rarely been reported with overdoses less than 7.5 g. In children, amounts less than 150 mg/kg are unlikely to produce hepatotoxicity. In both adults and children, toxicity associated with acetaminophen is usually caused by ingestion of quantities of the drug that are significantly above the recommended dosage range. Hepatotoxicity, ranging from transient sharp transaminase elevations to fatal, fulminant hepatic failure, is the most common result of clinically significant overdosage.

In a double-blind, placebo-controlled clinical study, healthy adults were given 4, 6 and 8 g/d of acetaminophen over 3 days. Plasma concentrations did not accumulate with repeat doses. Clinically all doses were well tolerated by the subjects and aminotransferase values stayed within normal limits throughout the study. These data provide information related to the margin of safety but are not intended to support dosing beyond the maximum recommended dose of 4 g/day.

A report has suggested that hepatotoxicity following greater than the recommended dose of acetaminophen may be enhanced by both prolonged fasting and/or chronic alcohol abuse.

Figure 1: TYLENOL Children's

Mean Data for a Standard (1 g, 15 mg/kg) and Higher (5.6 g, 75 mg/kg) Dose Relative to Risk and Treatment Lines of the Acetaminophen Nomogram

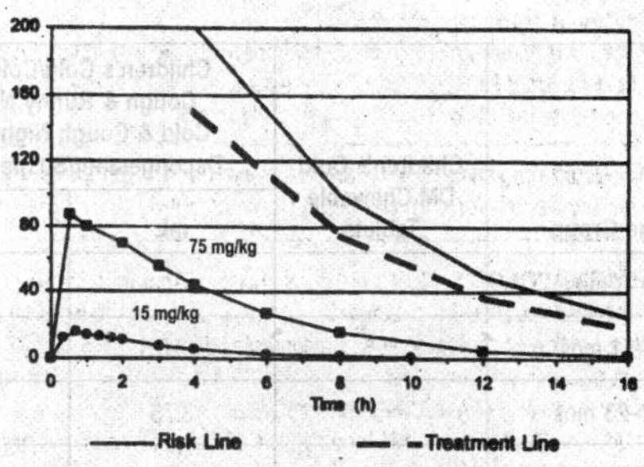

Acute Alcohol Use: Acute alcohol ingestion refers to the occasional or intermittent use of alcohol. When taken together, alcohol competes with acetaminophen for CYP2E1. CYP2E1 accepts alcohol more readily than acetaminophen; therefore, less NAPQI is produced. In the presence of alcohol, acetaminophen may be diverted to the glucuronidation and sulfation pathways. The overall result is that a smaller percentage of acetaminophen may be expected to be metabolized to the toxic intermediate, NAPQI, than would otherwise be the case. NAPQI production is increased above baseline for the period up to 18-24 hours post ethanol clearance from the body. In healthy adults, at normal labeled doses of acetaminophen, the temporary increase in NAPQI production is more than accommodated by normal glutathione stores in the liver.

Hypersensitivity: Sensitivity reactions are rare and may manifest as rash, urticaria, dyspnea, hypotension, laryngeal edema, angioedema, bronchospasm, or anaphylaxis. Cross-reactivity in ASA-sensitive persons has been rarely reported. If sensitivity is suspected, discontinue use of the drug.

Renal Effects: Acute nephrotoxicity has been reported following massive overdose either as a sequela of hepatic failure or, occasionally, in the absence of hepatic failure.

Clinical data have established that acetaminophen in recommended doses is not nephrotoxic.

Some studies suggest an association between the chronic long-term use of acetaminophen and renal effects. Results, however, are conflicting, limited by recall bias and confounded by the inability to determine whether analgesic use preceded or followed the onset of renal disease.

Case control studies have suggested a weak association between habitual acetaminophen use and prevalence of chronic renal failure and end stage renal disease. This National Kidney Foundation position paper concludes that acetaminophen has been preferentially recommended by physicians to patients with renal failure and that there is no evidence that occasional use of acetaminophen caused renal injury.

Special Populations: Pediatrics: Lesko and Mitchell enrolled more than 84 000 febrile children in a randomized, double blind, acetaminophen-controlled trial to assess the risks of rare but serious adverse events following use of pediatric ibuprofen. Of the children included in the analysis, 28 130 received acetaminophen and none experienced anaphylaxis, or serious hepatic, gastrointestinal or renal effects.

DRUG INTERACTIONS: Alcohol: Studies evaluating the metabolism of doses up to 20 mg/kg of acetaminophen in chronic alcohol abusers and a study evaluating the effects of 2 days of acetaminophen dosing at 4000 mg/day in chronic alcoholics undergoing detoxification, have yielded inconsistent results with regard to effects on acetaminophen pharmacokinetics and demonstrate no evidence of adverse effect on liver function tests.

Anticoagulants–Oral: Patients who concomitantly medicate with warfarin-type anticoagulants and regular doses of acetaminophen have occasionally been reported to have unforeseen elevations in their INR. Physicians should be cognizant of this potential interaction and monitor the INR in such patients closely while therapy is established. Many factors, including diet, medications, and environmental and physical states, may affect how a patient responds to anticoagulant therapy. There have been several reports that suggest that acetaminophen may produce hypoprothrombinemia (elevated international normalized ratio [INR] or prothrombin time) when administered with coumarin derivatives. In other studies, prothrombin time did not change. Reported changes have been generally of limited clinical significance, however, periodic evaluation of prothrombin time should be performed when these agents are administered concurrently.

In the period immediately following discharge from the hospital or whenever other medications are initiated, discontinued, or taken regularly, it is important to monitor patient response to anticoagulation therapy with additional prothrombin time or INR determinations. Despite the potential for interaction, acetaminophen is the least likely OTC analgesic to interfere with anticoagulant therapy.

Anticonvulsants: Some reports have suggested that patients taking long-term anticonvulsants, who overdose on acetaminophen, may be at increased risk of hepatotoxicity because of accelerated metabolism of acetaminophen. Available data are conflicting. A 7-year retrospective study of acetaminophen overdose admissions indicates that the overall mortality rate was not significantly different for patients taking concomitant anticonvulsant medications.

Hydantoins: Pharmacokinetic studies indicate that phenytoin primarily induces the glucuronidation pathway, whereas glutathione-derived metabolites are not increased in patients on chronic phenytoin therapy. Additionally, recent data demonstrate that phenytoin is metabolized primarily by CYP2C9 and CYP2C19, whereas acetaminophen is primarily metabolized by CYP2E1.

Carbamazepine: Carbamazepine is primarily metabolized by CYP3A4, whereas acetaminophen is metabolized primarily via CYP2E1. It is not known whether there is increased risk from an acetaminophen overdose in patients on chronic carbamazepine therapy.

Diflunisal: Professional literature from the manufacturer of diflunisal cautions that concomitant administration with acetaminophen produces an approximate 50% increase in plasma levels of acetaminophen in normal volunteers. Acetaminophen had no effect on diflunisal plasma levels. The clinical significance of these findings has not been established. However, caution should be used with concomitant administration of diflunisal and acetaminophen and patients should be monitored carefully.

Isoniazid: Some reports suggest that patients on chronic isoniazid therapy may be at risk for developing hepatotoxicity from an acetaminophen overdose. Since patients on isoniazid therapy may develop hepatic effects from isoniazid alone, data from individual case reports are unclear as to whether chronic administration of isoniazid may increase the risk of acetaminophen toxicity. Isoniazid is primarily metabolized by CYP2E1 and induces CYP2E1. Studies in healthy subjects demonstrate that isoniazid blocks the formation of the toxic metabolite NAPQI when administered concomitantly with acetaminophen, but increase NAPQI formation when acetaminophen is administered one day after discontinuation of isoniazid. Thus, concomitant use of isoniazid is unlikely to potentiate the risk of acetaminophen-induced hepatotoxicity at recommended doses. The isoniazid induction of CYP2E1 is short-lived, lasting only 12 to 48 hours after the discontinuation of isoniazid; it is during this period the toxicity of an acetaminophen overdose may be potentiated.

DOSAGE AND ADMINISTRATION: Children's and Junior Strength Cold DM, Children's Decongestant: Single dosage (see Table 1) may be repeated every 4 to 6 hours, as required, not to exceed 4 doses in 24 hours. (Note: For Children's Tylenol Cough & Runny Nose and Children's Cold & Cough Nighttime do not exceed 5 doses in 24 hours.) Whenever possible, use weight to dose; otherwise, use age. Parents should be counseled to discontinue use and consult a doctor to re-evaluate the dosage if child becomes nervous, dizzy or cannot sleep. Children's suspensions: Dose with dosage cup or measured teaspoon only.

OVERDOSAGE:

Symptoms and Treatment: Acetaminophen: Typical Toxidrome: Hepatic injury is the principal toxic effect of a substantial acetaminophen overdose. The physician should be mindful that there is no early presentation that is pathognomonic for the overdose. A high degree of clinical suspicion must always be maintained.

Untreated acetaminophen overdoses may produce hepatotoxicity. Acetaminophen hepatotoxicity occurs as a threshold effect and is characterized by a lack of toxicity at lower/therapeutic doses. Acetaminophen hepatotoxicity occurs after major depletion of glutathione, an endogenous detoxifying substance. Once the threshold is exceeded, increasing acetaminophen doses may produce increasing degrees of hepatotoxicity, unless N-acetylcysteine (NAC) is administered. Situations in which acetaminophen overdose and resultant hepatotoxicity may occur include acute intentional overdose and repeated supratherapeutic overdose in adults and acute accidental ingestion or overdose and repeated supratherapeutic overdose in children.

Table 1: TYLENOL Children's Dosage in Children

Weight (kg)	Age Group	Children's Cold DM Chewable Tablets	Children's Cold/Cold DM/ Cough & Runny Nose/ Cold & Cough Nighttime/ Decongestant/Suspensions		Junior Strength Cold DM Chewable Tablets
			mL	tsp	
2.5–5.4	0–3 mos				
5.5–7.9	4–11 mos	—[a]	2.5	½	—[a]
8–10.9	12–23 mos	—[a]	3.75	¾	—[a]
11–15.9	2–3 yrs	2	5	1	1
16–21.9	4–5 yrs	3	7.5	1½	1½
22–26.9	6–8 yrs	4	10	2	2
27–31.9	9–10 yrs	5	12.5	2½	2½
32–43.9	11–12 yrs		15	3	3

[a] Cold DM solid dosage forms may not be suitable for children under 2 years of age.

The clinical course of acetaminophen overdose generally occurs in a three-phase sequential pattern. The first phase begins shortly after ingestion and lasts for 12 to 24 hours. The patient may manifest signs of gastrointestinal irritability, nausea, vomiting, anorexia, diaphoresis, pallor and general malaise. If toxicity continues, there is a latent phase of up to 48 hours. During this second phase, initial symptoms abate and the patient may feel better. However, hepatic enzymes, bilirubin, and prothrombin time or INR values will progressively rise. Right upper quadrant pain may develop as the liver becomes enlarged and tender. Most patients do not progress beyond this phase, especially if given N-acetylcysteine (NAC) treatment early in the course. Signs and symptoms of the third phase depend on the severity of hepatic damage and usually occur from three to five days following overdose ingestion. Symptoms may be limited to anorexia, nausea, general malaise, and abdominal pain in less severe cases or may progress to confusion, stupor and sequelae of hepatic necrosis including jaundice, coagulation defects, hypoglycemia, and encephalopathy, as well as renal failure and cardiomyopathy. Death, if it occurs, is generally the result of complications associated with fulminant hepatic failure. Mortality rates in patients with toxic plasma levels who do not receive antidote therapy range from 3% to 4%.

Due to the wide availability of acetaminophen, it is commonly involved in single and mixed drug overdose situations and the practitioner should screen for its presence in a patient's serum. Acute toxicity after single dose overdoses of acetaminophen can be anticipated when the overdose exceeds 150 mg/kg. Chronic alcohol abusers, cachectic individuals, and persons taking pharmacologic inducers of the hepatic P450 microsomal enzyme system may be at risk with lower exposures.

Specific Antidote: Any individual presenting with a possible acetaminophen overdose should be treated with N-acetylcysteine (NAC), even if the amount of acetaminophen ingested is unknown or questionable. A blood sample for determination of the plasma acetaminophen concentration should be obtained as early as possible, but no sooner than four hours following ingestion. Do not await the results of assays for plasma acetaminophen levels before initiating treatment NAC. If the acetaminophen plasma level is found to plot above the treatment line on the acetaminophen overdose nomogram, NAC treatment should be continued for a full course of therapy. NAC is used clinically to treat acute acetaminophen overdose, and acts by interacting with the oxidative intermediate, NAPQI. NAC administered by either the i.v. or the oral route is known to be a highly effective antidote for acetaminophen poisoning. It is most effective when administered within 8 hours of a significant overdose but reports have indicated benefits to treatment initiated well beyond this time period. It is imperative to administer the antidote as early as possible in the time course of acute intoxication to reap the full benefits of the antidote's protective effects. For full prescribing information, consult the product monograph for NAC.

General Management: When the possibility of acetaminophen overdose exists, treatment should begin immediately and include appropriate decontamination of the gastrointestinal tract, proper supportive care, careful assessment of appropriately timed serum acetaminophen estimations evaluated against the Rumack-Matthew nomogram, timely administration of NAC as required and appropriate follow-up care. Liver function tests should be performed initially and repeated at 24-hour intervals.

Pseudoephedrine HCl: Typical Toxidrome: sympathomimetic/stimulant.

Specific Antidote: none.

General Management: Stabilize the patient (A, B, Cs), undertake appropriate gastrointestinal tract decontamination procedures, initiate supportive care, consult with a Regional Poison Control Centre regarding ongoing management, and arrange for appropriate follow-up care.

Dextromethorphan HBr: Typical Toxidrome: narcotic/opiate.

Specific Antidote: naloxone HCl.

General Management: Stabilize the patient (A, B, Cs), undertake appropriate gastrointestinal tract decontamination procedures, initiate supportive care, consult with a Regional Poison Control Centre regarding ongoing management, and arrange for appropriate follow-up care.

Chlorpheniramine Maleate or Diphenhydramine HCl: Typical Toxidrome: anticholinergic, CNS depressant (adult), CNS stimulant (child).

Specific Antidote: none.

General Management: Stabilize the patient (A, B, Cs), undertake appropriate gastrointestinal tract decontamination procedures, initiate supportive care, consult with a Regional Poison Control Centre regarding ongoing management, and arrange for appropriate follow-up care.

> For management of a suspected drug overdose, CPhA recommends that you contact your **regional Poison Control Centre**. See the *CPS* Directory section for a list of Poison Control Centres.

ACTION AND CLINICAL PHARMACOLOGY: Mechanism of Action: Acetaminophen is a centrally acting analgesic and antipyretic drug. Although the precise mechanism of action is not totally understood, work by Boutaud suggests acetaminophen is an inhibitor of the peroxidase portion of cyclooxygenase (prostaglandin H synthase inhibitor). Depending on the redox state and substrate concentrations surrounding the enzymes, acetaminophen may or may not have a significant inhibitory effect. This accounts for its selective activity on pain and fever with little anti-inflammatory effect.

It is postulated that the analgesic effect is produced by elevation of the pain threshold and the antipyretic effect is produced through action on the hypothalamic heat-regulating centre.

The optimal effective analgesic dose of acetaminophen was demonstrated in dental pain studies and is 1000 mg every four to six hours, up to 4000 mg daily. At least 500 published and unpublished controlled clinical trials in adults and children have evaluated acetaminophen for the relief of pain or fever. These studies include single and multiple dose treatments. Most studies were less than 14 days in duration, although the longest study duration was two years. No significant safety issues were reported in any of these studies.

Moreover, at recommended doses, acetaminophen has not been shown to increase the risk of developing renal diseases or upper gastrointestinal ulceration/bleeding. This observation is consistent with its minimal inhibitory effect on peripheral prostaglandin synthesis and on gastric prostaglandin synthesis.

* Container provided with a child-resistant closure.

Acetaminophen is considered equipotent to ASA and ibuprofen, within the recommended OTC dosing ranges, in its analgesic and antipyretic effects. Acetaminophen at recommended doses does not cause the type of gastrointestinal complications associated with NSAID-containing products, such as gastric irritation, gastric erosions, occult or overt gastrointestinal blood loss, or ulcers. Unlike these drugs, however, it has no anti-inflammatory effect at clinically relevant doses in humans.

Pharmacokinetics: Absorption: Oral acetaminophen is rapidly and almost completely absorbed from the gastrointestinal tract primarily in the small intestine. This absorption process occurs by passive transport. Peak plasma concentrations occur within 0.4 to 1 hour depending on the product formulation. Although high-fat foods delay the time to peak concentration for up to an hour, the dose is completely absorbed.

Distribution: Acetaminophen is uniformly distributed throughout most body fluids, but not in fatty tissue. As a result, the volume of distribution in adults ranges between 0.8 and 1.0 L/kg. Since acetaminophen has low protein binding in plasma of only 10% to 25%, it does not compete with drugs that are highly protein bound.

Metabolism: Acetaminophen is primarily metabolized by the liver via three principal separate pathways: conjugation with glucuronide; conjugation with sulfate; oxidation via the cytochrome P450 mixed function oxidase system.

Both the glucuronic and oxidative pathways adhere to a first-order rate process, which means the concentration of acetaminophen metabolized increases as the concentration in the liver increases. The sulfate pathway adheres to Michaelis-Menten kinetics, which means the concentration of acetaminophen metabolized remains constant once the concentration in the liver increases above a saturation level. A schematic of acetaminophen metabolism is shown in Figure 2.

The major metabolic pathway is glucuronidation, where 47% to 62% of the acetaminophen dose conjugates with glucuronide. These glucuronide conjugates are inactive and nontoxic, and are secreted in bile and eliminated in the urine.

The second major pathway is sulfation, where 25% to 36% of the dose conjugates with sulfate. These sulfate ester conjugates are also inactive and nontoxic and are excreted in the urine.

The third pathway is oxidation, where 5% to 8% of the dose is metabolized via the cytochrome P450 enzyme system. The cytochrome P450 isoenzyme that is primarily responsible is CYP2E1. When acetaminophen is metabolized by CYP2E1, it forms a highly reactive intermediate, N-acetyl-p-benzoquinoneimine (NAPQI). Since NAPQI is highly reactive, it cannot be measured outside the liver nor can it accumulate. This intermediate is rapidly inactivated by hepatocellular stores of glutathione to form cysteine and mercapturate conjugates, which are both inactive and nontoxic. These conjugates are excreted in the urine.

Figure 2: TYLENOL Children's Acetaminophen Metabolism

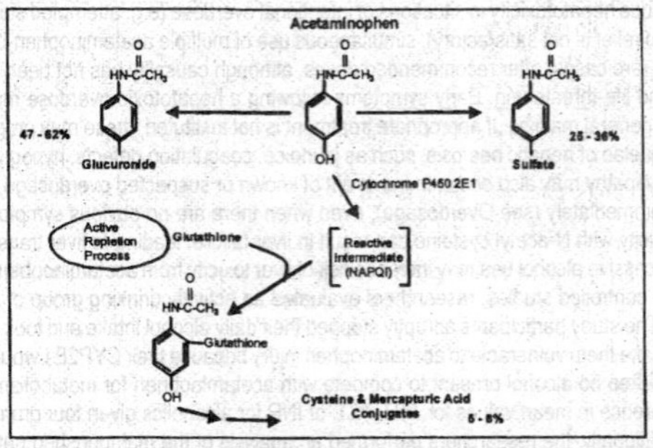

Excretion: Acetaminophen undergoes first-order elimination from the body, and has a short plasma half-life that ranges from 2 to 3 hours in healthy young and elderly adults and from 1.5 to 2.9 hours in children. Since acetaminophen clears rapidly from the body, repeated doses do not lead to accumulation of acetaminophen plasma concentrations.

DOSAGE FORMS, COMPOSITION AND PACKAGING: Children's Decongestant Suspension (bubblegum): Each 5 mL contains: acetaminophen 160 mg and pseudoephedrine HCl 15 mg in a red, bubblegum-flavoured liquid. Nonmedicinal ingredients: butylparaben, carboxymethylcellulose sodium, cellulose, citric acid, corn syrup, FD&C Red no. 40, flavour, glycerin, propylene glycol, purified water, sodium benzoate, sorbitol and xanthan gum. Energy: 76.6 kJ (18.3 kcal)/5 mL. Sodium: 1.6 mg/5 mL. Alcohol-, gluten-, lactose-, sucrose-, sulfite- and tartrazine-free. Plastic bottles of 100 mL*.

Children's Cold Suspension (bubblegum): Each 5 mL contains: acetaminophen 160 mg, chlorpheniramine maleate 1 mg and pseudoephedrine HCl 15 mg in a pink, bubblegum-flavoured vehicle. Nonmedicinal ingredients: butylparaben, carboxymethylcellulose sodium, cellulose, citric acid, corn syrup, FD&C Red no. 40, flavour, glycerin, polysorbate 60, propylene glycol, purified water, sodium benzoate, sorbitol and xanthan gum. Energy: 76.6 kJ (18.3 kcal)/5 mL. Sodium: 1.6 mg/5 mL. Alcohol-, gluten-, lactose-, sucrose- and tartrazine-free. Plastic bottles of 100 mL*.

Children's Cough and Runny Nose Suspension (cherry blast): Each 5 mL contains: acetaminophen 160 mg, dextromethorphan HBr 5 mg and chlorpheniramine maleate 1 mg in a cherry-red, fruit-flavoured suspension. Nonmedicinal ingredients: acesulfame potassium, carboxymethylcellulose sodium, cellulose, citric acid, corn syrup, D&C Red no. 33, FD&C Red no. 40, flavour, glycerin, purified water, sodium benzoate, sorbitol and xanthan gum. Alcohol-, gluten-, lactose-, sucrose-, sulfite- and tartrazine-free. Plastic bottles of 100 mL*.

Children's Cold and Cough Nighttime Suspension (soothing apple): Each 5 mL contains: acetaminophen 160 mg, diphenhydramine HCl 6.25 mg and dextromethorphan HBr 5 mg in a light green, apple-flavoured suspension. Nonmedicinal ingredients: carboxymethylcellulose sodium, cellulose, citric acid, corn syrup, D&C Yellow no. 10, FD&C Blue no. 1, flavour, glycerin, polysorbate 60, propylene glycol, purified water, sodium benzoate, sorbitol and xanthan gum. Alcohol-, gluten-, lactose-, sucrose-, sulfite- and tartrazine-free. Plastic bottles of 100 mL*.

Children's Cold DM Suspension (bubblegum): Each 5 mL contains: acetaminophen 160 mg, chlorpheniramine maleate 1 mg, pseudoephedrine HCl 15 mg and dextromethorphan HBr 7.5 mg in a pink, bubblegum-flavoured vehicle. Nonmedicinal ingredients: butylparaben, carboxymethylcellulose sodium, cellulose, citric acid, corn syrup, FD&C Red no. 40, flavour, glycerin, polysorbate 60, propylene glycol, purified water, sodium benzoate, sorbitol and xanthan gum. Energy: 76.6 kJ (18.3 kcal)/5 mL. Sodium: 1.6 mg/5 mL. Alcohol-, gluten-, lactose-, sucrose- and tartrazine-free. Plastic bottles of 100 mL*.

Children's Cold DM Tablets (bubblegum): Each pink, chewable tablet, engraved "TYLENOL COLD DM" on one side and "80" with a partial score on the other side, contains: acetaminophen 80 mg, chlorpheniramine maleate 0.5 mg, pseudoephedrine HCl 7.5 mg and dextromethorphan HBr 3.75 mg. Nonmedicinal ingredients: cellulose, corn starch, D&C Red no. 7, ethylcellulose, flavour, magnesium stearate, magnesium trisilicate, mannitol, sucralose and sucrose. Energy: 5.9 kJ (1.4 kcal). Sodium: 0 mg. Gluten-, lactose-, sodium- and tartrazine-free. Plastic bottles of 24*.

Junior Strength Cold DM Tablets (grape): Each round, purple tablet, engraved "TCM DM" on one side and "160" with a partial score on the other side, contains: acetaminophen 160 mg, chlorpheniramine maleate 1 mg, pseudoephedrine HCl 15 mg and dextromethorphan HBr 7.5 mg. Phenylketonurics: contains phenylalanine (aspartame). Nonmedicinal ingredients: aspartame, cellulose, citric acid, corn starch, D&C Red no. 7, ethylcellulose, FD&C Blue no. 1, flavour, magnesium stearate, magnesium trisilicate and mannitol. Energy: 8.4 kJ (2.0 kcal). Sodium: 0 mg. Gluten-, lactose-, sodium- and tartrazine-free. Plastic bottles of 20*.

All packages are safety sealed.

Tylenol® Cold Extra Strength Daytime

acetaminophen—dextromethorphan HBr—phenylephrine HCl

Analgesic—Antipyretic—Antitussive—Decongestant

McNeil Consumer Healthcare

Tylenol® Cold Extra Strength Nighttime

acetaminophen—dextromethorphan HBr—phenylephrine HCl—chlorpheniramine maleate

Analgesic—Antipyretic—Antitussive—Decongestant—Antihistamine

McNeil Consumer Healthcare

Tylenol® Cold Regular Strength Daytime

acetaminophen—dextromethorphan HBr—phenylephrine HCl

Analgesic—Antipyretic—Antitussive—Decongestant

McNeil Consumer Healthcare

Tylenol® Cold Regular Strength Nighttime

acetaminophen—dextromethorphan HBr—phenylephrine HCl—chlorpheniramine maleate

Analgesic—Antipyretic—Antitussive—Decongestant—Antihistamine

McNeil Consumer Healthcare

Date of Revision: October 30, 2009

SUMMARY PRODUCT INFORMATION:

Route of Administration	Dosage Form/ Strength	Clinically Relevant Nonmedicinal Ingredients
Oral	Extra Strength Daytime Tablet/500 mg acetaminophen, 10 mg dextromethorphan HBr and 5 mg phenylephrine HCl	Alcohol-, gluten-, lactose-, sulfite- and tartrazine-free For a complete listing of nonmedicinal ingredients, see Dosage Forms, Composition and Packaging.
	Extra Strength Nighttime Tablet/500 mg acetaminophen, 10 mg dextromethorphan HBr, 5 mg phenylephrine HCl and 2 mg chlorpheniramine maleate	Alcohol-, gluten-, lactose-, sulfite- and tartrazine-free For a complete listing of nonmedicinal ingredients, see Dosage Forms, Composition and Packaging.
	Regular Strength Daytime Caplet/ 325 mg acetaminophen, 10 mg dextromethorphan HBr and 5 mg phenylephrine HCl	Alcohol-, gluten-, lactose-, sulfite- and tartrazine-free For a complete listing of nonmedicinal ingredients, see Dosage Forms, Composition and Packaging.
	Regular Strength Nighttime Caplet/ 325 mg acetaminophen, 10 mg dextromethorphan HBr, 5 mg phenylephrine HCl and 2 mg chlorpheniramine maleate	Alcohol-, gluten-, lactose-, sulfite- and tartrazine-free For a complete listing of nonmedicinal ingredients, see Dosage Forms, Composition and Packaging.

INDICATIONS AND CLINICAL USE: Extra Strength and Regular Strength TYLENOL Cold Daytime: A non-drowsy formulation for the effective relief of nasal congestion, dry cough, fever, aches and pain due to common colds and other upper respiratory tract infections.

Extra Strength and Regular Strength TYLENOL Cold Nighttime: For the effective relief of nasal congestion, dry cough, fever, runny nose, sneezing, aches and pain due to common colds and other upper respiratory tract infections.

CONTRAINDICATIONS: Hypersensitivity to acetaminophen, pressor amines or to the ingredients of this formulation (see Dosage Forms, Composition and Packaging). Allergic reactions (primarily skin rash) or reports of hypersensitivity secondary to acetaminophen are rare and generally are controlled by discontinuation of the drug and, when necessary, symptomatic treatment.

In patients receiving or having received MAO inhibitors in the preceding 2 weeks. Although phenylephrine is virtually without pressor effect in normotensive patients, it should be used with caution in hypertensives.

WARNINGS AND PRECAUTIONS: General: Consumers should not exceed 4 g/day of acetaminophen or use two or more acetaminophen-containing products together. This includes combination products that contain acetaminophen. Do not use with other products containing salicylates or any other pain or fever medicine.

Acetaminophen-containing products should be kept out of the reach of children.

Physicians should be cognizant of and supervise the use of acetaminophen in patients with chronic alcoholism, serious kidney or serious liver disease. Physicians should alert their patients who regularly consume large amounts of alcohol not to exceed the recommended doses of acetaminophen. Chronic heavy alcohol abusers may be at increased risk of liver toxicity from excessive doses of acetaminophen.

Patients should be counseled to consult a physician if redness or swelling is present in an area of pain, if symptoms do not improve or if they worsen, or if new symptoms such as high fever, rash, itching, excessive mucus, persistent or recurring cough or persistent headache occur, as these may be signs of a condition which requires medical attention.

Acetaminophen should not be taken for pain for more than 5 days, for fever for more than 3 days or if new symptoms appear, without consulting a physician.

In patients with high blood pressure, heart disease, diabetes, thyroid disease, difficulty in urination due to enlargement of the prostate gland or who are taking a prescription drug for high blood pressure or depression, phenylephrine HCl should be used with caution and only under close medical supervision.

Patients with asthma, glaucoma, emphysema, chronic pulmonary disease or shortness of breath should not use this medication unless directed by a physician. This product should not be used for persistent or chronic cough such as occurs with smoking, asthma or emphysema unless directed by a physician.

Occupational Hazards: Preparations containing chlorpheniramine maleate may cause drowsiness. Alcoholic beverages, sedatives and tranquilizers may increase this effect and should be avoided. Advise caution when driving a motor vehicle or operating machinery or engaging in any activity requiring alertness. Patients taking tranquilizers or sedatives should not take this medication before consulting a physician.

Hepatic/Biliary/Pancreatic: Slower metabolism of acetaminophen, increased activity of the cytochrome P450 enzyme system, or depleted glutathione stores are cited as theoretical risk factors for acetaminophen hepatotoxicity in patients with chronic liver disease. However, acetaminophen has been studied in both adults and children with a wide variety of liver diseases including various types of cirrhosis, hepatitis (including hepatitis C), nodular transformation, congenital hepatic fibrosis, and α1-antitrypsin deficiency. In none of these conditions is there evidence of an increased risk for hepatotoxicity at currently recommended acetaminophen doses but the studies were insufficiently powered to definitely establish the extent of risk.

Forrest compared acetaminophen metabolism following a single 1500 mg dose in normal subjects, patients with mild liver disease, and patients with severe liver disease. There were no significant differences in overall 24-hour urinary excretion of acetaminophen and glucuronide, sulfate, cysteine, and mercapturic acid conjugates, evidence that acetaminophen metabolism was similar to that in normal subjects. However, the elimination half-life was significantly prolonged in patients with severe liver disease.

Acetaminophen has also been studied in pediatric patients with liver disease. Following a single (10 mg/kg) dose of acetaminophen, the pharmacokinetic profiles in pediatric patients with mild, moderate, or severe liver disease were not significantly different. Although the plasma half-life of acetaminophen was prolonged in patients with severe liver disease, there were no significant differences in the 36-hour (children) urinary excretion of acetaminophen or its conjugates.

Acetaminophen may cause hepatotoxicity in situations of intentional overdose (e.g. attempted suicide), unintentional overdose (e.g. overdosing when pain relief is not satisfactory), simultaneous use of multiple acetaminophen-containing preparations, accidental overdose or in very rare cases, after recommended doses, although causality has not been determined. The hepatotoxic reaction can be severe and life-threatening. Early symptoms following a hepatotoxic overdose may include nausea, vomiting, diaphoresis, lethargy, and general malaise. If appropriate treatment is not instituted, these may progress to upper quadrant pain, confusion, stupor, and sequelae of hepatic necrosis, such as jaundice, coagulation defects, hypoglycemia, and encephalopathy. Renal failure and cardiomyopathy may also occur. In the event of known or suspected overdosage, treatment with N-acetyl cysteine should be instituted immediately (see Overdosage), even when there are no obvious symptoms. Failure to promptly treat acetaminophen hepatotoxicity with N-acetyl cysteine can result in liver failure, leading to liver transplantation and/or death.

Chronic Alcohol Use: Excessive alcohol use may increase risk of liver toxicity from acetaminophen overdose (acute or chronic).

In prospective, placebo controlled studies, researchers evaluated an actively drinking group of alcoholics with a high prevalence of malnourishment. The study participants abruptly stopped their daily alcohol intake and took acetaminophen the next day. This should theoretically make them vulnerable to acetaminophen injury because their CYP2E1 would be maximally induced from the alcohol and there would be no alcohol present to compete with acetaminophen for metabolism by CYP2E1. There was no statistically significant difference in mean values for AST, ALT, or INR for alcoholics given four grams per day of acetaminophen compared to placebo. Additionally, the researchers performed an analysis of the malnourished patients that showed there was no increase in AST or ALT levels in these patients. Study limitations include a limited duration of 2 days and exclusion of patients with preexisting AST or ALT elevations greater than 120 U/L. Study results do not preclude the possibility of an idiosyncratic hepatic reaction.

Renal: Martin found that patients with chronic renal failure had higher plasma concentrations of acetaminophen and the inactive glucuronide and sulfate metabolites than healthy subjects during repeated dosing up to ten days.

Several single-dose studies demonstrate accumulation of acetaminophen metabolites in patients with moderate chronic renal failure and in anephric patients for whom hemodialysis appeared to be the major route of elimination.

The habitual consumption of acetaminophen should be discouraged. If indicated medically, the long-term use of acetaminophen should be supervised by a physician.

A National Kidney Foundation position paper notes that physicians preferentially recommend acetaminophen to patients with renal failure because of the bleeding complications associated with ASA in these individuals.

Special Populations: Geriatrics: In a comprehensive metabolic study by Miners, the formation and clearance of glucuronide and glutathione conjugates were the same in young and elderly adults, although clearance of the sulphate conjugate and unchanged acetaminophen were reduced. This finding provides prospective scientific data that the amount of acetaminophen metabolized via the oxidative pathway, from which the highly reactive intermediate, NAPQI, is generated, does not increase with age. Recently, Bannwarth evaluated the multiple-dose pharmacokinetics of acetaminophen in elderly patients. After seven days of repeat dosing, acetaminophen did not accumulate in the plasma, and the elimination half-life was the same as that reported for young adults.

Elderly patients who require therapy for longer than 5 days should consult their physician for condition monitoring.

Glucose-6-Phosphate Dehydrogenase (G6PD) Deficiency: In therapeutic doses, acetaminophen does not shorten the life-span of red blood cells and does not produce any clinically perceptible destruction of circulating red blood cells.

Obese Adults: O'Shea studied the pharmacokinetics of chlorzoxazone (a putative probe for CYP2E1 activity) to evaluate the effect of obesity on CYP2E1 activity. The authors concluded that CYP2E1 is induced in obese adults and that this could impact the metabolic pathway of a number of drugs metabolized by CYP2E1, including acetaminophen. However, acetaminophen pharmacokinetic data have been investigated in obese adults. In this prospective study, 650 mg acetaminophen was administered intravenously to obese men (297 lb), obese women (193 lb), control men (155 lb) and control women (121 lb). Acetaminophen distribution volume per total body weight was slightly lower in the obese adults but, more importantly, the half-life and metabolic clearance per total body weight did not differ among groups.

ADVERSE REACTIONS: Central Nervous System Effects: Acetaminophen at recommended doses has no obvious effects on central nervous system function. In an overdose situation, central nervous system effects are uncommon.

Chlorpheniramine maleate may cause excitability, especially in children.

Gastrointestinal Effects: Acetaminophen at recommended doses does not cause gastric irritation, gastric erosions, occult or overt gastrointestinal blood loss or ulcers

Blot and McLaughlin conducted an independent analysis of case-control data from a study conducted by the American College of Gastroenterology. The risk of gastrointestinal bleeding increased two to three-fold among recent users of ASA, ibuprofen and other NSAIDs at OTC doses, and the risk was also dose-related. In contrast, the use of acetaminophen was not associated with an increased risk of gastrointestinal bleeding.

Hematologic Effects: Acetaminophen does not have any immediate or delayed effects on small vessel hemostasis, as measured by bleeding time. In normal volunteers receiving a single dose of acetaminophen (975 or 1950 mg) or multiple doses of acetaminophen (1950 mg daily for 6 weeks), no change in bleeding time or platelet aggregation was observed. In another study, a single 1000 mg dose of acetaminophen was given to normal volunteers and did not affect bleeding time or platelet aggregation. Patients with hemophilia receiving multiple doses of acetaminophen showed no significant changes in bleeding time.

Haematological reactions including thrombocytopenia, leucopenia, pancytopenia, neutropenia, and agranulocytosis have been reported, although these are rare and causality has not been established.

Hepatic Effects: As an illustration of the margin of safety of acetaminophen at supratherapeutic doses, a comparison of serum concentrations of acetaminophen over time for a standard 15 mg/kg dose and for a dose exceeding the standard by a multiple of 5 (75 mg/kg) are shown in Figure 1. The serum concentrations are drawn relative to the risk line for hepatotoxicity and treatment line of the Rumack-Matthew nomogram used to manage acute overdoses. The mean plasma concentrations for this supratherapeutic dose are well below the risk and treatment lines of the nomogram at all times. However, to minimize the risk for adverse effects, the maximum recommended dose should not be exceeded.

Acetaminophen in overdosage may cause hepatotoxicity. In adults and adolescents, hepatotoxicity may occur following ingestion of greater than 150 mg/kg over a period of 8 hours or less. Fatalities are infrequent (less than 3% to 4% of untreated cases in which blood levels exceed the treatment line) and have rarely been reported with overdoses less than 7.5 g. In children, amounts less than 150 mg/kg are unlikely to produce hepatotoxicity. In both adults and children, toxicity associated with acetaminophen is usually caused by ingestion of quantities of the drug that are significantly above the recommended dosage range. Hepatotoxicity, ranging from transient sharp transaminase elevations to fatal, fulminant hepatic failure, is the most common result of clinically significant overdosage.

In a double-blind, placebo-controlled clinical study, healthy adults were given 4, 6 and 8 g/day of acetaminophen over 3 days. Plasma concentrations did not accumulate with repeat doses. Clinically all doses were well tolerated by the subjects and aminotransferase values stayed within normal limits throughout the study. These data provide information related to the margin of safety but are not intended to support dosing beyond the maximum recommended dose of 4 g/day.

A report has suggested that hepatotoxicity following greater than the recommended dose of acetaminophen may be enhanced by both prolonged fasting and/or chronic alcohol abuse.

Figure 1: TYLENOL Cold

Mean Data for a Standard (1 g, 15 mg/kg) and Higher (5.6 g, 75 mg/kg) Dose Relative to Risk and Treatment Lines of the Acetaminophen Nomogram

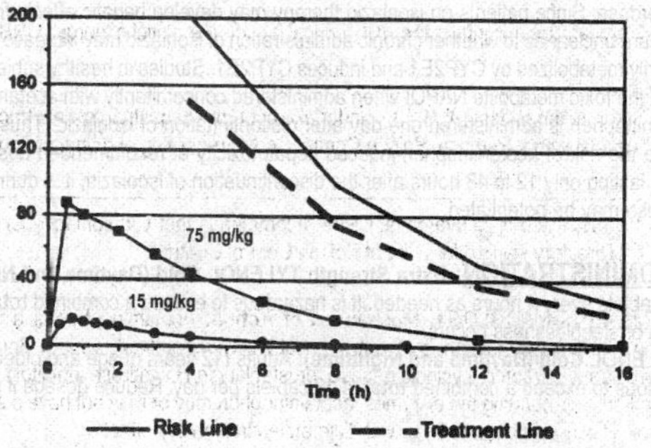

Acute Alcohol Use: Acute alcohol ingestion refers to the occasional or intermittent use of alcohol. When taken together, alcohol competes with acetaminophen for CYP2E1. CYP2E1 accepts alcohol more readily than acetaminophen; therefore, less NAPQI is produced. In the presence of alcohol, acetaminophen may be diverted to the glucuronidation and sulfation pathways. The overall result is that a smaller percentage of acetaminophen may be expected to be metabolized to the toxic intermediate, NAPQI, than would otherwise be the case. NAFQI production is increased above baseline for the period up to 18-24 hours post ethanol clearance from the body. In healthy adults, at normal labeled doses of acetaminophen, the temporary increase in NAPQI production is more than accommodated by normal glutathione stores in the liver.

Hypersensitivity: Sensitivity reactions are rare and may manifest as rash, urticaria, dyspnea, hypotension, laryngeal edema, angioedema, bronchospasm, or anaphylaxis. Cross-reactivity in ASA-sensitive persons has been rarely reported. If sensitivity is suspected, discontinue use of the drug.

Renal Effects: Acute nephrotoxicity has been reported following massive overdose either as a sequela of hepatic failure or, occasionally, in the absence of hepatic failure.

Clinical data have established that acetaminophen in recommended doses is not nephrotoxic.

Some studies suggest an association between the chronic long-term use of acetaminophen and renal effects. Results, however, are conflicting, limited by recall bias and confounded by the inability to determine whether analgesic use preceded or followed the onset of renal disease.

Case control studies have suggested a weak association between habitual acetaminophen use and prevalence of chronic renal failure and end stage renal disease. This National Kidney Foundation position paper concludes that acetaminophen has been preferentially recommended by physicians to patients with renal failure and that there is no evidence that occasional use of acetaminophen caused renal injury.

Special Populations: Pediatrics: Lesko and Mitchell enrolled more than 84 000 febrile children in a randomized, double blind, acetaminophen-controlled trial to assess the risks of rare but serious adverse events following use of pediatric ibuprofen. Of the children included in the analysis, 28 130 received acetaminophen and none experienced anaphylaxis, or serious hepatic, gastrointestinal or renal effects.

Pregnancy and Lactation: As with any drug, patients who are pregnant or nursing a baby should consult a physician before taking this product.

Pregnancy: Issues of risks in pregnancy are multifactorial. The information provided cannot be substituted for direct patient consultation. Acetaminophen is believed to be non-teratogenic in humans. However, existing studies have not assessed the effect of very high doses. The Motherrisk Collaborative Perinatal project monitored 50 282 mother-child pairs, of which 226 had first trimester exposure to acetaminophen and 781 had used acetaminophen at any time during their pregnancy. No evidence was found to suggest a relationship between acetaminophen use and major or minor malformations. In a surveillance study of Michigan Medicaid recipients conducted between 1985 and 1992 involving 229 101 completed pregnancies, 9146 newborns had been exposed to acetaminophen during the first trimester. This data do not support an association between acetaminophen use and the occurrence of birth defects. Another cohort study, using prescription monitoring, found no excess risk for malformation, and no evidence that acetaminophen influenced fetal growth. Finally, as part of a larger study, 697 women used acetaminophen with or without codeine in their first trimester. No teratogenic risk was found.

A prospective study investigated the outcome of pregnancy in 300 women who had self-administered an overdose of acetaminophen, either alone, or as part of a combined preparation. Exposure to overdose occurred in all trimesters. The majority of the pregnancies had normal outcomes. The malformation rate was within the expected range. There was no obvious relationship between the time of exposure and the time of delivery. The overall conclusion was that acetaminophen overdose is not an indication for termination of pregnancy.

In a long-term developmental follow-up study, acetaminophen did not adversely affect IQ or behavior measures at four years of age. Height, weight and head circumference were also not affected by exposure to acetaminophen in-utero.

Unlike ASA, which has been shown to profoundly affect platelet function, there does not seem to be a risk of hemorrhage associated with acetaminophen use at term.

Currently there is no evidence to suggest that acetaminophen is teratogenic when used as recommended. However, data for continuous high daily doses are not sufficient, and safety during pregnancy has not yet been established.

Lactation: Following a typical therapeutic dose, acetaminophen is excreted in breast milk in very low concentrations. Based on a number of published reports, infant exposure levels are at most 4.5% of a weight adjusted pediatric therapeutic dose. In addition, acetaminophen is considered compatible with breast-feeding by the American Academy of Pediatrics.

DRUG INTERACTIONS: Alcohol: Studies evaluating the metabolism of doses up to 20 mg/kg of acetaminophen in chronic alcohol abusers and a study evaluating the effects of 2 days of acetaminophen dosing at 4000 mg/day in chronic alcoholics undergoing detoxification, have yielded inconsistent results with regard to effects on acetaminophen pharmacokinetics and demonstrate no evidence of adverse effect on liver function tests.

Anticoagulants–Oral: Patients who concomitantly medicate with warfarin-type anticoagulants and regular doses of acetaminophen have occasionally been reported to have unforeseen elevations in their INR. Physicians should be cognizant of this potential interaction and monitor the INR in such patients closely while therapy is established. Many factors, including diet, medications, and environmental and physical states, may affect how a patient responds to anticoagulant therapy. There have been several reports that suggest that acetaminophen may produce hypoprothrombinemia (elevated international normalized ratio [INR] or prothrombin time) when administered with coumarin derivatives. In other studies, prothrombin time did not change. Reported changes have been generally of limited clinical significance, however, periodic evaluation of prothrombin time should be performed when these agents are administered concurrently.

In the period immediately following discharge from the hospital or whenever other medications are initiated, discontinued, or taken regularly, it is important to monitor patient response to anticoagulation therapy with additional prothrombin time or INR determinations. Despite the potential for interaction, acetaminophen is the least likely OTC analgesic to interfere with anticoagulant therapy.

Anticonvulsants: Some reports have suggested that patients taking long-term anticonvulsants, who overdose on acetaminophen, may be at increased risk of hepatotoxicity because of accelerated metabolism of acetaminophen. Available data are conflicting. A 7-year retrospective study of acetaminophen overdose admissions indicates that the overall mortality rate was not significantly different for patients taking concomitant anticonvulsant medications.

Hydantoins: Pharmacokinetic studies indicate that phenytoin primarily induces the glucuronidation pathway, whereas glutathione-derived metabolites are not increased in patients on chronic phenytoin therapy. Additionally, recent data demonstrate that phenytoin is metabolized primarily by CYP2C9 and CYP2C19, whereas acetaminophen is primarily metabolized by CYP2E1.

Carbamazepine: Carbamazepine is primarily metabolized by CYP3A4, whereas acetaminophen is metabolized primarily via CYP2E1. It is not known whether there is increased risk from an acetaminophen overdose in patients on chronic carbamazepine therapy.

Diflunisal: Professional literature from the manufacturer of diflunisal cautions that concomitant administration with acetaminophen produces an approximate 50% increase in plasma levels of acetaminophen in normal volunteers. Acetaminophen had no effect on diflunisal plasma levels. The clinical significance of these findings has not been established. However, caution should be used with concomitant administration of diflunisal and acetaminophen and patients should be monitored carefully.

Isoniazid: Some reports suggest that patients on chronic isoniazid therapy may be at risk for developing hepatotoxicity from an acetaminophen overdose. Since patients on isoniazid therapy may develop hepatic effects from isoniazid alone, data from individual case reports are unclear as to whether chronic administration of isoniazid may increase the risk of acetaminophen toxicity. Isoniazid is primarily metabolized by CYP2E1 and induces CYP2E1. Studies in healthy subjects demonstrate that isoniazid blocks the formation of the toxic metabolite NAPQI when administered concomitantly with acetaminophen, but increase NAPQI formation when acetaminophen is administered one day after discontinuation of isoniazid. Thus, concomitant use of isoniazid is unlikely to potentiate the risk of acetaminophen-induced hepatotoxicity at recommended doses. The isoniazid induction of CYP2E1 is short-lived, lasting only 12 to 48 hours after the discontinuation of isoniazid, it is during this period the toxicity of an acetaminophen overdose may be potentiated.

DOSAGE AND ADMINISTRATION: Extra Strength TYLENOL Cold (Daytime and Nighttime): Adults (12 years of age and older): 1 to 2 tablets every 4 hours as needed. It is hazardous to exceed a combined **total** of 8 tablets per day. Reduce dosage if nervousness or sleeplessness occurs.

Regular Strength TYLENOL Cold (Daytime and Nighttime): Adults (12 years of age and older): 1 to 2 caplets every 4 hours as needed. It is hazardous to exceed a combined **total** of 12 caplets per day. Reduce dosage if nervousness or sleeplessness occurs.

OVERDOSAGE:

Symptoms and Treatment: Acetaminophen: Typical Toxidrome: Hepatic injury is the principal toxic effect of a substantial acetaminophen overdose. The physician should be mindful that there is no early presentation that is pathognomic for the overdose. A high degree of clinical suspicion must always be maintained.

Untreated acetaminophen overdoses may produce hepatotoxicity. Acetaminophen hepatotoxicity occurs as a threshold effect and is characterized by a lack of toxicity at lower/therapeutic doses. Acetaminophen hepatotoxicity occurs after major depletion of glutathione, an endogenous detoxifying substance. Once the threshold is exceeded, increasing acetaminophen doses may produce increasing degrees of hepatotoxicity, unless N-acetylcysteine (NAC) is administered. Situations in which acetaminophen overdose and resultant hepatotoxicity may occur include acute intentional overdose and repeated supratherapeutic overdose in adults and acute accidental ingestion or overdose and repeated supratherapeutic overdose in children.

The clinical course of acetaminophen overdose generally occurs in a three-phase sequential pattern. The first phase begins shortly after ingestion and lasts for 12 to 24 hours. The patient may manifest signs of gastrointestinal irritability, nausea, vomiting, anorexia, diaphoresis, pallor and general malaise. If toxicity continues, there is a latent phase of up to 48 hours. During this second phase, initial symptoms abate and the patient may feel better. However, hepatic enzymes, bilirubin, and prothrombin time or INR values will progressively rise. Right upper quadrant pain may develop as the liver becomes enlarged and tender. Most patients do not progress beyond this phase, especially if given N-acetylcysteine (NAC) treatment early in the course. Signs and symptoms of the third phase depend on the severity of hepatic damage and usually occur from three to five days following overdose ingestion. Symptoms may be limited to anorexia, nausea, general malaise, and abdominal pain in less severe cases or may progress to confusion, stupor and sequelae of hepatic necrosis including jaundice, coagulation defects, hypoglycemia, and encephalopathy, as well as renal failure and cardiomyopathy. Death, if it occurs, is generally the result of complications associated with fulminant hepatic failure. Mortality rates in patients with toxic plasma levels who do not receive antidote therapy range from 3% to 4%.

Due to the wide availability of acetaminophen, it is commonly involved in single and mixed drug overdose situations and the practitioner should screen for its presence in a patient's serum. Acute toxicity after single dose overdoses of acetaminophen can be anticipated when the overdose exceeds 150 mg/kg. Chronic alcohol abusers, cachectic individuals, and persons taking pharmacologic inducers of the hepatic P450 microsomal enzyme system may be at risk with lower exposures.

Specific Antidote: Any individual presenting with a possible acetaminophen overdose should be treated with N-acetylcysteine (NAC), even if the amount of acetaminophen ingested is unknown or questionable. A blood sample for determination of the plasma acetaminophen concentration should be obtained as early as possible, but no sooner than four hours following ingestion. Do not await the results of assays for plasma acetaminophen levels before initiating treatment NAC. If the acetaminophen plasma level is found to plot above the treatment line on the acetaminophen overdose nomogram, NAC treatment should be continued for a full course of therapy. NAC is used clinically to treat acute acetaminophen overdose, and acts by interacting with the oxidative intermediate, NAPQI. NAC administered by either the i.v. or the oral route is known to be a highly effective antidote for acetaminophen poisoning. It is most effective when administered within 8 hours of a significant overdose but reports have indicated benefits to treatment initiated well beyond this time period. It is imperative to administer the antidote as early as possible in the time course of acute intoxication to reap the full benefits of the antidote's protective effects. For full prescribing information, consult the product monograph for NAC.

General Management: When the possibility of acetaminophen overdose exists, treatment should begin immediately and include appropriate decontamination of the gastrointestinal tract, proper supportive care, careful assessment of appropriately timed serum acetaminophen estimations evaluated against the Rumack-Matthew nomogram, timely administration of NAC as required and appropriate follow-up care. Liver function tests should be performed initially and repeated at 24-hour intervals.

Phenylephrine HCl: Typical Toxidrome: sympathomimetic/stimulant.

Specific Antidote: none.

General Management: Stabilize the patient (A, B, Cs), undertake appropriate gastrointestinal tract decontamination procedures, initiate supportive care, consult with a Regional Poison Control Centre regarding ongoing management, and arrange for appropriate follow-up care.

Dextromethorphan HBr: Typical Toxidrome: narcotic/opiate.

Specific Antidote: naloxone HCl.

General Management: Stabilize the patient (A, B, Cs), undertake appropriate gastrointestinal tract decontamination procedures, initiate supportive care, consult with a Regional Poison Control Centre regarding ongoing management, and arrange for appropriate follow-up care.

Chlorpheniramine maleate: Typical Toxidrome: anticholinergic, CNS depressant (adult), CNS stimulant (child).

Specific Antidote: none.

General Management: Stabilize the patient (A, B, Cs), undertake appropriate gastrointestinal tract decontamination procedures, initiate supportive care, consult with a Regional Poison Control Centre regarding ongoing management, and arrange for appropriate follow-up care.

Overdose During Pregnancy: Acetaminophen is one of the most common overdoses in pregnancy. Hepatic toxicity of acetaminophen follows the formation of the highly reactive metabolite N-acetyl-p-benzoquinoneimine produced by acetaminophen metabolism through the cytochrome P450 mixed-function oxidase system. Hepatic failure can be prevented by timely administration of NAC either orally for 72 hours, or intravenously (IV) for 20 hours.

Acetaminophen crosses the human placenta though the fetus is theoretically at risk when maternal overdose of acetaminophen occurs. Acetaminophen can be transformed to its toxic metabolite since the oxidative capacity of fetal microsomes is present in the fetus by 14 weeks gestation.

Studies on placental transfer of NAC in rats and sheep yielded conflicting results. Placental transfer of N-acetylcysteine in humans was demonstrated in 4 women treated with NAC for acetaminophen overdose during labour. NAC blood levels in the fetuses were within the range associated with therapeutic doses of NAC administered to adults with acetaminophen poisoning.

Fetal toxicity and stillbirth after a large (e.g. 30 g) acetaminophen overdose has been reported, but others observed a normal outcome for the offspring after acetaminophen overdose in pregnancy. A large case series investigated the pregnancy outcome in 300 women who had overdosed with acetaminophen. In this group, 118 cases occurred in the first trimester, 103 in the second trimester and 79 in the third trimester. Forty-nine of these mothers were treated with specific antidotes (33 with NAC and 16 with methionine). There were 219 live-born infants, 11 have malformations (including minor); none had been exposed to acetaminophen during the first trimester. Nine women were treated with NAC during the first trimester; there were two elective terminations; two spontaneous abortions, and five healthy babies in this group.

In summary, acetaminophen overdose during pregnancy should be treated according to regular protocols in order to prevent maternal and potentially fetal toxicity. Unless severe maternal toxicity develops, an acetaminophen overdose does not increase the risk for birth defects or adverse pregnancy outcomes.

Physicians unfamiliar with the current management of acetaminophen overdose should consult with a Poison Control Centre immediately. Telephone numbers for local Poison Control Centres are available in the local phone directory. Delays in initiation of appropriate therapy may jeopardize the patient's chances for full recovery.

> For management of a suspected drug overdose, CPhA recommends that you contact your **regional Poison Control Centre**. See the *CPS* Directory section for a list of Poison Control Centres.

ACTION AND CLINICAL PHARMACOLOGY: Mechanism of Action: Acetaminophen is a centrally acting analgesic and antipyretic drug. Although the precise mechanism of action is not totally understood, work by Boutaud suggests acetaminophen is an inhibitor of the peroxidase portion of cyclooxygenase (prostaglandin H synthase inhibitor). Depending on the redox state and substrate concentrations surrounding the enzymes, acetaminophen may or may not have a significant inhibitory effect. This accounts for its selective activity on pain and fever with little anti-inflammatory effect.

It is postulated that the analgesic effect is produced by elevation of the pain threshold and the antipyretic effect is produced through action on the hypothalamic heat-regulating centre.

The optimal effective analgesic dose of acetaminophen was demonstrated in dental pain studies and is 1000 mg every four to six hours, up to 4000 mg daily. At least 500 published and unpublished controlled clinical trials in adults and children have evaluated acetaminophen for the relief of pain or fever. These studies include single and multiple dose treatments. Most studies were less than 14 days in duration, although the longest study duration was two years. No significant safety issues were reported in any of these studies.

Moreover, at recommended doses, acetaminophen has not been shown to increase the risk of developing renal diseases or upper gastrointestinal ulceration/bleeding. This observation is consistent with its minimal inhibitory effect on peripheral prostaglandin synthesis and on gastric prostaglandin synthesis.

Acetaminophen is considered equipotent to ASA and ibuprofen, within the recommended OTC dosing ranges, in its analgesic and antipyretic effects. Acetaminophen at recommended doses does not cause the type of gastrointestinal complications associated with NSAID-containing products, such as gastric irritation, gastric erosions, occult or overt gastrointestinal blood loss, or ulcers. Unlike these drugs, however, it has no anti-inflammatory effect at clinically relevant doses in humans.

Pharmacokinetics: Absorption: Oral acetaminophen is rapidly and almost completely absorbed from the gastrointestinal tract primarily in the small intestine. This absorption process occurs by passive transport. Peak plasma concentrations occur within 0.4 to 1 hour depending on the product formulation. Although high-fat foods delay the time to peak concentration for up to an hour, the dose is completely absorbed.

Distribution: Acetaminophen is uniformly distributed throughout most body fluids, but not in fatty tissue. As a result, the volume of distribution in adults ranges between 0.8 and 1.0 L/kg. Since acetaminophen has low protein binding in plasma of only 10% to 25%, it does not compete with drugs that are highly protein bound.

Metabolism: Acetaminophen is primarily metabolized by the liver via three principal separate pathways: conjugation with glucuronide; conjugation with sulfate; oxidation via the cytochrome P450 mixed function oxidase system.

Both the glucuronic and oxidative pathways adhere to a first-order rate process, which means the concentration of acetaminophen metabolized increases as the concentration in the liver increases. The sulfate pathway adheres to Michaelis-Menten kinetics, which means the concentration of acetaminophen metabolized remains constant once the concentration in the liver increases above a saturation level. A schematic of acetaminophen metabolism is shown in Figure 2.

The major metabolic pathway is glucuronidation, where 47% to 62% of the acetaminophen dose conjugates with glucuronide. These glucuronide conjugates are inactive and nontoxic, and are secreted in bile and eliminated in the urine.

The second major pathway is sulfation, where 25% to 36% of the dose conjugates with sulfate. These sulfate ester conjugates are also inactive and nontoxic and are excreted in the urine.

The third pathway is oxidation, where 5% to 8% of the dose is metabolized via the cytochrome P450 enzyme system. The cytochrome P450 isoenzyme that is primarily responsible is CYP2E1. When acetaminophen is metabolized by CYP2E1, it forms a highly reactive intermediate, N-acetyl-p-benzoquinoneimine (NAPQI). Since NAPQI is highly reactive, it cannot be measured outside the liver nor can it accumulate. This intermediate is rapidly inactivated by hepatocellular stores of glutathione to form cysteine and mercapturate conjugates, which are both inactive and nontoxic. These conjugates are excreted in the urine.

Figure 2: TYLENOL Cold

Acetaminophen Metabolism

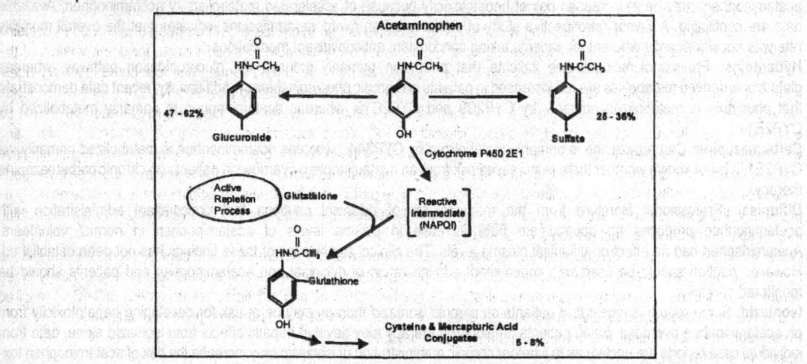

Excretion: Acetaminophen undergoes first-order elimination from the body, and has a short plasma half-life that ranges from 2 to 3 hours in healthy young and elderly adults and from 1.5 to 2.9 hours in children. Since acetaminophen clears rapidly from the body, repeated doses do not lead to accumulation of acetaminophen plasma concentrations.

STORAGE AND STABILITY: Store at room temperature (15 to 30°C). Protect from moisture.

DOSAGE FORMS, COMPOSITION AND PACKAGING: Caplets: Regular Strength Daytime: Each white, caplet-shaped tablet with "TY C1078" printed in black ink on one side, contains: acetaminophen 325 mg, dextromethorphan HBr 10 mg and phenylephrine HCl 5 mg. Nonmedicinal ingredients: carnauba wax, castor oil, cellulose, colloidal silicon dioxide, corn starch, flavour, hypromellose, iron oxide black, magnesium stearate, potassium sorbate, shellac glaze, sodium benzoate, sodium starch glycolate, stearic acid and sucralose. Energy: 1.3 kJ (0.3 kcal). Sodium: 0.4 mg. Alcohol, gluten-, lactose-, sulfite- and tartrazine-free. Blister packs of 10 in combination with blister packs of 10 Regular Strength TYLENOL Cold Nighttime caplets. All packages are safety sealed.

Regular Strength Nighttime: Each light blue, caplet-shaped tablet with "TY C1075" printed in black ink on one side, contains: acetaminophen 325 mg, dextromethorphan HBr 10 mg, phenylephrine HCl 5 mg and chlorpheniramine maleate 2 mg. Nonmedicinal ingredients: carnauba wax, cellulose, colloidal silicon dioxide, corn starch, FD&C Blue no. 1, flavor, hypromellose, iron oxide black, magnesium stearate, polyethylene glycol, polysorbate 80, potassium sorbate, shellac glaze, sodium benzoate, sodium starch glycolate, stearic acid, sucralose and titanium dioxide. Energy: 1.3 kJ (0.3 kcal). Sodium: 0.4 mg. Alcohol, gluten-, lactose-, sulfite- and tartrazine-free. Blister packs of 10 in combination with blister packs of 10 Regular Strength TYLENOL Cold Daytime caplets. All packages are safety sealed.

Tablets: Extra Strength Daytime: Each round, yellow coated tablet, with "TYLENOL" over "Cold DT" printed in black ink on one side, blank on the other side and with a characteristic mint odor, contains: acetaminophen 500 mg, dextromethorphan HBr 10 mg and phenylephrine HCl 5 mg. Nonmedicinal ingredients: carnauba wax, cellulose, corn starch, D&C Yellow no. 10, FD&C Yellow no. 6, flavor, hypromellose, iron oxide black, magnesium stearate, polydextrose, polyethylene glycol, sodium starch glycolate, sucralose, titanium dioxide and triacetin. Energy: 1.3 kJ (0.3 kcal). Sodium: 0.4 mg. Alcohol, gluten-, lactose-, sulfite- and tartrazine-free. Plastic bottles of 20* and 40*. Blister packs of 6 in combination with blister packs of 4 Extra Strength TYLENOL Cold Nighttime tablets. Blister packs of 10 in combination with blister packs of 10 Extra Strength TYLENOL Cold Nighttime tablets. Blister packs of 24 in combination with blister packs of 16 Extra Strength TYLENOL Cold Nighttime tablets. All packages are safety sealed.

Extra Strength Nighttime: Each round, blue coated tablet, with "TYLENOL" over "Cold NT" printed in black ink on one side, blank on the other side and with a characteristic mint odor, contains: acetaminophen 500 mg, dextromethorphan HBr 10 mg, phenylephrine HCl 5 mg and chlorpheniramine maleate 2 mg. Nonmedicinal ingredients: carnauba wax, cellulose, corn starch, FD&C Blue no. 1, flavor, hypromellose, iron oxide black, magnesium stearate, polydextrose, polyethylene glycol, sodium starch glycolate, sucralose, titanium dioxide and triacetin. Energy: 1.3 kJ (0.3 kcal). Sodium: 0.4 mg. Alcohol, gluten-, lactose-, sulfite- and tartrazine-free. Plastic bottles of 20* and 40*. Blister packs of 4 in combination with blister packs of 6 Extra Strength TYLENOL Cold Daytime tablets. Blister packs of 10 in combination with blister packs of 10 Extra Strength TYLENOL Cold Daytime tablets. Blister packs of 16 in combination with blister packs of 24 Extra Strength TYLENOL Cold Daytime tablets. All packages are safety sealed.

Tylenol® Cold & Flu Daytime Liquid

acetaminophen—dextromethorphan HBr—phenylephrine HCl

Analgesic—Antipyretic—Antitussive—Decongestant

McNeil Consumer Healthcare

Tylenol® Cold & Flu Nighttime Liquid

acetaminophen—dextromethorphan HBr—phenylephrine HCl—doxylamine succinate

Analgesic—Antipyretic—Antitussive—Decongestant—Antihistamine

McNeil Consumer Healthcare

Date of Revision: October 30, 2009

SUMMARY PRODUCT INFORMATION:

Route of Administration	Dosage Form/ Strength	Clinically Relevant Nonmedicinal Ingredients
Oral	Daytime Liquid/Per 30 mL: 650 mg acetaminophen, 10 mg phenylephrine HCl and 20 mg dextromethorphan HBr Nighttime Liquid/Per 30 mL: 650 mg acetaminophen, 10 mg phenylephrine HCl, 20 mg dextromethorphan HBr and 12.5 mg doxylamine succinate	Gluten-, lactose- and tartrazine-free For a complete listing of nonmedicinal ingredients, see Dosage Forms, Composition and Packaging.

INDICATIONS AND CLINICAL USE: TYLENOL Cold & Flu Daytime: A non-drowsy formulation for the temporary relief of aches, pain, sore throat and fever, dry cough and nasal congestion due to colds and flu.

TYLENOL Cold & Flu Nighttime: For the temporary relief of aches, pain, sore throat and fever, dry cough, nasal congestion, sneezing and runny nose due to colds and flu.

* Container provided with a child-resistant closure.

CONTRAINDICATIONS: Hypersensitivity to acetaminophen, pressor amines or to the ingredients of this formulation (see Dosage Forms, Composition and Packaging). Allergic reactions (primarily skin rash) or reports of hypersensitivity secondary to acetaminophen are rare and generally are controlled by discontinuation of the drug and, when necessary, symptomatic treatment.

In patients receiving or having received MAO inhibitors in the preceding 2 weeks. Although phenylephrine is virtually without pressor effect in normotensive patients, it should be used with caution in hypertensives.

WARNINGS AND PRECAUTIONS: General: Consumers should not exceed 4 g/day of acetaminophen or use two or more acetaminophen-containing products together. This includes combination products that contain acetaminophen. Do not use with other products containing salicylates or any other pain or fever medicine.

Acetaminophen-containing products should be kept out of the reach of children.

Physicians should be cognizant of and supervise the use of acetaminophen in patients with chronic alcoholism, serious kidney or serious liver disease. Physicians should alert their patients who regularly consume large amounts of alcohol not to exceed the recommended doses of acetaminophen. Chronic heavy alcohol abusers may be at increased risk of liver toxicity from excessive doses of acetaminophen.

Patients should be counseled to consult a physician if redness or swelling is present in an area of pain, if symptoms do not improve or if they worsen, or if new symptoms such as high fever, rash, itching, excessive mucus, persistent or recurring cough or persistent headache occur, as these may be signs of a condition which requires medical attention.

Acetaminophen should not be taken for pain for more than 5 days, for fever for more than 3 days or if new symptoms appear, without consulting a physician.

In patients with high blood pressure, heart disease, diabetes, thyroid disease, difficulty in urination due to enlargement of the prostate gland or who are taking a prescription drug for high blood pressure or depression, phenylephrine HCl should be used with caution and only under close medical supervision.

Patients with asthma, glaucoma, emphysema, chronic pulmonary disease or shortness of breath should not use this medication unless directed by a physician. This product should not be used for persistent or chronic cough such as occurs with smoking, asthma or emphysema unless directed by a physician.

Occupational Hazards: Preparations containing doxylamine succinate may cause marked drowsiness. Alcoholic beverages, sedatives and tranquilizers may increase this effect and should be avoided. Advise caution when driving a motor vehicle or operating machinery or engaging in any activity requiring alertness. Patients taking tranquilizers or sedatives should not take this medication before consulting a physician.

Hepatic/Biliary/Pancreatic: Slower metabolism of acetaminophen, increased activity of the cytochrome P450 enzyme system, or depleted glutathione stores are cited as theoretical risk factors for acetaminophen hepatotoxicity in patients with chronic liver disease. However, acetaminophen has been studied in both adults and children with a wide variety of liver diseases including various types of cirrhosis, hepatitis (including hepatitis C), nodular transformation, congenital hepatic fibrosis, and α1-antitrypsin deficiency. In none of these conditions is there evidence of an increased risk for hepatotoxicity at currently recommended acetaminophen doses but the studies were insufficiently powered to definitely establish the extent of risk.

Forrest compared acetaminophen metabolism following a single 1500 mg dose in normal subjects, patients with mild liver disease, and patients with severe liver disease. There were no significant differences in overall 24-hour urinary excretion of acetaminophen and glucuronide, sulfate, cysteine, and mercapturic acid conjugates, evidence that acetaminophen metabolism was similar to that in normal subjects. However, the elimination half-life was significantly prolonged in patients with severe liver disease.

Acetaminophen has also been studied in pediatric patients with liver disease. Following a single (10 mg/kg) dose of acetaminophen, the pharmacokinetic profiles in pediatric patients with mild, moderate, or severe liver disease were not significantly different. Although the plasma half-life of acetaminophen was prolonged in patients with severe liver disease, there were no significant differences in the 36-hour (children) urinary excretion of acetaminophen or its conjugates.

Acetaminophen may cause hepatotoxicity in situations of intentional overdose (e.g. attempted suicide), unintentional overdose (e.g. overdosing when pain relief is not satisfactory), simultaneous use of multiple acetaminophen-containing preparations, accidental overdose or in very rare cases, after recommended doses, although causality has not been determined. The hepatotoxic reaction can be severe and life-threatening. Early symptoms following a hepatotoxic overdose may include nausea, vomiting, diaphoresis, lethargy, and general malaise. If appropriate treatment is not instituted, these may progress to upper quadrant pain, confusion, stupor, and sequelae of hepatic necrosis, such as jaundice, coagulation defects, hypoglycemia, and encephalopathy. Renal failure and cardiomyopathy may also occur. In the event of known or suspected overdosage, treatment with N-acetyl cysteine should be instituted immediately (see Overdosage), even when there are no obvious symptoms. Failure to promptly treat acetaminophen hepatotoxicity with N-acetyl cysteine can result in liver failure, leading to liver transplantation and/or death.

Chronic Alcohol Use: Excessive alcohol use may increase risk of liver toxicity from acetaminophen overdose (acute or chronic).

In prospective, placebo controlled studies, researchers evaluated an actively drinking group of alcoholics with a high prevalence of malnourishment. The study participants abruptly stopped their daily alcohol intake and took acetaminophen the next day. This should theoretically make them vulnerable to acetaminophen injury because their CYP2E1 would be maximally induced from the alcohol and there would be no alcohol present to compete with acetaminophen for metabolism by CYP2E1. There was no statistically significant difference in mean values for AST, ALT, or INR for alcoholics given four grams per day of acetaminophen compared to placebo. Additionally, the researchers performed an analysis of the malnourished patients that showed there was no increase in AST or ALT levels in these patients. Study limitations include a limited duration of 2 days and exclusion of patients with preexisting AST or ALT elevations greater than 120 U/L. Study results do not preclude the possibility of an idiosyncratic hepatic reaction.

Renal: Martin found that patients with chronic renal failure had higher plasma concentrations of acetaminophen and the inactive glucuronide and sulfate metabolites than healthy subjects during repeated dosing up to ten days.

Several single-dose studies demonstrate accumulation of acetaminophen metabolites in patients with moderate chronic renal failure and in anephric patients for whom hemodialysis appeared to be the major route of elimination.

The habitual consumption of acetaminophen should be discouraged. If indicated medically, the long-term use of acetaminophen should be supervised by a physician.

A National Kidney Foundation position paper notes that physicians preferentially recommend acetaminophen to patients with renal failure because of the bleeding complications associated with ASA in these individuals.

Special Populations: Geriatrics: In a comprehensive metabolic study by Miners, the formation and clearance of glucuronide and glutathione conjugates were the same in young and elderly adults, although clearance of the sulphate conjugate and unchanged acetaminophen were reduced. This finding provides prospective scientific data that the amount of acetaminophen metabolized via the oxidative pathway, from which the highly reactive intermediate, NAPQI, is generated, does not increase with age. Recently, Bannwarth evaluated the multiple-dose pharmacokinetics of acetaminophen in elderly patients. After seven days of repeat dosing, acetaminophen did not accumulate in the plasma, and the elimination half-life was the same as that reported for young adults.

Elderly patients who require therapy for longer than 5 days should consult their physician for condition monitoring.

Glucose-6-Phosphate Dehydrogenase (G6PD) Deficiency: In therapeutic doses, acetaminophen does not shorten the lifespan of red blood cells and does not produce any clinically perceptible destruction of circulating red blood cells.

Obese Adults: O'Shea studied the pharmacokinetics of chlorzoxazone (a putative probe for CYP2E1 activity) to evaluate the effect of obesity on CYP2E1 activity. The authors concluded that CYP2E1 is induced in obese adults and that this could impact the metabolic pathway of a number of drugs metabolized by CYP2E1, including acetaminophen. However, acetaminophen pharmacokinetic data have been investigated in obese adults. In this prospective study, 650 mg acetaminophen was administered intravenously to obese men (297 lb), obese women (193 lb), control men (155 lb) and control women (121 lb). Acetaminophen distribution volume per total body weight was slightly lower in the obese adults but, more importantly, the half-life and metabolic clearance per total body weight did not differ among groups.

ADVERSE REACTIONS: Central Nervous System Effects: Acetaminophen at recommended doses has no obvious effects on central nervous system function. In an overdose situation, central nervous system effects are uncommon.

Doxylamine succinate may cause excitability, especially in children.

Gastrointestinal Effects: Acetaminophen at recommended doses does not cause gastric irritation, gastric erosions, occult or overt gastrointestinal blood loss or ulcers. Blot and McLaughlin conducted an independent analysis of case-control data from a study conducted by the American College of Gastroenterology. The risk of gastrointestinal bleeding increased two to three-fold among recent users of ASA, ibuprofen and other NSAIDs at OTC doses, and the risk was also dose-related. In contrast, the use of acetaminophen was not associated with an increased risk of gastrointestinal bleeding.

Hematologic Effects: Acetaminophen does not have any immediate or delayed effects on small vessel hemostasis, as measured by bleeding time. In normal volunteers receiving a single dose of acetaminophen (975 or 1950 mg) or multiple doses of acetaminophen (1950 mg daily for 6 weeks), no change in bleeding time or platelet aggregation was observed. In another study, a single 1000 mg dose of acetaminophen was given to normal volunteers and did not affect bleeding time or platelet aggregation. Patients with hemophilia receiving multiple doses of acetaminophen showed no significant changes in bleeding time.

Haematological reactions including thrombocytopenia, leucopenia, pancytopenia, neutropenia, and agranulocytosis have been reported, although these are rare and causality has not been established.

Hepatic Effects: As an illustration of the margin of safety of acetaminophen at supratherapeutic doses, a comparison of serum concentrations of acetaminophen over time for a standard 15 mg/kg dose and for a dose exceeding the standard by a multiple of 5 (75 mg/kg) are shown in Figure 1. The serum concentrations are drawn relative to the risk line for hepatotoxicity and treatment line of the Rumack-Matthew nomogram used to manage acute overdoses. The mean plasma concentrations for this supratherapeutic dose are well below the risk and treatment lines of the nomogram at all times. However, to minimize the risk for adverse effects, the maximum recommended dose should not be exceeded.

Figure 1: TYLENOL Cold & Flu

Mean Data for a Standard (1 g, 15 mg/kg) and Higher (5.6 g, 75 mg/kg) Dose Relative to Risk and Treatment Lines of the Acetaminophen Nomogram

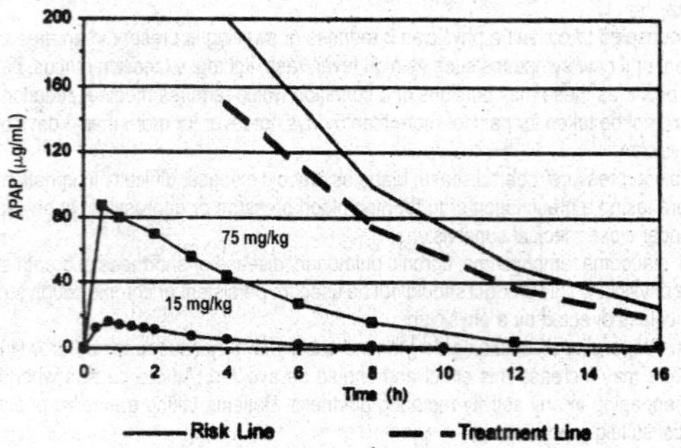

Acetaminophen in overdosage may cause hepatotoxicity. In adults and adolescents, hepatotoxicity may occur following ingestion of greater than 150 mg/kg over a period of 8 hours or less. Fatalities are infrequent (less than 3% to 4% of untreated cases in which blood levels exceed the treatment line) and have rarely been reported with overdoses less than 7.5 g. In children, amounts less than 150 mg/kg are unlikely to produce hepatotoxicity. In both adults and children, toxicity associated with acetaminophen is usually caused by ingestion of quantities of the drug that are significantly above the recommended dosage range. Hepatotoxicity, ranging from transient sharp transaminase elevations to fatal, fulminant hepatic failure, is the most common result of clinically significant overdosage.

In a double-blind, placebo-controlled clinical study, healthy adults were given 4, 6 and 8 g/day of acetaminophen over 3 days. Plasma concentrations did not accumulate with repeat doses. Clinically all doses were well tolerated by the subjects and aminotransferase values stayed within normal limits throughout the study. These data provide information related to the margin of safety but are not intended to support dosing beyond the maximum recommended dose of 4 g/day.

A report has suggested that hepatotoxicity following greater than the recommended dose of acetaminophen may be enhanced by both prolonged fasting and/or chronic alcohol abuse.

Acute Alcohol Use: Acute alcohol ingestion refers to the occasional or intermittent use of alcohol. When taken together, alcohol competes with acetaminophen for CYP2E1. CYP2E1 accepts alcohol more readily than acetaminophen; therefore, less NAPQI is produced. In the presence of alcohol, acetaminophen may be diverted to the glucuronidation and sulfation pathways. The overall result is that a smaller percentage of acetaminophen may be expected to be metabolized to the toxic intermediate, NAPQI, than would otherwise be the case. NAPQI production is increased above baseline for the period up to 18-24 hours post ethanol clearance from the body. In healthy adults, at normal labeled doses of acetaminophen, the temporary increase in NAPQI production is more than accommodated by normal glutathione stores in the liver.

Hypersensitivity: Sensitivity reactions are rare and may manifest as rash, urticaria, dyspnea, hypotension, laryngeal edema, angioedema, bronchospasm, or anaphylaxis. Cross-reactivity in ASA-sensitive persons has been rarely reported. If sensitivity is suspected, discontinue use of the drug.

Renal Effects: Acute nephrotoxicity has been reported following massive overdose either as a sequela of hepatic failure or, occasionally, in the absence of hepatic failure.

Clinical data have established that acetaminophen in recommended doses is not nephrotoxic.

Some studies suggest an association between the chronic long-term use of acetaminophen and renal effects. Results, however, are conflicting, limited by recall bias and confounded by the inability to determine whether analgesic use preceded or followed the onset of renal disease.

Case control studies have suggested a weak association between habitual acetaminophen use and prevalence of chronic renal failure and end stage renal disease. This National Kidney Foundation position paper concludes that acetaminophen has been preferentially recommended by physicians to patients with renal failure and that there is no evidence that occasional use of acetaminophen caused renal injury.

Special Populations: Pediatrics: Lesko and Mitchell enrolled more than 84 000 febrile children in a randomized, double blind, acetaminophen-controlled trial to assess the risks of rare but serious adverse events following use of pediatric ibuprofen. Of the children included in the analysis, 28 130 received acetaminophen and none experienced anaphylaxis, or serious hepatic, gastrointestinal or renal effects.

Pregnancy and Lactation: As with any drug, patients who are pregnant or nursing a baby should consult a physician before taking this product.

Pregnancy: Issues of risks in pregnancy are multifactorial. The information provided cannot be substituted for direct patient consultation. Acetaminophen is believed to be non-teratogenic in humans. However, existing studies have not assessed the effect of very high doses. The Motherrisk Collaborative Perinatal project monitored 50 282 mother-child pairs, of which 226 had first trimester exposure to acetaminophen and 781 had used acetaminophen at any time during their pregnancy. No evidence was found to suggest a relationship between acetaminophen use and major or minor malformations. In a surveillance study of Michigan Medicaid recipients conducted between 1985 and 1992 involving 229 101 completed pregnancies, 9146 newborns had been exposed to acetaminophen during the first trimester. This data do not support an association between acetaminophen use and the occurrence of birth defects. Another cohort study, using prescription monitoring, found no excess risk for malformation, and no evidence that acetaminophen influenced fetal growth. Finally, as part of a larger study, 697 women used acetaminophen with or without codeine in their first trimester. No teratogenic risk was found.

A prospective study investigated the outcome of pregnancy in 300 women who had self-administered an overdose of acetaminophen, either alone, or as part of a combined preparation. Exposure to overdose occurred in all trimesters. The majority of the pregnancies had normal outcomes. The malformation rate was within the expected range. There was no obvious relationship between the time of exposure and the time of delivery. The overall conclusion was that acetaminophen overdose is not an indication for termination of pregnancy.

In a long-term developmental follow-up study, acetaminophen did not adversely affect IQ or behavior measures at four years of age. Height, weight and head circumference were also not affected by exposure to acetaminophen in-utero.

Unlike ASA, which has been shown to profoundly affect platelet function, there does not seem to be a risk of hemorrhage associated with acetaminophen use at term.

Currently there is no evidence to suggest that acetaminophen is teratogenic when used as recommended. However, data for continuous high daily doses are not sufficient, and safety during pregnancy has not yet been established.

Lactation: Following a typical therapeutic dose, acetaminophen is excreted in breast milk in very low concentrations. Based on a number of published reports, infant exposure levels are at most 4.5% of a weight adjusted pediatric therapeutic dose. In addition, acetaminophen is considered compatible with breast-feeding by the American Academy of Pediatrics.

DRUG INTERACTIONS: Alcohol: Studies evaluating the metabolism of doses up to 20 mg/kg of acetaminophen in chronic alcohol abusers and a study evaluating the effects of 2 days of acetaminophen dosing at 4000 mg/day in chronic alcoholics undergoing detoxification, have yielded inconsistent results with regard to effects on acetaminophen pharmacokinetics and demonstrate no evidence of adverse effect on liver function tests.

Anticoagulants–Oral: Patients who concomitantly medicate with warfarin-type anticoagulants and regular doses of acetaminophen have occasionally been reported to have unforeseen elevations in their INR. Physicians should be cognizant of this potential interaction and monitor the INR in such patients closely while therapy is established. Many factors, including diet, medications, and environmental and physical states, may affect how a patient responds to anticoagulant therapy. There have been several reports that suggest that acetaminophen may produce hypoprothrombinemia (elevated international normalized ratio [INR] or prothrombin time) when administered with coumarin derivatives. In other studies, prothrombin time did not change. Reported changes have been generally of limited clinical significance, however, periodic evaluation of prothrombin time should be performed when these agents are administered concurrently.

In the period immediately following discharge from the hospital or whenever other medications are initiated, discontinued, or taken regularly, it is important to monitor patient response to anticoagulation therapy with additional prothrombin time or INR determinations. Despite the potential for interaction, acetaminophen is the least likely OTC analgesic to interfere with anticoagulant therapy.

Anticonvulsants: Some reports have suggested that patients taking long-term anticonvulsants, who overdose on acetaminophen, may be at increased risk of hepatotoxicity because of accelerated metabolism of acetaminophen. Available data are conflicting. A 7-year retrospective study of acetaminophen overdose admissions indicates that the overall mortality rate was not significantly different for patients taking concomitant anticonvulsant medications.

Hydantoins: Pharmacokinetic studies indicate that phenytoin primarily induces the glucuronidation pathway, whereas glutathione-derived metabolites are not increased in patients on chronic phenytoin therapy. Additionally, recent data demonstrate that phenytoin is metabolized primarily by CYP2C9 and CYP2C19, whereas acetaminophen is primarily metabolized by CYP2E1.

Carbamazepine: Carbamazepine is primarily metabolized by CYP3A4 , whereas acetaminophen is metabolized primarily via CYP2E1. It is not known whether there is increased risk from an acetaminophen overdose in patients on chronic carbamazepine therapy.

Diflunisal: Professional literature from the manufacturer of diflunisal cautions that concomitant administration with acetaminophen produces an approximate 50% increase in plasma levels of acetaminophen in normal volunteers. Acetaminophen had no effect on diflunisal plasma levels. The clinical significance of these findings has not been established. However, caution should be used with concomitant administration of diflunisal and acetaminophen and patients should be monitored carefully.

Isoniazid: Some reports suggest that patients on chronic isoniazid therapy may be at risk for developing hepatotoxicity from an acetaminophen overdose. Since patients on isoniazid therapy may develop hepatic effects from isoniazid alone, data from individual case reports are unclear as to whether chronic administration of isoniazid may increase the risk of acetaminophen toxicity. Isoniazid is primarily metabolized by CYP2E1 and induces CYP2E1. Studies in healthy subjects demonstrate that isoniazid blocks the formation of the toxic metabolite NAPQI when administered concomitantly with acetaminophen, but increase NAPQI formation when acetaminophen is administered one day after discontinuation of isoniazid. Thus, concomitant use of isoniazid is unlikely to potentiate the risk of acetaminophen-induced hepatotoxicity at recommended doses. The isoniazid induction of CYP2E1 is short-lived, lasting only 12 to 48 hours after the discontinuation of isoniazid, it is during this period the toxicity of an acetaminophen overdose may be potentiated.

DOSAGE AND ADMINISTRATION: Cold & Flu Daytime Liquid: Adults (12 years of age and older): 2 tablespoons (30 mL) every 4 hours as needed. It is hazardous to exceed 12 tablespoons (180 mL) per day unless advised by a doctor. Reduce dose if you feel nervous or cannot sleep.

Cold & Flu Nighttime Liquid: Adults (12 years of age and older): 2 tablespoons (30 mL) every 4 hours as needed. It is hazardous to exceed 12 tablespoons (180 mL) per day unless advised by a doctor. Reduce dose if you feel nervous or cannot sleep.

OVERDOSAGE:

Symptoms and Treatment: Acetaminophen: Typical Toxidrome: Hepatic injury is the principal toxic effect of a substantial acetaminophen overdose. The physician should be mindful that there is no early presentation that is pathognomic for the overdose. A high degree of clinical suspicion must always be maintained.

Untreated acetaminophen overdoses may produce hepatotoxicity. Acetaminophen hepatotoxicity occurs as a threshold effect and is characterized by a lack of toxicity at lower/therapeutic doses. Acetaminophen hepatotoxicity occurs after major depletion of glutathione, an endogenous detoxifying substance. Once the threshold is exceeded, increasing acetaminophen doses may produce increasing degrees of hepatotoxicity, unless N-acetylcysteine (NAC) is administered. Situations in which acetaminophen overdose and resultant hepatotoxicity may occur include acute intentional overdose and repeated supratherapeutic overdose in adults and acute accidental ingestion or overdose and repeated supratherapeutic overdose in children.

The clinical course of acetaminophen overdose generally occurs in a three-phase sequential pattern. The first phase begins shortly after ingestion and lasts for 12 to 24 hours. The patient may manifest signs of gastrointestinal irritability, nausea, vomiting, anorexia, diaphoresis, pallor and general malaise. If toxicity continues, there is a latent phase of up to 48 hours. During this second phase, initial symptoms abate and the patient may feel better. However, hepatic enzymes, bilirubin, and prothrombin time or INR values will progressively rise. Right upper quadrant pain may develop as the liver becomes enlarged and tender. Most patients do not progress beyond this phase, especially if given N-acetylcysteine (NAC) treatment early in the course. Signs and symptoms of the third phase depend on the severity of hepatic damage and usually occur from three to five days following overdose ingestion. Symptoms may be limited to anorexia, nausea, general malaise, and abdominal pain in less severe cases or may progress to confusion, stupor and sequelae of hepatic necrosis including jaundice, coagulation defects, hypoglycemia, and encephalopathy, as well as renal failure and cardiomyopathy. Death, if it occurs, is generally the result of complications associated with fulminant hepatic failure. Mortality rates in patients with toxic plasma levels who do not receive antidote therapy range from 3% to 4%.

Due to the wide availability of acetaminophen, it is commonly involved in single and mixed drug overdose situations and the practitioner should screen for its presence in a patient's serum. Acute toxicity after single dose overdoses of acetaminophen can be anticipated when the overdose exceeds 150 mg/kg. Chronic alcohol abusers, cachectic individuals, and persons taking pharmacologic inducers of the hepatic P450 microsomal enzyme system may be at risk with lower exposures.

Specific Antidote: Any individual presenting with a possible acetaminophen overdose should be treated with N-acetylcysteine (NAC), even if the amount of acetaminophen ingested is unknown or questionable. A blood sample for determination of the plasma acetaminophen concentration should be obtained as early as possible, but no sooner than four hours following ingestion. Do not await the results of assays for plasma acetaminophen levels before initiating treatment NAC. If the acetaminophen plasma level is found to plot above the treatment line on the acetaminophen overdose nomogram, NAC treatment should be continued for a full course of therapy. NAC is used clinically to treat acute acetaminophen overdose, and acts by interacting with the oxidative intermediate, NAPQI. NAC administered by either the i.v. or the oral route is known to be a highly effective antidote for acetaminophen poisoning. It is most effective when administered within 8 hours of a significant overdose but reports have indicated benefits to treatment initiated well beyond this time period. It is imperative to administer the antidote as early as possible in the time course of acute intoxication to reap the full benefits of the antidote's protective effects. For full prescribing information, consult the product monograph for NAC.

General Management: When the possibility of acetaminophen overdose exists, treatment should begin immediately and include appropriate decontamination of the gastrointestinal tract, proper supportive care, careful assessment of appropriately timed serum acetaminophen estimations evaluated against the Rumack-Matthew nomogram, timely administration of NAC as required and appropriate follow-up care. Liver function tests should be performed initially and repeated at 24-hour intervals.

Phenylephrine HCl: Typical Toxidrome: sympathomimetic/stimulant.

Specific Antidote: none.

General Management: Stabilize the patient (A, B, Cs), undertake appropriate gastrointestinal tract decontamination procedures, initiate supportive care, consult with a Regional Poison Control Centre regarding ongoing management and arrange for appropriate follow-up care.

Dextromethorphan HBr: Typical Toxidrome: narcotic/opiate.

Specific Antidote: naloxone HCl.

General Management: Stabilize the patient (A, B, Cs), undertake appropriate gastrointestinal tract decontamination procedures, initiate supportive care, consult with a Regional Poison Control Centre regarding ongoing management and arrange for appropriate follow-up care.

Doxylamine Succinate: Typical Toxidrome: anticholinergic, CNS depressant (adult), CNS stimulant (child).

Specific Antidote: none.

General Management: Stabilize the patient (A, B, Cs), undertake appropriate gastrointestinal tract decontamination procedures, initiate supportive care, consult with a Regional Poison Control Centre regarding ongoing management and arrange for appropriate follow-up care.

Overdose During Pregnancy: Acetaminophen is one of the most common overdoses in pregnancy. Hepatic toxicity of acetaminophen follows the formation of the highly reactive metabolite N-acetyl-p-benzoquinoneimine produced by acetaminophen metabolism through the cytochrome P450 mixed-function oxidase system. Hepatic failure can be prevented by timely administration of NAC either orally for 72 hours, or intravenously (IV) for 20 hours.

Acetaminophen crosses the human placenta though the fetus is theoretically at risk when maternal overdose of acetaminophen occurs. Acetaminophen can be transformed to its toxic metabolite since the oxidative capacity of fetal microsomes is present in the fetus by 14 weeks gestation.

Studies on placental transfer of NAC in rats and sheep yielded conflicting results. Placental transfer of N-acetylcysteine in humans was demonstrated in 4 women treated with NAC for acetaminophen overdose during labour. NAC blood levels in the fetuses were within the range associated with therapeutic doses of NAC administered to adults with acetaminophen poisoning.

Fetal toxicity and stillbirth after a large (e.g. 30 g) acetaminophen overdose has been reported, but others observed a normal outcome for the offspring after acetaminophen overdose in pregnancy. A large case series investigated the pregnancy outcome in 300 women who had overdosed with acetaminophen. In this group, 118 cases occurred in the first trimester, 103 in the second trimester and 79 in the third trimester. Forty-nine of these mothers were treated with specific antidotes (33 with NAC and 16 with methionine). There were 219 live-born infants, 11 have malformations (including minor); none had been exposed to acetaminophen during the first trimester. Nine women were treated with NAC during the first trimester; there were two elective terminations; two spontaneous abortions, and five healthy babies in this group.

In summary, acetaminophen overdose during pregnancy should be treated according to regular protocols in order to prevent maternal and potentially fetal toxicity. Unless severe maternal toxicity develops, an acetaminophen overdose does not increase the risk for birth defects or adverse pregnancy outcomes.

Physicians unfamiliar with the current management of acetaminophen overdose should consult with a Poison Control Centre immediately. Telephone numbers for local Poison Control Centres are available in the local phone directory. Delays in initiation of appropriate therapy may jeopardize the patient's chances for full recovery.

> For management of a suspected drug overdose, CPhA recommends that you contact your **regional Poison Control Centre**. See the *CPS* Directory section for a list of Poison Control Centres.

ACTION AND CLINICAL PHARMACOLOGY: Mechanism of Action: Acetaminophen is a centrally acting analgesic and antipyretic drug. Although the precise mechanism of action is not totally understood, work by Boutaud suggests acetaminophen is an inhibitor of the peroxidase portion of cyclooxygenase (prostaglandin H synthase inhibitor). Depending on the redox state and substrate concentrations surrounding the enzymes, acetaminophen may or may not have a significant inhibitory effect. This accounts for its selective activity on pain and fever with little anti-inflammatory effect.

It is postulated that the analgesic effect is produced by elevation of the pain threshold and the antipyretic effect is produced through action on the hypothalamic heat-regulating centre.

The optimal effective analgesic dose of acetaminophen was demonstrated in dental pain studies and is 1000 mg every four to six hours, up to 4000 mg daily. At least 500 published and unpublished controlled clinical trials in adults and children have evaluated acetaminophen for the relief of pain or fever. These studies include single and multiple dose treatments. Most studies were less than 14 days in duration, although the longest study duration was two years. No significant safety issues were reported in any of these studies.

Moreover, at recommended doses, acetaminophen has not been shown to increase the risk of developing renal diseases or upper gastrointestinal ulceration/bleeding. This observation is consistent with its minimal inhibitory effect on peripheral prostaglandin synthesis and on gastric prostaglandin synthesis.

Acetaminophen is considered equipotent to ASA and ibuprofen, within the recommended OTC dosing ranges, in its analgesic and antipyretic effects. Acetaminophen at recommended doses does not cause the type of gastrointestinal complications associated with NSAID-containing products, such as gastric irritation, gastric erosions, occult or overt gastrointestinal blood loss, or ulcers. Unlike these drugs, however, it has no anti-inflammatory effect at clinically relevant doses in humans.

Pharmacokinetics: Absorption: Oral acetaminophen is rapidly and almost completely absorbed from the gastrointestinal tract primarily in the small intestine. This absorption process occurs by passive transport. Peak plasma concentrations occur within 0.4 to 1 hour depending on the product formulation. Although high-fat foods delay the time to peak concentration for up to an hour, the dose is completely absorbed.

Distribution: Acetaminophen is uniformly distributed throughout most body fluids, but not in fatty tissue. As a result, the volume of distribution in adults ranges between 0.8 and 1.0 L/kg 32,95. Since acetaminophen has low protein binding in plasma of only 10% to 25%, it does not compete with drugs that are highly protein bound.

Metabolism: Acetaminophen is primarily metabolized by the liver via three principal separate pathways: conjugation with glucuronide; conjugation with sulfate; oxidation via the cytochrome P450 mixed function oxidase system.

Both the glucuronic and oxidative pathways adhere to a first-order rate process, which means the concentration of acetaminophen metabolized increases as the concentration in the liver increases. The sulfate pathway adheres to Michaelis-Menten kinetics, which means the concentration of acetaminophen metabolized remains constant once the concentration in the liver increases above a saturation level. A schematic of acetaminophen metabolism is shown in Figure 2.

The major metabolic pathway is glucuronidation, where 47% to 62% of the acetaminophen dose conjugates with glucuronide. These glucuronide conjugates are inactive and nontoxic, and are secreted in bile and eliminated in the urine.

The second major pathway is sulfation, where 25% to 36% of the dose conjugates with sulfate. These sulfate ester conjugates are also inactive and nontoxic and are excreted in the urine.

The third pathway is oxidation, where 5% to 8% of the dose is metabolized via the cytochrome P450 enzyme system. The cytochrome P450 isoenzyme that is primarily responsible is CYP2E1. When acetaminophen is metabolized by CYP2E1, it forms a highly reactive intermediate, N-acetyl-p-benzoquinoneimine (NAPQI). Since NAPQI is highly reactive, it cannot be measured outside the liver nor can it accumulate. This intermediate is rapidly inactivated by hepatocellular stores of glutathione to form cysteine and mercapturate conjugates, which are both inactive and nontoxic. These conjugates are excreted in the urine.

Figure 2: TYLENOL Cold & Flu
Acetaminophen Metabolism

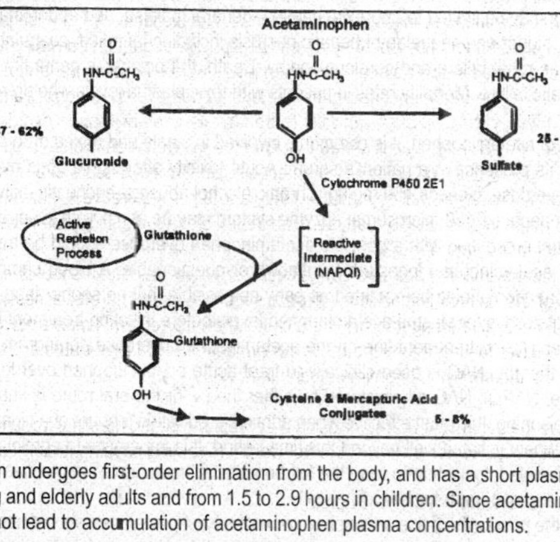

Excretion: Acetaminophen undergoes first-order elimination from the body, and has a short plasma half-life that ranges from 2 to 3 hours in healthy young and elderly adults and from 1.5 to 2.9 hours in children. Since acetaminophen clears rapidly from the body, repeated doses do not lead to accumulation of acetaminophen plasma concentrations.

STORAGE AND STABILITY: Store at room temperature (15 to 30°C).

DOSAGE FORMS, COMPOSITION AND PACKAGING: Cold & Flu Daytime Liquid: Each 30 mL (2 tablespoons) of clear, blue, slightly viscous liquid with a berry mint odour contains: acetaminophen 650 mg, phenylephrine HCl 10 mg and dextromethorphan HBr 20 mg. Nonmedicinal ingredients: citric acid, FD&C Blue no. 1, flavour, glycerin, propylene glycol, purified water, sodium benzoate, sorbitol and sucralose. Gluten-, lactose- and tartrazine-free. Bottles of 240 mL*. All packages are safety sealed.

Cold & Flu Nighttime Liquid: Each 30 mL (2 tablespoons) of clear, blue, slightly viscous liquid with a berry mint odour contains: acetaminophen 650 mg, phenylephrine HCl 10 mg, dextromethorphan HBr 20 mg and doxylamine succinate 12.5 mg. Nonmedicinal ingredients: citric acid, FD&C Blue no. 1, flavour, glycerin, propylene glycol, purified water, sodium benzoate, sorbitol and sucralose. Gluten-, lactose- and tartrazine-free. Bottles of 240 mL*. All packages are safety sealed.

* Container provided with a child-resistant closure.

Tylenol® Cough

acetaminophen—dextromethorphan HBr

Analgesic—Antipyretic—Antitussive

McNeil Consumer Healthcare

Date of Revision: June 2, 2008

SUMMARY PRODUCT INFORMATION:

Route of Administration	Dosage Form/Strength	Clinically Relevant Nonmedicinal Ingredients
Oral	Caplet/500 mg acetaminophen and 15 mg dextromethorphan HBr	Gluten-, lactose- and tartrazine-free For a complete listing of nonmedicinal ingredients, see Dosage Forms, Composition and Packaging.
	Liquid/Per 30 mL: 1000 mg acetaminophen and 30 mg dextromethorphan HBr	Gluten-, lactose- and tartrazine-free For a complete listing of nonmedicinal ingredients, see Dosage Forms, Composition and Packaging.

INDICATIONS AND CLINICAL USE: For the temporary relief of dry cough, sore throat pain, aches, pains and fever.

CONTRAINDICATIONS: Hypersensitivity to acetaminophen, pressor amines or to the ingredients of this formulation (see Dosage Forms, Composition and Packaging). Allergic reactions (primarily skin rash) or reports of hypersensitivity secondary to acetaminophen are rare and generally are controlled by discontinuation of the drug and, when necessary, symptomatic treatment.

In patients receiving or having received MAO inhibitors in the preceding 2 weeks.

WARNINGS AND PRECAUTIONS: General: Consumers should not exceed 4 g/day of acetaminophen or use two or more acetaminophen-containing products together. This includes combination products that contain acetaminophen. Do not use with other products containing salicylates or any other pain or fever medicine.

Acetaminophen-containing products should be kept out of the reach of children.

Physicians should be cognizant of and supervise the use of acetaminophen in patients with chronic alcoholism, serious kidney or serious liver disease. Physicians should alert their patients who regularly consume large amounts of alcohol not to exceed the recommended doses of acetaminophen. Chronic heavy alcohol abusers may be at increased risk of liver toxicity from excessive doses of acetaminophen.

Patients should be counseled to consult a physician if redness or swelling is present in an area of pain, if symptoms do not improve or if they worsen, or if new symptoms such as high fever, rash, itching, excessive mucus or persistent or recurring cough or persistent headache occur, as these may be signs of a condition which requires medical attention.

Acetaminophen should not be taken for pain for more than 5 days, for fever for more than 3 days or if new symptoms appear, without consulting a physician.

Patients with asthma, emphysema, chronic pulmonary disease or shortness of breath should not use this medication unless directed by a physician. This product should not be used for persistent or chronic cough such as occurs with smoking, asthma or emphysema unless directed by a physician.

Hepatic/Biliary/Pancreatic: Slower metabolism of acetaminophen, increased activity of the cytochrome P450 enzyme system, or depleted glutathione stores are cited as theoretical risk factors for acetaminophen hepatotoxicity in patients with chronic liver disease. However, acetaminophen has been studied in both adults and children with a wide variety of liver diseases including various types of cirrhosis, hepatitis (including hepatitis C), nodular transformation, congenital hepatic fibrosis, and α1-antitrypsin deficiency. In none of these conditions is there evidence of an increased risk for hepatotoxicity at currently recommended acetaminophen doses but the studies were insufficiently powered to definitely establish the extent of risk.

Forrest compared acetaminophen metabolism following a single 1500 mg dose in normal subjects, patients with mild liver disease, and patients with severe liver disease. There were no significant differences in overall 24-hour urinary excretion of acetaminophen and glucuronide, sulfate, cysteine, and mercapturic acid conjugates, evidence that acetaminophen metabolism was similar to that in normal subjects. However, the elimination half-life was significantly prolonged in patients with severe liver disease.

Acetaminophen has also been studied in pediatric patients with liver disease. Following a single (10 mg/kg) dose of acetaminophen, the pharmacokinetic profiles in pediatric patients with mild, moderate, or severe liver disease were not significantly different. Although the plasma half-life of acetaminophen was prolonged in patients with severe liver disease, there were no significant differences in the 36-hour (children) urinary excretion of acetaminophen or its conjugates.

Acetaminophen may cause hepatotoxicity in situations of intentional overdose (e.g. attempted suicide), unintentional overdose (e.g. overdosing when pain relief is not satisfactory), simultaneous use of multiple acetaminophen-containing preparations, accidental overdose or in very rare cases, after recommended doses, although causality has not been determined. The hepatotoxic reaction can be severe and life-threatening. Early symptoms following a hepatotoxic overdose may include nausea, vomiting, diaphoresis, lethargy, and general malaise. If appropriate treatment is not instituted, these may progress to upper quadrant pain, confusion, stupor, and sequelae of hepatic necrosis, such as jaundice, coagulation defects, hypoglycemia, and encephalopathy. Renal failure and cardiomyopathy may also occur. In the event of known or suspected overdosage, treatment with N-acetyl cysteine should be instituted immediately (see Overdosage), even when there are no obvious symptoms. Failure to promptly treat acetaminophen hepatotoxicity with N-acetyl cysteine can result in liver failure, leading to liver transplantation and/or death.

Chronic Alcohol Use: Excessive alcohol use may increase risk of liver toxicity from acetaminophen overdose (acute or chronic).

In prospective, placebo controlled studies, researchers evaluated an actively drinking group of alcoholics with a high prevalence of malnourishment. The study participants abruptly stopped their daily alcohol intake and took acetaminophen the next day. This should theoretically make them vulnerable to acetaminophen injury because their CYP2E1 would be maximally induced from the alcohol and there would be no alcohol present to compete with acetaminophen for metabolism by CYP2E1. There was no statistically significant difference in mean values for AST, ALT, or INR for alcoholics given four grams per day of acetaminophen compared to placebo. Additionally, the researchers performed an analysis of the malnourished patients that showed there was no increase in AST or ALT levels in these patients. Study limitations include a limited duration of 2 days and exclusion of patients with preexisting AST or ALT elevations greater than 120 U/L. Study results do not preclude the possibility of an idiosyncratic hepatic reaction.

Renal: Martin found that patients with chronic renal failure had higher plasma concentrations of acetaminophen and the inactive glucuronide and sulfate metabolites than healthy subjects during repeated dosing up to ten days.

Several single-dose studies demonstrate accumulation of acetaminophen metabolites in patients with moderate chronic renal failure and in anephric patients for whom hemodialysis appeared to be the major route of elimination.

The habitual consumption of acetaminophen should be discouraged. If indicated medically, the long-term use of acetaminophen should be supervised by a physician.

A National Kidney Foundation position paper notes that physicians preferentially recommend acetaminophen to patients with renal failure because of the bleeding complications associated with ASA in these individuals.

Special Populations: Geriatrics: In a comprehensive metabolic study by Miners, the formation and clearance of glucuronide and glutathione conjugates were the same in young and elderly adults, although clearance of the sulphate conjugate and unchanged acetaminophen were reduced. This finding provides prospective scientific data that the amount of acetaminophen metabolized via the oxidative pathway, from which the highly reactive intermediate, NAPQI, is generated, does not increase with age. Recently, Bannwarth evaluated the multiple-dose pharmacokinetics of acetaminophen in elderly patients. After seven days of repeat dosing, acetaminophen did not accumulate in the plasma, and the elimination half-life was the same as that reported for young adults.

Elderly patients who require therapy for longer than 5 days should consult their physician for condition monitoring.

Glucose-6-Phosphate Dehydrogenase (G6PD) Deficiency: In therapeutic doses, acetaminophen does not shorten the life-span of red blood cells and does not produce any clinically perceptible destruction of circulating red blood cells.

Obese Adults: O'Shea studied the pharmacokinetics of chlorzoxazone (a putative probe for CYP2E1 activity) to evaluate the effect of obesity on CYP2E1 activity. The authors concluded that CYP2E1 is induced in obese adults and that this could impact the metabolic pathway of a number of drugs metabolized by CYP2E1, including acetaminophen. However, acetaminophen pharmacokinetic data have been investigated in obese adults. In this prospective study, 650 mg acetaminophen was administered intravenously to obese men (297 lb), obese women (193 lb), control men (155 lb) and control women (121 lb). Acetaminophen distribution volume per total body weight was slightly lower in the obese adults but, more importantly, the half-life and metabolic clearance per total body weight did not differ among groups.

ADVERSE REACTIONS: Central Nervous System Effects: Acetaminophen at recommended doses has no obvious effects on central nervous system function. In an overdose situation, central nervous system effects are uncommon.

Gastrointestinal Effects: Acetaminophen at recommended doses does not cause gastric irritation, gastric erosions, occult or overt gastrointestinal blood loss or ulcers.

Blot and McLaughlin conducted an independent analysis of case-control data from a study conducted by the American College of Gastroenterology. The risk of gastrointestinal bleeding increased two to three-fold among recent users of ASA, ibuprofen and other NSAIDs at OTC doses, and the risk was also dose-related. In contrast, the use of acetaminophen was not associated with an increased risk of gastrointestinal bleeding.

Hematologic Effects: Acetaminophen does not have any immediate or delayed effects on small vessel hemostasis, as measured by bleeding time. In normal volunteers receiving a single dose of acetaminophen (975 or 1950 mg) or multiple doses of acetaminophen (1950 mg daily for 6 weeks), no change in bleeding time or platelet aggregation was observed. In another study, a single 1000 mg dose of acetaminophen was given to normal volunteers and did not affect bleeding time or platelet aggregation. Patients with hemophilia receiving multiple doses of acetaminophen showed no significant changes in bleeding time.

Haematological reactions including thrombocytopenia, leucopenia, pancytopenia, neutropenia, and agranulocytosis have been reported, although these are rare and causality has not been established.

Hepatic Effects: As an illustration of the margin of safety of acetaminophen at supratherapeutic doses, a comparison of serum concentrations of acetaminophen over time for a standard 15 mg/kg dose and for a dose exceeding the standard by a multiple of 5 (75 mg/kg) are shown in Figure 1. The serum concentrations are drawn relative to the risk line for hepatotoxicity and treatment line of the Rumack-Matthew nomogram used to manage acute overdoses. The mean plasma concentrations for this supratherapeutic dose are well below the risk and treatment lines of the nomogram at all times. However, to minimize the risk for adverse effects, the maximum recommended dose should not be exceeded.

Figure 1: TYLENOL Cough

Mean Data for a Standard (1 g, 15 mg/kg) and Higher (5.6 g, 75 mg/kg) Dose Relative to Risk and Treatment Lines of the Acetaminophen Nomogram

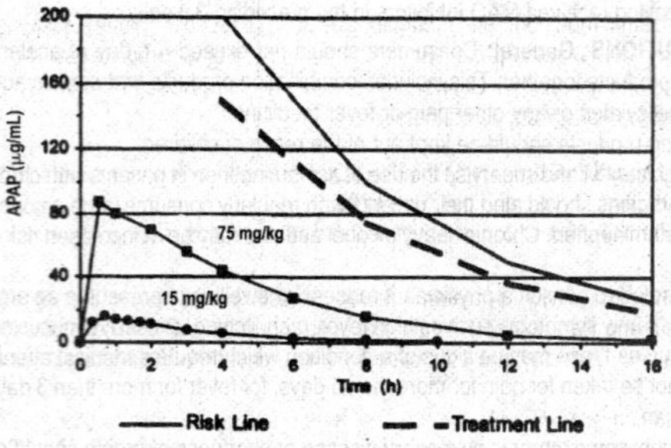

Acetaminophen in overdosage may cause hepatotoxicity. In adults and adolescents, hepatotoxicity may occur following ingestion of greater than 150 mg/kg over a period of 8 hours or less. Fatalities are infrequent (less than 3% to 4% of untreated cases in which blood levels exceed the treatment line) and have rarely been reported with overdoses less than 7.5 g. In children, amounts less than 150 mg/kg are unlikely to produce hepatotoxicity. In both adults and children, toxicity associated with acetaminophen is usually caused by ingestion of quantities of the drug that are significantly above the recommended dosage range. Hepatotoxicity, ranging from transient sharp transaminase elevations to fatal, fulminant hepatic failure, is the most common result of clinically significant overdosage.

In a double-blind, placebo-controlled clinical study, healthy adults were given 4, 6 and 8 g/day of acetaminophen over 3 days. Plasma concentrations did not accumulate with repeat doses. Clinically all doses were well tolerated by the subjects and aminotransferase values stayed within normal limits throughout the study. These data provide information related to the margin of safety but are not intended to support dosing beyond the maximum recommended dose of 4 g/day.

A report has suggested that hepatotoxicity following greater than the recommended dose of acetaminophen may be enhanced by both prolonged fasting and/or chronic alcohol abuse.

Acute Alcohol Use: Acute alcohol ingestion refers to the occasional or intermittent use of alcohol. When taken together, alcohol competes with acetaminophen for CYP2E1. CYP2E1 accepts alcohol more readily than acetaminophen; therefore, less NAPQI is produced. In the presence of alcohol, acetaminophen may be diverted to the glucuronidation and sulfation pathways. The overall result is that a smaller percentage of acetaminophen may be expected to be metabolized to the toxic intermediate, NAPQI, than would otherwise be the case. NAPQI production is increased above baseline for the period up to 18-24 hours post ethanol clearance from the body. In healthy adults, at normal labeled doses of acetaminophen, the temporary increase in NAPQI production is more than accommodated by normal glutathione stores in the liver.

Hypersensitivity: Sensitivity reactions are rare and may manifest as rash, urticaria, dyspnea, hypotension, laryngeal edema, angioedema, bronchospasm, or anaphylaxis. Cross-reactivity in ASA-sensitive persons has been rarely reported. If sensitivity is suspected, discontinue use of the drug.

Renal Effects: Acute nephrotoxicity has been reported following massive overdose either as a sequela of hepatic failure or, occasionally, in the absence of hepatic failure.

Clinical data have established that acetaminophen in recommended doses is not nephrotoxic.

Some studies suggest an association between the chronic long-term use of acetaminophen and renal effects. Results, however, are conflicting, limited by recall bias and confounded by the inability to determine whether analgesic use preceded or followed the onset of renal disease.

Case control studies have suggested a weak association between habitual acetaminophen use and prevalence of chronic renal failure and end stage renal disease. This National Kidney Foundation position paper concludes that acetaminophen has been preferentially recommended by physicians to patients with renal failure and that there is no evidence that occasional use of acetaminophen caused renal injury.

Special Populations: Pediatrics: Lesko and Mitchell enrolled more than 84 000 febrile children in a randomized, double blind, acetaminophen-controlled trial to assess the risks of rare but serious adverse events following use of pediatric ibuprofen. Of the children included in the analysis, 28 130 received acetaminophen and none experienced anaphylaxis, or serious hepatic, gastrointestinal or renal effects.

Pregnancy and Lactation: As with any drug, patients who are pregnant or nursing a baby should consult a physician before taking this product.

Pregnancy: Issues of risks in pregnancy are multifactorial. The information provided cannot be substituted for direct patient consultation. Acetaminophen is believed to be non-teratogenic in humans. However, existing studies have not assessed the effect of very high doses. The Motherrisk Collaborative Perinatal project monitored 50 282 mother-child pairs, of which 226 had first trimester exposure to acetaminophen and 781 had used acetaminophen at any time during their pregnancy. No evidence was found to suggest a relationship between acetaminophen use and major or minor malformations. In a surveillance study of Michigan Medicaid recipients conducted between 1985 and 1992 involving 229 101 completed pregnancies, 9146 newborns had been exposed to acetaminophen during the first trimester. This data do not support an association between acetaminophen use and the occurrence of birth defects. Another cohort study, using prescription monitoring, found no excess risk for malformation, and no evidence that acetaminophen influenced fetal growth. Finally, as part of a larger study, 697 women used acetaminophen with or without codeine in their first trimester. No teratogenic risk was found.

A prospective study investigated the outcome of pregnancy in 300 women who had self-administered an overdose of acetaminophen, either alone, or as part of a combined preparation. Exposure to overdose occurred in all trimesters. The majority of the pregnancies had normal outcomes. The malformation rate was within the expected range. There was no obvious relationship between the time of exposure and the time of delivery. The overall conclusion was that acetaminophen overdose is not an indication for termination of pregnancy.

In a long-term developmental follow-up study, acetaminophen did not adversely affect IQ or behavior measures at four years of age. Height, weight and head circumference were also not affected by exposure to acetaminophen in-utero.

Unlike ASA, which has been shown to profoundly effect platelet function, there does not seem to be a risk of hemorrhage associated with acetaminophen use at term.

Currently there is no evidence to suggest that acetaminophen is teratogenic when used as recommended. However, data for continuous high daily doses are not sufficient, and safety during pregnancy has not yet been established.

Lactation: Following a typical therapeutic dose, acetaminophen is excreted in breast milk in very low concentrations. Based on a number of published reports, infant exposure levels are at most 4.5% of a weight adjusted pediatric therapeutic dose. In addition, acetaminophen is considered compatible with breast-feeding by the American Academy of Pediatrics.

DRUG INTERACTIONS: Alcohol: Studies evaluating the metabolism of doses up to 20 mg/kg of acetaminophen in chronic alcohol abusers and a study evaluating the effects of 2 days of acetaminophen dosing at 4000 mg/day in chronic alcoholics undergoing detoxification, have yielded inconsistent results with regard to effects on acetaminophen pharmacokinetics and demonstrate no evidence of adverse effect on liver function tests.

Anticoagulants–Oral: Patients who concomitantly medicate with warfarin-type anticoagulants and regular doses of acetaminophen have occasionally been reported to have unforeseen elevations in their INR. Physicians should be cognizant of this potential interaction and monitor the INR in such patients closely while therapy is established. Many factors, including diet, medications, and environmental and physical states, may affect how a patient responds to anticoagulant therapy. There have been several reports that suggest that acetaminophen may produce hypoprothrombinemia (elevated international normalized ratio [INR] or prothrombin time) when administered with coumarin derivatives. In other studies, prothrombin time did not change. Reported changes have been generally of limited clinical significance, however, periodic evaluation of prothrombin time should be performed when these agents are administered concurrently.

In the period immediately following discharge from the hospital or whenever other medications are initiated, discontinued, or taken regularly, it is important to monitor patient response to anticoagulation therapy with additional prothrombin time or INR determinations. Despite the potential for interaction, acetaminophen is the least likely OTC analgesic to interfere with anticoagulant therapy.

Anticonvulsants: Some reports have suggested that patients taking long-term anticonvulsants, who overdose on acetaminophen, may be at increased risk of hepatotoxicity because of accelerated metabolism of acetaminophen. Available data are conflicting. A 7-year retrospective study of acetaminophen overdose admissions indicates that the overall mortality rate was not significantly different for patients taking concomitant anticonvulsant medications.

Hydantoins: Pharmacokinetic studies indicate that phenytoin primarily induces the glucuronidation pathway, whereas glutathione-derived metabolites are not increased in patients on chronic phenytoin therapy. Additionally, recent data demonstrate that phenytoin is metabolized primarily by CYP2C9 and CYP2C19, whereas acetaminophen is primarily metabolized by CYP2E1.

Carbamazepine: Carbamazepine is primarily metabolized by CYP3A4, whereas acetaminophen is metabolized primarily via CYP2E1. It is not known whether there is increased risk from an acetaminophen overdose in patients on chronic carbamazepine therapy.

Diflunisal: Professional literature from the manufacturer of diflunisal cautions that concomitant administration with acetaminophen produces an approximate 50% increase in plasma levels of acetaminophen in normal volunteers. Acetaminophen had no effect on diflunisal plasma levels. The clinical significance of these findings has not been established. However, caution should be used with concomitant administration of diflunisal and acetaminophen and patients should be monitored carefully.

Isoniazid: Some reports suggest that patients on chronic isoniazid therapy may be at risk for developing hepatotoxicity from an acetaminophen overdose. Since patients on isoniazid therapy may develop hepatic effects from isoniazid alone, data from individual case reports are unclear as to whether chronic administration of isoniazid may increase the risk of acetaminophen toxicity. Isoniazid is primarily metabolized by CYP2E1 and induces CYP2E1. Studies in healthy subjects demonstrate that isoniazid blocks the formation of the toxic metabolite NAPQI when administered concomitantly with acetaminophen, but increase NAPQI formation when acetaminophen is administered one day after discontinuation of isoniazid. Thus, concomitant use of isoniazid is unlikely to potentiate the risk of acetaminophen-induced hepatotoxicity at recommended doses. The isoniazid induction of CYP2E1 is short-lived, lasting only 12 to 48 hours after the discontinuation of isoniazid, it is during this period the toxicity of an acetaminophen overdose may be potentiated.

DOSAGE AND ADMINISTRATION:

Caplets: Adults (12 years of age and older): 2 caplets every 6 to 8 hours, as required. Do not exceed 8 caplets in any 24-hour period.

Liquid: Adults (12 years of age and older): 30 mL (2 tablespoons) every 6 to 8 hours as needed. It is hazardous to exceed 120 mL (8 tablespoons) per day.

OVERDOSAGE:

Symptoms and Treatment: Acetaminophen: Typical Toxidrome: Hepatic injury is the principal toxic effect of a substantial acetaminophen overdose. The physician should be mindful that there is no early presentation that is pathognomic for the overdose. A high degree of clinical suspicion must always be maintained.

Untreated acetaminophen overdoses may produce hepatotoxicity. Acetaminophen hepatotoxicity occurs as a threshold effect and is characterized by a lack of toxicity at lower/therapeutic doses. Acetaminophen hepatotoxicity occurs after major depletion of glutathione, an endogenous detoxifying substance. Once the threshold is exceeded, increasing acetaminophen doses may produce increasing degrees of hepatotoxicity, unless N-acetylcysteine (NAC) is administered. Situations in which acetaminophen overdose and resultant hepatotoxicity may occur include acute intentional overdose and repeated supratherapeutic overdose in adults and acute accidental ingestion or overdose and repeated supratherapeutic overdose in children.

The clinical course of acetaminophen overdose generally occurs in a three-phase sequential pattern. The first phase begins shortly after ingestion and lasts for 12 to 24 hours. The patient may manifest signs of gastrointestinal irritability, nausea, vomiting, anorexia, diaphoresis, pallor and general malaise. If toxicity continues, there is a latent phase of up to 48 hours. During this second phase, initial symptoms abate and the patient may feel better. However, hepatic enzymes, bilirubin, and prothrombin time or INR values will progressively rise. Right upper quadrant pain may develop as the liver becomes enlarged and tender. Most patients do not progress beyond this phase, especially if given N-acetylcysteine (NAC) treatment early in the course. Signs and symptoms of the third phase depend on the severity of hepatic damage and usually occur from three to five days following overdose ingestion. Symptoms may be limited to anorexia, nausea, general malaise, and abdominal pain in less severe cases or may progress to confusion, stupor and sequelae of hepatic necrosis including jaundice, coagulation defects, hypoglycemia, and encephalopathy, as well as renal failure and cardiomyopathy. Death, if it occurs, is generally the result of complications associated with fulminant hepatic failure. Mortality rates in patients with toxic plasma levels who do not receive antidote therapy range from 3% to 4%.

Due to the wide availability of acetaminophen, it is commonly involved in single and mixed drug overdose situations and the practitioner should screen for its presence in a patient's serum. Acute toxicity after single dose overdoses of acetaminophen can be anticipated when the overdose exceeds 150 mg/kg. Chronic alcohol abusers, cachectic individuals, and persons taking pharmacologic inducers of the hepatic P450 microsomal enzyme system may be at risk with lower exposures.

Specific Antidote: Any individual presenting with a possible acetaminophen overdose should be treated with N-acetylcysteine (NAC), even if the amount of acetaminophen ingested is unknown or questionable. A blood sample for determination of the plasma acetaminophen concentration should be obtained as early as possible, but no sooner than four hours following ingestion. Do not await the results of assays for plasma acetaminophen levels before initiating treatment NAC. If the acetaminophen plasma level is found to plot above the treatment line on the acetaminophen overdose nomogram, NAC treatment should be continued for a full course of therapy. NAC is used clinically to treat acute acetaminophen overdose, and acts by interacting with the oxidative intermediate, NAPQI. NAC administered by either the i.v. or the oral route is known to be a highly effective antidote for acetaminophen poisoning. It is most effective when administered within 8 hours of a significant overdose but reports have indicated benefits to treatment initiated well beyond this time period. It is imperative to administer the antidote as early as possible in the time course of acute intoxication to reap the full benefits of the antidote's protective effects. For full prescribing information, consult the product monograph for NAC.

General Management: When the possibility of acetaminophen overdose exists, treatment should begin immediately and include appropriate decontamination of the gastrointestinal tract, proper supportive care, careful assessment of appropriately timed serum acetaminophen estimations evaluated against the Rumack-Matthew nomogram, timely administration of NAC as required and appropriate follow-up care. Liver function tests should be performed initially and repeated at 24-hour intervals.

Dextromethorphan HBr: Typical Toxidrome: narcotic/opiate.

Specific Antidote: naloxone HCl.

General Management: Stabilize the patient (A, B, Cs), undertake appropriate gastrointestinal tract decontamination procedures, initiate supportive care, consult with a Regional Poison Control Centre regarding ongoing management and arrange for appropriate follow-up care.

Overdose During Pregnancy: Acetaminophen is one of the most common overdoses in pregnancy. Hepatic toxicity of acetaminophen follows the formation of the highly reactive metabolite N-acetyl-p-benzoquinoneimine produced by acetaminophen metabolism through the cytochrome P450 mixed-function oxidase system. Hepatic failure can be prevented by timely administration of NAC either orally for 72 hours, or intravenously (IV) for 20 hours.

Acetaminophen crosses the human placenta though the fetus is theoretically at risk when maternal overdose of acetaminophen occurs. Acetaminophen can be transformed to its toxic metabolite since the oxidative capacity of fetal microsomes is present in the fetus by 14 weeks gestation.

Studies on placental transfer of NAC in rats and sheep yielded conflicting results. Placental transfer of N-acetylcysteine in humans was demonstrated in 4 women treated with NAC for acetaminophen overdose during labour. NAC blood levels in the fetuses were within the range associated with therapeutic doses of NAC administered to adults with acetaminophen poisoning.

Fetal toxicity and stillbirth after a large (e.g. 30 g) acetaminophen overdose has been reported, but others observed a normal outcome for the offspring after acetaminophen overdose in pregnancy. A large case series investigated the pregnancy outcome in 300 women who had overdosed with acetaminophen. In this group, 118 cases occurred in the first trimester, 103 in the second trimester and 79 in the third trimester. Forty-nine of these mothers were treated with specific antidotes (33 with NAC and 16 with methionine). There were 219 live-born infants, 11 have malformations (including minor); none had been exposed to acetaminophen during the first trimester. Nine women were treated with NAC during the first trimester; there were two elective terminations; two spontaneous abortions, and five healthy babies in this group.

In summary, acetaminophen overdose during pregnancy should be treated according to regular protocols in order to prevent maternal and potentially fetal toxicity. Unless severe maternal toxicity develops, an acetaminophen overdose does not increase the risk for birth defects or adverse pregnancy outcomes.

Physicians unfamiliar with the current management of acetaminophen overdose should consult with a Poison Control Centre immediately. Telephone numbers for local Poison Control Centres are available in the local phone directory. Delays in initiation of appropriate therapy may jeopardize the patient's chances for full recovery.

> For management of a suspected drug overdose, CPhA recommends that you contact your **regional Poison Control Centre**. See the *CPS* Directory section for a list of Poison Control Centres.

ACTION AND CLINICAL PHARMACOLOGY: Mechanism of Action: Acetaminophen is a centrally acting analgesic and antipyretic drug. Although the precise mechanism of action is not totally understood, work by Boutaud suggests acetaminophen is an inhibitor of the peroxidase portion of cyclooxygenase (prostaglandin H synthase inhibitor). Depending on the redox state and substrate concentrations surrounding the enzymes, acetaminophen may or may not have a significant inhibitory effect. This accounts for its selective activity on pain and fever with little anti-inflammatory effect.

It is postulated that the analgesic effect is produced by elevation of the pain threshold and the antipyretic effect is produced through action on the hypothalamic heat-regulating centre.

The optimal effective analgesic dose of acetaminophen was demonstrated in dental pain studies and is 1000 mg every four to six hours, up to 4000 mg daily. At least 500 published and unpublished controlled clinical trials in adults and children have evaluated acetaminophen for the relief of pain or fever. These studies include single and multiple dose treatments. Most studies were less than 14 days in duration, although the longest study duration was two years. No significant safety issues were reported in any of these studies.

Moreover, at recommended doses, acetaminophen has not been shown to increase the risk of developing renal diseases or upper gastrointestinal ulceration/bleeding. This observation is consistent with its minimal inhibitory effect on peripheral prostaglandin synthesis and on gastric prostaglandin synthesis.

Acetaminophen is considered equipotent to ASA and ibuprofen, within the recommended OTC dosing ranges, in its analgesic and antipyretic effects. Acetaminophen at recommended doses does not cause the type of gastrointestinal complications associated with NSAID-containing products, such as gastric irritation, gastric erosions, occult or overt gastrointestinal blood loss, or ulcers. Unlike these drugs, however, it has no anti-inflammatory effect at clinically relevant doses in humans.

Pharmacokinetics: Absorption: Oral acetaminophen is rapidly and almost completely absorbed from the gastrointestinal tract primarily in the small intestine. This absorption process occurs by passive transport. Peak plasma concentrations occur within 0.4 to 1 hour depending on the product formulation. Although high-fat foods delay the time to peak concentration for up to an hour, the dose is completely absorbed.

Distribution: Acetaminophen is uniformly distributed throughout most body fluids, but not in fatty tissue. As a result, the volume of distribution in adults ranges between 0.8 and 1.0 L/kg. Since acetaminophen has low protein binding in plasma of only 10% to 25%, it does not compete with drugs that are highly protein bound.

Metabolism: Acetaminophen is primarily metabolized by the liver via three principal separate pathways: conjugation with glucuronide; conjugation with sulfate; oxidation via the cytochrome P450 mixed function oxidase system.

Both the glucuronic and oxidative pathways adhere to a first-order rate process, which means the concentration of acetaminophen metabolized increases as the concentration in the liver increases. The sulfate pathway adheres to Michaelis-Menten kinetics, which means the concentration of acetaminophen metabolized remains constant once the concentration in the liver increases above a saturation level. A schematic of acetaminophen metabolism is shown in Figure 2.

The major metabolic pathway is glucuronidation, where 47% to 62% of the acetaminophen dose conjugates with glucuronide. These glucuronide conjugates are inactive and nontoxic, and are secreted in bile and eliminated in the urine.

The second major pathway is sulfation, where 25% to 36% of the dose conjugates with sulfate. These sulfate ester conjugates are also inactive and nontoxic and are excreted in the urine.

The third pathway is oxidation, where 5% to 8% of the dose is metabolized via the cytochrome P450 enzyme system. The cytochrome P450 isoenzyme that is primarily responsible is CYP2E1. When acetaminophen is metabolized by CYP2E1, it forms a highly reactive intermediate, N-acetyl-p-benzoquinoneimine (NAPQI). Since NAPQI is highly reactive, it cannot be measured outside the liver nor can it accumulate. This intermediate is rapidly inactivated by hepatocellular stores of glutathione to form cysteine and mercapturate conjugates, which are both inactive and nontoxic. These conjugates are excreted in the urine.

Figure 2: TYLENOL Cough

Acetaminophen Metabolism

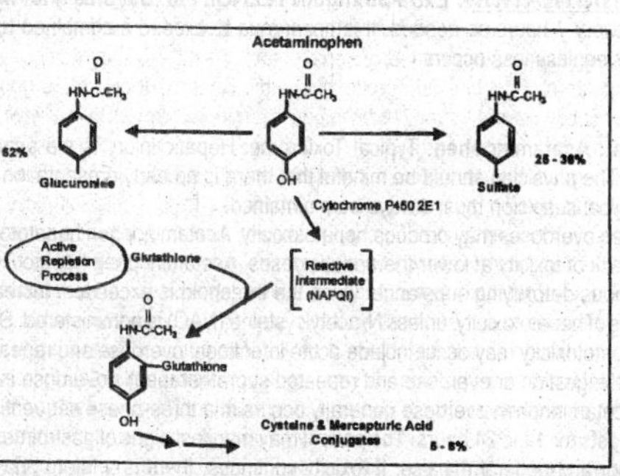

Excretion: Acetaminophen undergoes first-order elimination from the body, and has a short plasma half-life that ranges from 2 to 3 hours in healthy young and elderly adults and from 1.5 to 2.9 hours in children. Since acetaminophen clears rapidly from the body, repeated doses do not lead to accumulation of acetaminophen plasma concentrations.

STORAGE AND STABILITY: Store at room temperature (15 to 30°C).

DOSAGE FORMS, COMPOSITION AND PACKAGING: Caplets: Each extra strength, capsule-shaped, hard, red film-coated tablet, engraved "TYCOF" on one side and "500" on the other side, contains: acetaminophen 500 mg and dextromethorphan HBr 15 mg. Nonmedicinal ingredients: carnauba wax, cellulose, cornstarch, FD&C Red No. 40, FD&C Yellow No. 6, flavour, hypromellose, magnesium stearate, polyethylene glycol, polysorbate 80, sodium starch glycolate and titanium dioxide. Energy: 1.2 kJ (0.3 kcal). Sodium: 0.4 mg. Gluten-, lactose- and tartrazine-free. Plastic bottles of 20*.

Liquid: Each 30 mL (2 tablespoons) dose of clear, blue, slightly viscous liquid with a berry mint odour, contains: acetaminophen 1000 mg and dextromethorphan HBr 30 mg. Nonmedicinal ingredients: citric acid, FD&C Blue no. 1, flavour, polyethylene glycol, propylene glycol, purified water, sodium benzoate, sodium carboxymethylcellulose, sorbitol, sucralose and sucrose. Energy: 352.5 kJ (84.2 kcal)/30 mL. Sodium: 9.6 mg/30 mL. Gluten-, lactose- and tartrazine-free. Bottles of 240 mL*.

All packages are safety sealed.

* Container provided with a child-resistant closure.

Tylenol® Flu Extra Strength Daytime

acetaminophen—dextromethorphan HBr—phenylephrine HCl

Analgesic—Antipyretic—Antitussive—Decongestant

McNeil Consumer Healthcare

Tylenol® Flu Extra Strength Nighttime

acetaminophen—dextromethorphan HBr—phenylephrine HCl—chlorpheniramine maleate

Analgesic—Antipyretic—Antitussive—Decongestant—Antihistamine

McNeil Consumer Healthcare

Date of Revision: October 30, 2009

SUMMARY PRODUCT INFORMATION:

Route of Administration	Dosage Form/Strength	Clinically Relevant Nonmedicinal Ingredients
Oral	Daytime Tablet/ 500 mg acetaminophen, 10 mg dextromethorphan HBr and 5 mg phenylephrine HCl	Alcohol-, gluten-, lactose-, sulfite- and tartrazine-free For a complete listing of nonmedicinal ingredients, see Dosage Forms, Composition and Packaging.
	Nighttime Tablet/500 mg acetaminophen, 10 mg dextromethorphan HBr, 5 mg phenylephrine HCl and 2 mg chlorpheniramine maleate	Alcohol-, gluten-, lactose-, sulfite- and tartrazine-free For a complete listing of nonmedicinal ingredients, see Dosage Forms, Composition and Packaging.

INDICATIONS AND CLINICAL USE: Extra Strength TYLENOL Flu Daytime: A non-drowsy formulation for the effective relief of nasal congestion, dry cough, fever, aches and pain due to flu.

Extra Strength TYLENOL Flu Nighttime: For the effective relief of nasal congestion, dry cough, fever, runny nose, sneezing, aches and pain due to flu.

CONTRAINDICATIONS: Hypersensitivity to acetaminophen, pressor amines or to the ingredients of this formulation (see Dosage Forms, Composition and Packaging). Allergic reactions (primarily skin rash) or reports of hypersensitivity secondary to acetaminophen are rare and generally are controlled by discontinuation of the drug and, when necessary, symptomatic treatment.

In patients receiving or having received MAO inhibitors in the preceding 2 weeks. Although phenylephrine is virtually without pressor effect in normotensive patients, it should be used with caution in hypertensives.

WARNINGS AND PRECAUTIONS: General: Consumers should not exceed 4 g/day of acetaminophen or use two or more acetaminophen-containing products together. This includes combination products that contain acetaminophen. Do not use with other products containing salicylates or any other pain or fever medicine.

Acetaminophen-containing products should be kept out of the reach of children.

Physicians should be cognizant of and supervise the use of acetaminophen in patients with chronic alcoholism, serious kidney or serious liver disease. Physicians should alert their patients who regularly consume large amounts of alcohol not to exceed the recommended doses of acetaminophen. Chronic heavy alcohol abusers may be at increased risk of liver toxicity from excessive doses of acetaminophen.

Patients should be counseled to consult a physician if redness or swelling is present in an area of pain, if symptoms do not improve or if they worsen, or if new symptoms such as high fever, rash, itching, excessive mucus, persistent or recurring cough or persistent headache occur, as these may be signs of a condition which requires medical attention.

Acetaminophen should not be taken for pain for more than 5 days, for fever for more than 3 days or if new symptoms appear, without consulting a physician.

In patients with high blood pressure, heart disease, diabetes, thyroid disease, difficulty in urination due to enlargement of the prostate gland or who are taking a prescription drug for high blood pressure or depression, phenylephrine HCl should be used with caution and only under close medical supervision.

Patients with asthma, glaucoma, emphysema, chronic pulmonary disease or shortness of breath should not use this medication unless directed by a physician. This product should not be used for persistent or chronic cough such as occurs with smoking, asthma or emphysema unless directed by a physician.

Occupational Hazards: Preparations containing chlorpheniramine maleate may cause drowsiness. Alcoholic beverages, sedatives and tranquilizers may increase this effect and should be avoided. Advise caution when driving a motor vehicle or operating machinery or engaging in any activity requiring alertness. Patients taking tranquilizers or sedatives should not take this medication before consulting a physician.

Hepatic/Biliary/Pancreatic: Slower metabolism of acetaminophen, increased activity of the cytochrome P450 enzyme system, or depleted glutathione stores are cited as theoretical risk factors for acetaminophen hepatotoxicity in patients with chronic liver disease. However, acetaminophen has been studied in both adults and children with a wide variety of liver diseases including various types of cirrhosis, hepatitis (including hepatitis C), nodular transformation, congenital hepatic fibrosis, and α1-antitrypsin deficiency. In none of these conditions is there evidence of an increased risk for hepatotoxicity at currently recommended acetaminophen doses but the studies were insufficiently powered to definitely establish the extent of risk.

Forrest compared acetaminophen metabolism following a single 1500 mg dose in normal subjects, patients with mild liver disease, and patients with severe liver disease. There were no significant differences in overall 24-hour urinary excretion of acetaminophen and glucuronide, sulfate, cysteine, and mercapturic acid conjugates, evidence that acetaminophen metabolism was similar to that in normal subjects. However, the elimination half-life was significantly prolonged in patients with severe liver disease.

Acetaminophen has also been studied in pediatric patients with liver disease. Following a single (10 mg/kg) dose of acetaminophen, the pharmacokinetic profiles in pediatric patients with mild, moderate, or severe liver disease were not significantly different. Although the plasma half-life of acetaminophen was prolonged in patients with severe liver disease, there were no significant differences in the 36-hour (children) urinary excretion of acetaminophen or its conjugates.

Acetaminophen may cause hepatotoxicity in situations of intentional overdose (e.g. attempted suicide), unintentional overdose (e.g. overdosing when pain relief is not satisfactory), simultaneous use of multiple acetaminophen-containing preparations, accidental overdose or in very rare cases, after recommended doses, although causality has not been determined. The hepatotoxic reaction can be severe and life-threatening. Early symptoms following a hepatotoxic overdose may include nausea, vomiting, diaphoresis, lethargy, and general malaise. If appropriate treatment is not instituted, these may progress to upper quadrant pain, confusion, stupor, and sequelae of hepatic necrosis, such as jaundice, coagulation defects, hypoglycemia, and encephalopathy. Renal failure and cardiomyopathy may also occur. In the event of known or suspected overdosage, treatment with N-acetyl cysteine should be instituted immediately (see Overdosage), even when there are no obvious symptoms. Failure to promptly treat acetaminophen hepatotoxicity with N-acetyl cysteine can result in liver failure, leading to liver transplantation and/or death.

Chronic Alcohol Use: Excessive alcohol use may increase risk of liver toxicity from acetaminophen overdose (acute or chronic).

In prospective, placebo controlled studies, researchers evaluated an actively drinking group of alcoholics with a high prevalence of malnourishment. The study participants abruptly stopped their daily alcohol intake and took acetaminophen the next day. This should theoretically make them vulnerable to acetaminophen injury because their CYP2E1 would be maximally induced from the alcohol and there would be no alcohol present to compete with acetaminophen for metabolism by CYP2E1. There was no statistically significant difference in mean values for AST, ALT, or INR for alcoholics given four grams per day of acetaminophen compared to placebo. Additionally, the researchers performed an analysis of the malnourished patients that showed there was no increase in AST or ALT levels in these patients. Study limitations include a limited duration of 2 days and exclusion of patients with preexisting AST or ALT elevations greater than 120 U/L. Study results do not preclude the possibility of an idiosyncratic hepatic reaction.

Renal: Martin found that patients with chronic renal failure had higher plasma concentrations of acetaminophen and the inactive glucuronide and sulfate metabolites than healthy subjects during repeated dosing up to ten days.

Several single-dose studies demonstrate accumulation of acetaminophen metabolites in patients with moderate chronic renal failure and in anephric patients for whom hemodialysis appeared to be the major route of elimination.

The habitual consumption of acetaminophen should be discouraged. If indicated medically, the long-term use of acetaminophen should be supervised by a physician.

A National Kidney Foundation position paper notes that physicians preferentially recommend acetaminophen to patients with renal failure because of the bleeding complications associated with ASA in these individuals.

Special Populations: Geriatrics: In a comprehensive metabolic study by Miners, the formation and clearance of glucuronide and glutathione conjugates were the same in young and elderly adults, although clearance of the sulphate conjugate and unchanged acetaminophen were reduced. This finding provides prospective scientific data that the amount of acetaminophen metabolized via the oxidative pathway, from which the highly reactive intermediate, NAPQI, is generated, does not increase with age. Recently, Bannwarth evaluated the multiple-dose pharmacokinetics of acetaminophen in elderly patients. After seven days of repeat dosing, acetaminophen did not accumulate in the plasma, and the elimination half-life was the same as that reported for young adults.

Elderly patients who require therapy for longer than 5 days should consult their physician for condition monitoring.

Glucose-6-Phosphate Dehydrogenase (G6PD) Deficiency: In therapeutic doses, acetaminophen does not shorten the life-span of red blood cells and does not produce any clinically perceptible destruction of circulating red blood cells.

Obese Adults: O'Shea studied the pharmacokinetics of chlorzoxazone (a putative probe for CYP2E1 activity) to evaluate the effect of obesity on CYP2E1 activity. The authors concluded that CYP2E1 is induced in obese adults and that this could impact the metabolic pathway of a number of drugs metabolized by CYP2E1, including acetaminophen. However, acetaminophen pharmacokinetic data have been investigated in obese adults. In this prospective study, 650 mg acetaminophen was administered intravenously to obese men (297 lb), obese women (193 lb), control men (155 lb) and control women (121 lb). Acetaminophen distribution volume per total body weight was slightly lower in the obese adults but, more importantly, the half-life and metabolic clearance per total body weight did not differ among groups.

ADVERSE REACTIONS: Central Nervous System Effects: Acetaminophen at recommended doses has no obvious effects on central nervous system function. In an overdose situation, central nervous system effects are uncommon.

Chlorpheniramine maleate may cause excitability, especially in children.

Gastrointestinal Effects: Acetaminophen at recommended doses does not cause gastric irritation, gastric erosions, occult or overt gastrointestinal blood loss or ulcers. Blot and McLaughlin conducted an independent analysis of case-control data from a study conducted by the American College of Gastroenterology. The risk of gastrointestinal bleeding increased two to three-fold among recent users of ASA, ibuprofen and other NSAIDs at OTC doses, and the risk was also dose-related. In contrast, the use of acetaminophen was not associated with an increased risk of gastrointestinal bleeding.

Hematologic Effects: Acetaminophen does not have any immediate or delayed effects on small vessel hemostasis, as measured by bleeding time. In normal volunteers receiving a single dose of acetaminophen (975 or 1950 mg) or multiple doses of acetaminophen (1950 mg daily for 6 weeks), no change in bleeding time or platelet aggregation was observed. In another study, a single 1000 mg dose of acetaminophen was given to normal volunteers and did not affect bleeding time or platelet aggregation. Patients with hemophilia receiving multiple doses of acetaminophen showed no significant changes in bleeding time.

Haematological reactions including thrombocytopenia, leucopenia, pancytopenia, neutropenia, and agranulocytosis have been reported, although these are rare and causality has not been established.

Hepatic Effects: As an illustration of the margin of safety of acetaminophen at supratherapeutic doses, a comparison of serum concentrations of acetaminophen over time for a standard 15 mg/kg dose and for a dose exceeding the standard by a multiple of 5 (75 mg/kg) are shown in Figure 1. The serum concentrations are drawn relative to the risk line for hepatotoxicity and treatment line of the Rumack-Matthew nomogram used to manage acute overdoses. The mean plasma concentrations for this supratherapeutic dose are well below the risk and treatment lines of the nomogram at all times. However, to minimize the risk for adverse effects, the maximum recommended dose should not be exceeded.

Acetaminophen in overdosage may cause hepatotoxicity. In adults and adolescents, hepatotoxicity may occur following ingestion of greater than 150 mg/kg over a period of 8 hours or less. Fatalities are infrequent (less than 3% to 4% of untreated cases in which blood levels exceed the treatment line) and have rarely been reported with overdoses less than 7.5 g. In children, amounts less than 150 mg/kg are unlikely to produce hepatotoxicity. In both adults and children, toxicity associated with acetaminophen is usually caused by ingestion of quantities of the drug that are significantly above the recommended dosage range. Hepatotoxicity, ranging from transient sharp transaminase elevations to fatal, fulminant hepatic failure, is the most common result of clinically significant overdosage.

In a double-blind, placebo-controlled clinical study, healthy adults were given 4, 6 and 8 g/day of acetaminophen over 3 days. Plasma concentrations did not accumulate with repeat doses. Clinically all doses were well tolerated by the subjects and aminotransferase values stayed within normal limits throughout the study. These data provide information related to the margin of safety but are not intended to support dosing beyond the maximum recommended dose of 4 g/day.

A report has suggested that hepatotoxicity following greater than the recommended dose of acetaminophen may be enhanced by both prolonged fasting and/or chronic alcohol abuse.

Figure 1: TYLENOL Flu

Mean Data for a Standard (1 g, 15 mg/kg) and Higher (5.6 g, 75 mg/kg) Dose Relative to Risk and Treatment Lines of the Acetaminophen Nomogram

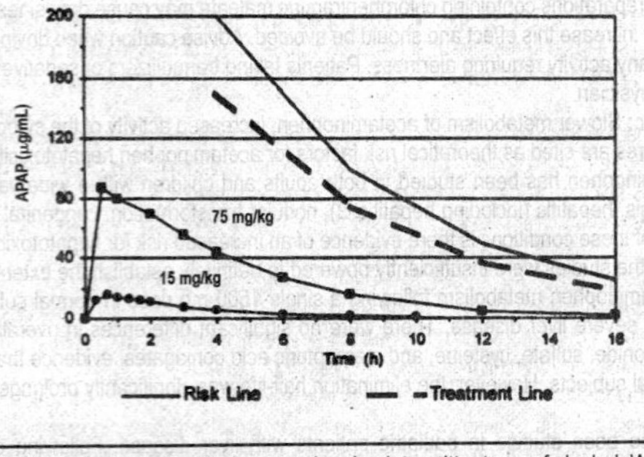

Acute Alcohol Use: Acute alcohol ingestion refers to the occasional or intermittent use of alcohol. When taken together, alcohol competes with acetaminophen for CYP2E1. CYP2E1 accepts alcohol more readily than acetaminophen; therefore, less NAPQI is produced. In the presence of alcohol, acetaminophen may be diverted to the glucuronidation and sulfation pathways. The overall result is that a smaller percentage of acetaminophen may be expected to be metabolized to the toxic intermediate, NAPQI, than would otherwise be the case. NAPQI production is increased above baseline for the period up to 18-24 hours post ethanol clearance from the body. In healthy adults, at normal labeled doses of acetaminophen, the temporary increase in NAPQI production is more than accommodated by normal glutathione stores in the liver.

Hypersensitivity: Sensitivity reactions are rare and may manifest as rash, urticaria, dyspnea, hypotension, laryngeal edema, angioedema, bronchospasm, or anaphylaxis. Cross-reactivity in ASA-sensitive persons has been rarely reported. If sensitivity is suspected, discontinue use of the drug.

Renal Effects: Acute nephrotoxicity has been reported following massive overdose either as a sequela of hepatic failure or, occasionally, in the absence of hepatic failure.

Clinical data have established that acetaminophen in recommended doses is not nephrotoxic.

Some studies suggest an association between the chronic long-term use of acetaminophen and renal effects. Results, however, are conflicting, limited by recall bias and confounded by the inability to determine whether analgesic use preceded or followed the onset of renal disease.

Case control studies have suggested a weak association between habitual acetaminophen use and prevalence of chronic renal failure and end stage renal disease. This National Kidney Foundation position paper concludes that acetaminophen has been preferentially recommended by physicians to patients with renal failure and that there is no evidence that occasional use of acetaminophen caused renal injury.

Special Populations: Pediatrics: Lesko and Mitchell enrolled more than 84 000 febrile children in a randomized, double blind, acetaminophen-controlled trial to assess the risks of rare but serious adverse events following use of pediatric ibuprofen. Of the children included in the analysis, 28 130 received acetaminophen and none experienced anaphylaxis, or serious hepatic, gastrointestinal or renal effects.

Pregnancy and Lactation: As with any drug, patients who are pregnant or nursing a baby should consult a physician before taking this product.

Pregnancy: Issues of risks in pregnancy are multifactorial. The information provided cannot be substituted for direct patient consultation. Acetaminophen is believed to be non-teratogenic in humans. However, existing studies have not assessed the effect of very high doses. The Motherrisk Collaborative Perinatal project monitored 50 282 mother-child pairs, of which 226 had first trimester exposure to acetaminophen and 781 had used acetaminophen at any time during their pregnancy. No evidence was found to suggest a relationship between acetaminophen use and major or minor malformations. In a surveillance study of Michigan Medicaid recipients conducted between 1985 and 1992 involving 229 101 completed pregnancies, 9146 newborns had been exposed to acetaminophen during the first trimester. This data do not support an association between acetaminophen use and the occurrence of birth defects. Another cohort study, using prescription monitoring, found no excess risk for malformation, and no evidence that acetaminophen influenced fetal growth. Finally, as part of a larger study, 697 women used acetaminophen with or without codeine in their first trimester. No teratogenic risk was found.

A prospective study investigated the outcome of pregnancy in 300 women who had self-administered an overdose of acetaminophen, either alone, or as part of a combined preparation. Exposure to overdose occurred in all trimesters. The majority of the pregnancies had normal outcomes. The malformation rate was within the expected range. There was no obvious relationship between the time of exposure and the time of delivery. The overall conclusion was that acetaminophen overdose is not an indication for termination of pregnancy.

In a long-term developmental follow-up study, acetaminophen did not adversely affect IQ or behavior measures at four years of age. Height, weight and head circumference were also not affected by exposure to acetaminophen in-utero.

Unlike ASA, which has been shown to profoundly effect platelet function, there does not seem to be a risk of hemorrhage associated with acetaminophen use at term.

Currently there is no evidence to suggest that acetaminophen is teratogenic when used as recommended. However, data for continuous high daily doses are not sufficient, and safety during pregnancy has not yet been established.

Lactation: Following a typical therapeutic dose, acetaminophen is excreted in breast milk in very low concentrations. Based on a number of published reports, infant exposure levels are at most 4.5% of a weight adjusted pediatric therapeutic dose. In addition, acetaminophen is considered compatible with breast-feeding by the American Academy of Pediatrics.

DRUG INTERACTIONS: Alcohol: Studies evaluating the metabolism of doses up to 20 mg/kg of acetaminophen in chronic alcohol abusers and a study evaluating the effects of 2 days of acetaminophen dosing at 4000 mg/day in chronic alcoholics undergoing detoxification, have yielded inconsistent results with regard to effects on acetaminophen pharmacokinetics and demonstrate no evidence of adverse effect on liver function tests.

Anticoagulants–Oral: Patients who concomitantly medicate with warfarin-type anticoagulants and regular doses of acetaminophen have occasionally been reported to have unforeseen elevations in their INR. Physicians should be cognizant of this potential interaction and monitor the INR in such patients closely while therapy is established. Many factors, including diet, medications, and environmental and physical states, may affect how a patient responds to anticoagulant therapy. There have been several reports that suggest that acetaminophen may produce hypoprothrombinemia (elevated international normalized ratio [INR] or prothrombin time) when administered with coumarin derivatives. In other studies, prothrombin time did not change. Reported changes have been generally of limited clinical significance, however, periodic evaluation of prothrombin time should be performed when these agents are administered concurrently.

In the period immediately following discharge from the hospital or whenever other medications are initiated, discontinued, or taken regularly, it is important to monitor patient response to anticoagulation therapy with additional prothrombin time or INR determinations. Despite the potential for interaction, acetaminophen is the least likely OTC analgesic to interfere with anticoagulant therapy.

Anticonvulsants: Some reports have suggested that patients taking long-term anticonvulsants, who overdose on acetaminophen, may be at increased risk of hepatotoxicity because of accelerated metabolism of acetaminophen. Available data are conflicting. A 7-year retrospective study of acetaminophen overdose admissions indicates that the overall mortality rate was not significantly different for patients taking concomitant anticonvulsant medications.

Hydantoins: Pharmacokinetic studies indicate that phenytoin primarily induces the glucuronidation pathway, whereas glutathione-derived metabolites are not increased in patients on chronic phenytoin therapy. Additionally, recent data demonstrate that phenytoin is metabolized primarily by CYP2C9 and CYP2C19, whereas acetaminophen is primarily metabolized by CYP2E1.

Carbamazepine: Carbamazepine is primarily metabolized by CYP3A4, whereas acetaminophen is metabolized primarily via CYP2E1. It is not known whether there is increased risk from an acetaminophen overdose in patients on chronic carbamazepine therapy.

Diflunisal: Professional literature from the manufacturer of diflunisal cautions that concomitant administration with acetaminophen produces an approximate 50% increase in plasma levels of acetaminophen in normal volunteers. Acetaminophen had no effect on diflunisal plasma levels. The clinical significance of these findings has not been established. However, caution should be used with concomitant administration of diflunisal and acetaminophen and patients should be monitored carefully.

Isoniazid: Some reports suggest that patients on chronic isoniazid therapy may be at risk for developing hepatotoxicity from an acetaminophen overdose. Since patients on isoniazid therapy may develop hepatic effects from isoniazid alone, data from individual case reports are unclear as to whether chronic administration of isoniazid may increase the risk of acetaminophen toxicity. Isoniazid is primarily metabolized by CYP2E1 and induces CYP2E1. Studies in healthy subjects demonstrate that isoniazid blocks the formation of the toxic metabolite NAPQI when administered concomitantly with acetaminophen, but increase NAPQI formation when acetaminophen is administered one day after discontinuation of isoniazid. Thus, concomitant use of isoniazid is unlikely to potentiate the risk of acetaminophen-induced hepatotoxicity at recommended doses. The isoniazid induction of CYP2E1 is short-lived, lasting only 12 to 48 hours after the discontinuation of isoniazid, it is during this period the toxicity of an acetaminophen overdose may be potentiated.

DOSAGE AND ADMINISTRATION: Extra Strength TYLENOL Flu (Daytime and Nighttime): Adults (12 years of age and older): 1 to 2 tablets every 4 hours as needed. It is hazardous to exceed a combined **total** of 8 tablets per day. Reduce dosage if nervousness or sleeplessness occurs.

OVERDOSAGE:

Symptoms and Treatment: Acetaminophen: Typical Toxidrome: Hepatic injury is the principal toxic effect of a substantial acetaminophen overdose. The physician should be mindful that there is no early presentation that is pathognomic for the overdose. A high degree of clinical suspicion must always be maintained.

Untreated acetaminophen overdoses may produce hepatotoxicity. Acetaminophen hepatotoxicity occurs as a threshold effect and is characterized by a lack of toxicity at lower/therapeutic doses. Acetaminophen hepatotoxicity occurs after major depletion of glutathione, an endogenous detoxifying substance. Once the threshold is exceeded, increasing acetaminophen doses may produce increasing degrees of hepatotoxicity, unless N-acetylcysteine (NAC) is administered. Situations in which acetaminophen overdose and resultant hepatotoxicity may occur include acute intentional overdose and repeated supratherapeutic overdose in adults and acute accidental ingestion or overdose and repeated supratherapeutic overdose in children.

The clinical course of acetaminophen overdose generally occurs in a three-phase sequential pattern. The first phase begins shortly after ingestion and lasts for 12 to 24 hours. The patient may manifest signs of gastrointestinal irritability, nausea, vomiting, anorexia, diaphoresis, pallor and general malaise. If toxicity continues, there is a latent phase of up to 48 hours. During this second phase, initial symptoms abate and the patient may feel better. However, hepatic enzymes, bilirubin, and prothrombin time or INR values will progressively rise. Right upper quadrant pain may develop as the liver becomes enlarged and tender. Most patients do not progress beyond this phase, especially if given N-acetylcysteine (NAC) treatment early in the course. Signs and symptoms of the third phase depend on the severity of hepatic damage and usually occur from three to five days following overdose ingestion. Symptoms may be limited to anorexia, nausea, general malaise, and abdominal pain in less severe cases or may progress to confusion, stupor and sequelae of hepatic necrosis including jaundice, coagulation defects, hypoglycemia, and encephalopathy, as well as renal failure and cardiomyopathy. Death, if it occurs, is generally the result of complications associated with fulminant hepatic failure. Mortality rates in patients with toxic plasma levels who do not receive antidote therapy range from 3% to 4%.

Due to the wide availability of acetaminophen, it is commonly involved in single and mixed drug overdose situations and the practitioner should screen for its presence in a patient's serum. Acute toxicity after single dose overdoses of acetaminophen can be anticipated when the overdose exceeds 150 mg/kg. Chronic alcohol abusers, cachectic individuals, and persons taking pharmacologic inducers of the hepatic P450 microsomal enzyme system may be at risk with lower exposures.

Specific Antidote: Any individual presenting with a possible acetaminophen overdose should be treated with N-acetylcysteine (NAC), even if the amount of acetaminophen ingested is unknown or questionable. A blood sample for determination of the plasma acetaminophen concentration should be obtained as early as possible, but no sooner than four hours following ingestion. Do not await the results of assays for plasma acetaminophen levels before initiating treatment NAC. If the acetaminophen plasma level is found to plot above the treatment line on the acetaminophen overdose nomogram, NAC treatment should be continued for a full course of therapy. NAC is used clinically to treat acute acetaminophen overdose, and acts by interacting with the oxidative intermediate, NAPQI. NAC administered by either the i.v. or the oral route is known to be a highly effective antidote for acetaminophen poisoning. It is most effective when administered within 8 hours of a significant overdose but reports have indicated benefits to treatment initiated well beyond this time period. It is imperative to administer the antidote as early as possible in the time course of acute intoxication to reap the full benefits of the antidote's protective effects. For full prescribing information, consult the product monograph for NAC.

General Management: When the possibility of acetaminophen overdose exists, treatment should begin immediately and include appropriate decontamination of the gastrointestinal tract, proper supportive care, careful assessment of appropriately timed serum acetaminophen estimations evaluated against the Rumack-Matthew nomogram, timely administration of NAC as required and appropriate follow-up care. Liver function tests should be performed initially and repeated at 24-hour intervals.

Phenylephrine HCl: Typical Toxidrome: sympathomimetic/stimulant.
Specific Antidote: none.
General Management: Stabilize the patient (A, B, Cs) undertake appropriate gastrointestinal tract decontamination procedures, initiate supportive care, consult with a Regional Poison Control Centre regarding ongoing management and arrange for appropriate follow-up care.

Dextromethorphan HBr: Typical Toxidrome: narcotic/opiate.
Specific Antidote: naloxone HCl.
General Management: Stabilize the patient (A, B, Cs), undertake appropriate gastrointestinal tract decontamination procedures, initiate supportive care, consult with a Regional Poison Control Centre regarding ongoing management and arrange for appropriate follow-up care.

Chlorpheniramine Maleate: Typical Toxidrome: anticholinergic, CNS depressant (adult), CNS stimulant (child).
Specific Antidote: none.
General Management: Stabilize the patient (A, B, Cs), undertake appropriate gastrointestinal tract decontamination procedures, initiate supportive care, consult with a Regional Poison Control Centre regarding ongoing management and arrange for appropriate follow-up care.

Overdose During Pregnancy: Acetaminophen is one of the most common overdoses in pregnancy. Hepatic toxicity of acetaminophen follows the formation of the highly reactive metabolite N-acetyl-p-benzoquinoneimine produced by acetaminophen metabolism through the cytochrome P450 mixed-function oxidase system. Hepatic failure can be prevented by timely administration of NAC either orally for 72 hours, or intravenously (IV) for 20 hours.

Acetaminophen crosses the human placenta though the fetus is theoretically at risk when maternal overdose of acetaminophen occurs. Acetaminophen can be transformed to its toxic metabolite since the oxidative capacity of fetal microsomes is present in the fetus by 14 weeks gestation.

Studies on placental transfer of NAC in rats and sheep yielded conflicting results. Placental transfer of N-acetylcysteine in humans was demonstrated in 4 women treated with NAC for acetaminophen overdose during labour. NAC blood levels in the fetuses were within the range associated with therapeutic doses of NAC administered to adults with acetaminophen poisoning.

Fetal toxicity and stillbirth after a large (e.g. 30 g) acetaminophen overdose has been reported, but others observed a normal outcome for the offspring after acetaminophen overdose in pregnancy. A large case series investigated the pregnancy outcome in 300 women who had overdosed with acetaminophen. In this group, 118 cases occurred in the first trimester, 103 in the second trimester and 79 in the third trimester. Forty-nine of these mothers were treated with specific antidotes (33 with NAC and 16 with methionine). There were 219 live-born infants, 11 have malformations (including minor); none had been exposed to acetaminophen during the first trimester. Nine women were treated with NAC during the first trimester; there were two elective terminations; two spontaneous abortions, and five healthy babies in this group.

In summary, acetaminophen overdose during pregnancy should be treated according to regular protocols in order to prevent maternal and potentially fetal toxicity. Unless severe maternal toxicity develops, an acetaminophen overdose does not increase the risk for birth defects or adverse pregnancy outcomes.

Physicians unfamiliar with the current management of acetaminophen overdose should consult with a Poison Control Centre immediately. Telephone numbers for local Poison Control Centres are available in the local phone directory. Delays in initiation of appropriate therapy may jeopardize the patient's chances for full recovery.

> For management of a suspected drug overdose, CPhA recommends that you contact your **regional Poison Control Centre**. See the *CPS* Directory section for a list of Poison Control Centres.

ACTION AND CLINICAL PHARMACOLOGY: Mechanism of Action: Acetaminophen is a centrally acting analgesic and antipyretic drug. Although the precise mechanism of action is not totally understood, work by Boutaud suggests acetaminophen is an inhibitor of the peroxidase portion of cyclooxygenase (prostaglandin H synthase inhibitor). Depending on the redox state and substrate concentrations surrounding the enzymes, acetaminophen may or may not have a significant inhibitory effect. This accounts for its selective activity on pain and fever with little anti-inflammatory effect.

It is postulated that the analgesic effect is produced by elevation of the pain threshold and the antipyretic effect is produced through action on the hypothalamic heat-regulating centre.

The optimal effective analgesic dose of acetaminophen was demonstrated in dental pain studies and is 1000 mg every four to six hours, up to 4000 mg daily. At least 500 published and unpublished controlled clinical trials in adults and children have evaluated acetaminophen for the relief of pain or fever. These studies include single and multiple dose treatments. Most studies were less than 14 days in duration, although the longest study duration was two years. No significant safety issues were reported in any of these studies.

Moreover, at recommended doses, acetaminophen has not been shown to increase the risk of developing renal diseases or upper gastrointestinal ulceration/bleeding. This observation is consistent with its minimal inhibitory effect on peripheral prostaglandin synthesis and on gastric prostaglandin synthesis.

Acetaminophen is considered equipotent to ASA and ibuprofen, within the recommended OTC dosing ranges, in its analgesic and antipyretic effects. Acetaminophen at recommended doses does not cause the type of gastrointestinal complications associated with NSAID-containing products, such as gastric irritation, gastric erosions, occult or overt gastrointestinal blood loss, or ulcers. Unlike these drugs, however, it has no anti-inflammatory effect at clinically relevant doses in humans.

Pharmacokinetics: Absorption: Oral acetaminophen is rapidly and almost completely absorbed from the gastrointestinal tract primarily in the small intestine. This absorption process occurs by passive transport. Peak plasma concentrations occur within 0.4 to 1 hour depending on the product formulation. Although high-fat foods delay the time to peak concentration for up to an hour, the dose is completely absorbed.

Distribution: Acetaminophen is uniformly distributed throughout most body fluids, but not in fatty tissue. As a result, the volume of distribution in adults ranges between 0.8 and 1.0 L/kg. Since acetaminophen has low protein binding in plasma of only 10% to 25%, it does not compete with drugs that are highly protein bound.

Metabolism: Acetaminophen is primarily metabolized by the liver via three principal separate pathways: conjugation with glucuronide; conjugation with sulfate; oxidation via the cytochrome P450 mixed function oxidase system.

Both the glucuronic and oxidative pathways adhere to a first-order rate process, which means the concentration of acetaminophen metabolized increases as the concentration in the liver increases. The sulfate pathway adheres to Michaelis-Menten kinetics, which means the concentration of acetaminophen metabolized remains constant once the concentration in the liver increases above a saturation level. A schematic of acetaminophen metabolism is shown in Figure 2.

The major metabolic pathway is glucuronidation, where 47% to 62% of the acetaminophen dose conjugates with glucuronide. These glucuronide conjugates are inactive and nontoxic, and are secreted in bile and eliminated in the urine.

The second major pathway is sulfation, where 25% to 36% of the dose conjugates with sulfate. These sulfate ester conjugates are also inactive and nontoxic and are excreted in the urine.

The third pathway is oxidation, where 5% to 8% of the dose is metabolized via the cytochrome P450 enzyme system. The cytochrome P450 isoenzyme that is primarily responsible is CYP2E1. When acetaminophen is metabolized by CYP2E1, it forms a highly reactive intermediate, N-acetyl-p-benzoquinoneimine (NAPQI). Since NAPQI is highly reactive, it cannot be measured outside the liver nor can it accumulate. This intermediate is rapidly inactivated by hepatocellular stores of glutathione to form cysteine and mercapturate conjugates, which are both inactive and nontoxic. These conjugates are excreted in the urine.

Excretion: Acetaminophen undergoes first-order elimination from the body, and has a short plasma half-life that ranges from 2 to 3 hours in healthy young and elderly adults and from 1.5 to 2.9 hours in children. Since acetaminophen clears rapidly from the body, repeated doses do not lead to accumulation of acetaminophen plasma concentrations.

* Container provided with a child-resistant closure.

Figure 2: TYLENOL Flu
Acetaminophen Metabolism

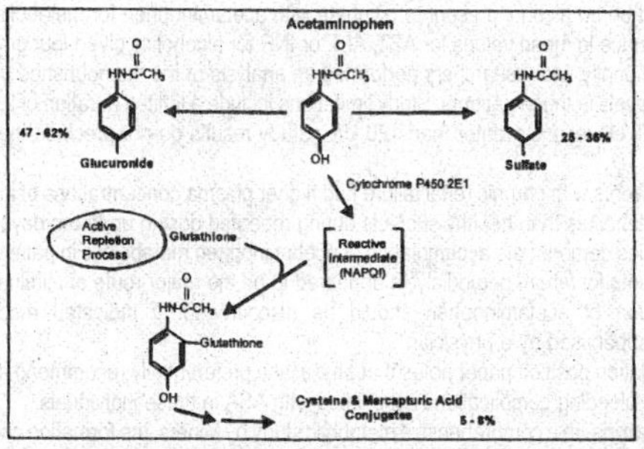

STORAGE AND STABILITY: Store at room temperature (15 to 30°C). Protect from moisture.

DOSAGE FORMS, COMPOSITION AND PACKAGING: Flu Extra Strength Daytime: Each round, yellow coated tablet, with "TYLENOL" over "Flu DT" printed in black ink on one side and blank on the other side, contains: acetaminophen 500 mg, dextromethorphan HBr 10 mg and phenylephrine HCl 5 mg. Nonmedicinal ingredients: carnauba wax, cellulose, cornstarch, D&C Yellow no. 10, FD&C Yellow no. 6, hypromellose, iron oxide black, magnesium stearate, polydextrose, polyethylene glycol, sodium starch glycolate, sucralose, titanium dioxide and triacetin. Energy: 1.3 kJ (0.3 kcal). Sodium: 0.4 mg. Alcohol-, gluten-, lactose-, sulfite- and tartrazine-free. Plastic bottles of 20*. Blister packs of 10 in combination with blister packs of 10 Flu Nighttime tablets. All packages are safety sealed.

Flu Extra Strength Nighttime: Each round, blue coated tablet, with "TYLENOL" over "Flu NT" printed in black ink on one side and blank on the other side, contains: acetaminophen 500 mg, dextromethorphan HBr 10 mg, phenylephrine HCl 5 mg and chlorpheniramine maleate 2 mg. Nonmedicinal ingredients: carnauba wax, cellulose, cornstarch, FD&C Blue no. 1, hypromellose, iron oxide black, magnesium stearate, polydextrose, polyethylene glycol, sodium starch glycolate, sucralose, titanium dioxide and triacetin. Energy: 1.3 kJ (0.3 kcal). Sodium: 0.4 mg. Alcohol-, gluten-, lactose-, sulfite- and tartrazine-free. Blister packs of 10 in combination with blister packs of 10 Flu Daytime tablets. All packages are safety sealed.

Tylenol® Menstrual Extra Strength

acetaminophen—pamabrom—pyrilamine maleate
Analgesic—Diuretic—Antihistamine

McNeil Consumer Healthcare

SUMMARY PRODUCT INFORMATION:

Route of Administration	Dosage Form/ Strength	Clinically Relevant Nonmedicinal Ingredients
Oral	Caplet/500 mg acetaminophen, 25 mg pamabrom and 15 mg pyrilamine maleate	Gluten-, lactose-, sucrose-, sulfite- and tartrazine-free For a complete listing of nonmedicinal ingredients, see Dosage Forms, Composition and Packaging.

INDICATIONS AND CLINICAL USE: For the temporary relief of premenstrual and menstrual symptoms, including backache, breast tenderness, bloating, swelling, cramps, headache, irritability, tension, mild to moderate aches and pains and the temporary water weight gain frequently associated with the premenstrual period.

CONTRAINDICATIONS: Hypersensitivity to acetaminophen, pamabrom, theophylline derivatives, pyrilamine maleate or to the ingredients of this formulation (see Dosage Forms, Composition and Packaging). Allergic reactions (primarily skin rash) or reports of hypersensitivity secondary to acetaminophen are rare and generally are controlled by discontinuation of the drug and, when necessary, symptomatic treatment.

WARNINGS AND PRECAUTIONS: General: Consumers should not exceed 4 g/day of acetaminophen or use two or more acetaminophen-containing products together. This includes combination products that contain acetaminophen. Do not use with other products containing salicylates or any other pain or fever medicine.

Acetaminophen-containing products should be kept out of the reach of children.

Physicians should be cognizant of and supervise the use of acetaminophen in patients with chronic alcoholism, serious kidney or serious liver disease. Physicians should alert their patients who regularly consume large amounts of alcohol not to exceed the recommended doses of acetaminophen. Chronic heavy alcohol abusers may be at increased risk of liver toxicity from excessive doses of acetaminophen.

Patients should be counseled to consult a physician if premenstrual or menstrual symptoms do not improve with use of this product or if they worsen, if other unusual symptoms develop, if redness or swelling is present in an area of pain or if new symptoms such as high fever, rash, itching or persistent headache occur, as these may be signs of a condition which requires medical attention. Acetaminophen should not be taken for pain for more than 5 days or if new symptoms appear, without consulting a physician.

Individuals with continuing severe or debilitating symptoms accompanying premenstrual syndrome should consult their doctor.

Patients with asthma, glaucoma, bladder-neck obstruction, peptic ulcer or pyloroduodenal obstruction, emphysema, chronic pulmonary disease or shortness of breath should not use this medication unless directed by a physician.

This product is not recommended for children under 12 years of age.

Occupational Hazards: May produce additive CNS effects when taken concomitantly with alcohol, hypnotics, anxiolytics, narcotic analgesics and neuroleptic drugs. Advise caution when driving a motor vehicle or operating machinery or engaging in any activity requiring alertness. Patients taking tranquilizers or sedatives should not take this mediation before consulting a physician.

Hepatic/Biliary/Pancreatic: Slower metabolism of acetaminophen, increased activity of the cytochrome P450 enzyme system, or depleted glutathione stores are cited as theoretical risk factors for acetaminophen hepatotoxicity in patients with chronic liver disease. However, acetaminophen has been studied in both adults and children with a wide variety of liver diseases including various types of cirrhosis, hepatitis (including hepatitis C), nodular transformation, congenital hepatic fibrosis, and α1-antitrypsin deficiency. In none of these conditions is there evidence of an increased risk for hepatotoxicity at currently recommended acetaminophen doses but the studies were insufficiently powered to definitely establish the extent of risk.

Forrest compared acetaminophen metabolism following a single 1500 mg dose in normal subjects, patients with mild liver disease, and patients with severe liver disease. There were no significant differences in overall 24-hour urinary excretion of acetaminophen and glucuronide, sulfate, cysteine, and mercapturic acid conjugates, evidence that acetaminophen metabolism was similar to that in normal subjects. However, the elimination half-life was significantly prolonged in patients with severe liver disease.

Acetaminophen has also been studied in pediatric patients with liver disease. Following a single (10 mg/kg) dose of acetaminophen, the pharmacokinetic profiles in pediatric patients with mild, moderate, or severe liver disease were not significantly different. Although the plasma half-life of acetaminophen was prolonged in patients with severe liver disease, there were no significant differences in the 36-hour (children) urinary excretion of acetaminophen or its conjugates.

Acetaminophen may cause hepatotoxicity in situations of intentional overdose (e.g. attempted suicide), unintentional overdose (e.g. overdosing when pain relief is not satisfactory), simultaneous use of multiple acetaminophen-containing preparations, accidental overdose or in very rare cases, after recommended doses, although causality has not been determined. The hepatotoxic reaction can be severe and life-threatening. Early symptoms following a hepatotoxic overdose may include nausea, vomiting, diaphoresis, lethargy, and general malaise. If appropriate treatment is not instituted, these may progress to upper quadrant pain, confusion, stupor, and sequelae of hepatic necrosis, such as jaundice, coagulation defects, hypoglycemia, and encephalopathy. Renal failure and cardiomyopathy may also occur. In the event of known or suspected overdosage, treatment with N-acetyl cysteine should be instituted immediately (see Overdosage), even when there are no obvious symptoms. Failure to promptly treat acetaminophen hepatotoxicity with N-acetyl cysteine can result in liver failure, leading to liver transplantation and/or death.

Chronic Alcohol Use: Excessive alcohol use may increase risk of liver toxicity from acetaminophen overdose (acute or chronic).

In prospective, placebo controlled studies, researchers evaluated an actively drinking group of alcoholics with a high prevalence of malnourishment. The study participants abruptly stopped their daily alcohol intake and took acetaminophen the next day. This should theoretically make them vulnerable to acetaminophen injury because their CYP2E1 would be maximally induced from the alcohol and there would be no alcohol present to compete with acetaminophen for metabolism by CYP2E1. There was no statistically significant difference in mean values for AST, ALT, or INR for alcoholics given four grams per day of acetaminophen compared to placebo. Additionally, the researchers performed an analysis of the malnourished patients that showed there was no increase in AST or ALT levels in these patients. Study limitations include a limited duration of 2 days and exclusion of patients with preexisting AST or ALT elevations greater than 120 U/L. Study results do not preclude the possibility of an idiosyncratic hepatic reaction.

Renal: Martin found that patients with chronic renal failure had higher plasma concentrations of acetaminophen and the inactive glucuronide and sulfate metabolites than healthy subjects during repeated dosing up to ten days.

Several single-dose studies demonstrate accumulation of acetaminophen metabolites in patients with moderate chronic renal failure and in anephric patients for whom hemodialysis appeared to be the major route of elimination.

The habitual consumption of acetaminophen should be discouraged. If indicated medically, the long-term use of acetaminophen should be supervised by a physician.

A National Kidney Foundation position paper notes that physicians preferentially recommend acetaminophen to patients with renal failure because of the bleeding complications associated with ASA in these individuals.

Special Populations: Geriatrics: In a comprehensive metabolic study by Miners, the formation and clearance of glucuronide and glutathione conjugates were the same in young and elderly adults, although clearance of the sulphate conjugate and unchanged acetaminophen were reduced. This finding provides prospective scientific data that the amount of acetaminophen metabolized via the oxidative pathway, from which the highly reactive intermediate, NAPQI, is generated, does not increase with age. Recently, Bannwarth evaluated the multiple-dose pharmacokinetics of acetaminophen in elderly patients. After seven days of repeat dosing, acetaminophen did not accumulate in the plasma, and the elimination half-life was the same as that reported for young adults.

Elderly patients who require therapy for longer than 5 days should consult their physician for condition monitoring.

Glucose-6-Phosphate Dehydrogenase (G6PD) Deficiency: In therapeutic doses, acetaminophen does not shorten the life-span of red blood cells and does not produce any clinically perceptible destruction of circulating red blood cells.

Obese Adults: O'Shea studied the pharmacokinetics of chlorzoxazone (a putative probe for CYP2E1 activity) to evaluate the effect of obesity on CYP2E1 activity. The authors concluded that CYP2E1 is induced in obese adults and that this could impact the metabolic pathway of a number of drugs metabolized by CYP2E1, including acetaminophen. However, acetaminophen pharmacokinetic data have been investigated in obese adults. In this prospective study, 650 mg acetaminophen was administered intravenously to obese men (297 lb), obese women (193 lb), control men (155 lb) and control women (121 lb). Acetaminophen distribution volume per total body weight was slightly lower in the obese adults but, more importantly, the half-life and metabolic clearance per total body weight did not differ among groups.

ADVERSE REACTIONS: Central Nervous System Effects: Acetaminophen at recommended doses has no obvious effects on central nervous system function. In an overdose situation, central nervous system effects are uncommon.

Other side effects are usually mild but may include drowsiness or listlessness.

Gastrointestinal Effects: Acetaminophen at recommended doses does not cause gastric irritation, gastric erosions, occult or overt gastrointestinal blood loss or ulcers.

Blot and McLaughlin conducted an independent analysis of case-control data from a study conducted by the American College of Gastroenterology. The risk of gastrointestinal bleeding increased two to three-fold among recent users of ASA, ibuprofen and other NSAIDs at OTC doses, and the risk was also dose-related. In contrast, the use of acetaminophen was not associated with an increased risk of gastrointestinal bleeding.

Hematologic Effects: Acetaminophen does not have any immediate or delayed effects on small vessel hemostasis, as measured by bleeding time. In normal volunteers receiving a single dose of acetaminophen (975 or 1950 mg) or multiple doses of acetaminophen (1950 mg daily for 6 weeks), no change in bleeding time or platelet aggregation was observed. In another study, a single 1000 mg dose of acetaminophen was given to normal volunteers and did not affect bleeding time or platelet aggregation. Patients with hemophilia receiving multiple doses of acetaminophen showed no significant changes in bleeding time.

Hematological reactions including thrombocytopenia, leucopenia, pancytopenia, neutropenia, and agranulocytosis have been reported, although these are rare and causality has not been established.

Hepatic Effects: As an illustration of the margin of safety of acetaminophen at supratherapeutic doses, a comparison of serum concentrations of acetaminophen over time for a standard 15 mg/kg dose and for a dose exceeding the standard by a multiple of 5 (75 mg/kg) are shown in Figure 1. The serum concentrations are drawn relative to the risk line for hepatotoxicity and treatment line of the Rumack-Matthew nomogram used to manage acute overdoses. The mean plasma concentrations for this supratherapeutic dose are well below the risk and treatment lines of the nomogram at all times. However, to minimize the risk for adverse effects, the maximum recommended dose should not be exceeded.

Figure 1: TYLENOL Menstrual

Mean Data for a Standard (1 g, 15 mg/kg) and Higher (5.6 g, 75 mg/kg) Dose Relative to Risk and Treatment Lines of the Acetaminophen Nomogram

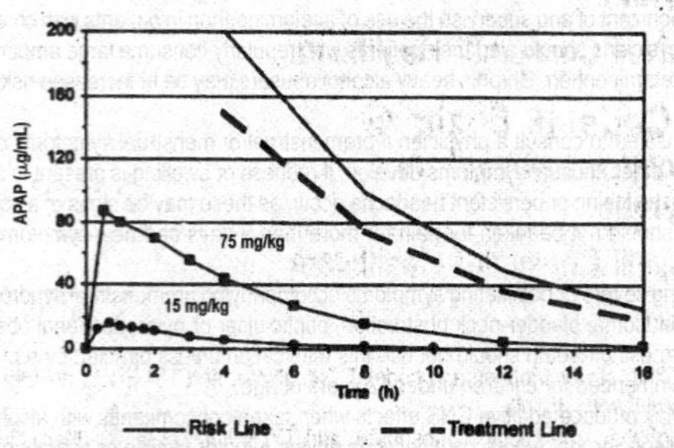

Acetaminophen in overdosage may cause hepatotoxicity. In adults and adolescents, hepatotoxicity may occur following ingestion of greater than 150 mg/kg over a period of 8 hours or less. Fatalities are infrequent (less than 3% to 4% of untreated cases in which blood levels exceed the treatment line) and have rarely been reported with overdoses less than 7.5 g. In children, amounts less than 150 mg/kg are unlikely to produce hepatotoxicity. In both adults and children, toxicity associated with acetaminophen is usually caused by ingestion of quantities of the drug that are significantly above the recommended dosage range. Hepatotoxicity, ranging from transient sharp transaminase elevations to fatal, fulminant hepatic failure, is the most common result of clinically significant overdosage.

In a double-blind, placebo-controlled clinical study, healthy adults were given 4, 6 and 8 g/d of acetaminophen over 3 days. Plasma concentrations did not accumulate with repeat doses. Clinically all doses were well tolerated by the subjects and aminotransferase values stayed within normal limits throughout the study. These data provide information related to the margin of safety but are not intended to support dosing beyond the maximum recommended dose of 4 g/day.

A report has suggested that hepatotoxicity following greater than the recommended dose of acetaminophen may be enhanced by both prolonged fasting and/or chronic alcohol abuse.

Acute Alcohol Use: Acute alcohol ingestion refers to the occasional or intermittent use of alcohol. When taken together, alcohol competes with acetaminophen for CYP2E1. CYP2E1 accepts alcohol more readily than acetaminophen; therefore, less NAPQI is produced. In the presence of alcohol, acetaminophen may be diverted to the glucuronidation and sulfation pathways. The overall result is that a smaller percentage of acetaminophen may be expected to be metabolized to the toxic intermediate, NAPQI, than would otherwise be the case. NAPQI production is increased above baseline for the period up to 18-24 hours post ethanol clearance from the body. In healthy adults, at normal labeled doses of acetaminophen, the temporary increase in NAPQI production is more than accommodated by normal glutathione stores in the liver.

Hypersensitivity: Sensitivity reactions are rare and may manifest as rash, urticaria, dyspnea, hypotension, laryngeal edema, angioedema, bronchospasm, or anaphylaxis. Cross-reactivity in ASA-sensitive persons has been rarely reported. If sensitivity is suspected, discontinue use of the drug.

Renal Effects: Acute nephrotoxicity has been reported following massive overdose either as a sequela of hepatic failure or, occasionally, in the absence of hepatic failure.

Clinical data have established that acetaminophen in recommended doses is not nephrotoxic.

Some studies suggest an association between the chronic long-term use of acetaminophen and renal effects. Results, however, are conflicting, limited by recall bias and confounded by the inability to determine whether analgesic use preceded or followed the onset of renal disease.

Case control studies have suggested a weak association between habitual acetaminophen use and prevalence of chronic renal failure and end stage renal disease. This National Kidney Foundation position paper concludes that acetaminophen has been preferentially recommended by physicians to patients with renal failure and that there is no evidence that occasional use of acetaminophen caused renal injury.

Special Populations: Pregnancy: This product should not be used by pregnant women. Issues of risks in pregnancy are multifactorial. The information provided cannot be substituted for direct patient consultation. Acetaminophen is believed to be non-teratogenic in humans. However, existing studies have not assessed the effect of very high doses. The Motherrisk Collaborative Perinatal project monitored 50 282 mother-child pairs, of which 226 had first trimester exposure to acetaminophen and 781 had used acetaminophen at any time during their pregnancy. No evidence was found to suggest a relationship between acetaminophen use and major or minor malformations. In a surveillance study of Michigan Medicaid recipients conducted between 1985 and 1992 involving 229 101 completed pregnancies, 9146 newborns had been exposed to acetaminophen during the first trimester. This data do not support an association between acetaminophen use and the occurrence of birth defects. Another cohort study, using prescription monitoring, found no excess risk for malformation, and no evidence that acetaminophen influenced fetal growth. Finally, as part of a larger study, 697 women used acetaminophen with or without codeine in their first trimester. No teratogenic risk was found.

A prospective study investigated the outcome of pregnancy in 300 women who had self-administered an overdose of acetaminophen, either alone, or as part of a combined preparation. Exposure to overdose occurred in all trimesters. The majority of the pregnancies had normal outcomes. The malformation rate was within the expected range.

There was no obvious relationship between the time of exposure and the time of delivery. The overall conclusion was that acetaminophen overdose is not an indication for termination of pregnancy.

In a long-term developmental follow-up study 46, acetaminophen did not adversely affect IQ or behavior measures at four years of age. Height, weight and head circumference were also not affected by exposure to acetaminophen in-utero.

Unlike ASA, which has been shown to profoundly effect platelet function, there does not seem to be a risk of hemorrhage associated with acetaminophen use at term.

Currently there is no evidence to suggest that acetaminophen is teratogenic when used as recommended. However, data for continuous high daily doses are not sufficient, and safety during pregnancy has not yet been established.

Lactation: As with any drug, patients who are nursing a baby should consult a physician before taking this product. Following a typical therapeutic dose, acetaminophen is excreted in breast milk in very low concentrations. Based on a number of published reports, infant exposure levels are at most 4.5% of a weight adjusted pediatric therapeutic dose. In addition, acetaminophen is considered compatible with breast-feeding by the American Academy of Pediatrics.

DRUG INTERACTIONS: Alcohol: Studies evaluating the metabolism of doses up to 20 mg/kg of acetaminophen in chronic alcohol abusers and a study evaluating the effects of 2 days of acetaminophen dosing at 4000 mg/day in chronic alcoholics undergoing detoxification, have yielded inconsistent results with regard to effects on acetaminophen pharmacokinetics and demonstrate no evidence of adverse effect on liver function tests.

Anticoagulants–Oral: Patients who concomitantly medicate with warfarin-type anticoagulants and regular doses of acetaminophen have occasionally been reported to have unforeseen elevations in their INR. Physicians should be cognizant of this potential interaction and monitor the INR in such patients closely while therapy is established. Many factors, including diet, medications, and environmental and physical states, may affect how a patient responds to anticoagulant therapy. There have been several reports that suggest that acetaminophen may produce hypoprothrombinemia (elevated international normalized ratio [INR] or prothrombin time) when administered with coumarin derivatives. In other studies, prothrombin time did not change. Reported changes have been generally of limited clinical significance, however, periodic evaluation of prothrombin time should be performed when these agents are administered concurrently.

In the period immediately following discharge from the hospital or whenever other medications are initiated, discontinued, or taken regularly, it is important to monitor patient response to anticoagulation therapy with additional prothrombin time or INR determinations. Despite the potential for interaction, acetaminophen is the least likely OTC analgesic to interfere with anticoagulant therapy.

Anticonvulsants: Some reports have suggested that patients taking long-term anticonvulsants, who overdose on acetaminophen, may be at increased risk of hepatotoxicity because of accelerated metabolism of acetaminophen. Available data are conflicting. A 7-year retrospective study of acetaminophen overdose admissions indicates that the overall mortality rate was not significantly different for patients taking concomitant anticonvulsant medications.

Hydantoins: Pharmacokinetic studies indicate that phenytoin primarily induces the glucuronidation pathway, whereas glutathione-derived metabolites are not increased in patients on chronic phenytoin therapy. Additionally, recent data demonstrate that phenytoin is metabolized primarily by CYP2C9 and CYP2C19, whereas acetaminophen is primarily metabolized by CYP2E1.

Carbamazepine: Carbamazepine is primarily metabolized by CYP3A4, whereas acetaminophen is metabolized primarily via CYP2E1. It is not known whether there is increased risk from an acetaminophen overdose in patients on chronic carbamazepine therapy.

Diflunisal: Professional literature from the manufacturer of diflunisal cautions that concomitant administration with acetaminophen produces an approximate 50% increase in plasma levels of acetaminophen in normal volunteers. Acetaminophen had no effect on diflunisal plasma levels. The clinical significance of these findings has not been established. However, caution should be used with concomitant administration of diflunisal and acetaminophen and patients should be monitored carefully.

Isoniazid: Some reports suggest that patients on chronic isoniazid therapy may be at risk for developing hepatotoxicity from an acetaminophen overdose. Since patients on isoniazid therapy may develop hepatic effects from isoniazid alone, data from individual case reports are unclear as to whether chronic administration of isoniazid may increase the risk of acetaminophen toxicity. Isoniazid is primarily metabolized by CYP2E1 and induces CYP2E1. Studies in healthy subjects demonstrate that isoniazid blocks the formation of the toxic metabolite NAPQI when administered concomitantly with acetaminophen, but increase NAPQI formation when acetaminophen is administered one day after discontinuation of isoniazid. Thus, concomitant use of isoniazid is unlikely to potentiate the risk of acetaminophen-induced hepatotoxicity at recommended doses. The isoniazid induction of CYP2E1 is short-lived, lasting only 12 to 48 hours after the discontinuation of isoniazid, it is during this period the toxicity of an acetaminophen overdose may be potentiated.

DOSAGE AND ADMINISTRATION:

Dosage: Adults and children over 12 years of age: 2 caplets every 4 hours, as required. It is hazardous to exceed 8 caplets per day. TYLENOL Menstrual caplets are most effective if taken at the first sign of menstrual discomfort.

OVERDOSAGE:

Symptoms and Treatment: Acetaminophen: Typical Toxidrome: Hepatic injury is the principal toxic effect of a substantial acetaminophen overdose. The physician should be mindful that there is no early presentation that is pathognomic for the overdose. A high degree of clinical suspicion must always be maintained.

Untreated acetaminophen overdoses may produce hepatotoxicity. Acetaminophen hepatotoxicity occurs as a threshold effect and is characterized by a lack of toxicity at lower/therapeutic doses. Acetaminophen hepatotoxicity occurs after major depletion of glutathione, an endogenous detoxifying substance. Once the threshold is exceeded, increasing acetaminophen doses may produce increasing degrees of hepatotoxicity, unless N-acetylcysteine (NAC) is administered. Situations in which acetaminophen overdose and resultant hepatotoxicity may occur include acute intentional overdose and repeated supratherapeutic overdose in adults and acute accidental ingestion or overdose and repeated supratherapeutic overdose in children.

The clinical course of acetaminophen overdose generally occurs in a three-phase sequential pattern. The first phase begins shortly after ingestion and lasts for 12 to 24 hours. The patient may manifest signs of gastrointestinal irritability, nausea, vomiting, anorexia, diaphoresis, pallor and general malaise. If toxicity continues, there is a latent phase of up to 48 hours. During this second phase, initial symptoms abate and the patient may feel better. However, hepatic enzymes, bilirubin, and prothrombin time or INR values will progressively rise. Right upper quadrant pain may develop as the liver becomes enlarged and tender. Most patients do not progress beyond this phase, especially if given N-acetylcysteine (NAC) treatment early in the course. Signs and symptoms of the third phase depend on the severity of hepatic damage and usually occur from three to five days following overdose ingestion. Symptoms may be limited to anorexia, nausea, general malaise, and abdominal pain in less severe cases or may progress to confusion, stupor and sequelae of hepatic necrosis including jaundice, coagulation defects, hypoglycemia, and encephalopathy, as well as renal failure and cardiomyopathy. Death, if it occurs, is generally the result of complications associated with fulminant hepatic failure. Mortality rates in patients with toxic plasma levels who do not receive antidote therapy range from 3% to 4%.

Due to the wide availability of acetaminophen, it is commonly involved in single and mixed drug overdose situations and the practitioner should screen for its presence in a patient's serum. Acute toxicity after single dose overdoses of acetaminophen can be anticipated when the overdose exceeds 150 mg/kg. Chronic alcohol abusers, cachectic individuals, and persons taking pharmacologic inducers of the hepatic P450 microsomal enzyme system may be at risk with lower exposures.

Specific Antidote: Any individual presenting with a possible acetaminophen overdose should be treated with N-acetylcysteine (NAC), even if the amount of acetaminophen ingested is unknown or questionable. A blood sample for determination of the plasma acetaminophen concentration should be obtained as early as possible, but no sooner than four hours following ingestion. Do not await the results of assays for plasma acetaminophen levels before initiating treatment NAC. If the acetaminophen plasma level is found to plot above the treatment line on the acetaminophen overdose nomogram, NAC treatment should be continued for a full course of therapy. NAC is used clinically to treat acute acetaminophen overdose, and acts by interacting with the oxidative intermediate, NAPQI. NAC administered by either the i.v. or the oral route is known to be a highly effective antidote for acetaminophen poisoning. It is most effective when administered within 8 hours of a significant overdose but reports have indicated benefits to treatment initiated well beyond this time period. It is imperative to administer the antidote as early as possible in the time course of acute intoxication to reap the full benefits of the antidote's protective effects. For full prescribing information, consult the product monograph for NAC.

General Management: When the possibility of acetaminophen overdose exists, treatment should begin immediately and include appropriate decontamination of the gastrointestinal tract, proper supportive care, careful assessment of appropriately timed serum acetaminophen estimations evaluated against the Rumack-Matthew nomogram, timely administration of NAC as required and appropriate follow-up care. Liver function tests should be performed initially and repeated at 24-hour intervals.

Pamabrom: Typical Toxidrome: xanthine group.

Specific Antidote: none.

General Management: Stabilize the patient (A, B, Cs), undertake appropriate gastrointestinal tract decontamination procedures, initiate supportive care, consult with a Regional Poison Control Centre regarding on-going management and arrange for appropriate follow-up care. Additionally, appropriate monitoring for seizures, arrhythmias and fluid and electrolyte imbalance should be employed.

Pyrilamine Maleate: Typical Toxidrome: anticholinergic, CNS depressant (adult), CNS stimulant (child).

Specific Antidote: none.

General Management: Stabilize the patient (A, B, Cs), undertake appropriate gastrointestinal tract decontamination procedures, initiate supportive care, consult with a Regional Poison Control Centre regarding on-going management and arrange for appropriate follow-up care.

Overdose During Pregnancy: Acetaminophen is one of the most common overdoses in pregnancy. Hepatic toxicity of acetaminophen follows the formation of the highly reactive metabolite N-acetyl-p-benzoquinoneimine produced by acetaminophen metabolism through the cytochrome P450 mixed-function oxidase system. Hepatic failure can be prevented by timely administration of NAC either orally for 72 hours, or intravenously (IV) for 20 hours.

Acetaminophen crosses the human placenta81 though the fetus is theoretically at risk when maternal overdose of acetaminophen occurs. Acetaminophen can be transformed to its toxic metabolite since the oxidative capacity of fetal microsomes is present in the fetus by 14 weeks gestation.

Studies on placental transfer of NAC in rats and sheep yielded conflicting results83. Placental transfer of N-acetylcysteine in humans was demonstrated in 4 women treated with NAC for acetaminophen overdose during labour. NAC blood levels in the fetuses were within the range associated with therapeutic doses of NAC administered to adults with acetaminophen poisoning.

Fetal toxicity and stillbirth after a large (e.g. 30 g) acetaminophen overdose has been reported, but others observed a normal outcome for the offspring after acetaminophen overdose in pregnancy. A large case series investigated the pregnancy outcome in 300 women who had overdosed with acetaminophen. In this group, 118 cases occurred in the first trimester, 103 in the second trimester and 79 in the third trimester. Forty-nine of these mothers were treated with specific antidotes (33 with NAC and 16 with methionine). There were 219 live-born infants, 11 have malformations (including minor); none had been exposed to acetaminophen during the first trimester. Nine women were treated with NAC during the first trimester; there were two elective terminations; two spontaneous abortions, and five healthy babies in this group.

In summary, acetaminophen overdose during pregnancy should be treated according to regular protocols in order to prevent maternal and potentially fetal toxicity. Unless severe maternal toxicity develops, an acetaminophen overdose does not increase the risk for birth defects or adverse pregnancy outcomes.

Physicians unfamiliar with the current management of acetaminophen overdose should consult with a Poison Control Centre immediately. Telephone numbers for local Poison Control Centres are available in the local phone directory. Delays in initiation of appropriate therapy may jeopardize the patient's chances for full recovery.

> For management of a suspected drug overdose, CPhA recommends that you contact your **regional Poison Control Centre**. See the *CPS* Directory section for a list of Poison Control Centres.

ACTION AND CLINICAL PHARMACOLOGY: Mechanism of Action: Acetaminophen is a centrally acting analgesic and antipyretic drug. Although the precise mechanism of action is not totally understood, work by Boutaud suggests acetaminophen is an inhibitor of the peroxidase portion of cyclooxygenase (prostaglandin H synthase inhibitor). Depending on the redox state and substrate concentrations surrounding the enzymes, acetaminophen may or may not have a significant inhibitory effect. This accounts for its selective activity on pain and fever with little anti-inflammatory effect.

It is postulated that the analgesic effect is produced by elevation of the pain threshold and the antipyretic effect is produced through action on the hypothalamic heat-regulating centre.

The optimal effective analgesic dose of acetaminophen was demonstrated in dental pain studies and is 1000 mg every four to six hours, up to 4000 mg daily. At least 500 published and unpublished controlled clinical trials in adults and children have evaluated acetaminophen for the relief of pain or fever. These studies include single and multiple dose treatments. Most studies were less than 14 days in duration, although the longest study duration was two years. No significant safety issues were reported in any of these studies.

Moreover, at recommended doses, acetaminophen has not been shown to increase the risk of developing renal diseases or upper gastrointestinal ulceration/bleeding. This observation is consistent with its minimal inhibitory effect on peripheral prostaglandin synthesis and on gastric prostaglandin synthesis.

Acetaminophen is considered equipotent to ASA and ibuprofen, within the recommended OTC dosing ranges, in its analgesic and antipyretic effects. Acetaminophen at recommended doses does not cause the type of gastrointestinal complications associated with NSAID-containing products, such as gastric irritation, gastric erosions, occult or overt gastrointestinal blood loss, or ulcers. Unlike these drugs, however, it has no anti-inflammatory effect at clinically relevant doses in humans.

Pyrilamine maleate is an antihistaminic agent of the ethylenediamine group. In addition, pyrilamine possesses local anesthetic activity and exerts a mild analgesic action.

Pamabrom, a xanthine derivative, is a safe and effective diuretic in relieving the water-accumulation symptoms of water-weight gain, bloating, swelling and/or full feeling associated with the premenstrual and menstrual periods.

Pharmacokinetics: Absorption: Oral acetaminophen is rapidly and almost completely absorbed from the gastrointestinal tract primarily in the small intestine. This absorption process occurs by passive transport. Peak plasma concentrations occur within 0.4 to 1 hour depending on the product formulation. Although high-fat foods delay the time to peak concentration for up to an hour, the dose is completely absorbed.

Distribution: Acetaminophen is uniformly distributed throughout most body fluids, but not in fatty tissue. As a result, the volume of distribution in adults ranges between 0.8 and 1.0 L/kg. Since acetaminophen has low protein binding in plasma of only 10% to 25%, it does not compete with drugs that are highly protein bound.

Metabolism: Acetaminophen is primarily metabolized by the liver via three principal separate pathways: conjugation with glucuronide; conjugation with sulfate; oxidation via the cytochrome P450 mixed function oxidase system.

Both the glucuronic and oxidative pathways adhere to a first-order rate process, which means the concentration of acetaminophen metabolized increases as the concentration in the liver increases. The sulfate pathway adheres to Michaelis-Menten kinetics, which means the concentration of acetaminophen metabolized remains constant once the concentration in the liver increases above a saturation level. A schematic of acetaminophen metabolism is shown in Figure 2.

The major metabolic pathway is glucuronidation, where 47% to 62% of the acetaminophen dose conjugates with glucuronide. These glucuronide conjugates are inactive and nontoxic, and are secreted in bile and eliminated in the urine.

The second major pathway is sulfation, where 25% to 36% of the dose conjugates with sulfate. These sulfate ester conjugates are also inactive and nontoxic and are excreted in the urine.

* Container provided with a child-resistant closure.

The third pathway is oxidation, where 5% to 8% of the dose is metabolized via the cytochrome P450 enzyme system. The cytochrome P450 isoenzyme that is primarily responsible is CYP2E1. When acetaminophen is metabolized by CYP2E1, it forms a highly reactive intermediate, N-acetyl-p-benzoquinoneimine (NAPQI). Since NAPQI is highly reactive, it cannot be measured outside the liver nor can it accumulate. This intermediate is rapidly inactivated by hepatocellular stores of glutathione to form cysteine and mercapturate conjugates, which are both inactive and nontoxic. These conjugates are excreted in the urine.

Figure 2: TYLENOL Menstrual Acetaminophen Metabolism

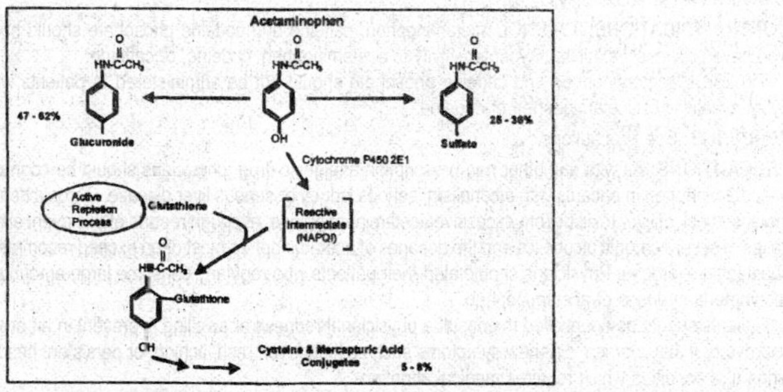

Excretion: Acetaminophen undergoes first-order elimination from the body, and has a short plasma half-life that ranges from 2 to 3 hours in healthy young and elderly adults and from 1.5 to 2.9 hours in children. Since acetaminophen clears rapidly from the body, repeated doses do not lead to accumulation of acetaminophen plasma concentrations.

STORAGE AND STABILITY: Store at room temperature (15 to 30°C).

DOSAGE FORMS, COMPOSITION AND PACKAGING: Each hard, salmon-coloured, coated, capsule-shaped tablet, engraved "TYME" on one side and "500" on the other side contains: acetaminophen 500 mg, pamabrom 25 mg and pyrilamine maleate 15 mg. Nonmedicinal ingredients: cellulose, citric acid, cornstarch, FD&C Red no. 40, FD&C Yellow no. 6, hypromellose, magnesium stearate, polydextrose, polyethylene glycol, sodium cyclamate, sodium starch glycolate, titanium dioxide and triacetin. Energy: 1.0 kJ (0.2 kcal). Sodium: 0.4 mg. Gluten-, lactose-, sucrose-, sulfite- and tartrazine-free. Plastic bottles of 16* and 32*. All packages are safety sealed.

Tylenol® No. 1 Ⓝ
acetaminophen—caffeine—codeine phosphate
Analgesic—Antipyretic

Janssen-Ortho/McNeil Consumer Healthcare

Tylenol® with Codeine No. 2 Ⓝ
acetaminophen—caffeine—codeine phosphate
Analgesic—Antipyretic

Janssen-Ortho/McNeil Consumer Healthcare

Tylenol® with Codeine No. 3 Ⓝ
acetaminophen—caffeine—codeine phosphate
Analgesic—Antipyretic

Janssen-Ortho/McNeil Consumer Healthcare

Tylenol® with Codeine No. 4 Ⓝ
acetaminophen—codeine phosphate
Analgesic—Antipyretic

Janssen-Ortho/McNeil Consumer Healthcare

Tylenol® with Codeine Elixir Ⓝ
acetaminophen—codeine phosphate
Analgesic—Antipyretic

Janssen-Ortho/McNeil Consumer Healthcare

Date of Revision: July 14, 2008

PHARMACOLOGY: TYLENOL acetaminophen and codeine phosphate, and TYLENOL acetaminophen, caffeine and codeine phosphate are analgesic, antipyretic agents.

Action: TYLENOL acetaminophen and codeine phosphate, and TYLENOL acetaminophen, caffeine and codeine phosphate combine the analgesic effects of the centrally acting analgesic codeine, with a peripherally acting analgesic, acetaminophen. Caffeine stimulates the CNS at all levels including the cerebral cortex. In addition, it acts on the kidney to produce mild diuresis, stimulates cardiac muscle, and depresses smooth muscle.

Acetaminophen, codeine phosphate and caffeine are well absorbed orally.

Acetaminophen is distributed throughout most tissues of the body. Acetaminophen is metabolized primarily in the liver. Little unchanged drug is excreted in the urine, but most metabolic products appear in the urine within 24 hours.

Codeine retains at least one-half of its analgesic activity when administered orally. A reduced first-pass metabolism of codeine by the liver accounts for the greater oral potency of codeine when compared to most other morphine-like narcotics. Following absorption, codeine is metabolized by the liver and metabolic products are excreted in the urine. Approximately 10% of the administered codeine is demethylated to morphine, which may account for its analgesic activity.

Caffeine is absorbed efficiently from the gastrointestinal tract, and peak plasma concentrations occur 15 to 120 minutes after ingestion. It is almost completely metabolized via oxidation, demethylation, and acetylation, with only about 1% of caffeine excreted via the urine. The principal metabolites in man are methyluric acid, 1-methylxanthine, paraxanthine, and theobromine.

Pharmacokinetics: Following oral administration of acetaminophen in combination with codeine, both drugs are rapidly absorbed with peak plasma levels occurring within 60 minutes. Given two tablets of TYLENOL with codeine No. 3, acetaminophen 600 mg produces a peak plasma level of 6.25 µg/mL within 40 minutes, codeine phosphate 60 mg produces a peak plasma level of 150 ng/mL within 60 minutes.

Following oral administration, caffeine is rapidly absorbed with a peak plasma level occurring within 15 to 120 minutes. Given an oral dose of 100 mg peak plasma caffeine concentrations of 1.5 to 1.8 µg/mL are reached within 60 minutes.

The plasma elimination half-life ($t_{1/2}$) ranges from 1.5 to 3.5 hours for acetaminophen, 1.5 to 4 hours for codeine, and from 2.5 to 4.5 hours for caffeine. Metabolism is rapid; the principal metabolites are conjugates of glucuronic acid which are excreted in the urine. Less than 1% of an administered dose of codeine or caffeine, and less than 4% of an administered dose of acetaminophen, is excreted unchanged in the urine.

INDICATIONS: TYLENOL with Codeine No. 1, 2 and 3: TYLENOL acetaminophen, caffeine and codeine phosphate tablets and caplets are indicated for the relief of mild to moderate pain associated with conditions such as headache, dental pain, myalgia, dysmenorrhea, pain following trauma, and pain following operative procedures. TYLENOL acetaminophen, caffeine and codeine phosphate may also be effective in relieving the pain associated with various forms of arthritis, but is **not** indicated as primary therapy for rheumatoid arthritis and similar inflammatory conditions.

TYLENOL with Codeine Elixir: TYLENOL acetaminophen and codeine phosphate oral solution is useful as an analgesic/antipyretic in the symptomatic treatment of mild to moderate pain and fever in children.

TYLENOL with Codeine No. 4: TYLENOL acetaminophen and codeine phosphate tablets are indicated for the relief of moderate to severe pain in adults only.

CONTRAINDICATIONS: TYLENOL acetaminophen, caffeine and codeine phosphate should not be administered to patients who have previously exhibited hypersensitivity to acetaminophen, codeine, or caffeine.

TYLENOL acetaminophen and codeine phosphate should not be administered to patients who have previously exhibited hypersensitivity to acetaminophen or codeine.

WARNINGS: See Precautions.

PRECAUTIONS: As with any other non-prescription analgesic drug, physicians should be cognizant of and supervise the use of acetaminophen in patients with alcoholism, serious kidney or serious liver disease. Chronic heavy alcohol abusers may be at increased risk of liver toxicity from excessive acetaminophen use, although reports of this event are rare. Reports usually involve cases of severe chronic alcoholics and the dosages of acetaminophen most often exceed recommended doses and often involve substantial overdose. Physicians should alert their patients who regularly consume large amounts of alcohol not to exceed the recommended doses of acetaminophen.

Patients should be counselled to consult a physician if redness or swelling is present in an area of pain, if symptoms do not improve or if they worsen, or if new symptoms such as high fever, rash, itching, or persistent headache occur, as these may be signs of a condition which requires medical attention.

Acetaminophen should not be taken for pain for more than 5 days or for fever for more than 3 days, unless directed by a physician. As with any drug, patients who are pregnant or nursing a baby should consult a physician before taking this product.

Do not use with other products containing acetaminophen, salicylates, or any other pain or fever medicine. Keep out of the reach of children.

In the presence of head injury or other intracranial lesions, the respiratory depressant effects of codeine and other narcotics may be markedly enhanced, as well as their capacity for elevating cerebrospinal fluid pressure. Narcotics also produce other CNS depressant effects, such as drowsiness, that may further obscure the clinical course of the patients with head injuries.

Codeine or other narcotics may obscure signs on which to judge the diagnosis or clinical course of patients with acute abdominal conditions.

Codeine is habit forming and potentially abusable. Consequently, the extended use of this product is not recommended.

General: TYLENOL with Codeine (acetaminophen and codeine phosphate) tablets should be prescribed with caution in certain special-risk patients, such as the elderly or debilitated, and those with severe impairment of renal or hepatic function, head injuries, elevated intracranial pressure, acute abdominal conditions, hypothyroidism, urethral stricture, Addison's disease, or prostatic hypertrophy.

Ultra-Rapid Metabolizers of Codeine: Some individuals may be ultra-rapid metabolizers due to a specific CYP2D6* 2×2 genotype. These individuals convert codeine into its active metabolite, morphine, more rapidly and completely than other people. This rapid conversion results in higher than expected serum morphine levels. Even at labeled dosage regimens, individuals who are ultra-rapid metabolizers may experience overdose symptoms such as extreme sleepiness, confusion, or shallow breathing.

The prevalence of this CYP2D6 phenotype varies widely and has been estimated at 0.5 to 1% in Chinese and Japanese, 0.5 to 1% in Hispanics, 1 to 10% in Caucasians, 3% in African Americans, and 16 to 28% in North Africans, Ethiopians, and Arabs. Data are not available for other ethnic groups.

When physicians prescribe codeine-containing drugs, they should choose the lowest effective dose for the shortest period of time and inform their patients about these risks and the signs of morphine overdose (see Precautions, Lactation).

Occupational Hazards: Codeine may impair the mental and/or physical abilities required for the performance of potentially hazardous tasks. Patients using this drug should be cautioned about driving a car or operating potentially hazardous machinery if they become drowsy or show impaired mental or physical abilities while taking this medication.

The patient should understand the single-dose and 24-hour dose limits, and the time interval between doses. Like other narcotic-containing medications, these drugs are subject to the Controlled Drugs and Substances Act.

Laboratory Tests: In patients with severe hepatic or renal disease, effects of therapy should be monitored with serial liver and/or renal function tests.

Drug Interactions: This drug may enhance the effects of other narcotic analgesics, alcohol, general anesthetics, tranquilizers such as chlordiazepoxide, sedative-hypnotics, or other CNS depressants, causing increased CNS depression.

Patients who concomitantly medicate with warfarin-type anticoagulants and regular doses of acetaminophen have occasionally been reported to have unforeseen elevations in their international normalized ratio [INR]. Physicians should be cognizant of this potential interaction and monitor the INR in such patients closely while therapy is established. Many factors, including diet, medications, and environmental and physical states, may affect how a patient responds to anticoagulant therapy. There have been several reports that suggest that acetaminophen may produce hypoprothrombinemia (elevated INR or prothrombin time) when administered with coumarin derivatives. In other studies, prothrombin time did not change. Reported changes have been generally of limited clinical significance, however, periodic evaluation of prothrombin time should be performed when these agents are administered concurrently.

In the period immediately following discharge from the hospital or whenever other medications are initiated, discontinued, or taken regularly, it is important to monitor patient response to anticoagulation therapy with additional prothrombin time of INR determinations.

Drug/Laboratory Test Interactions: Codeine may increase serum amylase levels.

Acetaminophen may produce false-positive test results for urinary 5-hydroxyindoleacetic acid.

Carcinogenesis, Mutagenesis, Impairment of Fertility: No adequate studies have been conducted in animals to whether acetaminophen or codeine have a potential for carcinogenesis or mutagenesis. No adequate studies have been conducted in animals to determine whether acetaminophen has a potential for impairment of fertility.

Acetaminophen and codeine have been found to have no mutagenic potential using the Ames Salmonella-Microsomal Activation test, the Basc test on Drosophila germ cells, and the Micronucleus test on mouse bone marrow.

Pregnancy: Teratogenic Effects: Codeine: A study in rats and rabbits reported no teratogenic effect of codeine administered during the period of organogenesis in doses ranging from 5 to 120 mg/kg. In the rat, doses at the 120 mg/kg level, in the toxic range for the adult animal, were associated with an increase in embryo resorption at the time of implantation. In another study, a single 100 mg/kg dose of codeine administered to pregnant mice reportedly resulted in delayed ossification in the offspring.

There are no adequate and well-controlled studies in pregnant women.

TYLENOL acetaminophen and codeine phosphate, and TYLENOL acetaminophen, caffeine and codeine phosphate should be used during pregnancy only if the potential benefit justifies the potential risk to the fetus.

Non-teratogenic Effects: Dependence and withdrawal signs have been reported in newborns whose mothers took opiates regularly during pregnancy. These signs include irritability, excessive crying, tremors, hyperreflexia, fever, vomiting and diarrhea. Signs usually appear during the first few days of life.

Labour and Delivery: Narcotic analgesics cross the placental barrier. The closer to delivery and the larger the dose used, the greater the possibility of respiratory depression in the newborn. Narcotic analgesics should be avoided during labour if delivery of a premature infant is anticipated. If the mother has received narcotic analgesics during labour, newborn infants should be observed closely for signs of respiratory depression. Resuscitation may be required (see Overdose). The effects of codeine, if any, on the later growth, development, and functional maturation of the child is unknown.

Lactation: Acetaminophen and codeine phosphate, and acetaminophen, caffeine and codeine phosphate products are not recommended during lactation because safety in nursing mothers has not been established.

Acetaminophen is excreted in breast milk in small amounts, but the significance of its effects on nursing infants is not known. Because of the potential for serious adverse reactions in nursing infants from acetaminophen, a decision should be made whether to discontinue the drug, taking into account the importance of the drug to the mother.

Codeine is secreted into human milk. In women with normal codeine metabolism (normal CYP2D6 activity), the amount of codeine secreted into human milk is low and dose-dependent. Despite the common use of codeine products to manage postpartum pain, reports of adverse events in infants are rare. However, some women are ultra-rapid metabolizers of codeine. These women achieve higher-than-expected serum levels of codeine's active metabolite, morphine, leading to higher-than-expected levels of morphine in breast milk and potentially dangerously high serum morphine levels in their breastfed infants. Therefore, maternal use of codeine can potentially lead to serious adverse reactions, including death, in nursing infants.

The prevalence of this CYP2D6 phenotype varies widely and has been estimated at 0.5 to 1% in Chinese and Japanese, 0.5 to 1% in Hispanics, 1 to 10% in Caucasians, 3% in African Americans, and 16 to 28% in North Africans, Ethiopians, and Arabs. Data are not available for other ethnic groups.

The risk of infant exposure to codeine and morphine through breast milk should be weighed against the benefits of breastfeeding for both the mother and baby. Caution should be exercised when codeine is administered to a nursing woman. If a codeine containing product is selected, the lowest dose should be prescribed for the shortest period of time to achieve the desired clinical effect. Mothers using codeine should be informed about when to seek immediate medical care and how to identify the signs and symptoms of neonatal toxicity, such as drowsiness or sedation, difficulty breastfeeding, breathing difficulties, and decreased tone, in their baby. Nursing mothers who are ultra-rapid metabolizers may also experience overdose symptoms such as extreme sleepiness, confusion, or shallow breathing. Prescribers should closely monitor mother-infant pairs and notify treating pediatricians about the use of codeine during breastfeeding (see Precautions, General, Ultra-Rapid Metabolizers of Codeine).

Caffeine is distributed into the milk of nursing women.

Children: These products contain codeine and should not be administered to children except on the advice of a physician. Tablets and caplets should not be administered to children below the age of 12 years. Safe dosage of the TYLENOL with Codeine Elixir has not been established in infants below the age of 2 years.

Drug Abuse and Dependence: Codeine can produce drug dependence of the morphine type and, therefore, has the potential for being abused. Psychic dependence, physical dependence, and tolerance may develop upon repeated administration of TYLENOL acetaminophen and codeine phosphate, and TYLENOL acetaminophen, caffeine and codeine phosphate. These drugs should be prescribed and administered with the same degree of caution appropriate to the use of other oral narcotic-containing medications.

ADVERSE EFFECTS: The most frequently observed adverse effects include drowsiness, lightheadedness, dizziness, sedation, shortness of breath, nausea, and vomiting. These effects seem to be more prominent in ambulatory patients than in non-ambulatory patients, and some of these adverse reactions may be alleviated if the patient lies down. Other adverse reactions include allergic reactions, euphoria, dysphoria, constipation, abdominal pain, pruritus, rash, thrombocytopenia, and agranulocytosis. The incidence and severity of gastrointestinal upset is less than that after salicylate administration.

The classic gastrointestinal irritation associated with non-steroidal anti-inflammatory drugs, including ASA, does not occur with acetaminophen. Sensitivity reactions are rare and may manifest as rash or urticaria. Cross-reactivity in ASA-sensitive persons has been rarely reported. If sensitivity is suspected, discontinue use of the drug.

Patients who concomitantly medicate with warfarin-type anticoagulants and regular doses of acetaminophen have occasionally been reported to have unforeseen elevations in their INR. Physicians should be cognizant of this potential interaction and monitor the INR in such patients closely while therapy is established (see Precautions, Drug Interactions).

At higher doses, codeine has most of the disadvantages of morphine, including respiratory depression.

Higher doses of caffeine lead to overstimulation of the higher centres of the CNS. Adverse CNS effects may include insomnia, restlessness, nervousness and mild delirium. Adverse gastrointestinal effects of caffeine may include nausea, vomiting, and gastric irritation. Although chronic administration of caffeine in animals has been associated with gastric ulceration, such a causal relationship in humans has not been adequately established to date.

OVERDOSE:

Symptoms: Acetaminophen: Typical Toxidrome: Significant overdoses of acetaminophen may result in potentially fatal hepatotoxicity. The physician should be mindful that there is no early presentation that is pathognomonic for the overdose. A high degree of clinical suspicion must always be maintained.

Due to the wide availability of acetaminophen, it is commonly involved in single and mixed drug overdose situations and the practitioner should have a low threshold for screening for its presence in a patient's serum. Acute toxicity after single dose overdoses of acetaminophen can be anticipated when the overdose exceeds 150 mg/kg. Chronic alcohol abusers, cachectic individuals, and persons taking pharmacologic inducers of the hepatic P450 microsomal enzyme system may be at risk with lower exposures. Chronic intoxication has rarely been reported in persons consuming in excess of 150 mg/kg of acetaminophen daily for several days.

Specific Antidote: NAC (N-acetylcysteine) administered by either the intravenous or the oral route is known to be a highly effective antidote for acetaminophen poisoning. It is most effective when administered within 8 hours of a significant overdose but reports have indicated benefits to treatment initiated well beyond this time period. It is imperative to administer the antidote as early as possible in the time course of acute intoxication to reap the full benefits of the antidote's protective effects.

General Management: When the possibility of acetaminophen overdose exists, treatment should begin immediately and include appropriate decontamination of the GI tract, proper supportive care, careful assessment of appropriately timed serum acetaminophen estimations evaluated against the Matthew-Rumack nomogram, timely administration of NAC as required and appropriate follow-up care. Physicians unfamiliar with the current management of acetaminophen overdose should consult with a poison control centre immediately. Telephone numbers for local poison control centres are available in the local phone directory. Delays in initiation of appropriate therapy may jeopardize the patient's chances for full recovery.

Codeine: Typical Toxidrome: Narcotic/opiate.

Specific Antidote: Naloxone HCl.

General Management: Stabilize the patient (A, B, C's), undertake appropriate gastrointestinal tract decontamination procedures, initiate supportive care, administer antidote as needed (see manufacturer's product monograph), consult with a Regional Poison Control Centre regarding ongoing management, and arrange for appropriate follow-up care.

Caffeine: Typical Toxidrome: Xanthine (theophylline-like picture), CNS excitation, skeletal muscle irritability.

Specific Antidote: None.

General Management: Stabilize the patient (A, B, C's), undertake appropriate gastrointestinal tract decontamination procedures, initiate supportive care, consult with a Regional Poison Control Centre regarding ongoing management, and arrange for appropriate follow-up care.

Treatment: See Symptoms.

For management of a suspected drug overdose, CPhA recommends that you contact your **regional Poison Control Centre**. See the *CPS* Directory section for a list of Poison Control Centres.

DOSAGE: Dosage should be adjusted according to severity of pain and response of the patient. However, it should be kept in mind that tolerance to codeine can develop with continued use and that the incidence of untoward effects is dose related. Adult doses of codeine, higher than 60 mg, fail to give commensurate relief of pain but merely prolong analgesia, and are associated with an appreciably increased incidence of undesirable side effects. Equivalently high doses in children would have similar effects.

TYLENOL acetaminophen, caffeine and codeine phosphate tablets and caplets, as well as TYLENOL acetaminophen and codeine phosphate tablets and oral solution are given orally.

TYLENOL No. 1: Adults: 1 to 2 caplets may be repeated up to every 4 hours as required, not to exceed 12 tablets in 24 hours. Children: When recommended by a physician or dentist: 12 to 14 years of age: 1 caplet 3 times daily. Not to exceed 1 caplet 4 times daily.

TYLENOL with Codeine No. 2 and No. 3: Adults: 1 or 2 tablets every 4 hours as required, not to exceed 12 tablets in 24 hours.

TYLENOL with Codeine No. 4: Adults: 1 tablet every 4 hours as required, not to exceed 6 tablets in 24 hours.

Based on the dosage guidance, the number of tablets per dose and the maximum number of tablets per 24 hours should be conveyed in the prescription.

TYLENOL with Codeine Elixir: Dosage should be adjusted according to severity of pain and response of the patient. As an analgesic-antipyretic, the dose is given every 4 hours as required. Not to exceed 5 doses in a 24-hour period.

Adults: 10 to 20 mL every 4 hours as required.

Children: 2 to 3 years: 3.75 to 5 mL; 4 to 5 years: 5 to 6.25 mL; 6 to 8 years: 6.25 to 8.75 mL; 9 to 10 years: 8.75 to 10 mL; 11 to 12 years: 10 to 12.5 mL.

Safe dosage of this elixir has not been established in children below the age of 2 years.

Note: The recommended dose of codeine in children is 0.5 mg/kg body weight.

SUPPLIED: TYLENOL No. 1: Each hard, white, capsule-shaped tablet imprinted with stylized "M" and "McNEIL" on one face and imprinted with "NO. 1" on the other face, contains: acetaminophen 300 mg, caffeine 15 mg and codeine phosphate 8 mg. Nonmedicinal ingredients: cellulose, cornstarch, magnesium stearate and sodium starch glycolate. Energy: 0.761 kJ (0.182 kcal). Sodium: <1 mmol (0.4 mg). Gluten-, lactose-, sodium metabisulfite- and tartrazine-free. Bottles of 30, 50 and 100 (supplied by McNeil Consumer Products). Keep bottles tightly closed. Store at 15-25°C.

TYLENOL with Codeine No. 2 and No. 3: Each round, hard, white tablet, flat-faced, bevelled, engraved with "2" or "3", respectively, on one side and has a flat-faced, special design, bevelled, engraved with "McNEIL" on the other side, contains: acetaminophen 300 mg and caffeine 15 mg, in combination with codeine phosphate 15 mg and 30 mg, respectively. Nonmedicinal ingredients: cellulose, magnesium stearate, microcrystalline cellulose, pregelatinized starch, sodium starch glycolate and starch NF. Gluten-, lactose-, sodium metabisulfite- and tartrazine-free. Bottles of 500 (supplied by Janssen-Ortho Inc.). Keep bottle tightly closed. Store at 15-30°C. Protect from light.

TYLENOL with Codeine No. 4: Each round, hard, white tablet, flat-faced, bevelled, engraved with "4" one side and has a flat-faced special design, bevelled, engraved with "McNEIL" on the other side, contains: acetaminophen 300 mg and codeine phosphate 60 mg. Nonmedicinal ingredients: cellulose, cornstarch, magnesium stearate, sodium lauryl sulfate, sodium starch glycolate and talc. Energy: 1.704 kJ (0.405 kcal). Sodium: <1 mmol (0.6 mg). Gluten-, lactose-, sodium metabisulfite- and tartrazine-free. Bottles of 100 (supplied by Janssen-Ortho Inc.). Keep bottle tightly closed. Store at 15-30°C. Protect from light.

TYLENOL with Codeine Elixir: Each 5 mL of elixir contains: acetaminophen 160 mg and codeine phosphate 8 mg in a slightly viscous, clear red liquid that tastes and smells like cherry. Nonmedicinal ingredients: alcohol, citric acid, D&C Red No. 33, flavour, polyethylene glycol, sodium benzoate, sodium cyclamate, sorbitol and sucrose. Alcohol: 6% w/v (7% v/v). Energy: 45.93 kJ (10.98 kcal)/5 mL. Sucrose: 31% w/v. Gluten-, lactose- and tartrazine-free. Dark amber plastic bottles of 500 mL (supplied by Janssen-Ortho Inc.). Dispense in tight and light-resistant containers. Keep bottle tightly closed. Store at 15-30°C. Protect from light.

(Shown in Product Identification Section)

Tylenol® Regular Strength Tablets, Caplets
acetaminophen
Analgesic—Antipyretic

McNeil Consumer Healthcare

Tylenol® Extra Strength Tablets, Caplets, Gelcaps
acetaminophen
Analgesic—Antipyretic

McNeil Consumer Healthcare

Tylenol® Arthritis Pain Extended Release Tablets
acetaminophen
Analgesic—Antipyretic

McNeil Consumer Healthcare

Tylenol® Muscle Aches & Body Pain Extended Release Tablets
acetaminophen
Analgesic—Antipyretic

McNeil Consumer Healthcare

Tylenol® Junior Strength Tablets "Meltaways"
acetaminophen
Analgesic—Antipyretic

McNeil Consumer Healthcare

Tylenol® Children's Tablets "Meltaways" and Suspension
acetaminophen
Analgesic—Antipyretic

McNeil Consumer Healthcare

Tylenol® Infants' Suspension Drops
acetaminophen
Analgesic—Antipyretic

McNeil Consumer Healthcare

Date of Preparation: September 2, 2005
Date of Revision: July 23, 2009

SUMMARY PRODUCT INFORMATION:

Route of Administration	Dosage Form/ Strength	Clinically Relevant Nonmedicinal Ingredients
Oral	Suspension/80 mg/mL	Alcohol-, gluten-, lactose-, sucrose-, sulfite- and tartrazine-free For a complete listing of nonmedicinal ingredients, see Dosage Forms, Composition and Packaging.
	Suspension/160 mg/5 mL	Alcohol-, gluten-, lactose-, sucrose-, sulfite- and tartrazine-free For a complete listing of nonmedicinal ingredients, see Dosage Forms, Composition and Packaging.
	Tablet/80 mg	Gluten-, lactose-, sucrose- and tartrazine-free For a complete listing of nonmedicinal ingredients, see Dosage Forms, Composition and Packaging.
	Tablet/160 mg	Gluten-, lactose-, sucrose- and tartrazine-free For a complete listing of nonmedicinal ingredients, see Dosage Forms, Composition and Packaging.
	Tablet and Caplet/325 mg	Gluten-, lactose- and tartrazine-free For a complete listing of nonmedicinal ingredients, see Dosage Forms, Composition and Packaging.
	Tablet, Caplet and Gelcap/500 mg	Gluten-, lactose- and tartrazine-free For a complete listing of nonmedicinal ingredients, see Dosage Forms, Composition and Packaging.
	Caplet/650 mg	Gluten-, lactose- and tartrazine-free For a complete listing of nonmedicinal ingredients, see Dosage Forms, Composition and Packaging.

INDICATIONS AND CLINICAL USE: As an analgesic-antipyretic for the temporary relief of mild to moderate pain in a wide variety of conditions involving musculoskeletal pain, as well as in other painful disorders such as headache pain (including mild to moderate migraine and tension headache), earache, low back pain, arthritis pain, dysmenorrhea, myalgias and neuralgias. Also indicated for the symptomatic reduction of fever due to the common cold, flu and other viral or bacterial infections.

CONTRAINDICATIONS: Hypersensitivity to acetaminophen or to the ingredients of this formulation (see Dosage Forms, Composition and Packaging). Allergic reactions (primarily skin rash) or reports of hypersensitivity secondary to acetaminophen are rare and generally are controlled by discontinuation of the drug and, when necessary, symptomatic treatment.

WARNINGS AND PRECAUTIONS: General: Consumers should not exceed 4 g/day of acetaminophen or use two or more acetaminophen-containing products together. This includes combination products that contain acetaminophen. Do not use with other products containing salicylates or any other pain or fever medicine.

Acetaminophen-containing products should be kept out of the reach of children.

Physicians should be cognizant of and supervise the use of acetaminophen in patients with chronic alcoholism, serious kidney or serious liver disease. Physicians should alert their patients who regularly consume large amounts of alcohol not to exceed the recommended doses of acetaminophen. Chronic heavy alcohol abusers may be at increased risk of liver toxicity from excessive doses of acetaminophen.

Patients should be counseled to consult a physician if redness or swelling is present in an area of pain, if symptoms do not improve or if they worsen, or if new symptoms such as high fever, rash, itching or persistent headache occur, as these may be signs of a condition which requires medical attention.

Acetaminophen should not be taken for pain for more than 5 days, for fever for more than 3 days or if new symptoms appear, without consulting a physician.

Hepatic/Biliary/Pancreatic: Slower metabolism of acetaminophen, increased activity of the cytochrome P450 enzyme system, or depleted glutathione stores are cited as theoretical risk factors for acetaminophen hepatotoxicity in patients with chronic liver disease. However, acetaminophen has been studied in both adults and children with a wide variety of liver diseases including various types of cirrhosis, hepatitis (including hepatitis C), nodular transformation, congenital hepatic fibrosis, and α1-antitrypsin deficiency. In none of these conditions is there evidence of an increased risk for hepatotoxicity at currently recommended acetaminophen doses but the studies were insufficiently powered to definitely establish the extent of risk.

Forrest compared acetaminophen metabolism following a single 1500 mg dose in normal subjects, patients with mild liver disease, and patients with severe liver disease. There were no significant differences in overall 24-hour urinary excretion of acetaminophen and glucuronide, sulfate, cysteine, and mercapturic acid conjugates, evidence that acetaminophen metabolism was similar to that in normal subjects. However, the elimination half-life was significantly prolonged in patients with severe liver disease.

Acetaminophen has also been studied in pediatric patients with liver disease. Following a single (10 mg/kg) dose of acetaminophen, the pharmacokinetic profiles in pediatric patients with mild, moderate, or severe liver disease were not significantly different. Although the plasma half-life of acetaminophen was prolonged in patients with severe liver disease, there were no significant differences in the 36-hour (children) urinary excretion of acetaminophen or its conjugates.

At the currently recommended doses acetaminophen is a suitable analgesic choice for use in patients with chronic stable liver disease when used under physician supervision.

Acetaminophen may cause hepatotoxicity in situations of intentional overdose (e.g. attempted suicide), unintentional overdose (e.g. overdosing when pain relief is not satisfactory), simultaneous use of multiple acetaminophen-containing preparations, accidental overdose or in very rare cases, after recommended doses, although causality has not been determined. The hepatotoxic reaction can be severe and life-threatening. Early symptoms following a hepatotoxic overdose may include nausea, vomiting, diaphoresis, lethargy, and general malaise. If appropriate treatment is not instituted, these may progress to upper quadrant pain, confusion, stupor, and sequelae of hepatic necrosis, such as jaundice, coagulation defects, hypoglycemia, and encephalopathy. Renal failure and cardiomyopathy may also occur. In the event of known or suspected overdosage, treatment with N-acetyl cysteine should be instituted immediately (see Overdosage), even when there are no obvious symptoms. Failure to promptly treat acetaminophen hepatotoxicity with N-acetyl cysteine can result in liver failure, leading to liver transplantation and/or death.

Chronic Alcohol Use: Excessive alcohol use may increase risk of liver toxicity from acetaminophen overdose (acute or chronic).

Prospective data from Kuffner demonstrate that chronic alcoholics can take recommended doses of acetaminophen without the added risk of liver injury. In these prospective, placebo controlled studies, the researchers evaluated an actively drinking group of alcoholics with a high prevalence of malnourishment. The study participants abruptly stopped their daily alcohol intake and took acetaminophen the next day. This should theoretically make them vulnerable to acetaminophen injury because their CYP2E1 would be maximally induced from the alcohol and there would be no alcohol present to compete with acetaminophen for metabolism by CYP2E1. There was no statistically significant difference in mean values for AST, ALT, or INR for alcoholics given four grams per day of acetaminophen compared to placebo. Additionally, the researchers performed an analysis of the malnourished patients that showed there was no increase in AST or ALT levels in these patients. Study limitations include a limited duration of 2 days and exclusion of patients with preexisting AST or ALT elevations greater than 120 U/L. Study results do not preclude the possibility of an idiosyncratic hepatic reaction.

Renal: Based on available clinical data, acetaminophen can be used in patients with chronic renal disease without dosage adjustment. Martin found that patients with chronic renal failure had higher plasma concentrations of acetaminophen and the inactive glucuronide and sulfate metabolites than healthy subjects during repeated dosing up to ten days. Several single-dose studies demonstrate accumulation of acetaminophen metabolites in patients with moderate chronic renal failure and in anephric patients for whom hemodialysis appeared to be the major route of elimination.

The habitual consumption of acetaminophen should be discouraged. If indicated medically, the long-term use of acetaminophen should be supervised by a physician.

A National Kidney Foundation position paper notes that physicians preferentially recommend acetaminophen to patients with renal failure because of the bleeding complications associated with ASA in these individuals. Acetaminophen was recommended as the non-narcotic analgesic of choice for episodic use in patients with underlying renal disease.

Special Populations: Notwithstanding appropriate precautions, acetaminophen is a suitable analgesic choice for the majority of sub-populations at increased risk of adverse events from analgesic use. This includes asthmatics, elderly, patients taking multiple prescription drugs, patients taking anti-coagulants, patients who are breast-feeding, as well as patients who may suffer from chronic alcoholism, serious kidney or liver disease.

Results of well-designed clinical studies indicate that a dose reduction of acetaminophen, to avoid potential increased risk for toxicity, is not necessary for elderly adults, and obese adults. Additionally, the weight of existing evidence does not indicate the need to adjust dosage in chronic renal disease or chronic stable liver disease.

Geriatrics: Acetaminophen at currently recommended doses can be used safely by elderly patients. Results of well-designed clinical studies indicate that a dose reduction of acetaminophen, to avoid potential increased risk for toxicity, is not necessary. In a comprehensive metabolic study by Miners, the formation and clearance of glucuronide and glutathione conjugates were the same in young and elderly adults, although clearance of the sulphate conjugate and unchanged acetaminophen were reduced. This finding provides prospective scientific data that the amount of acetaminophen metabolized via the oxidative pathway, from which the highly reactive intermediate, NAPQI, is generated, does not increase with age. Recently, Bannwarth evaluated the multiple-dose pharmacokinetics of acetaminophen in elderly patients. After seven days of repeat dosing, acetaminophen did not accumulate in the plasma, and the elimination half-life was the same as that reported for young adults.

Elderly patients who require therapy for longer than 5 days should consult their physician for condition monitoring; however, no reduction in recommended dosage is necessary. The American Geriatrics Society Clinical Practice Guidelines for the Management of Chronic Pain in Older Persons recommend acetaminophen as the drug of choice for relieving mild to moderate musculoskeletal pain, with the maximum dosage not to exceed 4000 mg daily. Acetaminophen is safe for use in the elderly population as currently labeled.

Glucose-6-Phosphate Dehydrogenase (G6PD) Deficiency: In therapeutic doses, acetaminophen does not shorten the life-span of red blood cells and does not produce any clinically perceptible destruction of circulating red blood cells.

Obese Adults: Results of well-designed clinical studies indicate that a dose reduction of acetaminophen, to avoid potential increased risk for toxicity, is not necessary. O'Shea studied the pharmacokinetics of chlorzoxazone (a putative probe for CYP2E1 activity) to evaluate the effect of obesity on CYP2E1 activity. The authors concluded that CYP2E1 is induced in obese adults and that this could impact the metabolic pathway of a number of drugs metabolized by CYP2E1, including acetaminophen. However, acetaminophen pharmacokinetic data have been investigated in obese adults. In this prospective study, 650 mg acetaminophen was administered intravenously to obese men (297 lb), obese women (193 lb), control men (155 lb) and control women (121 lb). Acetaminophen distribution volume per total body weight was slightly lower in the obese adults but, more importantly, the half-life and metabolic clearance per total body weight did not differ among groups.

ADVERSE REACTIONS: Central Nervous System Effects: Acetaminophen at recommended doses has no obvious effects on central nervous system function. In an overdose situation, central nervous system effects are uncommon.

Gastrointestinal Effects: Acetaminophen at recommended doses does not cause gastric irritation, gastric erosions, occult or overt gastrointestinal blood loss or ulcers.

Blot and McLaughlin conducted an independent analysis of case-control data from a study conducted by the American College of Gastroenterology. The risk of gastrointestinal bleeding increased two to three-fold among recent users of ASA, ibuprofen and other NSAIDs at OTC doses, and the risk was also dose-related. In contrast, the use of acetaminophen was not associated with an increased risk of gastrointestinal bleeding.

Hematologic Effects: Acetaminophen does not have any immediate or delayed effects on small vessel hemostasis, as measured by bleeding time. In normal volunteers receiving a single dose of acetaminophen (975 or 1950 mg) or multiple doses of acetaminophen (1950 mg daily for 6 weeks), no change in bleeding time or platelet aggregation was observed. In another study, a single 1000 mg dose of acetaminophen was given to normal volunteers and did not affect bleeding time or platelet aggregation. Patients with hemophilia receiving multiple doses of acetaminophen showed no significant changes in bleeding time.

Haematological reactions including thrombocytopenia, leucopenia, pancytopenia, neutropenia, and agranulocytosis have been reported, although these are rare and causality has not been established.

Hepatic Effects: As an illustration of the margin of safety of acetaminophen at supratherapeutic doses, a comparison of serum concentrations of acetaminophen over time for a standard 15 mg/kg dose and for a dose exceeding the standard by a multiple of 5 (75 mg/kg) are shown in Figure 1. The serum concentrations are drawn relative to the risk line for hepatotoxicity and treatment line of the Rumack-Matthew nomogram used to manage acute overdoses. The mean plasma concentrations for this supratherapeutic dose are well below the risk and treatment lines of the nomogram at all times. However, to minimize the risk for adverse effects, the maximum recommended dose should not be exceeded.

Figure 1: TYLENOL

Mean Data for a Standard (1 g, 15 mg/kg) and Higher (5.6 g, 75 mg/kg) Dose Relative to Risk and Treatment Lines of the Acetaminophen Nomogram

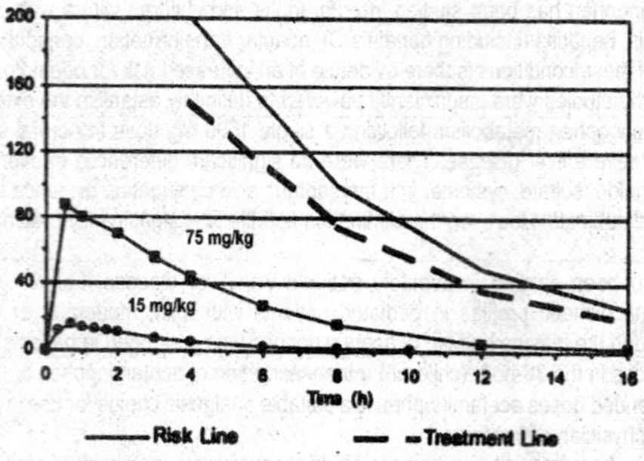

Acetaminophen in overdosage may cause hepatotoxicity. In adults and adolescents, hepatotoxicity may occur following ingestion of greater than 150 mg/kg over a period of 8 hours or less. Fatalities are infrequent (less than 3% to 4% of untreated cases in which blood levels exceed the treatment line) and have rarely been reported with overdoses less than 7.5 g. In children, amounts less than 150 mg/kg are unlikely to produce hepatotoxicity. In both adults and children, toxicity associated with acetaminophen is usually caused by ingestion of quantities of the drug that are significantly above the recommended dosage range. Hepatotoxicity, ranging from transient sharp transaminase elevations to fatal, fulminant hepatic failure, is the most common result of clinically significant overdosage.

In a double-blind, placebo-controlled clinical study, healthy adults were given 4, 6 and 8 g/day of acetaminophen over 3 days. Plasma concentrations did not accumulate with repeat doses. Clinically all doses were well tolerated by the subjects and aminotransferase values stayed within normal limits throughout the study. These data provide information related to the margin of safety but are not intended to support dosing beyond the maximum recommended dose of 4 g/day.

A report has suggested that hepatotoxicity following greater than the recommended dose of acetaminophen may be enhanced by both prolonged fasting and/or chronic alcohol abuse.

Acute Alcohol Use: Acute alcohol ingestion refers to the occasional or intermittent use of alcohol. When taken together, alcohol competes with acetaminophen for CYP2E1. CYP2E1 accepts alcohol more readily than acetaminophen; therefore, less NAPQI is produced. In the presence of alcohol, acetaminophen may be diverted to the glucuronidation and sulfation pathways. The overall result is that a smaller percentage of acetaminophen may be expected to be metabolized to the toxic intermediate, NAPQI, than would otherwise be the case. NAPQI production is increased above baseline for the period up to 18-24 hours post ethanol clearance from the body. In healthy adults, at normal labeled doses of acetaminophen, the temporary increase in NAPQI production is more than accommodated by normal glutathione stores in the liver.

Hypersensitivity: Sensitivity reactions are rare and may manifest as rash, urticaria, dyspnea, hypotension, laryngeal edema, angioedema, bronchospasm, or anaphylaxis. Cross-reactivity in ASA-sensitive persons has been rarely reported. If sensitivity is suspected, discontinue use of the drug.

Renal Effects: Acute nephrotoxicity has been reported following massive overdose either as a sequela of hepatic failure or, occasionally, in the absence of hepatic failure.

Clinical data have established that acetaminophen in recommended doses is not nephrotoxic.

Some studies suggest an association between the chronic long-term use of acetaminophen and renal effects. Results, however, are conflicting, limited by recall bias and confounded by the inability to determine whether analgesic use preceded or followed the onset of renal disease.

Case control studies have suggested a weak association between habitual acetaminophen use and prevalence of chronic renal failure and end stage renal disease. This National Kidney Foundation position paper concludes that acetaminophen has been preferentially recommended by physicians to patients with renal failure and that there is no evidence that occasional use of acetaminophen caused renal injury. In this position paper, acetaminophen was recommended as the non-narcotic analgesic of choice for episodic use in patients with underlying renal disease.

Special Populations: Pediatrics: Lesko and Mitchell enrolled more than 84 000 febrile children in a randomized, double blind, acetaminophen-controlled trial to assess the risks of rare but serious adverse events following use of pediatric ibuprofen. Of the children included in the analysis, 28 130 received acetaminophen and none experienced anaphylaxis, or serious hepatic, gastrointestinal or renal effects.

Pregnancy and Lactation: As with any drug, patients who are pregnant or nursing a baby should consult a physician before taking this product.

Pregnancy: Issues of risks in pregnancy are multifactorial. The information provided cannot be substituted for direct patient consultation. Acetaminophen is believed to be non-teratogenic in humans. However, existing studies have not assessed the effect of very high doses. The Motherisk Collaborative Perinatal project monitored 50 282 mother-child pairs, of which 226 had first trimester exposure to acetaminophen and 781 had used acetaminophen at any time during their pregnancy. No evidence was found to suggest a relationship between acetaminophen use and major or minor malformations. In a surveillance study of Michigan Medicaid recipients conducted between 1985 and 1992 involving 229 101 completed pregnancies, 9146 newborns had been exposed to acetaminophen during the first trimester. This data do not support an association between acetaminophen use and the occurrence of birth defects. Another cohort study, using prescription monitoring, found no excess risk for malformation, and no evidence that acetaminophen influenced fetal growth. Finally, as part of a larger study, 697 women used acetaminophen with or without codeine in their first trimester. No teratogenic risk was found.

A prospective study investigated the outcome of pregnancy in 300 women who had self-administered an overdose of acetaminophen, either alone, or as part of a combined preparation. Exposure to overdose occurred in all trimesters. The majority of the pregnancies had normal outcomes. The malformation rate was within the expected range. There was no obvious relationship between the time of exposure and the time of delivery. The overall conclusion was that acetaminophen overdose is not an indication for termination of pregnancy.

In a long-term developmental follow-up study, acetaminophen did not adversely affect IQ or behavior measures at four years of age. Height, weight and head circumference were also not affected by exposure to acetaminophen in-utero.

Unlike ASA, which has been shown to profoundly effect platelet function, there does not seem to be a risk of hemorrhage associated with acetaminophen use at term.

Currently there is no evidence to suggest that acetaminophen is teratogenic when used as recommended. However, data for continuous high daily doses are not sufficient, and safety during pregnancy has not yet been established.

Lactation: Following a typical therapeutic dose, acetaminophen is excreted in breast milk in very low concentrations. Based on a number of published reports, infant exposure levels are at most 4.5% of a weight adjusted pediatric therapeutic dose. In addition, acetaminophen is considered compatible with breast-feeding by the American Academy of Pediatrics.

DRUG INTERACTIONS: Alcohol: Studies evaluating the metabolism of doses up to 20 mg/kg of acetaminophen in chronic alcohol abusers and a study evaluating the effects of 2 days of acetaminophen dosing at 4000 mg/day in chronic alcoholics undergoing detoxification, have yielded inconsistent results with regard to effects on acetaminophen pharmacokinetics and demonstrate no evidence of adverse effect on liver function tests.

Anticoagulants–Oral: Patients who concomitantly medicate with warfarin-type anticoagulants and regular doses of acetaminophen have occasionally been reported to have unforeseen elevations in their INR. Physicians should be cognizant of this potential interaction and monitor the INR in such patients closely while therapy is established. Many factors, including diet, medications, and environmental and physical states, may affect how a patient responds to anticoagulant therapy. There have been several reports that suggest that acetaminophen may produce hypoprothrombinemia (elevated international normalized ratio [INR] or prothrombin time) when administered with coumarin derivatives. In other studies, prothrombin time did not change. Reported changes have been generally of limited clinical significance, however, periodic evaluation of prothrombin time should be performed when these agents are administered concurrently.

In the period immediately following discharge from the hospital or whenever other medications are initiated, discontinued, or taken regularly, it is important to monitor patient response to anticoagulation therapy with additional prothrombin time or INR determinations. Despite the potential for interaction, acetaminophen is the least likely OTC analgesic to interfere with anticoagulant therapy and thereby remains the OTC analgesic of choice for concomitant use.

Anticonvulsants: Some reports have suggested that patients taking long-term anticonvulsants, who overdose on acetaminophen, may be at increased risk of hepatotoxicity because of accelerated metabolism of acetaminophen. Available data are conflicting. A 7-year retrospective study of acetaminophen overdose admissions indicates that the overall mortality rate was not significantly different for patients taking concomitant anticonvulsant medications.

Hydantoins: At usual oral therapeutic doses of acetaminophen and hydantoins, no special dosage adjustment or monitoring is generally required. Pharmacokinetic studies indicate that phenytoin primarily induces the glucuronidation pathway, whereas glutathione-derived metabolites are not increased in patients on chronic phenytoin therapy. Additionally, recent data demonstrate that phenytoin is metabolized primarily by CYP2C9 and CYP2C19, whereas acetaminophen is primarily metabolized by CYP2E1. These data indicate that there is no increased risk of acetaminophen hepatotoxicity in patients on chronic hydantoin therapy who use the recommended dose of acetaminophen.

Carbamazepine: At usual oral therapeutic doses of acetaminophen and carbamazepine, no special dosage adjustment is generally required. Carbamazepine is primarily metabolized by CYP3A4, whereas acetaminophen is metabolized primarily via CYP2E1. It is not known whether there is increased risk from an acetaminophen overdose in patients on chronic carbamazepine therapy.

Diflunisal: Professional literature from the manufacturer of diflunisal cautions that concomitant administration with acetaminophen produces an approximate 50% increase in plasma levels of acetaminophen in normal volunteers. Acetaminophen had no effect on diflunisal plasma levels. The clinical significance of these findings has not been established. However, caution should be used with concomitant administration of diflunisal and acetaminophen and patients should be monitored carefully.

Isoniazid: Some reports suggest that patients on chronic isoniazid therapy may be at risk for developing hepatotoxicity from an acetaminophen overdose. Since patients on isoniazid therapy may develop hepatic effects from isoniazid alone, data from individual case reports are unclear as to whether chronic administration of isoniazid may increase the risk of acetaminophen toxicity. Isoniazid is primarily metabolized by CYP2E1 and induces CYP2E1. Studies in healthy subjects demonstrate that isoniazid blocks the formation of the toxic metabolite NAPQI when administered concomitantly with acetaminophen, but increase NAPQI formation when acetaminophen is administered one day after discontinuation of isoniazid. Thus, concomitant use of isoniazid is unlikely to potentiate the risk of acetaminophen-induced hepatotoxicity at recommended doses. The isoniazid induction of CYP2E1 is short-lived, lasting only 12 to 48 hours after the discontinuation of isoniazid, it is during this period the toxicity of an acetaminophen overdose may be potentiated.

DOSAGE AND ADMINISTRATION: Immediate Release: Adults and children over 12 years of age: 500 to 1000 mg every 4 to 6 hours, as required, not to exceed 4000 mg acetaminophen in 24 hours. Doses may be administered with or without food.

Children: 10 to 15 mg/kg every 4 to 6 hours, as required, not to exceed 75 mg/kg/24 hours and never to exceed the maximum adult daily dose of 4000 mg of acetaminophen. Alternatively, the following single doses (see Table 1) may be given every 4 to 6 hours not to exceed 5 doses in 24 hours. Doses may be given with or without food (i.e. milk, formula, juices, etc.).

Sustained Release: TYLENOL ARTHRITIS PAIN Extended Release Tablets: Adults and children over 12 years of age: 2 sustained release caplets (1300 mg) every 8 hours, not to exceed 6 caplets (4000 mg) in 24 hours. Swallow each caplet whole with water on an empty stomach. Do not crush, chew or dissolve the caplet.

TYLENOL Muscle Aches and Body Pain Extended Release Tablets: Adults and children over 12 years of age: 2 sustained release caplets (1300 mg) every 8 hours, not to exceed 6 caplets (4000 mg) in 24 hours. Swallow each caplet whole with water on an empty stomach. Do not crush, chew or dissolve the caplet.

OVERDOSAGE:

Symptoms and Treatment: Acetaminophen: Typical Toxidrome: Hepatic injury is the principal toxic effect of a substantial acetaminophen overdose. The physician should be mindful that there is no early presentation that is pathognomic for the overdose. A high degree of clinical suspicion must always be maintained.

Untreated acetaminophen overdoses may produce hepatotoxicity. Acetaminophen hepatotoxicity occurs as a threshold effect and is characterized by a lack of toxicity at lower/therapeutic doses. Acetaminophen hepatotoxicity occurs after major depletion of glutathione, an endogenous detoxifying substance. Once the threshold is exceeded, increasing acetaminophen doses may produce increasing degrees of hepatotoxicity, unless N-acetylcysteine (NAC) is administered. Situations in which acetaminophen overdose and resultant hepatotoxicity may occur include acute intentional overdose and repeated supratherapeutic overdose in adults and acute accidental ingestion or overdose and repeated supratherapeutic overdose in children.

The clinical course of acetaminophen overdose generally occurs in a three-phase sequential pattern. The first phase begins shortly after ingestion and lasts for 12 to 24 hours. The patient may manifest signs of gastrointestinal irritability, nausea, vomiting, anorexia, diaphoresis, pallor and general malaise. If toxicity continues, there is a latent phase of up to 48 hours. During this second phase, initial symptoms abate and the patient may feel better. However, hepatic enzymes, bilirubin, and prothrombin time or INR values will progressively rise. Right upper quadrant pain may develop as the liver becomes enlarged and tender. Most patients do not progress beyond this phase, especially if given N-acetylcysteine (NAC) treatment early in the course. Signs and symptoms of the third phase depend on the severity of hepatic damage and usually occur from three to five days following overdose ingestion. Symptoms may be limited to anorexia, nausea, general malaise, and abdominal pain in less severe cases or may progress to confusion, stupor and sequelae of hepatic necrosis including jaundice, coagulation defects, hypoglycemia, and encephalopathy, as well as renal failure and cardiomyopathy. Death, if it occurs, is generally the result of complications associated with fulminant hepatic failure. Mortality rates in patients with toxic plasma levels who do not receive antidote therapy range from 3% to 4%.

Due to the wide availability of acetaminophen, it is commonly involved in single and mixed drug overdose situations and the practitioner should screen for its presence in a patient's serum. Acute toxicity after single dose overdoses of acetaminophen can be anticipated when the overdose exceeds 150 mg/kg. Chronic alcohol abusers, cachectic individuals, and persons taking pharmacologic inducers of the hepatic P450 microsomal enzyme system may be at risk with lower exposures.

Specific Antidote: Any individual presenting with a possible acetaminophen overdose should be treated with N-acetylcysteine (NAC), even if the amount of acetaminophen ingested is unknown or questionable. A blood sample for determination of the plasma acetaminophen concentration should be obtained as early as possible, but no sooner than four hours following ingestion. Do not await the results of assays for plasma acetaminophen levels before initiating treatment NAC. If the acetaminophen plasma level is found to plot above the treatment line on the acetaminophen overdose nomogram, NAC treatment should be continued for a full course of therapy. NAC is used clinically to treat acute acetaminophen overdose, and acts by interacting with the oxidative intermediate, NAPQI. NAC administered by either the i.v. or the oral route is known to be a highly effective antidote for acetaminophen poisoning. It is most effective when administered within 8 hours of a significant overdose but reports have indicated benefits to treatment initiated well beyond this time period. It is imperative to administer the antidote as early as possible in the time course of acute intoxication to reap the full benefits of the antidote's protective effects. For full prescribing information, consult the product monograph for NAC.

General Management: When the possibility of acetaminophen overdose exists, treatment should begin immediately and include appropriate decontamination of the gastrointestinal tract, proper supportive care, careful assessment of appropriately timed serum acetaminophen estimations evaluated against the Rumack-Matthew nomogram, timely administration of NAC as required and appropriate follow-up care. Liver function tests should be performed initially and repeated at 24-hour intervals.

Table 1: TYLENOL

Dosage in Children

Weight (kg)	Age Group	Single Dose (mg)	Concentration of Available Products			
2.5–5.4	0–3 mos[a]	40	Infants' Suspension Drops (80 mg/mL)			
5.5–7.9	4–11 mos	80			Children's Suspension Liquid (160 mg/5 mL)	
8–10.9	12–23 mos	120				
11–15.9	2–3 yrs	160		Children's Tablets[b] (80 mg/tablet)		Junior Strength Tablets[b] (160 mg/tablet)
16–21.9	4–5 yrs	240				
22–26.9	6–8 yrs	320				
27–31.9	9–10 yrs	400				
32–43.9	11–12 yrs	480				

[a] Consumer labeling for Infants' and Children's TYLENOL acetaminophen does not offer dosing information for children less than 4 months of age; therefore, this dose is provided as a guideline for professional recommendations to the consumer. Note: Data not available to define appropriate adjustments, if any, needed for the immediate neonatal period. Use of antipyretics in the immediate neonatal period is extremely limited.

[b] TYLENOL solid dosage forms may not be appropriate for children under 2 years of age.

Overdose During Pregnancy: Acetaminophen is one of the most common overdoses in pregnancy. Hepatic toxicity of acetaminophen follows the formation of the highly reactive metabolite N-acetyl-p-benzoquinoneimine produced by acetaminophen metabolism through the cytochrome P450 mixed-function oxidase system. Hepatic failure can be prevented by timely administration of NAC either orally for 72 hours, or intravenously (IV) for 20 hours.

Acetaminophen crosses the human placenta though the fetus is theoretically at risk when maternal overdose of acetaminophen occurs. Acetaminophen can be transformed to its toxic metabolite since the oxidative capacity of fetal microsomes is present in the fetus by 14 weeks gestation.

Studies on placental transfer of NAC in rats and sheep yielded conflicting results. Placental transfer of N-acetylcysteine in humans was demonstrated in 4 women treated with NAC for acetaminophen overdose during labour. NAC blood levels in the fetuses were within the range associated with therapeutic doses of NAC administered to adults with acetaminophen poisoning.

Fetal toxicity and stillbirth after a large (e.g. 30 g) acetaminophen overdose has been reported, but others observed a normal outcome for the offspring after acetaminophen overdose in pregnancy. A large case series investigated the pregnancy outcome in 300 women who had overdosed with acetaminophen. In this group, 118 cases occurred in the first trimester, 103 in the second trimester and 79 in the third trimester. Forty-nine of these mothers were treated with specific antidotes (33 with NAC and 16 with methionine). There were 219 live-born infants, 11 have malformations (including minor); none had been exposed to acetaminophen during the first trimester. Nine women were treated with NAC during the first trimester; there were two elective terminations; two spontaneous abortions, and five healthy babies in this group.

In summary, acetaminophen overdose during pregnancy should be treated according to regular protocols in order to prevent maternal and potentially fetal toxicity. Unless severe maternal toxicity develops, an acetaminophen overdose does not increase the risk for birth defects or adverse pregnancy outcomes.

Physicians unfamiliar with the current management of acetaminophen overdose should consult with a Poison Control Centre immediately. Telephone numbers for local Poison Control Centres are available in the local phone directory. Delays in initiation of appropriate therapy may jeopardize the patient's chances for full recovery.

For management of a suspected drug overdose, CPhA recommends that you contact your **regional Poison Control Centre**. See the *CPS* Directory section for a list of Poison Control Centres.

ACTION AND CLINICAL PHARMACOLOGY: Mechanism of Action: Acetaminophen is a centrally acting analgesic and antipyretic drug. Although the precise mechanism of action is not totally understood, work by Boutaud suggests acetaminophen is an inhibitor of the peroxidase portion of cyclooxygenase (prostaglandin H synthase inhibitor). Depending on the redox state and substrate concentrations surrounding the enzymes, acetaminophen may or may not have a significant inhibitory effect. This accounts for its selective activity on pain and fever with little anti-inflammatory effect.

It is postulated that the analgesic effect is produced by elevation of the pain threshold and the antipyretic effect is produced through action on the hypothalamic heat-regulating centre.

The optimal effective analgesic dose of acetaminophen was demonstrated in dental pain studies and is 1000 mg every four to six hours, up to 4000 mg daily. At least 500 published and unpublished controlled clinical trials in adults and children have evaluated acetaminophen for the relief of pain or fever. These studies include single and multiple dose treatments. Most studies were less than 14 days in duration, although the longest study duration was two years. No significant safety issues were reported in any of these studies.

Moreover, at recommended doses, acetaminophen has not been shown to increase the risk of developing renal diseases or upper gastrointestinal ulceration/bleeding. This observation is consistent with its minimal inhibitory effect on peripheral prostaglandin synthesis and on gastric prostaglandin synthesis.

Acetaminophen is considered equipotent to ASA and ibuprofen, within the recommended OTC dosing ranges, in its analgesic and antipyretic effects. Acetaminophen at recommended doses does not cause the type of gastrointestinal complications associated with NSAID-containing products, such as gastric irritation, gastric erosions, occult or overt gastrointestinal blood loss, or ulcers. Unlike these drugs, however, it has no anti-inflammatory effect at clinically relevant doses in humans.

Pharmacokinetics: Absorption: Oral acetaminophen is rapidly and almost completely absorbed from the gastrointestinal tract primarily in the small intestine. This absorption process occurs by passive transport. Peak plasma concentrations occur within 0.4 to 1 hour depending on the product formulation. Although high-fat foods delay the time to peak concentration for up to an hour, the dose is completely absorbed.

Distribution: Acetaminophen is uniformly distributed throughout most body fluids, but not in fatty tissue. As a result, the volume of distribution in adults ranges between 0.8 and 1.0 L/kg. Since acetaminophen has low protein binding in plasma of only 10% to 25%, it does not compete with drugs that are highly protein bound.

Metabolism: Acetaminophen is primarily metabolized by the liver via three principal separate pathways: conjugation with glucuronide; conjugation with sulfate; oxidation via the cytochrome P450 mixed function oxidase system.

Both the glucuronic and oxidative pathways adhere to a first-order rate process, which means the concentration of acetaminophen metabolized increases as the concentration in the liver increases. The sulfate pathway adheres to Michaelis-Menten kinetics, which means the concentration of acetaminophen metabolized remains constant once the concentration in the liver increases above a saturation level. A schematic of acetaminophen metabolism is shown in Figure 2.

The major metabolic pathway is glucuronidation, where 47% to 62% of the acetaminophen dose conjugates with glucuronide. These glucuronide conjugates are inactive and nontoxic, and are secreted in bile and eliminated in the urine.

The second major pathway is sulfation, where 25% to 36% of the dose conjugates with sulfate. These sulfate ester conjugates are also inactive and nontoxic and are excreted in the urine.

The third pathway is oxidation, where 5% to 8% of the dose is metabolized via the cytochrome P450 enzyme system. The cytochrome P450 isoenzyme that is primarily responsible is CYP2E1. When acetaminophen is metabolized by CYP2E1, it forms a highly reactive intermediate, N-acetyl-p-benzoquinoneimine (NAPQI). Since NAPQI is highly reactive, it cannot be measured outside the liver nor can it accumulate. This intermediate is rapidly inactivated by hepatocellular stores of glutathione to form cysteine and mercapturic conjugates, which are both inactive and nontoxic. These conjugates are excreted in the urine.

* Container provided with a child-resistant closure.

† Easy-to-Open.

Figure 2: TYLENOL

Acetaminophen Metabolism

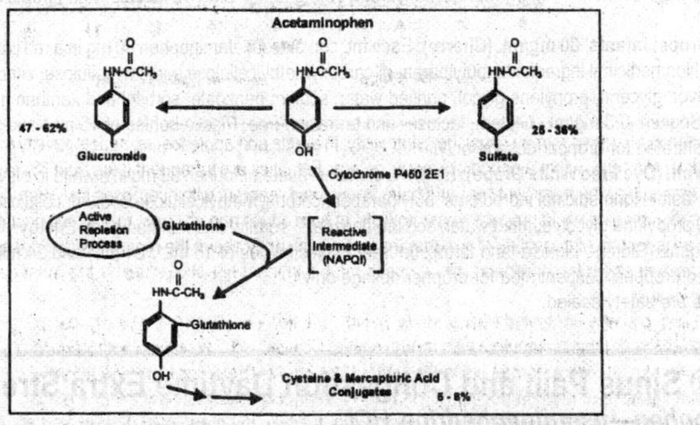

Excretion: Acetaminophen undergoes first-order elimination from the body, and has a short plasma half-life that ranges from 2 to 3 hours in healthy young and elderly adults and from 1.5 to 2.9 hours in children. Since acetaminophen clears rapidly from the body, repeated doses do not lead to accumulation of acetaminophen plasma concentrations.

STORAGE AND STABILITY: Store at room temperature (15 to 30°C). Extra Strength TYLENOL Gelcaps "Rapid Release" should additionally be protected from high heat and humidity.

DOSAGE FORMS, COMPOSITION AND PACKAGING: Adults: Caplets: Regular Strength 325 mg: Each elongated, capsule-shaped white tablet, engraved "TYLENOL" on one side and "325" on the other side, contains: acetaminophen 325 mg. Nonmedicinal ingredients: cellulose, cornstarch, hypromellose, magnesium stearate, polyethylene glycol and sodium starch glycolate. Energy: 0.7 kJ (0.2 kcal). Sodium: 0.3 mg. Gluten-, lactose- and tartrazine-free. Plastic bottles of 24*, 50*, 100* and 200†.

Extra Strength 500 mg: Each elongated, capsule-shaped white tablet, engraved "TYLENOL" on one side and "500" on the other side, contains: acetaminophen 500 mg. Nonmedicinal ingredients: cellulose, cornstarch, hypromellose, magnesium stearate, polyethylene glycol and sodium starch glycolate. Energy: 1.1 kJ (0.3 kcal). Sodium: 0.4 mg. Gluten-, lactose- and tartrazine-free. Vials of 10* and plastic bottles of 24*, 50*, 100* and 150†.

Gelcaps: Extra Strength 500 mg ("Rapid Release"): Each solid, capsule-shaped tablet, coated with red gelatin on one end, blue gelatin on the other end, a gray band between the two gelatin-coated ends, printed "TY" on one gelatin-coated end and "500" on the other gelatin-coated end, contains: acetaminophen 500 mg. Nonmedicinal ingredients: butylparaben, carboxymethylcellulose sodium, cellulose, cornstarch, D&C Yellow no. 10, edetate calcium disodium, FD&C Blue no. 1, FD&C Red no. 40, gelatin, hypromellose, iron oxide black, iron oxide red, iron oxide yellow, magnesium stearate, methylparaben, polyethylene glycol, polysorbate 80, propylparaben, sodium lauryl sulfate, sodium propionate, sodium starch glycolate and titanium dioxide. Energy: 1.2 kJ (0.3 kcal). Sodium: 0.8 mg. Gluten-, lactose- and tartrazine-free. Bottles of 20*, 40* and 80*.

Extended Release: ARTHRITIS PAIN Extended Release Tablet 650 mg: Each elongated, bilayer yellow and white, extended release tablet, engraved "TYLENOL ART" on one side, contains: acetaminophen 650 mg (325 mg immediate release acetaminophen and 325 mg delayed release acetaminophen in a slow dissolving matrix). Nonmedicinal ingredients: carnauba wax, cellulose, cornstarch, D&C Yellow no. 10, FD&C Yellow no. 6, hydroxyethyl cellulose, hypromellose, magnesium stearate, povidone, sodium starch glycolate and triacetin. Energy: 0.7 kJ (0.2 kcal). Sodium: 0.3 mg. Gluten-, lactose- and tartrazine-free. Bottles of 24*, 50* and 100†.

Muscle Aches & Body Pain 650 mg: Each elongated, white, extended release tablet, engraved "TYLENOL ER" on one side, contains: acetaminophen 650 mg (325 mg immediate release acetaminophen and 325 mg delayed release acetaminophen in a slow dissolving matrix). Nonmedicinal ingredients: carnauba wax, cellulose, cornstarch, hydroxyethyl cellulose, hypromellose, magnesium stearate, povidone, sodium starch glycolate, titanium dioxide and triacetin. Energy: 0.7 kJ (0.2 kcal). Sodium: 0.3 mg. Gluten-, lactose- and tartrazine-free. Bottles of 16* and 72.

Tablets: Regular Strength 325 mg: Each round, white tablet, engraved "TYLENOL" on one side and "325" on the other side, contains: acetaminophen 325 mg. Nonmedicinal ingredients: cellulose, cornstarch, magnesium stearate and sodium starch glycolate. Energy: 0.7 kJ (0.2 kcal). Sodium: 0.3 mg. Gluten-, lactose- and tartrazine-free. Vials of 12* and plastic bottles of 24*, 50* and 100.

Extra Strength 500 mg ("eZ TABS"): Each round, red, sweet-coated tablet, printed with "TYLENOL 500", contains: acetaminophen 500 mg. Nonmedicinal ingredients: carnauba wax, cellulose, cornstarch, FD&C Red no. 40, FD&C Yellow no. 6, hypromellose, iron oxide black, polyethylene glycol, polysorbate 80, povidone, sodium starch glycolate, stearic acid, sucralose and titanium dioxide. Energy: 1.1 kJ (0.3 kcal). Sodium: 0.4 mg. Gluten-, lactose- and tartrazine-free. Plastic bottles of 24*, 50, 100*, 150† and 200. See next entry for vials.

Extra Strength 500 mg ("eZ TABS"): Each round, red, sweet-coated tablet, printed "TYLENOL 500", contains: acetaminophen 500 mg. Nonmedicinal ingredients: carnauba wax, cellulose, corn starch, FD&C Red no. 40, FD&C Yellow no. 6, hypromellose, iron oxide black, magnesium stearate, polyethylene glycol, polysorbate 80, propylene glycol, sodium starch glycolate, sucralose and titanium dioxide. Energy: 1.1 kJ (0.3 kcal). Sodium: 0.4 mg. Gluten-, lactose- and tartrazine-free. Vials of 10*.

Children's: Tablets: Junior Strength 160 mg ("Meltaways" Bubblegum Burst): Each pink, 5/8" round troche tablet with characteristic bubblegum odor, debossed with "TY" over "160" on one side, contains: acetaminophen 160 mg. Nonmedicinal ingredients: cellulose acetate, citric acid, D&C Red no. 7, dextrose, flavor, magnesium stearate, povidone and sucralose. Energy: 15.4 kJ (3.7 kcal). Sodium: 0 mg. Gluten-, lactose- and tartrazine-free. Bottles of 20*.

Junior Strength 160 mg ("Meltaways" Grape Punch): Each purple, 5/8" round troche tablet with characteristic grape odor, debossed with "TY" over "160" on one side, contains: acetaminophen 160 mg. Nonmedicinal ingredients: cellulose acetate, citric acid, D&C Red no. 7, D&C Red no. 30, dextrose, FD&C Blue no. 1, flavor, magnesium stearate, povidone and sucralose. Energy: 15.4 kJ (3.7 kcal). Sodium: 0 mg. Gluten-, lactose- and tartrazine-free. Bottles of 20*.

Children's 80 mg ("Meltaways" Bubblegum Burst): Each pink, ½" round troche tablet with characteristic bubble gum odor, debossed with "TY" over "80" on one side, contains: acetaminophen 80 mg. Nonmedicinal ingredients: cellulose acetate, citric acid, D&C Red no. 7, dextrose, flavor, magnesium stearate, povidone and sucralose. Energy: 9.8 kJ (2.3 kcal). Sodium: 0 mg. Gluten-, lactose- and tartrazine-free. Plastic bottles of 24*.
Children's 80 mg ("Meltaways" Grape Punch): Each purple, ½" round troche tablet with characteristic grape odor, debossed with "TY" over "80" on one side, contains: acetaminophen 80 mg. Nonmedicinal ingredients: cellulose acetate, citric acid, D&C Red no. 7, D&C Red no. 30, dextrose, FD&C Blue no. 1, flavor, magnesium stearate, povidone and sucralose. Energy: 9.8 kJ (2.3 kcal). Sodium: 0 mg. Gluten-, lactose- and tartrazine-free. Plastic bottles of 24* and 50* (for institutional use only).
Suspension: Children's 160 mg/5 mL (Banana Berry Twist): Each 5 mL contains: acetaminophen 160 mg in a pink liquid vehicle with a strawberry-banana flavored taste. Nonmedicinal ingredients: butylparaben, carboxymethylcellulose sodium, cellulose, citric acid, corn syrup, FD&C Red no. 40, flavor, glycerin, propylene glycol, purified water, sodium benzoate, sorbitol and xanthan gum. Energy: 76.6 kJ/5 mL (18.3 kcal/5 mL). Sodium: 1.6 mg/5 mL. Gluten-, lactose- and tartrazine-free. Plastic bottles 100 mL*.
Children's 160 mg/5 mL (Bubblegum Burst): Each 5 mL contains: acetaminophen 160 mg in a dark pink liquid vehicle with a bubble gum-flavored taste. Nonmedicinal ingredients: butylparaben, carboxymethylcellulose sodium, cellulose, citric acid, corn syrup, D&C Red no. 33, FD&C Red no. 40, flavor, glycerin, propylene glycol, purified water, sodium benzoate, sorbitol and xanthan gum. Energy: 76.6 kJ/5 mL (18.3 kcal/5 mL). Sodium: 1.6 mg/5 mL. Gluten-, lactose- and tartrazine-free. Plastic bottles of 24* and 100 mL*.
Children's 160 mg/5 mL (Grape Punch): Each 5 mL contains: acetaminophen 160 mg in a purple liquid vehicle with a grape-flavored taste. Nonmedicinal ingredients: butylparaben, carboxymethylcellulose sodium, cellulose, citric acid, corn syrup, D&C Red no. 33, FD&C Blue no. 1, flavor, glycerin, propylene glycol, purified water, sodium benzoate, sorbitol and xanthan gum. Energy: 76.6 kJ/5 mL (18.3 kcal/5 mL). Sodium: 1.6 mg/5 mL. Gluten-, lactose- and tartrazine-free. Plastic bottles of 100 mL*.
Children's 160 mg/5 mL (Dye-Free Cherry): Each 5 mL contains: acetaminophen 160 mg in a pink liquid vehicle with a grape-flavored taste. Nonmedicinal ingredients: butylparaben, carboxymethylcellulose sodium, cellulose, flavors, glycerin, propylene glycol, propylparaben, purified water, sodium citrate, sorbitol, sucralose, sucrose and xanthan gum. Energy: 54 kJ/5 mL (12.9 kcal/5 mL). Sodium: <1 mg/5 mL. Carbohydrates: 3.5 g/5 mL. Gluten-, lactose- and tartrazine-free. Plastic bottles of 100 mL*.
Children's 160 mg/5 mL (Dye-Soothing Berry): Each 5 mL contains: acetaminophen 160 mg in a pink liquid vehicle with a grape-flavored taste. Nonmedicinal ingredients: butylparaben, carboxymethylcellulose sodium, cellulose, citric acid, flavors, glycerin, propylene glycol, propylparaben, purified water, sorbitol, sucralose powder, sucrose and xanthan gum. Energy: 54 kJ/5 mL (12.9 kcal/5 mL). Sodium: <1 mg/5 mL. Carbohydrates: 3.5 g/5 mL. Gluten-, lactose- and tartrazine-free. Plastic bottles of 100 mL*.
Suspension Drops: Infants' 80 mg/mL (Cherry): Each mL contains: acetaminophen 80 mg in a red liquid vehicle with a cherry-flavored taste. Nonmedicinal ingredients: butylparaben, carboxymethylcellulose sodium, cellulose, citric acid, corn syrup, FD&C Red no. 40, flavor, glycerin, propylene glycol, purified water, sodium benzoate, sorbitol and xanthan gum. Energy: 14.6 kJ/mL (3.5 kcal/mL). Sodium: 0.3 mg/mL. Gluten-, lactose- and tartrazine-free. Plastic bottles of 15 mL* and 24 mL* with a calibrated dropper. Concentrated for dropper dosage only.
Infants' 80 mg/mL (Dye Free White Grape): Each mL contains: acetaminophen 80 mg in a white to off-white liquid vehicle with a grape-flavored taste. Nonmedicinal ingredients: butylparaben, carboxymethylcellulose sodium, cellulose, citric acid, corn syrup, flavor, glycerin, propylene glycol, purified water, sodium benzoate, sorbitol and xanthan gum. Energy: 14.6 kJ/mL (3.5 kcal/mL). Sodium: 0.3 mg/mL. Gluten-, lactose- and tartrazine-free. Plastic bottles of 15 mL*, 24 mL* and 24 mL* (institutional use only) with a calibrated dropper. Concentrated for dropper dosage only.

All packages are safety sealed.

Tylenol® Sinus Pain and Congestion Daytime Extra Strength
acetaminophen—pseudoephedrine HCl
Analgesic—Decongestant

McNeil Consumer Healthcare

Tylenol® Sinus Pain and Congestion Nighttime Extra Strength
acetaminophen—pseudoephedrine HCl—chlorpheniramine maleate
Analgesic—Decongestant—Antihistamine

McNeil Consumer Healthcare

SUMMARY PRODUCT INFORMATION:

Route of Administration	Dosage Form/ Strength	Clinically Relevant Nonmedicinal Ingredients
Oral	Extra Strength Daytime Caplet/ 500 mg acetaminophen and 30 mg pseudoephedrine HCl	Gluten-, lactose- and tartrazine-free For a complete listing of nonmedicinal ingredients, see Dosage Forms, Composition and Packaging.
	Extra Strength Nighttime Caplet/ 500 mg acetaminophen, 30 mg pseudoephedrine HCl and 2 mg chlorpheniramine maleate	Gluten-, lactose- and tartrazine-free For a complete listing of nonmedicinal ingredients, see Dosage Forms, Composition and Packaging.

INDICATIONS AND CLINICAL USE: Extra Strength TYLENOL Sinus Pain and Congestion Daytime: A non-drowsy formulation for the temporary relief of sinus headache and sinus congestion caused by sinusitis and common colds.
Extra Strength TYLENOL Sinus Pain & Congestion Nighttime: For the temporary relief of sinus congestion, pain and pressure, headache, nasal congestion, runny nose and sneezing caused by sinusitis and common colds.
CONTRAINDICATIONS: Hypersensitivity to acetaminophen, pressor amines or to the ingredients of this formulation (see Dosage Forms, Composition and Packaging). Allergic reactions (primarily skin rash) or reports of hypersensitivity secondary to acetaminophen are rare and generally are controlled by discontinuation of the drug and, when necessary, symptomatic treatment.

In patients receiving or having received MAO inhibitors in the preceding 2 weeks. Although pseudoephedrine is virtually without pressor effect in normotensive patients, it should be used with caution in hypertensives.
WARNINGS AND PRECAUTIONS: General: Consumers should not exceed 4 g/day of acetaminophen or use two or more acetaminophen-containing products together. This includes combination products that contain acetaminophen. Do not use with other products containing salicylates or any other pain or fever medicine.

Acetaminophen-containing products should be kept out of the reach of children.

Physicians should be cognizant of and supervise the use of acetaminophen in patients with chronic alcoholism, serious kidney or serious liver disease. Physicians should alert their patients who regularly consume large amounts of alcohol not to exceed the recommended doses of acetaminophen. Chronic heavy alcohol abusers may be at increased risk of liver toxicity from excessive doses of acetaminophen.

Patients should be counseled to consult a physician if redness or swelling is present in an area of pain, if symptoms do not improve or if they worsen, or if new symptoms such as high fever, rash, itching or persistent headache occur, as these may be signs of a condition which requires medical attention.

Acetaminophen should not be taken for pain for more than 5 days or if new symptoms appear, without consulting a physician.

In patients with high blood pressure, heart disease, diabetes, thyroid disease, difficulty in urination due to enlargement of the prostate gland or who are taking a prescription drug for high blood pressure or depression, pseudoephedrine HCl should be used with caution and only under close medical supervision.

Patients with asthma, glaucoma, emphysema, chronic pulmonary disease or shortness of breath should not use this medication unless directed by a physician.
Occupational Hazards: Preparations containing chlorpheniramine maleate may cause drowsiness. Alcoholic beverages, sedatives and tranquilizers may increase this effect and should be avoided. Advise caution when driving a motor vehicle or operating machinery or engaging in any activity requiring alertness. Patients taking tranquilizers or sedatives should not take this medication before consulting a physician.

Hepatic/Biliary/Pancreatic: Slower metabolism of acetaminophen, increased activity of the cytochrome P450 enzyme system, or depleted glutathione stores are cited as theoretical risk factors for acetaminophen hepatotoxicity in patients with chronic liver disease. However, acetaminophen has been studied in both adults and children with a wide variety of liver diseases including various types of cirrhosis, hepatitis (including hepatitis C), nodular transformation, congenital hepatic fibrosis, and α1-antitrypsin deficiency. In none of these conditions is there evidence of an increased risk for hepatotoxicity at currently recommended acetaminophen doses but the studies were insufficiently powered to definitely establish the extent of risk.

Forrest compared acetaminophen metabolism following a single 1500 mg dose in normal subjects, patients with mild liver disease, and patients with severe liver disease. There were no significant differences in overall 24-hour urinary excretion of acetaminophen and glucuronide, sulfate, cysteine, and mercapturic acid conjugates, evidence that acetaminophen metabolism was similar to that in normal subjects. However, the elimination half-life was significantly prolonged in patients with severe liver disease.

Acetaminophen has also been studied in pediatric patients with liver disease. Following a single (10 mg/kg) dose of acetaminophen, the pharmacokinetic profiles in pediatric patients with mild, moderate, or severe liver disease were not significantly different. Although the plasma half-life of acetaminophen was prolonged in patients with severe liver disease, there were no significant differences in the 36-hour (children) urinary excretion of acetaminophen or its conjugates.

Acetaminophen may cause hepatotoxicity in situations of intentional overdose (e.g. attempted suicide), unintentional overdose (e.g. overdosing when pain relief is not satisfactory), simultaneous use of multiple acetaminophen-containing preparations, accidental overdose or in very rare cases, after recommended doses, although causality has not been determined. The hepatotoxic reaction can be severe and life-threatening. Early symptoms following a hepatotoxic overdose may include nausea, vomiting, diaphoresis, lethargy, and general malaise. If appropriate treatment is not instituted, these may progress to upper quadrant pain, confusion, stupor, and sequelae of hepatic necrosis, such as jaundice, coagulation defects, hypoglycemia, and encephalopathy. Renal failure and cardiomyopathy may also occur. In the event of known or suspected overdosage, treatment with N-acetyl cysteine should be instituted immediately (see Overdosage), even when there are no obvious symptoms. Failure to promptly treat acetaminophen hepatotoxicity with N-acetyl cysteine can result in liver failure, leading to liver transplantation and/or death.
Chronic Alcohol Use: Excessive alcohol use may increase risk of liver toxicity from acetaminophen overdose (acute or chronic).

In prospective, placebo controlled studies, researchers evaluated an actively drinking group of alcoholics with a high prevalence of malnourishment. The study participants abruptly stopped their daily alcohol intake and took acetaminophen the next day. This should theoretically make them vulnerable to acetaminophen injury because their CYP2E1 would be maximally induced from the alcohol and there would be no alcohol present to compete with acetaminophen for metabolism by CYP2E1. There was no statistically significant difference in mean values for AST, ALT, or INR for alcoholics given four grams per day of acetaminophen compared to placebo. Additionally, the researchers performed an analysis of the malnourished patients that showed there was no increase in AST or ALT levels in these patients. Study limitations include a limited duration of 2 days and exclusion of patients with preexisting AST or ALT elevations greater than 120 U/L. Study results do not preclude the possibility of an idiosyncratic hepatic reaction.
Renal: Martin found that patients with chronic renal failure had higher plasma concentrations of acetaminophen and the inactive glucuronide and sulfate metabolites than healthy subjects during repeated dosing up to ten days.

Several single-dose studies demonstrate accumulation of acetaminophen metabolites in patients with moderate chronic renal failure and in anephric patients 8-10 for whom hemodialysis appeared to be the major route of elimination.

The habitual consumption of acetaminophen should be discouraged. If indicated medically, the long-term use of acetaminophen should be supervised by a physician.

A National Kidney Foundation position paper notes that physicians preferentially recommend acetaminophen to patients with renal failure because of the bleeding complications associated with ASA in these individuals.
Special Populations: Geriatrics: In a comprehensive metabolic study by Miners, the formation and clearance of glucuronide and glutathione conjugates were the same in young and elderly adults, although clearance of the sulphate conjugate and unchanged acetaminophen were reduced. This finding provides prospective scientific data that the amount of acetaminophen metabolized via the oxidative pathway, from which the highly reactive intermediate, NAPQI, is generated, does not increase with age. Recently, Bannwarth evaluated the multiple-dose pharmacokinetics of acetaminophen in elderly patients. After seven days of repeat dosing, acetaminophen did not accumulate in the plasma, and the elimination half-life was the same as that reported for young adults.

Elderly patients who require therapy for longer than 5 days should consult their physician for condition monitoring.
Glucose-6-Phosphate Dehydrogenase (G6PD) Deficiency: In therapeutic doses, acetaminophen does not shorten the life-span of red blood cells and does not produce any clinically perceptible destruction of circulating red blood cells.
Obese Adults: O'Shea studied the pharmacokinetics of chlorzoxazone (a putative probe for CYP2E1 activity) to evaluate the effect of obesity on CYP2E1 activity. The authors concluded that CYP2E1 is induced in obese adults and that this could impact the metabolic pathway of a number of drugs metabolized by CYP2E1, including acetaminophen. However, acetaminophen pharmacokinetic data have been investigated in obese adults. In this prospective study, 650 mg acetaminophen was administered intravenously to obese men (297 lb), obese women (193 lb), control men (155 lb) and control women (121 lb). Acetaminophen distribution volume per total body weight was slightly lower in the obese adults but, more importantly, the half-life and metabolic clearance per total body weight did not differ among groups.
ADVERSE REACTIONS: Central Nervous System Effects: Acetaminophen at recommended doses has no obvious effects on central nervous system function. In an overdose situation, central nervous system effects are uncommon.

Chlorpheniramine maleate may cause excitability, especially in children.
Gastrointestinal Effects: Acetaminophen at recommended doses does not cause gastric irritation, gastric erosions, occult or overt gastrointestinal blood loss or ulcers.

Blot and McLaughlin conducted an independent analysis of case-control data from a study conducted by the American College of Gastroenterology. The risk of gastrointestinal bleeding increased two to three-fold among recent users of ASA, ibuprofen and other NSAIDs at OTC doses, and the risk was also dose-related. In contrast, the use of acetaminophen was not associated with an increased risk of gastrointestinal bleeding.
Hematologic Effects: Acetaminophen does not have any immediate or delayed effects on small vessel hemostasis, as measured by bleeding time. In normal volunteers receiving a single dose of acetaminophen (975 or 1950 mg) or multiple doses of acetaminophen (1950 mg daily for 6 weeks), no change in bleeding time or platelet aggregation was observed. In another study, a single 1000 mg dose of acetaminophen was given to normal volunteers and did not affect bleeding time or platelet aggregation. Patients with hemophilia receiving multiple doses of acetaminophen showed no significant changes in bleeding time.

Hematological reactions including thrombocytopenia, leucopenia, pancytopenia, neutropenia, and agranulocytosis have been reported, although these are rare and causality has not been established.
Hepatic Effects: As an illustration of the margin of safety of acetaminophen at supratherapeutic doses, a comparison of serum concentrations of acetaminophen over time for a standard 15 mg/kg dose and for a dose exceeding the standard by a multiple of 5 (75 mg/kg) are shown in Figure 1. The serum concentrations are drawn relative to the risk line for hepatotoxicity and treatment line of the Rumack-Matthew nomogram used to manage acute overdoses. The mean plasma concentrations for this supratherapeutic dose are well below the risk and treatment lines of the nomogram at all times. However, to minimize the risk for adverse effects, the maximum recommended dose should not be exceeded.

Acetaminophen in overdosage may cause hepatotoxicity. In adults and adolescents, hepatotoxicity may occur following ingestion of greater than 150 mg/kg over a period of 8 hours or less. Fatalities are infrequent (less than 3% to 4% of untreated cases in which blood levels exceed the treatment line) and have rarely been reported with overdoses less than 7.5 g. In children, amounts less than 150 mg/kg are unlikely to produce hepatotoxicity. In both adults and children, toxicity associated with acetaminophen is usually caused by ingestion of quantities of the drug that are significantly above the recommended dosage range. Hepatotoxicity, ranging from transient sharp transaminase elevations to fatal, fulminant hepatic failure, is the most common result of clinically significant overdosage.

In a double-blind, placebo-controlled clinical study, healthy adults were given 4, 6 and 8 g/day of acetaminophen over 3 days. Plasma concentrations did not accumulate with repeat doses. Clinically all doses were well tolerated by the subjects and aminotransferase values stayed within normal limits throughout the study. These data provide information related to the margin of safety but are not intended to support dosing beyond the maximum recommended dose of 4 g/day.

A report has suggested that hepatotoxicity following greater than the recommended dose of acetaminophen may be enhanced by both prolonged fasting and/or chronic alcohol abuse.
Acute Alcohol Use: Acute alcohol ingestion refers to the occasional or intermittent use of alcohol. When taken together, alcohol competes with acetaminophen for CYP2E1. CYP2E1 accepts alcohol more readily than acetaminophen; therefore, less NAPQI is produced. In the presence of alcohol, acetaminophen may be diverted to the glucuronidation and sulfation pathways. The overall result is that a smaller percentage of acetaminophen may be expected to be metabolized to the toxic intermediate, NAPQI, than would otherwise be the case. NAPQI production is increased above baseline for the period up to 18-24 hours post ethanol clearance from the body. In healthy adults, at normal labeled doses of acetaminophen, the temporary increase in NAPQI production is more than accommodated by normal glutathione stores in the liver.

Figure 1: TYLENOL Sinus

Mean Data for a Standard (1 g, 15 mg/kg) and Higher (5.6 g, 75 mg/kg) Dose Relative to Risk and Treatment Lines of the Acetaminophen Nomogram

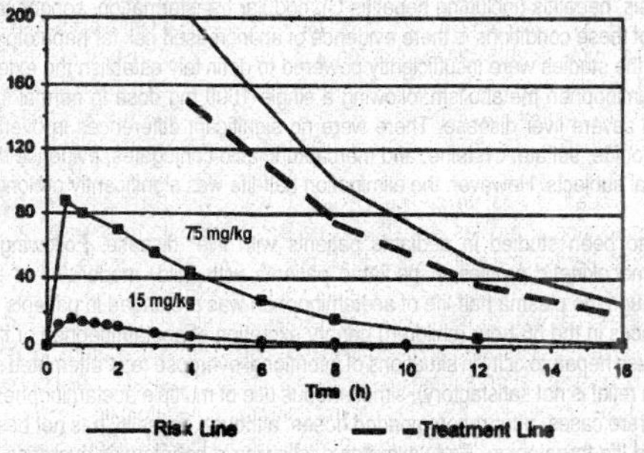

Hypersensitivity: Sensitivity reactions are rare and may manifest as rash, urticaria, dyspnea, hypotension, laryngeal edema, angioedema, bronchospasm, or anaphylaxis. Cross-reactivity in ASA-sensitive persons has been rarely reported. If sensitivity is suspected, discontinue use of the drug.

Renal Effects: Acute nephrotoxicity has been reported following massive overdose either as a sequela of hepatic failure or, occasionally, in the absence of hepatic failure.

Clinical data have established that acetaminophen in recommended doses is not nephrotoxic.

Some studies suggest an association between the chronic long-term use of acetaminophen and renal effects. Results, however, are conflicting, limited by recall bias and confounded by the inability to determine whether analgesic use preceded or followed the onset of renal disease.

Case control studies have suggested a weak association between habitual acetaminophen use and prevalence of chronic renal failure and end stage renal disease. This National Kidney Foundation position paper concludes that acetaminophen has been preferentially recommended by physicians to patients with renal failure and that there is no evidence that occasional use of acetaminophen caused renal injury.

Special Populations: Pregnancy and Lactation: As with any drug, patients who are pregnant or nursing a baby should consult a physician before taking this product.

Pregnancy: Issues of risks in pregnancy are multifactorial. The information provided cannot be substituted for direct patient consultation. Acetaminophen is believed to be non-teratogenic in humans. However, existing studies have not assessed the effect of very high doses. The Motherrisk Collaborative Perinatal project monitored 50 282 mother-child pairs, of which 226 had first trimester exposure to acetaminophen and 781 had used acetaminophen at any time during their pregnancy. No evidence was found to suggest a relationship between acetaminophen use and major or minor malformations. In a surveillance study of Michigan Medicaid recipients conducted between 1985 and 1992 involving 229 101 completed pregnancies, 9146 newborns had been exposed to acetaminophen during the first trimester. This data do not support an association between acetaminophen use and the occurrence of birth defects. Another cohort study, using prescription monitoring, found no excess risk for malformation, and no evidence that acetaminophen influenced fetal growth. Finally, as part of a larger study, 697 women used acetaminophen with or without codeine in their first trimester. No teratogenic risk was found.

A prospective study investigated the outcome of pregnancy in 300 women who had self-administered an overdose of acetaminophen, either alone, or as part of a combined preparation. Exposure to overdose occurred in all trimesters. The majority of the pregnancies had normal outcomes. The malformation rate was within the expected range. There was no obvious relationship between the time of exposure and the time of delivery. The overall conclusion was that acetaminophen overdose is not an indication for termination of pregnancy.

In a long-term developmental follow-up study, acetaminophen did not adversely affect IQ or behavior measures at four years of age. Height, weight and head circumference were also not affected by exposure to acetaminophen in-utero.

Unlike ASA, which has been shown to profoundly effect platelet function, there does not seem to be a risk of hemorrhage associated with acetaminophen use at term.

Currently there is no evidence to suggest that acetaminophen is teratogenic when used as recommended. However, data for continuous high daily doses are not sufficient, and safety during pregnancy has not yet been established.

Lactation: Following a typical therapeutic dose, acetaminophen is excreted in breast milk in very low concentrations. Based on a number of published reports, infant exposure levels are at most 4.5% of a weight adjusted pediatric therapeutic dose. In addition, acetaminophen is considered compatible with breast-feeding by the American Academy of Pediatrics.

DRUG INTERACTIONS: Alcohol: Studies evaluating the metabolism of doses up to 20 mg/kg of acetaminophen in chronic alcohol abusers and a study evaluating the effects of 2 days of acetaminophen dosing at 4000 mg/day in chronic alcoholics undergoing detoxification, have yielded inconsistent results with regard to effects on acetaminophen pharmacokinetics and demonstrate no evidence of adverse effect on liver function tests.

Anticoagulants–Oral: Patients who concomitantly medicate with warfarin-type anticoagulants and regular doses of acetaminophen have occasionally been reported to have unforeseen elevations in their INR. Physicians should be cognizant of this potential interaction and monitor the INR in such patients closely while therapy is established. Many factors, including diet, medications, and environmental and physical states, may affect how a patient responds to anticoagulant therapy. There have been several reports that suggest that acetaminophen may produce hypoprothrombinemia (elevated international normalized ratio [INR] or prothrombin time) when administered with coumarin derivatives. In other studies, prothrombin time did not change. Reported changes have been generally of limited clinical significance, however, periodic evaluation of prothrombin time should be performed when these agents are administered concurrently.

In the period immediately following discharge from the hospital or whenever other medications are initiated, discontinued, or taken regularly, it is important to monitor patient response to anticoagulation therapy with additional prothrombin time or INR determinations. Despite the potential for interaction, acetaminophen is the least likely OTC analgesic to interfere with anticoagulant therapy.

Anticonvulsants: Some reports have suggested that patients taking long-term anticonvulsants, who overdose on acetaminophen, may be at increased risk of hepatotoxicity because of accelerated metabolism of acetaminophen. Available data are conflicting. A 7-year retrospective study of acetaminophen overdose admissions indicates that the overall mortality rate was not significantly different for patients taking concomitant anticonvulsant medications.

Hydantoins: Pharmacokinetic studies indicate that phenytoin primarily induces the glucuronidation pathway, whereas glutathione-derived metabolites are not increased in patients on chronic phenytoin therapy. Additionally, recent data demonstrate that phenytoin is metabolized primarily by CYP2C9 and CYP2C19, whereas acetaminophen is primarily metabolized by CYP2E1.

Carbamazepine: Carbamazepine is primarily metabolized by CYP3A4, whereas acetaminophen is metabolized primarily via CYP2E1. It is not known whether there is increased risk from an acetaminophen overdose in patients on chronic carbamazepine therapy.

Diflunisal: Professional literature from the manufacturer of diflunisal cautions that concomitant administration with acetaminophen produces an approximate 50% increase in plasma levels of acetaminophen in normal volunteers. Acetaminophen had no effect on diflunisal plasma levels. The clinical significance of these findings has not been established. However, caution should be used with concomitant administration of diflunisal and acetaminophen and patients should be monitored carefully.

Isoniazid: Some reports suggest that patients on chronic isoniazid therapy may be at risk for developing hepatotoxicity from an acetaminophen overdose. Since patients on isoniazid therapy may develop hepatic effects from isoniazid alone, data from individual case reports are unclear as to whether chronic administration of isoniazid may increase the risk of acetaminophen toxicity. Isoniazid is primarily metabolized by CYP2E1 and induces CYP2E1. Studies in healthy subjects demonstrate that isoniazid blocks the formation of the toxic metabolite NAPQI when administered concomitantly with acetaminophen, but increase NAPQI formation when acetaminophen is administered one day after discontinuation of isoniazid. Thus, concomitant use of isoniazid is unlikely to potentiate the risk of acetaminophen-induced hepatotoxicity at recommended doses. The isoniazid induction of CYP2E1 is short-lived, lasting only 12 to 48 hours after the discontinuation of isoniazid, it is during this period the toxicity of an acetaminophen overdose may be potentiated.

DOSAGE AND ADMINISTRATION: Extra Strength TYLENOL Sinus Pain and Congestion (Daytime and Nighttime): Adults (12 years of age and older): 1 to 2 caplets every 4 to 6 hours as required. It is hazardous to exceed a combined **total** of 8 caplets in a 24-hour period. Reduce dosage if nervousness or sleeplessness occurs.

OVERDOSAGE:

Symptoms and Treatment: Acetaminophen: Typical Toxidrome: Hepatic injury is the principal toxic effect of a substantial acetaminophen overdose. The physician should be mindful that there is no early presentation that is pathognomic for the overdose. A high degree of clinical suspicion must always be maintained.

Untreated acetaminophen overdoses may produce hepatotoxicity. Acetaminophen hepatotoxicity occurs as a threshold effect and is characterized by a lack of toxicity at lower/therapeutic doses. Acetaminophen hepatotoxicity occurs after major depletion of glutathione, an endogenous detoxifying substance. Once the threshold is exceeded, increasing acetaminophen doses may produce increasing degrees of hepatotoxicity, unless N-acetylcysteine (NAC) is administered. Situations in which acetaminophen overdose and resultant hepatotoxicity may occur include acute intentional overdose and repeated supratherapeutic overdose in adults and acute accidental ingestion or overdose and repeated supratherapeutic overdose in children.

The clinical course of acetaminophen overdose generally occurs in a three-phase sequential pattern. The first phase begins shortly after ingestion and lasts for 12 to 24 hours. The patient may manifest signs of gastrointestinal irritability, nausea, vomiting, anorexia, diaphoresis, pallor and general malaise. If toxicity continues, there is a latent phase of up to 48 hours. During this second phase, initial symptoms abate and the patient may feel better. However, hepatic enzymes, bilirubin, and prothrombin time or INR values will progressively rise. Right upper quadrant pain may develop as the liver becomes enlarged and tender. Most patients do not progress beyond this phase, especially if given N-acetylcysteine (NAC) treatment early in the course. Signs and symptoms of the third phase depend on the severity of hepatic damage and usually occur from three to five days following overdose ingestion. Symptoms may be limited to anorexia, nausea, general malaise, and abdominal pain in less severe cases or may progress to confusion, stupor and sequelae of hepatic necrosis including jaundice, coagulation defects, hypoglycemia, and encephalopathy, as well as renal failure and cardiomyopathy. Death, if it occurs, is generally the result of complications associated with fulminant hepatic failure. Mortality rates in patients with toxic plasma levels who do not receive antidote therapy range from 3% to 4%.

Due to the wide availability of acetaminophen, it is commonly involved in single and mixed drug overdose situations and the practitioner should screen for its presence in a patient's serum. Acute toxicity after single dose overdoses of acetaminophen can be anticipated when the overdose exceeds 150 mg/kg. Chronic alcohol abusers, cachectic individuals, and persons taking pharmacologic inducers of the hepatic P450 microsomal enzyme system may be at risk with lower exposures.

Specific Antidote: Any individual presenting with a possible acetaminophen overdose should be treated with N-acetylcysteine (NAC), even if the amount of acetaminophen ingested is unknown or questionable. A blood sample for determination of the plasma acetaminophen concentration should be obtained as early as possible, but no sooner than four hours following ingestion. Do not await the results of assays for plasma acetaminophen levels before initiating treatment NAC. If the acetaminophen plasma level is found to plot above the treatment line on the acetaminophen overdose nomogram, NAC treatment should be continued for a full course of therapy. NAC is used clinically to treat acute acetaminophen overdose, and acts by interacting with the oxidative intermediate, NAPQI. NAC administered by either the i.v. or the oral route is known to be a highly effective antidote for acetaminophen poisoning. It's most effective when administered within 8 hours of a significant overdose but reports have indicated benefits to treatment initiated well beyond this time period. It is imperative to administer the antidote as early as possible in the time course of acute intoxication to reap the full benefits of the antidote's protective effects. For full prescribing information, consult the product monograph for NAC.

General Management: When the possibility of acetaminophen overdose exists, treatment should begin immediately and include appropriate decontamination of the gastrointestinal tract, proper supportive care, careful assessment of appropriately timed serum acetaminophen estimations evaluated against the Rumack-Matthew nomogram, timely administration of NAC as required and appropriate follow-up care. Liver function tests should be performed initially and repeated at 24-hour intervals.

Pseudoephedrine HCl: Typical toxidrome: sympathomimetic/stimulant.

Specific Antidote: none.

General Management: Stabilize the patient (A, B, Cs), undertake appropriate gastrointestinal tract decontamination procedures, initiate supportive care, consult with a Regional Poison Control Centre regarding ongoing management, and arrange for appropriate follow-up care.

Chlorpheniramine Maleate: Typical Toxidrome: anticholinergic, CNS depressant (adult), CNS stimulant (child).

Specific Antidote: none.

General Management: Stabilize the patient (A, B, Cs), undertake appropriate gastrointestinal tract decontamination procedures, initiate supportive care, consult with a Regional Poison Control Centre regarding ongoing management, and arrange for appropriate follow-up care.

Overdose During Pregnancy: Acetaminophen is one of the most common overdoses in pregnancy. Hepatic toxicity of acetaminophen follows the formation of the highly reactive metabolite N-acetyl-p-benzoquinoneimine produced by acetaminophen metabolism through the cytochrome P450 mixed-function oxidase system. Hepatic failure can be prevented by timely administration of NAC either orally for 72 hours, or intravenously (IV) for 20 hours.

Acetaminophen crosses the human placenta though the fetus is theoretically at risk when maternal overdose of acetaminophen occurs. Acetaminophen can be transformed to its toxic metabolite since the oxidative capacity of fetal microsomes is present in the fetus by 14 weeks gestation.

Studies on placental transfer of NAC in rats and sheep yielded conflicting results. Placental transfer of N-acetylcysteine in humans was demonstrated in 4 women treated with NAC for acetaminophen overdose during labour. NAC blood levels in the fetuses were within the range associated with therapeutic doses of NAC administered to adults with acetaminophen poisoning.

Fetal toxicity and stillbirth after a large (e.g. 30 g) acetaminophen overdose has been reported, but others observed a normal outcome for the offspring after acetaminophen overdose in pregnancy. A large case series investigated the pregnancy outcome in 300 women who had overdosed with acetaminophen. In this group, 118 cases occurred in the first trimester, 103 in the second trimester and 79 in the third trimester. Forty-nine of these mothers were treated with specific antidotes (33 with NAC and 16 with methionine). There were 219 live-born infants, 11 have malformations (including minor); none had been exposed to acetaminophen during the first trimester. Nine women were treated with NAC during the first trimester; there were two elective terminations; two spontaneous abortions, and five healthy babies in this group.

In summary, acetaminophen overdose during pregnancy should be treated according to regular protocols in order to prevent maternal and potentially fetal toxicity. Unless severe maternal toxicity develops, an acetaminophen overdose does not increase the risk for birth defects or adverse pregnancy outcomes.

Physicians unfamiliar with the current management of acetaminophen overdose should consult with a Poison Control Centre immediately. Telephone numbers for local Poison Control Centres are available in the local phone directory. Delays in initiation of appropriate therapy may jeopardize the patient's chances for full recovery.

For management of a suspected drug overdose, CPhA recommends that you contact your **regional Poison Control Centre**. See the *CPS* Directory section for a list of Poison Control Centres.

ACTION AND CLINICAL PHARMACOLOGY: Mechanism of Action: Acetaminophen is a centrally acting analgesic and antipyretic drug. Although the precise mechanism of action is not totally understood, work by Boutaud suggests acetaminophen is an inhibitor of the peroxidase portion of cyclooxygenase (prostaglandin H synthase inhibitor). Depending on the redox state and substrate concentrations surrounding the enzymes, acetaminophen may or may not have a significant inhibitory effect. This accounts for its selective activity on pain and fever with little anti-inflammatory effect.

It is postulated that the analgesic effect is produced by elevation of the pain threshold and the antipyretic effect is produced through action on the hypothalamic heat-regulating centre.

The optimal effective analgesic dose of acetaminophen was demonstrated in dental pain studies and is 1000 mg every four to six hours, up to 4000 mg daily. At least 500 published and unpublished controlled clinical trials in adults and children have evaluated acetaminophen for the relief of pain or fever. These studies include single and multiple dose treatments. Most studies were less than 14 days in duration, although the longest study duration was two years. No significant safety issues were reported in any of these studies.

Moreover, at recommended doses, acetaminophen has not been shown to increase the risk of developing renal diseases or upper gastrointestinal ulceration/bleeding. This observation is consistent with its minimal inhibitory effect on peripheral prostaglandin synthesis and on gastric prostaglandin synthesis.

Acetaminophen is considered equipotent to ASA and ibuprofen, within the recommended OTC dosing ranges, in its analgesic and antipyretic effects. Acetaminophen at recommended doses does not cause the type of gastrointestinal complications associated with NSAID-containing products, such as gastric irritation, gastric erosions, occult or overt gastrointestinal blood loss, or ulcers. Unlike these drugs, however, it has no anti-inflammatory effect at clinically relevant doses in humans.

Pharmacokinetics: Absorption: Oral acetaminophen is rapidly and almost completely absorbed from the gastrointestinal tract primarily in the small intestine. This absorption process occurs by passive transport. Peak plasma concentrations occur within 0.4 to 1 hour depending on the product formulation. Although high-fat foods delay the time to peak concentration for up to an hour, the dose is completely absorbed.

Distribution: Acetaminophen is uniformly distributed throughout most body fluids, but not in fatty tissue. As a result, the volume of distribution in adults ranges between 0.8 and 1.0 L/kg. Since acetaminophen has low protein binding in plasma of only 10% to 25%, it does not compete with drugs that are highly protein bound.

Metabolism: Acetaminophen is primarily metabolized by the liver via three principal separate pathways: conjugation with glucuronide; conjugation with sulfate; oxidation via the cytochrome P450 mixed function oxidase system.

Both the glucuronic and oxidative pathways adhere to a first-order rate process, which means the concentration of acetaminophen metabolized increases as the concentration in the liver increases. The sulfate pathway adheres to Michaelis-Menten kinetics, which means the concentration of acetaminophen metabolized remains constant once the concentration in the liver increases above a saturation level. A schematic of acetaminophen metabolism is shown in Figure 2.

The major metabolic pathway is glucuronidation, where 47% to 62% of the acetaminophen dose conjugates with glucuronide. These glucuronide conjugates are inactive and nontoxic, and are secreted in bile and eliminated in the urine.

The second major pathway is sulfation, where 25% to 36% of the dose conjugates with sulfate. These sulfate ester conjugates are also inactive and nontoxic and are excreted in the urine.

The third pathway is oxidation, where 5% to 8% of the dose is metabolized via the cytochrome P450 enzyme system. The cytochrome P450 isoenzyme that is primarily responsible is CYP2E1. When acetaminophen is metabolized by CYP2E1, it forms a highly reactive intermediate, N-acetyl-p-benzoquinoneimine (NAPQI). Since NAPQI is highly reactive, it cannot be measured outside the liver nor can it accumulate. This intermediate is rapidly inactivated by hepatocellular stores of glutathione to form cysteine and mercapturate conjugates, which are both inactive and nontoxic. These conjugates are excreted in the urine.

Figure 2: TYLENOL Sinus

Acetaminophen Metabolism

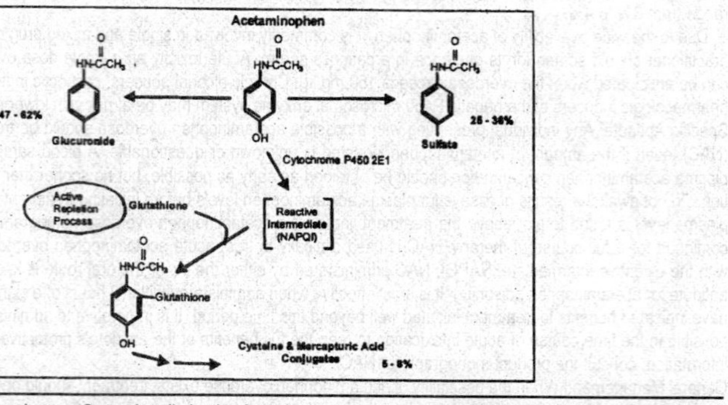

Excretion: Acetaminophen undergoes first-order elimination from the body, and has a short plasma half-life that ranges from 2 to 3 hours in healthy young and elderly adults and from 1.5 to 2.9 hours in children. Since acetaminophen clears rapidly from the body, repeated doses do not lead to accumulation of acetaminophen plasma concentrations.

STORAGE AND STABILITY: Store at room temperature (15 to 30°C). Protect from moisture.

DOSAGE FORMS, COMPOSITION AND PACKAGING: Sinus Pain and Congestion Daytime Extra Strength: Each green, film-coated caplet, engraved "MSTSM" on one side and "500" on the other side, contains: acetaminophen 500 mg and pseudoephedrine HCl 30 mg. Nonmedicinal ingredients: carnauba wax, cellulose, citric acid, corn starch, D&C Yellow no. 10, FD&C Blue no. 1, FD&C Yellow no. 6, flavour, hypromellose, magnesium stearate, mannitol, potassium sorbate, sodium benzoate, sodium citrate, sodium starch glycolate, sucralose and triacetin. Energy: 1.2 kJ (0.3 kcal). Sodium: 0.4 mg. Gluten-, lactose- and tartrazine-free. Plastic bottles 50*. Blister packs of 12 in combination with blister packs of 12 Extra Strength TYLENOL Sinus Pain & Congestion Nighttime caplets.

Sinus Pain and Congestion Nighttime Extra Strength: Each white, film-coated caplet, engraved "SNT" on one side and "500" on the other side, contains: acetaminophen 500 mg, pseudoephedrine HCl 30 mg and chlorpheniramine maleate 2 mg. Nonmedicinal ingredients: carnauba wax, cellulose, citric acid, corn starch, flavour, hypromellose, magnesium stearate, mannitol, potassium sorbate, sodium benzoate, sodium citrate, sodium starch glycolate and sucralose. Energy: 1.2 kJ (0.3 kcal). Sodium: 0.4 mg. Gluten-, lactose- and tartrazine-free. Blister packs of 12 in combination with blister packs of 12 Extra Strength TYLENOL Sinus Pain & Congestion Daytime caplets.

All packages are safety sealed.

Tylenol® Ultra Relief Migraine Pain

acetaminophen—caffeine

Analgesic—Antipyretic

McNeil Consumer Healthcare

SUMMARY PRODUCT INFORMATION:

Route of Administration	Dosage Form/ Strength	Clinically Relevant Nonmedicinal Ingredients
Oral	Tablet/500 mg acetaminophen and 65 mg caffeine	Gluten-, lactose- and tartrazine-free For a complete listing of nonmedicinal ingredients, see Dosage Forms, Composition and Packaging.

INDICATIONS AND CLINICAL USE: As an analgesic-antipyretic for the temporary relief of mild to moderate pain in a wide variety of conditions involving musculoskeletal pain, as well as in other painful disorders such as headache pain (including mild to moderate migraine and tension headache), earache, low back pain, arthritis pain, dysmenorrhea, myalgias, and neuralgias. Also indicated for the symptomatic reduction of fever due to the common cold, flu and other viral or bacterial infections.

The combination of acetaminophen and caffeine has been clinically proven to provide superior headache pain relief relative to acetaminophen alone.

CONTRAINDICATIONS: Hypersensitivity to acetaminophen, caffeine or to the ingredients of this formulation (see Dosage Forms, Composition and Packaging). Allergic reactions (primarily skin rash) or reports of hypersensitivity secondary to acetaminophen are rare and generally are controlled by discontinuation of the drug and, when necessary, symptomatic treatment.

WARNINGS AND PRECAUTIONS: General: Consumers should not exceed 4 g/day of acetaminophen or use two or more acetaminophen-containing products together. This includes combination products that contain acetaminophen. Do not use with other products containing salicylates or any other pain or fever medicine.

Acetaminophen-containing products should be kept out of the reach of children.

Physicians should be cognizant of and supervise the use of acetaminophen in patients with chronic alcoholism, serious kidney or serious liver disease. Physicians should alert their patients who regularly consume large amounts of alcohol not to exceed the recommended doses of acetaminophen. Chronic heavy alcohol abusers may be at increased risk of liver toxicity from excessive doses of acetaminophen.

Patients should be counseled to consult a physician if redness or swelling is present in an area of pain, if symptoms do not improve or if they worsen, or if new symptoms such as high fever, rash, itching or persistent headache occur, as these may be signs of a condition which requires medical attention.

* Container provided with a child-resistant closure.

Acetaminophen should not be taken for pain for more than 5 days, for fever for more than 3 days or if new symptoms appear, without consulting a physician.

Hepatic/Biliary/Pancreatic: Slower metabolism of acetaminophen, increased activity of the cytochrome P450 enzyme system, or depleted glutathione stores are cited as theoretical risk factors for acetaminophen hepatotoxicity in patients with chronic liver disease. However, acetaminophen has been studied in both adults and children with a wide variety of liver diseases including various types of cirrhosis, hepatitis (including hepatitis C), nodular transformation, congenital hepatic fibrosis, and α1-antitrypsin deficiency. In none of these conditions is there evidence of an increased risk for hepatotoxicity at currently recommended acetaminophen doses but the studies were insufficiently powered to definitely establish the extent of risk.

Forrest compared acetaminophen metabolism following a single 1500 mg dose in normal subjects, patients with mild liver disease, and patients with severe liver disease. There were no significant differences in overall 24-hour urinary excretion of acetaminophen and glucuronide, sulfate, cysteine, and mercapturic acid conjugates, evidence that acetaminophen metabolism was similar to that in normal subjects. However, the elimination half-life was significantly prolonged in patients with severe liver disease.

Acetaminophen has also been studied in pediatric patients with liver disease. Following a single (10 mg/kg) dose of acetaminophen, the pharmacokinetic profiles in pediatric patients with mild, moderate, or severe liver disease were not significantly different. Although the plasma half-life of acetaminophen was prolonged in patients with severe liver disease, there were no significant differences in the 36-hour (children) urinary excretion of acetaminophen or its conjugates.

Acetaminophen may cause hepatotoxicity in situations of intentional overdose (e.g. attempted suicide), unintentional overdose (e.g. overdosing when pain relief is not satisfactory), simultaneous use of multiple acetaminophen-containing preparations, accidental overdose or in very rare cases, after recommended doses, although causality has not been determined. The hepatotoxic reaction can be severe and life-threatening. Early symptoms following a hepatotoxic overdose may include nausea, vomiting, diaphoresis, lethargy, and general malaise. If appropriate treatment is not instituted, these may progress to upper quadrant pain, confusion, stupor, and sequelae of hepatic necrosis, such as jaundice, coagulation defects, hypoglycemia, and encephalopathy. Renal failure and cardiomyopathy may also occur. In the event of known or suspected overdosage, treatment with N-acetyl cysteine should be instituted immediately (see Overdosage), even when there are no obvious symptoms. Failure to promptly treat acetaminophen hepatotoxicity with N-acetyl cysteine can result in liver failure, leading to liver transplantation and/or death.

Chronic Alcohol Use: Excessive alcohol use may increase risk of liver toxicity from acetaminophen overdose (acute or chronic).

In prospective, placebo controlled studies, researchers evaluated an actively drinking group of alcoholics with a high prevalence of malnourishment. The study participants abruptly stopped their daily alcohol intake and took acetaminophen the next day. This should theoretically make them vulnerable to acetaminophen injury because their CYP2E1 would be maximally induced from the alcohol and there would be no alcohol present to compete with acetaminophen for metabolism by CYP2E1. There was no statistically significant difference in mean values for AST, ALT, or INR for alcoholics given four grams per day of acetaminophen compared to placebo. Additionally, the researchers performed an analysis of the malnourished patients that showed there was no increase in AST or ALT levels in these patients. Study limitations include a limited duration of 2 days and exclusion of patients with preexisting AST or ALT elevations greater than 120 U/L. Study results do not preclude the possibility of an idiosyncratic hepatic reaction.

Renal: Martin found that patients with chronic renal failure had higher plasma concentrations of acetaminophen and the inactive glucuronide and sulfate metabolites than healthy subjects during repeated dosing up to ten days.

Several single-dose studies demonstrate accumulation of acetaminophen metabolites in patients with moderate chronic renal failure and in anephric patients for whom hemodialysis appeared to be the major route of elimination.

The habitual consumption of acetaminophen should be discouraged. If indicated medically, the long-term use of acetaminophen should be supervised by a physician.

A National Kidney Foundation position paper notes that physicians preferentially recommend acetaminophen to patients with renal failure because of the bleeding complications associated with ASA in these individuals.

Special Populations: Geriatrics: In a comprehensive metabolic study by Miners, the formation and clearance of glucuronide and glutathione conjugates were the same in young and elderly adults, although clearance of the sulphate conjugate and unchanged acetaminophen were reduced. This finding provides prospective scientific data that the amount of acetaminophen metabolized via the oxidative pathway, from which the highly reactive intermediate, NAPQI, is generated, does not increase with age. Recently, Bannwarth evaluated the multiple-dose pharmacokinetics of acetaminophen in elderly patients. After seven days of repeat dosing, acetaminophen did not accumulate in the plasma, and the elimination half-life was the same as that reported for young adults.

Elderly patients who require therapy for longer than 5 days should consult their physician for condition monitoring.

Glucose-6-Phosphate Dehydrogenase (G6PD) Deficiency: In therapeutic doses, acetaminophen does not shorten the lifespan of red blood cells and does not produce any clinically perceptible destruction of circulating red blood cells.

Obese Adults: O'Shea studied the pharmacokinetics of chlorzoxazone (a putative probe for CYP2E1 activity) to evaluate the effect of obesity on CYP2E1 activity. The authors concluded that CYP2E1 is induced in obese adults and that this could impact the metabolic pathway of a number of drugs metabolized by CYP2E1, including acetaminophen. However, acetaminophen pharmacokinetic data have been investigated in obese adults. In this prospective study, 650 mg acetaminophen was administered intravenously to obese men (297 lb), obese women (193 lb), control men (155 lb) and control women (121 lb). Acetaminophen distribution volume per total body weight was slightly lower in the obese adults but, more importantly, the half-life and metabolic clearance per total body weight did not differ among groups.

ADVERSE REACTIONS: In recommended therapeutic doses, acetaminophen and caffeine are usually well tolerated.

Central Nervous System Effects: Acetaminophen at recommended doses has no obvious effects on central nervous system function. In an overdose situation, central nervous system effects are uncommon.

Higher doses of caffeine lead to overstimulation of the higher centres of the CNS.

Caffeine may cause CNS stimulation leading to symptoms such as restlessness, nervousness and insomnia.

Gastrointestinal Effects: Acetaminophen at recommended doses does not cause gastric irritation, gastric erosions, occult or overt gastrointestinal blood loss or ulcers.

Blot and McLaughlin conducted an independent analysis of case-control data from a study conducted by the American College of Gastroenterology. The risk of gastrointestinal bleeding increased two to three-fold among recent users of ASA, ibuprofen and other NSAIDs at OTC doses, and the risk was also dose-related. In contrast, the use of acetaminophen was not associated with an increased risk of gastrointestinal bleeding.

Long-term use of caffeine may cause gastric disturbances and subsequent development of gastric ulcers. Use with caution in patients with a history of peptic ulcer.

Hematologic Effects: Acetaminophen does not have any immediate or delayed effects on small vessel hemostasis, as measured by bleeding time. In normal volunteers receiving a single dose of acetaminophen (975 or 1950 mg) or multiple doses of acetaminophen (1950 mg daily for 6 weeks), no change in bleeding time or platelet aggregation was observed. In another study, a single 1000 mg dose of acetaminophen was given to normal volunteers and did not affect bleeding time or platelet aggregation. Patients with hemophilia receiving multiple doses of acetaminophen showed no significant changes in bleeding time.

Hematological reactions including thrombocytopenia, leucopenia, pancytopenia, neutropenia, and agranulocytosis have been reported, although these are rare and causality has not been established.

Hepatic Effects: As an illustration of the margin of safety of acetaminophen at supratherapeutic doses, a comparison of serum concentrations of acetaminophen over time for a standard 15 mg/kg dose and for a dose exceeding the standard by a multiple of 5 (75 mg/kg) are shown in Figure 1. The serum concentrations are drawn relative to the risk line for hepatotoxicity and treatment line of the Rumack-Matthew nomogram used to manage acute overdoses. The mean plasma concentrations for this supratherapeutic dose are well below the risk and treatment lines of the nomogram at all times. However, to minimize the risk for adverse effects, the maximum recommended dose should not be exceeded.

Acetaminophen in overdosage may cause hepatotoxicity. In adults and adolescents, hepatotoxicity may occur following ingestion of greater than 150 mg/kg over a period of 8 hours or less. Fatalities are infrequent (less than 3% to 4% of untreated cases in which blood levels exceed the treatment line) and have rarely been reported with overdoses less than 7.5 g. In children, amounts less than 150 mg/kg are unlikely to produce hepatotoxicity. In both adults and children, toxicity associated with acetaminophen is usually caused by ingestion of quantities of the drug that are significantly above the recommended dosage range. Hepatotoxicity, ranging from transient sharp transaminase elevations to fatal, fulminant hepatic failure, is the most common result of clinically significant overdosage.

In a double-blind, placebo-controlled clinical study, healthy adults were given 4, 6 and 8 g/d of acetaminophen over 3 days 30. Plasma concentrations did not accumulate with repeat doses. Clinically all doses were well tolerated by the subjects and aminotransferase values stayed within normal limits throughout the study. These data provide information related to the margin of safety but are not intended to support dosing beyond the maximum recommended dose of 4 g/day.

A report has suggested that hepatotoxicity following greater than the recommended dose of acetaminophen may be enhanced by both prolonged fasting and/or chronic alcohol abuse.

Figure 1: TYLENOL Ultra Relief Migraine Pain

Mean Data for a Standard (1 g, 15 mg/kg) and Higher (5.6 g, 75 mg/kg) Dose Relative to Risk and Treatment Lines of the Acetaminophen Nomogram

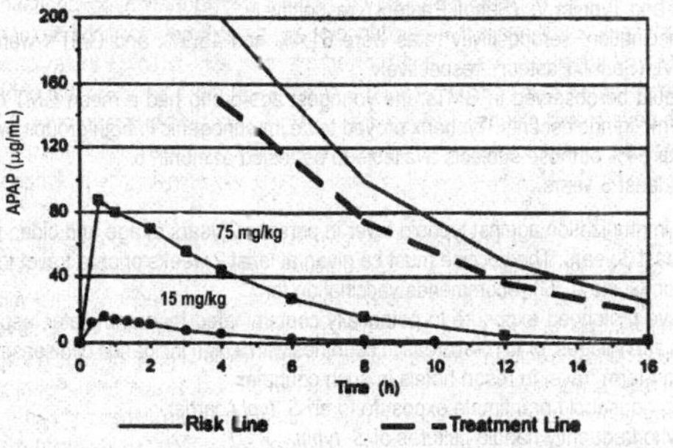

Acute Alcohol Use: Acute alcohol ingestion refers to the occasional or intermittent use of alcohol. When taken together, alcohol competes with acetaminophen for CYP2E1. CYP2E1 accepts alcohol more readily than acetaminophen; therefore, less NAPQI is produced. In the presence of alcohol, acetaminophen may be diverted to the glucuronidation and sulfation pathways. The overall result is that a smaller percentage of acetaminophen may be expected to be metabolized to the toxic intermediate, NAPQI, than would otherwise be the case. NAPQI production is increased above baseline for the period up to 18-24 hours post ethanol clearance from the body. In healthy adults, at normal labeled doses of acetaminophen, the temporary increase in NAPQI production is more than accommodated by normal glutathione stores in the liver.

Hypersensitivity: Sensitivity reactions are rare and may manifest as rash, urticaria, dyspnea, hypotension, laryngeal edema, angioedema, bronchospasm, or anaphylaxis. Cross-reactivity in ASA-sensitive persons has been rarely reported. If sensitivity is suspected, discontinue use of the drug.

Renal Effects: Acute nephrotoxicity has been reported following massive overdose either as a sequela of hepatic failure or, occasionally, in the absence of hepatic failure.

Clinical data have established that acetaminophen in recommended doses is not nephrotoxic.

Some studies suggest an association between the chronic long-term use of acetaminophen and renal effects. Results, however, are conflicting, limited by recall bias and confounded by the inability to determine whether analgesic use preceded or followed the onset of renal disease.

Case control studies have suggested a weak association between habitual acetaminophen use and prevalence of chronic renal failure and end stage renal disease. This National Kidney Foundation position paper concludes that acetaminophen has been preferentially recommended by physicians to patients with renal failure and that there is no evidence that occasional use of acetaminophen caused renal injury.

Special Populations: Pediatrics: Lesko and Mitchell enrolled more than 84 000 febrile children in a randomized, double blind, acetaminophen-controlled trial to assess the risks of rare but serious adverse events following use of pediatric ibuprofen. Of the children included in the analysis, 28 130 received acetaminophen and none experienced anaphylaxis, or serious hepatic, gastrointestinal or renal effects.

Pregnancy and Lactation: As with any drug, patients who are pregnant or nursing a baby should consult a physician before taking this product. Caffeine is found in breast milk following consumption of tea or coffee. About 1% of the caffeine in these beverages is recovered in approximately 100 mL of breast milk at 4 hours.

Pregnancy: Issues of risks in pregnancy are multifactorial. The information provided cannot be substituted for direct patient consultation. Acetaminophen is believed to be non-teratogenic in humans. However, existing studies have not assessed the effect of very high doses. The Motherisk Collaborative Perinatal project monitored 50 282 mother-child pairs, of which 226 had first trimester exposure to acetaminophen and 781 had used acetaminophen at any time during their pregnancy. No evidence was found to suggest a relationship between acetaminophen use and major or minor malformations. In a surveillance study of Michigan Medicaid recipients conducted between 1985 and 1992 involving 229 101 completed pregnancies, 9146 newborns had been exposed to acetaminophen during the first trimester. This data do not support an association between acetaminophen use and the occurrence of birth defects. Another cohort study, using prescription monitoring, found no excess risk for malformation, and no evidence that acetaminophen influenced fetal growth. Finally, as part of a larger study, 697 women used acetaminophen with or without codeine in their first trimester. No teratogenic risk was found.

A prospective study investigated the outcome of pregnancy in 300 women who had self-administered an overdose of acetaminophen, either alone, or as part of a combined preparation. Exposure to overdose occurred in all trimesters. The majority of the pregnancies had normal outcomes. The malformation rate was within the expected range. There was no obvious relationship between the time of exposure and the time of delivery. The overall conclusion was that acetaminophen overdose is not an indication for termination of pregnancy.

In a long-term developmental follow-up study, acetaminophen did not adversely affect IQ or behavior measures at four years of age. Height, weight and head circumference were also not affected by exposure to acetaminophen in-utero.

Unlike ASA, which has been shown to profoundly effect platelet function, there does not seem to be a risk of hemorrhage associated with acetaminophen use at term.

Currently there is no evidence to suggest that acetaminophen is teratogenic when used as recommended. However, data for continuous high daily doses are not sufficient, and safety during pregnancy has not yet been established.

Lactation: Following a typical therapeutic dose, acetaminophen is excreted in breast milk in very low concentrations. Based on a number of published reports, infant exposure levels are at most 4.5% of a weight adjusted pediatric therapeutic dose. In addition, acetaminophen is considered compatible with breast-feeding by the American Academy of Pediatrics.

DRUG INTERACTIONS: Alcohol: Studies evaluating the metabolism of doses up to 20 mg/kg of acetaminophen in chronic alcohol abusers and a study evaluating the effects of 2 days of acetaminophen dosing at 4000 mg/day in chronic alcoholics undergoing detoxification, have yielded inconsistent results with regard to effects on acetaminophen pharmacokinetics and demonstrate no evidence of adverse effect on liver function tests.

Anticoagulants–Oral: Patients who concomitantly medicate with warfarin-type anticoagulants and regular doses of acetaminophen have occasionally been reported to have unforeseen elevations in their INR. Physicians should be cognizant of this potential interaction and monitor the INR in such patients closely while therapy is established. Many factors, including diet, medications, and environmental and physical states, may affect how a patient responds to anticoagulant therapy. There have been several reports that suggest that acetaminophen may produce hypoprothrombinemia (elevated international normalized ratio [INR] or prothrombin time) when administered with coumarin derivatives. In other studies, prothrombin time did not change. Reported changes have been generally of limited clinical significance, however, periodic evaluation of prothrombin time should be performed when these agents are administered concurrently.

In the period immediately following discharge from the hospital or whenever other medications are initiated, discontinued, or taken regularly, it is important to monitor patient response to anticoagulation therapy with additional prothrombin time or INR determinations. Despite the potential for interaction, acetaminophen is the least likely OTC analgesic to interfere with anticoagulant therapy.

Anticonvulsants: Some reports have suggested that patients taking long-term anticonvulsants, who overdose on acetaminophen, may be at increased risk of hepatotoxicity because of accelerated metabolism of acetaminophen. Available data are conflicting. A 7-year retrospective study of acetaminophen overdose admissions indicates that the overall mortality rate was not significantly different for patients taking concomitant anticonvulsant medications.

Hydantoins: Pharmacokinetic studies indicate that phenytoin primarily induces the glucuronidation pathway, whereas glutathione-derived metabolites are not increased in patients on chronic phenytoin therapy. Additionally, recent data demonstrate that phenytoin is metabolized primarily by CYP2C9 and CYP2C19, whereas acetaminophen is primarily metabolized by CYP2E1.

Carbamazepine: Carbamazepine is primarily metabolized by CYP3A4, whereas acetaminophen is metabolized primarily via CYP2E1. It is not known whether there is increased risk from an acetaminophen overdose in patients on chronic carbamazepine therapy.

Diflunisal: Professional literature from the manufacturer of diflunisal cautions that concomitant administration with acetaminophen produces an approximate 50% increase in plasma levels of acetaminophen in normal volunteers. Acetaminophen had no effect on diflunisal plasma levels. The clinical significance of these findings has not been established. However, caution should be used with concomitant administration of diflunisal and acetaminophen and patients should be monitored carefully.

Isoniazid: Some reports suggest that patients on chronic isoniazid therapy may be at risk for developing hepatotoxicity from an acetaminophen overdose. Since patients on isoniazid therapy may develop hepatic effects from isoniazid alone, data from individual case reports are unclear as to whether chronic administration of isoniazid may increase the risk of acetaminophen toxicity. Isoniazid is primarily metabolized by CYP2E1 and induces CYP2E1. Studies in healthy subjects demonstrate that isoniazid blocks the formation of the toxic metabolite NAPQI when administered concomitantly with acetaminophen, but increase NAPQI formation when acetaminophen is administered one day after discontinuation of isoniazid. Thus, concomitant use of isoniazid is unlikely to potentiate the risk of acetaminophen-induced hepatotoxicity at recommended doses. The isoniazid induction of CYP2E1 is short-lived, lasting only 12 to 48 hours after the discontinuation of isoniazid, it is during this period the toxicity of an acetaminophen overdose may be potentiated.

DOSAGE AND ADMINISTRATION: Dosage: Adults and children over 12 years of age: 1 to 2 tablets every 4 hours as required, not to exceed 8 tablets in 24 hours. Doses may be administered with or without food.

OVERDOSAGE:

Symptoms and Treatment: Acetaminophen: Typical Toxidrome: Hepatic injury is the principal toxic effect of a substantial acetaminophen overdose. The physician should be mindful that there is no early presentation that is pathognomic for the overdose. A high degree of clinical suspicion must always be maintained.

Untreated acetaminophen overdoses may produce hepatotoxicity. Acetaminophen hepatotoxicity occurs as a threshold effect and is characterized by a lack of toxicity at lower/therapeutic doses. Acetaminophen hepatotoxicity occurs after major depletion of glutathione, an endogenous detoxifying substance. Once the threshold is exceeded, increasing acetaminophen doses may produce increasing degrees of hepatotoxicity, unless N-acetylcysteine (NAC) is administered. Situations in which acetaminophen overdose and resultant hepatotoxicity may occur include acute intentional overdose and repeated supratherapeutic overdose in adults and acute accidental ingestion or overdose and repeated supratherapeutic overdose in children.

The clinical course of acetaminophen overdose generally occurs in a three-phase sequential pattern. The first phase begins shortly after ingestion and lasts for 12 to 24 hours. The patient may manifest signs of gastrointestinal irritability, nausea, vomiting, anorexia, diaphoresis, pallor and general malaise. If toxicity continues, there is a latent phase of up to 48 hours. During this second phase, initial symptoms abate and the patient may feel better. However, hepatic enzymes, bilirubin, and prothrombin time or INR values will progressively rise. Right upper quadrant pain may develop as the liver becomes enlarged and tender. Most patients do not progress beyond this phase, especially if given N-acetylcysteine (NAC) treatment early in the course. Signs and symptoms of the third phase depend on the severity of hepatic damage and usually occur from three to five days following overdose ingestion. Symptoms may be limited to anorexia, nausea, general malaise, and abdominal pain in less severe cases or may progress to confusion, stupor and sequelae of hepatic necrosis including jaundice, coagulation defects, hypoglycemia, and encephalopathy, as well as renal failure and cardiomyopathy. Death, if it occurs, is generally the result of complications associated with fulminant hepatic failure. Mortality rates in patients with toxic plasma levels who do not receive antidote therapy range from 3% to 4%.

Due to the wide availability of acetaminophen, it is commonly involved in single and mixed drug overdose situations and the practitioner should screen for its presence in a patient's serum. Acute toxicity after single dose overdoses of acetaminophen can be anticipated when the overdose exceeds 150 mg/kg. Chronic alcohol abusers, cachectic individuals, and persons taking pharmacologic inducers of the hepatic P450 microsomal enzyme system may be at risk with lower exposures.

Specific Antidote: Any individual presenting with a possible acetaminophen overdose should be treated with N-acetylcysteine (NAC), even if the amount of acetaminophen ingested is unknown or questionable. A blood sample for determination of the plasma acetaminophen concentration should be obtained as early as possible, but no sooner than four hours following ingestion. Do not await the results of assays for plasma acetaminophen levels before initiating treatment NAC. If the acetaminophen plasma level is found to plot above the treatment line on the acetaminophen overdose nomogram, NAC treatment should be continued for a full course of therapy. NAC is used clinically to treat acute acetaminophen overdose, and acts by interacting with the oxidative intermediate, NAPQI. NAC administered by either the i.v. or the oral route is known to be a highly effective antidote for acetaminophen poisoning. It is most effective when administered within 8 hours of a significant overdose but reports have indicated benefits to treatment initiated well beyond this time period. It is imperative to administer the antidote as early as possible in the time course of acute intoxication to reap the full benefits of the antidote's protective effects. For full prescribing information, consult the product monograph for NAC.

General Management: When the possibility of acetaminophen overdose exists, treatment should begin immediately and include appropriate decontamination of the gastrointestinal tract, proper supportive care, careful assessment of appropriately timed serum acetaminophen estimations evaluated against the Rumack-Matthew nomogram, timely administration of NAC as required and appropriate follow-up care. Liver function tests should be performed initially and repeated at 24-hour intervals.

Caffeine: Typical Toxidrome: xanthine (theophylline-like picture), CNS excitation, skeletal muscle irritability.

Antidote: none.

General Management: Stabilize the patient, undertake appropriate gastrointestinal tract decontamination procedures, initiate supportive care and consult with a Poison Control Centre regarding ongoing management.

Overdose During Pregnancy: Acetaminophen is one of the most common overdoses in pregnancy. Hepatic toxicity of acetaminophen follows the formation of the highly reactive metabolite N-acetyl-p-benzoquinoneimine produced by acetaminophen metabolism through the cytochrome P450 mixed-function oxidase system. Hepatic failure can be prevented by timely administration of NAC either orally for 72 hours, or intravenously (IV) for 20 hours.

Acetaminophen crosses the human placenta though the fetus is theoretically at risk when maternal overdose of acetaminophen occurs. Acetaminophen can be transformed to its toxic metabolite since the oxidative capacity of fetal microsomes is present in the fetus by 14 weeks gestation.

Studies on placental transfer of NAC in rats and sheep yielded conflicting results. Placental transfer of N-acetylcysteine in humans was demonstrated in 4 women treated with NAC for acetaminophen overdose during labour. NAC blood levels in the fetuses were within the range associated with therapeutic doses of NAC administered to adults with acetaminophen poisoning.

Fetal toxicity and stillbirth after a large (e.g. 30 g) acetaminophen overdose has been reported, but others observed a normal outcome for the offspring after acetaminophen overdose in pregnancy. A large case series investigated the pregnancy outcome in 300 women who had overdosed with acetaminophen. In this group, 118 cases occurred in the first trimester, 103 in the second trimester and 79 in the third trimester. Forty-nine of these mothers were treated with specific antidotes (33 with NAC and 16 with methionine). There were 219 live-born infants, 11 have malformations (including minor); none had been exposed to acetaminophen during the first trimester. Nine women were treated with NAC during the first trimester; there were two elective terminations; two spontaneous abortions, and five healthy babies in this group.

In summary, acetaminophen overdose during pregnancy should be treated according to regular protocols in order to prevent maternal and potentially fetal toxicity. Unless severe maternal toxicity develops, an acetaminophen overdose does not increase the risk for birth defects or adverse pregnancy outcomes.

Physicians unfamiliar with the current management of acetaminophen overdose should consult with a Poison Control Centre immediately. Telephone numbers for local Poison Control Centres are available in the local phone directory. Delays in initiation of appropriate therapy may jeopardize the patient's chances for full recovery.

> For management of a suspected drug overdose, CPhA recommends that you contact your **regional Poison Control Centre**. See the *CPS* Directory section for a list of Poison Control Centres.

ACTION AND CLINICAL PHARMACOLOGY: Mechanism of Action: Acetaminophen is a centrally acting analgesic and antipyretic drug. Although the precise mechanism of action is not totally understood, work by Boutaud suggests acetaminophen is an inhibitor of the peroxidase portion of cyclooxygenase (prostaglandin H synthase inhibitor). Depending on the redox state and substrate concentrations surrounding the enzymes, acetaminophen may or may not have a significant inhibitory effect. This accounts for its selective activity on pain and fever with little anti-inflammatory effect.

It is postulated that the analgesic effect is produced by elevation of the pain threshold and the antipyretic effect is produced through action on the hypothalamic heat-regulating centre.

The optimal effective analgesic dose of acetaminophen was demonstrated in dental pain studies and is 1000 mg every four to six hours, up to 4000 mg daily. At least 500 published and unpublished controlled clinical trials in adults and children have evaluated acetaminophen for the relief of pain or fever. These studies include single and multiple dose treatments. Most studies were less than 14 days in duration, although the longest study duration was two years. No significant safety issues were reported in any of these studies.

Moreover, at recommended doses, acetaminophen has not been shown to increase the risk of developing renal diseases or upper gastrointestinal ulceration/bleeding. This observation is consistent with its minimal inhibitory effect on peripheral prostaglandin synthesis and on gastric prostaglandin synthesis.

Acetaminophen is considered equipotent to ASA and ibuprofen, within the recommended OTC dosing ranges, in its analgesic and antipyretic effects. Acetaminophen at recommended doses does not cause the type of gastrointestinal complications associated with NSAID-containing products, such as gastric irritation, gastric erosions, occult or overt gastrointestinal blood loss, or ulcers. Unlike these drugs, however, it has no anti-inflammatory effect at clinically relevant doses in humans.

Caffeine stimulates the CNS at all levels including the cortex. In addition, it acts on the kidney to produce diuresis, stimulates cardiac muscle and depresses smooth muscle.

Pharmacokinetics: Absorption: Oral acetaminophen is rapidly and almost completely absorbed from the gastrointestinal tract primarily in the small intestine. This absorption process occurs by passive transport. Peak plasma concentrations occur within 0.4 to 1 hour depending on the product formulation. Although high-fat foods delay the time to peak concentration for up to an hour, the dose is completely absorbed.

Caffeine is considered an effective analgesic adjuvant in combination with acetaminophen. It is thought to improve the rate of absorption of acetaminophen and enhance its analgesic effect. This adjuvancy effect has been demonstrated in a variety of pain states including headache.

Distribution: Acetaminophen is uniformly distributed throughout most body fluids, but not in fatty tissue. As a result, the volume of distribution in adults ranges between 0.8 and 1.0 L/kg. Since acetaminophen has low protein binding in plasma of only 10% to 25%, it does not compete with drugs that are highly protein bound.

Caffeine is rapidly distributed and appears in all tissues within 5 minutes with peak plasma levels being reached in 30 minutes.

Metabolism: Acetaminophen is primarily metabolized by the liver via three principal separate pathways: conjugation with glucuronide; conjugation with sulfate; oxidation via the cytochrome P450 mixed function oxidase system.

Both the glucuronic and oxidative pathways adhere to a first-order rate process, which means the concentration of acetaminophen metabolized increases as the concentration in the liver increases. The sulfate pathway adheres to Michaelis-Menten kinetics, which means the concentration of acetaminophen metabolized remains constant once the concentration in the liver increases above a saturation level. A schematic of acetaminophen metabolism is shown in Figure 2.

The major metabolic pathway is glucuronidation, where 47% to 62% of the acetaminophen dose conjugates with glucuronide. These glucuronide conjugates are inactive and nontoxic, and are secreted in bile and eliminated in the urine.

The second major pathway is sulfation, where 25% to 36% of the dose conjugates with sulfate. These sulfate ester conjugates are also inactive and nontoxic and are excreted in the urine.

The third pathway is oxidation, where 5% to 8% of the dose is metabolized via the cytochrome P450 enzyme system. The cytochrome P450 isoenzyme that is primarily responsible is CYP2E1. When acetaminophen is metabolized by CYP2E1, it forms a highly reactive intermediate, N-acetyl-p-benzoquinoneimine (NAPQI). Since NAPQI is highly reactive, it cannot be measured outside the liver nor can it accumulate. This intermediate is rapidly inactivated by hepatocellular stores of glutathione to form cysteine and mercapturate conjugates, which are both inactive and nontoxic. These conjugates are excreted in the urine.

Figure 2: TYLENOL Ultra Relief Migraine Pain Acetaminophen Metabolism

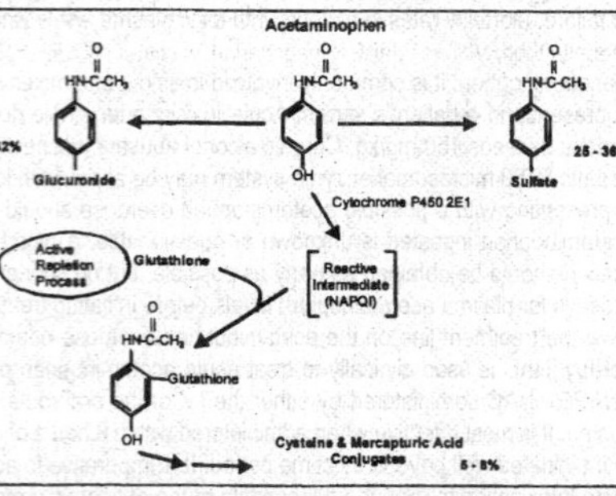

Caffeine is almost completely metabolized via oxidation, demethylation and acetylation, with only about 1% of caffeine excreted via the urine. The principle metabolites in humans are methyluric acid, 1-methylxanthine, paraxanthine and theobromine.

Excretion: Acetaminophen undergoes first-order elimination from the body, and has a short plasma half-life that ranges from 2 to 3 hours in healthy young and elderly adults and from 1.5 to 2.9 hours in children. Since acetaminophen clears rapidly from the body, repeated doses do not lead to accumulation of acetaminophen plasma concentrations.

STORAGE AND STABILITY: Store at room temperature (15 to 30°C).

DOSAGE FORMS, COMPOSITION AND PACKAGING: Each round, red, sweet-coated tablet, printed "TYLENOL Ultra" contains: acetaminophen 500 mg and caffeine 65 mg. Nonmedicinal ingredients: carnauba wax, cellulose, cornstarch, FD&C Blue no. 2, FD&C Red no. 40, hypromellose, iron oxide black, magnesium stearate, polydextrose, polyethylene glycol, propylene glycol, sodium starch glycolate, sucralose, titanium dioxide and triacetin. Energy: 1.1 kJ (0.3 kcal). Sodium: 0.4 mg. Gluten-, lactose- and tartrazine-free. Plastic bottles of 20*, 80* and 120†. All packages are safety sealed.

Typherix®

Salmonella typhi Vi capsular polysaccharide vaccine

Active Immunizing Agent

GlaxoSmithKline

Date of Revision: February 26, 2009

PHARMACOLOGY: Typhoid fever is an acute generalized infection caused by *S. typhi*, an organism for which humans are the only reservoir. The disease affects the reticuloendothelial system, intestinal lymphoid tissue and gall bladder.

The course of typhoid fever may be insidious, with fever that increases in stepwise fashion to reach 39-40°C, malaise, anorexia, myalgia, headache and abdominal discomfort. Without appropriate antimicrobial therapy, the fever remains for approximately 10-14 days. The most frequent serious complications, intestinal perforation and hemorrhage, occur in 0.5 to 1% of the infected population.

Typhoid fever is still a common disease and although its incidence is decreasing globally, it is still increasing in Asia, Africa and Latin America where more than 500 cases/100 000 people/year occur and where mortality is significant. In these developing countries, satisfactory control of drinking water, food, and sewage disposal has not yet been achieved. Infection is transmitted when susceptible hosts ingest fecally contaminated food or water; small numbers of organisms are ingested and many subclinical and mild infections occur for each fullblown clinical case of the disease.

In endemic areas, the majority of clinical infections occurs in 3- to 19-year-old children, the incidence decreases in adults from the age of 35 years. In contrast, common-source food outbreaks occur in more developed countries when chronic carriers contaminate food following a breakdown in personal and food hygiene; large numbers of organisms are present, attack rates are high and relatively few subclinical cases follow.

Although the incidence of typhoid fever is declining steadily in Canada, about 90 cases are still reported annually. Only a small number of these infections occur in Canada, with the vast majority occurring abroad. The decline in incidence of the disease has been primarily due to improved living conditions and to water and sewage treatment. Vaccine is not believed to have played a significant role. For travelers to areas where sanitation is likely to be poor, immunization is not a substitute for careful selection and handling of food and water.

* Container provided with a child-resistant closure.
† Easy-to-Open.

Clinical trials have been carried out in over 1570 subjects, to compare seropositivity (seroconversion is defined as an increase in anti-Vi antibody titres from <150 EL.U/mL pre vaccination to ≥150 EL.U/mL post vaccination) and geometric mean titres (GMT's) in subjects receiving either TYPHERIX (Salmonella typhi Vi Capsular Polysaccharide Vaccine) or TYPHIM Vi, (Sanofi Pasteur).

Two weeks after vaccination, seropositivity rates were at a maximum of 96.5% and 96.8% and GMTs were at 1554 and 1656 EL.U/mL in Typherix and Typhim Vi, (Sanofi Pasteur), respectively.

Two years following vaccination, seropositivity rates were 61.4% and 45.9%, and GMT's were 290 and 235 EL.U/mL in TYPHERIX and TYPHIM Vi, (Sanofi Pasteur), respectively.

An age-related trend could be observed in GMTs: the youngest age-group had a mean GMT of 3597 EL.U/mL compared with a mean of 1966 EL.U/mL in adolescents. Typherix proved to be immunogenic in both groups, with higher GMTs in children. Antibodies persisted in over 94% of those subjects available to be tested at month 6.

Immunity persists for at least 3 years.

INDICATIONS: For active immunization against typhoid fever in persons 2 years of age and older. One dose administered i.m. ensures protection for at least 3 years. The vaccine must be given at least 2 weeks prior to travel to endemic areas.

The Canadian Immunization Guide (CIG) recommends vaccination for:

1. Travelers who will have prolonged exposure to potentially contaminated food and water, especially those traveling to or working in small cities and villages, or to rural areas in countries with a high incidence of disease. Vaccination is not routinely recommended for short-term travel to resort hotels in such countries.
2. Persons with on-going household or intimate exposure to an *S. typhi* carrier.
3. Laboratory workers who frequently handle cultures of *S. typhi.*

CONTRAINDICATIONS: Should not be administered to subjects with known hypersensitivity to any component of the vaccine or to subjects having shown signs of hypersensitivity after previous administration.

As with other vaccines, the administration of Typherix should be postponed in subjects suffering from acute severe febrile illness.

WARNINGS: The vaccine protects against typhoid fever caused by *S. typhi*. Protection is not conferred against paratyphoid fever or illness caused by non-invasive Salmonellae.

The importance of scrupulous attention to personal, food and water hygiene must be emphasized for all persons at risk of typhoid fever.

Typherix should under no circumstances be administered intravascularly.

PRECAUTIONS: General: As with all injectable vaccines, appropriate medical treatment and supervision should always be readily available in case of a rare anaphylactic reaction following the administration of the vaccine.

Typherix should be administered with caution to subjects with thrombocytopenia or bleeding disorders since bleeding may occur following an i.m. administration to these subjects: following injection, firm pressure should be applied to the site (without rubbing) for at least 2 minutes.

Children: Typherix has not been evaluated in children under 2 years of age. Nevertheless, it is known that children under this age may show a suboptimal response to polysaccharide antigen vaccines. The decision to use the vaccine in this age group should be based upon the risk of exposure to disease.

Pregnancy: The effect of Typherix on fetal development has not been assessed. However, as with other purified polysaccharide vaccines, no effect is expected.

Typherix should only be used during pregnancy when there is a high risk of infection.

Lactation: The effect on breast-fed infants of the administration of Typherix to their mothers has not been evaluated in clinical studies. Typherix should therefore only be used in breast-feeding women, when there is a high risk of infection.

Drug Interactions: It may be expected that in patients receiving immunosuppressive treatment or patients with immunodeficiency, an adequate response may not be achieved.

In clinical studies in adults, Typherix has been administered simultaneously with Havrix 1440, GlaxoSmithKline Biologicals' inactivated hepatitis A vaccine. There was no adverse effect on either the reactogenicity or immunogenicity of the vaccines when they were administered simultaneously.

The concomitant administration of Typherix and vaccines other than Havrix 1440 has not specifically been studied.

ADVERSE EFFECTS: See Table 1, Table 2 and Table 3. The reactogenicity of Typherix was determined by systematic recording of local and general reactions to the vaccine. General symptoms occurred more frequently in adolescents and older children than in the adult and younger populations; it is not clear why this phenomenon was observed, but it can be said that the vast majority of symptoms reported were mild and transient in nature. The most frequent local symptom reported was soreness at the injection site, and headache and fever were the most frequent general symptoms.

In clinical studies, in the majority of instances, local reactions were usually reported only during the first 48 hours following immunization. The most common reaction, soreness, has been reported in approximately 7% of vaccinees.

In clinical studies, systemic reactions were also transient; the incidence of the most frequently reported symptoms, fever, headache, general aches, malaise, nausea and itching did not exceed 9%.

Anaphylaxis, allergic reactions, including anaphylactoid reactions and urticaria have been reported very rarely with Typherix.

Table 1: Typherix

Incidence of Solicited Local Symptoms in Healthy Adults

Symptom (N=551)		n	%
Soreness	All	52	9.4
	graded "3"	2	0.4
Redness	All	30	5.4
	>30 mm	1	0.2
Swelling	All	10	1.8
	>30 mm	0	—

Legend: N=total number of symptom sheets returned; n=number of symptom sheets with a report of a symptom.
Graded "3": severe: adverse experience which prevents normal everyday activities.

Table 2: Typherix

Incidence of Solicited General Symptoms in Healthy Adults

Symptom (N=400)		n	%
Fever	All	6	1.5
Headache	All	31	7.8
	graded "3"	2	0.5
General Aches	All	5	1.3
Malaise	All	16	4.0
Nausea	All	20	5.0
Itching	All	7	1.8
	graded "3"	1	0.3

No general aches, malaise or nausea graded "3" or temperature >39°C reported.
Graded "3": severe: adverse experience which prevents normal everyday activities.

Table 3: Typherix

Frequency of Solicited Symptoms in Adolescents and Children (Studies 003, 005, 006)

		005 (11–18 yrs) N=99		003 (5–15 yrs) N=199		006 (2–5 yrs) N=170	
		n	%	n	%	n	%
Local symptoms							
Soreness	All	16	16.2	1	0.5	0	—
Redness	All	1	1.0	1	0.5	9	5.3
Swelling	All	1	1.0	7	3.5	0	—
General Symptoms							
Fever	All >39°C	8 2	8.1 2.0	63 4	31.7 2.0	5 0	2.9 —
Headache	All	19	19.2	28	14.1	0	—
General Aches	All	13	13.1	6	3.0	1	0.6
Malaise	All	4	4.0	0	—	0	—
Nausea	All	3	3.0	7	3.5	0	—
Itching	All	8	8.1	0	—	0	—

Legend: N=total number of symptom sheets returned; n=number of symptom sheets with a report of a symptom.
Graded "3": severe: adverse experience which prevents normal everyday activities.

DOSAGE: Primary Immunization: A single dose of 0.5 mL containing 25 µg of the Vi polysaccharide of *S. typhi* is recommended.

Adults 19 years and older: Typherix can be co-administered with Havrix 1440 in opposite arms.

For other injectable vaccines, different syringes and different injection sites must be used.

Booster Dose: For individuals who remain at risk, or who may be re-exposed to risk of typhoid fever, it is recommended that they be revaccinated using a single dose of vaccine every 3 years.

Method of Administration: Typherix is for i.m. injection. Vaccines should be inspected for any foreign particulate matter and/or variation of physical aspect. In the event of either being observed, discard the vaccine.

Do not remove the white back-stop from the syringe. Prior to administration, ensure that the plunger rod is firmly attached to the rubber stopper by turning the plunger clockwise until slight resistance is felt. **Do not** over tighten. Remove syringe LUER Tip-cap and needle cap. Attach needle by pressing and twisting in a clockwise rotation until secured to the syringe.

Typherix should be administered with caution to subjects with thrombocytopenia or bleeding disorders, since bleeding may occur following an i.m. administration to these subjects: following injection, firm pressure should be applied to the site (without rubbing) for at least 2 minutes.

Typherix should under no circumstances be administered intravascularly.

SUPPLIED: Each 0.5 mL dose contains: Vi polysaccharide of *S. typhi* 25 µg. Single-dose prefilled syringes of 0.5 mL, in packages of 1, 10, 50 and 100.

Typherix is a clear colorless liquid containing the cell surface Vi polysaccharide extracted from *S. typhi* Ty2 strain.

The amount of Vi capsular polysaccharide (25 µg) complies with the European Pharmacopoeia and WHO recommendations for a Vi polysaccharide typhoid vaccine. The excipients present in the finished product are sodium chloride, sodium phosphate dihydrate, disodium phosphate dihydrate, phenol and water for injection.

The expiry date of the vaccine is indicated on the label and packaging. Store at 2 to 8°C. Protect from light. **Do not freeze; discard if vaccine has been frozen.**

Typhim Vi®

Salmonella typhi Vi capsular polysaccharide vaccine

Active Immunizing Agent

sanofi pasteur

Date of Revision: November 2005

PHARMACOLOGY: *S. typhi* is the etiological agent of typhoid fever, an acute, febrile enteric disease transmitted by contaminated water and food. The incidence of typhoid fever is very low in industrialized countries, with an average of 70 cases reported each year in Canada. The greatest risk of typhoid infection for Canadians occurs while they are travelling in countries or regions of countries where sanitation is likely to be poor.

Typhoid vaccination is not required for international travel, but it is recommended for travellers to areas where there is a recognized risk of exposure to *S. typhi. S. typhi* is prevalent in many countries of Africa and Asia, as well as Central and South America. Vaccination is particularly recommended for travellers who will have prolonged exposure (>4 weeks) to potentially contaminated food and water in smaller cities, villages, or rural areas in countries with a high incidence of disease. However, even travellers who have been vaccinated should use caution in selecting and handling food and water.

The fatality rate for untreated typhoid fever is approximately 16% but can be reduced to 1% with effective antibiotic therapy. Antibiotic resistance is increasing dramatically among *S. typhi* isolates complicating the treatment of this illness. Surveillance of US cases revealed that approximately 30% of isolates tested between 1990-1994 were resistant to at least one of the commonly used antibiotics. This compares to only 12% in the preceding five-year period. A Canadian study of samples isolated from travellers returning from South Asia and their contacts showed that 22% of specimens were resistant to at least 4 antibiotics.

An increase in specific serum antibodies is the predominant immune response elicited by injection of capsular polysaccharides. The Vi vaccine confers significant protection against typhoid fever based on the production of measurable antibodies, predominantly of the IgG class. The protective efficacy against typhoid fever of a single intramuscular injection of 25 µg of the TYPHIM Vi [Salmonella typhi Vi Capsular Polysaccharide Vaccine] was assessed in two randomized double-blind controlled trials.

A randomized, double-blind, controlled trial done in Nepal focused on a target population 5-44 years of age. There were 6907 vaccinated subjects, of whom 6438 were members of the target population; 3457 received Vi and 3450 received the control vaccine. There were 165 children under 5 years of age and 304 adults over 44. The protective efficacy of TYPHIM Vi is approximately 75% as shown in Table 1. The seroconversion rates (≥4-fold rise in serum antibodies), 76.9% in the 5-14 year age group, 79.1% in the 15-44 year age group and 62.5% in the over 45-55 year age group, were similar to the protective efficacy. This provides evidence that serum antibodies to the Vi antigen confer immunity to typhoid fever.

In a second double-blind, controlled efficacy trial conducted in South Africa 11 384 children ages 5-16 were immunized with TYPHIM Vi or a control vaccine, while a total of 23 075 children were followed. A total of 239 cases of blood-culture proven *S. typhi* infection occurred during the 21 month follow-up period among the 23 075 children participating (5.9 cases per annum, per 1000 children). There were 173 cases in the unvaccinated group (n=11 691) (8.5 cases per annum, per 1000 children), 47 cases in the children immunized with control vaccine (4.7 cases per annum, per 1000 children) and 19 cases in children immunized with the Vi vaccine (1.9 cases per annum, per 1000 children). The incidence of typhoid in the Vi immunized children was significantly lower than in the control vaccinated children (p <0.001). Estimates of vaccine efficacy after 21 months ranged from 60% (comparison to control group, all cases from date of immunization) to 81% (comparison to untreated group, all cases 6 weeks post immunization). Serology in a random sample of 0.5% of vaccinees showed an increase in anti-Vi antibodies as measured by radioimmunoassay and enzyme-linked immunosorbent assay. Antibody levels remained significantly elevated at 6 and 12 months post vaccination. Follow-up for 3 years following immunization showed a Vi vaccine efficacy of 50% in the third year.

Table 1: TYPHIM Vi

Efficacy of TYPHIM Vi Against Typhoid Fever in Nepal

Typhoid Fever Cases	Vaccine: Vi	Vaccine: Control	Efficacy %
Culture Positive	9	32	72
Clinically Suspected	5	25	80
Combined	14	57	75

A double-blind, controlled safety and immunogenicity trial of TYPHIM Vi involving 268 Indonesian children was designed to include younger children. The overall seroconversion rate was 98.7% one month after vaccination. The seroconversion rates for the different age groups were: 100% for 12-24 months, 98% for 24-60 months and 99% for children 60-144 months. Although antibody levels to Vi antigen are generally correlated with the protective levels, there are no specific data available to substantiate the efficacy in children 2 to 5 years old. No data are available on revaccination doses in children.

In the developed world, most individuals have not had previous exposure to *S. typhi*. Immunogenicity trials performed in Houston, Texas in a racially mixed adult American population (n=182) showed seroconversion rates and antibody levels equal to, or greater than, those seen in South Africa or Nepal. A four-fold rise in antibody level occurred by 1 week in 60%, by 2 weeks in 80% and by one month in 93% of those immunized with TYPHIM Vi. In a sub-group followed for nearly three years post-immunization (n=39), protective levels of antibody were still evident in 64% of individuals at 11 months and in 38% at 27 months. A second dose of Vi given at 27-34 months following initial immunization elicited antibody levels similar to those observed following the first dose.

French military experience suggests a high level of effectiveness when travellers from the developed world have been vaccinated with TYPHIM Vi. Between 1991-1995, more than 1.3 million members of the French military were vaccinated with TYPHIM Vi. Epidemiological surveillance was conducted through hospitalization and laboratory registries. Although 225 000 individuals travelled to endemic areas with an estimated exposure to *S. typhi* of 16 million person days, no cases of typhoid fever were reported.

A clinical trial involving 400 Belgian adults compared the tolerability and immunogenicity of a commercially available Vi polysaccharide vaccine to TYPHIM Vi. TYPHIM Vi produced a more immediate immune response with 86.4% of individuals who received TYPHIM Vi seroconverting by day 7 compared to only 65.6-76.7% of those receiving the other vaccine.

INDICATIONS: TYPHIM Vi [Salmonella typhi Vi Capsular Polysaccharide Vaccine] is indicated for active immunization against *S. typhi*, the organism which causes typhoid fever.

TYPHIM Vi is recommended for active immunization in persons 2 years of age and older in the following situations:

1. Travellers to endemic or epidemic areas or where sanitary conditions may be doubtful and where travellers may be exposed to potentially contaminated food and water, particularly when prolonged exposure is anticipated. (See Pharmacology and Warnings.)
2. Travellers with reduced or absent gastric acid secretion.
3. Persons with ongoing household or intimate exposure to a *S. typhi* carrier.
4. Laboratory workers who frequently handle cultures of *S. typhi*.

No data are available on the response to TYPHIM Vi in chronic carriers.

Human Immunodeficiency Virus (HIV) Infected Persons: HIV-infected persons may be safely immunized with TYPHIM Vi, but efficacy is significantly impaired in individuals with CD4 cell counts <200.

CONTRAINDICATIONS: Immunization with TYPHIM Vi [Salmonella typhi Vi Capsular Polysaccharide Vaccine] should be deferred in the presence of any acute illness, including febrile illness to avoid superimposing adverse effects from the vaccine on the underlying illness or mistakenly identifying a manifestation of the underlying illness as a complication of vaccine use. A minor illness such as mild upper respiratory infection is not reason to defer immunization.

Allergy to any component of TYPHIM Vi, or its container, or an anaphylactic or other allergic reaction to a previous dose of TYPHIM Vi is a contraindication to vaccination. (See components listed in Supplied.)

WARNINGS: As with any vaccine, immunization with TYPHIM Vi [Salmonella typhi Vi Capsular Polysaccharide Vaccine] may not protect 100% of susceptible individuals. This vaccine will not afford protection against species of Salmonella other than *S. typhi* or against other bacteria that cause enteric disease. Immunity may be overwhelmed by a large inoculum of *S. typhi*. Warn vaccinees that immunization is only one preventive measure and that care in selection of food and water is of primary importance.

If the vaccine is administered less than 2 weeks prior to departure, optimum antibody protection may not yet be reached. (See Pharmacology.)

Intramuscular injections should be given with care in persons suffering from coagulation disorders or on anticoagulant therapy because of the risk of hemorrhage.

TYPHIM Vi should not be administered into the buttocks due to the varying amount of fatty tissue in this region, nor by the intradermal route, since these methods of administration may induce a weaker immune response.

Immunocompromised persons (whether from disease or treatment) may not obtain the expected immune response. If possible, consideration should be given to delaying vaccination until after the completion of any immunosuppressive treatment.

PRECAUTIONS: The possibility of allergic reactions in persons sensitive to components of the vaccine should be evaluated. Epinephrine Hydrochloride Solution (1:1000) and other appropriate agents should be available for immediate use in case an anaphylactic or acute hypersensitivity reaction occurs. Health-care providers should be familiar with current recommendations for the initial management of anaphylaxis in non-hospital settings, including proper airway management.

For instructions on recognition and treatment of anaphylactic reactions, see the current edition of the Canadian Immunization Guide or visit the Health Canada Website.

Before administration, take all appropriate precautions to prevent adverse reactions. This includes a review of the patient's history concerning possible hypersensitivity to the vaccine or similar vaccine, previous immunization history, the presence of any contraindications to immunization and current health status.

Before administration of TYPHIM Vi, [Salmonella typhi Vi Capsular Polysaccharide Vaccine] health-care providers should inform the patient, parent or guardian of the benefits and risks of immunization, inquire about the recent health status of the patient and comply with any local requirements regarding information to be provided to the patient before immunization.

If a patient returns for revaccination, it is extremely important that the patient, parent or guardian be questioned concerning any symptoms and/or signs of an adverse reaction after a previous dose of vaccine. (See Contraindications and Adverse Effects.)

Do not inject into a blood vessel.

Use a separate sterile needle and syringe, or a sterile disposable unit, for each individual dose to prevent disease transmission.

There have been case reports of transmission of HIV and hepatitis by failure to scrupulously observe sterile technique. In particular, the same needle and/or syringe must never be used to re-enter a multidose vial to withdraw vaccine even when it is to be used for inoculation of the same patient. This may lead to contamination of the vial contents and infection of patients who subsequently receive vaccine from the vial.

Drug Interactions: There are no known interactions of TYPHIM Vi with drugs or foods.

TYPHIM Vi may be administered during the same patient visit with other vaccines commonly administered to international travellers, including vaccines which protect against meningococcus (groups A and C), hepatitis A and yellow fever. There is no known interaction between TYPHIM Vi and other live or inactivated vaccines. Vaccines should be administered at separate sites using separate syringes.

TYPHIM Vi should not be mixed in the same syringe with other vaccines, unless supplied as a combination product by the manufacturer.

Pregnancy: Animal reproduction studies have not been conducted with TYPHIM Vi. It is also not known whether TYPHIM Vi can cause fetal harm when administered to a pregnant woman or can affect reproductive capacity. Although the administration of typhoid vaccine would not be expected to have any adverse effects, its safety in pregnancy has not been directly studied. Therefore, the benefits of vaccination must be carefully weighed against the potential adverse effects before it is given to a pregnant women.

Lactation: The effect of administration of TYPHIM Vi during lactation has not been assessed. As TYPHIM Vi is inactivated, any risk to the mother or the infant is improbable. TYPHIM Vi should only be used in lactating women after careful consideration of the risk-benefit ratio.

Children: Safety and immunogenicity of TYPHIM Vi have been demonstrated in children 2 years of age and older. (See Pharmacology.)

ADVERSE EFFECTS: Adverse reactions reported after vaccination with TYPHIM Vi [Salmonella typhi Vi Capsular Polysaccharide Vaccine] are usually mild and short lasting. They consist mainly of local reactions at the site of injection (pain, edema, redness) and mild systemic reactions such as headache or malaise. Tolerance has been studied in more than 10 000 subjects both in countries of high and low endemicity.

Adverse reactions from trials in Houston, Texas (18-40 year old adults) are summarized in Table 2. No severe or unusual side effects were observed.

Table 2: TYPHIM Vi

Percentage of 18 to 40-Year-old Adults Presenting with Local or Systemic Reactions Within the First 24 to 48 Hours After Immunization with TYPHIM Vi

Reaction	TYPHIM Vi Trial 1 (%) (n=54)	TYPHIM Vi Trial 2 (%) (n=98)
General Disorders and Administration Site Conditions		
Injection site tenderness	98	96.9
Injection site pain	40.7	26.5
Induration	14.8	5.1
Erythema at injection site	3.7	5.1
Malaise	24	8.3
Fever	2	3.1
Nervous System Disorders		
Headache	20.3	16.3
Musculoskeletal, Connective and Bone Disorders		
Myalgia	7.4	3.1
Gastrointestinal Disorders		
Nausea	1.9	8.1
Vomiting	1.9	0
Diarrhea	0	3.0

Adults who received a booster dose of TYPHIM Vi 27 to 34 months following the initial dose were more likely to develop erythema and/or induration (10/55) than those given a first dose (13/182), but the rate of systemic reactions was not increased.

Adverse reactions from a trial in Indonesia in children 1 to 7 years old are summarized in Table 3. No severe or unusual side effects were observed.

Table 3: TYPHIM Vi

Percentage of Children 1 to 7 Years Presenting with Local or Systemic Reactions After Immunization with TYPHIM Vi

	Children (Age In Months)		
	12–24 (n=21)	24–60 (n=66)	60–144 (n=88)
General Disorders and Administration Site Conditions			
Soreness at the injection site	4.8	4.6	21
Pain at the injection site	9.6	9.1	19
Erythema at the injection site	0	4.6	10.2
Induration	4.8	3	2.3
Fever	0	3	3.4
Headache	0	0	0
Decreased activity	0	4.6	0
Rash	0	0	0

Adverse reactions associated with TYPHIM Vi are very rarely reported in post-market surveillance. From 1998-2002 the following adverse reactions were reported:

Gastrointestinal Disorders: Very rare (<1:10 000): nausea, vomiting, diarrhea.

General Disorders and Administration Site Conditions: Very rare (<1:10 000): injection site pain, injection site rash, abdominal pain, fever, malaise, asthenia.

Immune System Disorders: Very rare (<1:10 000): anaphylactic reaction, serum sickness.

Musculoskeletal and Connective Tissue Disorders: Very rare (<1:10 000): arthralgia, myalgia.

Respiratory, Thoracic and Mediastinal Disorders: Very rare (<1:10 000): asthma.

Nervous System Disorders: Very rare (<1:10 000): headache.

Skin and Subcutaneous Tissue Disorders: Very rare (<1:10 000): injection site inflammation, urticaria.

Physicians, nurses and pharmacists should report any adverse occurrences temporally associated with the administration of the product in accordance with local requirements and to the Global Pharmacovigilance Department, Sanofi Pasteur Limited, 1755 Steeles Avenue West, Toronto, ON, M2R 3T4, Canada. 1-888-621-1146 (phone) or 416-667-2435 (fax).

DOSAGE: The immunizing dose is a single injection of 0.5 mL given intramuscularly.

Inspect for extraneous particulate matter and/or discolouration before use. If these conditions exist, the product should not be administered. (See Supplied.)

For information on vaccine administration, see the current edition of the Canadian Immunization Guide or visit the Health Canada website.

Shake the vial/prefilled syringe well to uniformly distribute the solution before use.

When administering a dose from a prefilled syringe, remove the tip cap from the syringe. Select a needle of appropriate length to ensure that the vaccine will be delivered intramuscularly. Remove the selected needle from the blister pack and fix to the tip of the prefilled syringe.

When administering a dose from a stoppered vial, remove the plastic flip off cap. Do not remove either the stopper or the metal seal holding it in place. Aseptic technique must be used for withdrawal of each dose. (See Precautions.)

Administer the dose intramuscularly. The preferred site is into the deltoid muscle or into the anterolateral aspect of the mid thigh (vastus lateralis muscle).

Do not inject intravenously.

Needles should not be recapped and should be disposed of properly.

Revaccination every three years under conditions of repeated or continuous exposure to *S. typhi* is recommended.

Give the patient a permanent personal immunization record. In addition, it is essential that the physician or nurse record the immunization history in the permanent medical record of each patient. This permanent office record should contain the name of the vaccine, date given, dose, manufacturer and lot number.

SUPPLIED: TYPHIM Vi [Salmonella typhi Vi Capsular Polysaccharide Vaccine], produced by Sanofi Pasteur SA, is a sterile, clear, colourless solution ready for intramuscular injection. The Vi antigen contained in TYPHIM Vi is extracted from the bacterial capsule of *S. typhi* strain Ty2. TYPHIM Vi complies with the World Health Organization's requirements for Vi polysaccharide typhoid vaccine. Each dose (0.5 mL) contains: *Salmonella typhi* (Ty2 strain) purified Vi capsular polysaccharide 25 µg, phenol (as preservative) 0.25% w/v, isotonic buffer solution up to 0.5 mL.

Prefilled syringes of 0.5 mL with a choice of two needles (1×25G×16 mm and 1×25G×25 mm). Vials of 10 mL (20 doses). Neither the stopper of the vial nor the plunger stopper of the syringe for this product contains dry natural latex rubber. Store at 2 to 8°C. **Do not freeze.** Discard product if exposed to freezing. Do not use after expiration date.

Tysabri® Ⓟ

natalizumab

Selective Adhesion Molecule Inhibitor

Biogen Idec

Date of Revision: March 30, 2010

SUMMARY PRODUCT INFORMATION:

Route of Administration	Dosage Form/ Strength	Clinically Relevant Nonmedicinal Ingredients
Intravenous infusion	Concentrate for solution/300 mg per 15 mL	There are no clinically relevant nonmedicinal ingredients. For a complete listing of nonmedicinal ingredients see Dosage Forms, Composition and Packaging.

DESCRIPTION: TYSABRI (natalizumab) is a recombinant humanized IgG_{4k} monoclonal antibody selective for α4-integrin. Natalizumab is produced in murine myeloma cells. The molecular weight of natalizumab is 149 kilodaltons. TYSABRI is supplied as a sterile, colourless, clear to slightly opalescent concentrate for solution for intravenous (IV) infusion.

INDICATIONS AND CLINICAL USE: TYSABRI (natalizumab) is indicated as monotherapy (i.e. single disease-modifying agent) for the treatment of patients with the relapsing-remitting form of multiple sclerosis (MS) to reduce the frequency of clinical exacerbations, to decrease the number and volume of active brain lesions identified on magnetic resonance imaging (MRI) scans and to delay the progression of physical disability. TYSABRI is generally recommended in MS patients who have had an inadequate response to, or are unable to tolerate, other therapies for multiple sclerosis.

Safety and efficacy in patients with chronic progressive multiple sclerosis, and in geriatric and pediatric patients, have not been established.

The efficacy of TYSABRI for a treatment duration beyond 2 years has not been determined.

TYSABRI should be used by physicians who have sufficient knowledge of multiple sclerosis and who have familiarized themselves with the efficacy/safety profile of TYSABRI.

Geriatrics (>65 years of age): Clinical studies of TYSABRI did not include sufficient numbers of patients aged 65 years and over to determine whether they respond differently than younger patients.

Pediatrics (<18 years of age): Safety and effectiveness of TYSABRI in pediatric patients with multiple sclerosis have not been studied.

CONTRAINDICATIONS:

- Patients who are hypersensitive to this drug or to any ingredient in the formulation or component of the container. For a complete listing, see Dosage Forms, Composition and Packaging.
- Patients who have or have had progressive multifocal leukoencephalopathy (PML).
- Patients who are immunocompromised, including those immunocompromised due to immunosuppressant or antineoplastic therapies, or immunodeficiencies (HIV, leukemias, lymphomas, etc.).

WARNINGS AND PRECAUTIONS:

Serious Warnings and Precautions

- **Treatment with TYSABRI (natalizumab) has been associated with an increased risk of progressive multifocal leukoencephalopathy (PML). PML can cause disability or death (see Warnings and Precautions, Infections; Contraindications; and Adverse Reactions).**
- **Healthcare professionals should monitor patients on TYSABRI for any new sign or symptom that may be suggestive of PML. TYSABRI dosing should be withheld immediately at the first sign or symptom suggestive of PML.**

General: Before initiation of treatment with TYSABRI (natalizumab), a recent magnetic resonance image (MRI) should be available. This MRI may be helpful in differentiating subsequent MS symptoms from PML. For diagnosis of PML, an evaluation that includes a gadolinium-enhanced magnetic resonance imaging (MRI) scan of the brain and, when indicated, cerebrospinal fluid analysis for JC viral DNA are recommended (see Warnings and Precautions, Infections).

Patients who are prescribed TYSABRI are to be enrolled in the TYSABRI Care Program (TCP)—a registry of Canadian patients. To enroll, physicians fax an enrollment form to 1-877-827-2827. The TCP is a comprehensive program associated with the prescribing, administration and monitoring of patients who receive TYSABRI treatment. Prescribers and TCP healthcare professionals are educated regarding the appropriate use of TYSABRI. Prescribers are expected to educate patients on the benefits and risks of treatment, especially the risk of PML. Patients should remain under medical supervision while receiving TYSABRI and should be evaluated by the prescriber every six months.

At 24 months of treatment, physicians should inform patients again about the risks of TYSABRI, including that the risk of PML increases with longer treatment duration. Physicians should obtain consent from their patients for continuation of treatment. At 24 months of treatment, the patient, their partner and/or caregiver should be re-instructed about the early signs and symptoms of PML.

Carcinogenesis and Mutagenesis: No clastogenic or mutagenic effects of natalizumab were observed in the Ames human chromosomal aberration assays. Natalizumab showed no effects on in vitro assays of α4-integrin-positive human tumour line proliferation/cytotoxicity. Xenograft transplantation models in SCID and nude mice with two α4-integrin-positive human tumour lines (leukemia, melanoma) demonstrated no increase in tumour growth rates or metastasis resulting from natalizumab treatment.

Hematologic: TYSABRI induces increases in circulating lymphocytes, monocytes, eosinophils and nucleated red blood cells. During phase 3 clinical trials, cell counts were measured every 12 weeks. The largest cell increases were seen in lymphocytes, which were found to be elevated within 12 weeks after initiating TYSABRI treatment, reaching a plateau by 24 weeks. Although elevated, mean cell counts remained within the normal range. Observed increases persist during TYSABRI exposure, but are reversible, returning to baseline levels usually within 16 weeks after the last dose. Elevations of neutrophils were not observed. TYSABRI also induces mild decreases in hemoglobin levels that are frequently transient. These observations were not associated with clinical symptoms; therefore routine blood monitoring is not required.

Hepatic/Biliary/Pancreatic: In post-marketing experience there have been rare reports of clinically significant liver injury, including markedly elevated serum hepatic enzymes and elevated total bilirubin, as early as 6 days after the first dose. In some patients, liver injury recurred upon rechallenge. Some cases occurred in patients with pre-existing liver disease or in the presence of other drugs that have been associated with hepatic injury. Patients with history of liver disease, alcohol abuse, and/or treatment with other therapies that are known to cause liver injury should be carefully evaluated prior to commencement of treatment with TYSABRI and closely monitored for possible liver damage during and after treatment. TYSABRI should be discontinued in patients who develop jaundice or other evidence of clinically significant liver injury, e.g., 5-fold or greater elevation in serum hepatic enzymes, and the patient should be fully evaluated. In cases with no other identifiable cause, TYSABRI should be permanently discontinued.

Infections: Progressive Multifocal Leukoencephalopathy: Use of TYSABRI has been associated with an increased risk of progressive multifocal leukoencephalopathy (PML). PML can cause severe disability or death.

Clinical Trial Data: Cases of PML included patients who were treated with TYSABRI for over 2 years or who received intermittent doses of TYSABRI over an 18-month period. In clinical trials, two cases of PML were observed in 1869 patients with multiple sclerosis treated for a median of 120 weeks; the third case occurred among 1043 patients with Crohn's disease after the patient received 8 doses. These patients were concomitantly exposed to immunomodulators (e.g. interferon beta) or were immunocompromised due to treatment with immunosuppressants (e.g. azathioprine).

Post-Marketing Experience: There have been rare reports of PML in patients who received TYSABRI monotherapy.

In patients treated with TYSABRI for up to 3 years, the risk of PML appears to increase with longer treatment duration. For patients treated up to 24 months, the rate of PML is below that observed in pre-approval clinical trials. In patients treated for greater than 24 months in the post-marketing setting, the rate of PML is generally similar to the rates seen in clinical trials. There is limited experience beyond 3 years of treatment, therefore the risk of PML in these patients cannot currently be estimated.

The treating physician must inform the patient of the risks of TYSABRI, especially the increased risk of PML. The patient should remain under medical supervision while on TYSABRI. At 24 months of treatment, physicians should inform patients again about the risks of TYSABRI, including that the risk of PML increases with longer treatment duration. Physicians should obtain consent from their patients for continuation of treatment. At 24 months of treatment, the patient, their partner and/or caregiver should be re-instructed about the early signs and symptoms of PML.

TYSABRI should be suspended immediately at the first signs or symptoms suggestive of PML and an evaluation that includes a gadolinium-enhanced magnetic resonance imaging (MRI) scan of the brain should be performed. When indicated, cerebrospinal fluid analysis for JC viral DNA is recommended to confirm a diagnosis of PML. If initial investigations prove negative but clinical suspicion for PML still remains, TYSABRI should not be restarted and repeat investigations should be undertaken. Pretreatment investigations (e.g. magnetic resonance imaging) may be helpful in the evaluation of patients who may develop signs or symptoms suggestive of PML. Patients being treated with TYSABRI should be instructed to report any new neurological signs or symptoms to their physician.

In the postmarketing setting, early detection of PML and suspension of TYSABRI therapy may have contributed to improved survival rates from PML compared with the TYSABRI pre-approval clinical trial PML cases. Plasma exchange has been used to reduce the serum levels of TYSABRI.

In TYSABRI treated patients who developed PML, Immune Reconstitution Inflammatory Syndrome (IRIS) has been described following PML; this can lead to serious neurological complications. IRIS has been reported and occurred after discontinuation or removal of TYSABRI (by plasma exchange). In patients who have undergone plasma exchange, IRIS has occurred within days to several weeks. IRIS presents as a worsening in neurological status that may be rapid, as a result of the sudden reconstitution of immune function. It can lead to serious neurological complications and may be fatal. Monitoring for development of IRIS and appropriate treatment of the associated inflammatory reaction involving the brain should be undertaken.

There are no known interventions that can reliably prevent PML or adequately treat PML if it occurs. It is not known whether early detection of PML and discontinuation of TYSABRI will mitigate the disease.

It is unclear whether the risk of PML is increased in MS patients treated with TYSABRI in combination with interferon beta compared to TYSABRI alone. Until more is known, TYSABRI should not be used in combination with other immunosuppressive or immunomodulatory agents, regardless of their class.

Short courses of corticosteroids can be used in combination with TYSABRI. In phase 3 MS clinical trials, concomitant treatment of relapses with a short course of corticosteroids was not associated with an increased rate of infection in patients treated with TYSABRI as compared with those on placebo.

Healthcare professionals should be alert to any new signs or symptoms that may be suggestive of PML. Typical symptoms of PML are diverse, progress over days to weeks, and include progressive weakness on one side of the body or clumsiness of limbs, disturbance of vision, and changes in thinking, memory and orientation leading to confusion and personality changes.

Immune: Hypersensitivity Reactions: TYSABRI has been associated with hypersensitivity reactions, which occurred at an incidence of 4%, including serious systemic reactions (e.g. anaphylaxis), which occurred at an incidence of <1%. These reactions usually occurred within 2 hours of the start of the infusion. Symptoms associated with these reactions included urticaria, dizziness, fever, rash, rigors, pruritus, nausea, flushing, hypotension, dyspnea and chest pain. Generally, these reactions are associated with antibodies to TYSABRI. The risk for hypersensitivity was greatest with early infusions and in patients re-exposed to TYSABRI following an initial short exposure (up to three infusions) and extended period (three months or more) without treatment. If a hypersensitivity reaction occurs, discontinue administration of TYSABRI immediately and initiate appropriate therapy.

Physicians should inform patients about the importance of uninterrupted dosing, particularly in the early months of treatment.

Post-Marketing Experience: There have been reports of hypersensitivity reactions which have been associated with one or more of the following: hypotension, hypertension, chest pain, chest discomfort, and dyspnea.

Immunosuppression: The safety and efficacy of TYSABRI in combination with antineoplastic or immunosuppressive agents have not been established. Concurrent use of these agents with TYSABRI may increase the risk of infections, including opportunistic infections. In clinical studies for conditions other than MS, opportunistic infections (e.g. *P. carinii* pneumonia, pulmonary *M. avium*-intracellulare, bronchopulmonary aspergillosis and *B. cepacia*) have been uncommonly observed in patients receiving TYSABRI; some of these patients were receiving concurrent immunosuppressants (see Adverse Reactions). In pivotal clinical trials (1801 and 1802), concomitant treatment of relapses with a short course of corticosteroids was not associated with an increased rate of infection in patients treated with TYSABRI as compared with placebo.

Immunizations: No data are available on the effects of vaccination in patients receiving TYSABRI. Similarly, no data are available on the secondary transmission of infection by live vaccines in patients receiving TYSABRI.

Special Populations: Pregnant Women: There are no adequate and well-controlled studies of TYSABRI therapy in pregnant women. In premarketing clinical trials, the extent of exposure is very limited. Because animal reproduction studies are not always predictive of human response, this drug should only be used during pregnancy if clearly needed. If a woman becomes pregnant while taking TYSABRI, discontinuation of TYSABRI should be considered.

In reproductive studies in monkeys and guinea pigs, there was no evidence of teratogenic effects or effects on survival or growth of offspring at doses up to 30 mg/kg (7 times the human clinical dose based on body weight comparison). In one of five studies that exposed monkeys or guinea pigs during pregnancy, the number of abortions in treated (30 mg/kg) monkeys was 33% vs. 17% in controls. No effects on abortion rates were noted in any other study. A study in pregnant cynomolgus monkeys treated at 2.3-fold the clinical dose demonstrated natalizumab-related changes in the fetus. These changes included mild anemia, reduced platelet count, increased spleen weights, and reduced liver and thymus weights associated with increased splenic extramedullary hematopoiesis, thymic atrophy and decreased hepatic hematopoiesis. In offspring born to mothers treated with natalizumab at 7-fold the clinical dose, platelet counts were also reduced. This effect was reversed upon clearance of natalizumab. There was no evidence of anemia in these offspring.

Nursing Women: It is unknown if natalizumab is excreted in human milk. Because many drugs are excreted in human milk and the potential for serious adverse reactions is unknown, discontinuation of nursing or TYSABRI should be considered.

Pediatrics (<18 years): Safety and effectiveness of TYSABRI in pediatric MS patients have not been studied.

Geriatrics (>65 years): Clinical studies of TYSABRI did not include sufficient numbers of patients to determine whether they respond differently than younger patients.

ADVERSE REACTIONS: Adverse Drug Reaction Overview: Serious adverse drug reactions most frequently reported during treatment with TYSABRI (natalizumab) in clinical trials were infections (3.2% vs. 2.6% placebo, including urinary tract infection [0.8% vs. 0.3%] and pneumonia [0.6% vs. 0%]); acute hypersensitivity reactions (1.1% vs. 0.3%, including anaphylaxis/anaphylactoid reaction [0.8% vs. 0%]); depression (1.0% vs. 1.0%, including suicidal ideation [0.6% vs. 0.3%]); and cholelithiasis (1.0% vs. 0.3%) (see Warnings and Precautions, Immune, Hypersensitivity Reactions).

The most frequently reported adverse events leading to discontinuation of TYSABRI therapy were urticaria (1%) and other hypersensitivity reactions (1%) (see Warnings and Precautions, Immune, Hypersensitivity Reactions).

In clinical trials, cases of PML have been reported. PML can cause severe disability or death. Two cases occurred in MS patients who were being treated with concomitant interferon beta-1a for more than 2 years. One patient in other clinical trials who had a long history of treatment with immunosuppressants and associated leucopenia also developed PML (see Warnings and Precautions, Infections).

Clinical Trial Adverse Drug Reactions: Because clinical trials are conducted under very specific conditions the adverse reaction rates observed in the clinical trials may not reflect the rates observed in practice and should not be compared to the rates in the clinical trials of another drug. Adverse drug reaction information from clinical trials is useful for identifying drug-related adverse events and for approximating rates.

Summary Listing of Adverse Events: In placebo-controlled trials in 1617 patients with multiple sclerosis treated with TYSABRI, the incidence of common events was balanced between the TYSABRI-treated patients and those who received placebo. Adverse events leading to discontinuation of therapy occurred in 5.8% of patients receiving TYSABRI and in 4.8% of patients receiving placebo. Events are listed in Table 1 by body system and frequency of occurrence in the TYSABRI group.

Table 1: TYSABRI

All Adverse Events in Placebo-Controlled Studies of MS Occurring with Incidence ≥1.0% in TYSABRI Group and >0.5% in TYSABRI Group than Placebo Group

System Organ Class	Preferred Term	Placebo (n=1135)	TYSABRI (n=1617)
Infections and Infestations	Influenza	146 (12.9%)	225 (13.9%)
	Sinusitis	122 (10.7%)	184 (11.4%)
	Upper respiratory tract infection viral	88 (7.8%)	134 (8.3%)
	Pharyngitis	59 (5.2%)	125 (7.7%)
	Gastroenteritis	21 (1.9%)	56 (3.5%)
	Tonsillitis	23 (2.0%)	51 (3.2%)
	Bladder infection	16 (1.4%)	38 (2.4%)
	Herpes zoster	16 (1.4%)	33 (2.0%)
	Respiratory tract infection	15 (1.3%)	30 (1.9%)
	Gingival infection	6 (0.5%)	18 (1.1%)
Blood and Lymphatic System Disorders	Anemia	14 (1.2%)	30 (1.9%)
Immune System Disorders	Seasonal allergy	35 (3.1%)	58 (3.6%)
Psychiatric Disorders	Depressed mood	16 (1.4%)	37 (2.3%)
Nervous System Disorders	Headache	436 (38.4%)	634 (39.2%)
	Dysesthesia	23 (2.0%)	42 (2.6%)
	Sinus headache	19 (1.7%)	38 (2.4%)
Cardiac Disorders	Tachycardia	9 (0.8%)	23 (1.4%)
Vascular Disorders	Hematoma	6 (0.5%)	17 (1.1%)
Respiratory, Thoracic and Mediastinal Disorders	Cough	81 (7.1%)	130 (8.0%)
	Sinus congestion	22 (1.9%)	51 (3.2%)
	Epistaxis	13 (1.1%)	28 (1.7%)
Gastrointestinal Disorders	Abdominal pain	43 (3.8%)	75 (4.6%)
Musculoskeletal and Connective Tissue Disorders	Muscle cramp	42 (3.7%)	82 (5.1%)
	Joint swelling	13 (1.1%)	32 (2.0%)
Reproductive System and Breast Disorders	Menstruation irregular	12 (1.1%)	37 (2.3%)
General Disorders and Administration Site Conditions	Fatigue	305 (26.9%)	445 (27.5%)
	Oedema peripheral	25 (2.2%)	62 (3.8%)
	Chest pain	35 (3.1%)	58 (3.6%)
	Rigors	12 (1.1%)	55 (3.4%)
	Weight decreased	11 (1.0%)	27 (1.7%)
Injury, Poisoning, Procedural Complications	Limb injury	20 (1.8%)	38 (2.4%)
	Thermal burn	12 (1.1%)	29 (1.8%)

Additional Information: Hypersensitivity: The incidence of hypersensitivity reactions was based on the investigator assessment that the event was urticaria or an allergic reaction, which may have included terms such as urticaria, itch, flushing, hypersensitivity or anaphylactoid reaction. In controlled clinical trials in MS patients, hypersensitivity reactions occurred in up to 4% of patients. Serious systemic hypersensitivity reactions (e.g. anaphylactic/anaphylactoid) occurred in <1% (study 1801: 5/627) of MS patients. Hypersensitivity reactions usually occurred within two hours of the start of the infusion.

Immunogenicity: Persistent anti-natalizumab antibodies (detected on two occasions at least 6 weeks apart) were associated with decreased efficacy of TYSABRI and an increased incidence of hypersensitivity reactions. The majority of patients who became persistently antibody-positive had developed antibodies by 12 weeks.

In controlled clinical trials in MS patients, persistent anti-natalizumab antibodies developed in approximately 6% of patients. Antibodies were detected on only one occasion in 4% of patients. Additional infusion-related reactions associated with persistent antibodies included rigors, nausea, vomiting and flushing. Approximately 90% of patients who became persistently antibody-positive in 2-year clinical trials had developed antibodies by 12 weeks.

If, after 3 months of TYSABRI treatment, the presence of persistent antibodies is suspected, or in patients who have received an initial short exposure to TYSABRI and extended periods without treatment, antibody testing should be performed. Antibodies may be detected and confirmed with sequential serum antibody tests. Antibodies detected early in the treatment course (e.g. within 6 months) may be transient and disappear with continued dosing. Repeat testing between 6 weeks and 3 months after the initial positive result is recommended in patients in whom antibodies are detected to confirm that antibodies are persistent. In the presence of persistent antibodies, discontinuation of treatment with TYSABRI should be considered (see Figure 1).

Information regarding the availability and location of testing laboratories may be obtained by contacting Biogen Idec Canada at 1-888-827-2827.

Figure 1: TYSABRI

Subject Relapse Rate Prior to and After Antibody Detection—Persistent Positives—Study 1801

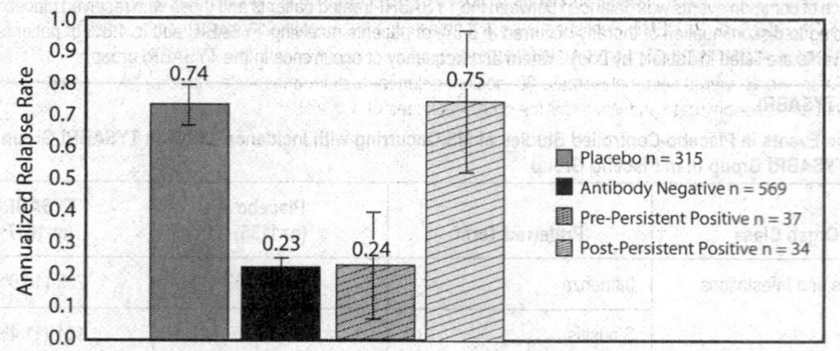

Infections: In controlled clinical trials in MS patients, the rate of infection was approximately 1.5 per patient year in both TYSABRI and placebo-treated patients. The nature of the infections was generally similar in TYSABRI and placebo-treated patients. The majority of patients did not interrupt TYSABRI therapy during infections, and recovery occurred with appropriate treatment.

In clinical trials, cases of PML have been reported (see Warnings and Precautions, Infections; and Adverse Drug Reaction Overview).

In other clinical trials, cases of opportunistic infections have been reported. While a causal role for natalizumab cannot be excluded, it is reasonable to conclude that comorbidities and concomitant medications played an important role in these infections. Should a serious opportunistic infection develop, TYSABRI therapy should be withheld until the infection has been successfully treated (see Warnings and Precautions, Immunosuppression).

In clinical trials, herpes infections occurred slightly more frequently in natalizumab-treated patients than in placebo-treated patients. During post-marketing experience, there have been rare reports of serious cases. Should a serious herpes infection occur, TYSABRI therapy should be withheld until the infection has been treated.

Infusion-Related Reactions: An infusion-related reaction was defined in clinical trials as any adverse event occurring within 2 hours of the start of an infusion. These events occurred in 23.1% of MS patients treated with TYSABRI (18.7% placebo). Events reported more commonly with TYSABRI than with placebo included headache, dizziness, fatigue, urticaria, pruritus and rigors.

Malignancies: No differences in incidence rates or the nature of malignancies between TYSABRI and placebo-treated patients were observed over 2 years of treatment. Should a malignancy develop, TYSABRI therapy should be withheld at least until appropriate treatment has been initiated for the malignancy and the benefit and risks of resuming TYSABRI therapy have been deemed to be acceptable by the treating physician.

Less Common Clinical Trial Adverse Drug Reactions: The incidence of adverse drug reactions experienced by <1% of subjects in natalizumab group and at least 0.1% higher in natalizumab compared to placebo are listed below:

Blood and Lymphatic System Disorders: anemia, thrombocytopenia, leukocytosis.

Cardiac Disorders: tachycardia, angina pectoris.

Ear and Labyrinth Disorders: vertigo.

Gastrointestinal Disorders: flatulence, upper abdominal pain, abdominal distention, epigastric discomfort.

General Disorders and Administration Site Conditions: feeling hot, peripheral edema, lethargy, feeling abnormal, infusion site erythema, pain, thirst, hyperpyrexia, infusion site pruritus.

Immune System Disorders: hypersensitivity, anaphylactoid reaction, anaphylactic reaction.

Infections and Infestations: progressive multifocal leukoencephalopathy, pharyngitis, sinusitis, herpes simplex, herpes zoster, rhinitis infective, bronchial infection, gastroenteritis, skin and subcutaneous tissue abscess, furuncle, pharyngitis streptococcal, bladder infection, breast abscess, dermatitis infected, herpes viral infection, oral infection, pharyngitis viral, tooth infection, urinary tract infection.

Injury, Poisoning and Procedural Complications: overdose.

Investigations: aspartate aminotransferase increased, neutrophil count increased, heart rate increased, neutrophil count decreased, white blood cell count increased, blood test abnormal.

Musculoskeletal and Connective Tissue Disorders: myalgia, muscle cramp, muscle spasms, sensation of heaviness, joint stiffness, muscle tightness, muscle weakness.

Neoplasms Benign, Malignant and Unspecified (incl cysts and polyps): cyst.

Nervous System Disorders: tremor, paresthesia oral, sensory disturbance, paresis, psychomotor hyperactivity, syncope.

Psychiatric Disorders: depression, agitation.

Reproductive System and Breast Disorders: irregular menstruation.

Respiratory, Thoracic and Mediastinal Disorders: cough, sinus congestion, wheezing, throat irritation.

Skin and Subcutaneous Tissue Disorders: erythema, rash pruritic, acne, pruritus, urticaria, dry skin, onychorrhexis, skin irritation.

Vascular Disorders: petechiae, poor venous access, thrombophlebitis, vasodilatation.

Post-Market Adverse Drug Reactions: The following adverse reactions have been identified during post-marketing use of TYSABRI. Because these reactions are reported voluntarily from a population of uncertain size, it is not always possible to reliably estimate their frequency or to establish a causal relationship to drug exposure.

Hypersensitivity: There have been reports of hypersensitivity reactions which have been associated with one or more of the following: hypotension, hypertension, chest pain, chest discomfort, and dyspnea.

Hepatic: There have been rare reports of clinically significant liver injury, including markedly elevated serum hepatic enzymes and elevated total bilirubin, as early as 6 days after the first dose. In some patients, liver injury recurred upon rechallenge. Some cases occurred in patients with pre-existing liver disease or in the presence of other drugs that have been associated with hepatic injury.

Infections: There have been rare reports of progressive multifocal leukoencephalopathy (PML) in patients with MS receiving TYSABRI monotherapy.

There have been rare reports of serious cases of herpes infections.

DRUG INTERACTIONS: Drug-Drug Interactions: If a decision is made to stop treatment with TYSABRI, the physician needs to be aware that TYSABRI has pharmacodynamic effects (e.g. increased lymphocyte counts) for approximately 12 weeks following the last dose. For drugs such as interferon and glatiramer acetate, concomitant exposure of this duration was not associated with safety risks in clinical trials. This should be carefully considered on a case-by-case basis and a washout period of TYSABRI might be appropriate.

Should TYSABRI therapy be administered after treatment with another immunosuppressive drug, physicians should consider the half-life of the drug and the potential for persistent immunosuppressive effects of these products when considering if a washout period is needed and, if so, its duration.

TYSABRI should not be diluted with anything other than 0.9% Sodium Chloride Injection, USP.

Drug-Food Interactions: No information is available.

Drug-Laboratory Test Interactions: TYSABRI induces increases in circulating lymphocytes, monocytes, eosinophils and nucleated red blood cells. Observed increases persist during TYSABRI exposure, but are reversible, returning to baseline levels usually within 16 weeks after the last dose. Elevations of neutrophils are not observed.

DOSAGE AND ADMINISTRATION: Dosing Considerations:

- TYSABRI (natalizumab) should be administered by a healthcare professional.
- Patients should be observed during the infusion and for 1 hour after the infusion is complete for signs and symptoms of infusion reactions. Promptly discontinue the infusion upon the first observation of any signs or symptoms consistent with a hypersensitivity reaction.
- Dilute only with 0.9% Sodium Chloride Injection, USP.

Recommended Dose and Dosage Adjustment: The recommended dose of TYSABRI is 300 mg IV infusion every 4 weeks. Do not administer TYSABRI as an IV push or bolus injection.

Administration: Dilution: Parenteral Products: Use aseptic technique when preparing TYSABRI solution for IV infusion. Each vial contains a single dose and is intended for single patient use only.

TYSABRI is a colourless, clear to slightly opalescent concentrate. Inspect the TYSABRI vial for particulate material prior to dilution and administration. If visible particulates are observed and/or the liquid in the vial is discoloured, the vial must not be used. Do not use TYSABRI beyond the expiration date on the carton or vial.

To prepare the solution, withdraw 15 mL of TYSABRI concentrate from the vial using a sterile needle and syringe. Inject the concentrate into 100 mL 0.9% Sodium Chloride Injection, USP. No other IV diluents may be used to prepare the TYSABRI solution.

Gently invert the TYSABRI solution to mix completely. Do not shake. Inspect for particulate material prior to administration.

Following dilution, intravenously infuse TYSABRI solution. If immediate infusion is not possible, store the diluted solution at 2 to 8°C. If stored at 2 to 8°C, allow the solution to warm to room temperature prior to infusion and complete the infusion within 8 hours of dilution. **Do not freeze.**

Vial Size	Volume of Diluent to be Mixed with Concentrate	Approximate Volume for Infusion	Diluted Solution Concentration
15 mL	100 mL 0.9% Sodium Chloride Injection, USP	115 mL	2.6 mg

Infuse over approximately 1 hour. Observe patients during the infusion and for 1 hour after the infusion is completed for signs and symptoms of infusion reactions.

After the infusion is complete, flush with 0.9% Sodium Chloride Injection, USP. Other medications should not be injected into infusion set side ports or mixed with TYSABRI.

OVERDOSAGE:

Safety of doses higher than 300 mg has not been adequately evaluated. The maximum amount of TYSABRI (natalizumab) that can be safely administered has not been determined.

For management of a suspected drug overdose, CPhA recommends that you contact your **regional Poison Control Centre**. See the *CPS* Directory section for a list of Poison Control Centres.

ACTION AND CLINICAL PHARMACOLOGY: Mechanism of Action: TYSABRI (natalizumab) is a selective adhesion molecule (SAM) inhibitor and binds to the α4-subunit of human integrin, which is highly expressed on the surface of all leukocytes, with the exception of neutrophils.

Specifically, natalizumab binds to the α4β1 integrin blocking the interaction with its cognate receptor, vascular cell adhesion molecule-1 (VCAM-1), and additional ligands such as osteopontin, and an alternatively spliced domain of fibronectin, connecting segment-1 (CS-1). Natalizumab blocks the interaction of α4β7 integrin with the mucosal addressin cell adhesion molecule-1 (MadCAM-1). Disruption of these molecular interactions prevents transmigration of mononuclear leukocytes across the endothelium into inflamed parenchymal tissue. A further mechanism of action of natalizumab may be to suppress ongoing inflammatory reactions in diseased tissues by inhibiting the interaction of α4-expressing leukocytes with their ligands in the extracellular matrix and on parenchymal cells. As such, natalizumab may act to suppress inflammatory activity present at the disease site, and inhibit further recruitment of immune cells into inflamed tissues.

In multiple sclerosis (MS), lesions are believed to occur when activated inflammatory cells, including T-lymphocytes, cross the blood-brain barrier (BBB). Leukocyte migration across the BBB involves interaction between adhesion molecules on inflammatory cells and endothelial cells of the vessel wall. The interaction between α4β1 and its targets is an important component of pathological inflammation in the brain, and disruption of these interactions leads to reduced inflammation. Under normal conditions, VCAM-1 is not expressed in the brain parenchyma. However, in the presence of pro-inflammatory cytokines, VCAM-1 is upregulated on endothelial cells, and possibly on glial cells near the sites of inflammation. In the setting of central nervous system (CNS) inflammation in MS, it is the interaction of α4β1 with VCAM-1, CS-1 and osteopontin that mediates the firm adhesion and transmigration of leukocytes into the brain parenchyma, and may perpetuate the inflammatory cascade in CNS tissue. Blockade of the molecular interactions of α4β1 with its targets reduces inflammatory activity present in the brain in MS and inhibits further recruitment of immune cells into inflamed tissue, thus reducing the formation or enlargement of MS lesions.

Pharmacodynamics: Treatment with TYSABRI (natalizumab) led to an increase in circulating white blood cells and total lymphocytes that was maintained throughout the treatment period. This is due to the ability of natalizumab to inhibit adhesion of leukocytes to endothelial cells and diminish transmigration of these cells from the vascular space into inflamed tissues. These increases were not clinically significant and once treatment was discontinued, counts returned to baseline levels. Consistent with the mechanism of action of natalizumab and the lack of α4 on the surface of this cell type, there was no change in the number of circulating neutrophils.

Pharmacokinetics: Pharmacokinetic values determined after a single 300 mg dose of TYSABRI in healthy subjects are provided in Table 2. Similar values observed in MS patients after a single dose and after 6 months of dosing as monotherapy are given in Table 3. Some accumulation occurs over the 6 month dosing period.

Table 2: TYSABRI

Pharmacokinetic Parameters, Single-Dose 300 mg Natalizumab as Intravenous Infusion of 60 Minutes

Median Values of Parameter	Study 1805	Study 1806
AUC_t (µg/mL·h)	19900	21500
C_{max} (µg/mL)	110	94
T_{max} (h)	2.98	3.00
$t_{½}$ (h)	224	249
Vdis (mL/kg)	66.6	67.4
CL (mL/h/kg)	0.212	0.179

Table 3: TYSABRI

Summary of Pharmacokinetic Parameters Following 60-Minute 300 mg Natalizumab Infusions Given Monthly in MS Patients (Mean +/− s.d.)

Dose Number	Study	C_{max} (µg/mL)	Minimum (Trough) Conc. (µg/mL)	$AUC_{(last)}$ (µg·h/mL)	Vd (mL/kg)	CL (mL/h/kg)	$t_{½}$ (h)
1	C-1801	84.8±22.3	none	17 884±9165	77±36	0.23±0.09	249±105
6	C-1801	94.7±34.2	21.3±15.3[a]	19 609 ± 5701	81±43	0.22±0.06	265±98

[a] Representative of concentration at the end of 6-months dosing (24-week measurement).

Clinical studies, 101MS101 and 101MS102, demonstrated that the pharmacokinetic, pharmacodynamic, immunogenicity and safety profiles of drug product produced from a high yield drug substance manufacturing process are comparable to the drug product produced from the original drug substance manufacturing process.

In study 101MS101, α4-integrin saturation levels were generally consistent with those observed in the phase 3 studies (C-1801 and C-1802). In these studies which demonstrated efficacy, α4-integrin saturation approximating 70% was observed, however there was a high degree of assay variability.

Special Populations and Conditions: Pediatrics: The pharmacokinetics of TYSABRI in pediatric MS patients have not been studied.

Geriatrics: The pharmacokinetics of TYSABRI in MS patients over 65 years of age have not been established.

Hepatic Insufficiency: The pharmacokinetics of TYSABRI in patients with hepatic insufficiency have not been studied.
Renal Insufficiency: The pharmacokinetics of TYSABRI in patients with renal insufficiency have not been studied.
Gender: Results of a population pharmacokinetics study demonstrated that gender did not influence natalizumab pharmacokinetics.
Race: The effects of race on the pharmacokinetics of TYSABRI have not been studied.
Duration of Effect: TYSABRI has pharmacodynamic effects (e.g. increased lymphocyte counts) for approximately 12 weeks following the last dose.

STORAGE AND STABILITY: TYSABRI (natalizumab) single-use vials must be stored in a refrigerator between 2 to 8°C. Do not use beyond the expiration date on the carton and vial label. Do not shake or freeze. Protect from light.

If not used immediately, store the TYSABRI solution for infusion at 2 to 8°C. The administration of TYSABRI solution for infusion must be completed within 8 hours of dilution.

SPECIAL HANDLING INSTRUCTIONS: TYSABRI (natalizumab) is for single use only. One vial of TYSABRI should be diluted only with 0.9% Sodium Chloride Injection, USP before use.

Any unused product or waste material should be disposed of in accordance with local requirements.

INFORMATION FOR THE PATIENT: Published in e-CPS, available by subscription at www.e-cps.ca.

DOSAGE FORMS, COMPOSITION AND PACKAGING: Each sterile, single-use vial, free of preservatives contains: natalizumab 300 mg. Nonmedicinal ingredients: polysorbate 80, sodium chloride, sodium phosphate, dibasic, heptahydrate, sodium phosphate, monobasic, monohydrate and Water for Injection. Packages of one vial.

U
V
W

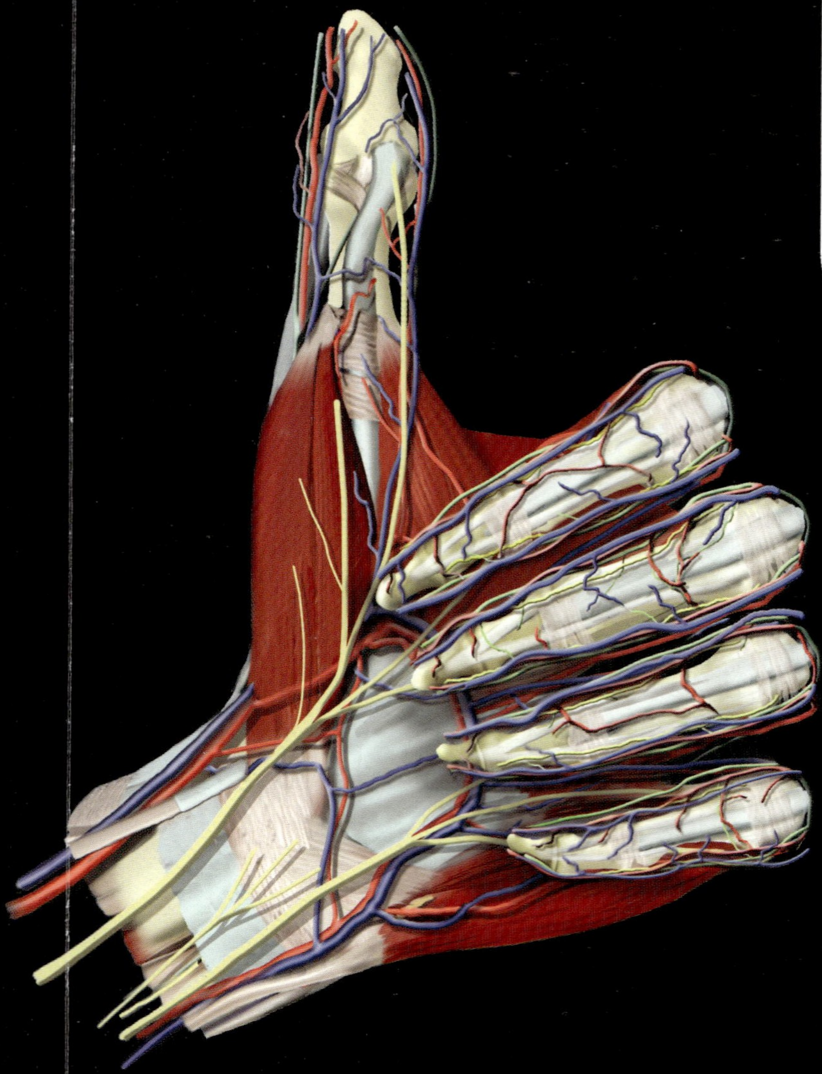

U

Ulone™
chlophedianol HCl
Antitussive

Graceway

PHARMACOLOGY: Chlophedianol, a nonopioid antitussive, shows cough suppressant potency comparable to that of the opioids but with a slower onset of maximum effect and a longer duration of action. Tolerance or addiction, respiratory depression and/or constipation have not been observed.

Chlophedianol exhibits moderate local anesthetic effects and some anticholinergic action. Analgesic, sedative-hypnotic, antihistaminic and antiemetic properties have not been demonstrated.

INDICATIONS: Symptomatic relief of cough.

CONTRAINDICATIONS: No data supplied by the manufacturer.

WARNINGS: No data supplied by the manufacturer.

PRECAUTIONS: *Pregnancy:* Safe use in pregnancy has not been established. Use of any drug in pregnancy or in women of childbearing potential requires that the possible risk to mother and/or fetus be weighed against the expected therapeutic benefit. Children: The safe use of chlophedianol in infants has not been established. Chlophedianol is not recommended in children under 2 years of age.

Use chlophedianol judiciously in sedated or debilitated patients. Patients with a productive cough should not have their cough reflex severely inhibited since this may lead to retention of secretions. Since chlophedianol is a centrally acting drug it should be used with caution in patients taking drugs that depress or stimulate the CNS.

ADVERSE EFFECTS: An occasional patient may develop excitation, hyperirritability and nightmares. The symptoms disappear within a few hours after the drug is discontinued. In a few patients in whom the drug was continued in large or even excessive amounts after stimulation was present, hallucinations developed. Upon withdrawal of the medication, the patients recovered rapidly within a few hours. Hypersensitivity reactions and urticaria are infrequent. When large doses are used, dry mouth, vertigo, visual disturbances, nausea, vomiting and drowsiness have occurred.

OVERDOSE:
No data supplied by the manufacturer.

> For management of a suspected drug overdose, CPhA recommends that you contact your **regional Poison Control Centre**. See the *CPS* Directory section for a list of Poison Control Centres.

DOSAGE: Adults: Adults, 25 mg 3 or 4 times daily as required.
Children: Children 6 to 12 years of age, 12.5 to 25 mg 3 or 4 times daily as required; 2 to 6 years of age, 12.5 mg 3 or 4 times daily as required.

SUPPLIED: Each 5 mL contains: chlophedianol HCl 25 mg in a flavored syrup base. Nonmedicinal ingredients: citric acid, ethyl alcohol, FD&C Yellow #6, flavoring, glycerin, menthol racemic, methyl- and propylparabens, sodium citrate, sucrose, water. Tartrazine-free. Bottles of 100 mL.

Uloric Pr
febuxostat
Xanthine Oxidase Inhibitor

Takeda Canada

Date of Preparation: September 21, 2010

SUMMARY PRODUCT INFORMATION:

Route of Administration	Dosage Form/ Strength	Clinically Relevant Nonmedicinal Ingredients
Oral	Tablet 80 mg	Lactose monohydrate For a complete listing, see Dosage Forms, Composition and Packaging.

INDICATIONS AND CLINICAL USE: ULORIC (febuxostat) is indicated to lower serum uric acid levels in patients with gout.
Geriatrics (>65 years of age): No clinically significant differences in safety or efficacy were observed in geriatric patients compared to younger patients in clinical studies.
Pediatrics (<18 years of age): Safety and efficacy in pediatric patients have not been established.
CONTRAINDICATIONS: ULORIC is contraindicated in patients being treated with azathioprine, mercaptopurine, or theophylline (see Drug Interactions).

ULORIC is contraindicated in patients with a history of hypersensitivity to febuxostat or to any other ingredient in the formulation. For a complete listing of ingredients, see Dosage Forms, Composition and Packaging.

WARNINGS AND PRECAUTIONS: General:

- **Gout Flare:** ULORIC treatment should not be started until an acute attack of gout has completely subsided. After initiation of ULORIC therapy, an increase in gout flares is frequently observed.
  In order to reduce the likelihood of gout flares when ULORIC is initiated, concurrent flare prophylactic treatment with drugs such as a non-steroidal anti-inflammatory drug (NSAID) or colchicine is recommended. Flare prophylactic therapy may be beneficial for up to six months. If a gout flare occurs during ULORIC treatment, ULORIC should not be discontinued. The gout flare should be managed concurrently, as appropriate for the individual patient.
- ULORIC is not recommended for use in patients with a greatly increased rate of urate formation (e.g., malignant disease and its treatment, Lesch-Nyhan syndrome). No studies have been conducted in these populations. ULORIC has not been studied in organ transplant recipients. The use of ULORIC in these patients with secondary hyperuricemia is not recommended.

Cardiovascular: In the randomized controlled studies, there was a higher rate of cardiovascular thromboembolic events (cardiovascular deaths, non-fatal myocardial infarctions, and non-fatal strokes) in patients treated with ULORIC 80 mg [1.09 per 100 P-Y (95% CI 0.44-2.24)] than allopurinol [0.60 per 100 P-Y (95% CI 0.16-1.53)] (see Adverse Reactions). Monitor for signs and symptoms of myocardial infarction (MI) and stroke.
Gastrointestinal: ULORIC tablets contain lactose. Patients with rare hereditary problems of galactose intolerance, the Lapp lactase deficiency or glucose-galactase malabsorption should not take ULORIC.

Hepatic/Biliary/Pancreatic: During randomized controlled studies, transaminase elevations greater than 3 times the upper limit of normal (ULN) were observed (AST: 2%, 2% and ALT: 3%, 2% in ULORIC and allopurinol-treated patients, respectively). No dose-effect relationship for these transaminase elevations was noted. Laboratory assessment of liver function is recommended prior to the initiation of ULORIC therapy and periodically thereafter (see Adverse Reactions, Abnormal Hematologic and Clinical Chemistry Findings).
Skin: There have been some post-marketing reports of serious skin reactions and hypersensitivity, and many, but not all of these patients reported previous hypersensitivity to allopurinol (see Adverse reactions, Post-Market Adverse Drug Reactions).
Special Populations: Pregnant Women: There are no adequate and well-controlled studies in pregnant women using ULORIC. ULORIC should not be used in pregnant women. Febuxostat was not teratogenic when orally administered to pregnant rats and rabbits during the period of organogenesis at doses up to 48 mg/kg. Febuxostat and febuxostat-derived metabolites do not readily cross the placenta of pregnant rats.
Nursing Women: It is not known whether ULORIC is excreted in human milk. ULORIC should not be used in nursing women.

Febuxostat is excreted in the milk of pregnant female rats and is associated with reduced neonatal body weight, increased neonatal mortality, and developmental delays at 48 mg/kg.
Geriatrics (>65 years of age): Of the total number of subjects in clinical studies of ULORIC, 16% were 65 and over, while 4% were 75 and over. Comparing subjects in different age groups, no clinically significant differences in safety or efficacy were observed but greater sensitivity of some older individuals can not be ruled out.
Pediatrics (<18 years of age): Safety and efficacy in pediatric patients have not been established. The use of ULORIC in the pediatric population is not recommended.
Renal Impairment: There are insufficient data in patients with severe renal impairment (Cl_{cr} less than 30 mL/min); and there are no data in end stage renal impairment patients who are on dialysis. The use of ULORIC in these populations is not recommended (see Action and Clinical Pharmacology).
Hepatic Impairment: No studies have been conducted in patients with severe hepatic impairment (Child-Pugh Class C). The use of ULORIC in this population is not recommended (see Action and Clinical Pharmacology).
Monitoring and Laboratory Tests: Cardiovascular: Signs and symptoms of myocardial infarction and strokes should be monitored during therapy with ULORIC (see Adverse Reactions, Adverse Drug Reaction Overview).
Hepatic: Laboratory assessment of liver function (serum transaminases) is recommended prior to the initiation of ULORIC therapy and periodically thereafter.
ADVERSE REACTIONS: Adverse Drug Reaction Overview: The most frequently reported Adverse Drug Reactions (ADRs) in Phase 3 randomized controlled studies with ULORIC 80 mg were: liver function abnormalities (4.6%), diarrhea (3.0%), rash (1.6%), nausea (1.3%), and dizziness (1.1%). The most frequently reported ADR in the long-term open label extension studies with ULORIC 80 mg was liver function abnormalities. The overall incidence of adverse reactions did not increase during long-term studies.

The most common adverse reaction leading to discontinuation from therapy in randomized, controlled studies was liver function abnormalities in 1.2% of ULORIC 80 mg and in 0.9% of allopurinol-treated subjects.

Cardiovascular events and deaths were adjudicated to one of the pre-defined endpoints from the Anti-Platelet Trialists' Collaboration (APTC) (cardiovascular death, non-fatal myocardial infarction, and non-fatal stroke) in the randomized controlled and long-term extension studies. In Phase 3 randomized controlled studies, the incidences of adjudicated APTC events per 100 patients-years of exposure were: Placebo 0 (95% CI 0.00-6.16), ULORIC 80 mg 1.09 (95% CI 0.44-2.24), and allopurinol 0.60 (95% CI 0.16-1.53).

In the long-term extension studies, the incidences of adjudicated APTC events were: ULORIC 80 mg 0.97 (95% CI 0.57-1.56) and allopurinol 0.58 (95% CI 0.02-3.24).

Overall, a non-statistically significant higher rate of APTC events was observed in patients treated with ULORIC than in allopurinol-treated patients. No causal relationship with ULORIC has been established.
Clinical Trial Adverse Drug Reactions: Because clinical trials are conducted under very specific conditions the adverse reaction rates observed in the clinical trials may not reflect the rates observed in practice and should not be compared to the rates in the clinical trials of another drug. Adverse drug reaction information from clinical trials is useful for identifying drug-related adverse events and for approximating rates.

In clinical studies, patients received ULORIC in doses ranging from 10 mg to 300 mg. The total exposure to ULORIC 80 mg in randomized controlled studies and long-term extension studies was greater than 2300 patient-years. For ULORIC 80 mg, 1377 subjects were treated for ≥6 months, 674 patients were treated for ≥1 year and 515 patients were treated for ≥2 years.

In three randomized, controlled clinical studies which were 6 to 12 months in duration, the following adverse reactions were reported by the treating physician as related to study drug. Table 1 summarizes the most common adverse reactions reported at a rate of at least 1% for ULORIC 80 mg and at an incidence at least 0.5% higher than placebo.

Table 1: ULORIC

Adverse Reactions Occurring in ≥1% of Patients Treated with ULORIC and at Least 0.5% Greater than Seen in Patients Receiving Placebo in Controlled Studies

Adverse Reactions	Placebo (N=134)	ULORIC 80 mg (N=1279)	Allopurinol[a] (N=1277)
Liver Function Abnormalities	0.7%	4.6%	4.2%
Nausea	0.7%	1.3%	0.8%
Rash	0.7%	1.6%	1.6%

[a] Of the subjects who received allopurinol, 10 received 100 mg, 145 received 200 mg and 1122 received 300 mg based on level of renal impairment.

In addition to the adverse reactions presented in Table 1, diarrhea and dizziness were reported in more than 1% of subjects treated with ULORIC although not at a rate more than 0.5% greater than placebo.
Less Common Clinical Trial Adverse Drug Reactions (<1%): In phase 2 and 3 clinical studies the following causally related adverse reactions occurred in less than 1% of subjects treated with 80 mg of ULORIC. This list also includes adverse reactions which occurred in at least one subject treated with doses ranging from 40 mg to 240 mg of ULORIC.
Blood and Lymphatic System Disorders: anemia, idiopathic thrombocytopenic purpura, leukocytosis/leukopenia, neutropenia, pancytopenia, splenomegaly, thrombocytopenia.
Cardiac Disorders: angina pectoris, atrial fibrillation/flutter, cardiac murmur, ECG abnormal, palpitations, sinus bradycardia, tachycardia.
Ear and Labyrinth Disorders: deafness, tinnitus, vertigo.
Eye Disorders: cataract, vision blurred.
Gastrointestinal Disorders: abdominal distention, abdominal pain, colitis, constipation, diarrhea, dry mouth, dyspepsia, esophageal stenosis, flatulence, frequent stools, gastritis, gastroenteritis, gastroesophageal reflux disease, gastrointestinal discomfort, gingival pain, haematemesis, hematochezia, hyperchlorhydria, mouth ulceration, pancreatitis, peptic ulcer, rectal hemorrhage, vomiting.
General Disorders and Administration Site Conditions: asthenia, chest pain/discomfort, edema, fatigue, feeling abnormal, gait disturbance, influenza-like symptoms, mass, pain, thirst.
Hepatobiliary Disorders: cholelithiasis/cholecystitis, hepatic steatosis, hepatitis, hepatomegaly.
Immune System Disorder: hypersensitivity.
Infections and Infestations: cellulitis, herpes zoster, sinusitis, tinea pedis.
Injury, Poisoning and Procedural Complications: contusion.
Metabolism and Nutrition Disorders: anorexia, appetite decreased/increased, cow's milk intolerance, dehydration, diabetes mellitus, dyslipidemia, gout, hypercholesterolemia, hyperglycemia, hyperlipidemia, hypertriglyceridemia, hypokalemia, weight decreased/increased.
Musculoskeletal and Connective Tissue Disorders: arthralgia, arthritis, bunion, bursitis, costochondritis, gouty tophus, joint stiffness, joint swelling, muscle spasms/twitching/tightness/weakness, musculoskeletal pain/stiffness, myalgia.
Neoplasms Benign, Malignant and Unspecified: malignant melanoma, myelodysplastic syndrome.
Nervous System Disorders: altered taste, amnesia, balance disorder, burning sensation, cerebrovascular accident, dizziness, Guillain-Barré syndrome, headache, hemiparesis, hypoesthesia, hyposmia, lacunar infarction, lethargy, mental impairment, migraine, paresthesia, peripheral neuropathy, somnolence, transient ischemic attack, tremor.

Psychiatric Disorders: agitation, anxiety, depression, insomnia, irritability, libido decreased, nervousness, panic attack, personality change.
Renal and Urinary Disorders: hematuria, incontinence, kidney infection, nephrolithiasis, pollakiuria, proteinuria, renal failure, renal insufficiency, urgency, urinary tract infection.
Reproductive System and Breast Changes: breast pain, erectile dysfunction, gynecomastia, mastitis.
Respiratory, Thoracic and Mediastinal Disorders: bronchitis, cough, dyspnea, epistaxis, nasal dryness, paranasal sinus hypersecretion, pharyngeal edema, respiratory tract congestion, sneezing, throat irritation, upper respiratory tract infection, wheezing.
Skin and Subcutaneous Tissue Disorders: alopecia, angio-edema, dermatitis, dermographism, ecchymosis, eczema, hair color changes, hair growth abnormal, hyperhidrosis, peeling skin, petechiae, photosensitivity, pruritus, purpura, skin discoloration/altered pigmentation, skin lesion, skin odor abnormal, urticaria.
Vascular Disorders: flushing, hot flush, hypertension, hypotension.
Laboratory Parameters: activated partial thromboplastin time prolonged, creatine increased, bicarbonate decreased, sodium increased, EEG abnormal, glucose increased, cholesterol increased, triglycerides increased, amylase increased, potassium increased, TSH increased, platelet count decreased, hematocrit decreased, hemoglobin decreased, MCV increased/decreased, RBC decreased, creatinine increased, blood urea increased, BUN/creatinine ratio increased, creatine phosphokinase (CPK) increased, alkaline phosphatase increased, LDH increased, PSA increased, urine output increased/decreased, lymphocyte count decreased, neutrophil count decreased, WBC increased/decreased, coagulation test abnormal, low density lipoprotein (LDL) increased, prothrombin time prolonged, urinary casts, urine positive for white blood cells and protein.
Abnormal Hematologic and Clinical Chemistry Findings: During the 3 randomized controlled studies, transaminase elevations greater than 3 times the upper limit of normal were observed. The clinically important abnormalities in liver function tests reported in the controlled studies are shown in Table 2.

Table 2: ULORIC

Incidence of Clinically Important Laboratory Abnormalities Reported in Controlled Studies

Laboratory Abnormality	Normal Values[a]	Treatment Group (%) Placebo (N=134)	ULORIC 80 mg (N=1279)	Allopurinol[b] (N=1277)
Alkaline Phosphatase ≥2×ULN	Males: 31–131 U/L Females: 31–135 U/L	0%	0.4%	0%
ALT ≥3×ULN	Males: 6–43 U/L Females: 6–34 U/L	0.8%	3.2%	1.9%
AST ≥3×ULN	Males: 11–36 U/L Females: 9–34 U/L	0.8%	1.3%	2.0%
Total Bilirubin ≥2.0 mg/dL	Both genders: 0.2–1.2 mg/dL	0.8%	0.5%	1.0%

[a] Normal values across age groups as reported by the central laboratory. ULN=upper limit of normal.
[b] Of the patients who received allopurinol, 10 received 100 mg, 145 received 200 mg, and 1122 received 300 mg based on the level of renal impairment.
Percentages are based on the number of patients with post-baseline laboratory data.

Post-Market Adverse Drug Reactions: The following adverse reactions have been identified during the post-approval use of ULORIC. Because these reactions are reported voluntarily from a population of uncertain size, it is not always possible to reliably estimate their frequency or establish a causal relationship.
Cardiac Disorders: myocardial infarction (some fatal).
Immune System Disorders: anaphylactic reaction/shock, tubulointerstitial nephritis.
Musculoskeletal and Connective Tissue Disorders: rhabdomyolysis.
Psychiatric Disorders: psychotic behavior including aggressive thoughts.
Skin and Subcutaneous Tissue Disorders: erythema, generalized rash.

There have been some reports of serious skin reactions and hypersensitivity, and many, but not all of these patients reported previous hypersensitivity to allopurinol.

DRUG INTERACTIONS:

> **Serious Drug Interactions**
> ULORIC is contraindicated in patients being treated with the following drugs. Inhibition of xanthine oxidase (XO) by ULORIC may cause increased plasma concentrations of these drugs leading to toxicity:
> - Azathioprine
> - Mercaptopurine
> - Theophylline

Overview: Febuxostat is unlikely to inhibit or induce CYP450 enzymes at clinically relevant concentrations and therefore, has low potential to be involved in drug-drug interactions with drugs that are substrates of CYP450. However, ULORIC is a xanthine oxidase (XO) inhibitor, and therefore, may cause increased plasma concentrations of drugs metabolized by XO when co-administered, potentially leading to toxicity by these other drugs.
Drug-Drug Interactions: Xanthine Oxidase (XO) Substrate Drugs Such as Azathioprine, Mercaptopurine, and Theophylline: Interaction studies of ULORIC with drugs that are metabolized by XO have not been conducted. Inhibition of XO is known to result in an increase in plasma concentrations of these drugs leading to toxicity. On the basis of the mechanism of action of ULORIC on XO inhibition, concomitant use is contraindicated (see Contraindications).

Drug interaction studies of ULORIC with cytotoxic chemotherapy have not been conducted. No data are available regarding the safety of ULORIC during cytotoxic chemotherapy.
Colchicine: Administration of ULORIC (40 mg QD) with colchicine (0.6 mg BID) resulted in an increase of 12% in C_{max} and 7% in AUC_{24} of febuxostat. Colchicine had no effect on the total exposure to febuxostat. In addition, administration of colchicine (0.6 mg BID) with ULORIC (120 mg QD) resulted in less than 11% change in C_{max} or AUC of colchicine for both AM and PM doses. These changes were not considered clinically significant. No dose adjustment is necessary for either ULORIC or colchicine when the two drugs are co-administered.
Naproxen: Febuxostat metabolism depends on uridine diphosphate glucuronosyltransferase (UGT) enzymes. Medicinal products that inhibit glucuronidation, such as NSAIDs, could in theory affect the elimination of febuxostat. In healthy subjects, administration of ULORIC (80 mg QD) with naproxen (500 mg BID) resulted in a 28% increase in C_{max} and a 40% increase in AUC of febuxostat. An increase in febuxostat plasma exposure following co-administration with naproxen is not expected to raise any safety concerns. In addition, there were no significant changes in the C_{max} or AUC of naproxen (less than 2%). ULORIC can be co-administered with naproxen with no dose adjustment of febuxostat or naproxen being necessary.
Indomethacin: Administration of ULORIC (80 mg QD) with indomethacin (50 mg BID) did not result in any significant changes in C_{max} or AUC of febuxostat or indomethacin (less than 7%). No dose adjustment is necessary for either ULORIC or indomethacin when these two drugs are co-administered.
Hydrochlorothiazide: Administration of ULORIC (80 mg single dose) with hydrochlorothiazide (50 mg single dose) did not result in any clinically significant changes in C_{max} or AUC of febuxostat (less than 4%), and serum uric acid concentrations were not substantially affected. No dose adjustment is necessary for ULORIC when co-administered with hydrochlorothiazide.
Warfarin: Administration of ULORIC (80 mg QD) with warfarin had no effect on the pharmacokinetics of warfarin in healthy subjects. INR and Factor VII activity were also not affected by the co-administration of ULORIC. No dose adjustment is necessary for warfarin when co-administered with ULORIC.
Desipramine: Febuxostat was shown to be a weak inhibitor of CYP2D6 in vitro. In healthy subjects, 120 mg ULORIC QD resulted in a mean 22% increase in AUC of desipramine (25 mg QD), a CYP2D6 substrate, indicating a potential weak inhibitory effect of febuxostat on the CYP2D6 enzyme in vivo. The increase of desipramine plasma exposure following co-administration with febuxostat was associated with a 17% decrease in the 2-hydroxydesipramine to desipramine metabolic ratio (based on AUC).

In combination with other weak inhibitors of CYP2D6, this increase of desipramine plasma exposure could be exacerbated. Co-administration of a drug that is CYP2D6 substrate with ULORIC is not expected to require any dose adjustment for those compounds.
Antacids: Concomitant ingestion of an antacid containing magnesium hydroxide and aluminum hydroxide with an 80 mg single dose of ULORIC has been shown to delay absorption of febuxostat (approximately 1 hour) and to cause a 31% decrease in C_{max} and a 15% decrease in AUC_{∞}. As AUC rather than C_{max} was related to drug effect, change observed in AUC was not considered clinically significant. ULORIC may be taken without regard to antacid use.
Drug-Food Interactions: No interactions with food have been observed with ULORIC (see Action and Clinical Pharmacology).
Drug-Herb Interactions: Interactions with herbal products have not been established.
Drug-Laboratory Test Interactions: Interactions with laboratory tests have not been established.
Drug-Lifestyle Interactions: No studies on the effects on the ability to drive or use machines have been performed. Caution should be exercised before driving or using machinery.

DOSAGE AND ADMINISTRATION: Dosing Considerations: After initiation of ULORIC therapy, an increase in gout flares is frequently observed.

In order to reduce the likelihood of gout flares when ULORIC is initiated, concurrent flare prophylactic treatment with drugs such as a non-steroidal anti-inflammatory drug (NSAID) or colchicine is recommended. Flare prophylactic therapy may be beneficial for up to six months. This can be determined by the physician. If a gout flare occurs during ULORIC treatment, ULORIC should not be discontinued. The gout flare should be managed concurrently, as appropriate for the individual patient.
Recommended Dose and Dosage Adjustment: The recommended oral dose of ULORIC is 80 mg once daily.

ULORIC can be taken without regard to food or antacid use (see Action and Clinical Pharmacology).

No dose adjustment is necessary in geriatric patients (>65 years of age) (see Action and Clinical Pharmacology).

No dose adjustment is necessary in patients with mild or moderate hepatic impairment (Child-Pugh Class A or B) (see Action and Clinical Pharmacology).

No dose adjustment is necessary in patients with mild or moderate renal impairment (Cl_{cr} 30-89 mL/min) (see Action and Clinical Pharmacology).
Missed Dose: If a dose of ULORIC is missed at its usual time, it should be taken as soon as possible. However if it is too close to the time of the next dose, the missed dose should be skipped and treatment should be resumed with the next scheduled dose.

OVERDOSAGE:
ULORIC was studied in healthy subjects in doses up to 300 mg daily for seven days without evidence of dose-limiting toxicities. No overdose of ULORIC was reported in clinical studies.

> For management of a suspected drug overdose, contact your regional Poison Control Centre. See the *CPS Directory* section for a list of Poison Control Centres.

ACTION AND CLINICAL PHARMACOLOGY: Mechanism of Action: Uric acid is the end product of purine metabolism in humans and is generated in the cascade of hypoxanthine → xanthine → uric acid. Both steps in the above transformations are catalyzed by xanthine oxidase (XO). Febuxostat is a 2-arylthiazole derivative that achieves its therapeutic effect of decreasing serum uric acid by selectively inhibiting XO with in vitro Ki values in the range of 0.6-10 nM. Febuxostat is a nonpurine selective inhibitor of XO (NP-SIXO) that potently inhibits both the oxidized and reduced forms of XO.
Pharmacodynamics: Effect on Uric Acid and Xanthine Concentrations: In healthy subjects, ULORIC resulted in a dose dependent decrease in 24-hour mean serum uric acid concentrations, and an increase in 24-hour mean serum xanthine concentrations. In addition, there was a decrease in the total daily urinary uric acid excretion and an increase in total daily urinary xanthine excretion. The percent reduction in 24-hour mean serum uric acid concentrations was approximately 55% following 80 mg daily doses.
Effect on Cardiac Repolarization: The effect of ULORIC on cardiac repolarization as assessed by the QTc interval was evaluated in normal healthy subjects and in patients with gout. ULORIC in doses up to 300 mg daily, at steady state, did not demonstrate an effect on the QTc interval.
Pharmacokinetics: In healthy subjects, maximum plasma concentrations (C_{max}) and AUC of febuxostat increased in a dose proportional manner following single and multiple doses of 10 mg to 120 mg. There is no accumulation when therapeutic doses are administered every 24 hours. Febuxostat has a mean terminal elimination half-life ($t_{½}$) of approximately 5 to 8 hours. Febuxostat pharmacokinetic parameters for patients with hyperuricemia and gout estimated by population pharmacokinetic analyses were similar to those estimated in healthy subjects.
Absorption: The absorption of radiolabeled febuxostat following oral dose administration was estimated to be at least 49% (based on total radioactivity recovered in urine). Maximum plasma concentrations of febuxostat occurred between 1 to 1.5 hours post-dose. After multiple oral 80 mg once daily doses, C_{max} is approximately 2.9±1.4 µg/mL (N=226). Absolute bioavailability of the febuxostat tablet has not been studied.

ULORIC may be taken without regard to food. Following multiple 80 mg once daily doses with a high fat meal, there was a 49% decrease in C_{max} and an 18% decrease in AUC, respectively. However, no clinically significant change in the percent decrease in serum uric acid concentration was observed (58% fed vs. 51% fasting).
Distribution: The mean apparent steady state volume of distribution (V_{ss}/F) of febuxostat was approximately 54 L (CV 49%). The plasma protein binding of febuxostat is approximately 99.2% (primarily to albumin).
Metabolism: Febuxostat is extensively metabolized by both conjugation via uridine diphosphate glucuronosyltransferase (UGT) enzymes including UGT1A1, UGT1A3, UGT1A9, and UGT2B7 and oxidation via cytochrome P450 (CYP) enzymes including CYP1A2, 2C8 and 2C9 and non-P450 enzymes. The relative contribution of each enzyme isoform in the metabolism of febuxostat is not clear. The oxidation of the isobutyl side chain leads to the formation of four pharmacologically active hydroxy metabolites, all of which occur in plasma of humans at a much lower extent than febuxostat.

In urine and feces, acyl glucuronide metabolites of febuxostat (~35% of the dose), and oxidative metabolites, 67M-1 (~10% of the dose), 67M-2 (~11% of the dose), and 67M-4, a secondary metabolite from 67M-1, (~14% of the dose) appeared to be the major metabolites of febuxostat in vivo.
Excretion: Febuxostat is eliminated by both hepatic and renal pathways. Following an 80 mg oral dose of ^{14}C-labeled febuxostat, approximately 49% of the dose was recovered in the urine as unchanged febuxostat (3%), the acyl glucuronide of the drug (30%), its known oxidative metabolites and their conjugates (13%), and other unknown metabolites (3%). In addition to the urinary excretion, approximately 45% of the dose was recovered in the feces as the unchanged febuxostat (12%), the acyl glucuronide of the drug (1%), its known oxidative metabolites and their conjugates (25%), and other unknown metabolites (7%).

The mean terminal elimination half-life ($t_{½}$) of febuxostat was approximately 5 to 8 hours.
Special Populations and Conditions: Geriatrics: The C_{max} and AUC of febuxostat and its metabolites following multiple oral doses of ULORIC in geriatric subjects (≥65 years) were similar to those in younger subjects (18-40 years). In addition, the percent decrease in serum uric acid concentration was similar between elderly and younger subjects.
Gender: Following multiple oral doses of ULORIC, the C_{max} and AUC_{24} of febuxostat were 30% and 14% higher in females than in males, respectively. However, weight-corrected C_{max} and AUC were similar between the genders. In addition, the percent decrease in serum uric acid concentrations was similar between genders.
Race: No specific pharmacokinetic study was conducted to investigate the effects of race.
Hepatic Impairment: No studies have been conducted in subjects with severe hepatic impairment (Child-Pugh Class C). The use of ULORIC in this population is not recommended. Following multiple 80 mg doses of ULORIC in patients with mild (Child-Pugh Class A) or moderate (Child-Pugh Class B) hepatic impairment, an average of 20-30% increase was observed for both C_{max} and AUC_{24} (total and unbound) in hepatic impairment groups compared to subjects with normal hepatic function. In addition, the percent decrease in serum uric acid concentration was comparable between different hepatic groups (62% in healthy group, 49% in mild hepatic impairment group, and 48% in moderate hepatic impairment group).
Renal Impairment: There are insufficient data in patients with severe renal impairment (Cl_{cr} less than 30 mL/min) and there are no data in end stage renal impairment patients who are on dialysis. The use of ULORIC in these populations is not recommended.

ULORIC has not been studied in end stage renal impairment patients who are on dialysis.

Following multiple 80 mg doses of ULORIC in healthy subjects with mild (Cl_{cr} 50 to 80 mL/min), moderate (Cl_{cr} 30 to 49 mL/min) or severe renal impairment (Cl_{cr} 10 to 29 mL/min), the C_{max} of febuxostat did not change relative to subjects with normal renal function (Cl_{cr} greater than 80 mL/min). AUC and half-life of febuxostat increased in subjects with renal impairment in comparison to subjects with normal renal function, but values were similar among the three renal impairment groups. Mean febuxostat AUC values were up to 1.8 times higher in subjects with renal impairment compared to those with normal renal function. However, the percent decrease in serum uric acid concentration for subjects with renal impairment was comparable to those with normal renal function (58% in normal renal function group and 55% in the severe renal function group).
STORAGE AND STABILITY: ULORIC should be protected from light. Store at 15-30°C.

INFORMATION FOR THE PATIENT: Published in e-CPS, available by subscription at www.e-cps.ca.

DOSAGE FORMS, COMPOSITION AND PACKAGING: Each light green to green in color, teardrop shaped tablet, debossed with "TAP" on one side and "80" on the other side, contains: febuxostat 80 mg. Nonmedicinal ingredients: hydroxypropyl cellulose, lactose monohydrate, magnesium stearate, microcrystalline cellulose, silicon dioxide and sodium croscarmellose; coating: Opadry II green (polyvinyl alcohol, talc, PEG 3000, titanium dioxide, D&C Yellow No. 10 Aluminum Lake, FD&C Blue No. 1 and FD&C Blue No. 2). High-density polyethylene (HDPE) bottles of 30.

Ultiva® Ⓝ

remifentanil HCl

Opioid Component to Anesthesia

Abbott

Date of Preparation: October 12, 1999
Date of Revision: January 8, 2009

SUMMARY PRODUCT INFORMATION:

Route of Administration	Dosage Form/ Strength	Clinically Relevant Nonmedicinal Ingredients
i.v.	1 mg, 2 mg vials of remifentanil base as the hydrochloride salt	Glycine, hydrochloric acid For a complete listing see Dosage Forms, Composition and Packaging.

INDICATIONS AND CLINICAL USE: ULTIVA (remifentanil hydrochloride) is indicated for i.v. administration as an analgesic agent for use during the induction and maintenance of general anesthesia for inpatient and outpatient procedures.

Due to insufficient safety and efficacy data, remifentanil is not recommended for use in spontaneous ventilation anesthesia, in monitored anesthesia care, for continuation as an analgesic in the immediate postoperative period, in neurosurgery, in cardiac surgery, or in paediatric anesthesia.

Geriatrics (>65 years of age) : For details, see Dosage and Administration, Recommended Dose and Dosage Adjustment.

Pediatrics: ULTIVA is not indicated in children.

CONTRAINDICATIONS: Due to the presence of glycine in the formulation, ULTIVA (remifentanil hydrochloride) is contraindicated for epidural or intrathecal administration.

Remifentanil is also contraindicated in patients with known hypersensitivity to the drug or any component of its formulation/preparation or to other fentanyl analogs.

WARNINGS AND PRECAUTIONS: General: Remifentanil is not recommended for use as the sole agent in general anesthesia because loss of consciousness cannot be assured and because of a high incidence of apnea, muscle rigidity and tachycardia.

Continuous infusions of remifentanil should be administered only by an infusion device. **I.V. bolus administration should only be used in intubated patients during the maintenance of general anesthesia.** For induction of anesthesia in nonintubated patients, a single dose of remifentanil, not exceeding 1 µg/kg, may be administered over 30 to 60 seconds.

Interruption of an infusion of remifentanil will result in rapid offset of effect. Rapid clearance and lack of drug accumulation result in rapid dissipation of respiratory depressant and analgesic effects upon discontinuation of remifentanil at recommended doses. However, delayed respiratory depression may occur in some patients up to 30 minutes after termination of remifentanil infusions due to residual effects of concomitant anesthetics. Discontinuation of an infusion of remifentanil should be preceded by the establishment of adequate postoperative analgesia (see Warnings and Precautions, Dosage and Administration).

Injections of remifentanil should be made into i.v. tubing at or close to the venous cannula. Upon discontinuation of remifentanil, the i.v. tubing should be removed or cleared to prevent the inadvertent administration of remifentanil at a later point in time. **Failure to adequately clear the i.v. tubing to remove residual remifentanil has been associated with the appearance of respiratory depression, apnea and muscle rigidity upon the administration of additional fluids or medications through the same i.v. tubing.**

Use of remifentanil is associated with apnea and respiratory depression. Remifentanil should be administered only in a setting fully equipped for the monitoring and support of respiratory and cardiovascular function. Resuscitative and intubation equipment, oxygen and an opioid antagonist must be readily available.

Remifentanil should be administered only by persons specifically trained in the use of anesthetic drugs and the recognition and management of the expected adverse effects of potent opioids, including respiratory and cardiac resuscitation of patients in the age-group being treated. Such training must include the establishment and maintenance of a patent airway and assisted ventilation.

Skeletal muscle rigidity can be caused by remifentanil and is related to the dose and speed of administration. Remifentanil may cause chest wall rigidity (inability to ventilate) after single doses >1 µg/kg administered over 30 to 60 seconds, or after infusion rates >0.1 µg/kg/min. Single doses <1 µg/kg may cause chest wall rigidity when given concurrently with a continuous infusion of remifentanil.

Muscle rigidity induced by remifentanil should be managed in the context of the patient's clinical condition. Muscle rigidity occurring during the induction of anesthesia should be treated by the administration of a neuromuscular blocking agent and the concurrent induction medications.

Remifentanil should not be administered into the same i.v. tubing with blood/serum/plasma due to potential inactivation by nonspecific esterases in blood products.

Vital signs and oxygenation must be continually monitored during the administration of remifentanil.

Intraoperative awareness has been reported in patients under 55 years of age when remifentanil has been administered with propofol infusion rates of ≤75 µg/kg/min. Therefore, propofol rates <100 µg/kg/min are not recommended for use with remifentanil for total intravenous anesthesia in patients <55 years of age.

Carcinogenesis and Mutagenesis: Remifentanil, with or without a rat liver enzyme fraction (S9), was not mutagenic in the 5 strains of *S. typhimurium* tested by gene mutation assay (Ames test) and did not produce chromosome aberrations in the Chinese hamster ovary cells. Remifentanil was also negative in the in vivo micronucleus test and the liver unscheduled DNA synthesis assay.

Remifentanil was found to be genotoxic in mammalian cells in vitro in the mouse lymphoma assay. Remifentanil concentrations over 4000 times greater than those seen with clinical use (50 ng/mL) were mutagenic only in the presence of metabolic activation.

Cardiovascular: Hypotension has been reported with remifentanil and is responsive to decreases in the administration of remifentanil or to i.v. fluids or catecholamine (ephedrine, epinephrine, norepinephrine, etc.) administration.

Dependence/Tolerance: As with other opioids, remifentanil can produce drug dependence of the morphine type and therefore has the potential of being abused.

Hepatic/Biliary/Pancreatic: Remifentanil pharmacokinetic/pharmacodynamic profile is not changed in patients with severe hepatic impairment. However, these patients may be slightly more sensitive to respiratory depressant effects of remifentanil. Therefore these patients should be closely monitored and the dose of remifentanil titrated to individual patient need.

Peri-Operative Considerations: Use in Cardiovascular Surgery: Clinical experience with remifentanil in patients undergoing cardiac surgery is limited to coronary artery bypass graft procedures (CABG). There are insufficient data to make a dosage recommendation.

Use in Neurosurgery: Due to the limited number of patients studied, there are insufficient data to make dosage recommendations.

Renal: The pharmacodynamic/pharmacokinetic profile of remifentanil is not changed in patients with end stage renal disease (creatinine clearance <10 mL/min). No dosage adjustment is necessary in this patient population.

In anephric patients, the half-life of the carboxylic acid metabolite increases from 90 minutes to approximately 30 hours. The metabolite is removed by haemodialysis with a dialysis extraction ratio of approximately 30%.

Respiratory: Within 5 to 10 minutes after the discontinuation of ULTIVA (remifentanil hydrochloride), no residual analgesic activity will be present. However, respiratory depression may occur in some patients up to 30 minutes after termination of infusion due to residual effects of concomitant anesthetics. Standard monitoring should be maintained in the postoperative period to ensure adequate recovery without stimulation. For patients undergoing surgical procedures where postoperative pain is generally anticipated, other analgesics should be administered prior to the discontinuation of remifentanil.

Bradycardia has been reported with remifentanil and is responsive to ephedrine or anticholinergic drugs, such as atropine and glycopyrrolate.

Special Populations: Pregnant Women, Labour and Delivery, and Nursing Women: There are insufficient clinical data to support safety, and therefore, remifentanil is not recommended for use in these populations.

Pediatrics (<12 years of age): Due to the limited number of patients studied, there are insufficient data to make dosage recommendations in the pediatric population.

Geriatrics (>65 years of age): The clearance of remifentanil is reduced (approximately 25%) in the elderly (>65 years of age) compared to young adults (average 25 years of age). However, remifentanil blood concentrations fall as rapidly after termination of administration in the elderly as in young adults. The pharmacodynamic activity of remifentanil (as measured by the EC_{50} for development of delta waves on the electroencephalogram [EEG]) increases with increasing age. The EC_{50} of remifentanil for this measure was 50% less in patients over 65 years of age when compared to healthy volunteers (25 years of age); therefore, the recommended starting dose of remifentanil should be decreased by 50% in elderly patients and then titrated to individual patient need (see Dosage and Administration).

Morbidly Obese Patients: As for all potent opioids, caution is required when used in morbidly obese patients because of alterations in cardiovascular and respiratory physiology (see Dosage and Administration).

ASA III/IV Patients: Limited data is available from 65 ASA III and 1 ASA IV patients. As the hemodynamic effects of potent opioids can be expected to be more pronounced in ASA III/IV patients, caution should be exercised in the administration of remifentanil in this population. Initial dosage reduction and subsequent titration to effect is therefore recommended.

ADVERSE REACTIONS: Adverse Drug Reaction Overview: ULTIVA (remifentanil hydrochloride) produces adverse events that are characteristic of µ-opioids, such as respiratory depression, bradycardia, hypotension, and skeletal muscle rigidity. These adverse events dissipate within minutes of discontinuing or decreasing the infusion rate of remifentanil (see Action and Clinical Pharmacology, Warnings and Precautions on the management of these events).

Clinical Trial Adverse Drug Reactions: Because clinical trials are conducted under very specific conditions the adverse reaction rates observed in the clinical trials may not reflect the rates observed in practice and should not be compared to the rates in the clinical trials of another drug. Adverse drug reaction information from clinical trials is useful for identifying drug-related adverse events and for approximating rates.

Adverse event information is derived from controlled clinical trials that were conducted in a variety of surgical procedures of varying duration, using a variety of premedications and other anesthetics, and in patient populations with diverse characteristics including underlying disease.

Approximately 2492 patients were exposed to remifentanil in controlled clinical trials. The frequencies of adverse events during general anesthesia with the recommended doses of ULTIVA are given in Table 1.

In the elderly population (>65 years), the incidence of hypotension is higher, whereas the incidence of nausea and vomiting is lower (see Warnings and Precautions).

Data from cardiac risk analysis in non-cardiac general anesthesia studies indicate the incidence of hypotension in patients with cardiac risk factors (i.e., >65 years of age, concomitant use of cardiac medication) is higher with remifentanil then comparator drugs (27% vs. 12%, respectively).

Table 1: ULTIVA

Adverse Events ≥1% of Patients in General Anesthesia Studies at the Recommended Doses of Remifentanil[a]

Adverse Event	Induction/Maintenance Remifentanil (n=921)	Induction/Maintenance Alfentanil/ Fentanyl (n=466)	After Discontinuation Remifentanil (n=929)	After Discontinuation Alfentanil/ Fentanyl (n=466)
Nausea	8 (<1%)	0	339 (36%)	202 (43%)
Hypotension	178 (19%)	30 (6%)	16 (2%)	9 (2%)
Vomiting	4 (<1%)	1 (<1%)	150 (16%)	91 (20%)
Muscle rigidity	98 (11%)[b]	37 (8%)	2 (<1%)	1 (<1%)
Bradycardia	62 (7%)	24 (5%)	11 (1%)	6 (1%)
Shivering	3 (<1%)	0	49 (5%)	10 (2%)
Fever	1 (<1%)	0	44 (5%)	9 (2%)
Dizziness	0	0	27 (3%)	9 (2%)
Visual disturbance	0	0	24 (3%)	14 (3%)
Headache	0	0	21 (2%)	8 (2%)
Respiratory depression	1 (<1%)	0	17 (2%)	20 (4%)
Apnea	0	1 (<1%)	2 (<1%)	1 (<1%)
Pruritus	2 (<1%)	0	22 (2%)	7 (2%)
Tachycardia	6 (<1%)	7 (2%)	10 (1%)	8 (2%)
Postoperative pain	0	0	4 (<1%)	5 (1%)
Hypertension	10 (1%)	7 (2%)	12 (1%)	8 (2%)
Agitation	2 (<1%)	0	6 (<1%)	1 (<1%)
Hypoxia	0	0	10 (1%)	7 (2%)

[a] **Not all doses of remifentanil were equipotent to the comparator opioid. Administration of remifentanil in excess of the recommended dose (i.e., doses >1 and up to 20 µg/kg) resulted in a higher incidence of some adverse events: muscle rigidity (37%), bradycardia (12%), hypertension (4%), and tachycardia (4%).**

[b] Included in the muscle rigidity incidence is chest wall rigidity (5%). The overall muscle rigidity incidence is reduced to <1% when remifentanil is administered concurrently with or after a hypnotic induction agent.

Less Common Clinical Trial Adverse Drug Reactions (<1%): Other adverse events reported less frequently (<1%) include constipation and sedation.

Post-Market Adverse Drug Reactions: Very rarely, allergic reactions including anaphylaxis have been reported in patients receiving ULTIVA in conjunction with one or more anesthetic agents.

DRUG INTERACTIONS: Overview: Drug-Drug Interactions: Remifentanil clearance is not altered by concomitant administration of thiopental, isoflurane, propofol or temazepam during anesthesia. In vitro studies with atracurium, mivacurium, esmolol, echothiophate, neostigmine, physostigmine and midazolam revealed no inhibition of remifentanil hydrolysis in whole human blood by these drugs. In animals the duration of muscle paralysis from succinylcholine is not prolonged by remifentanil.

Remifentanil is synergistic with other anesthetics and doses of thiopental, propofol, isoflurane and midazolam have been reduced by up to 75% with the coadministration of remifentanil. If doses of concomitantly administered CNS depressant drugs are not reduced, patients may experience an increased incidence of adverse effects associated with these agents.

DOSAGE AND ADMINISTRATION: Dosing Considerations: Due to insufficient safety and efficacy data, ULTIVA (remifentanil hydrochloride) is not recommended for use in spontaneous ventilation anesthesia, in monitored anesthesia care, for continuation as an analgesic in the immediate postoperative period, in neurosurgery, in cardiac surgery, or in pediatric anesthesia.

Remifentanil is not recommended as the sole agent in general anesthesia because loss of consciousness cannot be assured and because of a high incidence of apnea, muscle rigidity, and tachycardia.

Recommended Dose and Dosage Adjustment: Remifentanil is synergistic with other anesthetics and doses of thiopental, propofol, isoflurane and midazolam have been reduced by up to 75% with the coadministration of remifentanil. At the recommended doses shown in Table 2, remifentanil significantly reduces the amount of hypnotic agent required to maintain anesthesia. Therefore isoflurane and propofol should be administered as recommended below to avoid excessive depth of anesthesia.

Intraoperative awareness has been reported in patients under 55 years of age when remifentanil has been administered with propofol infusion rates of ≤75 μg/kg/min. Therefore, propofol rates <100 μg/kg/min are not recommended for use with remifentanil for total intravenous anesthesia in patients <55 years of age.

I.V. bolus administration should only be used in intubated patients during the maintenance of general anesthesia. For induction of anesthesia in nonintubated patients, a single dose of remifentanil, not exceeding 1 μg/kg, may be administered over 30 to 60 seconds.

Reconstituted solutions of remifentanil should be diluted prior to administration (see Dosage and Administration, Reconstitution, Parenteral Products).

The administration of remifentanil must be individualized based on the patient's response. Table 2 summarizes the recommended doses in adult patients, predominately ASA physical status I, II, or III.

Table 2: ULTIVA
Dosing Guidelines

Phase	Continuous I.V. Infusion of ULTIVA (μg/kg/min)	Infusion Dose Range of ULTIVA (μg/kg/min)	Supplemental I.V. Bolus Dose of ULTIVA (μg/kg)
Induction of Anesthesia (through intubation)	0.5–1[a]		
Maintenance of Anesthesia with:			
Nitrous oxide (66%)	0.4	0.1–2	0.5–1
Isoflurane (starting dose 0.5 MAC)	0.25	0.05–2	0.5–1
Propofol (starting dose 100 μg/kg/min)	0.25	0.05–2	0.5–1

[a] An initial dose of 1 μg/kg may be administered over 30 to 60 seconds.

During Induction of Anesthesia: Remifentanil should be administered at an infusion rate of 0.5 to 1 μg/kg/min with a hypnotic or volatile agent for the induction of anesthesia. If endotracheal intubation is to occur less than 8 minutes after the start of the infusion of remifentanil, then an initial dose of 1 μg/kg may be administered over 30 to 60 seconds.

During Maintenance of Anesthesia: After endotracheal intubation, the infusion rate of remifentanil should be decreased in accordance with the dosing guidelines in Table 2. Due to the fast onset and short duration of action of remifentanil, the rate of administration during anesthesia can be titrated upward in 25% to 100% increments or downward in 25% to 50% decrements every 2 to 5 minutes to attain the desired level of μ-opioid effect. In response to light anesthesia or transient episodes of intense surgical stress, supplemental bolus doses of 0.5 to 1 μg/kg may be administered every 2 to 5 minutes. At infusion rates >1 μg/kg/min, increases in the concomitant anesthetic agents should be considered to increase the depth of anesthesia.

Guidelines for Discontinuation: Upon discontinuation of remifentanil, the i.v. tubing should be cleared to prevent the inadvertent administration of remifentanil at a later time. Due to the rapid offset of action of remifentanil, no residual analgesic activity will be present within 5 to 10 minutes after discontinuation. However respiratory depression may occur in some patients up to 30 minutes after termination of infusion due to residual effects of concomitant anesthetics. Standard monitoring should be maintained in the postoperative period to ensure adequate recovery without stimulation. For those patients undergoing surgical procedures where postoperative pain is generally anticipated, alternative analgesics should be administered prior to discontinuation of remifentanil. Sufficient time must be allowed to reach the maximum effect of the longer acting analgesic. The choice of analgesic should be appropriate for the patient's surgical procedure and the level of follow-up care.

Use in Elderly Patients: Due to the increased sensitivity to the pharmacological effects of remifentanil in this population (>65 years), the starting doses of remifentanil should be decreased by 50% and then be titrated to individual patient need.

Use in Obese Patients: The starting doses of remifentanil should be based on ideal body weight in obese patients as the clearance and volume of distribution of remifentanil are better correlated with ideal body weight than actual body weight in this population.

Preanesthetic Medication: The need for premedication and the choice of anesthetic agents must be individualized. In clinical studies, patients who received remifentanil frequently received a benzodiazepine premedication.

Individualization of Infusion Rates: Infusion rates of ULTIVA can be individualized for each patient using Table 3.

Table 3: ULTIVA
Infusion Rates of ULTIVA (mL/kg/h)

Drug Delivery Rate (μg/kg/min)	Infusion Delivery Rate (mL/kg/h)		
	25 μg/mL	50 μg/mL	250 μg/mL
0.05	0.12	0.06	0.012
0.075	0.18	0.09	0.018
0.1	0.24	0.12	0.024
0.15	0.36	0.18	0.036
0.2	0.48	0.24	0.048
0.25	0.6	0.3	0.06
0.5	1.2	0.6	0.12
0.75	1.8	0.9	0.18
1.0	2.4	1.2	0.24
1.25	3.0	1.5	0.3
1.5	3.6	1.8	0.36
1.75	4.2	2.1	0.42
2.0	4.8	2.4	0.48

Table 4 is a guideline for milliliter-per-hour delivery for a solution of 25 μg/mL with an infusion device.

Table 4: ULTIVA
Infusion Rates of ULTIVA (mL/h) for a 25 μg/mL Solution

Infusion Rate (μg/kg/min)	Patient Weight (kg)							
	30	40	50	60	70	80	90	100
0.05	3.6	4.8	6.0	7.2	8.4	9.6	10.8	12.0
0.075	5.4	7.2	9.0	10.8	12.6	14.4	16.2	18.0
0.1	7.2	9.6	12.0	14.4	16.8	19.2	21.6	24.0
0.15	10.8	14.4	18.0	21.6	25.2	28.8	32.4	36.0
0.2	14.4	19.2	24.0	28.8	33.6	38.4	43.2	48.0

Table 5 is a guideline for milliliter-per-hour delivery for a solution of 50 μg/mL with an infusion device.

Table 5: ULTIVA
Infusion Rates of ULTIVA (mL/h) for a 50 μg/mL Solution

Infusion Rate (μg/kg/min)	Patient Weight (kg)							
	30	40	50	60	70	80	90	100
0.05	1.8	2.4	3.0	3.6	4.2	4.8	5.4	6.0
0.075	2.7	3.6	4.5	5.4	6.3	7.2	8.1	9.0
0.1	3.6	4.8	6.0	7.2	8.4	9.6	10.8	12.0
0.15	5.4	7.2	9.0	10.8	12.6	14.4	16.2	18.0
0.2	7.2	9.6	12.0	14.4	16.8	19.2	21.6	24.0
0.25	9.0	12.0	15.0	18.0	21.0	24.0	27.0	30.0
0.5	18.0	24.0	30.0	36.0	42.0	48.0	54.0	60.0
0.75	27.0	36.0	45.0	54.0	63.0	72.0	81.0	90.0
1.0	36.0	48.0	60.0	72.0	84.0	96.0	108.0	120.0
1.25	45.0	60.0	75.0	90.0	105.0	120.0	135.0	150.0
1.5	54.0	72.0	90.0	108.0	126.0	144.0	162.0	180.0
1.75	63.0	84.0	105.0	126.0	147.0	168.0	189.0	210.0
2.0	72.0	96.0	120.0	144.0	168.0	192.0	216.0	240.0

Table 6 is a guideline for milliliter-per-hour delivery for a solution of 250 μg/mL with an infusion device.

Table 6: ULTIVA
Infusion Rates of ULTIVA (mL/h) for a 250 μg/mL Solution

Infusion Rate (μg/kg/min)	Patient Weight (kg)							
	30	40	50	60	70	80	90	100
0.1	0.72	0.96	1.20	1.44	1.68	1.92	2.16	2.40
0.15	1.08	1.44	1.80	2.16	2.52	2.88	3.24	3.60
0.2	1.44	1.92	2.40	2.88	3.36	3.84	4.32	4.80
0.25	1.80	2.40	3.00	3.60	4.20	4.80	5.40	6.00
0.5	3.60	4.80	6.00	7.20	8.40	9.60	10.80	12.00
0.75	5.40	7.20	9.00	10.80	12.60	14.40	16.20	18.00
1.0	7.20	9.60	12.00	14.40	16.80	19.20	21.60	24.00
1.25	9.00	12.00	15.00	18.00	21.00	24.00	27.00	30.00
1.5	10.80	14.40	18.00	21.60	25.20	28.80	32.40	36.00
1.75	12.60	16.80	21.00	25.20	29.40	33.60	37.80	42.00
2.0	14.40	19.20	24.00	28.80	33.60	38.40	43.20	48.00

Missed Dose: Not applicable.

Administration: Remifentanil should be administered only in a setting fully equipped for the monitoring and support of respiratory and cardiovascular function. Resuscitative and intubation equipment, oxygen and an opioid antagonist must be readily available.

Remifentanil should only be administered by persons specifically trained in the use of anesthetic drugs and the recognition and management of the expected adverse effects of potent opioids, including respiratory and cardiac resuscitation of patients in the age-group being treated. Such training must include the establishment and maintenance of a patent airway and assisted ventilation.

Remifentanil is for i.v. use only and must not be administered by epidural or intrathecal injection. Continuous infusions of remifentanil should be administered only by an infusion device. The injection site should be close to the venous cannula and all i.v. tubing should be cleared at the time of discontinuation of infusion.

Reconstitution: Parenteral Products: Preparation for Administration: To reconstitute solution, add 1 mL of diluent per mg of remifentanil. Shake well to dissolve. When reconstituted as directed, the solution contains approximately 1 mg of remifentanil activity per 1 mL. ULTIVA should be reconstituted and diluted to a recommended final concentration of 25, 50, or 250 μg/mL prior to administration as indicated in Table 7 and Table 8. **ULTIVA should not be administered without dilution.** ULTIVA does not contain any antimicrobial preservatives and thus care must be taken to assure the sterility of prepared solutions.

ULTIVA can be reconstituted and diluted to concentrations of 20 to 250 μg/mL in any of the following i.v. fluids:

- Sterile Water for Injection, USP

- 5% Dextrose Injection, USP
- 5% Dextrose and 0.9% Sodium Chloride Injection, USP
- 0.9% Sodium Chloride Injection, USP
- 0.45% Sodium Chloride Injection, USP
- Lactated Ringer's and 5% Dextrose Injection, USP
- Lactated Ringer's Injection, USP

ULTIVA has been shown to be compatible with these i.v. fluids when coadministered into a running i.v. administration set.

Table 7: ULTIVA

Reconstitution of ULTIVA

Vial Size (mg of remifentanil base)	Volume of Diluent to be Added to Vial	Approximate[a] Available Volume	Nominal Concentration
1 mg	1 mL	1 mL	1 mg/mL
2 mg	2 mL	2 mL	1 mg/mL
5 mg	5 mL	5 mL	1 mg/mL

[a] Densities for water and reconstituted ULTIVA are not significantly different.

Table 8: ULTIVA

Dilution of ULTIVA

Final Concentration	Amount of Remifentanil in Each Vial	Volume to be Added to Dilute[a]	Final Volume after Dilution
25 µg/mL	1 mg	39 mL	40 mL
	2 mg	78 mL	80 mL
	5 mg	195 mL	200 mL
50 µg/mL	1 mg	19 mL	20 mL
	2 mg	38 mL	40 mL
	5 mg	95 mL	100 mL
250 µg/mL	5 mg	15 mL	20 mL

[a] Note amounts indicated are those to be added after ULTIVA has been reconstituted to a 1 mg/mL solution as indicated in Table 7.

Compatibility with Other Therapeutic Agents: ULTIVA has been shown to be compatible with Propofol Injection when coadministered into a running i.v. administration set. The compatibility of ULTIVA with other therapeutic agents has not been evaluated.

Incompatibilities: Nonspecific esterases in blood products may lead to the hydrolysis of remifentanil to its carboxylic acid metabolite. Therefore, administration of ULTIVA into the same i.v. tubing with blood/serum/plasma is not recommended.

Note: Parenteral drug products should be inspected visually for particulate matter and discoloration prior to administration whenever solution and container permit. Product should be a clear, colorless liquid after reconstitution and free of visible particulate matter.

OVERDOSAGE:

As with all potent opioid analgesics, overdosage would be manifested by an extension of the pharmacological actions of ULTIVA (remifentanil hydrochloride). Expected signs and symptoms of overdosage include: apnea, chest-wall rigidity, seizures, hypoxemia, hypotension, and bradycardia.

In case of overdosage or suspected overdosage, discontinue administration of remifentanil, maintain a patent airway, initiate assisted or controlled ventilation with oxygen, and maintain adequate cardiovascular function. If depressed respiration is associated with muscle rigidity, a neuromuscular blocking agent or a µ-opioid antagonist may be required to facilitate assisted or controlled respiration. Intravenous fluids and vasopressors for the treatment of hypotension and other supportive measures may be employed. Glycopyrrolate or atropine may be useful for the treatment of bradycardia and/or hypotension.

Intravenous administration of an opioid antagonist such as naloxone may be employed as a specific antidote to manage severe respiratory depression or muscle rigidity. Respiratory depression following overdosage with remifentanil is not expected to last longer than the opioid antagonist, naloxone. Reversal of the opioid effects may lead to acute pain and sympathetic hyperactivity.

For management of a suspected drug overdose, CPhA recommends that you contact your **regional Poison Control Centre**. See the *CPS* Directory section for a list of Poison Control Centres.

ACTION AND CLINICAL PHARMACOLOGY: Mechanism of Action: ULTIVA (remifentanil hydrochloride) is a µ-opioid agonist with rapid onset and peak effect, and ultra-short duration of action. The µ-opioid activity of remifentanil is antagonized by opioid antagonists such as naloxone.

The analgesic effects of remifentanil are rapid in onset and offset. Its effects and side effects are dose dependent and similar to other µ-opioids. Remifentanil in humans has a rapid blood-brain equilibration half-time of 1±1 minutes (mean±SD) and a rapid onset of action. The pharmacodynamic effects of remifentanil closely follow the measured blood concentrations, allowing direct correlation between dose, blood levels, and response. Blood concentration decreases 50% in 3 to 6 minutes after a 1-minute infusion or after prolonged continuous infusion due to rapid distribution and elimination processes and is independent of duration of drug administration. Recovery from the effects of remifentanil occurs rapidly (within 5 to 10 minutes). New steady-state concentrations occur within 5 to 10 minutes after changes in infusion rate. When used as a component of an anesthetic technique, remifentanil can be rapidly titrated to the desired depth of anesthesia/analgesia (e.g., as required by varying levels of intraoperative stress) by changing the continuous infusion rate or by administering an i.v. bolus injection.

Pharmacodynamics: Haemodynamics: In premedicated patients undergoing anesthesia, 1-minute infusions of <2 µg/kg of remifentanil caused dose-dependent hypotension and bradycardia. While additional doses >2 µg/kg (up to 30 µg/kg) do not produce any further decreases in heart rate or blood pressure, the duration of the hemodynamic change is increased in proportion to the blood concentrations achieved. Peak hemodynamic effects occur within 3 to 5 minutes of a single dose of remifentanil or an infusion rate increase. Glycopyrrolate, atropine, and vagolytic neuromuscular blocking agents attenuate the hemodynamic effects associated with remifentanil. When appropriate, bradycardia and hypotension can be reversed by reduction of the rate of infusion of remifentanil, or the dose of concurrent anesthetics, or by the administration of fluids or vasopressors.

Respiration: Remifentanil depresses respiration in a dose-related fashion. Unlike other fentanyl analogs, the duration of action of remifentanil at a given dose does not increase with increasing duration of administration, due to lack of drug accumulation. When remifentanil and alfentanil were dosed to equal levels of respiratory depression, recovery of respiratory drive after 3-hour infusions was more rapid and less variable with remifentanil (see Figure 1).

Spontaneous respiration occurs at blood concentrations of 4 to 5 ng/mL in the absence of other anesthetic agents; for example, after discontinuation of a 0.25-µg/kg/min infusion of remifentanil, these blood concentrations would be reached in 2 to 4 minutes. In patients undergoing general anesthesia, the rate of respiratory recovery depends upon the concurrent anesthetic; N_2O < propofol < isoflurane.

Muscle Rigidity: Skeletal muscle rigidity can be caused by remifentanil and is related to the dose and speed of administration. Remifentanil may cause chest wall rigidity (inability to ventilate) after single doses of >1 µg/kg administered over 30 to 60 seconds or infusion rates >0.1 µg/kg/min; peripheral muscle rigidity may occur at lower doses. Administration of doses <1 µg/kg may cause chest wall rigidity when given concurrently with a continuous infusion of remifentanil. Prior or concurrent administration of a hypnotic (propofol or thiopental) or a neuromuscular blocking agent may attenuate the development of muscle rigidity. Excessive muscle rigidity can be treated by decreasing the rate or discontinuing the infusion of remifentanil or by administering a neuromuscular blocking agent.

Figure 1: ULTIVA

Recovery of Respiratory Drive After Equipotent[a] Doses of Remifentanil and Alfentanil Using CO_2-Stimulated Minute Ventilation in Volunteers (±1.5 SEM)

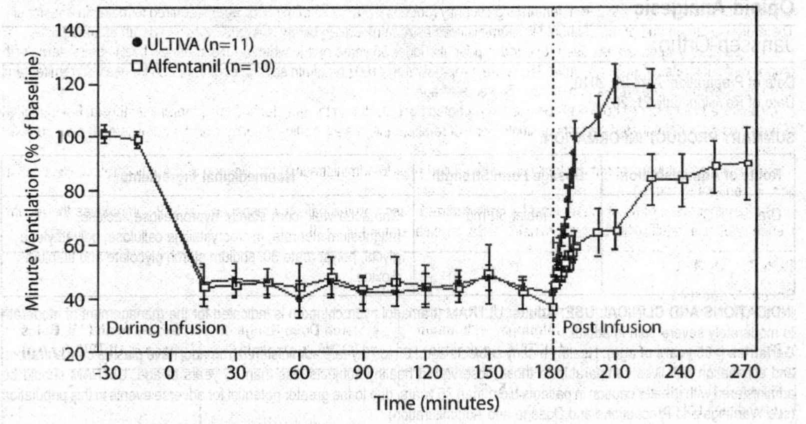

[a] Equipotent refers to level of respiratory depression.

Histamine Release: Assays of histamine in patients and normal volunteers have shown no elevation in plasma histamine levels after administration of remifentanil in doses up to 30 µg/kg over 60 seconds.

Anesthesia: Remifentanil is synergistic with the activity of hypnotics (propofol and thiopental), inhaled anesthetics, and benzodiazepines (see Warnings and Precautions, and Dosage and Administration).

Gender: No differences have been shown in the pharmacodynamic activity (as measured by the EEG) of remifentanil between men and women.

Pharmacokinetics: Absorption: After i.v. doses administered over 60 seconds, the pharmacokinetics of remifentanil fit a three-compartment model with a rapid distribution half-life of 1 minute, a slower distribution half-life of 6 minutes, and a terminal elimination half-life of 10 to 20 minutes. Since the terminal elimination component contributes less than 10% of the overall area under the concentration versus time curve (AUC), the effective biological half-life of remifentanil is 3 to 10 minutes. This is similar to the 3- to 10-minute half-life measured after termination of prolonged infusions (up to 4 hours; see Figure 2) and correlates with recovery times observed in the clinical setting after infusions up to 12 hours. Concentrations of remifentanil are proportional to the dose administered throughout the recommended dose range. The pharmacokinetics of remifentanil are unaffected by the presence of renal or hepatic impairment.

Distribution: The initial volume of distribution (V_d) of remifentanil is approximately 100 mL/kg and represents distribution throughout the blood and rapidly perfused tissues. Remifentanil subsequently distributes into peripheral tissues with a steady-state volume of distribution of approximately 350 mL/kg. These two distribution volumes generally correlate with total body weight (except in severely obese patients when they correlate better with ideal body weight [IBW]). Remifentanil is approximately 70% bound to plasma proteins of which two-thirds is binding to alpha-1-acid-glycoprotein.

Metabolism: Remifentanil is an esterase-metabolized opioid. A labile ester linkage renders this compound susceptible to hydrolysis by nonspecific esterases in blood and tissues. This hydrolysis results in production of the carboxylic acid metabolite (3-[4-methoxycarbonyl-4-[(1-oxopropyl)phenylamino]-1-piperidine]propanoic acid), and represents the principal metabolic pathway for remifentanil (>95%). The carboxylic acid metabolite is essentially inactive (1/4 600 as potent as remifentanil in dogs) and is excreted by the kidneys with an elimination half-life of approximately 90 minutes. Remifentanil is not metabolized by plasma cholinesterase (pseudocholinesterase) and is not appreciably metabolized by the liver or lung.

Excretion: The clearance of remifentanil in young, healthy adults is approximately 40 mL/min/kg. Clearance generally correlates with total body weight (except in severely obese patients when it correlates better with ideal body weight). The high clearance of remifentanil combined with a relatively small volume of distribution produces a short elimination half-life of approximately 3 to 10 minutes (see Figure 2). This value is consistent with the time taken for blood or effect site concentrations to fall by 50% (context-sensitive half-times), which is approximately 3 to 6 minutes. Unlike other fentanyl analogs, the duration of action does not increase with prolonged administration.

Figure 2: ULTIVA

Mean Concentration (SD) Versus Time

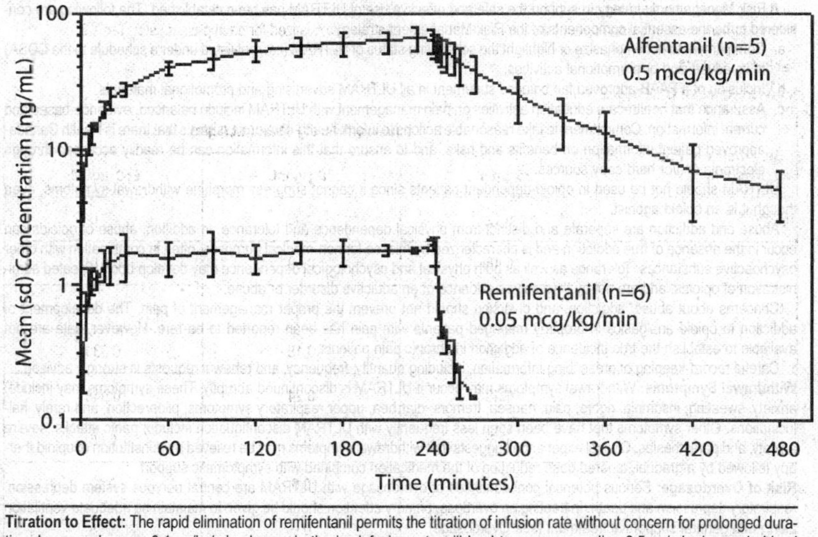

Titration to Effect: The rapid elimination of remifentanil permits the titration of infusion rate without concern for prolonged duration. In general, every 0.1-µg/kg/min change in the i.v. infusion rate will lead to a corresponding 2.5-ng/mL change in blood remifentanil concentration within 5 to 10 minutes. In intubated patients only, a more rapid increase (within 3 to 5 minutes) to a new steady state can be achieved with a 1.0-µg/kg bolus dose in conjunction with an infusion rate increase.

STORAGE AND STABILITY: ULTIVA for Injection should be stored between 2 to 25°C. Reconstituted and diluted solutions of ULTIVA (20 to 250 µg/mL) are stable for 24 hours at room temperature for all recommended i.v. fluids except those containing Lactated Ringer's Solution (stable for 4 hours).

INFORMATION FOR THE PATIENT: Published in e-CPS, available by subscription at www.e-cps.ca.

DOSAGE FORMS, COMPOSITION AND PACKAGING: 1 mg: Each vial of lyophilized powder contains: remifentanil base (as the HCl salt) 1 mg. Nonmedicinal ingredients: glycine and hydrochloric acid (adjust pH). Vials of 3 mL, cartons of 10.

2 mg: Each vial of lyophilized powder contains: remifentanil base (as the HCl salt) 2 mg. Nonmedicinal ingredients: glycine and hydrochloric acid (adjust pH). Vials of 5 mL, cartons of 10.

Ultram® ℞
tramadol HCl
Opioid Analgesic

Janssen-Ortho

Date of Preparation: April 21, 2010
Date of Revision: July 21, 2010

SUMMARY PRODUCT INFORMATION:

Route of Administration	Dosage Form/Strength	Nonmedicinal Ingredients
Oral	Tablet 50 mg	Carnauba wax, corn starch, hypromellose, lactose, magnesium stearate, microcrystalline cellulose, polyethylene glycol, polysorbate 80, sodium starch glycolate and titanium dioxide

INDICATIONS AND CLINICAL USE: Adults: ULTRAM (tramadol hydrochloride) is indicated for the management of moderate to moderately severe pain in adults.

Geriatrics (>65 years of age): Healthy elderly subjects aged 65 to 75 years administered tramadol have plasma concentrations and elimination half-lives comparable to those observed in healthy subjects less than 65 years of age. ULTRAM should be administered with greater caution in patients older than 75 years, due to the greater potential for adverse events in this population (see Warnings and Precautions and Dosage and Administration).

Pediatrics (<18 years of age): The safety and effectiveness of ULTRAM have not been studied in the pediatric population. Therefore, use of ULTRAM tablets is not recommended in patients under 18 years of age.

CONTRAINDICATIONS:

- ULTRAM should not be administered to patients who have previously demonstrated hypersensitivity to tramadol, opioids or to any component of this product.
- ULTRAM is contraindicated in any situation where opioids are contraindicated, including acute intoxication with any of the following: alcohol, hypnotics, centrally acting analgesics, opioids or psychotropic drugs. ULTRAM may worsen central nervous system and respiratory depression in these patients.
- The concomitant use of ULTRAM and MAO inhibitors (or within 14 days following discontinuation of such therapy) is contraindicated.

WARNINGS AND PRECAUTIONS: Seizure Risk: Seizures have been reported in patients receiving tramadol within the recommended dosage range. Spontaneous post-marketing reports indicate that seizure risk is increased with doses of ULTRAM above the recommended range. Concomitant use of ULTRAM increases the seizure risk in patients taking:

- selective serotonin reuptake inhibitors (SSRI antidepressants or anorectics) (see Use with Serotonin Reuptake Inhibitors);
- tricyclic antidepressants (TCAs) and other tricyclic compounds (e.g. cyclobenzaprine, promethazine, etc.); or
- other opioids.

Administration of tramadol may enhance the seizure risk in patients taking:

- MAO inhibitors (see Contraindications);
- neuroleptics; or
- other drugs that reduce the seizure threshold.

Risk of convulsions may also increase in patients with epilepsy, those with a history of seizures or in patients with a recognized risk for seizure (such as head trauma, metabolic disorders, alcohol and drug withdrawal, CNS infections). In ULTRAM overdose, naloxone administration may increase the risk of seizure.

Anaphylactoid Reactions: Serious and rarely, fatal anaphylactoid reactions have been reported in patients receiving therapy with tramadol. When these rare reactions do occur, it is often following the first dose. Other reported allergic reactions include pruritus, hives, bronchospasm, angioedema, toxic epidermal necrolysis and Stevens-Johnson syndrome. Patients with a history of anaphylactoid reactions to codeine and other opioids may be at increased risk and therefore should not receive ULTRAM tablets (see Contraindications).

Drug Abuse, Addiction and Dependence: ULTRAM has the potential to cause psychic and physical dependence of the morphine-type (μ-opioid). The drug has been associated with craving, drug-seeking behaviour and tolerance development. Cases of abuse and dependence on ULTRAM have been reported. ULTRAM tablets should not be used in opioid-dependent patients. ULTRAM can re-initiate physical dependence in patients who have been previously dependent or chronically using other opioids. In patients with a tendency to abuse drugs or a history of drug dependence, and in patients who are chronically using opioids, treatment with ULTRAM is not recommended.

Proper assessment of the patient, proper prescribing practices, periodic re-evaluation of therapy, and proper dispensing and storage are appropriate measures that help to limit abuse of opioid drugs.

A Risk Management strategy to support the safe and effective use of ULTRAM has been established. The following are considered to be the essential components of the Risk Management strategy:

a. Commitment to not emphasize or highlight the scheduling status of ULTRAM (i.e., not listed under a schedule to the CDSA) in its advertising or promotional activities.
b. Inclusion of a PAAB-approved fair balance statement in all ULTRAM advertising and promotional materials.
c. Assurance that health-care education activities on pain management with ULTRAM include balanced, evidence-based and current information. Commitment to take reasonable actions to inform health-care professionals that there is Health Canada-approved patient information on benefits and risks, and to ensure that this information can be readily accessed through electronic and/or hard copy sources.

ULTRAM should not be used in opioid-dependent patients since it cannot suppress morphine withdrawal symptoms, even though it is an opioid agonist.

Abuse and addiction are separate and distinct from physical dependence and tolerance. In addition, abuse of opioids can occur in the absence of true addiction and is characterized by misuse for non-medical purposes, often in combination with other psychoactive substances. Tolerance as well as both physical and psychological dependence may develop upon repeated administration of opioids, and are not by themselves evidence of an addictive disorder or abuse.

Concerns about abuse, addiction, and diversion should not prevent the proper management of pain. The development of addiction to opioid analgesics in properly managed patients with pain has been reported to be rare. However, data are not available to establish the true incidence of addiction in chronic pain patients.

Careful record-keeping of prescribing information, including quantity, frequency, and renewal requests is strongly advised.

Withdrawal Symptoms: Withdrawal symptoms may occur if ULTRAM is discontinued abruptly. These symptoms may include: anxiety, sweating, insomnia, rigors, pain, nausea, tremors, diarrhea, upper respiratory symptoms, piloerection, and rarely, hallucinations. Other symptoms that have been seen less frequently with ULTRAM discontinuation include: panic attacks, severe anxiety, and paresthesias. Clinical experience suggests that withdrawal symptoms may be relieved by reinstitution of opioid therapy followed by a gradual, tapered dose reduction of the medication combined with symptomatic support.

Risk of Overdosage: Serious potential consequences of overdosage with ULTRAM are central nervous system depression, respiratory depression and death. In treating an overdose, primary attention should be given to maintaining adequate ventilation along with general supportive treatment (see Overdosage).

Do not prescribe ULTRAM for patients who are suicidal or addiction-prone.

ULTRAM should not be taken in doses higher than those recommended by the physician. The judicious prescribing of tramadol is essential to the safe use of this drug. With patients who are depressed or suicidal, consideration should be given to the use of non-narcotic analgesics. Patients should be cautioned about the concomitant use of tramadol products and alcohol because of potentially serious CNS-additive effects of these agents. Because of its added depressant effects, tramadol should be prescribed with caution for those patients whose medical condition requires the concomitant administration of sedatives, tranquilizers, muscle relaxants, antidepressants, or other CNS-depressant drugs. Patients should be advised of the additive depressant effects of these combinations.

Intracranial Pressure or Head Trauma: ULTRAM should be used with caution in patients with increased intracranial pressure or head injury. The respiratory depressant effects of opioids include carbon dioxide retention and secondary elevation of cerebrospinal fluid pressure and may be markedly exaggerated in these patients. Additionally, pupillary changes (miosis) from ULTRAM may obscure the existence, extent, or course of intracranial pathology. Clinicians should also maintain a high index of suspicion for adverse drug reaction when evaluating altered mental status in these patients if they are receiving ULTRAM (see Respiratory, Respiratory Depression).

Respiratory: Respiratory Depression: Administer ULTRAM cautiously in patients at risk for respiratory depression. In these patients, alternative non-opioid analgesics should be considered. When large doses of ULTRAM are administered with anesthetic medications or alcohol, respiratory depression may result. Respiratory depression should be treated as an overdose. If naloxone is to be administered, use cautiously because it may precipitate seizures (see Seizure Risk and Overdosage).

Interaction with Central Nervous System (CNS) Depressants: ULTRAM should be used with caution and in reduced dosages when administered to patients receiving CNS depressants such as alcohol, opioids, anesthetic agents, narcotics, phenothiazines, tranquilizers or sedative hypnotics. ULTRAM increases the risk of CNS and respiratory depression in these patients.

ULTRAM may be expected to have additive effects when used in conjunction with alcohol, other opioids, or illicit drugs that cause central nervous system depression.

Use with Alcohol: ULTRAM should not be used concomitantly with alcohol consumption.

Use in Ambulatory Patients: ULTRAM may impair mental or physical abilities required for the performance of potentially hazardous tasks such as driving a car or operating machinery. The patient using this drug should be cautioned accordingly.

Use with MAO Inhibitors: Concomitant use of ULTRAM with MAO inhibitors is contraindicated (see Contraindications).

Animal studies have shown increased deaths with combined administration of MAO inhibitors and tramadol. Concomitant use of ULTRAM with MAO inhibitors increases the risk of adverse events, including seizure (see Seizure Risk and Drug Interactions) and serotonin syndrome.

Use with Serotonin Reuptake Inhibitors: Concomitant use of ULTRAM with SSRIs increases the risk of adverse events, including seizure (see Seizure Risk) and serotonin syndrome. When coadministration of ULTRAM and SSRIs is indicated, monitor the patient for seizures and possible early signs and symptoms of serotonin syndrome. Early symptoms of serotonin syndrome may include myoclonus, tremors, hyper-reflexia, diaphoresis, fever, tachycardia, tachypnoea, labile blood pressure, altered mental status (agitation, hallucinations, coma, excitement) and /or gastrointestinal symptoms (e.g., nausea, vomiting, diarrhea).

Gastrointestinal: Acute Abdominal Conditions: The administration of ULTRAM may complicate the clinical assessment of patients with acute abdominal conditions.

Use in Drug and Alcohol Addiction: ULTRAM is an opioid with no approved use in the management of addictive disorders.

Special Populations: Use in Renal and Hepatic Disease: Impaired renal function results in a decreased rate and extent of excretion of tramadol and its active metabolite, M1. In patients with creatinine clearances of less than 30 mL/min, a dose reduction is recommended (see Dosage and Administration). Metabolism of tramadol and M1 is reduced in patients with advanced cirrhosis of the liver. In cirrhotic patients, adjustment of the dosing regimen is recommended (see Dosage and Administration).

With the prolonged half-life in these conditions, achievement of steady-state is delayed, so that it may take several days for elevated plasma concentrations to develop.

Pregnant Women: There are no adequate and well-controlled studies in pregnant women. ULTRAM should be used during pregnancy only if the potential benefit justifies the potential risk to the fetus. Neonatal seizures, neonatal withdrawal syndrome, fetal death and stillbirth have been reported with tramadol hydrochloride during post-marketing.

ULTRAM should not be used in pregnant women prior to or during labour unless the potential benefits outweigh the risks. Safe use in pregnancy has not been established. Chronic use during pregnancy may lead to physical dependence and postpartum withdrawal symptoms in the newborn (see Drug Abuse, Addiction and Dependence). Tramadol has been shown to cross the placenta. The mean ratio of serum tramadol in the umbilical veins compared to maternal veins was 0.83 for 40 women given tramadol during labour.

The effect of ULTRAM, if any, on the later growth, development, and functional maturation of the child is unknown.

Nursing Women: ULTRAM is not recommended for obstetrical pre-operative medication or for post-delivery analgesia in nursing mothers because its safety in infants and newborns has not been studied.

Following a single 100 mg i.v. dose of tramadol, the cumulative excretion in breast milk within 16 hours post-dose was 100 μg of tramadol (0.1% of the maternal dose) and 27 μg of M1.

Pediatrics (<18 years of age): The safety and effectiveness of ULTRAM has not been studied in the pediatric population. Therefore, use of ULTRAM tablets is not recommended in patients under 18 years of age.

Geriatrics (>65 years of age): In general, dose selection for an elderly patient should be cautious, usually starting at the low end of the dosing range, reflecting the greater frequency of decreased hepatic, renal or cardiac function and of concomitant disease or other drug therapy. In patients over 75 years of age, daily doses in excess of 300 mg are not recommended (see Action and Clinical Pharmacology and Dosage and Administration).

A total of 455 elderly (65 years of age or older) subjects were exposed to ULTRAM in controlled clinical trials. Of those, 145 subjects were 75 years of age and older. In studies including geriatric patients, treatment-limiting adverse events were higher in subjects over 75 years of age compared to those under 65 years of age. Specifically, 30% of those over 75 years of age had gastrointestinal treatment-limiting adverse events compared to 17% of those under 65 years of age. Constipation resulted in discontinuation of treatment in 10% of those over 75.

ADVERSE REACTIONS: Adverse Drug Reaction Overview: The most commonly reported adverse reactions are dizziness, nausea, constipation, headache, somnolence and vomiting as presented in Table 1.

Clinical Trial Adverse Drug Reactions: Because clinical trials are conducted under very specific conditions the adverse reaction rates observed in the clinical trials may not reflect the rates observed in practice and should not be compared to the rates in the clinical trials of another drug. Adverse drug reaction information from clinical trials is useful for identifying drug-related adverse events and for approximating rates.

Incidence of Adverse Reactions for ULTRAM in Chronic Trials of Non-Malignant Pain (non titration trials): ULTRAM was administered to 550 patients during the double-blind or open-label extension periods in studies of chronic non-malignant pain. Of these patients, 375 were 65 years old or older. Table 1 reports the cumulative incidence rate of adverse reactions by 7, 30 and 90 days for the most frequent reactions (5% or more by 7 days). The most frequently reported events were in the central nervous system and gastrointestinal system. The overall incidence rates of adverse experiences in these trials were similar for ULTRAM and the active control groups, acetaminophen with codeine, and aspirin with codeine, however, the rates of withdrawals due to adverse events appeared to be higher in the ULTRAM group. In the tramadol treatment groups, 16.8-24.5% of patients withdrew due to an AE, compared to 9.6-11.6% for acetaminophen with codeine and 18.5% for aspirin with codeine.

Table 1: ULTRAM

Cumulative Incidence of Adverse Reactions for ULTRAM in Chronic Trials of Non-Malignant Pain

	Percentage of Patients with Adverse Reaction N=427		
	Up to 7 Days	**Up to 30 Days**	**Up to 90 Days**
Dizziness/Vertigo	26%	31%	33%
Nausea	24%	34%	40%
Constipation	24%	38%	46%
Headache	18%	26%	32%
Somnolence	16%	23%	25%
Vomiting	9%	13%	17%
Pruritus	8%	10%	11%
"CNS Stimulation"[a]	7%	11%	14%
Asthenia	6%	11%	12%
Sweating	6%	7%	9%

(cont'd)

Table 1: ULTRAM *(cont'd)*

Cumulative Incidence of Adverse Reactions for ULTRAM in Chronic Trials of Non-Malignant Pain

	Percentage of Patients with Adverse Reaction N=427		
	Up to 7 Days	Up to 30 Days	Up to 90 Days
Dyspepsia	5%	9%	13%
Dry Mouth	5%	9%	10%
Diarrhea	5%	6%	10%

[a] "CNS Stimulation" is a composite of nervousness, anxiety, agitation, tremor, spasticity, euphoria, emotional lability and hallucinations.

Two titration trials showed that the incidence of withdrawal due to AEs could be significantly reduced by using dose titration.

Incidence of Adverse Reactions for ULTRAM CAPSS-047 Titration Trial: In the double-blind phase of this pivotal trial, gastrointestinal complaints (primarily nausea and vomiting) and dizziness were the adverse events reported most frequently by tramadol treated subjects, Table 2. Most of the adverse events were assessed as mild or moderate in intensity and resolved.

Table 2: ULTRAM

Adverse Events in CAPSS-047—Double-Blind Phase—Frequently Reported (≥2%[a]) Adverse Events[b] and Total Incidence of AEs Summarized by WHOART Body System, Treatment Group and Preferred Term

	AEs in CAPSS-047 Double-Blind Phase ≥2% of Patients Tramadol Group/Titration Schedule					
Body System	10-days to 200 mg/day N=54		16-days to 200 mg/day N=59		13-days to 150 mg/day N=54	
Preferred Term	n	%	n	%	n	%
Any Adverse Event	41	75.9	41	69.5	33	61.1
Body as a Whole—General Disorders						
Influenza-like symptoms	0	0.0	2	3.4	0	0.0
Pain	1	1.9	2	3.4	0	0.0
Fatigue	0	0.0	0	0.0	2	3.7
Central & Peripheral Nervous System Disorders						
Dizziness	4	7.4	4	6.8	4	7.4
Headache	10	18.5	9	15.3	7	13.0
Gastrointestinal System Disorders						
Mouth Dry	0	0.0	1	1.7	3	5.6
Constipation	4	7.4	2	3.4	6	11.1
Diarrhea	4	7.4	3	5.1	1	1.9
Vomiting	10	18.5	7	11.9	4	7.4
Nausea	29	53.7	25	42.4	18	33.3
Psychiatric Disorders						
Insomnia	1	1.9	2	3.4	2	3.7
Somnolence	5	9.3	4	6.8	0	0.0
Reproductive Disorders, Female						
Menstrual Disorder	0	0.0	2	2.0	0	0.0
Reproductive Disorders, Male						
Epididymitis	0	0.0	0	0.0	1	11.1
Respiratory Systems Disorders						
Coughing	0	0.0	3	5.1	0	0.0
Sinusitis	1	1.9	2	3.4	2	3.7
Upper Resp Tract Infection	2	3.7	0	0.0	0	0.0
Skin and Appendages Disorders						
Pruritus	2	3.7	1	1.7	4	7.4
Rash	0	0.0	2	3.4	2	3.7

[a] Preferred terms reported by ≥2% of subjects in one or more treatment groups, intent-to-treat population.
[b] Number of patients with adverse event; numbers shown are all events regardless of relationship to study drug.

Incidence 1% to Less Than 5% Possibly Causally Related: The following lists adverse reactions that occurred with an incidence of 1% to less than 5% in clinical trials, and for which the possibility of a causal relationship with ULTRAM exists.

Body as a Whole: malaise.
Cardiovascular: vasodilation.
Central Nervous System: anxiety, confusion, coordination disturbance, euphoria, miosis, nervousness, sleep disorder.
Gastrointestinal: abdominal pain, anorexia, flatulence.
Musculoskeletal: hypertonia.
Skin: rash.
Special Senses: visual disturbance.
Urogenital: menopausal symptoms, urinary frequency, urinary retention.

Incidence Less Than 1%, Possibly Causally Related: The following lists adverse reactions that occurred with an incidence of less than 1% in clinical trials and/or reported in post-marketing experience.
Body as a Whole: accidental injury, allergic reaction, anaphylaxis, death, suicidal tendency, weight loss, serotonin syndrome (mental status change, hyperreflexia, fever, shivering, tremor, agitation, diaphoresis, seizures and coma).
Cardiovascular: orthostatic hypotension, syncope, tachycardia.
Central Nervous System: abnormal gait, amnesia, cognitive dysfunction, depression, difficulty in concentration, hallucinations, paresthesia, seizure (see Warnings and Precautions), tremor.
Respiratory: dyspnea.
Skin: Stevens-Johnson syndrome/toxic epidermal necrolysis, urticaria, vesicles.
Special Senses: dysgeusia.
Urogenital: dysuria, menstrual disorder.

Other Adverse Experiences, Causal Relationship Unknown: A variety of other adverse events were reported infrequently in patients taking ULTRAM during clinical trials and/or reported in post-marketing experience. A causal relationship between ULTRAM and these events has not been determined. However, the most significant events are listed below as alerting information to the physician.
Cardiovascular: abnormal ECG, hypertension, hypotension, myocardial ischemia, palpitations, pulmonary edema, pulmonary embolism.
Central Nervous System: migraine, speech disorders.
Gastrointestinal: gastrointestinal bleeding, hepatitis, stomatitis, liver failure.
Laboratory Abnormalities: creatinine increase, elevated liver enzymes, hemoglobin decrease, proteinuria.
Sensory: cataracts, deafness, tinnitus.

Other Adverse Experiences Previously Reported in Clinical Trials or Post-Marketing Reports with Tramadol Hydrochloride: Adverse events which have been reported with the use of tramadol products include: allergic reactions (including anaphylaxis, angioneurotic edema and urticaria), bradycardia, convulsions, drug dependence, drug withdrawal (including agitation, anxiety, gastrointestinal symptoms, hyperkinesia, insomnia, nervousness, tremors), hyperactivity, hypoactivity, hypotension and respiratory depression. Other adverse events which have been reported with the use of tramadol products and for which a causal association has not been determined include: difficulty concentrating, hepatitis, liver failure, pulmonary edema, Stevens-Johnson syndrome and suicidal tendency.

Serotonin syndrome (whose symptoms may include mental status change, hyperreflexia, fever, shivering, tremor, agitation, diaphoresis, seizures and coma) has been reported with tramadol when used concomitantly with other serotonergic agents such as SSRI's and MAOIs.

Drug Abuse, Addiction and Dependence: Tramadol may induce psychic and physical dependence of the morphine-type (μ-opioid) (see Warnings and Precautions, Drug Abuse, Addiction and Dependence). Dependence and abuse, including drug-seeking behaviour and taking illicit actions to obtain the drug are not limited to those patients with a prior history of opioid dependence. The risk in patients with substance abuse has been observed to be higher. Tramadol is associated with craving and tolerance development.

A Risk Management program to support the safe and effective use of ULTRAM has been established. The following are considered to be the essential components of the Risk Management program:

a. Commitment to not emphasize or highlight the scheduling status of ULTRAM (i.e., not listed under a schedule to the CDSA) in its advertising or promotional activities.
b. Inclusion of a PAAB-approved fair balance statement in all ULTRAM advertising and promotional materials.
c. Assurance that health-care education activities on pain management with ULTRAM include balanced, evidence-based and current information. Commitment to take reasonable actions to inform health-care professionals that there is Health Canada-approved patient information on benefits and risks, and to ensure that this information can be readily accessed through electronic and/or hard copy sources.

Withdrawal Symptoms: Withdrawal symptoms may occur if ULTRAM is discontinued abruptly. These symptoms may include: anxiety, sweating, insomnia, rigors, pain, nausea, tremors, diarrhea, upper respiratory symptoms, piloerection, and rarely, hallucinations. Other symptoms that have been seen less frequently with ULTRAM discontinuation include: panic attacks, severe anxiety, and paresthesias. Clinical experience suggests that withdrawal symptoms may be relieved by reinstitution of opioid therapy followed by a gradual, tapered dose reduction of the medication combined with symptomatic support.

DRUG INTERACTIONS: Overview: In vitro studies indicate that tramadol is unlikely to inhibit the CYP3A4-mediated metabolism of other drugs when tramadol is administered concomitantly at therapeutic doses. Tramadol does not appear to induce its own metabolism in humans, since observed maximal plasma concentrations after multiple oral doses are higher than expected based on single dose data. Tramadol is a mild inducer of selected drug metabolism pathways measured in animals.

Drug-Drug Interactions: Use with MAO Inhibitors: ULTRAM is contraindicated in patients receiving MAO inhibitors or who have used them within the previous 14 days (see Contraindications and Warnings and Precautions).

Drugs that Lower Seizure Threshold: Tramadol can increase the potential for selective serotonin re-uptake inhibitors (SSRIs), tricyclic antidepressants (TCAs), anti-psychotics and other seizure threshold lowering drugs to cause convulsions. If concomitant treatment of ULTRAM with a drug affecting the serotonergic neurotransmitter system is clinically warranted, careful observation of the patient is advised, particularly during treatment initiation and dose increases (see Warnings and Precautions, Use with Serotonin Reuptake Inhibitors).

CNS Depressants: Concurrent administration of tramadol with other centrally acting drugs, including alcohol, centrally acting analgesics, opioids and psychotropic drugs may potentiate CNS depressant effects (see Warnings and Precautions).

Use with Carbamazepine: Patients taking carbamazepine may have a significantly reduced analgesic effect of ULTRAM. Because carbamazepine increases tramadol metabolism and because of the seizure risk associated with tramadol, concomitant administration of ULTRAM and carbamazepine is not recommended.

Use with Quinidine: Tramadol is metabolized to M1 by the CYP2D6 P450 isoenzyme. Quinidine is a selective inhibitor of that isoenzyme, so that concomitant administration of quinidine and ULTRAM results in increased concentrations of tramadol and reduced concentrations of M1. The clinical consequences of these findings are unknown. In vitro drug interaction studies in human liver microsomes indicate that tramadol has no effect on quinidine metabolism.

Use with CYP2D6 and CYP3A4 Inhibitors: Concomitant administration of CYP2D6 and/or CYP3A4 inhibitors (see Action and Clinical Pharmacology, Pharmacokinetics), such as quinidine, fluoxetine, paroxetine, amitriptyline (CYP2D6 inhibitors), ketoconazole and erythromycin CYP3A4 inhibitors), may reduce metabolic clearance of tramadol increasing the risk for serious adverse events including seizures and serotonin syndrome.

Use with Cimetidine: Concomitant administration of ULTRAM and cimetidine does not result in clinically significant changes in tramadol pharmacokinetics. Therefore, no alteration of the ULTRAM dosage regimen is recommended.

Use with Digoxin: Post-marketing surveillance of tramadol has revealed rare reports of digoxin toxicity.

Use with Warfarin-like Compounds: Post-marketing surveillance of tramadol has revealed rare alterations of warfarin effect, including elevation of prothrombin times.

Periodic evaluation of prothrombin time should be performed when ULTRAM tablets and warfarin-like compounds are administered concurrently.

Triptans: Based on the mechanism of action of tramadol and the potential for serotonin syndrome, caution is advised when ULTRAM is coadministered with a triptan. If concomitant treatment of ULTRAM with a triptan is clinically warranted, careful observation of the patient is advised, particularly during treatment initiation and dose increases.

Drug-Food Interactions: Oral administration of ULTRAM with food does not significantly affect its rate or extent of absorption; therefore, ULTRAM can be administered without regard to food.

DOSAGE AND ADMINISTRATION: Dosing Considerations: ULTRAM is not recommended for minor pain that may be treated adequately through lesser means where benefit does not outweigh the possible opioid-related side effects.

ULTRAM can be administered without regard to food.

Do not coadminister ULTRAM tablets with other tramadol-containing products

Due to the differences in pharmacokinetic properties, ULTRAM tablets are not interchangeable with tramadol extended-release formulations.

The maximum recommended dose of ULTRAM should not be exceeded.

Recommended Dose and Dosage Adjustment: Good pain management practice dictates that the dose be individualized according to patient need using the lowest beneficial dose. Studies with tramadol in adults have shown that starting at the lowest possible dose and titrating upward will result in fewer discontinuations and increased tolerability.

Adults (18 years of age and over): For patients with moderate to moderately severe chronic pain not requiring rapid onset of analgesic effect, the tolerability of ULTRAM can be improved by initiating therapy with the following titration regimen: ULTRAM should be started at 25 mg/day (half ULTRAM scored tablet) qAM and titrated in 25 mg increments as separate doses every 3 days to reach 100 mg/day (25 mg q.i.d.). Thereafter the total daily dose may be increased by 50 mg as tolerated every 3 days to reach 200 mg/day (50 mg q.i.d.) as shown in Table 3.

Table 3: ULTRAM

Initiation Titration Dose of ULTRAM by Days

Days 1 to 3	Days 4 to 6	Days 7 to 9	Days 10 to 12	Days 13 to 15	Days 16 to 18
Initiate at 25 mg (AM) (half ULTRAM scored tablet)	25 mg b.i.d.	25 mg t.i.d.	25 mg q.i.d.	50 mg t.i.d.	50 mg q.i.d.

After titration, ULTRAM 50 to 100 mg can be administered as needed for pain relief every 4 to 6 hours **not to exceed 400 mg/day.**

For the subset of patients for whom rapid onset of analgesic effect is required and for whom the benefits outweigh the risk of discontinuation due to adverse events associated with higher initial doses, ULTRAM 50 mg to 100 mg can be administered as needed for pain relief every four to six hours, **not to exceed 400 mg per day.**

Use in Renal Impairment: In all patients **with creatinine clearance less than 30 mL/min**, it is recommended that the dosing interval of ULTRAM be increased to 12 hours, with a maximum daily dose of 200 mg. Since only 7% of an administered dose is removed by hemodialysis, **dialysis patients** can receive their regular dose on the day of dialysis.

Use in Hepatic Impairment: The recommended dose for adult patients with cirrhosis is 50 mg every 12 hours.

Elderly Patients (>65 years old): In general, dose selection for an elderly patient over 65 years old should be cautious, usually starting at the low end of the dosing range, reflecting the greater frequency of decreased hepatic, renal or cardiac function and of concomitant disease or other drug therapy. For elderly patients **over 75 years old**, total dose should not exceed 300 mg/day.

Pediatric Patients (<18 years old): The safety and effectiveness of ULTRAM has not been studied in the pediatric population. Therefore, use of ULTRAM tablets is not recommended in patients under 18 years of age.

Management of Patients Requiring Rescue Medication: If ULTRAM is used as rescue medication in conjunction with extended-release tramadol tablets, the total daily dose of tramadol should not exceed 400 mg. Fentanyl products should not be used as rescue medication in patients taking ULTRAM.

Missed Dose: If a patient misses a dose, they should take their next dose as soon as they remember. If it is almost time for their next dose, they should not take the missed dose. Instead, they should take the next scheduled dose. They should not make up for the missed dose by taking a double dose.

Discontinuation: Withdrawal symptoms may occur if ULTRAM is discontinued abruptly (see Warnings and Precautions, Drug Abuse, Addiction and Dependence). These symptoms may include: anxiety, sweating, insomnia, rigors, pain, nausea, tremors, diarrhea, upper respiratory symptoms, piloerection, and rarely, hallucinations. Other symptoms that have been seen less frequently with ULTRAM discontinuation include panic attacks, severe anxiety, and paresthesias. Clinical experience suggests that withdrawal symptoms may be avoided by tapering ULTRAM at the time of discontinuation.

OVERDOSAGE:

Symptoms: Symptoms of overdosage with ULTRAM are respiratory depression, somnolence progressing to stupor or coma, skeletal muscle flaccidity, cold and clammy skin, constricted pupils, seizures, bradycardia, hypotension, cardiac arrest, and death.

Deaths due to overdose have been reported with abuse and misuse of tramadol (see Warnings and Precautions, Drug Abuse, Addiction and Dependence). Review of case reports has indicated that the risk of fatal overdose is further increased when tramadol is abused concurrently with alcohol or other CNS depressants, including other opioids.

Treatment: A single or multiple overdose with ULTRAM may be a potentially lethal polydrug overdose, and consultation with a regional poison control centre is recommended.

In treating an overdose of ULTRAM, primary attention should be given to maintaining adequate ventilation along with general supportive treatment. Supportive measures (including oxygen and vasopressors) should be employed in the management of circulatory shock and pulmonary edema accompanying overdose as indicated. Cardiac arrest or arrhythmias may require cardiac massage or defibrillation.

While naloxone will reverse some, but not all, symptoms caused by overdosage with tramadol, the risk of seizures is also increased with naloxone administration. Seizures may be controlled with diazepam.

In animals, convulsions following the administration of toxic doses of tramadol could be suppressed with barbiturates or benzodiazepines but were increased with naloxone. Naloxone administration did not change the lethality of an overdose in mice.

Based on experience with tramadol, hemodialysis is not expected to be helpful in an overdose because it removes less than 7% of the administered dose in a 4-hour dialysis period.

Emptying of the gastric contents is useful to remove any unabsorbed drug.

> For management of a suspected drug overdose, contact your regional Poison Control Centre. See the *CPS* Directory section for a list of Poison Control Centres.

ACTION AND CLINICAL PHARMACOLOGY: Mechanism of Action: ULTRAM is a centrally acting synthetic opioid analgesic. Although its mode of action is not completely understood, from animal tests, at least two complementary mechanisms appear applicable: binding of parent and M1 metabolite to μ-opioid receptors and weak inhibition of reuptake of norepinephrine and serotonin.

Opioid activity is due to both low affinity binding of the parent compound and higher affinity binding of the O-demethylated metabolite M1 to μ-opioid receptors. In animal models, M1 is up to 6 times more potent than tramadol in producing analgesia and 200 times more potent in μ-opioid binding. Tramadol-induced analgesia is only partially antagonized by the opiate antagonist naloxone in several animal tests. The relative contribution of both tramadol and M1 to human analgesia is dependent upon the plasma concentrations of each compound (see Pharmacokinetics).

Tramadol has been shown to inhibit reuptake of norepinephrine and serotonin in vitro, as have some other opioid analgesics. These mechanisms may contribute independently to the overall analgesic profile of ULTRAM. Analgesia in humans begins approximately within one hour after administration and reaches a peak in approximately two to three hours.

Apart from analgesia, ULTRAM administration may produce a constellation of symptoms (including dizziness, somnolence, nausea, constipation, sweating and pruritus) similar to that of opioids. In contrast to morphine, tramadol has not been shown to cause histamine release. At therapeutic doses, ULTRAM has no effect on heart rate, left-ventricular function or cardiac index. Orthostatic hypotension has been observed.

Pharmacokinetics: The analgesic activity of ULTRAM is due to both parent drug and the M1 metabolite (see Mechanism of Action). Tramadol is administered as a racemate and both the [−] and [+] forms of both tramadol and M1 are detected in the circulation. Tramadol is well absorbed orally with an absolute bioavailability of 75%. Tramadol has a volume of distribution of approximately 2.7 L/kg and is only 20% bound to plasma proteins. Tramadol is extensively metabolized by a number of pathways, including CYP2D6 and CYP3A4, as well as by conjugation of parent and metabolites. One metabolite, M1, is pharmacologically active in animal models. The formation of M1 is dependent upon CYP2D6 and as such is subject to inhibition, which may affect the therapeutic response (see Drug Interactions). Tramadol and its metabolites are excreted primarily in the urine with observed plasma half-lives of 6.3 and 7.4 hours for tramadol and M1, respectively. Linear pharmacokinetics have been observed following multiple doses of 50 and 100 mg to steady-state.

Absorption: Racemic tramadol is rapidly and almost completely absorbed after oral administration. The mean absolute bioavailability of a 100 mg oral dose is approximately 75%. The mean peak plasma concentration of racemic tramadol and M1 occurs at two and three hours, respectively, after administration in healthy adults. In general, both enantiomers of tramadol and M1 follow a parallel time course in the body following single and multiple doses although small differences (~10%) exist in the absolute amount of each enantiomer present.

Steady-state plasma concentrations of both tramadol and M1 are achieved within two days with q.i.d. dosing. There is no evidence of self-induction (see Figure 1 and Table 4).

Figure 1: ULTRAM

Mean Tramadol and M1 Plasma Concentration Profiles after a Single 100 mg Oral Dose and after Twenty-Nine 100 mg Oral Doses of Tramadol HCl given q.i.d.

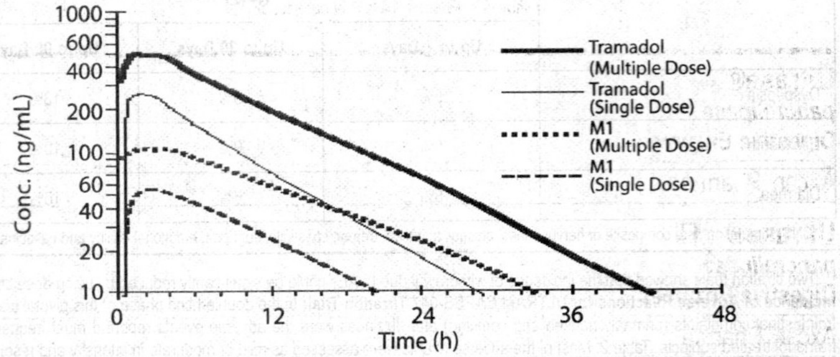

Table 4: ULTRAM

Mean (% CV) Pharmacokinetic Parameters for Racemic Tramadol and M1 Metabolite

Population/ Dosage Regimen[a]	Parent Drug/ Metabolite	C_{max} (ng/mL)	Time to Peak (hrs)	Clearance/F[b] (mL/min/Kg)	$t_{1/2}$ (hrs)
Healthy Adults, 100 mg qid, MD p.o.	Tramadol	592 (30)	2.3 (61)	5.90 (25)	6.7 (15)
	M1	110 (29)	2.4 (46)	[c]	7.0 (14)
Healthy Adults, 100 mg SD p.o.	Tramadol	308 (25)	1.6 (63)	8.50 (31)	5.6 (20)
	M1	55.0 (36)	3.0 (51)	[c]	6.7 (16)
Geriatric, (>75 yrs) 50 mg SD p.o.	Tramadol	208 (31)	2.1 (19)	6.89 (25)	7.0 (23)
	M1	[d]	[d]	[c]	[d]
Hepatic Impaired, 50 mg SD p.o.	Tramadol	217 (11)	1.9 (16)	4.23 (56)	13.3 (11)
	M1	19.4 (12)	9.8 (20)	[c]	18.5 (15)
Renal Impaired, CL_{cr} 10–30 mL/min 100 mg SD i.v.	Tramadol	[c]	[c]	4.23 (54)	10.6 (31)
	M1	[c]	[c]	[c]	11.5 (40)
Renal Impaired, CL_{cr} <5 mL/min 100 mg SD i.v.	Tramadol	[c]	[c]	3.73 (17)	11.0 (29)
	M1	[c]	[c]	[c]	16.9 (18)

[a] SD=single dose; MD=multiple dose; p.o.=oral administration; i.v.=intravenous administration; q.i.d.=four times daily.
[b] F represents the oral bioavailability of tramadol.
[c] Not applicable.
[d] Not measured.

Distribution: The volume of distribution of tramadol was 2.6 and 2.9 L/kg in male and female subjects, respectively, following a 100 mg intravenous dose. The binding of tramadol to human plasma proteins is approximately 20% and binding also appears to be independent of concentration up to 10 μg/mL. Saturation of plasma protein binding occurs only at concentrations outside the clinically relevant range.

Metabolism: Following oral administration, tramadol is extensively metabolized by a number of pathways, including CYP2D6 and CYP3A4, as well as by conjugation of parent and metabolites. Approximately 30% of the dose is excreted in the urine as unchanged drug, whereas 60% of the dose is excreted as metabolites. The major metabolic pathways appear to be N- and O-demethylation and glucuronidation or sulfation in the liver. Metabolite M1 (O-desmethyltramadol) is pharmacologically active in animal models. Formation of M1 is dependent on CYP2D6 and as such is subject to inhibition, which may affect the therapeutic response (see Drug Interactions).

Approximately 7% of the population has reduced activity of the CYP2D6 isoenzyme of cytochrome P450. These individuals are "poor metabolizers" of debrisoquine, dextromethorphan, and tricyclic antidepressants, among other drugs. Based on a population PK analysis of Phase I studies in healthy subjects, concentrations of tramadol were approximately 20% higher in "poor metabolizers" versus "extensive metabolizers", while M1 concentrations were 40% lower. In vitro drug interaction studies in human liver microsomes indicate that inhibitors of CYP2D6 such as fluoxetine and its metabolite norfluoxetine, amitriptyline and quinidine inhibit the metabolism of tramadol to various degrees. The full pharmacological impact of these alterations in terms of either efficacy or safety is unknown. Concomitant use of serotonin reuptake inhibitors and MAO inhibitors may enhance the risk of adverse events, including seizure (see Warnings and Precautions) and serotonin syndrome.

Excretion: Tramadol is eliminated primarily through metabolism by the liver and the metabolites are eliminated primarily by the kidneys. The mean terminal plasma elimination half-lives of racemic tramadol and racemic M1 are 6.3±1.4 and 7.4±1.4 hours, respectively. The plasma elimination half-life of racemic tramadol increased from approximately six hours to seven hours upon multiple dosing.

Special Populations and Conditions: Pediatrics: Pharmacokinetics of ULTRAM tablets have not been studied in pediatric patients below 18 years of age.

Geriatrics: Healthy elderly subjects aged 65 to 75 years have plasma tramadol concentrations and elimination half-lives comparable to those observed in healthy subjects less than 65 years of age. In subjects over 75 years, maximum serum concentrations are elevated (208 vs 162 ng/mL) and the elimination half-life is prolonged (7 vs 6 hours) compared to subjects 65 to 75 years of age. Adjustment of the daily dose is recommended for patients older than 75 years (see Dosage and Administration).

Gender: The absolute bioavailability of tramadol was 73% in males and 79% in females. The plasma clearance was 6.4 mL/min/kg in males and 5.7 mL/min/kg in females following a 100 mg IV dose of tramadol. Following a single oral dose, and after adjusting for body weight, females had a 12% higher peak tramadol concentration and a 35% higher area under the concentration-time curve compared to males. The clinical significance of this difference is unknown.

Hepatic Insufficiency: Metabolism of tramadol and M1 is reduced in patients with advanced cirrhosis of the liver, resulting in both a larger area under the concentration time curve for tramadol and longer tramadol and M1 elimination half-lives (13 hrs for tramadol and 19 hrs for M1). In cirrhotic patients, adjustment of the dosing regimen is recommended (see Warnings and Precautions and Dosage and Administration).

Renal Insufficiency: Excretion of tramadol and metabolite M1 is reduced in patients with creatinine clearance of less than 30 mL/min, adjustment of dosing regimen in this patient population is recommended. The total amount of tramadol and M1 removed during a 4-hour dialysis period is less than 7% of the administered dose (see Warnings and Precautions and Dosage and Administration).

STORAGE AND STABILITY: Dispense in a tight container. Store at 15-30°C.

INFORMATION FOR THE PATIENT: Published in e-CPS, available by subscription at www.e-cps.ca.

DOSAGE FORMS, COMPOSITION AND PACKAGING: Each white, capsule-shaped, coated tablet, imprinted "ULTRAM" on one side and "06 59" on the scored side, contains: tramadol hydrochloride 50 mg. Nonmedicinal ingredients: carnauba wax, corn starch, hypromellose, lactose, magnesium stearate, microcrystalline cellulose, polyethylene glycol, polysorbate 80, sodium starch glycolate and titanium dioxide. HDPE bottles of 100.

(Shown in Product Identification Section)

Ultrase®
pancrelipase
Digestive Enzymes

Axcan Pharma

Ultrase® MT
pancrelipase
Digestive Enzymes

Axcan Pharma

PHARMACOLOGY: ULTRASE and ULTRASE MT (pancrelipase) capsules are designed to prevent inactivation by gastric acid thereby resulting in the delivery of predictable, high levels of biologically active enzymes into the duodenum. The enzymes catalyze the hydrolysis of fats into glycerol and fatty acids, starch into dextrins and sugars, and protein into proteoses and derived substances.

INDICATIONS: For patients with partial or complete exocrine pancreatic insufficiency such as: cystic fibrosis, chronic pancreatitis, post-pancreatectomy, post-gastrointestinal bypass surgery (e.g., Billroth II gastroenterostomy), and ductal obstruction from neoplasm (e.g., of the pancreas or common bile duct).

Pancrelipase capsules are effective in controlling steatorrhea.

CONTRAINDICATIONS: In patients known to be hypersensitive to pork protein.

Pancrelipase capsules are contraindicated in patients with acute pancreatitis or with acute exacerbations of chronic pancreatic diseases.

WARNINGS: Should hypersensitivity occur, discontinue medication and treat symptomatically.

PRECAUTIONS: General: Individuals previously sensitized to trypsin, pancreatin or pancrelipase may have allergic manifestations.

To protect enteric coating, minitablets or microspheres must not be crushed or chewed. Where swallowing of capsules is difficult, they may be opened and the minitablets or microspheres added to a small quantity of a soft food (e.g., applesauce, gelatin, etc.), that does not require chewing, and swallowed immediately. Contact of the minitablets or microspheres with foods having a pH greater than 5.5 can dissolve the protective enteric shell.

Carcinogenesis, Mutagenesis, Impairment of Fertility: Long-term studies in animals have not been performed to evaluate carcinogenic potential. Methacrylic acid, a minor component of the methacrylic acid copolymer enteric-coating contained in ULTRASE capsules, has been reported to act as a teratogen in rat embryo cultures. However, ULTRASE capsules have been shown to contain <0.001% of methacrylic acid, and the mammalian teratology studies in the rat and rabbit were negative.

The copolymer enteric-coating of ULTRASE capsules was not mutagenic by the Ames test, and it did not produce chromosome damage in a test for unscheduled DNA synthesis in rat hepatocytes.

Pregnancy: Animal reproduction studies have not been conducted with ULTRASE and ULTRASE MT (pancrelipase) capsules. It is not known whether ULTRASE and ULTRASE MT (pancrelipase) capsules can cause fetal harm when administered to a pregnant woman or can affect reproduction capacity. ULTRASE and ULTRASE MT (pancrelipase) capsules should be given to a pregnant woman only if the potential benefit outweighs the potential risk to the fetus.

Lactation: It is not known whether ULTRASE and ULTRASE MT (pancrelipase) capsules are excreted in human milk. Because many drugs are excreted in human milk, caution should be exercised when ULTRASE and ULTRASE MT (pancrelipase) capsules are administered to a nursing mother.

ADVERSE EFFECTS: The most frequently reported adverse reactions to pancrelipase-containing products are gastrointestinal in nature. Less frequently, allergic-type reactions have also been observed.

Extremely high doses of exogenous pancreatic enzymes have been associated with hyperuricosuria and hyperuricemia when the preparations given were pancrelipase in powdered or capsule form, or pancreatin in tablet form.

In 2 clinical studies with ULTRASE MT in 193 patients with cystic fibrosis, the adverse events described were all gastrointestinal in nature and may actually represent symptoms of the underlying disease, such as abdominal pain/cramps (5.7%), diarrhea (3.6%), and greasy stools and flatulence (1.5%). In a postmarketing trial with another enteric-coated formulation, 160 adverse events occurred in the 15 711 patients (0.97%) evaluated. The most frequent events reported were diarrhea, skin reaction, and abdominal discomfort (0.2% each).

Colonic strictures have been reported in cystic fibrosis patients treated with both high- and lower-strength enzyme supplements. A causal relationship has not been established. The possibility of bowel stricture should be considered if symptoms suggestive of gastrointestinal obstruction occur. Since impaired fluid secretion may be a factor in the development of intestinal obstruction, care should be taken to maintain adequate hydration, particularly in warm weather.

"Fibrosing colonopathy" is a term used to describe a condition seen in patients with CF who have taken high amounts of pancreatic enzyme supplements (>6000 lipase U/kg/meal). At its most advanced, this condition leads to colonic strictures.

OVERDOSE:

No data supplied by the manufacturer.

For management of a suspected drug overdose, CPhA recommends that you contact your **regional Poison Control Centre**. See the *CPS* Directory section for a list of Poison Control Centres.

DOSAGE: The smallest effective dose should be used. Dosage should be adjusted according to the severity of the exocrine pancreatic insufficiency. Begin therapy with 1 or 2 capsules with meals or snacks and adjust dosage according to symptoms. The number of capsules or capsule strength given with meals and/or snacks should be estimated by assessing which dose minimizes steatorrhea and maintains good nutritional status.

Dosages should be adjusted according to the response of the patient. Where swallowing of capsules is difficult, they may be opened and the minitablets or microspheres added to a small quantity of a soft food (e.g., applesauce, gelatin, etc.), which does not require chewing, and swallowed immediately.

It is recommended that the total dose of pancrelipase being ingested for a meal or snack be dispersed equally (with fluids) before, during, and after the meal or snack.

SUPPLIED: ULTRASE and ULTRASE MT (pancrelipase) capsules are orally administered capsules containing enteric-coated minitablets of porcine pancreatic enzyme concentrate, predominantly pancreatic lipase, amylase, and protease.

ULTRASE: Each opaque white capsule, printed "ULTRASE" and "MS 4" of enteric-coated microspheres contains: lipase 4500 USP units, amylase 20 000 USP units and protease 25 000 USP units. Nonmedicinal ingredients: methacrylic acid copolymer (Type C), povidone, simethicone emulsion, sugar, talc and triethyl citrate. Bottles of 100.

ULTRASE MT12: Each white and yellow capsule, printed "ULTRASE" and "MT 12" of enteric-coated minitablets, contains: lipase 12 000 USP units, amylase 39 000 USP units and protease 39 000 USP units. Nonmedicinal ingredients: croscarmellose sodium, gelatin, hydrogenated castor oil, hydroxypropyl methylcellulose pthalate (HP55) (as dry substance), iron oxides, magnesium stearate, microcrystalline cellulose, silicone dioxide, talc, titanium dioxide and triethyl citrate. Bottles of 100.

ULTRASE MT20: Each light grey and yellow capsule, printed "ULTRASE" and "MT 20" of enteric-coated minitablets, contains: lipase 20 000 USP units, amylase 65 000 USP units and protease 65 000 USP units. Nonmedicinal ingredients: croscarmellose sodium, gelatin, hydrogenated castor oil, hydroxypropyl methylcellulose pthalate (HP55) (as dry substance), iron oxides, magnesium stearate, microcrystalline cellulose, silicone dioxide, talc, titanium dioxide and triethyl citrate. Bottles of 100.

Keep bottle tightly closed. Store at controlled room temperature (15-25°C) in a safe, dry place. Do not refrigerate. Dispense in a tight container.

(Shown in Product Identification Section)

The reader is invited to consult CPhA's monograph **Corticosteroids: Topical**.

Ultravate® Pr
halobetasol propionate
Topical Corticosteroid

Valeant

Date of Preparation: April 14, 2010

INDICATIONS: ULTRAVATE (halobetasol propionate) Cream and Ointment are high to super-high potency topical corticosteroids indicated for the relief of inflammatory manifestations of resistant or severe psoriasis and corticosteroid-responsive dermatoses. These products are not recommended for use in children.

CONTRAINDICATIONS: ULTRAVATE (halobetasol propionate) Cream and Ointment are contraindicated in patients who are hypersensitive to halobetasol propionate, to other corticosteroids, or to any of the ingredients in these products.

ULTRAVATE (halobetasol propionate) Cream and Ointment are contraindicated in viral diseases of the skin including herpes simplex, vaccinia and varicella. They are also contraindicated in untreated bacterial, tubercular and fungal infections involving the skin.

WARNINGS: *Pregnancy:* There are no clinical trials of ULTRAVATE in pregnant women. Therefore, this product should be used during pregnancy only if the potential benefit justifies the potential risk to the fetus.

Corticosteroids have been shown to be teratogenic and embryotoxic in laboratory animals at low doses when administered systemically. Some corticosteroids have been shown to be teratogenic after topical application. Halobetasol propionate has been shown to be teratogenic in rats and rabbits at low doses. The human topical dose of ULTRAVATE was embryotoxic in rabbits.

Lactation: Systemically administered corticosteroids appear in human milk and can suppress growth, interfere with endogenous corticosteroid production, or cause other adverse effects. It is not known whether topical administration of corticosteroids could result in sufficient systemic absorption to produce detectable quantities in human milk. Because many drugs are excreted in human milk, caution should be exercised when administering ULTRAVATE to a nursing woman.

ULTRAVATE (halobetasol propionate) Cream or Ointment are not to be used with occlusive dressing. These products are not formulated for ophthalmic use and should not be used in or near the eyes.

ULTRAVATE (halobetasol propionate) Cream or Ointment are for dermatological use only.

PRECAUTIONS: General: In the presence of bacterial infections of the skin, an appropriate antibacterial agent should be used as primary therapy. If it is considered necessary, the topical corticosteroid may be used as an adjunct to control inflammation, erythema, and itching. If a favourable response does not occur within a few days to a week, the steroid should be discontinued until the infection has been adequately controlled.

Significant systemic absorption may occur when steroids are applied over large areas of the body. To minimize this possibility, when long term therapy is anticipated, interrupt treatment periodically or treat one area of the body at a time.

ULTRAVATE Ointment produced HPA axis suppression when used at recommended doses of 7 g per day for one week in patients with psoriasis. These effects were reversible upon discontinuation of treatment.

Laboratory Tests: Patients receiving a large dose of a high potency topical steroid applied to a large surface area should be evaluated periodically for evidence of HPA axis suppression. This may be done by using the ACTH stimulation, A.M. plasma cortisol and urinary free-cortisol tests. Patients receiving super-potent corticosteroids should not be treated for more than 2 weeks at a time and it is recommended that only small areas be treated at any one time due to the increased risk of HPA suppression.

Prolonged use of topical corticosteroid products may produce atrophy of the skin and subcutaneous tissues. If this occurs, treatment should be discontinued.

Topical corticosteroids should be used with caution in patients with stasis dermatitis and other skin diseases associated with impaired circulation, hypersensitive patients and patients with glaucoma.

Patients should be advised to inform subsequent physician of the prior use of corticosteroids.

Carcinogenesis, Mutagenesis: Long-term animal studies have not been performed to evaluate the carcinogenic potential of halobetasol propionate. Positive mutagenicity studies were observed in two genotoxicity assays. Halobetasol was positive in a Chinese hamster micronucleus test in vivo and in a mouse lymphoma gene mutation assay in vitro. In other genotoxicity tests including Ames/Salmonella assay, sister chromatid exchange test, chromosome aberration studies of germinal and somatic cells of rodents and in a mammalian spot test for point mutations, halobetasol propionate was not found to be genotoxic.

Children: ULTRAVATE (halobetasol propionate) Cream or Ointment should not be used in children. Because of the higher ratio of skin surface area to body mass, children are at greater risk for HPA axis suppression, glucocorticoid insufficiency after withdrawal of treatment and Cushing's syndrome while on treatment.

Information to Be Provided to the Patient: Patients using ULTRAVATE (halobetasol propionate) Cream or Ointment should receive the following information:

1. This medication is to be used as directed by the physician and should not be used longer than the prescribed time period. It is for external use only. Avoid contact with eyes.
2. The medication should not be used for any disorder other than for which it was prescribed.
3. The treated skin area should not be bandaged or otherwise covered or wrapped so as to be occlusive.
4. Any signs of local adverse reactions should be reported to your physician.

ADVERSE EFFECTS: A total of 1018 patients have been studied in ULTRAVATE (halobetasol propionate) clinical trials, 596 received the ointment formulation, 341 received the cream formulation and 81 received both formulations. The incidence of adverse reactions with ULTRAVATE cream and ointment were those commonly observed with topical corticosteroids.

The most frequently reported adverse reaction across all clinical trials with ULTRAVATE Ointment was stinging (2%). Other adverse reactions related and probably related that were reported at less than 1% were: burning, erythema, acne, skin atrophy, pruritus, leukoderma, telangiectasia, pustulation, dry skin, bruise, rash, lichenified dermatitis, paraesthesia, urticaria, and fungal infection.

The most frequently reported adverse reaction across all clinical trials with ULTRAVATE Cream was also stinging (3%). Other adverse reactions related and probably related that were reported at less than 1% were: pruritus, burning skin, dry skin, leukoderma, erythema, skin atrophy, sore joint, and eye pressure.

The following adverse skin reactions have been reported with the use of topical corticosteroids and may occur more frequently with high potency corticosteroids such as ULTRAVATE Cream and Ointment. These reactions are listed in an approximately decreasing order of occurrence: burning, itching, irritation, dryness, folliculitis, hypertrichosis, acneiform eruptions, hypopigmentation, perioral dermatitis, allergic contact dermatitis, maceration of the skin, secondary infection, skin atrophy, striae and miliaria. Systemic absorption of topical corticosteroids has produced reversible HPA axis suppression, manifestations of Cushing's syndrome, hyperglycemia, and glucosuria in some patients. In rare instances, treatment (or withdrawal of treatment) of psoriasis with corticosteroids is thought to have provoked the pustular form of the disease.

OVERDOSE:

Symptoms: Topically applied ULTRAVATE (halobetasol propionate) Cream or Ointment can be absorbed in sufficient amounts to produce systemic effects including reversible HPA axis suppression with the potential for glucocorticosteroid insufficiency after withdrawal of treatment. If HPA axis suppression is noted, withdraw the drug gradually by reducing the amount and frequency of application. Recovery of HPA axis function is generally prompt and complete upon discontinuation of topical corticosteroids. Infrequently, signs and symptoms of glucocorticosteroid insufficiency may occur requiring supplemental systemic corticosteroids.

Treatment: See Symptoms.

For management of a suspected drug overdose, CPhA recommends that you contact your **regional Poison Control Centre**. See the *CPS* Directory section for a list of Poison Control Centres.

DOSAGE: Apply a thin layer of ULTRAVATE (halobetasol propionate) Cream or Ointment to the affected skin and rub in gently and completely. Apply twice daily, or as directed by your physician. Treatment is to be discontinued when the dermatologic disorder is controlled.

Treatment with ULTRAVATE (halobetasol propionate) Cream or Ointment should be limited to 50 g per week. The duration of therapy should not exceed two weeks without patient re-evaluation. ULTRAVATE (halobetasol propionate) Cream and Ointment are not to be used with occlusive dressing.

INFORMATION FOR THE PATIENT: Published in e-CPS, available by subscription at www.e-cps.ca.

SUPPLIED: Cream: Each g contains: halobetasol propionate 0.5 mg. Nonmedicinal ingredients: cetyl alcohol, diazolidinyl urea, glycerin, isopropyl isostearate, isopropyl palmitate, methylchloroisothiazolinone and methylisothiazolinone, steareth-21 and water. Aluminum tubes of 15 and 50 g. Store at controlled room temperature between 15 and 25°C.

Ointment: Each g contains: halobetasol propionate 0.5 mg. Nonmedicinal ingredients: beeswax, dehymuls E, petrolatum and propylene glycol. Aluminum tubes of 15 and 50 g. Store at controlled room temperature between 15 and 25°C.

Ultravist® 240
iopromide
Non-ionic Iodinated Radiographic Contrast Medium

Bayer

Ultravist® 300
iopromide
Non-ionic Iodinated Radiographic Contrast Medium

Bayer

Ultravist® 370
iopromide
Non-ionic Iodinated Radiographic Contrast Medium

Bayer

Date of Revision: March 18, 2009

PHARMACOLOGY: ULTRAVIST (iopromide) is a non-ionic iodinated radiographic contrast medium which is available in three stable, ready-to-use solutions of different concentrations. Following intravascular injection, iopromide provides radiographic opacification of the vasculature and extracellular space allowing diagnostic assessment of the limbs and internal organs. For example, after intravenous injection, opacification of the renal parenchyma begins within 1 minute. Excretion of the contrast agent becomes apparent in 1 to 3 minutes with optimal contrast in the calyces and collecting system occurring between 5 and 15 minutes. In nephropathic conditions, particularly when excretory capacity has been altered, the excretion rate varies unpredictably and opacification may be delayed for several hours after injection.

Pharmacokinetics: The pharmacokinetics of iopromide are similar to those of other ionic and non-ionic contrast media. Immediately following intravascular injection, iopromide reaches peak plasma concentrations and is then rapidly distributed throughout the extracellular fluid compartment. It is excreted unchanged by the kidneys mainly by glomerular filtration. About 90% of the injected dose is excreted unchanged by the kidneys during the first 24 hours with peak urine concentrations occurring in the first hour. In healthy volunteers, elimination half-life is approximately 2 hours and renal clearance is 93±14 mL/min.

Iopromide does not cross the intact blood-brain barrier. It displays little tendency to bind to serum or plasma proteins and there is no evidence of metabolism, deiodination or biotransformation in rats and humans.

In double-blind clinical trials ULTRAVIST has shown diagnostic efficacy comparable to other non-ionic and ionic radiographic contrast agents when studied in excretory urography (vs. iopamidol, ioxithalamate, and ioxaglate); renal arteriography (vs. amidotrizoate) cerebral arteriography (vs. iopamidol); peripheral arteriography of the leg (vs. ioxaglate); phlebography of the pelvis and leg (vs. ioglicinate); coronary arteriography and ventriculography (vs. iohexol and diatrizoate and amidotrizoate); and in computed tomography (vs. ioglicinate). In these studies ULTRAVIST has demonstrated properties comparable to other non-ionic compounds with respect to neuroangiographic and cardiovascular tolerance and has demonstrated superiority over ionic agents particularly in causing less pain and warmth following injection.

The influence of iopromide on clotting, fibrinolysis, complement activation and erythrocyte morphology has been minimal (see Warnings).

INDICATIONS: ULTRAVIST (iopromide) in its three strengths, is indicated for intravascular use to provide diagnostic information in a number of radiographic contrast procedures. It is also indicated for the visualization of various body cavities, e.g. arthrography and hysterosalpingography.

ULTRAVIST 240: computed tomography (CT); peripheral arteriography (bifemoral pelvis/leg); phlebography of the extremities; cerebral arteriography; arthrography; hysterosalpingography.

ULTRAVIST 300: computed tomography (CT); excretory urography; pediatric excretory urography; renal arteriography; peripheral arteriography (bifemoral pelvis/leg); cerebral arteriography; phlebography of the extremities; arthrography.

ULTRAVIST 370: computed tomography (CT); excretory urography; coronary arteriography (including PTCA), with or without left ventriculography; pediatric angiocardiography; arthrography.

CONTRAINDICATIONS: ULTRAVIST (iopromide) is not indicated for use in myelography, cerebral ventriculography, and cisternography.

ULTRAVIST should not be administered to patients with known hypersensitivity to the drug, anuria or severe oliguria, clinically significant impairment of both renal and hepatic function, or with manifest hyperthyroidism.

Hysterosalpingography must not be performed during pregnancy or in the presence of acute inflammatory process in the pelvic cavity.

WARNINGS: The use of renally excreted intravascular X-ray contrast media can lead to transient impairment of kidney function.

Non-ionic iodinated contrast media inhibit blood coagulation less than ionic contrast media. Clotting has been reported in vivo and in vitro when blood remains in contact with syringes, catheters or tubes containing non-ionic contrast media.

Serious, rarely fatal, thromboembolic events causing myocardial infarction and stroke have been reported during angiographic procedures with both non-ionic and ionic contrast media. Therefore, meticulous intravascular administration technique is necessary, particularly during angiographic procedures, to minimize thromboembolic events. Numerous factors, including length of procedure, number of injections, catheter and syringe material, underlying disease state, and concomitant medication may contribute to the development of thromboembolic events. For these reasons, meticulous angiographic techniques are recommended including close attention to keeping guidewires, catheters and all angiographic equipment free of blood; use of manifold systems and/or three way stopcocks; frequent catheter flushing with heparinized saline solution; and minimizing the length of the procedure. The use of plastic syringes in place of glass syringes has been reported to decrease but not eliminate the likelihood of in vitro clotting. Non-ionic contrast media are not suitable flush solutions.

ULTRAVIST (iopromide) is related chemically to other tri-iodinated benzoic acid derivatives which have been associated with serious and fatal reactions. Therefore, clear indication and evaluation of the benefit/risk ratio for every patient should precede each examination with contrast media. Also, it is of utmost importance that adequate facilities and appropriate personnel be readily available and a course of action be planned in advance for the immediate treatment of any serious untoward reaction. Diagnostic procedures utilizing a radiopaque contrast agent should be conducted only by a physician with the requisite training and a thorough knowledge of the particular procedure to be performed. The physician must also be thoroughly familiar with the emergency treatment of all adverse effects.

PRECAUTIONS: As with other iodinated contrast agents, the use of ULTRAVIST (iopromide) contrast enhancement may obscure some lesions which were seen on previously unenhanced CT scans.

Before any contrast medium is injected, the patient should be questioned for a history of allergy (e.g. shellfish), sensitivity to iodine or to radiographic media and bronchial asthma, as the reported incidence of adverse reactions to contrast media are higher in patients with these conditions. Most adverse reactions to contrast agents appear within 30 minutes after the start of their injection, but a delayed reaction may occur. If premedication is given to avoid or minimize possible allergic adverse reactions, a corticosteroid regimen is recommended. However, corticosteroids should not be mixed in the same syringe with any contrast medium because of potential chemical incompatibility. Patients who experience hypersensitivity reactions while taking beta blockers may be resistant to treatment effects of beta agonists (see Drug Interactions). In the event of a severe hypersensitivity reaction, patients with cardiovascular disease are more susceptible to serious or even fatal outcomes. Due to the possibility of severe hypersensitivity reactions after administration, post-procedure observation of the patient is recommended.

Caution is advised in patients with cardiac and circulatory insufficiency, hypertension, pheochromocytoma, cerebral arteriosclerosis, latent hyperthyroidism, severe impairment of hepatic or renal function, pulmonary emphysema, very poor general condition, diabetes with renal dysfunction requiring treatment, cerebral arterial spasm, bland nodular goiter and multiple myeloma, homocystinuria and other paraproteinemias, and renal transplant.

An intravenous test dose of 0.5-1 mL of the contrast agent before injection of the full dose has been employed to predict severe or fatal reactions. These provocative tests may themselves cause severe, even fatal, reactions and are unreliable in predicting patients at special risk.

Renal function should be assessed before injecting ULTRAVIST since the drug is excreted largely by the kidney and may accumulate in the absence of normal renal function.

In patients with myeloma, diabetes mellitus, polyuria, oliguria or gout, in newborns, small children, and in patients in poor general health, fluid intake should not be restricted even before the use of low-osmolar contrast media.

Assessment of thyroid function may be obscured for several weeks following the administration of ULTRAVIST.

Reports of thyroid storm after the intravascular use of iodinated radiopaque agents in patients with hyperthyroidism or with an autonomously functioning thyroid nodule suggest that this additional risk be evaluated in appropriate patients prior to the use of ULTRAVIST.

Administration of ULTRAVIST should be postponed in patients who have to undergo oral cholecystography.

Premedication with an alpha-blocker is recommended in patients having a pheochromocytoma because of the risk of hypertensive crises.

In patients with decreased renal function, 48 hours should elapse between 2 examinations. Special attention should be paid to patients with increased intracranial pressure, disrupted blood-brain barrier (tumour, subarachnoid hemorrhage, transient ischemic attack, cerebral thrombosis, ischemia) or any condition whereby the presence of contrast material in the vessels is prolonged. Serious neurological sequelae (stroke, aphasia, cortical blindness, convulsions) may occur following intraarterial or intravascular infusion of contrast media. The benefit/risk ratio of the procedure has to be evaluated and the amount of contrast medium necessary to obtain a diagnostic picture kept to a minimum.

ULTRAVIST should be administered intravascularly with caution to patients with known convulsive disorders.

The administration of iodinated contrast media may aggravate the symptoms of myasthenia gravis.

Pregnancy: The safe use of ULTRAVIST during pregnancy has not been established. Therefore, it should not be used unless the benefits outweigh the risks.

Lactation: If the use of ULTRAVIST is considered necessary in a nursing mother, it is suggested to discontinue breast feeding for 48 hours.

Geriatrics: Elderly patients may present a special risk in the use of radiographic contrast media. These patients may have compromised renal and cardiac function and may be taking medication (e.g. beta-blockers) which may make them more susceptible to the potentially harmful effects of procedures involving the use of contrast agents.

Intravascular Use: ULTRAVIST produces less circulatory osmotic load than ionic contrast agents; however, it can produce significant hemodynamic disturbances especially in patients with reduced cardiac reserve. The volume of injection should be minimized and the patient's vital signs should be continuously monitored for several hours following the procedure to detect delayed hemodynamic disturbances. Hypotension should be corrected promptly as it can lead to serious arrhythmias. Special care regarding dosage should be observed in patients with right ventricular failure, pulmonary emphysema, pulmonary hypertension or a stenotic pulmonary vascular bed because serious hemodynamic changes may occur in these individuals. There may be an increased risk of clinically relevant hemodynamic changes and arrhythmia in patients with significant cardiac disease or severe coronary artery disease.

Mesenteric necrosis, acute pancreatitis, renal shutdown and serious neurologic complications including spinal cord damage and hemiplegia have been reported following inadvertent injection of a large part of the aortic dose of an ionic contrast medium directly into an aortic branch or arterial trunk.

There are inherent dangers associated with catheter manipulation, contrast medium injection and angiographic procedures. Dislodging plaques or damaging, dissecting or perforating a vessel wall or causing injury to neighbouring organs can lead to embolization. The possibility of these occurrences should be borne in mind during the procedure. Fluoroscope guidance is to be used to place the catheter.

Pulsation must be present in the artery to be injected. Extreme caution is therefore advised for patients considered for angiography, particularly those suspected of having thromboangiitis obliterans (Buerger's disease), since vascular procedures may induce severe arterial spasm.

In intraarterial administration, caution is advisable in patients with suspected thrombosis, ischemic disease, local infection, a totally obstructed vascular system, or severe ischemia associated with ascending infection or advanced arteriosclerosis. With the use of conventional ionic contrast media, occasional serious neurologic complications, including paraplegia, have been reported in patients with aorto-iliac or femoral artery obstruction, abdominal compression, hypotension or hypertension, and following the injection of vasopressors.

When large individual doses are administered, an appropriate time interval should elapse between injections to allow any hemodynamic disturbances to subside. Hemodynamic changes are likely to be more pronounced following repeated injections given in rapid succession.

Following arterial catheterization and injection, pressure hemostasis is advisable with immobilization of the limb for several hours to prevent hemorrhage from the site of arterial puncture.

Drug Interactions: The prevalence of delayed reactions e.g. fever, rash, flu-like symptoms, joint pain and pruritus) to contrast media is higher in patients who received interleukins.

Treatment with beta-blockers or general anesthesia increases the incidence and may aggravate adverse reactions, particularly in people with asthma. Patients who experience hypersensitivity reactions while taking a beta blocker may be resistant to treatment effects of beta agonists (see Precautions).

Biguanides (metformin): Transient renal impairment associated with use of ULTRAVIST can lead to biguanide accumulation and the development of lactic acidosis in patients who are taking biguanides. As a precaution, biguanides should be discontinued 48 hours prior to the contrast medium examination until at least 48 hours after the administration of contrast medium and reinstated only after adequate renal function has been regained.

ADVERSE EFFECTS: Adverse Drug Reaction Overview: Adverse reactions reported with ULTRAVIST (iopromide) have generally been less frequent than with some commonly used iodinated compounds. However, all side effects and toxicity associated with this class of compound are possible during the use of ULTRAVIST, including severe and life-threatening reactions as well as death.

Careful patient observation for adverse reactions is recommended in the use of all contrast media. Reactions accompanying use may vary with the dosage, the technique of administration, the procedure and the underlying condition of the patient. Adverse reactions generally occur within 30 minutes after injection but some may be delayed or of long-lasting nature. These reactions include: laryngospasm, bronchospasm, wheezing, dyspnea, and status asthmaticus; angioedema, subglottic edema and signs of airway obstruction; anaphylactic shock; cardiovascular collapse with peripheral vasodilation, hypotension, tachycardia, dyspnea, cyanosis, sweating, pallor, ventricular fibrillation and cardiac arrest; CNS stimulation or depression with agitation, convulsions, coma and death. Severe life-threatening reactions to iodinated contrast media require appropriate emergency measures.

Many life-threatening reactions begin with only mild symptoms such as nasal congestion, sneezing, watery eyes, skin erythema, or a vague sense of discomfort. It is therefore extremely important that all patients be watched closely until their symptoms have abated. The symptoms, which occur regardless of the amount of contrast medium administered and the mode of administration, can indicate incipient shock. Administration of the contrast medium must then be interrupted immediately and, if necessary, specific therapy initiated intravenously. In the case of intravenous administration, use of a flexible indwelling catheter is therefore recommended.

The most common adverse event following intravenous injection of ULTRAVIST is a sensation of warmth and/or pain especially in peripheral arteriography. This is generally less severe with ULTRAVIST than with ionic contrast media.

Clinical Trial Adverse Drug Reactions: A clinical trial dataset of 2398 patients was used to generate the adverse drug reaction profile of ULTRAVIST prior to market authorization in Canada. The following list of adverse reactions and their incidence is based on this dataset (see Table 1).

Table 1: ULTRAVIST

Adverse Reactions

General Reactions	Incidence
Warmth	
(slight to moderate)	36.4%
(severe)	3.0%

(cont'd)

Table 1: ULTRAVIST *(cont'd)*

Adverse Reactions

General Reactions	Incidence
Pain	
(slight to moderate)	6.1%
(severe)	0.4%
Nausea/Vomiting/Diarrhea	2.3%

Adverse Reactions Having an Incidence of <1%: Allergic/Cutaneous Reactions: urticaria (0.8%); respiratory symptoms (0.3%): sneezing, coughing, bronchospasm; angioedema and lip swelling (0.1%); Quincke's edema (0.1%).
Cardiovascular Reactions: hypotension (0.4%); tachycardia (0.3%); unconsciousness/collapse (0.3%); hypertension (0.1%); bradycardia (0.1%); extrasystoles (0.1%); left bundle branch heart block (0.1%); anginal symptoms (0.1%); arrhythmia (0.1%).
CNS Reactions: restlessness/anxiety (0.3%); paresthesia (0.2%): arm or face; vertigo (0.1%); blurred vision (0.1%).
Other Reactions: taste sensation (0.4%); headache (0.3%); knee swelling/pain (0.1%); shoulder pain (0.1%); venous pressure (0.1%); numbness (0.1%); shivers (0.1%); popliteal region tension (0.1%); pressure over eyes (0.1%); vegetative dystonia (0.1%); sore throat (0.1%); septicemia (0.1%); dizziness (0.1%).
Postmarket Adverse Drug Reactions: Adverse drug reactions reported subsequent to market introduction in Canada are presented below.
Cardiac: cardiac arrest, cardiac rhythm or function disturbances, chest pain/tightness, cyanosis, heart failure, myocardial ischemia/infarction, palpitations.
Ear and Labyrinth: hearing disorders, hearing disturbances.
Endocrine: alteration in thyroid function, thyrotoxic crisis.
Eye: conjunctivitis, blurred/disturbed vision, lacrimation, photophobia, vision disturbances.
Gastrointestinal: abdominal pain, dysphagia, swelling of salivary glands, throat irritation.
General Disorders and Administration Site Conditions: body temperature alterations, chills, edema, inflammation and tissue injury in case of extravasation, malaise, pallor, sweating, vasovagal reactions, warmth (mild) with edema.
Immune System: anaphylactic reactions, anaphylactoid reactions / hypersensitivity, anaphylactoid shock (including fatal cases).
Musculoskeletal, Connective Tissue and Bone: hypertonia.
Nervous System: amnesia, cerebral ischemia/infarction, coma, convulsion, hypoesthesia, paresis/paralysis, somnolence, speech disorders, speech disturbances, stroke, transient cortical blindness*, tremor.
Psychiatric: agitation, confusion.
Renal and Urinary: renal failure*, renal impairment.
Respiratory, Thoracic and Mediastinal: asthma, dyspnea, hoarseness, laryngeal/pharyngeal/tongue/face edema, laryngeal/pharyngeal spasm, mucosal swelling, pulmonary edema, respiratory insufficiency, respiratory arrest, respiratory distress, rhinitis, transient disturbances in respiratory rate.
Skin and Subcutaneous Tissue: erythema, mucocutaneous syndrome (e.g. Stevens-Johnson's or Lyell syndrome), pruritus, rash.
Vascular: blood pressure disturbances, shock, thromboembolic events*, thrombophlebitis, vasculitis (severe), vasodilatation, vasospasm*, venous thrombosis.

ULTRAVIST is not indicated for use intrathecally or for use in Endoscopic Retrograde Cholangiopancreatography (see Indications). Based on experience with other nonionic contrast media, the following adverse drug reactions may occur if ULTRAVIST is administered intrathecally:
General Disorders and Administration Site Conditions: back pain, injection site pain, micturition difficulties, pain in extremities.
Nervous System: aseptic meningitis, EEG-changes, meningism, neuralgia, paraplegia.
Psychiatric: psychosis.

Headache, including severe prolonged cases, nausea and vomiting occur commonly. The majority of the reactions after myelography or use in body cavities occur some hours after the administration.

In addition to the adverse drug reactions listed above, the following have been reported when ULTRAVIST is used for ERCP: Endocrine: elevation of pancreatic enzyme levels, pancreatitis.

OVERDOSE:

Symptoms: An overdose of ULTRAVIST (iopromide) should be treated by support of vital functions and prompt institution of symptomatic therapy.

Treatment: ULTRAVIST is dialyzable. In the event of accidental intravascular overdose, water and electrolyte losses must be compensated by infusion. Renal function should be monitored for at least the next 3 days. If needed, hemodialysis can be used to eliminate the bulk of the contrast medium from the patient's system.

For management of a suspected drug overdose, CPhA recommends that you contact your **regional Poison Control Centre**. See the *CPS* Directory section for a list of Poison Control Centres.

DOSAGE: General Information: Solutions of ULTRAVIST (iopromide), like those of other radiopaque contrast agents, should be at or close to body temperature when injected. As with other sterile parenteral products, ULTRAVIST should not be withdrawn from the vial except immediately prior to use (see Warnings). ULTRAVIST should not be mixed with other drugs. Any unused portion should be discarded.

Vials containing contrast medium solutions are not intended for the withdrawal of multiple doses. The rubber stopper should never be pierced more than once. The use of a cannula or needle with a long tip and a maximum diameter of 18 G is recommended for piercing the stopper and drawing up the contrast medium.

Patients should be in a fasted state (when this can be safely achieved) and adequately hydrated on the day of the examination. Disturbances of water and electrolyte balance must be corrected prior to the administration of ULTRAVIST.

In the case of abdominal angiography and urography, the diagnostic yield is increased if the bowels are empty of fecal matter and gas. It may be necessary to administer an enema or laxative in the evening prior to examination, provided purging of the bowels is not contraindicated.

However, in infants and young children, prolonged fasting, restriction of fluids and the administration of a laxative before the examination are contraindicated.

Experience shows that pronounced states of excitement, anxiety and pain can be the cause of side effects or intensified contrast medium-related reactions. They can be counteracted by calm management of the patients and the use of suitable drugs.

Intravascular administration of contrast media should, if possible, be done with the patient lying down. After the administration, the patient should be kept under observation for at least 30 minutes, since experience shows that the majority of all severe incidents occur within this time.

The recommended dosages of ULTRAVIST should not be exceeded. The volume of each individual injection is a more important consideration than the total dose used. When large individual volumes are administered, as in cardiac ventriculography, sufficient time should be permitted to elapse between injections to allow any hemodynamic disturbances to subside.
Excretory Urography: Adults: Recommended doses for each concentration of ULTRAVIST:
ULTRAVIST 300: 40-70 mL.
ULTRAVIST 370: 30-55 mL.

The dose may be adjusted in special indications (e.g. obese patients, impaired renal function), if necessary.
Children: The physiologically poor concentrating ability of the immature nephron necessitates the administration of relatively high doses of contrast medium in children.

The doses of ULTRAVIST 300 should not exceed:
Neonates: 4 mL/kg of body weight equivalent to 1.2 g I/kg.
Infants: 3 mL/kg of body weight equivalent to about 1.0 g I/kg.
Small Children: 1.5 mL/kg of body weight equivalent to about 0.5 g I/kg.
Computerized Tomography (CT): Cranial CT: The following doses are recommended and should not be exceeded:
ULTRAVIST 240: 105-175 mL
ULTRAVIST 300: 70-140 mL
ULTRAVIST 370: 70-105 mL
Whole-body CT: In whole-body computerized tomography, the necessary doses of ULTRAVIST and the rates of administration depend on the organs under investigation, the diagnostic problem and, in particular, the different scan and image reconstruction times of the scanner. An infusion is preferred for slow scanners, and a bolus injection for fast scanners.
Recommended doses for each concentration of ULTRAVIST:
ULTRAVIST 240: 125-180 mL
ULTRAVIST 300: 100-150 mL
ULTRAVIST 370: 80-120 mL
Angiography: The dosage of ULTRAVIST depends on the age, weight, cardiac output and general condition of the patient, the clinical problem, examination technique, and the nature and volume of the vascular region to be investigated. The following dosages may serve as a guide: see Table 2.

* Intravascular use only.

Table 2: ULTRAVIST

Dosage

Procedure	ULTRAVIST Concentration (mg I/mL)	Usual Recommended Single Dose (mL/injection)
Cerebral Arteriography		
Aortic arch angiography	300	40–80
Retrograde carotid angiography	300	30–40
Common carotid	300	6–12
Internal carotid	300	5–12
External carotid	300	4–8
Vertebral artery	300	6–10
Aortography		
Thoracic aortography	300	50–80
Abdominal aortography	300	40–60
Peripheral Angiography		
Selective arteriography	300	8–12
Aorto-femoral runoffs	300	40–80
Phlebography	240	60–100
	300	60–90
Angiocardiography		
Left ventriculography	370	30–60
Coronary arteriography	370	5–8
Arthrography		
Intraarticular injections of contrast media should be monitored by fluoroscopy to ensure adequate injection technique and opacification while preventing over distention of the joint space. Excessive dilution of the contrast medium should be avoided.		
Knee	240	5–11
	300	5–11
	370	5–11
Hysterosalpingography		
Hysterosalpingography contrast media should be instilled into the uterine cavity under controlled pressure with fluoroscopic monitoring of the dose, to avoid excessive injection pressures and doses.		
	240	10–25

SUPPLIED:

Table 3: ULTRAVIST

Physical Properties

	ULTRAVIST 240	ULTRAVIST 300	ULTRAVIST 370
Iodine concentration (mg/mL)	240	300	370
Iopromide concentration (mg/mL)	499.0	623.0	769.0
Viscosity (mPa·s or cp)			
at 20°C	4.8	8.7	20.1
at 37°C	2.8	4.6	9.5
Osmotic pressure at 37°C			
(MPa)	1.22	1.59	2.02
(atm)	12.1	15.7	19.9
Osmolality at 37°C (osm/kg H_2O)	0.48	0.61	0.77
Specific gravity at 37°C	1.263	1.33	1.409

ULTRAVIST 240 (iopromide 49.9%): Each mL of sterile colourless to pale yellow aqueous solution contains: 499 mg of iopromide equivalent to 240 mg of organically bound iodine. Nonmedicinal ingredients: calcium disodium edetate (EDTA), hydrochloric acid and tromethamine. Preservative-free. pH has been adjusted to between 6.5 and 8.0 with hydrochloric acid. Vials of 50 and 200 mL.

ULTRAVIST 300 (iopromide 62.3%): Each mL of sterile colourless to pale yellow aqueous solution contains: 623 mg of iopromide equivalent to 300 mg of organically bound iodine. Nonmedicinal ingredients: calcium disodium edetate (EDTA), hydrochloric acid and tromethamine. Preservative-free. pH has been adjusted to between 6.5 and 8.0 with hydrochloric acid. Vials of 50, 100 and 150 mL.

ULTRAVIST 370 (iopromide 76.9%): Each mL of sterile colourless to pale yellow aqueous solution contains: 769 mg of iopromide equivalent to 370 mg of organically bound iodine. Nonmedicinal ingredients: calcium disodium edetate (EDTA), hydrochloric acid and tromethamine. Preservative-free. pH has been adjusted to between 6.5 and 8.0 with hydrochloric acid. Vials of 50, 100 and 200 mL.

Stability and Storage Recommendations: ULTRAVIST (iopromide) should be stored between 15°C and 30°C and protected from light.

ULTRAVIST should be visually inspected and used only if: it is clear and within the normal colourless to pale yellow range; it contains no particulate matter (including crystals); the container does not appear to be defective. Since ULTRAVIST is a highly concentrated solution, crystallization (milky-cloudy appearance and/or sediment at bottom, or floating crystals) may occur very rarely. Discard unused portions.

Uniphyl® Ⓟ

theophylline

Bronchodilator

Purdue Pharma

Date of Revision: March 11, 2009

PHARMACOLOGY: Theophylline relaxes bronchial smooth muscle (particularly when the muscles are constricted); produces vasodilation except in cerebral vessels; stimulates the CNS including the respiratory center; stimulates cardiac muscle; produces diuresis and increases gastric acid secretion. In addition to its activity as a bronchodilator, theophylline may also stimulate mucociliary clearance, inhibit anaphylactic mediator release, suppress mediator induced inflammation and improve contractility of the diaphragm.

Uniphyl (theophylline sustained release tablets) are a sustained release formulation of theophylline. The release system consists of a homogeneous matrix of aliphatic alcohol, cellulose, and active drug. The proportion of these components in the formulation has been chosen to provide gradual, measured release of theophylline by diffusion through the tablet matrix and dissolution. The rate of release of active drug is dependent upon the drug's partition coefficients between the components of the tablet matrix and the aqueous phase within the gastrointestinal tract. The controlled release of theophylline from Uniphyl tablets has been demonstrated by both dissolution and pharmacokinetic studies.

Theophylline's mechanism of action is not fully known and evidence exists indicating that phosphodiesterase inhibition, prostaglandin inhibition, effects on calcium flux and intracellular calcium distribution, and antagonism of endogenous adenosine may all contribute to its pharmacological effects.

Theophylline is usually well absorbed from the gastrointestinal tract, although there are some differences in the pharmacokinetic behavior of various sustained release formulations. Theophylline distributes to all body compartments and is approximately 50% protein bound. Elimination is primarily by hepatic biotransformation with approximately 50% excreted as 1,3-dimethyluric acid. Unchanged theophylline, 3-methylxanthine and 1-methyluric acid each account for 10% to 15% and 1-methylxanthine is excreted in smaller amounts.

The generally accepted optimal therapeutic serum theophylline concentrations are 10 to 20 mg/L (55 to 110 µmol/L). Levels above 20 mg/L (110 µmol/L) are usually associated with toxic reactions. The pharmacokinetics of theophylline are influenced by a number of variables such as age, concomitant medications, disease state and smoking (see Precautions). Therefore, each patient's optimal therapeutic maintenance dosage should be determined by individual titration.

At steady state, Uniphyl tablets taken once daily produce peak theophylline levels between 8 and 12 hours post-dose, and trough levels almost always occur at the time of dosing. During once-daily dosing, the mean fluctuation between peak and trough theophylline levels is 130%.

$$\% \text{ Fluctuation} = \frac{C_{max} - C_{min}}{C_{min}} \times 100$$

INDICATIONS: The symptomatic treatment of reversible bronchoconstriction associated with bronchial asthma, chronic obstructive pulmonary emphysema, chronic bronchitis and related bronchospastic disorders.

CONTRAINDICATIONS: Should not be administered to patients with hypersensitivity to xanthines, to patients with coronary artery disease where cardiac stimulation might prove harmful, or to patients with active peptic ulcer.

WARNINGS: In clinical situations where immediate bronchodilation is required, such as status asthmaticus, Uniphyl (theophylline sustained release tablets) are not appropriate.

Theophylline has a narrow therapeutic index, the margin of safety above therapeutic doses is small.

Whenever signs of intolerance to theophylline develop, the therapy should be reassessed.

Theophylline clearance can be affected by various disease states, the age of the patient, concomitant use of other medication and lifestyle habits (see Precautions).

A dosage schedule in the pediatric population has not been established. Use in children under 12 years of age is not recommended.

PRECAUTIONS: General: There is a marked variation in serum levels achieved in different patients given the same dose of theophylline. Therefore, high serum levels may occur in some patients receiving doses considered to be conventional. The possibility of theophylline overdose should always be considered. Overdoses of theophylline may cause serious side effects such as tachycardia, arrhythmias, seizures, vascular collapse and even death. These may occur without warning and may not be preceded by less severe side effects such as nausea or restlessness.

The variability in serum levels is primarily due to differences in the rate of metabolism. Therefore, it is advisable to individualize the dosage regimen. Ideally, all patients should have serum theophylline levels measured which would enable doses and dosing regimens to be tailored for each patient in order to maintain therapeutic levels, ensure optimal clinical response and avoid toxicity. The incidence of adverse reactions increases at theophylline levels greater than 15 mg/L (82.5 µmol/L) and levels above 20 mg/L (110 µmol/L) are usually quite toxic in most adults.

Although Uniphyl (theophylline sustained release) tablets have pharmacokinetic properties similar to other sustained release theophylline formulations, it is not possible to ensure interchangeability between different formulations. Careful clinical monitoring is required when changing from one formulation to another. The equivalent content of anhydrous theophylline is the active ingredient that determines the blood concentration and clinical response. If a change in theophylline product is made and it involves a change in anhydrous theophylline equivalence, the dose should be adjusted accordingly.

Patients with Special Diseases and Conditions: Theophylline clearance is decreased, which may result in increased serum levels and resultant toxicity in patients: with impaired liver or kidney function; over 55 years of age, particularly males and those with chronic lung disease; with cardiac failure from any cause; with active influenza or other viral disease or after influenza immunization; with a high carbohydrate, low protein diet; patients taking certain drugs such as cimetidine, ciprofloxacin, norfloxacin, erythromycin, troleandomycin and fluvoxamine; thyroid disease or associated treatment may alter theophylline plasma levels.

Laboratory monitoring of serum theophylline levels is especially appropriate in the above individuals in order to maintain the appropriate theophylline dosage.

Patients who are rapid metabolizers of theophylline, such as the young, smokers and some nonsmoking adults may not be suitable candidates for once-daily dosing. In rapid metabolizers, peak to trough fluctuations in theophylline levels may be greater than desirable or result in side effects at the time of maximum levels and/or the recurrence of symptoms toward the end of the 24 hour dose interval when levels are lowest. In such patients, dividing the total daily theophylline dose into 2 equal doses may be indicated.

Theophylline is known to stimulate gastric acid secretion and may also act as a local gastrointestinal irritant. Therefore, the drug should only be used with caution in patients with a history of peptic ulcer disease.

Theophylline may cause arrhythmia and/or worsen pre-existing arrhythmia. Any significant change in rate and/or rhythm warrants monitoring and further investigation.

Many patients who require theophylline may exhibit tachycardia due to their underlying disease process so that the cause/effect relationship to elevated serum theophylline concentrations may not be appreciated.

Use with caution in patients with severe cardiac disease, severe hypoxemia, hypertension, hyperthyroidism, acute myocardial injury, cor pulmonale, congestive heart failure, liver disease, in the elderly (especially males).

Drug Interactions: Theophylline pharmacokinetics are altered by the concurrent use of various drugs as listed in Table 1.

Table 1: Uniphyl

Effect of Various Drugs on Theophylline Pharmacokinetics

Drug	Effect on Theophylline Clearance and Elimination Half-Life
Allopurinol, carbimazole, cimetidine, diltiazem, disulfiram, fluconazole, interferon, isoniazid, quinolone antibacterials (ciprofloxacin, norfloxacin, ofloxacin), macrolide antibiotics (erythromycin, clarithromycin, troleandomycin), methotrexate, mexiletine, nizatidine, oral contraceptives, propafenone, propranolol, pentoxiphylline, selective serotonin re-uptake inhibitors (e.g., fluvoxamine), thiabendazole, verapamil, viloxazine hydrochloride	↑ t½, ↓ clearance
Alkalinizing agents	↑ t½, ↓ clearance
Influenza vaccine	↑ t½, ↓ clearance reported to be decreased or no change
Aminoglutethimide, barbiturates, carbamazepine, hypericum perforatum (St. John's Wort), isoproterenol, moracizine, phenytoin, rifampin, sulphinpyrazone	↓ t½, ↑ clearance
Tobacco, alcohol	↓ t½, ↑ clearance
Acidifying agents	↓ t½, ↑ clearance

Concurrent use of theophylline influences the actions of certain drugs (see Table 2).

Table 2: Uniphyl

Effect of Theophylline on Certain Drugs

Drug	Influence of Theophylline
Digitalis glycosides	↑ cardiac effect
Thiazides	↑ diuresis
Nephrotoxic drugs	↑ nephrotoxicity
Lithium	↑ ratio of lithium/creatinine clearance, thus a decrease in serum lithium levels
Sympathomimetic amines	↑ toxicity ↑ CNS stimulation
Coumarin anticoagulants	↓ anticoagulant activity ↓ prothrombin and fibrinogen blood concentrations ↓ prothrombin time
Allopurinol	↓ antihyperuricemic action
Probenecid and pyrazolone derivatives	↓ uricosuric action

There is also a pharmacological interaction with adenosine, benzediazepines, halothane and lomustine. Care should also be taken in its concomitant use with glucagon and other xanthine drugs.

Hypokalemia resulting from β_2 agonist therapy, steroids, diuretics and hypoxia may be potentiated by xanthines. Particular care is advised in patients suffering from severe asthma who require hospitalization. It is recommended that serum concentrations are monitored in such situations. Theophylline may decrease steady state phenytoin levels.

Pregnancy: Theophylline crosses the placental barrier and also passes freely into breast milk, where concentrations are similar to plasma levels. Safe use in pregnancy has not been established relative to possible adverse effects on fetal development. Therefore, use of theophylline in pregnant women and nursing mothers should be balanced against the risk of uncontrolled asthma.

Lactation: See Pregnancy.

Laboratory Test Interactions: When plasma levels are measured by spectrophotometric methods, coffee, tea, cola beverages, chocolate and acetaminophen contribute to falsely high values.

When high pressure liquid chromatography (HPLC) method is used, plasma theophylline concentration may be falsely increased by caffeine, some cephalosporins and sulfa medications.

Theophylline may cause elevation of urine catecholamines, plasma uric acid and free fatty acids.

Food Interaction: When immediate release theophylline formulations are administered with food, the rate of absorption is reduced but absorption remains complete. Various sustained release formulations, because of differences in their release mechanisms, may be affected in different ways by concomitant food intake.

Studies have shown that Uniphyl tablets are more completely absorbed when taken with food as opposed to under fasting conditions.

ADVERSE EFFECTS: The most common adverse reactions are gastric irritation, nausea, vomiting, epigastric pain, and tremor. These are usually early signs of toxicity, however, with high doses ventricular arrhythmias or seizures may be the first signs to appear.

Gastrointestinal: nausea, vomiting, epigastric pain, hematemesis, diarrhea, anorexia, intestinal bleeding and reactivation of peptic ulcer.

Central Nervous System: headache, irritability, restlessness, insomnia, twitching, convulsions and reflex hyperexcitability.

Cardiovascular: palpitations, tachycardia, hypotension, circulatory failure, ventricular arrhythmias, extrasystoles and flushing.

Renal: albuminuria, diuresis and hematuria.

Other: hyperglycemia, tachypnea and inappropriate ADH syndrome.

OVERDOSE:

Symptoms: Treat symptoms on appearance. Sustained release tablets may release medication for hours. Insomnia, restlessness, mild excitement or irritability and rapid pulse are the early symptoms, which may progress to mild delirium. Sensory disturbances such as tinnitus or flashes of light are common. Anorexia, nausea and vomiting are also frequently early observations of theophylline overdosage.

Fever, diuresis, dehydration and extreme thirst, acid/base disturbances, rhabdomyolysis, sinus tachycardia and ventricular arrhythmias may be seen. Severe overdosage results in bloody, syrup-like "coffeeground" vomitus, tremors, tonic extensor spasm interrupted by clonic convulsions, extrasystoles, quickened respiration, stupor and finally coma.

Cardiovascular disorders and respiratory collapse, leading to shock, cyanosis and death follow gross overdosages.

Treatment: Monitoring Serum Theophylline Levels: It is important to note that, following the intake of Uniphyl (theophylline sustained release) tablets, the peak theophylline levels may not occur until 8 to 12 hours post ingestion. Moreover, patients ingesting overdoses of sustained release theophylline formulations may also have, after the initial rise in the blood theophylline, a secondary increase in theophylline levels (1 report on lethal self-poisoning has attributed this to compacted tablets in the gastrointestinal tract). **Following initial treatment, longer careful clinical and laboratory monitoring, including electrocardiograms is advisable after patients' stabilization.**

If a potential oral overdose is established and a seizure has not occurred, induce emesis. Administer a cathartic (this is particularly important when a sustained release preparation has been taken). Administer activated charcoal.

If patient is having a seizure, establish an airway. Administer oxygen. Treat the seizure with i.v. diazepam, 0.1 to 0.3 mg/kg up to 10 mg. Monitor vital signs, maintain blood pressure and provide adequate hydration.

Post Seizure Coma: Maintain airway and oxygenation. If a result of oral medication, follow the above recommendations to prevent absorption of the drug, but intubation and lavage will have to be performed instead of inducing emesis and the cathartic and charcoal will need to be introduced via a large bore gastric lavage tube. Continue to provide full supportive care and adequate hydration while waiting for the drug to be metabolized. In general, the drug is metabolized sufficiently rapidly so as not to warrant consideration of dialysis. However, if serum levels exceed 50 mg/L (275 µmol/L) charcoal hemoperfusion may be indicated.

> For management of a suspected drug overdose, CPhA recommends that you contact your **regional Poison Control Centre**. See the *CPS* Directory section for a list of Poison Control Centres.

DOSAGE: Administration and dosing of theophylline should be individualized in respect of the patient's clinical response and serum theophylline levels. There is considerable patient-to-patient variation in the daily theophylline dose required to achieve therapeutic and safe levels. Ideally, all patients should have serum theophylline levels measured which would enable doses and dosing regimens to be tailored in order to maintain therapeutic levels, ensure optimal clinical response and avoid toxicity. Therapeutic serum levels are generally considered to be between 10 and 20 mg/L (55 and 110 µmol/L). Dosage calculations should be based on lean body mass (ideal body weight). A serum level of 20 mg/L (110 µmol/L) is an important reference point in terms of toxicity (see Precautions).

Initial Adult Dose: For patients not currently receiving oral theophylline, the recommended initial dose is 400 to 600 mg once daily.

In patients currently controlled on oral theophylline, Uniphyl (theophylline sustained release tablets) therapy should start at the same daily theophylline dosage (mg for mg basis) provided by the previous formulation. For example, a patient receiving 400 mg twice daily (800 mg daily dosage) would be given two 400 mg Uniphyl tablets once daily. A minimum of 12 hours should elapse between a patient's last dose of the previous oral theophylline formulation and the first dose of Uniphyl.

It is recommended that once daily Uniphyl be taken in the evening. Studies have demonstrated that while the bioavailability and pharmacokinetics of Uniphyl tablets were not significantly different between morning and evening dosing, a better clinical response was obtained with evening dosing. Subsequent studies indicate that the clinical advantages of evening dosing are likely a result of the maximum theophylline levels occurring in the early morning hours, a time of greatest bronchoconstriction and symptoms for many asthmatics.

It is advisable that Uniphyl be taken **with** food, or within 1 to 2 hours of mealtime, as studies have suggested that absorption may be incomplete if taken under conditions of prolonged fasting.

Overall, therefore, it is recommended that most patients should take once daily Uniphyl with, or shortly following, the evening meal.

Dose Titration: Dosage adjustments should be based on the patient's clinical response and/or serum theophylline levels, with increases of ½ tablet/day at 3 to 4 day intervals. Individual requirements vary considerably, therefore, the physician should be prepared to adjust each patient's dose. Do not attempt to maintain any dosage that is poorly tolerated.

Monitoring serum theophylline levels is important, especially during initiation of therapy and dosage adjustment. For serum levels to be most useful, it is important that the patient not have missed or added any doses during the previous 3 days and that the dose intervals remained relatively constant. At steady state, Uniphyl tablets produce peak theophylline levels between 8 and 12 hours post-dose, and trough levels almost always occur at the time of dosing. During once daily dosing, the mean fluctuation between peak and trough theophylline levels is 130%.

The generally accepted optimal therapeutic range is 10 to 20 mg/L (55 to 110 µmol/L), although some patients obtain a very good bronchodilator effect from serum levels less than 10 mg/L (55 µmol/L). In cases where it is not possible to monitor theophylline levels, patients should be closely observed for signs of toxicity and dosages greater than 13 mg/kg/day (or 900 mg/day, whichever is less) should not be given.

Uniphyl tablets should not be chewed, dissolved or crushed as this may lead to a rapid release of theophylline with the potential for toxicity. Tablets may be halved.

INFORMATION FOR THE PATIENT: Published in e-CPS, available by subscription at www.e-cps.ca.

SUPPLIED: 400 mg: Each round, flat-faced, white, scored, sustained release tablet, engraved U over 400 on one side and PF on the reverse, contains: theophylline 400 mg . Nonmedicinal ingredients: cetostearyl alcohol, hydroxyethyl cellulose, magnesium stearate, povidone and talc. Sodium- and tartrazine-free. Opaque plastic bottles of 50. Dispense in amber or opaque containers. Store at room temperature, below 30°C.

600 mg: Each capsule-shaped, concave-faced, white, scored, sustained release tablet, engraved U over 600 on one side and PF on the reverse, contains: theophylline 600 mg. Nonmedicinal ingredients: cetostearyl alcohol, hydroxyethyl cellulose, magnesium stearate, povidone and talc. Sodium- and tartrazine-free. Opaque plastic bottles of 50. Dispense in amber or opaque containers. Store at room temperature, below 30°C.

(Shown in Product Identification Section)

Unisom®
diphenhydramine HCl
Sleep Aid

Paladin

SUPPLIED: Capsules: Each liquid filled soft gelatine capsule contains: diphenhydramine HCl 50 mg. Nonmedicinal ingredients: FD&C Blue No. 1, gelatin, glycerin, Opacode WB (ammonium hydrochloride, ethanol, isopropyl alcohol, polyvinyl acetate phthalate, propylene glycol, titanium dioxide), polyethylene glycol 400, purified water and sorbitol. Boxes of 20, packaged in blister pack cards. Store between 15 and 30°C.

Tablets: Each pale blue, oval, score tablet contains: diphenhydramine HCl 50 mg. Nonmedicinal ingredients: dibasic calcium phosphate dihydrate, FD&C Blue No. 1 Lake, magnesium stearate, microcrystalline cellulose, Opadry YS-1-7006, purified water and sodium starch glycolate. Boxes of 20, packaged in blister pack cards. Store between 15 and 30°C.

(Shown in Product Identification Section)

Unisom-2®
doxylamine succinate
Nighttime Sleep Aid

Paladin

SUPPLIED: Each pale blue, oval, scored tablet contains: doxylamine succinate 25 mg. Nonmedicinal ingredients: dibasic calcium phosphate, FD&C Blue No. 1 Aluminum Lake, magnesium stearate, microcrystalline cellulose and sodium starch glycolate. Boxes of 20 and 40, packaged in blister pack cards. Store between 15 and 30°C.

(Shown in Product Identification Section)

Unitron™ PEG Ⓟ
peginterferon alfa-2b
Biological Response Modifier

Schering-Plough

Date of Preparation: January 26, 2005

PHARMACOLOGY: UNITRON PEG (peginterferon alfa-2b) is a covalent conjugate of recombinant interferon alfa-2b with monomethoxy polyethylene glycol (PEG, with an average molecular weight of 12 000 daltons). The average molecular weight of the molecule is approximately 31 000 daltons).

In vitro and in vivo studies suggest that the biological activity of peginterferon alfa-2b is derived from its interferon alfa-2b moiety.

Interferons exert their cellular activities by binding to specific membrane receptors on the cell surface. Studies with other interferons have demonstrated species specificity. However, certain monkey species, e.g., Rhesus monkeys, are susceptible to pharmacodynamic stimulation upon exposure to human type I interferons. The results of several studies suggest that, once bound to the cell membrane, interferon initiates a complex sequence of intracellular events that include the induction of certain enzymes. It is thought that this process, at least in part, is responsible for the various cellular responses to interferon, including inhibition of virus replication in virus-infected cells, suppression of cell proliferation and such immunomodulation activities as enhancement of the phagocytic activity of macrophages and augmentation of the specific cytotoxicity of lymphocytes for target cells. Any or all of these activities may contribute to interferon's therapeutic effects. Intron A (recombinant interferon alfa-2b) also inhibits viral replication in vitro and in vivo: Although the exact antiviral mode of action of Intron A is unknown, it appears to alter the host cell metabolism. This action inhibits viral replication or if replication occurs, the progeny virions are unable to leave the cell.

Pharmacokinetics: Peginterferon alfa-2b is a well-characterized polyethylene glycol-modified ("pegylated") derivative of interferon alfa-2b that is predominantly composed of monopegylated species with small amounts of dipegylated and free interferon alfa-2b. The plasma half-life of peginterferon alfa-2b is prolonged compared with non-pegylated interferon alfa-2b. Peginterferon alfa-2b has a potential to depegylate to free interferon alfa-2b. The biologic activity of the pegylated isomers is qualitatively similar to, but lower than that of free interferon alfa-2b.

Following s.c. administration, maximal serum concentrations occur between 15 and 44 hours post-dose, and are sustained for up to 48 to 72 hours postdose. Peginterferon alfa-2b C_{max} and AUC measurements increase in a dose-related manner. Mean apparent volume of distribution is 0.99 L/kg.

Upon multiple dosing, there is an accumulation of immunoreactive interferons. There is, however, only a modest increase in biologic activity as measured by a bioassay.

Mean peginterferon alfa-2b elimination half-life is approximately 40 hours , with apparent clearance of 22 mL/hrxkg. The mechanisms involved in clearance of interferons in man have not yet been fully elucidated. Based on a retrospective regression analysis of UNITRON PEG Cl/F and creatinine clearance, from an expanded database, it is estimated that renal clearance of UNITRON PEG may account for approximately 30% of the apparent clearance.

Special Populations: Renal Function: Renal clearance appears to account for 30% of total clearance of peginterferon alfa-2b. In a single dose study (1 µg/kg) in patients with impaired renal function, C_{max}, AUC, and half-life increased in relation to the degree of renal impairment (see Contraindications and Warnings). Because of marked intrasubject variability in interferon pharmacokinetics, it is recommended that patients be monitored closely during treatment with UNITRON PEG (see Warnings). Patients with severe renal dysfunction (creatinine clearance <50 mL/min) must not be treated with UNITRON PEG (see Contraindications).

Hepatic Function: The pharmacokinetics of peginterferon alfa-2b have not been evaluated in patients with severe hepatic dysfunction. Therefore, UNITRON PEG must not be used in these patients.

Elderly Patients (>65 years of age): In a single dose study using a subcutaneous dose of 1.0 µg/kg, the pharmacokinetics of peginterferon alfa-2b were not affected by age. The study was not powered to detect specified differences between the age groups (20-45 years and 65-80 years). However, as in younger patients, renal function must be determined prior to the administration of UNITRON PEG therapy.

Pediatric Patients: Specific pharmacokinetic evaluations in patients under 18 years of age were not performed. Safety and effectiveness of UNITRON PEG in these patients have not been evaluated. UNITRON PEG is indicated for the treatment of chronic hepatitis C only in patients 18 years of age or older.

INDICATIONS: UNITRON PEG (peginterferon alfa-2b) is indicated in monotherapy in case of intolerance or contraindication to ribavirin, for the treatment of adult patients with chronic hepatitis C without liver decompensation. This indication is based on a study in patients naive to prior therapy.

The optimal treatment for chronic hepatitis C is considered to be the administration of the combination of ribavirin plus peginterferon alfa-2b.

CONTRAINDICATIONS: UNITRON PEG (peginterferon alfa-2b) is contraindicated in patients with: hypersensitivity to the active substance, to any component of the injection, or to any interferons; autoimmune hepatitis or a history of autoimmune disease; pre-existing severe psychiatric condition or a history of severe psychiatric disorder, pre-existing thyroid abnormalities for which thyroid function cannot be maintained in the normal range by medication; epilepsy; decompensated liver disease; or severe renal dysfunction (creatinine clearance <50 mL/min).

WARNINGS: Alpha interferons cause or aggravate fatal or life-threatening neuropsychiatric, autoimmune, ischemic, and infectious disorders. Patients should be monitored closely with periodic clinical and laboratory evaluations. Patients with persistently severe or worsening signs or symptoms of these conditions should be withdrawn from therapy. In many cases, but not all cases, these disorders resolve after stopping interferon therapy.

Cardiovascular: Chest pain, hypertension, cardiac arrhythmia, cardiac ischemia, and myocardial infarction have been reported in patients with and without a history of cardiac disorder or abnormality in association with the use of alpha interferon therapies including UNITRON PEG (see Adverse Effects). UNITRON PEG should not be administered to patients with a history of severe pre-existing cardiac disease including unstable or uncontrolled cardiac disease in the previous 6 months. As with other alpha interferons, patients with a history of congestive heart failure, myocardial infarction and/or previous or current arrhythmic disorders receiving UNITRON PEG (peginterferon alfa-2b) therapy require close monitoring. It is recommended that patients who have pre-existing cardiac abnormalities have electrocardiograms taken prior to and during the course of treatment. Cardiac arrhythmias (primarily supraventricular) usually respond to conventional therapy but may require discontinuation of UNITRON PEG therapy.

Psychiatric and Central Nervous System (CNS): Severe CNS effects, particularly severe depression, suicidal behavior (suicidal ideation, attempted suicide and suicide), psychosis including hallucinations and aggressive behavior have been observed in some patients during UNITRON PEG therapy (see Adverse Effects). Other CNS effects including confusion and alterations of mental status have been observed with alpha interferons, including UNITRON PEG. More significant obtundation and coma, including cases of encephalopathy, have been observed in some patients, usually elderly, treated at higher doses. While these effects are generally reversible upon discontinuation of therapy, in a few patients full resolution took up to three weeks. Very rarely, seizures have occurred with high doses of UNITRON PEG. UNITRON PEG therapy should be used with extreme caution in patients with a history of pre-existing psychiatric disorders who report a history of severe depression. If patients develop psychiatric or CNS problems, including clinical depression, it is recommended that the patient be carefully monitored due to the potential seriousness of these undesirable effects. If such symptoms appear, the potential seriousness of these undesirable effects must be borne in mind by the prescribing physician. If symptoms persist or worsen, discontinue UNITRON PEG therapy.

UNITRON PEG therapy should not be used in patients with severe, debilitating medical conditions.

Renal Function: It is recommended that renal function be evaluated in all patients prior to initiation of UNITRON PEG therapy and that patients be monitored closely during treatment. Increases in serum creatinine levels have been observed in patients with renal insufficiency treated with interferons, including UNITRON PEG. Patients with impairment of renal function should be closely monitored for signs and symptoms of toxicity, including increases in serum creatinine, and, should have their weekly dose of UNITRON PEG reduced if medically appropriate. Patients with severe renal dysfunction (creatinine clearance <50 mL/min) must not be treated with UNITRON PEG, as the clearance of peginterferon alfa-2b is reduced in patients with significant renal impairment (see Pharmacology and Contraindications). If serum creatinine rises >2 mg/dL, UNITRON PEG must be discontinued.

Hepatic Function: Any patient developing liver function abnormalities or hepatopathy during treatment should be monitored closely. As with treatment with any interferon, discontinue treatment with UNITRON PEG in patients who develop prolongation of coagulation markers or other markers of hepatic function, which might indicate liver decompensation. The safety and efficacy of peginterferon alfa-2b have not been evaluated in patients with severe hepatic dysfunction. Therefore, UNITRON PEG must not be used for these patients. UNITRON PEG therapy should be discontinued for any patient developing signs and symptoms of liver failure. Patients should be tested for the presence of antibody to HCV. Other causes of chronic hepatitis including autoimmune hepatitis should be excluded.

Pulmonary Changes: As with other alpha interferons, pulmonary infiltrates, pneumonitis, and pneumonia, occasionally resulting in fatality, have been observed rarely in UNITRON PEG treated patients. Any patient developing fever, cough, dyspnea or other respiratory symptoms must have a chest X-ray taken. If the chest X-ray shows pulmonary infiltrates or there is evidence of pulmonary function impairment, the patient is to be monitored closely. If appropriate, discontinue UNITRON PEG therapy. Prompt discontinuation of therapy and treatment with corticosteroids appear to be associated with resolution of pulmonary adverse events. These symptoms have been reported more frequently when Shosaikoto (also known as Xiao-Chai-Hu-Tang), a Chinese herbal medication, has been administered concomitantly with alpha interferons. UNITRON PEG should not be administered to patients with chronic obstructive pulmonary disease (COPD).

Acute Hypersensitivity: Acute hypersensitivity reactions, (e.g. angioedema, bronchoconstriction and anaphylaxis), have been observed rarely during alpha interferon therapy. If such a reaction develops during treatment with UNITRON PEG, discontinue treatment and institute appropriate medical therapy immediately. As with other alpha interferons, urticaria has been observed rarely during UNITRON PEG therapy. Transient rashes do not necessitate interruption of treatment.

Hydration: Adequate hydration must be maintained in patients undergoing therapy with UNITRON PEG since hypotension related to fluid depletion has been seen in some patients treated with alpha interferons, including UNITRON PEG. Fluid replacement may be necessary.

Ocular Changes: As with other alpha interferons, ophthalmologic disorders, including retinopathies (including macular edema), retinal hemorrhages, retinal artery or vein obstruction, cotton wool spots, loss of visual acuity or visual field, optic neuritis, and papilledema have been reported in rare instances after treatment with UNITRON PEG (see Adverse Effects). All patients should have a baseline eye examination. Any patient complaining of ocular symptoms, including loss of visual acuity or visual field must have a prompt and complete eye examination. Because these ocular events may occur in conjunction with other disease states, periodic ocular examinations during UNITRON PEG therapy are recommended in patients with disorders that may be associated with retinopathy, such as diabetes mellitus or hypertension. Discontinuation of UNITRON PEG therapy should be considered in patients who develop new or worsening ophthalmological disorders.

Hearing disorders and hearing loss have been reported with the use of alpha interferons, including UNITRON PEG therapy.

Diabetes Mellitus and Hyperglycemia: As with other alpha interferons, diabetes mellitus and hyperglycemia have been observed in patients treated with UNITRON PEG therapy. Symptomatic patients should have their blood glucose measured and followed up accordingly. Patients with diabetes mellitus may require adjustment of their antidiabetic regimen.

Bone Marrow Toxicity: Alpha interferons, including UNITRON PEG, may suppress bone marrow function which may result in severe cytopenias. As with other alpha interferons, UNITRON PEG may be very rarely associated with aplastic anemia. UNITRON PEG dosing should be reduced or discontinued in patients developing decreases in neutrophil or platelet counts (see Dosage, Dose Modification).

Pancreatitis: Pancreatitis, sometimes life-threatening, has occurred in patients treated with alpha interferons, including UNITRON PEG. UNITRON PEG therapy should be suspended if symptoms or signs of pancreatitis are observed. UNITRON PEG should be discontinued in patients diagnosed with pancreatitis.

Colitis: As seen with other alpha interferons, ulcerative and ischemic colitis, sometimes serious, have been observed within 12 weeks of starting UNITRON PEG therapy. UNITRON PEG should be discontinued immediately if symptoms of colitis develop (typical manifestations include abdominal pain, bloody diarrhea and fever). The colitis usually resolves within 1 to 3 weeks of discontinuation of alpha interferon.

Special Populations: General: The safety and efficacy of UNITRON PEG have not been established in patients who have failed other alpha interferon treatments.

HCV/HIV/HBV Co-infection: The safety and efficacy of UNITRON PEG treatment have not been established for hepatitis C patients co-infected with human immunodeficiency virus (HIV) or hepatitis B virus (HBV).

Transplantation: The safety and efficacy of UNITRON PEG treatment have not been established for patients with liver or other organ transplants. Preliminary data indicates that interferon alpha therapy may be associated with an increased rate of kidney graft rejection. Liver graft rejection has also been reported but a causal association with interferon alpha therapy has not been established.

Effects on Fertility: Interferons, including peginterferon alfa-2b, may impair fertility. In studies of interferon administration in non-human primates, menstrual cycle abnormalities have been observed. Decreases in serum estradiol and progesterone concentrations have been reported in women treated with human leukocyte interferon. The effects of interferon on male fertility have not been studied. The genotoxicity of peginterferon alfa-2b was evaluated in bacterial (Ames) and mammalian cell clastogenicity (HPBL) assays, and was negative in both assays.

UNITRON PEG is recommended for use in fertile women only when they are using effective contraception during the treatment period. There are no adequate and well-controlled studies on the use of interferon alfa-2b or peginterferon alfa-2b in pregnant women.

Pregnancy: UNITRON PEG is not recommended for use during pregnancy, as reproductive studies with peginterferon alfa-2b have not been performed. Interferon alfa-2b has been shown to have abortifacient effects in Macaca mulatta (rhesus monkeys) at 15 and 30 million IU/kg (estimated human equivalent of 5 and 10 million IU/kg, based on body surface area adjustment for a 60 kg adult). This same effect is expected with peginterferon alfa-2b. High doses of other forms of interferon alpha and beta are known to produce dose-related anovulatory and abortifacient effects in rhesus monkeys.

Lactation: It is not known whether interferon alfa-2b and/or peginterferon alfa-2b are excreted in human milk. Because of the potential for serious adverse reactions from UNITRON PEG in nursing infants, nursing must be discontinued prior to the start of UNITRON PEG therapy.

Children: Safety and effectiveness of UNITRON PEG in these patients have not been evaluated (see Indications). UNITRON PEG is not recommended for use in children and adolescents under the age of 18 years.

PRECAUTIONS: Immunological Effects: A number of immune-mediated dermatological reactions associated with the use of alfa interferons have been reported ranging from erythema multiforme to more severe but very rare occurrences of Stevens-Johnson syndrome and toxic epidermal necrolysis.

Autoimmune Disease: As with other alpha interferons, the development of autoantibodies has been reported during treatment with UNITRON PEG. Clinical manifestations of autoimmune disease during interferon therapy may occur more frequently in patients predisposed to the development of autoimmune disorders.

Thyroid Changes: Infrequently, patients treated for chronic hepatitis C with alpha interferons including UNITRON PEG, have developed thyroid abnormalities, either hypothyroidism or hyperthyroidism. After discontinuation of therapy, thyroid dysfunction may or may not be reversed. Determine thyroid-stimulating hormone (TSH) levels if, during the course of therapy, a patient develops symptoms consistent with possible thyroid dysfunction. In the presence of thyroid dysfunction, UNITRON PEG (peginterferon alfa-2b) treatment may be initiated or continued only if TSH levels can be maintained in the normal range by medication.

Fever: While fever may be associated with the flu-like syndrome reported commonly during interferon therapy, other causes of persistent fever must be ruled out.

Hypertriglyceridemia: Hypertriglyceridemia and aggravation of hypertriglyceridemia, sometimes severe, have been observed with UNITRON PEG therapy. Monitoring of lipid levels is, therefore, recommended.

Psoriatic Disease and Sarcoidosis: Use of alpha interferons, including UNITRON PEG, has been associated with exacerbating pre-existing psoriatic disease and sarcoidosis. Use of UNITRON PEG in patients with psoriasis or sarcoidosis is recommended only if the potential benefit justifies the potential risk.

Drug Interactions: Results of a single-dose study with UNITRON PEG demonstrated no effect on the activity of cytochrome P450 isoenzymes CYP1A2, CYP2C8/9, CYP2D6, and CYP3A4 or hepatic N-acetyl transferase. The literature, however, reports up to a 50% reduction in clearance of CYP1A2 substrates (e.g., theophylline) when administered with other forms of interferon alpha and therefore caution should be exercised when UNITRON PEG is used with medications metabolized by CYP1A2.

A multi-dose probe study assessing P450 substrates was performed in 26 subjects with chronic hepatitis C, who received a once-weekly UNITRON PEG (1.5 µg/kg) for 4 weeks. There was no inhibition of CYP1A2, 3A4 or N-acetyltransferase. There was a 27% increase in activity of CYP2C8/9 and a 69% increase in CYP2D6. Caution should be used when administering peginterferon alfa-2b with medications metabolized by CYP2C8/9 and CYP2D6.

Laboratory Tests: Standard hematologic tests, blood chemistry and a test of thyroid function are recommended in all patients prior to initiating therapy. Acceptable baseline values that may be considered as a guideline prior to initiation of UNITRON PEG therapy are: platelets $\geq 100 \times 10^9$/L; neutrophil count $\geq 1.5 \times 10^9$/L; TSH levels must be within normal limits.

Lower baseline values may be considered acceptable (see Dosage).

Laboratory evaluations are to be conducted at weeks 2 and 4 of therapy, and periodically thereafter as clinically appropriate.

Occupational Hazards: Effects on Ability to Drive and Use Machines: Patients who develop fatigue, somnolence or confusion during treatment with UNITRON PEG therapy are cautioned to avoid driving or operating machinery.

Information to Be Provided to the Patient: Patients receiving UNITRON PEG treatment should be directed in its appropriate use, informed of the benefits and risks associated with treatment and referred to the patient information sheet. This information is intended to aid in the safe and effective use of this medication. It is not disclosure of all possible adverse or intended effects.

If home use is prescribed, a puncture-resistant container for the disposal of used syringes and needles should be supplied to the patient. Patients should be thoroughly instructed on the importance of proper disposal and cautioned against any reuse of needles and syringes. The full container should be disposed of according to the directions provided by the physician.

The most common adverse experiences occurring with UNITRON PEG therapy are "flu-like" symptoms such as headache, fatigue, myalgia, and fever (see Adverse Effects) and may decrease in severity as treatment continues. Some of these "flu-like" symptoms may be minimized by bedtime administration of UNITRON PEG. Antipyretics should be considered to prevent or partially alleviate the fever and headache. Another common adverse experience associated with peginterferon alfa-2b therapy is thinning of the hair.

Patients should be advised that laboratory evaluations are required prior to starting therapy and periodically thereafter (see Laboratory Tests). It is advised that patients be well hydrated especially during the initial stages of treatment.

ADVERSE EFFECTS: The safety of UNITRON PEG (peginterferon alfa-2b) was investigated in a phase III clinical trial in 1 219 previously untreated chronic hepatitis C patients. In the clinical trial the majority of adverse events were mild to moderate in severity and not treatment limiting. The majority of patients reported headache and myalgia.

The main categories of serious adverse events that were considered to be related to study drug included neutropenia (0.3%), thrombocytopenia (0.7%) and psychiatric events (1 to 3%).

The most common treatment emergent adverse events (≥10%) are presented in Table 1 by treatment group.

Table 1: UNITRON PEG

Most Common Treatment-emergent Adverse Events (≥10%)

	% of Subjects			
	UNITRON PEG 0.5 µg/kg (N=315)	**UNITRON PEG 1.0 µg/kg (N=297)**	**UNITRON PEG 1.5 µg/kg (N=304)**	**Interferon alfa-2b 3MIU (N=303)**
Application Site Disorders				
Injection Site Inflammation	44	42[a]	40	16
Injection Site Reaction	7	10[a]	10	5
Body as a Whole				
Headache	61	64[a]	64	58
Fatigue	43	51	45	50
Rigors	34	40[a]	44	33
Fever	31	45[a]	44	30
Influenza-like Symptoms	18	22	25	19
Asthenia	12	12	15	11
Right Upper Quadrant Pain	12	8	9	8
Weight Decrease	10	11	21	13
Gastrointestinal				
Nausea	21	26[a]	25	20
Anorexia	10	20	25	17
Diarrhea	16	18	20	16
Abdominal Pain	14	15	13	11
Musculoskeletal				
Myalgia	48	54	61	53
Arthralgia	26	25	31	27
Musculoskeletal Pain	19	28[a]	20	22
Psychiatric				
Depression	27	29	27	25
Irritability	19	18	17	24
Insomnia	17	23	20	23
Anxiety	10	9	7	10
Concentration Impaired	10	10	10	8
Skin and Appendages				
Alopecia	20	22	34	22
Pruritus	9	12	10	8
Skin Dry	7	11	10	9
Other				
Dizziness	8	12	14	10
Infection Viral	13	11	9	10
Pharyngitis	12	10	7	7
Sweating Increased	7	6	10	7

(cont'd)

Table 1: UNITRON PEG *(cont'd)*

Most Common Treatment-emergent Adverse Events (≥10%)

	% of Subjects			
	UNITRON PEG 0.5 µg/kg (N=315)	**UNITRON PEG 1.0 µg/kg (N=297)**	**UNITRON PEG 1.5 µg/kg (N=304)**	**Interferon alfa-2b 3MIU (N=303)**
Sinusitis	10	7	9	7

[a] ≥5% greater than interferon alfa-2b.

Commonly reported adverse events (≥2%) were malaise, neutropenia, rash, vomiting, dry mouth, emotional lability, nervousness, dyspnea, somnolence, thyroid disorders, chest pain, dyspepsia, flushing, paresthesia, coughing, agitation, hypertonia, hyperesthesia, blurred vision, confusion, flatulence, decreased libido, erythema, eye pain, apathy, hypoesthesia, loose stool, conjunctivitis, nasal congestion, constipation, vertigo, menorrhagia, menstrual disorder.

As with other alpha interferons, severe central nervous system effects, particularly severe depression, suicidal ideation, attempted suicide, suicide, psychosis including hallucinations and aggressive behavior have been rarely or very rarely reported during therapy with UNITRON PEG (see Warnings).

As with other alpha interferons, ophthalmological disorders including retinopathies (including macular edema), retinal hemorrhages, retinal artery or vein obstruction, cotton wool spots, loss of visual acuity or visual field, optic neuritis, and papilledema have been rarely reported during therapy with UNITRON PEG (see Warnings).

Adverse reactions of the cardiovascular system (CVS), particularly arrhythmia, appeared to be correlated mostly with preexisting CVS disease and prior cardiotoxic therapy. Cardiomyopathy was also observed in patients treated with peginterferon alfa and has been reported more frequently in patients with known risk factors for cardiovascular diseases. There are limited data to assess the reversibility of cardiomyopathy reported with the use of peginterferon alfa; however cases of reversible cardiomyopathy have been reported with the use of interferon alfa.

As with other alpha interferons seizures, pancreatitis, hypertriglyceridemia, arrhythmia, diabetes, peripheral neuropathy, colitis (including ischemic and ulcerative), aplastic anemia, hypertension, cardiac ischemia, myocardial infarction, cerebrovascular ischemia, cerebrovascular hemorrhage, encephalopathy (see Warnings), sarcoidosis or exacerbation of sarcoidosis, erythema multiforme, Stevens-Johnson syndrome, toxic epidermal necrolysis, injection site necrosis rhabdomyolysis, myositis, renal failure and renal insufficiency have been rarely or very rarely reported during therapy with UNITRON PEG.

Alpha interferons have been associated with altered lipid metabolism (including hypercholesterolemia and hyperlipemia) and pulmonary hypertension.

Laboratory Values: Granulocytopenia (<0.75×10⁹/L) occurred in 4% of patients receiving 0.5 µg/kg, and 7% of patients receiving 1 µg/kg of UNITRON PEG. Thrombocytopenia (<70×10⁹/L) occurred in 1% of patients receiving 0.5 µg/kg and 3% of patients receiving 1 µg/kg of UNITRON PEG.

OVERDOSE:

Symptoms: There is limited experience with overdosage. Serious adverse events reported in cases of UNITRON PEG overdose include cyanosis, diarrhea, fatigue, gastritis, headache, influenza-like illness, nausea, pyrexia, acute renal failure, suicide attempt, vomiting, and weight decreased.

Treatment: In cases of overdoses, symptomatic treatment and close observation of the patient are recommended (see Dosage, Dose Modification).

For management of a suspected drug overdose, CPhA recommends that you contact your **regional Poison Control Centre**. See the *CPS* Directory section for a list of Poison Control Centres.

DOSAGE: UNITRON PEG treatment should be initiated only by a physician experienced in the treatment of patients with hepatitis C.

UNITRON PEG is administered s.c. once weekly on the same day of the week for 48 weeks. Therapy should be discontinued in patients who do not respond by 24 weeks, i.e., those without loss of HCV-RNA. Based upon the results of the pivotal clinical trial, the following dose based on 1 µg/kg/week with a pre-specified amount per 4 body weight range categories is recommended. Each category is comprised of a lower weight range and a higher weight range with a pre-calculated dose as per Table 2.

Table 2: UNITRON PEG

Recommended Dosing

Patient Weight (kg)	Strength (µg/0.5 mL) After Reconstitution (with 0.7 mL of Sterile Water for Injection)	Amount of UNITRON PEG to be administered mL (µg)
37–45 46–57	50	0.4 (40) 0.5 (50)
58–72 73–89	80	0.4 (64) 0.5 (80)
90–107 108–136	120	0.4 (96) 0.5 (120)
137–160	150	0.5 (150)

In a large clinical trial, the most effective dose was determined to be 1 µg/kg.

There are no data on treatment for longer than 1 year.

Dose Modification: In general, the dosage may be adjusted according to the patient's tolerance to the medication. If severe adverse reactions or laboratory abnormalities develops during the course of treatment, the dosage should be modified or therapy should be temporarily discontinued until the adverse reactions abates. If persistent or recurrent intolerance develops despite adequate dosage adjustment, or if the disease progresses rapidly, treatment with UNITRON PEG should be discontinued. See Table 3.

Table 3: UNITRON PEG

Dose Modification Guidelines for UNITRON PEG

Laboratory Values	Reduce UNITRON PEG dose by 50% if:	Discontinue UNITRON PEG if:
Neutrophils	<0.75×10⁹/L	<0.50×10⁹/L
Platelets	<80×10⁹/L	<50×10⁹/L
White blood cell	<1.5×10⁹/L	<1.0×10⁹/L

Concomitant therapy: Acetaminophen has been used successfully to alleviate the symptoms of fever and headache, which can occur with peginterferon alfa-2b therapy. The recommended acetaminophen dosage is 500 mg to 1 g given 30 minutes before administration of UNITRON PEG. The maximum dosage of acetaminophen to be given is 1 g four times daily. In order to properly assess the source of fever, adjunctive acetaminophen should be limited to a maximum of 5 consecutive days unless otherwise specified by the prescribing physician.

Stability and Storage Recommendations: Before reconstitution, store in the refrigerator between 2 to 8°C.

After reconstitution with Sterile Water for Injection, the product is to be used immediately. Since no preservative is present, it is recommended that administration of the solution occur as soon as possible and within 3 hours of reconstitution. For reconstitution under controlled and validated aseptic conditions such as a hospital pharmacy, the chemical and physical in-use stability for the reconstituted solution has been demonstrated 24 hours at 2 to 8°C. Discard any unused portion.

Do not use past expiry date on the label.

Reconstituted Solution: Instructions for Use and Handling: Use a sterilized syringe and injection needle, inject 0.7 mL of Sterilized Water for Injection **slowly**, into the vial of UNITRON PEG. Powder for Solution for Injection aiming the stream of liquid at the glass wall of the vial. It is best not to aim the stream directly at the white solid or powder, or to inject the liquid quickly, as this causes a greater amount of bubbles. The solution may appear cloudy or bubbly for a few minutes. Swirl the vial gently to complete dissolution of powder. **Do not shake,** but gently turn the vial upside down. The content should now be completely dissolved. Once the solution has settled and all bubbles have risen to the top of the solution, you should have a clear solution with a small ring of tiny bubbles around the top. The appropriate dose can now be withdrawn with a sterilized injection syringe and injected.

A small volume is lost during preparation of UNITRON PEG solution when the dose is measured and injected. Thus, each unit contains an excess amount of diluent and UNITRON PEG powder to ensure delivery of the labeled dose in 0.5 mL of UNITRON PEG injection. **The labeled strength will be contained in 0.5 mL of the reconstituted solution.** The reconstituted solution for each of the available strengths will have a concentration of 50 µg/0.5 mL, 80 µg/0.5 mL, 120 µg/0.5 mL or 150 µg/0.5 mL.

As for all parenteral medicinal products, inspect visually the reconstituted solution prior to administration. Do not use if discoloration is present. UNITRON PEG Powder for Solution for Injection must not be mixed with other injectable products. Discard any unused material after opening.

Incompatibilities: UNITRON PEG should only be reconstituted with Sterile Water for Injection and must not be mixed with other medicinal products.

UNITRON PEG Powder for Solution for Injection vials are single dose vials. Once reconstituted, use immediately (see Stability and Storage Recommendations).

INFORMATION FOR THE PATIENT: Published in e-CPS, available by subscription at www.e-cps.ca.

SUPPLIED: UNITRON PEG (peginterferon alfa-2b) Powder for Solution for Injection is supplied as a white powder packaged in single-dose vials, which deliver either 50, 80, 120 or 150 µg in each 0.5 mL.

Deliverable Dose 50 µg/0.5 mL Vial—Patients ≥37 and ≤57 kg—(74 µg/vial prior to reconstitution): Each single-dose vial of white lyophilized powder contains: peg-interferon alfa-2b 74 µg. Nonmedicinal ingredients: polysorbate 80, sodium phosphate dibasic anhydrous, sodium phosphate monobasic dihydrate and sucrose. A box containing 2 vials of UNITRON PEG Powder for Solution for Injection, 4 syringes, 2 vials of diluent containing 10 mL Sterile Water for Injection and 4 alcohol swabs.

Deliverable Dose 80 µg/0.5 mL Vial—Patients >57 and ≤89 kg—(118.4 µg/vial prior to reconstitution): Each single-dose vial of white lyophilized powder contains: peg-interferon alfa-2b 118.4 µg. Nonmedicinal ingredients: polysorbate 80, sodium phosphate dibasic anhydrous, sodium phosphate monobasic dihydrate and sucrose. A box containing 2 vials of UNITRON PEG Powder for Solution for Injection, 4 syringes, 2 vials of diluent containing 10 mL Sterile Water for Injection and 4 alcohol swabs.

Deliverable Dose 120 µg/0.5 mL Vial—Patients >89 and ≤136 kg—(177.6 µg/vial prior to reconstitution): Each single-dose vial of white lyophilized powder contains: peg-interferon alfa-2b 177.6 µg. Nonmedicinal ingredients: polysorbate 80, sodium phosphate dibasic anhydrous, sodium phosphate monobasic dihydrate and sucrose. A box containing 2 vials of UNITRON PEG Powder for Solution for Injection, 4 syringes, 2 vials of diluent containing 10 mL Sterile Water for Injection and 4 alcohol swabs.

Deliverable Dose 150 µg/0.5 mL Vial—Patients >136 and ≤160 kg—(222 µg/vial prior to reconstitution): Each single-dose vial of white lyophilized powder contains: peg-interferon alfa-2b 222 µg. Nonmedicinal ingredients: polysorbate 80, sodium phosphate dibasic anhydrous, sodium phosphate monobasic dihydrate and sucrose. A box containing 2 vials of UNITRON PEG Powder for Solution for Injection, 4 syringes, 2 vials of diluent containing 10 mL Sterile Water for Injection and 4 alcohol swabs.

Each vial must be reconstituted with 0.7 mL of Sterile Water for Injection to give a final volume of 0.74 mL for administration of up to 0.5 mL of solution. The reconstituted solutions will have concentrations of 100, 160, 240 and 300 µg/mL respectively.

Uracyst®

sodium chondroitin sulfate

Replenishment of the Glycosaminoglycan (GAG) Layer

Stellar

DESCRIPTION: Chondroitin is an acidic mucopolysaccharide and is one of the glycosaminoglycans (GAGs). Its repeating disaccharide unit is made of a glucuronic acid and a galactosamine with one sulfate group in β (1-3') linkage.

This disaccharide unit is polymerized in β (1-4') linkage. The O-sulfation at C-4 is chondroitin sulfate A. O-sulfation at C-6 is chondroitin sulfate C.

The luminal surface of the bladder is coated with a layer of glycosaminoglycans (GAGs) that provide a protective impermeable barrier to the bladder. The highly charged poly anionic molecules of GAGs bind with water molecules thereby creating a molecular layer of water between the surface to which GAGs are bound and urine.

This layer inhibits adherence of bacteria, microcrystals, carcinogens and irons. Damage to this GAG layer may result in deficiencies to its protective barrier, inducing irritations in the bladder wall.

Chondroitin is an important component of the bladder GAGs that can replenish the deficient GAG layer on the bladder epithelium.

INDICATIONS: For replenishment of the glycosaminoglycan (GAG) layer in the bladder, for patients with damaged or GAG deficient bladder epithelium.

CONTRAINDICATIONS: Do not administer to patients with known hypersensitivity to the solution.

WARNINGS: For Bladder Instillation only. Uracyst contains neither preservatives nor antimicrobials; therefore, any unused portion must be discarded.

PRECAUTIONS: Bring to room temperature before use.

ADVERSE EFFECTS: No known adverse effects. Short term discomfort may be caused by the catheterization process. Some patients have experienced discomfort associated with sensitivity to catheter lubricants.

OVERDOSE:

For management of a suspected drug overdose, CPhA recommends that you contact your **regional Poison Control Centre**. See the *CPS* Directory section for a list of Poison Control Centres.

DOSAGE: Instill 20 mL into the bladder after any residual urine has been removed. For optimum results, Uracyst should be used full strength without dilution, and retained in the bladder as long as possible (not less than 30 minutes).

Repeat the instillation of 20 mL weekly for 4 to 6 weeks; then, monthly thereafter until symptoms are relieved. Most patients benefit from 6 weekly 20 mL instillations, then monthly instillations thereafter depending on their symptomatic response.

SUPPLIED: Each mL contains: sodium chondroitin sulfate 20 mg. Single dose glass vials of 20 mL, packages of 4. Only the contents of the vial are sterile. Store 2 to 25°C. **Do not freeze.** Bring the contents to room temperature before use.

Blister Pack Directions: To be opened immediately prior to use. To access vial, grip tab at top while supporting neighbouring strip and peel off one strip as needed. To separate individual blister packs, fold on perforation and bend back and forth several times prior to tearing.

Uremol® 10

urea

Emollient—Moisturizer—Antipruritic

Stiefel, a GSK company

SUPPLIED: Cream: Each tube or jar contains: urea 10% in a white emollient cream containing moisturizers and skin protectant. Nonmedicinal ingredients: cyclomethicone/dimethicone copolyol, germaben II, lauryl methicone copolyol, polyalpha olefin, polydimethyl cyclosiloxane, purified water and white petrolatum. Tubes of 75 g and jars of 120 g. Store between 15-30°C.

Lotion: Each bottle contains: urea 10% in an emollient lotion containing moisturizers and skin protectants. Nonmedicinal ingredients: carbomer 940, ceteareth-12, ceteareth-20, decanoic acid triglyceride, dibasic sodium anhydrous phosphate, germaben II, glyceryl stearate, glycerol, octyldodecanol, potassium phosphate, purified water and xanthan gum. Plastic bottles of 250 mL with fliptops. Store between 15-30°C.

Uremol® 20

urea

Emollient—Moisturizer—Antipruritic

Stiefel, a GSK company

SUPPLIED: Each tube or jar of cream contains: urea 20% in an emollient base. Nonmedicinal ingredients: carbomer 940, ceteareth-12, ceteareth-20, citric acid anhydrous, decanoic acid triglyceride, germaben II, glyceryl monostearate, octyl dodecanol, potassium phosphate monobasic, purified water, sodium hydroxide and sodium phosphate dibasic. Tubes of 100 g and jars of 225 g.

Uremol® HC ℞

hydrocortisone acetate—urea

Topical Corticosteroid—Emollient—Antipruritic

Stiefel, a GSK company

SUPPLIED: Cream: Each tube or jar contains: hydrocortisone acetate USP 1% in an aqueous emollient hydrating base consisting of urea USP 10%. Nonmedicinal ingredients: caprylic/capric triglyceride, ceteareth-12, ceteareth-20, cetyl alcohol, disodium EDTA, germaben II, glyceryl stearate, isopropyl myristate, mineral oil and lanolin alcohol, potassium phosphate monobasic, propylene glycol, purified water, sodium lauryl sulfate, sodium phosphate dibasic and xantham gum. Plastic tubes of 50 g and plastic jars of 225 g.

Lotion: Each bottle contains: hydrocortisone acetate USP 1% in an aqueous emollient hydrating base consisting of urea USP 10%. Nonmedicinal ingredients: cetyl acetate and acetylated lanolin alcohol, ceteareth-12, ceteareth-20, citric acid anhydrous, decanoic acid triglyceride, disodium edetate, germaben II, glycerin, glyceryl monostearate, isopropyl myristate, octyl dodecanol, purified water, sodium phosphate dibasic and xantham gum. Plastic bottles of 150 mL.

Unscented. Store between 15-30°C.

Urisec™

urea

Emollient—Moisturizer—Antipruritic

Odan

Urisec™-10

urea

Emollient—Moisturizer—Antipruritic

Odan

SUPPLIED: Urisec: Cream: Each tube or jar contains: urea USP 22% in an emollient base. Nonmedicinal ingredients: ceteareth-12, collagen, dimethicone, Germaben II, glyceryl stearate, menthyl lactate, octyldodecanol, perfume, propylene glycol, purified water, sodium laureth sulfate and xanthan gum. pH approximately 7. Tubes of 120 g. Jars of 225 and 454 g. Store at room temperature between 15 and 30°C.

Lotion: Each bottle contains: urea USP 12% in an emollient base. Nonmedicinal ingredients: ceteareth-12, ceteareth-20, cetearyl alcohol, collagen, dimethicone, glyceryl stearate, menthyl lactate, methylparaben, mineral oil, octyldodecanol, perfume, propylene glycol, propylparaben, purified water and xanthan gum. pH approximately 7. Plastic applicator bottles of 250 mL. Store at room temperature between 15 and 30°C.

Urisec-10: Each tube contains: urea USP 10% in an emollient base. Nonmedicinal ingredients: allantoin, aluminum starch octenylsuccinate, beta-glucan, caprylic/capric triglycerides, carbomer, cetyl alcohol, cetyl palmitate, chlorphenesin, dimethicone, edetate disodium, glycerin, menthyl lactate, polyethylene beeswax, purified water, safflower oil, stearic acid, triethanolamine, white petrolatum and xanthan gum. Contains no fragrance or artificial colors. Plastic tubes of 75 and 120 g. Store at room temperature between 15 and 30°C.

Urisec™-40

urea

Keratolytic Potent Tissue Softener

Odan

SUPPLIED: Each tube contains: urea USP 40 % in an emollient base. Nonmedicinal ingredients: carbomer, ceteth-20, cetyl alcohol, cyclomethicone, glycerin, glyceryl stearate, mineral oil, PEG-75 stearate, PEG/PPG 18/18 dimethicone, purified water, steareth-20, triethanolamine, white petrolatum and xanthan gum. Plastic tubes of 30 and 100 g. Store at room temperature between 15 and 30°C.

Uromax® ℞

oxybutynin chloride

Anticholinergic—Antispasmodic

Purdue Pharma

Date of Preparation: November 28, 2005
Date of Revision: June 16, 2010

SUMMARY PRODUCT INFORMATION:

Route of Administration	Dosage Form/ Strength	Clinically Relevant Nonmedicinal Ingredients
Oral	Controlled release tablets 10 mg, 15 mg	None For a complete listing of other ingredients see Dosage Forms, Composition and Packaging.

INDICATIONS AND CLINICAL USE: Uromax (oxybutynin chloride controlled release tablets) is indicated for:

- treatment of patients with symptoms of an overactive bladder including urge incontinence, urinary frequency, urgency or any combination of these symptoms

Geriatrics: Available data does not suggest a difference in the balance between efficacy and adverse event profile in patients over the age of 65 years and less than 65 years.

Pediatrics: No data is available on use in children.

CONTRAINDICATIONS:

- Patients who are hypersensitive to oxybutynin or to any ingredient in the formulation (for a complete listing, see the Dosage Forms, Composition and Packaging).
- Partial or complete obstruction of the gastrointestinal tract
- Paralytic ileus
- Intestinal atony of the elderly or debilitated patient
- Megacolon
- Toxic megacolon complicating ulcerative colitis
- Glaucoma
- Myasthenia gravis
- Obstructive uropathy
- Unstable cardiovascular status in acute haemorrhage

WARNINGS AND PRECAUTIONS: General: When oxybutynin is administered in the presence of high environmental temperature, it can cause heat prostration (fever and heat stroke due to decreased sweating).

Oxybutynin may produce drowsiness or blurred vision. Patients should be cautioned regarding activities requiring mental alertness, such as operating a motor vehicle or other machinery or performing hazardous work while taking this drug, until it is clear that their ability to do so is not impaired. Alcohol or other sedative drugs may enhance the drowsiness caused by oxybutynin.

Cardiovascular: The symptoms of coronary heart disease, congestive heart failure, cardiac arrhythmias, tachycardia and hypertension may be aggravated following administration of Uromax.

Although not reported for immediate-release or controlled-release oxybutynin formulations, newer antimuscarinic agents used in the treatment of urinary incontinence have been reported to prolong the QT/QTc interval of the electrocardiogram. Some drugs that cause QT/QTc prolongation may increase the risk of the rare, but serious ventricular arrhythmia—torsades de pointes. Patients at risk for QT/QTc prolongation, such as those with clinically relevant heart failure, long QT syndrome, recent significant hypokalemia, or receiving other drugs known to prolong QT/QTc, should be appropriately monitored when receiving oxybutynin. Patients who develop prolonged QT/QTc or symptoms of possible arrhythmia such as dizziness, palpitations, or fainting should be evaluated electrocardiographically and for electrolyte disturbances.

Endocrine and Metabolism: The symptoms of hyperthyroidism may be aggravated following administration of oxybutynin.

Gastrointestinal: Diarrhea may be an early symptom of incomplete intestinal obstruction, especially in patients with ileostomy or colostomy. In such cases, treatment with oxybutynin would be inappropriate and possibly harmful.

Administer with caution to patients with hiatal hernia associated with reflux esophagitis, since anticholinergic drugs may aggravate this condition.

Administration of oxybutynin in large doses to patients with ulcerative colitis may suppress intestinal motility to the point of producing a paralytic ileus and precipitate or aggravate toxic megacolon, a serious complication of the disease.

Genitourinary: The symptoms of prostatic hypertrophy may be aggravated following administration of oxybutynin.

Hepatic/Biliary/Pancreatic: Use with caution in patients with hepatic impairment.

Neurologic: Oxybutynin may cause drowsiness.

Use with caution in patients with autonomic neuropathy.

Ophthalmologic: Oxybutynin may produce blurred vision.

Renal: Use with caution in patients with renal impairment.

Special Populations: Pregnant Women: The safety of Uromax in pregnancy has not been established. Therefore, it should not be used in women of childbearing potential, unless, in the opinion of the physician, the expected benefit to the patient outweighs the possible risk to the fetus.

Nursing Women: It is not known whether oxybutynin is excreted in human milk. Because many drugs are excreted in human milk, caution should be exercised when Uromax is administered to a nursing woman.

Pediatrics (<18 years of age): Because the safety of Uromax tablets in children has not been evaluated, use of the drug in this age group should be with appropriate caution.

Geriatrics: Uromax should be used with caution in debilitated patients.

ADVERSE REACTIONS: Adverse Drug Reaction Overview: The most frequent adverse effects of oxybutynin are those related to its anticholinergic (antimuscarinic) effects, most notably dry mouth and pharyngitis. Although the incidence of dry mouth increased with increasing dose, in Uromax clinical trials, patient satisfaction also improved at higher doses because of correspong improvement in control of urinary incontinence.

Clinical Trial Adverse Drug Reactions: Because clinical trials are conducted under very specific conditions the adverse event rates observed in the clinical trials may not reflect the rates observed in practice and should not be compared to the rates in the clinical trials of another drug. Adverse event information from clinical trials is useful for identifying potential drug-related adverse reactions and for approximating their rates.

Table 1 includes spontaneously reported adverse events in three Canadian clinical trials of Uromax in patients with urinary incontinence: Study 018-004 was an open-label, sequential, crossover comparison with immediate-release (IR) oxybutynin (12 patients); Study 018-005 was a double-blind, randomized, parallel group comparison with IR oxybutynin (65 patients CR; 60 patients IR); and Study 018-009 was a double-blind, randomized, parallel group comparison of doses of 5, 10, and 15 mg per day (77, 77, and 83 patients respectively). Adverse events that were considered by the clinical investigator to be unrelated to the drug are excluded from this list.

Table 1: Uromax

Adverse Event Reports in Uromax Clinical Trials (1%)

	Uromax n=314 (%)	IR Oxybutynin N=72 (%)
Body as a Whole		
Headache	7.0	18.1
Halitosis	6.4	0
Asthenia	4.8	13.9
Abdominal Pain	4.5	9.7
Chest Pain	1.6	1.4
Pain	1.6	1.4
Back Pain	1.3	2.8
Cardiovascular		
Vasodilatation	2.9	5.6
Hypertension	1.3	0
Palpitation	1.3	0
Syncope	0.3	2.8
Central Nervous System		
Dry Mouth	64.0	72.2

(cont'd)

Table 1: Uromax *(cont'd)*

Adverse Event Reports in Uromax Clinical Trials (1%)

	Uromax n=314 (%)	IR Oxybutynin N=72 (%)
Dizziness	6.4	15.3
Insomnia	4.8	0
Somnolence	3.2	9.7
Increased Salivation	1.6	1.4
Sleep Disorder	1.6	0
Thinking Abnormal	1.6	0
Hypertonia	1.0	0
Amnesia	0	1.4
Depersonalization	0	1.4
Hyperkinesia	0	1.4
Hypesthesia	0	1.4
Digestive		
Nausea	6.4	12.5
Constipation	5.1	11.1
Dyspepsia	5.1	11.1
Diarrhea	4.8	1.4
Dysphagia	3.8	11.1
Flatulence	2.2	2.8
Stomatitis	1.3	0
Anorexia	1.0	5.6
Gastrointestinal Disorder	1.0	0
Glossitis	1.0	4.2
Vomiting	1.0	1.4
Eructation	0.6	2.8
Esophagitis	0	1.4
Tongue Discoloration	0	1.4
Metabolic and Nutritional		
Peripheral Edema	1.9	6.9
Thirst	1.9	5.6
Musculoskeletal		
Tenosynovitis	0	1.4
Respiratory		
Pharyngitis	28.7	30.6
Rhinitis	5.7	18.1
Cough Increased	3.2	6.9
Epistaxis	1.9	2.8
Voice Alteration	1.9	1.4
Increased Upper Airway Secretion	0.3	1.4
Sinusitis	0	1.4
Skin and Appendages		
Dry Skin	10.2	9.7
Rash	1.3	0
Pruritus	1.0	1.4
Skin Discoloration	0.3	2.8
Nail Disorder	0.3	1.4
Special Senses		
Taste Perversion	4.1	9.7

(cont'd)

Table 1: Uromax *(cont'd)*

Adverse Event Reports in Uromax Clinical Trials (1%)

	Uromax n=314 (%)	IR Oxybutynin N=72 (%)
Dry Eyes	2.5	12.5
Amblyopia	1.9	6.9
Eye Pain	0.3	1.4
Mydriasis	0.3	1.4
Taste Loss	0	1.4
Urogenital		
Urinary Retention	4.8	1.4
Urinary Tract Infection	4.5	4.2
Dysuria	1.9	2.8
Urinary Frequency	1.6	0
Urination Impaired	1.3	4.2
Urinary Urgency	0.3	1.4
Hematuria	0	1.4

During the first two or three days of overactive bladder symptom relief, patients may experience dry mouth, constipation, drowsiness or blurred vision. Provided these symptoms are not intolerable, patients should be encouraged to continue at the same dose for a few days since these symptoms tend to decrease in severity, or even disappear, over time. If excessive dry mouth, constipation, drowsiness or blurred vision persists, the dose should be reduced by 5 mg. If it is necessary to reduce the dose, it may be possible to carefully increase it again after three or four days if the symptoms of overactive bladder are not being well controlled.

Less Common Clinical Trial Adverse Drug Reactions (<1%): Body as a Whole: abdomen enlarged, allergic reaction, face edema, lack of drug effect, malaise.

Cardiovascular: migraine, syncope.

Central Nervous System: akathisia, anxiety, circumoral paresthesia, confusion, depression, libido decreased, nervousness, paresthesia.

Digestive: colitis, eructation, increased appetite, liver function tests abnormal, melena, mouth ulceration, tongue disorder.

Metabolic and Nutritional: creatinine increased, generalized edema.

Musculoskeletal: arthritis, joint disorder.

Respiratory: hiccup, increased upper airway secretion, lung disorder.

Skin and Appendages: hair disorder, nail disorder, skin discolouration, sweating decreased, urticaria, vesiculobullous rash.

Special Senses: abnormal vision, conjunctivitis, eye pain, iritis, mydriasis, tinnitus.

Urogenital: cystitis, nocturia, urethral pain, urethritis, urinary urgency.

Abnormal Hematologic and Clinical Chemistry Findings: See Table 2.

Table 2: Uromax

Abnormal Hematologic and Clinical Chemistry Findings

# Patients	Parameter	Unit	Value Recorded	Reference Range [Low-High]	Clinically Significant
1	ALT	U/L	201	5–42	2× upper limit
1	AST	U/L	80	10–40	2× upper limit

Post-Market Adverse Drug Reactions: Other adverse effects reported with other formulations of oxybutynin are: impotence, increased ocular tension, interference with normal heat regulation, mood changes, suppression of lactation, tachycardia, drug idiosyncrasies that may include dermal manifestations or paralysis of the ciliary muscles of the eye causing blurred vision.

DRUG INTERACTIONS: Overview: Oxybutynin is metabolized through the cytochrome P450 system, specifically the 3A4 enzymes. Inhibitors of these enzymes may alter the pharmacokinetics of Uromax. The clinical significance of this is unknown. Alcohol may increase drowsiness.

Drug-Drug Interactions: Interactions with other drugs have not been formally investigated.

Drug-Food Interactions: Interactions with foods have not been formally investigated.

Drug-Herb Interactions: Interactions with herbal products have not been formally investigated.

Drug-Laboratory Test Interactions: Interactions with laboratory tests have not been formally investigated.

DOSAGE AND ADMINISTRATION: Dosing Considerations:

- There is a dose-response relationship for the reduction in episodes of urinary incontinence, with the greatest reduction at a daily dose of Uromax 15 mg. This is also the dose associated with the highest level of patient satisfaction, even though anticholinergic side effects also increase with increasing dose.
- Although peak plasma concentrations are lower with Uromax, than with immediate-release oxybutynin preparations administered three times daily, at the same total daily dose, it is recommended that the daily dose of Uromax not be higher than the maximum recommended daily dose for the immediate-release preparation (20 mg).

Recommended Dose and Dosage Adjustment: The recommended initial dose of Uromax is 10-15 mg once a day. The dose may be adjusted in 5 mg increments according to individual efficacy and tolerability. The maximum recommended daily dose is 20 mg.

Uromax is designed to allow once daily dosing. If frequency, urgency or incontinence repeatedly occurs at the end of a dose interval, it is generally an indication for a dosage increase, not more frequent administration.

Dose adjustments should be based on the patient's clinical response. Because of the sustained release properties of Uromax, dose adjustments should generally be separated by 48 hours. Uromax may be taken with or without food. In debilitated patients or patients with impaired hepatic or renal function, it is advisable to initiate at the lowest dose and to increase carefully according to tolerance and response.

Missed Dose: If a patient forgets to take one or more doses, they should take their next dose at the normal time and in the normal amount.

Administration: Uromax tablets should be swallowed intact with the aid of liquids. The tablets should not be crushed, chewed or divided.

OVERDOSAGE:

The symptoms of overdose with oxybutynin may be any of those seen with other anticholinergic agents. Symptoms may include signs of CNS excitation (e.g., restlessness, tremor, irritability, delirium, hallucinations), flushing, fever, nausea, vomiting, tachycardia, hypotension or hypertension, respiratory failure, paralysis and coma.

In the event of overdose or exaggerated response, treatment should be symptomatic and supportive. Induce emesis or perform gastric lavage (emesis is contraindicated in precomatose, convulsive, or psychotic state) and maintain respiration. Activated charcoal may be administered as well as magnesium sulfate. Physostigmine may be considered to reverse symptoms of anticholinergic intoxication. Hyperpyrexia may be treated symptomatically with ice bags or other cold applications and alcohol sponges.

For management of a suspected drug overdose, CPhA recommends that you contact your **regional Poison Control Centre**. See the *CPS* Directory section for a list of Poison Control Centres.

ACTION AND CLINICAL PHARMACOLOGY: Mechanism of Action: Oxybutynin chloride is a tertiary amine ester with anticholinergic (antimuscarinic), as well as direct spasmolytic and local anesthetic properties. It depresses spontaneous activity of smooth muscle and inhibits contractions produced by non-cholinergic stimulation. It does not have blocking effects at skeletal neuromuscular junctions or autonomic ganglia (nicotinic effects).

In vitro studies of isolated detrusor muscle or intact bladder preparations from several animal species have demonstrated that oxybutynin competitively antagonizes smooth muscle contraction due to acetylcholine or parasympathetic nerve stimulation. In vitro studies of bladder homogenates demonstrate that oxybutynin binds to muscarinic receptor sites.

Oxybutynin also has a direct inhibitory effect on smooth muscle. In vitro studies using isolated detrusor or intact bladder preparations have demonstrated oxybutynin-induced reductions in spontaneous and non-cholinergically induced contractions of the detrusor, with a potency greater than that of atropine. Oxybutynin also demonstrates local anesthetic effects.

The combination of anticholinergic, spasmolytic and local anesthetic actions make oxybutynin a therapeutically useful agent in the treatment of urinary incontinence.

Pharmacodynamics: In patients with urinary incontinence, urodynamic studies have demonstrated that oxybutynin increases maximal bladder capacity, detrusor compliance, and volume at first bladder contraction and first desire to void, and decreases maximum detrusor pressure. These effects are associated with decreases in urgency, frequency of micturition and incontinence episodes.

In a steady-state pharmacokinetic study, stimulated saliva output over 24 hours, was greater with Uromax than immediate-release oxybutynin, and subjective evaluations of dry mouth severity were lower with Uromax than immediate-release oxybutynin, indicating less propensity for anticholinergic side effects with Uromax.

The pharmacodynamics (anticholinergic effects) of oxybutynin at steady state were assessed by measuring Stimulated Saliva Output (SSO), Dry Mouth Severity and Dry Mouth Symptom Score (DMSS) after administration of each treatment. The mean Stimulated Saliva Output was significantly greater for Uromax than IR oxybutynin at each observation time point (0-20 hours; $p \leq 0.05$ and at 24 hours; $p<0.06$) and as a cumulative amount (28.9 g and 21.6 g; $p=0.0001$). The mean Dry Mouth Severity was less for Uromax than IR oxybutynin at each observation time point (significantly at hours 8, 10, 12, 14 and 24; $p<0.05$) and as a cumulative measure (51.6 ±32.3 and 57.9 ±31.5; $p=0.0816$). The Mean DMSS Index for Uromax was significantly greater than for IR oxybutynin (0.58±0.26 and 0.46±0.28; $p=0.0064$) indicating less frequency and bother of dry mouth symptoms for Uromax.

The duration of effect of Uromax tablets is 24 hours. Once daily dosing with Uromax provides comparable reductions in micturition frequency, urgency and incontinence episodes to immediate-release oxybutynin, given three times per day. Uromax produced a significant reduction (62%) in night-time incontinence episodes but immediate-release oxybutynin did not. In a study comparing fixed doses of 5, 10 or 15 mg, the reduction in episodes of urinary incontinence was greatest at a daily dose of 15 mg. This was also the dose associated with the greatest level of overall control of urinary symptoms (urgency, frequency and incontinence) and with the highest rating of patient satisfaction, in consideration of both efficacy and side effects.

Pharmacokinetics: See Table 3.

Table 3: Uromax

Summary of Uromax Single-Dose Mean Pharmacokinetic Parameters in Healthy Subjects

	C_{max} (ng/mL)	T_{max} (h)	AUC_I (ng·h/mL)
Uromax (fasted)	5.22	11.6	89.22
IR Oxybutynin (fasted)	8.34	0.84	65.42
Uromax (fed)	3.64	10.8	74.54
IR Oxybutynin (fed)	9.87	1.35	81.47

Absorption: Oxybutynin is rapidly absorbed from the gastrointestinal tract when given orally. There is inter-individual variability in absorption and it is increased in the presence of food. The terminal plasma elimination half-life of oxybutynin ranges from 2 to 3 hours in healthy individuals to 5 hours in frail elderly individuals.

The rate of absorption of oxybutynin was lower with Uromax than with immediate-release oxybutynin tablets under both fasting and fed conditions, while the extent of absorption of Uromax and immediate-release oxybutynin are equivalent under fed and fasted conditions.

At steady-state, the maximum plasma oxybutynin concentration was lower and the minimum concentration higher with Uromax (15 mg once daily) than with immediate-release oxybutynin (5 mg q8h) (Relative C_{max} 75%; Relative C_{min} 220%). Fluctuation in plasma oxybutynin concentrations was lower with Uromax than with immediate-release oxybutynin (135% vs. 319%). Extent of absorption was higher with Uromax than with immediate-release oxybutynin (Relative AUC 136%) but concentrations of the metabolite N-desethyloxybutynin were lower (Relative AUC 76%; Relative C_{max} 54%) and fluctuation was less with Uromax than immediate-release oxybutynin (148% vs. 255%) (see Figure 1).

Figure 1: Uromax

Oxybutynin Plasma Concentration vs Time

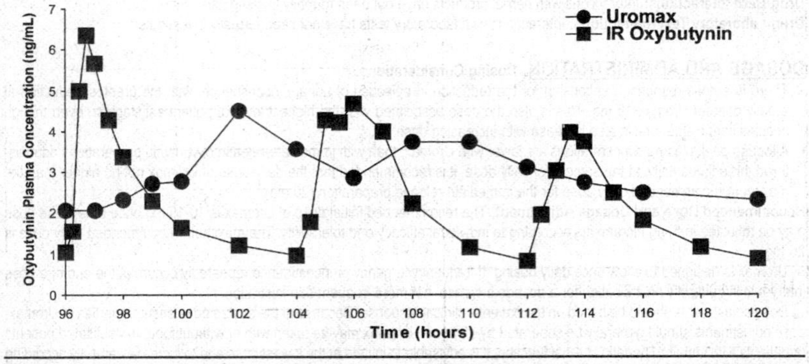

Distribution: Plasma concentrations of oxybutynin decline biexponentially following intravenous or oral administration. The volume of distribution is 193 L after intravenous administration of 5 mg oxybutynin chloride.

Metabolism: Oxybutynin is metabolized through the cytochrome P450 system, specifically the 3A4 enzymes. Oxybutynin is extensively metabolized in the liver and gut wall. The parent compound and the metabolite (N-desethyloxybutynin) are both active and are equipotent. The most abundant but inactive metabolite is phenylcyclohexylglycolic acid.

Excretion: Only negligible amounts of the parent compound are excreted renally.

STORAGE AND STABILITY: Temperature: Store at room temperature (15-30°C).

Light: Protect from exposure to light.

Moisture: Protect from moisture. Protect from high humidity.

Others: Keep in a safe place out of the reach of children.

INFORMATION FOR THE PATIENT: Published in e-CPS, available by subscription at www.e-cps.ca.

DOSAGE FORMS, COMPOSITION AND PACKAGING: 10 mg: Each yellow, round, film coated tablet, engraved with "U" on one side and a number corresponding to the mg strength on the other, contains: oxybutynin chloride 10 mg. Nonmedicinal ingredients: cetostearyl alcohol, dibasic calcium phosphate dihydrate, dye blend yellow, hydroxyethyl cellulose, magnesium stearate, methacrylic acid copolymer Type C, microcrystalline cellulose, sodium alginate, talc and triethyl citrate; film coating: hydroxypropyl methylcellulose, polyethylene glycol, polysorbate 80, synthetic yellow iron oxide and titanium dioxide. Opaque plastic bottles of 100.

15 mg: Each pink, oval, film coated tablet, engraved with "U" on one side and a number corresponding to the mg strength on the other, contains: oxybutynin chloride 15 mg. Nonmedicinal ingredients: cetostearyl alcohol, dibasic calcium phosphate dihydrate, dye blend yellow, hydroxyethyl cellulose, magnesium stearate, methacrylic acid copolymer Type C, microcrystalline cellulose, sodium alginate, talc and triethyl citrate; film coating: hydroxypropyl methylcellulose, polyethylene glycol, polysorbate 80, synthetic red iron oxide, titanium dioxide. Opaque plastic bottles of 100.

(Shown in Product Identification Section)

Uromitexan™ Pr

mesna

Uroprotector

Baxter

PHARMACOLOGY: Mesna is rapidly and easily converted by autooxidation to its only metabolite disodium 2,2-dithio-bis ethane sulfonate (mesna disulfide, dimesna), forming a disulfide link. Following i.v. injection, only a small portion of the administered dose is detected in the blood as a reactive thiol compound (mesna). Mesna disulfide remains in the intravascular space and is rapidly forwarded to the kidney. In the renal tubular epithelium a considerable proportion of mesna disulfide is again reduced to a free thiol compound, presumably by mediation of glutathione reductase. It is then capable of chemically reacting with acrolein or other urotoxic oxazaphosphorine metabolites in the urine, thereby developing its detoxifying activity.

The first and most important step towards detoxification is the addition of mesna to the double bond of acrolein, resulting in the formation of a stable thio ether which could be detected in the urine by chromatography. In the second step, mesna reduces the speed of degradation of the 4-hydroxy metabolite in the urine. A relatively stable, non-urotoxic condensation product from 4-hydroxy cyclophosphamide or 4-hydroxy ifosfamide and mesna is formed. By such stabilization mesna inhibits the degradation of 4-hydroxy cyclophosphamide or 4-hydroxy ifosfamide and hence the formation of acrolein. This intermediate deactivated product could also be detected by chromatographic urinalysis.

INDICATIONS: For the reduction and prevention of urinary tract toxicity (hemorrhagic cystitis) of oxazaphosphorines (see Adverse Effects sections of the Cytoxan and Ifex product monographs).

CONTRAINDICATIONS: In individuals with a known hypersensitivity to it.

WARNINGS: The protective effect of mesna applies only to the urotoxic effects of oxazaphosphorines. Additional prophylactic or accompanying measures recommended during treatment with oxazaphosphorines are thus not affected and should not be discontinued.

In vitro, mesna is incompatible with cisplatin. The combination of an oxazaphosphorine cytostatic agent with mesna and cisplatin in the same infusion solution is not stable and is not to be used.

PRECAUTIONS: Mesna treatment may cause false positive reactions in tests for ketone bodies in the urine. The color reaction is reddish purple rather than purple. The reddish purple color is less stable, and fades immediately by adding glacial acetic acid.

Children: Mesna has been administered to patients as young as 13 years of age.

Pregnancy: Although the use of mesna in pregnant women has not been established, animal studies have not revealed any embryotoxic or mutagenic effects. However, in view of the fact that oxazaphosphorines are not recommended during pregnancy, this would eliminate the need for mesna.

ADVERSE EFFECTS: At recommended doses, side effects are not usually observed.

The following adverse reactions have been reported in a phase I trial in healthy volunteers: diarrhea, abdominal pain, headache, pain in limbs and joints, transient drop in blood pressure, increase in pulse rate. These reactions occurred at doses of 60 mg/kg or more, given as a single bolus.

Venous irritation may occur in rare instances. This reaction may be attributed to the physical properties of mesna (i.e., pH 6, and hypertonic solution). No venous complications were observed when the solution was given diluted with Sterile Water for Injection USP (1 part mesna solution to 3 parts water).

OVERDOSE:

Symptoms: No specific antidote for mesna is known. Overdosage should be managed with supportive measures to sustain the patient through any period of toxicity. Mesna has been administered at doses from 70 to 100 mg/kg without any toxic effect on hematopoiesis, hepatic and renal function or the CNS.

Treatment: See Symptoms.

For management of a suspected drug overdose, CPhA recommends that you contact your **regional Poison Control Centre**. See the *CPS* Directory section for a list of Poison Control Centres.

DOSAGE: Mesna should be administered by i.v. injection, usually at 20% of the respective oxazaphosphorine dose at time 0 (=administration of the cytostatic agent), 4 hours and 8 hours. In the case of ifosfamide, the usual dose of mesna is 10 to 12 mg/kg i.v. at 0, 4 and 8 hours after the ifosfamide dose (see Dosage sections of Cytoxan and Ifex product monographs).

In the treatment of children, and particularly when administering very high doses, such as required when conditioning patients for bone-marrow transplantations, the mesna doses should be given at 0, 1, 3, 6, 9 and 12 hours or dosage increased to 30% of the respective oxazaphosphorine dose.

Oral administration of mesna, e.g., in patients with poor veins, is also feasible. Mesna is then given either at doses of 20% of the oxazaphosphorine dose at time 0 hours by the parenteral route, followed by oral doses of 40% of the oxazaphosphorine dose after 4 and 8 hours, taken in juice or cola, or in 3 oral doses of 40% of the oxazaphosphorine dose at time 0, 4 and 8 hours.

Solution for I.V. Infusion: 5% Dextrose Injection USP, 5% Dextrose Injection with 0.45% Sodium Chloride Injection USP, 0.9% Sodium Chloride Injection USP, Lactated Ringer's Injection USP. Solutions for infusion should be made up at a concentration of 1 mg/mL or greater.

Stability of Solution: Solutions for infusion should be used within 24 hours from the time of preparation.

SUPPLIED: Each mL of solution contains: mesna 100 mg. Nonmedicinal ingredients: disodium edetate, sodium hydroxide (for pH adjustments) and water for injection. Ampuls of 4 and 10 mL.

URSO® Pr

ursodiol

Cholestatic Liver Diseases

Axcan Pharma

URSO DS® Pr

ursodiol

Cholestatic Liver Diseases

Axcan Pharma

Date of Preparation: September 5, 2002

Date of Revision: September 10, 2008

SUMMARY PRODUCT INFORMATION:

Route of Administration	Dosage Form/ Strength	Clinically Relevant Nonmedicinal Ingredients
Oral	Tablet 250 mg, 500 mg	None

INDICATIONS AND CLINICAL USE: URSO and URSO DS (ursodiol, also known as ursodeoxycholic acid (UDCA)) are indicated for:

- the management of cholestatic liver diseases, such as primary biliary cirrhosis (PBC).

Cholestatic liver diseases are characterized by a decrease in bile secretion and bile flow.

The diagnosis of cholestatic liver diseases is based on the biochemical signs of cholestasis (such as an increase in alkaline phosphatase, γ-GT, bilirubin), and also an increase in IgM levels and the presence of antimitochondrial antibodies in PBC.

The monitoring of the efficacy of URSO and URSO DS in the management of cholestatic liver diseases should be based on the biochemical parameters of cholestasis, as described above, as well as on signs of hepatic cytolysis (such as AST, ALT) which are very often associated with cholestasis during the progression of the diseases.

Therefore, liver function tests (γ-GT, alkaline phosphatase, AST, ALT) and bilirubin level should be monitored every month for three months after start of therapy, and every six months thereafter. Serum levels of these parameters usually decrease rapidly, thus, demonstrating efficacy. Treatment should be discontinued if the levels of the above parameters increase (see Warnings and Precautions).

URSO and URSO DS are not indicated for the treatment of decompensated cirrhosis.

Geriatrics: Appropriate studies with URSO and URSO DS have not been performed in the geriatric population. However, geriatric-specific problems that would limit the use or usefulness of URSO and URSO DS in the elderly are not expected.

Pediatrics: The safety and effectiveness of URSO and URSO DS in children have not been established.

CONTRAINDICATIONS: Patients who are hypersensitive or intolerant to ursodiol or to any ingredient in the formulation. For a complete listing, see Dosage Forms, Composition and Packaging.

WARNINGS AND PRECAUTIONS: Carcinogenesis and Mutagenesis: URSO and URSO DS have no carcinogenic, mutagenic or teratogenic effects in laboratory animals treated at higher doses than those intended for therapy in humans, and after long-term treatment.

Hepatic/Biliary/Pancreatic: Patients with variceal bleeding, hepatic encephalopathy, ascites, or in need of an urgent liver transplant, should receive appropriate specific treatment.

Special Populations: Pregnant Women: There are no adequate or well-controlled studies in pregnant women. Because animal reproduction studies are not always predictive of human response, URSO and URSO DS should not be used in women who are or may become pregnant. If this drug is used during pregnancy or if the patient becomes pregnant while taking this drug, the patient should be apprised of the potential hazard to the fetus.

Nursing Women: It is not known whether ursodiol is excreted in human milk. Since many drugs are excreted in human milk, caution should be exercised when URSO or URSO DS is administered to a nursing mother.

Pediatrics: The safety and effectiveness of URSO and URSO DS in children have not been established.

Geriatrics: Appropriate studies with URSO and URSO DS have not been performed in the geriatric population. However, geriatric-specific problems that would limit the use or usefulness of URSO and URSO DS in the elderly are not expected.

Monitoring and Laboratory Tests: Lithocholic acid, one of the metabolites of ursodeoxycholic acid (URSO and URSO DS) is hepatotoxic unless it is effectively detoxified in the liver. Therefore, the following tests are important for patient monitoring:

Liver function tests (γ-GT, alkaline phosphatase, AST, ALT), and bilirubin levels should be monitored every month for three months after start of therapy, and every six months thereafter. Serum levels of these parameters usually decrease rapidly, thus, demonstrating efficacy. Treatment should be discontinued if the levels of the above parameters increase.

ADVERSE REACTIONS: Adverse Drug Reaction Overview: Adverse events observed in clinical trials are tabulated and described below. In a 130 patient placebo-controlled trial in primary biliary cirrhosis, the common adverse events (i.e. ≥1 %) included leukopenia, skin rash, diarrhea, blood creatinine increased, blood glucose increased, and peptic ulcer. In a second trial with 60 patients, the frequency of treatment-emergent adverse event reporting was higher with the most common (defined as ≥5%) being asthenia, dyspepsia, edema peripheral, hypertension, nausea, GI disorder, chest pain, and pruritus. In this second trial there were 4 serious adverse events: 1 patient with diabetes mellitus, 1 patient with breast nodule and 2 patients with fibrocystic breast disease. None of these events were considered related to the medication. At the recommended dosage, ursodiol is well-tolerated and has no significant adverse events.

Clinical Trial Adverse Drug Reactions: Because clinical trials are conducted under very specific conditions the adverse reaction rates observed in the clinical trials may not reflect the rates observed in practice and should not be compared to the rates in the clinical trials of another drug. Adverse drug reaction information from clinical trials is useful for identifying drug-related adverse events and for approximating rates.

The adverse reactions in Table 1 were observed in clinical trials in primary biliary cirrhosis with 180 patients (89 randomized to URSO treatment, 91 to placebo treatment). Adverse events are reported regardless of attribution to the test medication. Adverse reactions occurring at a rate of 1% or higher in the URSO group, and that are higher than placebo are included in Table 1. Diarrhea and thrombocytopenia at 12 months, nausea/vomiting, fever and other side effects are not included, because they occurred at the same rate or a lower rate than placebo.

Table 1: URSO

Adverse Events With a Frequency ≥1% Observed in a Clinical Trial of 180 Patients

Adverse event (ordered by MedDRA System Organ Class)		Visit at 12 Months		Visit at 24 Months	
		UDCA[a] n (%)	Placebo n (%)	UDCA[a] n (%)	Placebo n (%)
Blood and lymphatic system disorders	Leukopenia	—	—	2 (2.63)	—
Gastrointestinal disorders	Diarrhea	—	—	1 (1.32)	—
	Peptic ulcer	—	—	1 (1.32)	—
Investigations	Blood creatinine increased	—	—	1 (1.32)	—
	Blood glucose increased	1 (1.18)	—	1 (1.32)	—
Skin and subcutaneous tissue disorders	Rash	—	—	2 (2.63)	—

[a] UDCA=Ursodeoxycholic acid=Ursodiol =URSO.

Note: Those AEs occurring at the same or higher incidence in the placebo as in the UDCA group have been deleted from this table (this includes diarrhea and thrombocytopenia at 12 months, nausea/vomiting, fever and other toxicity).

In a randomized, cross over study in sixty PBC patients, four patients experienced one serious adverse event each (diabetes mellitus, breast nodule, and fibrocystic breast disease (2 patients)). No deaths occurred in the study. Forty-three patients (43/71.7%) experienced at least one treatment-emergent adverse event (TEAEs) during the study. The most common (defined as ≥5%) TEAEs were asthenia, (11.7%), dyspepsia (10%), edema peripheral (8.3%), hypertension (8.3%), nausea (8.3%), GI disorders (5%), chest pain (5%), and pruritus (5%). These nine TEAEs included abdominal pain and asthenia (1 patient), nausea (3 patients) dyspepsia (2 patients), and anorexia and esophagitis (1 patient each). One patient on the BID regimen (total dose 1000 mg) withdrew due to nausea. All of these nine TEAEs except esophagitis were observed with the BID regimen at a total daily dose of 1000 mg or greater.

Table 2: URSO

Treatment-Emergent Adverse Events (TEAEs) with a Frequency of ≥1 % Observed in a Clinical Trial of 60 PBC Patients

Adverse event (ordered by MedDRA System Organ Class)		TEAEs, n (%)
Blood and lymphatic system disorders	Anemia	1 (1.7)
	Lymphadenopathy	2 (3.3)
Cardiac disorders	Arrhythmia	2 (3.3)
	Cardiovascular disorder	2 (3.3)
Ear and labyrinth disorders	Deafness	1 (1.7)
	Vertigo	1 (1.7)
Eye disorders	Cataract	2 (3.3)
	Eye disorder	1 (1.7)
	Retinal disorder	1 (1.7)
Gastrointestinal disorders	Abdominal pain	2 (3.3)
	Diarrhea	2 (3.3)
	Dyspepsia	6 (10)
	Dysphagia	1 (1.7)
	Esophagitis	1 (1.7)
	Flatulence	1 (1.7)
	Gastrointestinal disorder	3 (5.0)
	Nausea	5 (8.3)
	Salivary gland enlargement	1 (1.7)
	Stomach ulcer	1 (1.7)
General disorders and administration site conditions	Asthenia	7 (11.7)
	Chest pain	3 (5.0)
	Chest pain substernal	1 (1.7)
	Cyst	1 (1.7)
	Edema	5 (8.3)
	Edema generalized	1 (1.7)
	Edema peripheral	5 (8.3)
	Granuloma	1 (1.7)
	Hemorrhagic ulcer	1 (1.7)
	Pain	1 (1.7)
Hepatobiliary disorders	Biliary pain	1 (1.7)
Immune system disorders	Amyloidosis	1 (1.7)
Infections and infestations	Bronchitis	1 (1.7)
	Cystitis	1 (1.7)
	Herpes simplex	1 (1.7)
	Infection	1 (1.7)
	Otitis media	1 (1.7)
	Pharyngitis	1 (1.7)
	Pneumonia	1 (1.7)
	Rhinitis	2 (3.3)
	Urinary tract infection	1 (1.7)
	Vaginitis	1 (1.7)
Metabolism and nutrition disorders	Anorexia	1 (1.7)
	Diabetes mellitus	2 (3.3)
Musculoskeletal and connective tissue disorders	Back pain	1 (1.7)
	Bone disorder	1 (1.7)
	Bone fracture spontaneous	1 (1.7)

(cont'd)

Table 2: URSO *(cont'd)*

Treatment-Emergent Adverse Events (TEAEs) with a Frequency of ≥1 % Observed in a Clinical Trial of 60 PBC Patients

Adverse event (ordered by MedDRA System Organ Class)		TEAEs, n (%)
Neoplasms benign, malignant and unspecified (incl cysts and polyps)	Breast neoplasm	1 (1.7)
	Lung nodule	1 (1.7)
	Plantar warts	1 (1.7)
Nervous system disorders	Dizziness	2 (3.3)
	Headache	1 (1.7)
	Migraine	1 (1.7)
	Paresthesia	1 (1.7)
Reproductive system and breast disorders	Breast nodule	1 (1.7)
	Fibrocystic breast disease	2 (3.3)
	Menorrhagia	1 (1.7)
Respiratory, thoracic and mediastinal disorders	Dyspnea	1 (1.7)
	Lung disorder	1 (1.7)
	Respiratory disorder	1 (1.7)
	Sore nose	2 (3.3)
Skin and subcutaneous tissue disorders	Acne	2 (3.3)
	Miliaria	1 (1.7)
	Pruritus	3 (5.0)
	Psoriasis	1 (1.7)
	Rash	1 (1.7)
	Skin disorder	2 (3.3)
	Skin hypertrophy	1 (1.7)
Vascular disorders	Hypertension	5 (8.3)

Less Common Clinical Trial Adverse Drug Reactions (<1%): Analysis of the data in the trial with 180 patients (Table 1) revealed no reports of adverse events at rates <1 % with the exception of those adverse events that occurred at the same or at a higher incidence in the treatment group than placebo. No data for TEAEs occurring at rates <1 % in the trial of 60 patients (Table 2) are available due to the small sample size.

Abnormal Hematologic and Clinical Chemistry Findings: In the placebo-controlled trial with 180 patients, change from baseline in hematologic parameters and non-hepatic clinical chemistry were analyzed. Statistically significant differences from baseline are reported in Table 3 and Table 4.

There was a significant decrease (p<0.01) in WBC and platelets in the UDCA-treated group from baseline and a significant (p<0.05) decrease in platelets in the placebo group. There was no significant change in haemoglobin.

Table 3: URSO

Hematologic Parameters: Changes from Baseline

		Baseline		Endpoint		Change from Baseline	
		UDCA	Placebo	UDCA	Placebo	UDCA (± SD)	Placebo (± SD)
WBC	Mean (±SD)	5.9 (2.0)	6.2 (4.1)	5.5 (1.6)	5.8 (2.4)	−0.5[b] (1.4)	−0.5 (4.3)
	n	88	87	83	75		
Platelets	Mean (±SD)	238.5 (92.5)	245.4 (112.4)	211.2 (87.2)	223.9 (94.3)	−29.4[b] (39.3)	−17.7[a] (58.0)
	n	86	86	82	74		

[a] Statistically different from zero, p<0.05.
[b] Statistically different from zero, p<0.01.

Table 4: URSO

Clinical Chemistries: Changes from Baseline

		Baseline		Endpoint		Change from Baseline	
		UDCA	Placebo	UDCA	Placebo	UDCA (±SD)	Placebo (±SD)
Calcium (mg/dL)	Mean (±SD)	9.49[c] (0.40)	9.47 (0.40)	9.39 (0.43)	9.30 (0.51)	−0.12[a,c] (0.37)	−0.19[a] (0.37)
	n	89	91	83	76		
Cholesterol (mg/dL)	Mean (±SD)	287.73[c] (121.12)	276.03 (105.22)	223.53 (56.80)	261.46 (83.53)	−67.39[a,d] (93.31)	−11.32[b] (47.70)
	n	89	91	83	76		

(cont'd)

All the non-hepatic clinical chemistries at baseline were not significantly different (p>0.05) between the UDCA- and placebo-treated groups. In the UDCA group there was a significant (p>0.05) decrease from baseline in calcium, cholesterol and total thyroxine and a significant increase (p>0.05) in creatinine and triglycerides. In the placebo group there was a significant (p>0.05) decrease in cholesterol and significant increase (p>0.05) in calcium and creatinine. There was no significant change seen for sodium, potassium, phosphorus, HDL, and AMA.

Post-Market Adverse Drug Reactions: Most of the serious adverse events were received from Japan. These adverse events occurred in patients taking ursodiol (ursodeoxycholic acid) with a different formulation, however, containing the same active ingredient as that contained in product marketed in North America (URSO). In Japan, ursodiol is indicated for PBC and other hepatic conditions. Interstitial pneumonia was included in the Japanese product labeling due to the frequency of its occurrence. There have been rare reports from Japan of hepatic function disorder, thrombocytopenia and hemolytic anemia. Very rare cases of melena and hip fracture have been reported in the U.S. It is not possible to determine the causality and frequency of reported events attributed to URSO due to the uncontrolled nature of post-marketing surveillance.

A review of the literature revealed specific findings of adverse events and drug interactions [see Drug Interactions]. This analysis listed abdominal pain in upper right quadrant, diarrhea, flatulence, nausea and vomiting as recorded adverse events. It also noted decompensation of liver cirrhosis in single cases of late-stage PBC during UCDA treatment.

DRUG INTERACTIONS: Overview: Bile acid sequestering agents may interfere with the action of URSO and URSO DS by reducing absorption. Aluminum based antacids adsorb bile acids in vitro and may act in the same manner as sequestering agents, thereby interfering with the action of URSO and URSO DS. Ursodiol has been shown to be an inducer of CYP3A however the clinical relevance is not known. Metabolic interactions with compounds metabolized by cytochrome P4503A are to be expected.

Drug-Drug Interactions: See Table 5.

Drug-Food Interactions: Interactions with food have not been established.

Drug-Herb Interactions: Interactions with herbal products have not been established.

Drug-Laboratory Test Interactions: Interactions with laboratory tests have not been established.

DOSAGE AND ADMINISTRATION: Dosing Considerations: Patient Monitoring: Liver function tests (γ-GT, alkaline phosphatase, AST, ALT) and bilirubin levels should be monitored every month for three months after start of therapy, and then every six months. Serum levels of these parameters usually decrease rapidly, thus, demonstrating efficacy. Treatment should be discontinued if the levels of the above parameters increase.

Recommended Dose and Dosage Adjustment: The recommended adult dosage for URSO and URSO DS (ursodiol) in the treatment of PBC is 13-15 mg/kg/day administered in two to four divided doses with food. The URSO DS scored tablet can be broken in halves to provide recommended dosage.

Missed Dose: If you miss a dose, take the missed dose as soon as you remember. If it is almost time for your next dose, skip the dose you missed and take your next regularly scheduled dose. Do not take a double dose.

OVERDOSAGE:

Accidental or intentional overdosage with ursodiol has not been reported. The most severe manifestation of overdosage would likely consist of diarrhea that should be treated symptomatically.

Symptoms of acute toxicity in animal studies were salivation and vomiting in dogs, and ataxia, dyspnea, ptosis, agonal convulsions and coma in hamsters.

For management of a suspected drug overdose, CPhA recommends that you contact your **regional Poison Control Centre**. See the *CPS* Directory section for a list of Poison Control Centres.

ACTION AND CLINICAL PHARMACOLOGY: Mechanism of Action: Ursodiol, a naturally occurring hydrophilic bile acid, derived from cholesterol, is present as a minor fraction of the total human bile acid pool. Oral administration of ursodiol increases this fraction in a dose related manner, to become the major biliary acid, replacing/displacing toxic concentrations of endogenous hydrophobic bile acids that tend to accumulate in cholestatic liver disease.

Multiple mechanisms of action at the cellular and molecular level in addition to the replacement and displacement of toxic bile acids include cytoprotection of the injured bile duct epithelial cells (cholangiocytes) against toxic effects of bile acids, inhibition of apoptosis of hepatocytes, immunomodulatory effects via a number of mechanisms including decreasing expression of MHC class I proteins on hepatocytes and cholangiocytes, and stimulation of bile secretion by hepatocytes and cholangiocytes.

The cholesterol-lowering effect observed following the administration of URSO and URSO DS in patients with primary biliary cirrhosis could be related to an improvement of cholestasis, modifications in cholesterol metabolism, or both. Changes in the endogenous bile acid composition induced by URSO and URSO DS might be the common denominator of these two mechanisms.

Pharmacodynamics: During chronic administration, ursodiol becomes a major biliary and plasma bile acid. At a chronic dose of 13-15 mg/kg/day, ursodiol constitutes 30-50% of biliary and plasma bile acids.

Table 4: URSO *(cont'd)*

Clinical Chemistries: Changes from Baseline

		Baseline		Endpoint		Change from Baseline	
		UDCA	**Placebo**	**UDCA**	**Placebo**	**UDCA (±SD)**	**Placebo (±SD)**
Creatinine (mg/dL)	Mean (±SD)	0.86 (0.19)	0.84 (0.21)	0.92 (0.19)	0.92 (0.26)	0.07[a,c] (0.18)	0.07[a] (0.23)
	n	89	91	83	76		
Total Thyroxine (µg/dL)	Mean (±SD)	8.66[c] (1.63)	8.60 (2.27)	7.96 (1.87)	8.27 (3.25)	−0.69[b,c] (1.52)	−0.49 (2.52)
	n	87	90	83	74		
Triglycerides (mg/dL)	Mean (±SD)	102.82[c] (49.25)	117.11 (70.57)	114.18 (55.13)	121.52 (57.56)	11.76[b,c] (44.38)	3.00 (56.74)
	n	88	89	83	75		

[a] Statistically different from zero, $p<0.01$.
[b] Statistically different from zero, $p<0.05$.
[c] p=ns, UDCA versus placebo.
[d] $p=0.0001$, UDCA versus placebo.

Table 5: URSO

Drug-Drug Interactions

	Effect	**Clinical comment**
Bile acid sequestrants (i.e. cholestyramine or cholestipol)	Reduces ursodiol absorption	May interfere with the action of URSO and URSO DS
Aluminum based antacids	Reduces ursodiol absorption Adsorbs bile acid in vitro	May be expected to interfere with URSO and URSO DS
Cytochrome P4503A substrates cyclosporine, nitrendipine and dapsone	Metabolic interaction.	Metabolic interactions with compounds metabolized by cytochrome P4503A are to be expected.

Pharmacokinetics: Absorption: Ursodiol (UDCA) is normally present as a minor fraction of the total bile acids in humans (about 5%). Following oral administration, the majority of ursodiol is absorbed by passive diffusion and its absorption is incomplete.

Distribution: In healthy subjects, at least 70% of ursodiol (unconjugated) is bound to plasma protein. No information is available on the binding of conjugated ursodiol to plasma protein in healthy subjects or primary biliary cirrhosis (PBC) patients. However, since the efficacy of ursodiol is related to its concentration in bile rather than in plasma, serum levels are not indicative of bioavailability in clinical settings. Its volume of distribution has not been determined, but is expected to be small since the drug is mostly distributed in the bile and small intestine. In bile, UDCA concentration reaches a peak in 1-3 hours.

Metabolism: Once absorbed, ursodiol undergoes hepatic extraction to the extent of about 70% in the absence of liver disease. This leads to low blood levels in the systemic circulation. As the severity of liver disease increases, the extent of extraction decreases. In the liver, ursodiol is conjugated with glycine or taurine, then secreted into bile. These conjugates of ursodiol are absorbed in the small intestine by passive and active mechanisms. The conjugates can also be deconjugated in the ileum by intestinal enzymes, leading to the formation of free ursodiol that can be reabsorbed and reconjugated in the liver. Nonabsorbed ursodiol passes into the colon where it is mostly 7-dehydroxylated to lithocholic acid. Some ursodiol is epimerized to chenodiol (CDCA) via a 7-oxo intermediate. Chenodiol also undergoes 7-dehydroxylation to form lithocholic acid. These metabolites are poorly soluble and excreted in the feces. A small portion of lithocholic acid is reabsorbed, conjugated in the liver with glycine or taurine, and sulfated at the 3 position. The resulting sulfated lithocholic acid conjugates are excreted in bile and then lost in feces.

Lithocholic acid, when administered chronically to animals, causes cholestatic liver injury that may lead to death from liver failure in certain species unable to form sulfate conjugates. Ursodiol is 7-dehydroxylated more slowly than chenodiol. For equimolar doses of ursodiol and chenodiol, steady state levels of lithocholic acid in biliary bile acids are lower during ursodiol administration than with chenodiol administration. Humans and chimpanzees can sulfate lithocholic acid. Although liver injury has not been associated with ursodiol therapy, a reduced capacity to sulfate may exist in some individuals. Nonetheless, such a deficiency has not yet been clearly demonstrated and must be extremely rare, given the several thousand patient-years of clinical experience with ursodiol.

Excretion: Ursodiol is excreted primarily in the feces. With treatment, urinary excretion increases, but remains less than 1%, except in severe cholestatic liver disease.

STORAGE AND STABILITY: URSO and URSO DS tablets should be stored at controlled room temperature (15-30°C) in a closed container.

Half-tablets (scored URSO DS tablets broken in half) maintain acceptable quality for up to 28 days when stored in the current packaging (bottles) at 15-30°C.

SPECIAL HANDLING INSTRUCTIONS: There are no special handling instructions.

INFORMATION FOR THE PATIENT: Published in e-CPS, available by subscription at www.e-cps.ca.

DOSAGE FORMS, COMPOSITION AND PACKAGING: URSO: Each white, elliptical, biconvex, film-coated tablet, engraved with "URS785" on one side, contains: ursodiol USP 250 mg. Nonmedicinal ingredients: carnauba wax, dibutyl sebacate, ethylcellulose aqueous (cetyl alcohol, ethylcellulose, hydrogen peroxide, sodium lauryl sulfate), hydroxypropyl methylcellulose, magnesium stearate, microcrystalline cellulose, polyethylene glycol, povidone and sodium starch glycolate. Bottles of 100.

URSO DS: Each white, elliptical, biconvex, scored, film-coated tablet, engraved with "URS790" on one side, contains: ursodiol USP 500 mg. Nonmedicinal ingredients: carnauba wax, dibutyl sebacate, ethylcellulose aqueous (cetyl alcohol, ethylcellulose, hydrogen peroxide, sodium lauryl sulfate), hydroxypropyl methylcellulose, magnesium stearate, microcrystalline cellulose, polyethylene glycol, povidone and sodium starch glycolate. Bottles of 100.

(Shown in Product Identification Section)

V

Vagifem® ℞
estradiol-17β
Estrogen

Novo Nordisk

Date of Revision: October 2, 2007

SUMMARY PRODUCT INFORMATION:

Route of Administration	Dosage Form/ Strength	Clinically Relevant Nonmedicinal Ingredients
Vaginal	Vaginal tablet with applicator/25 µg estradiol	Lactose, maize starch, methylhydroxypropylcellulose, magnesium stearate and polyethylene glycol 6000

INDICATIONS AND CLINICAL USE: Vagifem (estradiol vaginal tablet) is indicated for:
- The treatment of the symptoms of atrophic vaginitis due to estrogen deficiency. Addition of a progestin is not recommended.

Geriatrics (>65 years of age): Clinical studies of Vagifem did not include sufficient number of subjects aged 65 and over to determine if they responded differently from younger subjects.
Pediatrics (<18 years of age): Vagifem is not indicated for use in the pediatric population.

CONTRAINDICATIONS: Vagifem (estradiol vaginal tablet) is contraindicated in women with:
- Hypersensitivity to this drug or to any ingredient in the formulation or component of the container. For a complete listing, see Dosage Forms, Composition and Packaging.
- Known or suspected estrogen-dependent malignant neoplasia (e.g. endometrial cancer).
- Endometrial hyperplasia.
- Known, suspected, or past history of breast cancer.
- Undiagnosed abnormal genital bleeding.
- Known or suspected pregnancy.
- Active or past history of confirmed venous thromboembolism (such as deep vein thrombosis or pulmonary embolism) or active thrombophlebitis.
- Lactation

WARNINGS AND PRECAUTIONS: General: Risks and benefits of treatment with Vagifem should be re-assessed at least annually. Vagifem should only be continued as long as the benefits outweigh the risks.

Vagifem is a topical, low-dose vaginal estrogen therapy product (see Action and Clinical Pharmacology, Pharmacokinetics, Absorption). The following warnings and precautions associated with oral estrogen therapy should be considered in the absence of comparable data with other dosage forms of estrogens.

Carcinogenesis and Mutagenesis: Breast Cancer: There is a need for caution in prescribing estrogens of any kind to women with a strong family history (first degree relative) of breast cancer or women who have nodules, fibro cystic disease or abnormal mammograms and/or atypical hyperplasia at breast biopsy.

In the oral **estrogen-alone** arm of the WHI trial, there was no statistically significant difference in the rate of invasive breast cancer in hysterectomized women treated with conjugated equine estrogens versus women treated with placebo.

It is recommended that estrogens not be given to women with existing breast cancer or those with a previous history of the disease (see Contraindications).

Other known risk factors for the development of breast cancer such as nulliparity, obesity, early menarche, late age at first full term pregnancy and at menopause should also be evaluated.

It is recommended that women undergo mammography prior to the start of HT treatment and at regular intervals during treatment, as deemed appropriate by the treating physician and according to the perceived risks for each patient.

The overall benefits and possible risks of hormone therapy should be fully considered and discussed with patients.

Instructions for regular self-examination of the breasts should be included in this counseling.

Endometrial Hyperplasia & Endometrial Carcinoma: There is no systemic effect under local estrogen treatment with Vagifem, the addition of a progestin is not recommended.

Endometrial histology was evaluated in 5 clinical trials conducted in the USA and Canada. Endometrial biopsies were evaluated at the end of the study in nonhysterectomized subjects. Table 1 provides a summary of endometrial biopsies taken at the end of 3 short-term studies and Table 2 provides a summary of endometrial biopsies taken at the end of 2 long-term studies. Only one woman treated with Vagifem developed simple endometrial hyperplasia. There were two cases of endometrial hyperplasia in women treated with conjugated estrogen vaginal cream (2 g containing 625 µg/g of conjugated equine estrogen), and no cases of endometrial hyperplasia in women treated with placebo.

Table 1: Vagifem
Endometrial Biopsies Taken at the End of the Short-Term Studies, n (%)

	Vagifem	Conjugated Estrogen Vaginal Cream	Placebo
Treated	199	79	47
Biopsies	89	49	21
Insufficient Tissue	20 (22)	21 (43)	3 (14)
Results			
Normal			
Atrophic	64 (72)	15 (31)	18 (86)
Weakly Proliferative	0 (0)	4 (8)	0 (0)
Proliferative	3 (3)	7 (14)	0 (0)
Abnormal			
Endometrial hyperplasia			
-Simple	1 (1)	1 (2)	0 (0)
-Complex	0 (0)	1 (2)	0 (0)
Other			
Polyp	1 (1)	0 (0)	0 (0)

(cont'd)

Table 1: Vagifem *(cont'd)*

Table 2: Vagifem
Endometrial Biopsies Taken at the End of the Long-Term Studies, n (%)

Treated	**Vagifem 158**
Biopsies	79
Insufficient Tissue	23 (29)
Results	
Normal	
Atrophic	53 (68)
Weakly Proliferative	1 (1.3)
Proliferative	2 (2.6)
Abnormal	0 (0)

Ovarian Cancer: Recent epidemiologic studies have found the use of hormone therapy (estrogen-alone and estrogen plus progestin therapies), in particular for five or more years, has been associated with an increased risk of ovarian cancer.

Cardiovascular: The results of the Heart and Estrogen/progestin Replacement Studies (HERS and HERS II) and the Women's Health Initiative (WHI) trial indicate that the use of continuous combined oral conjugated estrogens (CEE) and medroxyprogesterone acetate (MPA) is associated with an increased risk of coronary heart disease (CHD) in postmenopausal women. The results of the WHI trial indicate that the use of oral **estrogen-alone** and oral **estrogen plus progestin** is associated with an increased risk of stroke in postmenopausal women.

Blood Pressure: Women using hormone therapy sometimes experience increased blood pressure. Blood pressure should be monitored with HT use. Elevation of blood pressure in previously normotensive or hypertensive patients should be investigated and HT may have to be discontinued.

Endocrine and Metabolism: Glucose and Lipid Metabolism: Although no effect of low dose vaginal estradiol supplementation has been seen on glucose tolerance, fluid retention, elevation of blood pressure or other liver or endocrine functions, women with predisposition to or signs indicating an effect on those variables could indicate caution.

Hyperlipidemia has been reported in women on other types of estrogen replacement therapy, but it has not been observed in women using Vagifem.

Genitourinary: Vaginal Bleeding: Abnormal vaginal bleeding, due to its prolongation, irregularity or heaviness, occurring during therapy should prompt appropriate diagnostic measures to rule out the possibility of uterine malignancy and the treatment should be re-evaluated.

Women should be advised to inform their physician if irritation, pain, discharge, unusual or unexpected bleeding occur during treatment.

Women with signs of ulceration or severe inflammation due to unresponsive atrophic vaginitis, withdrawal from treatment should be considered and appropriate investigations should be conducted.

Applicator Trauma: Trauma induced by the Vagifem applicator may occur, especially in patients with severely atrophic vaginal mucosa. After gynecological surgery, any vaginal applicator should be used with caution and only if clearly indicated.

Uterine Leiomyomata: Pre-existing uterine leiomyomata may increase in size during estrogen use. Growth, pain or tenderness of uterine leiomyomata requires discontinuation of medication and appropriate investigation.

Endometriosis: Symptoms and physical findings associated with a previous diagnosis of endometriosis may reappear or become aggravated with estrogen use.

Vaginal Infection: Vaginal infection is generally more common in postmenopausal women due to the lack of the normal flora seen in fertile women, especially lactobacillus, and the subsequent higher pH. Vaginal infections should be treated with appropriate antimicrobial therapy **before** initiation of Vagifem. If a vaginal infection develops during the maintenance phase of the treatment, appropriate therapy should be instituted. The next dose of Vagifem should be inserted once the therapy is completed.

Hematologic: Venous Thromboembolism: Available epidemiological data indicate that use of oral estrogen with or without progestin by postmenopausal women is associated with an increased risk of developing venous thromboembolism (VTE).

The benefits and risks of hormone therapy should be carefully weighed when prescribing Vagifem to women with a risk factor for thrombotic disorders. The physician should be alert to the earliest manifestations of thrombotic disorders. If these occur or are suspected, estrogen therapy should be discontinued immediately. Women with a positive family history and women with a history of thromboembolic disorders during pregnancy or in association with estrogen use should be kept under special observation.

Generally recognized risk factors for VTE include a personal history, a family history (the occurrence of VTE in a direct relative at a relatively early age may indicate genetic predisposition), severe obesity (body mass index >30 kg/m²) and systemic lupus erythematosus. The risk of VTE also increases with age and smoking.

The risk of VTE may be temporarily increased with prolonged immobilization, major surgery or trauma. In women on HT, attention should be given to prophylactic measures to prevent VTE following surgery. Also, patients with varicose veins should be closely supervised. The physician should be alert to the earliest manifestations of thrombotic disorders (thrombophlebitis, retinal thrombosis, cerebral embolism and pulmonary embolism). If these occur or are suspected, hormone therapy should be discontinued immediately, given the risks of long-term disability or fatality.

If feasible, estrogens should be discontinued at least 4 weeks before major surgery which may be associated with an increased risk of thromboembolism, or during periods of prolonged immobilization.

Hepatic/Biliary/Pancreatic: Gallbladder Diseases: A 2- to 4-fold increase in the risk of gallbladder disease requiring surgery in women receiving postmenopausal estrogens has been reported.

Neurologic: Cerebrovascular Insufficiency: Patients who develop visual disturbances, classical migraine, transient aphasia, paralysis or loss of consciousness should discontinue medication.

Patients with a previous history of classical migraine and who develop a recurrence or worsening of migraine symptoms should be reevaluated.

Dementia: Available epidemiological data indicate that the use of combined oral estrogen plus progestin in women age 65 and over may increase the risk of developing probable dementia.

Epilepsy: HT may cause an exacerbation of epilepsy.

Renal: Fluid Retention: Estrogens may cause fluid retention.

Therefore, particular caution is indicated in cardiac or renal dysfunction, epilepsy or asthma. If, in any of the above-mentioned conditions, a worsening of the underlying disease is diagnosed or suspected during treatment, the benefits and risks of treatment should be reassessed based on the individual case.

Special Populations: Pregnant Women: Estrogen should not be used in pregnancy. Any possibility of pregnancy must be ruled out before prescribing Vagifem. If pregnancy occurs during Vagifem treatment, the medication should be discontinued immediately.
Nursing Women: Estrogens should not be used during lactation. Vagifem should not be prescribed for nursing mothers.
Pediatrics (<18 years of age): Vagifem is not indicated for use in the pediatric population.
Geriatrics (>65 years of age): Clinical studies of Vagifem did not include sufficient number of subjects aged 65 and over to determine if they responded differently from younger subjects.
Conditions Which Need Supervision: Due to the local administration of low dose estradiol in Vagifem, the recurrence or aggravation of some conditions is less likely than with systemic estrogen treatment, such as:

- Leiomyomata (uterine fibroids) or endometriosis
- A history of, or risk factors for, thromboembolic disorders (see below)
- Hypertension
- Liver disorders (e.g. liver adenoma)
- Diabetes mellitus with or without vascular involvement
- Cholelithiasis
- Migraine or (severe) headache
- Systemic lupus erythematosus
- A history of endometrial hyperplasia (see below)
- Epilepsy
- Asthma
- Otosclerosis.

Therapy should be discontinued if any of the following situations is discovered:

- Jaundice or deterioration in liver function
- Significant increase in blood pressure
- New onset of migraine-type headache
- Pregnancy

Monitoring and Laboratory Tests: Before Vagifem is administered, the patient should have a complete physical examination including a blood pressure determination. Breasts and pelvic organs should be appropriately examined and a Papanicolaou smear should be performed. Endometrial biopsy should be done only when indicated. Baseline tests should include mammography, measurements of blood glucose, calcium, triglycerides and cholesterol, and liver function tests.

The first follow-up examination should be done within 3-6 months after initiation of treatment to assess response to treatment. Thereafter, examinations should be made at intervals at least once a year. Appropriate investigations should be arranged at regular intervals as determined by the physician.

The importance of regular self-examination of the breasts should be discussed with the patient.

Women treated with Vagifem should be advised to keep their regular medical checkups to assess the need for continuing therapy.

ADVERSE REACTIONS: Adverse Drug Reaction Overview: Reproductive System and Breast Disorders: Breakthrough bleeding; spotting; change in menstrual flow; dysmenorrhea; vaginal itching/discharge; dyspareunia; endometrial hyperplasia; pre-menstrual-like syndrome; reactivation of endometriosis; changes in cervical erosion and amount of cervical secretion; breast swelling and tenderness.
Clinical Trial Adverse Drug Reactions: Because clinical trials are conducted under very specific conditions the adverse reaction rates observed in the clinical trials may not reflect the rates observed in practice and should not be compared to the rates in the clinical trials of another drug. Adverse drug reaction information from clinical trials is useful for identifying drug-related adverse events and for approximating rates.
Comparative Studies: In an open-labelled, multi-centre, comparative clinical trial conducted in Canada, women were treated with either Vagifem (N=80) or conjugated estrogen vaginal cream (N=79) for up to 6 months. Vagifem (25 µg estradiol) was administered daily for 2 weeks, then twice weekly with at least 3 days between each application, for the remaining 22 weeks; 2 g of the comparator drug, containing approximately 1.25 mg conjugated estrogen, was given daily for 3 weeks, withheld for 1 week, then repeated cyclically (3 weeks on, 1 week off) for up to 24 weeks. Table 3 lists the percentage and reasons for discontinuation form the study.

Table 3: Vagifem

Reasons for Discontinuation/Study Duration—24 wks (%)

Reason	Vagifem N=80	Conjugated Estrogen Vaginal Cream N=79
Adverse Event	4 (5)	14 (18)
Non-compliance with protocol	2 (2.5)	8 (10)
Other	2 (2.5)	3 (4)
Total	8 (10%)	25 (32%)

Placebo Controlled Studies: A placebo-controlled comparison study was done in the U.S., in which 230 patient were randomized to receive either placebo, 17 β-estradiol 10 µg vaginal tablets, or Vagifem (25 µg estradiol). Patients inserted one tablet intra-vaginally each day for 14 days, then one tablet twice weekly for the remaining 10 weeks. All patients were assessed for vaginal symptoms.

Overall, Vagifem is well tolerated, is comparable to placebo in overall incidence of treatment-emergent adverse events, has not demonstrated a potential for causing adverse events associated with endogenous levels of estrogen that differs from other topical hormone therapies and has not demonstrated a potential for causing adverse events associated with cumulative dosing in long-term therapy extending to 64 weeks.

In 8 clinical trials, conducted in North America and Europe, involving 438 women treated with Vagifem for atrophic vaginitis, including 115 women treated for 52 weeks, approximately 21% of women experienced a treatment emergent adverse event that could possibly or probably be related to Vagifem.

Table 4 lists the treatment-emergent adverse events reported by 5% or greater of the women in short term (up to 24 weeks) studies conducted in Canada and the United States.

Table 4: Vagifem

Frequency of Treatment-Emergent Adverse Events (TEAE) Regardless of Drug Relationship

	Vagifem		Conjugated Estrogen Vaginal Cream		Placebo	
Events	**n**	**(%)**	**n**	**(%)**	**n**	**(%)**
No. Treated	199		79		47	
No. with TEAE	122	(61)	55	(70)	26	(55)
Female Reproductive						
Pruritus Genital	7	(4)	5	(6)	0	0
Candidiasis	9	(5)	1	(1)	1	(2)
Postmenopausal Bleeding	4	(2)	13	(16)	2	(4)
Breast Pain Female	5	(3)	7	(9)	0	0
Perineal Pain	2	(1)	6	(8)	0	0
Vaginitis	7	(4)	3	(4)	3	(6)
Respiratory						
URI	14	(7)	7	(9)	2	(4)
Influenza	3	(2)	4	(5)	0	0
Body as a Whole						
Headache	17	(9)	4	(5)	3	(6)
Abdominal Pain	9	(5)	4	(5)	2	(4)
Back Pain	8	(4)	0	0	3	(6)
Gastrointestinal						
Flatulence	3	(2)	4	(5)	1	(2)

Less Common Clinical Trial Adverse Drug Reactions (<5%): The following adverse events were reported at an incidence of <5% for Vagifem regardless of drug relationship.
Skin/Appendages: acne, dermatitis contact, nail disorder, pruritus, pruritus genital, rash, skin disorder, skin ulceration, urticaria.
Musculoskeletal: arthralgia, arthritis, arthritis aggravated, arthrosis, bone disorder, myalgia.
Central Nervous System: dizziness, hypertonia, hypoaesthesia, migraine, involuntary muscle contractions, paraesthesia.
Vision Disorders: blepharitis, conjunctivitis.
Psychiatric Disorders: agitation, anxiety, increased appetite, depression, insomnia, libido decrease, nervousness, somnolence.
Gastrointestinal: abdominal pain, constipation, diarrhea, diverticulitis, dyspepsia, flatulence, gastroesophageal reflux, nausea, tooth disorder, vomiting.
Endocrine Disorders: goiter.
Cardiovascular: hearth murmur, hypertension, palpitation.
Vascular Disorders (non-CVD): cerebrovascular disorder, thrombophlebitis leg superficial.
Respiratory System: bronchitis, bronchospasm, coughing, pharyngitis, rhinitis, sinusitis.
Urinary System: dysuria, haematuria, micturition frequency, urethral disorder, urinary incontinence, urinary tract infection.
Reproductive Disorders: abdominal pain, breast disorder (not otherwise specified), breast pain, endometrial hyperplasia, leukorrhea, perineal pain, postmenopausal bleeding, vaginitis, vaginitis ulcerative, vulva discomfort.
Foetal Disorders: spinal malformation.
Neoplasm: basal cell carcinoma, breast fibroadenomosis, renal carcinoma, uterine fibroid, vaginal neoplasm benign.
Hearing and Vestibular: ear disorder NOS, earache.
Liver and Biliary: gama-GT increased, hepatitis, AST and ALT increased.
Metabolic and Nutritional: LHD increased, oedema legs, phosphatase alkaline increased.
Platelet, Bleeding & Clotting: haematoma, purpura.
Immune System: herpes simplex, infection, fungal infection, candidiasis genital, lymphadenopathy.
Body as a Whole: allergic reaction, allergy, aesthenia, back pain, carpal tunnel syndrome, fatigue, fever, headache, hot flushes, influenza-like symptoms, leg pain, neck rigidity, oedema peripheral, pain.
Post-Market Adverse Drug Reactions: The following events have been spontaneously reported during Vagifem use in clinical practice. Because these reactions were reported voluntarily from a population of uncertain size, it is not possible to reliably estimate their frequency or establish a causal relationship to drug exposure.
Neoplasm Benign and Malignant: breast cancer, endometrial cancer.
Immune System Disorders: hypersensitivity.
Metabolism and Nutrition Disorders: fluid retention.
Psychiatric Disorders: insomnia, depression.
Nervous System Disorders: migraine aggravated.
Vascular Disorders: deep venous thrombosis.
Gastrointestinal Disorders: diarrhea.
Skin and Subcutaneous Disorders: urticaria, rash erythematous, rash pruritic.
Reproductive System and Breast Disorders: endometrial hyperplasia, vaginal irritation, vaginal pain, vaginismus, vaginal ulceration.
General Disorders and Administration Site Conditions: drug ineffective.
Investigations: weight increase, blood estrogen increase.

DRUG INTERACTIONS: Overview: Vagifem is a topical vaginal estrogen therapy product. The following drug-interactions are based on the experience of systematic estrogen treatment.

Enzyme inducers, (e.g. barbiturates, hydantoins, carbamazepine, meprobamates, or rifampicin) can enhance estrogen metabolism, resulting in breakthrough bleeding or vaginal spotting.

Estrogens may diminish the effectiveness of anticoagulant, antidiabetic and antihypertensive agents.
Drug-Drug Interactions: No Drug-Drug Interactions with Vagifem have been reported.

See Warnings and Precautions regarding potential induction of malignant neoplasms and adverse effects similar to those of oral contraceptives.
Drug-Food Interactions: No Drug-Food Interactions with Vagifem have been reported.
Drug-Herb Interactions: No Drug-Herb Interactions with Vagifem have been reported.

Physicians and other health care providers should be made aware of other non-prescription products concomitantly used by the patient, including herbal and natural products.
Drug-Laboratory Test Interactions: There are no studies investigating Drug-Laboratory interactions with Vagifem.

The pathologist should be informed that the patient is receiving hormone therapy (HT) when relevant specimens are submitted.

DOSAGE AND ADMINISTRATION: Dosing Considerations: For initiation and continuation of treatment of postmenopausal symptoms, the lowest effective dose for the shortest duration should be used.

Vagifem may be used in women with or without an intact uterus.

During treatment, especially during the first 2 weeks, minimal absorption may be seen however, as plasma estradiol levels after the first 2 weeks usually do not exceed postmenopausal levels; the addition of a progestin is not recommended.
Recommended Dose and Dosage Adjustment: Treatment may be started on any convenient day.

Initial dose:	1 vaginal tablet daily for 2 weeks
Maintenance dose:	1 vaginal tablet twice a week with a 3 or 4 day interval between doses

Missed Dose: If a patient misses a dose, it should be administered as soon as possible. If it is close to the patient's next scheduled dose, the missed dose should be skipped, and the patient should continue with her normal schedule. The patient should not take two doses at the same time.

Administration: Accidental injury during administration of Vagifem may occur if the applicator is introduced too high into the vagina. **Women should be shown how to administer Vagifem correctly.** No incidences of applicator injury were reported in the clinical trials of Vagifem.

Vagifem (estradiol vaginal tablet) is gently inserted into the vagina as far as it can comfortably go without force, using the supplied applicator. Detailed instructions for use are provided in Information for the Patient.

OVERDOSAGE:

No cases of overdose have been reported.

Numerous reports of ingestion of large doses of estrogen products and estrogen-containing oral contraceptives by young children have not revealed acute serious ill effects. In general, excessive doses of estrogen may result in nausea, vomiting, abdominal cramps, headache, dizziness and general malaise.

The dose of estradiol in Vagifem is very low compared with oral estrogen products. Treatment of overdose should be symptomatic.

For management of a suspected drug overdose, CPhA recommends that you contact your **regional Poison Control Centre**. See the *CPS* Directory section for a list of Poison Control Centres.

ACTION AND CLINICAL PHARMACOLOGY: Mechanism of Action: Vagifem (estradiol vaginal tablet) is a hydrophilic, cellulose-derived matrix tablet which hydrates upon contact with moisture, releasing 17β-estradiol (see Figure 1). The estradiol in Vagifem is chemically and biologically identical to the endogenous human estradiol and is therefore classified as a human estrogen. 17β-estradiol is the primary estrogen and the most active of the ovarian hormones.

Figure 1: Vagifem

Diffusion of Estradiol From a Dry Vaginal Tablet

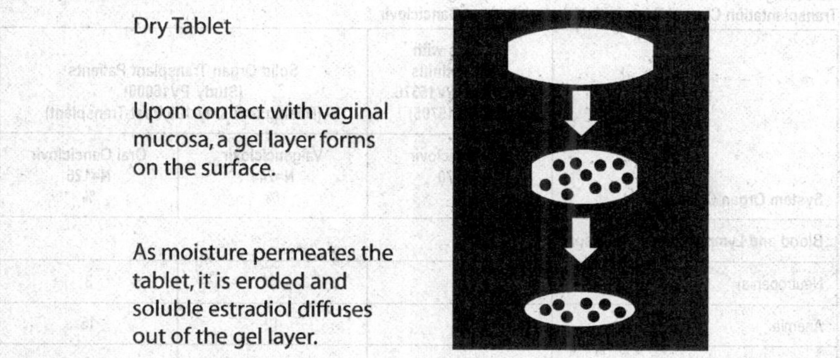

Pharmacodynamics: In vivo estrogens diffuse through cell membranes, distribute throughout the cell, bind to and activate the estrogen receptors, thereby eliciting their biological effects. Estrogen receptors have been identified in the tissue of the reproductive tract, breast, pituitary, hypothalamus, liver and bone of women. Estrogens regulate growth, differentiation and function of many different tissues within and outside of the reproductive system. Estrogens are intricately involved with other hormones, especially progesterone, and during the ovulatory phase of the menstrual cycle cause proliferation of the endometrium.

Endogenous 17β-estradiol induces and maintains the primary and secondary female sexual characteristics. Most of the activities of 17β-estradiol appear to be exerted via binding to specific estrogen receptors in target cells of tissue. The steroid-receptor complex is bound to the cell's DNA and induces synthesis of specific proteins.

The hormone deficient state associated with menopause leads to atrophic changes in the urogenital epithelial and subepithelial tissues. Vaginal blood flow is reduced, causing decreased lubrification during sexual arousal rendering the tissue more susceptible to trauma. Thinning of the vaginal mucosa occurs, cellular and glycogen production declines, decreasing the colonization of lactobacilli and thus lactic acid production. The usual acidity of the vagina, which serves as a potent defence mechanism, is lost. Symptoms associated with the atrophic changes are vaginal dryness, genital itching and burning and dyspareunia. The goal of local estrogen therapy is to provide sufficient estrogen to reverse atrophic changes in the local tissues and relieve associated symptoms.

Maturation of the vaginal epithelium is dependent on estrogen. Estrogen increases the number of superficial and intermediate cells as compared to basal cells.

Estrogen keeps pH in the vagina down to around 4.5 which enhances normal bacterial flora, *Lactobacillus Döderlein* predominating.

Pharmacokinetics: Absorption: Estrogens are well absorbed through skin, mucous membranes, and the gastrointestinal (GI) tract. The vaginal route of estrogen delivery avoids firs-pass metabolism. After administration of Vagifem, 17 β-estradiol is absorbed form the vaginal mucosa.

A single-centre, randomized, double-blind, comparison study was conducted in U.S. to investigate the effects of Vagifem treatment on serum hormone concentrations. Subjects were treated with Vagifem daily for 2 weeks followed by twice weekly administration for 10 weeks. Serum estradiol (E_2) and estrone (E_1) levels were measured after the first dose at 1, 2, 4, 5, 6, 7, 8, 10, 12 and 24 hours after administration at each study visit. E_1S (estrone sulfate) and FSH levels were determined after the first dose at 6, 12 and 24 hours after administration at each study visit. Study visits were scheduled on the first day of dosing after 1, 2, 4, 8, and 12 weeks of treatment. A total of 28 healthy women with atrophic vaginitis received Vagifem of which 22 completed the study.

Figure 2: Vagifem

Serum E_2 Levels (Mean ± 2× Standard Error) After Application of Vagifem at Weeks 0, 2, and 12

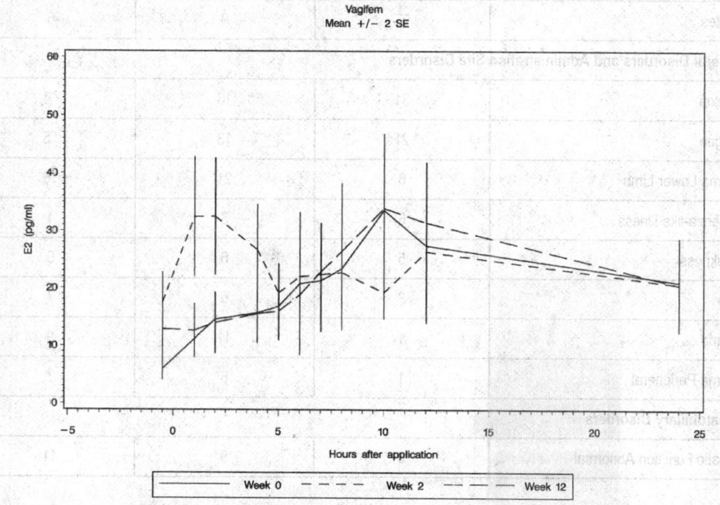

Figure 2 illustrates the serum E_2 levels following the first dose after 2 and 12 weeks of treatment. This study showed that the vaginal application of Vagifem over a 12-week period did not result in accumulation of estradiol as measured by the AUC_{0-24} (see Table 5). C_{max} of serum estradiol was constant from the first day of treatment (week 0) to the end of treatment (week 12). There was a small statistically significant increase in mean E_1S (estrone sulfate) concentrations during the 12 weeks of therapy. The mean concentrations over the 24-hour period after dosing at weeks 0, 2 and 12 ranged from 360-469 pg/mL, 572-673 pg/mL, and 470-556 pg/mL, respectively, for women treated with Vagifem. Mean FSH (averaged over the 24-hour sampling period) decreased significantly, with a median change of −9.0 IU/L at week 2 and −4.4 IU/L at week 12.

Table 5: Vagifem

Mean ± Standard Deviation for AUC, C_{max}, T_{max} for E_2 and E_1 at Weeks 0, 2 and 12 Following Vagifem Treatment

Parameter	Week	Vagifem Estradiol	Vagifem Estrone
AUC (pgh/mL)			
	0	538±265	649±230
	2	567±246	744±267
	12	563±341	681±271
C_{max} (pg/mL)			
	0	51±34	35±12
	2	47±21	39±13
	12	49±27	35±12
t_{max} (h)			
	0	15±9	14±9
	2	8±8	7±8
	12	13±6	12±11

Distribution: Circulating, unbound estrogens are known to modulate pharmacological response. Estrogens circulate in the blood bound to sex-hormone binding globulin (SHBG) and albumin.

Metabolism: Exogenously-derived or enogenously-derived estrogens are primarily metabolized in the liver to estrone and estradiol, which are also found in the systemic circulation. Vagifem intravaginal administration avoids first-pass metabolism that occurs with oral estrogens.

Excretion: Estrogen metabolites are primarily excreted in the urine as glucuronides and sulfates.

STORAGE AND STABILITY: Store in a dry place, protected from light. Store between 15- 30°C. Do not refrigerate. Store in original package.

Keep in a safe place out of the reach of children and pets.

INFORMATION FOR THE PATIENT: Published in e-CPS, available by subscription at www.e-cps.ca.

DOSAGE FORMS, COMPOSITION AND PACKAGING: Each small, white, film-coated tablet contains: estradiol hemihydrate 25.8 µg equivalent to estradiol 25 µg. Nonmedicinal ingredients: lactose monohydrate, magnesium stearate, maize starch, methylhydroxypropylcellulose polyethylene glycol 6000. Each white tablet is 6 mm in diameter and is contained in a single-use high density polyethylene/polypropylene applicator. Each tablet-filled applicator is packaged separately in a laminated blister package. Cartons of 15 pre-loaded applicators.

Valcyte® Ⓟ

valganciclovir HCl

Antiviral Agent

Roche

Date of Preparation: May 2, 2002
Date of Revision: May 11, 2010

SUMMARY PRODUCT INFORMATION:

Route of Administration	Dosage Form/ Strength	Clinically Relevant Nonmedicinal Ingredients
Oral	Tablet/450 mg valganciclovir (as valganciclovir hydrochloride)	None
Oral	Powder for oral solution/50 mg/mL valganciclovir (as valganciclovir hydrochloride) when reconstituted	None
For a complete listing of nonmedicinal ingredients see Dosage Forms, Composition and Packaging.		

INDICATIONS AND CLINICAL USE: VALCYTE (valganciclovir hydrochloride) is indicated for adult patients:

- For the treatment of cytomegalovirus (CMV) retinitis in patients with acquired immunodeficiency syndrome (AIDS).
- For the prevention of cytomegalovirus (CMV) disease in solid organ transplant patients who are at risk. This indication is based on a double-blind, double-dummy, active comparator study in heart, liver, kidney and kidney-pancreas transplant patients at high risk for CMV disease (donor CMV seropositive/recipient seronegative [D+/R-] (see Warnings and Precautions for information on specific solid organ transplant subgroups).

CONTRAINDICATIONS:

- VALCYTE (valganciclovir hydrochloride) is contraindicated in patients with known hypersensitivity to valganciclovir, ganciclovir or to any component of the product (see Dosage Forms, Composition and Packaging).
- Due to the similarity of the chemical structure of valganciclovir and that of acyclovir and valacyclovir, a cross-hypersensitivity reaction between these drugs is possible.

WARNINGS AND PRECAUTIONS: General: The clinical toxicity of VALCYTE (valganciclovir hydrochloride) includes granulocytopenia, anemia and thrombocytopenia. In animal and in-vitro studies ganciclovir was mutagenic, carcinogenic, teratogenic and caused aspermatogenesis. Therefore it should be considered a potential teratogen and carcinogen in humans. VALCYTE is indicated for use only in immunocompromised patients, where the potential benefit outweighs the risks. Safety and efficacy of VALCYTE have not been established for congenital or neonatal CMV disease; nor for the treatment of established CMV disease other than retinitis; nor for use in non-immunocompromised individuals.

Strict adherence to dosage recommendations is essential to avoid overdose.

Specific Solid Organ Transplant (SOT) Subgroups: Liver: In an unpowered subanalysis of the SOT study, PV16000, there was a higher incidence of tissue-invasive CMV disease in liver transplant patients treated with VALCYTE compared with the oral ganciclovir group. The clinical significance of this is unknown.

Other: The safety and efficacy of VALCYTE for the prevention of CMV disease in other SOT patients not mentioned in the Indications and Clinical Use section, such as lung transplant patients, have not been established.

Carcinogenesis and Mutagenesis: No long-term carcinogenicity studies have been conducted with valganciclovir. However, upon oral administration, valganciclovir is rapidly and extensively converted to ganciclovir. Therefore, like ganciclovir, valganciclovir is a potential carcinogen.

Hematologic: VALCYTE should not be administered if the absolute neutrophil count is less than 500 cells/µL, the platelet count is less than 25 000/µL, or the hemoglobin is less than 80 g/L. Severe leukopenia, neutropenia, anemia, thrombocytopenia, pancytopenia, bone marrow depression and aplastic anemia have been observed in patients treated with VALCYTE tablets (and ganciclovir) (see Warnings and Precautions, Monitoring and Laboratory Tests, Adverse Reactions and Dosage and Administration, Dosing Considerations).

VALCYTE should, therefore, be used with caution in patients with pre-existing cytopenias, or who have received or are receiving myelosuppressive drugs or irradiation. Cytopenia may occur at any time during treatment and may increase with continued dosing. Cell counts usually begin to recover within 3 to 7 days of discontinuing drug. Colony-stimulating factors have been shown to increase neutrophil counts in patients receiving ganciclovir for treatment of CMV retinitis.

Renal: Since ganciclovir is excreted by the kidneys, normal clearance depends on adequate renal function. **If renal function is impaired, dosage adjustments are required for VALCYTE.** Such adjustments should be based on measured or estimated creatinine clearance values (see Dosage and Administration, Recommended Dose and Dosage Adjustment, Renal Impairment).

Patients Undergoing Hemodialysis: Dosage adjustment is necessary for patients on hemodialysis (CrCl <10 mL/min) (see Dosage and Administration, Dosing Considerations, Recommended Dose and Dosage Adjustment and Action and Clinical Pharmacology, Special Populations and Conditions, Hemodialysis).

Sexual Function/Reproduction: Animal data indicate that administration of ganciclovir causes inhibition of spermatogenesis and subsequent infertility. These effects were reversible at lower doses and irreversible at higher doses. It is considered probable that in humans, valganciclovir at the recommended doses may cause temporary or permanent inhibition of spermatogenesis. Animal data also indicate that suppression of fertility in females may occur.

Because of the mutagenic and teratogenic potential of ganciclovir, women of childbearing potential should be advised to use effective contraception during treatment. Similarly, men should be advised to practice barrier contraception during, and for at least 90 days following, treatment with VALCYTE.

In animal studies, ganciclovir was found to be mutagenic and carcinogenic. Valganciclovir should, therefore, be considered a potential teratogen and carcinogen in humans with the potential to cause birth defects and cancers (see Special Handling Instructions).

Special Populations: Pregnant Women: There are no adequate and well-controlled studies in pregnant women. VALCYTE should be used during pregnancy only if the potential benefit justifies the potential risk to the fetus.

Nursing Women: It is not known whether ganciclovir or valganciclovir is excreted in human milk. However, many drugs are excreted in human milk and, because carcinogenic and teratogenic effects occurred in animals treated with ganciclovir, the possibility of serious adverse reactions from ganciclovir in nursing infants is considered likely. Mothers should be instructed to discontinue the drug or discontinue nursing if they are receiving VALCYTE.

Pediatrics: Safety and efficacy of VALCYTE in pediatric patients have not been established. The use of VALCYTE in children warrants extreme caution due to the probability of long-term carcinogenicity and reproductive toxicity. Administration to children should be undertaken only after careful evaluation and only if the potential benefits of treatment outweigh these considerable risks.

Geriatrics (>65 years of age): The pharmacokinetic profiles of VALCYTE in elderly patients have not been established. Since elderly individuals frequently have a reduced glomerular filtration rate, particular attention should be paid to assessing renal function before and during administration of VALCYTE (see Dosage and Administration).

Clinical studies of VALCYTE did not include sufficient numbers of subjects aged 65 and over to determine whether they respond differently from younger subjects. In general, dose selection for an elderly patient should be cautious, reflecting the greater frequency of decreased hepatic, renal, or cardiac function, and of concomitant disease or other drug therapy. VALCYTE is known to be substantially excreted by the kidney, and the risk of toxic reactions to this drug may be greater in patients with impaired renal function. Because elderly patients are more likely to have decreased renal function, care should be taken in dose selection. In addition, renal function should be monitored and dosage adjustments should be made accordingly (see Warnings and Precautions and Action and Clinical Pharmacology, Special Populations and Conditions, Renal Insufficiency and Dosage and Administration, Recommended Dose and Dosage Adjustment, Renal Impairment).

Monitoring and Laboratory Tests: Due to the frequency of neutropenia, anemia and thrombocytopenia in patients receiving VALCYTE (see Adverse Reactions), it is recommended that complete blood counts and platelet counts be performed frequently, especially in patients in whom ganciclovir or other nucleoside analogues have previously resulted in leukopenia, or in whom neutrophil counts are less than 1000 cells/µL at the beginning of treatment. In patients with severe leukopenia, neutropenia, anemia and/or thrombocytopenia, it is recommended that treatment with hematopoietic growth factors and/or dose interruption be considered. Increased serum creatinine levels have been observed in trials evaluating VALCYTE tablets. Patients should have serum creatinine or creatinine clearance values monitored carefully to allow for dosage adjustments in renally impaired patients (see Dosage and Administration, Recommended Dose and Dosage Adjustment, Renal Impairment).

ADVERSE REACTIONS: Clinical Trial Adverse Drug Reactions: Because clinical trials are conducted under very specific conditions the adverse reaction rates observed in the clinical trials may not reflect the rates observed in practice and should not be compared to the rates in the clinical trials of another drug. Adverse drug reaction information from clinical trials is useful for identifying drug-related adverse events and for approximating rates.

Adverse Drug Reaction Overview: Valganciclovir is a prodrug of ganciclovir, and is rapidly converted to ganciclovir after oral administration. The undesirable effects known to be associated with ganciclovir usage can therefore be expected to occur with VALCYTE (valganciclovir hydrochloride). All of the adverse events observed in clinical studies of VALCYTE have been previously observed with ganciclovir.

Treatment of CMV Retinitis in AIDS Patients: The safety profiles of valganciclovir and intravenous ganciclovir during 28 days of randomized study phase (21 days induction dose and 7 days maintenance) in 79 patients each were comparable. The most frequently reported events were diarrhea, neutropenia and pyrexia. More patients reported diarrhea, oral candidiasis, headache and fatigue in the oral valganciclovir arm, and nausea and injection site related events in the intravenous ganciclovir arm (see Table 1).

Table 1: VALCYTE

Percentage of Patients with Selected Adverse Events Occurring During the Randomized Study Phase

Adverse Event	Valganciclovir Arm N=79 %	Intravenous Ganciclovir Arm N=79 %
Diarrhea	19	10
Oral Candidiasis	14	6
Headache	9	5
Fatigue	8	5
Nausea	9	14
Venous Phlebitis and Thrombophlebitis	—	6
Pyrexia	14	13
Neutropenia	14	13

Table 2 shows the adverse events regardless of seriousness and drug relationship with an incidence of ≥ 5% obtained either from trials looking at the use of valganciclovir in patients with CMV retinitis or the use of valganciclovir in solid organ transplant patients.

The information in Table 2 pertaining to the patients with CMV retinitis is based on two clinical trials (n=370) where patients with CMV retinitis received VALCYTE at a dosage of 900 mg twice daily or once daily, corresponding to the induction or maintenance regimen, respectively. A total of 370 patients received maintenance therapy with VALCYTE tablets 900 mg once daily, with approximately 252 (68%) of these patients receiving VALCYTE tablets for more than nine months (maximum duration was 36 months).

The most frequently reported adverse events (% of patients), regardless of seriousness and drug relationship in patients taking VALCYTE reported from these two clinical trials (n=370) were diarrhea (41%), pyrexia (31%), nausea (30%), neutropenia (27%) and anemia (26%). The majority of the adverse events were of mild or moderate intensity. The most frequently reported adverse reactions (% of patients), regardless of seriousness that were considered related (remotely, possibly or probably) to VALCYTE by the investigator were neutropenia (23%), anemia (17%), diarrhea (13%) and nausea (10%).

Prevention of CMV Disease in Solid Organ Transplantation: Table 2 shows the adverse events regardless of seriousness and drug relationship with an incidence of ≥5% from a clinical trial, PV16000 (up to 28 days after study treatment) where heart, kidney, kidney-pancreas, and liver transplant patients received valganciclovir (N=244) or oral ganciclovir (N=126) starting within 10 days of transplantation until Day 100 post-transplant. The most frequently reported adverse events (% of patients), regardless of seriousness and drug relationship in patients taking VALCYTE reported in this clinical trial (n=244) were diarrhea (30%), tremors (28%), graft rejection (24%), nausea (23%), headache (22%), edema lower limb (21%), constipation (20%), back pain (20%), insomnia (20%), hypertension (18%) and vomiting (16%). These events were also seen with oral ganciclovir at a comparable incidence. The majority of adverse events were of mild or moderate intensity.

The most frequently reported adverse reactions (% of patients), regardless of seriousness, that were considered related (remotely, possibly or probably) to VALCYTE by the investigator in solid organ transplant patients treated until Day 100 post-transplant were leukopenia (9%), diarrhea (7%), nausea (6%), neutropenia (5%). Leukopenia and neutropenia were more common in patients taking VALCYTE compared to the oral ganciclovir arm (4% and 1%, respectively).

Table 2: VALCYTE

Percentage of Patients with Adverse Events Occurring in ≥5% of Patients in Either CMV Retinitis or Solid Organ Transplantation Clinical Trials with Valganciclovir or Ganciclovir

	Patients with CMV Retinitis (Studies WV15376 and WV15705)	Solid Organ Transplant Patients (Study PV16000) (Dosing until Day 100 Post-Transplant)	
System Organ Class	Valganciclovir N=370 %	Valganciclovir N=244 %	Oral Ganciclovir N=126 %
Blood and Lymphatic System Disorders			
Neutropenia	27	8	3
Anemia	26	12	15
Thrombocytopenia	6	5	5
Leukopenia	5	14	7
Lymphadenopathy	5	—	—
Eye Disorders			
Retinal Detachment	15	—	—
Vision Blurred	7	1	4
Vitreous Floaters	5	—	—
Macular Edema	5	—	—
Gastrointestinal Disorders			
Diarrhea	41	30	29
Nausea	30	23	23
Vomiting	21	16	14
Abdominal Pain	15	14	14
Constipation	8	20	20
Abdominal Pain Upper	6	9	6
Dyspepsia	4	12	10
Abdominal Distention	3	6	6
Ascites	—	9	6
General Disorders and Administration Site Disorders			
Pyrexia	31	13	14
Fatigue	21	13	15
Edema Lower Limb	6	21	16
Influenza-like Illness	6	3	1
Weakness	5	6	6
Pain	3	5	7
Edema	1	11	9
Edema Peripheral	1	6	7
Hepatobiliary Disorders			
Hepatic Function Abnormal	5	9	11

(cont'd)

Table 2: VALCYTE *(cont'd)*

Percentage of Patients with Adverse Events Occurring in ≥5% of Patients in Either CMV Retinitis or Solid Organ Transplantation Clinical Trials with Valganciclovir or Ganciclovir

System Organ Class	Patients with CMV Retinitis (Studies WV15376 and WV15705)	Solid Organ Transplant Patients (Study PV16000) (Dosing until Day 100 Post-Transplant)	
	Valganciclovir N=370 %	Valganciclovir N=244 %	Oral Ganciclovir N=126 %
Immune System Disorders			
Graft Rejection	—	24	30
Infections and Infestations			
Oral Candidiasis	24	3	3
Influenza	15	—	
Upper Respiratory Tract Infection	12	7	7
Pharyngitis/Nasopharyngitis	12	4	8
Sinusitis	12	3	—
Bronchitis	11	—	1
Pneumonia	9	4	2
P. carnii Pneumonia	6		
Urinary Tract Infection	6	11	9
Candida	5	1	1
Esophageal Candidiasis	5	—	—
Injury, Poisoning and Procedural Complications			
Wound Drainage Increased	—	5	9
Wound Dehiscence	<1	5	6
Investigations			
Weight Decrease	11	3	3
Blood Creatinine Increased	1	10	14
Metabolism and Nutrition Disorders			
Appetite Decreased	9	4	5
Dehydration	7	5	6
Cachexia	6	—	—
Anorexia	5	3	—
Hypokalemia	3	8	8
Hyperkalemia	1	14	14
Hypomagnesemia	1	8	8
Hyperglycemia	1	6	7
Hypocalcemia	1	4	6
Hypophosphatemia	<1	9	6
Musculoskeletal and Connective Tissue Disorders			
Back Pain	8	20	15
Arthralgia	8	7	7
Pain in Limb	4	5	7
Muscle Cramps	3	6	11
Neoplasms, Benign, Malignant and Unspecified			
Kaposi's Sarcoma	5	—	—
Nervous System Disorders			
Headache	22	22	27
Insomnia	16	20	16
Dizziness (excluding vertigo)	11	10	6
Peripheral Neuropathy	9	1	1
Paresthesia	8	5	5

(cont'd)

Table 2: VALCYTE *(cont'd)*

Percentage of Patients with Adverse Events Occurring in ≥5% of Patients in Either CMV Retinitis or Solid Organ Transplantation Clinical Trials with Valganciclovir or Ganciclovir

System Organ Class	Patients with CMV Retinitis (Studies WV15376 and WV15705)	Solid Organ Transplant Patients (Study PV16000) (Dosing until Day 100 Post-Transplant)	
	Valganciclovir N=370 %	Valganciclovir N=244 %	Oral Ganciclovir N=126 %
Anxiety	5	6	5
Tremors	2	28	25
Psychiatric Disorders			
Depression	11	7	6
Renal and Urinary Disorders			
Dysuria	2	7	6
Renal Impairment	1	7	12
Respiratory, Thoracic and Mediastinal Disorders			
Cough	19	6	8
Dyspnea	9	11	10
Productive Cough	6	2	2
Nasal Congestion	5	4	1
Sore Throat	5	3	5
Rhinorrhea	3	4	6
Pleural Effusion	<1	7	8
Skin and Subcutaneous Tissue Disorders			
Dermatitis	22	4	5
Pruritus	8	7	4
Night Sweats	8	3	4
Acne	<1	4	6
Surgical and Medical Procedures			
Postoperative Pain	2	13	7
Postoperative Wound Infection	2	11	6
Postoperative Complications	1	12	8
Vascular Disorders			
Hypertension	3	18	15
Hypotension	1	3	8

Serious adverse events considered related by the company to the use of VALCYTE reported from these three clinical trials (n=614) with a frequency of less than 5% and which are not mentioned in Table 1 and Table 2, are listed below:

Bleeding Complications: potentially life-threatening bleeding associated with thrombocytopenia.

Body as a Whole: valganciclovir hypersensitivity.

Central and Peripheral Nervous Systems: convulsion, psychotic disorder, hallucinations, confusion, agitation.

Hemic and Lymphatic System: pancytopenia, bone marrow depression, aplastic anemia.

Urogenital System: decreased creatinine clearance.

Experience with Ganciclovir: VALCYTE is rapidly converted to ganciclovir. Key adverse events reported with ganciclovir, and not mentioned above, are listed below. However, for a full listing of ganciclovir adverse reactions please refer to the current CYTOVENE product monograph.

Body as a Whole—General Disorders: asthenia, bacterial, fungal and viral infections, hemorrhage, malaise, mucous membrane disorder, photosensitivity reaction, rigors, sepsis.

Hepatic System Disorders: hepatitis, jaundice.

Cardiovascular System Disorders: arrhythmia (including ventricular arrhythmia), migraine, phlebitis, tachycardia, thrombophlebitis deep, vasodilatation.

Central and Peripheral Nervous System Disorders: abnormal dreams, amnesia, ataxia, coma, dry mouth, emotional disturbance, hyperkinetic syndrome, hypertonia, libido decreased, myoclonic jerks, nervousness, somnolence, thinking abnormal.

Gastrointestinal System Disorders: cholangitis, dysphagia, eructation, esophagitis, fecal incontinence, flatulence, gastritis, gastrointestinal disorder, gastrointestinal hemorrhage, mouth ulceration, pancreatitis, tongue disorder.

Hemic and Lymphatic: eosinophilia, leukocytosis, splenomegaly.

Hepatic System Disorders: hepatitis, jaundice.

Metabolic and Nutritional Disorders: blood alkaline phosphatase increased, blood creatine phosphokinase increased, blood glucose decreased, blood lactic dehydrogenase increased, diabetes mellitus, hypoproteinemia.

Musculoskeletal System Disorders: musculoskeletal pain, myasthenic syndrome.

Respiratory System Disorders: sinus congestion.

Skin and Appendages Disorders: alopecia, dry skin, sweating increased, urticaria.

Special Senses: amblyopia, blindness, earache, eye hemorrhage, eye pain, deafness, glaucoma, taste disturbance, tinnitus, vision abnormal, vitreous disorder.

Urogenital System Disorders: hematuria present, impotence, renal failure, urinary frequency.

Abnormal Hematologic and Clinical Chemistry Findings: Laboratory abnormalities reported with VALCYTE tablets in CMV retinitis studies and transplantation are listed in Table 3.

Table 3: VALCYTE

Laboratory Abnormalities Reported in Two Clinical Studies in the Treatment of CMV Retinitis and One Clinical Study in Transplantation

Laboratory Abnormalities	CMV Retinitis Patients (WV15376 and WV15705)	Solid Organ Transplant Patients (PV16000)	
	Valganciclovir N=370 (%)	Valganciclovir N=244 (%)	Oral ganciclovir N=126 (%)
Anemia: Hemoglobin g/L			
<65	7	1	2
65–<80	13	5	7
80–<95	16	31	25
Neutropenia: ANC/µL			
<500	19	5	3
500–<750	17	3	2
750–<1000	17	5	2
Serum Creatinine: mg/dL			
>2.5	3	14	21
>1.5–2.5	12	45	47
Thrombocytopenia: Platelets/µL			
<25 000	4	0	2
25 000–<50 000	6	1	3
50 000–<100 000	22	18	21

Severe neutropenia (ANC <500/µL) is seen more frequently in CMV retinitis patients (19%) undergoing treatment with valganciclovir than in solid organ transplant patients receiving valganciclovir (5%) or oral ganciclovir (3%) until Day 100 post-transplant. There was a greater increase in serum creatinine seen in solid organ transplant patients treated until Day 100 post-transplant with both valganciclovir and oral ganciclovir when compared to CMV retinitis patients. Impaired renal function is a feature common to solid organ transplantation patients.

Post-Market Adverse Drug Reactions: Adverse reactions from post-marketing spontaneous reports with intravenous and oral ganciclovir not mentioned in any section above, and for which a causal relationship cannot be excluded are listed below. As VALCYTE is rapidly and extensively converted to ganciclovir, such adverse events might also occur with VALCYTE.

- Anaphylaxis
- Decreased fertility in males

Adverse events that have been reported during the post-marketing period are consistent with those seen in clinical trials with VALCYTE and ganciclovir. For a full listing of ganciclovir post-marketing adverse events please refer to the current CYTOVENE product monograph.

DRUG INTERACTIONS: Overview: Drug Interaction Studies Conducted with Valganciclovir: Valganciclovir is rapidly and extensively converted to ganciclovir; therefore interactions associated with ganciclovir will be expected for VALCYTE (valganciclovir hydrochloride). In a rat in situ model of intestinal permeability, there was no interaction of valacyclovir, didanosine, nelfinavir, cyclosporine, omeprazole and mycophenolate mofetil with valganciclovir.

Drug Interaction Studies Conducted with Ganciclovir: Binding of ganciclovir to plasma proteins is only about 1% to 2%, and drug interactions involving binding site displacement are not anticipated.

Drug-drug interaction studies were conducted in patients with normal renal function. Patients with impaired renal function may have increased concentrations of ganciclovir and the coadministered drug following concomitant administration of VALCYTE and drugs excreted by the same pathway as ganciclovir. Therefore, these patients should be closely monitored for toxicity of ganciclovir and the coadministered drug.

Drug-Drug Interactions:

Table 4: VALCYTE

Results of Drug Interaction Studies with Ganciclovir: Effects of Coadministered Drug on Ganciclovir Plasma AUC and C_{max} Values

Coadministered Drug	Ganciclovir Dosage	n	Ganciclovir Pharmacokinetic (PK) Parameter	Clinical Comment
Zidovudine 100 mg every 4 hours	1000 mg every 8 hours	12	AUC ↓17±25% (range: –52% to 23%)	Zidovudine and VALCYTE each have the potential to cause neutropenia and anemia. Some patients may not tolerate concomitant therapy at full dosage.
Didanosine 200 mg every 12 hours administered 2 hours before ganciclovir	1000 mg every 8 hours	12	AUC ↓21±17% (range: –44% to 5%)	Effect not likely to be clinically significant.
Didanosine 200 mg every 12 hours simultaneously administered with ganciclovir	1000 mg every 8 hours	12	No effect on ganciclovir PK parameters observed	No effect expected.
	I.V. ganciclovir 5 mg/kg twice daily	11	No effect on ganciclovir PK parameters observed	No effect expected.
	I.V. ganciclovir 5 mg/kg once daily	11	No effect on ganciclovir PK parameters observed	No effect expected.
Probenecid 500 mg every 6 hours	1000 mg every 8 hours	10	AUC ↑53±91% (range: –14% to 299%) Ganciclovir renal clearance ↓22±20% (range: –54% to –4%)	Patients taking probenecid and VALCYTE should be monitored for evidence of ganciclovir toxicity.
Zalcitabine 0.75 mg every 8 hours administered 2 hours before ganciclovir	1000 mg every 8 hours	10	AUC ↑13%	Effect not likely to be clinically significant.
Trimethoprim 200 mg once daily	1000 mg every 8 hours	12	Ganciclovir renal clearance ↓16.3% Half-life ↑15%	Effect not likely to be clinically significant.
Mycophenolate mofetil 1.5 g single dose	I.V. ganciclovir 5 mg/kg single dose	12	No effect on ganciclovir PK parameters observed (patients with normal renal function)	Patients with renal impairment should be monitored carefully as levels of metabolites of both drugs may increase.

Table 5: VALCYTE

Results of Drug Interaction Studies with Ganciclovir: Effects of Ganciclovir on Plasma AUC and C_{max} Values of Coadministered Drug

Coadministered Drug	Ganciclovir Dosage	n	Coadministered Drug Pharmacokinetic (PK) Parameter	Clinical Comment
Zidovudine 100 mg every 4 hours	1000 mg every 8 hours	12	AUC_{0-4} ↑19±27% (range: –11% to 74%)	Zidovudine and VALCYTE each have the potential to cause neutropenia and anemia. Some patients may not tolerate concomitant therapy at full dosage.
Didanosine 200 mg every 12 hours when administered 2 hours prior to or concurrent with ganciclovir	1000 mg every 8 hours	12	AUC_{0-12} ↑111±114% (range: 10% to 493%)	Patients should be closely monitored for didanosine toxicity.
Didanosine 200 mg every 12 hours	I.V. ganciclovir 5 mg/kg twice daily	11	AUC_{0-12} ↑70±40% (range: 3% to 121%) C_{max} ↑49±48% (range: –28% to 125%)	Patients should be closely monitored for didanosine toxicity.
Didanosine 200 mg every 12 hours	I.V. ganciclovir 5 mg/kg once daily	11	AUC_{0-12} ↑50±26% (range: 22% to 110%) C_{max} ↑36±36% (range: –27% to 94%)	Patients should be closely monitored for didanosine toxicity.
Zalcitabine 0.75 mg every 8 hours administered 2 hours before ganciclovir	1000 mg every 8 hours	10	No clinically relevant PK parameter changes	No effect expected.
Trimethoprim 200 mg once daily	1000 mg every 8 hours	12	Increase (12%) in C_{min}	Effect not likely to be clinically significant.
Mycophenolate mofetil (MMF) 1.5 g single dose	I.V. ganciclovir 5 mg/kg single dose	12	No PK interaction observed (patients with normal renal function)	Patients with renal impairment should be monitored carefully as levels of metabolites of both drugs may increase.

Cyclosporine: There was no evidence that introduction of ganciclovir affects the pharmacokinetics of cyclosporine based on the comparison of cyclosporine trough concentrations. However, there was some evidence of increases in the maximum serum creatinine value observed following initiation of ganciclovir therapy.

Didanosine: Didanosine has been associated with pancreatitis. In three controlled trials, pancreatitis was reported in 2% of patients taking didanosine and CYTOVENE (ganciclovir sodium for injection) or ganciclovir capsules. The rates of pancreatitis were similar in the intravenous solution and capsule groups.

Other than laboratory abnormalities, concomitant treatment with zidovudine, didanosine, or zalcitabine did not appear to affect the type or frequency of reported adverse events, with the exception of moderately increased rates of diarrhea. Among patients taking CYTOVENE as ganciclovir sodium for injection or ganciclovir capsules, the diarrhea rates were 51% and 49% respectively with didanosine versus 39% and 35% respectively, without didanosine.

Imipenem-cilastatin: Convulsions have been reported in patients taking ganciclovir and imipenem-cilastatin concomitantly. VALCYTE should not be used concomitantly with imipenem-cilastatin unless the potential benefits outweigh the potential risks.

Stavudine: No statistically significant pharmacokinetic interaction was observed when stavudine and oral ganciclovir were given in combination.

Other Medications: It is possible that drugs that inhibit replication of rapidly dividing cell populations such as bone marrow, spermatogonia and germinal layers of skin and gastrointestinal mucosa may have additive toxicity when administered concomitantly with ganciclovir. In addition, toxicity may be enhanced when ganciclovir is coadministered with other drugs known to be associated with renal impairment. Therefore, drugs known to be myelosuppressive or associated with renal impairment, such as dapsone, pentamidine, flucytosine, vincristine, vinblastine, doxorubicin, amphotericin B, trimethoprim/sulfamethoxazole combinations, other nucleoside analogues, or hydroxyurea, should be considered for concomitant use with ganciclovir only if the potential benefits are judged to outweigh the risks.

DOSAGE AND ADMINISTRATION: Dosing Considerations:

- **Caution—Strict adherence to dosage recommendations is essential to avoid overdose.**

- VALCYTE (valganciclovir hydrochloride) is administered orally, and should be taken with food (see Action and Clinical Pharmacology, Pharmacokinetics, Absorption). After oral administration, valganciclovir is rapidly and extensively converted into the active ingredient ganciclovir. The bioavailability of ganciclovir from VALCYTE is significantly higher than from oral ganciclovir. The dosage and administration of VALCYTE tablets or oral solution as described below should be closely followed (see Warnings and Precautions, General and Overdosage).
- Dosage adjustment is necessary for patients on hemodialysis (CrCl <10 mL/min) (see Warnings and Precautions, General and Patients Undergoing Hemodialysis, Dosage and Administration, Recommended Dose and Dosage Adjustment and Action and Clinical Pharmacology, Special Populations and Conditions, Hemodialysis).
- The ganciclovir systemic exposure following administration of 900 mg valganciclovir oral solution is equivalent to a 900 mg valganciclovir dose administered as two 450 mg tablets.
- Severe leukopenia, neutropenia, anemia, thrombocytopenia, pancytopenia, bone marrow depression and aplastic anemia have been observed in patients treated with VALCYTE tablets (and ganciclovir). Therapy should not be initiated if the absolute neutrophil count is less than 500 cells/µL, or the hemoglobin is less than 80 g/L, or the platelet count is less than 25 000/µL (see Warnings and Precautions, Hematologic and Monitoring and Laboratory Tests and Adverse Reactions).
- Due to the frequency of leukopenia, granulocytopenia (neutropenia), anemia, thrombocytopenia, pancytopenia, bone marrow depression and aplastic anemia in patients taking VALCYTE, it is recommended that complete blood counts and platelet counts be performed frequently, especially in patients in whom ganciclovir or other nucleoside analogues have previously resulted in cytopenia, or in whom neutrophil counts are less than 1000 cells/µL at the beginning of treatment. Patients should have serum creatinine or creatinine clearance values followed carefully to allow for dosage adjustments in renally impaired patients (see Dosage and Administration, Renal Impairment).

Recommended Dose for the Treatment of CMV Retinitis in Adult Patients with Normal Renal Function: Induction Treatment: For patients with active CMV retinitis, the recommended dosage is 900 mg twice a day (with food) for 21 days. Prolonged induction treatment may increase the risk of bone marrow toxicity (see Warnings and Precautions, Hematologic).

Maintenance Treatment: Following induction treatment, or in patients with inactive CMV retinitis, the recommended dosage is 900 mg once daily (with food). Patients whose retinitis worsens may repeat induction treatment (see Induction Treatment).

Recommended Dose for the Prevention of CMV Disease in Adult Patients with Solid Organ Transplantation: For patients who have received a solid organ transplant, the recommended dose is 900 mg once daily (with food) starting within 10 days of transplantation and continuing until 100 days posttransplantation.

Evidence for safety and efficacy of VALCYTE for the prevention of CMV disease in solid organ transplant patients beyond the follow-up of 6 months post-transplant is not available.

Recommended Dose and Dosage Adjustment: Reduction of Dose: Dosage reductions in renally impaired patients are required for VALCYTE (see Renal Impairment). Dosage reductions should also be considered for those with neutropenia, anemia and/or thrombocytopenia (see Adverse Reactions). VALCYTE should not be administered in patients with severe neutropenia (ANC less than 500/µL), severe thrombocytopenia (platelets less than 25 000/µL), or severe anemia (hemoglobin less than 80 g/L).

Renal Impairment: Serum creatinine or creatinine clearance levels should be monitored carefully. Dosage adjustment is required for adult patients based on creatinine clearance as shown in Table 6 and Table 7 (see Warnings and Precautions, Renal and Action and Clinical Pharmacology, Special Populations and Conditions, Renal Insufficiency).

The dose-reduction algorithm was based on predicted ganciclovir exposures. The range of exposures in renally impaired patients may be greater than in renally sufficient patients. Thus, increased monitoring for cytopenias may be warranted in patients with renal impairment (see Warnings and Precautions, Monitoring and Laboratory Tests).

Patients Undergoing Hemodialysis: Dosage adjustment is necessary for patients on hemodialysis (CrCl <10 mL/min) and a dosing recommendation is given in Table 7 (see Warnings and Precautions, Patients Undergoing Hemodialysis, Dosage and Administration, Dosing Considerations and Action and Clinical Pharmacology, Special Populations and Conditions, Hemodialysis).

Table 6: VALCYTE

Valcyte Tablet Dose for Patients with Impaired Renal Function

CrCl[a] (mL/min)	Treatment of CMV Retinitis: Induction Dose VALCYTE Tablets	Treatment of CMV Retinitis: Maintenance Dose VALCYTE Tablets	Prophylaxis of CMV Disease in Solid Organ Transplantation VALCYTE Tablets
≥60	900 mg twice daily	900 mg once daily	900 mg once daily
40–59	450 mg twice daily	450 mg once daily	450 mg once daily
25–39	450 mg once daily	450 mg every 2 days	450 mg every 2 days
10–24	450 mg every 2 days	450 mg twice weekly	450 mg twice weekly
<10	not recommended	not recommended	not recommended

[a] Creatinine clearance is calculated from serum creatinine by the following formulas:

Table 7: VALCYTE

Valcyte Oral Solution Dose for Patients with Impaired Renal Function

CrCl[a] (mL/min)	Treatment of CMV Retinitis: Induction Dose VALCYTE Oral Solution	Treatment of CMV Retinitis: Maintenance Dose VALCYTE Oral Solution	Prophylaxis of CMV Disease in Solid Organ Transplantation VALCYTE Oral Solution
≥60	900 mg twice daily	900 mg once daily	900 mg once daily
40–59	450 mg twice daily	450 mg once daily	450 mg once daily
25–39	450 mg once daily	225 mg once daily	225 mg once daily
10–24	225 mg once daily	125 mg once daily	125 mg once daily
<10	200 mg (three times a week after dialysis)	100 mg (three times a week after dialysis)	100 mg (three times a week after dialysis)

[a] Creatinine clearance is calculated from serum creatinine by the following formulas:

$$\text{For males} = \frac{(140-\text{age [years]})\times(\text{body weight [kg]})}{(72)\times(0.011\times\text{serum creatinine [micromol/L]})}$$

$$\text{For females} = 0.85\times\text{male value}$$

Missed Dose: The missed dose should be taken as soon as remembered, then the regular dosing schedule should be continued. Two doses of VALCYTE should not be taken at the same time.

Administration: VALCYTE should be administered orally, and should be taken with food (see Action and Clinical Pharmacology, Absorption).

Reconstitution of Oral Solution: VALCYTE powder for oral solution requires reconstitution prior to oral administration. An oral dosing dispenser with 25 mg graduations up to 500 mg is provided with the powder for oral solution. It is recommended that this dispenser is used to measure and administer the dose.

Since VALCYTE is considered a potential teratogen and carcinogen in humans, caution should be observed in handling the powder and the reconstituted solution. Avoid direct contact of the powder and solution with skin and mucous membranes. If such contact occurs, wash thoroughly with soap and water. If the powder or solution gets into the eyes, rinse eyes thoroughly with sterile water or plain water if sterile water is not available (see Special Handling Instructions).

It is recommended that VALCYTE powder for oral solution be reconstituted by the pharmacist prior to dispensing to the patient.

Preparation of solution:

1. Measure 91 mL of purified water in a graduated cylinder.
2. Remove the child resistant cap and add the water to the bottle. Shake the closed bottle until the powder is dissolved.
3. Remove the child resistant cap and push the bottle adapter into the neck of the bottle.
4. Close bottle with child resistant cap tightly. This will assure the proper seating of the bottle adapter in the bottle and child resistant status of the cap.
5. Write the date of expiration of the reconstituted solution on the bottle label. The shelf-life of the reconstituted solution is 49 days when stored at 2 to 8°C (see Storage and Stability).

Several guidelines for the handling and disposal of hazardous pharmaceuticals (including cytotoxic drugs) are available (e.g. CSHP, 1997) (see Special Handling Instructions).

OVERDOSAGE:

Overdose Experience with VALCYTE (valganciclovir hydrochloride) Tablets: One adult developed fatal bone marrow depression (medullary aplasia) after several days of dosing that was at least 10-fold greater than recommended for the patient's estimated degree of renal impairment (decreased creatinine clearance).

It is expected that an overdose of VALCYTE could result in increased renal toxicity (see Warnings and Precautions, General and Dosage and Administration, Recommended Dose and Dosage Adjustment, Renal Impairment).

Since ganciclovir is dialyzable, dialysis may be useful in reducing serum concentrations in patients who have received an overdose of VALCYTE. Adequate hydration should be maintained. The use of hematopoietic growth factors should be considered (see Action and Clinical Pharmacology, Special Populations and Conditions, Hemodialysis).

Overdose Experience with Intravenous Ganciclovir: Reports of overdoses with intravenous ganciclovir have been received from clinical trials and during postmarketing experience. In some of these cases no adverse reactions were reported. The majority of patients experienced one or more of the following adverse reactions:

Gastrointestinal Toxicity: abdominal pain, diarrhea, vomiting.

Hematological Toxicity: pancytopenia, bone marrow depression, medullary aplasia, leukopenia, neutropenia, granulocytopenia.

Hepatotoxicity: hepatitis, liver function disorder.

Neurotoxicity: generalized tremor, convulsion.

Renal Toxicity: worsening of hematuria in a patient with pre-existing renal impairment, acute renal failure, elevated creatinine.

For management of a suspected drug overdose, contact your regional Poison Control Centre. See the *CPS* Directory section for a list of Poison Control Centres.

ACTION AND CLINICAL PHARMACOLOGY: Mechanism of Action: Valganciclovir is an L-valyl ester salt (prodrug) of ganciclovir that exists as a mixture of two diastereomers. After oral administration, both diastereomers are rapidly converted to ganciclovir by intestinal and hepatic esterases. Ganciclovir is a synthetic analogue of 2′-deoxyguanosine, which inhibits replication of herpes viruses in vitro and in vivo.

In CMV-infected cells, ganciclovir is initially phosphorylated to ganciclovir monophosphate by the viral protein kinase, UL97. Further phosphorylation occurs by cellular kinases to produce ganciclovir triphosphate, which is then slowly metabolized intracellularly. This has been shown to occur in CMV-infected cells (half-life 18 hours) and HSV-infected cells (half-life between 6 and 24 hours) after removal of extracellular ganciclovir. As the phosphorylation is largely dependent on the viral kinase, phosphorylation of ganciclovir occurs preferentially in virus-infected cells.

The virustatic activity of ganciclovir is due to inhibition of viral DNA synthesis by: (a) competitive inhibition of incorporation of deoxyguanosine-triphosphate into DNA by viral DNA polymerase, and (b) incorporation of ganciclovir triphosphate into viral DNA causing termination of, or very limited, further viral DNA elongation.

The median concentration of ganciclovir that inhibits CMV replication (IC_{50}) in vitro (laboratory strains or clinical isolates) has ranged from 0.02 to 3.58 µg/mL (0.08 to 14.32 µM). Ganciclovir inhibits mammalian cell proliferation (CIC_{50}) in vitro at higher concentrations ranging from 10.21 to >250 µg/mL (40 to >1000 µM). Bone marrow-derived colony-forming cells are more sensitive (CIC_{50} 0.69 to 3.06 µg/mL; 2.7 to 12 µM). The relationship of in vitro sensitivity of CMV to ganciclovir and clinical response has not been established.

Pharmacokinetics: Absorption: Valganciclovir, a prodrug of ganciclovir, is well absorbed from the gastrointestinal tract and rapidly metabolized in the intestinal wall and liver to ganciclovir. The absolute bioavailability of ganciclovir from VALCYTE tablets following food was approximately 60% (3 studies, n=18; n=16; n=28). Dose proportionality with respect to ganciclovir AUC following administration of VALCYTE tablets in the dose range 450 to 2625 mg was demonstrated only under fed conditions. Systemic exposure to the prodrug, valganciclovir, was transient and low, and the AUC_{24} and C_{max} values were approximately 1% and 3% of those of ganciclovir, respectively.

When VALCYTE tablets were administered with food at a dose of 900 mg, the area under the plasma concentration time curve (AUC) over 24 hours was 28.0±8.9 µg·h/mL (n=75), and the maximum plasma concentration (C_{max}) was 5.37±1.53 µg/mL (n=76).

Following the administration of valganciclovir as an oral solution, equivalent systemic ganciclovir exposures were obtained compared to the tablet formulation.

Food Effects: When VALCYTE tablets were administered with a meal containing 569 calories (31.1 g fat, 51.6 g carbohydrates, and 22.2 g protein) at a dosage of 875 mg once daily to 16 HIV-positive subjects, the steady-state ganciclovir AUC increased by 30% (95% CI: 12 to 51%), and the C_{max} increased by 14% (95% CI: −5 to 36%), without any prolongation in time to peak plasma concentrations (T_{max}). Therefore it is recommended that VALCYTE be administered with food (see Dosage and Administration).

Distribution: Due to the rapid conversion of valganciclovir to ganciclovir, plasma protein binding of valganciclovir was not determined. Plasma protein binding of ganciclovir was 1% to 2% over concentrations of 0.5 and 51 µg/mL. When ganciclovir was administered intravenously, the steady state volume of distribution of ganciclovir was 0.680±0.161 L/kg (n=114).

After administration of VALCYTE tablets, no correlation was observed between ganciclovir AUC and weight; oral dosing of VALCYTE according to weight is not required.

Metabolism: Valganciclovir is rapidly hydrolyzed to ganciclovir; no other metabolites have been detected. No metabolite of orally-administered radiolabeled ganciclovir (1000 mg single dose) accounted for more than 1% to 2% of the radioactivity recovered in the feces or urine.

Excretion: The major route of elimination of valganciclovir is by renal excretion as ganciclovir through glomerular filtration and active tubular secretion. Systemic clearance of intravenously administered ganciclovir was 3.05±0.81 mL/min/kg (n=86) while renal clearance was 2.40±0.93 mL/min/kg (n=46).

The terminal half-life ($t_{½}$) of ganciclovir following oral administration of VALCYTE tablets to either healthy or HIV-positive/CMV-positive subjects was 4.18±0.80 hours (n=244), and that following administration of intravenous ganciclovir was 3.85±0.74 hours (n=87). In liver transplant recipients, the $t_{½}$ of ganciclovir after oral administration of VALCYTE tablets (900 mg dose) was 5.10±1.10 hours (n=28), compared to 5.17±1.39 hours (n=27) after intravenous administration of ganciclovir.

Special Populations and Conditions: Pediatrics: The pharmacokinetic characteristics of VALCYTE in pediatric patients have not been well established (see Warnings and Precautions, Special Populations, Pediatrics).

Geriatrics: No studies of VALCYTE have been conducted in adults older than 65 years of age (see Warnings and Precautions, Special Populations, Geriatrics (>65 years of age)).

Gender: Insufficient data are available to demonstrate any effect of gender on the pharmacokinetics of valganciclovir.

Race: Insufficient data are available to demonstrate any effect of race on the pharmacokinetics of valganciclovir.

Renal Insufficiency: The pharmacokinetics of ganciclovir from a single oral dose of 900 mg VALCYTE tablets were evaluated in 24 otherwise healthy adult individuals with renal impairment. See Table 8.

Decreased renal function resulted in decreased clearance of ganciclovir from valganciclovir, and a corresponding increase in terminal half-life. Therefore, dosage adjustment is required for renally impaired patients (see Warnings and Precautions, Renal and Dosage and Administration, Recommended Dose and Dosage Adjustment, Renal Impairment).

Hemodialysis: For patients receiving hemodialysis (CrCl <10 mL/min) VALCYTE powder for oral solution is recommended to provide an individualized dose (see Warnings and Precautions, Patients Undergoing Hemodialysis and Dosage and Administration, Dosing Considerations and Recommended Dose and Dosage Adjustment).

Table 8: VALCYTE

Pharmacokinetics of Ganciclovir from a Single Oral Dose of 900 mg VALCYTE Tablets

Estimated Creatinine Clearance (mL/min)	N	Apparent Clearance (mL/min) Mean±SD	AUC_{last} (µg·h/mL) Mean±SD	Half-life (hours) Mean±SD
51–70	6	249±99	49.5±22.4	4.85±1.4
21–50	6	136±64	91.9±43.9	10.2±4.4
11–20	6	45±11	223±46	21.8±5.2
≤10	6	12.8±8	366±66	67.5±34

STORAGE AND STABILITY: VALCYTE tablets: Store in tightly closed container between temperatures of 15 and 30°C.
VALCYTE powder for oral solution: Do not store dry powder above 30°C. Store reconstituted solution in a refrigerator at 2 to 8°C. After reconstitution with purified water the solution should not be used for longer than 49 days. For preparation of the reconstituted medicinal product see Dosage and Administration, Reconstitution of Oral Solution.

SPECIAL HANDLING INSTRUCTIONS: Caution should be exercised in the handling of VALCYTE (valganciclovir hydrochloride) tablets or powder for oral solution. Tablets should not be broken or crushed. Since valganciclovir is considered a potential teratogen and carcinogen in humans, caution should be observed in handling broken tablets (see Warnings and Precautions, Sexual Function/Reproduction). Avoid direct contact of broken or crushed tablets, powder or reconstituted solution with skin or mucous membranes. If such contact occurs, wash thoroughly with soap and water, and rinse eyes thoroughly with sterile water or plain water if sterile water is not available.

Several guidelines for the handling and disposal of hazardous pharmaceuticals (including cytotoxic drugs) are available (e.g. CSHP, 1997). Disposal of VALCYTE should follow provincial, municipal, and local hospital guidelines or requirements.

INFORMATION FOR THE PATIENT: Published in e-CPS, available by subscription at www.e-cps.ca.

DOSAGE FORMS, COMPOSITION AND PACKAGING: Tablets: Each pink, convex, oval, film-coated tablet with "VGC" on one side and "450" on the other side contains: valganciclovir HCl 496.3 mg (corresponding to valganciclovir 450 mg). Nonmedicinal ingredients: crospovidone, microcrystalline cellulose, povidone K-30 and stearic acid powder; Opadry Pink film-coat: hydroxypropyl methylcellulose, polyethylene glycol 400/macrogol, polysorbate 80, synthetic red iron oxide and titanium dioxide. Plastic bottles of 60.
Powder for Oral Solution: Each bottle of white to slightly yellow powder (granulate) contains: valganciclovir hydrochloride 5.5 g (corresponding to valganciclovir 5 g), in 12 g powder for oral solution. Following reconstitution, 1 mL solution contains: valganciclovir hydrochloride 55 mg corresponding to valganciclovir 50 mg (free base). Nonmedicinal ingredients: fumaric acid, mannitol, povidone K30, sodium benzoate, sodium saccharin and tutti-frutti flavour (maltodextrins (maize), propylene glycol, arabic gum and natural identical flavouring substances mainly consisting of banana, pineapple, and peach flavour). Cartons containing an amber glass bottle with child-resistant plastic screw cap, a bottle adapter and a sealed bag containing 2 oral dispensers. Each bottle contains 12 g of powder for oral solution. When reconstituted, the volume of the solution is 100 mL, providing a minimal usable volume of 88 mL.

(Shown in Product Identification Section)

Valisone-G® Pr
betamethasone valerate—gentamicin sulfate
Topical Corticosteroid—Antibiotic

Valeo Pharma

Date of Revision: January 19, 2005

PHARMACOLOGY: Valisone-G provides the combined anti-inflammatory, anti-allergic, and anti-pruritic actions of betamethasone 17-valerate with the antibacterial topical effect of gentamicin.
Betamethasone 17-valerate: Clinical trials and extensive experience now available have established the effective activity of betamethasone 17-valerate in the suppression of inflammatory reactions, prompt and prolonged control of pruritus, erythema, swelling, and infiltration, which are common manifestations of allergic conditions. Reduction of scratching decreases the likehood of exacerbating the lesions of producing secondary infection. Clinical trials by numerous dermatologists who have used betamethasone 17-valerate in various localized and generalized corticosteroid-responsive diseases, indicated a high incidence of good to excellent results, either by inunction or under occlusive dressings.
Gentamicin sulfate: This wide spectrum antibiotic was proven to be very effective in the topical treatment of primary and secondary bacterial infections of the skin. In vitro, antibacterial activity of gentamicin shows this antibiotic to be bactericidal against a wide variety of gram-positive and gram-negative bacteria. At concentrations of 4 µg/mL or less, gentamicin inhibited 95% of the strains of *S. aureus* and 70 to 90% of the strains of *E. coli* and *A. aerogenes*. Bacteria sensitive to gentamicin include Streptococci (group A beta hemolytic, alpha hemolytic) *S. aureus* (coagulase postitive, coagulase negative, and some penicillinase-producing strains), and the gram-negative bacteria *P. aeruginosa*, *A. aerogenes*, *E. coli*, *P. vulgaris*, and *K. pneumoniae*. Clinically, gentamicin has proven to be effective in the treatment of Impetigo contagiosa, superficial folliculitis, ecthyma, furunculosis, sycosis barbae, and pyoderma gangrenosum; also secondary skin infections such as eczematoid dermatitis, pustular acne, pustular psoriasis, infected seborrheic dermatitis, infected contact dermatitis (including poison Ivy), infected excoriations, and bacterial superinfections of fungal or viral infections. Results of cutaneous patch tests in 100 patients demonstrated that the antibiotic was not a primary irritant.

INDICATIONS: Valisone-G is indicated in the topical management of secondarily infected allergic or inflammatory dermatoses responsive to corticosteroid therapy, such as contact dermatitis, seborrheic dermatitis, neurodermatitis, intertrigo, exfoliative dermatitis, stasis dermatitis and psoriasis.

It is also indicated for the treatment of the aforementioned conditions whenever the possibility of secondary infection is present by Gram-positive or Gram-negative bacteria including Streptococci, Staphylococcus and species of Pseudomonas, Aerobacter, Escherichia, and Klebsiella, which are susceptible organisms to the topical action of gentamicin.

The Valisone-G ointment may be preferred for the treatment of dry, scaling and fissured lesions.

CONTRAINDICATIONS: Valisone-G is contraindicated in most viral diseases including chicken pox, herpes simplex and vaccinia, and in tuberculosis of the skin. Application in or near the eyes must be avoided. Valisone-G is contraindicated in those patients with a history of sensitivity reactions to any of its components.

WARNINGS: Use of topical antibiotics occasionally allows overgrowth of nonsusceptible organisms, including fungi, yeasts or viruses. If this occurs or if irritation, sensitization or superinfection develops, treatment with Valisone-G should be discontinued and appropriate therapy instituted.

Corticosteroids and gentamicin are known to be absorbed percutaneously in patients under prolonged treatment, with extensive body surface treatment or particularly in those using the occlusive dressing technique on large areas of the body. In such cases, it is recommended that kidney function studies such as B.U.N. be carried out prior to treatment and regularly throughout the course of the treatment.

Causal factors should be sought and eliminated whenever possible and the sensitivity of an infecting organism to gentamicin should be verified.

Percutaneous absorption of the corticosteroid can produce systemic effects such as adrenal suppression, moon facies, striae, suppression of growth in children. When long-term topical treatment under occlusive dressings is necessary, small dosages, rotation of sites and intermittent therapy should be considered.

Systemic absorption of topical corticosteroids will be increased if extensive body surface areas are treated or if the occlusive technique is used. Suitable precautions should be taken under these conditions or when long-term use is anticipated, particularly in infants and children.

Systemic absorption of topically applied gentamicin may be increased if extensive body surface areas are treated, especially over prolonged time periods or in the presence of dermal disruption. In these cases, the undesirable effects, which occur following systemic use of gentamicin, may potentially occur. Cautious use is recommended under these conditions, particularly in infants and children.

Pediatric patients may demonstrate greater susceptibility to topical corticosteroid-induced HPA axis suppression and Cushing's syndrome than mature patients because of a larger skin surface area to body weight ratio.

Use of topical corticosteroids in children should be limited to the least amount compatible with an effective therapeutic regimen. Chronic corticosteroid therapy may interfere with growth and development of children. HPA axis suppression, Cushing's syndrome, linear growth retardation, delayed weight gain, and intracranial hypertension have been reported in children receiving topical corticosteroids. Manifestations of adrenal suppression in children include low plasma cortisol levels and absence of response to ACTH stimulation. Manifestations of intracranial hypertension include a bulging fontanelle, headaches and bilateral papilledema.

Patients should be advised to inform subsequent physicians of the prior use of corticosteroids.

While no systemic effects have been observed following the topical application of gentamicin, toxic systemic concentrations can cause permanent impairment of vestibular function in the presence of renal insufficiency or existing 8th cranial nerve damage.

Caution should be exercised if gentamicin is used in individuals who are known to be sensitive to topically applied antibacterials.

The possibility of sensitivity reactions to any of the product's components should be kept in mind.

Valisone-G Cream or Valisone-G Ointment are not for ophthalmic use.

Pregnancy: The use of any drug during pregnancy and the lactation period or in women of childbearing age requires that the potential benefits of the drug be weighed against the possible hazards to the foetus or infant. Although topical steroids have not been reported to have had an adverse effect on the foetus, the safety of their use in pregnant patients has not been definitively established.

Accordingly, they should not be used extensively or for prolonged periods of time in pregnant patients.

Lactation: Since it is not known whether topical administration of corticosteroids can result in sufficient systemic absorption to produce detectable quantities in breast milk, a decision should be made to discontinue nursing or to discontinue the drug, taking into account the importance of the drug to the mother.

Children: Any of the side effects that have been reported following systemic use of corticosteroids, including adrenal suppression, may also occur with topical corticosteroids, especially in infants and children.

PRECAUTIONS: See Warnings.

ADVERSE EFFECTS: The following local adverse reactions have been reported rarely with the use of topical corticosteroids: burning, itching, dryness, folliculitis, hypertrichosis, acneiform eruptions, hypopigmentation, perioral dermatitis and allergic contact dermatitis.

The following may occur more frequently with occlusive dressings: maceration of the skin, secondary infection, skin atrophy, striae, millaria.

In patients with dermatoses treated with gentamicin, mild irritation (erythema and pruritus) that did not usually require discontinuance of treatment, has been reported in a small percentage of cases. There was no evidence of irritation or sensitization, however, in any of these patients patch tested subsequently with gentamicin or normal skin.

Possible photosensitization has been reported in several patients but could not be elicited in these patients by reapplication of gentamicin followed by exposure to u.v. radiation.

OVERDOSE:

Symptoms: Excessive or prolonged use of topical corticosteroids can suppress pituitary-adrenal function, resulting in secondary adrenal insufficiency, and produce manifestations of hypercorticism, including Cushing's disease.

A single overdose of gentamicin would not be expected to produce symptoms.

Excessive prolonged use of topical gentamicin may lead to overgrowth of lesions by fungi or non-susceptible bacteria.

Treatment of Accidental Ingestion: There is no known antidote but gastric lavage should be performed.

Appropriate symptomatic treatment is indicated. Acute hypercorticoid symptoms are usually reversible. Treat electrolyte imbalance, if necessary. In case of chronic toxicity, slow withdrawal of corticosteroids is advised.

Appropriate antifungal or antibacterial therapy is indicated if overgrowth occurs.

For management of a suspected drug overdose, CPhA recommends that you contact your **regional Poison Control Centre**. See the *CPS* Directory section for a list of Poison Control Centres.

DOSAGE: A thin film of Valisone-G Cream or Valisone-G Ointment should be applied to cover completely the affected area two or three times daily.

Refractory lesions of psoriasis and deep-seated dermatoses which have been secondarily infected may respond better to topical corticosteroids and antibiotics when used with the hydration technique or occlusive dressing described below:

Occlusive Dressing Technique:
1. Apply a thick layer of medication over the entire surface of the lesion under a light gauze dressing and cover it with a pliable, transparent, impermeable, plastic material well beyond the edges of the treated area.
2. Seal the edges to the normal skin by adhesive tape or other means.
3. Leave the dressing in place one to three days and repeat the procedure three or four time as needed.

With this method of treatment, marked improvement often is seen in a few days. However, this technique requires closer supervision of the patient since occasionally miliary eruptions of folliculitis develop in the skin under and occlusive dressing, requiring removal of the plastic cover and/or discontinuance of this method of treatment.

SUPPLIED: Cream: Each g of cream contains: betamethasone valerate USP equivalent to 1 mg (0.1%) betamethasone alcohol and gentamicin sulfate USP equivalent to 1 mg (0.1%) of gentamicin base. The microdispersion of these active ingredients in a greaseless, odorless, non-staining, washable and cosmetically-pleasing cream insures effective contact with the skin and rapid onset of action of the steroid and the antibiotic. Nonmedicinal ingredients: cetostearyl alcohol, chlorocresol, mineral oil, monobasic sodium phosphate, phosphoric acid, polyethylene glycol 1000 monocetyl ether, purified water, sodium hydroxide and white petrolatum. Tubes of 30 g. Store at 15 to 30°C.
Ointment: Each g of ointment contains: betamethasone valerate USP equivalent to 1 mg (0.1%) betamethasone alcohol and gentamicin sulfate USP equivalent to 1 mg (0.1%) of gentamicin base. The microdispersion of these active ingredients in an odorless, nonstaining ointment base insures effective contact with the skin and rapid onset of action of the steroid and the antibiotic. Nonmedicinal ingredient: white petrolatum USP. Tubes of 30 g. Store at 15 to 30°C.

Valisone® Scalp Lotion Pr
betamethasone valerate
Glucocorticoid

Valeo Pharma

SUPPLIED: Each mL of lotion contains: betamethasone 1 mg (as valerate USP). Nonmedicinal ingredients: carbomer 934P, isopropanol, purified water and sodium hydroxide. Plastic squeeze bottles of 75 mL. Store between 2 to 30°C.

Valium® Roche® Oral
diazepam
Anxiolytic—Sedative

Roche

SUPPLIED: Each pale yellow cylindrical, biplane beveled-edged tablet, engraved ROCHE 5 on one side, single scored on one side, contains: diazepam 5 mg. Nonmedicinal ingredients: cornstarch, iron oxide yellow, lactose and magnesium stearate. Energy: 2.8 kJ (0.7 kcal). Gluten-, paraben-, sodium-, sulfite- and tartrazine-free. Cartons of 4 blister cards each with 25 tablets. Store between 15 and 30°C. Keep in a tightly closed, light-resistant container.

Valtrex®

valacyclovir HCl

Antiviral Agent

GlaxoSmithKline

Date of Revision: August 28, 2009

SUMMARY PRODUCT INFORMATION:

Route of Administration	Dosage Form/ Strength	Clinically Relevant Nonmedicinal Ingredients
Oral	Caplet 500 mg and 1000 mg	For a complete listing of ingredients see Dosage Forms, Composition and Packaging.

INDICATIONS AND CLINICAL USE: VALTREX (valacyclovir hydrochloride) caplets are indicated:

- For the treatment of herpes zoster (shingles).
- For the treatment or suppression of genital herpes in immunocompetent individuals and for the suppression of recurrent genital herpes in HIV infected individuals.
- To reduce the risk of transmission of genital herpes with the use of suppressive therapy. Safer sex practices should be used with suppressive therapy.
- For the treatment of cold sores (herpes labialis).

Geriatrics (>65 years of age): Use in the geriatric population may be associated with differences in safety due to age-related changes in renal function and a brief discussion can be found in the appropriate sections (see Warnings and Precautions).

Pediatrics (<12 years old): No data is available.

CONTRAINDICATIONS: VALTREX (valacyclovir hydrochloride) caplets are contraindicated in patients with a known hypersensitivity or intolerance to valacyclovir, acyclovir, or any component of the formulation. For a complete listing of ingredients, see Dosage Forms, Composition and Packaging.

WARNINGS AND PRECAUTIONS: General: Care should be taken to ensure adequate fluid intake in patients who are at risk of dehydration particularly in geriatric patients.

In patients with advanced HIV disease (CD4 cell counts <100 cells/mm³), allogenic bone marrow transplant and renal transplant recipients receiving VALTREX (valacyclovir hydrochloride) at a dose of 8000 mg per day, there have been reports of Thrombotic Thrombocytopenia Purpura/Hemolytic Uremic Syndrome (TTP/HUS), in some cases resulting in death.

The safety and efficacy of VALTREX have not been established for the treatment of disseminated herpes zoster.

The safety and efficacy of VALTREX have not been established in immunocompromised patients other than for the suppression of ano-genital herpes in HIV-infected patients. The safety and efficacy of VALTREX for the suppression of recurrent ano-genital herpes in patients with advanced HIV disease (CD4 cell count <100 cells/mm³) have not been established.

Patients should be informed that VALTREX is not a cure for genital herpes.

Safer sex practices should be used in combination with suppressive therapy. VALTREX alone should not be used for reducing the risk of transmitting genital herpes. Because genital herpes is a sexually transmitted infection, patients should, in order to further reduce the risk of infecting partners, avoid contact with lesions, damaged skin/mucosa, and also avoid intercourse when lesions and/or symptoms are present. Genital herpes is frequently transmitted in the absence of symptoms through asymptomatic viral shedding; therefore patients should be counselled to use safer sex practices. The effect of VALTREX on transmission of sexually transmitted infections other than herpes (including HIV, gonorrhea, syphilis and Chlamydia) is unknown.

The efficacy of VALTREX for reducing transmission of genital herpes has not been established in individuals with multiple partners, non-heterosexual couples, and couples not counselled to use safer sex practices.

Hepatic/Biliary/Pancreatic: Dose modification is not required in patients with mild or moderate cirrhosis (hepatic synthetic function maintained). Pharmacokinetic data in patients with advanced cirrhosis (impaired hepatic synthetic function and evidence of portal-systemic shunting) do not indicate the need for dosage adjustment. There are no data available on the use of higher doses of VALTREX (4 g or more per day) in patients with liver disease. Caution should therefore be exercised when administering higher doses of VALTREX to these patients.

Renal: Renal insufficiency or acute renal failure has been observed in patients taking VALTREX at the recommended dosage and/or with no previous renal conditions and may be associated with renal pain (see Adverse Reactions, Post-Market Adverse Drug Reactions).

Acyclovir, the active metabolite of valacyclovir, is eliminated by renal clearance, therefore the dose of VALTREX must be reduced in patients with renal impairment (see Dosage and Administration, Patients with Acute or Chronic Renal Impairment). Geriatric patients are likely to have reduced renal function and therefore the need for dose reduction must be considered in this group of patients. Both geriatric patients and patients with a history of renal impairment are at increased risk of developing neurological side effects and should be closely monitored for evidence of these effects. In the reported cases, these reactions were generally reversible on discontinuation of treatment (see Adverse Reactions).

Caution should be exercised when administering VALTREX to patients with significant renal impairment or those receiving potentially nephrotoxic agents, since this may increase the risk of renal dysfunction (see Dosage and Administration, Patients with Acute or Chronic Renal Impairment) and/or the risk of reversible central nervous system symptoms such as those that occur infrequently in patients treated with intravenous acyclovir.

Given the dosage recommendations for treatment of cold sores, special attention should be paid when prescribing VALTREX for cold sores in patients who are geriatric or who have impaired renal function (see Dosage and Administration, Patients with Acute or Chronic Renal Impairment, Table 9). Treatment should not exceed 1 day (2 doses of 2000 mg in 24 hours). Therapy beyond 1 day does not provide additional clinical benefit.

Special Populations: Pregnant Women: There are no adequate and well-controlled studies with either acyclovir or VALTREX in pregnant women. In a study of the pharmacokinetics of valacyclovir and acyclovir during late pregnancy, the steady-state daily acyclovir AUC (area under plasma concentration-time curve) following valacyclovir 1000 mg was approximately 2 times greater than that observed with oral acyclovir at 1200 mg daily. VALTREX caplets should be used during pregnancy only if the potential benefit justifies the potential risk to the fetus.

Pregnancy registries have documented the pregnancy outcomes in women exposed to VALTREX or to any formulation of acyclovir (the active metabolite of valacyclovir); 111 and 1246 outcomes (29 and 756 exposed during the first trimester of pregnancy), respectively, were obtained from women prospectively registered. The findings of the acyclovir pregnancy registry have not shown an increase in the number of birth defects amongst acyclovir-exposed subjects compared with the general population, and any birth defects showed no uniqueness or consistent pattern to suggest a common cause. Given the small number of women enrolled into the valacyclovir pregnancy registry, reliable and definitive conclusions could not be reached regarding the safety of VALTREX in pregnancy.

Valacyclovir hydrochloride was not teratogenic in rats or rabbits given 400 mg/kg (which results in 10 and 7 times human plasma levels, respectively) during the period of major organogenesis. However, in a non-standard test in rats given three subcutaneous doses of 100 mg/kg acyclovir (20 times human plasma levels) on gestation day 10, there were fetal abnormalities, such as head and tail anomalies, and maternal toxicity.

Nursing Women: Acyclovir, the principal metabolite of valacyclovir, is excreted in breast milk. Following oral administration of a 500 mg dose of valacyclovir, peak acyclovir concentrations (C_{max}) in breast milk ranged from 0.5 to 2.3 (median 1.4) times the corresponding maternal acyclovir serum concentrations. The acyclovir breast milk to maternal serum AUC ratios ranged from 1.4 to 2.6 (median 2.2).

The median acyclovir concentration in breast milk was 2.24 μg/mL (9.95 μM). With a maternal valacyclovir dosage of 500 mg twice daily, this level would expose a nursing infant to a daily oral acyclovir dosage of about 0.61 mg/kg/day. The elimination half-life of acyclovir from breast milk was similar to that for serum.

Unchanged valacyclovir was not detected in maternal serum, breast milk, or infant urine.

Caution should be exercised when VALTREX is administered to a nursing woman. Consideration should be given to temporary discontinuation of nursing, as the safety of VALTREX has not been established in infants.

Pediatrics: Safety and efficacy in children have not been established.

Geriatrics: Of the total number of patients included in clinical studies of VALTREX, more than 800 were age 65 or older, and more than 330 were age 75 or older. A total of 34 volunteers age 65 or older completed a pharmacokinetic trial of valacyclovir hydrochloride. The pharmacokinetics of acyclovir following single- and multiple-dose oral administration of VALTREX caplets in geriatric volunteers varied with renal function. The possibility of renal impairment in geriatric patients must be considered and the dosage should be adjusted accordingly (see Warnings and Precautions, Renal and Dosage and Administration, Patients with Acute or Chronic Renal Impairment). Adequate hydration should be maintained.

ADVERSE REACTIONS: Adverse Drug Reaction Overview: The most frequent adverse reactions associated with the use of VALTREX (valacyclovir hydrochloride) are headache and nausea.

Neurological side effects have also been reported in rare instances. Geriatric patients and patients with a history of renal impairment are at increased risk of developing these effects. In the reported cases, these reactions were generally reversible on discontinuation of treatment (see Warnings and Precautions and Adverse Reactions, Post-Market Adverse Drug Reactions).

Clinical Trial Adverse Drug Reactions: Because clinical trials are conducted under very specific conditions the adverse reaction rates observed in the clinical trials may not reflect the rates observed in practice and should not be compared to the rates in the clinical trials of another drug. Adverse drug reaction information from clinical trials is useful for identifying drug-related adverse events and for approximating rates.

Herpes Zoster: Adverse drug reactions were not significantly different in recipients of VALTREX compared to placebo or acyclovir in the two double-blind, randomized clinical trials of treatment of herpes zoster (shingles) in immunocompetent patients. The most frequent adverse drug reactions reported in recipients of VALTREX are listed in Table 1.

Table 1: VALTREX

Incidence (%) of Drug-Related Adverse Reactions Occurring in ≥1% of Patients Receiving VALTREX in Two Clinical Trials of Treatment of Herpes Zoster

	Herpes Zoster			
	18–50 Years		>50 Years	
Adverse Drug Reaction	VALTREX (n=202) (%)	Placebo (n=195) (%)	VALTREX (n=765) (%)	Acyclovir (n=376) (%)
Nausea	8	6	12	14
Headache	11	8	8	7
Diarrhea	4	4	4	4
Vomiting	2	2	4	3
Asthenia	1	3	3	2
Constipation	<1	<1	3	3
Abdominal Pain	<1	1	2	1
Anorexia	<1	2	2	2
Dizziness	1	1	2	2
Dry Mouth	<1	0	2	1
Dyspepsia	0	<1	2	1
Flatulence	0	0	1	1
Pruritus	1	0	<1	0

Genital Herpes: In two double-blind, randomized trials of treatment of recurrent genital herpes in immunocompetent patients, adverse drug reactions were not significantly different in recipients of VALTREX compared to placebo. The most frequent adverse reactions are listed in Table 2.

Table 2: VALTREX

Incidence (%) of Drug-Related Adverse Reactions Occurring in ≥1% of Patients Receiving VALTREX in Two Clinical Trials of Treatment of Recurrent Genital Herpes

Adverse Drug Reaction	VALTREX (n=1235) (%)	Placebo (n=439) (%)
Headache	11	9
Nausea	5	6
Diarrhea	4	4
Dizziness	2	2
Abdominal Pain	2	1
Asthenia	1	3

In two recurrent genital herpes suppression studies of immunocompetent patients, adverse drug reactions were not significantly different in recipients of VALTREX 1000 mg once daily or VALTREX 500 mg once daily, compared to placebo or ZOVIRAX (acyclovir) 400 mg twice daily. The most frequent adverse reactions are reported in Table 3.

Table 3: VALTREX

Incidence (%) of Drug-Related Adverse Reactions Occurring in ≥1% of Patients Receiving VALTREX in Two Clinical Trials for Suppression of Recurrent Genital Herpes

	Trial 123–026 (52 Weeks)				Trial 123–037 (16 Weeks)	
Adverse Drug Reaction	VALTREX 1000 mg q.d. (n=269) (%)	VALTREX 500 mg q.d. (n=266) (%)	ZOVIRAX 400 mg b.i.d. (n=267) (%)	Placebo (n=134) (%)	VALTREX 500 mg q.d. (n=288) (%)	Placebo (n=94) (%)
Headache	13	13	12	11	7	6
Nausea	8	8	6	5	6	9

(cont'd)

Table 3: VALTREX *(cont'd)*

Incidence (%) of Drug-Related Adverse Reactions Occurring in ≥1% of Patients Receiving VALTREX in Two Clinical Trials for Suppression of Recurrent Genital Herpes

	Trial 123–026 (52 Weeks)				Trial 123–037 (16 Weeks)	
Adverse Drug Reaction	**VALTREX 1000 mg q.d. (n=269) (%)**	**VALTREX 500 mg q.d. (n=266) (%)**	**ZOVIRAX 400 mg b.i.d. (n=267) (%)**	**Placebo (n=134) (%)**	**VALTREX 500 mg q.d. (n=288) (%)**	**Placebo (n=94) (%)**
Abdominal Pain	4	2	3	3	2	2
Diarrhea	4	3	5	7	2	0
Dyspepsia	3	<1	3	2	<1	0
Dizziness	2	2	1	1	<1	1
Pain	2	2	<1	<1	<1	1
Acne	1	<1	<1	0	<1	0
Arthralgia	1	0	0	0	0	0
Constipation	1	<1	1	0	<1	0
Flu Syndrome	1	<1	<1	<1	0	0
Vomiting	1	<1	1	0	<1	2
Depression	<1	1	<1	1	<1	0
Insomnia	<1	2	<1	<1	0	0
Migraine	<1	<1	<1	1	1	1
Paresthesia	<1	1	<1	<1	0	0
Rash	<1	2	1	1	1	0
Asthenia	0	2	1	<1	0	1
Dry Mouth	0	3	<1	<1	<1	1
Eczema	0	1	<1	0	<1	1
Pruritis	0	1	1	0	<1	0
Vasodilatation	0	<1	0	0	1	0

In one multicenter, double-blind, randomized study of immunocompetent patients for the treatment of an initial episode of genital herpes, the frequency of adverse events, regardless of attributability to study medication, was similar in both treatment groups: VALTREX 1000 mg twice daily (n=318) compared to acyclovir 200 mg five times a day (n=318). The most frequent adverse events were headache (13% with VALTREX versus 10% with ZOVIRAX) and nausea (6% with both treatments). All other adverse events were reported by 3% or less of patients.

In a 6-month study of suppression of recurrent genital herpes in HIV-infected patients, adverse drug reactions were similar in nature and incidence in the groups receiving VALTREX 500 mg twice daily and placebo when duration of exposure was considered. Adverse reactions reported with an incidence ≥1% during the double-blind phase are detailed in Table 4.

Table 4: VALTREX

Incidence (%) of Drug-Related Adverse Reactions Occurring in ≥1% of Patients Receiving VALTREX in a Clinical Trial for Suppression of Recurrent Genital Herpes in HIV-Infected Patients

Adverse Drug Reaction	**Valacyclovir 500 mg b.i.d. (n=194) (%)**	**Placebo (n=99) (%)**
Headache	5	3
Diarrhea	3	2
Nausea	2	5
Constipation	1	0
Dizziness	1	0

Adverse reactions reported by patients receiving VALTREX 500 mg once daily (n=743) or placebo once daily (n=741) in a clinical study for the reduction of transmission of genital herpes are listed below in Table 5.

Table 5: VALTREX

Incidence (%) of Drug-Related Adverse Reactions Occurring in ≥1% of Patients Receiving VALTREX in a Clinical Trial for the Reduction of Transmission of Genital Herpes

Adverse Drug Reaction	**VALTREX (n=743) (%)**	**Placebo (n=741) (%)**
Headache	6	4
Diarrhea	2	1
Nausea	2	2
Dyspepsia	1	1

Of the 1484 patients enrolled in the reduction of transmission study, 1018 entered the open-label phase of the study (≤12 months), 499 from the placebo group and 519 from the VALTREX group. The nature and incidence of events in the open-label phase were similar to those observed during the double-blind phase of the study (Table 6).

Table 6: VALTREX

Incidence (%) of Drug-Related Adverse Reactions Occurring in ≥1% of Patients Receiving VALTREX in the Double-Blind, Open-Label, and Combined Double-Blind + Open-Label Phases of a Clinical Trial for the Reduction of Transmission of Genital Herpes

	Double-Blind Phase (≤8 months)		Open-Label Phase (≤12 months)	Combined Double-Blind + Open-Label Phases (≤20 months)
Adverse Drug Reaction	**VALTREX (n=519[a]) (%)**	**Placebo (n=499[b]) (%)**	**VALTREX (n=1018[c]) (%)**	**VALTREX (n=519[d]) (%)**
Headache	5	4	2	6
Diarrhea	2	2	<1	2
Nausea	1	3	<1	1
Dyspepsia	1	<1	<1	2
Abdominal Pain, Upper	1	0	<1	1

[a] Number of patients from the VALTREX group of the double-blind phase who entered the open-label phase of the study.
[b] Number of patients from the placebo group of the double-blind phase who entered the open-label phase of the study.
[c] Total number of patients (VALTREX + placebo groups) from the double-blind phase who entered the open-label phase of the study. All patients in the open-label phase received VALTREX 500 mg once daily.
[d] Number of patients who received VALTREX during the double-blind phase followed by open-label VALTREX suppressive therapy.

Cold Sores: Adverse drug reactions reported by patients receiving VALTREX 2000 mg twice daily for one day (n=609) or placebo (n=609) in clinical studies for the treatment of cold sores are listed in Table 7.

Table 7: VALTREX

Incidence (%) of Drug-Related Adverse Reactions Occurring in ≥1% of Patients Receiving VALTREX in Two Clinical Trials for the Treatment of Cold Sores

Adverse Drug Reaction	**VALTREX (n=609) (%)**	**Placebo (n=609) (%)**
Headache	9	5
Nausea	4	5
Diarrhea	3	3
Dyspepsia	1	1

Abnormal Hematologic and Clinical Chemistry Findings: In herpes zoster trials, the frequencies of white blood cells abnormality (<0.75 times the lower limit of normal) were 1.3% for patients receiving VALTREX compared with 0.6% for patients receiving placebo. This difference was not clinically or statistically significant.

In studies of suppression of genital herpes in HIV-infected patients and of reduction of transmission of genital herpes, there were no clinically significant changes from baseline in laboratory parameters in patients receiving VALTREX compared to placebo.

In clinical studies for the treatment of cold sores, the frequencies of abnormal ALT values (>2 times the upper limit of normal) were 1.8% for patients receiving VALTREX at the recommended clinical dose and 0.8% for placebo. Other laboratory abnormalities (hemoglobin, white blood cells, alkaline phosphatase, and serum creatinine) occurred with similar frequencies in the 2 groups.

Post-Market Adverse Drug Reactions: The following events have been reported voluntarily during post-approval use of VALTREX in clinical practice. These events have been chosen for inclusion due to either their seriousness, frequency of reporting, causal connection to VALTREX, or a combination of these factors. Post-market adverse events are reported spontaneously from a population of unknown size, thus estimates of frequency cannot be made.

General: facial edema, hypertension, tachycardia.

Gastrointestinal: nausea, abdominal discomfort, vomiting and diarrhea.

Hematological: reports of thrombocytopenia, aplastic anemia, leukocytoclastic vasculitis, thrombotic thrombocytopenic purpura/hemolytic uremic syndrome (TTP/HUS). Leukopenia, mainly reported in immunocompromised patients.

Allergic: acute hypersensitivity reactions including anaphylaxis, angioedema, dyspnea, pruritus, rash and urticaria.

Skin: erythema multiforme, rashes including photosensitivity.

Renal: reports of renal impairment, elevated blood creatinine and blood urea nitrogen (BUN) acute renal failure, renal pain and hematuria. Renal pain may be associated with renal failure (see Warnings and Precautions).

Hepatobiliary Tract and Pancreas: reports of reversible increases in liver function test, hepatitis.

CNS Symptoms: headache. Reports of neurological reactions including dizziness, confusion, hallucinations (auditory and visual), aggressive behaviour, decreased consciousness, tremor, ataxia, dysarthria, convulsions, encephalopathy, coma. Agitation and psychotic symptoms have also been reported. These events are generally reversible and usually seen in patients with renal impairment or with other predisposing factors (see Warnings and Precautions).

Other: There have been reports of renal insufficiency, microangiopathic hemolytic anemia and thrombocytopenia (sometimes in combination) in severely immunocompromised patients, particularly those with advanced HIV disease, receiving high doses (8000 mg daily) of valacyclovir for prolonged periods in clinical trials. These findings have also been observed in patients not treated with valacyclovir who have the same underlying or concurrent conditions.

DRUG INTERACTIONS: Drug-Drug Interactions: No clinically significant interactions have been identified.

No dosage adjustment is recommended when VALTREX (valacyclovir hydrochloride) is coadministered with digoxin, antacids, thiazide diuretics, cimetidine, or probenecid in subjects with normal renal function.

Acyclovir is eliminated primarily unchanged in the urine via active renal tubular secretion. Any drugs administered concurrently that compete with this mechanism may increase acyclovir plasma concentrations following valacyclovir administration.

Following administration of valacyclovir 1000 mg, cimetidine and probenecid increase the area under the curve (AUC) of acyclovir by this mechanism, and reduce acyclovir renal clearance. However, no dosage adjustment is necessary at this dose because of the wide therapeutic index of acyclovir.

Care is also required (with monitoring for changes in renal function) if administering higher-doses of VALTREX (4 g or more/day) with drugs which affect other aspects of renal physiology (e.g., cyclosporin, tacrolimus).

Drug-Food Interactions: There is no known interaction with food.

Drug-Herb Interactions: Interactions with herbal products have not been established.

Drug-Laboratory Test Interactions: Interactions with laboratory tests have not been established.

DOSAGE AND ADMINISTRATION: Dosing Considerations:

- The dosage of VALTREX (valacyclovir hydrochloride) should be reduced in patients with impaired renal function (see Table 8).
- Therapy should be initiated as soon as possible after a diagnosis of herpes zoster, or at the first sign or symptoms of an outbreak of oral or genital herpes.
- The recommended dose and duration of use is dependent on the indication.
- The safety and tolerability of VALTREX 500 mg once daily has been established for up to 20 months (see Adverse Reactions).

Recommended Dose and Dosage Adjustment: VALTREX caplets may be given without regard to meals.

Herpes Zoster: The recommended dosage of VALTREX caplets for the treatment of herpes zoster is 1000 mg orally three times daily for 7 days. Treatment with VALTREX should be initiated within 72 hours of the onset of rash.

Initial Episode of Genital Herpes: The recommended dosage of VALTREX caplets for the treatment of an initial episode of genital herpes is 1000 mg orally twice daily for 10 days. There are no data on the effectiveness of treatment with VALTREX when initiated more than 72 hours after the onset of signs and symptoms. Therapy was most effective when administered within 48 hours of the onset of signs and symptoms.

Recurrent Episodes of Genital Herpes: The recommended dosage of VALTREX caplets for the treatment of recurrent episodes of genital herpes is 500 mg orally twice daily for 3 days. Therapy should be initiated at the earliest sign or symptom of recurrence. VALTREX can prevent lesion development when taken at the first signs and symptoms of a genital herpes recurrence.

Suppression of Genital Herpes: The recommended dosage of VALTREX caplets for chronic suppressive therapy of recurrent genital herpes is 1000 mg orally once daily in patients with normal immune function. The safety and efficacy of VALTREX 1000 mg once daily beyond 1 year have not been established. In patients with a history of 9 or fewer recurrences per year, an alternative dose is 500 mg orally once daily. The safety and tolerability of VALTREX 500 mg once daily have been established for up to 20 months (see Adverse Reactions).

In patients with HIV infection with CD4 cell count >100 cells/mm³, the recommended dosage of VALTREX caplets for chronic suppressive therapy of recurrent genital herpes is 500 mg orally twice daily. The safety and efficacy of therapy with VALTREX beyond 6 months in patients with HIV infection have not been established.

Reduction of Transmission of Genital Herpes: The recommended dosage of VALTREX caplets for reduction of transmission of genital herpes in patients with a history of 9 or fewer recurrences per year is 500 mg orally once daily for the source partner. The efficacy of reducing transmission beyond 8 months in couples discordant for HSV-2 infection has not been established. The safety and tolerability of VALTREX 500 mg once daily has been established for up to 20 months (see Adverse Reactions).

Cold Sores (Herpes Labialis): The recommended dosage of VALTREX for the treatment of cold sores (herpes labialis) is 2000 mg orally twice daily for 1 day (24-hour period). The second dose should be taken approximately 12 hours after the first dose, but not less than 6 hours after the first dose. Therapy should be initiated at the earliest symptom of a cold sore (e.g., tingling, itching, or burning). There are no data on the efficacy of treatment initiated after the development of clinical signs of a cold sore (e.g., papule, vesicle or ulcer).

Patients with Acute or Chronic Renal Impairment: Caution is advised when administering valacyclovir to patients with impaired renal function. Adequate hydration should be maintained.

Pharmacokinetic and safety evaluations following administration of oral valacyclovir hydrochloride have been performed in patients with renal impairment and volunteers with end-stage renal disease (ESRD) managed by hemodialysis. Based on these studies and extensive experience with acyclovir, the following dosage adjustments are recommended (see Table 8 and Table 9).

Table 8: VALTREX

Dosage Adjustments for Renal Impairment

Creatinine Clearance (mL/min)	Dosage for Herpes Zoster	Dosage for Recurrent Episodes of Genital Herpes	Dosage for Suppression of Genital Herpes: 500 mg (9 or fewer recurrences/year)	1000 mg (chronic suppressive therapy)	HIV-infected adults	Dosage for Initial Episode of Genital Herpes
>30	1000 mg every 8 hours[a]	500 mg every 12 hours[a]	500 mg every 24 hours[a]	1000 mg every 24 hours[a]	500 mg every 12 hours[a]	1000 mg every 12 hours[a]
15 to 30	1000 mg every 12 hours	500 mg every 12 hours[a]	500 mg every 24 hours[a]	500 mg every 24 hours[a]	500 mg every 24 hours	1000 mg every 24 hours
<15	1000 mg every 24 hours	500 mg every 24 hours	500 mg every 48 hours	500 mg every 24 hours	500 mg every 24 hours	500 mg every 24 hours

[a] Standard dose—adjustment not necessary.

Table 9: VALTREX

Dosage Adjustments for Renal Impairment

Creatinine Clearance (mL/min)	Dosage for Cold Sores (Herpes Labialis)[a]
>50	Two 2000 mg doses within 24 hours[b,c]
30 to 49	Two 1000 mg doses within 24 hours[c]
10 to 29	Two 500 mg doses within 24 hours[c]
<10	500 mg single dose

[a] Do not exceed one day of treatment.
[b] Standard dose—adjustment not necessary.
[c] Doses should be taken about 12 hours apart (not less than 6 hours apart).

Hemodialysis: During hemodialysis, the half-life of acyclovir after administration of valacyclovir is approximately 4 hours. About 1/3 of acyclovir in the body is removed by dialysis during a 4-hour hemodialysis session. These patients should receive the daily dose of VALTREX recommended for patients with creatinine clearance of <15 mL/min, with the dose administered after hemodialysis on the days it is performed.

Peritoneal Dialysis: There is no information specific to administration of VALTREX. The effect of continuous ambulatory peritoneal dialysis (CAPD) and continuous arteriovenous hemofiltration/dialysis (CAVHD) on acyclovir pharmacokinetics has been studied. The removal of acyclovir after CAPD and CAVHD is less pronounced than with hemodialysis, and the pharmacokinetic parameters closely resemble those observed in patients with ESRD not receiving hemodialysis. Therefore, supplemental doses of VALTREX should not be required following CAPD or CAVHD.

Missed Dose: If a dose of VALTREX is missed, the patient should be advised to take it as soon as he/she remembers, and then continue with the next dose at the proper time interval.

OVERDOSAGE:

Activated charcoal may be administered to aid in the removal of unabsorbed drug. General supportive measures are recommended.

Acute renal failure and neurological symptoms, including confusion, hallucinations, agitation, decreased consciousness and coma, have been reported in patients receiving overdoses of VALTREX (valacyclovir hydrochloride). Nausea and vomiting may also occur. Caution is required to prevent inadvertent overdose. Many of the reported cases involved renally impaired and geriatric patients receiving repeated overdoses, due to lack of appropriate dosage reduction (see Warnings and Precautions, Renal and Adverse Reactions).

Patients should be observed closely for signs of toxicity. Hemodialysis significantly enhances the removal of acyclovir from the blood and may, therefore be considered a management option in the event of symptomatic overdose. However, it is known that precipitation of acyclovir in renal tubules may occur when the solubility (2.5 mg/mL) is exceeded in the intratubular fluid. In the event of acute renal failure and anuria, the patient may benefit from hemodialysis until renal function is restored (see Dosage and Administration).

For management of a suspected drug overdose, contact your **regional Poison Control Centre**. See the *CPS* Directory section for a list of Poison Control Centres.

ACTION AND CLINICAL PHARMACOLOGY: Mechanism of Action: VALTREX (valacyclovir hydrochloride) is the L-valyl ester and a pro-drug of the antiviral drug acyclovir. Valacyclovir hydrochloride is rapidly converted to acyclovir, which has in vitro and in vivo inhibitory activity against human herpes viruses including herpes simplex virus types 1 (HSV-1) and 2 (HSV-2), and varicella-zoster virus (VZV).

The inhibitory activity of acyclovir is highly selective due to its unique affinity for the thymidine kinase (TK) encoded by HSV and VZV. This viral enzyme converts acyclovir into acyclovir monophosphate, a nucleotide analogue. The monophosphate is further converted into diphosphate by cellular guanylate kinase and into triphosphate by a number of cellular enzymes. In vitro, acyclovir triphosphate terminates growing chains of viral DNA. Once incorporated, acyclovir irreversibly binds to viral DNA polymerase, effectively inactivating the enzyme. Acyclovir triphosphate is a potent inhibitor of all of the human herpes virus DNA polymerases studied.

Acyclovir is virtually inactive in uninfected cells, since it is preferentially taken up and selectively converted to the active triphosphate form by herpes virus-infected cells. Additionally, the enzyme thymidine kinase of uninfected cells does not effectively use acyclovir as a substrate and cellular α-DNA polymerase is less sensitive than viral DNA polymerase to the effects of acyclovir.

A combination of the thymidine kinase specificity, competitive inhibition of DNA polymerase and incorporation and termination of the growing viral DNA chain results in inhibition of herpes virus replication. No effect on latent non-replicating virus has been demonstrated. Inhibition of viral replication reduces the period of viral shedding, limits the degree of spread and level of pathology, and thereby facilitates healing. The pain of shingles is related to viral damage to neurons which takes place during viral replication.

Pharmacokinetics: Acyclovir pharmacokinetics are unaltered after multiple-dose administration.

Absorption: After oral administration, valacyclovir hydrochloride is rapidly absorbed from the gastrointestinal tract. The absolute bioavailability of acyclovir after administration of valacyclovir hydrochloride is 54.5%±9.1% as determined following a 1000 mg oral dose of valacyclovir hydrochloride and a 350 mg intravenous acyclovir dose to 12 healthy volunteers.

Distribution: The binding of valacyclovir to human plasma proteins ranged from 13.5% to 17.9%.

Metabolism: Following absorption, valacyclovir is rapidly and nearly completely hydrolyzed to acyclovir and L-valine, an essential amino acid, by first-pass metabolism. This hydrolysis is mediated primarily by the enzyme valacyclovir hydrolase, and occurs predominantly in the liver.

Excretion: The pharmacokinetic disposition of acyclovir delivered by valacyclovir is consistent with previous experience from intravenous and oral acyclovir. Acyclovir is eliminated primarily by urinary excretion of unchanged drug. In all studies of valacyclovir hydrochloride, the half-life of acyclovir typically averages 2.5 to 3.3 hours in subjects with normal renal function.

Special Populations and Conditions: Pediatrics: The pharmacokinetics of valacyclovir hydrochloride have not been evaluated in pediatric patients.

Geriatrics: The pharmacokinetics of acyclovir following single- and multiple-dose oral administration of valacyclovir hydrochloride caplets in geriatric volunteers varied with renal function. Dosage reduction may be required in geriatric patients with reduced renal function (see Dosage and Administration).

Renal Insufficiency: The half-life and total body clearance of acyclovir are dependent on renal function. A dosage adjustment is recommended for patients with reduced renal function (see Dosage and Administration).

STORAGE AND STABILITY: VALTREX (valacyclovir hydrochloride) caplets should be stored between 15 and 30°C and protected from light.

INFORMATION FOR THE PATIENT: Published in e-CPS, available by subscription at www.e-cps.ca.

DOSAGE FORMS, COMPOSITION AND PACKAGING: 500 mg: Each blue, film-coated, capsule-shaped tablet (caplet), printed with edible white ink with "VALTREX 500 mg", contains: valacyclovir HCl equivalent to 500 mg valacyclovir. Nonmedicinal ingredients: carnauba wax, cellulose, crospovidone, hydroxypropyl methylcellulose, Indigotine Aluminum Lake, magnesium stearate, polyethylene glycol, polysorbate 80, povidone, silicon dioxide and titanium dioxide. Blister packs of 30.

1000 mg: Each white, film-coated, capsule-shaped tablet (caplet), printed with edible blue ink with "GX CF2", contains: valacyclovir HCl equivalent to 1000 mg valacyclovir. Nonmedicinal ingredients: carnauba wax, cellulose, crospovidone, hydroxypropyl methylcellulose, magnesium stearate, polyethylene glycol, polysorbate 80, povidone, silicon dioxide and titanium dioxide. Blister packs of 21.

(Shown in Product Identification Section)

Val-Vanco™ Ⓟ

vancomycin HCl

Antibiotic

Valeo Pharma

SUPPLIED: 500 mg: Each vial of sterile, lyophilized powder contains: vancomycin HCl equivalent to vancomycin base 500 mg. Single-dose glass vials of 20 mL, closed with rubber stoppers and flip-top caps, packages of 10.

1000 mg: Each vial of sterile, lyophilized powder contains: vancomycin HCl equivalent to vancomycin base 1000 mg. Single-dose glass vials of 20 mL, closed with rubber stoppers and flip-top caps, packages of 10.

Vancocin® Ⓟ

vancomycin HCl

Antibiotic

Iroko

Date of Preparation: October 1, 2007

PHARMACOLOGY: In vitro studies indicate that the bactericidal action of vancomycin hydrochloride against many gram-positive bacteria results from the inhibition of cell-wall synthesis. There is also evidence that vancomycin alters the permeability of the cell membrane and selectively inhibits RNA synthesis.

Microbiology: Cross-resistance has not been demonstrated between vancomycin and other classes of antibiotics. Laboratory-induced resistance has been reported to occur in a slow stepwise fashion. The development of resistance to vancomycin by staphylococci has not been reported in clinical use. Its activity is not significantly altered by changes in pH or by the presence of serum. Vancomycin is active against most strains of the following organisms in vitro and in clinical infections: *S. aureus* (including heterogeneous methicillin-resistant strains), *C. difficile*, *S. epidermidis* (including heterogeneous methicillin-resistant strains), *S. pneumoniae* (including multiple-resistant strains), *S. pyogenes* (group A beta-hemolytic), *S. agalactiae* (group B beta-hemolytic), *S. bovis*, Alpha-hemolytic streptococci (viridans groups), Enterococci (e.g., *E. faecalis*), Bacillus species, *L. monocytogenes*, Lactobacillus species, Neisseria species, Diphtheroids, Actinomyces species.

Note: Many strains of streptococci, staphylococci, *C. difficile* and other gram-positive bacteria are sensitive in vitro to concentrations of 0.5 to 5 μg/mL. Staphylococci are generally susceptible to less than 5 μg/mL, but a small proportion of *S. aureus* strains requires 10 to 20 μg/mL for inhibition.

In vitro resistance to vancomycin has been reported among some enterococcal and staphylococcal isolates.

Vancomycin is not effective in vitro against gram-negative bacilli, mycobacteria, or fungi.

Human Pharmacology: Adults: Renal Insufficiency: Infusions of 1 g vancomycin in 250 mL D5-W were given over 30 minutes to 29 anephric patients. After 18 days with intermittent dialysis at 3-day intervals, the serum concentration was still 3.5 μg/mL. The elimination half-life was about 7.5 days.

Oral Administration: Vancomycin is poorly absorbed after oral administration, only trace amounts being found in blood or urine. Following 125 mg orally 4 times daily, the mean concentration of vancomycin in stools was approximately 350 µg/g. Following up to 10 daily oral doses of 2 g, a mean level of 3100 µg/g with a range of 905 to 8760 µg/g was detected in feces of patients with pseudomembranous colitis.

Tissue Penetration and Distribution: Central Nervous System: Vancomycin does not readily diffuse across normal meninges into the spinal fluid; but, when the meninges are inflamed, penetration into the spinal fluid occurs.

Other Tissues and Fluids: Vancomycin concentration in human pericardial, pleural, bile, ascitic and synovial fluids reaches approximately one third of the equivalent serum level after single i.v. doses. A level of 7.6 µg/mL was achieved in the brain cyst of one infant following i.v. infusion of 40 mg/kg daily for 4 days.

INDICATIONS: VANCOCIN capsules may be used orally for the treatment of staphylococcal enterocolitis and antibiotic associated pseudomembranous colitis produced by *C. difficile*. **Parenteral administration of VANCOCIN is not effective for these indications, therefore VANCOCIN must be given orally.**

VANCOCIN is not effective by the oral route for the treatment of other types of infection. Vancomycin is not effective in vitro against gram-negative bacilli, mycobacteria, or fungi.

CONTRAINDICATIONS: VANCOCIN is contraindicated in patients with known hypersensitivity to this antibiotic.

WARNINGS: When given intravenously, toxic serum levels can occur. Vancomycin is excreted fairly rapidly by the kidney and blood levels increase markedly with decreased renal clearance. During parenteral therapy, the risk of toxicity appears appreciably increased by high blood concentrations or prolonged treatment. VANCOCIN is poorly absorbed orally. Toxic serum levels are therefore not attained from oral dosage.

Clinically significant serum concentrations have been reported in some patients who have taken multiple oral doses of vancomycin for active *C. difficile*-induced pseudomembranous colitis; therefore, monitoring of serum concentrations may be appropriate in these patients.

Ototoxicity has occurred when serum levels exceeded 80 µg/mL. Deafness may be preceded by tinnitus. The elderly are more susceptible to auditory damage. Experience with other antibiotics suggests that deafness may be progressive despite cessation of treatment.

Concurrent and sequential use of other neurotoxic and/or nephrotoxic agents, particularly ethacrynic acid, neuromuscular blocking agents, aminoglycoside antibiotics, polymixin B, colistin, viomycin, and cisplatin, requires careful monitoring.

If parenteral and oral vancomycin are administered concomitantly an additive effect can occur. This should be taken into consideration when calculating the total dose. In this situation serum levels of the antibiotic should be monitored.

PRECAUTIONS: Because of its ototoxicity and nephrotoxicity, VANCOCIN should be used with care in patients with renal insufficiency.

VANCOCIN should be avoided (if possible) in patients with previous hearing loss. If it is used in such patients, the dose of VANCOCIN should be regulated by periodic determination of drug levels in the blood. Patients with renal insufficiency and individuals over the age of 60 should be given serial tests of auditory function and of vancomycin blood levels. All patients receiving the drug should have periodic hematologic studies, urinalyses, and liver and renal function tests.

The prolonged use of VANCOCIN may result in overgrowth of non-susceptible organisms. If new infections due to bacteria or fungi appear during therapy with this product, appropriate measures should be taken, including withdrawal of VANCOCIN.

Some patients with inflammatory disorders of the intestinal mucosa may have significant systemic absorption of oral vancomycin and, therefore, may be at risk for the development of adverse reactions associated with the parenteral administration of vancomycin. The risk is greater if renal impairment is present. It should be noted that the total systemic and renal clearances of vancomycin are reduced in the elderly.

When patients with underlying renal dysfunction or those receiving concomitant therapy with an aminoglycoside are being treated, serial monitoring of renal function should be performed.

In vitro resistance to vancomycin has been reported among some enterococcal and staphylococcal isolates.

Pregnancy: VANCOCIN should be given to a pregnant woman only if clearly needed. In a controlled clinical study, VANCOCIN was administered to 10 pregnant women for serious staphylococcal infections complicating intravenous drug abuse to evaluate potential ototoxic and nephrotoxic effects on the infant. VANCOCIN levels of 13.2 and 16.6 µg/mL were measured in cord blood of two patients. No sensorineural hearing loss or nephrotoxicity attributable to VANCOCIN was noted. One infant whose mother received VANCOCIN in the third trimester experienced conductive hearing loss that was not attributed to the administration of VANCOCIN. Because the number of patients treated in this study was limited and VANCOCIN was administered only in the second and third trimesters, it is not known whether VANCOCIN causes fetal harm.

Lactation: VANCOCIN is excreted in human milk. Caution should be exercised if VANCOCIN is administered to a nursing woman. Because of the potential for adverse events, a decision should be made whether to discontinue nursing or discontinue administration of the drug, taking into account the importance of the drug to the mother.

Children: In premature neonates and young infants, it may be appropriate to confirm desired vancomycin serum concentrations. Concomitant administration of vancomycin and anesthetic agents has been associated with erythema and histamine-like flushing in children.

Geriatrics: The natural decrease of glomerular filtration with increasing age may lead to elevated vancomycin serum concentrations if dosage is not adjusted. Vancomycin dosage schedules should be adjusted in elderly patients.

ADVERSE EFFECTS: Nephrotoxicity: Rarely, renal failure, principally manifested by increased serum creatinine or BUN concentrations, especially in patients given large doses of VANCOCIN, has been reported. Rare cases of interstitial nephritis have been reported. Most of these have occurred in patients who were given aminoglycosides concomitantly or who had pre-existing kidney dysfunction. When VANCOCIN was discontinued, azotemia resolved in most patients.

Ototoxicity: A few dozen cases of hearing loss associated with VANCOCIN have been reported. Most of these patients had kidney dysfunction, pre-existing hearing loss, or concomitant treatment with an ototoxic drug. Vertigo, dizziness, and tinnitus have been reported rarely.

Hematopoietic: Reversible neutropenia, usually starting one week or more after onset of therapy with VANCOCIN or after a total dose of more than 25 g, has been reported in several dozen patients. Neutropenia appears to be promptly reversible when VANCOCIN is discontinued. Thrombocytopenia has rarely been reported. Although a causal relationship has not been established, reversible agranulocytosis (granulocyte count less than 500/mm³) has been reported rarely.

Miscellaneous: Anaphylaxis, drug fever, nausea, chills, eosinophilia, hypotension, wheezing, dyspnea, urticaria, pruritus flushing of the upper body ("red neck"), pain and muscle spasm of the chest and back, rashes, including exfoliative dermatitis, Stevens-Johnson syndrome, linear IgA bullous dermatosis and rare cases of vasculitis have been associated with the administration of VANCOCIN.

OVERDOSE:

Treatment: Other than general supportive treatment, no specific antidote is known. Dialysis does not remove significant amounts of vancomycin. Hemofiltration and hemoperfusion with polysulfone resin have been reported to result in increased vancomycin clearance.

In managing overdosage, consider the possibility of multiple drug overdoses, interaction among drugs, and unusual drug kinetics in your patient.

For management of a suspected drug overdose, CPhA recommends that you contact your **regional Poison Control Centre**. See the *CPS* Directory section for a list of Poison Control Centres.

DOSAGE: Adults: The usual daily dosage for antibiotic-associated pseudomembranous colitis produced by *C. difficile* and staphylococcal enterocolitis is 125 to 500 mg administered orally every 6 to 8 hours for 7 to 10 days. Vancomycin is not effective by the oral route for other types of infections.

Children: The usual daily dosage is approximately 40 mg/kg in 3 or 4 divided doses for 7 to 10 days. The total daily dosage should not exceed 2 g.

Note: VANCOCIN capsules are formulated in a matrix gel that prevents administration by a nasogastric tube; if this route of administration is being considered, the IV dosage form should be used.

SUPPLIED: 125 mg: Each peach and dark blue capsule, imprinted in white ink with "VANCOCIN HCL 125 mg" on one side and "3125" on the other side, contains: vancomycin HCl equivalent to vancomycin 125 mg. Nonmedicinal ingredients: FD&C Blue No. 2, gelatin, iron oxide, polyethylene glycol and titanium dioxide. Unit dose packages of 20.

250 mg: Each pale brown and dark blue capsule, imprinted in white ink with "VANCOCIN HCL 250 mg" on one side and "3126" on the other side, contains: vancomycin HCl equivalent to vancomycin 250 mg. Nonmedicinal ingredients: FD&C Blue No. 2, gelatin, iron oxide, polyethylene glycol and titanium dioxide. Unit dose packages of 20.

(Shown in Product Identification Section)

Vancomycin Hydrochloride, USP ℞

vancomycin HCl

Antibiotic

Hospira

SUPPLIED: 500 mg: Each vial of lyophilized, sterile powder contains: vancomycin base 500 mg (as HCl). Nonmedicinal ingredients: hydrochloric acid and/or sodium hydroxide (for pH adjustment). Single dose vials of 10 mL.

1 g: Each vial of lyophilized, sterile powder contains: vancomycin base 1 g (as HCl). Nonmedicinal ingredients: hydrochloric acid and/or sodium hydroxide (for pH adjustment). Single dose vials of 30 mL.

Store powder between 15 and 25°C. Reconstituted solutions and further diluted infusion mixtures should be used within 24 hours if kept at room temperature or within 96 hours if stored under refrigeration (5°C). Note: Parenteral drug products should be inspected visually for particulate matter and discoloration prior to administration, whenever solution or container permits.

Vaniqa® ℞

eflornithine HCl

Hair Growth Inhibitor

Triton Pharma

Date of Preparation: January 5, 2010

PHARMACOLOGY: VANIQA irreversibly inhibits ornithine decarboxylase in vitro and in vivo. This enzyme is integral in hair shaft production by the follicle. In preclinical and clinical studies, eflornithine administered topically has been shown to reduce the rate of hair growth.

Pharmacokinetics: The steady-state cutaneous penetration of eflornithine hydrochloride is minimal (less than 1%) after multiple-dose topical application of VANIQA to visibly intact facial skin of hirsute women. Absorption was determined under conditions of clinical use including shaving. Steady-state plasma levels are reached within four days of twice-daily application. The apparent plasma $t_{1/2}$ of eflornithine is approximately 8 hrs. The steady-state C_{max}, C_{trough} and $AUC_{12\ hr}$, expressed in terms of the anhydrous free base, following twice-daily topical application of 0.5 g of the VANIQA cream are approximately 10 ng/mL, 5 ng/mL, and 92 ng·hr/mL, respectively. Eflornithine is not known to be metabolized and is excreted unchanged in the urine.

INDICATIONS: VANIQA is indicated for slowing of the growth of unwanted facial hair in women. It is recommended as an adjunct to any hair removal technique.

VANIQA Cream has only been studied on the face and neck of affected women. Usage should be limited to those areas.

CONTRAINDICATIONS: Hypersensitivity to eflornithine or to any of the excipients of VANIQA.

WARNINGS: None.

PRECAUTIONS: General: VANIQA is for topical use only. Avoid contact with eyes or mucous membranes (e.g., nose or mouth). Discontinue use if hypersensitivity occurs. If skin irritation or intolerance develops, the patient should be directed to temporarily reduce the frequency of application to once per day. If irritation continues, the patient should discontinue use of VANIQA and consult their physician.

Transient stinging or burning may occur when applied to abraded or broken skin.

Geriatrics: Of the total number of patients in clinical trials with VANIQA (n=1370), approximately 6% were 65 years or older, while approximately 1% were 75 years or older. No overall differences in safety were observed between older and younger patients.

Children: The safety and effectiveness of this product in pediatric patients have not been established.

Adolescents: The safety and efficacy of this product in adolescent patients has not been established.

Pregnancy: There are no well-controlled studies of VANIQA Cream in pregnant women. Therefore, VANIQA should be used during pregnancy only if the physician considers the potential benefits to outweigh the potential risks to the fetus.

Lactation: It is not known whether or not eflornithine hydrochloride is excreted in human milk. Caution should be exercised when VANIQA cream is administered to a nursing woman.

Hepatic and Renal Impairment: Safety and efficacy of VANIQA Cream in patients with hepatic or renal impairment have not been established. Considering the low systemic exposure after topical application, problems would not be expected.

Drug Interactions: None known.

Information to Be Provided to the Patient: Patients using VANIQA cream should receive the following information and instructions:

1. This medication is not a depilatory, but rather appears to reduce hair growth to improve the condition and the patient's appearance. Patients will likely need to continue using a hair removal method (e.g. shaving, plucking, etc.) in conjunction with VANIQA.
2. Onset of improvement may be seen after as little as 4-8 weeks of treatment. Further improvement may be seen with continued use. The condition may return to pretreatment levels 8 weeks after discontinuing treatment.
3. If skin irritation or intolerance develops, direct the patient to temporarily reduce the frequency of application (e.g., once a day). If irritation continues, the patient should discontinue use of the product.

ADVERSE EFFECTS: Adverse reactions reported for most body systems occurred at similar frequencies in active and vehicle groups. The most frequent adverse reactions related to treatment with VANIQA Cream were skin related. Table 1 notes the skin-related adverse reactions that occurred in greater than 1% of patients treated with VANIQA or vehicle in controlled studies.

Table 1: VANIQA

Incidence Attributed to Therapy. Percentage (%) of Patients

Adverse Reaction	VANIQA 13.9% (N=395)	Vehicle (N=201)
Acne	21.3	21.4
Pseudofolliculitis barbae	16.2	15.4
Burning, stinging, tingling	14.2	5.0
Pruritus (itching)	3.8	4.0
Dry skin	1.8	3.0
Alopecia	1.5	2.5
Erythema (redness)	1.3	0
Skin irritation	1.3	1.0
Dermatitis	1.0	0.5
Rash	1.0	0

Treatment related skin adverse reactions that occurred in less than 1% of the subjects treated with VANIQA Cream are: bleeding skin, cheilitis, contact dermatitis, edema face, edema mouth, folliculitis, hair ingrown, herpes simplex, numbness and rosacea.

Adverse reactions were primarily mild in intensity and generally resolved without medical treatment or discontinuation of VANIQA Cream. No serious adverse reactions were related to treatment. Only 2% of subjects discontinued studies due to an adverse reaction related to use of VANIQA Cream. The drug was generally well tolerated.

Laboratory Test Abnormalities: No laboratory test abnormalities have been found to be associated with VANIQA Cream.

OVERDOSE: SYMPTOMS AND TREATMENT:
Dermal Administration: Given the minimal cutaneous penetration of this drug, overdosage via the topical route is not expected (see clinical pharmacology). However, should very high topical doses (e.g. multiple tubes per day) or oral ingestion be encountered (e.g., a 60 g tube contains 9 g of eflornithine HCl), the patient should be monitored, and appropriate supportive measures administered as necessary.
Intravenous Administration: Adverse effects and laboratory abnormalities have been noted with intravenous administration of high doses of eflornithine hydrochloride (400 mg/kg/day or approximately 24 g/day) for the treatment of Trypanosoma brucei gambiense infection (African sleeping sickness). Adverse events have included hair loss, facial swelling, seizures, hearing impairment, stomach upset, loss of appetite, headache, weakness and dizziness. A variety of hematological toxicities, including anemia, thrombocytopenia and leukopenia have also been observed, but these were usually reversible upon discontinuation of treatment.

For management of a suspected drug overdose, CPhA recommends that you contact your **regional Poison Control Centre**. See the *CPS* Directory section for a list of Poison Control Centres.

DOSAGE: Apply a thin layer of VANIQA Cream to affected areas of the face and neck and rub in thoroughly. The treated area should not be washed for at least 4 hours after application. VANIQA should be used twice daily at least 8 hours apart. The product may be used alone or in conjunction with other hair removal techniques. VANIQA may be applied 5 minutes after shaving or other hair removal techniques. Cosmetics or sunscreens may be applied over treated areas after cream has dried.
Geriatrics: No dosage adjustment is necessary.

INFORMATION FOR THE PATIENT: Published in e-CPS, available by subscription at www.e-cps.ca.
SUPPLIED: Each tube of smooth white to off-white, fragrance-free cream contains: 13.9% (139 mg/g) of anhydrous eflornithine hydrochloride. See tube crimp and carton end for expiration date and lot number. Nonmedicinal ingredients: ceteareth-20, cetearyl alcohol, dimethicone, glyceryl stearate, methylparaben, mineral oil, PEG-100 stearate, phenoxyethanol, propylparaben, stearyl alcohol and water. Flastic tubes of 30 g. Store between 15 to 25°C.

Vaqta®

hepatitis A vaccine, purified inactivated
Active Immunizing Agent Against Hepatitis A Virus

Merck Frosst

Date of Revision: July 21, 2010

SUMMARY PRODUCT INFORMATION:

Route of Administration	Dosage Form/ Strength	Clinically Relevant Nonmedicinal Ingredients
Intramuscular	Suspension for injection 25 U of hepatitis A virus protein/0.5 mL dose (pediatric/adolescent presentation) 50 U of hepatitis A virus protein/1.0 mL dose (adult presentation)	For a complete listing see Dosage Forms, Composition and Packaging.

INDICATIONS AND CLINICAL USE: VAQTA (hepatitis A vaccine, purified inactivated) is indicated for vaccination against infection caused by hepatitis A virus.

VAQTA is indicated for active pre-exposure prophylaxis against disease caused by hepatitis A virus. Vaccination is recommended in children 12 months of age and older, adolescents, and adults who are at risk of contracting or spreading infection or who are at risk of life-threatening disease if infected, including but not limited to:

A. **Travelers to Endemic or Outbreak Areas**
B. **Frequently Affected Communities:** Members residing in any community with one or more recorded outbreaks within the last five years.
C. **Day-Care:** Children and staff of day-care centers as well as their parents, siblings, and other contacts.
D. **Military Personnel Prior to Departure for Endemic or Outbreak Areas**
E. **Persons for whom Hepatitis A is an Occupational Hazard:** Health-care workers. Staff and residents of orphanages, chronic care hospitals and mental health care facilities. Sewage workers.
F. **Hemophiliacs and Other Recipients of Therapeutic Blood Products**
G. **People with Chronic Liver Disease (including chronic hepatitis C infection):** People with chronic liver disease who may not be at increased risk of infection but are at increased risk of fulminant hepatitis A.
H. **Food Handlers**
I. **Consumers of High-Risk Foods:** e.g. raw shellfish.
J. **Persons at Increased Risk of the Disease due to their Sexual Practices:** Homosexually-active males. Persons who repeatedly contract sexually transmitted diseases.
K. **Users of Illicit Injectable Drugs:** VAQTA will not prevent hepatitis caused by infectious agents other than hepatitis A virus.

Revaccination: See Dosage and Administration.

CONTRAINDICATIONS:

- Patients who are hypersensitive to this drug or to any ingredient in the formulation or component of the container. For a complete listing, see Dosage Forms, Composition and Packaging.

WARNINGS AND PRECAUTIONS: If VAQTA is used in individuals with malignancies or those receiving immunosuppressive therapy or who are otherwise immunocompromised, the expected immune response may not be obtained.

VAQTA is not recommended for use in infants younger than 12 months of age since data on use in this age group are not currently available.

General: Individuals who develop symptoms suggestive of hypersensitivity after an injection of VAQTA should not receive further injections of the vaccine (see Contraindications).

As with any vaccine, adequate treatment provisions, including epinephrine, should be available for immediate use should an anaphylactic or anaphylactoid reaction occur.

Since there is a possibility that the vaccine may contain trace amounts of neomycin, the possibility of an allergic reaction in individuals sensitive to this substance should be kept in mind when considering the use of this vaccine (see Dosage Forms, Composition and Packaging).

The vial stopper contains dry natural latex rubber. If a person reports a severe (anaphylactic) allergy to latex, products supplied in vials or syringes that contain natural rubber should not be administered, unless the benefit of administration outweighs the risk of an allergic reaction resulting from administration of the vaccine. A history of contact dermatitis to dry natural latex rubber is not a contraindication to receiving this vaccine.

As with any vaccine, vaccination with VAQTA may not result in a protective response in all susceptible vaccinees.

Any acute infection or febrile illness may be reason for delaying use of VAQTA except when, in the opinion of the physician, withholding the vaccine entails a greater risk.

VAQTA will not prevent hepatitis caused by infectious agents other than hepatitis A virus. Because of the long incubation period (approximately 20 to 50 days) for hepatitis A, it is possible for unrecognized hepatitis A infection to be present at the time the vaccine is given. The vaccine may not prevent hepatitis A in such individuals.

Carcinogenesis, Mutagenesis, Reproduction: VAQTA has not been evaluated for its carcinogenic or mutagenic potential, or its potential to impair fertility.

Special Populations: Pregnant Women: Animal reproduction studies have not been conducted with VAQTA. It is also not known whether VAQTA can cause fetal harm when administered to a pregnant woman or can affect reproductive capacity. VAQTA should be given to a pregnant woman only if clearly needed.

Nursing Women: It is not known whether VAQTA is excreted in human milk. Because many drugs are excreted in human milk, caution should be exercised when VAQTA is administered to a woman who is breast-feeding.

Pediatrics: VAQTA has been shown to be generally well-tolerated and highly immunogenic in individuals 12 months through 17 years of age See Dosage and Administration for the recommended dosage schedule.

Safety and effectiveness in infants below 12 months of age have not been established.

ADVERSE REACTIONS: Clinical Trial Adverse Drug Reactions: Children—12 Months Through 23 Months of Age: In combined clinical trials, 706 healthy children 12 through 23 months of age received one or more ~25 U doses of hepatitis A vaccine with or without other pediatric vaccines. Table 1 lists local complaints and fever reported during the first 5-days following vaccination, and other systemic complaints reported during the 14-day period postvaccination. Irritability and upper respiratory infection were the most frequently reported complaints.

Table 1: VAQTA
Local and Systemic Complaints (≥1%) in Healthy Children 12 Months Through 23 Months of Age from Combined Clinical Trials

	%
Localized Injection-site Reactions (generally mild and transient)	
Pain/Tenderness/Soreness	8.6
Erythema	5.9
Swelling	5.1
Warmth	3.2
Ecchymosis	1.0
Body as a Whole	
Fever ≥38.9°C, Oral	6.5
Digestive System	
Diarrhea	5.9
Vomiting	4.0
Anorexia	1.2
Nervous System/Psychiatric	
Irritability	10.8
Crying	1.8
Respiratory System	
Upper Respiratory Infection	10.1
Rhinorrhea	5.7
Cough	5.1
Respiratory Congestion	1.6
Nasal Congestion	1.2
Laryngotracheobronchitis	1.2
Skin and Skin Appendages	
Rash	4.5
Measles-like/rubella-like Rash	1.0
Viral Exanthema	1.0
Special Senses—Ear	
Otitis Media	7.6
Otitis	1.8
Special Senses—Eye	
Conjunctivitis	1.3

In more recent clinical trials involving 2453 healthy children 12 through 23 months of age who received two doses of hepatitis A vaccine (~25 U) 6 months apart with or without other vaccines, the incidence of adverse experiences appeared to be consistent with that reported in the prior trials with the exception of the following injection-site reactions: pain/tenderness/soreness (37.8%), erythema (19.7%), and swelling (12.7%).

In The Monroe Efficacy Study, 1037 healthy children and adolescents 2 to 16 years of age received either a primary dose of ~25 U of hepatitis A vaccine and a booster 6, 12, or 18 months later, or placebo. Subjects were observed during a 5-day period for fever and local complaints and during a 14-day period for systemic complaints. Injection-site complaints, generally mild and transient, were the most frequently reported complaints. Table 2 summarizes the local and systemic complaints (≥1%) reported in this study, without regard to causality. There were no significant differences in the rates of any complaint between vaccine and placebo recipients after Dose 1.

Table 2: VAQTA
Local and Systemic Complaints (≥1%) in Healthy Children and Adolescents From the Monroe Efficacy Study

Reaction	VAQTA Dose 1[a]	VAQTA Booster	Placebo[b]
Injection-site Complaints			
Pain	6.4% (33/515)	3.4% (16/475)	6.3% (32/510)
Tenderness	4.9% (25/515)	1.7% (8/475)	6.1% (31/510)

(cont'd)

Table 2: VAQTA *(cont'd)*

Local and Systemic Complaints (≥1%) in Healthy Children and Adolescents From the Monroe Efficacy Study

	VAQTA		
Reaction	**Dose 1**[a]	**Booster**	**Placebo**[b]
Erythema	1.9% (10/515)	0.8% (4/475)	1.8% (9/510)
Swelling	1.7% (9/515)	1.5% (7/475)	1.6% (8/510)
Warmth	1.7% (9/515)	0.6% (3/475)	1.6% (8/510)
Systemic Complaints			
Abdominal Pain	1.2% (6/519)	1.1% (5/475)	1.0% (5/518)
Pharyngitis	1.2% (6/519)	0% (0/475)	0.8% (4/518)
Headache	0.4% (2/519)	0.8% (4/475)	1.0% (5/518)

a No statistically significant differences between the two groups.
b Second injection of placebo not administered because code for the trial was broken.

Children/Adolescents—2 through 17 Years of Age: In combined clinical trials (including Monroe Efficacy Study participants) involving 2595 healthy children (≥2 years of age) and adolescents who received one or more ~25 U doses of hepatitis A vaccine, subjects were followed for fever and local complaints during a 5-day period postvaccination and systemic complaints during a 14-day period postvaccination. Injection-site complaints, generally mild and transient, were the most frequently reported complaints. Table 3 lists the complaints reported by ≥1% of subjects, without regard to causality, in decreasing order of frequency within each body system.

Table 3: VAQTA

Local and Systemic Complaints (≥1%) in Healthy Children and Adolescents from Combined Clinical Trials

	%
Localized Injection-site Reactions (generally mild and transient)	
Pain	18.7
Tenderness	16.8
Warmth	8.6
Erythema	7.5
Swelling	7.3
Ecchymosis	1.3
Body as a Whole	
Fever ≥38.9°C, Oral	3.1
Abdominal Pain	1.6
Digestive System	
Diarrhea	1.0
Vomiting	1.0
Nervous System/Psychiatric	
Headache	2.3
Respiratory System	
Pharyngitis	1.5
Upper Respiratory Infection	1.1
Cough	1.0

Laboratory Findings: Very few laboratory abnormalities were reported and included isolated reports of elevated liver function tests, eosinophilia, and increased urine protein.

Adults—18 Years of Age and Older: In combined clinical trials involving 1529 healthy adults who received one or more ~50 U doses of hepatitis A vaccine, subjects were followed for fever and local complaints during a 5-day period postvaccination and systemic complaints during a 14-day period postvaccination. Injection-site complaints, generally mild and transient, were the most frequently reported complaints. Table 4 lists the complaints reported by ≥1% of subjects without regard to causality, in decreasing order of frequency within each body system.

Table 4: VAQTA

Local and Systemic Complaints (≥1%) in Healthy Adults from Combined Clinical Trials

	%
Localized Injection-site Reactions (generally mild and transient)	
Tenderness	52.6
Pain	51.1
Warmth	17.3
Swelling	13.6
Erythema	12.9
Ecchymosis	1.5
Pain/Soreness	1.2
Body as a Whole	
Asthenia/Fatigue	3.9
Fever ≥38.3°C, Oral	2.6
Abdominal Pain	1.3
Digestive System	
Diarrhea	2.4
Nausea	2.3
Musculoskeletal System	
Myalgia	2.0
Arm Pain	1.3
Back Pain	1.1
Stiffness	1.0
Nervous System/Psychiatric	
Headache	16.1
Respiratory System	
Upper Respiratory Infection	2.8
Pharyngitis	2.7
Nasal Congestion	1.1
Urogenital System	
Menstruation Disorder	1.1

Local and/or systemic hypersensitivity reactions occurred in <1% of children, adolescents, or adults in clinical trials and included the following regardless of causality: pruritus, urticaria and rash.

As with any vaccine, there is the possibility that use of VAQTA in very large populations might reveal adverse experiences not observed in clinical trials.

Post-Market Adverse Drug Reactions: Post-Marketing Safety Study: In a post-marketing safety study, a total of 42,110 individuals ≥2 years of age received 1 or 2 doses of VAQTA. There was no serious, vaccine-related, adverse event identified. There was no nonserious, vaccine-related, adverse event resulting in outpatient visits, with the exception of diarrhea/gastroenteritis in adults at a rate of 0.5%.

Marketed Experience: The following additional adverse reactions have been reported with use of the marketed vaccine.

Nervous System: Very rarely, Guillain-Barré syndrome, cerebellar ataxia, encephalitis.

Hemic and Lymphatic System: Very rarely, thrombocytopenia.

DRUG INTERACTIONS: Use with Other Vaccines: VAQTA may be given concomitantly with measles, mumps, rubella, varicella, pneumococcal 7-valent conjugate, and oral or inactivated polio vaccines.

Adults—18 Years of Age and Older: VAQTA may be given concomitantly with yellow fever and typhoid vaccines.

Data on concomitant use with other vaccines are limited (see Dosage and Administration, Use with Other Vaccines).

Separate injection sites and syringes should be used for concomitant administration of injectable vaccines.

Vaccines administered simultaneously should be given using separate syringes at separate sites (unless otherwise specified by the manufacturer), consideration being given to the precautions that apply to each individual vaccine. Concomitant administration of other vaccines at other injection sites is unlikely to interfere with the immune response to hepatitis A vaccine.

The Advisory Committee on Immunization Practices, has stated that limited data from studies conducted among adults indicate that simultaneous administration of hepatitis A vaccine with diphtheria, poliovirus (oral and inactivated), tetanus, oral typhoid, cholera, Japanese encephalitis, rabies, or yellow fever vaccine does not decrease the immune response to either vaccine or increase the frequency of reported adverse events. Studies indicate that hepatitis B vaccine can be administered with VAQTA without affecting immunogenicity or increasing the frequency of adverse events.

Use with Immune Globulin: For individuals requiring either post exposure prophylaxis or combined immediate and longer-term protection (e.g. travelers departing on short notice to endemic areas), VAQTA may be administered concomitantly with immune globulin (IG) using separate sites and syringes.

DOSAGE AND ADMINISTRATION: Dosing Considerations: For intramuscular use only. The deltoid muscle is the preferred site for injection.

Do not inject intravascularly, intradermally, or subcutaneously.

Recommended Dose and Dosage Adjustment: The vaccination series consists of one primary dose and one booster dose given according to the following schedule:

Children/Adolescents—12 Months Through 17 Years of Age: Individuals 12 months through 17 years of age should receive a single 0.5 mL (~25 U) dose of vaccine at an elected date and a booster dose of 0.5 mL (~25 U) 6 to 18 months later.

Adults: Adults 18 years of age and older should receive a single 1.0 mL (~50 U) dose of vaccine at an elected date and a booster dose of 1.0 mL (~50 U) 6 months later.

Interchangeability of the Booster Dose: A booster dose of VAQTA may be given at 6 to 12 months following the initial dose of other inactivated hepatitis A vaccines.

Missed Dose: If a dose is missed, the physician will decide when to give it.

Administration: Use with Other Vaccines: Separate injection sites and syringes should be used for concomitant administration of injectable vaccines (see Drug Interactions, Use with Other Vaccines).

Known or Presumed Exposure to Hepatitis A Virus, Travel to Endemic Areas, and Use with Immune Globulin: VAQTA may be administered concomitantly with IG using separate sites and syringes. The vaccination regimen for VAQTA should be followed as stated above. Consult the manufacturers' Product Monograph for the appropriate dosage of IG. A booster dose of VAQTA should be administered at the appropriate time as outlined above (see Drug Interactions).

The vaccine should be used as supplied; no reconstitution is necessary.

Shake well before withdrawal and use. Thorough agitation is necessary to maintain suspension of the vaccine.

Parenteral drug products should be inspected visually for extraneous particulate matter and discoloration prior to administration whenever solution and container permit. After thorough agitation, VAQTA is a slightly opaque, white suspension.

It is important to use a separate, sterile syringe and needle for each individual to prevent transmission of infectious agents from one person to another.

OVERDOSAGE:
There are no data with regard to overdose.

> For management of a suspected drug overdose, contact your regional Poison Control Centre. See the *CPS* Directory section for a list of Poison Control Centres.

ACTION AND CLINICAL PHARMACOLOGY: Mechanism of Action: VAQTA is an inactivated whole virus vaccine which has been shown to induce antibody to hepatitis A virus protein.

Disease Epidemiology: Hepatitis A virus is one of several hepatitis viruses that cause a systemic infection with pathology in the liver. The incubation period ranges from approximately 20 to 50 days. While the course of the disease is generally benign and does not result in chronic hepatitis, infection with hepatitis A virus remains an important cause of morbidity and occasional fulminant hepatitis and death.

Hepatitis A is transmitted most often by the fecal-oral route, with infection occurring within private households, day-care centers, neonatal intensive care units, and chronic-care hospitals. Common-source outbreaks due to contaminated food and water supplies have occurred following consumption of certain foods such as raw shellfish, and uncooked foods prepared by an infected food-handler or otherwise contaminated prior to ingestion (salads, sandwiches, frozen raspberries, etc). Bloodborne transmission, while uncommon, is possible via blood transfusion, contaminated blood products, or from needles shared with an infected viremic individual. Sexual transmission has also been reported.

The disease burden due to hepatitis A as of 2006 in the United States has been estimated to be approximately 3579 cases of clinical hepatitis each year, resulting in 549 hospitalizations, and 5 deaths due to fulminant hepatitis. Worldwide, it has been estimated that 1.4 million cases occur annually. The clinical manifestations of hepatitis A infection often pass unrecognized in children <6 years of age whereas overt hepatitis develops in the majority of infected older children and adults. Symptoms and signs of hepatitis A infection are similar to those associated with other types of viral hepatitis and include anorexia, nausea, fever/chills, jaundice, dark urine, light-colored stools, abdominal pain, malaise, and fatigue.

STORAGE AND STABILITY: Store vaccine at 2-8°C.

Do not freeze since freezing destroys potency.

Stability studies with VAQTA show that the potency of unopened vaccine is not significantly affected after exposure at 37°C for up to 6 months. This is **not**, however, a storage recommendation.

INFORMATION FOR THE PATIENT: Published in e-CPS, available by subscription at www.e-cps.ca.

DOSAGE FORMS, COMPOSITION AND PACKAGING: VAQTA is a sterile, slightly opaque, white suspension for intramuscular injection.

The vaccine should be used as supplied; no reconstitution is necessary.

Manufacturing Process Residuals: Within the limits of current assay variability, the 50 unit (1 mL) dose of VAQTA contains less than 0.1 μg (less than 100 ng) of non-viral protein, less than 4×10^{-6} μg (less than 0.004 ng) of DNA, less than 10^{-4} μg (less than 0.1 ng) of bovine albumin, less than 0.8 μg (less than 800 ng) of formaldehyde and a trace of neomycin [≤0.002 μg (≤2 ng)]. Other process chemical residuals are less than 10 parts per billion (ppb). VAQTA meets the World Health Organization requirement for biological substances including those for final vaccine residual bovine serum albumin.

VAQTA is supplied in two presentations:

Pediatric/Adolescent Presentation: Each 0.5 mL dose contains approximately 25 U of hepatitis A virus protein. Nonmedicinal ingredients: aluminum (as amorphous aluminum hydroxyphosphate sulfate), sodium borate, sodium chloride and water for injection. Single-dose Type 1 glass 3 mL vials, containing one 0.5 mL dose, packages of 1. The vial stopper contains latex.

Adult Presentation: Each 1.0 mL dose contains approximately 50 U of hepatitis A virus protein. Nonmedicinal ingredients: aluminum (as amorphous aluminum hydroxyphosphate sulfate), sodium borate, sodium chloride and water for injection. Single-dose Type 1 glass 3 mL vials, containing one 1.0 mL dose, packages of 1. The vial stopper contains latex.

Varilrix®

varicella virus vaccine, live, attenuated (Oka-strain)

Active Immunizing Agent

GlaxoSmithKline

Date of Revision: September 10, 2010

SUMMARY PRODUCT INFORMATION:

Route of Administration	Dosage Form/ Strength	Clinically Relevant Nonmedicinal Ingredients
Subcutaneous Injection	Lyophilized vaccine for reconstitution/Not less than $10^{3.3}$ plaque-forming units of the varicella-zoster virus per 0.5 mL of reconstituted vaccine	Amino acids, human albumin, lactose, neomycin sulphate and polyalcohols

DESCRIPTION: VARILRIX (varicella virus vaccine, live, attenuated (Oka-strain)) is a live-attenuated varicella vaccine which contains the Oka-strain of the attenuated varicella-zoster virus. VARILRIX has been reformulated through the addition of a stabilizer, without modification of the viral strain, to permit storage at 2 to 8°C.

Epidemiology: Varicella is a very common and highly communicable disease of childhood which is experienced by most children. An epidemiological report of Chickenpox in Canada reported that at least 90% of the population will likely contract the infection by late adolescence. Therefore, at steady state conditions, the actual number of cases that occur annually should approximate the number of annual births. Approximately 50% of cases occur in children 5-9 years old, 20% in preschool children, 20% in children 10-14 years of age, 10% in children ≥15-19 years old and <2% in adults.

Based on epidemiological evidence, varicella-zoster virus (VZV) spreads by airborne droplets, however, the source of infectious virus remains controversial. Whether it originates primarily from skin or respiratory tract secretions is not clear but it is known that infectivity is maximal in the early stages of the illness. Among household contacts, 70-90% of susceptible individuals may become infected.

The symptoms of varicella in otherwise healthy children are usually mild and self limiting, however, complications such as secondary bacterial infections and otitis media have been reported in as many as 5-10% and 5% of children, respectively. More serious complications include pneumonia, encephalitis, Guillain-Barr Syndrome and Reye's Syndrome.

The severity of varicella and the potential for varicella-related complications increases substantially with age. Although less than 2% of all chickenpox cases occur in adults, a third of all varicella-zoster (VZ) deaths are in adults. In addition, in children with impaired immunity the disease is often severe and can be fatal. Children with a malignant disease who are receiving chemotherapy and/or radiotherapy appear to be at greatest risk.

INDICATIONS AND CLINICAL USE: VARILRIX (varicella virus vaccine, live, attenuated (Oka-strain)) is indicated for:

- the active immunization against varicella of healthy subjects from 12 months of age and up.
- the active immunization against varicella of susceptible high risk patients and their susceptible healthy close contacts.

Patients with Acute Leukemia: Patients suffering from leukemia have been recognized to be at special risk when they develop varicella, and should receive the vaccine if they have no history of the disease or are found to be seronegative.

When vaccinating patients in the acute phase of leukemia, maintenance chemotherapy should be withheld one week before and one week after immunization. Patients under radiotherapy should normally not be vaccinated during the treatment phase.

Generally patients are immunized when they are in complete hematological remission from the disease. It is advised that the total lymphocyte count should be at least 1200 per mm³, or that no other evidence of lack of cellular immune competence exists.

Patients Under Immunosuppressive Treatment: Patients under immunosuppressive treatment (including corticosteroid therapy) for malignant solid tumour or for serious chronic diseases (such as chronic renal failure, auto-immune diseases, collagen diseases, severe bronchial asthma) are predisposed to severe varicella.

It is advised that the total lymphocyte count should be at least 1200 per mm³, or that no other evidence of lack of cellular immune competence exists at the time of vaccination.

Patients with Planned Organ Transplantation: If organ transplantation (e.g. kidney transplant) is being considered, vaccination should be carried out 6-8 weeks before the administration of the immunosuppressive treatment.

Patients with Chronic Diseases: Other chronic disease, such as metabolic and endocrine disorders, chronic pulmonary and cardiovascular diseases, mucoviscidosis and neuromuscular abnormalities may also predispose to severe varicella.

Healthy Close Contacts: Susceptible healthy close contacts should be vaccinated in order to reduce the risk of the transmission of virus to high risk patients. These include parents and siblings of high risk patients, medical and paramedical personnel, and other people who are in close contact with varicella patients or high risk patients.

CONTRAINDICATIONS: VARILRIX (varicella virus vaccine, live, attenuated (Oka-strain)):

- should not be administered to subjects with known hypersensitivity to any component of the vaccine, or to subjects who developed an unacceptable reaction to a previous dose, including anaphylactic reaction.
- is contraindicated in subjects with known systemic hypersensitivity to neomycin, but a history of contact dermatitis to neomycin is not a contraindication.
- is contraindicated in subjects with primary or acquired immunodeficiency states with a total lymphocyte count less than 1200 per mm³ or presenting other evidence of lack of cellular immune competence, such as subjects with **active** leukemias, lymphomas, blood dyscrasias, clinically manifest HIV infection, or patients receiving immunosuppressive therapy (including high dose corticosteroids) (see Indications and Clinical Use).
- administration to pregnant women is contraindicated because the possible effects on fetal development are unknown. Furthermore, pregnancy should be avoided for three months after vaccination.
- as with other vaccines, administration of VARILRIX should be postponed in subjects suffering from acute severe febrile illness. In healthy subjects the presence of a minor infection, however, is not a contraindication for vaccination.

WARNINGS AND PRECAUTIONS: Salicylates should be avoided for 6 weeks after varicella vaccination, as Reye's Syndrome has been reported following the use of salicylates during natural varicella infection.

General: As with any parenteral vaccine, appropriate medication (e.g. epinephrine 1:1000) and supervision should be readily available for immediate use in case of anaphylaxis or anaphylactoid reactions following administration of the vaccine.

VARILRIX should not be administered intradermally. VARILRIX must under no circumstances be administered intravenously.

Transmission of the Oka vaccine virus has been shown to occur at a very low rate in seronegative contacts of vaccine recipients. However, transmission has not been confirmed to occur in the absence of vaccine-associated cutaneous lesions in the vaccinee.

VARILRIX (varicella virus vaccine, live, attenuated (Oka-strain)) can be administered at the same time as any other vaccine. Different injectable vaccines should be administered at different injection sites.

Inactivated vaccines can be administered in any temporal relationship to VARILRIX.

If a measles vaccine cannot be administered at the same time as VARILRIX, it is recommended that an interval of at least one month be allowed between the administration of the two vaccines as it is recognized that measles vaccination may lead to short lived suppression of the cell mediated immune response.

Skin: The mild nature of the rash in the healthy contacts indicates that the virus remains attenuated after passage through human hosts.

Special Populations: Pregnant Women: Administration to pregnant women is contraindicated because the possible effects on fetal development are unknown. Furthermore, pregnancy should be avoided for three months after vaccination.

Nursing Women: It is not known whether VARILRIX is excreted in human milk. Because many drugs are excreted in human milk, caution should be exercised when VARILRIX is administered to a nursing woman.

High Risk Patients: VARILRIX should not be administered at the same time as other live attenuated vaccines. Inactivated vaccines may be administered in any temporal relationship to VARILRIX given that no specific contraindication has been established.

Different injectable vaccines should always be administered at different injection sites.

ADVERSE REACTIONS: VARILRIX (varicella virus vaccine, live, attenuated (Oka-strain)) is a vaccine of low overall reactogenicity in all age groups.

Clinical Trial Adverse Drug Reactions: Because clinical trials are conducted under very specific conditions the adverse reaction rates observed in the clinical trials may not reflect the rates observed in practice and should not be compared to the rates in the clinical trials of another drug. Adverse drug reaction information from clinical trials is useful for identifying drug-related adverse events and for approximating rates.

Healthy Subjects: More than 7900 individuals have participated in clinical trials evaluating the reactogenicity profile of the vaccine administered alone or concomitantly with other vaccines.

The safety profile presented below is based on a total of 5369 doses of VARILRIX administered in monotherapy to children, adolescents and adults. See Table 1.

Table 1: VARILRIX
Safety Profile of VARILRIX

Very Common: ≥10%	
General Disorders and Administration Site Conditions	pain, redness
Common: ≥1% and <10%	
Skin and Subcutaneous Tissue Disorders	rash
General Disorders and Administration Site Conditions	swelling at the injection site[a], fever (oral/axillary temperature ≥37.5°C or rectal temperature ≥38.0°C)[a]
Uncommon: ≥0.1% and <1%	
Infections and Infestations	upper respiratory tract infection, pharyngitis
Blood and Lymphatic System Disorders	lymphadenopathy
Psychiatric Disorders	irritability
Nervous System Disorders	headache, somnolence
Respiratory, Thoracic and Mediastinal Disorders	cough, rhinitis
Gastrointestinal Disorders	nausea, vomiting
Skin and Subcutaneous Tissue Disorders	varicella-like rash, pruritus
Musculoskeletal and Connective Tissue Disorders	arthralgia, myalgia
General Disorders and Administration Site Conditions	fever (oral/axillary temperature >39.0°C or rectal temperature >39.5°C), fatigue, malaise
Rare: ≥0.01% and <0.1%	
Eye Disorders	conjunctivitis
Gastrointestinal Disorders	abdominal pain, diarrhea
Skin and Subcutaneous Tissue Disorders	urticaria

[a] Swelling at the injection site and fever were reported very commonly in studies conducted in adolescents and adults. Swelling was also reported very commonly after the second dose in children under 13 years of age.

A trend for a higher incidence of pain, redness, and swelling after the second dose was observed as compared to the first dose in children under 13 years of age.

The reactogenicity after the second dose in adolescents and adults was not higher than after the first dose. No difference was seen in the reactogenicity profile between initially seropositive and seronegative subjects.

High Rrisk Patients: Reactions at the site of injection (redness, swelling and pain) of VARILRIX are usually mild.

Papulo-vesicular eruptions, rarely accompanied by mild to moderate fever, have appeared a few days up to several weeks after immunization. Such reactions have occurred in less than a quarter of leukemic patients. These eruptions were generally mild and short lived.

Eruptions tend to occur in the more immunocompromised leukemic patients such as those still in the maintenance phase of chemotherapy. The appearance of these eruptions did not influence the clinical management of the patients. There is no evidence that immunization may have an adverse effect on the course of the disease.

Post-Market Adverse Drug Reactions: Following widespread use of the vaccine, the following events have been rarely reported in temporal association with VARILRIX vaccination.

Infections and Infestations: Herpes zoster*.

Immune System Disorders: hypersensitivity, anaphylactic reactions.

Nervous System Disorders: convulsions, cerebellar ataxia*.

DRUG INTERACTIONS: Drug-Drug Interactions: In subjects who have received immune globulins or a blood transfusion, vaccination should be delayed for at least three months because of the likelihood of vaccine failure due to passively acquired varicella antibodies.

DOSAGE AND ADMINISTRATION: Recommended Dose and Dosage Adjustment: One immunizing dose contains 0.5 mL of reconstituted vaccine.

Children (12 months to 12 years of age, inclusive) should receive 2 doses (0.5 mL each) of VARILRIX to ensure optimal protection against varicella with a minimum interval of 6 weeks between doses. If official recommendations prescribe, children in this age group may receive a single 0.5 mL dose of VARILRIX.

Adolescents and adults (13 years of age and older) should receive two 0.5 mL doses with a minimum interval of 6 weeks between doses.

For high risk patients additional doses of vaccine may be required.

Administration: VARILRIX (varicella virus vaccine, live, attenuated (Oka-strain)) should be administered by subcutaneous injection in the deltoid region.

VARILRIX should not be injected intradermally. **VARILRIX must under no circumstances be administered intravascularly.**

Reconstitution: Parenteral Products: VARILRIX is presented as a slightly cream to yellowish or pinkish coloured powder in a monodose glass vial. VARILRIX must be reconstituted by adding the contents of the supplied container of diluent (sterile water for injection) to the vial containing the pellet. After the addition of the diluent to the powder, the mixture should be well shaken until the powder is completely dissolved in the diluent.

Due to minor variations in pH, the colour of the reconstituted vaccine may vary from clear peach to pink coloured solution. The diluent (sterile water for injection) and the reconstituted vaccine should be inspected visually for any foreign particulate matter and/or variation of physical aspect prior to administration. In the event of either being observed, discard the diluent or the reconstituted vaccine.

Alcohol and other disinfecting agents must be allowed to evaporate from the skin before injection of the vaccine since they may inactivate the virus.

VARILRIX should not be mixed with other vaccines in the same syringe.

After reconstitution, it is recommended that the vaccine be injected as soon as possible. However, it has been demonstrated that the reconstituted vaccine may be kept for up to 90 minutes at room temperature (25°C) and up to 8 hours in the refrigerator (2 to 8°C). If not used within these timeframes, the reconstituted vaccine must be discarded.

OVERDOSAGE:

Cases of accidental administration of more than the recommended dose of VARILRIX have been reported. Amongst these cases, the following adverse events were reported: lethargy and convulsions. In the other cases reported as overdose there were no associated adverse events.

For management of a suspected drug overdose, contact your regional Poison Control Centre. See the *CPS* Directory section for a list of Poison Control Centres.

ACTION AND CLINICAL PHARMACOLOGY: Mechanism of Action: Varicella (chickenpox) is caused by primary infection with the varicella-zoster virus (VZV). VARILRIX (varicella virus vaccine, live, attenuated (Oka-strain)) produces an attenuated clinically inapparent varicella infection in susceptible subjects.

VARILRIX stimulates antibodies directed against varicella-zoster virus. Some protection may be obtained by immunization up to 72 hours after exposure to natural varicella. The presence of antibodies is accepted to be an indication of protection.

STORAGE AND STABILITY: The lyophilized vaccine should be stored in a refrigerator at 2 to 8°C. The diluent (sterile water for injection) may be stored in the refrigerator or at ambient temperature (maximum 25°C). The lyophilized vaccine is not affected by freezing.

The reconstituted vaccine may be kept for up to 90 minutes at room temperature (25°C) and up to 8 hours in the refrigerator (2 to 8°C). If not used within these timeframes, the reconstituted vaccine must be discarded.

Do not use beyond the expiry date printed on the label.

INFORMATION FOR THE PATIENT: Published in e-CPS, available by subscription at www.e-cps.ca.

DOSAGE FORMS, COMPOSITION AND PACKAGING: A 0.5 mL dose of the reconstituted vaccine contains not less than $10^{3.3}$ plaque-forming units (PFU) of the varicella-zoster virus. The reconstituted vaccine also contains amino acids, human albumin, lactose, neomycin sulfate, polyalcohols and water for injection. VARILRIX is supplied as a sterile powder and diluent (sterile water for injection) (prefilled syringe or ampoule) for subcutaneous injection. The vaccine must be reconstituted and shaken to ensure a uniform suspension before administration.

VARILRIX is presented as a slightly cream to yellowish or pinkish coloured powder and the diluent, sterile water for injection, presents as a clear and colourless solution.

Single monodose vial with diluent (sterile WFI) in prefilled syringe with separate needle and packages of 10 monodose vials. Diluent (sterile WFI) in ampoules in packages of 10 are available separately. Vials/prefilled syringes are made of neutral type I glass.

Varivax® III

varicella virus vaccine, live, attenuated (Oka/Merck)

Active Immunizing Agent Against Varicella

Merck Frosst

Date of Revision: February 27, 2009

SUMMARY PRODUCT INFORMATION:

Route of Administration	Dosage Form/ Strength	Clinically Relevant Nonmedicinal Ingredients
Subcutaneous injection	Lyophilized powder reconstituted for injection. Each 0.5 mL dose contains a minimum of 1350 PFU (plaque-forming units) of Oka/Merck varicella virus[a]	Hydrolyzed gelatin, neomycin For a complete listing see Dosage Forms, Composition and Packaging.

[a] Minimum potency remaining at expiry 90 minutes after reconstitution and storage at room temperature.

DESCRIPTION: VARIVAX III (varicella virus vaccine, live, attenuated [Oka/Merck]) is a live, attenuated virus vaccine (a lyophilized preparation of the Oka/Merck strain of varicella).

INDICATIONS AND CLINICAL USE: VARIVAX III (varicella virus vaccine, live, attenuated [Oka/Merck]) is indicated for vaccination against varicella in individuals 12 months of age and older.

* This reaction reported after vaccination is also a consequence of wild type varicella infection. There is no indication of an increased risk of its occurrence following vaccination compared with wild type disease.

Revaccination: The duration of protection of VARIVAX III is unknown at present and the need for booster doses is not defined. However, a boost in antibody levels has been observed in vaccinees following exposure to wild-type varicella as well as following a booster dose of varicella vaccine (Oka/Merck) administered four to six years postvaccination.

In a highly vaccinated population, immunity for some individuals may wane due to lack of exposure to wild-type varicella as a result of shifting epidemiology. Post-marketing surveillance studies are ongoing to evaluate the need and timing for booster vaccination. The National Advisory Committee on Immunization (NACI) does not recommend any booster dose(s) after the age-appropriate primary immunization (see Dosage and Administration).

Vaccination with VARIVAX III may not result in protection of all healthy, susceptible children, adolescents, and adults.

CONTRAINDICATIONS: VARIVAX III (varicella virus vaccine, live, attenuated [Oka/Merck]) should not be administered to:

- Individuals with a history of hypersensitivity to any component of the vaccine, including gelatin.
- Individuals with a history of anaphylactoid reaction to neomycin (each dose of reconstituted vaccine contains trace quantities of neomycin).
- Individuals with blood dyscrasias, leukemia, lymphomas of any type, or other malignant neoplasms affecting the bone marrow or lymphatic systems.
- Individuals receiving immunosuppressive therapy* (including high-dose corticosteroids); however, VARIVAX III is not contraindicated for use with topical corticosteroids or low-dose corticosteroids, as are commonly used for asthma prophylaxis. Individuals who are on immunosuppressant drugs are more susceptible to infections than healthy individuals. Vaccination with live attenuated varicella vaccine can result in a more extensive vaccine-associated rash or disseminated disease in individuals on immunosuppressant doses of corticosteroids.
- Individuals with primary and acquired immunodeficiency states, including immunosuppression in association with AIDS or other clinical manifestations of infection with human immunodeficiency virus, except immunosuppression in asymptomatic children with CD4 T-lymphocyte percentages ≥25%.
- Individuals with a family history of congenital or hereditary immunodeficiency, unless the immune competence of the potential vaccine recipient is demonstrated.
- Individuals with active untreated tuberculosis.
- Individuals with any active febrile illness with fever >38.5°C; however, low-grade fever itself is not a contraindication to vaccination.
- Women who are pregnant; the possible effects of the vaccine on fetal development are unknown at this time. However, wild-type varicella is known to sometimes cause fetal harm. If vaccination of postpubertal females is undertaken, pregnancy should be avoided for three months following vaccination (see Warnings and Precautions, Pregnant Women).

WARNINGS AND PRECAUTIONS: Vaccine recipients should avoid use of salicylates for 6 weeks after vaccination with VARIVAX III (varicella virus vaccine, live, attenuated [Oka/Merck]) as Reye's Syndrome has been reported following the use of salicylates during wild-type varicella infection.

General: Adequate treatment provisions, including epinephrine injection (1:1000), should be available for immediate use should an anaphylactoid reaction occur.

The duration of protection from varicella infection after vaccination with VARIVAX III is unknown.

The United States Advisory Committee on Immunization Practices (ACIP) and NACI recommend the vaccine for use in susceptible persons following exposure to varicella (if used within 3 days, and possibly up to 5 days of exposure).

There is an insufficient number of breakthrough chickenpox cases among vaccinated children, adolescents and adults to assess the rate of protection of VARIVAX III against the serious complications of chickenpox (e.g., encephalitis, hepatitis, pneumonia) and during pregnancy (congenital varicella syndrome).

Transmission: Post-marketing experience suggests that transmission of vaccine virus may occur rarely between healthy vaccinees who develop a varicella-like rash and healthy susceptible contacts. Transmission of vaccine virus from vaccinees without a varicella-like rash has been reported but has not been confirmed.

Therefore, vaccine recipients should attempt to avoid, whenever possible, close association with susceptible high-risk individuals for up to six weeks. In circumstances where contact with high-risk individuals is unavoidable, the potential risk of transmission of vaccine virus should be weighed against the risk of acquiring and transmitting wild-type varicella virus. Susceptible high-risk individuals include:

- immunocompromised individuals
- pregnant women without documented history of chickenpox or laboratory evidence of prior infection
- newborn infants of mothers without documented history of chickenpox or laboratory evidence of prior infection

Special Populations: Pregnant Women: There are no adequate and well controlled studies in pregnant women. It is not known whether VARIVAX III can cause fetal harm when administered to a pregnant woman or can affect reproduction capacity. Therefore, VARIVAX III should not be administered to pregnant females; furthermore, pregnancy should be avoided for three months following vaccination (see Contraindications).

A unique Oka/Merck Pregnancy Registry has been in place since 1995. Reporting to the Registry was voluntary. In the first 10 years of the Pregnancy Registry for varicella vaccine (Oka/Merck), of 138 seronegative women and 440 women of unknown serostatus who received varicella vaccine during pregnancy or within 3 months before pregnancy, none had newborns with abnormalities compatible with congenital varicella syndrome. In case of inadvertent use of the Oka/Merck varicella vaccine in a pregnant woman, please contact Merck Frosst Canada Ltd.

Nursing Women: It is not known whether varicella vaccine virus is secreted in human milk. Therefore, because some viruses are secreted in human milk, caution should be exercised if VARIVAX III is administered to a nursing woman.

Pediatrics: No clinical data are available on safety or efficacy of VARIVAX III in children less than one year of age. Administration to infants under twelve months of age is not recommended.

The safety and efficacy of VARIVAX III have not been established in children and young adults who are known to be infected with human immunodeficiency viruses with and without evidence of immunosuppression (see Contraindications).

ADVERSE REACTIONS: Clinical Trial Adverse Drug Reactions: Because clinical trials are conducted under very specific conditions the adverse reaction rates observed in the clinical trials may not reflect the rates observed in practice and should not be compared to the rates in the clinical trials of another vaccine. Adverse drug reaction information from clinical trials is useful for identifying vaccine-related adverse events and for approximating rates.

In clinical trials, varicella vaccine (Oka/Merck) was administered to approximately 17 000 healthy children, adolescents, and adults. Varicella vaccine (Oka/Merck) was generally well tolerated.

In a double-blind, placebo-controlled study among 956 healthy children and adolescents, 914 of whom were serologically confirmed to be susceptible to varicella, the only adverse reactions that occurred at a significantly (p<0.05) greater rate in vaccine recipients than in placebo recipients were pain and redness at the injection site and varicella-like rash.

Children 1 to 12 Years of Age: In clinical trials involving approximately 8900 healthy children monitored for up to 42 days after a single dose of varicella vaccine (Oka/Merck) the frequency of fever, injection-site complaints, or rashes were reported in Table 1.

Table 1: VARIVAX III
Fever, Local Reactions or Rashes (%) in Children 0 to 42 Days Postvaccination

Reaction	N	Postdose 1	Peak Occurrence in Postvaccination Days
Fever ≥39°C oral	8824	14.7%	0–42
Injection site complaints (pain/soreness, swelling and/or erythema, rash, pruritus, hematoma, induration, stiffness)	8913	19.3%	0–2
Varicella-like rash (injection site)	8913	3.4%	8–19
Median number of lesions		2	

* The National Advisory Committee on Immunization states that there is no additional or undue risk in vaccinating the following persons: Patients with nephrotic syndrome or those undergoing hemodialysis and peritoneal dialysis if they are not on immunosuppressive medication; Patients on low-dose steroid therapy (e.g., <2 mg prednisone/kg/day to a maximum of 20 mg/day for <2 weeks); Patients on inhaled or topical steroids.

(cont'd)

Table 1: VARIVAX III *(cont'd)*

Fever, Local Reactions or Rashes (%) in Children 0 to 42 Days Postvaccination

Reaction	N	Postdose 1	Peak Occurrence in Postvaccination Days
Varicella-like rash (generalized)	8913	3.8%	5–26
Median number of lesions		5	

In addition, the most frequently (≥1%) reported adverse experiences, without regard to causality, are listed in decreasing order of frequency: upper respiratory illness, cough, irritability/nervousness, fatigue, disturbed sleep, diarrhea, loss of appetite, vomiting, otitis, diaper rash/contact rash, headache, teething, malaise, abdominal pain, other rash, nausea, eye complaints, chills, lymphadenopathy, myalgia, lower respiratory illness, allergic reactions (including allergic rash, hives), stiff neck, heat rash/prickly heat, insect bites, arthralgia, eczema/dry skin/dermatitis, constipation, itching.

Pneumonitis has been reported rarely (<1%) in children vaccinated with varicella vaccine (Oka/Merck); a causal relationship has not been established.

Febrile seizures have occurred rarely (<0.1%) in children vaccinated with varicella vaccine (Oka/Merck); a causal relationship has not been established.

Adolescents and Adults 13 Years of Age and Older: In clinical trials involving approximately 1600 healthy adolescents and adults, the majority of whom received two doses of varicella vaccine (Oka/Merck) and were monitored for up to 42 days after any dose, the frequency of fever, injection-site complaints, or rashes were reported in Table 2.

Table 2: VARIVAX III

Fever, Local Reactions or Rashes (%) in Adolescents and Adults 0 to 42 Days Postvaccination

Reaction	N	Postdose 1	Peak Occurrence in Postvaccination Days	N	Postdose 2	Peak Occurrence in Postvaccination Days
Fever ≥37.7°C oral	1584	10.2%	14–27	956	9.5%	0–42
Injection site complaints (soreness, erythema, swelling, rash, pruritus, pyrexia, hematoma, induration, numbness)	1606	24.4%	0–2	955	32.5%	0–2
Varicella-like rash (injection site)	1606	3.1%	6–20	955	1.0%	0–6
Median number of lesions		2			2	
Varicella-like rash (generalized)	1606	5.5%	7–21	955	0.9%	0–23
Median number of lesions		5			5.5	

In addition, the most frequently (≥1%) reported adverse experiences, without regard to causality, are listed in decreasing order of frequency: upper respiratory illness, headache, fatigue, cough, myalgia, disturbed sleep, nausea, malaise, irritability/nervousness, diarrhea, stiff neck, lymphadenopathy, chills, eye complaints, abdominal pain, loss of appetite, arthralgia, otitis, itching, vomiting, other rashes, constipation, lower respiratory illness, allergic reactions (including allergic rash, hives), contact rash, cold/canker sore, dizziness, and insect bites.

Post-Marketing Clinical Studies: In a post-marketing study conducted to evaluate short-term safety (follow-up of 30 or 60 days) in approximately 86 000 children, 12 months to 12 years of age, and in approximately 3600 adolescents and adults, 13 years of age and older, varicella vaccine (Oka/Merck) was generally well tolerated. No serious vaccine-related adverse events were reported.

As with any vaccine, there is the possibility that broad use of the vaccine could reveal adverse reactions not observed in clinical trials.

Post-Market Adverse Drug Reactions: Since the vaccine has been marketed, the following additional adverse reactions have been reported regardless of causality:

Body as a Whole: anaphylaxis (including anaphylactic shock) and related phenomena such as angioneurotic edema, facial edema, and peripheral edema; anaphylaxis in individuals with or without allergic history.

Hemic and Lymphatic System: thrombocytopenia (including ITP); lymphadenopathy.

Nervous/Psychiatric: encephalitis; cerebrovascular accident; transverse myelitis; Guillain-Barré syndrome; Bell's palsy; ataxia; febrile and non-febrile seizures; aseptic meningitis; dizziness; paresthesia; irritability.

Respiratory: pharyngitis; pneumonia/pneumonitis.

Skin: Stevens-Johnson syndrome; erythema multiforme; Henoch-Schönlein purpura; secondary bacterial infections of skin and soft tissue, including impetigo and cellulitis; herpes zoster.

DRUG INTERACTIONS: Drug-Drug Interactions: Vaccination should be deferred for at least 5 months following blood or plasma transfusions, or administration of immune globulin or varicella zoster immune globulin (VZIG).

Following administration of VARIVAX III (varicella virus vaccine, live, attenuated [Oka/Merck]), any immune globulin including VZIG should not be given for 2 months thereafter unless its use outweighs the benefits of vaccination.

Results from clinical studies indicate that varicella vaccine (Oka/Merck) can be administered concomitantly with M-M-R II (measles, mumps and rubella virus vaccine, live, attenuated, Merck Frosst Std.) or Tetramune (diphtheria and tetanus toxoids and pertussis vaccine adsorbed and Haemophilus b conjugate vaccine). If varicella vaccine (Oka/Merck) is not given concomitantly with M-M-R II, a one month interval between the two live virus vaccines should be observed.

Limited data from an experimental product containing varicella vaccine suggest that varicella vaccine (Oka/Merck) can be administered concomitantly with DTaP (diphtheria, tetanus, acellular pertussis) and Liquid PedvaxHIB [Haemophilus b conjugate vaccine (meningococcal protein conjugate)] using separate sites and syringes and with OPV (oral poliovirus vaccine).

DOSAGE AND ADMINISTRATION: Recommended Dose and Dosage Adjustment: Pediatrics: Children 12 months to 12 years of age should receive a single 0.5 mL dose administered subcutaneously.

Adolescents/Adults: Adolescents and adults 13 years of age and older should receive a 0.5 mL dose administered subcutaneously at an elected date and a second 0.5 mL dose 4 to 8 weeks later.

Administration: For subcutaneous administration only.

The outer aspect of the upper arm (deltoid region) is the preferred site for injection.

Do not inject intradermally, intravenously, or intramuscularly.

VARIVAX III (varicella virus vaccine, live, attenuated [Oka/Merck]) is recommended for subcutaneous administration. However, during clinical trials, some children received varicella vaccine (Oka/Merck) intramuscularly resulting in seroconversion rates similar to those in children who received the vaccine by the subcutaneous route. Persistence of antibody and efficacy in those receiving intramuscular injections have not been defined.

Reconstitution: To reconstitute the vaccine, use only the diluent supplied (Sterile Diluent for Merck & Co., Inc., live, attenuated, virus vaccines), since it is free of preservatives or other anti-viral substances that might inactivate the vaccine virus.

Caution: A sterile syringe free of preservatives, antiseptics and detergents should be used for each injection and/or reconstitution of VARIVAX III because these substances may inactivate the vaccine virus.

It is important to use a separate sterile syringe and needle for each patient to prevent transmission of infectious agents from one individual to another.

To reconstitute the vaccine, first withdraw 0.7 mL of diluent into the syringe to be used for reconstitution. Inject all the diluent in the syringe into the vial of lyophilized vaccine and gently agitate to mix thoroughly.

Prior to Administration: Inspect the reconstituted solution for particulate matter and discoloration, whenever solution and container permit. VARIVAX III, when reconstituted, is a clear, colourless to pale yellow liquid.

Withdraw the entire contents into a syringe and inject the total volume (about 0.5 mL) of reconstituted vaccine subcutaneously, preferably into the outer aspect of the upper arm (deltoid) or the anterolateral thigh. **To minimize loss of potency, it is recommended that the vaccine be administered immediately after reconstitution. Discard if reconstituted vaccine is not used within 90 minutes. Do not refreeze reconstituted vaccine.**

OVERDOSAGE:

There are no data with regard to overdose.

> For management of a suspected drug overdose, CPhA recommends that you contact your **regional Poison Control Centre**. See the *CPS* Directory section for a list of Poison Control Centres.

ACTION AND CLINICAL PHARMACOLOGY: Varicella: Varicella is a highly communicable disease in children, adolescents, and adults caused by the varicella-zoster virus (VZV). The disease usually consists of 300 to 500 maculopapular and/or vesicular lesions accompanied by a fever [oral temperature ≥37.7°C] in up to 70% of individuals. In Canada, it is estimated that about 350 000 cases occur each year and that 1871 of them will require hospitalization (complicated cases). Approximately 3.5 million cases of varicella occurred annually from 1980-1994 in the United States with the peak incidence occurring in children five to nine years of age. The incidence rate of chickenpox was 8.3-9.1% per year in children one to nine years of age. The attack rate of wild-type varicella following household exposure among healthy susceptible children was shown to be 87%. Although it is generally a benign, self-limiting disease, varicella may be associated with serious complications (e.g., bacterial superinfection, pneumonia, encephalitis, Reye's Syndrome), and/or death. In Canada, during 1994 and 1995, a total of 24 deaths were reported to be caused by chickenpox.

Varicella-zoster virus infection is associated with a 58-fold (95% confidence interval [CI]: 40, 85) increased risk of acquiring invasive Group A Streptococcal (GAS) disease in children. Children with invasive GAS disease and recent chickenpox were more likely to have necrotizing fasciitis (NF) (RR: 6.3; 95% CI: 1.8, 22.3).

STORAGE AND STABILITY: During shipment, to ensure that there is no loss of potency, the vaccine must be maintained at a temperature of 2 to 8°C or colder.

Before reconstitution, VARIVAX III (varicella virus vaccine, live, attenuated [Oka/Merck])) has a shelf-life of 24 months and should be stored at a temperature of 2 to 8°C or colder. Vaccine may be stored at room temperature (23 to 27°C) for a maximum of 6 hours prior to reconstitution. The vaccine may also be stored in a freezer; if subsequently transferred to a refrigerator, **the vaccine should not be refrozen. Do not use past expiry date on the label. Protect from light.**

The vial of diluent should be stored separately at room temperature (20 to 25°C) or in the refrigerator (2 to 8°C).

All vaccines must be discarded after the expiration date.

VARIVAX III has a minimum potency level of approximately 1350 PFU 90 minutes after reconstitution at room temperature (20 to 25°C). **Discard if reconstituted vaccine is not used within 90 minutes. Do not refreeze reconstituted vaccine.**

For additional information regarding stability under conditions other than recommended, call at 1-800-567-2594.

INFORMATION FOR THE PATIENT: Published in e-CPS, available by subscription at www.e-cps.ca.

DOSAGE FORMS, COMPOSITION AND PACKAGING: When reconstituted as directed, each single dose (0.5 mL) contains: varicella virus, Oka/Merck strain (live, attenuated) ≥1350 PFU*. Nonmedicinal ingredients: hydrolyzed gelatin, monosodium L-glutamate, potassium chloride, potassium phosphate monobasic, sodium chloride, sodium phosphate dibasic, sucrose, urea and water for injection. Preservative-free. The diluent is sterile water for injection. Manufacturing process residuals: The product also contains residual components of MRC-5 cells including DNA and protein, and trace quantities of neomycin and fetal bovine serum from MRC-5 culture media. Three mL single-dose Type I glass vials. Each vial contains one dose of lyophilized vaccine (approximately 0.5 mL when reconstituted as directed). The diluent (0.7 mL) is supplied separately in 3 mL single-dose Type I glass vials. The container closure systems of VARIVAX III and the diluent are free of latex. VARIVAX III is available in packages of 1 and 10 single-dose vials. The diluent is also available in packages of 1 and 10 single-dose vials.

VariZIG™

varicella zoster immune globulin (human)

Passive Immunizing Agent

Cangene

Date of Preparation: November 24, 2005

SUMMARY PRODUCT INFORMATION:

Route of Administration	Dosage Form/ Strength	Clinically Relevant Nonmedicinal Ingredients
Intravenous or Intramuscular	Powder for Injection/125 IU	For a complete listing see Dosage Forms, Composition and Packaging.

DESCRIPTION: VariZIG (Varicella Zoster Immune Globulin (Human) Injection) is a sterile freeze-dried gamma globulin (IgG) fraction of human plasma containing antibodies to varicella zoster virus (anti-VZV). Varicella zoster virus (VZV) is the causative agent of chickenpox. VariZIG, is manufactured from plasma collected from healthy, screened donors with high titres of anti-VZV which is purified by an anion-exchange column chromatography method.

VariZIG is prepared from pools of human plasma that may contain the causative agents of hepatitis and other viral diseases. The manufacturing process includes both a Planova 35 nm virus filter that effectively removes lipid-enveloped and non-enveloped viruses based on size and a solvent/detergent treatment step (using tri-n-butyl phosphate and Triton X-1007) that effectively inactivates lipid-enveloped viruses. These two processes are designed to increase product safety by reducing the risk of viral transmission of several viruses including human immunodeficiency virus (HIV), hepatitis B and hepatitis C. However, despite these measures, such products can still potentially transmit disease. There is also the possibility that unknown infectious agents may be present in such products (see Warnings and Precautions).

The product potency is expressed in international units (IU) by comparison to the World Health Organization (WHO) international anti-varicella zoster immune globulin reference preparation. Each vial contains approximately 125 IU of anti-VZV. The final product formulation includes addition of sodium chloride to yield 0.04 M, glycine to yield 0.1 M and polysorbate 80 to yield 0.01%. The accompanying sterile diluent contains 0.8% sodium chloride and 10 mM sodium phosphate. The reconstituted product contains no preservative.

INDICATIONS AND CLINICAL USE: VariZIG is indicated for:

- Prevention or reduction in severity of maternal infections within 4 days of exposure to the varicella zoster virus.

Administration of VariZIG is recommended for prevention or reduction of severity of maternal infections within 4 days of exposure to the varicella zoster virus. Greatest effectiveness of treatment is expected when it is begun within 4 days of exposure; treatment after 4 days is of uncertain value.

Pregnant women may be at a higher risk of complications from chickenpox than healthy adults. The decision to administer VariZIG to a pregnant woman should be evaluated on an individual basis. The clinician should consider the patient's health status, type of exposure, and likelihood of previous unrecognized varicella infections before deciding whether to administer VariZIG. If after careful evaluation of all available information, which may include the use of reliable and sensitive tests for varicella antibody, a normal pregnant woman with significant exposure to varicella is believed susceptible, VariZIG may be administered.

Geriatrics: No data is available.

* Minimum potency remaining at expiry 90 minutes after reconstitution and storage at room temperature.

Pediatrics: Based on the efficacy of other varicella zoster immune globulins in at-risk pediatric populations, similar efficacy can be expected for VariZIG. However, no specific pediatric clinical data is available for VariZIG.

CONTRAINDICATIONS: VariZIG should **not** be administered to patients:

- With known immunity to varicella zoster virus; i.e. with previous varicella infections or varicella vaccination.
- Who are deficient in IgA. While VariZIG contains less than 40 µg/mL IgA, individuals who are deficient in IgA may have the potential to develop IgA antibodies and have an anaphylactoid reaction.
- With a history of anaphylactic or other severe systemic reaction to immune globulins.
- Who are hypersensitive to this drug or to any ingredient in the formulation or component of the container. For a complete listing, see Dosage Forms, Composition and Packaging.

WARNINGS AND PRECAUTIONS:

> **Serious Warnings and Precautions**
> VariZIG is prepared from pools of human plasma, which may contain the causative agents of hepatitis and other viral diseases. The risk that such products will transmit an infectious agent has been reduced by screening plasma donors for prior exposure to certain viruses, by testing for the presence of certain current virus infections, and by inactivating and/or removing certain viruses during manufacturing. Despite these measures, such products can still potentially transmit disease. There is also the possibility that unknown infectious agents may be present in such products.
>
> True hypersensitivity reactions are rare. These reactions can occur in very rare cases of IgA deficiency or hypersensitivity to human globulin. In case of allergic or anaphylactic reaction, the infusion should be stopped immediately. In case of shock, the current medical standards for treatment of shock should be observed.
>
> The physician should discuss the risks and benefits of this product with the patient, before prescribing or administrating to the patient (see Warnings and Precautions, General).

General: Following administration of VariZIG (IV or IM), patients should be kept under observation for at least 20 minutes for monitoring of potential adverse effects. This product should be administered under the supervision of a qualified health professional that is experienced in the use of passive immunizing agents and in the management of pregnant women exposed to varicella zoster virus. Appropriate management of therapy and complications is only possible when adequate diagnostic and treatment facilities are readily available.

Products made from human plasma may contain infectious agents, such as viruses, that can cause disease. The risk that such products will transmit an infectious agent has been reduced by screening plasma donors for prior exposure to certain viruses, by testing for the presence of certain current virus infections, and by inactivating and/or removing certain viruses. The manufacturing process includes both a Planova 35 nm virus filter that effectively removes lipid-enveloped and non-enveloped viruses based on size and a solvent/detergent treatment step (using tri-n-butyl phosphate and Triton X-1007) that effectively inactivates lipid-enveloped viruses by irreversibly destroying the lipid coat. These two processes are designed to increase product safety by reducing the risk of viral transmission of several viruses including human immunodeficiency virus (HIV), hepatitis B and hepatitis C. However, despite these measures, such products can still potentially transmit disease. There is also the possibility that unknown infectious agents may be present in such products. Individuals who receive infusions of blood or plasma products may develop signs and/or symptoms of some viral infections. All infections thought to have been possibly transmitted by this product should be reported by the physician or other health care provider to Cangene Corporation at 1-800-768-2304 (phone) or 1-800-768-2281 (fax).

Cardiovascular: Rare thrombotic events have been reported in association with immune globulin intravenous (Human) (IGIV). Patients at risk may include those with a history of atherosclerosis, multiple cardiovascular risk factors, advanced age, impaired cardiac output, hypercoagulable disorders, prolonged periods of immobilization, and/or known or suspected hyperviscosity. The potential risks of VariZIG to produce thrombotic events is significantly lower than IGIV due to the differences in amount of protein infused, the volume of product infused and the relative health of the patient populations. Although the risk of thrombotic adverse events following VariZIG is extremely low, care should be taken in patients at risk for hyperviscosity, including those with cryoglobulins, fasting chylomicronemia/markedly high triacylglycerols (triglycerides), or monoclonal gammopathies. In such patients, it may be preferable to administer VariZIG intramuscularly as thrombotic adverse events have only been reported following intravenous administration of immune globulins.

Renal: IGIV products have been reported to be associated with renal dysfunction, acute renal failure, osmotic nephrosis, proximal tubular nephropathy, and death. Although these reports of renal dysfunction and acute renal failure have been associated with the use of many licensed IGIV products, those that contained sucrose as a stabilizer and were administered at daily doses of 400 mg of sucrose (or greater) have accounted for a disproportionate share of the total number. **VariZIG does not contain sucrose** as a stabilizer, and the recommended dose of VariZIG contains significantly lower amounts of protein than IGIV products (i.e. <0.75 g per dose vs. >20 g per dose). Patients predisposed to acute renal failure include the following: patients with any degree of pre-existing renal insufficiency, diabetes mellitus, volume depletion, sepsis, or paraproteinemia, or patients who are receiving known nephrotoxic drugs.

Respiratory: There have been rare reports of noncardiogenic pulmonary edema [Transfusion-Related Acute Lung Injury (TRALI)] in patients administered IGIV. TRALI is characterized by severe respiratory distress, pulmonary edema, hypoxemia, normal left ventricular function, and fever and typically occurs within 1 to 6 hours after transfusion. Patients with TRALI may be managed using oxygen therapy with adequate ventilatory support. The potential risks of VariZIG to produce severe respiratory complications is significantly lower than IGIV due to the differences in amount of protein infused, the volume of product infused and the relative health of the patient populations. Although the risk of severe respiratory complications following VariZIG is extremely low, care should be taken in patients with pre-existing respiratory conditions. In such patients, it may be preferable to administer VariZIG intramuscularly as severe respiratory adverse events have only been reported following intravenous administration of immune globulins.

VariZIG recipients should be monitored for pulmonary adverse reactions. If TRALI is suspected, appropriate tests should be performed for the presence of anti-neutrophil antibodies in both the product and patient serum.

Sensitivity/Resistance: Although allergic reactions have not been reported following VariZIG administration (see Adverse Reactions, Adverse Drug Reaction Overview), epinephrine and diphenhydramine should be available for the treatment of any allergic reactions.

VariZIG (Varicella Zoster Immune Globulin (Human)) contains trace quantities of IgA. The physician must weigh the potential benefit of treatment with VariZIG against the potential for hypersensitivity reactions. Individuals deficient in IgA have a potential for development of IgA antibodies and anaphylactic reactions after administration of blood components containing IgA. It has been reported that as little as 15 µg IgA/mL of blood product may elicit an anaphylactic reaction in IgA deficient individuals.

Special Populations: Pregnant Women: Animal reproduction studies have not been conducted with VariZIG. VariZIG should be given to pregnant women only if clearly needed. No new risk in pregnancy was identified in a randomized trial of VariZIG to prevent or modify the course of varicella zoster virus infection in 60 pregnant women. Clinical use of other immune globulins, such as Rho (D) immune globulin, administered during pregnancy suggests that there are no known adverse effects on the fetus from the immune globulin itself.

Nursing Women: It is not known whether VariZIG is excreted in human milk. Because many drugs are excreted in human milk, caution should be exercised when VariZIG is administered to a nursing mother.

Pediatrics (<18 years of age): Safety and effectiveness in the pediatric population have not been established for VariZIG.

Geriatrics (>65 years of age): Safety and effectiveness in the geriatric population have not been adequately established for VariZIG.

Monitoring and Laboratory Tests: In the prevention of varicella zoster infections, the presence of passively administered varicella zoster antibody in the blood can lead to false-positive tests for immunity to VZV for 3 months after receiving VariZIG. Therefore, serodiagnostic tests to determine immunity to VZV should not be performed within 3 months of VariZIG administration.

Immune globulin administration may impair the efficacy of live attenuated vaccines such as measles, rubella, mumps and varicella. Vaccination with live virus vaccines should be deferred until approximately three months after administration of VariZIG. People, who received VariZIG shortly after live virus vaccination, should be revaccinated 3 months after the administration of the immune globulin.

ADVERSE REACTIONS: Adverse Drug Reaction Overview: Reactions to VariZIG (Varicella Zoster Immune Globulin (Human)) are rare and mild in intensity. In the intended patient population, the most frequent treatment related adverse events were pain at the injection site (17%), headache (7%), and rash (5%). Other less frequent adverse reactions were myalgia, rigors, fatigue, nausea and flushing. The adverse event profile of VariZIG is expected to be comparable to other commercially available varicella zoster immune globulin (human) and intravenous immune globulin (human) products. The most common expected adverse drug reactions are chills, fever, headaches, vomiting, allergic reactions, nausea, arthralgia and moderate low back pain.

As is the case with all drugs of this nature, there is a remote chance of an anaphylactic/anaphylactoid reaction with VariZIG in individuals with hypersensitivity to blood products. In the event of an immediate reaction (anaphylaxis) characterized by collapse, rapid pulse, wheezing, difficulty breathing, pallor, cyanosis, edema or generalized urticaria, epinephrine should be instituted followed by administration of hydrocortisone, if necessary.

Clinical Trial Adverse Drug Reactions: Because clinical trials are conducted under very specific conditions the adverse reaction rates observed in the clinical trials may not reflect the rates observed in practice and should not be compared to the rates in the clinical trials of another drug. Adverse drug reaction information from clinical trials is useful for identifying drug-related adverse events and for approximating rates.

A randomized, active controlled clinical trial was conducted in 60 pregnant women without immunity to varicella zoster virus confirmed by a latex agglutination test. Patients were stratified on the basis of time from first exposure to varicella (1-4 days and 5-14 days) and randomized to receive 125 IU/10 kg body weight to a maximum dose of 625 IU of VariZIG (IV or IM) or another commercially available varicella zoster immune globulin, VZIG (IM). The patients were followed for 42 days after administration of VariZIG or active VZIG control for adverse events. A total of 94 adverse events were reported by 31 of the 41 patients (76%) treated with either IM or IV VariZIG; 24 of the adverse events were considered related to the administration of VariZIG. The most frequent adverse drug reactions were pain at injection site (17%), headache (7%), and rash (5%). Similar incidences of adverse drug reactions were reported in the reference product arm of the study. See Table 1.

Table 1: VariZIG

Adverse Drug Reactions Reported by Pregnant Women Following VariZIG or VZIG Administration

		VariZIG (IV or IM; N=41)			VZIG (IM; N=19)		
System Organ Class	**Preferred Tern**	**# of events**	**# of subj**	**% of subj**	**# of events**	**# of subj**	**% of subj**
All Body Systems	All preferred Terns	24	14	34.1	16	12	63.2
Gastrointestinal Disorders	Nausea	1	1	2.4	1	1	5.3
General Disorders and Administration Site Conditions	Fatigue	1	1	2.4	0	0	0.0
	Injection site bruising	1	1	2.4	0	0	0.0
	Injection site pain	7	7	17.1	9	9	47.4
	Injection site pruritus	1	1	2.4	0	0	0.0
	Injection site tenderness	1	1	2.4	0	0	0.0
	Pain	0	0	0.0	1	1	5.3
	Pyrexia	0	0	0.0	1	1	5.3
	Chills	1	1	2.4	0	0	0.0
Musculoskeletal and Connective Tissue Disorders	Myalgia	1	1	2.4	0	0	0.0
	Neck pain	0	0	0.0	1	1	5.3
Nervous System Disorders	Dizziness	0	0	0.0	1	1	5.3
	Dysgeusia	1	1	2.4	0	0	0.0
	Headache	3	3	7.3	2	2	10.5
Psychiatric Disorders	Insomnia	1	1	2.4	0	0	0.0

(cont'd)

Table 1: VariZIG *(cont'd)*
Adverse Drug Reactions Reported by Pregnant Women Following VariZIG or VZIG Administration

System Organ Class	Preferred Term	VariZIG (IV or IM; N=41)			VZIG (IM; N=19)		
		# of events	# of subj	% of subj	# of events	# of subj	% of subj
Skin and Subcutaneous Tissue Disorders	Dermatitis	1	1	2.4	0	0	0.0
	Rash erythematous	1	1	2.4	0	0	0.0
	Rash	2	2	4.9	0	0	0.0
Vascular Disorders	Flushing	1	1	2.4	0	0	0.0

In addition to the VZ-006 clinical study, VariZIG safety data was also collected from two other clinical studies conducted in either normal healthy subjects (VZ-001)27 or geriatric patients with post-herpetic neuralgia (VZ-003)28. Similar incidences and types of adverse events were reported in these patient populations following administration of VariZIG.

Post-Market Adverse Drug Reactions: There is no post-marketing experience.

DRUG INTERACTIONS:

Serious Drug Interactions
- Live attenuated virus vaccines: immune globulin administration may impair the efficacy of live attenuated virus vaccines for a period of 3 months or more (see Drug Interactions, Overview).

Overview: Immune globulin administration may impair the efficacy of live attenuated vaccines such as measles, rubella, mumps and varicella. Vaccination with live virus vaccines should be deferred until approximately three months after administration of VariZIG. Patients who have received VariZIG shortly after live virus vaccination, should be revaccinated 3 months after the administration of the immune globulin.

Administration of VariZIG with other drugs has not been evaluated. It is recommended that VariZIG be administered separately from other drugs. Refer to Dosage and Administration for information on drug compatibility.

Drug-Drug Interactions: See Table 2.

Table 2: VariZIG
Established or Potential Drug-Drug Interactions

Varicella Zoster Immune Globulin (Human)	Reference	Effect	Clinical comment
Live attenuated virus vaccines (e.g. measles, rubella, mumps, varicella)	T	Immune globulin may impair efficacy	If VariZIG is given less than 14 days after vaccination, revaccination should be considered.

Legend: C=Case Study; CT=Clinical Trial; T=Theoretical.

Interactions with other drugs have not been established.

Drug-Food Interactions: Interactions with foods have not been established.

Drug-Herb Interactions: Interactions with herbs have not been established.

Drug-Laboratory Test Interactions: After administration of VariZIG, a transitory increase of passively transferred antibodies in the patient's blood may result in misleading positive results in serological testing (e.g. Coomb's test).

DOSAGE AND ADMINISTRATION: **Recommended Dose and Dosage Adjustment:** Dosing of VariZIG is based on body weight. The recommended dose is 125 IU/10 kg body weight up to a maximum of 625 IU. VariZIG should be given by intravenous or intramuscular administration. The minimum dose is 125 IU and the maximum dose of 625 IU should be sufficient to prevent or modify infection in at-risk patients. VariZIG should be administered within 96 hours of varicella exposure, preferably as soon as possible. The efficacy of varicella immune globulins in the reduction of incidence or severity of varicella infections in at-risk patients has not been demonstrated when administered more than 96 hours after exposure.

Reconstitution: See Table 3.

Table 3: VariZIG
Reconstitution

Route of Administration	Vial Size	Volume of Diluent to be added to vial	Approximate Available Volume	Nominal Concentration per mL
Intravenous	6 mL	2.5 mL	2.4 mL	50 IU/mL
Intramuscular	6 mL	1.25 mL	1.2 mL	100 IU/mL

VariZIG should be reconstituted only with the accompanying vial of Sterile Diluent. Use aseptic technique throughout. Reconstitute shortly before use. To reconstitute:

1. Remove caps from the diluent and product vials.
2. Wipe exposed central portion of each rubber stopper with suitable disinfectant.
3. Withdraw 2.5 mL of diluent for IV administration or 1.25 mL diluent for IM administration using a suitable syringe and needle.
4. Inject diluent slowly at an angle so that the liquid is directed onto the inside glass wall of the vial containing the freeze-dried pellet.
5. Wet pellet by gently tilting and inverting the vial. Avoid frothing. Gently swirl upright vial until dissolved (less than ten minutes). **Do not shake.**

Parenteral products such as VariZIG (Varicella Zoster Immune Globulin (Human)) should be inspected for particulate matter and discoloration prior to administration. Reconstituted product can be stored for up to 12 hours at 2-8°C prior to use.

Administration: If VariZIG is administered by an intravenous route, then reconstituted drug should be infused into a suitable vein over 3-5 minutes.

If VariZIG is administered by an intramuscular route, it should be given as an injection into the deltoid muscle or the anterolateral aspects of the upper thigh. Due to the risk of sciatic nerve injury, the gluteal region should not be used as a routine injection site. If the gluteal region is used, use only the upper, outer quadrant.

To prevent the transmission of infectious agents from one person to another, a separate sterile disposable syringe and needle should be used for each individual patient.

There are no available data on concomitant use of VariZIG and other medications. Admixtures of VariZIG with other drugs have not been evaluated. It is recommended that VariZIG be administered separately from other drugs or medications that the patient may be receiving. If a pre-existing catheter must be used for IV administration, the line should be flushed with 0.9% Sodium Chloride for injection USP before administering the product.

OVERDOSAGE:
In clinical studies, 15 patients were administered a VariZIG dose of 50 IU/kg of body weight (IV). This dose is approximately four times greater than the recommended dose for the immunoprophylaxis of varicella. Related adverse events were mostly mild in nature. All of the related adverse events of chills, nausea, pain at the injection site, rash, urticaria, asthenia, headache, back pain, arthralgia, dizziness and twitch have previously been reported with the use of immune globulins and are expected adverse events. No clinically significant changes in laboratory test results or vital signs were associated with VariZIG infusion.

For management of a suspected drug overdose, CPhA recommends that you contact your **regional Poison Control Centre**. See the *CPS* Directory section for a list of Poison Control Centres.

ACTION AND CLINICAL PHARMACOLOGY: Mechanism of Action: VariZIG is used for the passive immunization of pregnant women in the event of contact with varicella zoster virus. Administration of VariZIG prevents or reduces the severity of maternal infections with varicella zoster virus when administered within 4 days of initial contact. It is hypothesized that anti-VZV antibodies in VariZIG bind to proteins on the varicella virus; thereby, preventing or reducing the severity of varicella infections.

Upon absorption into the circulation, varicella zoster antibodies persist for 6 weeks or longer. The precise concentration of antibodies that must be achieved or maintained in order to attenuate varicella is not known. In a clinical study of pregnant women without immunity to varicella, the overall infection frequency of 29% observed in patients administered VariZIG was significantly lower than the expected rate of 89% in at-risk pregnant women exposed to varicella. In addition to decreasing the incidence of varicella infections, VariZIG decreased the severity of varicella infections compared to historical cases of varicella infections in at-risk patients.

Pharmacodynamics: No pharmacodynamic studies have been conducted with VariZIG.

Pharmacokinetics: The pharmacokinetic properties of immune globulin preparations manufactured by anion exchange chromatography and having the same formulation as VariZIG (Varicella Zoster Immune Globulin (Human)) have been determined. Peak levels (C_{max}) following IV were reached in less than three hours while C_{max} was reached 2 to 7 days after intramuscular administration. In the VariZIG clinical development program, higher levels of varicella zoster antibodies were detected in patients 2 days after IV administration than compared to patients receiving VariZIG IM. Based on non-compartmental analysis, the area under the curve (AUC) was similar in these studies regardless of the route of administration of the drug. The half-life of hyperimmune products is approximately 18-24 or 24-30 days following IV or IM administration, respectively. Upon absorption into the circulation, varicella zoster antibodies are expected to persist for at least 6 weeks. Thus, an intravenous administration is expected to lead to a higher peak passive antibody level that is achieved earlier than with an intramuscular route of administration. However, the levels of circulating antibodies over time are expected to be similar regardless of route of administration.

Absorption: Following IM administration of varicella immune globulin products, varicella antibodies are detectable within 2-3 days. The maximum concentration of varicella antibodies is expected to occur within 3-7 days of VariZIG administration.

Distribution: The bioavailability following IV administration of VariZIG is expected to be immediate and complete, with passive antibodies quickly distributed between plasma and extravascular spaces. Based on AUC comparisons from pharmacokinetic studies of other hyperimmune products, IM administration is expected to be nearly 100% bioavailable.

Metabolism: Immune globulins and immune complexes are metabolized in the reticuloendothelial system.

Excretion: Based on the studies with other immune globulin products, an elimination half-life of 18-24 or 24-30 days for VariZIG is expected following IV or IM administration, respectively. The half-life is expected to vary from patient to patient.

STORAGE AND STABILITY: VariZIG is stable at 2-8°C until the expiry date indicated on the label. Store VariZIG at 2-8°C. **Do not freeze. Do not use after expiration date.**

SPECIAL HANDLING INSTRUCTIONS: The product should be brought to room or body temperature immediately prior to use. Following reconstitution, the product should be clear or slightly opalescent. Do not use product that appears cloudy or contains deposits.

INFORMATION FOR THE PATIENT: Published in e-CPS, available by subscription at www.e-cps.ca.

DOSAGE FORMS, COMPOSITION AND PACKAGING: Each vial of sterile freeze-dried solution contains: approximately 125 IU of Varicella Zoster Immune Globulin (Human) (60-200 mg human immunoglobulin G). Nonmedicinal ingredients: glycine, polysorbate 80 and sodium chloride. Preservative-free. Six mL type 1 glass tubing vials fitted with a 20 mm lyophilization stopper of rubber formulation and a 20 mm flip-off seal, and one vial of 8.5 mL, Sterile Diluent (0.8% Sodium Chloride, 10mM Sodium Phosphate) for reconstitution of VariZIG.

The reader is invited to consult CPhA's monograph **ACE Inhibitors** and **Thiazide Diuretics**.

Vaseretic® Pr

enalapril—hydrochlorothiazide

Angiotensin Converting Enzyme Inhibitor—Diuretic

Merck Frosst

Date of Revision: December 24, 2009

SUMMARY PRODUCT INFORMATION:

Route of Administration	Dosage Form/Strength	Nonmedicinal Ingredients
Oral	Tablets[a] 10 mg/25 mg[b]	Corn starch, lactose, magnesium stearate, pregelatinized starch, sodium bicarbonate and the following colouring agent: red ferric oxide See Dosage Forms, Composition and Packaging.

[a] Each tablet is made with 10 mg of enalapril maleate that appears as 8 mg of enalapril sodium in the tablet and 25 mg of hydrochlorothiazide.

[b] The splitting of VASERETIC 10 mg/25 mg tablets is not advised.

INDICATIONS AND CLINICAL USE: VASERETIC (enalapril and hydrochlorothiazide) is indicated for:
- Treatment of essential hypertension in patients for whom this combination therapy is appropriate

In using VASERETIC consideration should be given to the risk of angioedema (see Warnings and Precautions).

VASERETIC is not indicated for initial therapy. Patients in whom enalapril and diuretic are initiated simultaneously can develop symptomatic hypotension (see Drug Interactions).

Patients should be titrated on individual drugs. If the fixed combination represents the dose and dosing frequency determined by this titration, the use of VASERETIC may be more convenient in the management of patients. If during maintenance therapy dosage adjustment is necessary it is advisable to use the individual drugs.

Geriatrics (>65 years of age): See Dosage and Administration.

Pediatrics (<18 years of age): VASERETIC is not recommended in this age group.

CONTRAINDICATIONS: VASERETIC is contraindicated in:
- Patients who are hypersensitive to this product or to any ingredient in the formulation. For a complete listing, see Dosage Forms, Composition and Packaging.
- Patients with a history of angioneurotic edema relating to previous treatment with an angiotensin converting enzyme inhibitor.
- Patients with hereditary or idiopathic angioedema.

Because of the hydrochlorothiazide component, this product is contraindicated in:
- Patients with anuria or hypersensitivity to other sulfonamide-derived drugs.

WARNINGS AND PRECAUTIONS:

> **Serious Warnings and Precautions**
> - When used in pregnancy, angiotensin converting enzyme (ACE) inhibitors can cause injury or even death of the developing fetus. When pregnancy is detected, VASERETIC should be discontinued as soon as possible.

General: Angioedema: Angioedema of the face, extremities, lips, tongue, glottis and/or larynx has been reported rarely in patients treated with VASERETIC. This may occur at any time during treatment and may be life threatening.

Very rarely, fatalities have been reported due to angioedema associated with laryngeal edema or tongue edema. Patients with involvement of the tongue, glottis or larynx are likely to experience airway obstruction, especially those with a history of airway surgery. However, where there is involvement of the tongue, glottis or larynx, likely to cause airway obstruction, appropriate therapy which may include subcutaneous adrenaline solution 1:1000 (0.3 mL to 0.5 mL) and/or measures to ensure a patent airway should be administered promptly when indicated.

If angioedema occurs, VASERETIC should be promptly discontinued and appropriate monitoring should be instituted to ensure complete resolution of symptoms prior to dismissing the patient. Even in those instances where swelling of only the tongue is involved, without respiratory distress, patients may require prolonged observation since this may be life threatening and treatment with antihistamines and corticosteroids may not be sufficient.

In patients who experience angioedema, future administration is contraindicated (see Contraindications).

The incidence of angioedema during ACE inhibitor therapy has been reported to be higher in black than in non-black patients.

Patients with a history of angioedema unrelated to ACE inhibitor therapy may be at increased risk of angioedema while receiving an ACE inhibitor (see Contraindications).

Anaphylactoid Reactions during Membrane Exposure: Anaphylactoid reactions have been reported in patients dialysed with high-flux membranes (e.g. polyacrylonitrile [PAN]) and treated concomitantly with an ACE inhibitor. Dialysis should be stopped immediately if symptoms such as nausea, abdominal cramps, burning, angioedema, shortness of breath and severe hypotension occur. Symptoms are not relieved by antihistamines. In these patients consideration should be given to using a different type of dialysis membrane or a different class of antihypertensive agent.

Anaphylactoid Reactions during Desensitization: There have been isolated reports of patients experiencing sustained life-threatening anaphylactoid reactions while receiving ACE inhibitors during desensitizing treatment with hymenoptera (bees, wasp) venom. In the same patients, these reactions have been avoided when ACE inhibitors were temporarily withheld for at least 24 hours, but they have reappeared upon inadvertent rechallenge.

Anaphylactoid Reactions during LDL Apheresis: Rarely, patients receiving ACE inhibitors during low-density lipoprotein (LDL)-apheresis with dextran sulfate have experienced life-threatening anaphylactoid reactions. These reactions were avoided by temporarily withholding ACE inhibitor therapy prior to each apheresis.

Cardiovascular: Hypotension: Symptomatic hypotension has occurred after administration of enalapril, usually after the first or second dose or when the dose was increased. It is more likely to occur in patients who are volume depleted by diuretic therapy, dietary salt restriction, dialysis, diarrhea, or vomiting. Therefore, VASERETIC should not be used to start therapy or when a dose change is needed. In patients with severe congestive heart failure, with or without associated renal insufficiency, excessive hypotension has been observed and may be associated with oliguria and/or progressive azotemia, and rarely with acute renal failure and/or death. Because of the potential fall in blood pressure in these patients, therapy with enalapril should be started under very close medical supervision, usually in a hospital. Such patients should be followed closely for the first two weeks of treatment and whenever the dose of enalapril and/or hydrochlorothiazide is increased. In patients with ischemic heart or cerebrovascular disease, an excessive fall in blood pressure could result in a myocardial infarction or cerebrovascular accident (see Adverse Reactions).

If hypotension occurs, the patient should be placed in supine position and, if necessary, receive an intravenous infusion of normal saline. A transient hypotensive response is not a contraindication to further doses which usually can be given without difficulty once the blood pressure has increased after volume expansion.

Valvular Stenosis: There is concern on theoretical grounds that patients with aortic stenosis might be at particular risk of decreased coronary perfusion when treated with vasodilators because they do not develop as much afterload reduction.

Ear/Nose/Throat: Cough: A dry, persistent cough, which usually disappears only after withdrawal or lowering of the dose of VASERETIC has been reported.

Such possibility should be considered as part of the differential diagnosis of the cough.

Endocrine and Metabolism: Metabolism: Hyperuricemia may occur or acute gout may be precipitated in certain patients receiving thiazide therapy.

Thiazides may decrease serum protein-bound iodine (PBI) levels without signs of thyroid disturbance.

Thiazides have been shown to increase excretion of magnesium; this may result in hypomagnesemia.

Thiazides may decrease urinary calcium excretion. Thiazides may cause intermittent and slight elevation of serum calcium in the absence of known disorders of calcium metabolism. Marked hypercalcemia may be evidence of hidden hyperparathyroidism. Thiazides should be discontinued before carrying out tests for parathyroid function.

Increases in cholesterol and triglyceride levels may be associated with thiazide diuretic therapy.

Hematologic: Neutropenia/Agranulocytosis: Agranulocytosis and bone marrow depression have been caused by angiotensin converting enzyme inhibitors. Several cases of agranulocytosis and neutropenia have been reported in which a causal relationship to enalapril cannot be excluded. Current experience with the drug shows the incidence to be rare. Periodic monitoring of white blood cell counts should be considered, especially in patients with collagen vascular disease and renal disease.

Hepatic/Biliary/Pancreatic: Patients with Impaired Liver Function: Hepatitis, jaundice (hepatocellular and/or cholestatic), elevations of liver enzymes and/or serum bilirubin have occurred during therapy with enalapril in patients with or without pre-existing liver abnormalities (see Adverse Reactions). In most cases the changes were reversed on discontinuation of the drug.

Should the patient receiving VASERETIC experience any unexplained symptoms (see Information for the Patient), particularly during the first weeks or months of treatment, it is recommended that a full set of liver function tests and any other necessary investigation be carried out. Discontinuation of VASERETIC should be considered when appropriate.

There are no adequate studies in patients with cirrhosis and/or liver dysfunction. VASERETIC should be used with particular caution in patients with pre-existing liver abnormalities. In such patients baseline liver function tests should be obtained before administration of the drug and close monitoring of response and metabolic effects should apply.

Thiazides should be used with caution in patients with impaired hepatic function or progressive liver disease, since minor alterations of fluid and electrolyte balance may precipitate hepatic coma.

Nitritoid Reactions—Gold: Nitritoid reactions (symptoms include facial flushing, nausea, vomiting and symptomatic hypotension) have been reported rarely in patients on therapy with injectable gold (sodium aurothiomalate) and concomitant ACE inhibitor therapy including enalapril (including VASERETIC) (see Drug Interactions).

Peri-Operative Considerations: Surgery/Anesthesia: In patients undergoing major surgery or during anesthesia with agents that produce hypotension, enalapril blocks angiotensin II formation, secondary to compensatory renin release. If hypotension occurs and is considered to be due to this mechanism, it can be corrected by volume expansion.

Thiazides may increase the responsiveness to tubocurarine.

Renal: Renal Impairment: As a consequence of inhibiting the renin-angiotensin-aldosterone system, changes in renal function have been seen in susceptible individuals. In patients whose renal function may depend on the activity of the renin-angiotensin-aldosterone system, such as patients with bilateral renal artery stenosis, unilateral renal artery stenosis to a solitary kidney, or severe congestive heart failure, treatment with agents that inhibit this system has been associated with oliguria, progressive azotemia, and rarely, acute renal failure and/or death. In susceptible patients, concomitant diuretic use may further increase risk.

Use of VASERETIC should include appropriate assessment of renal function.

Thiazides may not be appropriate diuretics for use in patients with renal impairment and are ineffective at creatinine clearance values of 30 mL/min or below (i.e., moderate or severe renal insufficiency).

Azotemia: Azotemia may be precipitated or increased by hydrochlorothiazide. Cumulative effects of the drug may develop in patients with impaired renal function. If increasing azotemia and oliguria occur during treatment of severe progressive renal disease the diuretic should be discontinued.

Hyperkalemia: Elevated serum potassium (greater than 5.7 mEq/L) was observed in approximately one percent of hypertensive patients in clinical trials with enalapril alone. In most cases these were isolated values which resolved despite continued therapy. Hyperkalemia was a cause of discontinuation of therapy in 0.28% of hypertensive patients. Risk factors for the development of hyperkalemia include renal insufficiency, diabetes mellitus, and concomitant use of potassium-sparing diuretics (e.g., spironolactone, eplerenone, triamterene, or amiloride), potassium supplements, or potassium-containing salt substitutes. The use of potassium supplements, potassium-sparing diuretics, or potassium-containing salt substitutes particularly in patients with impaired renal function should be given only for documented hypokalemia and with caution and frequent monitoring of serum potassium since they may lead to a significant increase in serum potassium. Hyperkalemia can cause serious, sometimes fatal, arrhythmias. If concomitant use of VASERETIC and any of the above-mentioned agents is deemed appropriate, they should be used with caution and with frequent monitoring of serum potassium (see Drug Interactions, Agents Increasing Serum Potassium).

Sensitivity/Resistance: Hypersensitivity Reactions: Sensitivity reactions to hydrochlorothiazide may occur in patients with or without a history of allergy or bronchial asthma.

The possibility of exacerbation or activation of systemic lupus erythematosus has been reported in patients treated with hydrochlorothiazide.

Special Populations: Pregnant Women: ACE inhibitors can cause fetal and neonatal morbidity and mortality when administered to pregnant women. Several dozen cases have been reported in the world literature. When pregnancy is detected, VASERETIC should be discontinued as soon as possible.

The use of ACE inhibitors during the second and third trimesters of pregnancy has been associated with fetal and neonatal injury including hypotension, neonatal skull hypoplasia, anuria, reversible or irreversible renal failure, and death. Oligohydramnios has also been reported, presumably resulting from decreased fetal renal function, associated with fetal limb contractures, craniofacial deformation, and hypoplastic lung development.

Prematurity, and patent ductus arteriosus and other structural cardiac malformations, as well as neurologic malformations, have also been reported following exposure in the first trimester of pregnancy.

Infants with a history of in utero exposure to ACE inhibitors should be closely observed for hypotension, oliguria, and hyperkalemia. If oliguria occurs, attention should be directed toward support of blood pressure and renal perfusion. Exchange transfusion or dialysis may be required as a means of reversing hypotension and/or substituting for impaired renal function; however, limited experience with those procedures has not been associated with significant clinical benefit.

Enalapril has been removed from the neonatal circulation by peritoneal dialysis with some clinical benefit and may, theoretically, be removed by exchange transfusion, although there is no experience with the latter procedure.

Animal Data: Maternal and fetal toxicity occurred in some rabbits given enalapril at doses of 1 mg/kg/day or more. Saline supplementation prevented the maternal and fetal toxicity seen at doses of 3 and 10 mg/kg/day, but not at 30 mg/kg/day (50 times the maximum human dose). Enalapril was not teratogenic in rabbits.

There was no fetotoxicity or teratogenicity in rats treated with enalapril at doses up to 200 mg/kg/day (333 times the maximum human dose). Fetotoxicity expressed as a decrease in average fetal weight, occurred in rats given 1200 mg/kg/day of enalapril, but did not occur when these animals were supplemented with saline. Enalapril crosses the placental barrier in rats and hamsters.

Nursing Women: Both enalapril and thiazides appear in human milk. Use of ACE inhibitors (VASERETIC) is not recommended during breast-feeding.

Pediatrics: VASERETIC has not been studied in children and, therefore, use in this age group is not recommended.

ADVERSE REACTIONS: Adverse Drug Reaction Overview: In clinical trials involving 1580 hypertensive patients, including over 300 patients treated for one year or more, the most severe adverse reactions were: angioedema (0.3%), syncope (1.3%) and renal failure (0.1%).

The most frequent clinical adverse experiences in controlled trials were: dizziness (8.6%), headache (5.5%), fatigue (3.9%) and cough (3.5%).

Adverse experiences that have occurred have been those that were previously reported with enalapril or hydrochlorothiazide when used separately for the treatment of hypertension.

Clinical Trial Adverse Drug Reactions: Because clinical trials are conducted under very specific conditions the adverse reaction rates observed in the clinical trials may not reflect the rates observed in practice and should not be compared to the rates in the clinical trials of another drug. Adverse drug reaction information from clinical trials is useful for identifying drug-related adverse events and for approximating rates.

Adverse reactions occurring in greater than one percent of patients treated with VASERETIC in controlled trials are shown in Table 1.

Table 1: VASERETIC

Hypertension

	Percent of Patients in Controlled Studies	
	VASERETIC (n=1580) Incidence (%)	**Placebo (n=230) Incidence (%)**
Body as a Whole		
Fatigue	3.9	2.6
Orthostatic Effects	2.3	0
Asthenia	2.4	0.9
Cardiovascular		
Chest Pain	1.1	—[a]
Syncope	1.3	—[a]
Orthostatic Hypotension	1.5	—[a]
Palpitations	1	—[a]
Dermatologic		
Rash	1.3	—[a]
Digestive		
Diarrhea	2.1	1.7
Nausea	2.5	1.7
Vomiting	1.6	—[a]
Abdominal Pain	1.1	—[a]
Musculoskeletal		
Muscle Cramps	2.7	0.9
Nervous/Psychiatric		
Headache	5.5	9.1
Dizziness	8.6	4.3
Paresthesia	1.1	—[a]
Respiratory		

(cont'd)

Table 1: VASERETIC *(cont'd)*

Hypertension

	Percent of Patients in Controlled Studies	
	VASERETIC (n=1580) Incidence (%)	**Placebo (n=230) Incidence (%)**
Cough	3.5	0.9
Urogenital		
Impotence	2.2	0.5

[a] No data available.

Less Common Clinical Trial Adverse Drug Reactions (<1%): Hypertension: Cardiovascular: hypotension, myocardial infarction, tachycardia.
Digestive: dysphagia, dyspepsia, constipation, flatulence, dry mouth.
Hearing: tinnitus.
Hematologic: anemia.
Hypersensitivity: angioedema.
Metabolic and Nutritional: gout.
Musculoskeletal: back pain, arthralgia.
Nervous System/Psychiatric: insomnia, nervousness, somnolence, vertigo.
Respiratory: dyspnea.
Skin: pruritus, hyperhidrosis, diaphoresis.
Special Senses: taste disturbance.
Urogenital: renal failure, oliguria, proteinuria, decreased libido, urinary tract infection.
Abnormal Hematologic and Clinical Chemistry Findings: Hyperkalemia: (see Warnings and Precautions).
Creatinine, Blood Urea Nitrogen (BUN): In controlled clinical trials minor increases in blood urea nitrogen and serum creatinine, reversible upon discontinuation of therapy, were observed in about 0.6% of patients with essential hypertension treated with VASERETIC.

In patients treated with enalapril alone, increases in serum creatinine and BUN were reported in about 20% of patients with renovascular hypertension and in about 0.2% of patients with essential hypertension.

Hemoglobin and Hematocrit: Decreases in hemoglobin and hematocrit (mean approximately 0.34 g% and 1.0 vol% respectively) occurred frequently in hypertensive patients treated with enalapril, but were rarely of clinical importance. In clinical trials, less than 0.1% of patients discontinued therapy due to anemia.
Others: Elevations of liver enzymes and/or serum bilirubin have occurred (see Warnings and Precautions).
Post-Market Adverse Drug Reactions: Adverse Reactions Reported in Uncontrolled Trials and/or Marketing Experience: VASOTEC: Other serious clinical adverse experiences occurring since the drug was marketed or adverse experiences occurring in 0.5 to 1.0 percent of patients in clinical trials are listed below and, within each category, are in order of decreasing severity.
Body as a Whole: anaphylactoid reactions (see Warnings and Precautions).
Cardiovascular: cardiac arrest; myocardial infarction or cerebrovascular accident, possibly secondary to excessive hypotension in high-risk patients (see Warnings and Precautions); pulmonary embolism and infarction; pulmonary edema; angina pectoris; arrhythmia including atrial tachycardia and bradycardia; atrial fibrillation; palpitation, Raynaud's phenomenon.
Digestive: ileus, pancreatitis, hepatic failure, hepatitis (hepatocellular or cholestatic jaundice), liver function abnormalities (see Warnings and Precautions), melena, anorexia, dyspepsia, constipation, glossitis, stomatitis, dry mouth.
Hematologic: rare cases of neutropenia, thrombocytopenia, hemolytic anemia and bone marrow depression.
Musculoskeletal: muscle cramps.
Nervous/Psychiatric: vertigo, depression, confusion, ataxia, somnolence, insomnia, nervousness, peripheral neuropathy (e.g., paresthesia, dysesthesia), dream abnormality.
Respiratory: bronchospasm, rhinorrhea, sore throat and hoarseness, asthma, upper respiratory infection, pulmonary infiltrates, eosinophilic pneumonitis.
Skin: exfoliative dermatitis, toxic epidermal necrolysis, Stevens-Johnson syndrome, pemphigus, herpes zoster, erythema multiforme, urticaria, pruritus, alopecia, flushing, diaphoresis, photosensitivity.
Special Senses: blurred vision, taste alteration, anosmia, tinnitus, conjunctivitis, dry eyes, tearing, hearing impairment.
Urogenital: renal failure, oliguria, renal dysfunction (see Warnings and Precautions and Dosage and Administration), flank pain, gynecomastia, impotence.

A symptom complex has been reported which may include some or all of the following: fever, serositis, vasculitis, myalgia/myositis, arthralgia/arthritis, a positive antinuclear antibody (ANA), elevated erythrocyte sedimentation rate, eosinophilia and leukocytosis. Rash, photosensitivity or other dermatologic manifestations may occur. These symptoms may be reversible upon discontinuation of therapy.

In very rare cases, intestinal angioedema has been reported with angiotensin converting enzyme inhibitors including enalapril.
Laboratory Test Findings: hyponatremia.
VASERETIC (Marketing Experience Only): arthralgia, asthenia, constipation, decreased libido, dry mouth, dyspepsia, flatulence, gout, hypotension, syndrome of inappropriate antidiuretic hormone secretion (SIADH), tachycardia, tinnitus, vertigo.

DRUG INTERACTIONS:

> **Serious Drug Interactions**
> - Concomitant use of lithium and VASERETIC is not recommended.

Drug-Drug Interactions: Hypotension—Patients on Diuretic Therapy: Patients on diuretics and especially those in whom diuretic therapy was recently instituted, may occasionally experience an excessive reduction of blood pressure after initiation of therapy with enalapril. The possibility of hypotensive effects with enalapril can be minimized by either discontinuing the diuretic or increasing the salt intake prior to initiation of treatment with enalapril (see Warnings and Precautions and Dosage and Administration).
Agents Increasing Serum Potassium: Since enalapril decreases aldosterone production, elevation of serum potassium may occur. Potassium-sparing diuretics such as spironolactone, eplerenone, triamterene or amiloride, or potassium supplements should be given only for documented hypokalemia and with caution and frequent monitoring of serum potassium particularly in patients with impaired renal function since they may lead to a significant increase in serum potassium. If concomitant use of VASERETIC and any of these agents is deemed appropriate, they should be used with caution and with frequent monitoring of serum potassium. Salt substitutes which contain potassium should also be used with caution (see Warnings and Precautions, Hyperkalemia).
Agents Causing Renin Release: The antihypertensive effect of VASERETIC is augmented by antihypertensive agents that cause renin release (e.g., diuretics).
Agents Affecting Sympathetic Activity: Agents affecting sympathetic activity (e.g., ganglionic blocking agents or adrenergic neuron blocking agents) may be used with caution. Beta-adrenergic blocking drugs add some further antihypertensive effect to enalapril.
Lithium: Diuretic agents and ACE inhibitors reduce the renal clearance of lithium and add a high risk of lithium toxicity. Concomitant use is not recommended.
d-Tubocurarine: Thiazide drugs may increase the responsiveness to tubocurarine.
Insulin: Insulin requirements in diabetic patients treated with thiazide diuretics may be increased. Diabetes mellitus which has been latent may become manifest during thiazide administration.
Alcohol, Barbiturates, or Narcotics: In the presence of thiazide diuretics, potentiation of orthostatic hypotension may occur.
Corticosteroids, ACTH: Intensified electrolyte depletion, particularly hypokalemia may occur when given concomitantly with thiazide diuretics.
Cholestyramine and Colestipol Resins: Absorption of hydrochlorothiazide is impaired in the presence of anionic exchange resins. Single doses of either cholestyramine or colestipol resins bind the hydrochlorothiazide and reduce its absorption from the gastrointestinal tract by up to 85 and 43%, respectively.
Pressor Amines (e.g., norepinephrine): In the presence of thiazide diuretics, possible decreased response to pressor amines may be seen but not sufficient to preclude their use.
Non-steroidal Anti-inflammatory Drugs (NSAIDs) Including Selective Cyclooxygenase-2 Inhibitors: In some patients, the administration of a non-steroidal anti-inflammatory agent can reduce the diuretic, natriuretic, and antihypertensive effects of loop, potassium-sparing and thiazide diuretics. Therefore, when VASERETIC and non-steroidal anti-inflammatory agents are used concomitantly, the patient should be observed closely to determine if the desired effect of the diuretic is obtained.

The antihypertensive effect of enalapril may be diminished with concomitant non-steroidal anti-inflammatory drug use including selective cyclooxygenase-2 inhibitors (COX-2 inhibitors). In some patients with compromised renal function (e.g., elderly patients or patients who are volume-depleted including those on diuretic therapy) who are being treated with NSAIDS including selective COX-2 inhibitors, the coadministration of ACE inhibitors or angiotensin II receptor antagonists may result in further deterioration of renal function. Cases of acute renal failure, usually reversible, have also been reported. This combination should therefore be administered with caution in this patient population.
Gold: Nitritoid reactions (symptoms include facial flushing, nausea, vomiting and symptomatic hypotension) have been reported rarely in patients on therapy with injectable gold (sodium aurothiomalate) and concomitant ACE inhibitor therapy including enalapril (including VASERETIC) (see Warnings and Precautions).
Probenecid: The rate of elimination of hydrochlorothiazide is decreased somewhat by the coadministration of probenecid without, however, an accompanying reduction in diuresis.

DOSAGE AND ADMINISTRATION: Dosing Considerations:

- **Dosage must be individualized.**
- **The fixed combination is not for initial therapy.**
- **The dose of VASERETIC should be determined by the titration of the individual components.**
- **Special attention for dialysis patients.**
- **The splitting of VASERETIC 10 mg/25 mg tablets is not advised.**

Recommended Dose and Dosage Adjustment: Once the patient has been successfully titrated with the individual components as described below, VASERETIC may be substituted if the titrated doses and dosing schedule can be achieved by the fixed combination (see Indications and Clinical Use and Warnings and Precautions).

Patients usually do not require doses in excess of 50 mg of hydrochlorothiazide daily, particularly when combined with antihypertensive agents. Therefore, since each tablet of VASERETIC contains 25 mg of hydrochlorothiazide (in combination with 10 mg of enalapril), the total daily dosage of VASERETIC should not exceed two tablets of VASERETIC 10 mg/25 mg. If further blood pressure control is indicated, additional doses of enalapril or other nondiuretic, antihypertensive agents should be considered.

For enalapril monotherapy the recommended initial dose in patients not on diuretics is 5 mg of enalapril once a day. Dosage should be adjusted according to blood pressure response. The usual dosage range of enalapril is 10 to 40 mg per day administered in a single dose or two divided doses. In some patients treated once daily, the antihypertensive effects may diminish toward the end of the dosing interval. In such patients an increase in dosage or twice-daily administration should be considered. If blood pressure is not controlled with enalapril alone, a diuretic may be added.

In patients who are currently being treated with a diuretic, symptomatic hypotension occasionally may occur following the initial dose of enalapril. The diuretic should, if possible, be discontinued for two to three days before beginning therapy with enalapril to reduce the likelihood of hypotension (see Warnings and Precautions). If the patient's blood pressure is not controlled with enalapril alone, diuretic therapy may be resumed.

If the diuretic cannot be discontinued, an initial dose of 2.5 mg of enalapril should be used to determine whether excessive hypotension occurs.
Geriatrics (>65 years of age): In the elderly the starting dose of enalapril should be 2.5 mg since some elderly patients may be more responsive to enalapril than younger patients.
Dosing Adjustment in Renal Impairment: In patients with mild to moderate renal impairment (creatinine clearance >30 mL/min), the usual dose titration of the individual components is required. The recommended initial dose of enalapril, when used alone in patients with mild renal impairment, is 5 mg. In patients with moderate renal impairment, the initial dose of enalapril, when used alone, is 2.5 mg.

When concomitant diuretic therapy is required in patients with severe renal impairment, a loop diuretic, rather than a thiazide diuretic is preferred for use with enalapril. Therefore, for patients with severe renal dysfunction, VASERETIC is not recommended (see Warnings and Precautions, Anaphylactoid Reactions during Membrane Exposure).

OVERDOSAGE:

No specific information is available on the treatment of overdosage with VASERETIC. Treatment is symptomatic and supportive. Therapy with VASERETIC should be discontinued and the patient observed closely. Suggested measures include induction of emesis and/or gastric lavage, and correction of dehydration, electrolyte imbalance and hypotension by established procedures.

Enalaprilat may be removed from the general circulation by hemodialysis (see Warnings and Precautions, Anaphylactoid Reactions during Membrane Exposure).
Enalapril: The most prominent feature of overdosage reported to date is marked hypotension, beginning some six hours after ingestion of tablets, concomitant with blockade of the renin-angiotensin system, and stupor. Serum enalaprilat levels 100 times and 200 times higher than usually seen after therapeutic doses have been reported after ingestion of 300 mg and 440 mg of enalapril, respectively.

The recommended treatment of overdosage is intravenous infusion of normal saline solution.
Hydrochlorothiazide: The most common signs and symptoms observed are those caused by electrolyte depletion (hypokalemia, hypochloremia, hyponatremia) and dehydration resulting from excessive diuresis. If digitalis has also been administered hypokalemia may accentuate cardiac arrhythmias.

> For management of a suspected drug overdose, contact your regional Poison Control Centre. See the *CPS* Directory section for a list of Poison Control Centres.

ACTION AND CLINICAL PHARMACOLOGY: Mechanism of Action: VASERETIC combines the action of an angiotensin converting enzyme inhibitor, enalapril, and that of a diuretic, hydrochlorothiazide.
Enalapril: Angiotensin converting enzyme (ACE) is a peptidyl dipeptidase which catalyses the conversion of angiotensin I to the pressor substance, angiotensin II. After absorption, enalapril, a pro-drug, is hydrolyzed to enalaprilat, its active metabolite, which inhibits ACE. Inhibition of ACE results in decreased plasma angiotensin II, which leads to increased plasma renin activity (due to removal of negative feedback of renin release) and decreased aldosterone secretion. Although the latter decrease is small, it results in a small increase in serum potassium. In patients treated with enalapril and a thiazide diuretic there was essentially no change in serum potassium (see Warnings and Precautions).

ACE is identical to kininase II. Thus, enalapril may also block the degradation of bradykinin, a potent vasodepressor peptide. However, the role that this plays in the therapeutic effects of enalapril is unknown.

While the mechanism through which enalapril lowers blood pressure is believed to be primarily the suppression of the renin-angiotensin-aldosterone system, enalapril also lowers blood pressure in patients with low-renin hypertension.
Hydrochlorothiazide: Hydrochlorothiazide is a diuretic and antihypertensive which interferes with the renal tubular mechanism of electrolyte reabsorption. It increases excretion of sodium and chloride in approximately equivalent amounts. Natriuresis may be accompanied by some loss of potassium and bicarbonate. While this compound is predominantly a saluretic agent, in vitro studies have shown that it has a carbonic anhydrase inhibitory action which seems to be relatively specific for the renal tubular mechanism. It does not appear to be concentrated in erythrocytes or the brain in sufficient amounts to influence the activity of carbonic anhydrase in those tissues.
Pharmacodynamics: Enalapril: Administration of enalapril to patients with hypertension results in a reduction of both supine and standing blood pressure. Abrupt withdrawal of enalapril has not been associated with a rapid increase in blood pressure. In most patients studied, after oral administration of an individual dose of enalapril, the onset of antihypertensive activity is seen at one hour with peak reduction of blood pressure achieved by 4-6 hours. At recommended doses, the antihypertensive effect has been shown to be maintained for at least 24 hours. In some patients the effect may diminish towards the end of the dosing interval (see Dosage and Administration). On occasion, achievement of optimal blood pressure reduction may require several weeks of therapy.

In hemodynamic studies in patients with essential hypertension, blood pressure reduction was accompanied by a reduction in peripheral arterial resistance with an increase in cardiac output and little or no change in heart rate. Following administration of enalapril, there was an increase in renal blood flow; glomerular filtration rate was usually unchanged.

When used in hypertensive, normolipidemic patients, enalapril had no effect on plasma lipoprotein fractions.

Studies in dogs indicate that enalapril crosses the blood brain barrier poorly, if at all; enalaprilat does not enter the brain.
Hydrochlorothiazide: Hydrochlorothiazide is useful in the treatment of hypertension. It may be used alone or as an adjunct to other antihypertensive drugs. Hydrochlorothiazide does not affect normal blood pressure.

Onset of the diuretic action following oral administration occurs in 2 hours and the peak action in about 4 hours. Diuretic activity lasts about 6 to 12 hours.

Pharmacokinetics: See Table 2 and Table 3.

Table 2: VASERETIC

Summary of Enalaprilat's Pharmacokinetic Parameters in Healthy Volunteers Further to a 10 mg Oral Dose of Enalapril

	C_{max} (ng/mL)	$t_{½}$ (h)[a]	$AUC_{0-\infty}$ (ng·h/mL)
Single dose mean	32.3	11	423

[a] Effective half-life of accumulation.

Table 3: VASERETIC

Summary of Hydrochlorothiazide's Pharmacokinetic Parameters in Healthy Volunteers Further to a 25 mg Oral Dose of Hydrochlorothiazide

	C_{max} (ng/mL)	$t_{½}$ (h)	AUC_{0-36} (ng·h/mL)	Renal Clearance (mL/min)	Volume of distribution (L/kg)
Single dose mean	127	5.6–14.8	978	257	0.83

Enalapril: Absorption: Following oral administration, enalapril is rapidly absorbed with peak serum concentrations of enalapril occurring within one hour. Based on urinary recovery the extent of absorption of enalapril is approximately 60%.

The absorption of enalapril is not influenced by the presence of food in the gastrointestinal tract.

Metabolism: Following absorption, enalapril is rapidly and extensively hydrolyzed to enalaprilat, a potent angiotensin converting enzyme inhibitor (which itself is poorly absorbed). Peak serum concentrations of enalaprilat occur 3 to 4 hours after an oral dose of enalapril. Except for conversion to enalaprilat, there is no evidence of significant metabolism of enalapril.

Excretion: Excretion of enalapril is primarily renal. Approximately 94% of the dose is recovered in the urine and feces as enalaprilat or enalapril. The principal components in urine are enalaprilat, accounting for about 40% of the dose, and intact enalapril.

The serum concentration profile of enalaprilat exhibits a prolonged terminal phase, apparently associated with binding to ACE. The effective half-life for accumulation of enalaprilat following multiple doses of enalapril is 11 hours.

Hydrochlorothiazide: Absorption: Hydrochlorothiazide is rapidly absorbed from the gastrointestinal tract with an oral bioavailability of about 65% to 75%. Peak concentrations of hydrochlorothiazide were reached approximately 2 hours after dosing.

Distribution: Hydrochlorothiazide crosses the placental but not the blood-brain barrier and is excreted in breast milk. Its apparent volume of distribution is 0.83 L/kg.

Metabolism: Hydrochlorothiazide is not metabolized.

Excretion: Hydrochlorothiazide is eliminated rapidly by the kidney. The plasma half-life is 5.6-14.8 hours when the plasma levels can be followed for at least 24 hours. At least 61% of the oral dose is eliminated unchanged within 24 hours.

Enalapril—Hydrochlorothiazide: Concomitant administration of enalapril and hydrochlorothiazide has little, or no effect on the bioavailability of either drug. The combination tablet is bioequivalent to concomitant administration of the separate entities.

Special Populations and Conditions: Pediatrics: Safety and effectiveness in pediatric patients have not been established.

Race: The antihypertensive effect of angiotensin converting enzyme inhibitors is generally lower in black than in non-black patients.

Renal Insufficiency: The disposition of enalapril and enalaprilat in patients with renal insufficiency is similar to that in patients with normal renal function until the glomerular filtration rate is 30 mL/min (0.50 mL/s) or less. With renal function ≤30 mL/min (≤0.50 mL/s), peak and trough enalaprilat levels increase, time to peak concentration increases and time to steady state may be delayed. The effective half-life of enalaprilat following multiple doses of enalapril is prolonged at this level of renal insufficiency (see Dosage and Administration). Enalaprilat is dialyzable at the rate of 62 mL/min (1.03 mL/s).

STORAGE AND STABILITY: Store at controlled room temperature (15-30°C). Protect from moisture.

INFORMATION FOR THE PATIENT: Published in e-CPS, available by subscription at www.e-cps.ca.

DOSAGE FORMS, COMPOSITION AND PACKAGING: Each rust, oval-shaped, scored tablet, with MSD 720 on one side, contains: enalapril maleate 10 mg that appears as enalapril sodium 8 mg and hydrochlorothiazide 25 mg. Nonmedicinal ingredients: cornstarch, lactose, magnesium stearate, pregelatinized starch, red ferric oxide and sodium bicarbonate. The splitting of VASERETIC 10 mg/25 mg tablets is not advised. Blister packages of 28.

(Shown in Product Identification Section)

The reader is invited to consult CPhA's monograph **ACE Inhibitors.**

Vasotec®

enalapril

Angiotensin Converting Enzyme Inhibitor

Merck Frosst

Date of Revision: December 24, 2009

SUMMARY PRODUCT INFORMATION:

Route of Administration	Dosage Form/ Strength	All Nonmedicinal Ingredients
Oral	Tablet[a] 2.5 mg, 5 mg, 10 mg, 20 mg	Corn starch, lactose, magnesium stearate, pregelatinized starch, sodium bicarbonate. Tablets 10 and 20 mg contain red and/or yellow iron oxidest. See Dosage Forms, Composition and Packaging.

[a] The splitting of VASOTEC tablets is not advised. Each tablet is made with 2.5, 5, 10 or 20 mg of enalapril maleate that appears as 2, 4, 8 or 16 mg of enalapril sodium in the tablets.

INDICATIONS AND CLINICAL USE: VASOTEC: VASOTEC (enalapril) is indicated for:

- essential or renovascular hypertension
- treatment of symptomatic congestive heart failure

Hypertension: VASOTEC is indicated in the treatment of essential or renovascular hypertension. It is usually administered in association with other drugs, particularly thiazide diuretics.

In using VASOTEC consideration should be given to the risk of angioedema (see Warnings and Precautions).

Geriatrics (>65 years of age): See Dosage and Administration.

Pediatrics (<16 years of age): VASOTEC may be used in children (see Dosage and Administration).

Congestive Heart Failure: VASOTEC is indicated in the treatment of symptomatic congestive heart failure usually in combination with diuretics and/or digitalis. In these patients, VASOTEC improves symptoms, increases survival, and decreases the frequency of hospitalization. Treatment with VASOTEC should be initiated under close medical supervision.

In clinically stable asymptomatic patients with left ventricular dysfunction (ejection fraction ≤35%), VASOTEC decreases the rate of development of overt heart failure and decreases the incidence of hospitalization for heart failure.

CONTRAINDICATIONS: VASOTEC is contraindicated in:

- Patients who are hypersensitive to these products or to any ingredient in their formulation. For a complete listing, see Dosage Forms, Composition and Packaging.
- Patients with a history of angioneurotic edema relating to previous treatment with an angiotensin converting enzyme inhibitor.
- Patients with hereditary or idiopathic angioedema.

WARNINGS AND PRECAUTIONS:

Serious Warnings and Precautions

- When used in pregnancy, angiotensin converting enzyme (ACE) inhibitors can cause injury or even death of the developing fetus. When pregnancy is detected, VASOTEC should be discontinued as soon as possible.

General: Angioedema: Angioedema of the face, extremities, lips, tongue, glottis and/or larynx has been reported rarely in patients treated with VASOTEC. This may occur at any time during treatment and may be life threatening.

Very rarely, fatalities have been reported due to angioedema associated with laryngeal edema or tongue edema. Patients with involvement of the tongue, glottis or larynx are likely to experience airway obstruction, especially those with a history of airway surgery. However, where there is involvement of the tongue, glottis or larynx, likely to cause airway obstruction, appropriate therapy which may include subcutaneous adrenaline solution 1:1000 (0.3 mL to 0.5 mL) and/or measures to ensure a patent airway should be administered promptly when indicated.

If angioedema occurs, VASOTEC should be discontinued promptly and appropriate monitoring should be instituted to ensure complete resolution of symptoms prior to dismissing the patient. Even in those instances where swelling of only the tongue is involved, without respiratory distress, patients may require prolonged observation since this may be life threatening and treatment with antihistamines and corticosteroids may not be sufficient.

In patients who experience angioedema, future administration is contraindicated (see Contraindications).

The incidence of angioedema during ACE inhibitor therapy has been reported to be higher in black than in non-black patients.

Patients with a history of angioedema unrelated to ACE inhibitor therapy may be at increased risk of angioedema while receiving an ACE inhibitor (see Contraindications).

Anaphylactoid Reactions during Membrane Exposure: Anaphylactoid reactions have been reported in patients dialysed with high-flux membranes (e.g., polyacrylonitrile [PAN]) and treated concomitantly with an ACE inhibitor. Dialysis should be stopped immediately if symptoms such as nausea, abdominal cramps, burning, angioedema, shortness of breath and severe hypotension occur. Symptoms are not relieved by antihistamines. In these patients consideration should be given to using a different type of dialysis membrane or a different class of antihypertensive agent.

Anaphylactoid Reactions during Desensitization: There have been isolated reports of patients experiencing sustained life-threatening anaphylactoid reactions while receiving ACE inhibitors during desensitizing treatment with hymenoptera (bees, wasp) venom. In the same patients, these reactions have been avoided when ACE inhibitors were temporarily withheld for at least 24 hours, but they have reappeared upon inadvertent rechallenge.

Anaphylactoid Reactions during LDL Apheresis: Rarely, patients receiving ACE inhibitors during low-density lipoprotein (LDL)-apheresis with dextran sulfate have experienced life-threatening anaphylactoid reactions. These reactions were avoided by temporarily withholding ACE inhibitor therapy prior to each apheresis.

Cardiovascular: Hypotension: Symptomatic hypotension has occurred after administration of VASOTEC, usually after the first or second dose or when the dose was increased. It is more likely to occur in patients who are volume depleted by diuretic therapy, dietary salt restriction, dialysis, diarrhea, or vomiting. In patients with severe congestive heart failure, with or without associated renal insufficiency, excessive hypotension has been observed and may be associated with oliguria and/or progressive azotemia, and rarely with acute renal failure and/or death. Because of the potential fall in blood pressure in these patients, therapy should be started under very close medical supervision, usually in a hospital. Such patients should be followed closely for the first two weeks of treatment and whenever the dose of enalapril and/or diuretic is increased. Similar considerations may apply to patients with ischemic heart or cerebrovascular disease in whom an excessive fall in blood pressure could result in a myocardial infarction or cerebrovascular accident (see Adverse Reactions).

If hypotension occurs, the patient should be placed in supine position and, if necessary, receive an intravenous infusion of normal saline. A transient hypotensive response is not a contraindication to further doses which usually can be given without difficulty once the blood pressure has increased after volume expansion.

Valvular Stenosis: There is concern on theoretical grounds that patients with aortic stenosis might be at particular risk of decreased coronary perfusion when treated with vasodilators because they do not develop as much afterload reduction.

Ear/Nose/Throat: Cough: A dry, persistent cough, which usually disappears only after withdrawal or lowering of the dose of VASOTEC has been reported.

Such possibility should be considered as part of the differential diagnosis of the cough.

Endocrine and Metabolism: Hypoglycemia: Rare cases of hypoglycemia in diabetic patients on oral antidiabetic agents or insulin have been reported. Diabetic patients treated with oral antidiabetic agents or insulin starting an ACE inhibitor should be told to closely monitor for hypoglycemia, especially during the first month of combined use. In addition, hypoglycemia appeared to be more likely to occur during the first weeks of combined treatment and in patients with renal impairment (see Adverse Reactions).

Hematologic: Neutropenia/Agranulocytosis: Agranulocytosis and bone marrow depression have been caused by angiotensin converting enzyme inhibitors. Several cases of agranulocytosis and neutropenia have been reported in which a causal relationship to enalapril cannot be excluded. Current experience with the drug shows the incidence to be rare. Periodic monitoring of white blood cell counts should be considered, especially in patients with collagen vascular disease and renal disease.

Hepatic/Biliary/Pancreatic: Patients with Impaired Liver Function: Hepatitis, jaundice (hepatocellular and/or cholestatic), elevations of liver enzymes and/or serum bilirubin have occurred during therapy with VASOTEC in patients with or without pre-existing liver abnormalities (see Adverse Reactions). In most cases the changes were reversed on discontinuation of the drug.

Should the patient receiving VASOTEC experience any unexplained symptoms (see Information for the Patient), particularly during the first weeks or months of treatment, it is recommended that a full set of liver function tests and any other necessary investigation be carried out. Discontinuation of VASOTEC should be considered when appropriate.

There are no adequate studies in patients with cirrhosis and/or liver dysfunction. VASOTEC should be used with particular caution in patients with pre-existing liver abnormalities. In such patients baseline liver function tests should be obtained before administration of the drug and close monitoring of response and metabolic effects should apply.

Nitritoid Reactions—Gold: Nitritoid reactions (symptoms include facial flushing, nausea, vomiting and symptomatic hypotension) have been reported rarely in patients on therapy with injectable gold (sodium aurothiomalate) and concomitant ACE inhibitor therapy including enalapril (see Drug Interactions).

Peri-Operative Considerations: Surgery/Anesthesia: In patients undergoing major surgery or during anesthesia with agents that produce hypotension, enalapril blocks angiotensin II formation, secondary to compensatory renin release. If hypotension occurs and is considered to be due to this mechanism, it can be corrected by volume expansion.

Renal: Renal Impairment: As a consequence of inhibiting the renin-angiotensin-aldosterone system, changes in renal function have been seen in susceptible individuals. In patients whose renal function may depend on the activity of the renin-angiotensin-aldosterone system, such as patients with bilateral renal artery stenosis, unilateral renal artery stenosis to a solitary kidney, or severe congestive heart failure, treatment with agents that inhibit this system has been associated with oliguria, progressive azotemia, and rarely, acute renal failure and/or death. In susceptible patients, concomitant diuretic use may further increase risk.

Use of VASOTEC should include appropriate assessment of renal function.

Hyperkalemia: Elevated serum potassium (greater than 5.7 mEq/L) was observed in approximately one percent of hypertensive patients in clinical trials with enalapril. In most cases these were isolated values which resolved despite continued therapy. Hyperkalemia was a cause of discontinuation of therapy in 0.28% of hypertensive patients. Risk factors for the development of hyperkalemia include renal insufficiency, diabetes mellitus, and concomitant use of potassium-sparing diuretics (e.g., spironolactone, eplerenone, triamterene, or amiloride), potassium supplements, or potassium-containing salt substitutes. The use of potassium supplements, potassium-sparing diuretics, or potassium-containing salt substitutes particularly in patients with impaired renal function should be given only for documented hypokalemia and with caution and frequent monitoring of serum potassium since they may lead to a significant increase in serum potassium. Hyperkalemia can cause serious, sometimes fatal, arrhythmias. If concomitant use of VASOTEC and any of the above-mentioned agents is deemed appropriate, they should be used with caution and with frequent monitoring of serum potassium (see Drug Interactions, Agents Increasing Serum Potassium).

Special Populations: Pregnant Women: ACE inhibitors can cause fetal and neonatal morbidity and mortality when administered to pregnant women. When pregnancy is detected, VASOTEC should be discontinued as soon as possible.

The use of ACE inhibitors during the second and third trimesters of pregnancy has been associated with fetal and neonatal injury including hypotension, neonatal skull hypoplasia, anuria, reversible or irreversible renal failure, and death. Oligohydramnios has also been reported, presumably resulting from decreased fetal renal function, associated with fetal limb contractures, craniofacial deformation, and hypoplastic lung development.

Prematurity, and patent ductus arteriosus and other structural cardiac malformations, as well as neurologic malformations, have also been reported following exposure in the first trimester of pregnancy.

Infants with a history of in utero exposure to ACE inhibitors should be closely observed for hypotension, oliguria, and hyperkalemia. If oliguria occurs, attention should be directed toward support of blood pressure and renal perfusion. Exchange transfusion or dialysis may be required as a means of reversing hypotension and/or substituting for impaired renal function; however, limited experience with those procedures has not been associated with significant clinical benefit.

Enalapril has been removed from the neonatal circulation by peritoneal dialysis with some clinical benefit and may, theoretically, be removed by exchange transfusion, although there is no experience with the latter procedure.

Animal Data: Maternal and fetal toxicity occurred in some rabbits given enalapril at doses of 1 mg/kg/day or more. Saline supplementation prevented the maternal and fetal toxicity seen at doses of 3 and 10 mg/kg/day, but not at 30 mg/kg/day (50 times the maximum human dose). Enalapril was not teratogenic in rabbits.

There was no fetotoxicity or teratogenicity in rats treated with enalapril at doses up to 200 mg/kg/day (333 times the maximum human dose). Fetotoxicity expressed as a decrease in average fetal weight, occurred in rats given 1200 mg/kg/day of enalapril, but did not occur when these animals were supplemented with saline. The drug crosses the placental barrier in rats and hamsters.

Nursing Women: Enalapril and enalaprilat are secreted in human milk in trace amounts. Use of ACE inhibitors (VASOTEC) is not recommended during breast-feeding.

Pediatrics (<16 years of age): The safety and antihypertensive effect have been studied short-term (one month) in patients aged 6 to 16 years (see Dosage and Administration and Action and Clinical Pharmacology, Pharmacokinetics).

VASOTEC is not recommended in neonates and in children with glomerular filtration rate <30 mL/min/1.73 m^2, as no data are available.

ADVERSE REACTIONS: VASOTEC: Adverse Drug Reaction Overview: In controlled clinical trials involving 2314 hypertensive patients and 363 patients with congestive heart failure, the most severe adverse reactions were: angioedema (0.2%), hypotension (2.3%) and renal failure (5 cases).

In hypertensive patients, hypotension occurred in 0.9% and syncope in 0.5%, with a discontinuation rate of 0.1%.

In congestive heart failure patients, hypotension occurred in 4.4% and syncope in 0.8%, with a discontinuation rate of 2.5%.

The most frequent clinical adverse reactions in controlled clinical trials were: headache (4.8%), dizziness (4.6%) and fatigue (2.8%). Discontinuation of therapy was required in 6.0% of the 2677 patients.

Clinical Trial Adverse Drug Reactions—Hypertension: Because clinical trials are conducted under very specific conditions the adverse reaction rates observed in the clinical trials may not reflect the rates observed in practice and should not be compared to the rates in the clinical trials of another drug. Adverse drug reaction information from clinical trials is useful for identifying drug-related adverse events and for approximating rates.

Adverse experiences occurring in greater than one percent of patients with hypertension treated with VASOTEC in controlled clinical trials are shown below. In patients treated with VASOTEC, the maximum duration of therapy was three years; in placebo treated patients the maximum duration of therapy was 12 weeks. See Table 1.

Table 1: VASOTEC

Hypertension

	VASOTEC n=2314	Placebo n=230
Body as a Whole		
Fatigue	3.0	2.6
Orthostatic Effects	1.2	0.0
Asthenia	1.1	0.9
Digestive		
Diarrhea	1.4	1.7
Nausea	1.4	1.7
Nervous/Psychiatric		
Headache	5.2	9.1
Dizziness	4.3	4.3
Respiratory		
Cough	1.3	0.9
Skin		
Rash	1.4	0.4

Less Common Clinical Trial Adverse Drug Reactions (<1%)—Hypertension: Cardiovascular: hypotension, chest pain, palpitations, acute myocardial infarction.
Digestive: vomiting, dysphagia, abdominal pain.
Hematologic: anemia, leukopenia.
Hypersensitivity: angioedema.
Musculoskeletal: muscle cramps.
Nervous System/Psychiatric: insomnia, nervousness, somnolence, paresthesia.
Respiratory: dyspnea.
Skin: pruritus, hyperhidrosis.
Special Senses: taste disturbance.
Urogenital: renal failure, proteinuria, oliguria, impotence.

Clinical Trial Adverse Drug Reactions—Heart Failure: Because clinical trials are conducted under very specific conditions the adverse reaction rates observed in the clinical trials may not reflect the rates observed in practice and should not be compared to the rates in the clinical trials of another drug. Adverse drug reaction information from clinical trials is useful for identifying drug-related adverse events and for approximating rates.

Adverse experiences occurring in greater than one percent of patients with heart failure treated with VASOTEC are shown in Table 2. The incidences represent the experiences from both controlled and uncontrolled clinical trials (maximum duration of therapy was approximately one year). In the placebo treated patients, the incidences reported are from the controlled trials (maximum duration of therapy is 12 weeks). The percentage of patients with severe heart failure [New York Heart Association (NYHA) Class IV] was 29 percent and 43 percent for patients treated with VASOTEC and placebo, respectively.

Table 2: VASOTEC

Congestive Heart Failure

	VASOTEC n=673	Placebo n=339
Body as a Whole		
Orthostatic Effects	2.2	0.3
Syncope	2.2	0.9
Chest Pain	2.1	2.1
Fatigue	1.8	1.8
Abdominal Pain	1.6	2.1
Asthenia	1.6	0.3
Cardiovascular		
Hypotension	6.7	0.6
Orthostatic Hypotension	1.6	0.3
Angina Pectoris	1.5	1.8
Myocardial Infarction	1.2	1.8
Digestive		
Diarrhea	2.1	1.2
Nausea	1.3	0.6
Vomiting	1.3	0.9
Nervous/Psychiatric		
Dizziness	7.9	0.6
Headache	1.8	0.9
Vertigo	1.6	1.2
Respiratory		
Cough	2.2	0.6
Bronchitis	1.3	0.9
Dyspnea	1.3	0.4
Pneumonia	1.0	2.4
Skin		
Rash	1.3	2.4
Urogenital		
Urinary Tract Infection	1.3	2.4

(cont'd)

Table 2: VASOTEC (cont'd)

Less Common Clinical Trial Adverse Drug Reactions (<1%)—Heart Failure: Cardiovascular: palpitations.
Musculoskeletal: muscle cramps.
Nervous System/Psychiatric: insomnia.
Skin: pruritus.
Special Senses: taste disturbance.
Urogenital: renal failure, impotence.

Abnormal Hematologic and Clinical Chemistry Findings: Hyperkalemia: (See Warnings and Precautions, Renal).

Creatinine, Blood Urea Nitrogen (BUN): Increases in serum creatinine and BUN were reported in about 20% of patients with renovascular hypertension and in about 0.2% of patients with essential hypertension treated with VASOTEC alone.

In patients with congestive heart failure, who were also receiving diuretics and/or digitalis, increases in BUN and serum creatinine, usually reversible upon discontinuation of VASOTEC and/or concomitant therapy, were observed in about 9.7% of patients.

Hemoglobin and Hematocrit: Decreases in hemoglobin and hematocrit (mean approximately 0.34 g% and 1.0 vol%, respectively) occurred frequently in either hypertensive or congestive heart failure patients treated with VASOTEC, but were rarely of clinical importance. In clinical trials, less than 0.1% of patients discontinued therapy due to anemia.

Hepatic: Elevations of liver enzymes and/or serum bilirubin have occurred (see Warnings and Precautions).

Pediatric Patients: In a four-week placebo-controlled clinical trial, 110 hypertensive pediatric patients (6-16 years of age) received medication for 14 days including 51 patients for a four-week period. The adverse experience profile was no different from that seen in adult patients.

Post-Market Adverse Drug Reactions: Adverse Reactions Reported in Uncontrolled Trials and/or Marketing Experience: Other serious clinical adverse experiences occurring since the drug was marketed or adverse experiences occurring in 0.5 to 1.0 percent of patients with hypertension or heart failure in clinical trials are listed below and, within each category, are in order of decreasing severity.

Body as a Whole: anaphylactoid reactions (see Warnings and Precautions).

Cardiovascular: cardiac arrest; myocardial infarction or cerebrovascular accident, possibly secondary to excessive hypotension in high-risk patients (see Warnings and Precautions); pulmonary embolism and infarction; pulmonary edema; angina pectoris; arrhythmia including atrial tachycardia and bradycardia; atrial fibrillation; palpitation, Raynaud's phenomenon.

Endocrine: syndrome of inappropriate antidiuretic hormone secretion (SIADH).

Digestive: ileus, pancreatitis, hepatic failure, hepatitis (hepatocellular or cholestatic jaundice), liver function abnormalities (see Warnings and Precautions), melena, anorexia, dyspepsia, constipation, glossitis, stomatitis, dry mouth.

Hematologic: rare cases of neutropenia, thrombocytopenia, hemolytic anemia and bone marrow depression.

Metabolic: Rare cases of hypoglycemia in diabetic patients on oral antidiabetic agents or insulin have been reported (see Warnings and Precautions).

Musculoskeletal: muscle cramps.

Nervous System/Psychiatric: vertigo, depression, confusion, ataxia, somnolence, insomnia, nervousness, peripheral neuropathy (e.g., paresthesia, dysesthesia), dream abnormality.

Respiratory: bronchospasm, rhinorrhea, sore throat and hoarseness, asthma, upper respiratory infection, pulmonary infiltrates, eosinophilic pneumonitis.

Skin: exfoliative dermatitis, toxic epidermal necrolysis, Stevens-Johnson syndrome, pemphigus, herpes zoster, erythema multiforme, urticaria, pruritus, alopecia, flushing, diaphoresis, photosensitivity.

Special Senses: blurred vision, taste alteration, anosmia, tinnitus, conjunctivitis, dry eyes, tearing, hearing impairment.

Urogenital: renal failure, oliguria, renal dysfunction (see Warnings and Precautions and Dosage and Administration), flank pain, gynecomastia, impotence.

A symptom complex has been reported which may include some or all of the following: fever, serositis, vasculitis, myalgia/myositis, arthralgia/arthritis, a positive antinuclear antibody (ANA), elevated erythrocyte sedimentation rate, eosinophilia and leukocytosis. Rash, photosensitivity or other dermatologic manifestations may occur. These symptoms may be reversible upon discontinuation of therapy.

In very rare cases, intestinal angioedema has been reported with angiotensin converting enzyme inhibitors including enalapril.

Laboratory Test Findings: hyponatremia

DRUG INTERACTIONS: Drug-Drug Interactions: Hypotension—Patients on Diuretic Therapy: Patients on diuretics and especially those in whom diuretic therapy was recently instituted, may occasionally experience an excessive reduction of blood pressure after initiation of therapy with enalapril. The possibility of hypotensive effects with enalapril can be minimized by either discontinuing the diuretic or increasing the salt intake prior to initiation of treatment with enalapril (see Warnings and Precautions and Dosage and Administration).

Agents Increasing Serum Potassium: Since enalapril decreases aldosterone production, elevation of serum potassium may occur. Potassium-sparing diuretics such as spironolactone, eplerenone, triamterene or amiloride, or potassium supplements should be given only for documented hypokalemia and with caution and frequent monitoring of serum potassium particularly in patients with impaired renal function since they may lead to a significant increase in serum potassium. Salt substitutes which contain potassium should also be used with caution (see Warnings and Precautions, Hyperkalemia).

Agents Causing Renin Release: The antihypertensive effect of VASOTEC is augmented by antihypertensive agents that cause renin release (e.g., diuretics).

Agents Affecting Sympathetic Activity: Agents affecting sympathetic activity (e.g., ganglionic blocking agents or adrenergic neuron blocking agents) may be used with caution. Beta-adrenergic blocking drugs add some further antihypertensive effect to enalapril.

Lithium Salts: As with other drugs which eliminate sodium, lithium clearance may be reduced. Therefore, the serum lithium levels should be monitored carefully if lithium salts are to be administered.

Non-Steroidal Anti-Inflammatory Drugs (NSAIDs) Including Selective Cyclooxygenase-2 Inhibitors: The antihypertensive effect of enalapril may be diminished with concomitant non-steroidal anti-inflammatory drug use including selective cyclooxygenase-2 inhibitors (COX-2 inhibitors). In some patients with compromised renal function (e.g., elderly patients or patients who are volume-depleted including those on diuretic therapy) who are being treated with NSAIDS including selective COX-2 inhibitors, the co-administration of ACE inhibitors or angiotensin II receptor antagonists may result in further deterioration of renal function. Cases of acute renal failure, usually reversible, have also been reported. This combination should therefore be administered with caution in this patient population.

Gold: Nitritoid reactions (symptoms include facial flushing, nausea, vomiting and symptomatic hypotension) have been reported rarely in patients on therapy with injectable gold (sodium aurothiomalate) and concomitant ACE inhibitor therapy including enalapril (see Warnings and Precautions).

Drug-Food Interactions: The absorption of enalapril is not influenced by the presence of food in the gastrointestinal tract.

DOSAGE AND ADMINISTRATION: VASOTEC for Oral Administration Only: Dosing Considerations:

- The absorption of VASOTEC is not affected by food.
- Dosage must be individualized.
- Special attention for dialysis patients.
- The splitting of VASOTEC tablets is not advised.

Recommended Dose and Dosage Adjustment: Hypertension: Initiation of therapy requires consideration of recent antihypertensive drug treatment, the extent of blood pressure elevation and salt restriction; the dosage of other antihypertensive agents being used with VASOTEC may need to be adjusted.

The recommended initial dose in patients not on diuretics is 5 mg once a day. Dosage should be adjusted according to blood pressure response. The usual dosage range is 10 to 40 mg per day administered in a single dose or two divided doses. In some patients treated once daily, the antihypertensive effect may diminish toward the end of the dosing interval. In such patients, an increase in dosage or twice-daily administration should be considered. If blood pressure is not controlled, a diuretic may be added.

The maximum daily dose is 40 mg. Raising the dose above that level is not recommended because of the possibility of increased adverse reactions.

Symptomatic hypotension occasionally may occur following the initial dose of VASOTEC and is more likely in patients who are currently being treated with a diuretic. The diuretic should, if possible, be discontinued for two to three days before beginning therapy with VASOTEC to reduce the likelihood of hypotension (see Warnings and Precautions).

If the diuretic cannot be discontinued, an initial dose of 2.5 mg should be used to determine whether excessive hypotension occurs.

To date there is insufficient experience with VASOTEC in the treatment of accelerated or malignant hypertension. VASOTEC, therefore, is not recommended in such situations.

Pediatrics (<16 years of age): The usual recommended starting dose is 0.08 mg/kg (up to 5 mg) once daily. Dosage should be adjusted according to blood pressure response. Doses above 0.58 mg/kg (or in excess of 40 mg) have not been studied in pediatric patients (see Action and Clinical Pharmacology). VASOTEC is not recommended in neonates and in pediatric patients with glomerular filtration rate <30 mL/min/1.73 m^2, as no data are available.

Geriatrics (>65 years of age): The starting dose should be 2.5 mg. Some elderly patients may be more responsive to VASOTEC than younger patients.

Dosing Adjustment in Renal Impairment: (See Warnings and Precautions, Anaphylactoid Reactions during Membrane Exposure.)

The doses should be reduced in patients with hypertension according to the following guidelines: See Table 3.

Table 3: VASOTEC

Dosing Adjustment in Renal Impairment

Renal Status	Creatinine Clearance mL/min (mL/s)	Initial Dose mg/day
Normal Renal Function	>80 mL/min (>1.33 mL/s)	5 mg
Mild Impairment	≤80 >30 mL/min (≤1.33 >0.50 mL/s)	5 mg
Moderate to Severe Impairment	≤30 mL/min (≤0.50 mL/s)	2.5 mg
Dialysis Patients	—	2.5 mg on dialysis days[a]

[a] Enalaprilat is dialyzable. Dosage on nondialysis days should be adjusted depending on the blood pressure response.

Congestive Heart Failure: VASOTEC is generally used in conjunction with a diuretic and/or digitalis. Blood pressure and renal function should be monitored, both before and during treatment with VASOTEC, because severe hypotension and, more rarely, consequent renal failure have been reported (see Warnings and Precautions).

Initiation of therapy requires consideration of recent diuretic therapy and the possibility of severe salt/volume depletion. If possible, the dose of diuretic should be reduced before beginning treatment to reduce the likelihood of hypotension. Serum potassium also should be monitored (see Drug interactions, Drug-Drug Interactions).

The recommended initial dose in patients with symptomatic heart failure or asymptomatic left ventricular dysfunction (ejection fraction ≤35%) is 2.5 mg once a day, to be administered under close medical supervision to determine the initial effect on blood pressure. After the initial dose, the patient should be observed for at least two hours or until the pressure has stabilized for at least one additional hour (see Warnings and Precautions, Hypotension).

In the absence of, or after effective management of symptomatic hypotension following initiation of therapy, the dose should be increased gradually depending on the patient's response. The usual therapeutic dosing range is 5 to 20 mg daily, given as a single dose or two divided doses.

This dose titration may be performed over a 2 to 4 week period, or more rapidly if indicated by the presence of residual signs and symptoms of heart failure. The dosage regimen, in patients with symptomatic heart failure, which was effective in reducing mortality and the need for hospitalization in multicentre studies ranged between 16.4 and 18.8 mg/day. The majority of patient experience in clinical studies has been with twice-daily dosage.

The maximum daily dose is 40 mg.

Dosage Adjustment in Patients with Congestive Heart Failure and Renal Impairment or Hyponatremia: In patients with heart failure who have hyponatremia (serum sodium less than 130 mEq/L) or with serum creatinine greater than 1.6 mg/dL, therapy should be initiated at 2.5 mg daily under close medical supervision (see Dosage and Administration, Congestive Heart Failure and Drug Interactions, Drug-Drug Interactions).

The dose may be increased to 2.5 mg b.i.d. then 5 mg b.i.d. and higher as needed, usually at intervals of four days or more if at the time of dosage adjustment there is not excessive hypotension or significant deterioration of renal function.

The maximum daily dose is 40 mg.

OVERDOSAGE:

Limited data are available for overdosage in humans. The most prominent features of overdosage reported to date are marked hypotension, beginning some six hours after ingestion of tablets, concomitant with blockade of the renin-angiotensin system, and stupor. Serum enalaprilat levels 100- and 200-fold higher than usually seen after therapeutic doses have been reported after ingestion of 300 mg and 440 mg of enalapril, respectively.

The recommended treatment of overdosage is intravenous infusion of normal saline solution. If ingestion is recent, induce emesis. Enalaprilat may be removed from the general circulation by hemodialysis (see Warnings and Precautions, Anaphylactoid Reactions during Membrane Exposure).

> For management of a suspected drug overdose, contact your regional Poison Control Centre. See the *CPS* Directory section for a list of Poison Control Centres.

ACTION AND CLINICAL PHARMACOLOGY: Mechanism of Action: VASOTEC is an ACE inhibitor which is used in the treatment of hypertension and heart failure.

Angiotensin converting enzyme (ACE) is a peptidyl dipeptidase which catalyzes the conversion of angiotensin I to the pressor substance, angiotensin II. After absorption, enalapril, a pro-drug, is hydrolyzed to enalaprilat, its active metabolite, which inhibits ACE. Inhibition of ACE results in decreased plasma angiotensin II, which leads to increased plasma renin activity (due to removal of negative feedback of renin release) and decreased aldosterone secretion. Although the latter decrease is small, it results in a small increase in serum potassium. In patients treated with VASOTEC and a thiazide diuretic there was essentially no change in serum potassium (see Warnings and Precautions).

ACE is identical to kininase II. Thus, VASOTEC may also block the degradation of bradykinin, a potent vasodepressor peptide. However, the role that this plays in the therapeutic effects of either drug is unknown.

While the mechanism through which VASOTEC lowers blood pressure is believed to be primarily the suppression of the renin-angiotensin-aldosterone system, VASOTEC also lowers blood pressure in patients with low-renin hypertension.

Pharmacodynamics: Administration of VASOTEC to patients with hypertension results in a reduction of both supine and standing blood pressure. Abrupt withdrawal of VASOTEC has not been associated with a rapid increase in blood pressure. In most patients studied, after oral administration of an individual dose of enalapril, the onset of antihypertensive activity is seen at one hour with peak reduction of blood pressure achieved by 4-6 hours. At recommended doses, the antihypertensive effect has been shown to be maintained for at least 24 hours. In some patients the effect may diminish towards the end of the dosing interval (see Dosage and Administration). On occasion, achievement of optimal blood pressure reduction may require several weeks of therapy.

In hemodynamic studies in patients with essential hypertension, blood pressure reduction was accompanied by a reduction in peripheral arterial resistance with an increase in cardiac output and little or no change in heart rate. Following administration of VASOTEC, there was an increase in renal blood flow; glomerular filtration rate was usually unchanged.

When VASOTEC is given together with thiazide-type diuretics, its blood pressure lowering effect is approximately additive.

Administration of enalapril to patients with congestive heart failure reduces afterload and preload of the heart, resulting in an increase in cardiac output, without reflex tachycardia.

When used in hypertensive, normolipidemic patients, enalapril had no effect on plasma lipoprotein fractions.

Studies in dogs indicate that enalapril crosses the blood brain barrier poorly, if at all; enalaprilat does not enter the brain.

Pharmacokinetics: See Table 4.

Table 4: VASOTEC

Summary of Enalaprilat's Pharmacokinetic Parameters in Healthy Volunteers Further to a 10 mg Oral Dose of Enalapril

	C_{max} (ng/mL)	$t_{½}$ (h)[a]	$AUC_{0-\infty}$ (ng·h/mL)
Single dose mean	32.3	11	423

[a] Effective half-life of accumulation.

Absorption: VASOTEC is rapidly absorbed with peak serum concentrations of enalapril occurring within one hour. Based on urinary recovery the extent of absorption of enalapril from VASOTEC is approximately 60%. The absorption of enalapril is not influenced by the presence of food in the gastrointestinal tract.

Metabolism: Following absorption, enalapril is rapidly and extensively hydrolyzed to enalaprilat, a potent angiotensin converting enzyme inhibitor (which itself is poorly absorbed). Peak serum concentrations of enalaprilat occur 3 to 4 hours after an oral dose of enalapril. Except for conversion to enalaprilat, there is no evidence of significant metabolism of enalapril.

Excretion: Excretion of enalapril is primarily renal. Approximately 94% of the dose is recovered in the urine and feces as enalaprilat or enalapril. The principal components in urine are enalaprilat, accounting for about 40% of the dose, and intact enalapril.

The serum concentration profile of enalaprilat exhibits a prolonged terminal phase, apparently associated with binding to ACE. The effective half-life for accumulation of enalaprilat following multiple doses of enalapril is 11 hours.

In hypertensive children aged 2 months to 15 years the kinetics of VASOTEC were approximately similar to adults (see Dosage and Administration).

Special Populations and Conditions: Pediatrics: In pediatric patients the antihypertensive effect of VASOTEC has been studied in hypertensive children aged 6-16 years (see Dosage and Administration and Action and Clinical Pharmacology, Pharmacokinetics).

Race: The antihypertensive effect of angiotensin converting enzyme inhibitors is generally lower in black than in non-black patients.

Renal Insufficiency: The disposition of enalapril and enalaprilat in patients with renal insufficiency is similar to that in patients with normal renal function until the glomerular filtration rate is 30 mL/min (0.50 mL/s) or less. With renal function ≤30 mL/min (≤0.50 mL/s), peak and trough enalaprilat levels increase, time to peak concentration increases and time to steady state may be delayed. The effective half-life of enalaprilat following multiple doses of enalapril is prolonged at this level of renal insufficiency (see Dosage and Administration). Enalaprilat is dialyzable at the rate of 62 mL/min (1.03 mL/s).

STORAGE AND STABILITY: Store at controlled room temperature (15-30°C). Keep container tightly closed. Protect from moisture.

Note: 100 and 500 tablet bottle: discard remaining tablets six months after opening bottle.

INFORMATION FOR THE PATIENT: Published in e-CPS, available by subscription at www.e-cps.ca.

DOSAGE FORMS, COMPOSITION AND PACKAGING: 2.5 mg: Each white, oval-shaped, engraved MSD 14 on one side, and scored on both sides, contains: enalapril maleate 2.5 mg, that appears as enalapril sodium 2 mg. Nonmedicinal ingredients: cornstarch, lactose, magnesium stearate, pregelatinized starch and sodium bicarbonate. The splitting of VASOTEC tablets is not advised. Blisters of 28. Polyethylene bottles of 100 and 500.

5 mg: Each white, rounded triangle-shaped tablet, engraved MSD 712 on one side and scored on the other, contains: enalapril maleate 5 mg, that appears as enalapril sodium 4 mg. Nonmedicinal ingredients: cornstarch, lactose, magnesium stearate, pregelatinized starch and sodium bicarbonate. The splitting of VASOTEC tablets is not advised. Blisters of 28. Polyethylene bottles of 500.

10 mg: Each rust red, rounded triangle-shaped tablet, engraved MSD 713 on one side and scored on the other, contains: enalapril maleate 10 mg, that appears as enalapril sodium 8 mg. Nonmedicinal ingredients: cornstarch, lactose, magnesium stearate, pregelatinized starch, red and/or yellow iron oxides and sodium bicarbonate. The splitting of VASOTEC tablets is not advised. Blisters of 28. Polyethylene bottles of 500.

20 mg: Each peach-colored, rounded triangle-shaped tablet, engraved MSD 714 on one side and scored on the other, contains: enalapril maleate 20 mg, that appears as enalapril sodium 16 mg. Nonmedicinal ingredients: cornstarch, lactose, magnesium stearate, pregelatinized starch, red and/or yellow iron oxides and sodium bicarbonate. The splitting of VASOTEC tablets is not advised. Blisters of 28. Polyethylene bottles of 100 and 500.

(Shown in Product Identification Section)

Vaxigrip®

inactivated influenza vaccine trivalent types A and B (split virion)

Active Immunizing Agent for the Prevention of Influenza

sanofi pasteur

Date of Revision: May 2010

SUMMARY PRODUCT INFORMATION:

Route of Administration	Dosage Form/ Strength	Clinically Relevant Nonmedicinal Ingredients
Intramuscular injection	Suspension for injection Each 0.5 mL dose is formulated to contain: 15 µg of hemagglutinin (HA) for each strain listed below (see Description). Each 0.25 mL dose is formulated to contain: 7.5 µg of hemagglutinin (HA) for each strain listed below (see Description).	thimerosal[a], formaldehyde, Triton X-100[b], neomycin. For a complete listing see Dosage Forms, Composition and Packaging.

[a] Multidose presentation only.
[b] Triton X-100—a registered trademark of Union Carbide, Co.

DESCRIPTION: VAXIGRIF [Inactivated Influenza Vaccine Trivalent Types A and B (Split Virion)] for intramuscular use, is a sterile suspension containing 3 strains of influenza virus cultivated on embryonated eggs, concentrated, purified by zonal centrifugation in a sucrose gradient, split by Triton X-100, inactivated by formaldehyde and then diluted in phosphate buffered saline solution. The type and amount of viral antigens contained in VAXIGRIP conform to the current requirements of the World Health Organization (WHO). The strains for the 2010-2011 season are: A/California/7/2009 (H1N1)—like strain, A/Perth/16/2009 (H3N2)—like strain and B/Brisbane/60/2008.

INDICATIONS AND CLINICAL USE: VAXIGRIP is indicated for active immunization against influenza caused by the specific strains of influenza virus contained in the vaccine in adults and children 6 months of age and older.

Although the current influenza vaccine can contain one or more of the antigens administered in previous years, annual vaccination using the current vaccine is necessary because immunity declines in the year following vaccination.

The National Advisory Committee on Immunization (NACI) encourages annual influenza vaccination for all Canadians who have no contraindications.

Vaccine should be offered to both children and adults up to and even after influenza virus activity is documented in a community.

CONTRAINDICATIONS: Hypersensitivity: VAXIGRIP should not be administered to anyone with a history of severe allergic reaction to egg protein or any component of the vaccine (see Dosage Forms, Composition and Packaging) or after previous administration of the vaccine or a vaccine containing the same components or constituents.

WARNINGS AND PRECAUTIONS: General: Before administration of VAXIGRIP, health-care providers should inform the recipient, or parent/guardian of the recipient of the benefits and risks of immunization, inquire about the recent health status of the recipient, review the recipient's history concerning possible hypersensitivity to the vaccine or similar vaccine, previous immunization history, the presence of any contraindications to immunization and comply with any local requirements regarding information to be provided to the recipient/guardian before immunization.

As with any vaccine, immunization with influenza vaccine may not protect 100% of individuals.

Influenza virus is remarkably unpredictable in that significant antigenic changes may occur from time to time. It is known that VAXIGRIP as now constituted is not effective against all possible strains of influenza virus. Protection is limited to those strains of virus from which the vaccine is prepared or against closely related strains.

Prophylactic acetaminophen may decrease the frequency of some adverse reactions in adults.

Administration-route Related Precautions: Do not administer by intravascular injection: ensure that the needle does not penetrate a blood vessel.

VAXIGRIP should not be administered into the buttocks.

Aseptic technique must be used for withdrawal of each dose from a multidose vial. Use a separate, sterile needle and syringe or a sterile disposable unit for each individual patient and for each entry into a multidose vial, to prevent disease transmission. In particular, the same needle and/or syringe must never be used to re-enter a multidose vial to withdraw vaccine even when it is to be used for inoculation of the same patient. This may lead to contamination of the vial contents and infection of patients who subsequently receive vaccine from the vial.

Febrile or Acute Disease: Vaccination should be postponed in case of febrile or acute disease.

Hematologic: Because any intramuscular injection can cause an injection site haematoma in persons with any bleeding disorders, such as haemophilia or thrombocytopenia, or in persons on anticoagulant therapy, intramuscular injections with VAXIGRIP should not be administered to such persons unless the potential benefits outweigh the risk of administration. If the decision is made to administer any product by intramuscular injection to such persons, it should be given with caution, with steps taken to avoid the risk of haematoma formation following injection.

NACI has recommendations for giving vaccinations to persons with bleeding disorders.

Immune: As with all products, epinephrine hydrochloride solution (1:1000) and other appropriate agents should be available for immediate use in case an anaphylactic or acute hypersensitivity reaction occurs. Health-care providers should be familiar with current recommendations for the initial management of anaphylaxis in non-hospital settings including proper airway management. For instructions on recognition and treatment of anaphylactic reactions see the current edition of the Canadian Immunization Guide or visit the Health Canada website.

As each dose may contain traces of formaldehyde, Triton X-100 and undetectable traces of neomycin, which are used during vaccine production, caution should be exercised when the vaccine is administered to subjects with hypersensitivity to any of these substances (see Contraindications). The multidose vial of this vaccine contains thimerosal as a preservative. Thimerosal has been associated with allergic reactions.

Immunocompromised persons (whether from disease or treatment) may not achieve the expected immune response. Nevertheless, as recommended by NACI, the possibility of lower efficacy should not prevent immunization in those at high risk of influenza-associated morbidity, since protection is still likely to occur.

Since the influenza vaccine is produced in eggs, persons with known IgE-mediated hypersensitivity should not be routinely vaccinated with influenza vaccine (see Contraindications). Egg-allergic individuals who are at risk of the complications of influenza should be evaluated by an allergy specialist, as vaccination might be possible after careful evaluation, skin-testing and graded challenge or desensitization. If such an evaluation is not possible, the risk of an allergic reaction to the vaccine must be weighed against the risk of influenza disease.

Neurologic: Immunization should be delayed in a patient with an active neurologic disorder, but should be considered when the disease process has been stabilized.

Guillain-Barré syndrome has been reported after influenza vaccination. However, it is not known whether influenza vaccination specifically might increase the risk for recurrence of GBS. Therefore, NACI and ACIP state it is prudent to avoid vaccinating persons who are known to have experienced GBS within 6 to 8 weeks after a previous influenza vaccination.

Respiratory: According to NACI, persons who have experienced oculorespiratory syndrome (ORS) symptoms including severe ORS consisting of non-lower respiratory symptoms (bilateral red eyes, cough, sore throat, hoarseness, facial swelling), may be safely reimmunized with influenza vaccine. Please refer to the most current NACI recommendations regarding revaccination of subjects who experienced more severe oculo-respiratory syndrome.

Special Populations: Pregnant Women: Animal reproduction studies have not been conducted with VAXIGRIP. It is not known whether VAXIGRIP can cause fetal harm when administered to a pregnant woman or can affect reproductive capacity.

Data on the use of this vaccine in pregnant women are limited. VAXIGRIP should be given to pregnant women only if clearly needed and following an assessment of the risks and benefits.

NACI states that influenza vaccination is recommended for all pregnant women.

Nursing Women: It is not known whether VAXIGRIP is excreted in human milk. Caution must be exercised when VAXIGRIP is administered to a nursing mother.

NACI states that influenza vaccination is considered safe for breastfeeding women.

Pediatrics: The use of VAXIGRIP in infants under 6 months of age is not recommended.

ADVERSE REACTIONS: Adverse Drug Reaction Overview: Adverse event information is derived from uncontrolled clinical trials and worldwide post-marketing experience.

Because VAXIGRIP does not contain infectious viral particles, it cannot cause influenza.

The most common reactions occurring after vaccine administration are injection site pain, erythema and edema. The most common systemic reactions observed after vaccine administration are asthenia, headache and myalgia. Most of the adverse event reported after influenza vaccination are mild to moderate in intensity, resolving within 3 days.

Clinical Trial Adverse Drug Reactions: Because clinical trials are conducted under very specific conditions, the adverse reaction rates observed in the clinical trials of a vaccine cannot be directly compared to the rates in the clinical trials of another vaccine and may not reflect rates observed in practice. The adverse reaction information from clinical trials does, however, provide a basis for identifying the adverse events that appear to be related to vaccine use and for approximating rates of those events.

The strain composition of the influenza virus vaccines is subject to annual changes and corresponding clinical studies, including at least 50 adults 18-60 years of age and at least 50 elderly aged 60 years or older, are conducted as annual update requirements in Europe to assess the safety and immunogenicity of VAXIGRIP.

For the purpose of cumulative analysis, five years of annual clinical safety data were considered (see Table 1). A total of 779 vaccinees received an intramuscular injection of VAXIGRIP. Table 1 summarizes the frequencies (range across individual trials) of the solicited adverse events that were recorded within 3 days following the vaccination.

Data are categorized by age group and by MedDRA system organ class.

Table 1: VAXIGRIF

Adverse Events Within 3 Days After Vaccination of 779 Patients with VAXIGRIP

Adverse Events	Adult 18–59 years (N=393)	Elderly >60 years (N=386)
General Disorders and Administration Site Conditions Local Injection Site Reactions		
Pain	27 to 57%	11.5 to 23.7%
Erythema	7.1 to 29.1%	7.1 to 29.9%
Induration	4.5 to 17.3%	3.8 to 10.5%
Edema	2.2 to 21.5%	5.8 to 14.5%[a]
Bruising	1.1 to 7.4%[a]	1.9 to 4.5%[a]
Pruritus	1.1 to 4.9%[a]	1.9 to 3%[a]
Systemic Reactions		
Asthenia	4.3 to 14.8%	1.4 to 7.9%
Pyrexia (oral temperature >38°C)	1.2 to 1.4%[a]	1 to 1.5%[a]
Rigors	1.4 to 6.7%	1 to 3%[a]
Malaise	1.1 to 1.3%[a]	1.3%[a]
Nervous System Disorders		
Headache	1.4 to 10%	2.9 to 6%[a]
Musculoskeletal and Connective Tissue Disorders		
Arthralgia	1.4 to 3.8%[a]	1.5 to 2.6%[a]
Myalgia	1.1 to 8.9%	1.4 to 3%[a]
Skin and Subcutaneous Tissue Disorders		
Sweating increased	1.4 to 4.9%[a]	6%[a]

[a] Adverse event not reported in all studies.

Data from Post-marketing Experience: The following additional adverse events have been spontaneously reported during the post-marketing use of VAXIGRIP. Because these events are reported voluntarily from a population of uncertain size, it is not possible to reliably estimate their frequency or establish a causal relationship to vaccine exposure.

Blood and Lymphatic System Disorders: transient thrombocytopenia, lymphadenopathy.

Immune System Disorders: Allergic reactions: pruritus, erythematous rash, urticaria, dyspnea, angioneurotic edema, or anaphylaxis (including shock).

Nervous System Disorders: paraesthesia, Guillain-Barré syndrome (GBS), neuritis, neuralgia, convulsions, encephalomyelitis.

Vascular Disorders: vasculitis, such as Henoch-Schonlein purpura, with transient renal involvement in certain cases.

Additional Adverse Reactions: The following adverse events not listed above have been reported with influenza vaccines:

During the 2000-2001 influenza season, the Public Health Agency of Canada (PHAC) received an increased number of reports of influenza vaccine-associated symptoms and signs that were subsequently described as oculorespiratory syndrome (ORS). The pathophysiologic mechanism underlying ORS remains unknown, but it is considered distinct from IgE-mediated allergy. Since the 2000-2001 influenza season fewer ORS cases have been reported to PHAC.

Neurological disorders temporally associated with influenza vaccination such as encephalopathy (with or without permanent neurological - motor and/or sensory - deficit and/or intellectual impairment), optic neuritis, facial paralysis, labyrinthitis and brachial plexus neuropathy have been reported. However, no cause-and-effect relationships have been established.

Physicians, nurses and pharmacists should report any adverse occurrences temporally related to the administration of the product in accordance with local requirements and to the Global Pharmacovigilance Department, Sanofi Pasteur Limited, 1755 Steeles Avenue West, Toronto, ON, M2R 3T4, Canada. 1-888-621-1146 (phone) or 416-667-2435 (fax).

DRUG INTERACTIONS: Concomitant Vaccine Administration: Clinical studies show that influenza vaccine may be administered with pneumococcal polysaccharide vaccine using separate syringes at different sites.

No studies regarding the concomitant administration of inactivated influenza vaccine and other childhood vaccines have been conducted.

NACI states that influenza vaccine may be given at the same time as other vaccines. The same limb may be used if necessary, but different sites on the limb should be chosen. Different administration sets (needle and syringe) must be used.

VAXIGRIP must not be mixed in the same syringe with other parenterals.

Vaccine-Drug Interactions: Immunosuppressive treatments may interfere with the development of the expected immune response (see Warnings and Precautions).

DOSAGE AND ADMINISTRATION: Recommended Dose: The recommended dosage schedule is presented in Table 2.

Table 2: VAXIGRIP
Recommended Influenza Vaccine Dosage, by Age

Age Group	Dose	No. of Doses
6 to 35 months	0.25 mL	1 or 2[a]
3 to 8 years	0.5 mL	1 or 2[a]
≥9 years	0.5 mL	1

[a] Previously unvaccinated children <9 years of age require 2 doses of influenza vaccine with an interval of 4 weeks. Eligible children <9 years of age who have properly received one or more doses of TIV in the past are recommended to receive one dose per season thereafter.

Fractional doses (doses of less volume than indicated for each age group in Table 2) should not be given. The effect of fractional doses on the safety and efficacy has not been determined.

Administration: Inspect for extraneous particulate matter and/or discolouration before use. If these conditions exist, the product should not be administered.

Administer the vaccine **intramuscularly**. The preferred site is into the deltoid muscle, in adults and children >1 year of age. The preferred site for infants and young children (<1 year of age) is the anterolateral aspect of the mid-thigh (vastus lateralis muscle).

Shake the pre-filled syringe well to uniformly distribute the suspension before administration.

If using a pre-filled syringe with two needles, select a needle of appropriate length to ensure that the vaccine will be delivered intramuscularly. Remove the tip cap from the syringe, take the chosen needle from the blister pack and fix to the tip of the pre-filled syringe.

For children, when a single dose 0.5 mL syringe is to be used for administration of a 0.25 mL dose, push the plunger exactly to the edge of the mark so that half of the volume is eliminated. The remaining volume should be injected.

If using a multidose vial, **shake the vial well** to uniformly distribute the suspension before withdrawing each dose. When administering a dose from a stoppered vial, do not remove either the stopper or the metal seal holding it in place. Aseptic technique must be used for withdrawal of each dose (see Warnings and Precautions).

If using an ampoule, **shake the ampoule well** to uniformly distribute the suspension before withdrawing each dose. Before withdrawing a dose from an ampoule, tap the container first to ensure that any vaccine in the ampoule neck falls to the lower portion of the ampoule. Once the ampoule has been opened, any of its contents not used immediately should be discarded. Aseptic technique must be used for withdrawal of each dose (see Warnings and Precautions).

Aseptic technique must be used. Use a separate sterile needle and syringe, or a sterile disposable unit for each individual recipient, to prevent disease transmission. Needles should not be recapped and should be disposed of according to biohazard waste guidelines.

Give the patient a permanent personal immunization record. In addition, it is essential that the physician or nurse record the immunization history in the permanent medical record of each patient. This permanent office record should contain the name of the vaccine, date given, dose, manufacturer and lot number.

OVERDOSAGE: Not applicable.

> For management of a suspected drug overdose, contact your regional Poison Control Centre. See the *CPS Directory* section for a list of Poison Control Centres.

ACTION AND CLINICAL PHARMACOLOGY: Mechanism of Action: The inoculation of antigen prepared from inactivated influenza virus stimulates the production of specific antibodies. Protection is afforded only against those strains of virus from which the vaccine is prepared or closely related strains.

Immunity to the surface antigens, particularly the haemagglutinin, reduces the likelihood of infection. Antibody against one influenza virus type or subtype confers limited or no protection against another type or subtype of influenza. Furthermore, antibody to one antigenic type or subtype of influenza virus might not protect against infection with a new antigenic variant of the same type or subtype. Frequent emergence of antigenic variants through antigenic drift is the virologic basis for seasonal epidemics and is the reason for the usual incorporation of one or more new strains in each year's influenza vaccine.

Each year's influenza vaccine contains three virus strains (usually two type A, and one type B) representing the influenza viruses that are believed likely to circulate in the coming winter. The antigenic characteristics of current and emerging influenza virus strains provide the basis for selecting the strains included in each year's vaccine.

Pharmacodynamics: Seroprotection is expected within 2 to 3 weeks following influenza vaccination.

Pharmacokinetics: No pharmacokinetic studies have been performed.

Duration of Effect: The duration of post-vaccinal immunity varies and is usually 6-12 months.

STORAGE AND STABILITY: Store at 2 to 8°C (35 to 46°F). **Do not freeze.** Discard product if exposed to freezing.

Protect from light. Do not use vaccine after expiration date.

SPECIAL HANDLING INSTRUCTIONS: A multidose vial of VAXIGRIP which has been entered must be stored at 2 to 8°C and used within 7 days. Seven days after first entry, it must be discarded.

INFORMATION FOR THE PATIENT: Published in e-CPS, available by subscription at www.e-cps.ca.

DOSAGE FORMS, COMPOSITION AND PACKAGING: For the 2010-2011 season, each 0.5 mL dose of VAXIGRIP contains: A/California/7/2009 (H1N1)—like strain [A/California/7/2009 (H1N1) (NYMC X-179A)] 15 µg HA; A/Perth/16/2009 (H3N2)—like strain [A/Victoria/210/2009 (NYMC X-187)] 15 µg HA; and B/Brisbane/60/2008 15 µg HA. Other ingredients: 2 µg thimerosal (added as a preservative in multidose presentation only), up to 0.5 mL sodium phosphate buffered, isotonic sodium chloride solution, formaldehyde (≤30 µg), Triton X-100, and trace amounts of sucrose and neomycin.

Each 0.25 mL dose of VAXIGRIP is formulated to contain: 7.5 µg of hemagglutinin for each strain listed above; Other ingredients: 1 µg thimerosal (added as a preservative in multidose presentation only), up to 0.25 mL sodium phosphate buffered, isotonic sodium chloride solution, formaldehyde (≤15 µg), Triton X-100, and trace amounts of sucrose and neomycin.

After shaking, VAXIGRIP is slightly whitish and opalescent in color.

Packages of: 1×5 mL (multidose) vial, 1×0.25 mL (single dose) syringe with an attached (25G, 16 mm) needle, 1×0.5 mL (single dose) syringe with an attached (25G, 16 mm) needle, 1×0.5 mL (single dose) syringe co-packaged with two 25G needles of different lengths (16 mm and 25 mm), 1×0.5 mL (single dose) ampoule, 5×0.5 mL (single dose) ampoule. The vials and syringes are made of Type 1 glass. The container closure system for all presentations of VAXIGRIP does not contain latex (natural rubber). The vial stopper, plunger stopper and the needle shield of the pre-filled syringe do not contain latex (natural rubber). Not all presentations may be marketed for this upcoming season (2010-2011).

Vectibix® Pr
panitumumab
Antineoplastic

Amgen

Date of Revision: February 26, 2010

> **Vectibix, indicated as monotherapy for the treatment of patients with EGFR-expressing metastatic colorectal carcinoma with non-mutated (wild-type) KRAS after failure of fluoropyrimidine-, oxaliplatin-, and irinotecan-containing chemotherapy regimens, has been issued marketing authorization with conditions, pending the results of studies to verify its clinical benefit. Patients should be advised of the nature of the authorization.**

SUMMARY PRODUCT INFORMATION:

Route of Administration	Dosage Form/ Strength	Clinically Relevant Nonmedicinal Ingredients
Intravenous (IV) Infusion See Dosage and Administration.	Sterile concentrate for solution for infusion/100, 200, 400 mg (20 mg/mL)	Not applicable For a complete listing see Dosage Forms, Composition and Packaging.

DESCRIPTION: Vectibix (panitumumab) is a recombinant, fully human IgG2 monoclonal antibody that binds specifically to the human epidermal growth factor receptor (EGFR). Vectibix consists of 2 gamma heavy chains and 2 kappa light chains and has an approximate molecular weight of 147 kDa. Vectibix is produced in a mammalian cell line (CHO) by recombinant DNA technology.

INDICATIONS AND CLINICAL USE: Vectibix (panitumumab) is indicated as monotherapy for the treatment of patients with EGFR-expressing metastatic colorectal carcinoma with non-mutated (wild-type) KRAS after failure of fluoropyrimidine-, oxaliplatin-, and irinotecan-containing chemotherapy regimens.

The effectiveness of Vectibix as a single agent for the treatment of EGFR-expressing, metastatic colorectal carcinoma is based on progression-free survival. Currently no data are available that demonstrate an increased survival with Vectibix.

Geriatrics (≥65 years of age): Fifty-two patients ≥65 years old and 71 <65 years old in the non-mutated (wild-type) KRAS stratum were treated with Vectibix plus best supportive care (BSC). The efficacy and qualitative safety results were similar between the geriatric patients (65 years or older) versus those patients who were younger.

Pediatrics: The safety and effectiveness of Vectibix in pediatric patients have not yet been established.

CONTRAINDICATIONS: Vectibix (panitumumab) is contraindicated in patients with a history of severe or life-threatening hypersensitivity reactions to panitumumab or any other component of the product. For a complete listing of the components, see Dosage Forms, Composition and Packaging.

WARNINGS AND PRECAUTIONS:

> **Serious Warnings and Precautions**
>
> **Dermatologic Toxicity:** Dermatologic toxicities, related to Vectibix (panitumumab) blockade of EGF receptor occurred in 91% (721/789) of patients and were severe (NCI-CTC grade 3 and higher) in 12% of patients receiving Vectibix monotherapy. The clinical manifestations included dermatitis acneiform, pruritus, erythema, rash, skin exfoliation, paronychia, dry skin, and skin fissures. Severe dermatologic toxicities were complicated by infection, including sepsis, in rare cases leading to death, and local abscesses requiring incision and drainage. Withhold or discontinue Vectibix and monitor for inflammatory or infectious sequelae in patients with severe dermatologic toxicities (see Dosage and Administration, Recommended Dose and Dosage Adjustment). It is recommended that patients wear sunscreen and a hat and limit sun exposure while receiving Vectibix as sunlight can exacerbate any skin reactions that may occur.
>
> **Infusion Reactions:** Infusion reactions, including anaphylactic reactions, bronchospasm, fever, chills, and hypotension, have been reported in the clinical trials and post-marketing experience. Across all clinical studies, severe infusion reactions (NCI-CTC grade 3 and grade 4) occurred with the administration of Vectibix in <1% of patients. In the post-marketing setting, serious infusion reactions have been reported in <1% of patients, very rarely with a fatal outcome (<0.01%). Fatal reactions have also been observed in patients with a history of hypersensitivity to Vectibix (see Other Hypersensitivity Reactions). Stop infusion if a severe or life-threatening infusion reaction occurs. Depending on the severity and/or persistence of the reaction, consider permanently discontinuing Vectibix (see Dosage and Administration, Recommended Dose and Dosage Adjustment).
>
> **Increased toxicity and decreased overall survival in combination with bevacizumab and chemotherapy:** Vectibix is not indicated for use in combination with chemotherapy with or without bevacizumab. In an interim analysis of a randomized, open-label, multicenter trial in the first-line treatment of metastatic colorectal cancer, the addition of Vectibix to the combination of bevacizumab and chemotherapy resulted in decreased overall survival and increased incidence of NCI-CTC grade 3-5 (87% vs. 72%) adverse reactions.
>
> **Gastrointestinal: Combination treatment with IFL regimen:** Administration of Vectibix in combination with IFL should be avoided due to an increase in grade 3-5 diarrhea.

Other Hypersensitivity Reactions: Hypersensitivity reactions have been reported, including a fatal case of angioedema that occurred more than 24 hours after the infusion. Depending on the severity (eg presence of bronchospasm, edema, angioedema, hypotension, need for parenteral medication, or anaphylaxis) and/or persistence (eg prolonged versus transient) of hypersensitivity reactions, permanently discontinue Vectibix (see Contraindications and Adverse Reactions). Hypersensitivity reactions should be treated immediately with appropriate medical therapy consistent with the treating physician's medical judgement.

It is recommended to warn patients of the possibility of a late onset hypersensitivity reaction and instruct them to contact their physician if symptoms occur.

Carcinogenesis and Mutagenesis: No carcinogenesis or mutagenesis studies were conducted with Vectibix.

Respiratory: As Interstitial Lung Disease (ILD) has been observed with EGFR inhibitors, in the event of acute onset or worsening of pulmonary symptoms, Vectibix treatment should be interrupted and a prompt investigation of these symptoms should occur. If pneumonitis or lung infiltrates are confirmed, Vectibix should be discontinued and the patient should be treated appropriately.

In patients with a history of, or evidence of interstitial pneumonitis or pulmonary fibrosis, the benefits of administration of Vectibix versus the risk of pulmonary complications in these patients must be carefully considered before administration. These patients were excluded from clinical studies.

Sexual Function/Reproduction: No studies evaluating sexual function or reproduction in humans were conducted with Vectibix. Animal studies have shown reversible effects on the menstrual cycle and reduced female fertility in monkeys. Vectibix may impair fertility in women of childbearing potential.

Special Populations: Pregnant Women: There are no data from the use of Vectibix in pregnant women. The potential risk for humans is unknown. However, EGFR has been implicated in the control of prenatal development and may be essential for normal organogenesis, proliferation, and differentiation in the developing embryo. Therefore Vectibix has the potential to cause fetal harm when administered to pregnant women. Vectibix should not be used in pregnant women. Studies in animals have shown reproductive toxicity.

Human IgG is known to cross the placental barrier; therefore Vectibix may be transmitted from the mother to the developing fetus. In women of childbearing potential, appropriate contraceptive measures must be used during treatment with Vectibix and for 6 months following the last dose. If Vectibix is used during pregnancy or if the patient becomes pregnant while receiving this drug, she should be advised of the potential risk for loss of the pregnancy and the potential hazard to the fetus.

Nursing Women: It is unknown whether Vectibix is excreted in human breast milk. Because human IgG is secreted into human milk, Vectibix may also be secreted. The potential for absorption and harm to the infant after ingestion is unknown. It is recommended that women do not breastfeed during treatment with Vectibix and for 2 months after the last dose.

Pediatrics (<18 years of age): The safety and effectiveness of Vectibix in pediatric patients have not been established.

Geriatrics (≥65 years of age): Fifty-two patients ≥65 years old and 71 <65 years old in the non-mutated (wild-type) KRAS stratum were treated with Vectibix plus best supportive care (BSC). The efficacy results and qualitative safety were similar between the geriatric patients (65 years or older) versus those patients who were younger. Differences in adverse reactions between the ≥65 year old patients and <65 were in the following system organ classes: eye disorders with growth of eyelashes (17% vs. 4%), ocular hyperemia (10% vs. 1%) and conjunctivitis (6% vs. 1%); gastrointestinal disorders with diarrhea (13% vs. 7%); general disorders and administrative site conditions with fatigue (8% vs. 3%) and mucosal inflammation (13% vs. 3%); skin and subcutaneous tissue disorders with dermatitis acneiform (65% vs. 56%) and nail disorders (15% vs. 7%), respectively. The incidence of adverse events leading to permanent discontinuation from Vectibix plus BSC in patients ≥65 years (10%) was higher compared to patients <65 years (6%).

Renal/Hepatic: The safety and effectiveness of Vectibix in patients with renal or hepatic impairment have not been established.

Acute Renal Failure: Acute renal failure has been observed in mCRC patients treated with Vectibix who develop severe diarrhea and dehydration (see Adverse Reactions, Post-Market Adverse Drug Reactions, Gastrointestinal Disorders).

Patients should be monitored for signs and symptoms of severe diarrhea and dehydration (such as decreased urine output, dizziness, low blood pressure, rapid heartbeat) and treated immediately with appropriate medical therapy consistent with the treating physician's medical judgement. Vectibix should be withheld until the patient is no longer experiencing severe diarrhea, dehydration or acute renal failure.

Monitoring and Laboratory Tests: Electrolyte Monitoring: Progressively decreasing serum magnesium levels leading to severe hypomagnesemia have been observed in some patients. Patients should be monitored for hypomagnesemia and accompanying hypocalcemia prior to initiating Vectibix treatment, and periodically during Vectibix treatment and for up to 8 weeks after the completion of treatment. Magnesium repletion is recommended, as appropriate.

Other electrolyte disturbances, including hypokalemia, have also been observed. Repletion of these electrolytes is also recommended, as appropriate.

KRAS Testing: Detection of non-mutated KRAS expression should be performed by an experienced laboratory using a validated test method.

ADVERSE REACTIONS: Adverse Drug Reaction Overview: Safety data are available from 15 clinical trials in which 1467 patients received Vectibix; of these, 1293 received Vectibix monotherapy and 174 received Vectibix in combination with chemotherapy. The most common adverse events observed in clinical studies of Vectibix (n=1467) were skin rash with variable presentations, hypomagnesemia, paronychia, fatigue, abdominal pain, nausea, and diarrhea, including diarrhea resulting in dehydration. The most serious adverse events observed were pulmonary fibrosis, pulmonary embolism, severe dermatologic toxicity complicated by infectious sequelae and septic death, infusion reactions, abdominal pain, hypomagnesemia, nausea, vomiting, and constipation. Adverse events requiring discontinuation of Vectibix were infusion reactions, severe skin toxicity, paronychia, and pulmonary fibrosis.

Clinical Trial Adverse Drug Reactions: Because clinical trials are conducted under very specific conditions, the adverse reaction rates observed in the clinical trials may not reflect the rates observed in practice and should not be compared to the rates in the clinical trials of another drug. Adverse drug reaction information from clinical trials is useful for identifying drug-related adverse events and for approximating rates.

Adverse Drug Reactions by KRAS Status Pivotal Clinical Trial: The safety profile of Vectibix in patients whose tumors express KRAS wild-type (n=123) was generally consistent with overall mCRC monotherapy set.

In the randomized controlled trial, all 123 patients (100%), with non-mutated (wild-type) KRAS status, treated with Vectibix experienced adverse reactions, of which 62% reported grade 3-4 events.

The most frequently (≥20% patients) reported adverse reactions were erythema (71%), pruritus (69%), dermatitis acneiform (60%), paronychia (33%), fatigue (33%), anorexia (30%), abdominal pain (27%), exfoliative rash (25%), constipation (24%), diarrhea (24%), skin fissures (24%), rash (20%) and cough (20%) of which the grade 3-4 reactions included dermatitis acneiform (9%), erythema (6%), abdominal pain (7%), anorexia (6%), constipation (5%), fatigue (5%), pruritus (4%), paronychia (3%), exfoliative rash (3%), skin fissures (2%), rash (2%), and diarrhea (2%).

Adverse drug reactions by KRAS status reported in ≥1% whose tumour express KRAS wild-type are shown in Table 1.

Table 1: Vectibix

Per-Patient Incidence of Adverse Events Occurring in ≥1% of KRAS Wild-Type Patients (N=123)

System Organ Class Preferred Term	Panitumumab Plus BSC (N=123)		BSC Alone (N=120)	
	All Grades	Grade 3-4	All Grades	Grade 3-4
Subjects with at least one adverse event–n (%)	123 (100)	76 (62)	108 (90)	36 (30)
Blood and Lymphatic System Disorders	10 (8)	4 (3)	5 (4)	1 (1)
Anemia	8 (7)	2 (2)	3 (3)	1 (1)
Ear and Labyrinth Disorders	3 (2)	0 (0)	1 (1)	0 (0)
Vertigo	2 (2)	0 (0)	1 (1)	0 (0)
Eye Disorders	29 (24)	1 (1)	4 (3)	0 (0)
Conjunctivitis	5 (4)	0 (0)	1 (1)	0 (0)
Eye irritation	2 (2)	0 (0)	0 (0)	0 (0)
Eyelid irritation	3 (2)	0 (0)	0 (0)	0 (0)
Growth of eyelashes	12 (10)	0 (0)	0 (0)	0 (0)
Lacrimation increased	5 (4)	0 (0)	1 (1)	0 (0)
Ocular hyperemia	7 (6)	0 (0)	0 (0)	0 (0)
Gastrointestinal Disorders	87 (71)	27 (22)	64 (53)	10 (8)
Abdominal distension	5 (4)	1 (1)	3 (3)	0 (0)
Abdominal pain	33 (27)	9 (7)	21 (18)	5 (4)
Abdominal pain lower	2 (2)	1 (1)	1 (1)	0 (0)
Abdominal pain upper	11 (9)	2 (2)	12 (10)	3 (3)
Aphthous stomatitis	3 (2)	0 (0)	1 (1)	0 (0)
Ascites	6 (5)	2 (2)	2 (2)	0 (0)
Constipation	30 (24)	6 (5)	11 (9)	0 (0)
Diarrhea	30 (24)	3 (2)	13 (11)	0 (0)
Dry mouth	6 (5)	1 (1)	0 (0)	0 (0)
Dyspepsia	5 (4)	0 (0)	3 (3)	0 (0)
Flatulence	4 (3)	0 (0)	2 (2)	0 (0)
Gastritis	2 (2)	0 (0)	0 (0)	0 (0)
Gastroesophageal reflux disease	2 (2)	0 (0)	1 (1)	0 (0)
Intestinal obstruction	9 (7)	4 (3)	3 (3)	1 (1)
Nausea	22 (18)	1 (1)	19 (16)	1 (1)
Proctalgia	2 (2)	1 (1)	0 (0)	0 (0)
Rectal hemorrhage	3 (2)	0 (0)	4 (3)	0 (0)
Stomatitis	9 (7)	0 (0)	2 (2)	0 (0)
Vomiting	18 (15)	4 (3)	8 (7)	1 (1)

(cont'd)

Table 1: Vectibix *(cont'd)*

Per-Patient Incidence of Adverse Events Occurring in ≥1% of KRAS Wild-Type Patients (N=123)

System Organ Class Preferred Term	Panitumumab Plus BSC (N=123)		BSC Alone (N=120)	
	All Grades	Grade 3-4	All Grades	Grade 3-4
General Disorders and Administration Site Conditions	83 (67)	24 (20)	50 (42)	15 (13)
Asthenia	18 (15)	8 (7)	12 (10)	3 (3)
Chills	4 (3)	0 (0)	1 (1)	0 (0)
Fatigue	40 (33)	6 (5)	15 (13)	4 (3)
General physical health deterioration	11 (9)	7 (6)	4 (3)	2 (2)
Mucosal inflammation	10 (8)	1 (1)	2 (2)	0 (0)
Edema	7 (6)	1 (1)	4 (3)	1 (1)
Edema peripheral	14 (11)	1 (1)	9 (8)	1 (1)
Pain	5 (4)	0 (0)	4 (3)	2 (2)
Pyrexia	22 (18)	1 (1)	14 (12)	3 (3)
Hepatobiliary Disorders	20 (16)	10 (8)	13 (11)	8 (7)
Hepatic failure	2 (2)	0 (0)	2 (2)	2 (2)
Hepatic pain	1 (1)	0 (0)	3 (3)	0 (0)
Hepatomegaly	7 (6)	2 (2)	4 (3)	3 (3)
Hyperbilirubinemia	1 (1)	1 (1)	2 (2)	1 (1)
Jaundice	9 (7)	4 (3)	5 (4)	1 (1)
Infections and Infestations	68 (55)	11 (9)	19 (16)	6 (5)
Bronchitis	3 (2)	0 (0)	3 (3)	1 (1)
Catheter related infection	2 (2)	0 (0)	0 (0)	0 (0)
Eye infection	4 (3)	0 (0)	0 (0)	0 (0)
Eyelid infection	2 (2)	0 (0)	0 (0)	0 (0)
Folliculitis	2 (2)	0 (0)	0 (0)	0 (0)
Fungal infection	2 (2)	0 (0)	0 (0)	0 (0)
Impetigo	2 (2)	0 (0)	0 (0)	0 (0)
Nasopharyngitis	7 (6)	0 (0)	0 (0)	0 (0)
Paronychia	41 (33)	4 (3)	0 (0)	0 (0)
Pharyngitis	1 (1)	0 (0)	2 (2)	0 (0)
Rash pustular	5 (4)	2 (2)	0 (0)	0 (0)
Respiratory tract infection	3 (2)	0 (0)	0 (0)	0 (0)
Septic shock	0 (0)	0 (0)	2 (2)	2 (2)
Upper respiratory tract infection	2 (2)	0 (0)	0 (0)	0 (0)
Urinary tract infection	2 (2)	1 (1)	3 (3)	0 (0)
Injury, Poisoning and Procedural Complications	10 (8)	6 (5)	2 (2)	1 (1)
Procedural pain	2 (2)	2 (2)	0 (0)	0 (0)
Investigations	15 (12)	6 (5)	5 (4)	1 (1)
Blood bilirubin increased	2 (2)	2 (2)	1 (1)	0 (0)
Blood magnesium decreased	2 (2)	1 (1)	0 (0)	0 (0)
Blood urine present	2 (2)	1 (1)	0 (0)	0 (0)
Cardiac murmur	0 (0)	0 (0)	2 (2)	0 (0)
Weight decreased	7 (6)	1 (1)	1 (1)	0 (0)
Metabolism and Nutrition Disorders	49 (40)	13 (11)	32 (27)	6 (5)
Anorexia	37 (30)	7 (6)	25 (21)	4 (3)
Cachexia	4 (3)	0 (0)	0 (0)	0 (0)
Decreased appetite	3 (2)	1 (1)	1 (1)	0 (0)
Dehydration	5 (4)	3 (2)	3 (3)	0 (0)

(cont'd)

Table 1: Vectibix *(cont'd)*

Per-Patient Incidence of Adverse Events Occurring in ≥1% of KRAS Wild-Type Patients (N=123)

System Organ Class Preferred Term	Panitumumab Plus BSC (N=123)		BSC Alone (N=120)	
	All Grades	Grade 3-4	All Grades	Grade 3-4
Gout	1 (1)	0 (0)	2 (2)	1 (1)
Hypocalcemia	2 (2)	0 (0)	0 (0)	0 (0)
Hypokalemia	5 (4)	1 (1)	1 (1)	0 (0)
Hypomagnesemia	2 (2)	1 (1)	0 (0)	0 (0)
Musculoskeletal and Connective Tissue Disorders	38 (31)	5 (4)	27 (23)	1 (1)
Arthralgia	7 (6)	2 (2)	3 (3)	1 (1)
Back pain	16 (13)	1 (1)	6 (5)	0 (0)
Bone pain	4 (3)	1 (1)	1 (1)	0 (0)
Groin pain	0 (0)	0 (0)	2 (2)	0 (0)
Muscle spasms	5 (4)	0 (0)	2 (2)	0 (0)
Muscular weakness	2 (2)	0 (0)	2 (2)	0 (0)
Musculoskeletal chest pain	5 (4)	0 (0)	4 (3)	0 (0)
Myalgia	2 (2)	0 (0)	1 (1)	0 (0)
Pain in extremity	6 (5)	1 (1)	4 (3)	0 (0)
Shoulder pain	4 (3)	1 (1)	5 (4)	0 (0)
Neoplasms Benign, Malignant and Unspecified (Incl Cysts and Polyps)	25 (20)	3 (2)	21 (18)	2 (2)
Cancer pain	2 (2)	1 (1)	0 (0)	0 (0)
Colorectal cancer	7 (6)	0 (0)	4 (3)	0 (0)
Colorectal cancer metastatic	14 (11)	0 (0)	13 (11)	0 (0)
Nervous System Disorders	25 (20)	7 (6)	19 (16)	5 (4)
Dizziness	2 (2)	0 (0)	1 (1)	0 (0)
Dysgeusia	2 (2)	0 (0)	1 (1)	0 (0)
Headache	5 (4)	1 (1)	4 (3)	0 (0)
Lethargy	2 (2)	1 (1)	0 (0)	0 (0)
Neuropathy	2 (2)	1 (1)	0 (0)	0 (0)
Paresthesia	4 (3)	0 (0)	4 (3)	1 (1)
Somnolence	0 (0)	0 (0)	3 (3)	0 (0)
Psychiatric Disorders	19 (15)	3 (2)	13 (11)	2 (2)
Agitation	1 (1)	1 (1)	2 (2)	1 (1)
Anxiety	4 (3)	0 (0)	3 (3)	1 (1)
Confusional state	2 (2)	1 (1)	1 (1)	1 (1)
Depression	6 (5)	1 (1)	1 (1)	0 (0)
Insomnia	6 (5)	1 (1)	6 (5)	0 (0)
Renal and Urinary Disorders	16 (13)	6 (5)	2 (2)	0 (0)
Dysuria	3 (2)	1 (1)	0 (0)	0 (0)
Hematuria	5 (4)	1 (1)	0 (0)	0 (0)
Oliguria	2 (2)	1 (1)	0 (0)	0 (0)
Renal failure	2 (2)	2 (2)	0 (0)	0 (0)
Renal pain	2 (2)	0 (0)	0 (0)	0 (0)
Urinary retention	2 (2)	0 (0)	0 (0)	0 (0)
Respiratory, Thoracic and Mediastinal Disorders	49 (40)	8 (7)	27 (23)	4 (3)
Cough	24 (20)	0 (0)	9 (8)	0 (0)
Dysphonia	2 (2)	0 (0)	0 (0)	0 (0)
Dyspnea	23 (19)	6 (5)	18 (15)	4 (3)

(cont'd)

Table 1: Vectibix *(cont'd)*

Per-Patient Incidence of Adverse Events Occurring in ≥1% of KRAS Wild-Type Patients (N=123)

System Organ Class Preferred Term	Panitumumab Plus BSC (N=123)		BSC Alone (N=120)	
	All Grades	Grade 3-4	All Grades	Grade 3-4
Epistaxis	6 (5)	0 (0)	0 (0)	0 (0)
Hemoptysis	2 (2)	0 (0)	0 (0)	0 (0)
Pharyngolaryngeal pain	2 (2)	0 (0)	0 (0)	0 (0)
Pleural effusion	2 (2)	0 (0)	1 (1)	1 (1)
Productive cough	2 (2)	0 (0)	1 (1)	0 (0)
Skin and Subcutaneous Tissue Disorders	112 (91)	24 (20)	10 (8)	0 (0)
Acne	21 (17)	2 (2)	0 (0)	0 (0)
Alopecia	3 (2)	0 (0)	0 (0)	0 (0)
Dermatitis acneiform	74 (60)	11 (9)	1 (1)	0 (0)
Dry skin	16 (13)	0 (0)	0 (0)	0 (0)
Ecchymosis	0 (0)	0 (0)	2 (2)	0 (0)
Erythema	87 (71)	10 (8)	1 (1)	0 (0)
Exfoliative rash	31 (25)	4 (3)	0 (0)	0 (0)
Hair disorder	2 (2)	0 (0)	0 (0)	0 (0)
Hyperhidrosis	3 (2)	0 (0)	2 (2)	0 (0)
Intertrigo	2 (2)	0 (0)	0 (0)	0 (0)
Nail disorder	13 (11)	0 (0)	0 (0)	0 (0)
Night sweats	2 (2)	0 (0)	1 (1)	0 (0)
Onychoclasis	2 (2)	0 (0)	0 (0)	0 (0)
Onychomadesis	2 (2)	0 (0)	0 (0)	0 (0)
Pain of skin	3 (2)	0 (0)	0 (0)	0 (0)
Palmar-plantar erythrodysesthesia syndrome	2 (2)	0 (0)	0 (0)	0 (0)
Pruritus	85 (69)	5 (4)	2 (2)	0 (0)
Rash	25 (20)	2 (2)	1 (1)	0 (0)
Rash erythematous	3 (2)	0 (0)	0 (0)	0 (0)
Rash papular	4 (3)	0 (0)	0 (0)	0 (0)
Rash pruritic	2 (2)	0 (0)	0 (0)	0 (0)
Scab	6 (5)	2 (2)	0 (0)	0 (0)
Skin exfoliation	14 (11)	2 (2)	0 (0)	0 (0)
Skin fissures	30 (24)	3 (2)	0 (0)	0 (0)
Skin toxicity	4 (3)	0 (0)	0 (0)	0 (0)
Skin ulcer	8 (7)	1 (1)	0 (0)	0 (0)
Vascular Disorders	12 (10)	4 (3)	3 (3)	0 (0)
Hypertension	6 (5)	3 (2)	2 (2)	0 (0)
Pallor	2 (2)	0 (0)	1 (1)	0 (0)

Vectibix mCRC Monotherapy Set: Except where indicated, the safety data described below reflect single agent exposure to Vectibix (panitumumab) in 789 patients with mCRC. Patients who received Vectibix at the dose schedule of 2.5 mg/kg given weekly had a median of 8 infusions; patients who received Vectibix at the dose schedule of 6 mg/kg given once every 2 weeks had a median of 4 infusions; patients who received Vectibix at the dose schedule of 9 mg/kg given once every 3 weeks had a median of 4 infusions. The population had a median age of 61 and was 60% male and 90% Caucasian. The number of doses of Vectibix received by patients ranged from 1 to 69 doses corresponding to 1 to 87 weeks of treatment. Thirty-four percent of patients received Vectibix for 3 months and longer.

Serious adverse reactions associated with Vectibix treatment included hypersensitivity occurring within 24 hours of the first dose (1%), hypomagnesemia (1%), dehydration (1%), pulmonary embolism and diarrhea (<1%). Three percent of patients receiving Vectibix discontinued treatment primarily due to adverse reactions that were predominantly skin-related.

The most commonly reported adverse reactions were dermatologic-related toxicities including, but not limited to, dermatitis acneiform, pruritus, erythema, rash, skin exfoliation, paronychia, dry skin, and skin fissures occurring in 91% of patients treated with Vectibix. These toxicities are related to the pharmacological effects of Vectibix and are primarily mild to moderate in nature with 13% reported as severe (≥grade 3).

In clinical studies with Vectibix as a single agent, diarrhea was reported in 13% of the patients. Most of these cases of diarrhea were mild to moderate in severity; <2% of patients treated with Vectibix had reported grade 3 or higher diarrhea.

The data described in Table 2 reflect exposure to Vectibix administered as a single agent at the recommended dose and schedule (6.0 mg/kg every 2 weeks) in 229 patients randomized to the Vectibix arm with mCRC in the controlled trial. The control arm consisted of 234 subjects randomized to BSC (total n=463).

Adverse drug reactions reported in ≥5% of Vectibix-treated patients in the randomized controlled trial of 463 patients with EGFR-expressing metastatic carcinoma of the colon or rectum (mCRC) are shown in Table 2.

Table 2: Vectibix

Per-Patient Incidence of Adverse Events Occurring in ≥5% of Patients with a Between Group Difference of ≥5% (Randomized Controlled Trial N=463)

System Organ Class Preferred Term	Panitumumab Plus BSC (N=229)		BSC Alone (N=234)	
	All Grades	Grade3-4	All Grades	Grade 3-4
Subjects with at least one adverse event–n (%)	229 (100)	128 (56)	204 (87)	67 (29)
Eye Disorders	36 (16)	0 (0)	7 (3)	0 (0)
Growth of eyelashes	13 (6)	0 (0)	0 (0)	0 (0)
Gastrointestinal Disorders	159 (69)	40 (17)	117 (50)	23 (10)
Abdominal pain	58 (25)	17 (7)	40 (17)	12 (5)
Constipation	48 (21)	7 (3)	21 (9)	2 (1)
Diarrhea	49 (21)	4 (2)	26 (11)	0 (0)
Nausea	52 (23)	2 (1)	37 (16)	1 (0)
Stomatitis	15 (7)	0 (0)	2 (1)	0 (0)
Vomiting	43 (19)	5 (2)	28 (12)	2 (1)
General Disorders and Administration Site Conditions	143 (62)	41 (18)	104 (44)	27 (12)
Fatigue	60 (26)	10 (4)	34 (15)	7 (3)
General physical health deterioration	26 (11)	19 (8)	9 (4)	6 (3)
Mucosal inflammation	14 (6)	1 (0)	2 (1)	0 (0)
Edema peripheral	27 (12)	2 (1)	13 (6)	1 (0)
Infections and Infestations	108 (47)	14 (6)	34 (15)	7 (3)
Paronychia	57 (25)	4 (2)	0 (0)	0 (0)
Metabolism and Nutrition Disorders	86 (38)	16 (7)	58 (25)	7 (3)
Anorexia	66 (29)	8 (3)	45 (19)	5 (2)
Respiratory, Thoracic and Mediastinal Disorders	81 (35)	15 (7)	50 (21)	9 (4)
Cough	32 (14)	1 (0)	17 (7)	0 (0)
Skin and Subcutaneous Tissue Disorders	205 (90)	33 (14)	20 (9)	1 (0)
Acne	30 (13)	3 (1)	0 (0)	0 (0)
Dermatitis acneiform	130 (57)	17 (7)	2 (1)	0 (0)
Dry skin	22 (10)	0 (0)	0 (0)	0 (0)
Erythema	149 (65)	12 (5)	2 (1)	0 (0)
Nail disorder	21 (9)	0 (0)	0 (0)	0 (0)
Pruritus	131 (57)	5 (2)	4 (2)	0 (0)
Rash	50 (22)	2 (1)	2 (1)	0 (0)
Skin exfoliation	58 (25)	5 (2)	0 (0)	0 (0)
Skin fissures	45 (20)	2 (1)	1 (0)	0 (0)

Less Common Clinical Trial Adverse Drug Reactions: The following adverse drug reactions were reported at an incidence of <1% in clinical studies and occurring in more than 1 patient treated with Vectibix:

Respiratory, Thoracic and Mediastinal Disorders: pulmonary embolism.

Infections and Infestations: cellulitis.

Dermatologic Toxicity and Related Disorders: Dermatologic toxicity and related disorders were observed in 91% of patients receiving Vectibix. Skin rash most commonly occurred on the face, upper back and chest, but could extend to the extremities and was characterized by multiple pustular-, macular-, or papular-appearing lesions. Skin drying and fissures were common and in some cases were associated with inflammatory and infectious sequelae, including sepsis, in rare cases leading to death, and local abscesses requiring incisions and drainage (see Warnings and Precautions).

Paronychia, occurring in 19% of patients (1% grade 3), was characterized as a paronychial inflammation with associated swelling of the lateral nail folds of the toes and fingers. The following were also observed in patients treated with Vectibix: exfoliative rash (14%)*, acne (10%)*, rash pustular (6%)*, nail disorder (8%)*, rash papular (5%)*, skin ulcer (5%)*, conjunctivitis (3%), rash erythematous (3%)*, rash macular (3%)*, scab (3%)*, growth of eyelashes (2%), rash maculo-papular (2%)*, rash pruritic (2%)*, increased lacrimation (1%), ocular hyperemia (1%), eye infection (1%)*, eye irritation (<1%), dry eye (<1%), eye pruritus (<1%), eyelid infection (<1%)*, and eyelid irritation (<1%)*.

The median time to first symptom of dermatologic toxicity was 10 days, and the median time to resolution after the last dose of Vectibix was 28 days. The subject incidence and duration of dermatologic and related disorders were correlated with Vectibix exposure.

Infusion Reactions: Across all clinical studies, potential infusion reactions (occurring within 24 hours of any infusion), which may include symptoms/signs such as chills, fever or dyspnea, were reported in 3% of Vectibix-treated patients, of which <1% were severe (NCI-CTC grade 3- grade 4). Most of the symptoms of potential infusion reactions were mild in intensity, resolved without treatment, were isolated occurrences and did not require alteration or interruption of Vectibix administration.

* n=1052.

† Doses higher than 1000 mg should be diluted in 150 mL 0.9% sodium chloride injection USP and should be infused over approximately 90 minutes via infusion pump.

Abnormal Hematologic and Clinical Chemistry Findings: Electrolyte Depletion: In clinical studies in which magnesium levels were collected at specified time intervals during treatment with Vectibix, hypomagnesemia (any grade) was observed in 39% of patients assessed (n=649) and occurred at various time points during treatment. Grade 3 or higher hypomagnesemia was reported in 5% of these patients, most of whom proceeded to receive IV electrolyte repletion. Serious cases of hypomagnesemia occurred 6 weeks or longer after the initiation of Vectibix. In <1% of patients, adverse reactions of hypomagnesemia were associated with adverse reactions of hypocalcemia. Patients' electrolytes should be periodically monitored prior to initiating Vectibix therapy, during, and for 8 weeks after, the completion of Vectibix therapy. Institute appropriate treatment, eg, oral or intravenous electrolyte repletion, as needed (see Warnings and Precautions).

Other Adverse Reactions: Combination with Anti-Tumour Therapies: In a study of 19 patients with mCRC treated with Vectibix in combination with the IFL regimen (bolus 5-fluorouracil, leucovorin, and irinotecan), the incidence of grade 3 or higher diarrhea was 58% (see Warnings and Precautions). In a study of 24 patients with mCRC treated with Vectibix plus FOLFIRI (infusional 5-fluorouracil, leucovorin, and irinotecan), the incidence of grade 3 or higher diarrhea was 25%.

A randomized, open-label, multicenter study of 1053 patients evaluated the efficacy of bevacizumab and oxaliplatin- or irinotecan-containing chemotherapeutic regimens with and without Vectibix in the first-line treatment of metastatic colorectal cancer. In an interim analysis based on 947 randomized patients, shortened progression-free survival time and increased deaths were observed in the patients receiving Vectibix in combination with bevacizumab and chemotherapy. A greater frequency of pulmonary embolism, infections (predominantly of dermatologic origin), diarrhea, and dehydration was also observed in the treatment arms using Vectibix in combination with bevacizumab and chemotherapy. The addition of Vectibix to the combination of bevacizumab and chemotherapy in first-line metastatic colorectal cancer is not indicated.

Immunogenicity: The immunogenicity of panitumumab has been evaluated using two different immunoassays (an ELISA which detects high-affinity antibodies, and a Biosensor Immunoassay which detects both high- and low-affinity antibodies). Pre-dose antibodies were detected in <1% (5/636) and 2.5% (16/635) of patients tested by the ELISA and Biosensor Immunoassay, respectively. The overall incidence of a post-dose anti-panitumumab antibody response was low. Post-dose neutralizing antibodies were detected in 0.2% (1/447) and 1.6% (7/447) of patients tested by the ELISA and Biosensor Immunoassay, respectively. Compared with patients who did not develop antibodies, no relationship between the presence of anti-panitumumab antibodies and pharmacokinetics, efficacy and safety has been observed.

The detection of antibody formation is dependent on the sensitivity and specificity of the assay. The observed incidence of antibody positivity in an assay may be influenced by several factors including sample handling, concomitant medications and underlying disease. Therefore, comparison of the incidence of antibodies to other products may be misleading.

Post-Market Adverse Drug Reactions: Gastrointestinal Disorders: There have been reports of severe diarrhea and dehydration in patients administered Vectibix. In some cases of severe diarrhea and dehydration patients have experienced reduction in renal function. Although there appeared to be confounding factors in some of the cases, such as underlying sepsis, diabetes or hypertension, a review of these cases suggests a risk of acute renal failure (secondary to diarrhea and or dehydration), primarily in the setting of combination chemotherapy, in patients administered Vectibix (see Warnings and Precautions).

Patients should be monitored for signs and symptoms of severe diarrhea and dehydration (such as decreased urine output, dizziness, low blood pressure, rapid heartbeat) and treated immediately with appropriate medical therapy consistent with the treating physician's medical judgement. Vectibix should be withheld until the patient is no longer experiencing severe diarrhea, dehydration or acute renal failure.

Angioedema: Angioedema has been identified during post-approval use of Vectibix. Because these reactions are reported in a population of uncertain size, it is not always possible to estimate reliably their frequency or establish a causal relationship to drug exposure.

Infusion Reactions: In the post-marketing setting, serious infusion reactions, including anaphylaxis, have been reported in <1% of patients, very rarely with a fatal outcome (<0.01%).

DRUG INTERACTIONS: Overview: No formal drug interaction studies between Vectibix (panitumumab) and other drugs have been performed. No evidence of pharmacokinetic interaction has been seen in clinical studies in which Vectibix was administered concurrently with paclitaxel- or irinotecan-containing chemotherapy regimens.

Drug-Drug Interactions: Interactions with other drugs have not been established.

Drug-Food Interactions: Interactions with food have not been established.

Drug-Herb Interactions: Interactions with herbal products have not been established.

Drug-Laboratory Test Interactions: Interactions with laboratory tests have not been established.

DOSAGE AND ADMINISTRATION

Dosing Considerations: The Vectibix (panitumumab) infusion should be prepared using appropriate aseptic technique. **Do not administer Vectibix as an IV push or bolus. Vectibix must be administered using an IV infusion pump and a low protein binding 0.2 µm or 0.22 µm in-line filter.**

Recommended Dose and Dosage Adjustment: The recommended dose of Vectibix is 6 mg/kg of body weight given once every 2 weeks.

Infusion Reactions: Reduce infusion rate by 50% in patients experiencing a mild or moderate (grade 1 or 2) infusion reaction for the duration of that infusion.

Stop infusion if a severe or life-threatening infusion reaction occurs. Depending on the severity and/or persistence of the reaction, consider permanently discontinuing Vectibix.

Dermatological Reactions: If a patient develops dermatologic toxicities related to Vectibix that are grade 3 or higher or are considered intolerable, temporarily withhold Vectibix administration until the toxicities have improved (≤grade 2). Once improved, reinstate Vectibix administration at 50% of the original dose. If toxicities do not worsen, escalate each additional dose of Vectibix by 25% increments of the original dose until the recommended starting dose is reached. If toxicity does not resolve to at least grade 2 after withholding 1 or 2 doses of Vectibix, or if toxicity worsens or becomes intolerable at 50% of the original dose level, the use of Vectibix should be permanently discontinued (see Warnings and Precautions).

Missed Dose: Every attempt should be made to administer Vectibix within 3 days before or 3 days after the scheduled dose (except as noted in the Recommended Dose and Dosage Adjustment, Dermatological Reactions). If this dose is missed, Vectibix should be administered as soon as possible. The next dose should be given on a new schedule, relative to the day the last dose was administered (i.e. every 2 weeks for doses of 6 mg/kg of Vectibix).

Administration: Vectibix is supplied as a sterile, colourless, preservative-free solution containing 20 mg/mL panitumumab in a single-use vial. The solution may contain a small amount of visible, amorphous, panitumumab particulates. Vectibix should not be shaken.

The Vectibix infusion should be prepared using appropriate aseptic technique. **Do not administer Vectibix as an IV push or bolus. Vectibix must be administered using an IV infusion pump:**

- Withdraw the necessary amount of Vectibix for a dose of 6 mg/kg as appropriate.
- Dilute in a total volume of 100 mL in 0.9% sodium chloride injection USP†. Final concentration should not exceed 10 mg/mL.
- Mix diluted solution by gentle inversion. **Do not shake.**
- **Administer using a low protein binding 0.2 µm or 0.22 µm in-line filter.**
- Infuse over approximately 60 minutes through a peripheral line or indwelling catheter†.
- Flush line before and after Vectibix administration with 0.9% sodium chloride injection USP to avoid mixing with other drug products or IV solutions.

Vectibix should not be mixed with, or administered as, an infusion with other medicinal products. No other medications should be added to solutions containing Vectibix, and Vectibix should be diluted with 0.9% sodium chloride injection USP.

The solution may contain a small amount of visible amorphous panitumumab particulates that will be removed during infusion by a low protein binding 0.2 µm or 0.22 µm in-line filter; the filtration does not impact the quality of the administered product.

Vectibix should not be administered if discolouration is observed.

No incompatibilities have been observed between Vectibix and 0.9% sodium chloride injection USP in polyvinyl chloride bags or polyolefin bags.

OVERDOSAGE:

Doses up to 9 mg/kg have been tested in clinical trials. There have been reports of overdosage at doses up to approximately twice the recommended therapeutic dose. Adverse events observed included skin toxicity, diarrhea, dehydration, and fatigue and were consistent with the safety profile at the recommended dose.

For management of a suspected drug overdose, CPhA recommends that you contact your **regional Poison Control Centre**. See the *CPS* Directory section for a list of Poison Control Centres.

ACTION AND CLINICAL PHARMACOLOGY: Mechanism of Action: Vectibix (panitumumab) is a recombinant, fully human IgG2 monoclonal antibody that binds with high affinity and specificity to the human EGFR. EGFR is a transmembrane glycoprotein that is a member of a subfamily of type I receptor tyrosine kinases including EGFR (HER1/c-ErbB-1), HER2, HER3, and HER4. EGFR promotes cell growth in normal epithelial tissues, including the skin and hair follicle, and is expressed on a variety of tumour cells (including colon, lung, breast, prostate, pancreatic, and head and neck carcinomas).

Vectibix binds to the ligand-binding domain of EGFR and competitively inhibits receptor autophosphorylation induced by all known EGFR ligands. Binding of Vectibix to EGFR results in the internalization of the receptor, inhibition of cell growth, induction of apoptosis, and decreased interleukin 8 and vascular endothelial growth factor production.

In vitro assays and in vivo animal studies have shown that Vectibix inhibits the growth and survival of tumour cells expressing EGFR. No anti-tumour effects of Vectibix were observed in human tumour xenografts lacking EGFR expression. The addition of Vectibix to chemotherapy and/or targeted therapeutic agents in animal studies resulted in an increase in anti-tumour effects compared to chemotherapy or targeted therapeutic agents alone.

The KRAS gene encodes a small, GTP-binding protein involved in signal transduction. A variety of stimuli, including that from the EGFR, activates KRAS, which in turn stimulates other intracellular proteins to promote cell proliferation, cell survival, and angiogenesis.

Activating mutations in the KRAS gene occur frequently in a variety of human tumours and have been implicated in both oncogenesis and tumour progression.

Pharmacokinetics: Absorption: In all clinical trials, Vectibix (panitumumab) was administered as an intravenous infusion. Therefore, panitumumab is 100% bioavailable to the blood circulation.

Distribution: After intravenous infusion, serum panitumumab declined bi-exponentially and was best described by a model with 2 compartments: central and peripheral compartments. Compartmental analysis suggested that the volume of distribution approximated the plasma volume (42 mL/kg) for the central compartment and was approximately 26 mL/kg for the peripheral compartment.

Elimination (Metabolism and Excretion): Over a wide range of clinical doses examined (0.75 to 9 mg/kg), panitumumab exhibited nonlinear pharmacokinetics; the time-averaged clearance (estimated by dose divided by area under the concentration time curve, AUC) decreased with increasing dose. The elimination of panitumumab is assumed to be mediated by two pathways: (1) via the reticuloendothelial system (RES), a common pathway for endogenous immunoglobulins, and (2) via the EGF receptor (EGFR). Since panitumumab that is bound to cell-surface EGFR can be internalized and degraded, the nonlinear clearance is probably related to saturable binding of panitumumab to EGFR.

At doses >2 mg/kg, the time-averaged clearance of panitumumab remains relatively constant, because at these higher doses the nonlinear clearance pathway is saturated and becomes relatively insignificant, leaving the overall clearance process being driven mainly by the linear pathway. When the clearance of panitumumab is relatively constant, the exposure to panitumumab (AUC) increases in a dose-proportional manner.

Pharmacokinetic steady-state is reached after 3 doses at 6 mg/kg given once every 2 weeks without a loading dose. The pharmacokinetic parameter of panitumumab at steady state is summarized in Table 3.

Table 3: Vectibix

Mean (SD) Panitumumab Pharmacokinetic Parameters at Steady State

Dose Regimen	N	C_{max} (μg/mL)	C_{min} (μg/mL)	AUC_{0-tau} (μg· day/mL)	$t_{1/2}$ (day)	CL (mL/day/kg)
6 mg/kg Q2W	14	219 (54)	47 (19)	1431 (412)	7.5 (1.8)	4.6 (1.4)

Legend: C_{max}=maximum serum concentration; C_{min}=minimum serum concentration; AUC_{0-tau}=area under the curve for the dosing interval; $t_{1/2}$=half-life during the dosing interval; CL=serum clearance.

Special Populations and Conditions: A population pharmacokinetic analysis was performed to explore the potential effects of selected covariates on Vectibix pharmacokinetics. Results suggest that age, gender, tumour type, race, hepatic function, renal function, chemotherapeutic agents, and EGFR membrane expression in tumour cells had no apparent impact on the pharmacokinetics of Vectibix.

No clinical studies have been conducted to examine the pharmacokinetics of Vectibix in patients with renal impairment or hepatic impairment. No age-related differences in the pharmacokinetics of Vectibix were observed in clinical studies in patients 26 to 85 years of age (see Warnings and Precautions, Special Populations, Geriatrics (≥65 years of age)).

STORAGE AND STABILITY: Store vials in the original carton under refrigeration at 2 to 8°C until time of use. Protect from light. **Do not freeze Vectibix (panitumumab).** Do not shake. Since Vectibix does not contain preservatives, any unused portion remaining in the vial must be discarded.

The diluted infusion solution of panitumumab should be used within 6 hours of preparation if stored at room temperature, or within 24 hours of dilution if stored at 2 to 8°C. **Do not freeze the diluted infusion solution of Vectibix.**

SPECIAL HANDLING INSTRUCTIONS: Vectibix (panitumumab) should not be shaken or frozen.

INFORMATION FOR THE PATIENT: Published in e-CPS, available by subscription at www.e-cps.ca.

DOSAGE FORMS, COMPOSITION AND PACKAGING: Each mL of sterile, colourless solution contains: panitumumab 20 mg. Nonmedicinal ingredients: sodium acetate USP, sodium chloride USP and water for injection USP. Preservative-free. pH 5.8. Single-use vials of 5, 10 and 20 mL, dispensing packs of 1.

Velcade™ Pr

bortezomib mannitol boronic ester

Antineoplastic

Janssen-Ortho

Date of Preparation: January 25, 2005
Date of Revision: August 13, 2009

SUMMARY PRODUCT INFORMATION:

Route of Administration	Dosage Form/ Strength	Clinically Relevant Nonmedicinal Ingredients
Intravenous	Sterile lyophilized powder for injection/3.5 mg	None

VELCADE (bortezomib mannitol boronic ester) for Injection will be referenced throughout the Product Monograph as either VELCADE (bortezomib) for Injection, VELCADE or bortezomib.

INDICATIONS AND CLINICAL USE: VELCADE (bortezomib) for Injection is indicated as follows:

- as part of combination therapy for the treatment of patients with previously untreated multiple myeloma who are unsuitable for stem cell transplantation.
- for the treatment of progressive multiple myeloma in patients who have received at least one prior therapy and who have already undergone or are unsuitable for stem cell transplantation.
- for the treatment of patients with mantle cell lymphoma who have relapsed or were refractory to at least 1 prior therapy.

Geriatrics (>65 years of age): No overall differences in safety or effectiveness of VELCADE were observed between younger patients and patients ≥65 years of age. Greater sensitivity of some older individuals cannot be ruled out (see Adverse Reactions and Action and Clinical Pharmacology).

Pediatrics and Adolescents (<18 years of age): The safety and effectiveness of VELCADE in children and adolescents have not been established.

CONTRAINDICATIONS: VELCADE (bortezomib) for Injection is contraindicated in patients with hypersensitivity to bortezomib, boron or any of the excipients.

WARNINGS AND PRECAUTIONS:

Serious Warnings and Precautions

- VELCADE must be administered under the supervision of a physician qualified in the use of antineoplastic agents.
- Twice the recommended dose has been fatal (see Warnings and Precautions, General)
- Hypotension and other serious cardiac disorders (see Warnings and Precautions, Cardiovascular, and Adverse Reactions, Randomized Open-Label Phase III Multiple Myeloma Clinical Study)
- Hemorrhage (gastrointestinal and intracerebral) (see Warnings and Precautions, Hematologic and Adverse Reactions, Post-Market Adverse Drug Reactions)
- Severe motor neuropathy, including fatalities (see Warnings and Precautions, Neurologic)
- Acute diffuse infiltrative pulmonary disease (see Warnings and Precautions, Respiratory)

General: Dose Preparation: VELCADE (bortezomib) for Injection has a narrow therapeutic window and has shown high acute toxicity in all animal species evaluated. Fatalities have been reported after accidental administration of at least twice the recommended dose in patients (see Overdosage). Careful attention is required to ensure the recommended dose is not exceeded.

Tumour Lysis Syndrome: Because VELCADE is a cytotoxic agent and can rapidly kill malignant plasma cells, the complications of tumour lysis syndrome may occur. The patients at risk of tumour lysis syndrome are those with high tumour burden prior to treatment. These patients should be monitored closely and appropriate precautions taken.

Carcinogenesis and Mutagenesis: Carcinogenicity studies have not been conducted. Bortezomib was clastogenic in mammalian cells in the in vitro chromosomal aberration assay. Bortezomib was not mutagenic in bacteria (Ames assay) and in the in vivo micronucleus assay in mice.

Cardiovascular: VELCADE treatment is commonly associated with orthostatic/postural hypotension which is not an acute reaction and is observed throughout treatment (see Adverse Reactions). In the Phase II and III relapsed multiple myeloma studies, the incidence of hypotension (postural, orthostatic, and hypotension NOS) was 11% and 12%, respectively. In the Phase II study, there was no prior history of orthostatic hypotension in these patients but half had pre-existing hypertension, one-third had evidence of peripheral neuropathy, and orthostatic hypotension was associated with syncope in some patients. In another Phase II study, there was evidence of autonomic nervous system abnormalities following VELCADE therapy. The mechanism is unknown although it may be due to bortezomib-induced autonomic neuropathy. Most cases required pharmacological treatment, including hydration and/or adjustment of antihypertensive medications. Administration of mineralocorticoids and/or sympathomimetics was infrequently required. Caution should be used when treating patients with a history of syncope, patients receiving medications known to be associated with hypotension, and patients who are dehydrated. Patients should be instructed to seek medical advice if they experience symptoms of dizziness, light-headedness or fainting spells.

Acute development or exacerbation of congestive heart failure and/or new onset of decreased left ventricular ejection fraction has been reported, including reports in patients with few or no risk factors for decreased left ventricular ejection fraction. Patients with risk factors for or existing heart disease should be closely monitored.

There have been isolated cases of QT-interval prolongation in clinical studies; causality has not been established.

Events of pericarditis (<1%) have been reported in clinical trials and during post-marketing use of VELCADE. New or worsening cases of pericarditis should be investigated promptly.

In the Phase III relapsed multiple myeloma study, the incidence of any treatment-emergent cardiac disorder was 15% and 13% in the VELCADE and dexamethasone groups, respectively. The incidence of heart failure events (acute pulmonary edema, cardiac failure, congestive cardiac failure, cardiogenic shock, pulmonary edema) was similar in the VELCADE and dexamethasone groups, 5% and 4%, respectively.

Gastrointestinal: Gastrointestinal events, including nausea, diarrhea, constipation, and vomiting occur frequently during VELCADE treatment (see Adverse Reactions). Events usually occur earlier in treatment (Cycles 1 and 2), and may persist for several cycles, sometimes requiring administration of antiemetics and antidiarrheals. Fluid and electrolyte replacement should be administered if the patient becomes dehydrated. Cases of ileus have been reported and patients who experience constipation should be closely monitored.

Hematologic: Although VELCADE treatment may be associated with hematological toxicities, significant myelosuppression is uncommon (see Adverse Reactions). The most common hematological toxicity is thrombocytopenia which is generally dose related, occurring during Days 1 to 11 of therapy, with a return to baseline in platelet count during the rest period (Days 12 to 21) in each treatment cycle. Onset is common in Cycles 1 and 2 but can continue throughout therapy. On average, the pattern of platelet count decrease and recovery remained consistent over the 8-cycle study period and there was no evidence of cumulative thrombocytopenia. The mean platelet count nadir measured was approximately 40% of baseline. The severity of thrombocytopenia related to pre-treatment platelet count is shown in Table 1. In the Phase III relapsed multiple myeloma study, the incidence of significant bleeding events (≥ Grade 3) was similar on both the VELCADE (4%) and dexamethasone (5%) arms. Platelet count should be monitored prior to each dose of VELCADE. VELCADE therapy should be held when the platelet count is $<25\times10^9$/L and re-initiated at a reduced dose. There have been reports of gastrointestinal and intracerebral hemorrhage in association with VELCADE induced thrombocytopenia (see Dosage and Administration and Adverse Reactions). Platelet transfusions, red blood cell transfusions and administration of growth factors may be utilized in the management of hematological toxicities.

Table 1: VELCADE

The Severity of Thrombocytopenia Related to Pre-Treatment Platelet Count in the Phase III Relapsed Multiple Myeloma Study

Pre-treatment Platelet Count[a]	Number of Patients (N=331)[b]	Number (%) of Patients with Platelet Count $<10\times10^9$/L	Number (%) of Patients with Platelet Count 10×10^9–25×10^9/L
$\geq75\times10^9$/L	309	8 (3%)	36 (12%)
$\geq50\times10^9$/L–$<75\times10^9$/L	14	2 (14%)	11 (79%)
$\geq10\times10^9$/L–$<50\times10^9$/L	7	1 (14%)	5 (71%)

[a] A baseline platelet count of 50×10^9/L was required for study eligibility.
[b] Data were missing at baseline for 1 patient.

Hepatic/Biliary: Bortezomib is metabolized by liver enzymes and bortezomib's clearance may decrease in patients with hepatic impairment. No formal studies evaluating the effect of liver dysfunction on the pharmacokinetics or pharmacodynamics of VELCADE have been completed. These patients should be treated with extreme caution and monitored for toxicity, and a dose reduction should be considered (see Dosage and Administration).

Rare cases of acute liver failure have been reported in VELCADE-treated patients receiving multiple concomitant medications and with serious underlying medical conditions. Other reported hepatic events include asymptomatic increases in liver enzymes, hyperbilirubinemia, and hepatitis. Such changes may be reversible upon discontinuation of VELCADE. There is limited re-challenge information in these patients.

Neurologic: Treatment with VELCADE is commonly associated with peripheral neuropathy that is predominantly sensory. However, cases of severe motor neuropathy with or without sensory peripheral neuropathy have been reported, including those with fatal outcomes. Rare cases of Guillain-Barré syndrome without established causal relationship to VELCADE and aspiration pneumonia in association with motor neuropathy have also been reported.

In clinical trials, of the patients who experienced treatment-emergent neuropathy, 70% had previously been treated with neurotoxic agents and 80% had signs or symptoms of peripheral neuropathy at baseline. Worsening of existing neuropathy is dose related and cumulative. Patients with pre-existing symptoms (numbness, pain or a burning feeling in the feet or hands) and/or signs of peripheral neuropathy (hyperesthesia, hypoesthesia, paresthesia, neuropathic pain or weakness) may experience worsening during treatment with VELCADE and it is recommended that all patients should be monitored for symptoms of neuropathy.

Complete resolution to baseline has been documented in 14% of patients with severe symptoms in the Phase II studies, with limited follow-up data available. In the Phase III relapsed multiple myeloma study, following dose adjustments, improvement in or resolution of peripheral neuropathy was reported in 51% of patients with ≥ Grade 2 peripheral neuropathy, and the median time to improvement or resolution was 107 days. VELCADE was discontinued because of peripheral neuropathy in 8% of patients in the Phase III study, and was the most common adverse event leading to treatment discontinuation. Improvement in or resolution of peripheral neuropathy was reported in 71% of patients who discontinued due to peripheral neuropathy or who had ≥ Grade 3 peripheral neuropathy in the Phase II multiple myeloma studies (see Adverse Reactions). The mechanism underlying VELCADE induced peripheral neuropathy is not known and the complete time-course of this toxicity has not been fully characterized. Full reversibility has not been demonstrated in preclinical studies.

Patients experiencing new or worsening peripheral neuropathy may require a change in the dose and schedule or cessation of VELCADE therapy (see Dosage and Administration).

Autonomic neuropathy may contribute to some adverse reactions, such as postural hypotension, diarrhea, constipation with ileus and pyrexia, but information on this is limited.

Seizures are uncommonly reported in patients without previous history of seizures. Caution should be exercised when treating patients with any risk factors.

There have been rare reports of reversible posterior leukoencephalopathy syndrome (RPLS) in patients receiving VELCADE. RPLS is a rare, reversible, neurological disorder which can present with seizure, hypertension, headache, lethargy, confusion, blindness, and other visual and neurological disturbances. Brain imaging, preferably MRI (Magnetic Resonance Imaging), is used to confirm the diagnosis. In patients developing RPLS, discontinue VELCADE. The safety of reinitiating VELCADE therapy in patients previously experiencing RPLS is not known.

Renal: Hypercalcemia and renal failure are complications of multiple myeloma most often associated with high tumour burden. Supportive treatments for these complications include bisphosphonates (for hypercalcemia and myeloma bone disease), hydration and other measures depending on the patient's status and the type and severity of the complications.

VELCADE has not been formally studied in patients with impaired renal function. Limited clinical information is available on the use of VELCADE in patients with varying degrees of impaired renal function. No clinical information is available on the use of VELCADE in patients on hemodialysis. Patients with renal impairment, especially if creatinine clearance is ≤30 mL/min, should be closely monitored for toxicities when treated with VELCADE (see Action and Clinical Pharmacology, Special Populations and Conditions).

Respiratory: There have been rare reports of acute diffuse infiltrative pulmonary disease of unknown etiology such as pneumonitis, interstitial pneumonia, lung infiltration and Acute Respiratory Distress Syndrome (ARDS) in patients receiving VELCADE. Some of these events have been fatal. A pre-treatment chest radiography should be done to determine if any additional diagnostic measures are necessary and to serve as a baseline for potential post-treatment pulmonary changes.

In the event of new or worsening pulmonary symptoms (e.g. cough, dyspnea), a prompt diagnostic evaluation should be performed and patients treated appropriately. The benefit/risk ratio should be considered prior to continuing VELCADE therapy.

In a clinical trial, two patients given high-dose cytarabine (2 g/m^2 per day) by continuous infusion over 24 hours with daunorubicin and VELCADE for relapsed acute myelogenous leukemia died of ARDS early in the course of therapy. Therefore, this specific regimen is not recommended.

Sexual Function/Reproduction: Fertility studies with bortezomib have not been performed. Degenerative effects in ovaries and testes in the general toxicity studies suggest a potential effect on male and female fertility.

Amyloidosis: The impact of proteasome inhibition by bortezomib on disorders associated with protein accumulation such as amyloidosis is unknown. Caution is advised in these patients.

Special Populations: Pregnant Women: Women of child-bearing potential should avoid becoming pregnant while being treated with VELCADE. Males and females of child-bearing capacity should use effective contraceptive measures during treatment and for 3 months following treatment.

Bortezomib was not teratogenic in rats and rabbits at the highest dose tested (0.45 and 0.55 mg/m^2, respectively) but caused post-implantation loss in rabbits.

No placental transfer studies have been conducted with bortezomib. There are no adequate and well-controlled studies in pregnant women. If VELCADE is used during pregnancy, or if the patient becomes pregnant while receiving this drug, the patient should be aware of the potential hazard to the fetus.

Nursing Women: It is not known whether bortezomib is excreted in milk. Because many drugs are excreted in milk and because of the potential for serious adverse reactions from VELCADE in nursing infants, women should be advised against breast-feeding while being treated with VELCADE.

Pediatrics (<18 years of age): The safety and effectiveness of VELCADE in children and adolescents have not been established.

Monitoring and Laboratory Tests: Complete blood counts including platelet counts should be frequently monitored throughout treatment with VELCADE.

Chest radiography should be done prior to initiating VELCADE therapy (see Warnings and Precautions, Respiratory).

ADVERSE REACTIONS: Adverse Drug Reaction Overview: Multiple Myeloma: Herpes Zoster Virus Reactivation: The administration of VELCADE has been associated with herpes zoster reactivation. In the randomized Phase 3 study in relapsed multiple myeloma, the incidence of herpes zoster occurring on treatment with VELCADE was 13% (42/331) versus 5% (15/332) in the high-dose dexamethasone group. In the randomized study in patients with previously untreated multiple myeloma, the overall incidence of herpes zoster reactivation was more common in subjects treated with VELCADE, melphalan and prednisone (VMP) than in the control group treated with melphalan and prednisone (14% vs. 4%, respectively). In this study, antiviral prophylaxis was administered to 26% (90/340) of patients in the VMP treatment group. In this treatment group, herpes zoster virus reactivation was less common in subjects receiving prophylactic antiviral therapy (3% [3/90]) than in subjects who did not receive prophylactic antiviral therapy (17% [43/250]). In the post-market setting, cases of herpes meningoencephalitis and ophthalmic herpes have been reported.

Clinical Trial Adverse Drug Reactions: Multiple Myeloma: Randomized Open-Label Combination Phase III Clinical Study in Patients with Previously Untreated Multiple Myeloma (Front-Line Therapy): In the VELCADE, melphalan, prednisone (VMP) and melphalan, prednisone (MP) treatment groups, respectively, 99% and 97% of subjects experienced at least 1 treatment-emergent adverse event. Seventy-eight percent of subjects in the VMP treatment group had Blood and Lymphatic System Disorders considered related to study drug, compared with 70% in the MP treatment group. The most commonly reported adverse events thrombocytopenia (52% vs 47%), neutropenia (49% vs 46%), and leukopenia (33% vs 30%) were comparable between the 2 treatment groups (VMP vs MP). The incidence of lymphopenia was higher in the VMP group (24% vs 17%). However, anemia was observed in only 43% of subjects in the VMP group compared to 55% in the MP group. The Gastrointestinal Disorders SOC Grades 3 and ≥4 were reported more frequently in the VMP treatment group as compared to the MP treatment group (nausea: 48% vs 28%; diarrhea: 46% vs 17%; constipation: 37% vs 16%; vomiting: 33% vs 16%). As well, the incidence of Nervous System Disorders was higher in the VMP group (VMP vs MP): peripheral neuropathy (47% vs 5%), neuralgia (36% vs 1%), and paraesthesia (13% vs 4%). The incidence of termination of all study treatment because of adverse events was similar for the VMP and MP treatment groups (15% vs 14%, respectively).

A total of 155 (46%) patients from the VMP treatment group experienced a serious adverse event (SAE) during the study compared with 121 (36%) patients from the MP treatment group. The most frequently reported serious adverse events in both treatment groups were in the Infections and Infestation SOC (VMP: 17%; MP: 15%), with pneumonia being the predominant serious adverse event in both treatment groups (VMP: 11%, MP: 7%). The incidence of serious adverse events belonging to the Nervous System Disorders was 5% in the VMP treatment group and 2% in the MP treatment group.

Drug related adverse events that led to death during the study occurred in 2% of subjects in both treatment groups (6 subjects in the VMP treatment group and 8 subjects in the MP treatment group). The most frequent drug-related adverse events leading to death were of infectious origin: drug-related pneumonia/bronchopneumonia led to death in 3 subjects in the VMP treatment group and 4 subjects in the MP treatment group and drug-related sepsis led to death in 1 subject in the VMP treatment group and 3 subjects in the MP treatment group.

Table 2 describes safety data from 340 patients with previously untreated multiple myeloma who received VELCADE (1.3 mg/m^2) in combination with melphalan (9 mg/m^2) and prednisone (60 mg/m^2) in a prospective Phase 3 study. Overall, the safety profile of VELCADE in combination with melphalan/prednisone is consistent with the known safety profiles of both VELCADE and melphalan/prednisone.

Randomized Open-Label Phase III Multiple Myeloma Clinical Study: The incidence of treatment-emergent adverse events during the study was 100% in VELCADE-treated patients and 98% in dexamethasone-treated patients. Among the 331 VELCADE treated patients, the most commonly reported adverse events overall were asthenic conditions (61%), diarrhea (58%), nausea (57%), constipation (42%), peripheral neuropathy (36%), vomiting, pyrexia, thrombocytopenia (each 35%), anorexia and decreased appetite (34%), anemia and headache (each 26%), dyspnea (25%), myalgia, muscle cramps, spasms and stiffness (24%), rash (24%), and cough and paresthesia (each 21%). The most commonly reported adverse events among the 332 patients in the dexamethasone group were psychiatric disorders (49%), asthenic conditions (45%), insomnia (27%), anemia (22%), and diarrhea (21%). Fourteen percent (14%) of patients in the VELCADE treatment arm experienced a Grade 4 adverse event; the most common Grade 4 toxicities were thrombocytopenia (4%), neutropenia (2%) and hypercalcemia (2%). Sixteen percent (16%) of dexamethasone-treated patients experienced a Grade 4 adverse event; the most common toxicity was hyperglycemia (2%).

Table 2: VELCADE

Most Commonly Reported Adverse Events (≥10% in VELCADE, Melphalan and Prednisone arm) with Grades 3 and ≥4 Intensity in the Previously Untreated Multiple Myeloma Study

MedDRA System Organ Class	VELCADE, Melphalan and Prednisone (N=340)			Melphalan and Prednisone (N=337)		
	Total	Toxicity Grade, n (%)		Total	Toxicity Grade, n (%)	
Preferred Term	n (%)	3	≥4	n (%)	3	≥4
Blood and Lymphatic System Disorders						
Thrombocytopenia	178 (52)	68 (20)	59 (17)	159 (47)	55 (16)	47 (14)
Neutropenia	165 (49)	102 (30)	35 (10)	155 (46)	79 (23)	49 (15)
Anemia	147 (43)	53 (16)	9 (3)	187 (55)	66 (20)	26 (8)
Leukopenia	113 (33)	67 (20)	10 (3)	100 (30)	55 (16)	13 (4)
Lymphopenia	83 (24)	49 (14)	18 (5)	58 (17)	30 (9)	7 (2)
Gastrointestinal Disorders						
Nausea	164 (48)	14 (4)	0	94 (28)	1 (<1)	0
Diarrhea	157 (46)	23 (7)	2 (1)	58 (17)	2 (1)	0
Constipation	125 (37)	2 (1)	0	54 (16)	0	0
Vomiting	112 (33)	14 (4)	0	55 (16)	2 (1)	0
Abdominal pain	49 (14)	7 (2)	0	22 (7)	1 (<1)	0
Abdominal pain upper	40 (12)	1 (<1)	0	29 (9)	0	0
Dyspepsia	39 (11)	0	0	23 (7)	0	0
Nervous System Disorders						
Peripheral neuropathy	159 (47)	43 (13)	2 (1)	18 (5)	0	0
Neuralgia	121 (36)	28 (8)	2 (1)	5 (1)	1 (<1)	0
Dizziness	56 (16)	7 (2)	0	37 (11)	1 (<1)	0
Headache	49 (14)	2 (1)	0	35 (10)	4 (1)	0
Paresthesia	45 (13)	6 (2)	0	15 (4)	0	0
General Disorders and Administration Site Conditions						
Pyrexia	99 (29)	8 (2)	2 (1)	64 (19)	6 (2)	2 (1)
Fatigue	98 (29)	23 (7)	2 (1)	86 (26)	7 (2)	0
Asthenia	73 (21)	20 (6)	1 (<1)	60 (18)	9 (3)	0
Edema peripheral	68 (20)	2 (1)	0	34 (10)	0	0
Infections and Infestations						
Pneumonia	56 (16)	16 (5)	13 (4)	36 (11)	13 (4)	9 (3)
Herpes Zoster	45 (13)	11 (3)	0	14 (4)	6 (2)	0
Bronchitis	44 (13)	4 (1)	0	27 (8)	4 (1)	0
Nasopharyngitis	39 (11)	1 (<1)	0	27 (8)	0	0
Musculoskeletal and Connective Tissue Disorders						
Back pain	58 (17)	9 (3)	1 (<1)	62 (18)	11 (3)	1 (<1)
Pain in extremity	47 (14)	8 (2)	0	32 (9)	3 (1)	1 (<1)
Bone pain	37 (11)	7 (2)	1 (<1)	35 (10)	7 (2)	0
Arthralgia	36 (11)	4 (1)	0	50 (15)	2 (1)	1 (<1)
Metabolism and Nutrition Disorders						
Anorexia	77 (23)	9 (3)	1 (<1)	34 (10)	4 (1)	0
Hypokalemia	44 (13)	19 (6)	3 (1)	25 (7)	8 (2)	2 (1)
Skin and Subcutaneous Tissue Disorders						
Rash	66 (19)	2 (1)	0	24 (7)	1 (<1)	0
Pruritus	35 (10)	3 (1)	0	18 (5)	0	0
Respiratory, Thoracic and Mediastinal Disorders						
Cough	71 (21)	0	0	45 (13)	2 (1)	0
Dyspnea	50 (15)	11 (3)	2 (1)	44 (13)	5 (1)	4 (1)

(cont'd)

Table 2: VELCADE *(cont'd)*

Most Commonly Reported Adverse Events (≥10% in VELCADE, Melphalan and Prednisone arm) with Grades 3 and ≥4 Intensity in the Previously Untreated Multiple Myeloma Study

	VELCADE, Melphalan and Prednisone (N=340)			Melphalan and Prednisone (N=337)		
MedDRA System Organ Class	Total	Toxicity Grade, n (%)		Total	Toxicity Grade, n (%)	
Preferred Term	n (%)	3	≥4	n (%)	3	≥4
Psychiatric Disorders						
Insomnia	69 (20)	1 (<1)	0	43 (13)	0	0
Vascular Disorders						
Hypertension	45 (13)	8 (2)	1 (<1)	25 (7)	2 (1)	0
Hypotension	41 (12)	4 (1)	3 (1)	10 (3)	2 (1)	2 (1)

A total of 144 (44%) patients from the VELCADE treatment arm experienced a serious adverse event (SAE) during the study, as did 144 (43%) dexamethasone-treated patients. An SAE is defined as any event, regardless of causality, that results in death, is life-threatening, requires hospitalization or prolongs a current hospitalization, results in a significant disability or is deemed to be an important medical event. The most commonly reported SAEs in the VELCADE treatment arm were pyrexia (6%), diarrhea (5%), dyspnea and pneumonia (4%), and vomiting (3%). In the dexamethasone treatment group, the most commonly reported SAEs were pneumonia (7%), pyrexia (4%), and hyperglycemia (3%).

A total of 145 patients, including 84 (25%) of 331 patients in the VELCADE treatment group and 61 (18%) of 332 patients in the dexamethasone treatment group were discontinued from treatment due to adverse events assessed as drug-related by the investigators. Among the 331 VELCADE treated patients, the most commonly reported drug-related event leading to discontinuation was peripheral neuropathy (8%). Among the 332 patients in the dexamethasone group, the most commonly reported drug-related events leading to treatment discontinuation were psychotic disorder and hyperglycemia (2% each).

Of the 669 patients enrolled in this study, 37% were 65 years of age or older. The incidence of Grade 3 and 4 events was 64%, 78% and 75% for VELCADE patients ≤50, 51-64 and ≥65 years of age, respectively.

Four deaths were considered to be VELCADE related in the Phase III multiple myeloma study: 1 case each of cardiogenic shock, respiratory insufficiency, congestive heart failure and cardiac arrest. Four deaths were considered dexamethasone-related: 2 cases of sepsis, 1 case of bacterial meningitis, and 1 case of sudden death at home.

Non-Randomized Phase II Relapsed Multiple Myeloma Clinical Studies: Two Phase II studies evaluated 228 patients with multiple myeloma receiving VELCADE (bortezomib) for Injection 1.3 mg/m²/dose twice weekly for 2 weeks followed by a 10-day rest period (21-day treatment cycle length) for a maximum of 8 treatment cycles.

The most commonly reported adverse events were asthenic conditions (65%), nausea (64%), diarrhea (55%), anorexia and decreased appetite (43%), constipation (43%), thrombocytopenia (43%), peripheral neuropathy (37%), pyrexia (36%), vomiting (36%), and anemia (32%). Fourteen percent (14%) of patients experienced at least one episode of Grade 4 toxicity, with the most common toxicity being thrombocytopenia (3%) and neutropenia (3%).

During the studies, a total of 113 (50%) of the 228 patients experienced SAEs. The most commonly reported SAEs included pyrexia (7%), pneumonia (7%), diarrhea (6%), vomiting (5%), dehydration (5%), and nausea (4%).

Adverse events thought by the investigator to be drug related and leading to discontinuation occurred in 18% of patients. The reasons for discontinuation included peripheral neuropathy (5%), thrombocytopenia (4%), diarrhea (2%), and fatigue (2%).

In the Phase II clinical study of 202 patients, 35% of whom were 65 years of age or older, the incidence of ≥ Grade 3 adverse events was 74%, 80% and 85% for VELCADE-treated patients ≤50, 51-64 and ≥65 years of age, respectively.

Two deaths were reported and considered by the investigator to be possibly related to study drug: one case of cardiopulmonary arrest and one case of respiratory failure.

Patients from the two Phase II studies who, in the investigators' opinion, would experience additional clinical benefit were allowed to receive VELCADE beyond 8 cycles on an extension study). Compared to the parent studies, patients in this extension study experienced a greater incidence of selected adverse events including edema overall (41% versus 29%), Grade 4 adverse events (22% versus 5%), and serious adverse events (48% versus 33%). As well, there was a greater incidence of lower limb edema (27% versus 10%), hyperglycemia (19% versus 5%), increased blood creatinine (13% versus 3%), productive cough (13% versus 2%), hypoproteinemia (10% versus 0%) and chest wall pain (10% versus 0%) in this extension study compared to the parent Phase II studies. Most of these adverse events were mild or moderate in intensity, and none was reported as an SAE. Of the commonly reported side effects attributable to VELCADE treatment, there was no evidence of their increase with cumulative dosing.

Mantle Cell Lymphoma: Non-Randomized Phase II Mantle Cell Lymphoma Study: Safety data for patients with mantle cell lymphoma were evaluated in a phase II study, which included 155 patients treated with VELCADE at the recommended dose of 1.3 mg/m² twice weekly on days 1, 4, 8 and 11 of a 21-day cycle. The most commonly reported adverse events were asthenic conditions (72%), peripheral neuropathy (55%), constipation (50%), diarrhea (47%), nausea (44%), decreased appetite (39%), vomiting (27%), rash (28%), edema (28%), anemia (17%), dizziness (excluding vertigo) (23%), dyspnea (23%), thrombocytopenia (21%), insomnia (21%). The safety profile of VELCADE in these patients was similar to that observed in patients with multiple myeloma. Notable differences between the two patient populations were that thrombocytopenia, neutropenia, anemia, nausea, vomiting and pyrexia were reported more often in the patients with multiple myeloma than in those with mantle cell lymphoma; whereas peripheral neuropathy, rash and pruritus were higher among patients with mantle cell lymphoma compared to patients with multiple myeloma. The most common adverse event leading to the discontinuation of VELCADE-treated patients was peripheral neuropathy (10%).

The most common treatment-emergent adverse drug reactions occurring at ≥10% incidence for Phase III and Phase II relapsed multiple myeloma studies are presented in Table 3 and Table 4, respectively, by System Organ Class. As well the most common treatment-emergent adverse drug reactions occurring at ≥10% incidence for the Phase II mantle cell lymphoma study is presented in Table 5 by System Organ Class.

Table 3: VELCADE

Most Commonly Reported Adverse Events (≥10% in VELCADE arm), with Grades 3 and 4 Intensity in the Phase III Multiple Myeloma Randomized Study (N=663)

	Treatment Group					
	VELCADE (n=331) [n (%)]			Dexamethasone (n=332) [n (%)]		
System Organ Class	All Events	Grade 3 Events	Grade 4 Events	All Events	Grade 3 Events	Grade 4 Events
Blood and Lymphatic System Disorders						
Thrombocytopenia	115 (35)	85 (26)	12 (4)	36 (11)	18 (5)	4 (1)
Anemia NOS	87 (26)	31 (9)	2 (<1)	74 (22)	32 (10)	3 (<1)
Neutropenia	62 (19)	40 (12)	8 (2)	5 (2)	4 (1)	0
Gastrointestinal Disorders						
Diarrhea NOS, loose stools	192 (58)	24 (7)	0	70 (21)	6 (2)	0
Nausea	190 (57)	8 (2)	0	46 (14)	0	0
Constipation	140 (42)	7 (2)	0	49 (15)	4 (1)	0
Vomiting NOS	117 (35)	11 (3)	0	20 (6)	4 (1)	0
Abdominal pain NOS	53 (16)	6 (2)	0	12 (4)	1 (<1)	0
Dyspepsia	32 (10)	2 (<1)	0	28 (8)	0	0
General Disorders and Administration Site Conditions						
Asthenia (fatigue, weakness, malaise, fatigue aggravated, lethargy)	201 (61)	39 (12)	1 (<1)	148 (45)	20 (6)	0
Pyrexia	116 (35)	6 (2)	0	54 (16)	4 (1)	1 (<1)
Edema lower limb, edema peripheral, peripheral swelling, edema NOS[a]	56 (17)	0	0	65 (20)	1 (<1)	0
Rigors	37 (11)	0	0	8 (2)	0	0
Pain NOS	33 (10)	7 (2)	0	12 (4)	2 (<1)	1 (<1)
Infections and Infestations						
Nasopharyngitis	45 (14)	1 (<1)	0	22 (7)	0	0
Herpes Zoster (including multi-dermatomal or disseminated)	42 (13)	6 (2)	0	15 (5)	4 (1)	1 (<1)
Metabolism and Nutrition Disorders						
Anorexia, appetite decreased NOS	112 (34)	9 (3)	0	31 (9)	1 (<1)	0
Musculoskeletal and Connective Tissue Disorders						
Bone pain, bone pain aggravated	54 (16)	12 (4)	0	53 (16)	11 (3)	0
Muscle cramps, muscle spasms, muscle stiffness, myalgia	78 (24)	2 (<1)	0	66 (20)	5 (2)	0
Arthralgia, joint stiffness	49 (15)	3 (<1)	0	35 (11)	5 (2)	0
Pain in the limb	50 (15)	5 (2)	0	24 (7)	2 (<1)	0
Back pain	46 (14)	10 (3)	0	33 (10)	4 (1)	0
Musculoskeletal pain	33 (10)	3 (<1)	0	11 (3)	3 (<1)	0
Nervous System Disorders						
Peripheral neuropathy NOS, peripheral neuropathy aggravated, peripheral sensory neuropathy	119 (36)	24 (7)	2 (<1)	28 (8)	1 (<1)	1 (<1)
Headache NOS	85 (26)	3 (<1)	0	43 (13)	2 (<1)	0
Paresthesia, burning sensation NOS	70 (21)	5 (2)	0	28 (8)	0	0
Dizziness (excluding vertigo)	45 (14)	3 (<1)	0	34 (10)	0	0
Psychiatric Disorders						
Insomnia	60 (18)	1 (<1)	0	90 (27)	5 (2)	0
Respiratory, Thoracic and Mediastinal Disorders						
Dyspnea NOS, dyspnea exertional	84 (25)	17 (5)	1 (<1)	65 (20)	9 (3)	2 (<1)
Cough	70 (21)	2 (<1)	0	35 (11)	1 (<1)	0

(cont'd)

Table 3: VELCADE *(cont'd)*

Most Commonly Reported Adverse Events (≥10% in VELCADE arm), with Grades 3 and 4 Intensity in the Phase III Multiple Myeloma Randomized Study (N=663)

	Treatment Group					
	VELCADE (n=331) [n (%)]			Dexamethasone (n=332) [n (%)]		
System Organ Class	All Events	Grade 3 Events	Grade 4 Events	All Events	Grade 3 Events	Grade 4 Events
Skin and Subcutaneous Tissue Disorders						
Rash NOS, rash pruritic, rash erythematous, rash generalized, rash macular, rash papular, erythema, urticaria NOS	79 (24)	6 (2)	0	28 (8)	0	0
Vascular Disorders						
Orthostatic hypotension, hypotension NOS, postural hypotension	38 (11)	3 (<1)	0	6 (2)	2 (<1)	1 (<1)

[a] Preferred terms mapped to General Disorders and Administration Site Conditions SOC or Musculoskeletal and Connective Tissue Disorders SOC.

Table 4: VELCADE

Most Commonly Reported (≥10% overall) Adverse Events Reported from 2 Phase II Clinical Trials in Multiple Myeloma Patients (N=228)

	VELCADE-Treated Patients at 1.3 mg/m²/dose (N=228)		
System Organ Class	All Events n (%)	Grade 3 Events n (%)	Grade 4 Events n (%)
Blood and Lymphatic System Disorders			
Thrombocytopenia	97 (43)	61 (27)	7 (3)
Anemia NOS or anemia NOS aggravated, hemoglobin decreased, red blood cell count decreased[a]	74 (32)	21 (9)	0
Neutropenia or neutropenia aggravated	54 (24)	29 (13)	6 (3)
Eye Disorders			
Vision blurred	25 (11)	1 (<1)	0
Gastrointestinal Disorders			
Nausea or nausea aggravated	145 (64)	15 (7)	0
Diarrhea NOS or loose stools	125 (55)	16 (7)	2 (1)
Constipation or constipation aggravated	99 (43)	5 (2)	0
Vomiting NOS	82 (36)	16 (7)	1 (<1)
Abdominal pain NOS, abdominal pain upper or abdominal discomfort	45 (20)	5 (2)	0
Dyspepsia	30 (13)	0	0
General Disorders and Administration Site Conditions			
Asthenia (fatigue, weakness, malaise, fatigue aggravated, lethargy)	149 (65)	42 (18)	1 (<1)
Pyrexia	82 (36)	9 (4)	0
Edema peripheral, edema lower limb, peripheral swelling[b]	48 (21)	2 (1)	0
Rigors	27 (12)	1 (<1)	0
Pain NOS	22 (10)	3 (1)	0
Infections and Infestations			
Upper respiratory tract infection NOS	41 (18)	0	0
Herpes zoster (including multidermatomal or disseminated)	26 (11)	2 (1)	0
Pneumonia NOS	23 (10)	12 (5)	0
Metabolism and Nutrition Disorders			
Anorexia, appetite decreased NOS	99 (43)	6 (3)	0
Dehydration	42 (18)	15 (7)	0
Weight decreased, failure to thrive[c]	26 (11)	2 (1)	0
Musculoskeletal and Connective Tissue Disorders			
Arthralgia, joint stiffness	63 (28)	11 (5)	0
Pain in the limb	59 (26)	16 (7)	0
Muscle cramps, muscle spasms, muscle stiffness, myalgia	60 (26)	8 (4)	0
Bone pain, bone pain aggravated	39 (17)	11 (5)	0
Back pain	31 (14)	9 (4)	0
Nervous System Disorders			
Peripheral neuropathy NOS, peripheral neuropathy aggravated, peripheral sensory neuropathy	84 (37)	31 (14)	0
Headache NOS	63 (28)	8 (4)	0
Dizziness (excluding vertigo)	48 (21)	3 (1)	0
Paresthesia, burning sensation NOS	32 (14)	5 (2)	0
Dysgeusia	29 (13)	1 (<1)	0
Hypoesthesia	26 (11)	1 (<1)	0
Psychiatric Disorders			
Insomnia	62 (27)	3 (1)	0
Anxiety NEC	32 (14)	0	0
Respiratory, Thoracic and Mediastinal Disorders			
Dyspnea NOS, dyspnea exertional, dyspnea exacerbated	66 (29)	8 (4)	1 (<1)
Cough	39 (17)	1 (<1)	0
Epistaxis	23 (10)	1 (<1)	0
Skin and Subcutaneous Tissue Disorders			
Rash NOS, rash pruritic, rash erythematous, rash generalized, rash macular, rash papular, erythema, urticaria NOS	63 (28)	1 (<1)	0
Pruritus NOS, pruritus generalized	28 (12)	0	0
Vascular Disorders			
Orthostatic hypotension, hypotension NOS, postural hypotension	27 (12)	8 (4)	0

[a] Preferred terms mapped to Blood and Lymphatic System Disorders System Organ Class (SOC) or Investigations SOC.
[b] Preferred terms mapped to General Disorders and Administration Site Conditions SOC or Musculoskeletal and Connective Tissue Disorders SOC.
[c] Preferred terms mapped to Investigations SOC or Metabolism and Nutrition Disorders SOC.

Table 5: VELCADE

Most Commonly Reported Adverse Events (≥10% overall) Reported in the Phase II Mantle Cell Lymphoma Study

	VELCADE-Treated Patients at 1.3 mg/m²/dose (N=155)	
System Organ Class	All Events n (%)	≥ Grade 3 n (%)
Blood and Lymphatic System Disorders		
Thrombocytopenia	33 (21)	17 (11)
Anemia	27 (17)	4 (3)
Gastrointestinal Disorders		
Constipation	77 (50)	4 (3)
Diarrhea	73 (47)	11 (7)
Nausea	68 (44)	4 (3)
Vomiting	42 (27)	4 (3)
Abdominal pain	24 (15)	8 (5)
General Disorders and Administration Site Conditions		

(cont'd)

Table 5: VELCADE *(cont'd)*

Most Commonly Reported Adverse Events (≥10% overall) Reported in the Phase II Mantle Cell Lymphoma Study

System Organ Class	VELCADE-Treated Patients at 1.3 mg/m²/dose (N=155) All Events n (%)	≥ Grade 3 n (%)
Asthenic conditions	112 (72)	29 (19)
Edema	44 (28)	4 (3)
Pyrexia	30 (19)	2 (1)
Infections and Infestations		
Upper respiratory tract infection	24 (15)	1 (<1)
Metabolism and Nutrition Disorders		
Appetite decreased	60 (39)	5 (3)
Musculoskeletal and Connective Tissue Disorders		
Arthralgia	20 (13)	2 (1)
Myalgia	15 (10)	0
Nervous System Disorders		
Peripheral neuropathy[a]	85 (55)	20 (13)
Dizziness (excluding vertigo)	36 (23)	5 (3)
Headache	26 (17)	0
Psychiatric Disorders		
Insomnia	33 (21)	1 (<1)
Respiratory, Thoracic and Mediastinal Disorders		
Dyspnea	35 (23)	7 (5)
Cough	30 (19)	0
Skin and Subcutaneous Tissue Disorders		
Rash	43 (28)	4 (3)
Vascular Disorders		
Hypotension	23 (15)	5 (3)

[a] Peripheral neuropathy includes all terms under peripheral neuropathy NEC (peripheral neuropathy NOS, peripheral neuropathy aggravated, peripheral sensory neuropathy, and peripheral motor neuropathy, and neuropathy NOS).

Serious Adverse Events from Other Clinical Studies (hematological malignancy and solid tumours): The following clinically important serious adverse events that are not described above have been reported in clinical trials in patients treated with VELCADE administered as monotherapy or in combination with other chemotherapeutics. These studies were conducted in patients with hematological malignancies and in solid tumours.

Blood and Lymphatic System Disorders: disseminated intravascular coagulation.

Cardiac Disorders: angina pectoris, atrial fibrillation aggravated, atrial flutter, bradycardia, sinus arrest, cardiac amyloidosis, cardiac arrest, congestive heart failure, myocardial ischemia, myocardial infarction, pericarditis, pericardial effusion, pulmonary edema, ventricular tachycardia.

One case of torsades de pointes (not described above) has been reported in a patient receiving VELCADE; causality has not been established.

Ear and Labyrinth Disorders: hearing impaired.

Eye Disorders: diplopia.

Gastrointestinal Disorders: ascites, dysphagia, fecal impaction, gastroenteritis, gastritis hemorrhagic, gastrointestinal hemorrhage, hematemesis, hemorrhagic duodenitis, ileus paralytic, large intestinal obstruction, paralytic intestinal obstruction, small intestinal obstruction, large intestinal perforation, stomatitis, melena, pancreatitis acute.

General Disorders and Administration Site Conditions: injection site erythema.

Hepatobiliary: cholestasis, hepatic hemorrhage, hyperbilirubinemia, portal vein thrombosis, hepatitis and liver failure.

Immune System Disorders: anaphylactic reaction, drug hypersensitivity, immune complex mediated hypersensitivity, acute renal failure (proliferative glomerulonephropathy), diffuse polyarthritis and rash.

Infections and Infestations: aspergillosis, bacteremia, urinary tract infection, herpes viral infection, listeriosis, septic shock, toxoplasmosis, oral candidiasis.

Injury, Poisoning and Procedural Complications: skeletal fracture, subdural hematoma.

Metabolism and Nutrition Disorders: hypocalcemia, hyperuricemia, hypokalemia, hyperkalemia, hypernatremia, hyponatremia, tumour lysis syndrome.

Nervous System: ataxia, coma, dizziness, dysarthria, dysautonomia, encephalopathy, cranial palsy, grand mal convulsion, hemorrhagic stroke, motor dysfunction, spinal cord compression, paraplegia, transient ischemic attack.

Psychiatric: agitation, confusion, mental status changes, psychotic disorder, suicidal ideation.

Renal and Urinary: calculus renal, bilateral hydronephrosis, bladder spasm, hematuria, hemorrhagic cystitis, urinary incontinence, urinary retention, renal failure—acute and chronic, glomerular nephritis proliferative.

Respiratory, Thoracic and Mediastinal: acute respiratory distress syndrome, aspiration pneumonia, atelectasis, chronic obstructive airways disease exacerbated, dysphagia, epistaxis, hemoptysis, hypoxia, lung infiltration, pleural effusion, pneumonitis, respiratory distress, respiratory failure.

Skin and Subcutaneous Tissue Disorders: urticaria, face edema.

Vascular: cerebrovascular accident, deep venous thrombosis, peripheral embolism, pulmonary embolism, pulmonary hypertension.

Abnormal Hematologic and Clinical Chemistry Findings: Hematological abnormalities are expected in patients with advanced multiple myeloma. With bortezomib, cyclical thrombocytopenia was seen, with a general progressive decrease in platelet count during the bortezomib dosing period (Days 1 to 11) and a return to baseline in platelet count during the rest period (Days 12 to 21) in each treatment cycle. A trend towards an increase in hemoglobin and absolute neutrophil count across treatment cycles was noted especially with an improvement in the underlying disease. A trend towards a decrease in the absolute lymphocyte count was noted across the 8 treatment cycles; however, no trend was noted by cycle. Effects on electrolytes and calcium (hyper- and hypokalemia, hyper- and hyponatremia, hyper- and hypocalcemia) and hypophosphatemia, hypochloremia and hypomagnesemia were noted.

Post-Market Adverse Drug Reactions: The following adverse events have been reported from post-marketing experience: central neurotoxicity/psychiatric events including seizures, mental status changes, encephalopathy, acute psychosis, bilateral hearing loss, dysautonomia, reversible posterior leukoencephalopathy syndrome; cardiovascular and pulmonary events including tachycardia, heart failure, cardiac tamponade, pericarditis, pulmonary hypertension, cardiac and cardiopulmonary arrest, complete heart block, pneumonitis, respiratory failure, pulmonary alveolar hemorrhage, pleural effusion, acute pulmonary edema, cardiogenic shock; serious bleeding events including subarachnoid hemorrhage, intracerebral hemorrhage, disseminated intravascular coagulation, ischemic stroke; hypersensitivity events including immune complex type diseases, angioedema; tumour lysis syndrome; amyloidosis; hepatic abnormalities including increased transaminases, alkaline phosphatase, gamma-glutamyl transferase, hepatocellular damage, hepatitis, pancreatitis; renal abnormalities including acute renal failure, nephrotic syndrome, renal tubular acidosis; sepsis and septic shock; gastrointestinal events including ischemic colitis and paralytic ileus; hyper- and hypocalcemia, hyper- and hypokalemia, severe hyponatremia, inappropriate ADH secretion; acute diffuse infiltrative pulmonary disease; Stevens-Johnson Syndrome and toxic epidermal necrolysis; herpes meningoencephalitis and ophthalmic herpes.

DRUG INTERACTIONS: Drug-Drug Interactions: No formal drug interaction studies have been conducted with bortezomib.

Bortezomib is a substrate for cytochrome P450 (CYP) 3A4, 2C19, 1A2, 2D6 and 2C9 in human liver microsomes and a weak inhibitor of CYP isozymes 1A2, 2C9, 2D6 and 3A4 (IC_{50} ≥30 μM or 11.5 μg/mL) and CYP2C19 (IC_{50} ≥18 μM or 6.9 μg/mL).

The effect of concomitant medicinal products that are potent CYP inhibitors and inducers on the pharmacokinetics of bortezomib is unknown at this time. With bortezomib's extensive metabolism, caution must be used in the co-administration of VELCADE with agents that are known to be potent inducers and inhibitors of the CYP3A4 and 2C19 isoforms.

A drug-drug interaction study assessing the effect of melphalan-prednisone on VELCADE showed a 17% increase in mean bortezomib AUC based on data from 21 patients.

During clinical trials, hypoglycemia and hyperglycemia were reported in diabetic patients receiving oral hypoglycemics. Patients on oral antidiabetic agents receiving VELCADE treatment may require close monitoring of their blood glucose levels and adjustment of the dose of their antidiabetic medication.

Drug-Food Interactions: Interactions with food have not been established.

Drug-Herb Interactions: Interactions with herbal products have not been established.

Drug-Laboratory Test Interactions: Interactions with results of laboratory tests have not been established.

Drug-Lifestyle Interactions: VELCADE may be associated with fatigue, dizziness, syncope, orthostatic/postural hypotension or blurred vision. Therefore, patients are advised to be cautious when operating machinery, or when driving.

DOSAGE AND ADMINISTRATION:

Dosing Considerations: Treatment must be administered under the supervision of a physician qualified and experienced in the use of antineoplastic agents.

VELCADE (bortezomib) for Injection has not been formally studied in patients with impaired renal function. Patients with compromised renal function should be monitored carefully, especially if creatinine clearance is ≤30 mL/minute (see Warnings and Precautions and Adverse Reactions).

VELCADE has not been studied in patients with impaired hepatic function. Patients with impaired liver function should be treated with extreme caution and a dose reduction should be considered (see Warnings and Precautions).

There is no evidence to suggest that dose adjustments are necessary in elderly patients (see Adverse Reactions).

The safety and effectiveness of VELCADE in children and adolescents have not been established.

Dosage in Previously Untreated Multiple Myeloma: VELCADE (bortezomib) is administered as a 3-5 second bolus IV injection in combination with oral melphalan and oral prednisone for nine 6-week treatment cycles as shown in Table 6. In Cycles 1-4, VELCADE is administered twice weekly (days 1, 4, 8, 11, 22, 25, 29 and 32). In Cycles 5-9, VELCADE is administered once weekly (days 1, 8, 22 and 29). At least 72 hours should elapse between consecutive doses of VELCADE.

Dose Modification Guidelines for Combination Therapy with VELCADE, Melphalan and Prednisone: Dose modification and re-initiation of therapy when VELCADE is administered in combination with melphalan and prednisone.

Prior to initiating a new cycle of therapy:

- Platelet count should be ≥70×10⁹/L and the ANC should be ≥1.0×10⁹/L
- Non-hematological toxicities should have resolved to Grade 1 or baseline

Table 6: VELCADE

Dosage Regimen for Patients with Previously Untreated Multiple Myeloma

Twice Weekly VELCADE (Cycles 1-4)												
Week	**1**				**2**		**3**	**4**		**5**		**6**
VELCADE (1.3 mg/m²)	Day 1	—	—	Day 4	Day 8	Day 11	rest period	Day 22	Day 25	Day 29	Day 32	rest period
Melphalan (9 mg/m²) Prednisone (60 mg/m²)	Day 1	Day 2	Day 3	Day 4	—		rest period	—	—	—	—	rest period
Once Weekly VELCADE (Cycles 5-9 when used in combination with Melphalan and Prednisone)												
Week	**1**				**2**		**3**	**4**		**5**		**6**
VELCADE (1.3 mg/m²)	Day 1	—	—	—	Day 8		rest period	Day 22		Day 29		rest period
Melphalan (9 mg/m²) Prednisone (60 mg/m²)	Day 1	Day 2	Day 3	Day 4	—		rest period	—		—		rest period

Table 7: VELCADE

Dose Modifications During Subsequent Cycles of Combination VELCADE, Melphalan and Prednisone Therapy

Toxicity	Dose Modification or Delay
Hematological toxicity during a cycle:	
If prolonged (≥5 days) Grade 4 neutropenia or thrombocytopenia, or thrombocytopenia with bleeding is observed in the previous cycle	Consider reduction of the melphalan dose by 25% in the next cycle.
If platelet count ≤30×10⁹/L or ANC ≤0.75×10⁹/L on a VELCADE dosing day (other than day 1)	VELCADE dose should be withheld.
If several VELCADE doses in a cycle are withheld (≥3 doses during twice weekly administration or ≥2 doses during weekly administration)	VELCADE dose should be reduced by 1 dose level (from 1.3 mg/m² to 1 mg/m², or from 1 mg/m² to 0.7 mg/m²).
Grade ≥3 non-hematological toxicities	VELCADE therapy should be withheld until symptoms of the toxicity have resolved to Grade 1 or baseline. Then, VELCADE may be reinitiated with one dose level reduction (from 1.3 mg/m² to 1 mg/m², or from 1 mg/m² to 0.7 mg/m²). For VELCADE-related neuropathic pain and/or peripheral neuropathy, hold and/or modify VELCADE as outlined in Table 8.

Please refer to the melphalan and prednisone Product Monographs for additional information.

Dosage in Relapsed Multiple Myeloma and Mantle Cell Lymphoma: The recommended starting dose of bortezomib is 1.3 mg/m² body surface area administered as a 3 to 5 second bolus intravenous injection twice weekly for two weeks (Days 1, 4, 8, and 11) followed by a 10-day rest period (Days 12-21). This 3-week period is considered a treatment cycle. For extended therapy beyond 8 cycles, VELCADE may be administered on a maintenance schedule of once weekly for 4 weeks (Days 1, 8, 15, and 22) followed by a 13-day rest period (Days 23 to 35). At least 72 hours should elapse between consecutive doses of VELCADE to minimize drug accumulation.

For tolerability reasons, dose reduction to 1.0 mg/m² has been found effective. VELCADE therapy should be withheld at the onset of any Grade 3 non-hematological or any Grade 4 hematological toxicities, excluding neuropathy as discussed below (see Warnings and Precautions). Once the symptoms of the toxicity have resolved, VELCADE treatment may be re-initiated at a 25% reduced dose (1.3 mg/m² reduced to 1.0 mg/m²; 1.0 mg/m² reduced to 0.7 mg/m²). If toxicity is not resolved or if it recurs at the lowest dose, discontinuation of VELCADE must be considered unless the benefit of treatment clearly outweighs the risk.

Treatment with VELCADE may be associated with a dose-related, transient decrease in platelet count. It is recommended that platelets be monitored before each dose, and that therapy be held if platelet counts are <25×10⁹/L and re-initiated at a reduced dose after resolution (see Warnings and Precautions).

In a supportive Phase 2 relapsed multiple myeloma study in which the majority of patients were not refractory and had received less than 2 prior lines of therapy, a dose of 1.0 mg/m² was investigated.

It is recommended that patients with a confirmed complete response receive 2 additional cycles of VELCADE beyond a confirmation. It is also recommended that responding patients who do not achieve a complete remission receive a total of 8 cycles of VELCADE therapy.

Currently there are limited data concerning retreatment with VELCADE.

Patients who experience VELCADE related neuropathic pain and/or peripheral sensory neuropathy are to be managed as presented in Table 8. Patients with pre-existing severe neuropathy may be treated with VELCADE only after careful risk/benefit assessment.

Table 8: VELCADE

Recommended Dose Modification for VELCADE-related Neuropathic Pain and/or Peripheral Sensory or Motor Neuropathy

Severity of Peripheral Neuropathy Signs and Symptoms	Modification of Dose and Regimen
Grade 1 (paresthesia, weakness and/or loss of reflexes) without pain or loss of function	No action
Grade 1 with pain or Grade 2 (interfering with function but not with activities of daily living)	Reduce VELCADE to 1.0 mg/m²
Grade 2 with pain or Grade 3 (interfering with activities of daily living)	Withhold VELCADE treatment until symptoms of toxicity have resolved. When toxicity resolves, re-initiate VELCADE treatment and reduce dose to 0.7 mg/m² and change treatment schedule to once per week.
Grade 4 (sensory neuropathy which is disabling or motor neuropathy that is life-threatening or leads to paralysis)	Discontinue VELCADE

NCI common toxicity criteria.

Missed Dose: A minimum of 72 hours is required between doses. In a Day 1, 4, 8 and 11 dose schedule, if Day 4, 8 or 11 dose is missed, that dose is not made up.

Administration: The reconstituted solution is administered as a 3-5 second bolus intravenous injection through a peripheral or central intravenous catheter followed by a flush with 0.9% Sodium Chloride Injection, USP.

VELCADE is a cytotoxic agent. Caution should be used during handling and preparation. Proper aseptic technique should be used since no preservative is present. Use of gloves and other protective clothing is recommended. In clinical trials, local skin irritation was reported in 5% of patients, but extravasation of VELCADE was not associated with tissue damage.

Reconstitution: Prior to use, the contents of each vial must be reconstituted with 3.5 mL of 0.9% Sodium Chloride Injection, USP. The reconstituted product should be a clear and colourless solution.

Parenteral drug products should be inspected visually for particulate matter and discolouration prior to administration whenever solution and container permit. If any discolouration or particulate matter is observed, the reconstituted product should not be used.

Vial Size	Volume of Diluent to be Added to Vial	Approximate Available Volume	Nominal Concentration per mL
10 mL	3.5 mL 0.9% Sodium Chloride Injection, USP	3.5 mL	1 mg/mL

Stability: VELCADE contains no antimicrobial preservative. When reconstituted as directed, VELCADE may be stored at 25°C. Reconstituted VELCADE should be administered within eight hours of preparation. The reconstituted material may be stored for up to eight hours in the original vial or in a syringe. The total storage time for the reconstituted material must not exceed eight hours when exposed to normal indoor lighting.

OVERDOSAGE:
Cardiovascular safety pharmacology studies in monkeys and dogs show that single IV doses approximately two to three times the recommended clinical dose on a mg/m² basis are associated with hypotension, increases in heart rate, decreases in contractility, altered temperature control and death. The decreased cardiac contractility and hypotension responded to acute intervention with positive inotropic or pressor agents. In dog studies, increases in the QT and corrected QT interval were observed at lethal doses.

Accidental overdosage of at least twice the recommended dose has been associated with the acute onset of symptomatic hypotension and thrombocytopenia with fatal outcomes.

There is no known specific antidote for VELCADE overdosage. In the event of an overdosage, the patient's vital signs should be monitored and appropriate supportive care given to maintain blood pressure (such as fluids, pressors, and/or inotropic agents) and body temperature (see Warnings and Precautions and Dosage and Administration).

For management of a suspected drug overdose, CPhA recommends that you contact your **regional Poison Control Centre**. See the *CPS* Directory section for a list of Poison Control Centres.

ACTION AND CLINICAL PHARMACOLOGY: Mechanism of Action: Bortezomib is a reversible inhibitor of the chymotrypsin-like activity of the 26S proteasome in mammalian cells. The 26S proteasome is a large protein complex that degrades ubiquitinated proteins. The ubiquitin-proteasome pathway plays an essential role in regulating the intracellular concentration of specific proteins, thereby maintaining homeostasis within cells. Inhibition of the 26S proteasome prevents this targeted proteolysis which can affect multiple signalling cascades within the cell. This disruption of normal homeostatic mechanisms can lead to cell death.

The mechanism of action of VELCADE suggests that it should be active in MCL. Proteasome inhibition blocks degradation of IkB and inhibits NFkB. NFkB activates transcription of many genes that inhibit apoptosis and promote proliferation in lymphoma cells. Proteasome inhibition also leads to accumulation of p27 and other cyclin D kinase inhibitors. Low levels of p27 correlate with poor survival in MCL.

Pharmacodynamics: Bortezomib is a selective, reversible proteasome inhibitor and experiments have demonstrated that bortezomib is cytotoxic to a variety of cancer cell types. Bortezomib causes a reduction of tumour growth in vivo in many preclinical tumour models, including multiple myeloma.

Pharmacokinetics: Following intravenous bolus administration of 1.0 mg/m² and 1.3 mg/m² doses to 24 patients with multiple myeloma (n=12 per each dose level), the mean first-dose maximum plasma concentrations of bortezomib were 57 and 112 ng/mL, respectively. In subsequent doses administered twice weekly, mean maximum observed plasma concentrations ranged from 67 to 106 ng/mL for the 1.0 mg/m² dose and 89 to 120 ng/mL for the 1.3 mg/m² dose. The mean elimination half-life of bortezomib upon multiple dosing ranged from 40 to 193 hours for the 1.0 mg/m² dose, and 49 to 109 hours for the 1.3 mg/m² dose. Bortezomib is eliminated more rapidly following the first dose compared to subsequent doses. Mean total body clearances were 102 and 112 L/h following the first dose for doses of 1.0 mg/m² and 1.3 mg/m², respectively, and ranged from 15 to 32 L/h following subsequent doses for doses of 1.0 mg/m² and 1.3 mg/m², respectively.

Absorption: VELCADE is administered intravenously and therefore has 100% bioavailability.

Distribution: The mean distribution volume of bortezomib ranged from 489 to 1884 L/m² following single- or repeat-dose administration of 1.0 mg/m² or 1.3 mg/m² to patients with multiple myeloma. This suggests that bortezomib distributes widely to peripheral tissues. In vitro bortezomib binding to human plasma protein averaged 83% over a concentration range of 10 to 1000 ng/mL.

Metabolism: Bortezomib is primarily metabolized via cytochrome P450-mediated deboronation to metabolites that subsequently are hydroxylated. In vitro studies indicate that CYP3A4 and 2C19 are quantitatively the major isoforms with CYP1A2, 2C9 and 2D6 having a minor contribution to the overall metabolism of bortezomib. Evaluated deboronated-bortezomib metabolites are inactive as 26S proteasome inhibitors. Pooled plasma data from 8 patients at 10 min and 30 min after dosing indicate that the plasma levels of metabolites are low compared to the parent drug.

Excretion: The pathway of elimination of bortezomib has not been characterized in humans. The predominant route of elimination is biliary excretion in the rat whereas in the monkey, renal elimination is higher than biliary/fecal elimination.

Special Populations and Conditions: Gender and Race, Pediatrics, Geriatrics, Hepatic Insufficiency and Renal Insufficiency: There are no data on effects of bortezomib on the pharmacokinetics in these special populations and conditions.

STORAGE AND STABILITY: Unopened vials may be stored between 15 and 30°C. Retain in original package to protect from light.

Single-use vials. Discard unused portion.

The product may be stored for up to eight hours in a syringe; however, total storage time for the reconstituted material must not exceed eight hours when exposed to normal indoor lighting.

SPECIAL HANDLING INSTRUCTIONS: VELCADE (bortezomib) for Injection is a cytotoxic agent. Caution should be used during handling and preparation. Proper aseptic technique should be used since no preservative is present. Use of gloves and other protective clothing to prevent skin contact is recommended.

INFORMATION FOR THE PATIENT: Published in e-CPS, available by subscription at www.e-cps.ca .

DOSAGE FORMS, COMPOSITION AND PACKAGING: Each vial of white to off-white cake or powder for injection contains: bortezomib 3.5 mg as a mannitol boronic ester. Nonmedicinal ingredients: mannitol. Vials of 10 mL, individually cartoned.

(Shown in Product Identification Section)

Ventolin® Diskus® P

salbutamol sulfate

Bronchodilator

GlaxoSmithKline

Date of Revision: October 3, 2007

SUMMARY PRODUCT INFORMATION:

Route of Administration	Dosage Form/Strength	Clinically Relevant Nonmedicinal Ingredients
Oral Inhalation	Powder for inhalation/200 µg/salbutamol	Lactose (which contains milk protein). For a complete listing see Dosage Forms, Composition and Packaging.

INDICATIONS AND CLINICAL USE: VENTOLIN (salbutamol sulfate) DISKUS inhalation powder is indicated for:

- the symptomatic relief and prevention of bronchospasm due to bronchial asthma, chronic bronchitis and other chronic bronchopulmonary disorders in which bronchospasm is a complicating factor.
- the prevention of exercise-induced bronchospasm.

Pediatrics (<4 years of age): The safety and efficacy in children below the age of 4 years has not been established.

CONTRAINDICATIONS:

- Patients with a known or suspected hypersensitivity to any of the ingredients. For a complete listing, see Dosage Forms, Composition and Packaging.
- Patients with IgE mediated allergic reactions to lactose (which contains milk protein) or milk.

WARNINGS AND PRECAUTIONS: General: Patients should always carry their VENTOLIN DISKUS inhalation powder to use immediately if an episode of asthma is experienced. If therapy does not produce a significant improvement or if the patient's condition worsens, medical advice must be sought to determine a new plan of treatment. In the case of acute or rapidly worsening dyspnea, a doctor should be consulted immediately.

Use of Anti-Inflammatory Agents: In accordance with the present practice for asthma treatment, concomitant anti-inflammatory therapy (eg. corticosteroids) should be part of the regimen if VENTOLIN (salbutamol sulfate) DISKUS inhalation powder needs to be used more than three times a week (not including its use to prevent exercise-induced bronchospasm). It is essential that the physician instruct the patient in the need for further evaluation if the patient's asthma becomes worse. (See Dosage and Administration.)

Cardiovascular: In individual patients, any beta$_2$-adrenergic agonist, including salbutamol sulfate, may have a clinically significant cardiac effect. Care should be taken with patients suffering from cardiovascular disorders, especially coronary insufficiency, cardiac arrhythmias and hypertension. Special care and supervision are required in patients with idiopathic hypertrophic subvalvular aortic stenosis, in whom an increase in the pressure gradient between the left ventricle and the aorta may occur, causing increased strain on the left ventricle.

Fatalities have been reported in association with excessive use of inhaled sympathomimetic drugs in patients with asthma. The exact cause of death is unknown, but cardiac arrest following an unexpected development of a severe acute asthmatic crisis and subsequent hypoxia is suspected.

Endocrine and Metabolism: Metabolic Effects: In common with other beta-adrenergic agents, salbutamol sulfate can induce reversible metabolic changes such as potentially serious hypokalemia, particularly following nebulised or especially infused administration. Particular caution is advised in acute severe asthma since hypokalemia may be potentiated by concomitant treatment with xanthine derivatives, steroids and diuretics and by hypoxia. Hypokalemia will increase the susceptibility of digitalis-treated patients to cardiac arrhythmias. It is recommended that serum potassium levels be monitored in such situations.

Care should be taken with patients with diabetes mellitus. Salbutamol can induce reversible hyperglycemia during nebulised administration or especially during infusions of the drug. The diabetic patient may be unable to compensate for this and the development of ketoacidosis has been reported. Concurrent administration of corticosteroids can exaggerate this effect.

Care should be taken with patients with hyperthyroidism.

Immune: Immediate hypersensitivity reactions may occur after administration of salbutamol sulfate, as demonstrated by rare cases of urticaria, angioedema, rash, bronchospasm, hypotension, anaphylaxis, and oropharyngeal edema.

Care should be taken with patients who are unusually responsive to sympathomimetic amines.

Neurologic: Care should be taken with patients with convulsive disorders.

Respiratory: VENTOLIN DISKUS inhalation powder can produce paradoxical bronchospasm, which may be life threatening. If paradoxical bronchospasm occurs, VENTOLIN DISKUS inhalation powder should be discontinued immediately and alternative therapy instituted.

Special Populations: Pregnant Women: Salbutamol has been in widespread use for many years in humans without apparent ill consequence. However, there are no adequate and well-controlled studies in pregnant women and there is little published evidence of its safety in the early stages of human pregnancy. Administration of any drug to pregnant women should only be considered if the anticipated benefits to the expectant woman are greater than any possible risks to the foetus.

During worldwide marketing experience, rare cases of various congenital anomalies, including cleft palate and limb defects have been reported in the offspring of patients being treated with salbutamol. Some of the mothers were taking multiple medications during their pregnancies. Because no consistent pattern of defects can be discerned, and baseline rate for congenital anomalies is 2-3%, a relationship with salbutamol use cannot be established.

Labour and Delivery: Because of the potential for beta-agonist interference with uterine contractility, use of VENTOLIN DISKUS inhalation powder for relief of bronchospasm during labour should be restricted to those patients in whom the benefits clearly outweigh the risk.

Nursing Women: It is not known whether salbutamol sulfate is excreted in breast milk after inhalation at recommended doses. Because of the potential for tumorigenicity shown in some animal studies, a decision should be made whether to discontinue nursing or to discontinue the drug, taking into account the benefit of the drug to the mother. It is not known whether salbutamol sulfate in breast milk has a harmful effect on the neonate.

Pediatrics: The application of this inhalation system in children depends on the ability of the individual child to learn the proper use of the device. During inhalation, children should be assisted or supervised by an adult who knows the proper use of the device.

Rarely, in children, hyperactivity occurs and occasionally, sleep disturbances, hallucination or atypical psychosis have been reported.

Safety and efficacy in children below 4 years of age have not been established.

Geriatrics: As with other beta$_2$-agonists, special caution should be observed when using VENTOLIN DISKUS in elderly patients who have concomitant cardiovascular disease that could be adversely affected by this class of drug.

Monitoring and Laboratory Tests: In accordance with the present practice for asthma treatment, patient response should be monitored clinically and by lung function tests.

Monitoring Control of Asthma: Failure to respond for at least three hours to a previously effective dose of VENTOLIN DISKUS inhalation powder indicates a deterioration of the condition and the physician should be contacted promptly. Patients should be warned not to exceed the recommended dose.

The increasing use of fast acting, short duration inhaled beta$_2$-adrenergic agonists to control symptoms indicates deterioration of asthma control and the patient's therapy plan should be reassessed. In worsening asthma it is inadequate to increase beta$_2$-agonist use only, especially over an extended period of time. In the case of acute or rapidly worsening dyspnea, a doctor should be consulted immediately. Sudden or progressive deterioration in asthma control is potentially life threatening; the treatment plan must be re-evaluated, and consideration be given to corticosteroid therapy (see Dosage and Administration).

ADVERSE REACTIONS: Adverse Drug Reaction Overview: As with other bronchodilator inhalation therapy, the potential for paradoxical bronchospasm should be kept in mind. If it occurs, the preparation should be discontinued immediately and alternative therapy instituted.

Potentially serious hypokalemia may result from β_2-agonist therapy primarily from parenteral and nebulised routes of administration (see Warnings and Precautions, Endocrine and Metabolism).

Peripheral vasodilation and a compensatory small increase in heart rate may occur in some patients. Cardiac arrhythmias (including atrial fibrillation, supraventricular tachycardia, extrasystoles) have been reported usually in susceptible patients.

The adverse reactions to salbutamol are similar in nature to reactions to other sympathomimetic agents, although the incidence of certain cardiovascular effects is lower with salbutamol.

Other adverse reactions associated with salbutamol are nervousness and tremor. In some patients, inhaled salbutamol may cause a fine tremor of skeletal muscle, particularly in the hands. This effect is common to all beta$_2$-adrenergic stimulants. Adaptation occurs during the first few days of dosing and the tremor usually disappears as treatment continues.

In addition, salbutamol, like other sympathomimetic agents, can cause adverse effects such as drowsiness, flushing, restlessness, irritability, chest discomfort, difficulty in micturition, hypertension, angina, vertigo, central nervous system stimulation, hyperactivity in children, unusual taste, drying or irritation of the oropharynx, palpitations, transient muscle cramps, insomnia, weakness and dizziness.

Immediate hypersensitivity reactions including angioedema, urticaria, bronchospasm, hypotension, rash, oropharyngeal oedema, anaphylaxis and collapse have been reported very rarely.

Clinical Trial Adverse Drug Reactions: Because clinical trials are conducted under very specific conditions the adverse reaction rates observed in the clinical trials may not reflect the rates observed in practice and should not be compared to the rates in the clinical trials of another drug. Adverse drug reaction information from clinical trials is useful for identifying drug-related adverse events and for approximating rates.

Clinical trials with VENTOLIN (salbutamol sulfate) DISKUS inhalation powder 200 µg in 268 adolescents and adults and 142 children aged 4 to 11 years demonstrated generally similar adverse event profiles in both patient populations. The most common adverse events were headache and throat irritation. Combined results are shown in Table 1.

Table 1: VENTOLIN DISKUS

Adverse Experiences with ≥3% Incidence in Two 4-Week Chronic Dosing Studies with Patients 4 Years of Age and Older

Adverse Experience	Placebo[a]	Ventolin Diskus[a] Inhalation Powder 200 µg 4 times daily	Ventolin Inhalation Aerosol[a] 200 µg 4 times daily
Number of Patients	136	139	135
Central Nervous System			
Headache	10%	13%	9%
Gastrointestinal			
Nausea and Vomiting	2%	4%	1%
General			
Fever	1%	3%	1%
Muscle Pain	<1%	3%	1%
Musculoskeletal Pain	1%	3%	0%
Oropharyngeal			
Throat Irritation	3%	6%	3%
Respiratory System			
Upper Respiratory Tract Infections	6%	6%	7%
Ear, Nose, and Throat Infections	1%	0%	3%

[a] Patients in all groups could use VENTOLIN Inhalation Aerosol 100 µg prn as rescue medication.

DRUG INTERACTIONS: Drug-Drug Interactions: See Table 2.

Table 2: VENTOLIN DISKUS

Established or Potential Drug-Drug Interactions

Proper Name	Ref	Effect	Clinical Comment
Monoamine oxidase inhibitors or tricyclic antidepressants	CS	May potentiate action of salbutamol on cardiovascular system.	Salbutamol should be administered with extreme caution to patients being treated with monoamine oxidase inhibitors or tricyclic antidepressants.
Other inhaled sympathomimetic bronchodilators or epinephrine	CS	May lead to deleterious cardiovascular effects.	Other inhaled sympathomimetic bronchodilators or epinephrine should not be used concomitantly with salbutamol sulfate. If additional adrenergic drugs are to be administered by any route to the patient using inhaled salbutamol sulfate, the adrenergic drugs should be used with caution. Such concomitant use must be individualized and not given on a routine basis. If regular coadministration is required then alternative therapy must be considered.
Beta-blockers	CS	May effectively antagonise the action of salbutamol.	Beta-adrenergic blocking drugs, especially the non-cardioselective ones, such as propranolol, should not usually be prescribed together.
Diuretics	CS	May lead to ECG changes and/or hypokalemia, although the clinical significance of these effects is not known.	The ECG changes and/or hypokalemia that may result from the administration of non-potassium sparing diuretics (such as loop or thiazide diuretics) can be acutely worsened by beta-agonists, especially when the recommended dose of the beta-agonist is exceeded. Caution is advised in the coadministration of beta-agonists with non-potassium sparing diuretics.
Digoxin	CS	May lead to decrease in serum digoxin levels. The clinical significance of these findings for patients with obstructive airways disease who are receiving salbutamol sulfate and digoxin on a chronic basis is unclear.	Mean decreases of 16-22% in serum digoxin levels were demonstrated after single dose intravenous and oral administration of salbutamol, respectively, to normal volunteers who had received digoxin for 10 days. It would be prudent to carefully evaluate serum digoxin levels in patients who are currently receiving digoxin and salbutamol sulfate.

Legend: C=case study; CT=clinical trial; T=theoretical.

DOSAGE AND ADMINISTRATION: Dosing Considerations: The dosage should be individualised, and the patient's response should be monitored by the prescribing physician on an ongoing basis.

In accordance with the current Canadian asthma guidelines, if salbutamol sulfate is required for relief of symptoms more than three times a week, (not including its use to prevent exercise induced bronchospasm), anti-inflammatory therapy (e.g. corticosteroids) should be part of the regimen.

Increasing demand for VENTOLIN (salbutamol sulfate) DISKUS inhalation powder in bronchial asthma is usually a sign of worsening asthma and indicates that the treatment plan should be reviewed.

If a previously effective dose fails to provide the usual relief, or the effects of a dose last for less than three hours, patients should seek prompt medical advice since this is usually a sign of worsening asthma.

As there may be adverse effects associated with excessive dosing, the dosage or frequency of administration should only be increased on medical advice. However, if a more severe attack has not been relieved by the usual dose, additional doses may be required. In these cases, patients should immediately consult their doctors or the nearest hospital.

Recommended Dose and Dosage Adjustment: See Table 3.

Missed Dose: If a single dose is missed, instruct the patient to take the next dose when it is due or if they become wheezy.

Administration: VENTOLIN DISKUS inhalation powder is administered by the inhaled route only. To ensure administration of the proper dose of the drug, the patient should be instructed by the physician or other health professional in the proper use of the DISKUS inhalation device.

OVERDOSAGE:

Symptoms and Signs: The most common signs and symptoms of overdose with salbutamol are transient beta agonist pharmacologically mediated events (see Warnings and Precautions and Adverse Reactions). Overdosage may cause tachycardia, cardiac arrhythmia, hypokalemia, hypertension and, in extreme cases, sudden death. Serum potassium levels should be monitored.

Treatment: Consideration should be given to discontinuation of treatment and appropriate symptomatic therapy. To antagonise the effect of salbutamol, the judicious use of a cardioselective beta-adrenergic blocking agent (e.g. metoprolol, atenolol) may be considered, bearing in mind the danger of inducing an asthmatic attack. There is insufficient evidence to determine if dialysis is beneficial for overdosage of VENTOLIN (salbutamol sulfate) DISKUS inhalation powder.

For management of a suspected drug overdose, CPhA recommends that you contact your **regional Poison Control Centre**. See the *CPS* Directory section for a list of Poison Control Centres.

ACTION AND CLINICAL PHARMACOLOGY: Mechanism of Action: Salbutamol produces bronchodilation through stimulation of $beta_2$-adrenergic receptors in bronchial smooth muscle, thereby causing relaxation of bronchial muscle fibres. This action is manifested by an improvement in pulmonary function as demonstrated by spirometric measurements. At therapeutic doses, salbutamol has little action on the $beta_1$-adrenergic receptors in cardiac muscle.

Table 3: VENTOLIN DISKUS

Recommended Dose and Dosage Adjustment

	Acute Symptoms[a]	Intermittent and Long term Treatment[b]	Prevention of Exercise-induced Asthma	Maximum Daily Dose (Total daily dose should not exceed)
Adults and Children (4 years and older)	One Inhalation (200 µg) as required	One Inhalation (200 µg) three to four times daily	One Inhalation (200 µg) 15 minutes before exercise.	Four Inhalations (800 µg)

[a] If a more severe attack has not been relieved by the usual dose, further inhalations may be required. In these cases, patients should immediately consult their doctors or the nearest hospital.

[b] If despite appropriate anti-inflammatory therapy (e.g. corticosteroids), regular daily use of the VENTOLIN DISKUS inhalation powder remains necessary for the control of bronchospasm.

In pediatric, adolescent and adult patients, the median onset of effect ranged from 3.0 to 3.6 minutes, and the median duration of effect ranged from 2.9 to 4.9 hours. In some patients, duration of effect was as long as 6 hours.

Pharmacokinetics: After inhalation of recommended doses of salbutamol, plasma drug levels are very low. When 100 µg of titrated salbutamol aerosol was administered to two normal volunteers, plasma levels of drug-radioactivity were insignificant at 10, 20 and 30 minutes following inhalation. The plasma concentration of salbutamol may be even less as the amount of plasma drug-radioactivity does not differentiate salbutamol from its principal metabolite, a sulfate ester. In a separate study, plasma salbutamol levels ranged from less than 0.5 ng/mL to 1.6 ng/mL in ten asthmatic children one hour after inhalation of 200 µg of salbutamol.

Approximately 10% of an inhaled salbutamol dose is deposited in the lungs. Eighty-five per cent of the remaining salbutamol administered from a metered-dose inhaler is swallowed, however, since the dose is low (100 to 200 µg), the absolute amount swallowed is too small to be of clinical significance. Salbutamol is only weakly bound to plasma proteins. Results of animal studies indicate that following systemic administration, salbutamol does not cross the blood-brain barrier but does cross the placenta using an in vitro perfused isolated human placenta model. It has been found that between 2% and 3% of salbutamol was transferred from the maternal side to the fetal side of the placenta.

Salbutamol is metabolized in the liver. The principal metabolite in humans is salbutamol-o-sulfate, which has negligible pharmacologic activity. Salbutamol may also be metabolized by oxidative deamination and/or conjugation with glucuronide.

Salbutamol is longer acting than isoprenaline in most patients by any route of administration because it is not a substrate for the cellular uptake processes for catecholamines nor for catechol-O-methyl transferase. Salbutamol and its metabolites are excreted in the urine (>80%) and the feces (5% to 10%). Plasma levels are insignificant after administration of aerosolized salbutamol; the plasma half-life ranges from 3.8 to 7.1 hours.

STORAGE AND STABILITY: Keep out of the reach of children. Do not store above 30°C. Keep in a dry place.

INFORMATION FOR THE PATIENT: Published in e-CPS, available by subscription at www.e-cps.ca.

DOSAGE FORMS, COMPOSITION AND PACKAGING: Each blister contains: salbutamol 200 µg (as sulfate). Nonmedicinal ingredients: lactose (milk sugar), including milk protein, which acts as a carrier. Disposable blue-colored plastic inhaler device containing a foil strip with 60 blisters.

Ventolin® HFA Ⓟ

salbutamol sulfate

Bronchodilator

GlaxoSmithKline

Date of Revision: October 3, 2007

SUMMARY PRODUCT INFORMATION:

Route of Administration	Dosage Form/ Strength	Clinically Relevant Nonmedicinal Ingredients
Oral Inhalation	Inhalation Aerosol/ 100 µg salbutamol	1,1,1,2-tetrafluoroethane (HFA-134a) For a complete listing see Dosage Forms, Composition and Packaging.

INDICATIONS AND CLINICAL USE: VENTOLIN HFA (salbutamol sulfate) inhalation aerosol is indicated for:

- the symptomatic relief and prevention of bronchospasm due to bronchial asthma, chronic bronchitis and other chronic bronchopulmonary disorders in which bronchospasm is a complicating factor.
- the prevention of exercise-induced bronchospasm.

Pediatrics (<4 years of age): The safety and efficacy in children below the age of 4 years has not been established.

CONTRAINDICATIONS:

- Patients who are hypersensitive to this drug or to any ingredient in the formulation or component of the container. For a complete listing, see Dosage Forms, Composition and Packaging.

WARNINGS AND PRECAUTIONS: General: Patients should always carry their VENTOLIN HFA (salbutamol sulfate) inhalation aerosol to use immediately if an episode of asthma is experienced. If therapy does not produce a significant improvement or if the patient's condition worsens, medical advice must be sought to determine a new plan of treatment. In the case of acute or rapidly worsening dyspnea, a doctor should be consulted immediately.

Use of Anti-inflammatory Agents: In accordance with the present practice for asthma treatment, concomitant anti-inflammatory therapy (e.g. corticosteroids) should be part of the regimen if VENTOLIN HFA needs to be used more than 3 times a week (not including its use to prevent exercise-induced bronchospasm) (see Dosage and Administration). It is essential that the physician instruct the patient in the need for further evaluation if the patient's asthma becomes worse.

Cardiovascular: In individual patients, any $beta_2$-adrenergic agonist, including salbutamol, may have a clinically significant cardiac effect. Care should be taken with patients suffering from cardiovascular disorders, especially coronary insufficiency, cardiac arrhythmias and hypertension. Special care and supervision are required in patients with idiopathic hypertrophic subvalvular aortic stenosis, in whom an increase in the pressure gradient between the left ventricle and the aorta may occur, causing increased strain on the left ventricle.

Fatalities have been reported in association with excessive use of inhaled sympathomimetic drugs in patients with asthma. The exact cause of death is unknown, but cardiac arrest following an unexpected development of a severe acute asthmatic crisis and subsequent hypoxia is suspected.

Endocrine and Metabolism: Metabolic Effects: In common with other beta-adrenergic agents, salbutamol sulfate can induce reversible metabolic changes such as potentially serious hypokalemia, particularly following nebulised or especially infused administration. Particular caution is advised in acute severe asthma since hypokalemia may be potentiated by concomitant treatment with xanthine derivatives, steroids and diuretics and by hypoxia. Hypokalemia will increase the susceptibility of digitalis-treated patients to cardiac arrhythmias. It is recommended that serum potassium levels be monitored in such situations.

Care should be taken with patients with diabetes mellitus. Salbutamol can induce reversible hyperglycemia during nebulised administration or especially during infusions of the drug. The diabetic patient may be unable to compensate for this and the development of ketoacidosis has been reported. Concurrent administration of corticosteroids can exaggerate this effect.

Care should be taken with patients with hyperthyroidism.

Immune: Immediate hypersensitivity reactions may occur after administration of salbutamol sulfate, as demonstrated by rare cases of urticaria, angioedema, rash, bronchospasm, hypotension, anaphylaxis and oropharyngeal edema.

Care should be taken in patients who are unusually responsive to sympathomimetic amines.

Neurologic: Care should be taken with patients with convulsive disorders.

Respiratory: VENTOLIN HFA can produce paradoxical bronchospasm, which may be life-threatening. If paradoxical bronchospasm occurs, VENTOLIN HFA should be discontinued immediately and alternative therapy instituted. It should be recognized that paradoxical bronchospasm, when associated with inhaled formulations, frequently occurs with the first use of a new canister.

Special Populations: Pregnant Women: Salbutamol has been in widespread use for many years in humans without apparent ill consequence. However, there are no adequate and well-controlled studies in pregnant women and there is little published evidence of its safety in the early stages of human pregnancy. Administration of any drug to pregnant women should only be considered if the anticipated benefits to the expectant woman are greater than any possible risks to the fetus.

During worldwide marketing experience, rare cases of various congenital anomalies, including cleft palate and limb defects have been reported in the offspring of patients being treated with salbutamol. Some of the mothers were taking multiple medications during their pregnancies. Because no consistent pattern of defects can be discerned, and baseline rate for congenital anomalies is 2-3%, a relationship with salbutamol use cannot be established.

Labour and Delivery: Because of the potential for beta-agonist interference with uterine contractility, use of VENTOLIN HFA for relief of bronchospasm during labour should be restricted to those patients in whom the benefits clearly outweigh the risks.

Nursing Women: Plasma levels of salbutamol sulfate and HFA-134a after inhaled therapeutic doses are very low in humans, but it is not known whether the components are excreted in human milk. Because of the potential for tumorigenicity shown for salbutamol in some animal studies, a decision should be made whether to discontinue nursing or to discontinue the drug, taking into account the benefit of the drug to the mother. It is not known whether salbutamol in breast milk has a harmful effect on the neonate.

Pediatrics: The use of metered-dose inhalers in children depends on the ability of the individual child to learn the proper use of this device. Metered-dose inhalers with spacers are recommended for children under 5 years of age, especially for administration of inhaled corticosteroids. Conversion from a face mask to a mouthpiece is strongly encouraged as soon as the age and the cooperation of the child permit.

During inhalation, children should be assisted or supervised by an adult who knows the proper use of the device.

Rarely, in children, hyperactivity occurs and occasionally, sleep disturbances, hallucination or atypical psychosis have been reported.

The safety and efficacy in children below the age of 4 years has not been established.

Geriatrics: As with other $beta_2$-agonists, special caution should be observed when using VENTOLIN HFA in elderly patients who have concomitant cardiovascular disease that could be adversely affected by this class of drug.

Monitoring and Laboratory Tests: In accordance with the present practice for asthma treatment, patient response should be monitored clinically and by lung function tests.

Monitoring Control of Asthma: Failure to respond for at least three hours to a previously effective dose of VENTOLIN HFA indicates a deterioration of the condition and the physician should be contacted promptly. Patients should be warned not to exceed the recommended dose.

The increasing use of fast-acting, short duration inhaled $beta_2$-adrenergic agonists to control symptoms indicates deterioration of asthma control and the patient's therapy plan should be reassessed. In worsening asthma it is inadequate to increase $beta_2$-agonist use only, especially over an extended period of time. In the case of acute or rapidly worsening dyspnea, a doctor should be consulted immediately. Sudden or progressive deterioration in asthma control is potentially life threatening; the treatment plan must be re-evaluated, and consideration be given to corticosteroid therapy (see Dosage and Administration).

ADVERSE REACTIONS: Adverse Drug Reaction Overview: As with other bronchodilator inhalation therapy, the potential for paradoxical bronchospasm should be kept in mind. If it occurs, the preparation should be discontinued immediately and alternative therapy instituted.

Potentially serious hypokalemia may result from $beta_2$-agonist therapy primarily from parenteral and nebulised routes of administration (see Warnings and Precautions, Endocrine and Metabolism).

Peripheral vasodilation and a compensatory small increase in heart rate may occur in some patients. Cardiac arrhythmias (including atrial fibrillation, supraventricular tachycardia, extrasystoles) have been reported usually in susceptible patients.

Other adverse reactions associated with salbutamol are nervousness and tremor. In some patients inhaled salbutamol may cause a fine tremor of skeletal muscle, particularly in the hands. This effect is common to all $beta_2$-adrenergic stimulants. Adaptation occurs during the first few days of dosing and the tremor usually disappears as treatment continues.

In addition, salbutamol, like other sympathomimetic agents, can cause adverse effects such as drowsiness, flushing, restlessness, irritability, chest discomfort, difficulty in micturition, hypertension, angina, vomiting, vertigo, central nervous system stimulation, hyperactivity in children, unusual taste and drying or irritation of the oropharynx, headache, palpitations, transient muscle cramps, insomnia, nausea, weakness and dizziness.

Clinical Trial Adverse Drug Reactions: Because clinical trials are conducted under very specific conditions the adverse reaction rates observed in the clinical trials may not reflect the rates observed in practice and should not be compared to the rates in the clinical trials of another drug. Adverse drug reaction information from clinical trials is useful for identifying drug-related adverse events and for approximating rates.

Adverse reaction information concerning VENTOLIN HFA (salbutamol sulfate) inhalation aerosol is derived from two 12-week, randomized, double-blind studies in 610 adolescent and adult asthmatic patients that compared VENTOLIN HFA, VENTOLIN inhalation aerosol (CFC formulation), and an HFA-134a placebo inhaler. See Table 1.

Overall, the incidence and nature of the adverse events reported for VENTOLIN HFA and VENTOLIN inhalation aerosol (CFC formulation) were similar. Results in a 2-week pediatric clinical study (n=35) showed that the adverse event profile was generally similar to that of the adult.

Adverse events reported by less than 3% of the adolescent and adult patients receiving VENTOLIN HFA and by a greater proportion of patients receiving VENTOLIN HFA than receiving HFA-134a placebo inhaler and that have the potential to be related to VENTOLIN HFA include diarrhea, laryngitis, cough, lung disorders, tachycardia, and extrasystoles. Palpitation and dizziness have also been observed with VENTOLIN HFA.

Immediate hypersensitivity reactions including angioedema, urticaria, bronchospasm, hypotension, rash, oropharyngeal oedema, anaphylaxis and collapse have been reported very rarely.

Table 1: VENTOLIN HFA

Adverse Experience Incidence (% of patients) in 2 Large 12-Week Adolescent and Adult Clinical Trials[a]

	VENTOLIN HFA n=202 (% Patients)	VENTOLIN (CFC formulation) n=207 (% Patients)	Placebo (HFA-134a) n=201 (% Patients)
Ear, Nose and Throat			
Throat Irritation	10	6	7
Upper Respiratory Inflammation	5	5	2
Lower Respiratory			
Viral Respiratory Infections	7	4	4

(cont'd)

Table 1: VENTOLIN HFA *(cont'd)*

Adverse Experience Incidence (% of patients) in 2 Large 12-Week Adolescent and Adult Clinical Trials[a]

	VENTOLIN HFA n=202 (% Patients)	VENTOLIN (CFC formulation) n=207 (% Patients)	Placebo (HFA-134a) n=201 (% Patients)
Cough	5	2	2
Musculoskeletal			
Musculoskeletal Pain	5	5	4

[a] Table 1 includes all adverse events (whether considered by the investigator to be drug-related or unrelated to drug) that occurred at an incidence rate of at least 3.0% in the group treated with VENTOLIN HFA and more frequently in the group treated with VENTOLIN HFA than in the HFA-134a placebo inhaler group.

DRUG INTERACTIONS: Drug-Drug Interactions: See Table 2.

Table 2: VENTOLIN HFA

Established or Potential Drug-Drug Interactions

Proper Name	Ref	Effect	Clinical Comment
Monoamine oxidase inhibitors or tricyclic antidepressants	CS	May potentiate action of salbutamol on cardiovascular system.	Salbutamol should be administered with extreme caution to patients being treated with monoamine oxidase inhibitors or tricyclic antidepressants.
Other inhaled sympathomimetic bronchodilators or epinephrine	CS	May lead to deleterious cardiovascular effects.	Other inhaled sympathomimetic bronchodilators or epinephrine should not be used concomitantly with salbutamol. If additional adrenergic drugs are to be administered by any route to the patient using inhaled salbutamol, the adrenergic drugs should be used with caution. Such concomitant use must be individualised and not given on a routine basis. If regular co-administration is required then alternative therapy must be considered.
Beta-blockers	CS	May effectively antagonize the action of salbutamol.	Beta-adrenergic blocking drugs, especially the non-cardioselective ones, such as propranolol, should not usually be prescribed together.
Diuretics	CS	May lead to ECG changes and/or hypokalemia although the clinical significance of these effects is not known.	The ECG changes and/or hypokalemia that may result from the administration of non-potassium sparing diuretics (such as loop or thiazide diuretics) can be acutely worsened by beta-agonists, especially when the recommended dose of the beta-agonist is exceeded. Caution is advised in the co-administration of beta-agonists with non-potassium sparing diuretics.
Digoxin	CS	May lead to a decrease in serum digoxin levels, although the clinical significance of these findings for patients with obstructive airways disease who are receiving salbutamol and digoxin on a chronic basis is unclear.	Mean decreases of 16-22% in serum digoxin levels were demonstrated after single dose intravenous and oral administration of salbutamol, respectively, to normal volunteers who had received digoxin for 10 days. It would be prudent to carefully evaluate serum digoxin levels in patients who are currently receiving digoxin and salbutamol.

Legend: CS=Class Statement.

DOSAGE AND ADMINISTRATION: Dosing Considerations: The dosage should be individualised, and the patient's response should be monitored by the prescribing physician on an ongoing basis.

In accordance with current Canadian asthma guidelines, if salbutamol is required more than three times a week (not including its use to prevent exercise-induced bronchospasm), anti-inflammatory therapy (eg. corticosteroids) should be part of the regimen.

Increasing demand for VENTOLIN HFA (salbutamol sulfate) inhalation aerosol in bronchial asthma is usually a sign of worsening asthma and indicates that the treatment plan should be reviewed.

If a previously effective dose fails to provide the usual relief, or the effects of a dose last for less than three hours, patients should seek prompt medical advice since this is usually a sign of worsening asthma.

As there may be adverse effects associated with excessive dosing, the dosage or frequency of administration should only be increased on medical advice. However, if a more severe attack has not been relieved by the usual dose, additional doses may be required. In these cases, patients should immediately consult their doctors or the nearest hospital.

Recommended Dose and Dosage Adjustment: See Table 3.

It is recommended to test spray VENTOLIN HFA into the air four times before using for the first time and in cases where the aerosol has not been used for more than 4 weeks.

Missed Dose: If a single dose is missed, instruct the patient to take the next dose when it is due or if they become wheezy.

Administration: VENTOLIN HFA is administered by the inhaled route only. To ensure administration of the proper dose of the drug, the patient should be instructed by the physician or other health professional in the proper use of the inhalation aerosol.

Inhaler actuation should be synchronised with inspiration to ensure optimum delivery of drug to the lungs.

The use of open mouth technique to administer VENTOLIN HFA has not been investigated in clinical trials.

OVERDOSAGE:

Symptoms and Signs: The most common signs and symptoms of overdose with salbutamol are transient beta agonist pharmacologically mediated events (see Warnings and Precautions and Adverse Reactions). Overdosage may cause tachycardia, cardiac arrhythmia, hypokalemia, hypertension and, in extreme cases, sudden death. Serum potassium levels should be monitored.

Treatment: Consideration should be given to discontinuation of treatment and appropriate symptomatic therapy. To antagonise the effect of salbutamol, the judicious use of a cardioselective beta-adrenergic blocking agent (e.g. metoprolol, atenolol) may be considered, bearing in mind the danger of inducing an asthmatic attack. There is insufficient evidence to determine if dialysis is beneficial for overdosage of VENTOLIN HFA (salbutamol sulphate) inhalation aerosol.

Fatalities have been reported in association with excessive use of inhaled sympathomimetic drugs in patients with asthma. The exact cause of death is unknown, but cardiac arrest following an unexpected development of a severe acute asthmatic crisis and subsequent hypoxia is suspected.

For management of a suspected drug overdose, CPhA recommends that you contact your **regional Poison Control Centre**. See the *CPS* Directory section for a list of Poison Control Centres.

ACTION AND CLINICAL PHARMACOLOGY: Mechanism of Action: Salbutamol produces bronchodilation through stimulation of beta$_2$-adrenergic receptors in bronchial smooth muscle, thereby causing relaxation of bronchial muscle fibres. This action is manifested by an improvement in pulmonary function as demonstrated by spirometric measurements. At therapeutic doses, salbutamol has little action on the beta$_1$-adrenergic receptors in cardiac muscle.

A measurable decrease in airway resistance is typically observed 5 to 15 minutes after inhalation of salbutamol. The maximum improvement in pulmonary function usually occurs 60 to 90 minutes after salbutamol treatment, and significant bronchodilator activity has been observed to persist for 3 to 6 hours.

Table 3: VENTOLIN HFA

Recommended Dose and Dosage Adjustment

	Acute Symptoms	Intermittent and Long-term Treatment[a]	Prevention of Exercise-induced Asthma	Maximum Daily Dose (Total daily dose should not exceed)
Adult	One to two puffs [100 to 200 µg salbutamol (as sulfate)]	One to two puffs [100 to 200 µg salbutamol (as sulfate)] four times daily	Two puffs [200 µg salbutamol (as sulfate)] before exercise	Eight puffs [800 µg salbutamol (as sulfate)]
Children (4 years and older)	One puff [100 µg salbutamol (as sulfate)]. May be increased to two puffs (200 µg salbutamol), if required.	One puff [100 µg salbutamol (as sulfate)] four times daily	One puff [100 µg salbutamol (as sulfate)] before exercise. May be increased to two puffs (200 µg salbutamol), if required.	Four puffs [400 µg salbutamol (as sulfate)]

[a] Despite appropriate anti-inflammatory therapy (e.g. Corticosteroids), regular daily use of the VENTOLIN HFA remains necessary for the control of bronchospasm.

Pharmacokinetics: After inhalation of recommended doses of salbutamol, plasma drug levels are very low. When 100 µg of tritiated salbutamol aerosol was administered to two normal volunteers, plasma levels of drug-radioactivity were insignificant at 10, 20 and 30 minutes following inhalation. The plasma concentration of salbutamol may be even less as the amount of plasma drug-radioactivity does not differentiate salbutamol from its principal metabolite, a sulfate ester. In a separate study, plasma salbutamol levels ranged from less than 0.5 ng/mL to 1.6 ng/mL in ten asthmatic children one hour after inhalation of 200 µg of salbutamol.

Approximately 10% of an inhaled salbutamol dose is deposited in the lungs. Eighty-five per cent of the remaining salbutamol administered from a metered-dose inhaler is swallowed, however, since the dose is low (100 to 200 µg), the absolute amount swallowed is too small to be of clinical significance. Salbutamol is only weakly bound to plasma proteins. Results of animal studies indicate that following systemic administration, salbutamol does not cross the blood-brain barrier but does cross the placenta using an in vitro perfused isolated human placenta model. It has been found that between 2% and 3% of salbutamol was transferred from the maternal side to the fetal side of the placenta.

Salbutamol is metabolized in the liver. The principal metabolite in humans is salbutamol-o-sulfate, which has negligible pharmacologic activity. Salbutamol may also be metabolized by oxidative deamination and/or conjugation with glucuronide.

Salbutamol is longer acting than isoprenaline in most patients by any route of administration because it is not a substrate for the cellular uptake processes for catecholamines nor for catechol-O-methyl transferase. Salbutamol and its metabolites are excreted in the urine (>80%) and the feces (5% to 10%). Plasma levels are insignificant after administration of aerosolized salbutamol; the plasma half-life ranges from 3.8 to 7.1 hours.

Propellant HFA-134a is devoid of pharmacological activity except at very high doses in animals (140 to 800 times the maximum human exposure based on comparisons of AUC values), primarily producing ataxia, tremors, dyspnea, or salivation. These are similar to effects produced by the structurally related CFCs, which have been used extensively in metered-dose inhalers.

In animals and humans, propellant HFA-134a was eliminated rapidly in the breath, with no evidence of metabolism or accumulation in the body. Time to maximum plasma concentration (t_{max}) and mean residence time are both extremely short, leading to a transient appearance of HFA-134a in the blood with no evidence of accumulation.

STORAGE AND STABILITY: Replace the mouthpiece cover firmly and snap it into position. Keep out of the reach of children. Store at a temperature between 15 and 25°C.

SPECIAL HANDLING INSTRUCTIONS: The contents of VENTOLIN HFA (salbutamol sulfate) inhalation aerosol are under pressure. The container may explode if heated. Do not place in hot water or near radiators, stoves or other sources of heat. Even when empty, do not puncture or incinerate container.

INFORMATION FOR THE PATIENT: Published in e-CPS, available by subscription at www.e-cps.ca.

DOSAGE FORMS, COMPOSITION AND PACKAGING: Each inhalation aerosol contains a microcrystalline suspension of salbutamol sulfate in propellant HFA-134a (1,1,1,2-tetrafluoroethane). Each inhalation aerosol is a pressurized metered-dose inhaler (MDI) consisting of an aluminum canister fitted with a metering valve. Each canister is fitted into the supplied blue plastic actuator. A blue dust cap is fitted over the actuator's mouthpiece when not in use. Each depression of the valve delivers 100 µg of salbutamol (as sulfate). Nonmedicinal ingredients: none. Chlorofluorocarbon-free. Formats of 200 doses.

(Shown in Product Identification Section)

Ventolin® I.V. Infusion Solution ℞

salbutamol sulfate

Bronchodilator

GlaxoSmithKline

Date of Revision: October 3, 2007

SUMMARY PRODUCT INFORMATION:

Route of Administration	Dosage Form/ Strength	Clinically Relevant Nonmedicinal Ingredients
Intravenous (I.V.)	salbutamol I.V. Infusion/ 1000 µg/mL	Not applicable For a complete listing see Dosage Forms, Composition and Packaging.

INDICATIONS AND CLINICAL USE: VENTOLIN (salbutamol sulfate) I.V. infusion solution is indicated for:

- the relief of severe bronchospasm associated with acute exacerbations of chronic bronchitis and bronchial asthma,
- the treatment of status asthmaticus.

In many patients, VENTOLIN infusion solution will be no more effective, and likely less well tolerated, than VENTOLIN HFA inhalation aerosol or VENTOLIN respirator solution. However, patients who are severely ill with airway inflammation and mucus plugging may respond well to parenteral salbutamol after failing to benefit from the inhaled drug.

This product should be administered under the supervision of a qualified health professional who is experienced in the use of parenteral preparations and in the management of asthma. Appropriate management of therapy and complications is only possible when adequate diagnostic and treatment facilities are readily available.

CONTRAINDICATIONS:

- Patients who are hypersensitive to this drug or to any ingredient in the formulation or component of the container.
- Patients with cardiac tachyarrhythmias.
- Patients at risk of threatened abortion during the first or second trimester.

WARNINGS AND PRECAUTIONS: General: VENTOLIN I.V. infusion solution may be diluted with Water for Injection BP, Sodium Chloride Injection BP, Dextrose Injection BP, or Sodium Chloride and Dextrose Injection BP (see Dosage and Administration). These are the only recommended diluents. Dextrose-containing solutions may not be suitable for patients with diabetes mellitus, due to the possible danger of glucose overload.

The use of VENTOLIN infusion solution in the treatment of severe bronchospasm or status asthmaticus does not obviate the requirement for glucocorticoid steroid therapy as appropriate. When practicable, administration of oxygen, concurrently with VENTOLIN infusion solution is recommended, particularly when salbutamol is given by intravenous infusion to hypoxic patients.

Cardiovascular: In individual patients, any beta$_2$-adrenergic agonist, including salbutamol, may have a clinically significant cardiac effect. Care should be taken with patients suffering from cardiovascular disorders, especially coronary insufficiency, cardiac arrhythmias and hypertension. Special care and supervision are required in patients with idiopathic hypertrophic subvalvular aortic stenosis, in whom an increase in the pressure gradient between the left ventricle and the aorta may occur, causing increased strain on the left ventricle.

Fatalities have been reported following excessive use of inhaled sympathomimetic drugs in patients with asthma. The exact cause of death is unknown, but cardiac arrest following an unexpected development of a severe acute asthmatic crisis and subsequent hypoxia is suspected.

Endocrine and Metabolism: Metabolic Effects: In common with other beta-adrenergic agents, salbutamol can induce reversible metabolic changes, such as potentially serious hypokalemia, particularly following nebulised or especially infused administration. Particular caution is advised in acute severe asthma since hypokalemia may be potentiated by concomitant treatment with xanthine derivatives, steroids and diuretics, and by hypoxia. Hypokalemia will increase the susceptibility of digitalis-treated patients to cardiac arrythmias. It is recommended that serum potassium levels be monitored in such situations.

Large doses of intravenous salbutamol have been reported to aggravate pre-existing diabetes mellitus. The diabetic patient may be unable to compensate for the increased blood glucose levels and the development of ketoacidosis has been reported. Concurrent administration of corticosteroids can exaggerate this effect. Diabetic patients and those concurrently receiving corticosteroids should be monitored frequently during intravenous infusion of VENTOLIN I.V. infusion solution so that remedial steps (e.g. an increase in insulin dosage) can be taken to counter any metabolic change that is occurring. For these patients, VENTOLIN I.V. infusion solution should be diluted with Sodium Chloride Injection BP, rather than Sodium Chloride and Dextrose Injection BP.

Lactic acidosis has been reported very rarely in association with high therapeutic doses of intravenous and nebulised short-acting beta-agonist therapy, mainly in patients being treated for an acute asthma exacerbation (see Adverse Reactions). Increase in lactate levels may lead to dyspnea and compensatory hyperventilation, which could be misinterpreted as a sign of asthma treatment failure and lead to inappropriate intensification of short-acting beta-agonist treatment. It is therefore recommended that patients are monitored for the development of elevated serum lactate and consequent metabolic acidosis in this setting.

Care should be taken with patients with hyperthyroidism.

Immune: Immediate hypersensitivity reactions may occur after administration of salbutamol, as demonstrated by rare cases of urticaria, angioedema, rash, bronchospasm, hypotension, anaphylaxis and oropharyngeal edema.

Care should be taken in patients who are unusually responsive to sympathomimetic amines.

Neurologic: Neurologic should be taken with patients with convulsive disorders.

Respiratory: Some patients have been reported to have developed severe paradoxical bronchospasm with repeated excessive use of sympathomimetic inhalation preparations. In this event, the use of the preparation should be discontinued immediately and alternate therapy instituted, since in the reported cases the patients did not respond to other forms of therapy until the drug was withdrawn.

Special Populations: Pregnant Women: Salbutamol, in common with other betamimetics, is not approved to stop or prevent premature labour.

Due to the risk of pulmonary edema and myocardial ischaemia that has been observed during the use of betamimetics in the treatment of premature labour, before VENTOLIN infusion solution is given to any patient with known heart disease, an adequate assessment of the patient's cardiovascular status should be made by a physician experienced in cardiology.

There are no adequate and well-controlled studies in pregnant women and there is little published evidence of its safety in the early stages of human pregnancy. Administration of any drug to pregnant women should only be considered if the anticipated benefits to the expectant woman are greater than any possible risks to the foetus.

During worldwide marketing experience, rare cases of various congenital anomalies including cleft palate and limb defects have been reported in the offspring of patients being treated with salbutamol. Some of the mothers were taking multiple medications during their pregnancies. Because no consistent pattern of defects can be discerned, and baseline rate for congenital anomalies is 2-3%, a relationship with salbutamol use cannot be established.

Labour and Delivery: It has been reported that high doses of salbutamol, administered intravenously, inhibit uterine contractions.

Therefore, cautious use of VENTOLIN infusion solution is required in pregnant patients when it is given for relief of bronchospasm so as to avoid interference with uterine contractibility. During I.V. infusion of salbutamol, the maternal pulse rate should be monitored and not normally allowed to exceed a steady rate of 140 beats per minute.

As maternal pulmonary edema and myocardial ischaemia have been reported during or following premature labour in patients receiving beta$_2$-agonists, careful attention should be given to fluid balance and cardio-respiratory function, including ECG, should be monitored. If signs of pulmonary edema or myocardial ischaemia develop, discontinuation of treatment should be considered (see Adverse Reactions).

Nursing Women: As salbutamol is probably secreted in breast milk and because of the potential for tumorigenicity of salbutamol shown in some animal studies, a decision should be made whether to discontinue nursing or to discontinue the drug, taking into account the importance of the drug to the mother. It is not known whether salbutamol has a harmful effect on the neonate.

Pediatrics: The dosage of VENTOLIN infusion solution in the pediatric age group has not been established. At present there are insufficient data to recommend a dosage regimen for use in children.

Monitoring and Laboratory Tests: In accordance with the present practice for asthma treatment, patient response should be monitored clinically and by lung function tests.

Electrocardiogram, and serum potassium and glucose should be monitored during continuous infusions of salbutamol.

Monitoring and Control of Asthma: Failure to respond to a previously effective dose of salbutamol indicates a deterioration of the condition and the physician should be contacted promptly.

In worsening asthma it is inadequate to increase beta$_2$-agonist use only, especially over an extended period of time. Instead, a reassessment of the patient's therapy plan is required and concomitant anti inflammatory therapy should be considered. Sudden or progressive deterioration in asthma control is potentially life threatening; the treatment plan must be re-evaluated, and consideration be given to corticosteroid therapy.

ADVERSE REACTIONS: Adverse Drug Reaction Overview: Fine muscle tremor is a common side effect of VENTOLIN infusion solution. This is due to direct beta$_2$-stimulation by salbutamol of skeletal muscle. There have been very rare reports of transient muscle cramps.

A dose-dependent increase in heart rate, secondary to a reduction in peripheral resistance, due to vasodilation, may occur with parenteral salbutamol, and may cause palpitations. This is most likely to occur in patients with normal heart rates. In patients with pre-existing sinus tachycardia, especially those in status asthmaticus, the heart rate tends to fall as the condition of the patient improves. Cardiac arrhythmias (including atrial fibrillation, supraventricular tachycardia and extrasystoles) have been reported, usually in susceptible patients.

In the management of pre-term labour, salbutamol solution for infusion has uncommonly been associated with pulmonary edema and myocardial ischaemia. Patients with predisposing factors including multiple pregnancies, fluid overload, maternal infection and pre-eclampsia may have an increased risk of developing pulmonary edema.

Paradoxical bronchospasm has been reported to occur following salbutamol inhalation therapy, requiring the immediate discontinuation of the drug and the institution of alternative forms of therapy. As with other beta$_2$-agonists, hyperactivity has been reported rarely in children.

Potentially serious hypokalemia may result from beta$_2$-agonist therapy, mainly from parenteral and nebulised administration.

Other side effects which may occur with salbutamol are sweating, headache, dizziness, flushing, nausea, vomiting, muscle cramps, insomnia, drowsiness, restlessness, irritability, chest discomfort, difficulty in micturition, hypertension, angina, vertigo, central nervous system stimulation, unusual taste and drying or irritation of the oropharynx.

Immediate hypersensitivity reactions including angioedema, urticaria, bronchospasm, hypotension, rash, oropharyngeal oedema, anaphylaxis and collapse have been reported very rarely.

Lactic acidosis has also been reported very rarely in patients receiving intravenous salbutamol therapy for the treatment of acute asthma exacerbation.

DRUG INTERACTIONS: Drug-Drug Interactions: See Table 1.

Table 1: VENTOLIN I.V. Infusion Solution

Established or Potential Drug-Drug Interactions

Salbutamol sulfate	Ref	Effect	Clinical comment
Monoamine oxidase inhibitors or tricyclic antidepressants	CS	May potentiate action of salbutamol on cardiovascular system.	Salbutamol should be administered with extreme caution to patients being treated with monoamine oxidase inhibitors or tricyclic antidepressants.
Other sympathomimetic bronchodilators or epinephrine.	CS	May lead to deleterious cardiovascular effects.	Other sympathomimetic bronchodilators or epinephrine should not be used concomitantly with salbutamol. If additional adrenergic drugs are to be administered by any route to the patient using salbutamol, the adrenergic drugs should be used with caution to avoid deleterious cardiovascular effects. Such concomitant use must be individualised and not given on a routine basis. If regular co-administration is required then alternative therapy must be considered.
Beta-blockers	CS	May effectively antagonise the action of salbutamol.	Beta-adrenergic blocking drugs, especially the non-cardioselective ones, such as propranolol, should not usually be prescribed together.
Diuretics	CS	May lead to ECG changes and/or hypokalemia, although the clinical significance of these effects is not known.	The ECG changes and/or hypokalemia that may result from the administration of non-potassium sparing diuretics (such as loop or thiazide diuretics) can be acutely worsened by beta-agonists, especially when the recommended dose of the beta-agonist is exceeded. Caution is advised in the co-administration of beta-agonists with non-potassium sparing diuretics.
Digoxin	CS	May lead to mean decrease in serum digoxin levels. The clinical significance of these findings for patients with obstructive airways disease who are receiving salbutamol and digoxin on a chronic basis is unclear.	Mean decreases of 16-22% in serum digoxin levels were demonstrated after single doses intravenous and oral administration of salbutamol, respectively, to normal volunteers who had received digoxin for 10 days. It would be prudent to carefully evaluate serum digoxin levels in patients who are currently receiving digoxin and salbutamol.

Legend:
CS=class statement.

DOSAGE AND ADMINISTRATION: Recommended Dose and Dosage Adjustment: Adults: In Severe Bronchospasm and Status Asthmaticus: Continuous Intravenous Infusion: 5 µg/min., increased to 10 µg/min., and 20 µg/min. at 15-30 minute intervals, if necessary. A suitable solution for infusion may be prepared by diluting 5 mL of VENTOLIN I.V. infusion solution (1 mg/mL) in 500 mL of a chosen i.v. solution to provide a salbutamol concentration of 10 µg/mL.

VENTOLIN I.V. infusion solution must not be injected undiluted. The concentration should be reduced 50% before administration. VENTOLIN infusion solution is compatible in PVC bags and in glass bottles with Water for Injection BP, Sodium Chloride Injection BP, Dextrose Injection BP, and Sodium Chloride and Dextrose Injection BP. Dextrose-containing solutions may not be suitable for patients with diabetes mellitus due to the possible danger of glucose overload (see Warnings and Precautions).

Children: The dosage of VENTOLIN infusion solution in the pediatric age group has not been established. At present, there are insufficient data to recommend a dosage regimen for children.

Administration: VENTOLIN infusion solution is not to be administered with other medication as part of the same infusion.

Continuous intravenous infusion, when practicable, is the preferred method of administration.

Reconstituted Solutions: VENTOLIN infusion solution may be diluted with Water for Injection BP, Sodium Chloride Injection BP, Sodium Chloride and Dextrose Injection BP or Dextrose Injection BP. These are the only recommended diluents.

As with all parenteral drug products, intravenous admixtures should be inspected visually for clarity, particulate matter, precipitate, discoloration and leakage prior to administration, whenever solution and container permit.

All unused admixtures of VENTOLIN infusion solution with infusion fluids should be discarded 24 hours after preparation.

OVERDOSAGE:

Symptoms and Signs: The most common signs and symptoms of overdose with salbutamol are transient beta agonist pharmacologically mediated events (see Warnings and Precautions and Adverse Reactions). Overdosage may cause tachycardia, cardiac arrhythmia, hypokalemia, hypertension and, in extreme cases, sudden death. Serum potassium levels should be monitored.

Nausea, vomiting and hyperglycaemia have been reported, predominantly in children and when salbutamol overdose has been taken via the oral route.

Treatment: Consideration should be given to discontinuation of treatment and appropriate symptomatic therapy. To antagonise the effect of salbutamol, the judicious use of a cardioselective beta-adrenergic blocking agent (e.g. metoprolol, atenolol) may be considered, bearing in mind the danger of inducing an asthmatic attack.

For management of a suspected drug overdose, CPhA recommends that you contact your **regional Poison Control Centre**. See the *CPS* Directory section for a list of Poison Control Centres.

ACTION AND CLINICAL PHARMACOLOGY: Mechanism of Action: Salbutamol produces bronchodilation through stimulation of beta$_2$-adrenergic receptors in bronchial smooth muscle, thereby causing relaxation of bronchial muscle fibers. This action is manifested by an improvement in pulmonary function as demonstrated by spirometric measurements.

STORAGE AND STABILITY: VENTOLIN infusion solution should be protected from light and stored at controlled room temperature (15-30°C).

INFORMATION FOR THE PATIENT: Published in e-CPS, available by subscription at www.e-cps.ca.

DOSAGE FORMS, COMPOSITION AND PACKAGING: Each mL of clear, colorless to pale straw-colored sterile, isotonic solution contains: salbutamol 1000 µg as salbutamol sulfate. Adjusted to pH 3.5 with sulfuric acid and/or sodium hydroxide. Clear neutral glass ampuls of 5 mL.

Ventolin® Respirator Solution ℞
salbutamol sulfate
Bronchodilator

GlaxoSmithKline

Ventolin Nebules® P.F. ℞
salbutamol sulfate
Bronchodilator

GlaxoSmithKline

Date of Revision: October 3, 2007

SUMMARY PRODUCT INFORMATION:

Route of Administration	Dosage Form/ Strength	Clinically Relevant Nonmedicinal Ingredients
Oral Inhalation	Respirator Solution/5 mg salbutamol base/mL	Not applicable For a complete listing see Dosage Forms, Composition and Packaging.
	Nebules/unit dose/2.5 or 5 mg salbutamol base/2.5 mL	Not applicable For a complete listing see Dosage Forms, Composition and Packaging.

INDICATIONS AND CLINICAL USE: VENTOLIN (salbutamol sulphate) Respirator Solutions are indicated for:

- the treatment of severe bronchospasm associated with exacerbations of chronic bronchitis and bronchial asthma. They can be used by "wet" nebulization. When administered through a nebulizer, salbutamol respirator solutions should be used with compressed air or oxygen.

Pediatrics (<5 years of age): Experience is insufficient for recommending the treatment of children under 5 years of age.

CONTRAINDICATIONS:

- Patients with a hypersensitivity to any of the ingredients and in patients with tachyarrythmias. For a complete listing, see Dosage Forms, Composition and Packaging.

WARNINGS AND PRECAUTIONS: General: Patients should always carry their salbutamol aerosol or dry powder to use immediately if an episode of asthma is experienced. If therapy does not produce a significant improvement or if the patient's condition worsens, medical advice must be sought to determine a new plan of treatment. In the case of acute or rapidly worsening dyspnea, a doctor should be consulted immediately.

The application of these inhalation systems in children depends on the ability of the individual child to learn the proper use of the devices. During inhalation, children should be assisted or supervised by an adult who knows the proper use of the devices.

VENTOLIN Respirator Solution and NEBULES P.F. must only be used by inhalation, to be breathed in through the mouth, and must not be injected or swallowed.

Use of Anti-inflammatory Agents: In accordance with the present practice for asthma treatment, concomitant anti-inflammatory therapy (eg. corticosteroid) should be part of the regimen if inhaled salbutamol needs to be used on a regular daily basis (see Dosage and Administration). It is essential that the physician instruct the patient in the need for further evaluation if the patient's asthma becomes worse.

Cardiovascular: In individual patients, any beta$_2$-adrenergic agonist, including salbutamol, may have a clinically significant cardiac effect. Care should be taken with patients suffering from cardiovascular disorders, especially coronary insufficiency, cardiac arrhythmias and hypertension. Special care and supervision are required in patients with idiopathic hypertrophic subvalvular aortic stenosis, in whom an increase in the pressure gradient between the left ventricle and the aorta may occur, causing increased strain on the left ventricle.

Fatalities have been reported in association with excessive use of inhaled sympathomimetic drugs in patients with asthma. The exact cause of death is unknown, but cardiac arrest following an unexpected development of a severe acute asthmatic crisis and subsequent hypoxia is suspected.

Endocrine and Metabolism: Metabolic Effects: In common with other beta-adrenergic agents, salbutamol can induce reversible metabolic changes such as potentially serious hypokalemia, particularly following nebulized or especially infused administration. Particular caution is advised in acute severe asthma since hypokalemia may be potentiated by concomitant treatment with xanthine derivatives, steroids and diuretics and by hypoxia. Hypokalemia will increase the susceptibility of digitalis-treated patients to cardiac arrhythmias. It is recommended that serum potassium levels be monitored in such situations.

Care should be taken with patients with diabetes mellitus. Salbutamol can induce reversible hyperglycemia during nebulized administration or especially during infusions of the drug. The diabetic patient may be unable to compensate for this and the development of ketoacidosis has been reported. Concurrent administration of corticosteroids can exaggerate this effect.

Lactic acidosis has been reported very rarely in association with high therapeutic doses of intravenous and nebulised short-acting beta-agonist therapy, mainly in patients being treated for an acute asthma exacerbation (see Adverse Reactions). Increase in lactate levels may lead to dyspnea and compensatory hyperventilation, which could be misinterpreted as a sign of asthma treatment failure and lead to inappropriate intensification of short-acting beta-agonist treatment. It is therefore recommended that patients are monitored for the development of elevated serum lactate and consequent metabolic acidosis in this setting.

Care should be taken with patients with hyperthyroidism.

Hypersensitivity: Immediate hypersensitivity reactions may occur after administration of salbutamol sulphate, as demonstrated by rare cases of urticaria, angioedema, rash, bronchospasm, anaphylaxis, and oropharyngeal edema.

Care should be taken with patients who are unusually responsive to sympathomimetic amines.

Neurologic: Care should be taken with patients with convulsive disorders.

Respiratory: With repeated excessive use of sympathomimetic inhalation preparations, some patients have been reported to have developed severe paradoxical bronchospasm, occasionally leading to death. The cause of either the refractory state or death is unknown. However, it is suspected in the fatal episodes that cardiac arrest occurred following the unexpected development of a severe acute asthmatic crisis and subsequent hypoxia. Several cases have been reported in which intermittent positive pressure ventilation in acute asthma attacks was related to lethal episodes of hypoxia and pneumothorax. This method of drug administration may be ineffective in patients with severe obstruction and greatly increased airway resistance, and it may induce severe hypercapnia and hypoxia. During intermittent ventilation therapy, the monitoring of arterial blood gases is highly desirable. It is advisable that in the event of either hypoxia and pneumothorax or paradoxical bronchospasm the use of the preparation should be discontinued immediately and alternate therapy instituted, since in the reported cases the patients did not respond to other forms of therapy until the drug was withdrawn.

Special Populations: Pregnant Women: Salbutamol has been in widespread use for many years in human beings without apparent ill consequence. However, there are no adequate and well-controlled studies in pregnant women and there is little published evidence of its safety in the early stages of human pregnancy. Administration of any drug to pregnant women should only be considered if the anticipated benefits to the expectant woman are greater than any possible risks to the foetus.

Labour and Delivery: Although there have been no reports concerning the use of inhaled VENTOLIN Respirator Solution during labour and delivery, intravenously administered salbutamol given at high doses may inhibit uterine contractions. While this effect is extremely unlikely as a consequence of using inhaled formulations, it should be kept in mind. Oral salbutamol has been shown to delay preterm labour in some reports but there are no well-controlled studies which demonstrate that it will stop preterm labour or prevent labour at term. When given to pregnant patients for relief of bronchospasm, cautious use of VENTOLIN Respirator Solution is required to avoid interference with uterine contractility.

Nursing Women: Since salbutamol is probably excreted in breast milk and because of its observed tumorigenicity in animal studies, a decision should be made whether to discontinue nursing or to discontinue the drug, taking into account the benefit of the drug to the mother. It is not known whether salbutamol in breast milk has a harmful effect on the neonate.

Pediatrics: VENTOLIN Respirator Solution and VENTOLIN NEBULES: VENTOLIN Respirator Solution and VENTOLIN NEBULES should be used under the supervision of an adult who understands the proper use of the nebulizer (and VENTOLIN NEBULES if applicable), and only as presented by the doctor.

Experience is insufficient for recommending the treatment of children under 5 years of age.

Monitoring and Laboratory Tests: The management of asthma should normally follow a stepwise program and patient response should be monitored clinically and by lung function tests.

Monitoring Control of Asthma: Failure to respond for at least three hours to a previously effective dose of salbutamol indicates a deterioration of the condition and the physician should be contacted promptly. Patients should be warned not to exceed the recommended dose.

The increasing use of fast acting, short duration inhaled beta$_2$-adrenergic agonists to control symptoms indicates deterioration of asthma control and the patient's therapy plan should be reassessed. In worsening asthma it is inadequate to increase beta$_2$-agonist use only, especially over an extended period of time. In the case of acute or rapidly worsening dyspnea, a doctor should be consulted immediately. Sudden or progressive deterioration in asthma control is potentially life threatening; the treatment plan must be re-evaluated, and consideration be given to corticosteroid therapy (see Dosage and Administration).

ADVERSE REACTIONS: Adverse Drug Reaction Overview: As with other bronchodilator inhalation therapy, the potential for paradoxical bronchospasm should be kept in mind. If it occurs, the preparation should be discontinued immediately and alternative therapy instituted.

Potentially serious hypokalemia may result from beta$_2$-agonist therapy, primarily from parenteral and nebulized routes of administration (see Warnings and Precautions, Endocrine and Metabolism).

Peripheral vasodilation and a compensatory small increase in heart rate may occur in some patients. Cardiac arrhythmias (including atrial fibrillation, supraventricular tachycardia and extrasystoles) have been reported, usually in susceptible patients.

The most frequent adverse reactions associated with salbutamol inhalation aerosol, dry powder or respirator solution formulations are nervousness and tremor. In some patients inhaled salbutamol may cause a fine tremor of skeletal muscle, particularly in the hands. This effect is common to all beta$_2$-adrenergic stimulants. Adaptation occurs during the first few days of dosing and the tremor usually disappears as treatment continues.

Headache, palpitations, transient muscle cramps, insomnia, nausea, weakness and dizziness have been reported as untoward effects following salbutamol administration.

Rarely reported adverse effects include drowsiness, flushing, restlessness, irritability, chest discomfort, difficulty in micturition, hypertension, angina, vomiting, vertigo, central nervous system stimulation, hyperactivity in children, unusual taste and drying or irritation of the oropharynx.

Immediate hypersensitivity reactions including angioedema, urticaria, bronchospasm, hypotension, rash, oropharyngeal oedema, anaphylaxis and collapse have been reported very rarely.

Lactic acidosis has been reported very rarely in patients receiving intravenous and nebulised salbutamol therapy for the treatment of acute asthma exacerbation.

DRUG INTERACTIONS: Drug-Drug Interactions: See Table 1.

Table 1: VENTOLIN Respirator Solution/VENTOLIN NEBULES P.F.
Established or Potential Drug-Drug Interactions

Proper Name	Ref	Effect	Clinical Comment
Monoamine oxidase inhibitors or tricyclic antidepressants	CS	May potentiate action of salbutamol on cardiovascular system.	Salbutamol should be administered with extreme caution to patients being treated with monoamine oxidase inhibitors or tricyclic antidepressants.
Other inhaled sympathomimetic bronchodilators or epinephrine	CS	May lead to deleterious cardiovascular effects.	Other inhaled sympathomimetic bronchodilators or epinephrine should not be used concomitantly with salbutamol. If additional adrenergic drugs are to be administered by any route to the patient using inhaled salbutamol, the adrenergic drugs should be used with caution. Such concomitant use must be individualized and not given on a routine basis. If regular coadministration is required then alternative therapy must be considered.
Beta-blockers	CS	May effectively antagonize the action of salbutamol.	Beta-adrenergic blocking drugs, especially the non-cardioselective ones, such as propranolol, should not usually be prescribed together.
Diuretics	CS	May lead to ECG changes and/or hypokalemia although the clinical significance of these effects is not known.	The ECG changes and/or hypokalemia that may result from the administration of non-potassium sparing diuretics (such as loop or thiazide diuretics) can be acutely worsened by beta-agonists, especially when the recommended dose of the beta-agonist is exceeded. Caution is advised in the coadministration of beta-agonists with non-potassium sparing diuretics.
Digoxin	CS	May lead to decrease in serum digoxin levels. The clinical significance of these findings for patients with obstructive airways disease who are receiving salbutamol and digoxin on a chronic basis is unclear.	Mean decreases of 16-22% in serum digoxin levels were demonstrated after single dose intravenous and oral administration of salbutamol, respectively, to normal volunteers who had received digoxin for 10 days. It would be prudent to carefully evaluate serum digoxin levels in patients who are currently receiving digoxin and salbutamol.
Ipratropium bromide	CS	Acute angle closure glaucoma has been reported with coadministration.	A small number of cases of acute angle closure glaucoma have been reported in patients treated with a combination of nebulized salbutamol and ipratropium bromide. Therefore, a combination of nebulized salbutamol with nebulized anticholinergics should be used cautiously. Patients should receive adequate instruction in correct administration and be warned not to let the solution or mist enter the eye.

Legend: CS=class statement.

DOSAGE AND ADMINISTRATION: **Dosing Considerations:** The dosage should be individualized, and the patient's response should be monitored by the prescribing physician on an ongoing basis.

In accordance with current Canadian asthma guidelines, if salbutamol is required for relief of symptoms more than twice a day on a regular daily basis or for an extended period of time anti-inflammatory therapy (eg. corticosteroid) should be part of the regimen.

Increasing demand for VENTOLIN (salbutamol sulphate) Respirator Solution in bronchial asthma is usually a sign of worsening asthma and indicates that the treatment plan should be reviewed.

If a previously effective dose fails to provide the usual relief, or the effects of a dose last for less than three hours, patients should seek prompt medical advice since this is usually a sign of worsening asthma.

As there may be adverse effects associated with excessive dosing the dosage or frequency of administration should only be increased on medical advice. However, if a more severe attack has not been relieved by the usual dose, additional doses may be required. In these cases, patients should immediately consult their doctors or the nearest hospital.

VENTOLIN Respirator Solution may be preferred in the treatment of severe bronchospasm associated with exacerbations of chronic bronchitis and bronchial asthma.

Recommended Dose and Dosage Adjustment: VENTOLIN Respirator Solution: Adults: In adults, VENTOLIN Respirator Solution 0.5 to 1 mL (2.5 to 5 mg of salbutamol) should be diluted in 2 to 5 mL or more of sterile normal saline. Treatment may be repeated four times a day if necessary.

Children (5-12 years): The average dose for a single treatment is 0.25 to 0.5 mL of VENTOLIN Respirator Solution (1.25 to 2.5 mg of salbutamol) diluted in 2 to 5 mL or more of sterile normal saline. For more refractory cases, the single dose of VENTOLIN Respirator Solution may be increased to 1 mL (5 mg of salbutamol). Treatment may be repeated four times a day if necessary.

VENTOLIN NEBULES P.F.: Adults: Patients requiring single doses of 2.5 mg or 5 mg may be administered the contents of a single VENTOLIN Respirator Solution unit dose (VENTOLIN NEBULES P.F. 2.5 or 5 mg of salbutamol). Treatment may be repeated 4 times a day if necessary.

Children (5-12 years): Children requiring a single dose of 2.5 mg may be administered the contents of a single VENTOLIN Respirator Solution unit dose (VENTOLIN NEBULES P.F. 2.5 mg of salbutamol). For more refractory cases children may use a 5 mg unit dose (see dosage above). Treatment may be repeated 4 times a day if necessary.

If a more severe attack has not been relieved by a treatment, further treatments may be required. In these cases, patients should immediately consult their doctor or the nearest hospital.

Missed Dose: If a single dose is missed, instruct the patient to take the next dose at the time when it is due or if they become wheezy.

Administration: To ensure administration of the proper dose of the drug, the patient should be instructed by the physician or other health professional in the proper use of the nebulizer system.

VENTOLIN Respirator Solution is to be used only under the direction of a physician employing either a respirator or nebulizer. VENTOLIN Respirator Solution can be taken by either the nebulization or intermittent positive pressure ventilation method. When used in a nebulizer, a mouthpiece or a face mask may be applied. The nebulizer should be connected to a compressed air or oxygen pump. Gas flow should be in the range of 6 to 10 L/minute. With an average volume of 3 mL, a single treatment lasts approximately 10 minutes. It is advisable to prepare one dose at a time or to utilize the Unit Dose (VENTOLIN NEBULES P.F.) presentation. When administered through intermittent positive pressure ventilation, the inspiratory pressure is usually 10-20 cm H_2O and the duration of administration varies from 5 to 20 minutes, depending upon the patient and the control of the apparatus. This length of administration provides a more gradual and more complete lysis of bronchospasm. In several cases it has been reported that the use of intermittent positive pressure ventilation in acute asthma attacks was related to lethal episodes of hypoxia and pneumothorax. This method of drug administration may be ineffective in patients with severe obstruction and may greatly increase airway resistance and possibly induce severe hypercapnia and hypoxia. It is highly desirable to monitor arterial blood gases during intermittent positive pressure ventilation therapy.

In hospitals VENTOLIN Respirator Solution, diluted (1:5 or 1:10) with sterile normal saline, should be used within 24 hours from time of dilution when stored at room temperature or within 48 hours when stored under refrigeration.

Cleansing and maintenance of the nebulizer must be carefully exercised by strict adherence to the manufacturer's instructions.

OVERDOSAGE:

Symptoms and Signs: The most common signs and symptoms of overdose with salbutamol are transient beta agonist pharmacologically mediated events (see Warnings and Precautions and Adverse Reactions). Overdosage may cause tachycardia, cardiac arrhythmia, hypokalemia, hypertension and, in extreme cases, sudden death. Serum potassium levels should be monitored.

Treatment: Consideration should be given to discontinuation of treatment and appropriate symptomatic therapy. To antagonise the effect of salbutamol, the judicious use of a cardioselective beta-adrenergic blocking agent (e.g. metoprolol, atenolol) may be considered, bearing in mind the danger of inducing an asthmatic attack.

During continuous administration of salbutamol Respirator Solution, any signs of overdosage can usually be counteracted by withdrawal of the drug.

For management of a suspected drug overdose, CPhA recommends that you contact your **regional Poison Control Centre**. See the *CPS* Directory section for a list of Poison Control Centres.

ACTION AND CLINICAL PHARMACOLOGY: Mechanism of Action: Salbutamol produces bronchodilation through stimulation of $beta_2$-adrenergic receptors in bronchial smooth muscle, thereby causing relaxation of bronchial muscle fibres. This action is manifested by an improvement in pulmonary function as demonstrated by spirometric measurements. At therapeutic doses, salbutamol has little action on the $beta_1$-adrenergic receptors in cardiac muscle.

A measurable decrease in airway resistance is typically observed 5 to 15 minutes after inhalation of salbutamol. The maximum improvement in pulmonary function usually occurs 60 to 90 minutes after salbutamol treatment, and significant bronchodilator activity has been observed to persist for 3 to 6 hours.

Pharmacokinetics: After inhalation of recommended doses of salbutamol, plasma drug levels are very low. When 100 µg of tritiated salbutamol aerosol was administered to two normal volunteers, plasma levels of drug-radioactivity were insignificant at 10, 20 and 30 minutes following inhalation. The plasma concentration of salbutamol may be even less as the amount of plasma drug-radioactivity does not differentiate salbutamol from its principal metabolite, a sulphate ester. In a separate study, plasma salbutamol levels ranged from less than 0.5 ng/mL to 1.6 ng/mL in ten asthmatic children one hour after inhalation of 200 µg of salbutamol.

Five asthmatic patients were given tritium-labelled salbutamol from the nebulizer of an intermittent positive pressure ventilator. In all patients, there was a rapid initial rise in plasma concentration of total radioactivity. In four of the five patients, there was a further rise in plasma concentration to a peak at 2 to 4 hours. All patients showed an improvement in FEV_1 with peak improvement at 30 minutes to 2 hours. An average of 12.5% of the initial dose was recovered in the urine. Of the radioactivity recovered, 88% was recovered in the first 24 hours. The metabolite in the urine was the same as that in the plasma. During the first 2 hours, the ratio of free salbutamol to metabolite average 2:1, whereas by 8 hours, the ratio was 9:11, and thereafter this reversed ratio was maintained.

Approximately 10% of an inhaled salbutamol dose is deposited in the lungs. Eighty-five per cent of the remaining salbutamol administered from a metered-dose inhaler is swallowed, however, since the dose is low (100 to 200 µg), the absolute amount swallowed is too small to be of clinical significance. Salbutamol is only weakly bound to plasma proteins. Results of animal studies indicate that following systemic administration, salbutamol does not cross the blood-brain barrier but does cross the placenta using an in vitro perfused isolated human placenta model. It has been found that between 2% and 3% of salbutamol was transferred from the maternal side to the fetal side of the placenta.

Salbutamol is metabolized in the liver. The principal metabolite in humans is salbutamol-o-sulphate, which has negligible pharmacologic activity. Salbutamol may also be metabolized by oxidative deamination and/or conjugation with glucuronide.

Salbutamol is longer acting than isoprenaline in most patients by any route of administration because it is not a substrate for the cellular uptake processes for catecholamines nor for catechol-O-methyl transferase. Salbutamol and its metabolites are excreted in the urine (>80%) and the feces (5% to 10%). Plasma levels are insignificant after administration of aerosolized salbutamol; the plasma half-life ranges from 3.8 to 7.1 hours.

STORAGE AND STABILITY: Keep out of the reach of children.

VENTOLIN Respirator Solution: Store between 15 to 25°C. Protect from light. Discard if not used within one month of opening.

Overwrapped VENTOLIN NEBULES: Store between 2 to 25°C.

VENTOLIN NEBULES Removed From Overwrap: Store between 2 to 25°C. Protect from light. Use within 3 months.

Reconstituted VENTOLIN Respirator Solution: In hospitals, VENTOLIN Respirator Solution, diluted (1:5 or 1:10), with sterile normal saline, should be used within 24 hours from time of dilution when stored at room temperature or within 48 hours when stored under refrigeration. Instructions for the dilution of VENTOLIN Respirator Solution are given in Table 2.

In the home, the unit dose preparation (VENTOLIN NEBULES P.F.), which is pre-diluted and ready to use, is the most convenient preparation. However, if the standard VENTOLIN Respirator Solution is used, it may be diluted with sterile normal saline immediately before use. Any unused solution in the nebulizer should be discarded.

Table 2: VENTOLIN Respirator Solution

Dilution Table for VENTOLIN Respirator Solution

Dose (mg) of Salbutamol (per treatment)	Volume (mL) of VENTOLIN Respirator Solution (per treatment)	Volume[a] (mL) of Sterile Normal Saline to Be Added as Diluent
1.25	0.25	2–5 mL or more
2.5	0.50	2–5 mL or more
5	1.00	2–5 mL or more

[a] Approximate volumes only are given. Actual volume of diluent used may vary according to the type of nebulizer and individual patient needs.

INFORMATION FOR THE PATIENT: Published in e-CPS, available by subscription at www.e-cps.ca.

DOSAGE FORMS, COMPOSITION AND PACKAGING: VENTOLIN Respirator Solution: Each mL of isotonic solution contains: salbutamol sulfate, equivalent to salbutamol base 5 mg. Nonmedicinal ingredients: benzalkonium chloride 0.01% w/v, dilute sulphuric acid and water for Injection. Adjusted to pH 3.4 to 4.4. Bottles of 10 mL.

VENTOLIN Respirator Solution Unit Dose (VENTOLIN NEBULES P.F.): Each unit dose of sterile, isotonic solution contains: salbutamol sulfate equivalent to salbutamol base 2.5 or 5 mg in 2.5 mL. Nonmedicinal ingredients: dilute sulphuric acid, sodium chloride and water for Injection. Adjusted to pH 3.5 to 4.5. Boxes of 20 ampoules.

Vepesid® Ⓟ

etoposide

Antineoplastic Agent

Bristol-Myers Squibb

Date of Preparation: May 15, 1981
Date of Revision: August 8, 2008

Caution: VEPESID (etoposide) is a potent drug and should be used only by qualified physicians experienced with cancer chemotherapeutic drugs (see Warnings and Precautions). Severe myelosuppression with resulting infection or bleeding may occur. Blood counts as well as renal and hepatic function tests should be taken regularly. Discontinue the drug if abnormal depression of bone marrow or abnormal renal or hepatic function is seen.

PHARMACOLOGY: VEPESID (etoposide) is a semisynthetic derivative of podophyllotoxin used in the treatment of certain neoplastic diseases.

In vitro, etoposide has cytostatic action, which prevents the cells from entering mitosis or destroys them in the premitotic phase. Etoposide interferes with the synthesis of DNA and has a secondary effect on arresting cells in resting (G_2) phase in experiments with human lymphoblastic cell lines.

Etoposide has a marked action on human hemopoietic cells causing leukopenia and thrombocytopenia. Animal experiments have shown evidence of teratogenicity.

An i.v. dose (259 mg/m²) of tritium-labelled etoposide given over 1 hour in man, showed the mean volume of distribution to be 32% of body weight. The plasma decay was biphasic with a beta half-life of 11.5 hours. Urinary recovery was 44% of which 67% was unchanged drug. Recovery in feces was variable (1.5 to 16%) over a 3-day period.

A plasma decay with a beta half-life of 6.8 hours was observed following oral administration of etoposide. The $T_{½}$ for oral absorption was 0.44 hour and peak plasma concentrations were noted 0.5 to 3 hours after oral administration.

In a limited number of children, VEPESID administered in a dose of 200 to 250 mg/m² produced a peak serum concentration between 17 and 88 µg/mL and showed a terminal half-life ($T_{½β}$) of 5.7±1.3 hours. Mean plasma clearance was 21.5 mL/min/m² and CSF concentrations 24 hours postinfusion ranged from less than 10 ng/mL to 45 µg/mL.

After either i.v. infusion or oral capsule administration of etoposide, the C_{max} and AUC values exhibit marked intra- and inter-subject variability. The overall mean value of oral capsule bioavailability is approximately 50% (range 25 to 75%).

Etoposide crosses the blood brain barrier in low concentrations.

Etoposide is cleared by both renal and nonrenal processes, i.e., metabolism and biliary excretion. Biliary excretion, however, appears to be a minor route of etoposide elimination.

INDICATIONS: VEPESID (etoposide) is indicated as follows:

For oral formulation: Small Cell Carcinoma of the Lung: First-line therapy in combination with other established antineoplastic agents. Second-line combination or single agent therapy in patients who have not responded or relapsed on other chemotherapeutic regimens.

Malignant Lymphoma (histiocytic type): First-line therapy in combination with other established antineoplastic agents.

Non-small Cell Carcinoma of the Lung: For patients considered ineligible for surgery, etoposide has been shown effective alone or in combination with cisplatin. For patients who require chemotherapy following surgery.

Testicular Malignancies (germ cell tumors including seminomas): In combination with other effective chemotherapeutic agents in patients who have already received appropriate therapy.

CONTRAINDICATIONS: VEPESID (etoposide) should not be given to individuals who have demonstrated a previous hypersensitivity to etoposide or to any component of the formulation. Also, it is contraindicated in patients having severe leukopenia, thrombocytopenia and severe hepatic and/or renal impairment.

WARNINGS: VEPESID (etoposide) is a potent drug and should be used only by qualified physicians experienced with cancer chemotherapeutic drugs (see Precautions). Severe myelosuppression with resulting infection or bleeding may occur. Blood counts as well as renal and hepatic function tests should be taken regularly. Discontinue the drug if abnormal depression of bone marrow or abnormal renal or hepatic function is seen.

Fatal myelosuppression has been reported following etoposide administration. Patients being treated with VEPESID (etoposide) must be frequently observed for myelosuppression both during and after therapy. Dose-limiting bone marrow suppression is the most significant toxicity associated with VEPESID therapy. The following studies should be obtained at the start of therapy and prior to each subsequent dose of VEPESID: platelet count, hemoglobin, white blood cell count and differential.

The occurrence of a platelet count below 50 000/mm³ or an absolute neutrophil count below 500/mm³ is an indication to withhold further therapy until the blood counts have sufficiently recovered. A white blood cell count of between 2000 to 3000 cells/mm³ suggests that the dose of VEPESID should be reduced by 50%. Platelet counts between 75 000 to 100 000 cells/mm³ require a dosage reduction of 50%.

Bacterial infection must be brought under control before the administration of VEPESID therapy because of the risk of septicemia.

Physicians should be aware of the possible occurrence of an anaphylactic reaction manifested by chills, fever, tachycardia, bronchospasm, dyspnea and/or hypotension (see Adverse Effects). Treatment is symptomatic. The administration of VEPESID should be terminated immediately, followed by the administration of pressor agents, corticosteroids, antihistamines, or volume expanders at the discretion of the physician.

Pregnancy: VEPESID can cause fetal harm when administered to pregnant women.

VEPESID has been shown to be embryotoxic in rats and teratogenic in mice and rats. There are no adequate and well-controlled studies in pregnant women. If the drug is used during pregnancy, or if the patient becomes pregnant while receiving this drug, the patient should be apprised of the potential hazard to the fetus. Women of childbearing potential should be advised to avoid becoming pregnant and should exercise adequate contraceptive control.

VEPESID has caused reduced or absent spermatogenesis and reduced testes weights at autopsy in rats and dogs, as well as reduced weight of ovaries in female rats. Chronic toxicity studies in rats have shown etoposide to have an oncogenic potential (see Adverse Effects, Hematologic Toxicity).

Lactation: There has been evidence of VEPESID being excreted in human milk.

Because of the potential for serious adverse reactions in nursing infants from etoposide, breast-feeding should be discontinued.

As with any potent antineoplastic drug, the benefit to patient versus the risk of toxicity must be carefully weighed.

PRECAUTIONS: General: The physician must evaluate the need and usefulness of the drug against the risk of adverse reactions. Most such adverse reactions are reversible if detected early. If severe reactions occur, the drug should be reduced in dosage or discontinued and appropriate corrective measures should be taken according to the clinical judgment of the physician. Reinstitution of VEPESID (etoposide) therapy should be carried out with caution, and with adequate consideration of the further need for the drug and **alertness** to the possible recurrence of toxicity. Patients with low serum albumin may be at increased risk for etoposide-associated toxicities.

VEPESID should be administered by individuals experienced in the use of antineoplastic therapy.

Myelosuppression is dose related and dose limiting, with granulocyte nadirs occurring 7 to 14 days and platelet nadirs occurring 9 to 16 days after drug administration. Bone marrow recovery is usually complete by day 20, and no cumulative toxicity has been reported.

Liver and renal function should be regularly monitored.

Professional staff administering VEPESID should exercise particular care to prevent spillage and self-contact with the drug. Skin reactions, at times severe, associated with accidental exposure to VEPESID may occur. Gloves should be worn by anyone handling the drug.

Carcinogenesis: Carcinogenicity tests with VEPESID have not been conducted in laboratory animals. Given its mechanism of action, it should be considered a possible carcinogen in humans.

The occurrence of acute leukemia, which can occur with or without a preleukemic phase, has been reported rarely in patients treated with VEPESID in association with other antineoplastic drugs. Neither the cumulative risk, nor the predisposing factors related to the development of secondary leukemia are known. The roles of both administration schedules and cumulative doses of etoposide have been suggested, but have not been clearly defined.

An 11q23 chromosome abnormality has been observed in some cases of secondary leukemia in patients who have received epipodophyllotoxins. This abnormality has also been seen in patients developing secondary leukemia after being treated with chemotherapy regimens not containing epipodophyllotoxins and in leukemia occurring de novo. Another characteristic that has been associated with secondary leukemia in patients who have received epipodophyllotoxins appears to be a short latency period, with average median time to development of leukemia being approximately 32 months.

Drug Interactions: High dose cyclosporine, resulting in concentrations above 2000 ng/mL, administered with oral etoposide has led to an 80% increase in etoposide exposure (AUC) with a 38% decrease in total body clearance of etoposide compared to etoposide alone. Severe cases of neuropathy have been reported in 0.7% of patients possibly due to an interaction of vincristine and VEPESID.

Children: Safety and effectiveness in pediatric patients have not been systematically studied. Clinical experience in childhood malignancies is very limited (see Warnings).

ADVERSE EFFECTS: The following data on adverse events are based on both oral and i.v. administration of VEPESID (etoposide) as a single agent, using several different dose schedules for treatment of a wide variety of malignancies.

Hematologic Toxicity: Since leukopenia and thrombocytopenia have been reported in patients on VEPESID (etoposide) therapy, platelets and white blood cell counts should be performed prior to each cycle (see Warnings).

Myelosuppression with fatal outcome has been reported following etoposide administration (see Warnings and Precautions).

The occurrence of acute leukemia with or without a preleukemic phase has been reported in patients treated with VEPESID in association with other antineoplastic agents.

Gastrointestinal Toxicity: Nausea and vomiting are the major gastrointestinal toxicities. The severity of such nausea and vomiting is generally mild to moderate with treatment discontinuation required in 1% of patients. Nausea and vomiting can usually be controlled with standard antiemetic therapy. Gastrointestinal toxicities are slightly more frequent after oral administration than after i.v. infusion. Mild to severe mucositis/esosphagitis may occur.

Hypotension: Transient hypotension following rapid i.v. administration has been reported in 1 to 2% of patients. It has not been associated with cardiac toxicity or ECG changes. No delayed hypotension has been noted. To prevent this occurrence, it is recommended that VEPESID injection be administered by slow i.v. infusion over a 30- to 60-minute period. Hypotension usually responds to cessation of the infusion and/or other supportive therapy as appropriate. When restarting the infusion, a slower administration rate should be used.

Allergic Reactions: Anaphylactic-like reactions characterized by chills, fever, tachycardia, bronchospasm, dyspnea and/or hypotension have been reported to occur in 0.7 to 2% of patients during or immediately after i.v. VEPESID administration. Higher rates of anaphylactic-like reactions have been reported in children who received VEPESID infusions at concentrations higher than those recommended. The role that concentration of infusion (or rate of infusion) plays in the development of anaphylactic-like reactions is uncertain. Reactions have occurred very rarely in patients treated with oral capsules. Anaphylactic-like reactions have usually responded promptly to the cessation of the infusion of VEPESID, and subsequent administration of pressor agents, corticosteroids, antihistamines or volume expanders as appropriate. Acute fatal reactions associated with bronchospasm have been reported. Hypertension and/or flushing and/or seizures have also been reported. Blood pressure usually normalizes within a few hours after cessation of the infusion. Anaphylactic-like reactions can occur with the initial dose of VEPESID. Apnea with spontaneous resumption of breathing following discontinuation has been described in patients receiving etoposide infusion.

Alopecia: Reversible alopecia, sometimes progressing to total baldness was observed in up to 66% of patients.

Neuropathy: Peripheral neuropathy has been reported in 0.7% of patients.

Other Toxicities: weakness (3%), mouth ulceration (2%). The following adverse events have been reported in less than 1%: hyperuricemia, sepsis, numbness and tingling, dizziness, depression, nail pigmentation and moniliasis. The following adverse reactions have been rarely reported: interstitial pneumonitis/pulmonary fibrosis, seizures (occasionally associated with allergic reactions), somnolence and fatigue, liver toxicity, fever, aftertaste, Stevens-Johnson syndrome, toxic epidermal necrolysis (1 fatal case has been reported), rash, pigmentation, pruritus, urticaria, constipation, dysphagia, asthenia, malaise, transient cortical blindness, optic neuritis, and radiation recall dermatitis.

Occasionally following extravasation, soft tissue irritation and inflammation has occurred; ulceration is generally not seen.

The incidences of adverse reactions in Table 1 are derived from multiple data bases from studies in patients when VEPESID was used either orally or by injection as a single agent.

Table 1: VEPESID

Adverse Reactions

Adverse Drug Effect	Range of Reported Incidence (%)
Hematologic Toxicity	
Leukopenia (less than 1000 WBC/mm³)	3–17
Leukopenia (less than 4000 WBC/mm³)	60–91
Thrombocytopenia (less than 50 000 platelets/mm³)	1–20
Thrombocytopenia (less than 100 000 platelets/mm³)	22–41
Anemia	0–33
Gastrointestinal Toxicity	
Nausea and Vomiting	31–43
Abdominal Pain	0–2
Anorexia	10–13
Diarrhea	1–13
Stomatitis	1–6
Other	
Alopecia	8–66
Peripheral Neurotoxicity	1–2
Hypotension	1–2
Allergic Reaction	1–2
Hepatic	0–3

Legend: WBC=white blood cell.

OVERDOSE:

Symptoms: The anticipated acute complications would be related to VEPESID's hematotoxicity.

Total doses of 2.4 g/m² to 3.5 g/m² administered i.v. over 3 days resulted in severe mucositis and myelotoxicity.

Metabolic acidosis and cases of serious hepatic toxicity have been reported in patients receiving higher than recommended i.v. doses of etoposide.

Treatment: There is no known antidote and therefore symptomatic measures should be taken to sustain the patient through any period of toxicity that might occur. Patients' renal and hepatic functions should be monitored for 3 to 4 weeks in case of delayed toxicity.

For management of a suspected drug overdose, CPhA recommends that you contact your **regional Poison Control Centre**. See the *CPS* Directory section for a list of Poison Control Centres.

DOSAGE: Oral: 100 to 200 mg/m² daily for 5 days.

The bioavailability also varies from patient to patient following any oral dose. This should be taken into consideration when prescribing this medication. In view of significant intra-patient variability, dose adjustment may be required to achieve the desired therapeutic effect. Daily doses greater than 200 mg should be given divided (b.i.d.).

Dosage should be modified to take into account the myelosuppressive effects of other drugs in the combination or the effects of prior x-ray therapy or chemotherapy which may have compromised bone marrow reserve.

Capsules should be taken on an empty stomach.

Oral: Renal Impairment: In patients with impaired renal function, the following initial dose modification should be considered based on measured creatinine clearance. See Table 2.

Table 2: VEPESID

Dosage in Renal Impairment

Measured Creatinine Clearance	Dose of Etoposide
>50 mL/min	100% of dose
15–50 mL/min	75% of dose

Subsequent dosing should be based on patient tolerance and clinical effect. Data are not available in patients with creatinine clearance <15 mL/min and further dose reduction should be considered in those patients.

Stability and Storage Recommendations: VEPESID capsules should be stored at room temperature (15-30°C).

Special Instructions: To minimize the risk of dermal exposure, always wear impervious gloves when handling bottles containing VEPESID capsules. This includes handling activities in clinical settings, pharmacies, storerooms, and home healthcare settings, including during unpacking and inspection, transport within a facility, and dose preparation and administration.

Procedures for proper handling and disposal of anticancer drugs should be considered. Several guidelines on this subject have been published. There is no general agreement that all of the procedures recommended in the guidelines are necessary or appropriate.

SUPPLIED: Each pink, liquid-filled, soft gelatin capsule contains: etoposide 50 mg. Nonmedicinal ingredients: citric acid, glycerol, polyethylene glycol 400 and water; capsule shell: gelatin, glycerol, iron oxide red, parabens (ethyl and propyl), purified water, sorbitol and titanium dioxide. The capsules are printed with edible ink. Bottles of 20. Store at room temperature (15 to 30°C).

(Shown in Product Identification Section)

Verapamil Ⓟ

CPhA Monograph

see *Calcium Channel Blockers*

Verapamil Hydrochloride Injection USP Ⓟ

verapamil HCl

Antiarrhythmic

Hospira

SUPPLIED: Each mL of sterile, nonpyrogenic solution contains: verapamil HCl 2.5 mg (equivalent to verapamil 2.3 mg) and sodium chloride in water for injection. The solution contains no bacteriostat or antimicrobial agent and is intended for single use only. May contain hydrochloric acid for pH adjustment; pH 4.9 (4.0 to 6.5). Ampoules of 2 mL, sleeves of 5. Store between 15 and 25°C. Discard unused portion. Protect from light and freezing. Retain in carton until ready for use.

Vermox® Ⓟ

mebendazole

Anthelmintic

Janssen-Ortho

Date of Preparation: July 8, 1975
Date of Revision: July 23, 2004

PHARMACOLOGY: VERMOX mebendazole induces in vitro and in vivo inhibition of the glucose uptake by parasitic helminths; this is associated with glycogen depletion and a decrease in the generation of ATP, leading to inhibition of larval development.

There is no evidence that VERMOX mebendazole is effective in the treatment of cysticercosis.

(cont'd)

Pharmacokinetics: Absorption: Following oral administration, approximately 20% of the dose reaches the systemic circulation, due to incomplete absorption and to extensive pre-systemic metabolism (first-pass effect). Maximum plasma concentrations are generally seen 2 to 4 hours after administration. Dosing with a high fat meal leads to a modest increase in the bioavailability of mebendazole.

Distribution: The plasma protein binding of mebendazole is 90 to 95%. The volume of distribution is 1 to 2 L/kg, indicating that mebendazole penetrates areas outside the vascular space. This is supported by data in patients on chronic mebendazole therapy (e.g. 40 mg/kg/day for 3-21 months) that show drug levels in tissue.

Metabolism: Orally administered mebendazole is extensively metabolized primarily by the liver. Plasma concentrations of its major metabolites (amino and hydroxylated amino forms of mebendazole) are substantially higher than those of mebendazole. Impaired hepatic function, impaired metabolism, or impaired biliary elimination may lead to higher plasma levels of mebendazole.

Elimination: Mebendazole, the conjugated forms of mebendazole, and its metabolites likely undergo some degree of enterohepatic recirculation and are excreted in the urine and bile. The apparent elimination half-life after an oral dose ranges from 3 to 6 hours in most patients.

Steady-state Pharmacokinetics: During chronic dosing (e.g. 40 mg/kg/day for 3-21 months), plasma concentrations of mebendazole and its major metabolites increase, resulting in approximately 3-fold higher exposure to steady-state compared to single dosing.

INDICATIONS: VERMOX mebendazole has a broad spectrum of anthelmintic activity and is effective in the treatment of single or mixed helminthic infestations. Clinical studies have shown it effective in the treatment of *Enterobius vermicularis* (pinworm); *Ascaris lumbricoides* (roundworm); *Trichuris trichiura* (whipworm); *Ankylostoma duodenale* and *Necator americanus* (hookworm). It has also been used to treat infections due to *Strongyloides stercoralis* and *Taenia solium* (large tapeworms).

CONTRAINDICATIONS: VERMOX mebendazole is contraindicated in persons who have shown hypersensitivity to the drug or its components.

WARNINGS: Results from a case-control study investigating an outbreak of Stevens-Johnson syndrome/toxic epidermal necrolysis (SJS/TEN) suggested a possible relationship between SJS/TEN and the concomitant use of mebendazole and metronidazole. Further data suggesting such a drug-drug interaction are not available. Therefore, concomitant use of mebendazole and metronidazole should be avoided.

Pregnancy: Animal trials conducted in a wide range of species revealed an embryotoxic and teratogenic effect in the rat. Also, the safety of use in pregnant women has not been established. Therefore, VERMOX mebendazole should not be administered during pregnancy, particularly in the first trimester, unless the potential benefit to the patient outweighs the possible risk to the fetus.

PRECAUTIONS: Patients should be carefully checked to detect any alteration in blood studies or hepatic or renal function tests following treatment with VERMOX mebendazole. Special attention should be given to patients with intestinal pathology (e.g. Crohn's ileitis, ulcerative colitis).

Lactation: Mebendazole is only absorbed to a small extent. It is not known whether mebendazole is excreted in human breast milk. Therefore, caution should be exercised when VERMOX mebendazole tablets are administered to nursing women.

Children Under 2 Years: Since VERMOX mebendazole has not been extensively studied in infants under 2 years of age, its use in such individuals should only be implemented in cases where the potential therapeutic effects outweigh the possible hazard to the patient. There have been very exceptional reports of convulsions in infants less than 1 year old. VERMOX mebendazole should only be given to very young children if their worm infestation interferes significantly with their nutritional status and their physical development.

Drug Interactions: Concomitant treatment with cimetidine may inhibit the metabolism of mebendazole in the liver, resulting in increased plasma concentrations of the drug, especially during prolonged treatment. In the latter case, determination of plasma concentrations is recommended in order to allow dose adjustments.

Concomitant use of mebendazole and metronidazole should be avoided.

ADVERSE EFFECTS: At the recommended dose, VERMOX mebendazole is generally well tolerated. However, patients with high parasitic burdens have manifested diarrhea, vomiting, and/or abdominal pain when treated with VERMOX mebendazole. Other adverse reactions reported were drowsiness, itching, headache, and dizziness. Reports from clinical trials also mentioned increased AST, ALT, alkaline phosphatase, and BUN.

Eosinophilia and decreased hemoglobin and/or white cell count, hematuria, and cylindruria have been reported.

Post-marketing Experience: Within each system organ class, the adverse drug reactions are ranked under the headings of reporting frequency, using the following convention: Very common (>1/10); Common (>1/100, <1/10); Uncommon (>1/1000, <1/100); Rare (>1/10 000, <1/1000); Very rare (<1/10 000) including isolated reports.

Blood and the lymphatic system disorders: Very rare: neutropenia (with prolonged use at dosages substantially above those recommended)

Immune system disorders: Very rare: hypersensitivity reactions such as anaphylactic and anaphylactoid reactions.

Nervous system disorders: Very rare: convulsions in infants.

Gastrointestinal disorders: Very rare: abdominal pain, diarrhea (these symptoms can also be the result of the worm infestation itself).

Hepato-biliary disorders: Very rare: hepatitis and abnormal liver function tests (with prolonged use at dosages substantially above those recommended).

Skin and subcutaneous tissue disorders: Very rare: toxic epidermal necrolysis, Stevens-Johnson syndrome, exanthema, angioedema, urticaria, rash.

Renal and urinary disorders: Very rare: glomerulonephritis (with prolonged use at dosages substantially above those recommended).

OVERDOSE:

Symptoms: In the event of accidental overdose, abdominal cramps, nausea, vomiting and diarrhea may occur. Although the recommended maximum treatment duration of VERMOX mebendazole is limited to three days, there have been rare reports of reversible liver function disturbances, hepatitis, and neutropenia in patients who were treated for hydatid disease with dosages substantially above those recommended for prolonged periods of time.

Treatment: There is no specific antidote. Within the first hour after ingestion, gastric lavage with aqueous potassium permanganate at 20 mg/100 mL may be performed. Activated charcoal may be given if considered appropriate.

For management of a suspected drug overdose, CPhA recommends that you contact your **regional Poison Control Centre**. See the *CPS* Directory section for a list of Poison Control Centres.

DOSAGE: Adults and Children 2 Years and Older: Enterobiasis: One tablet (100 mg) given as a single dose. Since reinfections by *Enterobius* are known to be very frequent, it is recommended that treatment be repeated after 2 or 4 weeks, especially in eradication programs.

Trichuriasis, ascariasis, ankylostomiasis, strongyloidiasis, taeniasis and mixed infections: One tablet (100 mg) in the morning and evening for 3 consecutive days.

If the patient is not cured 3 weeks after treatment, a second course of treatment is advised.

No special procedures such as fasting or purgation are required.

Children Under 2 Years: For use in children under 2 years see Precautions.

SUPPLIED: Each faintly orange, flat-faced, round tablet, inscribed with "JANSSEN" on one side and M/100 (scored) on the other, contains: mebendazole 100 mg. Nonmedicinal ingredients: colloidal anhydrous silica, cornstarch, FD&C Yellow #6 (orange yellow S), magnesium stearate, microcrystalline cellulose, orange flavor, saccharin sodium, sodium lauryl sulfate, sodium starch glycolate, talc and vegetable oil. Blister cards of 6 tablets, cartons of 1. Store between 15 and 30°C. Protect from light. Keep out of the reach of children.

Vesanoid® Ⓟ

tretinoin

Differentiation Inducing Agent

Roche

Date of Preparation: December 12, 1994
Date of Revision: August 20, 2007

All-trans retinoic acid should be administered to patients with Acute Promyelocytic Leukemia (APL) only under the supervision of a physician experienced in the treatment of hematological/oncological diseases (see Warnings).

PHARMACOLOGY: All-trans retinoic acid is a natural metabolite of retinol and belongs to the class of compounds known as retinoids, which are structurally related to vitamin A and comprise natural and synthetic analogs. In vitro studies with all-trans retinoic acid have demonstrated induction of differentiation and inhibition of cell proliferation in transformed hemopoietic cell lines, including human myeloid leukemia cell lines.

Acute promyelocytic leukemia (APL) is associated with a nonrandom chromosomal abnormality characterized by balanced and reciprocal translocations between the long arm of chromosomes 15 and 17 [t(15;17)(q22;q21)]. The gene encoding the retinoic acid receptor-alpha (RAR-α) is located on chromosome 17. A previously unidentified gene, PML, that may act as a transcription factor, is located on chromosome 15. The 15;17 translocation fuses the genes for PML and RAR-α, resulting in the synthesis of 2 reciprocal fusion transcripts, PML/RAR-α (found in all patients) and RAR-α/PML (found in about 2/3 of patients). PML/RAR-α may inhibit the differentiation of myeloid cells, resulting in carcinogenesis, an effect which may be overcome by the use of high doses of all-trans retinoic acid. Orally administered all-trans retinoic acid induces a high rate of complete remissions in patients with APL.

Pharmacokinetics: All-trans retinoic acid is an endogenous metabolite of vitamin A and is normally present in plasma at concentrations of 2 to 4 ng/mL. All-trans retinoic acid is transported directly via the portal system rather than through the lymphatics and thus absorption does not require specific transport mechanisms. All-trans retinoic acid is highly lipophilic with more than 95% of total drug concentration bound to plasma protein. All-trans retinoic acid is primarily metabolized by liver enzymes and is converted to the 13-cis isomer. Oxidation by P450 isoenzymes leads to the corresponding 4-hydroxy and 4-oxo-compounds. After glucuronidation, these metabolites are excreted in the urine and bile.

Following a single dose of radiolabelled all-trans retinoic acid, about 30% of the total radioactivity was recovered in the feces and about 60% in the urine. Nearly the entire dose was excreted within 3 to 6 days.

Single Dose: The pharmacokinetics of all-trans retinoic acid were investigated in healthy volunteers following a single oral dose of 40 mg of all-trans retinoic acid and in patients with acute promyelocytic leukemia (APL) treated with 45 mg/m². Maximum plasma concentrations of all-trans retinoic acid were reached within 1 to 2 hours in the APL patients and within 3 to 4 hours in the healthy volunteers. Large intersubject variability was observed. Plasma concentrations declined mono-exponentially with a mean elimination half-life of 0.71 hours. Endogenous levels (2 to 4 ng/mL) were reached 7 to 12 hours after dosing.

Multiple Doses: Multiple oral doses of all-trans retinoic acid were associated with a significant (about 2-fold) decrease in both the peak plasma levels and the AUC levels, after 2 to 6 weeks of treatment. These changes were associated with a 10-fold increase in urinary excretion of 4-oxo all-trans retinoic acid glucuronide.

The administration of ketoconazole, an inhibitor of the P450 enzyme system, after multiple doses of all-trans retinoic acid, resulted in a greater mean plasma all-trans retinoic acid AUC than after the administration of all-trans retinoic acid alone.

Pharmacokinetics in Pediatric Patients: A phase I trial of all-trans retinoic acid administered orally twice-daily for treatment courses of 28 days was performed in pediatrics. Cohorts of at least 3 patients were entered at successive all-trans retinoic acid dose levels (from 45 to 80 mg/m²/day, with a twice a day dosing regimen) until dose-limiting toxicity was consistently observed. Twenty-one patients with a median age of 14 years and various types of tumors including 2 patients with APL were entered into the trial.

Pharmacokinetics were determined in 18 patients on day 1 and in 7 patients on day 1 and day 28. Time to peak plasma concentrations was between 1 and 4 hours after dosing. Peak plasma concentrations of all-trans retinoic acid of 0.59, 0.62 and 1.64 μM (180, 190 and 490 ng/mL) were observed following doses of 22.5, 30 and 40 mg/m². AUC values for these doses were 1.29, 1.13 and 3.35 μM (387, 339 and 1005 ng·h/mL), respectively. Peak plasma concentrations and AUC values did not appear to increase in proportion to dose. A greater than 3-fold increase in AUC was observed following a 30% increase in dose (30 to 40 mg/m²). The average terminal half-life was 0.7 hours. The AUC on day 1 was significantly greater than the AUC on day 28 (mean decrease 78%±30 SD). Quantifiable concentrations of 4-oxo metabolites of all-trans retinoic acid were not observed.

Pharmacokinetics in Renal and Hepatic Impairment: The pharmacokinetics of all-trans retinoic acid in patients with compromised kidney or liver function have not been studied.

INDICATIONS: For the induction of remission in acute promyelocytic leukemia (APL; FAB classification AML-M3). Previously untreated patients, as well as patients who relapsed after, or were refractory to, standard chemotherapy (daunomycin and cytosine arabinoside or equivalent therapies) may be treated with all-trans retinoic acid. Upon achievement of complete remission, full-dose consolidation chemotherapy should be employed. Among patients maintained on all-trans retinoic acid, a loss of responsiveness to all-trans retinoic acid has been reported, with a median time to relapse of 4 to 6 months.

CONTRAINDICATIONS: *Pregnancy:* All-trans retinoic acid is highly teratogenic; therefore it is contraindicated during pregnancy and in nursing mothers. All-trans retinoic acid must not be used by women of childbearing potential unless effective contraception is practiced for at least 1 month before beginning therapy, during therapy and at least 1 month following discontinuation of therapy.

Lactation: See Contraindications, Pregnancy.

All-trans retinoic acid is contraindicated in patients with a known hypersensitivity to all-trans retinoic acid or related compounds.

The use of all-trans retinoic acid in combination with vitamin A is contraindicated (see Precautions, Drug Interactions).

WARNINGS: All-trans retinoic acid should be administered to patients with APL only under the strict supervision of a physician who is experienced in the treatment of hematological/oncological diseases.

Pregnancy:

Pregnancy: All-trans retinoic acid is highly teratogenic. Its use is contraindicated in pregnant women and women who might become pregnant during or within 1 month of the cessation of treatment. There is an extremely high risk that a deformed infant will result if pregnancy occurs while taking all-trans retinoic acid irrespective of the dose or duration of the treatment. Potentially all exposed fetuses can be affected. Therapy with all-trans retinoic acid should only be started in female patients if each of the following conditions is met:

- The patient is suffering from life-threatening malignancies. She is informed by her physicians of the hazards of becoming pregnant during and within 1 month after treatment with all-trans retinoic acid.
- She is willing to comply with the mandatory contraception measures.
- Every woman of childbearing potential who is to undergo treatment with all-trans retinoic acid uses effective contraception for 4 weeks before, during and for 1 month after discontinuation of treatment with all-trans retinoic acid.
- Therapy should not begin until the second or third day of the next normal menstrual period.
- A negative pregnancy test result must be obtained within the 2 weeks before commencement of treatment. It is advisable to perform additional pregnancy tests at monthly intervals during therapy.

Should pregnancy occur in spite of these precautions during treatment with all-trans retinoic acid or within 1 month after its discontinuation, there is a high risk of severe malformation of the fetus particularly when all-trans retinoic acid was given during the first trimester of pregnancy.

All these measures should be considered in relationship to the severity of the disease and the urgency of the treatment.

Lactation: Nursing should be discontinued if therapy with all-trans retinoic acid is initiated.

Retinoic Acid Syndrome: In many patients (20 to 25%) with acute promyelocytic leukemia (APL) treated with all-trans retinoic acid, a syndrome may occur characterized by some or all of the following symptoms: fever, dyspnea, acute respiratory distress, pulmonary infiltrates, hypotension, pleural and pericardial effusions, edema, weight gain, hepatic, renal and multiorgan failure (Retinoic Acid syndrome). RAS is frequently associated with hyperleukocytosis and may be fatal. If symptoms of the Retinoic Acid syndrome become apparent, treatment with a short course of high doses of corticosteroids (i.e., dexamethasone) should be initiated immediately particularly in patients where the syndrome is suspected but hyperleukocytosis is not observed.

During clinical trials hyperleukocytosis has been frequently observed (75%), sometimes associated with the RAS.

For those patients experiencing hyperleukocytosis when they receive all-trans retinoic acid (ATRA) alone, the RAS can be prevented by addition of full-dose anthracycline-based chemotherapy to the all-trans retinoic acid regimen based on the white blood cell (WBC) count. The current therapeutic treatment recommendations are the following:

- Immediate treatment of patients presenting with a WBC count of >5×10⁹/L at diagnosis or at any time with a combination of all-trans retinoic acid and chemotherapy.
- Addition of full-dose chemotherapy to ATRA therapy in patients with a WBC of <5×10⁹/L at day 0 of the treatment with ATRA and if WBC counts become: ≥6×10⁹/L at any time from day 1 to day 6 of treatment and/or ≥10×10⁹/L at any time from day 7 to day 10 of treatment and/or ≥15×10⁹/L at any time from day 11 to day 28 of treatment.
- Treatment with dexamethasone (10 mg every 12 hours for up to maximum 3 days or until resolution of the symptoms), if the patient presents early clinical signs of the syndrome.
- In cases of moderate and severe RAS, temporary interruption of all-trans retinoic acid therapy should be considered.

Mortality and morbidity is reduced by following these treatment recommendations in patients with this syndrome.

There is a risk of thrombosis (both venous and arterial) which may involve any organ system during the first month of treatment (see Adverse Effects). Therefore, caution should be exercised when treating patients with the combination of all-trans retinoic acid and antifibrinolytic agents such as tranexamic acid, aminocaproic acid or aprotinin (see Precautions, Drug Interactions).

Supportive care appropriate for patients with acute promyelocytic leukemia, for example, prophylaxis for bleeding and prompt therapy for infection, should be maintained during therapy with tretinoin. The patient's hematologic profile, coagulation profile, liver function test results, and triglyceride and cholesterol levels should be monitored frequently.

All-trans retinoic acid may cause intracranial hypertension/pseudotumor cerebri. The concomitant use of other agents known to cause intracranial hypertension/pseudotumor cerebri such as tetracyclines might increase the risk of this condition (see Precautions, Drug Interactions).

Occupational Hazards: The ability to drive or operate machinery might be impaired in patients treated with all-trans retinoic acid, particularly if they are experiencing dizziness or severe headache.

Micro-dosed progesterone preparations ("minipill") may be an inadequate method of contraception during treatment with all-trans retinoic acid.

PRECAUTIONS: *Drug Interactions*: As all-trans retinoic acid is metabolized by the hepatic P450 system, there is potential for alteration of pharmacokinetics parameters in patients administered concomitant medications that are also inducers or inhibitors of this system. Medications that generally induce hepatic P450 enzymes include rifampin, glucocorticoids, phenobarbital and pentobarbital. Medications that generally inhibit hepatic P450 enzymes include ketoconazole, cimetidine, erythromycin, verapamil, diltiazem and cyclosporine. There are no data to suggest that co-use with these medications increases or decreases either efficacy or toxicity of all-trans retinoic acid. There are no data on a possible pharmacokinetic interaction between all-trans retinoic acid and daunorubicin and cytosine arabinoside.

Antifibrinolytic agents such as tranexamic acid, aminocaproic acid, and aprotinin: Cases of fatal thrombotic complications have been reported rarely in patients concomitantly treated with all-trans retinoic acid and antifibrinolytic agents. Therefore, caution should be exercised when administering all-trans retinoic acid concomitantly with these agents (see Warnings).

Agents known to cause intracranial hypertension/pseudotumor cerebri such as tetracyclines: All-trans retinoic acid may cause intracranial hypertension/pseudotumor cerebri. Concomitant administration of all-trans retinoic acid and agents known to cause intracranial hypertension/pseudotumor cerebri as well might increase the risk of this condition (see Warnings).

Contraindicated Drug Associations (see Contraindications): Vitamin A: As with other retinoids, all-trans retinoic acid must not be administered in combination with vitamin A because symptoms of hypervitaminosis A could be aggravated.

Renal and Hepatic Impairment: The pharmacokinetics of all-trans retinoic acid in patients with compromised kidney or liver function have not been studied. As with other retinoids, the need for dosage adjustments in patients with renal or hepatic impairment is unknown, however, a reduction of dose to 25 mg/m² is recommended as a precautionary measure.

ADVERSE EFFECTS: Symptoms of the "Retinoic Acid Syndrome" in APL have been frequently reported and may be life-threatening unless treated (see Warnings).

The safety profile of all-trans retinoic acid has been evaluated retrospectively in a small number of patients.

In persons treated with the recommended daily doses of all-trans retinoic acid, the following adverse events were observed frequently (in about 1/4 of the patients or more): signs and symptoms of the hypervitaminosis A syndrome (including xeroderma, lip and mouth dryness, cheilitis, rash, edema, nausea, vomiting and bone pain). Headache, fever, shivering, fatigue, back pain, chest pain, dyspnea, coughing, abdominal pain, dermal bleeding, and elevation in serum triglycerides, cholesterol and transaminases may also be observed.

The following adverse events, considered remotely, possibly or probably related to drug treatment, have been reported in less than 1/4 of all APL patients treated with all-trans retinoic acid in the clinical trials:

Autonomic Nervous System: tachycardia, hypertension, hypotension, flushing, pallor, red extremities.

Body as a Whole: generalized pain, abdominal distention, post-traumatic pain, chest discomfort, hypothermia.

Cardiovascular System: cardiac failure, cyanosis, heart enlarged, arrhythmias. Cases of thrombosis (both venous and arterial) involving various sites (e.g. cerebrovascular accident, myocardial infarctions, renal infarct) have been reported uncommonly.

Central and Peripheral Nervous Systems: dizziness, confusion, intracranial hypertension, light-headed feeling, flank pain, numbness of extremities, abnormal gait, leg weakness, neurologic reaction, inguinal pain, visual field defects, hyporeflexia, paresthesia.

Dermatological: pruritus, increased sweating, alopecia, dry scalp, nasal dryness, nail disorder, photosensitivity reaction, xerophthalmia, erythemia.

Gastrointestinal: abdominal pain, diarrhea, constipation, blisters in the mouth, stomach upset, dysphagia, buccal mucosa ulceration, stomatitis, flatulence, ulcer, pancreatitis, diminished appetite.

Metabolic and Nutritional Disorders: weight changes, edema of extremities, acidosis, gout, dehydration, fluid overload, moonface, elevation in serum creatinine.

Musculoskeletal: musculoskeletal pain.

Platelet, Bleeding and Clotting: disseminated intravascular coagulation (DIC), nosebleed and other bleeding disorders, thrombosis.

Psychiatric: generalized weakness, anxiety, lethargy, depression, malaise, insomnia, anorexia, agitation, forgetfulness.

Resistance Mechanism Disorders: infection, septicemia, moniliasis.

Respiratory: pleural effusion, nasal congestion, pharyngitis, rale, respiratory insufficiency, asthma-like syndrome, pneumonia, respiratory distress, tachypnea, pharynx irritation, pulmonary infiltration, hypoxia, sinusitis, bronchial asthma.

Special Senses: blurred vision, visual disturbance, photophobia, conjunctivitis, decreased vision, changes in visual acuity, ear fullness, earache, ear buzzing.

Urinary: dysuria, kidney failure, urinary tract infection, micturition frequency, renal insufficiency, cystitis.

The decision to interrupt or continue therapy should be based on an evaluation of the benefit of the treatment versus the severity of the side effects.

Postmarketing Experience:

Metabolic and Nutritional Disorders: Occasional cases of hypercalcemia have been reported.

Dermatological: Sweet's syndrome has been reported uncommonly. Erythema nodosum has been reported rarely.

Hematologic: Thrombocytosis has been reported rarely. Marked basophilia with or without symptomatic hyperhistaminemia has been reported rarely, mainly in patients with the rare APL variant associated with basophilic differentiation.

Musculoskeletal: Myositis has been reported rarely.

Others: Vasculitis, predominantly involving the skin has been reported rarely.

Children: There is limited safety information on the use of all-trans retinoic acid in children. There have been some reports of increased toxicity in children treated with tretinoin, particularly increased pseudotumor cerebri.

OVERDOSE:

Symptoms: In cases of overdose with all-trans retinoic acid reversible signs of hypervitaminosis A (headache, nausea, vomiting, mucocutaneous symptoms) can appear. The recommended dose in acute promyelocytic leukemia is one quarter of the maximum tolerated dose in solid tumor patients and below the maximum tolerated dose in children.

Treatment: There is no specific treatment in the case of an overdose, however, it is important that the patient be treated in a special hematological unit.

> For management of a suspected drug overdose, CPhA recommends that you contact your **regional Poison Control Centre**. See the *CPS* Directory section for a list of Poison Control Centres.

DOSAGE: A total daily dose of 45 mg/m² body surface divided in 2 equal doses is recommended for oral administration to APL patients, including pediatric and geriatric patients.

This is approximately 8 capsules per adult dose. It is recommended that pediatric patients be treated with 45 mg/m² unless severe toxicity becomes apparent. Dose reduction should be particularly considered for children with intractable headache.

Treatment should be continued for 30 to 90 days until complete remission has been achieved.

After completion of remission, a course of consolidation chemotherapy including anthracycline and cytosine arabinoside should be initiated immediately; for example, 3 courses in 5- to 6-week intervals.

If there has been a remission with ATRA alone, it is not necessary to modify doses of ATRA if ATRA is used with chemotherapy.

The effect of food on the bioavailability of all-trans retinoic acid has not been characterized. Since the bioavailability of retinoids, as a class, is known to increase in the presence of food, it is recommended that all-trans retinoic acid be administered with a meal or shortly thereafter.

INFORMATION FOR THE PATIENT: Published in e-CPS, available by subscription at www.e-cps.ca.

SUPPLIED: Each oval-shaped, soft gelatin capsule, one half reddish-brown opaque and the other half brownish-yellow opaque, contains: tretinoin 10 mg. Nonmedicinal ingredients: gelatin, glycerol, hydrogenated hydrolyzed starch, hydrogenated soybean oil, iron oxide, mannitol, partially hydrogenated soybean oil, sorbitol, soybean oil, titanium dioxide and yellow beeswax. Bottles of 100. Keep the bottle tightly closed. Store at 15 to 30°C. Protect from light.

(Shown in Product Identification Section)

Vesicare® Ⓟ

solifenacin succinate

Urinary Antispasmodic

Astellas

Date of Revision: July 24, 2008

SUMMARY PRODUCT INFORMATION:

Route of Administration	Dosage Form/ Strength	Clinically Relevant Nonmedicinal Ingredients
Oral	Tablet, film coated 5 mg, 10 mg	Lactose monohydrate For a complete listing see Dosage Forms, Composition and Packaging.

INDICATIONS AND CLINICAL USE: VESICARE (solifenacin succinate) is indicated for:

- Treatment of overactive bladder in adults with symptoms of urge urinary incontinence, urinary urgency and urinary frequency.

Geriatrics: In placebo controlled clinical studies, similar safety and effectiveness were observed between older (623 patients ≥65 years and 189 patients ≥75 years) and younger patients (1188 patients <65 years) treated with VESICARE (see Action and Clinical Pharmacology).

Pediatrics: Safety and effectiveness in children have not yet been established.

CONTRAINDICATIONS:

- Patients with urinary retention, dependent on dialysis, gastroparesis or narrow angle glaucoma
- Patients who are hypersensitive to this drug or to any ingredient in the formulation or component of the container. For a complete listing, see Dosage Forms, Composition and Packaging.

WARNINGS AND PRECAUTIONS: General: VESICARE, like other anticholinergic drugs, should be administered with caution in patients with impaired ability to sweat, to reduce the risk of heat prostration, and in patients with clinically significant bladder outflow obstruction because of the risk of urinary retention.

VESICARE may cause blurred vision. Patients should be advised to exercise caution in driving or operating machinery until the drug's effect on vision has been determined.

Monitoring and Laboratory Tests: Monitoring of the QT/QTc interval and/or serum electrolyte levels may be appropriate in high risk patients who are being treated with VESICARE, such as: patients with known congenital or acquired QT/QTc interval prolongation or electrolyte disturbances; patients who are taking drugs that have been associated with QT/QTc interval prolongation and/or torsades de pointes such as Class IA (eg quinidine, procainamide) or Class III (eg amiodarone, sotalol) antiarrhythmic medications or those taking potent CYP3A4 inhibitors.

Carcinogenesis and Mutagenesis: Solifenacin succinate was not mutagenic in the in vitro *S. typhimurium* or *E. coli* microbial mutagenicity test or chromosomal aberration test in human peripheral blood lymphocytes, with or without metabolic activation, or in the in vivo micronucleus test in rats.

No increase in tumors was found following the administration of solifenacin succinate to male and female mice for 104 weeks at doses up to 200 mg/kg/day (5 and 9 times human exposure at the maximum recommended human dose [MRHD], respectively), and male and female rats for 104 weeks at doses up to 20 and 15 mg/kg/day, respectively (<1 times exposure at the MRHD).

Cardiovascular: A study of the effect of solifenacin on the QT interval was conducted in 76 healthy women. The QTc interval prolongation effect appeared greater for the 30 mg compared to the 10 mg dose of solifenacin. Although the effect of the highest solifenacin dose (three times the maximum therapeutic dose) studied did not appear as large as that of the positive control moxifloxacin at its therapeutic dose, the confidence interval overlapped. This study was not designed to draw direct statistical comparison between the drugs or the dose levels (see Action and Clinical Pharmacology). This observation should be considered in clinical decisions to prescribe VESICARE for patients with a known history of QT prolongation or patients who are taking medications known to prolong the QT interval.

The effect of solifenacin on QTc interval change in males has not been investigated, and caution should be taken in extrapolating the findings of this study to male subjects.

The effect of solifenacin on QTc interval change in elderly subjects with occult renal insufficiency, (in whom plasma concentration of solifenacin might be higher than those observed in younger subjects), has not been investigated.

Gastrointestinal: VESICARE, like other anticholinergics should be used with caution in patients with decreased gastrointestinal motility.

Hepatic: VESICARE should be used with caution in patients with reduced hepatic function. Doses of VESICARE greater than 5 mg are not recommended in patients with moderate hepatic impairment. (Child-Pugh B). VESICARE is not recommended for patients with severe hepatic impairment (Child-Pugh C) (see Action and Clinical Pharmacology, Dosage and Administration and Adverse Reactions).

Renal: Use with caution in patients with reduced renal function. Doses of VESICARE greater than 5 mg are not recommended in patients with severe renal impairment (CL_{cr} <30 mL/min) (see Action and Clinical Pharmacology, Dosage and Administration). VESICARE is contraindicated in dialysis dependent patients (see Contraindications).

Sexual Function/Reproduction: No clinical data are available from reproductively competent women who have received long-term treatment with VESICARE. The potential risk to such women is presently unknown. Therefore, VESICARE should be used during pregnancy only if the potential benefit for the mother justifies the potential risk for the fetus. Women of childbearing potential should be considered for treatment only if using adequate contraception.

In a 13-week toxicity study in mice treated with 400 mg/kg/day [15 times exposure at the maximum recommended human dose (MRHD)] of solifenacin succinate and in a 26-week toxicity study in rats treated with 30 mg/kg/day (<1 times exposure at the MRHD) or greater of solifenacin succinate, follicular degeneration/reduced corpora lutea in the ovaries and/or uterine atrophy were observed in female animals that died or were sacrificed in extremis. Low uterine weight and uterine immaturity were observed in female dogs treated with 3 mg/kg/day (<1 times exposure at the MRHD) or greater of solifenacin succinate in the 13-week toxicity study.

Solifenacin succinate had no effect on reproductive function, fertility or early embryonic development of the fetus in male and female mice treated with 250 mg/kg/day (13 times exposure at the MRHD) of solifenacin succinate for 4 weeks and 2 weeks, respectively, and in male rats treated with 50 mg/kg/day (<1 times exposure at the MRHD) for 4 weeks and female rats treated with 100 mg/kg/day (1.7 times exposure at the MRHD) for 2 weeks.

Special Populations: Pregnant Women: There are no adequate and well-controlled studies investigating the effects of solifenacin succinate in pregnant women. Animal reproduction studies are not always predictive of human response; therefore, VESICARE should be used during pregnancy only if the potential benefit justifies the potential risk to the fetus.

Women of childbearing potential should be considered for treatment only if using adequate contraception.

Reproduction studies have been performed in mice, rats and rabbits. After oral administration of ^{14}C-solifenacin succinate to pregnant mice, drug-related material has been shown to cross the placental barrier. No embryotoxicity or teratogenicity was observed in mice treated with 30 mg/kg/day (1.2 times exposure at the maximum recommended human dose [MRHD]). Administration of solifenacin succinate to pregnant mice, at doses of 100 mg/kg and greater (3.6 times exposure at the MRHD), during the major period of organ development resulted in reduced fetal body weights. Administration of 250 mg/kg/kg (7.9 times exposure at the MRHD) to pregnant mice resulted in an increased incidence of cleft palate. In utero and lactational exposures to maternal doses of solifenacin succinate of 100 mg/kg/day and greater (3.6 times exposure at the MRHD) resulted in reduced peripartum and postnatal survival, reductions in body weight gain, and delayed physical development (eye opening and vaginal patency). An increase in the percentage of male offspring was also observed in litters from offspring exposed to maternal doses of 250 mg/kg/day. No embryotoxic effects were observed in rats at up to 50 mg/kg/day (<1 times exposure at the MRHD) or in rabbits at up to 50 mg/kg/day (1.8 times exposure at the MRHD).

The effect of VESICARE on labor and delivery in humans has not been studied. There were no effects on natural delivery in mice treated with 30 mg/kg/day (1.2 times exposure at the MRHD). Administration of solifenacin succinate at 100 mg/kg/day (3.6 times exposure at the MRHD) or greater increased peripartum pup mortality.

Nursing Women: It is not known whether solifenacin is excreted in human milk. Because many drugs are excreted in human milk, VESICARE should not be administered during nursing. A decision should be made whether to discontinue nursing or to discontinue VESICARE in nursing mothers.

After oral administration of ^{14}C-solifenacin succinate to lactating mice, radioactivity was detected in maternal milk. There were no adverse observations in mice treated with 30 mg/kg/day (1.2 times exposure at the maximum recommended human dose [MRHD]). Pups of female mice treated with 100 mg/kg/day (3.6 times exposure at the MRHD) or greater revealed reduced body weights, postpartum pup mortality or delays in the onset of reflex and physical development during the lactation period.

ADVERSE REACTIONS: Adverse Drug Reaction Overview: Expected side effects of antimuscarinic agents are dry mouth, constipation, blurred vision (accommodation abnormalities), urinary retention, and dry eyes. The most common adverse events reported in patients treated with VESICARE were dry mouth and constipation and the incidence of these side effects was higher in the 10 mg compared to the 5 mg dose group. Compared to twelve weeks of treatment with VESICARE, the incidence and severity of adverse events were similar in patients who remained on drug for up to 12 months. The most frequent reason for discontinuation due to an adverse event was dry mouth, 1.5%.

Clinical Trial Adverse Drug Reactions: Because clinical trials are conducted under very specific conditions the adverse reaction rates observed in the clinical trials may not reflect the rates observed in practice and should not be compared to the rates in the clinical trials of another drug. Adverse drug reaction information from clinical trials is useful for identifying drug-related adverse events and for approximating rates.

VESICARE has been evaluated for safety in 1811 patients in randomized, placebo-controlled trials. In the four 12-week double-blind clinical trials, there were three intestinal serious adverse events in patients, all treated with VESICARE 10 mg (one fecal impaction, one colonic obstruction, and one intestinal obstruction). The overall rate of serious adverse events in the double-blind trials was 2%.

Table 1 lists adverse events, regardless of causality, that were reported in randomized, placebo-controlled trials at an incidence greater than placebo and in 1% or more of patients treated with VESICARE 5 or 10 mg once daily for up to 12 weeks.

Table 1: VESICARE

Percentages of Patients with Treatment-Emergent Adverse Events Exceeding Placebo Rate and Reported by 1% or More Patients for Combined Pivotal Studies

System Organ Class MedDRA Preferred Term	Placebo (%)	VESICARE 5 mg (%)	VESICARE 10 mg (%)
Number of Patients	1216	578	1233
Number of Patients with Treatment-emergent AE	634	265	773
Eye Disorders			
Vision Blurred	1.8	3.8	4.8
Dry Eyes NOS	0.6	0.3	1.6
Gastrointestinal Disorders			
Dry Mouth	4.2	10.9	27.6
Constipation	2.9	5.4	13.4
Nausea	2.0	1.7	3.3
Dyspepsia	1.0	1.4	3.9
Abdominal Pain Upper	1.0	1.9	1.2
Vomiting NOS	0.9	0.2	1.1
General Disorders And Administration Site Conditions			
Fatigue	1.1	1.0	2.1
Edema Lower Limb	0.7	0.3	1.1
Infections And Infestations			
Urinary Tract Infection NOS	2.8	2.8	4.8
Influenza	1.3	2.2	0.9
Pharyngitis NOS	1.0	0.3	1.1
Nervous System Disorders			
Dizziness	1.8	1.9	1.8
Psychiatric Disorders			
Depression NOS	0.8	1.2	0.8
Renal And Urinary Disorders			
Urinary Retention	0.6	0	1.4
Respiratory, Thoracic And Mediastinal Disorders			
Cough	0.2	0.2	1.1
Vascular Disorders			
Hypertension NOS	0.6	1.4	0.5

One young male subject developed a reversible increase in hepatic enzymes following a single dose of solifenacin during a Phase I study. Although causality has not been established, special attention should be paid to subjects who develop abnormal liver function tests after starting solifenacin and consideration given to discontinuing treatment.

Post-Market Adverse Drug Reactions: In addition to the adverse events observed in clinical trials, the following events have been reported in association with VESICARE (solifenacin succinate) use in worldwide post-marketing experience, although the frequency of events or a causal relationship with VESICARE could not always be confirmed: urinary retention; vomiting; peripheral edema; hypersensitivity reactions including rash, pruritus, and urticaria; dizziness; headache; and hallucination.

DRUG INTERACTIONS: Overview: Concomitant medication with other medicinal products with anticholinergic properties may result in more pronounced therapeutic effects and undesirable effects. An interval of approximately 1 week should be allowed after stopping treatment with VESICARE, before commencing other anticholinergic therapy.

The therapeutic effect of solifenacin may be reduced by concomitant administration of cholinergic receptor agonists. Solifenacin may reduce the effect of medicinal products that stimulate the motility of the gastrointestinal tract, such as metoclopramide.

Drugs Metabolized by Cytochrome P450: At therapeutic concentrations, solifenacin does not inhibit CYP1A1/2, 2C9, 2C19, 2D6 or 3A4 derived from human liver microsomes.

CYP 3A4 Inhibitors: In vitro drug metabolism studies have shown that solifenacin is a substrate of CYP3A4. Inducers or inhibitors of CYP3A4 may alter solifenacin pharmacokinetics. Therefore, the dose of solifenacin should be maintained at, or dropped to, 5 mg daily while patients are taking a potent CYP3A4 inhibitor such as ketoconazole, clarithromycin, erythromycin, diclofenac, nefazodone, verapamil and others.

Drug-Drug Interactions: Solifenacin is metabolised by CYP3A4. Simultaneous administration of ketoconazole (200 mg/day), a potent CYP3A4 inhibitor, resulted in a two-fold increase of the AUC of solifenacin, while ketoconazole at a dose of 400 mg/day resulted in a three-fold increase of the AUC of solifenacin. Therefore, the maximum dose of VESICARE should be restricted to 5 mg, when used simultaneously with ketoconazole or therapeutic doses of other potent CYP3A4 inhibitors. See Table 2 for investigated potential drug-drug interactions.

Table 2: VESICARE

Investigated Potential Drug-Drug Interactions

Drug Name	Ref	Effect	Clinical Comment
Digoxin	CT	No significant effect on pharmacokinetics of digoxin in healthy subjects.	
Ketoconazole	CT	↑ solifenacin The mean C_{max} and AUC of solifenacin increased by 1.5 and 2.7-fold, respectively.	It is recommended not to exceed a 5 mg daily dose of VESICARE when administered with therapeutic doses of ketoconazole or other potent CYP 3A4 inhibitors.
Oral Contraceptives (OCP)	CT	No significant effect on plasma concentration of combined OCPs (ethinyl estradiol/levonorgestrel)	
Warfarin	CT	No significant effect on pharmacokinetics of R-warfarin or S-warfarin	

Legend: CT=Clinical Trial.

Drug-Food Interactions: Co-ingestion of grapefruit juice with VESICARE may increase the serum level of solifenacin.

Drug-Herb Interactions: Interactions with herbal products have not been established and caution should be taken if such agents are used by patients.

Drug-Laboratory Test Interactions: Interactions with laboratory tests have not been investigated.

DOSAGE AND ADMINISTRATION: Dosing Considerations: Dose Adjustment in Renal Impairment: For patients with severe renal impairment (CL_{cr} <30 mL/min), a daily dose of VESICARE greater than 5 mg is not recommended. VESICARE is contraindicated in dialysis dependent patients (see Contraindications).

Dose Adjustment in Hepatic Impairment: For patients with moderate hepatic impairment (Child-Pugh B), a daily dose of VESICARE greater than 5 mg is not recommended. Use of VESICARE in patients with severe hepatic impairment (Child Pugh C) is not recommended.

Dose Adjustment with CYP3A4 Inhibitors: When administered with therapeutic doses of ketoconazole or other potent CYP3A4 inhibitors, a daily dose of VESICARE should be maintained at, or dropped to, 5 mg daily.

Recommended Dose and Dosage Adjustment: The recommended dose of VESICARE is 5 mg once daily. If the 5 mg dose is well tolerated, the dose may be increased to 10 mg once daily.

VESICARE should be taken with liquids and swallowed whole. VESICARE can be administered with or without food, without regard to meals.

The maximum effect can be determined after 4 weeks at the earliest.

Missed Dose: If a dose is missed, the next tablet should be taken as planned. Doses should not be doubled to make up for a missed dose.

OVERDOSAGE:

Acute: Overdosage with VESICARE can potentially result in severe anticholinergic effects and should be treated accordingly. The highest dose of solifenacin succinate accidentally given to a single patient was 280 mg in a 5-hour period, resulting in mental status changes. The patient was given charcoal treatment and recovered without sequelae.

Chronic: Intolerable anticholinergic side effects (fixed and dilated pupils, blurred vision, failure of heel-to-toe exam, tremors and dry skin) occurred on day 3 in normal volunteers taking 50 mg daily (5 times the maximum recommended therapeutic dose) and resolved within 7 days following discontinuation of drug.

Treatment of Overdosage: In the event of overdose with VESICARE treat with gastric lavage and appropriate supportive measures. ECG monitoring is also recommended.

For management of a suspected drug overdose, CPhA recommends that you contact your **regional Poison Control Centre**. See the *CPS* Directory section for a list of Poison Control Centres.

ACTION AND CLINICAL PHARMACOLOGY: Mechanism of Action: Muscarinic receptors play an important role in several major cholinergically mediated functions, including contractions of urinary bladder smooth muscle and stimulation of salivary secretion. Solifenacin is a competitive muscarinic receptor antagonist with selectivity for the urinary bladder over salivary glands in vitro and in vivo (mice, rats and monkeys). In cells isolated from rats and monkeys, solifenacin inhibited carbachol-induced intracellular calcium mobilization more potently in bladder smooth muscle cells than in salivary gland cells. The bladder selectivity of solifenacin in monkeys is significantly greater than those of other antimuscarinics as illustrated by selectivity ratios (bladder/salivary gland) of 2.1, 0.51, 0.65, 0.46 and 0.61 for solifenacin, oxybutynin, tolterodine, darifenacin and atropine, respectively. In anesthetized rats, solifenacin is also more potent in inhibiting carbachol-induced increases in intravesical pressure than in inhibiting salivary secretion. Although other antimuscarinics also showed some tissue selectivity, the selectivity ratio of solifenacin (6.5) estimated from its potency to inhibit urinary bladder and salivary gland was the greatest among all antimuscarinics tested (1.0 to 2.4).

Pharmacokinetics: See Table 3.

Absorption: After oral administration of VESICARE to healthy volunteers, peak plasma levels (C_{max}) of solifenacin are reached within 3 to 8 hours after administration, and at steady state ranged from 32.3 to 62.9 ng/mL for the 5 and 10 mg VESICARE tablets, respectively. The absolute bioavailability of solifenacin is approximately 90%, and plasma concentrations of solifenacin are proportional to the dose administered.

Table 3: VESICARE

Summary of Pharmacokinetic Parameters in the Normal Population

Solifenacin Dose	C_{max} (ng/mL)	$t_{½}$ (h)	AUC_{0-24h} (ng·h/mL)
5 mg od	32.3 (11.2)	64.4 (18.6)	637 (239)
10 mg od	62.9 (23.1)	60.9 (17.1)	1236 (459)

Data are expressed as mean (SD).

Effect of Food: There is no significant effect of food on the pharmacokinetics of solifenacin.
Distribution: Solifenacin is approximately 98% (in vivo) bound to human plasma proteins, principally to α_1-acid glycoprotein. Solifenacin is highly distributed to non-CNS tissues, having a mean steady-state volume of distribution of 600 L.
Metabolism: Solifenacin is extensively metabolized in the liver. The primary pathway for elimination is by way of CYP3A4; however, alternate metabolic pathways exist. The primary metabolic routes of solifenacin are through N-oxidation of the quinuclidin ring and 4R-hydroxylation of tetrahydroisoquinoline ring. One pharmacologically active metabolite (4R-hydroxy solifenacin), occurring at low concentrations and unlikely to contribute significantly to clinical activity, and three pharmacologically inactive metabolites (N-glucuronide and the N-oxide and 4R-hydroxy-N-oxide of solifenacin) have been found in human plasma after oral dosing.
Excretion: Following the administration of 10 mg of ^{14}C-solifenacin succinate to healthy volunteers, 69.2 % of the radioactivity was recovered in the urine and 22.5 % in the feces over 26 days. Less than 15% (as mean value) of the dose was recovered in the urine as intact solifenacin. The major metabolites identified in urine were N-oxide of solifenacin, 4R-hydroxy solifenacin and 4R-hydroxy-N-oxide of solifenacin, and in feces 4R-hydroxy solifenacin. The elimination half-life of solifenacin following chronic dosing is approximately 45-68 hours.
Special Populations and Conditions: Geriatrics: Multiple dose studies of VESICARE in elderly volunteers (65 to 80 years) showed that C_{max}, AUC and $t_{1/2}$ values were 20-25% higher as compared to the younger volunteers (18 to 55 years) (see Indications and Clinical Use).
Pediatrics: The pharmacokinetics of solifenacin have not been established in pediatric patients.
Gender: The pharmacokinetics of solifenacin are not significantly influenced by gender.
Renal Insufficiency: VESICARE should be used with caution in patients with renal impairment. There is a 2.1-fold increase in AUC and 1.6-fold increase in $t_{1/2}$ of solifenacin in patients with severe renal impairment. Doses of VESICARE greater than 5 mg are not recommended in patients with severe renal impairment (CL_{cr} <30 mL/min) (see Warnings and Precautions, Dosage and Administration). VESICARE is contraindicated in dialysis dependent patients (see Contraindications).
Hepatic Insufficiency: VESICARE should be used with caution in patients with reduced hepatic function. There is a 2-fold increase in the $t_{1/2}$ and 35% increase in AUC of solifenacin in patients with moderate hepatic impairment. Doses of VESICARE greater than 5 mg are not recommended in patients with moderate hepatic impairment (Child-Pugh B). VESICARE is not recommended for patients with severe hepatic impairment (Child-Pugh C) (see Warnings and Precautions, Dosage and Administration).
Cardiac Electrophysiology: The effect of 10 mg and 30 mg solifenacin succinate on the QT interval was evaluated at the time of peak plasma concentration of solifenacin in a multi-dose, randomized, double-blind, placebo and positive-controlled (moxifloxacin 400 mg) trial. Patients were randomized to one of two treatment groups after receiving placebo and moxifloxacin sequentially. One group (n=51) went on to complete 3 additional sequential periods of dosing with solifenacin 10, 20 and 30 mg while the second group (n=25) in parallel completed a sequence of placebo and moxifloxacin. Study subjects were female volunteers aged 19 to 79 years. The 30 mg dose of solifenacin succinate (three times the highest recommended dose) was chosen for use in this study because this dose results in a solifenacin exposure that covers those observed upon coadministration of 10 mg VESICARE with potent CYP3A4 inhibitors (e.g., ketoconazole, 400 mg). Due to the sequential dose escalating nature of the study, baseline EKG measurements were separated from the final QT assessment (of the 30 mg dose level) by 33 days.

The median difference from baseline in heart rate associated with the 10 and 30 mg doses of solifenacin succinate compared to placebo was −2 and 0 beats/minute, respectively. Because a significant period effect on QTc was observed, QTc effects were analyzed utilizing the parallel placebo control arm rather than the pre-specified intra-patient analysis. Representative results are shown in Table 4.

Table 4: VESICARE

QTc Changes in msec (90% CI) from Baseline at T_{max} (relative to placebo)

Drug/Dose	Fridericia Method (using median difference)
Solifenacin 10 mg	0 (−5,5)
Solifenacin 30 mg	7 (2,12)

Results displayed are those derived from the parallel design portion of the study and represent the comparison of Group 1 to time-matched placebo effects in Group 2.

The effect of moxifloxacin on the QT interval was evaluated in 3 different sessions of the trial. All subjects received moxifloxacin in Session 1 while only those subjects in the placebo/moxifloxacin group received moxifloxacin in Sessions 3 and 5. The placebo subtracted mean changes (90% CI) for moxifloxacin in the three sessions (1, 3 and 5) were 11 (7, 14), 12 (8, 17), and 16 (12, 21), respectively.

The QT interval prolonging effect appeared greater for the 30 mg compared to the 10 mg dose of solifenacin. The lower limit of the 90% confidence interval was greater than zero in the 30 mg dose of solifenacin. This study was not designed to draw direct statistical conclusions between the drugs or the dose levels.

The effect of solifenacin on QTc interval change in male has not been investigated, and caution should be taken in extrapolating the findings of this study to males.

STORAGE AND STABILITY: Store between 15-30°C.
INFORMATION FOR THE PATIENT: Published in e-CPS, available by subscription at www.e-cps.ca.
DOSAGE FORMS, COMPOSITION AND PACKAGING: 5 mg: Each light yellow, round, film-coated tablet, debossed with logo 150, contains: solifenacin succinate 5 mg (equivalent to solifenacin 3.8 mg). Nonmedicinal ingredients: corn starch, hypromellose 2910, lactose monohydrate, magnesium stearate, polyethylene glycol 8000, talc, titanium dioxide and yellow ferric oxide. Bottles and unit dose blister packages.
10 mg: Each light pink, round, film-coated tablet, debossed with logo 151, contains: solifenacin succinate 10 mg (equivalent to solifenacin 7.5 mg). Nonmedicinal ingredients: corn starch, hypromellose 2910, lactose monohydrate, magnesium stearate, polyethylene glycol 8000, red ferric oxide, talc and titanium dioxide. Bottles and unit dose blister packages.

(Shown in Product Identification Section)

The reader is invited to consult CPhA's monograph **Corticosteroids: Eye, Ear, Nose.**

Vexol® Ⓟ

rimexolone

Corticosteroid

Alcon

SUPPLIED: Each mL of sterile, multidose topical ophthalmic suspension, contains: rimexolone 1%. Preservative: benzalkonium chloride 0.01%. Nonmedicinal ingredients: carbomer 974P, edetate disodium, polysorbate 80, purified water, sodium chloride, sodium hydroxide and/or hydrochloric acid to adjust pH. Plastic Drop-Tainer dispensers of 5 mL. Store upright between 2 and 30°C.

Vfend™ Ⓟ

voriconazole

Antifungal

Pfizer

Date of Revision: March 22, 2010

SUMMARY PRODUCT INFORMATION:

Route of Administration	Dosage Form/ Strength	Clinically Relevant Nonmedicinal Ingredients
Oral	Tablet: 50 mg/200 mg	Lactose For complete listing see Dosage Forms, Composition and Packaging.
	Powder for oral suspension: 3 g/vial (40 mg/mL when reconstituted)	Sucrose For complete listing see Dosage Forms, Composition and Packaging.
Intravenous injection	Lyophilized powder for reconstitution: 200 mg/vial, 10 mg/mL reconstituted	SBECD (sulfobutylether-β-cyclodextrin) For complete listing see Dosage Forms, Composition and Packaging.

INDICATIONS AND CLINICAL USE: VFEND (voriconazole) is indicated in the treatment of:
- Invasive aspergillosis;
- Candidemia in non-neutropenic patients and the following Candida infections: disseminated infections in skin and infections in abdomen, kidney, bladder wall and wounds.

Geriatrics: Evidence from clinical studies and experience suggests that safety and effectiveness of VFEND are similar in geriatric and adult subjects (see Warnings and Precautions, Dosage and Administration).
Pediatrics: Safety and effectiveness of VFEND in pediatric subjects below the age of twelve years have not been established (see Warnings and Precautions).
CONTRAINDICATIONS: VFEND (voriconazole) is contraindicated in patients with known hypersensitivity to voriconazole or its excipients. For a complete listing see Dosage Forms, Composition and Packaging. There is no information regarding cross-sensitivity between voriconazole and other azole antifungal agents. Caution should be used when prescribing VFEND to patients with hypersensitivity to other azoles.

VFEND is a substrate and inhibitor of cytochrome P450 isozymes CYP2C19, CYP2C9 and CYP3A4. Thus, coadministration of voriconazole is contraindicated with drugs that are highly dependent on these isozymes for clearance and for which elevated plasma concentrations are associated with serious and/or life threatening events. In addition, coadministration of voriconazole is contraindicated with drugs that significantly decrease voriconazole plasma concentrations due to induction of these isozymes (see Drug Interactions).

Drugs That Are Contraindicated with VFEND Due to Potential CYP450-Mediated Interactions (See Drug Interactions for more detailed information)

CYP450 substrates—voriconazole significantly increases plasma concentrations of these drugs which may lead to serious or life threatening events	terfenadine[a], astemizole[a], cisapride[a], pimozide, quinidine, sirolimus, efavirenz (standard dose), rifabutin, ergot alkaloids (ergotamine. dihydroergotamine)
CYP450 inducers—coadministration significantly decreases plasma concentrations of voriconazole	rifampicin, carbamazepine, long-acting barbiturates, ritonavir (400 mg Q12h), efavirenz (standard dose), rifabutin, St John's Wort[b]

[a] Not marketed in Canada.
[b] Also P-gp inducer.

WARNINGS AND PRECAUTIONS:

Serious Warnings and Precautions
- **Drug Interactions (see Contraindications and Drug Interactions)**
- **Cardiovascular effects—QT interval prolongation (see Cardiovascular)**
- **Visual disturbances (see Ophthalmologic)**
- **Hepatic toxicity (see Hepatic)**
- **Dermatological reactions (see Skin)**
- **Teratogenic in the rat (see Pregnant Woman)**

General: VFEND tablets contain lactose and should not be given to patients with rare hereditary problems of galactose intolerance.

VFEND for Oral Suspension contains sucrose and is not recommended for patients with rare hereditary problems of fructose intolerance, sucrase-isomaltase deficiency or glucose-galactose malabsorption.
Cardiovascular: QT Interval Prolongation: VFEND (voriconazole) has been associated with prolongation of the QT interval of the electrocardiogram in some patients. Prolongation of QT interval may increase the risk of arrhythmia. During clinical development and post-marketing surveillance, there have been rare cases of arrhythmias (including ventricular arrhythmias such as torsades de pointes), cardiac arrests and sudden deaths in patients taking voriconazole. These cases usually involved patients with risk factors such as history of cardiotoxic chemotherapy, cardiomyopathy, hypokalemia and concomitant medications that may have been contributory.

Due to limited clinical experience, voriconazole should be administered with caution to patients with potentially proarrhythmic conditions such as hypokalemia, clinically significant bradycardia, acute myocardial ischemia, congestive heart failure or congenital prolongation of QT.

Caution should be exercised if voriconazole is used in patients taking other drugs that may prolong the QT interval, such as antipsychotics, tricyclic antidepressants, erythromycin, Class IA (e.g. procainamide, quinidine) Class III (e.g. amiodarone, sotalol) antiarrhythmic agents.

There is a report of a life-threatening syncopal episode in a patient receiving concomitant voriconazole and methadone (see Drug Interactions, Effect of Voriconazole on Pharmacokinetics of Other Drugs).

Drugs metabolized by the hepatic cytochrome P450 isoenzymes CYP2C19, CYP2C9 and CYP3A4 may also affect, or be affected by, voriconazole levels, with possible resulting QT effects. Such drugs include tacrolimus, HIV protease inhibitors, and macrolide antibiotics.

See Drug Interactions.
Ophthalmologic: Voriconazole may cause visual symptoms including photophobia altered/enhanced visual perception, blurred vision and/or color vision change. The majority of visual symptoms appeared to spontaneously resolve within 60 minutes. **The effect of VFEND (voriconazole) on visual function is not known if treatment continues beyond 28 days.** If treatment continues beyond 28 days, visual function including visual acuity, visual field and color perception should be monitored.

There has been a small number of post-marketing reports of vision loss (including decreased visual acuity or visual fields) where a relationship to voriconazole could not be excluded. These events mostly occurred in medically complex patients, where underlying disease processes and the primary infections themselves confound interpretation (see Adverse Reactions).

There have been post-marketing reports of prolonged visual adverse events, including optic neuritis and papilledema. These events occurred primarily in severely ill patients who had underlying conditions and/or concomitant medications which may have caused or contributed to these events (see Adverse Reactions, Post-Market Adverse Drug Reactions).

Effects on Ability to Drive and Operating Machines: Voriconazole may cause visual symptoms including blurring and/or photophobia. The majority of visual symptoms appeared to spontaneously resolve within 60 minutes. Patients on voriconazole must avoid potentially hazardous tasks, such as driving or operating machinery if they perceive any change in vision. Patients should not drive at night while taking voriconazole.

Hepatic: In clinical trials, there have been uncommon cases of serious hepatic reactions during treatment with VFEND (including clinical hepatitis, cholestasis, and fulminant hepatic failure, including fatalities). Instances of hepatic reactions were noted to occur primarily in patients with serious underlying medical conditions (predominantly hematological malignancy). Hepatic reactions, including hepatitis and jaundice, have occurred among patients with no other identifiable risk factors. Liver dysfunction has usually been reversible on discontinuation of therapy.

Patients who develop abnormal liver function tests during voriconazole therapy should be monitored for the development of more severe hepatic injury. Discontinuation of voriconazole must be considered if clinical signs and symptoms consistent with liver disease develop that may be attributable to voriconazole (see Patients with Hepatic Impairment, Adverse Reactions, Dosage and Administration).

Infusion Related Reactions: During infusion of the intravenous formulation of voriconazole in healthy subjects, anaphylactoid type reactions, including flushing, fever, sweating, tachycardia, chest tightness, dyspnea, faintness, nausea, pruritus and rash, have occurred uncommonly. Symptoms appeared immediately upon initiating the infusion. Consideration should be given to stopping the infusion should these reactions occur. Other symptoms, including hypotension, were considered to be infusion related in the clinical trial setting.

Pancreatic: Adults and children with risk factors for acute pancreatitis (e.g. recent chemotherapy, hematopoietic stem cell transplantation [HSCT]), should be monitored for development of pancreatitis during voriconazole treatment.

Renal: Acute renal failure has been observed in severely ill patients undergoing treatment with voriconazole. Patients being treated with voriconazole are likely to be treated concomitantly with nephrotoxic medications and have concurrent conditions that may result in decreased renal function.

Sensitivity and Resistance: Voriconazole does not have activity against Zygomycete spp in vitro. Cases of breakthrough zygomycosis, most fatal, have been reported in patients who had received voriconazole.

Skin: There have been cases of exfoliative cutaneous reactions, such as Stevens-Johnson Syndrome (uncommon), toxic epidermal necrolysis (rare) and erythema multiforme (rare) during treatment with voriconazole (see Adverse Reactions). Stevens-Johnson Syndrome and toxic epidermal necrolysis should be considered as a differential diagnosis if patients develop prodromal flu-like symptoms (fever, malaise, rhinitis, chest pain. vomiting, sore throat, cough, diarrhea, headache, myalgia and arthralgia). Patients should be closely monitored at the first appearance of a skin rash and voriconazole should be discontinued if lesions progress.

Photosensitivity reactions have been observed. It is recommended that patients avoid strong sunlight.

There was a small number of post-marketing reports of squamous cell carcinoma, all of which were preceded by episodes of photosensitivity and/or phototoxicity.

Special Populations: Women of Child-Bearing Potential: Women of child-bearing potential should always use effective contraception during treatment with voriconazole.

Pregnant Woman: Voriconazole can cause fetal harm when administered to a pregnant woman. If this drug is used in pregnancy, or if the patient becomes pregnant while taking this drug, the patient should be apprized of the potential hazard to the fetus.

In reproduction studies in rats, voriconazole was teratogenic (cleft palate, hydronephrosis/hydroureter) from 10 mg/kg (0.3 times the human exposure based on body surface area comparisons) and above. Plasma estradiol in pregnant rats was reduced at all dose levels. Voriconazole treatment in rats produced increased gestational length and dystocia which was associated with increased perinatal pup mortality at the 10 mg/kg dose. In rabbits, voriconazole increased embryolethality, and reduced fetal weight.

Nursing Woman: The excretion of voriconazole in breast milk has not been investigated. Voriconazole should not be used by nursing mothers unless the potential benefit to the patient clearly outweighs the potential risks to the nursing infant.

Pediatrics (<12 years): Safety and effectiveness in pediatric subjects below the age of twelve years have not been established. A limited number of pediatric subjects have received voriconazole at doses comparable to those used in adults on a per kilogram body weight basis. There were no apparent differences in safety or efficacy of voriconazole compared to adults although post-marketing data suggest there might be a higher occurrence of skin reactions in the pediatric population compared to adults. A total of 22 patients aged 12-18 years with invasive aspergillosis were included in the therapeutic studies. Twelve out of 22 (55%) patients had successful response after treatment with a maintenance dose of voriconazole 4 mg/kg twice daily.

Geriatrics (>65 years): In multiple-dose therapeutic trials of voriconazole, 9.2% of patients were >65 years of age and 1.8% of patients were >75 years of age. In a clinical pharmacology study in healthy volunteers, some differences were seen in the pharmacokinetic parameters of elderly males compared to young males, and a relationship between plasma concentrations and age was observed in the patients in therapeutic studies. However, the overall safety profile of the elderly patients appeared similar to that of the young. Therefore dosage adjustment does not appear to be required (see Dosage and Administration).

Patients with Hepatic Impairment: It is recommended that the standard loading dose regimens be used but that the maintenance dose be halved in patients with mild to moderate hepatic cirrhosis (Child-Pugh A and B) receiving voriconazole (see Hepatic, Adverse Reactions, Dosage and Administration).

Safety and efficacy of reduced voriconazole dosing in this setting is not established.

Due to the small number of subjects studied, close clinical monitoring is advised.

Voriconazole has not been studied in patients with severe cirrhosis (Child-Pugh Class C). Voriconazole has been associated with elevations in liver function tests and clinical signs of liver damage, such as jaundice, and should only be used in patients with severe hepatic insufficiency if the benefit outweighs the potential risk. Patients with hepatic insufficiency must be carefully monitored for drug toxicity.

Patients with Renal Impairment: In patients with moderate to severe renal dysfunction (creatinine clearance <50 mL/min), accumulation of the intravenous vehicle, SBECD, occurs. Oral voriconazole should be administered to these patients, unless an assessment of the benefit/risk to the patient justifies the use of intravenous voriconazole. Renal function (including serum creatinine levels and creatinine clearance) should be closely monitored in these patients, and if significant changes occur, consideration should be given to changing to oral voriconazole therapy (see Dosage and Administration).

Monitoring and Laboratory Tests: Patient management should include periodic laboratory evaluation of renal (particularly serum creatinine) and hepatic function (particularly liver function tests and bilirubin).

Electrolyte disturbances such as hypokalemia, hypomagnesemia and hypocalcemia should be corrected prior to initiation of voriconazole therapy (see Dosage and Administration).

Carcinogenesis and Mutagenesis: Voriconazole demonstrated clastogenic activity in human lymphocyte cultures in vitro. Voriconazole did not display mutagenic activity in bacterial or mammalian cells in vitro, or clastogenic activity in vivo.

ADVERSE REACTIONS: Adverse Drug Reaction Overview: The most frequently reported adverse events (all causalities) in the therapeutic trials were visual disturbances, fever, rash, vomiting, nausea, diarrhea, headache, sepsis, peripheral edema, abdominal pain, and respiratory disorder. The treatment-related adverse events which most often led to discontinuation of voriconazole therapy were elevated liver function tests, rash, and visual disturbances (see Warnings and Precautions).

Clinical Trial Adverse Drug Reactions: Because clinical trials are conducted under very specific conditions the adverse reaction rates observed in the clinical trials may not reflect the rates observed in practice and should not be compared to the rates in the clinical trials of another drug. Adverse drug reaction information from clinical trials is useful for identifying drug-related adverse events and for approximating rates.

The data described in the table below reflect exposure to voriconazole in 1655 patients in the therapeutic studies. This represents a heterogeneous population, including immunocompromised patients with hematological malignancy or HIV and non neutropenic patients. This subgroup does not include healthy volunteers and patients treated in the compassionate use and non therapeutic studies. This patient population was 62% male, had a mean age of 46 years (range 11-90, including 51 patients aged 12-18 years), and was 78% white and 10% black. Five hundred sixty one patients had a duration of voriconazole therapy of greater than 12 weeks, with 136 patients receiving voriconazole for over six months. Table 1 includes all adverse events which were reported at an incidence of >2% during voriconazole therapy in all therapeutic studies population, studies 307/602 and 608 combined, or study 305, as well as events of concern which occurred at an incidence of <2%.

In studies 307/602, 381 patients (196 on voriconazole, 185 on amphotericin B) were treated to compare voriconazole to amphotericin B followed by other licensed antifungal therapy in the primary treatment of patients with acute invasive aspergillosis. In study 608, 403 non-neutropenic patients with candidemia were treated to compare voriconazole (272 patients) to the regimen of amphotericin B followed by fluconazole (131 patients). Study 305 evaluated the effects of oral voriconazole (200 patients) and oral fluconazole (191 patients) for another indication in immunocompromised (primarily HIV) patients. Laboratory test abnormalities are discussed under Clinical Laboratory Values.

Table 1: VFEND

Treatment-Emergent Adverse Events. Rate ≥2% on Voriconazole or Adverse Events of Concern in all Therapeutic Studies Population, Studies 307/602-608 Combined, or Study 305. Possibly Related to Therapy or Causality Unknown

	All Therapeutic Studies	Studies 307/602 and 608 (iv/oral therapy)			Study 305 (oral therapy)	
	Voriconazole N=1655	Voriconazole N=468	Ampho B[a] N=185	Ampho B→ Fluconazole N= 131	Voriconazole N=200	Fluconazole N=191
	N (%)	N (%)	N (%)	N (%)	N (%)	N (%)
Special Senses						
Abnormal vision	310 (18.7)	63 (13.5)	1 (0.5)	0	31 (15.5)	8 (4.2)
Photophobia	37 (2.2)	8 (1.7)	0	0	5 (2.5)	2 (1.0)
Chromatopsia	20 (1.2)	2 (0.4)	0	0	2 (1.0)	0
Body as a Whole						
Fever	94 (5.7)	8 (1.7)	25 (13.5)	5 (3.8)	0	0
Chills	61 (3.7)	1 (0.2)	36 (19.5)	8 (6.1)	1 (0.5)	0
Headache	49 (3.0)	9 (1.9)	8 (4.3)	1 (0.8)	0	1 (0.5)
Cardiovascular System						
Tachycardia	39 (2.4)	6 (1.3)	5 (2.7)	0	0	0
Digestive System						
Nausea	89 (5.4)	18 (3.8)	29 (15.7)	2 (1.5)	2 (1.0)	3 (1.6)
Vomiting	72 (4.4)	15 (3.2)	18 (9.7)	1 (0.8)	2 (1.0)	1 (0.5)
Liver function tests abnormal	45 (2.7)	15 (3.2)	4 (2.2)	1 (0.8)	6 (3.0)	2 (1.0)
Cholestatic jaundice	17 (1.0)	8 (1.7)	0	1 (0.8)	3 (1.5)	0
Metabolic and Nutritional Systems						
Alkaline phosphatase increased	59 (3.6)	19 (4.1)	4 (2.2)	3 (2.3)	10 (5.0)	3 (1.6)
Hepatic enzymes increased	30 (1.8)	11 (2.4)	5 (2.7)	1 (0.8)	3 (1.5)	0
AST increased	31 (1.9)	9 (1.9)	0	1 (0.8)	8 (4.0)	2 (1.0)
ALT increased	29 (1.8)	9 (1.9)	1 (0.5)	2 (1.5)	6 (3.0)	2 (1.0)
Hypokalemia	26 (1.6)	3 (0.6)	36 (19.5)	16 (12.2)	0	0
Billrubinemia	15 (0.9)	5 (1.1)	3 (1.6)	2 (1.5)	1 (0.5)	0
Creatinine increased	4 (0.2)	0	59 (31.9)	10 (7.6)	1 (0.5)	0
Nervous System						
Hallucinations	39 (2.4)	13 (2.8)	1 (0.5)	0	0	0
Skin and Appendages						
Rash	88 (5.3)	20 (4.3)	7 (3.8)	1 (0.8)	3 (1.5)	1 (0.5)
Urogenital						
Kidney function abnormal	10 (0.6)	6 (1.3)	40 (21.6)	9 (6.9)	1 (0.5)	1 (0.5)
Acute kidney failure	7 (0.4)	2 (0.4)	11 (5.9)	7 (5.3)	0	0

[a] Amphotericin B followed by other licensed antifungal therapy.

Visual Disturbances: In clinical trials, Voriconazole treatment-related visual disturbances were common. In these studies, approximately 21% of patients experienced altered/enhanced visual perception, blurred vision, color vision change and/or photophobia. These visual disturbances were generally mild and rarely resulted in discontinuation. Visual disturbances may be associated with higher plasma concentrations and/or doses.

The mechanism of action of the visual disturbance is unknown, although the site of action is most likely to be within the retina. The majority of visual symptoms appeared to spontaneously resolve within 60 minutes. The serious conditions of the patients treated in Phase 3 studies did not generally allow rigorous testing of visual function. In a study in healthy volunteers investigating the effect of 28 days treatment with voriconazole on retinal function, voriconazole caused a decrease in the electroretinogram (ERG) waveform amplitude, a decrease in the visual field and an alteration in colour perception. The effects were noted early in administration and continued through the course of study drug dosing. Fourteen days after the end of dosing, ERG, visual fields and colour perception returned to normal (see Warnings and Precautions).

Dermatological Reactions: Dermatological reactions were common in the patients treated with voriconazole. The mechanism underlying these dermatologic adverse events remains unknown. In clinical trials, rashes considered related to therapy were reported by 7% (110/1655) of voriconazole-treated patients. The majority of rashes were of mild to moderate severity. Cases of photosensitivity reactions appear to be more likely to occur with long term treatment. Patients have developed serious cutaneous reactions, including Stevens-Johnson syndrome (uncommon), toxic epidermal necrolysis (rare) and erythema multiforme (rare) during treatment with voriconazole. Stevens-Johnson Syndrome and toxic epidermal necrolysis should be considered as a differential diagnosis if patients develop prodromal flu-like symptoms (fever, malaise, rhinitis, chest pain. vomiting, sore throat, cough, diarrhea, headache, myalgia and arthralgia).

Patients should be closely monitored at the first appearance of a skin rash and voriconazole should be discontinued if lesions progress. It is recommended that patients avoid strong, direct sunlight during voriconazole therapy (see Warnings and Precautions).

Less Common Clinical Trial Adverse Drug Reactions: The following adverse events occurred in <2% of all voriconazole treated patients, in all therapeutic studies (N=1655). This listing includes events where a causal relationship to voriconazole cannot be ruled out or those which may help the physician in managing the risks to the patients. The list does not include events included in Table 1 above and does not include every event reported in the voriconazole clinical program.

Body as a Whole: abdomen enlarged, abdominal pain, allergic reaction, anaphylactoid reaction (see Contraindications), ascites, asthenia, back pain, chest pain, cellulitis, edema, face edema, flank pain, flu syndrome, graft versus host reaction, granuloma, infection, bacterial infection, fungal infection, injection site pain, injection site infection/inflammation, mucous membrane disorder, multi organ failure, pain, pelvic pain, peritonitis, sepsis, substernal chest pain.

Cardiovascular: A fatal case of ventricular fibrillation occurred where a relationship to voriconazole could not be ruled out. There have been rare cases of torsades de pointes in which a causal relationship to voriconazole could not be excluded.

Atrial arrhythmia, atrial fibrillation, AV block complete, bigeminy, bradycardia, bundle branch block, cardiomegaly, cardiomyopathy, cerebral hemorrhage, cerebral ischemia, cerebrovascular accident, congestive heart failure, deep thrombophlebitis, endocarditis, extrasystoles, heart arrest, hypertension, hypotension, myocardial infarction, nodal arrhythmia, palpitation, phlebitis, postural hypotension, pulmonary embolus, QT interval prolonged, supraventricular extrasystoles, supraventricular tachycardia, syncope, thrombophlebitis, vasodilatation, ventricular arrhythmia, ventricular fibrillation, ventricular tachycardia (including torsades de pointes).

Digestive: anorexia, cheilitis, cholecystitis, cholelithiasis, constipation, diarrhea, dry mouth, duodenal ulcer perforation, duodenitis, dyspepsia, dysphagia, esophageal ulcer, esophagitis, flatulence, gastroenteritis, gastrointestinal hemorrhage, GGT/LDH elevated, gingivitis, glossitis, gum hemorrhage, gum hyperplasia, hematemesis, hepatic coma, hepatic failure, hepatitis, intestinal perforation, intestinal ulcer, jaundice, enlarged liver, melena, mouth ulceration, pancreatitis, parotid gland enlargement, periodontitis, proctitis, pseudomembranous colitis, rectal disorder, rectal hemorrhage, stomach ulcer, stomatitis, tongue edema.

Endocrine: adrenal cortex insufficiency, diabetes insipidus, hyperthyroidism, hypothyroidism.

Hemic and Lymphatic: agranulocytosis, anemia (macrocytic, megaloblastic, microcytic, normocytic), aplastic anemia, hemolytic anemia, bleeding time increased, cyanosis, DIC, ecchymosis, eosinophilia, hypervolemia, leukopenia, lymphadenopathy, lymphangitis, marrow depression, pancytopenia, petechia, purpura, enlarged spleen, thrombocytopenia, thrombotic thrombocytopenic purpura.

Metabolic and Nutritional: albuminuria, BUN increased, creatine phosphokinase increased, edema, glucose tolerance decreased, hypercalcemia, hypercholesteremia, hyperglycemia, hyperkalemia, hypermagnesemia, hypernatremia, hyperuricemia, hypocalcemia, hypoglycemia, hypomagnesemia, hyponatremia, hypophosphatemia, peripheral edema, uremia.

Musculoskeletal: arthralgia, arthritis, bone necrosis, bone pain, leg cramps, myalgia, myasthenia, myopathy, osteomalacia, osteoporosis.

Nervous System: abnormal dreams, acute brain syndrome, agitation, akathisia, amnesia, anxiety, ataxia, brain edema, coma, confusion, convulsion, delirium, dementia, depersonalization, depression, diplopia, dizziness, encephalitis, encephalopathy, euphoria, Extrapyramidal Syndrome, grand mal convulsion, Guillain-Barré syndrome, hypertonia, hypesthesia, insomnia, intracranial hypertension, libido decreased, neuralgia, neuropathy, nystagmus, oculogyric crisis, paresthesia, psychosis, somnolence, suicidal ideation, tremor, vertigo.

Respiratory System: cough increased, dyspnea, epistaxis, hemoptysis, hypoxia, lung edema, pharyngitis, pleural effusion, pneumonia, respiratory disorder, respiratory distress syndrome, respiratory tract infection, rhinitis, sinusitis, voice alteration.

Skin and Appendages: alopecia, angioedema, contact dermatitis, discoid lupus erythematosis, eczema, erythema multiforme, exfoliative dermatitis, fixed drug eruption, furunculosis, herpes simplex, maculopapular rash, melanosis, photosensitivity skin reaction, psoriasis, pruritus, skin discoloration, skin disorder, skin dry, sweating, toxic epidermal necrolysis, urticaria.

Special Senses: abnormality of accommodation, blepharitis, color blindness, conjunctivitis, corneal opacity, deafness, ear pain, eye pain, eye hemorrhage, hypoacusis, dry eyes, keratitis, keratoconjunctivitis, mydriasis, night blindness, optic atrophy, optic neuritis, otitis externa, papilledema, retinal hemorrhage, retinitis, scleritis, taste loss, taste perversion, tinnitus, uveitis, visual field defect.

Urogenital: anuria, blighted ovum, creatinine clearance decreased, dysmenorrhea, dysuria, epididymitis, glycosuria, hemorrhagic cystitis, hematuria, hydronephrosis, impotence, kidney pain, kidney tubular necrosis, metrorrhagia, nephritis, nephrosis, oliguria, scrotal edema, urinary incontinence, urinary retention, urinary tract infection, uterine hemorrhage, vaginal hemorrhage.

Clinical Laboratory Values: The overall incidence of clinically significant transaminase abnormalities in all therapeutic studies was 12.4% (206/1655) of patients treated with voriconazole. Increased incidences of liver function test abnormalities may be associated with higher plasma concentrations and/or doses. The majority of abnormal liver function tests either resolved during treatment without dose adjustment or following dose adjustment, including discontinuation of therapy.

In clinical trials, there have been uncommon cases of serious hepatic reactions during treatment with VFEND (including clinical hepatitis, cholestasis, and fulminant hepatic failure, including fatalities). Instances of hepatic reactions were noted to occur primarily in patients with serious underlying medical conditions (predominantly hematological malignancy). Hepatic reactions, including hepatitis and jaundice, have occurred among patients with no other identifiable risk factors. Liver dysfunction has usually been reversible on discontinuation of therapy.

Liver function tests should be evaluated at the start of and during the course of voriconazole therapy. Patients who develop abnormal liver function tests should be monitored for the development of more severe hepatic injury. Patient management should include laboratory evaluation of hepatic function (particularly liver function tests and bilirubin). Discontinuation of voriconazole must be considered if clinical signs and symptoms consistent with liver disease develop that may be attributable to voriconazole (see Warnings and Precautions).

Acute renal failure has been observed in severely ill patients undergoing treatment with voriconazole. Patients being treated with voriconazole are likely to be treated concomitantly with nephrotoxic medications and have concurrent conditions that may result in decreased renal function. It is recommended that patients are monitored for the development of abnormal renal function. This should include laboratory evaluation, particularly serum creatinine.

Table 2, Table 3 and Table 4 show the number of patients with hypokalemia and clinically significant changes in renal and liver function tests in three randomized, comparative multicenter studies. In Study 305, patients were randomized to either oral voriconazole or oral fluconazole to evaluate an indication other than invasive aspergillosis in immunocompromised patients. In protocol 307/602, patients with definite or probable invasive aspergillosis were randomized to either voriconazole or amphotericin B therapy. In study 608, patients with candidemia were randomized to either voriconazole or the regimen of amphotericin B followed by fluconazole.

Table 2: VFEND

Protocol 305—Clinically Significant Laboratory Test Abnormalities

	Criteria[a]	VORICONAZOLE n/N (%)	FLUCONAZOLE n/N (%)
T. Bilirubin	>1.5×ULN	8/185 (4.3)	7/186 (3.8)
AST	>3.0×ULN	38/187 (20.3)	15/186 (8.1)
ALT	>3.0×ULN	20/187 (10.7)	12/186 (6.5)
Alk phos	>3.0×ULN	19/187 (10.2)	14/186 (7.5)

[a] Without regard to baseline value.

Legend: n=number of patients with a clinically significant abnormality while on study therapy; N=total number of patients with at least one observation of the given lab test while on study therapy; ULN=upper limit of normal.

Table 3: VFEND

Protocol 307/602—Clinically Significant Laboratory Test Abnormalities

	Criteria[a]	VORICONAZOLE n/N (%)	AMPHOTERICIN B[b] n/N (%)
T. Bilirubin	>1.5×ULN	35/180 (19.4)	46/173 (26.6)
AST	>3.0×ULN	21/180 (11.7)	18/174 (10.3)
ALT	>3.0×ULN	34/180 (18.9)	40/173 (23.1)
Alk phos	>3.0×ULN	29/181 (16.0)	38/173 (22.0)
Creatinine	>1.3×ULN	39/182 (21.4)	102/177 (57.6)
Potassium	<0.9×LLN	30/181 (16.6)	70/178 (39.3)

[a] Without regard to baseline value.

[b] Amphotericin B followed by other licensed antifungal therapy.

Legend: n=number of patients with a clinically significant abnormality while on study therapy; N=total number of patients with at least one observation of the given lab test while on study therapy; ULN=upper limit of normal; LLN=lower limit of normal.

Table 4: VFEND

Protocol 608—Clinically Significant Laboratory Test Abnormalities

	Criteria[a]	VORICONAZOLE n/N (%)	AMPHOTERICIN B followed by FLUCONAZOLE n/N (%)
T. Bilirubin	>1.5×ULN	50/261 (19.2)	31/115 (27.0)
AST	>3.0×ULN	40/261 (15.3)	16/116 (13.8)
ALT	>3.0×ULN	22/261 (8.4)	15/116 (12.9)
Alk phos	>3.0×ULN	59/261 (22.6)	26/115 (22.6)
Creatinine	>1.3×ULN	39/260 (15.0)	32/118 (27.1)
Potassium	<0.9×LLN	43/258 (16.7)	35/118 (29.7)

[a] Without regard to baseline value.

Legend: n=number of patients with a clinically significant abnormality while on study therapy; N=total number of patients with at least one observation of the given lab test while on study therapy; ULN=upper limit of normal; LLN=lower limit of normal.

Post-Market Adverse Drug Reactions: During post-marketing surveillance, cases of severe hypoglycemia have been reported in patients receiving voriconazole and glipizide (see Drug Interactions).

During post-marketing surveillance, there have been rare cases of arrhythmias (including ventricular arrhythmias such as torsades de pointes), cardiac arrests and sudden deaths in patients taking voriconazole. These cases usually involved patients with risk factors such as history of cardiotoxic chemotherapy, cardiomyopathy, hypokalemia and concomitant medications that may have been contributory (see Warnings and Precautions).

There have been post-marketing reports of pancreatitis in pediatric patients (see Warnings and Precautions).

There has been a small number of post-marketing reports of vision loss (including decreased visual acuity or visual fields) where a relationship to voriconazole could not be excluded. These events mostly occurred in medically complex patients, where underlying disease processes and the primary infections themselves confound interpretation (see Warnings and Precautions).

There have been post-marketing reports of prolonged visual adverse events (see Warnings and Precautions).

DRUG INTERACTIONS:

Serious Drug Interactions
- See Contraindications.

Effect of Other Drugs on Voriconazole Pharmacokinetics: See Table 5.

Table 5: VFEND

Effect of Other Drugs on Voriconazole Pharmacokinetics

Drug/Drug Class (Mechanism of Interaction by the Drug)	Voriconazole Plasma Exposure (C_{max} and AUC_τ after 200 mg Q12h)	Recommendations for Voriconazole Dosage Adjustment/Comments
	Contraindications	
Rifampin[a] and Rifabutin[a] (CYP450 Induction)	Significantly reduced	**Contraindicated**
Efavirenz (CYP450 Induction)	Significantly reduced	**Coadministration of standard doses of efavirenz with voriconazole is contraindicated.** When voriconazole is coadministered with efavirenz, voriconazole maintenance dose should be increased to 400 mg every 12 hours and that of efavirenz should be decreased to 300 mg once daily. When treatment with voriconazole is stopped, the initial dosage of efavirenz should be restored.
Other NNRTIs[c] (CYP3A4 Inhibition or CYP450 Induction)	In vitro studies demonstrated potential for inhibition of voriconazole metabolism by delavirdine and other NNRTIs (increased plasma exposure)	Frequent monitoring for adverse events and toxicity related to voriconazole

(cont'd)

Table 5: VFEND *(cont'd)*

Effect of Other Drugs on Voriconazole Pharmacokinetics

Drug/Drug Class (Mechanism of Interaction by the Drug)	Voriconazole Plasma Exposure (C_{max} and AUC_t after 200 mg Q12h)	Recommendations for Voriconazole Dosage Adjustment/Comments
	A voriconazole-efavirenz drug interaction study demonstrated the potential for the metabolism of voriconazole to be induced by efavirenz and other NNRTIs (decreased plasma exposure)	Careful assessment of voriconazole effectiveness
High-dose ritonavir (400 mg Q12h HIV Protease Inhibitor)[b] (CYP450 Induction)	Significantly reduced	**Contraindicated**
Low-dose ritonavir (100 mg Q12h HIV Protease Inhibitor) (CYP450 Induction)	Significantly reduced	Coadministration of voriconazole and low-dose ritonavir (100 mg twice daily Q12h) should be avoided unless an assessment of the benefit/risk justifies the use of voriconazole.
St John's Wort (CYP450 Induction and P-gp induction)	Significantly reduced	**Contraindicated**
Carbamazepine and Long Acting Barbiturates (CYP450 Induction)	Not studied in vivo or in vitro, but likely to result in significant reduction	**Contraindicated**
	Drug Interactions	
Oral Contraceptives containing ethinyl estradiol and norethindrone (CYP2C19 Inhibition)	Increased	Monitoring for adverse events and toxicity related to voriconazole is recommended when coadministered with oral contraceptives.
Phenytoin[a] (CYP450 Induction)	Significantly reduced	There is insufficient data to make specific dosing recommendations. Frequent monitoring of phenytoin plasma concentrations and frequent monitoring of adverse effects related to phenytoin.
Other HIV Protease Inhibitors (CYP3A4 Inhibition)	In vivo studies showed no significant effects of indinavir on voriconazole exposure	No dosage adjustment in the voriconazole dosage needed when coadministered with indinavir
	In vitro studies demonstrated potential for inhibition of voriconazole metabolism (increased plasma exposure)	Frequent monitoring for adverse events and toxicity related to voriconazole when coadministered with other HIV protease inhibitors

[a] Results based on in vivo clinical studies generally following repeat oral dosing with 200 mg Q12h voriconazole to healthy subjects.
[b] Results based on in vivo clinical study following repeat oral dosing with 400 mg Q12h for 1 day, then 200 mg Q12h for 8 days voriconazole to healthy subjects.
[c] Non-Nucleoside Reverse Transcriptase Inhibitors.

Effect of Voriconazole on Pharmacokinetics of Other Drugs: See Table 6.

Table 6: VFEND

Effect of Voriconazole on Pharmacokinetics of Other Drugs

Drug/Drug Class (Mechanism of Interaction by Voriconazole)	Drug Plasma Exposure (C_{max} and AUC_t)	Recommendations for Drug Dosage Adjustment/Comments
	Contraindications	
Sirolimus[a] (CYP3A4 Inhibition)	Significantly increased	**Contraindicated**
Rifabutin[a] (CYP3A4 Inhibition)	Significantly increased	**Contraindicated**
Efavirenz (CYP3A4 Inhibition)	Significantly increased	**Coadministration of standard doses of efavirenz with voriconazole is contraindicated.** When voriconazole is coadministered with efavirenz, voriconazole maintenance dose should be increased to 400 mg every 12 hours and that of efavirenz should be decreased to 300 mg once daily. When treatment with voriconazole is stopped, the initial dosage of efavirenz should be restored.
Other NNRTIs[c] (CYP3A4 Inhibition or CYP450 Induction)	In vitro studies demonstrated potential for inhibition of voriconazole metabolism by delavirdine and other NNRTIs (increased plasma exposure)	Frequent monitoring for adverse events and toxicity related to voriconazole

(cont'd)

Table 6: VFEND *(cont'd)*

Effect of Voriconazole on Pharmacokinetics of Other Drugs

Drug/Drug Class (Mechanism of Interaction by Voriconazole)	Drug Plasma Exposure (C_{max} and AUC_t)	Recommendations for Drug Dosage Adjustment/Comments
	A voriconazole-efavirenz drug interaction study demonstrated the potential for the metabolism of voriconazole to be induced by efavirenz and other NNRTIs (decreased plasma exposure)	Careful assessment of voriconazole effectiveness
High-dose ritonavir (400 mg Q12h HIV Protease Inhibitor)[b] (CYP3A4 Inhibition)	No significant effect of voriconazole on ritonavir C_{max} or AUC_t	**Contraindicated** because of significant reduction of voriconazole C_{max} and AUC_t
Low-dose ritonavir (100 mg Q12h HIV Protease Inhibitor) (CYP3A4 Inhibition)	Slight decrease in Ritonavir C_{max} or AUC_t	Coadministration of voriconazole and low-dose ritonavir (100 mg Q12h) should be avoided (due to the reduction in voriconazole C_{max} and AUC_t) unless an assessment of the benefit/risk justifies the use of voriconazole.
Terfenadine[e], Astemizole[e], Cisapride[e], Pimozide, Quinidine (CYP3A4 Inhibition)	Not studied in vivo or in vitro, but drug plasma exposure likely to be increased	**Contraindicated** because of potential for QT prolongation and rare occurrence of torsades de pointes
Ergot Alkaloids (CYP450 Inhibition)	Not studied in vivo or in vitro, but drug plasma exposure likely to be increased	**Contraindicated**
	Drug Interactions	
Benzodiazepines (CYP3A4 Inhibition)	In vitro studies demonstrated potential for voriconazole to inhibit metabolism (increased plasma exposure)	Frequent monitoring for adverse events and toxicity (i.e., prolonged sedation) related to benzodiazepines metabolized by CYP3A4 (e.g., midazolam, triazolam, alprazolam). Adjustment of benzodiazepine dosage may be needed.
Cyclosporine[a] (CYP3A4 Inhibition)	AUC_t significantly increased; no significant effect on C_{max}	When initiating therapy with VFEND in patients already receiving cyclosporine, reduce the cyclosporine dose to one-half of the starting dose and follow with frequent monitoring of cyclosporine blood levels. Increased cyclosporine levels have been associated with nephrotoxicity. When VFEND is discontinued, cyclosporine concentrations must be frequently monitored and the dose increased as necessary.
Dihydropyridine Calcium Channel Blockers (CYP3A4 Inhibition)	In vitro studies demonstrated potential for voriconazole to inhibit metabolism (increased plasma exposure)	Frequent monitoring for adverse events and toxicity related to calcium channel blockers. Adjustment of calcium channel blocker dosage may be needed.
HMG-CoA Reductase Inhibitors (Statins) (CYP3A4 Inhibition)	In vitro studies demonstrated potential for voriconazole to inhibit metabolism (increased plasma exposure)	Frequent monitoring for adverse events and toxicity related to statins. Increased statin concentrations in plasma have been associated with rhabdomyolysis. Adjustment of the statin dosage may be needed.
Methadone[c] (CYP3A4 Inhibition)	Increased	Increased plasma concentrations of methadone have been associated with toxicity including QT prolongation. Frequent monitoring for adverse events and toxicity related to methadone is recommended during coadministration. Dose reduction of methadone may be needed
Omeprazole[a] (CYP2C19/3A4 Inhibition)	Significantly increased	When initiating therapy with VFEND in patients already receiving omeprazole doses of 40 mg or greater, reduce the omeprazole dose by one-half. The metabolism of other proton pump inhibitors that are CYP2C19 substrates may also be inhibited by voriconazole and may result in increased plasma concentrations of other proton pump inhibitors.
Oral contraceptives containing ethinyl estradiol and norethindrone (CYP2C19 Inhibition)	Increased	Monitoring for adverse events related to oral contraceptives is recommended during coadministration.
Phenytoin[a] (CYP2C9 Inhibition)	Significantly increased	Frequent monitoring of phenytoin plasma concentrations and frequent monitoring of adverse effects related to phenytoin.

(cont'd)

Table 6: VFEND *(cont'd)*

Effect of Voriconazole on Pharmacokinetics of Other Drugs

Drug/Drug Class (Mechanism of Interaction by Voriconazole)	Drug Plasma Exposure (C_{max} and AUC_t)	Recommendations for Drug Dosage Adjustment/Comments
Short acting opiates (CYP3A4 Inhibition)	Significantly increased	Reduction in the dose of alfentanil and other opiates metabolized by CYP3A4 (e. g., sufentanil) should be considered when coadministered with VFEND. A longer period for monitoring respiratory and other opiate-associated adverse events may be necessary.
NSAIDs[f] (including. ibuprofen and diclofenac) (CYP2C9 Inhibition)	Increased	Frequent monitoring for adverse events and toxicity related to NSAIDs is recommended. Dosage adjustment of NSAIDs may be needed.
Sulfonylurea Oral Hypoglycemics (CYP2C9 Inhibition)	Not studied in vivo or in vitro, but drug plasma exposure likely to be increased	Frequent monitoring of blood glucose and for signs and symptoms of hypoglycemia. During post-marketing surveillance, cases of severe hypoglycemia have been reported in patients receiving voriconazole and glipizide. Adjustment of oral hypoglycemic drug dosage may be needed.
Tacrolimus[a] (CYP3A4 Inhibition)	Significantly increased	When initiating therapy with VFEND in patients already receiving tacrolimus, reduce the tacrolimus dose to one-third of the starting dose and follow with frequent monitoring of tacrolimus blood levels. Increased tacrolimus levels have been associated with nephrotoxicity. When VFEND is discontinued, tacrolimus concentrations must be frequently monitored and the dose increased as necessary.
Vinca Alkaloids (CYP3A4 Inhibition)	Not studied in vivo or in vitro, but drug plasma exposure likely to be increased	Frequent monitoring for adverse events and toxicity (i.e., neurotoxicity) related to vinca alkaloids. Adjustment of vinca alkaloid dosage may be needed.
Warfarin[a] (CYP2C9 Inhibition)	Prothrombin time significantly increased	Monitor PT or other suitable anti-coagulation tests. Adjustment of warfarin dosage may be needed.
Other HIV Protease Inhibitors (CYP3A4 Inhibition)	In vivo studies showed no significant effects on indinavir exposure	No dosage adjustment for indinavir when coadministered with VFEND
	In vitro studies demonstrated potential for voriconazole to inhibit metabolism (increased plasma exposure)	Frequent monitoring for adverse events and toxicity related to other HIV protease inhibitors

[a] Results based on in vivo clinical studies generally following repeat oral dosing with 200 mg BID voriconazole to healthy subjects.
[b] Results based on in vivo clinical study following repeat oral dosing with 400 mg Q12h for 1 day, then 200 mg Q12h for 8 days voriconazole to healthy subjects.
[c] Results based on in vivo clinical study following repeat oral dosing with 400 mg Q12h for 1 day, then 200 mg Q12h for 4 days voriconazole to subjects receiving a methadone maintenance dose (30-100 mg QD).
[d] Non-Nucleoside Reverse Transcriptase Inhibitors.
[e] Not marketed in Canada.
[f] Non-Steroidal Anti-Inflammatory Drug

Drug-Food Interactions: Interactions with food have not been established.
Drug-Herb Interactions: Interactions with herbal products have not been established.
Drug-Laboratory Test Interactions: Interactions with laboratory tests have not been established.

DOSAGE AND ADMINISTRATION: Dosing Considerations:

- **Therapy should be initiated with the specified loading dose regimen.**
- **Dosage is based on weight.**
- **Dose can be adjusted if patient response is inadequate or patient is unable to tolerate treatment.**
- **In patients with mild to moderate hepatic impairment, the maintenance dose should be halved.**
- **In patients with moderate to severe renal insufficiency (CrCl <50 mL/min), oral voriconazole should be used because accumulation of the intravenous vehicle SBECD occurs.**
- **When VFEND is taken concomitantly with other drugs, the dosage of VFEND or the concomitant drugs may need to be adjusted (see Drug Interactions).**

Recommended Dose and Dosage Adjustment: Dosage: Use in Adults: Therapy must be initiated with the specified loading dose regimen of either intravenous or oral VFEND to achieve plasma concentrations on Day 1 that are close to steady state. On the basis of high oral bioavailability (96%), switching between intravenous and oral administration is appropriate when clinically indicated. Once the patient can tolerate medication given by mouth, the oral tablet or oral suspension of VFEND may be utilized.

Cumulative dosing of the IV formulation should not extend beyond 6 months. Detailed information on dosage recommendations is provided in Table 7.

Dosage Adjustment: If patient response is inadequate, the oral maintenance dose may be increased from 200 mg every twelve hours to 300 mg every 12 hours. For patients weighing less than 40 kg, the oral dose may be increased from 100 mg every twelve hours to 150 mg every 12 hours. If patients are unable to tolerate 300 mg orally every 12 hours, reduce the oral maintenance dose by 50 mg steps to a minimum of 200 mg every 12 hours (or to 100 mg every 12 hours for adult patients weighing less than 40 kg).

If patients are unable to tolerate 4 mg/kg IV, reduce the intravenous maintenance dose to 3 mg/kg every 12 hours.

Treatment duration depends upon the patient's clinical and mycological response. Patients with candidemia should be treated for at least 14 days following resolution of symptoms or following last positive culture, whichever is longer.

Administration: VFEND Tablets: VFEND (voriconazole) Tablets should be taken at least one hour before, or two hours following, a meal.

VFEND Powder for Oral Suspension: VFEND Powder for Oral Suspension should be taken at least one hour before or following a meal.

VFEND Powder for Oral Suspension requires reconstitution with water prior to administration (see Reconstitution).

Table 7: VFEND

Voriconazole Dosage and Administration

	Loading Dose Regimen (first 24 hours)			Maintenance Dose (after first 24 hours)		
	IV	Oral		IV	Oral	
		Patients ≥40 kg	Patients <40 kg		Patients ≥40 kg	Patients <40 kg
Invasive Aspergillosis	6 mg/kg BID	400 mg BID (two 200 mg tablets or 10 mL of suspension)	200 mg BID (one 200 mg tablets or 5 mL of suspension)	4 mg/kg BID	200 mg BID (one 200 mg tablets or 5 mL of suspension)	100 mg BID (two 50 mg tablets or 2.5 mL of suspension)
Candidemia and invasive candidiasis	6 mg/kg BID	400 mg BID (two 200 mg tablets or 10 mL of suspension)	400 mg BID (two 200 mg tablets or 10 mL of suspension)	3–4 mg/kg BID[a]	200 mg BID (one 200 mg tablets or 5 mL of suspension)	100 mg BID (two 50 mg tablets or 2.5 mL of suspension)

[a] In clinical trials, patients with candidemia received 3 mg/kg every 12 hours as primary therapy, while patients with invasive candidiasis received 4 mg/kg as salvage therapy. Appropriate dose should be based on the severity and nature of the infection.
Legend: BID=twice daily.

VFEND for Injection: VFEND for Injection requires reconstitution and dilution prior to administration as an infusion at a maximum rate of 3 mg/kg per hour over 1-2 hours (see Reconstitution).

Not for IV bolus injection.

Electrolyte disturbances such as hypokalemia, hypomagnesemia and hypocalcemia should be corrected prior to initiation of voriconazole therapy (see Warnings and Precautions, Monitoring and Laboratory Tests).

Missed Dose: Patients who miss taking a dose should take their regular dose next time it is due. Patients should not take a double dose to make up for the forgotten dose.

VFEND Powder for Oral Suspension: Reconstitution: Tap the bottle to release the powder. Add 46 mL of water to the bottle, to provide 75 mL of suspension with a 70 mL usable volume. Shake the closed bottle vigorously for about 1 minute. Remove child-resistant cap and push bottle adaptor into the neck of the bottle. Replace the cap. Write the date of expiration of the reconstituted suspension on the bottle label (the shelf-life of the reconstituted suspension is 14 days at 15 to 30°C). Discard any unused portion after 14 days. Do not refrigerate or freeze. Keep the container tightly closed.

Incompatibilities: VFEND Powder for Oral Suspension and the 40 mg/mL reconstituted oral suspension should not be mixed with any other medication or additional flavoring agent. The suspension should not be further diluted with water or other vehicles.

Instructions for Use: Shake the closed bottle of reconstituted suspension for approximately 10 seconds before each use. The reconstituted oral suspension should only be administered using the oral dispenser supplied with each pack.

VFEND for Injection: Reconstitution: The powder is reconstituted with 19 mL of "Water For Injection" to obtain an extractable volume of 20 mL of clear concentrate containing 10 mg/mL of voriconazole. It is recommended that a standard 20 mL (non automated) syringe be used to ensure that the exact amount (19.0 mL) of water for injection is dispensed. Discard the vial if a vacuum does not pull the diluent into the vial. Shake the vial until all the powder is dissolved.

Dilution for Infusion: VFEND must be infused over 1 2 hours, at a concentration of 5 mg/mL or less. Therefore, the required volume of the 10 mg/mL VFEND concentrate should be further diluted as follows (appropriate diluents listed below):

1. Calculate the volume of 10 mg/mL VFEND concentrate required based on the patient's weight (Table 8)
2. In order to allow the required volume of VFEND concentrate to be added, withdraw and discard at least an equal volume of diluent from the infusion bag or bottle to be used. The volume of diluent remaining in the bag or bottle should be such that when the 10 mg/mL VFEND concentrate is added, the final concentration is not less than 0.5 mg/mL or greater than 5 mg/mL.
3. **Using a suitable size syringe and aseptic technique, withdraw the required volume of VFEND concentrate from the appropriate number of vials and add to the infusion bag or bottle. Discard partially used vials.**

The final VFEND solution must be infused over 1-2 hours at a maximum rate of 3 mg/kg per hour.

Table 8: VFEND

Required Volumes of 10 mg/mL VFEND Concentrate

Body Weight (kg)	Volume of VFEND Concentrate 10 mg /mL Required for: 3 mg/kg dose (number of vials)		4 mg/kg dose (number of vials)		6 mg/kg dose (number of vials)	
30	9.0 mL	1	12 mL	1	18 mL	1
35	10.5 mL	1	14 mL	1	21 mL	2
40	12.0 mL	1	16 mL	1	24 mL	2
45	13.5 mL	1	18 mL	1	27 mL	2
50	15.0 mL	1	20 mL	1	30 mL	2
55	16.5 mL	1	22 mL	2	33 mL	2
60	18.0 mL	1	24 mL	2	36 mL	2
65	19.5 mL	1	26 mL	2	39 mL	2
70	21.0 mL	2	28 mL	2	42 mL	3
75	22.5 mL	2	30 mL	2	45 mL	3
80	24.0 mL	2	32 mL	2	48 mL	3
85	25.5 mL	2	34 mL	2	51 mL	3
90	27.0 mL	2	36 mL	2	54 mL	3
95	28.5 mL	2	38 mL	2	57 mL	3
100	30.0 mL	2	40 mL	2	60 mL	3

VFEND I.V. for Injection is a single dose unpreserved sterile lyophile. Therefore, from a microbiological point of view, once reconstituted, the product should be used immediately. If not used immediately, in use storage times and conditions prior to use are the responsibility of the user and should not be longer than 24 hours at 2 to 8°C. This medicinal product is for single use only and any unused solution should be discarded.

The reconstituted solution can be diluted with: 0.9% Sodium Chloride USP; Lactated Ringers USP; 5% Dextrose and Lactated Ringers USP; 5% Dextrose and 0.45% Sodium Chloride USP; 5% Dextrose USP; 5% Dextrose and 20 mEq Potassium Chloride USP; 0.45% Sodium Chloride USP; 5% Dextrose and 0.9% Sodium Chloride USP.

The compatibility of VFEND for Injection with diluents other than those described above is unknown (see Incompatibilities).

Parenteral drug products should be inspected visually for particulate matter and discoloration prior to administration, whenever solution and container permit.

Incompatibilities:

- **Blood products and concentrated electrolytes:** Voriconazole must not be infused concomitantly with any blood product or any short-term infusion of concentrated electrolytes, even if the two infusions are running in separate intravenous lines (or cannulas).

Electrolyte disturbances such as hypokalemia, hypomagnesemia and hypocalcemia should be corrected prior to initiation of voriconazole therapy (see Warnings and Precautions, Monitoring and Laboratory Tests).

- **Intravenous solutions containing (non-concentrated) electrolytes:** Voriconazole can be infused at the same time as other intravenous solutions containing (nonconcentrated) electrolytes, but must be infused through a separate line.
- **Total Parenteral Nutrition (TPN):** Voriconazole can be infused at the same time as total parenteral nutrition, but must be infused in a separate line. If infused through a multiple-lumen catheter, TPN needs to be administered using a different port from the one used for voriconazole.
- VFEND for Injection must not be diluted with 4.2% Sodium Bicarbonate Infusion. Compatibility with other concentrations is unknown.

As with all parenteral drug products, intravenous admixtures should be inspected visually for clarity, particulate matter, precipitate, discoloration and leakage prior to administration, whenever solution and container permit. Solutions showing haziness, particulate matter, precipitate, discoloration or leakage should not be used. Discard unused portion.

Special Populations: Pediatrics: (See Warnings and Precautions.)

Geriatrics: Dosage adjustment does not appear to be required for elderly patients (see Warnings and Precautions).

Hepatic Insufficiency: Hepatic impairment is likely to result in increased voriconazole plasma levels in patients with mild to moderate hepatic cirrhosis (Child-Pugh A and B).

It is recommended that the standard loading dose regimens be used but that the maintenance dose be halved in patients with mild to moderate hepatic cirrhosis (Child-Pugh A and B).

Safety and efficacy of reduced voriconazole dosing in this setting is not established.

Due to the small number of subjects studied, close clinical monitoring is advised.

VFEND has not been studied in patients with severe hepatic cirrhosis (Child-Pugh C). VFEND should be used only if the benefit outweighs the potential risk. Patients should be carefully monitored for drug toxicity (see Warnings and Precautions).

Renal Insufficiency: The pharmacokinetics of orally administered VFEND do not appear to be affected by renal insufficiency. Therefore, no dosage adjustment is necessary for **oral** dosing in patients with mild to severe renal impairment.

Due to the small number of subjects studied, close clinical monitoring is advised.

In patients with moderate or severe renal insufficiency (creatinine clearance <50 mL/min), accumulation of the intravenous vehicle, SBECD, occurs. Oral voriconazole should be administered to these patients, unless an assessment of the benefit risk to the patient justifies the use of intravenous voriconazole. Renal function (including serum creatinine levels and creatinine clearance) should be closely monitored in these patients, and, if significant changes occur, consideration should be given to changing to oral voriconazole therapy (see Warnings and Precautions).

Voriconazole is hemodialyzed with clearance of 121 mL/min. The intravenous vehicle, SBECD, is hemodialyzed with clearance of 55 mL/min. The mean amount of voriconazole removed during 4 hour hemodialysis session (8%, range 1-16%) is not enough to warrant dose adjustment.

OVERDOSAGE:

There is no known antidote to voriconazole; it is recommended that treatment of overdose is symptomatic and supportive. Administration of activated charcoal may be used to aid in removal of unabsorbed drug.

EKG monitoring is recommended due to the possible prolongation of the QT interval and ensuing risk of arrhythmia.

Voriconazole is hemodialyzed with clearance of 121 mL/min. The intravenous vehicle, SBECD, is hemodialyzed with clearance of 55 mL/min. In an overdose, hemodialysis may assist in the removal of voriconazole and SBECD from the body.

In clinical trials, there were three cases of accidental overdose with VFEND (voriconazole). All occurred in pediatric patients who received up to five times the recommended intravenous dose of voriconazole. A single adverse event of photophobia of 10 minutes duration was reported.

> For management of a suspected drug overdose, contact your regional Poison Control Centre. See the *CPS* Directory section for a list of Poison Control Centres.

ACTION AND CLINICAL PHARMACOLOGY: Mechanism of Action: VFEND (voriconazole) is a triazole antifungal agent, which exhibits broad-spectrum in vitro activity and fungicidal activity against Aspergillus spp. as well as a range of other filamentous fungi. The primary mode of action of voriconazole is the inhibition of fungal cytochrome P450-mediated 14α-sterol demethylation, an essential step in ergosterol biosynthesis. The subsequent loss of normal sterols correlates with the accumulation of 14α-methyl sterols in fungi and may be responsible for its fungistatic/fungicidal activity.

The voriconazole clinical program included a total of 38 patients with Scedosporium spp. and 21 patients with Fusarium spp. This limited clinical data suggest that voriconazole may be effective against infections caused by these rare pathogens in patients intolerant of or refractory to other therapies.

Absorption: Voriconazole is rapidly and almost completely absorbed following oral administration, with maximum plasma concentrations (C_{max}) achieved 1-2 hours after dosing.

Distribution: The volume of distribution at steady state for voriconazole is estimated to be 4.6 L/kg, suggesting extensive distribution into tissues. Plasma protein binding is estimated to be 58%.

Metabolism: In vitro studies showed that voriconazole is metabolised by the hepatic cytochrome P450 isoenzymes, CYP2C19, CYP2C9 and CYP3A4.

The interindividual variability of voriconazole pharmacokinetics is high. Greater than proportional increase in exposure is observed with increasing dose. It is estimated that, on average, increasing the oral dose in healthy subjects from 200 mg Q12h to 300 mg Q12h leads to a 2.5 fold increase in exposure (AUC) while increasing the intravenous dose from 3 mg/kg Q12h to 4 mg/kg Q12h produces a 2.3 fold increase in exposure (see Table 9).

Table 9: VFEND

Population Pharmacokinetic Parameters of Voriconazole in Volunteers

	200 mg Oral Q12h	300 mg Oral Q12h	3 mg/kg IV Q12h	4 mg/kg IV Q12h
AUC_t[a] (μg·h/mL)	19.86	50.32	21.81	50.40
CV (%)	94%	74%	100%	83%

[a] Mean AUC_t are predicted values from population pharmacokinetic analysis of data from 236 volunteers.

The major metabolite of voriconazole is the N-oxide, which accounts for 72% of the circulating radiolabelled metabolites in plasma.

Elimination: Voriconazole is eliminated primarily by hepatic metabolism with less than 2% of the dose excreted unchanged in the urine. The terminal half-life ($T_{1/2}$) depends on the dose and is approximately 6 hours at 3 mg/kg (intravenously) or 200 mg (oral). Because of non-linear pharmacokinetics, the terminal half-life is not useful in predicting the accumulation or elimination of voriconazole.

STORAGE AND STABILITY: VFEND Tablets: VFEND Tablets should be stored at controlled room temperature, 15-30°C.

VFEND Powder for Oral Suspension: Unreconstituted Powder: Store at 2 to 8°C.

Reconstituted Suspension: Store at 15 to 30°C for up to 14 days. Keep the container tightly closed. Discard remaining suspension 14 days after constitution.

VFEND for Injection: Unreconstituted Vials: Store at controlled room temperature, 15-30°C.

Reconstituted Solution: VFEND for Injection is a single dose unpreserved sterile lyophile. From a microbiological point of view, following reconstitution of the lyophile with Water for Injection, the reconstituted solution should be used immediately. If not used immediately, in-use storage times and conditions prior to use are the responsibility of the user and would normally not be longer than 24 hours at 2-8°C, unless reconstitution has taken place in controlled and validated aseptic conditions. Single dose vials. Discard unused portion.

INFORMATION FOR THE PATIENT: Published in e-CPS, available by subscription at www.e-cps.ca.

DOSAGE FORMS, COMPOSITION AND PACKAGING: Injection: Each single use vial of white, sterile lyophilized powder contains: voriconazole 200 mg and SBECD 3200 mg. Preservative-free. Type I clear glass single dose vials of 30 mL. VFEND for Injection is intended for administration by intravenous infusion. Vials containing 200 mg lyophilized voriconazole are intended for reconstitution with Water for Injection to produce a solution containing 10 mg/mL voriconazole and 160 mg/mL of sulphobutylether-β-cyclodextrin sodium (SBECD) as a molecular inclusion complex. The resultant solution is further diluted prior to administration as an intravenous infusion (see Dosage and Administration).

Powder for Oral Suspension: White to off-white powder providing a white to off-white orange-flavored suspension when reconstituted. Bottles containing 3 g voriconazole in 45 g powder for oral suspension (40 mg/mL when reconstituted). Nonmedicinal ingredients: anhydrous citric acid, colloidal silicon dioxide, natural orange flavor, sodium benzoate, sodium citrate dihydrate, sucrose, titanium dioxide and xanthan gum.

Tablets: 50 mg: Each white, film-coated, round tablet, debossed with "Pfizer" on one side and "VOR50" on the reverse, contains: voriconazole 50 mg. Nonmedicinal ingredients: croscarmellose sodium, lactose monohydrate, magnesium stearate, povidone, pregelatinized starch; coating: hypromellose, lactose monohydrate, titanium dioxide and triacetin. HDPE bottles of 30.

200 mg: Each white, film-coated, capsule-shaped tablet, debossed with "Pfizer" on one side and "VOR200" on the reverse, contains: voriconazole 200 mg. Nonmedicinal ingredients: croscarmellose sodium, lactose monohydrate, magnesium stearate, povidone, pregelatinized starch; coating: hypromellose, lactose monohydrate, titanium dioxide and triacetin. HDPE bottles of 30.

(Shown in Product Identification Section)

Viaderm-K.C. ℞

triamcinolone acetonide—neomycin sulfate—nystatin—gramicidin

Topical Dermatoses Therapy

Taro

SUPPLIED: Cream: Each g contains: triamcinolone acetonide 1 mg, neomycin base (as sulfate) 2.5 mg, gramicidin 0.25 mg, nystatin 100 000 units. It is formulated in a perfumed aqueous vanishing cream base which permits its use even in most intertriginous areas. Nonmedicinal ingredients: cetomacrogol emulsifying wax, citric acid, ethyl alcohol, liquid paraffin, methylparaben, perfume, propylparaben, propylene glycol, purified water, sodium phosphate dibasic and white petrolatum. Tubes of 15, 30 and 60 g. Jars of 454 g. Store at room temperature (15-30°C).

Ointment: Each g contains: triamcinolone acetonide 1 mg, neomycin base (as sulfate) 2.5 mg, gramicidin 0.25 mg, nystatin 100 000 units. It is formulated in a protective emollient ointment base of mineral oil and white petrolatum. Tubes of 15 and 30 g. Store at room temperature (15-30°C).

Viagra™ ℞

sildenafil citrate

Treatment of Erectile Dysfunction

Pfizer

Date of Revision: March 31, 2009

SUMMARY PRODUCT INFORMATION:

Route of Administration	Dosage Form/ Strength	Clinically Relevant Nonmedicinal Ingredients
Oral	Tablets 25 mg, 50 mg and 100 mg	The tablets also contain the following nonmedicinal ingredients: microcrystalline cellulose, anhydrous dibasic calcium phosphate, croscarmellose sodium, magnesium stearate, hypromellose, titanium dioxide, lactose, triacetin, and FD&C Blue #2 aluminum lake.

INDICATIONS AND CLINICAL USE: VIAGRA (sildenafil citrate) is indicated for:

- the treatment of erectile dysfunction, which is the inability to achieve or maintain a penile erection sufficient for satisfactory sexual performance.

CONTRAINDICATIONS: VIAGRA (sildenafil citrate) has been shown to potentiate the hypotensive effects of nitrates in healthy volunteers and in patients, and is therefore contraindicated in patients who are taking any type of nitrate drug therapy, or who utilize short-acting nitrate-containing medications, due to the risk of developing potentially life-threatening hypotension. The use of organic nitrates, either regularly and/or intermittently, in any form (e.g. oral, sublingual, transdermal, by inhalation) is absolutely contraindicated (see Action and Clinical Pharmacology, Dosage and Administration).

After patients have taken VIAGRA, it is unknown when nitrates, if necessary, can be safely administered. Plasma levels of sildenafil at 24 hours post-dose are much lower (2 ng/mL) than at peak concentration (440 ng/mL). In the following patients: age >65, hepatic impairment (e.g. cirrhosis), severe renal impairment (e.g. CLcr <30 mL/min), and concomitant use of potent cytochrome P-450 3A4 inhibitors (erythromycin), plasma levels of sildenafil at 24 hours post-dose have been found to be 3 to 8 times higher than those seen in healthy volunteers. Although plasma levels of sildenafil at 24 hours post-dose are much lower than at peak concentration, it is unknown whether nitrates can be safely coadministered at this time point.

Treatments for erectile dysfunction should not be generally used in men for whom sexual activity is inadvisable (see also Warnings and Precautions).

VIAGRA is contraindicated in patients with a known hypersensitivity to any component of the tablet.

WARNINGS AND PRECAUTIONS: General: The evaluation of erectile dysfunction should include a determination of potential underlying causes and the identification of appropriate treatment following a complete medical assessment.

Cardiovascular: As with all treatments for erectile dysfunction, there is a potential cardiac risk of sexual activity in patients with pre-existing cardiovascular disease, including hypertension (BP>140/90). Therefore, treatments for erectile dysfunction, including VIAGRA (sildenafil citrate), should not be generally administered in men for whom sexual activity is inadvisable because of their underlying cardiovascular status.

There are no controlled clinical data on the safety or efficacy of VIAGRA in the following groups, if prescribed, this should be done with caution.

- Patients who have suffered a myocardial infarction, stroke, or life-threatening arrhythmia within the last 6 months
- Patients with resting hypotension (BP <90/50 at rest) or hypertension (BP >170/110 at rest)
- Patients with cardiac failure or coronary artery disease causing unstable angina (See Action and Clinical Pharmacology).

Caution is advised when sildenafil is administered to patients taking an alpha-blocker, as the coadministration may lead to symptomatic hypotension in a few susceptible individuals (see Drug Interactions). In order to minimize the potential for developing postural hypotension, patients should be hemodynamically stable on alpha-blocker therapy prior to initiating sildenafil treatment. Initiation of sildenafil at lower doses should be considered. In addition, physicians should advise patients what to do in the event of postural hypotensive symptoms.

Hematologic: In clinical trials, sildenafil has been shown to have systemic vasodilatory properties that result in transient decreases in blood pressure. This is of little or no consequence in most patients. However, prior to prescribing sildenafil, physicians should carefully consider whether their patients with certain underlying conditions could be adversely affected by such vasodilatory effects, especially in combination with sexual activity. Patients with increased susceptibility to vasodilators include those with left ventricular outflow obstruction (e.g., aortic stenosis, hypertrophic obstructive cardiomyopathy), or those with the rare syndrome of multiple system atrophy manifesting as severely impaired autonomic control of blood pressure.

In humans, VIAGRA (sildenafil citrate) has no effect on bleeding time when taken alone or with acetylsalicylic acid. In vitro studies with human platelets indicate that sildenafil potentiates the antiaggregatory effect of sodium nitroprusside (a nitric oxide donor). The combination of heparin and VIAGRA had an additive effect on bleeding time in the anesthetized rabbit, but this interaction has not been studied in humans (see Action and Clinical Pharmacology).

There is no safety information on the administration of VIAGRA to patients with bleeding disorders or active peptic ulceration. Therefore, VIAGRA should be administered with caution to these patients.

Hepatic/Biliary/Pancreatic: In volunteers with hepatic cirrhosis (Child-Pugh A and B), sildenafil clearance was reduced, resulting in increases in AUC (84%) and C_{max} (47%) compared to age-matched volunteers with no hepatic impairment.

A starting dose of 25 mg should be considered in patients with hepatic impairment (see Action and Clinical Pharmacology, Dosage and Administration).

Ophthalmologic: Postmarketing reports of sudden loss of vision have occurred rarely, in temporal association with the use of PDE5 inhibitors. It is not clear whether these are related directly to the use of PDE5 inhibitors or to other factors. There may be an increased risk to patients who have already experienced Non-Arteritic Anterior Ischemic Optic Neuropathy (NAION).

There are no controlled clinical data on the safety or efficacy of VIAGRA in patients with retinitis pigmentosa (a minority of these patients have genetic disorders of retinal phosphodiesterases). If prescribed, this should be done with caution (see Action and Clinical Pharmacology).

A small percentage of patients experience visual effects (e.g. impairment of colour discrimination, increased perception to light, blurred vision, eye pain, ocular redness) after taking VIAGRA. If this happens, then the patient should not operate a motor vehicle or any heavy machinery until the adverse effects disappear (see Action and Clinical Pharmacology).

Otologic: Sudden decrease or loss of hearing has been reported in a few number of postmarketing and clinical trial cases with the use of PDE5 inhibitors, including VIAGRA. These events, which may be accompanied by tinnitus and dizziness, have been reported in temporal association to the intake of PDE5 inhibitors, including VIAGRA. In some of the cases, medical conditions and other factors were reported that may have also played a role in the otologic adverse events. In many cases, medical follow-up information was limited. It is not possible to determine whether these events are related directly to the use of PDE5 inhibitors or to other factors (see Adverse Reactions, Post-Market Adverse Drug Reactions and Information for the Patient). Physicians should advise patients to stop taking VIAGRA and seek prompt medical attention in case of sudden decrease or loss of hearing.

Renal: In volunteers with mild (CLcr=50-80 mL/min) and moderate (CLcr=30-49 mL/min) renal impairment, the pharmacokinetics of a single oral dose of VIAGRA (50 mg) was not altered. In volunteers with severe (CLcr <30 mL/min) renal impairment, sildenafil clearance was reduced, resulting in increases in AUC (100%) and C_{max} (88%) compared to age-matched volunteers with no renal impairment.

A starting dose of 25 mg should be considered in patients with severe renal impairment (see Action and Clinical Pharmacology, Dosage and Administration).

Sexual Function/Reproduction: Although **priapism** had not been reported during clinical trials, prolonged erection greater than 4 hours and priapism (painful erections greater than 6 hours in duration) have been reported infrequently during the postmarketing surveillance of VIAGRA. In the event of an erection that persists longer than 4 hours, the patient should seek immediate medical assistance. If priapism is not treated immediately, penile tissue damage and permanent loss of potency could result (see Adverse Reactions).

Agents for the treatment of erectile dysfunction should be used with caution in patients with anatomical deformation of the penis (such as angulation, cavernosal fibrosis or Peyronie's disease) or in patients who have conditions which may predispose them to priapism (such as sickle cell anemia, multiple myeloma or leukemia).

The safety and efficacy of combinations of VIAGRA with other agents for the treatment of erectile dysfunction have not been studied. Therefore, the use of such combinations is not recommended.

Special Populations: Pregnant Women: VIAGRA is not indicated for use in women.

Nursing Women: VIAGRA is not indicated for use in women.

Pediatrics: VIAGRA is not indicated for use in children.

Geriatrics (>65 years of age): Healthy elderly volunteers had a reduced clearance of sildenafil, with free plasma concentrations approximately 40% greater than those seen in younger volunteers (18 to 45 years). Since higher plasma levels may increase both the pharmacological action and incidence of some adverse events, a starting dose of 25 mg should be considered (see Action and Clinical Pharmacology, Dosage and Administration).

Information to Be Provided to the Patient: Physicians should discuss with patients the increased risk of Non-Arteritic Anterior Ischemic Optic Neuropathy (NAION) in individuals who have already experienced NAION in one eye, including whether such individuals could be adversely affected by use of vasodilators, such as PDE5 inhibitors. Patients should stop taking VIAGRA and consult their physician if they experience a decrease in, or loss of, vision in one or both eyes.

ADVERSE REACTIONS: Adverse Drug Reaction Overview: Pre-Marketing Experience: VIAGRA (sildenafil citrate) was administered to over 3700 patients (aged 19-87 years) during clinical trials worldwide. Over 550 patients were treated for longer than one year.

In placebo-controlled clinical studies, the discontinuation rate due to adverse events for VIAGRA (2.5%) was not significantly different from placebo (2.3%). The adverse events were generally transient and mild to moderate in nature.

Clinical Trial Adverse Drug Reactions: Because clinical trials are conducted under very specific conditions the adverse reaction rates observed in the clinical trials may not reflect the rates observed in practice and should not be compared to the rates in the clinical trials of another drug. Adverse drug reaction information from clinical trials is useful for identifying drug-related adverse events and for approximating rates.

In trials of all designs, adverse events reported by patients receiving VIAGRA were generally similar. In fixed-dose studies, the incidence of some adverse events increased with dose. The nature of the adverse events in flexible-dose studies, which more closely reflect the recommended dosage regimen, was similar to that for fixed-dose studies.

When VIAGRA was taken as recommended (on an as-needed basis) in flexible-dose, placebo-controlled clinical trials, the following adverse events were reported: (see Table 1).

Table 1: VIAGRA

Adverse Events Reported by ≥2% of Patients Treated with VIAGRA or Placebo in PRN Flexible-dose Phase II/III Studies

	Percentage of Patients Reporting Event	
Adverse Event	**VIAGRA (n=734) (%)**	**Placebo (n=725) (%)**
Headache	15.8	3.9
Flushing	10.5	0.7
Dyspepsia	6.5	1.7
Nasal Congestion	4.2	1.5
Respiratory Tract Infection	4.2	5.4
Flu Syndrome	3.3	2.9
Urinary Tract Infection	3.1	1.5
Abnormal Vision[a]	2.7	0.4
Diarrhea	2.6	1.0
Dizziness	2.2	1.2
Rash	2.2	1.4
Back Pain	2.2	1.7
Arthralgia	2.0	1.5

[a] Abnormal Vision: Mild and transient changes, predominantly impairment of color discrimination (blue/green), but also increased perception to light or blurred vision.

At doses above the recommended dose range, adverse events were similar to those detailed above but generally were reported more frequently.

Less Common Clinical Trial Adverse Drug Reactions (<2%): The following events occurred in <2% of patients in controlled clinical trials where a causal relationship is uncertain:

Autonomic: sweating, dry mouth.

Cardiovascular: abnormal electrocardiogram, angina pectoris, arrhythmia, AV block, cardiac arrest, cardiomyopathy, heart failure, hypertension, hypotension, palpitation, postural hypotension, myocardial ischemia, syncope, tachycardia, varicose vein, vascular anomaly.

Central & Peripheral Nervous System: tremor, abnormal dreams, anxiety, agitation, ataxia, depression, insomnia, nervousness, somnolence, paresthesia, vertigo, speech disorder, reflexes decreased, hyperesthesia, neuropathy, migraine, myasthenia, oculogyric crisis, neuralgia, hypertonia.

Gastrointestinal: vomiting, gastritis, gastrointestinal disorder, flatulence, increased appetite, gastroenteritis, stomatitis, eructation, dysphagia, colitis, glossitis, constipation, rectal hemorrhage, mouth ulceration, esophagitis, rectal disorder, gingivitis, tooth disorder.

Hematopoietic: anemia and leukopenia.

Liver/Biliary: liver function tests abnormal, ALT increased.

Metabolic/Nutritional: edema, thirst, gout, hyperuricemia, hypoglycemic reaction, unstable diabetes, hyperglycemia, hyperlipidemia, hypernatremia.

Musculoskeletal: myalgia, bone disorder, arthrosis, arthritis, tendon rupture, tenosynovitis, bone pain, joint disorder, synovitis.

Respiratory: asthma, dyspnea, laryngitis, pharyngitis, sinusitis, bronchitis, respiratory disorder, carcinoma of lung, sputum increased, cough increased.

Skin/Appendages: skin carcinoma, skin disorder, skin hypertrophy, skin ulcer, contact dermatitis, exfoliative dermatitis, pruritus, urticaria, photosensitivity reaction, nail disorder, acne, herpes simplex, furunculosis.

Special Senses: sudden decrease or loss of hearing, mydriasis, conjunctivitis, photophobia, eye pain, tinnitus, ear pain, lacrimation disorder, eye disorder, eye hemorrhage, ear disorder, cataract, dry eyes.

Urogenital: penile erection, other sexual dysfunction, cystitis, nocturia, balanitis, urinary frequency, breast enlargement, prostatic disorder, testis disorder, urinary incontinence, urinary tract disorder, urine abnormality, abnormal ejaculation, genital edema and anorgasmia.

Vascular Disorders: cerebrovascular disorder, cerebral thrombosis.

General: face edema, peripheral edema, chills, allergic reaction, asthenia, pain, infection, shock, hernia, accidental fall, abdominal pain, chest pain, accidental injury, intentional overdose.

In an analysis of double blind placebo controlled clinical trials encompassing over 700 person-years of observation on placebo and over 1300 person-years on sildenafil, there were no differences in the incidence rate of myocardial infarction (MI) or in the rate of cardiovascular mortality for patients receiving sildenafil compared to those receiving placebo. The rates of MI were 1.1 per 100 person-years for men receiving sildenafil and for those receiving placebo. The rates of cardiovascular mortality were 0.3 per 100 person-years for men receiving sildenafil and those receiving placebo.

Post-Market Adverse Drug Reactions: Reports of adverse events temporally associated with VIAGRA during post-marketing surveillance that are not listed above and for which the causal relationship is unknown, include the following:

Cardiovascular: Epistaxis; serious cardiovascular events—including myocardial infarction, sudden cardiac death, ventricular arrhythmia, cerebrovascular hemorrhage, and transient ischemic attack—have been reported. Most of these patients had pre-existing cardiovascular risk factors. Many of these events were reported to occur during or shortly after sexual activity, and a few were reported to occur shortly after the use of VIAGRA without sexual activity. Others were reported to have occurred hours to days after the use of VIAGRA with sexual activity. It is not possible to determine whether these events are related directly to VIAGRA, to sexual activity, to the patient's underlying cardiovascular disease, to combination of these factors, or to other factors (see Warnings and Precautions).

Central & Peripheral Nervous System: seizure, seizure recurrence, transient global amnesia.

Gastrointestinal: vomiting.

Urogenital: prolonged erection, priapism (see Warnings and Precautions) and hematuria.

Special Senses: diplopia, temporary vision loss/decreased vision, blurred vision, Non Arteritic Anterior Ischemic Optic Neuropathy (NAION), retinal vein occlusion, visual field defect, eye pain, ocular redness or bloodshot appearance, ocular burning, ocular swelling/pressure, increased intraocular pressure, retinal vascular disease of bleeding, vitreous detachment/traction and paramacular edema.

Cases of sudden decrease or loss of hearing have been reported post-marketing in temporal association with the use of PDE5 inhibitors, including VIAGRA. In some of the cases, medical conditions and other factors were reported that may have also played a role in the otologic adverse events. In many cases, medical follow-up information was limited. It is not possible to determine whether these events are related directly to the use of VIAGRA, to the patient's underlying risk factors for hearing loss, a combination of these factors, or to other factors (see Warnings and Precautions, Adverse Reactions and Information for the Patient).

DRUG INTERACTIONS:

Serious Drug Interactions

- Use of organic nitrates in any form is absolutely contraindicated (see Contraindications)

Overview: In vitro studies: Sildenafil metabolism is principally mediated by the cytochrome P-450 (CYP) isoforms 3A4 (major route) and 2C9 (minor route) (see Action and Clinical Pharmacology). Therefore, inhibitors of these isoenzymes may reduce sildenafil clearance and inducers of these isoenzymes may increase sildenafil clearance.

Sildenafil is a weak inhibitor of the cytochrome P-450 isoforms 1A2, 2C9, 2C19, 2D6, 2E1 and 3A4 (IC_{50}>150 μM). Given sildenafil peak plasma concentrations of approximately 1 μM after recommended doses, it is unlikely that VIAGRA will alter the clearance of the substrates of these isoenzymes.

In vivo studies: Sildenafil (50 mg) did not potentiate the hypotensive effect of alcohol in healthy volunteers with mean maximum blood alcohol levels of 0.08%.

Drug-Drug Interactions: Effects of Other Drugs on VIAGRA: Pharmacokinetic data from patients in clinical trials showed no effect on sildenafil pharmacokinetics of CYP2C9 inhibitors (such as tolbutamide, warfarin), CYP2D6 inhibitors (such as selective serotonin reuptake inhibitors, tricyclic antidepressants), thiazide and related diuretics, angiotensin converting enzyme (ACE) inhibitors, and calcium channel blockers. The AUC of the active metabolite, N desmethyl sildenafil, was increased 62% by loop and potassium sparing diuretics and 102% by nonspecific beta blockers. These effects on the metabolite are not expected to be of clinical consequence.

In normal healthy male volunteers, there was no evidence of an effect of azithromycin (500 mg daily for 3 days) on the AUC, C_{max}, T_{max}, elimination rate constant, or subsequent half-life of sildenafil or its principle circulating metabolite.

CYP3A4 Inhibitors: The concomitant use of potent cytochrome P-450 3A4 inhibitors (e.g. erythromycin, saquinavir, ritonavir, ketoconazole, itraconazole) as well as the non-specific CYP inhibitor, cimetidine, is associated with increased plasma levels of sildenafil (see Dosage and Administration).

When a single 100 mg dose of VIAGRA was administered with erythromycin, a specific CYP3A4 inhibitor, at steady state (500 mg b.i.d. for 5 days), there was a 182% increase in sildenafil systemic exposure (AUC).

When the dose of sildenafil for subjects receiving potent CYP3A4 inhibitors was administered as recommended, the maximum free plasma sildenafil concentration did not exceed 200 nM for any individual and was consistently well tolerated.

Cimetidine (800 mg), a cytochrome P450 inhibitor and a non-specific CYP3A4 inhibitor, caused a 56% increase in plasma sildenafil concentrations when co-administered with VIAGRA (50 mg) to healthy volunteers.

Population pharmacokinetic analysis of clinical trial data indicated a reduction in sildenafil clearance when co-administered with CYP3A4 inhibitors (such as ketoconazole, erythromycin, cimetidine). However, there was no increased incidence of adverse events in these patients.

HIV Protease Inhibitor: In addition, coadministration of the HIV protease inhibitor saquinavir, also CYP3A4 inhibitor, at steady state (1200 mg t.i.d) with sildenafil (100 mg single dose) resulted in a 140% increase in sildenafil C_{max} and a 210% increase in sildenafil AUC. Sildenafil had no effect on saquinavir pharmacokinetics. Stronger CYP3A4 inhibitors such as ketoconazole, itraconazole would be expected to have still greater effects (see Dosage and Administration).

Coadministration with the HIV protease inhibitor ritonavir, which is a highly potent P-450 inhibitor, at steady state (500 mg b.i.d) with sildenafil (100 mg single dose) resulted in a 300% (4-fold) increase in sildenafil C_{max} and a 1000% (11-fold) increase in sildenafil plasma AUC. At 24 hours the plasma levels of sildenafil were still approximately 200 ng/mL, compared to approximately 5 ng/mL when sildenafil was dosed alone. This is consistent with the marked effects of ritonavir on a broad range of P-450 substrates. Sildenafil had no effect on ritonavir pharmacokinetics (see Dosage and Administration).

CYP3A4 Inducers: It can be expected that concomitant administration of CYP3A4 inducers, such as rifampin, will decrease plasma levels of sildenafil.

CYP2C9 Substrate: No significant interactions were shown with tolbutamide (single 250 mg dose) or warfarin (single 40 mg dose), both of which are metabolized by CYP2C9, when co-administered with 50 mg sildenafil.

Antacids: In normal healthy male volunteers, co-administration of single doses of antacid (magnesium hydroxide/aluminium hydroxide) with sildenafil did not affect the AUC, C_{max}, elimination rate constant, or subsequent half-life of sildenafil. The T_{max} was reduced by 0.42 hours.

Effect of VIAGRA on Other Drugs: Alpha-blockers: In three specific drug-drug interaction studies, the alpha-blocker doxazosin (4 mg and 8 mg) and sildenafil (25 mg, 50 mg, or 100 mg) were administered simultaneously to patients with benign prostatic hyperplasia (BPH) stabilized on doxazosin therapy. In these study populations, mean additional reductions of supine blood pressure of 7/7 mmHg, 9/5 mmHg, and 8/4 mmHg, and mean additional reductions of standing blood pressure of 6/6 mmHg, 11/4 mmHg, and 4/5 mmHg, for 25 mg, 50 mg, or 100 mg respectively, were observed. When sildenafil and doxazosin were administered simultaneously to patients stabilized on doxazosin therapy, there were infrequent reports of patients who experienced symptomatic postural hypotension. These reports included dizziness and lightheadedness, but not syncope. Concomitant administration of sildenafil to patients taking alpha-blocker therapy may lead to symptomatic hypotension in a few susceptible individuals (see Warnings and Precautions).

Some alpha-blockers and antidepressants have reported priapism or prolonged/painful erections in their labels.

Bleeding Time: VIAGRA (50 mg) did not potentiate the increase in bleeding time, measured using a standard simplate method, caused by acetylsalicylic acid (150 mg).

Use with Other Concomitant Therapies: Antihypertensives: When VIAGRA (100 mg) was co-administered with amlodipine, 5 mg or 10 mg, in hypertensive patients, the mean additional reduction of supine blood pressure was 8 mm Hg systolic and 7 mm Hg diastolic (see Action and Clinical Pharmacology).

Patients on multiple antihypertensive medications were included in the pivotal clinical trials for VIAGRA (sildenafil citrate). Analysis of the safety database was carried out after pooling of the following classes of antihypertensive medication: diuretics, beta-blockers, ACE inhibitors, angiotensin II antagonists, antihypertensive medicinal products (vasodilator and centrally-acting), adrenergic neurone blockers, calcium channel blockers and alpha-adrenoceptor blockers. The analysis showed no differences in the adverse effect profile of patients taking VIAGRA with and without antihypertensive medication.

A large controlled study was performed in men with erectile dysfunction and arterial hypertension who were taking combinations of diuretics, beta blockers, ACE inhibitors and calcium channel blockers. The incidence rate of all adverse events, including those possibly related to hypotensive episodes, was consistent with observations in other patient populations. Also, there was no evidence of an increased incidence rate of any adverse event in the subgroups taking 2 antihypertensive agents and 3 or more antihypertensive agents. There was no indication of additional safety risk of sildenafil use in this subject population.

Drug-Food Interactions: Grapefruit juice being a weak inhibitor of CYP3A4 gut wall metabolism may give rise to modest increases in plasma levels of sildenafil.

VIAGRA (sildenafil citrate) can be taken with or without food. However, when VIAGRA is taken with a high-fat meal, the rate of absorption is reduced with a mean delay in T_{max} of 60 minutes and a mean reduction in C_{max} of 29%. AUC is decreased by 11%. The patient may find that it takes longer to work if taken with a high-fat meal (see Action and Clinical Pharmacology).

DOSAGE AND ADMINISTRATION:

Dosing Considerations: The following factors are associated with increased plasma levels (AUC) of sildenafil:

- age 65 years or over (40%)
- hepatic impairment (e.g. cirrhosis: 84%)
- severe renal impairment (e.g. creatinine clearance <30 mL/min: 100%)
- concomitant use of potent cytochrome P-450 3A4 inhibitors (e.g. erythromycin: 182%; saquinavir: 210%; ritonavir: 1000%). It can also be expected that more potent cytochrome P-450 3A4 inhibitors such as ketoconazole and intraconazole would result in increased levels of sildenafil.

(See Recommended Dose and Dosage Adjustment, Action and Clinical Pharmacology, Warnings and Precautions).

VIAGRA (sildenafil citrate) has been shown to potentiate the hypotensive effects of nitrates in healthy volunteers and in patients, and is therefore contraindicated in patients who are taking any type of nitrate drug therapy, or who utilize short-acting nitrate-containing medications, due to the risk of developing potentially life-threatening hypotension. The use of organic nitrates, either regularly and/or intermittently, in any form (e.g. oral, sublingual, transdermal, by inhalation) is absolutely contraindicated (see Action and Clinical Pharmacology, Contraindications).

Recommended Dose and Dosage Adjustment: For most patients, the recommended dose of VIAGRA is 50 mg taken as needed. The maximum recommended dose is 100 mg. Dosage may be decreased to 25 mg if necessary.

Since higher plasma levels may increase both efficacy and the incidence of adverse events, a starting dose of 25 mg should be considered in patients, age 65 years or over, on concomitant CYPA4 inhibitors, with severe renal impairment, with hepatic impairment and on ritonavir (see Dosing Considerations above, Action and Clinical Pharmacology, Warnings and Precautions).

The concomitant use of the potent cytochrome P-450 3A4 inhibitor, ritonavir is associated with a 1000% (11-fold) increase in plasma levels (AUC) of sildenafil. Given the extent of the interaction with patients receiving concomitant therapy with ritonavir, it is recommended not to exceed a maximum single dose of 25 mg of sildenafil in a 48-hour period (see Warnings and Precautions).

Administration: To be taken as needed approximately 30-60 minutes before sexual activity. However, VIAGRA may be taken anywhere from 0.5 hour to 4 hours before sexual activity. The maximum recommended dosing frequency is once per day.

OVERDOSAGE:

In studies with healthy volunteers of single doses of up to 800 mg, adverse events were similar to those seen at lower doses but incidence rates and severities were increased. In cases of overdose, standard supportive measures should be adopted as required. Renal dialysis is not expected to accelerate clearance as sildenafil is highly bound to plasma proteins and not eliminated in the urine.

Treatment of Priapism: Patients should be instructed to report any erections persisting for more than 4 hours to a physician. The treatment of priapism/prolonged erection should be according to established medical practice. Physicians may refer to two suggested protocols for detumescence presented below.

Detumescence Protocols:

1. Aspirate 40 to 60 mL blood from either left or right corpora using vacutainer and holder for drawing blood. Patient will often detumesce while aspirating. Apply ice for 20 minutes post aspiration if erection remains.

If procedure 1) is unsuccessful, then try procedure 2).

2. Put patient in supine position. Dilute 10 mg phenylephrine into 20 mL distilled water for injection (0.05%). With an insulin syringe, inject 0.1 to 0.2 mL (50-100 µg) into the corpora every 2 to 5 minutes, until the detumescence occurs. The occasional patient may experience transient bradycardia and hypertension when given phenylephrine injections, therefore monitor patient's blood pressure and pulse every 10 minutes. Patients at risk include those with cardiac arrhythmias and diabetes. Refer to the prescribing information for phenylephrine before use. **Do not give phenylephrine to patients on MAO inhibitors.** When phenylephrine is used within the first 12 hours of erection, the majority of patients will respond.

If procedure 2) is unsuccessful, then try procedure 3).

3. If the above measures fail to detumesce the patient, a urologist should be consulted as soon as possible, especially if the erection has been present for many hours. If priapism is not treated immediately, penile tissue damage and/or permanent loss of potency may result.

> For management of a suspected drug overdose, contact your **regional Poison Control Centre**. See the *CPS* Directory section for a list of Poison Control Centres.

ACTION AND CLINICAL PHARMACOLOGY: Mechanism of Action: VIAGRA (sildenafil citrate) is a cGMP-specific phosphodiesterase type 5 (PDE5) inhibitor, used for the treatment of male erectile dysfunction.

The physiological mechanism responsible for erection of the penis involves the release of nitric oxide (NO) in the corpus cavernosum in response to sexual stimulation. Nitric oxide then activates the enzyme guanylate cyclase, which results in increased levels of cyclic guanosine monophosphate (cGMP), producing smooth muscle relaxation in the corpus cavernosum and allowing inflow of blood.

Sildenafil has no direct relaxant effect on isolated human corpus cavernosum, but enhances the effect of NO by inhibiting PDE5, which is responsible for the biodegradation of cGMP in the corpus cavernosum. When sexual stimulation causes local release of NO, inhibition of PDE5 by sildenafil produces increased levels of cGMP in the corpus cavernosum, resulting in smooth muscle relaxation and increased inflow of blood to the corpus cavernosum. Sildenafil, at recommended doses, has no effect in the absence of sexual stimulation.

Studies in vitro have shown that sildenafil has between 10 and 10,000-fold greater selectivity for PDE5 than for other phosphodiesterase isoforms namely PDEs 1, 2, 3, 4, and 6 and greater than 700-fold effect on PDE7-PDE11. In particular, sildenafil has greater than 4,000-fold selectivity for PDE5 over PDE3, the cAMP-specific phosphodiesterase isoform involved in the control of cardiac contractility. Sildenafil is about 10-fold as potent for PDE5 compared to PDE6, an isoenzyme found in the retina; this lower selectivity is thought to be the basis for colour vision abnormalities observed with higher doses or plasma levels of sildenafil (see Warnings and Precautions).

PDE5 is also found in lower concentrations in platelets, vascular and visceral smooth muscles, and skeletal muscle. The sildenafil-induced inhibition of PDE5 in these tissues appears to be the basis for the enhanced platelet antiaggregatory activity of nitric oxide observed in vitro, and inhibition of platelet thrombus formation in vivo, and peripheral arterial-venous dilation in vivo (see Warnings and Precautions).

Pharmacodynamics: Effects of VIAGRA on Blood Pressure (BP): Single oral doses of sildenafil (100 mg) administered to healthy volunteers produced decreases in supine blood pressure (mean maximum decrease of 8.3/5.3 mm Hg). The decrease in blood pressure was most notable approximately 1-2 hours after dosing. The effects are not related to dose or plasma levels. Larger effects were recorded among patients receiving concomitant nitrates (see Contraindications).

Effects of VIAGRA on Cardiac Parameters: Single oral doses of VIAGRA up to 100 mg in healthy volunteers produced no clinically relevant effects on ECG.

Effects of VIAGRA on Erectile Response: VIAGRA was studied in clinical trials of various designs. In fixed-dose clinical trials, 62%, 74%, and 82% of patients on 25 mg, 50 mg and 100 mg of VIAGRA, respectively, reported an improvement in their erections, compared to 25% on placebo (p <0.0001).

In eight double-blind, placebo-controlled, cross-over studies using RigiScan (a device used to objectively measure penile rigidity and duration of erections), erections during sexual stimulation improved significantly on VIAGRA compared to placebo. These studies included patients with organic etiologies (such as spinal cord injury and diabetes mellitus), and patients without an established organic cause. Most studies assessed the efficacy of VIAGRA approximately 60 minutes post-dose.

All eight studies investigating the effects of sildenafil on penile plethysmography (RigiScan) after visual sexual stimulation (VSS) under laboratory conditions, consistently showed that doses of up to 100 mg resulted in statistically significant improvements in duration of erections of 60% rigidity (considered hard enough for penetrative sexual intercourse), compared with placebo. In patients who respond, the median time to onset of erections (60% rigidity) in response to VSS, was 25 minutes after an oral dose of 50 mg sildenafil. The mean total duration of erections 60% rigidity at the base of the penis was 3, 24 and 32 minutes for subjects receiving placebo, 25 mg and 50 mg doses, respectively, when exposed to VSS for 2 hours.

VIAGRA increases couples' ability to have sexual intercourse.

Pharmacokinetics: Absorption: Sildenafil is rapidly absorbed. Maximum observed plasma concentrations are reached within 30 to 120 minutes (median 60 minutes) of oral dosing in the fasted state. The mean absolute bioavailability is 41% (range 25%-63%). The oral pharmacokinetics of VIAGRA is proportional over the recommended dose range studied (25 mg to 100 mg).

Sildenafil inhibits the human PDE5 enzyme in vitro by 50% at a concentration of 3.5 nM. In man, the mean maximum free plasma concentration of sildenafil following a single oral dose of 100 mg is approximately 18 ng/mL, or 38 nM.

When VIAGRA was administered with a high-fat meal, the rate of absorption was significantly decreased, with a 29% reduction in C_{max} and a 60-minute delay in T_{max}. The patient may find that it takes longer to work if taken with a high-fat meal. However, although it was statistically significant (AUC decreased by 11%), the decrease in the extent of absorption was not clinically relevant. The relative bioavailability fed/fasted was 89% (90% CI; 84-94%) (see Drug Interactions).

Distribution: The mean steady state volume of distribution (V_{ss}) for sildenafil is 105 litres, indicating distribution into the tissues. Sildenafil and its major circulating N desmethyl metabolite are both approximately 96% bound to plasma proteins. Protein binding is independent of total drug concentrations.

Based upon measurements of sildenafil in the semen of healthy volunteers, less than 0.001% of the ingested dose may appear in the semen of patients 90 minutes after drug intake.

Metabolism: Sildenafil is cleared predominantly by the CYP3A4 (major route) and CYP2C9 (minor route) hepatic microsomal isoenzymes. The major circulating metabolite results from N-demethylation of sildenafil at the N-methyl piperazine moiety. This metabolite has a PDE selectivity profile similar to sildenafil and an in vitro potency against PDE5 approximately 50% that of the parent drug. Plasma concentrations of this metabolite are approximately 40% of those seen for sildenafil. The N-desmethyl metabolite is further metabolised, with a terminal half-life of approximately 4 hours.

Excretion: The total body clearance of sildenafil is 41 L/h with a resultant terminal phase half-life of 3-5 hours. After either oral or intravenous administration, sildenafil is excreted as metabolites predominantly in the feces (approximately 80% of administered dose) and to a lesser extent in the urine (approximately 13% of the administered dose).

Special Populations and Conditions: Geriatrics: Healthy elderly subjects (65 years or older) had a reduced clearance of sildenafil, resulting in approximately 90% higher plasma concentrations of sildenafil and the active N-desmethyl metabolite compared to those seen in healthy younger volunteers (18-45 years). Due to age-differences in plasma protein binding, the corresponding increase in free sildenafil plasma concentration was approximately 40%.

Hepatic Insufficiency: In volunteers with hepatic cirrhosis (Child-Pugh A and B), sildenafil clearance was reduced, resulting in increases in AUC (85%) and C_{max} (47%) compared to age-matched volunteers with no hepatic impairment. The pharmacokinetics of sildenafil in patients with severe hepatic impairment (Child-Pugh class C) have not been studied.

Since sildenafil clearance is reduced in geriatric patients (65 years or older), patients with renal impairment or patients with hepatic impairment, a starting dose of 25 mg should be considered. Based on efficacy and toleration, the dose may be increased to 50 mg or 100 mg (see Warnings and Precautions, Dosage and Administration).

Renal Insufficiency: In volunteers with mild (CLcr=50-80 mL/min) and moderate (CLcr=30-49 mL/min) renal impairment, the pharmacokinetics of a single oral dose of VIAGRA (50 mg) were not altered. In volunteers with severe (CLcr <30 mL/min) renal impairment, sildenafil clearance was reduced, resulting in increases in AUC (100%) and C_{max} (88%) compared to age-matched volunteers with no renal impairment.

In addition, N-desmethyl metabolite AUC and C_{max} values were significantly increased by 200% and 79% respectively in subjects with severe renal impairment compared to subjects with normal renal function.

STORAGE AND STABILITY: Store at controlled room temperature between 15 and 30°C.

SPECIAL HANDLING INSTRUCTIONS: Not applicable.

INFORMATION FOR THE PATIENT: Published in e-CPS, available by subscription at www.e-cps.ca.

DOSAGE FORMS, COMPOSITION AND PACKAGING: 25 mg: Each blue, round, diamond-shaped tablet marked "PFIZER" on one side and "VGR 25" on the other side, contains: sildenafil citrate equivalent to 25 mg of sildenafil. Nonmedicinal ingredients: anhydrous dibasic calcium phosphate, croscarmellose sodium, FD&C Blue #2 aluminum lake, hypromellose, lactose, magnesium stearate, microcrystalline cellulose, titanium dioxide and triacetin. Blister packs of 4.

50 mg: Each blue, round, diamond-shaped tablet marked "PFIZER" on one side and "VGR 50" on the other side, contains: sildenafil citrate equivalent to 50 mg of sildenafil. Nonmedicinal ingredients: anhydrous dibasic calcium phosphate, croscarmellose sodium, FD&C Blue #2 aluminum lake, hypromellose, lactose, magnesium stearate, microcrystalline cellulose, titanium dioxide and triacetin. Blister packs of 4 and 8.

100 mg: Each blue, round, diamond-shaped tablet marked "PFIZER" on one side and "VGR 100" on the other side, contains: sildenafil citrate equivalent to 100 mg of sildenafil. Nonmedicinal ingredients: anhydrous dibasic calcium phosphate, croscarmellose sodium, FD&C Blue #2 aluminum lake, hypromellose, lactose, magnesium stearate, microcrystalline cellulose, titanium dioxide and triacetin. Blister packs of 4 and 8.

(Shown in Product Identification Section)

Vibramycin Ⓟ

doxycycline hyclate

Antibiotic

Pfizer

Vibra-Tabs™ Ⓟ

doxycycline hyclate

Antibiotic

Pfizer

Date of Revision: March 30, 2010

PHARMACOLOGY: Doxycycline hyclate is a broad-spectrum antibiotic and is active against a wide range of Gram-negative and Gram-positive organisms. Doxycycline exerts its bacteriostatic effect by the inhibition of protein synthesis.

INDICATIONS: VIBRAMYCIN/VIBRA-TABS (doxycycline hyclate) may be indicated for the treatment of:

Pneumonia: Single and multilobe pneumonia and bronchopneumonia due to susceptible strains of *S. pneunomiae* and other Streptococcus spp., Staphylococcus spp., *H. influenzae* and *K. pneumoniae*.
Other Respiratory Tract Infections: Pharyngitis, tonsillitis, sinusitis, otitis media, bronchitis caused by susceptible strains of β-hemolytic Streptococcus, Staphylococcus spp., *S. pneunomiae* and *H. influenzae*.
Genitourinary Tract Infections: Pyelonephritis, cystitis, urethritis caused by susceptible strains of Klebsiella spp., *E. aerogenes*, *E. coli*, Enterococcus spp., Staphylococcus spp., Streptococcus spp. and gonococcal urethritis caused by *N. gonorrhoeae*.

In adult patients with urethritis, cervicitis and vaginitis with a positive test for *C. trachomatis* and/or *U. urealyticum*, clinical resolution and absence of detectable organisms have only been observed at completion of **oral** therapy with VIBRAMYCIN/VIBRA-TABS. Relapses or reinfection can occur. In these cases, limited data suggest that some patients may derive clinical benefit from an alternative therapy. The effect on long term morbidity has not been established.
Skin and Soft Tissue Infections: Impetigo, furunculosis, cellulitis, abscess, wound infections, paronychia, caused by susceptible strains of *S. aureus* and *S. epidermidis*, Streptococcus spp., *E. coli*, Klebsiella spp. and *E. aerogenes*.
Gastro-intestinal Infections: Caused by susceptible strains of Shigella spp., Salmonella spp. and *E. coli*.

Up to 44 percent of strains of *S. pyogenes* and 74 percent of *S. faecalis* have been found to be resistant to tetracycline drugs.

Appropriate culture and susceptibility studies should be carried out prior to initiation of therapy with VIBRAMYCIN/VIBRA-TABS and if clinically indicated during treatment. Consideration may be given to the initiation of therapy before obtaining results of these tests, however modification of such treatment may be required once the results become available.

CONTRAINDICATIONS: VIBRAMYCIN/VIBRA-TABS (doxycycline hyclate) is contraindicated in individuals who have shown hypersensitivity to VIBRAMYCIN/VIBRA-TABS (doxycycline hyclate), and to any of its inert ingredients or to any other tetracycline, and in patients with myasthenia gravis.

WARNINGS: General: VIBRAMYCIN/VIBRA-TABS (doxycycline hyclate) like other tetracyclines, may form a stable calcium complex in any bone-forming tissue, though in vitro it binds calcium less strongly than other tetracyclines. It should be anticipated that the use of VIBRAMYCIN/VIBRA-TABS during tooth development (last trimester of pregnancy, during lactation, neonatal period and early childhood to the age of 8 years) may cause permanent discoloration of the teeth (yellow-gray-brown). Though more commonly associated with long term use of tetracyclines, this effect has also been known to occur after short courses. Enamel hypoplasia has also been reported.

VIBRAMYCIN/VIBRA-TABS should, therefore, not be used in these age groups unless other drugs are unlikely to be effective or are contraindicated.
Carcinogenesis and Mutagenesis: Long-term studies in animals to evaluate carcinogenic potential of doxycycline have not been conducted. However, there has been evidence of oncogenic activity in rats in studies with the related antibiotics, oxytetracycline (adrenal and pituitary tumors) and minocycline (thyroid tumors).

Likewise, although mutagenicity studies of doxycycline have not been conducted, positive results in in-vitro mammalian cell assays have been reported for related antibiotics (tetracycline).
Gastrointestinal: Instances of esophageal lesions (esophagitis and ulcerations), sometimes severe, have been reported in patients receiving doxycycline. The patients must be instructed to take VIBRAMICIN/VIBRA-TABS with a full glass of water, to keep in orthostatic position after the administration and not to go to bed within 1-2 hours after the intake. If symptoms such as dysphagia and retrosternal pain occur, VIBRAMYCIN/VIBRA-TABS should be discontinued and an esophagic lesion must be investigated (see Precautions, Adverse Effects, Dosage and Information for the Patient).

VIBRAMYCIN/VIBRA-TABS should not be prescribed to patients with obstructive esophagic pathology, such as stenosis and achalasia.

C. difficile-associated disease (CDAD) has been reported with use of many antibacterial agents, including VIBRAMYCIN/VIBRA-TABS. CDAD may range in severity from mild diarrhea to fatal colitis. It is important to consider this diagnosis in patients who present with diarrhea, or symptoms of colitis, pseudomembranous colitis, toxic megacolon, or perforation of colon subsequent to the administration of any antibacterial agent. CDAD has been reported to occur over 2 months after the administration of antibacterial agents.

Treatment with antibacterial agents may alter the normal flora of the colon and may permit overgrowth of *C. difficile*. *C. difficile* produces toxins A and B, which contribute to the development of CDAD. CDAD may cause significant morbidity and mortality. CDAD can be refractory to antimicrobial therapy.

If the diagnosis of CDAD is suspected or confirmed, appropriate therapeutic measures should be initiated. Mild cases of CDAD usually respond to discontinuation of antibacterial agents not directed against *C. difficile*. In moderate to severe cases, consideration should be given to management with fluids and electrolytes, protein supplementation, and treatment with an antibacterial agent clinically effective against *C. difficile*. Surgical evaluation should be instituted as clinically indicated, as surgical intervention may be required in certain severe cases. (See Adverse Effects.)
Skin: Photosensitivity manifested by an exaggerated sunburn reaction has been observed in some individuals taking tetracyclines. Patients apt to be exposed to direct sunlight or ultraviolet light should be advised that this reaction can occur with VIBRAMYCIN/VIBRA-TABS, and treatment should be discontinued at the first evidence of skin erythema (see Precautions, Adverse Effects and Information for the Patient). The use of sunscreen or sunblock prior to sun or UV light exposure should be considered in patients taking VIBRAMYCIN/VIBRA-TABS.
Immune: Hypersensitivity adverse drug reactions that included, but not limited to anaphylactic shock, angioneurotic edema, dyspnea, tachycardia, hypotension, pericarditis, urticaria, rash, erythema multiforme, Stevens-Johnson and toxic epidermal necrolysis have been reported with VIBRAMYCIN/VIBRA-TABS use. Some of these reactions were serious. If an allergic reaction occurs, administration of VIBRAMYCIN/VIBRA-TABS should be discontinued and appropriate therapy should be initiated.

VIBRAMYCIN/VIBRA-TABS has been associated with the development of autoimmune adverse drug reactions including exacerbation of systemic lupus erythematosus, rash, peripheral edema, arthralgia, myalgia, serum sickness. If patients with autoimmune reactions are suspected, administration of VIBRAMYCIN/VIBRA-TABS should be discontinued and liver function tests, ANA, CBC, and other appropriate tests should be performed to evaluate the patients.
Renal: The anti-anabolic action of tetracyclines may cause an increase in BUN. Studies to date indicate that this anti-anabolic effect does not occur with the use of doxycycline in patients with impaired renal function.
Pregnancy: VIBRAMYCIN/VIBRA-TABS should not be administered to pregnant women, unless in the judgment of the physician the potential benefit to the mother outweighs the risk to the fetus (see above Warnings about use during tooth development).

Results of animal studies indicate that tetracyclines cross the placenta, are found in fetal tissues, and can have toxic effects on the developing fetus (often related to retardation of skeletal development). Evidence of embryotoxicity has also been noted in animals treated early in pregnancy.
Lactation: Tetracyclines are excreted in the milk of lactating women. Accordingly the use of VIIBRAMYCIN/VIBRA-TABS is not recommended in women while they are breast feeding (see above Warnings about use during tooth development).
Use in Newborns, Infants and Children: The use of VIBRAMYCIN/VIBRA-TABS in children under 8 years is not recommended because safe conditions for its use have not been established (see above Warnings about use during tooth development).

Doxycycline hyclate like other tetracyclines forms a stable calcium complex in any bone-forming tissue. A decrease in the fibula growth rate has been observed in prematures given oral tetracycline in doses of 25 mg/kg every six hours. This reaction was shown to be reversible when the drug was discontinued.

PRECAUTIONS: In clinical studies to date, administration of VIBRAMYCIN/VIBRA-TABS (doxycycline hyclate) did not lead to increased serum levels nor to an increase in the serum half-life of doxycycline in patients with impaired renal function. Modification of VIBRAMYCIN/VIBRA-TABS dosage for these patients is not necessary. Although no evidence of increased toxicity has been observed in such patients, the potential for increased hepatic or other toxicity should be considered until further data on the metabolic fate of doxycycline under these conditions become available.

Concurrent administration of VIBRAMYCIN/VIBRA-TABS with agents known to be hepatotoxic should be avoided.

The use of antibiotics may occasionally result in overgrowth of non-susceptible organisms including fungi; thus, observation of the patient is essential.

Patients should be advised that the use of doxycycline might increase the incidence of vaginal candidiasis (see Adverse Effects and Information for the Patient).

Bulging fontanels in infants and benign intracranial hypertension in adults have been reported in individuals receiving full therapeutic dosages. Although the mechanism of this phenomenon is unknown the signs and symptoms have disappeared rapidly upon cessation of treatment with no sequelae (see Adverse Effects).

Cases of esophageal injury consisting of esophagitis and esophageal ulceration have been reported in patients receiving VIBRAMYCIN/VIBRA-TABS orally. Most of these patients took medication immediately before going to bed and/or without adequate amount of fluid (see Dosage). If this should occur, VIBRAMYCIN/VIBRA-TABS should be discontinued until healing occurs. Administration of antacids and/or cimetidine has provided relief in the treatment of such cases. **To reduce the risk of esophageal injury, patients should be advised to take VIBRAMYCIN capsules or VIBRA-TABS film coated tablets with an adequate amount of fluid while standing or sitting upright.** VIBRAMYCIN/VIBRA-TABS should not be given at bedtime.

In long term therapy with VIBRAMYCIN/VIBRA-TABS, periodic laboratory evaluation of organ systems, including hematopoietic, renal and hepatic studies should be performed. Liver function tests should be carried out at regular intervals on patients receiving high doses for prolonged periods of time.
Drug Interactions: VIBRAMYCIN/VIBRA-TABS should be given with caution to patients receiving oral anticoagulants. Because the tetracyclines have been shown to depress plasma prothrombin activity, patients who are on anticoagulant therapy may require downward adjustment of their anticoagulant dosage.

Antacids containing aluminum, calcium or magnesium impair absorption and should not be given to patients taking VIBRAMYCIN/VIBRA-TABS.

The concurrent use of VIBRAMYCIN/VIBRA-TABS (doxycycline hyclate) with alcohol, barbiturates, phenytoin and carbamazepine (hepatic enzyme inducers) has been reported to result in a reduction of plasma half-life of doxycycline, thereby reducing the antimicrobial effectiveness of VIBRAMYCIN/VIBRA-TABS. This effect may last for several days after discontinuation of therapy with the interacting agent. Therefore, consideration should be given to re-adjustment of the daily dose of VIBRAMYCIN/VIBRA-TABS when administered concomitantly with alcohol and with drugs known to be enzyme inducers.

It has been reported that concurrent administration of ferrous sulphate (iron) lowered serum concentrations of doxycycline given orally and shortened the serum half-life after a single intravenous injection. In the event that iron and iron-containing products have to be given during treatment with VIBRAMYCIN/VIBRA-TABS, the interval between administration of each drug should be as wide as possible.

It has been reported that when subsalicylate bismuth was given simultaneously and as a multiple-dose regimen before oral VIBRAMYCIN/VIBRA-TABS there was a reduced bioavailability of doxycycline. Also peak serum concentrations of doxycycline were significantly decreased when subsalicylate bismuth was given 2 hours before oral VIBRAMYCIN/VIBRA-TABS but not when given 2 hours after oral VIBRAMYCIN/VIBRA-TABS. Therefore subsalicylate bismuth should not be taken during therapy with oral VIBRAMYCIN/VIBRA-TABS.

Since bacteriostatic drugs may interfere with the bactericidal action of penicillin, it is advisable to avoid giving VIBRAMYCIN/VIBRA-TABS, or any other tetracycline, in conjunction with penicillin.

There have been anecdotal reports that concurrent use of tetracyclines may render oral contraceptives less effective.

The concurrent use of tetracycline and Penthrane (methoxyflurane) has been reported to result in fatal renal toxicity.
Drug Laboratory Test Interactions: False elevations of urinary catecholamine levels may occur due to interference with the fluorescence test.

ADVERSE EFFECTS: Gastrointestinal: As with other broad spectrum antibiotics administered orally and parenterally, gastrointestinal disturbances such as anorexia, nausea, vomiting, diarrhea, glossitis, dysphagia, stomatitis, proctitis and enterocolitis, may occur, but have rarely been sufficiently troublesome to warrant discontinuation of therapy with VIBRAMYCIN/VIBRA-TABS (doxycycline hyclate). Abdominal pain, dyspepsia, pseudomembranous colitis, *C. difficile* diarrhea and inflammatory lesions (with monilial overgrowth) in the anogenital region have also been reported. Due to oral doxycycline's virtually complete absorption, side effects of the lower bowel, particularly diarrhea, have been infrequent.

Cases of esophagitis and esophageal ulcerations, sometimes severe, in patients receiving capsule and tablet form of VIBRAMYCIN/VIBRA-TABS (doxycycline hyclate) have been reported (see Warnings, Precautions, Dosage and Information for the Patient).
Autonomic Nervous System: flushing.
Hypersensitivity: Hypersensitivity reactions consisting of urticaria, angioneurotic edema, anaphylaxis, anaphylactic shock, anaphylactoid reaction, anaphylactoid purpura, dyspnea, hypotension, pericarditis, peripheral edema, serum sickness, tachycardia and exacerbation of systemic lupus erythematosus have been reported.
Skin: Maculopapular and erythematous rashes, photosensitivity skin reactions, photo-onycholysis, erythema multiforme, Stevens-Johnson syndrome and Toxic Epidermal Necrolysis have been reported. Exfoliative dermatitis has also been reported but is uncommon (see Warnings).
Musculoskeletal: arthralgia and myalgia.
Central Nervous System: headache, bulging fontanels in infants and benign intracranial hypertension in adults. In relation to benign intracranial hypertension, symptoms included blurring of vision, scotomata and diplopia. Permanent visual loss has been reported (see Precautions).
Liver/Biliary: There have been reports of hepatotoxicity (including hepatic failure, autoimmune hepatitis and cholestasis). As with other tetracyclines, hepatitis, elevation of AST or ALT values have been reported, the significance of which is not known.
Hematologic: hemolytic anemia, thrombocytopenia, neutropenia, eosinophilia, leukopenia.
Hearing/Vestibular: tinnitus.
Investigations (Renal Function Analyses): Elevated BUN (apparently dose related) has been reported.
Urogenital: vaginal candidiasis (see Precautions).
Others: When given over prolonged periods tetracyclines have been reported to produce brown-black microscopic discolouration of the thyroid gland. Abnormalities of thyroid function have not been shown to date.

OVERDOSE:

Symptoms: Specific information on symptoms or treatment of overdosage with VIBRAMYCIN/VIBRA-TABS (doxycycline hyclate) is not available. In case of overdosage, discontinue medication.

Treatment: Treatment, therefore, should be symptomatic and gastric lavage may be considered for overdosage with the oral preparation. Dialysis does not alter serum half-life and thus would not be of benefit in treating cases of overdosage.

> For management of a suspected drug overdose, contact your regional Poison Control Centre. See the *CPS* Directory section for a list of Poison Control Centres.

DOSAGE: Exceeding the recommended dosage may result in an increased incidence of side effects.
Adults: The recommended dosage of oral VIBRAMYCIN/VIBRA-TABS for the majority of susceptible infections is a single loading dose of 200 mg on the first day of treatment followed by a maintenance dosage of 100 mg once daily at the same time each day thereafter.

In the management of more severe infections (particularly chronic infections of the urinary tract), 200 mg should be given daily throughout the treatment period.

Therapy should be continued for at least 24-48 hours after symptoms and fever have subsided. It should be noted, however, that effective antibacterial levels are usually present 24 to 36 hours following discontinuance of VIBRAMYCIN/VIBRA-TABS therapy.

When used in streptococcal infections, therapy should be continued for 10 days to prevent the development of rheumatic fever or glomerulonephritis.

For treatment of uncomplicated acute gonococcal infections, the recommended dosage is 200 mg starting and 100 mg in the evening, the first day, followed by 100 mg b.i.d. for 3 days.

For treatment of uncomplicated urethral, endocervical, or vaginal infections in adults associated with *C. trachomatis* and *U. urealyticum*: 100 mg, by mouth, twice a day for at least 10 days.

No alteration in recommended dosage schedule need be made when treating patients with impaired renal function.
Administration: VIBRAMYCIN Capsules and VIBRA-TABS Film Coated Tablets should be given with or after a meal in order to minimize the possibility of gastric upset. Antacids and iron preparations impair absorption and should not be given concomitantly to patients taking oral VIBRAMYCIN/VIBRA-TABS.

Patients should be advised to take VIBRAMYCIN Capsules and VIBRA-TABS Film Coated Tablets with a full glass of water, to keep in orthostatic position after the administration and not to go to bed within 1-2 hours after the intake.

INFORMATION FOR THE PATIENT: Published in e-CPS, available by subscription at www.e-cps.ca.

SUPPLIED: Vibra-Tabs: Each orange, film-coated tablet contains: doxycycline hyclate equivalent to doxycycline 100 mg. Nonmedicinal ingredients: aluminum hydroxide, ethylcellulose, FD&C Yellow #6, hypromellose, magnesium stearate/sodium lauryl sulfate, microcrystalline cellulose, propylene glycol, talc and titanium dioxide. Plastic bottles (high density polyethylene) of 100. Store at a temperature 15 to 30°C. Protect from light. Dispense in a light resistant container.
Vibramycin Capsules: Each blue, hard gelatin capsule contains: doxycycline hyclate equivalent to doxycycline 100 mg. Nonmedicinal ingredients: magnesium stearate/sodium lauryl sulfate, microcrystalline cellulose; capsule shell: FD&C Blue #1, gelatin, sulfur dioxide and titanium dioxide. Plastic bottles (high density polyethylene) of 50. Store at a temperature 15 to 30°C. Protect from light. Dispense in a light resistant container.

(Shown in Product Identification Section)

Vicks® Children's NyQuil®
chlorpheniramine maleate—dextromethorphan HBr
Antihistamine—Cough Suppressant

Procter & Gamble

SUPPLIED: Each 15 mL contains: chlorpheniramine maleate 2 mg and dextromethorphan hydrobromide 15 mg. Nonmedicinal ingredients: citric acid, FD&C Red No. 40, flavour, potassium sorbate, propylene glycol, purified water, sodium citrate and sucrose. Bottles of 115 mL.

Vicks® Custom Care Body Aches
acetaminophen
Pain Reliever—Fever Reducer

Procter & Gamble

SUPPLIED: Each 15 mL contains: acetaminophen 650 mg. Nonmedicinal ingredients: acesulfame K, carboxymethylcellulose sodium, citric acid, FD&C Red No. 40, flavour, high fructose corn syrup, polyethylene glycol, propylene glycol, purified water, saccharin sodium, sodium benzoate, sodium citrate and sucralose. Bottles of 170 mL.

Vicks® Custom Care Dry Cough
dextromethorphan HBr
Cough Suppressant

Procter & Gamble

SUPPLIED: Each 15 mL contains: dextromethorphan hydrobromide 30 mg. Nonmedicinal ingredients: carboxymethylcellulose sodium, citric acid, FD&C Red No. 40, flavour, high fructose corn syrup, propylene glycol, purified water, saccharin sodium, sodium benzoate and sodium citrate. Bottles of 170 mL.

Vicks® Custom Care Nasal Congestion/Cough
dextromethorphan HBr—phenylephrine HCl
Cough Suppressant—Nasal Decongestant

Procter & Gamble

SUPPLIED: Each 15 mL contains: dextromethorphan hydrobromide 20 mg and phenylephrine hydrochloride 10 mg. Nonmedicinal ingredients: citric acid, FD&C Red No. 40, flavour, glycerin, propylene glycol, purified water, sodium benzoate, sodium carboxymethylcellulose, sodium chloride, sodium saccharin, sorbitol and sucrose. Bottles of 170 mL.

Vicks® DayQuil® Cough
dextromethorphan hydrobromide
Cough Suppressant

Proctor & Gamble

SUPPLIED: Each 30 mL of citrus blend flavoured liquid contains: dextromethorphan hydrobromide 30 mg. Nonmedicinal ingredients: citric acid, D&C Yellow No. 10, FD&C Yellow No. 6, flavour, high fructose corn syrup, polyethylene glycol 400, propylene glycol, purified water, saccharin sodium and sodium citrate. Bottles 295 mL.

Vicks® DayQuil® Liquicaps
dextromethorphan HBr—phenylephrine HCl—acetaminophen
Cough Suppressant—Nasal Decongestant—Pain Reliever—Fever Reducer

Procter & Gamble

Vicks® DayQuil® Liquid
acetaminophen—dextromethorphan HBr—phenylephrine HCl
Pain Reliever—Fever Reducer—Dry Cough Suppressant—Nasal Decongestant

Procter & Gamble

SUPPLIED: Vicks DayQuil Liquicaps: Each liquid-filled capsule contains: dextromethorphan hydrobromide 10 mg, phenylephrine hydrochloride 5 mg and acetaminophen 325 mg. Nonmedicinal ingredients: FD&C Red No. 40, FD&C Yellow No. 6, gelatin, glycerin, polyethylene glycol, povidone, propylene glycol, purified water, sorbitol and titanium dioxide. Cartons of 12 and 20. DayQuil/NyQuil combopacks of 24 and 40.
Vicks DayQuil Liquid: Each 30 mL contains: acetaminophen 650 mg, dextromethorphan hydrobromide 20 mg and phenylephrine hydrochloride 10 mg. Nonmedicinal ingredients: carboxymethylcellulose sodium, citric acid, disodium EDTA, FD&C Yellow No. 6, flavour, glycerin, propylene glycol, purified water, saccharin sodium, sodium benzoate, sodium chloride, sodium citrate, sorbitol and sucralose. Bottles of 175 mL.

Vicks® DayQuil® Mucus Control
guaifenesin
Expectorant

Procter & Gamble

Vicks® DayQuil® Mucus Control DM
guaifenesin—dextromethorphan HBr
Expectorant—Cough Suppressant

Procter & Gamble

Vicks® Custom Care Chest Congestion/Cough
dextromethorphan HBr—guaifenesin
Cough Suppressant—Expectorant

Procter & Gamble

SUPPLIED: Vicks DayQuil Mucus Control: Each 15 mL contains: guaifenesin 200 mg. Nonmedicinal ingredients: carboxymethylcellulose sodium, citric acid, D&C Yellow No. 10, FD&C Yellow No. 6, flavour, high fructose corn syrup, propylene glycol, purified water, saccharin sodium, sodium benzoate and sodium citrate. Bottles of 295 mL.
Vicks DayQuil Mucus Control DM: Each 15 mL contains: guaifenesin 200 mg and dextromethorphan hydrobromide 10 mg. Nonmedicinal ingredients: carboxymethylcellulose sodium, citric acid, D&C Yellow No. 10, FD&C Yellow No. 6, flavor, high fructose corn syrup, propylene glycol, purified water, saccharin sodium, sodium benzoate and sodium citrate. Bottles of 295 mL.
Vicks Custom Care Chest Congestion/Cough: Each 15 mL contains: dextromethorphan hydrobromide 20 mg and guaifenesin 200 mg. Nonmedicinal ingredients: carboxymethylcellulose sodium, citric acid, FD&C Red No. 40, flavour, high fructose corn-syrup, propylene glycol, purified water, saccharin sodium, sodium benzoate and sodium citrate. Bottles of 170 mL.

Vicks® DayQuil® Sinus LiquiCaps
acetaminophen—phenylephrine HCl
Relieves Sinus Pain and Headache—Relieves Nasal and Sinus Congestion

Procter & Gamble

SUPPLIED: Each liquid-filled capsule contains: acetaminophen 325 mg and phenylephrine hydrochloride 5 mg. Nonmedicinal ingredients: FD&C Yellow No. 6, gelatin, glycerin, polyethylene glycol, povidone, propylene glycol, purified water, sorbitol and titanium dioxide. Cartons of 12 and 20. DayQuil/NyQuil combopacks of 24 and 40.

Vicks® NyQuil® Cough Liquid
dextromethorphan hydrobromide—doxylamine succinate
Antihistamine—Cough Suppressant

Proctor & Gamble

SUPPLIED: Each 15 mL of cherry flavour liquid contains: dextromethorphan hydrobromide 15 mg and doxylamine succinate 6.25 mg. Nonmedicinal ingredients: alcohol, citric acid, FD&C Blue No. 1, FD&C Red No. 40, flavour, high fructose corn syrup, polyethylene glycol 400, propylene glycol, purified water, saccharin sodium and sodium citrate. Bottles of 295 mL.

Vicks® NyQuil® Liquicaps
dextromethorphan HBr—doxylamine succinate—acetaminophen
Antihistamine—Cough Suppressant—Pain Reliever—Fever Reducer

Procter & Gamble

Vicks® NyQuil® Liquid
dextromethorphan HBr—doxylamine succinate—acetaminophen
Antihistamine—Cough Suppressant—Pain Reliever—Fever Reducer

Procter & Gamble

SUPPLIED: Vicks NyQuil Liquicaps: Each liquid-filled capsule contains: dextromethorphan hydrobromide 15 mg, doxylamine succinate 6.25 mg and acetaminophen 325 mg. Nonmedicinal ingredients: D&C Yellow No. 10, FD&C Blue No. 1, gelatin, glycerin, polyethylene glycol, povidone, propylene glycol, purified water, sorbitol and titanium dioxide. Cartons of 12 and 20. DayQuil/NyQuil combopacks of 24 and 40.
Vicks NyQuil Liquid: Original: Each 30 mL contains: dextromethorphan hydrobromide 30 mg, doxylamine succinate 12.5 mg and acetaminophen 1000 mg. Nonmedicinal ingredients: alcohol, anethole, citric acid, D&C Yellow No. 10, FD&C Green No. 3, FD&C Yellow No. 6, high fructose corn syrup, polyethylene glycol, propylene glycol, purified water, saccharin sodium and sodium citrate. Bottles of 175 mL.
Cherry: Each 30 mL contains: dextromethorphan hydrobromide 30 mg, doxylamine succinate 12.5 mg and acetaminophen 1000 mg. Nonmedicinal ingredients: alcohol, citric acid, FD&C Blue No. 1, FD&C Red No. 40, flavour, high fructose corn syrup, polyethylene glycol, propylene glycol, purified water, saccharin sodium and sodium citrate. Bottles of 175 mL.

Vicks® NyQuil® Sinus LiquiCaps
acetaminophen—doxylamine succinate—phenylephrine HCl
Relieves Sinus Pain and Headache—Relieves Nasal and Sinus Congestion—Relieves Runny Nose and Sneezing

Procter & Gamble

SUPPLIED: Each liquid-filled capsule contains: acetaminophen 325 mg, doxylamine succinate 6.25 mg and phenylephrine hydrochloride 5 mg. Nonmedicinal ingredients: FD&C Blue No. 1, gelatin, glycerine, polyethylene glycol, povidone, propylene glycol, purified water, sorbitol and titanium dioxide. Cartons of 12 and 20. DayQuil/NyQuil combopacks of 24 and 40.

Vicks® VapoDrops
menthol
Throat Irritations

Procter & Gamble

SUPPLIED: Menthol: Each drop contains: 0.163% menthol. Nonmedicinal ingredients: ascorbic acid, caramel, corn syrup, eucalyptus oil and sucrose. Cartons of 20.
Lemon: Each drop contains: 0.064% menthol. Nonmedicinal ingredients: ascorbic acid, citric acid, corn syrup, FD&C Yellow No. 5 (contains tartrazine), flavour and sucrose. Cartons of 20.
Cherry: Each drop contains: 0.0834% menthol. Nonmedicinal ingredients: ascorbic acid, citric acid, corn syrup, eucalyptus oil, FD&C Blue No. 1, FD&C Red No. 40, flavour and sucrose. Cartons of 20.

Vicks® VapoRub®
camphor—menthol—eucalyptus
Nasal Decongestant—Cough Suppressant

Procter & Gamble

Vicks® Vapour Inhaler
camphor—menthol
Nasal Decongestant

Procter & Gamble

SUPPLIED: Vicks VapoRub: Each mL of ointment contains: 4.73% camphor, 2.6% menthol and 1.2% eucalyptus. Nonmedicinal ingredients: cedarleaf oil, myristica oil, special petrolatum, thymol and turpentine oil. Jars of 57, 115 and 190 mL.
Vicks Vapour Inhaler: Each mL of vapour contains: 41.53% camphor and 41.53% menthol. Nonmedicinal ingredients: abies sibirica oil and methyl salicylate. Tubes of 0.20 mL.

Vicks® Vitamin C Orange Drops
ascorbic acid
Vitamin

Procter & Gamble

SUPPLIED: Each vitamin C drop contains: ascorbic acid 25 mg. Nonmedicinal ingredients: citric acid, corn syrup, FD&C Yellow No. 6, flavour and sucrose. Cartons of 20.

Victoza® Ⓟ
liraglutide
Human Glucagon Like Peptide-1 (GLP-1)

Novo Nordisk

Date of Preparation: May 21, 2010
SUMMARY PRODUCT INFORMATION:

Route of Administration	Dosage Form/ Strength	Clinically Relevant Nonmedicinal Ingredients
Subcutaneous	Injectable, 6 mg/mL	Disodium phosphate dihydrate, propylene glycol, phenol and water for injections. For a complete listing see Dosage Forms, Composition and Packaging.

DESCRIPTION: VICTOZA contains liraglutide, an analog of human GLP-1 and acts as a GLP-1 receptor agonist. The peptide precursor of liraglutide, produced by a process that includes expression of recombinant DNA in *S. cerevisiae*, has been engineered to be 97% homologous to native human GLP-1 by substituting arginine for lysine at position 34. Liraglutide is made by attaching a C-16 fatty acid (palmitic acid) with a glutamic acid spacer on the remaining lysine residue at position 26 of the peptide precursor.

VICTOZA is a clear, colorless solution. Each 1 mL of VICTOZA solution contains 6 mg of liraglutide. Each pre-filled pen contains a 3 mL solution of VICTOZA equivalent to 18 mg liraglutide (free-base, anhydrous).

INDICATIONS AND CLINICAL USE: VICTOZA is indicated for once-daily administration for the treatment of adults with type 2 diabetes to improve glycemic control in combination with:
- Metformin, when diet and exercise plus maximal tolerated dose of metformin do not achieve adequate glycemic control.
- Metformin and a sulfonylurea, when diet and exercise plus dual therapy with metformin and a sulfonylurea do not achieve adequate glycemic control.

VICTOZA should not be used in Type 1 diabetes (formerly known as insulin-dependent diabetes mellitus or IDDM).

Geriatrics (>65 years of age): No difference in effectiveness was observed in clinical trial subjects ≥65 years of age. Patients >70 years may experience more gastrointestinal side effects when treated with VICTOZA. Therapeutic experience in patients ≥75 years of age is limited. (See Warnings and Precautions, Special Populations, Geriatrics (>65 years of age); Adverse Reactions, Adverse Drug Reaction Overview; Clinical Trial Adverse Drug Reactions, Gastrointestinal Adverse Events; and Dosage and Administration, Recommended Dose and Dosage Adjustment, Geriatrics (>65 years of age).)

Pediatrics (<18 years of age): The safety and efficacy of VICTOZA have not been studied in pediatric populations. VICTOZA is not indicated for use in pediatric patients (see Warnings and Precautions, Special Populations, Pediatrics (<18 years of age)).

CONTRAINDICATIONS:
- In patients with a personal or family history of medullary thyroid carcinoma or in patients with Multiple Endocrine Neoplasia syndrome type 2 (MEN 2).
- VICTOZA is contraindicated in patients who are hypersensitive to liraglutide or to any ingredient in the formulation. For a complete listing, see Dosage Forms, Composition and Packaging.
- In pregnancy or breast-feeding women.

WARNINGS AND PRECAUTIONS:

Serious Warnings and Precautions
Risk of Thyroid C-cell Tumours:
- Liraglutide causes dose-dependent and treatment-duration-dependent thyroid C-cell tumours at clinically relevant exposures in both genders of rats and mice. It is unknown whether VICTOZA causes thyroid C-cell tumours, including medullary thyroid carcinoma (MTC), in humans, as human relevance could not be ruled out by clinical or nonclinical studies.
- VICTOZA is contraindicated in patients with a personal or family history of MTC and in patients with Multiple Endocrine Neoplasia syndrome type 2 (MEN 2). Based on the findings in rodents, monitoring with serum calcitonin or thyroid ultrasound was performed during clinical trials, but this may have increased the number of unnecessary thyroid surgeries. It is unknown whether monitoring with serum calcitonin or thyroid ultrasound will mitigate human risk of thyroid C-cell tumours. Patients should be counselled regarding the risk and symptoms of thyroid tumours (see Contraindications, Warnings and Precautions and Adverse Reactions).

Carcinogenesis and Mutagenesis: Risk of Thyroid C-Cell Tumors: VICTOZA causes dose-dependent and treatment-duration-dependent thyroid C-cell tumors (adenomas and/or carcinomas) at clinically relevant exposures in both genders of rats and mice. Malignant thyroid C-cell carcinomas were detected in rats and mice. A statistically significant increase in cancer was observed in rats receiving liraglutide at 8-times clinical exposure compared to controls. It is unknown whether VICTOZA will cause thyroid C-cell tumors, including medullary thyroid carcinoma (MTC), in humans, as the human relevance of liraglutide-induced rodent thyroid C-cell tumors could not be determined by clinical or nonclinical studies.

In the clinical trials, there have been 4 reported cases of thyroid C-cell hyperplasia among VICTOZA treated patients and 1 case in a comparator-treated patient (1.3 vs 0.6 cases per 1000 subject-years). Two additional cases of thyroid C-cell hyperplasia in VICTOZA treated patients and 1 case of MTC in a comparator-treated patient have subsequently been reported. This comparator-treated patient with MTC had pre-treatment serum calcitonin concentrations >1000 ng/L suggesting pre-existing disease. All of these cases were diagnosed after thyroidectomy, which was prompted by abnormal results on routine, protocol-specified measurements of serum calcitonin. Four of the five liraglutide-treated patients had elevated calcitonin concentrations at baseline and throughout the trial. One liraglutide and one nonliraglutide-treated patient developed elevated calcitonin concentrations while on treatment. (See Adverse Reactions, Clinical Trial Adverse Drug Reactions.)

Counsel patients regarding the risk for MTC and the symptoms of thyroid tumors (e.g. a mass in the neck, dysphagia, dyspnea or persistent hoarseness). It is unknown whether monitoring with serum calcitonin or thyroid ultrasound will mitigate the potential risk of MTC, and such monitoring may increase the risk of unnecessary procedures, due to low test specificity for serum calcitonin and a high background incidence of thyroid disease. Patients with thyroid nodules noted on physical examination or neck imaging obtained for other reasons should be referred to an endocrinologist for further evaluation. Although routine monitoring of serum calcitonin is of uncertain value in patients treated with VICTOZA, if serum calcitonin is measured and found to be elevated, the patient should be referred to an endocrinologist for further evaluation. (See Adverse Reactions, Adverse Drug Reaction Overview and Clinical Trial Adverse Drug Reactions.)

Cardiovascular: Increase in Heart Rate: A 24 h time-averaged increase in mean heart rate of 7-8 bpm was reported with VICTOZA treatment in a clinical trial in healthy volunteers undergoing serial ECG monitoring (see Action and Clinical Pharmacology, Cardiac Electrophysiology). In patients with diabetes, a 2-4 bpm increase in mean pulse rate was observed in long term clinical trials. Because of limited clinical experience in patients who have cardiac conditions that might be worsened by an increase in heart rate, such as ischemic heart disease and tachyarrhythmia, caution should be observed in these patients (see Drug Interactions). The incidence of a composite endpoint for all tachyarrhythmia in pooled clinical trials in diabetic patients was higher for VICTOZA than for placebo (see Adverse Reactions, Cardiovascular).

PR Interval Prolongation: A prolongation of the mean PR interval of up to 10 ms was reported with VICTOZA treatment in a clinical trial in healthy volunteers (see Action and Clinical Pharmacology, Cardiac Electrophysiology). In healthy volunteers and in patients with diabetes, the incidence of first degree atrioventricular (AV) block was higher with VICTOZA than with placebo (see Action and Clinical Pharmacology, Cardiac Electrophysiology; Adverse Reactions, Cardiovascular). The clinical significance of these changes is not fully known; however, because of limited clinical experience in patients with pre-existing conduction system abnormalities (e.g., marked first-degree AV block or second- or third-degree AV block) and heart rhythm disturbances (e.g., tachyarrhythmia), caution should be observed in these patients (see Drug Interactions).

General: VICTOZA should not be used in patients with type 1 diabetes mellitus or for the treatment of diabetic ketoacidosis. VICTOZA should not be administered intravenously or intramuscularly.

Endocrine and Metabolism: Hypoglycemia: Patients receiving VICTOZA in combination with a sulfonylurea may have an increased risk of hypoglycemia. In the clinical trials of at least 26 weeks duration, major hypoglycemia requiring the assistance of another person for treatment occurred in 7 VICTOZA treated patients and in no comparator-treated patients. Six of these 7 patients treated with VICTOZA were also taking a sulfonylurea (see Adverse Reaction, Hypoglycemia). The risk of hypoglycemia can be lowered by reducing the dose of sulfonylurea.

Pancreatitis: In clinical trials conducted in adult patients with type 2 diabetes, very rare cases of pancreatitis were reported more frequently in the VICTOZA treated group than in the comparator treated group (2.2 vs 0.6 cases per 1000 subject-years). In the VICTOZA treated group one fatal case of necrotizing pancreatitis was observed (see Adverse Reactions, Pancreatitis). The causality relationship to VICTOZA is unclear. After initiation of VICTOZA and after dose increases, observe patients carefully for signs and symptoms of pancreatitis (including persistent severe abdominal pain, sometimes radiating to the back and which may or may not be accompanied by vomiting). If pancreatitis is suspected, VICTOZA and other potentially suspect medications should be discontinued promptly, confirmatory tests should be performed and appropriate management should be initiated. If pancreatitis is confirmed, VICTOZA should not be restarted. Use with caution in patients with a history of pancreatitis.

Special Populations: Pregnant Women: There have been no studies conducted in pregnant women with VICTOZA. Studies in animals have shown reproductive and developmental toxicity, including teratogenicity, at or above 0.8 times the clinical exposure.

VICTOZA should not be used during pregnancy (see Contraindications). If a patient wishes to become pregnant, or pregnancy occurs, treatment with liraglutide should be discontinued.

Nursing Women: It is not known whether VICTOZA is excreted in human milk. In lactating animals VICTOZA was excreted unchanged in milk. Because many drugs are excreted in human milk and because of the potential for tumorigenicity shown for liraglutide in animal studies, women who are nursing should discontinue VICTOZA treatment.

Pediatrics (<18 years of age): The safety and efficacy of VICTOZA in pediatric patients has not been studied. VICTOZA is not indicated in pediatric type 2 diabetes patients.

Geriatrics (>65 years of age): In the VICTOZA clinical trials, a total of 797 (20%) of the patients were 65 years of age and over, of which 113 (2.8%) were 75 years of age and over. No differences in effectiveness were observed between subjects 65 years and over and younger subjects in the clinical studies. Patients >70 years experienced more gastrointestinal side effects when treated with VICTOZA. (See Adverse Reactions, Adverse Drug Reaction Overview; Clinical Trial Adverse Drug Reactions, Gastrointestinal Adverse Events; Dosage and Administration, Recommended Dose and Dosage Adjustment, Geriatrics (>65 years of age) and Action and Clinical Pharmacology, Special Populations and Conditions, Geriatrics (>65 years of age).)

Cardiovascular—Patients with Recent MI, Unstable Angina and Congestive Heart Failure: In clinical trials of VICTOZA, subjects with clinically significant heart disease, acute myocardial infarction within 6 months, unstable angina pectoris and congestive heart failure (NYHA, class III to IV) were not studied. Therefore, VICTOZA should be used with caution in this population.

Hepatic Insufficiency: The safety and efficacy of VICTOZA in patients with hepatic insufficiency has not been studied. The use of VICTOZA in patients with hepatic insufficiency is not recommended.

Renal Insufficiency: There is limited clinical experience with VICTOZA in patients with mild renal insufficiency. There is very limited or no clinical experience in patients with moderate and severe renal insufficiency, including end-stage renal disease; use of VICTOZA in these patients is not recommended (see Dosage and Administration, Recommended Dose and Dosage Adjustment, Renal Insufficiency and Action and Clinical Pharmacology, Special Populations and Conditions, Renal Insufficiency).

Patients treated with VICTOZA should be advised of the potential risk of dehydration in relation to gastrointestinal side effects and take precautions to avoid fluid depletion.

Gastrointestinal Disease: The use of VICTOZA is associated with transient gastrointestinal adverse reactions, including nausea, vomiting and diarrhea (see Adverse Reactions, Adverse Drug Reaction Overview and Clinical Trial Adverse Drug Reactions, Gastrointestinal Adverse Events). The safety of VICTOZA in subjects with inflammatory bowel disease and diabetic gastroparesis has not been studied. VICTOZA should not be used in this population.

Monitoring and Laboratory Tests: Regular self-monitoring of blood glucose is not needed in order to adjust the dose of VICTOZA. However, when initiating treatment with VICTOZA in combination with a sulfonylurea blood glucose self-monitoring may become necessary to reduce the dose of the sulfonylurea in order to reduce the risk of hypoglycemia.

However, patients should be informed that response to all diabetic therapies should be monitored by periodic measurement of A1C levels, with a goal of decreasing these levels towards the normal range. A1C is especially useful for evaluating long-term glycemic control.

ADVERSE REACTIONS: Adverse Drug Reaction Overview: In long term clinical trials, the most common adverse drug reactions were gastrointestinal disorders, infections and nervous system disorders. Discontinuation of treatment due to adverse events was most common with VICTOZA (7.8%) as compared to comparator treatments (3.4%). The difference was driven by withdrawals due to gastrointestinal disorders.

Serious adverse events occurred in a similar proportion of patients treated with VICTOZA (5.7%) as compared to other study treatments (5.6%), most commonly cardiac disorders (19.6 vs 18.9 events per 1000 patient years respectively).

Clinical Trial Adverse Drug Reactions: Because clinical trials are conducted under very specific conditions the adverse drug reaction rates observed in the clinical trials may not reflect the rates observed in practice and should not be compared to the rates in the clinical trials of another drug. Adverse drug reaction information from clinical trials is useful for identifying drug-related adverse events and for approximating rates.

Table 1 provides a listing of the treatment-emergent adverse events with frequency ≥1% from two 26 week combination trials 1572 and 1697 regardless of investigator assessment of causality. The two 26 week controlled clinical studies of VICTOZA were LEAD 2-1572 for add on combination therapy with metformin and LEAD 5-1697 for add on combination therapy with metformin + sulfonylurea.

Medullary Thyroid Cancer: Calcitonin was measured throughout the clinical development program. The serum calcitonin assay used in the VICTOZA clinical trials had a lower limit of quantification (LLOQ) of 0.7 ng/L and the upper normal limit of the reference range was 5.0 ng/L for women and 8.4 ng/L for men. At Weeks 26 and 52 in the clinical trials, adjusted mean serum calcitonin concentrations were higher in patients treated with VICTOZA compared to patients treated with placebo but not compared to patients receiving active comparator. At these timepoints, the adjusted mean serum calcitonin values (~1.0 ng/L) were just above the LLOQ with between-group differences in adjusted mean serum calcitonin values of approximately 0.1 ng/L or less. Among patients with pre-treatment serum calcitonin below the upper limit of the reference range, shifts to above the upper limit of the reference range which persisted in subsequent measurements occurred most frequently among patients treated with VICTOZA 1.8 mg/day.

In trials with on-treatment serum calcitonin measurements up to 5-6 months, 1.9% of patients treated with VICTOZA 1.8 mg/day developed new and persistent calcitonin elevations above the upper limit of the reference range compared to 0.8-1.1% of patients treated with control medication or the 0.6 and 1.2 mg doses of VICTOZA. In trials with on-treatment serum calcitonin measurements up to 12 months, 1.3% of patients treated with VICTOZA 1.8 mg/day had new and persistent elevations of calcitonin from below or within the reference range to above the upper limit of the reference range, compared to 0.6%, 0% and 1.0% of patients treated with VICTOZA 1.2 mg, placebo and active control, respectively. VICTOZA did not produce consistent dose-dependent or time-dependent increases in serum calcitonin.

Table 1: VICTOZA

Treatment-Emergent Adverse Events from Two 26 Week Combination Trials 1572 and 1697

	Trial 1572 (LEAD 2)					Trial 1697 (LEAD 5)		
	VICTOZA 0.6 mg + metformin	VICTOZA 1.2 mg + metformin	VICTOZA 1.8 mg + metformin	Placebo + metformin	Active Comparator (metformin + glimepiride)	VICTOZA 1.8 mg + metformin + glimepiride	Placebo + metformin + glimepiride	Active Comparator (insulin glargine + metformin + glimepiride)
	N (%)	N (%)	N (%)	N (%)	N (%)	N (%)	N (%)	N (%)
Safety Analysis Set	242	240	242	121	242	230	114	232
Blood and Lymphatic System Disorders								
Anemia	4 (1.7)	1 (0.4)	1 (0.4)	0 (0.0)	2 (0.8)	1 (0.4)	0 (0.0)	0 (0.0)
Ear and Labyrinth Disorders								
Vertigo	1 (0.4)	1 (0.4)	3 (1.2)	0 (0.0)	2 (0.8)	3 (1.3)	0 (0.0)	1 (0.4)
Motion sickness	1 (0.4)	1 (0.4)	0 (0.0)	0 (0.0)	2 (0.8)	0 (0.0)	2 (1.8)	0 (0.0)
Eye Disorders								
Diabetic retinopathy	5 (2.1)	4 (1.7)	5 (2.1)	1 (0.8)	8 (3.3)	2 (0.9)	3 (2.6)	4 (1.7)
Cataract	3 (1.2)	2 (0.8)	3 (1.2)	2 (1.7)	1 (0.4)	1 (0.4)	0 (0.0)	2 (0.9)
Conjunctivitis	0 (0.0)	3 (1.3)	2 (0.8)	1 (0.8)	0 (0.0)	0 (0.0)	0 (0.0)	0 (0.0)
Arteriosclerotic retinopathy	0 (0.0)	1 (0.4)	0 (0.0)	2 (1.7)	2 (0.8)	0 (0.0)	0 (0.0)	0 (0.0)
Injury, Poisoning and Procedural Complications								
Soft tissue injury	0 (0.0)	0 (0.0)	0 (0.0)	0 (0.0)	3 (1.2)	0 (0.0)	0 (0.0)	0 (0.0)
Fall	1 (0.4)	1 (0.4)	0 (0.0)	0 (0.0)	2 (0.8)	0 (0.0)	2 (1.8)	1 (0.4)
Gastrointestinal Disorders								
Nausea	26 (10.7)	39 (16.3)	45 (18.6)	5 (4.1)	8 (3.3)	32 (13.9)	4 (3.5)	3 (1.3)
Diarrhea	23 (9.5)	20 (8.3)	36 (14.9)	5 (4.1)	9 (3.7)	23 (10.0)	6 (5.3)	3 (1.3)
Vomiting	13 (5.4)	16 (6.7)	18 (7.4)	1 (0.8)	1 (0.4)	15 (6.5)	4 (3.5)	1 (0.4)
Dyspepsia	9 (3.7)	5 (2.1)	17 (7.0)	1 (0.8)	3 (1.2)	15 (6.5)	1 (0.9)	4 (1.7)
Gastritis	8 (3.3)	6 (2.5)	12 (5.0)	1 (0.8)	2 (0.8)	3 (1.3)	0 (0.0)	1 (0.4)
Abdominal pain upper	5 (2.1)	7 (2.9)	8 (3.3)	0 (0.0)	3 (1.2)	10 (4.3)	2 (1.8)	2 (0.9)
Toothache	2 (0.8)	6 (2.5)	3 (1.2)	5 (4.1)	2 (0.8)	5 (2.2)	0 (0.0)	3 (1.3)
Abdominal pain	2 (0.8)	4 (1.7)	6 (2.5)	2 (1.7)	1 (0.4)	2 (0.9)	1 (0.9)	1 (0.4)
Constipation	5 (2.1)	11 (4.6)	6 (2.5)	2 (1.7)	4 (1.7)	5 (2.2)	0 (0.0)	2 (0.9)
Abdominal discomfort	3 (1.2)	2 (0.8)	3 (1.2)	0 (0.0)	2 (0.8)	3 (1.3)	2 (1.8)	1 (0.4)
Abdominal distension	2 (0.8)	2 (0.8)	2 (0.8)	0 (0.0)	4 (1.7)	3 (1.3)	1 (0.9)	1 (0.4)
Epigastric discomfort	2 (0.8)	2 (0.8)	3 (1.2)	0 (0.0)	0 (0.0)	0 (0.0)	0 (0.0)	0 (0.0)
Gastrointestinal disorder	2 (0.8)	2 (0.8)	3 (1.2)	0 (0.0)	0 (0.0)	2 (0.9)	0 (0.0)	0 (0.0)
Gastroesophageal reflux disease	4 (1.7)	2 (0.8)	1 (0.4)	0 (0.0)	0 (0.0)	1 (0.4)	0 (0.0)	0 (0.0)
General Disorders and Administration Site Conditions								
Fatigue	3 (1.2)	5 (2.1)	6 (2.5)	2 (1.7)	3 (1.2)	1 (0.4)	0 (0.0)	0 (0.0)
Asthenia	2 (0.8)	2 (0.8)	3 (1.2)	0 (0.0)	3 (1.2)	1 (0.4)	1 (0.9)	0 (0.0)
Influenza like illness	2 (0.8)	0 (0.0)	0 (0.0)	1 (0.8)	3 (1.2)	1 (0.4)	1 (0.9)	0 (0.0)
Early satiety	1 (0.4)	3 (1.3)	1 (0.4)	0 (0.0)	0 (0.0)	1 (0.4)	0 (0.0)	0 (0.0)
Chest pain	0 (0.0)	3 (1.3)	0 (0.0)	0 (0.0)	2 (0.8)	0 (0.0)	1 (0.9)	1 (0.4)
Pyrexia	1 (0.4)	3 (1.3)	0 (0.0)	0 (0.0)	1 (0.4)	5 (2.2)	1 (0.9)	5 (2.2)
Hepatobiliary Disorders								
Hepatic steatosis	6 (2.5)	2 (0.8)	1 (0.4)	0 (0.0)	4 (1.7)	0 (0.0)	0 (0.0)	0 (0.0)
Immune System Disorders								
Seasonal allergy	2 (0.8)	3 (1.3)	0 (0.0)	0 (0.0)	2 (0.8)	0 (0.0)	0 (0.0)	0 (0.0)
Infections and Infestations								
Nasopharyngitis	27 (11.2)	21 (8.8)	21 (8.7)	11 (9.1)	30 (12.4)	21 (9.1)	10 (8.8)	26 (11.2)
Influenza	5 (2.1)	1 (0.4)	8 (3.3)	2 (1.7)	8 (3.3)	2 (0.9)	5 (4.4)	8 (3.4)

(cont'd)

Table 1: VICTOZA *(cont'd)*

Treatment-Emergent Adverse Events from Two 26 Week Combination Trials 1572 and 1697

	Trial 1572 (LEAD 2)					Trial 1697 (LEAD 5)		
	VICTOZA 0.6 mg + metformin	VICTOZA 1.2 mg + metformin	VICTOZA 1.8 mg + metformin	Placebo + metformin	Active Comparator (metformin + glimepiride)	VICTOZA 1.8 mg + metformin + glimepiride	Placebo + metformin + glimepiride	Active Comparator (insulin glargine + metformin + glimepiride)
	N (%)	N (%)	N (%)	N (%)	N (%)	N (%)	N (%)	N (%)
Pharyngitis	2 (0.8)	2 (0.8)	2 (0.8)	0 (0.0)	1 (0.4)	2 (0.9)	5 (4.4)	2 (0.9)
Upper respiratory tract infection	4 (1.7)	8 (3.3)	5 (2.1)	3 (2.5)	3 (1.2)	2 (0.9)	0 (0.0)	2 (0.9)
Acute tonsillitis	1 (0.4)	0 (0.0)	0 (0.0)	0 (0.0)	1 (0.4)	1 (0.4)	0 (0.0)	3 (1.3)
Lower respiratory tract infection	0 (0.0)	0 (0.0)	0 (0.0)	1 (0.8)	1 (0.4)	1 (0.4)	1 (0.9)	3 (1.3)
Bronchitis	5 (2.1)	9 (3.8)	4 (1.7)	1 (0.8)	9 (3.7)	7 (3.0)	1 (0.9)	3 (1.3)
Respiratory tract infection	0 (0.0)	0 (0.0)	4 (1.7)	0 (0.0)	1 (0.4)	0 (0.0)	1 (0.9)	1 (0.4)
Gastroenteritis	6 (2.5)	4 (1.7)	3 (1.2)	2 (1.7)	4 (1.7)	3 (1.3)	1 (0.9)	3 (1.3)
Urinary tract infection	3 (1.2)	5 (2.1)	3 (1.2)	3 (2.5)	3 (1.2)	3 (1.3)	2 (1.8)	3 (1.3)
Tooth abscess	0 (0.0)	0 (0.0)	3 (1.2)	1 (0.8)	1 (0.4)	0 (0.0)	0 (0.0)	1 (0.4)
Pneumonia	1 (0.4)	3 (1.3)	2 (0.8)	1 (0.8)	3 (1.2)	0 (0.0)	2 (1.8)	3 (1.3)
Onychomycosis	3 (1.2)	1 (0.4)	1 (0.4)	0 (0.0)	1 (0.4)	0 (0.0)	0 (0.0)	0 (0.0)
Sinusitis	4 (1.7)	4 (1.7)	1 (0.4)	0 (0.0)	2 (0.8)	0 (0.0)	2 (1.8)	3 (1.3)
Viral infection	2 (0.8)	1 (0.4)	1 (0.4)	0 (0.0)	1 (0.4)	3 (1.3)	1 (0.9)	2 (0.9)
Investigations								
Weight decreased	0 (0.0)	2 (0.8)	4 (1.7)	0 (0.0)	0 (0.0)	0 (0.0)	0 (0.0)	0 (0.0)
Blood creatine phosphokinase increased	2 (0.8)	3 (1.3)	2 (0.8)	1 (0.8)	4 (1.7)	2 (0.9)	0 (0.0)	0 (0.0)
Blood calcitonin increased	3 (1.2)	1 (0.4)	1 (0.4)	3 (2.5)	2 (0.8)	3 (1.3)	0 (0.0)	0 (0.0)
Urine albumin/creatinine ratio increased	2 (0.8)	1 (0.4)	0 (0.0)	2 (1.7)	1 (0.4)	1 (0.4)	0 (0.0)	0 (0.0)
Blood pressure increased	0 (0.0)	1 (0.4)	0 (0.0)	2 (1.7)	0 (0.0)	0 (0.0)	0 (0.0)	0 (0.0)
Metabolism and Nutrition Disorders								
Anorexia	6 (2.5)	10 (4.2)	14 (5.8)	1 (0.8)	1 (0.4)	10 (4.3)	1 (0.9)	0 (0.0)
Decreased appetite	4 (1.7)	14 (5.8)	10 (4.1)	0 (0.0)	0 (0.0)	2 (0.9)	1 (0.9)	0 (0.0)
Dyslipidemia	2 (0.8)	2 (0.8)	2 (0.8)	2 (1.7)	2 (0.8)	3 (1.3)	3 (2.6)	1 (0.4)
Hyperlipidaemia	1 (0.4)	1 (0.4)	1 (0.4)	3 (2.5)	3 (1.2)	1 (0.4)	1 (0.9)	2 (0.9)
Hyperglycaemia	1 (0.4)	0 (0.0)	1 (0.4)	3 (2.5)	0 (0.0)	2 (0.9)	0 (0.0)	0 (0.0)
Musculoskeletal and Connective Tissue Disorders								
Back pain	7 (2.9)	5 (2.1)	6 (2.5)	4 (3.3)	9 (3.7)	7 (3.0)	3 (2.6)	8 (3.4)
Arthralgia	6 (2.5)	0 (0.0)	3 (1.2)	3 (2.5)	7 (2.9)	4 (1.7)	3 (2.6)	6 (2.6)
Muscle spasms	5 (2.1)	0 (0.0)	2 (0.8)	3 (2.5)	3 (1.2)	2 (0.9)	3 (2.6)	3 (1.3)
Pain in extremity	0 (0.0)	2 (0.8)	7 (2.9)	1 (0.8)	2 (0.8)	1 (0.4)	1 (0.9)	0 (0.0)
Musculoskeletal pain	3 (1.2)	1 (0.4)	3 (1.2)	3 (2.5)	1 (0.4)	3 (1.3)	2 (1.8)	4 (1.7)
Osteoarthritis	3 (1.2)	1 (0.4)	1 (0.4)	2 (1.7)	2 (0.8)	0 (0.0)	1 (0.9)	2 (0.9)
Myalgia	1 (0.4)	3 (1.3)	4 (1.7)	2 (1.7)	4 (1.7)	0 (0.0)	1 (0.9)	3 (1.3)
Neck pain	1 (0.4)	1 (0.4)	0 (0.0)	1 (0.8)	3 (1.2)	3 (1.3)	0 (0.0)	1 (0.4)
Nervous System Disorders								
Headache	13 (5.4)	22 (9.2)	30 (12.4)	8 (6.6)	23 (9.5)	22 (9.6)	9 (7.9)	13 (5.6)
Dizziness	5 (2.1)	7 (2.9)	5 (2.1)	1 (0.8)	2 (0.8)	3 (1.3)	2 (1.8)	1 (0.4)
Sciatica	3 (1.2)	2 (0.8)	1 (0.4)	0 (0.0)	1 (0.4)	0 (0.0)	0 (0.0)	1 (0.4)
Psychiatric Disorders								
Anxiety	0 (0.0)	1 (0.4)	4 (1.7)	0 (0.0)	0 (0.0)	1 (0.4)	3 (2.6)	0 (0.0)
Depression	0 (0.0)	4 (1.7)	3 (1.2)	0 (0.0)	3 (1.2)	2 (0.9)	3 (2.6)	0 (0.0)
Insomnia	0 (0.0)	2 (0.8)	3 (1.2)	1 (0.8)	0 (0.0)	1 (0.4)	0 (0.0)	0 (0.0)
Respiratory, Thoracic and Mediastinal Disorders								
Pharyngolaryngeal pain	3 (1.2)	4 (1.7)	2 (0.8)	1 (0.8)	3 (1.2)	2 (0.9)	2 (1.8)	1 (0.4)

(cont'd)

Table 1: VICTOZA *(cont'd)*

Treatment-Emergent Adverse Events from Two 26 Week Combination Trials 1572 and 1697

	Trial 1572 (LEAD 2)				Trial 1697 (LEAD 5)			
	VICTOZA 0.6 mg + metformin	VICTOZA 1.2 mg + metformin	VICTOZA 1.8 mg + metformin	Placebo + metformin	Active Comparator (metformin + glimepiride)	VICTOZA 1.8 mg + metformin + glimepiride	Placebo + metformin + glimepiride	Active Comparator (insulin glargine + metformin + glimepiride)
	N (%)	N (%)	N (%)	N (%)	N (%)	N (%)	N (%)	N (%)
Cough	4 (1.7)	3 (1.3)	2 (0.8)	1 (0.8)	5 (2.1)	4 (1.7)	1 (0.9)	7 (3.0)
Skin and Subcutaneous Tissue Disorders								
Pruritus	2 (0.8)	3 (1.3)	1 (0.4)	0 (0.0)	3 (1.2)	0 (0.0)	0 (0.0)	1 (0.4)
Rash	0 (0.0)	1 (0.4)	1 (0.4)	1 (0.8)	3 (1.2)	3 (1.3)	0 (0.0)	2 (0.9)
Hyperhidrosis	1 (0.4)	0 (0.0)	1 (0.4)	2 (1.7)	1 (0.4)	1 (0.4)	0 (0.0)	0 (0.0)
Vascular Disorders								
Hypertension	5 (2.1)	7 (2.9)	5 (2.1)	2 (1.7)	6 (2.5)	7 (3.0)	3 (2.6)	5 (2.2)
Vascular calcification	2 (0.8)	2 (0.8)	1 (0.4)	1 (0.8)	3 (1.2)	0 (0.0)	0 (0.0)	0 (0.0)
Aortic calcification	2 (0.8)	0 (0.0)	1 (0.4)	0 (0.0)	3 (1.2)	0 (0.0)	0 (0.0)	0 (0.0)
Arteriosclerosis	3 (1.2)	0 (0.0)	1 (0.4)	0 (0.0)	0 (0.0)	0 (0.0)	0 (0.0)	1 (0.4)
Hematoma	3 (1.2)	0 (0.0)	1 (0.4)	0 (0.0)	1 (0.4)	0 (0.0)	0 (0.0)	0 (0.0)

Patients with MTC usually have calcitonin values >50 ng/L. In VICTOZA clinical trials, among patients with pre-treatment serum calcitonin <50 ng/L, one patient treated with VICTOZA and no comparator-treated patients developed serum calcitonin >50 ng/L. The patient treated with VICTOZA who developed serum calcitonin >50 ng/L had an elevated pre-treatment serum calcitonin of 10.7 ng/L that increased to 30.7 ng/L at Week 12 and 53.5 ng/L at the end of the 6-month trial. Follow-up serum calcitonin was 22.3 ng/L more than 2.5 years after the last dose of VICTOZA.

The largest increase in serum calcitonin in a comparator-treated patient was seen with glimepiride in a patient whose serum calcitonin increased from 19.3 ng/L at baseline to 44.8 ng/L at Week 65 and 38.1 ng/L at Week 104.

Among patients who began with serum calcitonin <20 ng/L, calcitonin elevations to >20 ng/L occurred in 0.7% of patients treated with VICTOZA 0.3% of placebo-treated patients, and 0.5% of active-comparator-treated patients, with an incidence of 1.1% among patients treated with 1.8 mg/day of VICTOZA The clinical significance of these findings is unknown (see Warnings and Precautions, Boxed Serious Warnings and Precautions and Carcinogenesis and Mutagenesis).

Papillary Thyroid Cancer: In the completed trials the rates of papillary thyroid carcinoma were 1.9 and 0.6 (liraglutide vs non-liraglutide) events per 1000 subjects-years of exposure. Papillary (follicular) thyroid cancers occurred at a higher frequency in the liraglutide clinical development programme than in the general Canadian population. Subjects included in the liraglutide clinical trial program underwent thyroid related assessments, leading to a high number of thyroidectomies. The majority of papillary carcinomas were incidental findings arising from thyroidectomies performed as a result of elevations in serum calcitonin; all but one of the papillary carcinomas were microcarcinomas of less than 1.0 cm. In subjects with pre-existing thyroid disease, the rates of thyroid neoplasms were comparable for liraglutide and placebo (28.8 per 1000 subject-years and 29.3 per 1000 subject-years; none in active comparator).

Neoplasms: In the intermediate and long-term trials, 115 treatment emergent neoplasm adverse events were reported and of these, 45 events were classified as malignant neoplasms. The proportion and rate (shown in brackets) of subjects with neoplasm adverse events (benign and malignant) was 1.8% (26.9 cases per 1000 subject-years), 1.2% (17.0 per cases 1000 subject-years) and 1.3% (25.3 cases per 1000 subject-years) for liraglutide, active comparator and placebo, respectively. The proportion and rate of subjects with malignant neoplasm adverse events was 0.8% (10.9 cases per 1000 subject-years), 0.5% (7.2 cases per 1000 subject-years) and 0.3% (6.3 cases per 1000 subject-years) for liraglutide, active comparator and placebo, respectively.

Thyroid neoplasms were the most common neoplasm adverse events. The proportion and rate of subjects with benign thyroid neoplasms were higher for subjects treated with liraglutide compared to subjects treated with active comparator and placebo [liraglutide: 1.1% (16.0 cases per 1000 subject-years); active comparator: 0.6% (9.8 cases per 1000 subject-years); placebo: 1.0% (19.0 cases per 1000 subject-years)]. With regard to malignant neoplasms which are of more clinical relevance, prostate cancer, breast cancer, thyroid cancer, basal cell carcinoma, rectal cancer, renal cell carcinoma and colon cancer were the most commonly reported across treatment groups. The proportion of subjects with malignant prostate cancer, breast cancer, renal cell carcinoma and colon cancer were similar for subjects treated with liraglutide and either one of the comparators. No cases of rectal cancer or basal cell carcinoma were reported with comparators. The remaining malignant neoplasms occurred at low rates with no apparent pattern in type of neoplasms.

Cardiovascular: Adverse events identified using a composite endpoint for all tachyarrhythmias in pooled intermediate and long term trials, including open label arms, occurred at rates of 16.5, 6.1, and 15.3 per 1000 subject-years in the liraglutide, placebo and active comparator groups respectively. The respective proportions were 0.7, 0.2 and 0.7 per cent. The most commonly reported episodes of tachyarrhythmia were extrasystoles. The rate of pooled events of atrial fibrillation, atrial flutter, supraventricular tachycardia and supraventricular arrhythmia was 6.4 per 1000 subject-years in the liraglutide group and 5.6 per 1000 subject-years in the active comparator group; no events were reported in the placebo group. Rates of adverse events related to tachyarrhythmia reported as Serious Adverse Events were 2.7, 0 and 2.8 per 1000 subject-years in the VICTOZA, placebo and active comparator groups respectively.

In pooled long term trials, the rate of first-degree AV block was reported to be 2.6, 0 and 1.4 per 1000 subject-years in the liraglutide, placebo and active comparator groups.

In the above trials patients were excluded in case of known clinically significant active cardiovascular disease including history of myocardial infarction within the past 6 months and/or heart failure, at the discretion of the Investigator, and uncontrolled treated/untreated hypertension (systolic blood pressure =180 mmHg and/or diastolic blood pressure =100 mmHg). (See also Warnings and Precautions, Special Populations, Cardiovascular—Patients with Recent MI, Unstable Angina and Congestive Heart Failure; Drug Interactions, Drug-Drug Interactions, Drugs that Increase Heart Rate and Drugs that Cause PR Interval Prolongation; Action and Clinical Pharmacology, Cardiac Electrophysiology.)

Pancreatitis: In clinical trials of VICTOZA there were 7 cases of pancreatitis among VICTOZA treated patients and 1 case among comparator-treated patients (2.2 vs 0.6 cases per 1000 subject-years). Five cases with VICTOZA were reported as acute pancreatitis and two cases with VICTOZA were reported as chronic pancreatitis. All events were serious except for one case of chronic pancreatitis in a patient treated with VICTOZA. One fatal case of pancreatitis with necrosis was observed, in a VICTOZA treated patient.

Five additional cases of pancreatitis have subsequently been reported in clinical trials of VICTOZA. One of these was a case of acute pancreatitis in a patient whose treatment remains blinded. The remaining 4 cases occurred in VICTOZA treated patients; 2 cases were acute pancreatitis, 1 case was chronic pancreatitis and 1 case was reported as "not acute". (See Warnings and Precautions, Pancreatitis.)

Hypoglycemia: Major hypoglycemic episodes in the long-term phase 3 trials were rare (10 episodes in 9 subjects) and seven of these major episodes were reported when liraglutide was used in combination with glimepiride. When liraglutide was used in combination with a sulfonylurea, an increased rate of hypoglycemia was observed (see also Warnings and Precautions, Endocrine and Metabolism, Hypoglycemia and Dosage and Administration, Dosing Considerations).

In trial 1572 (LEAD 2) the rate of minor hypoglycemic episodes was 0.14, 0.03, 0.09, 0.13 and 1.23 events/subject year in the liraglutide 0.6 mg + metformin, liraglutide 1.2 mg + metformin, liraglutide 1.8 mg + metformin, placebo + metformin and glimepiride + metformin groups respectively; the corresponding proportion of affected subjects was 3.3%, 0.8%, 2.5%, 2.5% and 16.9%, respectively. Rates of minor nocturnal hypoglycemia were 0.00, 0.02, 0.00, 0.02 and 0.05 events/subject year, respectively.

In trial 1697 (LEAD 5) the rate of minor hypoglycemic episodes was 1.16, 0.95 and 1.29 events/subject year in the liraglutide 1.8 mg + metformin + glimepiride, placebo + metformin + glimepiride and insulin glargine + glimepiride + metformin groups respectively; the corresponding proportion of affected subjects was 27.4%, 16.7% and 28.9% respectively. Major hypoglycemic episodes were only reported in the liraglutide group where 6 events were reported in 5 subjects. Rates of major hypoglycemia were 0.06, 0.00, 0.00 events/subject year and rates of nocturnal hypoglycemia were 0.16, 0.19, 0.23 events/subject year, in the liraglutide 1.8 mg + metformin + glimepiride, placebo + metformin + glimepiride and insulin glargine + glimepiride + metformin groups respectively.

Gastrointestinal Adverse Events: In pooled long term clinical trials, gastrointestinal adverse events were reported in 41% of VICTOZA treated patients and were dose related. Gastrointestinal adverse events occurred in 17% of comparator-treated patients. Events that occurred more commonly among VICTOZA treated patients included nausea, vomiting, diarrhea, dyspepsia and constipation. Approximately 13% of VICTOZA treated patients and 2% of comparator-treated patients reported nausea during the first 2 weeks of treatment. Most episodes of nausea were mild or moderate in severity and declined over time (see Figure 1). Withdrawals due to gastrointestinal adverse events occurred in 5.0% of VICTOZA treated patients and 0.5% of comparator-treated patients, mainly during the first 2-3 months of the trials.

Figure 1: VICTOZA

Observed Proportion of Patients Experiencing Nausea by Treatment Over Time in LEAD-2 †††p<0.0001, ††p<0.01, †p<0.5 vs Placebo

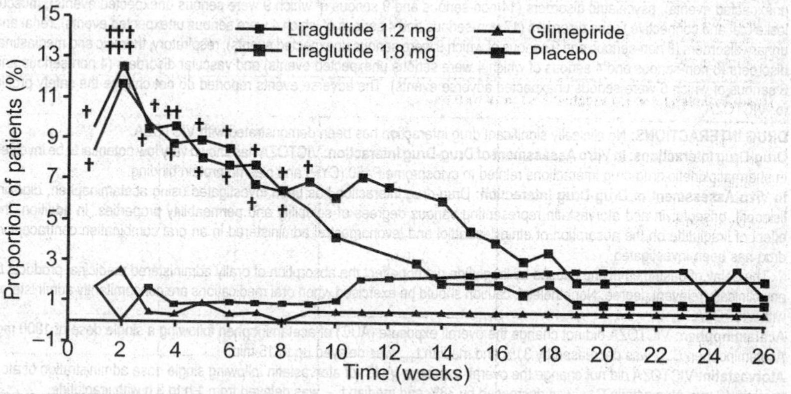

The rate of gastrointestinal disorders in VICTOZA treated subjects increased with age, especially at the 1.8 mg dose of VICTOZA. (See also Indications and Clinical Use, Geriatrics (>65 years of age); Warnings and Precautions, Special Populations, Gastrointestinal Disease; Dosage and Administration, Dosing Considerations; Action and Clinical Pharmacology, Pharmacodynamics, Gastric Emptying.)

Immunogenicity: Approximately 50-70% of VICTOZA treated patients in pooled clinical trials of 26 weeks or longer were tested for the presence of anti-liraglutide antibodies at the end of treatment. Anti-liraglutide antibodies were detected in 8.6% of these VICTOZA treated patients. Sampling was not performed uniformly across all patients in the clinical trials, and this may have resulted in an underestimated percentage of patients who developed antibodies. Cross reacting antibodies to native GLP-1 occurred in 6.9% of VICTOZA treated patients in a 52 week monotherapy trial and 4.8% of VICTOZA treated patients in 26 week combination therapy trials. The antibodies cross-reacting with native GLP-1 were not tested for neutralizing effect against native GLP-1, and thus the potential for clinically significant neutralization of native GLP-1 was not assessed. Antibodies that had a neutralizing effect on liraglutide in an in vitro assay occurred in 2.3% of VICTOZA treated patients in a 52 week monotherapy trial and 1.0% of VICTOZA treated patients in 26 week combination therapy trials.

Antibody formation was not associated with reduced efficacy of VICTOZA when comparing mean HbA1c of all antibody-positive and all antibody-negative patients. However, the 3 patients with the highest titers of anti-liraglutide antibodies had no reduction in HbA1c with VICTOZA treatment.

The most frequent adverse event categories for subjects without antibodies were gastrointestinal disorders (35.7%), infections and infestations (36.1%) and nervous system disorders (13.6%). The most frequent adverse event categories for subjects with antibodies were infections and infestations (40%), gastrointestinal disorders, (36.9%) and musculoskeletal and connective tissue disorders (20.6%). Two (2) subjects with liraglutide antibodies reported 4 events of hypersensitivity (rate: 33.6 events per 1000 subject-years of exposure), whereas 10 subjects without liraglutide antibodies reported 10 events (rate: 5.5 events per 1000 subject-years of exposure). Drug hypersensitivity was reported by 1 subjects with liraglutide antibodies (rate: 8.4 events per 1000 subject-years of exposure), whereas 4 subjects without antibodies reported 5 events (rate: 2.8 events per 1000 subject-years of exposure).

Figure 2: VICTOZA

Rate of Events with Gastrointestinal Disorders by Treatment and Age Group—All Long-term Trials—Safety Analysis Set

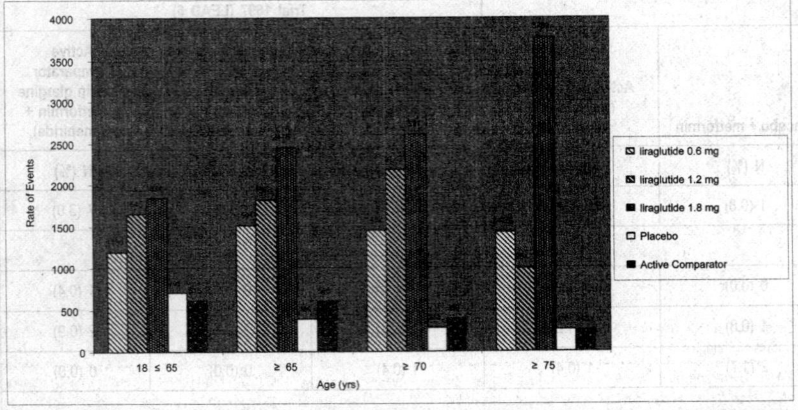

In clinical trials of VICTOZA, events from a composite of adverse events potentially related to immunogenicity (e.g. urticaria, angioedema) occurred among 0.8% of VITOZA treated patients (rate 12.2 events per 1000 subject-years of exposure with total liraglutide) and among 0.4% of total comparator-treated patients (rate 6.3 events per 1000 subject-years of exposure.) Patients who developed anti-liraglutide antibodies were not more likely to develop events from the immunogenicity events composite than were patients who did not develop anti-liraglutide antibodies.

Injection Site Reactions: Overall injection site reactions have been reported in approximately 2% of subjects receiving VICTOZA in long-term controlled trials, most frequently bruising and pain. The rate of injection site disorders was 18.1, 27.6 and 37.6 events per 1000 subject-years of exposure for patients treated with liraglutide 0.6, 1.2 and 1.8 mg as compared to 34.0 and 14.9 events per 1000 subject-years of exposure for patients treated with placebo and active comparator.

Less than 0.2% of VICTOZA treated patients discontinued due to injection site reactions. None of these patients were tested positive for liraglutide antibodies.

Less Common Clinical Trial Serious Adverse Drug Reactions (SAEs) and Rare Adverse Drug Reactions of interest ≥0.1% and <1% from Long Term Clinical Trials: Blood and Lymphatic System Disorders: thrombocytopenia.

Cardiac Disorders: angina pectoris, acute myocardial infarction, myocardial infarction coronary artery disease, atrial fibrillation, cardiac failure congestive, supraventricular tachycardia.

Eye Disorders: cataract.

GI Disorders: appendicitis perforated, gastritis, inguinal hernia, pancreatitis.

Infections and Infestations: upper respiratory tract infection, bronchitis, gastroenteritis, osteomyelitis.

Neoplasms Benign, Malignant and Unspecified (Incl Cysts and Polyps): papillary thyroid cancer, prostate cancer, breast cancer.

Musculoskeletal and Connective Tissue Disorders: intervertebral disc potrusion, osteoarthritis.

Nervous System Disorders: cerebrovascular accident, syncope.

Injury, Poisoning and Procedural Complications: fall.

General Disorders and Administration Site Conditions: chest pain.

Metabolism and Nutrition Disorders: hypoglycemia.

Respiratory, Thoracic and Mediastinal Disorders: pulmonary embolism.

Post-Market Adverse Drug Reactions: VICTOZA has been marketed since July 2009. As of 31 March 2010, Novo Nordisk has received 367 adverse drug reaction reports from market use of VICTOZA comprising 767 adverse drug reactions of which 303 were non-serious reports and 64 were serious reports. Most adverse reactions were reported in the category of gastrointestinal disorders (235 non-serious, 62 serious of which 21 were serious unexpected events), general disorders and administrative site conditions (114 non-serious and 12 serious of which 9 were serious unexpected events), investigations (56 non-serious and 20 serious events of which 20 were serious unexpected events), nervous system disorders (57 non-serious and 10 serious of which 10 were serious unexpected events), skin and subcutaneous tissue disorder (31 non-serious and 5 serious of which 5 were serious unexpected events), metabolism and nutrition disorders (28 non-serious and 14 serious of which 14 were serious unexpected events), psychiatric disorders (14 non-serious and 9 serious of which 9 were serious unexpected events), musculoskeletal and connective tissue disorders (17 non-serious and 4 serious of which 4 were serious unexpected events), renal and urinary disorders (8 non-serious and 9 serious of which 9 were serious unexpected events), respiratory, thoracic and mediastinal disorders (8 non-serious and 4 serious of which 4 were serious unexpected events) and vascular disorders (4 non-serious and 6 serious of which 6 were serious unexpected adverse events). The adverse events reported do not change the safety profile for VICTOZA.

DRUG INTERACTIONS: No clinically significant drug interaction has been demonstrated with VICTOZA.

Drug-Drug Interactions: In Vitro Assessment of Drug-Drug Interaction: VICTOZA has shown very low potential to be involved in pharmacokinetic drug-drug interactions related to cytochrome P450 (CYP) and plasma protein binding.

In Vivo Assessment of Drug-Drug Interaction: Drug-drug interaction has been investigated using acetaminophen, digoxin, lisinopril, griseofulvin and atorvastatin representing various degrees of solubility and permeability properties. In addition, the effect of liraglutide on the absorption of ethinylestradiol and levonorgestrel administered in an oral combination contraceptive drug has been investigated.

The delay of gastric emptying caused by liraglutide did not affect the absorption of orally administered medicinal products to any clinically relevant degree. Nonetheless, caution should be exercised when oral medications are concomitantly administered with VICTOZA.

Acetaminophen: VICTOZA did not change the overall exposure (AUC) of acetaminophen following a single dose of 1000 mg. Acetaminophen C_{max} was decreased by 31% and median t_{max} was delayed up to 15 min.

Atorvastatin: VICTOZA did not change the overall exposure (AUC) of atorvastatin following single dose administration of atorvastatin 40 mg. Atorvastatin C_{max} was decreased by 38% and median t_{max} was delayed from 1 h to 3 h with liraglutide.

Griseofulvin: VICTOZA did not change the overall exposure (AUC) of griseofulvin following administration of a single dose of griseofulvin 500 mg. Griseofulvin C_{max} increased by 37% while median t_{max} did not change.

Lisinopril and Digoxin: Single dose administration of lisinopril 20 mg or digoxin 1mg with liraglutide showed a reduction of lisinopril and digoxin AUC by 15% and 16%, respectively; C_{max} decreased by 27% and 31%, respectively. Lisinopril median t_{max} was delayed from 6 h to 8 h with liraglutide; whereas digoxin median t_{max} was delayed from 1 h to 1.5 h.

Oral Contraceptives: VICTOZA lowered ethinylestradiol and levonorgestrel C_{max} by 12 and 13%, respectively, following administration of a single dose of an oral contraceptive product. t_{max} was 1.5 h later with liraglutide for both compounds. There was no clinically relevant effect on the overall exposure (AUC) of either ethinylestradiol or levonorgestrel. The contraceptive effect is therefore anticipated to be unaffected when co-administered with liraglutide.

Warfarin: No interaction study has been performed. A clinically relevant interaction with active substances with poor solubility or with narrow therapeutic index such as warfarin cannot be excluded. Upon initiation of liraglutide treatment in patients on warfarin more frequent monitoring of INR (International Normalized Ratio) is recommended.

Insulin: Combination of liraglutide with insulin has not been evaluated and is therefore not recommended.

Drugs that Increase Heart Rate: VICTOZA causes an increase in heart rate (see Actions and Clinical Pharmacology, Cardiac Electrophysiology). The impact on the heart rate of co-administration of VICTOZA with other drugs that increase heart rate, (e.g., sympathomimetic drugs) has not been evaluated in drug-drug interaction studies. As a result, co-administration of VICTOZA with these drugs should be undertaken with caution.

Drugs that Cause PR Interval Prolongation: VICTOZA causes an increase in the PR interval (see Actions and Clinical Pharmacology, Cardiac Electrophysiology). The impact on the PR interval of co-administration of VICTOZA with other drugs that prolong the PR interval (including calcium channel blockers, beta-adrenergic blockers, digitalis glycosides, and HIV protease inhibitors) has not been evaluated in drug-drug interaction studies. As a result, co-administration of VICTOZA with these drugs should be undertaken with caution.

Drug-Food Interactions: There are no known interactions with food.

Drug-Herb Interactions: Interactions with herbal products have not been established.

DOSAGE AND ADMINISTRATION: Dosing Considerations: For all patients VICTOZA is administered once daily at any time, independent of meals. VICTOZA should be initiated with a dose of 0.6 mg once daily for at least one week. The 0.6 mg dose is a starting dose intended to reduce gastrointestinal symptoms during initial titration. After one week at 0.6 mg per day, the dose should be increased to 1.2 mg once daily. Based on clinical response and after at least one week the dose can be increased to 1.8 mg once daily to achieve maximum efficacy for glycemic control.

VICTOZA can be added to existing metformin therapy. The current dose of metformin can be continued unchanged at the discretion of the physician.

VICTOZA can be added to combined metformin and sulfonylurea therapy. During clinical trials physicians were advised, at their discretion, to lower the dose of sulfonylurea to minimize the risk of unacceptable hypoglycemia.

Recommended Dose and Dosage Adjustment: Renal Insufficiency: No dose adjustment is required for patients with mild renal insufficiency. There is limited clinical experience with VICTOZA in patients with mild renal insufficiency. There is very limited or no clinical experience with VICTOZA in patients with moderate and severe renal insufficiency, including end-stage renal disease; use of VICTOZA in these patients is not recommended. (See Warnings and Precautions, Special Populations; and Action and Clinical Pharmacology, Special Populations and Conditions.)

Hepatic Insufficiency: The safety and efficacy of VICTOZA in patients with hepatic insufficiency have not been studied. The use of VICTOZA in patients with hepatic insufficiency is not recommended. (See Warnings and Precautions, Special Populations; and Action and Clinical Pharmacology, Special Populations and Conditions.)

Geriatrics (>65 years of age): In the VICTOZA clinical trials, a total of 797 (20%) of the patients were 65 years of age and over and 113 (2.8%) were 75 years of age and over. No overall differences in safety or effectiveness were observed between these patients and younger patients, but greater sensitivity of some older individuals cannot be ruled out. (See Warnings and Precautions, Special Populations; Adverse Reactions, Clinical Trial Adverse Drug Reactions, Gastrointestinal Adverse Events; and Action and Clinical Pharmacology, Special Populations and Conditions.)

Pediatrics (<18 years of age): The safety and efficacy of VICTOZA have not been studied in pediatric populations. VICTOZA is not indicated for use in pediatric patients.

Missed Dose: If a dose of VICTOZA is missed take your dose on the next day as usual. Do not take an extra dose or increase the dose on the following day to make up for the missed dose.

Administration: VICTOZA is administered once daily at anytime, independent of meals, and can be injected subcutaneously in the abdomen, in the thigh or in the upper arm. The injection site and timing can be changed if needed without dose adjustment.

OVERDOSAGE:

In a clinical study of VICTOZA, one patient with type 2 diabetes experienced a single overdose of 17.4 mg subcutaneous (10 times the maximum recommended dose). Effects of the overdose included severe nausea and vomiting. No hypoglycemia was reported. The patient recovered without complication. In the event of overdosage, appropriate supportive treatment should be initiated according to the patient's clinical signs and symptoms.

For management of a suspected drug overdose, contact your regional Poison Control Centre. See the *CPS Directory* section for a list of Poison Control Centres.

ACTION AND CLINICAL PHARMACOLOGY: Mechanism of Action: VICTOZA (liraglutide) is an acylated human Glucagon-Like Peptide-1 (GLP-1) receptor agonist with 97% amino acid sequence homology to endogenous human GLP-1(7-37). GLP-1(7-37) represents <20% of total circulating endogenous GLP-1. Like GLP-1(7-37), liraglutide activates the GLP-1 receptor, a membrane-bound cell-surface receptor coupled to adenylyl cyclase by the stimulatory G-protein, Gs, in pancreatic beta cells. Liraglutide increases intracellular cyclic AMP (cAMP) leading to insulin release in the presence of elevated glucose concentrations. This insulin secretion subsides as blood glucose concentrations decrease and approach euglycemia. Liraglutide also decreases glucagon secretion in a glucose-dependent manner. The mechanism of blood glucose lowering also involves a delay in gastric emptying.

GLP-1(7-37) has a half-life of 1.5-2 minutes due to degradation by the ubiquitous endogenous enzymes, dipeptidyl peptidase IV (DPP-IV) and neutral endopeptidases (NEP). Unlike native GLP-1, liraglutide is stable against metabolic degradation by both peptidases and has a plasma half-life of 13 hours after subcutaneous administration. The pharmacokinetic profile of liraglutide, which makes it suitable for once daily administration, is a result of self-association that delays absorption, plasma protein binding and stability against metabolic degradation by DPP-IV and NEP.

Pharmacodynamics: VICTOZA has 24-hour duration of action and improves long-term glycemic control by lowering fasting and postprandial blood glucose in patients with type 2 diabetes mellitus. Inadequately controlled hyperglycemia is associated with an increased risk of diabetic complications, including cardiovascular disorders and diabetic nephropathy, retinopathy and neuropathy.

VICTOZA 1.8 mg and 1.2 mg reduced the mean fasting glucose by 3.90 mmol/L and 3.33 mmol/L, respectively, when compared to placebo (Figure 3). Following a standard meal, the difference versus placebo in mean 2-hour postprandial glucose concentration was 6.02 mmol/L and 5.63 mmol/L. In addition, VICTOZA 1.8 mg and 1.2 mg decreased the incremental postprandial glucose (defined as the difference between blood glucose values 90 minutes post and immediately before the meal across all three meals) on average by 1.1 mmol/L and 1.08 mmol/L, respectively.

Figure 3: VICTOZA

Mean Absolute (left) and Incremental (right) Postprandial Plasma Glucose Concentrations in Patients with Type 2 Diabetes Treated with Liraglutide 1.8 mg or Placebo in a Cross-over Design (N=18) (Trial 1698)

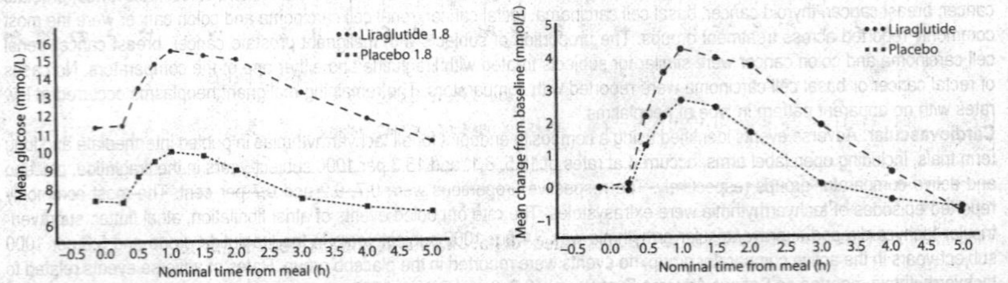

Glucose Dependent Insulin Secretion: VICTOZA increased insulin secretion in relation to increasing glucose concentrations. Using a stepwise graded glucose infusion, the insulin secretion rate was increased following a single dose of liraglutide in patients with type 2 diabetes to a level comparable to that observed in healthy subjects (Figure 4).

Glucagon Secretion: VICTOZA lowered blood glucose by stimulating insulin secretion and lowering glucagon secretion. A single dose of VICTOZA of ~0.7 mg did not impair glucagon response to low glucose concentrations. Furthermore, due to increased insulin and lower glucagon secretion, a lower endogenous glucose release has been observed with VICTOZA.

Gastric Emptying: VICTOZA caused a delay of gastric emptying, thereby reducing the rate at which postprandial glucose appeared in the circulation.

Cardiac Electrophysiology: A randomised, double-blind, 2-period crossover, placebo-controlled trial was performed in 51 healthy volunteers (25 M/26 F, 18-44 years). Following randomisation, subjects in the liraglutide treatment arm received 0.6 mg s.c. liraglutide daily for the first week of treatment, 1.2 mg s.c. daily for the second week of treatment, and 1.8 mg s.c. daily for the third week of treatment according to an upward titration design. At the end of the second and third weeks, immediately following the seventh and final doses of 1.2 and 1.8 mg liraglutide, respectively, subjects had 24 hours of serial ECG monitoring. Subjects randomised to the placebo arm had an identical schedule of treatment and assessments with a placebo s.c. injection.

Heart Rate: Liraglutide was associated with statistically significant increases in heart rate at all time points during treatment with the 1.2 mg dose on day 14 and the 1.8 mg dose on day 21. The incidence of subjects with heart rate values greater than 90 bpm was 20.0% for liraglutide 1.2 mg versus 8.0% for placebo and 23.5% for liraglutide 1.8 mg versus 3.9% for placebo.

PR Interval: Liraglutide at a dose of 1.2 mg caused statistically significant increases in the PR interval at all time points on day 14. The 1.8 mg dose of liraglutide resulted in statistically significant PR interval prolongation at 10 of 12 post-dose time points on day 21. The maximum placebo- and baseline-adjusted mean PR interval prolongation was 10.0 ms (90% CI: 6.9, 13.1) for the 1.2 mg dose and 9.0 ms (90% CI: 6.1, 12.0) for the 1.8 mg dose. Treatment-emergent PR values >200 ms were reported for 4% of subjects in the liraglutide arm and 2% of subjects in the placebo arm. The incidence of subjects who had PR values >200 ms at baseline that increased in magnitude and/or frequency during treatment was 6% for the liraglutide arm and 2% for the placebo arm.

QT Interval: Liraglutide at 1.2 mg and 1.8 mg doses was associated with statistically significant shortening of the QTc interval at most post-dose time points. The clinical significance of an acquired, drug-induced QTc shortening of this magnitude is not known.

Pharmacokinetics: Absorption: The absorption of VICTOZA following subcutaneous administration is slow, reaching maximum concentration 8-12 hours post dosing. Estimated maximum liraglutide concentration was 9.4 nmol/L for a subcutaneous single dose of liraglutide 0.6 mg. At 1.8 mg liraglutide, the average steady state concentration of liraglutide ($AUC_τ/24$) reached approximately 34 nmol/L. VICTOZA exposure (AUC) increased approximately linearly with the dose (μg/kg) with increasing slope due to accumulation between days 1 and 11. The intra-subject coefficient of variation for liraglutide AUC was 11% following single dose administration. VICTOZA can be administered subcutaneously in the abdomen, thigh, or upper arm.

The absolute bioavailability of VICTOZA following subcutaneous administration is approximately 55%.

Distribution: The apparent volume of distribution after subcutaneous administration is 11-17 L. The mean volume of distribution after intravenous administration of VICTOZA is 0.07 L/kg. VICTOZA is extensively bound to plasma protein (>98%).

Metabolism: During 24 h following administration of a single [^{3}H]-liraglutide dose to healthy subjects, the major component in plasma was intact liraglutide. Two minor plasma metabolites were detected (≤9 % and ≤5% of total plasma radioactivity exposure). VICTOZA is endogenously metabolized in a similar manner to large proteins without a specific organ as major route of elimination.

Excretion: Following a [^{3}H]-liraglutide dose, intact liraglutide was not detected in urine or feces. Only a minor part of the administered radioactivity was excreted as liraglutide-related metabolites in urine or feces (6% and 5%, respectively). The urine and feces radioactivity was mainly excreted during the first 6-8 days, and corresponded to three minor metabolites, respectively.

The mean clearance following s.c. administration of a single dose of VICTOZA is approximately 1.2 L/h with an elimination half-life of approximately 13 hours.

Figure 4: VICTOZA

Mean Insulin Secretion Rate (ISR) Versus Glucose Concentration Following Single Dose 7.5 μg/kg (~0.66 mg) or Placebo in Subjects with Type 2 Diabetes (N=10) and Untreated Healthy Subjects (N=10) During Graded Glucose Infusion (Trial 2063)

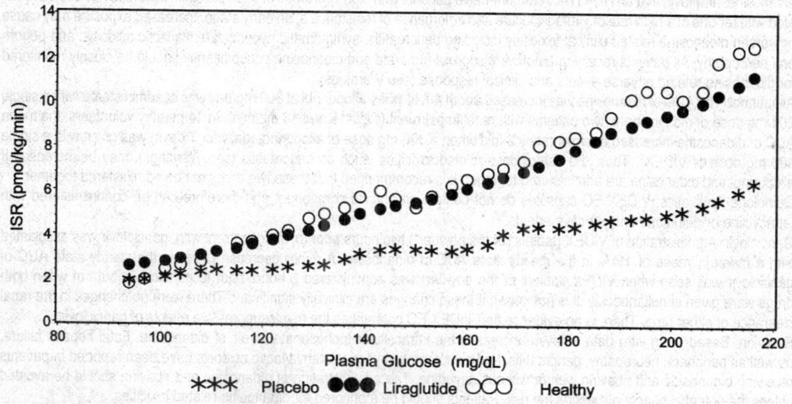

Figure 5: VICTOZA

Time-Matched Difference Between Baseline Subtracted (Delta) Liraglutide and Placebo HR (bpm)

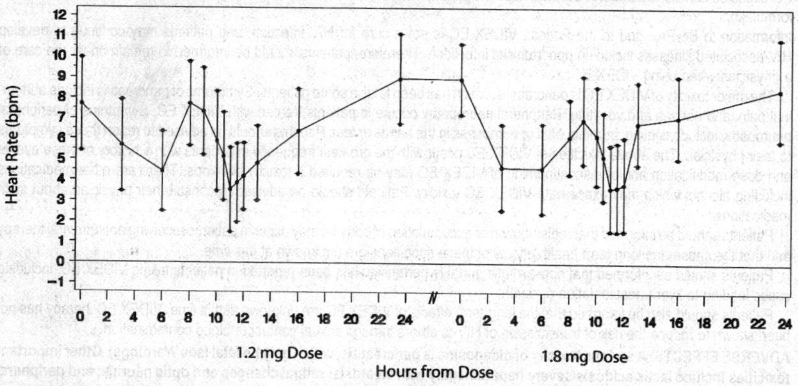

Legend: Delta=The difference between HR at current time and HR at baseline for each patient; LCL=Lower Confidence Limit; UCL=Upper Confidence Limit.

Figure 6: VICTOZA

Time-Matched Difference Between Baseline Subtracted (Delta) Liraglutide and Placebo PR (msec)

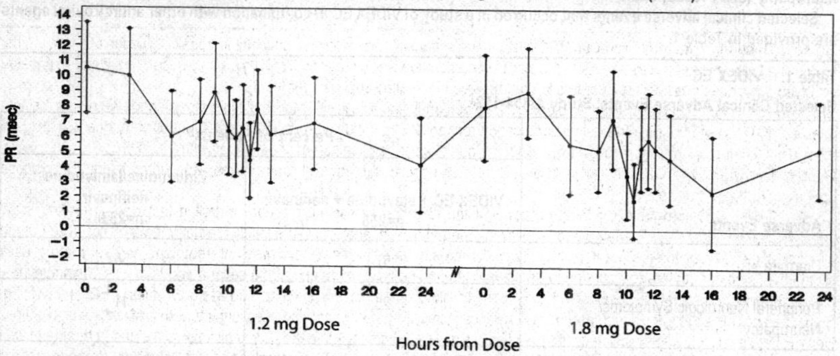

Legend: Delta=The difference between PR at current time and PR at baseline for each patient; LCL=Lower Confidence Limit; UCL=Upper Confidence Limit.

Special Populations and Conditions: Pediatrics (<18 years of age): VICTOZA has not been studied in pediatric patients.

Geriatrics (>65 years of age): Exposure (AUC) to VICTOZA is independent of age (see Dosage and Administration and Action and Clinical Pharmacology).

Gender: After adjusting for body weight, AUC(0-t), C_{max}, t_{max}, AUC(0-∞), CL/F, Vz/F, and $t_{½}$ appeared to be comparable between male and female subjects after administration of a single dose of liraglutide. A pharmacokinetic study in healthy subjects indicated that gender has no clinically meaningful effect on the pharmacokinetics of VICTOZA.

Figure 7: VICTOZA

Time-Matched Difference Between Baseline Subtracted (Delta) Liraglutide and Placebo QTcl (msec)

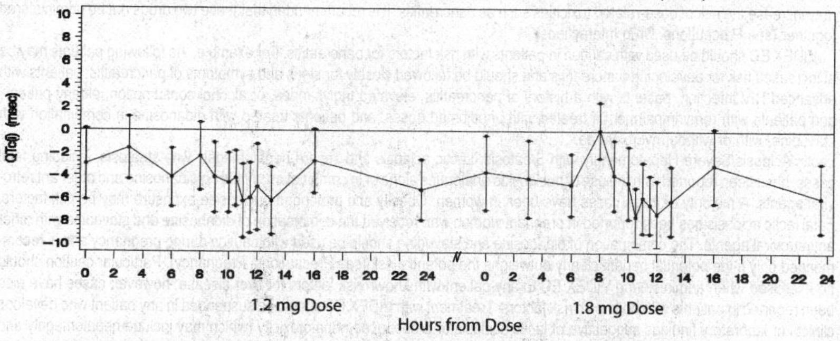

Legend: Delta=The difference between QTcl at current time and QTcl at baseline for each patient; LCL=Lower Confidence Limit; UCL=Upper Confidence Limit.

Race: There seems to be no clinically relevant effect on the pharmacokinetics of VICTOZA based on the results of a population pharmacokinetic analysis which included subjects of White, Black, Asian and Hispanic groups.

Hepatic Insufficiency: Subjects with varying degrees of hepatic insufficiency displayed a reduced exposure to VICTOZA. After a single-dose, the AUC in mild (Child Pugh score 5-6), moderate, and severe (Child Pugh score >9) compared to healthy subjects was lower on average by 23%, 13% and 44% respectively.

Renal Insufficiency: Subjects with varying degrees of renal insufficiency displayed a reduced exposure to VICTOZA. After a single-dose, the AUC in mild (CrCL 50-80 mL/min), moderate (CrCL 30-50 mL/min), severe (CrCL <30 mL/min) and end-stage renal disease requiring dialysis compared to healthy subjects was lower on average by 33%, 14%, 27% and 26%, respectively.

Obesity: Body weight significantly affects the pharmacokinetics of VICTOZA based on results of ANCOVA analyses. The exposure of VICTOZA decreases with an increase in baseline body weight. However, the 1.2 mg and 1.8 mg daily doses of VICTOZA provided adequate systemic exposures over the body weight range of 40-160 kg evaluated in the clinical trials. VICTOZA was not studied in patients with body weight >160 kg.

STORAGE AND STABILITY: VICTOZA should be stored in a refrigerator (2-8°C). Do not store in the freezer or directly adjacent to the refrigerator cooling element. Do not freeze VICTOZA and do not use VICTOZA if it has been frozen.

After initial use of the VICTOZA pen, the product can be stored for 30 days at room temperature (not above 30°C) or in a refrigerator (2-8°C).

SPECIAL HANDLING INSTRUCTIONS: VICTOZA should be kept with the pen cap on when pen is not in use in order to protect from light. VICTOZA should be protected from excessive heat and sunlight. Always remove the injection needle after each injection and store the VICTOZA pen without an injection needle attached. This prevents contamination, infection, and leakage. It also ensures that the dosing is accurate.

INFORMATION FOR THE PATIENT: Published in e-CPS, available by subscription at www.e-cps.ca.

DOSAGE FORMS, COMPOSITION AND PACKAGING: Each mL of clear, colorless solution contains: liraglutide 6 mg. Nonmedicinal ingredients: disodium phosphate dihydrate, propylene glycol, phenol and water for injections. Pre-filled disposable pens, comprising of a pen injector assembled with a cartridge (3 mL). The cartridge is made of glass (type 1), containing a bromobutyl rubber closure shaped as a plunger and closed with a bromobutyl/polyisoprene rubber closure. The pen injector is made of polyolefin and polyacetal. When incinerated these materials only result in non-toxic waste products (carbon dioxide and water). VICTOZA multidose pen can deliver 30 doses of 0.6 mg, 15 doses of 1.2 mg or 10 doses of 1.8 mg. VICTOZA Pen multidose (0.6, 1.2 or 1.8 mg): 1 pen (total supply 10 days), 2 pens (total supply 20 days) or 3 pens (total supply 30 days).

Videx™ EC ℞

didanosine

Antiretroviral Agent

Bristol-Myers Squibb

Date of Preparation: September 21, 2001
Date of Revision: May 12, 2010

PHARMACOLOGY: VIDEX EC (didanosine) capsules contain enteric-coated didanosine beadlets. Didanosine is a synthetic, purine nucleoside analogue of deoxyadenosine, active against the Human Immunodeficiency Virus (HIV).

Didanosine inhibits the in vitro replication of HIV in human primary cells cultures and in established cell lines. The active antiviral metabolite, dideoxyadenosine-triphosphate (ddATP), is formed in several steps by phosphorylation of didanosine by cellular enzymes. Inhibition of HIV reverse transcriptase by ddATP is through competition with endogenous deoxyadenosine triphosphate (dATP) for binding to the active site of the enzyme. In addition, ddATP is a substrate for reverse transcriptase and is incorporated into the growing DNA chain. The resulting nucleoside, dideoxyadenosine (ddA) lacks a 3'-hydroxyl group, which normally is the acceptor for covalent attachment of subsequent nucleoside 5'-monophosphates in DNA chain extension. Thus, ddA incorporated in the DNA prevents further chain extension and aborts proviral DNA synthesis.

Pharmacokinetics: In VIDEX EC, the active ingredient, didanosine, is protected against degradation by stomach acid by the use of an enteric coating on the beadlets in the capsule. The enteric coating dissolves when the beadlets empty into the small intestine, the site of drug absorption.

Effect of Food on Absorption of Didanosine: VIDEX EC should be taken on an empty stomach, at least 1.5 hours before or 2 hours after a meal. Compared to the fasting condition, the administration of VIDEX EC capsules with a high-fat meal significantly decreased the didanosine C_{max} (46%) and AUC (19%). Coadministering VIDEX EC capsules with a light meal, 1.5 hours before a light meal, or 2 hours after a light meal resulted in significant decrease in both C_{max} (22%, 15%, and 15% respectively) and AUC of didanosine (27%, 24%, and 10% respectively) compared to the fasting condition. Administration of VIDEX EC capsules 1.5, 2 or 3 hours before a light meal resulted in equivalent C_{max} and AUC values compared to those obtained under fasting conditions. Compared to the intact capsule administered in the fasting condition, coadministration of VIDEX EC beadlets with yogurt or apple sauce resulted in a significant decrease in C_{max} (30% and 24% respectively) and AUC of didanosine (20% and 18% respectively).

INDICATIONS: VIDEX EC (didanosine) in combination with other antiretroviral agents, is indicated for the treatment of HIV-1 infection in adults.

The duration of clinical benefit from antiretroviral therapy may be limited. Alteration in antiretroviral therapy should be considered if disease progression occurs while receiving VIDEX EC.

CONTRAINDICATIONS: VIDEX EC (didanosine) is contraindicated in patients with previously demonstrated hypersensitivity to any of the components of the formulations.

WARNINGS: The major clinical toxicity of didanosine is pancreatitis (see Adverse Effects).

Pancreatitis: **Fatal and nonfatal pancreatitis have occurred during therapy with didanosine used alone or in combination regimens in both treatment-naive and treatment-experienced patients, regardless of degree of immunosupression. VIDEX EC should be suspended in patients with signs or symptoms of pancreatitis and discontinued in patients with confirmed pancreatitis. Suspension of treatment should also be considered when biochemical markers of pancreatitis have increased to clinically significant levels, even in the absence of symptoms. Patients treated with VIDEX EC in combination with stavudine, with or without hydroxyurea, may be at increased risk for pancreatitis.**

Positive relationships have been found between the risk of pancreatitis and daily dose. Pancreatitis is also a complication of HIV infection alone.

Signs or symptoms of pancreatitis include abdominal pain and nausea, vomiting, or elevated biochemical markers for pancreatitis.

When treatment with other drugs known to cause pancreatic toxicity is required (for example, IV pentamidine), or known to increase exposure or activity of didanosine (e.g., hydroxyurea or allopurinol), suspension of didanosine therapy is recommended. Allopurinol was observed to increase exposure to didanosine in renally impaired patients and healthy volunteers and may increase the risk of dose-related toxicities such as pancreatitis. It is recommended that these two drugs not be administered together (see Precautions, Drug Interactions).

VIDEX EC should be used with caution in patients with risk factors for pancreatitis. For example, the following patients may be at increased risk for developing pancreatitis and should be followed closely for signs and symptoms of pancreatitis: patients with advanced HIV infection, patients with a history of pancreatitis, elevated triglycerides, or alcohol consumption; elderly patients and patients with renal impairment if treated with unadjusted doses; and patients treated with didanosine in combination with stavudine, with or without hydroxyurea.

Lactic Acidosis/Severe Hepatomegaly with Steatosis: Lactic acidosis and severe hepatomegaly with steatosis, including fatal cases, have been reported with the use of nucleoside analogues alone or in combination, including didanosine and other antiretroviral agents. A majority of these cases have been in women. Obesity and prolonged nucleoside exposure may be risk factors. Fatal lactic acidosis has been reported in pregnant women who received the combination of didanosine and stavudine with other antiretroviral agents. The combination of didanosine and stavudine should be used with caution during pregnancy and is recommended only if the potential benefit clearly outweighs the potential risk (see Precautions, Pregnancy). Particular caution should be exercised when administering VIDEX EC to any patient with known risk factors for liver disease; however, cases have also been reported in patients with no known risk factors. Treatment with VIDEX EC should be suspended in any patient who develops clinical or laboratory findings suggestive of lactic acidosis or pronounced hepatotoxicity (which may include hepatomegaly and steatosis even in the absence of marked transaminase elevations).

Liver Disease: Hepatotoxicity and hepatic failure resulting in death were reported during postmarketing surveillance in HIV-infected patients treated with antiretroviral agents in combination with hydroxyurea. Fatal hepatic events were reported most often in patients treated with the combination of hydroxyurea, didanosine, and stavudine. This combination should be avoided.

The safety and efficacy of VIDEX EC have not been established in patients with significant underlying liver disorders. During combination antiretroviral therapy, patients with preexisting liver dysfunction, including chronic active hepatitis, have an increased frequency of liver function abnormalities, including severe and potentially fatal hepatic adverse events, and should be monitored according to standard practice. If there is evidence of worsening liver disease in such patients, discontinuation of treatment must be considered. In case of concomitant antiviral therapy for hepatitis B or C, please refer also to the relevant product information for these medicinal products (see Precautions and Dosage).

Liver Failure: Liver failure, of unknown etiology, has occured in patients receiving didanosine and may be fatal. Patients should be observed for liver enzyme elevations and didanosine should be suspended if enzymes rise to a clinically significant level. Rechallenge should be considered only if the potential benefits clearly outweigh the potential risks.

Non-cirrhotic Portal Hypertension: Postmarketing cases of non-cirrhotic portal hypertension have been reported, including cases leading to liver transplantation or death. Cases of didanosine-associated non-cirrhotic portal hypertension were confirmed by liver biopsy in patients with no evidence of viral hepatitis. Onset of signs and symptoms ranged from months to years after start of didanosine therapy. Common presenting features included elevated liver enzymes, esophageal varices, hematemesis, ascites, and splenomegaly.

Patients receiving VIDEX EC should be monitored for early signs of portal hypertension (eg, thrombocytopenia and splenomegaly) during routine medical visits. Appropriate laboratory testing including liver enzymes, serum bilirubin, albumin, complete blood count, and international normalized ratio (INR) and ultrasonography should be considered. VIDEX EC should be discontinued in patients with evidence of non-cirrhotic portal hypertension.

Peripheral Neuropathy: **Peripheral neuropathy occurs in patients treated with didanosine and the frequency appears to be related to dose and/or stage of disease.** Lower rates were seen in patients with less advanced disease. Patients should be monitored for the development of a neuropathy that is usually characterized by bilateral symmetrical distal numbness, tingling, and pain in feet and, less frequently, hands. In controlled clinical trials, neuropathy has occurred more frequently in patients with a history of neuropathy or neurotoxic drug therapy, including stavudine, and these patients may be at increased risk of neuropathy during didanosine therapy.

Peripheral neuropathy, which was severe in some cases, has been reported in HIV-infected patients receiving hydroxyurea in combination with antiretroviral agents, including didanosine, with or without stavudine.

Neuropathy has been reported rarely in children treated with didanosine. However, because signs and symptoms of neuropathy are difficult to assess in children, physicians should be alerted to the possibility of this event.

Retinal Depigmentation and Vision: There have been rare (<1%) reports of retinal depigmentation and optic neuritis in adult patients (see Adverse Effects). Periodic retinal examinations should be considered for patients receiving didanosine. Consideration should be given to modifying treatment based on the physician's assessment of benefit to risk.

Opportunistic Infections and Other Complications of HIV Infection: Patients receiving VIDEX EC or any antiretroviral therapy may continue to develop opportunistic infections and other complications of HIV infection, and therefore should remain under close clinical observation by physicians experienced in the treatment of patients with HIV-associated diseases.

PRECAUTIONS: Frequency of Dosing: VIDEX EC should only be administered once daily. There are no data on the use of VIDEX EC dosed more frequently than once daily.

Fat Redistribution: Redistribution accumulation of body fat including central obesity, dorsocervical fat enlargement (buffalo hump), peripheral wasting, facial wasting, breast enlargement and "cushingoid appearance" have been observed in patients receiving antiretroviral therapy. The mechanism and long-term consequences of these events are currently unknown. A causal relationship has not been established.

Immune Reconstitution: During the initial phase of treatment, patients responding to antiretroviral therapy may develop an inflammatory response to indolent or residual opportunistic infections (such as MAC, CMV, PCP, and TB), which may necessitate evaluation and treatment.

Food Interaction: Ingestion of VIDEX EC with food significantly reduces the amount of didanosine absorbed. VIDEX EC should be administered at least 1.5 hours before or 2 hours after eating (see Dosage).

Children: VIDEX EC capsules have not been studied in pediatric patients.

Pregnancy: There are no adequate and well-controlled studies of didanosine in pregnant women. VIDEX EC should be used during pregnancy only if the potential benefit justifies the potential risk.

Fatal lactic acidosis has been reported in pregnant women who received the combination of didanosine and stavudine with other antiretroviral agents. It is not known if pregnancy augments the risk of lactic acidosis/hepatic steatosis syndrome reported in nonpregnant individuals receiving nucleoside analogues (see Warnings, Lactic Acidosis/Severe Hepatomegaly with Steatosis). The combination of didanosine and stavudine should be used with caution during pregnancy and is recommended only if the potential benefit clearly outweighs the potential risk. Health care providers caring for HIV-infected pregnant women receiving didanosine should be alert for early diagnosis of lactic acidosis/hepatic steatosis syndrome.

Reproduction studies have been performed in rats and rabbits at doses up to 12 and 14.2 times the estimated human exposure (based upon plasma levels) respectively, and have revealed no evidence of impaired fertility or harm to the fetus due to didanosine. At approximately 12 times the estimated human exposure, didanosine was slightly toxic to female rats and their pups during mid and late lactation. These rats showed reduced food intake and body weight gains but the physical and functional development of the offspring was not impaired and there were no major changes in the F_2 generation. A study in rats showed that didanosine and/or its metabolites are transferred to the fetus through the placenta.

Because animal reproduction studies are not always predictive of human response, this drug should be used during pregnancy only if clearly needed.

Lactation: HIV-Infected mothers should not breast-feed their infants to avoid risking postnatal transmission of HIV. It is not known whether VIDEX is excreted in human milk. A study in rats showed that, following oral administration, didanosine and/or its metabolites were excreted into the milk of lactating rats.

Geriatrics: In an Expanded Access Program using a buffered formulation of didanosine for the treatment of advanced HIV infection, patients aged 65 years and older had a higher frequency of pancreatitis (10%) than younger patients (5%) (see Warnings). Clinical studies of didanosine, including those for VIDEX EC, did not include sufficient numbers of subjects aged 65 years and over to determine whether they respond differently than younger subjects. Didanosine is known to be substantially excreted by the kidney, and the risk of toxic reactions to this drug may be greater in patients with impaired renal function. Because elderly patients are more likely to have decreased renal function, care should be taken in dose selection. In addition renal function should be monitored and dosage adjustments should be made accordingly (see Dosage, Dose Adjustment).

Patients with Special Diseases and Conditions: Patients on Sodium-Restricted Diets: VIDEX EC Capsules: Sodium contents are minimal, 0.53 mg for the 125 mg capsule formulation, 0.85 mg for the 200 mg capsules formulation, 1.06 mg for the 250 mg capsule formulation, and 1.70 mg for the 400 mg formulation.

* Videx tablets and powder are no longer marketed in Canada.

Patients with Renal Impairment: Patients with renal impairment (serum creatinine >1.5 mg/dL or creatinine clearance <60 mL/min) may be at greater risk for toxicity from VIDEX EC due to decreased drug clearance. The risk of pancreatitis (see Warnings), may be increased if allopurinol and didanosine are administered together in this patient population; it is recommended that these 2 drugs not be administered together (see Drug Interactions).

The elimination half-life of didanosine is increased in anuric patients requiring hemodialysis (see Pharmacokinetics, Pharmacology). Because of the potential for drug removal, VIDEX EC should be administered after dialysis. Dose reductions should be considered in patients with renal impairment (see Warnings and Dosage).

Patients with Hepatic Impairment: Patients with hepatic impairment may be at greater risk for toxicity related to VIDEX EC treatment due to altered metabolism (see Warnings and Dosage).

Hyperuricemia: Didanosine has been associated with asymptomatic hyperuricemia; treatment suspension may be necessary if clinical measures aimed at reducing uric acid levels fail.

Diabetes Mellitus: The VIDEX EC capsule formulation does not contain sucrose.

Drug Interactions: **Coadministration of VIDEX EC with drugs that are known to cause peripheral neuropathy or pancreatitis may increase the risk of these toxicities (see Warnings, Pancreatitis, Peripheral Neuropathy) and should be done only with extreme caution.**

Methadone: When VIDEX tablets* were administered to opiate-dependent patients (n=16) chronically treated with methadone, didanosine exposure, as measured by AUC, was decreased by 57% compared to untreated controls (n=10). There was no clinically significant impact on methadone exposure. No studies have been conducted with VIDEX EC.

Tenofovir disoproxil fumarate: Exposure to VIDEX EC is increased when coadministered with tenofovir. When VIDEX EC was administered (in the fasting state) 2 hours before tenofovir disoproxil fumarate with a light meal, the AUC of didanosine increased by 48% relative to VIDEX EC alone in the fasted state. When VIDEX EC was administered together with tenofovir disoproxil fumarate and a light meal, the AUC of didanosine increased by 60% relative to VIDEX EC alone in the fasted state. Administration of reduced doses of VIDEX EC with tenofovir and a light meal resulted in didanosine exposures (AUC) similar to the recommended doses of VIDEX EC given alone in the fasted state. Therefore, a dose reduction of VIDEX EC is recommended when coadministered with tenofovir (see Dosage, Concomitant Therapy). Caution should be used when coadministering reduced-dose didanosine, tenofovir, and an NNRTI in treatment-naive patients with high viral loads at baseline since such use has been associated with reports of a high rate of virologic failure and emergence of resistance at an early stage. Increased exposure may cause or worsen didanosine-related clinical toxicities including pancreatitis, symptomatic hyperlactatemia/lactic acidosis, and peripheral neuropathy. All patients receiving tenofovir disoproxil fumarate and didanosine concomitantly should be closely monitored for didanosine-related adverse events and clinical response (see Warnings).

Allopurinol: The AUC of didanosine was increased about 4-fold when allopurinol at 300 mg/day was coadministered with a single 200-mg dose of didanosine to two patients with renal impairment (CL_{cr}=15 and 18 mL/min). In 14 healthy volunteers, the mean AUC of didanosine increased approximately 2-fold when a 300-mg dose of allopurinol (daily for 7 days) was given with a single 400 mg dose of VIDEX*. Thus, the risk of dose-related toxicities, such as pancreatitis (see Warnings), may be increased if allopurinol and didanosine are administered together. It is recommended that these two drugs not be administered together.

Quinolone Antibiotics: VIDEX EC capsules do not contain an antacid component and therefore can be coadministered with tetracycline or quinolone anti-infective agents.

Ganciclovir: Administration of VIDEX (tablets* or the powder*) two hours prior to, or concurrent with, ganciclovir was associated with a mean increase of 111% in the steady state AUC of didanosine. A minor decrease (21%) in the steady state AUC of ganciclovir was seen when VIDEX (tablets or the powder) was administered 2 hours prior to ganciclovir, but not when both drugs were given simultaneously. It is not known if these changes are clinically significant. There were no changes in the renal clearance of either drug. There is no evidence that VIDEX EC potentiates the myelosuppressive effects of ganciclovir.

Ribavirin: Based on in vitro data, ribavirin increases the intracellular triphosphate levels of didanosine. Fatal hepatic failure, as well as peripheral neuropathy, pancreatitis, and symptomatic hyperlactatemia/lactic acidosis have been reported in patients receiving didanosine and ribavirin with or without stavudine. The administration of didanosine and ribavirin should be avoided unless the potential benefit outweighs the risk. Patients should be monitored for didanosine-related toxicities.

Interactions with Other Antiretroviral Drugs: There is no drug-drug interaction between VIDEX EC capsules and indinavir, therefore, these two products can be given together.

Drugs whose absorption can be affected by the level of acidity in the stomach (e.g., ketoconazole, dapsone, itraconazole): VIDEX EC capsules can be coadministered with these drugs, due to the absence of the antacid component in the VIDEX EC capsule formulation.

Information to Be Provided to the Patient: VIDEX EC is not a cure for HIV infection, and patients may continue to develop HIV-associated illnesses including opportunistic infections. Therefore, patients should be informed to remain under the care of a physician when using VIDEX EC.

The major toxicity of VIDEX EC is pancreatitis, which has been fatal in some patients. Symptoms of pancreatitis include abdominal pain, and nausea and vomiting. Peripheral neuropathy occurs in patients treated with VIDEX EC. Symptoms of peripheral neuropathy include tingling, burning, pain or numbness in the hands or feet. Patients should be advised to report these symptoms to their physician. The above toxicities of VIDEX EC occur with the greatest frequency in patients with a history of these events and dose modification and/or discontinuation of VIDEX EC may be required if toxicity develops. There are other medications including alcohol which may exacerbate VIDEX EC toxicity. Patients should be advised to consult their physician about such medications.

Patients should be informed that redistribution or accumulation of body fat may occur in patients receiving antiretroviral therapy and that the cause and long term health effects of these conditions are not known at this time.

Patients should be informed that non-cirrhotic portal hypertension has been reported in patients taking VIDEX EC, including cases leading to liver transplantation or death.

Patients should also be informed that the long-term effects of VIDEX EC are unknown at this time. VIDEX EC therapy has not been shown to reduce the risk of transmission of HIV to others through sexual contact or blood contamination.

ADVERSE EFFECTS: A serious toxicity of didanosine is pancreatitis, which may be fatal (see Warnings). Other important toxicities include lactic acidosis/severe hepatomegaly with steatosis; retinal changes and optic neuritis; and peripheral neuropathy (see Warnings and Precautions).

When didanosine is used in combination with other agents with similar toxicities, the incidence of these toxicities may be higher than when didanosine is used alone. Thus, patients treated with VIDEX EC in combination with stavudine, with or without hydroxyurea, may be at increased risk for pancreatitis, which may be fatal, and hepatotoxicity (see Warnings). Patients treated with VIDEX EC in combination with stavudine may also be at increased risk for peripheral neuropathy (see Precautions).

Selected clinical adverse events that occurred in a study of VIDEX EC in combination with other antiretroviral agents are provided in Table 1.

Table 1: VIDEX EC

Selected Clinical Adverse Events, Study AI454-152[a]

Adverse Events	Percent of Patients[b]	
	VIDEX EC + stavudine + nelfinavir n=258	Zidovudine/lamivudine[c] + nelfinavir n=253
Diarrhea	57	58
Peripheral Neurologic Symptoms/ Neuropathy	25	11
Nausea	24	36
Headache	22	17
Rash	14	12
Vomiting	14	19

(cont'd)

Table 1: VIDEX EC *(cont'd)*

Selected Clinical Adverse Events, Study AI454-152[a]

Adverse Events	Percent of Patients[b]	
	VIDEX EC + stavudine + nelfinavir n=258	Zidovudine/lamivudine[c] + nelfinavir n=253
Pancreatitis (see below)	<1	[d]

[a] Median duration of treatment was 62 weeks in the VIDEX EC + stavudine + nelfinavir group and 61 weeks in the zidovudine/lamivudine + nelfinavir group.
[b] Percentages based on treated patients.
[c] Zidovudine/lamivudine combination tablet.
[d] This event was not observed in this study arm.

In clinical trials using a buffered formulation of didanosine, pancreatitis resulting in death was observed in one patient who received didanosine plus stavudine plus nelfinavir, one patient who received didanosine plus stavudine plus indinavir, and 2 of 68 patients who received didanosine plus stavudine plus indinavir plus hydroxyurea. In an early access program, pancreatitis resulting in death was observed in one patient who received VIDEX EC plus stavudine plus hydroxyurea plus ritonavir plus indinavir plus efavirenz (see Warnings).

The frequency of pancreatitis is dose related. In phase 3 studies with buffered formulations of didanosine, incidence ranged from 1% to 10% with doses higher than are currently recommended and 1% to 7% with recommended dose. Selected laboratory abnormalities that occurred in a study of VIDEX EC in combination with other antiretroviral agents are shown in Table 2.

Table 2: VIDEX EC

Selected Laboratory Abnormalities, AI454-152[a]

Parameter	Percent of Patients[b]			
	VIDEX EC + stavudine + nelfinavir n=258		Zidovudine/lamivudine[c] + nelfinavir n=253	
	Grades 3-4[d]	All Grades	Grades 3-4[d]	All Grades
AST	5	46	5	19
ALT	6	44	5	22
Lipase	5	23	2	13
Bilirubin	<1	9	<1	3

[a] Median duration of treatment was 62 weeks in the VIDEX EC + stavudine + nelfinavir group and 61 weeks in the zidovudine/lamivudine + nelfinavir group.
[b] Percentages based on treated patients.
[c] Zidovudine/lamivudine combination tablet.
[d] >5×ULN for AST and ALT, ≥2.1×ULN for lipase, and ≥2.6×ULN for bilirubin (ULN=upper limit of normal).

Adverse Events Observed During Clinical Practice: The following events have been identified during postapproval use of didanosine buffered formulations. Because they are reported voluntarily from a population of unknown size, estimates of frequency cannot be made. These events have been chosen for inclusion due to their seriousness, frequency of reporting, causal connection to didanosine, or a combination of these factors.
Body as a Whole: abdominal pain, alopecia, anaphylactoid reaction, asthenia, chills/fever, and pain, redistribution/accumulation of body fat (see Precautions, Fat Redistribution).
Digestive Disorders: anorexia, dyspepsia, and flatulence.
Exocrine Gland Disorders: pancreatitis (including fatal cases) (see Warnings), sialoadenitis, parotid gland enlargement, dry mouth, and dry eyes.
Hematologic Disorders: anemia, leukopenia, granulocytopenia and thrombocytopenia.
Liver: lactic acidosis and hepatic steatosis (see Warnings and Precautions); non-cirrhotic portal hypertension (see Warnings, Non-cirrhotic Portal Hypertension); hepatitis and liver failure.
Metabolic Disorders: diabetes mellitus, elevated serum alkaline phosphatase level, elevated serum amylase level, elevated serum gamma-glutamyltransferase level, elevated serum uric acid level, hypoglycemia, and hyperglycemia.
Musculoskeletal Disorders: myalgia (with or without increases in creatine kinase), rhabdomyolysis including acute renal failure and hemodialysis, arthralgia, and myopathy.
Ophthalmologic Disorders: Retinal depigmentation and optic neuritis (see Warnings).

OVERDOSE:

Symptoms: Although no data with didanosine are available, activated charcoal should be administered to aid in the removal of unabsorbed drug, as recommended in American College of Emergency Physicians guidelines. General supportive measures are also recommended.

There is no known antidote for didanosine overdosage. Experience in the Phase I studies in which didanosine was initially administered at doses ten times the currently recommended doses indicates that the complications of chronic overdosage would include pancreatitis, peripheral neuropathy, diarrhea, hyperuricemia and, and hepatic dysfunction. Didanosine is not dialyzable by peritoneal dialysis, although there is some clearance by hemodialysis (see Pharmacology, Pharmacokinetics). The fractional removal of didanosine during an average hemodialysis session of 3 to 4 hours is approximately 20-35% of the amount present in the body at the start of dialysis.

Treatment: See Symptoms.

For management of a suspected drug overdose, contact your regional Poison Control Centre. See the *CPS* Directory section for a list of Poison Control Centres.

DOSAGE: Adults: VIDEX EC (didanosine) should be administered once daily on an empty stomach at least 1.5 hours before or 2 hours after eating (see Precautions).

VIDEX EC Capsules should be swallowed intact. The recommended daily dose is dependent on body weight and is usually administered as one capsule given on a once-daily schedule as outlined in Table 3.

Table 3: VIDEX EC

Adult Dosing

Patient Weight	VIDEX EC Capsules
≥60 kg	400 mg once daily
<60 kg	250 mg once daily

Children: The safety and efficacy of VIDEX EC in pediatric patients have not been established.
Dose Adjustment: Clinical and laboratory signs suggestive of pancreatitis should prompt dose suspension and careful evaluation of the possibility of pancreatitis. VIDEX EC use should be discontinued in patients with confirmed pancreatitis (see Warnings).

Patients who have presented with symptoms of neuropathy may tolerate a reduced dose of VIDEX EC after resolution of these symptoms upon drug discontinuation.

In adult patients with impaired renal function, the dose of VIDEX EC should be adjusted to compensate for the slower rate of elimination (see Table 4).

Table 4: VIDEX EC

Dose in Adult Patients with Renal Impairment

Creatinine Clearance (mL/min/1.73 m²)	EC Capsule
Patient Weight ≥60 kg	
≥60 (normal dose)	400 mg QD
30–59	200 mg QD
10–29	125 mg QD
<10	125 mg QD
Patient Weight <60 kg	
≥60 (normal dose)	250 mg QD
30–59	125 mg QD
10–29	125 mg QD
<10	[a]

[a] EC capsules are not suitable for use in patients <60 kg with creatinine clearance <10 mL/min.

For patients undergoing dialysis, the daily dose of VIDEX EC should be administered after dialysis. It is not necessary to administer a supplemental dose of VIDEX EC following hemodialysis.
Geriatrics: Because elderly patients are more likely to have decreased renal function, care should be taken in dose selection. In addition, renal function should be monitored and dosage adjustment should be made accordingly.
Hepatic Impairment: There were no substantial alterations in didanosine pharmacokinetics in patients with moderate or severe (Child-Pugh class B or C) hepatic impairment compared with healthy subjects. No dose adjustment of VIDEX EC is necessary for patients with moderate (Child-Pugh class B) hepatic impairment. There is insufficient data to recommend a specific dose of adjustment in patients with severe (Child-Pugh class C) hepatic impairment.

During treatment with VIDEX EC, patients should be observed for liver enzyme elevations and VIDEX EC suspended if enzymes rise to a clinically significant level (see Warnings and Precautions).
Concomitant Therapy: Tenofovir disoproxil fumarate: A dose reduction of VIDEX EC is recommended when coadministered with tenofovir (see Precautions, Drug Interactions).
VIDEX EC: 250 mg (adults weighing ≥60 kg with creatinine clearance ≥60 mL/min) or 200 mg (adults weighing <60 kg with creatinine clearance ≥60 mL/min) once daily together with tenofovir and a light meal (≤400 kcalories, ≤20% fat).

The appropriate dose of VIDEX EC coadministered with tenofovir in patients with creatinine clearance <60 mL/min has not been established.

INFORMATION FOR THE PATIENT: Published in e-CPS, available by subscription at www.e-cps.ca.

SUPPLIED: 125 mg: Each white, opaque enteric coated beadlet capsule, printed in tan with "BMS 125 mg" and "6671", contains: didanosine 125 mg. Nonmedicinal ingredients: carboxymethylcellulose sodium, diethyl phthalate, methacrylic acid copolymer, sodium hydroxide, sodium starch glycolate and talc; capsule shell: gelatin, sodium lauryl sulfate and titanium dioxide. Capsules are imprinted with edible ink. Bottles of 30. Store in tightly closed bottles at room temperature (15 to 30°C).
200 mg: Each white, opaque enteric coated beadlet capsule, printed in green with "BMS 200 mg" and "6672", contains: didanosine 200 mg. Nonmedicinal ingredients: carboxymethylcellulose sodium, diethyl phthalate, methacrylic acid copolymer, sodium hydroxide, sodium starch glycolate and talc; capsule shell: gelatin, sodium lauryl sulfate and titanium dioxide. Capsules are imprinted with edible ink. Bottles of 30. Store in tightly closed bottles at room temperature (15 to 30°C).
250 mg: Each white, opaque, enteric coated beadlet capsule, printed in blue with "BMS 250 mg" and "6673", contains: didanosine 250 mg. Nonmedicinal ingredients: carboxymethylcellulose sodium, diethyl phthalate, methacrylic acid copolymer, sodium hydroxide, sodium starch glycolate and talc; capsule shell: gelatin, sodium lauryl sulfate and titanium dioxide. Capsules are imprinted with edible ink. Bottles of 30. Store in tightly closed bottles at room temperature (15 to 30°C).
400 mg: Each white, opaque, enteric coated beadlet capsule, printed in red with "BMS 400 mg" and "6674", contains: didanosine 400 mg. Nonmedicinal ingredients: carboxymethylcellulose sodium, diethyl phthalate, methacrylic acid copolymer, sodium hydroxide, sodium starch glycolate and talc; capsule shell: gelatin, sodium lauryl sulfate and titanium dioxide. Capsules are imprinted with edible ink. Bottles of 30. Store in tightly closed bottles at room temperature (15 to 30°C).

(Shown in Product Identification Section)

The reader is invited to consult CPhA's monograph **Fluoroquinolones.**

Vigamox® Pr

moxifloxacin HCl

Antibacterial (Ophthalmic)

Alcon

Date of Preparation: May 4, 2004

PHARMACOLOGY: Moxifloxacin is a synthetic fluoroquinolone antibacterial agent active in vitro against a broad spectrum of Gram-positive and Gram-negative ocular pathogens, atypical microorganisms and anaerobes.

The antibacterial action of moxifloxacin results from inhibition of topoisomerase II (DNA gyrase) and topoisomerase IV. DNA gyrase is an essential enzyme that is involved in the replication, transcription and repair of bacterial DNA. Topoisomerase IV is an enzyme known to play a key role in the partitioning of the chromosomal DNA during bacterial cell division.
Pharmacokinetics/Pharmacodynamics: Following topical ocular administration of VIGAMOX (moxifloxacin hydrochloride) ophthalmic solution, moxifloxacin was absorbed into the systemic circulation. Plasma concentrations of moxifloxacin were measured in 21 male and female adult subjects who received bilateral topical ocular doses of VIGAMOX solution every 8 hours for a total of 13 doses. The mean steady-state C_{max} and AUC were 2.7 ng/mL and 41.9 ng·hr/mL, respectively. These systemic exposure values were at least 1600 and 1000 times lower than the mean C_{max} and AUC reported after therapeutic 400 mg oral doses of moxifloxacin. The plasma half-life of moxifloxacin was estimated to be 13 hours. Moxifloxacin is widely distributed in the body and is excreted in feces or urine either unchanged or as glucuronide or sulfate conjugates.

Tear film concentrations were studied in 31 healthy male and female adult volunteers who were administered 1 drop of VIGAMOX solution to both eyes every 8 hours for a total of 10 doses. Mean tear concentrations at 5 minutes following the first and last topical dose were 46.0 and 55.2 µg/mL, respectively. Thereafter, they decline rapidly in a biphasic manner with the means ranging approximately 1 to 4 µg/mL over the 1 to 8 hour sampling period. Pre-dose morning tear concentrations on Days 2 to 4 averaged over 4 µg/mL. Studies conducted in animals indicate penetration into the conjunctiva and ocular tissues with prolonged binding to melanin.

INDICATIONS: VIGAMOX (moxifloxacin hydrochloride) ophthalmic solution is indicated for the treatment of patients 1 year of age and older with bacterial conjunctivitis caused by susceptible strains of the following organisms:
Aerobic, Gram-Positive: *S. aureus, S. epidermidis, S. haemolyticus, S. hominis, S. pneumoniae, S. viridans* group.
Aerobic, Gram-Negative: Acinetobacter species, *H. influenzae.*

CONTRAINDICATIONS: VIGAMOX (moxifloxacin hydrochloride) ophthalmic solution is contraindicated in patients with a history of hypersensitivity to moxifloxacin, to other quinolones, or to any of the components in this medication (see Supplied).

WARNINGS: VIGAMOX (moxifloxacin hydrochloride) ophthalmic solution is not for injection into the eye.

VIGAMOX solution should not be injected subconjunctivally, nor should it be introduced directly into the anterior chamber of the eye.

In patients receiving systemically administered quinolones, serious and occasionally fatal hypersensitivity (anaphylactic) reactions have been reported, some following the first dose. Some reactions were accompanied by cardiovascular collapse, loss of consciousness, angioedema (including laryngeal, pharyngeal or facial edema), airway obstruction, dyspnea, urticaria, and itching. If an allergic reaction to moxifloxacin occurs, discontinue use of the drug. Serious acute hypersensitivity reactions may require immediate emergency treatment. Oxygen and airway management should be administered as clinically indicated.

Serious and sometimes fatal events, some due to hypersensitivity and some due to uncertain etiology, have been reported in patients receiving therapy with all oral antibiotics. These events may be severe and generally occur following the administration of multiple doses. Clinical manifestations may include one or more of the following: fever, rash or severe dermatologic reactions (e.g. toxic epidermal necrolysis, Stevens-Johnson Syndrome), vasculitis, arthralgia, myalgia, serum sickness, allergic pneumonitis, interstitial nephritis, acute renal insufficiency or failure, hepatitis, jaundice, acute hepatic necrosis or failure, anemia including hemolytic and aplastic, thrombocytopenia including thrombotic thrombocytopenic purpura, leukopenia, agranulocytosis, pancytopenia, and/or other hematologic abnormalities.

PRECAUTIONS: General: As with other anti-infectives, prolonged use may result in overgrowth of non-susceptible organisms, including fungi. If superinfection occurs, discontinue use and institute alternative therapy. Whenever clinical judgment dictates, the patient should be examined with the aid of magnification, such as slit-lamp biomicroscopy, and, where appropriate, fluorescein staining.

In general, patients with signs and symptoms of bacterial conjunctivitis should be advised not to wear contact lenses.

Information to Be Provided to the Patient: Avoid contaminating the applicator tip with material from the eye, fingers or other source.

Systemically administered quinolones have been associated with hypersensitivity reactions, even following a single dose. Discontinue use immediately and contact your physician at the first sign of a rash or allergic reaction.

The potential of VIGAMOX (moxifloxacin hydrochloride) ophthalmic solution to produce arthropathy in animals has not been studied. Moxifloxacin and other members of the quinolone class have been shown to cause arthropathy in immature Beagle dogs following oral administration.

Drug Interactions: Drug-drug interaction studies have not been conducted with VIGAMOX solution. Moxifloxacin can be chelated by polyvalent ions such as Mg^{++}, Al^{+++}, Fe^{++} and Zn^{++}. There is limited information available on the concurrent use of VIGAMOX solution and other ophthalmic products.

Following oral administration, no clinically significant drug-drug interactions between theophylline, warfarin, digoxin, oral contraceptives or glyburide have been observed with moxifloxacin. Theophylline, digoxin, probenecid, and ranitidine have been shown not to alter the pharmacokinetics of moxifloxacin. In vitro studies indicate that moxifloxacin does not inhibit CYP3A4, CYP2D6, CYP2C9, CYP2C19 or CYP1A2 indicating that moxifloxacin is unlikely to alter the pharmacokinetics of drugs metabolized by these cytochrome P450 isozymes.

Pregnancy: Since there are no adequate and well-controlled studies in pregnant women VIGAMOX solution should only be used during pregnancy if the potential benefit justifies the potential risk to the fetus.

VIGAMOX solution has not been studied in pregnant animals. Oral and IV studies in pregnant animals indicated that moxifloxacin is not teratogenic. Decreased fetal birth weights and slightly delayed fetal skeletal development were observed in rats and rabbits following oral and intravenous administration of moxifloxacin, respectively. An increased incidence of smaller fetuses was observed in monkeys following oral dosing. When ^{14}C-moxifloxacin was administered orally to pregnant rats, radioactivity penetrated the placenta and was absorbed to a moderate extent by the fetus.The ratio for AUC (0-24 h) for fetal plasma to maternal plasma was 0.656.

As with other members of the quinolone class, moxifloxacin has caused arthropathy in immature Beagle dogs following oral administration. The significance of these findings to humans is unknown.

Lactation: Moxifloxacin is excreted in the breast milk of rats following oral and intravenous administration. Because of the potential for unknown effects from moxifloxacin in infants being nursed by mothers taking VIGAMOX solution, a decision should be made to either discontinue nursing or discontinue the administration of VIGAMOX solution, taking into account the importance of VIGAMOX solution therapy to the mother and the possible risk to the infant.

Children: The safety and efficacy of VIGAMOX solution in patients less than one year of age has not been established.

The effect of VIGAMOX solution on weight bearing joints has not been assessed. Oral administration of some quinolones, including moxifloxacin, has been shown to cause arthropathy in immature animals.

Geriatrics: No overall differences in safety and effectiveness have been observed between elderly and other adult patients.

ADVERSE EFFECTS: In clinical trials involving 1068 subjects/patients, VIGAMOX (moxifloxacin hydrochloride) ophthalmic solution was administered twice-daily for three days, three-times-daily for four to fourteen days and eight-times-daily for fourteen days. During treatment with VIGAMOX solution, 6.6% (71 out of 1068) subjects/patients experienced treatment-related adverse drug reactions and of these only two (0.2%) discontinued study participation. No serious ophthalmic or systemic adverse reactions related to VIGAMOX solution were reported.

Clinical Trial Adverse Drug Reactions: The most frequently reported treatment-related adverse drug reactions were transient eye irritation (3.9%) (burning and/or stinging) and eye pruritus (1.1%).

Treatment-related adverse drug reactions that occurred at an incidence of 0.1% to less than 1.0% included the following:

Eye Disorders: ocular hyperaemia, keratoconjunctivitis sicca, abnormal sensation in eye, ocular discomfort, corneal epithelium defect, conjunctivitis, conjunctival hemorrhage, visual acuity reduced, eyelid oedema, eye pain.

General Disorders and Administration Site Conditions: sensation of foreign body.

Investigations: corneal staining, alanine aminotransferase increased.

Nervous System Disorders: dysgeusia, headache.

Respiratory, Thoracic, and Mediastinal Disorders: pharyngolaryngeal pain.

Post-Market Adverse Drug Reactions: All adverse drug reactions with VIGAMOX solution based on post-marketing reports (from more than 1.1 million units sold) have been reported at an incidence of less than 0.01%. The most frequently reported adverse reactions with VIGAMOX solution based on post-marketing reports include:

Eye Disorders: endophthalmitis, eye irritation, corneal infiltrates, anterior chamber cells, corneal deposits.

Immune System Disorders: hypersensitivity NOS.

Skin and Subcutaneous Disorders: erythema.

OVERDOSE:

Symptoms: No information is available on overdose of VIGAMOX (moxifloxacin hydrochloride) ophthalmic solution in humans. A topical overdose of VIGAMOX solution may be flushed from the eye(s) with warm tap water.

In an oral (gavage) monkey study, doses of moxifloxacin hydrochloride up to 15 mg/kg/day did not produce any toxicity. This dose is at least 10 times higher than the accidental ingestion of the contents of a 3 mL bottle of VIGAMOX solution by a 10 kg child.

For management of a suspected drug overdose, CPhA recommends that you contact your **regional Poison Control Centre**. See the *CPS* Directory section for a list of Poison Control Centres.

DOSAGE: The recommended dosage regimen for patients one year of age and older is one drop in the affected eye(s) 3 times a day for 7 days.

INFORMATION FOR THE PATIENT: Published in e-CPS, available by subscription at www.e-cps.ca.

SUPPLIED: Each mL of ophthalmic solution contains: moxifloxacin HCl 5.45 mg equivalent to moxifloxacin base 5 mg. Nonmedicinal ingredients: boric acid, purified water and sodium chloride. May also contain hydrochloric acid/sodium hydroxide to adjust pH. Preservative-free. Product is self-preserved. Solution is isotonic and formulated at pH 6.8 with an osmolality of approximately 290 mOsm/kg. Supplied as a 3 mL sterile ophthalmic solution in the Alcon DROP-TAINER dispensing system consisting of a natural low density polyethylene bottle and dispensing plug and tan polypropylene closure. Tamper evidence is provided with a shrink band around the closure and neck area of the package. Store at 4-25°C. Discard 28 days after opening.

Vimpat™ Ⓟ

lacosamide

Antiepileptic

UCB

Date of Preparation: September 23, 2010

SUMMARY PRODUCT INFORMATION:

Route of Administration	Dosage Form/ Strength	Nonmedicinal Ingredients
Oral	Film-coated tablets/ 50 mg, 100 mg, 150 mg and 200 mg	Colloidal silicon dioxide, crospovidone, hydroxypropylcellulose, hypromellose, lecithin, magnesium stearate, microcrystalline cellulose, polyethylene glycol, polyvinyl alcohol, talc, titanium dioxide, and dye pigments: 50 mg tablets: red iron oxide, black iron oxide, FD&C Blue #2/indigo carmine Aluminum Lake 100 mg tablets: yellow iron oxide 150 mg tablets: yellow iron oxide, red iron oxide, black iron oxide 200 mg tablets: FD&C Blue #2/indigo carmine Aluminum Lake

INDICATIONS AND CLINICAL USE: Adults (≥18 years of age): VIMPAT (lacosamide) is indicated as adjunctive therapy in the management of partial-onset seizures in adult patients with epilepsy who are not satisfactorily controlled with conventional therapy.

Geriatrics (≥65 years of age): The clinical experience with VIMPAT in elderly patients with epilepsy is limited (n=18). Caution should be exercised during dose titration and age-associated decreased renal clearance should be considered in elderly patients (see Warnings and Precautions, Special Populations, Geriatrics (≥65 years of age); Dosage and Administration and Action and Clinical Pharmacology, Special Populations and Conditions, Geriatrics (≥65 years of age)).

Pediatrics (<18 years of age): The safety and efficacy of VIMPAT in pediatric patients (<18 years of age) have not been established and its use in this patient population is not indicated (see Warnings and Precautions, Special Populations, Pediatrics (<18 years of age)). Only ten pediatric patients (16 to 17 years of age) participated in controlled trials of partial-onset seizures.

CONTRAINDICATIONS:

- Patients who are hypersensitive to the active substance or to any of the excipients. For a complete listing, see Dosage Forms, Composition and Packaging.
- Patients with a history of, or presence of, second-or third-degree atrioventricular (AV) block.
- Patients with hypersensitivity to peanuts or soya should not take VIMPAT (lacosamide) film-coated tablets.

WARNINGS AND PRECAUTIONS: General: Withdrawal of Antiepileptic Drugs (AEDs): As with all AEDs, VIMPAT (lacosamide) should be withdrawn gradually (over a minimum of 1 week) to minimize the potential of increased seizure frequency (see Dosage and Administration, Recommended Dose and Dosage Adjustment).

Cardiac Conduction: PR Interval Prolongation: VIMPAT should be used with caution in patients with known conduction problems [e.g. marked first-degree atrioventricular (AV) block, sick sinus syndrome without pacemaker], or with severe cardiac disease such as myocardial ischemia or heart failure. In such patients, obtaining an ECG before beginning VIMPAT, and after VIMPAT is titrated to steady-state, is recommended.

Caution should be exercised when VIMPAT is given with other drugs that prolong the PR interval (e.g. carbamazepine, pregabalin, lamotrigine or beta-blockers), as further PR prolongation is possible (see Drug Interactions).

In clinical trials of healthy subjects and patients with epilepsy, VIMPAT treatment was associated with PR interval prolongation in a dose-dependent manner (see Action and Clinical Pharmacology, Pharmacodynamics). Patients with significant electrocardiographic (ECG) abnormalities were systematically excluded from these trials. The mean PR interval increase (at t_{max}) in a clinical pharmacology ECG trial of healthy subjects was 13.6 ms for the 400 mg/day VIMPAT group, 18.2 ms for the 800 mg/day VIMPAT group, and 6.3 ms for the placebo group. The mean increase in PR interval at the end of 12 weeks maintenance treatment for patients with partial-onset seizures who participated in the controlled trials was 1.4 ms, 4.4 ms, and 6.6 ms for the VIMPAT 200, 400, and 600 mg/day groups, respectively, and −0.3 ms for the placebo group. The mean maximum increase in PR interval in these controlled trials was 12.7 ms, 14.3 ms, and 15.7 ms in the VIMPAT 200, 400, and 600 mg/day groups and 11.2 ms in the placebo group. Among patients who participated in these controlled trials, asymptomatic first-degree atrioventricular (AV) block was detected on ECG and reported as an adverse reaction for 0.4% (4/944 patients) in the VIMPAT group and 0% (0/364 patients) in the placebo group (see Adverse Reactions).

VIMPAT administration may predispose to atrial arrhythmias (atrial fibrillation or flutter), especially in patients with diabetic neuropathy and/or cardiovascular disease.

Atrial Fibrillation and Atrial Flutter: In the short-term investigational trials of VIMPAT in epilepsy patients, there were no cases of atrial fibrillation or flutter. In patients with diabetic neuropathy, 0.6% of patients treated with VIMPAT experienced an adverse reaction of atrial fibrillation or atrial flutter, compared to 0% of placebo-treated patients. VIMPAT administration may predispose to atrial arrhythmias (atrial fibrillation or flutter), especially in patients with diabetic neuropathy and/or cardiovascular disease. Patients should be made aware of the symptoms of atrial fibrillation and flutter (e.g., palpitations, rapid pulse, shortness of breath) and told to contact their physician should any of these symptoms occur.

Syncope: In the short-term controlled trials of VIMPAT in epilepsy patients with no significant system illnesses, there was no increase in syncope compared to placebo. In the short-term controlled trials of VIMPAT in patients with diabetic neuropathy, 1.0% of patients who were treated with VIMPAT reported an adverse reaction of syncope or loss of consciousness, compared to 0% of placebo-treated patients with diabetic neuropathy. Most of the cases of syncope were observed in patients receiving doses above 400 mg/day. The cause of syncope was not determined in most cases. However, several were associated with either changes in orthostatic blood pressure, atrial flutter/fibrillation (and associated tachycardia), or bradycardia (see Adverse Reactions).

Immune: Multiorgan hypersensitivity reactions (also known as Drug Rash with Eosinophilia and Systemic Symptoms, or DRESS), Stevens-Johnson Syndrome (SJS) and Toxic Epidermal Necrolysis (TEN) have been reported with other anticonvulsants. Typically, although not exclusively, DRESS presents with fever and rash associated with other organ system involvement, that may or may not include eosinophilia, hepatitis, nephritis, lymphadenopathy, and/or myocarditis. Because these disorders are variable in their expression, other organ system signs and symptoms not noted here may also occur. If any of these hypersensitivity reactions are suspected, VIMPAT should be discontinued and alternative treatment started.

Neurologic: Dizziness and Ataxia: Treatment with VIMPAT has been associated with dizziness and ataxia which could increase the occurrence of accidental injury or falls.

In controlled clinical trials, dizziness was experienced by 25% of patients with partial-onset seizures taking 1 to 3 concomitant AEDs randomized to the recommended doses (200 to 400 mg/day) of VIMPAT (compared with 8% of placebo patients) and was the adverse event most frequently leading to discontinuation (3%). Ataxia was experienced by 6% of patients randomized to the recommended doses (200 to 400 mg/day) of VIMPAT (compared to 2% of placebo patients) (see Adverse Reactions, Clinical Trial Adverse Drug Reactions). There was a substantial increase in the frequency of occurrence of these events when patients received VIMPAT doses greater than 400 mg/day.

Accordingly, patients should be advised not to drive a car or to operate other complex machinery or perform hazardous tasks until they are familiar with the effects of VIMPAT on their ability to perform such activities (see Information for the Patient).

Ophthalmologic: In controlled trials in patients with partial-onset seizures, VIMPAT treatment was associated with vision-related adverse events such as blurred vision (VIMPAT, 8%; placebo, 3%) and diplopia (VIMPAT, 11%; placebo, 2%). Three percent of patients randomized to VIMPAT discontinued treatment due to vision-related adverse events (primarily diplopia) (see Adverse Reactions).

Patients should be informed that if visual disturbances occur, they should notify their physician promptly. If visual disturbance persists, further assessment, including dose reduction and possible discontinuation of VIMPAT, should be considered. More frequent assessments should be considered for patients with known vision-related issues or those who are already routinely monitored for ocular conditions.

Psychiatric: Suicidal Ideation and Behavior: Suicidal ideation and behaviour have been reported in patients treated with antiepileptic agents in several indications.

All patients treated with antiepileptic drugs, irrespective of indication, should be monitored for signs of suicidal ideation and behaviour and appropriate treatment should be considered. Patients (and caregivers of patients) should be advised to seek medical advice should signs of suicidal ideation or behaviour emerge.

An FDA meta-analysis of randomized placebo controlled trials, in which antiepileptic drugs were used for various indications, has shown a small increased risk of suicidal ideation and behaviour in patients treated with these drugs. The mechanism of this risk is not known.

There were 43 892 patients treated in the placebo controlled clinical trials that were included in the meta-analysis. Approximately 75% of patients in these clinical trials were treated for indications other than epilepsy and, for the majority of non-epilepsy indications the treatment (antiepileptic drug or placebo) was administered as monotherapy. Patients with epilepsy represented approximately 25% of the total number of patients treated in the placebo controlled clinical trials and, for the majority of epilepsy patients, treatment (antiepileptic drug or placebo) was administered as adjunct to other antiepileptic agents (i.e., patients in both treatment arms were being treated with one or more antiepileptic drug). Therefore, the small increased risk of suicidal ideation and behaviour reported from the meta-analysis (0.43% for patients on antiepileptic drugs compared to 0.24% for patients on placebo) is based largely on patients that received monotherapy treatment (antiepileptic drug or placebo) for non-epilepsy indications. The study design does not allow an estimation of the risk of suicidal ideation and behaviour for patients with epilepsy that are taking antiepileptic drugs, due both to this population being the minority in the study, and the drug-placebo comparison in this population being confounded by the presence of adjunct antiepileptic drug treatment in both arms.

Special Populations: Women of Childbearing Potential/Contraception: There was no clinically relevant interaction between lacosamide and oral contraceptives (ethinylestradiol and levonorgestrel) in clinical studies (see Drug Interactions, Drug-Drug Interactions, Oral Contraceptives).

Pregnant Women: There are no studies with lacosamide in pregnant women. Studies in animals did not indicate any teratogenic effects in rats or rabbits, but embryotoxicity was observed in rats and rabbits at maternal toxic doses.

Since the potential risk for humans is unknown, VIMPAT should not be used during pregnancy unless the benefit to the mother clearly outweighs the potential risk to the foetus. If women decide to become pregnant while taking VIMPAT, the use of this product should be carefully re-evaluated.

Pregnancy Registry: Physicians are advised to recommend that pregnant patients taking VIMPAT enroll in the North American Antiepileptic Drug Pregnancy Registry. This can be done by calling the toll free number 1-888-233-2334, and must be done by patients themselves. Information on the registry can also be found at the following website: http://www.aedpregnancyregistry.org/.

Nursing Women: It is unknown whether lacosamide is excreted in human breast milk. Animal studies have shown excretion of lacosamide in breast milk. Because many drugs are excreted into human milk, a decision should be made whether to discontinue nursing or to discontinue lacosamide, taking into account the importance of the drug to the mother.

Fertility: No adverse effects on male or female fertility or reproduction were observed in rats at doses producing plasma exposures (AUC) up to approximately 2 times the plasma AUC in humans at the maximum recommended human dose (MRHD) of 400 mg/day.

Pediatrics (<18 years of age): VIMPAT is not indicated for use in pediatrics (<18 years of age) as there is insufficient data on safety and efficacy of the drug in this population (see Indications and Clinical Use and Dosage and Administration).

Geriatrics (≥65 years of age): The experience with VIMPAT in elderly patients with epilepsy is limited (n=18). Although no dose reduction is necessary in elderly patients, caution should be exercised during dose titration and age-associated decreased renal clearance with an increase in AUC levels should be considered in elderly patients (see Dosage and Administration and Action and Clinical Pharmacology, Special Populations and Conditions, Geriatrics (≥65 years of age)).

Monitoring and Laboratory Tests: See Warnings and Precautions, Cardiac Conduction.

ADVERSE REACTIONS: Adverse Drug Reaction Overview: In controlled clinical trials in patients with partial-onset seizures, 924 patients received VIMPAT (lacosamide).

Some of the most frequently reported adverse reactions in controlled clinical trials with lacosamide treatment were dizziness, nausea, and vision-related events (e.g, diplopia, blurred vision). They were dose-related and usually mild to moderate in intensity.

Clinical Trial Adverse Drug Reactions: Because clinical trials are conducted under very specific conditions, the adverse reaction rates observed in the clinical trials may not reflect the rates observed in practice and should not be compared to the rates in the clinical trials of another drug. Adverse drug reaction information from clinical trials is useful for identifying drug-related adverse events and for approximating rates.

Table 1 gives the incidence of treatment-emergent adverse events that occurred in ≥1% of adult patients with partial-onset seizures in the total VIMPAT group (N=944) and for which the frequency was greater than placebo, in controlled clinical trials. The majority of adverse events were reported with a maximum intensity of "mild" or "moderate".

Table 1: VIMPAT

Treatment-Emergent Adverse Event Incidence in Double-Blind, Placebo-Controlled Partial-Onset Seizure Trials (Events ≥1% of Patients in the total VIMPAT group and More Frequent Than in the Placebo Group)

MedDRA System Organ Class/Preferred Term	Placebo N=364 %	200 mg/day N=270 %	400 mg/day N=471 %	600 mg/day N=203 %
Ear and Labyrinth Disorders				
Vertigo	1	5	3	4
Tinnitus	1	0	2	2
Eye Disorders				
Diplopia	2	6	10	16
Vision blurred	3	2	9	16
Conjunctivitis	<1	2	<1	0
Gastrointestinal Disorders				
Nausea	4	7	11	17
Vomiting	3	6	9	16
Diarrhoea	3	3	5	4
Constipation	1	1	2	4
Flatulence	0	3	2	1
Dyspepsia	1	1	2	2
Toothache	1	2	2	1
Dry mouth	1	1	1	2
Hypoaesthesia oral	0	0	1	1
General Disorders and Administration Site Conditions				
Fatigue	6	7	7	15
Gait disturbance	<1	<1	2	4

(cont'd)

Table 1: VIMPAT *(cont'd)*

Treatment-Emergent Adverse Event Incidence in Double-Blind, Placebo-Controlled Partial-Onset Seizure Trials (Events ≥1% of Patients in the total VIMPAT group and More Frequent Than in the Placebo Group)

MedDRA System Organ Class/Preferred Term	Placebo N=364 %	200 mg/day N=270 %	400 mg/day N=471 %	600 mg/day N=203 %
Asthenia	1	2	2	4
Irritability	1	1	2	2
Chest pain	1	2	1	2
Pyrexia	1	2	1	1
Feeling drunk	0	0	1	3
Oedema peripheral	0	1	<1	2
Feeling abnormal	<1	0	1	2
Infections and Infestations				
Nasopharyngitis	6	6	8	4
Bronchitis	0	2	1	1
Rhinitis	<1	<1	1	1
Ear infection	<1	1	1	0
Cystitis	<1	1	<1	1
Gastroenteritis	0	1	<1	0
Injury, Poisoning and Procedural Complications				
Skin laceration	2	2	3	3
Fall	<1	1	2	1
Head injury	<1	2	1	1
Joint sprain	0	1	1	2
Investigations				
Positive rombergism	0	1	1	2
Gamma-glutamyltransferase increased	<1	2	<1	1
White blood cell count decreased	<1	0	<1	2
Metabolism and Nutrition Disorders				
Decreased appetite	<1	<1	2	3
Hypercholesterolaemia	<1	1	1	1
Musculoskeletal and Connective Tissue Disorders				
Muscle spasms	<1	1	1	2
Neck pain	<1	1	1	1
Nervous System Disorders				
Dizziness	8	16	30	53
Headache	9	11	14	12
Ataxia	2	4	7	15
Somnolence	5	5	8	8
Tremor	4	4	6	12
Nystagmus	4	2	5	10
Balance disorder	0	1	5	6
Memory impairment	2	1	2	6
Cognitive disorder	<1	<1	2	2
Hypoaesthesia	1	2	2	2
Dysarthria	<1	<1	1	3
Disturbance in attention	1	0	1	2
Psychiatric Disorders				
Depression	1	2	2	2
Insomnia	1	2	2	1

(cont'd)

Table 1: VIMPAT *(cont'd)*

Treatment-Emergent Adverse Event Incidence in Double-Blind, Placebo-Controlled Partial-Onset Seizure Trials (Events ≥1% of Patients in the total VIMPAT group and More Frequent Than in the Placebo Group)

MedDRA System Organ Class/Preferred Term	Placebo N=364 %	200 mg/day N=270 %	400 mg/day N=471 %	600 mg/day N=203 %
Confusional state	1	0	2	3
Mood altered	<1	1	1	2
Respiratory, Thoracic and Mediastinal Disorders				
Dyspnoea	<1	0	1	1
Epistaxis	0	1	1	0
Skin and Subcutaneous Tissue Disorders				
Pruritus	1	3	2	3
Hyperhidrosis	<1	0	1	2

Table 2: VIMPAT

Incidence of Most Common Dose-Related Treatment-Emergent Adverse Events in Double-Blind, Placebo-Controlled Partial-Onset Seizure Trials (Events ≥1% of Patients in the total VIMPAT group and More Frequent Than in the Placebo Group)

MedDRA Preferred Term	Placebo N=364 %	200 mg/day N=270 %	400 mg/day N=471 %	600 mg/day N=203 %
Diplopia	2	6	10	16
Vision blurred	3	2	9	16
Nausea	4	7	11	17
Vomiting	3	6	9	16
Dizziness	8	16	30	53
Ataxia	2	4	7	15
Tremor	4	4	6	12
Nystagmus	4	2	5	10

Less Common Clinical Trial Adverse Drug Reactions (<1%): Other adverse events reported by <1% of patients with partial-onset seizures in the total VIMPAT group in placebo-controlled clinical trials that occurred more frequently than in the placebo group were:
Eye Disorders: eye irritation.
Nervous System Disorders: hypokinesia.
Vascular Disorders: hot flush.
Cardiac: Dose-dependent prolongations in PR interval with VIMPAT have been observed in clinical studies in patients and in healthy subjects (see Action and Clinical Pharmacology). In clinical trials in patients with partial-onset seizures, asymptomatic first-degree AV block was observed as an adverse reaction in 0.4% (4/944) of patients randomized to receive VIMPAT and 0% (0/364) of patients randomized to receive placebo. In clinical trials in patients with diabetic neuropathy, asymptomatic first-degree AV block was observed as an adverse reaction in 0.6% (8/1393) of patients receiving VIMPAT and 0% (0/470) of patients receiving placebo. No second or higher degree AV block was seen in lacosamide treated epilepsy patients in controlled clinical trials. In clinical trials in patients with diabetic neuropathic pain, second-degree AV block has been rarely reported (<0.1%) (see Warnings and Precautions). However, cases with second and third degree AV block associated with lacosamide treatment have been reported in post-marketing experience (see Post-Market Adverse Drug Reactions).
Discontinuation Due to Adverse Events in Pre-Marketing Controlled Clinical Studies: In controlled clinical trials in patients with partial-onset seizures, the rate of discontinuation as a result of an adverse event was 8% and 17% in patients randomized to receive VIMPAT at doses of 200 and 400 mg/day, respectively (placebo: 5%). At VIMPAT doses of 600 mg/day, 29% of the patients discontinued the trials due to adverse events. The adverse events most commonly (≥1% in the VIMPAT total group and greater than placebo) leading to discontinuation were dizziness, coordination abnormal, vomiting, diplopia, nausea, vertigo, and vision blurred. Other adverse events that led to discontinuation (<1% in the VIMPAT total group and greater than placebo) were typically CNS related and included tremor, nystagmus, fatigue, balance disorder, and disturbance in attention.
Comparison of Gender and Race: The overall adverse event rate was similar in male and female patients. Although there were few non-Caucasian patients, no differences in the incidences of adverse events compared to Caucasian patients were observed.
Abnormal Hematologic and Clinical Chemistry Findings: Abnormalities in liver function tests have been observed in controlled trials with VIMPAT in adult patients with partial-onset seizures who were taking 1 to 3 concomitant anti-epileptic drugs. Elevations of ALT to ≥3×ULN (upper limit of normal) occurred in 0.7% (7/935) of VIMPAT patients and 0% (0/356) of placebo patients. One case of hepatitis with transaminases >20×ULN was observed in one healthy subject 10 days after VIMPAT treatment completion, along with nephritis (proteinuria and urine casts). Serologic studies were negative for viral hepatitis. Transaminases returned to normal within one month without specific treatment. At the time of this event, bilirubin was normal. The hepatitis/nephritis was interpreted as a delayed hypersensitivity reaction to VIMPAT.
Drug Abuse and Dependence/Liability: Lacosamide showed no signs of abuse potential in three rat models. After prolonged administration to rats and dogs, there was no tolerance to lacosamide's pharmacological actions and abrupt cessation of treatment did not produce symptoms of psychological or physical dependence.

In a human abuse potential study, single doses of 200 mg and 800 mg lacosamide produced euphoria-type subjective responses that differentiated statistically from placebo; at 800 mg, these euphoria-type responses were statistically indistinguishable from those produced by alprazolam. The duration of the euphoria-type responses following lacosamide was less than that following alprazolam. A high rate of euphoria was also reported as an adverse event in the human abuse potential study following single doses of 800 mg lacosamide (15% [5/34]) compared to placebo (0%) and in two pharmacokinetic studies following single and multiple doses of 300-800 mg lacosamide (ranging from 6% [2/33] to 25% [3/12]) compared to placebo (0%). However, the rate of euphoria reported as an adverse event in the VIMPAT development program at therapeutic doses was less than 1%.

Abrupt termination of lacosamide in clinical trials with diabetic neuropathic pain patients produced no signs or symptoms that are associated with a withdrawal syndrome indicative of physical dependence. However, psychological dependence cannot be excluded due to the ability of lacosamide to produce euphoria-type adverse events in humans.
Post-Market Adverse Drug Reactions: Since the first global approval of VIMPAT on 29 August 2008 through 28 February 2010, there are approximately 25 899 patient-years of exposure to VIMPAT. In addition to the adverse reactions reported during clinical studies and listed above, the following adverse reactions have been reported in post-marketing experience. Data are insufficient to support an estimate of their incidence in the population to be treated.
Immune System Disorders: drug hypersensitivity reactions, potential cases of multiorgan hypersensitivity reactions have been reported rarely with lacosamide.
Cardiac Disorders: bradycardia.
Metabolism and Nutrition Disorders: hyponatremia.
Nervous System Disorders: ataxia, syncope.
Psychiatric Disorders: euphoric mood, suicide attempt and suicidal ideation.
Skin and Subcutaneous Tissue Disorders: rash.
Cardiac Disorders: Second and third degree AV block associated with lacosamide treatment has been reported in post-marketing experience (see Warnings and Precautions, Cardiac Conduction).

DRUG INTERACTIONS: VIMPAT (lacosamide) should be used with caution in patients treated with medicinal products known to be associated with PR prolongation (e.g. carbamazepine, lamotrigine, pregabalin, beta-blockers) and in patients treated with class I antiarrhythmic drugs (see Warnings and Precautions, Cardiac Conduction).
In Vitro Assessment of Drug Interactions: In vitro metabolism studies indicate that lacosamide does not induce the enzyme activity of drug metabolizing cytochrome P450 isoforms CYP1A2, 2B6, 2C9, 2C19 and 3A4 at concentrations (12.5 μg/mL) close to the human peak plasma concentration (10.9 μg/mL, C_{max}, steady state at maximum recommended human dose (MRHD) of 400 mg/day). At concentrations 10 times higher (125 μg/mL), enzyme activities were less than 2-fold increased. Lacosamide did not inhibit CYP 1A1, 1A2, 2A6, 2B6, 2C8, 2C9, 2D6, 2E1, 3A4/5 at concentrations up to 1000-fold greater than the C_{max} for 400 mg/day. The inhibitory concentrations (IC_{50}) of CYP3A4, 3A5, 2C9 and 1A1 by lacosamide are at least 70-fold higher than the C_{max} for 400 mg/day.

In vitro data suggest that lacosamide has the potential to inhibit CYP2C19 at therapeutic concentrations (60% inhibition at 25 μg/mL). However, an in vivo evaluation in healthy subjects showed no inhibitory effect of lacosamide (600 mg/day administered as 300 mg BID dosing) on the single dose pharmacokinetics of omeprazole (40 mg).

Lacosamide is a CYP2C19 substrate. The relative contribution of other CYP isoforms or non-CYP enzymes in the metabolism of lacosamide is not clear.

Lacosamide was not a substrate or inhibitor for P-glycoprotein.

Since <15% of lacosamide is bound to plasma proteins, a clinically relevant interaction with other drugs through competition for protein binding sites is unlikely.
In Vivo Assessment of Drug Interactions: Drug-drug interaction studies in healthy subjects showed no pharmacokinetic interactions between VIMPAT and carbamazepine, valproic acid, digoxin, metformin, omeprazole, or an oral contraceptive containing ethinylestradiol and levonorgestrel. There was no evidence for any relevant drug-drug interaction of VIMPAT with common AEDs in the placebo-controlled clinical trials in patients with partial-onset seizures.

The lack of pharmacokinetic interaction does not rule out the possibility of pharmacodynamic interactions, particularly among drugs that affect the heart conduction system.
Drug-Drug Interactions: Drug-Interaction Studies with AEDs: Effect of VIMPAT on Concomitant AEDs: VIMPAT 400 mg/day had no influence on the pharmacokinetics of 600 mg/day valproic acid and 400 mg/day carbamazepine in healthy subjects.

The placebo-controlled clinical studies in patients with partial-onset seizures showed that steady-state plasma concentrations of levetiracetam, carbamazepine, carbamazepine epoxide, lamotrigine, topiramate, oxcarbazepine monohydroxy derivative (MHD), phenytoin, valproic acid, phenobarbital, gabapentin, clonazepam, and zonisamide were not affected by concomitant intake of VIMPAT at 200 to 600 mg/day.
Effect of Concomitant AEDs on VIMPAT: Drug-drug interaction studies in healthy subjects showed that 600 mg/day valproic acid had no influence on the pharmacokinetics of 400 mg/day VIMPAT. Likewise, 400 mg/day carbamazepine had no influence on the pharmacokinetics of VIMPAT (400 mg/day) in a healthy subject study. Population pharmacokinetics results in patients with partial-onset seizures showed small reductions (approximately 25% lower) in lacosamide plasma concentrations when VIMPAT (200 to 600 mg/day) was coadministered with carbamazepine, phenobarbital or phenytoin.
Drug-Drug Interaction Studies with Other Drugs: Digoxin: VIMPAT (400 mg/day) did not affect pharmacokinetics of digoxin (0.5 mg once daily) in a study in healthy subjects. There was no effect of digoxin on the pharmacokinetics of VIMPAT.
Metformin: There were no clinically relevant changes in metformin levels following co-administration of VIMPAT (400 mg/day). Metformin (500 mg three times a day) had no effect on the pharmacokinetics of VIMPAT (400 mg/day) in healthy subjects.
Omeprazole: Omeprazole (40 mg once daily) increased the AUC of lacosamide by 19% (300 mg, single dose), which is unlikely to be clinically significant. Lacosamide (600 mg/day) did not affect the single-dose pharmacokinetics of omeprazole (40 mg) in healthy subjects.
Oral Contraceptives: In an interaction trial in healthy subjects, there was no clinically relevant interaction between lacosamide (400 mg/day) and the oral contraceptives ethinylestradiol (0.03 mg) and levonorgestrel (0.15 mg). Progesterone concentrations were not affected when the medicinal products were co-administered (see Warnings and Precautions, Special Populations, Women of Childbearing Potential/Contraception).
Drug-Food Interactions: VIMPAT is completely absorbed after oral administration. Food does not affect the rate or extent of absorption.
Drug-Herb Interactions: Interactions with herbal products have not been evaluated.
Drug-Laboratory Test Interactions: Interactions with laboratory tests have not been observed.

DOSAGE AND ADMINISTRATION: Dosing Considerations: VIMPAT (lacosamide) may be taken with or without food.
Film-Coated Tablets: On the first day of treatment the patient starts with VIMPAT 50 mg tablets twice a day. During the second week, the patient takes VIMPAT 100 mg tablets twice a day. Depending on response and tolerability, VIMPAT 150 mg tablets may be taken twice a day during the third week and VIMPAT 200 mg tablets twice a day during the fourth week.
Recommended Dose and Dosage Adjustment: Adults: The recommended starting dose for VIMPAT is 50 mg twice a day, with or without food, which should be increased to an initial therapeutic dose of 100 mg twice a day after one week. Depending on patient response and tolerability, the maintenance dose can be further increased by 50 mg twice a day every week, to a maximum recommended daily dose of 400 mg (200 mg twice a day). Doses above 400 mg/day do not confer additional benefit, are associated with more severe and substantially higher frequency of adverse reactions and are not recommended.

In accordance with current clinical practice, if VIMPAT has to be discontinued, it is recommended this be done gradually (e.g. taper the daily dose by 200 mg/week).
Patients with Renal Impairment: No dose adjustment is necessary in patients with mild or moderate renal impairment (creatinine clearance (CL_{CR}) >30 mL/min). A maximum dose of 300 mg/day is recommended for patients with severe renal impairment (CL_{CR} ≤30 mL/min) and in patients with end-stage renal disease. In all patients with any degree of renal impairment, the dose titration should be performed with caution (see Action and Clinical Pharmacology, Special Populations and Conditions, Renal Insufficiency).

Following a 4-hour hemodialysis treatment, AUC of VIMPAT was reduced by approximately 50%. Thus, dosage supplementation of up to 50% following hemodialysis may be considered. Treatment of patients with end-stage renal disease should be made with caution as there is limited clinical experience in subjects (N=8) and no experience in patients, and there is accumulation of a metabolite (with no known pharmacological activity).
Patients with Hepatic Impairment: The dose titration should be performed with caution in patients with mild to moderate hepatic impairment. A maximum dose of 300 mg/day is recommended for patients with mild or moderate hepatic impairment. The pharmacokinetics of VIMPAT have not been evaluated in severe hepatic impairment. VIMPAT is not recommended in patients with severe hepatic impairment (see Action and Clinical Pharmacology, Special Populations and Conditions, Hepatic Insufficiency).
Geriatrics (≥65 years of age): Clinical experience with VIMPAT in elderly patients with epilepsy is limited (n=18). Although no dose reduction is necessary in elderly patients, caution should be exercised during dose titration and age-associated decreased renal clearance with an increase in AUC levels should be considered in elderly patients (see Action and Clinical Pharmacology, Special Populations and Conditions, Geriatrics (≥65 years of age)).
Pediatrics (<18 years of age): The safety and effectiveness of VIMPAT in pediatric patients <18 years has not been established, and therefore its use in this patient population is not indicated (see Indications and Clinical Use and Warnings and Precautions, Special Populations, Pediatrics (<18 years of age)).
Missed Dose: If the patient misses a dose by a few hours, they should be instructed to take VIMPAT as soon as they remember. If it is close to their next dose, they should be instructed to take their medication at the next regular time. Patients should not take two doses at the same time.

OVERDOSAGE:
Signs, Symptoms, and Laboratory Findings of Acute Overdose in Humans: There is limited clinical experience with VIMPAT (lacosamide) overdose in humans. Clinical symptoms (dizziness and nausea) following doses of 1200 mg/day were mainly related to the central nervous system and the gastrointestinal system.

There has been a single case of intentional overdose by a patient who self-administered 12 g VIMPAT along with large doses of zonisamide, topiramate, and gabapentin. The patient presented in a coma and was hospitalized. An EEG revealed epileptic waveforms. The patient recovered 2 days later.

During pre-marketing controlled clinical studies, no intentional overdose of VIMPAT resulted in death.

Treatment or Management of Overdose: There is no specific antidote for overdose with VIMPAT. Standard decontamination procedures should be followed. General supportive care of the patient is indicated including monitoring of vital signs and observation of the clinical status of patient. A Poison Control Centre should be contacted for up to date information on the management of overdose with VIMPAT. Standard hemodialysis procedures result in significant clearance of VIMPAT (reduction of systemic exposure by 50% in 4 hours). Hemodialysis has not been performed in the few known cases of overdose, but may be helpful based on the patient's clinical state or in patients with significant renal impairment.

For management of a suspected drug overdose, contact your regional Poison Control Centre. See the *CPS* Directory section for a list of Poison Control Centres.

ACTION AND CLINICAL PHARMACOLOGY: Mechanism of Action: The precise mechanism by which lacosamide exerts its antiepileptic effect in humans is unknown.

Pharmacodynamics: A pharmacokinetic-pharmacodynamic (efficacy) analysis was performed based on the pooled data from the 3 efficacy trials for partial-onset seizures. Lacosamide exposure is correlated with the reduction in seizure frequency. However, in group analyses, doses above 400 mg/day do not appear to confer additional benefit and are associated with more severe and substantially higher frequency of adverse reactions.

Cardiac Electrophysiology: Electrocardiographic effects of VIMPAT (lacosamide) were determined in a double-blind, randomized clinical pharmacology ECG trial of 247 healthy subjects. Chronic oral doses of 400 and 800 mg/day were compared with placebo and a positive control (400 mg moxifloxacin). VIMPAT did not prolong QTc interval and did not have a dose-related or clinically important effect on QRS duration. VIMPAT produced a dose-related increase in mean PR interval. At steady-state, the time of the maximum observed mean PR interval corresponded with t_{max}. The placebo-subtracted maximum increase in PR-interval (at t_{max}) was 7.3 ms for the 400 mg/day group and 11.9 ms for the 800 mg/day group.

For patients with partial-onset seizures who participated in the controlled trials, the placebo-subtracted maximum increase in PR interval for a 400 mg/day VIMPAT dose was 3.1 ms. For patients with diabetic neuropathic pain who participated in controlled trials, the placebo-subtracted maximum increase in PR-interval for a 400 mg/day VIMPAT dose was 8.3 ms (see Warnings and Precautions and Adverse Reactions).

Pharmacokinetics: The pharmacokinetics of VIMPAT has been studied in healthy adult subjects (age range 18 to 87), adults with partial-onset seizures, adults with diabetic neuropathy, and subjects with renal and hepatic impairment. A summary of lacosamide's pharmacokinetic parameters in healthy subjects is provided in Table 3.

Lacosamide is completely absorbed after oral administration with negligible first-pass effect with a high absolute bioavailability of approximately 100%. The maximum lacosamide plasma concentrations occur approximately 0.25 to 4 hours post-dose after oral dosing, and elimination half-life is approximately 13 hours. Steady state plasma concentrations are achieved after 3 days of twice daily repeated administration. Pharmacokinetics of lacosamide is dose proportional (100-800 mg) and time invariant, with low inter- and intra-subject variability. Compared to lacosamide, the major metabolite, O-desmethyl metabolite, has a longer T_{max} (0.5 to 12 hours) and elimination half-life (15-23 hours) but has no known pharmacologic activity.

Table 3: VIMPAT

Summary of Lacosamide's Pharmacokinetic Parameters in Healthy Subjects

	C_{max} (µg/mL) Arithmetic Mean	$t_{1/2}$ (h) Arithmetic Mean	AUC_T (µg/mL·h) Arithmetic Mean	t_{max} (h) Median (range)
Oral Tablet 200 mg	5.03	13.96	88.61	0.75 (0.25–4.00)

Absorption: Lacosamide is rapidly and completely absorbed after oral administration. The oral bioavailability of lacosamide tablets is approximately 100%. Following oral administration, the plasma concentration of unchanged lacosamide increases rapidly and reaches C_{max} about 0.25 to 4 hours post-dose. Food does not affect the rate and extent of absorption.

After intravenous administration (30-60 minutes), C_{max} is reached at the end of infusion. The plasma concentration increases proportionally with dose after oral (100-800 mg) and intravenous (50-300 mg) administration.

Distribution: The volume of distribution is approximately 0.6 L/kg. Lacosamide is less than 15% bound to plasma proteins.

Metabolism: The metabolism of lacosamide has not been completely characterized. Approximately 95% of the dose is excreted in the urine as drug and metabolites. The major compounds excreted in urine are unchanged lacosamide (approximately 40% of the dose) and its O-desmethyl metabolite, which has no known pharmacological activity (less than 30%). A structurally unknown polar fraction (about 20%) was also found in urine, but was detected only in small amounts (0-2%) in human plasma of some subjects. Small amounts (0.5-2%) of additional metabolites were also found in the urine. The plasma exposure of the major human metabolite (AUC), O-desmethyl-lacosamide, is approximately 15% of the drug product, lacosamide.

CYP2C19 is mainly responsible for the formation of the O-desmethyl metabolite. However, no clinically relevant difference in lacosamide exposure was observed comparing its pharmacokinetics in extensive metabolisers (EMs, with a functional CYP2C19) and poor metabolisers (PMs, lacking a functional CYP2C19). Furthermore, an interaction trial with omeprazole (CYP2C19-inhibitor) demonstrated no clinically relevant changes in lacosamide plasma concentrations indicating that the importance of this pathway is minor. No other enzymes have been identified to be involved in the metabolism of lacosamide.

Excretion: Lacosamide is primarily eliminated from the systemic circulation by renal excretion and biotransformation. After oral administration of 100 mg radiolabeled lacosamide, approximately 95% of radioactivity administered was recovered in the urine and less than 0.5% in the feces. The elimination half-life of the unchanged drug is approximately 13 hours and is not altered by different doses; or multiple dosing. The pharmacokinetics are dose-proportional and time-invariant, with low intra- and inter-subject variability. Following twice daily dosing, steady state plasma concentrations are achieved after a 3 day period. The plasma concentration increases with an accumulation factor of approximately 2.

Special Populations and Conditions: Pediatrics (<18 years of age): Pharmacokinetics of lacosamide have not been established in pediatric patients.

Geriatrics (≥65 years of age): In a study in elderly men and women, the AUC was about 30 and 50% increased compared to young men, respectively. This is partly related to lower body weight. The body weight normalized difference is 26 and 23%, respectively. An increased variability in exposure was also observed. The renal clearance of lacosamide was only slightly reduced in elderly subjects in this study.

Gender: VIMPAT clinical trials indicate that gender does not have a clinically relevant influence on the pharmacokinetics of VIMPAT.

Race: Approximately 90% of the patient population in epilepsy trials was Caucasian. There are no clinically relevant differences in the pharmacokinetics of VIMPAT between Asian, Black, and Caucasian subjects.

Hepatic Insufficiency: Lacosamide undergoes metabolism. Subjects with moderate hepatic impairment (Child-Pugh B) showed higher plasma concentrations of lacosamide (approximately 50-60% higher AUC compared to healthy subjects). A maximum dose of 300 mg/day is recommended for patients with mild to moderate hepatic impairment. Patients with mild to moderate hepatic impairment should be titrated with caution and observed closely during dose titration. Patients with co-existing hepatic and renal impairment of any degree should also be monitored closely during dose titration.

The pharmacokinetics of lacosamide have not been evaluated in patients with severe hepatic impairment. VIMPAT use in patients with severe hepatic impairment is not recommended (see Dosage and Administration and Action and Clinical Pharmacology, Special Populations and Conditions, Renal Insufficiency).

Renal Insufficiency: Lacosamide and its major metabolite are eliminated from the systemic circulation primarily by renal excretion.

The AUC of lacosamide was increased approximately 25% in mildly (CL_{CR} 50-80 mL/min) and moderately (CL_{CR} 30-50 mL/min), and 60% in severely (CL_{CR} ≤30 mL/min) renally impaired patients compared to subjects with normal renal function (CL_{CR} >80 mL/min), whereas C_{max} was unaffected. No dose adjustment is considered necessary in mildly and moderately renal impaired subjects. A maximum dose of 300 mg/day is recommended for patients with severe renal impairment (CL_{CR} ≤30 mL/min) and in patients with endstage renal disease.

Hemodialysis: Lacosamide is effectively removed from plasma by hemodialysis. Following a 4-hour hemodialysis treatment, AUC of VIMPAT is reduced by approximately 50%. Therefore dosage supplementation of up to 50% following hemodialysis should be considered. In all renal impaired patients, the dose titration should be performed with caution.

CYP2C19 Genetic Polymorphism: There are no clinically relevant differences in the pharmacokinetics of lacosamide between CYP2C19 poor metabolizers and extensive metabolizers. Results from a trial in poor metabolizers (PM) (N=4) and extensive metabolizers (EM) (N=8) of cytochrome P450 (CYP) 2C19 showed that lacosamide plasma concentrations were similar in PMs and EMs, but plasma concentrations and the amount excreted into urine of the O-desmethyl metabolite were about 70% reduced in PMs compared to EMs.

STORAGE AND STABILITY: Store at room temperature (15-30°C).

INFORMATION FOR THE PATIENT: Published in e-CPS, available by subscription at www.e-cps.ca.

DOSAGE FORMS, COMPOSITION AND PACKAGING: 50 mg: Each pink, oval, film-coated tablet, debossed with "SP" on one side and "50" on the other, contains: lacosamide 50 mg. Nonmedicinal ingredients: black iron oxide, colloidal silicon dioxide, crospovidone, FD&C Blue #2/indigo carmine Aluminum Lake, hydroxypropylcellulose, hypromellose, lecithin, magnesium stearate, microcrystalline cellulose, polyethylene glycol, polyvinyl alcohol, red iron oxide, talc and titanium dioxide. HDPE bottles of 60.

100 mg: Each dark yellow, oval, film-coated tablet, debossed with "SP" on one side and "100" on the other, contains: lacosamide 100 mg. Nonmedicinal ingredients: colloidal silicon dioxide, crospovidone, hydroxypropylcellulose, hypromellose, lecithin, magnesium stearate, microcrystalline cellulose, polyethylene glycol, polyvinyl alcohol, talc, titanium dioxide and yellow iron oxide. HDPE bottles of 60.

150 mg: Each salmon, oval, film-coated tablet, debossed with "SP" on one side and "150" on the other, contains: lacosamide 150 mg. Nonmedicinal ingredients: black iron oxide, colloidal silicon dioxide, crospovidone, hydroxypropylcellulose, hypromellose, lecithin, magnesium stearate, microcrystalline cellulose, polyethylene glycol, polyvinyl alcohol, red iron oxide, talc, titanium dioxide and yellow iron oxide. HDPE bottles of 60.

200 mg: Each blue, oval, film-coated tablet, debossed with "SP" on one side and "200" on the other, contains: lacosamide 200 mg. Nonmedicinal ingredients: colloidal silicon dioxide, crospovidone, FD&C Blue #2/indigo carmine Aluminum Lake, hydroxypropylcellulose, hypromellose, lecithin, magnesium stearate, microcrystalline cellulose, polyethylene glycol, polyvinyl alcohol, talc and titanium dioxide. HDPE bottles of 60.

(Shown in Product Identification Section)

Vinblastine ℞

Antineoplastic

CPhA Monograph

Date of Preparation: January 2004
Date of Revision: March 2009

This monograph has been compiled by CPhA and reviewed by experts. It may contain information different from that found in Health Canada-approved Product Monographs. The reader is referred to the *CPS* Editorial Policy for more information.

SUMMARY PRODUCT INFORMATION:

Route of Administration	Dosage Form	Strength
Intravenous	Single use vial: 10 mL	Vinblastine sulphate 1 mg/mL

INDICATIONS AND CLINICAL USE: Vinblastine (also known as vinca leukoblastine, VLB, VBL) is indicated for treatment of breast cancer, Hodgkin's disease and Kaposi's sarcoma. It is also used in the treatment of choriocarcinoma, histiocytosis X, mycosis fungoides, non-Hodgkin's lymphoma.

Other uses not approved by Health Canada include bladder cancer, germ cell cancer, immune thrombocytopenic purpura, metastatic melanoma, renal cell cancer and non-small cell lung cancer.

Although effective as a single agent, vinblastine is usually used in combination with other antineoplastics depending on the type of cancer being treated.

Pediatrics: Vinblastine has been used in children.

CONTRAINDICATIONS: Vinblastine is contraindicated in patients with significant bone marrow suppression (that is not a result of the disease being treated). It should not be used in patients with bacterial infections. These infections should be treated prior to starting vinblastine. Intrathecal administration of vinblastine is absolutely contraindicated. Accidental intrathecal administration could be fatal. Vinblastine is contraindicated in patients who are hypersensitive to the drug or to any ingredient in the formulation.

WARNINGS AND PRECAUTIONS:

Serious Warnings and Precautions
Vinblastine is fatal if given intrathecally and is intended for iv use only. Syringes containing this drug should carry the label: "Warning: For iv use only. Do not remove this covering until time of injection. Fatal if given intrathecally."

General: Vinblastine should only be used by physicians familiar with the use of cancer chemotherapy.

Local: Vinblastine is a vesicant; avoid extravasation which can result in pain and cellulitis or tissue necrosis. Properly position the needle in the vein before injecting the drug. As a general caution, administer in a large vein not adjacent to joints or tendons. The insertion site should not be in an arm with compromised circulation or distal to a recent puncture. If leakage into the surrounding tissue occurs, stop the injection immediately and administer any remaining drug into another vein. Delayed reactions are possible so monitor patients in the weeks following the injection. If extravasation does occur follow local extravasation procedures.

Carcinogenesis and Mutagenesis: Vinblastine is potentially carcinogenic and mutagenic.

Cardiovascular: Cases of unexpected myocardial infarction, cerebrovascular accidents and Raynaud's phenomenon have occurred in patients receiving combination chemotherapy with vinblastine, bleomycin and cisplatin. Use caution when treating patients with ischemic cardiovascular disease with vinblastine.

Endocrine and Metabolism: Hyperuricemia secondary to the active cell lysis that occurs when patients with highly proliferative tumours are given cytotoxic chemotherapy may be minimized by using allopurinol. Hydration can also be used in those who are not fluid restricted. Sodium bicarbonate can be added to iv fluids of hospitalized patients to alkalinize urine when tumour lysis is anticipated.

Gastrointestinal: Nausea and vomiting caused by vinblastine usually begins within hours to days of administration and lasts less than 24 hours. It is most often easily managed by administration of antiemetics.

Hematologic: Vinblastine can cause bone marrow toxicity that can be dose-limiting. Leukopenia is the most common adverse effect and is usually the dose-limiting factor. Discontinue or decrease dose of vinblastine if bone marrow is suppressed. The nadir in the leukocyte count usually occurs 4 to 10 days after vinblastine administration with recovery after 7 to 14 days, but can take up to 21 days or more with high doses. When doses higher than usually recommended are used, leukopenia (granulocytopenia) may be severe. In cases of leukopenia below 2000 WBC/mm^3, monitor for infection until counts return to a safe level. With malignant cell infiltration of bone marrow, even moderate doses of vinblastine have led to unexpectedly large falls in leukocyte and platelet counts. Vinblastine should be discontinued in these patients. Patients who have had therapy with radiation or other chemotherapeutic agents may experience thrombocytopenia. Recovery is usually within a few days.

Effects on red blood cell counts and hemoglobin are usually not complications with vinblastine; however, any patient with malignant disease may suffer from anemia.

Hepatic/Biliary/Pancreatic: Hepatic insufficiency may enhance toxicity.

Immune: Increased frequency of infections and hemorrhagic complications as the drug is myelosuppressive. Fever, chills, sore throat, sore mouth or unusual bruising or bleeding should be reported to the physician.

Neurologic: Neurotoxicity can be dose-limiting and disabling. Risk of neurologic toxicity may increase if small amounts of drug are used daily for long periods. These effects often occur in the first days to weeks of vinblastine therapy. The risk of neurotoxicity is less than with some other vinca alkaloids (vincristine>vindesine>vinblastine).

Eighth cranial nerve damage leading to a variety of manifestations including hearing impairment may occur. Use caution if vinca alkaloids are given with other potentially ototoxic drugs such as platinum-containing antineoplastics, furosemide and aminoglycosides.

Vocal cord paresis/paralysis and bilateral facial nerve palsies are usually bilateral and reversible when vinblastine is discontinued. Severe jaw or parotid gland pain occurring within hours of vinblastine administration can be treated with analgesics and should not be a dose-limiting toxicity. High doses (>20 mg) can be associated with autonomic neuropathy including urinary retention, orthostatic hypotension and constipation.

Ophthalmologic: Avoid accidental contamination of the eye with vinblastine because of the risk of severe irritation. Wash the eye with water immediately and thoroughly.

Respiratory: Vinca alkaloids have caused acute shortness of breath and severe bronchospasm (usually when used with mitomycin C). This can occur within minutes or hours after vinblastine injection. Aggressive and even chronic therapy may be necessary. Do not readminister vinblastine. Those with preexisting pulmonary dysfunction may be more likely to experience respiratory adverse effects associated with vinblastine.
Sexual Function/Reproduction: Gonadal dysfunction has been reported in men and women receiving vinblastine in combination with other antineoplastics (e.g., alkylating agents). In some cases, aspermia has reversed and ovarian function has returned.
Skin: Leukopenic response is more pronounced in those with ulcerated skin areas. Alopecia is very common (e.g., >10%) with the use of vinblastine. It presents as slow thinning of the hair usually in the days to weeks following administration. Sometimes hair regrows to its pretreatment extent with continued maintenance therapy.
Special Populations: Pregnancy: Data is limited but vinblastine may cause fetal toxicity when administered to pregnant women. However, in a small number of cases the drug has been used in pregnancy without resulting malformations. Animal studies suggest teratogenicity. Advise women of child-bearing age not to become pregnant.
Lactation: Breastfeeding is not recommended in women receiving vinblastine; it may be excreted in breast milk.
Geriatrics: Elderly/cachectic patients may suffer more marked myelosuppressive effects (see Warnings and Precautions).
Monitoring and Laboratory Tests: Blood count monitoring (i.e., CBC with differential) should be performed once or twice per week. Counts should be taken just before administration of a vinblastine dose. With leukopenia below 2000 WBC/mm^3 monitor for infection until counts return to a safe level. Modify dose accordingly. Patients should have baseline liver function tests if there is a suspicion of liver failure. Because of the risk of neurologic toxicity patients should undergo neurologic toxicity ratings at each visit. Monitor electrolytes and uric acid (if indicated). Monitor injection sites for phlebitis or delayed tissue necrosis. Vinblastine or its metabolites are not known to interfere with clinical laboratory tests.
Occupational Hazards: The literature provides inconclusive evidence of long-term effects of occupational exposure to cytotoxic agents. Caution should be exercised during the preparation and handling of vinblastine to minimize any potential hazards. Procedures for the safe handling of cytotoxic and hazardous materials should be used when handling vinblastine.

ADVERSE REACTIONS: Adverse Drug Reaction Overview: In general, adverse events seen in patients treated with vinblastine appear to be related to dose administered (see Table 1).

Table 1: Vinblastine

More Common Adverse Reactions (1 to >10%)

Adverse Reaction by Body System	%
Cardiovascular	
Hypertension	1–10
Raynaud's Phenomenon	1–10
CNS	
Depression	1–10
Headache	1–10
Malaise	1–10
Seizures	1–10
Dermatologic	
Alopecia	> 10
Rash	1–10
Photosensitivity	1–10
Dermatitis	1–10
Endocrine and Metabolism	
Hyperuricemia	1–10
Gastrointestinal	
Nausea	>10
Vomiting	>10
Constipation	>10
Stomatitis	>10
Abdominal Cramps	>10
Anorexia	>10
Metallic Taste	>10
Diarrhea	1–10
Paralytic Ileus	1–10
Hematologic	
Leukopenia	>10
Myelosuppression	>10
Musculoskeletal	
Jaw Pain	1–10
Myalgia	1–10

(cont'd)

Table 1: Vinblastine *(cont'd)*

More Common Adverse Reactions (1 to >10%)

Adverse Reaction by Body System	%
Renal	
Urinary Retention	1–10
Respiratory	
Bronchospasm	1–10
Miscellaneous	
Cellulitis/Phlebitis due to Extravasation	1–10

Less Common Adverse Drug Reactions (<1%): Autonomic: autonomic neuropathy with symptoms such as constipation, abdominal pain, urinary retention, paralytic ileus and tender parotid glands associated with dry mouth.
Cardiovascular: angina pectoris, transient ECG abnormalities.
CNS: neurotoxicity including peripheral neuropathy, loss of deep tendon reflexes and weakness; vocal cord paresis or paralysis, oculomotor nerve dysfunction and bilateral facial nerve palsies.
Digestive: rectal bleeding, bleeding from old peptic ulcers, hemorrhagic colitis, vesiculation of the mouth.
Ear/Nose/Throat: eighth cranial nerve damage leading to vestibular symptoms such as dizziness, nystagmus and vertigo or auditory manifestations such as hearing impairment (temporary or permanent).
Hematologic: anemia.
Musculoskeletal: bone, muscle and tumour pain.
Renal: syndrome of inappropriate secretion of ADH (SIADH).
Miscellaneous: pain on injection, pain in tumour containing tissue (possibly because of swelling of tumour tissue during response to treatment).

DRUG INTERACTIONS: Drug-Drug Interactions: See Table 2.

Table 2: Vinblastine

Drug-Drug Interactions

Interacting Drug	Effect	Clinical Comment
Aprepitant	Aprepitant may inhibit or induce CYP3A4	Monitor response to vinblastine
Carbamazepine	Vinblastine plasma concentration and efficacy may be decreased probably as a result of increased metabolism through CYP3A4	Monitor clinical response when initiating or discontinuing carbamazepine
Erythromycin	Risk of vinblastine toxicity (e.g., myalgia, constipation, neutropenia) may be increased possibly through inhibition of vinblastine metabolism	Best to avoid this combination. When combined, administer conservative vinblastine dose and monitor carefully for vinblastine adverse effects
Itraconazole (and other azole antifungals)	Risk of vinblastine toxicity (e.g., myalgia, constipation, neutropenia) may be increased possibly through inhibition of vinblastine metabolism	Best to avoid this combination. When combined, monitor carefully for vinblastine adverse effects
Mitomycin C	In patients previously or simultaneously treated with mitomycin C, vinblastine administration has been associated with acute bronchospasm and dyspnea within minutes to hours of vinblastine administration. This reaction may occur up to 2 wks after mitomycin dosing	Avoid this combination if possible. When the combination is necessary, patients should seek medical advice if they experience difficulty breathing. The reaction appears to recur on rechallenge, so future use of the combination should be avoided in those who experience dyspnea. Mitomycin alone is known to cause pulmonary toxicity, but the reaction associated with vinblastine and mitomycin is more abrupt
Ototoxic Medications	Vinblastine neurotoxicity may include eighth cranial nerve damage resulting in varying degrees of permanent or temporary hearing impairment. This risk may be increased when used with other potentially ototoxic drugs (e.g., cisplatin, furosemide, aminoglycosides)	Use ototoxic drug combinations with extreme caution
Phenytoin	Decreased serum concentrations of phenytoin have led to loss of effect possibly because of decreased absorption or increased metabolism of phenytoin.	Monitor phenytoin serum levels and adjust dose as necessary
Tolterodine	Tolterodine plasma concentrations increased due to CYP3A4 inhibition by vinblastine	Reduce tolterodine dose by 50%

Drug-Herb Interactions: See Table 3.

Table 3: Vinblastine

Drug-Herb Interactions

Interacting Herb	Effect	Clinical Comment
St. John's Wort	St. John's wort may decrease vinblastine levels	Avoid this combination

DOSAGE AND ADMINISTRATION: Dosing Considerations: Refer to individual protocols. Dose will vary depending on previous or concomitant chemotherapy and/or radiation therapy. Dose may need to be reduced or delayed depending on clinical and hematologic response. The dose of vinblastine is usually titrated by increments of about 1.8 mg/m^2 for adults, and about 1.25 mg/m^2 for children. See Table 4. Dose should not be increased above the dose which reduces white cell count to approximately 3000 cells/mm^3. When a dose is given that decreases white cell counts to 3000 cells/mm^3, a maintenance dose of one increment (about 1.8 mg/m^2 in adults) **less than this amount** should be given weekly.

Although dosing is usually weekly, the next dose of vinblastine should not be given until white cell count has returned to at least 4000/mm^3. Usual dose is 5.5–7.4 mg/m^2 and maximum dose is 18.5 mg/m^2.

A simplified, conservative incremental dosing at **weekly** intervals is shown below:

Table 4: Vinblastine

Simplified Incremental Dosing

	Adult Dose (BSA)	Pediatric Dose (BSA)
First Dose	3.7 mg/m²	2.5 mg/m²
Second Dose	5.5 mg/m²	3.75 mg/m²
Third Dose	7.4 mg/m²	5 mg/m²
Fourth Dose	9.25 mg/m²	6.25 mg/m²
Fifth Dose	11.1 mg/m²	7.5 mg/m²

The duration of maintenance therapy depends on a variety of factors including disease being treated, patient status and combination of therapies being employed. Shorter periods of maintenance may lead to longer survival in some patients; however, shorter maintenance may result in relapse. Risks of prolonged maintenance include infections, secondary cancers (as a result of immune suppression), neurologic deficits and sterility.

Hepatic Impairment: See Table 5. Dosage should be adjusted in the presence of hepatic insufficiency as follows:

Table 5: Vinblastine

Dosage in Hepatic Failure

Bilirubin (µmol/L)	% usual dose
25–50	50%
>50	25%

Renal Impairment: No dosage adjustment suggested with renal dysfunction.

Administration: Vinblastine should be administered only by iv injection by those experienced with use of the drug.

Intermittent infusion: Causes less pain on injection than when administered by direct intravenous. Give vinblastine dose in 100 mL over 20 to 30 minutes. Volumes greater than 250 mL are given over 3 to 8 hours. Central venous access is best. Vinblastine is compatible with NS and D5W. Do not admix with solutions that could change the pH (e.g., lactate-containing solutions) Direct intravenous: Administer via a small gauge needle (e.g., 21 or 23) into the tubing of a running iv push slowly to not stop or reverse drip of iv solution. Check for blood return before administration and regularly during injection (e.g., after every 2 to 3 mL of drug). Immediately stop the injection and assess the site if there is no blood return. Flush any remaining drug from tubing with 20 mL of NS or D5W. Syringe and needle can be rinsed with venous blood before withdrawing the needle to further decrease the risk of extravasation. Continuous infusion—only by central line—has also been used as per individual protocols. Great care must be taken to avoid extravasation.

Vinblastine is not given sc or im because it is a vesicant. Intrathecal administration is absolutely contraindicated. Syringes containing this drug should carry the label: "Warning: For iv use only. Do not remove this covering until time of injection. Fatal if given intrathecally." Management of patients inadvertently given intrathecal vinblastine is a medical emergency.

OVERDOSAGE:

Signs and Symptoms of Overdose: Administration of a dose higher than that recommended will lead to the greater adverse effects (e.g., bone marrow suppression, mental depression, paresthesias, neurotoxicity), but to a greater magnitude. Neurotoxicity more similar to that seen with vincristine may be seen. Toxicity may be further exaggerated in the presence of hepatic impairment.

Management of Overdose: Patients receiving an inadvertent overdose of vinblastine should be admitted to a monitored bed for at least 24 hours. Though treatment is largely supportive, glutamic acid may prevent neurologic sequelae and should be considered. Leucovorin may also be of some benefit. Seizures should be treated with either lorazepam, diazepam and/or phenobarbital. Hypertension can be treated with nifedipine. Patients should be monitored for bone marrow suppression and SIADH.

For management of a suspected drug overdose, CPhA recommends that you contact your **regional Poison Control Centre**. See the *CPS* Directory section for a list of Poison Control Centres.

ACTION AND CLINICAL PHARMACOLOGY: Vinblastine disrupts the formation of the mitotic spindle arresting the cell at metaphase by binding to tubulin and inhibiting microtubule formation. The vinca alkaloids are cell cycle phase-specific (i.e., M and S phases). Vinblastine also has some immunosuppressant effect.

Pharmacokinetics: Absorption: Oral absorption is erratic.

Distribution: Vinblastine distributes to the liver and binds extensively to protein (43 to 99%) and other tissues. The drug does not penetrate the CNS or other fatty tissues.

Metabolism: Vinblastine undergoes hepatic metabolism to an active (desacetylvinblastine) and inactive metabolites. Dose modification is required with hepatic insufficiency.

Metabolism is mediated by the CYP3A subfamily including CYP3A4. Vinblastine is thought to inhibit CYP3A4 and CYP2D6.

Excretion: The major route of excretion is the feces (95%) with less than 1% excreted in the urine as unchanged drug. Tissue sequestration is high. Vinblastine is slowly excreted with triphasic serum decay. The initial half-life is 3.7 minutes; middle half-life is 1.6 hours and terminal half-life is 19 to 25 hours.

Vinblastine Sulfate Injection Pr

vinblastine sulfate

Antineoplastic

Hospira

SUPPLIED: Each mL of sterile aqueous solution contains: vinblastine sulfate 1 mg. Nonmedicinal ingredients: sodium chloride 9 mg. Sulfuric acid or sodium hydroxide may be added as pH adjusters. Preservative-free. Single use vials of 10 mL, cartons of 1. Store between 2 and 8°C. Protect from light and freezing. Discard unused portion.

Vincristine Pr

Antineoplastic

CPhA Monograph

Date of Preparation: November 2004

Date of Revision: March 2009

This monograph has been compiled by CPhA and reviewed by experts. It may contain information different from that found in Health Canada-approved Product Monographs. The reader is referred to the *CPS* Editorial Policy for more information.

SUMMARY PRODUCT INFORMATION:

Route of Administration	Dosage Form	Product Strength
Intravenous	Single use vials: 1 and 2 mL Pharmacy bulk vial: 5 mL	Vincristine sulfate 1 mg/mL and mannitol 100 mg/mL as stabilizer

INDICATIONS AND CLINICAL USE: Vincristine (also known as LCR, leurocristine, VCR) is indicated for:

- Treatment of acute lymphocytic leukemia, breast cancer, cervical cancer, colorectal cancer, Ewing's sarcoma, Hodgkin's disease, melanoma, neuroblastoma, non-Hodgkin's lymphoma, osteosarcoma, ovarian cancer, rhabdomyosarcoma, small cell lung cancer, soft tissue sarcoma, Wilm's tumour and refractory idiopathic thrombocytopenic purpura

  Other uses not approved by Health Canada include treatment of acute myeloid leukemia, autoimmune hemolytic anemia, brain tumours, hepatoblastoma, choriocarcinoma, chronic leukemia, Kaposi's sarcoma, multiple myeloma, mycosis fungoides, pheochromocytoma, retinoblastoma, gestational trophoblastic neoplasms, testicular cancer, thrombotic thrombocytopenic purpura and Waldenstrom's macroglobulinemia.

Although effective as a single agent, vincristine is usually used in combination with other antineoplastics depending on the type of cancer being treated.

Pediatrics: Vincristine has been used in children as part of a chemotherapeutic regimen to treat a variety of cancers including leukemia, multiple myeloma, acute lymphocytic leukemia, Wilm's tumour, Ewing's sarcoma and rhabdomyosarcoma.

CONTRAINDICATIONS:

- Patients who are hypersensitive to vincristine or vinca alkaloids or to any ingredient in the formulation or component of the container.
- Vincristine can worsen underlying neurological diseases. Patients with the demyelinating form of Charcot-Marie Tooth Syndrome or childhood poliomyelitis should not receive vincristine.
- Patients receiving radiation therapy that may involve the liver.
- Intrathecal administration is fatal; vincristine is for intravenous use only.

WARNINGS AND PRECAUTIONS:

Serious Warnings and Precautions

- Vincristine is fatal if given intrathecally and is intended for intravenous use only. Syringes containing the drug should carry the label: "Warning: For intravenous use only. Do not remove this covering until time of injection. Fatal if given intrathecally."

General: Vincristine has a low therapeutic index and should be used by physicians experienced with the use of cancer chemotherapy. Use with caution in patients receiving other neurotoxic drugs or those with pre-existing neuromuscular disease (e.g., Guillain-Barré syndrome).

Local: Vincristine is a vesicant; avoid extravasation, which can result in pain and cellulitis or tissue necrosis. Properly position the needle in the vein before injecting the drug. As a general caution, administer into a large vein not adjacent to joints or tendons. The injection site should not be in an arm with compromised circulation or distal to recent puncture. If leakage into the surrounding tissue occurs, stop the injection immediately and administer any remaining drug into another vein. Delayed reactions are possible so monitor patients in the weeks following injection. If extravasation does occur apply warm compresses to the extravasation site for one hour to disperse the drug and minimize discomfort and tissue damage.

Carcinogenesis and Mutagenesis: Vincristine is potentially carcinogenic but has not been shown to be mutagenic in bacterial or mammalian cells.

Cardiovascular: Hypertension and hypotension have been reported. Rare and unexpected cases of coronary artery disease and myocardial infarction have occurred in patients receiving vincristine in combination with other antineoplastic drugs. Causality has not been established.

Endocrine and Metabolism: A syndrome of inappropriate antidiuretic hormone secretion (SIADH) has occurred rarely in patients receiving vincristine. Fluid restriction improves sodium balance and facilitates completion of vincristine therapy. Hyperuricemia secondary to active cell lysis can occur when patients with highly proliferative tumors (e.g., non-Hodgkin's lymphomas, leukemia) are given cytotoxic chemotherapy. Uric acid nephropathy can develop in some patients. These effects may be minimized by using allopurinol, and/or hydration (in those not fluid restricted) and alkalinizing urine by using sodium bicarbonate added to iv fluids of hospitalized patients when tumour lysis is anticipated.

Gastrointestinal: Gastrointestinal autonomic neuropathy presents as severe constipation and abdominal cramps. Adynamic ileus occurs frequently, especially in young children. Constipation may be treated with enemas and laxatives. Patients receiving vincristine should receive a routine prophylactic regimen of laxatives. Mild nausea and vomiting are commonly reported after vincristine administration.

Genitourinary: Polyuria, dysuria and urinary retention can occur with vincristine as a manifestation of autonomic neuropathy.

Hematologic: Vincristine produces less hematological toxicity than most other chemotherapeutic agents. Occasionally mild leukopenia, mild anemia and thrombocytopenia occur.

Hepatic/Biliary/Pancreatic: Hepatic insufficiency may enhance toxicity; dosage reduction may be required. (See Dosage and Administration.) Vincristine should not be administered to patients receiving radiation that may involve the liver.

Immune: Vincristine, unlike other vinca alkaloids, causes negligible myelosuppression.

Neurologic: Neurotoxicity is the primary dose-limiting toxic effect of vincristine and is related to cumulative dose. It presents as peripheral, autonomic or central neuropathy. Previous neurotoxicity or neurological disorders may contribute to increased sensitivity or decreased tolerance. In adults, neurotoxic effects may be observed with cumulative doses of as little as 5 to 6 mg. The only treatment for vincristine neurotoxicity is discontinuation of drug therapy or reduction of the dose or frequency of administration. (See Dosage and Administration.)

Peripheral (mixed sensorimotor) neuropathy is most common and develops in most patients. Early signs include depression of the Achilles reflex followed by loss of deep tendon reflexes commonly accompanied by peripheral paresthesias (numbness, pain and tingling). With prolonged or high dose therapy, wrist drop, foot drop, cranial nerve palsy, atrophy and ataxia may occur. If stair climbing or picking up small objects becomes impaired (motor neuropathy) subsequent doses of vincristine should be held until symptoms disappear. Cranial nerve neuropathy manifests as facial nerve palsies, jaw pain (occurring within 24 hours of first or second dose and rarely recurring) and headache. Cranial nerve neuropathy involving the larynx produces hoarseness and vocal cord paralysis. Those involving the eye may cause ptosis, double vision and optic neuropathy. Optic atrophy with blindness or transient cortical blindness has been reported.

Eighth cranial nerve damage causing vestibular impairment (dizziness, nystagmus and vertigo) as well as hearing impairment may occur. Use caution if vinca alkaloids are given with other potentially ototoxic drugs such as platinum-containing antineoplastics, furosemide and aminoglycosides.

Less frequently, vincristine causes autonomic and CNS toxicity. Urinary tract disturbances include bladder atony, incontinence, retention, nocturia, dysuria and polyuria. If bladder atony occurs, vincristine should be held until symptoms subside. CNS toxicity includes depression, agitation, insomnia and hallucinations. Seizures (accompanied by hypertension), progressive encephalopathy, respiratory difficulties and coma have been reported.

Ophthalmologic: Avoid accidental contact with eyes because of the risk of severe irritation. Wash eyes with water immediately and thoroughly and seek medical attention immediately. See Precautions, Neurologic for cranial nerve neuropathies.

Renal: Urinary retention, bladder atony with polyuria and dysuria has been reported as a manifestation of autonomic neuropathy. See Precautions, Neurologic.

Respiratory: Vinca alkaloids (vinblastine, vindesine) have caused acute shortness of breath and severe bronchospasm (primarily when used with mitomycin C). Aggressive or even chronic therapy may be required. Vinca alkaloids should not be re-administered. Those with pre-existing pulmonary dysfunction may be more likely to experience respiratory adverse effects.

Sensitivity/Resistance: Acute anaphylactic type reactions to vincristine sulfate have been reported rarely.

Sexual Function/Reproduction: Gonadal dysfunction has been reported in men and women receiving vincristine in combination with other antineoplastics. Recovery occurred in some but not all patients post therapy. Irreversible azoospermia and amenorrhea is less likely when treatment that includes vincristine is administered in prepubertal patients.

Skin: Alopecia is common and occurs in 20 to 50% of patients receiving vincristine. Alopecia is reversible upon discontinuation of the drug and hair regrowth may occur during continued therapy. Rash occurs occasionally.

Special Populations: Pregnant Women: Data are limited but vincristine can cause fetal toxicity when administered to pregnant women. However there are individual case reports of normal infants being born to patients receiving vincristine alone or in combination with other drugs. Animal studies suggest vincristine is embryotoxic and teratogenic. Advise women of childbearing age not to become pregnant while receiving the drug.

Nursing Women: It is not known if vincristine is distributed into breast milk; breast-feeding is not recommended in women receiving vincristine.
Pediatrics (birth to 16 years old): Infants weighing 10 kg or less are especially susceptible to neurotoxicity and dose should be based on body weight rather than surface area in this group. Infants are also more susceptible to ileus, SIADH and hematologic toxicities from vincristine.
Geriatrics: Geriatric patients may be more susceptible to neurotoxic effects of vincristine.
Monitoring and Laboratory Tests: Laboratory parameters: monitor hematocrit/hemoglobin, platelet count, and differential leukocyte count to detect development of leukopenia or thrombocytopenia. Measure serum uric acid for possible hyperuricemia during the first 3 to 4 weeks of treatment. Perform baseline liver function tests on initiation of therapy with vincristine and repeat periodically to monitor for hepatotoxicity. Monitor serum sodium for SIADH. Physical exam: monitor patients for development of neuropathy (e.g., blurred vision, difficulty in walking, pain in fingers or jaw, numbness or tingling of fingers/toes) and neurotoxicity (e.g., constipation, abdominal pain, urinary retention, loss of deep tendon reflexes) at each visit to detect the need or dosage modification. Monitor injection sites for phlebitis or delayed tissue necrosis.
Occupational Hazards: The literature provides inconclusive evidence of long-term effects of occupational exposure to cytotoxic agents. Caution should be exercised during the preparation and handling of vincristine to minimize any potential hazards. Procedures for the safe handling of cytotoxic and hazardous materials should be used when handling vincristine.

ADVERSE REACTIONS: Adverse Drug Reaction Overview: In general, adverse reactions are dose related and reversible. Neurotoxicity is the primary dose-limiting adverse effect of vincristine. Recovery is often slow but complete.
More Common Adverse Drug Reactions: Dermatologic: reversible alopecia (20 to 50%).
Gastrointestinal: mild nausea and vomiting; GI autonomic dysfunction (bloating, constipation, abdominal pain, and adynamic ileus).
Neurologic: loss of deep tendon reflexes (after 3 or more weekly doses), peripheral paresthesia (numbness, pain, tingling), jaw pain (occurs within 24 hours after first or second dose and rarely recurs), ataxia.
Ophthamologic: blurred vision, droopy eyelids.
Renal: urinary retention (autonomic neuropathy).
Less Common Adverse Drug Reactions: Cardiovascular: hypotension, hypertension (autonomic neuropathy).
CNS: confusion, depression, agitation, insomnia, seizures (rare), hallucinations (rare, associated with high doses); cranial nerves rarely affected manifested as hoarseness, diplopia and facial palsies.
Dermatologic: rash, pain or redness at injection site.
Ear/Nose/Throat: rare occurrences of vestibular and auditory damage to the eight cranial nerve.
Hematologic: leukopenia, anemia and thrombocytopenia.
Neurologic: foot drop, wrist drop, motor dysfunction, ataxia, paralysis (more often associated with prolonged or high-dose therapy).
Ophthalmologic: transient blindness, optic atrophy (cranial nerve neuropathy).
Renal: syndrome of inappropriate secretion of antidiuretic hormone (SIADH-rare, symptom of central neurotoxicity).

DRUG INTERACTIONS:

Serious Drug Interactions
- Potent inhibitors of cytochrome P450 isoenzyme CYP3A4 may impair vincristine metabolism and cause increased neurotoxicity.
- Asparaginase reduces vincristine clearance resulting in increased neuropathy. Administer vincristine 12 to 24 hours before asparaginase.

Overview: Vincristine is metabolized via the cytochrome P450 isoenzyme CYP3A4. Administration of erthromycin and other inhibitors of CYP3A4 may lead to severe toxicity. Administering drugs that induce CYP3A4 like phenobarbital may result in a decrease in the vincristine serum level.
Drug-Drug Interactions: See Table 1.

Table 1: Vincristine
Drug-Drug Interactions

Interacting Drug	Effect	Clinical Comment
Aprepitant	Aprepitant may inhibit or induce CYP3A4	Monitor response to vincristine
Asparaginase	Hepatic clearance of vincristine may be reduced resulting in increased neuropathy and disturbances of erythropoiesis	Give vincristine 12-24 hours before asparaginase
Carbamazepine	Vincristine plasma concentration and efficacy may be decreased probably as a result of increased metabolism through CYP3A4	Monitor clinical response when initiating or discontinuing carbamazepine
Ciprofloxacin	Decrease in antimicrobial effect of ciprofloxacin due to decreased oral absorption	Monitor for clinical response to ciprofloxacin therapy
Digoxin	Decreased serum concentration of digoxin. Possible alteration in intestinal mucosa may decrease absorption of digoxin	Monitor for signs of decreased effect of digoxin and adjust dose as necessary
Erythromycin	Risk of vincristine toxicity may be increased possibly through inhibition of metabolism (CYP3A4) of vincristine	Avoid combination. When combined, monitor for vincristine toxicity. Azithromycin may be substituted
Isoniazid	Risk of vincristine toxicity may be increased possibly through inhibition of metabolism (CYP3A4) of vincristine	Best to avoid combination; if combined monitor for vincristine toxicity
Itraconazole and other azole antifungals	Risk of vincristine toxicity may be increased possibly through inhibition of metabolism (CYP3A4) of vincristine	Best to avoid combination; if combined monitor for vincristine toxicity
Mitomycin C	Acute bronchospasm has occurred minutes to hours after administration of a vinca alkaloid (vinblastine, vinorelbine) in some patients previously or simultaneously treated with mitomycin	Use with caution. Bronchodilators, corticosteroids and oxygen have produced symptomatic relief
Nifedipine	Probable increase in half-life of vincristine resulting in increased toxicity. Mechanism unknown	Best to avoid combination; if combined, monitor for vincristine toxicity
Ototoxic medications	Vincristine neurotoxicity may include eighth cranial nerve damage resulting in varying degrees of permanent or temporary hearing loss. Risk may be increased when used with other ototoxic drugs (e.g., cisplatin, furosemide, aminoglycosides)	Use ototoxic drug combinations with extreme caution

(cont'd)

Table 1: Vincristine *(cont'd)*
Drug-Drug Interactions

Interacting Drug	Effect	Clinical Comment
Phenytoin	Decreased phenytoin serum concentrations and loss of effect possibly because of decreased absorption or increased metabolism	Monitor phenytoin serum levels and adjust dose as necessary
Verapamil	Potential increase in vincristine toxicity possibly because of competition for plasma protein binding sites	Best to avoid combination; if combined, monitor for vincristine toxicity

DOSAGE AND ADMINISTRATION: Dosing Considerations:
- Refer to individual protocols for the dosage of vincristine and other chemotherapeutic agents and the method and sequence of administration. Numerous dosing schedules exist and depend on disease, response and concomitant therapy. The therapeutic index is narrow and individual patients' responses vary. The dosage must be carefully adjusted according to the needs of the patient.

Recommended Dose and Dosage Adjustment: Vincristine Dose in Adult Patients: The usual adult dose is 1.4 mg/m² body surface area administered weekly. Some regimens may limit the total single dose of vincristine to 2 mg to minimize neurotoxicity. However, current protocols are often written with no upper limit on the vincristine dose. Single doses greater than 3 mg or administered more frequently than once per week should be questioned.
Vincristine Dose in Pediatric Patients: The usual dose in children weighing more than 10 kg is 1 to 2 mg/m² weekly. In infants, vincristine doses are calculated according to body weight. The usual dose for children weighing less than 10 kg is 0.03 to 0.05 mg/kg weekly .
Renal Impairment: No dose adjustment required in renal impairment.
Dosage in Dialysis: Vincristine is not significantly removed by hemodialysis; small quantities appear in dialysate.
Hepatic Impairment: See Table 2. Dosage should be adjusted in the presence of hepatic insufficiency as follows:

Table 2: Vincristine
Dosage Adjustment in Hepatic Failure

Bilirubin (µmol/L)	% usual dose
25–50	50%
>50	25%

Neurotoxicity: See Table 3.

Table 3: Vincristine
Dosage Adjustment for Neurotoxicity

Symptom	% Usual Dose
Areflexia only	100%
Abnormal buttoning, writing	67%
Moderate motor neuropathy	50%
Severe motor neuropathy	Omit dose

Administration: Vincristine should be administered only by intravenous injection by those experienced with the use of the drug. Administer vincristine push through the sidearm of free flowing iv (5% dextrose or normal saline); inject over at least 1 minute. May be given direct iv push, followed by normal saline flush. May be mixed in 50 mL minibag (5% dextrose or normal saline); infuse over 15 minutes.

Vincristine is not given subcutaneously or intramuscularly because it is a vesicant. Intrathecal administration is absolutely contraindicated. Syringes containing this drug should carry the label: "Warning: For iv use only. Do not remove this covering until time of injection. Fatal if given intrathecally." Management of patients inadvertently given vincristine intrathecally is a medical emergency. No successful antidote has been described.

OVERDOSAGE:
Signs and Symptoms: Toxic effects of vincristine are dose related, therefore exaggerated adverse effects will be seen in those administered an overdose. Doses 10 times the usual recommended dose have been lethal in children under 13 years of age. In adults single doses of 3 mg/m² BSA can produce severe toxic effects.
Recommended Management: Patients receiving an inadvertent overdose of vincristine should be admitted to a monitored bed for at least 24 hours. Seizures should be treated with intravenous benzodiazepines and, if prolonged, phenobarbital. Monitor bowel function for constipation, blood counts for anemia and neutropenia, and electrolytes for SIADH for up to ten days. Case reports suggest that leucovorin calcium may be useful in treating vincristine overdose. A suggested regimen is to administer leucovorin calcium 100 mg iv every 3 hours for 24 hours, then every 6 hours for 48 hours. Glutamic acid may prevent neurologic sequelae and should also be considered.

For management of a suspected drug overdose, CPhA recommends that you contact your **regional Poison Control Centre**. See the *CPS* Directory section for a list of Poison Control Centres.

STORAGE AND STABILITY: Store in refrigerator between 2 and 8°C. Protect from light. Vincristine sulfate may be further diluted with 0.9% sodium chloride injection or 5% dextrose in water injection. Diluted solutions should be used within 6 hours if stored at room temperature and 24 hours if refrigerated and protected from light.

SPECIAL HANDLING INSTRUCTIONS: Trained personnel should prepare vincristine sulfate injection. Preparation should be done in a biological safety cabinet. Personnel should wear protective gown, mask, gloves and appropriate eye protection. If accidental skin contact occurs wash skin thoroughly. All used syringes, needles and sharps should not be crushed, clipped or recapped, but placed directly into an approved sharps container. Dispose of any cleanup materials and waste residue according to applicable laws and regulations. If disposed of by incineration a temperature of at least 850°C for solids and 950°C for liquids is required.

Vincristine Sulfate Pharmacy Bulk Vials are only supplied to hospitals with a recognized intravenous admixture program.

Vincristine Sulfate Injection USP Ⓟ

vincristine sulfate
Antineoplastic

Hospira

SUPPLIED: Each mL of sterile aqueous solution contains: vincristine sulfate 1 mg. Nonmedicinal ingredients: 100 mg mannitol. May contain sulfuric acid or sodium hydroxide as pH adjusters. Preservative-free. Single use vial of 2 mL and pharmacy bulk vials of 5 mL, cartons of 1. Store between 2 and 8°C. Protect from light. Discard unused portion.

Vinorelbine Tartrate for Injection Pr
vinorelbine tartrate
Antineoplastic

Hospira

SUPPLIED: Each mL of solution for injection contains: vinorelbine tartrate equivalent to 10 mg vinorelbine base. Nonmedicinal ingredients: none. Preservative-free. Single use vials of 1 mL and 5 mL, cartons of 1. Store between 2 and 8°C. Protect from light and freezing. Must be diluted before use. Discard unused portion.

Vioform® Hydrocortisone Pr
clioquinol—hydrocortisone
Antibacterial—Antifungal—Topical Corticosteroid

Paladin

SUPPLIED: Each tube of off-white water soluble cream contains: clioquinol 3% and hydrocortisone 1%. Nonmedicinal ingredients: cetyl alcohol, cetyl palmitate, glycerin, petrolatum, phenoxyethanol, sodium lauryl sulfate, stearyl alcohol and water. Sodium: <1 mmol (0.8 mg)/g. Bisulfite- and tartrazine-free. Tubes of 30 g. Protect from heat (store between 15 and 30°C) and freezing. May turn yellow when exposed to air and may cause staining of the skin, nails, hair or fabrics.

Viokase®
pancrelipase
Oral Enzyme Therapy

Axcan Pharma

PHARMACOLOGY: The natural digestive enzymes in VIOKASE hydrolyze fats into fatty acids and glycerol, split protein into amino acids, and convert carbohydrates to dextrins and short chain sugars. Under conditions of the USP test method (in vitro), VIOKASE has the following total digestive capacity: See Table 1.

Table 1: VIOKASE

Total Digestive Capacity

	VIOKASE 8 Tablet	VIOKASE 16 Tablet	Each 0.7 g VIOKASE Powder (¼ Teaspoonful)
Dietary Fat (g)	28	56	59
Dietary Protein (g)	30	60	70
Dietary Starch (g)	30	60	70

VIOKASE 8 and 16 tablets are immediate release and are not enteric coated.

The digestive capacity of a pancreatic enzyme concentrate depends on the amount that passes through the stomach unchanged and is available at the site of action in the small intestine.

INDICATIONS: In the treatment of exocrine pancreatic insufficiency as associated with but not limited to cystic fibrosis, chronic pancreatitis, pancreatectomy, or obstruction of the pancreatic ducts.

CONTRAINDICATIONS: Should not be used in patients hypersensitive to pork protein.

In patients with acute pancreatitis or with acute exacerbation of chronic pancreatic diseases.

WARNINGS: Should hypersensitivity occur, discontinue medication and treat symptomatically.

PRECAUTIONS: General: Individuals previously sensitized to trypsin, pancreatin or pancrelipase may have allergic manifestations.

Information to Be Provided to the Patient: VIOKASE should not be held in the mouth as the proteolytic action may cause irritation of the mucosa.

Avoid inhalation of the powder when administering VIOKASE.

Carcinogenesis, Mutagenesis, Impairment of Fertility: Long-term studies in animals have not been performed to evaluate the carcinogenic or mutagenic potential of pancrelipase.

Pregnancy: Animal reproduction studies have not been conducted with VIOKASE. It is also not known whether VIOKASE can cause fetal harm when administered to a pregnant woman or can affect reproduction capacity. VIOKASE should be given to a pregnant woman only if clearly needed.

Lactation: It is not known whether this drug is excreted in human milk. Because many drugs are excreted in human milk, caution should be exercised when pancrelipase is administered to a nursing mother.

ADVERSE EFFECTS: The dust or finely powdered pancreatic enzyme concentrate is irritating to the nasal mucosa and the respiratory tract. It has been documented that inhalation of the airborne powder can precipitate an asthma attack. The literature also contains several references to asthma due to inhalation in patients sensitized to pancreatic enzyme concentrates. Extremely high doses of exogenous pancreatic enzymes have been associated with hyperuricemia and hyperuricosuria.

Overdosage of pancreatic enzyme concentrate may cause diarrhea or transient intestinal upset.

OVERDOSE:

Symptoms: Acute toxicity determinations in animals have not been possible since the maximum dose that could be given orally produced no toxic reaction. In chronic feeding tests, rats developed swollen salivary glands. This is believed due to the proteolytic activity and the mucosal irritation caused by tissue digestion.

No acute toxic reactions have been reported.

> For management of a suspected drug overdose, CPhA recommends that you contact your **regional Poison Control Centre**. See the *CPS* Directory section for a list of Poison Control Centres.

DOSAGE: Powder: Dosage for patients with cystic fibrosis: ¼ teaspoonful (0.7 g) with meals.

Tablets: Dosage range for patients with cystic fibrosis or chronic pancreatitis is from 8000 to 32 000 lipase USP units taken with meals, i.e., 1 to 4 VIOKASE 8 tablets or 1 to 2 VIOKASE 16 tablets with meals or as directed by a physician.

In patients with pancreatectomy or obstruction of pancreatic ducts: 1 to 2 VIOKASE 8 tablets or 1 VIOKASE 16 tablet taken at 2-hour intervals or as directed by a physician.

SUPPLIED: Powder: Tan-colored, each 0.7 g contains: lipase 16 800 USP units, protease 70 000 USP units and amylase 70 000 USP units. Nonmedicinal ingredients: lactose and sodium chloride. Bottles of 114 g.

Tablets: VIOKASE 8: Each tan-colored, round, compressed tablet, engraved VIOKASE on one side and 9111 on the other side, contains: lipase 8000 USP units, protease 30 000 USP units and amylase 30 000 USP units. Nonmedicinal ingredients: croscarmellose sodium, lactose, microcrystalline cellulose, silicon dioxide, stearic acid and talc. Bottles of 100.

VIOKASE 16: Each tan, oval, biconvex tablet, engraved "V[16]" on one side and 9116 on the other side, contains: lipase 16 000 USP units, protease 60 000 USP units and amylase 60 000 USP units. Nonmedicinal ingredients: croscarmellose sodium, lactose, microcrystalline cellulose, silicon dioxide, stearic acid and talc. Bottles of 100.

Store at controlled room temperature (15 to 25°C). Protect from heat and moisture. Dispense tablets and powder in a tight container, preferably with a desiccant.

(Shown in Product Identification Section)

Viracept® Pr
nelfinavir mesylate
HIV Protease Inhibitor

Pfizer

Date of Revision: February 4, 2010

SUMMARY PRODUCT INFORMATION:

Route of Administration	Dosage Form/Strength	Clinically Relevant Nonmedicinal Ingredients
Oral	Film-coated tablets, 250, 625 mg nelfinavir Powder, nelfinavir 50 mg/g	Not applicable For a complete listing see Dosage Forms, Composition and Packaging.

INDICATIONS AND CLINICAL USE: VIRACEPT (nelfinavir mesylate) is indicated for the treatment of HIV infection in combination with other antiretroviral agents. This indication is based on analyses of surrogate endpoints in studies of up to 48 weeks.

Geriatrics (>65 years of age): Clinical studies of VIRACEPT did not include sufficient numbers of subjects aged 65 and over to determine whether they respond differently from younger subjects (see Warnings and Precautions; Dosage and Administration, Recommended Dose and Dosage Adjustment).

Pediatrics (<13 years of age): The safety and effectiveness of VIRACEPT have been established in patients from 2 to 13 years of age. In patients less than 2 years of age, VIRACEPT was found to be safe at the doses studied but a reliably effective dose could not be established. Therefore, VIRACEPT should be used in children below the age of 2 years only when the potential benefit clearly outweighs the potential risks (see Warnings and Precautions; Dosage and Administration, Recommended Dose and Dosage Adjustment, Children (2-13 years)).

CONTRAINDICATIONS: VIRACEPT (nelfinavir mesylate) is contraindicated in patients with clinically significant hypersensitivity to any of its components. For a complete listing, see Dosage Forms, Composition and Packaging.

Coadministration of VIRACEPT is contraindicated with drugs that are highly dependent on CYP3A for clearance and for which elevated plasma concentrations are associated with serious and/or life-threatening events. These drugs are listed in Table 1.

Table 1: VIRACEPT

Drugs That Are Contraindicated with VIRACEPT

Drug Class	Drugs Within Class That Are Contraindicated with VIRACEPT
Gastrointestinal Prokinetic	Cisapride[a]
Antiarrhythmics	Amiodarone, quinidine
Ergot Derivatives	Dihydroergotamine, ergonovine, ergotamine, methylergonovine
Neuroleptic	Pimozide
Sedative/hypnotics	Midazolam, triazolam
HMG-CoA Reductase Inhibitors	Lovastatin, simvastatin
Herbal Products	St. John's Wort (hypericum perforatum)

[a] Is no longer marketed in Canada.

WARNINGS AND PRECAUTIONS: General: VIRACEPT (nelfinavir mesylate) is an inhibitor of the P450 isoform CYP3A. In vitro data indicates that nelfinavir is unlikely to be an inhibitor of CYP2C19 (Ki=68 µM or 39 mg/L). Coadministration of VIRACEPT (nelfinavir mesylate) and drugs primarily metabolized by CYP3A may result in increased plasma concentrations of the other drug that could increase or prolong its therapeutic and adverse effects. Caution should be exercised when inhibitors of CYP3A, including VIRACEPT, are coadministered with drugs that are metabolized by CYP3A and that prolong the QT interval. (See Adverse Reactions, Post-Market Adverse Drug Reactions.) Nelfinavir is metabolized by CYP3A and CYP2C19. Coadministration of VIRACEPT and drugs that induce CYP3A or CYP2C19 may decrease nelfinavir plasma concentrations and reduce its therapeutic effect. Coadministration of VIRACEPT and drugs that inhibit CYP3A or CYP2C19 may increase nelfinavir plasma concentrations (see Drug Interactions).

Patients with Phenylketonuria: VIRACEPT Oral Powder contains 11.2 mg phenylalanine per gram of powder.

Diabetes Mellitus/Hyperglycemia: New onset diabetes mellitus, exacerbation of pre-existing diabetes mellitus and hyperglycemia have been reported during post-marketing surveillance in HIV-infected patients receiving protease inhibitor therapy. Some patients required either initiation or dose adjustments of insulin or oral hypoglycemic agents for treatment of these events. In some cases diabetic ketoacidosis has occurred. In those patients who discontinued protease inhibitor therapy, hyperglycemia persisted in some cases. Because these events have been reported voluntarily during clinical practice, estimates of frequency cannot be made and a causal relationship between protease inhibitor therapy and these events has not been established.

Hepatic/Biliary/Pancreatic: VIRACEPT (nelfinavir mesylate) is principally metabolized by the liver. Therefore, caution should be exercised when administering this drug to patients with hepatic impairment (see Action and Clinical Pharmacology, Hepatic Insufficiency).

Resistance/Cross-Resistance: HIV cross-resistance between protease inhibitors has been observed.

Hemophilia: There have been reports of increased bleeding including spontaneous skin hematomas and hemarthrosis in patients with hemophilia type A and B treated with protease inhibitors. In some patients, additional factor VIII was given. In more than half of the reported cases, treatment with protease inhibitors was continued or re-introduced. A causal relationship between protease inhibitors and these events has not been established, however, the frequency of bleeding episodes should be closely monitored in patients on nelfinavir mesylate.

Redistribution/Accumulation of Body Fat: Redistribution/accumulation of body fat including central obesity, dorsocervical fat enlargement (buffalo hump), peripheral wasting, facial wasting, breast enlargement, and "cushingoid appearance" have been observed in patients receiving antiretroviral therapy. The mechanism and long-term consequences of these events are currently unknown. A causal relationship has not been established.

Immune Reconstitution Syndrome: During the initial phase of treatment, patients responding to antiretroviral therapy may develop an inflammatory response to indolent or residual opportunistic infections (such as MAC, CMV, PCP and TB), which may necessitate further evaluation and treatment.

Special Populations: Pregnant Women (Pregnancy, Fertility and Reproduction): Clinical experience in pregnant women is lacking. Until additional data become available, VIRACEPT (nelfinavir mesylate) is not recommended for use in pregnant women.

No treatment-related effects were demonstrated in nonclinical developmental and reproductive toxicity studies when nelfinavir was administered to pregnant rats at systemic exposures (AUC) comparable to that observed in humans at the recommended therapeutic doses of VIRACEPT. Administration of nelfinavir to pregnant rabbits resulted in no fetal development effects up to a dose at which a slight maternal decrease was observed; however even at the highest dose evaluated, systemic exposure in rabbits was appreciably lower than that achieved in humans administered therapeutic doses of nelfinavir.

Antiretroviral Pregnancy Registry: To monitor maternal-fetal outcomes of pregnant women exposed to nelfinavir and other antiretroviral agents, an Antiretroviral Pregnancy Registry has been established. Physicians are encouraged to register patients by calling (800) 258-4263 or via email at http://www.apregistry.com.

A prospective review of first trimester exposures to VIRACEPT reported that there was no increased risk (at least two-fold increase) of overall birth defects including the more common classes, cardiovascular and genitourinary systems. To date, fifteen birth defects out of 416 live births of first trimester exposure have been reported.

Nursing Women: It is recommended that HIV-infected women not breastfeed their infants under any circumstances to avoid the transmission of HIV. Studies in lactating rats have demonstrated that nelfinavir is excreted in milk. It is not known whether nelfinavir is excreted in human milk. Mothers should be instructed not to breast-feed if they are receiving VIRACEPT because of both the potential for HIV transmission and the potential for serious adverse reactions in nursing infants.

Pediatrics: The safety and effectiveness of VIRACEPT have been established in patients from 2 to 13 years of age. In patients less than 2 years of age, VIRACEPT was found to be safe at the doses studied but a reliably effective dose could not be established. Response rates in children <2 years of age appeared to be poorer than those in patients ≥2 years of age in some studies. Therefore, nelfinavir should be used in children below the age of 2 years only when the potential benefits clearly outweigh the potential risks.

Highly variable drug exposure remains a significant problem in the use of VIRACEPT in pediatric patients. Unpredictable drug exposure may be exacerbated in pediatric patients because of increased clearance compared to adults and difficulties with compliance and adequate food intake with dosing (see Adverse Reactions, Pediatric Population, Dosage and Administration, Recommended Dose and Dosage Adjustment, Children (2-13 years)).

Renal Insufficiency: The pharmacokinetics of nelfinavir have not been studied in patients with renal insufficiency. Less than 2% of nelfinavir mesylate is excreted in the urine, so the impact of renal impairment on nelfinavir elimination should be minimal.

Geriatrics: Clinical studies of nelfinavir did not include sufficient numbers of subjects aged 65 and over to determine whether they respond differently from younger subjects (see Dosage and Administration, Recommended Dose and Dosage Adjustment).

Gender and Race: No significant pharmacokinetic differences have been detected between males and females. Pharmacokinetic differences due to race have not been evaluated; however, pivotal trials have revealed no significant differences between races for efficacy or safety.

ADVERSE REACTIONS: Adverse Drug Reaction Overview: The safety of VIRACEPT (nelfinavir mesylate) was studied in over 5000 patients who received drug either alone or in combination with antiretroviral agents. The majority of adverse events were of mild intensity. The most frequently reported adverse event among patients receiving VIRACEPT was diarrhea, which was generally of mild to moderate intensity. The frequency of nelfinavir-associated diarrhea may be increased in patients receiving the 625 mg tablet because of the increased bioavailability of this formulation.

Clinical Trial Adverse Drug Reactions: Drug-related clinical adverse experiences of moderate or severe intensity in ≥2% of patients treated with VIRACEPT coadministered with d4T and lamivudine (Study 542) for up to 48 weeks or with ZDV + lamivudine (Study 511) for up to 24 weeks are presented in Table 2.

Table 2: VIRACEPT

Percentage of Patients with Treatment-Emergent[a] Adverse Events of Moderate or Severe Intensity Reported in ≥2% of Patients

	Study 511 (24 weeks)			Study 542 (48 weeks)	
Adverse Events	**Placebo+ ZDV/3TC (n=101) %**	**500 mg TID VIRACEPT+ ZDV/3TC (n=97) %**	**750 mg TID VIRACEPT+ ZDV/3TC (n=100) %**	**1250 mg BID VIRACEPT+ d4T/3TC (n=296) %**	**750 mg TID VIRACEPT+ d4T/3TC (n=159) %**
Body as a Whole					
Asthenia	2	1	1	1	1
Digestive System					
Diarrhea	3	14	20	18	14
Nausea	4	3	7	1	3
Flatulence	0	5	2	0	0
Skin/Appendages					
Rash	1	1	3	2	2

[a] Includes those adverse events at least possibly related to study drug or of unknown relationship and excludes concurrent HIV conditions.

Less Common Clinical Trial Adverse Drug Reactions: Adverse events occurring in less than 2% of patients receiving VIRACEPT in all phase II/III clinical trials and considered at least possibly related or of unknown relationship to treatment and of at least moderate severity are listed below.

Body as a Whole: abdominal pain, accidental injury, allergic reaction, back pain, fever, headache, malaise, pain and redistribution/accumulation of body fat (see Warning and Precautions, Redistribution/Accumulation of Body Fat).

Digestive System: anorexia, dyspepsia, epigastric pain, gastrointestinal bleeding, hepatitis, mouth ulceration, pancreatitis and vomiting.

Hemic/Lymphatic System: anemia, leukopenia and thrombocytopenia.

Metabolic/Nutritional System: increases in alkaline phosphatase, amylase, creatinine phosphokinase, lactic dehydrogenase, AST, ALT and gamma glutamyl transpeptidase; hyperlipemia, hyperuricemia, hyperglycemia, hypoglycemia, dehydration and liver function tests abnormal.

Musculoskeletal System: arthralgia, arthritis, cramps, myalgia, myasthenia and myopathy.

Nervous System: anxiety, depression, dizziness, emotional lability, hyperkinesia, insomnia, migraine, paresthesia, seizures, sleep disorder, somnolence and suicide ideation.

Respiratory System: dyspnea, pharyngitis, rhinitis and sinusitis.

Skin/Appendages: dermatitis, folliculitis, fungal dermatitis, maculopapular rash, pruritus, sweating and urticaria.

Special Senses: acute iritis and eye disorder.

Urogenital System: kidney calculus, sexual dysfunction and urine abnormality.

Abnormal Hematologic and Clinical Chemistry Findings: The percentage of patients with marked laboratory abnormalities in Studies 542 and 511 are presented in Table 3. Marked laboratory abnormalities are defined as a Grade 3 or 4 abnormality in a patient with a normal baseline value or a Grade 4 abnormality in a patient with a Grade 1 abnormality at baseline.

Table 3: VIRACEPT

Percentage of Patients by Treatment Group with Marked Laboratory Abnormalities[a] in ≥2% of Patients

	Study 511 (24 Weeks)			Study 542 (48 Weeks)	
	Placebo +ZDV/3TC (n=101) %	**500 mg TID VIRACEPT +ZDV/3TC (n=97) %**	**750 mg TID VIRACEPT +ZDV/3TC (n=100) %**	**1250 mg BID VIRACEPT +d4T/3TC (n=296) %**	**750 mg TID VIRACEPT +d4T/3TC (n=159) %**
Hematology					
Hemoglobin	6	3	2	0	0
Neutrophils	4	3	5	2	1
Lymphocytes	1	6	1	1	0
Chemistry					
ALT	6	1	1	3	0
AST	4	1	0	2	1
Creatine Kinase	7	2	2	—	—

[a] Marked laboratory abnormalities are defined as a shift from Grade 0 at baseline to at least Grade 3 or from Grade 1 to Grade 4.

Pediatric Population: VIRACEPT has been studied in over 400 pediatric patients in clinical trials from birth to 13 years of age. The adverse event profile seen during five pediatric clinical trials was similar to that for adults.

Drug-related, treatment-emergent adverse events of all grades in ≥2% of patients treated with VIRACEPT TID with 2 NRTIs for up to 48 weeks in two pediatric studies (Study 524 and Study 556) are presented in Table 4, by age range. In Study 524, diarrhea, leukopenia, abdominal pain and rash were the most commonly reported drug-related adverse events in pediatric patients older than 2 years of age. In the group less than 2 years of age, rash, diarrhea, anorexia and leukopenia were the most commonly reported drug-related adverse events. In Study 556, no drug-related adverse events were reported in children less than 2 years of age; in children older than 2 years of age, two instances of Grade 2 diarrhea and one instance of Grade 4 rash were reported as drug related.

Table 4: VIRACEPT

Number (%) of Drug-related Treatment-emergent Adverse Events Reported in >2% Pediatric Patients

	Children			
	Study 524 VIRACEPT 20 mg/kg TID+NRTI[a]		Study 556 VIRACEPT 25–35 mg/kg TID+ZDV/ddI	
Body System COSTART Adverse Event Term	**<2 Yrs n=25**	**≥2 Yrs n=39**	**<2 Yrs n=47**	**≥2 Yrs n=94**
Body as a Whole				
Fever	0 (0)	1 (3)	0 (0)	0 (0)
Pain abdomen	0 (0)	2 (5)	0 (0)	0 (0)
Digestive				
Anorexia	1 (4)	0 (0)	0 (0)	0 (0)
Diarrhea	1 (4)	15 (38)	0 (0)	2 (2)
Flatulence	0 (0)	1 (3)	0 (0)	0 (0)
Nausea	0 (0)	1 (3)	0 (0)	0 (0)
Hemic and Lymphatic				
Anemia	0 (0)	1 (3)	0 (0)	0 (0)
Leukopenia	1 (4)	2 (5)	0 (0)	0 (0)
Respiratory				
Epistaxis	0 (0)	1 (3)	0 (0)	0 (0)
Skin and Skin Structures				
Rash	2 (8)	2 (5)	0 (0)	1 (1)

[a] "NRTI" indicates the subjects were also treated with a nucleoside reverse transcriptase inhibitor.

Although no drug-related events were reported in Study PACTG 377, treatment emergent adverse events included neutropenia and gastrointestinal events in 33% (7/21 each) of children less than 2 years of age treated with VIRACEPT (27-33 mg/kg TID) in the presence of NRTIs+/−NNRTIs. Neutropenia occurred in all treatment groups including the arm that did not include VIRACEPT (three grade 2, three grade 3, and one grade 4). In the majority of cases, the neutropenia was reported as mild in nature and often resolved without discontinuation from study.

In neonates, Study PENTA 7 (20 subjects, VIRACEPT at 75 mg/kg BID) reported one treatment-emergent, drug-related adverse event of Grade 2 rash/erythema in the ddI+d4T+VIRACEPT arm; this event resolved without discontinuation of treatment.

Adverse Events from Pre/Postnatal Exposure: In neonates, Study PACTG 353 (31 subjects, VIRACEPT at 40 mg/kg BID) indicates that the drug-related adverse events include neutropenia (two Grade 3 and one Grade 4) and decreased hemoglobin (seven Grade 3).

Post-Market Adverse Drug Reactions: The following additional adverse experiences have been reported from postmarketing surveillance as at least possibly related or of unknown relationship to VIRACEPT:

Body as a Whole: hypersensitivity reactions (including bronchospasm, moderate to severe rash, fever and edema).

Cardiovascular System: QT prolongation, torsades de pointes.

Digestive System: jaundice.

Metabolic/Nutritional System: bilirubinemia, metabolic acidosis.

DRUG INTERACTIONS: Overview: Nelfinavir is an inhibitor of CYP3A (cytochrome P450 3A). Coadministration of VIRACEPT and drugs primarily metabolized by CYP3A (e.g., dihydropyridine, calcium channel blockers, HMG-CoA reductase inhibitors, immunosuppressants and sildenafil) may result in increased plasma concentrations of the other drugs that could increase or prolong both its therapeutic and adverse effects see Table 7 and Table 8. Nelfinavir is metabolized via CYP3A and CYP2C19. Coadministration of VIRACEPT and drugs that induce CYP3A or CYP2C19, such as rifampin, may decrease nelfinavir plasma concentrations and reduce its therapeutic effect. Coadministration of VIRACEPT and drugs that inhibit CYP3A or CYP2C19 may increase nelfinavir plasma concentrations. Caution should therefore be exercised when coadministering drugs that induce CYP3A or CYP2C19 or potentially toxic drugs which are themselves metabolized by CYP3A or CYP2C19. Based on in vitro data, nelfinavir is unlikely to inhibit other cytochrome P450 isoforms at concentrations in the therapeutic range.

Drug-Drug Interactions: Specific drug interaction studies were performed with nelfinavir and a number of drugs. Table 5 summarizes the effect of nelfinavir on the geometric mean AUC and C_{max} of coadministered drugs. Table 6 shows the effects of coadministered drugs on the geometric mean AUC and C_{max} of nelfinavir.

Table 5: VIRACEPT

Drug Interactions: Changes in Pharmacokinetic Parameters for Coadministered Drug in the Presence of Nelfinavir

			Coadministered Drug	
Coadministered Drug	**Nelfinavir Dose**	**N**	**AUC (95% CI)**	**C_{max} (95% CI)**
HIV-Protease Inhibitors				
Indinavir 800 mg Single Dose	750 mg q8h × 7 days	6	↑51% (25–83%)	↔
Ritonavir 500 mg Single Dose	750 mg q8h × 5 doses	10	↔	↔
Saquinavir 1200 mg Single Dose[a]	750 mg tid × 4 days	14	↑392% (271–553%)	↑179% (105–280%)
Amprenavir 800 mg tid × 14 days	750 mg tid × 14 days	6	↔	↔
Nucleoside Reverse Transcriptase Inhibitors				
Lamivudine 150 mg single dose	750 mg q8h × 7–10 days	11	↑10% (1–20%)	↑31% (5–62%)
Zidovudine 200 mg single dose	750 mg q8h × 7–10 days	11	↓35% (28–41%)	↓31% (8–49%)
Stavudine 30–40 mg bid × 56 days	750 mg tid × 56 days	8	↔	↔
Non-Nucleoside Reverse Transcriptase Inhibitors				
Efavirenz 600 mg once daily × 7 days	750 mg q8h × 7 days	10	↔	↔
Delavirdine 400 mg q8h × 14 days	750 mg q8h × 7 days	7	↓31% (62–25%)	↓27% (53–14%)
Anti-infective Agents				
Rifabutin 150 mg once daily × 8 days[b]	750 mg q8h × 7–8 days[c]	12	↑83% (69–99%)	↑19% (9–30%)
Rifabutin 300 mg once daily × 8 days	750 mg q8h × 7–8 days	10	↑207% (151–276%)	↑146% (112–186%)
Azithromycin 1200 mg single dose	750 mg tid × 11 days	12	↑112% (73–160%)	↑136% (66–237%)
HMG-CoA Reductase Inhibitors				
Atorvastatin 10 mg once daily × 28 days	1250 mg bid × 14 days	15	↑74% (34–126%)	↑122% (58–211%)
Simvastatin 20 mg once daily × 28 days	1250 mg bid × 14 days	16	↑505% (372–675%)	↑517% (340–764%)
Other Agents				
Ethinyl estradiol 35 µg once daily × 15 days	750 mg q8h × 7 days	12	↓47% (41–63%)	↓28% (14–39%)
Norethindrone 0.4 mg once daily × 15 days	750 mg q8h × 7 days	12	↓18% (12–27%)	↔
Methadone 80 mg +/−21 mg once daily[d] >1 month	1250 mg bid × 8 days	13	↓47% (41–52%)	↓46% (42–49%)
Phenytoin 300 mg once daily × 14 days	1250 mg bid × 7 days	12	↓29% (15–35%)	↓21% (12–29%)

[a] Using the soft gelatin capsule formulation of saquinavir 1200 mg.
[b] Rifabutin 150 mg (od) changes are relative to Rifabutin 300 mg od×8 days without coadministration with nelfinavir.
[c] Comparable changes in Rifabutin concentrations were observed with VIRACEPT 1250 mg q12h×7 days.
[d] Changes are reported for total plasma methadone; changes for the individual R-enantiomer and S-enantiomer were similar.
Legend: ↑ Indicates increase. ↓ Indicates decrease. ↔ Indicates no change (p value>0.05).

Table 6: VIRACEPT

Drug Interactions: Changes in Pharmacokinetic Parameters for Nelfinavir in the Presence of the Coadministered Drug

			Nelfinavir	
Coadministered Drug	**Nelfinavir Dose**	**N**	**AUC (95% CI)**	**C_{max} (95% CI)**
HIV-Protease Inhibitors				
Indinavir 800 mg q8h × 7 days	750 mg single dose	6	↑83% (34–150%)	↑31% (13–52%)
Ritonavir 500 mg q12 h × 3 doses	750 mg single dose	10	↑152% (86–242%)	↑44% (25–67%)
Saquinavir 1200 mg tid × 4 days[a]	750 mg single dose	14	↑18% (5–33%)	↔
Nucleoside Reverse Transcriptase Inhibitors				
Zidovudine 200 mg + Lamivudine 150 mg single dose	750 mg q8h × 7–10 days	11	↔	↔
Didanosine 200 mg single dose	750 mg single dose	9	↔	↔
Non-Nucleoside Reverse Transcriptase Inhibitors				
Efavirenz 600 mg once daily × 7 days	750 mg q8h × 7 days	10	↑20% (5–38%)	↑21% (8–36%)
Nevirapine 200 mg once daily × 14 days followed by 200 mg bid × 14 days	750 mg tid × 36 days	23	↔[b]	↔[b]
Delavirdine 400 mg q8h × 7 days	750 mg q8h × 14 days	12	↑107% (78–142%)	↑88% (61–119%)
Anti-infective Agents				
Ketoconazole 400 mg once daily × 7 days	500 mg q8h × 5-6 days	12	↑35% (21–49%)	↑25% (8–44%)
Rifampin 600 mg once daily × 7 days	750 mg q8h × 5–6 days	12	↓82% (77–86%)	↓76% (67–83%)
Rifabutin 150 mg once daily × 8 days	750 mg q8h × 7–8 days	11	↓23% (12–33%)	↓18% (6–29%)
	1250 mg q12h × 7–8 days	11	↔	↔
Rifabutin 300 mg once daily × 8 days	750 mg q8h × 7–8 days	10	↓32% (10–48%)	↓25% (6–38%)
Azithromycin 1200 mg single dose	750 mg tid × 9 days	12	↓15% (6–24%)	↔
Other Agents				
Phenytoin 300 mg once daily × 7 days	1250 mg bid × 14 days	15	↔	↔
Omeprazole 40 mg qd x 4 days	1250 mg bid x 4 days	19	↓36% (15–52%)	↓37% (20-51%)

[a] Using the soft gelatin capsule formulation of saquinavir 1200 mg.
[b] The overall effect of nevirapine on [NFV+M8 metabolite] was an 11±35% (median −15%) reduction in the [NFV+M8 metabolite] area under the plasma concentration-time curve.
Legend: ↑ Indicates increase. ↓ Indicates decrease. ↔ Indicates no change (p value>0.05).

Drug interaction studies reveal no clinically significant drug interactions between nelfinavir and didanosine, lamivudine, stavudine, zidovudine, efavirenz, nevirapine or ketoconazole and no dose adjustments are needed. In the case of didanosine, it is recommended that didanosine be administered on an empty stomach; therefore, nelfinavir should be administered with a meal one hour after or more than 2 hours before didanosine.

Based on known metabolic profiles, clinically significant drug interactions are not expected between VIRACEPT and dapsone, itraconazole, trimethoprim/sulfamethoxazole.

Drug-Food Interactions: Food increases nelfinavir exposure and decreases nelfinavir pharmacokinetic variability relative to the fasted state. VIRACEPT should be taken with a meal.

Drug-Herb Interactions: St. John's Wort: Concomitant use of St. John's Wort (Hypericum perforatum) or St. John's Wort-containing products is not recommended. Coadministration of St. John's Wort with protease inhibitors, including nelfinavir, is expected to substantially decrease protease inhibitor concentrations and may result in sub-optimal levels of nelfinavir and lead to loss of virologic response and possible resistance to nelfinavir or the class of protease inhibitors (see Warnings and Precautions).

Table 7: VIRACEPT

Drugs That Should Not Be Coadministered with VIRACEPT

Drug Class: Drug Name	Clinical Comment
Antiarrhythmics: amiodarone, quinidine	**Contraindicated** due to potential for serious and/or life-threatening reactions such as cardiac arrhythmias.
Antimycobacterial: rifampin	May lead to loss of virologic response and possible resistance to VIRACEPT or other coadministered antiretroviral agents.
Ergot Derivatives: dihydroergotamine, ergonovine, ergotamine, methylergonovine	**Contraindicated** due to potential for serious and/or life-threatening reactions such as acute ergot toxicity characterized by peripheral vasospasm and ischemia of the extremities and other tissues.
HMG-CoA Reductase Inhibitors (statins): lovastatin, simvastatin	Potential for serious reactions such as risk of myopathy including rhabdomyolysis.
Neuroleptic: pimozide	**Contraindicated** due to potential for serious and/or life-threatening reactions such as cardiac arrhythmias.
Proton Pump Inhibitors: omeprazole	Can result in a decrease in nelfinavir concentrations that may lead to a loss of virologic response and possible resistance to VIRACEPT.
Sedative/Hypnotics: midazolam, triazolam	**Contraindicated** due to potential for serious and/or life-threatening reactions such as prolonged or increased sedation or respiratory depression.

Drug-Laboratory Test Interactions: Interactions with laboratory tests have not been established.

DOSAGE AND ADMINISTRATION: Recommended Dose and Dosage Adjustment: Adults: The recommended dose of VIRACEPT (nelfinavir mesylate) tablets is 1250 mg (as free base; five 250 mg tablets or two 625 mg tablets) twice daily or 750 mg (three 250 mg tablets) three times daily orally. VIRACEPT should be taken with a meal. It is recommended that VIRACEPT be used in combination with other antiretroviral agents.

Geriatrics (>65 years of age): Clinical studies of nelfinavir did not include sufficient numbers of subjects aged 65 and over to determine whether they respond differently from younger subjects (see Warnings and Precautions, Geriatrics).

(cont'd)

Table 8: VIRACEPT

Established and Other Potentially Significant Drug Interactions: Alteration in Dose or Regimen May Be Recommended Based on Drug Interaction Studies (See Table 5 and Table 6 for Magnitude of Interaction)

Concomitant Drug Class: Drug Name	Effect on Concentration	Clinical Comment
	HIV-Antiviral Agents	
Protease Inhibitors: indinavir	↑nelfinavir ↑indinavir	Appropriate doses for this combination, with respect to safety and efficacy, have not been established.
ritonavir	↑nelfinavir	
saquinavir (sgc)[a]	↑saquinavir	
Non-nucleoside Reverse Transcriptase Inhibitor: delavirdine	↑nelfinavir ↓delavirdine	Appropriate doses for this combination, with respect to safety and efficacy, have not been established.
Nucleoside Reverse Transcriptase Inhibitor: didanosine	NA[b]	It is recommended that didanosine be administered on an empty stomach; therefore, didanosine should be given 1 hour before or 2 hours after VIRACEPT (given with a meal).
	Other Agents	
Anticonvulsants: carbamazepine, phenobarbital	NA[c]	May decrease nelfinavir plasma concentrations: VIRACEPT may not be effective due to decreased nelfinavir plasma concentrations in patients taking these agents concomitantly.
Anticonvulsant: phenytoin	↓phenytoin	Phenytoin plasma/serum concentrations should be monitored; phenytoin dose may require adjustment to compensate for altered phenytoin concentration.
Antidepressant: trazodone	↑trazodone	Concomitant use of trazodone and VIRACEPT may increase plasma concentrations of trazodone. Adverse events of nausea, dizziness, hypotension and syncope have been observed following coadministration of trazodone and ritonavir. If trazodone is used with CYP3A4 inhibitor such as VIRACEPT, the combination should be used with caution and a lower dose of trazodone should be considered.
Antimycobacterial: rifabutin	↑rifabutin ↓nelfinavir (750 mg tid) ↔ nelfinavir (1250 mg bid)	It is recommended that the dose of rifabutin be reduced to one-half the usual dose when administered with VIRACEPT; 1250 mg bid is the preferred dose of VIRACEPT when coadministered with rifabutin.
PDE-5 Inhibitor: sildenafil	↑sildenafil	Concomitant use of PDE-5 inhibitors with protease inhibitors, such as nelfinavir, should be done with caution. Co-administration of nelfinavir with a PDE-5 inhibitor is expected to substantially increase the PDE-5 concentration and may result in an increase in PDE-5 inhibitor-associated adverse events including hypotension, visual changes and priapism. If concomitant use of VIRACEPT with sildenafil is required, sildenafil at a single dose not exceeding 25 mg in 48 hours is recommended. Drug interaction studies have not been conducted between nelfinavir and other PDE-5 inhibitors.
HMG-CoA Reductase Inhibitor: atorvastatin	↑atorvastatin	Use lower possible dose of atorvastatin with careful monitoring, or consider other HMG-CoA reductase inhibitors such as pravastatin or fluvastatin in combination with VIRACEPT.
Immunosuppressants: cyclosporine, tacrolimus	↑immunosuppressants	Plasma concentrations may be increased by VIRACEPT.
Inhaled/Nasal Steroid: fluticasone	↑fluticasone	Concomitant use of fluticasone propionate and VIRACEPT may increase plasma concentrations of fluticasone propionate. Caution should be undertaken for usage. Consider alternatives to fluticasone propionate, particularly for long-term use.
Narcotic Analgesic: methadone	↓methadone	Dosage of methadone may need to be increased when coadministered with VIRACEPT.
Oral Contraceptive: ethinyl estradiol	↓ethinyl estradiol	Alternative or additional contraceptive measures should be used when oral contraceptives and VIRACEPT are coadministered.
Macrolide Antibiotic: azithromycin	↑azithromycin	Dose adjustment of azithromycin is not recommended, but close monitoring for known side effects such as liver enzyme abnormalities and hearing impairment is warranted.

[a] Using the soft gelatin capsule (sgc) formulation of saquinavir.
[b] Not applicable.
[c] Not available.

Children (2-13 years): The recommended oral dose of VIRACEPT for pediatric patients 2 to 13 years of age is 25-30 mg/kg per dose, three times daily with a meal. The pharmacokinetics of twice daily dosing of VIRACEPT in pediatric patients has not been sufficiently established to recommend a BID dosing regimen.

Overall, use of VIRACEPT in the pediatric population is associated with highly variable drug exposure. The high variability may be due to increased clearance compared to adults and difficulties with compliance and adequate food intake with dosing (see Warnings and Precautions, Pediatrics).

For children unable to take tablets, VIRACEPT Oral Powder may be administered (see Administration). The maximum recommended dose is 2500 mg per day. The healthcare provider should assess appropriate formulation and dosage for each patient. Crushed tablets can be used in lieu of powder.

The recommended pediatric dose of VIRACEPT to be administered three times daily is described in Table 9.

Table 9: VIRACEPT

Pediatric Dose to Be Administered Three Times Daily

Body Weight Kg	Number of Level 1 g Scoops	Number of Level Teaspoons	Number of 250 mg Tablets
7 to <8.5	4	1	—
8.5 to <10.5	5	1¼	1
10.5 to <12	6	1½	—
12 to <14	7	1¾	—
14 to <16	8	2	—
16 to <18	9	2¼	—
18 to <23	10	2½	2
≥23	15	3¾	3

Missed Dose: If a dose is missed, patients should take the next dose as soon as possible. A dose should not be doubled.

Administration: Tablets: Patients unable to swallow tablets may place whole tablets or crushed tablets in a small amount of water to disperse before ingestion or they may mix crushed tablets in a small amount of food. Once mixed with food or dispersed in water, the entire contents must be consumed in order to obtain the full dose. It is recommended that the entire contents be consumed immediately after mixing with food or dispersing in water. The drinking glass should be rinsed and the rinse swallowed to insure the entire dose is consumed. Acidic food or juice (i.e., orange juice, apple juice or apple sauce) are not recommended to be used in combination with VIRACEPT because the combination may result in a bitter taste.

Reconstitution of Oral Powder: The oral powder may be mixed with a small amount of water, milk, formula, soy formula, soy milk or nutritional preparations; once mixed, the entire contents must be consumed in order to obtain the full dose. The recommended use period for storage of the product in these media is 6 hours under refrigeration (2-8°C). Dosing media not recommended include any acidic food or juice (e.g., orange juice, apple juice or apple sauce) because the combination may result in a bitter taste. VIRACEPT Oral Powder should not be reconstituted with water in its original container.

OVERDOSAGE:

Human experience of acute overdose with VIRACEPT (nelfinavir mesylate) is limited. There is no specific antidote for overdose with VIRACEPT. Administration of activated charcoal should be used to aid removal of unabsorbed drug. Since nelfinavir mesylate is highly protein bound, dialysis is unlikely to significantly remove drug from blood.

For management of a suspected drug overdose, contact your regional Poison Control Centre. See the *CPS Directory* section for a list of Poison Control Centres.

ACTION AND CLINICAL PHARMACOLOGY: Mechanism of Action: Nelfinavir is an inhibitor of the human immunodeficiency virus (HIV) protease. The HIV protease is an enzyme required for the proteolytic cleavage of the viral polyprotein precursors to the individual proteins found in infectious HIV. Nelfinavir reversibly binds to the active site of the HIV protease and prevents it from cleaving the gag-pol polyprotein resulting in the formation of immature non-infectious viral particles.

Pharmacodynamics: Antiretroviral Activity In vitro: The antiretroviral activity of nelfinavir in vitro has been demonstrated in both acute and/or chronic HIV infections in lymphoblastoid cell lines, peripheral blood lymphocytes and monocytes/macrophages. Nelfinavir was found to be active against several laboratory strains and clinical isolates of HIV-1 and the HIV-2 strain ROD. The EC_{95} (95% effective concentration) of nelfinavir ranged from 7 to 111 nM. Drug combination studies with protease inhibitors showed nelfinavir has antagonistic interactions with indinavir, additive interactions with ritonavir or saquinavir and synergistic interactions with amprenavir and lopinavir. Minimal to no cellular cytotoxicity was observed with any of these protease inhibitors alone or in combination with nelfinavir. When nelfinavir was combined with reverse transcriptase inhibitors in vitro, nelfinavir demonstrated additive (didanosine or stavudine) to synergistic (zidovudine, lamivudine, zalcitabine, abacavir, tenofovir, delavirdine, efavirenz or nevirapine) antiviral activity without enhanced cytotoxicity.

HIV isolates with reduced susceptibility to nelfinavir have been selected in vitro. Genotypic analysis of a variant which exhibited a nine-fold decrease in sensitivity showed a unique substitution of an aspartic acid (D) to an asparagine (N) in HIV protease at amino acid residue 30 (D30N). Consistent with the in vitro results, the predominant genotypic change in clinical HIV isolates with reduced susceptibility to nelfinavir is the D30N substitution.

Pharmacokinetics: Absorption: Administration of a single 1250 mg dose of VIRACEPT (nelfinavir mesylate) 250 mg tablets (total of 5 tablets) to normal, healthy volunteers with a meal containing 125 to 1000 kilocalories and 20% to 50% calories from fat was associated with a 2.2 to 5.2 and 2.0 to 3.3 fold increase in nelfinavir AUC and C_{max}, respectively, relative to fasting. In healthy volunteers receiving a single 1250 mg dose, the 625 mg tablet was not bioequivalent to the 250 mg tablet formulation. Under fasted conditions (n=27), the AUC and C_{max} were 34% and 24% higher, respectively, for the 625 mg tablets. In a relative bioavailability assessment under fed conditions (n=28), the AUC was 24% higher for the 625 mg tablet; the C_{max} was comparable for both formulations (see Adverse Reactions). To enhance bioavailability and minimize pharmacokinetic variability, nelfinavir should be taken with a meal.

Distribution: The apparent volume of distribution (VD_{area}/F) for nelfinavir to adult humans was approximately 150 L, i.e. 2 L/kg. Nelfinavir in serum is extensively protein-bound (>98%). In both humans and animals, the estimated distribution volumes exceed total body water, suggesting extensive penetration of nelfinavir into tissues.

Metabolism: Unchanged nelfinavir comprised 82-86% of the total plasma radioactivity after a single oral 750 mg dose of ^{14}C-nelfinavir. In vitro, multiple cytochrome P-450 isoforms including CYP3A and CYP2C19 are responsible for metabolism of nelfinavir. One major and several minor oxidative metabolites were found in plasma. The major oxidative metabolite has in vitro antiviral activity equal to the parent drug.

Excretion: Oral clearance estimates after single doses (24-33 L/h) and multiple doses (26-61 L/h) indicate that nelfinavir is a drug with medium to high hepatic bioavailability. The terminal half-life in plasma was typically 2.5 to 5 hours. The majority (87%) of an oral 750 mg dose containing ^{14}C-nelfinavir was recovered in the feces; fecal radioactivity consisted of nelfinavir (22%) and numerous oxidative metabolites. Only 1-2% of the dose was recovered in urine, of which unchanged nelfinavir was the major component.

Special Populations and Conditions: Pediatrics: The pharmacokinetics of nelfinavir have been investigated in 5 studies in pediatric patients from birth to 13 years of age either receiving VIRACEPT three times or twice daily.

Hepatic Insufficiency: Pharmacokinetics of nelfinavir after a single dose of 750 mg VIRACEPT was studied in patients with liver impairment and healthy volunteers. A 49%-69% increase was observed in AUC of nelfinavir in the hepatically impaired groups (Child-Turcotte-Pugh Classes A to C) compared to the healthy group. The single, oral 750 mg dose of VIRACEPT was safe and well tolerated by the healthy and hepatically impaired subjects participating in this study. Specific dosage recommendations for VIRACEPT cannot be made based on the results of this study; it is recommended to monitor liver function tests in patients who are hepatically impaired.

STORAGE AND STABILITY: VIRACEPT Tablets and Oral Powder should be stored at 15 to 30°C in a USP tight container. Exposure to temperature as low as −20°C for periods of up to 24 hours will not adversely affect VIRACEPT Tablets stability.

INFORMATION FOR THE PATIENT: Published in e-CPS, available by subscription at www.e-cps.ca.

DOSAGE FORMS, COMPOSITION AND PACKAGING: Oral Powder: Each level scoopful (1 g) of off-white, sweetened powder contains: 50 mg nelfinavir (from nelfinavir mesylate). Nonmedicinal ingredients: aspartame, crospovidone, dibasic potassium phosphate, hypromellose, maltodextrin, microcrystalline cellulose, natural and artificial flavors and sucrose palmitate. Multiple use bottles containing 144 g of powder with scoop.

Tablets: 250 mg: Each light blue, capsule-shaped, clear film-coated tablet, engraved with "VIRACEPT" on one side and "250 mg" on the other, contains: nelfinavir 250 mg (as nelfinavir mesylate). Nonmedicinal ingredients: calcium silicate, crospovidone, FD&C Blue #2 powder, hypromellose, magnesium stearate and triacetin. Plastic bottles of 300.
625 mg: Each white, oval-shaped, clear film-coated tablet, engraved with "V" on one side and "625" on the other, contains: nelfinavir 625 mg (as nelfinavir mesylate). Nonmedicinal ingredients: calcium silicate, colloidal silicon dioxide, crospovidone, hypromellose, magnesium stearate and triacetin. Plastic bottles of 120.

(Shown in Product Identification Section)

Viramune® Ⓟ

nevirapine

Antiretroviral Agent—Non-Nucleoside Reverse Transcriptase Inhibitor with Activity Against Human Immunodeficiency Virus Type 1 (HIV-1)

Boehringer Ingelheim

Date of Revision: June 7, 2010

SUMMARY PRODUCT INFORMATION:

Route of Administration	Dosage Form/ Strength	Clinically Relevant Nonmedicinal Ingredients
Oral	Tablet, 200 mg	Lactose For a complete listing see Dosage Forms, Composition and Packaging.

INDICATIONS AND CLINICAL USE: VIRAMUNE (nevirapine) is indicated as an alternative for:
- treatment of HIV-1 infection in combination with other antiretroviral agents.

The decision to use VIRAMUNE should take into account liver and skin toxicity, potentially fatal, especially in patients with higher CD4 counts and in women (see Warnings and Precautions). Clinical trials have not established equivalence of nevirapine to protease inhibitors or to other NNRTIs.

Based on serious and life-threatening hepatotoxicity observed in controlled and uncontrolled studies, VIRAMUNE should not be initiated in adult females with CD4+ cell counts greater than 250 cells/mm³ or in adult males with CD4+ cell counts greater than 400 cells/mm³ unless the benefit outweighs the risk.

Geriatrics (>65 years of age): Clinical studies of VIRAMUNE did not include sufficient numbers of subjects aged 65 and older to determine whether elderly subjects respond differently from younger subjects. In general, dose selection for an elderly patient should be cautious, reflecting the greater frequency of decreased hepatic, renal or cardiac function, and of concomitant disease or other drug therapy.

Pediatrics (<15 years of age): Safety and effectiveness of VIRAMUNE in HIV-1 infected pediatric patients younger than 15 years of age has not been established. Nevirapine is metabolized more rapidly in pediatric patients than in adults.

CONTRAINDICATIONS:
- VIRAMUNE (nevirapine) is contraindicated in patients with clinically significant hypersensitivity to any of its components. For a complete listing, see Dosage Forms, Composition and Packaging.
- VIRAMUNE should not be administered to patients with severe hepatic dysfunction or pre-treatment AST or ALT >5×Upper Limit of Normality (ULN).
- VIRAMUNE should not be readministered to patients who have been discontinued for severe rash, rash accompanied by constitutional symptoms, hypersensitivity reactions, or clinical hepatitis due to nevirapine.
- VIRAMUNE should not be readministered in patients who previously had AST or ALT> 5×Upper Limit of Normality (ULN) during nevirapine therapy (see Warnings and Precautions).
- VIRAMUNE should not be administered to patients with rare hereditary conditions of galactose intolerance e.g. galactosaemia, the Lapp lactase deficiency or glucose/galactose malabsorption.
- Herbal preparations containing St. John's Wort (hypericum perforatum) must not be used while taking VIRAMUNE due to the risk of potentially significant decreases of plasma concentrations and reduced clinical effects of nevirapine (see Drug Interactions).

WARNINGS AND PRECAUTIONS:

> **Serious Warnings and Precautions**
> Severe, life-threatening, and in some cases fatal hepatotoxicity, particularly in the first 18 weeks, has been reported in patients treated with VIRAMUNE. Female gender and higher CD4 counts (women with CD4 counts >250 cells/mm³, including pregnant women), at the initiation of therapy place patients at increased risk of hepatic adverse events (see General and Hepatic/Biliary/Pancreatic).
> Severe, life-threatening skin reactions, including fatal cases, have been reported with VIRAMUNE treatment, occurring almost exclusively during the first 6 weeks of therapy. These have included cases of Stevens-Johnson syndrome (SJS), toxic epidermal necrolysis (TEN), and hypersensitivity syndrome characterized by rash, constitutional findings, and organ dysfunction (see Adverse Reactions). Patients should be carefully monitored during the first 18 weeks of treatment. Patients developing signs or symptoms of severe skin reactions or hypersensitivity reactions (including, but not limited to, severe rash or rash accompanied by fever, general malaise, fatigue, muscle or joint aches, blisters, oral lesions, conjunctivitis, facial edema, and/or hepatitis, eosinophilia, granulocytopenia, lymphadenopathy, and renal dysfunction) must permanently discontinue VIRAMUNE and seek medical evaluation immediately (see Guideline for the Management of Rash Events, Warnings and Precautions and Adverse Reactions).

General: Women and patients with higher CD4 counts are at increased risk of hepatic adverse events. The first 18 weeks of therapy with VIRAMUNE (nevirapine) are a critical period during which intensive monitoring of patients is required to detect potentially life-threatening hepatic events and skin reactions. The optimal frequency of monitoring during this time period has not been established, however it may be prudent to conduct clinical and laboratory monitoring more often than once per month; for example, liver function tests at baseline, prior to dose escalation and at two weeks post dose escalation. After the initial 18 week period, frequent clinical and laboratory monitoring should continue throughout treatment. The greatest risk of hepatic events and skin reactions occurs in the first 6 weeks of therapy. However, the risk of any hepatic event continues past this period and monitoring should continue at frequent intervals.

Resistant virus emerges rapidly and uniformly when VIRAMUNE is administered as monotherapy. Therefore, VIRAMUNE should always be administered in combination with other antiretroviral agents for the treatment of HIV-1 infection.

When discontinuing an antiretroviral regimen containing VIRAMUNE, the longer half-life of nevirapine should be taken into account; if antiretrovirals with shorter half-lives than VIRAMUNE are stopped concurrently, low plasma concentrations of nevirapine alone may persist for a week or longer and virus resistance may subsequently develop.

When administering VIRAMUNE as part of a multi-drug antiretroviral treatment regimen, the complete product information for each therapeutic component should be consulted before initiation of treatment.

Patients receiving VIRAMUNE or any other antiretroviral therapy may continue to develop opportunistic infections and other complications of HIV infection, and therefore should remain under close clinical observation by physicians experienced in the treatment of patients with associated HIV diseases. VIRAMUNE therapy has not been shown to reduce the risk of horizontal transmission of HIV-1 to others.

Hepatic/Biliary/Pancreatic: Severe, life-threatening, and in some cases fatal hepatotoxicity, including fulminant and cholestatic hepatitis, hepatic necrosis and hepatic failure, have been reported in patients treated with VIRAMUNE. In some cases, patients presented with non-specific prodromal signs or symptoms of hepatitis and progressed to hepatic failure. These events are often associated with rash. Female gender and higher CD4 counts at the initiation of therapy place patients at greater risk of hepatic adverse events. Based on serious and life-threatening hepatotoxicity observed in controlled and uncontrolled studies, VIRAMUNE should not be initiated in adult females with CD4+ cell counts greater than 250 cells/mm³, including pregnant women receiving chronic treatment for HIV infection, or in adult males with CD4+ cell counts greater than 400 cells/mm³ unless the benefit outweighs the risk. In some cases, hepatic injury has progressed despite discontinuation of treatment. Patients developing signs or symptoms of hepatitis, severe skin reaction or hypersensitivity reactions must discontinue VIRAMUNE and seek medical evaluation immediately. VIRAMUNE should not be restarted following severe hepatic, skin or hypersensitivity reactions.

In clinical trials, the risk of hepatic events regardless of severity was greatest in the first 6 weeks of therapy. The risk continued to be greater in the VIRAMUNE groups compared to controls through 18 weeks of treatment. However, hepatic events may occur at any time during treatment. In some cases, patients presented with non-specific, prodromal signs or symptoms of fatigue, malaise, anorexia, nausea, jaundice, liver tenderness or hepatomegaly, with or without initially abnormal serum transaminase levels. Some of these events have progressed to hepatic failure with transaminase elevation, with or without hyperbilirubinemia, prolonged partial thromboplastin time, or eosinophilia. Rash and fever accompanied some of these hepatic events. Patients with signs or symptoms of hepatitis must be advised to discontinue VIRAMUNE and immediately seek medical evaluation, which should include liver function tests.

In rare instances rhabdomyolysis has been observed in patients experiencing skin and/or liver reactions associated with VIRAMUNE use.

Increased AST or ALT levels and/or co-infection with hepatitis B and C at the start of antiretroviral therapy are associated with a greater risk of hepatic adverse events.

In general, women have a three fold higher risk than men for symptomatic, often rash-associated, hepatic events (5.8% versus 2.2%), and patients with higher CD4 counts at initiation of VIRAMUNE therapy are at higher risk for symptomatic hepatic events with VIRAMUNE. In a retrospective review, women with CD4 counts >250 cells/mm³ had a 12 fold higher risk of symptomatic hepatic adverse events compared to women with CD4 counts <250 cells/mm³ (11.0% versus 0.9%). An increased risk was also observed in men with CD4 counts >400 cells/mm³ (6.3% versus 2.3% for men with CD4 counts <400 cells/mm³).

Intensive clinical and laboratory monitoring, including liver function tests, is essential at baseline and during the first 18 weeks of treatment (see Warnings and Precautions, General). Monitoring should continue at frequent intervals thereafter, depending on the patient's clinical status. Liver function tests should be performed immediately if a patient experiences signs or symptoms suggestive of hepatitis and/or hypersensitivity reaction. Liver function tests should also be obtained for all patients who develop a rash in the first 18 weeks of treatment. Physicians and patients should be vigilant for the appearance of signs or symptoms of hepatitis, such as fatigue, malaise, anorexia, nausea, jaundice, bilirubinuria, acholic stools, liver tenderness or hepatomegaly. The diagnosis of hepatic injury should be considered in this setting, even if liver function tests are initially normal or alternative diagnoses are possible (see Warnings and Precautions; Adverse Reactions; and Dosage and Administration).

If clinical hepatitis occurs, VIRAMUNE should be permanently discontinued and not restarted after recovery. If either AST or ALT increase to >5×ULN, VIRAMUNE should be immediately stopped. VIRAMUNE should not be readministered to patients who have been discontinued for severe rash, rash accompanied by constitutional symptoms, hypersensitivity reactions, or clinical hepatitis due to VIRAMUNE (see Guideline for the Management of Hepatic Events). In some cases hepatic injury progresses despite the discontinuation of treatment.

With AST or ALT values >2×ULN, liver tests should be monitored more frequently.

Asymptomatic elevation of liver enzymes occurs frequently in patients infected with HIV and is not necessarily a contraindication to initiating therapy with VIRAMUNE. Asymptomatic GGT elevations are not a contraindication to continuing therapy.

VIRAMUNE is extensively metabolised by the liver and nevirapine metabolites are eliminated largely by the kidney. Increased nevirapine levels and nevirapine accumulation may be observed in patients with serious liver disease. Single dose pharmacokinetic results suggest caution should be exercised when VIRAMUNE is administered to patients with moderate hepatic dysfunction. VIRAMUNE should not be administered to patients with severe hepatic dysfunction (see Contraindications).

> **Management of Hepatic Events with VIRAMUNE*:**
> **Risk Factors for Symptomatic Hepatic Events:**
> - Elevated pretreatment ALT or AST
> - HBV and/or HCV coinfection†
> - Higher CD4+ cell count at initiation of VIRAMUNE therapy
> - Female gender
> - **Women with CD4+ cell counts >250 cells/mm³, including pregnant women receiving chronic treatment for HIV infection, are at considerably higher risk of hepatotoxicity, including fatal events**
>
> **Patient Management:**
> - Counsel patients that if signs or symptoms of hepatitis,‡ severe skin reactions, or hypersensitivity occur, then discontinue VIRAMUNE and seek medical evaluation immediately
> - Frequent clinical and laboratory monitoring is essential, especially during the first 18 weeks of treatment—extra vigilance is warranted during the first 6 weeks
> - Baseline assessments should include LFTs and HBV/HCV status
> - If hepatic symptoms occur:
>   - Permanently discontinue VIRAMUNE
>   - Consider stopping all potential hepatotoxins, including concomitant antiretrovirals
>   - Evaluate patient for other causes, including HBV/HCV coinfection, alcohol use, and coadministered medications
>   - Continue to monitor patient until symptoms resolve
> - In some cases, hepatic injury has progressed despite discontinuation of treatment
>
> See Figure 1.
>
> **Figure 1: VIRAMUNE**
> **Hepatic Event Management**
>
> 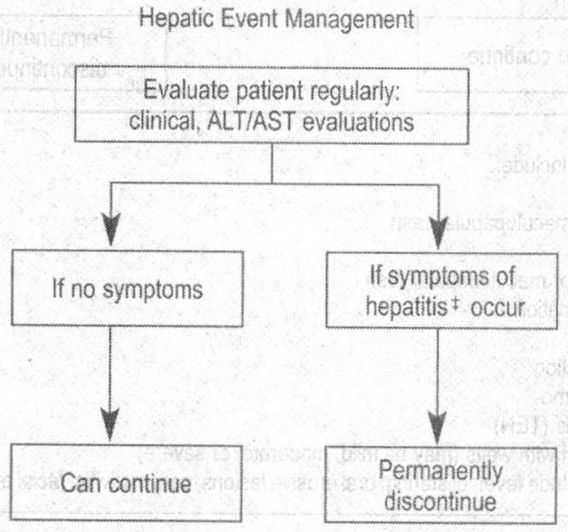
>
>
> **Other Important Information:**
> - The 14-day lead-in period with VIRAMUNE 200 mg daily must be strictly followed§
> - VIRAMUNE should not be used for multiple-dose postexposure prophylaxis. Serious hepatotoxicity, including hepatic failure, has occurred in this setting
>
> **Severe, life-threatening, and in some cases fatal, hepatotoxicity, including fulminant and cholestatic hepatitis, hepatic necrosis, and hepatic failure, has been reported in patients treated with VIRAMUNE. In some cases, patients presented with nonspecific prodromal signs or symptoms of hepatitis and progressed to hepatic failure. Patients with signs and symptoms of hepatitis must seek medical evaluation immediately and should be advised to discontinue VIRAMUNE.**

† Risk factors associated with regimens with and without VIRAMUNE.
‡ Signs and symptoms of hepatitis may include anorexia, malaise, jaundice, nausea/vomiting, bilirubinemia, acholic stools, hepatomegaly, and hepatic tenderness. Other constitutional symptoms may include fever, arthralgia, fatigue, and other findings of generalized organ dysfunction. The presence of one or more of these findings does not necessarily indicate hepatitis. Diagnosis should be based on sound clinical judgment.
§ If VIRAMUNE has been interrupted for >7 days, reintroduce with 200-mg once-daily lead-in dose.

* Hepatic events include symptomatic hepatitis and/or ALT/AST >5×ULN.

Skin: Severe, life-threatening skin reactions, including fatal cases, have been reported with VIRAMUNE treatment, occurring almost exclusively during the first 6 weeks of therapy. These have included cases of Stevens-Johnson syndrome (SJS), toxic epidermal necrolysis (TEN), and hypersensitivity syndrome characterized by rash, constitutional findings, and organ dysfunction (see Adverse Reactions). Patients should be carefully monitored during the first 18 weeks of treatment. Patients developing signs or symptoms of severe skin reactions or hypersensitivity reactions (including, but not limited to, severe rash or rash accompanied by fever, general malaise, fatigue, muscle or joint aches, blisters, oral lesions, conjunctivitis, facial edema, and/or hepatitis, eosinophilia, granulocytopenia, lymphadenopathy, and renal dysfunction) must permanently discontinue VIRAMUNE and seek medical evaluation immediately (see Guideline for the Management of Rash Events, Warnings and Precautions and Adverse Reactions). VIRAMUNE should not be restarted following severe skin rash or hypersensitivity reaction (see Guideline for the Management of Rash Events). Some of the risk factors for developing serious cutaneous reactions include failure to follow the initial dosing of 200 mg daily during the 14-day lead-in period and delay in stopping the VIRAMUNE treatment after the onset of the initial symptoms.

Therapy with VIRAMUNE must be initiated with a 14-day lead-in period of 200 mg/day which has been shown to reduce the frequency of rash. If rash is observed during this lead-in period, dose escalation should not occur until the rash has resolved (see Guideline for the Management of Rash Events, and Dosage and Administration). Patients should be monitored closely if an isolated rash of any severity occurs. The risk of development of resistance to VIRAMUNE is unknown when the 200 mg once daily dosing regimen is continued beyond 14 days.

If patients present with a suspected VIRAMUNE-associated rash, liver function tests should be performed. Patients with rash-associated AST or ALT elevations should be permanently discontinued from VIRAMUNE.

In rare instances rhabdomyolysis has been observed in patients experiencing skin and/or liver reactions associated with VIRAMUNE use.

Women appear to be at higher risk than men of developing rash with VIRAMUNE.

In a clinical trial, the concomitant use of prednisone was associated with an increase in the incidence and severity of rash during the first 6 weeks of VIRAMUNE therapy. Therefore, the use of prednisone to prevent VIRAMUNE-associated rash is not recommended.

Management of Rash Events with VIRAMUNE¶:

Patient Management: The recommended 14-day, 200 mg once-daily lead-in dose, prior to escalation to 200 mg twice daily, has been shown to reduce the frequency of rash and must be strictly followed.

Do not increase the dose of VIRAMUNE in the presence of rash.

If VIRAMUNE is interrupted for >7 days, reintroduce with the 14-day, 200 mg once-daily lead-in dose.

It is suggested that VIRAMUNE and other medications that often cause rash should not be started simultaneously.

Prednisone should not be used to prevent rash. Prednisone administration during the first 2 weeks of therapy with VIRAMUNE appears to increase the incidence of rash.

Antihistamines do not appear to be effective in preventing rash with VIRAMUNE.

See Figure 2.

Figure 2: VIRAMUNE

Rash Management Algorithm

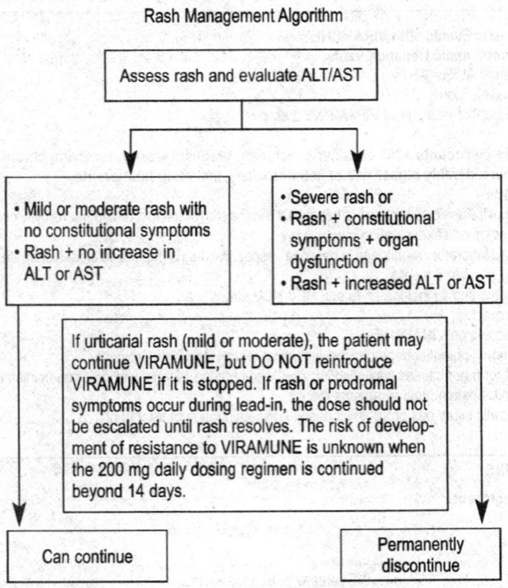

Definitions:

- Mild or moderate rash may include:
  - Erythema
  - Diffuse erythematous or maculopapular rash
- Severe rash may include:
  - Extensive erythematous or maculopapular rash
  - Rash with moist desquamation
  - Rash with angioedema
  - Serum sickness-like reaction
  - Stevens-Johnson syndrome
  - Toxic epidermal necrolysis (TEN)
- Urticaria: pruritic raised rash with welts (may be mild, moderate, or severe)
- Constitutional symptoms include fever, blistering, oral erosive lesions, conjunctivitis, facial edema, and myalgia/arthralgia

Post-Exposure Prophylaxis: VIRAMUNE is not recommended for post-exposure prophylaxis. In the setting of post-exposure prophylaxis, an unapproved use, serious hepatotoxicity, including one instance of liver failure requiring transplantation, and serious skin rash including Stevens-Johnson syndrome, have been reported in HIV-uninfected individuals receiving multiple doses of VIRAMUNE in combination with other antiretroviral agents.

Carcinogenesis and Mutagenesis: In long-term carcinogenicity studies, the incidence of hepatocellular adenomas and carcinomas in mice increased at all doses in males and at the two high doses in females. In rats an increase in hepatocellular adenomas was seen in males at all doses and in females at the high dose. The systemic exposure (based on AUCs) at all doses in the two animal studies were lower than that measured in humans at the recommended daily dose.

In genetic toxicology assays, nevirapine showed no evidence of mutagenic activity in a battery of in vitro and in vivo assays including microbial assays for gene mutation (Ames test in Salmonella strains and *E. coli*), mammalian cell gene mutation (HGRPT) assays in Chinese hamster ovary (CHO) cell line, cytogenetic assays using a CHO cell line and mouse bone marrow micronucleus assay following oral administration. In reproductive toxicology studies, evidence of impaired fertility was seen in female rats at doses providing systemic exposure, based on AUC, approximately equivalent to that observed following a human clinical dosage of 400 mg/day.

¶ **Severe, life-threatening skin reactions, including fatal cases, have occurred in patients treated with VIRAMUNE. These have included severe cases of SJS, TEN, and hypersensitivity reactions characterized by rash, constitutional findings, and organ dysfunction. Patients developing signs and symptoms of severe skin reactions or hypersensitivity reactions must discontinue VIRAMUNE as soon as possible.**

Renal: VIRAMUNE is extensively metabolised by the liver and nevirapine metabolites are eliminated largely by the kidney. In renal dysfunction, a single dose study suggested that patients with a creatinine clearance ≥20 mL/min do not require an adjustment in VIRAMUNE dosing.

Fat Redistribution: Redistribution/accumulation of body fat including central obesity, dorsocervical fat enlargement (buffalo hump), peripheral wasting, facial wasting, breast enlargement, and "cushingoid appearance" have been observed in patients receiving antiretroviral therapy. The mechanism and long-term consequences of these events are currently unknown. A causal relationship has not been established.

Immune Reconstitution: During the initial phase of treatment, patients responding to antiretroviral therapy may develop an inflammatory response to indolent or residual opportunistic infections (such as MAC, CMV, PCP and TB), which may necessitate further evaluation and treatment.

Concomitant Use with Other Drugs: VIRAMUNE can alter plasma exposure of other drugs, and other drugs can alter plasma exposure of VIRAMUNE. Combining the following compounds with VIRAMUNE is not recommended: efavirenz, rifampicin (rifampin), ketoconazole; if not coadministered with low dose ritonavir: fosamprenavir and saquinavir (see Drug Interactions).

Birth Control Methods: Depo Medroxyprogesterone Acetate (DMPA): Hormonal methods of birth control other than DMPA should not be used as the sole method of contraception in women taking VIRAMUNE. Nevirapine may lower the plasma concentrations of these medications (see Drug Interactions). Therefore, when postmenopausal hormone therapy is used during administration of VIRAMUNE, its therapeutic effect should be monitored.

Special Populations: Pregnant Women: VIRAMUNE should be used during pregnancy only if the potential benefit justifies the potential risk to the fetus. There have been no adequate and well-controlled studies of nevirapine in pregnant women, nor are there reports of infants born to women who conceived while receiving nevirapine chronic dosing in clinical trials. The Antiretroviral Pregnancy Registry, which has been surveying pregnancy outcomes since January 1989, has not found an increased risk of birth defects following first trimester exposures to nevirapine. The prevalence of birth defects after any trimester exposure to nevirapine is comparable to the prevalence observed in the general population.

Severe hepatic events, including fatalities, have been reported in pregnant women receiving chronic VIRAMUNE therapy as part of combination treatment for HIV infection. Regardless of pregnancy status, women with CD4 counts >250 $cells/mm^3$ should not initiate VIRAMUNE unless the benefit outweighs the risk. It is unclear if pregnancy augments the risk observed in non-pregnant women (see Warnings and Precautions).

Antiretroviral Pregnancy Registry: To monitor maternal-fetal outcomes of pregnant women exposed to VIRAMUNE, an Antiretroviral Pregnancy Registry has been established. Physicians are encouraged to register patients by calling 1-800-258-4263.

Nursing Women: It is currently recommended that HIV-1 infected women should not breast feed infants regardless of the use of antiretroviral agents, to avoid post-natal transmission of HIV-1.

Preliminary results from a pharmacokinetic study (ACTG 250) of 10 HIV-1-infected pregnant women who were administered a single oral dose of 100 or 200 mg VIRAMUNE at a median of 5.8 hours before delivery, indicated that nevirapine readily crosses the placenta and is found in breast milk (breast milk samples taken from 3 out of 10 mothers).

Pediatrics (<15 years of age): Safety and effectiveness of VIRAMUNE in HIV-1-infected pediatric patients younger than 15 years of age have not been established. Nevirapine is metabolized more rapidly in pediatric patients than in adults.

Geriatrics (>65 years of age): Clinical studies of VIRAMUNE did not include sufficient numbers of subjects aged 65 and older to determine whether elderly subjects respond differently from younger subjects. In general, dose selection for an elderly patient should be cautious, reflecting the greater frequency of decreased hepatic, renal or cardiac function, and of concomitant disease or other drug therapy.

Ethnic Origin: An evaluation of nevirapine plasma concentrations (pooled data from several clinical trials) from HIV-1-infected patients (27 Black, 24 Hispanic, 189 Caucasian) revealed no marked difference in nevirapine steady-state trough concentrations (median C_{minss}=4.7 µg/mL Black, 3.8 µg/mL Hispanic, 4.3 µg/mL Caucasian) with long-term nevirapine treatment at 400 mg/day. However, the pharmacokinetics of nevirapine have not been evaluated specifically for the effects of ethnicity.

Gender: In general, women have a three fold higher risk than men for symptomatic, often rash-associated, hepatic events (5.8% versus 2.2%), and patients with higher CD4 counts at initiation of VIRAMUNE therapy are at higher risk for symptomatic hepatic events with VIRAMUNE. In a retrospective review, women with CD4 counts >250 $cells/mm^3$ had a 12 fold higher risk of symptomatic hepatic adverse events compared to women with CD4 counts <250 $cells/mm^3$ (11.0% versus 0.9%). An increased risk was also observed in men with CD4 counts >400 $cells/mm^3$ (6.3% versus 2.3% for men with CD4 counts <400 $cells/mm^3$) (see Adverse Reactions).

ADVERSE REACTIONS: Adverse Drug Reaction Overview: The most serious adverse reactions associated with VIRAMUNE (nevirapine) are clinical hepatitis/hepatic failure, Stevens-Johnson syndrome, toxic epidermal necrolysis, and hypersensitivity reactions. Clinical hepatitis/hepatic failure may be isolated or associated with signs of hypersensitivity which may include, severe rash or rash accompanied by fever, general malaise, fatigue, muscle or joint aches, blisters, oral lesions, conjunctivitis, facial edema, and/or hepatitis, eosinophilia, granulocytopenia, lymphadenopathy and renal dysfunction. Severe and life-threatening hepatic injury, and fatal fulminant hepatitis, have been reported in patients treated with VIRAMUNE. The first 18 weeks of treatment is a critical period, but such events may also occur later. The risk of hepatic events is greatest in the first 6 weeks of therapy. However the risk continues past this period and monitoring should continue at frequent intervals throughout treatment (see Warnings and Precautions).

Hepato-Biliary: In controlled clinical trials, clinical hepatic events regardless of severity occurred in 4.0% (range 2.5% to 11.0%) of patients who received VIRAMUNE and 1.2% of patients in control groups. Transaminase elevations (ALT or AST >5×ULN) were observed in 8.8% of patients receiving VIRAMUNE and 6.2% of patients in control groups in clinical trials. In a retrospective analysis of controlled and uncontrolled clinical trials, patients with higher CD4 counts at initiation of VIRAMUNE therapy, particularly women, were at greater risk for acute symptomatic hepatic events, including death, especially in the first six weeks of therapy.

Patients with chronic hepatitis B or C infection were at higher risk for later hepatic events (see Warnings and Precautions).

Skin and Subcutaneous Tissues: The most common clinical toxicity of nevirapine is rash. In placebo-controlled trials involving 1374 patients treated with VIRAMUNE (see Table 1), rash, of all grades and causality occurred in 14-20% of patients treated with VIRAMUNE. Severe or life-threatening rash occurred in approximately 2% of VIRAMUNE-treated patients, almost exclusively within the first 6 weeks of therapy.

Rashes were usually mild to moderate, maculopapular erythematous cutaneous eruptions, with or without pruritus, located on the trunk, face and extremities. Allergic reactions (anaphylaxis, angio-oedema and urticaria) have been reported. Severe and life-threatening skin reactions have occurred in patients treated with nevirapine, including Stevens-Johnson syndrome (SJS) and toxic epidermal necrolysis (TEN). Fatal cases of SJS, TEN and hypersensitivity reactions have been reported. Based on a denominator of 2861 nevirapine-treated clinical trial patients, the overall incidence of SJS was 0.3% (9/2861).

Rashes occur alone or in the context of a hypersensitivity syndrome characterised by rash with constitutional symptoms such as fever, arthralgia, myalgia and lymphadenopathy plus visceral involvement, such as hepatitis, eosinophilia, granulocytopenia and renal dysfunction.

Table 1: VIRAMUNE

Risk of Rash (%) in Adult Placebo-Controlled Trials[a]—Regardless of Causality

		VIRAMUNE	Placebo
		n=1374 %	n=1331 %
Through 6 Weeks of Treatment[b]			
Rash events of all grades[c]		14.8	5.9
Grade 1	Erythema, pruritus	8.5	4.2
Grade 2	Diffuse maculopapular rash, dry desquamation	4.8	1.6

(cont'd)

Table 1: VIRAMUNE *(cont'd)*

Risk of Rash (%) in Adult Placebo-Controlled Trials[a]—Regardless of Causality

		VIRAMUNE n=1374 %	Placebo n=1331 %
Grade 3 or 4	Grade 3: vesiculation, moist desquamation, ulceration; Grade 4: erythema multiforme, Stevens-Johnson syndrome, toxic epidermal necrolysis, necrosis requiring surgery, exfoliative dermatitis	1.5	0.1
Through 52 Weeks of Treatment[b]			
Rash events of all grades[c]		24.0	14.9
Grade 1	See above	15.5	10.8
Grade 2	See above	7.1	3.9
Grade 3 or 4	See above	1.7	0.2
Proportion of Patients who Discontinued Treatment Due to Rash		4.3	1.2

[a] Trials 1037, 1038, 1046 and 1090.
[b] % based on Kaplan-Meier probability estimates.
[c] NCI grading system.

Clinical Trial Adverse Drug Reactions: Because clinical trials are conducted under very specific conditions the adverse reaction rates observed in the clinical trials may not reflect the rates observed in practice and should not be compared to the rates in the clinical trials of another drug. Adverse drug reaction information from clinical trials is useful for identifying drug-related adverse events and for approximating rates.

Adverse Events in Controlled Clinical Trials: Treatment related, adverse experiences of moderate or severe intensity observed in >2% of patients receiving VIRAMUNE in placebo-controlled trials are shown in Table 2.

Table 2: VIRAMUNE

Percentage of Patients With Moderate or Severe Drug Related Events in Adult Placebo-Controlled Trials

	Trial 1090[a]		Trials 1037, 1038, 1046[b]	
	VIRAMUNE (n=1121)	Placebo (n=1128)	VIRAMUNE (n=253)	Placebo (n=203)
Median exposure (weeks)	58	52	28	28
Any adverse event	14.5%	11.1%	31.6%	13.3%
Rash	5.1	1.8	6.7	1.5
Abnormal LFTs	1.2	0.9	6.7	1.5
Nausea	0.5	1.1	8.7	3.9
Granulocytopenia	1.8	2.8	0.4	0
Headache	0.7	0.4	3.6	0.5
Fatigue	0.2	0.3	4.7	3.9
Diarrhea	0.2	0.8	2.0	0.5
Abdominal pain	0.1	0.4	2.0	0
Myalgia	0.2	0	1.2	2.0

[a] Background therapy included 3TC for all patients and combinations of NRTIs and PIs. Patients had CD4+ counts <200 cells/mm³.
[b] Background therapy included ZDV and ZDV+ddI; VIRAMUNE monotherapy was administered in some patients. Patients had CD4+ >200 cells/mm³.

Abnormal Hematologic and Clinical Chemistry Findings: The most frequently observed laboratory test abnormalities are elevations in liver function tests (LFTs), including ALT, AST, GGT, total bilirubin and alkaline phosphatase. Asymptomatic elevations of GGT levels are the most frequent. Cases of jaundice have been reported. Cases of hepatitis, severe and life-threatening hepatotoxicity, and fatal fulminant hepatitis, have been reported in patients treated with nevirapine.

Liver function test abnormalities (AST, ALT) were observed more frequently in patients receiving VIRAMUNE than in controls (Table 3). Asymptomatic elevations in GGT occur frequently but are not a contraindication to continue VIRAMUNE therapy in the absence of elevations in other liver function tests. Other laboratory abnormalities (bilirubin, anemia, neutropenia, thrombocytopenia) were observed with similar frequencies in clinical trials comparing VIRAMUNE and control regimens (see Table 3).

Table 3: VIRAMUNE

Percentage of Adult Patients with Marked Laboratory Abnormalities

Laboratory Abnormality	Trial 1090[a] VIRAMUNE n=1121	Trial 1090[a] Placebo n=1128	Trials 1037, 1038, 1046[b] VIRAMUNE n=253	Trials 1037, 1038, 1046[b] Placebo n=203
Hematology				
Hemoglobin 80 g/L	3.2%	4.1%	0%	0%
Platelets <50×10⁹/L	1.3	1	0.4	1.5
Neutrophils <750×10⁶/L	13.3	13.5	3.6	1
Blood Chemistry				
AST >250 U/L	3.7	2.5	7.6	1.5
ALT >250 U/L	5.3	4.4	14	4
Bilirubin >42.5 μm/L	1.7	2.2	1.7	1.5

(cont'd)

Table 3: VIRAMUNE *(cont'd)*

Percentage of Adult Patients with Marked Laboratory Abnormalities

[a] Background therapy included 3TC for all patients and combinations of NRTIs and PIs. Patients had CD4+ counts <200 cells/mm³.
[b] Background therapy included ZDV and ZDV+ddI; VIRAMUNE monotherapy was administered in some patients. Patients had CD4+ ≥200 cells/mm³.

Because clinical hepatitis has been reported in VIRAMUNE-treated patients, intensive clinical and laboratory monitoring, including liver function tests, is essential at baseline and during the first 18 weeks of treatment. Monitoring should continue at frequent intervals thereafter, depending on the patient's clinical status (see Warnings and Precautions).

Post-Market Adverse Drug Reactions: In addition to the adverse events identified during clinical trials, the following events have been reported with the use of VIRAMUNE in clinical practice:

Body as a Whole: fever, somnolence, drug withdrawal (see Warnings and Precautions; Drug Interactions), redistribution/accumulation of body fat (see Warnings and Precautions, Fat Redistribution).

Gastrointestinal: vomiting.

Liver and Biliary: jaundice, fulminant and cholestatic hepatitis, hepatic necrosis, hepatic failure.

Hematology: anemia (more commonly observed in children), eosinophilia, neutropenia.

Musculoskeletal: arthralgia.

Neurologic: paraesthesia.

Skin and Appendages: allergic reactions including anaphylaxis, angioedema, bullous eruptions, ulcerative stomatitis and urticaria have all been reported. In addition, hypersensitivity reactions with rash associated with constitutional findings such as fever, blistering, oral lesions, conjunctivitis, facial edema, muscle or joint aches, general malaise or significant hepatic abnormalities (see Warnings and Precautions) plus one or more of the following: hepatitis, eosinophilia, granulocytopenia and/or renal dysfunction have been reported with the use of VIRAMUNE.

Apart from rash and abnormal LFTs, the most frequently reported adverse events related to VIRAMUNE therapy across all clinical trials were nausea, fatigue, fever, headache, vomiting, diarrhea, abdominal pain and myalgia. In very rare instances, cases of anaemia and neutropenia may be associated with VIRAMUNE therapy. Arthralgia has been reported as a stand-alone event in rare instances in patients receiving VIRAMUNE containing regimens.

The following events have also been reported when VIRAMUNE has been used in combination with other antiretroviral agents: pancreatitis, peripheral neuropathy and thrombocytopenia. These events are commonly associated with other antiretroviral agents and may be expected to occur when VIRAMUNE is used in combination with other agents.

In summary the list of side effects, which can be expected with VIRAMUNE treatment, includes: rash (including severe and life-threatening skin reactions including fatal cases of SJS/TEN); hypersensitivity syndrome characterised by rash associated with constitutional symptoms such as fever, arthalgia, myalgia and lymphadenopathy plus one or more of the following: hepatitis, eosinophilia, granulocytopenia, renal dysfunction or other visceral involvement has also been reported; abnormal LFTs (AST, ALT, GGT, total bilirubin, alkaline phosphatase); jaundice; hepatitis, including severe and life-threatening hepatotoxicity and fatal fulminant hepatitis; nausea; fatigue; fever; headache; vomiting; diarrhea; abdominal pain; myalgia; arthralgia; granulocytopenia; allergic reaction (anaphylaxis, angio-edema, urticaria); anemia.

DRUG INTERACTIONS:

Serious Drug Interactions
- See Table 4 for drugs that may need a dose adjustment.
- See Table 5 for the changes in pharmacokinetic parameters of nevirapine in the presence of coadministered drugs.
- See Table 6 for the changes in pharmacokinetic parameters of coadministered drugs.

Overview: Cytochrome P450: Nevirapine induces hepatic cytochrome P450 metabolic isoenzymes 3A4 and 2B6. Coadministration of VIRAMUNE and drugs primarily metabolized by CYP3A4 or CYP2B6 may result in decreased plasma concentrations of these drugs and attenuate their therapeutic effects.

Nevirapine does not appear to affect the plasma concentrations of drugs that are substrates of other CYP450 enzyme systems, such as 1A2, 2D6, 2A6, 2E1, 2C9 or 2C19.

Table 4 contains the results of drug interaction studies performed with VIRAMUNE and other drugs likely to be coadministered. Alterations in dose or regimen may also be recommended based on these drug interaction studies conducted in HIV-1 seropositive subjects unless otherwise indicated.

Table 4: VIRAMUNE

Established and Other Potential Significant Drug Interactions; Alteration in Dose or Regimen May Be Recommended Based on Drug interaction Studies or Predicted Interactions

Concomitant Drug Class: Drug Name	Effect on Concentration of Nevirapine or Concomitant Drug	Clinical Comment
Anti-Infectives		
Antiretrovirals		
NRTIs		
Didanosine	↔ didanosine	In one crossover study, nevirapine had no effect on the steady-state pharmacokinetics of ddI (n=18). No significant effect on didanosine PK parameters seen. Didanosine and VIRAMUNE can be used without dose adjustments.
Lamivudine	↔ lamivudine	A population pharmacokinetic study of 90 patients assigned to receive lamivudine with VIRAMUNE or placebo revealed no changes to lamivudine apparent clearance and volume of distribution, suggesting no induction effect of VIRAMUNE on lamivudine clearance. Lamivudine and VIRAMUNE can be used without dose adjustments.
Stavudine	↔ nevirapine ↔ stavudine	Results from a 36 day study in HIV infected patients administered VIRAMUNE, nelfinavir and stavudine showed no statistically significant changes in the AUC or C_{max} of stavudine. Nevirapine: compared to historical controls, levels appeared to be unchanged. Stavudine and VIRAMUNE can be used without dose adjustments.

(cont'd)

Table 4: VIRAMUNE *(cont'd)*

Established and Other Potential Significant Drug Interactions; Alteration in Dose or Regimen May Be Recommended Based on Drug interaction Studies or Predicted Interactions

Concomitant Drug Class: Drug Name	Effect on Concentration of Nevirapine or Concomitant Drug	Clinical Comment
Tenofovir	↔ nevirapine ↔ tenofovir	Tenofovir plasma levels remain unchanged when coadministered with nevirapine. Tenofovir does not have an effect on nevirapine plasma levels. Tenofovir and VIRAMUNE can be used without dose adjustments.
Zalcitabine[a]	↔ zalcitabine	In one crossover study, nevirapine had no effect on the steady-state pharmacokinetics of ddC (n=6). Zalcitabine and VIRAMUNE can be used without dose adjustments.
Zidovudine	↔ nevirapine ↓ zidovudine	Zidovudine had no effect on the pharmacokinetics of nevirapine. No significant effect on zidovudine PK parameters is seen. Zidovudine and VIRAMUNE can be used without dose adjustments.
NNRTIs		
Efavirenz	↓ efavirenz	It is not recommended to co-administer efavirenz and VIRAMUNE because of the EFV pharmacokinetic changes and the higher risk for side effects associated with their coadministration. Moreover this coadministration does not improve efficacy over either NNRTI alone. There has been no determination of appropriate doses for the safe and effective use of this combination.
PIs		
Darunavir/ritonavir	↑ nevirapine ↑ darunavir	No significant effect on darunavir PK parameters is seen when administered concomitantly with nevirapine. Exposure to nevirapine increased when administered in combination with darunavir and ritonavir. Darunavir and VIRAMUNE can be used without dose adjustments.
Fosamprenavir	↑ nevirapinert ↓ amprenavir	It is not recommended to co-administer fosamprenavir and VIRAMUNE if fosamprenavir is not coadministered with ritonavir.
Fosamprenavir/ritonavir	↑ nevirapine ↓ amprenavir	No significant alteration of plasma pharmacokinetic parameters of amprenavir. Plasma trough concentrations of nevirapine were increased. Fosamprenavir/ritonavir and VIRAMUNE can be used without dose adjustments.
Indinavir	↔ nevirapine ↓ indinavir	Results from a clinical trial with HIV infected patients administered nevirapine and indinavir indicated that their coadministration leads to a decrease in indinavir AUC and C_{min}. There was no significant change in nevirapine plasma levels. A dose increase of indinavir to 1000 mg q8h should be considered when indinavir is given with VIRAMUNE 200 mg BID; however, there are no data currently available to establish that the short term or long term antiviral activity of indinavir 1000 mg q8h with VIRAMUNE 200 mg BID will differ from that of indinavir 800 mg q8h with VIRAMUNE 200 mg BID. No clinically relevant change in nevirapine plasma levels was found.
Lopinavir/ritonavir	Adult patients: ↓ lopinavir	In HIV positive adults, nevirapine used in combination with lopinavir/ritonavir 400/100 mg (3 capsules) twice daily resulted in a decline in the mean lopinavir AUC and C_{min}. Although the clinical relevance of this observation has not been fully established, an increase in the dose of lopinavir/ritonavir to 533/133 mg (4 capsules) twice daily with food is recommended in combination with VIRAMUNE. Dose adjustment of VIRAMUNE is not required when coadministered with lopinavir.
Lopinavir[b]/ritonavir	Paediatric patients: ↓ lopinavir	For children, increase of the dose of lopinavir/ritonavir to 300/75 mg/m² twice daily with food should be considered when used in combination with VIRAMUNE, particularly for patients in whom reduced susceptibility to lopinavir/ritonavir is suspected. Results from a pharmacokinetic study in paediatric patients were consistent with the findings in adults. During nevirapine coadministration, mean lopinavir AUC and C_{min} decreased. In children 6 months to 12 years of age, consideration should be given to increasing the dose of lopinavir/ritonavir to 13/3.25 mg/kg for those 7 to <15 kg; 11/2.75 mg/kg for those 15 to 45 kg; and up to a maximum dose of 533/133 mg for those >45 kg twice daily when used in combination with nevirapine, particularly for patients in whom reduced susceptibility to lopinavir/ritonavir is suspected.

(cont'd)

Table 4: VIRAMUNE *(cont'd)*

Established and Other Potential Significant Drug Interactions; Alteration in Dose or Regimen May Be Recommended Based on Drug interaction Studies or Predicted Interactions

Concomitant Drug Class: Drug Name	Effect on Concentration of Nevirapine or Concomitant Drug	Clinical Comment
Nelfinavir	↔ nevirapine ↓ nelfinavir C_{min} ↓ nelfinavir-M8 metabolite	Results from a 28 day study in HIV infected patients administered VIRAMUNE, nelfinavir showed no statistically significant changes in nelfinavir pharmacokinetic parameters after the addition of VIRAMUNE. Compared to historical controls VIRAMUNE levels appeared to be unchanged. The major metabolite of nelfinavir (M8) which has comparable activity to the parent compound, however, has a decrease in AUC, C_{max} and C_{min}. The appropriate dose for nelfinavir in combination with nevirapine, with respect to safety and efficacy, has not been established. Nelfinavir and VIRAMUNE can be used without dose adjustments.
Ritonavir	↔ nevirapine ↔ ritonavir	Results from a clinical trial with HIV infected patients administered nevirapine and ritonavir indicated that their coadministration leads to no significant change in ritonavir or nevirapine plasma concentrations. Ritonavir and VIRAMUNE can be used without dose adjustments.
Saquinavir	↔ nevirapine ↓ saquinavir	Results from a clinical trial with HIV infected patients administered nevirapine and saquinavir hard gelatine capsule indicated that their coadministration leads to a mean reduction in saquinavir AUC and no significant change in nevirapine plasma levels. This decrease is not thought to be clinically significant and no dose adjustments of saquinavir or nevirapine are recommended. The safety and efficacy of the combination of nevirapine and saquinavir/ritonavir have not been established.
Tipranavir/ritonavir	↓ nevirapine ↓ tipranavir	No specific drug-drug interaction study has been performed. The limited data available from a phase IIa study in HIV-infected patients have shown a clinical non significant 20% decrease of TPV C_{min}. No significant effect on tipranavir and VIRAMUNE PK parameters is expected. Tipranavir and VIRAMUNE can be used without dose adjustments.
Entry Inhibitors		
Enfuvirtide	↔ nevirapine ↔ enfuvirtide	No clinically significant pharmacokinetic interactions are expected between enfuvirtide and concomitantly given medicinal products metabolised by CYP450 enzymes. No significant effect on enfurtivide and VIRAMUNE PK parameters is expected. Enfuvirtide and VIRAMUNE can be used without dose adjustments.
Maraviroc	↑ maraviroc	Nevirapine concentrations not measured, no effect is expected. No significant effect on maraviroc and VIRAMUNE PK parameters is expected. The combination of maraviroc and VIRAMUNE, lamivudine and tenofovir can he administered without dose adjustment.
Integrase Inhibitors		
Raltegravir	↔ nevirapine ↔ raltegravir	No clinical data available. Due to the metabolic pathway of raltegravir no interaction is expected. No significant effect on raltegravir and VIRAMUNE PK parameters is expected. Raltegravir and VIRAMUNE can be used without dose adjustments.
Antibiotics		
Clarithromycin	↑ nevirapine ↓ clarithromycin ↑ clarithromycin-14-OH Metabolite	Results of a VIRAMUNE-clarithromycin drug-drug interaction study resulted in a significant reduction in clarithromycin AUC, C_{max} and C_{min} but a significant increase in AUC and C_{max} of the active metabolite 14-OH clarithromycin. There was a significant increase in the nevirapine C_{min} and a non-significant increase in nevirapine AUC and C_{max}. Alternatives to clarithromycin, such as azithromycin should be considered. Close monitoring of hepatic abnormalities is recommended.
Rifabutin	↔ nevirapine ↑ rifabutin ↑ Metabolite 25-O-desacetylrifabutin	In an open label pharmacokinetic study the concomitant administration of rifabutin following full induction with nevirapine resulted in an increase in the steady-state AUC, C_{max}, and C_{min} of rifabutin. There was also an increase in the 25-O-desacetyl-rifabutin metabolite exposure in extent and rate. Due to the high intersubject variability some patients may experience large increases in rifabutin exposure and may be at higher risk for rifabutin toxicity. Therefore, caution should be used in concomitant administration. A clinically not relevant increase in the apparent clearance of nevirapine (by 9%) compared to historical pharmacokinetic data was reported. Rifabutin and VIRAMUNE can be used without dose adjustments.

(cont'd)

Table 4: VIRAMUNE *(cont'd)*

Established and Other Potential Significant Drug Interactions; Alteration in Dose or Regimen May Be Recommended Based on Drug interaction Studies or Predicted Interactions

Concomitant Drug Class: Drug Name	Effect on Concentration of Nevirapine or Concomitant Drug	Clinical Comment
Rifampicin (Rifampin)	↓ nevirapine ↔ rifampicin	It is not recommended to co-administer rifampicin and VIRAMUNE. Limited clinical data exist with a dose adjustment for VIRAMUNE when coadministered with rifampicin. Physicians needing to treat patients coinfected with tuberculosis and using a VIRAMUNE containing regimen may consider use of rifabutin instead. (see Warnings and Precautions).
Antifungals		
Fluconazole	↑ nevirapine ↔ fluconazole	Nevirapine exposure: ↑ 100% compared with historical data where nevirapine was administered alone. Because of the risk of increased exposure to VIRAMUNE, caution should be exercised if the medicinal products are given concomitantly and patients should be monitored closely. Fluconazole may only be added to a stable nevirapine containing regimen when the benefits clearly outweigh the risks. There was no clinically relevant effect of nevirapine on fluconazole.
Itraconazole	↔ nevirapine ↓ itraconazole	There was no significant difference in nevirapine pharmacokinetic parameters. A dose adjustment for itraconazole should be considered when these two agents are administered concomitantly; however, a higher dosage of itraconazole might have an inhibitory effect on nevirapine plasma concentration.
Ketoconazole	↑ nevirapine ↓ ketoconazole	Administration of nevirapine with ketoconazole resulted in a significant reduction in ketoconazole AUC and C_{max}. In the same study, ketoconazole administration resulted in an increase in the plasma levels of nevirapine compared to historical controls. It is not recommended to co-administer ketoconazole and VIRAMUNE. A dose adjustment for ketoconazole should be considered when these two agents are administered concomitantly.
Antacids		
Cimetidine	↑ nevirapine C_{min}	The median nevirapine trough for patients on cimetidine was 7% higher than the control group. The limited data suggest no dose adjustment when cimetidine is coadministered with VIRAMUNE.
Antithrombotics		
Warfarin	↑ or ↓ warfarin	The interaction between nevirapine and the antithrombotic agent warfarin is complex with the potential for both increases and decreases in coagulation time when used concomitantly. The net effect of the interaction may change during the first weeks of coadministration, during the re-establishment of therapeutic effect only after dose adjustment, or upon discontinuation of VIRAMUNE. Close monitoring of anticoagulation levels is therefore warranted.
Contraceptives		
Depo medroxy-progesterone acetate (DMPA)	↑ nevirapine ↔ DMPA	No significant effect on DMPA and VIRAMUNE PK parameters is seen. DMPA and VIRAMUNE can be used without dose adjustments. VIRAMUNE coadministration did not alter the ovulation suppression effects of DMPA as measured by progesterone levels.
Ethinyl estradiol (EE)/Norethindrone (NET)	↓ ethinyl estradiol (EE) ↓ norethindrone (NET)	Oral hormonal contraceptives should not be used as the sole method of contraception in women taking VIRAMUNE. Appropriate doses for hormonal contraceptives (oral or other forms of application) other than DMPA in combination with VIRAMUNE have not been established with respect to safety and efficacy.
Drug Abuse		
Methadone	↓ methadone	Results from a study with HIV-infected patients in the presence of nevirapine, steady state plasma methadone concentrations have been shown to be reduced at C_{max} and in extent of methadone exposure (AUC). Narcotic withdrawal syndrome has been reported in patients treated with VIRAMUNE and methadone concomitantly. Methadone-maintained patients beginning VIRAMUNE therapy should be monitored for evidence of withdrawal and methadone dose should be adjusted accordingly.
Herbal Products		
St. John's Wort	↓ nevirapine	Concomitant use of VIRAMUNE and St. John's wort (Hypericum perforatum) or St. John's wort-containing products is not recommended. Coadministration of non-nucleoside reverse transcriptase inhibitors including VIRAMUNE, with St. John's Wort is expected to decrease NNRTI concentrations and may result in sub-optimal levels of VIRAMUNE and lead to loss of virologic response and possible resistance to VIRAMUNE or to the class of NNRTIs. This is due to induction of drug metabolism enzymes and/or transport proteins by St. John's Wort. If a patient is already taking St. John's Wort check nevirapine and, if possible, viral levels and stop St. John's Wort. Nevirapine levels may increase on stopping St. John's Wort. The dose of VIRAMUNE may need adjusting. The inducing effect may persist for at least 2 weeks after cessation of treatment with St. John's Wort.

[a] Discontinued in Canada.
[b] Pediatric subjects ranging in age from 6 months to 12 years.
§=C_{min} below detectable level of the assay.
Legend: ↑=Increase; ↓=Decrease; ↔=No Effect.

The effects of Nevirapine on the pharmacokinetics of coadministered drugs and the coadministered drugs on Nevirapine are summarized in Table 5 and Table 6, respectively. This data is based on the results of drug interaction studies conducted in HIV-1 seropositive subjects unless otherwise indicated.

Table 5: VIRAMUNE

Drug Interactions: Pharmacokinetic Parameters for Nevirapine in the Presence of Coadministered Drug (See Table 4 for Recommended Alterations in Dose or Regimen)

Coadministered Drug	Dose of Coadministered Drug	Dose Regimen of VIRAMUNE	n	Ratio Change of Nevirapine Pharmacokinetic Parameters (90% CI) No Effect=1.00		
Anti-Infectives				AUC	C_{max}	C_{min}
Antiretrovirals						
PIs						
Darunavir/ritonavir[a]	400/100 mg BID	200 mg BID	8	1.27 (1.12–1.44)	1.18 (1.02–1.37)	1.47 (1.20–1.82)
Fosamprenavir	1400 mg BID	200 mg BID	17	1.29 (1.19–1.40)	1.25 (1.14–1.37)	1.34 (1.21–1.49)
Fosamprenavir/ritonavir	700/100 mg BID	200 mg BID	17	1.14 (1.05–1.24)	1.13 (1.03–1.24)	1.22 (1.10–1.35)
Antibiotics						
Clarithromycin[b]	500 mg BID	200 mg daily×14 days; 200 mg BID×14 days	15	1.26	1.24	1.28
Rifampin[b]	600 mg daily	200 mg daily×14 days; 200 mg BID×14 days	14	0.42	0.50	0.32
Antifungals						
Itraconazole[a]	200 mg daily	200 mg daily	12	1.02[c] (1.00–1.06)	1.05[c] (1.04–1.06)	1.14 (1.08–1.27)[c]
Contraceptives						
Depo medroxy-progesterone acetate (DMPA)	150 mg every 3 months	200 mg daily×14 days; 200 mg BID×14 days)	16	1.17 (1.03–1.33)	1.19 (1.05–1.33)	—

[a] Studies reported from healthy subjects.
[b] For information regarding clinical recommendations see Table 4.
[c] Mean ratio measured at 95% confidence interval.
Legend: ↑=Increase; ↓=Decrease.

Table 6: VIRAMUNE

Drug Interactions: Pharmacokinetic Parameters for Coadministered Drug in the Presence of Nevirapine (See Table 4 for Recommended Alterations in Dose or Regimen)

Coadministered Drug	Dose of Coadministered Drug	Dose Regimen of VIRAMUNE	n	Ratio Change of Nevirapine Pharmacokinetic Parameters (90% CI) No Effect=1.00		
Anti-Infectives				AUC	C_{max}	C_{min}
Antiretrovirals						
NRTIs						

(cont'd)

Table 6: VIRAMUNE *(cont'd)*

Drug Interactions: Pharmacokinetic Parameters for Coadministered Drug in the Presence of Nevirapine (See Table 4 for Recommended Alterations in Dose or Regimen)

Coadministered Drug	Dose of Coadministered Drug	Dose Regimen of VIRAMUNE	n	Ratio Change of Nevirapine Pharmacokinetic Parameters (90% CI) No Effect=1.00		
Anti-Infectives				**AUC**	**C_{max}**	**C_{min}**
Antiretrovirals						
Didanosine	100-150 mg BID	200 mg daily×14 days; 200 mg BID×14 days	18	1.08 (0.92–1.27)	0.98 (0.79–1.21)	[a]
Stavudine/ nelfinavir	30–40 mg BID 750 mg TID	200 mg daily×14 days; 200 mg BID×14 days	22	0.96 (0.89–1.03)	0.94 (0.86–1.03)	[a]
Zalcitabine[b] Zidovudine	0.125–0.25 mg TID 100–200 mg TID	200 mg daily×14 days; 200 mg BID×14 days	6	1.14 (0.87–1.52)	0.97 (0.75–1.25)	[a]
Zidovudine	100–200 mg TID	200 mg daily×14 days; 200 mg BID×14 days	11	0.72 (0.60–0.96)	0.70 (0.49–1.14)	[a]
NNRTIs						
Efavirenz[c]	600 mg daily	200 mg daily×14 days; 400 mg daily×14 days	17	0.72 (0.66–0.86)	0.88 (0.77–1.01)	0.68 (0.65–0.81)
PIs						
Darunavir/ ritonavir[d]	400/100 mg BID	200 mg BID	8	1.24 (0.97–1.57)	1.40 (1.14–1.73)	1.02 (0.79–1.32)
Fosamprenavir	1400 mg BID	200 mg BID	17	0.67 (0.55–0.80)	0.75 (0.63–0.89)	0.65 (0.49–0.85)
Fosamprenavir/ ritonavir	700/100 mg BID	200 mg BID	17	0.89 (0.77–1.03)	0.97 (0.85–1.10)	0.81 (0.69–0.96)
Indinavir[c]	800 mg q8H	200 mg daily×14 days; 200 mg BID×14 days	19	0.69 (0.61–0.78)	0.85 (0.76–0.96)	0.56 (0.47–0.67)
Lopinavir[c,e]	300/75 mg/m^2 BID (lopinavir/ritonavir)[e]	7 mg/kg or 4 mg/kg daily×2 weeks; BID×1 week	12, 15[f]	0.78 (0.56–1.09)	0.86 (0.64–1.16)	0.45 (0.25–0.81)
Lopinavir[c]	400/100 mg BID (lopinavir/ritonavir)	200 mg daily×14 days; 200 mg BID >1 year	22, 19[f]	0.73 (0.53–0.98)	0.81 (0.62–0.95)	0.54 (0.28–0.74)
Nelfinavir[c]	750 mg TID	200 mg daily×14 days; 200 mg BID×14 days	23	0.94 (0.78–1.14)	1.06 (0.92–1.22)	0.68 (0.50–1.05)
Nelfinavir-M8 metabolite				0.38 (0.30–0.47)	0.41 (0.32–0.52)	0.34 (0.26–0.45)
Ritonavir	600 mg BID	200 mg daily×14 days; 200 mg BID×14 days	18	0.92 (0.79–1.07)	0.91 (0.78–1.07)	0.93 (0.76–1.14)
Saquinavir[c]	600 mg TID	200 mg daily×14 days; 200 mg BID×21 days	23	0.62 (0.53–0.89)	0.68 (0.56–0.94)	[a]
Entry Inhibitors						
Maraviroc/ Lamivudine/ Tenofovir DF	300 mg Single Dose/300 mg daily/ 300 mg daily	200 mg BID	8	1.01 (0.65–1.55)	1.54 (0.94–2.51)	[a]
Antibiotics						
Clarithromycin[c]	500 mg BID	200 mg daily×14 days; 200 mg BID×14 days	15	0.69 (0.62–0.76)	0.77 (0.69–0.86)	0.44 (0.30–0.64)
Metabolite 14-OH-clarithromycin				1.42 (1.16–1.73)	1.47 (1.21–1.80)	0 (0.68–1.49)
Rifabutin[c]	150 or 300 mg daily	200 mg daily×14 days; 200 mg BID×14 days	19	1.17 (0.98–1.40)	1.28 (1.09–1.51)	1.07 (0.84–1.37)
Metabolite 25-O-desacetylrifabutin				1.24 (0.84–1.84)	1.29 (0.98–1.68)	1.22 (0.86–1.74)
Rifampicin (Rifampin)[c]	600 mg daily	200 mg daily×14 days; 200 mg BID×14 days	14	1.11 (0.96–1.28)	1.06 (0.91–1.22)	[a]
Antifungals						

(cont'd)

Table 6: VIRAMUNE *(cont'd)*

Drug Interactions: Pharmacokinetic Parameters for Coadministered Drug in the Presence of Nevirapine (See Table 4 for Recommended Alterations in Dose or Regimen)

Coadministered Drug	Dose of Coadministered Drug	Dose Regimen of VIRAMUNE	n	Ratio Change of Nevirapine Pharmacokinetic Parameters (90% CI) No Effect=1.00		
Anti-Infectives				**AUC**	**C_{max}**	**C_{min}**
Antiretrovirals						
Fluconazole	200 mg daily	200 mg daily×14 days; 200 mg BID×14 days	19[0]	0.94 (0.88–1.01)	0.92 (0.85–0.99)	0.93 (0.86–1.01)
Itraconazole[d]	200 mg daily[1]	200 mg daily	12	0.39[g]	0.62[g]	0.13[g]
Ketoconazole[c]	400 mg daily	200 mg daily×14 days; 200 mg BID×14 days	21	0.28 (0.20–0.40)	0.56 (0.42–0.73)	[a]
Contraceptives						
Ethinyl estradiol (EE)[c]	0.035 mg (as Ortho-Novum 1/35)	200 mg daily×14 days; 200 mg BID×14 days	10	0.80 (0.67–0.97)	0.94 (0.79–1.12)	[a]
Norethindrone[c] (NET)	1 mg (as Ortho-Novum 1/35)			0.81 (0.70–0.93)	0.84 (0.73–0.97)	[a]
Drug Abuse						
Methadone	Individual Patient Dosing	200 mg daily×14 days; 200 mg BID ≥7 days	8	0.40 (0.31–0.51)	0.58 (0.50–0.67)	[a]

[a] C_{min} below detectable level of the assay.
[b] Discontinued in Canada.
[c] For information regarding clinical recommendations see Table 4.
[d] Studies reported from healthy subjects.
[e] Pediatric subjects ranging in age from 6 months to 12 years.
[f] Parallel group design; n for VIRAMUNE +lopinavir/ritonavir, n for lopinavir/ritonavir alone.
[g] Mean ratio measured at 95% confidence interval.
Legend: ↑=Increase; ↓=Decrease; ↔=No Effect.

In addition to established drug interactions, there may be potential pharmacokinetic interactions between nevirapine and other drug classes that are metabolized by the cytochrome P450 system. These potential drug interactions are listed in Table 7. Although specific drug interaction studies in HIV-1 seropositive subjects have not been conducted for the classes of drugs listed in Table 7, additional clinical monitoring may be warranted when co-administering these drugs.

Table 7: VIRAMUNE

Potential Drug Interactions: Use with Caution, Dose Adjustment of Coadministered Drug may be Needed due to Possible Decrease in Clinical Effect

Drug Class	Examples of Drugs	Clinical Comment
Antiarrhythmics	Amiodarone, disopyramide, lidocaine	Plasma concentrations may be decreased.
Anticonvulsants	Carbamazepine, clonazepam, ethosuximide	Plasma concentrations may be decreased.
Calcium channel blockers	Diltiazem, nifedipine, verapamil	Plasma concentrations may be decreased.
Calcium channel blockers	Diltiazem, nifedipine, verapamil	Plasma concentrations may be decreased.
Cancer chemotherapy	Cyclophosphamide	Plasma concentrations may be decreased.
Ergot alkaloids	Ergotamine	Plasma concentrations may be decreased.
Immunosuppressants	Cyclosporin, tacrolimus, sirolimus	Plasma concentrations may be decreased.
Motility agents	Cisapride[a]	Plasma concentrations may be decreased.
Opiate agonists	Fentanyl	Plasma concentrations may be decreased.

[a] Cisapride is no longer marketed in Canada

Other Drugs Metabolized By CYP3A: Biotransformation of nevirapine involves extensive cytochrome P450 metabolism (CYP3A>CYP2B6) and glucuronidation with maximal induction occurring within 2-4 weeks of initiating multiple-dose therapy. Available data on the potential interaction between nevirapine and other drugs that are extensively metabolized by CYP3A are limited and preliminary; therefore, careful monitoring of the therapeutic effectiveness of CYP3A-metabolized drugs is recommended when taken in combination with nevirapine.

In Vitro Studies: Studies using human liver microsomes indicated that the formation of nevirapine hydroxylated metabolites was not affected by the presence of dapsone, rifabutin, rifampin and trimethoprim/sulphamethoxazole. Ketoconazole and erythromycin significantly inhibited the formation of nevirapine hydroxylated metabolites.

Drug-Lifestyle Interactions: Occupational Hazards—Psychomotor Performance: Psychomotor Performance: There are no specific studies assessing psychomotor performance in patients using VIRAMUNE. Somnolence has been reported in association with VIRAMUNE therapy; if this occurs during VIRAMUNE administration, patients should be advised to refrain from driving a motor vehicle or operating potentially hazardous machinery.

DOSAGE AND ADMINISTRATION: Recommended Dose and Dosage Adjustment: The recommended dose for VIRAMUNE (nevirapine) is one 200 mg tablet daily for the first 14 days (this lead-in period should be used because it has been found to lessen the frequency of rash), followed by one 200 mg tablet twice daily, as part of a multi-drug antiretroviral treatment regimen. The manufacturer's recommended dosage and monitoring for the concomitantly administered antiretroviral therapy should be used.

Dosing Considerations: Monitoring of Patients: Intensive clinical and laboratory monitoring, including liver function tests, is essential at baseline and during the first 18 weeks of treatment with VIRAMUNE. The optimal frequency of monitoring during this period has not been established, however it may be prudent to conduct clinical and laboratory monitoring more often than once per month; for example, liver function tests at baseline, prior to dose escalation and at two weeks post-dose escalation. After the initial 18 week period, frequent clinical and laboratory monitoring should continue throughout VIRAMUNE treatment (see Warnings and Precautions).

VIRAMUNE should be discontinued if patients experience severe rash or a rash accompanied by constitutional findings (see Warnings and Precautions). Patients experiencing rash during the 14-day lead-in period of 200 mg/day should not have their VIRAMUNE dose increased until the rash has resolved (see Warnings and Precautions). The risk of development of resistance to VIRAMUNE is unknown when the 200 mg once daily dosing regimen is continued beyond 14 days.

VIRAMUNE administration should be interrupted in patients experiencing moderate or severe liver function test abnormalities (>5×ULN) (excluding GGT), until the liver function test elevations have returned to baseline. VIRAMUNE may then be restarted at the lead-in dose of 200 mg/day. Increasing the daily dose to 200 mg twice daily (400 mg/day) should be done with caution, after extended observation. Patients should be aware that this may not prevent serious adverse reactions. VIRAMUNE should be permanently discontinued if moderate or severe liver function test abnormalities recur (see Warnings and Precautions).

Patients with Renal Impairment: In End Stage Renal Disease (ESRD) appropriate doses of VIRAMUNE with respect to safety and efficacy have not been established. Subjects with ESRD requiring dialysis exhibited a 43.5% reduction in VIRAMUNE AUC over a one week exposure period with an accumulation of nevirapine hydroxy-metabolites in plasma. An additional 200 mg dose of VIRAMUNE following each dialysis treatment is recommended in patients requiring dialysis. In renal dysfunction, a single dose study suggested that patients with a creatinine clearance ≥20 mL/min do not require an adjustment in VIRAMUNE dosing.

Patients with Hepatic Impairment: Patients with mild hepatic impairment do not require an adjustment in VIRAMUNE dosing; however, caution should be exercised when VIRAMUNE is administered to patients with moderate hepatic impairment. VIRAMUNE should not be administered to patients with severe hepatic dysfunction.

Patients with Lactose Intolerance: VIRAMUNE tablets contain 636 mg of lactose per maximum recommended daily dose. Patients with rare hereditary conditions of galactose intolerance e.g. galactosaemia, the Lapp lactase deficiency or glucose-galactose malabsorption should not take this medicine.

Missed Dose: Patients who miss a dose should take it as soon as they remember and then continue as before. Do not double the next dosage.

Patients who interrupt VIRAMUNE dosing for more than 7 days should restart the recommended dosing, using one 200 mg tablet daily for the first 14 days (lead-in) followed by one 200 mg tablet twice daily.

OVERDOSAGE:

There is no known antidote for VIRAMUNE (nevirapine) overdosage. The use of activated charcoal may be helpful.

Cases of VIRAMUNE overdose at doses ranging from 800 to 6000 mg per day for up to 15 days have been reported. Patients have experienced edema, erythema nodosum, fatigue, fever, headache, insomnia, nausea, pulmonary infiltrates, rash, vertigo, vomiting, increase in transaminases, and weight decrease. All subsided following discontinuation of VIRAMUNE.

In one case, a patient accidentally ingested VIRAMUNE 1200 mg daily for three days, and then 1800 mg for a fourth day. The patient suffered fever, generalized rash, nausea, vomiting, headache, chills, and facial swelling, and was admitted to hospital for 5 days. The event resolved without sequelae.

In another case, a patient ingested 9 tablets of VIRAMUNE (1800 mg) per day for 10 days. The patient presented with rash (erythema nodosum), pulmonary infiltrate, and bilateral edema of hands and feet. He was hospitalized for 2 weeks during which time he was aggressively diuresed. The events resolved over 3 weeks.

No acute toxicities or sequelae were reported for one patient who ingested 800 mg of VIRAMUNE for one day.

For management of a suspected drug overdose, contact your regional Poison Control Centre. See the *CPS* Directory section for a list of Poison Control Centres.

ACTION AND CLINICAL PHARMACOLOGY: Mechanism of Action: VIRAMUNE (nevirapine) is a highly selective, non-nucleoside reverse transcriptase inhibitor (NNRTI) of Human Immunodeficiency Virus Type 1 (HIV-1). The enzymatic activity of reverse transcriptase (RT) is required for replication of HIV. Nevirapine binds directly to RT and blocks the RNA-dependent and DNA-dependent DNA polymerase activities by causing a disruption of the enzyme's catalytic site. The inhibitory activity of nevirapine is not competitive with respect to template or nucleoside triphosphates. Reverse transcriptase from HIV-2 and eukaryotic DNA polymerases (such as human DNA polymerases α, β, γ, or δ) are not inhibited by nevirapine.

Pharmacodynamics: Nevirapine is a non-nucleoside RT inhibitor which exhibits selective antiviral activity against HIV-1. Nevirapine inhibits the replication of a wide variety of HIV-1 strains in a number of cellular assays. HIV-1 isolates exhibiting reduced susceptibility to nevirapine were selected in cell culture experiments and during in vivo clinical studies.

The in vitro antiviral activity of nevirapine has been measured in a variety of cell lines including peripheral blood mononuclear cells, monocyte derived macrophages, and lymphoblastoid cell lines. In recent studies using human cord blood lymphocytes and human embryonic kidney 293 cells, EC50 values (50% inhibitory concentration) ranged from 14->400 nM against laboratory and clinical isolates of HIV-1. Some isolates of HIV-1 group M clade A demonstrated reduced susceptibility to nevirapine in vitro. The antiviral activity of nevirapine against HIV-1, group M, clade E is unknown.

Nevirapine exhibited antiviral activity in vitro against group M HIV-1 isolates from clades A, B, C, D, F, G, and H, and circulating recombinant forms (CRF), CRF01_AE, CRF02_AG and CRF12_BF (median EC50 value of 63 nM). Nevirapine had no antiviral activity in vitro against isolates from group O HIV-1 and HIV-2. Some isolates of HIV-1 group M clade A demonstrated reduced susceptibility to nevirapine in vitro. The antiviral activity of nevirapine against HIV-1, group M, clade E is unknown.

Nevirapine in combination with efavirenz exhibited a strong antagonistic anti-HIV-1 activity in vitro and was additive to antagonistic with the protease inhibitor ritonavir or the fusion inhibitor enfuvirtide. Nevirapine exhibited additive to synergistic anti-HIV-1 activity in combination with the protease inhibitors amprenavir, atazanavir, indinavir, lopinavir, nelfinavir, saquinavir and tipranavir, and the NRTIs abacavir, didanosine, emtricitabine, lamivudine, stavudine, tenofovir and zidovudine. The anti-HIV-1 activity of nevirapine was antagonized by the anti-HBV drug adefovir and by the anti-HCV drug ribavirin in vitro.

Resistance: HIV isolates with reduced susceptibility (100-250 fold) to nevirapine emerge in vitro. Genotypic analysis showed mutations in the HIV-1 RT gene Y181C and/or V106A depending upon the virus strain and cell line employed. Time to emergence of nevirapine resistance in vitro was not altered when selection included nevirapine in combination with several other NRTIs.

Phenotypic or genotypic changes in HIV-1 isolates from treatment-naïve patients treated with either nevirapine (n=24) or nevirapine and ZDV (n=14) were monitored in Phase I/II trials over 1 to ≥12 weeks. After 1 week of nevirapine monotherapy, isolates from 3/3 patients had decreased susceptibility to nevirapine in vitro; one or more of the RT mutations at amino acid positions 103, 106, 108, 181, 188, and 190 were detected in some patients as early as 2 weeks after therapy initiation. By week eight of nevirapine monotherapy, 100% of the patients tested (n=24) had HIV isolates with a >100 fold decrease in susceptibility to nevirapine in vitro compared to baseline, and had one or more of the nevirapine-associated RT resistance mutations; 19 of 24 patients (80%) had isolates with a position 181 mutation regardless of dose.

The prevalence of phenotypic drug resistance was assessed in 60 patients with a viral rebound after they received a protease inhibitor (PI) or nevirapine containing regimen. Resistance testing was done within 36 weeks of viral rebound classified as a subsequent increase to >500 copies/mL following an initial viral load decrease to <500 copies/mL or a viral rebound of ≥0.5 $\log_{10}$ following an initial drop of ≥1.0 $\log_{10}$. In total, 88.9% given nevirapine had strains with reduced susceptibility to the drug. Overall, 46 patients (76.7%) harboured a strain resistant to ≥1 drug of their initial PI or nevirapine containing regimen. Of 53 patients who remained on treatment at the time of the study (40 had switched to a different combination from that at baseline), 6 harboured isolates susceptible to all drugs they had ever received.

Genotypic analysis of isolates from antiretroviral naïve patients with virologic rebound (n=71) receiving nevirapine once daily (n=25) or twice daily (n=46) in combination with lamivudine and stavudine (study 2NN) for 48 weeks showed that isolates from 8/25 and 23/46 patients, respectively, contained one or more of the following NNRTI resistance-associated mutations: Y181C, K101E, G190A/S, K103N, V106A/M, V108I, Y188C/L, A98G, F227L and M230L.

Cross-Resistance: Rapid emergence of HIV strains which are cross-resistant to NNRTI's has been observed in vitro. Data on cross-resistance between the NNRTI nevirapine and nucleoside analogue RT inhibitors are very limited. In four patients, ZDV-resistant isolates tested in vitro retained susceptibility to nevirapine and in six patients, nevirapine-resistant isolates were susceptible to ZDV and ddI. One case of double resistance to ZDV and nevirapine including transmission has been reported.

Cross-resistance between nevirapine and HIV protease inhibitors is unlikely because the enzyme targets involved are different.

Cross-resistance among the currently registered NNRTIs is broad. Some genotypic resistance data indicate that in most patients failing NNRTIs, viral strains express cross-resistance to the other NNRTIs.

Nevirapine must not be used as a single agent to treat HIV or added on as a sole agent to a failing regimen. As with all other non-nucleoside reverse transcriptase inhibitors, resistant virus emerges rapidly when nevirapine is administered as monotherapy. The choice of new antiretroviral agents to be used in combination with nevirapine should take into consideration the potential for cross resistance. When discontinuing an antiretroviral regimen containing nevirapine, the long half-life of nevirapine should be taken into account; if antiretrovirals with shorter half-lives than nevirapine are stopped concurrently, low plasma concentrations of nevirapine alone may persist for a week or longer and virus resistance may subsequently develop.

Absorption: Nevirapine is readily absorbed (>90%) after oral administration in healthy volunteers and in adults with HIV-1 infection. Absolute bioavailability in 12 healthy adults following single-dose administration was 93±9% (mean±SD) for the 50 mg tablet and 91.8% for the oral solution. Peak plasma nevirapine concentrations of 2±0.4 µg/mL are attained by 4 hours following a single 200 mg dose. Following multiple doses, nevirapine peak concentrations appear to increase linearly in the dose range of 200 to 400 mg/day. Steady state trough nevirapine concentrations of 4.5±1.9 µg/mL (17±7 µM), (n=242) were attained at 400 mg/day.

When VIRAMUNE (200 mg) was administered to 24 healthy adults (12 male, 12 female), with either a high fat breakfast (857 kcal, 50 g fat, 53% of calories from fat) or antacid (Maalox 30 mL), the extent of nevirapine absorption (AUC) was comparable to that observed under fasting conditions. In a separate study in HIV-1-infected patients (n=6), nevirapine steady-state systemic exposure (AUC_τ) was not significantly altered by ddI, which is formulated with an alkaline buffering agent. VIRAMUNE may be administered with or without food, antacid or ddI.

Distribution: Nevirapine is highly lipophilic and is essentially nonionized at physiologic pH. Animal studies have shown that nevirapine is widely distributed to nearly all tissues and readily crosses the blood-brain barrier. Following intravenous administration in healthy adults, the apparent volume of distribution (Vdss) of nevirapine was 1.21±0.09 L/kg, suggesting that nevirapine also is widely distributed in humans. Nevirapine is approximately 57-61% bound to plasma proteins in the plasma concentration range of 1-10 µg/mL. Nevirapine concentrations in human cerebrospinal fluid (n=6) were 45% (±5%) of the concentrations in plasma; this ratio is approximately equal to the fraction not bound to plasma protein.

Metabolism: In vivo studies in humans and in vitro studies with human liver microsomes have shown that nevirapine is extensively biotransformed via cytochrome P-450 (oxidative) metabolism to several hydroxylated metabolites. In vitro studies with human liver microsomes suggest that oxidative metabolism of nevirapine is mediated primarily by cytochrome P-450 isozymes from the CYP3A4 and CYP2B6 families, although other isozymes may have a secondary role. In a mass balance/excretion study in eight healthy male volunteers dosed to steady state with nevirapine 200 mg b.i.d. followed by a single dose of 50 mg ^{14}C-nevirapine, approximately 91.4%±10.5% of the radiolabeled dose was recovered, with urine (81.3%±11.1%) representing the primary route of excretion compared to feces (10.1%±1.5%). Greater than 80% of the radioactivity in urine was made up of glucuronide conjugates of hydroxylated metabolites. Thus cytochrome P-450 metabolism, glucuronide conjugation, and urinary excretion of glucuronidated metabolites represent the primary route of nevirapine biotransformation and elimination in humans. Only a small fraction (<5%) of the radioactivity in urine (representing <3% of the total dose) was made up of parent compound; therefore, renal excretion of nevirapine plays a minor role in elimination of the parent compound.

Excretion: Nevirapine is an inducer of hepatic cytochrome P450 (CYP) metabolic enzymes 3A4 and 2B6. Nevirapine induces CYP3A4 and CYP2B6 by approximately 20-25%, as indicated by erythromycin breath test results and urine metabolites. Autoinduction of CYP3A4 and CYP2B6 mediated metabolism leads to an approximately 1.5 to 2 fold increase in the apparent oral clearance of nevirapine as treatment continues from a single dose to two-to-four weeks of dosing with 200-400 mg/day. Autoinduction also results in a corresponding decrease in the terminal phase half-life of nevirapine in plasma, from approximately 45 hours (single dose) to approximately 25-30 hours following multiple dosing with 200-400 mg/day.

Special Populations and Conditions: Pediatrics: Safety and effectiveness of VIRAMUNE in HIV-1 infected pediatric patients younger than 15 years of age has not been established.

Age: Nevirapine pharmacokinetics in HIV-1-infected adult males and females do not appear to change with age (range 18-68 years); however, nevirapine has not been extensively evaluated in patients beyond the age of 65 years. Nevirapine is metabolized more rapidly in pediatric patients than in adults.

Gender: In one Phase I study in healthy volunteers (15 females, 15 males), the weight-adjusted apparent volume of distribution (Vdss/F) of nevirapine was higher in the female subjects (1.54 L/kg) compared to the males (1.38 L/kg), suggesting that nevirapine was distributed more extensively in the female subjects. However, this difference was offset by a slightly shorter terminal-phase half-life in the females resulting in no significant gender difference in nevirapine oral clearance (24.6±7.7 mL/kg/hr in females vs. 19.9±3.9 mL/kg/hr in males after single dose) or plasma concentrations following either single- or multiple-dose administration(s).

An evaluation of nevirapine plasma concentrations (pooled data from several clinical trials) from HIV-1-infected patients (37 females, 205 males) revealed no clinically significant difference in nevirapine steady-state trough concentrations (median C_{minss}=4.6 µg/mL females, 4.2 µg/mL males) with long-term nevirapine treatment at 400 mg/day.

Race: The pharmacokinetics of nevirapine have not been evaluated specifically for the effects of ethnicity. However, an evaluation of nevirapine plasma concentrations (pooled data from several clinical trials) from HIV-1-infected patients (27 Black, 24 Hispanic, 189 Caucasian) revealed no marked difference in nevirapine steady-state trough concentrations (median C_{minss}=4.7 µg/mL Black, 3.8 µg/mL Hispanic, 4.3 µg/mL Caucasian) with long-term nevirapine treatment at 400 mg/day.

Hepatic Insufficiency: The single-dose pharmacokinetics of VIRAMUNE have been compared in 10 subjects with hepatic impairment and 8 subjects with normal hepatic function. Overall, the results suggest that mild to moderate hepatic impairment, had no significant effect on the pharmacokinetics of VIRAMUNE. However, the pharmacokinetics of VIRAMUNE in one subject with a Child-Pugh score of 8 and moderate to severe ascites suggests that patients with worsening hepatic function may be at risk of accumulating nevirapine in the systemic circulation (see Dosage and Administration).

In a 200 mg nevirapine single dose pharmacokinetic study of HIV-negative patients with mild and moderate hepatic impairment, a significant increase in the AUC of nevirapine was observed in one patient with moderate hepatic impairment and ascites suggesting that patients with worsening hepatic function and ascites may be at risk of accumulating nevirapine in the systemic circulation.

Renal Insufficiency: The single dose pharmacokinetics of VIRAMUNE have been compared in 23 subjects with either mild (50 ≤Cl_{cr} <80 mL/min), moderate (30 ≤Cl_{cr} <50 mL/min) or severe (Cl_{cr} <30 mL/min) renal impairment or end stage renal disease (ESRD) requiring dialysis and 8 subjects with normal renal function (CL_{cr} >80 mL/min). Renal impairment (mild, moderate and severe) resulted in no significant change in the pharmacokinetics of VIRAMUNE. Subjects with ESRD requiring dialysis exhibited a 43.5% reduction in VIRAMUNE AUC over a one week exposure period with an accumulation of nevirapine hydroxy-metabolites in plasma (see Dosage and Administration).

STORAGE AND STABILITY: Solid substance stability studies have shown nevirapine bulk drug to be extremely stable. Tablets are packaged in bottles of 60 tablets and should be stored at 15-30°C. The bottles should be kept tightly closed.

INFORMATION FOR THE PATIENT: Published in e-CPS, available by subscription at www.e-cps.ca.

DOSAGE FORMS, COMPOSITION AND PACKAGING: Each white, oval, biconvex, 9.3×19.1 mm tablet, one side embossed with "54 193", with a single bisect separating the "54" and "193", the opposite side with a single bisect, contains: nevirapine 200 mg. Nonmedicinal ingredients: colloidal silicon dioxide, lactose, magnesium stearate, microcrystalline cellulose, povidone and sodium starch glycolate. Bottles of 60. The bottles should be kept tightly closed.

(Shown in Product Identification Section)

Virazole® (Lyophilized) Ⓟ

ribavirin

Antiviral Agent

Valeant

PHARMACOLOGY: Ribavirin is active against respiratory syncytial virus (RSV). In cell cultures, the inhibitory activity of ribavirin for RSV is selective. The mechanism(s) of action is unknown, although evidence exists that inhibition of other RNA and DNA viruses may be due to ribavirin competition with guanosine in formation of viral mRNA cap structures and/or interference with enzymes responsible for functional methylation of these molecules which are critical for production of structural viral proteins.

INDICATIONS: RSV infection should be documented by a rapid diagnostic method such as demonstration of viral antigen in respiratory tract secretions by immunofluorescence or ELISA before or during the first 24 hours of treatment. Ribavirin aerosol is indicated only for lower respiratory tract infection due to RSV. Treatment may be initiated while awaiting rapid diagnostic test results. However, treatment should not be continued without documentation of RSV infection.

Limited clinical data indicate that ribavirin administered as a small particle aerosol may be beneficial in the treatment of severe respiratory syncytial virus infection in neonates and infants when associated with underlying cardiovascular, pulmonary or immune deficiency. Treatment should be confined to hospitalized patients and administration should be continuous during the period of therapy apart from the time required for ancillary care of the patient. Only severe RSV lower respiratory tract infection is to be treated with ribavirin aerosol.

Ribavirin aerosol treatment must be accompanied by and does not replace standard supportive respiratory and fluid management for infants and children with severe respiratory tract infection.

CONTRAINDICATIONS: Ribavirin aerosol is contraindicated in women or girls who are or may become pregnant during exposure to the drug. Ribavirin may cause fetal harm, and respiratory syncytial virus infection is self-limited in this population. Ribavirin is not completely cleared from human blood even 4 weeks after administration. Although there are no pertinent human data, ribavirin has been found to be teratogenic and/or embryolethal in nearly all species in which it has been tested; however, pregnant baboons given up to 120 mg/kg/day of ribavirin over a 4 day period within the 20 days of organogenesis during gestation failed to exhibit any teratogenic effect.

WARNINGS: Close monitoring of patients and respiratory equipment must be guaranteed when ribavirin is used in infants requiring assisted ventilation. Precipitation of ribavirin powder in respiratory equipment may interfere with safe and effective patient ventilation.

Bronchospasm was observed in a tolerance study with ribavirin aerosol in adults with chronic obstructive pulmonary disease and asthma.

Respiratory function should be carefully monitored during treatment. If initiation of ribavirin aerosol treatment appears to produce sudden deterioration of respiratory function, treatment should be stopped and only reinstituted with caution and continuous monitoring.

Pregnancy: Although ribavirin is not indicated in adults, the physician should be aware that it is teratogenic in animals (see Contraindications).

Ribavirin administered by aerosol produced cardiac lesions in mice and rats after 30 and 36 mg/kg, respectively, for 4 weeks, and after oral administration in monkeys at 120 mg/kg and rats at 154 to 200 mg/kg for 1 to 6 months. Ribavirin aerosol administered to developing ferrets at 60 mg/kg for 10 or 30 days resulted in inflammatory and possibly emphysematous changes in the lungs. Proliferative changes were seen at 131 mg/kg for 30 days. The significance of these findings to human administration is unknown.

Ribavirin lyophilized in 6 g vials is intended for use as an aerosol only.

It has been noted that ribavirin has shown some evidence of mutagenesis in some in vitro test systems. Carcinogenicity studies are incomplete and inconclusive. Some evidence for the production of benign tumors has been shown.

PRECAUTIONS: Ribavirin has been in use for many years in human beings without any reported adverse effects in human fetuses. However, there are no adequate and well-controlled studies in pregnant women, and there is little published evidence of its safety in the early stages of human pregnancy. Since ribavirin is delivered in aerosolized form and because of known teratogenic effects in animals, pregnant women should not care for patients receiving ribavirin, although human teratogenic effects have not been proven.

Patients with lower respiratory tract infections due to respiratory syncytial virus require optimum monitoring and attention to respiratory and fluid status.

Drug Interactions: Interactions of ribavirin with other drugs such as digoxin, bronchodilators, other antiviral agents, antibiotics, or antimetabolites have not been evaluated. Interference by ribavirin with laboratory tests has not been evaluated. Appropriate attention should be given to the possibility of such interactions.

ADVERSE EFFECTS: The safety data from patients treated with ribavirin aerosol has been carefully evaluated in 26 studies. Bronchospasm was observed in a tolerance study with ribavirin aerosol (20 mg/mL) in adults. One of 6 adult patients with chronic obstructive pulmonary disease and 2 of 6 asthmatic adults became dyspneic during the period of ribavirin aerosol administration. These patients required chronic administration of bronchodilators which were discontinued 24 hours prior to ribavirin treatment. An inhalation of a bronchodilator by puffer produced symptomatic relief and return to baseline conditions.

Several serious adverse events occurred in severely ill infants with life-threatening underlying diseases, many of whom required assisted ventilation. These events include: worsening of respiratory status, bacterial pneumonia and pneumothorax. The role of ribavirin in these events is indeterminate.

There were 19 deaths during or shortly after treatment with ribavirin aerosol. No death was attributed to ribavirin aerosol by the investigators.

Some subjects requiring assisted ventilation have experienced serious difficulties, which may jeopardize adequate ventilation and gas exchange. Precipitation of drug within the ventilatory apparatus, including the endotracheal tube, has resulted in increased positive end expiratory pressure and increased positive inspiratory pressure. Accumulation of fluid in tubing "rain out" has also been noted.

Although anemia has not been reported with use of the aerosol, it occurs frequently with oral and i.v. ribavirin, and most infants treated with the aerosol have not been evaluated 1 to 2 weeks post-treatment when anemia is likely to occur. Reticulocytosis has been reported with aerosol use.

Conjunctivitis has been reported in controlled studies with ribavirin aerosol, however, no significant difference was observed between ribavirin treated and control groups.

OVERDOSE:

No overdosage with ribavirin by aerosol administration has been reported in the human. In man, ribavirin is sequestered in red blood cells for weeks after dosing.

For management of a suspected drug overdose, CPhA recommends that you contact your **regional Poison Control Centre**. See the *CPS* Directory section for a list of Poison Control Centres.

DOSAGE: Before use, read thoroughly the ICN Small Particle Aerosol Generator (SPAG) Model SPAG-2 Operator's Manual for small particle aerosol generator operating instructions.

Treatment should be instituted as early as possible within the first 3 days of respiratory syncytial virus lower respiratory tract infection. Treatment early in the course of severe lower respiratory tract infection may be necessary to achieve efficacy. Treatment is carried out continuously, apart from the time required for ancillary care, for at least 3 and no more than 7 days, and is part of a total treatment program.

The aerosol is delivered to an infant oxygen hood from the SPAG-2 aerosol generator. Administration by face mask or oxygen tent may be necessary if a hood cannot be employed (see SPAG-2 manual). However, the volume of distribution and condensation area are larger in a tent and efficacy of this method of administering the drug has been evaluated in only a small number of patients. Ribavirin aerosol is not to be administered with any other aerosol generating device or from the same reservoir with other aerosolized medications.

Aerosolized bronchodilators, when clinically indicated, should be administered with the ribavirin SPAG-2 generator shut down.

Using the recommended drug concentration of 20 mg/mL ribavirin as the starting solution in the drug reservoir of the SPAG unit, the average aerosol concentration for a 12 hour period is 190 µg/L (0.19 mg/L) of air.

Reconstitution: By sterile technique, reconstitute drug with a minimum of 70 mL sterile water USP for injection or inhalation in the original 100 mL glass vial. Shake well. Transfer to the clean, sterilized 500 mL widemouth Erlenmeyer flask (SPAG-2 Reservoir) and further dilute to a final volume of 300 mL with sterile USP water for injection or inhalation. The final concentration should be 20 mg/mL.

Important: This water should not have **any antimicrobial agent or other substance added.** The solution should be inspected visually for particulate matter and discoloration prior to administration. When the liquid level in the SPAG-2 unit is low, it should be discarded before adding newly reconstituted solution. Solutions that have been placed in the SPAG-2 unit should be discarded at least every 24 hours.

Stability and Storage of Solution: Reconstituted solutions should be prepared immediately before use or may be stored in 100 mL glass vials under sterile conditions at 2 to 6°C for 24 hours. Further diluted solutions should not be stored.

SUPPLIED: Each 100 mL glass vial of sterile, lyophilized powder contains: ribavirin 6 g. The drug is administered only by a small particle aerosol generator (SPAG-2). Store in a dry place at 15 to 25°C. Packs of 4.

Viread® Ⓟ

tenofovir disoproxil fumarate

Antiretroviral Agent

Gilead Sciences

Date of Revision: August 11, 2010

SUMMARY PRODUCT INFORMATION:

Route of Administration	Dosage Form/ Strength	Clinically Relevant Nonmedicinal Ingredients
Oral	Tablet 300 mg	Lactose monohydrate, pregelatinized starch (gluten free) For a complete listing, see Dosage Forms, Composition and Packaging.

INDICATIONS AND CLINICAL USE: HIV-1 Infection: VIREAD (tenofovir disoproxil fumarate) is indicated for the treatment of HIV-1 infection in combination with other antiretroviral agents in patients 12 years of age and older.

Chronic Hepatitis B: VIREAD is indicated for the treatment of chronic hepatitis B infection in patients 18 years of age and older. This indication is based on:

- The results from two phase 3 trials in nucleoside naïve (n=375) and nucleoside-experienced (n=51) adult patients with HBeAg negative (presumed pre-core mutant) and HBeAg positive chronic hepatitis B virus infection with compensated liver function and evidence of active viral replication. The primary end point in both studies was a composite endpoint which included virological and histological markers.
- The results from a small (N=45 patients treated with VIREAD) phase 2 trial in nucleoside naïve and nucleoside experienced adult patients with HBeAg negative and HBeAg positive chronic hepatitis B infection with primarily Child-Pugh-Turcotte Class A or B decompensated liver disease. Hepatobiliary and renal parameters should be closely monitored in this patient population. The number of patients with Child-Pugh-Turcotte Class C at baseline was too small (N=6) to reach conclusions regarding safety and efficacy. Patients with a history of solid organ or bone marrow transplant and patients with a diagnosis of proximal tubulopathy were not studied and therefore the safety and efficacy of VIREAD in this population have not been demonstrated.

Geriatrics (>65 years of age): Clinical studies of VIREAD did not include sufficient numbers of subjects aged 65 and over to determine whether they respond differently from younger subjects.

Pediatrics (12 to <18 years of age): The safety and efficacy of VIREAD in adolescent patients aged 12 to <18 years is supported by data from one randomized study in which VIREAD was administered to HIV-1 infected treatment experienced subjects. In this study, the pharmacokinetic profile of VIREAD was similar to that found to be safe and effective in adult populations.

Safety and effectiveness in pediatric patients less than 12 years of age have not been established.

CONTRAINDICATIONS: VIREAD (tenofovir disoproxil fumarate) is contraindicated in patients with previously demonstrated hypersensitivity to any of the components of the product.

For a complete listing, see Dosage Forms, Composition and Packaging.

VIREAD should not be used in combination with the fixed-dose combination products TRUVADA or ATRIPLA since it is a component of these products.

VIREAD should not be administered in combination with HEPSERA (adefovir dipivoxil).

WARNINGS AND PRECAUTIONS:

Serious Warnings and Precautions

- **Lactic Acidosis and Severe Hepatomegaly with Steatosis:** Lactic acidosis and severe hepatomegaly with steatosis, including fatal cases, have been reported with the use of nucleoside analogs, including VIREAD, alone or in combination with other antiretrovirals (see Warnings and Precautions).
- **Post-Treatment Exacerbation of Hepatitis:** Severe acute exacerbations of hepatitis have been reported in HBV-infected patients who have discontinued anti-hepatitis B therapy, including VIREAD. Hepatic function should be monitored closely with both clinical and laboratory follow-up for at least several months in patients who discontinue anti-hepatitis B therapy, including VIREAD. If appropriate, resumption of anti-hepatitis B therapy may be warranted (see Warnings and Precautions).
- **Nephrotoxicity:** Renal impairment, including cases of acute renal failure and Fanconi syndrome (renal tubular injury with severe hypophosphatemia) has been reported with the use of VIREAD during clinical practice (see Warnings and Precautions).

General: For the effect of co-administered drugs, see Drug Interactions.

Clinical studies in HIV-infected patients have demonstrated that certain regimens that only contain three nucleoside reverse transcriptase inhibitors (NRTI) are generally less effective than triple drug regimens containing two NRTIs in combination with either a non-nucleoside reverse transcriptase inhibitor or a HIV-1 protease inhibitor. In particular, early virological failure and high rates of resistance mutations have been reported. Triple nucleoside regimens should therefore be used with caution. Patients on a therapy utilizing a triple nucleoside-only regimen should be carefully monitored and considered for treatment modification.

Bone Effects: In HIV-infected patients treated with VIREAD in Study 903 through 144 weeks, decreases from baseline in bone mineral density (BMD) were seen at the lumbar spine and hip in both VIREAD and stavudine treatment arms of the study and significantly greater decreases were seen in the lumbar spine measurement in the VIREAD group relative to the stavudine group. Clinically relevant fractures were reported in both treatment groups. Increases in biochemical markers of bone metabolism (serum bone-specific alkaline phosphatase, serum osteocalcin, serum C-telopeptide, and urinary N-telopeptide) were observed, suggesting increased bone turnover. Except for bone specific alkaline phosphatase, these changes resulted in values that remained within the normal range (see Adverse Reactions, Study 903—Treatment-Emergent Adverse Events). In a clinical study of HIV-1 infected adolescent subjects (Study 321), bone effects were similar to adult subjects. Under normal circumstances, BMD increases rapidly in adolescents. In this study, the mean rate of bone gain was less in the VIREAD-treated group compared to the placebo group. Six VIREAD treated adolescents and one placebo treated adolescent had significant (>4%) lumbar spine BMD loss in 48 weeks. Among 28 subjects receiving 96 weeks of VIREAD, Z-scores declined by −0.341 for lumbar spine and −0.458 for total body. Skeletal growth (height) appeared to be unaffected. Markers of bone turnover in VIREAD-treated adolescents increased bone turnover, consistent with the effects observed in adults. The effects of VIREAD-associated changes in BMD and biochemical markers on long-term bone health and future fracture risk are unknown.

Cases of osteomalacia (associated with proximal renal tubulopathy and infrequently contributing to fractures) have been reported in association with the use of VIREAD (see Adverse Reactions, Post-Market Adverse Drug Reactions).

Bone monitoring should be considered for patients who have a history of pathologic bone fracture or are at risk for osteopenia. Although the effect of supplementation with calcium and vitamin D was not studied, such supplementation may be beneficial for all patients. If bone abnormalities are suspected then appropriate consultation should be obtained.

Carcinogenesis, Mutagenesis, Impairment of Fertility: Tenofovir DF did not show any carcinogenic potential in a long-term oral carcinogenicity study in rats. A long-term oral carcinogenicity study in mice showed a low incidence of duodenal tumors, considered likely related to high local concentrations in the gastrointestinal tract at the high dose of 600 mg/kg/day. The mechanism of tumor formation in mice and potential relevance for humans are uncertain.

Tenofovir disoproxil fumarate was mutagenic in the in vitro mouse lymphoma assay and negative in an in vitro bacterial mutagenicity test (Ames test). In an in vivo mouse micronucleus assay, tenofovir disoproxil fumarate was negative at doses up to 2000 mg/kg when administered orally to male mice.

There were no effects on fertility, mating performance or early embryonic development when tenofovir disoproxil fumarate was administered at 600 mg/kg/day to male rats for 28 days prior to mating and to female rats for 15 days prior to mating through day seven of gestation. There was, however, an alteration of the estrous cycle in female rats. A dose of 600 mg/kg/day is equivalent to 19 times the human dose based on body surface area comparisons.

Endocrine and Metabolism: Fat Redistribution: In HIV-infected patients, redistribution/accumulation of body fat (lipodystrophy) including central obesity, dorsocervical fat enlargement (buffalo hump), peripheral wasting, facial wasting, breast enlargement, and "cushingoid appearance" have been observed in patients receiving combination antiretroviral therapy. The mechanism and long-term consequences of these events are currently unknown. A causal relationship has not been established.

Hepatic/Biliary/Pancreatic: Lactic Acidosis/Severe Hepatomegaly with Steatosis: Lactic acidosis and severe hepatomegaly with steatosis, including fatal cases, have been reported with the use of antiretroviral nucleoside analogues, including tenofovir disoproxil fumarate, alone or in combination with other antiretrovirals in the treatment of HIV infection. A majority of these cases have been reported in women. Obesity and prolonged nucleoside exposure may be risk factors. Caution should be exercised when administering nucleoside analogs to any patient, and particularly to those with known risk factors for liver disease; however, cases have also been reported in patients with no known risk factors. Treatment with VIREAD should be suspended in any patient who develops clinical or laboratory findings suggestive of lactic acidosis or pronounced hepatotoxicity (which may include hepatomegaly and steatosis even in the absence of marked transaminase levels).

Pancreatitis: Pancreatitis has occurred during therapy with combination regimens that included VIREAD. Caution should be used when administering nucleoside analogues (including VIREAD) to patients with a history of pancreatitis or risk factors for the development of pancreatitis. Therapy should be suspended in patients with suspected pancreatitis.

Hepatic Impairment: Tenofovir and tenofovir disoproxil are not metabolized by liver enzymes. Clinically relevant pharmacokinetic changes in patients with hepatic impairment are not observed. Therefore, no dose adjustment is required in patients with hepatic impairment. The safety and efficacy of tenofovir DF has not been established or specifically studied in patients with underlying liver disorders. Patients with chronic hepatitis B or C and treated with antiretroviral therapy are at increased risk for severe and potentially fatal hepatic adverse events. In case of concomitant antiviral therapy for hepatitis B or C, please refer also to the relevant product information for these medicinal products.

Exacerbation of Hepatitis After Discontinuation of Treatment: Discontinuation of anti-HBV therapy, including VIREAD, may be associated with severe acute exacerbations of hepatitis. Patients infected with HBV who discontinue VIREAD should be closely monitored with both clinical and laboratory follow-up for at least several months after stopping treatment. If appropriate, resumption of anti-hepatitis B therapy may be warranted. In patients with advanced liver disease or cirrhosis, post-treatment exacerbation of hepatitis may lead to hepatic decompensation. Therefore, in these patients, discontinuation of treatment without initiation of alternative anti-hepatitis B therapy is not recommended.

Immune: Immune Reconstitution Syndrome: During the initial phase of treatment, HIV-infected patients responding to antiretroviral therapy may develop an inflammatory response to indolent or residual opportunistic infections (such as MAC, CMV, PCP, and TB), which may necessitate further evaluation and treatment.

Angioedema: Cases of angioedema have been reported in patients taking tenofovir DF (see Adverse Reactions, Post-Market Adverse Drug Reactions).

Renal: Nephrotoxicity: Tenofovir is principally eliminated by the kidney. Renal impairment, including cases of acute renal failure and Fanconi syndrome (renal tubular injury with severe hypophosphatemia) has been reported with the use of VIREAD in clinical practice (see Adverse Reactions, Post-Market Adverse Drug Reactions and Drug Interactions). The majority of these cases occurred in patients with underlying systemic or renal disease, or in patients taking nephrotoxic agents, however, some cases occurred in patients without identified risk factors.

It is recommended that creatinine clearance be calculated in all patients prior to initiating therapy and as clinically appropriate during therapy with VIREAD. Routine monitoring of calculated creatinine clearance and serum phosphorus should be performed in patients at risk for renal impairment, including patients who have previously experienced renal events while receiving HEPSERA.

Particular caution should be exercised when administering VIREAD to patients with known risk factors for renal disease and a history of renal dysfunction; however, cases of renal failure have also been reported in patients with no known risk factors. VIREAD should be avoided with concurrent or recent use of a nephrotoxic agent.

Dosing interval adjustment is required in all patients with creatinine clearance <50 mL/min (see Dosage and Administration). The safety and effectiveness of these dosing interval adjustment recommendations have not been clinically evaluated, therefore, clinical response to treatment and renal function should be closely monitored in these patients. The potential benefit of VIREAD therapy should be assessed against the potential risk for renal toxicity.

Special Populations: Patients with HIV and Hepatitis B Virus Co-infection: Due to the risk of development of HIV resistance, VIREAD should only be used in HIV and HBV co-infected patients as part of an appropriate antiretroviral combination therapy.

HIV antibody testing should be offered to all HBV-infected patients before initiating therapy with VIREAD. It is also recommended that all patients with HIV be tested for the presence of chronic hepatitis B before initiating treatment with VIREAD.

Pregnant Women: There are no adequate and well-controlled studies in pregnant women. Reproduction studies have been performed in rats and rabbits at doses up to 14 and 19 times the human dose based on body surface area comparisons and revealed no evidence of impaired fertility or harm to the fetus due to tenofovir. Reduced pup body weights, survival, and delay in sexual maturation was observed in a peri- and postnatal toxicity study in rats at the maternally toxic doses of 450 and 600 mg/kg (approximately 14 and 19 times the human dose based on body surface area comparisons). Because animal reproduction studies are not always predictive of human response, tenofovir disoproxil fumarate should be used in pregnant women only if the potential benefits outweigh the potential risks to the fetus.

Antiretroviral Pregnancy Registry: To monitor fetal outcomes of pregnant women exposed to ART including VIREAD, an Antiretroviral Pregnancy Registry has been established. Healthcare providers are encouraged to register patients by calling 1-800-258-4263.

Nursing Women: It is currently recommended that HIV- and HBV-infected women should not breast-feed to avoid postnatal transmission of HIV-1 and HBV. Studies in rats and rhesus monkeys have demonstrated that tenofovir is secreted in milk. It is not known whether tenofovir is excreted in human milk. Mothers should be instructed not to breast-feed if they are receiving VIREAD.

Pediatrics: The safety and efficacy of VIREAD in HIV adolescent patients aged 12 to <18 years is supported by data from one randomized study in which VIREAD was administered to HIV-1 infected treatment experienced subjects. In this study, the pharmacokinetic profile of VIREAD was similar to that found to be safe and effective in adult populations.

Safety and effectiveness in patients less than 12 years of age have not been established.

Geriatrics: Clinical studies of VIREAD did not include sufficient numbers of subjects aged 65 and over to determine whether they respond differently than younger subjects. In general, dose selection for the elderly patient should be cautious, keeping in mind the greater frequency of decreased hepatic, renal, or cardiac function, and of concomitant disease or other drug therapy.

ADVERSE REACTIONS: Clinical Trial Adverse Drug Reactions: Because clinical trials are conducted under very specific conditions the adverse reaction rates observed in the clinical trials may not reflect the rates observed in practice and should not be compared to the rates in the clinical trials of another drug. Adverse drug reaction information from clinical trials is useful for identifying drug-related adverse events and for approximating rates.

HIV-1 Infection: Clinical Trials: More than 12 000 patients have been treated with VIREAD alone or in combination with other antiretroviral medicinal products for periods of 28 days to 215 weeks in Phase I-III clinical trials and expanded access studies. A total of 1544 patients have received VIREAD 300 mg once daily in Phase I-III clinical trials; over 11 000 patients have received VIREAD in expanded access studies.

Treatment-Experienced Adult Patients: Study 907—Treatment-Emergent Adverse Events: The most common adverse events that occurred in patients receiving VIREAD with other antiretroviral agents in clinical trials were mild to moderate gastrointestinal events, such as nausea, diarrhea, vomiting and flatulence. Less than 1% of patients discontinued participation in the clinical studies due to gastrointestinal adverse events (Study 907).

A summary of treatment-emergent adverse events that occurred during the first 48 weeks of Study 907 is provided in Table 1.

Table 1: VIREAD

Selected Treatment-Emergent Adverse Events (Grades 2-4) Reported in ≥3% in Any Treatment Group in Study 907 (0–48 weeks)

	VIREAD (N=368) (Week 0-24) (%)	Placebo (N=182) (Week 0-24) (%)	VIREAD (N=368) (Week 0-48) (%)	Placebo Crossover to VIREAD (N=170) (Week 24-48) (%)
Body as a Whole				
Asthenia	7	6	11	1
Pain	7	7	12	4
Headache	5	5	8	2
Abdominal Pain	4	3	7	6
Back Pain	3	3	4	2
Chest Pain	3	1	3	2
Fever	2	2	4	2
Digestive System				
Diarrhea	11	10	16	11
Nausea	8	5	11	7
Vomiting	4	1	7	5
Anorexia	3	2	4	1
Dyspepsia	3	2	4	2
Flatulence	3	1	4	1
Respiratory				
Pneumonia	2	0	3	2
Nervous System				
Depression	4	3	8	4
Insomnia	3	2	4	4
Peripheral Neuropathy[a]	3	3	5	2
Dizziness	1	3	3	1
Skin and Appendages				
Rash Event[b]	5	4	7	1
Sweating	3	2	3	1
Musculoskeletal				
Myalgia	3	3	4	1
Metabolic				
Weight Loss	2	1	4	2

[a] Peripheral neuropathy includes peripheral neuritis and neuropathy.
[b] Rash event includes rash, pruritus, maculopapular rash, urticaria, vesiculobullous rash and pustular rash.

Laboratory Abnormalities: Laboratory abnormalities observed in this study occurred with similar frequency in the VIREAD and placebo-treated groups. A summary of Grade 3 and 4 laboratory abnormalities is provided in Table 2.

Table 2: VIREAD

Grade 3/4 Laboratory Abnormalities Reported in ≥1% of VIREAD-Treated Patients in Study 907 (0-48 weeks)

	VIREAD (N=368) (Week 0-24) (%)	Placebo (N=182) (Week 0-24) (%)	VIREAD (N=368) (Week 0-48) (%)	Placebo Crossover to VIREAD (N=170) (Week 24-48) (%)
Any ≥Grade 3 Laboratory Abnormality	25	38	35	34
Triglycerides (>750 mg/dL)	8	13	11	9
Creatine Kinase (M:>990 U/L) (F:>845 U/L)	7	14	12	12
Serum Amylase (>175 U/L)	6	7	7	6
Urine Glucose (≥3+)	3	3	3	2
AST (M:>180 U/L) (F:>170 U/L)	3	3	4	5
ALT (M:>215 U/L) (F:>170 U/L)	2	2	4	5
Serum Glucose (>250 U/L)	2	4	3	3
Neutrophils (<750/mm³)	1	1	2	1

Treatment-Naïve Adult Patients: Study 903—Treatment-Emergent Adverse Events: The adverse reactions seen in a double-blind active controlled study in which 600 treatment-naïve patients received VIREAD (N=299) or stavudine (N=301) in combination with lamivudine and efavirenz for 144 weeks (Study 903) were generally consistent, with the addition of dizziness, with those seen in treatment-experienced patients (see Table 3).

Mild adverse events (Grade 1) were common with a similar incidence in both arms, and included dizziness, diarrhea and nausea.

Laboratory Abnormalities: With the exception of triglyceride elevations that were more common in the stavudine group (14%) compared with VIREAD (3%), laboratory abnormalities observed in this study occurred with similar frequency in the VIREAD and stavudine treatment arms. A summary of Grade 3 and 4 laboratory abnormalities is provided in Table 4.

Table 3: VIREAD

Selected Treatment-Emergent Adverse Events (Grades 2-4) Reported in ≥5% in Any Treatment Group in Study 903 (0-144 weeks)

	VIREAD + 3TC + EFV N=299 (%)	d4T + 3TC + EFV N=301 (%)
Body as a Whole		
Headache	14	17
Pain	13	12
Back Pain	9	8
Fever	8	7
Abdominal Pain	7	12
Asthenia	6	7
Digestive System		
Diarrhea	11	13
Nausea	8	9
Vomiting	5	9
Dyspepsia	4	5
Metabolic Disorders		
Lipodystrophy	1	8
Musculoskeletal		
Arthralgia	5	7
Myalgia	3	5
Nervous System		
Depression	11	10
Anxiety	6	6
Insomnia	5	8
Dizziness	3	6
Peripheral Neuropathy[a]	1	5
Respiratory		
Pneumonia	5	5
Skin and Appendages		
Rash Event[b]	18	12

[a] Peripheral neuropathy includes peripheral neuritis and neuropathy.
[b] Rash event includes rash, pruritus, maculopapular rash, urticaria, vesiculobullous rash and pustular rash.

Table 4: VIREAD

Grade 3/4 Laboratory Abnormalities Reported in ≥1% of VIREAD-Treated Patients in Study 903 (0-144 weeks)

	VIREAD + 3TC + EFV N=299 (%)	d4T + 3TC + EFV N=301 (%)
Any ≥Grade 3 Laboratory Abnormality	36	42
Fasting Cholesterol (>240 mg/dL)	19	40
Creatine Kinase (M:>990 U/L) (F:>845 U/L)	12	12
Serum Amylase (>175 U/L)	9	8
AST (M:>180 U/L) (F:>170 U/L)	5	7
ALT (M:>215 U/L) (F:>170 U/L)	4	5
Hematuria (>100 RBC/HPF)	7	7
Neutrophil (<750/mm^3)	3	1
Fasting Triglyceride (>750 mg/dL)	1	9

In Study 903 through 144 weeks, decreases from baseline in bone mineral density (BMD) were seen at the lumbar spine and hip in both arms of the study. At Week 144, there was a significantly greater mean percentage decrease from baseline in BMD at the lumbar spine in patients in the VIREAD group compared with patients in the stavudine group (see Table 5). In both groups, the majority of the reduction in BMD occurred in the first 24-48 weeks of the study and this reduction was sustained through Week 144. Twenty-eight percent of VIREAD-treated patients vs 21% of the stavudine-treated patients lost at least 5% of BMD at the spine or 7% of BMD at the hip. Clinically relevant fractures (excluding fingers and toes) were reported in 4 patients in the VIREAD group and 6 patients in the stavudine group. In addition, there were significant increases in biochemical markers of bone metabolism (serum bone-specific alkaline phosphatase, serum osteocalcin, serum C-telopeptide, and urinary N-telopeptide) in the VIREAD group relative to the stavudine group, suggesting increased bone turnover. Serum parathyroid hormone levels and 1,25 Vitamin D levels were also higher in the VIREAD group. Except for bone specific alkaline phosphatase, these changes resulted in values that remained within the normal range. The effects of VIREAD-associated changes in BMD and biochemical markers on long-term bone health and future fracture risk are unknown.

Table 5: VIREAD

Changes in Bone Mineral Density Study 903

	Mean Percent Change (±SD) to Week 144 in BMD	
	VIREAD + 3TC + EFV	d4T + 3TC + EFV
Lumbar Spine	−2.2%±3.9	−1.0%±4.6
Hip	−2.8%±3.5	−2.4%±4.5

Study 934—Treatment-Emergent Adverse Events: Study 934 was an open-label active-controlled study in which 511 antiretroviral-naïve patients received either VIREAD + EMTRIVA (emtricitabine) administered in combination with efavirenz (N=257) or Combivir (lamivudine/zidovudine) administered in combination with efavirenz (N=254). Adverse events observed in this study were generally consistent with those seen in other studies in treatment experienced or treatment-naïve patients (Table 6).

Table 6: VIREAD

Selected Treatment-Emergent Adverse Events (Grades 2-4) Reported in ≥3% in Any Treatment Group in Study 934 (0-48 weeks)

	VIREAD + FTC + EFV N=257 %	AZT/3TC + EFV N=254 %
Blood and Lymphatic System Disorders		
Anemia	<1	5
Gastrointestinal Disorder		
Diarrhea	7	4
Nausea	8	6
Vomiting	1	4
General Disorders and Administration Site Condition		
Fatigue	7	6
Infections and Infestations		
Sinusitis	4	2
Upper Respiratory Tract Infections	3	3
Nasopharyngitis	3	1
Nervous System Disorders		
Somnolence	3	2
Headache	5	4
Dizziness	8	7
Psychiatric Disorders		
Depression	4	7
Insomnia	4	5
Abnormal Dreams	4	3
Skin and Subcutaneous Tissue Disorders		
Rash	5	4

Patients who received treatment up to 144 weeks in Study 934 reported adverse events similar in nature and severity to those reported in the first 48 weeks.

Through 48 weeks, 7 patients in the EMTRIVA + VIREAD group and 5 patients in the lamivudine/zidovudine group experienced a new CDC Class C event (10 and 6 patients, respectively, through 144 weeks). Renal safety assessed by laboratory abnormalities was similar in the two groups and no patient discontinued study drug due to renal events. At Week 48 and 144, total limb fat (as measured by dual-energy x ray absorptiometry) was significantly less in a subgroup of patients in the lamivudine/zidovudine group compared to the tenofovir/emtricitabine subgroup (see Table 7).

Table 7: VIREAD

Study 934 Total Limb Fat at Week 48 and 144 (Dual-Energy X-Ray Absorptiometry)

	VIREAD + FTC + EFV	AZT/3TC + EFV
Week 48[a]	**N=51**	**N=49**
Total Limb Fat (kg) (Mean±S.D.)	8.9±5.4	6.9±3.9
Week 144[b]	**N=145**	**N=124**

(cont'd)

Table 7: VIREAD *(cont'd)*

Study 934 Total Limb Fat at Week 48 and 144 (Dual-Energy X-Ray Absorptiometry)

	VIREAD + FTC + EFV	AZT/3TC + EFV
Total Limb Fat (kg) (Mean±S.D.)	9.2±5.4	6.5±4.3

[a] P=0.03 for the comparison between arms.
[b] P<0.001 for the comparison between arms.

Laboratory Abnormalities: Laboratory abnormalities observed in this study were generally consistent with those seen in other studies (see Table 8).

Table 8: VIREAD

Grade 3/4 Laboratory Abnormalities Reported in ≥1% in Any Treatment Group in Study 934 (0-48 weeks)

	EMTRIVA + VIREAD + EFV N=257 %	AZT/3TC + EFV N=254 %
Any ≥Grade 3 Laboratory Abnormality	25	22
Fasting Cholesterol (>240 mg/dL)	15	17
Creatine Kinase (M:>990 U/L) (F:>845 U/L)	7	6
Serum Amylase (>175 U/L)	7	3
Alkaline Phosphatase (>550 U/L)	1	0
AST (M:>180 U/L) (F:>170 U/L)	3	2
ALT (M:>215 U/L) (F:>170 U/L)	2	2
Hemoglobin (<8.0 mg/dL)	0	3
Hyperglycemia (>250 mg/dL)	1	1
Hematuria (>75 RBC/HPF)	2	2
Neutrophil (>750/mm³)	3	4
Fasting Triglycerides (>750 mg/dL)	4	2

Laboratory abnormalities in patients who received treatment up to 144 weeks in Study 934 were consistent with those observed in the first 48 weeks of treatment.

Adolescent Patients with HIV-1 Infection: Assessment of adverse reactions is based on one randomized study (Study 321) in 87 HIV-1 infected adolescent patients (12 to <18 years of age) who received treatment with VIREAD (N=45) or placebo (N=42) in combination with other antiretroviral agents for 48 weeks. The adverse reactions observed in adolescent patients who received treatment with VIREAD were consistent with those observed in clinical studies in adults.

Chronic Hepatitis B: Adult Patients: Patients with chronic hepatitis B and compensated liver function received double-blind treatment with VIREAD (n=426) or HEPSERA (n=215) for 48 weeks in studies 0102 (HBeAg−) and 0103 (HBeAg+).

The most common adverse events in tenofovir DF treated patients (incidence ≥5%) identified during the 48-week double-blind period of these studies, at any severity and regardless of causality are presented in Table 9.

Table 9: VIREAD

Treatment-Emergent Adverse Events[a] (≥5% in tenofovir DF-treated patients) in Pooled Studies GS-US-174-0102 and GS-US-174-0103 (0-48 weeks)

	VIREAD (N=426) (%)	HEPSERA (N=215) (%)
Body as a Whole		
Abdominal Pain Upper	7	5
Back Pain	7	5
Gastrointestinal Disorders		
Nausea	9	3
Diarrhea	7	5
General Disorders		
Fatigue	9	7
Infections and Infestations		
Nasopharyngitis	10	11
Nervous System Disorders		
Headache	13	14
Dizziness	6	3

[a] Regardless of causality and severity.

No change in the tolerability profile (nature or severity of adverse events) was observed in patients continuing treatment with VIREAD for up to 96 weeks in Studies 0102 and 0103.

Adverse events observed in a double-blind, randomized, controlled study (Study 0106) in which 105 patients previously treated with HEPSERA were treated with tenofovir DF for 48 weeks were similar in nature to those observed in Studies 0102 and 0103.

No new adverse events causally associated with tenofovir DF were identified from a double-blind active controlled study (Study 0108) in which patients with decompensated liver disease received treatment containing tenofovir DF (N=90) for up to 48 weeks. This study was not large enough to detect rare or unexpected adverse events in this patient population. In this study, 7 of 90 patients (8%) receiving a tenofovir DF-containing regimen, including 4 of 45 patients (9%) receiving VIREAD, experienced a confirmed increase in serum creatinine of ≥0.5 mg/dL or confirmed decrease in serum phosphorus of <2 mg/dL through Week 48.

Laboratory Abnormalities: In Studies 0102 and 0103, the most frequently occurring Grade 3 or 4 laboratory abnormality during the 48-week double-blind period in the VIREAD treatment group was ALT increased. All patients with treatment-emergent Grade 3 or 4 ALT increases had elevated ALT at baseline. A summary of Grade 3 and 4 laboratory abnormalities is provided in Table 10.

Table 10: VIREAD

Grade 3/4 Laboratory Abnormalities Reported in ≥1% in Any Treatment Group in Pooled Studies GS-US-174-0102 and GS-US-174-0103 (0-48 weeks)

	VIREAD N=426 (%)	HEPSERA N=215 (%)
Any ≥Grade 3 Laboratory Abnormality	19	13
ALT (>5.00×ULN)	10	6
AST (>5.00×ULN)	4	4
Serum Amylase (>2.0×ULN)	4	1
Urine Glucose (≥3+)	3	1
Creatine Kinase (≥10.0×ULN)	2	3
Hyperglycemia (>250 mg/dL)	1	2

Grade 3/4 laboratory abnormalities were similar in nature and frequency in patients continuing treatment for up to 96 weeks in these studies. Overall, the following grade 3-4 laboratory abnormalities were reported in ≥1% of subjects (Weeks 48-96 of Studies 0102 and 0103): serum amylase (2%), creatine kinase (1%), prothrombin time (2%), ALT (1%), AST (1%) and urine glucose (3%).

Post-Market Adverse Drug Reactions: The following adverse reactions have been identified during post-approval use of VIREAD. Because these events have been reported voluntarily from a population of unknown size, estimates of frequency cannot be made. These events have been considered possible adverse reactions due to a combination of their seriousness, frequency of reporting or potential causal relationship with VIREAD.

Immune System Disorders: allergic reaction (including angioedema).

Metabolism and Nutrition Disorders: lactic acidosis, hypokalemia, hypophosphatemia.

Respiratory, Thoracic and Mediastinal Disorders: dyspnea.

Gastrointestinal Disorders: pancreatitis, increased amylase, abdominal pain.

Blood and Lymphatic System: thrombocytopenia.

Hepatobiliary Disorders: hepatic steatosis, hepatitis, increased liver enzymes (most commonly AST, ALT, GGT).

Skin and Subcutaneous Tissue Disorders: rash.

Musculoskeletal and Connective Tissue Disorders: rhabdomyolysis, osteomalacia (manifested as bone pain and infrequently contributing to fractures), muscular weakness, myopathy.

Renal and Urinary Disorders: acute renal failure, renal failure, acute tubular necrosis, Fanconi syndrome, proximal renal tubulopathy, interstitial nephritis (including acute cases), nephrogenic diabetes insipidus, renal insufficiency, increased creatinine, proteinuria, polyuria.

General Disorders and Administrative Site Conditions: asthenia.

The following adverse reactions, listed under the body system headings above, sometimes appeared to be concurrent with proximal renal tubulopathy: rhabdomyolysis, osteomalacia (manifested as bone pain and infrequently contributing to fractures), hypokalemia, muscular weakness, myopathy, hypophosphatemia.

There have been three post-marketing reports of acute renal failure in patients on concomitant NSAIDs therapy where a relationship to VIREAD could not be excluded. These events mostly occurred in medically complex patients, where underlying disease processes confound interpretation.

In HIV-infected patients with severe immune deficiency at the time of initiation of antiretroviral therapy an inflammatory reaction to infectious pathogens (active or inactive) may arise (see Warnings and Precautions).

In HBV-infected patients, clinical and laboratory evidence of exacerbations of hepatitis have occurred after discontinuation of HBV therapy (see Warnings and Precautions, Exacerbation of Hepatitis After Discontinuation of Treatment).

DRUG INTERACTIONS:

Serious Drug Interactions

- **Atazanavir and lopinavir/ritonavir increase tenofovir disoproxil fumarate concentrations which may lead to tenofovir-associated adverse events (see Warnings and Precautions).**
- **Tenofovir disoproxil fumarate decreases atazanavir concentrations—administer atazanavir with ritonavir (see below).**
- **Tenofovir disoproxil fumarate increases didanosine (ddI) concentrations—the dose of ddI may be reduced but use with caution and monitor for ddI-related adverse events and clinical response (see below).**

Drug-Drug Interactions: At concentrations substantially higher (~300-fold) than those observed in vivo, tenofovir did not inhibit in vitro drug metabolism mediated by any of the following human CYP450 isoforms: CYP3A4, CYP2D6, CYP2C9 or CYP2E1. However, a small (6%) but statistically significant reduction in metabolism of CYP1A substrate was observed. Based on the results of in vitro experiments and the known elimination pathway of tenofovir, the potential for CYP450 mediated interactions involving tenofovir with other medicinal products is low (see Action and Clinical Pharmacology, Pharmacokinetics).

Tenofovir is primarily excreted by the kidneys by a combination of glomerular filtration and active tubular secretion. Coadministration of VIREAD with drugs that are eliminated by active tubular secretion may increase serum concentrations of either tenofovir or the coadministered drug, due to competition for this elimination pathway. Some examples include, but are not limited to cidofovir, acyclovir, valacyclovir, ganciclovir, and valganciclovir. Drugs that decrease renal function may also increase serum concentrations of tenofovir.

VIREAD should not be administered in combination with HEPSERA (adefovir dipivoxil).

VIREAD has been evaluated in healthy volunteers in combination with abacavir, atazanavir, didanosine, efavirenz, emtricitabine, entecavir, indinavir, lamivudine, lopinavir/ritonavir, methadone, nelfinavir, oral contraceptives, ribavirin, saquinavir/ritonavir and tacrolimus (see below). No clinically significant drug interactions have been observed between tenofovir disoproxil fumarate and abacavir, efavirenz, emtricitabine, entecavir, indinavir, lamivudine, methadone, nelfinavir, oral contraceptives, ribavirin, saquinavir/ritonavir and tacrolimus. Table 11 and Table 12 summarize pharmacokinetic effects of coadministered drug on tenofovir pharmacokinetics and effects of tenofovir on the pharmacokinetics of coadministered drug.

Didanosine: Pharmacokinetic studies have shown that coadministration of didanosine and tenofovir DF results in 40-60% increase in C_{max} and AUC of didanosine (see Table 13). The mechanism of this interaction is unknown. **Increases in didanosine concentrations of this magnitude could potentiate didanosine-associated adverse events, including pancreatitis, lactic acidosis, and neuropathy.** In addition, suppression of CD4 counts has been observed in patients receiving tenofovir DF with didanosine at a dose of 400 mg daily.

A reduced dose of Videx EC (ddI-EC) is recommended when coadministered with VIREAD. When coadministered with VIREAD, the Videx EC Product Monograph recommends a reduced dose of 250 mg ddI-EC for HIV-infected adults with body weight ≥60 kg and creatinine clearance ≥60 mL/min. For adult patients with body weight <60 kg, and creatinine clearance ≥60 mL/min, the recommended dose of ddI-EC is 200 mg. Data are not available to recommend a dose adjustment for patients with creatinine clearance <60 mL/min or for the buffered tablet formulation of didanosine (Videx).

Caution should be used when coadministering reduced-dose didanosine, tenofovir, and an NNRTI in treatment-naïve patients with high viral loads at baseline since such use has been associated with reports of a high rate of virologic failure and emergence of resistance at an early stage. All patients receiving tenofovir disoproxil fumarate and didanosine concomitantly should be closely monitored for didanosine-related adverse events and clinical response.

Atazanavir and Lopinavir/Ritonavir: Atazanavir and lopinavir/ritonavir have been shown to increase tenofovir concentrations (see Table 11). The mechanism of this interaction is unknown. Higher tenofovir concentrations could potentiate tenofovir-associated adverse events, including renal disorders. Patients receiving atazanavir, lopinavir/ritonavir and tenofovir disoproxil fumarate should be monitored for tenofovir-associated adverse events.

Tenofovir decreases atazanavir concentrations (see Table 12). Although safety and efficacy data are limited, it is recommended that atazanavir, without ritonavir, should not be coadministered with tenofovir disoproxil fumarate. The recommended regimen is atazanavir 300 mg given with ritonavir 100 mg when used in combination with tenofovir disoproxil fumarate 300 mg (all as a single daily dose with food).

Table 11: VIREAD

Drug Interactions: Changes in Pharmacokinetic Parameters for Tenofovir[a] in the Presence of the Coadministered Drug

Coadministered Drug	Dose of Coadministered Drug (mg)	N	% Change of Tenofovir Pharmacokinetic Parameters[b] (90% CI)		
			C_{max}	AUC	C_{min}
Abacavir	300 once	8	↔	↔	NC
Atazanavir Sulfate[c]	400 once daily×14 days	33	↑ 14 (↑ 8 to ↑ 20)	↑ 24 (↑ 21 to ↑ 28)	↑ 22 (↑ 15 to ↑ 30)
Didanosine (enteric-coated)	400 once	25	↔	↔	↔
Didanosine (buffered)[d]	250 or 400 once daily×7 days	14	↔	↔	↔
Efavirenz	600 once daily×14 days	29	↔	↔	↔
Emtricitabine	200 once daily×7 days	17	↔	↔	↔
Entecavir	1 mg once daily×10 days	28	↔	↔	↔
Indinavir	800 three times daily×7 days	13	↑ 14 (↓ 3 to ↑ 33)	↔	↔
Lamivudine	150 twice daily×7 days	15	↔	↔	↔
Lopinavir/Ritonavir	400/100 twice daily×14 days	24	↔	↑ 32 (↑ 25 to ↑ 38)	↑ 51 (↑ 37 to ↑ 66)
Nelfinavir	1250 twice daily×14 days	29	↔	↔	↔
Saquinavir/ Ritonavir	1000/100 twice daily×14 days	35	↔	↔	↑ 23 (↑ 16 to ↑ 30)
Tacrolimus	0.05 mg/kg twice daily×7 days	21	↑ 13 (↑ 1 to ↑ 27)	↔	↔

[a] Patients received VIREAD 300 mg once daily.
[b] Increase=↑; Decrease=↓; No Effect=↔, NC=Not Calculated.
[c] REYATAZ prescribing information (Bristol-Myers Squibb).
[d] Includes 4 subjects weighing <60 kg receiving ddI 250 mg.

Table 12: VIREAD

Drug Interactions: Changes in Pharmacokinetic Parameters for Coadministered Drug in the Presence of VIREAD

Coadministered Drug	Dose of Coadministered Drug (mg)	N	% Change of Coadministered Drug Pharmacokinetic Parameters[a] (90% CI)		
			C_{max}	AUC	C_{min}
Abacavir	300 once	8	↑ 12 (↓ 1 to ↑ 26)	↔	NA
Atazanavir	400 once daily×14 days	34	↓ 21 (↓ 27 to ↓ 14)	↓ 25 (↓ 30 to ↓ 19)	↓ 40 (↓ 48 to ↓ 32)
Atazanavir[b]	Atazanavir/Ritonavir 300/100 once daily×42 days	10	↓ 28 (↓ 50 to ↑ 5)	↓ 25[c] (↓ 42 to ↓ 3)	↓ 23[c] (↓ 46 to ↑ 10)
Efavirenz	600 once daily×14 days	30	↔	↔	↔
Emtricitabine	200 once daily×7 days	17	↔	↔	↑ 20 (↑ 12 to ↑ 29)
Entecavir	1 mg once daily×10 days	28	↔	↑ 13 (↑ 11 to ↑ 15)	↔
Indinavir	800 three times daily×7 days	12	↓ 11 (↓ 30 to ↑ 12)	↔	↔
Lamivudine	150 twice daily×7 days	15	↓ 24 (↓ 34 to ↓ 12)	↔	↔
Lopinavir Ritonavir	Lopinavir/Ritonavir 400/100 twice daily×14 days	24	↔	↔	↔
Methadone[d]	40–110 once daily×14 days[e]	13	↔	↔	↔
Nelfinavir M8 metabolite	1250 twice daily×14 days	29	↔ ↔	↔ ↔	↔ ↔
Oral Contraceptives[f]	Ethinyl Estradiol/Norgestimate (Ortho-Tricyclen) once daily×7 days	20	↔	↔	↔
Ribavirin	600 once	22	↔	↔	NA
Saquinavir	1000/100 twice daily×14 days	32	↑ 22 (↑ 6 to ↑ 41)	↑ 29[g] (↑ 12 to ↑ 48)	↑ 47[g] (↑ 23 to ↑ 76)
Ritonavir			↔	↔	↑ 23 (↑ 3 to ↑ 46)
Tacrolimus	0.05 mg/kg twice daily×7 days	21	↔	↔	↔

(cont'd)

Table 12: VIREAD *(cont'd)*

Drug Interactions: Changes in Pharmacokinetic Parameters for Coadministered Drug in the Presence of VIREAD

[a] Increase=↑; Decrease=↓; No Effect=↔; NA=Not Applicable.
[b] REYATAZ prescribing information (Bristol-Myers Squibb).
[c] In HIV-infected patients, addition of tenofovir DF to atazanavir 300 mg plus ritonavir 100 mg, resulted in AUC and C_{min} values of atazanavir that were 2.3- and 4-fold higher than the respective values observed for atazanavir 400 mg when given alone.
[d] R-(active), S- and total methadone exposures were equivalent when dosed alone or with VIREAD.
[e] Individual subjects were maintained on their stable methadone dose. No pharmacodynamic alterations (opiate toxicity or withdrawal signs or symptoms) were reported.
[f] Ethinyl estradiol and 17-deacetyl norgestimate (pharmacologically active metabolite) exposures were equivalent when dosed alone or with VIREAD.
[g] Increase in AUC and C_{min} are not expected to be clinically relevant; hence no dose adjustments are required when tenofovir DF and ritonavir-boosted saquinavir are coadministered.

Table 13: VIREAD

Drug Interactions: Pharmacokinetic Parameters for Didanosine in the Presence of VIREAD

Didanosine[a] Dose (mg)/ Method of Administration[b]	VIREAD Method of Administration[b]	N	% Difference (90% CI) vs Didanosine 400 mg Alone, Fasted[c]	
			C_{max}	AUC
Buffered Tablets				
400 once daily[d] ×7 days	Fasted 1 h after didanosine	14	↑ 28 (↑ 11 to ↑ 48)	↑ 44 (↑ 31 to ↑ 59)
Enteric Coated Capsules				
400 once, fasted	With food, 2 h after didanosine	26	↑ 48 (↑ 25 to ↑ 76)	↑ 48 (↑ 31 to ↑ 67)
400 once, with food	Simultaneously with didanosine	26	↑ 64 (↑ 41 to ↑ 89)	↑ 60 (↑ 44 to ↑ 79)
250 once, fasted	With food, 2 h after didanosine	28	↓ 10 (↓ 22 to ↑ 3)	↔
250 once, fasted	Simultaneously with didanosine	28	↔	↑ 14 (0 to ↑ 31)
250 once, with food	Simultaneously with didanosine	28	↓ 29 (↓ 39 to ↓ 18)	↓ 11 (↓ 23 to ↑ 2)

[a] See Warnings and Precautions regarding use of didanosine with VIREAD.
[b] Administration with food was with a light meal (~373 kcal, 20% fat).
[c] Increase=↑; Decrease=↓; No Difference=↔.
[d] Includes 4 subjects weighing <60 kg receiving ddI 250 mg.

Drug-Food Interactions: Interactions of VIREAD with food have not been established (see Action and Clinical Pharmacology, Pharmacokinetics, Effects of Food on Oral Absorption).
Drug-Herb Interactions: Interactions of VIREAD with herbs have not been established.
Drug-Laboratory Interactions: Interactions of VIREAD with laboratory tests have not been established.

DOSAGE AND ADMINISTRATION: **Adults:** For the Treatment of HIV or Chronic Hepatitis B: The dose of VIREAD (tenofovir disoproxil fumarate) is 300 mg once daily taken orally without regard to food.

In the treatment of chronic hepatitis B, the optimal duration of treatment is unknown. VIREAD may be discontinued if there is HBsAg loss or HBsAg seroconversion.

Adolescent Patients with HIV-1 Infection (12 Years of Age and Over): Body weight ≥35 kg: Take one 300 mg VIREAD tablet once daily orally, without regard to food.

Dose Adjustment for Renal Impairment: Significantly increased drug exposures occurred when VIREAD was administered to patients with moderate to severe renal impairment (see Action and Clinical Pharmacology, Pharmacokinetics, Renal Insufficiency). Therefore, the dosing interval of VIREAD should be adjusted in patients with baseline creatinine clearance <50 mL/min using the recommendations in Table 14. These dosing interval recommendations are based on modeling of single-dose pharmacokinetic data in non-HIV and non-HBV infected subjects with varying degrees of renal impairment, including end-stage renal disease requiring hemodialysis. The safety and effectiveness of these dosing interval adjustment recommendations have not been clinically evaluated in moderate to severe renal impairment, therefore, clinical response to treatment and renal function should be closely monitored in these patients. Routine monitoring of creatinine clearance and serum phosphorus should be performed in patients with mild renal impairment (creatinine clearance 50-80 mL/min) (see Warnings and Precautions).

The pharmacokinetics of tenofovir have not been evaluated in non-hemodialysis patients with creatinine clearance <10 mL/min; therefore, no dosing recommendation is available for these patients.

No data are available to make dose recommendations in adolescent patients with renal impairment.

Missed Dose: If a patient misses a dose at the regularly scheduled time, but then remembers it that same day, the patient should take the missed dose immediately. The next dose should be taken at the regularly scheduled time the following day. The patient should not take two doses of VIREAD at once to make up for missing a dose.

Table 14: VIREAD

Dosage Adjustment for Patients with Altered Creatinine Clearance

	Creatinine Clearance (mL/min)[a]			Hemodialysis Patients
	≥50	30–49	10–29	
Recommended 300 mg Dosing Interval	Every 24 hours	Every 48 hours	Every 72 to 96 hours	Every 7 days or after a total of approximately 12 hours of dialysis[b]

[a] Calculated using ideal (lean) body weight.
[b] Generally once weekly assuming three hemodialysis sessions a week of approximately 4 hours duration. VIREAD should be administered following completion of dialysis.

OVERDOSAGE:
Limited clinical experience at doses higher than the therapeutic dose of VIREAD 300 mg is available. In study 901 tenofovir disoproxil fumarate 600 mg was administered to 8 patients orally for 28 days. No severe adverse reactions were reported. The effects of higher doses are not known.

If overdose occurs the patient must be monitored for evidence of toxicity, and standard supportive treatment applied as necessary. Administration of activated charcoal may also be used to aid in removal of unabsorbed drug.

Tenofovir is efficiently removed by hemodialysis with an extraction coefficient of approximately 54%. Following a single 300 mg dose of VIREAD, a four-hour hemodialysis session removed approximately 10% of the administered tenofovir dose.

> For management of a suspected drug overdose, contact your regional Poison Control Centre. See the *CPS* Directory section for a list of Poison Control Centres.

ACTION AND CLINICAL PHARMACOLOGY: VIREAD (tenofovir disoproxil fumarate) is an acyclic nucleotide diester analog of adenosine monophosphate. Tenofovir disoproxil fumarate requires initial diester hydrolysis (by non-specific esterases in blood and tissues) for conversion to tenofovir and subsequent phosphorylations by cellular enzymes to form tenofovir diphosphate, an obligate chain terminator. Tenofovir diphosphate inhibits the activity of HIV reverse transcriptase and HBV polymerase by competing with the natural substrate deoxyadenosine 5'-triphosphate and, after incorporation into DNA, by DNA chain termination.

Tenofovir diphosphate is a weak inhibitor of mammalian DNA polymerases α, β, and mitochondrial DNA polymerase γ.

VIREAD is a water soluble diester prodrug of the active ingredient tenofovir. Following oral administration of a single dose of VIREAD 300 mg to HIV-infected patients in the fasted state, maximum serum concentrations (C_{max}) of tenofovir are achieved in 1.0±0.4 hours. The oral bioavailability of tenofovir from VIREAD in fasted patients is approximately 25%. Administration of VIREAD following a high-fat meal increases the oral bioavailability, with an increase in tenofovir AUC_{∞} of approximately 40% and an increase in C_{max} of approximately 14% (see Dosage and Administration).

Tenofovir is eliminated by a combination of glomerular filtration and active tubular secretion. There may be competition with other compounds that are also renally eliminated.

Pharmacodynamics: Activity in HIV-1: The in vitro antiviral activity of tenofovir against laboratory and clinical isolates of HIV-1 was assessed in lymphoblastoid cell lines, primary monocyte/macrophage cells and peripheral blood lymphocytes. The IC_{50} values for tenofovir were in the range of 0.04-8.5 μM. In drug combination studies of tenofovir with nucleoside reverse transcriptase inhibitors (abacavir, didanosine, lamivudine, stavudine, zalcitabine, and zidovudine), non-nucleoside reverse transcriptase inhibitors (delavirdine, efavirenz, and nevirapine), and protease inhibitors (amprenavir, indinavir, nelfinavir, ritonavir, and saquinavir), additive to synergistic effects were observed. Most of these drug combinations have not been studied in humans. Tenofovir displayed antiviral activity in vitro against HIV-1 clades A, B, C, D, E, F, G, and O (IC_{50} values ranged from 0.5-2.2 μM).

The antiviral effects of tenofovir disoproxil fumarate monotherapy in reducing HIV-1 viral load and the relationship with dose were assessed in clinical phase 1 studies in treatment-naive and treatment-experienced HIV infected patients. Doses of tenofovir disoproxil fumarate ranging from 75 mg to 600 mg once daily resulted in statistically significant decreases in plasma HIV-1 RNA levels compared with placebo. In a mixed population of treatment-naive and treatment-experienced patients who received 28 days of repeat daily dosing with tenofovir disoproxil fumarate 300 mg QD (Study GS-97-901) the median decrease in plasma $\log_{10}$ HIV-1 RNA level was 1.22 $\log_{10}$ copies/mL.

Activity in HBV: The in vitro antiviral activity of tenofovir against HBV was assessed in the HepG2 2.2.15 cell line. The EC_{50} values for tenofovir were in the range of 0.14 to 1.5 μM, with CC_{50} (50% cytotoxicity concentration) values >100 μM. Tenofovir diphosphate inhibits recombinant HBV polymerase with a Ki (inhibition constant) of 0.18 μM. In in vitro drug combination studies of tenofovir with nucleoside anti-HBV reverse transcriptase inhibitors lamivudine, telbivudine, and entecavir, additive anti-HBV activity was observed. Additive to slightly synergistic effects were observed with the combination of tenofovir and emtricitabine.

Pharmacokinetics: Pharmacokinetics of intravenous tenofovir were evaluated in Study GS-96-701 (N=16). Following intravenous administration of tenofovir 1.0 and 3.0 mg/kg, pharmacokinetics were dose-proportional with the exception of the estimated terminal half-life (5.3 and 7.8 hours, respectively). The pharmacokinetics of tenofovir were not affected by repeated dosing in the 1.0 mg/kg/day group, with the exception of half-life (5.3 on Day 1 vs 7.7 on Day 14) and volume of distribution (763 vs 1320 mL/kg). At the 3.0 mg/kg/day, there was an approximate 27% decrease in serum clearance of tenofovir following 7 days of once daily administration; renal clearance and estimated terminal half-life were also significantly different.

The pharmacokinetics of tenofovir following administration of tenofovir disoproxil fumarate were evaluated in the fasted state in Study GS-97-901 (HIV-infected patients) and Study GS-00-914 (healthy volunteers). The pharmacokinetics in HIV-infected patients and healthy volunteers were similar. The estimated terminal half-life in HIV-infected patients measured over 24 hours was ~12-13 h. The terminal elimination half-life in healthy subjects assessed over 48 hours was ~17 hours. There were no significant differences in the dose-normalized steady-state pharmacokinetics of tenofovir over the dose range of 75 to 600 mg. Tenofovir exposure following 8 and 28 days was slightly higher than those observed following the first dose.

Absorption: VIREAD is a water soluble diester prodrug of the active ingredient tenofovir. The oral bioavailability of tenofovir from VIREAD in fasted patients is approximately 25%. Following oral administration of a single dose of VIREAD 300 mg to HIV-infected patients in the fasted state, maximum serum concentrations (C_{max}) are achieved in 1.0±0.4 hours. C_{max} and AUC values are 296±90 ng/mL and 2287±685 ng·h/mL, respectively.

Distribution: In vitro binding of tenofovir to human plasma or serum proteins is less than 0.7 and 7.2%, respectively, over the tenofovir concentration range 0.01-25 μg/mL. The volume of distribution at steady-state is 1.3±0.6 L/kg and 1.2±0.4 L/kg, following intravenous administration of tenofovir 1.0 mg/kg and 3.0 mg/kg.

Metabolism: In vitro studies indicate that neither tenofovir disoproxil nor tenofovir are substrates of CYP450 enzymes.

Following IV administration of tenofovir, approximately 70-80% of the dose is recovered in the urine as unchanged tenofovir within 72 hours of dosing. After multiple oral doses of VIREAD 300 mg once daily (under fed conditions), 32±10% of the administered dose is recovered in urine over 24 hours.

Excretion: Tenofovir is eliminated by a combination of glomerular filtration and active tubular secretion. There may be competition for elimination with other compounds that are also renally eliminated.

Effects of Food on Oral Absorption: Administration of VIREAD following a high-fat meal (~700 to 1000 kcal containing 40-50% fat) increases the oral bioavailability, with an increase in tenofovir $AUC_{0-\infty}$ of approximately 40% and an increase in C_{max} of approximately 14%. Food delays the time to tenofovir C_{max} by approximately 1 hour. C_{max} and AUC of tenofovir are 326±119 ng/mL and 3324±1370 ng·h/mL following multiple doses of VIREAD 300 mg once daily in the fed state, when meal content was not controlled.

Special Populations and Conditions: Pediatric: Steady-state pharmacokinetics of tenofovir were evaluated in 8 HIV-1 infected adolescent patients (12 to <18 years). All pediatric patients were receiving VIREAD with a ritonavir-boosted protease inhibitor. Mean (±SD) C_{max} and AUC_{tau} are 0.38±0.13 μg/mL and 3.39±1.22 μg·h/mL, respectively. Tenofovir exposure achieved in adolescent patients receiving oral daily doses of VIREAD 300 mg was similar to exposures achieved in adults receiving once-daily doses of VIREAD 300 mg.

Geriatrics: Pharmacokinetic studies have not been performed in the elderly.

Race: There were insufficient numbers from racial and ethnic groups other than Caucasian to adequately determine potential pharmacokinetic differences among these populations.

Gender: Limited data on the pharmacokinetics of tenofovir in women indicate no major gender effect.

Hepatic Insufficiency: The pharmacokinetics of tenofovir following a 300 mg single dose of VIREAD have been studied in 8 non-HIV, non-HBV infected subjects with moderate hepatic impairment and 8 non-HIV infected subjects with severe hepatic impairment. There were no substantial alterations in tenofovir pharmacokinetics in subjects with hepatic impairment compared with unimpaired subjects. No change in VIREAD dosing is required in patients with hepatic impairment.

Renal Insufficiency: The pharmacokinetics of tenofovir are altered in subjects with renal impairment (see Warnings and Precautions, Renal, Nephrotoxicity). In non-HIV, non-HBV infected subjects with creatinine clearance <50 mL/min or with end stage renal disease (ESRD) requiring dialysis, C_{max}, and $AUC_{0-\infty}$ of tenofovir were increased (see Table 15). It is recommended that the dosing interval for VIREAD be modified in patients with creatinine clearance <50 mL/min or in patients with ESRD who require dialysis (see Dosage and Administration).

Table 15: VIREAD

Pharmacokinetic Parameters (Mean±SD) of Tenofovir[a] in Patients with Varying Degrees of Renal Function

Baseline Creatinine Clearance (mL/min)	>80 (N=3)	50–80 (N=10)	30–49 (N=8)	12–29 (N=11)
C_{max} (ng/mL)	335.5±31.8	330.4±61.0	372.1±156.1	601.6±185.3
AUC_{∞} (ng·h/mL)	2184.5±257.4	3063.8±927.0	6008.5±2504.7	15984.7± 7223.0
CL/F (mL/min)	1043.7±115.4	807.7±279.2	444.4±209.8	177.0±97.1
CL_{renal} (mL/min)	243.5±33.3	168.6±27.5	100.6±27.5	43.0±31.2

[a] 300 mg, single dose of VIREAD.

Tenofovir is efficiently removed by hemodialysis with an extraction coefficient of approximately 54%. Following a single 300 mg dose of VIREAD, a four-hour hemodialysis session removed approximately 10% of the administered tenofovir dose.

STORAGE AND STABILITY: Store at 25°C, excursions permitted to 15-30°C.

SPECIAL HANDLING INSTRUCTIONS: There are no special handling instructions.

INFORMATION FOR THE PATIENT: Published in e-CPS, available by subscription at www.e-cps.ca.

DOSAGE FORMS, COMPOSITION AND PACKAGING: Each almond-shaped, light blue film-coated tablet, debossed with "GILEAD" and "4331" on one side and with "300" on the other side, contains: tenofovir disoproxil fumarate 300 mg, which is equivalent to 245 mg of tenofovir disoproxil. Nonmedicinal ingredients: croscarmellose sodium, lactose monohydrate, magnesium stearate, microcrystalline cellulose and pregelatinized starch. The tablets are coated with a blue colored film (Opadry II Y-30-10671-A) that is made of FD&C Blue #2 Aluminum Lake, hydroxypropyl methylcellulose 2910, lactose monohydrate, titanium dioxide and triacetin. Bottles of 30, with a desiccant (silica gel canister or sachet) and closed with child-resistant closure.

Viroptic® Ⓟ

trifluridine

Topical Antiviral Agent

Theramed

PHARMACOLOGY: Trifluridine is phosphorylated by a cellular thymidine kinase to its nucleotide monophosphate. Trifluridine monophosphate is an inhibitor of thymidylate synthetase, the target enzyme for the action of monofluorinated pyrimidines. Trifluridine has been demonstrated to combine slowly and irreversibly with thymidylate synthetase in a reaction that requires ATP.

Trifluridine monophosphate is further phosphorylated by cellular enzymes to the triphosphate which is incorporated into DNA (but not RNA) by competitively inhibiting the incorporation of the natural nucleotide, thymidine triphosphate (dTTP).

The inhibition of viral replication can be reversed by the addition of thymidine (thymidine rescue).

Viral DNA polymerase has a higher affinity for trifluridine triphosphate than does the DNA polymerase of uninfected cells, resulting in the preferential incorporation of the analogue into viral DNA.

Trifluridine is active against the following DNA viruses: herpes simplex types 1 and 2, varicella zoster, adenovirus and vaccinia virus.

Intraocular penetration of trifluridine was evaluated in 5 patients undergoing intraocular surgery. One drop of 1% trifluridine was instilled into the affected eye 4 times at 10 minute intervals, the last dose being administered 5 minutes before sterile preparation for surgery. Penetration of the drug was demonstrated in 4 of the 5 patients in concentrations ranging from 3.1 to 43.9 μM with a mean value of 16.75 μM which exceeds the ED_{50}'s for most clinical isolates of HSV-1. There appeared to be a correlation between the degree of corneal integrity and the degree of penetration of trifluridine into the aqueous humor as evidenced by the fact that patients with corneal thinning had higher drug levels (mean 21.3 μM) than did the single patient with an intact cornea (3.1 μM). The major metabolite of trifluridine (5-carboxy-2'-deoxyuridine) was not detected in any of the eyes.

Pharmacokinetics: The pharmacokinetics of trifluridine in humans is similar to that of animals. The plasma half-life in human cancer patients following i.v. administration of the drug is short and dose-independent. In 3 patients, doses of 5, 15 and 27 mg/kg produced half-lives of 14, 28 and 18 minutes, respectively.

Following i.v. administration trifluridine is excreted in the urine largely as 5-carboxy-2'-deoxyuridine, with trace amounts of its intermediates and unchanged drug. Evidence indicates minimal tissue protein binding both in animals and man.

Samples from 12 volunteers who received topical 1% trifluridine did not reveal detectable serum levels of the drug, indicating that systemic absorption from the eye is minimal.

INDICATIONS: For the treatment of primary keratoconjunctivitis and recurrent epithelial keratitis due to herpes simplex viruses, types 1 and 2.

Trifluridine is also effective in the treatment of epithelial keratitis that has not responded clinically to the topical administration of idoxuridine or when ocular toxicity or hypersensitivity to idoxuridine has occurred. In a smaller number of patients found to be resistant to topical vidarabine, trifluridine was also effective.

Note: Trifluridine is not indicated for the treatment of keratitis with deep stromal invasion and uveitis, ocular vaccinia, adenoviral ocular disease, prophylaxis of keratoconjunctivitis and/or recurrent epithelial keratitis, Epstein Barr virus keratitis, or ocular bacterial, fungal, or chlamydial infections.

CONTRAINDICATIONS: For patients who are known to be hypersensitive or intolerant to trifluridine or any of its nonmedicinal ingredients.

WARNINGS: The recommended dosage and frequency of administration should not be exceeded (see Dosage).

Pregnancy: Trifluridine should not be administered to pregnant women or nursing mothers unless the anticipated benefits outweigh the potential risks. The teratogenic potential of this compound in humans is unknown.

The topical application of trifluridine to the eyes of rabbits on days 6 to 18 of gestation produced no teratogenic effects. When administered s.c. to rabbits and rats, fetal toxicity has been observed at doses above 1 mg/kg/day.

Lactation: See Pregnancy.

The maximum dose anticipated in a human being based on the recommended dosage is approximately 0.1 mg/kg/day, assuming a body weight of 45 kg.

PRECAUTIONS: General: Trifluridine should be prescribed only for patients who have a clinical diagnosis of herpetic keratitis.

Trifluridine may cause mild local irritation of the conjunctiva and cornea when instilled, but these effects are usually transient.

Caution should be exercised in the use of trifluridine in the treatment of infections caused by strains of herpes simplex virus resistant to other antivirals. Conflicting evidence has been presented on the issue of cross-resistance to other antiviral agents. Resistance of herpes simplex virus type 1 to trifluridine has been produced in vitro and these strains are able to produce trifluridine-resistant infections in vivo. HSV-1 strains insensitive to trifluridine were also resistant to idoxuridine and vidarabine (adenine arabinoside). On the other hand, it has been shown that viruses lacking thymidine kinase and/or DNA polymerase activity may retain complete or reduced sensitivity to trifluridine in vitro and that trifluridine is still of some benefit in rabbit eyes infected with acyclovir-resistant strains of HSV-1. Early work showed that rabbits infected with HSV-1 strains made resistant to idoxuridine could still be treated successfully with trifluridine.

Following re-epithelialization, trifluridine should not be used in an attempt to reduce the rate of recurrence of herpetic keratitis, as supporting experimental and clinical data are lacking, and toxicity may occur with prolonged use.

Children: There is no specific experience respecting efficacy and safety of use in children.

Drug Interactions: Trifluridine should not be applied to the eye simultaneously with other medications. However, the following ophthalmic drugs have been administered topically and concurrently with trifluridine in a limited number of patients without apparent evidence of adverse interaction: antibiotics: chloramphenicol, erythromycin, polymyxin B sulfate, bacitracin, gentamicin sulfate, tetracycline HCl, sodium sulfacetamide, neomycin sulfate; steroids: dexamethasone sodium phosphate, dexamethasone, prednisolone acetate, prednisolone sodium phosphate, hydrocortisone, fluorometholone; and other ophthalmic drugs: atropine sulfate, scopolamine HBr, naphazoline HCl, cyclopentolate HCl, homatropine HBr, pilocarpine, l-epinephrine HCl and sodium chloride.

Pregnancy: There are no adequate and well-controlled studies in pregnant women. The product should be used during pregnancy only if the potential benefit justifies the potential risk to the fetus.

Lactation: It is unlikely that trifluridine is excreted in human milk after ophthalmic instillation because of the relatively small dosage (≤5.0 mg/day), its dilution in body fluids and its extremely short half-life (approximately 12 minutes). The drug should not be prescribed for nursing mothers unless the potential benefit justifies the potential risk.

ADVERSE EFFECTS: The following adverse reactions were noted in controlled and open studies during the administration of trifluridine: 54 of 297 (18%) patients experienced adverse reactions: burning upon instillation (12%); superficial punctate keratitis (2%); and eyelid edema, irritation, epithelial keratopathy, allergic reaction, increased intraocular pressure, keratitis sicca, stromal edema, blurred vision and nausea each occurred in less than 1% of the patients.

OVERDOSE:

Symptoms: Overdosage by ocular instillation is unlikely because any excess solution should be quickly expelled from the conjunctival sac.

Acute overdosage by accidental oral ingestion has not been reported. However, should such ingestion occur, the 75 mg of trifluridine in a single bottle of solution would not be expected to produce adverse effects.

Single i.v. doses of 1.5 to 30 mg/kg/day in children and adults with neoplastic disease produce reversible bone marrow depression as the only potentially serious toxic effect and only after at least 5 doses. The acute oral LD_{50} in the mouse and rat was 4 379 mg/kg or higher.

For management of a suspected drug overdose, CPhA recommends that you contact your **regional Poison Control Centre**. See the *CPS* Directory section for a list of Poison Control Centres.

DOSAGE: Adults: Instill 1 drop onto the cornea of the affected eye every 2 hours while awake. The maximum daily dosage is 9 drops.

This therapeutic regimen should be continued until the herpetic lesion has completely re-epithelialized. At this time the dosage should be reduced to 1 drop every 4 hours for a maximum daily dosage of 5 drops. This regimen should be continued for 7 days post-re-epithelialization.

If there are no signs of improvement after 7 days of full therapy or complete re-epithelialization has not occurred after 14 days of full therapy, other forms of therapy should be considered.

Administration of a full dosage regimen for periods exceeding 21 days should be avoided because of potential ocular toxicity.

Children: There is no specific information relating to use in children.

SUPPLIED: Each bottle of sterile, aqueous, ophthalmic solution contains: trifluridine 1%. Nonmedicinal ingredients: acetic acid, benzalkonium chloride (as preservative), sodium acetate and sodium chloride. Plastic drop-dose dispenser bottle of 7.5 mL. Store under refrigeration at 2 to 8°C.

Visine® Advance True Tears
glycerin—hypromellose
Artificial Tears

Johnson & Johnson

Visine® Contact Lens Eye Drops
glycerin—hypromellose
Artificial Tears

Johnson & Johnson

SUPPLIED: Visine Advance True Tears: Sterile isotonic solution containing: glycerin 0.2% v/v and hypromellose 0.2% w/v. Nonmedicinal ingredients: ascorbic acid, benzalkonium chloride, boric acid, dextrose, disodium phosphate, glycine, magnesium chloride, polyethylene glycol 400, potassium chloride, sodium borate, sodium chloride, sodium citrate, sodium lactate and water. Plastic dispenser bottles of 15 mL. Store between 15 and 30°C.

Visine Contact Lens Eye Drops: Sterile isotonic solution containing: glycerin 0.2% v/v and hypromellose 0.2% w/v. Nonmedicinal ingredients: boric acid, edetate disodium, potassium sorbate, sodium borate and water. Plastic dispenser bottles of 15 mL. Store between 15 and 30°C.

Visine® Allergy Eye Drops
tetrahydrozoline HCl—zinc sulfate
Ophthalmic Decongestant—Astringent

Johnson & Johnson

Visine® Advance Allergy
pheniramine maleate—naphazoline HCl
Antihistamine—Ophthalmic Decongestant

Johnson & Johnson

Visine® Advance Triple Action
tetrahydrozoline HCl—polyethylene glycol 400—dextran—povidone
Ophthalmic Decongestant—Lubricant

Johnson & Johnson

Visine® Cool Eye Drops
tetrahydrozoline HCl—polyethylene glycol
Ophthalmic Decongestant—Lubricant

Johnson & Johnson

Visine® Original Eye Drops
tetrahydrozoline HCl
Ophthalmic Decongestant

Johnson & Johnson

Visine® Workplace Eye Drops
oxymetazoline HCl
Ophthalmic Decongestant

Johnson & Johnson

SUPPLIED: Visine Allergy Eye Drops: Sterile isotonic solution containing: tetrahydrozoline HCl 0.05% w/v and zinc sulfate 0.25% w/v. Nonmedicinal ingredients: benzalkonium chloride, boric acid, edetate disodium, sodium chloride, sodium citrate and water. Plastic dispenser bottles of 15 mL. Store between 15 and 30°C.

Visine Advance Allergy: Sterile isotonic solution containing: pheniramine maleate 0.3% w/v, naphazoline HCl 0.025% w/v. Nonmedicinal ingredients: benzalkorium chloride, boric acid, edetate disodium, sodium borate and water. Plastic dispenser bottles of 15 mL. Store between 15 and 30°C.

Visine Advance Triple Action: Sterile isotonic solution containing: tetrahydrozoline HCl 0.05% w/v, polyethylene glycol 400 1.0% w/v, dextran 70 0.1% w/v, povidone 1.0 % w/v. Nonmedicinal ingredients: benzalkonium chloride, boric acid, edetate disodium, sodium borate, sodium chloride and water. Plastic dispenser bottles of 15 mL. Store between 15 and 30°C.

Visine Cool Eye Drops: Sterile isotonic solution containing: polyethylene glycol 400 1.0% w/v and tetrahydrozoline HCl 0.05% w/v. Nonmedicinal ingredients: benzalkonium chloride, boric acid, edetate disodium, sodium borate, sodium chloride and water. Plastic dispenser bottles of 15 mL. Store between 15 and 30°C.

Visine Original Eye Drops: Sterile isotonic solution containing: tetrahydrozoline HCl 0.05 % w/v. Nonmedicinal ingredients: benzalkonium chloride, boric acid, edetate disodium, sodium borate, sodium chloride and water. Plastic dispenser bottles of 15 mL and 30 mL. Store between 15 and 30°C.

Visine Workplace Eye Drops: Sterile isotonic solution containing: oxymetazoline HCl 0.025% w/v. Nonmedicinal ingredients: benzalkonium chloride, boric acid, edetate disodium, sodium borate, sodium chloride and water. Plastic dispenser bottles of 15 mL. Store between 15 and 30°C.

Visionex™
bilberry—lutein—zeaxanthin
Vitamin and Mineral Supplement

USANA Health Sciences

SUPPLIED: Each tablet contains: vitamin C (calcium, magnesium, potassium and zinc ascorbates; ascorbyl palmitate) 250 mg, zinc (citrate, ascorbate) 5 mg, bilberry fruit extract (Vaccinium myrtillus, 100:1, equiv. to 2.5 g fresh fruit) 25 mg, marigold flower extract (Tagetes erecta, standardized to 5 mg lutein and 0.17 mg zeaxanthin) 100 mg, and zeaxanthin 0.83 mg. Nonmedicinal ingredients: ascorbyl palmitate, croscarmellose sodium, dextrine, dextrose, microcrystalline cellulose, silicon dioxide, soybean lecithin and starch. Bottles of 56. Safety seal under cap. Store below 25°C.

(Shown in Product Identification Section)

Viskazide® Ⓟ
pindolol—hydrochlorothiazide
Antihypertensive

Novartis Pharmaceuticals

PHARMACOLOGY: Viskazide contains the antihypertensive activity of 2 agents: a beta-adrenergic receptor blocking agent (pindolol) and a diuretic (hydrochlorothiazide).

Pindolol is a nonselective beta-adrenergic receptor blocking agent which possesses partial agonist activity (intrinsic sympathomimetic activity-ISA).

The mechanism of the antihypertensive effect of beta-adrenergic receptor blocking agents has not been established. Among the factors that may be involved are: (a) competitive ability to antagonize catecholamine induced tachycardia at the beta-receptor sites in the heart, thus decreasing cardiac output; (b) a reduction in total peripheral resistance; (c) inhibition of the vasomotor centres; (d) inhibition of renin release by the kidneys.

Hydrochlorothiazide increases excretion of sodium and chloride in approximately equivalent amounts, and may cause a simultaneous, usually minimal, loss of bicarbonate. Natriuresis is usually accompanied by some loss of potassium. The mechanism of the antihypertensive effect of thiazides may be related to the excretion and redistribution of body sodium. Hydrochlorothiazide usually does not decrease normal blood pressure.

The combination of pindolol with thiazide-like diuretics has been shown to be compatible and generally more effective than either of the drugs used alone in reducing elevated blood pressure.

In humans, orally administered pindolol is rapidly and completely absorbed. Because of negligible hepatic first pass effect, the bioavailability of oral pindolol is high and approaches 90% of the oral dose. Maximum plasma concentrations are reached within 2 hours after oral administration and the plasma half-life is approximately 3.5 hours. The elimination of pindolol is not dose dependent.

In man, pindolol is partially metabolized with approximately 40% of an oral dose being excreted unchanged in the urine. The principal metabolites of pindolol consist of the conjugated glucuronide and phenolic derivatives of pindolol conjugated with sulfuric or glucuronic acid.

Approximately 80% of an oral dose is accounted for in the urine within 24 hours.

The onset of the diuretic action of hydrochlorothiazide occurs in 2 hours and the peak action in about 4 hours. Diuretic activity lasts about 6 to 12 hours. Hydrochlorothiazide is eliminated rapidly by the kidney.

INDICATIONS: This fixed combination is not indicated for initial therapy of hypertension. Hypertension requires therapy titrated to the individual patient. It is always better to adjust the dosage of each antihypertensive drug separately, but when the fixed combination corresponds to the optimum drug and dose requirements of the patient, its use may be more convenient in patient management. For further adjustment of dosage, however, it is best to use the individual drugs again. The treatment of hypertension is not static, but must be re-evaluated as conditions in each patient warrant.

Viskazide is indicated for the maintenance therapy of patients with hypertension who require pindolol and hydrochlorothiazide in the dosage and ratios present in Viskazide.

CONTRAINDICATIONS: The presence of: congestive heart failure (see Warnings); right ventricular failure secondary to pulmonary hypertension; significant cardiomegaly; sinus bradycardia, second and third degree AV block; cardiogenic shock; bronchospasm (including bronchial asthma), or severe chronic obstructive pulmonary disease (see Precautions); anesthesia with agents that produce myocardial depression, e.g., ether; anuria; hypersensitivity to pindolol, hydrochlorothiazide, or to sulfonamide derived drugs.

WARNINGS: Cardiac Failure: Special caution should be exercised when administering Viskazide to patients with a history of heart failure. Sympathetic stimulation is a vital component supporting circulatory function in congestive heart failure, and inhibition with beta-blockade always carries the potential hazard of further depressing myocardial contractility and precipitating cardiac failure.

In patients without a history of cardiac failure, continued depression of the myocardium over a period of time can, in some cases, lead to cardiac failure. Therefore, at the first sign or symptom of impending cardiac failure occurring during therapy, patients should be fully digitalized and/or given additional diuretic therapy, and the response observed closely.

Pindolol acts selectively without blocking the inotropic action of digitalis on heart muscle. However, the positive inotropic action of digitalis may be reduced by the negative inotropic effect of pindolol when the 2 drugs are used concomitantly. The effects of pindolol and digitalis are additive in depressing AV conduction. If cardiac failure persists, therapy with Viskazide should be discontinued (see below).

Abrupt Cessation of Therapy in Angina Pectoris: Patients with angina should be warned against abrupt discontinuation of Viskazide. There have been reports of severe exacerbation of angina, and of myocardial infarction or ventricular arrhythmias occurring in patients with angina pectoris, following abrupt discontinuation of beta-blocker therapy. The last 2 complications may occur with or without preceding exacerbation of angina pectoris. Therefore, when discontinuation of Viskazide is planned in patients with angina pectoris, the dosage should be reduced over a period of about 2 weeks and the patient should continue to be observed. The same frequency of administration should be maintained.

In situations of greater urgency, therapy should be discontinued step-wise and under conditions of closer observation. If angina markedly worsens or acute coronary insufficiency develops, it is recommended that treatment be reinstituted promptly, at least temporarily.

Since ischemic heart disease may be unrecognized, the above advice should be followed in patients considered to be at risk of having asymptomatic ischemic heart disease.

Various skin rashes and conjunctival xerosis have been reported with beta-blockers, including pindolol. A severe syndrome (oculo-mucocutaneous syndrome) whose signs include conjunctivitis sicca and psoriasiform rashes, otitis, and sclerosing serositis has occurred with the chronic use of one beta-adrenergic blocking agent (practolol). This syndrome has not been observed with pindolol, however, physicians should be alert to the possibility of such reactions and should discontinue treatment in the event that they occur.

Sinus bradycardia may occur with the use of pindolol due to unopposed vagal activity remaining after blockade of $beta_1$-adrenergic receptors. Due to its intrinsic sympathomimetic activity (ISA), pindolol causes less bradycardia at rest than some other beta-adrenergic blocking agents. If excessive bradycardia occurs, the dosage should be reduced.

In patients with thyrotoxicosis, pindolol may give a false impression of improvement by diminishing peripheral manifestations of hyperthyroidism without improving thyroid function. Special considerations should be given to the potential of pindolol to aggravate congestive heart failure. Pindolol does not alter thyroid function tests. Patients suspected of developing thyrotoxicosis should be managed carefully to avoid abrupt withdrawal of beta-blockade which might precipitate a thyroid storm. Thiazides may decrease serum PBI levels without signs of thyroid disturbance.

In patients with renal disease, thiazides may precipitate azotemia, and cumulative effects may develop in the presence of impaired renal function. If progressive renal impairment becomes evident, Viskazide should be discontinued.

In patients with impaired hepatic function or progressive liver disease, even minor alterations in fluid and electrolyte balance may precipitate hepatic coma. Hepatic encephalopathy, manifested by tremors, confusion, and coma, has been reported in association with diuretic therapy including hydrochlorothiazide.

In patients receiving thiazides, sensitivity reactions may occur with or without a history of allergy or bronchial asthma.

The possible exacerbation or activation of systemic lupus erythematosus has been reported with thiazides.

PRECAUTIONS: Viskazide should be administered with caution to patients prone to non allergic bronchospasm (e.g., chronic bronchitis, emphysema) since beta-blockade may block bronchodilatation produced by endogenous and exogenous catecholamine stimulation of beta receptors.

Elective or Emergency Surgery: Beta-adrenergic receptor blockade impairs the ability of the heart to respond to beta-adrenergically mediated reflex stimuli. Some patients receiving beta-adrenergic receptor blocking agents have been subject to protracted severe hypotension during anesthesia. Difficulty in restarting and maintaining the heartbeat has also been reported.

For these reasons, in patients with angina pectoris undergoing elective surgery, some authorities recommend gradual withdrawal of beta-adrenergic receptor blocking agents (see recommendations given under Warnings, Abrupt Cessation of Therapy).

In emergency surgery, since pindolol is a competitive inhibitor of beta-adrenergic receptor agonists its effects may be reversed, if necessary, by sufficient doses of such agonists as isoproterenol or levarterenol.

Viskazide should be administered with caution to patients with allergic rhinitis prone to bronchospasm.

Beta-adrenergic receptor blocking agents may mask the premonitory signs and symptoms of acute hypoglycemia. Therefore, Viskazide should be administered with caution to patients subject to spontaneous hypoglycemia, or to diabetic patients (especially those with labile diabetes) who are receiving insulin or oral hypoglycemic agents. Insulin requirements in diabetic patients may be increased, decreased, or unchanged by thiazides. Diabetes mellitus which has been latent may become manifest during administration of thiazide diuretics.

Epinephrine and Beta-blockers: There may be increased difficulty in treating an allergic type reaction in patients on beta-blockers. In these patients, the reaction may be more severe due to pharmacologic effects of the beta-blockers and problems with fluid changes. Epinephrine should be administered with caution since it may not have its usual effects in the treatment of anaphylaxis. On the one hand, larger doses of epinephrine may be needed to overcome the bronchospasm, while on the other hand, these doses can be associated with excessive alpha adrenergic stimulation with consequent hypertension, reflex bradycardia and heart block and possible potentiation of bronchospasm. Alternatives to the use of large doses of epinephrine include vigorous supportive care such as fluids and the use of beta agonists including parenteral salbutamol or isoproterenol to overcome bronchospasm and norepinephrine to overcome hypotension.

Patients receiving catecholamine depleting drugs, such as reserpine or guanethidine, should be closely monitored because the added beta-adrenergic blocking action of Viskazide may produce an excessive reduction of sympathetic activity. Viskazide should not be combined with other beta-blockers.

Patients receiving thiazides should be carefully observed for clinical signs of fluid and electrolyte imbalance (hyponatremia, hypochloremic alkalosis and hypokalemia). Periodic determination of serum electrolytes should be performed at appropriate intervals. Serum and urine electrolyte determinations are particularly important when the patient is vomiting excessively or receiving parenteral fluids. Warning signs or symptoms of fluid and electrolyte imbalance include dryness of the mouth, thirst, weakness, lethargy, drowsiness, restlessness, muscle pains or cramps, muscular fatigue, hypotension, oliguria, tachycardia, and gastrointestinal disturbances such as nausea and vomiting.

Hypokalemia may develop, especially with brisk diuresis, when severe cirrhosis is present, or during concomitant use of corticosteroids or ACTH. Interference with adequate oral electrolyte intake will also contribute to hypokalemia. Hypokalemia can sensitize or exaggerate the response of the heart to the toxic effects of digitalis (e.g., increased ventricular irritability). Hypokalemia may be avoided or treated by use of potassium supplements, potassium sparing agents or foods with a high potassium content.

Any chloride deficit during thiazide therapy is generally mild and usually does not require specific treatment except under extraordinary circumstances (as in liver disease or renal disease). Dilutional hyponatremia may occur in edematous patients in hot weather; appropriate therapy is water restriction rather than administration of salt, except in rare instances, when the hyponatremia is life threatening. In actual salt depletion, appropriate replacement is the therapy of choice.

Because calcium excretion is decreased by thiazides, Viskazide should be discontinued before carrying out tests for parathyroid function. Pathologic changes in the parathyroid glands, with hypercalcemia and hypophosphatemia, have been observed in a few patients on prolonged thiazide therapy; however, the common complications of hyperparathyroidism such as renal lithiasis, bone resorption, and peptic ulceration have not been seen.

The antihypertensive effects of thiazides may be enhanced in the postsympathectomy patient.

Hyperuricemia may occur or acute gout may be precipitated in certain patients receiving thiazide therapy.

The combination of Viskazide with an antihypertensive peripheral vasodilator produces a greater fall in blood pressure than either drug alone. The same degree of blood pressure control can be achieved by lower than usual doses of each drug. Therefore, when using such combined therapy, careful monitoring of the dosages is required until the patient is stabilized.

Thiazides may decrease arterial responsiveness to norepinephrine. This diminution is not sufficient to preclude the therapeutic effectiveness of the pressor agent in therapy.

Thiazides may increase the responsiveness to tubocurarine.

Lithium generally should not be given with diuretics because they reduce its renal clearance and add a high risk of lithium toxicity. Read prescribing information for lithium preparations before use of such preparations with Viskazide.

Orthostatic hypotension may occur and may be potentiated by alcohol, barbiturates or narcotics.

Pregnancy: Thiazides cross the placental barrier and appear in cord blood. The use of Viskazide in pregnancy or in women of child bearing potential requires that the anticipated benefit be weighed against possible risk to mother and/or fetus. These hazards include fetal or neonatal jaundice, thrombocytopenia, and possibly, other adverse reactions which have occurred in the adult.

Lactation: Thiazides appear in human milk. If use of Viskazide is deemed essential, the patient should stop nursing.

Children: The safety for use of pindolol in children has not been established; therefore, Viskazide is not recommended in the pediatric age group.

ADVERSE EFFECTS: Cardiovascular: congestive heart failure (see Warnings), severe bradycardia (see Warnings) may occur as may syncope, lightheadedness, and postural hypotension. Lengthening of PR interval, second degree AV block, palpitation, chest pains, cold extremities, Raynaud's phenomenon, claudication, hot flushes, very rarely arrhythmia, coronary insufficiency. Orthostatic hypotension may be potentiated by alcohol, barbiturates or narcotics.

Central Nervous System: insomnia, nightmares, vivid dreams, fatigue, drowsiness, weakness, paresthesias, dizziness, vertigo, tinnitus, headache, mental depression, nervousness. Rarely have the following adverse reactions been reported: aggressiveness, motor disorders, confusion, xanthopsia.

Gastrointestinal: anorexia, gastric irritation, cramping, diarrhea, constipation, flatulence, heartburn, nausea and vomiting, abdominal pain, dry mouth, jaundice (intrahepatic, cholestatic), pancreatitis, sialoadenitis.

Respiratory: shortness of breath and/or dyspnea, wheezing, bronchospasm (see Contraindications and Precautions).

Hematologic: leukopenia, agranulocytosis, thrombocytopenia, aplastic anemia, hemolytic anemia.

Urogenital: impotence.

Hypersensitivity: exanthema, sweating, pruritus, purpura, photosensitivity, urticaria, exfoliative dermatitis, psoriasiform rash, necrotizing angiitis vasculitis, cutaneous vasculitis, fever, respiratory distress, including pneumonitis, anaphylactic reactions.

Special Senses: visual disturbances, including xanthopsia and transient blurred vision, dry eyes, conjunctivitis, itching and/or burning eyes, tinnitus, vestibular disorder.

Other: hyperglycemia, glycosuria, hyperuricemia, muscle cramps, weakness, restlessness, weight gain or loss, urinary frequency, appetite stimulation.

Clinical Laboratory Test Findings: On rare occasions, changes in the following parameters were noted: elevations in transaminases, alkaline phosphate, LDH, serum uric acid; a reduction in bilirubin. The most common changes associated with the thiazide component are increases in uric acid and decreases in serum potassium and chloride.

OVERDOSE:

Symptoms: The pindolol component may cause bradycardia, hypotension, bronchospasm, hypoglycemia or acute cardiac failure.

The hydrochlorothiazide component may cause excessive diuresis with electrolyte depletion and dehydration. Signs are dry mouth, thirst, weakness, lethargy, drowsiness, restlessness, muscle pains or cramps, muscular fatigue, hypotension, oliguria, tachycardia, gastrointestinal disturbances, mental confusion, delirium, convulsions, shock and coma.

If digitalis has also been administered, hypokalemia may accentuate myocardial abnormalities (e.g., cardiac arrhythmias).

Hydrochlorothiazide may precipitate hepatic coma in cirrhotics, potentiate other antihypertensive agents and decrease responsiveness to norepinephrine.

Treatment: Discontinue Viskazide. There is no specific antidote. If ingestion is, or may have been, recent, gastric lavage or emesis may reduce absorption; when ingestion has been earlier, infusions may be helpful to promote urinary excretion.

If required the following therapeutic measures are suggested: Bradycardia: Atropine or another anticholinergic drug. Heart block: (second or third degree) Isoproterenol or transvenous cardiac pacemaker. Congestive heart failure: Conventional therapy. Hypotension: (depending on associated factors) Epinephrine rather than isoproterenol or norepinephrine may be useful in addition to atropine and digitalis. Bronchospasm: Aminophylline or isoproterenol. Hypoglycemia: I.V. glucose. Stupor or Coma: Supportive therapy as clinically warranted. Gastrointestinal Effects: Though usually of short duration, these may require symptomatic treatment.

Abnormalities in BUN and/or Serum Electrolytes: Monitor serum electrolyte levels and renal function; institute supportive measures as required individually to maintain hydration, electrolyte balance, respiration and cardiovascular-renal function.

It should be remembered that pindolol is a competitive antagonist of isoproterenol and hence large doses of isoproterenol can be expected to reverse many of the effects of excessive doses of Viskazide. However, the complications of excess isoproterenol should not be overlooked.

For management of a suspected drug overdose, CPhA recommends that you contact your **regional Poison Control Centre**. See the *CPS* Directory section for a list of Poison Control Centres.

DOSAGE: Dosage must be determined for individual patients by titration of each component separately. Where the fixed combination in Viskazide supplies the dosage so determined, the combination product may be used for maintenance therapy. 1 or 2 Viskazide tablets once daily in the morning can be used to administer up to 20 mg pindolol and 100 mg hydrochlorothiazide.

If higher doses of either ingredient are needed, the individual components should be used.

When necessary, another antihypertensive agent may be added gradually, beginning with 50% of the usual recommended starting dose to avoid excessive reduction in blood pressure.

If dosage adjustment is necessary during maintenance therapy, it is advisable to use the individual drugs.

SUPPLIED: Viskazide 10/25: Each peach, round, compressed tablet, 9 mm diameter, one side slope-faced and bisected with "10/25" embossed on each side of the bisect, reverse side flat-faced with beveled edge and embossed with "VISKAZIDE" around the circumference and "△" centered, contains: pindolol 10 mg and hydrochlorothiazide 25 mg. Nonmedicinal ingredients: D&C Red #21 Aluminium Lake, D&C Yellow #10 Lake, magnesium stearate, microcrystalline cellulose, pregelatinized starch and silicon dioxide. Calendar packs of 35.

Viskazide 10/50: Each orange, round, compressed tablet, 9 mm diameter, one side slope-faced and bisected with "10/50" embossed on each side of the bisect, reverse side flat-faced with beveled edge and embossed with "VISKAZIDE" around the circumference and "△" centered, contains: pindolol 10 mg and hydrochlorothiazide 50 mg. Nonmedicinal ingredients: D&C Red #21 Aluminium Lake, D&C Yellow #10 Lake, magnesium stearate, microcrystalline cellulose, pregelatinized starch and silicon dioxide. Calendar packs of 35.

(Shown in Product Identification Section)

Visken® Ⓟ

pindolol

Antihypertensive—Antianginal

Novartis Pharmaceuticals

PHARMACOLOGY: Pindolol is a beta-adrenergic-receptor-blocking agent which possesses partial agonist activity (intrinsic sympathomimetic activity—I.S.A.).

Hypertension: The mechanism of the antihypertensive effect of pindolol has not been established. Among the factors that may be involved are: competitive ability to antagonize catecholamine-induced tachycardia at the beta-receptor sites in the heart, thus decreasing cardiac output; a reduction in total peripheral resistance; inhibition of the vasomotor centres; inhibition of renin release by the kidneys.

Angina Pectoris: The mechanism of the antianginal effect of pindolol has not been established. Pindolol may reduce the oxygen requirement of the heart at any level of effort by blocking catecholamine-induced increases in the heart rate, systolic blood pressure, and the velocity and extent of myocardial contraction. However, oxygen requirements may be increased by such actions as increases in left ventricular fibre length, end diastolic pressure and the systolic ejection period. When the net effect is beneficial in anginal patients, it manifests itself during exercise or stress by delaying the onset of pain and reducing the incidence and severity of anginal attacks.

In humans, orally-administered pindolol is rapidly and almost completely absorbed (≥ 95%). Because of negligible hepatic first pass effect, the bioavailability of oral pindolol is high and approaches 90% of the oral dose. Maximum plasma concentrations are reached 1 to 2 hours after oral administration and the plasma half-life is approximately 3.5 hours. The elimination rate of pindolol is not dose dependent. Forty percent of pindolol is bound to plasma proteins. Pindolol has a volume of distribution of 2 to 3L/kg and a total clearance of 500 mL/min.

Pindolol is partially metabolized with approximately 40% of an oral dose being excreted unchanged in the urine. The remaining 60% is excreted in the urine and feces as inactive metabolites. The principle metabolites of pindolol consist of the conjugated glucuronide, and phenolic derivatives of pindolol conjugated with sulfuric or glucuronic acid.

Approximately 80% of an oral dose is accounted for in the urine within 24 hours.

INDICATIONS: a) Mild to moderate hypertension. Pindolol is usually used in combination with other drugs, particularly a thiazide diuretic. However, it may be used alone as an initial agent in those patients in whom, in the judgment of the physician, treatment should be started with a beta-blocker rather than a diuretic.

The combination of pindolol with a diuretic and/or peripheral vasodilator has been found to be compatible and generally more effective than pindolol alone. Limited experience with other antihypertensive agents, including methyldopa, has not shown evidence of incompatibility with pindolol.

Not recommended for the emergency treatment of hypertensive crises.

b) The prophylaxis of angina pectoris.

CONTRAINDICATIONS: Sinus bradycardia; second and third degree AV block; right ventricular failure secondary to pulmonary hypertension; congestive heart failure (see Warnings); cardiogenic shock; anesthesia with agents that produce myocardial depression, e.g., ether; bronchospasm, including bronchial asthma or severe chronic obstructive pulmonary disease (see Precautions).

WARNINGS: Cardiac Failure: Special caution should be exercised when administering pindolol to patients with a history of heart failure. Sympathetic stimulation is a vital component supporting circulatory function in congestive heart failure, and inhibition with beta-blockade always carries the potential hazard of further depressing myocardial contractility and precipitating cardiac failure. Pindolol may reduce but does not abolish the inotropic action of digitalis on the heart muscle. However, the positive inotropic action of digitalis may be reduced by pindolol's negative inotropic effect when the 2 drugs are used concomitantly. The effects of beta-blockers and digitalis are additive in depressing AV conduction. In patients without a history of cardiac failure, continued depression of the myocardium over a period of time can, in some cases, lead to cardiac failure. Therefore, at the first sign or symptom of impending cardiac failure, patients should be fully digitalized and/or given a diuretic and the response observed closely. If cardiac failure continues, despite adequate digitalization and diuretic therapy, pindolol should be immediately withdrawn.

Abrupt Cessation of Therapy: Warn patients with angina against abrupt discontinuation of pindolol. There have been reports of severe exacerbation of angina, and of myocardial infarction or ventricular arrhythmias occurring in patients with angina pectoris, following abrupt discontinuation of beta-blocker therapy. The last 2 complications may occur with or without preceding exacerbation of angina pectoris. Therefore, when discontinuation of pindolol is planned in patients with angina pectoris, the dosage should be gradually reduced over a period of about 2 weeks and the patient should be observed carefully. The same frequency of administration should be maintained. In situations of greater urgency, discontinue pindolol therapy step-wise and under conditions of very close observation. If angina markedly worsens or acute coronary insufficiency develops, it is recommended that treatment with pindolol be reinstituted promptly, at least temporarily.

Various skin rashes and conjunctival xerosis have been reported with beta-blockers, including pindolol. A severe oculo-mucocutaneous syndrome whose signs include conjunctivitis sicca and psoriasiform rashes, otitis and sclerosing serositis has occurred with the chronic use of one beta-adrenergic-blocking agent (practolol). This syndrome has not been observed with pindolol. However, physicians should be alert to the possibility of such reactions and should discontinue treatment in the event that they occur.

Sinus bradycardia may occur with the use of pindolol due to unopposed vagal activity remaining after blockade of $beta_1$-adrenergic receptors. Due to its intrinsic sympathomimetic activity, pindolol causes less bradycardia at rest than some other beta-adrenergic-blocking agents. If excessive bradycardia occurs, reduce the dosage.

In patients with thyrotoxicosis, possible deleterious effects from long-term use of pindolol have not been adequately appraised. Beta-blockade may mask the clinical signs of continuing hyperthyroidism or complications, and give a false impression of improvement. Therefore, abrupt withdrawal of pindolol may be followed by an exacerbation of the symptoms of hyperthyroidism, including thyroid storm.

PRECAUTIONS: Caution should be exercised in patients prone to nonallergic bronchospasm (e.g., chronic bronchitis, emphysema) since pindolol may block bronchodilation produced by endogenous and exogenous catecholamine stimulation of beta receptors.

Pindolol should be administered with caution to patients with allergic rhinitis prone to bronchospasm.

Epinephrine and Beta-blockers: There may be increased difficulty in treating an allergic type reaction in patients on beta-blockers. In these patients, the reaction may be more severe due to pharmacologic effects of the beta-blockers and problems with fluid changes. Epinephrine should be administered with caution since it may not have its usual effects in the treatment of anaphylaxis. On the one hand, larger doses of epinephrine may be needed to overcome the bronchospasm, while on the other hand, these doses can be associated with excessive alpha adrenergic stimulation with consequent hypertension, reflex bradycardia and heart block and possible potentiation of bronchospasm. Alternatives to the use of large doses of epinephrine include vigorous supportive care such as fluids and the use of beta agonists including parenteral salbutamol or isoproterenol to overcome bronchospasm and norepinephrine to overcome hypotension.

Pindolol should be administered with caution to patients subject to spontaneous hypoglycemia, or to diabetic patients (especially those with labile diabetes) who are receiving insulin or oral hypoglycemic agents. Beta-adrenergic-blockers may mask the premonitory signs and symptoms (tachycardia, tremor) of acute hypoglycemia.

Pindolol dosage should be individually adjusted when used concomitantly with other antihypertensive agents (see Dosage).

Patients receiving catecholamine depleting drugs, such as reserpine of guanethidine, should be closely monitored because the added beta-adrenergic-blocking action of pindolol may produce an excessive reduction of sympathetic activity. Do not combine pindolol with other beta-blockers.

Appropriate laboratory tests should be performed at regular intervals during long-term treatment.

Patients Undergoing Elective or Emergency Surgery: The management of patients being treated with beta-blockers and undergoing elective or emergency surgery is controversial. Although beta-adrenergic -receptor blockade impairs the ability of the heart to respond to beta-adrenergically-mediated reflex stimuli, abrupt discontinuation of pindolol therapy may be followed by severe complications (see Warnings). Some patients receiving beta-adrenergic-blocking agents have been subject to protracted severe hypotension during anesthesia. Difficulty in restarting and maintaining the heartbeat has also been reported.

For these reasons, in patients with angina undergoing elective surgery, withdraw pindolol gradually following the recommendation given under "Abrupt cessation of therapy" (see Warnings). According to available evidence, all clinical and physiological effects of beta-blockade are no longer present 48 hours after cessation of medication.

In emergency surgery, since pindolol is a competitive inhibitor of beta-adrenergic-receptor agonists, its effects may be reversed, if necessary, by sufficient doses of such agonists as isoproterenol or levarterenol.

Impaired Renal or Hepatic Function: β-blocking agents should be used with caution in patients with impaired hepatic or renal function. Poor renal function has only minor effects on pindolol clearance, but poor hepatic function may cause blood levels of pindolol to increase substantially.

Pregnancy: Since pindolol has not been studied in human pregnancy, it should not be given to pregnant women. The use of any drug in patients of child-bearing potential requires that the anticipated benefit be weighed against possible hazards. Pindolol crosses the placental barrier.

Lactation: Pindolol passes in small quantities into breast milk.

Children: There is no experience with pindolol in the treatment of pediatric age groups.

Occupational Hazards: Because dizziness or fatigue may occur during initiation of treatment with β-adrenoreceptor blocking drugs, patients driving vehicles or operating machinery should exercise caution until they have determined their individual response to treatment.

ADVERSE EFFECTS: Cardiovascular: Congestive heart failure, severe bradycardia (see Warnings) may occur. Syncope, lightheadedness and postural hypotension. Lengthening of PR interval, second degree AV block, palpitation, chest pains, cold extremities, Raynaud's phenomenon, claudication, hot flushes. Very rarely: arrhythmia, coronary insufficiency.

Central Nervous System: insomnia, nightmares, vivid dreams, fatigue, drowsiness, weakness, dizziness, vertigo, tinnitus, headache, mental depression, nervousness. Rarely have the following adverse reactions been reported: aggressiveness, motor disorders, confusion.

Gastrointestinal: diarrhea, constipation, flatulence, heartburn, nausea and vomiting, abdominal pain and dry mouth.

Respiratory: shortness of breath and/or dyspnea, wheezing, bronchospasm.

Allergic, Dermatological (see Warnings): exanthema, sweating, pruritus, psoriasiform rash.

Eyes: itching, burning, grittiness, dryness.

Miscellaneous: muscle cramps, appetite stimulation, weight gain, urinary frequency.

Clinical Laboratory: The following parameters have been rarely elevated: transaminases, alkaline phosphatase, LDH, serum uric acid. Rarely reduction in bilirubin.

OVERDOSE:

Symptoms: The most common signs to be expected with overdosage of a beta-adrenergic-blocking agent are bradycardia, congestive heart failure, hypotension, bronchospasm, or hypoglycemia.

Treatment: If overdosage occurs, in all cases therapy with pindolol should be discontinued and the patient observed closely. In addition, if required, the following therapeutic measures are suggested:

1. Bradycardia: Atropine or another anticholinergic drug.
2. Heart block (second or third degree): Isoproterenol or transvenous cardiac pacemaker.
3. Congestive heart failure: Conventional therapy.
4. Hypotension: (depending on associated factors) Epinephrine rather than isoproterenol or norepinephrine may be useful in addition to atropine and digitalis (see Precautions concerning the use of epinephrine).
5. Bronchospasm: Aminophylline or isoproterenol.
6. Hypoglycemia: I.V. glucose.

It should be remembered that pindolol is a competitive antagonist of isoproterenol and hence large doses of isoproterenol can be expected to reverse many of the effects of excessive doses of pindolol. However, the complications of excess isoproterenol should not be overlooked.

For management of a suspected drug overdose, CPhA recommends that you contact your **regional Poison Control Centre**. See the *CPS* Directory section for a list of Poison Control Centres.

DOSAGE: Hypertension: Pindolol is usually used in conjunction with other antihypertensive agents, particularly a thiazide diuretic but may be used alone (see Indications). Pindolol should be taken with meals.

The dosage of pindolol must always be adjusted to the individual requirements of the patients in accordance with the following guidelines: therapy should be initiated with doses of 5 mg in the morning with breakfast and 5 mg with the evening meal. If an adequate response is not achieved after 1 to 2 weeks, the dose should be increased to 10 mg twice daily.

If after 1 to 2 additional weeks an adequate response is not observed, dosage may be increased to 30 mg daily with 15 mg given in the morning with breakfast and 15 mg with the evening meal.

Doses greater than 30 mg daily must be given on a t.i.d. schedule.

Patients who show a satisfactory response to pindolol at daily doses of 10 to 20 mg may be maintained by giving the required total dose once daily in the morning with breakfast.

The usual maintenance dose is within the range of 15 to 45 mg daily which should not be exceeded. However, during long-term therapy, some patients may be maintained on smaller doses.

Angina Pectoris: The dosage must always be adjusted to the individual requirements of the patient.

In angina, pindolol should be administered on a 3 or 4 times per day dosing regimen. Therapy should be initiated with doses of 5 mg 3 times a day with meals. If after 1 to 2 weeks an adequate response is not observed dosage may be increased. The usual maintenance dose is 15 mg up to the maximum of 40 mg/day.

SUPPLIED: 5 mg: Each whitish, compressed tablet, 7 mm diameter, slope faced, bisected with "LB" embossed on one side and flat faced, beveled edge with "VISKEN 5" embossed on reverse side, contains: pindolol 5 mg. Nonmedicinal ingredients: magnesium stearate, microcrystalline cellulose, silicon dioxide and starch. Bottles of 100.

10 mg: Each whitish, compressed tablet, 8 mm diameter, slope faced, bisected on one side and flat-faced, beveled edge with "VISKEN 10" embossed on reverse side, contains: pindolol 10 mg. Nonmedicinal ingredients: magnesium stearate, microcrystalline cellulose, silicon dioxide and starch. Bottles of 100.

15 mg: Each whitish, compressed tablet, 9 mm diameter, slope faced, bisected with "JU" embossed on one side and flat faced, beveled edge with "VISKEN 15" embossed on reverse side, contains: pindolol 15 mg. Nonmedicinal ingredients: magnesium stearate, microcrystalline cellulose, silicon dioxide and starch. Bottles of 100.

Protect from light.

(Shown in Product Identification Section)

Visudyne® Ⓟ

verteporfin

Photosensitizing Agent for Photodynamic Therapy of Choroidal Neovascularization

Novartis Pharmaceuticals

Date of Preparation: May 31, 2000
Date of Revision: April 30, 2008

SUMMARY PRODUCT INFORMATION:

Route of Administration	Dosage Form/ Strength	Clinically Relevant Nonmedicinal Ingredients
Intravenous infusion	Lyophylized powder for injection containing 15 mg verteporfin per vial.	Ascorbyl palmitate, butylated hydroxytoluene, egg phosphatidylglycerol, dimyristoyl phosphatidylcholine, lactose. This is a complete listing.

INDICATIONS AND CLINICAL USE: VISUDYNE Therapy is indicated for the treatment of predominantly classic subfoveal choroidal neovascularization in patients with:

- age-related macular degeneration (AMD),
- pathologic myopia,
- presumed ocular histoplasmosis.

Geriatrics: Approximately 90% of the patients treated with VISUDYNE in the clinical efficacy trials were over the age of 65. A reduced treatment effect was seen with increasing age.

Pediatrics: No data is available.

CONTRAINDICATIONS:

- Patients who are hypersensitive to this drug or to any ingredient in the formulation or component of the container. For a complete listing, see Dosage Forms, Composition and Packaging.
- Porphyria.
- Severe hepatic impairment.

WARNINGS AND PRECAUTIONS: VISUDYNE (verteporfin) is a drug to be used in Visudyne Therapy. Visudyne Therapy is a two-stage process requiring administration of both verteporfin for injection and nonthermal red light.

Caution: Visudyne Therapy should only be used by physicians trained in the treatment of predominantly classic subfoveal choroidal neovascularization using photodynamic therapy with verteporfin for injection and specified lasers. Following VISUDYNE injection, residual photosensitivity for 48 hours or more may result in erythema and blistering of the skin when exposed to sunlight or brightly focused indoor light.

Use of incompatible lasers that do not provide the required characteristics of light for the photoactivation of VISUDYNE could result in incomplete treatment due to partial photoactivation of VISUDYNE, overtreatment due to overactivation of VISUDYNE, or damage to surrounding normal tissue.

Appropriate facilities and personnel must be available to treat any complications of the procedure, as well as for the emergency treatment of allergic reactions to the agent itself (see Cardiovascular and Immune).

General: Following injection with VISUDYNE, care should be taken to avoid exposure of skin or eyes to direct sunlight or bright indoor light for 2 days. If emergency surgery is necessary within 48 hours after treatment, as much of the internal tissue as possible should be protected from intense light.

Extravasation of VISUDYNE, especially if the affected area is exposed to light, can cause severe pain, inflammation, swelling or discoloration at the injection site.

If extravasation does occur, the infusion should be stopped immediately. The extravasation area must be thoroughly protected from direct light until the swelling and discoloration have faded in order to prevent the occurrence of a local burn which could be severe. Cold compresses should be applied to the injection site. The relief of pain may require analgesic treatment.

Standard precautions should be taken during infusion of VISUDYNE to avoid extravasation. Examples of standard precautions include, but are not limited to the following:

- a free-flowing intravenous (IV) line should be established before starting VISUDYNE infusion and the line should be carefully monitored,
- due to the possible fragility of vein walls of some elderly patients, it is strongly recommended that the largest arm vein possible, preferably antecubital, be used for injection,
- small veins in the back of the hand should be avoided.

Carcinogenesis and Mutagenesis: No studies have been conducted to evaluate the carcinogenic potential of verteporfin.

Verteporfin was not mutagenic, in the absence or presence of light, when studied in microbial mutagenicity, unscheduled DNA synthesis, mammalian point mutation, chromosome aberration, and mouse micronucleus assays.

Photodynamic therapy (PDT) as a class has been reported to result in DNA damage including DNA strand breaks, alkali-labile sites, DNA degradation, and DNA-protein cross links which may result in chromosomal aberrations, sister chromatid exchanges (SCE), and mutations. In addition, other photodynamic therapeutic agents have been shown to increase the incidence of SCE in Chinese hamster ovary (CHO) cells irradiated with visible light and in Chinese hamster lung fibroblasts irradiated with near UV light, increase mutations and DNA-protein cross-linking in mouse L5178 cells, and increase DNA-strand breaks in malignant human cervical carcinoma cells, but not in normal cells. Verteporfin was not evaluated in these latter systems. It is not known how the potential for DNA damage with PDT agents translates into human risk.

No effect on male or female reproduction has been observed in rats following intravenous administration of verteporfin for injection up to 10 mg/kg/day (approximately 60- and 40-fold human exposure at 6 mg/m² based on AUC_{inf} in male and female rats, respectively). Males were dosed 28 days prior to and during mating until necropsy (approximately 60 days). Females were dosed for 14 days prior to and during mating until Gestation Day 7.

Cardiovascular: Chest pain, vaso-vagal reactions and hypersensitivity reactions, which on rare occasions can be severe, have been reported. Both vaso-vagal and hypersensitivity reactions are associated with general symptoms such as syncope, sweating, dizziness, rash, dyspnea, flushing, and changes in blood pressure and heart rate. This may be related to complement activation (see Immune).

Hepatic/Biliary/Pancreatic: Visudyne Therapy should be considered carefully in patients with moderate hepatic impairment or biliary obstruction since there is no clinical experience with verteporfin in such patients.

Immune: VISUDYNE at >5 times the expected maximum plasma concentration in treated patients caused a low level of complement activation in human blood in vitro. VISUDYNE resulted in a concentration-dependent increase in complement activation in human blood in vitro. At 10 µg/mL (approximately 5 times the expected plasma concentration in human patients), there was mild to moderate complement activation. At ≥100 µg/mL, there was significant complement activation. Signs (chest pain, syncope, dyspnea, and flushing, see the information under Cardiovascular) consistent with complement activation have been observed in <1% of patients administered VISUDYNE. Patients should be supervised during VISUDYNE infusion and observed for at least 30 minutes after infusion.

Fluorescein Angiography: Standard precautions for fluorescein angiography should be observed. Certain medical conditions (such as pregnancy or allergy to fluorescein) may make the injection of fluorescein dye for a particular patient inadvisable in the opinion of the ophthalmologist. Approximately 1/225 000 patients may experience a severe reaction resulting in a heart attack, stroke, or death. Most reactions are mild, such as temporary nausea or vomiting in a few patients and a rash, hives, or wheezing in about 1%.

Ophthalmologic: Patients who experience severe decrease of vision of 4 lines or more within 1 week after treatment should not be retreated, at least until their vision completely recovers to pretreatment levels and the potential benefits and risks of subsequent treatment are carefully considered by the treating physician.

Following Visudyne Therapy, patients may develop transient visual disturbances such as abnormal vision, vision decrease, or visual field defects that may interfere with their ability to drive or use machines. Patients should be advised to not drive or use machines as long as these symptoms persist.

Patients will become temporarily photosensitive for 2 days after the infusion should avoid exposure of unprotected eyes to direct sunlight or bright indoor light. See the information under Skin.

Peri-Operative Considerations: Caution should be exercised when Visudyne Treatment under general anesthesia is considered. There is no clinical data related to the use of VISUDYNE in anesthetized patients. At a >10-fold higher dose given by bolus injection to sedated or anesthetized pigs, verteporfin caused severe hemodynamic effects, including death, probably as a result of complement activation. These effects were diminished or abolished by pretreatment with antihistamine and they were not seen in conscious non-sedated pigs or in any other species, whether conscious or under general anesthesia. Caution should be exercised when Visudyne Treatment under general anesthesia is considered.

Sexual Function/Reproduction: No effect on male or female reproduction has been observed in rats following intravenous administration of verteporfin for injection up to 10 mg/kg/day (approximately 60- and 40- fold human exposure at 6 mg/m² based on AUC_{inf} in male and female rats, respectively). Males were dosed 28 days prior to and during mating until necropsy (approximately 60 days). Females were dosed for 14 days prior to and during mating until Gestation Day 7.

Skin: Patients who receive VISUDYNE will become temporarily photosensitive for 2 days after the infusion. During that period, patients should avoid exposure of unprotected skin, eyes or other body organs to direct sunlight or bright indoor light. This includes, but is not limited to, tanning salons, bright halogen lighting and high power lighting used in surgical operating rooms or dental offices. Prolonged exposure to light from light-emitting medical devices such as pulse oximeters should also be avoided for 48 hours following VISUDYNE administration.

If treated patients must go outdoors in daylight during the first 2 days after treatment, they should protect all parts of their skin and their eyes by wearing protective clothing and dark sunglasses. UV sunscreens are not effective in protecting against photosensitivity reactions because photoactivation of the residual drug in the skin can be caused by visible light.

Patients should not stay in the dark and should be encouraged to expose their skin to ambient indoor light, as it will help inactivate the drug in the skin through a process called photobleaching.

Special Populations: Pregnant Women: There are no adequate and well-controlled studies in pregnant women. VISUDYNE should be used during pregnancy only if the benefit justifies the potential risk to the fetus.

Teratogenic Effects: Rat fetuses of dams administered verteporfin for injection intravenously at ≥10 mg/kg/day during organogenesis (approximately 40-fold the human exposure at 6 mg/m² based on AUC_{inf} in female rats) exhibit an increase in the incidence of anophthalmia/microphthalmia. Rat fetuses of dams administered 25 mg/kg/day (approximately 125-fold the human exposure at 6 mg/m² based on AUC_{inf} in female rats) had an increased incidence of wavy ribs and fetal alterations.

In pregnant rabbits, a decrease in body weight gain and food consumption was observed in animals that received verteporfin for injection intravenously at 10 mg/kg/day during organogenesis. The no observed adverse effect level (NOAEL) for maternal toxicity was 3 mg/kg/day (approximately 7-fold the human exposure at 6 mg/m² based on body surface area). There were no teratogenic effects observed in rabbits at doses up to 10 mg/kg/day.

Nursing Women: Verteporfin and its diacid metabolite have been found in the breast milk of one woman after a 6 mg/m² infusion. The verteporfin breast milk levels were up to 66% of the corresponding plasma levels and declined below the limit of quantification (2 ng/mL) within 24 hours. The diacid metabolite had lower peak concentrations but persisted up to at least 48 hours. Because the effects of verteporfin and its metabolite on neonates are unknown, either nursing should be interrupted or treatment postponed, taking into account the risks of delayed treatment to the mother. Women should not nurse for 96 hours after Visudyne Therapy.

Pediatrics: Safety and effectiveness in pediatric patients have not been established.

Geriatrics: Approximately 90% of the patients treated with VISUDYNE in the clinical efficacy trials were over the age of 65. A reduced treatment effect was seen with increasing age.

ADVERSE REACTIONS: Adverse Drug Reaction Overview: Because clinical trials are conducted under very specific conditions the adverse drug reaction rates observed in the clinical trials may not reflect the rates observed in practice and should not be compared to the rates in the clinical trials of another drug. Adverse drug reaction information from clinical trials is useful for identifying drug-related adverse events and for approximating rates.

In randomized clinical trials in choroidal neovascularization, mainly in patients with agerelated macular degeneration (AMD), the most frequently reported adverse events to VISUDYNE (verteporfin for injection) are injection site reactions (including pain, edema, inflammation, extravasation, rashes, and less commonly, hemorrhage and discoloration) and visual disturbances (including blurred vision, flashes of light, decreased visual acuity and visual field defects such as grey or dark haloes, scotoma and black spots). These events occurred in approximately 10-30% of AMD patients.

Severe vision decrease, equivalent of 4 lines or more, within 7 days has been reported in approximately 1-5% of AMD patients. At least partial recovery of vision, defined as more than one line improvement of vision following the event, occurred in most patients (approximately 75% of patients).

Photosensitivity reactions usually occurred in the form of skin sunburn following exposure to sunlight during the first 2 days after treatment usually within 24 hours of VISUDYNE infusion. The higher incidence of back pain in the VISUDYNE group occurred primarily during infusion and was not associated with any evidence of hemolysis or allergic reaction and usually resolved by the end of the infusion.

Vaso-vagal and hypersensitivity reactions can occur, which on rare occasions can be severe. See information under Warnings and Precautions, Cardiovascular, and Immune.

Clinical Trial Adverse Drug Reactions: Table 1 describes adverse events associated with treatment (Adverse Drug Reactions) that occurred with a frequency equal to or greater than 1 percent, in the pivotal 24-month study populations supporting the three indications.

Less Common Clinical Trial Adverse Drug Reactions (<1%): The following describes adverse events associated with treatment (Adverse Drug Reactions) that occurred with a frequency of less than one percent, in the pivotal 24-Month study predominantly classic study population. No ADRs <1% occurred in patients with pathologic myopia and ocular histoplasmosis. The ADRs with an asterisk (*) are those that also occurred in patients who received placebo.

In patients with AMD treated with VISUDYNE, systemic ADRs that occurred in one patient only (<1%) were abdominal pain*, accidental injury, chest pain, chills, chills and fever, flu syndrome*, abnormal lab test*, tachycardia, diarrhea*, dyspepsia*, gastrointestinal carcinoma, hepatomegaly, stomach ulcer hemorrhage, tongue disorder, hypothyroidism, basophilia, blood dyscrasia, leukocytosis, leukopenia, lymphocytosis, diabetes mellitus, gout, hyperglycemia*, hypoglycemia, hypokalemia*, arthralgia*, depression*, hypertonia, neuralgia, vertigo, increased cough*, pharyngitis*, eczema, skin discoloration, dysuria, metrorrhagia, and frequent urination.

ADRs <1% occurring in the ocular treatment site were AMD progression*, dry eyes*, lacrimation disorder, subretinal hemorrhage, and vitreous disorder.

ADRs <1% occurring in the other eye were cataract, lacrimation disorder, photophobia*, and decreased vision.

The following have also been reported in other clinical trials: retinal detachment (nonrhegmatogenous), retinal or choroidal vessel nonperfusion, severe vision decrease with or without subretinal or vitreous hemorrhage, and severe vision decrease with retinal hemorrhage.

Clinical Trial Adverse Events (AEs): Table 2 describes all adverse events, whether or not considered related to the treatment that occurred with a frequency equal to or greater than one percent, in the pooled pivotal 24-month study populations.

Table 1: VISUDYNE

Summary of Associated Treatment-Emergent Adverse Events Occurring with Incidence ≥1% (Predominantly Classic CNV due to AMD from the TAP Studies, CNV due to PM from the VIP PM Study, and CNV due to OHS from the VOH Study)

	% of Patients				
	BPD OCR 002 A+B (AMD)		BPD OCR 003 (PM)		BPD OCR 004 (OHS)
Body System: Preferred Term	VISUDYNE (N=159) %	Placebo (N=83) %	VISUDYNE (N=81) %	Placebo (N=39) %	VISUDYNE (N=26) %
Any Associated Event	49.1	37.3	30.9	33.3	34.6
Body as a Whole					
Allergic reaction			1.2		
Asthenia	2.5		4.9		
Body odor			1.2		
Fever	1.3				
Headache	5.7	10.8	4.9	7.7	3.8
Infusion related back pain	3.1		1.2		
Injection site discoloration	1.3		1.2		
Injection site edema	8.2		2.5		
Injection site extravasation	8.2	4.8	2.5	2.6	11.5
Injection site hemorrhage	2.5		1.2		
Injection site hypersensitivity	1.3				
Injection site inflammation	3.8		2.5		
Injection site pain	9.4		6.2	2.6	
Injection site reaction					3.8
Pain	3.1				3.8
Photosensitivity reaction	2.5		3.7		
Cardiovascular System					
Hypertension	1.9		1.2		
Syncope					3.8
Digestive System					
Constipation	1.9				
Nausea	1.9	2.4	1.2		
Hemic and Lymphatic System					
Anemia	1.3	1.2			
Eosinophilia	1.3				
Metabolic and Nutritional Disorders					
Creatinine Increased	1.3	1.2			
Glycosuria	1.9				
Hypercholesteremia	1.9				
Ketosis	1.3	2.4			
Musculoskeletal System					
Arthralgia					3.8
Nervous System					
Dizziness	1.3	1.2			
Hypesthesia	1.9				
Respiratory System					
Dyspnea	1.3		1.2		
Skin and Appendages					
Pruritus			2.5	2.6	3.8
Rash	1.3				

(cont'd)

Table 1: VISUDYNE *(cont'd)*

Summary of Associated Treatment-Emergent Adverse Events Occurring with Incidence ≥1% (Predominantly Classic CNV due to AMD from the TAP Studies, CNV due to PM from the VIP PM Study, and CNV due to OHS from the VOH Study)

Body System: Preferred Term	% of Patients				
	BPD OCR 002 A+B (AMD)		BPD OCR 003 (PM)		BPD OCR 004 (OHS)
	VISUDYNE (N=159) %	Placebo (N=83) %	VISUDYNE (N=81) %	Placebo (N=39) %	VISUDYNE (N=26) %
Skin disorder			1.2		
Urticaria			1.2		
Special Senses[a]					
Eye disorder			1.2		
Photophobia			2.5		
Vision abnormal			1.2		
Vision decreased			1.2		
Treatment Site Ocular[b]					
Cataract	1.3				
Conjunctivitis	2.5	3.6	2.5		
Dry eyes			1.2		
Eye disorder			1.2		
Eye pain	3.8	2.4			
Face edema			1.2	2.6	
Photophobia	1.3	1.2	2.5		
Retinal disorder					3.8
Vision abnormal	3.1	3.6	3.7		7.7
Vision decreased	5.0	1.2	11.1	10.3	3.8
Visual field defect	4.4	1.2	3.7	5.1	3.8

[a] Special Senses includes events in the untreated ("other") eye.
[b] Treatment Site-Ocular includes ocular treatment site (study eye) events.

Table 2: VISUDYNE

Summary of Not Associated Treatment-Emergent Adverse Events Occurring with Incidence ≥1% (Predominantly Classic CNV due to AMD from the TAP Studies, CNV due to PM from the VIP PM Study, and CNV due to OHS from the VOH Study)

Body System: Preferred Term	VISUDYNE (N=266) %	Placebo (N=122) %
Any Not Associated Event	84.2	81.1
Body As a Whole		
Infection	12.8	9.0
Flu syndrome	10.2	2.5
Pain	8.6	6.6
Accidental injury	7.5	10.7
Headache	5.6	11.5
Back pain	4.9	6.6
Chest pain	3.8	2.5
Abdominal pain	3.4	4.1
Asthenia	3.0	2.5
Allergic reaction	2.6	4.1
Fever	2.6	1.6
Viral infection	1.5	0.8
Cyst	1.1	
Hernia	1.1	
Cardiovascular System		
Hypertension	7.1	8.2

(cont'd)

Table 2: VISUDYNE *(cont'd)*

Summary of Not Associated Treatment-Emergent Adverse Events Occurring with Incidence ≥1% (Predominantly Classic CNV due to AMD from the TAP Studies, CNV due to PM from the VIP PM Study, and CNV due to OHS from the VOH Study)

Body System: Preferred Term	VISUDYNE (N=266) %	Placebo (N=122) %
Cardiovascular disorder	2.6	0.8
Syncope	2.3	
Myocardial infarct	1.9	1.6
Angina pectoris	1.5	1.6
Arrhythmia	1.5	0.8
Arteriosclerosis	1.5	1.6
Coronary artery disorder	1.5	1.6
Peripheral vascular disorder	1.5	0.8
Pulmonary embolus	1.1	
Digestive System		
Nausea	3.8	5.7
Gastrointestinal disorder	2.6	3.3
Diarrhea	2.3	3.3
Cholecystitis	1.9	0.8
Gastrointestinal carcinoma	1.5	
Cholelithiasis	1.1	
Constipation	1.1	
Gastroenteritis	1.1	1.6
Tooth disorder	1.1	0.8
Endocrine System		
Hypothyroidism	1.9	0.8
Hyperthyroidism	1.1	0.8
Metabolic and Nutritional Disorders		
Hypercholesteremia	6.4	7.4
Creatinine increased	3.4	1.6
Peripheral edema	3.4	4.1
Glycosuria	2.6	1.6
Albuminuria	2.3	1.6
Ketosis	1.9	4.1
AST increased	1.5	
Alkaline phosphatase increased	1.1	2.5
Hyperkalemia	1.1	0.8
Musculoskeletal System		
Arthritis	4.5	4.9
Arthralgia	3.0	6.6
Myalgia	1.9	3.3
Arthrosis	1.1	1.6
Bone disorder	1.1	2.5
Nervous System		
Depression	4.9	3.3
Dizziness	4.5	3.3
Insomnia	2.6	0.8
Anxiety	2.3	0.8
Sleep disorder	2.3	
Vertigo	1.5	1.6
Cerebrovascular accident	1.1	0.8

(cont'd)

Table 2: VISUDYNE *(cont'd)*

Summary of Not Associated Treatment-Emergent Adverse Events Occurring with Incidence ≥1% (Predominantly Classic CNV due to AMD from the TAP Studies, CNV due to PM from the VIP PM Study, and CNV due to OHS from the VOH Study)

Body System: Preferred Term	VISUDYNE (N=266) %	Placebo (N=122) %
Respiratory System		
Bronchitis	6.8	3.3
Sinusitis	4.9	4.9
Pharyngitis	4.5	3.3
Cough increased	4.1	1.6
Rhinitis	3.4	2.5
Dyspnea	1.9	2.5
Lung disorder	1.9	1.6
Pneumonia	1.9	1.6
Emphysema	1.1	1.6
Skin and Appendages		
Rash	3.8	0.8
Skin ulcer	1.5	1.6
Skin disorder	1.1	0.8
Sweating	1.1	
Special Senses[a]		
Conjunctivitis	6.4	4.1
Cataract	5.6	4.9
Vision decreased	4.1	0.8
AMD progression	3.4	7.4
Vision abnormal	3.0	3.3
Corneal lesion	2.3	0.8
Eye disorder	2.3	2.5
Eye pain	2.3	
Glaucoma	2.3	4.1
Dry eyes	1.9	0.8
Eye itching	1.9	0.8
Blepharitis	1.5	1.6
Otitis media	1.5	1.6
Corneal opacity	1.1	
Diplopia	1.1	
Vitreous disorder	1.1	0.8
Treatment Site Ocular[b]		
Cataract	12.0	9.0
Vision abnormal	8.6	7.4
Vision decreased	5.6	4.9
Conjunctivitis	5.3	4.1
Corneal lesion	3.4	0.8
Visual field defect	3.0	1.6
Eye itching	2.6	0.8
Eye pain	2.3	1.6
Glaucoma	2.3	3.3
Blepharitis	1.9	1.6
Dry eyes	1.9	0.8
Vitreous disorder	1.9	1.6
Eye disorder	1.5	0.8

(cont'd)

Table 2: VISUDYNE *(cont'd)*

Summary of Not Associated Treatment-Emergent Adverse Events Occurring with Incidence ≥1% (Predominantly Classic CNV due to AMD from the TAP Studies, CNV due to PM from the VIP PM Study, and CNV due to OHS from the VOH Study)

Body System: Preferred Term	VISUDYNE (N=266) %	Placebo (N=122) %
AMD progression	1.1	
Keratitis	1.1	
Lacrimation disorder	1.1	2.5
Urogenital System		
Cystitis	3.8	1.6
Prostatic disorder	3.8	0.8
Prostatic carcinoma	1.1	
Prostatic specific antigen increase	1.1	
Urinary tract infection	1.1	6.6
Vaginal hemorrhage	1.1	0.8

[a] Special Senses includes events in the untreated ("other") eye.
[b] Treatment Site-Ocular includes ocular treatment site (study eye) events.

Based on long-term experience in patients receiving open-label Visudyne treatment beyond the 24-month placebo-controlled phase (TAP 60-Months extension study), no additional safety concern was identified.

Based on long-term experience in patients receiving open-label Visudyne treatment beyond the 24-month placebo-controlled phase for pathologic myopia (VIP-60-Month extension study where 54 of 67 patients completed the study, or presumed ocular histoplasmosis (VOH 48-Month extension study where 15 of 17 patients completed the study), no additional safety concern was identified.

Post-Market Adverse Drug Reactions: Other adverse drug reactions that have been reported include chest and back pain (which may radiate to other areas including but not limited to pelvis, shoulder girdle or rib cage) and other musculoskeletal pain during infusion. Vaso-vagal and hypersensitivity reactions have occurred, which on rare occasions have been severe. General symptoms can include headache, malaise, syncope, sweating, dizziness, rash, urticaria, pruritus, dyspnea, flushing and changes in blood pressure or heart rate.

Rare cases of retinal pigment epithelial tear have been reported.

Rare cases of complete retinal tear, including complete retinal tear have been reported.

DRUG INTERACTIONS: Overview: Drug interaction studies in humans have not been conducted with VISUDYNE (verteporfin for injection).

Verteporfin is rapidly eliminated by the liver, mainly as unchanged drug. Metabolism is limited and occurs by liver and plasma esterases. Microsomal cytochrome P450 does not appear to play a role in verteporfin metabolism.

Drug-Drug Interactions: Based on the mechanism of action of verteporfin, many drugs used concomitantly could influence the effect of Visudyne Therapy. Possible examples include the following: calcium channel blockers, polymyxin B or radiation therapy. These could enhance the rate of VISUDYNE uptake by the vascular endothelium. Other photosensitizing agents (e.g., tetracyclines, sulfonamides, phenothiazines, sulfonylurea hypoglycemic agents, thiazide diuretics and griseofulvin) could increase the potential for skin photosensitivity reactions.

Compounds that quench active oxygen species or scavenge radicals, such as dimethyl sulfoxide, β-carotene, ethanol, formate and mannitol, would be expected to decrease VISUDYNE activity. Drugs that decrease clotting, vasoconstriction or platelet aggregation, e.g., thromboxane A2 inhibitors, could also decrease the efficacy of Visudyne Therapy.

Drug-Food Interactions: Interactions with food have not been established.

Drug-Herb Interactions: Interactions with herbal products have not been established.

Drug-Laboratory Test Interactions: Interactions with laboratory tests have not been established.

DOSAGE AND ADMINISTRATION: Dosing and Treatment Considerations:

- A course of Visudyne Therapy is a two-step process requiring administration of both drug and light.
- The first step is the intravenous infusion of VISUDYNE (verteporfin for injection).
- The second step is the activation of VISUDYNE with light from a nonthermal diode laser.
- The physician should re-evaluate the patient every 3 months and if choroidal neovascular leakage is detected on fluorescein angiography, therapy should be repeated.
- The average number of treatments needed declines over time.

Concurrent Bilateral Treatment: The controlled trials only allowed treatment of one eye per patient. In patients who present with eligible lesions in both eyes, physicians should evaluate the potential benefits and risks of treating both eyes concurrently. If the patient has already received previous Visudyne Therapy in one eye with an acceptable safety profile, both eyes can be treated concurrently after a single administration of VISUDYNE. The more aggressive lesion should be treated first, at 15 minutes after the start of infusion. Immediately at the end of light application to the first eye, the laser settings should be adjusted to introduce the treatment parameters for the second eye, with the same light dose and intensity as for the first eye, starting no later than 20 minutes from the start of infusion.

In patients who present for the first time with eligible lesions in both eyes without prior Visudyne Therapy, it is prudent to treat only one eye (the most aggressive lesion) at the first course. One week after the first course, if no significant safety issues were identified, the second eye can be treated using the same treatment regimen after a second VISUDYNE infusion. Approximately 3 months later, both eyes can be evaluated and concurrent treatment following a new VISUDYNE infusion can be started if both lesions still show evidence of leakage.

Lesion Size Determination: The greatest linear dimension (GLD) of the lesion is estimated by fluorescein angiography and color fundus photography. All classic and occult CNV, blood and/or blocked fluorescence, and any serous detachments of the retinal pigment epithelium should be included for this measurement. Fundus cameras with magnification within the range of 2.4-2.6× are recommended. The GLD of the lesion on the fluorescein angiogram must be corrected for the magnification of the fundus camera to obtain the GLD of the lesion on the retina.

Spot Size Determination: The treatment spot size should be 1000 microns larger than the GLD of the lesion on the retina to allow a 500 micron border, ensuring full coverage of the lesion. The maximum spot size used in the clinical trials was 6400 microns.

The nasal edge of the treatment spot must be positioned at least 200 microns from the temporal edge of the optic disc, even if this will result in lack of photoactivation of CNV within 200 microns of the optic nerve. For treatment of lesions that are larger than the maximum treatment spot size, apply the light to the greatest possible area of active lesion.

Recommended Dose and Dosage Adjustment: The Visudyne dose is 6 mg/m² body surface area, diluted in 30 mL infusion solution, given by a 10-minute intravenous infusion.

Administration: Drug Administration: VISUDYNE should be reconstituted according to the directions given under Reconstitution.

The volume of reconstituted VISUDYNE required to achieve the desired dose of 6 mg/m² body surface area is withdrawn from the vial and diluted with 5% Dextrose for Injection to a total infusion volume of 30 mL. The full infusion volume is administered intravenously over 10 minutes at a rate of 3 mL/minute, using an appropriate syringe pump and in-line filter. The clinical studies were conducted using a standard infusion line filter of 1.2 microns.

Precautions should be taken to prevent extravasation at the injection site. If extravasation occurs, protect the site from light (see Warnings and Precautions, General).

Light Administration: Initiate 689 nm wavelength laser light delivery to the patient 15 minutes after the start of the 10-minute infusion with VISUDYNE.

Photoactivation of VISUDYNE is controlled by the total light dose delivered. In the treatment of choroidal neovascularization, the recommended light dose is 50 J/cm² of neovascular lesion administered at an intensity of 600 mW/cm². This dose is administered over 83 seconds.

Light dose, light intensity, ophthalmic lens magnification factor and zoom lens setting are important parameters for the appropriate delivery of light to the predetermined treatment spot. Follow the laser system manuals for procedure set up and operation.

The laser system must be acceptable for the delivery of a stable power output at a wavelength of 689±3 nm. Light is delivered to the retina as a single circular spot via a fiber optic and a slit lamp, using a suitable ophthalmic magnification lens.

The following laser systems have been tested for compatibility with VISUDYNE and are acceptable for the delivery of a stable power output at a wavelength of 689±3 nm:

- Lumenis Opal Photoactivator laser console and modified LaserLink adapter, distributed by Coherent-AMT, 15-550 Trillium Drive, Kitchener, Ontario, Canada N2R 1K3,
- Zeiss VISULAS 690s laser and VISULINK PDT adapter, distributed by Carl Zeiss Canada Ltd., 45 Valleybrook Drive, Toronto, Ontario M3B 2S6.

Reconstitution: Parenteral Products:

Vial Size	Volume of Diluent to be Added to Vial	Approximate Available Volume	Nominal Concentration per mL
15 mg	Sterile Water for Injection, 7.0 mL	7.5 mL	2 mg/mL

Reconstituted VISUDYNE must be stored at 20-25EC, protected from light and used within 4 hours. It is recommended that reconstituted VISUDYNE be inspected visually for particulate matter and discoloration prior to administration. Reconstituted VISUDYNE is an opaque dark green solution. Discard the unused portion.

Incompatibilities: VISUDYNE should only be reconstituted with sterile Water for Injection. Do not mix VISUDYNE in the same solution with other drugs. VISUDYNE may precipitate in saline solutions. Do not use normal saline or other parenteral solutions.

Dilution for Intravenous Infusion: Once reconstituted VISUDYNE is diluted with 5% Dextrose Injection, it should preferably be used immediately, but not exceeding 4 hours. As with all parenteral drug products, intravenous admixtures should be inspected visually for clarity, particulate matter, precipitate, discoloration, and leakage prior to administration whenever solution and container permit. Solutions showing haziness, particulate matter, precipitate, discoloration, or leakage should not be used.

OVERDOSAGE:

Overdose of drug and/or light in the treated eye may result in nonperfusion of normal retinal vessels with the possibility of severe decrease in vision that could be permanent. An overdose of drug will also result in the prolongation of the period during which the patient remains photosensitive to bright light. In such cases, it is recommended to extend the photosensitivity precautions for a time proportional to the overdose.

> For management of a suspected drug overdose, CPhA recommends that you contact your **regional Poison Control Centre**. See the *CPS* Directory section for a list of Poison Control Centres.

ACTION AND CLINICAL PHARMACOLOGY: Pharmacodynamics: Verteporfin is transported in the plasma primarily by lipoproteins. Once verteporfin is activated by light in the presence of oxygen, highly reactive, short-lived singlet oxygen and reactive oxygen radicals are generated. Light activation of verteporfin results in local damage to neovascular endothelium, resulting in vessel occlusion. Damaged endothelium is known to release procoagulant and vasoactive factors through the lipo-oxygenase (leukotriene) and cyclo-oxygenase (eicosanoids such as thromboxane) pathways, resulting in platelet aggregation, fibrin clot formation and vasoconstriction. Verteporfin appears to preferentially accumulate in neovasculature, including choroidal neovasculature. However, animal models indicate that the drug is also present in the retina. Therefore, there may be collateral damage to retinal structures following photoactivation including the retinal pigmented epithelium and outer nuclear layer of the retina. The temporary occlusion of choroidal neovascularization (CNV) following Visudyne Therapy has been confirmed in humans by fluorescein angiography.

Pharmacokinetics: Following intravenous infusion, verteporfin exhibits bi-exponential elimination with a terminal elimination half-life of approximately 5-6 hours. The extent of exposure and the maximal plasma concentration are proportional to the dose between 6 and 20 mg/m².

Metabolism: Verteporfin is metabolized to a small extent to its diacid metabolite by liver and plasma esterases. NADPH dependent liver enzyme systems (including the cytochrome P450 isozymes) do not appear to play a role in the metabolism of verteporfin.

Excretion: Elimination is by the fecal route, with less than 0.01% of the dose recovered in urine.

Special Populations and Conditions: Gender: At the intended dose, pharmacokinetic parameters are not significantly affected by gender.

Hepatic Insufficiency: In a study of patients with mild hepatic insufficiency (defined as having two abnormal hepatic function tests at enrolment), AUC and C_{max} were not significantly different from the control group, half-life however was significantly increased by approximately 20%.

Renal Insufficiency: No data is available. Elimination is by the fecal route, with less than 0.01% of the dose recovered in urine.

STORAGE AND STABILITY: Store VISUDYNE between 20 and 25°C.

SPECIAL HANDLING INSTRUCTIONS: Spills and Disposal: Spills of VISUDYNE should be wiped up with a damp cloth. Skin and eye contact should be avoided due to the potential for photosensitivity reactions upon exposure to light. Use of rubber gloves and eye protection is recommended. All materials should be disposed of properly.

Accidental Exposure: Because of the potential to induce photosensitivity reactions, it is important to avoid contact with the eyes and skin during preparation and administration of VISUDYNE. Any exposed person must be protected from bright light (see Warnings and Precautions).

INFORMATION FOR THE PATIENT: Published in e-CPS, available by subscription at www.e-cps.ca.

DOSAGE FORMS, COMPOSITION AND PACKAGING: Each vial of dark green to black lyophilized cake contains: verteporfin 15 mg. After reconstitution, each mL of solution for i.v. use contains: verteporfin 2 mg. The product is intended for i.v. injection only. Nonmedicinal ingredients: ascorbyl palmitate, butylated hydroxytoluene, dimyristoyl phosphatidylcholine, egg phosphatidylglycerol and lactose. Single-use glass vial of 15 mg, with a gray bromobutyl stopper and aluminum flip-off cap.

Vita 3B

vitamin B complex

Vitamin Supplement

Riva

Vita 3B+C

vitamin B complex—ascorbic acid

Vitamin Supplement

Riva

SUPPLIED: Vita 3B: Each red, film-coated tablet contains: thiamine HCl (B_1) 250 mg, pyridoxine HCl (B_6) 125 mg and cyanocobalamin (B_{12}) 250 µg. Nonmedicinal ingredients: carnauba wax, cellulose, colloidal silicone, FD&C Red, FD&C Yellow, hydroxypropyl methylcellulose, magnesium stearate, polyethylene glycol, polysorbate 80, polyvinylpyrrolidone, starch, stearic acid and titanium dioxide. Gluten-, sucrose-, tartrazine-free. Bottles of 50 and 300.

Vita 3B+C: Each yellow, film-coated tablet contains: thiamine HCl (B_1) 250 mg, pyridoxine HCl (B_6) 125 mg, cyanocobalamin (B_{12}) 250 µg and ascorbic acid (C) 250 mg. Nonmedicinal ingredients: carnauba wax, cellulose, colloidal silicone, D&C Yellow, hydroxypropyl methylcellulose, iron oxide, magnesium stearate, polyethylene glycol, polysorbate 80, polyvinylpyrrolidone, starch and titanium dioxide. Gluten-, sucrose-, tartrazine-free. Bottles of 50 and 300.

Vitalux® AREDS

multiple vitamins and minerals

Multivitamin—Multimineral Supplement

Novartis Pharmaceuticals

SUPPLIED: Each time-release tablet contains: beta-carotene (provitamin A) 12 500 IU (7.5 mg), vitamin C (ascorbic acid) 250 mg, vitamin E (d-alpha tocopheryl acetate) 200 IU, zinc (gluconate) 40 mg, copper (HVP: Hydrolyzed Vegetable Protein chelate) 1 mg, in a nonmedicinal base containing lutein 3 mg (supplying 132 µg of zeaxanthin), calcium silicate, caramel colour, carnauba wax, diacetylated monoglycerides, dicalcium phosphate, ethyl vanillin, hydroxypropyl cellulose, hydroxypropyl methylcellulose, microcrystalline cellulose, polyethylene glycol, polysorbate 80, stearic acid, titanium dioxide, vegetable magnesium stearate, xanthan gum. Bottles of 50.

Vitalux®-S

multiple vitamins and minerals

Multivitamin—Multimineral Supplement

Novartis Pharmaceuticals

SUPPLIED: Each time-release tablet contains: vitamin C (ascorbic acid) 250 mg, vitamin E (d-alpha tocopheryl acetate) 200 IU, zinc (gluconate) 40 mg, copper (HVP: Hydrolyzed Vegetable Protein chelate) 1 mg, in a nonmedicinal base containing lutein 3 mg (supplying 132 µg of zeaxanthin), hypromellose, cellulose, vegetable magnesium stearate, calcium silicate. Bottles of 50.

Vitalux® Time Release

multiple vitamins and minerals

Multivitamin—Multimineral Supplement

Novartis Pharmaceuticals

SUPPLIED: Each time-release tablet contains: beta-carotene (provitamin A) 10 000 IU, vitamin C (ascorbic acid) 300 mg, vitamin E (d-alpha tocopheryl acetate) 100 IU, vitamin B_2 (riboflavin) 20 mg, selenium (HVP: Hydrolyzed Vegetable Protein chelate) 50 µg, zinc (gluconate) 40 mg, copper (HVP chelate) 2 mg, in a nonmedicinal base containing lutein 4 mg (supplying 176 µg of zeaxanthin), acetylated monoglycerides, calcium silicate, caramel color, ethyl vanillin, hydroxypropyl cellulose, hydroxypropyl methylcellulose, microcrystalline cellulose, montan wax, polyethylene glycol, polysorbate 80, purified stearic acid, purified water, silicon dioxide, titanium dioxide, vegetable magnesium stearate and xanthan powder. Ethanol-, gluten-, lactose-, sulfite- and tartrazine-free. Bottles of 50.

Vitamin A

Vitamin

CPhA Monograph

Date of Revision: October 2009

> This monograph has been compiled by CPhA and reviewed by experts. It may contain information different from that found in Health Canada-approved Product Monographs. The reader is referred to the *CPS* Editorial Policy for more information.

SUMMARY PRODUCT INFORMATION:

Drug	Route of Administration	Dosage Form	Strength
Vitamin A	Oral	Capsule	1000 units, 5000 units, 10 000 units
Beta-Carotene	Oral	Capsule or Tablet	10 000 units, 25 000 units

PHARMACOLOGY: The term vitamin A is applied to a number of substances with similar structure and activity. The principal and most active substance is all-trans retinol (vitamin A alcohol), but beta-carotene and retinal (vitamin A aldehyde) also possess effective and reliable vitamin A activity. Plant-based carotenoids (e.g., beta-carotene, alpha-carotene, beta-cryptoxanthin) are less easily absorbed by the body than retinol; thus, a higher dietary intake of these substances is needed to provide equivalent vitamin A activity. Vitamin A activity is assayed biologically and is measured in retinol activity equivalents (RAE). One RAE is equivalent to 1 µg retinol, 2 µg of beta-carotene in supplement form, 12 µg of dietary beta-carotene or 24 µg of other dietary carotenoids. Supplement dosages are usually expressed in units: 1 unit = 0.3 µg RAE.

Exogenous sources of vitamin A are required for growth and bone development, vision, immune function, reproduction, and maintenance of the integrity of mucosal and epithelial surfaces. Vitamin A also plays a role in the regulation of gene expression.

Retinal and retinol are in chemical equilibrium in the body and possess equivalent antixerophthalmic activity. Dietary vitamin A deficiency is a major cause of blindness in children in some developing countries. In developed areas, deficiency is rare in the absence of concurrent illness such as liver disease or intestinal malabsorption. Night blindness is the earliest symptom of deficiency, followed by degenerative changes in the retina such as xerophthalmia and keratomalacia. Vitamin A deficiency is a known risk factor for severe measles infections.

Pharmacokinetics: Vitamin A is a fat-soluble vitamin and is readily absorbed from the normal gastrointestinal tract. Absorption is impaired in the presence of hepatic or pancreatic disease or in patients with low protein intake. Plasma concentrations peak within 3 to 5 hours. Beta-carotene is converted to retinal, which is mostly reduced to retinol. Some retinol is esterified, mainly to retinyl palmitate which is stored in the liver along with small amounts of retinol and retinal. Normal plasma concentration is approximately 1.4 µmol/L (130 units/100 mL). Retinyl esters are released from the liver bound to retinol-binding protein. Body stores of vitamin A are normally sufficient to meet the body's needs for up to 2 years. Retinol in the circulation is conjugated with glucuronic acid, further oxidized and excreted in the urine and feces.

INDICATIONS: Prophylaxis and treatment of vitamin A deficiency.

Vitamin A has been used to measure fat absorption. Fasting serum vitamin A levels are measured before and 4 hours after an oral dose of 2100 RAE/kg of oil-soluble vitamin A. Patients with normal fat absorption will have an increase of 1 µg/mL or more in their fasting vitamin A level.

Vitamin A has been used to treat rare forms of retinitis pigmentosa associated with abetalipoproteinemia (Bassen-Kornzweig syndrome).

A review of vitamin A treatment in children with measles found that two high doses of vitamin A reduced overall and pneumonia-specific mortality in children less than 2 years of age. Some experts recommend vitamin A be given to children aged 6 months to 2 years who are hospitalized with measles and its complications, and in children with measles who show ophthalmic signs of vitamin A deficiency.

There is no conclusive evidence to support use of vitamin A in the prevention of cancer. High doses of beta-carotene supplements have been associated with increased incidence of lung cancer in men (see Warnings).

Synthetic retinoid analogues are used orally (isotretinoin, acitretin) or topically (tretinoin, adapalene, tazarotene) to treat acne and certain other skin disorders. Oral tretinoin is also used for induction of remission in acute promyelocytic leukemia.

CONTRAINDICATIONS: Hypervitaminosis A; hypersensitivity to vitamin A or any component of a vitamin A-containing pharmaceutical preparation. Doses exceeding the recommended daily allowance (RDA) are contraindicated in pregnancy.

WARNINGS: See Precautions.

Some studies have shown an increased incidence of lung cancer in men taking high-dose beta-carotene supplements, with or without vitamin A.

PRECAUTIONS: In physiologic doses, vitamin A is relatively nontoxic. Prolonged use of dosages greater than 7500 µg RAE (25 000 units) may lead to symptoms of chronic toxicity such as bone and joint pain, hair loss, anorexia and hepatosplenomegaly.

Excessive consumption of vitamin A supplements or foods rich in beta-carotene such as carrots may cause carotenemia and yellow discoloration of the skin. The same effect may result from defective utilization of vitamin A precursors in patients with diabetes mellitus or myxedema.

Retinol consumption ≥10 000 units from fish has been associated with lower bone density and a higher hip fracture rate.

Drug Interactions: Vitamin A should not be used concurrently with oral retinoids (e.g., tretinoin, isotretinoin, acitretin) because of possible additive toxicity.

Significant increases in plasma vitamin A concentrations have been demonstrated in women taking oral contraceptives.

Excessive use of mineral oil as a laxative may reduce the utilization of the provitamin by carrying away large amounts in the feces.

Cholestyramine can bind to and impair absorption of fat-soluble vitamins including vitamin A.

Orlistat decreases the absorption of fat-soluble vitamins including vitamin A. Supplementation with a standard multiple vitamin preparation is sometimes recommended during orlistat therapy. To avoid interference with vitamin absorption, doses of orlistat and fat-soluble vitamins should be separated by at least 2 hours.

Large doses of vitamin A may increase the hypoprothrombinemic effect of warfarin.

Pregnancy: Vitamin A is teratogenic in animals. Although pregnant women require adequate vitamin A, they should not exceed a daily supplement of 3300 units. Excessive intake of vitamin A during pregnancy may be a potential hazard to the mother and fetus. Effective measures to avoid pregnancy are necessary with high dose vitamin A therapy.

Oral retinoids (isotretinoin, tretinoin, acitretin) are contraindicated during pregnancy. There is an extremely high risk that major fetal abnormalities will result if pregnancy occurs during treatment with these drugs.

Lactation: Vitamin A is distributed into milk. Hypervitaminosis is a theoretical possibility, but this normally does not occur with normal maternal daily doses.

ADVERSE EFFECTS: See Overdose.

OVERDOSE:

Symptoms: The amount required to cause toxicity will vary among individuals. The manifestations of toxicity will depend on the patient's age and hepatic function, and on the dose and duration of administration.

Acute toxicity, i.e., single ingestion of 7500 µg RAE/kg (25 000 units/kg) or more: Signs and symptoms may be delayed for 8 to 24 hours and include: increased intracranial pressure, headache, irritability, drowsiness, dizziness, lethargy, vomiting, diarrhea, bulging fontanels in infants, diplopia, papilledema. Peeling of skin around mouth may be observed from 1 to several days after ingestion and may spread to the rest of the body. Hepatotoxicity has been reported with acute ingestion of > 600 000 units.

Chronic, excessive ingestion (1200 µg RAE/kg or 4000 units/kg daily in adults for 6 to 15 months) may produce symptoms of pseudotumor cerebri, anorexia, weakness, arthralgias, bone pain, bone demineralization, dry skin, cracked lips, brittle nails, hair loss, splenomegaly, hepatomegaly, hypoplastic anemia, leukopenia, optic neuropathy, and blindness. Increased plasma concentrations of vitamin A occur but do not necessarily correlate with toxicity.

Treatment: For an acute overdose, activated charcoal should be used to achieve gastrointestinal decontamination. Treat symptomatically.

Intracranial pressure may be reduced with iv dexamethasone or iv mannitol. In untreated patients, increased intracranial pressure may persist for 4 weeks after discontinuation of vitamin A.

For chronic toxicity, discontinue vitamin A. Toxicity is slowly reversible but may persist for several weeks. Monitor blood pressure, fluids, electrolytes, CNS status, complete blood count and hepatic function.

> For management of a suspected drug overdose, CPhA recommends that you contact your **regional Poison Control Centre**. See the *CPS* Directory section for a list of Poison Control Centres.

DOSAGE: In preventing vitamin deficiency, adequate dietary intake is preferred over supplementation, whenever possible. Preformed vitamin A is found in animal products (e.g., liver, oily fish, whole eggs, dairy products) as well as in fortified foods such as cereals and margarine. Beta-carotene and other carotenoids are plant-derived and found in deep yellow and orange fruits and vegetables (e.g., apricots, cantaloupe, papaya, mangoes, carrots, sweet potatoes, pumpkin) and dark green leafy vegetables (e.g., kale, spinach).

Table 1 presents daily recommendations for vitamin A intake [*Dietary reference intakes for vitamin A, vitamin K, arsenic, boron, chromium, copper, iodine, iron, manganese, molybdenum, nickel, silicon, vanadium and zinc.* Washington (DC): National Academy Press; 2001]. There is no distinct RDA for beta-carotene and other carotenoids. Evaluate and consider vitamin A intake from dietary sources when determining appropriate supplement doses. Patients taking >25 000 units daily should be closely monitored for evidence of toxicity.

Table 1: Vitamin A

Recommended Dietary Allowance (RDA)[a] for Vitamin A

Life-Stage Group	RDA (µg Retinol Activity Equivalents per Day)
Birth to 6 months	400 µg (AI)[b]
7 to 12 months	500 µg (AI)[b]
1 to 3 years	300 µg
4 to 8 years	400 µg
9 to 13 years	600 µg
≥14 years	
Men	900 µg
Women	700 µg
Pregnancy	
≤18 years	750 µg
19 to 50 years	770 µg
Lactation	
≤18 years	1200 µg
19 to 50 years	1300 µg

[a] The RDA is the average daily dietary nutrient intake sufficient to meet the nutrient needs of nearly all healthy individuals (97 to 98%) in a particular life-stage and gender group.
[b] For all healthy infants, the Adequate Intake (AI) is used and is based on estimated mean intakes of human milk.

Treatment of Xerophthalmia: The World Health Organization suggests the following for individuals with all stages of active xerophthalmia: Children less than 6 months of age: 50 000 units immediately on diagnosis; repeat dose of 50 000 units the next day and again at least 2 weeks later. Children 6-12 months of age: 100 000 units immediately on diagnosis; repeat dose of 100 000 units the next day and again at least 2 weeks later. Patients older than 1 year: 200 000 units immediately on diagnosis; repeat dose of 200 000 units the next day and again at least 2 weeks later.

Deficiency without Corneal Changes: Infants <1 year: 10 000 units/kg/day for 5 days, then 7500 to 15 000 units/day for 10 days. Children 1 to 8 years: 5000 to 10 000 units/kg/day for 5 days, then 17 000 to 35 000 units per day for 10 days. Children >8 years and Adults: 100 000 units/day for 3 days, then 25 000 to 50 000 units per day for 14 days.

As a Supplement in Children Hospitalized with Measles and Complications: 6 months to 1 year of age, 100 000 units as a single dose; 1 to 2 years of age, 200 000 units as a single dose. If there is ophthalmologic evidence of vitamin A deficiency the dose should be repeated the next day and again after 4 weeks.

It has been suggested that persons with chronic intestinal malabsorption be given vitamin A in a water-miscible preparation as follows: Infants and children <8 years 2000 units daily; Children >8 years and Adults 10 000 to 50 000 units daily. Monitor patients for signs of toxicity.

Vitamin A Acid ℞

tretinoin

Topical Acne Therapy

sanofi-aventis

Date of Revision: October 15, 2009

PHARMACOLOGY: The interest in oral vitamin A in the treatment of acne started some 30 years ago following publication of a report by Straumfjord and theoretical support for the use of the vitamin in the reduction of hyperkeratosis came from basic science investigations. Hunter and Pinkus showed a reduction in the number of keratinocytes in the human stratum corneum during oral vitamin A therapy. Fell and Mellanby noticed a suppression of keratinization by excessive vitamin A in tissue culture. This led to the opinion that vitamin A is antikeratinizing.

Topical use of vitamin A was suggested as a means of reducing systemic toxicity from vitamin A taken orally and a number of topical forms of vitamin A were tried. Topical tretinoin was found to be the most potent because of its greater peeling action.

Topical tretinoin has a very pronounced keratolytic action according to both Von Beer and Von Stuttgen. This action has led to its use in a number of dermatological conditions. It was tried successfully by Kligman et al in the treatment of acne vulgaris since follicular hyperkeratosis is considered as being an initial stage of acne.

INDICATIONS: For topical application in the treatment of acne vulgaris, primarily Grades I, II and III in which comedones, papules and pustules predominate.

CONTRAINDICATIONS: Use should be discontinued if hypersensitivity to any of the ingredients is noted.

WARNINGS: *Pregnancy:* **Topical tretinoin should be used by women of childbearing years only after contraceptive counseling. It is recommended that topical tretinoin not be used by pregnant women.** There have been rare reports of birth defects among babies born to women exposed to topical tretinoin during pregnancy. However, there are no well controlled prospective studies of the use of topical tretinoin in pregnant women. A retrospective study of mothers exposed to topical tretinoin during the first trimester of pregnancy found no increase in the incidence of birth defects. Topical retinoid teratology studies in rats and rabbits have been inconclusive. As with all retinoids, tretinoin administered orally at high doses is teratogenic.

When applying topical tretinoin, care should be taken not to apply near the eyes, mouth, angles of the nose and mucous membranes. Topical use may cause severe local redness and peeling at the site of the application. If the degree of local irritation warrants, use the medication less frequently, discontinue use temporarily, or discontinue use completely, and consult your physician.

PRECAUTIONS: Concomitant topical medications and particularly other peeling agents should be used with caution. In case of a change of medications to topical tretinoin, it would be advisable to wait until peeling from previous medications has subsided.

Because of an increased susceptibility to sunlight in patients with sunburn, the use of a topical tretinoin is not advisable until the skin has fully recovered. Exposure to sunlight and sunlamps should be avoided or minimized during treatment with topical tretinoin because of heightened susceptibility to UV radiation as a result of the use of tretinoin.

Use of sunburn protectant products with a sun protection factor (SPF) of at least 15 and protective clothing over treated areas is recommended when exposure cannot be avoided.

ADVERSE EFFECTS: In certain very sensitive patients, the skin may get to be very erythematous, edematous, blistered or crusted. In such cases, application of topical tretinoin should be discontinued until the skin has fully recovered; further application should be at a level that the individual can tolerate. Temporary hyper- or hypopigmentation can occur with repeated application of topical tretinoin. Increased susceptibility to sunlight has been reported. All adverse reactions seem to be reversible when treatment is discontinued.

OVERDOSE:

Symptoms: Topical tretinoin if used excessively, may cause marked erythema, severe peeling of the skin and discomfort; on the other hand, excessive application may not bring more rapid or better results. Amount or frequency of application should be reduced if undesirable reactions occur.

Inadvertent oral ingestion of topical tretinoin may lead to the same adverse effects as those associated with excessive oral intake of vitamin A including teratogenesis in women of childbearing years. Therefore, in such cases, pregnancy testing should be carried out in women of childbearing years.

> For management of a suspected drug overdose, CPhA recommends that you contact your **regional Poison Control Centre**. See the *CPS* Directory section for a list of Poison Control Centres.

DOSAGE: Apply daily, preferably before retiring, where acne lesions are present, using enough of the gel to lightly cover the affected area. An exacerbation of the inflammatory lesions may take place during the early weeks of application. These result from the action of the topical tretinoin on deep and previously unseen comedones and papules. Therapeutic results should be seen after 2 to 4 weeks of treatment. Results may take 6 to 8 weeks before reaching optimal degree. Once the acne lesions have responded satisfactorily, improvement can be maintained with less frequent application.

In cases of severe erythema at an early stage of treatment, the frequency of application and amount may be reduced at the beginning of treatment and then increased progressively.

INFORMATION FOR THE PATIENT: Published in e-CPS, available by subscription at www.e-cps.ca.

SUPPLIED: Each g of gel contains: tretinoin USP 0.01%, 0.025% or 0.05%. Also contains methylparaben and propylparaben. Tubes of 25 g. Store at controlled room temperature (15 to 30°C).

Vitamin B_1

thiamine HCl

Vitamin

CPhA Monograph

Date of Revision: November 2007

> This monograph has been compiled by CPhA and reviewed by experts. It may contain information different from that found in Health Canada-approved Product Monographs. The reader is referred to the *CPS* Editorial Policy for more information.

SUMMARY PRODUCT INFORMATION:

Route of Administration[a]	Dosage Form[a]	Strength[a]
Oral	Caplet	100 mg
	Tablet	50 mg, 100 mg, 500 mg

Route of Administration[a]	Dosage Form[a]	Strength[a]
Parenteral	Injectable solution	100 mg/mL

[a] Table includes single entity vitamin B_1 products only. For specific product information consult Health Canada's Drug Product Database http://www.hc-sc.gc.ca/dhp-mps/prodpharma/databasdon/index_e.html

PHARMACOLOGY: Vitamin B_1 is a water soluble B complex vitamin. In vivo, vitamin B_1 combines with adenosine triphosphate (ATP) to form thiamine pyrophosphate, also known as cocarboxylase, a coenzyme. Its role in carbohydrate metabolism is the decarboxylation of pyruvic acid and alpha-ketoacids to acetaldehyde and carbon dioxide. Increased levels of pyruvic acid in the blood indicate vitamin B_1 deficiency.

Vitamin B_1 requirements are usually satisfied by dietary sources in patients with normal gastrointestinal absorption. Deficiency can occur in patients with malabsorption (e.g., alcoholics, GI disease, cirrhosis, diarrhea) or inadequate intake (e.g., alcoholics, severe nausea and vomiting, anorexia). Increased requirements are associated with pregnancy, increased carbohydrate intake, increased physical activity, hyperthyroidism, hepatic disease and infection.

Deficiency of vitamin B_1 eventually leads to beriberi and Wernicke's encephalopathy. The cardiovascular or nervous system, or both, may be affected. Cardiovascular involvement is manifested by high output, biventricular heart failure and edema. Neurologic symptoms include peripheral neuropathy and an encephalopathy syndrome characterized by nystagmus, ophthalmoplegia, fever, ataxia and progressive mental deterioration that can ultimately result in coma and death.

Pharmacokinetics: Orally administered vitamin B_1 is absorbed mainly from the duodenum, by both active and passive processes. The total amount that can be absorbed following administration of a large dose is 4 to 8 mg. Body stores are approximately 30 mg, with a 1 mg daily turnover. Storage of vitamin B_1 is mainly in skeletal muscle, heart, liver, kidneys and brain.

Vitamin B_1 is metabolized in the liver and renally excreted. When large doses are administered, body stores may become saturated and unchanged vitamin B_1 may be renally excreted.

INDICATIONS: Prophylaxis and treatment of vitamin B_1 deficiency states including beriberi and Wernicke's encephalopathy. Studies do not support the use of oral vitamin B_1 as a mosquito repellent.

CONTRAINDICATIONS: Hypersensitivity to vitamin B_1 or any component of a product containing vitamin B_1.

WARNINGS: See Precautions.

PRECAUTIONS: Serious sensitivity reactions can occur. Deaths have resulted from iv use. Some manufacturers recommend an intradermal test dose prior to iv administration in patients with suspected hypersensitivity.

Simple vitamin B_1 deficiency is rare. Multiple vitamin deficiencies should be suspected in any case of dietary inadequacy.

Pregnancy: No adverse effects have been reported with intake of normal daily requirements. Severe nausea and vomiting of pregnancy may lead to thiamine deficiency that could present as Wernicke's encephalopathy.

Lactation: No adverse effects have been reported with intake of normal daily requirements.

ADVERSE EFFECTS: Feeling of warmth, pruritus, urticaria, weakness, sweating, nausea, restlessness, tightness of the throat, angioneurotic edema, cyanosis, pulmonary edema, hemorrhage into the gastrointestinal tract, collapse and death have been rarely reported, mainly following repeated iv administration of the drug.

OVERDOSE:

> For management of a suspected drug overdose, CPhA recommends that you contact your **regional Poison Control Centre**. See the *CPS* Directory section for a list of Poison Control Centres.

DOSAGE: In preventing vitamin deficiencies, adequate dietary intake is preferred over supplementation whenever possible. Vitamin B_1 is found in whole-grain and enriched cereals and breads, meat (especially pork), brewer's yeast, beans and Brazil nuts.

In the treatment of deficiency, vitamin B_1 is usually administered orally. When oral administration is not feasible, when malabsorption is suspected, or in patients with Wernicke's encephalopathy or high output heart failure secondary to beriberi, vitamin B_1 may be administered im or iv Improvement in neuritis, ocular signs, ataxia, edema and heart failure should be seen a few hours after administration of vitamin B_1 and should disappear in a few days. Confusion and psychosis will respond more slowly or not at all if nerves are damaged.

Oral: Usual adult dose to treat deficiency is 5 to 30 mg daily given as a single dose or in 3 divided doses for 1 month.

Usual dose for thiamine deficiency in children who are not critically ill is 10 to 50 mg daily in divided doses.

Parenteral: Wernicke's encephalopathy and high output cardiac failure secondary to beriberi must be treated as emergencies. Critically ill patients or those with malabsorption syndromes should also be treated by the iv or im route.

The treatment of beriberi is usually 10 to 30 mg 3 times daily im or iv for 2 weeks followed by 5 to 10 mg po daily for 1 month.

In Wernicke's encephalopathy 100 mg iv is given initially followed by 50 to 100 mg im or iv daily until the patient is eating a well-balanced diet. IV dextrose solutions increase thiamine requirements and 100 mg thiamine should be given parenterally before administering these solutions to the patient with Wernicke's. Following clinical improvement and resumption of a regular diet, oral therapy may be instituted.

Vitamin B_2

riboflavin

Vitamin

CPhA Monograph

Date of Revision: October 2007

> This monograph has been compiled by CPhA and reviewed by experts. It may contain information different from that found in Health Canada-approved Product Monographs. The reader is referred to the *CPS* Editorial Policy for more information.

SUMMARY PRODUCT INFORMATION:

Route of Administration[a]	Dosage Form[a]
Oral	Component of oral multivitamin preparations
Parenteral	Component of injectable multivitamin preparations
	50 mg/mL single-entity product

[a] For specific product information consult Health Canada's Drug Product Database http://www.hc-sc.gc.ca/dhp-mps/prodpharma/databasdon/index_e.html

PHARMACOLOGY: Vitamin B_2 is a water-soluble, B complex vitamin, required for tissue respiration and indirectly involved in maintaining erythrocyte integrity.

Vitamin B_2 deficiency is associated with conditions such as alcoholism, malignancy, cardiac disease, infection, chronic diarrhea, malabsorption syndrome, diabetes mellitus and chronic debilitating diseases. Deficiency is manifested by angular stomatitis, magenta tongue, fissuring of the lips and desquamation of mucous membranes, redness and scaling of the scrotum, normocytic and normochromic anemia and neuropathy.

Pharmacokinetics: Vitamin B_2 is readily absorbed from the upper gastrointestinal tract, except in the presence of malabsorption syndromes. The extent of gastrointestinal absorption is increased when the drug is administered with food and is decreased in patients with hepatitis, cirrhosis or biliary obstruction.

Vitamin B_2 is inactive until phosphorylated to flavin mononucleotide (FMN) in gastrointestinal mucosal cells, erythrocytes and the liver; FMN is converted to another coenzyme, flavin adenine dinucleotide (FAD). Free vitamin B_2 is present in the retina. In blood, about 60% of FAD and FMN is protein bound.

The biologic half-life is about 66 to 84 minutes following oral or im administration of a single large dose in healthy individuals.

Only about 9% of the drug is excreted unchanged; the fate of the remainder is unknown. Excretion appears to involve renal tubular secretion as well as glomerular filtration. Amounts in excess of the body's needs are excreted in urine.

INDICATIONS: Prophylaxis and treatment of vitamin B_2 deficiency.

Other uses: Oral riboflavin has shown some efficacy in migraine prophylaxis but more trials are needed.

CONTRAINDICATIONS: Patients hypersensitive to any component of vitamin B_2 formulations.

WARNINGS: See Precautions.

PRECAUTIONS: *Drug Interactions:* Alcohol impairs intestinal absorption of vitamin B_2.

Phenothiazines, Tricyclic Antidepressants: These drugs may inhibit the conversion of vitamin B_2 to the active coenzyme form. Requirements for vitamin B_2 may be increased in patients receiving these drugs.

Probenecid: The extent of gastrointestinal absorption of vitamin B_2 is decreased when it is used concomitantly with probenecid.

Pregnancy: Vitamin B_2 crosses the placenta. Adverse effects have not been reported with intake of normal requirements.

Lactation: Vitamin B_2 is distributed into breast milk. The American Academy of Pediatrics considers maternal consumption of riboflavin to be compatible with breast-feeding.

ADVERSE EFFECTS: Vitamin B_2 is usually well tolerated and nontoxic. Because of its fluorescent yellow color, vitamin B_2 may cause yellow discoloration of urine. Diarrhea and gastrointestinal upset have been reported with higher doses.

OVERDOSE:

> For management of a suspected drug overdose, CPhA recommends that you contact your **regional Poison Control Centre**. See the *CPS* Directory section for a list of Poison Control Centres.

DOSAGE: In preventing vitamin deficiencies, adequate dietary intake is preferred over supplementation whenever possible. Vitamin B_2 is found in milk, meat, eggs, nuts, enriched flour and green vegetables.

Vitamin B_2 is usually given orally as a component of multivitamin preparations. It may also be given by im injection or iv infusion as a component of multivitamin injections. It is recommended that vitamin B_2 deficiency be treated with multivitamin preparations since it is often associated with other vitamin deficiencies.

The usual oral dose in the treatment of deficiency is 5 to 30 mg daily in divided doses for adults and 3 to 10 mg daily in divided doses for children. Ocular and dermatologic symptoms should improve after several days. Reticulocyte count should begin to increase within a few days in patients with normocytic or normochromic anemia.

The dose that has been used in migraine prophylaxis is 400 mg orally daily.

Vitamin B_3

CPhA Monograph

see *Niacin/Niacinamide*

Vitamin B_5

CPhA Monograph

see *Pantothenic Acid*

Vitamin B_6

pyridoxine HCl

Vitamin

CPhA Monograph

Date of Revision: October 2007

> This monograph has been compiled by CPhA and reviewed by experts. It may contain information different from that found in Health Canada-approved Product Monographs. The reader is referred to the *CPS* Editorial Policy for more information.

SUMMARY PRODUCT INFORMATION:

Route of Administration[a,b]	Dosage Form[a,b]	Strength[a,b]
Oral	Capsules	100 mg, 250 mg
	Tablets	8.3 mg, 10 mg, 20 mg, 25 mg, 50 mg, 100 mg, 200 mg, 250 mg
Parenteral	Injectable solution	100 mg/mL

[a] Table includes single-entity vitamin B_6 products only. For specific product information consult Health Canada's Drug Product Database http://www.hc-sc.gc.ca/dhp-mps/prodpharma/databasdon/index_e.html

[b] Does not include homeopathic products

PHARMACOLOGY: Vitamin B_6 is a water-soluble B complex vitamin which is present in many foods as pyridoxine, pyridoxal and pyridoxamine. These forms of vitamin B_6 are converted in vivo to pyridoxal phosphate and pyridoxamine phosphate, which are essential coenzymes in the metabolism of certain amino acids, carbohydrates and lipids and the synthesis of heme and GABA, an inhibitory neurotransmitter.

Deficiency of vitamin B_6 is associated with conditions such as uremia, alcoholism, cirrhosis, hyperthyroidism, malabsorption syndromes and heart failure. Deficiency may also be seen in those receiving isoniazid, hydralazine, pyrazinamide and penicillamine. Vitamin B_6 deficiency is characterized by seizures, seborrheic dermatitis, glossitis, dizziness, depression, confusion and urinary excretion of xanthurenic acid (an intermediary metabolite of tryptophan which may be measured to aid in diagnosing vitamin B_6 deficiency).

Vitamin B_6 requirements are increased in pregnancy and lactation and in patients taking estrogens (e.g., oral contraceptives). Certain hereditary conditions have been identified that are unrelated to deficiency, but may respond to high doses of vitamin B_6. These include xanthurenic aciduria, cystathioninuria, hyperoxaluria, primary homocystinuria, hereditary sideroblastic anemia and vitamin B_6-dependent seizures in neonates and infants.

Pharmacokinetics: Pyridoxine, pyridoxal and pyridoxamine are readily absorbed from the gastrointestinal tract, converted to the active forms of vitamin B_6 and stored in the liver and brain. Total body stores amount to 16 to 27 mg. Vitamin B_6 is metabolized in the liver and excreted in the urine.

Vitamin B_6 crosses the placenta and is excreted in breast milk.

INDICATIONS: In the prevention and treatment of vitamin B_6 deficiency and in the management of acute isoniazid overdosage. Vitamin B_6 has also been used in the treatment and prevention of isoniazid-induced neurotoxicity, in the management of acute toxicity caused by hydrazine-containing mushrooms of the genus *Gyromitra* and in the treatment of pyridoxine-responsive sideroblastic anemia associated with high serum iron concentration.

More study is needed to determine whether vitamin B_6 is of clear benefit in the treatment of premenstrual syndrome or nausea and vomiting of pregnancy.

CONTRAINDICATIONS: Hypersensitivity to vitamin B_6 or any component of a vitamin B_6-containing pharmaceutical preparation.

WARNINGS: See Precautions.

PRECAUTIONS: Vitamin B_6 is relatively nontoxic in usual doses. However, chronic administration of high doses (e.g., 2 g or more daily for several months) has led to sensory neuropathy with associated ataxia and numbness of hands and feet. Symptoms will lessen upon discontinuation of vitamin B_6, but may take up to 6 months to normalize.

Drug Interactions: Vitamin B_6 increases the peripheral metabolism of levodopa. When levodopa is combined with carbidopa, this effect is prevented.

Patients taking estrogens (e.g., oral contraceptives) have higher vitamin B_6 requirements.

Pregnancy: No adverse effects have been reported with the use of physiologic doses of vitamin B_6 during pregnancy. However, the use of high doses during pregnancy has been implicated in some cases of vitamin B_6 dependent syndrome in infants (see Pharmacology).

Lactation: Vitamin B_6 is excreted in breast milk; however, adverse effects have not been reported with the use of physiologic doses of vitamin B_6 during lactation.

ADVERSE EFFECTS: Nausea, headache, paresthesia, somnolence and low serum folic acid concentrations have been reported. Sensory neuropathy can occur following long-term administration of large doses (2 g or more daily for 2 months or longer).

Transient dependency symptoms have occurred upon withdrawal of vitamin B_6 therapy at a dose of 200 mg/day for 33 days. The significance of this is unknown; however, for patients on large doses for long periods of time, withdrawal of vitamin B_6 should probably be gradual.

Temporary burning or stinging and pain may be experienced at the site of sc or im injection.

OVERDOSE:

For management of a suspected drug overdose, CPhA recommends that you contact your **regional Poison Control Centre**. See the *CPS* Directory section for a list of Poison Control Centres.

DOSAGE: In the prevention of vitamin deficiencies, adequate dietary intake is preferred over supplementation whenever possible. Vitamin B_6 is found in meat, poultry, fish (e.g., salmon, trout, tuna), liver, legumes (e.g., garbanzo beans, lima beans), bananas, potatoes, fortified cereals and whole grains.

Patients taking isoniazid, hydralazine, pyrazinamide, penicillamine or oral contraceptives may require higher daily intake. Requirements are also higher during pregnancy and lactation.

Vitamin B_6 is usually administered orally; however, it can be given by iv, im, or sc injection when the oral route is not possible.

Treatment of Deficiency: 2.5 to 10 mg daily in adults. Once the clinical signs of deficiency have been corrected, the dose may be reduced to 2 to 5 mg daily for several weeks. A multivitamin preparation should be used since vitamin B_6 deficiency rarely occurs alone and is usually associated with multiple vitamin deficiencies. Children: 5 to 25 mg/day for 3 weeks then 1.5 to 2.5 mg/day.

Metabolic Disorders: Usual dose for xanthurenic aciduria, cystathioninuria, hyperoxaluria or homocystinuria is 100 to 500 mg daily. If the patient responds, this dose should be continued indefinitely.

Vitamin B_6 Dependency in Infants: For the treatment of seizures in these infants, a single dose of 10 to 100 mg vitamin B_6 im or iv has been recommended. Seizures usually stop within 2 to 3 minutes. Some infants may require maintenance supplementation with oral doses of 2 to 100 mg daily.

Hereditary Sideroblastic Anemia: An oral dose of 200 to 600 mg daily has been suggested. Lifelong supplementation may be required to prevent recurrence.

Treatment of Isoniazid Overdosage: For the treatment or prevention of seizures or coma following isoniazid poisoning, a dose of vitamin B_6 equal to the amount of isoniazid ingested is given by iv injection. Alternatively, if the amount ingested is unknown, a dose of 5 g vitamin B_6 may be given iv initially and repeated at 30-minute intervals until seizures are controlled.

Prevention of Isoniazid-induced Neurotoxicity: Adults: An oral dose of 10 to 50 mg daily has been recommended. A higher dose of 25 to 50 mg daily or 50 to 100 mg twice weekly is recommended for HIV patients since they are more prone to isoniazid-induced neurotoxicity. Children: 1 to 2 mg/kg/day orally.

Mushroom Poisoning (see Indications): Initial dose of vitamin B_6 in management of neurologic symptoms is 25 mg/kg iv. May be repeated if necessary to control seizures to a maximum cumulative dose of 15 to 20 g daily. Seizures associated with this mushroom poisoning may be controlled with lower doses of pyridoxine if diazepam is also administered.

Vitamin B_{12}

cyanocobalamin
hydroxocobalamin

Hematopoietic Agent

CPhA Monograph

Date of Revision: October 2007

This monograph has been compiled by CPhA and reviewed by experts. It may contain information different from that found in Health Canada-approved Product Monographs. The reader is referred to the *CPS* Editorial Policy for more information.

SUMMARY PRODUCT INFORMATION:

Route of Administration[a]	Dosage Form[a]	Strength[a]
Oral	Capsules	100 µg
	Drops	1000 µg/drop
	Fast-dissolving strips	1000 µg/strip
	Liquid	10 µg/mL, 50 µg/mL, 1000 µg/mL
	Tablets	100 µg, 250 µg, 1000 µg
Parenteral	Injectable solution	100 µg/mL, 1 mg/mL

[a] Table includes single-entity vitamin B_{12} products only. For specific information consult Health Canada's Drug Product Database http://www.hc-sc.gc.ca/dhp-mps/prodpharma/databasdon/index_e.html

PHARMACOLOGY: Vitamin B_{12}, also known as cyanocobalamin or hydroxocobalamin, is a group of cobalt-containing B complex vitamins, also known as cobalamins, synthesized by microorganisms. Food sources of vitamin B_{12} (mainly as adenosylcobalamin and methylcobalamin) include liver, fish, shellfish, meat and dairy products. Cyanocobalamin and hydroxocobalamin are synthetic forms of vitamin B_{12} and are used clinically. They have equivalent vitamin B_{12} activity. An exogenous source of vitamin B_{12} is required for nucleoprotein and myelin synthesis, cell production, normal growth, and for the maintenance of normal erythropoiesis. Coenzyme B_{12} results from the conversion of synthetic vitamin B_{12}. This coenzyme is essential for the synthesis of methionine from homocysteine.

Deficiency of vitamin B_{12} may be caused by dietary deficiency, malabsorption, or lack of sufficient intrinsic factor, and results in megaloblastic anemia, gastrointestinal lesions and neurologic damage characterized by demyelination and progressive axonal degeneration. Therapy with vitamin B_{12} reverses the anemia and gastrointestinal manifestations of deficiency, and halts the progression of neurologic damage. However, the existing nerve damage may not be completely reversible.

Vitamin B_{12} is essential for folate utilization with functional folate deficiency resulting from its absence.

Pharmacokinetics: Vitamin B_{12} is irregularly absorbed from the distal small intestine following oral administration. Vitamin B_{12} absorption is an active process that requires gastric intrinsic factor. Intrinsic factor is a glycoprotein secreted by the gastric mucosa. Approximately 1% of an oral dose of cyanocobalamin is absorbed by simple diffusion (without intrinsic factor) through the intestinal wall but large amounts of B_{12} are required to meet the daily recommended intake (i.e., >1 mg). It is rapidly absorbed from im and sc sites of injection; peak plasma concentrations are reached within 1 hour after im injection.

Vitamin B_{12} is distributed into the liver, bone marrow, and other tissues, including the placenta. At birth, the serum concentration of vitamin B_{12} in neonates is 3 to 5 times that of the mother.

Total body stores of vitamin B_{12} in healthy individuals are estimated to range from 1 to 11 mg, with an average of 5 mg; 50 to 90% is stored in the liver. Vitamin B_{12} is believed to be converted to coenzyme form in the liver and is probably stored in tissues in this form.

Following iv or im administration of 0.1 to 1 mg of cyanocobalamin, 50 to 90% of the dose may be excreted in urine by glomerular filtration within 48 hours, with the major portion being excreted in the first 8 hours. Hydroxocobalamin is more highly protein bound and is retained in the body longer than cyanocobalamin.

INDICATIONS: Vitamin B_{12} is used in the treatment of pernicious anemia and other vitamin B_{12} deficiency states such as those seen in strict vegetarians who consume no animal products. Vitamin B_{12} is also used to treat other macrocytic, megaloblastic anemias, in cases where malabsorption of vitamin B_{12} is suspected, e.g., gastric carcinoma, gastrectomy, sprue, ileal resection, strictures, or anastomoses involving the ileum.

Vitamin B_{12} deficiency requiring therapy may also be caused by an insufficiency of intrinsic factor which could have many causes, or by bacteria (blind loop syndrome), the fish tapeworm, or by certain drug therapies that may impair vitamin B_{12} absorption (see Precautions, Drug Interactions).

Vitamin B_{12} is used in conjunction with radiolabelled vitamin B_{12} in the study of vitamin B_{12} absorption and diagnosis of pernicious anemia (Schilling test).

CONTRAINDICATIONS: Hypersensitivity to cobalamins.

WARNINGS: See Precautions.

PRECAUTIONS: An intradermal sensitivity test may be performed in patients with suspected hypersensitivity to cobalamins.

In the treatment of megaloblastic anemia, erythrocyte potassium requirements may be increased as erythropoiesis normalizes, and potassium administration may be required.

It is important to accurately diagnose anemias prior to treatment, to ensure that appropriate therapy is initiated. If folic acid is used to treat pernicious anemia, for example, hematologic improvement may occur while neurologic complications continue to progress.

Cyanocobalamin (specifically) has been associated with accelerated optic nerve atrophy in patients with early Leber's disease (hereditary optic nerve atrophy) and its use should be avoided in these patients.

Drug Interactions: Chloramphenicol may antagonize the hematopoietic response to vitamin B_{12}.

Colchicine, aminoglycosides, certain anticonvulsants (e.g., phenytoin, phenobarbital, primidone), para-aminosalicylic acid or excessive alcohol intake for longer than 2 weeks may impair the absorption of vitamin B_{12}. Long-term ingestion of metformin and antacids may also contribute to food-cobalamin malabsorption especially in elderly patients.

Histamine$_2$-Receptor (H_2) Antagonists (e.g., cimetidine, ranitidine, nizatidine, famotidine) and proton pump inhibitors (e.g., omeprazole, esomeprazole, lansoprazole, pantoprazole, rabeprazole) may potentially cause vitamin B_{12} deficiency by decreasing gastric acid cleavage of vitamin B_{12} from food sources. This may be important in patients with low stores of vitamin B_{12} or in patients taking H_2-antagonists or proton pump inhibitors for extended periods of time (>2 years).

Drug-Laboratory Interactions: Most antibiotics, methotrexate and pyrimethamine invalidate folic acid and vitamin B_{12} diagnostic microbiological blood assays.

Pregnancy: No adverse effects have been reported with ingestion of normal daily requirements during pregnancy.

Lactation: Vitamin B_{12} is distributed into the milk of nursing women in concentrations that approximate the maternal blood vitamin B_{12} concentration. No adverse effects have been reported with intake of normal daily requirements during lactation.

ADVERSE EFFECTS: Vitamin B_{12} is usually nontoxic even in large doses. However, some adverse effects have been reported such as mild, transient diarrhea, itch, urticaria. Hypersensitivity reactions have occurred.

OVERDOSE:

For management of a suspected drug overdose, CPhA recommends that you contact your **regional Poison Control Centre**. See the *CPS* Directory section for a list of Poison Control Centres.

DOSAGE: In the prevention of deficiency of any nutrient, adequate dietary intake is preferred over supplementation whenever possible. Vitamin B_{12} is found in liver, fish (e.g., haddock, salmon, tuna), shellfish, meat, dairy products (e.g., cheese, milk, yogurt), fortified cereals and eggs.

Parenteral: Vitamin B_{12} should be administered either im or deep sc (avoiding the dermis and upper subcutaneous tissue).

Treatment of Vitamin B_{12} Deficiency: Confirmatory diagnostic tests should be performed prior to initiation of therapy. Adults: The usual im or sc dose is 30 to 100 µg daily for 5 to 10 days. A maintenance dose of 100 to 200 µg monthly is usually sufficient to maintain normal erythrocyte count.

Oral: Oral vitamin B_{12} is effective in many cobalamin-deficient patients. Parenteral therapy is often used in complicated deficiency especially with severe neurologic involvement or in those with vomiting, diarrhea or bowel resection. Oral doses of 1000 to 2000 µg daily have been used for initial treatment followed by a 1000 µg daily maintenance dose. In some cases, vitamin B_{12} stores are replenished with appropriate doses of parenteral therapy then patients are switched to oral maintenance.

Children: 100 µg im or sc daily until a total dose of 1 to 5 mg is given. The maintenance dose is at least 60 µg monthly. Smaller doses may be used when treating deficiencies other than pernicious anemia.

It is important that patients understand their need for lifelong, regular maintenance therapy.

Vitamin B_{12} Injection

cyanocobalamin

Hematopoietic Agent

Sandoz

SUPPLIED: 100 µg/mL: Each mL contains: cyanocobalamin 100 µg. Nonmedicinal ingredients: sodium chloride (for isotonicity), sodium acetate and acetic acid (as buffers), sodium hydroxide and/or hydrochloric acid (to adjust pH) and water for injection. Preservative-free. Discard unused portion. Ampoules of 1 mL, boxes of 10.

1000 µg/mL: Each mL contains: cyanocobalamin 1000 µg. Nonmedicinal ingredients: benzyl alcohol 1.5% (as preservative), sodium acetate and acetic acid (as buffers), sodium chloride (for isotonicity), sodium hydroxide and/or hydrochloric acid (to adjust pH) and water for injection. Ampoules of 1 mL, boxes of 10. Multidose vials of 10 and 30 mL, boxes of 1.

Store between 15 and 30°C. Protect from light.

Vitamin C

ascorbic acid

Vitamin

CPhA Monograph

Date of Revision: October 2007

This monograph has been compiled by CPhA and reviewed by experts. It may contain information different from that found in Health Canada-approved Product Monographs. The reader is referred to the *CPS* Editorial Policy for more information.

SUMMARY PRODUCT INFORMATION:

Route of Administration[a]	Dosage Form[a]	Strength[a]
Oral	Capsule	500 mg, 1000 mg

Route of Administration[a]	Dosage Form[a]	Strength[a]
	Lozenge	25 mg, 60 mg
	Powder	1 g/1.25 mL
	Tablet	100 mg, 125 mg, 250 mg, 500 mg, 1000 mg, 1500 mg
	Tablet, chewable	40 mg, 100 mg, 250 mg, 500 mg, 1000 mg
Parenteral	Injectable solution	500 mg/mL

[a] Table includes single-entity vitamin C products only. For specific product information consult Health Canada's Drug Product Database http://www.hc-sc.gc.ca/dhp-mps/prodpharma/databasdon/index_e.html

PHARMACOLOGY: Vitamin C, also known as ascorbic acid, is a water-soluble vitamin, essential for the formation of collagen and intercellular material. Vitamin C influences the formation of hemoglobin, erythrocyte maturation, and certain immunologic and biochemical reactions in the body. Vitamin C deficiency results in scurvy, which is characterized by degenerative changes in capillaries, bone and connective tissues. Symptoms include rash, muscle weakness, joint pain, fatigue, gingivitis and loose teeth. Vitamin C also has antioxidant properties.

Requirements for vitamin C may be increased in pregnancy, lactation, the elderly, hyperthyroidism, fever, cold exposure, stress, infection, trauma, burns, smoking and exposure to certain drugs (see Precautions, Drug Interactions).

Pharmacokinetics: Vitamin C is readily absorbed from the gastrointestinal tract by an active mechanism. It is widely distributed, with higher concentrations in liver, brain, leukocytes, platelets, glandular tissue and the lens of the eye. Normal plasma concentrations range from 10 to 20 µg/mL; levels of 1 to 1.5 µg/mL are associated with scurvy.

Vitamin C is approximately 25% bound to plasma proteins. Its metabolism involves oxidation to dehydroascorbic acid and other inactive compounds, all of which are renally excreted. With large doses, saturation occurs and unchanged vitamin C is excreted renally.

Vitamin C is removable by hemodialysis.

INDICATIONS: Vitamin C is used to prevent or treat scurvy.

Vitamin C supplementation is required in total parenteral nutrition.

As part of a regimen to slow the progression of age-related macular degeneration some clinicians support the use of vitamin C supplements.

Although large doses of vitamin C have been advocated for the prevention of the common cold, the results of most controlled studies do not support this use in the general population.

CONTRAINDICATIONS: Patients hypersensitive to any component of vitamin C preparations.

WARNINGS: See Precautions.

PRECAUTIONS: Large doses of vitamin C may lead to hyperoxaluria, or precipitation of urate, cystine, oxalate or certain drugs in the urinary tract.

Vitamin C may cause transient mild pain at the site of sc or im injection. Rapid iv injection may cause temporary faintness or dizziness.

The acidity of chewable vitamin C may break down tooth enamel when used as a lozenge. Vitamin C tablets and capsules should be given with a glass of water. Patients should be instructed not to lie down immediately after taking a dose because prolonged contact of ascorbic acid with the esophageal mucosa may cause localized esophagitis.

Drug Interactions: Salicylates inhibit uptake of vitamin C into leukocytes and platelets. The clinical significance of this effect is variable. Patients on high dose salicylate therapy should be evaluated for possible vitamin C deficiency if they exhibit the related signs or symptoms.

Because vitamin C is a urinary acidifier in large doses, the excretion of drugs that are weak acids or bases may be decreased or increased respectively.

Drug-Laboratory Test Interactions: Because vitamin C is a potent reducing agent, it can interfere with the results of tests that are based on oxidation-reduction reactions (e.g., false-negative urine glucose test results with glucose-oxidase method; false-positive results with cupric sulfate reagent). Because the degree of interference depends on many factors, specialized references should be consulted.

Pregnancy: Vitamin C crosses the placenta. It is considered safe for use in pregnancy if normal daily doses are used. Ingestion of large doses of vitamin C during pregnancy has resulted in scurvy in neonates.

Lactation: Vitamin C is excreted in breast milk. Adverse effects have not been reported with intake of normal daily requirements.

ADVERSE EFFECTS: Vitamin C is generally well tolerated. Reported adverse effects include nausea, vomiting, heartburn, abdominal cramps, fatigue, flushing, headache, insomnia and sleepiness. Dosages of >1 g daily may be associated with diarrhea and may increase the risk of renal stones in predisposed individuals.

OVERDOSE:

For management of a suspected drug overdose, CPhA recommends that you contact your **regional Poison Control Centre**. See the *CPS* Directory section for a list of Poison Control Centres.

DOSAGE: In preventing vitamin deficiencies, adequate dietary intake is preferred over supplementation whenever possible. Vitamin C is present in some fresh vegetables and fruits, like sweet peppers (green, red, yellow), cantaloupe, kiwi fruit, mangos, papayas, citrus fruits (e.g., grapefruits, oranges) and citrus fruit juices.

Vitamin C is usually administered orally. When the oral route is not feasible, it may be given by sc, im or iv injection.

Treatment of Scurvy: Adults: An oral or parenteral dose of 100 to 250 mg once or twice daily will successfully reverse the skeletal and vascular changes associated with scurvy within 2 days to 3 weeks.

Children: 100 to 300 mg daily in divided doses, orally or parenterally.

Age-related Macular Degeneration: Based on results of a clinical study in adults with age-related macular degeneration, some clinicians recommend vitamin C 500 mg as part of a high-dose antioxidant regimen which also includes beta-carotene, vitamin E, zinc and copper. However, smokers who take supplemental beta-carotene have an increased risk of lung cancer and should not take this combination.

Vitamin D

alfacalcidol
calcitriol
cholecalciferol
doxercalciferol
ergocalciferol
paricalcitol

Vitamin

CPhA Monograph

Date of Revision: October 2007

This monograph has been compiled by CPhA and reviewed by experts. It may contain information different from that found in Health Canada-approved Product Monographs. The reader is referred to the *CPS* Editorial Policy for more information.

SUMMARY PRODUCT INFORMATION:

Drug[a]	Route of Administration	Dosage Form	Strength
Alfacalcidol	Oral	Capsule	0.25 µg, 1 µg
		Drops	2 µg/mL
	Parenteral	Injectable solution	2 µg/mL
Calcitriol	Oral	Capsule	0.25 µg, 0.5 µg
		Solution	1 µg/mL
	Parenteral	Injectable solution	1 µg/mL, 2 µg/mL
Cholecalciferol	Oral	Capsule	10 000 IU
		Drops	400 IU/mL
		Tablet	400 IU, 1000 IU
Doxercalciferol	Oral	Capsule	2.5 µg
Ergocalciferol	Oral	Drops	approximately 207 IU/drop
Paricalcitol	Parenteral	Injectable solution	5 µg/mL

[a] Table includes single-entity products only. For specific product information consult Health Canada's Drug Product Database http://www.hc-sc.gc.ca/dhp-mps/prodpharma/databasdon/index_e.html

PHARMACOLOGY: Vitamin D analogs are fat-soluble vitamins that help regulate serum calcium and phosphorus concentrations, mainly by enhancing their absorption from the small intestine. Vitamin D is essential for normal mineralization of bone.

Vitamin D deficiency results in abnormal bone metabolism. Inadequate vitamin D results in decreased serum calcium concentrations which stimulates parathyroid hormone secretion. This ultimately leads to mobilization of calcium from bone, to correct the hypocalcemia. In children, the resultant inadequate mineralization of skeletal bone causes rickets, characterized by abnormal long bone development and other skeletal deformities. In adults, the result is osteomalacia, with bone pain and fractures.

Vitamin D analogs are split sterols that occur in nature or are produced synthetically. The biologic activity is expressed as International Units (IU), with 1 µg of either ergocalciferol (vitamin D_2) or cholecalciferol (vitamin D_3) equivalent to 40 IU of vitamin D activity, although cholecalciferol appears to be more effective in raising serum 25–hydroxyvitamin D [25(OH)D] levels. Both of these vitamin D analogs are metabolized by the liver to form calcifediol (25-hydroxycholecalciferol) which is then metabolized by the kidney to form calcitriol (1,25-dihydroxycholecalciferol), the most biologically active form of vitamin D. Other vitamin D analogs include alfacalcidol (1α-hydroxycholecalciferol, which is converted in the liver to calcitriol) and dihydrotachysterol (produced by synthetic reduction of ergocalciferol). Doxercalciferol is a synthetic vitamin D analog which is the 1–hydroxylated form of ergocalciferol. Paricalcitol is a synthetic analog of calcitriol. Vitamin D supplements usually contain cholecalciferol. Calcitriol, alfacalcidol, doxercalciferol and paricalcitol have specific therapeutic uses (see Indications and Dosage).

Humans synthesize cholecalciferol from cutaneous 7-dehydrocholesterol, on exposure to ultraviolet B (UVB) light. Cholecalciferol can be stored in fat cells for use during periods of decreased exposure to UVB light. Sunscreens that absorb UVB light, protective clothing, high melanin pigmentation and age-related skin changes can significantly limit cutaneous vitamin D synthesis. Lack of access to adequate sunlight, as well as active avoidance of it because of the associated risks, presents a challenge in terms of meeting the body's need for this essential nutrient.

There are very few natural food sources of vitamin D. Cholecalciferol is found in fatty fish, fish liver oils, in the livers of animals that eat fish and in eggs produced by chickens that have been fed fortified feed. In many countries, certain foods are fortified with vitamin D to address concerns over inadequate cutaneous synthesis and dietary intake of vitamin D. In Canada, vitamin D is added to cow's and goat's milk, margarine, infant formulas, fortified liquid diets, meal replacements and nutritional supplements.

Pharmacokinetics: Vitamin D analogs are readily absorbed from the small intestine if fat absorption is normal. The presence of bile is required for the absorption of ergocalciferol. Ergocalciferol and cholecalciferol are activated by a 2-step metabolic process (see Pharmacology). Because alfacalcidol, calcitriol and doxercalciferol do not require metabolic conversion by the kidney to become activated, they are useful in patients with chronic renal failure who require vitamin D therapy. Table 1 lists half-lives of some vitamin D analogs.

The metabolites of vitamin D analogs are excreted primarily in the bile and feces.

Table 1: Vitamin D Pharmacokinetics

Drug	t½ (hours)
Alfacalcidol	3
Calcitriol	3 to 6
Doxercalciferol	32 to 37
Ergocalciferol	19 to 48
Paricalcitol	14 to 15[a]

[a] In patients with kidney disease on dialysis.

INDICATIONS: Cholecalciferol and ergocalciferol are used in the treatment and prevention of vitamin D deficiency and in the management and prevention of primary and corticosteroid-induced osteoporosis, in conjunction with calcium. Cholecalciferol is more potent than ergocalciferol. Certain vitamin D analogs are used to treat vitamin D-resistant (or refractory) rickets, familial hypophosphatemia and hypoparathyroidism, tetany and hypocalcemia and osteodystrophy in dialysis patients (see Dosage).

The Canadian Paediatric Society recommends that all breast-fed full-term infants receive supplementary vitamin D (see Dosage).

Doxercalciferol and paricalcitol are used for secondary hyperparathyroidism in patients with chronic renal failure.

Some experts advocate the use of vitamin D supplements for the prevention of cancer (see Dosage).

CONTRAINDICATIONS: Known hypersensitivity to vitamin D or any of its analogs and derivatives. Vitamin D analogs should not be administered to patients with hypercalcemia, abnormal sensitivity to the toxic effects of vitamin D or hypervitaminosis D.

WARNINGS: See Precautions.

PRECAUTIONS: Chronic or acute administration of excessive doses may lead to hypervitaminosis D, manifested by hypercalcemia and its sequelae.

The therapeutic index of vitamin D analogs is narrow, and there is great interindividual variation in the dose that will lead to chronic toxicity. Daily doses of cholecalciferol or ergocalciferol ranging from 1.25 to 2.5 mg (50 000 to 100 000 IU) in adults and 25 µg (1000 IU) in children may result in hypervitaminosis. Other vitamin D analogs with shorter duration of action may have a lower propensity to accumulate and to cause hypercalcemia.

Early symptoms of hypercalcemia may include weakness, fatigue, somnolence, headache, anorexia, dry mouth, metallic taste, nausea, vomiting, vertigo, tinnitus, ataxia, hypotonia. Later and possibly more serious manifestations include nephrocalcinosis, renal dysfunction (resulting in excessive thirst and polyuria), osteoporosis in adults, impaired growth in children, anemia, metastatic calcification, pancreatitis, generalized vascular calcification, seizures and rarely, confusion and psychosis (see Overdose).

Periodic monitoring of serum calcium, phosphate, Ca x P product, magnesium, alkaline phosphatase is recommended for patients taking vitamin D analogs. Serum calcium should be maintained in the range of 2.25 to 2.5 mmol/L and not allowed to exceed 2.75 mmol/L (serum albumin must be considered).

Drug Interactions: Antacids (Aluminum-containing): Increased intestinal absorption of aluminum may lead to increased aluminum levels. Avoid this combination if possible.
Antacids (Magnesium-containing): Hypermagnesemia may develop when these agents are used concurrently with vitamin D. Monitor magnesium levels particularly in patients with chronic renal failure.
Anticonvulsants (Phenytoin, Phenobarbital): Decreased vitamin D effects may occur when certain anticonvulsants are administered. One theory is that they may induce hepatic microsomal enzymes and accelerate the conversion of vitamin D to inactive metabolites. Prophylactic administration of calcium and vitamin D is recommended.
Cholestyramine, Colestipol, Mineral Oil, Orlistat: Intestinal absorption of vitamin D may be impaired. Patients on cholestyramine or colestipol should be advised to allow as much time as possible between the ingestion of these drugs and vitamin D.
Digoxin: Vitamin D should be used with caution in patients taking digoxin as hypercalcemia (which may result from vitamin D use) may precipitate cardiac arrhythmias.

For specific drug interactions of doxercalciferol and paricalcitol see the individual product monographs.

Pregnancy: The Health Canada recommended dietary allowance of vitamin D for pregnant women is 200 IU daily. The Canadian Paediatric Society currently advocates much higher doses (see Dosage). Maternal hypercalcemia, possibly caused by excessive vitamin D intake during pregnancy, has been associated with hypercalcemia in neonates, which may lead to supravalvular aortic stenosis syndrome, the features of which may include retinopathy, mental or growth retardation, strabismus and other effects. Hypercalcemia during pregnancy may also lead to suppression of parathyroid hormone release in the neonate, resulting in hypocalcemia, tetany and seizures.

However, very high doses of vitamin D have been used to treat hypoparathyroidism during pregnancy resulting in normal children (n=27). Severe deficiency of vitamin D during pregnancy can result in maternal osteomalacia and lead to significant morbidity in both mother and fetus.

Lactation: Vitamin D is distributed into breast milk in small amounts. Breast-fed infants require supplementation. The Canadian Paediatric Society recommends vitamin D 400 IU daily for full-term breast-fed infants and 800 IU daily for infants living in northern communities.

If a lactating mother is receiving pharmacologic doses of vitamin D, calcium levels should be monitored in the infant.

ADVERSE EFFECTS: Vitamin D analogs are well tolerated in normal daily doses. Chronic excessive dosing can lead to toxicity (see Precautions).

OVERDOSE:

Symptoms: Acute intoxication with vitamin D rarely causes symptoms. Chronic ingestion of excessive doses can cause hypercalcemia, with symptoms such as anorexia, nausea, vomiting, fatigue, confusion, headache, weakness, renal impairment, arrhythmias, hypertension, calcification of soft tissues and hyperphosphatemia.

Treatment: Treatment of acute or chronic intoxication includes withdrawal of the vitamin D analog and any calcium supplements, monitoring of serum and urine electrolytes, renal function and ECG, and maintaining fluid balance. In addition, the following measures may be required: iv normal saline plus furosemide to enhance urinary excretion of calcium; calcitonin, corticosteroid or bisphosphonate therapy; hemodialysis or peritoneal dialysis.

For management of a suspected drug overdose, CPhA recommends that you contact your **regional Poison Control Centre**. See the *CPS* Directory section for a list of Poison Control Centres.

DOSAGE: Controversy currently surrounds the recommended dosing of vitamin D for the general population especially as it concerns the prevention of certain conditions such as cancer, osteoporosis, autoimmune diseases and neuromuscular disorders. It should be noted that expert groups are now recommending a total daily intake (for adults) of 400 to 800 IU vitamin D to optimize calcium absorption and prevent primary or corticosteroid-induced osteoporosis. The 2006 Canadian Consensus Conference on Osteoporosis recommends routine supplementation with vitamin D 800 IU/day in conjunction with calcium and other measures in the treatment of osteoporosis. Higher doses of vitamin D have been studied and are sometimes used for this indication.

The Canadian Paediatric Society recommends that breast-fed full-term infants receive supplementary vitamin D 10 µg (400 IU) daily. For infants living in northern communities, 20 µg (800 IU) daily is recommended. For breast-fed infants, supplementation should begin at birth and continue until the infant's diet includes at least 400 IU/day from other dietary sources or until the breast-fed infant reaches one year of age. For formula-fed babies they suggest a supplement of 400 IU/day during the winter for those living in communities north of the 55° parallel. The Canadian Pediatric Society has also suggested that consideration should be given to administering higher doses of vitamin D to pregnant and lactating women especially during the winter months (i.e., 2000 IU daily). They suggest the effectiveness of this regimen and possible side effects be checked with periodic assays for 25(OH)D and calcium.

The Canadian Cancer society now recommends a vitamin D supplement of 1000 IU daily for adults during the fall and winter months. They suggest those at risk of having lower levels of vitamin D such as the elderly, those with dark skin or those with minimal sun exposure take a vitamin D supplement of 1000 IU/day year round. Additional research is required to clarify the role of vitamin D supplements in the prevention of cancer. The few studies supporting this possible use of vitamin D had a number of limitations, e.g., long-term safety was not assessed. As a result, Health Canada has not changed their recommendations for vitamin D intake.

Dosage of vitamin D analogs must be individualized with careful monitoring of serum calcium levels. Careful titration is necessary to avoid overdosage. Dietary and other sources of vitamin D must be taken into consideration. Fortified dairy products (e.g., margarine, milk), fatty fish (e.g., cod, eel, salmon) and fish liver oils contain vitamin D. Appropriate calcium intake should be maintained.

Cholecalciferol: For vitamin D deficiency: 5000 IU (125 µg) daily until a biochemical and radiographic response is achieved.
For vitamin D-resistant rickets: 12 000 to 500 000 IU (0.3 to 12.5 mg) daily.
For hypoparathyroidism: 50 000 to 200 000 IU (1.25 to 5 mg) daily.

Alfacalcidol: For hypocalcemia and osteodystrophy in patients with chronic renal failure undergoing dialysis: Initial: 1 µg daily, the dosage being increased in increments of 0.5 µg every 2 to 4 weeks as necessary, up to 2 µg daily. Rarely, a dose of 3 µg/day is required. Maintenance: 0.25 µg to 1 µg/day.

Alfacalcidol is usually administered with food once daily. For information on dosage in patients with chronic renal failure who are not yet on dialysis, see the product monograph.

Calcitriol: Adults: For management of hypocalcemia and osteodystrophy in patients with chronic renal failure on dialysis: Initial: 0.25 µg daily; the daily dose may be increased by 0.25 µg every 4 to 8 weeks as necessary.
Maintenance: 0.5 to 1 µg daily. Patients with normal or only slightly reduced serum calcium levels may respond to 0.25 µg every other day.

For hypoparathyroidism and vitamin D resistant rickets, initially, 0.25 µg daily; the dosage may be increased by 0.25 µg/day at 2- to 4-week intervals if necessary.

Children: Initiation of Treatment: For x-linked hypophosphatemic rickets, 0.01 to 0.02 µg/kg/day (mean 0.018 µg/kg/day). For vitamin D dependency rickets type I, 0.010 to 0.025 µg/kg/day (mean 0.017 µg/kg/day). For hypoparathyroidism, 0.03 to 0.05 µg/kg/day (mean 0.04 µg/kg/day). If biochemical improvement has not occurred in 2 weeks, the dose is increased by 25% and re-evaluated in 2 weeks. Maintenance: For x-linked hypophosphatemic rickets, 0.01 to 0.05 µg/kg/day (mean 0.022 µg/kg/day). For vitamin D dependency rickets type I, 0.0046 to 0.015 µg/kg/day. For hypoparathyroidism, 0.014 to 0.04 µg/kg/day (mean 0.025 µg/kg/day).

Doxercalciferol: For reduction of elevated iPTH levels in the management of secondary hyperparathyroidism in patients undergoing chronic renal dialysis the recommended initial adult dose is 10 µg administered 3 times weekly after dialysis. For more detailed dosing information see the product monograph.

Paricalcitol: For the prevention and treatment of secondary hyperparathyroidism associated with chronic renal failure the recommended initial dose is 0.04 µg/kg to 0.1 µg/kg administered as a bolus dose no more frequently than every other day at any time during dialysis. For more detailed dosing information see the product monograph.

Vitamin D
vitamin D
Vitamin Supplement

USANA Health Sciences

SUPPLIED: Each tablet contains: vitamin D 25 µg. Nonmedicinal ingredients: ascorbyl palmitate, cellulose, corn starch, croscarmellose sodium, dextrose, lecithin, silica and sodium citrate.

(Shown in Product Identification Section)

Vitamin E
Vitamin

CPhA Monograph

Date of Revision: October 2009

This monograph has been compiled by CPhA and reviewed by experts. It may contain information different from that found in Health Canada-approved Product Monographs. The reader is referred to the *CPS* Editorial Policy for more information.

SUMMARY PRODUCT INFORMATION:

Route of Administration	Dosage Form[a]	Strength
Oral	Capsule	100 IU, 200 IU, 400 IU, 800 IU
	Chewable Tablet	200 IU
	Drops	50 IU/mL

[a] Table includes single entity Vitamin E products only. For specific product information consult Health Canada's Drug Product Database [www.hc-sc.gc.ca/dhp-mps/prodpharma/databasdon/index_e.html].

PHARMACOLOGY: Vitamin E is a fat-soluble vitamin that occurs naturally in 8 forms with varying biologic activity: four tocopherols and four tocotrienols (alpha, beta, delta and gamma). Of these, α-tocopherol is the most active natural form and the only one that is maintained in the plasma. The other tocopherols and the tocotrienols do not convert to α-tocopherol and thus do not contribute to fulfilling the body's Vitamin E requirements; their role in the body remains unclear.

Alpha-tocopherol has 8 possible stereoisomers (2R configurations RRR-, RRS-, RSR-, RSS-; and 2S configurations SSS-, SRS-, SSR-, and SRR). Only the 2R- stereoisomers are maintained in the plasma and are thus the only ones included in the definition for Vitamin E activity. RRR-α-tocopherol (formerly called d-α-tocopherol) is the only form that occurs naturally in food. Synthetic or all-racemic alpha-tocopherol (formerly called dl-α-tocopherol), contains an equal mixture of all 8 stereoisomers and is found in fortified foods and vitamin supplements.

Although the exact biological function of vitamin E in humans is unknown, it is considered an essential element of human nutrition. Vitamin E is thought to function as an antioxidant that prevents free-radical formation and thus the destruction of lipids by peroxidation. It has been postulated that vitamin E promotes wound healing and inhibits platelet aggregation.

Vitamin E deficiency rarely causes clinical symptoms in adults; in premature neonates, irritability, edema, thrombosis and hemolytic anemia may result from vitamin E deficiency. Low serum tocopherol concentrations in adults and children have been associated with creatinuria, ceroid deposition, muscle weakness, and increased erythrocyte susceptibility to in vitro hemolysis by oxidizing agents. Administration of vitamin E completely reverses these signs.

Table 1 presents recommendations for daily Vitamin E intake [*Dietary reference intakes for vitamin C, vitamin E, selenium and carotenoids*. Washington (DC): National Academy Press; 2000].

Table 1: Vitamin E

Recommended Dietary Allowance (RDA)[a] for Vitamin E

Life Stage Group	RDA (mg/day)[b]
0–6 mo	4[c]
7–12 mo	5[c]
1–3 yr	6
4–8 yr	7
9–13 yr	11
>13 yr	15
Pregnant Women	15
Lactating Women	19

[a] The RDA is the average daily dietary nutrient intake sufficient to meet the nutrient needs of nearly all healthy individuals (97 to 98%) in a particular life-stage and gender group.
[b] Values are expressed in mg of α-tocopherol (2R stereoisomeric forms); 1 mg α-tocopherol = 1.49 IU RRR-α-tocopherol (natural form) or 2.22 IU all-rac (synthetic) form.
[c] For all healthy infants, the Adequate Intake (AI) is used and is based on the estimated mean intakes of human milk.

Pharmacokinetics: Absorption of vitamin E from the gastrointestinal tract depends on the presence of bile and only 20 to 60% of vitamin E obtained from dietary sources is absorbed. As the dosage increases, the fraction of vitamin E absorbed decreases. Chylomicrons and lipoproteins are involved in transporting vitamin E to the general circulation.

Plasma concentrations of the tocopherols vary widely among individuals but are highly correlated with plasma lipoprotein and total lipid concentrations. After large doses of vitamin E, plasma tocopherol concentrations may be elevated for 1 to 2 days.

Vitamin E is widely distributed after absorption and stored mainly in adipose tissue. It is believed that normal body stores, estimated to be 3 to 8 g, are sufficient to meet the body's needs for 4 years or more.

Vitamin E is metabolized in the liver and excreted primarily in the bile.

INDICATIONS: In the prevention and treatment of vitamin E deficiency.

Vitamin E has been used as part of an antioxidant vitamin and mineral combination to slow the progression of age-related macular degeneration (AMD). In the AREDS trial, a formulation of vitamin E, vitamin C, beta-carotene, zinc and copper significantly reduced vision loss in generally well-nourished patients 55-80 years of age with intermediate or advanced AMD. Further trials are needed to determine whether the results of this study can be generalized to other patient populations [*Cochrane Database Syst Rev* 2006;(2):CD000254].

Current evidence does not support the use of vitamin E supplements to prevent cardiovascular or cerebrovascular disease, cancer, dementia, or infections.

CONTRAINDICATIONS: Hypersensitivity to components of vitamin E formulations.

WARNINGS: See Precautions.

PRECAUTIONS: Vitamin E is usually nontoxic; however, prolonged use of high doses has caused symptoms and metabolic disturbances (see Adverse Effects).

While not conclusive, results of a pooled analysis suggest that vitamin E in doses ≥ 400 IU/day for one year or longer in patients with chronic disease may increase all-cause mortality [*Ann Intern Med* 2005;142(1):37-46].

Drug Interactions: Vitamin A absorption, utilization and storage may be increased.

Vitamin E may increase the hypoprothrombinemic response to oral anticoagulants. Doses in excess of recommended daily nutrient intakes should be avoided in patients taking oral anticoagulants.

In dosages greater than 10 IU/kg daily, vitamin E may delay the response to iron therapy in children with iron-deficiency anemia, and low birth-weight infants treated with iron supplements may develop vitamin E-deficiency hemolytic anemia.

Cholestyramine and colestipol may reduce vitamin E absorption.

Excessive use of mineral oil may decrease the absorption of vitamin E.

Orlistat may decrease the absorption of fat-soluble vitamins, including vitamin E. It is recommended that at least 2 hours elapse between doses of orlistat and vitamin E.

Pregnancy: Neither deficiency nor excess of vitamin E has been associated with fetal complications during pregnancy. There is insufficient evidence to determine whether vitamin E supplementation is effective in reducing pre-eclampsia in pregnancy [*Cochrane Database Syst Rev* 2005;(2):CD004069].

Lactation: Vitamin E is excreted in breast milk. Human milk is 5 times richer in vitamin E than is cow's milk. Vitamin E applied topically to the nipples of breast-feeding women should be avoided as it can lead to a significant rise in infant serum levels.

ADVERSE EFFECTS: Large doses (greater than 300 IU/day) have rarely caused nausea, diarrhea, intestinal cramps, fatigue, weakness, headache, blurred vision, rash, gonadal dysfunction, creatinuria, increased serum creatinine kinase, increased serum cholesterol and triglycerides, increased urinary estrogens and androgens, and decreased serum thyroxine and triiodothyronine. These effects disappear after discontinuing the vitamin.

OVERDOSE:

> For management of a suspected drug overdose, CPhA recommends that you contact your **regional Poison Control Centre**. See the *CPS* Directory section for a list of Poison Control Centres.

DOSAGE: To prevent nutrient deficiencies, adequate dietary intake is preferred over supplementation whenever possible. Food sources include vegetable oils, cereal grains (especially wheat germ and wheat germ oil), egg yolks, meats (particularly the fat), nuts, fruits and vegetables.

It is important to consider biologic activity when comparing dosages of vitamin E; while natural source vitamin E may be more potent on a mg (weight) basis, IU of synthetic vitamin E are equivalent to IU of natural source vitamin E, as IU are an expression of the actual biologic activity of the dosage form.

Vitamin E is usually administered orally, but is also available parenterally as a component of a multiple vitamin preparation. Because of its purported wound-healing properties, vitamin E is also available in many different topical formulations with varying strengths.

Treatment of Deficiency: Adults: 60 to 75 IU orally, daily.

Age-Related Macular Degeneration: Based on results of a clinical study in adults with age-related macular degeneration, some clinicians recommend vitamin E 400 IU as part of a high-dose antioxidant regimen which also includes beta-carotene, vitamin C, zinc and copper. However, smokers who take supplemental beta-carotene have an increased risk of lung cancer and should not take this combination.

To Convert From IU to mg of α-tocopherol: For natural source Vitamin E (RRR form), multiply IU × 0.67. For all-racemic (synthetic) Vitamin E, multiply IU × 0.45.

Vitamin K_1 Pr

phytonadione

Hypoprothrombinemia Therapy

CPhA Monograph

Date of Revision: March 2010

> This monograph has been compiled by CPhA and reviewed by experts. It may contain information different from that found in Health Canada-approved Product Monographs. The reader is referred to the *CPS* Editorial Policy for more information.

SUMMARY PRODUCT INFORMATION:

Route of Administration	Dosage Form	Strength
Parenteral (im, iv, sc)	Solution	2 mg/mL, 10 mg/mL

PHARMACOLOGY: Phytonadione (vitamin K_1) is a fat-soluble naphthoquinone. It is one of the naturally occurring vitamin K compounds. These compounds share similar pharmacologic actions. Phytonadione is found in food (see Dosage), however, commercially prepared phytonadione is synthetically produced. Phytonadione possesses essentially the same type and degree of activity as naturally occurring vitamin K_1.

Vitamin K compounds are necessary for synthesis of active factor II (prothrombin), factor VII, factor IX and factor X in the liver. Deficiency of vitamin K or disturbances of liver function may lead to deficiencies of these factors. When the prothrombin level falls to about 10% to 15% of normal, even slight trauma may cause bleeding; when the level is below 10%, spontaneous hemorrhage may occur, in the form of hematoma, hematemesis, hematuria or melena.

Vitamin K deficiency may occur in patients with biliary obstruction or other conditions such as celiac disease, ulcerative colitis, sprue, regional enteritis, cystic fibrosis or intestinal resection that limit absorption of vitamin K compounds, and in patients receiving drugs that may affect liver function or intestinal flora.

Pharmacokinetics: Phytonadione is absorbed from the gastrointestinal tract only in the presence of bile salts and pancreatic lipase. Once absorbed, it accumulates in the liver, spleen and lungs, but significant amounts are not stored in the body for long periods.

The action of phytonadione, when administered parenterally, is generally detectable within 1 or 2 hours and hemorrhage is usually controlled within 3 to 8 hours. A normal prothrombin level may often be obtained in 12 to 14 hours.

INDICATIONS: Health Canada-approved indications include:

- prevention of coagulation disorders resulting from vitamin K deficiency or impaired action; including hemorrhagic disease of the newborn and malabsorption syndromes.
- treatment of coagulation disorders resulting from vitamin K deficiency or impaired action; including hypoprothrombinemia due to vitamin K antagonist oral anticoagulants and hemorrhagic disease of the newborn.

CONTRAINDICATIONS: Hypersensitivity to phytonadione or any of the ingredients in the formulation.

WARNINGS: Severe reactions, including fatalities, have occurred during and immediately after iv phytonadione injection even when precautions have been taken to dilute the phytonadione solution and to avoid rapid infusion. These severe reactions, which may occur in patients receiving phytonadione for the first time, resemble hypersensitivity or anaphylaxis, including shock and cardiac or respiratory arrest. Therefore, use of the iv route should be restricted to those situations where other routes are not feasible and the serious risk involved is considered justified.

Benzyl alcohol contained in some products has been associated with toxicity in newborns. Toxicity appears to have resulted from administration of large amounts (100 to 400 mg/kg daily) of benzyl alcohol in these neonates. Products containing benzyl alcohol should be used cautiously in newborns who are also receiving other benzyl alcohol-containing medications. In each case, the attending physician must weigh the potential benefits against the possible risks.

PRECAUTIONS: Because the liver is the site of prothrombin biosynthesis, hypoprothrombinemia resulting from hepatocellular damage is not corrected by administration of vitamin K compounds such as phytonadione. Repeated large doses of vitamin K compounds are not warranted in liver disease if the response to initial use of the vitamin is unsatisfactory. Failure to respond may indicate that a coagulation defect exists or that the condition is unresponsive to vitamin K administration.

Vitamin K compounds such as phytonadione do not counteract the anticoagulant effect of heparin. Dietary supplements high in vitamin K (≥0.7 mg/day) can block the effect of oral anticoagulants.

Vitamin K compounds such as phytonadione promote the activation of prothrombin in the liver but do not directly reverse the effects of oral anticoagulants. Immediate coagulant effects should not be expected. It takes up to 2 hours for a measurable improvement in the prothrombin time. Whole blood or component therapy may also be necessary if bleeding is severe or if there is no response to phytonadione.

Newborns should be observed for vitamin K deficiency. The incidence of vitamin K deficiency is higher in breast-fed infants. This increase may be partly due to lower concentrations of vitamin K in human milk than in cow's milk formula or it may be due to the smaller volume of milk infants may receive in their first few days of life, especially those exclusively breast-fed. Therefore, because an infant's milk intake cannot be predicted at birth, it is recommended that vitamin K prophylaxis be given to all newborns (see Indications and Dosage).

Drug Interactions: Anticoagulants (coumarin): Anticoagulant effects are antagonized by phytonadione. Temporary resistance to vitamin K antagonist anticoagulants may result from phytonadione administration, especially when relatively large doses have been given. Therefore, when reinstituting anticoagulant therapy, it may be necessary to use larger doses of the vitamin K antagonist anticoagulant or to use one that acts by a different mechanism, such as heparin.

Broad Spectrum Antibiotics, Quinidine, Quinine and High Dose Salicylates: Requirements for vitamin K compounds may be increased.

Cholestyramine: Vitamin K absorption may be reduced. Give phytonadione 1 hour before or 4 to 6 hours after cholestyramine dose.

Mineral Oil: Vitamin K absorption may be reduced. Doses of phytonadione should be separated from mineral oil by several hours.

Children: In newborns, particularly premature infants, hyperbilirubinemia and hemolytic anemia have been reported rarely. The risk is much less with phytonadione than other vitamin K preparations unless high doses (e.g., 10 to 20 mg) are given.

Pregnancy: Vitamin K compounds cross the placenta in small amounts. Limited data suggest that phytonadione in daily doses <20 mg is safe in pregnancy. Phytonadione is the treatment of choice for maternal hypoprothrombinemia.

Lactation: Vitamin K compounds may appear in human breast milk. There are no published reports of adverse effects on nursing infants associated with maternal vitamin K intake. The American Academy of Pediatrics considers maternal use of phytonadione compatible with breast-feeding.

ADVERSE EFFECTS: Deaths have occurred following iv administration of phytonadione (see Warnings).

Transient flushing sensations and peculiar sensations of taste have been observed following phytonadione injection as well as rare instances of dizziness, rapid and weak pulse, profuse sweating, brief hypotension, dyspnea and cyanosis. Bronchospasm, shock, cardiac and/or respiratory arrest may also occur.

Pain, swelling and tenderness at the injection site may occur. The potential for a hypersensitivity reaction, including rash, urticaria or anaphylaxis, should be borne in mind.

Large doses of vitamin K compounds may further depress liver function in patients with severe hepatic disease and thereby further decrease the concentration of prothrombin.

Neonates: In infants (particularly premature babies), excessive doses of vitamin K compounds such as phytonadione during the first few days of life rarely cause hyperbilirubinemia, severe hemolytic anemia, hemoglobinuria, kernicterus, leading to brain damage or even death. Immaturity is apparently an important factor in toxic reactions to vitamin K compounds, as full term and larger premature infants show greater tolerance than smaller premature infants.

OVERDOSE:

> For management of a suspected drug overdose, CPhA recommends that you contact your **regional Poison Control Centre**. See the *CPS* Directory section for a list of Poison Control Centres.

DOSAGE: Health Canada provides Adequate Intake values for vitamin K (Table 1). The abundance of phytonadione in the average diet of older children and adults normally satisfies daily requirements. Food sources include dark green leafy vegetables (e.g., lettuce, spinach), broccoli, cauliflower, dairy products and meat. Infants require exogenous vitamin K at birth and may require further doses (see Hemorrhagic Disease of the Newborn). Pregnancy and lactation are not considered to alter a woman's vitamin K requirements.

Table 1: Vitamin K

Health Canada Recommendations for Adequate Intake of Vitamin K

Age Group	Adequate Intake (μg/day)
Infants	
0 to 6 months	2.0
7 to 12 months	2.5
Children	
1 to 3 years	30
4 to 8 years	55
Males & Females	
9 to 13 years	60
14 to 18 years	75
Males 19 to >70 years	120
Females 19 to >70 years	90

Dose, frequency of administration and duration of treatment with phytonadione depend on the severity of the prothrombin deficiency and the response of the patient.

At present only an injectable form of phytonadione is available commercially. It is approved for sc, im or iv administration. Oral phytonadione 5 mg tablets are available through the Special Access Programme, Health Canada (see Appendix 2). The injectable formulation can be withdrawn from the vial and used orally. It can be given undiluted or diluted in water or juice just prior to administration. For more information on the risks of iv administration see Warnings. Oral absorption of phytonadione requires the presence of bile salts. Supplementation of bile salts should be considered in patients with decreased bile secretion who receive phytonadione.

In older children and adults, im injection should be made in the upper outer quadrant of the buttocks. In infants and young children, the anterolateral aspect of the thigh or the deltoid region is preferred.

When iv administration must be used, phytonadione should be injected very slowly, at a rate not exceeding 1 mg/minute.

Anticoagulant-induced Hypoprothrombinemia: The American College of Chest Physicians (ACCP) suggest that in patients with mild to moderately elevated INRs with no major bleeding, phytonadione be given orally. They do not discuss the use of the im route because of erratic absorption and increased risk of hematoma. Use of the subcutaneous route of administration is also not recommended by these guidelines. To limit the development of "warfarin resistance" the lowest necessary dose of phytonadione should be used. Dose recommendations for adults are as follows: [*Chest* 2008;133(6 Suppl):160S-198S]

For patients with INR ≥5 but <9 with no significant bleeding, clinicians may choose to treat with phytonadione. Omit a dose of warfarin and give phytonadione, 1 to 2.5 mg orally, especially for patients at increased risk of bleeding. In patients who will be undergoing urgent surgery requiring more rapid reversal, phytonadione (≤5 mg orally) can be given with the expectation that a reduction of the INR will occur in 24 hours. Additional phytonadione (usually 1 to 2 mg orally) can be given if the INR is still high.

For patients with INR ≥9 with no significant bleeding, hold warfarin and administer a higher dose of phytonadione (2.5 to 5 mg orally). This is given with the expectation that the INR will be reduced substantially in 24 to 48 hours. Monitor more frequently using additional phytonadione if necessary. When INR is in the therapeutic range, resume therapy at a lower dose.

For patients with serious bleeding and elevated INRs, hold warfarin and give phytonadione (10 mg by slow iv infusion) supplemented by other necessary measures (e.g., fresh frozen plasma). Administration of phytonadione can be repeated every 12 hours.

For patients with life-threatening bleeding and elevated INR, hold warfarin and give prothrombin complex concentrate (or recombinant factor VIIa as alternative) supplemented with phytonadione (10 mg by slow iv infusion). Repeat if necessary depending on INR.

Infants and Children: Limited data are available in children. Patients with no bleeding requiring reversal for invasive procedures: 0.5 to 2 mg po or iv for those who require further anticoagulant therapy; 2 to 5 mg po or iv for patients who do not require further anticoagulant therapy.

Infants and Children with Non-life-threatening Significant Bleeding: 2 to 5 mg po or iv.

Infants and Children with Life-threatening Significant Bleeding: 5 mg iv over 10 to 20 minutes. Oral dosing may be used in some situations.

Hemorrhagic Disease of the Newborn (HDNB): Prophylaxis: The Canadian Paediatric Society recommends that phytonadione be given as a single im injection to all newborns within 6 hours of birth, at a dose of 1 mg for infants with a birth weight of >1500 g and 0.5 mg if birth weight is ≤1500 g. Vitamin K administration at birth may not provide complete protection from HDNB, especially for breast-fed infants whose oral intake of vitamin K is low. The possibility of vitamin K deficiency should be considered if bleeding occurs in the first 6 months of life. It is reasonable to consider further prophylactic doses of phytonadione to infants at high risk of HDNB, such as those who fail to thrive, have liver disease or long-term diarrhea.

The guidelines recommend the oral route only when the parents refuse an im injection for the newborn. The recommended oral dose is 2 mg, given at the time of first feeding, and again at 2 to 4 weeks and 6 to 8 weeks of age, for a total of 3 doses. The importance of the follow-up doses should be stressed with the parents.

At present, oral phytonadione 5 mg tablets are available only through the Special Access Programme, Health Canada (see Appendix 2); however, the injectable formulation has been used orally.

Treatment: Phytonadione 1 mg im or iv.

Hypoprothrombinemia from Other Causes: When other drug therapy is the cause, discontinuation or reduction of the dosage of drug is suggested as an alternative to administering phytonadione. The severity of the coagulation disorder should determine whether the immediate administration of vitamin K is required in addition to discontinuation or reduction of dose of interfering drug(s).

Adults: A dosage of 2.5 to 25 mg or more (rarely up to 50 mg) is recommended; the dose and route of administration should be based on the severity of the condition and patient response.

Children: For the treatment of hypoprothrombinemia, the dose for infants is 1 to 2 mg and for older children, 5 to 10 mg.

Vivaglobin®

immune globulin subcutaneous (human)

Passive Immunizing Agent

CSL Behring

Date of Revision: April 7, 2010

SUMMARY PRODUCT INFORMATION:

Route of Administration	Dosage Form/ Strength	Clinically Relevant Nonmedicinal Ingredients
Subcutaneous	Solution for subcutaneous infusion ≥96% IgG	Glycine, sodium chloride For a complete listing of the nonmedicinal ingredients, see Dosage Forms, Composition and Packaging.

DESCRIPTION: Vivaglobin Immune Globulin Subcutaneous (Human), is a pasteurized, polyvalent human normal immunoglobulin for subcutaneous infusion. Vivaglobin consists of a 16% protein solution in 22.5 mg/mL glycine, 0.3% sodium chloride, and water for injection U.S.P. Vivaglobin is manufactured from large pools of human plasma by cold alcohol fractionation and is not chemically altered or enzymatically degraded. Vivaglobin contains no preservative.

INDICATIONS AND CLINICAL USE: Vivaglobin, Immune Globulin Subcutaneous (Human), is indicated for the treatment of adult and pediatric patients with primary immune deficiency (PID) who require immune globulin replacement therapy.

Geriatrics (>65 years of age): No specific studies in elderly patients have been conducted.

Pediatrics (2-16 years of age): See Warnings and Precautions, Pediatrics (2-16 years of age).

CONTRAINDICATIONS: As with all immune globulin products, Vivaglobin, Immune Globulin Subcutaneous (Human), is contraindicated in individuals with a history of anaphylactic or severe systemic response to immune globulin preparations, in persons with IgA deficiency who have known antibody against IgA and in patients who are hypersensitive to this drug or to any ingredient in the formulation or component of the container.

WARNINGS AND PRECAUTIONS:

Serious Warnings and Precautions
- Products made from human plasma may contain infectious agents such as viruses, and theoretically, the Creutzfeldt-Jacob (CJD) agent (see General)
- Immune Globulin (human) products have been reported to be associated with the following events:
  - aseptic meningitis syndrome
  - thrombo-embolism
  - renal impairment
  - hemolysis/hemolytic anemia
  - TRALI

General: Administer Vivaglobin, Immune Globulin Subcutaneous (Human), subcutaneously. **Do not administer this product intravenously.** The recommended infusion rate and amount per injection site stated under Dosage and Administration should be followed. When initiating therapy with Vivaglobin, patients should be monitored for any adverse events during and after the infusion.

Patients who receive immune globulin therapy for the first time, who are switched from another brand of immune globulin, or who have not received immune globulin therapy within the preceding eight weeks may be at risk for developing reactions including fever, chills, nausea, and vomiting. On rare occasions these reactions may lead to shock. Such patients should be monitored for these reactions in a clinical setting during the initial administration of Vivaglobin.

If anaphylactic or anaphylactoid reactions are suspected, discontinue administration immediately. Treat any acute anaphylactoid reactions as medically appropriate.

Vivaglobin is made from human plasma. Products made from human plasma may contain infectious agents, such as viruses, that can cause disease. Because Vivaglobin is made from human blood, it may carry a risk of transmitting infectious agents, e.g., viruses, and theoretically, the CJD agent. The risk that such plasma-derived products will transmit an infectious agent has been reduced by screening plasma donors for prior exposure to certain viruses, by testing for the presence of certain current virus infections, and by inactivating and/or removing certain viruses during manufacture. Stringent procedures utilized at plasma collection centers, plasma-testing laboratories and fractionation facilities are designed to reduce the risk of virus transmission. The primary virus reduction steps of the Vivaglobin manufacturing process are inactivation by pasteurization (heat treatment of the aqueous solution at 60°C for 10 hours) and alcohol/pH precipitation. Additional purification procedures used in the manufacture of Vivaglobin also potentially provide virus reduction. Despite these measures, such products may still potentially contain human pathogenic agents, including those not yet known or identified. Thus, the risk of transmission of infectious agents cannot be totally eliminated. Any infections thought by a physician to have been possibly transmitted by this product should be reported by the physician or other healthcare professional to CSL Behring at 1-613-783-1892. The physician should discuss the risks and benefits of this product with the patient.

During clinical trials, no cases of hepatitis A, B, C virus or HIV infections were reported with the use of Vivaglobin.

Special Populations: Pregnant Women: Animal reproduction studies have not been conducted with Vivaglobin, Immune Globulin Subcutaneous (Human). It is also not known whether Vivaglobin can cause fetal harm when administered to a pregnant woman, or can affect reproduction capacity. Vivaglobin should only be used in pregnant women when the benefits outweigh the risks associated with its use.

Nursing Women: Vivaglobin should only be used in nursing woman when the benefits outweigh the risks associated with its use.

Pediatrics (2-16 years of age): Vivaglobin was evaluated in 6 children and 4 adolescents in the US and Canada study and in 16 children and 6 adolescents in the European study. There were no apparent differences in the safety and efficacy profiles as compared to adult subjects. No pediatric-specific dose requirements were necessary to achieve the desired serum IgG levels. The safety and efficacy of Vivaglobin have not been studied in pediatric subjects under two years of age.

Geriatrics: Clinical studies of Vivaglobin, Immune Globulin Subcutaneous (Human), did not include sufficient numbers of subjects aged 65 and over to determine whether they respond differently from younger subjects.

Monitoring and Laboratory Tests: After injection of immunoglobulins, the transitory rise of the various passively transferred antibodies in the patient's blood may yield misleading positive serological testing results such as positive direct or indirect antiglobulin (Coomb's test) and anti-HBs/anti-HBc results in absence of viral transmission.

Periodic monitoring of renal function and urine output is particularly important in patients judged to have a potential increased risk for developing acute renal failure. Renal function, including measurements of blood urea nitrogen (BUN)/serum creatinine, should be assessed prior to initial infusion of Vivaglobin and again at appropriate intervals thereafter.

If signs or symptoms of hemolysis are present after Vivaglobin infusion, appropriate confirmatory laboratory testing, such as unconjugated serum bilirubin, serum haptoglobulin, Direct Antiglobulin Test (DAT) and serum LDH, should be done.

ADVERSE REACTIONS: Adverse Drug Reaction Overview with Post-Marketing Data: Immunoglobulins as a class of products manufactured by CSL Behring have been widely used clinically, by the intramuscular (i.m.) route, starting in the early 1950s. The subcutaneous (s.c.) use of CE 1200 in the treatment of antibody deficiency syndromes has been approved in Europe, starting in 1994. Post-marketing surveillance of product administered i.m. or s.c., showed that the Immunoglobulins are well tolerated. The following undesirable effects have been reported in rare cases:
- allergic reactions including fall in blood pressure, dyspnea, cutaneous reactions, and in isolated cases reaching as far as anaphylactic shock, even when the patients have shown no hypersensitivity to previous administration.
- generalized reactions such as chills, fever, headache (headaches may also be caused by increased blood pressure), malaise, nausea, vomiting, arthralgia and moderate back pain.
- cardiovascular reactions particularly if the product is inadvertantly infused intravascularly.
- local reactions at the injection or infusion site: swelling, soreness, redness, induration, local heat, itching, bruising or rash.
- nervous system disorders—migraine, aseptic meningitis.

Clinical Trial Adverse Drug Reactions: In clinical studies, administration of Vivaglobin, Immune Globulin Subcutaneous (Human), has been shown to be safe and well tolerated in both adult and pediatric subjects. Reactions similar to those reported with administration of other immune globulin products may also occur with Vivaglobin. Rarely, immediate anaphylactoid and hypersensitivity reactions may occur. In exceptional cases, sensitization to IgA may result in an anaphylactic reaction (see Contraindications and Warnings and Precautions). Because clinical trials are conducted under very specific conditions, the adverse drug reaction rates observed in the clinical trials may not reflect the rates observed in practice and should not be compared to the rates in the clinical trials of another drug. Adverse drug reaction information from clinical trials is useful for identifying drug related adverse events and for approximating rate. Should evidence of an acute hypersensitivity reaction be observed, the infusion should be stopped promptly and appropriate treatment and supportive therapy should be administered.

In two clinical studies, Vivaglobin was evaluated in 125 patients diagnosed with PID. The most frequent adverse reaction was local reaction at the injection site. Table 1 summarizes the most frequent adverse events by subject reported in the two clinical studies, and Table 2 summarizes the most frequent adverse events by infusion.

Table 1: Vivaglobin

Most Frequent Adverse Events by Subject[a] Irrespective of Causality

	US/Canada Clinical Study (65 subjects)	Europe/Brazil Clinical Study (60 subjects)
Adverse Events	**No. of Subjects (% of total)**	**No. of Subjects (% of total)**
Adverse Events at the Injection Site	60 (92%)	44 (73%)
Non-Injection Site Reactions		
Headache	31 (48%)	21 (35%)
Gastrointestinal disorder	24 (37%)	26 (43%)
Fever	16 (25%)	25 (42%)
Nausea	12 (18%)	0 (0%)
Sore throat	11 (17%)	5 (8%)
Rash	11 (17%)	2 (3%)
Allergic reaction	7 (11%)	5 (8%)
Skin disorder	5 (8%)	8 (13%)
Pain	6 (9%)	1 (2%)
Diarrhea	6 (9%)	1 (2%)
Cough increased	6 (9%)	1 (2%)

[a] Excluding infections.

Table 2: Vivaglobin

Most Frequent Adverse Events by Infusion[a] Irrespective of Causality

	US/Canada Clinical Study (3656 infusions)	Europe/Brazil Clinical Study (2297 infusions)	Both Studies (5953 infusions)
Adverse Events (≥1% of infusions)	**No. of AEs (Rate[b])**	**No. of AEs (Rate[b])**	**No. of AEs (Rate[b])**
Adverse Events at the Injection Site	1789 (49%)	641 (28%)	2430 (41%)
Mild	1112 (30%)	626 (27%)	1738 (29%)
Moderate	601 (16%)	14 (1%)	615 (10%)
Severe	65 (2%)	0	65 (1%)
Unknown Severity	11 (<1%)	1 (<1%)	12 (<1%)
Non-Injection Site Reactions			
Headache	159 (4%)	49 (2%)	208 (3%)
Gastrointestinal disorder	36 (1%)	46 (2%)	82 (1%)

(cont'd)

Table 2: Vivaglobin *(cont'd)*

Most Frequent Adverse Events by Infusion[a] Irrespective of Causality

	US/Canada Clinical Study (3656 infusions)	Europe/Brazil Clinical Study (2297 infusions)	Both Studies (5953 infusions)
Adverse Events (≥1% of infusions)	**No. of AEs (Rate[b])**	**No. of AEs (Rate[b])**	**No. of AEs (Rate[b])**
Fever	28 (1%)	78 (3%)	106 (2%)

[a] Excluding infections.
[b] Rate=number of reactions/infusion.

Table 3 summarizes the most frequent related adverse events by subject reported in the two clinical studies, and Table 4 summarizes the most frequent related adverse events by infusion.

Table 3: Vivaglobin

Most Frequent Related Adverse Events by Subject[a]

	US/Canada Clinical Study (65 subjects)	Europe/Brazil Clinical Study (60 subjects)
Related Adverse Event (≥2 subjects in at least one study)	**No. of Subjects (% of total)**	**No. of Subjects (% of total)**
Adverse Events at the Injection Site	60 (92%)	44 (73%)
Non-Injection Site Reactions		
Headache	21 (32%)	0
Fever	2 (3%)	7 (12%)
Nausea	7 (11%)	0
Rash	4 (6%)	1 (2%)
Skin disorder	2 (3%)	2 (3%)
Asthenia	3 (5%)	0
Gastrointestinal disorder	3 (5%)	0
Tachycardia	2 (3%)	0
Urine abnormality	2 (3%)	0

[a] Excluding infections.

Table 4: Vivaglobin

Most Frequent Related Adverse Events by Infusion[a]

	US/Canada Clinical Study (3656 infusions)	Europe/Brazil Clinical Study (2297 infusions)	Both Studies (5953 infusions)
Related Adverse Event (≥2 AEs in at least one study)	**No. of AEs (Rate[b])**	**No. of AEs (Rate[b])**	**No. of AEs (Rate[b])**
Adverse Events at the Injection Site	1787 (49%)	633 (28%)	2420 (41%)
Non-Injection Site Reactions			
Headache	59 (1.6%)	0	59 (1%)
Fever	2 (0.1%)	18 (0.8%)	20 (0.3%)
Rash	9 (0.2%)	2 (0.1%)	11 (0.2%)
Nausea	9 (0.2%)	0	9 (0.2%)
Skin disorder	3 (0.1%)	3 (0.1%)	6 (0.1%)
Nervousness	4 (0.1%)	0	4 (0.1%)
Asthenia	3 (0.1%)	0	3 (0.1%)
Chills	1 (<0.1%)	2 (0.1%)	3 (0.1%)
Gastrointestinal disorder	3 (0.1%)	0	3 (0.1%)
Syncope	1 (<0.1%)	2 (0.1%)	3 (0.1%)
Urine abnormality	3 (0.1%)	0	3 (0.1%)
Dyspnea	2 (0.1%)	0	2 (<0.1%)
Gastrointestinal pain	2 (0.1%)	0	2 (<0.1%)
Tachycardia	2 (0.1%)	0	2 (<0.1%)

[a] Excluding infections.
[b] Rate=number of reactions/infusion.

Local (Injection Site) Reactions: Local injection site reactions consisting of mostly mild or moderate swelling, redness and itching, have been observed with the use of Vivaglobin. Furthermore, the majority of injection site reactions resolved within four days. No serious local site reactions were observed. Four subjects discontinued Immune Globulin Subcutaneous (IGSC) therapy due to local site reactions.

Additionally, the number of subjects reporting local injection site reactions decreased substantially after repeated use (see Figure 1).

Figure 1: Vivaglobin

Subjects Reporting Local Site Reactions By Infusion

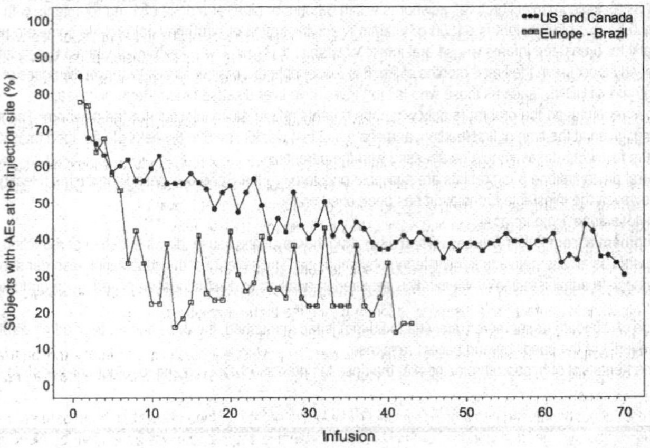

Note: Analysis is confined to 70 infusions.

Abnormal Hematologic and Clinical Chemistry Findings: No clinically significantly abnormal hematologic or clinical chemistry findings were observed in the clinical studies.

Small fluctuations of the safety laboratory results are commonly observed in routine safety laboratory testing, irrespectively of departures from the normal range values. To overcome the interpretation of natural variations within small study populations, a pre-defined changes analyses from baseline values was conducted using the following validated pre-defined changes parameters for the respective analytes: See Table 5.

Table 5: Vivaglobin

Summary of Pre-Defined Changes for Selected Laboratory Parameters Study CE1200_3001

Parameter	Pre-defined change (PC)	N[a]	No. (%) of subjects with PC
Hemoglobin	Decrease ≥1.2 mmol/L	62	3 (5%)
Hematocrit	Decrease ≥0.07	62	2 (3%)
Red blood cells	Decrease $\geq 0.7^a$ 10^{12}/L	62	4 (6%)
Platelet count	Decrease $\geq 93^a$ 10^9/L	62	6 (10%)
Potassium	Decrease ≥1.1 mmol/L	64	1 (2%)
Glucose	Increase ≥4.2 mmol/L	64	3 (5%)

[a] N=number of subjects with values at baseline and post-baseline.

DRUG INTERACTIONS: Overview: Immunoglobulin administration can transiently impair the efficacy of live attenuated virus vaccines such as measles, mumps, rubella. The immunizing physician should be informed of recent therapy with Vivaglobin, Immune Globulin Subcutaneous (Human), so that appropriate precautions may be taken.

Vivaglobin should not be mixed with other medicinal products.

Drug-Drug Interactions: Please refer to Overview.
Drug-Food Interactions: Interaction with food has not been established.
Drug-Herb Interactions: Interaction with herbal products has not been established.
Drug-Laboratory Test Interactions: See Warning and Precautions, Monitoring and Laboratory Tests.

DOSAGE AND ADMINISTRATION: Vivaglobin, Immune Globulin Subcutaneous (Human), contains no preservative. Therefore, discard unused product immediately after use.

Vivaglobin must not be mixed with other products.

Vivaglobin is to be injected subcutaneously, preferentially in the abdomen, thighs, upper arms, and/or lateral hip.

Do not inject into a blood vessel.

Recommended Dose and Dosage Adjustment: All subjects who received Vivaglobin in the clinical trials had previously been treated with immune globulin. It is recommended that the patient starts treatment with Vivaglobin one week after receiving a regularly scheduled IGIV infusion.

The initial weekly Vivaglobin dose can be calculated by multiplying the previous IGIV dose by 1.37, then dividing this dose into weekly doses based on the patient's previous IGIV treatment interval; for example, if IGIV was administered every three weeks, divide by 3. This dose of Vivaglobin will provide a systemic IgG exposure (AUC) comparable to that of the previous IGIV treatment. Weekly administration of this dose will lead to stable steady-state serum IgG levels with lower IgG peak levels and higher IgG trough levels compared to monthly IGIV treatment.

The recommended weekly dose of Vivaglobin is 100 to 200 mg/kg body weight administered subcutaneously. Doses may be adjusted over time to achieve the desired clinical response and serum IgG levels. As there can be differences in the half-life of IgG among patients with primary immune deficiencies, the dose and dosing interval of immunoglobulin therapy may vary.

Doses and Associated IgG Levels: The minimum serum concentration of IgG necessary for protection has not been established in randomized and controlled clinical studies. However, based on clinical experience, a target serum IgG trough level (i.e., prior to the next infusion) of at least 500 mg/dL has been proposed in the literature for IGIV therapy (*Roifman CM and al. 1987*).

Table 6 shows the resulting serum trough IgG levels after Vivaglobin treatment in the two clinical studies, which can be used as a dosing guide. Vivaglobin administered at mean doses of 136% in the United States and Canada clinical study (158 mg/kg) and 101% in the European and Brazil clinical study (89 mg/kg) of the subject's immune globulin resulted in a mean increase in serum IgG levels of 255 and 86 mg/dL, respectively, over previous immune globulin-derived serum IgG trough levels before starting Vivaglobin therapy.

Table 6: Vivaglobin

Weekly Vivaglobin Doses And Resulting Serum IgG Trough Levels Compared With Previous Immune Globulin Therapy In Two Clinical Studies

Clinical Studies (number of subjects)	Mean IGSC Dose (mg/kg b.w.)	Mean IGSC Dose (as % of previous IgG dose)	Mean (range) Serum IgG Trough Levels (mg/dL IgG)	Mean Increase Over Baseline Serum IgG Trough Levels[a] (mg/dL IgG)
US/Canada (n=51)	158	136	1040 (568 to 1810)	255
Europe/Brazil (n=47)	89	101	922 (650 to 1684)	86

[a] Over previous immune globulin-derived serum IgG trough levels before starting Vivaglobin therapy.

Serum IgG levels can be sampled at any time during routine weekly treatment. Subjects on IGSC therapy maintained relatively constant IgG levels, rather than the peak and trough pattern observed with monthly IGIV therapy.

Missed Dose: A missed dose should be administered as soon as possible to ensure an adequate IgG serum level.

Administration: Do not inject intravenously.

In clinical studies with Vivaglobin, a volume of 15 mL per injection site at a rate of 20 mL per hour per site was not exceeded. Doses over 15 mL were divided and infused simultaneously into several sites using an infusion pump with a splitter to enable multiple simultaneous injections (CADD-Legacy pumps were used in the study conducted in the U.S. and Canada). Injection sites were at least two inches apart.

The following areas were used for subcutaneous injection of Vivaglobin: abdomen, thighs, upper arms, and/or lateral hip. The actual point of injection was changed with each weekly administration.

Prior to use, allow the solution to reach ambient room temperature. Parenteral drug products should be inspected visually for particulate matter and discoloration prior to administration whenever solution and container permit. Do not use if the solution is cloudy or has particulates. The color of Vivaglobin can vary from colorless to light brown.

1. Use aseptic technique when preparing and administering Vivaglobin for injection.
2. Remove the cap from the vial to expose the central portion of the rubber stopper.
3. Wipe the rubber stopper of the vial with antiseptic solution and allow to dry.
4. **Do not shake.** Withdraw the appropriate amount of Vivaglobin by injecting air into the vial and withdraw the appropriate volume. Follow the manufacturer's instructions for preparing the pump and tubing.
5. Select the number of injection sites depending on the volume of the total dose.
6. Cleanse the injection site(s) with antiseptic solution followed by povidone-iodine using a circular motion from the inside to the outside of the injection site. The injection site should be clean, dry, and at least five centimeters (two inches) away from other injection sites.
7. Vivaglobin must not be infused into a blood vessel. To make sure that no blood vessel has been entered, slightly pull back the plunger of the syringe. If a blood vessel has been accidentally entered, this will be evident by blood flowing into the tubing of the catheter. An alternative injection site must then be chosen.
8. Inject Vivaglobin following the manufacturer's instructions for using the infusion pump.
9. After administration, any unused solution and administration equipment should be discarded in accordance with biohazard procedures.

Home Treatment: If the physician believes that home administration is appropriate, the physician or health professional should provide the patient with instructions on subcutaneous infusion for home treatment. This should include the type of equipment to be used along with its maintenance, proper infusion techniques, selection of appropriate infusion sites (e.g., abdomen, thighs, upper arms, and/or lateral hip), maintenance of a treatment diary, and measures to be taken in case of adverse reactions.

Reconstitution: Not applicable. Vivaglobin is a ready to use solution of human immunoglobulin for subcutaneous infusion.

OVERDOSAGE:

Consequences of an overdose are not known.

For management of a suspected drug overdose, CPhA recommends that you contact your **regional Poison Control Centre**. See the *CPS* Directory section for a list of Poison Control Centres.

ACTION AND CLINICAL PHARMACOLOGY: Mechanism of Action: Immune Globulin Subcutaneous (Human), Vivaglobin supplies a broad spectrum of opsonizing and neutralizing IgG antibodies against a wide variety of bacterial and viral agents.

Pharmacodynamics: See Mechanism of Action.

Pharmacokinetics: Vivaglobin is to be administered by injection into the subcutaneous tissue. Subcutaneous administration of immune globulin decreases bioavailability compared to intravenous administration (Smith and al.1972). The bioavailability of Vivaglobin is approximately 73% compared to IGIV. Various factors, such as the site of administration and IgG catabolism, can affect absorption (Smith and al.1972, Waniewski and al.1993). With Vivaglobin administration, peak serum IgG levels are lower than those achieved with immune globulin intravenous (IGIV). Subcutaneous administration results in relatively stable steady-state serum IgG levels when administered on a weekly basis (Waniewski and al.1993, Data on file). This serum IgG profile is representative of that seen in a normal population.

The pharmacokinetics (PK) of Vivaglobin was evaluated in the PK phase of a pivotal 12-month clinical study conducted in the United States and Canada in subjects with primary immune deficiency (PID). Subjects who were previously treated with IGIV were switched over to weekly Vivaglobin subcutaneous treatment and, after a 3-month wash-in/wash-out period, doses were individually adjusted to provide an IgG systemic exposure (area under the curve; AUC) that was not inferior to the AUC of the previous weekly-equivalent IGIV dose. For the 19 per-protocol subjects completing the wash-in/wash-out period, the average Vivaglobin dose adjustment was 137% (range: 103 to 192%) of the previous weekly-equivalent IGIV dose. Following 10 to 12 weeks of treatment with Vivaglobin at this adjusted dose, the final steady-state AUC determinations were made. The geometric mean ratio of the steady-state AUCs, standardized to a weekly treatment period, for Vivaglobin versus IGIV treatment was 94.5% (range: 71.4 to 110.1%) with a lower 95% confidence limit of 89.8% for the per-protocol population (n=17). Table 7 summarizes additional pharmacokinetic parameters for this study including dosing and serum IgG peak and trough levels following treatment with IGIV and Vivaglobin.

Table 7: Vivaglobin

Summary of Additional Pharmacokinetics Parameters—US and Canada PK Sub-study—Per-protocol Subjects

	IGIV	Vivaglobin
Number of Subjects	**17**	**17**
Dose[a]		
Mean Range	120 mg/kg 55–243 mg/kg	165 mg/kg 63–319 mg/kg
IgG peak levels		
Mean Range	1735 mg/dL 1110–3230 mg/dL	1163 mg/dL 743–2240 mg/dL
IgG trough levels		
Mean Range	883 mg/dL 430–1600 mg/dL	1064 mg/dL 547–2140 mg/dL

[a] For IGIV: weekly-equivalent dose.

A non-IND 6-month clinical study was conducted in Europe and Brazil in 60 subjects with PID. After the subjects had reached steady state with weekly Vivaglobin administration, peak serum IgG levels were observed after a mean of 2.5 days (range 0 to 7 days) in 41 subjects. Table 8 summarizes additional PK parameters including C_{max}, t_{max}, AUC, and clearance for Vivaglobin from a supplementary analysis.

In contrast to serum IgG levels observed with monthly IGIV treatment (rapid peaks followed by a slow decline), the serum IgG levels in subjects receiving weekly subcutaneous Vivaglobin therapy were relatively stable in both studies.

Duration of Effect: In two studies (one was conducted in North America and the other in Europe and Brazil), subcutaneous weekly treatment with Vivaglobin at doses between 50 and 200 mg/kg b.w. resulted in stable IgG trough levels between 900 and 1000 mg/dL at steady state (after 4 month of treatment) without major variations.

STORAGE AND STABILITY: Store Vivaglobin in the refrigerator at 2-8°C. Vivaglobin may be stored at room temperature (not to exceed 25°C) for up to 5 months within an overall storage period of 36 months at 2-8°C. If the product is stored outside the refrigerator, please add the date removed from refrigeration and note a new expiry date on the carton on the space provided. The new expiry date should be 5 months from the date the product is removed from the regigerator, or the previously stamped expiry date, whichever is shorter. Once the product is removed from refrigeration, it cannot be returned to the refrigerator. Immune Globulin Subcutaneous (Human), Immune Globulin Subcutaneous (Human), Vivaglobin, is stable for the period indicated by the expiration date on its label. Do not freeze. Keep vials in storage box until use.

Since the product contains no antimicrobial preservative, do not begin administration more than 4 hours after the vial has been opened. Destroy unused portions to prevent the possibility of subsequent use of a solution that may have become contaminated.

Table 8: Vivaglobin

Summary of Additional Pharmacokinetics Parameters—European and Brazilian PK Sub-study—Per-protocol Subjects

	Vivaglobin
Number of Subjects	**41**
Dose	
Mean Range	96 mg/kg 51–147 mg/kg
IgG trough levels	
Mean Range	871 mg/dL 604–1401 mg/dL
C_{max}	
Mean Range	949 mg/dL 637–1517 mg/dL
t_{max}	
Mean Range	2.46 d 0–6.95 d
AUC_{last}	
Mean Range	62.25 g/L[a] d 39.91–102.24 g/L[a] d
[a]CLss/F:	
Mean Range	1.54 mL/d/kg 0.83–2.60 mL/d/kg

[a] These results are based on 32 subjects only.

SPECIAL HANDLING INSTRUCTIONS: Vivaglobin, Immune Globulin Subcutaneous (Human), is a ready-for-use solution and should be administered at room temperature.

Vivaglobin is a clear solution. The color can vary from colorless to pale-yellow up to light-brown during shelf-life. Do not use solutions that are cloudy or contain residues (deposits/particles).

Any unused product or waste material should be disposed of in accordance with local authorities' requirements.

INFORMATION FOR THE PATIENT: Published in e-CPS, available by subscription at www.e-cps.ca.

DOSAGE FORMS, COMPOSITION AND PACKAGING: Each mL contains: immune globulin subcutaneous (human) 160 mg. Single-use vials of 3, 10 and 20 mL, boxes of 2 (10 mL vials), and 20.

ViVAXIM®

combined purified Vi polysaccharide typhoid and inactivated hepatitis A vaccine

Active Immunizing Agent

sanofi pasteur

Date of Revision: August 2008

PHARMACOLOGY: Hepatitis A is an infection of the liver caused by the hepatitis A virus (HAV), an RNA virus genus Hepatovirus, and a member of the Picornaviridae family. While 1.4 million cases are reported worldwide every year, the true incidence may be three to 10 times greater. The virus is almost always spread through the fecal-oral route either by direct contact with infected persons or indirectly through ingestion of contaminated food or water, especially raw or undercooked shellfish. A small number of cases (<5%) is acquired through sexual activity or contaminated blood products. The virus can survive in a dried state for at least a week in ambient conditions and can survive in water for as long as 10 months. Hepatitis A is the most frequent vaccine-preventable disease in travellers, and has the highest mortality and morbidity rates for any vaccine-preventable infection in travellers.

In adults, the average duration of illness is 1 month, but lethargy and weakness can last up to 12 months. More serious disease with liver necrosis, fulminant liver failure, and death is rare, and the estimated mortality rate is 0.14%. Disease severity is age-related with mortality rates for adults >40 years of age up to 20 times higher than those for younger age groups.

The risk for non-immune travellers to developing countries is estimated to be 3 to 5/1000 per month with cases in males being 1.5 times higher than in females. The risk is up to 6 times higher for low-budget travellers eating in poorer hygienic conditions.

S. typhi is the etiological agent of typhoid fever, an acute, febrile enteric disease transmitted by contaminated water and food. The fatality rate ranges from 16% in untreated cases to less than 1% in those given appropriate antibiotic therapy. Recently there has been increasing resistance to antibiotics. The risk of severe illness is increased in persons with depressed immunity or decreased gastric acid levels.

The incidence of typhoid fever is very low in industrialized countries, with an average of 70 cases reported each year in Canada. Typhoid vaccination is not required for international travel, but it is recommended for travellers to areas where there is a recognized risk of exposure to *S. typhi*, the organism which causes typhoid fever. *S. typhi* is prevalent in many countries of Africa, Asia and Central and South America. Vaccination is particularly recommended for travellers with reduced or absent gastric acid secretion; or those who will have prolonged (>4 weeks) exposure to potentially contaminated food and water, especially those travelling to or working in smaller cities and villages, or rural areas with a high incidence of disease. However, even travellers who have been vaccinated should use caution in selecting food and water.

TYPHIM Vi [Salmonella typhi Vi Capsular Polysaccharide Vaccine] confers significant protection against typhoid fever based on the production of measurable antibodies, predominantly of the IgG class.

AVAXIM [Hepatitis A Vaccine Inactivated] confers immunity against hepatitis A virus (HAV) infection by inducing the production of specific anti-hepatitis A virus antibodies.

In a clinical trial conducted in adults aged 16-65 years, 179 persons received ViVAXIM [Combined Purified Vi Polysaccharide Typhoid and Inactivated Hepatitis A Vaccine] and 181 received AVAXIM in one arm and TYPHIM Vi in the other arm. Equivalent seroconversion rates were seen, both at 14 and 28 days after vaccine administration. In another clinical trial conducted in adults aged 16-59 years, 610 persons received one dose of ViVAXIM. Antibody responses are in Table 1 and Table 2.

To assess the persistence of antibody, individuals in the comparative trial were followed for 3 years. During the three-year follow-up period, antibody trends for both valences were similar in both groups as shown in Table 3 and Table 4. The anti-Vi titres and percentage of subjects seroconverted gradually declined over the three years in both groups. Regarding anti-HAV titres, whether the group had initially received ViVAXIM or AVAXIM and TYPHIM Vi more than 99% of subjects were still seroconverted 3 years later.

Three years after the initial immunization, a sub-group of 102 individuals was reimmunized with ViVAXIM. Complete serology results were available for 47 individuals who had initially received ViVAXIM and 37 individuals who had initially received AVAXIM and TYPHIM Vi concomitantly at separate sites. Comparison of geometric mean titres (GMTs) 28 days after ViVAXIM injection at year 3, indicated that, for both valences, the GMTs obtained for the ViVAXIM group are non-inferior to the GMTs obtained for the group receiving AVAXIM and TYPHIM Vi.

INDICATIONS: ViVAXIM [Combined Purified Vi Polysaccharide Typhoid and Inactivated Hepatitis A Vaccine] is indicated for simultaneous active immunization against infection caused by *S. typhi*, the organism that causes typhoid fever, and hepatitis A virus (HAV) in persons 16 years of age or older. ViVAXIM can be used for hepatitis A primary immunization or booster.

ViVAXIM is recommended for pre-exposure prophylaxis of individuals at increased risk of infection.

Potential candidates for the vaccine are:

- travellers to countries where hepatitis A and typhoid fever are endemic or epidemic, or where sanitary conditions may be doubtful and where travellers may be exposed to potentially contaminated food and water.
- members of the armed forces, emergency relief workers and others likely to be posted abroad at short notice to areas with high rates of HAV and *S. typhi* infection.

The vaccine should be administered at least 14 days before risk of exposure to both typhoid fever and hepatitis A.

There is no contraindication to administering ViVAXIM to someone who is already immune to hepatitis A.

Table 1: ViVAXIM

Antibody Response to Vi 14 and 28 Days Post Vaccination with ViVAXIM

	D0	**D14**	**D28**
Anti-Vi titre (µg/mL)			
n	787	177	785
Geometric mean (95% CI[a])	**0.206** (0.196–0.217)	**2.98** (2.61–3.40)	**2.83** (2.67–3.01)
≥1 µg/mL			
n	35	158	702
% (95% CI)	**4.4** (3.1–6.1)	**89.3** (83.7–93.4)	**89.4** (87.1–91.5)
≥4-fold rise			
n		153	707
% (95% CI)		**86.4** (80.5–91.1)	**90.3** (88.0–92.3)

[a] 95% CI: 95% confidence interval.

Table 2: ViVAXIM

Antibody Response to HAV 14 and 28 Days Post Vaccination with ViVAXIM in Initially Anti-HAV Seronegative Subjects

	D0	**D14**	**D28**
Anti-HAV titre (mIU/mL)			
n	743	160	740
Geometric mean (95% CI[a])	**6.14** (5.93–6.35)	**232** (188–285)	**858** (799–921)
≥20 mIU/mL			
n	0	153	738
% (95% CI)	**0.0** (0.0–0.5)	**95.6** (91.2–98.2)	**99.7** (99.0–100)

[a] 95% CI: 95% confidence interval.

Table 3: ViVAXIM

Antibody Response to Vi

	ViVAXIM			**TYPHIM Vi and AVAXIM**		
	Year 1 (n=139)	**Year 2 (n=124)**	**Year 3 (n=112)**	**Year 1 (n=140)**	**Year 2 (n=117)**	**Year 3 (n=104)**
Anti-Vi titre (µg/mL)						
GMT	**0.85**	**0.698**	**0.641**	**0.944**	**0.704**	**0.662**
95% CI[a]	0.716–1.01	0.585–0.834	0.530–0.776	0.769–1.16	0.564–0.878	0.520–0.843
≥1 µg/mL						
%	**44.6**	**40.3**	**32.1**	**44.3**	**41**	**35.6**
95% CI	36.2–53.3	31.6–49.5	23.6–41.6	35.9–52.9	32.0–50.5	26.4–45.6

[a] 95% CI: 95% confidence interval.

Table 4: ViVAXIM

Antibody Response to HAV

	ViVAXIM			**TYPHIM Vi and AVAXIM**		
	Year 1 (n=140)	**Year 2 (n=124)**	**Year 3 (n=112)**	**Year 1 (n=139)**	**Year 2 (n=116)**	**Year 3 (n=103)**
Anti-HAV titre (mIU/mL)						
GMT	**548**	**419**	**425**	**321**	**257**	**258**
95% CI[a]	443–678	340–518	345–524	265–390	204–324	202–329
≥20 mIU/mL						
%	**99.3**	**98.4**	**99.1**	**99.3**	**98.3**	**99**
95% CI	96.1–100	94.3–99.8	95.1–100	96.1–100	93.9–99.8	94.7–100

[a] 95% CI: 95% confidence interval.

CONTRAINDICATIONS: Immunization with ViVAXIM [Combined Purified Vi Polysaccharide Typhoid and Inactivated Hepatitis A Vaccine] should be deferred in the presence of any acute illness, including febrile illness to avoid superimposing adverse effects from the vaccine on the underlying illness or mistakenly identifying a manifestation of the underlying illness as a complication of vaccine use. A minor afebrile illness such as mild upper respiratory infection is not usually reason to defer immunization.

Allergy to any component of ViVAXIM (see components listed in Supplied) or an anaphylactic or other allergic reaction to a previous dose of ViVAXIM, AVAXIM or TYPHIM Vi are contraindications to vaccination.

WARNINGS: Immunocompromised persons (from disease or treatment) may not obtain the expected immune response. If possible, consideration should be given to delaying vaccination until the completion of any immunosuppressive treatment. Subjects with chronic immunodeficiency such as HIV infection may be vaccinated if the underlying pathology permits the induction of an antibody response, even if limited. If ViVAXIM [Combined Purified Vi Polysaccharide Typhoid and Inactivated Hepatitis A Vaccine] is used in these persons, hepatitis A seroconversion should be confirmed by antibody testing.

ViVAXIM will not provide protection against species of Salmonella other than *S. typhi* or against other bacteria that cause enteric disease; it does not provide protection against infection caused by hepatitis B virus, hepatitis C virus, delta virus, hepatitis E virus or by other liver pathogens, other than hepatitis A virus.

Because of the incubation period of hepatitis A disease, infection may be present but not clinically apparent at the time of vaccination. It is not known whether ViVAXIM will prevent hepatitis A in this case.

ViVAXIM should not be administered into the buttocks because of the varying amount of fatty tissue in this region nor by the intradermal route, since these methods of administration may induce a weaker immune response.

Intramuscular injections should be given with care in persons suffering from coagulation disorders or on anticoagulant therapy because of the risk of hemorrhage.

ViVAXIM may be administered by the subcutaneous route in patients with thrombocytopenia or in those at risk of hemorrhage; however, this may be associated with a higher risk of local reactions including injection site nodule.

As with any vaccine, immunization with ViVAXIM may not protect 100% of susceptible individuals. Travellers should take all necessary precautions to avoid contaminated food and water. This is of particular concern when the vaccine is administered less than 2 weeks before departure as optimum antibody protection may not yet be achieved.

Drug Interactions: If indicated, ViVAXIM may be administered simultaneously with immune globulin at separate sites with separate syringes. Hepatitis A seroconversion rates are not modified, but hepatitis A antibody titres could be lower than after vaccination using the vaccine alone.

As the vaccine is inactivated, concomitant administration of other vaccine(s) given at other injection sites is unlikely to interfere with immune responses. Based on data obtained from the concomitant administration of the monovalent vaccines [Purified Vi Polysaccharide Typhoid Vaccine and Inactivated Hepatitis A Vaccine] with yellow fever vaccine, no interference with the immune response is expected when ViVAXIM is administered concurrently at a different site with yellow fever vaccine. No interaction with other medication is currently known.

If any other vaccines are administered at the same visit, they must be given at separate sites and using separate syringes.

PRECAUTIONS: General: The possibility of allergic reactions in persons sensitive to components of the vaccine should be evaluated. Epinephrine Hydrochloride Solution (1:1000) and other appropriate agents should be available for immediate use in case an anaphylactic or acute hypersensitivity reaction occurs. Health-care providers should be familiar with current recommendations for the initial management of anaphylaxis in non-hospital settings, including proper airway management.

Before administration, take all appropriate precautions to prevent adverse reactions. This includes a review of the patient's history concerning possible hypersensitivity to the vaccine or similar vaccines, asking about previous immunization history, and the presence of any contraindications to immunization, current health status, and a current knowledge of the literature concerning the use of the vaccine under consideration.

Do not inject into a blood vessel.

Use a separate sterile needle and syringe, or a sterile disposable unit, for each individual patient to prevent disease transmission.

Needles should not be recapped and should be disposed of properly.

Before administration of ViVAXIM [Combined Purified Vi Polysaccharide Typhoid and Inactivated Hepatitis A Vaccine], health-care personnel should inform the parent or guardian or the patient to be immunized of the benefits and risks of immunization, inquire about the recent health status of the patient and comply with any local requirements with respect to information to be provided to the patient before immunization.

Pregnancy: On theoretic grounds, any purified polysaccharide vaccine or inactivated viral vaccine should not pose a risk to a human fetus. However, because animal reproduction studies have not been conducted with ViVAXIM, AVAXIM, or TYPHIM Vi, it is unknown whether these vaccines can cause fetal harm when administered to a pregnant woman or can affect reproductive capacity. Therefore, ViVAXIM is not recommended for pregnant women, particularly during the first trimester. The potential risks of vaccination in pregnancy should be considered and weighed against the risks of acquiring hepatitis A and/or typhoid fever. Administering ViVAXIM during pregnancy should only be done where the benefit clearly outweighs the risk.

Lactation: The effect of administration of ViVAXIM during lactation has not been assessed. On theoretic grounds, a purified polysaccharide vaccine or inactivated viral vaccine, like ViVAXIM, should not pose risk to the mother or the infant; however, ViVAXIM is not recommended for use in lactating women except where careful consideration of the potential risks and benefits of vaccination are carefully assessed and where the benefit clearly outweighs the risk.

ADVERSE EFFECTS: In controlled clinical studies using ViVAXIM [Combined Purified Vi Polysaccharide Typhoid and Inactivated Hepatitis A Vaccine], the most commonly reported reactions were those occurring at the injection site.

In a clinical trial comparing ViVAXIM with the two monovalent vaccines given simultaneously at separate sites, pain at the injection site was reported by 89.9% of subjects (4.5% severe) following administration of ViVAXIM compared with 84.9% of subjects (5% severe) who received monovalent Vi polysaccharide typhoid vaccine and inactivated hepatitis A vaccine at separate injection sites.

During clinical trials, the following adverse events were observed:

Nervous System Disorders: Very common (≥1:10): headache. Uncommon (≥1:1000 and <1:100): dizziness.

Gastrointestinal Disorders: Common (≥1:100 and <1:10): nausea; diarrhea.

Skin and Subcutaneous Tissue Disorders: Uncommon (≥1:1000 and <1:100): pruritus; rash.

Musculoskeletal, Connective Tissue and Bone Disorders: Common (≥1:100 and <1:10): myalgia; arthralgia.

General Disorders and Administration Site Conditions: Very common (≥1:10): pain, induration/oedema, and erythema at the injection site; asthenia. Common (≥1:100 and <1:10): malaise; fever.

In post market surveillance of the two vaccines that comprise ViVAXIM, adverse reactions are very rarely reported. The frequencies listed below are based on spontaneous reporting rates and have been calculated using the number of reports and estimated number of patients.

The following adverse reactions have been reported in association with TYPHIM Vi:

Gastrointestinal Disorders: Very rare (<1:10 000): nausea; vomiting; diarrhea.

General Disorders and Administration Site Conditions: Very rare (<1:10 000): injection site pain; injection site rash; abdominal pain; fever; malaise; asthenia.

Immune System Disorders: Very rare (<1:10 000): anaphylactic reaction; serum sickness.

Musculoskeletal and Connective Tissue Disorders: Very rare (<1:10 000): arthralgia; myalgia.

Respiratory, Thoracic and Mediastinal Disorders: Very rare (<1:10 000): asthma.

Nervous System Disorders: Very rare (<1:10 000): headache.

Skin and Subcutaneous Tissue Disorders: Very rare (<1:10 000): injection site inflammation; urticaria.

The following adverse reactions have been reported in association with AVAXIM:

Gastrointestinal Disorders: Very rare (<1:10 000): gastrointestinal disorders.

General Disorders and Administration Site Conditions: Very rare (<1:10 000): injection site pain; injection site rash; injection site nodule; fever; asthenia.

Investigation: Very rare (<1:10 000): transaminases increased.

Musculoskeletal and Connective Tissue Disorders: Very rare (<1:10 000): arthralgia; myalgia.

Nervous System Disorders: Very rare (<1:10 000): headache.

Skin and Subcutaneous Tissue Disorders: Very rare (<1:10 000): urticaria.

Physicians, nurses, and pharmacists should report any adverse occurrences temporally related to the administration of the product in accordance with local requirements and to the Global Pharmacovigilance Department, Sanofi Pasteur Limited, 1755 Steeles Avenue West, Toronto, ON, M2R 3T4, Canada. 1-888-621-1146 (phone) or 416-667-2435 (fax).

DOSAGE: Primary immunization is achieved with one single dose of ViVAXIM [Combined Purified Vi Polysaccharide Typhoid and Inactivated Hepatitis A Vaccine]. The recommended dosage is 1 mL of the mixed vaccine.

To provide long-term protection against infection caused by the hepatitis A virus, a booster injection of inactivated hepatitis A vaccine (such as AVAXIM) should be given 6 to 12 months later. It is predicted that HAV antibodies persist for many years (at least 10 years) after the booster.

Revaccination against typhoid fever should be carried out with a single dose of purified Vi polysaccharide typhoid vaccine (such as TYPHIM Vi) every 3 years in subjects who remain at risk.

ViVAXIM may be used as a booster vaccine in subjects who have received an inactivated hepatitis A vaccine 6 to 12 months earlier and who require protection against typhoid fever.

Inspect for extraneous particulate matter and/or discolouration before use.

The Purified Vi Polysaccharide Typhoid Vaccine (solution for injection) is contained in the chamber of the syringe closest to the syringe tip and the Inactivated Hepatitis A Vaccine (suspension for injection) in the chamber closest to the plunger.

The two vaccine components should only be mixed **immediately** before injection. The final volume to be injected is 1 mL.

Instructions for Use—Dual Chamber Syringe (see package insert for illustrations):

1. Remove the tip-cap.
2. Attach needle and needle shield to the syringe.
3. Screw the plunger rod into the plunger stopper (stopper 2).
4. Shake the syringe; then mix the vaccine components by slowly pushing the plunger, keeping the needle upwards. The vaccine in the lower chamber moves into the upper chamber by means of the by-pass channel.
5. Shake vigorously until a homogeneous suspension is achieved.
6. Holding the needle shield at the tip, remove by pulling upwards without twisting.
7. Proceed immediately with the injection. A vein test may be carried out by pulling back slightly on the plunger. The stoppers may separate but ensure that stopper 2 does not reach the 'by-pass channel' in order to avoid any leakage of liquid. If a blood vessel has been penetrated, blood will be pulled back into the syringe.

ViVAXIM should be administered by slow intramuscular injection in the deltoid region. Do not administer in the buttocks.

Do not inject intravenously.

Give the patient a permanent personal immunization record. In addition, it is essential that the physician or nurse record the immunization history in the permanent medical record of each patient. This permanent office record should contain the name of the vaccine, date given, dose, manufacturer and lot number.

SUPPLIED: ViVAXIM [Combined Purified Vi Polysaccharide Typhoid and Inactivated Hepatitis A Vaccine] is a combination vaccine consisting of purified Vi Polysaccharide Typhoid and Inactivated Hepatitis A supplied in a dual chamber syringe.

TYPHIM Vi is a sterile, clear, colorless, solution. The Vi antigen contained in TYPHIM Vi vaccine is extracted from the bacterial capsule of *Salmonella typhi* strain Ty2. Each human dose of purified Vi polysaccharide typhoid vaccine contains 25 µg.

AVAXIM is a cloudy whitish suspension. The active ingredient is a purified and formaldehyde-inactivated hepatitis A virus obtained from the GBM strain cultured on MRC-5 human diploid cells. Each human dose (0.5 mL) of inactivated hepatitis A vaccine contains: 160 antigen units (in the absence of an international standardized reference, the antigen content is expressed using an in-house reference).

The dual chamber syringe contains: 0.5 mL of purified Vi polysaccharide typhoid vaccine and 0.5 mL of inactivated hepatitis A vaccine which are mixed immediately before administration.

Each 1 mL dose of vaccine contains: first chamber: *S. typhi* (Ty2 strain) purified Vi capsular polysaccharide 25 µg, phosphate buffer solution containing: sodium chloride 4.150 mg, disodium phosphate dihydrate 0.065 mg, sodium dihydrogen phosphate dihydrate 0.023 mg, water for injection qs to 0.5 mL; second chamber: inactivated hepatitis A virus* 160 antigen units†, 2-phenoxyethanol 2.5 µL, formaldehyde 12.5 µg, aluminum hydroxide (expressed as aluminum) 0.3 mg, medium 199 Hanks/water for injection‡ qs to 0.5 mL, neomycin—(may contain residual traces from the production process).

ViVAXIM [Combined Purified Vi Polysaccharide Typhoid and Inactivated Hepatitis A Vaccine] meets the WHO requirements for production of biological substances.

Packages containing one prefilled single-dose, dual chamber syringe. Store at 2 to 8°C. **Do not freeze.** Discard product if exposed to freezing temperatures. The vaccine must be administered immediately after mixing. Do not use vaccine after expiration date on the label.

* GBM strain cultured on MRC-5 human diploid cells.

† In the absence of an international standardized reference, the antigen content is expressed using an in-house reference.

‡ Medium 199 Hanks (without phenol red) is a mixture of amino acids, mineral salts, vitamins and other components supplemented with polysorbate 80.

Volibris® Ⓟ

ambrisentan

Endothelin Receptor Antagonist

GlaxoSmithKline

Date of Revision: May 27, 2010

SUMMARY PRODUCT INFORMATION:

Route of Administration	Dosage Form/Strength	Nonmedicinal Ingredients
Oral	Tablet, 5 mg and 10 mg	Microcrystalline cellulose, lactose monohydrate, croscarmellose sodium, magnesium stearate, polyvinyl alcohol, talc, titanium dioxide and macrogol/polyethylene glycol 3350, lecithin and FD&C Red #40 Aluminum Lake

INDICATIONS AND CLINICAL USE: VOLIBRIS (ambrisentan) is indicated for:

- treatment of idiopathic ('primary') pulmonary arterial hypertension and pulmonary arterial hypertension associated with connective tissue disease in patients with WHO functional class II or III symptoms who have not responded to conventional therapy.

CONTRAINDICATIONS:

- Patients with a known or suspected hypersensitivity to VOLIBRIS or any of its components (see Dosage Forms, Composition and Packaging).
- Pregnancy (see Warnings and Precautions, Special Populations, Pregnant Women).

WARNINGS AND PRECAUTIONS: General: There have been no studies to investigate the effect of VOLIBRIS on driving performance or the ability to operate machinery. Further, a detrimental effect on such activities cannot be predicted from the pharmacology of the active substance.

Hematologic: The development of drug-related decreases in hemoglobin concentration and hematocrit has been associated with administration of endothelin receptor antagonists and was observed in clinical studies with VOLIBRIS and there have been cases where this has resulted in anemia (see Adverse Reactions). These decreases were generally observed within the first few weeks of treatment with VOLIBRIS, and stabilized thereafter.

Initiation of VOLIBRIS is not recommended for patients with clinically significant anemia (see Monitoring and Laboratory Tests).

Hepatic/Biliary/Pancreatic: Liver Function: Liver function abnormalities have been associated with pulmonary arterial hypertension. Hepatic enzyme elevations potentially related to therapy have been observed with endothelin receptor antagonists (ERAs). Therefore, hepatic function should be evaluated prior to initiation of VOLIBRIS. If aminotransferase (alanine aminotransferase, ALT or aspartate aminotransferase, AST) concentrations are greater than 3 times upper limit of normal (>3×ULN), initiation of VOLIBRIS is not recommended.

Although the incidence of aminotransferase abnormalities was low, the possibility of serum aminotransferase elevations associated with VOLIBRIS administration cannot be excluded. Therefore monthly monitoring of ALT and AST is recommended (see Monitoring and Laboratory Tests; Action and Clinical Pharmacology, Special Populations and Conditions, Hepatic Insufficiency).

Fluid Retention: Peripheral edema has been observed with ERAs including VOLIBRIS. Peripheral edema may also be a clinical consequence of PAH. VOLIBRIS induced a dose-dependent increase of occurrence of mild to moderate peripheral edema, although in elderly patients the severity and frequency were higher (see Adverse Reactions).

Fluid retention has been reported occurring within weeks after starting ambrisentan and, in some cases, has required intervention with a diuretic or hospitalization for fluid management or decompensated heart failure. If patients have pre-existing fluid overload, this should be managed as clinically appropriate prior to starting VOLIBRIS.

If clinically significant peripheral edema develops during therapy with VOLIBRIS, with or without associated weight gain, further evaluation should be undertaken to determine the cause, such as ambrisentan or underlying heart failure, and the possible need for specific treatment or discontinuation of ambrisentan therapy.

Pulmonary Veno-Occlusive Disease: If patients develop acute pulmonary edema during initiation of therapy with vasodilating agents such as an endothelin receptor antagonist, the possibility of pulmonary veno-occlusive disease should be considered.

Renal: VOLIBRIS has not been studied in individuals with renal impairment. Ambrisentan does not undergo significant renal metabolism or renal clearance (excretion), and therefore dose adjustment is unlikely to be required in patients with renal impairment (see Action and Clinical Pharmacology, Pharmacokinetics).

Sexual Function/Reproduction: The development of testicular tubular atrophy that was not reversible after 13 or 20 weeks has been observed in male rats at dose levels of 10 to 300 mg/kg/day, although reduced fertility and morphologic effects on sperm only occurred at 300 mg/kg/day and were reversible. The effect on male human fertility is not known.

Special Populations: Pregnant Women: The use of VOLIBRIS is contraindicated in pregnant women. Animal studies have reported increased incidences of fetal malformations and abnormalities following administration of ERAs including ambrisentan during pregnancy.

Women of child bearing potential should be advised of the risk of fetal harm if VOLIBRIS is taken during pregnancy. Pregnancy must be excluded before the start of treatment with VOLIBRIS and prevented thereafter by reliable contraception. Pregnancy tests during treatment with ambrisentan are recommended as clinically indicated.

Women of child bearing potential should be advised to contact their physician immediately if they become pregnant or suspect they may be pregnant. If pregnancy is to be continued, VOLIBRIS should be discontinued and alternative treatment should be initiated (see Contraindications).

Nursing Women: It is not known whether ambrisentan is excreted in human or animal milk. VOLIBRIS is not recommended for use by nursing mothers.

Pediatrics (<18 years of age): There are no data available on the use of VOLIBRIS in patients under 18 years of age, and therefore its use in this age group is not recommended.

Geriatrics (>65 years of age): No dose adjustment is required (see Action and Clinical Pharmacology, Pharmacokinetics).

Monitoring and Laboratory Tests: Hemoglobin: VOLIBRIS has been associated with reductions in hemoglobin concentrations and hematocrit (see Adverse Reactions).

Initiation of VOLIBRIS is not recommended for patients with clinically significant anemia. It is recommended that hemoglobin and/or hematocrit levels are measured prior to the initiation of VOLIBRIS, again at one month, and periodically thereafter as clinically indicated. If a clinically significant decrease in hemoglobin or hematocrit is observed, and other causes have been excluded, dose reduction or discontinuation of treatment should be considered.

Liver Function Tests: Liver transaminase levels should be measured prior to initiation of treatment and subsequently at monthly intervals.

If patients develop sustained unexplained significant elevations of transaminases accompanied by signs or symptoms of hepatic injury (such as nausea, vomiting, fever, abdominal pain, jaundice or unusual lethargy or fatigue) or increases in bilirubin 2×ULN, treatment with VOLIBRIS should be stopped.

In patients without clinical symptoms of hepatic injury or jaundice, re-initiation of VOLIBRIS may be considered following resolution of hepatic enzyme abnormalities.

ADVERSE REACTIONS: Adverse Drug Reaction Overview: The safety of VOLIBRIS has been evaluated in Phase II and Phase III clinical studies totalling 483 patients with PAH who were treated with doses of 1, 2.5, 5, or 10 mg once daily, ranging in exposure from 1 day to 3.5 years. Overall, VOLIBRIS was well tolerated.

In placebo-controlled 12-week studies, the most commonly reported adverse drug reactions (ADRs) with VOLIBRIS were peripheral edema, headache, nasal congestion, sinusitis and palpitations.

The adverse events reported during long-term therapy with VOLIBRIS were consistent with those observed in the 12-week, placebo-controlled studies. The incidence of adverse events was generally greater during the first 12 weeks of therapy.

In placebo-controlled phase III studies, the proportion of subjects who prematurely discontinued for any reason was higher in the placebo group (15.9%) than in the combined VOLIBRIS group (7.6%). The proportion of subjects who discontinued because of adverse events was similar across all treatment groups: 3.0% in the placebo group and 2.3% in the combined VOLIBRIS group.

In the combined placebo-controlled studies, six (4.5%) subjects in the placebo group died and 4 (1.5 %) subjects in the ambrisentan groups died. A higher proportion of subjects in the placebo group had at least 1 non-fatal SAE compared to the combined VOLIBRIS group. The most frequent SAEs for both the placebo and combined ambrisentan groups were right ventricular failure (placebo, 6.1%; ambrisentan, 1.9%) and (worsening) pulmonary hypertension (placebo, 3.8%; ambrisentan, 1.1%). Treatment-related SAEs occurred with a similar frequency across all ambrisentan treatment groups.

Clinical Trial Adverse Drug Reactions: Because clinical trials are conducted under very specific conditions the adverse reaction rates observed in the clinical trials may not reflect the rates observed in practice and should not be compared to the rates in the clinical trials of another drug. Adverse drug reaction information from clinical trials is useful for identifying drug-related adverse events and for approximating rates.

The following safety data for VOLIBRIS were obtained from two Phase III 12-week placebo controlled studies in subjects with PAH (ARIES-1 and ARIES-2). A total of 261 patients received VOLIBRIS at doses of 2.5, 5, or 10 mg once daily and 132 patients received placebo.

Table 1 presents adverse events with a >3% incidence in the combined ambrisentan treatment group and that were more frequent than placebo from the combined analysis of ARIES-1 and ARIES-2. AEs are summarized by randomized treatment assignment.

Table 1: VOLIBRIS

Adverse Events in >3% of PAH Patients Receiving VOLIBRIS and More Frequent than Placebo (ARIES-1 and ARIES-2, Population: Safety)

Treatment group, n (%) Preferred Term	Placebo (N=132)	5 mg Ambrisentan (N=130)	10 mg Ambrisentan (N=67)	Combined Ambrisentan[a] (N=261)
Peripheral edema	14 (10.6)	24 (18.5)	19 (28.4)	45 (17.2)
Headache	18 (13.6)	20 (15.4)	13 (19.4)	38 (14.6)
Nasal congestion	2 (1.5)	7 (5.4)	7 (10.4)	15 (5.7)
Palpitations	3 (2.3)	5 (3.8)	3 (4.5)	12 (4.6)
Dyspnea	4 (3.0)	7 (5.4)	3 (4.5)	11 (4.2)
Constipation	2 (1.5)	4 (3.1)	4 (6.0)	10 (3.8)
Flushing	1 (0.8)	5 (3.8)	1 (1.5)	10 (3.8)
Nasopharyngitis	1 (0.8)	7 (5.4)	2 (3.0)	9 (3.4)
Abdominal pain	1 (0.8)	4 (3.1)	2 (3.0)	8 (3.1)
Sinusitis	0	4 (3.1)	3 (4.5)	8 (3.1)

[a] Combined ambrisentan treatment group includes 2.5 mg dose group.

Note: This table includes all adverse events >3% incidence in combined ambrisentan treatment group and more frequent than in the placebo group, with a difference of ≥1% between the ambrisentan and placebo groups.

Adverse drug reactions were generally mild to moderate. The higher dose (10 mg) is associated with a higher incidence of peripheral edema, headache, nasal congestion, palpitations, constipation and sinusitis. Peripheral edema was the most common adverse event observed with VOLIBRIS.

All adverse events >1% and ≤3% incidence in the combined ambrisentan treatment group and more frequent than in the placebo group in Phase III clinical studies are as follows:

Blood and Lymphatic Disorders: anemia.

Cardiac Disorders: angina pectoris, tachycardia.
Gastrointestinal Disorders: diarrhea, gastritis, abdominal pain—upper.
General Disorders and Administration Site Conditions: chest discomfort, chest pain, edema, non-cardiac chest pain, pyrexia.
Infections and Infestations: pharyngitis, influenza, pneumonia.
Injury, Poisoning, and Procedural Complications: contusion.
Investigations: hemoglobin decreased.
Metabolism and Nutritional Disorders: anorexia, fluid retention, hypokalemia.
Musculoskeletal and Connective Tissue Disorders: muscle cramp, myalgia.
Psychiatric Disorders: insomnia, sleep disorder.
Renal and Urinary tract Disorders: nocturia.
Reproductive System and Breast Disorders: vaginal hemorrhage.
Respiratory, Thoracic and Mediastinal Disorders: lung crackles, pleural effusion, rhinitis, wheezing.
Skin and Subcutaneous Tissue Disorder: pruritus, skin ulcer.
Miscellaneous: a number of patients (19%) showed an increase of γGT (>3×ULN). The clinical significance is not known.

The common adverse events observed during long-term treatment with VOLIBRIS were similar to those reported during the 12 week placebo-controlled periods. During long-term studies, commonly reported events (≥10%) in the combined VOLIBRIS group—peripheral edema, headache, upper respiratory tract infection, dizziness, cough, arthralgia, right ventricular failure, pulmonary hypertension, dyspnea exacerbated, palpitations, diarrhea, nausea, nasopharyngitis, nasal congestion and anemia—were generally reported at a higher frequency in the 10 mg group.

Immune System Disorders: Hypersensitivity: Events suggestive of hypersensitivity to ambrisentan including descriptions of rash and angioedema have been reported uncommonly.

Abnormal Hematologic and Clinical Chemistry Findings: Hematologic Changes: In the placebo-controlled Phase III studies in patients with PAH, a decrease from baseline in mean hemoglobin (−0.84 g/dL) and hematocrit (−3% units) was observed in patients receiving VOLIBRIS. Marked decreases in hemoglobin (>15% decrease from baseline resulting in a value below the lower limit of normal) were observed in 7% of patients receiving VOLIBRIS and 4% of patients receiving placebo. Similar decreases in hemoglobin/hematocrit have been observed with other ERAs; the cause of the decrease is not fully understood, but it is not due to hemorrhage or hemolysis. The mean decrease was slightly greater with 10 mg (1.1 g/dL) than with 5 mg VOLIBRIS (0.76 g/dL). There were few events related to anemia, low hemoglobin or low hematocrit (n=8). These events appeared to be more frequent with 10 mg VOLIBRIS than lower doses or placebo.

Post-Market Adverse Drug Reactions: In addition to adverse reactions identified from clinical studies, the following adverse reactions were identified during post-approval use of VOLIBRIS. Because these events have been reported voluntarily from a population of unknown size, estimates of frequency cannot be made.

Post-marketing reports of fluid retention and heart failure associated with fluid retention have been reported occurring within weeks after starting ambrisentan and in some cases, have required intervention with a diuretic or hospitalization for fluid management or decompensated heart failure.

Cases of worsening dyspnea of unclear etiology have been reported shortly after starting VOLIBRIS therapy.

Post-marketing reports of nausea and vomiting have been reported during VOLIBRIS therapy.

DRUG INTERACTIONS: Overview: Studies with human liver tissue indicate that ambrisentan is metabolized by uridine 5′-diphosphate glucuronosyltransferases (UGTs) 1A9S, 2B7S, and 1A3S, CYP3A4 and CYP2C19. In vitro studies suggest that ambrisentan is a substrate of Organic Anion Transport Protein (OATP). In vitro studies show ambrisentan is a substrate but not an inhibitor of P-gp.

The drug interaction potential of ambrisentan is not well characterized because in vivo drug interaction studies were not conducted with the following types of drugs: strong inhibitors of CYP2C19 (omeprazole), strong inducers of CYP3A and 2C19 (rifampin), strong inhibitors of the transporters P-gp (cyclosporine A) and OATP (cyclosporine A, rifampin); and inducers of CYPs, UGTs and P-gp (rifampin). The impact of co-administration of such drugs on ambrisentan exposure is therefore unknown. Regarding inhibition of CYP3A4, the only data available were obtained with ketoconazole (see Drug-Drug Interactions, Ketoconazole).

Drug-Drug Interactions: Cyclosporine A: Cyclosporine A is known to inhibit P-gp, Organic Anion Transport Protein and CYP3A4 which in vitro studies indicate ambrisentan is a substrate. Since drug-drug interaction studies with cyclosporine A have not been completed, caution is advised when VOLIBRIS is co-administered with cyclosporine A.

Inducers of P-gp, CYPs, and UGTs: Caution is advised when VOLIBRIS is co-administered with inducers of P-gp, CYPs, and UGTs. The impact of co-administration of such drugs on ambrisentan exposure is unknown.

Oral Contraceptives: VOLIBRIS is contraindicated in pregnancy. In a clinical study in healthy volunteers, steady-state dosing with ambrisentan 10 mg once daily did not significantly affect the single-dose pharmacokinetics of the ethinyl estradiol and norethindrone components of a combined oral contraceptive. Based on this pharmacokinetic study, ambrisentan would not be expected to significantly affect exposure to oestrogen- or progestogen-based contraceptives.

The effects of 12 days dosing with ambrisentan (10 mg once daily) on the pharmacokinetics of a single dose of oral contraceptive containing ethinyl estradiol (35 μg) and norethindrone (1 mg) were studied in healthy female volunteers. The C_{max} and $AUC_{(0-\infty)}$ were slightly decreased for ethinyl estradiol (8% and 4%, respectively), and slightly increased for norethindrone (13% and 14 %, respectively). These changes in exposure to ethinyl estradiol or norethindrone were small and are unlikely to be clinically significant.

Phosphodiesterase Inhibitors: Co-administration of ambrisentan with a phosphodiesterase inhibitor, either sildenafil or tadalafil (both substrates of CYP3A4) in healthy volunteers did not significantly affect the pharmacokinetics of the phosphodiesterase inhibitor or ambrisentan.

Sildenafil: In healthy volunteers receiving a single dose of sildenafil (20 mg), daily doses of VOLIBRIS (10 mg) did not have a clinically relevant effect on the pharmacokinetics of sildenafil or the active metabolite, n-desmethyl sildenafil. Similarly, daily doses of sildenafil (20 mg tid) did not have a clinically relevant effect on the pharmacokinetics of a single dose of VOLIBRIS (10 mg) (see Action and Clinical Pharmacology, Pharmacokinetics). Nonetheless, co-administration of the two drugs could result in a drop of blood pressure. The combination should therefore be used with caution.

Tadalafil: The effects of steady-state ambrisentan (10 mg once daily) on the pharmacokinetics of a single dose of tadalafil, and the effects of steady-state tadalafil (40 mg once daily) on the pharmacokinetics of a single dose of ambrisentan were studied in 23 healthy volunteers. Ambrisentan did not have any clinically relevant effects on the pharmacokinetics of tadalafil. Similarly, co-administration with tadalafil did not affect the pharmacokinetics of ambrisentan. Nonetheless, co-administration of the two drugs could result in a drop of blood pressure. The combination should therefore be used with caution.

Ketoconazole: Data indicate that steady state administration of ketoconazole increases the AUC_{∞} and C_{max} of ambrisentan by 35 and 20%, respectively. The clinical significance of these changes is not known. Patients on 10 mg of ambrisentan while on ketoconazole should be monitored closely for any signs of adverse effects.

Strong 2C19 Inhibitor: In clinical studies of patients with PAH, co-administration of ambrisentan and omeprazole (an inhibitor of CYP2C19) did not significantly affect the pharmacokinetics of ambrisentan.

Warfarin: In healthy volunteers receiving warfarin, daily doses of VOLIBRIS (10 mg) did not have a clinically relevant effect on prothrombin time (PT), International Normalized Ratio (INR), or the pharmacokinetics of S-warfarin (CYP2C9 substrate) or R-warfarin (CYP3A4 substrate).

In patients with PAH receiving warfarin-type anticoagulants, concomitant administration of VOLIBRIS did not result in a clinically relevant change in PT, INR or anticoagulant dose (see Action and Clinical Pharmacology, Pharmacokinetics).

Drug-Food Interactions: VOLIBRIS can be taken with or without food (see Action and Clinical Pharmacology, Pharmacokinetics).

Drug-Herb Interactions: Interactions with herbal products have not been established.

DOSAGE AND ADMINISTRATION: Dosing Considerations:

- Treatment should only be initiated by a physician experienced in the treatment of PAH.
- VOLIBRIS treatment should only be initiated in women of childbearing potential following a negative pregnancy test and providing they are using a reliable method of contraception (see Contraindications; Warnings and Precautions, Special Populations, Pregnant Women).
- VOLIBRIS is not recommended in patients with severe hepatic impairment and should be used with caution in patients with moderate hepatic impairment (see Warnings and Precautions; Action and Clinical Pharmacology, Pharmacokinetics and Special Populations and Conditions, Hepatic Insufficiency).

Recommended Dose and Dosage Adjustment: VOLIBRIS should be initiated at a dose of 5 mg once daily. Additional benefit may be obtained by increasing the dose to 10 mg once daily. Patients with PAH associated with connective tissue disease may require 10 mg VOLIBRIS for optimal efficacy. Consider increasing the dose to 10 mg VOLIBRIS providing the 5 mg dose is well tolerated (see Adverse Reactions).

The maximum recommended daily dose is 10 mg.

VOLIBRIS can be administered with or without food.

Missed Dose: If a dose of VOLIBRIS is missed, the patient should be advised to take it as soon as they remember, and then continue with the next dose at the regular interval. Two doses should not be taken at the same time to make up for a missed dose.

OVERDOSAGE:

There is currently no experience with overdosage of VOLIBRIS. No specific antidote is available. In healthy volunteers, single doses of 50 and 100 mg (5 to 10 times the maximum recommended dose) were associated with headache, flushing, dizziness, nausea, and nasal congestion.

Due to the mechanism of action of ambrisentan, an overdosage of VOLIBRIS could potentially result in hypotension. In the case of pronounced hypotension, active cardiovascular support may be required.

> For management of a suspected drug overdose, contact your regional Poison Control Centre. See the *CPS* Directory section for a list of Poison Control Centres.

ACTION AND CLINICAL PHARMACOLOGY: Mechanism of Action: Ambrisentan is an orally active, propanoic acid-class, endothelin receptor antagonist (ERA) that is selective for the endothelin type A (ET_A) receptor. Selective inhibition of the ET_A receptor inhibits phospholipase C-mediated vasoconstriction and protein kinase C-mediated cell proliferation, while preserving nitric oxide and prostacyclin production, cyclic GMP- and cyclic AMP-mediated vasodilation, and endothelin-1 (ET-1) clearance that is associated with the endothelin type B (ET_B) receptor.

Pharmacodynamics: Cardiopulmonary Hemodynamics: Invasive hemodynamic parameters were assessed in patients with pulmonary arterial hypertension (PAH) at baseline and after 12 weeks (n=29) in a Phase II study. Treatment with ambrisentan resulted in a significant increase in mean cardiac index (+0.3 L/min/m²; 95% CI: 0.15 to 0.51; p<0.001), and a decrease in mean pulmonary artery pressure (−5.2 mmHg; 95% CI: −7.6 to −2.9; p<0.001), and mean pulmonary vascular resistance (−2.8 mmHg/L/min; 95% CI: −3.8 to −1.8; p<0.001) for the combined ambrisentan group. There was also a trend toward a reduction in mean right atrial pressure (−0.5 mmHg).

B-type Natriuretic Peptide: In patients with PAH, reductions in B-type natriuretic peptide (BNP) have been shown to parallel improvements in hemodynamics and 6-minute walk distance. Combined analysis of results from two Phase III placebo-controlled studies demonstrated that plasma concentrations of BNP decreased in patients who received ambrisentan for 12 weeks. The geometric mean plasma concentration of BNP increased by 11% in the placebo group, and decreased by 29% in the 2.5 mg, 30% in the 5 mg, and 45% in the 10 mg group (p<0.001 for each dose group). A positive association was observed between change in BNP and improvement in WHO class at Week 12.

Cardiac Electrophysiology: In a randomized, positive- and placebo-controlled, parallel-group study, healthy subjects received either VOLIBRIS 10 mg daily followed by a single dose of 40 mg, placebo followed by a single dose of moxifloxacin 400 mg, or placebo alone. VOLIBRIS 10 mg daily had no significant effect on the QTc interval. The 40 mg dose of VOLIBRIS increased mean QTc at t_{max} by 5 ms with an upper 95% confidence limit of 9 ms. For patients receiving VOLIBRIS 5-10 mg daily and not taking metabolic inhibitors, no significant QT prolongation is expected.

Pharmacokinetics: Absorption: Ambrisentan is absorbed rapidly in humans. The absolute bioavailability of ambrisentan is not known. After oral administration, maximum plasma concentrations (C_{max}) of ambrisentan typically occurs between 1 and 2 hours post dose under both fasted and fed conditions. C_{max} and area under the plasma concentration-time curve (AUC) increase dose proportionally over the therapeutic dose range. Steady-state is generally achieved following 4 days of repeat dosing.

A food-effect study involving administration of ambrisentan to healthy volunteers under fasting conditions and with a high-fat meal indicated that the C_{max} was decreased 12% while the AUC remained unchanged. This decrease in peak concentration is not clinically significant, and therefore ambrisentan can be taken with or without food.

Distribution: Ambrisentan is highly plasma protein bound. The in vitro plasma protein binding of ambrisentan was, on average, 99% and independent of concentration over the range of 0.2-20 μg/mL. Ambrisentan is primarily bound to albumin (96.5%) and to a lesser extent to alpha$_1$-acid glycoprotein.

The distribution of ambrisentan into red blood cells is low, with a mean blood:plasma ratio of 0.57 and 0.61 in males and females, respectively.

Metabolism: Ambrisentan is glucuronidated via several UGT isoenzymes (UGT1A9S, UGT2B7S, and UGT1A3S) to form ambrisentan glucuronide (13%). Ambrisentan also undergoes oxidative metabolism mainly by CYP3A4 and to a lesser extent by CYP3A5 and CYP2C19 to form 4-hydroxymethyl ambrisentan (21%) which is further glucuronidated to 4-hydroxymethyl ambrisentan glucuronide (5%). The binding affinity of 4-hydroxymethyl ambrisentan for the human endothelin receptor is 65-fold less than ambrisentan. Therefore at concentrations observed in the plasma (approximately 20% relative to parent ambrisentan), 4-hydroxymethyl ambrisentan is not expected to contribute to pharmacological activity of ambrisentan.

Using human liver microsome, in vitro data have shown that at therapeutic concentrations, ambrisentan does not inhibit UGT1A1, UGT1A6, UGT1A9, UGT2B7 or cytochrome P450 enzymes 1A2, 2A6, 2B6, 2C8, 2C9, 2C19, 2D6, 2E1, 3A4. Additional in vitro studies showed that ambrisentan is a substrate for the organic anion export pump (OATP); the interaction between strong inhibitors of this transporter and ambrisentan is possible (see Drug Interactions). Furthermore, ambrisentan does not affect biliary/xenobiotic transporters NTCP, OATP, multi-drug resistance protein isoform-2 (MRP2), P-glycoprotein (P-gp), or BSEP.

Excretion: Ambrisentan and its metabolites are primarily found in the feces following hepatic and/or extra-hepatic metabolism. Approximately 22% of the administered dose is recovered in the urine following oral administration with 3.3% being unchanged ambrisentan. The half-life after multiple dosing is approximately 15 hours (range 13.6 to 16.5 hours) in healthy volunteers and 9 to 15 hours in PAH patients. The mean oral clearance of ambrisentan is 38 mL/min and 19 mL/min in healthy subjects and in PAH patients, respectively.

Special Populations and Conditions: Pediatrics: There are no data available on the use of ambrisentan in patients under 18 years of age.

Geriatrics: Based on the results of a population pharmacokinetic analysis in healthy volunteers and patients with PAH, the pharmacokinetics of ambrisentan were not significantly influenced by age (see Dosage and Administration).

Gender: Based on the results of a population pharmacokinetic analysis in healthy volunteers and patients with PAH, the pharmacokinetics of ambrisentan were not significantly influenced by gender.

Hepatic Insufficiency: The pharmacokinetics of ambrisentan in patients with severe hepatic impairment or with clinically significant elevated hepatic transaminases has not been studied. However, since the main routes of metabolism of ambrisentan are glucuronidation and oxidation with subsequent elimination in the bile, moderate to severe hepatic impairment would be expected to increase exposure (C_{max} and AUC) of ambrisentan, however the magnitude of this and any effect on safety and efficacy has not been evaluated. Therefore ambrisentan should be used with caution in patients with moderate to severe hepatic impairment (see Warnings and Precautions, and Action and Clinical Pharmacology, Pharmacokinetics).

Renal Insufficiency: No pharmacokinetic studies have been conducted in renally impaired patients. However, the renal excretion of ambrisentan is minimal, therefore renal impairment should not significantly increase exposure to ambrisentan.

STORAGE AND STABILITY: Store between 15-30°C.

INFORMATION FOR THE PATIENT: Published in e-CPS, available by subscription at www.e-cps.ca.

DOSAGE FORMS, COMPOSITION AND PACKAGING: 5 mg: Each square, pale pink, film-coated tablet, engraved with "GS" on one side and "K2C" on the other, contains: ambrisentan 5 mg. Nonmedicinal ingredients: croscarmellose sodium, FD&C Red #40 Aluminum Lake, lactose monohydrate, lecithin, macrogol/polyethylene glycol 3350, magnesium stearate, microcrystalline cellulose, polyvinyl alcohol, talc and titanium dioxide. Blister packs of 30.

10 mg: Each oval, deep pink, film-coated tablet, engraved with "GS" on one side and "KE3" on the other, contains: ambrisentan 10 mg. Nonmedicinal ingredients: croscarmellose sodium, FD&C Red #40 Aluminum Lake, lactose monohydrate, lecithin, macrogol/polyethylene glycol 3350, magnesium stearate, microcrystalline cellulose, polyvinyl alcohol, talc and titanium dioxide. Blister packs of 30.

(Shown in Product Identification Section)

Voltaren® ℞

diclofenac sodium

Nonsteroidal Anti-inflammatory Drug (NSAID)

Novartis Pharmaceuticals

Voltaren® SR Pr
diclofenac sodium
Nonsteroidal Anti-inflammatory Drug (NSAID)

Novartis Pharmaceuticals

Date of Preparation: July 5, 1989
Date of Revision: April 8, 2010

SUMMARY PRODUCT INFORMATION:

Route of Administration	Dosage Form/ Strength	Clinically Relevant Nonmedicinal Ingredients
Oral	Enteric Coated Tablets, 50 mg	Lactose For a complete listing see Dosage Forms, Composition and Packaging.
	Slow-release Tablets, 75 mg, 100 mg	Sucrose For a complete listing see Dosage Forms, Composition and Packaging.
Rectal	Suppositories, 50 mg, 100 mg	For a complete listing see Dosage Forms, Composition and Packaging.

INDICATIONS AND CLINICAL USE: VOLTAREN (diclofenac sodium) and VOLTAREN SR (diclofenac sodium) are indicated for the following:

- the symptomatic treatment of rheumatoid arthritis and osteoarthritis, including degenerative joint disease of the hip.

Throughout this document, the term NSAIDs refers to both non-selective NSAIDs and selective COX-2 inhibitor NSAIDs, unless otherwise indicated.

For patients with an increased risk of developing CV and/or GI adverse events, other management strategies that do NOT include the use of NSAIDs should be considered first. (See Contraindications and Warnings and Precautions.)

Use of VOLTAREN or VOLTAREN SR should be limited to the lowest effective dose for the shortest possible duration of treatment in order to minimize the potential risk for cardiovascular or gastrointestinal adverse events. (See Contraindications and Warnings and Precautions.)

VOLTAREN and VOLTAREN SR, as NSAIDs, do **not** treat clinical disease or prevent its progression.

VOLTAREN and VOLTAREN SR, as NSAIDs, only relieve symptoms and decrease inflammation for as long as the patients continues to take them.

Patients Subsets: Geriatrics: Evidence from clinical studies and post-market experience suggests that use in the geriatric population is associated with differences in safety (see Warnings and Precautions).

Pediatrics (<16 years of age): Safety and efficacy have not been established in the pediatric population.

CONTRAINDICATIONS: VOLTAREN and VOLTAREN SR are contraindicated in:

- the peri-operative setting of coronary artery bypass graft surgery (CABG). Although VOLTAREN and VOLTAREN SR have **not** been studied in this patient population, a selective COX-2 inhibitor NSAID studied in such a setting has led to an increased incidence of cardiovascular/thromboembolic events, deep surgical infections and sternal wound complications.
- the third trimester of pregnancy, because of risk of premature closure of the ductus arteriosus and prolonged parturition
- women who are breastfeeding, because of the potential for serious adverse reactions in nursing infants
- severe uncontrolled heart failure
- known hypersensitivity to VOLTAREN or VOLTAREN SR or to any of the components/excipients
- history of asthma, urticaria, or allergic-type reactions after taking ASA or other NSAIDs (i.e. complete or partial syndrome of ASA-intolerance—rhinosinusitis, urticaria/angioedema, nasal polyps, asthma). Fatal anaphylactoid reactions have occurred in such individuals. Individuals with the above medical problems are at risk of a severe reaction even if they have taken NSAIDs in the past without any adverse reaction. The potential for cross-reactivity between different NSAIDs must be kept in mind (see Warnings and Precautions, Hypersensitivity Reactions, Anaphylactoid Reactions).
- active gastric/duodenal/peptic ulcer, active GI bleeding or perforation, regional ulcer, gastritis or ulcerative colitis
- cerebrovascular bleeding or other bleeding disorders
- inflammatory bowel disease
- severe liver impairment or active liver disease
- severe renal impairment (creatinine clearance <30 mL/min or 0.5 mL/sec) or deteriorating renal disease (individuals with lesser degrees of renal impairment are at risk of deterioration of their renal function when prescribed NSAIDs and must be monitored) (see Warnings and Precautions, Renal)
- known hyperkalemia (see Warnings and Precautions, Renal, Fluid and Electrolyte Balance)
- children and adolescents less than 16 years of age
- suppositories are contraindicated in patients with inflammatory lesions of the rectum or anus and in patients with a recent history of rectal or anal bleeding.

WARNINGS AND PRECAUTIONS:

Risk of Cardiovascular (CV) Adverse Events: Ischemic Heart Disease, Cerebrovascular Disease, Congestive Heart Failure (NYHA II-IV) (see Warnings and Precautions, Cardiovascular): VOLTAREN and VOLTAREN SR are non-steroidal anti-inflammatory drug (NSAID). Use of some NSAIDs is associated with an increased incidence of cardiovascular adverse events (such as myocardial infarction, stroke or thrombotic events) which can be fatal. The risk may increase with duration of use. Patients with cardiovascular disease or risk factors for cardiovascular disease may be at greater risk.

Caution should be exercised in prescribing VOLTAREN or VOLTAREN SR to any patient with ischemic heart disease (including but NOT limited to acute myocardial infarction, history of myocardial infarction and/or angina), cerebrovascular disease (including but NOT limited to stroke, cerebrovascular accident, transient ischemic attacks and/or amaurosis fugax) and/or congestive heart failure (NYHA II-IV).

Use of NSAIDs, such as VOLTAREN and VOLTAREN SR, can promote sodium retention in a dose-dependent manner, through a renal mechanism, which can result in increased blood pressure and/or exacerbation of congestive heart failure. (See also Warnings and Precautions, Renal, Fluid and Electrolyte Balance.)

Randomized clinical trials with VOLTAREN and VOLTAREN SR have not been designed to detect differences in cardiovascular events in a chronic setting. Therefore, caution should be exercised when prescribing VOLTAREN or VOLTAREN SR.

Risk of Gastrointestinal (GI) Adverse Events (see Warnings and Precautions, Gastrointestinal (GI)): Use of NSAIDs, such as VOLTAREN and VOLTAREN SR, is associated with an increased incidence of gastrointestinal adverse events (such as peptic/duodenal ulceration, perforation, obstruction and gastrointestinal bleeding).

General: Frail or debilitated patients may tolerate side effects less well and therefore special care should be taken in treating this population. **To minimize the potential risk for an adverse event, the lowest effective dose should be used for the shortest possible duration.** As with other NSAIDs, caution should be used in the treatment of elderly patients who are more likely to be suffering from impaired renal, hepatic or cardiac function. For high risk patients, alternate therapies that do not involve NSAIDs should be considered.

VOLTAREN and VOLTAREN SR are **not** recommended for use with other NSAIDs, with the exception of low-dose ASA for cardiovascular prophylaxis, because of the absence of any evidence demonstrating synergistic benefits and the potential for additive adverse reactions. (See Drug Interactions, Drug-Drug Interactions, Acetylsalicylic acid (ASA) or other NSAIDs.)

Diclofenac sodium should not be used concomitantly with diclofenac potassium (VOLTAREN RAPIDE) since both exist in plasma as the same active organic ion.

Cardiovascular: VOLTAREN and VOLTAREN SR are non-steroidal anti-inflammatory drugs (NSAIDs). Use of some NSAIDs is associated with an increased incidence of cardiovascular adverse events (such as myocardial infarction, stroke or thrombotic events) which can be fatal. Large population-based observational studies, meta-analyses and systematic reviews suggest an increased risk of myocardial infarction and stroke also in association with the use of diclofenac. The risk may increase with the dose and duration of use. Patients with cardiovascular disease or risk factors for cardiovascular disease may be at greater risk.

Caution should be exercised in prescribing VOLTAREN and VOLTAREN SR to patients with risk factors for cardiovascular disease, cerebrovascular disease or renal disease, such as any of the following (NOT an exhaustive list): hypertension; dyslipidemia/hyperlipidemia; diabetes mellitus; congestive heart failure (NYHA I); coronary artery disease (atherosclerosis); peripheral arterial disease; smoking; creatinine clearance <60 mL/min or 1 mL/sec.

Use of NSAIDs, such as VOLTAREN and VOLTAREN SR, can lead to new hypertension or can worsen pre-existing hypertension, either of which may increase the risk of cardiovascular events as described above. Thus blood pressure should be monitored regularly. Consideration should be given to discontinuing VOLTAREN and VOLTAREN SR should hypertension either develop or worsen with its use.

Use of NSAIDs, such as VOLTAREN and VOLTAREN SR, can induce fluid retention and edema, and may exacerbate congestive heart failure, through a renally-mediated mechanism. (See Warnings and Precautions, Renal, Fluid and Electrolyte Balance.)

For patients with a high risk of developing an adverse CV event, other management strategies that do **not** include the use of NSAIDs should be considered first. **To minimize the potential risk for an adverse CV event, the lowest effective dose should be used for the shortest possible duration.**

Endocrine and Metabolism: Corticosteroids: VOLTAREN and VOLTAREN SR (diclofenac sodium) are **not** a substitute for corticosteroids. They do **not** treat corticosteroid insufficiency. Abrupt discontinuation of corticosteroids may lead to exacerbation of corticosteroid-responsive illness. Patients on prolonged corticosteroid therapy should have their therapy tapered slowly if a decision is made to discontinue corticosteroids. (See Drug Interactions, Drug-Drug Interactions, Glucocorticoids.)

Gastrointestinal (GI): Serious GI toxicity (sometimes fatal), such as peptic/duodenal ulceration, inflammation, perforation, obstruction and gastrointestinal bleeding, can occur at any time, with or without warning symptoms, in patients treated with NSAIDs, such as VOLTAREN or VOLTAREN SR. Minor upper GI problems, such as dyspepsia, commonly occur at any time. Health care providers should remain alert for ulceration and bleeding in patients treated with VOLTAREN or VOLTAREN SR, even in the absence of previous GI tract symptoms. Most spontaneous reports of fatal GI events are in elderly or debilitated patients and therefore special care should be taken in treating this population. **To minimize the potential risk for an adverse GI event, the lowest effective dose should be used for the shortest possible duration.** For high risk patients, alternate therapies that do not involve NSAIDs should be considered. (See Warnings and Precautions, Special Populations, Geriatrics.)

Patients should be informed about the signs and/or symptoms of serious GI toxicity and instructed to discontinue using VOLTAREN or VOLTAREN SR and seek emergency medical attention if they experience any such symptoms. The utility of periodic laboratory monitoring has **not** been demonstrated, nor has it been adequately assessed. Most patients who develop a serious upper GI adverse event on NSAID therapy have no symptoms. Upper GI ulcers, gross bleeding or perforation, caused by NSAIDs, appear to occur in approximately 1% of patients treated for 3-6 months, and in about 2-4% of patients treated for one year. These trends continue, thus increasing the likelihood of developing a serious GI event at some time during the course of therapy. Even a short-term therapy has its risks.

Caution should be taken if prescribing VOLTAREN or VOLTAREN SR to patients with a prior history of peptic/duodenal ulcer disease or gastrointestinal bleeding as these individuals have a greater than 10-fold higher risk for developing a GI bleed when taking a NSAID than patients with neither of these risk factors. Other risk factors for GI ulceration and bleeding include the following: *H. pylori* infection, increased age, prolonged use of NSAID therapy, excess alcohol intake, smoking, poor general health status or concomitant therapy with any of the following: anti-coagulants (e.g. warfarin); anti-platelet agents (e.g. ASA, clopidogrel); oral corticosteroids (e.g. prednisone); Selective Serotonin Reuptake Inhibitors (SSRIs) (e.g. citalopram, fluotexine, paroxetine, sertraline).

There is no definitive evidence that the concomitant administration of histamine H_2-receptor antagonists and/or antacids will either prevent or reduce the occurrence of gastrointestinal adverse events associated with the use of VOLTAREN SR or the enteric-coated or suppository formulation of VOLTAREN. Concurrent administration of histamine H_2-receptor antagonists and/or antacids with the enteric-coated version of VOLTAREN might results in altered absorption.

Genitourinary: Some NSAIDs are associated with persistent urinary symptoms (bladder pain, dysuria, urinary frequency), hematuria or cystitis. The onset of these symptoms may occur at any time after the initiation of therapy with an NSAID. Should urinary symptoms occur, in the absence of an alternate explanation, treatment with VOLTAREN or VOLTAREN SR should be stopped to ascertain if symptoms disappear. This should be done before urological investigations or treatments are carried out.

Hematologic: NSAIDs inhibiting prostaglandin biosynthesis interfere with platelet function to varying degrees; patients who may be adversely affected by such an action, such as those on anti-coagulants or suffering from hemophilia or platelet disorders should be carefully observed when VOLTAREN or VOLTAREN SR is administered.

Anti-coagulants: Numerous studies have shown that the concomitant use of NSAIDs and anti-coagulants increases the risk of bleeding. Concurrent therapy of VOLTAREN or VOLTAREN SR with warfarin requires close monitoring of the international normalized ratio (INR).

Even with therapeutic INR monitoring, increased bleeding may occur.

Anti-platelet Effects: NSAIDs inhibit platelet aggregation and have been shown to prolong bleeding time in some patients. Unlike acetylsalicylic acid (ASA), their effect on platelet function is quantitatively less, or of shorter duration, and is reversible.

VOLTAREN, VOLTAREN SR and other NSAIDs have no proven efficacy as anti-platelet agents and should **not** be used as a substitute for ASA or other anti-platelet agents for prophylaxis of cardiovascular thromboembolic diseases. Anti-platelet therapies (e.g. ASA) should **not** be discontinued. There is some evidence that use of NSAIDs with ASA can markedly attenuate the cardioprotective effects of ASA. (See Drug Interactions, Drug-Drug Interactions, Acetylsalicylic Acid (ASA) or other NSAIDs).

Concomitant administration of VOLTAREN or VOLTAREN SR with low dose ASA increases the risk of GI ulceration and associated complications.

Blood Dyscrasias: Blood dyscrasias (such as neutropenia, leukopenia, thrombocytopenia, aplastic anemia and agranulocytosis) associated with the use of NSAIDs are rare, but could occur with severe consequences.

Anemia is sometimes seen in patients receiving NSAIDs, including VOLTAREN and VOLTAREN SR. This may be due to fluid retention, GI blood loss, or an incompletely described effect upon erythropoiesis. Patients on long-term treatment with NSAIDs, including VOLTAREN and VOLTAREN SR, should have their hemoglobin or hematocrit checked if they exhibit any signs or symptoms of anemia or blood loss.

Hepatic/Biliary/Pancreatic: As with other NSAIDs, including VOLTAREN or VOLTAREN SR, borderline elevations of one or more liver enzyme tests (AST, ALT, alkaline phosphatase) may occur in up to 15% of patients. These abnormalities may progress, may remain essentially unchanged, or may be transient with continued therapy.

A patient with symptoms and/or signs suggesting liver dysfunction, or in whom an abnormal liver test has occurred, should be evaluated for evidence of the development of a more severe hepatic reaction, while on therapy with VOLTAREN or VOLTAREN SR. Severe hepatic reactions including jaundice and cases of fatal hepatitis, liver necrosis and hepatic failure, some of them with fatal outcomes, have been reported with VOLTAREN or VOLTAREN SR.

Although such reactions are rare, if abnormal liver function tests persist or worsen, if clinical signs and symptoms consistent with liver disease develop (e.g. jaundice), or if systemic manifestations occur (e.g. eosinophilia, associated with rash etc.), this drug should be discontinued.

If there is a need to prescribe this drug in the presence of impaired liver function, it must be done under strict observation.

Caution is advised when using VOLTAREN or VOLTAREN SR in patients with hepatic porphyria, since VOLTAREN or VOLTAREN SR may trigger an attack.

Hypersensitivity Reactions: Anaphylactoid Reactions: As with NSAIDs in general, anaphylactoid reactions have occurred in patients without known prior exposure to VOLTAREN or VOLTAREN SR. In post-marketing experience, rare cases of anaphylactic/anaphylactoid reactions and angioedema have been reported in patients receiving VOLTAREN or VOLTAREN SR. VOLTAREN or VOLTAREN SR should **not** be given to patients with the ASA-triad. This symptom complex typically occurs in asthmatic patients who experience rhinitis with or without nasal polyps, or who exhibit severe, potentially fatal bronchospasm after taking ASA or other NSAIDs (see Contraindications).

ASA-intolerance: VOLTAREN or VOLTAREN SR should **not** be given to patients with complete or partial syndrome of ASA-intolerance (rhinosinusitis, urticaria/angioedema, nasal polyps, asthma) in whom asthma, anaphylaxis, urticaria/angioedema, rhinitis or other allergic manifestations are precipitated by ASA or other NSAIDs. Fatal anaphylactoid reactions have occurred in such individuals. As well, individuals with the above medical problems are at risk of a severe reaction even if they have taken NSAIDs in the past without any adverse reaction (see Contraindications).

Cross-sensitivity: Patients sensitive to any one of the NSAIDs may be sensitive to any of the other NSAIDs as well.

Serious Skin Reactions: (See Warnings and Precautions, Skin.)

Immune: (See Warnings and Precautions, Infection, Aseptic Meningitis.)

Infection: VOLTAREN and VOLTAREN SR, in common with other NSAIDs, may mask signs and symptoms of an underlying infectious disease.

Aseptic Meningitis: Rarely, with some NSAIDs, the symptoms of aseptic meningitis (stiff neck, severe headaches, nausea and vomiting, fever or clouding of consciousness) have been observed. Patients with autoimmune disorders (systemic lupus erythematosus, mixed connective tissue diseases, etc.) seem to be pre-disposed. Therefore, in such patients, the health care provider must be vigilant to the development of this complication.

Neurologic: Some patients may experience drowsiness, dizziness, blurred vision, vertigo, insomnia, depression, tinnitus or hearing loss with the use of NSAIDs, such as VOLTAREN and VOLTAREN SR. If patients experience such adverse reaction(s) they should exercise caution in carrying out activities that require alertness.

Ophthalmologic: Blurred and/or diminished vision has been reported with the use of NSAIDs. If such symptoms develop, VOLTAREN or VOLTAREN SR should be discontinued and an ophthalmologic examination performed. Ophthalmologic examination should be carried out at periodic intervals in any patient receiving VOLTAREN or VOLTAREN SR for an extended period of time.

Sun exposure in patients using VOLTAREN or VOLTAREN SR might cause photosensitivity and vision changes. Patients should be advised to contact their physician for assessment and advice if this occurs.

Peri-Operative Considerations: (See Contraindications, Coronary Artery Bypass Graft Surgery.)

Psychiatric: (See Warnings and Precautions, Neurologic.)

Renal: Long term administration of NSAIDs to animals has resulted in renal papillary necrosis and other abnormal renal pathology. In humans, there have been reports of acute interstitial nephritis, hematuria, low grade proteinuria and occasionally nephrotic syndrome.

During long-term therapy, kidney function should be monitored periodically. (See Action and Clinical Pharmacology, Special Populations and Conditions, Renal Insufficiency.)

Renal insufficiency due to NSAID use is seen in patients with pre-renal conditions leading to reduction in renal blood flow or blood volume. Under these circumstances, renal prostaglandins help maintain renal perfusion and glomerular filtration rate (GFR). In these patients, administration of a NSAID may cause a reduction in prostaglandin synthesis leading to impaired renal function. Patients at greatest risk of this reaction are those with pre-existing renal insufficiency (GFR <60 mL/min or 1 mL/s), dehydrated patients, patients on salt restricted diets, those with congestive heart failure, cirrhosis, liver dysfunction, taking angiotensin-converting enzyme inhibitors, angiotensin-II receptor blockers, cyclosporin, diuretics, and those who are elderly. Serious or life-threatening renal failure has been reported in patients with normal or impaired renal function after short term therapy with NSAIDs. Even patients at risk who demonstrate the ability to tolerate a NSAID under stable conditions may decompensate during periods of added stress (e.g. dehydration due to gastroenteritis). Discontinuation of NSAIDs is usually followed by recovery to the pre-treatment state.

Caution should be used when initiating treatment with NSAIDs, such as VOLTAREN or VOLTAREN SR, in patients with considerable dehydration. Such patients should be rehydrated prior to initiation of therapy. Caution is also recommended in patients with pre-existing kidney disease.

(See Warning and Precautions, Monitoring and Laboratory Tests, Renal.)

Advanced Renal Disease: (See Contraindications.)

Fluid and Electrolyte Balance: Use of NSAIDs, such as VOLTAREN or VOLTAREN SR, can promote sodium retention in a dose-dependant manner, which can lead to fluid retention and edema, and consequences of increased blood pressure and exacerbation of congestive heart failure. Thus, caution should be exercised in prescribing VOLTAREN or VOLTAREN SR in patients with a history of congestive heart failure, compromised cardiac function, hypertension, increased age or other conditions predisposing to fluid retention. (See Warnings and Precautions, Cardiovascular.)

Use of NSAIDs, such as VOLTAREN or VOLTAREN SR, can increase the risk of hyperkalemia, especially in patients with diabetes mellitus, renal failure, increased age, or those receiving concomitant therapy with adrenergic blockers, angiotensin-converting enzyme inhibitors, angiotensin-II receptor antagonists, cyclosporin, or some diuretics. Electrolytes should be monitored periodically. (See Contraindications.)

Respiratory: ASA-induced asthma is an uncommon but very important indication of ASA and NSAIDs sensitivity. It occurs more frequently in patients with asthma who have nasal polyps.

Pre-existing Asthma: In patients with asthma, seasonal allergic rhinitis, swelling of the nasal mucosa (i.e. nasal polyps), chronic obstructive pulmonary diseases or chronic infections of the respiratory tract (especially if linked to allergic rhinitis-like symptoms), reactions on NSAIDs like asthma exacerbations (so-called intolerance to analgesics/analgesics-asthma), Quincke's oedema or urticaria are more frequent than in other patients. Therefore, special precaution is recommended in such patients (readiness for emergency). This is applicable as well for patients who are allergic to other substances, e.g. with skin reactions, pruritus or urticaria.

Sexual Function/Reproduction: The use of VOLTAREN or VOLTAREN SR, as with any drug known to inhibit cyclooxygenase/prostaglandin synthesis, may impair fertility and is not recommended in women attempting to conceive. Therefore, in women who have difficulties conceiving, or who are undergoing investigation of infertility, withdrawal of VOLTAREN or VOLTAREN SR should be considered.

Skin: In rare cases, serious skin reactions such as Stevens-Johnson syndrome, toxic epidermal necrolysis, exfoliative dermatitis and erythema multiforme have been associated with the use of some NSAIDs. Because the rate of these reactions is low, they have usually been noted during post-marketing surveillance in patients taking other medications also associated with the potential development of these serious skin reactions. Thus, causality is **not** clear. These reactions are potentially life threatening but may be reversible if the causative agent is discontinued and appropriate treatment instituted. Patients should be advised that if they experience a skin rash they should discontinue their NSAID and contact their physician for assessment and advice, including which additional therapies to discontinue.

Use of VOLTAREN or VOLTAREN SR may cause photosensitivity upon exposure to sunlight or UV light causing symptoms such as sunburn, skin rash, skin blisters, pruritus, erythema and discolouration.

Special Populations: Pregnant Women: VOLTAREN or VOLTAREN SR are CONTRAINDICATED for use during the third trimester of pregnancy because of risk of premature closure of the ductus arteriosus and the potential to prolong parturition.

Caution should be exercised in prescribing VOLTAREN and VOLTAREN SR during the first and second trimesters of pregnancy.

Inhibition of prostaglandin synthesis may adversely affect pregnancy and/or the embryofoetal development. Data from epidemiological studies suggest an increased risk of miscarriage and of cardiac malformation after use of a prostaglandin synthesis inhibitor in early pregnancy.

In animals, administration of a prostaglandin synthesis inhibitor has been shown to result in increased pre- and post-implantation loss and embryo-foetal lethality. In addition, increased incidences of various malformations, including cardiovascular, have been reported in animals given a prostaglandin synthesis inhibitor during the organogenetic period. Diclofenac sodium readily crosses the placental barrier.

Nursing Women: (See Contraindications.)

Pediatrics: (See Contraindications.)

Geriatrics: Patients older than 65 years (referred to in this document as older or elderly) and frail or debilitated patients are more susceptible to a variety of adverse reactions from NSAIDs; the incidence of these adverse reactions increases with dose and duration of treatment. In addition, these patients are less tolerant to ulceration and bleeding. Most reports of fatal GI events are in this population. Older patients are also at risk of lower esophageal injury including ulceration and bleeding.

For such patients, consideration should be given to a starting dose lower than the one usually recommended, with individual adjustment when necessary and under close supervision.

Monitoring and Laboratory Tests: Cardiovascular: (Hypertension): Blood pressure should be monitored regularly during therapy with VOLTAREN or VOLTAREN SR.

Hematologic: Patients on long-term treatment with VOLTAREN or VOLTAREN SR should have their hemoglobin, hematocrit, red blood cells (RBC), white blood cells (WBC), and platelets checked if they exhibit any signs or symptoms of anemia or blood loss or blood dyscrasia.

Hepatic: Hepatic function (e.g.serum transaminases, bilirubine) should be monitored regularly during therapy with VOLTAREN or VOLTAREN SR.

Ophthalmologic: Patients on long-term treatment with VOLTAREN or VOLTAREN SR should have an ophthalmologic examination performed periodically, and if they experience blurred and/or diminished vision.

Renal: Patients with pre-existing renal insufficiency (GFR <60 mL/min or 1 mL/s), dehydrated patients, patients on salt restricted diets, those with congestive heart failure, cirrhosis, liver dysfunction, taking angiotensin-converting enzyme inhibitors, angiotensin-II receptor blockers, cyclosporin, diuretics, and the elderly should have their renal function monitored (e.g. urine output, serum creatinine, creatinine clearance and serum urea) during therapy with VOLTAREN or VOLTAREN SR.

Electrolytes, including serum potassium, should be monitored periodically, especially in patients with diabetes mellitus, renal failure, increased age, or those receiving concomitant therapy with adrenergic blockers, angiotensin-converting enzyme inhibitors, angiotensin-II receptor antagonists, cyclosporin, or some diuretics.

ADVERSE REACTIONS: Adverse Drug Reaction Overview: Although not all adverse drug reactions have been reported with VOLTAREN or VOLTAREN SR (diclofenac sodium), the types of adverse drug reactions are expected to be similar to those of VOLTAREN RAPIDE (diclofenac potassium) since both formulations exist in the plasma as the same active organic anion.

Gastrointestinal, dermatological, CNS and hepatic adverse reactions are the most commonly seen with diclofenac. The most severe gastrointestinal adverse reactions observed were ulceration and bleeding, while the most severe dermatological albeit rare reactions observed with diclofenac were erythema multiforme (Stevens-Johnson Syndrome and Lyell Syndrome). Fatalities have occurred on occasion, particularly in the elderly.

This section summarizes adverse drug reaction data pooled from clinical trials, published investigations and post-marketing experience with diclofenac potassium and diclofenac sodium.

Frequency estimate: Very common: ≥10%. Common: ≥1% and <10%. Uncommon: ≥0.01% and <1%. Very rare: <0.01%, including isolated reports. See Table 1 and Table 2.

Table 1: VOLTAREN/VOLTAREN SR

Most Common Adverse Drug Reactions (≥1%)

Gastrointestinal Disorders	Very common	Nausea, vomiting, diarrhea, dyspepsia, abdominal pain, flatulence, anorexia
Nervous System	Common	Dizziness, headache, vertigo
Hepatic	Common	Elevations (≥3 times the upper normal limit) of serum aminotransferase enzymes (AST or ALT)
Skin and Subcutaneous Disorders	Common	Rash, pruritus

Table 2: VOLTAREN/VOLTAREN SR

Less Common Adverse Drug Reactions (<1%)

Gastrointestinal Disorders	Uncommon	Gastritis, gastrointestinal hemorrhage, hemorrhagic diarrhea, melena, hematemesis gastric and intestinal ulcerations (with or without bleeding or perforation)
	Very rare	Lower gut disorders (including hemorrhagic colitis and exacerbation of ulcerative colitis or Crohn's disease), diaphragm-like intestinal strictures, hyperacidity, stomatitis, glossitis, coated tongue, esophageal lesions, constipation, pancreatitis
Nervous System	Uncommon	Drowsiness, malaise, impaired concentration, tiredness
	Very rare	Sensory disturbances including paresthesia, memory disturbance, convulsions, anxiety, tremor, aseptic meningitis, cerebrovascular accident (including transient ischemic attack, cerebral hemorrhage)
Special Senses	Very rare	Vision disturbances (blurred vision, diplopia), impaired hearing, tinnitus, taste alteration disorders
Cardiac Disorders	Uncommon	Palpitation, angina, arrhythmias
	Very rare	Exacerbation of cardiac failure, hypertension, myocardial infarction
Skin and Subcutaneous Disorders	Uncommon	Urticaria
	Very rare	Bullous eruption, erythema, eczema, erythema multiforme, Stevens-Johnson Syndrome, Lyell Syndrome (toxic epidermal necrolysis), erythroderma (exfoliative dermatitis), loss of hair, photosensitivity reactions, purpura, allergic purpura
Renal and Urinary Disorders	Uncommon	Edema (facial, general, peripheral)
	Very rare	Acute renal failure, nephrotic syndrome, urinary abnormalities (e.g., hematuria and proteinuria), interstitial nephritis, renal papillary necrosis
Hematologic	Very rare	Thrombocytopenia, leukopenia, agranulocytosis, hemolytic anemia, aplastic anemia, anemia secondary to gastrointestinal bleeding
Hepatic	Uncommon	Liver function disorders including hepatitis, jaundice
	Very rare	Fulminant hepatitis
Immune System Disorders	Uncommon	Hypersensitivity anaphylactic/anaphylactoid systemic reactions (including hypotension and shock)
	Very rare	Angioneurotic edema, (including face edema)
Psychiatric Disorders	Very rare	Disorientation, depression, insomnia, nightmare, irritability, psychotic disorder
Respiratory Disorders	Uncommon	Asthma
	Very rare	Pneumonitis
Other		Administration of the suppositories may occasionally give rise to local irritation, proctitis, rarely local bleeding and exacerbation of hemorrhoids.

Post-Market Adverse Drug Reactions: Hepatic: hepatic necrosis, hepatic failure.

DRUG INTERACTIONS: Drug-Drug Interactions: See Table 3.

Table 3: VOLTAREN/VOLTAREN SR
Established Potential Drug-Drug Interactions

VOLTAREN or VOLTAREN SR	Clinical Comment
Acetaminophen	There may be an increased risk of adverse renal effects when administered concomitantly with NSAIDs.
Acetylsalicylic Acid (ASA) or Other NSAIDs	The use of VOLTAREN or VOLTAREN SR in addition to any other NSAID, including over the counter ones (such as ASA and ibuprofen) for analgesic and/or anti-inflammatory effects is **not** recommended because of the absence of any evidence demonstrating synergistic benefits and the potential for additive adverse reactions. The exception is the use of low dose ASA for cardiovascular protection when another NSAID is being used for its analgesic/anti-inflammatory effect, keeping in mind that combination NSAID therapy is associated with additive adverse reactions. Some NSAIDs (e.g. ibuprofen) may interfere with the anti-platelet effects of low dose ASA, possibly by competing with ASA for access to the active site of cyclooxygenase-1. Diclofenac sodium should not be used concomitantly with diclofenac potassium (VOLTAREN RAPIDE) since both exist in plasma as the same active organic ion. Concomitant administration of diclofenac and other systemic NSAIDs or corticosteroids may increase the frequency of gastrointestinal undesirable effects.
Alcohol	There may be an increased risk of gastrointestinal side effects, including ulceration or hemorrhage, when administered concomitantly with NSAIDs.
Antacids	Concomitant administration of antacids with NSAIDs may affect the rate, but generally not the extent of the absorption of the NSAID.
Anticoagulants	(See Warnings and Precautions, Hematologic, Anti-coagulants.)
Anti-hypertensives	NSAIDs may diminish the anti-hypertensive effect of Angiotensin Converting Enzyme (ACE) inhibitors. Combinations of ACE inhibitors, angiotensin-II antagonists, or diuretics with NSAIDs might have an increased risk for acute renal failure and hyperkalemia. Blood pressure and renal function (including electrolytes) should be monitored more closely in this situation, as occasionally there can be a substantial increase in blood pressure (see Warnings and Precautions, Renal). Therefore the combination should be administered with caution, especially in the elderly (see Warnings and Precautions, Monitoring and Laboratory Tests).
Anti-platelet Agents (including ASA)	There is an increased risk of bleeding, via inhibition of platelet function, when anti-platelet agents are combined with NSAIDs, such as VOLTAREN and VOLTAREN SR (see Warnings and Precautions, Hematologic, Anti-platelet Effects).
Cyclosporin or Tacrolimus	Nephrotoxicity of cyclosporin and tacrolimus may be increased because of the effect of NSAIDs on renal prostaglandins. Therefore, it should be given at doses lower than those that would be used in patients not receiving cyclosporin or tacrolimus.
Digoxin	Diclofenac may increase the plasma concentration of digoxin. Dosage adjustment may be required. Monitoring of serum digoxin level is recommended.
Diuretics	Clinical studies as well as post-marketing observations have shown that NSAIDs can reduce the effect of diuretics (see Warnings and Precautions, Renal). **Class Statement** Concomitant treatment with potassium-sparing diuretics may be associated with increased serum potassium, thus making it necessary to monitor levels (see Warnings and Precautions, Monitoring and Laboratory Tests, Renal).
Glucocorticoids	Some studies have shown that concomitant use of NSAIDs and oral glucocorticoids increases the risk of GI adverse events such as ulceration and bleeding. This is especially the case in older (>65 years of age) individuals.
Lithium	Monitoring of plasma lithium concentrations is advised when stopping or starting a NSAID, as increased lithium concentrations can occur in patients taking lithium. Dosage adjustment of lithium may be required.
Methotrexate	Caution should be exercised when NSAIDs, including VOLTAREN or VOLTAREN SR, are administered less than 24 hours before or after treatment with methotrexate. Elevated blood concentrations of methotrexate may occur, increasing toxicity.
Oral Hypoglycemics	Pharmacodynamic studies have shown no potentiation of effect with concurrent administration with diclofenac; however, there are isolated reports of both hypoglycemic and hyperglycemic effects in the presence of diclofenac, which necessitated changes in the dosage of hypoglycemic agents. For this reason, monitoring of the blood glucose level is recommended as a precautionary measure during concomitant therapy.
Probenecid	May decrease the excretion and increase serum concentrations of NSAIDs possibly enhancing efficacy and/or increasing potential for toxicity. Concurrent therapy of NSAIDs with probenecid requires close monitoring to be certain that no change in dosage is necessary.
Quinolone Antibacterials	There have been isolated reports of convulsions which may have been due to concomitant use of quinolones and NSAIDs.
Selective Serotonin Reuptake Inhibitors (SSRIs)	Concomitant administration of NSAIDs, including VOLTAREN or VOLTAREN SR, and SSRIs may increase the risk of gastrointestinal ulceration and bleeding (see Warnings and Precautions, Gastrointestinal (GI)).

Drug-Food Interactions: Interactions with food have not been established.
Drug-Herb Interactions: Interactions with herbal products have not been established.
Drug-Laboratory Test Interactions: Diclofenac increases platelet aggregation time but does not affect bleeding time, plasma thrombin clotting time, plasma fibrinogen, or factors V and VII to XII. Statistically significant changes in prothrombin and partial thromboplastin times have been reported in normal volunteers. The mean changes were observed to be less than 1 second in both instances, and are unlikely to be clinically important.

Persistently abnormal or worsening renal, hepatic or hematological test values should be followed up carefully since they may be related to therapy.

Drug-Lifestyle Interactions: Patients experiencing visual disturbances, dizziness, vertigo, somnolence or other central nervous system disturbances while taking VOLTAREN or VOLTAREN SR should refrain from driving or using machines.

DOSAGE AND ADMINISTRATION: Dosing Considerations: Geriatrics: For such patients, consideration should be given to a starting dose lower than the one usually recommended, with individual adjustment when necessary and under close supervision. (See Warnings and Precautions, Special Populations, Geriatrics.)
Renal Insufficiency: Lower doses of VOLTAREN or VOLTAREN SR should be considered in patients with impaired renal function. (See Warnings and Precautions, Renal.)
Hepatic Impairment: Lower doses of VOLTAREN or VOLTAREN SR should be considered in patients with impaired hepatic function. (See Warnings and Precautions, Hepatic/Biliary/Pancreatic.)
Recommended Dose and Dosage Adjustment: VOLTAREN and VOLTAREN SR are to be used for maintenance therapy only.

As a general recommendation, the dose should be individually adjusted and the lowest effective dose given for the shortest possible duration.

VOLTAREN Tablets 50 mg (enteric-coated): Rheumatoid arthritis and osteoarthritis patients may use VOLTAREN (diclofenac sodium) enteric-coated tablets if:

- They were previously initiated at the lowest dose of 75 mg (enteric-coated) per day in 3 divided doses and required up-titration because they did not respond to that dose.
- The maximum recommended daily dose is 100 mg.
- For patients experiencing an inflammatory flare, who do not achieve control of symptoms with 100 mg of diclofenac, the dosage may be increased to a maximum of 150 mg per day in divided doses (50 mg TID), for the shortest possible duration and under close monitoring (see Warnings and Precautions, Cardiovascular).

In elderly patients, and patients with renal insufficiency, hepatic impairment or with a cardiovascular risk, the maximum daily dose should not exceed 100 mg of diclofenac (see Dosing Considerations).

VOLTAREN should be taken with food and the tablets should be swallowed whole.

VOLTAREN SR 75 mg and 100 mg (slow-release tablets):

- Patients with rheumatoid arthritis or osteoarthritis on a maintenance dose of 75 mg diclofenac sodium per day may be changed to a once daily dose of VOLTAREN SR 75 mg administered morning or evening.
- Patients on a maintenance dose of 100 mg diclofenac sodium per day may be changed to a once daily dose of VOLTAREN SR 100 mg, administered morning or evening.
- The maximum recommended daily dose is 100 mg.
- For patients experiencing an inflammatory flare, who do not achieve control of symptoms with 100 mg of diclofenac, the dosage may be increased to a maximum of 150 mg per day in divided doses (75 mg administered morning and evening), for the shortest possible duration and under close monitoring (see Warnings and Precautions, Cardiovascular).

In elderly patients, and patients with renal insufficiency, hepatic impairment or with a cardiovascular risk, the maximum daily dose should not exceed 100 mg of diclofenac (see Dosing Considerations).

VOLTAREN SR tablets should be swallowed whole with liquid, preferably at mealtime.

VOLTAREN Suppositories:

- VOLTAREN suppositories, 50 or 100 mg, may be given as substitute for the last oral daily doses.
- The maximum recommended daily dose is 100 mg.
- For patients experiencing an inflammatory flare, who do not achieve control of symptoms with 100 mg of diclofenac, the dosage may be increased to a maximum of 150 mg per day in divided doses, for the shortest possible duration and under close monitoring (see Warnings and Precautions, Cardiovascular).

In elderly patients, and patients with renal insufficiency, hepatic impairment or with a cardiovascular risk, the maximum daily dose should not exceed 100 mg of diclofenac (see Dosing Considerations).

Missed Dose: Patients who miss one or more doses of VOLTAREN (diclofenac sodium) 50 mg tablets, 50 mg or 100 mg suppositories or VOLTAREN SR (diclofenac sodium) 75 and 100 mg tablets should not increase the dose of VOLTAREN (diclofenac sodium) or VOLTAREN SR to compensate for the missed dose or doses, but should continue with their therapy as soon as possible.

OVERDOSAGE:
Symptoms: There is no typical clinical picture resulting from diclofenac overdosage. Overdosage can cause symptoms such as vomiting, gastrointestinal haemorrhage, diarrhoea, dizziness, tinnitus or convulsions. In the event of significant poisoning, acute renal failure and liver damage are possible.
Therapeutic Measures: Management of acute poisoning with NSAIDs, including VOLTAREN or VOLTAREN SR, essentially consists of supportive measures and symptomatic treatment. Supportive measures and symptomatic treatment should be given for complications such as hypotension, renal failure, convulsions, gastrointestinal disorder, and respiratory depression. Special measures such as forced diuresis, dialysis or haemoperfusion are probably of no help in eliminating NSAIDs, including VOLTAREN or VOLTAREN SR, due to the high protein binding and extensive metabolism. Activated charcoal may be considered after ingestion of a potentially toxic overdose, and gastric decontamination (e.g. vomiting, gastric lavage) after ingestion of a potentially life threatening overdose.

> For management of a suspected drug overdose, contact your regional Poison Control Centre. See the *CPS* Directory section for a list of Poison Control Centres.

ACTION AND CLINICAL PHARMACOLOGY: Mechanism of Action: Diclofenac sodium is a non-steroidal anti-inflammatory drug (NSAID). The mode of action is not fully known but it does not act through the pituitary-adrenal axis. Diclofenac sodium inhibits prostaglandin synthesis by interfering with the action of prostaglandin synthetase. This inhibitory effect may partially explain its actions.
Pharmacodynamics: The effects of VOLTAREN and VOLTAREN SR are largely mediated by inhibition of cyclooxygenases (COXs, COX-1, COX-2). These enzymes are found throughout the body and produce prostaglandins, which are important mediators of pain, fever, and adaptive and protective reactions in many organs and (inflamed) tissues.
Pharmacokinetics: Absorption: In humans, orally-administered diclofenac sodium is rapidly and almost completely absorbed and distributed to blood, liver, and kidneys. The plasma concentrations show a linear relationship to the amount of drug administered. No accumulation occurs provided the recommended dosage intervals are observed.

Enteric coating may delay the onset of absorption from 50 mg tablets. Absorption occurs more rapidly when the drug is administered on an empty stomach (T_{max} 2.5 hours), than with meals (T_{max} 6 hours). The bioavailability remains the same under both conditions. The mean peak plasma concentration of 1.5 µg/mL (5 µmol/L) is attained, on average, 2 hours after ingestion of one 50 mg enteric-coated tablet.

Following administration of slow-release (SR) diclofenac sodium, C_{max} is reached at approximately 4 hours or later. Significant drug plasma concentrations persist when levels would have dropped almost to baseline values following enteric-coated tablet administration. Mean plasma concentrations of 13 ng/mL (40 nmol/L) were produced 24 hours after VOLTAREN SR 100 mg, or 16 hours after VOLTAREN SR 75 mg (single dose). Trough levels are approximately 22-25 ng/mL (70-80 nmol/L) during treatment with VOLTAREN SR 100 once daily or VOLTAREN SR 75 twice daily. In pharmacokinetic studies no accumulation of diclofenac sodium was found following repeated once daily administration of VOLTAREN SR 100 mg tablets or repeated twice daily administration of VOLTAREN SR 75 mg tablets.

Suppositories have a more rapid onset, but slower rate of absorption than oral enteric-coated tablets. C_{max} is approximately 2/3 of that produced by an equivalent 50 mg enteric-coated tablet oral dose. T_{max} occurs within 1 hour. The unchanged diclofenac plasma AUC values for rectal administration are within the range of values produced by equivalent oral enteric-coated tablet doses. Since about half the active substance is metabolised during its first passage through the liver ("first pass" effect), the area under the concentration curve (AUC) following oral or rectal administration is about half as large as it is following a parenteral dose of equal size.
Distribution: Diclofenac sodium is extensively bound (99%) to serum albumin. The apparent volume of distribution is 0.12 to 0.17 L/kg. Single-dose (P.O. or I.M). studies in rheumatoid patients with joint effusions have shown that diclofenac is distributed to the synovial fluid, where T_{max} occurs 2 to 4 hours after plasma T_{max}. Synovial fluid concentrations exceed plasma levels within 4 to 6 hours of administration. This elevation above plasma concentrations can be maintained for up to 12 hours. The synovial fluid elimination half-life is at least 3 times greater than that for plasma.
Metabolism: Diclofenac undergoes single and multiple hydroxylation and methoxylation, producing 3'-, 4'-, 5-hydroxy, 4'-5-hydroxy and 3'-hydroxy-4'-methoxy derivatives of diclofenac. These phenolic metabolites are largely inactive, and (along with the parent compound) are mostly converted to glucuronide conjugates.
Excretion: Plasma clearance of diclofenac is 263±56 mL/min. The mean terminal drug half-life in plasma is 1.8 hours after oral doses. In humans about 60% of the drug and its metabolites are eliminated in the urine and the balance through bile in the feces. More than 90% of an oral dose is accounted for in elimination products within 72 hours. About 1% of an oral dose is excreted unchanged in urine.
Special Populations and Conditions: Pediatrics: VOLTAREN and VOLTAREN SR are contraindicated in children and adolescents less than 16 years of age (see Contraindications).

Geriatrics: The ability of elderly subjects to absorb, metabolize and excrete VOLTAREN or VOLTAREN SR does not appear to differ significantly from those of younger subjects.
Hepatic Insufficiency: In a study of ten patients with impaired hepatic function (chronic hepatitis and non-decompensated cirrhosis) receiving a single oral dose of 100 mg diclofenac sodium, the kinetics and metabolism of diclofenac, were the same as in patients without liver disease.
Renal Insufficiency: In patients suffering from renal impairment, no accumulation of the unchanged active substance can be inferred from the single-dose kinetics when applying the usual dosage schedule. At a creatinine clearance of <10 mL/min, the calculated steady-state plasma levels of the hydroxy metabolites are about 4 times higher than in normal subjects. However, the metabolites are ultimately cleared through the bile. Although no accumulation of pharmacologically active substance seem to occur, caution is advised while administering VOLTAREN or VOLTAREN SR to patients with impaired kidney function (ie GFR <60 mL/min or 1 mL/sec) (see Warnings and Precautions, Renal). VOLTAREN and VOLTAREN SR are contraindicated in patients with severely impaired or deteriorating renal function (creatinine clearance <30 mL/min (0.5 mL/s) (see Contraindications).

STORAGE AND STABILITY: Protect the tablets from heat (i.e., store between 15-30°C) and humidity.
Protect suppositories from heat (i.e., store between 15-30°C).

INFORMATION FOR THE PATIENT: Published in e-CPS, available by subscription at www.e-cps.ca.

DOSAGE FORMS, COMPOSITION AND PACKAGING: VOLTAREN Tablets: Each light brown, round, slightly biconvex, enteric-coated tablet, printed VOLTAREN on one side and 50 on the other, contains: diclofenac sodium 50 mg. Nonmedicinal ingredients: black ink, castor oil derivatives, colloidal silicon dioxide, corn starch, hypromellose, iron oxides, lactose, magnesium stearate, microcrystalline cellulose, polyethylene glycol, povidone, sodium starch glycolate, talc and titanium dioxide. Energy: 1.6 kJ (0.39 kcal). Sodium: <1 mmol (4.06 mg). Alcohol-, bisulfite-, gluten-, parabens- and tartrazine-free. Bottles of 100.
VOLTAREN SR Tablets: 75 mg: Each light pink, triangular, biconvex, film-coated, slow-release tablet, printed VOLTAREN on one side and SR/75 on the other, contains: diclofenac sodium 75 mg. Nonmedicinal ingredients: black ink, carnauba wax, cellulose compounds, cetyl alcohol, colloidal silicon dioxide, hypromellose, magnesium stearate, polysorbate 80, povidone, red iron oxide, sucrose, talc and titanium dioxide. Energy: 1.56 kJ (0.37 kcal). Sodium: <1 mmol (6.1 mg). Alcohol-, bisulfite-, gluten-, lactose-, parabens- and tartrazine-free. Bottles of 100.
100 mg: Each pink, round, biconvex, film-coated, slow-release tablet, printed VOLTAREN SR on one side and 100 on the other, contains: diclofenac sodium 100 mg. Nonmedicinal ingredients: black ink, carnauba wax, cellulose compounds, cetyl alcohol, colloidal silicon dioxide, hypromellose, magnesium stearate, polysorbate 80, povidone, red iron oxide, sucrose, talc and titanium dioxide. Energy: 2.04 kJ (0.49 kcal). Sodium: <1 mmol (8.13 mg). Alcohol-, bisulfite-, gluten-, lactose-, parabens- and tartrazine-free. Bottles of 100.
VOLTAREN Suppositories: 50 mg: Each bullet shaped suppository, white to yellowish-white in colour, with a smooth surface with a fat like odour, contains: diclofenac sodium 50 mg. Nonmedicinal ingredients: semi-synthetic glycerides. Sodium: <1 mmol (4.06 mg). Cartons of 30.
100 mg: Each bullet shaped suppository, white to yellowish-white in colour, with a smooth surface with a fat like odour, contains: diclofenac sodium 100 mg. Nonmedicinal ingredients: semi-synthetic glycerides. Sodium: <1 mmol (8.13 mg). Cartons of 30.

(Shown in Product Identification Section)

Voltaren® Emulgel™

diclofenac diethylamine

Nonsteroidal Anti-inflammatory (NSAID)—Analgesic Agent for Topical Use

Novartis Consumer Health

Voltaren® Emulgel™ Joint Pain

diclofenac diethylamine

Nonsteroidal Anti-inflammatory (NSAID)—Analgesic Agent for Topical Use

Novartis Consumer Health

Date of Revision: August 16, 2010

SUMMARY PRODUCT INFORMATION:

Route of Administration	Dosage Form/ Strength	Clinically Relevant Nonmedicinal Ingredients
Topical	Gel/11.6 mg/g diclofenac diethylamine (1.16% w/w)	None. For a complete listing see Dosage Forms, Composition and Packaging.

INDICATIONS AND CLINICAL USE: Voltaren Emulgel (diclofenac diethylamine gel) is indicated for:
- Relief of pain associated with recent (acute), localized muscle or joint injuries such as sprains, strains or sports injuries (e.g. sprain of ankle, strain of shoulder or back muscles). This is typically as an adjunct to other measures such as rest for the relief of discomfort associated with such injuries.

Voltaren Emulgel should be applied over the affected area 3 or 4 times daily and rubbed gently into the skin. The amount needed depends on the size of the painful area: 2 g to 4 g Voltaren Emulgel (1 g equals a strip approx. 2 cm long) is sufficient to treat an area of about 400-800 cm^2. After application, the hands should be washed, unless they are the site being treated.

The duration of treatment will depend on the natural course of healing, rest and also on clinical response. The gel should not be used for more than 7 days for muscle and joint injuries, unless recommended by a doctor. Consumers should consult their doctor if the condition does not improve within 7 days, or if it gets worse.
Geriatrics (>65 years of age): The usual adult dosage may be used.
Pediatrics (<16 years of age): Not for use in children under 16 years of age.

CONTRAINDICATIONS:
- Patients who are hypersensitive to this drug or to any ingredient in the formulation or component of the container. For a complete listing, see the Dosage Forms, Composition and Packaging.
- Hypersensitivity to diclofenac, acetylsalicylic acid or other non-steroidal anti-inflammatory drugs.
- Patients with or without chronic asthma in whom attacks of asthma, urticaria or acute rhinitis are precipitated by acetylsalicylic acid or other non-steroidal anti-inflammatory agents.
- Concomitant use of other products containing diclofenac.
- Concomitant use of oral non-steroidal anti-inflammatory drugs (NSAIDs).

WARNINGS AND PRECAUTIONS: General: Voltaren Emulgel is for topical use only and should be applied only to intact, non-diseased skin and not to skin wounds or open injuries. It should not be used with occlusion. It should not be allowed to come into contact with the eyes or mucous membranes, and should never be taken by mouth.

Systemic availability of diclofenac diethylamine through percutaneous absorption is low compared with plasma levels obtained following oral forms of diclofenac. Nevertheless, the possibility of systemic side effects cannot be completely excluded. Chances of this may be increased where Voltaren Emulgel is applied to a relatively large area of skin and/or over an extended period of time (e.g., especially if this goes beyond the maximum duration recommended for use).

Some possibility of gastro-intestinal bleeding in patients with a significant history of peptic ulceration has been reported in isolated cases. Voltaren Emulgel should therefore be used with caution by patients under medication for active peptic ulcers in the stomach or duodenum (e.g., proton pump inhibitors or histamine H_2 receptor antagonists). If the patient is uncertain, they should be advised to consult their doctor or pharmacist.

Like other drugs that inhibit prostaglandin synthetase activity, diclofenac and other NSAIDs can precipitate bronchospasm if administered to patients suffering from or with a previous history of bronchial asthma.

Asthma has been rarely reported in patients using topical NSAID preparations.

Local irritation, erythema, pruritus or dermatitis may occasionally occur with topical diclofenac diethylamine. Skin photosensitivity, desquamation, discoloration and bullous or vesicular eruptions have been reported in isolated cases. Patients should be warned against excessive exposure to sunlight in order to reduce the incidence of photosensitivity.

The following additional side effects have been observed with **oral** forms of diclofenac sodium.
Cardiovascular: Isolated cases: palpitation, chest pain, hypertension.
Gastrointestinal: Occasional: epigastric pain, other gastro-intestinal disorders (e.g. nausea, vomiting, diarrhoea, abdominal cramps, dyspepsia, flatulence, anorexia). Rare: gastro-intestinal bleeding, peptic ulcer (with or without bleeding or perforation), bloody diarrhoea. In isolated cases: lower gut disorders (e.g. non-specific haemorrhagic colitis and exacerbations of ulcerative colitis or Crohn's proctocolitis, colonic damage and stricture formation), pancreatitis, aphthous stomatitis, glossitis, oesophageal lesions, constipation.
Hematologic: In isolated cases: thrombocytopenia, leucopenia, agranulocytosis, haemolytic anaemia, aplastic anaemia.
Hepatic/Biliary/Pancreatic: Occasional: elevation of serum aminotransferase enzymes (ALT, AST). Rare: liver function disorders including hepatitis (in isolated cases fulminant) with or without jaundice.
Immune: Hypersensitivity reactions have been reported following treatment with NSAIDs. These may consist of rare cases of anaphylactic/anaphylactoid systemic reactions including hypotension, and respiratory tract reactivity comprising asthma, aggravated asthma, bronchospasm or dyspnoea. (See also Skin.)
Neurologic: Occasional: headache, dizziness, or vertigo. Rare: drowsiness, tiredness. In isolated cases: disturbances of sensation, paraesthesia, memory disturbance, disorientation, disturbance of vision (blurred vision, diplopia), impaired hearing. Tinnitus, insomnia, irritability, convulsions, depression, anxiety, nightmares, tremor, psychotic reactions. Taste alteration disorders.
Renal: In isolated cases: acute renal failure, urinary abnormalities (e.g. haematuria, proteinuria), interstitial nephritis, nephrotic syndrome, papillary necrosis.
Sexual Function/Reproduction: Isolated cases: impotence (association with diclofenac is doubtful).
Skin: Occasional: rashes or skin eruptions. Rare: urticaria. In isolated cases: eczema, erythema multiforme, Stevens-Johnson syndrome, Lyell's syndrome, (acute toxic epidermolysis), photosensitivity reactions, erythroderma (exfoliative dermatitis), loss of hair, purpura including allergic purpura.
Special Populations: Pregnant Women: Since no experience has been acquired with diclofenac diethylamine gel in pregnancy, it is not recommended for use in these circumstances.

During the last trimester of pregnancy the use of prostaglandin synthetase inhibitors may result in premature closure of the ductus arteriosus, or in uterine inertia.

Animal data has shown an increased incidence of dystonia and delayed parturition when drug administration is continued into late pregnancy.
Nursing Women: Since no experience has been acquired with diclofenac diethylamine gel in lactation, it is not recommended for use in these circumstances.

Following oral doses of 50 mg diclofenac administered every 8 hours, diclofenac passes into breast milk in quantities so small that no undesirable effects on the infant are to be expected.
Pediatrics (<16 years of age): Not for use in children under 16 years of age.
Geriatrics (>65 years of age): No specific hazards are associated with geriatric use of diclofenac diethylamine gel.
Monitoring and Laboratory Tests: No monitoring parameters or laboratory tests are required to monitor response to therapy or possible adverse reactions.

ADVERSE REACTIONS: Adverse Drug Reaction Overview: The adverse event incidence in the clinical studies was very low. The benign safety profile documented in the clinical studies is confirmed in the post-marketing experience in over 200 million patients worldwide. The adverse events occurring in studies were usually either moderate or mild. Five serious adverse events occurred in all the studies (all unrelated, one fatal) and led to withdrawal, or interruption of treatment, of the affected subjects.

In post-marketing surveillance, cutaneous or application site adverse events constitute about two thirds of all adverse events reported. The most common type of serious systemic event is gastrointestinal bleeding; however, in more than half of these cases patients were known to be taking concomitant systemic medications that may precipitate gastrointestinal bleeding, such as NSAIDs, salicylates, corticosteroids and/or anticoagulants.
Clinical Trial Adverse Drug Reactions: Because clinical trials are conducted under very specific conditions the adverse reaction rates observed in the clinical trials may not reflect the rates observed in practice and should not be compared to the rates in the clinical trials of another drug. Adverse drug reaction information from clinical trials is useful for identifying drug-related adverse events and for approximating rates.

The clinical data set includes data obtained in approximately 4926 patients with either the target indication of soft-tissue injuries (e.g. sprains, strains, bruises), osteoarthritis or soft-tissue rheumatism, 2728 of whom received Voltaren Emulgel, 1267 of whom received an active comparator, and 931 of whom received placebo. Patients were treated from 3-28 days as befitted the nature of the conditions under study.

Data from the safety population with the target indication investigated, who received short term exposure to Voltaren Emulgel in controlled trials and uncontrolled trials, confirm that a dose of 2-4 g of Voltaren Emulgel applied topically 3-4 times a day is safe and that the systemic adverse event profile observed for systemic NSAIDs is not seen with the topical formulation.

No subgroup analyses were performed. Long-term safety data from patients was not obtained in these studies as this is not relevant to a product intended for only short-term use up to 1 week. The safety of Voltaren Emulgel was demonstrated in the safety population in clinical trials, which all showed that the incidence and type of rare or serious events resembles those of active controls or placebo.

The adverse events (AEs) whether or not drug related reported in 33 clinical trials are summarized in Table 1 (WHO-ART coding).

Table 1: Voltaren Emulgel

Adverse events (AEs) Reported in Clinical Trials (WHO-ART coding) with a Frequency of ≥1%

	Voltaren Emulgel n=2258 (100)	<Placebo> n=633 (100)	Reference[a,b] n=112 (100)
Local skin AEs	76 (3.4)	35 (5.5)	29 (2.6)

[a] Topical reference drugs (number of patients): felbinac (195), piroxicam (306), etofenamate (140), Mobilat containing adrenocortical extract, mucopolysaccharide, salicylic acid (113), Movelat containing mucopolysaccharide polysulphate, salicylic acid (78), ketoprofen (15), naproxen (15), benzydamine HCl (52), indomethacin (55), Dolobene containing dimethylsulfoxid heparin (39), monosalicylic acid (15-20).
[b] Oral reference drug: ibuprofen (155).

Similar percentages of local skin reactions including mostly itching, burning, erythema, local allergy and blistering were reported after both Voltaren Emulgel (3.4%) and placebo (5.5%). Most of the local AEs were mild to moderate. There were no reports of photosensitivity, although one case report referred to exposure to the sun. Approximately 0.3% of patients were withdrawn due to local skin AEs after applying Voltaren Emulgel or placebo.

In conclusion, the absolute numbers of reported adverse events were relatively small and there are no clinically significant differences in the incidence of adverse events in the Voltaren Emulgel, placebo and reference drug treatment groups. Most of the AEs are local, mild to moderate and reversible.
Less Common Clinical Trial Adverse Drug Reactions (<1%): WHO-ART-coded Clinical Trials: Digestive: Dyspepsia was observed in 0.58, 0.32, and 0.18% of Voltaren Emulgel, Placebo, and Reference groups, respectively.
Body as a Whole: Allergic events were observed in 0.04, 0.16, and 0.09% of Voltaren Emulgel, Placebo, and Reference groups, respectively.
CNS: CNS events were observed in 0.09, 0.32, and 0.45% of Voltaren Emulgel, Placebo, and Reference groups, respectively.
Abnormal Hematologic and Clinical Chemistry Findings: Clinical laboratory evaluations were not routinely performed in the studies undertaken for the indication of muscle and joint soft tissue injuries. The treatments were given for short periods only.
Post-Market Adverse Drug Reactions: Voltaren Emulgel was first approved for marketing in 1985 and now is marketed worldwide in over 100 countries. Since first launch to the end of October 2005 it is estimated by Novartis that over 200 million patients have been exposed to the product, based on kg of substance sold and the assumption that there is an average usage of two 100 g tubes per patient.

Voltaren Emulgel worldwide spontaneous adverse event reporting from first marketing launch 1985 to the end of October 2005 included a total of 1359 spontaneous case report forms (one congenital case reported twice). There were 195 serious spontaneous adverse event reports. The remaining spontaneous adverse event reports were not considered serious in nature. Occurrence of adverse events (AEs) and serious adverse events (SAEs), whether or not drug related, are presented in Table 2. AEs are broken down into Unlisted AEs (including case reports where relation to list was not reported) and Listed AEs.

Cutaneous or application site adverse events constituted approximately two thirds of all adverse events reported. Only 49 people had cutaneous adverse events considered to be serious in nature (see Table 3). The most common type of serious systemic event was gastrointestinal bleeding (39 cases); however, in more than half of these cases, patients were known to be taking concomitant systemic medications that may precipitate gastrointestinal bleeding, such as NSAIDs, salicylates, corticosteroids and/or anticoagulants.

Table 2: Voltaren Emulgel

Voltaren Emulgel Safety Database: Occurrence of AE and SAE Case Reports

Body System	All AEs	Serious Unlisted[a]		Serious Listed		Total SAEs
		SR	CT	SR	CT	
Blood and lymphatic system disorders	14	3	1	2		6
Cardiac disorders	9	2				2
Congenital, familial and genetic disorders	1	1				1
Ear and labyrinth disorders	5	1				1
Eye disorders	17	1				1
Gastro-intestinal disorders	89	26	5	15		46
General disorders and administration site conditions	249	7				7
Hepatobiliary disorders	5	4		1		5
Immune system disorders	84	1		9		10
Infections and infestations	29	3				3
Injury, poisoning and procedural complications	49	5				5
Investigations	35	4	1	1		6
Metabolism and nutrition disorders	6	4				4
Musculoskeletal and connective tissue disorders	25	4	1	1		6
Nervous system disorders	27	9				9
Neoplasma	3	1				1
Pregnancy, puerperium and perinatal conditions	7	4				4
Psychiatric disorders	8	3				3
Renal and urinary disorders	19	12		1		13
Reproductive system and breast disorders	2					
Respiratory, thoracic and mediastinal disorders	30	3		5		8
Skin and subcutaneous tissue disorders	617	16	3	29	1	49
Social circumstances	2					
Surgical and Medical Procedures						
Vascular disorders	12	5				5
CT AEs reported to safety database	16					
Total	1359	119	11	64	1	195

[a] SAEs unlisted or unknown, SR: spontaneous report, CT: clinical trials.

Table 3: Voltaren Emulgel

Voltaren Emulgel Safety Database: Most Frequently Reported SAEs

	N	Deaths
Number of Reports	1359	
Number of SAEs (%)	195 (100%)	9
Local SAEs	61 (31.3%)	
• Skin and subcutaneous tissue disorders	49 (25.1%)	3
• General disorders and administration site conditions	7 (3.6%)	
• Injury, poisoning and procedural complications	5 (2.6%)	
Systemic SAEs	133 (68.2%)	
• Gastro-intestinal disorders	46 (23.6%)	1
• Immune system disorders	10 (5.1%)	
• Blood and lymphatic system disorders	6 (3.1%)	
• Renal and urinary disorders	13 (6.7%)	1
• Other systems/disorders	58 (29.7%)	4

(cont'd)

Table 3: Voltaren Emulgel (cont'd)

Voltaren Emulgel Safety Database: Most Frequently Reported SAEs

DRUG INTERACTIONS: Overview: No drug and substance interaction studies have been performed as part of the clinical development of Voltaren Emulgel 11.6 mg/g (1.16%) gel.

From the pharmacokinetic point of view, diclofenac is extensively (>99.7%) protein bound, mainly to albumin (99.4%). Binding to serum albumin is characterised by 2 classes of binding sites: the high affinity sites are likely to be shared with benzodiazepines and the low affinity site with warfarin. Diclofenac does not modify other strongly protein bound drugs but may, in vitro, be displaced by salicylic acid (Davies and Anderson, 1997).

There is a considerable body of literature regarding interactions of oral NSAIDs, and diclofenac in particular, with other medicinal products. No interactions with other drugs are to be expected due to very low plasma levels observed after topical application of Voltaren Emulgel.

Drug-Drug Interactions: No drug-drug interactions were noted in the clinical studies presented. Isolated interaction cases have been reported for topical Voltaren Emulgel from the marketplace.

Only 22 cases of possible drug interactions with Voltaren Emulgel over 200 million patients exposed have been made to the Novartis world-wide safety database since first marketing:

- Twelve cases with oral anticoagulant therapy (3 with acenocoumarol, 3 with warfarin, 2 with phenprocoumon, 2 with fluindione, and 2 unknown).
- Four cases with blood pressure increase (with anti-hypertensive product of different classes).
- Three case with blood glucose increase (in insulin-dependent and in non-insulin dependent diabetes mellitus).
- One case of a psychiatric disorder (with concomitant ofloxacin use).
- One case of a rash and vascular bleeding associated with acetylsalicylic acid. The patient was also taking heparin and a topical herbal product containing camphor, methanol and ethanol.
- One case of gastric ulcer associated with concomitant acetylsalicylic acid use.

The customary drug-drug interactions between oral NSAIDs and anticoagulants, oral antidiabetic agents and certain other classes are usually based on the high protein-binding nature of the NSAID. With significantly lower amounts of active substance in circulation following topical application compared with after oral administration, such interactions may be predicted to be very unlikely with use of Voltaren Emulgel.

DOSAGE AND ADMINISTRATION: Recommended Dose and Dosage Adjustment: Adults and adolescents 16 years and older: Voltaren Emulgel should be rubbed gently into the skin. Depending on the size of the affected site to be treated, 2-4 g (1 g equals a strip approx. 2 cm long) should be applied 3-4 times a day. After application, the hands should be washed unless they are the site being treated.

The duration of treatment depends on the natural course of healing, rest and also on clinical response. The gel should not be used for more than 7 days for muscle and joint injuries, unless recommended by a doctor. Consumers should consult their doctor if the condition does not improve within 7 days, or if it gets worse.

Missed Dose: If a dose of Voltaren Emulgel is missed, it should be applied when the consumer remembers and then again at the next scheduled time. A double quantity should not be applied.

OVERDOSAGE:

The low systemic absorption of topical diclofenac renders overdosage extremely unlikely. In the event of accidental ingestion, resulting in significant systemic side effects, general therapeutic measures normally adopted to treat poisoning with non-steroidal anti-inflammatory drugs should be used.

Management of overdosage with NSAIDs essentially consists of supportive and symptomatic measures. Supportive and symptomatic treatment should be given for complications such as hypotension, renal failure, convulsions, gastro-intestinal irritation, and respiratory depression; specific therapies such as forced diuresis, dialysis or haemoperfusion are probably of no help in eliminating NSAIDs due to their high rate of protein binding and extensive metabolism.

Twenty times the oral dose of 200 mg of diclofenac in overdose produced only somnolence with no signs of toxicity (AHFS Drug Information 1999). This would represent about 65 tubes of Voltaren Emulgel. In case of accidental ingestion of one tube of product, the amount of diclofenac ingested would be less than one tablet of diclofenac 50 mg (which is the most common oral unit dose).

There are five cases of overdose in the paediatric population with Voltaren Emulgel listed on the Novartis Safety Database. A 2-year-old girl swallowed a "soup spoonful". Assuming that a spoon contains 15 mL (or grams) and that 100% of the dose was absorbed, the amount of available diclofenac would have been approximately 150 mg. No details of the other overdose are available. A 1-year-old girl and a 3-year-old boy were also reported to have swallowed unknown quantities of Voltaren Emulgel with no apparent adverse events. There are 2 cases of accidental topical exposure to Voltaren Emulgel in children, one to a 2-year-old boy and another to a 2-year-old child (gender not reported). No adverse events were reported in either case.

In the adult population, there is one case of an adult swallowing an unknown quantity of Voltaren in the database. No adverse events were reported. One report of a patient applying 1.5 tubes of Voltaren Emulgel per day on his legs resulted in skin changes and "thin skin" (skin atrophy). Additionally, there is a consumer report of a patient with a history of cerebrovascular accident with left paralysis, hypertension, diabetes and epilepsy that used half a tube at the site of application in a single dose and experienced an increase in pain at the site. The database also includes a case report stated as serious where the patient became 'intoxicated', but there is no additional information.

The database contains a report of accidental exposure to haemorrhoids, resulting in a burning sensation. Finally, there were 3 consumer reports of accidental exposure in the eyes resulting in eye redness, eye discharge, eye irritation, and a feeling of increased intraocular pressure.

For management of a suspected drug overdose, CPhA recommends that you contact your **regional Poison Control Centre**. See the *CPS* Directory section for a list of Poison Control Centres.

ACTION AND CLINICAL PHARMACOLOGY: Mechanism of Action: Diclofenac is a well characterized, potent nonsteroidal anti-inflammatory drug (NSAID) with clinically proven anti-inflammatory, analgesic and antipyretic properties (Davies & Anderson 1997). NSAIDs, including diclofenac, reduce pain principally by inhibiting formation of prostaglandins, leukotrienes and free oxygen radicals.

All non-salicylate NSAIDs reversibly block cyclooxygenase activity, which is responsible for converting arachidonic acid to prostaglandins. Diclofenac is a potent, non-selective inhibitor of COX-1 and COX-2 (preferentially COX-2), which may underlie both its therapeutic efficacy and potential side effects (Giuliano & Warner 1999). In addition, diclofenac, when compared to NSAIDs such as ibuprofen, also blocks the lipoxygenase pathway of the arachidonic acid cascade, thereby inhibiting the formation of leukotriene B4 (LTB4), which is a known pain mediator and has been shown to stimulate pain receptors in the peripheral nerves. The inhibition of lipoxygenase also prevents the pro-inflammatory and gastrointestinal damaging effects of leukotrienes (Bertolini, Ottani & Sandrini 2001). Prostaglandins, along with thromboxanes and LTB4, are responsible for several inflammatory effects. The lipoxygenase inhibition produced by diclofenac may therefore play a significant role in its efficacy as an analgesic and anti-inflammatory agent (Amadio, Cummings & Amadio, 1993; Todd & Sorkin 1988).

Pharmacodynamics: As with other NSAIDs, the ability of diclofenac to inhibit prostaglandin synthesis is instrumental in the anti-inflammatory response. Data from in vitro studies show that most topical NSAIDs are able to inhibit prostaglandin synthesis to a significant degree. In this respect, diclofenac has a high intrinsic activity, as demonstrated in vitro in human rheumatoid synovial microsomes (Dreiser 1994).

The pharmacodynamic properties of diclofenac have been demonstrated for each of the sodium, potassium and diethylamine salts administered either orally or topically in standard animal models of acute and chronic inflammation (Hiramatsu et al 1990, Kyuki et al 1983).

It has also been reported that topically applied diclofenac diethylamine 1.16% actively inhibited methyl nicotinate induced skin inflammation, which is known to involve prostaglandins and free arachidonic acid. Topical diclofenac was shown to exhibit a prolonged potent anti-inflammatory effect, even 48 hours after application (Duteil et al 1990).

The anti-inflammatory properties of Voltaren Emulgel were demonstrated in two placebo-controlled, double-blind, randomized trials, one in healthy volunteers using the urate crystal induced inflammation model (NGB5) and the other in patients with chronic synovitis of the knee (NGB 8855). Voltaren Emulgel proved to be superior to placebo in significantly reducing the diameter of erythema at 24 hours in study NGB 5 ($p<0.05$), and significantly reducing the thermal index in study NGB 8855 ($p<0.04$). Due to the small size of the studies, only objective parameters of erythema and thermal index could be evidenced.

Pharmacokinetics: Absorption: The quantity of diclofenac absorbed systemically from Voltaren Emulgel is proportional to the size of the treated area, and depends on both the total dose applied and the degree of skin hydration. Absorption amounts to about 6% of the applied dose of diclofenac after topical application of 2.5 g Voltaren Emulgel on 500 cm^2 skin, determined by the total renal elimination, compared with Voltaren tablets. A 10-hour occlusion leads to a 3-fold increase in the amount of diclofenac absorbed.

Distribution: Diclofenac concentrations have been measured from plasma, synovial tissue and synovial fluid after topical administration of Voltaren Emulgel to hand and knee joints. Maximum plasma concentrations are approximately 100 times lower than after oral administration of the same quantity of diclofenac. 99.7% of diclofenac is bound to serum proteins, mainly albumin (99.4%).

Metabolism: Biotransformation of diclofenac involves partly glucuronidation of the intact molecule, but mainly single and multiple hydroxylation resulting in several phenolic metabolites, most of which are converted to glucuronide conjugates. Two of the phenolic metabolites are biologically active, however, to a much smaller extent than diclofenac.

Excretion: The total systemic clearance of diclofenac from plasma is 263±56 mL/min. The terminal plasma half-life is 1-2 hours. Four of the metabolites, including the two active ones, also have short plasma half-lives of 1-3 hours. One metabolite, 3'-hydroxy-4'-methoxy-diclofenac, has a longer half-life but is virtually inactive. Diclofenac and its metabolites are excreted mainly in the urine.

Special Populations and Conditions: There are no gender differences in the pharmacokinetics of diclofenac. No safety or efficacy concerns relating to ethnicity have been identified from the marketplace. Davies and Anderson (1997) discuss the influence of age on diclofenac pharmacokinetics with relevance in the very young and elderly. Also, changes to the skin in the elderly will affect absorption in some patients. However, as plasma levels will be very low after topical application these factors are not a clinical concern. For similar reasons, any effect of hepatic or renal impairment on the pharmacokinetics of diclofenac is unlikely to be clinically significant.

STORAGE AND STABILITY: Voltaren Emulgel should be stored between 15 and 30°C.

SPECIAL HANDLING INSTRUCTIONS: There are no special handling instructions for Voltaren Emulgel.

INFORMATION FOR THE PATIENT: Published in e-CPS, available by subscription at www.e-cps.ca.

DOSAGE FORMS, COMPOSITION AND PACKAGING: Each tube of white to practically white, soft, homogenous, cream-like oil-in-water topical emulsion contains: diclofenac diethylamine 1.16% w/w. Nonmedicinal ingredients: carbomer, cocoyl caprylocaprate, diethylamine, isopropyl alcohol, liquid paraffin, macrogol cetostearyl ether, perfume, propylene glycol and purified water. Packaged in an aluminium laminated tube [low density polyethylene/aluminium/high density polyethylene (internal layer)] fitted with a high density polyethylene shoulder and closed by a moulded seal. The tube is closed with a polypropylene screw cap, incorporating a moulded feature used to insert, twist and remove the seal before first use. Voltaren Emulgel: Tubes of 20, 50, 100 and 150 g. Voltaren Emulgel Joint Pain: Tubes of 75 g.

Voltaren Ophtha® Ⓟ

diclofenac sodium

Anti-inflammatory—Analgesic

Novartis Pharmaceuticals

Date of Revision: June 1, 2010

SUMMARY PRODUCT INFORMATION:

Route of Administration	Dosage Form/ Strength	Clinically Relevant Nonmedicinal Ingredients
Topical Ophthalmic	Ophthalmic solution diclofenac sodium 0.1%	**Multi-dose bottles:** sorbic acid 0.2% preservative For a complete listing see Dosage Forms, Composition and Packaging.

INDICATIONS AND CLINICAL USE: VOLTAREN OPHTHA (diclofenac sodium 0.1%) ophthalmic solution is indicated for the following conditions of the eye:

- Post-operative inflammation after cataract surgery
- Non-chronic post-traumatic inflammation in non-penetrating wounds

Pediatrics (under 18 years of age): The safety and dosage ranges of VOLTAREN OPHTHA have not been established in children under 18 years of age. VOLTAREN OPHTHA is not indicated for use in children.

CONTRAINDICATIONS: Known hypersensitivity to (diclofenac sodium) or any component of the medication.

Since there exists the potential for cross-sensitivity, VOLTAREN OPHTHA should not be used in patients in whom acute asthmatic attacks, urticaria, rhinitis or other allergic manifestations are precipitated by ASA or other nonsteroidal anti-inflammatory agents.

WARNINGS AND PRECAUTIONS: General: The anti-inflammatory and analgesic effects of VOLTAREN OPHTHA may mask signs of infection and physicians should be alert to the development of infection and closely monitor patients receiving the drug.

In the presence of infection or if there is a risk of infection, appropriate therapy (antibiotics) should be given concurrently with VOLTAREN OPHTHA.

Hematologic: Although there have been no reported adverse events, there is a theoretical possibility that patients receiving other medications which may prolong bleeding time, or with known hemostatic defects may experience exacerbation with VOLTAREN OPHTHA.

With some nonsteroidal anti-inflammatory drugs, there exists the potential for increased bleeding time due to interference with thrombocyte aggregation. There have been reports that ocularly applied nonsteroidal anti-inflammatory drugs may cause increased bleeding of ocular tissues (including hyphema) in conjunction with ocular surgery.

Ophthalmologic: All topical nonsteroidal anti-inflammatory drugs (NSAIDs) may slow or delay healing. Topical corticosteroids are also known to slow or delay healing. Concomitant use of topical NSAIDs such as VOLTAREN OPHTHA and topical steroids may increase the potential for healing problems. It should also be noted that concomitant use of VOLTAREN OPHTHA and topical corticosteroids in patients with significant pre-existing corneal inflammation may increase the risk of developing corneal complications. The concomitant use of diclofenac sodium with topical corticosteroids should be undertaken with caution. (See Drug-Drug Interactions.)

Post-marketing experience with topical NSAIDs suggests that patients experiencing complicated ocular surgeries, corneal denervation, corneal epithelial defects, diabetes mellitus, ocular surface disease (e.g., dry eye syndrome), rheumatoid arthritis, or repeat ocular surgeries within a short period of time may be at increased risk for corneal adverse events (keratitis, epithelial breakdown, corneal thinning, corneal infiltrates, corneal erosion, corneal ulceration, and corneal perforation), these events may be sight threatening. Patients with evidence of corneal epithelial breakdown should immediately discontinue use of topical NSAIDs and should be closely monitored for corneal health. Topical NSAIDs such as VOLTAREN OPHTHA should be used with caution in these patients. Post-marketing experience with topical NSAIDs also suggest that use more than 24 hours prior to surgery or use beyond 14 days post surgery may increase patient risk for occurrence and severity of corneal adverse events.

It is recommended that physicians conduct periodic examinations of the eye, including measurement of intraocular pressure. A slight and transient elevation in the intraocular pressure (IOP) has been observed in some patients, following surgery, even with the use of VOLTAREN OPHTHA.

Soft contact lenses should not be worn during treatment. The lenses must be removed before application of the drops and not reinserted earlier than 15 minutes after use.

Special Populations: Pregnant Women: The safety of VOLTAREN OPHTHA (diclofenac sodium) in pregnancy has not been established and its use is therefore not recommended in pregnant women, unless the potential benefit to the mother outweighs the possible risk to the child.

Nursing Women: The safety of VOLTAREN OPHTHA (diclofenac sodium) in lactation has not been established and its use is therefore not recommended in lactating women, unless the potential benefit to the mother outweighs the possible risk to the child.

Pediatrics (under 18 years of age): The safety and dosage ranges of VOLTAREN OPHTHA have not been established in children under 18 years of age. VOLTAREN OPHTHA is not indicated for use in children.

Geriatrics (over 65 years of age): VOLTAREN OPHTHA was well tolerated by patients presenting with post-traumatic ocular inflammatory conditions and inflammatory responses of the eye resulting from surgical intervention for cataracts, including elderly patients with senile cataracts requiring lens extraction and re-implantation.

ADVERSE REACTIONS: Adverse Drug Reaction Overview: The most frequently observed adverse reaction is a transient, mild to moderate eye irritation in the eye.

Other less frequently observed reactions are eye pain, eye pruritus, ocular hyperemia and blurred vision immediately after instillation of the eye drops.

Punctate keratitis or corneal disorders have been observed, usually after frequent application.

In rare cases dyspnoea and exacerbation of asthma have been reported.

Clinical Trial Adverse Drug Reactions: Because clinical trials are conducted under very specific conditions the adverse reaction rates observed in the clinical trials may not reflect the rates observed in practice and should not be compared to the rates in the clinical trials of another drug. Adverse drug reaction information from clinical trials is useful for identifying drug-related adverse events and for approximating rates.

When instilled into the eye, VOLTAREN OPHTHA has been associated with a mild to moderate burning sensation in 5 to 15% of patients studied. This symptom was transient in nature and almost never necessitated discontinuation of treatment. In addition, there has been one report each of the following symptoms: sensitivity to light, bad taste, feeling of pressure and a stainable cornea. There have also been 2 reports of an allergic reaction. The incidence of these latter five symptoms was 0.2 to 0.3% of all patients studied.

In cataract surgery studies, keratitis was reported in up to 28% of patients receiving VOLTAREN OPHTHA, although in many of these cases keratitis was initially noted prior to the initiation of treatment.

Elevated intraocular pressure following cataract surgery was reported in approximately 15% of patients undergoing cataract surgery.

Lacrimation complaints were reported in approximately 30% of cases studies undergoing incisional refractive surgery.

The following adverse reactions were reported in approximately 5% or less of the patients: abnormal vision, acute elevated IOP, blurred vision, conjunctivitis, corneal deposits, corneal edema, corneal opacity, corneal lesions, discharge, eyelid swelling, injection, iritis, irritation, itching, lacrimation disorder and ocular allergy.

The following adverse reactions were reported in 3% or less of the patients: Abdominal pain, asthenia, chills, dizziness, facial edema, fever, headache, insomnia, nausea, pain, rhinitis, viral infection, and vomiting.

Post-Market Adverse Drug Reactions: In patients with risk factors for corneal disorders such as during the use of corticosteroids or with concomitant diseases such as infections, rheumatoid arthritis, diclofenac has been associated, in rare cases, with ulcerative keratitis, corneal thinning, punctuate keratitis, corneal ephitelium defect and corneal edema, which might become sight-threatening.

Allergic conditions has been reported such as conjunctival hyperaemia, conjunctivitis allergic, erythema of eyelid, eye allergy, eyelid oedema, eyelid pruritus, urticaria, rash, eczema, erythema, pruritus, hypersensitivity, cough and rhinitis.

DRUG INTERACTIONS: Drug-Drug Interactions: Concomitant use of topical NSAIDs such as VOLTAREN OPHTHA and topical steroids may increase the potential for healing problems. It should also be noted that concomitant use of VOLTAREN OPHTHA and topical corticosteroids in patients with significant pre-existing corneal inflammation may increase the risk of developing corneal complications. The concomitant use of diclofenac sodium with topical corticosteroids should be undertaken with caution.

DOSAGE AND ADMINISTRATION: Recommended Dose and Dosage Adjustment: Cataract Surgery Procedures: Pre-operatively: Instill 1 drop in the conjunctival sac up to 5 times during the 3 hours preceding surgery.

Post-operatively: Instill 1 drop in the conjunctival sac 15, 30 and 45 minutes following surgery, then 3 to 5 times daily, for up to 4 weeks.

Non-Chronic Post-Traumatic Inflammation in Non-Penetrating Wounds: Instill 1 drop in the conjunctival sac 4 to 5 times daily, depending upon the severity of the disease. Eye swab for culture should be taken before initiation of therapy.

Administration: In surgery, VOLTAREN OPHTHA has been combined with such standard pretreatment measures as mydriatics and topical antibiotics.

To prevent the active substances from being washed out when additional ophthalmic medication is used, leave an interval of at least 5 minutes between each application.

OVERDOSAGE:

There has been limited experience with diclofenac sodium overdosage, even when given systemically. The risk of an acute toxic response is highly remote, as a 5 mL bottle of VOLTAREN OPHTHA contains a total of only 5 mg diclofenac sodium, equivalent to just 3% of the normal recommended oral adult dose.

If VOLTAREN OPHTHA is accidentally ingested, fluids should be taken to dilute the medication.

For management of a suspected drug overdose, contact your regional Poison Control Centre. See the *CPS* Directory section for a list of Poison Control Centres.

ACTION AND CLINICAL PHARMACOLOGY: Mechanism of Action: Diclofenac sodium is a nonsteroidal anti-inflammatory drug with analgesic properties. The mode of action is not fully known, but it does not act through the pituitary-adrenal axis, even when given systemically. Diclofenac sodium inhibits prostaglandin synthesis by interfering with the action of prostaglandin synthetase. Prostaglandins play a critical role in many inflammatory processes of the eye and appear to play a role in the miotic response during ocular surgery. Topically applied diclofenac sodium significantly reduces prostaglandin-synthetase activity in inflamed eyes, but does not appear to suppress the immune system.

Pharmacodynamics: In clinical studies VOLTAREN OPHTHA has been found to inhibit miosis during cataract surgery, to reduce inflammation following surgical interventions, trauma, and in other non-infected inflammatory conditions. VOLTAREN OPHTHA reduced the frequency and intensity of cystoid macular edema when administered prophylactically to patients undergoing cataract lens extraction with intraocular lens implantation.

Epithelialization was not adversely affected or delayed. A slight and transient elevation in the intraocular pressure (IOP) has been observed in some patients, following surgery, even with the use of VOLTAREN OPHTHA.

Pharmacokinetics: In man, the drug promptly passed into the aqueous humour following the topical application of 3-16 drops of 0.1% diclofenac sodium to the eye. Levels of unchanged diclofenac in the aqueous humour were highly variable, ranging from 10 to 505 ng/g. There were no detectable levels of drug in plasma, indicating that no measurable systemic absorption occurs following a single instillation of the ophthalmic drops.

STORAGE AND STABILITY: Storage: VOLTAREN OPHTHA (diclofenac sodium) 0.1% ophthalmic solution in bottles should be stored at 15 to 30°C and protected from light. Single-dose units should be stored at 25°C.

Others: Keep in a safe place out of reach of children.

SPECIAL HANDLING INSTRUCTIONS: Not applicable.

INFORMATION FOR THE PATIENT: Published in e-CPS, available by subscription at www.e-cps.ca.

DOSAGE FORMS, COMPOSITION AND PACKAGING: Each mL of ophthalmic solution contains: diclofenac sodium 0.1%. Nonmedicinal ingredients: preserved multi-dose bottles: boric acid, cremophor EL, edetate disodium, purified water, sorbic acid and tromethamine (TRIS); unpreserved single dose units: boric acid, cremophor EL, purified water and tromethamine (TRIS). Dropper bottles (preserved with sorbic acid) of 2.5, 5 and 10 mL. Single dose units (unpreserved) of 0.3 mL.

Voltaren Rapide® Pr

diclofenac potassium

Nonsteroidal Anti-inflammatory Drug (NSAID)

Novartis Pharmaceuticals

Date of Preparation: February 25, 1993
Date of Revision: April 8, 2010

SUMMARY PRODUCT INFORMATION:

Route of Administration	Dosage Form/ Strength	Clinically Relevant Nonmedicinal Ingredients
Oral	Sugar coated tablets/50 mg	Corn starch, sodium carboxymethyl starch, sucrose For a complete listing see Dosage Forms, Composition and Packaging.

INDICATIONS AND CLINICAL USE: VOLTAREN RAPIDE (diclofenac potassium) is indicated for the following:

- the short-term (up to one week) treatment of acute, mild to moderately severe pain that may be accompanied by inflammation, in conditions such as: musculoskeletal and/or soft tissue trauma including sprains, post-operative pain following dental extraction, episiotomy, or dysmenorrhea.

Throughout this document, the term NSAIDs refers to both non-selective NSAIDs and selective COX-2 inhibitor NSAIDs, unless otherwise indicated.

For patients with an increased risk of developing CV and/or GI adverse events, other management strategies that do NOT include the use of NSAIDs should be considered first (see Contraindications and Warnings and Precautions).

Use of VOLTAREN RAPIDE should be limited to the lowest effective dose for the shortest possible duration of treatment in order to minimize the potential risk for cardiovascular or gastrointestinal adverse events (see Contraindications and Warnings and Precautions).

VOLTAREN RAPIDE, as a NSAID, does **not** treat clinical disease or prevent its progression.

VOLTAREN RAPIDE, as a NSAID, only relieves symptoms and decreases inflammation for as long as the patient continues to take it.

Patient Subsets: Geriatrics: Evidence from clinical studies and post-market experience suggests that use in the geriatric population is associated with differences in safety (see Warnings and Precautions).

Pediatrics (<16 years of age): Safety and efficacy have not been established in the pediatric population.

CONTRAINDICATIONS: VOLTAREN RAPIDE is contraindicated in:

- the peri-operative setting of coronary artery bypass graft surgery (CABG). Although VOLTAREN RAPIDE has **not** been studied in this patient population, a selective COX-2 inhibitor NSAID studied in such a setting has led to an increased incidence of cardiovascular/thromboembolic events, deep surgical infections and sternal wound complications
- the third trimester of pregnancy, because of risk of premature closure of the ductus arteriosus and prolonged parturition
- women who are breastfeeding, because of the potential for serious adverse reactions in nursing infants
- severe uncontrolled heart failure
- known hypersensitivity to VOLTAREN RAPIDE or to any of the components/excipients
- history of asthma, urticaria, or allergic-type reactions after taking ASA or other NSAIDs (i.e. complete or partial syndrome of ASA-intolerance—rhinosinusitis, urticaria/angioedema, nasal polyps, asthma). Fatal anaphylactoid reactions have occurred in such individuals. Individuals with the above medical problems are at risk of a severe reaction even if they have taken NSAIDs in the past without any adverse reaction. The potential for cross-reactivity between different NSAIDs must be kept in mind (see Warnings and Precautions, Hypersensitivity Reactions, Anaphylactoid Reactions)
- active gastric/duodenal/peptic ulcer, active GI bleeding or perforation, gastritis or ulcerative colitis, regional enteritis, recurrent ulceration
- cerebrovascular bleeding or other bleeding disorders
- inflammatory bowel disease
- severe liver impairment or active liver disease
- severe renal impairment (creatinine clearance <30 mL/min or 0.5 mL/sec) or deteriorating renal disease (individuals with lesser degrees of renal impairment are at risk of deterioration of their renal function when prescribed NSAIDs and must be monitored) (see Warnings and Precautions, Renal)
- known hyperkalemia (see Warnings and Precautions, Renal, Fluid and Electrolyte Balance)
- children and adolescents less than 16 years of age

WARNINGS AND PRECAUTIONS:

Risk of Cardiovascular (CV) Adverse Events: Ischemic Heart Disease, Cerebrovascular Disease, Congestive Heart Failure (NYHA II-IV) (see Warnings and Precautions, Cardiovascular): VOLTAREN RAPIDE is a non-steroidal anti-inflammatory drug (NSAID). Use of some NSAIDs is associated with an increased incidence of cardiovascular adverse events (such as myocardial infarction, stroke or thrombotic events) which can be fatal. The risk may increase with duration of use. Patients with cardiovascular disease or risk factors for cardiovascular disease may be at greater risk.

Caution should be exercised in prescribing VOLTAREN RAPIDE to any patient with ischemic heart disease (including but NOT limited to acute myocardial infarction, history of myocardial infarction and/or angina), cerebrovascular disease (including but NOT limited to stroke, cerebrovascular accident, transient ischemic attacks and/or amaurosis fugax) and/or congestive heart failure (NYHA II-IV).

Use of NSAIDs, such as VOLTAREN RAPIDE, can promote sodium retention in a dose-dependent manner, through a renal mechanism, which can result in increased blood pressure and/or exacerbation of congestive heart failure. (See also Warnings and Precautions, Renal, Fluid and Electrolyte Balance.)

Randomized clinical trials with VOLTAREN RAPIDE have not been designed to detect differences in cardiovascular events in a chronic setting. Therefore, caution should be exercised when prescribing VOLTAREN RAPIDE.

Risk of Gastrointestinal (GI) Adverse Events (see Warnings and Precautions, Gastrointestinal (GI)): Use of NSAIDs, such as VOLTAREN RAPIDE, is associated with an increased incidence of gastrointestinal adverse events (such as peptic/duodenal ulceration, perforation, obstruction and gastrointestinal bleeding).

General: Frail or debilitated patients may tolerate side effects less well and therefore special care should be taken in treating this population. **To minimize the potential risk for an adverse event, the lowest effective dose should be used for the shortest possible duration.** As with other NSAIDs, caution should be used in the treatment of elderly patients who are more likely to be suffering from impaired renal, hepatic or cardiac function. For high risk patients, alternate therapies that do not involve NSAIDs should be considered.

VOLTAREN RAPIDE is **not** recommended for use with other NSAIDs, with the exception of low-dose ASA for cardiovascular prophylaxis, because of the absence of any evidence demonstrating synergistic benefits and the potential for additive adverse reactions. (See Drug Interactions, Drug-Drug Interactions, Acetylsalicylic acid (ASA) or other NSAIDs.)

Diclofenac potassium should not be used concomitantly with diclofenac sodium (e.g. VOLTAREN or VOLTAREN SR) since both exist in plasma as the same active organic anion.

Cardiovascular: VOLTAREN RAPIDE is a non-steroidal anti-inflammatory drug (NSAID). Use of some NSAIDs is associated with an increased incidence of cardiovascular adverse events (such as myocardial infarction, stroke or thrombotic events) which can be fatal. Large population-based observational studies, meta-analyses and systematic reviews suggest an increased risk of myocardial infarction and stroke also in association with the use of diclofenac. The risk may increase with the dose and duration of use. Patients with cardiovascular disease or risk factors for cardiovascular disease may be at greater risk.

Caution should be exercised in prescribing VOLTAREN RAPIDE to patients with risk factors for cardiovascular disease, cerebrovascular disease or renal disease, such as any of the following (NOT an exhaustive list):

- **Hypertension**
- **Dyslipidemia/Hyperlipidemia**
- **Diabetes Mellitus**
- **Congestive Heart Failure (NYHA I)**
- **Coronary Artery Disease (Atherosclerosis)**
- **Peripheral Arterial Disease**
- **Smoking**
- **Creatinine Clearance <60 mL/min or 1 mL/sec**

Use of NSAIDs, such as VOLTAREN RAPIDE, can lead to new hypertension or can worsen pre-existing hypertension, either of which may increase the risk of cardiovascular events as described above. Thus blood pressure should be monitored regularly. Consideration should be given to discontinuing VOLTAREN RAPIDE should hypertension either develop or worsen with its use.

Use of NSAIDs, such as VOLTAREN RAPIDE, can induce fluid retention and edema, and may exacerbate congestive heart failure, through a renally-mediated mechanism. (See Warnings and Precautions, Renal, Fluid and Electrolyte Balance.)

For patients with a high risk of developing an adverse CV event, other management strategies that do **not** include the use of NSAIDs should be considered first. **To minimize the potential risk for an adverse CV event, the lowest effective dose should be used for the shortest possible duration.**

Endocrine and Metabolism: Corticosteroids: VOLTAREN RAPIDE (diclofenac potassium) is **not** a substitute for corticosteroids. It does **not** treat corticosteroid insufficiency. Abrupt discontinuation of corticosteroids may lead to exacerbation of corticosteroid-responsive illness. Patients on prolonged corticosteroid therapy should have their therapy tapered slowly if a decision is made to discontinue corticosteroids (see Drug Interactions, Drug-Drug Interactions, Glucocorticoids).

Gastrointestinal (GI): Serious GI toxicity (sometimes fatal), such as peptic/duodenal ulceration, inflammation, perforation, obstruction and gastrointestinal bleeding, can occur at any time, with or without warning symptoms, in patients treated with NSAIDs, such as VOLTAREN RAPIDE. Minor upper GI problems, such as dyspepsia, commonly occur at any time. Health care providers should remain alert for ulceration and bleeding in patients treated with VOLTAREN RAPIDE, even in the absence of previous GI tract symptoms. Most spontaneous reports of fatal GI events are in elderly or debilitated patients and therefore special care should be taken in treating this population. **To minimize the potential risk for an adverse GI event, the lowest effective dose should be used for the shortest possible duration.** For high risk patients, alternate therapies that do not involve NSAIDs should be considered (see Warnings and Precautions, Special Populations, Geriatrics).

Patients should be informed about the signs and/or symptoms of serious GI toxicity and instructed to discontinue using VOLTAREN RAPIDEand seek emergency medical attention if they experience any such symptoms. The utility of periodic laboratory monitoring has **not** been demonstrated, nor has it been adequately assessed. Most patients who develop a serious upper GI adverse event on NSAID therapy have no symptoms. Upper GI ulcers, gross bleeding or perforation, caused by NSAIDs, appear to occur in approximately 1% of patients treated for 3-6 months, and in about 2-4% of patients treated for one year. These trends continue, thus increasing the likelihood of developing a serious GI event at some time during the course of therapy. Even a short-term therapy has its risks.

Caution should be taken if prescribing VOLTAREN RAPIDE to patients with a prior history of peptic/duodenal ulcer disease or gastrointestinal bleeding as these individuals have a greater than 10-fold higher risk for developing a GI bleed when taking a NSAID than patients with neither of these risk factors. Other risk factors for GI ulceration and bleeding include the following: *H. pylori* infection, increased age, prolonged use of NSAID therapy, excess alcohol intake, smoking, poor general health status or concomitant therapy with any of the following: anti-coagulants (e.g. warfarin); anti-platelet agents (e.g. ASA, clopidogrel); oral corticosteroids (e.g. prednisone); Selective Serotonin Reuptake Inhibitors (SSRIs) (e.g. citalopram, fluotexine, paroxetine, sertraline).

There is no definitive evidence that the concomitant administration of histamine H_2-receptor antagonists and/or antacids will either prevent or reduce the occurrence of gastrointestinal adverse events associated with the use of VOLTAREN RAPIDE.

Genitourinary: Some NSAIDs are associated with persistent urinary symptoms (bladder pain, dysuria, urinary frequency), hematuria or cystitis. The onset of these symptoms may occur at any time after the initiation of therapy with an NSAID. Should urinary symptoms occur, in the absence of an alternate explanation, treatment with VOLTAREN RAPIDE should be stopped to ascertain if symptoms disappear. This should be done before urological investigations or treatments are carried out.

Hematologic: NSAIDs inhibiting prostaglandin biosynthesis interfere with platelet function to varying degrees; patients who may be adversely affected by such an action, such as those on anti-coagulants or suffering from hemophilia or platelet disorders should be carefully observed when VOLTAREN RAPIDE is administered.

Anti-coagulants: Numerous studies have shown that the concomitant use of NSAIDs and anti-coagulants increases the risk of bleeding. Concurrent therapy of VOLTAREN RAPIDE with warfarin requires close monitoring of the international normalized ratio (INR).

Even with therapeutic INR monitoring, increased bleeding may occur.

Anti-platelet Effects: NSAIDs inhibit platelet aggregation and have been shown to prolong bleeding time in some patients. Unlike acetylsalicylic acid (ASA), their effect on platelet function is quantitatively less, or of shorter duration, and is reversible.

VOLTAREN RAPIDE and other NSAIDs have no proven efficacy as anti-platelet agents and should **not** be used as a substitute for ASA or other anti-platelet agents for prophylaxis of cardiovascular thromboembolic diseases. Anti-platelet therapies (e.g. ASA) should **not** be discontinued. There is some evidence that use of NSAIDs with ASA can markedly attenuate the cardioprotective effects of ASA (see Drug Interactions, Drug-Drug Interactions, Acetylsalicylic Acid (ASA) or other NSAIDs).

Concomitant administration of VOLTAREN RAPIDE with low dose ASA increases the risk of GI ulceration and associated complications.

Blood Dyscrasias: Blood dyscrasias (such as neutropenia, leukopenia, thrombocytopenia, aplastic anemia and agranulocytosis) associated with the use of NSAIDs are rare, but could occur with severe consequences.

Anemia is sometimes seen in patients receiving NSAIDs, including VOLTAREN RAPIDE. This may be due to fluid retention, GI blood loss, or an incompletely described effect upon erythropoiesis. Patients on long-term treatment with NSAIDs, including VOLTAREN RAPIDE, should have their hemoglobin or hematocrit checked if they exhibit any signs or symptoms of anemia or blood loss.

Hepatic/Biliary/Pancreatic: As with other NSAIDs, borderline elevations of one or more liver enzyme tests (AST, ALT, alkaline phosphatase) may occur in up to 15% of patients. These abnormalities may progress, may remain essentially unchanged, or may be transient with continued therapy.

A patient with symptoms and/or signs suggesting liver dysfunction, or in whom an abnormal liver test has occurred, should be evaluated for evidence of the development of a more severe hepatic reaction, while on therapy with VOLTAREN RAPIDE. Severe hepatic reactions including jaundice and cases of fatal hepatitis, liver necrosis and hepatic failure, some of them with fatal outcomes, have been reported with VOLTAREN RAPIDE.

Although such reactions are rare, if abnormal liver tests persist or worsen, if clinical signs and symptoms consistent with liver disease develop (e.g. jaundice), or if systemic manifestations occur (e.g. eosinophilia, associated with rash, etc.), this drug should be discontinued.

If there is a need to prescribe this drug in the presence of impaired liver function, it must be done under strict observation.

Caution is advised when using VOLTAREN RAPIDE in patients with hepatic porphyria, since VOLTAREN RAPIDE may trigger an attack.

Hypersensitivity Reactions: Anaphylactoid Reactions: As with NSAIDs in general, anaphylactoid reactions have occurred in patients without known prior exposure to VOLTAREN RAPIDE. In post-marketing experience, rare cases of anaphylactic/anaphylactoid reactions and angioedema have been reported in patients receiving VOLTAREN RAPIDE. VOLTAREN RAPIDE should **not** be given to patients with the ASA-triad. This symptom complex typically occurs in asthmatic patients who experience rhinitis with or without nasal polyps, or who exhibit severe, potentially fatal bronchospasm after taking ASA or other NSAIDs (see Contraindications).

ASA-intolerance: VOLTAREN RAPIDE should **not** be given to patients with complete or partial syndrome of ASA-intolerance (rhinosinusitis, urticaria/angioedema, nasal polyps, asthma) in whom asthma, anaphylaxis, urticaria/angioedema, rhinitis or other allergic manifestations are precipitated by ASA or other NSAIDs. Fatal anaphylactoid reactions have occurred in such individuals. As well, individuals with the above medical problems are at risk of a severe reaction even if they have taken NSAIDs in the past without any adverse reaction (see Contraindications).

Cross Sensitivity: Patients sensitive to any one of the NSAIDs may be sensitive to any of the other NSAIDs as well.

Serious Skin Reactions: (See Warnings and Precautions, Skin.)

Immune: (See Warnings and Precautions, Infection, Aseptic Meningitis.)

Infection: VOLTAREN RAPIDE, in common with other NSAIDs, may mask signs and symptoms of an underlying infectious disease.

Aseptic Meningitis: Rarely, with some NSAIDs, the symptoms of aseptic meningitis (stiff neck, severe headaches, nausea and vomiting, fever or clouding of consciousness) have been observed. Patients with autoimmune disorders (systemic lupus erythematosus, mixed connective tissue diseases, etc.) seem to be pre-disposed. Therefore, in such patients, the health care provider must be vigilant to the development of this complication.

Neurologic: Some patients may experience drowsiness, dizziness, blurred vision, vertigo, tinnitus, hearing loss, insomnia or depression with the use of NSAIDs, such as VOLTAREN RAPIDE. If patients experience such adverse reaction(s) they should exercise caution in carrying out activities that require alertness.

Ophthalmologic: Blurred and/or diminished vision has been reported with the use of NSAIDs. If such symptoms develop, VOLTAREN RAPIDE should be discontinued and an ophthalmologic examination performed. Ophthalmologic examination should be carried out at periodic intervals in any patient receiving VOLTAREN RAPIDE for an extended period of time.

Sun exposure in patients using VOLTAREN RAPIDE might cause photosensitivity and vision changes. Patients should be advised to contact their physician for assessment and advice if this occurs.

Peri-Operative Considerations: (See Contraindications, Coronary Artery Bypass Graft Surgery.)

Psychiatric: (See Warnings and Precautions, Neurologic.)

Renal: Long term administration of NSAIDs to animals has resulted in renal papillary necrosis and other abnormal renal pathology. In humans, there have been reports of acute interstitial nephritis, hematuria, low grade proteinuria and occasionally nephrotic syndrome.

During long-term therapy, kidney function should be monitored periodically. (See Action and Clinical Pharmacology, Special Populations and Conditions, Renal Insufficiency.)

Renal insufficiency due to NSAID use is seen in patients with pre-renal conditions leading to reduction in renal blood flow or blood volume. Under these circumstances, renal prostaglandins help maintain renal perfusion and glomerular filtration rate (GFR). In these patients, administration of a NSAID may cause a reduction in prostaglandin synthesis leading to impaired renal function. Patients at greatest risk of this reaction are those with pre-existing renal insufficiency (GFR <60 mL/min or 1 mL/s), dehydrated patients, patients on salt restricted diets, those with congestive heart failure, cirrhosis, liver dysfunction, taking angiotensin-converting enzyme inhibitors, angiotensin-II receptor blockers, cyclosporin, diuretics, and those who are elderly. Serious or life-threatening renal failure has been reported in patients with normal or impaired renal function after short term therapy with NSAIDs. Even patients at risk who demonstrate the ability to tolerate a NSAID under stable conditions may decompensate during periods of added stress (e.g. dehydration due to gastroenteritis). Discontinuation of NSAIDs is usually followed by recovery to the pre-treatment state.

Caution should be used when initiating treatment with NSAIDs, such as VOLTAREN RAPIDE, in patients with considerable dehydration. Such patients should be rehydrated prior to initiation of therapy. Caution is also recommended in patients with pre-existing kidney disease. (See Warning and Precautions, Monitoring and Laboratory Tests, Renal.)

Advanced Renal Disease: (See Contraindications.)

Fluid and Electrolyte Balance: Use of NSAIDs, such as VOLTAREN RAPIDE, can promote sodium retention in a dose-dependant manner, which can lead to fluid retention and edema, and consequences of increased blood pressure and exacerbation of congestive heart failure. Thus, caution should be exercised in prescribing VOLTAREN RAPIDE in patients with a history of congestive heart failure, compromised cardiac function, hypertension, increased age or other conditions predisposing to fluid retention (see Warnings and Precautions, Cardiovascular).

Use of NSAIDs, such as VOLTAREN RAPIDE, can increase the risk of hyperkalemia, especially in patients with diabetes mellitus, renal failure, increased age, or those receiving concomitant therapy with adrenergic blockers, angiotensin-converting enzyme inhibitors, angiotensin-II receptor antagonists, cyclosporin, or some diuretics. Electrolytes should be monitored periodically (see Contraindications).

Respiratory: ASA-induced asthma is an uncommon but very important indication of ASA and NSAID sensitivity. It occurs more frequently in patients with asthma who have nasal polyps.

Pre-existing Asthma: In patients with asthma, seasonal allergic rhinitis, swelling of the nasal mucosa (i.e. nasal polyps), chronic obstructive pulmonary diseases or chronic infections of the respiratory tract (especially if linked to allergic rhinitis-like symptoms), reactions on NSAIDs like asthma exacerbations (so-called intolerance to analgesics/analgesics-asthma), Quincke's oedema or urticaria are more frequent than in other patients. Therefore, special precaution is recommended in such patients (readiness for emergency). This is applicable as well for patients who are allergic to other substances, e.g. with skin reactions, pruritus or urticaria.

Sexual Function/Reproduction: The use of VOLTAREN RAPIDE, as with any drug known to inhibit cyclooxygenase/prostaglandin synthesis, may impair fertility and is not recommended in women attempting to conceive. Therefore, in women who have difficulties conceiving, or who are undergoing investigation of infertility, withdrawal of VOLTAREN RAPIDE should be considered.

Skin: In rare cases, serious skin reactions such as Stevens-Johnson syndrome, toxic epidermal necrolysis, exfoliative dermatitis and erythema multiforme have been associated with the use of some NSAIDs. Because the rate of these reactions is low, they have usually been noted during post-marketing surveillance in patients taking other medications also associated with the potential development of these serious skin reactions. Thus, causality is **not** clear. These reactions are potentially life threatening but may be reversible if the causative agent is discontinued and appropriate treatment instituted. Patients should be advised that if they experience a skin rash they should discontinue their NSAID and contact their physician for assessment and advice, including which additional therapies to discontinue.

Use of VOLTAREN RAPIDE may cause photosensitivity upon exposure to sunlight or UV light causing symptoms such as sunburn, skin rash, skin blisters, pruritus, erythema and discolouration.

Special Populations: Pregnant Women: VOLTAREN RAPIDE is CONTRAINDICATED for use during the third trimester of pregnancy because of risk of premature closure of the ductus arteriosus and the potential to prolong parturition.

Caution should be exercised in prescribing VOLTAREN RAPIDE during the first and second trimesters of pregnancy.

Inhibition of prostaglandin synthesis may adversely affect pregnancy and/or the embryofoetal development. Data from epidemiological studies suggest an increased risk of miscarriage and of cardiac malformation after use of a prostaglandin synthesis inhibitor in early pregnancy.

In animals, administration of a prostaglandin synthesis inhibitor has been shown to result in increased pre- and post-implantation loss and embryo-foetal lethality. In addition, increased incidences of various malformations, including cardiovascular, have been reported in animals given a prostaglandin synthesis inhibitor during the organogenetic period. Diclofenac potassium readily crosses the placental barrier.

Nursing Women: (See Contraindications.)

Pediatrics: (See Contraindications.)

Geriatrics: Patients older than 65 years (referred to in this document as older or elderly) and frail or debilitated patients are most susceptible to a variety of adverse reactions from NSAIDs. The incidence of these adverse reactions increases with dose and duration of treatment. In addition, these patients are less tolerant to ulceration and bleeding. Most reports of fatal GI events are in this population. Older patients are also at risk of lower esophageal injury including ulceration and bleeding.

For such patients, the dosage should be given to a starting dose lower than the one usually recommended, with individual adjustment when necessary and under close supervision.

Monitoring and Laboratory Tests: Cardiovascular: (Hypertension): Blood pressure should be monitored regularly during therapy with VOLTAREN RAPIDE.

Hematologic: Patients on long-term treatment with VOLTAREN RAPIDE should have their hemoglobin, hematocrit, red blood cells (RBC), white blood cells (WBC), and platelets checked if they exhibit any signs or symptoms of anemia or blood loss or blood dyscrasia.

Hepatic: Hepatic function (e.g. serum transaminases, bilirubine) should be monitored regularly during therapy with VOLTAREN RAPIDE.

Ophthalmologic: Patients on long-term treatment with VOLTAREN RAPIDE should have an ophthalmologic examination performed periodically, and if they experience blurred and/or diminished vision.

Renal: Patients with pre-existing renal insufficiency (GFR <60 mL/min or 1 mL/s), dehydrated patients, patients on salt restricted diets, those with congestive heart failure, cirrhosis, liver dysfunction, taking angiotensin-converting enzyme inhibitors, angiotensin-II receptor blockers, cyclosporin, diuretics, and the elderly should have their renal function monitored (e.g. urine output, serum creatinine, creatinine clearance and serum urea) during therapy with VOLTAREN RAPIDE.

Electrolytes, including serum potassium, should be monitored periodically, especially in patients with diabetes mellitus, renal failure, increased age, or those receiving concomitant therapy with adrenergic blockers, angiotensin-converting enzyme inhibitors, angiotensin-II receptor antagonists, cyclosporin, or some diuretics.

ADVERSE REACTIONS: Adverse Drug Reaction Overview: Although not all adverse drug reactions have been reported with VOLTAREN RAPIDE (diclofenac potassium), the types of adverse drug reactions are expected to be similar to those of VOLTAREN and VOLTAREN SR (diclofenac sodium) since both formulations exist in the plasma as the same active organic anion.

Gastrointestinal, dermatological, CNS and hepatic adverse reactions are the most commonly seen with diclofenac. The most severe gastrointestinal adverse reactions observed were ulceration and bleeding, while the most severe dermatological, albeit rare, reactions observed with diclofenac were erythema multiforme (Stevens-Johnson Syndrome and Lyell Syndrome). Fatalities have occurred on occasion, particularly in the elderly.

This section summarizes adverse drug reaction data pooled from clinical trials, published investigations and post-marketing experience with diclofenac potassium and diclofenac sodium.

Frequency estimate: Very common: ≥10%. Common: ≥1% and <10%. Uncommon: ≥0.01% and <1%. Very rare: <0.01%, including isolated reports. See Table 1 and Table 2.

Table 1: VOLTAREN RAPIDE

Most Common Adverse Drug Reactions (≥1%)

Gastrointestinal Disorders	Very common	Nausea, vomiting, diarrhea, dyspepsia, abdominal pain, flatulence, anorexia
Nervous System	Common	Dizziness, headache, vertigo
Hepatic	Common	Elevations (≥3 times the upper normal limit) of serum aminotransferase enzymes (AST or ALT)
Skin and Subcutaneous Disorders	Common	Rash, pruritus

Table 2: VOLTAREN RAPIDE

Less Common Adverse Drug Reactions (<1%)

Gastrointestinal Disorders	Uncommon	Gastritis, gastrointestinal hemorrhage, hemorrhagic diarrhea, melena, hematemesis, gastric and intestinal ulcerations (with or without bleeding or perforation)
	Very rare	Lower gut disorders (including hemorrhagic colitis and exacerbation of ulcerative colitis or Crohn's disease), diaphragm-like intestinal strictures, hyperacidity, stomatitis, glossitis, coated tongue, esophageal lesions, constipation, pancreatitis
Nervous System	Uncommon	Drowsiness, malaise, impaired concentration, tiredness.
	Very rare	Sensory disturbances including paresthesia, memory disturbance, convulsions, anxiety, tremor, aseptic meningitis, cerebrovascular accident (including transient ischemic attack, cerebral hemorrhage)
Special Senses	Very rare	Vision disturbances (blurred vision, diplopia), impaired hearing, tinnitus, taste alteration disorders.
Cardiac Disorders	Uncommon	Palpitation, angina, arrhythmias
	Very rare	Exacerbation of cardiac failure, hypertension, myocardial infarction
Skin and Subcutaneous Disorders	Uncommon	Urticaria
	Very rare	Bullous eruption, erythema, eczema, erythema multiforme, Stevens-Johnson Syndrome, Lyell Syndrome (toxic epidermal necrolysis), erythroderma (exfoliative dermatitis), loss of hair, photosensitivity reactions, purpura, allergic purpura
Renal and Urinary Disorders	Uncommon	Edema (facial, general, peripheral)
	Very rare	Acute renal failure, nephrotic syndrome, urinary abnormalities (e.g. hematuria and proteinuria), interstitial nephritis, renal papillary necrosis
Hematologic	Very rare	Thrombocytopenia, leukopenia, agranulocytosis, hemolytic anemia, aplastic anemia, anemia secondary to gastrointestinal bleeding
Hepatic	Uncommon	Liver function disorders including hepatitis, jaundice
	Very rare	Fulminant hepatitis
Immune System Disorders	Uncommon	Hypersensitivity, anaphylactic/anaphylactoid systemic reactions (including hypotension and shock)
	Very rare	Angioneurotic edema, (including face edema)
Psychiatric Disorders	Very rare	Disorientation, depression, insomnia, nightmare, irritability, psychotic disorder
Respiratory Disorders	Uncommon	Asthma
	Very rare	Pneumonitis

Post-Market Adverse Drug Reactions: Hepatic: hepatic necrosis, hepatic failure.

DRUG INTERACTIONS: Drug-Drug Interactions: See Table 3.

Drug-Food Interactions: Interactions with food have not been established.

Drug-Herb Interactions: Interactions with herbal products have not been established.

Drug-Laboratory Test Interactions: Diclofenac increases platelet aggregation time but does not affect bleeding time, plasma thrombin clotting time, plasma fibrinogen, or factors V and VII to XII. Statistically significant changes in prothrombin and partial thromboplastin times have been reported in normal volunteers. The mean changes were observed to be less than 1 second in both instances, and are unlikely to be clinically important.

Persistently abnormal or worsening renal, hepatic or hematological test values should be followed up carefully since they may be related to therapy.

Drug-Lifestyle Interactions: Patients experiencing visual disturbances, dizziness, vertigo, somnolence or other central nervous system disturbances while taking VOLTAREN RAPIDE should refrain from driving or using machines.

DOSAGE AND ADMINISTRATION: Dosing Considerations: Geriatrics: In the elderly, frail and debilitated, the dosage should be reduced to the lowest level providing control of symptoms, and adjusted when necessary (see Warnings and Precautions, Special Populations, Geriatrics).

Renal Insufficiency: Lower doses of VOLTAREN RAPIDE should be considered in patients with impaired renal function (see Warnings and Precautions, Renal).

Hepatic Impairment: Lower doses of VOLTAREN RAPIDE should be considered in patients with impaired hepatic function (see Warnings and Precautions, Hepatic/Biliary/Pancreatic).

Recommended Dose and Dosage Adjustment: As a general recommendation, the dose should be individually adjusted and the lowest effective dose given for the shortest possible duration.

VOLTAREN RAPIDE (diclofenac potassium) 50 mg sugar-coated tablets:

VOLTAREN RAPIDE is indicated for short-term (up to one week) treatment only.

Table 3: VOLTAREN RAPIDE
Established Potential Drug-Drug Interactions

VOLTAREN RAPIDE	Clinical comment
Acetaminophen	There may be an increased risk of adverse renal effects when administered concomitantly with NSAIDs.
Acetylsalicylic Acid (ASA) or Other NSAIDs	The use of VOLTAREN RAPIDE in addition to any other NSAID, including over the counter ones (such as ASA and ibuprofen) for analgesic and/or anti-inflammatory effects is **not** recommended because of the absence of any evidence demonstrating synergistic benefits and the potential for additive adverse reactions. The exception is the use of low dose ASA for cardiovascular protection, when another NSAID is being used for its analgesic/anti-inflammatory effect, keeping in mind that combination NSAID therapy is associated with additive adverse reactions. Some NSAIDs (e.g. ibuprofen) may interfere with the anti-platelet effects of low dose ASA, possibly by competing with ASA for access to the active site of cyclooxygenase-1 **Diclofenac potassium should not be used concomitantly with diclofenac sodium (e.g. VOLTAREN) since both exist in plasma as the same active organic anion.** Concomitant administration of diclofenac and other systemic NSAIDs or corticosteroids may increase the frequency of gastrointestinal undesirable effects.
Alcohol	There may be an increased risk of gastrointestinal side effects, including ulceration or hemorrhage, when administered concomitantly with NSAIDs.
Antacids	Concomitant administration of antacids with NSAIDs may affect the rate, but generally not the extent of the absorption of the NSAID
Anti-coagulants	(See Warnings and Precautions, Hematologic, Anti-coagulants)
Anti-hypertensives	NSAIDs may diminish the anti-hypertensive effect of Angiotensin Converting Enzyme (ACE) inhibitors. Combinations of ACE inhibitors, angiotensin-II antagonists or diuretics with NSAIDs might have an increased risk for acute renal failure and hyperkalemia. Blood pressure and renal function (including electrolytes) should be monitored more closely in this situation, as occasionally there can be a substantial increase in blood pressure (see Warnings and Precautions, Renal). Therefore the combination should be administered with caution especially in the elderly (see Warnings and Precautions, Monitoring and Laboratory Tests).
Anti-platelet Agents (including ASA)	There is an increased risk of bleeding, via inhibition of platelet function, when anti-platelet agents are combined with NSAIDs, such as VOLTAREN RAPIDE (see Warnings and Precautions, Hematologic, Anti-platelet Effects).
Cyclosporin or Tacrolimus	Nephrotoxicity of cyclosporin and tacrolimus may be increased because of the effect of NSAIDs on renal prostaglandins. Therefore, patients treated with cyclosporine or tacrolimus should receive doses of diclofenac lower than the regular doses.
Digoxin	Diclofenac may increase the plasma concentration of digoxin. Dosage adjustment may be required. Monitoring of serum digoxin level is recommended.
Diuretics	Clinical studies as well as post-marketing observations have shown that NSAIDs can reduce the effect of diuretics (see Warnings and Precautions, Renal). (See Warnings and Precautions, Monitoring and Laboratory Tests, Renal.)
Glucocorticoids	Some studies have shown that the concomitant use of NSAIDs and oral glucocorticoids increases the risk of GI adverse events such as ulceration and bleeding. This is especially the case in older (>65 years of age) individuals.
Lithium	Monitoring of plasma lithium concentrations is advised when stopping or starting a NSAID, as increased lithium concentrations can occur in patients taking lithium. Dosage adjustment of lithium may be required.
Methotrexate	Caution should be exercised when NSAIDs, including VOLTAREN RAPIDE, are administered less than 24 hours before or after treatment with methotrexate.
Oral Hypoglycemics	Pharmacodynamic studies have shown no potentiation of effect with concurrent administration with diclofenac; however, there are isolated reports of both hypoglycemic and hyperglycemic effects in the presence of diclofenac, which necessitated changes in the dosage of hypoglycemic agents. For this reason, monitoring of the blood glucose level is recommended as a precautionary measure during concomitant therapy.
Probenecid	May decrease the excretion and increase serum concentrations of NSAIDs possibly enhancing effectiveness and/or increasing potential for toxicity. Concurrent therapy of NSAIDs with probenicid requires close monitoring to be certain that no change in dosage is necessary.
Quinolone Antibacterials	There have been isolated reports of convulsions which may have been due to concomitant use of quinolones and NSAIDs.
Selective Serotonin Reuptake Inhibitors (SSRIs)	Concomitant administration of NSAIDs, including VOLTAREN RAPIDE and SSRIs may increase the risk of gastrointestinal ulceration and bleeding (see Warnings and Precautions, Gastrointestinal (GI)).

VOLTAREN RAPIDE should be taken with food.

The recommended daily dose for VOLTAREN RAPIDE is one 50 mg tablet, every 6-8 hours as required for a total daily maximum amount of 150 mg. For primary dysmenorrhea, treatment may be initiated with a loading dose of 100 mg, followed by 50 mg every six to eight hours, when required. When a loading dose is necessary, the first day maximum total amount is 200 mg.

Patients should be maintained on the lowest effective dose.

Missed Dose: Patients who miss one or more doses of VOLTAREN RAPIDE (diclofenac potassium) should not increase the dose of VOLTAREN RAPIDE to compensate for the missed dose or doses, but should continue with their therapy as soon as possible.

OVERDOSAGE:
Symptoms: There is no typical clinical picture resulting from diclofenac overdosage. Overdosage can cause symptoms such as vomiting, gastrointestinal haemorrhage, diarrhoea, dizziness, tinnitus or convulsions. In the event of significant poisoning, acute renal failure and liver damage are possible.

Therapeutic Measures: Management of acute poisoning with NSAIDs, including VOLTAREN RAPIDE essentially consists of supportive measures and symptomatic treatment. Supportive measures and symptomatic treatment should be given for complications such as hypotension, renal failure, convulsions, gastrointestinal disorder, and respiratory depression. Special measures such as forced diuresis, dialysis or haemoperfusion are probably of no help in eliminating NSAIDs, including VOLTAREN RAPIDE due to the high protein binding and extensive metabolism. Activated charcoal may be considered after ingestion of a potentially toxic overdose, and gastric decontamination (e.g. vomiting, gastric lavage) after ingestion of a potentially life threatening overdose.

For management of a suspected drug overdose, contact your regional Poison Control Centre. See the *CPS* Directory section for a list of Poison Control Centres.

ACTION AND CLINICAL PHARMACOLOGY: Mechanism of Action: Diclofenac, the active substance of VOLTAREN RAPIDE (diclofenac potassium), is a non-steroidal anti-inflammatory (NSAID) drug with analgesic properties. Diclofenac inhibits prostaglandin synthesis by interfering with the action of prostaglandin synthetase. This inhibitory effect may partially explain its actions. It is considered to be a peripherally acting analgesic.

Diclofenac potassium tablets have a rapid onset of action, making them particularly suitable for the treatment of acute painful inflammatory conditions.

Pharmacodynamics: The effects of VOLTAREN RAPIDE are largely mediated by inhibition of cyclooxygenases (COXs, COX-1, COX-2). These enzymes are found throughout the body and produce prostaglandins, which are important mediators of pain, fever, and adaptive and protective reactions in many organs and (inflamed) tissues.

Pharmacokinetics: Absorption: In humans, diclofenac can be detected in the plasma within 10 minutes of oral administration of diclofenac potassium tablets. Absorption is virtually complete. The area under the plasma curve (AUC) is dose proportional. A 50 mg tablet produces a mean peak plasma concentration of 3.8 µmol/L, 20-60 min post dose. The amount of diclofenac absorbed from VOLTAREN RAPIDE is the same as that obtained from an equivalent VOLTAREN enteric-coated tablet dose. Since diclofenac undergoes extensive first pass metabolism, only half of an orally administered dose is systemically available. The rate and extent of absorption of diclofenac are insignificantly affected (slightly delayed) when diclofenac potassium tablets are taken with food. When given in a regimen of 50 mg TID for 8 days, diclofenac potassium did not produce plasma accumulation of diclofenac.

Distribution: Diclofenac sodium is extensively bound (99%) to serum albumin. The apparent volume of distribution is 0.12 to 0.17 L/kg. Single-dose (P.O. or I.M.) studies in rheumatoid patients with joint effusions have shown that diclofenac is distributed to the synovial fluid, where T_{max} occurs 2 to 4 hours after plasma T_{max}. Synovial fluid concentrations exceed plasma levels within 4 to 6 hours of administration. This elevation above plasma concentrations can be maintained for up to 12 hours. The synovial fluid elimination half-life is at least 3 times greater than that for plasma.

Metabolism: The potassium salt of diclofenac in VOLTAREN RAPIDE yields the same active organic anion produced by the sodium salt found in VOLTAREN enteric coated tablets. Therefore, the fate of the systemically available anion is the same for both formulations.

Diclofenac undergoes single and multiple hydroxylation and methoxylation, producing 3'-, 4'-, 5-hydroxy, 4'- 5-hydroxy and 3'-hydroxy-4'-methoxy derivatives of diclofenac. These phenolic metabolites are largely inactive, and (along with the parent compound) are mostly converted to glucuronide conjugates.

Excretion: Plasma clearance of diclofenac is 263±56 mL/min. The mean terminal drug half-life in plasma is 1.8 hr after oral doses. In humans about 60% of the drug and its metabolites are eliminated in the urine and the balance through the bile in the feces. About 1% of an oral dose is excreted unchanged in urine.

Special Populations and Conditions: Pediatrics: VOLTAREN RAPIDE is contraindicated in children and adolescents less than 16 years of age (see Contraindications).

Geriatrics: No relevant age-dependant differences in the absorption, metabolism, or excretion of diclofenac have been observed.

Hepatic Insufficiency: In a study of ten patients with impaired hepatic function (chronic hepatitis and non-decompensated cirrhosis) receiving a single 100 mg oral dose of diclofenac sodium, the kinetics and metabolism of diclofenac were similar to patients without liver disease.

Renal Insufficiency: In patients suffering from renal impairment, no accumulation of the unchanged active substance can be inferred from the single-dose kinetics when applying the usual dosage schedule. At a creatinine clearance of <10 mL/min, the calculated steady-state plasma levels of the hydroxy metabolites are about 4 times higher than in normal subjects. However, the metabolites are ultimately cleared through the bile. Although no accumulation of pharmacologically active substance seems to occur, caution is advised while administering VOLTAREN RAPIDE to patients with impaired kidney function (i.e. GFR <60 mL/min or 1 mL/sec) (see Warnings and Precautions, Renal). VOLTAREN RAPIDE is contraindicated in patients with severely impaired or deteriorating renal function (creatinine clearance <30 mL/min (0.5 mL/s) (see Contraindications).

STORAGE AND STABILITY: Protect the tablets from heat (i.e. store between 15-30°C) and humidity.

INFORMATION FOR THE PATIENT: Published in e-CPS, available by subscription at www.e-cps.ca.

DOSAGE FORMS, COMPOSITION AND PACKAGING: Each reddish-brown, round, biconvex, sugar-coated tablet, contains: diclofenac potassium 50 mg. Nonmedicinal ingredients: cellulose, colloidal silicon dioxide, corn starch, ferric oxide, magnesium stearate, polyethylene glycol, povidone, sodium carboxymethyl starch, sucrose, talc, titanium dioxide and tribasic calcium phosphate. Bottles of 100.

(Shown in Product Identification Section)

Voluven®
hydroxyethyl starch
Plasma Volume Expander

Fresenius Kabi

Date of Revision: October 28, 2008

SUMMARY PRODUCT INFORMATION:

Route of Administration	Dosage Form/ Strength	Clinically Relevant Nonmedicinal Ingredients
Intravenous	Solution for infusion	Sodium chloride pH adjusted with Sodium hydroxide or hydrochloric acid

For complete information see Dosage Forms, Composition and Packaging.

INDICATIONS AND CLINICAL USE: VOLUVEN (6% HES 130/0.4) is indicated for the treatment of hypovolemia when plasma volume expansion is required.

It is not a substitute for red blood cells or coagulation factors in plasma.

CONTRAINDICATIONS: VOLUVEN is contraindicated in patients with fluid overload (hyperhydration) and especially in cases of pulmonary edema and congestive cardiac failure.

VOLUVEN should not be used in renal failure with oliguria or anuria not related to hypovolemia.

VOLUVEN should not be administered in patients receiving dialysis treatment.

Solutions containing VOLUVEN should not be administered to patients with severe hypernatremia or severe hyperchloremia.

VOLUVEN is contraindicated in patients with known hypersensitivity to hydroxyethyl starch.

VOLUVEN is contraindicated in patients with intracranial bleeding.

WARNINGS AND PRECAUTIONS: Fluid overload caused by overdose should be avoided in general. Particularly, for patients with cardiac insufficiency or severe kidney dysfunctions the increased risk of hyperhydration must be taken into consideration; posology must be adapted.

In case of severe dehydration a crystalloid should be given first.

Caution should be observed before administering VOLUVEN to patients with severe liver disease or severe bleeding disorders (e.g. severe cases of von Willebrand's disease).

Administration of large volumes of hydroxyethyl starch may transiently alter the coagulation mechanism and decrease hematocrit and plasma proteins due to hemodilution.

Elevated serum amylase levels may be observed temporarily following administration of VOLUVEN and can interfere with the diagnosis of pancreatitis.

It is important to supply sufficient fluid and to regularly monitor kidney function and fluid balance.

Serum electrolytes should be monitored.

Regarding the occurrence of anaphylactoid reactions please refer to Adverse Reactions.

Carcinogenesis and Mutagenesis: No mutagenic effects were observed with HES 130/0.4 10% solution according to the following tests on mutagenic activity: Salmonella typhimurium reverse mutation assay (in vitro), mammalian cells in the in vitro gene mutation assay (HPRT), assessment of the clastogenic activity in cultured human peripheral lymphocytes (in vitro), bone marrow cytogenetic test in Sprague-Dawley rats.

Special Populations: Pregnant Women: There are no adequate and well-controlled studies using VOLUVEN in pregnant women. Reproduction studies performed in rats and rabbits have revealed no evidence of harm to the fetus due to VOLUVEN. Embryotoxic effects were observed in rabbits at 50 mL/kg BW/day.

VOLUVEN should be used during pregnancy only if the potential benefit justifies the potential risk to the fetus.

Nursing Women: It is not known whether HES 130/0.4 is excreted in human milk. Because many drugs are excreted in human milk, caution should be exercised when VOLUVEN is administered to a nursing mother.

Pediatrics: There is limited experience on the use of VOLUVEN in children. In non-cardiac surgery of children below 2 years of age, the tolerability of VOLUVEN administered perioperatively was comparable to 5% albumin. VOLUVEN may be given to premature infants and newborns only after careful risk/benefit evaluation.

Geriatrics: Of the total number of patients in clinical trials of VOLUVEN (N=390), 26% were 65 years old or older. Other reported experience has not identified specific risks for the application of VOLUVEN in this patient group.

ADVERSE REACTIONS: Adverse reactions with VOLUVEN reported spontaneously, from clinical trials and in the literature include:

Anaphylactoid reactions (mild influenza-like symptoms, bradycardia, tachycardia, bronchospasm, non-cardiac pulmonary edema) have been reported rarely with solutions containing hydroxyethyl starch. If a hypersensitivity reaction occurs, administration of the drug should be discontinued immediately and the appropriate treatment and supportive measures should be undertaken until symptoms have resolved.

The concentration of serum amylase can rise commonly during administration of hydroxyethyl starch and can interfere with the diagnosis of pancreatitis.

Pruritus (itching) is a known complication of administration of hydroxyethyl starches, though is typically more common with prolonged use of high doses. In the pivotal study, with patients monitored to 28 days post-operatively, pruritus occurred in 10.2% of cases in the VOLUVEN group and 9.8% of cases in the hetastarch group. In both groups, pruritus was mild and self-limiting.

However, HES-induced pruritus may be delayed in onset, typically one to six weeks after exposure, may be severe and may be of protracted (weeks and months) persistence. It is generally unresponsive to therapy. The decreased molecular weight, lower degree of substitution, decreased tissue storage and intra-vascular persistence in conjunction with a shorter plasma half-life of VOLUVEN may result in a lower incidence of pruritus related to its use.

At high dosages the dilution effects may commonly result in a corresponding dilution of blood components such as coagulation factors and other plasma proteins and in a decrease of hematocrit.

With the administration of hydroxyethyl starches, disturbances of blood coagulation can occur rarely depending on the dosage.

Table 1: VOLUVEN
Frequency of Occurrence of Adverse Drug Reactions

System Organ Class	Adverse Drug Reaction	Frequency of Occurrence
Blood and Lymphatic System Disorders	Coagulation disorders	Rare (in high doses) (>0.01%–≤0.1%)
Immune System Disorders	Anaphylactoid reactions	Rare (>0.01%–≤0.1%)
Skin and Subcutaneous Tissue Disorders	Pruritus	Common (dose dependent) (≥1%–<10%)
Investigations	Increase of serum amylase	Common (dose dependent) (≥1%–<10%)
	Decrease of hematocrit	Common (dose dependent) (≥1%–<10%)
	Decrease of plasma proteins	Common (dose dependent) (≥1%–<10%)

DRUG INTERACTIONS: Based on limited studies interactions are not known, however, mixing with other drugs should be avoided.

DOSAGE AND ADMINISTRATION: VOLUVEN (6% HES 130/0.4) is **administered by intravenous infusion only**.

Total volume and rate of infusion are dependent on the clinical situation and the individual patient. As with any intravenous fluid, VOLUVEN should be administered in accordance with accepted clinical practices for fluid and electrolyte management.

In clinical trials, infusions up to 33 mL/kg/day were most commonly used. There is limited experience with infusions up to 50 mL/kg/day.

The initial 10-20 mL are to be infused slowly, keeping the patient under close observation (due to possible anaphylactoid reactions).

VOLUVEN can be administered repetitively over several days. The dosage and duration of treatment should be individualized according to the duration and extent of hypovolemia, the hemodynamic status and on the resultant hemodilution.

Children: Limited clinical data on the use of VOLUVEN in children is available. In 41 children including newborns to infants (<2 years), a mean dose of 16±9 mL/kg was administered safely and well tolerated for stabilization of hemodynamics.

The dosage in children should be adapted to the individual patient colloid needs, taking into account the disease state, as well as the hemodynamic and hydration status.

OVERDOSAGE:

As with all volume substitutes, overdose can lead to overloading of the circulatory system (e.g. pulmonary edema). In this case the infusion should be stopped immediately and if necessary, a diuretic should be administered.

For management of a suspected drug overdose, CPhA recommends that you contact your **regional Poison Control Centre**. See the *CPS* Directory section for a list of Poison Control Centres.

ACTION AND CLINICAL PHARMACOLOGY: VOLUVEN, 6% hydroxyethyl starch (HES 130/0.4), tetrastarch, is an artificial colloid, third generation starch, for volume replacement whose effect on intravascular volume expansion and hemodilution depends on the molar substitution by hydroxyethyl groups (0.4), the mean molecular weight (130 000 Da), the concentration (6%), the degree of substitution (C_2/C_6 ratio) of approx. 9:1 as well as the dosage and infusion rate. Hydroxyethyl starch 130/0.4 is a derivative of thin boiling waxy maize starch, which mainly consists of a glucose polymer (amylopectin) predominately consisting of α-1.4-connected glucose units with several α-1.6-branches. The medium molecular weight (130 000 Da), low degree of substitution (0.4) and narrow molecular weight distribution of hydroxyethyl starch (HES 130/0.4) contained in VOLUVEN contribute to its beneficial effects on pharmacokinetics, intravascular volume effect and hemodilution.

Pharmacodynamics: Infusion of 500 mL VOLUVEN over 30 minutes in healthy volunteers results in a plateau-like non-expansive volume increase of approximately 100% of the infused volume which lasts for approximately 4 to 6 hours. Isovolemic exchange of blood with VOLUVEN maintains blood volume for at least 6 hours.

Pharmacokinetics: The pharmacokinetic profile of HES is complex and largely dependent on its molar substitution as well as its molecular weight. When administered intravenously, molecules smaller than the renal threshold (60 000-70 000 Da) are readily and rapidly excreted in the urine, while molecules with higher molecular weights are metabolised by plasma amylase prior to excretion via the renal route.

The mean in vivo molecular weight of VOLUVEN in plasma is 70 000-80 000 Da immediately following infusion and remains above the renal threshold throughout the treatment period.

The volume of distribution of VOLUVEN after intravenous administration of 500 mL to healthy volunteers is about 5.9 L. Plasma levels of VOLUVEN remain at 75% of peak concentration at 30 minutes post-infusion and decrease rapidly to 14% at 6 hours post-infusion. Plasma levels of VOLUVEN return to baseline levels 24 hours following infusion.

Plasma clearance of VOLUVEN following intravenous administration of 500 mL was 31.4 mL/min with an AUC of 14.3 mg/mL/h, following non-linear pharmacokinetics. A single dose of 500 mL of VOLUVEN results in elimination in the urine of approximately 62% within 72 hours. VOLUVEN is eliminated from systemic circulation with a $t_{½}$ of 1.4 h and a terminal half-life ($t_{½β}$) of 12.1 h following administration of a single dose of 500 mL.

The kinetics of VOLUVEN are similar following single and multiple dose administration. No significant plasma accumulation occurred after daily administration of 500 mL of a 10% solution containing HES 130/0.4 over a period of 10 days. Elimination rates in the urine were approximately 70% within 72 hours.

In an experimental model in rats using repetitive doses of 0.7 g/kg BW per day of HES 130/0.4 over 18 days, 52 days after the last administration tissue storage was 0.6% of the total administered dose.

Special Populations and Conditions: Renal Insufficiency: Single intravenous administration of VOLUVEN (500 mL) in subjects with mild to severe renal impairment resulted in a moderate increase in AUC by a factor of 1.7 (95% confidence limits 1.44 and 2.07) only in subjects with Cl_{Cr} <50 mL/min compared to ≥50 mL/min. However, terminal half-life and peak HES concentration were not affected by renal impairment. Plasma levels of VOLUVEN return to baseline levels 24 hours following infusion.

59% of HES 130/0.4 was recovered in the urine of subjects with Cl_{Cr} ≥30 mL/min versus 51% in those with Cl_{Cr} between 15 to 30 mL/min.

There is no data available on the use of VOLUVEN in dialysis.

Hepatic Insufficiency: Pharmacokinetic data of patients with hepatic insufficiency are not available.

Age: Pharmacokinetic data of elderly or children are not available.

STORAGE AND STABILITY: To be used immediately after the bag is opened.

The solution is intended for intravenous administration using sterile equipment.

Use only clear solutions and undamaged containers.

Parenteral drug products should be inspected visually for clarity, particulate matter, precipitate, discoloration and leakage prior to administration. Solutions showing haziness, particulate matter, precipitate, discoloration or leakage should not be used. Discard unused portion.

Do not use VOLUVEN after expiry date.

freeflex bag storage: at 15-25°C.

The product should be used immediately after opening.

Do not freeze.

SPECIAL HANDLING INSTRUCTIONS: Before administering the product in plastic bags to patient, review these directions:

Freeflex IV Solution Container: These instructions are only intended as guidelines for product use. Please refer to your own departmental guidelines.

1. (See package insert for illustrations.)

Preparation for Administration:

2. • Check the **free**flex IV container solution composition, lot number and expiry date.
   • Inspect the container for damage or solution leakage. If damaged, do not use!
   • Check the **free**flex solution for visible particles or cloudiness. Do not use unless the solution is clear.
3. • Turn the **free**flex IV container over so that the text is face down. Using the pre-cut corner tabs peel open the overwrap to remove the primary bag. The overwrap adheres slightly to the primary bag to improve handling even when wearing disposable gloves.
4. • Identify the blue infusion port. Check the **free**flex IV container solution for visible particles or cloudiness. Do not administer unless the solution is clear.
5. • Flip off the blue tamper-evident cover from the **free**flex IV container infusion port.
6. • Use a non-vented giving set or, if using a vented set, close the air inlet. Grip the base of the infusion port with your fingers behind the guard. Push and twist the giving set firmly into the port. A slight resistance should be felt, as the port membrane is broken. To prevent leaks, insert the spike until the clear plastic collar of the port meets the shoulder of the spike.

Warnings:

1. Do not remove the **free**flex IV container from its overwrap until immediately before use.
2. Do not administer unless the solution is clear, free from particles and the **free**flex IV container is undamaged.
3. Discontinue the infusion if adverse reaction occurs.
4. Do not vent.
5. It is recommended that administration sets are changed at least once every 24 hours.
6. Partially used **free**flex IV container must be discarded.

Incompatibilities: The mixing with other drugs should be avoided. If, in exceptional cases, a mixture with other drugs is required, care should be taken with the compatibility (clouding or precipitation), hygienic injection and a good admixture.

INFORMATION FOR THE PATIENT: Published in e-CPS, available by subscription at www.e-cps.ca.

DOSAGE FORMS, COMPOSITION AND PACKAGING: Each 100 mL of sterile and pyrogen-free solution contains: poly (O-2-hydroxyethyl) starch 6 g (molar substitution: 0.4) (mean molecular weight: 130 000 Da), sodium chloride 0.9 g, water for injection qs, pH adjusted with sodium hydroxide or hydrochloric acid qs. Approximate concentration of electrolytes per litre: sodium (Na^+) 154 mmol, chloride (Cl^-) 154 mmol, theoretical osmolarity: 308 mosmol/L, pH: 4.0-5.5, titratable acidity: <1.0 mmol NaOH/L. Polyolefine bags (**free**flex) with overwrap: 30×250 mL; 20×500 mL.

(Shown in Product Identification Section)

Votrient™ Ⓟ

pazopanib HCl

Antineoplastic

GlaxoSmithKline

Date of Preparation: May 27, 2010

SUMMARY PRODUCT INFORMATION:

Route of Administration	Dosage Form/ Strength	Clinically Relevant Nonmedicinal Ingredients
Oral	Tablets/200 mg	None. For a complete listing see Dosage Forms, Composition and Packaging.

INDICATIONS AND CLINICAL USE: VOTRIENT (pazopanib hydrochloride) is indicated for:

- the treatment of patients with metastatic renal cell (clear cell) carcinoma (mRCC) who have received no prior systemic therapies or who have received prior treatment with cytokines for metastatic disease.

Approval of VOTRIENT is based on significant progression-free survival benefit in patients with mRCC of good performance status (ECOG 0-1). Prolongation of overall survival was not demonstrated nor were quality-of-life differences shown between patients receiving VOTRIENT versus placebo in the pivotal phase III trial.

Geriatrics (65 years of age and over): In clinical trials with VOTRIENT for the treatment of mRCC, 196 subjects (33%) were aged ≥65 years, and 34 subjects (6%) were aged >75 years. No overall differences in safety or effectiveness of VOTRIENT were observed between these subjects and younger subjects but a greater sensitivity of some older individuals cannot be ruled out.

Pediatrics (less than 18 years of age): The safety and efficacy of pazopanib in children have not been established. Toxicology studies in rodents showed hypertrophy of epiphyseal growth plates and abnormalities in growing incisors. VOTRIENT is not recommended for use in children.

CONTRAINDICATIONS:

- Patients who are hypersensitive to this drug or to any ingredient in the formulation or component of the container. For a complete listing, see Dosage Forms, Composition and Packaging.

WARNINGS AND PRECAUTIONS:

Serious Warnings and Precautions
VOTRIENT tablets should be prescribed by a physician experienced in the administration of anti-cancer agents.
Monitor hepatic function and interrupt, reduce or discontinue dosing as recommended.
VOTRIENT is not recommended for patients that have baseline plasma bilirubin concentrations >1.5×ULN (with direct bilirubin >35%) and ALT elevations of >2×ULN, or who have moderate or severe hepatic impairment (Child Pugh B and C).
The following are clinically significant adverse events:
- Hepatotoxicity, including fatalities (see Hepatic)
- Hypertension (see Cardiovascular)
- QT/QTc prolongation (see Cardiovascular)
- Arterial Thrombotic Events (see Cardiovascular)
- Hemorrhage (see Hemorrhagic)
- Gastrointestinal Perforation and Fistula (see Gastrointestinal)

General: Drug-Drug Interactions: Coadministration of VOTRIENT with strong inhibitors of CYP3A4 or P-glycoprotein (PgP) is not recommended as this may increase pazopanib concentrations (see Dosage and Administration and Drug Interactions) and drug toxicity. Coadministration with inducers of CYP3A4 or PgP should be avoided due to the risk of reduced effectiveness of the drug.
Carcinogenesis and Mutagenesis: Carcinogenicity studies with VOTRIENT have not been conducted. However, proliferative lesions were found in mice treated with VOTRIENT. Genotoxicity studies showed no evidence of clastogenic or mutagenic activity.
Cardiovascular: Hypertension: Hypertension is a common adverse event in patients treated with VOTRIENT (see Adverse Reactions) and blood pressure should be well controlled prior to initiating treatment with VOTRIENT. Patients were required to have diastolic BP ≤90 mm Hg and systolic BP ≤140 mm Hg for entry into the controlled phase III trial. During therapy patients should be monitored for hypertension and treated as needed with standard anti-hypertensive therapy (see Adverse Reactions). In clinical studies, hypertension occurred early in the course of treatment (88% occurring in first 18 weeks). In the case of persistent hypertension despite anti-hypertensive therapy, the VOTRIENT dose should be reduced (see Dosage and Administration). VOTRIENT should be discontinued if hypertension is severe and persists despite anti-hypertensive therapy and VOTRIENT dose reduction.
Hypertensive crisis has been reported in mRCC clinical trials (1/586) with VOTRIENT.
Patients with hypertension that is not controlled by medications should not be treated with VOTRIENT.
QT Prolongation and Torsade de Pointes: In clinical studies for VOTRIENT, events of QT prolongation or Torsade de Pointes have occurred (see Adverse Reactions). VOTRIENT should be used with caution in patients with a history of QT interval prolongation, patients taking antiarrythmics or other medications that may potentially prolong QT interval, or those with relevant pre-existing cardiac disease (including myocardial ischemia and congestive heart failure). Other risk factors for Torsade de Pointes include diabetes mellitus, autonomic neuropathy and electrolyte disturbances (hypokalemia, hypomagnesemia, hypocalcemia). When using VOTRIENT, baseline and periodic monitoring of electrocardiograms and maintenance of electrolytes within normal range is recommended.
Arterial Thrombotic Events: In clinical studies for VOTRIENT, myocardial infarctions, angina, ischemic stroke and transient ischemic attack were observed, some of which were fatal (see Adverse Reactions). In the controlled phase III study, these events were observed more frequently with VOTRIENT compared to placebo. VOTRIENT should be used with caution in patients who are at increased risk of thrombotic events or who have had a history of thrombotic events. VOTRIENT has not been studied in patients who have had an event within the previous 6 months and should not be used in these patients.
Cardiac Dysfunction: VOTRIENT has been associated with decreases in left ventricular ejection fraction (LVEF) and cardiac failure in clinical studies with various cancers, including mRCC (see Warnings and Precautions). In the controlled phase III study, the rates of cardiac dysfunction were similar between the placebo and pazopanib arms. LVEF was not monitored in clinical studies of mRCC.
Endocrine and Metabolism: Hypothyroidism: In clinical studies with VOTRIENT, events of hypothyroidism have occurred (see Adverse Reactions). Proactive monitoring of thyroid function tests is recommended.
Gastrointestinal: Gastrointestinal Perforations and Fistula: In clinical studies for VOTRIENT, events of gastrointestinal (GI) perforation or fistula have occurred, some of which were fatal (see Adverse Reactions). VOTRIENT should be used with caution in patients at risk for GI perforation or fistula.
Hemorrhagic: In clinical studies with VOTRIENT hemorrhagic events have been reported, some of which were fatal (see Adverse Reactions). VOTRIENT has not been studied in patients who had a history of hemoptysis, cerebral, or clinically significant gastrointestinal hemorrhage in the past 6 months. Treatment with VOTRIENT is not recommended if there is a history of hemoptysis, cerebral or clinically significant gastrointestinal bleeding in the past 6 months, and VOTRIENT should be used with caution in patients with a significant risk of hemorrhage.
Hepatic: Hepatic Effects: Cases of hepatic failure (including fatalities) have been reported during use of VOTRIENT. In a phase I hepatic impairment study, patients with moderate hepatic impairment at baseline experienced dose limiting toxicity at 400 mg (half the recommended daily dose). VOTRIENT should not be used in patients with baseline plasma bilirubin concentrations >1.5×ULN (with direct bilirubin >35%) and ALT elevations of >2×ULN, or who have moderate or severe hepatic impairment (Child Pugh B and C). VOTRIENT should be used with caution in patients with mild hepatic impairment as no formal studies have been carried out in this patient population.
In clinical trials with VOTRIENT, increase in serum transaminases (ALT, AST) and bilirubin were observed (see Adverse Reactions). In the majority of the cases, isolated increases in ALT and AST have been reported, without concomitant elevations of alkaline phosphatase or bilirubin. The vast majority (92.5 %) of all transaminase elevations of any grade occurred in the first 18 weeks. Grades are based on the National Cancer Institute Common Terminology Criteria for Adverse Events, Version 3 (NCI CTCAE).
Monitor serum liver tests before initiation of treatment with VOTRIENT and at least once every 3-4 weeks for at least the first 4 months of treatment, and as clinically indicated. Periodic monitoring should then continue after this time period. Physicians should inform patients on the possible signs and symptoms of hepatic dysfunction (including jaundice, unusual darkening of the urine, anorexia, nausea, fatigue, right upper abdominal discomfort and vomiting) so appropriate management can be implemented to minimize this impact.
The following guidelines are provided for patients with baseline values of total bilirubin ≤1.5×ULN and AST and ALT ≤2×ULN.
- Patients with isolated ALT elevations between 3×ULN and ≤8×ULN may be continued on VOTRIENT with weekly monitoring of liver function until ALT returns to Grade 1 (NCI CTCAE) or baseline.
- Patients with ALT of >8×ULN should have VOTRIENT interrupted until they return to Grade 1 (NCI CTCAE) or baseline. If the potential benefit for reinitiating VOTRIENT treatment is considered to outweigh the risk for hepatotoxicity, then reintroduce VOTRIENT at a reduced dose of 400 mg once daily and measure serum liver tests weekly for 8 weeks (see Dosage and Administration). Following reintroduction of VOTRIENT, if ALT elevations >3×ULN recur, then VOTRIENT should be permanently discontinued.
- If ALT elevations >3×ULN occur concurrently with bilirubin elevations >2×ULN, VOTRIENT should be permanently discontinued. Patients should be monitored until return to Grade 1 (NCI CTCAE) or baseline. VOTRIENT is a UGT1A1 inhibitor. Mild, indirect (unconjugated) hyperbilirubinaemia may occur in patients with Gilbert's syndrome. Patients with only a mild indirect hyperbilirubinaemia, known or suspected Gilbert's syndrome, and elevation in ALT >3×ULN should be managed as per the recommendations outlined for isolated ALT elevations.

Peri-Operative Considerations: Wound Healing: No formal studies on the effect of VOTRIENT on wound healing have been conducted. Since Vascular Endothelial Growth Factor (VEGF) inhibitors may impair wound healing, treatment with VOTRIENT should be stopped at least 7 days prior to scheduled surgery. The decision to resume VOTRIENT after surgery should be based on clinical judgement of adequate wound healing. VOTRIENT should be discontinued in patients with wound dehiscence.
Renal: Proteinuria: In clinical studies with VOTRIENT, proteinuria has been reported (see Adverse Reactions). Baseline and periodic urinalyses during treatment are recommended and patients should be monitored for worsening proteinuria. Patients with >1 g protein (24 h collection) at baseline were excluded from clinical studies. VOTRIENT should be discontinued if the patient develops nephrotic syndrome.
Reproduction: VOTRIENT may impair fertility in human males and females. In female reproductive toxicity studies in rats, reduced female fertility has been observed.
Special Populations: Pregnant Women: Pre-clinical studies in animals have shown that pazopanib was teratogenic, embryotoxic, fetotoxic and abortifacient.

* see Warnings and Precautions for additional information.

VOTRIENT may cause fetal harm when administered to pregnant women. If VOTRIENT is used during pregnancy, or if the patient becomes pregnant while receiving VOTRIENT, the potential hazard to the fetus should be explained to the patient. Women of childbearing potential should be advised to avoid becoming pregnant while receiving treatment with VOTRIENT and for up to 8 weeks after ending treatment.
Nursing Women: The safe use of pazopanib during lactation has not been established. It is not known whether VOTRIENT is excreted in human milk. Breastfeeding should be discontinued during treatment with VOTRIENT.
Pediatrics: The safety and efficacy of VOTRIENT in children less than 18 years of age have not been established. Toxicology studies in rodents showed hypertrophy of epiphyseal growth plates and abnormalities in growing incisors. VOTRIENT is not recommended for use in children less than 18 years of age.
Monitoring and Laboratory Tests: Prior to treatment and during the course of therapy with VOTRIENT patients should be monitored for hypertension and standard anti-hypertensive therapy should be initiated as required (see Adverse Reactions). Normal blood pressure (diastolic ≤90 mm Hg and systolic ≤140 mm Hg), confirmed by two measurements separated by 24 hours, should be recorded for patients prescribed anti-hypertensive medication prior to treatment with VOTRIENT.
When using VOTRIENT, complete blood counts (CBC), clinical chemistries [including blood glucose, lipase/amylase, creatinine and electrolytes (calcium, magnesium, potassium, phosphate and sodium)], urinalyses and electrocardiograms should be measured at baseline and periodically during treatment.
Proactive monitoring of thyroid function tests is recommended.
Monitor serum liver tests before initiation of treatment with VOTRIENT and at least once every 3-4 weeks for at least the first 4 months of treatment, and as clinically indicated. Periodic monitoring should then continue after this time period (see Warnings and Precautions, Hepatic, Hepatic Effects).

ADVERSE REACTIONS: Adverse Drug Reaction Overview: The safety of VOTRIENT has been evaluated in more than 1600 subjects in clinical trials including 977 patients in the monotherapy studies which include 586 mRCC patients. The data described below reflect exposure to VOTRIENT in 290 mRCC patients who participated in a randomized, double-blind, placebo-controlled study. The median duration of treatment was 7.4 months for patients who received VOTRIENT and 3.8 months for the placebo arm. Forty-two percent (42%) of patients on VOTRIENT required a dose interruption and thirty-six percent (36%) required a dose reduction.
Clinical Trial Adverse Drug Reactions: Potentially serious adverse reactions with VOTRIENT included hepatic effects, hypertension, QT prolongation and Torsade de Pointes, arterial thrombotic events, cardiac dysfunction, hemorrhagic events, and gastrointestinal perforation and fistula (see Warnings and Precautions).
Table 1 presents the most common adverse reactions occurring in ≥10 % of patients who received VOTRIENT.

Table 1: VOTRIENT

Adverse Reactions Occurring in ≥10% of Patients who Received VOTRIENT

Reactions	VOTRIENT (N=290) All Grades[a] %	VOTRIENT (N=290) Grade 3 %	VOTRIENT (N=290) Grade 4 %	Placebo (N=145) All Grades[a] %	Placebo (N=145) Grade 3 %	Placebo (N=145) Grade 4 %
Gastrointestinal Disorders						
Diarrhea	52	3	<1	9	<1	0
Nausea	26	<1	0	9	0	0
Vomiting	21	2	<1	8	2	0
Abdominal pain	11	2	0	1	0	0
Vascular Disorders						
Hypertension	40	4	0	10	<1	0
General Disorders and Administrative Site Conditions						
Fatigue	19	2	0	8	1	1
Asthenia	14	3	0	8	0	0
Skin and Subcutaneous Tissue Disorders						
Hair colour changes	38	<1	0	3	0	0
Metabolism and Nutrition Disorders						
Anorexia	22	2	0	10	<1	0
Nervous System Disorder						
Headache	10	0	0	5	0	0

[a] National Cancer Institute Common Terminology Criteria for Adverse Events, version 3.

Other notable treatment-emergent adverse reactions observed more commonly in patients treated with VOTRIENT than placebo but with an incidence <10% (all grades) include:
Renal and Urinary Disorders: proteinuria* (9%), dysuria (2%).
Investigations: weight decreased (9%).
Skin and Subcutaneous Disorders: alopecia (8%), rash (8%), palmar-plantar erythrodysesthesia (hand-foot syndrome 6%), skin depigmentation (3%), hyperhidrosis (3%).
Blood and Lymphatic System Disorders: thrombocytopenia (8%), neutropenia (5%), leucopenia (3%), lymphopenia (2%).
Nervous System Disorders: dysguesia (altered taste 8%), paraesthesia (3%).
General Disorders and Administration Site Conditions: chest pain (5%).
Gastrointestinal Disorders: dyspepsia (5%), stomatitis (4%).
Hepatobiliary Disorders: hyperbilirubinemia (4%), abnormal hepatic function (3%), hepatotoxicity (2%).
Infections and Infestations: urinary tract infection (4%).
Metabolism and Nutrition Disorders: hyperkalemia (3%).
Respiratory, Thoracic and Mediastinal Disorders: epistaxis (2%).
Cardiac Disorders: myocardial ischaemia (1%).
Abnormal Hematologic and Clinical Chemistry Findings: Table 2 presents the most common laboratory abnormalities occurring in ≥15% of patients who received pazopanib and more commonly than in the placebo arm.
Hepatic Effects: In the controlled phase III clinical study with VOTRIENT for the treatment of mRCC, ALT >3×ULN was reported in 18% and 3% of patients who received VOTRIENT and placebo, respectively. ALT >10×ULN was reported in 4% of patients who received VOTRIENT and in <1% of placebo patients. Concurrent elevation in ALT >3×ULN and bilirubin >2×ULN in the absence of significant alkaline phosphatase elevation occurred in 1% of patients on VOTRIENT and <1% on placebo. In patients who discontinued study treatment due to an adverse event, hepatic related effects were the most common reasons for study discontinuation in the phase III controlled clinical trial (4%) and in the phase II single-arm study (4%). Across all monotherapy studies with VOTRIENT, ALT >3×ULN was reported in 138/977 (14%) and ALT >10×ULN was reported in 27/977 (3%) of patients who received VOTRIENT (see Warnings and Precautions, Hepatic, Hepatic Effects).

Table 2: VOTRIENT

Selected Laboratory Abnormalities in ≥15% of Patients who Received Pazopanib and More Commonly than in the Placebo Arm

	VOTRIENT (N=290)			Placebo (N=145)		
Parameters	All Grades[a] %	Grade 3 %	Grade 4 %	All Grades[a] %	Grade 3 %	Grade 4 %
Hematologic						
Leukopenia	37	0	0	6	0	0
Neutropenia	34	1	<1	6	0	0
Thrombocytopenia	32	<1	<1	5	0	<1
Lymphocytopenia	31	4	<1	24	1	0
Chemistry						
Gastrointestinal						
ALT increased	53	10	2	22	1	0
AST increased	53	7	<1	19	<1	0
Glucose increased	41	<1	0	33	1	0
Total bilirubin increased	36	3	<1	10	1	<1
Phosphorus decreased	34	4	0	11	0	0
Calcium decreased	33	1	1	26	1	<1
Sodium decreased	31	4	1	24	4	1
Potassium increased	27	4	<1	23	5	0
Creatinine increased	26	0	<1	25	<1	0
Magnesium decreased	26	<1	1	14	0	0
Glucose decreased	17	0	<1	3	0	0

[a] National Cancer Institute Common Terminology Criteria for Adverse Events, version 3. Grades 1-4.

Hypertension: In the controlled phase III clinical study with VOTRIENT for the treatment of mRCC, 115/290 patients (40%) receiving VOTRIENT compared with 15/145 patients (10%) on placebo experienced hypertension. Grade 3 hypertension was reported in 13/290 patients (4%) receiving VOTRIENT compared with 1/145 patients (0.7%) on placebo. The majority of cases of hypertension were manageable with anti-hypertensive agents or dose reductions with 2/290 patients (0.7%) permanently discontinuing treatment with VOTRIENT. In the overall safety population for mRCC (N=586), one patient had hypertensive crisis on VOTRIENT (see Warnings and Precautions, Cardiovascular).

QT Prolongation and Torsade de Pointes: In the controlled phase III clinical study with VOTRIENT, QT prolongation (≥500 msec) was identified on routine electrocardiogram monitoring in 3/290 (1.0%) patients treated with VOTRIENT compared with no patients on placebo. Torsade de Pointes occurred in 2/586 (0.3%) patients who received VOTRIENT in the mRCC clinical studies (see Warnings and Precautions, Cardiovascular).

Arterial Thrombotic Events: In the controlled phase III clinical study with VOTRIENT, the incidences of arterial thrombotic events such as myocardial infarction/ischemia 5/290 (1.7%), cerebral vascular accident 1/290 (0.3%), and transient ischemic attack 4/290 (1.4%) were higher in patients treated with VOTRIENT compared to the placebo arm (0/145 for each event) (see Warnings and Precautions, Cardiovascular).

Hemorrhagic Events: In the controlled clinical study with VOTRIENT, 37/290 patients (13%) treated with VOTRIENT and 7/145 patients (5%) on placebo experienced at least 1 hemorrhagic event. The most common hemorrhagic events in the patients treated with VOTRIENT were hematuria (4%), epistaxis (2%), hemoptysis (2%), and rectal hemorrhage (1%). Nine (9/37) patients treated with VOTRIENT who had hemorrhagic events experienced serious events including pulmonary, gastrointestinal, and genitourinary hemorrhage (see Warnings and Precautions, Hemorrhagic). In the overall safety populations in mRCC (N=586), cerebral hemorrhage was observed in <1% of patients treated with VOTRIENT.

Hypothyroidism: In the controlled phase III clinical study with VOTRIENT, more patients had a shift from thyroid stimulating hormone (TSH) within the normal range at baseline to above the normal range at any post-baseline visit in VOTRIENT compared with the placebo arm (31% compared with 5%, respectively). Hypothyroidism was reported as an adverse reaction in 19 patients (7%) treated with VOTRIENT and no patients (0%) in the placebo arm (see Warnings and Precautions, Endocrine and Metabolism).

Diarrhea: Diarrhea occurred frequently and was predominantly mild to moderate in severity. Patients should be advised how to manage mild diarrhea and instructed to notify their healthcare provider if moderate to severe diarrhea occurs so appropriate management can be implemented to minimize this impact.

Proteinuria: In the controlled phase III clinical study with VOTRIENT, proteinuria has been reported as an adverse reaction in 27 patients (9%) treated with VOTRIENT. In 2 patients, proteinuria led to discontinuation of treatment with VOTRIENT.

Amylase/Lipase Elevations: In a single-arm phase II clinical study, increases in amylase values were observed for 42/184 patients (23%) and increases in lipase values were observed for 48/181 patients (27%). Increased blood amylase as an adverse reaction was reported for 6/225 patients (3%), all were Grade 1 or Grade 2 in severity. Elevations in lipase as an adverse reaction were reported for 10 patients (4%) and were Grade 3 for 6 patients and Grade 4 for 1 patient. In clinical mRCC studies of VOTRIENT, clinical pancreatitis was observed in 4/586 patients (0.7%).

Cardiac Dysfunction: VOTRIENT has been associated with cardiac dysfunction (such as a decrease in ejection fraction and congestive heart failure) in patients with various cancer types, including mRCC. In the overall safety population for mRCC (N=586), cardiac dysfunction was observed in 4/586 patients (0.7%).

DRUG INTERACTIONS: Overview: Pazopanib is a substrate of CYP3A4 and the multidrug efflux pump P-glycoprotein (PgP). Therefore, absorption and subsequent elimination of pazopanib may be influenced by products that affect CYP3A4 and/or PgP.

Pazopanib is a potent in vitro inhibitor of proteins UDP glucuronsyltransferase 1 family, polypeptide A1 (UGT1A1) and the organic anion transporter polypeptide 1B1 (OATP1B1). Concomitant administration of pazopanib with UGT1A1 substrates (e.g. irinotecan) should be undertaken with caution. It cannot be excluded that pazopanib will affect the pharmacokinetics of substrates of OATP1B1 (eg. rosuvastatin).

Pazopanib is a weak inhibitor of CYP3A4, CYP2D6 and CYP2C8 based on results from clinical pharmacology studies.

Drug-Drug Interactions: Drugs that Inhibit or Induce Cytochrome P450 3A4 Enzymes: In vitro studies suggested that the oxidative metabolism of pazopanib in human liver microsomes is mediated primarily by CYP3A4, with minor contributions from CYP1A2 and CYP2C8. Therefore, inhibitors and inducers of CYP3A4 may alter the metabolism of pazopanib.

CYP3A4 Inhibitors: Coadministration of strong CYP3A4 inhibitors (e.g. ketoconazole, itraconazole, clarithromycin, atazanavir, indinavir, nefazodone, nelfinavir, ritonavir, saquinavir, telithromycin, voriconazole) with VOTRIENT (pazopanib hydrochloride) is not recommended because they may increase pazopanib concentrations. An alternate concomitant medication with no or minimal potential to inhibit CYP3A4 should be chosen (see Dosage and Administration).

Administration of 1500 mg lapatinib a substrate and weak inhibitor of CYP3A4, PgP and BCRP with 800 mg pazopanib resulted in an approximately 50% to 60% increase in mean pazopanib $AUC_{(0-24)}$ and C_{max} compared to administration of 800 mg pazopanib alone. Coadministration of VOTRIENT with a CYP3A4, PgP and BCRP inhibitor, such as lapatinib, will result in an increase in plasma pazopanib concentrations.

CYP3A4 Inducers: CYP3A4 inducers such as rifampin may decrease plasma pazopanib concentrations and are not recommended due to the potential for reduced effectiveness of the drug. Selection of an alternate concomitant medication with no or minimal enzyme induction potential is recommended.

Effects of Pazopanib on CYP Substrates: In vitro studies with human liver microsomes showed that pazopanib inhibited CYP enzymes 1A2, 3A4, 2B6, 2C8, 2C9, 2C19, and 2E1. Potential induction of human CYP3A4 was demonstrated in an in vitro human PXR assay. Clinical pharmacology studies, using VOTRIENT 800 mg once daily, have demonstrated that VOTRIENT does not have a clinically relevant effect on the pharmacokinetics of caffeine (CYP1A2 probe substrate), warfarin (CYP2C9 probe substrate), or omeprazole (CYP2C19 probe substrate) in cancer patients. VOTRIENT resulted in an increase of approximately 30% in the mean AUC and C_{max} of midazolam (CYP3A4 probe substrate) and increases of 33% to 64% in the ratio of dextromethorphan to dextrorphan concentrations in the urine after oral administration of dextromethorphan (CYP2D6 probe substrate). Coadministration of VOTRIENT 800 mg once daily and paclitaxel 80 mg/m² (CYP3A4 and CYP2C8 substrate) once weekly resulted in a mean increase of 26% and 31% in paclitaxel AUC and C_{max}, respectively. Coadministration of VOTRIENT with agents with a narrow therapeutic window that are substrates for CYP3A4, CYP2C8 and CYP2D6 should be avoided.

Effects of Pazopanib on Transporters: In vitro studies also showed that pazopanib is a potent inhibitor of UGT1A1 and OATP1B1 with IC_{50} of 1.2 and 0.79 μM, respectively. Pazopanib may increase concentrations of drugs primarily eliminated through UGT1A1 (e.g. irinotecan) and OATP1B1 (e.g. rosuvastatin).

Drug-Food Interactions: Grapefruit, grapefruit juice and other foods that are known to affect CYP3A4 and PgP activity should be avoided during treatment.

Administration of VOTRIENT with a high-fat or low-fat meal results in an approximately 2-fold increase in AUC and C_{max}. Therefore, pazopanib should be administered at least 1 hour before or 2 hours after a meal.

Drug-Herb Interactions: Interactions with herbal products have not been established. St. John's wort (Hypericum perforatum) is an inducer of CYP3A4 that may increase the metabolism of pazopanib and decrease pazopanib blood levels.

Drug-Laboratory Test Interactions: Interactions between VOTRIENT and laboratory tests have not been studied.

DOSAGE AND ADMINISTRATION:

The recommended dose of VOTRIENT is 800 mg orally once daily.

VOTRIENT should be taken without food (at least one hour before or two hours after a meal) (see Action and Clinical Pharmacology, Pharmacokinetics).

Dosing Considerations: Initial dose reduction should be from 800 mg to 400 mg daily. Subsequent dose modification, either an increase or decrease in dose, should be in 200 mg increments in a stepwise fashion based on individual tolerability in order to manage adverse reactions. The dose of VOTRIENT should not exceed 800 mg.

Hepatic Impairment: VOTRIENT is not recommended in patients with baseline plasma bilirubin concentrations >1.5×ULN (with direct bilirubin >35%) and ALT elevations >2×ULN, or who have moderate or severe hepatic impairment (Child-Pugh B and C). No formal studies have been carried out in patients with mild hepatic impairment and caution is recommended in these patients (see Action and Clinical Pharmacology, Pharmacokinetics, Special Populations and Conditions).

Renal Impairment: No dose adjustments are recommended for patients with mild or moderate renal impairment. VOTRIENT is not recommended for patients with severe renal impairment (see Action and Clinical Pharmacology, Pharmacokinetics, Special Populations and Conditions).

CYP3A4 inhibitors: The concomitant use of strong CYP3A4 inhibitors may increase pazopanib concentrations and is not recommended (e.g., ketoconazole, itraconazole, clarithromycin, atazanavir, indinavir, nefazodone, nelfinavir, ritonavir, saquinavir, telithromycin, voriconazole) (see Drug Interactions).

No alteration of dosage, dosing frequency or route of administration is required in patients over 65 years.

Missed Dose: If a dose is missed, VOTRIENT should not be taken if it is less than 12 hours until the next dose.

Administration: For oral use.

VOTRIENT should be taken whole with a glass of water and must not be broken or crushed (see Action and Clinical Pharmacology, Pharmacokinetics).

OVERDOSAGE:

Pazopanib doses up to 2000 mg have been evaluated in clinical trials. Grade 3 fatigue (dose limiting toxicity) and Grade 3 hypertension were each observed in 1 of 3 patients dosed at 2000 mg and 1000 mg daily, respectively.

Treatment of overdoses with VOTRIENT should consist of general supportive measures. There is no specific antidote for overdosage of VOTRIENT.

Hemodialysis is not expected to enhance the elimination of VOTRIENT because pazopanib is not significantly renally excreted and is highly bound to plasma proteins.

> For management of a suspected drug overdose, contact your regional Poison Control Centre. See the *CPS* Directory section for a list of Poison Control Centres.

ACTION AND CLINICAL PHARMACOLOGY: Mechanism of Action: Pazopanib is an orally administered, small molecule, multi-target tyrosine kinase inhibitor (TKI). It is a potent inhibitor of vascular endothelial growth factor (VEGF) receptors (VEGFR)-1, -2, and -3, platelet-derived growth factor (PDGFR)-α and -β, and stem cell factor receptor (c-KIT), with IC_{50} values of 10, 30, 47, 71, 84 and 74 nM, respectively. In preclinical experiments, pazopanib dose-dependently inhibited ligand-induced auto-phosphorylation of VEGFR-2, c-Kit and PDGFR-β receptors in cells. In vivo, pazopanib inhibited VEGF-induced VEGFR-2 phosphorylation in mouse lungs, angiogenesis in various animal models, and the growth of multiple human tumour xenografts in mice.

Pharmacokinetics:

Table 3: VOTRIENT

Pazopanib Pharmacokinetic Parameters After Administration of 800 mg Pazopanib Once Daily for 17 Days (N=18)

	$AUC_{(0-24)}$ (μg·h/mL)	C_{max} (μg/mL)	t_{max}[a] (h)
Geometric mean	1037	58.1	3.13
CVb%	34.3	33.3	1.0–8.0

[a] t_{max} reported as median and range.

Results from a population pharmacokinetic analysis suggest that the coefficients of variation for inter-subject variability in pazopanib oral clearance and volume of distribution were 52.3% and 67.1%, respectively.

Absorption: Pazopanib is absorbed orally with median time to achieve peak concentrations of 2.0 to 4.0 hours after the dose. Daily dosing results in 1.23- to 4-fold increase in AUC. Bioavailability differences accounts for non-linear kinetics between 200 to 800 mg (400 mg is approximately 1.4× more bioavailable than 800 mg). No consistent increases in AUC and C_{max} were observed when the oral dose was increased above 800 mg (plateau was reached). The oral bioavailability of pazopanib reflects absorption that is limited by solubility and reaches saturation at doses above 800 mg once daily.

Systemic exposure to pazopanib is increased when administered with food. Administration of pazopanib with a high-fat or low-fat meal results in an approximately 2-fold increase in AUC and C_{max}. Therefore, pazopanib should be administered at least 1 hour before or 2 hours after a meal (see Dosage and Administration).

Administration of a single pazopanib 400 mg crushed tablet increased $AUC_{(0-72)}$ by 46% and C_{max} by approximately 2 fold and decreased t_{max} by approximately 1.5 hours compared to administration of the whole tablet. These results indicate that the bioavailability and the rate of pazopanib oral absorption are increased after administration of the crushed tablet relative to administration of the whole tablet. Therefore, due to this potential for increased exposure, tablets should not be crushed (see Dosage and Administration).

Distribution: Binding of pazopanib to human plasma protein in vivo was greater than 99% with no concentration dependence over the range of 10-100 μg/mL. In vitro studies suggest that pazopanib is a substrate for P-glycoprotein (PgP) and breast cancer resistant protein (BCRP).
Metabolism: Results from in vitro studies demonstrated that the metabolism of pazopanib is mediated primarily by CYP3A4, with minor contributions from CYP1A2 and CYP2C8.
Excretion: Pazopanib is eliminated slowly with mean half-life of 30.9 hours after administration of the recommended dose of 800 mg. Most of the oral dose (60-70%) is not metabolized and excreted unmodified in the feces. Approximately 7-15% of the administered dose is recovered as metabolites in the feces, with renal elimination accounting for <4% of the administered dose.
Special Populations and Conditions: Hepatic Insufficiency: The safety and pharmacokinetics of pazopanib in patients with pre-existing hepatic impairment have not been fully established (see Warnings and Precautions). Pharmacokinetic data from patients with normal hepatic function (n=12) and moderate (n=7) hepatic impairment indicate that pazopanib clearance was decreased by approximately 50 % in those with moderate hepatic impairment [total bilirubin >1.5 to 3× Upper Limit of Normal (ULN)]. However, patients with moderate hepatic impairment experienced dose-limiting toxicity at the 400 mg dose. There are no data in patients with severe hepatic impairment (total bilirubin >3×ULN). There are no data to support dosing recommendation in patients with mild hepatic impairment (see Warnings and Precautions).
Renal Insufficiency: Patients with renal cell cancer and mild/moderate renal impairment (creatinine clearance ≥30 mL/min) were included in clinical studies for VOTRIENT.

Renal impairment is not expected to have a clinically relevant effect on pazopanib pharmacokinetics given the low renal excretion of pazopanib and metabolites (see Pharmacokinetics, Excretion). In a population pharmacokinetic analysis using 408 subjects with various cancers, creatinine clearance (30-150 mL/min) did not influence clearance of pazopanib. Therefore, renal impairment is not expected to influence pazopanib exposure, and dose adjustment is not necessary. There is no experience of pazopanib in patients with severe renal impairment or in patients undergoing peritoneal dialysis or haemodialysis; therefore, use of pazopanib is not recommended in these patients.
STORAGE AND STABILITY: Store between 15-30°C.
INFORMATION FOR THE PATIENT: Published in e-CPS, available by subscription at www.e-cps.ca.
DOSAGE FORMS, COMPOSITION AND PACKAGING: Each modified capsule shaped, grey, film coated tablet with GS JT debossed on one side contains: pazopanib as pazopanib hydrochloride 200 mg. Nonmedicinal ingredients: tablet core: magnesium stearate, microcrystalline cellulose, povidone (K30) and sodium starch glycolate; coating: hypromellose, iron oxide black (E172), macrogol, polysorbate 80 and titanium dioxide (E171). Bottles of 30, 90 and 120.

(Shown in Product Identification Section)

Vumon® Parenteral Pr

teniposide

Antineoplastic

Bristol-Myers Squibb

Date of Preparation: March 9, 1984
Date of Revision: October 26, 2004

Caution: VUMON (teniposide) is a potent drug and should be used only by physicians experienced with cancer chemotherapeutic drugs (see Warnings and Precautions). Blood counts as well as renal and hepatic function tests must be done regularly. Discontinue the drug if abnormal depression of bone marrow or abnormal renal or hepatic function is seen.

PHARMACOLOGY: VUMON (teniposide) is a semi-synthetic derivative of podophyllotoxin used in the treatment of neoplastic diseases.

VUMON is a phase-specific cytotoxic drug, acting in the late S_2 or G_2 phase of the cell cycle preventing cells from entering mitosis. VUMON also produces single and double-strand breaks in DNA. The mechanism of action appears to be due to inhibition of type II topoisomerases.

Teniposide produces a dose dependent inhibition of thymidine uptake after 2.5 hours. This, however, is not accompanied by a comparable reduction in DNA synthesis.
Pharmacokinetics: The pharmacokinetics of teniposide appear to be linear over a range of doses. Drug accumulation does not occur after daily administration for 3 days. No major differences in the disposition of the drug in adults and children have been identified.

Following i.v. infusion, initial clearance from the central compartment is rapid with a distribution half-life of approximately 1 hour. Teniposide is highly protein bound, >99%. Levels of teniposide in CSF are low relative to simultaneously measured plasma levels. Mean terminal half-life has ranged from approximately 6 to 20 hours with renal clearance accounting for only about 10% of total clearance. While metabolic pathways for teniposide have not been characterized, agents such as phenobarbital and phenytoin that induce hepatic metabolism, have been shown to increase the clearance of teniposide (see Precautions, Drug Interactions).
INDICATIONS: VUMON (teniposide) is indicated as follows:
Neuroblastoma: Second-line single agent or combination therapy in patients who have not responded or who have relapsed on other chemotherapeutic regimens.
Non-Hodgkin's Lymphoma: Second-line combination or as a single agent in patients who are or have become refractory to other chemotherapeutic regimens.
Acute Lymphocytic Leukemia: Second-line combination therapy with cytosine arabinoside in patients who have not responded or relapsed on other chemotherapeutic regimens.
CONTRAINDICATIONS: VUMON (teniposide) should not be given to individuals who have demonstrated a previous hypersensitivity to teniposide or to any component of the formulation. Also, it is contraindicated in patients having severe leukopenia, thrombocytopenia and severe hepatic and/or renal impairment.
WARNINGS: Life-threatening anaphylactic reactions have occurred following initial teniposide administration or after repeated exposure.

VUMON (teniposide) should be given cautiously to individuals with pre-existing hepatic and/or renal impairment.

Bacterial infection must be brought under control before the administration of teniposide therapy because of the risk of septicemia. Near fatal anaphylactic reactions have occurred following teniposide administration.
Pregnancy: VUMON may cause fetal harm when administered to a pregnant woman. Embryotoxic and teratogenic effects have been seen in pregnant rats given teniposide. No studies in pregnant women have been conducted. If this drug is used during pregnancy or if the patient becomes pregnant while taking this drug, the patient should be apprised of the potential hazard to the fetus. Women of childbearing potential should be advised to avoid becoming pregnant.
PRECAUTIONS: VUMON (teniposide) should be administered only by individuals experienced with cancer chemotherapeutic drugs. Severe myelosuppression with resultant infection or bleeding may occur. Blood counts as well as renal and hepatic function tests must be done regularly.

VUMON (teniposide) should be administered with care to patients with marrow involvement by tumor and to patients with impaired renal or hepatic function.

Regular monitoring of white blood cell and platelet counts should be performed during treatment with VUMON. If the white blood cell count is below 2000 cells/mm^3 or the platelet count is below 75 000 cells/mm^3, unless caused by malignant disease, treatment should be postponed until bone marrow recovery is complete.

Care should be taken to ensure that VUMON infusions are given i.v. with indwelling catheter in proper position prior to infusion as extravasation, necrosis and/or thrombophlebitis may result with improper administration.

Instances of hypotension have been reported during VUMON infusion. Therefore, vital signs should be monitored carefully during the first 30 to 60 minutes after the start of the infusion.
Drug Interactions: Anticonvulsants such as phenobarbital and phenytoin increase the clearance rate of teniposide resulting in lower systemic exposure for a given teniposide dose. An increase in dose may be required in patients receiving anticonvulsant therapy.

Tolbutamide, sodium salicylate and sulfamethiazole have been shown in vitro to displace teniposide from plasma proteins. Because of extremely high binding of teniposide to proteins, small decreases in binding could result in substantial increases in free drug with associated increased drug effect and toxicity.
Carcinogenesis, Mutagenesis, Impairment of Fertility: The occurrence of acute nonlymphocytic leukemia has been reported in patients treated with VUMON in association with other antineoplastic agents. Teniposide should be considered a potential carcinogen in humans.

Teniposide has been shown to be mutagenic in various bacterial and mammalian genetic toxicity tests. Teniposide has caused gene mutations in murine cell lines and DNA damage in human cell lines. Chromosome aberrations have been demonstrated in several human and murine tissue cultures.

Teniposide has caused reduced spermatogenesis in monkeys and dogs, and reduced testicular and ovarian weights in dogs.
Lactation: It is not known whether this drug is excreted in human milk. Because many drugs are excreted in human milk and because of the potential for serious adverse reactions in nursing infants from VUMON, a decision should be made whether to discontinue nursing or to discontinue the drug, taking into account the importance of the drug to the mother.
Children: VUMON contains benzyl alcohol. Benzyl alcohol has been associated with toxicity in newborns. A syndrome characterized by gasping respirations, kernicterus, metabolic acidosis, neurologic deterioration, hematologic abnormalities and death have been reported to occur following administration of benzyl alcohol containing flush solutions to low birth weight, preterm infants.

Acute CNS depression, hypotension and metabolic acidosis have been observed in patients who were receiving higher than recommended doses of VUMON, and who were also pretreated with antiemetic drugs.
ADVERSE EFFECTS: Hematologic: Myelosuppression is often dose-limiting, with leukopenia and thrombocytopenia occurring 7 to 14 days after VUMON treatment. Bone marrow recovery is usually complete within 2 to 3 weeks. Leukopenia is more frequent and more severe than thrombocytopenia. Anemia also occurs and immune hemolytic anemia has been reported.

The occurrence of acute nonlymphocytic leukemia has been reported in patients treated with VUMON in association with other antineoplastic agents.
Gastrointestinal: Nausea and vomiting are the major gastrointestinal toxicities. The nausea and vomiting can usually be controlled by antiemetic therapy. Stomatitis/mucositis, anorexia, diarrhea, abdominal pain and hepatic dysfunction may occur.
Alopecia: A high incidence of alopecia has been reported, especially in patients receiving multiple courses of therapy.
Hypotension: Transient hypotension may occur following rapid i.v. administration of VUMON (see Dosage). Sudden death due to probable arrhythmia and hypotension has been reported.
Hypersensitivity: Anaphylactic-like reactions characterized by chills, fever, tachycardia, bronchospasm, dyspnea and hypotension have been reported to occur during or immediately after VUMON administration. They may be due to the Cremophor EL component of the vehicle or to teniposide itself. These reactions may occur on the first dose and may occur more commonly in patients with brain tumors or in patients with neuroblastoma. The risk of having a reaction may be related to repeated exposure and cumulative dose. These reactions have usually responded promptly to cessation of the infusion and administration of pressor agents, corticosteroids, antihistamines or volume expanders as appropriate. Flushing, sweating, hypertension and edema have also been reported.
Dermatologic: Urticaria, with or without pruritus, has been reported.
Neurotoxicity: Neurotoxicity has been reported, including severe cases of neuropathy in patients due to an interaction of vincristine sulfate and VUMON. CNS depression has been observed in patients receiving higher than recommended doses (see Overdose, Symptoms and Treatment).
Other: The following reactions also have been reported: infection, renal dysfunction, hypertension, headache, confusion and asthenia.

OVERDOSE:

Symptoms: Acute CNS depression, hypotension and metabolic acidosis have been observed in patients who were receiving higher than recommended doses of VUMON, and who were also pretreated with antiemetic drugs.
Treatment: No proven antidotes have been established for VUMON overdosage. The anticipated complications of overdosage are secondary to bone marrow suppression.

> For management of a suspected drug overdose, CPhA recommends that you contact your **regional Poison Control Centre**. See the *CPS* Directory section for a list of Poison Control Centres.

DOSAGE: VUMON is administered **after dilution** with a suitable parenteral vehicle, by i.v. infusion.

The following Table 1 is given to provide a guideline for dosage schedules in neuroblastoma, non-Hodgkin's lymphoma, and acute lymphocytic leukemia.

To avoid the possibility of hypotensive reactions, VUMON should not be administered by bolus injection or rapid infusion.

The current literature should be consulted for specific doses and regimens for particular indications.
Monotherapy: Total dose per course is 300 mg/m^2, given over a 3- to 5-day period. Cycles may be repeated every 3 weeks or upon recovery of bone marrow.

Dosage should be adjusted according to individual patient variability and toxicity, when employed as a single agent or in combination with other antineoplastic agents.
Combination Therapy: VUMON has been used in combination with several other approved chemotherapeutic agents as shown in Table 2, Table 3, Table 4 and Table 5. When it is used in combination with other myelosuppressive drugs, the dose should be appropriately reduced.
Note: Patients with Down's Syndrome may be especially sensitive to myelosuppressive chemotherapy, therefore, dose modification may need to be considered in these patients.

Table 1: VUMON Parenteral

Guidelines for Dosage Schedules

Indication	VUMON Dose and Schedule
Neuroblastoma	
Single Agent	130 to 180 mg/m^2/day once weekly given in normal saline or 5% dextrose in water i.v. at a concentration of 0.2 mg/mL over a minimum of 30 minutes.
Combination	100 mg/m^2/day every 21 days given in normal saline or 5% dextrose in water i.v. at a concentration of 0.2 mg/mL over a minimum of 30 minutes.
Non-Hodgkin's Lymphoma	
Single Agent	The following regimens have been used: 30 mg/m^2/day for 10 days given in normal saline or 5% dextrose in water i.v. at a concentration of 0.2 mg/mL over a minimum of 30 minutes. 30 mg/m^2/day every 5 days given in normal saline or 5% dextrose in water i.v. at a concentration of 0.2 mg/mL over a minimum of 30 minutes. 50 to 100 mg/m^2/day once weekly given in normal saline or 5% dextrose in water i.v. at a concentration of 0.2 mg/mL over a minimum of 30 minutes.
Combination	60 to 70 mg/m^2/day once weekly given in normal saline or 5% dextrose in water i.v. at a concentration of 0.2 mg/mL over a minimum of 30 minutes.
Acute Lymphocytic Leukemia	
Combination	165 mg/m^2/day twice weekly given in normal saline or 5% dextrose in water i.v. at a concentration of 0.2 mg/mL over a minimum of 30 minutes.

Table 2: VUMON Parenteral
Neuroblastoma (Journal Articles)

Investigator	Combination	Dose mg/m²	Days on Treatment	Frequency
Hayes (1981)	Teniposide	100 i.v.	On day 1	Every 21 days
	Cisplatin	90 i.v.	On day 1	Every 21 days

Table 3: VUMON Parenteral
Non-Hodgkin's Lymphoma (Journal Articles)

Investigator	Single Therapy	Dose mg/m²	Days of Treatment	Frequency
Single Therapy				
Broc (1972)	Teniposide	30 i.v.	On days 1–5	Repeat every 10–15 days
Mathe (1974)	Teniposide	30 i.v.	On days 1–10	Repeat every 5 days
		30 i.v.	On day 1	
		50–100 i.v.	Once weekly	
Combination				
Missett (1977)	Adriamycin	40 i.v.	On day 1	Repeat every 15 to 21 days
	Teniposide	60 i.v.	On day 2	
	Cyclophosphamide	300 i.m.	On day 3 and 4	
	Prednisone	40 p.o.	On days 3 to 7	
Lawkowicz (1975)	Teniposide	50 i.v.		Twice weekly
Durand (1978)	Prednisone	40	On days 1-15	Only one cycle was given
	Vincristine	0.7	On days 1, 8 and 15	
	Cyclophosphamide	400	On days 3, 10 and 17	
	Teniposide	70	On days 5, 12 and 19	

Table 4: VUMON Parenteral
Treatment Schedule for Patients on Combination Therapy-Literature Reports

Investigator	Combination	Dose mg/m²	Days on Treatment	Frequency
Data on file[a] (Patient 643296)	Teniposide	200 mg i.v.	0nce weekly	For 5 weeks
	Methotrexate	480 mg i.v.	On day 36	1 week rest period
	L-asparaginase	10 000 IU i.v.	On day 37 and 51	
	Methotrexate	400 mg i.v.	On day 50	2 weeks rest period
	Cytosine arabinoside	100 mg i.v.	On day 71	3 weeks rest period
		150 mg i.v.	On day 71	
	Teniposide	200 mg i.v.	On days 1 and 14	Repeat, alternating with MTX/L-asp cycle
	Cytosine arabinoside	200 mg i.v.	On days 1 and 14	
	Methotrexate	450 mg i.v.	On days 28 and 42	
	L-asparaginase	10 000 IU i.v.	On days 29 and 43	
Data on file (Patient 372366)	Teniposide	247 i.v.	On days 1 and 2	One cycle was given
	Prednisone	31	On days 2-6 and 23-29	
	Methotrexate	432 i.v.	On days 15 and 36	
	Methotrexate	12 i.t.	On day 36	
	Vincristine	1.5	On day 1	
	Vincristine	1.8	On days 22, 29, 62 and 69	
	Adriamycin	60	On days 23 and 63	
	6-mercaptopurine	185	On days 38, 40 and 42	
	6-mercaptopurine	216	On days 29, 41	

[a] Patient's response occurred after day 71.

Table 5: VUMON Parenteral
Acute Lymphocytic Leukemia-Literature Report

Investigator	Combination	Dose mg/m²	Days on Treatment	Frequency
Data on file	Teniposide	165 i.v.	Twice weekly	
	Cytosine arabinoside	300 i.v.	Twice weekly	
Data on file	Teniposide	175 i.v.	Twice weekly	
	Cytosine arabinoside	300 i.v.	Twice weekly	
Data on file	Teniposide	300 i.v.	Twice weekly	
	Cytosine arabinoside	500 i.v.	Twice weekly	
Data on file	Teniposide	125 i.v.	Twice weekly	
	Vincristine	1.5	Once weekly	For 2 weeks
	Prednisone	50 mg	Daily	For 14 days
	Cytosine arabinoside	165 i.v.	Once weekly during week 4	
Data on file	Teniposide	150 i.v.	On days 1, 5, 8 & 14	
	Cytosine arabinoside	290 i.v.	On days 1, 5, 8 & 14	
Rivera (1980)	Teniposide	165 i.v.	Twice weekly	For 4 weeks
	Cytosine arabinoside	300 i.v.	Twice weekly	

Preparation of I.V. Solutions: Note: Hard plastic devices made of ABS (a polymer composed of acronitrile, butadine and styrene) have been reported to decompose when exposed to N,N-dimethylacetamide, one of the solvents present in the VUMON formulation. This effect has not been reported for VUMON itself, or for diluted solutions of VUMON.

In order to prevent extraction of the plasticizer DEHP (di(2-ethylhexyl)phthalate) from polyvinyl chloride (PVC) containers, solutions of VUMON should be prepared in non-DEHP containing large volume parenteral containers such as glass or polyolefin containers. VUMON solutions should be administered with non-DEHP-containing administration sets.

Immediately before administration, each 5 mL ampul of VUMON containing 50 mg of teniposide must be diluted with 50, 125, 250 or 500 mL of either 5% Dextrose Injection or 0.9% Sodium Chloride Injection. Such dilution provides final teniposide concentrations of 1, 0.4, 0.2 and 0.1 mg/mL, respectively. The diluted solution should then be administered by i.v. infusion over a minimum of 30 minutes. To reduce the possibility of hypotensive reactions, **VUMON should not be administered by bolus injection or rapid infusion**. Greatest care should be taken to insure that the catheter tip remains in the vein during administration, to avoid extravasation and possible tissue irritation.

When diluted as recommended above, solutions that contain teniposide 0.1 mg, 0.2 mg, or 0.4 mg/mL are stable under normal fluorescent lighting for 24 hours in the recommended large volume glass or polyolefin parenteral containers. Refrigeration is not recommended. VUMON solutions prepared at a final teniposide concentration of 1 mg/mL and stored at room temperature under normal fluorescent lighting are less stable, and should be administered within 4 hours of preparation to reduce the potential for precipitation.

Note: This product may precipitate when diluted in any manner, with any diluent or to any concentration other than those described above. If evidence of precipitation does appear, the solution should not be administered. Likewise, precipitation has occurred when prolonged infusions of teniposide (24 hour) were administered through a variety of infusion devices. These infusions, and their delivery systems, should be inspected frequently during administration. Heparin solution can cause precipitation of teniposide, therefore, administration sets/tubing, etc., should be flushed thoroughly with 5% Dextrose Injection or 0.9% Sodium Chloride Injection, before and after administration of VUMON. Diluted VUMON solutions should be subjected to as little agitation as is necessary to prepare the solution, since excessive agitation can result in precipitation. No other drugs should be mixed with VUMON infusion.

Handling and Disposal: Caution should be exercised in handling and preparing solutions of VUMON. If VUMON contacts the skin, immediately wash thoroughly with soap and water. If VUMON contacts mucous membranes, flush thoroughly with water.

Procedures for proper handling and disposal of anticancer drugs should be considered. Several guidelines on this subject have been published. There is no general agreement that all of the procedures recommended in these guidelines are necessary or appropriate.

1. Preparation of VUMON should be done in a vertical laminar flow hood (Biological Safety Cabinet—Class II).
2. Personnel preparing VUMON should wear PVC gloves, safety glasses, disposable gowns, and masks.
3. All needles, syringes, vials and other materials which have come in contact with VUMON should be segregated and incinerated at 1000°C or more. Sealed containers may explode. Intact vials should be returned to the manufacturer for destruction. Proper precautions should be taken in packaging these materials for transport.
4. Personnel regularly involved in the preparation and handling of VUMON should have bi-annual blood examinations.

Stability: When stored at room temperature (25°C), VUMON packaged in flint glass ampuls will remain stable until expiration date indicated on package.

SUPPLIED: Each 5 mL clear, glass ampul contains: teniposide 50 mg (10 mg/mL) dissolved in 5 mL of a nonaqueous solution. Nonmedicinal ingredients: benzyl alcohol, dehydrated ethanol 42.7% (v/v), maleic acid to adjust pH to approximately 5, N.N.-dimethylacetamide and polyoxyethylated castor oil (Cremophor EL).

Vyvanse® Ⓒ

lisdexamfetamine dimesylate

Central Nervous System Stimulant for Attention Deficit Hyperactivity Disorder

Shire

Date of Revision: August 31, 2010

SUMMARY PRODUCT INFORMATION:

Route of Administration	Dosage Form/ Strength	Nonmedicinal Ingredients
Oral	Capsule 20 mg, 30 mg, 40 mg, 50 mg, 60 mg	Inactive ingredients consist of croscarmellose sodium, magnesium stearate, microcrystalline cellulose and capsule shells which contain gelatin, titanium dioxide, and one or more of the following: FD&C Yellow #6, FD&C Blue #1, and FD&C Red #3, FDA/E172 Black Iron Oxide, FDA/E172 Yellow Iron Oxide.

INDICATIONS AND CLINICAL USE: Pediatrics: VYVANSE (lisdexamfetamine dimesylate capsules) is indicated for the treatment of Attention Deficit Hyperactivity Disorder (ADHD) in children aged 6 to 12 years.

Adolescents, Adults and Geriatrics: VYVANSE is not currently indicated for use in adolescents (13 to 17 years of age) or in adults (over 18 years of age). VYVANSE has not been systematically studied in, and is therefore not indicated for use in, the geriatric population (>65 years of age).

A diagnosis of ADHD (DSM-IV-TR) implies the presence of hyperactive-impulsive or inattentive symptoms that cause impairment and were present before the age of 7 years. The symptoms must be persistent, must be more severe than is typically observed in individuals at a comparable level of development, must cause clinically significant impairment, e.g., in social, academic, or occupational functioning, and be present in two or more settings, e.g., school (or work), and at home. The symptoms must not be better accounted for by another mental disorder. For the Inattentive Type, at least six of the following symptoms must have persisted for at least 6 months: lack of attention to details/careless mistakes, lack of sustained attention, poor listener, failure to follow through on tasks, poor organization, avoids tasks requiring sustained mental effort, loses things, easily distracted, forgetful. For the Hyperactive-Impulsive Type, at least six of the following symptoms must have persisted for at least 6 months: fidgeting/squirming, leaving seat, inappropriate running/climbing, difficulty with quiet activities, "on the go", excessive talking, blurting answers, can't wait turn, intrusive. For a Combined Type diagnosis, both inattentive and hyperactive-impulsive criteria must be met.

Special Diagnostic Considerations: The specific etiology of ADHD is unknown, and there is no single diagnostic test. Adequate diagnosis requires the use not only of medical but also of special psychological, educational, and social resources. Learning may or may not be impaired. The diagnosis must be based upon a complete history and evaluation of the patient and not solely on the presence of the required number of DSM-IV characteristics.

Need for Comprehensive Treatment Program: VYVANSE is indicated as an integral part of a total treatment program for ADHD that may include other measures (psychological, educational/vocational, social) for patients with this syndrome. Drug treatment may not be indicated for all patients with this syndrome. Drug treatment is not intended for use in patient who exhibits symptoms secondary to environmental factors and/or other primary psychiatric disorders, including psychosis. Appropriate educational/vocational placement is essential patients with this diagnosis and psychosocial intervention is often helpful. When remedial measures alone are insufficient, the decision to prescribe drug treatment will depend upon the physician's assessment of the chronicity and severity of the child's symptoms and on the level of functional impairment.

Long-Term Use: The effectiveness of VYVANSE for long-term use, i.e., for more than 4 weeks, has not been systematically evaluated in controlled trials. Therefore, the physician who elects to use VYVANSE for extended periods should periodically re-evaluate the long-term usefulness of the drug for the individual patient (see Dosage and Administration).

Pediatrics (<6 years of age): Amphetamines are not recommended for use in children under 6 years of age.

CONTRAINDICATIONS:

- Advanced arteriosclerosis, symptomatic cardiovascular disease, moderate to severe hypertension, hyperthyroidism, known hypersensitivity or idiosyncrasy to the sympathomimetic amines, glaucoma, allergy to amphetamines or to components of VYVANSE (lisdexamfetamine dimesylate capsules) or its container.
- Agitated states.
- Patients with a history of drug abuse.
- Administration of VYVANSE during or within 14 days following the administration of monoamine oxidase inhibitors may result in hypertensive crises (see Drug Interactions).

WARNINGS AND PRECAUTIONS: General: The least amount of amphetamine feasible should be prescribed or dispensed at one time in order to minimize the possibility of overdosage. VYVANSE should be used with caution in patients who use other sympathomimetic drugs.

Cardiovascular: Misuse and Serious Cardiovascular Adverse Events: The misuse of amphetamines may cause serious cardiovascular adverse events and sudden death.

Pre-Existing Structural Cardiac Abnormalities or Other Serious Heart Problems and Sudden Death: Sudden death has been reported with sympathomimetic drugs used for ADHD treatment at therapeutic doses in children/adolescents with structural cardiac abnormalities or other serious heart problems. Although some serious heart problems alone carry an increased risk of sudden death, sympathomimetic drugs generally should not be used in children/adolescents with known serious structural cardiac abnormalities or other serious cardiac problems (e.g., cardiomyopathy, serious heart rhythm abnormalities), that may place them at increased vulnerability to the sympathomimetic effects of ADHD drugs (see also Contraindications).

Adults: Sudden deaths, stroke, and myocardial infarction have been reported in adults taking stimulant drugs at usual doses for ADHD. Although the role of stimulants in these adult cases is also unknown, adults have a greater likelihood than children of having serious structural cardiac abnormalities, cardiomyopathy, serious heart rhythm abnormalities, coronary artery disease, or other serious cardiac problems. Adults with such abnormalities should also generally not be treated with stimulant drugs (see Contraindications).

Hypertension and Other Cardiovascular Conditions: Sympathomimetic medications can cause a modest increase in average blood pressure and average heart rate and individuals may have larger increases. While the mean changes alone would not be expected to have short-term consequences, all patients should be monitored for larger changes in heart rate and blood pressure. Caution is indicated in treating patients whose underlying medical conditions might be compromised by increases in blood pressure or heart rate, e.g., those with pre-existing hypertension, heart failure, recent myocardial infarction, or ventricular arrhythmia (see also Contraindications). Blood pressure and pulse should be monitored at appropriate intervals in patients taking VYVANSE (lisdexamfetamine dimesylate capsules), especially patients with hypertension.

Assessing Cardiovascular Status in Patients Being Treated with Sympathomimetic Medications: Theoretically there exists a pharmacological potential for all ADHD drugs to increase the risk of sudden/cardiac death. Although confirmation of an incremental risk for adverse cardiac events arising from treatment with ADHD medications is lacking, prescribers should consider this potential risk.

All drugs with sympathomimetic effects prescribed in the management of ADHD should be used with caution in patients who: a) are involved in strenuous exercise or activities b) use other sympathomimetic drugs or c) have a family history of sudden/cardiac death. Patients who are being considered for treatment with sympathomimetic medications should have a careful history (including assessment for a family history of sudden death or ventricular arrhythmia) and physical exam to assess for the presence of cardiac disease, and should receive further cardiac evaluation if findings suggest such disease (e.g. electrocardiogram and echocardiogram). Patients who develop symptoms such as exertional chest pain, unexplained syncope, or other symptoms suggestive of cardiac disease during stimulant treatment should undergo a prompt cardiac evaluation.

Effects on Weight and Long-Term Suppression of Growth: Children in VYVANSE Clinical Trials: In a controlled trial of lisdexamfetamine in children ages 6 to 12 years, mean weight loss from baseline after 4 weeks of therapy was −0.9, −1.9, and −2.5 lb, respectively, for patients receiving 30 mg, 50 mg, and 70 mg of lisdexamfetamine, compared to a 1 lb weight gain for patients receiving placebo. Higher doses were associated with greater weight loss with 4 weeks of treatment. Careful follow-up for weight in children ages 6 to 12 years who received lisdexamfetamine over 12 months suggests that consistently medicated children (i.e., treatment for 7 days per week throughout the year) have a slowing in growth rate measured by body weight as demonstrated by an age- and sex-normalized mean change from baseline in percentile of −13.4 over 1 year (average percentile at baseline and 12 months, were 60.6 and 47.2, respectively). Therefore, growth should be monitored during treatment with stimulants, and patients who are not growing or gaining weight as expected may need to have their treatment interrupted.

Stimulant Use in Adolescents and Children: Published data for other stimulants report that in children aged 7-10 years there is a temporary slowing in growth rate without evidence of growth rebound during this period of development. In a controlled trial of amphetamine (d to l enantiomer ratio of 3:1) in adolescents, mean weight change from baseline within the initial 4 weeks of therapy was −1.1 lbs. and −2.8 lbs., respectively, for patients receiving 10 mg and 20 mg of amphetamine (d to l enantiomer ratio of 3:1). Higher doses were associated with greater weight loss within the initial 4 weeks of treatment. Published data are inadequate to determine whether the chronic use of amphetamines in children may be causally associated with suppression of growth.

Dependence Liability: VYVANSE is a Schedule III drug under the Controlled Drugs and Substances Act (CDSA).

Amphetamines have been extensively abused. Tolerance, extreme psychological dependence, and severe social disability have occurred. There are reports of patients who have increased the dosage to levels many times higher than recommended. Abrupt cessation following prolonged high dosage administration results in extreme fatigue and mental depression; changes are also noted on the sleep EEG. Careful supervision is therefore recommended during drug withdrawal. Manifestations of chronic intoxication with amphetamines may include severe dermatoses, marked insomnia, irritability, hyperactivity, and personality changes. The most severe manifestation of chronic intoxication is psychosis, often clinically indistinguishable from schizophrenia.

Human Studies: In a human abuse liability study, when equivalent oral doses of 100 mg VYVANSE and 40 mg immediate release d-amphetamine sulfate were administered to individuals with a history of drug abuse, VYVANSE 100 mg produced subjective responses on a scale of "Drug Liking Effects" (primary endpoint) that were significantly less than d-amphetamine immediate release 40 mg. However, oral administration of 150 mg VYVANSE produced increases in positive subjective responses on this scale that were statistically indistinguishable from the positive subjective responses produced by 40 mg of oral immediate-release d-amphetamine and 200 mg of diethylpropion.

Intravenous administration of 50 mg lisdexamfetamine to individuals with a history of drug abuse produced positive subjective responses on scales measuring "Drug Liking", "Euphoria", "Amphetamine Effects", and "Benzedrine Effects" that were not significantly different from placebo. Administration of a dose of 20 mg of intravenous d-amphetamine produced significant positive subjective responses on these scales.

Animal Studies: In animal studies, lisdexamfetamine produced behavioral effects qualitatively similar to those of the CNS stimulant d-amphetamine. In monkeys trained to self-administer cocaine, intravenous lisdexamfetamine maintained self-administration at a rate that was statistically less than that for cocaine, but greater than that of placebo.

Psychiatric: Pre-existing Psychosis: Clinical experience suggests that in psychotic patients, administration of stimulants may exacerbate symptoms of behavior disturbance and thought disorder.

Bipolar Illness: Particular care should be taken in using stimulants to treat ADHD in patients with comorbid bipolar disorder because of concern for possible induction of a mixed/manic episode in such patients. Prior to initiating treatment with a stimulant, patients with comorbid depressive symptoms should be adequately screened to determine if they are at risk for bipolar disorder; such screening should include a detailed psychiatric history, including a family history of suicide, bipolar disorder, and depression.

Emergence of New Psychotic or Manic Symptoms: Treatment emergent psychotic or manic symptoms, e.g., hallucinations, delusional thinking, or mania in children/adolescents without a prior history of psychotic illness or mania can be caused by stimulants at therapeutic doses. If such symptoms occur, consideration should be given to a possible causal role of the stimulant, and discontinuation of treatment may be appropriate (see also Contraindications). In a pooled analysis of multiple short-term, placebo-controlled studies, such symptoms occurred in about 0.1% (4 patients with events out of 3482 exposed to methylphenidate or amphetamine for several weeks at usual doses) of stimulant-treated patients compared to 0 in placebo-treated patients.

Aggression: Aggressive behavior or hostility is often observed in children/adolescents with ADHD, and has been reported in clinical trials and the post marketing experience of some medications indicated for the treatment of ADHD. Although there is no systematic evidence that stimulants cause aggressive behavior or hostility, patients beginning treatment of ADHD should be monitored for the appearance of or worsening of aggressive behavior or hostility.

Neurologic: Seizures: There is some clinical evidence that stimulants may lower the convulsive threshold in patients with prior history of seizures, in patients with prior EEG abnormalities in absence of seizures, and, very rarely, in patients without a history of seizures and no prior EEG evidence of seizures. In the presence of seizures, the drug should be discontinued.

Tics: Amphetamines have been reported to exacerbate motor and phonic tics in Tourette's syndrome. Therefore, careful clinical evaluation for tics in Tourette's syndrome in patients and their families should precede use of stimulant medications.

Ophthalmologic: Difficulties with accommodation and blurring of vision have been reported with stimulant treatment (see also Contraindications).

Special Populations: Pregnant Women: VYVANSE had no apparent effects on embryofetal development or survival when administered orally to pregnant rats and rabbits throughout the period of organogenesis at doses up to 40 and 120 mg/kg/day respectively. These doses are approximately 2.7 and 16 times respectively the maximum recommended dose of 70 mg/day on a mg/m² body surface area basis.

The effects of VYVANSE on labor and delivery in humans is unknown.

There are no adequate and well-controlled studies in pregnant women. There has been one report of severe congenital bony deformity, tracheoesophageal fistula, and anal atresia (VATER association) in a baby born to a woman who took d-amphetamine sulfate with lovastatin during the first trimester of pregnancy.

Non-Teratogenic Effects: Infants born to mothers dependent on amphetamines have an increased risk of premature delivery and low birth weight. Also, these infants may experience symptoms of withdrawal as demonstrated by dysphoria, including agitation, and significant lassitude.

Amphetamines should be used during pregnancy only if the potential benefit justifies the potential risk to the fetus.

Nursing Women: Amphetamines are excreted in human milk. Mothers taking amphetamines should be advised to refrain from nursing.

Pediatrics (<6 years of age): Amphetamines are not recommended for use in children under 6 years of age. Long-term effects of amphetamines in children have not been well established.

A study was conducted in which juvenile rats received oral doses of 4, 10, or 40 mg/kg/day of lisdexamfetamine from day 7 to day 63 of age. These doses are approximately 0.3, 0.7, and 3 times the maximum recommended human daily dose of 70 mg on a mg/m² basis. Dose-related decreases in food consumption, bodyweight gain, and crown-rump length were seen; after a four week drug-free recovery period bodyweights and crown-rump lengths had significantly recovered in females but were still substantially reduced in males. Time to vaginal opening was delayed in females at the highest dose, but there were no drug effects on fertility when the animals were mated beginning on day 85 of age.

In a study in which juvenile dogs received lisdexamfetamine for 6 months beginning at 10 weeks of age, decreased bodyweight gain was seen at all doses tested (2, 5, and 12 mg/kg/day, which are approximately 0.5, 1, and 3 times the maximum recommended human daily dose on a mg/m² basis). This effect partially or fully reversed during a four week drug-free recovery period.

ADVERSE REACTIONS: Adverse Drug Reaction Overview: The premarketing pediatric development program for VYVANSE included exposures in a total of 401 participants in clinical trials (345 pediatric patients and 56 healthy adult subjects). Of these, 345 pediatric patients (ages 6 to 12) were evaluated in two controlled clinical studies (one parallel-group and one crossover), one open-label extension study, and one single-dose clinical pharmacology study.

The information included in this section is based on data from the 4-week parallel-group controlled clinical trial in pediatric patients with ADHD. Adverse reactions were assessed by collecting adverse events, results of physical examinations, vital signs, weights, laboratory analyses, and ECGs.

Adverse events during exposure were obtained primarily by general inquiry and recorded by clinical investigators using terminology of their own choosing. Consequently, it is not possible to provide a meaningful estimate of the proportion of individuals experiencing adverse events without first grouping similar types of events into a smaller number of standardized event categories. In the tables and listings that follow, MedDRA terminology has been used to classify reported adverse events.

The stated frequencies of adverse events represent the proportion of individuals who experienced, at least once, a treatment-emergent adverse event of the type listed.

Adverse drug reactions observed with VYVANSE treatment mainly reflect side effects commonly associated with amphetamine use. In clinical trials, approximately a third of pediatric subjects treated with VYVANSE reported decreased appetite and insomnia. Other very common adverse drug reactions include dry mouth, headache and upper abdominal pain. Stimulant side effects generally occur early in treatment and tend to decrease over time.

Adverse Events Associated with Discontinuation of Treatment: Nine percent (20/218) of VYVANSE-treated patients discontinued due to adverse events compared to 1% (1/72) who received placebo. The most frequent adverse events leading to discontinuation and considered to be drug-related (i.e., leading to discontinuation in at least 1% of VYVANSE-treated patients and at a rate at least twice that of placebo) were ECG voltage criteria for ventricular hypertrophy, tic, vomiting, psychomotor hyperactivity, insomnia, and rash (2/218 each; 1%).

Clinical Trial Adverse Drug Reactions: Because clinical trials are conducted under very specific conditions the adverse reaction rates observed in the clinical trials may not reflect the rates observed in practice and should not be compared to the rates in the clinical trials of another drug. Adverse drug reaction information from clinical trials is useful for identifying drug-related adverse events and for approximating rates.

Adverse events reported in a 4-week clinical trial in pediatric patients treated with VYVANSE (incidence of 1% or greater) and greater than that observed in placebo-treated patients are presented in Table 1.

The pediatric clinical trial was a phase 3, randomized, multi-center, double-blind, parallel-group, placebo-controlled study in 290 children aged 6-12 years with ADHD. Adverse drug reactions with the highest subject incidence rates in VYVANSE treatment group combined were decreased appetite, insomnia, upper abdominal pain, headache, irritability, vomiting, weight decreased, and nausea. All of these adverse drug reactions are typical side effects of amphetamine products. Fifty percent of these adverse drug reactions occurred within the first week of treatment with VYVANSE, when all of the active-treated subjects received VYVANSE 30 mg.

Small increases in heart rate were observed with VYVANSE use. These changes were small in magnitude and are known effects of amphetamine use.

Effect on Body Weight: In the pediatric study, VYVANSE demonstrated a dose-response effect on subjects' body weight over 4 weeks. No significant differences were observed among the treatment groups in systolic blood pressure and diastolic blood pressure (see Warnings and Precautions, Effects on Weight and Long-Term Suppression of Growth).

Table 1: VYVANSE

Adverse Drug Reactions Reported by 1% or More of Pediatric Patients Taking VYVANSE in a 4 Week Clinical Trial

Body System	Preferred Term	VYVANSE (n=218) %	Placebo (n=72) %
Metabolism and Nutrition Disorders	Decreased appetite	39.0	4.2
	Anorexia	1.8	0
Psychiatric Disorders	Affect lability	3.2	0
	Agitation	1.4	0
	Aggression	1.4	0
	Initial insomnia	4.1	0
	Insomnia	18.8	2.8
	Irritability	9.6	0
	Tic	2.3	0
Nervous System Disorders	Dizziness	5.0	0
	Headache	11.9	9.7
Gastrointestinal Disorders	Abdominal pain upper	11.9	5.6
	Vomiting	8.7	4.2
	Nausea	6.0	2.8
	Dry mouth	4.6	0
Skin and Subcutaneous Tissue Disorders	Rash	2.8	0
General Disorder and Administration Site Conditions	Pyrexia	2.3	1.4
Investigations	Weight decreased	9.2	1.4

Note: This table includes those events for which the incidence in patients taking VYVANSE was greater than the incidence in patients taking placebo.

Uncommon adverse drug reactions (reported by ≥0.1% to <1% of pediatric patients taking VYVANSE) in a 4-week clinical trial include: Immune System Disorders: hypersensitivity.
Psychiatric Disorders: dysphoria, logorrhea.
Eye Disorders: vision blurred.
Cardiac Disorders: palpitation and tachycardia.
Gastrointestinal Disorders: diarrhea.
General Disorders and Administration Site Conditions: feeling jittery.
Investigations: blood pressure increased.
Post-Market Adverse Drug Reactions: See Table 2.

Table 2: VYVANSE

Post-Market Adverse Drug Reactions

Body System	Preferred Term
Psychiatric Disorders	Anxiety Euphoria Depression Hallucination Mania Psychotic episodes Suicidal behavior
Nervous System Disorders	Dyskinesia Restlessness Seizure Tremor
Eye Disorders	Mydriasis
Skin and Subcutaneous Tissue Disorders	Angioedema Hyperhidrosis Stevens-Johnson Syndrome Urticaria
Immune System Disorders	Anaphylactic reaction

DRUG INTERACTIONS: Drug-Drug Interactions: Agents that Lower Blood Levels of Amphetamines: Urinary Acidifying Agents: These agents (ammonium chloride, sodium acid phosphate, etc.) increase the concentration of the ionized species of the amphetamine molecule, thereby increasing urinary excretion.
Methenamine Therapy: Urinary excretion of amphetamines is increased, and efficacy is reduced, by acidifying agents used in methenamine therapy.
Agents that Increase Blood Levels of Amphetamines: Urinary Alkalinizing Agents: These agents (acetazolamide, some thiazides) increase the concentration of the non-ionized species of the amphetamine molecule, thereby decreasing urinary excretion.
Monoamine Oxidase Inhibitors: MAOI antidepressants, as well as a metabolite of furazolidone, slow amphetamine metabolism. This slowing potentiates amphetamines, increasing their effect on the release of norepinephrine and other monoamines from adrenergic nerve endings; this can cause headaches and other signs of hypertensive crisis. A variety of toxic neurological effects and malignant hyperpyrexia can occur, sometimes with fatal results.
Agents Whose Effects May be Reduced by Amphetamines: Adrenergic Blockers: Adrenergic blockers are inhibited by amphetamines.
Antihistamines: Amphetamines may counteract the sedative effect of antihistamines.
Antihypertensives: Amphetamines may antagonize the hypotensive effects of antihypertensives.
Veratrum Alkaloids: Amphetamines inhibit the hypotensive effect of veratrum alkaloids.
Ethosuximide: Amphetamines may delay intestinal absorption of ethosuximide.

Agents Whose Effects May be Potentiated by Amphetamines: Antidepressants, Tricyclic: Amphetamines may enhance the activity of tricyclic antidepressants or sympathomimetic agents; d-amphetamine with desipramine or protriptyline and possibly other tricyclics cause striking and sustained increases in the concentration of d-amphetamine in the brain; cardiovascular effects can be potentiated.
Meperidine: Amphetamines potentiate the analgesic effect of meperidine.
Phenobarbital: Amphetamines may delay intestinal absorption of phenobarbital; co-administration of phenobarbital may produce a synergistic anticonvulsant action.
Phenytoin: Amphetamines may delay intestinal absorption of phenytoin; co-administration of phenytoin may produce a synergistic anticonvulsant action.
Agents that May Reduce the Effects of Amphetamines: Chlorpromazine: Chlorpromazine blocks dopamine and norepinephrine receptors, thus inhibiting the central stimulant effects of amphetamines, and can be used to treat amphetamine poisoning.
Haloperidol: Haloperidol blocks dopamine receptors, thus inhibiting the central stimulant effects of amphetamines.
Lithium Carbonate: The anorectic and stimulatory effects of amphetamines may be inhibited by lithium carbonate.
Agents that May Potentiate the Effects of Amphetamines: Norepinephrine: Amphetamines enhance the adrenergic effect of norepinephrine.
Propoxyphene Overdosage: In cases of propoxyphene overdosage, amphetamine CNS stimulation is potentiated and fatal convulsions can occur.
Drug-Food Interactions: Food does not affect the observed AUC and C_{max} of d-amphetamine in healthy adults after single-dose oral administration of 70 mg of VYVANSE (lisdexamfetamine dimesylate) capsules but prolongs T_{max} by approximately 1 hour (from 3.8 hrs at fasted state to 4.7 hrs after a high fat meal). After an 8-hour fast, the AUC for d-amphetamine following oral administration of lisdexamfetamine dimesylate in solution and as intact capsules were equivalent.
Drug-Laboratory Test Interactions: Amphetamines can cause a significant elevation in plasma corticosteroid levels. This increase is greatest in the evening. Amphetamines may interfere with urinary steroid determinations.

DOSAGE AND ADMINISTRATION:

Dosing Considerations: Dosage should be individualized according to the therapeutic needs and response of the patient. VYVANSE (lisdexamfetamine dimesylate capsules) should be administered orally starting at the lowest possible effective dosage.

VYVANSE should not be used in patients with symptomatic cardiovascular disease including coronary artery disease and should generally not be used in patients with known serious structural cardiac abnormalities or other serious heart problems (e.g., cardiomyopathy, serious heart rhythm abnormalities) that may place them at increased vulnerability to the sympathomimetic effects of ADHD drugs (see Contraindications and Warnings and Precautions).

Theoretically there exists a pharmacological potential for all ADHD drugs to increase the risk of sudden/cardiac death. Although confirmation of an incremental risk for adverse cardiac events arising from treatment with ADHD medications is lacking, prescribers should consider this potential risk.

All drugs with sympathomimetic effects prescribed in the management of ADHD should be used with caution in patients who: a) are involved in strenuous exercise or activities b) use other sympathomimetic drugs or c) have a family history of sudden/cardiac death. Prior to the initiation of treatment with sympathomimetic medications, a personal and family history (including assessment for a family history of sudden death or ventricular arrhythmia) and physical exam should be obtained to assess for the presence of cardiac disease. In patients with relevant risk factors and based on the clinician's judgment, further cardiovascular evaluation may be considered (e.g., electrocardiogram and echocardiogram). Patients who develop symptoms such as exertional chest pain, unexplained syncope, or other symptoms suggestive of cardiac disease during ADHD treatment should undergo a prompt cardiac evaluation.

Patients who are considered to need extended treatment with VYVANSE should undergo periodic evaluation of their cardiovascular status (see Warnings and Precautions).

Recommended Dose and Dosage Adjustment: Children (6 to 12 years of age): In children with ADHD who are either starting treatment for the first time or switching from another medication, 30 mg once daily in the morning is the usual starting dose. When in the judgment of the clinician a lower dose is appropriate, patients may begin treatment with 20 mg once daily in the morning. In clinical studies, doses of 20-70 mg/day were shown to be effective, although no additional benefit was demonstrated at doses greater than 30 mg/day, and adverse events and discontinuations were more frequent at higher doses. Doses greater than 70 mg/day of VYVANSE have not been studied. If the physician, based on clinical judgment, decides a dose increase is warranted for an individual patient, the maximum dose should not exceed 60 mg/day; dosage may be adjusted at approximately weekly intervals. VYVANSE has not been studied, and is not recommended for use in patients under 6 years or over 12 years of age.

VYVANSE should be taken in the morning. Afternoon doses should be avoided because of the potential for insomnia.

VYVANSE may be taken with or without food.

VYVANSE capsules may be taken whole, or the capsule may be opened and the entire contents dissolved in a glass of water. If the patient is using the solution administration method, the solution should be consumed immediately; it should not be stored. The dose of a single capsule should not be divided. The contents of the entire capsule should be taken, and patients should not take anything less than one capsule per day.

Where possible, drug administration should be interrupted occasionally to determine if there is a recurrence of behavioral symptoms sufficient to require continued therapy.

OVERDOSAGE:
Individual patient response to amphetamines varies widely. Toxic symptoms may occur idiosyncratically at low doses.
Symptoms: Manifestations of acute overdosage with amphetamines include restlessness, tremor, hyperreflexia, rapid respiration, confusion, assaultiveness, hallucinations, panic states, hyperpyrexia and rhabdomyolysis. Fatigue and depression usually follow the central nervous system stimulation. Cardiovascular effects include arrhythmias, hypertension or hypotension and circulatory collapse. Gastrointestinal symptoms include nausea, vomiting, diarrhea, and abdominal cramps. Fatal poisoning is usually preceded by convulsions and coma.
Treatment: Treatment of overdosage consists of appropriate supportive measures. Consult with a Certified Poison Control Center for up to date guidance and advice. Management of acute amphetamine intoxication is largely symptomatic and includes gastric lavage, administration of activated charcoal, administration of a cathartic and sedation. Experience with hemodialysis or peritoneal dialysis is inadequate to permit its recommendation in this regard. Acidification of the urine increases amphetamine excretion, but is believed to increase risk of acute renal failure if myoglobinuria is present. If acute severe hypertension complicates amphetamine overdosage, administration of intravenous phentolamine has been suggested. However, a gradual drop in blood pressure will usually result when sufficient sedation has been achieved. Chlorpromazine antagonizes the central stimulant effects of amphetamines and can be used to treat amphetamine intoxication.

The prolonged release of VYVANSE (lisdexamfetamine dimesylate capsules) should be considered when treating patients with overdose.
Animal Toxicology: Acute administration of high doses of amphetamine (d- or d,l-) has been shown to produce long-lasting neurotoxic effects, including irreversible nerve fiber damage, in rodents. The significance of these findings to humans is unknown.

> For management of a suspected drug overdose, contact your regional Poison Control Centre. See the *CPS* Directory section for a list of Poison Control Centres.

ACTION AND CLINICAL PHARMACOLOGY: Mechanism of Action: VYVANSE (lisdexamfetamine dimesylate capsules) is a prodrug of dextroamphetamine. After oral administration, lisdexamfetamine dimesylate is rapidly absorbed from the gastrointestinal tract and converted to dextroamphetamine, which is responsible for the drug's activity.
Pharmacodynamics: Amphetamines are non-catecholamine sympathomimetic amines with CNS stimulant activity. The mode of therapeutic action of amphetamine in Attention-Deficit/Hyperactivity Disorder (ADHD) is not fully established, however, it is thought to be due to its ability to block the reuptake of norepinephrine and dopamine into the presynaptic neuron and increase the release of these monoamines into the extraneuronal space. The parent drug, lisdexamfetamine, does not bind to the sites responsible for the reuptake of norepinephrine and dopamine in vitro.
Pharmacokinetics: Absorption: Pharmacokinetic studies of dextroamphetamine after oral administration of lisdexamfetamine dimesylate have been conducted in healthy adult and pediatric (6-12 yrs) patients with ADHD.

In 18 pediatric patients (6-12 yrs) with ADHD, the T_{max} of dextroamphetamine was approximately 3.5 hours following single-dose oral administration of lisdexamfetamine dimesylate either 30 mg, 50 mg, or 70 mg after an 8-hour overnight fast. The T_{max} of lisdexamfetamine dimesylate was approximately 1 hour. Linear pharmacokinetics of dextroamphetamine after single-dose oral administration of lisdexamfetamine dimesylate was established over the dose range of 30 mg to 70 mg in children aged 6 to 12 years.

There is no unexpected accumulation of dextroamphetamine AUC at steady state in healthy adults and no accumulation of lisdexamfetamine dimesylate after once-daily dosing for 7 consecutive days.

Food does not affect the observed AUC and C_{max} of dextroamphetamine in healthy adults after single-dose oral administration of 70 mg of VYVANSE capsules but prolongs T_{max} by approximately 1 hour (from 3.8 hrs at fasted state to 4.7 hrs after a high fat meal). After an 8-hour fast, the AUC for dextroamphetamine following oral administration of lisdexamfetamine dimesylate in solution and as intact capsules were equivalent.

Weight/dose normalized AUC and C_{max} were 22% and 12% lower, respectively, in adult females than in males on day 7 following a 70 mg/day dose of lisdexamfetamine for 7 days. Weight/Dose normalized AUC and C_{max} values were the same in girls and boys following single doses of 30-70 mg.

Metabolism and Excretion: After oral administration, lisdexamfetamine dimesylate is rapidly absorbed from the gastrointestinal tract. Lisdexamfetamine dimesylate is converted to d-amphetamine and L-lysine, which is believed to occur by first-pass intestinal and/or hepatic metabolism. Lisdexamfetamine is not metabolized by cytochrome P450 enzymes. Following the oral administration of a 70 mg dose of radiolabeled lisdexamfetamine dimesylate to 6 healthy subjects, approximately 96% of the oral dose radioactivity was recovered in the urine and only 0.3% recovered in the feces over a period of 120 hours. Of the radioactivity recovered in the urine 42% of the dose was related to amphetamine, 25% to hippuric acid, and 2% intact lisdexamfetamine. Plasma concentrations of unconverted lisdexamfetamine are low and transient, generally becoming non-quantifiable by 8 hours after administration. The plasma elimination half-life of lisdexamfetamine typically averaged less than one hour in studies of lisdexamfetamine dimesylate in volunteers.

D-amphetamine is known to inhibit monoamine oxidase. The ability of d-amphetamine and its metabolites to inhibit various P450 isozymes and other enzymes has not been adequately elucidated. In vitro experiments with human microsomes indicate minor inhibition of CYP2D6 by amphetamine and minor inhibition of CYP1A2, 2D6, and 3A4 by one or more metabolites, but there are no in vivo studies of P450 enzyme inhibition.

Special Populations and Conditions: The pharmacokinetics of dextroamphetamine is similar in pediatric (6-12 years) and adolescent (13-17 years) ADHD patients, and healthy adult volunteers. Any differences in kinetics seen after oral administration are a result of differences in mg/kg dosing.

Gender: Systemic exposure to dextroamphetamine is similar for men and women given the same mg/kg dose.

Race: Formal pharmacokinetic studies for race have not been conducted.

STORAGE AND STABILITY: Dispense in a tight, light-resistant container as defined in the USP.

Store at 25°C. Excursions permitted to 15-30°C.

INFORMATION FOR THE PATIENT: Published in e-CPS, available by subscription at www.e-cps.ca.

DOSAGE FORMS, COMPOSITION AND PACKAGING: 20 mg: Each capsule with ivory body/ivory cap, imprinted S489 20 mg, for once-a-day oral administration, contains: lisdexamfetamine dimesylate 20 mg. Nonmedicinal ingredients: croscarmellose sodium, magnesium stearate and microcrystalline cellulose; capsule shell: gelatin, titanium dioxide, and one or more of the following: FD&C Yellow #6, FD&C Blue #1, FD&C Red #3, FDA/E172 Black Iron Oxide and FDA/E172 Yellow Iron Oxide. Bottles of 100.

30 mg: Each capsule with white body/orange cap, imprinted S489 30 mg, for once-a-day oral administration, contains: lisdexamfetamine dimesylate 30 mg. Nonmedicinal ingredients: croscarmellose sodium, magnesium stearate and microcrystalline cellulose; capsule shell: gelatin, titanium dioxide, and one or more of the following: FD&C Yellow #6, FD&C Blue #1, FD&C Red #3, FDA/E172 Black Iron Oxide and FDA/E172 Yellow Iron Oxide. Bottles of 100.

40 mg: Each capsule with white body/dark green cap, imprinted S489 40 mg, for once-a-day oral administration, contains: lisdexamfetamine dimesylate 40 mg. Nonmedicinal ingredients: croscarmellose sodium, magnesium stearate and microcrystalline cellulose; capsule shell: gelatin, titanium dioxide, and one or more of the following: FD&C Yellow #6, FD&C Blue #1, FD&C Red #3, FDA/E172 Black Iron Oxide and FDA/E172 Yellow Iron Oxide. Bottles of 100.

50 mg: Each capsule with white body/blue cap, imprinted S489 50 mg for once-a-day oral administration, contains: lisdexamfetamine dimesylate 50 mg. Nonmedicinal ingredients: croscarmellose sodium, magnesium stearate and microcrystalline cellulose; capsule shell: gelatin, titanium dioxide, and one or more of the following: FD&C Yellow #6, FD&C Blue #1, and FD&C Red #3. Bottles of 100.

60 mg: Each capsule with aqua blue body/aqua blue cap, imprinted S489 60 mg for once-a-day oral administration, contains: lisdexamfetamine dimesylate 60 mg. Nonmedicinal ingredients: croscarmellose sodium, magnesium stearate and microcrystalline cellulose; capsule shell: gelatin, titanium dioxide, and one or more of the following: FD&C Yellow #6, FD&C Blue #1, and FD&C Red #3. Bottles of 100.

(Shown in Product Identification Section)

W

Wake Ups
caffeine
Helps Prevent Drowsiness

Adrem

INDICATIONS: Wake Ups help to temporarily restore wakefulness when experiencing drowsiness.
CONTRAINDICATIONS : No data supplied by the manufacturer.
WARNINGS: No data supplied by the manufacturer.
PRECAUTIONS: No data supplied by the manufacturer.
ADVERSE EFFECTS: No data supplied by the manufacturer.
OVERDOSE:
No data supplied by the manufacturer.

> For management of a suspected drug overdose, CPhA recommends that you contact your **regional Poison Control Centre**. See the *CPS* Directory section for a list of Poison Control Centres.

DOSAGE: Adults: Take 100 mg-200 mg every 4 hours as required. Not to exceed 1000 mg in any 24 hour period. For best results take before eating or on an empty stomach.

Not to be given to children. Do not use if pregnant or breastfeeding.

Caution: For occasional use only. Not intended for use as a substitute for sleep. Do not take within 1½ hours of the time you plan to sleep. Caffeine intake is not advisable in cases of high blood pressure. Consult your physician before using this product if you are taking other medication or under a doctor's care. The recommended dose of this product contains about as much caffeine as a cup of coffee. Limit the amount of caffeine containing medications, beverages (coffee, tea, colas) or foods (chocolate) as too much caffeine may cause nervousness, irritability, sleeplessness and, occasionally, rapid heart rate.

Not to be given to children. Not advisable during pregnancy or breastfeeding.

SUPPLIED: 100 mg: Each round, pink, monogrammed tablet contains: caffeine alkaloid (synthetic) 100 mg. Nonmedicinal ingredients: alcohol SDAG 1-G (95%), calcium phosphate dibasic dihydrate, colloidal silicon dioxide, cornstarch, FD&C Red No. 3, lactose anhydrous, magnesium stearate, povidone, sodium starch glycolate and water. Bottles of 100 (cap is safety sealed). Cartons of 12 and 36. Store at room temperature.
200 mg: Each round, white, monogrammed tablet contains: caffeine alkaloid (synthetic) 200 mg. Nonmedicinal ingredients: calcium phosphate dibasic dihydrate, colloidal silicon dioxide, magnesium stearate and microcrystalline cellulose. Bottles of 50 (cap is safety sealed). Store at room temperature.

Wellbutrin® SR Pr
bupropion HCl
Antidepressant

Biovail Pharmaceuticals

Date of Preparation: November 20, 2008
Date of Revision: February 4, 2009

SUMMARY PRODUCT INFORMATION:

Route of Administration	Dosage Form/ Strength	Clinically Relevant Nonmedicinal Ingredients
Oral	Tablets: 150 mg	Tablet components: carnauba wax, cysteine hydrochloride, hydroxypropyl methylcellulose, magnesium stearate, microcrystalline cellulose, polyethylene glycol, titanium dioxide, edible black ink, FD&C Blue No. 2 Lake, FD&C Red No. 40 lake, and polysorbate 80. For complete information see Dosage Forms, Composition and Packaging.

INDICATIONS AND CLINICAL USE: Adults: WELLBUTRIN SR is indicated for the symptomatic relief of major depressive illness. The effectiveness of WELLBUTRIN SR in long-term use (greater than 8 weeks) has not been evaluated in controlled trials. Therefore, the physician who elects to use WELLBUTRIN SR for extended periods should periodically re-evaluate the long-term usefulness of the drug for the individual patient.
Pediatrics (<18 years of age): WELLBUTRIN SR is not indicated for use in patients below the age of 18 years (see Warnings and Precautions, General, Potential Association with Behavioural and Emotional Changes, Including Self-harm).
CONTRAINDICATIONS: To reduce the risk of seizures, WELLBUTRIN SR (bupropion hydrochloride) is contraindicated in patients:

- receiving WELLBUTRIN XL, ZYBAN or any other medications that contain bupropion hydrochloride because the incidence of seizure is dose dependent (see Warnings and Precautions).
- with a current seizure disorder (see Warnings and Precautions).
- with a current or prior diagnosis of bulimia or anorexia nervosa because of a higher incidence of seizures (see Warnings and Precautions) noted in patients treated for bulimia with the immediate release formulation of bupropion.
- undergoing abrupt withdrawal from alcohol or benzodiazepines or other sedatives.

To reduce risks due to drug interaction, the concomitant use of WELLBUTRIN SR is contraindicated in patients currently taking:

- Monoamine oxidase (MAO) inhibitors.
- The antipsychotic thioridazine, since bupropion may inhibit thioridazine metabolism, thus causing an increase in thioridazine levels and a potential increased risk of thioridazine-related serious ventricular arrhythmias and sudden death.

At least 14 days should elapse between discontinuation of one drug and the start of another.

WELLBUTRIN SR is contraindicated in patients with known hypersensitivity to bupropion or to any of the components of the formulation.

WARNINGS AND PRECAUTIONS: Potential Association with Behavioural and Emotional Changes, Including Self-harm: Pediatrics: Placebo-Controlled Clinical Trial Data:

- **Recent analyses of placebo-controlled clinical trial safety databases from SSRIs and other newer antidepressants suggests that use of these drugs in patients under the age of 18 may be associated with behavioural and emotional changes, including an increased risk of suicidal ideation and behaviour over that of placebo.**
- **The small denominators in the clinical trial database, as well as the variability in placebo rates, preclude reliable conclusions on the relative safety profiles among these drugs.**

Adults and Pediatrics: Additional Data:

- **There are clinical trial and post-marketing reports with SSRIs and other newer antidepressants, in both pediatrics and adults, of severe agitation-type adverse events coupled with self-harm or harm to others. The agitation-type events include: akathisia, agitation, disinhibition, emotional lability, hostility, aggression, depersonalization. In some cases, the events occurred within several weeks of starting treatment.**

Rigorous clinical monitoring for suicidal ideation or other indicators of potential for suicidal behaviour is advised in patients of all ages given an antidepressant drug. This includes monitoring for agitation-type emotional and behavioural changes.

Seizures: Patients should be made aware that WELLBUTRIN SR contains the same active ingredient (bupropion hydrochloride) as ZYBAN and WELLBUTRIN XL. WELLBUTRIN SR should **not** be administered to patients already receiving a product containing bupropion hydrochloride (see Contraindications).

Data for WELLBUTRIN SR Tablets revealed a seizure incidence of approximately 0.1% (3 of 3100 patients followed prospectively) in patients treated at the recommended dose range of 100 to 300 mg/day. The incidence of seizures increased to 0.4% (4/1000), above the recommended dose, at 400 mg/day. Data for the immediate release bupropion revealed a seizure incidence of approximately 0.4% (13 of 3,200 patients followed prospectively) in patients treated at doses of 300 to 450 mg/day. Additional data accumulated for the immediate release formulation of bupropion suggests that the estimated seizure incidence increases almost tenfold between 450 and 600 mg/day. Given the wide variability among individuals and their capacity to metabolize and eliminate drugs, the disproportionate increase in seizure incidence with dose incrementation calls for caution in dosing.

Predisposing Risk Factors for Seizures: The risk of seizure occurring with bupropion use appears to be associated with the presence of predisposing risk factors. Therefore extreme caution should be used when treating patients with predisposing factors which increase the risk of seizures, including: history of head trauma or prior seizure; central nervous system (CNS) tumour; the presence of severe hepatic impairment; excessive use of alcohol; addiction to opiates, cocaine, or stimulants; use of concomitant medications that lower seizure threshold, including but not limited to: antipsychotics, antidepressants, lithium, amantadine, theophylline, systemic steroids, quinolone antibiotics, and anti-malarials; use of over-the-counter stimulants or anorectics; diabetes treated with oral hypoglycemics or insulin.

The above group of risk factors, including medications, should not be considered exhaustive; for each patient, all potential predisposing factors must be carefully considered.

In Order to Minimize the Risk of Seizure: The total daily dose of WELLBUTRIN SR must not exceed 300 mg (the maximum recommended dose); no single dose of WELLBUTRIN SR may exceed 150 mg, in order to avoid high peak concentrations of bupropion and/or its metabolites.

If a Seizure Occurs: Patients should be warned that if they experience a seizure while taking WELLBUTRIN SR, they should contact their doctor or be taken to a hospital emergency ward immediately, and should stop taking WELLBUTRIN SR. Treatment should not be restarted if a patient has experienced a seizure while taking WELLBUTRIN SR, WELLBUTRIN XL or ZYBAN.

Hepatic Impairment: The results of two single dose pharmacokinetic studies indicate that the clearance of bupropion is reduced in all subjects with Child-Pugh Grades C hepatic impairment, and in some subjects with milder forms of liver impairment. Given the risks associated with both peak bupropion levels and drug accumulation, WELLBUTRIN SR is not recommended for use in patients with severe hepatic impairment. However, should clinical judgement deem it necessary, it should be used only with extreme caution at a reduced dose, to a maximum dose of 150 mg every other day.

All patients with hepatic impairment should be closely monitored for possible adverse effects (e.g., insomnia, dry mouth, seizures) that could indicate high drug or metabolite levels (see Dosage and Administration; Action and Clinical Pharmacology and Warnings and Precautions).

Potential for Hepatotoxicity: In rats receiving large doses of bupropion chronically, there was an increase in incidence of hepatic hyperplastic nodules and hepatocellular hypertrophy. In dogs receiving large doses of bupropion chronically, various histologic changes were seen in the liver, and laboratory tests suggesting mild hepatocellular injury were noted.

Clinical Worsening and Suicide: The possibility of a suicide attempt in seriously depressed patients is inherent to the illness and may persist until significant remission occurs. Patients with depression may experience worsening of their depressive symptoms and/or the emergence of suicidal ideation and behaviours (suicidality) whether or not they are taking antidepressant medications. As improvement may not occur during the first few weeks or more of treatment, patients should be closely monitored for clinical worsening (including development of new symptoms) and suicidality, especially at the beginning of a course of treatment, or at the time of dosage changes, either increases or decreases. Close supervision of high risk patients should accompany initial drug therapy, and consideration should be given to the need for hospitalization. (See Warnings and Precautions, Potential Association with Behavioural and Emotional Changes, Including Self-harm.)

It should be noted that a causal role for SSRIs and other newer antidepressants in inducing self-harm or harm to others has not been established.

In order to reduce the risk of overdose, prescriptions for WELLBUTRIN SR (bupropion hydrochloride) should be written for the smallest number of tablets consistent with good patient management.

Allergic Reactions: Anaphylactoid/anaphylactic reactions characterized by symptoms such as pruritus, urticaria, angioedema, and dyspnea requiring medical treatment have been reported in clinical trials with bupropion at a rate of 1-3 per thousand. In addition, there have been rare spontaneous postmarketing reports of erythema multiforme, Stevens-Johnson syndrome, and anaphylactic shock associated with bupropion. In uncontrolled and controlled clinical trials, skin disorders, primarily rashes, pruritus, and urticaria, lead to discontinuation of 1.5% and 1.9%, respectively of bupropion-treated subjects. A patient should stop taking WELLBUTRIN SR and consult a doctor if experiencing allergic or anaphylactoid/anaphylactic reactions (e.g., skin rash, pruritus, hives, chest pain, edema, and shortness of breath) during treatment.

Arthralgia, myalgia and fever have also been reported in association with rash and other symptoms suggestive of delayed hypersensitivity. These symptoms may resemble serum sickness.

Bupropion should be discontinued immediately if any hypersensitivity reactions are experienced. Symptoms of hypersensitivity should be treated in accordance with established medical practice. Clinicians should be aware that symptoms may persist beyond the discontinuation of bupropion, and clinical management should be provided accordingly. In post-market experience, there have been reports of hypersensitivity reactions in patients who consumed alcohol while taking bupropion. As the contribution of alcohol to these reactions has been established, patients should avoid alcohol when they are taking bupropion (see Drug Interactions, Alcohol Interactions).

Agitation and Insomnia: In placebo controlled trials patients receiving WELLBUTRIN SR Tablets experienced an increased incidence of insomnia and anxiety relative to those receiving placebo (see Adverse Reactions and Warnings and Precautions, Potential Association with Behavioural and Emotional Changes, Including Self-harm). These symptoms were sometimes of sufficient magnitude to require discontinuation of WELLBUTRIN SR, or concurrent treatment with sedative/hypnotic drugs. Insomnia may be minimized by avoiding bedtime doses and, if necessary, reduction in dose.

Psychosis, Confusion, and Other Neuropsychiatric Phenomena: Patients treated with WELLBUTRIN SR have been reported to show a variety of neuropsychiatric signs and symptoms including delusions, hallucinations, psychosis, concentration disturbance, paranoia and confusion. In some cases these abated upon dose reduction and/or withdrawal of treatment.

Activation of Psychosis and/or Mania: Antidepressants can precipitate manic episodes in bipolar patients during the depressed phase of their illness and may activate latent psychosis in other susceptible patients. WELLBUTRIN SR is expected to pose similar risks.

Altered Appetite and Weight: In clinical trials WELLBUTRIN SR was associated with dose-related weight loss. In eight week controlled trials mean weight loss for trial completers was 0.1 kg for placebo, 0.8 kg for WELLBUTRIN SR 100 mg/day, 1.4 kg at 150 mg/ day, and 2.3 kg at 300 mg/day. If weight loss is a major presenting sign of a patient's depressive illness, the potential anorectic and/or weight reducing effect of bupropion hydrochloride should be considered.

Cardiovascular Effects: In clinical practice, hypertension, in some cases severe, requiring acute treatment, has been reported in patients receiving bupropion alone and in combination with nicotine replacement therapy. These events have been observed in both patients with and without evidence of pre-existing hypertension.

Data from a comparative study of the sustained-release formulation of bupropion (ZYBAN Sustained-Release Tablets), nicotine transdermal system (NTS), the combination of sustained-release bupropion plus NTS, and placebo as an aid to smoking cessation suggest a higher incidence of treatment-emergent hypertension in patients treated with the combination of sustained-release bupropion and NTS. In this study, 6.1% of patients treated with the combination of sustained- release bupropion and NTS had treatment-emergent hypertension compared to 2.5%, 1.6%, and 3.1% of patients treated with sustained-release bupropion, NTS, and placebo, respectively. The majority of these patients had evidence of pre-existing hypertension. Three patients (1.2%) treated with the combination of ZYBAN and NTS and one patient (0.4%) treated with NTS had study medication discontinued due to hypertension compared to none of the patients treated with ZYBAN or placebo. Monitoring of blood pressure is recommended in patients who receive the combination of bupropion and nicotine replacement.

There is no clinical experience establishing the safety of bupropion in patients with a recent history of myocardial infarction or unstable heart disease. Therefore, care should be exercised if it is used in these groups. In a study of depressed inpatients with stable heart failure, bupropion was associated with a rise in supine blood pressure, resulting in discontinuation of two patients for exacerbation of baseline hypertension.

Hepatic Impairment: Based on the variability reported for individual pharmacokinetic (PK) values of patients with mild hepatic impairment in a single dose pharmacokinetic study, patients with mild or moderate hepatic impairment should be initiated on the lowest recommended dose. Bupropion is not recommended for patients with severe hepatic impairment (see Warnings and Precautions, and also Dosage and Administration). All patients with hepatic impairment should be closely monitored for possible adverse effects that could indicate high drug and metabolite levels (see Action and Clinical Pharmacology; Warnings and Precautions and Dosage and Administration).

Renal Impairment: Bupropion is extensively metabolized in the liver to active metabolites, which are largely further metabolised before being excreted by the kidneys. WELLBUTRIN SR treatment of patients with renal impairment should be initiated at a reduced dosage regimen, as metabolites may accumulate in such patients to a greater extent than usual. The patient should be closely monitored for possible adverse effects (e.g., insomnia, dry mouth, seizures) that could indicate high drug or metabolite levels.

Occupational Hazards: Any psychoactive drug may impair judgement, thinking or motor skills. Therefore patients should be cautioned about operating hazardous machinery, including automobiles, until they are reasonably certain that the drug treatment does not affect their performance adversely.

Special Populations: Pregnancy: Pregnancy, Labour and Delivery: There are no adequate and well-controlled studies of WELLBUTRIN SR in pregnant women. WELLBUTRIN SR should thus not be used during pregnancy unless the potential benefit is judged to outweigh the potential risk.

Post-marketing reports indicate that some neonates exposed to SSRIs (Selective Serotonin Reuptake Inhibitors), or other newer antidepressants, such as WELLBUTRIN SR, late in the third trimester have developed complications requiring prolonged hospitalization, respiratory support, and tube feeding. Such complications can arise immediately upon delivery. Reported clinical findings have included respiratory distress, cyanosis, apnea, seizures, temperature instability, feeding difficulty, vomiting, hypoglycemia, hypotonia, hyperreflexia, tremor, jitteriness, irritability, and constant crying. The frequency of symptoms may vary with each drug. These features are consistent with either a direct toxic effect of SSRIs and other newer antidepressants, or, possibly, a drug discontinuation syndrome. When treating a pregnant woman with WELLBUTRIN SR during the third trimester, the physician should carefully consider the potential risks and benefits of treatment. (See Dosage and Administration.)

Nursing Women: Like many other drugs, bupropion and its metabolites are secreted in human milk. Because of the potential for serious adverse reactions in nursing infants from WELLBUTRIN SR, a decision should be made whether to discontinue nursing or to discontinue the drug, taking into account the importance of the drug to the mother.

Pediatrics (<18 years of age): WELLBUTRIN SR is not indicated for use in patients below the age of 18 years (see Warnings and Precautions, Potential Association with Behavioural and Emotional Changes, Including Self-harm). See also Indications and Clinical Use, Pediatrics (<18 years of age) and Dosage and Administration, Special Patient Populations, Pediatrics.

Geriatrics: Of the approximately 6000 patients who participated in clinical trials with bupropion sustained-release tablets (depression and smoking cessation studies), 275 were 65 and over and 47 were 75 and over. In addition, several hundred patients 65 and over participated in clinical trials using the immediate-release formulation of bupropion (depression studies). No overall differences in safety or effectiveness were observed between these subjects and younger subjects, and other reported clinical experience has not identified differences in responses between the elderly and younger patients, but greater sensitivity of some older individuals cannot be ruled out.

A single-dose pharmacokinetic study demonstrated that the disposition of bupropion and its metabolites in elderly subjects was similar to that of younger subjects; however, another single and multiple dose pharmacokinetic study, has suggested that the elderly are at increased risk for accumulation of bupropion and its metabolites (see Action and Clinical Pharmacology, Pharmacokinetics).

Bupropion is extensively metabolized in the liver to active metabolites, of which some are eliminated by the kidney, while others are further metabolized before being excreted in urine. The risk of toxic reaction to this drug may be greater in patients with impaired renal function. Because elderly patients are more likely to have decreased renal function, care should be taken in dose selection, and it may be useful to monitor renal function (see Warnings and Precautions, Hepatic Impairment or Renal Impairment).

ADVERSE REACTIONS: Adverse Drug Reaction Overview: The information included under Adverse Reactions is based on data from clinical trials with WELLBUTRIN SR (bupropion hydrochloride), the sustained release formulation of bupropion in the treatment of depression. Information on additional adverse events associated with the sustained release formulation of bupropion as well as the immediate release formulation of bupropion, is included in a separate subsection (see Events Observed During Development and Post-Marketing Experience of Bupropion with Other Formulations or Indications).

Incidence of Commonly Observed Adverse Events in Controlled Clinical Trials: Adverse events commonly encountered during the clinical development of WELLBUTRIN SR (incidence of 5% or greater; and higher incidence in WELLBUTRIN SR-treated, than placebo-treated patients) were headache, constipation, dry mouth, nausea, dizziness, insomnia, tremor and tinnitus.

Adverse Events Associated with Discontinuation of Treatment: In placebo controlled studies of depression (987 patients treated with WELLBUTRIN SR, and 385 treated with placebo), adverse events caused discontinuation in 7% of WELLBUTRIN SR-treated patients and 3% of placebo-treated patients. The more common events leading to discontinuation of WELLBUTRIN SR included nervous system disturbances (2.2%), primarily agitation, anxiety and insomnia; skin disorders (1.9%), primarily rashes, pruritus, and urticaria; general body complaints (1.0%), primarily headaches, and digestive system disturbances (1.0%), primarily nausea. Two patients in WELLBUTRIN SR treatment groups discontinued due to hallucinations (auditory or visual). The rates of premature discontinuation due to an adverse event were dose-related in these studies.

In an open label, uncontrolled (acute treatment and continuation) study of WELLBUTRIN SR, 11% patients (361 out of 3100) discontinued treatment due to an adverse event. Adverse events leading to premature discontinuation in 1% or more of patients were: headache (1.1%), nausea (1.0%), and insomnia (1.0%). Adverse events leading to premature discontinuation in 0.5% to 1% of patients were: anxiety (0.8%), rash (0.8%), agitation (0.7%), irritability (0.5%), and dizziness (0.5%). In those patients (n=1577) who went into the continuation phase after 8 weeks of treatment, 6 (0.4%) discontinued due to alopecia. Because this study was uncontrolled, it is not possible to reliably assess the causal relationship of these events to treatment with WELLBUTRIN SR.

Clinical Trial Adverse Drug Reactions: Because clinical trials are conducted under very specific conditions the adverse reaction rates observed in the clinical trials may not reflect the rates observed in practice and should not be compared to the rates in the clinical trials of another drug. Adverse drug reaction information from clinical trials is useful for identifying drug-related adverse events and for approximating rates.

Table 1 enumerates treatment-emergent adverse events that occurred at an incidence of 1% or more in placebo-controlled trials, and were more frequent in the WELLBUTRIN SR group than the placebo group. Reported adverse events were classified using a COSTART-based Dictionary.

Less Common WELLBUTRIN SR Clinical Trial Adverse Drug Reactions (<1%): Events Observed During Development and Post-Marketing Experience of Bupropion with Other Formulations or Indications: In addition to the events noted above, the following adverse events have been reported in clinical trials and post-marketing experience with the sustained release formulation of bupropion in depressed patients and in non-depressed smokers, as well as in clinical trials and post-marketing experience with the immediate release formulation of bupropion.

The frequencies represent the proportion of patients who experienced a treatment-emergent adverse event on at least one occasion in placebo-controlled studies for depression (n=987) or smoking cessation (n=1013), or patients who experienced an adverse event requiring discontinuation of treatment in an open-label surveillance study with WELLBUTRIN SR Tablets (n=3100). All treatment-emergent adverse events are included except those listed in Table 1, those events listed in other safety-related sections, those adverse events subsumed under COSTART terms that are either overly general or excessively specific so as to be uninformative, those events not reasonably associated with the use of the drug, and those events that were not serious and occurred in fewer than two patients.

Events of major clinical importance are described in the Warnings and Precautions sections.

Events are further categorized by body system and listed in order of decreasing frequency according to the following definitions of frequency: Frequent adverse events are defined as those occurring in at least 1/100 patients. Infrequent adverse events are those occurring in 1/100 to 1/1000 patients, while rare events are those occurring in less than 1/1000 patients.

Adverse events for which frequencies are not provided occurred in clinical trials or postmarketing experience with bupropion. Only those adverse events not previously listed for sustained-release bupropion are included. The extent to which these events may be associated with WELLBUTRIN SR is unknown.

Table 1: WELLBUTRIN SR

Adverse Event (%) Placebo-Controlled Studies: Treatment-Emergent Adverse Experiences Occurring in ≥1% of Patients in Any BUP SR Group for Studies 203, 205, and 212

Body System	Adverse Experience	% AEs BUP SR 100–150 (n=382)	% AEs BUP SR 200–300 (n=491)	% AEs PBO (n=385)
Body (General)	Asthenia	1.8	1.6	1.6
	Flu Syndrome	6.2	2.4	3.1
	Headache	27.5	26.9	23.4
	Infection	4.7	7.5	6.5
	Accidental Injury	1.8	1.8	1.8
	Pain	1.3	2.4	2.1
	Abdominal Pain	3.9	3.5	1.6
	Back Pain	1.8	4.5	3.1
	Chest Pain	1	2.9	0.8
	Neck Pain	1.3	2	1.3
Cardiovascular	Hot Flashes	1.3	1	0.8
	Migraine	0.8	1.4	1
	Palpitations	2.9	2	1.6
	Tachycardia	1.6	0.6	0.5
Digestive	Anorexia	3.1	4.5	1.6
	Constipation	6.5	10.8	6.8
	Diarrhea	3.9	5.9	5.7
	Dry Mouth	13.1	16.5	7
	Dyspepsia	4.2	4.7	4.4
	Flatulence	1.8	3.1	2.1
	Nausea	10.7	12.6	7.5
	Vomiting	1.8	3.9	1.6
Musculoskeletal	Arthralgia	2.6	0.8	0.5
	Leg Cramps	1	0.2	0.5
	Myalgia	1.6	3.3	2.9
	Twitch	0.8	1	0.3
Nervous System	Agitation	1.6	3.5	1.8
	Anxiety	4.5	4.3	3.1
	CNS Stimulation	0	1.2	0.5
	Dizziness	7.1	8.6	5.5
	Hypertonia	1	1.2	0.5
	Insomnia	7.9	11.4	6.5
	Irritability	2.4	3.9	1.6
	Decreased Libido	1	0.6	0.5
	Nervousness	4.5	4.1	2.6
	Somnolence	2.6	2.0	2.1
	Tremor	3.1	6.1	0.8
Respiratory	Pharyngitis	1.3	2.9	1.8
	Rhinitis	9.9	6.7	9.6
	Sinusitis	1.6	2.4	2.1
Skin	Pruritus	2.4	2.2	1.6
	Rash	2.1	4.1	1.3
	Sweating	2.4	5.1	1.6
	Urticaria	0.8	1.4	0

(cont'd)

Table 1: WELLBUTRIN SR *(cont'd)*

Adverse Event (%) Placebo-Controlled Studies: Treatment-Emergent Adverse Experiences Occurring in ≥1% of Patients in Any BUP SR Group for Studies 203, 205, and 212

Body System	Adverse Experience	% AEs BUP SR 100–150 (n=382)	% AEs BUP SR 200–300 (n=491)	% AEs PBO (n=385)
Special Senses	Amblyopia	2.9	2.4	1.8
	Taste Perversion	1	1.4	0.3
	Tinnitus	3.9	5.1	1.8
Urogenital	Urinary Tract Infection	1	1.8	0.3
	Urinary Frequency	1.3	2.4	1.6

Body (General): Infrequent were chills, facial edema, musculoskeletal chest pain, and photosensitivity. Rare was malaise.
Cardiovascular: Infrequent were postural hypotension, stroke and vasodilation. Rare was syncope. Also observed were complete atrioventricular block, extrasystoles, hypotension, hypertension (in some cases severe, see Warnings and Precautions, Cardiovascular Effects), myocardial infarction, phlebitis, and pulmonary embolism.
Digestive: Infrequent were abnormal liver function, bruxism, gastric reflux, gingivitis, glossitis, increased salivation, jaundice, mouth ulcers, stomatitis, and thirst. Rare was edema of tongue. Also observed were colitis, esophagitis, gastrointestinal hemorrhage, gum hemorrhage, hepatitis, intestinal perforation, liver damage, pancreatitis, and stomach ulcer.
Endocrine: Also observed were hyperglycemia, hypoglycemia, and syndrome of inappropriate antidiuretic hormone.
Hemic and Lymphatic: Infrequent was ecchymosis. Also observed were anemia, leukocytosis, leukopenia, lymphadenopathy, pancytopenia, and thrombocytopenia.
Metabolic and Nutritional: Infrequent were edema and peripheral edema. Also observed was glycosuria.
Musculoskeletal: Also observed were arthritis, muscle rigidity/fever/ rhabdomyolysis and muscle weakness.
Nervous System: Infrequent were abnormal coordination, depersonalization, dysphoria, emotional lability, hostility, hyperkinesia, hypesthesia, suicidal ideation, and vertigo. Rare were amnesia, ataxia, derealization, and hypomania. Also observed were abnormal electroencephalogram (EEG), akinesia, aphasia, coma, delirium, dysarthria, dyskinesia, dystonia, euphoria, extrapyramidal syndrome, hallucinations, hypokinesia, increased libido, manic reaction, neuralgia, neuropathy, paranoid reaction, and unmasking tardive dyskinesia.
Respiratory: Rare was bronchospasm/dyspnea. Also observed was pneumonia and epistaxis.
Skin/Hypersensitivity: Rare was maculopapular rash. Also observed were alopecia, hirsutism, angioedema, exfoliative dermatitis, erythema multiforme, and Stevens-Johnson syndrome. Arthralgia, myalgia and fever have also been reported in association with rash and other symptoms suggestive of delayed hypersensitivity. These symptoms may resemble serum sickness.
Special Senses: Infrequent were accommodation abnormality and dry eye. Also observed were deafness, diplopia, and mydriasis.
Urogenital: Infrequent were impotence, polyuria, and prostate disorder. Also observed were abnormal ejaculation, cystitis, dyspareunia, dysuria, gynecomastia, menopause, painful erection, salpingitis, urinary incontinence, urinary retention, and vaginitis.
Seizures: Post-marketing reports suggest that the reintroduction of WELLBUTRIN SR in patients who experienced a seizure is associated with a risk of seizure reoccurrence in some cases. Thus, patients should not restart WELLBUTRIN SR therapy if they have had a seizure on a bupropion formulation (WELLBUTRIN SR, WELLBUTRIN XL, or ZYBAN). See Warnings and Precautions.
Drug Abuse and Dependence: WELLBUTRIN SR is likely to have a low abuse potential. There have been few reported cases of drug dependence and withdrawal symptoms associated with the immediate release formulation of bupropion. In human studies of abuse liability, individuals experienced with drugs of abuse reported that bupropion produced a feeling of euphoria and desirability. In these a single dose of 400 mg (1.33 times the recommended daily dose) of the immediate release formulation of bupropion produced mild amphetamine-like effects compared to placebo on the Morphine-Benzedrine Subscale of the Addiction Research Center Inventories (ARCI), which is indicative of euphorigenic properties and a score intermediate between placebo and amphetamine on the Liking Scale of the ARCI. Higher doses could not be tested because of the risk of seizure.
DRUG INTERACTIONS: Overview: In vitro studies indicate that bupropion is primarily metabolized to hydroxybupropion by the CYP2B6 isoenzyme (see Action and Clinical Pharmacology, Pharmacokinetics). Therefore, the potential exists for a drug interaction between WELLBUTRIN SR and drugs that affect the CYP2B6 isoenzyme (e.g., orphenadrine, and cyclophosphamide). The threohydrobupropion metabolite of bupropion does not appear to be produced by the cytochrome P450 isoenzymes. Few systematic data have been collected on the metabolism of WELLBUTRIN SR following concomitant administration with other drugs or alternatively, the effect of concomitant administration of WELLBUTRIN SR on the metabolism of other drugs.

Following chronic administration of bupropion, 100 mg t.i.d. to 8 healthy male volunteers for 14 days, there was no evidence of induction of its own metabolism.

Because bupropion is extensively metabolized, the coadministration of other drugs may affect its clinical activity. In particular, certain drugs may induce the metabolism of bupropion (e.g., carbamazepine, phenobarbital, phenytoin).
Drug-Drug Interactions: Drugs Metabolized by CYP2D6: Many drugs, including most antidepressants (SSRIs, many tricyclics), beta-blockers, antiarrhythmics, and antipsychotics are metabolized by the CYP2D6 isoenzyme. Although bupropion is not metabolized by this isoenzyme, bupropion and hydroxybupropion are inhibitors of CYP2D6 isoenzyme in vitro. In a study of 15 male subjects (ages 19 to 35 years) who were extensive metabolizers of the CYP2D6 isoenzyme, daily doses of bupropion given as 150 mg twice daily, followed by a single dose of 50 mg desipramine, increased the C_{max}, AUC, and $t_{1/2}$ of desipramine by an average of approximately two-, five- and two-fold, respectively. The effect was present for at least 7 days after the last dose of bupropion. Concomitant use of bupropion with other drugs metabolized by CYP2D6 has not been formally studied.
Co-Administration of Thioridazine Contraindicated: Administration of the antipsychotic thioridazine alone produces prolongation of the QTc interval, which is associated with serious ventricular arrhythmias such as torsades de pointes, and sudden death. As this effect appears to be dose-related, it is anticipated that risk increases with inhibition of thioridazine metabolism. An in-vivo study suggests that drugs which inhibit CYP2D6 will elevate plasma levels of thioridazine. Therefore concomitant use of thioridazine with WELLBUTRIN SR is contraindicated (see Contraindications).
Co-Administration of Other Drugs Metabolized by CYP2D6 Isoenzyme: Co-administration of bupropion with other drugs that are metabolized by CYP2D6 isoenzyme including certain antidepressants (e.g., nortriptyline, imipramine, desipramine, paroxetine, fluoxetine, sertraline), antipsychotics (e.g., haloperidol, risperidone), beta-blockers (e.g., metoprolol), and Type 1C antiarrhythmics (e.g., propafenone, flecainide), should be approached with caution and should be initiated at the lower end of the dose range of the concomitant medication. If bupropion is added to the treatment regimen of a patient already receiving a drug metabolized by CYP2D6, the need to decrease the dose of the original medication should be considered, particularly for those concomitant medications with a narrow therapeutic index.
MAO Inhibitors: Studies in animals demonstrate that the acute toxicity of bupropion is enhanced by the MAO inhibitor, phenelzine (see Contraindications).
Cimetidine: The effects of concomitant administration of cimetidine on the pharmacokinetics of bupropion and its active metabolites were examined in a crossover study in 24 healthy young male volunteers, following oral administration of two 150 mg WELLBUTRIN SR tablets with and without 800 mg of cimetidine. A single dose of cimetidine had no effect on single dose pharmacokinetic parameter estimates for bupropion, or hydroxybupropion, but caused a small statistically significant increase in the combined threohydro-erythrobupropion AUC (16%) and C_{max} (32%).
Levodopa and Amantadine: Limited clinical data suggest a higher incidence of neuropsychiatric adverse experiences, such as confusion, agitation and delirium, in patients receiving bupropion, concurrently with either levodopa or amantadine. Tremor, ataxia and dizziness were also reported. Administration of WELLBUTRIN SR to patients receiving either levodopa or amantadine concurrently should be undertaken with caution, using small initial doses and gradual dose increases.
Clopidogrel and Ticlopidine: Both clopidogrel and ticlopidine have been shown to significantly inhibit CYP2B6-catalysed bupropion hydroxylation. The mean area under the plasma concentration-time curve (AUC) of hydroxybupropion was reduced by 52% by clopidogrel and by 84% by ticlopidine. The AUC of bupropion was increased by 60% with clopidogrel and by 85% with ticlopidine. Therefore, concomitant administration of bupropion and either clopidogrel or ticlopidine may result in increased plasma concentrations of bupropion and reduced concentrations of hydroxybupropion. This may affect the efficacy of bupropion and may also increase the risk of concentration-dependent adverse events of bupropion, such as seizures (see Warnings and Precautions, Seizures). Patients receiving drugs used to reduce blood clots (such as either clopidogrel and/or ticlopidine) are likely to require dose adjustments of bupropion.
Use of WELLBUTRIN SR with Drugs that Predispose Patients to Seizures: Concurrent administration of WELLBUTRIN SR Tablets with agents that lower seizure threshold (e.g., antipsychotics, other antidepressants, theophylline, lithium, systemic steroids etc) should be undertaken only with extreme caution (see Warnings and Precautions). Low initial dosing and gradual dose increases should be employed.
Other Drugs with CNS Activity: The risk of using WELLBUTRIN SR in combination with other CNS-active drugs has not been systematically evaluated. Consequently, caution is advised if the concomitant administration of WELLBUTRIN SR and such drugs is required.
Transdermal Nicotine Interaction: (See Warnings and Precautions, Cardiovascular Effects.)
Alcohol Interactions: In post-marketing experience, there have been reports of adverse neuropsychiatric events, or reduced alcohol tolerance, in patients who were drinking alcohol during treatment with bupropion. Rarely, reports of fatal outcomes with this combination have been received; however, a causal relationship has not been established. The consumption of alcohol during treatment with bupropion should be avoided (also see Warnings and Precautions, Predisposing Risk Factors for Seizures).

DOSAGE AND ADMINISTRATION: WELLBUTRIN SR (bupropion hydrochloride) is not indicated for use in children under 18 years of age (See Warnings and Precautions, Potential Association with Behavioural and Emotional Changes, Including Self-harm).
Recommended Dose and Dosage Adjustment: The usual recommended dose of sustained release bupropion hydrochloride is 100 to 150 mg/day given once daily. As with all antidepressants, the full antidepressant effect of WELLBUTRIN SR may not be evident until several weeks of treatment. In patients who are not responding to a dose of 150 mg/day, the dose may be increased up to a maximum of 300 mg/day. Dose increases should occur at intervals of at least one week. **In order to minimize the risk of seizures (see Warnings and Precautions), single doses of WELLBUTRIN SR must not exceed 150 mg.** Doses of WELLBUTRIN SR greater than 150 mg/day should be administered b.i.d. preferably with at least 8 hours between successive doses.
Missed Dose: WELLBUTRIN SR should be taken at the same time each day and no more than the recommended dose should be taken each day. If the normal administration time has been missed, the dose should be skipped and administration resumed at the normal administration time of the following day.
Administration: Patients should be advised to swallow WELLBUTRIN SR Tablets whole with fluids, and **not** to chew, divide, crush or otherwise tamper with the tablets in any way that might affect the release rate of bupropion.
Treatment of Pregnant Women During the Third Trimester : Post-marketing reports indicate that some neonates exposed to WELLBUTRIN SR, SSRIs, or other newer antidepressants late in the third trimester have developed complications requiring prolonged hospitalization, respiratory support, and tube feeding (see Warnings and Precautions). When treating pregnant women with WELLBUTRIN SR during the third trimester, the physician should carefully consider the potential risks and benefits of treatment. The physician may consider tapering WELLBUTRIN SR in the third trimester.
Geriatrics or Debilitated Patients: No pharmacokinetic or therapeutic trials have been conducted to systematically investigate dose requirements in patients who are elderly or debilitated (see Warnings and Precautions). As such patients may have reduced clearance of bupropion and its metabolites, and/or increased sensitivity to the side-effects of CNS active drugs, treatment with sustained release bupropion hydrochloride should be initiated at the lowest recommended dose (100 mg/day).
Hepatic Impairment: Mild and Moderate Hepatic Impairment: Given the variable pharmacokinetics of bupropion in patients with either mild or moderate hepatic impairment (Child-Pugh Grade A or B), treatment with WELLBUTRIN SR should be initiated at the lowest recommended dose. Maintenance dose may be adjusted according to clinical response and tolerance. Caution should be exercised as there is no clinical experience with WELLBUTRIN SR in hepatically impaired patients (see also Warnings and Precautions).
Severe Impairment: Given the risks associated with both peak bupropion levels and drug accumulation, WELLBUTRIN SR is not recommended for use in patients with severe hepatic impairment. However, should clinical judgement deem it necessary, the drug should be used only with extreme caution (see also Warnings and Precautions). The dose should not exceed 150 mg every day or every other day in these patients. Any theoretical dose reduction for this patient population based on the findings of the pharmacokinetic studies may result in toxic drug levels in these patients (see Action and Clinical Pharmacology and Warnings and Precautions).
Renal Impairment: WELLBUTRIN SR should be used with caution in patients with renal impairment due to the potential for drug accumulation, and a reduced frequency and/or dose should be considered (see Action and Clinical Pharmacology and Warnings and Precautions).

All patients with hepatic or renal impairment should be closely monitored for possible adverse effects (e.g., insomnia, dry mouth, seizures) that could indicate high drug or metabolite levels.
Pediatrics: WELLBUTRIN SR is not indicated for use in children under 18 years of age (see Indications and Clinical Use and Warnings and Precautions, Potential Association with Behavioural and Emotional Changes, Including Self-harm).

OVERDOSAGE:
Human Overdose Experience: In addition to those events reported under Adverse Reactions, overdose has resulted in symptoms including drowsiness, loss of consciousness and ECG changes such as conduction disturbances (including QRS prolongation) or arrhythmias. Three overdoses with WELLBUTRIN SR (bupropion hydrochloride) occurred during clinical trials. One patient ingested 3000 mg of WELLBUTRIN SR tablets and vomited quickly after the overdose; the patient experienced blurred vision and lightheadedness. A second patient ingested a "handful" of WELLBUTRIN SR tablets and experienced confusion, lethargy, nausea, jitteriness, and seizure. A third patient ingested 3600 mg of WELLBUTRIN SR tablets and a bottle of wine; the patient experienced nausea, visual hallucinations, and "grogginess". None of the patients experienced further sequelae.

The information included in the remainder of this section is based on the clinical experience with overdosage of the immediate release formulation of bupropion. Thirteen overdoses occurred during clinical trials. Twelve patients ingested 850 to 4200 mg and recovered without significant sequelae. Another patient who ingested 9000 mg of WELLBUTRIN and 300 mg of tranylcypromine experienced a grand mal seizure and recovered without further sequelae.

Since introduction, overdoses of up to 17 500 mg of WELLBUTRIN, the immediate release formulation of bupropion, have been reported. Seizure was reported in approximately one-third of all cases. Other serious reactions reported with overdoses of WELLBUTRIN alone included hallucinations, loss of consciousness, and sinus tachycardia. Fever, muscle rigidity, rhabdomyolysis, hypotension, stupor, coma, and respiratory failure have been reported when WELLBUTRIN was part of multiple drug overdoses.

Although most patients recovered without sequelae, deaths associated with overdoses of WELLBUTRIN alone have been reported rarely in patients ingesting massive doses of WELLBUTRIN Tablets. Multiple uncontrolled seizures, bradycardia, cardiac failure, and cardiac arrest prior to death were reported in these patients.
Management of Overdose: In the event of overdose, hospitalization is advised. Ensure an adequate airway, oxygenation, and ventilation. Monitor cardiac rhythm (ECG) and vital signs EEG monitoring is also recommended for the first 48 hours post-ingestion. General supportive and symptomatic measures are also recommended. Induction of emesis is not recommended. Gastric lavage with a large-bore orogastric tube with appropriate airway protection, if needed, may be indicated if performed soon after ingestion or in symptomatic patients.

Activated charcoal should be administered. There is no experience with the use of forced diuresis, dialysis, hemoperfusion, or exchange transfusion in the management of bupropion overdoses. No specific antidotes for bupropion are known.

Due to the dose-related risk of seizures with WELLBUTRIN SR, hospitalization following suspected overdose should be considered. Based on studies in animals, it is recommended that seizures be treated with intravenous benzodiazepine administration and other supportive measures, as appropriate.

In managing overdosage, consider the possibility of multiple drug involvement. The physician should consider contacting a poison control center for additional information on the treatment of any overdose. Telephone numbers for certified poison control centers are listed in the *Compendium of Pharmaceuticals and Specialties* (CPS).

For management of a suspected drug overdose, CPhA recommends that you contact your **regional Poison Control Centre**. See the *CPS* Directory section for a list of Poison Control Centres.

ACTION AND CLINICAL PHARMACOLOGY: WELLBUTRIN SR (bupropion hydrochloride) is an antidepressant of the aminoketone class. It is chemically unrelated to tricyclic, tetracyclic, selective serotonin re-uptake inhibitors or other known antidepressant agents. Its structure closely resembles that of diethylpropion. It is related to the phenylethylamines.

Mechanism of Action: The mechanism of bupropion's antidepressant activity is unknown but appears to be mediated by noradrenergic (and possibly dopaminergic), rather than serotonergic mechanisms. Preclinical studies have shown that bupropion blocks norepinephrine (NE) reuptake and dopamine (DA) reuptake. Its major metabolite (hydroxybupropion), which in man is present at blood levels 10-20-fold higher than bupropion, blocks only NE reuptake.

The non-serotonergic mechanism of action of bupropion likely contributes to a distinct side effect profile that includes low rates of sexual dysfunction and somnolence.

Pharmacodynamics: In vitro, bupropion and its major metabolites had essentially no affinity for β-adrenergic, dopaminergic, GABA, benzodiazepine, 5HT1A, glycine and adenosine receptors, and only weakly inhibited α-adrenergic receptors in rat brain, α2-adrenergic, 5HT2, and muscarinic cholinergic receptors. High concentrations of bupropion and its major metabolites did not inhibit MAO-A or MAO-B activity. Bupropion and its major metabolites had no significant affinity for the 5HT transport system.

Pharmacokinetics: Absorption: Bupropion has not been administered intravenously to humans; therefore, the absolute bioavailability of WELLBUTRIN SR Tablets in humans has not been determined. In rat and dog studies, the bioavailability of bupropion ranged from 5% to 20%. Following oral administration of WELLBUTRIN SR to healthy volunteers, peak plasma concentrations of bupropion are achieved within 3 hours. In two single-dose (150 mg) studies the mean peak concentration (C_{max}) values were 91 and 143 ng/mL. At steady state, the mean C_{max} following a 150 mg dose every 12 hours was 136 ng/mL.

Three studies in healthy volunteers suggest that exposure to bupropion may be increased when sustained release bupropion tablets are taken with food. When taken following food, peak plasma concentration of bupropion (C_{max}) increased by 11%, 16% and 35% in three studies. The overall exposure to bupropion (AUC) increased by 17%, 17% and 19% in these three studies.

Distribution: In vitro tests show that bupropion is 84% bound to human plasma proteins at concentrations up to 200 μg/mL. The extent of protein binding of hydroxybupropion is similar to that of bupropion, whereas the extent of protein binding of the threohydrobupropion metabolite is about half that seen with bupropion. The volume of distribution (V_{ss}/F) estimated from a single 150 mg dose given to 17 subjects is 1950 L (20% CV).

Metabolism: Bupropion is extensively metabolized in humans. There are three active metabolites: hydroxybupropion and the amino-alcohol isomers threohydrobupropion and erythrohydrobupropion, which are formed via hydroxylation of the tert-butyl group of bupropion and/or reduction of the carbonyl group. Oxidation of the bupropion side chain results in the formation of a glycine conjugate of meta-chlorobenzoic acid, which is then excreted as the major urinary metabolite. In preclinical tests used to predict antidepressant activity, it has been observed that hydroxybupropion is comparable in potency to bupropion, while the other metabolites are one half to one tenth as potent. This may be of clinical importance because the plasma concentrations of the metabolites are higher than those of bupropion.

In vitro results indicate that biotransformation of bupropion to hydroxybupropion is catalyzed primarily by CYP2B6, and to a much lesser extent by CYP1A2, 2A6, 2C9, 2E1 and 3A4 isozymes. Detectable levels of hydroxybupropion are not observed with CYP1A1 and CYP2D6 isozymes. Cytochrome P450 isoenzymes are not involved in the formation of threohydrobupropion. Following a single 150 mg dose of bupropion in humans, peak plasma concentrations of hydroxybupropion occur approximately 6 hours after administration. Peak plasma concentrations of hydroxybupropion are approximately 10 times the peak level of the parent drug at steady state. The AUC of hydroxybupropion at steady state is about 17 fold higher than that of bupropion. The times to peak concentrations for the erythrohydrobupropion and threohydrobupropion metabolites are similar to that of hydroxybupropion, and steady-state AUCs are 1.5 and 7 times that of bupropion, respectively.

Because bupropion is extensively metabolized, there is the potential for drug-drug interactions, particularly with those agents that are metabolized by the CYP2B6 isoenzyme. Although bupropion is not metabolized by CYP2D6, there is the potential for drug-drug interactions when bupropion is co-administered with drugs metabolized by this isoenzyme (see Drug Interactions).

Excretion: In two single-dose (150 mg) studies the mean (±% CV) apparent clearance (Cl/F) of bupropion was 135 (±20%) and 209 L/h (±21%). Following chronic dosing of 150 mg of WELLBUTRIN SR every 12 hours for 14 days (n=34), the mean Cl/F at steady state was 160 L/h (±23%). The mean elimination half-life of bupropion (estimated from a series of studies) is approximately 21 hours. Estimates of the half-lives of the metabolites determined from a multiple-dose study were 20 hours (25%) for hydroxybupropion, 37 hours (35%) for threohydrobupropion, and 33 hours (30%) for erythrohydrobupropion. Steady-state plasma concentrations of bupropion and metabolites are reached within 5 and 8 days, respectively. Following oral administration of 200 mg of ^{14}C-bupropion in humans, 87% and 10% of the radioactive dose were recovered in the urine and feces, respectively. The fraction of the oral dose of bupropion excreted unchanged was only 0.5%. Bupropion and its metabolites exhibit linear kinetics following chronic administration of 150 to 300 mg/day.

Special Populations and Conditions: Factors or conditions altering metabolic capacity (e.g., liver disease, congestive heart failure, age, concomitant medications, etc.) or elimination may be expected to influence the degree and extent of accumulation of the active metabolites of bupropion. The elimination of the major metabolites of bupropion may be affected by reduced renal or hepatic function because they are moderately polar compounds and are likely to undergo further metabolism or conjugation in the liver prior to urinary excretion.

Pediatrics: The pharmacokinetics of WELLBUTRIN SR in individuals under 18 years old has not been evaluated.

Geriatrics: The effects of age on the pharmacokinetics of bupropion and its metabolites have not been fully characterized, but an exploration of steady state bupropion concentrations from several depression efficacy studies involving patients dosed in a range of 300 to 750 mg/day, on a three times a day schedule, revealed no relationship between age (18 to 83 years) and plasma concentration of bupropion. A single-dose pharmacokinetic study demonstrated that the disposition of bupropion and its metabolites in elderly subjects was similar to that of younger subjects. These data suggest there is no prominent effect of age on bupropion concentration: however, another single and multiple dose pharmacokinetic study, has suggested that the elderly are at increased risk for accumulation of bupropion and its metabolites (see Warnings and Precautions and Dosage and Administration).

Race: The influence of race (Asian, Black and Caucasian) on the pharmacokinetics of bupropion (bupropion hydrochloride immediate release tablets) was evaluated based on dose normalized data pooled from five healthy volunteer studies. A comparison of pharmacokinetic parameter values did not detect any important differences in race with respect to AUC (p=0.5564) and C_{max} (p=0.8184).

Hepatic Insufficiency: The effect of hepatic impairment on the pharmacokinetics of bupropion was characterized in two single-dose studies, one in subjects with alcoholic liver disease and one in subjects with mild to severe liver cirrhosis.

The first study involved 8 subjects with alcoholic liver disease, and 8 healthy matched controls. While mean AUC values were not significantly different, individual AUC values for both the parent drug bupropion and the primary metabolite hydroxybupropion were more variable in subjects with alcoholic liver disease, and increased by approximately 50% over those of healthy volunteers. The mean half-life of the primary metabolite hydroxybupropion was significantly longer by approximately 40% in subjects with alcoholic liver disease than in healthy volunteers (32±14 hours versus 21±5 hours, respectively). For all other pharmacokinetic values, for both parent drug and metabolites, there were minimal differences between the two groups.

The second study involved 17 subjects with hepatic impairment (n=9 mild/Grade A child-Pugh rating; n=8 severe/Grade C Child-Pugh rating) and 8 healthy matched controls. In the severe group, the mean value for bupropion AUC was increased threefold over control values, with mean clearance decreased proportionately. Mean C_{max} and plasma half-life were increased by approximately 70% and 40% respectively. For the primary metabolites, mean AUC was increased by approximately 30%-50%, with mean clearance decreased proportionately. Mean C_{max} was lower by approximately 30% to 70%, and mean plasma half life increased threefold.

In the mild group, while mean values were not statistically increased from those of controls, the variability in the pharmacokinetic values was higher in the subjects with impairment; a sub-group of 1 to 3 subjects (dependent on pharmacokinetic parameter examined) showed individual values which were in the range of the severely impaired subjects. For the primary metabolites, the differences between groups in pharmacokinetic parameters were minimal.

In patients with hepatic impairment, treatment should be initiated at reduced dosage (see Warnings and Precautions and Dosage and Administration).

Effect of Smoking: In a single dose study, there were no significant differences in the pharmacokinetics of bupropion or its major metabolites in smokers compared with non-smokers.

STORAGE AND STABILITY: Store at room temperature (15-25°C).

INFORMATION FOR THE PATIENT: Published in e-CPS, available by subscription at www.e-cps.ca.

DOSAGE FORMS, COMPOSITION AND PACKAGING: Each purple, round, biconvex, film-coated, sustained-release tablet, printed "WELLBUTRIN SR 150", contains: bupropion HCl 150 mg. Nonmedicinal ingredients: carnauba wax, cysteine HCl, edible black ink, FD&C Blue No. 2 Lake, FD&C Red No. 40 Lake, hydroxypropyl methylcellulose, magnesium stearate, microcrystalline cellulose, polyethylene glycol, polysorbate 80 and titanium dioxide. Bottles of 60.

(Shown in Product Identification Section)

For assistance in the visual identification of drug dosage forms, refer to the PRODUCT IDENTIFICATION SECTION.

Wellbutrin® XL ℞

bupropion HCl

Antidepressant

Biovail Pharmaceuticals

Date of Preparation: August 22, 2008
Date of Revision: February 4, 2009

SUMMARY PRODUCT INFORMATION:

Route of Administration	Dosage Form/ Strength	Clinically Relevant Nonmedicinal Ingredients
Oral	Tablets: 150 mg and 300 mg	Tablet components: denatured ethyl alcohol, ethylcellulose, glyceryl behenate, isopropyl alcohol, methylacrylic acid co-polymer dispersion, polyethylene glycol, polyvinyl alcohol, povidone, silicon dioxide, triethyl citrate, N-butyl alcohol, propylene glycol, shellac glaze, titanium dioxide, and red and blue FDC dyes (150 mg), iron oxide black (300 mg). For complete information see Dosage Forms, Composition and Packaging.

INDICATIONS AND CLINICAL USE: Adults: Major Depressive Disorder: WELLBUTRIN XL is indicated for the symptomatic relief of major depressive illness. The efficacy of WELLBUTRIN XL for the treatment of major depressive episode was established in three, double-blind, 8 week, placebo-controlled trials, in adult outpatients with a history of major depressive illness. The effectiveness of WELLBUTRIN XL in long-term use (greater than 8 weeks) has not been evaluated in controlled trials. Therefore, the physician who elects to use WELLBUTRIN XL for extended periods should periodically re-evaluate the long-term usefulness of the drug for the individual patient.

Prevention of Seasonal Major Depressive Episodes: WELLBUTRIN XL is indicated for the prevention of major depressive illness with an autumn-winter seasonal pattern.

The efficacy of WELLBUTRIN XL for the prevention of seasonal major depressive episodes was established in three double-blind, placebo-controlled trials in adult outpatients with a history of major depressive disorder with an autumnal-winter seasonal pattern as defined by Diagnostic and Statistical Manual of Mental Disorders, 4th edition (DSM-IV) criteria. Treatment duration was approximately 4 to 6 months.

The efficacy of WELLBUTRIN XL in preventing seasonal depressive episodes has not been compared to light therapy.

Pediatrics (<18 years of age): WELLBUTRIN XL is not indicated for use in patients below the age of 18 years (see Warnings and Precautions, Potential Association with Behavioural and Emotional Changes, Including Self-Harm).

CONTRAINDICATIONS: To reduce the risk of seizures, WELLBUTRIN XL (bupropion hydrochloride) is contraindicated in patients:

- receiving other medications that contain bupropion hydrochloride such as WELLBUTRIN SR, and ZYBAN, because the incidence of seizure is dose dependent (see Warnings and Precautions)
- with a current seizure disorder (see Warnings and Precautions)
- with a current or prior diagnosis of bulimia or anorexia nervosa because of a higher incidence of seizures (see Warnings and Precautions) noted in patients treated for bulimia with the immediate release formulation of bupropion
- undergoing abrupt withdrawal from alcohol or benzodiazepines or other sedatives

To reduce risks due to drug interaction, the concomitant use of WELLBUTRIN XL is contraindicated in patients currently taking:

- Monoamine oxidase (MAO) inhibitors.
- the antipsychotic thioridazine, since bupropion may inhibit thioridazine metabolism, thus causing an increase in thioridazine levels and a potential increased risk of thioridazine-related serious ventricular arrhythmias and sudden death.

  At least 14 days should elapse between discontinuation of one drug and the start of another.

WELLBUTRIN XL is contraindicated in patients with known hypersensitivity to bupropion or to any of the components of the formulation.

WARNINGS AND PRECAUTIONS: Potential Association with Behavioural and Emotional Changes, Including Self-Harm:
Pediatrics: Placebo-Controlled Clinical Trial Data:

- **Recent analyses of placebo-controlled clinical trial safety databases from SSRIs and other newer antidepressants suggests that use of these drugs in patients under the age of 18 may be associated with behavioural and emotional changes, including an increased risk of suicidal ideation and behaviour over that of placebo.**
- **The small denominators in the clinical trial database, as well as the variability in placebo rates, preclude reliable conclusions on the relative safety profiles among these drugs.**

Adults and Pediatrics: Additional Data:

- **There are clinical trial and post-marketing reports with SSRIs and other newer antidepressants, in both pediatrics and adults, of severe agitation-type adverse events coupled with self-harm or harm to others. The agitation-type events include: akathisia, agitation, disinhibition, emotional lability, hostility, aggression, depersonalization. In some cases, the events occurred within several weeks of starting treatment.**

Rigorous clinical monitoring for suicidal ideation or other indicators of potential for suicidal behaviour is advised in patients of all ages given an antidepressant drug. This includes monitoring for agitation-type emotional and behavioural changes.

Seizures: Patients should be made aware that WELLBUTRIN XL contains the same active ingredient (bupropion hydrochloride) as ZYBAN and WELLBUTRIN SR. WELLBUTRIN XL should **not** be administered to patients already receiving a product containing bupropion hydrochloride (see Contraindications).

The recommended dose of extended release bupropion tablets should not be exceeded, since bupropion is associated with a dose-related risk of seizure. The overall incidence of seizure with WELLBUTRIN XL in clinical trials at doses up to 450 mg/day was approximately 0.1% (2 of 2146 subjects/patients). Seizure incidence in clinical trials with doses of 450 mg/day was approximately 0.39% (2 of 537 subjects). There were no seizures in clinical trials where subjects (n=1638) were treated up to the maximum recommended dose of 300 mg/day. In post marketing data however, seizures have been observed across all doses and formulations of WELLBUTRIN.

Predisposing Risk Factors for Seizures: The risk of seizure occurring with bupropion use appears to be associated with the presence of predisposing risk factors. Therefore extreme caution should be used when treating patients with predisposing factors which increase the risk of seizures, including: history of head trauma or prior seizure; central nervous system (CNS) tumour; the presence of severe hepatic impairment; excessive use of alcohol; addiction to opiates, cocaine, or stimulants; use of concomitant medications that lower seizure threshold, including but not limited to: antipsychotics, antidepressants, lithium, amantadine, theophylline systemic steroids, quinolone antibiotics, and anti-malarials; use of over-the-counter stimulants or anorectics; diabetes treated with oral hypoglycemics or insulin.

The above group of risk factors, including medications, should not be considered exhaustive; for each patient, all potential predisposing factors must be carefully considered.

In Order to Minimize the Risk of Seizure: The total daily dose of WELLBUTRIN XL must not exceed 300 mg (the maximum recommended dose).

If a Seizure Occurs: Patients should be warned that if they experience a seizure while taking WELLBUTRIN XL, they should contact their doctor or be taken to a hospital emergency ward immediately, and should stop taking WELLBUTRIN XL. Treatment should not be restarted if a patient has experienced a seizure while taking WELLBUTRIN XL, WELLBUTRIN SR or ZYBAN.

Potential for Hepatotoxicity: In rats receiving large doses of bupropion chronically, there was an increase in incidence of hepatic hyperplastic nodules and hepatocellular hypertrophy. In dogs receiving large doses of bupropion chronically, various histologic changes were seen in the liver, and laboratory tests suggesting mild hepatocellular injury were noted.

Clinical Worsening and Suicide: The possibility of a suicide attempt in seriously depressed patients is inherent to the illness and may persist until significant remission occurs. Patients with depression may experience worsening of their depressive symptoms and/or the emergence of suicidal ideation and behaviours (suicidality) whether or not they are taking antidepressant medications. As improvement may not occur during the first few weeks or more of treatment, patients should be closely monitored for clinical worsening (including development of new symptoms) and suicidality, especially at the beginning of a course of treatment, or at the time of dosage changes, either increases or decreases. Close supervision of high risk patients should accompany initial drug therapy, and consideration should be given to the need for hospitalization. (See Warnings and Precautions, Potential Association with Behavioural and Emotional Changes, Including Self-Harm.)

It should be noted that a causal role for SSRIs and other newer antidepressants in inducing self-harm or harm to others has not been established. In order to reduce the risk of overdose, prescriptions for WELLBUTRIN XL (bupropion hydrochloride) should be written for the smallest number of tablets consistent with good patient management.

Allergic Reactions: Anaphylactoid/anaphylactic reactions characterized by symptoms such as pruritus, urticaria, angioedema, and dyspnea requiring medical treatment have been reported in clinical trials with bupropion at a rate of 1-3 per thousand. In addition, there have been rare spontaneous postmarketing reports of erythema multiforme, Stevens-Johnson syndrome, and anaphylactic shock associated with bupropion. In uncontrolled and controlled clinical trials, skin disorders, primarily rashes, pruritus, and urticaria, lead to discontinuation of 1.5% and 1.9 %, respectively of bupropion-treated subjects. A patient should stop taking WELLBUTRIN XL and consult a doctor if experiencing allergic or anaphylactoid/anaphylactic reactions (e.g., skin rash, pruritus, hives, chest pain, edema, and shortness of breath) during treatment.

Arthralgia, myalgia and fever have also been reported in association with rash and other symptoms suggestive of delayed hypersensitivity. These symptoms may resemble serum sickness.

Bupropion should be discontinued immediately if any hypersensitivity reactions are experienced. Symptoms of hypersensitivity should be treated in accordance with established medical practice. Clinicians should be aware that symptoms may persist beyond the discontinuation of bupropion, and clinical management should be provided accordingly. In post-market experience, there have been reports of hypersensitivity reactions in patients who consumed alcohol while taking bupropion. As the contribution of alcohol to these reactions has been established, patients should avoid alcohol when they are taking bupropion (see Drug Interactions, Alcohol Interactions).

Agitation and Insomnia: In placebo controlled trials patients receiving WELLBUTRIN SR Tablets experienced an increased incidence of insomnia and anxiety relative to those receiving placebo (see Adverse Reactions and Warnings and Precautions, Potential Association with Behavioural and Emotional Changes, Including Self-Harm). These symptoms were sometimes of sufficient magnitude to require discontinuation of WELLBUTRIN SR, or concurrent treatment with sedative/hypnotic drugs. Insomnia may be minimized by avoiding bedtime doses and, if necessary, reduction in dose.

Psychosis, Confusion, and Other Neuropsychiatric Phenomena: Patients treated with WELLBUTRIN SR have been reported to show a variety of neuropsychiatric signs and symptoms including delusions, hallucinations, psychosis, concentration disturbance, paranoia and confusion. In some cases these abated upon dose reduction and/or withdrawal of treatment.

Activation of Psychosis and/or Mania: Antidepressants can precipitate manic episodes in bipolar patients during the depressed phase of their illness and may activate latent psychosis in other susceptible patients. WELLBUTRIN XL is expected to pose similar risks.

Altered Appetite and Weight: In clinical trials WELLBUTRIN SR was associated with dose-related weight loss. In eight week controlled trials mean weight loss for trial completers was 0.1 kg for placebo, 0.8 kg for WELLBUTRIN SR 100 mg/day, 1.4 kg at 150 mg/day, and 2.3 kg at 300 mg/day.

In 3 placebo-controlled clinical trials of seasonal depression using WELLBUTRIN XL (up to 6 months of treatment), 23% of subjects who received WELLBUTRIN XL lost >5 lbs, compared to 11% of subjects who received placebo. The mean weight change from baseline to the subject's last visit was −0.9 kg in the WELLBUTRIN XL group and 0.8 kg in the placebo group.

If weight loss is a major presenting sign of a patient's depressive illness, the potential anorectic and/or weight reducing effect of bupropion hydrochloride should be considered.

Cardiovascular: In clinical practice, hypertension, in some cases severe, requiring acute treatment, has been reported in patients receiving bupropion alone and in combination with nicotine replacement therapy. These events have been observed in both patients with and without evidence of preexisting hypertension.

Data from a comparative study of the sustained-release formulation of bupropion (ZYBAN Sustained-Release Tablets), nicotine transdermal system (NTS), the combination of sustained-release bupropion plus NTS, and placebo as an aid to smoking cessation suggest a higher incidence of treatment-emergent hypertension in patients treated with the combination of sustained-release bupropion and NTS. In this study, 6.1% of patients treated with the combination of sustained-release bupropion and NTS had treatment-emergent hypertension compared to 2.5%, 1.6%, and 3.1% of patients treated with sustained-release bupropion, NTS, and placebo, respectively. The majority of these patients had evidence of preexisting hypertension. Three patients (1.2%) treated with the combination of ZYBAN and NTS and one patient (0.4%) treated with NTS had study medication discontinued due to hypertension compared to none of the patients treated with ZYBAN or placebo. Monitoring of blood pressure is recommended in patients who receive the combination of bupropion and nicotine replacement.

There is no clinical experience establishing the safety of bupropion in patients with a recent history of myocardial infarction or unstable heart disease. Therefore, care should be exercised if it is used in these groups. In a study of depressed inpatients with stable heart failure, bupropion was associated with a rise in supine blood pressure, resulting in discontinuation of two patients for exacerbation of baseline hypertension.

Hepatic Impairment: The results of two single dose pharmacokinetic studies indicate that the clearance of bupropion is reduced in all subjects with Child-Pugh Grades C hepatic impairment, and in some subjects with milder forms of liver impairment. Given the risks associated with both peak bupropion levels and drug accumulation, WELLBUTRIN XL is not recommended for use in patients with severe hepatic impairment. However, should clinical judgement deem it necessary, it should be used only with extreme caution at a reduced dose, to a maximum dose of 150 mg every other day.

All patients with hepatic impairment should be closely monitored for possible adverse effects (e.g., insomnia, dry mouth, seizures) that could indicate high drug or metabolite levels (see Dosage and Administration and Action and Clinical Pharmacology).

Renal Impairment: Bupropion is extensively metabolized in the liver to active metabolites, which are largely further metabolised before being excreted by the kidneys. WELLBUTRIN XL treatment of patients with renal impairment should be initiated at a reduced dosage regimen, as metabolites may accumulate in such patients to a greater extent than usual. The patient should be closely monitored for possible adverse effects (eg., insomnia, dry mouth, seizures) that could indicate high drug or metabolite levels.

Occupational Hazards: Any psychoactive drug may impair judgement, thinking or motor skills. Therefore patients should be cautioned about operating hazardous machinery, including automobiles, until they are reasonably certain that the drug treatment does not affect their performance adversely.

Special Populations: Pregnant Women: Pregnancy, Labour and Delivery: There are no adequate and well-controlled studies of WELLBUTRIN XL in pregnant women. WELLBUTRIN XL should thus not be used during pregnancy unless the potential benefit is judged to outweigh the potential risk.

Post-marketing reports indicate that some neonates exposed to SSRIs (Selective Serotonin Reuptake Inhibitors), or other newer antidepressants, such as WELLBUTRIN SR, late in the third trimester have developed complications requiring prolonged hospitalization, respiratory support, and tube feeding. Such complications can arise immediately upon delivery. Reported clinical findings have included respiratory distress, cyanosis, apnea, seizures, temperature instability, feeding difficulty, vomiting, hypoglycemia, hypotonia, hyperreflexia, tremor, jitteriness, irritability, and constant crying. The frequency of symptoms may vary with each drug. These features are consistent with either a direct toxic effect of SSRIs and other newer antidepressants, or, possibly, a drug discontinuation syndrome. When treating a pregnant woman with WELLBUTRIN XL during the third trimester, the physician should carefully consider the potential risks and benefits of treatment. (See Dosage and Administration.)

Nursing Women: Like many other drugs, bupropion and its metabolites are secreted in human milk. Because of the potential for serious adverse reactions in nursing infants from WELLBUTRIN XL, a decision should be made whether to discontinue nursing or to discontinue the drug, taking into account the importance of the drug to the mother.

Pediatrics (<18 years of age): WELLBUTRIN XL is not indicated for use in patients below the age of 18 years (see Warnings and Precautions, Potential Association with Behavioural and Emotional Changes, Including Self-Harm). See also Indications and Clinical Use, Pediatrics (<18 years of age) and Dosage and Administration, Special Patient Populations, Pediatrics.

Geriatrics: Of the approximately 6000 patients who participated in clinical trials with bupropion sustained-release tablets (depression and smoking cessation studies), 275 were 65 and over and 47 were 75 and over. In addition, several hundred patients 65 and over participated in clinical trials using the immediate-release formulation of bupropion (depression studies). No overall differences in safety or effectiveness were observed between these subjects and younger subjects, and other reported clinical experience has not identified differences in responses between the elderly and younger patients, but greater sensitivity of some older individuals cannot be ruled out.

A single-dose pharmacokinetic study demonstrated that the disposition of bupropion and its metabolites in elderly subjects was similar to that of younger subjects; however, another single and multiple dose pharmacokinetic study, has suggested that the elderly are at increased risk for accumulation of bupropion and its metabolites (see Action and Clinical Pharmacology, Pharmacokinetics).

Bupropion is extensively metabolized in the liver to active metabolites, of which some are eliminated by the kidney, while others are further metabolized before being excreted in urine. The risk of toxic reaction to this drug may be greater in patients with impaired renal function. Because elderly patients are more likely to have decreased renal function, care should be taken in dose selection, and it may be useful to monitor renal function (see Warnings and Precautions, Hepatic Impairment or Renal Impairment).

ADVERSE REACTIONS: Adverse Drug Reaction Overview: The information included under Adverse Reactions is based on data from clinical trials with WELLBUTRIN XL (bupropion hydrochloride), the once daily extended release formulation of bupropion in the treatment of major depressive disorder (MDD) and prevention of seasonal major depressive episodes. Information on additional adverse events associated with the sustained release formulation of bupropion as well as the immediate release formulation of bupropion, is included in a separate subsection (see Events Observed During Development and Post-Marketing Experience of Bupropion with Other Formulations or Indications).

Incidence of Commonly Observed Adverse Events in Controlled Clinical Trials: Major Depressive Disorder: The most common adverse events encountered in WELLBUTRIN XL MDD clinical trials (incidence of ≥5% and higher incidence in WELLBUTRIN XL treated than placebo treated) were, dry mouth, nausea, constipation, insomnia, dizziness, anxiety, decreased appetite.

Prevention of Seasonal Major Depressive Episodes: The most common adverse events encountered in WELLBUTRIN XL seasonal depression clinical trials (incidence of ≥5% and higher incidence with WELLBUTRIN XL than placebo) were , dry mouth, nausea, constipation, flatulence, headache, dizziness, insomnia, anxiety, nasopharyngitis, upper respiratory infection, and sinusitis.

Adverse Events Associated with Discontinuation of Treatment: Major Depressive Disorder: In placebo controlled studies in depression (411 patients treated with WELLBUTRIN XL, and 412 treated with placebo), adverse events caused discontinuation in 6% of WELLBUTRIN XL-treated patients and 3% of placebo-treated patients. All adverse events leading to discontinuation of WELLBUTRIN XL occurred with an incidence of less than 1%.

Prevention of Seasonal Major Depression: In placebo-controlled clinical trials, 9% of patients treated with WELLBUTRIN XL and 5% of patients treated with placebo discontinued treatment due to adverse events. The adverse events in these trials that led to discontinuation in at least 1% of patients treated with WELLBUTRIN XL and at a rate numerically greater than the placebo rate were insomnia (2% vs <1%) and headache (1% vs <1%).

Prospective Studies in Major Depressive Disorder Trials to Assess Drug-related Adverse Events on Sexual Function: Using identical protocols, studies AK130926 and AK130927 set orgasm dysfunction as a primary outcome measure, in addition to the HAMD-17 score. The studies compared the effects of WELLBUTRIN XL, placebo and a representative SSRI as a positive control, in a sample of depressed subjects with normal orgasmic function at baseline. Orgasm dysfunction, as defined by presence of orgasm delay, orgasm failure, or both, was based on investigator interview at the 0, 2, 4, 6 and 8 week points in the study.

In each of the two studies, AK130926 and AK130927, the percentage of subjects with orgasm dysfunction in the WELLBUTRIN XL groups (16% and 13%) were not significantly different from the placebo groups (8% and 11%). Statistically, these observed rates in both the placebo groups and the WELLBUTRIN XL groups were significantly lower as compared to the SSRI positive control groups (29% and 32%).

Clinical Trial Adverse Drug Reactions: Because clinical trials are conducted under very specific conditions the adverse reaction rates observed in the clinical trials may not reflect the rates observed in practice and should not be compared to the rates in the clinical trials of another drug. Adverse drug reaction information from clinical trials is useful for identifying drug-related adverse events and for approximating rates.

Major Depressive Disorder (MDD): Table 1 enumerates treatment-emergent adverse events that occurred at an incidence of 1% or more in placebo-controlled trials, and were more frequent in the WELLBUTRIN XL group than the placebo group. Reported adverse events were classified using MedDRA. (Treatment-Emergent adverse events related to sexual function were assessed using specific outcome measures in two placebo-controlled studies—see Adverse Reactions, Prospective Studies in Major Depressive Disorder Trials to Assess Drug-related Adverse Events on Sexual Function).

Table 1: WELLBUTRIN XL

Adverse Events in MDD Placebo-Controlled Studies: Treatment-Emergent Adverse Experiences Occurring in ≥1% of Patients taking WELLBUTRIN XL (with an incidence greater than placebo)

System Organ Class	Preferred Term	Pooled Results	
		Placebo n=412	WELLBUTRIN XL n=411
Cardiac Disorders	Palpitations	10 (2%)	13 (3%)
Ear and Labyrinth Disorders	Tinnitus	3 (<1%)	11 (3%)
Eye Disorders	Vision Blurred	4 (<1%)	8 (2%)
Gastrointestinal Disorders	Nausea	42 (10%)	63 (15%)
	Dry Mouth	38 (9%)	79 (19%)
	Constipation	27 (7%)	41 (10%)
	Abdominal Upper Pain	7 (2%)	17 (4%)
	Vomiting	8 (2%)	10 (2%)
	Abdominal Pain	5 (1%)	6 (1%)
General Disorders	Feeling Jittery	6 (1%)	9 (2%)
	Pyrexia	4 (<1%)	5 (1%)
	Chest Pain	2 (<1%)	5 (1%)
	Chest Discomfort	0	5 (1%)
Infections & Infestations	Nasopharyngitis	11 (3%)	16 (4%)
	Influenza	6 (1%)	8 (2%)
Investigations	Weight Decreased	1 (<1%)	8 (2%)
	Heart Rate Increased	0	6 (1%)
Metabolism and Nutrition	Decreased Appetite	14 (3%)	19 (5%)
Musculoskeletal Disorders	Myalgia	7 (2%)	10 (2%)
Nervous System Disorders	Dizziness	15 (4%)	32 (8%)
	Tremor	4 (<1%)	17 (4%)
	Dysgeusia	2 (<1%)	12 (3%)
Psychiatric Disorders	Insomnia	17 (4%)	40 (10%)
	Irritability	16 (4%)	17 (4%)
	Anxiety	8 (2%)	21 (5%)

(cont'd)

Table 1: WELLBUTRIN XL *(cont'd)*

Adverse Events in MDD Placebo-Controlled Studies: Treatment-Emergent Adverse Experiences Occurring in ≥1% of Patients taking WELLBUTRIN XL (with an incidence greater than placebo)

System Organ Class	Preferred Term	Pooled Results	
		Placebo n=412	WELLBUTRIN XL n=411
	Restlessness	8 (2%)	11 (3%)
	Initial Insomnia	4 (<1%)	5 (1%)
	Middle Insomnia	3 (<1%)	5 (1%)
	Panic Attack	1 (<1%)	5 (1%)
Respiratory Disorders	Cough	6 (1%)	10 (2%)
Skin & Subcutaneous Tissue	Hyperhidrosis	5 (1%)	9 (2%)
	Rash	5 (1%)	11 (3%)
	Pruritus	5 (1%)	6 (1%)
Vascular Disorders	Hot Flush	2 (<1%)	5 (1%)
	Hypertension	3 (<1%)	5 (1%)

Prevention of Seasonal Major Depression: Table 2 enumerates treatment-emergent adverse events that occurred at an incidence of 1% or more in placebo-controlled trials, and were more frequent in the WELLBUTRIN XL group than the placebo group.

Table 2: WELLBUTRIN XL

Adverse Events Seasonal Depression Placebo-Controlled Studies: Treatment-Emergent Adverse Experiences Occurring in ≥1% of Patients taking WELLBUTRIN XL (with an incidence greater than placebo)

System Organ Class	Preferred Term	Pooled Results	
		Placebo n=511	WELLBUTRIN XL n=537
Gastrointestinal Disorders	Dry Mouth	79 (15%)	137 (26%)
	Nausea	39 (8%)	68 (13%)
	Constipation	10 (2%)	47 (9%)
	Flatulence	17 (3%)	30 (6%)
	Abdominal Pain	2 (<1%)	11 (2%)
	Toothache	5 (<1%)	8 (1%)
Vascular Disorders	Hypertension	0	10 (2%)
	Hot Flush	1 (<1%)	7 (1%)
Metabolism and Nutrition	Decreased Appetite	6 (1%)	20 (4%)
Respiratory Disorders	Cough	16 (3%)	21 (4%)
	Dyspnoea	2 (<1%)	8 (1%)
Nervous System Disorders	Headache	138 (27%)	182 (34%)
	Dizziness	23 (5%)	31 (6%)
	Tremor	6 (1%)	18 (3%)
	Dysgeusia	3 (<1%)	8 (1%)
	Memory Impairment	0	6 (1%)
General Disorders	Feeling Jittery	8 (2%)	17 (3%)
	Thirst	3 (<1%)	6 (1%)
	Chest Pain	2 (<1%)	6 (1%)
Psychiatric Disorders	Insomnia	58 (11%)	84 (16%)
	Anxiety	22 (4%)	28 (5%)
	Middle Insomnia	7 (1%)	12 (2%)
	Abnormal Dreams	5 (<1%)	11 (2%)
	Agitation	4 (<1%)	11 (2%)
	Initial Insomnia	3 (<1%)	11 (2%)
	Disturbance in Attention	4 (<1%)	7 (1%)
Infections & Infestations	Nasopharyngitis	62 (12%)	71 (13%)
	Upper Respiratory Tract Infection	43 (8%)	47 (9%)
	Sinusitis	20 (4%)	27 (5%)

(cont'd)

Table 2: WELLBUTRIN XL *(cont'd)*

Adverse Events Seasonal Depression Placebo-Controlled Studies: Treatment-Emergent Adverse Experiences Occurring in ≥1% of Patients taking WELLBUTRIN XL (with an incidence greater than placebo)

System Organ Class	Preferred Term	Pooled Results	
		Placebo n=511	WELLBUTRIN XL n=537
	Urinary Tract Infection	5 (<1%)	8 (1%)
	Pharyngitis Streptococcal	3 (<1%)	6 (1%)
Skin & Subcutaneous Tissue	Rash	11 (2%)	14 (3%)
	Acne	1 (<1%)	8 (1%)
	Pruritus	4 (<1%)	7 (1%)
	Urticaria	0	7 (1%)
Musculoskeletal Disorders	Myalgia	11 (2%)	14 (3%)
	Pain in Extremity	10 (2%)	14 (3%)
	Muscle Cramp	1 (<1%)	7 (1%)
Ear and Labyrinth Disorders	Tinnitus	3 (<1%)	18 (3%)
Reproductive Disorders	Dysmenorrhoea	2 (<1%)	11 (2%)
Eye Disorders	Vision Blurred	3 (<1%)	7 (1%)

Less Common Clinical Trial Adverse Drug Reactions (<1%): The following treatment-emergent adverse drug reactions were reported with <1% incidence in the three pooled MDD, and the three pooled seasonal depression WELLBUTRIN XL clinical trials. The extent to which these events may be associated with WELLBUTRIN XL is unknown.

Blood and Lymphatic System Disorders: lymphadenopathy, anaemia.

Cardiovascular Disorders: cardiac flutter, tachycardia, supraventricular tachycardia.

Ear and Labyrinth Disorders: ear pain, motion sickness, vertigo, hyperacusis.

Eye Disorders: eye pruritus, conjunctivitis, eye pain, keratoconjunctivitis sicca, acquired dacryostenosis, lacrimation decreased, lacrimation increased, photophobia, vitreous floaters.

Gastrointestinal Disorders: loose stools, stomach discomfort, gastroesophageal reflux disease, frequent bowel movements, gastrointestinal discomfort, lower abdominal pain, eructation, gastritis, halitosis, gastric irritation, hyperacidity, oral hypoaesthesia, lip dry, pancreatitis, abdominal distension, food poisoning, defaecation urgency, duodenal ulcer haemorrhage, gastrointestinal pain, gingival pain, gingivitis, infrequent bowel movements, mouth ulceration, oral pain.

General Disorders and Administration Site Conditions: pain, oedema peripheral, asthenia, feeling abnormal, feeling hot, influenza like illness, thirst, energy increased, hunger, malaise, rigors, respiratory sighs, energy increased, feeling cold, impaired healing, injection site joint pain, temperature tolerance.

Immune System Disorders: seasonal allergy, drug hypersensitivity, latex allergy, hypersensitivity, food allergy.

Infections and Infestations: bronchitis, fungal infection, ear infection, gastroenteritis, bacterial vaginitis, cystitis, herpes zoster, pharyngitis, vaginal mycosis, wound infection, infective conjunctivitis, dental caries, herpes virus infection, hordeolum, localized infection, viral upper respiratory tract infection, respiratory tract infection, rhinitis, tooth infection, laryngitis, tooth abscess, pneumonia, folliculitis, viral gastritis, hepatitis C, prostate infection, tinea pedis, tonsillitis.

Injury, Poisoning and Procedural Complications: contusion, joint sprain, muscle strain, skin laceration, excoriation, post procedural pain, limb injury, sunburn, accidental overdose, arthropod bite, facial bones fracture, mouth injury, soft tissue injury, wrist fracture, back injury, joint injury, epicondylitis, concussion, fall, animal scratch, laceration, lower limb fracture.

Investigations: blood pressure increased, weight increased, heart rate irregular.

Metabolism and Nutrition Disorders: anorexia, food craving, increased appetite, dehydration, hypercholesterolaemia.

Musculoskeletal and Connective Tissue Disorders: muscle tightness, neck pain, muscle twitching, pain in jaw, musculoskeletal stiffness, muscle spasms, sensation of heaviness, tendonitis, chest wall pain, musculoskeletal pain, bursitis, flank pain, joint stiffness, joint swelling, muscular weakness, musculoskeletal chest pain, osteoporosis, tendon disorder.

Neoplasms (benign, malignant incl. cysts and polyps): basal cell carcinoma, cyst, breast cancer.

Nervous System Disorders: amnesia, depressed level of consciousness, disturbance in attention, dyslexia, sinus headache, hypersomnia, hypoaesthesia, lethargy, migraine, muscle contractions involuntary, myoclonus, paraesthesia, oral paraesthesia, parosmia, sedation, tension headache, psychomotor hyperactivity, somnolence, carpel tunnel syndrome, nerve compression, sensory disturbance, hypotonia, sciatica.

Psychiatric Disorders: aggression, affect lability, anger, bruxism, confusional state, crying, depersonalization, depressed mood, depressive symptom, disturbance in sexual arousal, early morning awakening, euphoric mood, feeling of despair, feelings of worthlessness, hallucination, auditory hallucination, altered mood, mood swings, nervousness, abnormal orgasm, paranoia, sleep disorder, tension, thinking abnormal, trichotillomania, libido decreased, nightmare, restlessness, panic reaction, disorientation, hostility, psychomotor agitation, stress symptoms, apathy, delusion, mood altered, perseveration, sleep walking, social avoidant behaviour.

Renal and Urinary Disorders: micturition urgency, urethral pain, dysuria, hypertonic bladder, micturition disorder, polyuria, renal pain, urinary incontinence.

Reproductive System and Breast Disorders: metrorrhagia, menstruation irregular, amenorrhoea, genital rash, premenstrual syndrome, erectile dysfunction, menstrual disorder, breast tenderness, testicular pain, breast microcalcification, breast hypertrophy, nipple pain, ovarian cyst, vaginal haemorrhage.

Respiratory, Thoracic, and Mediastinal Disorders: asthma, dyspnoea, epistaxis, increased upper airway secretion, respiratory tract congestion, rhinorrhoea, sinus disorder, sneezing, throat irritation, vocal cord disorder, yawning, sinus pain, hyperventilation, snoring, nasal dryness, pleuritic pain, pulmonary congestion, wheezing.

Skin and Subcutaneous Tissue Disorders: alopecia, cold sweat, dermal cyst, dry skin, increased tendency to bruise, night sweats, photosensitivity reaction, rash erythematous, skin irritation, urticaria, eczema, facial oedema, hypotrichosis, pruritus generalized, swelling face, circumoral oedema, allergic dermatitis, rash pruritic, sebaceous gland disorder.

Vascular Disorders: flushing, peripheral coldness.

Events Observed During Development and Post-Marketing Experience of Bupropion with Other Formulations or Indications: In addition to the events noted above for WELLBUTRIN XL, the following adverse events have been reported in clinical trials and post-marketing experience with the sustained release formulation of bupropion in depressed patients and in non-depressed smokers, as well as in clinical trials and post-marketing experience with the immediate release formulation of bupropion.

Seizures: Post-marketing reports suggest that the reintroduction of WELLBUTRIN SR in patients who experienced a seizure is associated with a risk of seizure reoccurrence in some cases. Thus, patients should not restart WELLBUTRIN SR therapy if they have had a seizure on either bupropion formulation (WELLBUTRIN SR or ZYBAN). See Warnings and Precautions.

At doses of WELLBUTRIN SR up to a dose of 300 mg/day, the incidence of seizure is approximately 0.1% (1/1000) and increases to approximately 0.4% (4/1000) at a dose of 400 mg/day. Data for the immediate release bupropion revealed a seizure incidence of approximately 0.4% (13 of 3200 patients followed prospectively) in patients treated at doses of 225 to 450 mg/day. Additional data accumulated for the immediate release formulation of bupropion suggests that the estimated seizure incidence increases almost tenfold between 450 and 600 mg/day. The 600 mg dose is twice the adult dose of WELLBUTRIN XL tablets. This disproportionate increase in seizure incidence with dose incrementation calls for caution in dosing.

Adverse Events Associated with Discontinuation of Treatment with Other Formulations: In placebo-controlled studies of depression with WELLBUTRIN SR (987 patients treated, and 385 treated with placebo) adverse events caused discontinuation in 7% of WELLBUTRIN SR-treated patients and 3% of placebo-treated patients. The more common events leading to discontinuation of WELLBUTRIN SR included nervous system disturbances (2.2%), primarily agitation, anxiety and insomnia; skin disorders

(1.9%), primarily rashes, pruritus, and urticaria; general body complaints (1.0%), primarily headaches, and digestive system disturbances (1.0%), primarily nausea. Two patients in WELLBUTRIN SR treatment groups discontinued due to hallucinations (auditory or visual). The rates of premature discontinuation due to an adverse event were dose-related in these studies.

Adverse Events Occurring at an Incidence of 1% or More Among Patients Treated with WELLBUTRIN SR in Placebo Controlled Trials: Table 3 enumerates treatment-emergent adverse events that occurred at an incidence of 1% or more and were more frequent than in the placebo group, in patients participating in placebo-controlled clinical trials. Reported adverse events were classified using a COSTART-based Dictionary.

Table 3: WELLBUTRIN XL

Adverse Events (%): Treatment-Emergent Adverse Experiences Occurring in ≥1% of Patients in Any BUP SR Group for Studies 203, 205, and 212

Body System	Adverse Experience	% AEs BUP SR 100–150 (n=382)	% AEs BUP SR 200–300 (n=491)	% AEs PBO (n=385)
Body (General)	Asthenia	1.8	1.6	1.6
	Flu Syndrome	6.2	2.4	3.1
	Headache	27.5	26.9	23.4
	Infection	4.7	7.5	6.5
	Accidental Injury	1.8	1.8	1.8
	Pain	1.3	2.4	2.1
	Abdominal Pain	3.9	3.5	1.6
	Back Pain	1.8	4.5	3.1
	Chest Pain	1	2.9	0.8
	Neck Pain	1.3	2	1.3
Cardiovascular	Hot Flashes	1.3	1	0.8
	Migraine	0.8	1.4	1
	Palpitations	2.9	2	1.6
	Tachycardia	1.6	0.6	0.5
Digestive	Anorexia	3.1	4.5	1.6
	Constipation	6.5	10.8	6.8
	Diarrhoea	3.9	5.9	5.7
	Dry Mouth	13.1	16.5	7
	Dyspepsia	4.2	4.7	4.4
	Flatulence	1.8	3.1	2.1
	Nausea	10.7	12.6	7.5
	Vomiting	1.8	3.9	1.6
Musculoskeletal	Arthralgia	2.6	0.8	0.5
	Leg Cramps	1	0.2	0.5
	Myalgia	1.6	3.3	2.9
	Twitch	0.8	1	0.3
Nervous System	Agitation	1.6	3.5	1.8
	Anxiety	4.5	4.3	3.1
	CNS Stimulation	0	1.2	0.5
	Dizziness	7.1	8.6	5.5
	Hypertonia	1	1.2	0.5
	Insomnia	7.9	11.4	6.5
	Irritability	2.4	3.9	1.6
	Decreased Libido	1	0.6	0.5
	Nervousness	4.5	4.1	2.6
	Somnolence	2.6	2.0	2.1
	Tremor	3.1	6.1	0.8
Respiratory	Pharyngitis	1.3	2.9	1.8
	Rhinitis	9.9	6.7	9.6
	Sinusitis	1.6	2.4	2.1
Skin	Pruritus	2.4	2.2	1.6
	Rash	2.1	4.1	1.3

(cont'd)

Table 3: WELLBUTRIN XL *(cont'd)*

Adverse Events (%): Treatment-Emergent Adverse Experiences Occurring in ≥1% of Patients in Any BUP SR Group for Studies 203, 205, and 212

Body System	Adverse Experience	% AEs BUP SR 100–150 (n=382)	% AEs BUP SR 200–300 (n=491)	% AEs PBO (n=385)
	Sweating	2.4	5.1	1.6
	Urticaria	0.8	1.4	0
Special Senses	Amblyopia	2.9	2.4	1.8
	Taste Perversion	1	1.4	0.3
	Tinnitus	3.9	5.1	1.8
Urogenital	Urinary Tract Infection	1	1.8	0.3
	Urinary Frequency	1.3	2.4	1.6

In an open label, uncontrolled (acute treatment and continuation) study of WELLBUTRIN SR, 11% patients (361 out of 3100) discontinued treatment due to an adverse event. Adverse events leading to premature discontinuation in 1% or more of patients were: headache (1.1%), nausea (1.0%), and insomnia (1.0%). Adverse events leading to premature discontinuation in 0.5% to 1% of patients were: anxiety (0.8%), rash (0.8%), agitation (0.7%), irritability (0.5%), and dizziness (0.5%). In those patients (n=1577) who went into the continuation phase after 8 weeks of treatment, 6 (0.4%) discontinued due to alopecia. Because this study was uncontrolled, it is not possible to reliably assess the causal relationship of these events to treatment with WELLBUTRIN SR.

Adverse events for which frequencies are provided below occurred in clinical trials with the sustained-release formulation of bupropion. The frequencies represent the proportion of patients who experienced a treatment-emergent adverse event on at least one occasion in placebo-controlled studies for depression (n=987) or smoking cessation (n=1013), or patients who experienced an adverse event requiring discontinuation of treatment in an open-label surveillance study with WELLBUTRIN SR Tablets (n=3100). All treatment-emergent adverse events are included except those listed in Table 3, those events listed in other safety-related sections, those adverse events subsumed under COSTART terms that are either overly general or excessively specific so as to be uninformative, those events not reasonably associated with the use of the drug, and those events that were not serious and occurred in fewer than two patients.

Events of major clinical importance are described in the Warnings and Precautions sections.

Events are further categorized by body system and listed in order of decreasing frequency according to the following definitions of frequency: Frequent adverse events are defined as those occurring in at least 1/100 patients. Infrequent adverse events are those occurring in 1/100 to 1/1000 patients, while rare events are those occurring in less than 1/1000 patients.

Adverse events for which frequencies are not provided occurred in clinical trials or postmarketing experience with bupropion. Only those adverse events not previously listed for sustained-release bupropion are included. The extent to which these events may be associated with WELLBUTRIN SR is unknown.

Body (General): Infrequent were chills, facial edema, musculoskeletal chest pain, and photosensitivity. Rare was malaise.

Cardiovascular: Infrequent were postural hypotension, stroke and vasodilation. Rare was syncope. Also observed were complete atrioventricular block, extrasystoles, hypotension, hypertension (in some cases severe, see Warnings and Precautions, Cardiovascular), myocardial infarction, phlebitis, and pulmonary embolism.

Digestive: Infrequent were abnormal liver function, bruxism, gastric reflux, gingivitis, glossitis, increased salivation, jaundice, mouth ulcers, stomatitis, and thirst. Rare was edema of tongue. Also observed were colitis, esophagitis, gastrointestinal haemorrhage, gum haemorrhage, hepatitis, intestinal perforation, liver damage, pancreatitis, and stomach ulcer.

Endocrine: Also observed were hyperglycemia, hypoglycemia, and syndrome of inappropriate antidiuretic hormone.

Hemic and Lymphatic: Infrequent was ecchymosis. Also observed were anemia, leukocytosis, leukopenia, lymphadenopathy, pancytopenia, and thrombocytopenia.

Metabolic and Nutritional: Infrequent were edema and peripheral edema. Also observed was glycosuria.

Musculoskeletal: Also observed were arthritis, muscle rigidity/fever/ rhabdomyolysis and muscle weakness.

Nervous System: Infrequent were abnormal coordination, depersonalization, dysphoria, emotional lability, hostility, hyperkinesia, hypesthesia, suicidal ideation, and vertigo. Rare were amnesia, ataxia, derealization, and hypomania. Also observed were abnormal electroencephalogram (EEG), akinesia, aphasia, coma, delirium, dysarthria, dyskinesia, dystonia, euphoria, extrapyramidal syndrome, hallucinations, hypokinesia, increased libido, manic reaction, neuralgia, neuropathy, paranoid reaction, and unmasking tardive dyskinesia.

Respiratory: Rare was bronchospasm/dyspnea. Also observed was pneumonia and epistaxis.

Skin/Hypersensitivity: Rare was maculopapular rash. Also observed were alopecia, hirsutism, angioedema, exfoliative dermatitis, erythema multiforme, and Stevens-Johnson syndrome. Arthralgia, myalgia and fever have also been reported in association with rash and other symptoms suggestive of delayed hypersensitivity. These symptoms may resemble serum sickness.

Special Senses: Infrequent were accommodation abnormality and dry eye. Also observed were deafness, diplopia, and mydriasis.

Urogenital: Infrequent were impotence, polyuria, and prostate disorder. Also observed were abnormal ejaculation, cystitis, dyspareunia, dysuria, gynecomastia, menopause, painful erection, salpingitis, urinary incontinence, urinary retention, and vaginitis.

Post-marketing reports suggest that the reintroduction of WELLBUTRIN SR in patients who experienced a seizure is associated with a risk of seizure reoccurrence in some cases. Thus, patients should not restart WELLBUTRIN SR therapy if they have had a seizure on either bupropion formulation (WELLBUTRIN SR or ZYBAN). See Warnings and Precautions.

Drug Abuse and Dependence: WELLBUTRIN XL is likely to have a low abuse potential. There have been few reported cases of drug dependence and withdrawal symptoms associated with the immediate release formulation of bupropion. In human studies of abuse liability, individuals experienced with drugs of abuse reported that bupropion produced a feeling of euphoria and desirability. In these a single dose of 400 mg (1.33 times the recommended daily dose) of the immediate release formulation of bupropion produced mild amphetamine-like effects compared to placebo on the Morphine-Benzedrine Subscale of the Addiction Research Center Inventories (ARCI), which is indicative of euphorigenic properties and a score intermediate between placebo and amphetamine on the Liking Scale of the ARCI. Higher doses could not be tested because of the risk of seizure.

DRUG INTERACTIONS: Overview: In vitro studies indicate that bupropion is primarily metabolized to hydroxybupropion by the CYP2B6 isoenzyme (see Action and Clinical Pharmacology, Pharmacokinetics). Therefore, the potential exists for a drug interaction between WELLBUTRIN XL and drugs that affect the CYP2B6 isoenzyme (e.g., orphenadrine, and cyclophosphamide). The threohydrobupropion metabolite of bupropion does not appear to be produced by the cytochrome P450 isoenzymes. Few systematic data have been collected on the metabolism of WELLBUTRIN SR following concomitant administration with other drugs or alternatively, the effect of concomitant administration of WELLBUTRIN SR on the metabolism of other drugs.

Following chronic administration of bupropion, 100 mg t.i.d. to 8 healthy male volunteers for 14 days, there was no evidence of induction of its own metabolism.

Because bupropion is extensively metabolized, the coadministration of other drugs may affect its clinical activity. In particular, certain drugs may induce the metabolism of bupropion (e.g., carbamazepine, phenobarbital, phenytoin).

Drug-Drug Interactions: Drugs Metabolized by CYP2D6: Many drugs, including most antidepressants (SSRIs, many tricyclics), beta-blockers, antiarrhythmics, and antipsychotics are metabolized by the CYP2D6 isoenzyme. Although bupropion is not metabolized by this isoenzyme, bupropion and hydroxybupropion are inhibitors of CYP2D6 isoenzyme in vitro. In a study of 15 male subjects (ages 19 to 35 years) who were extensive metabolizers of the CYP2D6 isoenzyme, daily doses of bupropion given as 150 mg twice daily, followed by a single dose of 50 mg desipramine, increased the C_{max}, AUC, and $t_{½}$ of desipramine by an average of approximately two-, five- and two-fold, respectively. The effect was present for at least 7 days after the last dose of bupropion. Concomitant use of bupropion with other drugs metabolized by CYP2D6 has not been formally studied.

Coadministration of Thioridazine Contraindicated: Administration of the antipsychotic thioridazine alone produces prolongation of the QTc interval, which is associated with serious ventricular arrhythmias such as torsades de pointes, and sudden death. As this effect appears to be dose-related, it is anticipated that risk increases with inhibition of thioridazine metabolism. An in-vivo study suggests that drugs which inhibit CYP2D6 will elevate plasma levels of thioridazine. Therefore concomitant use of thioridazine with WELLBUTRIN XL is contraindicated (see Contraindications).

Coadministration of Other Drugs Metabolized by CYP2D6 Isoenzyme: Coadministration of bupropion with other drugs that are metabolized by CYP2D6 isoenzyme including certain antidepressants (e.g., nortriptyline, imipramine, desipramine, paroxetine, fluoxetine, sertraline), antipsychotics (e.g., haloperidol, risperidone), beta-blockers (e.g., metoprolol), and Type 1C antiarrhythmics (e.g., propafenone, flecainide), should be approached with caution and should be initiated at the lower end of the dose range of the concomitant medication. If bupropion is added to the treatment regimen of a patient already receiving a drug metabolized by CYP2D6, the need to decrease the dose of the original medication should be considered, particularly for those concomitant medications with a narrow therapeutic index.

MAO Inhibitors: Studies in animals demonstrate that the acute toxicity of bupropion is enhanced by the MAO inhibitor, phenelzine (see Contraindications).

Cimetidine: The effects of concomitant administration of cimetidine on the pharmacokinetics of bupropion and its active metabolites were examined in a crossover study in 24 healthy young male volunteers, following oral administration of two 150 mg WELLBUTRIN SR tablets with and without 800 mg of cimetidine. A single dose of cimetidine had no effect on single dose pharmacokinetic parameter estimates for bupropion, or hydroxybupropion, but caused a small statistically significant increase in the combined threohydro and erythrohydrobupropion AUC (16%) and C_{max} (32%).

Levodopa and Amantadine: Limited clinical data suggest a higher incidence of neuropsychiatric adverse experiences, such as confusion, agitation and delirium, in patients receiving bupropion, concurrently with either levodopa or amantadine. Tremor, ataxia and dizziness were also reported. Administration of WELLBUTRIN XL to patients receiving either levodopa or amantadine concurrently should be undertaken with caution, using small initial doses and gradual dose increases.

Clopidogrel and Ticlopidine: Both clopidogrel and ticlopidine have been shown to significantly inhibit CYP2B6-catalysed bupropion hydroxylation. The mean area under the plasma concentration-time curve (AUC) of hydroxybupropion was reduced by 52% by clopidogrel and by 84% by ticlopidine. The AUC of bupropion was increased by 60% with clopidogrel and by 85% with ticlopidine. Therefore, concomitant administration of bupropion and either clopidogrel or ticlopidine results in increased plasma concentrations of bupropion and reduced concentrations of hydroxybupropion. This may affect the efficacy of bupropion and may also increase the risk of concentration-dependent adverse events of bupropion, such as seizures (see Warnings and Precautions, Seizures). Patients receiving either clopidogrel or ticlopidine are likely to require dose adjustments of bupropion.

Use of WELLBUTRIN XL with Drugs that Predispose Patients to Seizures: Concurrent administration of WELLBUTRIN XL Tablets with agents that lower seizure threshold (e.g., antipsychotics, other antidepressants, theophylline, lithium, systemic steroids etc) should be undertaken only with extreme caution (see Warnings and Precautions). Low initial dosing and gradual dose increases should be employed.

Other Drugs with CNS Activity: The risk of using WELLBUTRIN XL in combination with other CNS-active drugs has not been systematically evaluated. Consequently, caution is advised if the concomitant administration of WELLBUTRIN XL and such drugs is required.

Transdermal Nicotine Interaction: (See Warnings and Precautions, Cardiovascular.)

Alcohol Interactions: In post-marketing experience, there have been reports of adverse neuropsychiatric events, or reduced alcohol tolerance, in patients who were drinking alcohol during treatment with bupropion. Rarely, reports of fatal outcomes with this combination have been received, however a causal relationship has not been established. The consumption of alcohol during treatment with bupropion should be avoided (also see Warnings and Precautions, Predisposing Risk Factors for Seizures).

DOSAGE AND ADMINISTRATION: **WELLBUTRIN XL (bupropion hydrochloride) is not indicated for use in children under 18 years of age. (See Warnings and Precautions, Potential Association with Behavioural and Emotional Changes, Including Self-Harm.)**

Recommended Dose and Dosage Adjustment: Major Depressive Disorder: Dosing with WELLBUTRIN XL Tablets should begin at 150 mg/day given as a single daily dose in the morning. The dose of WELLBUTRIN XL may be increased to the 300 mg/day maximum dose as early as 1 week after initiation of treatment. The usual adult target dose for WELLBUTRIN XL Tablets is 300 mg/day, given once daily in the morning. The dose can be reduced to, or maintained at 150 mg daily if the patient is unable to tolerate the 300 mg/day dose.

Prevention of Seasonal Major Depressive Episodes: WELLBUTRIN XL should be initiated in the autumn prior to the onset of depressive symptoms. Treatment should continue through the winter season and should be tapered and discontinued in early spring. The timing of initiation and duration of treatment should be individualized based on the patient's historical pattern of seasonal major depressive episodes. Patients whose seasonal depressive episodes are infrequent or not associated with significant impairment should generally not be treated prophylactically.

Dosing with WELLBUTRIN XL Tablets should begin at 150 mg/day given as a single daily dose in the morning. The dose of WELLBUTRIN XL may be increased to the 300 mg/day maximum dose after 1 week. The usual adult target dose for WELLBUTRIN XL Tablets is 300 mg/day, given once daily in the morning. The dose can be reduced to, or maintained at 150 mg daily if the patient is unable to tolerate the 300 mg/day dose. For patients taking 300 mg/day during the autumn-winter season, the dose should be tapered to 150 mg/day for 2 weeks prior to discontinuation.

Doses of WELLBUTRIN XL above 300 mg/day have not been studied for the prevention of seasonal major depressive episodes.

Missed Dose: WELLBUTRIN XL should be taken at the same time each day and no more than one dose should be taken each day. If the normal administration time has been missed, the dose should be skipped and administration resumed at the normal administration time of the following day.

Administration: Patients should be advised to swallow WELLBUTRIN XL Tablets whole with fluids, and **not** to chew, divide, crush or otherwise tamper with the tablets in any way that might affect the release rate of bupropion.

When switching patients from WELLBUTRIN SR (WSR) sustained-release tablets to WELLBUTRIN XL (WXL), give the same total daily dose when possible (for example 150 mg WSR twice a day may be switched to 300 mg WXL once daily). WELLBUTRIN XL should never be taken concurrently with WELLBUTRIN SR, ZYBAN or other medications containing bupropion.

Treatment of Pregnant Women During the Third Trimester: Post-marketing reports indicate that some neonates exposed to WELLBUTRIN SR, SSRIs, or other newer antidepressants late in the third trimester have developed complications requiring prolonged hospitalization, respiratory support, and tube feeding (see Warnings and Precautions). When treating pregnant women with WELLBUTRIN XL during the third trimester, the physician should carefully consider the potential risks and benefits of treatment. The physician may consider tapering WELLBUTRIN XL in the third trimester.

Geriatrics or Debilitated Patients: No pharmacokinetic or therapeutic trials have been conducted to systematically investigate dose requirements in patients who are elderly or debilitated (see Warnings and Precautions). As such patients may have reduced clearance of bupropion and its metabolites, and/or increased sensitivity to the side-effects of CNS active drugs, treatment with WELLBUTRIN XL should be initiated at the lowest recommended dose (150 mg/day).

Hepatic Impairment: Mild and Moderate Hepatic Impairment: Given the variable pharmacokinetics of bupropion in patients with either mild or moderate hepatic impairment (Child-Pugh Grade A or B), treatment with WELLBUTRIN XL should be initiated at the lowest recommended dose. Maintenance dose may be adjusted according to clinical response and tolerance. Caution should be exercised as there is no clinical experience with WELLBUTRIN XL in hepatically impaired patients (see also Warnings and Precautions).

Severe Impairment: Given the risks associated with both peak bupropion levels and drug accumulation, WELLBUTRIN XL is not recommended for use in patients with severe hepatic impairment. However, should clinical judgement deem it necessary, the drug should be used only with extreme caution (see also Warnings and Precautions). The dose should not exceed 150 mg every day or every other day in these patients. Any theoretical dose reduction for this patient population based on the findings of the pharmacokinetic studies may result in toxic drug levels in these patients (see Action and Clinical Pharmacology and Warnings and Precautions).

Renal Impairment: WELLBUTRIN XL should be used with caution in patients with renal impairment due to the potential for drug accumulation, and a reduced frequency and/or dose should be considered (see Action and Clinical Pharmacology and Warnings and Precautions).

All patients with hepatic or renal impairment should be closely monitored for possible adverse effects (e.g., insomnia, dry mouth, seizures) that could indicate high drug or metabolite levels.

Pediatrics: WELLBUTRIN XL is not indicated for use in children under 18 years of age (see Indications and Clinical Use and Warnings and Precautions, Potential Association with Behavioural and Emotional Changes, Including Self-Harm).

OVERDOSAGE:

Human Overdose Experience: In addition to those events reported under Adverse Reactions, overdose has resulted in symptoms including drowsiness, loss of consciousness and ECG changes such as conduction disturbances (including QRS prolongation) or arrhythmias. No overdoses occurred during WELLBUTRIN XL clinical trials. Three overdoses with WELLBUTRIN SR (bupropion hydrochloride) occurred during clinical trials. One patient ingested 3000 mg of WELLBUTRIN SR tablets and vomited quickly after the overdose; the patient experienced blurred vision and lightheadedness. A second patient ingested a "handful" of WELLBUTRIN SR tablets and experienced confusion, lethargy, nausea, jitteriness, and seizure. A third patient ingested 3600 mg of WELLBUTRIN SR tablets and a bottle of wine; the patient experienced nausea, visual hallucinations, and "grogginess". None of the patients experienced further sequelae.

The information included in the remainder of this section is based on the clinical experience with overdosage of the immediate release formulation of bupropion. Thirteen overdoses occurred during clinical trials. Twelve patients ingested 850 to 4200 mg and recovered without significant sequelae. Another patient who ingested 9000 mg of WELLBUTRIN and 300 mg of tranylcypromine experienced a grand mal seizure and recovered without further sequelae.

Since introduction, overdoses of up to 17 500 mg of the immediate release formulation of WELLBUTRIN, and up to 10 500 mg of WELLBUTRIN XL have been reported. Seizure was reported in approximately one-third of all cases. Other serious reactions reported with overdoses of WELLBUTRIN or WELLBUTRIN XL alone included hallucinations, loss of consciousness, respiratory arrest, amnesia, and sinus tachycardia. Fever, muscle rigidity, rhabdomyolysis, hypotension, stupor, coma, respiratory failure, delirium, and cerebral edema have been reported when WELLBUTRIN or WELLBUTRIN XL was part of multiple drug overdoses.

Although most patients recovered without sequelae, deaths associated with overdoses of WELLBUTRIN alone have been reported rarely in patients ingesting large doses of WELLBUTRIN Tablets. Multiple uncontrolled seizures, bradycardia, cardiac failure, and cardiac arrest prior to death were reported in these patients.

Management of Overdose: In the event of overdose, hospitalization is advised. Ensure an adequate airway, oxygenation, and ventilation. Monitor cardiac rhythm (ECG) and vital signs. EEG monitoring is also recommended for the first 48 hours post-ingestion. General supportive and symptomatic measures are also recommended. Induction of emesis is not recommended. Gastric lavage with a large-bore orogastric tube with appropriate airway protection, if needed, may be indicated if performed soon after ingestion or in symptomatic patients.

Activated charcoal should be administered. There is no experience with the use of forced diuresis, dialysis, hemoperfusion, or exchange transfusion in the management of bupropion overdoses. No specific antidotes for bupropion are known.

Due to the dose-related risk of seizures with WELLBUTRIN XL, hospitalization following suspected overdose should be considered. Based on studies in animals, it is recommended that seizures be treated with intravenous benzodiazepine administration and other supportive measures, as appropriate.

In managing overdosage, consider the possibility of multiple drug involvement. The physician should consider contacting a poison control centre for additional information on the treatment of any overdose. Telephone numbers for certified poison control centres are listed in the *Compendium of Pharmaceuticals and Specialties* (CPS).

> For management of a suspected drug overdose, CPhA recommends that you contact your **regional Poison Control Centre**. See the *CPS* Directory section for a list of Poison Control Centres.

ACTION AND CLINICAL PHARMACOLOGY: WELLBUTRIN XL (bupropion hydrochloride) is an antidepressant of the aminoketone class. It is chemically unrelated to tricyclic, tetracyclic, selective serotonin re-uptake inhibitors or other known antidepressant agents. Its structure closely resembles that of diethylpropion. It is related to the phenylethylamines.

Mechanism of Action: The mechanism of bupropion's antidepressant activity is unknown but appears to be mediated by noradrenergic (and possibly dopaminergic), rather than serotonergic mechanisms. Preclinical studies have shown that bupropion blocks norepinephrine (NE) reuptake and dopamine (DA) reuptake. Its major metabolite (hydroxybupropion), which in man is present at blood levels 10-20-fold higher than bupropion, blocks only NA reuptake.

The non-serotonergic mechanism of action of bupropion likely contributes to a distinct side effect profile that includes low rates of sexual dysfunction and somnolence (see Adverse Reactions).

Pharmacodynamics: In vitro, bupropion and its major metabolites had essentially no affinity for β-adrenergic, dopaminergic, GABA, benzodiazepine, 5HT1A, glycine and adenosine receptors, and only weakly inhibited α-adrenergic receptors in rat brain, α2-adrenergic, 5HT2, and muscarinic cholinergic receptors. High concentrations of bupropion and its major metabolites did not inhibit MAO-A or MAO-B activity. Bupropion and its major metabolites had no significant affinity for the 5HT transport system.

Pharmacokinetics: Absorption: Bupropion has not been administered intravenously to humans; therefore, the absolute bioavailability of WELLBUTRIN XL Tablets in humans has not been determined. In rat and dog studies, the bioavailability of bupropion ranged from 5% to 20%. Following oral administration of WELLBUTRIN SR to healthy volunteers, peak plasma concentrations of bupropion are achieved within 3 hours. In two single-dose (150 mg) studies the mean peak concentration (C_{max}) values were 91 and 143 ng/mL. At steady state, the mean C_{max} following a 150 mg dose every 12 hours was 136 ng/mL.

In a single-dose study, food increased the C_{max} of bupropion by 11% and the extent of absorption as defined by area under the plasma concentration-time curve (AUC) by 17%. The mean time to peak concentration (t_{max}) was prolonged by 1 hour. This effect was of no clinical significance.

Distribution: In vitro tests show that bupropion is 84% bound to human plasma proteins at concentrations up to 200 µg/mL. The extent of protein binding of hydroxybupropion is similar to that of bupropion, whereas the extent of protein binding of the threohydrobupropion metabolite is about half that seen with bupropion. The volume of distribution (V_{ss}/F) estimated from a single 150 mg dose given to 17 subjects is 1950 L (20% CV).

Metabolism: Bupropion is extensively metabolized in humans. There are three active metabolites: hydroxybupropion and the amino-alcohol isomers threohydrobupropion and erythrohydrobupropion, which are formed via hydroxylation of the tert-butyl group of bupropion and/or reduction of the carbonyl group. Oxidation of the bupropion side chain results in the formation of a glycine conjugate of meta-chlorobenzoic acid, which is then excreted as the major urinary metabolite. In preclinical tests used to predict antidepressant activity, it has been observed that hydroxybupropion is comparable in potency to bupropion, while the other metabolites are one half to one tenth as potent. This may be of clinical importance because the plasma concentrations of the metabolites are higher than those of bupropion.

In vitro results indicate that biotransformation of bupropion to hydroxybupropion is catalyzed primarily by CYP2B6, and to a much lesser extent by CYP1A2, 2A6, 2C9, 2E1 and 3A4 isozymes. Detectable levels of hydroxybupropion are not observed with CYP1A1 and CYP2D6 isozymes. Cytochrome P450 isoenzymes are not involved in the formation of threohyrobupropion. Following a single 150 mg dose of bupropion in humans, peak plasma concentrations of hydroxybupropion occur approximately 6 hours after administration. Peak plasma concentrations of hydroxybupropion are approximately 10 times the peak level of the parent drug at steady state. The AUC of hydroxybupropion at steady state is about 17 fold higher than that of bupropion. The times to peak concentrations for the erythrohydrobupropion and threohydrobupropion metabolites are similar to that of hydroxybupropion, and steady-state AUCs are 1.5 and 7 times that of bupropion, respectively.

Because bupropion is extensively metabolized, there is the potential for drug-drug interactions, particularly with those agents that are metabolized by the CYP2B6 isoenzyme. Although bupropion is not metabolized by CYP2D6, there is the potential for drug-drug interactions when bupropion is coadministered with drugs metabolized by this isoenzyme (see Drug Interactions).

Excretion: In two single-dose (150 mg) studies the mean (±% CV) apparent clearance (Cl/F) of bupropion was 135 (±20%) and 209 L/h (±21%). Following chronic dosing of 150 mg of WELLBUTRIN SR every 12 hours for 14 days (n=34), the mean Cl/F at steady state was 160 L/h (±23%). The mean elimination half-life of bupropion (estimated from a series of studies) is approximately 21 hours. Estimates of the half-lives of the metabolites determined from a multiple-dose study were 20 hours (25%) for hydroxybupropion, 37 hours (35%) for threohydrobupropion, and 33 hours (30%) for erythrohydrobupropion. Steady-state plasma concentrations of bupropion and metabolites are reached within 5 and 8 days, respectively. Following oral administration of 200 mg of ^{14}C-bupropion in humans, 87% and 10% of the radioactive dose were recovered in the urine and faeces, respectively. The fraction of the oral dose of bupropion excreted unchanged was only 0.5%. Bupropion and its metabolites exhibit linear kinetics following chronic administration of 150 to 300 mg/day.

Dose Proportionality: A randomized, two-way, single-dose, crossover bioavailability study with 35 healthy adult male and female volunteers was conducted under fasting conditions to determine the dose proportionality of the two strengths of WELLBUTRIN XL (2×150 mg versus 1×300 mg). A summary of the pharmacokinetic parameters obtained from the study is provided in Table 4. WELLBUTRIN XL 150 mg and 300 mg tablets are dose proportional with respect to blood levels.

Special Populations and Conditions: Factors or conditions altering metabolic capacity (e.g., liver disease, congestive heart failure, age, concomitant medications, etc.) or elimination may be expected to influence the degree and extent of accumulation of the active metabolites of bupropion. The elimination of the major metabolites of bupropion may be affected by reduced renal or hepatic function because they are moderately polar compounds and are likely to undergo further metabolism or conjugation in the liver prior to urinary excretion.

Pediatrics: The pharmacokinetics of WELLBUTRIN XL in individuals under 18 years old has not been evaluated.

Geriatrics: The effects of age on the pharmacokinetics of bupropion and its metabolites have not been fully characterized, but an exploration of steady state bupropion concentrations from several depression efficacy studies involving patients dosed in a range of 300 to 750 mg/day, on a three times a day schedule, revealed no relationship between age (18 to 83 years) and plasma concentration of bupropion. A single-dose pharmacokinetic study demonstrated that the disposition of bupropion and its metabolites in elderly subjects was similar to that of younger subjects. These data suggest there is no prominent effect of age on bupropion concentration: however, another single and multiple dose pharmacokinetic study, has suggested that the elderly are at increased risk for accumulation of bupropion and its metabolites (see Warnings and Precautions and Dosage and Administration).

Table 4: WELLBUTRIN XL

WELLBUTRIN XL Tablet Dose Proportionality

	Bupropion 2×150 mg Versus 1×300 mg Arithmetic Mean (CV%)	
Parameter	WELLBUTRIN XL 2×150 mg	WELLBUTRIN XL 1×300 mg
AUC_T (ng·h/mL)	1648.85±475.34	1676.61±474.09
AUC_I (ng·h/mL)	1702.69±489.30	1728.34±478.43
C_{max} (ng/mL)	150.11±7.22	146.88±47.61
T_{max} (h)	4.99±0.76	5.20±0.88
$T_{½}$ (h)	22.70±7.42	21.84±7.35

Race: The influence of race (Asian, Black and Caucasian) on the pharmacokinetics of bupropion (bupropion hydrochloride immediate release tablets) was evaluated based on dose normalized data pooled from five healthy volunteer studies. A comparison of pharmacokinetic parameter values did not detect any important differences in race with respect to AUC (p=0.5564) and C_{max} (p=0.8184).

Hepatic Insufficiency: The effect of hepatic impairment on the pharmacokinetics of bupropion was characterized in two single-dose studies, one in subjects with alcoholic liver disease and one in subjects with mild to severe liver cirrhosis.

The first study involved 8 subjects with alcoholic liver disease, and 8 healthy matched controls. While mean AUC values were not significantly different, individual AUC values for both the parent drug bupropion and the primary metabolite hydroxybupropion were more variable in subjects with alcoholic liver disease, and increased by approximately 50% over those of healthy volunteers. The mean half-life of the primary metabolite hydroxybupropion was significantly longer by approximately 40% in subjects with alcoholic liver disease than in healthy volunteers (32±14 hours versus 21±5 hours, respectively). For all other pharmacokinetic values, for both parent drug and metabolites, there were minimal differences between the two groups.

The second study involved 17 subjects with hepatic impairment (n=9 mild/Grade A child-Pugh rating; n=8 severe/Grade C Child-Pugh rating) and 8 healthy matched controls. In the **severe group**, the mean value for bupropion AUC was increased threefold over control values, with mean clearance decreased proportionately. Mean C_{max} and plasma half-life were increased by approximately 70% and 40% respectively. For the primary metabolites, mean AUC was increased by approximately 30%-50%, with mean clearance decreased proportionately. Mean C_{max} was lower by approximately 30% to 70%, and mean plasma half life increased threefold.

In the mild group, while mean values were not statistically increased from those of controls, the variability in the pharmacokinetic values was higher in the subjects with impairment; a sub-group of 1 to 3 subjects (dependent on pharmacokinetic parameter examined) showed individual values which were in the range of the severely impaired subjects. For the primary metabolites, the differences between groups in pharmacokinetic parameters were minimal.

In patients with hepatic impairment, treatment should be initiated at reduced dosage (see Warnings and Precautions and Dosage and Administration).

Effect of Smoking: In a single dose study, there were no significant differences in the pharmacokinetics of bupropion or its major metabolites in smokers compared with non-smokers.

STORAGE AND STABILITY: Store at room temperature (15-30°C)

INFORMATION FOR THE PATIENT: Published in e-CPS, available by subscription at www.e-cps.ca.

DOSAGE FORMS, COMPOSITION AND PACKAGING: 150 mg: Each creamy-white to pale yellow, round, extended-release tablet, printed with "WXL 150" in purple ink contains: bupropion HCl 150 mg. Nonmedicinal ingredients: n-butyl alcohol, denatured ethyl alcohol, ethylcellulose, glyceryl behenate, isopropyl alcohol, methylacrylic acid co-polymer dispersion, polyethylene glycol, polyvinyl alcohol, povidone, red and blue FD&C dyes, silicon dioxide, triethyl citrate, propylene glycol, shellac glaze and titanium dioxide. Bottles of 90.

300 mg: Each creamy-white to pale yellow, round, extended-release tablet, printed with "WXL 300" in gray ink contains: bupropion HCl 300 mg. Nonmedicinal ingredients: n-butyl alcohol, denatured ethyl alcohol, ethylcellulose, glyceryl behenate, iron oxide black, isopropyl alcohol, methylacrylic acid co-polymer dispersion, polyethylene glycol, polyvinyl alcohol, povidone, silicon dioxide, triethyl citrate, propylene glycol, shellac glaze and titanium dioxide. Bottles of 90.

(Shown in Product Identification Section)

wilate®

human coagulation factor VIII (FVIII)—human von Willebrand factor (VWF)
Blood Coagulation Factor

Octapharma

Date of Preparation: July 8, 2009

SUMMARY PRODUCT INFORMATION:

Route of Administration	Dosage Form/ Strength	Clinically Relevant Nonmedicinal Ingredients
Injection	Powder and solvent for solution for injection/450 IU/900 IU FVIII and 400 IU/800 IU VWF per vial	Sodium chloride, glycine, sucrose, sodium citrate and calcium chloride, solvent (Water for Injection with 0.1% polysorbate 80) For a complete listing see Dosage Forms, Composition and Packaging.

DESCRIPTION: wilate is a plasma-derived, stable, highly purified concentrate of freeze-dried active human coagulation factor VIII (FVIII) and von Willebrand factor (VWF). It is prepared from cryoprecipitate. wilate is supplied as a powder for reconstitution and intravenous injection.

The medicinal products contain per vial 450 IU/900 IU human coagulation factor VIII (FVIII) and 400 IU/800 IU human von Willebrand factor (VWF) prepared from human plasma for fractionation.

Solvent: 5 mL/10 mL Water for Injections with 0.1% polysorbate 80.

The reconstituted solution, which is prepared with the enclosed solvent, contains 90 IU/mL FVIII and 80 IU/mL VWF.

The potency of FVIII (FVIII:C) is determined by using the current "International Standard for Human Coagulation Factor VIII Concentrate". The determination of the VWF potency is carried out by determination of the Ristocetin Cofactor potency (VWF:RCo) by using the current "International standard for von Willebrand Factor Concentrate". The determinations are carried out according to European Pharmacopoeia (Ph.Eur.).

The specific activity of wilate is ≥60 IU FVIII:C/mg and ≥53 IU VWF:RCo/mg of total protein.

This product is prepared from large pools of human plasma, which may contain the causative agents of hepatitis and other viral diseases. Two effective virus inactivation steps provide a significant assurance in terms of viral safety. These are a solvent/detergent (S/D) virus inactivation step and a dry heat treatment in the final container at +100°C for 120 minutes. The efficacy of these two viral inactivation steps has been validated in accordance with international guidelines. (Refer to Warnings and Precautions.)

For list of excipients, see Summary Product Information.

INDICATIONS AND CLINICAL USE: wilate is indicated for:

- Treatment and prophylaxis of bleeding in patients with hemophilia A (congenital or acquired FVIII deficiency) and for the prevention and treatment of bleeding in minor surgical procedures.

Clinical trials to evaluate the safety and efficacy of wilate in major surgeries are ongoing. Therefore, limited data are presently available on which to evaluate or to base dosing recommendations. Thus, in the case of major surgical interventions, a precise monitoring of the substitution therapy by means of coagulation analysis (FVIII:C) is indispensable.

Geriatrics (>65 years of age): Although some of the patients who participated in the wilate studies were >65 years of age, no appropriate subgroup analyses were performed and therefore no data regarding use of wilate in the geriatric population are available at this point.

Pediatrics (<12 years of age): There are insufficient data to recommend the use of wilate in children below 12 years of age and in previously untreated hemophilia A patients.

Studies are being conducted in children with severe hemophilia A and VWD.

CONTRAINDICATIONS: wilate is contraindicated for patients who are hypersensitive to this drug or to any ingredient in the formulation or component of the container. For a complete listing, see Dosage Forms, Composition and Packaging.

WARNINGS AND PRECAUTIONS:

Serious Warnings and Precautions

This product is prepared from large pools of human plasma, which may contain the causative agents of hepatitis and other viral diseases. The physician should discuss the risks and benefits of this product with the patient before prescribing or administering to the patient (see Warnings, General).

General: Products made from human plasma may contain infectious agents such as viruses that can cause disease. Standard measures to prevent infections resulting from the use of medicinal products prepared from human blood or plasma include selection of donors, screening of individual donations and plasma pools for specific markers of infection and the inclusion of effective manufacturing steps for the inactivation/removal of viruses. Despite this, when medicinal products prepared from human blood or plasma are administered, the possibility of transmitting infective agents cannot be totally excluded. This also applies to unknown or emerging viruses and other pathogens. Like other plasma products, wilate carries the possibility for transmission of blood-borne viral agents, and theoretically, the variant Creutzfeldt-Jakob disease (vCJD) agent.

The measures taken are considered effective for enveloped viruses such as HIV, HBV and HCV, and for the non-enveloped virus HAV. The measures taken are of limited value against non-enveloped viruses such as parvovirus B19. Parvovirus B19 infection may be serious for pregnant women (fetal infection) and for individuals with immunodeficiency or increased erythropoiesis (e.g. hemolytic anemia). Eight patients in clinical studies were found to have seroconverted to parvovirus B19 antibody positive. In some cases the implicated lots of wilate were found to be parvovirus B19 positive (PCR).

The plasma used for wilate will be US-source plasma from FDA licensed donation centres, which is routinely tested for parvovirus B19 by PCR in minipools.

It is strongly recommended that every time that wilate is administered to a patient, the name and batch number of the product are recorded in order to maintain a link between the patient and the batch of the product.

Appropriate vaccination (hepatitis A and B) should be considered for patients in regular/repeated receipt of human plasma-derived FVIII/VWF concentrates.

Immune: The formation of neutralizing antibodies (inhibitors) to FVIII is a known complication in the management of individuals with hemophilia A. These inhibitors are usually IgG immunoglobulins directed against the FVIII procoagulant activity, which are quantified in Modified Bethesda Units (BU) per mL of plasma using the modified assay. The risk of developing inhibitors is correlated to the exposure to anti-hemophilic FVIII, this risk being highest within the first 20 exposure days. Rarely, inhibitors may develop after the first 100 exposure days. Patients treated with FVIII should be carefully monitored for the development of inhibitors by appropriate clinical observations and laboratory test. If such inhibitors occur, the condition will manifest as an insufficient clinical response. Management of such patients should be directed by physicians with experience in the care of patients with haemostatic disorders.

In previously untreated patients the inhibitor rate is estimated to be about <25%. Data, on which the rate is based, is from an on-going clinical study, therefore final results may differ.

In previously treated patients there is insufficient data to estimate the rate of inhibitor development in patients commencing treatment with wilate. Published data, based on treatment with other factor VIII products estimate the rate of inhibitor development to be in the range of 2 to 3%. Data from on-going and future studies with wilate and from post-marketing reviews will provide more accurate information on the rate of inhibitor development associated with the transfer of patients to treatment with wilate.

(See also Adverse Reactions.)

Peri-Operative Considerations: See Dosage and Administration for instructions for prevention of bleeding in case of surgery or severe trauma.

Sensitivity/Resistance: As with any intravenous protein product, allergic type hypersensitivity reactions are possible. Patients must be closely monitored and carefully observed for any symptoms throughout the infusion period.

Patients should be informed of the early signs of hypersensitivity reactions including hives, generalized urticaria, tightness of the chest, wheezing, hypotension, and anaphylaxis. If allergic symptoms occur, patients should discontinue the administration immediately and contact their physician. If patients develop inhibitors to FVIII, the condition will manifest itself as an inadequate clinical response. Such antibodies may precipitate and may occur concomitantly to anaphylactic reactions. Therefore, patients experiencing an anaphylactic reaction should be evaluated for the presence of inhibitors.

In case of shock, the current medical standards for treatment of shock are to be observed.

Skin: See Sensitivity/Resistance.

Special Populations: Pregnant Women: Animal reproduction studies have not been conducted with FVIII/VWF.

Based on the rare occurrence of hemophilia A in women, experience regarding the treatment during pregnancy and breast-feeding is not available. Therefore, wilate should be used during pregnancy and breastfeeding only if clearly indicated.

Nursing Women: See Pregnant Women.

Pediatrics (<12 years of age): There are insufficient data to recommend the use of wilate in children below 12 years of age and in previously untreated hemophilia A patients.

Studies are being conducted in children with severe hemophilia A and VWD.

Geriatrics (>65 years of age): Although some of the patients who participated in the wilate studies were >65 years of age, no appropriate subgroup analyses were performed and therefore no safety or tolerability data regarding a geriatric population can be presented at this point.

Monitoring and Laboratory Tests: The formation of inhibitors to FVIII in patients with hemophilia A treated with FVIII should be monitored. If the expected FVIII activity plasma levels are not attained, or if bleeding is not controlled with an appropriate dose, an assay should be performed (Bethesda test) to determine if FVIII inhibitors are present. In patients with high levels of inhibitors, FVIII therapy may not be effective and other therapeutic options should be considered. Management of such patients should be directed by physicians with experience in the care of patients with haemostatic disorders.

ADVERSE REACTIONS: Adverse Drug Reaction Overview: Hypersensitivity or allergic reactions (which may include angioedema, burning and stinging at the infusion site, chills, flushing, generalized urticaria, headache, hives, hypotension, lethargy, nausea, restlessness, tachycardia, tightness of the chest, tingling, vomiting, wheezing) have been observed infrequently, and may in some cases progress to severe anaphylaxis (including shock). In rare occasions, fever has been observed.

Patients with hemophilia A may develop neutralizing antibodies (inhibitors) to FVIII. If such inhibitors occur, the condition will manifest as an insufficient clinical response. In such cases, it is recommended that a specialized hemophilia centre be contacted.

In previously untreated patients the inhibitor rate is estimated to be about <25%. Data, on which the rate is based, is from an on-going clinical study, therefore final results may differ.

In previously treated patients there is insufficient data to estimate the rate of inhibitor development in patients commencing treatment with wilate. Published data, based on treatment with other factor VIII products estimate the rate of inhibitor development to be in the range of 2 to 3%. Data from on-going and future studies with wilate and from post-marketing reviews will provide more accurate information on the rate of inhibitor development associated with the transfer of patients to treatment with wilate.

Clinical Trial Adverse Drug Reactions: To present as much safety data as available from clinical studies with wilate, data from 4 completed studies in hemophilia A and 2 completed studies in VWD are summarized in this section. In total 116 individual patients (68 hemophilia patients and 48 VWD patients) received wilate on about 6567 occasions (4142 and 2425, respectively). See Table 1.

Less Common Clinical Trial Adverse Drug Reactions (<1%): Not applicable.

Abnormal Hematologic and Clinical Chemistry Findings: Standard clinical laboratory evaluations were performed in all the studies. There were no particular issues raised for any laboratory parameters in any of the studies.

Post-Market Adverse Drug Reactions: In February 2005, wilate received marketing approval for the treatment of all types of VWD and hemophilia A from the Paul Ehrlich Institute (PEI) in Germany. Since then 3.2 Mio IU of wilate have been sold. Eight patients in clinical studies were found to have seroconverted to parvovirus B19 antibody positive. In some cases the implicated lots of wilate were found to be parvovirus B19 positive (PCR).

The plasma used for wilate will be US-source plasma from FDA licensed donation centres, which is routinely tested for parvovirus B19 by PCR in minipools.

Table 1: wilate
Clinical Trial Adverse Drug Reactions

	wilate n=116 (%)
Immune System Disorders	
Allergic reactions	0.9
Allergic exanthema	0.9
Drug induced pruritus	0.9
Psychiatric Disorders	
Sleep disorder	0.9
Nervous System Disorders	
Dizziness	1.7
Vertigo	0.9
Headache	1.7
Respiratory, Thoracic and Mediastinal Disorders	
Shortness of breath	0.9
Gastrointestinal Disorders	
Nausea	0.9
Abdominal discomfort	0.9
General Disorders & Administration Site Conditions	
Fever	1.7

See: Medical Dictionary for Regulatory Activities (MedDRA) Maintenance and Support Services Organization (MSSO), Medical Regulatory Terminology March 2005.

DRUG INTERACTIONS: Overview: No interactions with other medicinal products are known.
Drug-Food Interactions: Interactions with food have not been established.
Drug-Herb Interactions: No interactions with other medicinal products are known.
Drug-Laboratory Test Interactions: There are no particular issues raised for any laboratory parameters in any of the studies.
Drug-Lifestyle Interactions: No effects on ability to drive and use machines have been observed.

DOSAGE AND ADMINISTRATION: Dosing Considerations: After 24-48 hours of treatment, in order to avoid an excessive rise in FVIII:C, reduced doses and/or prolongation of the dose interval should be considered.
Recommended Dose and Dosage Adjustment: Treatment should be initiated under the supervision of a physician experienced in the treatment of coagulation disorders.

The number of units of FVIII administered is expressed in International Units (IU), which are related to the current WHO standard for FVIII products. FVIII activity in plasma is expressed either as a percentage (relative to normal human plasma) or in IU (relative to the International Standards for FVIII in plasma).

The dosage and duration of the substitution therapy depend on the severity of the FVIII deficiency, on the location and extent of the bleeding and on the patient's clinical condition.

One IU of FVIII activity is equivalent to that quantity of FVIII in one mL of normal human plasma.

The calculation of the required dosage of FVIII is based on the empirical finding that 1 IU FVIII:C/kg BW raises the plasma level by 1.5-2% of normal activity. The required dosage is determined using the following formula:
Required IU = BW (kg)×desired FVIII rise (%)×0.5 IU/kg

The amount to be administered and the frequency of administration should always be oriented to the clinical effectiveness in the individual case. Table 2 can be used to guide dosing in bleeding episodes and surgery in adult patients and children older than 6 years.

In the case of the following hemorrhagic events, the FVIII:C should not fall below the given plasma level in the corresponding period.

Table 2: wilate
Hemophilia A—Treatment Scheme for Hemorrhages and Surgery

Degree of Hemorrhage/Type of Surgical Procedure	FVIII Level Required (%) (IU/dl)	Frequency of Doses (hours)/Duration of Therapy (days)
Hemorrhage		
Mild hemorrhage: Early hemarthrosis, muscle bleed, nosebleed, oral bleed and other minor injuries	20–40	Repeat every 12 to 24 hours. At least 1 day, until the bleeding episode as indicated by pain is resolved or healing is achieved.
More extensive hemarthrosis, muscle bleed or hematoma	30–60	Repeat infusion every 12 to 24 hours for 3 to 4 days or more until pain and disability are resolved.
Life threatening hemorrhage: cerebral hemorrhage, blunt trauma without visible bleeding site, severe abdominal bleed resp. internal bleeding, throat bleed	60–100	Repeat infusion every 8 to 24 hours until threat is resolved.
Surgery		
Minor including tooth extraction	30–60	Every 24 hours, at least 1 day, until healing is achieved.
Major	80–100 (pre- and postoperative)	Repeat infusion every 8 to 24 hours until adequate wound healing, then therapy for at least another 7 days to maintain a FVIII activity of 30% to 60%.

During the course of treatment, appropriate determination of FVIII:C levels is advised to guide the dose to be administered and the frequency of repeated infusions. In the case of major surgical interventions in particular, precise monitoring of the substitution therapy by means of coagulation analysis (FVIII:C) is indispensable. Individual patients may vary in their response to FVIII treatment, achieving different levels of in vivo recovery and demonstrating different half-lives.
Prophylaxis: For long-term prophylaxis against bleedings in patients with severe hemophilia A, doses of about 20 IU wilate/kg BW should be given at intervals of 2 to 3 days. In some cases, especially in younger patients, shorter dosage intervals or higher doses may be necessary.

There are insufficient data to recommend the use of wilate in children below 12 years of age and in previously untreated haemophilia A patients.

Studies are being conducted in children with severe hemophilia A and VWD.
Missed Dose: If a patient on prophylactic treatment missed a dose, the missed dose should be taken as soon as possible, and then treatment should continue as before. If a dose is skipped, the next dose must usually not be doubled.

In the unlikely event that a patient who is actively bleeding is missing a dose, it may be appropriate to adopt the next dosage depending on the extent of the bleeding and on the patient's clinical condition.
Administration: wilate is administered via intravenous infusion.
Instructions for Reconstitution:

1. Warm the wilate powder and solvent in the closed vials up to room temperature (maximum 37°C). This temperature should be maintained during reconstitution.
2. Remove the flip caps from the wilate vial and the solvent vial and clean the rubber stoppers with an alcohol swab.
3. Peel away the lid of the outer package of the Mix2Vial transfer set. Place the solvent vial on an even surface and hold the vial firmly. Take the Mix2Vial together with its outer package and invert it. Push the blue plastic cannula of the Mix2Vial firmly through the rubber stopper of the solvent vial. While holding onto the solvent vial, carefully remove the outer package from the Mix2Vial, being careful to leave the Mix2Vial attached firmly to the solvent vial.
4. With the wilate vial held firmly on an even surface, quickly invert the solvent vial (with the Mix2Vial attached) and push the transparent plastic cannula end of the Mix2Vial firmly through the stopper of the wilate vial. The solvent will be drawn into the wilate vial by vacuum.
5. With both vials still attached, slowly rotate the wilate vial to ensure the product is fully dissolved, giving a clear or slightly opalescent, colourless or slightly yellow solution. Once the contents of the wilate vial are dissolved, firmly hold both the transparent and blue parts of the Mix2Vial. Unscrew the Mix2Vial into two separate pieces with the vials still attached and discard the empty solvent vial and the blue part of the Mix2Vial.

Instructions for Injection: As a precautionary measure, the patients pulse rate should be measured before and during the injection. If a marked increase in the pulse rate occurs the injection speed must be reduced or the administration must be interrupted.

1. Attach a plastic sterile disposable syringe to the transparent part of Mix2Vial. Invert the system and draw the reconstituted wilate into the syringe.
2. Once the wilate solution has been transferred into the syringe, firmly hold the barrel of the syringe (keeping it facing down) and detach the Mix2Vial from the syringe. Discard the Mix2Vial (transparent plastic part) and the empty wilate vial.
3. Clean the intended injection site with an alcohol swab.
4. Attach a suitable infusion needle to the syringe.
5. Inject the solution intravenously at a slow speed of 2-3 mL/minute.

Incompatibilities: wilate must not be mixed with other medicinal products or administered simultaneously with other intravenous preparation in the same infusion set.
Shelf-life: wilate has a shelf-life of 3 years. The powder should be reconstituted only directly before injection. After reconstitution the solution should be used immediately.
Special Precautions for Storage: wilate and solvent can be stored at between +2 and +8°C until the indicated expiry date. Within this period wilate and solvent may be stored for a single block of up to 6 months at room temperature (max. +25°C). If stored at room temperature (max. +25°C) wilate must either be used within 6 months or discarded. Protect from light.

Do not freeze. The reconstituted solution should be used on one occasion only. Any solution remaining should be discarded.

OVERDOSAGE:
No symptoms of overdose with human FVIII or VWF have been reported.

For management of a suspected drug overdose, CPhA recommends that you contact your **regional Poison Control Centre**. See the *CPS* Directory section for a list of Poison Control Centres.

ACTION AND CLINICAL PHARMACOLOGY: Mechanism of Action: VWF is a multimeric protein with two key functions. It is an adhesive molecule, which mediates the binding between platelets and damaged sub-endothelial tissues. It is also a carrier protein, involved in the transport and stabilization of FVIII. Patients suffering from VWD have a deficiency or abnormality of VWF. A reduction in VWF concentration in the bloodstream results in low FVIII activity and abnormal platelet function, as the platelets are prevented from adhering to sub-endothelial tissue. As a result, excessive bleeding will occur.

In human plasma, the FVIII/VWF circulates as protein complex consisting of a small molecule with coagulant activity (FVIII), which is non-covalently bound to a larger carrier protein (VWF). FVIII is involved in the intrinsic pathway of blood coagulation, functioning as the co-factor for the factor IXa mediated activation of factor X. Patients with hemophilia A are deficient in factor VIII, and are therefore predisposed to episodes of recurrent bleeding.

The coagulation factors FVIII and VWF in wilate are normal constituents of human plasma and act like the endogenous FVIII and VWF. Therefore, wilate is a suitable treatment option for the prophylaxis and treatment of bleeding episodes in patients with hemophilia A.
Pharmacodynamics: Pharmacotherapeutic group: Von Willebrand factor and coagulation factor VIII in combination.

The FVIII/VWF complex consists of two molecules (FVIII and VWF) with different physiological functions. When infused into a hemophilia patient, FVIII binds to VWF in the patient's circulation. Activated FVIII (FVIIIa) acts as a cofactor for activated factor IX (FIXa), accelerating the conversion of factor X to activated factor X (FXa). FXa converts prothrombin into thrombin. Thrombin then converts fibrinogen into fibrin and a clot can be formed.

Hemophilia A is a sex-linked hereditary disorder of blood coagulation due to decreased levels of FVIII:C and results in profuse bleeding into joints, muscles or internal organs, either spontaneously or as a result of accidental or surgical trauma. By replacement therapy the plasma levels of FVIII are increased, thereby enabling a temporary correction of the factor deficiency and correction of the bleeding tendencies.

In addition to its role as a FVIII-protecting protein, VWF mediates platelet adhesion to sites of vascular injury and plays a role in platelet aggregation.
Pharmacokinetics: FVIII (from the concentrate) is a normal constituent of the human plasma and acts like the endogenous FVIII. After injection of the product, approximately two thirds to three quarters of the FVIII remain in the circulation. The level of FVIII:C reached in the plasma should be between 80-120% of the predicted FVIII:C.

FVIII:C decreases by a two-phase exponential decay. In the initial phase, distribution between the intravascular and other compartments (body fluids) occurs with a half-life of elimination from the plasma of 3 to 6 hours. In the subsequent slower phase, the half-life varies between 8 to 18 hours, with an average of 15 hours. This corresponds to the true biological half-life.

The following results were observed in one clinical study in 12 patients (one-stage clotting assay, single measurement): see Table 3.

Table 3: wilate
Pharmacokinetics of wilate (FVIII:C) in Hemophilia A Patients

Parameter	Mean	SD
Recovery %/IU/kg	2.04	1.15
AUC_{norm} % * h/IU/kg	37.8	10.0
Half-life (h)	14.8	3.1
MRT (h)	20.4	4.5

(cont'd)

Table 3: wilate *(cont'd)*

Pharmacokinetics of wilate (FVIII:C) in Hemophilia A Patients

Parameter	Mean	SD
Clearance mL/h/kg	2.9	1.0

Key: AUC=area under the curve; MRT=mean residence time; SD=standard deviation.

STORAGE AND STABILITY: wilate and solvent can be stored at between +2 and +8°C until the indicated expiry date. Within this period wilate and solvent may be stored for a single block of up to 6 months at room temperature (max. +25°C). If stored at room temperature (max. +25°C) wilate must either be used within 6 months or discarded. Protect from light.

Do not freeze. The reconstituted solution should be used on one occasion only. Any solution remaining should be discarded.

SPECIAL HANDLING INSTRUCTIONS: Any unused product or waste material should be disposed of in accordance with local requirements.

INFORMATION FOR THE PATIENT: Published in e-CPS, available by subscription at www.e-cps.ca.

DOSAGE FORMS, COMPOSITION AND PACKAGING: 450 in 5 mL: Each vial of powder contains: human coagulation factor VIII (FVIII) 450 IU and human von Willebrand factor (VWF) 400 IU prepared from human plasma for fractionation. Nonmedicinal ingredients: calcium chloride, glycine, sodium citrate, sodium chloride, solvent (water for injection with 0.1% polysorbate 80) and sucrose. One package contains: 1 vial with powder, 1 vial with solvent (5 mL Water for Injections with 0.1% polysorbate 80), Mix2Vial transfer set with integrated filter.

900 in 10 mL: Each vial of powder contains: human coagulation factor VIII (FVIII) 900 IU and human von Willebrand factor (VWF) 800 IU prepared from human plasma for fractionation. Nonmedicinal ingredients: calcium chloride, glycine, sodium citrate, sodium chloride, solvent (water for injection with 0.1% polysorbate 80) and sucrose. One package contains: 1 vial with powder, 1 vial with solvent (10 mL Water for Injections with 0.1% polysorbate 80), Mix2Vial transfer set with integrated filter.

Winpred™ Pr

prednisone

Glucocorticoid

Valeant

SUPPLIED: Each white, flat, compressed tablet imprinted ICN W1 contains: prednisone USP 1 mg. Nonmedicinal ingredients: lactose, magnesium stearate, maltodextrin, starch and talc. Bottles of 100.

WinRho® SDF

immune globulin, Rho (D) human

Passive Immunizing Agent

Cangene

Date of Revision: November 15, 2007

SUMMARY PRODUCT INFORMATION:

Route of Administration	Dosage Form/ Strength	Clinically Relevant Nonmedicinal Ingredients
Intravenous or Intramuscular	Lyophilized 600 IU (120 µg), 1500 IU (300 µg), 5000 IU (1000 µg) Liquid 600 IU (120 µg), 1500 IU (300 µg), 5000 IU (1000 µg)	For a complete listing see Dosage Forms, Composition and Packaging.

DESCRIPTION: WinRho SDF, Rh_o (D) Immune Globulin (Human), is available as a sterile lyophilized or liquid gamma globulin (IgG) fraction of human plasma containing antibodies to the Rh_o (D) antigen (D antigen). WinRho SDF is prepared from human plasma by using an anion-exchange column chromatography method.

WinRho SDF is prepared from pools of human plasma that may contain the causative agents of hepatitis and other viral diseases. The manufacturing process includes both a Planova 20N virus filter that effectively removes lipid-enveloped and non-enveloped viruses based on size and a solvent/detergent treatment step (using tri-n-butyl phosphate and Triton X-100) that effectively inactivates lipid-enveloped viruses. These two processes are designed to increase product safety by reducing the risk of viral transmission of several viruses including human immunodeficiency virus (HIV), hepatitis B and hepatitis C. However, despite these measures, such products can still potentially transmit disease. There is also the possibility that unknown infectious agents may be present in such products.

The product potency is expressed in International Units (IU) by comparison to the World Health Organization (WHO) second anti-D immune globulin international standard. A 1500 International Unit [IU]* (300 µg) vial contains sufficient anti-Rh_o (D) to effectively suppress the immunizing potential of approximately 17 mL of Rh_o (D) (D-positive) red blood cells (RBCs).

The final lyophilized product formulation is stabilized with 0.04M sodium chloride, 0.1M glycine and 0.01% (w/w) polysorbate 80. The accompanying sterile diluent contains 0.8% sodium chloride and 10mM sodium phosphate. The final liquid product formulation is stabilized with 10% maltose and 0.03% (w/w) polysorbate 80. There are no preservatives in either formulation. WinRho SDF contains not more than 40 µg/mL IgA when reconstituted as described below.

INDICATIONS AND CLINICAL USE: Pregnancy and Other Obstetric Conditions: WinRho SDF, Rh_o (D) Immune Globulin (Human) is recommended for prevention of Rh immunization of Rh_o (D) negative women at risk of developing Rh antibodies. Rh_o (D) Immune Globulin (Human) prevents the development of Rh antibodies in the Rh_o (D) negative and previously not sensitized mother carrying a Rh_o (D) positive fetus, thus preventing the occurrence of hemolytic disease in the fetus or the newborn.

WinRho SDF is indicated for the prevention of Rh immunization in Rh_o (D) negative mothers who had not been previously sensitized to the Rh_o (D) factor.

The administration of WinRho SDF to women satisfying the above conditions should be done at about 28 weeks gestation when the child's father is either Rh_o (D) positive or unknown.

WinRho SDF should be administered within 72 hours after delivery if the baby is Rh_o (D) positive or unknown.

WinRho SDF administration is also recommended in these same women within 72 hours after spontaneous or induced abortion, amniocentesis, chorion villus sampling, ruptured tubal pregnancy, abdominal trauma or transplacental hemorrhage, unless the blood type of the fetus or father are confirmed to be Rh_o (D) negative. It should be administered as soon as possible in the case of maternal bleeding due to threatened abortion.

Transfusion: WinRho SDF is recommended to prevent alloimmunization in Rh_o (D) negative individuals transfused with Rh_o (D) positive RBCs or blood components with Rh_o (D) positive RBCs. Treatment is indicated if the individual who has received the transfusion is a female child or adult in her child-bearing years. Treatment should only then be carried out (without preceding exchange transfusion), if the transfused Rh_o (D) positive blood represents less than 20% of the total circulating red cells.

Immune Thrombocytopenic Purpura (ITP): WinRho SDF, Rh_o (D) Immune Globulin (Human) is recommended in the treatment of destructive thrombocytopenia of an immune etiology in situations where platelet counts must be increased to control bleeding. Clinical studies have shown that the peak platelet counts occur about seven days after IV anti-Rh_o (D) treatment. The effect is not curative but is transient; platelet counts are usually elevated from several days to several weeks. For individuals with chronic ITP, a maintenance dosage is recommended with the dosage schedule determined on an individual basis.

* In the past, a full dose of Rh_o (D) Immune Globulin (Human) has traditionally been referred to as a "300 µg" dose. Potency and dosing recommendations are now expressed in IU by comparison to the WHO anti-D standard. The conversion of "µg" to "IU" is 1 µg=5 IU.

WinRho SDF, Rh_o (D) Immune Globulin (Human), is recommended for the treatment of non-splenectomized Rh_o (D) positive 1) children with chronic or acute ITP, 2) adults with chronic ITP, or 3) children and adults with ITP secondary to HIV infection in clinical situations requiring an increase in platelet count to prevent excessive hemorrhage. The safety and efficacy of WinRho SDF have not been evaluated in clinical trials for patients with non-ITP causes of thrombocytopenia or in previously splenectomized patients.

Geriatrics (>65 years of age): WinRho SDF has been evaluated for the treatment of chronic ITP and ITP secondary to HIV infection in adults >65 years of age. The recommended dose is the same as in adults <65 years of age (see Dosage and Administration).

Pediatrics (<16 years of age): WinRho SDF has been evaluated for the treatment of chronic or acute ITP and in children with ITP secondary to HIV infection in children <16 years of age. The dosing recommendation in the treatment of children with ITP is the same as in adults (see Dosage and Administration).

CONTRAINDICATIONS: Prophylaxis of Rh Immunization: WinRho SDF should **not** be administered to patients:

- Who are Rh_o (D) positive (including babies)
- Specifically Rh_o (D) negative women who are Rh immunized as evidenced by standard Rh antibody screening tests
- With a history of anaphylactic or other severe systemic reaction to immune globulins
- Who are hypersensitive to this drug or to any ingredient in the formulation or component of the container. For a complete listing, see Dosage Forms, Composition and Packaging.

Treatment of ITP: WinRho SDF should **not** be administered to patients:

- Who are Rh_o (D) negative
- Who are splenectomized
- With a history of anaphylactic or other severe systemic reaction to immune globulins
- Who are hypersensitive to this drug or to any ingredient in the formulation or component of the container. For a complete listing, see Dosage Forms, Composition and Packaging.

WARNINGS AND PRECAUTIONS:

Serious Warnings and Precautions

WinRho SDF, prepared from pools of human plasma, may contain infectious agents such as viruses (see General).

The rare serious adverse events of intravascular hemolysis (IVH) and its complications have been reported following treatment with WinRho SDF (see Hematologic). Physicians should discuss the risks and benefits of WinRho SDF and alert patients who are being treated for ITP, about the signs and/or symptoms.

Hypersensitivity reactions can occur in very rare cases of IgA deficiency or hypersensitivity to human globulin (see Sensitivity/Resistance).

The liquid formulation of WinRho SDF contains maltose. Maltose in IVIG products has been shown to give falsely high blood glucose levels in certain types of blood glucose testing systems (see Monitoring and Laboratory Tests).

General: Proper care should be taken when calculating the dose of WinRho SDF to be administered. A confusion between International Units (IU) and Micrograms (µg) of product or between Pounds (lbs) and Kilograms (kg) for the patient's body weight could result in either an overdose that could lead to a severe hemolytic reaction (see Overdosage).

Following administration of WinRho SDF (IV or IM), patients should be kept under observation for at least 20 minutes for monitoring of potential adverse effects. This product should be administered under the supervision of a qualified health professional that is experienced in the use of passive immunizing agents and in the management of non-sensitized Rh_o (D) negative individuals who receive Rh_o (D) positive RBCs and patients diagnosed with Immune Thrombocytopenic Purpura. Appropriate management of therapy and complications is only possible when adequate diagnostic and treatment facilities are readily available.

Products made from human plasma may contain infectious agents, such as viruses, that can cause disease. The risk that such products will transmit an infectious agent has been reduced by screening plasma donors for prior exposure to certain viruses, by testing for the presence of certain current virus infections, and by inactivating and/or removing certain viruses. The manufacturing process includes both a Planova 20N virus filter that effectively removes lipid-enveloped and non-enveloped viruses based on size and a solvent/detergent treatment step (using tri-n-butyl phosphate and Triton X-100) that effectively inactivates lipid-enveloped viruses by irreversibly destroying the lipid coat. These two processes are designed to increase product safety by reducing the risk of viral transmission of several viruses including human immunodeficiency virus (HIV), hepatitis B and hepatitis C. However, despite these measures, such products can still potentially transmit disease. The product may theoretically contain the Creutzfeldt-Jacob Disease (CJD) causing agent or Creutzfeldt-Jacob Disease variant (vCJD) agents. There is also the possibility that unknown infectious agents may be present in such products. Individuals who receive infusions of blood or plasma products may develop signs and/or symptoms of some viral infections. All infections thought to have been possibly transmitted by this product should be reported by the physician or other health care provider to Cangene Corporation at 1-800-768-2304 (phone) or 1-800-768-2281 (fax).

Prophylaxis of Rh Immunization: A large fetomaternal hemorrhage late in pregnancy or following delivery may cause a weak mixed field positive D^u test result. Such an individual should be screened for a large fetomaternal hemorrhage and the WinRho SDF (Rh_o (D) Immune Globulin (Human)) dose adjusted accordingly. WinRho SDF should be administered if there is any doubt about the mother's blood type.

Treatment of ITP: WinRho SDF **must be administered via the intravenous route** for the treatment of ITP as its efficacy has not been established by the intramuscular or subcutaneous routes.

WinRho SDF should not be administered to Rh_o (D) negative or splenectomized individuals as its efficacy in these patients has not been demonstrated.

Cardiovascular: Rare thrombotic events have been reported in association with immune globulin intravenous (Human) (IGIV). Patients at risk may include those with a history of atherosclerosis, multiple cardiovascular risk factors, advanced age, impaired cardiac output, hypercoagulable disorders, prolonged periods of immobilization, and/or known or suspected hyperviscosity. Although the risk of thrombotic adverse events following WinRho SDF is extremely low, care should be taken in patients at risk for hyperviscosity, including those with cryoglobulins, fasting chylomicronemia/markedly high triacylglycerols (triglycerides), or monoclonal gammopathies.

Hematologic: Although the mechanism of action of WinRho SDF in the treatment of ITP is not completely understood, it is postulated that anti-D binds to the Rh_o (D) RBC resulting in formation of antibody-coated RBC complexes. Immune-mediated clearance of the antibody-coated RBC complexes would spare the antibody-coated platelets because of the preferential destruction of antibody-coated RBC complexes by the macrophages located in the reticuloendothelial system. The side effect of this action is a decrease in hemoglobin levels (extravascular hemolysis). The pooled data from ITP clinical studies demonstrated a maximum decrease from baseline in hemoglobin levels of 1.2 g/dL within 7 days after administration of WinRho SDF.

Among patients treated for ITP, there have been rare post-marketing reports of signs and symptoms consistent with intravascular hemolysis that included back pain, discoloured urine occurring, in most cases, within four hours of administration. The expected maximum decrease in hemoglobin levels (extravascular hemolysis) following WinRho SDF is usually <3.0 g/dL and occurs within 7-14 days after administration. The decrease in hemoglobin levels in patients experiencing intravascular hemolysis is typically ≥3.0 g/dL and usually occurs within 72 hours following WinRho SDF administration. Potentially serious complications of intravascular hemolysis that have also been reported include clinically compromising anemia, acute renal insufficiency or disseminated intravascular coagulation (DIC) that have, in some cases, been fatal. The extent of risk of intravascular hemolysis and its complications is not known but is reported to be rare (<1/1000), especially for DIC, which is very rare (<1/10 000). In the rare cases reported following anti-D administration, there was no discernible contribution of age, gender, pre-treatment renal function, pre-treatment hemoglobin, concomitantly administered blood/blood products, co-morbid conditions or previous treatment with WinRho SDF to the development of intravascular hemolysis and its complications (see Adverse Reactions, Post-Market Adverse Drug Reactions).

Following administration of WinRho SDF, Rh_o (D) positive ITP patients should be monitored for signs and/or symptoms of intravascular hemolysis and its complications, which include:

- Hemoglobinuria
- Pallor
- Hypotension
- Tachycardia
- Oliguria or anuria
- Edema
- Dyspnea
- Increased bruising and prolongation of bleeding time and clotting time which may be difficult to detect in the ITP population

Patients should be **instructed to immediately report** symptoms of back pain, discolored urine, decreased urine output, sudden weight gain, fluid retention/edema and/or shortness of breath to their physicians.

The diagnosis of a serious complication of an intravascular hemolysis is dependent on laboratory testing (see Monitoring and Laboratory Tests).

If patients are to be transfused, Rh_o (D) negative red blood cells (PRBCs) should be used so as not to exacerbate ongoing IVH. Platelet products may contain up to 9% of RBCs, thus caution should likewise be exercised if platelets from Rh_o (D) positive donors are transfused.

If the patient has a lower than normal hemoglobin level (less than 10 g/dL), a reduced dose of 125 to 200 IU/kg (25 to 40 μg/kg) body weight should be given to minimize the risk of increasing the severity of anemia in the patient. WinRho SDF, Rh_o (D) Immune Globulin (Human), must be used with extreme caution in patients with a hemoglobin level that is less than 8 g/dL due to the risk of increasing the severity of the anemia. (See Dosage and Administration, Treatment of ITP.)

Renal: IGIV products have been reported to be associated with renal dysfunction, acute renal failure, osmotic nephrosis, proximal tubular nephropathy, and death. Although these reports of renal dysfunction and acute renal failure have been associated with the use of many licensed IGIV products, those that contained sucrose as a stabilizer and were administered at daily doses of 400 mg of sucrose (or greater) have accounted for a disproportionate share of the total number. **WinRho SDF does not contain sucrose** as a stabilizer. Patients predisposed to acute renal failure include the following: patients with any degree of pre-existing renal insufficiency, diabetes mellitus, volume depletion, sepsis, or paraproteinemia, or patients who are receiving known nephrotoxic drugs.

Respiratory: There have been rare reports of noncardiogenic pulmonary edema [Transfusion-Related Acute Lung Injury (TRALI)] in patients administered IGIV. TRALI is characterized by severe respiratory distress, pulmonary edema, hypoxemia, normal left ventricular function, and fever and typically occurs within 1 to 6 hours after transfusion. Patients with TRALI may be managed using oxygen therapy with adequate ventilatory support. The possibility of the rare occurrence of TRALI after WinRho SDF administration cannot be ruled out. Care should be taken in patients with pre-existing respiratory conditions.

WinRho SDF recipients should be monitored for pulmonary adverse reactions. If TRALI is suspected, appropriate tests should be performed for the presence of anti-neutrophil antibodies in both the product and patient serum.

Sensitivity/Resistance: Allergic reactions have been reported following WinRho SDF administration (see Adverse Reactions, Adverse Drug Reaction Overview). In the event of an allergic or anaphylactoid reaction to WinRho SDF subcutaneous injection of epinephrine hydrochloride should be instituted followed by intravenous administration of hydrocortisone if necessary.

WinRho SDF, Rh_o (D) Immune Globulin (Human) contains trace quantities of IgA. Although WinRho SDF has been used successfully to treat selected IgA deficient individuals, the physician must weigh the potential benefit of treatment with WinRho SDF against the potential for hypersensitivity reactions. Individuals deficient in IgA have a potential for development of IgA antibodies and anaphylactic reactions after administration of blood components containing IgA; Burks et al. (1986) have reported that as little as 15 μg IgA/mL of blood product has elicited an anaphylactic reaction in IgA deficient individuals. Individuals known to have had an anaphylactic or severe systemic reaction to human globulin should not receive WinRho SDF or any other Immune Globulin (Human).

Special Populations: Pregnant Women: Animal reproduction studies have not been conducted with WinRho SDF. Clinical use of WinRho SDF in the prophylaxis of Rh immunization in pregnant women has not resulted in any fetal harm. WinRho SDF, is not indicated for the treatment of ITP in pregnancy. WinRho SDF should be given to a pregnant woman only if clearly needed based on a risk: benefit assessment.

Nursing Women: It is unknown if WinRho SDF is excreted in human milk. Because many drugs are excreted in human milk precaution should be exercised.

Pediatrics (<16 years of age): WinRho SDF has been administered safely to children <16 years of age. The safety profile of WinRho SDF in children is similar to adults.

Geriatrics (>65 years of age): WinRho SDF has been administered safely to adults >65 years of age. The safety profile of WinRho SDF in geriatrics is similar to adults <65 years of age.

Monitoring and Laboratory Tests: The liquid formulation of WinRho SDF contains maltose. Maltose in IVIG products has been shown to give falsely high blood glucose levels in certain types of blood glucose testing systems (for example, by systems based on glucose dehydrogenase pyrroloquinolinequinone (GDH-PQQ) or glucose-dye-oxidoreductase methods). Due to the potential for falsely elevated glucose readings, only testing systems that are glucose-specific should be used to test or monitor blood glucose levels in patients receiving maltose-containing parenteral products, including WinRho SDF Liquid.

The product information of the blood glucose testing system, including that of the test strips, should be carefully reviewed to determine if the system is appropriate for use with maltose-containing parenteral products. If any uncertainty exists, contact the manufacturer of the testing system to determine if the system is appropriate for use with maltose-containing parenteral products.

In addition to anti-D antibody, WinRho SDF contains trace amounts of anti-C, E, A and B. These antibodies may be detected by laboratory screening tests.

The presence of passively administered anti-Rh_o (D) can lead to positive direct antiglobulin and indirect antiglobulin (Coombs') test. Interpretation of direct and indirect antiglobulin tests must be made in the context of the patient's underlying clinical condition and supporting laboratory data.

Prophylaxis of Rh Immunization: The presence of passively administered Rh antibody in maternal or fetal blood can lead to a positive direct antiglobulin (Coombs') test. In case of doubt as to the individual's Rh group or immune status, WinRho SDF, Rh_o (D) Immune Globulin (Human), should be administered.

Treatment of ITP: ITP patients presenting with signs and/or symptoms of intravascular hemolysis and its complications after anti-D administration should have confirmatory laboratory testing that may include, but is not limited to, CBC (i.e. hemoglobin, platelet counts), haptoglobin, plasma hemoglobin, urine dipstick and microscopic urinalysis, assessment of renal function (i.e. BUN, serum creatinine), liver function (i.e. LDH, direct and indirect bilirubin) and DIC specific tests such as D-dimer or Fibrin Degradation products (FDP) or Fibrin Split Products (FSP).

ADVERSE REACTIONS: The most serious adverse reactions have been observed in patients receiving WinRho SDF for treatment of ITP. These include: intravascular hemolysis, clinically compromising anemia, acute renal insufficiency and DIC, leading in some cases to death (see Warnings and Precautions).

Adverse Drug Reaction Overview: In addition to the adverse reactions described above, the following have been reported infrequently in clinical trials and/or post-marketing experience, in patients treated for ITP and/or the prevention of Rh immunization, and are thought to be temporally associated with WinRho SDF use: asthenia, abdominal or back pain, hypotension, pallor, diarrhea, increased LDH, arthralgia, myalgia, dizziness, nausea, vomiting, hypertension, hyperkinesia, somnolence, vasodilation, pruritus, rash and sweating.

As is the case with all drugs of this nature, there is a remote chance of an allergic or anaphylactoid reaction with WinRho SDF in individuals with hypersensitivity to blood products. An immediate reaction (anaphylaxis) characterized by collapse, rapid pulse, shallow respiration, pallor, cyanosis, edema or generalized urticaria.

Prophylaxis of Rh Immunization: Reactions to Rh_o (D) Immune Globulin (Human) are rare in Rh_o (D) negative individuals. Discomfort and light swelling at the site of injection and slight elevation in temperature have been reported in a small number of cases.

Treatment of ITP: WinRho SDF, Rh_o (D) Immune Globulin (Human), is administered to Rh_o (D) positive patients with ITP. Therefore, side effects related to the destruction of Rh_o (D) positive red blood cells, most notably a decreased hemoglobin, can be expected.

Clinical Trial Adverse Drug Reactions: Because clinical trials are conducted under very specific conditions the adverse reaction rates observed in the clinical trials may not reflect the rates observed in practice and should not be compared to the rates in the clinical trials of another drug. Adverse drug reaction information from clinical trials is useful for identifying drug-related adverse events and for approximating rates.

Prophylaxis of Rh Immunization: The safety of WinRho SDF was evaluated in clinical trials (n=2062) in pregnant Rh_o (D)-negative whose baby's father's Rh_o (D) serotype was either positive or unknown. Only 1 adverse reaction was reported during the clinical studies. The adverse reaction was an anaphylactic type reaction due to a considerably large dose administered within a short time period (12×600 IU).

In a clinical study with 5 healthy Rh_o (D) negative males, Rh_o (D) positive fetal red cells were administered to volunteers by IV infusion and then 1-2 days later the fetal red cells were cleared by IV administration of 600 IU (120 μg) WinRho SD. At 6-8 hours after administration of WinRho SD to these subjects, there was an elevation in mean levels of granulocytes from 4.25 to 7.88×10^9/L (p <0.01) and monocytes from 0.38 to 0.64×10^9/L (p <0.02). Levels of phagocytic leucocytes returned to pretreatment levels by 24 hours after WinRho SD treatment. This effect of WinRho SD is believed to result from the anti-Rh_o (D) mediated clearance of Rh_o (D) positive fetal red cells as it was not observed at much higher dosages of WinRho SD when no Rh_o (D) positive red cells were present in the circulation.

Treatment of ITP: The safety of WinRho SDF was evaluated in clinical trials (n=161) in children and adults with acute and chronic ITP and adults and children with ITP secondary to HIV. Overall 417 adverse events were reported by 91 patients (57%). The most common adverse events were headache (14% of the patients), fever (11% of the patients), and asthenia (11% of the patients). A total of 117 adverse drug reactions were reported by 46 patients (29%) Headache, chills, and fever were the most common related adverse events (see Table 1). With respect to safety profile per administration, 60 of 848 (7%) of infusions in the clinical trials were associated with at least one adverse event that was considered to be related to the study medication. The most common adverse events were headache (19 infusions; 2%), chills (14 infusions; <2%), and fever (nine infusions; 1%). All are expected adverse events associated with immunoglobulin infusion.

Table 1: WinRho SDF

Adverse Drug Reactions with an Incidence ≥5%

Body System	Adverse Event	# of Patients (%)		
		All Studies	**Children**	**Adults**
All Body Systems	Overall	46 (29)	19 (26)	27 (31)
Body as a Whole	Overall	40 (25)	19 (26)	21 (24)
	Asthenia	6 (4)	2 (3)	4 (5)
	Chills	13 (8)	4 (5)	9 (10)
	Fever	9 (6)	5 (7)	4 (5)
	Headache	18 (11)	8 (11)	10 (12)
	Infection	4 (3)	4 (5)	0 (0)
Nervous System	Overall	9 (6)	4 (5)	5 (6)
	Dizziness	6 (4)	2 (3)	4 (5)

Less common adverse drug reactions (<5%) include:
Body as a Whole: abdominal pain, asthenia, back pain, infection, malaise, pain.
Cardiovascular System: hypertension, palpitation.
Digestive System: anorexia, diarrhea, gastroenteritis, gastrointestinal disorder, glossitis, ulcerative stomatitis, vomiting.
Hematic and Lymphatic System: anemia, hypochromic anemia.
Metabolic and Nutritional System: weight gain.
Musculoskeletal System: arthralgia.
Nervous System: anxiety, dizziness, hypertonia, hypesthesia, somnolence, tremor.
Respiratory System: asthma, dyspnea, pharyngitis, rhinitis.
Skin and Appendages: urticaria.

The safety of WinRho was compared to high dose IVIG (2.0 g/kg), low dose IVIG (0.8 g/kg), and prednisone in children with acute ITP. The most common related adverse events in the WinRho group were chills, fever, and headache (see Table 2), similar to the related adverse events reported in all ITP studies (see Table 1). The most common related adverse events after high dose and low dose IVIG administrations were headache and vomiting and after prednisone administration was increased appetite.

Table 2: WinRho SDF

Adverse Drug Reaction with an Incidence ≥5% in Children With Acute ITP

Body System Preferred Term	No. of Patients (%)			
	High Dose IVIG (2.0 g/kg) N=35	**Low Dose IVIG (0.8 g/kg) N=34**	**Prednisone (4.0 mg/kg/day) N=39**	**WinRho (250 IU/kg IV) N=38**
All Body System	21 (60%)	14 (41%)	15 (39%)	10 (26%)
Body as a Whole	19 (54%)	10 (29%)	5 (13%)	10 (26%)
Abdominal Pain	0	3 (9%)	3 (8%)	2 (5%)
Chills	5 (14%)	1 (3%)	0	3 (8%)
Fever	9 (26%)	3 (9%)	1 (3%)	3 (8%)
Headache	12 (34%)	8 (24%)	2 (5%)	3 (8%)
Digestive System	10 (29%)	5 (15%)	9 (23%)	3 (8%)
Anorexia	0	0	0	2 (5%)
Diarrhea	0	0	2 (5%)	1 (3%)
Dyspepsia	0	0	2 (5%)	0
Increased Appetite	0	0	5 (13%)	0
Vomiting	10 (30%)	5 (15%)	3 (8%)	1 (3%)
Nervous System	4 (11%)	1 (3%)	6 (15%)	0
Emotional Liability	0	0	3 (8%)	0
Nervousness	0	0	2 (5%)	0
Tremor	2 (6%)	0	1 (3%)	0
Respiratory System	0	2 (6%)	1 (3%)	2 (5%)
Skin & Appendages	1 (3%)	0	2 (5%)	0
Acne	0	0	2 (5%)	0

Due to the proposed mechanism of action (i.e. Fc blockade, platelet sparing via anti-RBC antibodies), it is anticipated that administration of WinRho SDF to Rh_o (D)-positive patients will produce some degree of extravascular hemolysis. The mean decrease in hemoglobin within 7 days after WinRho SDF administration was 1.2 g/dL in all ITP studies. In a clinical study in normal healthy Rh_o (D)-positive subjects, the decrease in hemoglobin levels following WinRho SDF administration appeared to be dose-dependent.

In 4 clinical trials of patients treated with the recommended initial intravenous dose of 250 IU/kg (50 μg/kg), the mean maximum decrease in hemoglobin was 1.70 g/dL (range +0.40 to −6.1 g/dL). At a reduced dose, ranging from 125 to 200 IU/kg (25 to 40 μg/kg), the mean maximum decrease in hemoglobin was 0.81 g/dL (range +0.65 to −1.9 g/dL). Only 5 of 137 patients (3.7%)

had a maximum decrease in hemoglobin of greater than 4 g/dL (range 4.2 to 6.1 g/dL). In most cases, the RBC destruction is believed to occur in the spleen. However, signs and symptoms consistent with IVH, including back pain, shaking chills, and/or hemoglobinuria, have been reported, occurring within minutes and up to a few days after WinRho SDF administration.

Post-Market Adverse Drug Reactions: In addition to the adverse events experienced by the subjects during clinical trials, the following additional adverse events have been reported during the post-marketing use of WinRho SDF, they are based on spontaneous reporting. Because these events have been reported voluntarily from a population of uncertain size; the exact frequency rates cannot be precisely calculated; however, they have been rarely or very rarely reported.

Evaluation and interpretation of the post-marketing events is confounded by underlying diagnosis, concomitant medications, pre-existing conditions and inherent limitations of passive surveillance. Due to the complexity of the clinical reports and the minimal amount of pre- and post-WinRho SDF data provided, causation has not been described for the cases below.

IVH-related complications that have been reported between January 1995 and December 2005 include death (9 cases), acute onset or exacerbation of anemia (11 cases), acute onset or exacerbation of renal insufficiency (21 cases) and DIC (6 cases). One patient died of viral myocarditis after the administration of WinRho SDF for treatment of ITP. The other eight deaths had history of serious underlying disease; the extent to which IVH-related clinical complications exacerbated their conditions and contributed to their deaths is unknown.

The mean maximum decrease in hemoglobin in patients who were not transfused with PRBCs was 3.7 g/dL (range: 0.1-7.6 g/dL). Transfusions for treatment-associated anemia were administered within hours to days of the onset of IVH and consisted of between 1-6 units of RBCs. Acute renal insufficiency was noted within 2 to 48 hours of the onset of IVH. The mean maximum increase in serum creatinine was 3.5 mg/dL (range: 0.1-10.3 mg/dL) and occurred within 2-9 days. The renal insufficiency in all surviving patients resolved with medical management, including dialysis, within 4-32 days. This information is subject to changes as new cases may be reported in the future.

The etiology of IVH following WinRho SDF administration is unknown. No known risk factors associated with this adverse event have yet been identified from among those examined, which included age, gender, pre-treatment renal function, pre-treatment hemoglobin, concomitantly administered PRBCs, or WinRho SDF dose. However, it is noted that about half of the reported cases occurred in children and most of these cases had a diagnosis of acute ITP. The number of reported cases appears to indicate that the IVH event, while still an uncommon occurrence, may not be as rare as initially believed.

Post-marketing surveillance has noted reports of respiratory distress, possibly leading to death in elderly patients, following the administration of WinRho SDF. Seven cases of respiratory distress or Acute Respiratory Distress Syndrome (ARDS), six of which resulted in death, have been reported post-marketing between 1995 and 2004. These patients all had underlying disease that may have been the cause or contributed to the death of these individuals. The role of WinRho SDF in these deaths is unknown.

Prophylaxis of Rh Immunization: General Disorders and Administration Site Condition: injection site reaction (include induration, pruritus or swelling at injection site).

Immune Disorders: hypersensitivity, anaphylactic reaction.

Skin and Subcutaneous Tissue Disorders: pruritus, rash.

Treatment of ITP: In addition to the above very rare adverse events experienced after WinRho SDF administration in prophylaxis of Rh immunization, the following rare and very rare adverse events were reported after WinRho SDF treatment in patients with ITP during the post-marketing surveillance.

Blood and Lymphatic System Disorders: intravascular hemolysis, hemolysis, disseminated intravascular coagulation, jaundice.

Cardiovascular Disorders: tachycardia.

Gastrointestinal Disorders: nausea.

General Disorders and Administration Site Conditions: chest tightness, fatigue.

Investigation: hemoglobin decreased.

Musculoskeletal and Connective Tissue Disorders: back pain, myalgia.

Renal and Urinary Disorders: acute renal insufficiency, renal failure, hematuria.

Respiratory, Thoracic and Mediastinal Disorders: acute respiratory distress syndrome (ARDS), transfusion-related acute lung injury (TRALI).

Skin and Subcutaneous Tissue Disorders: sweating.

Vascular Disorders: hypotension pallor, vasodilation.

The signs and symptoms of intravascular hemolysis and its complications may include disseminated intravascular coagulation (DIC), discoloration of the urine, hemoglobinemia, hemoglobinuria, pallor, hypotension, tachycardia, oliguria or anuria, edema, dyspnea, increased bruising and prolongation of bleeding time and clotting time.

DRUG INTERACTIONS:

Serious Drug Interactions
Live attenuated virus vaccines: immune globulin administration may impair the efficacy of live attenuated virus vaccines for a period of 3 months or more (see Overview).

Overview: Immune globulin administration may impair the efficacy of live attenuated vaccines such as measles, rubella, mumps and varicella (see Table 3). Vaccination with live virus vaccines should be deferred until approximately three months after administration of WinRho SDF. Patients who have received WinRho SDF shortly after live virus vaccination, should be revaccinated 3 months after the administration of the immune globulin.

Administration of WinRho SDF, Rh_o (D) Immune Globulin (Human) concomitantly with other drugs has not been evaluated. It is recommended that WinRho SDF be administered separately from other drugs (see Dosage and Administration).

Drug-Drug Interactions:

Table 3: WinRho SDF

Established or Potential Drug-drug Interactions

Rh_o (D) Immune Globulin (Human)	Ref	Effect	Clinical Comment
Live attenuated virus vaccines (e.g. measles, rubella, mumps, varicella)	T	Immune globulin may impair efficacy	If WinRho SDF is given less than 14 days after vaccination, revaccination should be considered.

Legend:C=case study; CT=clinical trial; T=theoretical.

Interactions with other drugs have not been established.

Drug-Food Interactions: Interactions with foods have not been established.

Drug-Herb Interactions: Interactions with herbal products have not been established.

Drug-Laboratory Test Interactions: After administration of WinRho SDF, a transitory increase of passively transferred antibodies in the patient's blood may result in misleading positive results in serological testing (e.g. Coomb's test).

DOSAGE AND ADMINISTRATION: Recommended Dose and Dosage Adjustment: Prophylaxis of Rh Immunization: Pregnancy and Other Obstetric Conditions: A 1500 IU (300 µg) dose of WinRho SDF, Rh_o (D) Immune Globulin (Human) should be given by intravenous or intramuscular administration at 28 weeks gestation. A 600 IU (120 µg) dose of WinRho SDF, Rh_o (D) Immune Globulin (Human) should be given by intravenous or intramuscular administration as soon after delivery of a confirmed Rh_o (D) positive baby as possible and no later than 72 hours after delivery. In the event that the Rh status of the baby is not known at 72 hours, WinRho SDF should be administered to the mother at 72 hours after delivery.

If more than 72 hours have elapsed, WinRho SDF, should not be withheld but administered as soon as possible up to 28 days after delivery.

A 600 IU (120 µg) dose of WinRho SDF, Rh_o (D) Immune Globulin (Human) should be given by intravenous or intramuscular administration immediately after therapeutic abortion, amniocentesis (after 34 weeks gestation) or other manipulation late in pregnancy (after 34 weeks gestation) associated with increased risk of Rh_o (D) immunization and, in any event, no later than 72 hours after the event.

A 1500 IU (300 µg) dose of WinRho SDF should be given by intravenous or intramuscular administration immediately after amniocentesis before 34 weeks gestation or after chorion villus sampling, and this dosage should be repeated every 12 weeks while the woman is pregnant. In the case of threatened abortion, WinRho SDF should be administered as soon as possible. See Table 4.

Table 4: WinRho SDF

Obstetric Indications and Recommended Dose

Indication	Dose (Administer IM or IV)
Pregnancy:	—
• 28 weeks gestation	1500 IU (300 µg)
• Postpartum (if newborn Rh positive)	600 IU (120 µg)
Obstetric Conditions:	—
• Threatened abortion at any time	1500 IU (300 µg)
• Amniocentesis and chorionic villus sampling before 34 weeks gestation	1500 IU (300 µg)
• Abortion, amniocentesis, or any other manipulation after 34 weeks gestation	600 IU (120 µg)

Transfusion: WinRho SDF, Rh_o (D) Immune Globulin (Human) should be administered for treatment of incompatible blood transfusions or massive fetal hemorrhage as outlined in Table 5.

Table 5: WinRho SDF

Transfusion Indication and Recommended Dose

Route of Administration	WinRho SDF Dose: If Exposed to Rh_o (D) Positive Whole Blood	WinRho SDF Dose: If Exposed to Rh_o (D) Positive Red Blood Cells
Intravenous	45 IU (9 µg)/mL Blood	90 IU (18 µg)/mL Cells
Intramuscular	60 IU (12 µg)/mL Blood	120 IU (24 µg)/mL Cells

Administer 3000 IU (600 µg) every 8 hours **via the intravenous route**, until the total dose, calculated from Table 5, is administered.

Administer 6000 IU (1200 µg) every 12 hours **via the intramuscular route**, until the total dose, calculated from Table 5, is administered.

Treatment of ITP: WinRho SDF, Rh_o (D) Immune Globulin (Human), **must be given by intravenous administration** for the treatment of ITP. An intravenous dose of 125 to 300 IU/kg (25 to 60 µg/kg) body weight is recommended for individuals with ITP.

Initial Dosing: After confirming that the patient is Rh_o (D) positive, an initial dose of 250 IU/kg (50 µg/kg) body weight is recommended for the treatment of ITP. If the patient has a hemoglobin level that is less than 10 g/dL, a reduced dose of 125 to 200 IU/kg (25 to 40 µg/kg) should be given to minimize the risk of increasing the severity of anemia in the patient (see Warnings and Precautions, Hematologic). The initial dose may be administered in two divided doses given on separate days, if desired.

Subsequent Dosing: If subsequent therapy is required to elevate platelet counts, an intravenous dose of 125 to 300 IU/kg (25 to 60 µg/kg) body weight of WinRho SDF, Rh_o (D) Immune Globulin (Human), is recommended. The frequency and dose used should be administered by the patient's clinical response by assessing platelet counts, red cell counts, hemoglobin, and reticulocyte levels.

Administration: WinRho SDF, Lyophilized Formulation, should be reconstituted only with the accompanying vial of **Sterile Diluent**. If reconstituted product is not used immediately, then it should be stored at room temperature for no longer than four hours. It should not be administered concurrently with other products. There is no reconstitution required for the Liquid Formulation of WinRho SDF.

Parenteral products such as WinRho SDF, Rh_o (D) Immune Globulin (Human) should be inspected for particulate matter and discoloration prior to administration.

Aseptically administer the product intravenously in a suitable vein with a rate of injection of 1500 IU (300 µg)/5 to 15 seconds. Intramuscular injections are made into the deltoid muscle of the upper arm or the anterolateral aspects of the upper thigh. Due to the risk of sciatic nerve injury, the gluteal region should not be used as a routine injection site. If the gluteal region is used, use only the upper, outer quadrant. Discard any unused portion.

Lyophilized Formulation: Reconstitution: WinRho SDF should be reconstituted only with the accompanying vial of **sterile diluent**. Use aseptic technique throughout.

1. Reconstitute shortly before use.
2. Remove caps from the diluent and product vials.
3. Wipe exposed central portion of the rubber stopper with suitable disinfectant.
4. Withdraw diluent using a suitable syringe and needle. Use 1.25 to 2.5 mL of **sterile diluent** for intravenous injection or 1.25 mL for intramuscular injection for 600 IU (120 µg) and 1500 IU (300 µg). Use 8.5 mL of **sterile diluent** for intravenous and intramuscular injection for 5000 IU (1000 µg)s (see Table 6). Discard any unused diluent.
5. Inject diluent slowly at an angle so that the liquid is directed onto the inside glass wall of the vial containing the freeze-dried pellet.
6. Wet pellet by gently tilting and inverting the vial. **Do not shake.** Avoid frothing. Gently swirl upright vial until dissolved (less than ten minutes).

Table 6: WinRho SDF

Reconstitution

Vial Size	Volume of Diluent to be Added to Vial	Approximate Available Volume	Nominal Concentration/mL
Intravenous Injection			
600 IU (120 µg)	2.5 mL	2.4 mL	240 IU (48 µg)/mL
1500 IU (300 µg)	2.5 mL	2.4 mL	600 IU (120 µg)/mL
5000 IU (1000 µg)	8.5 mL	8.2 mL	588 IU (118 µg)/mL
Intramuscular Injection			
600 IU (120 µg)	1.25 mL	1.2 mL	480 IU (96 µg)/mL
1500 IU (300 µg)	1.25 mL	1.2 mL	1200 IU (240 µg)/mL
5000 IU (1000 µg)	8.5 mL	8.2 mL[a]	588 IU (118 µg)/mL

[a] To be administered into several sites.

Liquid Formulation: Table 7 describes the target fill volumes for each of the dosage sizes for the liquid presentation of WinRho SDF.

Table 7: WinRho SDF

Target Fill Volumes

Vial Size	Target Fill Volume
600 IU (120 µg)	0.5 mL
1500 IU (300 µg)	1.3 mL
2500 IU (500 µg)	2.2 mL
5000 IU (1000 µg)	4.4 mL
15 000 IU (3000 µg)	13.0 mL

Note: The entire contents of the vial should be removed to obtain the labeled dosage of WinRho SDF, Rh_o (D) Immune Globulin Intravenous (Human). If partial vials are required for dosage calculation, then calculation should be based on the target fill volume.

OVERDOSAGE:

If an Rh_o (D) positive individual is treated with large doses of WinRho SDF, a mild anemia may develop. However, this is normally compensated for by elevated red cell production. Normally, medical intervention other than discontinuation of WinRho SDF treatment would not be required.

In the post-marketing surveillance, a case of accidental overdose due to an error in calculating the dose, resulted in a severe hemolytic reaction and ultimately death in a patient with ITP.

> For management of a suspected drug overdose, CPhA recommends that you contact your **regional Poison Control Centre**. See the *CPS* Directory section for a list of Poison Control Centres.

ACTION AND CLINICAL PHARMACOLOGY: Mechanism of Action: Prophylaxis of Rh Immunization: WinRho SDF, Rh_o (D) Immune Globulin (Human), is used to suppress the immune response of non-sensitized Rh_o (D)-negative individuals who receive Rh_o (D) positive RBCs either by fetomaternal hemorrhage during delivery of an Rh_o (D) positive infant, abortion (either spontaneous or induced), following amniocentesis, abdominal trauma or mismatched transfusion. Administration of anti-Rh_o (D) antibody to the Rh_o (D) negative mother prevents an immune response with subsequent anti-Rh_o (D) antibody formation. The exact mechanism of action has yet to be determined.

WinRho SDF, when administered within 72 hours of a full-term delivery of an Rh_o (D)-positive infant by an Rh_o (D)-negative mother, will reduce the incidence of Rh alloimmunization from 12-13% to 1-2%. The 1-2% is, for the most part, due to alloimmunization during the last trimester of pregnancy. When treatment is given both antenatally at 28 weeks gestation and postpartum the Rh immunization rate drops to about 0.1%.

Treatment of ITP: In a clinical study of WinRho therapy of children with chronic ITP (duration of ITP >6 months), administration of anti-Rh_o (D) increased platelet counts from 36±14×10⁹/L to 263±138×10⁹/L; peak platelet levels were recorded at about one week after WinRho therapy; the effect of WinRho on platelet levels lasted a median of 29 days from the start of therapy. Comparable results were obtained in a clinical study of both adult and children with ITP of varying etiologies including ITP secondary to HIV infection. However, larger increases in platelet levels were seen in children than in adults.

WinRho SDF is used to increase platelet counts in nonsplenectomized Rh_o (D) positive patients with ITP and to alleviate clinical signs of bleeding in this patient population. The mechanism of action is not completely understood, but is thought to be due to binding of anti-Rh_o (D) (anti-D) to the Rh_o (D) RBC resulting in production of anti-D coated RBC complexes. This results in Fc receptor blockade, thus sparing antibody-coated platelets because of the preferential destruction of antibody-coated RBC complexes by the macrophages located in the reticuloendothelial system.

Pharmacodynamics: Two pharmacodynamic studies (WR-002 and 5696-2) measuring the clearance of Rh_o (D)-positive RBCs from the bloodstream after injection of WinRho and WinRho SD have been conducted. These 15 Rh_o (D)-negative subjects received fetal Rh_o (D)-positive erythrocytes followed by WinRho, given either IM (n=10) or IV (n=5). Clearance of Rh_o (D)-positive RBCs was complete within 24 hours. Six months later 5 subjects were re-challenged with Rh_o (D)-positive RBCs and none of them had evidence of a secondary immune response after having received a second administration of WinRho. Up to 102 days after the second injection, no demonstrable anti-D antibodies were present in the sera of any of the subjects. These pharmacodynamic results are consistent with the prophylaxis of Rh alloimmunization in Rh_o (D)-negative females exposed to Rh_o (D)-positive blood.

Pharmacokinetics: Pharmacokinetics of IV and IM administrations of WinRho SDF were evaluated (WS-031). The area under the curve (AUC_{0-t}) was similar after administration of IV and IM WinRho SDF which suggests IM administration is nearly 100% bioavailable. Peak levels (C_{max}) following IV administration was higher than the IM administration. The half-life ($t_{½}$) after IM administration was longer than the IV administration.

The pharmacokinetics of the freeze-dried and the liquid formulations of WinRho SDF were compared in 2 clinical studies (WS-029 and WS-038). In WS-029 the pharmacokinetic parameters of IV administration of the 2 formulations were evaluated. The measured mean of AUC_{0-t} and the C_{max} were similar after IV administrations of freeze-dried and liquid WinRho SDF. However, the 90% Confidence interval fell outside the predefined range of 80 to 125 % for the ratio of AUC_{0-t} after correction for actual product potency. The $t_{½}$ after IV administration of the 2 formulations was similar. The pharmacokinetics of the IM administrations of freeze-dried and the liquid formulations of WinRho SDF were also compared (WS-038). The AUC_{0-t} and the C_{max} appeared to be comparable after IM administrations of the 2 formulations, but a number of subjects were excluded in order to show comparability. Data from this trial was insufficient to demonstrate bioequivalence, based on the predefined criteria. The $t_{½}$ was the same after IM administration of the freeze-dried and liquid WinRho SDF (26 days).

Absorption: Following WinRho SDF administration by an IV route, peak levels are achieved within two hours, while the mean time to peak is 5-10 days when the drug is administered by an IM route. When 600 IU (120 µg) of product was administered to non-pregnant volunteers, the peak levels of passive anti-Rh_o (D) antibody were about 20 ng/mL and 40 ng/mL when the product was administered by IV and IM routes, respectively.

Distribution: When only 600 IU (120 µg) of drug is administered to pregnant women, passive anti-Rh_o (D) antibodies are not detectable in the circulation for more than six weeks and therefore a dose of 1500 IU (300 µg) should be used for antenatal administration.

The bioavailability following IV administration of WinRho SDF is expected to be immediate and complete, with passive antibodies quickly distributed between plasma and extravascular spaces. Based on AUC comparisons from pharmacokinetic studies of WinRho SDF and other hyperimmune products, IM administration is expected to be nearly 100% bioavailable.

Metabolism: Immune globulins and immune complexes are metabolized in the reticuloendothelial system.

Excretion: Based on numerous pharmacokinetic studies, in normal healthy individuals, WinRho SDF has typically an elimination half-life of 18-24 or 24-30 days following IV or IM administration, respectively. The half-life is expected to vary from patient to patient.

Duration of Effect: WinRho SDF, Rho (D) Immune Globulin (Human), has been shown to increase platelets in ITP patients. Platelet counts usually rise within one to two days and peak within seven to 14 days after initiation of therapy. The duration of response is variable; however, the average duration is approximately 30 days.

STORAGE AND STABILITY: WinRho SDF, Rh_o (D) Immune Globulin (Human) is stable at 2-8°C until the expiry date indicated on the label. Store WinRho SDF, Rh_o (D) Immune Globulin (Human) at 2-8°C. **Do not freeze. Do not use after expiration date.**

SPECIAL HANDLING INSTRUCTIONS: The product should be brought to room or body temperature immediately prior to use. Following reconstitution of freeze-dried WinRho SDF, the product should be clear or slightly opalescent. **Do not use solutions that appear cloudy or contain deposits.**

INFORMATION FOR THE PATIENT: Published in e-CPS, available by subscription at www.e-cps.ca.

DOSAGE FORMS, COMPOSITION AND PACKAGING: Lyophilized: 600 IU (120 µg): A carton box containing approximately 600 IU (120 µg) of anti-Rho (D), supplied freeze-dried in a 3 mL type 1 glass tubing vial fitted with a 13 mm lyophilization stopper of rubber formulation and a 13 mm flip-off seal, one single dose vial of sterile diluent, non-pyrogenic for reconstitution of WinRho SDF and a package insert. The final product formulation includes the addition of sodium chloride to yield 0.04 M, glycine to yield 0.1 M and polysorbate 80 to yield 0.01% (w/w). The accompanying sterile diluent contains 0.8 % sodium chloride and 10 mM sodium phosphate.

1500 IU (300 µg): A carton box containing approximately 1500 IU (300 µg) of anti-Rho (D), supplied freeze-dried in a 3 mL type 1 glass tubing vial fitted with a 13 mm lyophilization stopper of rubber formulation and a 13 mm flip-off seal, one single dose vial of sterile diluent, non-pyrogenic for reconstitution of WinRho SDF and a package insert. The final product formulation includes the addition of sodium chloride to yield 0.04 M, glycine to yield 0.1 M and polysorbate 80 to yield 0.01% (w/w). The accompanying sterile diluent contains 0.8 % sodium chloride and 10 mM sodium phosphate.

5000 IU (1000 µg): A carton box containing approximately 5000 IU (1000 µg) of anti-Rho (D), supplied freeze-dried in a 6 mL type 1 glass tubing vial fitted with a 20 mm lyophilization stopper of rubber formulation and a 20 mm flip-off seal, one single dose vial of sterile diluent, non-pyrogenic for reconstitution of WinRho SDF. The final product formulation includes the addition of sodium chloride to yield 0.04 M, glycine to yield 0.1 M and polysorbate 80 to yield 0.01% (w/w). The accompanying sterile diluent contains 0.8 % sodium chloride and 10 mM sodium phosphate.

Liquid: 600 IU (120 µg): A carton box containing a 0.5 mL single dose vial of 600 IU (120 µg) of anti-Rho(D) in a 3 mL type 1 glass tubing vial fitted with a 13 mm stopper of rubber formulation and a 13 mm flip-off seal and a package insert. The final liquid product formulation is stabilized with 10% maltose and 0.03% (w/w) polysorbate 80.

1500 IU (300 µg): A carton box containing a 1.3 mL single dose vial of 1500 IU (300 µg) of anti-Rho(D) in a 3 mL type 1 glass tubing vial fitted with a 13 mm stopper of rubber formulation and a 13 mm flip-off seal and a package insert. The final liquid product formulation is stabilized with 10% maltose and 0.03% (w/w) polysorbate 80.

5000 IU (1000 µg): A carton box containing a 4.4 mL single dose vial of 5000 IU (1000 µg) of anti-Rho(D) in a 6 mL type 1 glass tubing vial fitted with a 20 mm stopper of rubber formulation and a 20 mm flipoff seal and a package insert. The final liquid product formulation is stabilized with 10% maltose and 0.03% (w/w) polysorbate 80.

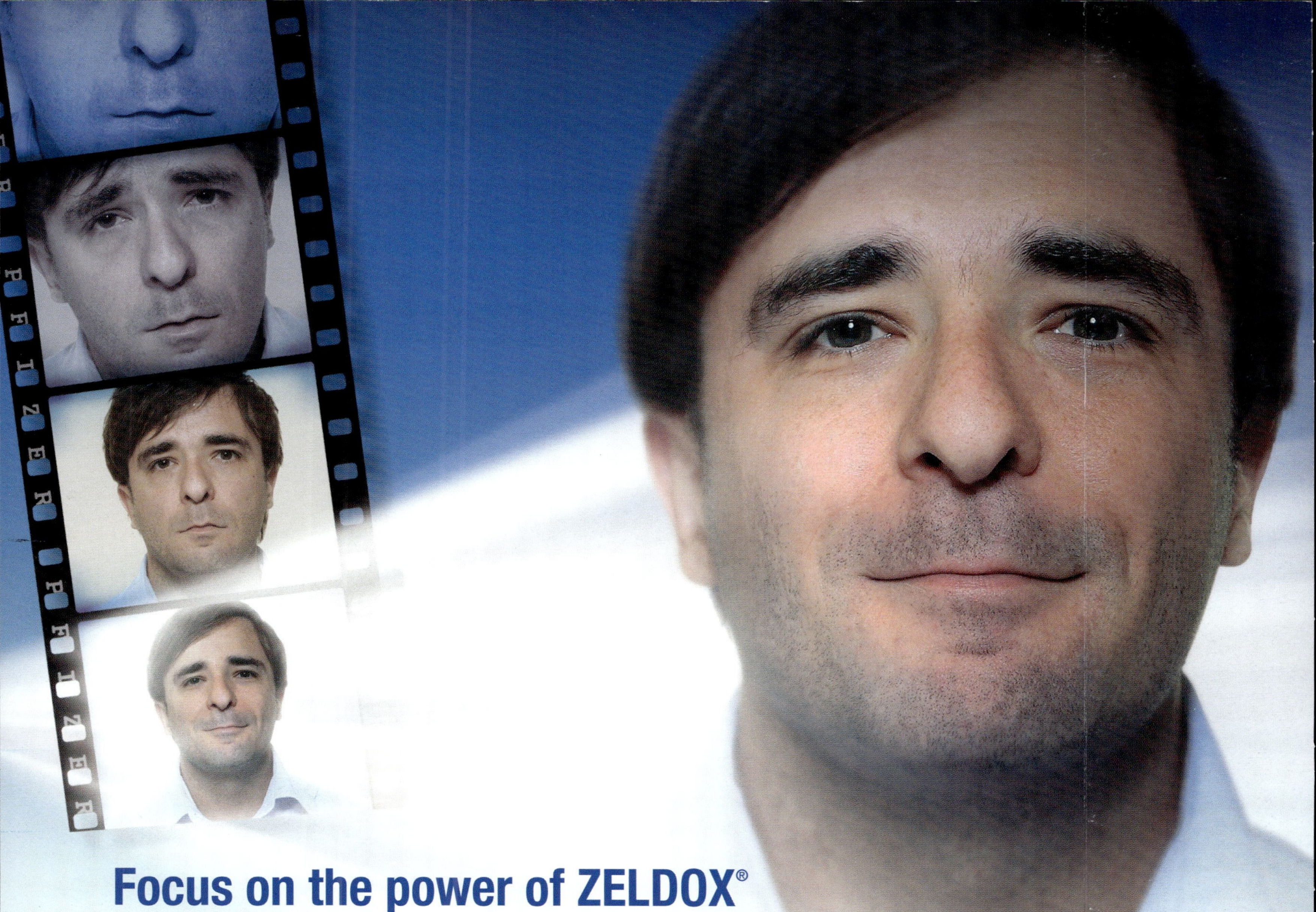

X
Y
Z

X Y Z

X

Xalacom™ [P]

latanoprost—timolol maleate

Elevated Intraocular Pressure Therapy

Pfizer

PHARMACOLOGY: XALACOM consists of two components: latanoprost and timolol maleate. Each mL of XALACOM contains latanoprost 50 micrograms and timolol maleate 6.8 mg equivalent to 5 mg timolol. These two components decrease elevated intraocular pressure (IOP) by different mechanisms of action.

Latanoprost is a prostanoid selective FP receptor agonist which reduces the IOP by increasing the outflow of aqueous humor. The main mechanism of action is increased uveoscleral outflow. In addition, some increase in outflow facility (decrease in trabecular outflow resistance) has been reported in man. Timolol maleate is a $beta_1$ and $beta_2$ (non-selective) adrenergic receptor blocking agent that does not have significant intrinsic sympathomimetic, direct myocardial depressant, or local anesthetic (membrane-stabilizing) activity. Timolol lowers the IOP by decreasing the formation of aqueous humor in the ciliary epithelium. The precise mechanism of action is not clearly established. The combined effect of these two agents administered as XALACOM once daily results in additional intraocular pressure reduction compared to either component administered alone separately.

Pharmacokinetics/Pharmacodynamics: Latanoprost: Latanoprost is an isopropyl ester prodrug which is inactive but becomes biologically active after hydrolysis to the acid of latanoprost. The prodrug is well absorbed through the cornea and all drug that enters the aqueous humor is hydrolysed by esterases during the passage through the cornea. Studies in man indicate that the maximum concentration in the aqueous humor, approximately 30 ng/mL, is reached about 2 hours after topical administration of latanoprost alone. The acid of latanoprost has a plasma clearance of 0.40 L/h/kg and a small volume of distribution, 0.16 L/kg, resulting in a rapid half-life in plasma (17 minutes). After topical ocular administration, the systemic bioavailability of the acid of latanoprost is 45%. The acid of latanoprost has a plasma protein binding of 87%. The main metabolism occurs in the liver. There is practically no metabolism of the acid of latanoprost in the eye. The main metabolites, 1,2-dinor and 1,2,3,4-tetranor metabolites, exert no or weak biological activity in animal studies and are excreted primarily in the urine.

Timolol: The maximum concentration of timolol in the aqueous humor is reached about one hour after topical ocular administration. Part of the dose is absorbed systemically and a maximum plasma concentration of 1 ng/mL is reached 10-20 minutes after topical ocular administration of one drop to each eye once daily (300 µg/day). The half-life of timolol in plasma is about 6 hours. Timolol is extensively metabolized in the liver. The metabolites, and unchanged timolol, are excreted in the urine.

XALACOM: No pharmacokinetic interactions between latanoprost and timolol have been observed although the aqueous humor concentrations of the acid of latanoprost tended to be higher 1 to 4 hours after administration of the combination product compared to monotherapy with either latanoprost or timolol.

Special Populations, Elderly, Gender, Pediatric and Race: Differences in the pharmacokinetics of XALACOM in these populations has not been investigated.

Diseases and Demographic Characteristics: No studies have been performed to investigate the influence of other diseases or demographic characteristics on the pharmacokinetics of XALACOM due to the inherit difficulties in measuring the drug concentrations after topical administration on the eyes.

INDICATIONS: XALACOM (latanoprost and timolol maleate) is indicated for the reduction of intraocular pressure (IOP) in patients with open-angle glaucoma or ocular hypertension who are insufficiently responsive to beta-blockers, prostaglandins, or other IOP lowering agents AND when the use of XALACOM (the combination drug) is considered appropriate.

XALACOM should not be used to initiate therapy.

For details of information obtained from Clinical Trials with XALACOM, please see Dosage.

CONTRAINDICATIONS: XALACOM (latanoprost and timolol maleate) is contraindicated in patients with:

- reactive airway disease including bronchial asthma, a history of bronchial asthma, or severe chronic obstructive pulmonary disease.
- sinus bradycardia, second or third degree atrioventricular block, overt cardiac failure, or cardiogenic shock.
- known hypersensitivity to latanoprost, timolol, benzalkonium chloride or any other ingredient in the product.

WARNINGS: Systemic Effects: Cardiac and Respiratory Reactions: Like other topically applied ophthalmic agents, XALACOM (latanoprost and timolol maleate) may be absorbed systemically. Due to the beta-adrenergic component timolol, the same types of adverse reactions as seen with systemic beta-blockers may occur including aggravation of Prinzmetal's angina, aggravation of peripheral and central circulatory disorders, bradycardia, and hypotension.

Severe respiratory reactions including death due to bronchospasm in patients with asthma and rarely death associated with cardiac failure have been reported following administration of timolol. Cardiac failure should be adequately controlled before beginning treatment. Patients with a history of severe cardiac disease should be watched for signs of cardiac failure and have their pulse rates checked.

Anaphylactic Reactions: While taking beta-blockers, patients with a history of atopy or severe anaphylactic reaction to a variety of allergens may be more active to repeated challenge with such allergens, either accidental, diagnostic or therapeutic. Such patients may be unresponsive to the usual doses of adrenaline used to treat anaphylactic reactions.

Additional Effects of Beta-adrenergic Blockade: Diabetes Mellitus: Beta-blockers should be administered with caution in patients subjected to spontaneous hypoglycemia or to diabetic patients (especially those with labile diabetes) who are receiving insulin or oral hypoglycemic agents. Beta-blockers may mask the signs and symptoms of acute hypoglycemia.

Thyrotoxicosis: Therapy with beta-blockers may mask certain symptoms of hyperthyroidism. Abrupt withdrawal of beta-blocker therapy may precipitate a worsening of symptoms.

Therapy with beta-blockers may aggravate symptoms of myasthenia gravis.

Concomitant Therapy: Timolol may interact with other drugs (see also Precautions, Drug Interactions). The effect on intraocular pressure or the known effects of systemic beta-blockers may be exaggerated when XALACOM is given to patients already receiving an oral beta-blocking agent. The use of two local beta-blockers or two local prostaglandins is not recommended.

Ocular Effects: **Changes to Pigmented Tissues: Latanoprost, the prostaglandin component contained in XALACOM, may gradually change the eye color, by increasing the amount of brown pigment in the iris. The color change is due to increased melanin content in stromal melanocytes on the iris rather than to an increase in the number of melanocytes. Typically the brown pigmentation around the pupil spreads concentrically towards the periphery in affected eyes, but the entire iris or parts of it may become more brownish. The change in iris colour occurs slowly and may not be noticeable for several months to years. The long term effects on the melanocytes and the consequences of potential injury to the melanocytes and/or deposition of pigment granules to other areas of the eye is currently unknown. Patients should be examined regularly and, depending on the clinical situation, treatment may be stopped if increased iris pigmentation ensues.**

This effect has predominantly been seen in patients with mixed colored irides (i.e. blue/gray-brown, green-brown, or yellow-brown). In patients with homogeneously blue, gray, green or brown eyes, the change has only rarely been seen during two years of treatment in clinical trials. The change in iris color occurs slowly, and may not be noticeable for several months to years. Patients should be informed of the possibility of iris color change. Patients who are expected to receive treatment in only one eye should be informed about the potential for increased brown pigmentation in the treated eye and thus, permanent heterochromia between the eyes. The increased pigmentation is permanent.

There is no evidence of melanin from iris melanocytes in trabecular meshwork in clinical studies which supports the lack of hyperpigmentation of the trabecular meshwork as a result of latanoprost treatment. In addition, no difference in iridial pigment epithelial melanin content has been observed between the latanoprost-treated eyes with increased iris pigmentation and untreated eyes from quantitative morphologic investigation of iridial specimens following colour change. Histopathologically, the increase in pigmentation was limited to a minor increase in the size of the melanin granules in the iris stroma.

Latanoprost has been reported to cause darkening, thickening and lengthening of eye lashes (see Adverse Effects).

Based on spontaneous reports, very rare cases of darkening of the palpebral skin have been reported with the administration of latanoprost ophthalmic solution (see Adverse Effects).

Pregnancy: No reproduction toxicity studies have been conducted with XALACOM. Embryofetal development studies with latanoprost have been performed in rats and rabbits. Latanoprost and/or its metabolites cross the placenta of rats. In rabbits, latanoprost caused embryofetal toxicity characterized by increased incidences of late resorption and reduced fetal weight at 5 µg/kg/day IV and total litter resorption at ≥50 µg/kg/day IV. No embryofetal effects were seen in rabbits at 1 µg/kg/day IV and in rats at up to 250 µg/kg/day IV.

Timolol maleate was not teratogenic in mice, rats and rabbits. Embryofetal development studies with timolol maleate in mice and rabbits showed no evidence of embryofetal toxicity at oral doses up to 50 µg/kg/day. At higher doses, increases in resorptions and fetal variations (14 ribs and hypoplastic sternebrae) were noticed in mice (1000 µg/kg/day) and increased resorption in rabbits (≥90 µg/kg/day). In rats, delayed ossification was seen ≥50 µg/kg/day and a decreased number of caudal vertebral bodies and arches and an increase in hypoplastic sternebrae were noted at 500 µg/kg/day.

XALACOM should be used during pregnancy only if the potential benefit justifies the potential risk to the fetus.

Lactation: There are limited experimental animal and no human data available on the pharmacokinetics of latanoprost lactation. Latanoprost and its metabolites may pass into breast milk. Timolol maleate has been detected in human milk following oral and ocular administration. Because of the potential for serious adverse reactions from XALACOM in nursing infants, XALACOM should be used with caution in nursing women.

Children: XALACOM is not recommended for use in children. The safety and efficacy of the use of XALACOM in children has not been established.

XALACOM has not been studied in patients with renal or hepatic impairment and therefore should be used with caution in such patients.

PRECAUTIONS: General: There have been reports of bacterial keratitis associated with the use of multiple-dose containers of topical ophthalmic products. These containers had been inadvertently contaminated by patients who, in most cases, had a concurrent corneal disease or a disruption of ocular epithelial surface (see Information for the Patient).

There is no or limited experience with latanoprost in inflammatory, neovascular, chronic angle closure or congenital glaucoma, open angle glaucoma in pseudophakic patients and pigmentary glaucoma. Latanoprost has no or little effect on the pupil but there is no experience in acute attacks of closed angle glaucoma. Therefore, it is recommended that XALACOM (latanoprost and timolol maleate) is used with caution in these conditions until more experience is obtained.

Macular edema, including cystoid macular edema, has been reported during treatment with latanoprost ophthalmic solution. These reports have mainly occurred in aphakic patients, in pseudophakic patients with a torn posterior lens capsule, or in patients with known risk factors for macular edema. XALACOM should be used with caution in these patients.

Choroidal detachment after filtration procedures has been reported with the administration of ocular hypotensive agents.

Drug Interactions: No specific interaction studies have been performed with XALACOM. Patients who are receiving treatment with XALACOM and an oral beta-adrenergic blocking agent should be observed for potential additive effects of beta-blockade, both systemic and on intraocular pressure. The concomitant use of two topical beta-adrenergic blocking agents is not recommended.

The potential exists for additive effects resulting in hypotension, and/or marked bradycardia when timolol ophthalmic drops are administered with oral calcium channel blockers, catecholamine-depleting drugs or beta-adrenergic blocking agents, antiarrhythmics (including amiodarone and quinidine), digitalis glycosides, parasympathomimetics, narcotics and monoamine oxidase (MAO) inhibitors.

Although XALACOM alone has little or no effect on pupil size, mydriasis has occasionally been reported when timolol is given with epinephrine.

Beta-blockers may increase the hypoglycemic effect of antidiabetic agents.

In vitro studies have shown that precipitation occurs when eye drops containing thimerosal are mixed with benzalkonium chloride, the preservative used in XALACOM. If such drugs are used they should be administered with an interval of at least 5 minutes between applications. Similarly, several contact lens soaking solutions contain thimerosal (see Use of Contact Lenses).

Occupational Hazards: Effects on ability to drive and use of machines: In common with other eye preparations, installation of eye drops may cause transient blurring of vision.

Use of Contact Lenses: XALACOM contains benzalkonium chloride which may be absorbed by contact lenses. Several contact lens soaking solutions contain thimerosal which may also form a precipitate with benzalkonium chloride (see Precautions, Drug Interactions). Therefore, contact lenses should be removed before installation of the eye drops and may be reinserted after 15 minutes.

ADVERSE EFFECTS: XALACOM (latanoprost and timolol maleate) was generally well tolerated. No adverse events specific to XALACOM have been observed in clinical studies. The adverse events have been limited to those that were reported previously with latanoprost and/or timolol maleate.

XALACOM was evaluated for safety in 394 patients with open-angle glaucoma or ocular hypertension in three long-term studies. Two percent (2%) of patients discontinued therapy with XALACOM due to adverse events.

Adverse events from clinical trials: Adverse events occurring at a frequency of ≥1% in three randomized, double blind comparative trials (004, 005 and 053) are presented in Table 1 and Table 2.

Table 1: XALACOM

Ocular Adverse Events (AE) that Occurred in ≥1% of Patients[a], in any Treatment Group, by Preferred Term[c]

Body System/Preferred Term	Number (%) Of Patients Per Treatment Group		
	XALACOM N=394	**Latanoprost N=414**	**Timolol N=415**
Vision			
Blepharitis	10 (2.5)	10 (2.4)	7 (1.7)
Cataract	11 (2.8)	18 (4.3)	10 (2.4)
Conjunctival disorder	4 (1.0)	3 (0.7)	4 (1.0)
Conjunctivitis	12 (3.0)	11 (2.7)	13 (3.1)
Corneal disorder	12 (3.0)	11 (2.7)	14 (3.4)
Corneal ulceration	1 (0.3)[a]	1 (0.2)[a]	—
Cystoid macular oedema	1 (0.3)[b]	1 (0.2)[a]	—
Epiphora	3 (0.8)	5 (1.2)	7 (1.7)
Errors of refraction	7 (1.8)	13 (3.1)	12 (2.9)
Eye hyperaemia	29 (7.4)	40 (9.7)	12 (2.9)
Eye pain	9 (2.3)	6 (1.4)	8 (1.9)
Increased intraocular pressure	1 (0.3)	5 (1.2)	7 (1.7)

(cont'd)

Table 1: XALACOM *(cont'd)*

Ocular Adverse Events (AE) that Occurred in ≥1% of Patients[a], in any Treatment Group, by Preferred Term[c]

	Number (%) Of Patients Per Treatment Group		
Body System/Preferred Term	**XALACOM N=394**	**Latanoprost N=414**	**Timolol N=415**
Iris pigmentation increased	6 (1.5)	13 (3.1)	4 (1.0)
Iritis	—	1 (0.2)[a]	2 (0.5)[a]
Irritation eye	49 (12.4)	54 (13.0)	29 (7.0)
Keratitis	4 (1.0)	3 (0.7)	1 (0.2)
Oedema eyelid	2 (0.5)	4 (1.0)	2 (0.5)
Photophobia	6 (1.5)	1 (0.2)	3 (0.7)
Retinal disorder	1 (0.3)	3 (0.7)	6 (1.4)
Uveitis	1 (0.3)[a]	—	—
Vision abnormal	26 (6.6)	29 (7.0)	22 (5.3)
Skin & Appendages			
Hypertrichosis[d]	9 (2.3)	6 (1.4)	2 (0.5)
Pigmentation abnormal	1 (0.3)[a]	—	—
Seborrhoea	2 (0.5)	4 (1.0)	—
Skin discolouration	1 (0.3)[a]	—	—
Skin disorder	8 (2.0)	4 (1.0)	—
Central & Peripheral Nervous System			
Optic atrophy	2 (0.5)	3 (0.7)	6 (1.4)
Visual field defect	18 (4.6)	19 (4.6)	18 (4.3)

[a] Despite a low frequency of reports, some AEs are included in the listing due to the implication of a potentially sight-threatening condition.
[b] A patient is counted only once per preferred term.
[c] Studies 004 and 005 included a 6 month and 053 a 12 month double-blinded period.
[d] Includes darkening, lengthening and growing of eye lashes.

Table 2: XALACOM

Systemic Adverse Events (AE) that Occurred in ≥1% of Patients[a], in any of the Treatment Groups, by Body System/Preferred Term[b]

	Number (%) Of Patients Per Treatment Group		
Body System/Preferred Term	**XALACOM N=394**	**Latanoprost N=414**	**Timolol N=415**
Respiratory			
Bronchitis	3 (0.8)	4 (1.0)	1 (0.2)
Coughing	1 (0.3)[a]	—	2 (0.5)[a]
Dyspnoea	2 (0.5)[a]	2 (0.5)[a]	2 (0.5)[a]
Pneumonia	1 (0.3)	3 (0.7)	4 (1.0)
Sinusitis	6 (1.5)	11 (2.7)	3 (0.7)
Upper respiratory tract infection	24 (6.1)	18 (4.3)	22 (5.3)
General			
Back pain	4 (1.0)	6 (1.4)	4 (1.0)
Chest pain	4 (1.0)	1 (0.2)	2 (0.5)
Influenza-like symptoms	10 (2.5)	4 (1.0)	3 (0.7)
Cardiovascular			
Hypertension	15 (3.8)	6 (1.4)	10 (2.4)
Hypertension aggravated	2 (0.5)[a]	1 (0.2)[a]	1 (0.2)[a]
Metabolic & Nutrition			
Diabetes mellitus	5 (1.3)	2 (0.5)	1 (0.2)
Diabetes mellitus aggravated	—	1 (0.2)	—
Glycosuria	2 (0.5)	1 (0.2)	—
Hyperglycaemia	1 (0.3)[a]	2 (0.5)[a]	2 (0.5)[a]
Hypercholesterolaemia	6 (1.5)	4 (1.0)	1 (0.2)
Central & Peripheral Nervous System			

(cont'd)

Table 2: XALACOM *(cont'd)*

Systemic Adverse Events (AE) that Occurred in ≥1% of Patients[a], in any of the Treatment Groups, by Body System/Preferred Term[b]

	Number (%) Of Patients Per Treatment Group		
Body System/Preferred Term	**XALACOM N=394**	**Latanoprost N=414**	**Timolol N=415**
Dizziness	2 (0.5)	4 (1.0)	1 (0.2)
Headache	9 (2.3)	15 (3.6)	5 (1.2)
Musculoskeletal			
Arthritis	8 (2.0)	5 (1.2)	4 (1.0)
Psychiatric			
Depression	6 (1.5)	7 (1.7)	4 (1.0)
Insomnia	1 (0.3)[a]	1 (0.2)[a]	1 (0.2)[a]
Sleep disorder	1 (0.3)	—	4 (1.0)
Skin & Appendages			
Bullous eruption	—	1 (0.2)	—
Rash	5 (1.3)	3 (0.7)	2 (0.5)
Resistance Mechanisms			
Infection	4 (1.0)	6 (1.4)	(1.4)
Gastrointestinal			
Dyspepsia	2 (0.5)	4 (1.0)	1 (0.2)
Urinary			
Cystitis	1 (0.3)	5 (1.2)	—
Urinary tract infection	1 (0.3)	2 (0.5)	4 (1.0)

[a] A patient is counted only once per preferred term. AEs that occurred in <1 % of the patients but were very similar to an event that did occur in ≥1% of the patients (such as "hypertension" and "hypertension aggravated") are listed. Also, groups of mutually related AEs, where each AE may be reported in <1%, but together they sum up to ≥1% (such as "diabetes mellitus aggravated" and "hyperglycaemia" together with "glucosuria") are summarised.
[b] Studies 004 and 005 included a 6 month- and 053 a 12 month double-blinded period.

Based on evidence from consecutive photographs, increased iris pigmentation was observed in 16-20% of patients treated with XALACOM for up to one year. The most frequent findings of increased iris pigmentation were in the known high-risk eye color groups, i.e. those with green-brown, yellow-brown, and blue/gray-brown irises. In patients with homogeneously blue, grey, green or brown eyes, the change was rarely observed. Darkening, thickening and lengthening of eye lashes were observed in 37.4% of patients.

The following additional adverse events that have been reported with latanoprost and timolol eye drops:

Latanoprost:

Ocular: foreign body sensation, punctate epithelial erosions, macular edema/cystoid macular edema, iritis/uveitis, corneal edema and erosions.

Respiratory: asthma, asthma exacerbation and dyspnea.

Skin: darkening of the palpebral skin.

Timolol Maleate (topical formulation):

Special Senses: signs and symptoms of ocular irritation including keratitis, decreased corneal sensitivity, dry eyes, visual disturbances including refractive changes (due to withdrawal of miotic therapy in some cases), diplopia, ptosis, choroidal detachment (following filtration surgery), tinnitus.

Cardiovascular: bradycardia, arrhythmia, hypotension, syncope, heart block, cerebrovascular accident, cerebral ischemia, congestive heart failure, palpitation, cardiac arrest, edema, claudication, Raynaud's phenomenon, cold hands and feet.

Respiratory: bronchospasm (predominantly in patients with pre-existing bronchospastic disease), respiratory failure, dyspnea, cough.

Body as Whole: asthenia, fatigue, chest pain.

Skin: alopecia, psoriasiform rash or exacerbation of psoriasis.

Hypersensitivity: symptoms of allergic reactions including angioedema, urticaria, localized and generalized rash.

Nervous System/Psychiatric: dizziness, depression, insomnia, nightmares, memory loss, increase in signs and symptoms of myasthenia gravis, parasthenia.

Digestive: nausea, diarrhea, dyspepsia, dry mouth.

Urogenital: decreased libido, Peyronie's disease.

Immunologic: systemic lupus erythematosus.

OVERDOSE:

There is no human data available on overdosage with XALACOM (latanoprost and timolol maleate).

Symptoms: Symptoms of systemic timolol overdosage are: bradycardia, hypotension, bronchospasm, and cardiac arrest. If such symptoms occur, treatment should be symptomatic and supportive. Studies have shown that timolol is not readily dialyzable.

Apart from ocular irritation and conjunctival or episcleral hyperemia, the ocular effects of latanoprost administered at high doses are not known. Intravenous infusion of up to 3 µg/kg in healthy volunteers induced no symptoms, but a dose of 5.5-10 µg/kg caused nausea, abdominal pain, dizziness, fatigue, hot flashes, and sweating. These events were mild to moderate in severity and resolved without treatment within 4 hours after terminating the infusion.

In monkeys, latanoprost has been infused intravenously to doses up to 500 µg/kg without major effects on the cardiovascular system. Intravenous administration of latanoprost in monkeys has been associated with transient bronchoconstriction.

Treatment: If overdose with XALACOM occurs, treatment should be symptomatic.

If XALACOM is accidentally ingested the following information may be useful: one bottle contains 125 µg latanoprost and 12.5 mg timolol. Both timolol and latanoprost are extensively metabolized in the liver. In fact, more than 90% of latanoprost is metabolized during the first pass through the liver.

For management of a suspected drug overdose, CPhA recommends that you contact your **regional Poison Control Centre**. See the *CPS* Directory section for a list of Poison Control Centres.

DOSAGE: The recommended adult (including the elderly) dosage of XALACOM (latanoprost and timolol maleate) is one drop in the affected eye(s) once daily. If one dose is missed, treatment should continue with the next dose as normal.

The use of XALACOM may be considered in patients who require both timolol and latanoprost. Whether patients who are adequately controlled with timolol given twice daily plus latanoprost given once daily, will be as well controlled with XALACOM given once daily has not been fully investigated. The IOP lowering effect of Xalacom once daily may be less than that seen with the concomitant administration of timolol twice daily and latanoprost once daily based on the results from a short term clinical trial.

INFORMATION FOR THE PATIENT: Published in e-CPS, available by subscription at www.e-cps.ca.

SUPPLIED: Each mL of sterile, isotonic, buffered, clear and colorless aqueous solution, for topical administration on the eye, contains: 50 µg of latanoprost and 5 mg of timolol (6.83 mg timolol maleate). One drop contains approximately 1.5 µg of latanoprost and 150 µg of timolol. Nonmedicinal ingredients: disodium hydrogen phosphate anhydrous, sodium chloride, sodium dihydrogen phosphate monohydrate and water for injection. Benzalkonium chloride 0.02% is added as a preservative. If required, the pH of the solution is adjusted with hydrochloric acid and/or sodium hydroxide. pH: approximately 6.0. Osmolality: approximately 290 mOsmol/kg. Plastic ophthalmic dispenser bottles of 5 mL with a dropper tip, screw cap and tamper proof polyethylene overcap. Each bottle contains 2.5 mL of XALACOM corresponding to approximately 80 drops of solution. Store unopened bottle under refrigeration (2 to 8°C). Protect from light. Once opened, the 2.5 mL container may be stored at room temperature up to 25°C for 10 weeks. Protect from light.

Xalatan™ Ⓟ

latanoprost

Prostaglandin F2α Analogue

Pfizer

PHARMACOLOGY: Latanoprost, a prostaglandin $F_{2\alpha}$ (13,14-dihydro-17-phenyl-18,19,20-trinor-PGF2α isopropyl ester) analogue, is a selective prostanoid FP receptor agonist which reduces the intraocular pressure by increasing the outflow of aqueous humor. Studies in animals and man indicate that the main mechanism of action is increased uveoscleral outflow.

Glaucoma is a disease with characteristic optic nerve damage and a corresponding visual field defect. Increased intraocular pressure (IOP) is one of the main risk factors. However, disturbances in blood flow may also play a role in some cases. In ocular hypertension, patients may have increased IOP but without changes in the visual field or corresponding optic nerve damage.

Xalatan is a sterile, isotonic, buffered aqueous solution with a pH of approximately 6.7.

Each mL contains 50 µg of latanoprost, a colorless to slightly yellow oil. Latanoprost is an isopropyl ester prodrug which is well absorbed through the cornea and upon entering the aqueous humor is rapidly and completely hydrolyzed to the biologically active acid. Studies in humans indicate that the peak concentration in the aqueous humor is reached about 2 hours after topical administration.

Following topical administration in monkeys, latanoprost is primarily distributed in the anterior segment, conjunctiva and eyelids with only minute quantities reaching the posterior segment. Reduction of IOP following a single dose in humans starts about 3 to 4 hours following topical administration, and the maximum effect is reached after 8 to 12 hours. Pressure reduction is maintained for at least 24 hours.

There is practically no metabolism of the acid of latanoprost in the eye. The plasma clearance is rapid and occurs in the liver. In humans, the half-life of the biologically active acid in plasma is approximately 17 minutes. In animal studies, the main metabolites were the 1,2-dinor and the 1,2,3,4-tetranor metabolites which exerted only weak or no biologic activity, and were excreted primarily in urine.

Clinical Studies: In five controlled clinical trials of up to 6 months' duration, reduction of IOP was evaluated in patients with open-angle glaucoma or ocular hypertension treated with either latanoprost dosed once a day or timolol dosed twice a day. The mean baseline IOP (mmHg) in these studies ranged from 23.1 to 29.9 and 23.1 to 28.7 for the groups treated with latanoprost and timolol, respectively. The results are in Table 1.

Table 1: Xalatan

Reduction of IOP (mmHg) in Patients Treated with Xalatan as Compared to Timolol[a]

Study (ref. #)	No. of Patients		Baseline IOP mmHg		Change from Baseline mmHg (%)[b]		Between Group Comparison (p-Value)
	Xalatan	Timolol	Xalatan	Timolol	Xalatan	Timolol	
Study 1 (5)	128	140	24.4	24.1	−6.2 (25.4)	−4.5 (17.8)	<0.001
Study 2 (24)	149	145	25.2	25.4	−7.9 (30.9)	−7.4 (29.1)	0.2
Study 3 (2)	183	84	25.1	24.6	−7.8 (30.7)	−6.6 (26.0)	0.002
Study 4 (34)	30	30	29.9	28.7	−11.7 (39.1)	−8.5 (29.6)	0.045
Study 5 (35)	76	78	23.1	23.1	−6.2 (26.8)	−4.4 (19.0)	<0.001

a Intent-to-treat (ITT) analysis, except for Study 5, which evaluated data for patients who completed the study.
b Mean diurnal IOPs (mean of 3 different daytime readings) used in Studies 1-4. Mean morning IOPs, representing trough values for both treatments, used in Study 5.

In latanoprost studies of up to 24 months' duration, there was no evidence of long-term drift in IOP reduction; the mean diurnal IOP reduction remained constant in patients treated up to 24 months.

Similar results were obtained from a 3 month phase III clinical trial in Asian patients with chronic angle closure glaucoma. In this study, 137 patients received latanoprost once daily and 138 patients received timolol twice daily. Latanoprost reduced IOP by 30% from the untreated baseline of 25.2 mmHg. Timolol reduced IOP by 20% from a baseline of 25.9 mmHg. The p-value for the difference between the IOP reduction by latanoprost versus timolol was p<0.001. The benefit to patients from latanoprost was irrespective of their degree of angle closure.

A 3-year open-label prospective safety study with a 2-year extension phase was conducted to evaluate the progression of increased iris pigmentation with continuous use of latanoprost once-daily as adjunctive therapy in 519 patients with open-angle glaucoma. The analysis was based on observed-cases population of the 380 patients who continued in the extension phase.

Results showed that the onset of noticeable increased iris pigmentation occurred within the first year of treatment for the majority of the patients who developed noticeable increased iris pigmentation. Patients continued to show signs of increasing iris pigmentation throughout the five years of the study. Observation of increased iris pigmentation did not affect the incidence, nature or severity of adverse events (other than increased iris pigmentation) recorded in the study. In the study, IOP reduction was similar regardless of the development of increased iris pigmentation during the study.

Clinical trials have shown that latanoprost has no significant effect on production of aqueous humour and no effect on the blood-aqueous barrier. At clinical dose levels, latanoprost has negligible or no effects on intraocular blood circulation when studied in monkeys. However, mild to moderate conjunctival or episcleral hyperemia may occur as a result of topical administration.

Latanoprost has not induced fluorescein leakage in the posterior segment of pseudophakic human eyes during short term treatment.

Phase II clinical trials have also demonstrated that latanoprost is effective in combination with other drugs used for treatment of glaucoma. The IOP reducing effect of latonoprost is additive to that of beta-adrenergic antagonists (timolol), adrenergic agonists (dipivefrin, epinephrine), cholinergic agonists (pilocarpine) and carbonic anhydrase inhibitors (acetazolamide).

INDICATIONS: For the reduction of intraocular pressure in patients with open-angle glaucoma and ocular hypertension. Latanoprost may be used for the reduction of intraocular pressure in patients with chronic angle-closure glaucoma who underwent peripheral iridotomy or laser iridoplasty.

See information in sections of Pharmacology, Warnings, Precautions and Adverse Effects.

CONTRAINDICATIONS: Known hypersensitivity to benzalkonium chloride or any other ingredient in this product.

WARNINGS: Latanoprost has been reported to cause changes to pigmented tissues. The most frequently reported changes have been increased pigmentation of the iris, periorbital tissue (eyelid) and eyelashes, and growth of eyelashes. Pigmentation is expected to increase as long as latanoprost is administered. After discontinuation of latanoprost, pigmentation of the iris is likely to be permanent while pigmentation of the periorbital tissue and eyelash changes have been reported to be reversible in some patients. Patients who receive treatment should be informed of the possibility of increased pigmentation. **The effects of increased pigmentation beyond 5 years are not known.** Patients who are expected to receive treatment in only one eye should be informed about the potential for increased pigmentation in the treatment eye and thus, heterochromia between the eyes.

Pregnancy: Reproduction studies have been performed in rats and rabbits. In rabbits an incidence of 4 of 16 dams had no viable fetuses at a dose that was approximately 80 times the maximum human dose, and the highest nonembryocidal dose in rabbits was approximately 15 times the maximum human dose. Latanoprost should be used during pregnancy only if the potential benefit justifies the potential risk to the fetus.

Lactation: The active substance in latanoprost and its metabolites may pass into breast milk, and latanoprost should therefore be used with caution in nursing women.

Children: The safety and efficacy of the use of latanoprost in children has not been established.

PRECAUTIONS: General: Latanoprost may gradually increase the pigmentation of the iris. This effect has predominantly been seen in patients with mixed coloured irides, i.e., blue-brown, grey-brown, green-brown or yellow-brown. The eye colour change is due to increased melanin content in the stromal melanocytes rather than to an increase in the number of melanocytes. This change may not be noticeable for several months to years (see Warnings). Typically, the brown pigmentation around the pupil spreads concentrically towards the periphery of the iris and the entire iris or parts of the iris become more brownish. Neither nevi nor freckles of the iris appear to be affected by treatment. While treatment with latanoprost can be continued in patients who develop noticeably increased pigmentation, these patients should be examined regularly.

During clinical trials, the increase in brown iris pigment has not been shown to progress further upon discontinuation of treatment, but the resultant colour change may be permanent. Eyelid skin darkening, which may be reversible, has been reported in association with the use of latanoprost (see Warnings).

Latanoprost may gradually change eyelashes and vellus hair in the treated eye; these changes include increased length, thickness, pigmentation, the number of lashes or hairs, and misdirected growth of eyelashes. Eyelash changes are usually reversible upon discontinuation of treatment.

Macular edema, including cystoid macular edema, has been reported during treatment with latanoprost. These reports have mainly occurred in aphakic patients, in pseudophakic patients with torn posterior lens capsule, or in patients with known risk factors for macular edema. Latanoprost should be used with caution in patients who do not have an intact posterior capsule or who have known risk factors for macular edema.

There is no experience with latanoprost in patients with inflammatory ocular conditions, inflammatory glaucoma, neovascular glaucoma or congenital glaucoma, and only limited experience with pseudophakic patients and in patients with pigmentary glaucoma.

Latanoprost should be used with caution in patients with a history of intraocular inflammation (iritis/uveitis) and should generally not be used in patients with active intraocular inflammation.

There is no experience in patients with severe or uncontrolled asthma. Such patients should therefore be treated with caution until there is sufficient experience (see Adverse Effects and Pharmacology for experience in patients with mild to moderate asthma).

Latanoprost has not been studied in patients with renal or hepatic impairment and should, therefore, be used with caution in such patients.

There have been reports of bacterial keratitis associated with the use of multiple-dose containers of topical ophthalmic products. These containers had been inadvertently contaminated by patients who, in most cases, had a concurrent corneal disease or a disruption of ocular epithelial surface (see Information for the Patient).

Contact lenses should be removed prior to the administration of latanoprost, and may be reinserted 15 minutes after administration (see Information for the Patient).

Drug Interactions: In vitro studies have shown that precipitation occurs when eye drops containing thimerosal are mixed with latanoprost. If such drugs are used, they should be administered with an interval of at least 5 minutes between applications.

ADVERSE EFFECTS: The ocular adverse events and ocular signs and symptoms reported in 5 to 15% of the patients on latanoprost in the 6 month, multicenter, double-masked, active-controlled trials were blurred vision, burning and stinging, conjunctival hyperemia, foreign body sensation, itching, increased iris pigmentation and punctate epithelial keratopathy.

Local conjunctival hyperemia was observed; however, less than 1% of the latanoprost treated patients required discontinuation of therapy because of intolerance to conjunctival hyperemia.

In addition to the above listed ocular events/signs and symptoms, the following were reported in 1 to 4% of the patients: dry eye, excessive tearing, eye pain, lid crusting, lid edema, lid erythema, lid discomfort/pain and photophobia.

The following events were reported in less than 1% of the patients: conjunctivitis, diplopia and discharge from the eye.

During clinical studies, there were extremely rare reports of the following: retinal artery embolus, retinal detachment, and vitreous hemorrhage from diabetic retinopathy.

The most common systemic adverse events seen with latanoprost were upper respiratory tract infection/cold/flu which occurred at a rate of approximately 4%. Pain in muscle/joint/back, chest pain/angina pectoris and rash/allergic skin reaction each occurred at a rate of 1 to 2%.

Macular edema, including cystoid macular edema, has been reported during treatment with latanoprost. These reports have mainly occurred in aphakic patients, in pseudophakic patients with a torn posterior lens capsule, or in patients with known risk factors for macular edema. Latanoprost should be used with caution in these patients. Upon discontinuation of latanoprost treatment, visual acuity has improved, in some cases with concurrent treatment with topical steroidal and nonsteroidal anti-inflammatory drugs.

Latanoprost has been reported to cause darkening, thickening and lengthening of eye lashes.

Based on spontaneous reports, rare cases of iritis/uveitis and very rare cases of darkening of the palpebral skin have been reported.

The following events, which have been chosen for inclusion due to either their seriousness, frequency of reporting, possible causal connection to latanoprost, or a combination of these factors, have been reported during postmarketing use of latanoprost in clinical practice and in the literature: eyelash changes (increased length, thickness, pigmentation of eyelashes, increased number of eyelashes and vellus hairs on the eyelid, curling of eyelashes, misdirected eyelashes sometimes resulting in eye irritation); eyelid skin darkening; intraocular inflammation (iritis/uveitis); macular edema, including cystoid macular edema; corneal edema and erosions; localized skin reaction on the eyelid; and toxic epidermal necrolysis. Those events are reported voluntarily from a population of unknown size; therefore, estimates of frequency cannot be made. Rare cases of asthma, asthma aggravation, acute asthma attack and dyspnea have been reported. There is limited experience from patients with asthma but latanoprost neither was found to affect pulmonary function when studied in a small number of steroid treated patients suffering from moderate asthma nor was it found to affect the pulmonary function, airway reactivity or β_2-responsiveness when studied in a small number of non-steroid treated asthma patients.

OVERDOSE:

Symptoms: Apart from ocular irritation and conjunctival or episcleral hyperemia, no other ocular side effects of latanoprost administered at high doses are known. I.V. infusion of up to 3 µg/kg in healthy volunteers produced mean plasma concentrations 200 times higher than during clinical treatment and no adverse reactions were observed. I.V. doses of 5.5 to 10 µg/kg caused abdominal pain, dizziness, fatigue, hot flushes, nausea and sweating.

In monkeys, latanoprost has been infused i.v. in doses of up to 500 µg/kg without major effects on the cardiovascular system. I.V. administration in monkeys has been associated with transient bronchoconstriction. However, in patients with bronchial asthma, bronchoconstriction was not induced by latanoprost when administered topically to the eyes at a dose 7 times the recommended clinical dose.

Treatment: If overdosage with latanoprost occurs, treatment should be symptomatic.

For management of a suspected drug overdose, CPhA recommends that you contact your **regional Poison Control Centre**. See the *CPS* Directory section for a list of Poison Control Centres.

DOSAGE: The recommended dose for adults including the elderly (over 60 years of age), is 1 drop in the affected eye(s) once daily. Optimal effect is obtained if latanoprost is administered in the evening.

The dose of latanoprost should not exceed once daily as it has been shown that more frequent administration decreases the IOP lowering effect. Reduction of IOP in humans starts about 3 to 4 hours after treatment and maximum effect is reached after 8 to 12 hours. Pressure reduction is maintained for at least 24 hours.

If 1 dose is missed, treatment should continue with the next dose the following day.

Use in Combination with Other Drugs: Latanoprost may be used concomitantly with other topical ophthalmic products to further lower intraocular pressure. If more than 1 topical ophthalmic drug is being used, the drugs should be administered at least 5 minutes apart.

INFORMATION FOR THE PATIENT: Published in e-CPS, available by subscription at www.e-cps.ca.

SUPPLIED: Each mL of a sterile, isotonic, buffered aqueous solution, for topical ophthalmic administration, contains: latanoprost 50 µg. One drop contains approximately 1.5 µg of latanoprost. Nonmedicinal ingredients: benzalkonium chloride as a preservative, disodium hydrogen phosphate anhydrous, sodium chloride, sodium dihydrogen phosphate monohydrate and water for injection. Buffered to a pH of approximately 6.7 and is isotonic with lacrimal fluid. Plastic ophthalmic dispenser bottles of 5 mL with a dropper tip, screw cap and tamper proof polyethylene overcap. Each bottle contains 2.5 mL of latanoprost corresponding to approximately 80 drops. Store unopened bottle under refrigeration (2 to 8°C). Protect from light. Once opened, bottle may be stored at room temperature up to 25°C, for up to 6 weeks.

Xamiol® Ⓟ

calcipotriol—betamethasone dipropionate

Topical Antipsoriatic Agent—Vitamin D Analogue—Corticosteroid

LEO Pharma

Date of Preparation: November 5, 2008

SUMMARY PRODUCT INFORMATION:

Route of Administration	Dosage Form/ Strength	Clinically Relevant Nonmedicinal Ingredients
Topical	Gel: 50 µg/g calcipotriol (as monohydrate) and 0.5 mg/g betamethasone (as dipropionate)	None For a complete listing see Dosage Forms, Composition and Packaging.

INDICATIONS AND CLINICAL USE: XAMIOL (calcipotriol and betamethasone dipropionate) gel is indicated for the topical treatment of moderate to severe scalp psoriasis for up to 4 weeks.

CONTRAINDICATIONS:

- known hypersensitivity to XAMIOL (calcipotriol and betamethasone dipropionate), to any ingredient in the formulation or to components of the tube. For a complete listing, see Dosage Forms, Composition and Packaging.
- **ophthalmic use**
- patients with known disorders of calcium metabolism
- viral (e.g. herpes or varicella) lesions of the skin, fungal or bacterial skin infections, parasitic infections, skin manifestations in relation to tuberculosis or syphilis, perioral dermatitis, atrophic skin, striae atrophicae, fragility of skin veins, ichthyosis, acne vulgaris, acne rosacea, rosacea, ulcers and wounds
- guttate, erythrodermic, exfoliative and pustular psoriasis
- patients with severe renal insufficiency or severe hepatic disorders.

WARNINGS AND PRECAUTIONS: General: Due to the content of calcipotriol, hypercalcaemia may occur if the maximum weekly dose (100 g) is exceeded. Serum calcium is quickly normalised when treatment is discontinued. The risk of hypercalcaemia is minimal when the recommendations relevant to calcipotriol are followed (see Monitoring and Laboratory Tests).

Carcinogenesis and Mutagenesis: Calcipotriol when used in combination with ultraviolet radiation (UVR) may enhance the known skin carcinogenic effect of UVR. This potential risk is based on the pre-clinical finding in mice of a reduced time to tumor formation from long term exposure of UVR and topically applied calcipotriol.

Endocrine and Metabolism: XAMIOL (calcipotriol and betamethasone dipropionate) contains a potent group III steroid and concurrent treatment with other steroids on the scalp must be avoided.

Application on large areas of broken skin or under occlusive dressings should be avoided since it increases systemic absorption of corticosteroids and the risk of adverse effects such as adrenocortical suppression with the potential for glucocorticosteroid insufficiency after withdrawal of treatment. Manifestations of Cushing's syndrome, and affects on the metabolic control of diabetes mellitus (e.g. hyperglycaemia, glucosuria) can also be produced in some patients by systemic absorption of topical corticosteroids.

In a study in patients with both extensive scalp and extensive body psoriasis using a combination of high doses of XAMIOL gel (scalp application) and high doses of DOVOBET ointment* (body application), 5 of 32 patients (15.6%) showed a borderline decrease in cortisol response to adrenocorticotropic hormone (ACTH) challenge after 4 weeks of treatment (see Action and Clinical Pharmacology).

Skin: Facial skin is very sensitive to corticosteroids and XAMIOL is not indicated for use in this area. The face should only be treated with weaker corticosteroids. Uncommon local adverse reactions (such as eye irritation or irritation of facial skin) were observed when the drug was accidentally administered in the area of the face, or accidentally to the eyes or conjunctiva (see Adverse Reactions). The patient must be instructed in the correct use of XAMIOL (for e.g. washing their hands after each application) to avoid accidental transfer or application to the face, mouth and eyes. Should facial dermatitis develop in spite of these precautions, XAMIOL therapy should be discontinued.

When lesions become secondarily infected, they should be treated with antimicrobiological therapy. However, if the infection worsens, treatment with corticosteroids should be stopped.

When treating psoriasis with topical corticosteroids, it is recommended that treatment be interrupted periodically. There may be a risk of generalised pustular psoriasis or of rebound psoriasis when discontinuing corticosteroids after prolonged periods of use. Medical supervision should therefore continue in the post-treatment period.

There is a risk of local and systemic corticosteroid adverse effects with XAMIOL, including striae or atrophy of the skin and adrenal suppression. Treatment should be discontinued in the case of corticosteroid adverse effects related to the use of XAMIOL.

Patients who apply XAMIOL to exposed skin (e.g. a bald scalp) should avoid both natural and artificial sunlight (e.g. phototherapy, tanning beds, sun lamps, etc.).

Special Populations: Pregnant Women: The safety of calcipotriol and/or topical corticosteroids for use during pregnancy has not been established. The use of XAMIOL is not recommended in pregnant women.

Nursing Women: The safety of calcipotriol and/or topical corticosteroids for use in nursing women has not been established. It is not known whether calcipotriol can be excreted in breast milk. Betamethasone passes into breast milk, but it is not known if topical application of corticosteroids can lead to sufficient systemic absorption to produce detectable quantities in breast milk. The use of XAMIOL is not recommended in nursing women.

Pediatrics (<18 years of age): There is no clinical trial experience with the use of XAMIOL in children, use is therefore not recommended. Children may demonstrate greater susceptibility to systemic steroid related adverse effects due to a larger skin surface area to body weight ratio as compared to adults.

Monitoring and Laboratory Tests: Treatment with XAMIOL in the recommended amounts (see Dosage and Administration) does not generally result in changes in laboratory values. However, in patients at risk of hypercalcaemia it is recommended that baseline serum calcium levels be obtained before starting treatment with subsequent monitoring of serum calcium levels at suitable intervals. If serum calcium becomes elevated, XAMIOL administration should be discontinued and serum calcium levels should be measured once weekly until they return to normal.

ADVERSE REACTIONS: Adverse Drug Reaction Overview: The clinical trial programme for XAMIOL (calcipotriol and betamethasone dipropionate) has included more than 1900 patients with scalp psoriasis treated with XAMIOL gel. Approximately 8% of patients treated with XAMIOL experienced an adverse reaction. Based on data from clinical trials, the most common adverse reaction is pruritus.

The following adverse reactions led to discontinuation of treatment with XAMIOL in 0.1-0.2% of patients: pruritus, skin pain or irritation, dermatitis, eye irritation, rash, burning sensation, face oedema, folliculitis and dry skin.

* DOVOBET ointment (50 µg/g calcipotriol and 0.5 mg/g betamethasone, as dipropionate).

Clinical Trial Adverse Drug Reactions: Because clinical trials are conducted under very specific conditions the adverse reaction rates observed in the clinical trials may not reflect the rates observed in practice and should not be compared to the rates in the clinical trials of another drug. Adverse drug reaction information from clinical trials is useful for identifying drug-related adverse events and for approximating rates.

Two pivotal and 4 supporting controlled clinical studies were conducted in scalp psoriasis. Table 1 summarizes adverse drug reactions reported by at least 1% of patients in any treatment group in the pivotal scalp studies. Overall, the incidence of patients with at least one ADR was lowest in the XAMIOL gel group.

Less Common Clinical Trial Adverse Drug Reactions: From clinical trials conducted in scalp psoriasis, the uncommon adverse reactions are listed by MeDRA SOC from most to least frequent.

Eye Disorders: eye irritation.

Infections: otitis externa.

Investigations: elevated blood calcium.

Skin and Subcutaneous Tissue Disorders: burning sensation of the skin, skin pain or irritation, folliculitis, dermatitis, contact dermatitis, erythema, acne, dry skin, exacerbations of psoriasis, rash and pustular rash, and face oedema.

Other Adverse Drug Reactions: Adverse reactions observed for the individual drug substances calcipotriol and betamethasone dipropionate are described below.

Calcipotriol: Adverse reactions include application site reactions, pruritus, skin irritation, burning and stinging sensation, dry skin, erythema, rash, dermatitis, eczema, aggravated psoriasis, photosensitivity and hypersensitivity reactions. There have been infrequent reports of angioedema and facial oedema. Isolated cases of hypercalcaemia or hypercalciuria have been reported (see Warnings and Precautions).

Betamethasone Dipropionate: Local reactions can occur after topical use especially during prolonged application including, skin atrophy, telangiectasia, striae, folliculitis, hypertrichosis, perioral dermatitis, allergic contact dermatitis, depigmentation and colloid milia. When treating psoriasis, there may be a risk of generalised pustular psoriasis.

Systemic effects due to topical use of corticosteroids in adults occur infrequently but can be severe. Adrenocortical suppression, cataract, infections, impact on the metabolic control of diabetes mellitus and increase of intra-ocular pressure can occur, especially after long-term treatment. Application of XAMIOL under occlusion or for prolonged treatment periods may result in an increased risk of systemic adverse events, and is therefore not recommended (see Warnings and Precautions).

Table 1: XAMIOL

Adverse Drug Reactions Occurring in ≥1% of Patients for the Pivotal Scalp Studies: Safety Analysis Set

Primary System Organ Class[a] Preferred Term[a]	XAMIOL Gel (n=1093)		Betamethasone Gel (n=1104)		Calcipotriol Gel (n=548)		Gel Vehicle (n=135)	
	Number of Patients	%	Number of Patients	%	Number of Patients	%	Number of Patients	%
Nervous System Disorders								
Headache	6	0.5	11	1.0	1	0.2	1	0.7
Burning sensation	2	0.2	6	0.5	10	1.8	0	0.0
Skin and Subcutaneous Tissue Disorders								
Pruritus	25	2.3	18	1.6	45	8.2	7	5.2
Skin irritation	5	0.5	5	0.5	15	2.7	3	2.2
Alopecia	4	0.4	6	0.5	3	0.5	2	1.5
Erythema	4	0.4	4	0.4	16	2.9	1	0.7
Dry skin	1	0.1	3	0.3	6	1.1	0	0
General Disorders and Administration Site Conditions								
Pain	1	0.1	0	0	3	0.5	3	2.2

[a] Coded according to MedDRA version 6.1.

DRUG INTERACTIONS: There is no experience of concomitant therapy with other antipsoriatic drugs.

DOSAGE AND ADMINISTRATION: Dosing Considerations:

- XAMIOL (calcipotriol and betamethasone dipropionate) is not recommended for use in children and adolescents below the age of 18 years.
- XAMIOL is **for topical use only** and not for ophthalmic use.

Recommended Dose and Dosage Adjustment: XAMIOL should be applied to affected areas of the scalp once daily for up to 4 weeks. After satisfactory improvement has occurred, the drug can be discontinued. If recurrence takes place after discontinuation, treatment may be reinstituted.

The maximum daily dose including other calcipotriol-containing products on the body should not exceed 15 g and the maximum weekly dose should not exceed 100 g.

All affected scalp areas may be treated with XAMIOL gel. Up to 30% of the total surface area of the body may be treated with calcipotriol and betamethasone (XAMIOL gel on the scalp + DOVOBET ointment on the body).

Missed Dose: If a dose is missed, the patient should apply XAMIOL when he/she remembers, but only once on a given day and then continue on as usual.

Administration: Application under occlusive dressings should be avoided since it increases systemic absorption of corticosteroids.

Patients should shake the product prior to use.

OVERDOSAGE:

Use of XAMIOL (calcipotriol and betamethasone dipropionate) above the recommended dose may cause elevated serum calcium which should rapidly subside when treatment is discontinued. In such cases, it is recommended to monitor serum calcium levels once weekly until they return to normal. Excessive prolonged use of topical corticosteroids may suppress the pituitary-adrenal functions, resulting in secondary adrenal insufficiency which is usually reversible. If this occurs, symptomatic treatment is indicated. In cases of chronic toxicity, treatment with XAMIOL must be discontinued gradually.

> For management of a suspected drug overdose, CPhA recommends that you contact your **regional Poison Control Centre**. See the *CPS* Directory section for a list of Poison Control Centres.

ACTION AND CLINICAL PHARMACOLOGY: Mechanism of Action: XAMIOL is a combination of the vitamin D analogue calcipotriol and the corticosteroid betamethasone dipropionate.

Calcipotriol is a non-steroidal antipsoriatic agent, derived from the naturally occurring vitamin D. Calcipotriol exhibits a vitamin D-like effect by competing for the $1,25(OH)_2D_3$ receptor. Calcipotriol is as potent as $1,25(OH)_2D_3$, the naturally occurring active form of vitamin D, in regulating cell proliferation and cell differentiation, but much less active than $1,25(OH)_2D_3$ in its effect on calcium metabolism. Calcipotriol induces differentiation and suppresses proliferation of keratinocytes (without any evidence of a cytotoxic effect), thus reversing the abnormal keratinocyte changes in psoriasis. The therapeutic goal envisaged with calcipotriol is thus a normalization of epidermal growth.

Topical corticosteroids such as betamethasone dipropionate have anti-inflammatory, anti-pruritic, vasoconstrictive and immunosuppressive properties. Through occlusion the effect can be enhanced due to increased penetration of the stratum corneum. As a result, the incidence of adverse events will increase. In general, the mechanism of the anti-inflammatory activity of topical steroids is unclear. Corticosteroids are thought to induce phospholipase A_2 inhibitor proteins, preventing arachidonic acid release and the biosynthesis of potent mediators of inflammation.

Pharmacodynamics: Adrenal response to ACTH was determined by measuring serum cortisol levels in patients with both extensive scalp and body psoriasis, using up to 106 g per week combined XAMIOL gel and DOVOBET ointment. A borderline decrease in cortisol response at 30 minutes post ACTH challenge was seen in 5 of 32 patients (15.6%) after 4 weeks of treatment and in 2 of 11 patients (18.2%) who continued treatment until 8 weeks. In all cases, the serum cortisol levels were normal at 60 minutes post ACTH challenge. There was no evidence of change of calcium metabolism observed in these patients.

A study was conducted to evaluate the atrophogenic potential of betamethasone dipropionate in XAMIOL gel compared with marketed betamethasone dipropionate ointment and gel vehicle. The study was conducted as an intra-individual comparison of once daily application for 4 weeks in 48 healthy volunteers. Skin thickness was measured by sonography performed before treatment, weekly during the 4-week treatment period and 2 weeks after the end of treatment. XAMIOL gel induced reversible skin thinning, which was similar to that induced by betamethasone dipropionate ointment.

Pharmacokinetics: Absorption: The systemic exposure to calcipotriol and betamethasone dipropionate from topically applied XAMIOL gel is comparable to DOVOBET ointment in rats and minipigs. Clinical studies with radiolabelled ointment indicate that the systemic absorption of calcipotriol and betamethasone dipropionate from the DOVOBET ointment formulation is less than 1% of the dose (2.5 g) when applied to normal skin (625 cm^2) for 12 hours. Application to psoriasis plaques and under occlusive dressings may increase the absorption of topical corticosteroids.

Calcipotriol and betamethasone dipropionate were below the lower limit of quantification in all blood samples of 34 patients treated for 4 or 8 weeks with XAMIOL gel and DOVOBET ointment for extensive psoriasis involving the scalp and body. One metabolite of calcipotriol and one metabolite of bethamethasone dipropionate were quantifiable in some of the patients. While the biological activity of the calcipotriol metabolite is less than that of calcipotriol, the activity of the betamethasone dipropionate metabolite cannot be distinguished from the activity of the parent compound.

Metabolism: Calcipotriol metabolism following systemic uptake is rapid and occurs in the liver. Calcipotriol is metabolized to MC1046 (the α,β-unsaturated ketone analog of calcipotriol), which is metabolized further to MC1080 (a saturated ketone analog). MC1080 is the major metabolite in plasma. MC1080 is slowly metabolized to calcitroic acid.

Betamethasone dipropionate is metabolized to betamethasone 17-propionate and betamethasone, including the 6β-hydroxy derivatives of those compounds by hydrolysis. Betamethasone 17-propionate (B17P) is the primary metabolite.

STORAGE AND STABILITY: Store at 15-30°C. Do not refrigerate. Shake before use. Protect from light, keep the bottle in the outer carton. Use within 3 months of first opening the bottle.

INFORMATION FOR THE PATIENT: Published in e-CPS, available by subscription at www.e-cps.ca.

DOSAGE FORMS, COMPOSITION AND PACKAGING: Each g of clear, colourless to slightly off-white lipophilic gel contains: calcipotriol (as monohydrate) 50 µg plus betamethasone (as dipropionate) 0.5 mg. Nonmedicinal ingredients: α-tocopherol, butylhydroxytoluene, hydrogenated castor oil, liquid paraffin and polyoxypropylene-15-stearyl ether. Polyethylene bottles of 60 g.

Xanax®
alprazolam
Anxiolytic—Antipanic

Pfizer

Xanax TS®
alprazolam
Anxiolytic—Antipanic

Pfizer

PHARMACOLOGY: Alprazolam, a triazolo 1,4 benzodiazepine analog, binds with high affinity to the GABA benzodiazepine receptor complex. Considerable evidence suggest that the central pharmacologic/therapeutic actions of alprazolam are mediated via interaction with this receptor complex.

Pharmacokinetics: Orally administered alprazolam is readily absorbed in man. Plasma levels are proportional to the dose given; over the dose range of 0.5 to 3 mg, peak levels of 8.0 to 37 ng/mL were observed. The mean elimination half-life of alprazolam is about 11 hours in healthy adults. With multiple doses, given 3 times daily, steady state is reached within 7 days. Alprazolam and its metabolites are excreted primarily in the urine. Degradation of alprazolam occurs mainly by oxidation yielding the primary metabolites α hydroxy-alprazolam and a benzophenone derivative. The α-hydroxy-metabolite is further transformed to demethylalprazolam. Both α-hydroxy-alprazolam and demethylalprazolam are active and appear to have half-lives similar to alprazolam but their plasma levels are low.

Table 1 summarizes some pharmacokinetic parameters in healthy adults and healthy elderly subjects (mean age 70 years, range 62 to 78 years), as well as in obese subjects and in patients with impaired hepatic or renal function. Clearance was decreased and half-lives were increased in all special patient populations except in patients on hemodialysis. Time to peak plasma concentration was increased in patients with liver disease and CAPD.

Cimetidine: Cimetidine significantly impaired the clearance of alprazolam and prolonged its half-life. In healthy volunteers, a single 1 mg dose of alprazolam was administered with and without concurrent administration of cimetidine (300 mg) every 6 hours. Cimetidine significantly reduced total metabolic clearance (1.05 versus 1.66 mL/min/kg) and significantly prolonged elimination half-life (16.6 hours versus 12.4 hours). Similar results were observed during repeated administration of both drugs.

Oral contraceptives: The effect of oral contraceptives on the pharmacokinetics of a single 1 mg dose of alprazolam was studied in healthy women. Alprazolam clearance was lower in subjects taking oral contraceptives (0.95 mL/min/kg) than in the control group (1.21 mL/min/kg) while its half-life was prolonged (12.4 hours versus 9.6 hours).

Anticoagulant: Alprazolam, 0.5 mg, administered 3 times a day for 14 days, did not affect prothrombin times or plasma warfarin levels in male volunteers administered sodium warfarin orally.

Clinical Trial: In a placebo-controlled, 8-week trial, which included 526 patients with diagnoses of panic disorder with or without agoraphobia, alprazolam in a dosage range of 1 to 10 mg/day (with a mean daily dosage of 5.7±2.27 mg at the end of the treatment period) was found effective in blocking or attenuating panic attacks and reducing phobic avoidance.

Table 1: Xanax

Alprazolam Pharmacokinetics in Special Patient Populations Following the Administration of Single Oral Doses[a]

Parameter	Patient Population					
	Adults	Elderly	Obese	Alcoholic Liver Disease	End Stage Renal Disease: Hemodialysis	End Stage Renal Disease: CAPD[b]
No.	16	16	12	17	7	5
Dose (mg)	1.0	1.0	1.0	1.0	0.5	0.5
C_{max} (ng/mL)	17.9 (8.5–29.5)	22.9 (12.4–36.3)	not reported	17.3 (8.6–26.0)	8.1 (5.9–14.4)	8.6 (6.8–10.5)
T_{max} (hr)	1.6 (0.25–6.0)	0.9 (0.5–2.0)	not reported	3.3 (0.5–8.0)	1.1 (0.5–2.0)	3.0 (0.5–6.0)
Cl (mL/min/kg)	1.33 (0.90–2.23)	0.86 (0.40–1.84)	0.59 (not available)	0.56 (0.17-1.46)	not reported	not reported
t½ (hr)	11.0 (6.3–15.8)	16.3 (9.0–26.9)	21.8 (9.9–40.5)	19.7 (5.8–65.3)	11.2 (7.1–19.1)	19.2 (8.8–33.8)
Unbound fraction in plasma (%)	29.0 (25.0–32.8)	29.8 (25.0–35.4)	30.3 (26.4–35.4)	23.2 (16.9–32.8)	27.6 (22.7–30.7)	30.9 (28.0–34.2)

[a] Values are means with the ranges in parentheses.
[b] CAPD: continuous ambulatory peritoneal dialysis.

Legend:
C_{max}: peak plasma concentration.
T_{max}: time of peak concentration.
Cl: total clearance.
t½: elimination half-life.

INDICATIONS: For the management of anxiety disorders or the short-term symptomatic relief of symptoms of excessive anxiety. Anxiety or tension associated with the stress of everyday life usually does not require treatment with an anxiolytic.

Generalized Anxiety Disorder: Alprazolam is indicated for the treatment of Generalized Anxiety Disorder (GAD). GAD is characterized by unrealistic or excessive anxiety and worry (apprehensive expectation) about two or more life circumstances, for a period of 6 months or longer, during which the person has been bothered more days than not by these concerns. At least 6 of the following 18 symptoms are often present in these patients: motor tension (trembling, twitching, or feeling shaky; muslce tension, aches, or soreness; restlessness; easy fatigability); autonomic hyperactivity (shortness of breath or smothering sensations; palpitations or accelerated heart rate; sweating, or cold clammy hands; dry mouth; dizziness or lightheadedness; nausea, diarrhea, or other abdominal distress; flushes or chills; frequent urination; trouble swallowing or "lump in throat"); vigilance and scanning (feeling keyed up or on edge; exaggerated startle response; difficulty concentrating or "mind going blank" because of anxiety; trouble falling or staying asleep; irritability). These symptoms must not be secondary to another psychiatric disorder or caused by some organic factor.

Panic disorder with/without Agoraphobia: Also indicated for the management of panic disorder with or without agoraphobia. Panic disorder is an illness characterized by recurrent panic attacks.

Panic attacks are discrete periods of intense fear or discomfort, with at least 4 of the following symptoms: dyspnea; dizziness, unsteady feelings, or faintness; tachycardia; trembling or shaking; sweating; choking; nausea or abdominal distress; depersonalization or derealization; paresthesias; flushes or chills; chest pain or discomfort, fear of dying; fear of going crazy or of doing something uncontrolled.

Attacks are usually of a few minutes duration but can, more rarely, last up to a few hours.

The diagnosis of panic disorders requires that either 4 attacks must have occurred within a 4 week period, or 1 or more attacks must have been followed by a period of at least 1 month of persistent fear of having another attack. The symptoms must not be attributable to known organic factors.

The panic attacks, at least initially, are unexpected. Later in the course of this disturbance certain situations, e.g., driving a car or being in a crowded place, may become associated with having a panic attack. These panic attacks are not triggered by situations in which the person is the focus of others' attention (as in social phobia).

During the natural course of the illness, the patient often develops symptoms of agoraphobia. Agoraphobia is a fear of being in situations from which escape might be difficult or in which help might not be available in the event of an unexpected panic attack. As a result of this fear, the patient either restricts travel or needs a companion when away from home, or else endures agoraphobic situations despite intense anxiety. The severity varies from mild (able to travel to work or to shop), to severe (completely housebound).

Demonstrations of the effectiveness of alprazolam by systematic clinical studies are limited to 4 months' duration for anxiety disorder and 4 to 10 weeks' duration for panic disorder; however, patients with panic disorder have been treated on an open basis for up to 8 months without apparent loss of benefit. The physician should periodically reassess the usefulness of drug treatment in all patients.

CONTRAINDICATIONS: Hypersensitivity to alprazolam or to any component of the product's formulation, or other benzodiazepines and in patients with myasthenia gravis and acute narrow angle glaucoma. However, alprazolam may be used in patients with open angle glaucoma who are receiving appropriate treatment.

WARNINGS: Alprazolam is not effective in patients with personality disorders. Alprazolam is not recommended for the management of mood or psychotic disorders.

Dependence and Withdrawal Reactions, Including Seizures: Physical dependence with withdrawal symptoms may occur with benzodiazepine discontinuation and can be severe (e.g., seizures) if benzodiazepines are suddenly discontinued or upon rapid decrease. Even after relatively short-term use at the doses recommended for the treatment of transient anxiety and anxiety disorder (i.e., 0.75 to 3 mg/day), there is some risk of dependence. Post-marketing surveillance data suggest that the risk of dependence and its severity appear to be greater in patients treated with relatively high doses (above 4 mg/day) and for long periods (more than 8 to 12 weeks).

The Importance of Dose and the Risks of Alprazolam as a Treatment for Panic Disorder: Because the management of panic disorder often requires the use of average daily doses of alprazolam above 3 mg, the risk of dependence among panic disorder patients may be higher than that among those treated for less severe anxiety. Randomized placebo-controlled discontinuation studies showed a high rate of rebound and withdrawal symptoms in patients treated with alprazolam compared to placebo-treated patients.

Relapse or return of illness was defined as a return of symptoms characteristic of panic disorder (primarily panic attacks) to levels approximately equal to those seen at baseline before active treatment was initiated. Rebound refers to a return of symptoms of panic disorder to a level substantially greater in frequency, or more severe in intensity, than seen at baseline. Withdrawal symptoms were identified as those which were generally not characteristic of panic disorder and which occurred for the first time more frequently during discontinuation than at baseline.

In a controlled clinical trial in which 63 patients were randomized to alprazolam and where withdrawal symptoms were specifically sought, the following were identified as symptoms of withdrawal: heightened sensory perception, impaired concentration, dysosmia, clouded sensorium, paresthesias, muscle cramps, muscle twitch, diarrhea, blurred vision, appetite decrease and weight loss. Other symptoms, such as anxiety and insomnia, were frequently seen during discontinuation, but it could not be determined if they were due to return of illness, rebound or withdrawal.

In a larger database comprised of both controlled and uncontrolled studies in which 641 patients received alprazolam, discontinuation-emergent symptoms which occurred at a rate of over 5% in patients treated with alprazolam and at a greater rate than the placebo-treated group are listed in Table 2.

Table 2: Xanax

Discontinuation-Emergent Symptom Incidence

Body System	Event	Percentage of Alprazolam Treated Patients Reporting Event (N=641)
Neurologic	insomnia	29.5
	lightheadedness	19.3
	abnormal involuntary movement	17.3
	headache	17.0

(cont'd)

Table 2: Xanax *(cont'd)*

Discontinuation-Emergent Symptom Incidence

Body System	Event	Percentage of Alprazolam Treated Patients Reporting Event (N=641)
	muscular twitching	6.9
	impaired coordination	6.6
	muscle tone disorders	5.9
	weakness	5.8
Psychiatric	anxiety	19.2
	fatigue and tiredness	18.4
	irritability	10.5
	cognitive disorder	10.3
	memory impairment	5.5
	depression	5.1
	confusional state	5.0
Gastrointestinal	nausea/vomiting	16.5
	diarrhea	13.6
	decreased salivation	10.6
Metabolic-Nutritional	weight loss	13.3
	decreased appetite	12.8
Dermatological	sweating	14.4
Cardiovascular	tachycardia	12.2
Special Senses	blurred vision	10.0

From the studies cited, it has not been determined whether these symptoms are clearly related to the dose and duration of therapy with alprazolam in patients with panic disorder. In 2 controlled trials of 6 to 8 weeks' duration where the ability of patients to discontinue medication was measured, 71 to 93% of patients treated with alprazolam tapered completely off therapy compared to 89 to 96% of placebo treated patients. The ability of patients to completely discontinue therapy with alprazolam after long-term therapy has not been reliably determined.

Seizures attributable to alprazolam were seen after drug discontinuance or dose reduction in 8 of 1 980 patients with panic disorder or in patients participating in clinical trials where doses of alprazolam greater than 4 mg daily for over 3 months were permitted. Five of these cases clearly occurred during abrupt dose reduction, or discontinuation from daily doses of 2 to 10 mg. Three cases occurred in situations where there was not a clear relationship to abrupt dose reduction or discontinuation. In one instance, seizure occurred after discontinuation from a single dose of 1 mg after tapering at a rate of 1 mg every 3 days, from 6 mg daily. In two other instances, the relationship to taper is indeterminate; in both of these cases the patients had been receiving doses of 3 mg daily prior to seizure. The duration of use in the above 8 cases ranged from 4 to 22 weeks. There have been occasional voluntary reports of patients developing seizures while apparently tapering gradually from alprazolam. The risk of seizure seems to be greatest 24 to 72 hours after discontinuation. In post-marketing surveillance, 128 cases of alprazolam withdrawal seizures were reported, 52 of which occurred in patients taking alprazolam alone. The dose range was 0.5 to 16 mg/day (median dose=4 mg/day). The duration of treatment was 1 to 365 days (median=35 days). There are no reports of fatalities associated with alprazolam withdrawal (see Dosage for recommended tapering and discontinuation schedule).

Status Epilepticus and its Treatment: The medical event voluntary reporting system shows that withdrawal seizures have been reported in association with the discontinuation of alprazolam. In most cases, only a single seizure was reported; however, multiple seizures and status epilepticus were reported as well. Ordinarily, the treatment of status epilepticus of any etiology involves use of i.v. benzodiazepines plus phenytoin or barbiturates, maintenance of a patent airway and adequate hydration. For additional details regarding therapy, consultation with an appropriate specialist may be considered.

Depression: Panic-related disorders have been associated with primary and secondary major depressive disorders and increased reports of suicide among untreated patients. Therefore, the same precaution must be exercised when using the higher doses of alprazolam in treating patients with panic-related disorders as is exercised with the use of any psychotropic drug in treating depressed patients or those in whom there is reason to expect concealed suicidal ideation or plans.

Interdose Symptoms: Early morning anxiety and emergence of anxiety symptoms between doses of alprazolam have been reported in patients with panic disorder taking prescribed maintenance doses of alprazolam. These symptoms may reflect the development of tolerance or a time interval between doses which is longer than the duration of clinical action of the administered dose. In either case, it is presumed that the prescribed dose is not sufficient to maintain plasma levels above those needed to prevent relapse, rebound or withdrawal symptoms over the entire course of the interdosing interval. In these situations, it is recommended that the same total daily dose be given, divided as more frequent administrations (see Dosage).

Risk of Dose Reduction: Withdrawal reactions may occur when dosage reduction occurs for any reason. This includes purposeful tapering, but also includes inadvertent reduction of dose (e.g., the patient forgets, the patient is admitted to a hospital, etc.). Therefore, the dosage of alprazolam should be reduced or discontinued gradually (see Dosage).

Pregnancy: The safety of the use of alprazolam in pregnancy has not been established. Therefore, alprazolam is not recommended for use during pregnancy.

Teratogenic effects: The data concerning teratogenicity and effects on postnatal development and behavior following benzodiazepine treatment are inconsistent. Several studies have suggested an increased risk of congenital malformations associated with the use of benzodiazepines during the first trimester of pregnancy. Later studies with the benzodiazepine class of drugs have provided no clear evidence of any type of defect. Since alprazolam is also a benzodiazepine derivative, the administration of alprazolam is rarely justified in women of childbearing potential. Women of childbearing potential should be warned to consult their physician regarding the discontinuation of the drug due to the potential hazard to the fetus if they are pregnant or intend to become pregnant.

Nonteratogenic effects: It should be considered that the child born of a mother who is receiving benzodiazepines may be at some risk for withdrawal symptoms from the drug during the postnatal period. Also, neonatal flaccidity and respiratory problems have been reported in children born of mothers who have been receiving benzodiazepines during late third trimester of pregnancy or during labor.

Labor and Delivery: Alprazolam has no established use in labor or delivery.

Lactation: Studies in rats have indicated that alprazolam and its metabolites are secreted into the milk. Levels of benzodiazepines, including alprazolam, in breast milk are low. Therefore, nursing should not be undertaken while a patient is receiving alprazolam.

Children and Adolescents: The safety and efficacy of alprazolam in patients under the age of 18 years have not been established.

Occupational Hazards: Driving and Hazardous Activities: Because of its CNS depressant effect, patients receiving alprazolam should be cautioned not to undertake activities requiring mental alertness, judgment and physical coordination such as driving or operating machinery. This is particularly true in the early phases of dose adjustment, and until it has been established that they do not become drowsy or dizzy while taking alprazolam. Alcohol or CNS depressant drugs should not be ingested during treatment with alprazolam.

PRECAUTIONS: Geriatrics: Elderly and debilitated patients have been found to be prone to the CNS depressant activity of benzodiazepines, even after low doses. Manifestations of this CNS depressant activity include ataxia, oversedation and hypotension. Therefore, medication should be administered with caution to these patients, particularly if a drop in blood pressure might lead to cardiac complications. Initial doses should be low and increments should be made gradually, depending on the response of the patient, in order to avoid oversedation, neurological impairment and other possible adverse reactions (see Pharmacology and Dosage).

Impaired Renal or Hepatic Function: If treatment is necessary in patients with impaired hepatic or renal function, therapy should be initiated at a very low dose and the dosage increased only to the extent that it is compatible with the degree of residual function of these organs. Such patients should be followed closely and have periodic laboratory assessments (see Pharmacology and Dosage).

Dependence Liability: Physical and psychological dependence may occur with benzodiazepines, including alprazolam. The risk of dependence increases with higher doses and long-term use. Patients who are prone to abuse drugs should be under careful surveillance when receiving alprazolam. Patients with a history of alcohol or drug abuse are at higher risk for developing psychological dependence.

Withdrawal symptoms can range from mild dysphoria and insomnia to a major syndrome that may include irritability, nervousness, insomnia, agitation, diarrhea, abdominal cramps, vomiting, sweating, tremors and convulsions. Since symptoms may be similar to those for which the patient is being treated, it may be difficult to differentiate between relapse and withdrawal upon discontinuation. Consequently, dosage must be gradually tapered to minimize withdrawal reactions. To discontinue treatment in patients taking alprazolam, the dosage should be reduced slowly in keeping with good medical practice. It is suggested that the daily dosage of alprazolam be decreased by no more than 0.5 mg every 3 days. Some patients may require an even slower dosage reduction. A decrease of 0.5 mg every 2 to 3 weeks is more appropriate when a dose of 6 mg daily or more has been administered even for only a few months. Once a dose of 2 mg daily is achieved, the dose should be decreased by 0.25 mg per 2 to 3 weeks (see Dosage).

Laboratory Tests: If alprazolam is administered for repeated cycles of therapy, periodic blood counts and liver function tests are advisable.

Drug Interactions: Benzodiazepines, including alprazolam, may potentiate or produce additive CNS depressant effects when combined with other psychotropic medication, alcohol, narcotics, barbiturates, antihistamines or anticonvulsants. Therefore, if alprazolam is to be combined with other drugs acting on the CNS, careful consideration should be given to the pharmacology of the agents involved because of the possible additive or potentiating effects. Patients should also be advised against the simultaneous use of other CNS depressant drugs and should be cautioned not to take alcohol during the administration of alprazolam.

Pharmacokinetic interactions can occur when alprazolam is administered along with drugs that interfere with its metabolism. Compounds which inhibit certain hepatic enzymes (particularly cytochrome P450IIIA4) may increase the concentration of alprazolam and enhance its activity. Data from clinical studies with alprazolam, in vitro studies with alprazolam, and clinical studies with drugs metabolized similarly to alprazolam provide evidence for varying degrees of interaction and possible interaction with alprazolam for a number of drugs.

Based on the degree of interaction and the type of data available, the following recommendations are made: The coadministration of alprazolam with ketoconazole, itraconazole, or other azole-type antifungals is not recommended. This is based on results of drug interaction studies of triazolam and midazolam, benzodiazepines metabolized similarly to alprazolam, with ketoconazole and itraconazole. In addition, an in vitro study showed ketoconazole to be a potent inhibitor of alprazolam metabolism.

Caution and consideration of dose reduction is recommended when alprazolam is coadministered with nefazodone, fluvoxamine and cimetidine.

When alprazolam (1 mg b.i.d.) and nefazodone (200 mg b.i.d.) were coadministered to steady state, peak concentrations, AUC and half-life values for alprazolam increased by approximately 2 fold. Nefazodone plasma concentrations were unaffected by alprazolam, although levels of the mCPP metabolite were increased. The concomitant use of alprazolam and nefazodone was also associated with an increase in psychomotor impairment presumably due to increased alprazolam plasma concentrations. If alprazolam is coadministered with nefazodone, a reduction in the alprazolam dosage may be appropriate; no dosage adjustment is required for nefazodone. The interactive effects of higher doses of these agents, such as the dosage levels of alprazolam used in panic disorder, have not been studied.

When alprazolam 1 mg and fluvoxamine (50 mg once daily for 3 days followed by 100 mg once daily for 7 days) were coadministered the AUC of alprazolam was approximately doubled, the C_{max} of alprazolam increased by about 50% and the half-life of alprazolam increased from 19.8 hours to 33.9 hours. C_{max} and AUC of fluvoxamine were decreased by about 25%. Psychomotor performance tests on day 10 showed significant decreases in performance.

Coadministration of alprazolam and cimetidine results in an approximate doubling of the C_{max} of alprazolam and a statistically significant increase in the AUC of alprazolam. The half-life of alprazolam increased from 12.2 hours to 14.2 hours.

Caution is recommended when alprazolam is coadministered with fluoxetine, propoxyphene, oral contraceptives, sertraline, diltiazem, or macrolide antibiotics such as erythromycin and troleandomycin.

A pharmacokinetic interaction has been noted between alprazolam and carbamazepine; significant reductions in alprazolam concentration have been noted after carbamazepine treatment has been initiated. Pharmacokinetic interactions between alprazolam and phenytoin have not been observed.

The steady-state plasma concentrations of imipramine and desipramine have been reported to be increased an average of 31% and 20%, respectively, by the concomitant administration of alprazolam tablets in doses up to 4 mg/day. The clinical significance of these changes is unknown.

Interactions involving HIV protease inhibitors (eg, ritonavir) and alprozolam are complex and time dependent. Low doses of ritonavir resulted in a large impairment of alprazolam clearance, prolonged its elimination half-life and enhanced clinical effects. However, upon extended exposure to ritonavir, CYP3A induction offset this inhibition. This interaction will require a dose-adjustment or discontinuation of alprazolam.

Alprazolam 0.5 mg, administered 3 times a day for 14 days, did not affect prothrombin times or plasma warfarin levels in male volunteers administered sodium warfarin orally.

ADVERSE EFFECTS: Side effects to alprazolam if they occur, are generally observed at the beginning of therapy and usually disappear upon continued medication or decreased dosage.

The data cited in Table 3 and Table 4 are estimates of untoward clinical event incidence among patients who participated under the following clinical conditions: relatively short duration (i.e., 4 weeks) placebo-controlled clinical studies with dosages up to 4 mg/day of alprazolam (for the management of anxiety disorders or for the short-term relief of the symptoms of anxiety) and short-term (up to 10 weeks) placebo-controlled clinical studies with dosages up to 10 mg/day of alprazolam in patients with panic disorder, with or without agoraphobia.

In addition to the relatively common (i.e., greater than 1%) untoward events listed in Table 3 and Table 4, the following events have been reported to occur with alprazolam and other benzodiazepines: seizures, loss of coordination, concentration difficulties, memory impairment/transient amnesia, dystonia, irritability, anorexia, fatigue, sedation, slurred speech, musculoskeletal weakness, changes in libido, menstrual irregularities, incontinence, urinary retention, abnormal liver function, jaundice, pruritus, diplopia and hyperprolactinemia. Increased intraocular pressure has been rarely reported.

As with all benzodiazepines, paradoxical reactions such as stimulation, agitation, rage, aggressive or hostile behavior, increased muscle spasticity, sleep disturbances, hallucinations and other adverse behavioral effects may occur in rare instances and in a random fashion. Should these occur, use of the drug should be discontinued.

In some of the spontaneous case reports of adverse behavioral effects such as stimulation, agitation, concentration difficulties, confusion and hallucinations, patients were receiving other CNS drugs concomitantly and/or were described as having underlying psychiatric conditions. Patients with borderline personality disorder, a prior history of violent or aggressive behavior, or alcohol or substance abuse may be at risk for such events. Instances of irritability, hostility and intrusive thoughts have been reported during discontinuance of alprazolam in patients with post-traumatic stress disorder.

Table 3: Xanax
Anxiety Disorders: Treatment-Emergent Symptom Incidence (% of Patients Reporting)

Body System	Event	Alprazolam (N=565)	Placebo (N=505)
CNS	drowsiness	41.0	21.6
	lightheadedness	20.8	19.3
	depression	13.9	18.1
	headache	12.9	19.6
	confusion	9.9	10.0
	insomnia	8.9	18.4
	nervousness	4.1	10.3
	syncope	3.1	4.0
	dizziness	1.8	0.8
	akathisia	1.6	1.2
Gastrointestinal	dry mouth	14.7	13.3
	constipation	10.4	11.4
	diarrhea	10.1	10.3
	nausea/vomiting	9.6	12.8
	increased salivation	4.2	2.4
Cardiovascular	tachycardia/palpitations	7.7	15.6
	hypotension	4.7	2.2
Sensory	blurred vision	6.2	6.2
Musculoskeletal	rigidity	4.2	5.3
	tremor	4.0	8.8
Cutaneous	dermatitis/allergy	3.8	3.1
Other	nasal congestion	7.3	9.3
	weight gain	2.7	2.7
	weight loss	2.3	3.0

Table 4: Xanax
Panic Disorders: Treatment-Emergent Symptom Incidence (% of patients reporting)

Body System	Event	Xanax (N=1 388)	Placebo (N=1 231)
CNS	drowsiness	76.8	42.7
	fatigue and tiredness	48.6	42.3
	impaired coordination	40.1	17.9
	irritability	33.1	30.1
	memory impairment	33.1	22.1
	lightheadedness/ dizziness	29.8	36.9
	insomnia	29.4	41.8
	headache	29.2	35.6
	cognitive disorder	28.8	20.5
	dysarthria	23.3	6.3
	anxiety	16.6	24.9
	abnormal involuntary movement	14.8	21.0
	decreased libido	14.4	8.0
	depression	13.8	14.0
	confusional state	10.4	8.2
	muscular twitching	7.9	11.8
	increased libido	7.7	4.1
	change in libido (not specified)	7.1	5.6

(cont'd)

Table 4: Xanax *(cont'd)*
Panic Disorders: Treatment-Emergent Symptom Incidence (% of patients reporting)

Body System	Event	Xanax (N=1 388)	Placebo (N=1 231)
	weakness	7.1	8.4
	muscle tone disorders	6.3	7.5
	syncope	3.8	4.8
	akathisia	3.0	4.3
	agitation	2.9	2.6
	disinhibition	2.7	1.5
	paresthesia	2.4	3.2
	talkativeness	2.2	1.0
	vasomotor disturbances	2.0	2.6
	derealization	1.9	1.2
	dream abnormalities	1.8	1.5
	fear	1.4	1.0
	feeling warm	1.3	0.5
Gastrointestinal	decreased salivation	32.8	34.2
	constipation	26.2	15.4
	nausea/vomiting	22.0	31.8
	diarrhea	20.6	22.8
	abdominal distress	18.3	21.5
	increased salivation	5.6	4.4
Cardiorespiratory	nasal congestion	17.4	16.5
	tachycardia	15.4	26.8
	chest pain	10.6	18.1
	hyperventilation	9.7	14.5
	upper respiratory infection	4.3	3.7
Sensory	blurred vision	21.0	21.4
	tinnitus	6.6	10.4
Musculoskeletal	muscular cramps	2.4	2.4
	muscle stiffness	2.2	3.3
Cutaneous	sweating	15.1	23.5
	rash	10.8	8.1
Other	increased appetite	32.7	22.8
	decreased appetite	27.8	24.1
	weight gain	27.2	17.9
	weight loss	22.6	16.5
	micturition difficulties	12.2	8.6
	menstrual disorders	10.4	8.7
	sexual dysfunction	7.4	3.7
	edema	4.9	5.6
	incontinence	1.5	0.6
	infection	1.3	1.7

OVERDOSE:

Symptoms: Manifested as an extension of alprazolam's pharmacologic activity. Thus, varying degrees of CNS depressant effects such as somnolence, confusion, drowsiness, slurred speech, impaired coordination, diminished reflexes, respiratory depression and coma may ensue. As in the management of overdose with any drug, it should be remembered that multiple agents may have been ingested.

Serious sequela are rare unless other drugs and/or ethanol are concomitantly ingested.

Death has been reported in association with overdoses of alprazolam by itself, as it has with other benzodiazepines. In addition, fatalities have been reported in patients who have overdosed with a combination of a single benzodiazepine, including alprazolam, and alcohol; alcohol levels seen in some of these patients have been lower than those usually associated with alcohol-induced fatality.

Treatment: Vomiting may be induced if the patient is fully awake. Vital signs should be monitored and general supportive measures should be employed as indicated. Gastric lavage should be instituted as soon as possible. I.V. fluids may be administered and an adequate airway should be maintained.

Experiments in animals have indicated that cardiopulmonary collapse can occur with massive i.v. doses of alprazolam. This could be reversed with positive mechanical respiration and the i.v. infusion of norepinephrine. Animal experiments with alprazolam and related compounds have suggested that hemodialysis and forced diuresis are probably of little value.

Treatment of overdosage is primarily supportive of respiratory and cardiovascular function.

Flumazenil may be used as an adjunct to the management of respiratory and cardiovascular function associated with overdose.

For management of a suspected drug overdose, CPhA recommends that you contact your **regional Poison Control Centre**. See the *CPS* Directory section for a list of Poison Control Centres.

DOSAGE: Should be individualized for maximal benefit. The lowest possible effective dose should be administered and the need for continued treatment reassessed frequently. The risk of dependence may increase with dose and duration of treatment. In general, patients who have not previously received psychotropic medication will require somewhat lower doses than those previously treated with minor tranquilizers, antidepressants, or hypnotics.

Anxiety Disorders: Adult: The initial adult dosage of alprazolam is 0.25 mg given 2 or 3 times daily. If required, increases may be made in 0.25 mg increments according to the severity of symptoms and patient response. It is recommended that the evening dose be increased before the daytime doses. Very severe manifestations of anxiety may require larger initial daily doses. The optimal dosage is one that permits symptomatic control of excessive anxiety without impairment of mental and motor function. Exceptionally, it may be necessary to increase dosage to a maximum of 3 mg daily, given in divided doses.

Elderly or Debilitated Patients: It is recommended that the general principle of using the lowest effective dose be followed in elderly or debilitated patients to preclude the development of ataxia or oversedation. The initial dosage is 0.125 mg given 2 or 3 times daily. If necessary, this dosage may be increased gradually depending on patient tolerance and response. The elderly may be especially sensitive to the effects of benzodiazepines.

Patients with Impaired Hepatic or Renal Function: In patients with advanced liver or renal disease, the usual dose is 0.125 to 0.25 mg, given 2 or 3 times daily. This may be gradually increased if needed and tolerated.

Panic Disorders: The usual starting dose is 0.5 to 1 mg at bedtime or 0.5 mg 3 times daily. The dose should be adjusted until the patient is free of attacks. Dosage adjustments should be in increments no greater than 1 mg every 3 to 4 days. Interdose symptoms may be lessened by using a schedule that provides for administration 3 or 4 times/day.

In controlled trials conducted to establish the efficacy of alprazolam in panic disorders, doses in the range of 1 to 10 mg daily were used. The mean dosage employed was approximately 5 to 6 mg daily. Among the approximately 1700 patients participating in the panic disorder development program, about 300 received maximum alprazolam doses of greater than 7 mg/day, including approximately 100 patients who received maximum dosages of greater than 9 mg/day. Occasional patients required as much as 10 mg/day to receive a successful response.

The necessary duration of treatment for panic disorder is unknown at this time. After a period of extended freedom from panic attacks, a supervised tapered discontinuation may be attempted.

Discontinuation: To discontinue treatment in patients taking alprazolam, the dosage should be reduced slowly in keeping with good medical practice. It is suggested that the daily dosage of alprazolam be decreased by no more than 0.5 mg every 3 days. Some patients may require an even slower dosage reduction. A decrease of 0.5 mg every 2 to 3 weeks is more appropriate when a dose of 6 mg daily or more has been administered even for only a few months. Once a dose of 2 mg daily is achieved, the dose should be decreased by 0.25 mg per 2 to 3 weeks.

INFORMATION FOR THE PATIENT: Published in e-CPS, available by subscription at www.e-cps.ca.

SUPPLIED: Xanax: 0.25 mg: Each white, single score tablet, embossed with "Upjohn 29," contains: alprazolam 0.25 mg. Nonmedicinal ingredients: cornstarch, docusate sodium, lactose, magnesium stearate, microcrystalline cellulose and silicon dioxide. Gluten-free. Bottles of 100 and 1000.

0.5 mg: Each peach, single score tablet, embossed "Upjohn 55," contains: alprazolam 0.5 mg. Nonmedicinal ingredients: cornstarch, docusate sodium, FD&C Yellow #6, lactose, magnesium stearate, microcrystalline cellulose and silicon dioxide. Gluten-free. Bottles of 100 and 1000.

1 mg: Each lavender, single score tablet, embossed "Upjohn 90", contains: alprazolam 1 mg. Nonmedicinal ingredients: cornstarch, docusate sodium, erythrosin sodium, FD&C Blue #2, lactose, magnesium stearate, microcrystalline cellulose and silicon dioxide. Gluten-free. Bottles of 100 and 1000.

Xanax TS: Each white, triscored tablet (3 scores), with the number "2" on one side and "Xanax" on the other side, contains: alprazolam 2 mg. The tablets can be broken into 4 equal parts of 0.5 mg. Nonmedicinal ingredients: cornstarch, docusate sodium, lactose, magnesium stearate, microcrystalline cellulose and silicon dioxide. Gluten-free. Bottles of 100.

Store at controlled room temperature (15 to 30°C).

(Shown in Product Identification Section)

Xarelto® ℞

rivaroxaban

Anticoagulant—Direct Factor Xa Inhibitor

Bayer

Date of Preparation: September 10, 2008

SUMMARY PRODUCT INFORMATION:

Route of Administration	Dosage Form/ Strength	Clinically Relevant Nonmedicinal Ingredients
Oral	Film-coated tablet, 10 mg	Lactose monohydrate For a complete listing see Dosage Forms, Composition and Packaging.

INDICATIONS AND CLINICAL USE: XARELTO (rivaroxaban tablet) is indicated for the prevention of venous thromboembolic events (VTE) in patients who have undergone elective total hip replacement or total knee replacement surgery.

Geriatrics (>65 years of age): In phase III clinical studies, 53% (n=2486) of the patients treated with XARELTO were aged ≥65 years, and 15% (n=694) were aged >75 years (see Warnings and Precautions, Geriatrics (>65 years of age) and Renal, and Dosage and Administration, Renal Impairment and Geriatrics (>65 years of age)).

Pediatrics (<18 years of age): The safety and efficacy of XARELTO have not been established in children less than 18 years of age; therefore, XARELTO is not recommended in this patient population.

CONTRAINDICATIONS:

- Hepatic disease (including Child-Pugh Class B and C) associated with coagulopathy and a clinically relevant bleeding risk (see Warnings and Precautions, Hepatic/Biliary/Pancreatic)
- Clinically significant active bleeding, including hemorrhagic manifestations and bleeding diathesis
- Lesions at increased risk of clinically significant bleeding, eg, cerebral infarction (hemorrhagic or ischemic) within the last 6 months, and patients with spontaneous impairment of hemostasis
- Concomitant **systemic** treatment with strong inhibitors of both CYP3A4 and P-gp (see Warnings and Precautions, General)
- Pregnancy
- Nursing women
- Hypersensitivity to XARELTO or to any ingredient in the formulation. (For a complete listing, see Dosage Forms, Composition and Packaging.)

WARNINGS AND PRECAUTIONS: General: The use of XARELTO is contraindicated in patients receiving concomitant **systemic** treatment with strong inhibitors of both CYP3A4 and P-gp such as ketoconazole, itraconazole, voriconazole, posaconazole, or ritonavir). These drugs may increase XARELTO plasma concentrations to a clinically relevant degree, which may lead to an increased bleeding risk (see Drug Interactions).

Strong CYP3A4 inducers should be administered with caution in combination with XARELTO (see Drug Interactions, Drug-Drug Interactions).

Care should be taken if patients are treated concomitantly with drugs affecting hemostasis such as nonsteroidal anti-inflammatory drugs (NSAIDs) and platelet aggregation inhibitors (see Drug Interactions). Coadministration of XARELTO with other anticoagulants or antithrombotic therapy has not been adequately studied in clinical trials and is not recommended, as it may lead to an increased bleeding risk.

Any unexplained fall in hemoglobin or blood pressure should lead to a search for a bleeding site.

Cardiovascular: No QTc prolonging effects were observed with XARELTO.

Hematologic: Hemorrhage: XARELTO, like other anticoagulants, should be used with caution in patients with an increased bleeding risk such as congenital or acquired bleeding disorders, uncontrolled severe arterial hypertension, vascular retinopathy, or concomitant use of drugs affecting hemostasis.

Due to the pharmacological mode of action, XARELTO may be associated with an increased risk of occult or overt bleeding which may result in posthemorrhagic anemia. The signs, symptoms, and severity will vary according to the location and degree, or extent, of the bleeding. The possibility of a hemorrhage should be considered in evaluating the condition of any anticoagulated patient. Hemorrhagic complications may present as weakness, asthenia, paleness, dizziness, headache, or unexplained swelling.

Hepatic/Biliary/Pancreatic: Patients with significant hepatic disease (eg, acute clinical hepatitis, chronic active hepatitis, liver cirrhosis) were excluded from clinical trials. Therefore, XARELTO is contraindicated in patients with hepatic disease (including Child-Pugh Class B and C) associated with coagulopathy and a clinically relevant bleeding risk.

The limited data available for patients with mild hepatic impairment without coagulopathy indicate that there is no difference in pharmacodynamic response or pharmacokinetics as compared to healthy subjects.

Peri-Operative Considerations: Neuraxial (Epidural/Spinal) Anesthesia: When neuraxial (epidural/spinal) anesthesia or spinal puncture is performed, patients treated with antithrombotics for prevention of thromboembolic complications are at risk for developing an epidural or spinal hematoma that may result in long-term neurological injury or permanent paralysis.

The risk of these events is increased by the use of indwelling epidural catheters or the concomitant use of drugs affecting hemostasis. The risk may also be increased by traumatic or repeated epidural or spinal puncture. If traumatic puncture occurs, the administration of XARELTO should be delayed for 24 hours.

Patients who have undergone epidural puncture and who are receiving XARELTO should be frequently monitored for signs and symptoms of neurological impairment (eg, numbness or weakness of the legs, bowel or bladder dysfunction). If neurological deficits are noted, urgent diagnosis and treatment is necessary.

The physician should consider the potential benefit versus the risk before neuraxial intervention in patients anticoagulated or to be anticoagulated for thromboprophylaxis and use XARELTO only when the benefits clearly outweigh the possible risks. An epidural catheter should not be withdrawn earlier than 18 hours after the last administration of XARELTO. XARELTO should be administered not earlier than 6 hours after the removal of the catheter.

Renal: Following oral dosing with XARELTO, there is a direct relationship between the pharmacodynamic effects and the degree of renal impairment (see Action and Clinical Pharmacology, Renal Insufficiency).

There are insufficient safety data in patients with severe renal impairment (CrCl <30 mL/min) as these patients were excluded from pivotal phase III trials. **Therefore, the use of XARELTO is not recommended in patients with severe renal impairment.** Patients who develop acute renal failure while on XARELTO should discontinue such treatment.

XARELTO should be used with caution in patients with moderate renal impairment (CrCl 30-49 mL/min) concomitantly receiving other drugs which increase rivaroxaban plasma concentrations (see Dosage and Administration, Renal Impairment and Drug Interactions, Drug-Drug Interactions).

Physicians should consider the benefit/risk of anticoagulant therapy before administering XARELTO to patients with moderate renal impairment with a creatinine clearance close to the severe renal impairment category (CrCl <30 mL/min) or with a potential to have deterioration of renal function during therapy.

Sensitivity/Resistance: XARELTO contains lactose. Patients with rare hereditary problems of lactose or galactose intolerance (eg, the Lapp lactase deficiency or glucose-galactose malabsorption) should not take XARELTO.

Special Populations: Pregnant Women: No data are available on the use of XARELTO in pregnant women.

Based on animal data, use of XARELTO is contraindicated throughout pregnancy (see Contraindications).

If XARELTO is to be used in women of childbearing potential, pregnancy should be avoided.

Nursing Women: No data are available on the use of XARELTO in nursing mothers. In rats, XARELTO is secreted into breast milk. Therefore, XARELTO may only be administered after breastfeeding is discontinued (see Contraindications).

Pediatrics (<18 years of age): The safety and efficacy of XARELTO have not been established in children less than 18 years of age; therefore, XARELTO is not recommended in this patient population.

Geriatrics (>65 years of age): No dose adjustment is required for the elderly (>65 years of age). Increasing age may be associated with declining renal and hepatic function (see Contraindications; Warnings and Precautions, Renal and Hepatic/Biliary/Pancreatic; and Dosage and Administration, Renal Impairment and Hepatic Impairment). Physicians should take into consideration that elderly patients exhibited higher plasma concentrations than younger patients with mean AUC values being approximately 1.5 fold higher, mainly due to reduced (apparent) total and renal clearance.

Monitoring and Laboratory Tests: Prothrombin and Activated Partial Thromboplastin Time: XARELTO, at recommended doses, prolongs several global (prothrombin time, activated partial thromboplastin time, Heptest) and specific (inhibition of factor Xa activity) clotting tests. Prothrombin time (PT) is influenced by XARELTO in a dose-dependent way if Neoplastin is used for the assay. In patients undergoing elective total hip replacement or total knee replacement surgery, the 5/95 percentiles for PT (Neoplastin) 2 to 4 hours after tablet intake (ie, at the time of maximum effect) ranged from 13 to 25 sec. In case of excessive doses, the PT is expected to be outside of this range.

Although the activated partial thromboplastin time (aPTT) and HepTest are also both prolonged dose-dependently, neither test is recommended for the assessment of the pharmacodynamic effects of XARELTO. Similarly, antifactor Xa activity as well as inhibition of factor Xa activity are influenced by XARELTO but, as for aPTT and Heptest, neither test is recommended to follow the effects of XARELTO (see Action and Clinical Pharmacology, Pharmacodynamics).

Hemoglobin: Any unexplained fall in hemoglobin or blood pressure should lead to a search for a bleeding site.

ADVERSE REACTIONS: Adverse Drug Reaction Overview: The safety of XARELTO 10 mg has been evaluated in three randomized, double-blind, active-control phase III studies (RECORD 1, RECORD 2, and RECORD 3). In the phase III studies, 4657 patients undergoing total hip replacement or total knee replacement surgery were randomized to XARELTO, with 4571 patients actually receiving XARELTO.

In RECORD 1 and 2, a total of 2209 and 1228 THR patients, respectively, were randomized to XARELTO 10 mg od. In RECORD 1, the treatment period for both groups was 35±4 days postoperatively. In RECORD 2, patients randomized to XARELTO were treated for 35±4 days postoperatively, and patients randomized to enoxaparin received placebo after day 12±2 until day 35±4 postoperatively. In RECORD 3, a total of 1220 TKR patients were randomized to XARELTO 10 mg od, and both groups received study drug until day 12±2 postoperatively.

The safety profile of XARELTO with regard to adverse events (AE) and serious adverse events (SAE) is similar to that of the active comparator in the RECORD 1, 2, and 3 studies.

Clinical Trial Adverse Drug Reactions: Because clinical trials are conducted under very specific conditions, the adverse reaction rates observed in the clinical trials may not reflect the rates observed in practice and should not be compared to the rates in the clinical trials of another drug. Adverse drug reaction information from clinical trials is useful for identifying drug-related adverse events and for approximating rates.

The database of RECORD 1, 2, and 3 comprised 4657 patients randomized to treatment with XARELTO 10 mg od and 4692 patients randomized to enoxaparin 40 mg od. Analysis of this pooled database showed that there was no statistically significant difference in bleeding (P >0.05) between XARELTO and the active comparator (see Table 1).

Due to the pharmacological mode of action, XARELTO may be associated with an increased risk of occult or overt bleeding which may result in posthemorrhagic anemia (see Warnings and Precautions, Hematologic).

The most common treatment-emergent adverse events reported by patients valid for safety analysis in the 3 phase III studies are presented in Table 2.

Less Common Clinical Trial Adverse Drug Reactions: Incidence is ≥0.1% to <1% unless specified.

Blood and the Lymphatic System Disorders: thrombocythemia (including platelet count increased).

Cardiac Disorders: tachycardia.

Gastrointestinal Disorders: abdominal and gastrointestinal pain (including upper abdominal pain, stomach discomfort), constipation, diarrhea, dry mouth, dyspepsia (including epigastric discomfort), vomiting.

General Disorders and Administration Site Conditions: edema peripheral, feeling unwell (including fatigue, asthenia), fever, localized edema.

Hepatobiliary Disorders: abnormal hepatic function (≥0.01% to <0.1%).

Immune System Disorders: allergic dermatitis (≥0.01% to <0.1%).

Injury, Poisoning, and Procedural Complications: wound secretion.

Table 1: XARELTO

RECORD 1, 2, and 3—Treatment-Emergent Bleeding Events[a] (Safety Population with Central Adjudication) in Patients Randomized to XARELTO (First Dose 6 to 8 Hours Postoperatively) or Enoxaparin (First Dose 12 Hours Preoperatively)

		Major Bleeding[b] n (%)	Major Bleeding Including Surgical Site Bleeding Events Associated with Hemoglobin Drops or Transfusions[c] n (%)	Any Bleeding (Major or Nonmajor)[d] n (%)
RECORD 1 (THR)	XARELTO (N=2209) 10 mg od po for 35±4 days	6 (0.3)	40 (1.8)	133 (6.0)
	Enoxaparin (N=2224) 40 mg od SC for 36±4 days	2 (0.1)	33 (1.5)	131 (5.9)
	P Value[e]	0.18	0.41	0.9
RECORD 2 (THR)	XARELTO (N=1228) 10 mg od po for 35±4 days	1 (0.1)	23 (1.9)	81 (6.6)
	Enoxaparin (N=1229) 40 mg od SC for 12±2 days	1 (0.1)	19 (1.6)	68 (5.5)
	P Value[e]	1.00	0.54	0.273
RECORD 3 (TKR)	XARELTO (N=1220) 10 mg od po for 12±2 days	7 (0.6)	21 (1.7)	60 (4.9)
	Enoxaparin (N=1239) 40 mg od SC for 13±2 days	6 (0.5)	17 (1.4)	60 (4.8)
	P Value[e]	0.79	0.52	1.00
Pooled Analysis[f] (RECORD 1, 2, 3)	XARELTO (N=4657)	14 (0.3)	84 (1.8)	274 (5.9)
	Enoxaparin (N=4692)	9 (0.2)	69 (1.5)	259 (5.5)
	P Value[e]	0.31	0.22	0.48

[a] Starts with administration of the first (placebo) tablet or (placebo) injection. Active XARELTO treatment started after surgery. Active enoxaparin treatment started on the day before surgery.
[b] Major bleeding events included: (1) fatal, (2) bleeding into a critical organ (eg, retroperitoneal, intracranial, intraocular or intraspinal bleeding/hemorrhagic puncture), (3) bleeding requiring reoperation, (4) clinically overt extra-surgical site bleeding associated with ≥2 g/dL fall in hemoglobin or leading to infusion of ≥2 units of whole blood or packed cells.
[c] Surgical-site bleeding events associated with a decrease in hemoglobin were based on a determination by the investigator. Surgical-site bleeding events requiring transfusion were based on an algorithmic assessment of blood transfusions given within 48 hours of the bleeding event. In addition, both types of surgical-site bleeding events must have been based on bleeding events confirmed by the adjudication committee and reported as overt surgical-site bleeding events by the investigator.
[d] Nonmajor bleeding events were bleeding events that did not fulfill the criteria of major bleeding.
[e] P value calculated as Fishers two-sided exact test.
[f] Note that pooling was done despite the shorter duration of therapy with enoxaparin in RECORD 2.
Legend: od=once daily; po=oral; SC=subcutaneous.

Table 2: XARELTO

Treatment-Emergent Drug-Related Adverse Events Occurring in >1% of Any Treatment Group—Pooled Data of RECORD 1, 2, 3 (Patients Valid for Safety Analysis[a])

Medical Entity	XARELTO (N=4571) n	(%)	Enoxaparin (N=4601) n	(%)
Gastrointestinal Disorders				
Nausea	57	(1.25)	70	(1.52)
Injury, Poisoning, and Procedural Complications				
Anemia (including laboratory parameter)	49	(1.07)	51	(1.11)
Post procedural hemorrhage	71	(1.55)	64	(1.39)
Investigations				
Increase in transaminases	91	(1.99)	128	(2.78)
Increase in Gamma-glutamyltransferase	51	(1.12)	72	(1.56)

[a] Started after administration of oral study medication (XARELTO or matching placebo tablet).
Note: Incidence=number of events/number at risk, where: number of events=number of patients reporting the event; number at risk=number of patients in reference population.
Only treatment emergent adverse events which occurred up to 2 days after the last dose of study medication are included.

Investigations: bilirubin conjugated increased (with or without concomitant increase of ALT) (≥0.01% to <0.1%), blood bilirubin increased, increased alkaline phosphatase, increased amylase, increased LDH, increased lipase.
Musculoskeletal, Connective Tissue, and Bone Disorders: pain in extremity.
Nervous System Disorders: dizziness, headache, syncope (including loss of consciousness).
Renal and Urinary Disorders: renal impairment (including serum creatinine increased, blood urea increased).
Skin and Subcutaneous Tissue Disorders: contusion, pruritus (including rare cases of generalized pruritus), rash, urticaria (including rare cases of generalized urticaria).
Vascular Disorders: gastrointestinal tract hemorrhage (including gingival bleeding, rectal hemorrhage, hematemesis), genital tract hemorrhage (including menorrhagia), hematuria (including blood urine present), hemorrhage (including hematoma and rare cases of muscle hemorrhage), hypotension (including blood pressure decreased, procedural hypotension), nose bleed.

In other clinical studies with XARELTO, single cases of adrenal hemorrhage and conjunctival hemorrhage, and fatal gastrointestinal ulcer hemorrhage were reported; jaundice and hypersensitivity were rare and hemoptysis was uncommon. Intracranial bleeding (especially in patients with arterial hypertension and/or on concomitant antihemostatic agents) which in single cases may be potentially life-threatening has been reported.

Abnormal Hematologic and Clinical Chemistry Findings: The incidence rates of laboratory abnormalities in the XARELTO and enoxaparin treatment groups were generally similar. In the RECORD 1, 2, and 3 studies, drug-related increases in transaminases were reported in 2.0% of XARELTO- and 2.8% of enoxaparin-treated patients and drug-related increases in gamma-glutamyltransferase occurred in 1.1% of XARELTO- and 1.6% of enoxaparin-treated patients.

DRUG INTERACTIONS: Overview: CYP Inhibition: XARELTO does not inhibit CYP3A4 or any other major CYP isoenzymes.
CYP Induction: XARELTO does not induce CYP3A4 or any other major CYP isoenzymes.

Drug-Drug Interactions: The use of XARELTO is contraindicated in patients receiving concomitant systemic treatment with strong inhibitors of both CYP3A4 and P-gp such as (ketoconazole, itraconazole, voriconazole, posaconazole, or ritonavir). These drugs may increase XARELTO plasma concentrations to a clinically relevant degree which may lead to an increased bleeding risk (see Contraindications and Warnings and Precautions, General).

Drugs strongly inhibiting only one of the XARELTO elimination pathways, either CYP3A4 or P gp, potentially increase XARELTO plasma concentrations. The expected increase is considered not clinically relevant.

Table 3: XARELTO

Established or Potential Drug-Drug Interactions

Concomitant Drug Class: Drug Name	Reference	Effect on Concentration of XARELTO	Clinical Comment
Azole antimycotic: ketoconazole	CT	↑ XARELTO	Coadministration of XARELTO with the azole-antimycotic ketoconazole (400 mg od) a strong CYP3A4 and P-gp inhibitor, led to a 2.6-fold increase in mean XARELTO steady state AUC and a 1.7-fold increase in mean XARELTO C_{max}, with significant increases in its pharmacodynamic effects. The use of XARELTO is contraindicated in patients receiving **systemic** treatment with ketoconazole (see Contraindications and Warnings and Precautions, General and Renal).
Protease inhibitor: ritonavir	CT	↑ XARELTO	Coadministration of XARELTO with the HIV protease inhibitor ritonavir (600 mg bid), a strong CYP3A4 and P-gp inhibitor, led to a 2.5-fold increase in mean XARELTO AUC and a 1.6-fold increase in mean XARELTO C_{max}, with significant increases in its pharmacodynamic effects. The use of XARELTO is contraindicated in patients receiving **systemic** treatment with ritonavir (see Contraindications and Warnings and Precautions, General and Renal).
Anti-infectives: erythromycin	CT	↑ XARELTO	Erythromycin (500 mg tid), which inhibits CYP3A4 and P-gp moderately, led to a 1.3-fold increase in mean XARELTO AUC and C_{max}. This increase is within the magnitude of the normal variability of AUC and C_{max} and is considered not clinically relevant.
rifampicin	CT	↓ XARELTO	Coadministration of XARELTO with the strong CYP3A4 and P-gp inducer rifampicin led to an approximate 50% decrease in mean XARELTO AUC, with parallel decreases in its pharmacodynamic effects. Strong CYP3A4 inducers should be administered with caution in combination with XARELTO.
Antithrombotic: enoxaparin	CT	No effect on XARELTO	After combined administration of enoxaparin (40 mg single dose) with XARELTO (10 mg single dose), an additive effect on antifactor Xa activity was observed, without any additional effects on clotting tests (PT, aPTT). Enoxaparin did not affect the bioavailability and pharmacokinetics of XARELTO (see Warnings and Precautions, General).
Nonsteroidal Anti-inflammatory Drugs (NSAIDS): naproxen	CT	No effect on XARELTO	Coadministration with naproxen did not affect XARELTO bioavailability and pharmacokinetics. No clinically relevant prolongation of bleeding time was observed after concomitant administration of XARELTO and 500 mg naproxen. Nevertheless there may be individuals with more pronounced pharmacodynamic response (see Warnings and Precautions, General).
acetylsalicylic acid (ASA)	CT	No effect on XARELTO	No clinically significant pharmacokinetic or pharmacodynamic interactions were observed when XARELTO was coadministered with 500 mg acetylsalicylic acid (see Warnings and Precautions, General).
Anticonvulsants: phenytoin carbamazepine phenobarbitone	T	↓ XARELTO	The concomitant use of XARELTO with strong CYP3A4 inducers (eg, phenytoin, carbamazepine, or phenobarbitone) may also lead to a decreased XARELTO plasma concentration. Strong CYP3A4 inducers should be administered with caution in combination with XARELTO.
Antiplatelet drugs: clopidogrel	CT	No effect on XARELTO	Clopidogrel (300 mg loading dose followed by 75 mg maintenance dose) did not affect XARELTO bioavailability and pharmacokinetics, but a relevant increase in bleeding times was observed in a subset of patients which was not correlated to platelet aggregation, P-selectin, or GPIIb/IIIa receptor levels (see Warnings and Precautions, General).

Legend: C=case study; CT=clinical trial; T=theoretical.

Interactions Shown Not to Exist: There were no mutual pharmacokinetic interactions between XARELTO and midazolam (substrate of CYP3A4), digoxin (substrate of P gp), or atorvastatin (substrate of CYP3A4 and P gp).

Coadministration of the H_2-receptor antagonist ranitidine, the antacid aluminum hydroxide/magnesium hydroxide, naproxen, clopidogrel, or enoxaparin did not affect XARELTO bioavailability and pharmacokinetics.

Drug-Food Interactions: XARELTO can be taken with or without food (see Action and Clinical Pharmacology).

Grapefruit juice is a moderate CYP3A4 inhibitor. Therefore, increase in XARELTO exposure upon grapefruit juice consumption is not expected to be clinically relevant.

Drug-Herb Interactions: The concomitant use of XARELTO with other strong CYP3A4 inducers (eg, St. John's Wort) may lead to a decreased XARELTO plasma concentration. Strong CYP3A4 inducers should be administered with caution in combination with XARELTO.

Drug-Laboratory Test Interactions: Clotting parameter tests (PT, aPTT, HepTest) are affected as expected by the mode of action of XARELTO (see Action and Clinical Pharmacology, Pharmacodynamics).

DOSAGE AND ADMINISTRATION: Recommended Dose and Dosage Adjustment: The recommended dose of XARELTO for VTE prevention in patients following elective total hip replacement or elective total knee replacement surgery is one tablet (10 mg) once daily (see also Special Populations below). XARELTO may be taken with or without food. The initial dose should be taken within 6 to 10 hours after surgery, provided that hemostasis has been established. If hemostasis is not established, treatment should be delayed.
The duration of treatment depends on the type of surgery:

- After elective total hip replacement surgery, patients should be treated for 35 days.
- After elective total knee replacement surgery, patients should be treated for 14 days.

Special Populations: Hepatic Impairment: XARELTO is contraindicated in patients with hepatic disease (including Child-Pugh Class B and C) associated with coagulopathy and a clinically relevant bleeding risk.

The limited clinical data for patients with moderate hepatic impairment indicate a significant increase in the pharmacological activity. No clinical data are available for patients with severe hepatic impairment (see Contraindications; Warnings and Precautions, Hepatic/Biliary/Pancreatic; and Action and Clinical Pharmacology, Hepatic Insufficiency).

The limited data available for patients with mild hepatic impairment without coagulopathy indicate that there is no difference in pharmacodynamic response or pharmacokinetics as compared to healthy subjects.

Renal Impairment: The use of XARELTO is not recommended in patients with severe renal impairment. Patients who develop acute renal failure while on XARELTO should discontinue such treatment.

XARELTO should be used with caution in patients with **moderate** renal impairment (CrCl 30-49 mL/min) concomitantly receiving other medicinal products which increase rivaroxaban plasma concentrations (see Warnings and Precautions, Renal and Drug Interactions, Drug-Drug Interactions).

Physicians should consider the benefit/risk of anticoagulant therapy before administering XARELTO to patients with moderate renal impairment with a creatinine clearance close to the severe renal impairment category (CrCl <30 mL/min) or with a potential to have deterioration of renal function during therapy. Consideration should be given to follow the renal function in these patients. Creatinine clearance can be estimated using the Cockcroft-Gault Formula as follows:

Creatinine Clearance (mL/min):

$$\text{Males} = \frac{(140\text{-age})\ (\text{years}) \times \text{weight (kg)}}{72 \times \text{serum creatinine (mg/100 mL)}}$$

$$\text{Females} = \frac{0.85 \times (140\text{-age})\ (\text{years}) \times \text{weight (kg)}}{72 \times \text{serum creatinine (mg/100 mL)}}$$

Sex, Ethnicity, or Body Weight: Body Weight: The exposure of 10 mg XARELTO in the extreme underweight group (<50 kg) resulted in a larger C_{max} by 24%, as compared to the normal subjects. The maximal effect of PT prolongation was approximately 20% higher at lower body weight. In overweight subjects with body weight higher than 120 kg, the PT maximal prolongation was less pronounced.

Sex: Sex effect was not observed.

Ethnicity: Ethnicity effect was not observed.

Pediatrics (<18 years of age): The safety and efficacy of XARELTO have not been established in children less than 18 years of age; therefore, XARELTO is not recommended in this patient population.

Geriatrics (>65 years of age): No dose adjustment is required for the elderly (>65 years of age). Increasing age may be associated with declining renal and/or liver function (see Contraindications; Warnings and Precautions, Renal and Hepatic/Biliary/Pancreatic; and Dosage and Administration, Renal Impairment and Hepatic Impairment).

Missed Dose: If a dose is missed, the patient should take XARELTO immediately and continue on the following day with the once daily intake as before. A double dose should not be taken to make up for a forgotten tablet.

OVERDOSAGE:

Overdose following administration of XARELTO may lead to hemorrhagic complications due to its pharmacodynamic properties.

The use of activated charcoal to reduce absorption in case of XARELTO overdose may be considered. Administration of activated charcoal up to 8 hours after overdose may reduce the absorption of XARELTO.

Due to the high plasma protein binding, XARELTO is not expected to be removed by dialysis.

Should bleeding occur, management of the hemorrhage may include the following steps:

Delay of next XARELTO administration or discontinuation of treatment as appropriate. XARELTO has a half-life of approximately 5 to 13 hours (see Action and Clinical Pharmacology).

Appropriate symptomatic treatment, eg, mechanical compression (eg, for severe epistaxis), surgical interventions, fluid replacement and hemodynamic support, or blood product or component transfusion should be considered.

If bleeding cannot be controlled by the above measures, consider administration of one of the following procoagulants:

- activated prothrombin complex concentrate (APCC)
- prothrombin complex concentrate (PCC)
- recombinant factor VIIa (rFVIIa)

However, there is currently no experience with the use of these products in individuals receiving XARELTO.

Protamine sulfate and vitamin K are not expected to affect the anticoagulant activity of XARELTO. There is no scientific rationale for benefit or experience with systemic hemostatics (eg, desmopressin, aprotinin, tranexamic acid, aminocaproic acid) in individuals receiving XARELTO.

> For management of a suspected drug overdose, CPhA recommends that you contact your **regional Poison Control Centre**. See the *CPS* Directory section for a list of Poison Control Centres.

ACTION AND CLINICAL PHARMACOLOGY: Mechanism of Action: Rivaroxaban is a highly selective, direct, antithrombin independent factor Xa inhibitor with high oral bioavailability.

Activation of factor X to factor Xa (FXa) via the intrinsic and extrinsic pathway plays a central role in the cascade of blood coagulation. FXa directly converts prothrombin to thrombin through the prothrombinase complex and, ultimately, this reaction leads to fibrin clot formation and activation of platelets by thrombin. One molecule of FXa is able to generate more than 1000 molecules of thrombin due to the amplification nature of the coagulation cascade. In addition, the reaction rate of prothrombinase-bound FXa increases 300 000-fold compared to that of free FXa and causes an explosive burst of thrombin generation. Selective inhibitors of FXa can terminate the amplified burst of thrombin generation, thereby diminishing thrombin-mediated activation of coagulation.

Pharmacodynamics: There is a clear correlation between plasma rivaroxaban concentration and the degree of anticoagulant effect. The maximal effect (E_{max}) of rivaroxaban on pharmacodynamic parameters occurs at the same time as C_{max}.

- A dose-dependent inhibition of factor Xa activity was observed over the complete dose range closely following the pharmacokinetic profiles which provides the 'proof of mechanism' in humans. Inhibition of factor Xa activity versus rivaroxaban plasma concentration follows a maximum effect (E_{max}) model. There is a close correlation between FXa inhibition and plasma concentrations with an r value of 0.97.
- Prothrombin time (PT) is influenced by rivaroxaban in a dose-dependent way with a close correlation to plasma concentrations (r=0.98) if Neoplastin is used for the assay. Other reagents would provide different results. The INR (International Normalized Ratio) is only calibrated and validated for coumarins and cannot be used for any other anticoagulant. In patients undergoing hip replacement surgery or knee replacement surgery, the 5/95 percentiles for PT (Neoplastin) 2 to 4 hours after tablet intake (ie, at the time of maximum effect) ranged from 13 to 25 sec.
- The activated partial thomboplastin time (aPTT) is also prolonged dose-dependently; however, the slope is rather flat and does not allow a sufficient discrimination at the relevant plasma concentrations. Therefore, aPTT is not considered to be adequate for following the pharmacodynamic effects. The r value for aPTT is 0.99.
- HepTest is also prolonged dose-dependently and correlates closely with plasma concentrations, following a curvilinear model. Despite the r value of 0.99 for the relation to plasma concentrations, the HepTest is not considered optimal to assess the pharmacodynamic effects due to the curvilinear relationship.
- Antifactor Xa activity is also influenced by rivaroxaban; however, no standard for calibration is available.

Pharmacokinetics: Absorption: The absolute bioavailability of rivaroxaban is approximately 100% for the 10 mg dose. Rivaroxaban is rapidly absorbed with maximum concentrations (C_{max}) appearing 2 to 4 hours after tablet intake.

Rivaroxaban 10 mg dose can be taken with or without food. Administration of the 10 mg rivaroxaban tablet with food (high-calorie/high-fat meal) showed no significant food effects (see Dosage and Administration).

Rivaroxaban pharmacokinetic parameters behave in a linear fashion; no evidence of bioaccumulation was seen after multiple doses.

Variability in rivaroxaban pharmacokinetics is moderate with interindividual variability (CV%) ranging from 30% to 40%.

Table 4: XARELTO

Summary of PK Parameters After Oral Administration of 10 mg of Rivaroxaban in Humans

	C_{max} [µg/L]	$t_{½}$ [h]	AUC [µg*h/L]	Clearance, Urinary Excretion	Volume of Distribution
Healthy (Young) Subjects	~114[a]	5–9	~817	CL_{sys}=~10 L/h CL_R =3–4 L/h Ae_{ur}=30%–40%	V_{ss}=~50 L
Patients	~125	7–11	~1170	N/A (no IV data)[b] Ae_{ur}=22%	N/A (no IV data)

[a] 2–4 hours after drug administration (t_{max}).

[b] Not available.

Legend: AUC=area under the plasma-concentration time curve; Ae_{ur}=amount of drug excreted unchanged into urine; CL_{sys}=systemic clearance (after intravenous administration); CL_R=renal clearance; C_{max}=maximum plasma concentration; $t_{½}$=terminal elimination half-life; t_{max}=time to reach C_{max}; V_{ss}=volume of distribution at steady state.

Distribution: Plasma protein binding in humans is high at approximately 92% to 95%, with serum albumin being the main binding component. The volume of distribution is moderate with V_{ss} being approximately 50 L.

Metabolism: Rivaroxaban is eliminated by metabolic degradation (approximately 2/3 of the administered dose) as well as by direct renal excretion of unchanged compound (approximately 1/3). Rivaroxaban is metabolized via CYP3A4, CYP2J2, and CYP-independent mechanisms. Oxidative degradation of the morpholinone moiety and hydrolysis of the amide bonds are the major sites of biotransformation.

Excretion: Rivaroxaban and metabolites have a dual route of elimination (via renal and fecal routes).

The clearance and excretion of rivaroxaban are as follows:

- 1/3 of the active drug is cleared as unchanged drug by the kidneys
- 1/3 of the active drug is metabolized to inactive metabolites and then excreted by the kidneys
- 1/3 of the active drug is metabolized to inactive metabolites and then excreted by the fecal route

Based on in vitro investigations, rivaroxaban is a substrate of the transporter proteins P-gp (P-glycoprotein) and Bcrp (breast cancer resistance protein).

Unchanged rivaroxaban is the most important compound in human plasma with no major or active circulating metabolites being present. With a systemic clearance of about 10 L/h rivaroxaban can be classified as low-clearance drug. Elimination of rivaroxaban from plasma occurred with terminal half-lives of 5 to 9 hours in young individuals and with terminal half-lives of 11 to 13 hours in the elderly.

Special Populations and Conditions: Pediatrics (<18 years of age): The safety and efficacy of XARELTO have not been established in children less than 18 years of age; therefore XARELTO is not recommended in this patient population.

Geriatrics (>65 years of age): Clinical studies have been conducted in older ages, with results of prolonged terminal half-lives (11 to 13 hours in elderly versus 5 to 9 hours in young subjects) accompanied by increases of XARELTO exposure (approximately 50%) compared to young healthy subjects. This difference may be due to reduced renal function in the elderly (see Contraindications; Warnings and Precautions, Renal; and Dosage and Administration, Renal Impairment).

Gender: There were no clinically relevant differences in pharmacokinetics between male and female patients.

Race: No clinically relevant interethnic differences among Caucasian, African-American, Hispanic, Japanese or Chinese patients were observed regarding pharmacokinetics and pharmacodynamics.

Hepatic Insufficiency: A phase I study investigated the influence of impaired hepatic function in cirrhotic patients (Child-Pugh Class A or B, number of patients 8 per group) on the pharmacodynamics and pharmacokinetics of a single dose of rivaroxaban.

In patients with mild hepatic impairment (Child-Pugh Class A), there was no difference as compared to healthy volunteers with respect to either pharmacodynamics (inhibition of factor Xa activity [1.08-fold for AUC and 0.98-fold for E_{max}]), prolongation of prothrombin time (1.02-fold for AUC and 1.06-fold for E_{max}), or pharmacokinetics (both total and unbound AUC [1.15 for total and 0.91-fold increase for unbound] and C_{max} [0.97 for total and 0.78-fold for unbound]).

Child-Pugh Class B patients had lower baseline factor Xa activity levels (0.64 U/mL) compared to healthy subjects and Child-Pugh Class A patients (0.85 U/mL, for both patient populations). Inhibition of factor Xa activity was more pronounced in Child-Pugh Class B patients compared to both healthy subjects and Child-Pugh Class A patients. The increase of inhibition was 2.6-fold $AUC_{(0\text{-}tn)}$ and 1.2-fold maximal effect (E_{max}). The group difference was statistically significant, both for $AUC_{(0\text{-}tn)}$ (P <0.01) as well as for E_{max} (P <0.05) of inhibition of factor Xa activity. In line with these results, a relevant difference in prolongation of PT was observed between healthy subjects and Child-Pugh Class B patients. The increase of prolongation was 2.1-fold ($AUC_{(0\text{-}tn)}$) and 1.4-fold (E_{max}). A statistically significant group-difference was observed for $AUC_{(0\text{-}tn)}$ (P <0.0004) as well as E_{max} (P <0.0001).

Pharmacokinetic parameters also indicated a significant increase in Child-Pugh Class B patients as compared to healthy volunteers both on AUC pharmacokinetics (both total and unbound AUC [2.27-fold for total and 2.57-fold increase for unbound]) and C_{max} (1.27-fold for total and 1.38-fold for unbound).

A PK/PD analysis showed that the slope of the prothrombin time/plasma concentration correlation is increased by more than 2-fold for Child-Pugh Class B patients as compared to healthy volunteers. Since the global clotting test PT assesses the coagulation factors VII, X, V, II which are synthesized in the liver, impaired liver function can also result in prolongations of PT in the absence of anticoagulant therapy.

The PK/PD changes observed in Child-Pugh Class B patients are markers for the severity of the underlying hepatic disease which is expected to lead to a subsequent increased bleeding risk in this patient group.

XARELTO is contraindicated in patients with hepatic disease (including Child-Pugh Class B and C) associated with coagulopathy and a clinically relevant bleeding risk (see Contraindications and Warnings and Precautions, Hepatic/Biliary/Pancreatic).

Renal Insufficiency: As active rivaroxaban is partially cleared via the kidneys (30% to 40% of the dose), there is a direct but moderate correlation of systemic exposure to rivaroxaban with degree of renal impairment.

In a phase I study, following oral single dosing with rivaroxaban 10 mg in subjects with mild (CrCl 50-79 mL/min), moderate (CrCl 30-49 mL/min), or severe (CrCl 15-29 mL/min) renal impairment, rivaroxaban plasma concentrations (AUC) were increased 1.4-, 1.5-, and 1.6-fold, respectively compared to healthy subjects with normal renal function (CrCl ≥80 mL/min).

The overall inhibition of factor Xa activity ($AUC_{(0\text{-}48h)}$ of effect versus time) was increased in these groups by a factor of 1.5, 1.9, and 2.0, respectively. The relative prolongation of prothrombin time (PT) was also affected by renal impairment and showed even more pronounced effects. $AUC_{(0\text{-}48h)}$ of effect versus time was increased by a factor of 1.3, 2.2, and 2.4, respectively.

In phase II, rivaroxaban plasma concentrations (AUC) were increased 1.2- and 1.5-fold in subjects with mild and moderate renal impairment respectively compared to healthy subjects with normal renal function and the peak inhibition of factor Xa activity ($AUC_{(0\text{-}48h)}$ of effect versus time) was increased in these groups by a factor of 1.0 and 1.3 respectively. In a pooled analysis of phase III subjects with mild and moderate renal impairment, the peak PT was increased by 1.0-, and 1.1-fold compared to subjects with normal renal function.

There was no evidence of substantial drug accumulation in patients with mild or moderate renal impairment. The phase III trials also showed that the bleeding rate with rivaroxaban in patients with renal impairment was not significantly different than that in patients with normal renal function.

The use of XARELTO is not recommended in patients with severe renal impairment. XARELTO should be used with caution in patients with moderate renal impairment (CrCl 30-49 mL/min) concomitantly receiving other medicinal products which increase rivaroxaban plasma concentrations (see Warnings and Precautions, Renal).

Different Weight Categories: Extremes in body weight (<50 kg or >120 kg) caused less than a 25% change in the plasma concentration of rivaroxaban.

STORAGE AND STABILITY: Store at 15 to 30°C.

INFORMATION FOR THE PATIENT: Published in e-CPS, available by subscription at www.e-cps.ca.

DOSAGE FORMS, COMPOSITION AND PACKAGING: Each film-coated, round, biconvex, light red, immediate release tablet of 6 mm diameter, for oral use, marked with the Bayer Cross on one side and 10 and a triangle on the other side, contains: rivaroxaban 10 mg. Nonmedicinal ingredients: croscarmellose sodium, hypromellose 5 cP, lactose monohydrate, magnesium stearate, microcrystalline cellulose and sodium lauryl sulfate; film-coating: ferric oxide red, hypromellose 15 cP, polyethylene glycol and titanium dioxide. HDPE bottles of 50.

(Shown in Product Identification Section)

Xatral® ℞

alfuzosin HCl

Symptomatic Treatment of Benign Prostatic Hyperplasia (BPH)—Adjunctive Therapy in Acute Urinary Retention (AUR)

sanofi-aventis

Date of Revision: July 30, 2010

SUMMARY PRODUCT INFORMATION:

Route of Administration	Dosage Form/ Strength	Clinically Relevant Nonmedicinal Ingredients
Oral	Prolonged-Release Tablet 10 mg	For a complete listing see Dosage Forms, Composition and Packaging.

INDICATIONS AND CLINICAL USE: XATRAL (alfuzosin hydrochloride) is indicated for:

- **Benign Prostatic Hyperplasia:** XATRAL is indicated for the treatment of the signs and symptoms of benign prostatic hyperplasia (BPH).
- **Acute Urinary Retention:** XATRAL is indicated as adjunctive therapy with urethral catheterization for Acute Urinary Retention related to BPH and management following catheter removal.

Geriatrics (>65 years of age): XATRAL has been found to be safe and effective when administered at the therapeutic dose (10 mg once-daily) to patients over the age of 65 years.

Women: XATRAL is not indicated nor recommended for use in women.

Pediatrics (<18 years): XATRAL is not indicated for use in children.

CONTRAINDICATIONS: XATRAL is contraindicated in:

- Patients with a known hypersensitivity to XATRAL or to any ingredient in the formulation. For a complete listing, see Dosage Forms, Composition and Packaging.
- Patients with moderate to severe hepatic insufficiency, since alfuzosin blood levels are increased in these patients (see Action and Clinical Pharmacology, Pharmacokinetics, Special Populations and Conditions, Hepatic Insufficiency).
- Combination with other alpha1-blockers.
- Combination with potent CYP3A4 inhibitors such as ketoconazole, ritonavir and itroconazole, because alfuzosin blood levels and exposure (AUC) are increased (see Drug Interactions, Overview).

WARNINGS AND PRECAUTIONS: General: Prostatic Carcinoma: Carcinoma of the prostate and BPH cause many of the same symptoms. These two diseases frequently coexist. Therefore, patients thought to have BPH should be examined prior to starting therapy with XATRAL to rule out the presence of carcinoma of the prostate.

Patients with known hypersensitivity to alpha1-blockers should be closely monitored while on XATRAL.

There are no data available on the effect on driving vehicles. Adverse reactions such as vertigo, dizziness and asthenia may occur essentially at the beginning of treatment. This has to be taken into consideration when driving vehicles and operating machines.

Patient should be warned that the tablet should be swallowed whole. Any other mode of administration, such as crunching, crushing, chewing, grinding or pounding to powder should be prohibited. These actions may lead to inappropriate release and absorption of the drug and therefore possible early adverse reactions (see Dosage and Administration, Administration).

Cardiovascular: XATRAL is not indicated for the treatment of hypertension.

As with all alpha1-blockers in some patients, in particular, patients receiving antihypertensive medications, postural hypotension with or without dizziness or other symptoms may develop within a few hours following administration of XATRAL. However, these effects are usually transient, occur at the beginning of treatment and do not usually prevent the continuation of treatment. In such cases, the patients should lie down until the symptoms have completely disappeared. **As with other alpha1-blockers (alpha1-adrenergic blocking agents), there is a potential for syncope. Patients beginning treatment should be warned of the possible occurrence of such events.**

Care should be taken when XATRAL is administered to patients with symptomatic orthostatic hypotension or patients who have had a pronounced hypotensive response to another alpha1-blocker.

As with all alpha1-blockers, alfuzosin has been observed to increase heart rate. Caution should be taken in patients with histories of tachyarrhythmia or with certain cardiovascular conditions, such as myocardial ischemia. The heart rate increasing effects of alfuzosin are additive to those of other heart rate increasing drugs (see Drug Interactions).

Coronary Insufficiency: Specific treatment for coronary insufficiency should be continued; however, if angina pectoris reappears or becomes worse, XATRAL should be discontinued.

Patients with congenital QTc prolongation, with a known history of acquired QTc prolongation or who are taking drugs known to increase the QTc interval should be evaluated before and during the administration of alfuzosin.

Co-administration of alfuzosin with a drug known to be a QTc prolonging drug should be evaluated by the physician based on individual patient's condition (see Action and Clinical Pharmacology, Pharmacodynamics, Electrocardiography).

Ophthalmologic: Intraoperative Floppy Iris Syndrome (IFIS, a variant of small pupil syndrome) has been observed during cataract surgery in some patients on or previously treated with some alpha-1-blockers. Cases of IFIS have been observed with XATRAL use. Ophthalmic surgeons should be informed in advance of cataract surgery of current or past use of alpha-1-blockers, as IFIS may lead to increased procedural complications. The ophthalmologists should be prepared for possible modifications to their surgical technique.

Special Populations: Pregnant Women: XATRAL is not indicated nor recommended for use in women. No embryotoxic and/or teratogenic effects in the rat and rabbit were observed with XATRAL. Parameters of male and female fertility, parturition, lactation and pup development were not modified by XATRAL.

Nursing Women: XATRAL is not indicated nor recommended for use in women. It is unknown if the drug is excreted in human milk.

Pediatrics (<18 years): XATRAL is not indicated for use in children.

Geriatrics (>65 years of age): The pharmacokinetic parameters (C_{max} and AUC) are not increased in elderly patients when compared to healthy male volunteers. XATRAL has been found to be a safe and effective alpha1-blockers when administered at the therapeutic dose (10 mg once-daily) to patients over the age of 65 years.

ADVERSE REACTIONS: Adverse Drug Reaction Overview: Dizziness and headache are the most frequent adverse drug reactions with XATRAL.

XATRAL was associated with a low incidence of postural symptoms. As with all alpha1-blockers, there is also a potential for syncope.

XATRAL was not associated with deleterious effects on sexual function.

Clinical Trial Adverse Drug Reactions: Because clinical trials are conducted under very specific conditions the adverse reaction rates observed in the clinical trials may not reflect the rates observed in practice and should not be compared to the rates in the clinical trials of another drug. Adverse drug reaction information from clinical trials is useful for identifying drug-related adverse events and for approximating rates.

Safety information was derived from placebo-controlled clinical trials involving 1608 men with BPH. The safety profile of XATRAL in the ALFAUR study which included 363 patients with Acute Urinary Retention due to BPH was similar to the safety profile reported in previous BPH studies.

In the BPH studies, 4% of patients taking XATRAL 10 mg tablets withdrew from the study due to adverse events, compared with 3% in the placebo group. Dizziness and headache were the most frequent cause in each of the groups, although no single symptom was predominant. The withdrawal rate was similar in the XATRAL group following long-term use in open-label extension studies for up to 1 year.

Table 1 summarizes the treatment-emergent adverse events that occurred in ≥2% of patients receiving XATRAL and placebo, in three 3-month trials. In general, the adverse events seen in long-term use were similar in type and frequency to the events described below for the 3-month trials.

Less Common Clinical Trial Adverse Drug Reactions: The following adverse events, reported by between 1% and 2% of patients receiving XATRAL and placebo are listed and are as follows: see Table 2.

Table 1: XATRAL

Treatment-Emergent Adverse Events Occurring in ≥2% of Patients with BPH Treated with XATRAL and with Placebo in 3-Month Placebo-Controlled Clinical Studies

Adverse Event	Placebo (N=678)	XATRAL (N=473)
General Disorders and Administration Site Conditions		
Fatigue[a]	12 (1.8%)	13 (2.7%)
Musculoskeletal and Connective Tissue Disorders		
Joint Disorders[b]	15 (2.2%)	10 (2.1%)
Infection and Infestations		
Upper Respiratory Tract Infection[c]	23 (3.4%)	29 (6.1%)
Nervous System Disorders		
Dizziness[d]	19 (2.8%)	27 (5.7%)
Headache	12 (1.8%)	14 (3.0%)

[a] Includes: fatigue and asthenia.
[b] Includes: arthritis, arthrosis, arthropathy, arthritis aggravated, arthralgia, and bursitis.
[c] Includes: upper respiratory tract infection, rhinitis, sinusitis, laryngitis, pharyngitis.
[d] Includes: dizziness and malaise.

Table 2: XATRAL

Treatment-Emergent Adverse Events Occurring Between 1% and 2% of Patients with BPH Treated with XATRAL and Placebo in 3-Month Placebo-Controlled Clinical Studies

Adverse Event	Placebo (N=678)	XATRAL (N=473)
Gastrointestinal Disorders		
Abdominal Pain	7 (1.0)	7 (1.5)
Dyspepsia	7 (1.0)	6 (1.3)
Constipation	3 (0.4)	5 (1.1)
Nausea	4 (0.6)	5 (1.1)
General Disorders and Administration Site Conditions		
Influenza-like Symptoms	14 (2.1)	9 (1.9)
Pain	4 (0.6)	7 (1.5)
Infection and Infestations		
Bronchitis	5 (0.7)	7 (1.5)
Injury, Poisoning and Procedural Complications		
Inflicted Injury[a]	3 (0.4)	6 (1.3)
Musculoskeletal and Connective Tissue Disorders		
Back Pain[b]	11 (1.6)	7 (1.5)
Reproductive System and Breast Disorders		
Impotence	4 (0.6)	7 (1.5)

[a] Includes: bite and inflicted injury.
[b] Includes: ischial neuralgia, neuralgia, neuropathy, back pain, and lumbar disc lesion.

Reproductive System and Breast Disorders: Impotence and other events related to sexual function are commonly associated with other alpha1-blockers, however, with XATRAL, there were minimal effects regarding sexual function and ejaculatory disorders/abnormalities with no reports of priapism. Also, no patient discontinued treatment with XATRAL due to ejaculation disorders. The reported incidence of ejaculation disorders was not associated with the study drug and is consistent with that reported in the untreated population.

Cardiac Disorders: Atrial Arrhythmias: A total of 47 cases of potential atrial arrhythmia were reported with alfuzosin whatever the formulation. Twenty nine cases of these arrhythmias were atrial fibrillations. In 13 double-blind clinical studies, 2881 patients were treated with alfuzosin (any formulation) and 15 (0.5%) cases of potential atrial arrhythmias have been detected. Six (0.2%) of these cases of arrhythmias were atrial fibrillations. Because atrial fibrillation has also been observed with other alpha1-blocker users, it may suggest that atrial fibrillation observed among the alfuzosin users may be possibly related to a class effect of alpha1-blockers.

Vascular Disorders: Signs and Symptoms of Orthostasis in Clinical Studies: The number of patients with symptoms of orthostasis are summarized in Table 3.

Table 3: XATRAL

Number (%) of Patients with BPH with Symptoms Possibly Associated with Orthostasis in 3-Month Placebo-Controlled Clinical Studies

Symptoms	Placebo (N=678)	XATRAL (N=473)
Dizziness	19 (2.8%)	27 (5.7%)
Hypotension or Postural Hypotension	0	2 (0.4%)
Syncope	0	1 (0.2%)

Multiple testing for blood pressure changes or orthostatic hypotension was conducted in the three controlled studies. These tests were considered positive for blood pressure decrease if (1) supine systolic blood pressure was ≤90 mmHg, with a decrease ≥20 mmHg versus baseline, and/or (2) supine diastolic blood pressure was ≤50 mmHg, with a decrease ≥15 mmHg versus baseline. The tests were considered positive for orthostatic hypotension if there was a decrease in systolic blood pressure of ≥20 mmHg upon standing from the supine position during the orthostatic tests. The percentage of patients with a positive test at any visit was 7.7% for placebo and 6.6% for XATRAL, as shown in Table 4.

Table 4: XATRAL

Number (%) of Patients with BPH with Clinically Meaningful Decreases in Blood Pressure at any Visit in 3-Month Placebo-Controlled Clinical Studies

Clinically Meaningful Change	Placebo (N=674)	XATRAL (N=469)
Decreased Systolic Blood Pressure	0	1 (0.2%)
Decreased Diastolic Blood Pressure	3 (0.4%)	4 (0.9%)
Positive Orthostatic Test	52 (7.7%)	31[a] (6.6%)

a N=471.

A subset of patients from Study 1 had blood pressure measurements 12 to 16 hours after the first dose to assess the potential to produce orthostatic hypotension. None of the 35 XATRAL treated patients showed a positive test for systolic, diastolic, or orthostatic blood pressure change.

No age effect on the overall incidence of patients reporting adverse events was observed in the XATRAL group; elderly patients (≥65 years) did not experience more vasodilatory adverse events than the younger patients.

Post-Market Adverse Drug Reactions: The following adverse events have also been reported in postmarketing experience: The following frequency rating is used; very common (≥10%), Common (≥1% and <10%), Uncommon (≥0.1% and <1%), Rare (≥0.01% and <0.1%), Very rare (<0.01%).

Cardiac Disorders: Uncommon: tachycardia. Very Rare: angina pectoris in patients with pre-existing coronary artery disease (see also Warnings and Precautions, Cardiovascular). Isolated spontaneous cases of QT interval prolongation, ventricular arrhythmias, including torsades de pointes, ventricular tachycardia and fibrillation have been reported particularly in patients with preexisting cardiovascular diseases; however, a relationship between these adverse events and the XATRAL treatment was not clearly established due to concomitant cardiac disorders, concomitant medications or absence of pre-treatment ECG measurement.

Cases of atrial fibrillation have been reported.

Vascular Disorders: Uncommon: flushing.

Gastrointestinal Disorders: Uncommon: diarrhea.

General Disorders and Administration Site Conditions: Uncommon: edema, chest pain.

Ear and Labyrinth Disorders: Uncommon: vertigo.

Eye Disorders: Cases of intraoperative floppy iris syndrome have been reported (see Warnings and Precautions, Ophthalmologic).

Hepato-biliary Disorders: Cases of hepatocellular injury and cholestatic liver disease have been reported.

Respiratory, Thoracic and Mediastinal Disorders: Uncommon: rhinitis.

Reproductive System and Breast Disorders: Cases of priapism have been reported.

Skin and Subcutaneous Tissue Disorders: Uncommon: rash, pruritus. Very rare: urticaria, angioedema.

DRUG INTERACTIONS: Overview: XATRAL is not an inducer or an inhibitor of any of the principal hepatic enzymes involved in the metabolism of other drugs.

CYP3A4 is the principal hepatic enzyme isoform involved in the metabolism of XATRAL.

Potent CYP3A4 inhibitors, such as ketoconazole, itraconazole and ritonavir, increased XATRAL blood levels and exposure (AUC). Therefore, XATRAL should not be co-administered with potent inhibitors of CYP3A4 (see Contraindications). **See Drug-Drug Interactions for details of increased XATRAL blood levels. As this is only a partial list, the physician is advised to consult current scientific literature regarding other CYP 3A4 competitive inhibitors prior to prescribing XATRAL if other concomitant medications are used as high blood levels of XATRAL can result.**

It is not known how combined exposure of any medications metabolized by the CYP3A4 hepatic enzyme isoform (such as modern alpha1-blockers), herbal remedies (particularly St. John's Wort, Milk thistle) and grapefruit juice may influence the overall efficacy and unwanted side effects of these medications, therefore, caution should be exercised.

XATRAL should be prescribed carefully in combination with antihypertensive drugs. (see Warnings and Precautions, Cardiovascular and Drug-Drug Interactions, Cardiovascular Drugs).

Drug-Drug Interactions: Anti-Infectious Drugs: Imidazole: Ketoconazole: CYP3A4 is the principal hepatic enzyme involved in the metabolism of XATRAL. Ketoconazole is a strong-potency inhibitor of CYP3A4. Repeated 200 mg daily dosing of ketoconazole, for seven days **increased XATRAL C_{max} 2.11-fold and AUC_{last} 2.46-fold following a single 10 mg dose of XATRAL** under fed condition. Other parameters such as t_{max} and $t_{1/2}$ were not modified. The 8-day repeated administration of ketoconazole 400 mg daily **increased C_{max} of XATRAL by 2.3-fold, AUC_{last} and AUC by 3.2 and 3.0 respectively.**

Cardiovascular Drugs: Alpha1-Blocker: XATRAL should not be used in combination with other alpha1-blockers (see Contraindications).

Anticoagulant: Warfarin: The potential drug interactions of XATRAL with warfarin was studied in clinical trials. The results showed that XATRAL can be prescribed without risk of interactions in combination with warfarin.

Beta-Blocker: Atenolol: The potential drug interactions of XATRAL with atenolol was studied in clinical trials. The results showed that XATRAL may be used with atenolol taking into account the hypotensive effects specific to drugs in this group.

Calcium Channel Blocker: Diltiazem: Repeated coadministration of 240 mg/day of diltiazem, a moderate-potency inhibitor of CYP3A4, with 7.5 mg/day alfuzosin (equivalent to the exposure with XATRAL) increased the C_{max} and AUC_{0-24} of alfuzosin 1.5- and 1.3-fold, respectively. Alfuzosin increased the C_{max} and AUC_{0-12} of diltiazem 1.4-fold. No changes in blood pressure were observed.

Cardiotonic Glycoside: Digoxin: Repeated coadministration of XATRAL and digoxin for 7 days did not influence the steady-state pharmacokinetics of either drug.

Diuretic: Hydrochlorothiazide: The potential drug interactions of XATRAL with hydrochlorothiazide was studied in clinical trials. The results showed that XATRAL can be prescribed without risk of interactions in combination with hydrochlorothiazide.

Nitrates: XATRAL should be prescribed carefully in combination with nitrates.

Gastrointestinal Drugs: Histamine H_2 Receptor Antagonist: Cimetidine: The potential drug interactions of XATRAL with cimetidine was studied in clinical trials. The results showed that XATRAL can be prescribed without risk of interactions in combination with cimetidine.

Sexual Function Drugs: Inhibitor of Cyclic Guanosine Monophosphate (cGMP)-Specific Phosphodiesterase Type 5 (PDE5): Because of the vasodilatory effects of alpha-blockers and PDE5-inhibitors, patients treated with alpha-blocker therapy should be hemodynamically stable before treatment with PDE5-inhibitors is initiated.

Tadalafil: The potential drug interaction of XATRAL with tadalafil was studied in a clinical trial. The results showed that there is no clinically significant hemodynamic interaction between XATRAL 10 mg once daily and tadalafil 20 mg. XATRAL can be prescribed in combination with tadalafil.

Sildenafil: The effect on QT/QTc interval of the combination of XATRAL 10 mg and sildenafil 100 mg has been studied in an electrophysiology trial (see Action and Clinical Pharmacology, Pharmacodynamics, Electrocardiography).

Vardenafil: The potential drug interaction of XATRAL with vardenafil was not studied in a clinical trial.

Drug-Food Interactions: XATRAL should be taken after a meal.

It is not known how combined exposure of grapefruit juice may influence the overall efficacy and unwanted side effects of these type of medications, therefore, caution should be exercised.

Drug-Herb Interactions: Interactions with herbal products have not been established. It is not known how combined exposure of herbal remedies (particularly St. John's Wort, Milk thistle) may influence the overall efficacy and unwanted side effects of these medications, therefore, caution should be exercised when taking herbal remedies with these types of medications.

Drug-Laboratory Test Interactions: Treatment with XATRAL for up to 12 months produced no clinically significant changes in urinalysis, the routine biochemical and hematologic tests as well as in prostate specific antigen (PSA).

DOSAGE AND ADMINISTRATION: Recommended Dose and Dosage Adjustment: Benign Prostatic Hyperplasia:

The recommended dosage is one 10 mg XATRAL tablet daily to be taken after the same meal each day.

Acute Urinary Retention: The recommended dosage is one 10 mg XATRAL tablet daily after a meal to be taken from the first day of catheterization and continued beyond catheter removal unless there is a relapse of acute urinary retention or disease progression.

Administration: The tablet should be swallowed whole. Any other mode of administration, such as crunching, crushing, chewing, grinding or pounding to powder should be prohibited. These actions may lead to an inappropriate release and absorption of the drug and therefore possible early adverse reactions.

OVERDOSAGE:

Should overdose of XATRAL lead to hypotension, support of the cardiovascular system is of first importance. Restoration of blood pressure and normalization of heart rate may be accomplished by keeping the patient in the supine position. If this measure is inadequate, then the administration of intravenous fluids should be considered. If necessary, vasopressor should then be used and the renal function should be monitored and supported as needed. XATRAL is 87% (82-90%) protein-bound, therefore, dialysis may not be of benefit.

> For management of a suspected drug overdose, contact your regional Poison Control Centre. See the *CPS* Directory section for a list of Poison Control Centres.

ACTION AND CLINICAL PHARMACOLOGY: Mechanism of Action: XATRAL, indicated for the treatment of benign prostatic hyperplasia (BPH) and as adjunctive therapy with urethral catheterization for acute urinary retention related to BPH and management following catheter removal, is a uroselective antagonist of post-synaptic α_1-adrenoceptors located in the prostate, bladder base, bladder neck, prostatic capsule, and prostatic urethra.

Pharmacodynamics: The clinical manifestations of benign prostatic hyperplasia are due to bladder outlet obstruction caused by anatomical (static) and functional (dynamic) factors. The static component is related to an increase in prostate size which may not cause symptoms. The dynamic component is related primarily to an increase in smooth muscle tone in the prostate, prostatic capsule, bladder base, bladder neck, and prostatic urethra. This increased tone is mediated by the activation of α_1-adrenoceptors and leads to an increased resistance to urinary voiding and the symptoms of BPH such as a hesitant, interrupted, weak stream; urgency and leaking or dribbling; and/or more frequent urination, especially at night. XATRAL blocks α_1-adrenoceptors leading to a relaxation of the smooth muscle in the bladder neck and prostate.

In animal studies, alfuzosin was shown to be functionally uroselective by preferentially decreasing urethral blood pressure over arterial blood pressure. In human tissue, in vitro, alfuzosin has induced preferential α_1-adrenoceptor antagonist activity on prostatic cells relative to renal artery cells. This is illustrated in Figure 1.

Figure 1: XATRAL

Prostatic Selectivity Score

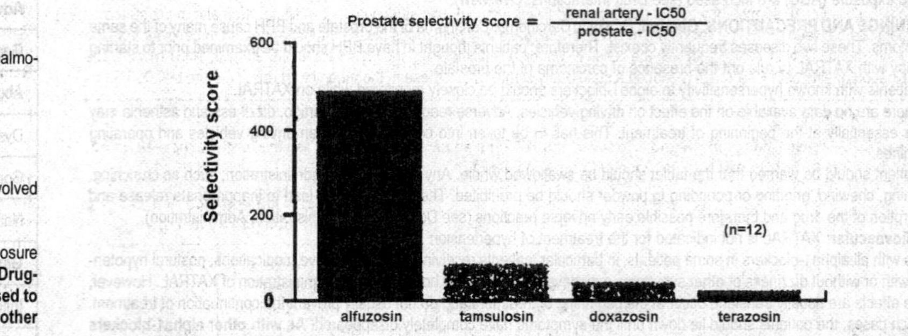

In placebo-controlled clinical studies in patients with BPH, XATRAL was shown to:

- significantly increase urine peak flow rate (Qmax) by 30% which is observed after the first dose.
- significantly reduce detrusor pressure and increase bladder capacity.
- significantly reduce residual urine volume.

These favourable urodynamic effects lead to an improvement of lower tract irritative and obstructive symptoms without any deleterious effect on sexual function. The Quality of Life Index was also significantly improved by 33% in the XATRAL-treated patients.

In addition, the efficacy of alfuzosin 10 mg OD on peak flow rate and the limited effect on blood pressure have been demonstrated to be related to its pharmacokinetic profile. Moreover, the efficacy on peak flow rate is maintained up to 24 hours after intake.

A lower frequency of acute urinary retention was observed in the alfuzosin treated patient than in the untreated patient.

Electrocardiography: The effect of 10 mg and 40 mg alfuzosin on QT interval was evaluated in a double-blind, randomized, placebo and active-controlled (moxifloxacin 400 mg), 4-way crossover single dose study in 45 healthy white male subjects aged 19 to 45 years. The 40 mg dose of alfuzosin was chosen because this dose achieves higher blood levels than those achieved with the co-administration of XATRAL and ketoconazole 400 mg (CYP3A4 inhibitor). QT interval, obtained with 12-lead ECGs, was measured from 2h to 12h post treatment administration. Table 5 summarizes the mean effect and the maximum mean effect on heart rate (HR) and corrected QT interval (QTc) with different methods of correction [Bazett (QTcB), Fridericia (QTcF) and population-specific (QTcN) correction methods]. There is a trend to lower values for QTc interval changes from QTcB → QTcF → QTcN, demonstrating the critical role of the correction formula used to minimize the biased overestimation linked to the heart rate increase. The maximum mean change of heart rate associated with a 10 mg dose of alfuzosin in this study was 3.69 beats/minute and 5.45 beats/minute with 40 mg alfuzosin. The change in heart rate with moxifloxacin was 2.85 beats/minute.

Table 5: XATRAL

12-Lead ECG—Mean Change in HR And QTc Data From T7–T11h and Maximum Mean Baseline- and Placebo-Adjusted HR and QTc Interval Changes Over the Observation Period T2-T12h

		Mean Difference		Largest Time-Matched Analysis (bootstrap adjusted)	
Parameter	Treatment	Mean Change From Baseline vs Placebo	95% CI (upper bound)	Estimation Of Largest Time-Matched Mean Difference	95% CI (upper bound)
HR (bpm)	Alfuzosin 10 mg	1.5	3	3.69	5.83
	Alfuzosin 40 mg	3.7	5.2	5.45	7.06
	Moxifloxacin[a]	1.5	3	2.85	4.26
QTcB (msec)	Alfuzosin 10 mg	3.3	6.9	6.08	9.59
	Alfuzosin 40 mg	10.8	14.4	13.27	16.71
	Moxifloxacin[a]	11.9	15.6	12.57	16.12

(cont'd)

Table 5: XATRAL *(cont'd)*

12-Lead ECG—Mean Change in HR And QTc Data From T7–T11h and Maximum Mean Baseline- and Placebo-Adjusted HR and QTc Interval Changes Over the Observation Period T2-T12h

Parameter	Treatment	Mean Difference: Mean Change From Baseline vs Placebo	Mean Difference: 95% CI (upper bound)	Largest Time-Matched Analysis (bootstrap adjusted): Estimation Of Largest Time-Matched Mean Difference	Largest Time-Matched Analysis (bootstrap adjusted): 95% CI (upper bound)
QTcF (msec)	Alfuzosin 10 mg	1.6	4.3	4.01	6.68
	Alfuzosin 40 mg	6.9	9.5	10.73	13.49
	Moxifloxacin[a]	10.3	13	11.17	14.06
QTcN (msec)	Alfuzosin 10 mg	0.5	3	2.74	5.27
	Alfuzosin 40 mg	4.6	7	9.3	12.14
	Moxifloxacin[a]	9.4	11.9	10.78	13.67

[a] Active control.

The maximum mean effect on QTcN appeared greater for 40 mg compared to 10 mg alfuzosin. The effect of the highest alfuzosin dose (four times the therapeutic dose) studied did not appear as large as that of the active control moxifloxacin at its therapeutic dose.

A separate post-marketing study evaluated the effect of the co-administration of 10 mg alfuzosin and a drug with similar QT effect size. It was a double-blind, randomized, placebo and active-controlled (moxifloxacin 400 mg), 5-way crossover study conducted in 39 healthy white male subjects aged 19 to 46 years. QT interval, obtained with 12-lead ECGs, was measured from 4 h to 12 h post treatment administration. Maximum mean effect on HR and QT interval were extracted from a time-matched placebo adjusted analysis. In this study, the maximum mean placebo-substracted QTcN increase of alfuzosin 10 mg alone was 4.41 msec (upperbound 95% CI, 7.09 msec), shown in Table 6. The concomitant administration of the two drugs (alfuzosin and sildenafil) showed an increased QT effect when compared with either drug alone. This maximum mean QTcN increase [8.27 msec (UB 95% CI, 10.90 msec)] was not more than additive. Although this study was not designed to make direct statistical comparisons between drugs, the maximum mean QTcN increase with both drugs given together appeared to be lower than the maximum mean QTcN increase seen with the positive control moxifloxacin 400 mg [11.44 msec (UB 95% CI, 14.01 msec)]. The combination of alfuzosin + sildenafil produced a statistically significant increase in the mean heart rate [+4 bpm, p<0.0001].

Table 6: XATRAL

12-Lead ECG—Mean Change in HR and QTc Data From T7-T10h and Maximum Mean Baseline- and Placebo-Adjusted HR and QT Interval Changes Over the Observation Period T4-T12h

Parameter	Treatment	Mean Difference: Mean Change from Baseline vs Placebo	Mean Difference: 95% CI (upper bound)	Largest Time-Matched Analysis (bootstrap adjusted): Estimation of Largest Time-Matched Mean Difference	Largest Time-Matched Analysis (bootstrap adjusted): 95% CI (upper bound)
HR (bpm)	Alfuzosin 10 mg	1.1	2.9	3.78	5.54
	Alfuzosin + Sildenafil	4	5.8	5.53	7.25
	Sildenafil 100 mg	1.4	3.2	2.13	3.82
	Moxifloxacin[a]	1.3	3.2	2.8	4.39
QTcB (msec)	Alfuzosin 10 mg	5	8.8	7.49	10.68
	Alfuzosin + Sildenafil	13.3	17.1	14.99	18.35
	Sildenafil 100 mg	6.3	10.1	7.85	11.3
	Moxifloxacin[a]	9.4	13.2	17.18	20.72
QTcF (msec)	Alfuzosin 10 mg	3.7	6.6	5.72	8.19
	Alfuzosin + Sildenafil	9.5	12.4	10.47	12.97
	Sildenafil 100 mg	4.8	7.7	6.4	8.97
	Moxifloxacin[a]	7.8	10.7	13.8	16.48
QTcN (msec)[b]	Alfuzosin 10 mg	2.2	5.1	4.41	7.09
	Alfuzosin + Sildenafil	7	10	8.27	10.9
	Sildenafil 100 mg	3.5	6.4	5.26	7.87
	Moxifloxacin[a]	6.5	9.4	11.44	14.01

[a] Active control.
[b] For the analysis of the mean difference, only QTcNi data are available (QT interval corrected by a subject specific formula).

QT interval prolongation has not been studied in patients with BPH, therefore similar data is not available. This population may suffer from other conditions and have a higher risk to develop QT interval prolongation due to concomitant risk factors or pre-existing cardiovascular disorders. Based on individual patient's condition, monitoring for ECG abnormalities should be considered by the physician during treatment.

Pharmacokinetics: The XATRAL tablet is based on the GEOMATRIX System, a patented prolonged-release technology designed to provide a sustained and continuous delivery of the active ingredient consistent with a once-daily administration. The pharmacokinetic properties of this system have been evaluated in healthy adult volunteers after single and/or multiple administrations with daily doses ranging from 7.5 mg to 30 mg, and in patients with BPH at doses from 7.5 mg to 15 mg.

Absorption: Bioavailability is reduced when XATRAL is administered under fasting conditions. A consistent pharmacokinetic profile is obtained when XATRAL is administered following a meal. A mean peak plasma concentration of 12.3±6.6 ng/mL is reached in 6 to 14 hours after a single dose.

Under fed conditions and after repeated doses, mean C_{max} and $C_{through}$ values are 13.6 (SD=5.6) and 3.1 (SD=1.6) ng/mL respectively. Mean AUC_{0-24} is 194 (SD=75) mg.h/mL. A plateau of concentration is observed from 3 to 14 hours with concentrations above 8.1 ng/mL (Cav) for 11 hours.

Figure 2: XATRAL

Mean (SEM) Alfuzosin Plasma Concentration-Time Profiles After a Repeated Administration of Alfuzosin 10 mg OD Tablet in Healthy Middle-Aged Male Volunteers (N=42)

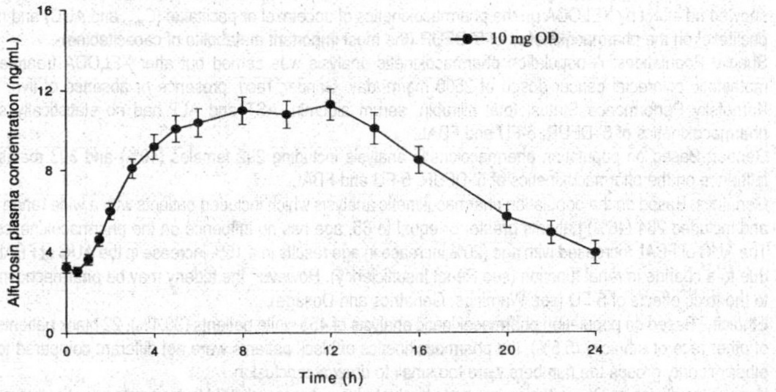

Distribution: The volume of distribution calculated following intravenous administration is 2.5 L/kg which indicates a distribution into extracellular fluids of the body. XATRAL is moderately bound to plasma proteins with the free fraction accounting for 13.3% in healthy volunteers. Fractions bound to serum albumin and α_1-glycoproteins are 68.2 and 52.5%, respectively. Salicylic acid, hydrochlorothiazide, diltiazem, digoxin and indomethacin does not affect the binding of XATRAL to human plasma proteins. Based on in vivo data, it is not likely that XATRAL will affect the extent of binding of these drugs to human plasma proteins. There is an increase in free fraction in renal insufficiency patients (16.8%) and in patients with hepatic disease (20.8%).

Metabolism: XATRAL undergoes metabolism by the liver, with only 11% of the parent compound being excreted as unchanged in the urine. The metabolites which are all inactive are eliminated in the urine (15-30%) and feces (75-91%). XATRAL is metabolized by three metabolic pathways (oxidation, O-demethylation, N-dealkylation) which are qualitatively identical to those observed in the animal (rat and dog).

CYP3A4 is the principal hepatic enzyme isoform involved in its metabolism.

Excretion: Following intravenous or oral administration, the elimination of XATRAL is characterized, in healthy young subjects and in the target population, by a terminal half-life of about 4.8 hours and a total clearance of 0.3 L/h/kg.

The apparent half-life of XATRAL is increased to 9.1 hours in healthy middle-aged volunteers and to 10.1 hours in elderly volunteers.

Special Populations and Conditions: Geriatrics: Compared to healthy middle-aged volunteers, the pharmacokinetic parameters of XATRAL (C_{max} and AUC) are not increased in elderly patients.

Renal Insufficiency: Compared to subjects with normal renal function, the mean C_{max} and AUC values of XATRAL are moderately increased (1.5- to 1.6-fold) in patients with various stages of renal impairment, with no change in the apparent elimination half-life. This change in the pharmacokinetic profile is not considered clinically relevant; and therefore, does not necessitate a dosing adjustment.

XATRAL has not been evaluated in patients with end-stage renal disease.

Hepatic Insufficiency: After a single oral administration of XATRAL in patients with severe hepatic insufficiency, the elimination half-life is prolonged. A two-fold increase in C_{max} values and a three-fold increase in the AUC is observed. Bioavailability is increased in comparison with that in healthy volunteers (see Contraindications).

Chronic Cardiac Insufficiency: The pharmacokinetic profile of XATRAL administered intravenously is not affected by chronic cardiac insufficiency.

STORAGE AND STABILITY: Store at room temperature (15-30°C). Keep in a safe place out of the reach of children.

SPECIAL HANDLING INSTRUCTIONS: There are no special handling instructions.

INFORMATION FOR THE PATIENT: Published in e-CPS, available by subscription at www.e-cps.ca.

DOSAGE FORMS, COMPOSITION AND PACKAGING: Each once-daily, prolonged-release, three-layer, round and biconvex tablet, contains: alfuzosin hydrochloride 10 mg in a white matrix layer between two inactive yellow layers. Nonmedicinal ingredients: colloidal hydrated silica, ethylcellulose, hydrogenated castor oil, hydroxypropyl methylcellulose (hypromellose), magnesium stearate, mannitol, microcrystalline cellulose, povidone and yellow ferric oxide. High Density Polyethylene (HDPE) bottles of 100.

(Shown in Product Identification Section)

Xeloda® ℞

capecitabine

Antineoplastic

Roche

Date of Preparation: August 24, 1998
Date of Revision: November 30, 2009

PHARMACOLOGY:

Caution: XELODA (capecitabine) is a potent drug and should be prescribed only by physicians experienced with cancer chemotherapeutic drugs (see Warnings). If toxicity on therapy occurs, XELODA should be interrupted until the event resolves, or the severity decreases when the following toxicities occur at a severity of grade 2 or greater: diarrhea, hand-foot syndrome, nausea, hyperbilirubinemia, vomiting or stomatitis (see Warnings, Precautions and Dosage).

Capecitabine is a tumor-activated antineoplastic agent (antimetabolite) belonging to the novel fluoropyrimidine carbamate class. It was rationally designed as an orally administered precursor of 5'-deoxy-5-fluorouridine (5'-DFUR). Capecitabine is selectively activated to the cytotoxic moiety, 5-fluorouracil (5-FU), by thymidine phosphorylase in tumors.

Bioactivation: Capecitabine is absorbed unchanged from the gastrointestinal tract, metabolized primarily in the liver by the 60kDa carboxylesterase to 5'-Deoxy-5-fluorocytidine (5'-DFCR) which is then converted to 5'-DFUR by cytidine deaminase, principally located in the liver and tumor tissue. Further metabolism of 5'-DFUR to the pharmacologically-active agent 5-FU occurs mainly at the site of the tumor by thymidine phosphorylase (dThdPase), which has levels considerably higher in tumor tissues compared to normal tissues. Healthy liver tissues also contain a relatively high activity of dThdPase. In human cancer xenograft models, capecitabine demonstrated a synergistic effect in combination with docetaxel which may be related to the upregulation of thymidine phosphorylase by docetaxel.

Mechanism of Action: Within normal and tumor cells, 5-FU is further metabolized to 5-fluoro-2'-deoxyuridine monophosphate (FdUMP) and 5-fluorouridine triphosphate (FUTP) which cause cell injury by both DNA and RNA-derived mechanisms.

Pharmacokinetics: In Colorectal Tumors and Adjacent Healthy Tissue: Following oral administration of capecitabine (1255 mg/m² b.i.d. 5 to 7 days) in patients with colorectal cancer, concentrations of 5-FU were significantly greater in primary tumor than in adjacent healthy tissue (geometric mean ratio 2.5; CI: 1.5 to 4.1) and in plasma (geometric mean ratio 14).

Pharmacokinetics: The pharmacokinetics of capecitabine and its metabolites have been evaluated in 11 studies in a total of 213 cancer patients at a dosage range of 502 to 3514 mg/m²/day. The parameters of capecitabine, 5'DFCR and 5'DFUR measured on days 1 and 14 were similar. AUC of 5-FU was 30% higher on day 14, but did not increase subsequently (day 22). At therapeutic doses, the pharmacokinetics of capecitabine and its metabolites were dose proportional, except for 5-FU. The elimination half-life of both capecitabine and 5-FU were about 45 minutes.

Absorption, Distribution, Metabolism and Excretion: Capecitabine reached peak blood levels in about 1.5 hours (T_{max}) with peak 5-FU blood levels occurring slightly later, at 2 hours. Administration with food decreases the rate of capecitabine absorption but only results in a minor decrease in the AUC's of 5'-DFUR and 5-FU (see Precautions and Dosage). Plasma protein binding of capecitabine and its metabolites is low (less than 60%) and is not concentration dependent. Capecitabine was primarily bound to human albumin (approximately 35%). Capecitabine is extensively metabolized to 5-FU. The enzyme dihydropyrimidine dehydrogenase hydrogenates 5-FU, the product of capecitabine metabolism, to the much less toxic, 5-fluoro-5,6-dihydro-fluorouracil

(FUH_2). Dihydropyrimidinase cleaves the pyrimidine ring to yield 5-fluoro-ureido-propionic acid (FUPA). Finally, β-ureido-propionase cleaves FUPA to α-fluoro-β-alanine (FBAL) which is cleared in the urine. Over 70% of the administered capecitabine dose is recovered in urine as drug-related material, about 50% of it as FBAL.

Phase I studies evaluating the effect of XELODA on the pharmacokinetics of either docetaxel or paclitaxel and vice versa showed no effect by XELODA on the pharmacokinetics of docetaxel or paclitaxel (C_{max} and AUC) and no effect by docetaxel or paclitaxel on the pharmacokinetics of 5'-DFUR (the most important metabolite of capecitabine).

Special Populations: A population pharmacokinetic analysis was carried out after XELODA treatment of 505 patients with metastatic colorectal cancer dosed at 2500 mg/m²/day. Gender, race, presence or absence of liver metastasis at baseline, Karnofsky Performance Status, total bilirubin, serum albumin, AST and ALT had no statistically significant effect on the pharmacokinetics of 5'-DFUR, 5-FU and FBAL.

Gender: Based on population pharmacokinetic analysis including 202 females (40%) and 303 males (60%), gender has no influence on the pharmacokinetics of 5'-DFUR, 5-FU and FBAL.

Geriatrics: Based on the population pharmacokinetic analysis which included patients with a wide range of ages (27 to 86 years) and included 234 (46%) patients greater or equal to 65, age has no influence on the pharmacokinetics of 5'-DFUR and 5-FU. The AUC of FBAL increased with age (20% increase in age results in a 15% increase in the AUC of FBAL). This increase is likely due to a change in renal function (see Renal Insufficiency). However, the elderly may be pharmacodynamically more sensitive to the toxic effects of 5-FU (see Warnings, Geriatrics and Dosage).

Ethnicity: Based on population pharmacokinetic analysis of 455 white patients (90.1%), 22 black patients (4.4%) and 28 patients of other race or ethnicity (5.5%), the pharmacokinetics of black patients were not different compared to white patients. For the other minority groups the numbers were too small to draw a conclusion.

Hepatic Insufficiency: Capecitabine has been evaluated in patients with mild to moderate hepatic dysfunction due to liver metastases. Both C_{max} and $AUC_{0-\infty}$ of capecitabine, 5'-DFUR and 5-FU were increased by 49%, 33% and 28% and by 48%, 20% and 15%, respectively. Conversely, C_{max} and AUC of 5'-DFCR decreased by 29% and 35%, respectively. Therefore, bioactivation of capecitabine is not affected. There are no pharmacokinetic data on patients with severe hepatic impairment (see Warnings and Dosage).

Renal Insufficiency: Based on a pharmacokinetic study in cancer patients with mild to severe renal impairment, there is no evidence for an effect of creatinine clearance on the pharmacokinetics of intact drug and 5-FU. Creatinine clearance was found to influence the systemic exposure to 5'-DFUR (35% increase in AUC when creatinine clearance decreases by 50%) and to FBAL (114% increase in AUC when creatinine clearance decreases by 50%). FBAL is a metabolite without antiproliferative activity; 5'-DFUR is the direct precursor of 5-FU.

As seen with 5-FU, the incidence of related grade 3 or 4 adverse events is higher in patients with moderate renal impairment (creatinine clearance 30 to 50 mL/min) (see Contraindications, Warnings and Dosage).

Clinical Studies: In a phase I study with XELODA, the maximum-tolerated dose as a single agent in the treatment of patients with solid tumors was 3000 mg/m² when administered daily for 2 weeks, followed by a 1-week rest period. The dose-limiting toxicities were diarrhea and leucopenia.

Combination Therapy—Second-Line Treatment of Metastatic Colorectal Cancer: Data from a multicenter, randomized, controlled phase III clinical study (NO16967) support the use of XELODA in combination with oxaliplatin for the second-line treatment of metastatic colorectal cancer. In this trial, 627 patients with metastatic colorectal carcinoma who have received prior treatment with irinotecan in combination with a fluoropyrimidine regimen as first-line therapy were randomized to treatment with XELOX or FOLFOX-4. For the dosing schedule of XELOX and FOLFOX-4, refer to Table 1.

Table 1: XELODA

Treatment Regimens in Study NO16967

Treatment		Starting Dose	Schedule
FOLFOX-4	Oxaliplatin	85 mg/m² IV 2 h	Oxaliplatin on Day 1, every 2 weeks
	Leucovorin	200 mg/m² IV 2 h	Leucovorin on Day 1 and 2, every 2 weeks
	5-Fluorouracil	400 mg/m² IV bolus, 600 mg/ m² IV 22 h	5-fluorouracil IV bolus/infusion, each on Days 1 and 2 , every 2 weeks
XELOX	Oxaliplatin	130 mg/m² IV 2 h	Oxaliplatin on Day 1, every 3 weeks
	Capecitabine	1000 mg/m² oral bid	Capecitabine oral bid for 2 weeks (followed by 1 week off treatment)

5-Fluorouracil: IV bolus injection immediately after leucovorin.

XELOX is at least equivalent to FOLFOX-4 in terms of progression-free survival in the per protocol population and intent-to-treat population in the investigator assessments. Progression-free survival by the IRC assessment also met the NI margin of 1.23 (HR=0.93; 95% CI [0.74; 1.17]).

Exploratory subgroup analyses for PFS (EP population) and OS (ITT population) for age suggest that XELOX may be less effective than FOLFOX-4 in patients ≥65 years of age (HR 1.32, 95% CI, 0.98-1.78 and HR 1.34, 95% CI, 1.00-1.80, respectively).

No quality of life data was collected. The median follow up at the time of the primary analyses in the intent-to-treat population was 2.1 years; data from analyses following an additional 6 months of follow up are also included in Table 2.

Table 2: XELODA

Key Non-Inferiority Efficacy Results for the Primary Analysis and 6-Month Follow-Up Data (PPP and ITT populations, Study NO16967)

	Primary Analysis PFS by Investigator Assessment[a]				
	XELOX		FOLFOX-4		
Population	# Events	Median Time to Event (Days)	# Events	Median Time to Event (Days)	HR (97.5% CI)
PPP	244	154	247	168	1.03 (0.87; 1.24)
ITT	301	144	301	146	0.97 (0.83; 1.14)
	OS Additional 6-Months of Follow-Up				
ITT	270	363	270	382	1.02 (0.86; 1.21)

[a] PFS by IRC assessment (PPP) met the NI margin of 1.23 (HR=0.93; 95% CI [0.74; 1.17]).

Metastatic Colorectal Cancer: Data from two multicentre, randomized, controlled phase III clinical trials involving 603 patients and one randomized phase II trial of 34 patients support the use of XELODA in the first-line treatment of patients with metastatic colorectal carcinoma (refer to Table 3).

XELODA was superior to 5-FU/LV for objective response rate in Study 1 and Study 2. The response rate observed in patients receiving the Mayo regimen was consistent with the published literature. It was also observed that in patients who received prior adjuvant chemotherapy the objective response rate was 15.3% and 14.5% for capecitabine and 5.5% and 4.4% (Study 1 and 2, respectively) for 5-FU/LV. There was no difference in time to disease progression and survival as compared to 5-FU/LV for both studies.

Table 3: XELODA

Clinical Studies in Metastatic Colorectal Carcinoma—Monotherapy

Design Diagnosis	Drug/Dosage	No. of Patients Enrolled Demographic Data	Results
Pivotal Phase III Studies **Study 1:** randomized, controlled, multicentre US, Canada, Mexico, Brazil	capecitabine 2500 mg/m²/day for 2 weeks with a 1-week rest period (given as 3-week cycles)	N=302 Age (yrs)-Md: 64; range: 23–86 M/F: 181(60%)/121(40%) Karnofsky PS-Md: 90%; range: 70–100 Colon/Rectum: 222 (74%)/79 (26%) Prior radiation therapy: 52 (17%) Prior adjuvant 5-FU: 84 (28%)	overall response rate: capecitabine-21% 5-FU/LV-11% (p=0.0014) median time to progression: capecitabine-128 days 5-FU/LV-131 days (p=0.90)
	5-FU/leucovorin (LV) Mayo regimen[a]	N=303 Age (yrs)-Md: 63; range: 24–87 M/F: 197(65%)/106(35%) Karnofsky PS-Md: 90%; range: 70–100 Colon/Rectum: 232 (77%)/70 (23%) Prior radiation therapy: 62 (21%) Prior adjuvant 5-FU: 110 (36%)	median survival: capecitabine-380 days 5-FU/LV-407 days (p=0.24)
Study 2: randomized, controlled, multicentre Europe, Israel, Australia, New Zealand, Taiwan	capecitabine 2500 mg/m²/day for 2 weeks with a 1-week rest period (given as 3-week cycles)	N=301 Age (yrs)-Md: 64; range: 29–84 M/F: 172(57%)/129(43%) Karnofsky PS-Md: 90%; range: 70–100 Colon/Rectum: 199 (66%)/101 (34%) Prior radiation therapy: 42 (14%) Prior adjuvant 5-FU: 56 (19%)	overall response rate: capecitabine-21% 5-FU/LV-14% (p=0.027) median time to progression: capecitabine-137 days 5-FU/LV-131 days (p=0.68)
	5-FU/leucovorin (LV) Mayo regimen[a]	N=301 Age (yrs)-Md: 64; range: 36–86 M/F: 173(57%)/128(43%) Karnofsky PS-Md: 90%; range: 70–100 Colon/Rectum: 196 (65%)/105 (35%) Prior radiation therapy: 42 (14%) Prior adjuvant 5-FU: 41 (14%)	median survival: capecitabine-404 days 5-FU/LV-379 days (p=0.30)
Phase II Study randomized, open label	capecitabine 1331 mg/m²/day (continuous)	39	objective response rate: 22%
	capecitabine 2510 mg/m²/day (intermittent)	34	25%
	capecitabine 1657 mg/m²/day/leucovorin 60 mg/day (intermittent)	35 Patients with advanced and/or metastatic colorectal carcinoma	24%

[a] 20 mg/m² leucovorin i.v. followed by 425 mg/m² i.v. bolus 5-FU on days 1 to 5, every 28 days.

Colorectal Carcinoma: Adjuvant Colon Cancer: Data from one open-label, multicenter, randomized, controlled, non-inferiority, phase III clinical trial in patients with stage III (Dukes C) colon cancer supports the use of XELODA for the adjuvant treatment of patients with stage III colon cancer (X-ACT Study: M66001). In this trial, 1987 patients were randomized to treatment with monotherapy XELODA (1250 mg/m² twice daily for 2 weeks followed by a 1-week rest period and given as 3-week cycles for 24 weeks) (N=1004) or 5 FU and leucovorin (Mayo regimen: 20 mg/m² leucovorin i.v. followed by 425 mg/m² i.v. bolus 5 FU, on days 1 to 5, every 28 days for 24 weeks) (N=983). Although this trial used bolus 5-FU in the control arm, infusional 5-FU has been shown to be superior to bolus 5-FU.

The primary efficacy endpoint was disease-free survival. The original conditional approval was based on primary analysis at a median follow-up time of 3.8 years which showed XELODA was at least equivalent to i.v. 5-FU/LV in disease-free survival (p=0.0001, non-inferiority margin 1.2) with a trend towards superiority in disease-free survival. The full approval was based on an updated analysis at a median follow-up time of 6.9 years which confirmed XELODA to be at least equivalent to 5-FU/LV in disease-free survival although there was no longer a trend toward superiority in disease-free survival (p=0.06). A summary of the results is provided in Table 4. Compared with 5-FU/LV, XELODA was associated with lower incidence of stomatitis, neutropenia and febrile neutropenia but with a considerably higher incidence of hand-and-foot syndrome and hyperbilirubinemia in the adjuvant treatment of patients with Dukes Stage C colon cancer. See Figure 1.

Figure 1: XELODA

Kaplan-Meier Estimates of Disease-Free Survival (All Randomized Population)

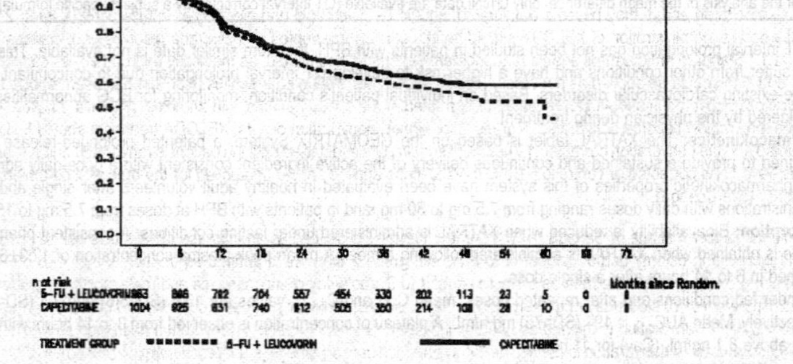

Table 4: XELODA
Efficacy of XELODA vs 5-FU/LV in Adjuvant Treatment of Stage III (Dukes Stage C) Colon Cancer

Design	Drug/Dosage	No. of Patients Enrolled Demographic Data	Results of Primary Analysis—Median Follow-Up 3.8 Years	Results of Updated Analysis—Median Follow-Up 6.9 Years
Pivotal Phase III Study (X-ACT Study) randomized, controlled, multicenter patients with stage III (Dukes' stage C) colon cancer US, Canada, Europe, Argentina, Australia, Brazil, Israel, Thailand, Uruguay	capecitabine 2500 mg/m²/day for 2 weeks with a 1 week rest period [given as 3 week cycles for a total of 8 cycles (24 weeks)] 5-FU/leucovorin (LV) Mayo regimen - 20 mg/m² leucovorin i.v. followed by 425 mg/m² i.v. bolus 5-FU on days 1 to 5, every 28 days [given as 4 week cycles for a total of 6 cycles (24 weeks)]	N=1004 Age (yrs) - Md: 62; range: 25–80 M/F: 542 (54%)/ 461(46%) ECOG Score: 0 (%) 849 (85) 1 (%) 152 (15) Node Status[a]: N1 (%) 695 (69) N2 (%) 305 (30) Other (%) 4 (0.4) N=983 Age (yrs) - Md: 63; range: 22–82 M/F: 532 (54%)/ 451 (46%) ECOG Score: 0 (%) 830 (85) 1 (%) 147 (15) Node Status[a]: N1 (%) 694 (71) N2 (%) 288 (29) Other (%) 1 (0.1)	**All Randomized Population:** Disease-Free Survival Hazard Ratio[b]=0.87 (95% C.I. 0.75–1.00); p[c]=0.053 3-year disease-free survival rate capecitabine - 64% 5-FU/LV - 61% Overall Survival Hazard Ratio[b]=0.84 (95% C.I. 0.69–1.01; p[c]=0.071) 3-year overall survival rate capecitabine - 81% 5-FU/LV - 78% **Per Protocol Population:** Disease-Free Survival Hazard Ratio[b]=0.89 (95% C.I. 0.76–1.04); p[c]=0.157 3-year overall survival rate capecitabine - 65% 5-FU/LV - 63% Overall Survival Hazard Ratio[b]=0.90 (95% C.I. 0.73–1.10); p[c]=0.298 3-year overall survival rate capecitabine – 83% 5-FU/LV – 80%	**All Randomized Population:** Disease-Free Survival Hazard Ratio[b]=0.88 (95% C.I. 0.77–1.01); p[c]=0.068 5-year disease-free survival rate capecitabine - 60.8% 5-FU/LV - 56.7% Overall Survival Hazard Ratio[b]=0.86 (95% C.I. 0.69–1.01; p[c]=0.060) 5-year overall survival rate capecitabine - 71.4% 5-FU/LV - 68.4% **Per Protocol Population:** Disease-Free Survival Hazard Ratio[b]=0.92 (95% C.I. 0.80–1.06); p[c]=0.2743 5-year disease free-survival rate capecitabine - 60.9% 5-FU/LV - 58.4% Overall Survival Hazard Ratio[b]=0.93 (95% C.I. 0.73–1.09); p[c]=0.357 5-year overall survival rate capecitabine – 72% 5-FU/LV – 70.5%

[a] N1- tumor in 1-3 regional lymph nodes; N2- tumor in ≥4 regional lymph nodes.
[b] Capecitabine versus 5-FU/LV; Non-inferiority margin of 1.20 corresponds to the retention by XELODA of approx. 75% of the 5-FU/LV effect on DFS.
[c] Wald chi square test for differences of XELODA vs 5-FU/LV.

Breast Carcinoma: XELODA has been evaluated in breast cancer clinical trials in combination with docetaxel and as monotherapy. Table 5 summarizes data from a pivotal combination trial as well as from 1 pivotal and 2 supportive monotherapy phase II clinical trials.

XELODA in Combination with Docetaxel: The dose of XELODA used in combination with docetaxel in the phase III clinical trial was based on the results of a phase I study, where a range of doses of docetaxel given every 3 weeks in combination with an intermittent regimen of XELODA were evaluated. The combination dose regimen was selected based on the tolerability profile of the 75 mg/m² every 3 weeks of docetaxel in combination with 1250 mg/m² twice daily for 14 days of XELODA administered every 3 weeks. The approved dose of 100 mg/m² of docetaxel administered every 3 weeks was the control arm of the phase III study.

As shown in Table 5, XELODA in combination with docetaxel resulted in statistically significant improvement in time to disease progression, overall survival and objective response rate compared to monotherapy with docetaxel.

Health Related Quality of Life (HRQoL) was assessed using EORTC QLQ-C30 (version 2) and Breast Cancer Module of the EORTC (BR23). HRQoL was similar in the two treatment groups. Approximately 11% of patients in the combination arm and 10% in the monotherapy arm did not complete a quality of life questionnaire at least once either at baseline or during the treatment phase.

INDICATIONS: Colorectal Cancer: Monotherapy: XELODA (capecitabine) is indicated for the adjuvant treatment of patients with stage III (Dukes' stage C) colon cancer.

XELODA is indicated for first-line treatment of patients with metastatic colorectal cancer.

Combination Therapy: XELODA in combination with oxaliplatin is indicated for the treatment of metastatic colorectal cancer following failure of irinotecan-containing combination chemotherapy. In second-line metastatic disease, subgroup analyses for PFS and OS for age suggest that XELODA in combination with oxaliplatin may be less effective in patients over the age of 65. Clinical studies suggest an increase in the incidence of adverse events. See Warnings.

Breast Cancer: Combination Therapy: XELODA in combination with docetaxel is indicated for the treatment of patients with advanced or metastatic breast cancer after failure of prior anthracycline-containing chemotherapy.

Monotherapy: XELODA is also indicated for the treatment of advanced or metastatic breast cancer after failure of standard therapy including a taxane, unless therapy with a taxane is clinically contraindicated.

CONTRAINDICATIONS: XELODA (capecitabine) is contraindicated in patients who have a known hypersensitivity to capecitabine or to any of its components, or to 5-fluorouracil and in patients with severe renal impairment (calculated creatinine clearance below 30 mL/min, or 0.5 mL/s). As with other fluoropyrimidines, XELODA is contraindicated in patients with known dihydropyrimidine dehydrogenase (DPD) deficiency. If contraindications exist to any of the agents in a combination regimen, that agent should not be used.

WARNINGS: General: Patients receiving therapy with XELODA (capecitabine) should be monitored by a physician experienced in the use of cancer chemotherapeutic agents. Most adverse reactions are reversible and do not require discontinuation, although doses may need to be withheld or reduced (see Dosage).

Diarrhea: XELODA very frequently induces diarrhea, which can sometimes be severe. Patients with severe diarrhea should be carefully monitored and, if they become dehydrated, should be given fluid and electrolyte replacement. If grade 2 (or higher) diarrhea occurs, administration of XELODA should be immediately interrupted until diarrhea resolves or decreases in intensity to grade 1.* Standard antidiarrheal agents (e.g. loperamide) should be initiated, as medically appropriate, as early as possible. Dose reduction should be applied as necessary (see Dosage). Necrotizing enterocolitis (typhlitis) has been reported.

Dehydration: Dehydration should be prevented or corrected at the onset. Patients with anorexia, asthenia, nausea, vomiting or diarrhea may rapidly become dehydrated. If grade 2 (or higher) dehydration occurs, XELODA treatment should be immediately interrupted and the dehydration corrected.† Treatment should not be restarted until the patient is rehydrated and any precipitating causes have been corrected or controlled. Dose modifications applied should be applied for the precipitating adverse event as necessary (see Dosage).

* National Cancer Institute of Canada (NCIC) grade 1 diarrhea is defined as an increase of <4 stools per day over baseline, mild increase in ostomy output compared to baseline, grade 2 diarrhea is defined as an increase of 4 to 6 stools/day or nocturnal stools, grade 3 diarrhea as an increase of 7 to 9 stools/day or incontinence and malabsorption, grade 4 diarrhea as an increase of 10 stools/day or grossly bloody diarrhea or the need for parenteral support, and grade 5 diarrhea as death.

† NCIC grade 2 dehydration is defined as IV fluids indicated <24 hours, grade 3 dehydration is defined as IV fluids indicated ≥24 hours, grade 4 dehydration is defined as life-threatening consequences (e.g. hemodynamic collapse), and grade 5 dehydration as death.

Table 5: XELODA
Clinical Studies in Breast Carcinoma

Design/Diagnosis	Drug/Dosage	No. Women Enrolled	Results
Pivotal Study—Combination Therapy			
-open label, randomized, parallel group -females with advanced and/or metastatic breast cancer resistant to or recurring during or after anthracycline-containing therapy or relapsing during or recurring within 2 years of completing anthracycline-containing adjuvant therapy	-capecitabine 2500 mg/m²/day for 2 weeks with a 1 week rest period in combination with docetaxel 75 mg/m² every 3 weeks	255	**Response Rate** Combination therapy: 41.6% Docetaxel monotherapy: 29.7% (p=0.0058) **Time to Disease Progression** Combination therapy: 186 days Docetaxel monotherapy: 128 days (p=0.0001) Hazard Ratio: 0.643 **Overall Survival** Combination therapy: 442 days Docetaxel monotherapy: 352 days (p=0.0126) Hazard Ratio: 0.775
	-docetaxel 100 mg/m² every 3 weeks	256	
Pivotal Study—Monotherapy			
-open label -females with advanced or metastatic breast cancer refractory to previous paclitaxel therapy: (77% resistant, 23% failed paclitaxel; 41% resistant, 26% failed anthracycline therapy; 82% prior 5-FU exposure).	-capecitabine 2510 mg/m²/day for 2 weeks with a 1-week rest period (given as 3-week cycles)	162 (135 measurable disease)	-overall response rate (ORR) intent-to-treat (n=135): 20% (95% CI:13.6-27.8); 3 complete responses -ORR (standard population, n=117): 23% (min. 6 weeks therapy) -median duration of response: 241 days -median time to progression: 93 days -median survival: 384 days -clinical benefit response: positive 29 pts. (20%); stable 45 pts. (31%). In 51 pts. with baseline pain ≥20 mm (visual analogue scale), 24 pts. (47%) positive response in pain intensity (≥50% decrease)
Supportive Studies—Monotherapy			
-open label, randomized, parallel group -females ≥55 with advanced or metastatic breast cancer without previous chemotherapy (other than adjuvant treatment)	-capecitabine 2510 mg/m²/day for 2 weeks with a 1-week rest period (given as 3-week cycles) -Cytoxan, methotrexate, 5FU (CMF) 600/40/600 mg/m² iv q3 weeks.	95	-capecitabine response rate: 25% (95%CI: 14%–37%) -CMF response rate: 16% (95% CI: 5%–33%) -median time to disease progression: capecitabine-132 days; CMF-94 days
-open-label, randomized parallel group -females with disease progression within 12 months of previous anthracycline treatment	-capecitabine 1331 mg/m²/day (continuous) for 6 weeks -capecitabine 2510 mg/m²/day for 2 weeks with a 1-week rest period (given as 3-week cycles) (intermittent) -paclitaxel 175 mg/m²/q 3 weeks	44	-capecitabine response rate (intermittent arm): 36% (95%CI: 17–59%); 3 complete responses -paclitaxel response rate: 21% (95% CI: 6–46%). -median time to disease progression: capecitabine 92 days; paclitaxel 95 days.

Coagulopathy: Altered coagulation parameters and/or bleeding have been reported in patients taking XELODA concomitantly with coumarin-derived anticoagulants such as warfarin. These events occurred within several days and up to several months after initiating XELODA therapy, and, in a few cases, within 1 month after stopping XELODA. These events occurred in patients with and without liver metastases. In a drug interaction study with single-dose warfarin administration, there was a significant increase in the mean AUC (+57%) of S-warfarin. These results suggest an interaction, probably due to an inhibition of the cytochrome P450 2C9 isoenzyme system by capecitabine. Patients taking coumarin-derivative anticoagulants concomitantly with XELODA should be monitored regularly for alterations in their coagulation parameters (PT or INR) and the anticoagulant dose adjusted accordingly (see Precautions, Coumarin Anticoagulants).

Geriatrics: XELODA in Combination with Docetaxel: An analysis of safety data in patients equal to or greater than 60 years of age showed an increase in the incidence of treatment-related grade 3 and 4 adverse events, treatment-related serious adverse events and early withdrawals from treatment due to adverse events compared to patients less than 60 years of age. The incidence of grade 3 or 4 stomatitis was greater in the 60 to 70 year old patient group (30%) than the general population (13%) (see Dosage).

XELODA in Combination with Oxaliplatin: In the second-line setting, subgroup analyses for PFS (EP population) and OS (ITT population) for age suggest that XELOX may be less effective than FOLFOX-4 in patients ≥65 years of age (HR 1.32, 95% CI, 0.98-1.78 and HR 1.34, 95% CI, 1.00-1.80, respectively). Physicians are advised to assess risks and benefits in these patients.

In the second-line setting, an analysis of safety data in patients equal to or greater than 65 years of age showed an increase in the incidence of treatment related serious adverse events, treatment related grade 3 and 4 adverse events, gastrointestinal grade 3/4 events (particularly diarrhea), and patients who discontinued trial treatment. In addition, deaths up to 60 days after treatment start and deaths up to 28 days after last dose were slightly higher in older patients. Careful monitoring of elderly patients is advisable.

XELODA Monotherapy: Patients ≥80 years old may experience a greater incidence of gastrointestinal grade 3/4 events.

Hepatic Insufficiency: Patients with hepatic impairment should be carefully monitored when capecitabine is administered. However, the effect of hepatic impairment not due to liver metastases or of severe hepatic impairment on the disposition of XELODA is not known.

Renal Insufficiency: In patients with moderate renal impairment (calculated creatinine clearance 30-50 mL/min [Cockroft and Gault])* at baseline, a dose reduction to 75% of the XELODA starting dose when used as monotherapy or in combination with docetaxel is recommended based upon pharmacokinetic and safety data. Careful monitoring and prompt treatment interruption is recommended if the patient develops a grade 2, 3, or 4 adverse event, with subsequent dose adjustment as outlined in Table 15 in the Dosage section.

Physicians should exercise caution when XELODA is administered to patients with impaired renal function. As seen with 5-FU, the incidence of treatment-related grade 3 or 4 adverse events was higher in patients with moderate renal impairment (calculated creatinine clearance 30 to 50 mL/min).

*Cockroft-Gault Formula for males:

Creatinine clearance (mL/min)=	$\frac{(140-\text{age})\times\text{weight (kg)}}{72\times\text{serum creatinine (mg/dL)}}$
Cockroft-Gault Formula for females:	Creatinine clearance (mL/min)=0.85×male value
Creatinine clearance in SI units (mL/s)=0.01667×value obtained from above formula in mL/min.	

Lactation: In a study of single oral administration of capecitabine in lactating mice, it was found that a significant amount of the capecitabine metabolites is transferred to the milk. Because of the potential for serious adverse reactions in nursing infants, it is recommended that nursing be discontinued when receiving XELODA therapy.

Children: The safety and effectiveness of XELODA in persons <18 years of age have not been established.

Pregnancy: There are no adequate and well-controlled studies in pregnant women using XELODA. If the drug is used during pregnancy, or if the patient becomes pregnant while receiving this drug, the patient should be apprised of the potential hazard to the fetus. Women of childbearing potential should be advised to avoid becoming pregnant while receiving treatment with XELODA. XELODA was found to be teratogenic and embryolethal in mice and embryolethal in monkeys.

Carcinogenesis and Mutagenesis: Although there was no evidence for oncogenic potential of capecitabine in a two-year carcinogenicity study in mice, capecitabine was clastogenic in vitro in human lymphocytes (similar to other nucleoside analogues such as 5-FU). There was also a positive trend in the in vivo mouse micronucleus assay. Women of childbearing potential should be advised to avoid becoming pregnant while receiving treatment with XELODA (see Warnings) and be provided with appropriate counselling if not currently using contraceptives. Males are advised not to father a child during treatment.

PRECAUTIONS: Hand-and-Foot Syndrome: Hand-and-foot syndrome (palmar-plantar erythrodysesthesia or chemotherapy induced acral erythema) is a cutaneous toxicity which can occur in patients receiving XELODA either as monotherapy or in combination therapy. For patients receiving XELODA monotherapy in the metastatic setting, median time to onset was 79 days (range from 11 to 360 days) with a severity range of grades 1 to 3‡. If grade 2 or 3 hand-and-foot syndrome occurs, administration of capecitabine should be interrupted until the event resolves or decreases in intensity to grade 1. Following grade 3 hand-and-foot syndrome, subsequent doses of XELODA should be decreased (see Dosage). For XELODA in combination with docetaxel, hand-and-foot syndrome was more common in patients in the combination therapy arm than in the monotherapy arm (63% vs 8%).

Cardiac: The spectrum of cardiotoxicity observed with XELODA is similar to that of other fluorinated pyrimidines. This includes myocardial infarction, angina, dysrhythmias, cardiac arrest, cardiac failure, and electrocardiograph changes. These adverse events may be more common in patients with a prior history of coronary artery disease. A thorough QT interval prolongation assessment study of XELODA has never been conducted.

Hematologic: In 251 patients with metastatic breast cancer who received XELODA in combination with docetaxel, 68% had grade 3 or 4 neutropenia, 2.8% had grade 3 or 4 thrombocytopenia and 9.6% had grade 3 or 4 anemia.

In 875 patients with either metastatic breast or colorectal cancer who received XELODA monotherapy, 3.2%, 1.7%, and 2.4% of patients had grade 3/4 neutropenia, thrombocytopenia and decreases in hemoglobin, respectively.

Hyperbilirubinemia: In 251 patients with metastatic breast cancer who received a combination of XELODA and docetaxel, grade 3 and 4 hyperbilirubinemia occurred in 6.8% (n=17) and 2% (n=5), respectively.

In 875 patients with either metastatic breast or colorectal cancer treated with XELODA monotherapy, grade 3 hyperbilirubinemia occurred in 133 (15.2%) and grade 4 hyperbilirubinemia occurred in 34 (3.9%) patients with either metastatic breast or colorectal cancer. If drug-related grade 2, 3 or 4§ elevations in bilirubin occur, administration of XELODA should be immediately interrupted until the hyperbilirubinemia resolves or decreases in intensity to grade 1. Following grade 3 or 4 hyperbilirubinemia, subsequent doses of XELODA should be decreased (see Dosage).

Information to Be Provided to the Patient: Patients and patients' caregivers should be informed of the expected adverse effects of XELODA, particularly of diarrhea, nausea, vomiting, and hand-and-foot syndrome and stomatitis. The frequent oral administration of XELODA allows patient specific dose adaptations during therapy (see Dosage). Patients should be taught to recognize and report the common grade 2 toxicities associated with XELODA treatment (see Information for the Patient).

If XELODA is prescribed in combination with docetaxel, patients and patients' caregivers should be informed of the expected adverse effects of the combination of XELODA and docetaxel (see Table 10).

Diarrhea: Patients experiencing grade 2 diarrhea (an increase of 4 to 6 stools/day or nocturnal stools) or greater should be instructed to stop taking XELODA immediately. Standard antidiarrheal agents (e.g., loperamide) should be prescribed for symptom control (see Dosage).

Nausea: Patients experiencing grade 2 nausea (food intake significantly decreased but able to eat intermittently) or greater should be instructed to stop taking XELODA immediately. Standard anti-nausea agents should be prescribed for symptom control (see Dosage).

Vomiting: Patients experiencing grade 2 vomiting (2 to 5 episodes in a 24-hour period) or greater should be instructed to stop taking XELODA immediately. Standard antiemetic agents should be prescribed for symptom control (see Dosage).

Hand-and-Foot Syndrome: Patients experiencing grade 2 hand-and-foot syndrome (painful erythema and swelling of the hands and/or feet and/or discomfort affecting the patients' activities of daily living) or greater should be instructed to stop taking XELODA immediately.

Stomatitis: Patients experiencing grade 2 stomatitis or greater (painful erythema, edema or ulcers, but are able to eat) should be instructed to stop taking XELODA immediately. Symptomatic treatment should be prescribed (see Dosage).

Drug-Food Interactions: The effect of food on the pharmacokinetics of capecitabine was investigated in 11 cancer patients. The rate and extent of absorption of capecitabine is decreased when administered with food. The effect on $AUC_{0-\infty}$ of the 3 main metabolites in plasma (5'DFUR, 5-FU, FBAL) is minor. In all clinical trials, patients were instructed to take XELODA within 30 minutes after a meal. Therefore, since current safety and efficacy data are based upon administration with food, it is recommended that XELODA be administered with food.

Drug Interactions: Phenytoin and Fosphenytoin: Increased phenytoin plasma concentrations have been reported during concomitant use of XELODA with phenytoin, suggesting a potential interaction. Formal drug-drug interaction studies with phenytoin have not been conducted, but the mechanism of interaction is presumed to be inhibition of the CYP 2C9 isoenzyme system by capecitabine (see Cytochrome P450 2C9 Substrates). Patients taking phenytoin or fosphenytoin concomitantly with XELODA should be regularly monitored for increased phenytoin plasma concentrations and associated clinical symptoms.

Coumarin Anticoagulants: Altered coagulation parameters and/or bleeding have been reported in patients taking XELODA concomitantly with coumarin-derivative anticoagulants such as warfarin and phenprocoumon. These events occurred within several days and up to several months after initiating XELODA therapy and, in a few cases, within 1 month after stopping XELODA. In a clinical interaction study, after a single 20 mg dose of warfarin, XELODA treatment increased the AUC of S-warfarin by 57% with a 91% increase in INR value. Patients taking coumarin-derivative anticoagulants concomitantly with XELODA should be monitored regularly for alterations in their coagulation parameters (PT or INR) and the anticoagulant dose adjusted accordingly.

Cytochrome P450 2C9 Substrates: No formal drug-drug interaction studies with capecitabine and other drugs known to be metabolized by the cytochrome P450 2C9 isoenzyme have been conducted. Care should be exercised when XELODA is coadministered with these drugs.

Antacid: The effect of an aluminum hydroxide and magnesium hydroxide-containing antacid (Maalox) on the pharmacokinetics of capecitabine was investigated in 12 cancer patients. There was a small increase in plasma concentrations of capecitabine and 1 metabolite (5'DFCR); there was no effect on the 3 major metabolites (5'DFUR, 5-FU and FBAL).

Leucovorin: A phase I study evaluating the effect of leucovorin on the pharmacokinetics of capecitabine was conducted in 22 cancer patients. Leucovorin has no effect on the pharmacokinetics of capecitabine and its metabolites; however, the toxicity of capecitabine may be enhanced by leucovorin.

Oxaliplatin: No clinically significant differences in exposure to capecitabine or its metabolites, free platinum or total platinum occurred when capecitabine and oxaliplatin were administered in combination.

‡ Grade 1 hand-and-foot syndrome is defined by numbness, dysesthesia/paresthesia, tingling, or erythema of the hands and/or feet and/or discomfort which does not disrupt normal activities. Grade 2 hand-and-foot syndrome is defined as painful erythema and swelling of the hands and/or feet that results in discomfort affecting the patient's activities of daily living and grade 3 hand-and-foot syndrome is defined as moist desquamation, ulceration, blistering or severe pain of the hands and/or feet that results in severe discomfort that causes the patient to be unable to work or perform activities of daily living.

§ NCIC grade 2 hyperbilirubinemia is defined as 1.5×normal, grade 3 hyperbilirubinemia as 1.5 to 3×normal and grade 4 hyperbilirubinemia as >3×normal.

Pregnancy: Women of childbearing potential should be advised to avoid becoming pregnant while receiving treatment with XELODA (see Warnings) and be provided with appropriate counselling if not currently using contraceptives.

Geriatrics: See Warnings and Dosage.

ADVERSE EFFECTS: Adverse drug reactions (ADRs) considered by the investigator to be possibly, probably, or remotely related to the administration of XELODA have been obtained from clinical studies conducted with XELODA monotherapy (in adjuvant therapy of colon cancer, in metastatic colorectal cancer and metastatic breast cancer), and clinical studies conducted with XELODA in combination with docetaxel (metastatic breast cancer) or in combination with oxaliplatin (metastatic colorectal cancer).

Metastatic Colorectal Cancer, Combination Therapy: XELODA in Combination with Oxaliplatin: Table 6 shows the most frequent ADRs (≥5%) reported in patients with metastatic colorectal cancer who received second-line (Study NO16967) treatment with XELODA in combination with oxaliplatin (XELOX). The intensity of adverse events was graded according to the toxicity categories of the NCI CTCAE Grading System Version 3.0.

Table 6: XELODA

Summary of ADRs in ≥5% of Patients who Received Second-Line Treatment with XELODA and Oxaliplatin for Metastatic Colorectal Cancer (Study NO16967)

	XELOX[a] (N=311)		**FOLFOX-4[b] (N=308)**	
Body System Adverse Drug Reaction	**All %**	**Grade 3/4 %**	**All %**	**Grade 3/4 %**
Gastrointestinal Disorders				
Nausea	60	4	56	3
Diarrhea	57	20	49	5
Vomiting	43	3	34	3
Stomatitis	14	<1	30	1
Abdominal pain	30	5	24	5
Constipation	16	2	26	3
Dyspepsia	11	<1	7	—
Abdominal pain upper	6	<1	6	<1
Nervous System Disorders				
Paraesthesia	33	4	32	3
Neuropathy peripheral	13	<1	10	—
Peripheral sensory neuropathy	13	<1	16	2
Dysgeusia	7	<1	11	—
Neuropathy	12	<1	9	<1
Dysaesthesia	10	<1	11	2
Dizziness	10	<1	9	—
Headache	10	<1	11	<1
Lethargy	6	2	6	<1
Hypoaesthesia	7	<1	6	<1
General Disorders and Administration Site Conditions				
Fatigue	41	7	42	9
Asthenia	19	3	18	5
Oedema peripheral	5	<1	9	<1
Pyrexia	21	—	23	<1
Temperature intolerance	5	—	6	—
Chills	3	—	6	—
Blood and Lymphatic System Disorders				
Neutropenia	18	5	48	35
Thrombocytopenia	13	3	17	2
Anaemia	6	1	8	2
Metabolism and Nutrition Disorders				
Anorexia	32	4	27	2
Hypokalemia	8	4	5	3
Dehydration	6	3	5	2
Skin and Subcutaneous Tissue Disorders				
Palmar-plantar erythrodysaesthesia syndrome	23	4	6	<1
Rash	10	—	7	<1
Alopecia	1	—	6	—

(cont'd)

Table 6: XELODA *(cont'd)*

Summary of ADRs in ≥5% of Patients who Received Second-Line Treatment with XELODA and Oxaliplatin for Metastatic Colorectal Cancer (Study NO16967)

	XELOX[a] (N=311)		FOLFOX-4[b] (N=308)	
Body System Adverse Drug Reaction	**All %**	**Grade 3/4 %**	**All %**	**Grade 3/4 %**
Respiratory, Thoracic and Mediastinal Disorders				
Cough	7	<1	15	
Dysaesthesia pharynx	11	2	4	<1
Epistaxis	3	—	7	<1
Dyspnea	9	1	10	2
Pharyngolaryngeal pain	3	—	5	—
Musculoskeletal and Connective Tissue Disorders				
Pain in extremity	6	<1	5	<1
Pain in jaw	5	<1	4	—
Pain in back	10	2	14	3
Myalgia	4	—	7	<1
Investigations				
Weight decreased	6	<1	6	<1
Psychiatric Disorders				
Insomnia	7	<1	12	—
Infections and Infestations				
Nasopharyngitis	4	—	6	<1
Vascular Disorders				
Flushing	3	—	6	
Immune System Disorders				
Hypersensitivity	2	<1	6	4

[a] XELOX: XELODA (1000 ^{2} twice daily for 2 weeks followed by a 7-day rest period) and oxaliplatin (130 mg/m² as a 2-hour infusion on day 1 every three weeks).

[b] FOLFOX-4: leucovorin (200 mg/m² as a 2-hour infusion on days 1 and 2 every two weeks), 5-FU (400 mg/m² as a bolus injection, 600 mg/m² as a 22-hour infusion on days 1 and 2 every two weeks), and oxaliplatin (85 mg/m² as a 2-hour infusion on day 1 every two weeks).

Rare or uncommon clinically relevant adverse reactions reported in <5% of metastatic colorectal cancer patients treated with XELODA in combination with oxaliplatin (second-line), that were considered at least remotely related to treatment are shown below. Occurrences of each grade 3 and 4 adverse event are provided in parentheses.

Gastrointestinal: intestinal obstruction (2%).
Nervous: peripheral motor neuropathy (<1%), encephalopathy (<1%).
Blood and Lymphatic: febrile neutropenia (<1%), pancytopenia (<1%).
Respiratory: pulmonary embolism (<1%), laryngospasm (<1%), bronchospasm (<1%).
Vascular: thrombosis (<1%), deep vein thrombosis (<1%), embolism (<1%).
Psychiatric: anxiety (<1%).
Renal and Urinary: renal failure acute (<1%).
Hepatobiliary: hepatic failure (<1%).
Cardiac: myocardial infarction (<1%).

Colorectal Cancer, Monotherapy: Adjuvant Colon Cancer: Safety data of XELODA monotherapy were reported from one phase III trial in adjuvant colon cancer (995 patients treated with XELODA and 974 treated with i.v. 5-FU/LV). The most frequently reported treatment related adverse events (≥10%) for XELODA in this trial were gastrointestinal disorders, especially diarrhea, stomatitis, nausea, vomiting, hand-foot syndrome, fatigue and lethargy. The most frequent treatment-related undesirable effects (≥5%) reported in this trial are presented in Table 7.

Table 7: XELODA

Summary of ADRs Reported in ≥5% of Patients with Colon Cancer Treated with XELODA Monotherapy or IV 5-FU/LV in the Adjuvant Setting

Adverse Event	XELODA 1250 mg/m²/bid (n=995)		IV 5-FU/LV[a] (n=974)	
Body System/ Adverse Event	**Total %**	**Grade 3/4 %**	**Total %**	**Grade 3/4 %**
Gastrointestinal				
Diarrhea	46	11	64	13
Stomatitis	22	2	60	14
Nausea	33	2	47	2
Vomiting	14	2	20	1
Abdominal pain	10	2	13	1
Constipation	6	—	7	<1
Abdominal pain upper	6	<1	5	<1
Dyspepsia	5	<1	4	—
Skin and Subcutaneous				
Hand-foot syndrome	60	17	9	
Alopecia	6	—	22	<1
Rash	6	—	8	—
Erythema	6	1	5	<1
General Disorders				
Fatigue	15	<1	15	1
Lethargy	10	<1	9	<1
Asthenia	9	<1	9	1
Pyrexia	4	<1	6	<1
Nervous System Disorders				
Dysgeusia	6	—	9	—
Dizziness	5	<1	4	—
Metabolism and Nutrition Disorders				
Anorexia	9	<1	10	<1
Eye				
Conjunctivitis	5	<1	5	<1
Blood and Lymphatic System				
Neutropenia	2	<1	8	5

[a] Mayo Clinic regimen.

Table 8 displays laboratory abnormalities observed in 995 patients, regardless of relationship to treatment, with XELODA in the adjuvant treatment of colon cancer.

Table 8: XELODA

Laboratory Abnormalities[a]: XELODA Monotherapy in Adjuvant Colon Cancer

	XELODA 1250 mg/m² Twice Daily Intermittent N=995			
Parameter	**Patients with Grade 3/4 Abnormality (%)**	**Patients with Worsening From Baseline of Any Grade (%)**	**Patients with Worsening From Baseline by 1 or 2 Grades (%)**	**Patients with Worsening From Baseline by 3 or 4 Grades (%)**
Increased ALAT	1.6	27.2	25.9	1.3
Increased ASAT	0.7	28.7	28	0.7
Increased alkaline phosphatase	0.1	26.0	25.9	0.1
Increased calcium	1.1	5.2	4.8	0.4
Decreased calcium	2.3	13.2	12.4	0.8
Decreased granulocytes	0.3	2.0	1.7	0.3
Decreased hemoglobin	1.1	27.8	27.7	0.1
Decreased lymphocytes	13	51.3	49.2	2.1
Decreased neutrophils	2.2	30.3	28.4	1.9
Decreased neutrophils/granulocytes	2.4	31.0	28.9	2.1
Decreased platelets	1.0	17.3	16.8	0.5
Decreased potassium	0.3	19.9	19.7	0.2
Increased serum creatinine	0.1	13.8	13.8	0
Decreased sodium	0.4	17.5	17.1	0.4
Increased bilirubin	20	50.3	31.7	18.6

[a] Laboratory abnormalities were graded according to the categories of the NCIC CTC Grading System.

The incidence of grade 3/4 white blood cell abnormalities was 1.3% in the XELODA arm and 4.9% in the I.V. 5-FU/LV arm.

Metastatic Colorectal Cancer: Presented in Table 9 are the most frequent adverse reactions (≥5%) with intensity reported as related (remotely, possibly or probably) to the administration of XELODA or 5-FU/leucovorin (LV). Rates are rounded to the nearest whole number. The data shown are from pooled phase III metastatic colorectal cancer trials, in which a total of 605 patients with metastatic colorectal cancer were treated with 2500 mg/m²/day of XELODA administered for 2 weeks followed by a 1-week rest period and 604 patients were administered 5-FU and leucovorin in the Mayo regimen (20 mg/m² leucovorin i.v. followed by 425 mg/m² i.v. bolus 5-FU, on days 1 to 5, every 28 days. The adverse event profile of 5-FU/LV in this study was consistent with the published literature. In the pooled colorectal database the median duration of treatment was 139 days for capecitabine treated patients and 140 days for 5-FU/LV treated patients. A total of 78 (13%) and 63 (11%) capecitabine and 5-FU/LV-treated patients, respectively, discontinued treatment because of adverse event/intercurrent illness.

Table 9: XELODA

Pooled Phase III Metastatic Colorectal Trials of XELODA Monotherapy vs 5-FU/LV: Percent Incidence of Adverse Reactions in ≥5% of Patients

Adverse Event	XELODA (n=596)			5-FU/LV (n=593)		
	NCIC Grade					
Body System/ Adverse Event	**1 to 4**	**3**	**4**	**1 to 4**	**3**	**4**
Gastrointestinal						
Diarrhea all	49	12	2	59	10	2
Nausea	38	3	—	47	2	—
Vomiting	23	3	—	27	3	—
Stomatitis all	25	2	—	62	14	1
Abdominal pain	17	4	—	16	2	—
Gastrointestinal motility disorder	10	—	—	11	1	—
Constipation	7	—	—	8	—	—
Oral discomfort	9	—	—	9	—	—
Skin and Subcutaneous						
Hand-and-foot syndrome	53	17	—	6	1	—
Dermatitis	24	1	—	23	1	—
Skin discoloration	7	—	—	5	—	—
Alopecia	6	—	—	21	—	—
General						
Fatigue/weakness	32	3	—	38	3	—
Pyrexia	9	—	—	12	1	—
Neurological						
Paresthesia	9	—	—	5	—	—
Sensory disturbance	6	—	—	11	—	—
Dizziness[a]	5	—	—	5	—	—
Metabolism						
Appetite decreased	20	1	—	25	2	—
Dehydration	4	2	—	6	2	—
Eye						
Eye irritation	11	—	—	8	—	—
Respiratory						
Dyspnea	6	—	—	4	—	—
Cardiac						
Edema	5	—	—	3	—	—
Blood and Lymphatic						
Neutropenia	21	0.7	2	55	8	13
Thrombocytopenia	20	0.5	0.5	28	0.2	0.2
Anemia	80	2	0.2	82	1	0.3
Lymphopenia	93	29	8	92	30	8
Hepatobiliary						
Hyperbilirubinemia	49	18	5	25	3	3

[a] Excluding vertigo.
Legend: —Not observed or applicable.

In the pooled phase III metastatic colorectal studies, dose reductions occurred in 34% of patients treated with capecitabine and in 42% with 5-FU. Dose reductions also occurred later with capecitabine than 5-FU/LV (median time to dose reduction was 76 and 36 days, respectively).

The hospitalization rate for the treatment-related adverse events was 11.6% for capecitabine-treated patients and 18.0% for 5-FU/LV-treated patients. The predominant treatment-related adverse events leading to hospitalization in capecitabine and 5-FU/LV-treated patients, respectively, were diarrhea (4.2% vs 3.7%), dehydration (2.2% vs 1.5%), and stomatitis (0.2% vs 3.7%).

Breast Cancer, Combination with Docetaxel: The following data are shown for the combination study with XELODA and docetaxel in patients with locally advanced and/or metastatic breast cancer in Table 10 and Table 11. In the XELODA-docetaxel combination arm, the treatment was XELODA administered orally 1250 mg/m² twice daily as intermittent therapy (2 weeks of treatment followed by 1 week without treatment) for at least 6 weeks and docetaxel administered as a 1-hour i.v. infusion at a dose of 75 mg/m² on the first day of each 3-week cycle for at least 6 weeks. In the monotherapy arm, docetaxel was administered as a 1-hour i.v. infusion at a dose of 100 mg/m² on the first day of each 3-week cycle for at least 6 weeks. The mean duration of treatment was 129 days in the combination arm and 98 days in the monotherapy arm. A total of 66 patients (26%) in the combination arm and 49 (19%) in the monotherapy arm withdrew from the study because of adverse events. The percentage of patients requiring dose reductions due to adverse events were 65% in the combination arm and 36% in the monotherapy arm. The hospitalization rate for treatment-related adverse events was 28.7% in the combination arm and 26.3% in the monotherapy arm.

Table 10: XELODA

Percent Incidence of Adverse Reactions in ≥5% of Patients Participating in the Combination Study of XELODA and Docetaxel in Metastatic Breast Cancer

Adverse Event	XELODA 1250 mg/m²/b.i.d. (Intermittent Regimen) with Docetaxel 75 mg/m²/3 Weeks (n=251)			Docetaxel 100 mg/m²/3 Weeks (n=255)		
	NCIC Grade					
Body System/ Adverse Event	**Total %**	**Grade 3 %**	**Grade 4 %**	**Total %**	**Grade 3 %**	**Grade 4 %**
Gastrointestinal						
Stomatitis	67	17.1	0.4	43	4.7	—
Diarrhea	64	13.5	0.4	45	5.4	0.4
Nausea	43	6.4	—	35	2.0	—
Vomiting	33	3.6	0.8	22	0.8	—
Constipation	14	1.2	—	12	—	—
Abdominal pain	14	2.0	—	9	0.8	—
Dyspepsia	12	—	—	5	0.4	—
Abdominal pain upper	9	—	—	6	—	—
Dry mouth	5	0.4	—	4	—	—
Skin and Subcutaneous						
Hand-and-foot syndrome	63	24.3	—	8	1.2	—
Alopecia	41	6.0	—	42	6.7	—
Nail disorder	14	2.0	—	15	—	—
Dermatitis	8	—	—	9	0.8	—
Rash erythematous	8	0.4	—	4	—	—
Nail discoloration	6	—	—	4	0.4	—
Onycholysis	5	1.2	—	5	0.8	—
Pruritus	2	—	—	5	—	—
General						
Pyrexia	21	0.8	—	29	0.4	—
Asthenia	23	3.2	0.4	22	5.5	—
Fatigue	21	4.4	—	25	5.1	—
Weakness	13	1.2	—	9	2.0	—
Pain in limb	9	0.4	—	8	0.4	—
Lethargy	6	—	—	5	1.2	—
Pain	6	—	—	2	—	—
Neurological						
Taste disturbance	15	0.4	—	14	0.4	—
Headache	7	0.4	—	8	—	—
Paresthesia	11	0.4	—	15	0.8	—
Dizziness[a]	9	—	—	6	0.4	—
Insomnia	4	—	—	5	0.4	—
Peripheral neuropathy	5	—	—	10	0.8	—
Hypoesthesia	4	—	—	7	0.4	—
Metabolism						
Anorexia	12	0.8	—	10	0.8	—
Appetite decreased	10	—	—	4	—	—
Dehydration	8	2.0	—	5	0.4	0.4

(cont'd)

Table 10: XELODA *(cont'd)*

Percent Incidence of Adverse Reactions in ≥5% of Patients Participating in the Combination Study of XELODA and Docetaxel in Metastatic Breast Cancer

Adverse Event	XELODA 1250 mg/m²/b.i.d. (Intermittent Regimen) with Docetaxel 75 mg/m²/3 Weeks (n=251)			Docetaxel 100 mg/m²/3 Weeks (n=255)		
	NCIC Grade					
Body System/ Adverse Event	**Total %**	**Grade 3 %**	**Grade 4 %**	**Total %**	**Grade 3 %**	**Grade 4 %**
Eye						
Lacrimation increased	12	—	—	5	—	—
Musculoskeletal						
Arthralgia	11	1.2	—	18	2.4	—
Myalgia	14	1.6	—	24	2.0	—
Back pain	7	0.8	—	6	0.8	—
Cardiac						
Edema lower limb	14	0.8	—	12	1.2	—
Edema NOS	4	—	—	5	—	0.8
Edema peripheral	4	—	—	5	0.4	—
Hematologic						
Neutropenia	17	4.8	10.8	16	2.7	11.8
Neutropenic fever	16	2.8	13.1	21	4.7	16.1
Anemia	13	2.8	0.8	11	3.9	
Respiratory						
Dyspnea	7	0.8	—	9	0.4	—
Cough	6	0.4	—	9	—	—
Sore throat	11	1.6	—	7	0.4	—
Epistaxis	5	0.4	—	5	—	—
Infections and Infestations						
Oral candidiasis	6	0.4	—	7	0.4	—

[a] Excluding vertigo.
Legend: —Not observed or applicable.

Shown below by body system are the adverse events in <5% of patients in the overall clinical trial safety database of 251 patients reported as related to the administration of capecitabine in combination with docetaxel and that were clinically at least remotely relevant. In parentheses is the incidence of grade 3 and 4 occurrences of each adverse event.

Gastrointestinal: hemorrhoids (0.39), ileus (0.39), necrotizing enterocolitis (0.39), esophageal ulcer (0.39), hemorrhagic diarrhea (0.80).
General: rigors (0.39), injection site infection (0.39), neuralgia (0.39).
Neurological: ataxia (0.39), syncope (1.20), taste loss (0.80), polyneuropathy (0.39), migraine (0.39).
Cardiac: supraventricular tachycardia (0.39).
Infection: neutropenic sepsis (2.39), lower respiratory tract infection NOS (0.39), pharyngitis (0.39), otitis media (0.39), sepsis (0.39), bronchopneumonia (0.39).
Blood and Lymphatic: agranulocytosis (0.39), prothrombin decreased (0.39).
Vascular: hypotension (1.20), venous phlebitis and thrombophlebitis (0.39), blood pressure increase (0.39), postural hypotension (0.80).
Renal: renal failure (0.39).
Hepatobiliary: jaundice (0.39), abnormal liver function tests (0.39), hepatic failure (0.39), hepatic coma (0.39), hepatotoxicity (0.39).
Immune System: hypersensitivity (1.20).

Breast Cancer, XELODA Monotherapy: The following data (see Table 11) are shown for the study in stage IV breast cancer patients who received a dose of 2500 mg/m² administered daily for 2 weeks followed by a 1-week rest period. The mean duration of treatment was 121 days. A total of 71 patients (13%) discontinued treatment because of adverse events/intercurrent illness.

Table 11: XELODA

XELODA Monotherapy: Percent Incidence of Adverse Reactions in ≥5% of Patients Participating in the Phase II Trial in Stage IV Breast Cancer

Body System/ Adverse Event	NCIC Grade		
	1 to 4	**3**	**4**
Gastrointestinal			
Diarrhea	57	12	3
Nausea	53	4	—
Vomiting	37	4	—
Stomatitis	24	7	—
Abdominal pain	20	4	—
Constipation	15	1	—
Dyspepsia	8	—	—
Skin and Subcutaneous			
Hand-and-foot syndrome	57	11	—
Dermatitis	37	1	—
Nail disorder	7	—	—
General			
Fatigue	41	8	—
Pyrexia	12	1	—
Pain in limb	6	1	—
Neurological			
Paresthesia	21	1	—
Headache	9	1	—
Dizziness	8	—	—
Insomnia	8	—	—
Metabolism			
Anorexia	23	3	—
Dehydration	7	4	1
Eye			
Eye irritation	15	—	—
Musculoskeletal			
Myalgia	9	—	—
Cardiac			
Edema	9	1	—
Blood			
Neutropenia	26	2	2
Thrombocytopenia	24	3	1
Anemia	72	3	1
Lymphopenia	94	44	15
Hepatobiliary			
Hyperbilirubinemia	22	9	2

XELODA Monotherapy Metastatic Breast and Colorectal Cancer: Shown below by body system are the clinical adverse events in <5% of 875 patients (phase III colorectal studies—596 patients, phase II colorectal study—34 patients, phase II breast cancer monotherapy studies—245 patients) reported as related to the administration of XELODA and that were clinically at least remotely relevant.

In parentheses is the incidence of grade 3 or 4 occurrences of each adverse event.

Gastrointestinal: abdominal distention, esophagitis (0.2), intestinal obstruction (0.3), dysphagia, proctalgia, hemorrhoids, fecal abnormality, tongue disorder, ascites (0.1), gastric ulcer (0.1), gastrointestinal hemorrhage (0.2), ileus (0.3), incisional hernia, rectal disorder, swallowing painful, toxic dilation of intestine, melena, gastroenteritis (0.1).
Skin and Subcutaneous: nail disorder (0.1), sweating increased (0.1), face edema, photosensitivity reaction (0.1), urticaria, skin ulcer, genital pruritus, skin lesion, ecchymoses, hyperkeratosis, intertrigo, leg ulcer (excluding varicose), localized skin reaction, red face, rosacea, scab, foot ulcer (0.1).
General: shivering, chest pain (0.2), influenza-like illness, hot flushes, palmar erythema, hiccups, pain (0.1), hoarseness, fluid retention, irritability, difficulty in walking, thirst, chest mass, collapse, fibrosis (0.1), hemorrhage, neck edema, sedation, sudden death unexplained (0.1), swelling, ulcer (0.1).
Neurological: insomnia, ataxia (0.5), sedation, syncope (0.1), tremor, dysphasia, encephalopathy (0.1), coordination abnormal, dysarthria, facial palsy, loss of consciousness (0.2), mental impairment, myoclonic jerks, peroneal nerve palsy (0.1), headache (0.5).
Metabolism: weight increase, malnutrition (0.2), appetite increased, food intolerance (0.1), hypertriglyceridemia (0.1), hypokalemia, diabetes control impaired (0.1), hypomagnesemia.
Eye: vision abnormal, cataract.
Respiratory: cough (0.1), epistaxis (0.1), sore throat, chest tightness, rhinitis, increased sputum production, bronchospasm (0.2), hemoptysis, nasal ulcer, pneumothorax, crackles, orthopnea, pharyngeal disorder, pleural disorder, respiratory distress (0.1), sneezing.
Cardiac: tachycardia (0.1), bradycardia, arrhythmia, chest pain (cardiac) (0.2), atrial fibrillation, cardiac failure, cardiomyopathy, extrasystoles, myocardial infarction (0.1), myocarditis (0.1), pericardial effusion.
Infection: herpes simplex, upper respiratory tract infection (0.1), urinary tract infection (0.2), localized infection, sepsis (0.3), bronchitis (0.1), lower respiratory tract infection, cellulitis, fungal infection (0.3), pneumonia (0.1), bronchopneumonia (0.1), herpes zoster, infection (0.1), influenza, keratoconjunctivitis, laryngitis (0.1), superinfection.
Musculoskeletal: myalgia, back pain, arthralgia (0.1), bone pain (0.1), neck pain, arthritis (0.1), calcaneal spur, muscle weakness.
Blood and Lymphatic: leucopenia (0.2), coagulation disorder (0.1), bone marrow depression (0.1), idiopathic thrombocytopenia purpura (1.0), pancytopenia (0.1).

(cont'd)

Vascular: hypotension (0.2), hypertension (0.1), flushing, lymphoedema (0.1), hematoma, pulmonary embolism (0.2), cerebrovascular accident (0.1), transient ischemic attack, varicose veins, venous thrombosis (0.8).
Psychiatric: depression, confusion (0.1), amnesia, libido decreased, loss of confidence, mood alteration, personality change, psychogenic disorder.
Renal: dysuria, urinary incontinence, hematuria, hydronephrosis (0.1), nocturia (0.1), urinary tract disorder, urine discoloration, polyuria, renal impairment (0.1), urinary retention.
Reproductive System: intermenstrual bleeding, balanoposthitis, vaginal pain, nipple disorder, premenstrual tension syndrome.
Ear: vertigo, earache, deafness, sensation of block in ear.
Hepatobiliary: jaundice (0.3), hepatomegaly, hepatic pain, fatty liver, bile duct stone (0.1), hepatic fibrosis (0.1), hepatitis (0.1), hepatic cholestatic (0.1).
Injury and Poisoning: radiation recall syndrome (0.1), bruising, overdose, scratch.
Surgical: paronychia drainage, postoperative complications, wound drainage increased.
Immune System: food allergy, hypersensitivity (0.1).
Endocrine: cushingoid, hypothyroidism, hirsutism.
Neoplasms: lipoma, solar keratosis (0.1).

Table 12 displays laboratory abnormalities observed in 949 patients, regardless of relationship to treatment with XELODA in metastatic breast and colorectal cancer.

Table 12: XELODA

Laboratory Abnormalities[a]: XELODA Monotherapy in Metastatic Breast and Colorectal Cancer

Parameter[a]	XELODA 1250 mg/m² Twice Daily Intermittent N=949 Patients with Grade 3/4 Abnormality (%)	Patients with Worsening From Baseline of any Grade (%)	Patients with Worsening From Baseline by 1 or 2 Grades (%)	Patients with Worsening From Baseline by 3 or 4 Grades (%)
Decreased hemoglobin	3.1	41.4	40.7	0.7
Decreased neutrophils	3.6	18.7	15.6	3.1
Decreased granulocytes	0.2	1.9	1.7	0.2
Decreased lymphocytes	44.4	58.2	53.1	5.1
Decreased platelets	2.0	20.4	18.8	1.6
Increased bilirubin	17.7	36.9	21.6	15.3
Increased ALAT	0.5	16.7	16.3	0.4
Increased ASAT	1.1	25.1	24.8	0.3
Increased serum creatinine	0.5	9.8	9.4	0.4
Increased alkaline phosphatase	3.5	27.2	27.2	0.0
Hyperglycemia	4.4	40.1	39.2	0.9

[a] Laboratory abnormalities were graded according to the categories of the NCIC CTC Grading System.

Postmarketing Reports of Adverse Events: Reports of adverse events in patients taking XELODA received after market introduction are of similar incidence and severity as reported in the Adverse Effects section.

The following additional adverse events have been identified during post-marketing use of XELODA. Because these events are reported voluntarily from a population of uncertain size, it is not possible to reliably estimate their frequency or establish a causal relationship to XELODA exposure. The occurrence of these events in individuals receiving XELODA does not establish a casual relationship.

Serious gastro-intestinal disorders have been reported in patients exposed to XELODA and include but are not limited to: necrotizing enterocolitis, ileus paralytic, gastrointestinal perforation and intestinal obstruction.

Thromboembolic events such as deep vein thrombosis, thrombophlebitis and pulmonary embolism have been reported.
Hepatobiliary: hepatic failure and cholestatic hepatitis have been reported during clinical trials and post-marketing exposure.
Other: lacrimal duct stenosis NOS.

Adverse events occurring in special patient populations in clinical trials with XELODA monotherapy in the metastatic setting are summarized below:
Geriatrics: Among the 21 patients (80 years of age and greater) with either metastatic breast or colorectal cancer who received XELODA monotherapy (N=875), 6 (28.6%), 3 (14.3%), and 2 (9.5%) patients experienced reversible grade 3/4 diarrhea, nausea and vomiting, respectively. Among the 496 patients aged 60 to 79 years old, the incidence of gastrointestinal toxicity was similar to that in the overall population. Patients 70 to 79 years old (22%) had a higher incidence of hand-and-foot syndrome.
Hyperbilirubinemia: In 875 patients with either metastatic breast or colorectal cancer who received at least one dose of capecitabine 2500 mg/m² daily for 2 weeks followed by a 1-week rest period, grade 3 hyperbilirubinemia occurred in 133 (15.2%) and grade 4 hyperbilirubinemia occurred in 34 (3.9%) patients. Grade 3/4 hyperbilirubinemia occurred in 22.8% of the 566 patients with hepatic metastases and in 12.3% of the 309 patients without hepatic metastases at baseline. Of the 167 patients with grade 3 or 4 hyperbilirubinemia, 31 (18.6%) also had post-baseline elevations (grades 1 to 4, without elevations at baseline) in alkaline phosphatase and 46 (27.5%) had post-baseline elevations in transaminases at any time (not necessarily concurrent). The majority of these patients, 20 (64.5%) and 33 (71.7%), had liver metastases at baseline. In addition, 96 (57.5%) and 59 (35.3%) of the 167 patients had elevations (grades 1 to 4) at both pre- and post-baseline in alkaline phosphatase or transaminases, respectively. Only 13 (7.8%) and 5 (3.0%) had grade 3 or 4 elevations in alkaline phosphatase or transaminases.

OVERDOSE:

Symptoms: The manifestations of acute overdose include: nausea, vomiting, diarrhea, mucositis, gastrointestinal irritation and bleeding, and bone marrow depression.

Treatment: Management of overdose should include customary therapeutic and supportive medical interventions aimed at correcting the presenting clinical manifestations and preventing their possible complications.

For management of a suspected drug overdose, CPhA recommends that you contact your **regional Poison Control Centre**. See the *CPS* Directory section for a list of Poison Control Centres.

DOSAGE: XELODA is intended for long-term administration unless clinically inappropriate. XELODA tablets should be swallowed with water within 30 minutes after a meal.
Recommended Dose and Dose Adjustment: Monotherapy: The recommended dose of XELODA (capecitabine) is 1250 mg/m² administered twice daily (morning and evening; equivalent to 2500 mg/m² total daily dose) for 14 days followed by a 7-day rest period.

For adjuvant treatment of stage III colon cancer, XELODA is intended to be given for a total of 8 cycles (or 24 weeks).
Colorectal Cancer, Combination Therapy with Oxaliplatin: In combination with oxaliplatin the recommended dose of XELODA is 1000 mg/m² twice daily for 2 weeks followed by a 7-day rest period. The first dose of XELODA is given on the evening of day 1 and the last dose is given on the morning of day 15. Given as a 3-weekly schedule, oxaliplatin is administered as a 130 mg/m² intravenous infusion over 2 hours.

Premedication to maintain adequate anti-emesis according to the oxaliplatin Product Monograph should be started prior to oxaliplatin administration for patients receiving the XELODA plus oxaliplatin combination.

Breast Cancer, Combination Therapy with Docetaxel: In combination with docetaxel, the recommended starting dose of XELODA is 1250 mg/m² twice daily for 2 weeks followed by a 7-day rest period combined with docetaxel 75 mg/m² administered as a 1-hour i.v. infusion every 3 weeks (see Pharmacology, Clinical Studies, Breast Carcinoma). Premedication according to the docetaxel labelling, should be started prior to docetaxel administration for patients receiving the capecitabine plus docetaxel combination.

XELODA dose is calculated according to body surface area. Table 13 and Table 14 show examples of the standard and reduced dose calculations for a XELODA starting dose of either 1250 mg/m² or 1000 mg/m².

Table 13: XELODA

Standard and Reduced Dose Calculations According to Body Surface Area for a Starting XELODA Dose of 1250 mg/m²

	Dose Level 1250 mg/m² (twice daily)				
	Full Dose 1250 mg/m²	Number of 150 mg Tablets and/or 500 mg Tablets Per Administration (each administration to be given morning and evening)		Reduced Dose (75%) 950 mg/m²	Reduced Dose (50%) 625 mg/m²
Body Surface Area (m²)	Dose Per Administration (mg)	150 mg	500 mg	Dose Per Administration (mg)	Dose Per Administration (mg)
≤1.26	1500	—	3	1150	800
1.27–1.38	1650	1	3	1300	800
1.39–1.52	1800	2	3	1450	950
1.53–1.66	2000	—	4	1500	1000
1.67–1.78	2150	1	4	1650	1000
1.79–1.92	2300	2	4	1800	1150
1.93–2.06	2500	—	5	1950	1300
2.07–2.18	2650	1	5	2000	1300
≥2.19	2800	2	5	2150	1450

Table 14: XELODA

Standard and Reduced Dose Calculations According to Body Surface Area for a Starting XELODA Dose of 1000 mg/m²

	Dose Level 1000 mg/m² (twice daily)				
	Full Dose 1000 mg/m²	Number of 150 mg Tablets and/or 500 mg Tablets Per Administration (each administration to be given morning and evening)		Reduced Dose (75%) 750 mg/m²	Reduced Dose (50%) 500 mg/m²
Body Surface Area (m²)	Dose Per Administration (mg)	150 mg	500 mg	Dose Per Administration (mg)	Dose Per Administration (mg)
≤1.26	1150	1	2	800	600
1.27–1.38	1300	2	2	1000	600
1.39–1.52	1450	3	2	1100	750
1.53–1.66	1600	4	2	1200	800
1.67–1.78	1750	5	2	1300	800
1.79–1.92	1800	2	3	1400	900
1.93–2.06	2000	—	4	1500	1000
2.07–2.18	2150	1	4	1600	1050
≥2.19	2300	2	4	1750	1100

Dose Modification Guidelines: Patients should be carefully monitored for toxicity. Toxicity due to XELODA administration may be managed by symptomatic treatment, dose interruptions and adjustment of XELODA dose. Once the dose has been reduced it should not be increased at a later time.

For those toxicities considered by the treating physician to be unlikely to become serious or life-threatening, treatment can be continued at the same dose without reduction or interruption.

Dose modifications for the use of XELODA monotherapy are shown in Table 15.

Table 15: XELODA

Recommended Dose Modifications for XELODA

Toxicity NCIC Grade[a]	During a Course of Therapy	Dose Adjustment for Next Cycle (% of starting dose)
Grade 1	Maintain dose level	Maintain dose level
	Grade 2	
1st appearance	Interrupt until resolved to grade 0-1	100%
2nd appearance	Interrupt until resolved to grade 0-1	75%
3rd appearance	Interrupt until resolved to grade 0-1	50%
4th appearance	Discontinue treatment permanently	
	Grade 3	

(cont'd)

Table 15: XELODA *(cont'd)*

Recommended Dose Modifications for XELODA

Toxicity NCIC Grade[a]	During a Course of Therapy	Dose Adjustment for Next Cycle (% of starting dose)
1st appearance	Interrupt until resolved to grade 0-1	75%
2nd appearance	Interrupt until resolved to grade 0-1	50%
3rd appearance	Discontinue treatment permanently	
Grade 4		
1st appearance	Discontinue permanently **or** If physician deems it to be in the patient's best interest to continue, interrupt until resolved to grade 0-1	50%
2nd appearance Discontinue permanently	Discontinue permanently	

[a] According to the National Cancer Institute of Canada Clinical Trial Group (NCIC CTG) Common Toxicity Criteria (Version 1 or the Common Terminology Criteria for Adverse Events (CTCAE) of the Cancer Therapy Evaluation Program, US National Cancer Institute, version 3.0. For Hand-and-Foot Syndrome and hyperbilirubinemia (see Precautions).

Dosage modifications are not recommended for grade 1 events. Therapy with XELODA should be interrupted upon the occurrence of a grade 2 or 3 adverse experience. Once the adverse event has resolved or decreased in intensity to grade 1, then XELODA therapy may be restarted at full dose or as adjusted according to Table 15 for XELODA monotherapy. If a grade 4 experience occurs, therapy should be discontinued or interrupted until resolved or decreased to grade 1, and therapy should be restarted at 50% of the original dose. Patients taking XELODA should be informed of the need to interrupt treatment immediately if moderate or severe toxicity occurs. Doses of XELODA omitted for toxicity are not replaced.

Haematology: Patients with baseline neutrophil counts of $<1.5\times10^9$/L and/or thrombocyte counts of $<100\times10^9$/L should not be treated with XELODA. If unscheduled laboratory assessments during a treatment cycle show grade 3 or 4 haematologic toxicity, treatment with XELODA should be interrupted.

Combination Therapy: Dose modifications for toxicity when XELODA is used in combination with other therapies should be made according to Table 15 for XELODA and according to the appropriate Product Monograph for the other agent(s).

At the beginning of a treatment cycle, if a treatment delay is indicated for either XELODA or the other agent(s), then administration of all agents should be delayed until the requirements for restarting all drugs are met.

During a treatment cycle for those toxicities considered by the treating physician not to be related to XELODA, XELODA should be continued and the dose of the other agent adjusted according to the appropriate Product Monograph.

If the other agent(s) have to be discontinued permanently, XELODA treatment can be resumed when the requirements for restarting XELODA are met.

This advice is applicable to all indications and to all special populations.

Adjustment of Starting Dose in Special Populations: Hepatic Impairment: In patients with mild to moderate hepatic dysfunction due to liver metastases, no dose adjustment is necessary; however, such patients should be carefully monitored. Patients with severe hepatic dysfunction have not been studied (see Warnings).

Renal Impairment: In patients with moderate renal impairment (calculated creatinine clearance 30-50 mL/min [Cockroft and Gault]) at baseline, a dose reduction to 75% from a starting dose of 1250 mg/m² is recommended based upon pharmacokinetic and safety data (see Pharmacology, Pharmacokinetics, Renal Insufficiency and Warnings). In patients with mild renal impairment (calculated creatinine clearance 51-80 mL/min) no adjustment in starting dose is recommended. In patients with severe renal impairment, XELODA should not be administered (see Contraindications). Careful monitoring and prompt treatment interruption is recommended if the patient develops a grade 2, 3, or 4 adverse event, with subsequent dose adjustment as outlined in Table 13 and Table 14. If the calculated creatinine clearance decreases during treatment to a value below 30 mL/min, XELODA should be discontinued. The dose adjustment recommendation for patients with moderate renal impairment apply both to monotherapy and combination use. For dosage calculations, see Table 13 and Table 14.

Geriatrics: No adjustment of the starting dose is needed for XELODA. However for XELODA monotherapy in the metastatic setting, severe grade 3 or 4 treatment-related adverse events were more frequent in patients over 80 years of age compared to younger patients. Careful monitoring of elderly patients is advisable.

When XELODA was used in combination with other agents, elderly patients (≥65 years) experienced more grade 3 and grade 4 adverse drug reactions (ADRs) and ADRs that led to discontinuation, than younger patients. Careful monitoring of elderly patients is advisable.

For treatment with XELODA in combination with docetaxel, an increased incidence of grade 3 or 4 treatment related adverse events and treatment related serious adverse events was observed in patients 60 years of age or more.

INFORMATION FOR THE PATIENT: Published in e-CPS, available by subscription at www.e-cps.ca.

SUPPLIED: 150 mg: Each light peach-colored, biconvex, film-coated, oblong shaped tablet with "XELODA" engraved on one side and "150" on the reverse, contains: capecitabine 150 mg. Nonmedicinal ingredients: croscarmellose sodium, hydroxypropyl methylcellulose, lactose anhydrous, magnesium stearate, microcrystalline cellulose, synthetic red iron oxide, synthetic yellow iron oxide, talc and titanium dioxide. HDPE bottles of 60. Store between 15 and 30°C.

500 mg: Each peach-colored, biconvex, film-coated, oblong shaped tablet with "XELODA" engraved on one side and "500" on the reverse, contains: capecitabine 500 mg. Nonmedicinal ingredients: croscarmellose sodium, hydroxypropyl methylcellulose, lactose anhydrous, magnesium stearate, microcrystalline cellulose, synthetic red iron oxide, synthetic yellow iron oxide, talc and titanium dioxide. HDPE bottles of 120. Store between 15 and 30°C.

(Shown in Product Identification Section)

Xenical® 🄿

orlistat

Antiobesity—Gastrointestinal Lipase Inhibitor

Roche

Date of Preparation: May 28, 1999
Date of Revision: October 6, 2009

SUMMARY PRODUCT INFORMATION:

Route of Administration	Dosage Form/ Strength	Clinically Relevant Nonmedicinal Ingredients
Oral	120 mg capsule	None For a complete listing of nonmedicinal ingredients, see Dosage Forms, Composition and Packaging.

INDICATIONS AND CLINICAL USE: XENICAL (orlistat), when used in conjunction with a mildly hypocaloric diet, is indicated for:

- obesity management including weight loss and weight maintenance
- reducing the risk of weight regain in obese patients after prior weight loss.

* The BMI is calculated by dividing weight in kilograms by height in metres squared.

These indications for the use of XENICAL apply to obese patients with a BMI* ≥30 kg/m² or a BMI ≥27 kg/m² in the presence of other risk factors (e.g., hypertension, type 2 diabetes, dyslipidemia, excess visceral fat).

The weight loss induced by the combination of XENICAL and a mildly hypocaloric diet results in an improvement of risk factors and comorbidities including hypercholesterolemia, impaired glucose tolerance, hyperinsulinemia, hypertension, reduction of visceral fat and waist circumference.

The weight loss induced by XENICAL improves glycemic control in diabetic patients and reduces the risk of developing type 2 diabetes in obese patients (BMI* ≥30 kg/m²) with impaired glucose tolerance. The effect of XENICAL on weight loss is adjunctive to that of diet and exercise.

XENICAL can be used in combination with anti-diabetic agents (sulphonylureas, metformin, insulin) to improve blood glucose control in overweight or obese type 2 diabetes patients who are inadequately controlled on diet, exercise, and one or more of a sulphonylurea, metformin, or insulin.

CONTRAINDICATIONS: XENICAL (orlistat) is contraindicated in patients with chronic malabsorption syndrome, cholestasis and in patients with known hypersensitivity to XENICAL or to any component of this product (for a complete listing of components, see Dosage Forms, Composition and Packaging).

WARNINGS AND PRECAUTIONS: General: Patient Counselling Information: Patients should be advised to adhere to dietary guidelines (see Dosage and Administration).

No serious adverse reactions or safety hazards related to the use of XENICAL (orlistat) have been reported to date during large, long-term clinical trials (up to 4 years) (see Adverse Reactions).

As with any weight-loss agent, the potential exists for misuse of XENICAL in inappropriate patient populations (e.g. patients with anorexia nervosa or bulimia). See the Indications and Clinical Use for appropriate prescribing guidelines.

When using XENICAL in combination with insulin or oral hypoglycemic agents in the treatment of type 2 diabetes, the risks of hypoglycemia, its symptoms and treatment, and conditions that predispose to its development should be explained to the patient, family members, caregiver or others.

For warnings and precautions involving drug interactions, see Drug Interactions.

Endocrine and Metabolism: Hypothyroidism and/or reduced control of hypothyroidism may occur. The mechanism may involve a decreased absorption of iodine salts and/or levothyroxine. Patients treated concomitantly with XENICAL and levothyroxine should be monitored for changes in thyroid function (see Drug Interactions).

Gastrointestinal: XENICAL should be used with caution in patients with pre-existing disease of the large bowel or rectum.

The possibility of experiencing gastrointestinal events (see Adverse Reactions) may increase when XENICAL is taken with a diet high in fat (e.g. in a 2000 Calorie/day diet, a diet high in fat would contain >30% calories from fat, which equates to >67g fat). The daily intake of fat should be distributed over three main meals. If XENICAL is taken with any one meal very high in fat, the possibility of gastrointestinal effects may increase. XENICAL only inhibits the absorption of dietary fat. Patients should be advised that if the resulting caloric reduction is compensated by an increase in calories from protein or carbohydrates, the expected weight loss will not occur.

Cases of rectal bleeding have been reported with XENICAL. Prescribers should investigate further in case of severe and/or persistent symptoms.

See also Warnings and Precautions, Sexual Function/Reproduction.

Neurologic: Anticonvulsants: Convulsions have been reported in patients treated concomitantly with orlistat and antiepileptic drugs. These patients should be monitored for possible changes in the frequency and/or severity of convulsions (see Drug Interactions).

Renal: Renal Calculi: Some patients may develop increased levels of urinary oxalate following treatment with XENICAL. Caution should be exercised when prescribing XENICAL to patients with a history of hyperoxaluria or calcium oxalate nephrolithiasis.

Sexual Function/Reproduction: The use of an additional contraceptive method is recommended to prevent possible failure of oral contraception that could occur in case of severe diarrhea (see Drug Interactions).

Special Populations: Pregnant Women: Teratogenicity studies were conducted in rats and rabbits at doses up to 800 mg/kg/day. Neither study showed embryotoxicity or teratogenicity. This dose is 22 and 43 times the daily human dose calculated, on a body surface area (mg/m²) basis, for rats and rabbits, respectively.

There are no adequate and well-controlled studies of orlistat in pregnant women. Because animal reproductive studies are not always predictive of human response, XENICAL should be used during pregnancy only if the benefit clearly outweighs any potential harm, and iodine supplementation should be considered as XENICAL may impair absorption of iodine salts.

Nursing Women: It is not known if orlistat is secreted in human milk. Therefore, XENICAL should not be used by nursing women unless the benefit to the mother clearly outweighs any potential for harm to the nursing infant, and iodine supplementation should be considered as XENICAL may impair absorption of iodine salts.

Pediatrics (<12 years of age): XENICAL has not been studied in pediatric patients below the age of 12 years.

Monitoring and Laboratory Tests: Diabetic patients treated with orlistat should have tests for fasting glucose and HbA1c as required.

The patient should be on a nutritionally balanced, mildly hypocaloric diet that contains no more than 30% of calories from fat. The daily intake of fat, carbohydrate and protein should be distributed over three main meals (see Drug Interactions, Drug-Drug Interactions, Fat-Soluble Vitamin Supplements and Analogues).

ADVERSE REACTIONS: Clinical Trial Adverse Drug Reactions: Because clinical trials are conducted under very specific conditions the adverse reaction rates observed in the clinical trials may not reflect the rates observed in practice and should not be compared to the rates in the clinical trials of another drug. Adverse drug reaction information from clinical trials is useful for identifying drug-related adverse events and for approximating rates.

Treatment of Obesity: Commonly Observed: (based on first year and second year data—120 mg versus placebo):

Gastrointestinal symptoms are the most commonly observed treatment-emergent adverse events associated with the use of XENICAL (orlistat) in double-blind, placebo-controlled clinical trials and are primarily a manifestation of the mechanism of action. (Commonly observed is defined as an incidence of ≥5% and an incidence in the XENICAL 120 mg group that is at least twice that of placebo.) (See Warnings and Precautions). See Table 1.

Table 1: XENICAL

Percentage of Patients with Commonly Observed GI Adverse Events (based on first and second year data) Which Occurred with a Frequency of ≥5% in XENICAL 120 mg or Placebo

	Year One		Year Two	
Adverse Event	**XENICAL (% Patients) (n=1913)**	**Placebo (% Patients) (n=1466)**	**XENICAL (% Patients) (n=613)**	**Placebo (% Patients) (n=524)**
Oily Spotting	26.6	1.3	4.4	0.2
Flatus with Discharge	23.9	1.4	2.1	0.2
Fecal Urgency	22.1	6.7	2.8	1.7
Fatty/Oily Stool	20.0	2.9	5.5	0.6
Oily Evacuation	11.9	0.8	2.3	0.2
Increased Defecation	10.8	4.1	2.6	0.8
Fecal Incontinence	7.7	0.9	1.8	0.2

These and other commonly observed adverse reactions were generally mild and transient, and decreased during the second year of treatment. Events occurred early in treatment (within 3 months) and most patients experienced only one episode. Only 3% experienced more than two episodes of any one adverse event. The incidence of these effects is directly related to the amount of dietary fat ingested and increases or decreases with the fat content of the diet. Patients should be counselled as to the possibility of the occurrence of gastrointestinal effects and how to minimize them, such as reinforcing the diet, particularly the percentage of fat it contains. Consumption of a diet low in fat (<30%) will decrease the likelihood of experiencing the gastrointestinal effects. The occurrence of gastrointestinal effects may actually help demonstrate to patients that the medication is working and help them monitor and regulate their fat intake.

In the 4-year double-blind, placebo-controlled XENDOS study, the incidence and duration of the commonly observed adverse reactions were comparable to those observed in the 1- and 2- year studies shown above.

Discontinuation of Treatment: In controlled obesity management clinical trials of 1-, and 2- year duration, 8.8% of patients treated with XENICAL discontinued treatment due to adverse events, compared to 5.0% of placebo treated patients. Similarly, in the 4-year XENDOS clinical trial, 8.0% and 4.0% of patients treated with XENICAL and placebo, respectively, discontinued treatment due to adverse events. For XENICAL, the most common adverse events resulting in discontinuation of treatment were gastrointestinal.

Incidence in Controlled Obesity Management Clinical Trials: The following Table 2 and Table 3 list other treatment-emergent adverse events from seven Phase III, multicenter, double-blind, placebo-controlled clinical trials that occurred at a frequency of ≥1% among patients treated with XENICAL 120 mg tid and with an incidence that was greater than placebo during year 1 and year 2, regardless of relationship to study medication.

Table 2: XENICAL

Other Treatment-Emergent Adverse Events From Phase III Placebo-Controlled Obesity Management Clinical Trials—Year One Treatment

Body System/Adverse Event	XENICAL % Patients (n=1913)	Placebo % Patients (n=1466)
Gastrointestinal System		
Abdominal Pain/Discomfort	25.5	21.4
Flatulence	16.0	13.1
Liquid Stools	15.8	11.4
Stools Soft	8.8	6.8
Nausea	8.1	7.3
Infectious Diarrhea	5.3	4.4
Rectal Pain/Discomfort	5.2	4.0
Tooth Disorder	4.3	3.1
Gingival Disorder	4.1	2.9
Vomiting	3.8	3.5
Oral Mucosa Disorder	1.5	0.5
Feces Discolored	1.1	0.3
Respiratory System Disorders		
Upper Respiratory Infection	38.1	32.8
Lower Respiratory Infection	7.8	6.6
Ear, Nose and Throat Symptoms	2.0	1.6
Asthma	1.8	0.8
Resistance Mechanism		
Influenza	39.7	36.2
Musculoskeletal System		
Back Pain	13.9	12.1
Arthritis	5.4	4.8
Myalgia	4.2	3.3
Joint Disorder	2.3	2.2
Tendonitis	1.9	1.7
Injury (Nonspecific)	1.0	0.5
Central Nervous System		
Headache	30.6	27.6
Dizziness	5.2	5.0
Paresthesia	1.2	0.8
Body as a Whole		
Fatigue	7.2	6.4
Surgical Procedure	5.5	4.9
Sleep Disorder	3.9	3.3
Body Temperature Abnormal	2.1	1.5
Anxiety	1.2	0.8
Skin and Appendages		
Rash	4.3	4.0
Dry Skin	2.1	1.4

(cont'd)

Table 2: XENICAL *(cont'd)*

Other Treatment-Emergent Adverse Events From Phase III Placebo-Controlled Obesity Management Clinical Trials—Year One Treatment

Body System/Adverse Event	XENICAL % Patients (n=1913)	Placebo % Patients (n=1466)
Hair Thinning	1.8	1.4
Infection	1.8	1.2
Acne	1.6	1.2
Nail Disorder	1.4	1.1
Insect Bites	1.2	1.0
Urticaria	1.1	0.9
Reproductive Disorders, Female		
Menstrual Irregularity	9.8	7.5
Vaginitis	3.8	3.6
Urinary System		
Urinary Tract Infection	7.5	7.3
Psychiatric Disorders		
Psychiatric Anxiety	4.7	2.9
Hearing and Vestibular Disorders		
Otitis	4.3	3.4
Cardiovascular Disorders		
Pedal Edema	1.2	1.1
Vascular (Extracardiac)		
Vein Disorder	1.3	1.0

Table 3: XENICAL

Other Treatment-Emergent Adverse Events From Phase III Placebo-Controlled Obesity Management Clinical Trials—Year Two Treatment

Body System/Adverse Event	XENICAL % Patients (n=613)	Placebo % Patients (n=524)
Gastrointestinal System		
Flatulence	4.4	3.2
Rectal Pain/Discomfort	3.3	1.9
Stools Soft	2.9	2.5
Nausea	3.6	2.7
Tooth Disorder	2.9	2.3
Gingival Disorder	2.0	1.5
Respiratory System		
Upper Respiratory Infection	26.1	25.8
Musculoskeletal System		
Pain Lower Extremities	10.8	10.3
Tendonitis	2.0	1.9
Muscle Cramps	1.1	0.8
Bone Fracture	1.0	0.8
Body as a Whole		
Fatigue	3.1	1.7
Body Temperature Abnormal	1.5	1.1
Injury	1.6	1.1
Pain	1.5	1.3
Allergic Reaction	1.1	1.0
Skin and Appendages		
Pruritus	1.1	0.8
Reproductive, Female		

(cont'd)

Table 3: XENICAL *(cont'd)*

Other Treatment-Emergent Adverse Events From Phase III Placebo-Controlled Obesity Management Clinical Trials—Year Two Treatment

Body System/Adverse Event	XENICAL % Patients (n=613)	Placebo % Patients (n=524)
Vaginitis	2.6	1.9
Breast Disorder	1.6	1.0
Menopausal Syndrome	1.3	1.0
Urinary System Disorders		
Urinary Tract Infection	5.9	4.8
Psychiatric Disorders		
Psychiatric Anxiety	2.8	2.1
Depression	3.4	2.5
Hearing and Vestibular Disorders		
Otitis	2.9	2.5
Cardiovascular Disorders		
Pedal Edema	2.8	1.9

In the 4-year XENDOS study, the pattern and distribution of adverse events was similar to that reported for the 1 and 2 year studies. The total incidence of gastrointestinal related adverse events occurring in year 1 decreased progressively with each additional year of treatment, over the four year period.

Pediatric Patients: In clinical trials with XENICAL in adolescent patients ages 12 to 16 years, the profile of adverse reactions was generally similar to that observed in adults.

Trials in Patients with Type 2 Diabetes: Commonly observed adverse events: Mild and transient gastrointestinal effects of the same type as those seen in the obesity management trials were observed in the double-blind, placebo-controlled clinical trials for type 2 diabetes management. However, the overall difference in incidence of these adverse events between patients treated with XENICAL and patients receiving placebo was generally less than in the overall obesity trials. Marked decreases were seen in the trials in patients with type 2 diabetes in the incidence of oily spotting, fecal urgency and flatus with discharge (15.8%, 10.5%, 9.4%)†, compared to those for obesity management (25.3%, 15.4% and 22.5% respectively)†. Recurrence also decreased in the diabetes trials: 4% of the patients experienced more than one episode of each gastrointestinal event compared to 6% in the obesity trials. The 2 sets of trials were not run concurrently and thus may not be directly comparable.

Of the other treatment-emergent adverse events reported in the diabetes trials, all were similar in type and generally occurred at a lower incidence compared to those of the obesity management trials, with the exception of cough (2.8% in XENICAL vs 2.4% in placebo), abdominal distension (5.8% vs 4.1%) and hypoglycemia (13.2% vs 9.5%). The majority of hypoglycemic events were mild to moderate in intensity and most patients could control the symptoms themselves. Only two patients in the placebo treatment group and three patients in the orlistat treatment group had hypoglycemic events that would be considered severe.

Weight loss induced by XENICAL is accompanied by improved metabolic control in type 2 diabetics which might allow or require reduction in the dose of hypoglycemic medication (see Warnings and Precautions and Drug Interactions, Diabetes Agents).

Post-Market Adverse Drug Reactions: Post-Marketing Experience: Rare cases of hypersensitivity have been reported. The main clinical symptoms were pruritus, rash, urticaria, angioedema, bronchospasm and anaphylaxis. Very rare cases of bullous eruption, increase in transaminases and in alkaline phosphatase, and exceptional cases of hepatitis that may be serious have been reported during the post-marketing. No causal relationship or physicopathological mechanism between hepatitis and orlistat therapy have been established.

Reports of decreased prothrombin, increased INR and unbalanced anticoagulant treatment resulting in change of haemostatic parameters have been reported in patients treated concomitantly with orlistat and anticoagulants.

Convulsions have been reported in patients treated concomitantly with orlistat and antiepileptic drugs (see Drug Interactions, Drug-Drug Interactions, Anticonvulsants).

Cases of rectal bleeding have been reported with XENICAL. Prescribers should investigate further in case of severe and/or persistent symptoms.

Cases of hypothyroidism and/or reduced control of hypothyroidism have been reported in patients with no history of hypothyroidism and in patients treated concomitantly with levothyroxine.

DRUG INTERACTIONS: Drug-Drug Interactions: Cyclosporine: A reduction in cyclosporine plasma levels has been observed when XENICAL (orlistat) is co-administered. Therefore, it is recommended to monitor cyclosporine plasma levels more frequently than usual if XENICAL is co-administered.

Fat-Soluble Vitamin Supplements and Analogues: A pharmacokinetic interaction study with β-carotene showed a 30% reduction in β-carotene supplement absorption when concomitantly administered with XENICAL. XENICAL inhibited absorption of a vitamin E acetate supplement by approximately 60%. The effect of orlistat on the absorption of supplemental vitamin D, vitamin A and nutritionally derived vitamin K is not known at this time. Obesity management studies indicated that some patients required vitamin D supplementation with a multivitamin to achieve desirable blood levels. The decreases in vitamin D were modest (measured by 25-OH-D) and were not associated with any changes in vitamin D metabolism, as evidenced by total or ionized calcium and parathyroid levels. Clinical studies did not reveal any interference with blood coagulation that would indicate vitamin K deficiency.

During obesity management studies, there were decreases in the levels of some fat soluble vitamins and β-carotene based on the pharmacologic action of the drug. The vast majority of patients in up to four full years of treatment had vitamin levels (vitamins A, D, E, and K, and beta-carotene) that stayed well within normal range, and there was no evidence of clinical sequelae.

The vitamin status of obese patients in general and patients on a weight control regimen, including pharmacotherapy with XENICAL, may be low. Therefore patients should be counselled to take a multivitamin which includes fat-soluble vitamins and β-carotene to ensure adequate nutrition. Pediatric patients should be instructed to take a multivitamin. The supplement should be taken at least two hours before or after the administration of XENICAL, or at bedtime.

Anticoagulants: As treatment with orlistat may potentially impair the GI absorption of vitamin K, close monitoring of the coagulation parameters is recommended when oral anticoagulants are co-administered.

Anticonvulsants: Convulsions have been reported in patients treated concomitantly with orlistat and antiepileptic drugs. XENICAL may unbalance anticonvulsive treatment by decreasing the absorption of antiepileptic drugs. A causal relationship has not been established, however patients should be monitored for possible changes in the frequency and/or severity of convulsions.

Cardiovascular Agents: Nifedipine : (Extended-Release Tablets): In 17 normal weight subjects receiving XENICAL 120 mg tid for 6 days, XENICAL did not alter the bioavailability of nifedipine extended-release tablets.

At 50 mg tid for 7-8 days, orlistat did not significantly alter the pharmacokinetics of atenolol, captopril, furosemide and nifedipine retard.

Amiodarone: In a pharmacokinetic (PK) study, oral administration of amiodarone during orlistat treatment demonstrated a 25-30% reduction in the systemic exposure to amiodarone and desethylamiodarone. Due to the complex pharmacokinetics of amiodarone, the clinical effects of this are unclear. The effect of commencing orlistat treatment in patients on stable amiodarone therapy has not been studied. A potential reduced therapeutic effect of amiodarone is possible.

No interactions based on specific drug-drug interaction studies have been observed with losartan, fibrates, or atorvastatin.

Diabetes Agents: Weight loss induced by XENICAL is accompanied by improved metabolic control in non-insulin dependent diabetics, which might allow or require reduction in dose of oral hypoglycemic medication (e.g. sulfonylureas).

† These values are the treatment difference between XENICAL and placebo.

Glyburide: In 12 normal weight subjects receiving XENICAL 80 mg tid for 4 1/3 days, XENICAL did not alter the pharmacokinetics or pharmacodynamics (blood-glucose-lowering) of glyburide.

Metformin: In 20 normal weight subjects receiving XENICAL 120 mg tid for 6 days in a two way crossover study, XENICAL did not alter the pharmacokinetics of metformin.

Narrow Therapeutic Index Drugs: Drug interaction studies were performed with XENICAL and a number of drugs with a narrow therapeutic index. XENICAL had no inhibitory effects on pharmacokinetic or pharmacodynamic parameters of the following drugs:

Phenytoin: In 12 normal weight subjects receiving XENICAL 120 mg tid for 7 days, XENICAL did not alter the pharmacokinetics of a single 300-mg dose of phenytoin.

Warfarin: In 12 normal weight subjects, administration of XENICAL 120 mg tid for 16 days did not result in any change in either warfarin pharmacokinetics (both R- and S-enantiomers) or pharmacodynamics (prothrombin time and serum Factor VII). Although Vitamin K nutritional status parameters (ratios of vitamin K_1 epoxide to vitamin K_1 and undercarboxylated osteocalcin to osteocalcin) were also unaltered by orlistat, treatment with orlistat may potentially impair the GI absorption of vitamin K. Close monitoring of the coagulation parameters, including international normalised ratio (INR) values, is recommended when oral anticoagulants are co-administered.

Digoxin: In 12 normal weight subjects receiving XENICAL 120 mg tid for 6 days, XENICAL did not alter the pharmacokinetics of a single dose of digoxin.

Other: Alcohol: In a multiple-dose study in 30 normal weight subjects, coadministration of orlistat and 40 grams of alcohol (e.g. approximately 3 glasses of wine) did not result in alteration of alcohol pharmacokinetics, orlistat pharmacodynamics (fecal fat excretion), and systemic exposure to orlistat.

Cyclosporine: A reduction in cyclosporine plasma levels has been observed when XENICAL is co-administered. Therefore, it is recommended to monitor cyclosporine plasma levels more frequently than usual if XENICAL is co-administered.

Oral Contraceptives: (various ethinyl estradiol and gestagen combinations commercially available): In 20 normal weight female subjects, the treatment of XENICAL 120 mg tid for 23 days resulted in no changes in the ovulation-suppressing action of oral contraceptives. Although the absence of an interaction between oral contraceptives and orlistat has been demonstrated, orlistat may indirectly reduce the availability of oral contraceptives and lead to unexpected pregnancies in some individual cases. An additional contraceptive method is recommended in case of severe diarrhea (see Warnings and Precautions, Sexual Function/Reproduction).

Pravastatin: In 24 normal weight, mildly hypercholesterolemic subjects receiving XENICAL 120 mg tid for 6 days in a two way cross-over study, XENICAL did not affect the pharmacokinetics or pharmacodynamics of pravastatin.

Levothyroxine: Hypothyroidism and/or reduced control of hypothyroidism may occur. The mechanism, although not proven, may involve a decreased absorption of iodine salts and/or levothyroxine. Patients treated concomitantly with XENICAL and levothyroxine should be monitored for changes in thyroid function.

No interactions based on specific drug-drug interaction studies have been observed with amitryptyline, fluoxetine, sibutramine, or phentermine.

DOSAGE AND ADMINISTRATION: Dosing Considerations:

- The patient should be on a nutritionally balanced, mildly hypocaloric diet that contains no more than 30% of calories from fat. The daily intake of fat, carbohydrate and protein should be distributed over three main meals (see Drug Interactions, Drug-Drug Interactions, Fat-Soluble Vitamin Supplements and Analogues).
- For patients with type 2 diabetes, the reduced calorie diet should be consistent with the dietary recommendations of the Canadian Diabetes Association Guidelines for the Nutritional Management of Diabetes Mellitis in the New Millennium.

Recommended Dose and Dosage Adjustment: The recommended dose of XENICAL (orlistat) is one 120 mg capsule three times daily with each main meal (during or up to 1 hour after the meal). If a meal is occasionally missed or contains no fat, the dose of XENICAL may be omitted.

Doses above 120 mg three times daily have not been shown to provide additional benefit. No dose adjustment is necessary for the geriatric patient.

Based on fecal fat measurements, the effect of XENICAL is seen as soon as 24 to 48 hours after dosing. Upon discontinuation of therapy, fecal fat content usually returns to pretreatment levels within 48 to 72 hours.

OVERDOSAGE:

Single doses of 800 mg XENICAL (orlistat) and multiple doses of up to 400 mg tid for 15 days have been studied in normal weight and obese subjects without significant adverse findings. In addition, doses of 240 mg tid have been administered to obese patients for 6 months without a significant increase in adverse findings.

Orlistat overdose cases received during post-marketing reported either no adverse events or adverse events that are similar to those reported with the recommended dose.

Should a significant overdose of XENICAL occur, it is recommended that the patient be observed for 24 hours. Based on human and animal studies, any systemic effects attributable to the lipase-inhibiting properties of orlistat should be rapidly reversible.

> For management of a suspected drug overdose, contact your **regional Poison Control Centre**. See the *CPS Directory* section for a list of Poison Control Centres.

ACTION AND CLINICAL PHARMACOLOGY: Mechanism of Action: XENICAL (orlistat) is a reversible inhibitor of lipases. It exerts its therapeutic activity non-systemically in the lumen of the stomach and small intestine by forming a covalent bond with the active serine site of gastric and pancreatic lipases. The inactivated enzymes are thus unavailable to hydrolyze dietary fat in the form of triglycerides into absorbable free fatty acids and monoglycerides. As undigested triglycerides are not absorbed, the resulting caloric deficit has a positive effect on weight loss, maintenance and prevention of weight regain. Systemic absorption of the drug is therefore not needed for activity. At the recommended dose of 120 mg three times a day, orlistat inhibits dietary fat absorption by approximately 30%.

Pharmacokinetics: Absorption: Systemic exposure to orlistat is negligible. Following oral dosing with 360 mg ^{14}C- orlistat, plasma radioactivity peaked at approximately 8 hours; plasma concentrations of intact orlistat were nonmeasurable (<5 ng/mL). In therapeutic studies involving monitoring of plasma samples, detection of intact orlistat in plasma was sporadic and concentrations were extremely low (<10 ng/mL or 0.02 µM), without evidence of accumulation, and consistent with negligible absorption.

Studies in rats and dogs indicated that the absolute bioavailability of orlistat in plasma is <2% at oral doses up to 1000 mg/kg/day.

Distribution: In vitro orlistat was >99% bound to plasma proteins (lipoproteins and albumin were major binding proteins). Orlistat minimally partitioned into erythrocytes.

Metabolism: Based on animal data, it is likely that the metabolism of orlistat occurs mainly within the gastrointestinal wall. Based on a ^{14}C -orlistat mass balance study in obese patients, of the minute fraction of the radio-labelled dose that was absorbed systemically, the presence of two metabolites, M1 (4-member lactone ring hydrolyzed) and M3 (M1 with N-formyl leucine moiety cleaved), accounted for approximately 42% of total radioactivity in plasma. M1 and M3 have an open β-lactone ring and extremely weak systemic lipase inhibitory activity (1000- and 2500- fold less than orlistat, respectively). In view of this low inhibitory activity and the low plasma levels at the therapeutic dose (average of 26 ng/mL and 108 ng/mL for M1 and M3, respectively), these metabolites are considered pharmacologically inconsequential. The primary metabolite M1 had a short half-life (approximately 3 hours) whereas the secondary metabolite M3 disappeared at a slower rate (half-life approximately 13.5 hours). In obese patients, steady state plasma levels of M1, but not M3, increased in proportion to orlistat doses.

Excretion: Following a single oral dose of 360 mg ^{14}C-orlistat in both normal weight and obese subjects, fecal excretion of the unabsorbed drug was found to be the major route of elimination. Approximately 97% of the administered radioactivity was excreted in feces and 83% of that was found to be unchanged orlistat. The cumulative renal excretion of total radioactivity was <2% of the given dose of 360 mg ^{14}C-orlistat.

The time to reach complete excretion (fecal plus urinary) was 3 to 5 days. The disposition of orlistat appeared to be similar between normal weight and obese subjects. Based on limited data, the half-life of the absorbed orlistat is in the range of 1 to 2 hours. Orlistat, M1 and M3 metabolites were also subject to biliary excretion.

Special Populations and Conditions: Special Populations: Because the drug is minimally absorbed, with no defined pharmacokinetics, studies in special populations (geriatric, pediatric, different races, patients with renal and hepatic insufficiency) were not conducted.

Pediatrics: Plasma concentrations of orlistat and its metabolites M1 and M3 were similar to those found in adults at the same dose level. Daily fecal fat excretions were 27% and 7% of dietary intake in orlistat and placebo treatment groups, respectively.

Hepatic and Renal Insufficiency: Clinical investigations in patients with hepatic and/or renal impairment have not been undertaken

Effect of Orlistat on Gastrointestinal and Systemic Physiological Processes: Adults: In several studies of up to 6-weeks duration, the effects of orlistat on gastrointestinal and systemic physiological processes were assessed in normal weight and obese subjects. Postprandial cholecystokinin plasma concentrations were lowered after multiple doses of orlistat in two studies

but not significantly different from placebo in two other experiments. There were no clinically significant changes observed in gallbladder motility, bile composition or lithogenicity or colonic cell proliferation rate, and no clinically significant reduction of gastric emptying time or gastric acidity. In addition, no effect on plasma triglyceride levels, systemic lipases or balance of six minerals (calcium, magnesium, phosphorus, zinc, copper and iron) were observed with administration of orlistat in these studies.
Pediatrics: In a 3-week study of 32 obese adolescents aged 12 to 16 years, XENICAL (120 mg, three times a day) did not significantly affect the balance of calcium, magnesium, phosphorous, zinc, or copper. The iron balance was decreased by 64.7 µmol/24 hours and 40.4 µmol/24 hours in orlistat and placebo treatment groups, respectively.

STORAGE AND STABILITY: XENICAL should be stored in its original package between 15-25°C. Protect from moisture. This medicine should not be used after the expiry date shown on the pack.

INFORMATION FOR THE PATIENT: Published in e-CPS, available by subscription at www.e-cps.ca.

DOSAGE FORMS, COMPOSITION AND PACKAGING: Each turquoise cap and turquoise body capsule, with "ROCHE XENICAL 120" printed in black ink, contains: orlistat 120 mg. Nonmedicinal ingredients: gelatin, indigo carmine, microcrystalline cellulose, povidone K30, sodium lauryl sulfate, sodium starch glycolate, talc and titanium dioxide. Blister packages, cartons of 84.

(Shown in Product Identification Section)

Xeomin® Ⓟ

Clostridium botulinum neurotoxin type A (150 kD), free from complexing proteins

Muscle Relaxant, Peripherally Acting Agent

Merz Pharma

Date of Preparation: March 27, 2009

SUMMARY PRODUCT INFORMATION:

Route of Administration	Dosage Form/ Strength	Clinically Relevant Nonmedicinal Ingredients
Intramuscular injection	Powder for solution for injection, 100 LD_{50} units per vial	None For a complete listing see Dosage Forms, Composition and Packaging.

DESCRIPTION: XEOMIN (Clostridium Botulinum Neurotoxin Type A (150 kD), free from complexing proteins) is produced by the anaerobic bacterial fermentation process from the Hall strain of *C. botulinum*. It consists of the purified neurotoxin which has been separated from protective complexing proteins (hemagglutinins and a non-toxic non-hemagglutinating protein) during production. It is a polypeptide comprised of a heavy chain, with a molecular weight of approximately 100 kD, and a light chain, with a molecular weight of approximately 50 kD. These separated chains are covalently linked via a disulphide bond. The light chain is associated with a zinc ion and functions as a zinc-dependent endopeptidase. The heavy chain comprises two functional domains: the N-terminal section is the translocation domain and the C-terminal section is the binding domain.

XEOMIN is supplied as a sterile, white, preservative free powder for solution for injection (lyophilisate) packed under nitrogen in glass vials. The vials are closed with rubber stoppers and aluminum caps. Each vial contains 100 mouse LD_{50} units of Clostridium Botulinum Neurotoxin Type A (150 kD), free from complexing proteins, 4.7 mg of sucrose and 1.0 mg of human serum albumin. Prior to use XEOMIN is reconstituted with commercially available 0.9 % physiological saline (not supplied in the pack) to form a clear, and colorless solution. The size of the vials allows different concentrations (i.e. doses) to be prepared.

INDICATIONS AND CLINICAL USE: XEOMIN is indicated in adults for the symptomatic management of:

- Blepharospasm
- Cervical dystonia of a predominantly rotational form (spasmodic torticollis)
- Post-stroke spasticity of the upper limb

XEOMIN as a treatment for focal spasticity has been studied in association with usual standard care regimens and is not intended as a replacement for these treatment modalities. XEOMIN is not likely to be effective at a joint affected by a fixed contracture.

XEOMIN may only be used by physicians with suitable qualifications and proven experience in the application of Botulinum toxin type A and in the use of the necessary equipment, e.g. EMG (electromyography).

Geriatrics (>65 years of age): Although clinical studies included a number of patients over the age of 65, no clinical trials specifically designed for elderly patients have been performed. Initial dosing should begin at the lowest recommended dose for the specific indication and be cautiously titrated within the recommended range for optimal patient outcome.

Pediatrics (<18 years of age): XEOMIN has not been studied in the pediatric population and is therefore not currently recommended in this age group.

CONTRAINDICATIONS:

- Hypersensitivity to Botulinum neurotoxin type A or to any of the excipients.
- Generalised disorders of muscle activity (e.g. myasthenia gravis, Lambert-Eaton syndrome).
- Presence of infection at the proposed injection site.

WARNINGS AND PRECAUTIONS:

Serious Warnings and Precautions

- The term "unit" or "U" upon which dosing is based, is a specific measurement of toxin activity that is unique to XEOMIN. Therefore, the "unit" or "U" used to describe XEOMIN activity are different from those used to describe that of other botulinum toxin preparations and the units representing XEOMIN activity are not interchangeable with other products.
- Follow the recommended dosage and frequency of administration for XEOMIN (see Dosage and Administration).

General: Patients and caregivers should be advised to seek immediate medical consultation if swallowing, speech, or respiratory disorders arise.

In very rare cases severe adverse events like muscle weakness, dysphagia or aspiration pneumonia with a suspected causal relationship to toxin spread have been reported with the use of botulinum toxin. Also very rare cases of adverse events with a fatal outcome have been reported. Patients with a neurological underlying disease or swallowing, speech or respiratory difficulties have an increased risk for these adverse drug reactions and should be treated and supervised very carefully.

An anaphylactic reaction may occur rarely after injection of Botulinum neurotoxin type A (see Adverse Reactions). Adrenaline and other medical aids for treating anaphylaxis should be available.

Prior to administering XEOMIN, the physician must familiarise himself/herself with the patient's anatomy and any alterations to the anatomy due to prior surgical procedures. Extra caution is required when injecting at sites close to sensitive structures such as the carotid artery and lung apices.

There were no clinical data available in long-term repeat dose treatment and in treatment-naïve patients for cervical dystonia and blepharospasm. However, there is information available with repeat dose treatment and in treatment-naive patients for post-stroke spasticity of the upper limb.

XEOMIN should be used with caution:

- In patients suffering from amyotrophic lateral sclerosis or other diseases which result in peripheral neuromuscular dysfunction
- In targeted muscles which display pronounced weakness or atrophy.

Clinical effects of XEOMIN may increase or decrease with repeated injections. Possible reasons for change in clinical effect are different techniques of reconstitution, the chosen injection intervals, the injected muscles and marginally varying toxin activity resulting from the biological testing procedure employed or secondary non-response.

Previously akinetic or sedentary patients should be reminded to gradually resume activities following the injection of XEOMIN.

XEOMIN as a treatment for focal spasticity has been studied in association with usual standard care regimens and is not intended as a replacement for these treatment modalities. XEOMIN is not likely to be effective at a joint affected by a fixed contracture.

XEOMIN contains albumin, a derivative of human blood. Standard measures to prevent infections resulting from the use of medicinal products prepared from human blood or plasma include careful selection of donors, screening of individual donations and plasma pools for specific markers of infection and the inclusion of effective manufacturing steps for the inactivation/removal of viruses. Despite this, when medicinal products prepared from human blood or plasma are administered, the possibility of transmitting infective agents cannot be totally excluded. This also applies to unknown or emerging viruses and other pathogens. There are no reports of viral transmissions with albumin manufactured to European Pharmacopoeia specifications by established processes.

Gastrointestinal: Spasmodic Torticollis: Patients should be informed that injections of XEOMIN for the management of spasmodic torticollis may cause mild to severe dysphagia with the risk of aspiration and dyspnoea. Medical intervention may be necessary (e.g. in the form of a gastric feeding tube) (see Adverse Reactions). Dysphagia can last for up to two to three weeks after injection, but a duration of up to five months has been reported in one case. Patients with smaller neck muscle mass, or patients who require bilateral injections into the sternocleidomastoid muscles are at greater risk. The occurrence of dysphagia is attributable to the spread of the pharmacological effect of Botulinum toxin as the result of the neurotoxin spread into the oesophageal musculature.

Hematologic: XEOMIN should be used with caution if bleeding disorders of any type occur. It should be used with caution in patients receiving anticoagulant therapy.

Immune: The risks for development of neutralizing antibodies to Botulinum toxins are related to high dosage, too frequent injections, young age at disease onset, and higher total dosage received of Botulinum toxin. Antibody development may lead to treatment resistance (see Dosage and Administration).

Ophthalmologic: Blepharospasm: Because of the anticholinergic effect of Botulinum toxin type A, XEOMIN should be used with caution in patients at risk of developing an angle closure glaucoma.

In order to prevent ectropion, injections into the lower lid area should be avoided, and vigorous treatment of any epithelial defect is necessary. This may require protective drops, ointments, soft bandage contact lenses, or closure of the eye by patching or similar means.

Reduced blinking following XEOMIN injection into the orbicularis muscle can lead to corneal exposure, persistent epithelial defects and corneal ulceration, especially in patients with cranial nerve disorders (facial nerve). Careful testing of corneal sensation should be performed in patients with previous eye operations.

Ecchymosis easily occurs in the soft tissues of the eyelid. Immediate gentle pressure at the injection site can limit that risk.

Special Populations: Pregnant Women: There have been no studies in pregnant women. Studies in animals have shown reproductive toxicity. The potential risk for humans is unknown.

XEOMIN should not be used during pregnancy unless clearly necessary and unless the potential benefit justifies the risk.

Nursing Women: It is not known whether Botulinum toxin type A is excreted into the breast milk. Therefore, the use of XEOMIN during lactation is not recommended.

Pediatrics (<18 years of age): No data is available on the use of XEOMIN in children and it is therefore not currently recommended in this age group.

Geriatrics (>65 years of age): Although clinical studies included a number of patients over the age of 65, no clinical trials specifically designed for elderly patients have been performed. Initial dosing should begin at the lowest recommended dose for the specific indication and be cautiously titrated within the recommended range for optimal patient outcome.

ADVERSE REACTIONS: Adverse Drug Reaction Overview: Undesirable effects associated with the therapeutic use of Botulinum toxin type A are mainly related to the diffusion of Botulinum neurotoxin type A from the target muscle to adjacent muscles. Such undesirable effects are rare, and most are localized in close proximity to the injection site; systemic side effects are uncommon. Intramuscular injection into neck muscles for treatment of cervical dystonia occasionally results in transient dysphagia and a general weakness in the neck muscles. Treatment of blepharospasm by periocular injection can result in ptosis and diplopia. Intramuscular injections of Botulinum toxin type A for upper limb spasticity were reported to be commonly associated with local reactions like hypertonia, ecchymosis, purpura, pain in shoulder, arm or hand, muscle weakness, bleeding and itching after administration at the injection site.

Side effects related to spread of toxin distant from the site of administration have been reported very rarely (exaggerated muscle weakness, dysphagia, and aspiration pneumonitis with fatal outcome in some cases). Dysphagia has been reported following injection to sites other than the cervical musculature. The following other adverse events have been reported following administration of conventional Botulinum toxin type A complex: dysarthria, abdominal pain, hyperhidrosis, anorexia, hypoacusis, tinnitus, radiculopathy, and syncope.

There have been rare reports of undesirable effects related to the cardiovascular system, such as arrhythmia and myocardial infarction, some with fatal outcomes. It remains unclear whether these deaths were induced by conventional preparations containing the Botulinum toxin type A complex or whether these were caused by pre-existing cardiovascular disease. Serious and/or immediate hypersensitivity reactions have been rarely reported, including anaphylaxis, serum sickness, urticaria, soft tissue oedema, and dyspnoea. Some of these reactions have been reported following the use of conventional Botulinum toxin type A complex either alone or in combination with other agents known to cause similar reactions.

QT interval prolongation has been reported in 2 out of 366 patients following administration of XEOMIN in clinical studies with blepharospasm and cervical dystonia patients. However, these findings were not considered clinically relevant in the opinion of the treating cardiologist and the exact relationship of these events to XEOMIN is unknown.

Clinical Trial Adverse Drug Reactions: Because clinical trials are conducted under very specific conditions the adverse reaction rates observed in the clinical trials may not reflect the rates observed in practice and should not be compared to the rates in the clinical trials of another drug. Adverse drug reaction information from clinical trials is useful for identifying drug-related adverse events and for approximating rates.

In the 6 studies conducted to provide data on the safety of XEOMIN 1082 subjects were treated with trial medications (XEOMIN, active comparator or placebo). In these studies 611 subjects received XEOMIN (46 healthy male volunteers, 272 patients with cervical dystonia, 148 blepharospasm patients and 145 patients with post-stroke spasticity of the upper limb). The duration of observation was 130 days in the phase II study in cervical dystonia. For the phase III trials, patients were observed for up to 16 weeks in the focal dystonia trials and for up to 69 weeks in the spasticity trial. In the phase 1 trials volunteers were followed for up to 90 days or up to 52 weeks.

In all active-controlled trials subjects received 1 dose of either XEOMIN and/or active comparator with doses ranging from 2-32 U in healthy volunteers, 30-300 U in cervical dystonia patients and 15-100 U in blepharospasm patients. In the placebo-controlled study in post-stroke spasticity of the upper limb doses administered ranged from 80-435 U. In the subsequent Open-Label Extension (OLEX) Period doses administered over up to a maximum of 5 injection intervals ranged between 95 U and 500 U XEOMIN. Overall the mean dose delivered was 122.4 units in the XEOMIN population and 92.6 U in the active comparator population. Table 1, Table 2, Table 3 and Table 4 summarize adverse drug reactions reported in ≥1% for each indication.

Less Common Clinical Trial Adverse Drug Reactions (<1%): Cervical Dystonia: eye pain, diarrhoea, dry mouth, vomiting, colitis, asthenia, injection site inflammation, injection site tenderness, skeletal pain, myalgia, headache, tremor, dysphonia skin rash, erythema, pruritus, sweating increased.

Blepharospasm: conjunctivitis, dry mouth, inflicted injury, muscle weakness, paraesthesia, headache, skin rash.

Post-stroke Spasticity of the Upper Limb: dry mouth, peripheral oedema, myalgia, cough.

Abnormal Hematologic and Clinical Chemistry Findings: In all clinical trials, there were no findings indicative of underlying pathological changes as a result of trial medication, both with regard to the incidence of abnormal hematologic and clinical chemistry values and with regard to the mean change in laboratory values for either treatment group.

Post-Market Adverse Drug Reactions: The following adverse reactions have been reported since XEOMIN has been marketed: eye swelling, eyelid edema, madarosis, vision blurred; injection site reactions; asthenia, fatigue; dysphagia, nausea, abdominal distension; hypersensitivity including allergic dermatitis, skin rash, erythema, drug eruptions, lymphadenopathy, alopecia; dysphonia, cough, dyspnoea, asthma; herpes zoster; muscular weakness, muscle spasm, myalgia, trismus; dysarthria, headache, somnolence; cardiovascular insufficiency, circulatory collapse; abnormal dreams.

Because these reactions are reported voluntarily from a population of uncertain size, it is not always possible to reliably estimate their frequency or establish a causal relationship to drug exposure.

Table 1: XEOMIN

Adverse Drug Reactions Reported in ≥1% of Cervical Dystonia Patients

System Organ Class Preferred Term	Number of Subjects (%)	
	XEOMIN N=272	**Active Comparator 1 (Botulinum toxin type A-complex) N=244**
Gastrointestinal Disorders	**24 (8.8)**	**15 (6.1)**
Dysphagia	24 (8.8)	15 (6.1)

(cont'd)

Table 1: XEOMIN *(cont'd)*

Adverse Drug Reactions Reported in ≥1% of Cervical Dystonia Patients

System Organ Class Preferred Term	Number of Subjects (%) XEOMIN N=272	 Active Comparator 1 (Botulinum toxin type A-complex) N=244
Musculoskeletal & Connective Tissue Disorders	**9 (3.3)**	**2 (≤1)**
Muscular weakness	4 (1.5)	1 (≤1)
Neck pain	5 (1.8)	1 (≤1)

Table 2: XEOMIN

Adverse Drug Reactions Reported in ≥1% of Blepharospasm Patients

System Organ Class Preferred Term	Number of Subjects (%) XEOMIN N=148	 Active Comparator 1 (Botulinum toxin type A- complex) N=152
Eye Disorders	**12 (8.1)**	**12 (7.9)**
Dry eye	3 (2.0)	0 (0.0)
Eyelid oedema	0 (0.0)	2 (1.3)
Eyelid ptosis	9 (6.1)	7 (4.6)
Vision blurred	0 (0.0)	3 (2.0)

Table 3: XEOMIN

Adverse Drug Reactions Reported in ≥1% of Patients with Post-stroke Spasticity of the Upper Limb (Double-blind Period)

System Organ Class Preferred Term	Number of Subjects (%) XEOMIN N=73	 Placebo N=75
Gastrointestinal Disorders	**0 (0.0)**	**1 (1.3)**
Dysphagia	0 (0.0)	1 (1.3)
General Dis. & Admin. Site Conditions	**0 (0.0)**	**1 (1.3)**
Injection site pain	0 (0.0)	1 (1.3)
Nervous System Dis.	**1 (1.4)**	**0 (0.0)**
Headache	1 (1.4)	0 (0.0)

Table 4: XEOMIN

Adverse Drug Reactions Reported in ≥1% of Patients with Post-Stroke Spasticity of the Upper Limb (Open-Label Extension Period)

System Organ Class Preferred Term	XEOMIN Number of Subjects (%) N=145
Gastrointestinal Disorders	
Dysphagia	2 (1.4)
General Dis. & Admin. Site Conditions	
Injection site pain	4 (2.8)
Musculoskeletal and Connective Tissue Disorders	
Muscular weakness	5 (3.4)
Pain in extremity	2 (1.4)

DRUG INTERACTIONS: Drug-Drug Interactions: Theoretically, the effects of Botulinum toxin may be potentiated by aminoglycoside antibiotics or other medicinal products that interfere with neuromuscular transmission, e.g. tubocurarine-type muscle relaxants.

Therefore, the concomitant use of XEOMIN with aminoglycosides, polymyxins, tetracyclines, linomycin, spectinomycin or any other drugs that interfere with neuromuscular transmission requires special care. Peripheral muscle relaxants should be used with caution, if necessary reducing the starting dose of relaxant, or using an intermediate-acting substance such as vecuronium or atracurium rather than substances with longer lasting effects.

4-Aminochinolines may reduce the effect of XEOMIN.

Drug-Food Interactions: Interactions with food are not relevant.

Drug-Herb Interactions: Interactions with herbal products have not been established.

Drug-Laboratory Test Interactions: Interactions with results of laboratory tests have not been established.

Drug-Lifestyle Interactions: XEOMIN has minor or moderate influence on the ability to drive and use machines. Due to the nature of the diseases being treated, the ability to drive and to operate machines may be reduced. This can be compounded by some of the therapeutic and/or adverse effects of XEOMIN, which may also interfere with the ability to drive and operate machinery. Consequently affected persons should avoid these tasks until their faculties are fully recovered.

DOSAGE AND ADMINISTRATION: Dosing Considerations:

- **Unit doses recommended for XEOMIN are not interchangeable with those for other preparations of Botulinum toxin.**
- XEOMIN may only be used by physicians with suitable qualifications and proven experience in the application of Botulinum toxin and in the use of the necessary equipment, e.g. EMG (electromyography).
- Reconstituted XEOMIN is intended for intramuscular injection. After reconstitution, XEOMIN should be used for only one injection session and for only one patient.
- The minimal injection intervals and the maximum doses of XEOMIN should be as recommended for the specific indication.
- The optimum dosage and number of injection sites in the treated muscle should be determined by the physician individually for each patient. A titration of the dose should be performed.
- A decrease or increase in the XEOMIN dose is possible by administering a smaller or larger injection volume. Initial dosing should begin at the lowest recommended dose for the specific indication and be cautiously titrated within the recommended range for optimal patient outcome. The smaller the injection volume the less pressure sensation and the less spread of Botulinum neurotoxin type A in the injected muscle occurs. This is of benefit in reducing effects on nearby muscles when small muscle groups are being injected.
- If no treatment effect occurs within one month after the initial injection, the following measures should be taken:
  - Clinical verification of the neurotoxin effect on the injected muscle: e.g. an electromyographic investigation in a specialised facility
  - Analysis of the reason for non-response, e.g. poor isolation of the muscles intended to be injected, too low dose, poor injection technique, fixed contracture, too weak antagonist, possible development of antibodies
  - Review of Botulinum neurotoxin type A treatment as an adequate therapy
  - If no adverse reactions have occurred during the initial treatment, an additional course of treatment can be performed under the following conditions: 1) dose adjustment with regard to analysis of the most recent therapy failure, 2) EMG-guidance, 3) the recommended minimum interval between the initial and repeat treatment is followed:
- A treatment-naïve patient should be regarded as a primary non-responder in cases of first injection failure. It has not been investigated whether secondary non-response due to the development of antibodies is less frequent under XEOMIN therapy than under treatment with conventional preparations containing the Botulinum toxin type A complex. In cases of non-response, alternative therapies should be considered.
- XEOMIN has not been studied in the paediatric population and is therefore not recommended in the paediatric age group until further data become available.

Recommended Dose and Dosage Adjustment: Blepharospasm: The initial recommended dose is 1.25 to 2.5 U (0.05-0.1 mL volume) per injection site. The initial dose should not exceed 25 U per eye. In the management of blepharospasm, total dosing should not exceed 70 U and the period between each treatment session is recommended to be at least every 12 weeks.

The median time to first onset of effect is observed within four days after injection. The effect of each treatment generally lasts approximately 3-4 months; however, it may last significantly longer or shorter. The treatment can be repeated if required. There is limited experience in treatment naïve patients and in long-term repeat dose treatment.

At repeat treatment sessions, the dose may be increased up to two-fold (as long as the total dose of 70 U is not exceeded) if the response to the initial treatment is considered insufficient—usually defined as an effect that does not last longer than two months. However, there appears to be no additional benefit obtainable from injecting more than 5.0 U per site. Normally, no additional benefit is conferred by treating more frequently than every three months.

Spasmodic Torticollis: In the management of spasmodic torticollis, XEOMIN dosing must be tailored to the individual patient, based on the patient's head and neck position, location of possible pain, muscle hypertrophy, patient's body weight, and response to the injection. A suitable sterile needle (e.g. 25-30 gauge/0.30-0.50 mm) is used for injections into superficial muscles, and an e.g. 22 gauge/0.70 mm needle may be used for injections into deeper musculature. An injection volume of approximately 0.1 to 0.5 mL per injection site is recommended.

In practice, the usual total dose does not exceed 200 U. Doses of up to 300 U may be given. No more than 50 U should be given at any one injection site.

The median first onset of effect is observed within seven days after injection. The effect of each treatment generally lasts approximately 3-4 months; however, it may last significantly longer or shorter. The period between each treatment session is recommended to be at least 12 weeks. There is limited experience in treatment naïve patients and in long-term repeat dose treatment.

Post-stroke Spasticity of the Upper Limb: Reconstituted XEOMIN is injected using a suitable sterile needle (e.g. 26 gauge/0.45 mm diameter/37 mm length, for superficial muscles and a longer needle, e.g. 22 gauge/0.7 mm diameter/75 mm length, for deeper musculature). An injection volume of approximately 0.2 to 1 mL per injection site is recommended, but it can be exceeded to 1.5 mL in selected cases.

The doses (units) usually administered in the management of post-stroke spasticity of the upper limb are presented in Table 5.

Table 5: XEOMIN

Dosage Guide for the Management of Post-Stroke Spasticity of the Upper Limb

Clinical Pattern Muscle	Units
Flexed Wrist (Total)	90
Flexor carpi radialis	50
Flexor carpi ulnaris	40
Clenched Fist (Total)	80
Flexor digitorum superficialis	40
Flexor digitorum profundus	40
Flexed Elbow (Total)	130–190
Brachioradialis	60
Biceps	80
Brachialis	50
Pronated Forearm (Total)	25–65
Pronator quadratus	25
Pronator teres	40
Thumb-in-Palm (Total)	10–40
Flexor pollicis longus	20
Adductor pollicis	10
Flexor pollicis brevis/Opponens pollicis	10

Total dosing should not exceed 400 units per treatment session involving different muscles.

Initial dosing should begin at the lowest recommended dose for the specific indication and be cautiously titrated within recommended dose range for optimal patient outcome.

The median time to first onset of effect is observed within four days after injection. The effect of each treatment generally lasts approximately 3 months; however, it may last significantly longer or shorter. The period between each treatment session is recommended to be at least 12 weeks.

Administration: The multiple point injection technique into target muscles with disperse innervation zones can reduce undesirable effects and, at the same time, may reach more intrafusal fibres.

Blepharospasm: After reconstitution, the XEOMIN solution is injected using a suitable sterile needle (e.g. 27-30 gauge/0.30-0.40 mm). Electromyographic guidance is not necessary. An injection volume of approximately 0.05 to 0.1 mL is recommended.

XEOMIN is injected into the medial and lateral orbicularis oculi of the upper lid and the lateral orbicularis oculi of the lower lid. Additional sites in the brow area, the lateral orbicularis and in the upper facial area may also be injected if spasms here interfere with vision.

Injections near the levator palpebrae superioris should be avoided to reduce the occurrence of ptosis. Diplopia may develop as a result of Botulinum neurotoxin type A diffusion into the inferior oblique. Avoiding medial injections into the lower lid may reduce this adverse reaction.

Spasmodic Torticollis: In the management of spasmodic torticollis, XEOMIN is usually injected into the sternocleidomastoid, levator scapulae, scalenus, splenius capitis, and/or the trapezius muscle(s). This list is not exhaustive as any of the muscles responsible for controlling head position may be involved and therefore require treatment. If difficulties arise isolating single muscles, injections should be performed using electromyographic guidance. The muscle mass and the degree of hypertrophy or atrophy are factors to be taken into consideration when selecting the appropriate dose.

Multiple injection sites permit XEOMIN more uniform coverage of the innervated areas of the dystonic muscle and are especially useful in larger muscles. The optimum number of injection sites is dependent upon the size of the muscle to be chemically denervated.

The sternocleidomastoid should not be injected bilaterally as there is an increased risk of adverse reactions (in particular dysphagia) when bilateral injections or doses in excess of 100 U are administered into this muscle.

Post-stroke Spasticity of the Upper Limb: Localisation of the involved muscles with electromyographic guidance or nerve stimulation techniques may be necessary. Multiple injection sites may allow XEOMIN to have more uniform contact with the innervation areas of the muscle and are especially useful when larger muscles are injected.

The exact dosage and number of injection sites should be tailored to the individual patient based on the size, number and location of muscles to be treated, the severity of spasticity, and the presence of local muscle weakness. Initial dosing should begin at the lowest recommended dose and be cautiously titrated within the recommended dose range for optimal patient outcome.

Reconstitution: This medicinal product must not be mixed with other medicinal products except those mentioned below.

XEOMIN is reconstituted prior to use with sterile unpreserved sodium chloride 9 mg/mL (0.9%) solution for injection. Reconstitution and dilution should be performed in accordance with good clinical practice guidelines, particularly with respect to asepsis.

It is good practice to perform vial reconstitution and syringe preparation over plastic-lined paper towels to catch any spillage. An appropriate amount of solvent (Table 6) is drawn up into a syringe. The exposed portion of the rubber stopper of the vial is cleaned with alcohol (70%) prior to insertion of the needle. The solvent must be injected gently into the vial. The vial must be discarded, if the vacuum does not pull the solvent into the vial. Reconstituted XEOMIN is a clear colourless solution free of particulate matter.

XEOMIN should not be used if the reconstituted solution (prepared as above) has a cloudy appearance or contains floccular or particulate matter.

Table 6: XEOMIN

Possible Dilutions of XEOMIN in the Reconstituted Solution

Solvent Added (sodium chloride 9 mg/mL (0.9%) solution for injection)	Resulting Dose in Units per 0.1 mL
0.5 mL	20.0 U
1.0 mL	10.0 U
2.0 mL	5.0 U
4.0 mL	2.5 U
8.0 mL	1.25 U

Any solution for injection that has been stored for more than 24 hours as well as any unused solution for injection should be discarded. For safe disposal of the reconstituted solution, see Special Handling Instructions.

OVERDOSAGE:

Increased doses of Botulinum neurotoxin type A may result in pronounced neuromuscular paralysis distant from the injection site. Symptoms of overdose are not immediately apparent post-injection. These typically occur 12 to 72 hours after exposure. Signs of overdose may include general weakness, ptosis, diplopia, swallowing and speech difficulties, or paralysis of the respiratory muscles resulting in an aspiration pneumonia.

In case of an overdose, the patient must be monitored medically for several days. If signs of intoxication appear, hospitalisation with general supportive measures is necessary. Intubation and assisted ventilation will become necessary until improvement if paralysis of the respiratory muscles occurs.

The lethal amount of crystalline Botulinum toxin Type A for a 70 kg human is calculated to be approximately 0.09 to 0.15 μg applied intravenously or intramuscularly, and 70 μg applied orally. A vial with 100 Units XEOMIN contains 0.6 ng Botulinum Neurotoxin Type A, i.e. less than 1/100 of the estimated human lethal dose following intravenous or intramuscular application.

For management of a suspected drug overdose, CPhA recommends that you contact your **regional Poison Control Centre**. See the *CPS* Directory section for a list of Poison Control Centres.

ACTION AND CLINICAL PHARMACOLOGY: Mechanism of Action: The mechanism of action of Botulinum neurotoxin type A is well characterized. It involves a 3 step process resulting in a reduction in muscular contractions.

The C-terminal end of the heavy chain of Botulinum neurotoxin type A binds to binding sites (SV2C and gangliosides) on presynaptic acetylcholinergic axon terminals with very high specificity and affinity (picomolar range). Binding is facilitated by the presence of polysialoganglioside, but the actual protein binding site of Botulinum neurotoxin type A has not yet been fully characterised.

After binding, the Botulinum neurotoxin type A molecule is taken up by endocytosis so that it resides in an endocytic vesicle in the cytosol of the nerve terminal. Internalisation is mediated by the 50 kD N-terminal domain of the heavy chain which undergoes a configuration change to form a transmembrane hydrophilic cleft in the vesicle, through which the light chain, a zinc-dependent endopeptidase, protrudes into the cytosol. Internalization is detectable in vitro within 20 minutes of binding, and reaches a peak after 90 minutes.

After internalization into the nerve terminal, the light chain of the neurotoxin specifically cleaves a component (SNAP 25) of the vesicle fusion machinery, which is essential for the release of acetylcholine. By inhibiting acetylcholine release Botulinum neurotoxin type A reduces muscular contractions. The blockade of transmission at the neuromuscular junction leads to retraction of the endplate nerve terminals and subsequent loss of endplate organization.

Extensive compensatory sprouting by the affected terminal nerve membrane begins within 4 days, leading to the formation of temporary functional synapses and partial recovery of muscle function within approximately 28 days of treatment. Within approximately 2 months, the affected nerve terminals begin to recover their ability to release acetylcholine and the original endplate connections are progressively restored. Sprouting stops and the temporary synapses begin to lose their functionality. Within approximately 3 months, the original nerve endings recover full functionality, leading to the normalization of the original motor endplates. This induces retraction and regression of the sprouts and a complete functional repair of the original terminals.

In addition, cholinergic, autonomic, parasympathetic, and postganglionic sympathetic nerve synapses are also potential targets of therapeutic intervention, e.g. the intradermal application of Botulinum neurotoxin type A leads to denervation of eccrine glands. It is therefore conceivable that systematic autonomic side effects of local Botulinum neurotoxin type A injections may include dryness of the mouth and eyes and ocular accommodation difficulties.

Pharmacodynamics: The pharmacodynamics of locally injected Botulinum neurotoxin type A are well established, with dose-related muscle weakness resulting from the irreversible blockade of acetylcholine release from presynaptic vesicles.

The desired pharmacological effect of Botulinum neurotoxin type A relates to reduced muscle contraction in the target muscle, whereas undesirable effects appear to relate to the diffusion of toxin from the target muscle to adjacent muscles and/or nerves. Relief of dystonic involuntary spasm generally occurs within 2 to 5 days after intramuscular injection, with an expected maximum effect after 2 weeks and a duration of effect for an average of 9 to 16 weeks.

The diffusion of Botulinum neurotoxin type A from intramuscular injection sites into surrounding tissue is dose-dependent. Limiting the dose of Botulinum neurotoxin type A in critical anatomical areas is therefore helpful in preventing complications (e.g. limiting dose administered to the orbicularis oculi to prevent ptosis, or limiting the dose administered to the sternocleidomastoid to prevent dysphagia in cervical dystonia). The multiple point injection technique into target muscles with disperse innervation zones (e.g., sternocleidomastoid, orbicularis oculi) can reduce undesirable effects in Botulinum neurotoxin type A -treated patients and, at the same time, may reach more intrafusal fibres.

Two pharmacodynamic studies were conducted with XEOMIN (Botulinum Neurotoxin Type A (150 kD), free from complexing proteins) in healthy volunteers. The studies were active-control (Botulinum toxin type A-complex) studies conducted in a small foot muscle [extensor digitorum brevis (EDB)] model. Active control studies showed a reduction in compound muscle action potential (CMAP) in all subjects with similar effects between treatments. No significant difference was seen between preparations with respect to degree of paralysis, onset of paralysis, and duration of effect. In a dose-response study overall, a dose-response relationship was observed when the highest dose (32 Unit) and the lowest dose (2 Unit) groups were compared with similar effects for XEOMIN (Botulinum Neurotoxin Type A (150 kD), free from complexing proteins) and the conventional Botulinum toxin type A preparation containing the Botulinum toxin type A complex observed in all dose groups. No local diffusion of either preparation was observed in adjacent muscles at tested doses.

Pharmacokinetics: Classic kinetic and distribution studies cannot be conducted with Botulinum neurotoxin type A because the active substance is applied in very small quantities (picograms per injection), and because it binds so rapidly and irreversibly to cholinergic nerve terminals.

Like many other proteins of its size, Botulinum neurotoxin type A has been shown to undergo retrograde axonal transport after intramuscular injection. Retrograde transsynaptic passage of active Botulinum neurotoxin type A into the central nervous system however has not been found. Proteolysed Botulinum neurotoxin type A yields amino acids which will enter the normal physiological metabolic pathways, being recycled or catabolised, according to the needs of the cell.

Duration of Effect: See Dosage and Administration.

STORAGE AND STABILITY: XEOMIN, unreconstituted is stored at room temperature (up to 25°C) and should not be used after the expiry date stated on the outer package.

Reconstituted Solution: This product does not contain any antimicrobial preservatives and should ideally be used immediately after reconstitution. Reconstituted solution is stable for up to 24 hours at 2 to 8°C.

SPECIAL HANDLING INSTRUCTIONS: For safe disposal, unused vials should be reconstituted with a small amount of water and then autoclaved. Any used vials, syringes, and spillage etc. should be autoclaved and any residual XEOMIN should be inactivated using diluted sodium hydroxide solution (0.1 N NaOH).

INFORMATION FOR THE PATIENT: Published in e-CPS, available by subscription at www.e-cps.ca.

DOSAGE FORMS, COMPOSITION AND PACKAGING: Each type 1 glass vial, with a latex-free rubber stopper (bromobutyl rubber) and tamper-proof seal (aluminum), of sterile, white, preservative free powder for solution for injection (lyophilisate) contains: 100 LD_{50} units of Clostridium Botulinum neurotoxin type A (150 kD), free from complexing proteins [where one unit corresponds to the median lethal dose (LD_{50}) when the reconstituted product is injected intraperitoneally into mice under defined conditions], 4.7 mg of sucrose and 1.0 mg of human serum albumin. Pack sizes of 1 (single unit pack). Prior to use XEOMIN is reconstituted with commercially available 0.9 % physiological saline (not supplied in the pack) to form a clear, and colorless solution.

Due to differences in the LD_{50} assay, these units are specific to XEOMIN and are not interchangeable with other Botulinum toxin preparations.

Xigris® 🅿

drotrecogin alfa (activated)

Antithrombotic Profibrinolytic Anti-inflammatory Enzyme

Lilly

Date of Revision: August 20, 2009

SUMMARY PRODUCT INFORMATION:

Route of Administration	Dosage Form/ Strength	Clinically Relevant Nonmedicinal Ingredients
Intravenous Injection	5 mg or 20 mg per vial	Sucrose For a complete listing, see Dosage Forms, Composition and Packaging.

DESCRIPTION: XIGRIS [drotrecogin alfa (activated)] is a recombinant form of human Activated Protein C with the same amino acid sequence as human plasma-derived Activated Protein C. Drotrecogin alfa (activated) is secreted into the fermentation medium by an established human cell line modified by recombinant DNA technology. Human Protein C is enzymatically activated by cleavage with thrombin and subsequently purified.

INDICATIONS AND CLINICAL USE: XIGRIS [drotrecogin alfa (activated)] is indicated for reduction of mortality in adult patients with severe sepsis (sepsis associated with acute organ dysfunction) who have a high risk of death (e.g. as determined by APACHE II, or multiple acute organ dysfunctions), when added to current best practice.

Efficacy has not been established in adult patients with severe sepsis and lower risk of death. XIGRIS should not be used in this category of patients.

This product should be administered under the supervision of a qualified health professional who is experienced in the use of drugs used in the treatment and in the management of severe sepsis. Appropriate management of therapy and complications is only possible when adequate diagnostic and treatment facilities are readily available.

Geriatrics (>65 years of age): In clinical studies evaluating 1821 adult patients with severe sepsis, approximately 50% of the patients were 65 years or older. No overall differences in safety or effectiveness were observed between these patients and younger patients (see Adverse Reactions).

Pediatrics (<18 years of age): Safety and efficacy have not been established in pediatric patients with severe sepsis. Therefore XIGRIS is not recommended for use in pediatric patients (see Warnings and Precautions and Adverse Reactions).

CONTRAINDICATIONS: XIGRIS [drotrecogin alfa (activated)] increases the risk of bleeding. XIGRIS is contraindicated in the following situations:

- Active internal bleeding
- Recent (within 3 months) hemorrhagic stroke
- Recent (within 2 months) intracranial or intraspinal surgery, or severe head trauma requiring hospitalization
- Trauma with an increased risk of life-threatening bleeding
- Presence of an epidural catheter
- Intracranial neoplasm or mass lesion or evidence of cerebral herniation.

XIGRIS is contraindicated in patients with known hypersensitivity to drotrecogin alfa (activated) or any component of this product. (For a complete listing of ingredients, see Dosage Forms, Composition and Packaging.)

WARNINGS AND PRECAUTIONS: Carcinogenesis and Mutagenesis: Long-term studies in animals to evaluate potential carcinogenicity of XIGRIS [drotrecogin alfa (activated)] have not been performed.

XIGRIS was not mutagenic in an in vivo micronucleus study in mice or in an in vitro chromosomal aberration study in human peripheral blood lymphocytes, with or without rat liver metabolic activation.

Hematologic: Bleeding is the most common serious adverse event associated with XIGRIS therapy. Serious bleeding includes intracranial hemorrhage (also described as central nervous system [CNS] bleeding), which has been reported in patients receiving XIGRIS in clinical trials (see Adverse Reactions, Bleeding Events). Each patient being considered for therapy with XIGRIS should be carefully evaluated and anticipated benefits weighed against potential risks associated with therapy.

Certain conditions increase the risk of bleeding with XIGRIS therapy. Post-marketing information confirms this possibility (Kanji et al., 2007 and Gentry et al., 2009). For patients with severe sepsis who have one or more of the following conditions, the increased risk of bleeding should be carefully considered when deciding whether to use XIGRIS therapy:

- Concurrent therapeutic heparin (≥15 units/kg/h) (see Drug Interactions).
- Heparin doses above those recommended for prophylaxis should not be used.
- Platelet count <30 000×10^6/L, even if the platelet count is increased after transfusions.
- Prothrombin time—International Normalized Ratio (INR) >3.0.
- Recent (within 6 weeks) gastrointestinal bleeding (unless definitive intervention has been performed).
- Recent administration (within 3 days) of thrombolytic therapy.
- Recent administration (within 7 days) of glycoprotein IIb/IIIa inhibitors or oral anticoagulants.
- Recent administration (within 7 days) of ASA >650 mg per day or other platelet inhibitors.

- Recent (within 3 months) ischemic stroke (see Contraindications).
- Intracranial arteriovenous malformation or aneurysm.
- Raised intracranial pressure.
- Known bleeding diathesis except for acute coagulopathy related to sepsis.
- Any other condition in which bleeding constitutes a significant hazard or would be particularly difficult to manage because of its location.
- Chronic severe hepatic disease.

For procedures with an inherent bleeding risk, XIGRIS should be discontinued for 2 hours prior to the start of the procedure. Once adequate hemostasis has been achieved, XIGRIS may be restarted immediately after uncomplicated less invasive procedures and XIGRIS may be restarted 12 hours after major invasive procedures or surgery.

As a component of routine care, measures of hemostasis (e.g., APTT, PT or platelet count) should be obtained during the infusion of XIGRIS. If during the infusion of XIGRIS, routine sequential tests of hemostasis indicate an uncontrolled or worsening coagulopathy that significantly increases the risk of bleeding, the benefits of continuing the infusion must be weighed against the potential increased risk of bleeding for that patient.

Most patients with severe sepsis have a coagulopathy that is commonly associated with prolongation of the activated partial thromboplastin time (APTT) and the prothrombin time (PT). XIGRIS may variably prolong the APTT. Therefore, the APTT cannot be reliably used to assess the status of the coagulopathy during XIGRIS infusion. XIGRIS has minimal effect on the PT and the PT can be used to monitor the status of the coagulopathy in these patients (see Warnings and Precautions, Monitoring and Laboratory Tests).

Unless considered medically necessary, prophylactic low-dose heparin should not be discontinued when drotrecogin alfa (activated) is added to the treatment of patients with severe sepsis. In a randomized study of prophylactic low-dose heparin versus placebo in 1935 adult severe sepsis patients treated with drotrecogin alfa (activated), discontinuation of prophylactic low-dose heparin was associated with increased mortality and risk of serious adverse events, including cardiac, gastrointestinal, and venous thrombotic events. The combination of prophylactic low-dose heparin and drotrecogin alfa (activated) did not affect mortality. In addition, the co-administration of prophylactic low-dose heparin and drotrecogin alfa (activated) was associated with a statistically significant increase in nonserious study-drugrelated adverse events and in any bleeding events, primarily gastrointestinal or renal bleeding events, which occurred during Study Days 0 through 6 (see Drug Interactions and Adverse Reactions).

Hepatic: In patients with severe sepsis, the plasma clearance of XIGRIS was significantly decreased by hepatic dysfunction, but the magnitude of the differences in clearance (<30%) does not warrant any dosage adjustment (see Warnings and Precautions, Special Populations).

Immune: As with all therapeutic proteins, there is a potential for an immune response following treatment with XIGRIS. In patients with severe sepsis, the formation of anti-Activated Protein C antibodies was uncommon (<1%) after a single course of therapy. These antibodies were not capable of neutralizing the effect of either human plasma derived or recombinant human Activated Protein C on the activated partial thromboplastin time (APTT) assay. No anti-Activated Protein C antibody formation was detected in healthy subjects, even after repeat administration up to 6 times.

Peri-Operative Considerations: Patients with Single Organ Dysfunction and Recent Surgery: In the randomized, placebo-controlled PROWESS (PROtein C Worldwide Evaluation in Severe Sepsis) trial, analysis showed that among the small number of patients with single organ dysfunction and surgery (within 30 days of study treatment), those treated with XIGRIS had numerically higher 28-day and in-hospital mortality rates than those treated with placebo (non-statistically significant) (see Table 1).

In the randomized, placebo-controlled ADDRESS [ADministration of DRotrecogin alfa (activated) in Early stage Severe Sepsis] trial, post-hoc analyses showed that for the surgical subpopulation of the single organ dysfunction subgroup, the 28-day mortality rate was higher in the XIGRIS treatment arm compared to placebo, which was statistically significant (p-value unadjusted for multiple comparisons). For this same subpopulation of patients, those treated with XIGRIS had a numerically higher in-hospital mortality rate than placebo treated patients (non-statistically significant) (see Table 1).

In surgical patients, particularly those with single organ dysfunction, it may be difficult to distinguish between a patient with systemic inflammatory response syndrome (SIRS) and a patient with severe sepsis, thus patients with single organ dysfunction and recent surgery may not be at high risk of death irrespective of APACHE II score, and therefore XIGRIS should not be used in these patients.

Table 1: XIGRIS

28 Day All Cause Mortality and In-Hospital Mortality for Surgical Patients With Single Organ Dysfunction in PROWESS and ADDRESS

	28-Day Mortality		In-Hospital Mortality Placebo	
	XIGRIS	Placebo	XIGRIS	Placebo
PROWESS	10/49	8/49	14/48	8/47
	p=0.60[a]		p=0.16[a]	
ADDRESS	67/323	44/313	76/325	62/314
	p=0.03[a]		p=0.26[a]	

[a] Chi-square test without adjustment for multiple comparisons.

Renal: In patients with severe sepsis, the plasma clearance of XIGRIS was significantly decreased by renal impairment, but the magnitude of the differences in clearance (<30%) does not warrant any dosage adjustment (see Warnings and Precautions, Special Populations).

Sexual Function/Reproduction: The potential of XIGRIS to impair fertility has not been evaluated in male or female animals.

Special Populations: Pregnant Women: Animal reproductive studies have not been conducted with XIGRIS. It is not known whether XIGRIS can cause foetal harm when administered to a pregnant woman or whether it can affect reproduction capacity. XIGRIS should be given to pregnant women only if clearly needed.

Nursing Women: It is not known whether XIGRIS is excreted in human milk or absorbed systemically after ingestion. Because many drugs are excreted in human milk, and because of the potential for adverse effects on the nursing infant, a decision should be made whether to discontinue nursing or discontinue the drug, taking into account the importance of the drug to the mother.

Pediatrics (<18 years of age): Data from a placebo-controlled clinical trial in 477 patients (where the median age of patients enrolled was 2.6 years) did not establish the safety or efficacy of XIGRIS in pediatric patients. Therefore XIGRIS is not recommended for use in pediatric patients (see Indications and Clinical Use and Adverse Reactions).

Analysis of the data from this trial showed that while the rate of serious bleeding events (over the infusion period and over the 28-day study period) between the XIGRIS and placebo groups were similar, the rate of serious bleeding defined as central nervous system (CNS) bleeding was higher in the XIGRIS versus the placebo group. Over the infusion period (study days 0-6) the number of patients experiencing CNS bleeding was 5 versus 1 for the XIGRIS versus placebo groups, with 4 of the 5 events in the XIGRIS group occurring in patients ≤60 days or ≤3kg. Fatal CNS bleeding events, overall 28-day mortality, serious adverse events, and major amputations were similar in the XIGRIS and placebo groups.

Geriatrics (>65 years of age): In clinical studies evaluating 1821 adult patients with severe sepsis, approximately 50% of the patients were 65 years or older. No overall differences in safety or effectiveness were observed between these patients and younger patients (see Indications and Clinical Use and Adverse Reactions).

Monitoring and Laboratory Tests: XIGRIS has minimal effect on the PT. Prolongation of the APTT in patients with severe sepsis receiving XIGRIS may be due to the underlying coagulopathy, the pharmacodynamic effect of XIGRIS, and/or the effect of other concurrent medications. The pharmacodynamic effect of XIGRIS on the APTT assay is dependent on the reagent and instrument used to perform the assay and the time that elapses between sample acquisition and assay performance. XIGRIS present in a plasma sample will be gradually neutralized by endogenous inhibitors. Virtually no measurable activity of XIGRIS is present 2 hours after obtaining the blood sample. Due to these biological and analytical variables, the APTT should not be used to assess the pharmacodynamic effect of XIGRIS. Similarly, approximately 2 hours after terminating the infusion of the drug, there is virtually no measurable activity of XIGRIS remaining in the circulation of the patient; blood samples drawn for APTT determination after this point are no longer affected by the drug. The interpretation of sequential determination of the PT and/or APTT should take these variables into consideration.

Because XIGRIS may affect the APTT assays, XIGRIS present in plasma samples may interfere with one-stage coagulation assays based on the APTT (such as factor VIII, IX, and XI assays). This interference may result in an apparent factor concentration that is lower than the true concentration. XIGRIS present in plasma samples does not interfere with one-stage factor assays based on the PT (such as factor II, V, VII and X assays).

ADVERSE REACTIONS: Clinical Trial Adverse Drug Reactions: Because clinical trials are conducted under very specific conditions the adverse reaction rates observed in the clinical trials may not reflect the rates observed in practice. Adverse drug reaction information from clinical trials is useful for identifying drug-related adverse events and for approximating rates.

In two placebo-controlled trials (the dose-ranging Phase 2 trial and pivotal Phase 3 trial [PROWESS]), 1821 adult patients with severe sepsis were evaluated. Patients ranged in age from 18 to 96 years (mean age of 60.5 years). Women and caucasians comprised 42% and 82% of the patient population, respectively. A total of 940 patients were randomized to and received XIGRIS [drotrecogin alfa (activated)]. Most patients (80%) received a dose of 24 μg/kg/h administered as a constant rate infusion for 96 hours.

An additional 2378 adult patients with severe sepsis received XIGRIS in the Phase 3b multi-country, single-arm, open-label trial (ENHANCE).

The following adverse events have occurred in patients with severe sepsis who received XIGRIS:

Bleeding Events: Bleeding events are common in patients with severe sepsis. In the placebo-controlled Phase 2 and PROWESS trials, the percentage of patients experiencing at least one bleeding event in the XIGRIS and placebo treatment groups was 23.9% and 17.3%, respectively. In both treatment groups, the majority of bleeding events were gastrointestinal tract bleeding or ecchymosis. Bleeding events were more frequent in the XIGRIS treatment group at all levels of severity, as shown in Table 2.

Table 2: XIGRIS

Maximum Severity of Bleeding Events Reported as Treatment-emergent Adverse Events (One Severity Per Patient) During Infusion or Within Close Proximity to the End of Infusion

Severity of Bleeding	XIGRIS (N=940)	Placebo (N=881)
Mild	95 (10.1%)	65 (7.4%)
Moderate	48 (5.1%)	16 (1.8%)
Severe	25 (2.7%)	11 (1.2%)

Table 3 lists the percentage of patients in clinical trials who experienced serious bleeding events by site of hemorrhage during the study drug infusion period and during the 28-day study period. In the Phase 2, PROWESS and ENHANCE trials, serious bleeding events included any intracranial hemorrhage [also described as central nervous system (CNS) bleeding], any life threatening or fatal bleed, any bleeding event requiring the administration of ≥3 units of packed red blood cells per day for 2 consecutive days, or any bleeding event assessed as serious by the investigator. The difference in the incidence of serious bleeding events between the two treatment groups occurred primarily during study drug administration.

CNS bleeding includes any bleed in the central nervous system including the following types of hemorrhage—petechial, parenchymal, subarachnoid, subdural, and stroke with hemorrhagic transformation. In the PROWESS study, there was a 0.2% incidence rate of CNS bleeding that occurred during the infusion period for XIGRIS-treated patients. There were no CNS bleeds in the placebo group during the infusion period. The incidence of CNS bleeding during the 28-day study period was 0.2% and 0.1% for XIGRIS-treated and placebo-treated patients, respectively. All cases of CNS bleeds that occurred during infusion and at 28-days were fatal. No CNS bleeds were reported during the Phase 2 study.

In the single-arm trial (ENHANCE), the incidence of CNS bleeding during the infusion period was 0.6% (0.2% fatal) and during the 28-day study period was 1.5% (0.5% fatal).

Although the majority of CNS bleeding occurred in patients with risk factors for bleeding such as severe coagulopathy, severe thrombocytopenia and/or meningitis, the risk of CNS bleeding in all patients with these risk factors and treated with XIGRIS is unknown (see Warnings and Precautions). The observed mortality rate for placebo-treated patients who had a platelet count <30 000/mm³ prior to or during infusion in the Phase 3 PROWESS study was very high (16 of 19 patients died) while similar patients in the XIGRIS treatment arm had a lower mortality rate (5 of 15 died). A thorough risk/benefit assessment must be performed for patients with severe coagulopathy, severe thrombocytopenia and/or meningitis.

Bleeding Events in ADDRESS Trial: In ADDRESS, the randomized, placebo-controlled trial in adult severe sepsis patients determined to be at low risk of death (the non-indicated population), the percentage of patients experiencing at least one bleeding event in XIGRIS-treated and placebo-treated patients was 10.9% and 6.4%, respectively (p<0.001). Bleeding events included serious bleeding events, bleeding events assessed as possibly study-drug related by the investigator, bleeding events associated with the need for a red blood cell transfusion, and bleeding events that led to permanent discontinuation of the study drug.

Table 4 lists the percent of patients experiencing serious bleeding events and CNS bleeding events in ADDRESS. The percent of patients experiencing a serious bleeding event by site of hemorrhage was similar to that observed in the Phase 2 and PROWESS trials.

Bleeding Events in Pediatric Patients: Safety and efficacy have not been established in pediatric patients. In an uncontrolled, safety and pharmacokinetic study of XIGRIS, in pediatric patients with severe sepsis, the percentage of patients experiencing at least one bleeding event was 20.5% (17 of 83). The most common bleeding events were hemorrhage, ecchymosis, hemoptysis, lung hemorrhage, and hematuria. In addition, 4.8% of patients (4 of 83) experienced a serious bleeding event reported as a serious adverse event. The 4 patients each experienced one serious bleeding event (nasopharyngeal hemorrhage caused by the attempted placing of a nasogastric tube [Part 1]; cerebral petechial hemorrhage, gastrointestinal bleeding, and intracranial hemorrhage [Part 2]). The intracranial hemorrhage was considered by the investigator to be possibly related to study drug administration.

The mortality rate for this study was 9.6% (8 of 83); there were no patient deaths in Part 1 (0 of 21 patients) of the study and eight in Part 2 (8 of 62 patients).

Non-Bleeding Events in Pediatric Patients: The safety profile for non-bleeding adverse events in pediatric patients is similar to that seen in adults. Nearly all of the adverse events reported were expected clinical manifestations of severe sepsis (i.e. agitation, edema, oliguria, etc.).

Adverse Events by Body System: Table 5 summarizes adverse events (excluding bleeding events) that occurred at an incidence of ≥5% among XIGRIS-treated patients during infusion and during the 28-day study period.

Except for increased bleeding events, which may relate to the pharmacologic action of XIGRIS, the incidence of all other adverse events (Table 4, Table 5 and Table 6) was comparable between the XIGRIS and placebo-treated groups. There were no types of non-bleeding adverse events suggesting a causal association with XIGRIS.

Post-Market Adverse Drug Reactions: Bleeding Events in XPRESS Trial: In a randomized study comparing heparin and placebo in 1935 adult severe sepsis patients treated with drotrecogin alfa (activated) (see Warnings and Precautions), prophylactic low-dose heparin did not affect mortality, adversely affect the efficacy of drotrecogin alfa (activated) or increase the risk of serious haemorrhagic events, including central nervous system bleeding. The incidence of nonserious bleeding events was increased by low-dose heparin.

Table 6 lists bleeding rates from a randomized study (XPRESS) of low-dose heparin versus placebo in 1935 adult severe sepsis patients treated with drotrecogin alfa (activated). Serious bleeding rates were consistent with those observed in previous studies of drotrecogin alfa (activated). Low-dose heparin did not increase the risk of serious bleeding, including central nervous system bleeding. Low-dose heparin increased the risk of nonserious bleeding compared with placebo over the treatment period of 0-6 days.

DRUG INTERACTIONS: Drug-Drug Interactions: Caution should be employed when XIGRIS is used with other drugs that affect hemostasis. Low-dose heparin for venous thrombotic event (VTE) prophylaxis may be coadministered with drotrecogin alfa (activated).

In a randomized study comparing heparin and placebo in 1935 adult severe sepsis patients treated with drotrecogin alfa (activated), prophylactic low-dose heparin did not affect mortality, adversely affect the efficacy of drotrecogin alfa (activated) or increase the risk of serious haemorrhagic events, including central nervous system bleeding. The incidence of nonserious bleeding events was increased by prophylactic low-dose heparin. Prophylactic low-dose heparin, if already used, should not be discontinued when XIGRIS [drotrecogin alfa (activated)] is added to the treatment of patients with severe sepsis (see Warnings and Precautions and Adverse Reactions, Clinical Trial Adverse Drug Reactions).

Drug-Food Interactions: Interactions with food have not been established.

Drug-Herb Interactions: Interactions with herbal products have not been established.

Drug-Laboratory Interactions: For interactions between XIGRIS and laboratory tests, see Warnings and Precautions, Monitoring and Laboratory Tests.

Table 3: XIGRIS
Number of Patients Experiencing a Serious Bleeding Event by Site of Hemorrhage During Study Drug Infusion[a] and 28-day Study Period

	Infusion Period			28-day Study Period		
	Phase 2 and PROWESS Trials (placebo-controlled)		ENHANCE (single-arm trial)	Phase 2 and PROWESS Trials (placebo-controlled)		ENHANCE (single-arm trial)
Site of Hemorrhage	XIGRIS (N=940)	Placebo (N=881)	XIGRIS (N=2378)	XIGRIS (N=940)	Placebo (N=881)	XIGRIS (N=2378)
Gastrointestinal	7 (0.7%)	4 (0.5%)	19 (0.8%)	12 (1.3%)	10 (1.1%)	37 (1.6%)
Intra-abdominal	2 (0.2%)	3 (0.3%)	18 (0.8%)	3 (0.3%)	4 (0.5%)	28 (1.2%)
Intra-thoracic	4 (0.4%)	0	11 (0.5%)	6 (0.6%)	1 (0.1%)	20 (0.8%)
Retroperitoneal	3 (0.3%)	0	4 (0.2%)	4 (0.4%)	0	5 (0.2%)
CNS[b]	2 (0.2%)	0	15 (0.6%)	2 (0.2%)	1 (0.1%)	35 (1.5%)
Genitourinary	2 (0.2%)	0	0	2 (0.2%)	0	0
Skin/Soft Tissue	2 (0.2%)	0	16 (0.7%)	3 (0.3%)	0	23 (1.0%)
Nasopharyngeal	0	0	4 (0.2%)	0	0	5 (0.2%)
Joint/Bone	0	0	1 (0.04%)	0	0	3 (0.1%)
Site Unknown[c]	1 (0.1%)	1 (0.1%)	6 (0.3%)	2 (0.2%)	2 (0.2%)	10 (0.4%)
Total	23 (2.4%)[e]	8 (0.9%)	85[d] (3.6%)	34 (3.6%)	18 (2.0%)	155 (6.5%)

[a] Study drug infusion period is defined as the date of initiation of study drug to the date of study drug discontinuation plus the next calendar day.
[b] CNS bleeding includes any bleed in the central nervous system including the following types of hemorrhage—petechial, parenchymal, subarachnoid, subdural, and stroke with hemorrhagic transformation.
[c] Patients requiring the administration of ≥3 units of packed red blood cells per day for 2 consecutive days without an identified site of bleeding.
[d] In ENHANCE six patients experienced multiple serious bleeding events during the study drug infusion period (94 events observed in 85 patients).
[e] Statistically significantly different from placebo.

Table 4: XIGRIS
Serious Bleeding Event Rates in ADDRESS

	Study Drug Infusion Period[b]		28-Day Study Period	
	XIGRIS N=1317	Placebo N=1293	XIGRIS N=1317	Placebo N=1293
Serious bleeding events[a]	31 (2.4%)[d]	15 (1.2%)	51 (3.9%)[d]	28 (2.2%)
CNS bleeding events[c]	4 (0.3%)	3 (0.2%)	6 (0.5%)	5 (0.4%)
Fatal CNS bleeding events	0	1 (0.1%)	2 (0.2%)	1(0.1%)

[a] Serious bleeding events included any fatal bleed, any life threatening bleed, any CNS bleed, or any bleeding event assessed as serious by the investigator.
[b] Study drug infusion period is defined as study Day 0 through study Day 6.
[c] CNS bleeding includes any bleed in the central nervous system, including the following types of hemorrhage—petechial, parenchymal, subarachnoid, subdural, and stroke with hemorrhagic transformation.
[d] Statistically significantly different from placebo.

DOSAGE AND ADMINISTRATION: **Dosing Considerations:**

- In adult patients with severe sepsis, differences were detected in the plasma clearance of XIGRIS [drotrecogin alfa (activated)] with regard to age, gender, obesity, hepatic and renal dysfunction, or co-administration of low-dose heparin. However, the magnitude of these changes is not considered to be clinically significant and therefore dose adjustment is not required based on these factors alone or in combination.
- The pharmacokinetics of XIGRIS has not been studied in patients with severe sepsis and pre-existing end-stage renal disease or chronic hepatic disease.
- If the infusion is interrupted for any reason, XIGRIS should be restarted at the 24 µg/kg/h infusion rate and continued to complete the recommended duration of infusion. Dose adjustments or bolus doses of XIGRIS are not recommended.
- **In the event of serious bleeding, immediately stop the infusion.**

Recommended Dose and Dosage Adjustment: XIGRIS should be administered intravenously at an infusion rate of 24 µg/kg/h (based on actual body weight) for a total duration of infusion of 96 hours.

Administration: XIGRIS must be administered with an IV infusion pump or syringe pump.

Re-administration: There have been no Lilly-sponsored clinical trials in severe sepsis specifically studying drotrecogin alfa (activated) re-administration. There is very limited information regarding re-administration of drotrecogin alfa (activated) in severe sepsis patients. (See Warnings and Precautions and Action and Clinical Pharmacology.)

Reconstitution: Prior to administration, XIGRIS must be reconstituted with Sterile Water for Injection. The solution of reconstituted XIGRIS must be further diluted into an infusion bag containing sterile 0.9% Sodium Chloride Injection.

Co-administration of XIGRIS solution with other IV crystalloid solutions (0.9% Sodium Chloride Injection (isotonic saline), Lactated Ringer's Injection, or Dextrose and Saline mixtures) is acceptable.

Preparation and Administration: Use aseptic technique.

1. Use appropriate aseptic technique during the preparation of XIGRIS for intravenous administration.
2. Calculate the dose and the number of XIGRIS vials needed. Each XIGRIS vial delivers 5 mg or 20 mg of XIGRIS. The vial contains an excess XIGRIS to facilitate delivery of the label amount.
3. Prior to administration, 5 mg vials of XIGRIS must be reconstituted with 2.5 mL Sterile Water for Injection, USP, and 20 mg vials of XIGRIS must be reconstituted with 10 mL of Sterile Water for Injection, USP. The resulting concentration of the solution is approximately 2 mg/mL of XIGRIS. Slowly add the Sterile Water for Injection to the vial and avoid inverting or shaking the vial. Gently swirl each vial until the powder is completely dissolved.
4. The solution of reconstituted XIGRIS must be further diluted with sterile 0.9% Sodium Chloride Injection. Slowly withdraw the appropriate amount of reconstituted XIGRIS solution from the vial. Add the reconstituted XIGRIS into a prepared infusion bag of sterile 0.9% Sodium Chloride Injection. When adding the XIGRIS into the infusion bag, direct the stream to the side of the bag to minimize the agitation of the solution. Gently invert the infusion bag to obtain a homogeneous solution. Do not transport the infusion bag between locations using mechanical delivery systems. For a summary of the reconstitution and dilution details, refer to Table 7 and Table 8.
5. Because XIGRIS contains no antibacterial preservatives, the intravenous solution should be prepared **immediately** upon reconstitution of the XIGRIS in the vial(s). If the vial of reconstituted XIGRIS is not used immediately, it may be kept at controlled room temperature 15 to 30°C, but must be used within 3 hours. After preparation in an IV bag, the intravenous solution must be used at controlled room temperature within 12 hours. If the intravenous solution is not administered immediately, the solution should be refrigerated for up to 12 hours; the total in-use time for the intravenous infusion bag solution, including dilution, refrigeration, and administration, should not exceed 24 hours.
6. Parenteral drug products should be inspected visually for particulate matter and discoloration prior to administration.
7. When using an intravenous infusion pump to administer the drug the solution of reconstituted XIGRIS is typically diluted into an infusion bag containing sterile 0.9% Sodium Chloride Injection to a final concentration of between 100 µg/mL and 200 µg/mL.
8. Confirm that the intended bag volume will result in an acceptable final concentration.
   Final concentration, mg/mL = (actual XIGRIS amount, mg) ÷ (bag volume, mL)
   If the calculated final concentration is not between 0.1 mg/mL and 0.2 mg/mL, select a different bag volume and recalculate the final concentration.
9. Calculate the actual duration of the infusion period for the diluted XIGRIS.
   Infusion period, hours = [(actual XIGRIS amount, mg)] × 1000 ÷ (patient weight, kg) ÷ 24 µg/kg/hr.
   Account for the added volume of reconstituted XIGRIS (0.5 mL per mg of XIGRIS used) and the volume of bag saline solution removed (if saline solution is removed prior to adding the reconstituted XIGRIS). Final bag volume, mL= starting bag volume, mL + reconstituted XIGRIS volume, mL − saline volume removed (if any), mL
   Calculate the actual infusion rate of the diluted XIGRIS. Infusion rate, mL/hr = final bag volume, mL ÷ infusion period, hours
   Note: After preparation in an IV bag, the intravenous solution must be used at controlled room temperature within 12 hours.
10. When using a syringe pump to administer the drug, the solution of reconstituted XIGRIS should be diluted with sterile 0.9% Sodium Chloride Injection to a final concentration of between 100 µg/mL and 200 µg/mL. Invert and/or rotate the syringe to obtain a homogeneous solution, but avoid excessive agitation. When administering XIGRIS at low flow rates (less than approximately 5 mL/hr), the infusion set must be primed for approximately 15 minutes at a flow rate of approximately 5 mL/hr.
11. Confirm that the intended solution volume will result in an acceptable final concentration.
    Final concentration, mg/mL = (actual XIGRIS amount, mg) ÷ (solution volume, mL)
    If the calculated final concentration is not between 0.1 mg/mL and 0.2 mg/mL, select a different volume and recalculate the final concentration.
12. Calculate the actual duration of the infusion period for the diluted XIGRIS
    Infusion period, hours = [(actual XIGRIS amount, mg)] × 1000 ÷ (patient weight, kg) ÷ 24 µg/kg/hr.
13. After preparation in a syringe, the intravenous solution should be used at room temperature (15 to 30°C) within 12 hours. If the intravenous solution is not administered immediately, the solution should be refrigerated at 2 to 8ºC for up to 12 hours. If the prepared solution is refrigerated prior to administration, the maximum time limit for use of the intravenous solution, including dilution, refrigeration, and administration, is 24 hours.
14. XIGRIS should be administered via a dedicated intravenous line or a dedicated lumen of a multilumen central venous catheter. The **ONLY** other solutions that can be administered through the same line are 0.9% Sodium Chloride Injection, Lactated Ringer's Injection, Dextrose, or Dextrose and Saline mixtures.
15. Avoid exposing XIGRIS solutions to heat and/or direct sunlight. No incompatibilities have been observed between XIGRIS and glass infusion bottles or infusion bags and syringes made of polyvinylchloride, polyethylene, polypropylene, or polyolefin.

Table 5: XIGRIS
Adverse Events Occurring in ≥5% of XIGRIS-Treated Patients[a]

	Study Drug Infusion Period[b]		28-Day Study Period	
Body System/ Adverse Event	XIGRIS (N=940)	Placebo (N=881)	XIGRIS (N=940)	Placebo (N=881)
Body as a Whole				
Infection	—	—	99 (10.5%)	99 (11.2%)
Sepsis	—	—	49 (5.2%)	43 (4.9%)
Pain	—	—	50 (5.3%)	40 (4.5%)
Cardiovascular				
Atrial Fibrillation	54 (5.7%)	56 (6.4%)	75 (8.0%)	75 (8.5%)
Digestive System				
Diarrhea	69 (7.3%)	54 (6.1%)	140 (14.9%)	115 (13.1%)
Vomiting	—	—	52 (5.5%)	41 (4.7%)

(cont'd)

Table 5: XIGRIS *(cont'd)*

Adverse Events Occurring in ≥5% of XIGRIS-Treated Patients[a]

Body System/ Adverse Event	Study Drug Infusion Period[b] XIGRIS (N=940)	Placebo (N=881)	28-Day Study Period XIGRIS (N=940)	Placebo (N=881)
Nausea	—	—	49 (5.2%)	39 (4.4%)
Hematologic and Lymphatic System				
Anemia	53 (5.6%)	42 (4.8%)	70 (7.4%)	61 (6.9%)
Metabolic				
Generalized Edema	—	—	49 (5.2%)	44 (5.0%)
Hypokalemia	—	—	47 (5.0%)	43 (4.9%)
Nervous System				
Confusion	—	—	68 (7.2%)	52 (5.9%)
Agitation	—	—	51 (5.4%)	68 (7.7%)
Respiratory System				
Pleural Effusion	—	—	72 (7.7%)	84 (9.5%)
Pneumonia	—	—	73 (7.8%)	63 (7.2%)
Skin and Appendages				
Rash	—	—	112 (11.9%)	121 (13.7%)
Skin Ulcer	—	—	68 (7.2%)	54 (6.1%)
Urogenital System				
Urinary Tract Infection	—	—	51 (5.4%)	52 (5.9%)

[a] None of the differences in event rates between XIGRIS and Placebo treatment were statistically significant.
[b] There were only three non-bleeding events that occurred in >5% of patients treated with XIGRIS during the study drug infusion period.

Table 6: XIGRIS

Bleeding Event Rates in XPRESS

	Study Drug Infusion Period		28-Day Study Period	
	Heparin plus XIGRIS N=976	Placebo plus XIGRIS N=959	Heparin plus XIGRIS N=976	Placebo plus XIGRIS N=959
Overall bleeding (serious and non-serious) events	105 (10.8%)[c]	78 (8.1%)	121 (12.4%)	105 (10.9%)
Serious bleeding events[a]	22 (2.3%)	24 (2.5%)	38 (3.9%)	50 (5.2%)
CNS bleeding events[b]	3 (0.3%)	3 (0.3%)	10 (1.0%)	7 (0.7%)

[a] Serious bleeding events included any fatal bleed, any life threatening bleed, any CNS bleed, or any bleeding event assessed as serious by the investigator.
[b] CNS bleeding includes any bleed in the central nervous system, including the following types of hemorrhage—petechial, parenchymal, subarachnoid, subdural, and stroke with hemorrhagic transformation.
[c] Statistically significantly different from placebo.

Table 7: XIGRIS

Dilution Table for Use with Infusion Pump

Vial Size (mg)	Volume of Sterile Water for Injection to be Added to Vial (mL)	Approximate Available Volume for Withdrawal (mL)	Diluents to be Used for Reconstitution	Solutions Which Can Be Administrated via the Same IV Line	Recommended Final Concentration per mL[a]
5	2.5	2.5	Sterile Water for Injection	0.9% Sodium Chloride for Injection; Lactated Ringer's Solution; Dextrose; Dextrose-saline mixtures	100–200 µg/mL
20	10	10			

[a] Refer to steps 8 & 9 for detailed instructions.

Table 8: XIGRIS

Dilution Table for Use with Syringe Pump

Vial Size (mg)	Volume of Sterile Water to be Added to Vial (mL)	Approximate Available Volume for Withdrawal (mL)	Diluents to be Used for Reconstitution	Solutions Which Can Be Administrated via the Same IV Line	Recommended Final Concentration per mL[a]
5	2.5	2.5	Sterile Water for Injection	0.9% Sodium Chloride for Injection; Lactated Ringer's Solution; Dextrose; Dextrose-saline mixtures	100–200 µg/mL
20	10	10			

[a] Refer to steps 11 & 12 for detailed instructions.

OVERDOSAGE:
In the post-marketing experience, accidental overdoses have been reported. Adverse events associated with the overdose have been observed. The observed adverse events were consistent with known effects of the drug and/or sequelae of the underlying condition of sepsis.

There is no known antidote for XIGRIS. In case of overdose, immediately stop the infusion and monitor closely for hemorrhagic complications (see Action and Clinical Pharmacology).

For management of a suspected drug overdose, CPhA recommends that you contact your **regional Poison Control Centre**. See the *CPS* Directory section for a list of Poison Control Centres.

ACTION AND CLINICAL PHARMACOLOGY: Mechanism of Action: Drotrecogin alfa (activated) is a recombinant version of Activated Protein C and is produced by genetic engineering from an established human cell line.

Severe sepsis, defined as sepsis associated with acute organ dysfunction, results from the activation of multiple inflammatory pathways recognized clinically as the systemic inflammatory response syndrome (SIRS). More specifically, sepsis induces a procoagulant, inflammatory and antifibrinolytic state; both the procoagulant and antifibrinolytic responses to infection are tightly linked to inflammation; proinflammatory cytokines (e.g., tumour necrosis factor, interleukin-1) are capable of activating coagulation and impairing fibrinolysis.

The specific mechanisms by which Activated Protein C exerts its effect on survival in patients with severe sepsis are not completely understood. Microcirculation is dependent on a homeostatic balance between procoagulant and anticoagulant pathways, and interactions between leukocytes and the endothelium. It is hypothesized that Activated Protein C adjusts this balance by affecting several pathways. In vivo, thrombin binds to endothelial thrombomodulin, which converts Protein C to Activated Protein C. Thrombin is also one of many factors capable of stimulating multiple inflammatory and antifibrinolytic pathways. Activated Protein C exerts an antithrombotic effect by inhibiting Factors Va and VIIIa, key factors in the coagulation cascade. In vitro data also indicate that therapeutic concentrations of Activated Protein C exert an anti-inflammatory effect by limiting the chemotactic response of leukocytes to inflammatory cytokines, an inhibitory process mediated by the leukocyte cell surface Activated Protein C receptor. In addition, in vivo data using therapeutic doses of Activated Protein C show reduced interactions between leukocytes and the microvascular endothelium while other leukocyte functions, such as bacterial phagocytosis, are not affected. At supra-therapeutic concentrations, in vitro data also indicate that Activated Protein C has indirect profibrinolytic activity due to its ability to inhibit plasminogen activator inhibitor-1 (PAI-1). In sepsis, Protein C concentrations decrease rapidly; observational studies have shown that decreased Protein C is associated with increased morbidity and mortality.

Pharmacodynamics: In two placebo-controlled trials by Derhaschnig et al. and Kalil et al., in a total of 42 healthy subjects receiving a single dose of intravenous endotoxin, drotrecogin alfa (activated) did not inhibit the early cytokine response (as measured by TNF, IL-1, IL-6, IL-8) to endotoxin. In the study by Kalil et al. (n=17), drotrecogin alfa (activated) prevented the development of endotoxin-induced hypotension. In another placebo-controlled trial by Nick et al., in 16 healthy subjects receiving a single dose of intra-pulmonary endotoxin, drotrecogin alfa (activated) did not inhibit the early cytokine response to endotoxin, but decreased neutrophil accumulation in the alveolar space. Drotrecogin alfa (activated) did not reduce the endotoxin-induced elevation of PAI-1 levels in these three placebo-controlled studies in healthy subjects.

In placebo controlled clinical trials in patients with severe sepsis, drotrecogin alfa (activated) exerted an antithrombotic effect by limiting thrombin generation and improved sepsis-associated coagulopathy, as shown by a more rapid improvement in markers of coagulation and fibrinolysis. Compared to placebo, drotrecogin alfa (activated) caused a more rapid decline in thrombotic markers such as D-dimer, prothrombin F1.2, and thrombin-antithrombin levels and a more rapid increase in Protein C and antithrombin levels. Drotrecogin alfa (activated) also restored endogenous fibrinolytic potential, as evidenced by a more rapid trend toward normalization in plasminogen levels and a more rapid decline in PAI-1 levels. Additionally, patients with severe sepsis treated with drotrecogin alfa (activated) had a more rapid decline in IL-6 levels indicating a reduction in the inflammatory response. Drotrecogin alfa (activated) had no effect on TNF, IL-1, IL-8, and IL-10 levels compared to placebo.

In healthy subjects, administration of drotrecogin alfa (activated) produced a dose-proportional increase in the bedside whole blood activated partial thromboplastin time (APTT). Following cessation of a 24 µg/kg/h infusion of drotrecogin alfa (activated), the average time for the APTT response to fall to within 25% of the pre-dose (baseline) value was 53 minutes. Administration of drotrecogin alfa (activated) to healthy subjects was associated with a prolongation of less than 3 seconds in the bedside whole blood prothrombin time (PT).

Pharmacokinetics: Drotrecogin alfa (activated) and endogenous human Activated Protein C are inactivated by endogenous plasma protease inhibitors; the mechanism by which these are cleared from plasma is unknown in humans. Plasma concentrations of endogenous Activated Protein C in healthy subjects and patients with severe sepsis are usually below detection limits and do not influence the pharmacokinetics of drotrecogin alfa (activated).

Absorption and Distribution: In healthy subjects, greater than 90% of the steady-state plasma concentration is attained within 2 hours following the start of a constant-rate intravenous infusion of drotrecogin alfa (activated). Plasma Activated Protein C steady-state concentrations (C_{ss}) are proportional to the infusion rate over a range of infusion rates from 12 µg/kg/h to 48 µg/kg/h. The mean steady-state plasma concentration of drotrecogin alfa (activated) in healthy subjects receiving 24 µg/kg/h is 72 ng/mL.

In patients with severe sepsis, drotrecogin alfa (activated) infusions of 12 µg/kg/h to 30 µg/kg/h rapidly produce steady state concentrations that are proportional to infusion rates. The median C_{ss} of 45 ng/mL (interquartile range of 35 to 62 ng/mL) was attained within 2 hours after starting infusion. The mean C_{ss} (±standard deviation), after censoring of the data to remove abnormally high outlier values, was 53.7±34.1 ng/mL.

Metabolism: For healthy patients, following the completion of an infusion, the decline in plasma Activated Protein C concentration is biphasic and is comprised of a rapid initial phase ($t_{1/2\alpha}$=13 minutes) and a slower second phase ($t_{1/2\beta}$=1.6 hours). The short half-life of 13 minutes accounts for approximately 80% of the area under the plasma concentration curve and governs the initial rapid accrual of plasma Activated Protein C concentrations towards the steady-state.

Excretion: In the Phase 3 trial, in patients with severe sepsis, the median clearance of drotrecogin alfa (activated) was 40 L/h (interquartile range of 27 to 52 L/h). In the majority of patients, plasma concentrations of drotrecogin alfa (activated) fell below the assay's quantitation limit of 10 ng/mL within 2 hours after stopping the infusion. Plasma clearance of drotrecogin alfa (activated) in patients with severe sepsis is approximately 50% higher than that in healthy subjects. This may reflect the higher levels of endogenous plasma protease inhibitors associated with sepsis, although this has not been confirmed.

Additional Information on Immunogenicity: In adult patients in severe sepsis clinical studies, the frequency of anti-human Activated Protein C IgA/IgG/IgM antibodies or neutralizing antibodies is low and is similar between drotrecogin alfa (activated)- and placebo-treated patients tested. No apparent correlation of antibody development to adverse reactions was observed. There was no evidence that the antibodies detected represented a specific immune response to drotrecogin alfa (activated) therapy.

Samples available from six adult severe sepsis patients who had received a prior course of drotrecogin alfa (activated) were subsequently tested and all were negative for anti-human Activated Protein C antibody (see Warnings and Precautions and Dosage and Administration).

Special Populations and Conditions: In adult patients with severe sepsis, differences were detected in the plasma clearance of drotrecogin alfa (activated) with regard to age, gender, obesity and hepatic and renal dysfunction. However, the magnitude of these changes is not considered to be clinically significant and therefore dose adjustment is not required based on these factors alone or in combination (see Dosage and Administration).

Pediatrics: Safety and efficacy have not been established in pediatric patients. Therefore XIGRIS is not recommended for use in pediatric patients. The limited data available in pediatric patients indicate that the pharmacokinetics of an infusion of drotrecogin alfa (activated) at a rate of 24 µg/kg/h appear to be similar to that in adult patients with severe sepsis (see Indications and Clinical Use, Warnings and Precautions and Adverse Reactions).

Geriatrics: In clinical studies evaluating 1821 adult patients with severe sepsis, approximately 50% of the patients were 65 years or older. No overall differences in safety or effectiveness were observed between these patients and younger patients (see Adverse Reactions).

Hepatic Insufficiency: The pharmacokinetics of drotrecogin alfa (activated) has not been studied in patients with severe sepsis and pre-existing end-stage chronic hepatic disease (see Warnings and Precautions, Hepatic).

Renal Insufficiency: The pharmacokinetics of drotrecogin alfa (activated) has not been studied in patients with severe sepsis and pre-existing end-stage renal disease (see Warnings and Precautions, Renal).

Patients with end-stage renal disease requiring chronic renal replacement therapy were excluded from the Phase 3 study. In patients without sepsis undergoing hemodialysis (n=6), plasma clearance (mean±SD) of drotrecogin alfa (activated) administered on non-dialysis days was 30±8 L/h. Plasma clearance of drotrecogin alfa (activated) was 23±4 L/h in patients without sepsis undergoing peritoneal dialysis (n=5). These clearance rates did not meaningfully differ from those in normal healthy subjects (28±9 L/h) (n=190).

STORAGE AND STABILITY: XIGRIS [drotrecogin alfa (activated)] should be stored in a refrigerator (2 to 8°C). Do not freeze. Protect unreconstituted vials of XIGRIS from light by retaining the vial in the carton until time of use.

SPECIAL HANDLING INSTRUCTIONS: Avoid exposing XIGRIS [drotrecogin alfa (activated)] solutions to heat and/or direct sunlight. Because XIGRIS contains no antibacterial preservatives, the IV solution should be prepared **immediately** upon reconstitution of the XIGRIS in the vial(s). If the vial of reconstituted XIGRIS is not used immediately, it may be stored at room temperature (15 to 30°C), but must be used within 3 hours. After preparation in an IV bag, the intravenous solution must be used at controlled room temperature within 12 hours. If the intravenous solution is not administered immediately, the solution should be refrigerated for up to 12 hours; the total in-use time for the infusion bag solution, including dilution, refrigeration, and administration, should not exceed 24 hours. After preparation in a syringe, the intravenous solution must be used at controlled room temperature within 12 hours.

INFORMATION FOR THE PATIENT: Published in e-CPS, available by subscription at www.e-cps.ca.

DOSAGE FORMS, COMPOSITION AND PACKAGING: 5 mg: Each single-use vial of sterile, preservative-free, lyophilized white to practically-white powder for intravenous infusion contains: drotrecogin alfa (activated) 5 mg. Other ingredients include sucrose, sodium chloride, citrate (buffer system composed of citric acid, sodium citrate, hydrochloric acid and sodium hydroxide), hydrochloric acid, if necessary, and sodium hydroxide, if necessary.

20 mg: Each single-use vial of sterile, preservative-free, lyophilized white to practically-white powder for intravenous infusion contains: drotrecogin alfa (activated) 20 mg. Other ingredients include sucrose, sodium chloride, citrate (buffer system composed of citric acid, sodium citrate, hydrochloric acid and sodium hydroxide), hydrochloric acid, if necessary, and sodium hydroxide, if necessary.

Xolair® Ⓟ

omalizumab

IgE-Neutralizing Antibody (Anti-IgE)

Novartis Pharmaceuticals

Date of Preparation: November 18, 2004
Date of Revision: February 5, 2010

SUMMARY PRODUCT INFORMATION:

Route of Administration	Dosage Form/ Strength	Clinically Relevant Nonmedicinal Ingredients
Subcutaneous	Sterile powder for reconstitution 150 mg vial	Sucrose, L-histidine hydrochloride monohydrate, L-histidine and polysorbate 20

INDICATIONS AND CLINICAL USE: XOLAIR (omalizumab) is indicated for adults and adolescents (12 years of age and above) with moderate to severe persistent asthma who have a positive skin test or in vitro reactivity to a perennial aeroallergen and whose symptoms are inadequately controlled with inhaled corticosteroids. Xolair has been shown to significantly decrease the incidence of asthma exacerbations and improve control of asthma symptoms in these patients. Safety and efficacy have not been established in other allergic conditions.

CONTRAINDICATIONS: XOLAIR (omalizumab) should not be administered to patients with known hypersensitivity to omalizumab or any component of the formulation (see Summary Product Information), or patients who have experienced a severe hypersensitivity reaction to XOLAIR (see Warnings and Precautions, Anaphylaxis).

WARNINGS AND PRECAUTIONS:

Serious Warnings and Precautions

Anaphylaxis, presenting as angioedema of the throat or tongue, bronchospasm, hypotension, syncope, and/or urticaria has been reported to occur after administration of XOLAIR. Anaphylaxis has occurred as early as after the first dose of XOLAIR, but also has occurred beyond 1 year after beginning regularly administered treatment. Because of the risk of anaphylaxis, patients should be closely observed for an appropriate period of time after XOLAIR administration, and health care providers administering XOLAIR should be prepared to manage anaphylaxis that can be life-threatening. Patients should also be informed of the signs and symptoms of anaphylaxis and instructed to seek immediate medical care should symptoms occur (see Warnings and Precautions, Information to Be Provided to the Patient).

General: XOLAIR (omalizumab) has not been shown to alleviate asthma exacerbations acutely and should not be used for the treatment of acute bronchospasm or status asthmaticus.

Patients with diabetes mellitus, the glucose-galactose malabsorption syndrome, fructose intolerance or sucrose-isomaltase deficiency should be warned that XOLAIR contains 145 mg of sucrose (0.5 calories or 2.3 Joules) per vial.

Anaphylaxis: Anaphylaxis has been reported to occur after administration of XOLAIR in premarketing clinical trials and in post-marketing spontaneous reports. Signs and symptoms in these reported cases have included angioedema of the throat or tongue, bronchospasm, hypotension, syncope, and/or urticaria. Some of these events have been life-threatening. In premarketing clinical trials the frequency of anaphylaxis attributed to XOLAIR use was estimated to be 0.1%. In postmarketing spontaneous reports, the frequency of anaphylaxis attributed to XOLAIR use was estimated to be at least 0.2% of patients based on an estimated exposure of about 57 300 patients from June 2003 through December 2006. Anaphylaxis and anaphylactoid reactions have been reported following the first or subsequent administrations of XOLAIR. Although most of these reactions occurred within 2 hours, some occurred beyond 2 hours. Anaphylaxis has occurred as early as after the first dose of XOLAIR, but also has occurred beyond one year after beginning regularly scheduled treatment.

XOLAIR should only be administered in a healthcare setting by healthcare providers prepared to manage anaphylaxis that can be life-threatening. Patients should be closely observed for an appropriate period of time after administration of XOLAIR, taking into account the time to onset of anaphylaxis seen in premarketing clinical trials and postmarketing spontaneous reports (see Adverse Reactions). Patients should be informed of the signs and symptoms of anaphylaxis, and instructed to seek immediate medical care should signs or symptoms occur (see Information to Be Provided to the Patient).

XOLAIR should be discontinued in patients who experience a severe hypersensitivity reaction (see Contraindications).

Cerebrovascular Disorders: In controlled clinical trials in adults and adolescents 12 years of age and older, cerebrovascular events including transient ischaemic attack and ischaemic stroke were observed in patients treated with XOLAIR. (See Adverse Reactions).

Corticosteroid Reduction: Systemic or inhaled corticosteroids should not be abruptly discontinued upon initiation of XOLAIR therapy. Decreases in corticosteroids should be performed under the direct supervision of a physician and may need to be performed gradually.

Immune: Churg-Strauss Syndrome and Hypereosinophilic Syndrome : Patients with severe asthma may rarely present systemic hypereosinophilic syndrome or allergic eosinophilic granulomatous vasculitis (Churg-Strauss syndrome), both of which are usually treated with systemic corticosteroids. In rare cases, patients on therapy with anti-asthma agents, including omalizumab, may present or develop systemic eosinophilia and vasculitis. These events are commonly associated with the reduction of oral corticosteroid therapy. In these patients, physicians should be alert to the development of marked eosinophilia, vasculitic rash, worsening pulmonary symptoms, paranasal sinus abnormalities, cardiac complications, and/or neuropathy.

Serum Sickness: Serum sickness and serum sickness-like reactions, which are delayed allergic type III reactions, have rarely been seen in patients treated with humanized monoclonal antibodies including omalizumab. The onset has typically been 1-5 days after administration of the first or subsequent injections, also after long duration of treatment. Symptoms suggestive of serum sickness include arthritis/arthralgia, rash (urticaria or other forms), fever and lymphadenopathy. Antihistamines and corticosteroids may be useful for preventing or treating this disorder, and patients should be advised to report any suspected symptoms.

Immunogenicity: As with all DNA derived humanized monoclonal antibodies patients may rarely (1 out of 1723 patients, <0.1%) develop antibodies to omalizumab.

Discontinuation of omalizumab should be considered in all severe cases of Churg-Strauss syndrome, hypereosinophilic syndrome and serum sickness.

Information to Be Provided to the Patient: Patients should be advised of the risk of life-threatening anaphylaxis with XOLAIR and that there have been reports of anaphylaxis up to 4 days after administration of XOLAIR. XOLAIR should only be administered in a healthcare setting by healthcare providers. Patients should be closely observed following its administration. Patients should be informed of the signs and symptoms of anaphylaxis. Patients should be instructed to seek immediate medical care should such signs or symptoms occur. (see Warnings and Precautions, Anaphylaxis).

Patients receiving XOLAIR should be instructed not to decrease the dose of or stop taking any other asthma medications unless otherwise instructed by their physician. Patients should be told that they may not see immediate improvement in their asthma after beginning XOLAIR therapy.

Patients receiving XOLAIR should be informed that if they experience dizziness, fatigue, syncope or somnolence, they should not drive or use machines.

Malignancy: During clinical trials, there was a numerical imbalance in malignancies arising in the active treatment group, compared with the control group. The frequency of observed cases was uncommon (less than 1 out of 100) in both the active and the control group (see Adverse Reactions). The diversity in the type of cancers observed, the relatively short duration of exposure and the clinical features of the individual cases render a causal relationship unlikely. The overall observed incidence rate of malignancy in the XOLAIR clinical trial program was comparable to that reported in the general population.

Other IgE-associated Disorders: XOLAIR has not been studied in patients with hyperimmunoglobulin E syndrome, allergic bronchopulmonary aspergillosis, or for the prevention of anaphylactic reactions. XOLAIR has not been adequately studied in food allergy, atopic dermatitis, allergic rhinitis, or parasitic infestations.

Parasitic (Helminth) Infections: IgE may be involved in the immunological response to some helminth infections. In patients at chronic high risk of helminth infection, a placebo-controlled trial showed a slight increase in infection rate with omalizumab, although the course, severity, and response to treatment of infection were unaltered. The helminth infection rate in the overall clinical programme, which was not designed to detect such infections, was less than 1 in 1000 patients. However, caution may be warranted in patients at high risk of helminth infection, in particular when travelling to areas where helminthic infections are endemic. If patients do not respond to recommended anti-helminth treatment, discontinuation of XOLAIR should be considered.

Special Populations: Pregnant Women: IgG molecules are known to cross the placental barrier. The safety and efficacy of XOLAIR in pregnant women has not been established. Because animal reproduction studies are not always predictive of human response, XOLAIR should be used during pregnancy only if clearly needed.

Reproduction studies in cynomolgus monkeys have been conducted with omalizumab. Subcutaneous doses up to 75 mg/kg (12-fold the maximum clinical dose) of omalizumab did not elicit maternal toxicity, embryotoxicity, or teratogenicity when administered throughout organogenesis and did not elicit adverse effects on fetal or neonatal growth when administered throughout late gestation, delivery, and nursing.

Nursing Women: While XOLAIR presence in human milk has not been studied, IgG is excreted in human milk and therefore it is expected that XOLAIR will be present in human milk. The potential for XOLAIR absorption or harm to the infant are unknown; caution should be exercised when administering XOLAIR to a nursing woman.

The excretion of omalizumab in milk was evaluated in female cynomolgus monkeys receiving s.c. doses of 75 mg/kg/week. Neonatal plasma levels of omalizumab after in utero exposure and 28 days of nursing were between 11% and 94% of the maternal plasma level. Milk levels of omalizumab were 1.5% of maternal blood concentration.

Although no clinically significant effects on platelets have been observed in patients, doses of omalizumab in excess of the clinical dose have been associated with age-dependent decreases in blood platelets in non-human primates, with a greater relative sensitivity in juvenile animals. In reproduction studies in cynomolgus monkeys, there was no clinical evidence of thrombocytopenia in neonatal monkeys from mothers treated up to 75 mg/kg omalizumab; however, platelet counts were not measured in these offspring.

Pediatrics (<12 years of age): The safety and efficacy of XOLAIR in children below the age of 12 have not been established and use of XOLAIR in such patients is therefore not recommended.

Geriatrics (>65 years of age): In clinical trials 145 patients 65 years of age or older were treated with XOLAIR. Although there were no apparent age-related differences observed in these studies, the number of patients aged 65 and over is not sufficient to determine whether they respond differently from younger patients.

Monitoring and Laboratory Tests: There has been no evidence of clinically significant abnormalities in laboratory tests following treatment with XOLAIR.

Serum total IgE levels increase following administration of XOLAIR due to formation of omalizumab:IgE complexes (see Action and Clinical Pharmacology and Dosage and Administration). Elevated serum total IgE levels may persist for up to 1 year following discontinuation of XOLAIR. Serum total IgE levels obtained less than 1 year following discontinuation may not reflect steady state free IgE levels and should not be used to reassess the dosing regimen.

ADVERSE REACTIONS: Adverse Drug Reaction Overview: The adverse reactions most commonly observed among patients treated with XOLAIR (omalizumab) in pre-marketing clinical studies included injection site reaction (45%), viral infections (24%), upper respiratory tract infection (19%), sinusitis (16%), headache (15%), and pharyngitis (10%). These events were observed at similar rates in XOLAIR-treated patients and control patients.

The occurrence of adverse events resulting in clinical intervention (e.g. discontinuation of XOLAIR, or the need for concomitant medication to treat an adverse reaction) was extremely small; 0.1 % or less.

The data described above reflect XOLAIR exposure for 2285 adult and adolescent patients ages 12 and older, including 1891 patients exposed for six months and 555 exposed for one year or more, in either placebo-controlled or other controlled asthma studies. The mean age of patients receiving XOLAIR was 41 years, 59% were women, and 86% Caucasian. Patients received XOLAIR 150 to 375 mg every 2 or 4 weeks or, for patients assigned to control groups, standard therapy with or without a placebo.

The frequency of adverse events was comparable between the XOLAIR and placebo groups (85.1% vs. 84.0%, respectively). The majority of these adverse events were regarded as mild or moderate in intensity. Treatment discontinuation due to an adverse event occurred more frequently in the placebo group compared with the XOLAIR-treated group (1.4% vs. 0.5%, respectively).

Table 1 shows adverse events that occurred ≥1% more frequently in patients receiving XOLAIR than in those receiving placebo in the placebo controlled asthma studies. Adverse events were classified using preferred terms from the International Medical Nomenclature (IMN) dictionary. Injection site reactions were recorded separately from the reporting of other adverse events and are described following the table.

Clinical Trial Adverse Drug Reactions:

Table 1: XOLAIR

All Adverse Events Occurring ≥1% More Frequently in XOLAIR-treated Asthma Patients 12 to 75 years of Age Compared with Placebo, Regardless of Causality Assessment

Adverse Event	XOLAIR (n=947) Number (%) of Patients Reporting the Event	Placebo (n=913) Number (%) of Patients Reporting the Event
Any Adverse Event	806 (85.1)	767 (84.0)
Body as a Whole		
Pain	51 (5.4)	40 (4.4)
Musculoskeletal System		
Fracture	20 (2.1)	10 (1.1)
Leg pain	26 (2.7)	14 (1.5)
Nervous System		
Dizziness	24 (2.5)	15 (1.5)

Less Common Adverse Drug Reactions (<1%): Allergic Events: As with any protein, local or systemic allergic reactions can occur (see Warnings and Precautions). Allergic symptoms, including urticaria, dermatitis, and pruritus were observed in patients treated with XOLAIR. There were 3 cases out of 3854 (<0.1%) of anaphylaxis observed within 2 hours of XOLAIR administration in which there were no other identifiable allergic triggers. Anaphylaxis occurred with the first dose of XOLAIR in two patients, and with the fourth dose in one patient. The time to onset of anaphylaxis was 90 minutes after administration in two patients and 2 hours after administration in one patient. These events included urticaria and throat and/or tongue edema. In the clinical studies the frequencies of all allergic-type events including anaphylaxis were similar in XOLAIR-treated patients and control patients.

Cerebrovascular: In controlled clinical trials in adults and adolescents 12 years of age and older, cerebrovascular events including transient ischaemic attack and ischaemic stroke were observed. There were 9 cerebrovascular events in 6 patients among 3605 patients treated with XOLAIR and one cerebrovascular event in a patient among 2383 patients receiving placebo. These 9 events in the XOLAIR treated patients were ischaemic strokes (n=2), dysarthria (n=1), paresis (n=4), amaurosis fugax (n=1), transient ischaemic attack (n=1); one of these patient had three episodes of paresis followed by an ischaemic stroke. The observed incidence rate of cerebrovascular events in the XOLAIR controlled clinical trials was comparable to that reported in the general asthma population.

Malignancies: During clinical trials, there was a numerical imbalance in malignancies arising in the active treatment group, compared with the control group. The number of observed cases was uncommon (<1/100) in both the active and the control group. Malignant neoplasms were observed in 25 of 5015 (0.5%) XOLAIR-treated patients compared with 5 of 2854 (0.2%) control patients in clinical studies of asthma and other allergic disorders. The diversity in the type of cancers observed, the relatively short duration of exposure and the clinical features of the individual cases render a causal relationship unlikely. The overall observed incidence rate of malignancy in the XOLAIR clinical trial program was comparable to that reported in the general population. The observed malignancies in XOLAIR-treated patients were a variety of types, with breast, non-melanoma skin, prostate, melanoma, and parotid occurring more than once, and five other types occurring once each.

Injection Site Reactions: Injection site reactions of any severity occurred at a rate of 45% in XOLAIR-treated patients compared with 43% in placebo-treated patients. The types of injection site reactions included: bruising, redness, warmth, burning, stinging, itching, hive formation, pain, indurations, mass, and inflammation. Most were regarded as mild or moderate in intensity and did not require discontinuation of therapy. Severe injection site reactions occurred more frequently in XOLAIR treated patients compared with patients in the placebo group (12% versus 9%).

The majority of injection site reactions occurred within 1 hour post injection, lasted less than 8 days, and generally decreased in frequency at subsequent dosing visits.

Asthma Exacerbations Leading to Hospitalizations: In the pivotal asthma studies, a statistically significant (six-fold) reduction in the number of hospitalizations due to serious asthma exacerbation was observed in the XOLAIR treated group compared to placebo group (13 vs 2, respectively, p=0.004).

Long-term Adverse Effects (Up to 1 Year): With long-term treatment, the adverse event profile did not significantly change and patients continued to tolerate XOLAIR well.

Post-Market Adverse Drug Reactions: The following reactions have been identified through spontaneous reportings.

Immune System Disorders: Anaphylaxis and anaphylactoid reactions have uncommonly been reported following the first or subsequent administrations; serum sickness has been rarely reported.

Anaphylaxis: Based on spontaneous reports and an estimated exposure of about 57 300 patients from June 2003 through December 2006, the frequency of anaphylaxis attributed to XOLAIR use was estimated to be at least 0.2% of patients. Diagnostic criteria of anaphylaxis were skin or mucosal tissue involvement, and, either airway compromise, and/or reduced blood pressure with or without associated symptoms, and a temporal relationship to XOLAIR administration with no other identifiable cause. Signs and symptoms in these reported cases included angioedema of the throat or tongue, bronchospasm, chest tightness, cough, cutaneous angioedema, dyspnea, hypotension, syncope, and/or urticaria. Pulmonary involvement was reported in 89% of the cases. Hypotension or syncope was reported in 14% of cases. A previous history of anaphylaxis unrelated to XOLAIR was reported in 24% of the cases.

Of the reported cases of anaphylaxis attributed to XOLAIR, 39% occurred with the first dose, 19% occurred with the second dose, 10% occurred after the third dose, and the rest after subsequent doses. One case occurred after 39 doses (after 19 months of continuous therapy followed by a 3 month gap, anaphylaxis occurred upon restarting). The time to onset of anaphylaxis in these cases was 30 minutes or less in 35%, 30 to less than 60 minutes in 16%, 60 to less than 90 minutes in 2%, 90 to less than 120 minutes in 6%, 2 hours to 6 hours in 5%, 6 to 12 hours in 14%, 12 to 24 hours in 8%, 24 hours to 48 hours in 2% and 48 hours to 4 days in 2%. In 9% of cases the times to onset were unknown.

Fifteen percent of the reported cases resulted in hospitalization. Twenty-three patients who experienced anaphylaxis were re-challenged with XOLAIR and 18 had a recurrence of similar symptoms of anaphylaxis. Four patients who received XOLAIR, from all reported anaphylaxis cases, experienced urticaria and upon re-exposure developed anaphylaxis.

Blood and Lymphatic System Disorders: idiopathic severe thrombocytopenia.

Musculoskeletal and Connective Tissue Disorders: arthralgia, myalgia, joint swelling.

Respiratory, Thoracic and Mediastinal Disorders: allergic granulomatous angiitis (i.e. Churg-Strauss syndrome).

Skin and Subcutaneous Disorders: alopecia.

DRUG INTERACTIONS: Overview: Cytochrome P450 enzymes, efflux pumps and protein binding mechanisms are not involved in the clearance of omalizumab; thus, there is little potential for drug-drug interactions. No formal drug interaction studies have been performed with XOLAIR (omalizumab). There is no pharmacological reason to expect that commonly prescribed medications used in the treatment of asthma will interact with omalizumab. In clinical studies XOLAIR was commonly used in conjunction with inhaled and oral corticosteroids, inhaled short-acting and long-acting beta agonists, leukotriene modifiers, theophyllines and oral antihistamines. There was no indication that safety of XOLAIR was altered with these other commonly used asthma medications. The concomitant use of XOLAIR and allergen immunotherapy has not been evaluated.

DOSAGE AND ADMINISTRATION:

Dosing Considerations: XOLAIR (omalizumab) 150 to 375 mg is administered s.c. every 2 or 4 weeks. See Table 2 and Table 3 for appropriate dose assignment. Doses (mg) and dosing frequency are determined by serum total IgE level (IU/mL), measured before the start of treatment, and body weight (kg). Doses of more than 150 mg are divided among more than one injection site to limit injections to not more than 150 mg per site. Because the solution is slightly viscous, the injection may take 5-10 seconds to administer.

The need for continued therapy should be periodically reassessed based upon the patient's disease severity and level of asthma control.

Recommended Dose and Dosage Adjustment: See Table 2 and Table 3.

Dosing Adjustments: Total IgE levels are elevated during treatment and remain elevated for up to one year after the discontinuation of treatment. Therefore, re testing of IgE levels during XOLAIR treatment cannot be used as a guide for dose determination. Dose determination after treatment interruptions lasting less than 1 year should be based on serum IgE levels obtained at the initial dose determination. Total serum IgE levels may be re tested for dose determination if treatment with XOLAIR has been interrupted for one year or more.

Doses should be adjusted for significant changes in body weight (See dosing charts under Recommended Dose and Dosage Adjustment).

Table 2: XOLAIR

Administration Every 4 weeks. XOLAIR Doses (mg per dose) Administered by Subcutaneous Injection Every 4 weeks

	Body Weight (kg)								
Baseline IgE[a]	**>20–30**	**>30–40**	**>40–50**	**>50–60**	**>60–70**	**>70–80**	**>80–90**	**>90–125**	**>125–150**
≥30–100 IU/mL or ≥72–240 ng/mL	150	150	150	150	150	150	150	300	300
>100–200 IU/mL or >240–480 ng/mL	150	150	300	300	300	300	300		
>200–300 IU/mL or >480–720 ng/mL	150	300	300	300					
>300–400 IU/mL or >720–960 ng/mL	300	300				See Table 3			
>400–500 IU/mL or >960–1200 ng/mL	300								
>500–600 IU/mL or >1200–1440 ng/mL	300								
>600–700 IU/mL or >1440–1680 ng/mL									

[a] 1 IU/mL=2.4 ng/mL=2.4 µg/L.

Table 3: XOLAIR

Administration Every 2 Weeks. XOLAIR Doses (mg per dose) Administered by Subcutaneous Injection Every 2 weeks

	Body Weight (kg)								
Baseline IgE[a]	**>20–30**	**>30–40**	**>40–50**	**>50–60**	**>60–70**	**>70–80**	**>80–90**	**>90-125**	**>125–150**
≥30–100 IU/mL or ≥72–240 ng/mL									
>100–200 IU/mL or >240–480 ng/mL				See Table 2				225	300
>200–300 IU/mL or >480–720 ng/mL					225	225	225	300	375
>300–400 IU/mL or >720–960 ng/mL			225	225	225	300	300		
>400–500 IU/mL or >960–1200 ng/mL		225	225	300	300	375	375		
>500–600 IU/mL or >1200–1440 ng/mL		225	300	300	375		Do not dose		
>600–700 IU/mL or >1440–1680 ng/mL	225	225	300	375					

[a] 1 IU/mL=2.4 ng/mL=2.4 µg/L.

Administration: Reconstitution: Parenteral Products:

Vial Size	Volume of Diluent to be Added to Vial	Approximate Available Volume	Nominal Concentration per mL
5 mL	1.4 mL	1.2 mL	150 mg per 1.2 mL (125 mg/mL)

Please read carefully before reconstitution. Failure to do so may result in unusable product.

XOLAIR for subcutaneous administration should be prepared using sterile water for injection (SWFI), **USP only**.

XOLAIR is for single use only. It is recommended that XOLAIR be used immediately following reconstitution (i.e. within 4 hours) as there is no preservative in the formulation. Physicochemical stability studies have shown that the reconstituted product may be stored at 2-8°C for up to 8 hours, if the recommended reconstitution procedures are followed.

The lyophilized product takes 15-20 minutes to dissolve. The fully reconstituted product will appear clear or slightly opalescent and may have a few small bubbles or foam around the edge of the vial. The reconstituted product is somewhat viscous; in order to obtain the full 1.2 mL dose **all of the product must be withdrawn** from the vial before expelling any air or excess solution from the syringe.

Step 1: Draw 1.4 mL of SWFI, USP into a 3-cc syringe equipped with a 2.5 cm, 18 gauge needle.

Step 2: Place the vial upright on a flat surface and using standard aseptic technique, insert the needle and inject the SWFI, USP directly onto the product.

Step 3: Keeping the vial upright, gently swirl the upright vial for approximately 1 minute to evenly wet the powder. Do not shake.

Step 4: After completing Step 3, gently swirl the vial for 5-10 seconds approximately every 5 minutes in order to dissolve any remaining solids. There should be no visible gel like particles in the solution. Do not use if foreign particles are present.

Note: Some vials may take longer than 20 minutes to dissolve completely. If this is the case, repeat Step 4 until there are no visible gel like particles in the solution. It is acceptable to have small bubbles or foam around the edge of the vial. Do not use if the contents of the vial do not dissolve completely by 40 minutes.

Step 5: Invert the vial for 15 seconds in order to allow the solution to drain toward the stopper. Using a new 3-cc syringe equipped with a 2.5 cm, 18 gauge needle, insert the needle into the inverted vial. Position the needle tip at the very bottom of the solution in the vial stopper when drawing the solution into the syringe. Before removing the needle from the vial, pull the plunger all the way back to the end of the syringe barrel in order to remove all of the solution from the inverted vial.

Step 6: Replace the 18 gauge needle with a 25 gauge needle for subcutaneous injection.

Step 7: Expel air, large bubbles, and any excess solution in order to obtain the required 1.2 mL dose. A thin layer of small bubbles may remain at the top of the solution in the syringe. Because the solution is slightly viscous, the injection may take 5 to 10 seconds to administer.

A vial delivers 1.2 mL (150 mg) of XOLAIR. For a 75 mg dose, draw up 0.6 mL into the syringe and discard the remaining product (see Table 4).

As with all parenteral admixtures, the constituted product should be examined for the presence of foreign particles, agglomeration or discolouration. Any defective units should be discarded.

Table 4: XOLAIR

Number of Injections and Total Injection Volumes

Dose (mg)	Number of Injections (vials needed)	Total Volume Injected (mL)[a]
150	1	1.2
225	2	1.8
300	2	2.4
375	3	3

[a] 1.2 mL maximum delivered volume per 150 mg vial.

OVERDOSE:

The maximum tolerated dose of XOLAIR has not been determined. Single intravenous doses up to 4000 mg have been administered to patients without evidence of dose-limiting toxicities. The highest cumulative dose administered to patients was 44 000 mg over a 20-week period, which was not associated with toxicities.

> For management of a suspected drug overdose, CPhA recommends that you contact your regional Poison Control Centre. See the *CPS* Directory section for a list of Poison Control Centres.

ACTION AND CLINICAL PHARMACOLOGY: XOLAIR (omalizumab), an IgE blocker, is a breakthrough recombinant DNA-derived humanized monoclonal antibody that selectively binds to human immunoglobulin E (IgE). The antibody is an IgG1 kappa that contains human framework regions with the complementarity-determining regions of a murine antibody that binds to IgE.

XOLAIR is produced by a Chinese Hamster Ovary cell suspension culture in a nutrient medium containing the antibiotic gentamicin. Gentamicin is not detectable in the final product.

Mechanism of Action: Omalizumab binds to IgE and prevents binding of IgE to the high-affinity FcεRI receptor, thereby reducing the amount of free IgE that is available to trigger the allergic-inflammatory cascade. Treatment of atopic subjects with omalizumab resulted in a significant (p=0.0022) marked down-regulation of FcεRI receptors on basophils. Furthermore, the in-vitro histamine release from basophils isolated from omalizumab treated subjects was reduced by approximately 90% following stimulation with an allergen compared to pre-treatment values.

Pharmacodynamics: In clinical studies, serum free IgE levels (i.e. unbound IgE) were reduced in a dose dependent manner within 1 hour following the first dose and maintained between doses. Mean serum free IgE decrease was greater than 96% using recommended doses. Serum total IgE levels (i.e., bound and unbound) increased after the first dose due to the formation of omalizumab:IgE complexes which have a slower elimination rate compared with free IgE. At 16 weeks after the first dose, average serum total IgE levels were five-fold higher compared with pre-treatment when using standard assays. After discontinuation of XOLAIR dosing, the XOLAIR induced increase in total IgE and decrease in free IgE were reversible with no observed rebound in IgE levels after drug washout. Total IgE levels returned to pre-treatment levels within one year after discontinuation of XOLAIR.

Pharmacokinetics: After s.c. administration, omalizumab is absorbed with an average absolute bioavailability of 62%. Following a single s.c. dose in adult and adolescent patients with asthma, omalizumab was absorbed slowly, reaching peak serum concentrations after an average of 7-8 days. The pharmacokinetics of omalizumab are linear at doses greater than 0.5 mg/kg. Following multiple doses of omalizumab, areas under the serum concentration-time curve from Day 0 to Day 14 at steady state were up to 6-fold of those observed after the first dose.

In vitro, omalizumab forms complexes of limited size with IgE. Precipitating complexes and complexes larger than 1 million daltons in molecular weight are not observed in vitro or in vivo. Tissue distribution studies in cynomolgus monkeys showed no specific uptake of ^{125}I-Omalizumab by any organ or tissue. The apparent volume of distribution in patients following s.c. administration was 78±32 mL/kg.

Clearance of omalizumab involves IgG clearance processes as well as clearance via specific binding and complex formation with its target ligand, IgE. Liver elimination of IgG includes degradation in the liver reticuloendothelial system (RES) and endothelial cells. Intact IgG is also excreted in bile. In studies with mice and monkeys, omalizumab:IgE complexes were eliminated by interactions with Fcγ receptors within the RES at rates that were generally faster than IgG clearance. In asthma patients omalizumab serum elimination half life averaged 26 days, with apparent clearance averaging 2.4±1.1 mL/kg/day. In addition, doubling body weight approximately doubled apparent clearance.

Special Populations and Conditions: The population pharmacokinetics of XOLAIR were analyzed to evaluate the effects of demographic characteristics. Analyses of these limited data suggest that no dose adjustments are necessary for age (12-76 years), race, ethnicity or gender.

STORAGE AND STABILITY: XOLAIR (omalizumab) should be stored under refrigerated conditions 2-8°C. Do not freeze. Do not use beyond the expiration date stamped on carton.

XOLAIR is for single use only. It is recommended that XOLAIR be used immediately following reconstitution (i.e. within 4 hours), as there is no preservative in the formulation. Physico-chemical stability studies have shown that the reconstituted product may be stored at 2-8°C for up to 8 hours, if the recommended reconstitution procedures are followed.

Reconstituted XOLAIR vials should be protected from direct sunlight.

INFORMATION FOR THE PATIENT: Published in e-CPS, available by subscription at www.e-cps.ca.

DOSAGE FORMS, COMPOSITION AND PACKAGING: Each single use vial of sterile, white, preservative-free, lyophilized powder, contains omalizumab 202.5 mg. Nonmedicinal ingredients: L-histidine, L-histidine hydrochloride monohydrate, polysorbate 20 and sucrose 145.5 mg (0.5 calories or 2.3 Joules). It is designed to deliver 150 mg omalizumab, in 1.2 mL, after reconstitution with 1.4 mL SWFI, USP. Single use vials of 5 mL

(Shown in Product Identification Section)

Xylocaine® Endotracheal

lidocaine

Topical Anesthetic

AstraZeneca

Date of Preparation: June 16, 1992
Date of Revision: April 2, 2008

SUMMARY PRODUCT INFORMATION:

Route of Administration	Dosage Form/ Strength	Clinically Relevant Nonmedicinal Ingredients
Oral	Non-aerosol spray, 10 mg/Metered Dose	Ethanol, methanol For a complete listing see Dosage Forms, Composition and Packaging.

INDICATIONS AND CLINICAL USE: Adults (>18 years of age): Xylocaine Endotracheal (lidocaine) is indicated for surface anesthesia associated with:

- nasal procedures, e.g. puncture of the maxillary sinus;
- procedures in the oropharynx, e.g. gastrointestinal endoscopy;
- procedures in the respiratory tract, e.g. insertion of instruments and tubes;
- procedures in the larynx, trachea and bronchi.

Geriatrics (>65 years of age): Elderly patients should be given reduced doses commensurate with their age and physical condition (see Dosage and Administration, Special Populations).

Pediatrics (<18 years of age): Children should be given reduced doses commensurate with their age, weight and physical condition (see Dosage and Administration, Special Populations).

Lidocaine should be used with caution in children younger than two years of age as there are insufficient data to support the safety and efficacy of this product in this patient population at this time (see Warnings and Precautions, Special Populations).

CONTRAINDICATIONS: XYLOCAINE Endotracheal (lidocaine) is contraindicated in:

- patients with a known history of hypersensitivity to local anesthetics of the amide type or to other components in the formulation (see Dosage Forms, Composition and Packaging).

WARNINGS AND PRECAUTIONS: General: Excessive dosage, or short intervals between doses, can result in high plasma levels of lidocaine or its metabolites and serious adverse effects. Absorption from the mucous membranes is variable but is especially high from the bronchial tree. Such applications may therefore result in rapidly rising or excessive plasma concentrations, with an increased risk for toxic symptoms, such as convulsions. This is especially important in children where doses vary with weight. The management of serious adverse reactions may require the use of resuscitative equipment, oxygen and other resuscitative drugs (see Overdosage).

The lowest dosage that results in effective anesthesia should be used to avoid high plasma levels and serious adverse effects. Tolerance to elevated blood levels varies with the status of the patient.

Lidocaine should be used with caution in patients with sepsis and/or traumatized mucosa at the area of application, since under such conditions there is the potential for rapid systemic absorption.

XYLOCAINE Endotracheal (lidocaine) should be used with caution in children under the age of 2 as there is insufficient data to support the safety and efficacy of this product in this patient population at this time.

In patients under general anesthesia who are paralyzed, higher plasma concentrations may occur than in spontaneously breathing patients. Unparalyzed patients are more likely to swallow a large proportion of the dose which then undergoes considerable first-pass hepatic metabolism following absorption from the gut.

Avoid contact with eyes.

Many drugs used during the conduct of anesthesia are considered potential triggering agents for familial malignant hyperthermia. It has been shown that the use of amide local anesthetics in malignant hyperthermia is safe. However, there is no guarantee that neural blockade will prevent the development of malignant hyperthermia during surgery. It is also difficult to predict the need for supplemental general anesthesia. Therefore a standard protocol for the management of malignant hyperthermia should be available.

When topical anesthetics are used in the mouth, the patient should be aware that the production of topical anesthesia may impair swallowing and thus enhance the danger of aspiration. Numbness of the tongue or buccal mucosa may enhance the danger of unintentional biting trauma. Food or chewing gum should not be taken while the mouth or throat area is anesthetized. See also Information for the Patient.

XYLOCAINE Endotracheal is ineffective when applied to intact skin.

Lidocaine has been shown to be porphyrinogenic in animal models. XYLOCAINE Endotracheal should only be prescribed to patients with acute porphyria on strong or urgent indications, when they can be closely monitored. Appropriate precautions should be taken for all porphyric patients.

Cardiovascular: Lidocaine should be used with caution in patients with bradycardia or impaired cardiovascular function since they may be less able to compensate for functional changes associated with the prolongation of A-V conduction produced by amide-type local anesthetics.

Lidocaine should be used with caution in patients with severe shock.

Neurologic: Epilepsy: The risk of central nervous system side effects when using lidocaine in patients with epilepsy is very low, provided that the dose recommendations are followed (see Dosage and Administration).

Locomotion and Coordination: Topical lidocaine formulations generally result in low plasma concentrations because of a low degree of systemic absorption. However, depending on the dose, local anesthetics may have a very mild effect on mental function and coordination even in the absence of overt CNS toxicity and may temporarily impair locomotion and alertness.

Renal: Lidocaine is metabolized primarily by the liver to monoethylglycinexylidine (MEGX, which has some CNS activity), and then further to metabolites glycinexylidine (GX) and 2,6-dimethylaniline (see Action and Clinical Pharmacology). Only a small fraction (2%) of lidocaine is excreted unchanged in the urine. The pharmacokinetics of lidocaine and its main metabolite were not altered significantly in haemodialysis patients (n=4) who received an intravenous dose of lidocaine. Therefore, renal impairment is not expected to significantly affect the pharmacokinetics of lidocaine when XYLOCAINE Endotracheal is used for short treatment durations, according to dosage instructions (see Dosage and Administration). Caution is recommended when lidocaine is used in patients with severely impaired renal function because lidocaine metabolites may accumulate during long term treatment (see Dosage and Administration).

Hepatic/Biliary/Pancreatic: Because amide-type local anesthetics such as lidocaine are metabolized by the liver, these drugs, especially repeated doses, should be used cautiously in patients with hepatic disease. Patients with severe hepatic disease, because of their inability to metabolize local anesthetics normally, are at greater risk of developing toxic plasma concentrations.

Sensitivity/Resistance: Lidocaine should be used with caution in persons with known drug sensitivities.

Special Populations: Debilitated patients, acutely ill patients and patients with sepsis should be given reduced doses commensurate with their age, weight and physical condition because they may be more sensitive to systemic effects due to increased blood levels of lidocaine following repeated doses.

Pregnant Women: There are no adequate and well-controlled studies in pregnant women on the effect of lidocaine on the developing fetus.

It is reasonable to assume that a large number of pregnant women and women of child-bearing age have been given lidocaine. No specific disturbances to the reproductive process have so far been reported, e.g. no increased incidence of malformations. However, care should be given during early pregnancy when maximum organogenesis takes place.

Labour and Delivery: Should XYLOCAINE Endotracheal be used concomitantly with other products containing lidocaine during labour and delivery, the total dose contributed by all formulations must be kept in mind.

Nursing Women: Lidocaine and its metabolites are excreted in the breast milk. At therapeutic doses the quantities of lidocaine and its metabolites in breast milk are small and generally are not expected to be a risk for the infant.

Pediatrics: Children should be given reduced doses commensurate with their age, weight and physical condition because they may be more sensitive to systemic effects due to increased blood levels of lidocaine following repeated doses (see Dosage and Administration).

XYLOCAINE Endotracheal should be used with caution in children under the age of 2 as there is insufficient data to support the safety and efficacy of this product in this patient population at this time.

Geriatrics: Elderly patients may be more sensitive to systemic effects due to increased blood levels of lidocaine following repeated doses and may require dose reductions.

Carcinogenesis and Mutagenesis: Genotoxicity tests with lidocaine showed no evidence of mutagenic potential. A metabolite of lidocaine, 2,6-dimethylaniline, showed weak evidence of activity in some genotoxicity tests. A chronic oral toxicity study of the metabolite 2,6-dimethylaniline (0, 14, 45, 135 mg/kg) administered in feed to rats showed that there was a significantly greater incidence of nasal cavity tumors in male and female animals that had daily oral exposure to the highest dose of 2,6-dimethylaniline for 2 years. The lowest tumor-inducing dose tested in animals (135 mg/kg) corresponds to approximately 45 times the amount of 2,6-dimethylaniline to which a 50 kg subject would be exposed following the application of 40×10 mg/metered dose of lidocaine non-aerosol spray for 24 hours on the mucosa, assuming the highest theoretical extent of absorption of 100%, and 80% conversion to 2,6-dimethylaniline. Based on a yearly exposure (once daily dosing with 2,6-dimethylaniline in animals and 5 treatment sessions with 40×10 mg/metered dose of lidocaine non-aerosol spray in humans), the safety margins would be approximately 3400 times when comparing the exposure in animals to man.

ADVERSE REACTIONS: Adverse experiences following the administration of lidocaine are similar in nature to those observed with other amide local anesthetic agents. These adverse experiences are, in general, dose-related and may result from high plasma levels caused by overdosage or rapid absorption, eg, application to areas below the vocal cords, or may result from a hypersensitivity, idiosyncrasy or diminished tolerance on the part of the patient.

Serious adverse experiences are generally systemic in nature. The following types are those most commonly reported:

Central Nervous System: CNS manifestations are excitatory and/or depressant and may be characterized by the following signs and symptoms of escalating severity: circumoral paresthesia, light-headedness, nervousness, apprehension, euphoria, confusion, dizziness, drowsiness, hyperacusis, tinnitus, blurred vision, vomiting, sensations of heat, cold or numbness, twitching, tremors, convulsions, unconsciousness, respiratory depression and arrest. The excitatory manifestations (e.g., twitching, tremors, convulsions) may be very brief or may not occur at all, in which case the first manifestation of toxicity may be drowsiness merging into unconsciousness and respiratory arrest.

Drowsiness following the administration of lidocaine is usually an early sign of a high lidocaine plasma level and may occur as a consequence of rapid absorption.

Cardiovascular System: Cardiovascular manifestations are usually depressant and are characterized by bradycardia, hypotension, arrhythmia, and cardiovascular collapse, which may lead to cardiac arrest.

Allergic: Allergic reactions are characterized by cutaneous lesions, urticaria, edema or, in the most severe cases, anaphylactic shock. Allergic reactions of the amide type are rare (<0.1%) and may occur as a result of sensitivity either to the local anesthetic agent or to other components in the formulation (see Dosage Forms, Composition and Packaging).

Local Reactions: Local irritation at the application site has been described. Following application to laryngeal mucosa before endotracheal intubation, reversible symptoms such as "sore throat", "hoarseness", and "loss of voice" have been reported. The use of XYLOCAINE Endotracheal provides surface anaesthesia during an endotracheal procedure but does not prevent post-intubation soreness.

DRUG INTERACTIONS: Overview: Lidocaine is mainly metabolized in the liver by CYP1A2 and CYP3A4 to its two major metabolites, monoethylglycinexylidine (MEGX) and glycinexylidine (GX), both of which are pharmacologically active. Lidocaine has a high hepatic extraction ratio. Only a small fraction (2%) of lidocaine is excreted unchanged in the urine. The hepatic clearance of lidocaine is expected to depend largely on blood flow.

Strong inhibitors of CYP1A2, such as fluvoxamine, given concomitantly with lidocaine, can cause a metabolic interaction leading to an increased lidocaine plasma concentration. Therefore, prolonged administration of lidocaine should be avoided in patients treated with strong inhibitors of CYP1A2, such as fluvoxamine. When co-administered with intravenous lidocaine, two strong inhibitors of CYP3A4, erythromycin and itraconazole, have each been shown to have a modest effect on the pharmacokinetics of intravenous lidocaine. Other drugs such as propranolol and cimetidine have been reported to reduce intravenous lidocaine clearance, probably through effects on hepatic blood flow and/or metabolism.

When lidocaine is used topically, plasma concentrations are of importance for safety reasons (see Warnings and Precautions, General and Adverse Reactions). However, with the low systemic exposure and short duration of topical application, the above-mentioned metabolic drug-drug interactions are not expected to be of clinical significance when XYLOCAINE Endotracheal is used according to dosage recommendations.

Clinically relevant pharmacodynamic drug interactions may occur with lidocaine and other local anesthetics or structurally related drugs, and Class I and Class III antiarrhythmic drugs due to additive effects.

Drug-Drug Interactions: Local Anesthetics and Agents Structurally Related to Amide-Type Local Anesthetics: Lidocaine should be used with caution in patients receiving other local anesthetics or agents structurally related to amide-type local anesthetics, e.g. antiarrhythmics such as mexiletine, since the toxic effects are additive.

Antiarrhythmic Drugs : Class I Antiarrhythmic Drugs : Class I antiarrhythmic drugs (such as mexiletine) should be used with caution since toxic effects are additive and potentially synergistic.

Class III Antiarrhythmic Drugs: Caution is advised when using Class III antiarrhythmic drugs concomitantly with lidocaine due to potential pharmacodynamic or pharmacokinetic interactions with lidocaine, or both. A drug interaction study has shown that the plasma concentration of lidocaine may be increased following administration of a therapeutic dose of intravenous lidocaine to patients treated with amiodarone (n=6). Case reports have described toxicity in patients treated concomitantly with lidocaine and amiodarone. Patients treated with Class III antiarrhythmic drugs (e.g. amiodarone) should be kept under close surveillance and ECG monitoring should be considered, since cardiac effects of these drugs and lidocaine may be additive.

Strong Inhibitors of CYP1A2 and CYP3A4: Cytochrome CYP1A2 and CYP3A4 are involved in the formation of the pharmacologically active lidocaine metabolite MEGX.

Fluvoxamine: Strong inhibitors of CYP1A2, such as fluvoxamine, given during prolonged administration of lidocaine to areas with a high extent of systemic absorption (e.g., mucous membranes) can cause a metabolic interaction leading to an increased lidocaine plasma concentration. The plasma clearance of a single intravenous dose of lidocaine was reduced by 41 to 60% during co-administration of fluvoxamine, a selective and potent CYP1A2 inhibitor, to healthy volunteers.

Erythromycin and Itraconazole: Erythromycin and itraconazole, which are strong inhibitors of CYP3A4, have been shown to reduce clearance of lidocaine by 9 to 18%, following a single intravenous dose of lidocaine to healthy volunteers.

During combined co-administration with fluvoxamine and erythromycin the plasma clearance of lidocaine was reduced by 53%.

β-blockers and Cimetidine: Following a single intravenous dose of lidocaine, administered to healthy volunteers, the clearance of lidocaine has been reported to be reduced up to 47% when co-administered with propanolol and up to 30% when co-administered with cimetidine. Reduced clearance of lidocaine when co-administered with these drugs is probably due to reduced liver blood flow and/or inhibition of microsomal liver enzymes. The potential for clinically significant interactions with these drugs should be considered during long-term treatment with high doses of lidocaine.

Drug-Food Interactions: Interactions of lidocaine with food have not been established.

Drug-Herb Interactions: Interactions of lidocaine with herbal products have not been established.

Drug-Laboratory Tests Interactions: Interactions of lidocaine with laboratory tests have not been established.

Drug-Lifestyle Interactions: Interactions of lidocaine with lifestyle have not been established.

DOSAGE AND ADMINISTRATION: Dosing Considerations: General: When XYLOCAINE Endotracheal (lidocaine) is used concomitantly with other products containing lidocaine, the total dose contributed by all formulations must be kept in mind.

Since absorption is variable and especially high in the trachea and bronchi, the maximum recommended doses vary depending on the area of application. Application to areas below the vocal cords may result in excessive plasma concentrations because of less transfer to the intestine and less first-pass loss.

Each actuation of the metered dose valve delivers 10 mg lidocaine.

Special Populations: Lidocaine should be used with caution in patients with epilepsy, impaired cardiac conduction, bradycardia, impaired hepatic or renal function and in severe shock (see Warnings and Precautions).

Debilitated, elderly patients, acutely ill patients, patients with sepsis and children should be given reduced doses commensurate with their age, weight and physical condition.

XYLOCAINE Endotracheal should be used with caution in children under the age of 2 as there is insufficient data to support the safety and efficacy of this product in this patient population at this time.

Administration: XYLOCAINE Endotracheal : When using the spray for the first time, after attaching the nozzle, the pump must be primed by pressing downwards on the actuator five to ten times. When changing to a new nozzle, the pump need not be re-primed but the air in the nozzle must be voided before a full dose is delivered. This usually requires two actuations.

The spray nozzle is already bent to its final configuration for use. No further manipulations should be made to the spray nozzle before use. The nozzle must not be shortened, otherwise the spray function will be destroyed. XYLOCAINE Endotracheal should be used in the upright position to ensure proper function.

XYLOCAINE Endotracheal should not be used on cuffs or endotracheal tubes made of plastic. Lidocaine base in contact with PVC and non-PVC cuffs or endotracheal tubes can damage the cuff (pinholes), which may cause leakage that could lead to pressure loss in the cuff.

Recommended Dose and Dosage Adjustment: Adults: See Table 1.

Table 1: XYLOCAINE Endotracheal

Dose Recommendations for Adults

Area	Recommended Dose (mg)	Maximum Dose for Short[a] Procedures (mg)	Maximum Dose for Prolonged[b] Procedures (mg)
Nasal procedures, e.g. puncture of the maxillary sinus	20–60	500	600
Procedures in the oropharynx, e.g. gastrointestinal endoscopy	20–200	500	600
Procedures in the respiratory tract, e.g. insertion of instruments and tubes	50–400	400	600
Procedures in the larynx, trachea and bronchi	50–200	200[c]	400

[a] For short procedures the drug is given for less than one minute.
[b] For prolonged procedures, the duration of application is more than 5 minutes.
[c] During controlled ventilation the dose should be reduced.

Children (Under 12 Years): For laryngotracheal use, the dose should not exceed 3 mg/kg. For nasal and oropharyngeal use, the dose should not exceed 4-5 mg/kg. In neonates and infants, less concentrated lidocaine solutions are recommended.

For children over 12 years of age doses should be commensurate with weight and physical condition.

OVERDOSAGE:
Acute systemic toxicity from local anesthetics is generally related to high plasma levels encountered during therapeutic use of local anesthetics and originates mainly in the central nervous and the cardiovascular systems (see Adverse Reactions and Warnings and Precautions). It should be kept in mind that clinically relevant pharmacodynamic drug interactions (i.e., toxic effects) may occur with lidocaine and other local anesthetics or structurally related drugs, and Class I and Class III antiarrhythmic drugs due to additive effects (see Drug Interactions).

Symptoms: Central nervous system toxicity is a graded response, with symptoms and signs of escalating severity. The first symptoms are circumoral paresthesia, numbness of the tongue, light-headedness, hyperacusis and tinnitus. Visual disturbance and muscular tremors are more serious and precede the onset of generalized convulsions. Unconsciousness and grand mal convulsions may follow, which may last from a few seconds to several minutes. Hypoxia and hypercarbia occur rapidly following convulsions due to the increased muscular activity, together with the interference with normal respiration. In severe cases apnea may occur. Acidosis, hyperkalaemia, hypocalcaemia and hypoxia increase and extend the toxic effects of local anesthetics.

Recovery is due to redistribution and metabolism of the local anesthetic drug. Recovery may be rapid unless large amounts of the drug have been administered.

Cardiovascular effects may be seen in cases with high systemic concentrations. Severe hypotension, bradycardia, arrhythmia and cardiovascular collapse may be the result in such cases.

Cardiovascular toxic effects are generally preceded by signs of toxicity in the central nervous system, unless the patient is receiving a general anesthetic or is heavily sedated with drugs such as a benzodiazepine or barbiturate.

Treatment: The first consideration is prevention, best accomplished by careful and constant monitoring of cardiovascular and respiratory vital signs and the patient's state of consciousness after each local anesthetic administration. At the first sign of change, oxygen should be administered.

The first step in the management of systemic toxic reactions consists of immediate attention to the maintenance of a patent airway and assisted or controlled ventilation with oxygen and a delivery system capable of permitting immediate positive airway pressure by mask. This may prevent convulsions if they have not already occurred.

If convulsions occur, the objective of the treatment is to maintain ventilation and oxygenation and support circulation. Oxygen must be given and ventilation assisted if necessary (mask and bag or tracheal intubation). Should convulsions not stop spontaneously after 15-20 seconds, an anticonvulsant should be given iv to facilitate adequate ventilation and oxygenation. Thiopental sodium 1-3 mg/kg iv is the first choice. Alternatively diazepam 0.1 mg/kg bw iv may be used, although its action will be slow. Prolonged convulsions may jeopardise the patient's ventilation and oxygenation. If so, injection of a muscle relaxant (e.g. succinylcholine 1 mg/kg bw) will facilitate ventilation, and oxygenation can be controlled. Early endotracheal intubation is required when succinylcholine is used to control motor seizure activity.

If cardiovascular depression is evident (hypotension, bradycardia), ephedrine 5-10 mg i.v. should be given and may be repeated, if necessary, after 2-3 minutes.

Should circulatory arrest occur, immediate cardiopulmonary resuscitation should be instituted. Optimal oxygenation and ventilation and circulatory support as well as treatment of acidosis are of vital importance, since hypoxia and acidosis will increase the systemic toxicity of local anesthetics. Epinephrine (0.1-0.2 mg as intravenous or intracardial injections) should be given as soon as possible and repeated, if necessary.

Children should be given doses of epinephrine commensurate with their age and weight.

For management of a suspected drug overdose, CPhA recommends that you contact your **regional Poison Control Centre**. See the *CPS* Directory section for a list of Poison Control Centres.

ACTION AND CLINICAL PHARMACOLOGY: Mechanism of Action: Lidocaine stabilizes the neuronal membrane by inhibiting the ionic fluxes required for the initiation and conduction of impulses, thereby effecting local anesthetic action. Local anesthetics of the amide type are thought to act within the sodium channels of the nerve membrane.

Onset of Action: XYLOCAINE Endotracheal (lidocaine), when applied topically to the oral cavity, acts on mucous membranes to produce local anesthesia. Anesthesia occurs usually within 1-5 minutes and persists for approximately 10-15 minutes. XYLOCAINE Endotracheal is ineffective when applied to intact skin.

Hemodynamics: Lidocaine, like other local anesthetics, may also have effects on excitable membranes in the brain and myocardium. If excessive amounts of drug reach systemic circulation rapidly, symptoms and signs of toxicity will appear, emanating from the central nervous and cardiovascular systems.

Central nervous system toxicity (see Overdosage) usually precedes the cardiovascular effects since it occurs at lower plasma concentrations. Direct effects of local anesthetics on the heart include slow conduction, negative inotropism and eventually cardiac arrest.

Pharmacokinetics: Absorption: The rate and extent of absorption depends upon concentration and total dose administered, the specific site of application and duration of exposure. In general, the rate of absorption of local anesthetic agents, following topical application to wound surfaces and mucous membranes is high, and occurs most rapidly after intratracheal and bronchial administration. Lidocaine is also well absorbed from the gastrointestinal tract, although little intact drug may appear in the circulation because of biotransformation in the liver.

Distribution: Lidocaine has a total plasma clearance of 0.95 L/min and a volume of distribution at steady state of 91 L.

Lidocaine readily crosses the placenta, and equilibrium in regard to free, unbound drug will be reached. Because the degree of plasma protein binding in the fetus is less than in the mother, the total plasma concentration will be greater in the mother, but the free concentrations will be the same.

The plasma binding of lidocaine is dependent on drug concentration, and the fraction bound decreases with increasing concentration. At concentrations of 1 to 4 μg of free base per mL, 60 to 80 percent of lidocaine is protein bound. Binding is also dependent on the plasma concentration of the alpha-1-acid glycoprotein.

Metabolism: Lidocaine is metabolized rapidly by the liver, and metabolites and unchanged drug are excreted by the kidneys. Biotransformation includes oxidative N-dealkylation, ring hydroxylation, cleavage of the amide linkage, and conjugation. Only 2% of lidocaine is excreted unchanged. Most of it is metabolized first to monoethylglycinexylidide (MEGX) and then to glycinexylidide (GX) and 2,6-dimethylaniline. Up to 70% appears in the urine as 4-hydroxy-2,6-dimethylaniline.

Excretion: Lidocaine has an elimination half-life of 1.6 h and an estimated hepatic extraction ratio of 0.65. The clearance of lidocaine is almost entirely due to liver metabolism, and depends both on liver blood flow and the activity of metabolizing enzymes.

The elimination half-life following an intravenous bolus injection is typically 1.5 to 2.0 hours. The elimination half-life in neonates (3.2 h) is approximately twice that of adults. The half-life may be prolonged two-fold or more in patients with liver dysfunction. Renal dysfunction does not affect lidocaine kinetics but may increase the accumulation of metabolites.

Special Populations and Conditions: Acidosis increases the systemic toxicity of lidocaine while the use of CNS depressants may increase the levels of lidocaine required to produce overt CNS effects. Objective adverse manifestations become increasingly apparent with increasing venous plasma levels above 6.0 mg free base per mL.

STORAGE AND STABILITY: Store at controlled room temperature (15-30°C). Protect from freezing.

INFORMATION FOR THE PATIENT: Published in e-CPS, available by subscription at www.e-cps.ca.

DOSAGE FORMS, COMPOSITION AND PACKAGING: Each metered dose contains: lidocaine 10 mg. Nonmedicinal ingredients: essence of banana, ethanol, menthol (natural), polyethylene glycol 400, purified water and saccharin. Nonaerosol spray bottles of 50 mL with a metered dose valve and a 12 cm plastic nozzle. Additional 12 cm plastic nozzles are available in packages of 50 nozzles.

Xylocaine® Jelly 2%

lidocaine HCl

Topical Anesthetic

AstraZeneca

Date of Revision: April 2, 2008

SUMMARY PRODUCT INFORMATION:

Route of Administration	Dosage Form/ Strength	Clinically Relevant Nonmedicinal Ingredients
Topical	Jelly syringe, 20 mg/mL	None
Topical	Jelly tube, 20 mg/mL	Methylparaben, propylparaben For a complete listing see Dosage Forms, Composition and Packaging.

INDICATIONS AND CLINICAL USE: Adults (>18 years of age): XYLOCAINE Jelly 2% (lidocaine hydrochloride) is indicated for:

Surface anesthesia and lubrication for:

- The male and female urethra during cystoscopy, catheterization, exploration by sound and other endourethral operations;
- Nasal and pharyngeal cavities in endoscopic procedures such as gastroscopy and bronchoscopy;
- Proctoscopy and rectoscopy;
- Tracheal intubation.

Symptomatic treatment of pain in connection with cystitis and urethritis.

Geriatrics (>65 years of age): Elderly patients should be given reduced doses commensurate with their age and physical condition (see Dosage and Administration, Special Populations).

Pediatrics (<18 years of age): Children should be given reduced doses commensurate with their age, weight and physical condition (see Dosage and Administration, Special Populations).

Lidocaine should be used with caution in children younger than two years of age as there are insufficient data to support the safety and efficacy of this product in this patient population at this time (see Warnings and Precautions, Special Populations).

CONTRAINDICATIONS: XYLOCAINE Jelly 2% (lidocaine hydrochloride) is contraindicated in:

- patients with a known history of hypersensitivity to local anesthetics of the amide type or to other components in the formulation (see Dosage Forms, Composition and Packaging).
- patients with a known hypersensitivity to methylparaben and/or propylparaben (preservatives used in the tube format of XYLOCAINE Jelly 2%), or to their metabolite para amino benzoic acid (PABA).

Formulations of lidocaine containing parabens should also be avoided in patients with a history of allergic reactions to ester local anesthetics, which are metabolized to PABA.

WARNINGS AND PRECAUTIONS: General: Excessive dosage, or short intervals between doses, can result in high plasma levels of lidocaine or its metabolites and serious adverse effects. Absorption from the mucous membranes is variable but is especially high from the bronchial tree. Such applications may therefore result in rapidly rising or excessive plasma concentrations, with an increased risk for toxic symptoms, such as convulsions. **Patients should be instructed to strictly adhere to the recommended dosage.** This is especially important in children where doses vary with weight. The management of serious adverse reactions may require the use of resuscitative equipment, oxygen and other resuscitative drugs (see Overdosage).

The lowest dosage that results in effective anesthesia should be used to avoid high plasma levels and serious adverse effects. Tolerance to elevated blood levels varies with the status of the patient.

Lidocaine should be used with caution in patients with sepsis and/or traumatized mucosa at the area of application, since under such conditions there is the potential for rapid systemic absorption.

XYLOCAINE Jelly 2% should be used with caution in children under the age of 2 as there is insufficient data to support the safety and efficacy of this product in this patient population at this time.

In patients under general anesthesia who are paralyzed, higher plasma concentrations may occur than in spontaneously breathing patients. Unparalyzed patients are more likely to swallow a large proportion of the dose, which then undergoes considerable first-pass hepatic metabolism following absorption from the gut.

Avoid contact with eyes.

Many drugs used during the conduct of anesthesia are considered potential triggering agents for familial malignant hyperthermia. It has been shown that the use of amide local anesthetics in malignant hyperthermia patients is safe. However, there is no guarantee that neural blockade will prevent the development of malignant hyperthermia during surgery. It is also difficult to predict the need for supplemental general anesthesia. Therefore, a standard protocol for the management of malignant hyperthermia should be available.

When used for endotracheal tube lubrication, care should be taken to avoid introduction of the jelly into the lumen of the tube. If allowed into the inner lumen, the jelly may dry on the inner surface leaving a residue which tends to clump with flexion, narrowing the lumen. There have been rare reports in which this residue has caused the lumen to occlude. Similarly, do not use the jelly to lubricate the endotracheal stylettes.

When topical anesthetics are used in the mouth, the patient should be aware that the production of topical anesthesia may impair swallowing and thus enhance the danger of aspiration. Numbness of the tongue or buccal mucosa may enhance the danger of unintentional biting trauma. Food or chewing gum should not be taken while the mouth or throat area is anesthetized. See also Information for the Patient.

XYLOCAINE Jelly 2% is ineffective when applied to intact skin.

Lidocaine has been shown to be porphyrinogenic in animal models. XYLOCAINE Jelly 2% should only be prescribed to patients with acute porphyria on strong or urgent indications, when they can be closely monitored. Appropriate precautions should be taken for all porphyric patients.

Cardiovascular: Lidocaine should be used with caution in patients with bradycardia or impaired cardiovascular function since they may be less able to compensate for functional changes associated with the prolongation of A-V conduction produced by amid-type local anesthetics.

Lidocaine should be used with caution in patients in severe shock.

Hepatic/Biliary/Pancreatic: Because amide-type local anesthetics such as lidocaine are metabolized by the liver, these drugs, especially repeated doses, should be used cautiously in patients with hepatic disease. Patients with severe hepatic disease, because of their inability to metabolize local anesthetics normally, are at greater risk of developing toxic plasma concentrations.

Neurologic: Epilepsy: The risk of central nervous system side effects when using lidocaine in patients with epilepsy is very low, provided that the dose recommendations are followed. (See Dosage and Administration.)

Locomotion and Coordination: Topical lidocaine formulations generally result in low plasma concentrations because of a low degree of systemic absorption. However, depending on the dose, local anesthetics may have a very mild effect on mental function and coordination even in the absence of overt CNS toxicity and may temporarily impair locomotion and alertness.

Renal: Lidocaine is metabolized primarily by the liver to monoethylglycinexylidine (MEGX, which has some CNS activity), and then further to metabolites glycinexylidine (GX) and 2,6-dimethylaniline (see Action and Clinical Pharmacology). Only a small fraction (2%) of lidocaine is excreted unchanged in the urine. The pharmacokinetics of lidocaine and its main metabolite were not altered significantly in haemodialysis patients (n=4) who received an intravenous dose of lidocaine. Therefore, renal impairment is not expected to significantly affect the pharmacokinetics of lidocaine when XYLOCAINE Jelly 2% is used for short treatment durations, according to dosage instructions (see Dosage and Administration). Caution is recommended when lidocaine is used in patients with severely impaired renal function because lidocaine metabolites may accumulate during long term treatment (see Dosage and Administration).

Sensitivity/Resistance: Lidocaine should be used with caution in persons with known drug sensitivities.

XYLOCAINE Jelly 2% is contraindicated in patients with known hypersensitivities to local anesthetics of the amide type, to other components in the formulation, methylparaben and/or propylparaben (preservatives of the tube) and their metabolite para amino benzoic acid (PABA). The use of paraben-containing lidocaine preparations should also be avoided in patients who are allergic to ester local anesthetics (see Contraindications).

Special Populations: Debilitated patients, acutely ill patients, and patients with sepsis should be given reduced doses commensurate with their age, weight and physical condition because they may be more sensitive to systemic effects due to increased blood levels of lidocaine following repeated doses.

Pregnant Women: There are no adequate and well-controlled studies in pregnant women on the effect of lidocaine on the developing fetus.

It is reasonable to assume that a large number of pregnant women and women of child-bearing age have been given lidocaine. No specific disturbances to the reproductive process have so far been reported, e.g. no increased incidence of malformations. However, care should be given during early pregnancy when maximum organogenesis takes place.

Labour and Delivery: Lidocaine is not contraindicated in labour and delivery. Should XYLOCAINE Jelly 2% be used concomitantly with other products containing lidocaine during labour and delivery, the total dose contributed by all formulations must be kept in mind.

Nursing Women: Lidocaine and its metabolites are excreted in the breast milk. At therapeutic doses, the quantities of lidocaine and its metabolites in breast milk are small and generally are not expected to be a risk for the infant.

Pediatrics: Children should be given reduced doses commensurate with their age, weight and physical condition because they may be more sensitive to systemic effects due to increased blood levels of lidocaine following repeated doses (see Dosage and Administration).

Xylocaine Jelly 2% should be used with caution in children under the age of 2 as there is insufficient data to support the safety and efficacy of this product in this patient population at this time.

Geriatrics: Elderly patients may be more sensitive to systemic effects due to increased blood levels of lidocaine following repeated doses and may require dose reductions.

Carcinogenesis and Mutagenesis: Genotoxicity tests with lidocaine showed no evidence of mutagenic potential. A metabolite of lidocaine, 2,6-dimethylaniline, showed weak evidence of activity in some genotoxicity tests. A chronic oral toxicity study of the metabolite 2,6-dimethylaniline (0, 14, 45, 135 mg/kg) administered in feed to rats showed that there was a significantly greater incidence of nasal cavity tumors in male and female animals that had daily oral exposure to the highest dose of 2,6-dimethylaniline for 2 years. The lowest tumor-inducing dose tested in animals (135 mg/kg) corresponds to approximately 50 times the amount of 2,6-dimethylaniline to which a 50 kg subject would be exposed following the application of 20 g of lidocaine jelly 2% for 24 hours on the mucosa, assuming the highest theoretical extent of absorption of 100% and 80% conversion to 2,6-dimethylaniline. Based on a yearly exposure (once daily dosing with 2,6-dimethylaniline in animals and 5 treatment sessions with 20 g lidocaine jelly 2% in humans), the safety margins would be approximately 3400 times when comparing the exposure in animals to man.

ADVERSE REACTIONS: Adverse experiences following the administration of lidocaine are similar in nature to those observed with other amide local anesthetic agents. These adverse experiences are, in general, dose-related and may result from high plasma levels caused by overdosage or rapid absorption, or may result from a hypersensitivity, idiosyncrasy or diminished tolerance on the part of the patient.

An increased incidence of postoperative sore throat has been reported following endotracheal tube lubrication with lidocaine jelly.

Serious adverse experiences are generally systemic in nature. The following types are those most commonly reported:

Central Nervous System: CNS manifestations are excitatory and/or depressant and may be characterized by the following signs and symptoms of escalating severity: circumoral paresthesia, light-headedness, nervousness, apprehension, euphoria, confusion, dizziness, drowsiness, hyperacusis, tinnitus, blurred vision, vomiting, sensations of heat, cold or numbness, twitching, tremors, convulsions, unconsciousness, respiratory depression and arrest. The excitatory manifestations (e.g., twitching, tremors, convulsions) may be very brief or may not occur at all, in which case the first manifestation of toxicity may be drowsiness merging into unconsciousness and respiratory arrest.

Drowsiness following the administration of lidocaine is usually an early sign of a high lidocaine plasma level and may occur as a consequence of rapid absorption.

Cardiovascular System: Cardiovascular manifestations are usually depressant and are characterized by bradycardia, hypotension, arrhythmia and cardiovascular collapse, which may lead to cardiac arrest.

Allergic: Allergic reactions are characterized by cutaneous lesions, urticaria, edema or, in the most severe instances, anaphylactic shock. Allergic reactions of the amide type are rare (<0.1%) and may occur as a result of sensitivity either to the local anesthetic agent or to other components in the formulation (see Dosage Forms, Composition and Packaging).

DRUG INTERACTIONS: Overview: Lidocaine is mainly metabolized in the liver by CYP1A2 and CYP3A4 to its two major metabolites, monoethylglycinexylidide (MEGX) and glycinexylidide (GX), both of which are pharmacologically active. Lidocaine has a high hepatic extraction ratio. Only a small fraction (2%) of lidocaine is excreted unchanged in the urine. The hepatic clearance of lidocaine is expected to depend largely on blood flow.

Strong inhibitors of CYP1A2, such as fluvoxamine, given concomitantly with lidocaine, can cause a metabolic interaction leading to an increased lidocaine plasma concentration. Therefore, prolonged administration of lidocaine should be avoided in patients treated with strong inhibitors of CYP1A2, such as fluvoxamine. When co-administered with intravenous lidocaine, two strong inhibitors of CYP3A4, erythromycin and itraconazole, have each been shown to have a modest effect on the pharmacokinetics of intravenous lidocaine. Other drugs such as propranolol and cimetidine have been reported to reduce intravenous lidocaine clearance, probably through effects on hepatic blood flow and/or metabolism.

When lidocaine is used topically, plasma concentrations are of importance for safety reasons (see Warnings and Precautions, General and Adverse Reactions). However, with the low systemic exposure and short duration of topical application, the above-mentioned metabolic drug-drug interactions are not expected to be of clinical significance when XYLOCAINE Jelly 2% is used according to dosage recommendations.

Clinically relevant pharmacodynamic drug interactions may occur with lidocaine and other local anesthetics or structurally related drugs, and Class I and Class III antiarrhythmic drugs due to additive effects.

Drug-Drug Interactions: Local Anesthetics and Agents Structurally Related To Amide-Type Local Anesthetics: Lidocaine should be used with caution in patients receiving other local anesthetics or agents structurally related to amide-type local anesthetics (e.g. antiarrhythmics such as mexiletine), since the toxic effects are additive.

Antiarryhythmic Drugs: Class I Antiarrhythmic Drugs: Class I antiarrhythmic drugs (such as mexiletine) should be used with caution since toxic effects are additive and potentially synergistic.

Class III Antiarrhythmic Drugs: Caution is advised when using Class III antiarrhythmic drugs concomitantly with lidocaine due to potential pharmacodynamic or pharmacokinetic interactions with lidocaine, or both. A drug interaction study has shown that the plasma concentration of lidocaine may be increased following administration of a therapeutic dose of intravenous lidocaine to patients treated with amiodarone (n=6). Case reports have described toxicity in patients treated concomitantly with lidocaine and amiodarone. Patients treated with Class III antiarrhythmic drugs (e.g. amiodarone) should be kept under close surveillance and ECG monitoring should be considered, since cardiac effects of these drugs and lidocaine may be additive.

Strong Inhibitors of CYP1A2 and CYP3A4: Cytochrome CYP1A2 and CYP3A4 are involved in the formation of the pharmacologically active lidocaine metabolite MEGX.

Fluvoxamine: Strong inhibitors of CYP1A2, such as fluvoxamine, given during prolonged administration of lidocaine to areas with a high extent of systemic absorption (e.g., mucous membranes) can cause a metabolic interaction leading to an increased lidocaine plasma concentration. The plasma clearance of a single intravenous dose of lidocaine was reduced by 41 to 60% during co-administration of fluvoxamine, a selective and potent CYP1A2 inhibitor, to healthy volunteers.

Erythromycin and Itraconazole: Erythromycin and itraconazole, which are strong inhibitors of CYP3A4, have been shown to reduce clearance of lidocaine by 9 to 18%, following a single intravenous dose of lidocaine to healthy volunteers.

During combined co-administration with fluvoxamine and erythromycin the plasma clearance of lidocaine was reduced by 53%.

β-blockers and Cimetidine: Following a single intravenous dose of lidocaine, administered to healthy volunteers, the clearance of lidocaine has been reported to be reduced up to 47% when co-administered with propranolol and up to 30% when co-administered with cimetidine. Reduced clearance of lidocaine when co-administered with these drugs is probably due to reduced liver blood flow and/or inhibition of microsomal liver enzymes. The potential for clinically significant interactions with these drugs should be considered during long-term treatment with high doses of lidocaine.

Drug-Food Interactions: Interactions of lidocaine with food have not been established.

Drug-Herb Interactions: Interactions of lidocaine with herbal products have not been established.

Drug-Laboratory Test Interactions: Interactions of lidocaine with laboratory tests have not been established.

Drug-Lifestyle Interactions: Interactions of lidocaine with lifestyle have not been established.

DOSAGE AND ADMINISTRATION:

Dosing Considerations: General: When XYLOCAINE Jelly 2% (lidocaine hydrochloride) is used concomitantly with other products containing lidocaine, the total dose contributed by all formulations must be kept in mind.

- XYLOCAINE Jelly 2% in the plastic syringe is preservative-free, and intended for single use only. The syringe is graduated, i.e., a 3 mm line of jelly is equivalent to approximately 1 mL of jelly (20 mg lidocaine hydrochloride).
- The tube presentation of XYLOCAINE Jelly 2% contains preservatives.

The absorption of lidocaine jelly from the nasopharynx is usually lower than with other lidocaine products. Blood concentrations of lidocaine after instillation of the jelly in the intact urethra and bladder in doses up to 800 mg are fairly low and below toxic levels.

Special Populations: Lidocaine should also be used with caution in patients with epilepsy, impaired cardiac conduction, bradycardia, impaired hepatic or renal function and in severe shock (see Warnings and Precautions).

Debilitated patients, elderly patients, acutely ill patients, patients with sepsis, and children should be given reduced doses commensurate with their age, weight and physical condition (see Warnings and Precautions).

XYLOCAINE Jelly 2% should be used with caution in children under the age of 2 as there is insufficient data to support the safety and efficacy of this product in this patient population at this time (see Warnings and Precautions).

Recommended Dose and Dosage Adjustment: Urethral Anesthesia: Surface Anesthesia of the Male Adult Urethra: For adequate analgesia in males, 20 mL (400 mg lidocaine hydrochloride) jelly is usually required. The jelly is instilled slowly until the patient has a feeling of tension (approximately 10 mL) (200 mg). A penile clamp is then applied for several minutes at the corona, after which the rest of the jelly is instilled.

When anesthesia is especially important, e.g., during sounding or cystoscopy, a larger quantity of jelly (e.g., 30-40 mL) may be instilled in 3-4 portions and allowed to act for 10-12 minutes before insertion of the instrument. The jelly instilled into the bladder is also effective for procedures in this region.

To anesthetize only the anterior male urethra, e.g., for catheterization, small volumes (5-10 mL, i.e., 100-200 mg lidocaine HCl) are usually adequate for lubrication.

For Surface Anesthesia of the Female Adult Urethra: Instill 5-10 mL of jelly in small portions to fill the whole urethra. If desired, some jelly may be deposited on the orifice and covered with a cotton swab. In order to obtain adequate anesthesia, several minutes should be allowed prior to performing urological procedures.

Endoscopy: The instillation of 10-20 mL is recommended for adequate analgesia and a small amount may be applied to the lubricating instrument. When combined with other lidocaine products (e.g., for bronchoscopy), the total dose of lidocaine should not exceed 400 mg.

Proctoscopy and Rectoscopy: Up to 20 mL can be used for anal and rectal procedures. The total dose should not exceed 400 mg lidocaine.

Lubrication for Endotracheal Intubation: Apply approximately 2 mL of jelly to the external surface of the endotracheal tube just prior to insertion. Care should be taken to avoid introducing the product into the lumen of the tube (see Warnings and Precautions). Do not use the jelly to lubricate endotracheal stylettes. It is also recommended that the use of endotracheal tubes with dried jelly on the external surface be avoided for lack of lubricating effect.

Maximum Dosage: Adults: The dose of XYLOCAINE Jelly 2% depends on the application site. A safe dose for oral use is 400 mg (20 mL). A safe dose for use in the urethra and bladder is 800 mg (40 mL). A maximum single dosage for XYLOCAINE Jelly 2% is not established. No more than four doses should be given during a 24-hour period.

Children (Under 12 Years): It is difficult to recommend a maximum dose of any drug for children since this varies as a function of age and weight. The maximum amount per dose of XYLOCAINE Jelly 2% should not exceed 6 mg/kg of body weight or 3 mL per 10 kg weight. No more than four doses should be given during a 24-hour period.

For children over 12 years of age doses should be commensurate with weight and physical condition.

OVERDOSAGE:

Acute systemic toxicity from local anesthetics is generally related to high plasma levels encountered during therapeutic use of local anesthetics and originates mainly in the central nervous and the cardiovascular systems (see Adverse Reactions and Warnings and Precautions). It should be kept in mind that clinically relevant pharmacodynamic drug interactions (i.e., toxic effects) may occur with lidocaine and other local anesthetics or structurally related drugs, and Class I and Class III antiarrhythmic drugs due to additive effects (see Drug Interactions).

Symptoms: Central nervous system toxicity is a graded response, with symptoms and signs of escalating severity. The first symptoms are circumoral paresthesia, numbness of the tongue, lightheadedness, hyperacusis and tinnitus. Visual disturbance and muscular tremors are more serious and precede the onset of generalized convulsions. Unconsciousness and grand mal convulsions may follow, which may last from a few seconds to several minutes. Hypoxia and hypercarbia occur rapidly following convulsions due to the increased muscular activity, together with the interference with normal respiration. In severe cases apnea may occur. Acidosis, hyperkalaemia, hypocalcaemia and hypoxia increase and extend the toxic effects of local anesthetics.

Recovery is due to redistribution and metabolism of the local anesthetic drug. Recovery may be rapid unless large amounts of the drug have been administered.

Cardiovascular effects may be seen in cases with high systemic concentrations. Severe hypotension, bradycardia, arrhythmia and cardiovascular collapse may be the result in such cases.

Cardiovascular toxic effects are generally preceded by signs of toxicity in the central nervous system, unless the patient is receiving a general anesthetic or is heavily sedated with drugs such as a benzodiazepine or barbiturate.

Treatment: The first consideration is prevention, best accomplished by careful and constant monitoring of cardiovascular and respiratory vital signs and the patient's state of consciousness after each local anesthetic administration. At the first sign of change, oxygen should be administered.

The first step in the management of systemic toxic reactions consists of immediate attention to the maintenance of a patent airway and assisted or controlled ventilation with oxygen and a delivery system capable of permitting immediate positive airway pressure by mask. This may prevent convulsions if they have not already occurred.

If convulsions occur, the objective of the treatment is to maintain ventilation and oxygenation and support circulation. Oxygen must be given and ventilation assisted if necessary (mask and bag or tracheal intubation). Should convulsions not stop spontaneously after 15-20 seconds, an anticonvulsant should be given iv to facilitate adequate ventilation and oxygenation. Thiopental sodium 1-3 mg/kg iv is the first choice. Alternatively diazepam 0.1 mg/kg bw iv may be used, although its action will be slow. Prolonged convulsions may jeopardise the patient's ventilation and oxygenation. If so, injection of a muscle relaxant (e.g. succinylcholine 1 mg/kg bw) will facilitate ventilation, and oxygenation can be controlled. Early endotracheal intubation is required when succinylcholine is used to control motor seizure activity.

If cardiovascular depression is evident (hypotension, bradycardia), ephedrine 5-10 mg i.v. should be given and may be repeated, if necessary, after 2-3 minutes.

Should circulatory arrest occur, immediate cardiopulmonary resuscitation should be instituted. Continual oxygenation and ventilation and circulatory support as well as treatment of acidosis are of vital importance, since hypoxia and acidosis will increase the systemic toxicity of local anesthetics. Epinephrine (0.1-0.2 mg as intravenous or intracardial injections) should be given as soon as possible and repeated, if necessary.

Children should be given doses of epinephrine commensurate with their age and weight.

For management of a suspected drug overdose, CPhA recommends that you contact your **regional Poison Control Centre**. See the *CPS* Directory section for a list of Poison Control Centres.

ACTION AND CLINICAL PHARMACOLOGY: Mechanism of Action: Lidocaine stabilizes the neuronal membrane by inhibiting the ionic fluxes required for the initiation and conduction of impulses, thereby effecting local anesthetic action. Local anesthetics of the amide type are thought to act within the sodium channels of the nerve membrane.

Onset of Action: Anesthesia is achieved within 5 minutes, depending on the area of application. Duration of anesthesia is approximately 20-30 minutes. XYLOCAINE Jelly 2% (lidocaine hydrochloride) is ineffective when applied to intact skin.

Hemodynamics: Lidocaine, like other local anesthetics, may also have effects on excitable membranes in the brain and myocardium. If excessive amounts of drug reach systemic circulation rapidly, symptoms and signs of toxicity will appear, emanating from the central nervous and cardiovascular systems.

Central nervous system toxicity (see Overdosage) usually precedes the cardiovascular effects since it occurs at lower plasma concentrations. Direct effects of local anesthetics on the heart include slow conduction, negative inotropism and eventually cardiac arrest.

Pharmacokinetics: Absorption: The rate and extent of absorption depends upon concentration and total dose administered, the specific site of application and duration of exposure. In general, the rate of absorption of local anesthetic agents following topical application to wound surfaces and mucous membranes is high, and occurs most rapidly after intratracheal and bronchial administration. The absorption of lidocaine jelly from the nasopharynx is usually lower than with other lidocaine products. Blood concentrations of lidocaine after instillation of the jelly in the intact urethra and bladder in doses up to 800 mg are fairly low and below toxic levels. Lidocaine is also well absorbed from the gastrointestinal tract, although little intact drug may appear in the circulation because of biotransformation in the liver.

Distribution: Lidocaine has a total plasma clearance of 0.95 L/min and a volume of distribution at steady state of 91 L.

Lidocaine readily crosses the placenta, and equilibrium in regard to free, unbound drug will be reached. Because the degree of plasma protein binding in the fetus is less than in the mother, the total plasma concentration will be greater in the mother, but the free concentrations will be the same.

The plasma binding of lidocaine is dependent on drug concentration, and the fraction bound decreases with increasing concentration. At concentrations of 1 to 4 μg of free base per mL, 60 to 80 percent of lidocaine is protein bound. Binding is also dependent on the plasma concentration of the alpha-1-acid glycoprotein. Lidocaine crosses the blood-brain and placental barriers, presumably by passive diffusion.

Metabolism: Lidocaine is metabolized rapidly by the liver, and its metabolites and the unchanged drug are excreted by the kidneys. Biotransformation includes oxidative N-dealkylation, ring hydroxylation, cleavage of the amide linkage, and conjugation. Only 2% of lidocaine is excreted unchanged. Most of it is metabolized first to monoethylglycinexylidide (MEGX) and then to glycinexylidide (GX) and 2,6-dimethylaniline. Up to 70% appears in the urine as 4-hydroxy-2,6-dimethylaniline. The pharmacological/toxicological actions of MEGX and GX are similar to, but less potent than those of lidocaine. GX has a longer half-life (about 10 h) than lidocaine and may accumulate during long-term administration.

Excretion: Lidocaine has an elimination half-life of 1.6 h and an estimated hepatic extraction ratio of 0.65. The clearance of lidocaine is almost entirely due to liver metabolism, and depends both on liver blood flow and the activity of metabolizing enzymes. Approximately 90% of the lidocaine administrated intravenously is excreted in the form of various metabolites, and less than 10% is excreted unchanged in the urine. The primary metabolite in urine is a conjugate of 4-hydroxy-2,6-dimethylaniline, accounting for about 70-80% of the dose excreted in the urine.

The elimination half-life of lidocaine following an intravenous bolus injection is typically 1.5 to 2.0 hours. The elimination half-life in neonates (3.2 h) is approximately twice that of adults. The half-life may be prolonged two-fold or more in patients with liver dysfunction. Renal dysfunction does not affect lidocaine kinetics but may increase the accumulation of metabolites.

Special Populations and Conditions: Acidosis increases the systemic toxicity of lidocaine while the use of CNS depressants may increase the levels of lidocaine required to produce overt CNS effects. Objective adverse manifestations become increasingly apparent with increasing venous plasma levels above 6.0 μg free base per mL.

STORAGE AND STABILITY: Store at 15-30°C. Protect from freezing.

SPECIAL HANDLING INSTRUCTIONS: Instructions for Use—Jelly Syringe:

1. Tear off the paper cover.
2. Screw plunger rod clockwise into grey rubber until rubber rotates.
3. Twist the protective tab and **then, without bending, pull slightly** to break the seal.
4. **Extrude a small amount (i.e. 1 cm) of Jelly. Inspect the syringe to ensure that there is no plastic fragment present in the Jelly.**
   Note: Upon visual inspection, a clear plastic fragment in clear jelly may be difficult to detect and may look like an air pocket.
   If the protective tab is broken, do not use the syringe.
5. **The syringe must not be used and must be discarded if there is any suspicion of a broken plastic fragment.**
6. **If the protective tab is intact and no plastic fragment is found in the Jelly, the syringe is ready for use.**

For further assistance please contact AstraZeneca Canada at 1-800-668-6000.

INFORMATION FOR THE PATIENT: Published in e-CPS, available by subscription at www.e-cps.ca.

DOSAGE FORMS, COMPOSITION AND PACKAGING: Each mL of a clear to almost clear, slightly colored jelly contains: lidocaine HCl 20 mg. Nonmedicinal ingredients: hydroxypropyl methylcellulose, methyl- and propylparabens (30 mL tube only), sodium hydroxide and/or hydrochloric acid to adjust pH 6.0 to 7.0 and water for injection. The vehicle of the active ingredient consists of water, thickened with hydroxypropyl methylcellulose. Its water-miscible base, characterized by high viscosity and low surface tension, allows close and prolonged contact with mucous membrane. Prefilled single-use plastic syringes of 10 mL. Aluminum tubes of 30 mL with an applicator cone. The jelly syringe contains no preservatives and is intended for single use only.

Xylocaine® Ointment 5%

lidocaine

Topical Anesthetic

AstraZeneca

Date of Preparation: October 1954
Date of Revision: December 21, 2006

SUMMARY PRODUCT INFORMATION:

Route of Administration	Dosage Form/ Strength	Clinically Relevant Nonmedicinal Ingredients
Topical	Ointment, 50 mg/g	Propylene glycol For a complete listing see Dosage Forms, Composition and Packaging.

INDICATIONS AND CLINICAL USE: XYLOCAINE Ointment 5% (lidocaine) is indicated for:

- Temporary relief of pain associated with minor burns and abrasions of the skin, e.g. sunburn, herpes zoster and labialis, pruritus, sore nipples, insect bites;
- Anesthesia of mucous membranes, e.g. various anal conditions such as hemorrhoids and fissures;
- The alleviation of pain during examination and instrumentation, e.g. proctoscopy, sigmoidoscopy, cystoscopy, endotracheal intubation.

CONTRAINDICATIONS: XYLOCAINE Ointment 5% (lidocaine) is contraindicated in:

- patients with a known history of hypersensitivity to local anesthetics of the amide type or to other components of the ointment (see Dosage Forms, Composition and Packaging).

WARNINGS AND PRECAUTIONS: General: Excessive dosage, or short intervals between doses, can result in high plasma levels of lidocaine or its metabolites and serious adverse effects. Absorption from wound surfaces and the mucous membranes is variable but is especially high from the bronchial tree. Such applications may therefore result in rapidly rising or excessive plasma concentrations, with an increased risk for toxic symptoms, such as convulsions. **Patients should be instructed to strictly adhere to the recommended dosage.** This is especially important in children where doses vary with weight. The management of serious adverse reactions may require the use of resuscitative equipment, oxygen and other resuscitative drugs (see Overdosage).

The lowest dosage that results in effective anesthesia should be used to avoid high plasma levels and serious adverse effects. Tolerance to elevated blood levels varies with the status of the patient.

Lidocaine should be used with caution in patients with sepsis and/or traumatized mucosa at the area of application, since under such conditions there is the potential for rapid systemic absorption.

XYLOCAINE Ointment 5% (lidocaine) should be used with caution in children under the age of 2 as there is insufficient data to support the safety and efficacy of this product in this patient population at this time.

In patients under general anesthesia who are paralyzed, higher plasma concentrations may occur than in spontaneously breathing patients. Unparalyzed patients are more likely to swallow a large proportion of the dose, which then undergoes considerable first-pass hepatic metabolism following absorption from the gut.

Avoid contact with eyes.

Many drugs used during the conduct of anesthesia are considered potential triggering agents for familial malignant hyperthermia. It has been shown that the use of amide local anesthetics in malignant hyperthermia patients is safe. However, there is no guarantee that neural blockade will prevent the development of malignant hyperthermia during surgery. It is also difficult to predict the need for supplemental general anesthesia. Therefore, a standard protocol for the management of malignant hyperthermia should be available.

When topical anesthetics are used in the mouth, the patient should be aware that the production of topical anesthesia may impair swallowing and thus enhance the danger of aspiration. Numbness of the tongue or buccal mucosa may enhance the danger of unintentional biting trauma. Food or chewing gum should not be taken while the mouth or throat area is anesthetized. See also Information for the Patient.

XYLOCAINE Ointment 5% is ineffective when applied to intact skin.

Carcinogenesis and Mutagenesis: Genotoxicity tests with lidocaine showed no evidence of mutagenic potential. A metabolite of lidocaine, 2,6-xylidine, showed weak evidence of activity in some genotoxicity tests. A chronic oral toxicity study of the metabolite 2,6-xylidine (0, 14, 45, 135 mg/kg) administered in feed to rats showed that there was a significantly greater incidence of nasal cavity tumors in male and female animals that had daily oral exposure to the highest dose of 2,6-xylidine for 2 years. The lowest tumor-inducing dose tested in animals (135 mg/kg) corresponds to approximately 40 times the amount of 2,6-xylidine to which a 50 kg subject would be exposed following the application of 8 g of lidocaine ointment 5% for 24 hours on the mucosa, assuming the highest theoretical extent of absorption of 100% and 80% conversion to 2,6-xylidine. Based on a yearly exposure (once daily dosing with 2,6-xylidine in animals and 5 treatment sessions with 8 g lidocaine ointment 5% in humans), the safety margins would be approximately 3000 times when comparing the exposure in animals to man.

Cardiovascular: Lidocaine should be used with caution in patients with bradycardia or impaired cardiovascular function since they may be less able to compensate for functional changes associated with the prolongation of A-V conduction produced by amide-type local anesthetics.

Lidocaine should be used with caution in patients in severe shock.

Neurologic: Epilepsy: The risk of central nervous system side effects when using lidocaine in patients with epilepsy is very low, provided that the dose recommendations are followed (see Dosage and Administration).

Locomotion and Coordination: Topical lidocaine formulations generally result in low plasma concentrations because of a low degree of systemic absorption. However, depending on the dose, local anesthetics may have a very mild effect on mental function and coordination even in the absence of overt CNS toxicity and may temporarily impair locomotion and alertness.

Renal: Lidocaine is metabolized primarily by the liver to monoethylglycinexylidine (MEGX, which has some CNS activity), and then further to metabolites glycinexylidine (GX) and 2,6-xylidine (see Action and Clinical Pharmacology). Only a small fraction (2%) of lidocaine is excreted unchanged in the urine. The pharmacokinetics of lidocaine and its main metabolite were not altered significantly in hemodialysis patients (n=4) who received an intravenous dose of lidocaine. Therefore, renal impairment is not expected to significantly affect the pharmacokinetics of lidocaine when XYLOCAINE Ointment 5% is used for short treatment durations, according to dosage instructions (see Dosage and Administration). Caution is recommended when lidocaine is used in patients with severely impaired renal function because lidocaine metabolites may accumulate during long term treatment (see Dosage and Administration).

Hepatic/Biliary/Pancreatic: Because amide-type local anesthetics such as lidocaine are metabolized by the liver, these drugs, especially repeated doses, should be used cautiously in patients with hepatic disease. Patients with severe hepatic disease, because of their inability to metabolize local anesthetics normally, are at greater risk of developing toxic plasma concentrations.

Sensitivity/Resistance: Lidocaine should be used with caution in persons with known drug sensitivities. Patients allergic to para-aminobenzoic acid derivates (procaine, tetracaine, benzocaine, etc.) have not shown cross sensitivity to lidocaine.

Special Populations: Debilitated patients, acutely ill patients, and patients with sepsis should be given reduced doses commensurate with their age, weight and physical condition because they may be more sensitive to systemic effects due to increased blood levels of lidocaine following repeated doses.

Lidocaine should be used with caution in patients with epilepsy or impaired renal function.

Pregnant Women: There are no adequate and well-controlled studies in pregnant women on the effect of lidocaine on the developing fetus.

It is reasonable to assume that a large number of pregnant women and women of child-bearing age have been given lidocaine. No specific disturbances to the reproductive process have so far been reported, e.g. no increased incidence of malformations. However, care should be given during early pregnancy when maximum organogenesis takes place.

Labour and Delivery: Should XYLOCAINE Ointment 5% be used concomitantly with other products containing lidocaine during labour and delivery, the total dose contributed by all formulations must be kept in mind.

Nursing Women: Lidocaine and its metabolites are excreted in the breast milk. At therapeutic doses the quantities of lidocaine and its metabolites in breast milk are small and generally are not expected to be a risk for the infant.

Pediatrics: Children should be given reduced doses commensurate with their age, weight and physical condition because they may be more sensitive to systemic effects due to increased blood levels of lidocaine following repeated doses (see Dosage and Administration).

XYLOCAINE Ointment 5% should be used with caution in children under the age of 2 as there is insufficient data to support the safety and efficacy of this product in this patient population at this time.

Geriatrics: Elderly patients may be more sensitive to systemic effects due to increased blood levels of lidocaine following repeated doses and may require dose reductions.

ADVERSE REACTIONS: Adverse experiences following the administration of lidocaine are similar in nature to those observed with other amide local anesthetic agents. These adverse experiences are, in general, dose-related and may result from high plasma levels caused by overdosage or rapid absorption, or may result from a hypersensitivity, idiosyncrasy or diminished tolerance on the part of the patient.

Serious adverse experiences are generally systemic in nature. The following types are those most commonly reported:

Central Nervous System: CNS manifestations are excitatory and/or depressant and may be characterized by the following signs and symptoms of escalating severity: circumoral paresthesia, lightheadedness, nervousness, apprehension, euphoria, confusion, dizziness, drowsiness, hyperacusis, tinnitus, blurred vision, vomiting, sensations of heat, cold or numbness, twitching, tremors, convulsions, unconsciousness, respiratory depression and arrest. The excitatory manifestations (e.g., twitching, tremors, convulsions) may be very brief or may not occur at all, in which case the first manifestation of toxicity may be drowsiness merging into unconsciousness and respiratory arrest.

Drowsiness following the administration of lidocaine is usually an early sign of a high lidocaine plasma level and may occur as a consequence of rapid absorption.

Cardiovascular System: Cardiovascular manifestations are usually depressant and are characterized by bradycardia, hypotension, arrhythmia and cardiovascular collapse, which may lead to cardiac arrest.

Allergic: Allergic reactions are characterized by cutaneous lesions, urticaria, edema or, in the most severe instances, anaphylactic shock. Allergic reactions of the amide type are rare (<0.1%) and may occur as a result of sensitivity either to the local anesthetic agent or to other components in the formulation (see Dosage Forms, Composition and Packaging).

Skin Irritation: Topical products that contain propylene glycol ay cause skin irritation.

DRUG INTERACTIONS: Overview: Lidocaine is mainly metabolized in the liver by CYP1A2 and CYP3A4 to its two major metabolites, monoethylglycinexylidine (MEGX) and glycinexylidine (GX), both of which are pharmacologically active. Lidocaine has a high hepatic extraction ratio. Only a small fraction (2%) of lidocaine is excreted unchanged in the urine. The hepatic clearance of lidocaine is expected to depend largely on blood flow.

Strong inhibitors of CYP1A2, such as fluvoxamine, given concomitantly with lidocaine, can cause a metabolic interaction leading to an increased lidocaine plasma concentration. Therefore, prolonged administration of lidocaine should be avoided in patients treated with strong inhibitors of CYP1A2, such as fluvoxamine. When coadministered with intravenous lidocaine, two strong inhibitors of CYP3A4, erythromycin and itraconazole, have each been shown to have a modest effect on the pharmacokinetics of intravenous lidocaine. Other drugs such as propranolol and cimetidine have been reported to reduce intravenous lidocaine clearance, probably through effects on hepatic blood flow and/or metabolism.

When lidocaine is used topically, plasma concentrations are of importance for safety reasons (see Warnings and Precautions, General and Adverse Reactions). However, with the low systemic exposure and short duration of topical application, the above-mentioned metabolic drug-drug interactions are not expected to be of clinical significance when XYLOCAINE Ointment 5% is used according to dosage recommendations.

Clinically relevant pharmacodynamic drug interactions may occur with lidocaine and other local anesthetics or structurally related drugs, and Class I and Class III antiarrhythmic drugs due to additive effects.

Drug-Drug Interactions: Local Anesthetics and Agents Structurally Related to Amide-type Local Anesthetics: Lidocaine should be used with caution in patients receiving other local anesthetics or agents structurally related to amide-type local anesthetics (e.g. antiarrhythmics such as mexiletine), since the toxic effects are additive.

Antiarrhythmic Drugs: Class I Antiarrhythmic Drugs: Class I antiarrhythmic drugs (such as mexiletine) should be used with caution since toxic effects are additive and potentially synergistic.

Class III Antiarrhythmic Drugs: Caution is advised when using Class III antiarrhythmic drugs concomitantly with lidocaine due to potential pharmacodynamic or pharmacokinetic interactions with lidocaine, or both. A drug interaction study has shown that the plasma concentration of lidocaine may be increased following administration of a therapeutic dose of intravenous lidocaine to patients treated with amiodarone (n=6). Case reports have described toxicity in patients treated concomitantly with lidocaine and amiodarone. Patients treated with Class III antiarrhythmic drugs (e.g. amiodarone) should be kept under close surveillance and ECG monitoring should be considered, since cardiac effects of these drugs and lidocaine may be additive.

Strong Inhibitors of CYP1A2 and CYP3A4: Cytochrome CYP1A2 and CYP3A4 are involved in the formation of the pharmacologically active lidocaine metabolite MEGX.

Fluvoxamine: Strong inhibitors of CYP1A2, such as fluvoxamine, given during prolonged administration of lidocaine to areas with a high extent of systemic absorption (e.g., mucous membranes) can cause a metabolic interaction leading to an increased lidocaine plasma concentration. The plasma clearance of a single intravenous dose of lidocaine was reduced by 41 to 60% during coadministration of fluvoxamine, a selective and potent CYP1A2 inhibitor, to healthy volunteers.

Erythromycin and Itraconazole: Erythromycin and itraconazole, which are strong inhibitors of CYP3A4, have been shown to reduce clearance of lidocaine by 9 to 18%, following a single intravenous dose of lidocaine to healthy volunteers.

During combined coadministration with fluvoxamine and erythromycin the plasma clearance of lidocaine was reduced by 53%.

β-blockers and Cimetidine: Following a single intravenous dose of lidocaine, administered to healthy volunteers, the clearance of lidocaine has been reported to be reduced up to 47% when coadministered with propanolol and up to 30% when coadministered with cimetidine. Reduced clearance of lidocaine when coadministered with these drugs is probably due to reduced liver blood flow and/or inhibition of microsomal liver enzymes. The potential for clinically significant interactions with these drugs should be considered during long-term treatment with high doses of lidocaine.

Drug-Food Interactions: Interactions of lidocaine with food have not been established.

Drug-Herb Interactions: Interactions of lidocaine with herbal products have not been established.

Drug-Laboratory Test Interactions: Interactions of lidocaine with laboratory tests have not been established.

Drug-Lifestyle Interactions: Interactions of lidocaine with lifestyle have not been established.

DOSAGE AND ADMINISTRATION: Dosing Considerations: General: When XYLOCAINE Ointment 5% (lidocaine) is used concomitantly with other products containing lidocaine, the total dose contributed by all formulations must be kept in mind.

Special Populations: Lidocaine should also be used with caution in patients with epilepsy, impaired cardiac conduction, bradycardia, impaired hepatic or renal function and in severe shock (see Warnings and Precautions).

Debilitated, elderly patients, acutely ill patients, patients with sepsis, and children should be given reduced doses commensurate with their age, weight and physical condition.

XYLOCAINE Ointment 5% should be used with caution in children under the age of 2 as there is insufficient data to support the safety and efficacy of this product in this patient population at this time.

Administration: XYLOCAINE Ointment 5%: The ointment should be applied in a thin layer for adequate control of symptoms. A sterile gauze pad is recommended for application to broken and burned tissue.

For sore nipples, apply on a small piece of gauze; the ointment must be washed away before the next feeding.

For endotracheal intubation, apply 1-2 g of ointment to the tube prior to intubation.

Recommended Dose and Dosage Adjustment: Maximum Dosage: Adults: No more than 2 g (100 mg lidocaine base) in a single dose for endotracheal intubation.

No more than 10 g (500 mg lidocaine base) in a single dose for other indications.

After a maximum endotracheal dose or application to mucous membranes the next dose should not be applied until 4 hours later. After a maximal dose given rectally or to burns the minimum dosing interval should be 8 hours.

The total maximum dose administered in a 24 hour period to healthy adults should not exceed 20 g (1000 mg lidocaine base).

Children (Under 12 Years): It is difficult to recommend a maximum dose of any drug for children since this varies as a function of age and weight. Hence, for safety reasons, in children less than 12 years of age 100% bioavailability should be assumed following application to mucous membranes and broken skin, and the maximum amount of XYLOCAINE Ointment 5% administered to children should not exceed 0.1 g ointment/kg body weight (corresponding to 5 mg lidocaine/kg of body weight). The minimum dosing interval in children should be 8 hours.

For children over 12 years of age doses should be commensurate with weight and physical condition.

OVERDOSAGE:
Acute systemic toxicity from local anesthetics is generally related to high plasma levels encountered during therapeutic use of local anesthetics and originates mainly in the central nervous and the cardiovascular systems (see Adverse Reactions and Warnings and Precautions). It should be kept in mind that clinically relevant pharmacodynamic drug interactions (i.e., toxic effects) may occur with lidocaine and other local anesthetics or structurally related drugs, and Class I and Class III antiarrhythmic drugs due to additive effects (see Drug Interactions).

Symptoms: Central nervous system toxicity is a graded response, with symptoms and signs of escalating severity. The first symptoms are circumoral paresthesia, numbness of the tongue, lightheadedness, hyperacusis and tinnitus. Visual disturbance and muscular tremors are more serious and precede the onset of generalized convulsions. Unconsciousness and grand mal convulsions may follow, which may last from a few seconds to several minutes. Hypoxia and hypercarbia occur rapidly following convulsions due to the increased muscular activity, together with the interference with normal respiration. In severe cases apnea may occur. Acidosis increases the toxic effects of local anesthetics.

Recovery is due to redistribution and metabolism of the local anesthetic drug. Recovery may be rapid unless large amounts of the drug have been administered.

Cardiovascular effects may be seen in cases with high systemic concentrations. Severe hypotension, bradycardia, arrhythmia and cardiovascular collapse may be the result in such cases.

Cardiovascular toxic effects are generally preceded by signs of toxicity in the central nervous system, unless the patient is receiving a general anesthetic or is heavily sedated with drugs such as a benzodiazepine or barbiturate.

Treatment: The first consideration is prevention, best accomplished by careful and constant monitoring of cardiovascular and respiratory vital signs and the patient's state of consciousness after each local anesthetic administration. At the first sign of change, oxygen should be administered.

The first step in the management of systemic toxic reactions consists of immediate attention to the maintenance of a patent airway and assisted or controlled ventilation with oxygen and a delivery system capable of permitting immediate positive airway pressure by mask. This may prevent convulsions if they have not already occurred.

If convulsions occur, the objective of the treatment is to maintain ventilation and oxygenation and support circulation. Oxygen must be given and ventilation assisted if necessary (mask and bag or tracheal intubation). Should convulsions not stop spontaneously after 15-20 seconds, an anticonvulsant should be given iv to facilitate adequate ventilation and oxygenation. Thiopental sodium 1-3 mg/kg iv is the first choice. Alternatively diazepam 0.1 mg/kg bw iv may be used, although its action will be slow. Prolonged convulsions may jeopardize the patient's ventilation and oxygenation. If so, injection of a muscle relaxant (e.g. succinylcholine 1 mg/kg bw) will facilitate ventilation, and oxygenation can be controlled. Early endotracheal intubation is required when succinylcholine is used to control motor seizure activity.

If cardiovascular depression is evident (hypotension, bradycardia), ephedrine 5-10 mg i.v. should be given and may be repeated, if necessary, after 2-3 minutes.

Should circulatory arrest occur, immediate cardiopulmonary resuscitation should be instituted. Continual oxygenation and ventilation and circulatory support as well as treatment of acidosis are of vital importance, since hypoxia and acidosis will increase the systemic toxicity of local anesthetics. Epinephrine (0.1-0.2 mg as intravenous or intracardial injections) should be given as soon as possible and repeated, if necessary.

Children should be given doses of epinephrine commensurate with their age and weight.

For management of a suspected drug overdose, CPhA recommends that you contact your **regional Poison Control Centre**. See the *CPS* Directory section for a list of Poison Control Centres.

ACTION AND CLINICAL PHARMACOLOGY: Mechanism of Action: Lidocaine stabilizes the neuronal membrane by inhibiting the ionic fluxes required for the initiation and conduction of impulses, thereby effecting local anesthetic action. Local anesthetics of the amide type are thought to act within the sodium channels of the nerve membrane.

Onset of Action: Anesthesia usually occurs within 3-5 minutes when applied to mucous membrane. The duration of analgesia for burn wound pain is about 4 hours. The application of gauze over the cream may prolong duration of analgesia in burn wounds. XYLOCAINE Ointment 5% (lidocaine) is ineffective when applied to intact skin.

Hemodynamics: Lidocaine, like other local anesthetics, may also have effects on excitable membranes in the brain and myocardium. If excessive amounts of drug reach systemic circulation rapidly, symptoms and signs of toxicity will appear, emanating from the central nervous and cardiovascular systems.

Central nervous system toxicity (see Overdosage) usually precedes the cardiovascular effects since it occurs at lower plasma concentrations. Direct effects of local anesthetics on the heart include slow conduction, negative inotropism and eventually cardiac arrest.

Pharmacokinetics: Absorption: The rate and extent of absorption depends upon concentration and total dose administered, the specific site of application and duration of exposure. In general, the rate of absorption of local anesthetic agents following topical application to wound surfaces and mucous membranes is high, and occurs most rapidly after intratracheal and bronchial administration. Lidocaine is also well absorbed from the gastrointestinal tract, although little intact drug may appear in the circulation because of biotransformation in the liver.

Distribution: Lidocaine has a total plasma clearance of 0.95 L/min and a volume of distribution at steady state of 91 L.

Following insertion of an endotracheal tube lubricated with a mean of 1.26 g (range 0.49-2.45) XYLOCAINE Ointment 5% in patients 18 to 80 years old, the mean peak venous plasma concentration of lidocaine was 0.45 (range 0.2-0.9) µg/mL and was usually observed within 15 min. A dose increase of 1 g ointment resulted in an average increase of 0.22 µg/mL.

Lidocaine readily crosses the placenta, and equilibrium in regard to free, unbound drug will be reached. Because the degree of plasma protein binding in the fetus is less than in the mother, the total plasma concentration will be greater in the mother, but the free concentrations will be the same.

The plasma binding of lidocaine is dependent on drug concentration, and the fraction bound decreases with increasing concentration. At concentrations of 1 to 4 µg of free base per mL, 60 to 80 percent of lidocaine is protein bound. Binding is also dependent on the plasma concentration of the alpha-1-acid glycoprotein.

Metabolism: Lidocaine is metabolized rapidly by the liver, and metabolites and unchanged drug are excreted by the kidneys. Biotransformation includes oxidative N-dealkylation, ring hydroxylation, cleavage of the amide linkage, and conjugation. Only 2% of lidocaine is excreted unchanged. Most of it is metabolized first to monoethylglycinexylidide (MEGX) and then to glycinexylidide (GX) and 2,6-xylidine. Up to 70% appears in the urine as 4-hydroxy- 2,6-xylidine.

Excretion: Lidocaine has an elimination half-life of 1.6 h and an estimated hepatic extraction ratio of 0.65. The clearance of lidocaine is almost entirely due to liver metabolism, and depends both on liver blood flow and the activity of metabolizing enzymes.

The elimination half-life of lidocaine following an intravenous bolus injection is typically 1.5 to 2.0 hours. The elimination half-life in neonates (3.2 h) is approximately twice that of adults. The half-life may be prolonged two-fold or more in patients with liver dysfunction. Renal dysfunction does not affect lidocaine kinetics but may increase the accumulation of metabolites.

Special Populations and Conditions: Acidosis increases the systemic toxicity of lidocaine while the use of CNS depressants may increase the levels of lidocaine required to produce overt CNS effects. Objective adverse manifestations become increasingly apparent with increasing venous plasma levels above 6.0 µg free base per mL.

STORAGE AND STABILITY: Store at 15-30°C. Protect from freezing.

SPECIAL HANDLING INSTRUCTIONS: On initial opening, do not use if the protective membrane of the tube is punctured.

INFORMATION FOR THE PATIENT: Published in e-CPS, available by subscription at www.e-cps.ca.

DOSAGE FORMS, COMPOSITION AND PACKAGING: Each g of white to greyish-white ointment contains: lidocaine (base) 50 mg. Nonmedicinal ingredients: polyethylene glycol, propylene glycol and purified water. Aluminum tubes of 35 g.

Xylocaine® Parenteral with Epinephrine

lidocaine HCl—epinephrine

Local Anesthetic

AstraZeneca

Xylocaine® Parenteral Without Epinephrine

lidocaine HCl

Local Anesthetic

AstraZeneca

Date of Revision: April 17, 2008

SUMMARY PRODUCT INFORMATION:

Route of Administration	Dosage Form/ Strength	Clinically Relevant Nonmedicinal Ingredients
Parenteral	Sterile solution: 5, 10, 15 and 20 mg/mL lidocaine hydrochloride 10, 15 and 20 mg/mL lidocaine hydrochloride solutions with epinephrine contain 0.010 mg/mL (1:100 000) or 0.005 mg/mL (1:200 000) epinephrine	**Multidose vials:** All multidose vials of lidocaine hydrochloride and lidocaine hydrochloride with epinephrine contain methylparaben **Solutions with Epinephrine:** sodium metabisulfite and citric acid (certain vial presentations, please refer to the product label) For a complete listing see Dosage Forms, Composition and Packaging.

INDICATIONS AND CLINICAL USE: Adults (>18 years of age): XYLOCAINE Parenteral Solutions (lidocaine hydrochloride) are indicated for production of local or regional anesthesia by:

- infiltration techniques including percutaneous injection,
- peripheral nerve block techniques such as brachial plexus and intercostal blocks, and
- central neural techniques including epidural and caudal blocks,

when the accepted procedures for these techniques, as described in standard textbooks, are observed.

Geriatrics (>65 years of age): Elderly patients should be given reduced doses commensurate with their age and physical condition (see Dosage and Administration, Special Populations).

Pediatrics (<18 years of age): Children should be given reduced doses commensurate with their age, weight and physical condition (see Dosage and Administration, Special Populations).

Lidocaine should be used with caution in children younger than two years of age as there are insufficient data to support the safety and efficacy of this product in this patient population at this time.

CONTRAINDICATIONS: XYLOCAINE Parenteral Solutions (lidocaine hydrochloride) are contraindicated in:

- Patients with a known history of hypersensitivity to local anesthetics of the amide type or to other components of the solution (see Dosage Forms, Composition and Packaging).
- Patients with a known history of hypersensitivity to sodium metabisulfite and/or citric acid (stabilizers used in solutions containing epinephrine).
- Patients with a known history of hypersensitivity to methylparaben and/or propylparaben (preservatives used in multidose solutions), or to their metabolite para amino benzoic acid (PABA).

Solutions of lidocaine containing parabens should also be avoided in patients with a history of allergic reactions to ester local anesthetics, which are metabolized to PABA.

XYLOCAINE Parenteral Solutions containing antimicrobial preservatives (e.g. methylparaben) should not be used for epidural or spinal anesthesia, or for any route of administration that would introduce solution into the cerebrospinal fluid because the safety of these agents has not been established with regard to intrathecal injection, either intentional or accidental. These solutions should not be administered intra-ocularly or retro-ocularly.

XYLOCAINE Parenteral Solutions containing antimicrobial preservatives should not be used in doses greater than 15 mL for other types of blockades.

WARNINGS AND PRECAUTIONS: General: Local anesthetics should only be employed by clinicians who are well versed in diagnosis and management of dose-related toxicity and other acute emergencies that might arise from the block to be employed and then only after ensuring the immediate availability of oxygen, other resuscitative drugs, cardiopulmonary equipment and the personnel needed for proper management of toxic reactions and related emergencies (see also Adverse Reactions and Overdosage). Delay in proper management of dose-related toxicity, underventilation from any cause, and/or altered sensitivity may lead to the development of acidosis, cardiac arrest and possibly, death.

An intravenous cannula must be inserted before the local anaesthetic is injected for nerve blocks which may result in hypotension or bradycardia, or where acute systemic toxicity may develop following inadvertent intravascular injection.

The lowest dosage of local anaesthetic that results in effective anaesthesia or analgesia should be used to avoid high plasma levels and serious adverse reactions. Injections should be made slowly or in incremental doses, with frequent aspirations before and during the injection to avoid intravascular injection.

Major peripheral nerve blocks may imply the administration of a large volume of local anaesthetic in areas of high vascularity, often close to large vessels where there is an increased risk of intravascular injection and/or rapid systemic absorption which can lead to high plasma concentrations.

Repeated doses of XYLOCAINE Parenteral Solutions (lidocaine hydrochloride) may cause significant increases in blood levels with each repeated dose because of slow accumulation of the drug or its metabolites. Tolerance to elevated blood levels varies with the status of the patient. Debilitated, elderly patients, acutely ill patients and children should be given reduced doses commensurate with their age and physical condition (see Dosage and Administration, Special Populations).

XYLOCAINE Parenteral Solutions containing epinephrine should not be used in areas of the body supplied by end arteries, such as digits, nose, ears or penis, or otherwise having a compromised blood supply (see also Drug Interactions).

Local anesthetic procedures should not be used when there is inflammation and/or sepsis in the region of the proposed injection.

Many drugs used during the conduct of anesthesia are considered potential triggering agents for familial malignant hyperthermia. It has been shown that the use of amide local anesthetics in malignant hyperthermia patients is safe. However, there is no guarantee that neural blockade will prevent the development of malignant hyperthermia during surgery. It is also difficult to predict the need for supplemental general anesthesia. Therefore, a standard protocol for the management of malignant hyperthermia should be available.

Lidocaine has been shown to be porphyrinogenic in animal models. XYLOCAINE Parenteral Solutions should only be used in patients with acute porphyria when no safer alternative is available. Appropriate precautions should be taken for all porphyric patients.

Cardiovascular: Lidocaine should be used with caution in patients with bradycardia or impaired cardiovascular function since they may be less able to compensate for functional changes associated with the prolongation of A-V conduction produced by amide-type local anesthetics.

Patients with partial or complete heart block require special attention since local anaesthetics may depress myocardial conduction. To reduce the risk of potentially serious adverse reactions, attempts should be made to optimize the patient's condition before major blocks are performed. Dosage should be adjusted accordingly.

Lidocaine should be used with caution in patients in severe shock.

Lumbar and caudal epidural anesthesia should be used with extreme caution in persons with severe hypertension.

Central nerve blocks may cause cardiovascular depression, especially in the presence of hypovolemia. Epidural anesthesia should be used with caution in patients with impaired cardiovascular function.

Epidural anesthesia may lead to hypotension and bradycardia. This risk can be reduced by preloading the circulation with crystalloidal or colloidal solutions. Hypotension should be treated promptly with e.g., ephedrine 5-10 mg intravenously and repeating as necessary.

Solutions containing epinephrine should be used with caution in patients whose medical history and physical evaluation suggest the existence of untreated hypertension, ischemic heart disease, heart block, cerebral vascular insufficiency, peripheral vascular disorder, and any other pathological condition that may be aggravated by the effects of epinephrine.

Patients treated with antiarrhythmic drugs (e.g., amiodarone, mexiletine) should be under close surveillance and ECG monitoring, since cardiac effects of these drugs and lidocaine may be additive (see Drug Interactions).

Peri-Operative Considerations: It is essential that aspiration for blood or cerebrospinal fluid (where applicable) be done prior to injecting any local anesthetics, both the original and all subsequent doses, to avoid intravascular or subarachnoid injection. However, a negative aspiration does not ensure against an intravascular or subarachnoid injection.

The safety and effectiveness of XYLOCAINE Parenteral Solutions (lidocaine hydrochloride) depend on proper dosage, correct technique, adequate precautions and readiness for emergencies. Standard textbooks should be consulted for specific techniques and precautions for various regional anesthetic procedures.

Resuscitative equipment, oxygen, and other resuscitative drugs should be available for immediate use (see Overdosage). During major regional nerve blocks or using large doses, the patient should be in an optimal condition and should have i.v. fluids running via an indwelling catheter to assure a functioning intravenous pathway. The clinician responsible should have adequate and appropriate training in the procedure to be performed, should take the necessary precautions to avoid intravascular injection (see Dosage and Administration), and should be familiar with the diagnosis and treatment of side effects, systemic toxicity and other complications (see Adverse Reactions and Overdosage). **The lowest dosage that results in effective anesthesia should be used to avoid high plasma levels and serious adverse effects. Injections should be made slowly, with frequent aspirations before and during the injection to avoid intravascular injection.**

Careful and constant monitoring of cardiovascular and respiratory (adequacy of ventilation) vital signs and the patient's state of consciousness should be performed after each local anesthetic injection. It should be kept in mind at such times that restlessness, anxiety, incoherent speech, lightheadedness, numbness and tingling of the mouth and lips, metallic taste, tinnitus, dizziness, blurred vision, tremors, twitching, depression or drowsiness may be early warning signs of central nervous system toxicity.

Head/Neck: Small doses of local anesthetics injected into the head and neck area, including retrobulbar, dental and stellate ganglion blocks, may produce adverse reactions caused by inadvertent injection to an artery. These reactions may be similar to systemic toxicity seen with unintentional intravascular injections of larger doses. Inadvertent injections into an artery can cause cerebral symptoms even at low doses. Confusion, convulsions, respiratory depression and/or respiratory arrest, and cardiovascular stimulation or depression leading to cardiac arrest have been reported. Patients receiving these blocks should have their circulation and respiration monitored and be constantly observed. Resuscitative equipment and personnel for treating adverse reactions should be immediately available. Dosage recommendations should not be exceeded (see Dosage and Administration).

Ophthalmic Surgery: Retrobulbar injections may very occasionally reach the cranial subarachnoid space causing temporary blindness, cardiovascular collapse, apnea, convulsions, etc. These reactions, which may be due to intra-arterial injection or direct injection into the central nervous system via the sheaths of the optic nerve, must be diagnosed and treated promptly.

Retrobulbar and peribulbar injections of local anesthetics carry a low risk of persistent ocular muscle dysfunction. The primary causes include trauma and/or local toxic effects on muscles and/or nerves. The severity of such tissue reactions is related to the degree of trauma, the concentration of the local anesthetic and the duration of exposure of the tissue to the local anesthetic. For this reason, as with all local anesthetics, the lowest effective concentration and dose of local anesthetic should be used. Vasoconstrictors and other additives may aggravate tissue reactions and should be used only when indicated.

Clinicians who perform retrobulbar blocks should be aware that there have been reports of respiratory arrest following local anaesthetic injection. Prior to retrobulbar block, as with all other regional procedures, the immediate availability of equipment, drugs, and personnel to manage respiratory arrest or depression, convulsions, and cardiac stimulation or depression should be assured (see also Warnings and Precautions, Injection in Head/Neck).

Epidural Anesthesia: During the administration of epidural anesthesia, it is recommended that a test dose be administered initially and that the patient be monitored for central nervous system toxicity and cardiovascular toxicity, as well as for signs of unintended intrathecal administration, before proceeding (see Dosage and Administration). When clinical conditions permit, consideration should be given to employing local anesthetic solutions that contain epinephrine for the test dose because circulatory changes compatible with epinephrine may also serve as a warning sign of unintended intravascular injection. An intravascular injection is still possible even if aspirations for blood are negative. Patients on beta-blockers may not manifest changes in heart rate, but blood pressure monitoring can detect an evanescent rise in systolic blood pressure.

Endocrine and Metabolism: Solutions containing epinephrine should be used with caution in patients whose medical history and physical evaluation suggest the existence of poorly controlled hyperthyroidism or diabetes.

Hepatic/Biliary/Pancreatic: Because amide-type local anesthetics such as lidocaine are metabolized by the liver, these drugs, especially repeated doses, should be used cautiously in patients with hepatic disease. Patients with severe hepatic disease, because of their inability to metabolize local anesthetics normally, are at greater risk of developing toxic plasma concentrations.

Neurologic: Lumbar and caudal epidural anesthesia should be used with extreme caution in persons with existing neurological disease or spinal deformities.

Epilepsy: Lidocaine should be used with caution in patients with epilepsy. The risk of central nervous system side effects when using lidocaine in patients with epilepsy is very low, provided that the dose recommendations are followed.

Locomotion and Coordination: When appropriate, patients should be informed in advance that they may experience temporary loss of sensation and motor activity, usually in the lower half of the body, following proper administration of epidural anesthesia.

Besides the direct anesthetic effect, local anesthetics may have a very mild effect on mental function and co-ordination even in the absence of overt CNS toxicity and may temporarily impair locomotion and alertness.

Renal: Lidocaine is metabolized primarily by the liver to monoethylglycinexylidine (MEGX, which has some CNS activity), and then further to metabolites glycinexylidine (GX) and 2,6-dimethylaniline (see Action and Clinical Pharmacology). Only a small fraction (3%) of lidocaine is excreted unchanged in the urine. The pharmacokinetics of lidocaine and its main metabolite were not altered significantly in haemodialysis patients (n=4) who received an intravenous dose of lidocaine. Therefore, renal impairment is not expected to significantly affect the pharmacokinetics of lidocaine when XYLOCAINE Parenteral Solutions are used for short treatment durations, according to dosage instructions (see Dosage and Administration). Caution is recommended when lidocaine is used in patients with severely impaired renal function because lidocaine metabolites may accumulate during long term treatment.

Sensitivity/Resistance: Lidocaine should be used with caution in persons with known drug sensitivities. Lidocaine solutions are contraindicated in patients with known hypersensitivities to local anesthetics of the amide type, to other components in the formulation, parabens and their metabolite para amino benzoic acid (PABA). The use of paraben-containing lidocaine preparations should also be avoided in patients who are allergic to ester local anesthetics (see Contraindications).

XYLOCAINE with epinephrine solutions contain sodium metabisulfite, a sulfite that may cause allergic reactions including anaphylactic symptoms and life-threatening or less severe asthmatic episodes in certain susceptible people. Sulfite sensitivity is seen more frequently in asthmatic than in non-asthmatic people.

Special Populations: Debilitated patients, acutely ill patients and patients with sepsis should be given reduced doses commensurate with their age, weight and physical condition because they may be more sensitive to systemic effects due to increased blood levels of lidocaine following repeated doses.

Lumbar and caudal epidural anesthesia should be used with extreme caution in persons with septicemia.

Pregnant Women: There are no adequate and well-controlled studies in pregnant women on the effect of lidocaine on the developing fetus.

It is reasonable to assume that a large number of pregnant women and women of child-bearing age have been given lidocaine. No specific disturbances to the reproductive process have so far been reported, e.g. no increased incidence of malformations. However, care should be given during early pregnancy when maximum organogenesis takes place.

The use of lidocaine solutions containing epinephrine may potentially decrease uterine blood flow and contractility, especially after inadvertent injection into maternal blood vessels.

Paracervical block can sometimes cause fetal bradycardia/tachycardia, and careful monitoring of the fetal heart rate is necessary.

Labour and Delivery: Local anesthetics rapidly cross the placenta and when used for epidural, paracervical, pudendal or caudal block anesthesia, can cause varying degrees of maternal, fetal and neonatal toxicity. The potential for toxicity depends upon the procedure performed, the type and amount of drug used, and the technique of drug administration. Adverse reactions in the parturient, fetus and neonate involve alterations of the central nervous system, peripheral vascular tone and cardiac function.

Maternal hypotension has resulted from regional anesthesia. Local anesthetics produce vasodilation by blocking sympathetic nerves. Elevating the patient's legs and positioning her on her left side will help prevent decreases in blood pressure. A vasopressor, such as ephedrine, may be indicated (see Warnings and Precautions, Cardiovascular). The fetal heart rate also should be monitored continuously, and electronic fetal monitoring is highly advisable.

Epidural, spinal, paracervical, or pudendal anesthesia may alter the forces of parturition through changes in uterine contractility or maternal expulsive efforts. In one study, paracervical block anesthesia was associated with a decrease in the mean duration of first stage labour and facilitation of cervical dilation. However, spinal and epidural anesthesia have also been reported to prolong the second stage of labour by removing the parturient's reflex urge to bear down or by interfering with motor function. The use of obstetrical anesthesia may increase the need for forceps assistance.

Case reports of maternal convulsions and cardiovascular collapse following use of some local anesthetics for paracervical block in early pregnancy (as anesthesia for elective abortion) suggest that systemic absorption under these circumstances may be rapid. Fetal bradycardia may occur in 20 to 30 percent of patients receiving paracervical nerve block anesthesia with the amide-type local anesthetics and may be associated with fetal acidosis. Fetal heart rate should always be monitored during paracervical anesthesia. The physician should weigh the possible advantages against risks when considering paracervical block in prematurity, toxemia of pregnancy, and fetal distress. Careful adherence to recommended dosage is of the utmost importance in obstetrical paracervical block. The recommended maximum dose of each drug should not be exceeded. Injection should be made slowly and with frequent aspiration. Allow a 5-minute interval between sides. Failure to achieve adequate analgesia with recommended doses should arouse suspicion of intravascular or fetal intracranial injection. Cases compatible with unintended fetal intracranial injection of local anesthetic solution have been reported following intended paracervical or pudendal block or both. Babies so affected, present with unexplained neonatal depression at birth, which correlates with high local anesthetic serum levels, and often manifest seizures within six hours. Prompt use of supportive measures combined with forced urinary excretion of the local anesthetic has been used successfully to manage this complication.

Nursing Women: Lidocaine and its metabolites are excreted in the breast milk. At therapeutic doses, the quantities of lidocaine and its metabolites in breast milk are small and generally are not expected to be a risk for the infant. It is not known whether epinephrine enters breast milk, but is unlikely to affect the breast-fed infant.

Pediatrics: Children should be given reduced doses commensurate with their age, weight and physical condition because they may be more sensitive to systemic effects due to increased blood levels of lidocaine following repeated doses (see Dosage and Administration).

In children, the dosage should be calculated on a weight basis up to 5 mg/kg. With the addition of epinephrine, up to 7 mg/kg can be used (see Dosage and Administration).

Lidocaine should be used with caution in children under the age of 2 as there is insufficient data to support the safety and efficacy of this product in this patient population at this time.

Geriatrics: Elderly patients may be more sensitive to systemic effects due to increased blood levels of lidocaine following repeated doses and may require dose reductions.

Carcinogenesis and Mutagenesis: Genotoxicity tests with lidocaine showed no evidence of mutagenic potential. A metabolite of lidocaine 2,6-dimethylaniline, showed weak evidence of activity in some genotoxicity tests. A chronic oral toxicity study of the metabolite 2,6-dimethylaniline (0, 14, 45, 135 mg/kg) administered in feed to rats showed that there was a significantly greater incidence of nasal cavity tumors in male and female animals that had daily oral exposure to the highest dose of 2,6-dimethylaniline for 2 years. The lowest tumor-inducing dose tested in animals (135 mg/kg) corresponds to approximately 11 times the amount of 2,6-dimethylaniline to which a 50 kg subject would be exposed following a single injection of 600 mg of lidocaine for injection, assuming 80% conversion to 2,6-dimethylaniline. Based on a yearly exposure (once daily dosing with 2,6-dimethylaniline in animals and 5 treatment sessions with 600 mg lidocaine for injection in humans), the safety margins would be approximately 1000 times when comparing the exposure in animals to man.

ADVERSE REACTIONS: Adverse experiences following the administration of lidocaine are similar in nature to those observed with other amide local anesthetic agents. These adverse experiences are, in general, dose-related and may result from high plasma levels caused by overdosage, rapid absorption, or inadvertent intravascular injection, or may result from a hypersensitivity, idiosyncrasy or diminished tolerance on the part of the patient. See Table 1.

Serious adverse experiences are generally systemic in nature. The following types are those most commonly reported:

Central Nervous System: CNS manifestations are excitatory and/or depressant and may be characterized by the following signs and symptoms of escalating severity: circumoral paresthesia, lightheadedness, nervousness, apprehension, euphoria, confusion, dizziness, drowsiness, hyperacusis, tinnitus, blurred vision, vomiting, sensations of heat, cold or numbness, twitching, tremors, convulsions, unconsciousness, respiratory depression and arrest. The excitatory manifestations (e.g., twitching, tremors, convulsions) may be very brief or may not occur at all, in which case the first manifestation of toxicity may be drowsiness merging into unconsciousness and respiratory arrest.

Drowsiness following the administration of lidocaine is usually an early sign of a high lidocaine plasma level and may occur as a consequence of rapid absorption.

Table 1: XYLOCAINE Parenteral Adverse Drug Reaction Frequencies

Common (≥1% and <10%)	Vascular Disorders: hypotension, hypertension Gastrointestinal Disorders: nausea, vomiting Nervous System Disorders: parethesia, dizziness Cardiac Disorders: bradycardia
Uncommon (≥0.1% and <1%)	Nervous System Disorders: Signs and symptoms of CNS toxicity (convulsions, paresthesia circumoral, numbness of the tongue, hyperacusis, visual disturbances, tremor, tinnitus, dysarthria, CNS depression)
Rare (≥0.01% and <0.1%)	Cardiac Disorders: cardiac arrest, cardiac arrhythmias Immune system disorders: allergic reactions, anaphylactic reaction/shock Respiratory Disorders: respiratory depression Nervous System Disorders: neuropathy, peripheral nerve injury, arachnoiditis Eye Disorders: diplopia

Cardiovascular System: Cardiovascular manifestations are usually depressant and are characterized by bradycardia, hypotension, arrhythmia and cardiovascular collapse, which may lead to cardiac arrest.

Allergic: Allergic reactions are characterized by cutaneous lesions, urticaria, edema or, in the most severe instances, anaphylactic shock. Allergic reactions of the amide type are rare (<0.1%) and may occur as a result of sensitivity either to the local anesthetic agent or to other components in the formulation (see Dosage Forms, Composition and Packaging).

Neurologic: The incidences of adverse reactions may be related to the total dose of local anesthetic administered but is also dependent upon the particular drug used, the route of administration and the physical status of the patient. Neuropathy and spinal cord dysfunction (e.g. anterior spinal artery syndrome, arachnoiditis, cauda equina syndrome), have been associated with regional anesthesia. Neurological effects may be related to local anesthetic techniques, with or without a contribution from the drug.

In the practice of lumbar epidural block, occasional unintentional penetration of the subarachnoid space by the catheter or needle may occur. For example, a high spinal is characterized by paralysis of the legs, loss of consciousness, respiratory paralysis and bradycardia.

Neurologic effects following unintentional subarachnoid administration during epidural anesthesia may include spinal block by varying magnitude (including total or high spinal block), hypotension secondary to spinal block, urinary retention, fecal and urinary incontinence, loss of perineal sensation and sexual function, persistent anesthesia, paresthesia, weakness, paralysis of the lower extremities and loss of sphincter control, all of which may have slow, incomplete or no recovery; headache, backache, septic meningitis, meningismus, slowing of labour, increased incidence of forceps delivery, or cranial nerve palsies due to traction on nerves from loss of cerebrospinal fluid.

DRUG INTERACTIONS: Overview: Lidocaine is mainly metabolized in the liver by CYP1A2 and CYP3A4 to its two major metabolites, monoethylglycinexylidine (MEGX) and glycinexylidine (GX), both of which are pharmacologically active. Lidocaine has a high hepatic extraction ratio. Only a small fraction (3%) of lidocaine is excreted unchanged in the urine. The hepatic clearance of lidocaine is expected to depend largely on blood flow.

Strong inhibitors of CYP1A2, such as fluvoxamine, given concomitantly with lidocaine, can cause a metabolic interaction leading to an increased lidocaine plasma concentration. Therefore, prolonged administration of lidocaine should be avoided in patients treated with strong inhibitors of CYP1A2, such as fluvoxamine. When co-administered with intravenous lidocaine, two strong inhibitors of CYP3A4, erythromycin and itraconazole, have each been shown to have a modest effect on the pharmacokinetics of intravenous lidocaine. Other drugs such as propranolol and cimetidine have been reported to reduce intravenous lidocaine clearance, probably through effects on hepatic blood flow and/or metabolism.

Clinically relevant pharmacodynamic drug interactions may occur with lidocaine and other local anesthetics or structurally related drugs, and Class I and Class III antiarrhythmic drugs due to additive effects.

Drug-Drug Interactions: Local Anesthetics and Agents Structurally Related to Amide-type Local Anesthetics: Lidocaine should be used with caution in patients receiving other local anesthetics or agents structurally related to amide-type local anesthetics (e.g. antiarrhythmics such as mexiletine), since the toxic effects are additive.

Antiarrhythmic Drugs: Class I Antiarrhythmic Drugs: Class I antiarrhythmic drugs (such as mexiletine) should be used with caution since toxic effects are additive and potentially synergistic.

Class III Antiarrhythmic Drugs: Caution is advised when using Class III antiarrhythmic drugs concomitantly with lidocaine due to potential pharmacodynamic or pharmacokinetic interactions with lidocaine, or both. A drug interaction study has shown that the plasma concentration of lidocaine may be increased following administration of a therapeutic dose of intravenous lidocaine to patients treated with amiodarone (n=6). Case reports have described toxicity in patients treated concomitantly with lidocaine and amiodarone. Patients treated with Class III antiarrhythmic drugs (e.g. amiodarone) should be kept under close surveillance and ECG monitoring should be considered, since cardiac effects of these drugs and lidocaine may be additive.

Strong Inhibitors of CYP1A2 and CYP3A4: Cytochrome CYP1A2 and CYP3A4 are involved in the formation of the pharmacologically active lidocaine metabolite MEGX.

Fluvoxamine: Strong inhibitors of CYP1A2, such as fluvoxamine, given during prolonged administration of lidocaine to areas with a high extent of systemic absorption can cause a metabolic interaction leading to an increased lidocaine plasma concentration. The plasma clearance of a single intravenous dose of lidocaine was reduced by 41 to 60% during co-administration of fluvoxamine, a selective and potent CYP1A2 inhibitor, to healthy volunteers.

Erythromycin and Itraconazole: Erythromycin and itraconazole, which are strong inhibitors of CYP3A4, have been shown to reduce clearance of lidocaine by 9 to 18%, following a single intravenous dose of lidocaine to healthy volunteers.

During combined co-administration with fluvoxamine and erythromycin the plasma clearance of lidocaine was reduced by 53%.

β-blockers and Cimetidine: Following a single intravenous dose of lidocaine, administered to healthy volunteers, the clearance of lidocaine has been reported to be reduced up to 47% when co-administered with propanolol and up to 30% when co-administered with cimetidine. Reduced clearance of lidocaine when co-administered with these drugs is probably due to reduced liver blood flow and/or inhibition of microsomal liver enzymes. The potential for clinically significant interactions with these drugs should be considered during long-term treatment with high doses of lidocaine.

Non-cardioselective betablockers such as propranolol enhance the pressor effects of epinephrine, which may lead to severe hypertension and bradycardia.

Ergot-Containing Drugs: XYLOCAINE with Epinephrine or other vasopressors should not be used concomitantly with ergot-type oxytocic drugs, because a severe persistent hypertension may occur and cerebrovascular and cardiac accidents are possible.

Monoamine Oxidase (MAO) Inhibitors: XYLOCAINE with Epinephrine or solutions containing XYLOCAINE and another vasoconstrictor should be used with extreme caution in patients receiving monoamine oxidase inhibitors (MAO) because severe prolonged hypertension may result. In situations when concurrent therapy is necessary, careful patient monitoring is essential.

Antidepressants (triptyline, imipramine): XYLOCAINE with Epinephrine or solutions containing XYLOCAINE and another vasoconstrictor should be used with extreme caution in patients receiving antidepressants of the triptyline or imipramine types because severe prolonged hypertension may result. In situations when concurrent therapy is necessary, careful patient monitoring is essential.

Antipsychotics (phenothiazines, butyrophenones): XYLOCAINE with Epinephrine or solutions containing XYLOCAINE and another vasoconstrictor should be used with extreme caution in patients receiving phenothiazines and butyrophenones. Phenothiazines and butyrophenone may oppose the vasoconstrictor effects of epinephrine giving rise to hypotensive responses and tachycardia. In situations when concurrent therapy is necessary, careful patient monitoring is essential.

Sedatives: If sedatives are employed to reduce patient apprehension, they should be used in reduced doses, since local anesthetic agents, like sedatives, are central nervous system depressants which in combination may have an additive effect.

General Anesthetics—Inhalation Agents (halothane, enflurane): Solutions containing epinephrine should be used with caution in patients undergoing general anesthesia with inhalation agents such as halothane and enflurane, due to the risk of serious cardiac arrhythmias.

Drug-Food Interactions: Interactions of lidocaine with food have not been established.

Drug-Herb Interactions: Interactions of lidocaine with herbal products have not been established.

Drug-Laboratory Test Interactions: The intramuscular injection of lidocaine may result in an increase in creatine phosphokinase levels. Thus, the use of this enzyme determination, without isoenzyme separation, as a diagnostic test for the presence of acute myocardial infarction may be compromised by the intramuscular injection of lidocaine.

Drug-Lifestyle Interactions: Interactions of lidocaine with lifestyle have not been established.

DOSAGE AND ADMINISTRATION: Dosing Considerations: General: XYLOCAINE Parenteral Solutions should only be used by or under the supervision of clinicians experienced in regional anesthesia.

Parenteral drug products should be inspected visually for particulate matter and discolouration prior to administration, whenever solution and container permit. Solutions which are discoloured or which contain particulate matter should not be administered.

Recommended doses serve only as a guide to the amount of anesthetic required for most routine procedures. The actual volumes and concentrations to be used depend on a number of factors such as type and extent of surgical procedure, depth of anesthesia and degree of muscular relaxation required, duration of anesthesia required, and the physical condition of the patient (see Special Populations).

The lowest concentration of anaesthetic and the lowest dosage needed to provide effective anaesthesia should be administered. The rapid injection of a large volume of local anaesthetic solution should be avoided and fractional doses should be used when feasible.

The use of lidocaine with epinephrine will prolong the anaesthetic action.

When XYLOCAINE Parenteral Solutions (lidocaine hydrochloride) are used concomitantly with other products containing lidocaine, the total dose contributed by all formulations must be kept in mind.

Special Populations: Lidocaine should be used with caution in patients with epilepsy, impaired cardiac conduction, bradycardia, impaired hepatic or renal function and in severe shock (see Warnings and Precautions).

Debilitated patients, elderly patients, acutely ill patients patients with sepsis and children should be given reduced doses commensurate with their age, weight and physical condition (see Warnings and Precautions).

Recommended Dose and Dosage Adjustment: Careful aspiration before and during injection is recommended to prevent intravascular injection. The main dose should be injected slowly or in incremental doses, while closely observing the patient's vital functions and maintaining verbal contact.

Adults: Table 2 (Recommended Dosages) summarizes the recommended volumes and concentrations of XYLOCAINE Parenteral Solutions for various types of anesthetic procedures. The dosages suggested in this table are for normal healthy adults and refer to the use of epinephrine-free solutions. When larger volumes are required, only solutions containing epinephrine should be used except in those cases where vasopressor drugs may be contraindicated.

Children: In children the dosage should be calculated on a weight basis up to 5 mg/kg. With the addition of epinephrine, up to 7 mg/kg can be used. Individual variations occur. In children with a high body weight a gradual reduction of the dosage is often necessary and should be based on the ideal body weight. Standard textbooks should be consulted for factors affecting specific block techniques and for individual patient requirements.

The onset of anesthesia, the duration of anesthesia and the degree of muscular relaxation are proportional to the volume and concentration (i.e. total dose) of local anesthetic used. Thus, an increase in volume and concentration of XYLOCAINE will decrease the onset of anesthesia, prolong the duration of anesthesia, provide a greater degree of muscular relaxation and increase the segmental spread of anesthesia. However, increasing the volume and concentration of XYLOCAINE may result in a more profound fall in blood pressure when used in epidural anesthesia. Although the incidence of side effects with lidocaine is quite low, caution should be exercised when employing large volumes and concentrations since the incidence of side effects is directly proportional to the total dose of local anesthetic agent injected. The risk of reaching a toxic plasma concentration or inducing a local neural injury must be considered when prolonged blocks and/or repeated administration are employed.

In general, complete block of all nerve fibres in large nerves requires the higher concentrations of drug. In smaller nerves, or when a less intense block is required (e.g., in the relief of labour pain), the lower concentrations are indicated. The volume of drug used will affect the extent of spread of anesthesia.

The duration of effect can be increased by using solutions containing epinephrine (see Table 2). The risk of epinephrine systemic effects with solutions containing large volumes of epinephrine should be considered.

Epidural Anesthesia: The lowest dosage that will produce the desired effect should be given. The amount varies with the number of dermatomes to be anesthetized (generally 2-3 mL of the indicated concentration per dermatome). Solutions with preservatives (methylparaben) should not be used since their safety has not been established.

Caudal and Lumbar Epidural Block: Test Dose: As a precaution against the adverse experience sometimes observed following unintentional penetration of the subarachnoid space, a test dose such as 3-5 mL of 1.5% lidocaine should be administered at least 5 minutes prior to injecting the total volume required for a lumbar or caudal epidural block. During the administration of a test dose, it is recommended that constant electrocardiographic (ECG) monitoring occur. The test dose should be repeated if the patient is moved in a manner that may have displaced the catheter. Epinephrine, if contained in the test dose (10-15 μg have been suggested), may serve as a warning of unintentional intravascular injection. If injected into a blood vessel, this amount of epinephrine is likely to produce a transient "epinephrine response" within 45 seconds, consisting of an increase in heart rate and systolic blood pressure, circumoral pallor, palpitations and nervousness in the unsedated patient. The sedated patient may exhibit only a pulse rate increase of 20 or more beats per minute for 15 or more seconds.

Patients on beta blockers may not manifest changes in heart rate, but blood pressure monitoring can detect an evanescent rise in systolic blood pressure. Adequate time should be allowed for onset of anesthesia after administration of each test dose. The rapid injection of a large volume of XYLOCAINE through the catheter should be avoided and when feasible, fractional doses should be administered.

The main dose should be injected slowly at a rate of 100-200 mg/min, or in incremental doses, while keeping in constant verbal contact with the patient. If toxic symptoms occur, the injection should be stopped immediately.

In the event of the known injection of a large volume of local anesthetic solution into the subarachnoid space, after suitable resuscitation and if the catheter is in place, consider attempting the recovery of drug by draining a moderate amount of cerebrospinal fluid (such as 10 mL) through the epidural catheter.

Table 2: XYLOCAINE Parenteral

Dosage Recommendations in Adults

Type of Block	Conc. (%)	Each Dose[a] mL	Each Dose[a] mg	Onset (min)	Duration (h) Without Epinephrine	Indication
Local infiltration	0.5	≤80	≤400	1–2	1.5–2	Surgical operations.
	1	≤40	≤400	1–2	2–3	
Digital[b]	1	1–5	10–50	2–5	1.5–2	Surgical operations.
Intercostal (per nerve)	1	2–5	20–50	3–5	1–2	Surgical operations, postoperative pain and fractured ribs.
	1.5	2–4	30–60	3–5	2–3	
Paracervical[c] (each side)	1	10	100	3–5	1–1.5	Surgical operations and dilation of cervix. Obstetric pain relief.
Paravertebral (per segment)	1	3–5	30–50	5–10	1–1.5	Pain management, diagnostic.
	2	3–5	60–100	5–10	1.5–2	
Pudendal (each side)	1	10	100	5–10	1.5–2	Instrumental delivery.
Intra-articular block	0.5	≤60	≤300	5–10	0.5–1	Arthroscopy and surgical operations.
	1	≤40	≤400	5–10	after washout	
Retrobulbar[c]	2	4	80	3–5	1.5–2	Ocular surgery.
Peribulbar[c]	1	10–15	100–150	3–5	1.5-2	Ocular surgery.
Brachial plexus:						
Axillary	1.0	40–50	400–500	15–30	1.5–2	Surgical operations.
	1.5	30–50	450–600	15–30	1.5–3	
Supraclavicular interscalene and subclavian perivascular	1.0	30–40	300–400	15–30	1.5–2	
	1.5	20–30	300–450	15–30	1.5–3	
Sciatic	1.5	15–20	225–300	15–30	2–3	Surgical operations.
	2	15–20	300–400	15–30	2–3	
3-in-1 (Femoral, obturator and lateral cutaneous)	1	30–40	300–400	15–30	1.5–2	Surgical operations.
	1.5	30	450	15–30	2–3	
Epidural	1.5	3–5	45–75			Test dose.
Lumbar epidural	2	15–25	300–500	15–20	1.5–2	Surgical operations.
Thoracic epidural	1.5	10–15	150–225	10–20	1–1.5	Surgical operations and pain relief.
	2	10–15	200–300	10–20	1.5–2	Surgical operations.
Caudal epidural	1	20–30	200–300	15–30	1–1.5	Surgical operations and pain relief.
	2	15–25	300–500	15–30	1.5–2	Surgical operations.

[a] For epidural blocks, dose includes test dose.
[b] Without epinephrine.
[c] See Warnings and Precautions.

Preservative containing solutions (i.e. those supplied in multidose vials) should not be used for epidural or spinal anaesthesia or for any route of administration that would introduce solution into the cerebrospinal fluid. Local anesthetic solutions containing antimicrobial preservatives solutions should not be administered intra-ocularly or retro-ocularly. These solutions should not be used in doses greater than 15 mL for other types of blockades (see Contraindications).

OVERDOSAGE:

Acute systemic toxicity from local anesthetics is generally related to high plasma levels encountered during therapeutic use of local anesthetics and originates mainly in the central nervous and the cardiovascular systems (see Adverse Reactions and Warnings and Precautions). It should be kept in mind that clinically relevant pharmacodynamic drug interactions (i.e., toxic effects) may occur with lidocaine and other local anesthetics or structurally related drugs, and Class I and Class III antiarrhythmic drugs due to additive effects (see Drug Interactions).

Symptoms: With accidental intravascular injections, the toxic effect will be obvious within 1-3 min, while with overdosage, peak plasma concentrations may not be reached for 20-30 min depending on the site of injection, with signs of toxicity thus being delayed.

Central nervous system toxicity is a graded response, with symptoms and signs of escalating severity. The first symptoms are circumoral paresthesia, numbness of the tongue, lightheadedness, hyperacusis and tinnitus. Visual disturbance and muscular tremors are more serious and precede the onset of generalized convulsions. Unconsciousness and grand mal convulsions may follow, which may last from a few seconds to several minutes. Hypoxia and hypercarbia occur rapidly following convulsions due to the increased muscular activity, together with the interference with normal respiration. In severe cases apnea may occur. Acidosis, hyperkalaemia, hypocalcaemia and hypoxia increase and extend the toxic effects of local anaesthetics.

Recovery is due to redistribution and metabolism of the local anesthetic drug. Recovery may be rapid unless large amounts of the drug have been administered.

Cardiovascular effects may be seen in cases with high systemic concentrations. Severe hypotension, bradycardia, arrhythmia and cardiovascular collapse may be the result in such cases.

Cardiovascular toxic effects are generally preceded by signs of toxicity in the central nervous system, unless the patient is receiving a general anesthetic or is heavily sedated with drugs such as a benzodiazepine or barbiturate.

Treatment: The first consideration is prevention, best accomplished by careful and constant monitoring of cardiovascular and respiratory vital signs and the patient's state of consciousness after each local anesthetic administration. At the first sign of change, oxygen should be administered. **If signs of acute systemic toxicity appear, injection of the local anesthetic should be immediately stopped.**

The first step in the management of systemic toxic reactions, as well as underventilation or apnea due to unintentional subarachnoid injection consists of immediate attention to the establishment and maintenance of a patent airway and assisted or controlled ventilation with oxygen and a delivery system capable of permitting immediate positive airway pressure by mask. This may prevent convulsions if they have not already occurred.

If convulsions occur, the objective of the treatment is to maintain ventilation and oxygenation and support circulation. Oxygen must be given and ventilation assisted if necessary (mask and bag or tracheal intubation). Should convulsions not stop spontaneously after 15-20 seconds, an anticonvulsant should be given iv to facilitate adequate ventilation and oxygenation. Thiopental sodium 1-3 mg/kg iv is the first choice. Alternatively diazepam 0.1 mg/kg bw iv may be used, although its action will be slow. Prolonged convulsions may jeopardise the patient's ventilation and oxygenation. If so, injection of a muscle relaxant (e.g. succinylcholine 1 mg/kg bw) will facilitate ventilation, and oxygenation can be controlled. Early endotracheal intubation is required when succinylcholine is used to control motor seizure activity.

If cardiovascular depression is evident (hypotension, bradycardia), ephedrine 5-10 mg i.v. should be given and may be repeated, if necessary, after 2-3 minutes.

Should circulatory arrest occur, immediate cardiopulmonary resuscitation should be instituted. Continual oxygenation and ventilation and circulatory support as well as treatment of acidosis are of vital importance, since hypoxia and acidosis will increase the systemic toxicity of local anesthetics. Epinephrine (0.1-0.2 mg as intravenous or intracardial injections) should be given as soon as possible and repeated, if necessary.

Children should be given doses of epinephrine commensurate with their age and weight.

For management of a suspected drug overdose, CPhA recommends that you contact your **regional Poison Control Centre**. See the *CPS* Directory section for a list of Poison Control Centres.

ACTION AND CLINICAL PHARMACOLOGY: Mechanism of Action: Lidocaine stabilizes the neuronal membrane by inhibiting the ionic fluxes required for the initiation and conduction of impulses, thereby effecting local anesthetic action. Local anesthetics of the amide type are thought to act within the sodium channels of the nerve membrane.

Onset of Action: The onset of action is 1-5 minutes following infiltration and 5-15 minutes following other types of administration. The duration of anesthesia depends on the concentration of lidocaine used, the dose, and the type of block. The 2% solution will last 1½-2 h when given epidurally, and up to 5 hours with peripheral nerve blocks. With the 1% concentration, there is less effect on motor nerve fibres and the duration of action is shorter. The addition of epinephrine decreases the rate of absorption, reducing toxicity and increasing the duration of effect.

Hemodynamics: Lidocaine, like other local anesthetics, may also have effects on other excitable membranes (e.g. brain and myocardium). If excessive amounts of drug reach systemic circulation, symptoms and signs of toxicity may appear, emanating from the central nervous and cardiovascular systems.

Central nervous system toxicity (see Overdosage) usually precedes the cardiovascular effects since it occurs at lower plasma concentrations. Direct effects of local anesthetics on the heart include slow conduction, negative inotropism and eventually cardiac arrest.

Indirect cardiovascular effects (hypotension, bradycardia) may occur after epidural administration depending on the extent of the concomitant sympathetic block.

Pharmacokinetics: Absorption: Lidocaine is completely absorbed following parenteral administration. The rate of absorption depends on the dose, route of administration, and the vascularity of the injection site. The highest peak plasma levels are obtained following intercostal nerve block (approximately 1.5 µg/mL per 100 mg injected) while abdominal subcutaneous injections give the lowest (approximately 0.5 µg/mL per 100 mg injected). Epidural and major nerve blocks are intermediate.

Absorption is considerably slowed by the addition of epinephrine, although it also depends on the site of injection. Peak plasma concentrations are reduced by 50% following subcutaneous injection, by 30% following epidural injection and by 20% following intercostal block if epinephrine 5 µg/mL is added.

Lidocaine shows complete and biphasic absorption from the epidural space with half lives of the two phases in the order of 9.3 min and 82 min respectively. The slow absorption is the rate limiting factor in the elimination of lidocaine, which explains why the apparent terminal half-life is longer after epidural administration. Absorption of lidocaine from the subarachnoid space is monophasic with an absorption half-life of 71 min.

Distribution: Lidocaine has a total plasma clearance of 0.95 L/min and a volume of distribution at steady state of 91 L.

Lidocaine readily crosses the placenta, and equilibrium with regard to the unbound concentration is rapidly reached. The degree of plasma protein binding in the fetus is less than in the mother, which results in lower total plasma concentrations in the fetus.

The plasma binding of lidocaine is dependent on drug concentration, and the fraction bound decreases with increasing concentration. At concentrations of 1 to 4 µg of free base per mL, 60 to 80 percent of lidocaine is protein bound. Binding is also dependent on the plasma concentration of the alpha-1-acid glycoprotein.

Metabolism: Lidocaine is metabolized rapidly by the liver, and metabolites and unchanged drug are excreted by the kidneys. The main metabolites formed from lidocaine are monoethylglycine xylidide (MEGX), glycinexylidide (GX), 2,6-dimethylaniline and 4-hydroxy-2,6-dimethylaniline. The N-dealkylation to MEGX, is considered to be mediated by both CYP1A2 and CYP3A4. The metabolite 2,6-dimethylaniline is converted to 4-hydroxy-2,6-dimethylaniline by CYP2A6, and the latter is the major urinary metabolite in man. Only 3% of lidocaine is excreted unchanged. About 70% appears in the urine as 4-hydroxy-2,6-dimethylaniline.

Excretion: Lidocaine has a terminal half-life of 1.6 h and an estimated hepatic extraction ratio of 0.65. The clearance of lidocaine is almost entirely due to liver metabolism, and depends both on liver blood flow and the activity of metabolizing enzymes.

The pharmacological/toxicological actions of MEGX and GX are similar to, but less potent than those of lidocaine. GX has a longer half-life (about 10 h) than lidocaine and may accumulate during long-term administration.

The elimination half-life of lidocaine following intravenous bolus injection is typically 1.5 to 2.0 hours. The terminal half-life in neonates (3.2 h) is approximately twice that of adults, whereas clearance is similar (10.2 mL/min·kg). The half-life may be prolonged two-fold or more in patients with liver dysfunction. Renal dysfunction does not affect lidocaine kinetics but may increase the accumulation of metabolites.

Special Populations and Conditions: Acidosis increases the systemic toxicity of lidocaine while the use of CNS depressants may increase the levels of lidocaine required to produce overt CNS effects. Objective adverse manifestations become increasingly apparent with increasing venous plasma levels above 6.0 µg free base per mL.

STORAGE AND STABILITY: XYLOCAINE Parenteral Solutions (lidocaine hydrochloride) should be stored at controlled room temperature (15-30°C). XYLOCAINE Parenteral Solutions containing epinephrine should be protected from light. Protect from freezing.

SPECIAL HANDLING INSTRUCTIONS: Sterilization, and Technical Procedures: Adequate precautions should be taken to avoid prolonged contact between local anesthetic solutions containing epinephrine (low pH) and metal surfaces (e.g. needles or metal parts of syringes), since dissolved metal ions, particularly copper ions, may cause severe local irritation (swelling, edema) at the site of injection and accelerate the degradation of epinephrine.

When chemical disinfection of multidose vials is desired, either isopropyl alcohol (70%) or ethyl alcohol (70%) is recommended. Many commercially available brands of rubbing alcohol, as well as solutions of ethyl alcohol not of USP grade, contain denaturants which are injurious to rubber and therefore are not to be used.

The solubility of lidocaine is limited at pH >6.5. This must be taken into consideration when alkaline solutions, i.e. carbonates, are added, since precipitation might occur. In the case of epinephrine-containing solutions, mixing with alkaline solutions may cause rapid degradation of epinephrine.

XYLOCAINE (lidocaine hydrochloride) plain solutions in glass vials may be autoclaved for 15-20 minutes at 121°C. Due to the nature of the Polyamp system, the plastic ampoules must not be autoclaved. Due to the heat sensitivity of epinephrine, products containing epinephrine should not be autoclaved.

Do not use if solution is coloured or if it contains a precipitate.

XYLOCAINE Parenteral Solutions without preservative are for single use only. Discard unused portion. The multidose vials should not be used for more than three days after the container has been opened for the first time.

There is a greater risk of microbial contamination with multidose vials than with single dose vials. Single-dose vials should therefore be used whenever possible. If a multidose vial is used, appropriate control procedures to prevent contamination should be employed, including the following: use of single-use sterile injecting equipment; use of a sterile needle and syringe for each insertion into the vial; rule out the introduction of contaminated material or fluid into a multidose vial.

INFORMATION FOR THE PATIENT: Published in e-CPS, available by subscription at www.e-cps.ca.

DOSAGE FORMS, COMPOSITION AND PACKAGING: 0.5%: Each mL contains: lidocaine HCl 5 mg. Nonmedicinal ingredients: methylparaben (1 mg/mL), sodium chloride, sodium hydroxide and/or hydrochloric acid to adjust pH between 5.0 and 7.0 and water for injection. Glass multidose vials of 50 mL.

1%: Each mL contains: lidocaine HCl 10 mg. Nonmedicinal ingredients: sodium chloride, sodium hydroxide and/or hydrochloric acid to adjust pH between 5.0 and 7.0 and water for injection. The multidose vials also contain methylparaben (1 mg/mL). Plastic Polyamp Duofit ampuls of 2, 5 and 10 mL. Glass multidose vials of 20 and 50 mL.

1% with Epinephrine: Each mL contains: lidocaine HCl 10 mg and epinephrine 1:100 000. Nonmedicinal ingredients: methylparaben (1 mg/mL), sodium chloride, sodium hydroxide and/or hydrochloric acid to adjust pH between 3.3 and 5.5, sodium metabisulfite and water for injection. May contain citric acid. Glass multidose vials of 20 and 50 mL.

Each mL contains: lidocaine HCl 10 mg and epinephrine 1:200 000. Nonmedicinal ingredients: methylparaben (1 mg/mL), sodium chloride, sodium hydroxide and/or hydrochloric acid to adjust pH between 3.3 and 5.5, sodium metabisulfite and water for injection. Glass multidose vials of 20 mL.

1.5% with Epinephrine: Each mL contains: lidocaine HCl 15 mg and epinephrine 1:200 000. Nonmedicinal ingredients: sodium chloride, sodium hydroxide and/or hydrochloric acid to adjust pH between 3.3 and 5.5, sodium metabisulfite and water for injection. May contain citric acid. Glass single use ampuls of 5 mL (Test Dose) and single use vials of 30 mL.

2%: Each mL contains: lidocaine HCl 20 mg. Nonmedicinal ingredients: sodium chloride, sodium hydroxide and/or hydrochloric acid to adjust pH between 5.0 and 7.0 and water for injection. The multidose vials also contain methylparaben (1 mg/mL). Plastic Polyamp Duofit ampuls of 2, 5 and 10 mL. Glass multidose vials of 20 and 50 mL.

2% with Epinephrine: Each mL contains: lidocaine HCl 20 mg and epinephrine 1:100 000. Nonmedicinal ingredients: methylparaben (1 mg/mL), sodium chloride, sodium hydroxide and/or hydrochloric acid to adjust pH between 3.3 and 5.5, sodium metabisulfite and water for injection. May contain citric acid. Glass multidose vials of 20 and 50 mL.

Each mL contains: lidocaine HCl 20 mg and epinephrine 1:200 000. Nonmedicinal ingredients: sodium chloride, sodium hydroxide and/or hydrochloric acid to adjust pH between 3.3 and 5.5, sodium metabisulfite and water for injection. Glass single use vials of 20 mL.

Plastic Polyamp Duofit ampuls and glass single-use vials are preservative-free.

Polyamp Duofit ampuls are suitable for Luer fit and Luer lock syringes.

Xylocaine® Topical 4%

lidocaine HCl

Oral Topical Anesthetic

AstraZeneca

Date of Preparation: June 1955
Date of Revision: April 2, 2008

SUMMARY PRODUCT INFORMATION:

Route of Administration	Dosage Form/ Strength	Clinically Relevant Nonmedicinal Ingredients
Topical	Solution, 40 mg/mL	Methylparaben For a complete listing see Dosage Forms, Composition and Packaging.

INDICATIONS AND CLINICAL USE: Adults (>18 years of age): XYLOCAINE Topical 4% (lidocaine hydrochloride) is indicated to:

- provide topical anesthesia of the oropharyngeal, tracheal and bronchial areas to reduce reflex activity, attenuate hemodynamic responses and facilitate insertion of the tube or the passage of instruments during endotracheal intubation and endoscopic procedures, e.g. bronchography, bronchoscopy, laryngoscopy, and esophagoscopy.

Geriatrics (>65 years of age): Elderly patients should be given reduced doses commensurate with their age and physical condition (see Dosage and Administration, Special Populations).

Pediatrics (<18 years of age): Children should be given reduced doses commensurate with their age, weight and physical condition (see Dosage and Administration, Special Populations).

Lidocaine should be used with caution in children younger than two years of age as there are insufficient data to support the safety and efficacy of this product in this patient population at this time (see Warnings and Precautions, Special Populations).

CONTRAINDICATIONS: XYLOCAINE Topical 4% (lidocaine hydrochloride) is contraindicated in:

- patients with a known history of hypersensitivity to local anesthetics of the amide type or to other components of the solution (see Dosage Forms, Composition and Packaging).
- patients with a known hypersensitivity to methylparaben and/or propylparaben (preservatives used in XYLOCAINE Topical 4%), or to their metabolite para amino benzoic acid (PABA).

Formulations of lidocaine containing parabens should also be avoided in patients with a history of allergic reactions to ester local anesthetics, which are metabolized to PABA.

WARNINGS AND PRECAUTIONS: General: Excessive dosage, or short intervals between doses, can result in high plasma levels of lidocaine or its metabolites and serious adverse effects. Absorption from the mucous membranes is variable but is especially high from the bronchial tree. Such applications may therefore result in rapidly rising or excessive plasma concentrations, with an increased risk for toxic symptoms, such as convulsions. This is especially important in children where doses vary with weight. The management of serious adverse reactions may require the use of resuscitative equipment, oxygen and other resuscitative drugs (see Overdosage).

The lowest dosage that results in effective anesthesia should be used to avoid high plasma levels and serious adverse effects. Tolerance to elevated blood levels varies with the status of the patient.

XYLOCAINE Topical 4% (lidocaine hydrochloride) is for topical use only and must not be used for injection.

XYLOCAINE Topical 4% must not be used as a gargle. The use of concentrated Xylocaine Topical 4% for gargling increases the risk of systemic toxicity due to overdosing and rapid uptake over the mucosa and/or ingestion.

Lidocaine should be used with caution in patients with sepsis and/or traumatized mucosa at the area of application, since under such conditions there is the potential for rapid systemic absorption.

XYLOCAINE Topical 4% should be used with caution in children under the age of 2 as there is insufficient data to support the safety and efficacy of this product in this patient population at this time.

In patients under general anesthesia who are paralyzed, higher plasma concentrations may occur than in spontaneously breathing patients. Unparalyzed patients are more likely to swallow a large proportion of the dose, which then undergoes considerable first-pass hepatic metabolism following absorption from the gut.

Avoid contact with eyes.

Many drugs used during the conduct of anesthesia are considered potential triggering agents for familial malignant hyperthermia. It has been shown that the use of amide local anesthetics in malignant hyperthermia patients is safe. However there is no guarantee that neural blockade will prevent the development of malignant hyperthermia during surgery. It is also difficult to predict the need for supplemental general anesthesia. Therefore, a standard protocol for the management of malignant hyperthermia should be available.

When topical anesthetics are used in the mouth, the patient should be aware that the production of topical anesthesia may impair swallowing and thus enhance the danger of aspiration. Numbness of the tongue or buccal mucosa may enhance the danger of unintentional biting trauma. Food or chewing gum should not be taken while the mouth or throat area is anesthetized. See also Information for the Patient.

XYLOCAINE Topical 4% is ineffective when applied to intact skin.

Lidocaine has been shown to be porphyrinogenic in animal models. XYLOCAINE Topical 4% should only be prescribed to patients with acute porphyria on strong or urgent indications, when they can be closely monitored. Appropriate precautions should be taken for all porphyric patients.

Cardiovascular: Lidocaine should be used with caution in patients with bradycardia or impaired cardiovascular function since they may be less able to compensate for functional changes associated with the prolongation of A-V conduction produced by amide-type local anesthetics.

Lidocaine should be used with caution in patients with severe shock.

Neurologic: Epilepsy: The risk of central nervous system side effects when using lidocaine in patients with epilepsy is very low, provided that the dose recommendations are followed (see Dosage and Administration).

Locomotion and Coordination: Topical lidocaine formulations generally result in low plasma concentrations because of a low degree of systemic absorption. However, depending on the dose, local anesthetics may have a very mild effect on mental function and coordination even in the absence of overt CNS toxicity and may temporarily impair locomotion and alertness.

Renal: Lidocaine is metabolized primarily by the liver to monoethylglycinexylidine (MEGX, which has some CNS activity), and then further to metabolites glycinexylidine (GX) and 2,6-dimethylaniline (see Action and Clinical Pharmacology). Only a small fraction (2%) of lidocaine is excreted unchanged in the urine. The pharmacokinetics of lidocaine and its main metabolite were not altered significantly in haemodialysis patients (n=4) who received an intravenous dose of lidocaine. Therefore, renal impairment is not expected to significantly affect the pharmacokinetics of lidocaine when XYLOCAINE Topical 4% is used for short treatment durations, according to dosage instructions (see Dosage and Administration). Caution is recommended when lidocaine is used in patients with severely impaired renal function because lidocaine metabolites may accumulate during long term treatment (see Dosage and Administration).

Hepatic/Biliary/Pancreatic: Because amide-type local anesthetics such as lidocaine are metabolized by the liver, these drugs, especially repeated doses, should be used cautiously in patients with hepatic disease. Patients with severe hepatic disease, because of their inability to metabolize local anesthetics normally, are at greater risk of developing toxic plasma concentrations.

Sensitivity/Resistance: Lidocaine should be used with caution in persons with known drug sensitivities.

XYLOCAINE Topical 4% is contraindicated in patients with known hypersensitivities to local anesthetics of the amide type, to other components in the formulation, methylparaben and/or propylparaben (preservatives) and their metabolite para amino benzoic acid (PABA). The use of paraben-containing lidocaine preparations should also be avoided in patients who are allergic to ester local anesthetics (see Contraindications).

Special Populations: Debilitated patients, acutely ill patients and patients with sepsis should be given reduced doses commensurate with their age, weight and physical condition because they may be more sensitive to systemic effects due to increased blood levels of lidocaine following repeated doses.

Pregnant Women: There are no adequate and well-controlled studies in pregnant women on the effect of lidocaine on the developing fetus.

It is reasonable to assume that a large number of pregnant women and women of child-bearing age have been given lidocaine. No specific disturbances to the reproductive process have so far been reported, e.g. no increased incidence of malformations. However, care should be given during early pregnancy when maximum organogenesis takes place.

Labour and Delivery: Should XYLOCAINE Topical 4% be used concomitantly with other products containing lidocaine during labour and delivery, the total dose contributed by all formulations must be kept in mind.

Nursing Women: Lidocaine and its metabolites are excreted in the breast milk. At therapeutic doses the quantities of lidocaine and its metabolites in breast milk are small and generally are not expected to be a risk for the infant.

Pediatrics: Children should be given reduced doses commensurate with their age, weight and physical condition because they may be more sensitive to systemic effects due to increased blood levels of lidocaine following repeated doses (see Dosage and Administration).

XYLOCAINE Topical 4% should be used with caution in children under the age of 2 as there is insufficient data to support the safety and efficacy of this product in this patient population at this time.

Geriatrics: Elderly patients may be more sensitive to systemic effects due to increased blood levels of lidocaine following repeated doses and may require dose reductions.

Carcinogenesis and Mutagenesis: Genotoxicity tests with lidocaine showed no evidence of mutagenic potential. A metabolite of lidocaine, 2,6-dimethylaniline, showed weak evidence of activity in some genotoxicity tests. A chronic oral toxicity study of the metabolite 2,6-dimethylaniline (0, 14, 45, 135 mg/kg) administered in feed to rats showed that there was a significantly greater incidence of nasal cavity tumors in male and female animals that had daily oral exposure to the highest dose of 2,6-dimethylaniline for 2 years. The lowest tumor-inducing dose tested in animals (135 mg/kg) corresponds to approximately 45 times the amount of 2,6-dimethylaniline to which a 50 kg subject would be exposed following the application of 10 g of lidocaine topical 4% for 24 hours on the mucosa, assuming the highest theoretical extent of absorption of 100%, and 80% conversion to 2,6-dimethylaniline. Based on a yearly exposure (once daily dosing with 2,6-dimethylaniline in animals and 5 treatment sessions with 10 g lidocaine topical 4% in humans), the safety margins would be approximately 3400 times when comparing the exposure in animals to man.

ADVERSE REACTIONS: Adverse experiences following the administration of lidocaine are similar in nature to those observed with other amide local anesthetic agents. These adverse experiences are, in general, dose-related and may result from high plasma levels caused by overdosage or rapid absorption, or may result from a hypersensitivity, idiosyncrasy or diminished tolerance on the part of the patient.

Serious adverse experiences are generally systemic in nature. The following types are those most commonly reported:

Central Nervous System: CNS manifestations are excitatory and/or depressant and may be characterized by the following signs and symptoms of escalating severity: circumoral paresthesia, lightheadedness, nervousness, apprehension, euphoria, confusion, dizziness, drowsiness, hyperacusis, tinnitus, blurred vision, vomiting, sensations of heat, cold or numbness, twitching, tremors, convulsions, unconsciousness, respiratory depression and arrest. The excitatory manifestations (e.g., twitching, tremors, convulsions) may be very brief or may not occur at all, in which case the first manifestation of toxicity may be drowsiness merging into unconsciousness and respiratory arrest.

Drowsiness following the administration of lidocaine is usually an early sign of a high lidocaine plasma level and may occur as a consequence of rapid absorption.

Cardiovascular System: Cardiovascular manifestations are usually depressant and are characterized by bradycardia, hypotension, arrhythmia and cardiovascular collapse, which may lead to cardiac arrest.

Allergic: Allergic reactions are characterized by cutaneous lesions, urticaria, edema or, in the most severe cases, anaphylactic shock. Allergic reactions of the amide type are rare (<0.1%) and may occur as a result of sensitivity either to the local anesthetic agent or to other components in the formulation (see Dosage Forms, Composition and Packaging).

DRUG INTERACTIONS: Overview: Lidocaine is mainly metabolized in the liver by CYP1A2 and CYP3A4 to its two major metabolites, monoethylglycinexylidine (MEGX) and glycinexylidine (GX), both of which are pharmacologically active. Lidocaine has a high hepatic extraction ratio. Only a small fraction (2%) of lidocaine is excreted unchanged in the urine. The hepatic clearance of lidocaine is expected to depend largely on blood flow.

Strong inhibitors of CYP1A2, such as fluvoxamine, given concomitantly with lidocaine, can cause a metabolic interaction leading to an increased lidocaine plasma concentration. Therefore, prolonged administration of lidocaine should be avoided in patients treated with strong inhibitors of CYP1A2, such as fluvoxamine. When co-administered with intravenous lidocaine, two strong inhibitors of CYP3A4, erythromycin and itraconazole, have each been shown to have a modest effect on the pharmacokinetics of intravenous lidocaine. Other drugs such as propranolol and cimetidine have been reported to reduce intravenous lidocaine clearance, probably through effects on hepatic blood flow and/or metabolism.

When lidocaine is used topically, plasma concentrations are of importance for safety reasons (see Warnings and Precautions, General and Adverse Reactions). However, with the low systemic exposure and short duration of topical application, the above-mentioned metabolic drug-drug interactions are not expected to be of clinical significance when XYLOCAINE Topical 4% is used according to dosage recommendations.

Clinically relevant pharmacodynamic drug interactions may occur with lidocaine and other local anesthetics or structurally related drugs, and Class I and Class III antiarrhythmic drugs due to additive effects.

Drug-Drug Interactions: Local Anesthetics and Agents Structurally Related to Amide-Type Local Anesthetics: Lidocaine should be used with caution in patients receiving other local anesthetics or agents structurally related to amide-type local anesthetics (e.g. antiarrhythmics such as mexiletine), since the toxic effects are additive.

Antiarrhythmic Drugs: Class I Antiarrhythmic Drugs: Class I antiarrhythmic drugs (such as mexiletine) should be used with caution since toxic effects are additive and potentially synergistic.

Class III Antiarrhythmic Drugs: Caution is advised when using Class III antiarrhythmic drugs concomitantly with lidocaine due to potential pharmacodynamic or pharmacokinetic interactions with lidocaine, or both. A drug interaction study has shown that the plasma concentration of lidocaine may be increased following administration of a therapeutic dose of intravenous lidocaine to patients treated with amiodarone (n=6). Case reports have described toxicity in patients treated concomitantly with lidocaine and amiodarone. Patients treated with Class III antiarrhythmic drugs (e.g. amiodarone) should be kept under close surveillance and ECG monitoring should be considered, since cardiac effects of these drugs and lidocaine may be additive.

Strong Inhibitors of CYP1A2 and CYP3A4: Cytochrome CYP1A2 and CYP3A4 are involved in the formation of the pharmacologically active lidocaine metabolite MEGX.

Fluvoxamine: Strong inhibitors of CYP1A2, such as fluvoxamine, given during prolonged administration of lidocaine to areas with a high extent of systemic absorption (e.g., mucous membranes) can cause a metabolic interaction leading to an increased lidocaine plasma concentration. The plasma clearance of a single intravenous dose of lidocaine was reduced by 41 to 60% during co-administration of fluvoxamine, a selective and potent CYP1A2 inhibitor, to healthy volunteers.

Erythromycin and Itraconazole: Erythromycin and itraconazole, which are strong inhibitors of CYP3A4, have been shown to reduce clearance of lidocaine by 9 to 18%, following a single intravenous dose of lidocaine to healthy volunteers.

During combined co-administration with fluvoxamine and erythromycin the plasma clearance of lidocaine was reduced by 53%.

β-blockers and Cimetidine: Following a single intravenous dose of lidocaine, administered to healthy volunteers, the clearance of lidocaine has been reported to be reduced up to 47% when co-administered with propranolol and up to 30% when co-administered with cimetidine. Reduced clearance of lidocaine when co-administered with these drugs is probably due to reduced liver blood flow and/or inhibition of microsomal liver enzymes. The potential for clinically significant interactions with these drugs should be considered during long-term treatment with high doses of lidocaine.

Drug-Food Interactions: Interactions of lidocaine with food have not been established.

Drug-Herb Interactions: Interactions of lidocaine with herbal products have not been established.

Drug-Laboratory Tests Interactions: Interactions of lidocaine with laboratory tests have not been established.

Drug-Lifestyle Interactions: Interactions of lidocaine with lifestyle have not been established.

DOSAGE AND ADMINISTRATION:

Dosing Considerations: General: When XYLOCAINE Topical 4% (lidocaine hydrochloride) is used concomitantly with other products containing lidocaine, the total dose contributed by all formulations must be kept in mind.

The degree of absorption from mucous membranes is variable but especially high from the bronchial tree. Application only to areas below the vocal cords may result in excessive plasma concentrations because of less transfer to the intestine and less first-pass loss. When inhaled from a nebulizer, the resulting plasma concentrations are lower than following spray (atomizer) applications.

Special Populations: Lidocaine should be used with caution in patients with epilepsy, impaired cardiac conduction, bradycardia, impaired hepatic or renal function and in severe shock (see Warnings and Precautions).

Debilitated, elderly patients, acutely ill patients, patients with sepsis, and children should be given reduced doses commensurate with their age, weight and physical condition.

XYLOCAINE Topical 4% should be used with caution in children under the age of 2 as there is insufficient data to support the safety and efficacy of this product in this patient population at this time.

Administration: XYLOCAINE Topical 4%: XYLOCAINE Topical 4% is for topical use only and must not be administered by injection or used as a gargle. Injection or gargling with concentrated Xylocaine Topical 4% increases the risk of systemic toxicity due to overdosing and/or rapid uptake over the mucosa and/or ingestion (see Warnings and Precautions).

Topical anesthesia may be achieved by spraying, e.g. using an atomizer or nebulizer. XYLOCAINE Topical 4% may also be applied with cotton applicators or by instillation into a cavity or onto a surface.

Recommended Dose and Dosage Adjustment: Adults: The recommended dose of XYLOCAINE Topical 4% is 2-7.5 mL (80-300 mg lidocaine hydrochloride). During prolonged procedures (>5 minutes), up to 400 mg may be administered. In addition, when combined with other lidocaine products, the total dose should not exceed 400 mg.

With applications mainly to the larynx, trachea, and bronchi, the dose should not exceed 5 mL (200 mg).

When inhaled from a nebulizer, 5-10 mL (200-400 mg) may be used.

Children (Under 12 Years): It is difficult to recommend a maximum dose of any drug for children since this varies as a function of age and weight. The maximum amount of XYLOCAINE Topical 4% administered should not exceed 3 mg/kg of body weight.

For children over 12 years of age doses should be commensurate with weight and physical condition.

OVERDOSAGE:

Acute systemic toxicity from local anesthetics is generally related to high plasma levels encountered during therapeutic use of local anesthetics and originates mainly in the central nervous and the cardiovascular systems (see Adverse Reactions and Warnings and Precautions). It should be kept in mind that clinically relevant pharmacodynamic drug interactions (i.e., toxic effects) may occur with lidocaine and other local anesthetics or structurally related drugs, and Class I and Class III antiarrhythmic drugs due to additive effects (see Drug Interactions).

Symptoms: Central nervous system toxicity is a graded response, with symptoms and signs of escalating severity. The first symptoms are circumoral paresthesia, numbness of the tongue, lightheadedness, hyperacusis and tinnitus. Visual disturbance and muscular tremors are more serious and precede the onset of generalized convulsions. Unconsciousness and grand mal convulsions may follow, which may last from a few seconds to several minutes. Hypoxia and hypercarbia occur rapidly following convulsions due to the increased muscular activity, together with the interference with normal respiration. In severe cases apnea may occur. Acidosis, hyperkalaemia, hypocalcaemia and hypoxia increase and extend the toxic effects of local anesthetics.

Recovery is due to redistribution and metabolism of the local anesthetic drug. Recovery may be rapid unless large amounts of the drug have been administered.

Cardiovascular effects may be seen in cases with high systemic concentrations. Severe hypotension, bradycardia, arrhythmia and cardiovascular collapse may be the result in such cases.

Cardiovascular toxic effects are generally preceded by signs of toxicity in the central nervous system, unless the patient is receiving a general anesthetic or is heavily sedated with drugs such as a benzodiazepine or barbiturate.

Treatment: The first consideration is prevention, best accomplished by careful and constant monitoring of cardiovascular and respiratory vital signs and the patient's state of consciousness after each local anesthetic administration. At the first sign of change, oxygen should be administered.

The first step in the management of systemic toxic reactions consists of immediate attention to the maintenance of a patent airway and assisted or controlled ventilation with oxygen and a delivery system capable of permitting immediate positive airway pressure by mask. This may prevent convulsions if they have not already occurred.

If convulsions occur, the objective of the treatment is to maintain ventilation and oxygenation and support circulation. Oxygen must be given and ventilation assisted if necessary (mask and bag or tracheal intubation). Should convulsions not stop spontaneously after 15-20 seconds, an anticonvulsant should be given iv to facilitate adequate ventilation and oxygenation. Thiopental sodium 1-3 mg/kg iv is the first choice. Alternatively diazepam 0.1mg/kg bw iv may be used, although its action will be slow. Prolonged convulsions may jeopardise the patient's ventilation and oxygenation. If so, injection of a muscle relaxant (e.g. succinylcholine 1mg/kg bw) will facilitate ventilation, and oxygenation can be controlled. Early endotracheal intubation is required when succinylcholine is used to control motor seizure activity.

If cardiovascular depression is evident (hypotension, bradycardia), ephedrine 5-10 mg i.v. should be given and may be repeated, if necessary, after 2-3 minutes.

Should circulatory arrest occur, immediate cardiopulmonary resuscitation should be instituted. Optimal oxygenation and ventilation and circulatory support as well as treatment of acidosis are of vital importance, since hypoxia and acidosis will increase the systemic toxicity of local anesthetics. Epinephrine (0.1-0.2 mg as intravenous or intracardial injections) should be given as soon as possible and repeated, if necessary.

Children should be given doses of epinephrine commensurate with their age and weight.

> For management of a suspected drug overdose, CPhA recommends that you contact your **regional Poison Control Centre**. See the *CPS* Directory section for a list of Poison Control Centres.

ACTION AND CLINICAL PHARMACOLOGY: Mechanism of Action: Lidocaine stabilizes the neuronal membrane by inhibiting the ionic fluxes required for the initiation and conduction of impulses, thereby effecting local anesthetic action. Local anesthetics of the amide type are thought to act within the sodium channels of the nerve membrane.

Onset of Action: Anesthesia usually occurs within 1-5 minutes depending on the area of application. The duration of anesthesia is approximately 15-30 minutes. XYLOCAINE Topical 4% (lidocaine hydrochloride) is ineffective when applied to intact skin.

Hemodynamics: Lidocaine, like other local anesthetics, may also have effects on excitable membranes in the brain and myocardium. If excessive amounts of drug reach systemic circulation rapidly, symptoms and signs of toxicity will appear, emanating from the central nervous and cardiovascular systems.

Central nervous system toxicity (see Overdosage) usually precedes the cardiovascular effects since it occurs at lower plasma concentrations. Direct effects of local anesthetics on the heart include slow conduction, negative inotropism and eventually cardiac arrest.

Pharmacokinetics: Absorption: The rate and extent of absorption depends upon concentration and total dose administered, the specific site of application and duration of exposure. In general, the rate of absorption of local anesthetic agents, following topical application to wound surfaces and mucous membranes is high, and occurs most rapidly after intratracheal and bronchial administration. Lidocaine is also well absorbed from the gastrointestinal tract, although little of the intact drug may appear in the circulation because of biotransformation in the liver.

Distribution: Lidocaine has a total plasma clearance of 0.95 L/min and a volume of distribution at steady state of 91 L.

Lidocaine readily crosses the placenta, and equilibrium in regard to free, unbound drug will be reached. Because the degree of plasma protein binding in the fetus is less than in the mother, the total plasma concentration will be greater in the mother, but the free concentrations will be the same.

The plasma binding of lidocaine is dependent on drug concentration, and the fraction bound decreases with increasing concentration. At concentrations of 1 to 4 μg of free base per mL, 60 to 80 percent of lidocaine is protein bound. Binding is also dependent on the plasma concentration of the alpha-1-acid glycoprotein.

Metabolism: Lidocaine is metabolized rapidly by the liver, and metabolites and unchanged drug are excreted by the kidneys. Biotransformation includes oxidative N-dealkylation, ring hydroxylation, cleavage of the amide linkage, and conjugation. Only 2% of lidocaine is excreted unchanged. Most of it is metabolized first to monoethylglycinexylidide (MEGX) and then to glycinexylidide (GX) and 2,6-dimethylaniline. Up to 70% appears in the urine as 4-hydroxy-2,6-dimethylaniline.

Excretion: Lidocaine has an elimination half-life of 1.6 h and an estimated hepatic extraction ratio of 0.65. The clearance of lidocaine is almost entirely due to liver metabolism, and depends both on liver blood flow and the activity of metabolizing enzymes.

The elimination half-life of lidocaine following an intravenous bolus injection is typically 1.5 to 2.0 hours. The elimination half-life in neonates (3.2 h) is approximately twice that of adults. The half-life may be prolonged two-fold or more in patients with liver dysfunction. Renal dysfunction does not affect lidocaine kinetics but may increase the accumulation of metabolites.

Special Populations and Conditions: Acidosis increases the systemic toxicity of lidocaine while the use of CNS depressants may increase the levels of lidocaine required to produce overt CNS effects. Objective adverse manifestations become increasingly apparent with increasing venous plasma levels above 6.0 μg free base per mL.

STORAGE AND STABILITY: Store at 15-30°C. Protect from freezing.

Incompatibilities: The solubility of lidocaine is limited at pH >6.5. This must be taken into consideration when alkaline solutions, i.e. carbonates, are added since precipitation might occur.

INFORMATION FOR THE PATIENT: Published in e-CPS, available by subscription at www.e-cps.ca.

DOSAGE FORMS, COMPOSITION AND PACKAGING: Each mL of clear colorless solution contains: lidocaine HCl 40 mg. Nonmedicinal ingredients: methylparaben, sodium hydroxide and/or hydrochloric acid to adjust pH to 6.0-7.0 and water for injection. Bottles of 50 mL.

Xylocaine® Viscous 2%
lidocaine HCl
Topical Anesthetic

AstraZeneca

Date of Preparation: December 1986
Date of Revision: April 2, 2008

SUMMARY PRODUCT INFORMATION:

Route of Administration	Dosage Form/ Strength	Clinically Relevant Nonmedicinal Ingredients
Topical	Liquid, 20 mg/mL	Methylparaben, propylparaben For a complete listing see Dosage Forms, Composition and Packaging.

INDICATIONS AND CLINICAL USE: Adults (>18 years of age): XYLOCAINE Viscous 2% (lidocaine hydrochloride) is indicated to provide relief of pain and discomfort in connection with:
- irritated or inflamed mucous membranes of the mouth and pharynx, e.g. lesions following tonsillectomy;
- introduction of instruments and catheters into the respiratory and digestive tracts, e.g. bronchoscopy, esophagoscopy;
- painful diseases of the upper gastrointestinal tract e.g. esophagitis.

Geriatrics (>65 years of age): Elderly patients should be given reduced doses commensurate with their age and physical condition (see Dosage and Administration, Special Populations).
Pediatrics (<18 years of age): Children should be given reduced doses commensurate with their age, weight and physical condition (see Dosage and Administration, Special Populations).

Lidocaine should be used with caution in children younger than two years of age as there are insufficient data to support the safety and efficacy of this product in this patient population at this time (see Warnings and Precautions, Special Populations).

CONTRAINDICATIONS: XYLOCAINE Viscous 2% (lidocaine hydrochloride) is contraindicated in:
- patients with a known history of hypersensitivity to local anesthetics of the amide type or to other components of the solution (see Dosage Forms, Composition and Packaging).
- patients with a known hypersensitivity to methylparaben and/or propylparaben (preservatives used in XYLOCAINE Viscous 2% format), or to their metabolite para amino benzoic acid (PABA).

Formulations of lidocaine containing parabens should also be avoided in patients with a history of allergic reactions to ester local anesthetics, which are metabolized to PABA.

WARNINGS AND PRECAUTIONS: General: Excessive dosage, or short intervals between doses, can result in high plasma levels of lidocaine or its metabolites and serious adverse effects. Following too high or repeated doses of viscous lidocaine in children under the age of three, serious side effects have been reported. Absorption from the wound surfaces and mucous membranes is variable but is especially high from the bronchial tree. Such applications may therefore result in rapidly rising or excessive plasma concentrations, with an increased risk for toxic symptoms, such as convulsions. **Patients should be instructed to strictly adhere to the recommended dosage.** This is especially important in children where doses vary with weight. The management of serious adverse reactions may require the use of resuscitative equipment, oxygen and other resuscitative drugs (see Overdosage).

The lowest dosage that results in effective anesthesia should be used to avoid high plasma levels and serious adverse effects. Tolerance to elevated blood levels varies with the status of the patient.

XYLOCAINE Viscous 2% (lidocaine hydrochloride) **is for topical use only and must not be used for injection**.

Lidocaine should be used with caution in patients with sepsis and/or traumatized mucosa at the area of application, since under such conditions there is the potential for rapid systemic absorption.

XYLOCAINE Viscous 2% should be used with caution in children under the age of 2 as there is insufficient data to support the safety and efficacy of this product in this patient population at this time.

In patients under general anesthesia who are paralyzed, higher plasma concentrations may occur than in spontaneously breathing patients. Unparalyzed patients are more likely to swallow a large proportion of the dose, which then undergoes considerable first-pass hepatic metabolism following absorption from the gut.

Avoid contact with eyes.

Many drugs used during the conduct of anesthesia are considered potential triggering agents for familial malignant hyperthermia. It has been shown that the use of amide local anesthetics in malignant hyperthermia patients is safe. However there is no guarantee that neural blockade will prevent the development of malignant hyperthermia during surgery. It is also difficult to predict the need for supplemental general anesthesia. Therefore a standard protocol for the management of malignant hyperthermia should be available.

When topical anesthetics are used in the mouth, the patient should be aware that the production of topical anesthesia may impair swallowing and thus enhance the danger of aspiration. Numbness of the tongue or buccal mucosa may enhance the danger of unintentional biting trauma. Food or chewing gum should not be taken while the mouth or throat area is anesthetized. See also Information for the Patient.

XYLOCAINE Viscous 2% is ineffective when applied to intact skin.

Lidocaine has been shown to be porphyrinogenic in animal models. XYLOCAINE Viscous 2% should only be prescribed to patients with acute porphyria on strong or urgent indications, when they can be closely monitored. Appropriate precautions should be taken for all porphyric patients.
Cardiovascular: Lidocaine should be used with caution in patients with bradycardia or impaired cardiovascular function since they may be less able to compensate for functional changes associated with the prolongation of A-V conduction produced by amide-type local anesthetics.

Lidocaine should be used with caution in patients in severe shock.
Neurologic: Epilepsy: The risk of central nervous system side effects when using lidocaine in patients with epilepsy is very low, provided that the dose recommendations are followed (see Dosage and Administration).
Locomotion and Coordination: Topical lidocaine formulations generally result in low plasma concentrations because of a low degree of systemic absorption. However, depending on the dose, local anesthetics may have a very mild effect on mental function and coordination even in the absence of overt CNS toxicity and may temporarily impair locomotion and alertness.
Renal: Lidocaine is metabolized primarily by the liver to monoethylglycinexylidine (MEGX, which has some CNS activity), and then further to metabolites glycinexylidine (GX) and 2,6-dimethylaniline (see Action and Clinical Pharmacology). Only a small fraction (2%) of lidocaine is excreted unchanged in the urine. The pharmacokinetics of lidocaine and its main metabolite were not altered significantly in haemodialysis patients (n=4) who received an intravenous dose of lidocaine. Therefore, renal impairment is not expected to significantly affect the pharmacokinetics of lidocaine when XYLOCAINE Viscous 2% is used for short treatment durations, according to dosage instructions (see Dosage and Administration). Caution is recommended when lidocaine is used in patients with severely impaired renal function because lidocaine metabolites may accumulate during long term treatment (see Dosage and Administration).
Hepatic/Biliary/Pancreatic: Because amide-type local anesthetics such as lidocaine are metabolized by the liver, these drugs, especially repeated doses, should be used cautiously in patients with hepatic disease. Patients with severe hepatic disease, because of their inability to metabolize local anesthetics normally, are at greater risk of developing toxic plasma concentrations.
Sensitivity/Resistance: Lidocaine should be used with caution in persons with known drug sensitivities.

XYLOCAINE Viscous 2% is contraindicated in patients with known hypersensitivities to local anesthetics of the amide type, to other components in the formulation, methylparaben and/or propylparaben (preservatives) and their metabolite para amino benzoic acid (PABA). The use of paraben-containing lidocaine preparations should also be avoided in patients who are allergic to ester local anesthetics (see Contraindications).
Special Populations: Debilitated patients, acutely ill patients and patients with sepsis should be given reduced doses commensurate with their age, weight and physical condition because they may be more sensitive to systemic effects due to increased blood levels of lidocaine following repeated doses.
Pregnant Women: There are no adequate and well-controlled studies in pregnant women on the effect of lidocaine on the developing fetus.

It is reasonable to assume that a large number of pregnant women and women of child-bearing age have been given lidocaine. No specific disturbances to the reproductive process have so far been reported, e.g. no increased incidence of malformations. However, care should be given during early pregnancy when maximum organogenesis takes place.
Labour and Delivery: Should XYLOCAINE Viscous 2% be used concomitantly with other products containing lidocaine during labour and delivery, the total dose contributed by all formulations must be kept in mind.
Nursing Women: Lidocaine and its metabolites are excreted in the breast milk. At therapeutic doses the quantities of lidocaine and its metabolites in breast milk are small and generally are not expected to be a risk for the infant.
Pediatrics: Children should be given reduced doses commensurate with their age, weight and physical condition because they may be more sensitive to systemic effects due to increased blood levels of lidocaine following repeated doses (see Dosage and Administration).

XYLOCAINE Viscous 2% should be used with caution in children under the age of 2 as there is insufficient data to support the safety and efficacy of this product in this patient population at this time.
Geriatrics: Elderly patients may be more sensitive to systemic effects due to increased blood levels of lidocaine following repeated doses and may require dose reductions.
Carcinogenesis and Mutagenesis: Genotoxicity tests with lidocaine showed no evidence of mutagenic potential. A metabolite of lidocaine, 2,6-dimethylaniline, showed weak evidence of activity in some genotoxicity tests. A chronic oral toxicity study of the metabolite 2,6-dimethylaniline (0, 14, 45, 135 mg/kg) administered in feed to rats showed that there was a significantly greater incidence of nasal cavity tumors in male and female animals that had daily oral exposure to the highest dose of 2,6-dimethylaniline for 2 years. The lowest tumor-inducing dose tested in animals (135 mg/kg) corresponds to approximately 50 times the amount of 2,6-dimethylaniline to which a 50 kg subject would be exposed following the application of 20 g of lidocaine viscous 2% for 24 hours on the mucosa, assuming the highest theoretical extent of absorption of 100% and 80% conversion to 2,6-dimethylaniline. Based on a yearly exposure (once daily dosing with 2,6-dimethylaniline in animals and 5 treatment sessions with 20 g lidocaine viscous 2% in humans), the safety margins would be approximately 3400 times when comparing the exposure in animals to man.

ADVERSE REACTIONS: Adverse experiences following the administration of lidocaine are similar in nature to those observed with other amide local anesthetic agents. These adverse experiences are, in general, dose-related and may result from high plasma levels caused by overdosage or rapid absorption, or may result from a hypersensitivity, idiosyncrasy or diminished tolerance on the part of the patient.

Serious adverse experiences are generally systemic in nature. The following types are those most commonly reported:
Central Nervous System: CNS manifestations are excitatory and/or depressant and may be characterized by the following signs and symptoms of escalating severity: circumoral paresthesia, lightheadedness, apprehension, euphoria, confusion, dizziness, drowsiness, hyperacusis, tinnitus, blurred vision, vomiting, sensations of heat, cold or numbness, twitching, tremors, convulsions, unconsciousness, respiratory depression and arrest. The excitatory manifestations (e.g., twitching, tremors, convulsions) may be very brief or may not occur at all, in which case the first manifestation of toxicity may be drowsiness merging into unconsciousness and respiratory arrest.

Drowsiness following the administration of lidocaine is usually an early sign of a high lidocaine plasma level and may occur as a consequence of rapid absorption.
Cardiovascular System: Cardiovascular manifestations are usually depressant and are characterized by bradycardia, hypotension, arrhythmia and cardiovascular collapse, which may lead to cardiac arrest.
Allergic: Allergic reactions are characterized by cutaneous lesions, urticaria, edema or, in the most severe instances, anaphylactic shock. Allergic reactions of the amide type are rare (<0.1%) and may occur as a result of sensitivity either to the local anesthetic agent or to other components in the formulation (see Dosage Forms, Composition and Packaging).

DRUG INTERACTIONS: Overview: Lidocaine is mainly metabolized in the liver by CYP1A2 and CYP3A4 to its two major metabolites, monoethylglycinexylidine (MEGX) and glycinexylidine (GX), both of which are pharmacologically active. Lidocaine has a high hepatic extraction ratio. Only a small fraction (2%) of lidocaine is excreted unchanged in the urine. The hepatic clearance of lidocaine is expected to depend largely on blood flow.

Strong inhibitors of CYP1A2, such as fluvoxamine, given concomitantly with lidocaine, can cause a metabolic interaction leading to an increased lidocaine plasma concentration. Therefore, prolonged administration of lidocaine should be avoided in patients treated with strong inhibitors of CYP1A2, such as fluvoxamine. When coadministered with intravenous lidocaine, two strong inhibitors of CYP3A4, erythromycin and itraconazole, have each been shown to have a modest effect on the pharmacokinetics of intravenous lidocaine. Other drugs such as propranolol and cimetidine have been reported to reduce intravenous lidocaine clearance, probably through effects on hepatic blood flow and/or metabolism.

When lidocaine is used topically, plasma concentrations are of importance for safety reasons (see Warnings and Precautions, General and Adverse Reactions). However, with the low systemic exposure and short duration of topical application, the abovementioned metabolic drug-drug interactions are not expected to be of clinical significance when XYLOCAINE Viscous 2% is used according to dosage recommendations.

Clinically relevant pharmacodynamic drug interactions may occur with lidocaine and other local anesthetics or structurally related drugs, and Class I and Class III antiarrhythmic drugs due to additive effects.
Drug-Drug Interactions: Local Anesthetics and Agents Structurally Related to Amide-type Local Anesthetics: Lidocaine should be used with caution in patients receiving other local anesthetics or agents structurally related to amide-type local anesthetics (e.g. antiarrhythmics such as mexiletine), since the toxic effects are additive.
Antiarrhythmic Drugs: Class I Antiarrhythmic Drugs: Class I antiarrhythmic drugs (such as mexiletine) should be used with caution since toxic effects are additive and potentially synergistic.
Class III Antiarrhythmic Drugs: Caution is advised when using Class III antiarrhythmic drugs concomitantly with lidocaine due to potential pharmacodynamic or pharmacokinetic interactions with lidocaine, or both. A drug interaction study has shown that the plasma concentration of lidocaine may be increased following administration of a therapeutic dose of intravenous lidocaine to patients treated with amiodarone (n=6). Case reports have described toxicity in patients treated concomitantly with lidocaine and amiodarone. Patients treated with Class III antiarrhythmic drugs (e.g. amiodarone) should be kept under close surveillance and ECG monitoring should be considered, since cardiac effects of these drugs and lidocaine may be additive.
Strong Inhibitors of CYP1A2 and CYP3A4: Cytochrome CYP1A2 and CYP3A4 are involved in the formation of the pharmacologically active lidocaine metabolite MEGX.
Fluvoxamine: Strong inhibitors of CYP1A2, such as fluvoxamine, given during prolonged administration of lidocaine to areas with a high extent of systemic absorption (e.g., mucous membranes) can cause a metabolic interaction leading to an increased lidocaine plasma concentration. The plasma clearance of a single intravenous dose of lidocaine was reduced by 41 to 60% during coadministration of fluvoxamine, a selective and potent CYP1A2 inhibitor, to healthy volunteers.
Erythromycin and Itraconazole: Erythromycin and itraconazole, which are strong inhibitors of CYP3A4, have been shown to reduce clearance of lidocaine by 9 to 18%, following a single intravenous dose of lidocaine to healthy volunteers.

During combined coadministration with fluvoxamine and erythromycin the plasma clearance of lidocaine was reduced by 53%.
β-blockers and Cimetidine: Following a single intravenous dose of lidocaine, administered to healthy volunteers, the clearance of lidocaine has been reported to be reduced up to 47% when coadministered with propanolol and up to 30% when coadministered with cimetidine. Reduced clearance of lidocaine when coadministered with these drugs is probably due to reduced liver blood flow and/or inhibition of microsomal liver enzymes. The potential for clinically significant interactions with these drugs should be considered during long-term treatment with high doses of lidocaine.
Drug-Food Interactions: Interactions of lidocaine with food have not been established.
Drug-Herb Interactions: Interactions of lidocaine with herbal products have not been established.
Drug-Laboratory Test Interactions: Interactions of lidocaine with laboratory tests have not been established.
Drug-Lifestyle Interactions: Interactions of lidocaine with lifestyle have not been established.

DOSAGE AND ADMINISTRATION: **Dosing Considerations: General:** When XYLOCAINE Viscous 2% (lidocaine hydrochloride) is used concomitantly with other products containing lidocaine, the total dose contributed by all formulations must be kept in mind.

The degree of absorption from mucous membranes is variable but especially high from the bronchial tree. The degree of systemic absorption depends on whether the lidocaine viscous is swallowed or expectorated. It is therefore important to expectorate in order to avoid unnecessary absorption. After a swallowed single dose of 300 mg (15 mL) of lidocaine viscous, the resulting blood concentrations are low.
Special Populations: Lidocaine should also be used with caution in patients with epilepsy, impaired cardiac conduction, bradycardia, impaired hepatic or renal function and in severe shock (see Warnings and Precautions).

Debilitated, elderly patients, acutely ill patients, patients with sepsis, and children should be given reduced doses commensurate with their age, weight and physical condition.

XYLOCAINE Viscous 2% should be used with caution in children under the age of 2 as there is insufficient data to support the safety and efficacy of this product in this patient population at this time.
Administration: XYLOCAINE Viscous 2%: XYLOCAINE Viscous 2% is for topical use only and must not be used for injection (see Warnings and Precautions).

For oral analgesia, the solution should be swished around in the mouth and spat out or swallowed slowly.

For use in the pharynx, the solution should be gargled and may be swallowed.

Recommended Dose and Dosage Adjustment: Adults:

- For treatment of pain from irritated or inflamed mucous membranes of the mouth and throat, 5-10 mL of lidocaine viscous (100-200 mg lidocaine) is recommended. Six doses may be given in 24 hours. Total dosage of XYLOCAINE Viscous 2% in 24 hours should not exceed 60 mL or 1200 mg lidocaine.
- For topical anesthesia before introduction of instruments and catheters into the upper respiratory or digestive tracts, 10-15 mL of lidocaine viscous (200-300 mg lidocaine) is recommended. When combined with other lidocaine products (e.g. for bronchoscopy), the total dosage of lidocaine should not exceed 400 mg.
- For diseases of the upper gastrointestinal tract, 5-15 mL of lidocaine viscous (100-300 mg of lidocaine) should be swallowed quickly in one gulp. Six doses may be given in 24 hours. Total dosage of XYLOCAINE Viscous 2% in 24 hours should not exceed 60 mL or 1200 mg lidocaine.

Children (Under 12 Years): In children under the age of 12, for treatment of irritated or inflamed mucous membranes of the mouth and throat, the dose should not exceed 4 mg/kg. It is recommended that excess lidocaine viscous solution is spat out. No more than four doses should be given during 24 hours.

For children over 12 years of age doses should be commensurate with weight and physical condition.

Children (Under 3 Years): In children under the age of 3, the dose should be accurately measured and applied to the affected area with a cotton tip applicator. The same procedure is also recommended for older children having problems in expectorating. No more than four doses should be given during 24 hours.

At the present time there is not enough documentation to allow recommendations for a more prolonged use of viscous lidocaine in children under the age of 3.

OVERDOSAGE:

Acute systemic toxicity from local anesthetics is generally related to high plasma levels encountered during therapeutic use of local anesthetics and originates mainly in the central nervous and the cardiovascular systems (see Adverse Reactions and Warnings and Precautions). It should be kept in mind that clinically relevant pharmacodynamic drug interactions (i.e., toxic effects) may occur with lidocaine and other local anesthetics or structurally related drugs, and Class I and Class III antiarrhythmic drugs due to additive effects (see Drug Interactions).

Symptoms: Central nervous system toxicity is a graded response with symptoms and signs of escalating severity. The first symptoms are circumoral paresthesia, numbness of the tongue, lightheadedness, hyperacusis and tinnitus. Visual disturbance and muscular tremors are more serious and precede the onset of generalized convulsions. Unconsciousness and grand mal convulsions may follow, which may last from a few seconds to several minutes. Hypoxia and hypercarbia occur rapidly following convulsions due to the increased muscular activity, together with the interference with normal respiration. In severe cases apnea may occur. Acidosis, hyperkalaemia, hypocalcaemia and hypoxia increase and extend the toxic effects of local anesthetics.

Recovery is due to redistribution and metabolism of the local anesthetic drug. Recovery may be rapid unless large amounts of the drug have been administered.

Cardiovascular effects may be seen in cases with high systemic concentrations. Severe hypotension, bradycardia, arrhythmia and cardiovascular collapse may be the result in such cases.

Cardiovascular toxic effects are generally preceded by signs of toxicity in the central nervous system, unless the patient is receiving a general anesthetic or is heavily sedated with drugs such as a benzodiazepine or barbiturate.

Treatment: The first consideration is prevention, best accomplished by careful and constant monitoring of cardiovascular and respiratory vital signs and the patient's state of consciousness after each local anesthetic administration. At the first sign of change, oxygen should be administered.

The first step in the management of systemic toxic reactions consists of immediate attention to the maintenance of a patent airway and assisted or controlled ventilation with oxygen and a delivery system capable of permitting immediate positive airway pressure by mask. This may prevent convulsions if they have not already occurred.

If convulsions occur, the objective of the treatment is to maintain ventilation and oxygenation and support circulation. Oxygen must be given and ventilation assisted if necessary (mask and bag or tracheal intubation). Should convulsions not stop spontaneously after 15-20 seconds, an anticonvulsant should be given iv to facilitate adequate ventilation and oxygenation. Thiopental sodium 1-3 mg/kg iv is the first choice. Alternatively diazepam 0.1 mg/kg bw iv may be used, although its action will be slow. Prolonged convulsions may jeopardize the patient's ventilation and oxygenation. If so, injection of a muscle relaxant (e.g. succinylcholine 1mg/kg bw) will facilitate ventilation, and oxygenation can be controlled. Early endotracheal intubation is required when succinylcholine is used to control motor seizure activity.

If cardiovascular depression is evident (hypotension, bradycardia), ephedrine 5-10 mg i.v. should be given and repeated, if necessary, after 2-3 minutes.

Should circulatory arrest occur, immediate cardiopulmonary resuscitation should be instituted. Optimal oxygenation and ventilation and circulatory support as well as treatment of acidosis are of vital importance, since hypoxia and acidosis will increase the systemic toxicity of local anesthetics. Epinephrine (0.1-0.2 mg as intravenous or intracardial injections) should be given as soon as possible and repeated, if necessary.

Children should be given doses of epinephrine commensurate with their age and weight.

> For management of a suspected drug overdose, CPhA recommends that you contact your **regional Poison Control Centre**. See the *CPS* Directory section for a list of Poison Control Centres.

ACTION AND CLINICAL PHARMACOLOGY: Mechanism of Action: Lidocaine stabilizes the neuronal membrane by inhibiting the ionic fluxes required for the initiation and conduction of impulses thereby, effecting local anesthetic action. Local anesthetics of the amide type are thought to act within the sodium channels of the nerve membrane.

Onset of Action: After application of XYLOCAINE Viscous 2% (lidocaine hydrochloride), local anesthesia is achieved within 5 minutes. Duration of anesthesia is approximately 20-30 minutes. XYLOCAINE Viscous 2% is ineffective when applied to intact skin.

Hemodynamics: Lidocaine, like other local anesthetics, may also have effects on excitable membranes in the brain and myocardium. If excessive amounts of drug reach the systemic circulation rapidly, symptoms and signs of toxicity will appear, emanating from the central nervous and cardiovascular systems.

Central nervous system toxicity (see Overdosage) usually precedes the cardiovascular effects since it occurs at lower plasma concentrations. Direct effects of local anesthetics on the heart include slow conduction, negative inotropism and eventually cardiac arrest.

Pharmacokinetics: Absorption: The rate and extent of absorption depends upon concentration and total dose administered, the specific site of application and duration of exposure. In general, the rate of absorption of local anesthetic agents, following topical application to wound surfaces and mucous membranes is high, and occurs most rapidly after intratracheal and bronchial administration. Lidocaine is also well absorbed from the gastrointestinal tract, although little of the intact drug may appear in the circulation because of biotransformation in the liver.

Distribution: Lidocaine has a total plasma clearance of 0.95 L/min and a volume of distribution at steady state of 91 L.

Lidocaine readily crosses the placenta, and equilibrium in regard to free, unbound drug will be reached. Because the degree of plasma protein binding in the fetus is less than in the mother, the total plasma concentration will be greater in the mother, but the free concentrations will be the same.

The plasma binding of lidocaine is dependent on drug concentration, and the fraction bound decreases with increasing concentration. At concentrations of 1 to 4 μg of free base per mL, 60 to 80 percent of lidocaine is protein bound. Binding is also dependent on the plasma concentration of the alpha-1-acid glycoprotein.

Metabolism: Lidocaine is metabolized rapidly by the liver, and metabolites and unchanged drug are excreted by the kidneys. Biotransformation includes oxidative N-dealkylation, ring hydroxylation, cleavage of the amide linkage, and conjugation. Only 2% of lidocaine is excreted unchanged. Most of it is metabolized first to monoethylglycinexylidide (MEGX) and then to glycinexylidide (GX) and 2,6-dimethylaniline. Up to 70% appears in the urine as 4-hydroxy-2,6-dimethylaniline.

Excretion: Lidocaine has an elimination half-life of 1.6 h and an estimated hepatic extraction ratio of 0.65. The clearance of lidocaine is almost entirely due to liver metabolism, and depends both on liver blood flow and the activity of metabolizing enzymes.

The elimination half-life of lidocaine following an intravenous bolus injection is typically 1.5 to 2.0 hours. The elimination half-life in neonates (3.2 h) is approximately twice that of adults. The half-life may be prolonged two-fold or more in patients with liver dysfunction.

Renal dysfunction does not affect lidocaine kinetics but may increase the accumulation of metabolites.

Special Populations and Conditions: Acidosis increases the systemic toxicity of lidocaine while the use of CNS depressants may increase the levels of lidocaine required to produce overt CNS effects. Objective adverse manifestations become increasingly apparent with increasing venous plasma levels above 6.0 mg free base per mL.

STORAGE AND STABILITY: Store at 15-30°C. Protect from freezing.

INFORMATION FOR THE PATIENT: Published in e-CPS, available by subscription at www.e-cps.ca.

DOSAGE FORMS, COMPOSITION AND PACKAGING: Each mL of clear to almost clear slightly coloured viscous liquid with an odour of cherries contains: lidocaine HCl 20 mg. Nonmedicinal ingredients: cherry essence, methylparaben, propylparaben, purified water, saccharin sodium, sodium carboxymethylcellulose to adjust viscosity, sodium hydroxide to adjust pH to 6.0-7.0. Plastic bottles of 100 mL.

XYLOCAINE Viscous 2% has a low surface tension which provides for an even film over the mucous membrane. Prolonged contact is possible due to its high viscosity.

Xylocard®

lidocaine HCl

Antiarrhythmic

AstraZeneca

Date of Preparation: April 12, 2000
Date of Revision: September 20, 2007

PHARMACOLOGY: Mechanism of Action: The mode of action of the antiarrhythmic effect of lidocaine appears to be similar to that of procaine, procainamide, and quinidine. Ventricular excitability is depressed and the stimulation threshold of the ventricle is increased during diastole. The sinoatrial node is, however, unaffected. In contrast to the latter 3 drugs, lidocaine in therapeutic doses does not produce a significant decrease in arterial pressure or in cardiac contractile force. In larger doses, lidocaine may produce circulatory depression, but the magnitude of the change is less than that found with comparable doses of procainamide. Neither drug appreciably affects the duration of the absolute refractory period.

Onset of Action: The onset of action following a single i.v. injection varies from 45 to 90 seconds. Duration of action is 10 to 20 minutes.

INDICATIONS: The treatment of ventricular tachycardia occurring during cardiac manipulation, such as surgery or catheterization, or which may occur during acute myocardial infarction, digitalis toxicity, or other cardiac diseases.

CONTRAINDICATIONS: Lidocaine is contraindicated in patients with:

1. Known hypersensitivity to local anesthetics of the amide type, such as prilocaine, mepivacaine or bupivacaine, or to other components of the solution;
2. Adams-Stokes syndrome, or severe degrees of sinoatrial, atrioventricular or intraventricular block.

The safety of lidocaine in the treatment of arrhythmias in children has not been established.

WARNINGS: Constant ECG monitoring is essential for the proper administration of lidocaine i.v.. Signs of excessive depression of cardiac conductivity, such as prolongation of PR interval and QRS complex, and the appearance of aggravation of arrhythmias, should be followed by prompt cessation of the i.v. infusion.

It is mandatory to have emergency resuscitative equipment and drugs immediately available to manage possible adverse reactions involving the cardiovascular, respiratory, or central nervous systems.

In emergency situations, when a ventricular rhythm disorder is suspected, and ECG equipment is not available, a single dose may be administered when the physician in attendance has determined that the potential benefits outweigh the possible risks. If possible, emergency resuscitative equipment and drugs should be available.

PRECAUTIONS: Lidocaine should be used with caution in patients with bradycardia, severe digitalis intoxication, first or second degree heart block in the absence of a pacemaker, or hypokalaemia (see Contraindications and Warnings).

In unconscious patients, circulatory collapse should be watched for, since CNS effects may not be apparent as an initial manifestation of toxicity.

Caution should be observed in patients with cardiac decompensation and hypotension or posterior diaphragmal infarction with a tendency towards development of heart block.

I.V. administration of lidocaine is sometimes accompanied by a hypotensive response, and, in overdosage, this may be precipitous. For this reason the i.v. dose should not exceed 100 mg in a single injection, and no more than 200 to 300 mg in a 1 hour period (see Dosage).

When high doses are used and the patient's myocardial function is impaired, combination with other drugs which reduce the excitability of cardiac muscle requires caution.

Repeated doses of lidocaine may cause significant increases in blood levels with each repeated dose because of slow accumulation of the drug or its metabolites. Tolerance to elevated blood levels varies with the status of the patient. Debilitated, elderly patients and acutely ill patients should be given reduced doses commensurate with their age and physical condition. Lidocaine should also be used with caution in patients with epilepsy, impaired cardiac conduction, bradycardia, impaired hepatic function or renal function and in severe shock.

Geriatrics: A reduction in dosage may be necessary for elderly patients, particularly those with compromised cardiovascular and/or hepatic function and/or prolonged infusion. Elderly patients should be given reduced doses commensurate to their age and physical status.

Impaired Renal Function: Caution should be employed in the repeated use of lidocaine in patients with severe renal disease, since possible accumulation of lidocaine or its metabolites may lead to toxic phenomena.

Impaired Hepatic Function: Caution should be employed in the repeated use of lidocaine in patients with severe liver disease, since possible accumulation of lidocaine or its metabolites may lead to toxic phenomena.

Pregnancy: It is reasonable to assume that lidocaine has been used, mainly as a local anesthetic, by a large number of pregnant women and women of childbearing age. No specific disturbances to the reproductive process have so far been reported, e.g., no increased incidence of malformations. However, care should be taken during early pregnancy when maximum organogenesis takes place.

There are no adequate and well-controlled studies with i.v. administration of lidocaine in pregnant women.

Lactation: Lidocaine is excreted in the breast milk, but in such small quantities that there is generally no risk of affecting the infant at therapeutic dose levels.

Neonates: Through their lower enzyme capacity, **very rarely**, neonates are at risk of methaemoglobinaemia. Methaemoglobinaemia can become clinically overt (cyanosis), and treatment with methylene blue may be considered necessary.

Use in Patients with Acute Porphyria: Theoretical evidence suggests that lidocaine may have porphyrogenic properties. The clinical significance of this is unknown. Caution should be exercised if intravenous lidocaine is administered to patients with acute porphyria.

Drug Interactions: Potential for the influence of lidocaine on the plasma levels/effect of other drugs: Lidocaine is metabolized by cytochromes P4501A2 (CYP1A2) and P4503A4 (CYP3A4) and thus has the potential to inhibit the metabolism of other drugs metabolized by these isoenzymes, resulting in increased plasma levels of these. This has so far not been reported for any CYP1A2 or CYP3A4 substrate.

Potential for the influence of other drugs on the plasma levels/effect of lidocaine: Concomitant treatment with drugs that are substrates, inhibitors, or inducers of CYP1A2 or CYP3A4 has the potential to influence the metabolism and hence the plasma levels and effect of lidocaine. Concomitant administration with the substrate amiodarone has resulted in increased plasma levels of lidocaine resulting in toxic effects.

During concomitant administration with carbamazepine, phenobarbital, and phenytoin which are inducers of CYP3A4, decreased plasma levels of lidocaine have been reported. Primidone has also been reported to induce the metabolism of lidocaine.

Cimetidine has an unspecific inhibitory effect on CYP (including CYP 3A4) mediated metabolism. It reduces liver blood flow and thus systemic clearance of drugs that are highly extracted by the liver. Clinical experiments showed that the concomitant administration of cimetidine reduces the systemic clearance of lidocaine and increases lidocaine serum concentration by as much as 50%. Thus, therapeutic serum levels of lidocaine may rise to toxic levels when cimetidine is used concomitantly. Ranitidine has not displayed this effect.

Coadministration with inhibitors of CYP1A2, such as fluvoxamine, drastically reduced the elimination of lidocaine in healthy subjects.

CYP1A2 is the isoenzyme shown most consistently to be decreased in human cirrhosis and hence makes smaller contribution in lidocaine metabolism than in patients with normal liver function.

Concomitant treatment with metoprolol, nadolol, and propranolol have also been reported to increase the plasma levels of lidocaine resulting in toxic effects. Administration of propranolol during infusion of lidocaine may increase the plasma concentration of lidocaine by about 30%. Patients already receiving propranolol tend to have higher lidocaine levels than controls. The combination should be avoided.

Carcinogenesis, Mutagenesis, Impairment of Fertility: Studies of lidocaine in animals to evaluate the carcinogenic and mutagenic potential or the effect on fertility have not been conducted.

ADVERSE EFFECTS: Adverse experiences following the administration of lidocaine are similar in nature to those observed with other amide type agents. These adverse experiences are, in general, dose-related and may result from high plasma levels caused by excessive dosage or rapid absorption, or may result from a hypersensitivity, idiosyncrasy or diminished tolerance on the part of the patient.

Common adverse reactions are those from the central and peripheral nervous system. They occur in 5 to 10% of the patients and are mostly dose-related. The following definitions of frequencies are used: very common (≥10%), common (1-9.9%), uncommon (0.1-0.9%), rare (0.01-0.09%) and very rare (<0.01%).

Systemic reactions of the following types have been reported:

Central Nervous System: CNS manifestations are excitatory and/or depressant. Common adverse reactions are circumoral paresthesia, dizziness and drowsiness. Rare adverse reactions would include persistent dizziness, lightheadedness, nervousness, apprehension, euphoria, confusion, dizziness, drowsiness, hyperacusis, tinnitus, blurred vision, vomiting, sensations of heat, cold or numbness, twitching, tremors, convulsions, unconsciousness, apnea, respiratory depression and arrest. The excitatory manifestations may be very brief or may not occur at all, in which case the first manifestation of toxicity may be drowsiness merging into unconsciousness and respiratory arrest.

Drowsiness following the administration of lidocaine is usually an early sign of a high lidocaine plasma level and may occur as a consequence of rapid absorption.

Cardiovascular: Rare cardiovascular manifestations are usually depressant and are characterized by bradycardia, hypotension, asystole and cardiovascular collapse which may lead to cardiac arrest. Arrhythmias, including ventricular tachycardia/ventricular fibrillation have also been reported.

Hematologic System: Very rarely, neonatal methaemoglobinaemia can occur (see Precautions).

Immune System: Allergic reactions are characterized by cutaneous lesions, urticaria, edema, or in the most severe and very rare instances, hypersensitivity including anaphylactic shock. Allergic reactions of the amide type are rare and may occur as a result of sensitivity either to the drug itself, or to other components of the formulation.

Idiosyncratic reactions have been reported at low doses in some patients. Cross-sensitivity between lidocaine and procainamide or lidocaine and quinidine have not been reported.

OVERDOSE:

Symptoms of overdose or idiosyncratic reactions are described under Adverse Effects.

Symptoms: CNS toxicity is a graded response, with symptoms and signs of escalating severity. The first symptoms are circumoral paresthesia, numbness of the tongue, lightheadedness, hyperacusis and tinnitus. Visual disturbance and muscular tremors are more serious and precede the onset of generalized convulsions. Unconsciousness and grand mal convulsions may follow, which may last from a few seconds to several minutes. Hypoxia and hypercarbia occur rapidly following convulsions due to the increased muscular activity, together with the interference with normal respiration. In severe cases apnea may occur. Acidosis increases the toxic effects.

Recovery is due to redistribution and metabolism of the drug. Recovery may be rapid unless large amounts of the drug have been administered.

Cardiovascular effects may be seen in cases with high systemic concentrations. Severe hypotension, bradycardia, arrhythmia and cardiovascular collapse may be the result in such cases.

Cardiovascular toxic effects are generally preceded by signs of toxicity in the CNS, unless the patient is receiving a general anesthetic or is heavily sedated with drugs such as a benzodiazepine or barbiturate.

Treatment: The first consideration is prevention, best accomplished by careful and constant monitoring of cardiovascular and respiratory vital signs and the patient's state of consciousness. At the first sign of change, oxygen should be administered.

The first step in the management of convulsions consists of immediate attention to the maintenance of a patent airway and assisted or controlled ventilation with oxygen and a delivery system capable of permitting immediate positive airway pressure by mask. Immediately after the institution of these ventilatory measures, the adequacy of the circulation should be evaluated, keeping in mind that drugs used to treat convulsions sometimes depress the circulation when administered i.v.

An anticonvulsant should be given i.v. if the convulsions do not stop spontaneously in 15 to 20 seconds. Thiopental 100 to 150 mg i.v. will abort the convulsions rapidly. Alternatively, diazepam 5 to 10 mg i.v. may be used, although its action is slower. Succinylcholine will stop the muscle convulsions rapidly, but will require tracheal intubation and controlled ventilation, and should only be used by those familiar with these procedures.

Hypotension may be counteracted by giving sympathicomimetic drugs (e.g., adrenaline). Adrenergic agents of both α-adrenoceptor stimulating (e.g., metaraminol) and β-adrenoceptor stimulating type (e.g., isoprenaline) are generally effective. The bradycardia may be treated with parasympatholytic agents (e.g., atropine).

Should circulatory arrest occur, immediate cardiopulmonary resuscitation should be instituted. Optimal oxygenation and ventilation and circulatory support as well as treatment of acidosis are of vital importance, since hypoxia and acidosis will increase the systemic toxicity of local anesthetics. Epinephrine (0.1 to 0.2 mg as i.v. or intracardial injections) should be given as soon as possible and repeated, if necessary.

> For management of a suspected drug overdose, CPhA recommends that you contact your **regional Poison Control Centre**. See the *CPS* Directory section for a list of Poison Control Centres.

DOSAGE: **Single I.V. injection:** The usual dose is 50 to 100 mg administered under ECG and blood pressure monitoring. This dose may be administered at the rate of approximately 25 to 50 mg/min. Sufficient time should be allowed to enable a slow circulation to carry the drug to the site of action. If the initial injection of 50 to 100 mg does not produce a desired response, a second dose may be repeated after 10 minutes. **No more than 200 to 300 mg of lidocaine should be administered during a 1 hour period.**

Continuous I.V. infusion: Following i.v. injection, lidocaine may be administered by i.v. infusion at a rate of 1 to 2 mg/min (approximately 15 to 30 µg/kg/min in the average 70 kg patient) in those patients in whom the arrhythmia tends to recur, and who are incapable of receiving oral antiarrhythmic therapy.

I.V. infusion of lidocaine must be administered under constant ECG and blood pressure monitoring, and with meticulous regulation of infusion rate, in order to avoid potential overdosage and toxicity.

I.V. infusions should be terminated as soon as the patient's basic cardiac rhythm appears to be stable or at the earliest signs of toxicity. It should rarely be necessary to continue i.v. infusion beyond 24 hours. As soon as possible, and when indicated, patients should be changed to an oral antiarrhythmic agent for maintenance therapy.

Solution for i.v. infusion may be prepared by the addition of 1 g of Xylocard (i.e., contents of ten 5 mL ampoules) to 1 L of an appropriate infusion solution. Approximately a 0.1% solution will result from this procedure; that is, each mL will contain approximately 1 mg of lidocaine.

In those cases in which fluid restriction is medically desirable a more concentrated solution may be prepared by adding 1 g of Xylocard (i.e., contents of ten 5 mL ampoules) to 500 mL of diluent. Approximately a 0.2% solution will result from this procedure; that is, each mL will contain approximately 2 mg of lidocaine.

Solutions should be prepared using aseptic technique. As with all i.v. admixtures, dilution should be made just prior to administration. Prepared solutions should be used within 12 hours.

SUPPLIED: I.V. Injection: Each mL of 2% solution contains: lidocaine HCl 20 mg. Nonmedicinal ingredients: sodium chloride, sodium hydroxide and/or hydrochloric acid to adjust to pH 5.0 to 7.0 and water for injection. Preservative-free. Single use glass ampoules of 5 mL (100 mg). Discard unused portion. Store at room temperature (15 to 30°C).

I.V. Infusion: 5% dextrose in water is the preferred diluent. See Dosage for instructions regarding preparation of solutions for continuous intravenous infusion. Discard unused portion. Store at room temperature (15 to 30°C).

Xylometazoline
Nasal Decongestant

CPhA Monograph

Date of Preparation: November 2004
Date of Revision: November 2008

> This monograph has been compiled by CPhA and reviewed by experts. It may contain information different from that found in Health Canada-approved Product Monographs. The reader is referred to the *CPS* Editorial Policy for more information.

SUMMARY PRODUCT INFORMATION:

Route of Administration	Dosage Form	Product Strength
Nasal	Spray with or without moisturizers; metered dose spray with or without moisturizers	0.05%; 0.1%
Nasal	Drops	0.1%

INDICATIONS AND CLINICAL USE:

- Topical xylometazoline may be used for short-term relief of nasal congestion in adults with allergic rhinitis, common cold or sinusitis; however, it is not recommended to be used regularly on a daily basis because of potential development of rhinitis medicamentosa.
- Topical xylometazoline has also been used to unblock obstructed eustachian ostia in patients with ear inflammation and to facilitate rhinoscopic or surgical procedures by reducing edema in the nasal and pharyngeal membranes; however, recent data suggests that use of topical decongestants is not helpful in this setting [*Laryngoscope* 2002;112(6):1115-8].

CONTRAINDICATIONS:

- Hypersensitivity to xylometazoline or to any ingredient in the formulation or component of the container.
- Angle-closure glaucoma.
- Concurrent therapy with MAO inhibitors.
- Patients with known sensitivity to adrenergic effects of drugs.
- Should not be used for irrigation following surgical procedures in which the dura mater may have been entered, e.g., sinus and transnasal procedures.

WARNINGS AND PRECAUTIONS: Ear/Nose/Throat: Xylometazoline should not be used for self-care for more than 3 to 7 days because of the risk of rhinitis medicamentosa (rebound congestion), characterized by persistent nasal congestion despite frequent use of a topical decongestant, or when it is abruptly discontinued. Rhinitis medicamentosa occurs more frequently with shorter acting topical decongestants (e.g., phenylephrine) than with longer acting agents such as xylometazoline. If the condition occurs, one approach to treatment is to slowly withdraw the use of the decongestant, from one nostril at a time, using nasal saline preparations if necessary to soothe irritated nasal mucosae. Intranasal corticosteroids may be required.

Excessive dosage can cause irritation of the nasal mucosa and, particularly in children, can lead to systemic effects including profound CNS depression that may require supportive care.

Special Populations: Pregnant Women: Safety of topical xylometazoline has not been studied in pregnancy. If used to relieve symptoms of allergic rhinitis during pregnancy, the lowest effective dose should be used for the shortest possible time. A normal saline nasal preparation is the treatment of choice during pregnancy.

Nursing Women: Safe use of topical decongestants during breastfeeding has not been established. See also Pregnant Women.

Pediatrics: Excessive dosage can cause irritation to the nasal mucosa and, particularly in children, can lead to systemic effects such as profound CNS depression that may require supportive care. Xylometazoline is not indicated in children under the age of 2 years. Little evidence exists for effectiveness of xylometazoline in the management of nasal congestion related to common cold, allergic rhinitis, sinusitis or acute otitis media, in children under the age of 12 years [Cochrane Database Syst Rev. 2007;(1):CD001953].

Geriatrics: Elderly patients may be more susceptible to the systemic adverse effects of decongestants (see Adverse Reactions).

ADVERSE REACTIONS: See also Warnings and Precautions. When topical xylometazoline is used appropriately for 3 to 7 days, the incidence of adverse effects is low.

Rarely, transient burning, stinging or dryness of the nasal mucosa, sneezing and rebound congestion have been reported.

Occasionally, the use of intranasal xylometazoline may result in systemic sympathomimetic effects such as hypertension, restlessness, nausea, dizziness, headache, insomnia or palpitations. Children and elderly patients may be more susceptible to these effects.

Chronic use of a related, nasally administered alpha(2A) agonist, oxymetazoline, has reportedly caused thunderclap headache in association with reversible cerebral vasoconstriction. This possible effect should be considered if a chronic user of nasal xylometazoline presents with severe headache.

DRUG INTERACTIONS: Drug-Drug Interactions: See Table 1.

Table 1: Xylometazoline

Established or Predicted Drug-Drug Interactions

Drug Name	Effect	Clinical Comment
MAO Inhibitors	Risk of severe hypertensive reactions.	Avoid combination. Risk persists for 2 weeks following discontinuation of nonselective MAO inhibitors, e.g., phenelzine, tranylcypromine.
Sympathomimetics, e.g., formoterol, pseudoephedrine	Concomitant use may increase adverse/toxic effects, e.g., increase in blood pressure.	Less likely to occur with topical decongestants than systemic agents. Caution and monitoring for signs of increased sympathomimetic effects are advised.
Tricyclic Antidepressants	May potentiate the pressor effects of direct acting sympathomimetic agents.	Less likely to occur with topical decongestants than systemic agents. Caution and monitoring for signs of increased sympathomimetic effects are advised.

Drug-Herb Interactions: See Table 2.

Table 2: Xylometazoline

Drug-Herb Interactions

Interacting Herb	Effect	Clinical Comment
Ma huang/ephedra	Possible additive sympathomimetic effects if xylometazoline is absorbed.	Theoretical interaction; monitor for signs of systemic sympathomimetic effects.
Indian snakeroot	Possibility of hypertensive response if xylometazoline is absorbed.	Theoretical interaction; monitor for increased blood pressure.

DOSAGE AND ADMINISTRATION: Dosing Considerations: Generally, xylometazoline nasal spray formulations are preferable to drops because the drug is less likely to be swallowed and absorbed when delivered as a spray. However, in young children, drops may be easier to use.

See also Administration.

Recommended Dose and Dosage Adjustment: See Table 3 and Table 4.

Table 3: Xylometazoline

Dose in Adult Patients

Indication	Route	Usual Dose	Maximum Dose	Duration of Treatment	Detailed Information
Nasal Congestion	Nasal	1–3 drops or sprays of 0.1% solution in each nostril every 8–10 hours as needed	3 doses in 24 hours	Maximum of 3 to 7 days	See Administration.

Table 4: Xylometazoline

Dose in Pediatric Patients

Indication	Route	Age	Usual Dose	Maximum Dose	Duration of Treatment	Detailed Information
Nasal Congestion	Nasal	2–12 years	1–3 drops or sprays of 0.05% solution in each nostril every 8–10 hours	3 doses in 24 hours	Maximum of 3–7 days. Little evidence exists demonstrating benefit in relief of congestion related to common cold, allergic rhinitis, sinusitis or acute otitis media in children under the age of 12 years.	See Administration. In children younger than 12 years, saline nose drops are preferred over decongestants for nasal congestion.

Administration: In younger children, drops may be easier to use than spray formulations. Otherwise, sprays are preferred.

To instill nose drops, adults and older children should gently blow the nose, tilt the head backward, insert the dropper approximately 1/3 inch (0.8 cm) into the nostril, instill the drop(s), then tilt the head forward and hold the position for a few seconds. For younger children, lie the child on their back on a bed with their head hanging slightly over the edge. Insert the dropper 1/3 inch (0.8 cm) into the nostril and instill the drop(s). The child should remain in this position for 2 to 3 minutes, tilting the head from one side to the other every 30 seconds. Avoid touching the nostril with the dropper when administering nose drops and blow the nose about 3 to 5 minutes after each dose. Rinse the dropper with hot water before placing it into the bottle.

For spray formulations, start by gently blowing the nose. Tilt the head slightly forward to direct the spray towards the back of the nose. Close one nostril by pressing on the side of the nose. Spray the medication into the open nostril while breathing in through the nose. Repeat on the opposite side. Blow the nose after 3 to 5 minutes. This procedure can be repeated if an additional spray is required. Rinse the tip of the spray bottle with hot water before replacing the cap. Do not use the spray bottle upside down as this can lead to a large volume being squirted out, with risk of systemic absorption and toxicity.

OVERDOSAGE:

For management of a suspected drug overdose, CPhA recommends that you contact your **regional Poison Control Centre**. See the *CPS* Directory section for a list of Poison Control Centres.

Xyntha™

antihemophilic factor (recombinant) [BDDrFVIII], plasma/albumin free (moroctocog alfa)

Antihemorrhagic Blood Coagulation Factor VIII

Pfizer

Date of Preparation: April 14, 2008

SUMMARY PRODUCT INFORMATION:

Route of Administration	Dosage Form/ Strength	Clinically Relevant Nonmedicinal Ingredients
Intravenous Infusion	Available as 250, 500, 1000, or 2000 IU in single-use vials	Polysorbate 80 (0.4 mg/vial), sucrose (12 mg/vial), L-histidine (6 mg/vial), calcium chloride dihydrate (1 mg/vial), sodium chloride (72 mg/vial) [after reconstitution with diluent]

Xyntha is prepared by a modified process that eliminates any exogenous human- or animal-derived protein in the cell culture process, purification, or final formulation. The purification process uses a series of chromatography steps, one of which is based on affinity chromatography using a synthetic peptide affinity ligand. The process also includes a solvent-detergent viral inactivation step and a virus-retaining nanofiltration step.

The labelled potency of Xyntha is based on the European Pharmacopoeial chromogenic substrate assay, in which the Wyeth In-House Recombinant Factor VIII Potency Reference Standard has been calibrated to the WHO 7th International Standard using the one-stage clotting assay. This method of potency assignment is intended to harmonize Xyntha with clinical monitoring using a one-stage clotting assay.

INDICATIONS AND CLINICAL USE: Xyntha, Antihemophilic Factor (Recombinant) [BDDrFVIII], Plasma/Albumin-free, indicated for the control and prevention of hemorrhagic episodes and for routine and surgical prophylaxis in patients with hemophilia A (congenital factor VIII deficiency or classic hemophilia). Xyntha does not contain von Willebrand factor and hence is not indicated in von Willebrand's disease.

Geriatrics (≥65 years of age): Clinical studies of Xyntha did not include sufficient numbers of subjects aged 65 and over to determine whether they respond differently from younger subjects. Other reported clinical experience has not identified differences in responses between the elderly and younger patients. As with any patient receiving Xyntha, dose selection for an elderly patient should be individualized.

Pediatrics: Xyntha is appropriate for use in children of all ages, including newborns.

CONTRAINDICATIONS: Xyntha may be contraindicated in patients with a known hypersensitivity to any of the constituents of the preparation.

Xyntha has not been studied in patients with a known history of hypersensitivity to hamster proteins and may be contraindicated in these patients.

WARNINGS AND PRECAUTIONS:

Serious Warnings and Precautions

- Anaphylaxis and severe hypersensitivity reactions are possible as with any intravenous protein product. Should such reactions occur, treatment with the product should be discontinued and appropriate treatment should be administered.
- Development of activity-neutralizing antibodies has been detected in patients receiving factor VIII-containing products. If expected plasma factor VIII activity levels are not attained, or if bleeding is not controlled with an appropriate dose, an assay that measures factor VIII inhibitor concentration should be performed.

General: It is recommended that, whenever possible, every time that Xyntha is administered to patients the lot number of the product is documented.

Effects on Ability to Drive and Use Machines: No studies on the ability to drive and use machines have been performed.

Carcinogenesis and Mutagenesis: Xyntha has been shown to be nonmutagenic in the mouse micronucleus assay. No other mutagenicity studies and no investigations on carcinogenesis, impairment of fertility or fetal development have been conducted.

Drug-Drug Interactions: No formal drug interaction studies have been conducted with Xyntha. No interactions with other medicinal products are known.

Immune: The occurrence of neutralizing antibodies (inhibitors) is well known in patients receiving factor VIII-containing products. Inhibitors most commonly occur early in the treatment course of previously untreated patients, but have also been observed in patients who have previously received large amounts of factor VIII products. All patients using coagulation factor VIII products, including Xyntha, should be monitored periodically for the development of factor VIII inhibitors. In addition, if expected factor VIII activity plasma levels are not attained, or if bleeding is not controlled with an appropriate dose, an assay should be performed to determine if a factor VIII inhibitor is present. In patients with factor VIII inhibitors, factor VIII therapy may not be effective and other therapeutic options should be considered. Management of such patients should be directed by physicians with experience in the care of patients with hemophilia.

Sensitivity/Resistance: As with any intravenous protein product, allergic type hypersensitivity reactions are possible. Patients should be informed of the early signs or symptoms of hypersensitivity reactions including hives (rash with itching), generalized urticaria, tightness of the chest, wheezing, and hypotension.

If allergic or anaphylactic reactions occur, administration of Xyntha should be stopped immediately, and appropriate medical management should be given, which may include treatment for shock. Patients should be advised to discontinue use of the product and contact their hemophilia physicians and/or seek immediate emergency care, depending on the type and severity of the reaction, if any of these symptoms occur.

Special Populations: Pregnant Women and Nursing Women: No animal reproduction and lactation studies have been conducted with Xyntha. Based on the rare occurrence of hemophilia A in women, experience regarding the use of factor VIII during pregnancy is not available. Xyntha should be administered to pregnant and lactating women only if the benefit outweighs the risk.

Pediatrics: Xyntha is appropriate for use in children of all ages, including newborns. Safety and efficacy studies have been performed both in previously treated children and adolescents (N=98, ages 7-18 years) and in previously untreated neonates, infants, and children (N=101, ages 0-52 months). An additional ongoing clinical study is evaluating the use of Xyntha in previously treated subjects under 6 years of age with moderately severe to severe hemophilia A.

Geriatrics (≥65 years of age): Clinical studies of Xyntha did not include sufficient numbers of subjects aged 65 and over to determine whether they respond differently from younger subjects. Other reported clinical experience with factor VIII products has not identified differences in responses between the elderly and younger patients. As with any patient receiving Xyntha, dose selection for an elderly patient should be individualized.

ADVERSE REACTIONS: See Table 1.

Table 1: Xyntha

Adverse Reactions for Body System

Body System Frequency per Infusion	Adverse Reactions
Blood and Lymphatic System Disorders	
Rare (≥0.01% and <0.1%)	Factor VIII inhibition[a]
Body as a Whole	
Rare (≥0.01% and <0.1%)	Asthenia, pyrexia
Very rare (<0.01%)	Chills, cold sensation
Cardiac Disorders	
Very rare (<0.01%)	Angina pectoris, tachycardia
Nervous System Disorders	
Very rare (<0.01%)	Dizziness, perspiration increased, somnolence, flushing, neuropathy
Uncommon (≥0.1% and <1%)	Headache
Metabolism and Nutrition Disorders	
Very rare (<0.01%)	Hypotension, palpitations, anorexia, increased amino transferase, CPK increased
Musculoskeletal Disorders	
Rare (≥0.01% and <0.1%)	Myalgia
Vascular Disorders	
Rare (≥0.01% and <0.1%)	Vasodilation
Very rare (<0.01%)	Bleeding/hematoma, thrombophlebitis
Respiratory, Thoracic and Mediastinal Disorders	
Very rare (<0.01%)	Coughing, dyspnea
Gastrointestinal Disorders	
Rare (≥0.01% and <0.1%)	Diarrhea, nausea, vomiting
Very rare (<0.01%)	Abdominal pain
Hepato-biliary Disorders	
Very rare (<0.01%)	Increased bilirubin
Skin	
Rare (≥0.01% and <0.1%)	Hives
Very rare (<0.01%)	Pruritus, rash, urticaria
Special Senses	
Very rare (<0.01%)	Taste perversion (altered taste)
General Disorders and Administration Site Disorders	
Very rare (<0.01%)	Injection site reaction, permanent venous access catheter complications, injection site inflammation, injections site pain

[a] This table reports the frequency of factor VIII inhibitors per infusion. The incidence of factor VIII inhibitors per patient is described in the individual study narratives below.

The most frequently reported treatment-emergent adverse reaction was headache. Most adverse reactions reported were considered mild or moderate in severity.

In addition, as with any intravenous protein product, allergic type hypersensitivity reactions are possible. Manifestations of hypersensitivity reactions may include hives, generalized urticaria, tightness of the chest, wheezing, hypotension, and anaphylaxis.

Patients with hemophilia A may develop neutralizing antibodies (inhibitors) to factor VIII. If such inhibitors occur, the condition may manifest itself as an insufficient clinical response or an unexpectedly low yield of plasma factor VIII activity. In such cases, it is recommended that a specialized hemophilia center be contacted.

Reports of lack of effect, mainly in prophylaxis patients, have been received during the clinical trials and post-marketing setting. The lack of effect and/or low factor VIII recovery has been reported in patients with inhibitors but also in patients who had no evidence of inhibitors. The lack of effect has been described as bleeding into target joints, bleeding into new joints, other bleeding or a subjective feeling by the patient of a new onset bleeding. In order to ensure an adequate therapeutic response, it is important **to individually titrate and monitor** each patient's dose of Xyntha, particularly when initiating treatment with Xyntha (see Warnings and Precautions and Dosage and Administration).

If any reaction takes place that is thought to be related to the administration of Xyntha, the rate of infusion should be decreased or the infusion stopped, as dictated by the response of the patient.

In a clinical trial, 32 out of 101 (32%) previously untreated patients treated with Xyntha manufactured by the previous process developed inhibitors: 16 out of 101 (16%) with a titer >5 Bethesda Units (BU) and 16 out of 101 (16%) with a titer ≤5 BU. The median number of exposure days prior to inhibitor development in these patients was 12 days (range 3-49 days). Of the 16 high responder patients, 15 received immune tolerance (IT) treatment. Eleven (11) of the high responders had a titer of <0.6 BU at their latest available test after IT. In addition, IT treatment was started in 10 of the 16 low titer (≤5 BU) patients, 9 of whom had titer <0.6 BU for their latest value. Therefore, IT had an overall efficacy of 80% (20/25), 73% for high-responders and 90% for low-responders. Five (5) of the 6 remaining low-responder patients who did not receive IT also had a titer <0.6 BU for their latest value.

In a clinical trial of Xyntha manufactured by the previous process, one of 113 (0.9%) previously heavily treated patients who were evaluated for efficacy in bleeding episodes developed a high titer inhibitor. Inhibitor development in this patient occurred in the same time frame as the development of monoclonal gammopathy of uncertain significance. The patient was noted initially at a local laboratory to have a treatment-emergent low titer inhibitor at 98 exposure days, which was confirmed at 2 BU at the central laboratory at 113 exposure days. After 18 months on continued treatment with Xyntha, the inhibitor level rose to nearly 13 BU and a bleeding episode failed to respond to Xyntha treatment.

In a pivotal phase 3 study, in which previously treated patients (PTPs) with hemophilia A received Xyntha for routine prophylaxis and on-demand treatment, 94 subjects received at least one dose of Xyntha resulting in a total of 6775 infusions. In this study, the incidence of FVIII inhibitors to Xyntha was the primary safety endpoint. Two patients with low titer, transient inhibitors were observed in these 94 patients (2.1%). In a Bayesian statistical analysis, results from this study were used to update PTP results from prior supporting studies of Xyntha. This Bayesian analysis indicates that the population (true) inhibitor rate for Xyntha was below a predefined acceptable value of 4.4%; the estimate of the 95% upper limit of the true inhibitor rate was 4.07%.

There have been spontaneous postmarketing reports of high titer inhibitors developing in previously treated patients.

Twenty of 113 (18%) previously treated patients (PTPs) had an increase in anti-CHO (Chinese hamster ovary, the cell line which is the source of factor VIII for Xyntha) antibody titer, without any apparent clinical effect.

DRUG INTERACTIONS: No interactions with other medicinal products are known.

DOSAGE AND ADMINISTRATION:

Treatment with Xyntha should be initiated under the supervision of a physician experienced in the treatment of hemophilia A.

Xyntha is appropriate for use in adults and children including newborns.

Dosage and duration of treatment depend on the severity of the factor VIII deficiency, the location and extent of bleeding, and the patient's clinical condition. Individual patients may vary in their response to factor VIII, achieving different levels of in vivo recovery and demonstrating different half-lives. Doses administered should be titrated to the patient's clinical response. In the presence of an inhibitor, higher doses or appropriate alternative treatment may be required. Dosage adjustment for patients with renal or hepatic impairment has not been studied in clinical trials.

The number of units of factor VIII administered is expressed in International Units (IU), which are related to the current World Health Organization (WHO) international standard for factor VIII activity. Factor VIII activity in plasma is expressed either as a percentage (relative to normal human plasma) or in IU (relative to an International Standard for factor VIII in plasma).

One IU of factor VIII activity corresponds approximately to the quantity of factor VIII in one mL of normal human plasma. The calculation of the required dosage of factor VIII is based upon the empirical finding that, on average, 1 IU of factor VIII per kg body weight raises the plasma factor VIII activity by 2 IU/dL. The required dosage is determined using the following formula:

Required units = body weight (kg) × desired factor VIII rise (IU/dL or % of normal) × 0.5 (IU/kg per IU/dL)

Clinical data support the use of the one-stage clotting assay for monitoring Xyntha therapy.

The labeled potency of Xyntha is based on the European Pharmacopoeia chromogenic substrate assay in which the Wyeth In-House Recombinant Factor VIII Potency Reference Standard has been calibrated using a one-stage clotting assay. This method of potency assignment is intended to harmonize Xyntha with clinical monitoring using a one-stage clotting assay.

Precise monitoring of the replacement therapy by means of plasma factor VIII activity assay should be considered, particularly for surgical intervention.

Dosing for Bleeding and Surgery: In the case of the following hemorrhagic events, consideration should be given to maintaining the factor VIII activity at or above the plasma levels (in % of normal or in IU/dL) for the indicated period, as outlined in Table 2.

Table 2: Xyntha

Maintenance of Factor VIII Activity for Various Hemorrhagic Events

Type of Hemorrhage	Factor VIII Level Required (% or IU/dL)	Frequency of Doses (h)/ Duration of Therapy (d)
Minor Early hemarthrosis, superficial muscle or soft tissue and oral bleeds	20–40	Repeat every 12 to 24 hours as necessary until resolved. At least 1 day, depending upon the severity of the hemorrhage.
Moderate Hemorrhages into muscles. Mild head trauma capitus. Minor operations including tooth extraction. Hemorrhages into the oral cavity.	30–60	Repeat infusion every 12–24 hours for 3–4 days or until adequate hemostasis is achieved. For tooth extraction a single infusion plus oral antifibrinolytic therapy within 1 hour may be sufficient.
Major Gastrointestinal bleeding. Intracranial, intra-abdominal or intrathoracic hemorrhages. Fractures. Major operations.	60–100	Repeat infusion every 8–24 hours until threat is resolved or in the case of surgery, until adequate local hemostasis is achieved, then continue therapy for at least another 7 days.

Dosage for Prophylaxis: Xyntha has been administered prophylactically in a pivotal clinical trial in adolescent and adult previously treated patients at a dose of 30±5 IU/kg given 3 times weekly.

Inhibitors: Patients using factor VIII replacement therapy should be monitored for the development of factor VIII inhibitors. If expected factor VIII activity plasma levels are not attained, or if bleeding is not controlled with an appropriate dose, an assay should be performed to determine if a factor VIII inhibitor is present. In patients with factor VIII inhibitors, factor VIII therapy may not be effective and other therapeutic options should be considered. Management of such patients should be directed by physicians with experience in the care of patients with hemophilia.

Administration: Xyntha is administered by IV infusion after reconstitution of the lyophilized powder with the supplied pre-filled diluent (0.9% Sodium Chloride solution) syringe.

Reconstitution: Always wash your hands before performing the following procedures. Use germ-free methods during the preparation procedures. Use only the materials provided in the Xyntha kit for dissolving the Xyntha powder with the sodium chloride diluent. All components used in the mixing and injection of Xyntha should be used as soon as possible after opening their sterile containers to minimize unnecessary exposure to room air. Xyntha is administered by intravenous injection after dissolving with the supplied diluent (0.9% sodium chloride) in the pre-filled syringe.

Note: If you use more than one vial of Xyntha per injection, each vial should be dissolved according to the following instructions. The empty syringe should be removed leaving the vial adapter in place, and a separate large luer lock syringe may be used to draw back the dissolved contents of each vial. Do not detach the diluent syringes or the large luer lock syringe until you are ready to attach the large luer lock syringe to the next vial adapter.

1. Allow the vial of freeze-dried Xyntha powder and the pre-filled diluent syringe to reach room temperature.
2. Remove the plastic flip-top cap from the Xyntha vial to expose the central portions of the rubber stopper.
3. Wipe the top of the vial with the alcohol swab provided, or use another antiseptic solution, and allow to dry. After cleaning, do not touch the rubber stopper with your hand or allow it to touch any surface.
4. Peel back the cover from the clear plastic vial adapter package. **Do not remove the adapter from the package.**
5. Place the vial on a flat surface. While holding the adapter in the package, place the vial adapter over the vial. Press down firmly on the package until the adapter snaps into place on top of the vial, with the adapter spike penetrating the vial stopper.
6. Grasp the plunger rod as shown in the diagram. Avoid contact with the shaft of the plunger rod. Attach the threaded end of the plunger rod to the diluent syringe by pushing and turning firmly.
7. Break off the tamper-resistant, plastic-tip cap from the diluent syringe by snapping the perforation of the cap. This is done by bending the cap up and down until the perforation is broken. Do not touch the inside of the cap or the syringe tip. The diluent syringe may need to be recapped (if the dissolved Xyntha is not used immediately), so place the cap on its top on a clean surface in a spot where it would be least likely to become contaminated.
8. Lift the package away from the adapter and discard the package.
9. Place the vial on a flat surface. Connect the diluent syringe to the vial adapter by inserting the tip of the syringe into the adapter opening while firmly pushing and turning the syringe clockwise until the connection is secured.
10. Slowly depress the plunger rod to inject all the diluent into the Xyntha vial.
11. With the syringe still connected to the adapter, gently swirl the contents of the vial until the powder is dissolved.
    Note: The final solution should be inspected visually for particulate matter before administration. The solution should be clear to slightly opalescent and colorless. If it is not, the solution should be discarded and a new kit should be used.
12. Ensuring that the syringe plunger rod is still fully depressed, invert the vial. Slowly draw the solution into the syringe.
    Note: If you prepared more than one vial of Xyntha, remove the diluent syringe from the vial adapter, leaving the vial adapter attached to the vial. Quickly attach a separate large luer lock syringe and draw back the dissolved contents as instructed above. Repeat this procedure with each vial in turn. Do not detach the diluent syringes or the large luer lock syringe until you are ready to attach the large luer lock syringe to the next vial adapter.
13. Detach the syringe from the vial adapter by gently pulling and turning the syringe counterclockwise. Discard the vial with the adapter attached.
    Note: If the solution is not to be used immediately, the syringe cap should be carefully replaced. Do not touch the syringe tip or the inside of the cap.

Xyntha should be infused within 3 hours after dissolving. The dissolved solution may be stored at room temperature prior to infusion.

Infusion (Intravenous Injection): You should inject Xyntha as instructed by your hemophilia doctor or nurse. Once you learn how to self-infuse, you can follow the instructions in this insert. Always wash your hands before doing the following procedures. Germ-free methods should be used during injection. Xyntha should be administered using the pre-filled diluent syringe provided or a single sterile disposable plastic luer-lock syringe. In addition, the solution should be withdrawn from the vial using the vial adapter.

1. Attach the syringe to the luer end of the provided infusion set tubing and perform venipuncture as instructed by your hemophilia doctor or nurse.
2. Apply a tourniquet and prepare the injection site by wiping the skin well with an alcohol swab provided in the kit.
3. Insert the needle on the infusion set tubing into the vein, and remove the tourniquet. Infuse the reconstituted Xyntha product over several minutes. Your comfort level should determine the rate of infusion.
4. After injecting Xyntha, remove the infusion set and discard. The amount of drug product left in the infusion set will not affect your treatment. Dispose of all unused solution, the empty vial(s), and the used needles and syringes in an appropriate sharps container used for throwing away waste that might hurt others if not handled properly.

You should record the lot number of the product every time you use Xyntha. The lot number can be found on the vial label. The peel-off label on the vial may be used to record the lot number.

In the absence of incompatibility studies, reconstituted Xyntha should not be administered in the same tubing or container with other medicinal products. Infusion kit components supplied in this carton are compatible with Xyntha for administration.

The reconstituted Xyntha solution does not contain a preservative and should be used within 3 hours of reconstitution.

Xyntha, when reconstituted, contains polysorbate-80, which is known to increase the rate of di-(2-ethylhexyl) phthalate (DEHP) extraction from polyvinyl chloride (PVC). This should be considered during the preparation and administration of Xyntha, including storage time elapsed in a PVC container following reconstitution. It is important that the recommendations in Dosage and Administration be followed closely.

OVERDOSAGE:

No symptoms case of overdose have been reported with recombinant coagulation factor VIII products.

For management of a suspected drug overdose, CPhA recommends that you contact your **regional Poison Control Centre**. See the *CPS Directory* section for a list of Poison Control Centres.

ACTION AND CLINICAL PHARMACOLOGY: Mechanism of Action: Xyntha is a glycoprotein with an approximate molecular mass of 170 000 Da consisting of 1438 amino acids. Xyntha is a recombinant DNA-based substance which has functional characteristics comparable to those of endogenous factor VIII. Activated factor VIII acts as a cofactor for activated factor IX accelerating the conversion of factor X to activated factor X. Activated factor X converts prothrombin into thrombin. Thrombin then converts fibrinogen into fibrin which forms an insoluble clot.

Pharmacodynamics: Factor VIII is the specific clotting factor deficient in patients with hemophilia A (classical hemophilia). The administration of Xyntha, Antihemophilic Factor (Recombinant) [BDDrFVIII] increases plasma levels of factor VIII and can temporarily correct the coagulation defect in these patients.

Pharmacokinetics: One Stage Assay: In a pivotal cross-over pharmacokinetic study, Xyntha was shown to be bioequivalent to another recombinant factor VIII product (rFVIII, Advate) in 30 previously treated patients (PTPs) (≥12 years) using the one-stage clotting assay. The ratios of geometric least square means of Xyntha-to-Advate were 100%, 89.8% and 88.0% for K-value, AUC_t and AUC_∞, respectively. The corresponding 90% confidence intervals about the ratios of Xyntha to Advate geometric means were within the bioequivalence window of 80% to 125%, demonstrating bioequivalence of Xyntha to Advate. See Figure 1.

Figure 1: Xyntha

Xyntha vs. Advate

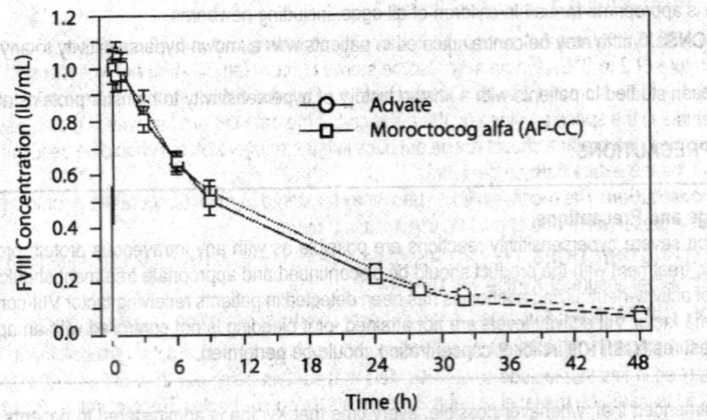

In the same study, the pharmacokinetic parameters for Xyntha were determined at baseline and followed-up in 25 PTPs (≥12 years) after repeated administration of Xyntha for six months. At baseline, following a single 2-minute intravenous infusion of 50 IU/kg dose of Xyntha, plasma FVIII:C increased sharply with a mean (±SD) C_{max} of 1.12 (±0.19) IU/mL. Thereafter, the decline of FVIII:C exhibited biphasic disposition characteristics. In the initial phase, the activity dropped at a rate consistent with relatively rapid but limited distribution into extravascular space. The mean (±SD) steady-state volume of distribution was 65.1 (±35.1)

Table 4: Xyntha

Mean Factor VIII Pharmacokinetic Parameters for 37 PTPS with Both Baseline and Month 12 Pharmacokinetic Profiles Following a Rapid Infusion of Xyntha Manufactured by the Previous Process at a Dose of 50 IU/kg

Parameter	C_{max} (IU/mL)	AUC_T (hr*IU/mL)	Half-life (hr)	AUC_∞ (hr*IU/mL)	Clearance (mL/hr/kg)	Mean Residence Time (hr)	V_{ss} (mL/kg)	K-value (IU/dL/IU/kg)
Baseline								
Mean	1.17	13.6	10.6	15.4	3.53	15.0	50.9	2.34
SD	0.24	3.4	2.5	4.5	1.03	3.4	13.0	0.49
Min	0.55	6.0	6.8	7.6	1.78	9.8	36.9	1.10
Max	1.90	21.1	17.2	28.1	6.60	24.7	99.0	3.80
Month 12								
Mean	1.20	14.0	11.4	16.5	3.37	16.1	51.1	2.40
SD	0.29	4.7	3.5	5.7	1.08	4.6	11.4	0.58
Min	0.84	7.8	6.6	8.8	1.49	9.7	21.3	1.67
Max	2.31	32.4	20.1	33.5	5.66	27.8	83.2	4.61

mL/kg. During the terminal phase, the rate of decline in FVIII:C was slower than the initial phase with a mean (±SD) terminal elimination half-life of 11.8 (±5.1) hours. A comparable pharmacokinetic profile was obtained after repeated use for six months. The ratios of geometric least square means of month 6-to-baseline pharmacokinetic were 107%, 100% and 104% for K-value, AUC_t and AUC_∞, respectively. The corresponding 90% confidence intervals about the ratios of month 6 to baseline for the above pharmacokinetic parameters were within the equivalence window of 80% to 125%. This indicates no time-dependent changes in the pharmacokinetic properties of Xyntha. See Table 3.

Table 3: Xyntha

Pharmacokinetic Parameter Estimates for Xyntha at Baseline and Month 6 in Previously Treated Patients (PTPs) with Hemophilia A

Visit	C_{max} (IU/mL)	AUC_t (IU·hr/mL)	AUC_∞ (IU·hr/mL)	K-value (IU/dL per IU/kg)	In vivo Recovery (%)
Baseline					
Mean±SD	1.12±0.19	13.3±5.2	14.2±5.5	2.23±0.39	105±19
(Min, Max)	(0.59, 1.41)	(4.1, 23.6)	(4.7, 25.0)	(1.19, 2.83)	(53.4, 132)
n	25	25	25	25	25
Month 6					
Mean±SD	1.24±0.42	13.3±6.7	15.0±7.5	2.47±0.84	116±40
(Min, Max)	(0.65, 2.60)	(5.0, 41.0)	(5.3, 42.0)	(1.29, 5.20)	(59.3, 256)
n	25	25	25	25	25

Legend: AUC_∞=area under the plasma concentration-time curve from time zero to infinity; AUC_t=area under the plasma concentration-time curve from zero to the last measurable concentration; C_{max}=peak concentration; K-value=incremental recovery; SD=standard deviation.

Chromogenic Assay: The labeled potency of Xyntha manufactured by the previous process is based on the European Pharmacopoeia chromogenic substrate assay in which the Wyeth In-House Recombinant Factor VIII Potency Reference Standard has been calibrated to the WHO 6th International Standard using the chromogenic substrate assay.

In a crossover pharmacokinetic study of eighteen (18) previously treated patients using the chromogenic assay, the circulating mean half-life for Xyntha manufactured by the previous process was 14.8±5.6 hours (ranged from 7.6-28.5 hours), which was not statistically significantly different from plasma-derived Antihemophilic Factor (Human), (pdAHF), which had a mean half-life of 13.7±3.7 hours (ranged from 8.8-25.1 hours). Mean incremental recovery (K-value) of Xyntha manufactured by the previous process in plasma was 2.4±0.4 IU/dL per IU/kg (ranged from 1.9-3.3 IU/dL per IU/kg). This was comparable to the mean incremental recovery observed in plasma for pdAHF which was 2.3±0.3 IU/dL per IU/kg (ranged from 1.7-2.9 IU/dL per IU/kg).

In additional clinical studies using Xyntha manufactured by the previous process, pharmacokinetic parameters measured using the chromogenic assay were determined for previously treated patients (PTPs) and previously untreated patients (PUPs). In PTPs (n=101; median age 26±12 years), Xyntha manufactured by the previous process had a recovery at Week 0 of 2.4±0.4 IU/dL per IU/kg (range 1.1 to 3.8 IU/dL per IU/kg). In measurements over 4 years of use (Month 3 [n=90], Month 6 [n=87], Month 12 [n=88], Month 24 [n=70], Month 36 [n=64] and Month 48 [n=52]), the mean incremental recovery was reproducible and ranged from 2.3 to 2.5 IU/dL per IU/kg. A subset of 37 study subjects had evaluable pharmacokinetic profiles at both baseline and Month 12. The 90% confidence intervals for the ratios of the mean values of Month 12-to-baseline AUC_T, AUC_∞, and K-value were well within the bioequivalence window of 80% to 125%, demonstrating the stability of these pharmacokinetic parameters over 1 year. In PUPs (n=59; median age 10±8.3 months), Xyntha manufactured by the previous process had a mean recovery at Week 0 of 1.5±0.6 IU/dL per IU/kg (range 0.2 to 2.8 IU/dL per IU/kg). The mean incremental recovery for PUPs was stable over time (5 visits during a 2-year period) and ranged from 1.5 to 1.8 IU/dL per IU/kg of Xyntha manufactured by the previous process. Population pharmacokinetic modeling using data from 44 PUPs led to a mean estimated half-life of Xyntha manufactured by the previous process in PUPs of 8.0±2.2 hours. See Table 4.

STORAGE AND STABILITY: Xyntha Antihemophilic Factor (Recombinant), Plasma/Albumin-Free should be stored under refrigeration at a temperature of 2 to 8°C. Xyntha may also be stored at room temperature not to exceed 25°C for up to 3 months. The diluent syringe should be stored at 2 to 25°C and should not be used subsequent to expiration of the Xyntha drug product. The patient should write in the space provided on the outer carton the date the product was placed at room temperature. At the end of the 3-month period, the product should not be put back into the refrigerator, but should be used immediately or discarded. Do not use Xyntha after the expiry date on the label.

Product After Reconstitution: The reconstituted solution may be stored at room temperature prior to administration. The product does not contain a preservative and should be used within 3 hours.

SPECIAL HANDLING INSTRUCTIONS: Freezing should be avoided to prevent damage to the pre-filled diluent syringe. During storage, avoid prolonged exposure of Xyntha vial to light.

INFORMATION FOR THE PATIENT: Published in e-CPS, available by subscription at www.e-cps.ca.

DOSAGE FORMS, COMPOSITION AND PACKAGING: Xyntha, Antihemophilic Factor (Recombinant), Plasma/Albumin-Free (freeze-dried) is supplied in kits that include single-use vials that contain nominally 250, 500, 1000, or 2000 IU per vial. Actual factor VIII activity in IU is stated on the label of each Xyntha Antihemophilic Factor (Recombinant), Plasma/Albumin-Free vial.

In addition, each Xyntha Antihemophilic Factor (Recombinant), Plasma/Albumin-Free kit contains: one pre-filled diluent syringe containing 4 mL 0.9% Sodium Chloride with plunger rod for assembly, one vial adapter, one sterile infusion set, two alcohol swabs, one bandage, one gauze, and one package insert.

Xyrem® Ⓒ

sodium oxybate

CNS Depressant

Valeant

Date of Revision: September 14, 2009

Warning: Central nervous system depressant with abuse potential. Should not be used with alcohol or other CNS depressants.

Sodium oxybate is gamma-hydroxybutyrate (GHB), a known drug of abuse that has been associated with some important central nervous system (CNS) adverse events, including death in abuse situations. Even at recommended doses, use has been associated with confusion, depression and other neuropsychiatric events. Reports of respiratory depression, occurred in clinical trials. Most patients receiving sodium oxybate during clinical trials maintained concomitant stimulant use.

Important CNS adverse events associated with abuse of GHB include seizure, respiratory depression, and profound decreases in level of consciousness, with instances of coma and death. For events that occurred outside of clinical trials in people taking GHB for recreational purposes, the circumstances surrounding the events are often unclear (e.g., dose of GHB taken, the nature and amount of alcohol or any concomitant drugs).

Under the Xyrem Success Program, Xyrem is made available to prescribers and pharmacists through a single wholesaler. Educational materials for physicians and pharmacists are available through the wholesaler (1-866-5XYREM5 (1-866-599-7365)). Physicians are required to read the materials prior to prescribing Xyrem. Educational materials are also available for patients, who should confirm that they have read and understood the materials.

The Xyrem Success Program includes recommendations for educating patients and information to help minimize the risks of inadvertent use by others. These recommendations encourage physicians to see their patients every 3 months during the course of therapy and to report all serious adverse events to the manufacturer.

Xyrem is approved for use only in the treatment of cataplexy in patients with narcolepsy.

PHARMACOLOGY: Mechanism of Action: The mechanism by which sodium oxybate (also known as gamma-hydroxybutyrate; GHB) produces its anti-cataplectic effects is unknown. Gamma-hydroxybutyrate is a CNS depressant that produces dose-dependent sedation and anesthesia. GHB is also an endogenous compound that is widely found throughout the body although its function outside of the CNS is essentially unknown. Endogenous GHB appears to fulfill the criteria necessary to be considered a neurotransmitter or neuromodulator.

Pharmacokinetics: Sodium oxybate is rapidly but incompletely absorbed after oral administration; absorption is delayed and decreased by a high fat meal. It is eliminated mainly by metabolism with a half-life of 0.5 to 1 hour. Pharmacokinetics are non-linear with blood levels increasing 3.7-fold as dose is doubled from 4.5 to 9 grams (g). The pharmacokinetics are not altered with repeat dosing.

Absorption: Sodium oxybate is absorbed rapidly following oral administration with an absolute bioavailability of about 25%. The average peak plasma concentrations (1st and 2nd peak) following administration of a 9 g daily dose divided into two equivalent doses given four hours apart were 78 and 142 µg/mL, respectively. The average time to peak plasma concentration (T_{max}) ranged from 0.5 to 1.25 hours in eight pharmacokinetic studies. Following oral administration, the plasma levels of sodium oxybate increased more than proportionally with increasing dose.

Single doses greater than 4.5 g have not been studied. Administration of sodium oxybate immediately after a high fat meal resulted in delayed absorption (average T_{max} increased from 0.75 hr to 2.0 hr) and a reduction in peak plasma level (C_{max}) by a mean of 58% and of systemic exposure (AUC) by 37%.

Distribution: Sodium oxybate is a hydrophilic compound with an apparent volume of distribution averaging 190 to 384 mL/kg. At sodium oxybate concentrations ranging from 3 to 300 µg/mL, less than 1% is bound to plasma proteins.

Metabolism: Animal studies indicate that metabolism is the major elimination pathway for sodium oxybate, producing carbon dioxide and water via the tricarboxylic acid (Krebs) cycle and secondarily by beta-oxidation. The primary pathway involves a cytosolic $NADP^+$-linked enzyme, GHB dehydrogenase, that catalyses the conversion of sodium oxybate to succinic semialdehyde, which is then biotransformed to succinic acid by the enzyme succinic semialdehyde dehydrogenase. Succinic acid enters the Krebs cycle where it is metabolized to carbon dioxide and water. A second mitochondrial oxidoreductase enzyme, a transhydrogenase, also catalyses the conversion to succinic semialdehyde in the presence of α-ketoglutarate. An alternate pathway of biotransformation involves β-oxidation via 3,4-dihydroxybutyrate to carbon dioxide and water. No active metabolites have been identified.

Studies in vitro with pooled human liver microsomes indicate that sodium oxybate does not significantly inhibit the activities of the human isoenzymes: CYP1A2, CYP2C9, CYP2C19, CYP2D6, CYP2E1, or CYP3A up to the concentration of 3 mM (378 µg/mL). These levels are considerably higher than levels achieved with therapeutic doses.

Elimination: The clearance of sodium oxybate is almost entirely by biotransformation. On average, less than 5% of unchanged drug appears in human urine within 6 to 8 hours after dosing. Fecal excretion is negligible.

Sodium oxybate is a hydrophilic compound with an apparent volume of distribution (Vz/F) averaging 190-384 mL/kg. The wide intersubject variation (CV 16-84%) could be influenced by dose-dependent kinetics of sodium oxybate, and by the variability at which kinetic non-linearity occurs. Absolute bioavailability of oral sodium oxybate was measured at 0.27 in a human subject, indicating substantial distribution into extravascular tissues. Less than 1% of sodium oxybate is bound to plasma proteins, at concentrations from 3 to 300 µg/mL (Borgen 2000a; 2000b; Palatini 1993).

Pharmacodynamics: The pharmacodynamic response to sodium oxybate dosing (4.5 to 9 g/night) in terms of sleep architecture was characterized in 21 patients with narcolepsy. A dose-related increase in Stages 3 and 4 (slow-wave) sleep and delta power was noted, with improved sleep continuity represented by a dose-related decrease in the number of nighttime awakenings, without significant changes in total sleep time. Also noted were dose-related decreases in total REM sleep and a decrease in Stage 1 sleep. No significant changes were seen in Stage 2 sleep nor the duration of wake after sleep onset. Measurement of daytime wakefulness utilizing the Maintenance of Wakefulness Test showed dose-related increases in sleep latency and a dose-related decrease in the percentage of patients with sleep-onset REM periods. A dose-related decrease in the Epworth Sleepiness Score was also seen (Mamelak 2004).

Special Populations: Geriatrics: The pharmacokinetics of sodium oxybate in patients greater than the age of 65 years have not been studied.

Pediatrics: The pharmacokinetics of sodium oxybate in patients under the age of 18 years have not been studied.

Gender: In a study of 18 female and 18 male healthy adult volunteers, no gender differences were detected in the pharmacokinetics of sodium oxybate following a single oral dose of 4.5 g.

Race: There are insufficient data to evaluate any pharmacokinetic differences among races.

Renal Disease: Because the kidney does not have a significant role in the excretion of sodium oxybate, no pharmacokinetic study in patients with renal dysfunction has been conducted; no effect of renal function on sodium oxybate pharmacokinetics would be expected. The sodium load associated with the administration of sodium oxybate should be considered in patients with renal insufficiency.

Hepatic Disease: Sodium oxybate undergoes significant presystemic (hepatic first-pass) metabolism. The kinetics of sodium oxybate in 16 cirrhotic patients, half without ascites, (Child's Class A) and half with ascites (Child's Class C) were compared to the kinetics in 8 healthy adults after a single oral dose of 25 mg/kg. AUC values were double in the cirrhotic patients, with apparent oral clearance reduced from 9.1 mL/min/kg in healthy adults to 4.5 and 4.1 mL/min/kg in Class A and Class C patients, respectively. Elimination half-life was significantly longer in Class C and Class A patients than in control subjects (mean $t_{1/2}$ of 59 and 32 versus 22 minutes). It is prudent to reduce the starting dose of Xyrem by one-half in patients with liver dysfunction (see Dosage).

Drug Interactions: Drug interaction studies in healthy adults demonstrated no pharmacokinetic interactions between sodium oxybate and protriptyline hydrochloride, zolpidem tartrate, and modafinil. However, pharmacodynamic interactions with these drugs cannot be ruled out. Nonetheless, sodium oxybate should not be used in combination with sedative hypnotics or other CNS depressants.

Clinical Trials: The effectiveness of sodium oxybate as an anti-cataplectic agent was established in two randomized, double-blind, placebo-controlled trials (Trials 1 and 2) in patients with narcolepsy, 85% and 80%, respectively, of whom were also being treated with CNS stimulants. The high percentages of concomitant stimulant use make it impossible to assess the efficacy and safety of Xyrem independent of stimulant use. In each trial, the treatment period was 4 weeks and the total daily doses ranged from 3 to 9 g, with the daily dose divided into two equal doses. The first dose each night was taken at bedtime and the second dose was taken 2.5 to 4 hours later. There were no restrictions on the time between food consumption and dosing.

Trial 1 was a multi-center, double-blind, placebo-controlled, parallel-group trial that enrolled 136 narcoleptic patients with moderate to severe cataplexy (median of 21 cataplexy attacks per week) at baseline. Prior to randomization, medications with possible effects on cataplexy were withdrawn, but stimulants were continued at stable doses. Patients were randomized to receive placebo, sodium oxybate 3 g/night, sodium oxybate 6 g/night, or sodium oxybate 9 g/night.

Trial 2 was a multi-center, double-blind, placebo-controlled, parallel-group, randomized withdrawal trial that enrolled 55 narcoleptic patients who had been taking open-label sodium oxybate for 7 to 44 months. To be included, patients were required to have a history of at least 5 cataplexy attacks per week prior to any treatment for cataplexy. Patients were randomized to continued treatment with sodium oxybate at their stable dose or to placebo. Trial 2 was designed specifically to evaluate the continued efficacy of sodium oxybate after long-term use.

The primary efficacy measure in each clinical trial was the frequency of cataplexy attacks. See Table 1.

Table 1: Xyrem

Summary of Outcomes in Clinical Trials Supporting the Efficacy of Sodium Oxybate

Trial/Dosage Group g/night (n)	Baseline	Median Change From Baseline	Comparison to Placebo p-value
Cataplexy Attacks			
Trial 1		(median attacks/week)	
Placebo (33)	20.5	−4	—
3.0 (33)	20.0	−7	0.5541
6.0 (31)	23.0	−10	0.0451
9.0 (33)	23.5	−16	0.0016
Trial 2		(median attacks/two weeks)	
Placebo (29)	4.0	21.0	—
Sodium oxybate (26)	1.9	0	<0.001

In Trial 1, both the 6 g/night and 9 g/night doses gave statistically significant reductions in the frequency of cataplexy attacks. The 3 g/night dose had little effect. In Trial 2, following the discontinuation of long-term open-label sodium oxybate therapy, patients randomized to placebo experienced a significant increase in cataplexy ($p<0.001$), providing evidence of long-term efficacy of sodium oxybate. In Trial 2, the response was numerically similar for patients treated with doses of 6 to 9 g/night, but there was no effect seen in patients treated with doses less than 6 g/night, suggesting little effect at these doses.

Results from two open-label trials (Trial 3 and Trial 4) provide further information regarding dosing of sodium oxybate (see Dosage, Clinical Experience).

INDICATIONS: Xyrem (sodium oxybate) oral solution is indicated for the treatment of cataplexy in patients with narcolepsy.

In Xyrem clinical trials, approximately 80% of patients maintained concomitant stimulant use (see Black Box Warning).

Xyrem should only be prescribed by physicians who meet the following requirements: i) Experience in treating cataplexy in patients with narcolepsy; ii) Completion of the Xyrem Physician Success Program.

The Xyrem Success Program is a Risk Management Program founded on the following core components that provide for the safe and effective use of the drug, and limit the potential for drug diversion and abuse: i) Implementation of a program to educate physicians, pharmacists, and patients about the risks and benefits of Xyrem, including critical information necessary for the safe use, storage, and handling of the drug. ii) Implementation of a restricted distribution program for Xyrem through a single wholesale distribution company that will ship the drug directly to pharmacies on an as-needed basis after patients have presented with an initial legitimate prescription. iii) Filling of the initial prescription only after the prescriber, pharmacist, and patient have received and read the educational materials. iv) Maintenance of a registry of Xyrem Success Program trained physicians, pharmacies, and patients.

Xyrem is not recommended for use in other indications as safety and efficacy has not been established outside of cataplexy.

Physicians may obtain more information about the Xyrem Success Program by calling the following toll-free phone number: 1-866-5XYREM5 (1-866-599-7365).

CONTRAINDICATIONS: Concurrent use of Xyrem (sodium oxybate) with sedative hypnotic agents or alcohol is contraindicated.

Xyrem is contraindicated in patients with succinic semialdehyde dehydrogenase deficiency. This rare disorder is an inborn error of metabolism variably characterized by mental retardation, hypotonia, and ataxia.

WARNINGS: See Boxed Warning.

Xyrem (sodium oxybate) should only be ingested at bedtime. For at least 6 hours after ingesting sodium oxybate, patients must not engage in hazardous occupations or activities requiring complete mental alertness or motor coordination, such as operating machinery, driving a motor vehicle, or flying an airplane. When patients first start taking Xyrem or any other sleep medicine, until they know whether the medicine will still have some carryover effect on them the next day, they should use extreme caution while performing any task that could be dangerous or requires full mental alertness.

The combined use of alcohol (ethanol) with sodium oxybate may result in potentiation of the central nervous system depressant effects of sodium oxybate. Therefore, patients should be warned to avoid the use of any alcoholic beverage in conjunction with sodium oxybate (see Contraindications). Sodium oxybate should not be used in combination with sedative hypnotics or other CNS depressants.

Central Nervous System Depression/Respiratory Depression: Sodium oxybate is a CNS depressant with the potential to impair respiratory drive, especially in patients with already-compromised respiratory function. In overdoses, life-threatening respiratory depression has been reported (see Overdose). In clinical trials, two subjects had profound CNS depression. A 39 year-old woman, a healthy volunteer received a single 4.5 g dose of sodium oxybate after fasting for 10 hours. An hour later, while asleep, she developed decreased respiration and was treated with an oxygen mask. An hour later, this event recurred. She also vomited and had fecal incontinence. In another case, a 64 year-old narcoleptic man was found unresponsive on the floor on Day 170 of treatment with sodium oxybate at a total daily dose of 4.5 g/night. Two other patients discontinued sodium oxybate because of severe difficulty breathing and an increase in obstructive sleep apnea.

The respiratory depressant effects of Xyrem, at recommended doses, were assessed in 21 patients with narcolepsy, and no dose-related changes in oxygen saturation were demonstrated in the group as a whole. One of these patients had significant concomitant pulmonary illness, and 4 of the 21 had moderate-to-severe sleep apnea. One of the 4 patients with sleep apnea had significant worsening of the apnea/hypopnea index during treatment, but worsening did not increase at higher doses. Another patient discontinued treatment because of a perceived increase in clinical apnea events. Caution should be observed if Xyrem is prescribed to patients with compromised respiratory function. Prescribers should be aware that sleep apnea has been reported with a high incidence (even 50%) in some cohorts of narcoleptic patients.

Confusion/Neuropsychiatric Adverse Events: During clinical trials, 7% of patients treated with sodium oxybate experienced confusion. Fewer than 1% of patients discontinued the drug because of confusion. In all cases, the confusion resolved soon after termination of treatment. In the majority of cases, confusion resolved with continued treatment. Patients treated with Xyrem who become confused should be evaluated fully, and appropriate intervention considered on an individual basis.

Other neuropsychiatric events included psychosis, paranoia, hallucinations, and agitation. The emergence of thought disorders and/or behaviour abnormalities when patients are treated with sodium oxybate requires careful and immediate evaluation.

Depression: In clinical trials, 6% of patients treated with sodium oxybate reported adverse events of depressive symptoms. In the majority of cases, no change in sodium oxybate treatment was required. Three patients (<1%) discontinued because of depressive symptoms. There was no dose relationship in depression reported during clinical trials.

Among patients with a previous history of depressive psychiatric disorder, there were two suicides and one attempted suicide recorded in the 448 patient dataset. Of the two suicides, one patient used multiple drugs, including sodium oxybate. Sodium oxybate was not involved in the second suicide. Sodium oxybate was the only drug involved in the attempted suicide. A fourth patient without a previous history of depression attempted suicide by taking an overdose of a drug other than sodium oxybate.

The emergence of depression when patients are treated with Xyrem requires careful and immediate evaluation. Patients with a previous history of a depressive illness and/or suicide attempt should be monitored especially carefully for the emergence of depressive symptoms while taking Xyrem.

Geriatrics: There is very limited experience with sodium oxybate in the elderly. Therefore, elderly patients should be monitored closely for impaired motor and/or cognitive function when taking sodium oxybate.

PRECAUTIONS: General: Incontinence: During clinical trials, 9% of narcoleptic patients treated with sodium oxybate experienced either a single episode or sporadic nocturnal urinary incontinence and <1% experienced a single episode of nocturnal fecal incontinence. Less than 1% of patients discontinued as a result of incontinence. Nocturnal urinary incontinence has been reported at all doses tested.

In a controlled clinical trial where patients were randomized to fixed total daily doses of 3, 6, and 9 g/night or placebo, a dose-response relationship for urinary incontinence was demonstrated with 14% of patients at 9 g/night experiencing urinary incontinence. In the same trial, one patient experienced fecal incontinence at a dose of 9 g/night and discontinued treatment as a result.

If a patient experiences urinary or fecal incontinence during Xyrem therapy, the prescriber should consider pursuing investigations to rule out underlying etiologies, including worsening sleep apnea or nocturnal seizures, although there is no evidence to suggest that incontinence has been associated with seizures in patients being treated with Xyrem.

Sleepwalking: The term "sleepwalking" in this section refers to confused behaviour occurring at night and, at times, associated with wandering. It is unclear if some or all of these episodes correspond to true somnambulism, which is a parasomnia occurring during non-REM sleep, or to any other specific medical disorder. Sleepwalking was reported in 7% of 448 patients treated in clinical trials with sodium oxybate. In sodium oxybate-treated patients <1% discontinued due to sleepwalking. In controlled trials of up to 4 weeks in duration, the incidence of sleepwalking was 1% in both placebo and sodium oxybate-treated patients. Sleepwalking was reported by 32% of patients treated with sodium oxybate for periods up to 16 years in one independent uncontrolled trial. Fewer than 1% of the patients discontinued due to sleepwalking. Five instances of significant injury or potential injury were associated with sleepwalking during a clinical trial of sodium oxybate over 16 years, including a fall, clothing set on fire while attempting to smoke, attempted ingestion of nail polish remover, and overdose of sodium oxybate. Therefore, episodes of sleepwalking should be fully evaluated and appropriate interventions considered.

Sodium Intake: Each mL of Xyrem (sodium oxybate) oral solution contains 91 mg of sodium (refer to Table 2). Sodium content should be considered when prescribing Xyrem for patients with salt restrictions such as hypertension, congestive heart failure, or compromised renal function.

Table 2: Xyrem

Sodium Content per Total Nightly Xyrem Dose

Total Nightly Dose (g)	Total Nightly Dose (mL)	Sodium Content/Total Nightly Dose
3	6	546 mg
4.5	9	819 mg
6	12	1092 mg
7.5	15	1365 mg
9	18	1638 mg

Drug Interactions: Interactions between sodium oxybate and three drugs commonly used in patients with narcolepsy (zolpidem tartrate, protriptyline hydrochloride, and modafinil) have been evaluated in formal studies. Sodium oxybate, in combination with these drugs, produced no significant pharmacokinetic changes for either drug (see Pharmacology, Pharmacokinetics). However, pharmacodynamic interactions cannot be ruled out. Nonetheless, sodium oxybate should not be used in combination with sedative hypnotics or other CNS depressants.

In animal models, sodium oxybate and depressant drug combinations generally gave greater central depressant effects than did either drug alone. Concomitant administration to animals of sodium oxybate and benzodiazepines, barbiturates, or ethanol increases sleep duration. In primates, sodium oxybate blood levels were elevated with phenytoin pretreatment and reduced with L-Dopa, ethosuximide, and trimethadione.

Geriatrics: There is very limited experience with sodium oxybate in patients greater than 65 years of age. Therefore, elderly patients should be monitored closely for impaired motor and/or cognitive function when taking Xyrem.

Children: The effects of sodium oxybate on early growth, development, and maturation in children are unknown. Xyrem is therefore not recommended for use in children under the age of 18 unless clearly needed.

Race and Gender Effects: There were too few non-Caucasian patients to permit evaluation of racial effects on safety or efficacy. More than 90% of the subjects in clinical trials were Caucasian.

The database was 58% female. No important differences in safety or efficacy of Xyrem were noted between men and women. The overall percentage of patients with at least one adverse event was higher in women (80%) than in men (69%). The incidence of serious adverse events and discontinuations due to adverse events were similar in both men and women.

Pregnancy: Reproduction studies conducted in pregnant rats at doses up to 1000 mg/kg (approximately equal to the maximum recommended human daily dose on a mg/m^2 basis) and in pregnant New Zealand White rabbits at doses up to 1200 mg/kg (approximately 3 times the maximum recommended human daily dose on a mg/m^2 basis) revealed no evidence of teratogenicity. In a study in which rats were given sodium oxybate from Day 6 of gestation through Day 21 post-partum, slight decreases in pup and maternal weight gains were seen at 1000 mg/kg; there were no drug effects on other developmental parameters.

There are, however, no adequate and well-controlled studies in pregnant women. Because animal reproduction studies are not always predictive of human response, this drug should be used during pregnancy only if clearly needed.

Obstetrics: Sodium oxybate has not been studied in labour or delivery. In obstetric anesthesia using an injectable formulation of sodium oxybate, newborns had stable cardiovascular and respiratory measures but were very sleepy, causing a slight decrease in Apgar scores. There was a fall in the rate of uterine contractions 20 minutes after injection. Placental transfer is rapid, but umbilical vein levels of sodium oxybate were no more than 25% of the maternal concentration. No sodium oxybate was detected in the infant's blood 30 minutes after delivery. Elimination curves of sodium oxybate between a 2-day old infant and a 15-year old patient were similar. Subsequent effects of sodium oxybate on later growth, development, and maturation in humans are unknown. Therefore, use of Xyrem in obstetrics is not recommended unless clearly needed.

Lactation: It is not known whether sodium oxybate is excreted in human milk. Because many drugs are excreted in human milk, caution should be exercised when Xyrem is administered to a nursing woman.

Patients with Special Diseases and Conditions: Hepatic Insufficiency: Patients with compromised liver function will have an increased elimination half-life and systemic exposure to sodium oxybate (see Pharmacology, Pharmacokinetics). Decrease the starting dose by one-half in such patients, and closely monitor the response to any dose increments (see Dosage).

Renal Insufficiency: No studies have been conducted in patients with renal failure. Because less than 5% of sodium oxybate is excreted via the kidney, no dose adjustment should be necessary in patients with renal impairment. The sodium load associated with administration of sodium oxybate should be considered in patients with renal insufficiency.

Dependence Liability: Xyrem (sodium oxybate or gamma-hydroxybutyrate (GHB)), is classified as a Schedule III controlled substance by Federal law.

Drug Abuse: While sodium oxybate has not been systematically studied in clinical trials for its potential for abuse, illicit use and abuse of GHB have been reported. Sodium oxybate is a psychoactive drug that produces a wide range of pharmacological effects. It is a sedative-hypnotic that produces dose and concentration dependent central nervous system effects in humans. The onset of effect is rapid, enhancing its desirability as a drug of abuse or misuse. The rapid onset of sedation, coupled with the amnestic features of sodium oxybate, particularly when combined with alcohol, has proven to be dangerous for the voluntary and involuntary (assault victim) user.

Illicit GHB has been abused in social settings primarily by young adults. Illicit GHB has some commonalities with ethanol over a limited dose range and some cross-tolerance with ethanol has been reported. Some of the doses reported during abuse may have been similar to the dose range studied for therapeutic treatment of cataplexy.

Dependence: There have been case reports of dependence after illicit use of GHB at frequent repeated doses in excess of the therapeutic dose range (18 to 250 g/day). In these cases, the discontinuation resulted in an abstinence syndrome consisting of insomnia, restlessness, anxiety, psychosis, lethargy, nausea, tremor, sweating, muscle cramps, and tachycardia, generally abating in 3 to 14 days. The effects of sodium oxybate discontinuation have not been systematically evaluated in controlled clinical trials. Neither a withdrawal nor an abstinence syndrome has been reported during clinical investigations, although, two patients reported anxiety and one reported insomnia following abrupt discontinuation at the termination of the clinical trial. In the two patients with anxiety, the frequency of cataplexy had markedly increased.

Tolerance: Tolerance to sodium oxybate has not been systematically studied in controlled clinical trials. Open-label, long-term (≥6 months) clinical trials did not demonstrate development of tolerance. There have been some case reports of symptoms of tolerance developing after illicit GHB use at dosages far in excess of the recommended Xyrem dosage regimen. Clinical studies of sodium oxybate in the treatment of alcohol withdrawal suggest a potential cross-tolerance with alcohol. Because illicit use and abuse of GHB have been reported, physicians should carefully evaluate patients for a history of drug abuse and follow such patients closely, observing them for signs of misuse or abuse of sodium oxybate (e.g., increase in size or frequency of dosing, drug-seeking behaviour). Physicians should document the diagnosis and indication for Xyrem, being alert to drug-seeking behaviour and/or feigned cataplexy.

Laboratory Tests: Laboratory tests are not required to monitor patient response or adverse events resulting from Xyrem administration.

Information to Be Provided to the Patient: The Xyrem Patient Information section includes information about the safe and proper use of Xyrem, and information to help prevent accidental use or abuse of Xyrem by others. Physicians and pharmacists should discuss the details of treatment with their patients, including the procedure for dose preparation, prior to the initiation of treatment. Patient educational materials are available, and patients should confirm that they have read and understood these materials. Patients should also be encouraged to read the Patient Package Insert for information regarding the proper use of Xyrem. Physicians should encourage their patients to be seen every 3 months during the course of Xyrem therapy and notify them that an account of the adverse reactions they may have experienced will be taken.

Specifically, the patient should be counseled on the following points:

- Xyrem has twice nightly dosing: the first dose is taken at bedtime and the second 2½-4 hours later.
- Xyrem is rapidly absorbed. Therefore, Xyrem should be taken only at bedtime, and patients should not walk around after taking their dose of Xyrem.
- Xyrem should not be taken with alcohol or other sedative hypnotics.
- Food significantly decreases the bioavailability of sodium oxybate. Whether Xyrem is taken in the fed or fasted state may affect both the efficacy and safety of Xyrem for a given patient. Patients should be made aware of this and take the first dose at least two hours after their last meal prior to bedtime.
- Xyrem may cause side effects including headache, dizziness, and nausea. Patients should also be made aware of the potential for enuresis and sleepwalking.
- Xyrem is a controlled substance. It is illegal to sell, distribute, or give Xyrem to anyone else, or to use Xyrem for purposes other than for what it was prescribed.

For additional information, see Information for the Patient.

ADVERSE EFFECTS: A total of 448 narcoleptic patients were exposed to sodium oxybate in clinical trials. The most commonly observed adverse events associated with the use of sodium oxybate were:

Headache 25%, nausea 21%, dizziness 17%, pain (unspecified) 16%, somnolence 13%, pharyngitis 11%, infection 10%, viral infection 10%, flu syndrome 9%, accidental injury 9%, diarrhea 8%, urinary incontinence 8%, vomiting 8%, rhinitis 8%, asthenia 8%, sinusitis 7%, nervousness 7%, back pain 7%, confusion 7%, sleepwalking 7%, depression 6%, dyspepsia 6%, abdominal pain 6%, abnormal dreams 6%, and insomnia 5%.

Two deaths occurred in these clinical trials, both from intentional drug overdoses. Both of these deaths resulted from ingestion of multiple drugs, including sodium oxybate in one patient.

In these clinical trials, 13% of patients discontinued because of adverse events. The most frequent reasons for discontinuation (>1%) were nausea (2%) and headache (1%).

Approximately 6% of patients receiving sodium oxybate in 3 controlled clinical trials (n=147) withdrew due to an adverse event, compared to 1% receiving placebo (n=79). The reasons for discontinuation that occurred more frequently in sodium oxybate-treated patients than in placebo-treated patients were: nausea (3%), somnolence (2%) and confusion (1%). Amnesia, asthenia, chest pain, dizziness, dyspnea, fecal incontinence, hallucinations, headache, hyperkinesia, paranoid reaction, thinking abnormal, vertigo, and vomiting, caused discontinuation in a single patient each.

Incidence in Controlled Clinical Trials: Table 3 lists the most commonly reported adverse events from controlled clinical trials associated with the use of sodium oxybate.

Table 3: Xyrem

Most Common Adverse Events in Controlled Clinical Trials

Adverse Event Costart Term	Placebo (n=79)	Sodium Oxybate (n=147)
Dizziness	3%	23%
Headache	15%	20%
Nausea	5%	16%
Somnolence	9%	12%
Pain (unspecified)	4%	12%
Sleep disorder	3%	9%
Confusion	1%	7%
Infection	1%	7%
Dyspepsia	6%	6%

(cont'd)

Table 3: Xyrem *(cont'd)*

Most Common Adverse Events in Controlled Clinical Trials

Adverse Event Costart Term	Placebo (n=79)	Sodium Oxybate (n=147)
Vomiting	1%	6%
Urinary incontinence	0%	5%
Nervousness	8%	5%

Table 4 lists the incidence of treatment emergent adverse events in Trial 1 (see Pharmacology). Events have been included for which there are at least two episodes in the considered drug group and for which the incidence in at least one dosage group is greater on drug than placebo.

Because clinical trials are conducted under widely varying conditions, adverse reaction rates observed in the clinical trials of a drug cannot be directly compared to rates in the clinical trials of another drug and may not reflect the rates observed in practice. The adverse reaction information from clinical trials does, however, provide a basis for identifying the adverse events that appear to be related to drug use and for approximating incidence rates.

Table 4: Xyrem

Incidence (%) of Treatment-Emergent Adverse Events in Trial 1

Body System COSTART Term	Placebo (n=34)	Sodium Oxybate Dose 3 g (n=34)	6 g (n=33)	9 g (n=35)
Body as a Whole				
Asthenia	1 (3%)	0 (0%)	2 (6%)	0 (0%)
Flu Syndrome	0 (0%)	1 (3%)	0 (0%)	2 (6%)
Headache	7 (21%)	3 (9%)	5 (15%)	11 (31%)
Infection	1 (3%)	3 (9%)	5 (15%)	0 (0%)
Infection Viral	1 (3%)	1 (3%)	3 (9%)	0 (0%)
Pain	2 (6%)	3 (9%)	4 (12%)	7 (20%)
Digestive System				
Diarrhea	0 (0%)	0 (0%)	2 (6%)	2 (6%)
Dyspepsia	2 (6%)	0 (0%)	3 (9%)	2 (6%)
Nausea	2 (6%)	2 (6%)	5 (15%)	12 (34%)
Nausea and Vomiting	0 (0%)	0 (0%)	2 (6%)	2 (6%)
Vomiting	0 (0%)	0 (0%)	2 (6%)	4 (11%)
Musculoskeletal System				
Myasthenia	0 (0%)	2 (6%)	1 (3%)	0 (0%)
Nervous System				
Amnesia	0 (0%)	1 (3%)	0 (0%)	2 (6%)
Anxiety	1 (3%)	1 (3%)	0 (0%)	2 (6%)
Confusion	1 (3%)	3 (9%)	1 (3%)	5 (14%)
Dizziness	2 (6%)	8 (24%)	10 (30%)	12 (34%)
Dream Abnormal	0 (0%)	0 (0%)	3 (9%)	1 (3%)
Hypertension	1 (3%)	0 (0%)	2 (6%)	0 (0%)
Hypoesthesia	0 (0%)	2 (6%)	0 (0%)	0 (0%)
Sleep Disorder	1 (3%)	2 (6%)	4 (12%)	5 (14%)
Somnolence	4 (12%)	5 (15%)	4 (12%)	5 (14%)
Thinking Abnormal	0 (0%)	1 (3%)	0 (0%)	2 (6%)
Skin				
Increased Sweating	0 (0%)	1 (3%)	1 (3%)	4 (11%)
Special Senses				
Amblyopia	1 (3%)	2 (6%)	0 (0%)	0 (0%)
Tinnitus	0 (0%)	2 (6%)	0 (0%)	0 (0%)
Urogenital System				
Dysmenorrhea	1 (3%)	1 (3%)	0 (0%)	2 (6%)
Incontinence Urine	0 (0%)	0 (0%)	2 (6%)	5 (14%)

Other Adverse Events Observed During All Clinical Trials: During clinical trials sodium oxybate was administered to 448 patients with narcolepsy, and 125 healthy volunteers. A total of 150 patients received 9 g/night, the maximum recommended dose. A total of 223 patients received sodium oxybate for at least one year. To establish the rate of adverse events, data from all subjects

receiving any dose of sodium oxybate were pooled. All adverse events reported by at least two people are included except for those already listed elsewhere in the labeling, terms too general to be informative, or events unlikely to be drug induced. These events are not necessarily related to sodium oxybate treatment.
Body as Whole: >1%: allergic reaction, chills; 1%-0.1%: abdomen enlarged, hangover effect, neck rigidity.
Cardiovascular: 1%-0.1%: syncope.
Digestive: >1%: anorexia, constipation; 1%-0.1%: mouth ulceration, stomatitis.
Hemic and lymphatic system: 1%-0.1%: anemia, ecchymosis, leukocytosis, lymphadenopathy, polycythemia.
Metabolic and nutritional: >1%: alkaline phosphatase increased, edema, hypercholesteremia, hypocalcemia, weight gain; 1%-0.1%: bilirubinemia, creatinine increased, dehydration, hyperglycemia, hypernatremia, hyperuricemia, AST increased, ALT increased, thirst.
Musculoskeletal: >1%: arthritis, leg cramps, myalgia.
Nervous System: >1%: agitation, ataxia, convulsion, stupor, tremor; 1%-0.1%: akathisia, apathy, coma, depersonalization, euphoria, hypertonia, libido decreased, myoclonus, neuralgia, paralysis.
Respiratory: >1%: dyspnea; 1%-0.1%: apnea, epistaxis, hiccup.
Skin and appendages: >1%: acne, alopecia, rash; 1%-0.1%: contact dermatitis, urticaria.
Special senses: 1%-0.1%: taste loss.
Urogenital system: >1%: albuminuria, cystitis, hematuria, metrorrhagia, urinary frequency; 1%-0.1%: urinary urgency.
Post-Market Adverse Drug Reactions: In addition to the adverse drug reactions reported during clinical studies and listed above, the following adverse events have been identified post-approval use of XYREM (sodium oxybate) oral solution. Because these events are reported voluntarily from a population of uncertain size, it is not always possible to reliably estimate their frequency or establish causal relationship to drug exposure. Events that have been reported during post-marketing experience include: fatigue, nightmares, and weight loss.
United States Post-Marketing Experience: Between the period of July 2002 through September 30, 2004, a total of 5869 patients have received Xyrem. Of those patients, 853 have discontinued Xyrem therapy, due to a wide range of reasons. Table 5 summarizes the most commonly reported adverse events (≥20 occurrences) during this time period. These adverse events are consistent with those identified in clinical studies.

Table 5: Xyrem

Summary of Post-Market Common Adverse Event Reports

System Organ Class, MedDRA Preferred Term	Number of Reports
Gastrointestinal Disorders	
Nausea	76
Vomiting	40
General Disorders and Administration Site Conditions	
Feeling abnormal	27
Nervous System Disorders	
Headache	40
Dizziness	28
Somnolence	33
Tremor	22
Psychiatric Disorders	
Confusion/confusional	47
Insomnia	43
Depression	22
Anxiety	21
Renal and Urinary Disorders	
Enuresis/incontinence	30

A U.S. Post-Marketing Evaluation Program (PMEP) was designed to capture solicited safety data on 1000 additional patients receiving Xyrem therapy. The PMEP specifically queried for the adverse events, vomiting, incontinence, sleepwalking, confusion, and convulsions. Through September 30, 2004, a total of 695 PMEP reports had been received. No adverse event was reported in 467 of these reports. The number of reports received for the adverse events listed above is as follows: vomiting (17/695), incontinence (24/695), sleepwalking (9/695), confusion (28/695), and convulsions (1/695).

OVERDOSE:

Symptoms: Information regarding overdose with sodium oxybate is extrapolated from literature reports of toxicity from illicit GHB. The co-ingestion of other drugs and alcohol is common, and may influence the presentation and severity of clinical manifestations of overdose. Therefore, literature reports of GHB overdose must be interpreted cautiously because overdose may be indistinguishable from other drug overdoses or medical conditions.

Patient presentation following overdose is influenced by the dose ingested, the time since ingestion, the co-ingestion of other drugs and alcohol, and the fed or fasted state. Patients have exhibited varying degrees of depressed consciousness that may fluctuate rapidly between a confusional, agitated combative state with ataxia and coma. Emesis (even when obtunded), diaphoresis, headache, and impaired psychomotor skills may be observed. No typical pupillary changes have been described to assist in diagnosis; pupillary reactivity to light is maintained. Blurred vision has been reported. An increasing depth of coma has been observed at higher doses. Myoclonus and tonic-clonic seizures have been reported. Respiration may be unaffected or compromised in rate and depth. Cheyne-Stokes respiration and apnea have been observed. Bradycardia and hypothermia may accompany unconsciousness, as well as muscular hypotonia, but tendon reflexes remain intact.

In clinical trials, two cases of overdose with Xyrem (sodium oxybate) oral solution were reported. In the first case, an estimated dose of 150 g, more than 15 times the maximum recommended dose, caused a patient to be unresponsive with brief periods of apnea and to experience urinary and fecal incontinence. This individual recovered without sequelae. In the second case, death was reported following a multiple drug overdose consisting of Xyrem and numerous other drugs.

Treatment: General symptomatic and supportive care should be instituted immediately, and gastric decontamination may be considered if co-ingestants are suspected. Because emesis may occur in the presence of obtundation, appropriate posture (left lateral recumbent position) or protection of the airway by intubation may be warranted. Although the gag reflex may be absent in deeply comatose patients, even unconscious patients may become combative to intubation, and rapid-sequence induction (without the use of sedative) should be considered. Vital signs and consciousness should be closely monitored. The bradycardia reported with GHB overdose has been responsive to intravenous atropine administration. No reversal of the central depressant effects of sodium oxybate can be expected from naloxone or flumazenil administration. The use of hemodialysis and other forms of extracorporeal drug removal have not been studied in GHB overdose. However, due to the rapid metabolism of sodium oxybate, these measures are not warranted.

As with the management of all cases of drug overdosage, the possibility of multiple drug ingestion should be considered. The physician is encouraged to collect urine and blood samples for routine toxicologic screening, and to consult with a regional poison control center for current treatment recommendations.

For management of a suspected drug overdose, CPhA recommends that you contact your **regional Poison Control Centre**. See the *CPS* Directory section for a list of Poison Control Centres.

DOSAGE: Xyrem should only be prescribed by physicians who meet the following requirements: i) Experience in treating cataplexy in patients with narcolepsy; ii) Completion of the Xyrem Physician Success Program.

The Xyrem Success Program is a Risk Management Program founded on the following core components that provide for the safe and effective use of the drug, and limit the potential for drug diversion and abuse:

i. **Implementation of a program to educate physicians, pharmacists, and patients about the risks and benefits of Xyrem, including critical information necessary for the safe use, storage, and handling of the drug.**
ii. **Implementation of a restricted distribution program for Xyrem through a single wholesale distribution company that will ship the drug directly to pharmacies on an as-needed basis after patients have presented with an initial legitimate prescription.**
iii. **Filling of the initial prescription only after the prescriber, pharmacist, and patient have received and read the educational materials.**
iv. **Maintenance of a registry of Xyrem Success Program trained physicians, pharmacies, and patients.**

Xyrem is not recommended for use in other indications as safety and efficacy have not been established outside of cataplexy.

Physicians may obtain more information about the Xyrem Success Program by calling the following toll-free phone number: 1-866-5XYREM5 (1-866-599-7365).

Xyrem (sodium oxybate) should be titrated to effect. The recommended starting dose is 4.5 g/night divided into two equal doses of 2.25 grams. The first dose should be taken at bedtime, and the second dose should be taken 2.5 to 4 hours later. The starting dosage can be increased or decreased in increments of 1.5 g/night (0.75 g per dose) to a maximum of 9 g/night while evaluating clinical response and adverse effects. Two-week intervals are recommended between dose titration. Xyrem is effective at doses of 6 to 9 g/night. The efficacy and safety of Xyrem at doses higher than 9 g/night have not been investigated, and doses greater than 9 g/night are not recommended. Eight to 10 weeks of therapy may be necessary before a maximal cataplexy response to sodium oxybate is seen (see Clinical Experience).

Xyrem is an oral solution with a concentration of 500 mg/mL sodium oxybate. Table 6 provides a conversion scale of total nightly Xyrem dose(s) from grams to mL.

Table 6: Xyrem

Total Nightly Dose: Conversion Scale

Total Nightly Dose (g)	Total Nightly Dose (mL)	Single Dose (taken twice nightly) (g)	Single Dose (taken twice nightly) (mL)
3 g	6 mL	1.5 g	3 mL
4.5 g	9 mL	2.25 g	4.5 mL
6 g	12 mL	3 g	6 mL
7.5 g	15 mL	3.75 g	7.5 mL
9 g	18 mL	4.5 g	9 mL

Because food significantly reduces the bioavailability of sodium oxybate, the patient should try to eat at least two hours before going to sleep and taking the first dose of Xyrem. Patients should try to minimize variability in the timing of dosing in relation to meals.
Clinical Experience: In Trial 3, an open-label trial, 117 patients with narcolepsy entered at a sodium oxybate starting dose of 6 g/night (3 g twice per night) and were titrated to optimum clinical response between the doses of 3 and 9 g/night. The nadir in cataplexy occurred 8 to 10 weeks later. This response was maintained across the remainder of the treatment period in general without dose escalation (U.S. Xyrem Multicenter Study Group 2003). Maintained treatment and appropriate dose titration is important for clinical response. In the majority of approximately 77% (90/117) of patients, maintenance doses were between 6 to 9 g/night.

Trial 4 was an open-label trial in 185 patients with narcolepsy in which sodium oxybate was added to existing treatments. Patients were entered at a starting dose of 4.5 g/night (2.25 g twice per night) followed by dose titration in 1.5 g increments over two week periods to optimize clinical response. Anti-depressant medications were then down-titrated. Seventy-two percent (31/43) of patients taking tricyclic antidepressants and 53% (19/36) of patients taking selective serotonin reuptake inhibitors for cataplexy reduced or discontinued use of these concomitant medications. In general, sodium oxybate dosing remained unchanged, with only 9 of these patients requiring an increase in dosage following discontinuation of prior medications.
Preparation and Administration: Prepare both doses of Xyrem prior to bedtime. Each dose of Xyrem must be diluted with approximately 60 mL (2 oz) of water or enough to fill ¾ of the supplied dosing cups provided prior to ingestion and sealed with the child-resistant cap. The first dose is to be taken at bedtime, and the second dose is to be taken 2.5 to 4 hours later while sitting in bed. Patients may need to set an alarm to awaken for the second dose. The second dose must be prepared prior to ingesting the first dose, and should be placed in close proximity to the patient's bed. After ingesting each dose, the patient should lie down and remain in bed.
Hepatic Insufficiency: Patients with compromised liver function will have a longer elimination half-life and greater systemic exposure along with reduced clearance. (See Special Populations in Pharmacology and Precautions.) As a result, the starting dose should be decreased by one-half and dose increments should be titrated to effect while closely monitoring potential adverse events.

Each bottle of Xyrem is provided with a child-resistant cap and two dosing cups with child-resistant caps.

INFORMATION FOR THE PATIENT: Published in e-CPS, available by subscription at www.e-cps.ca.

SUPPLIED: Each mL of clear to slightly opalescent oral solution USP contains: sodium oxybate 500 mg in purified water, neutralized to pH 7.5 with malic acid. Amber oval polyethylene teraphtalate (PET) bottles of 180 mL sealed with a child-resistant cap. The pharmacist places the PIBA in the bottle prior to dispensing Xyrem to the patient. Tamper evident single unit cartons containing one bottle of Xyrem, a press-in-bottle-adapter (PIBA), a 10 mL oral measuring device (plastic syringe), a Patient Package Insert, and two 90 mL dosing cups with child-resistant caps. Store between 15-30°C.

Following dilution, solutions prepared should be consumed within 24 hours to minimize bacterial growth and contamination.
Special Instructions: Any unused Xyrem should be returned to the pharmacy for proper disposal. Do not pour it down the drain.
Care should be taken to prevent access to this medication by children and pets.

Y

Yasmin® 21 ℞

drospirenone—ethinyl estradiol

Oral Contraceptive—Acne Therapy

Bayer

Yasmin® 28 ℞

drospirenone—ethinyl estradiol

Oral Contraceptive—Acne Therapy

Bayer

Date of Revision: June 4, 2010

SUMMARY PRODUCT INFORMATION:

Route of Administration	Dosage Form/ Strength	Clinically Relevant Nonmedicinal Ingredients
Oral	Tablet/3.0 mg drospirenone and 0.030 mg ethinyl estradiol	Lactose monohydrate For a complete listing see Dosage Forms, Composition and Packaging.

INDICATIONS AND CLINICAL USE: YASMIN (drospirenone and ethinyl estradiol) is indicated for:

- Conception control
- Treatment of moderate acne vulgaris in women ≥16 years of age who have no known contraindications to oral contraceptive therapy, desire contraception, and have achieved menarche

CONTRAINDICATIONS: YASMIN should not be used in women with:

- a history of or actual thrombophlebitis or thromboembolic disorders
- a history of or actual cerebrovascular disorders
- a history of or actual myocardial infarction or coronary artery disease
- valvular heart disease with complications
- history of or actual prodromi of a thrombosis (eg, transient ischemic attack, angina pectoris)
- presence of severe or multiple risk factor(s) for arterial or venous thrombosis:
  - severe hypertension (persistent values of ≥160/100 mmHg)
  - hereditary or acquired predisposition for venous or arterial thrombosis, such as Factor V Leiden mutation and activated protein C (APC-) resistance, antithrombin-III-deficiency, protein C deficiency, protein S deficiency, hyperhomocysteinemia and antiphospholipid antibodies (anticardiolipin antibodies, lupus anticoagulant)
  - severe dyslipoproteinemia
  - heavy smoking (>15 cigarettes per day) and over age 35
  - diabetes mellitus with vascular involvement
  - major surgery associated with an increased risk of postoperative thromboembolism
  - prolonged immobilization
- active liver disease or history of or actual benign or malignant liver tumors
- known or suspected carcinoma of the breast
- carcinoma of the endometrium or other known or suspected estrogen-dependent neoplasia
- undiagnosed abnormal vaginal bleeding
- steroid-dependent jaundice, cholestatic jaundice, history of jaundice in pregnancy
- any ocular lesion arising from ophthalmic vascular disease, such as partial or complete loss of vision or defect in visual fields
- known or suspected pregnancy
- current or history of migraine with focal aura
- history of or actual pancreatitis if associated with severe hypertriglyceridemia
- renal insufficiency
- hepatic dysfunction
- adrenal insufficiency
- hypersensitivity to this drug or to any ingredient in the formulation or component of the container. For a complete listing, see Dosage Forms, Composition and Packaging.

WARNINGS AND PRECAUTIONS:

> **Serious Warnings and Precautions**
> Cigarette smoking increases the risk of serious adverse effects on the heart and blood vessels. This risk increases with age and becomes significant in oral contraceptive users older than 35 years of age. Women should be counselled not to smoke (see Warnings and Precautions, Cardiovascular).
> Hormonal contraceptives **do not protect** against sexually transmitted infections (STIs) including HIV/AIDS. While using hormonal contraceptives, it is advisable to use latex or polyurethane condoms **in combination with** hormonal contraceptives to protect against STIs.

General: Discontinue Medication at the Earliest Manifestation of:

A. **Thromboembolic and cardiovascular disorders** such as thrombophlebitis, pulmonary embolism, cerebrovascular disorders, myocardial ischemia, mesenteric thrombosis, and retinal thrombosis.
B. **Conditions that predispose to venous stasis and to vascular thrombosis** (eg, immobilization after accidents or confinement to bed during long-term illness). Other nonhormonal methods of contraception should be used until regular activities are resumed. For use of oral contraceptives when surgery is contemplated, see Warnings and Precautions, Peri-operative Considerations.
C. **Visual defects—partial or complete.**
D. **Papilledema, or ophthalmic vascular lesions.**
E. **Severe headache of unknown etiology or worsening of preexisting migraine headache.**
F. **Increase in epileptic seizures.**

The following information is provided from studies of combination oral contraceptives (COCs).

The use of combination hormonal contraceptives is associated with increased risks of several serious conditions including myocardial infarction, thromboembolism, stroke, hepatic neoplasia, and gallbladder disease, although the risk of serious morbidity and mortality is small in healthy women without underlying risk factors. The risk of morbidity and mortality increases significantly if associated with the presence of other risk factors such as hypertension, hyperlipidemias, obesity, and diabetes. Other medical conditions which have been associated with adverse circulatory events include systemic lupus erythematosus, hemolytic uremic syndrome, chronic inflammatory bowel disease (Crohn's disease or ulcerative colitis), sickle cell disease, valvular heart disease and atrial fibrillation.

The following conditions have been reported to occur or deteriorate with both pregnancy and COC use, although a direct association with COCs has not been firmly established: porphyria, systemic lupus erythematosus, hemolytic uremic syndrome, Sydenham's chorea, herpes gestationis, and otosclerosis-related hearing loss.

The information contained in this section is principally from studies carried out in women who used combination oral contraceptives with higher formulations of estrogens and progestogens than those in common use today. The effect of long-term use of combination hormonal contraceptives with lower doses of both estrogen and progestogen administered orally remains to be determined.

YASMIN contains 3 mg of the progestogen drospirenone (DRSP) that has antimineralocorticoid activity, including the potential for hyperkalemia in high-risk patients, comparable to a 25 mg dose of spironolactone. YASMIN should not be used in patients with conditions that predispose to hyperkalemia (ie, renal insufficiency, hepatic dysfunction, and adrenal insufficiency). Women receiving daily, long-term treatment for chronic conditions or diseases with medications that may increase serum potassium should have their serum potassium level checked during the first treatment cycle. Drugs that may increase serum potassium include ACE inhibitors, angiotensin-II receptor antagonists, potassium-sparing diuretics, heparin, aldosterone antagonists, and NSAIDs.

Carcinogenesis and Mutagenesis: Breast Cancer: Increasing age and a strong family history are the most significant risk factors for the development of breast cancer. Other established risk factors include obesity, nulliparity, and late age for first full-term pregnancy. The identified groups of women that may be at increased risk of developing breast cancer before menopause are long-term users of oral contraceptives (more than eight years) and starters at early age. In a few women, the use of oral contraceptives may accelerate the growth of an existing but undiagnosed breast cancer. Since any potential increased risk related to oral contraceptive use is small, there is no reason to change prescribing habits at present.

Women receiving oral contraceptives should be instructed in self-examination of their breasts. Their physicians should be notified whenever any masses are detected. A yearly clinical breast examination is also recommended, because, if a breast cancer should develop, drugs that contain estrogen may cause a rapid progression.

Cervical Cancer: The most important risk factor for cervical cancer is persistent human papillomavirus infection. Some epidemiological studies have indicated that long-term use of COCs may further contribute to this increased risk but there continues to be controversy about the extent to which this finding is attributable to confounding effects, eg, cervical screening and sexual behaviour including use of barrier contraceptives.

Hepatocellular Carcinoma: Hepatocellular carcinoma may be associated with oral contraceptives. The risk appears to increase with duration of hormonal contraceptive use. However, the attributable risk (the excess incidence) of liver cancers in oral contraceptive users is extremely small. A liver tumor should be considered in the differential diagnosis when severe upper abdominal pain, liver enlargement, or signs of intra-abdominal hemorrhage occur in women taking COCs.

Cardiovascular: Predisposing Factors for Coronary Artery Disease: Cigarette smoking increases the risk of serious cardiovascular side effects and mortality. Birth control pills increase this risk, especially with increasing age. Convincing data are available to support an upper age limit of 35 years for oral contraceptive use by women who smoke.

Other women who are independently at high risk for cardiovascular disease include those with diabetes, hypertension, abnormal lipid profile, or a family history of these. Whether oral contraceptives accentuate this risk is unclear.

In low-risk, nonsmoking women of any age, the benefits of oral contraceptive use outweigh the possible cardiovascular risks associated with low-dose formulations. Consequently, oral contraceptives may be prescribed for these women up to the age of menopause.

Hypertension: Patients with essential hypertension, whose blood pressure is well-controlled, may be given hormonal contraceptives, but only under close supervision. If a significant elevation of blood pressure in previously normotensive or hypertensive subjects occurs at any time during the administration of the drug, cessation of medication is necessary.

Endocrine and Metabolism: Diabetes: Current low-dose oral contraceptives exert minimal impact on glucose metabolism. Diabetic patients, or those with a family history of diabetes, should be observed closely to detect any worsening of carbohydrate metabolism. Patients predisposed to diabetes who can be kept under close supervision may be given oral contraceptives. Young diabetic patients whose disease is of recent origin, well-controlled, and not associated with hypertension or other signs of vascular disease such as ocular fundal changes should be monitored more frequently while using oral contraceptives.

Lipid and Other Metabolic Effects: A small proportion of women will have adverse lipid changes while on oral contraceptives. Alternative contraception should be used in women with uncontrolled dyslipidemia (see also Contraindications). Elevations of plasma triglycerides may lead to pancreatitis and other complications.

Gastrointestinal: Published epidemiological studies indicate a possible association of COC use and the development of Crohn's disease and ulcerative colitis, although this has not been firmly established.

Genitourinary: Vaginal Bleeding: Persistent irregular vaginal bleeding requires assessment to exclude underlying pathology.

Fibroids: Patients with fibroids (leiomyomata) should be carefully observed. Sudden enlargement, pain, or tenderness requires discontinuation of the use of oral contraceptives.

Hematologic: Epidemiological studies have suggested an association between the use of COCs and an increased risk of arterial and venous thrombotic and thromboembolic diseases such as myocardial infarction, deep venous thrombosis, pulmonary embolism, and of cerebrovascular accidents. These events occur rarely.

The use of any combined oral contraceptive carries an increased risk of VTE compared with no use. The excess risk of VTE is highest during the first year a woman ever uses a combined oral contraceptive or restarts (following a 4-week or greater pill-free interval) the same or a different COC. Data from a large, prospective 3-armed cohort study suggest that this increased risk is mainly present during the first 3 months. VTE is fatal in 1% to 2% of cases.

A large, prospective 3-armed cohort study has shown that the frequency of VTE diagnosis ranges from about 8 to 10 per 10 000 woman-years in users of oral contraceptives with low estrogen content (<50 μg ethinyl estradiol). The most recent data suggest that the frequency of VTE diagnosis is approximately 4.4 per 10 000 woman-years in nonpregnant, non-COC users and ranges from 20 to 30 per 10 000 pregnant women or postpartum.

Overall the risk for venous thromboembolism (VTE) in users of oral contraceptives with low estrogen content (<50 μg ethinyl estradiol) is two- to three-fold higher than for nonusers of COCs who are not pregnant and remains lower than the risk associated with pregnancy and delivery.

Venous thromboembolism (VTE), manifesting as deep venous thrombosis and/or pulmonary embolism, may occur during the use of all COCs.

Extremely rarely, thrombosis has been reported to occur in other blood vessels (eg, hepatic, mesenteric, renal, cerebral, or retinal veins and arteries) in COC users. There is no consensus as to whether the occurrence of these events is associated with the use of COCs.

Symptoms of deep venous thrombosis (DVT) can include: unilateral swelling of the leg or along a vein in the leg; pain or tenderness in the leg, which may be felt only when standing or walking; increased warmth in the affected leg; red or discolored skin on the leg.

Symptoms of pulmonary embolism (PE) can include: sudden onset of unexplained shortness of breath or rapid breathing; sudden coughing which may bring up blood; sharp chest pain which may increase with deep breathing; sense of anxiety; severe light headedness or dizziness; rapid or irregular heartbeat. Some of these symptoms (eg, "shortness of breath", "coughing") are nonspecific and might be misinterpreted as more common or less severe events (eg, respiratory tract infections).

The risk for arterial thromboembolism (ATE) in users of oral contraceptives with low estrogen content (<50 μg ethinyl estradiol) ranges from about 1 to 3 cases per 10 000 woman-years. An arterial thromboembolic event (ATE) can include cerebrovascular accident, vascular occlusion, or myocardial infarction (MI). Symptoms of a cerebrovascular accident can include: sudden numbness or weakness of the face, arm, or leg, especially on one side of the body; sudden confusion, trouble speaking or understanding; sudden trouble seeing in one or both eyes; sudden trouble walking, dizziness, loss of balance or coordination; sudden, severe or prolonged headache with no known cause; loss of consciousness or fainting with or without seizure. Other signs of vascular occlusion can include: sudden pain, swelling, and slight blue discoloration of an extremity; acute abdomen.

Symptoms of MI can include: pain, discomfort, pressure, heaviness, sensation of squeezing or fullness in the chest, arm, or below the breastbone; discomfort radiating to the back, jaw, throat, arm, stomach; fullness, indigestion or choking feeling; sweating, nausea, vomiting, or dizziness; extreme weakness, anxiety, or shortness of breath; rapid or irregular heartbeats.

Arterial thromboembolic events may be fatal.

Other Risk Factors for Venous or Arterial Thromboembolism or of a Cerebrovascular Accident: Other generalized risk factors for venous or arterial thromboembolism include but are not limited to age, severe obesity (body mass index >30 kg/m²), a personal history, a positive family history (the occurrence of VTE/ATE in a direct relative at a relatively early age may indicate genetic predisposition) and systemic lupus erythematosus.

If a hereditary or acquired predisposition for venous or arterial thromboembolism is suspected, the woman should be referred to a specialist for advice before deciding on any COC use. The risk of VTE/ATE may be temporarily increased with prolonged immobilization, major surgery, or trauma. In these situations, it is advisable to discontinue COC use (in the case of elective surgery at least four weeks in advance) and not to resume COC use until two weeks after complete remobilization. Also, patients with varicose veins and leg cast should be closely supervised. Other risk factors may include smoking (with heavier smoking and increasing age, the risk further increases, especially in women over 35 years of age), dyslipoproteinemia, hypertension, migraine, valvular heart disease, and atrial fibrillation.

Biochemical factors that may be indicative of hereditary or acquired predisposition for venous or arterial thrombosis include Activated Protein C (APC) resistance, hyperhomocysteinemia, antithrombin-III deficiency, protein C deficiency, protein S deficiency, antiphospholipid antibodies (anticardiolipin antibodies, lupus anticoagulant).

When considering risk/benefit, the physician should take into account that adequate treatment of a condition may reduce the associated risk of thrombosis and that the risk associated with pregnancy is higher than that associated with low-dose COCs (<0.05 mg ethinyl estradiol).

Hepatic/Biliary/Pancreatic: In some cases of elevated liver enzymes reported during clinical trials with YASMIN, a contributory role of YASMIN could not be ruled out. YASMIN is contraindicated in patients with active liver disease (see Contraindications and Drug Interactions, Drug-Laboratory Test Interactions).

Acute or chronic disturbances of liver function may necessitate the discontinuation of COC use until markers of liver function return to normal.

Jaundice: Patients who have had jaundice should be given oral contraceptives with great care and under close observation. Oral contraceptive-related cholestasis has been described in women with a history of pregnancy-related cholestasis. Women with a history of cholestasis may have the condition recur with subsequent hormonal contraceptive use.

The development of severe generalized pruritus or icterus requires that the medication be withdrawn until the problem is resolved.

If a patient develops jaundice that proves to be cholestatic in type, the use of oral contraceptives should not be resumed. In patients taking hormonal contraceptives, changes in the composition of the bile may occur and an increased incidence of gallstones has been reported.

Gallbladder Disease: Patients taking oral contraceptives have a greater risk of developing gallbladder disease requiring surgery with the first year of use. The risk may double after 4 or 5 years.

Hepatic Nodules: Hepatic nodules (adenoma and focal nodular hyperplasia) have been reported, particularly in long-term users of oral contraceptives. Although these lesions are extremely rare, they have caused fatal intra-abdominal hemorrhage and should be considered in women presenting with an abdominal mass, acute abdominal pain, or evidence of intra-abdominal bleeding.

Immune: Angioedema: Exogenous estrogens may induce or exacerbate symptoms of angioedema, in particular, in women with hereditary angioedema.

Neurologic: Migraine and Headache: The onset or exacerbation of migraine or the development of headache with a new pattern that is recurrent, persistent, or severe requires discontinuation of hormonal contraceptives and evaluation of the cause. Women with migraine headaches who take oral contraceptives may be at increased risk of stroke (see Contraindications).

Ophthalmologic: Patients who are pregnant or are taking oral contraceptives may experience corneal edema that may cause visual disturbances and changes in tolerance to contact lenses, especially of the rigid type. Soft contact lenses usually do not cause disturbances. If visual changes or alterations in tolerance to contact lenses occur, temporary or permanent cessation of wear may be advised.

Peri-operative Considerations: There is an increased risk of thromboembolic complications in oral contraceptive users after major surgery. If feasible, oral contraceptives should be discontinued and an alternative method substituted at least one month prior to **major** elective surgery. Oral contraceptive use should not be resumed until the first menstrual period after hospital discharge following surgery.

Psychiatric: Patients with a history of emotional disturbances, especially the depressive type, may be more prone to have a recurrence of depression while taking oral contraceptives. In cases of a serious recurrence, a trial of an alternate method of contraception should be made, which may help to clarify the possible relationship. Women with premenstrual syndrome (PMS) may have a varied response to oral contraceptives, ranging from symptomatic improvement to worsening of the condition.

Renal: Fluid Retention: Hormonal contraceptives may cause some degree of fluid retention. They should be prescribed with caution and only with careful monitoring in patients with conditions which might be aggravated by fluid retention.

Sexual Function/Reproduction: Return to Fertility: After discontinuing oral contraceptive therapy, the patient should delay pregnancy until at least one normal spontaneous menstrual cycle has occurred in order to date the pregnancy. An alternate contraceptive method should be used during this time.

Amenorrhea: In some women, withdrawal bleeding may not occur during the tablet-free interval. If the COC has been taken according to directions, it is unlikely that the woman is pregnant. However, if the COC has not been taken according to directions prior to the first missed withdrawal bleed, or if two withdrawal bleeds are missed, pregnancy must be ruled out before COC use is continued.

Women having a history of oligomenorrhea, secondary amenorrhea, or irregular cycles may remain anovulatory or become amenorrheic following discontinuation of estrogen-progestin combination therapy.

Amenorrhea, especially if associated with breast secretion that continues for six months or more after withdrawal, warrants a careful assessment of hypothalamic-pituitary function.

Reduced Efficacy: The efficacy of COCs may be reduced in the event of missed tablets, gastro-intestinal disturbances, or concomitant medication (see Drug Interactions).

Skin: Chloasma may occasionally occur with use of COCs, especially in women with a history of chloasma gravidarum. Women with a tendency to chloasma should avoid exposure to the sun or ultraviolet radiation while taking COCs.

Special Populations: Pregnant Women: Oral contraceptives should not be taken by pregnant women. If pregnancy occurs during treatment with YASMIN, further intake must be stopped. However, if conception accidentally occurs while taking the pill, there is no conclusive evidence that the estrogen and progestin contained in the oral contraceptive will damage the developing child. One infant was born with esophageal atresia. A causal association with YASMIN is unknown.

Nursing Women: In breast-feeding women, the use of oral contraceptives results in the hormonal components being excreted in breast milk and may reduce its quantity and quality. If the use of oral contraceptives is initiated after the establishment of lactation, there does not appear to be any effect on the quantity and quality of the milk. There is no evidence that low-dose oral contraceptives are harmful to the nursing infant.

If possible, the nursing mother should be advised not to use oral contraceptives but to use other forms of contraception, until she has completely weaned her child.

After oral administration of YASMIN, about 0.02% of the drospirenone dose was excreted into the breast milk of postpartum women within 24 hours. This results in a maximal daily dose of about 3 μg drospirenone in an infant.

Pediatrics: The safety and efficacy of YASMIN has not been established in women under the age of 16 years. Use of this product before menarche is not indicated.

Geriatrics: YASMIN is not indicated for use in postmenopausal women.

Monitoring and Laboratory Tests: Physical Examination and Follow-up: Before oral contraceptives are used, a thorough history and physical examination should be performed, including a blood pressure determination and the family case history carefully noted. In addition, disturbances of the clotting system must be ruled out if any members of the family have suffered from thromboembolic diseases (eg, deep vein thrombosis, stroke, myocardial infarction) at a young age. Breasts, liver, extremities, and pelvic organs should be examined, and a Papanicolaou (PAP) smear should be taken if the patient has been sexually active.

The first follow-up visit should be done three months after oral contraceptives are prescribed. Thereafter, examinations should be performed at least once a year, or more frequently if indicated. At each annual visit, examination should include those procedures that were done at the initial visit as outlined above or per recommendations of the Canadian Task Force on the Periodic Health Examination.

ADVERSE REACTIONS: Adverse Drug Reaction Overview: An increased risk of the following serious adverse reactions has been associated with the use of oral contraceptives: thrombophlebitis; pulmonary embolism; mesenteric thrombosis; neuro-ocular lesions (eg, retinal thrombosis); myocardial infarction; cerebral thrombosis; cerebral hemorrhage; hypertension; benign hepatic tumors; gallbladder disease; congenital anomalies.

The following other adverse reactions also have been reported in patients receiving oral contraceptives: Nausea and vomiting, usually the most common adverse reaction, occurs in approximately 10% or fewer of patients during the first cycle. The following other reactions, as a general rule, are seen less frequently or only occasionally: gastrointestinal symptoms (such as abdominal cramps and bloating); breakthrough bleeding; spotting; change in menstrual flow; dysmenorrhea; amenorrhea during and after treatment; temporary infertility after discontinuation of treatment; edema; chloasma or melasma which may persist; breast changes (tenderness, enlargement, and secretion); change in weight (increase or decrease); endocervical hyperplasia; possible diminution in lactation when given immediately postpartum; cholestatic jaundice; migraine; increase in size of uterine leiomyomata; rash (allergic); mental depression; reduced tolerance to carbohydrates; vaginal candidiasis; premenstrual-like syndrome; intolerance to contact lenses; change in corneal curvature (steepening); cataracts; optic neuritis; retinal thrombosis; changes in libido; chorea; changes in appetite; cystitis-like syndrome; rhinitis; headache; nervousness; dizziness; hirsutism; loss of scalp hair; erythema multiforme; erythema nodosum; hemorrhagic eruption; vaginitis; porphyria; impaired renal function; Raynaud's phenomenon; auditory disturbances; hemolytic uremic syndrome; pancreatitis; abdominal pain; diarrhea; hypersensitivity; vaginal discharge; urticaria.

Clinical Trial Adverse Drug Reactions: Because clinical trials are conducted under very specific conditions the adverse reaction rates observed in the clinical trials may not reflect the rates observed in practice and should not be compared to the rates in the clinical trials of another drug. Adverse drug reaction information from clinical trials is useful for identifying drug-related adverse events and for approximating rates.

The following are the most common adverse events reported with use of YASMIN during clinical trials, occurring in >1% of subjects and which may or may not be drug related: headache, menstrual disorder, breast pain, abdominal pain, nausea, leukorrhea, flu syndrome, acne, vaginal moniliasis, depression, diarrhea, asthenia, dysmenorrhea, back pain, infection, pharyngitis, intermenstrual bleeding, migraine, vomiting, dizziness, nervousness, vaginitis, sinusitis, cystitis, bronchitis, gastroenteritis, allergic reaction, urinary tract infection, pruritus, emotional lability, surgery, rash, upper respiratory infection.

Less Common Clinical Trial Adverse Drug Reactions: Other reactions to oral contraceptives, as a general rule, are seen less frequently or only occasionally, as follows: gastrointestinal symptoms (such as abdominal cramps and bloating), breakthrough bleeding, spotting, change in menstrual flow, dysmenorrhea, amenorrhea during and after treatment, temporary infertility after discontinuation of treatment, edema, chloasma or melasma which may persist, breast changes (tenderness, enlargement, secretion), change in weight (increase or decrease), endocervical hyperplasias, possible diminution in lactation when given immediately postpartum, cholestatic jaundice, migraine, increase in size of uterine leiomyomata, rash (allergic), mental depression, reduced tolerance to carbohydrates, vaginal candidiasis, premenstrual-like syndrome, intolerance to contact lenses, change in corneal curvature (steepening), cataracts, optic neuritis, retinal thrombosis, changes in libido, chorea, changes in appetite, cystitis-like syndrome, rhinitis, headache, nervousness, dizziness, hirsutism, loss of scalp hair, erythema multiforme, erythema nodosum, hemorrhagic eruption, vaginitis, porphyria, impaired renal function, Raynaud's phenomenon, auditory disturbances, hemolytic uremic syndrome, pancreatitis.

Post-Market Adverse Drug Reactions: Cumulative postmarketing experience with YASMIN indicates a spontaneous reporting rate of venous thromboembolism of 5.1 events per 100 000 woman-years.

The following serious and unexpected adverse reactions have also been reported very rarely in users of YASMIN, but a causal relationship has not been established: pancytopenia, thrombocytopenia, arrhythmia, palpitations, tachycardia, ventricular extrasystoles, sudden hearing loss, ocular hypertension, visual disturbance, vitreous opacities, ischaemic colitis, hepatitis, hyperbilirubinemia, abnormal liver function test, decreased blood sodium, bone pain, pain in extremity, fibroadenoma of breast, seizure, dysarthria, facial paresis, hemiparesis, hypoesthesia, syncope, anxiety, nervousness, panic reaction, breast cyst, hematometra due to cervical polyp, asthma, erythema nodosum, leukocytoclastic vasculitis, lichen planus and petechiae.

Post-Market Adverse Events: The following unexpected adverse events have also been reported very rarely in users of YASMIN; but a causal relationship has not been established: hot/cold sensations, muscle spasms, and muscle twitching.

Post-Market Active Surveillance Study: A prospective, controlled, noninterventional, active surveillance cohort study (EURAS) was conducted in Europe to compare risks of adverse cardiovascular and other events associated with the use of DRSP-containing OCs (YASMIN) and other OCs. In this study, 58 674 OC users were actively followed for a total of 142 475 woman-years. Loss to follow-up was 2.4%. The hazard ratios for venous thromboembolic (VTE) and for all thromboembolic (TE) events were close to 1 and thus do not suggest a higher risk for YASMIN users. The results exclude a 1.5-fold thromboembolic risk of YASMIN users compared to users of LNG-containing OCs and a 1.2-fold thromboembolic risk compared to users of other OCs. Arrhythmic events that could be suggestive of an increased serum potassium level (eg, because of the antimineralocorticoid activity of DRSP) were not observed in this Post-Market Surveillance study.

Hazard ratios and confidence limits for VTE, ATE and TE are presented below in Table 1.

Table 1: YASMIN

Adjusted Hazard Ratios (HR) and Confidence Limits for VTE, ATE and TE (as Treated Analysis)

	YASMIN vs					
	LNG-containing OCs		Other OCs		LNG and Other OCs	
	HR	95% CI	HR	95% CI	HR	95% CI
VTE	1.05	0.61–1.81	0.77	0.48 –1.26	0.87	0.55–1.37
ATE	0.25	0.05–1.17	0.34	0.08–1.52	0.3	0.07–1.29
TE[a]	0.85	0.51–1.42	0.69	0.44–1.12	0.76	0.49–1.17

[a] All thromboembolic events (VTE and ATE combined).

Legend: ATE=arterial thromboembolism; CI=confidence interval; LNG=levonorgestrel; OC=oral contraception; TE=thromboembolic event; VTE=venous thromboembolism.

DRUG INTERACTIONS: Overview: The concurrent administration of oral contraceptives with other drugs may lead to breakthrough bleeding and/or may result in an altered response to either agent (see Table 2 and Table 3). Reduced effectiveness of the oral contraceptive, should it occur, is more likely with the low-dose formulations. It is important to ascertain all drugs that a patient is taking, both prescription and non-prescription, before oral contraceptives are prescribed.

Drug-Drug Interactions:

Table 2: YASMIN

Drugs Which May Decrease the Efficacy of Oral Contraceptives

Class of Compound	Drug	Proposed Mechanism	Suggested Management
Antacids		Decreased intestinal absorption of progestins.	Dose two hours apart.
Antibiotics	Ampicillin Cotrimoxazole Penicillin	Enterohepatic circulation disturbance, intestinal hurry.	For short course, use additional method or use another drug. For long course, use another method.
	Rifabutin Rifampin	Increased metabolism of progestins. Suspected acceleration of estrogen metabolism.	Use another method.
	Chloramphenicol Metronidazole Neomycin Nitrofurantoin Sulfonamides Tetracyclines	Induction of hepatic microsomal enzymes. Also disturbance of enterohepatic circulation.	For short course, use additional method or use another drug. For long course, use another method.
	Troleandomycin	May retard metabolism of oral contraceptives, increasing the risk of cholestatic jaundice.	

(cont'd)

Table 2: YASMIN *(cont'd)*

Drugs Which May Decrease the Efficacy of Oral Contraceptives

Class of Compound	Drug	Proposed Mechanism	Suggested Management
Anticonvulsants	Carbamazepine Ethosuximide Felbamate Lamotrigine Oxcarbazepine Phenobarbital Phenytoin Primidone Topiramate	Induction of hepatic microsomal enzymes. Rapid metabolism of estrogen and increased binding of progestin and ethinyl estradiol to SHBG.	Use higher dose oral contraceptives (50 µg ethinyl estradiol), another drug, or another method.
Antifungals	Griseofulvin	Stimulation of hepatic metabolism of contraceptive steroids may occur.	Use another method.
Cholesterol-lowering agents	Clofibrate	Reduces elevated serum triglycerides and cholesterol; this reduces oral contraceptive efficacy.	Use another method.
HIV protease inhibitors	Ritonavir	Induction of hepatic microsomal enzymes.	Use another drug or another method.
Non-nucleoside reverse transcriptase inhibitors	Nevirapine	Induction of hepatic microsomal enzymes.	Use another drug or another method.
Sedatives and hypnotics	Barbiturates Benzodiazepines Chloral hydrate Glutethimide Meprobamate	Induction of hepatic microsomal enzymes.	For short course, use additional method or another drug. For long course, use another method or higher dose oral contraceptives.
Other drugs	Analgesics Antihistamines Antimigraine preparations Phenylbutazone preparations Vitamin E	Reduced oral contraceptive efficacy has been reported. Remains to be confirmed.	

Oral contraceptives may interfere with the metabolism of other drugs. Accordingly, plasma and tissue concentrations may either increase (eg, cyclosporine) or decrease (eg, lamotrigine).

Table 3: YASMIN

Modification of Other Drug Action by Oral Contraceptives

Class of Compound	Drug	Modification of Drug Action	Suggested Management
Alcohol		Possible increased levels of ethanol or acetaldehyde	Use with caution.
Alpha-II adrenoreceptor agents	Clonidine	Sedation effect increased.	Use with caution.
Anticoagulants	All	Oral contraceptives increase clotting factors, decrease efficacy. However, oral contraceptives may potentiate action in some patients.	Use another method.
Anticonvulsants	All	Fluid retention may increase risk of seizures.	Use another method.
	Lamotrigine	Decreased lamotrigine levels, may lead to breakthrough seizures.	Use another method.
Antidiabetic drugs	Oral hypoglycemics and insulin	Oral contraceptives may impair glucose tolerance and increase blood glucose.	Use low-dose estrogen and progestin oral contraceptive or another method. Monitor blood glucose.
Antihypertensive agents	Guanethidine and methyldopa	Estrogen component causes sodium retention, progestin has no effect.	Use low-dose estrogen oral contraceptive or use another method.
	Beta blockers	Increased drug effect (decreased metabolism).	Adjust dose of drug if necessary. Monitor cardiovascular status.
Antipyretics	Acetaminophen	Increased metabolism and renal clearance.	Dose of drug may have to be increased.
	Antipyrine	Impaired metabolism.	Decrease dose of drug.
	ASA	Effects of ASA may be decreased by the short-term use of oral contraceptives.	Patients on chronic ASA therapy may require an increase in ASA dosage.
Aminocaproic acid		Theoretically, a hypercoagulable state may occur because oral contraceptives augment clotting factors.	Avoid concomitant use.

(cont'd)

Table 3: YASMIN *(cont'd)*

Modification of Other Drug Action by Oral Contraceptives

Class of Compound	Drug	Modification of Drug Action	Suggested Management
Betamimetic agents	Isoproterenol	Estrogen causes decreased response to these drugs.	Adjust dose of drug as necessary. Discontinuing oral contraceptives can result in excessive drug activity.
Caffeine		The actions of caffeine may be enhanced as oral contraceptives may impair the hepatic metabolism of caffeine.	Use with caution.
Cholesterol-lowering agents	Clofibrate	Its action may be antagonized by oral contraceptives. Oral contraceptives may also increase metabolism of clofibrate.	May need to increase dose of clofibrate.
Corticosteroids	Prednisone	Markedly increased serum levels.	Possible need for decrease in dose.
Cyclosporine		May lead to an increase in cyclosporine levels and hepatotoxicity.	Monitor hepatic function. The cyclosporine dose may have to be decreased.
Folic acid		Oral contraceptives have been reported to impair folate metabolism.	May need to increase dietary intake, or supplement.
Meperidine		Possible increased analgesia and CNS depression due to decreased metabolism of meperidine.	Use combination with caution.
Phenothiazine tranquilizers	All phenothiazines, reserpine and similar drugs	Estrogen potentiates the hyperprolactinemia effect of these drugs.	Use other drugs or lower-dose oral contraceptives. If galactorrhea or hyperprolactinemia occurs, use other method.
Sedatives and hypnotics	Chlordiazepoxide Lorazepam Oxazepam Diazepam	Increased effect (increased metabolism).	Use with caution.
Theophylline	All	Decreased oxidation, leading to possible toxicity.	Use with caution. Monitor theophylline levels.
Tricyclic antidepressants	Clomipramine (possibly others)	Increased side effects: e.g., depression	Use with caution.
Vitamin B_{12}		Oral contraceptives have been reported to reduce serum levels of Vitamin B_{12}	May need to increase dietary intake, or supplement.

Several of the anti-HIV protease inhibitors (eg, ritonavir) and non-nucleoside reverse transcriptase inhibitors (eg, nevirapine) have been studied with coadministration of oral combination hormonal contraceptives; significant changes (increase and decrease) in the mean AUC of the estrogen and progestogen and the potential to affect hepatic metabolism have been noted in some cases. The efficacy and safety of oral contraceptive products may be affected. Healthcare providers should refer to the label of the individual anti-HIV protease inhibitor for further drug-drug interaction information.

Interactions with Drugs That Have the Potential to Increase Serum Potassium: There is a potential for an increase in serum potassium in women taking YASMIN with other drugs (see Warnings and Precautions). Of note, occasional or chronic use of NSAID medication was not restricted in any of the YASMIN clinical trials.

A drug-drug interaction study of DRSP 3 mg/estradiol (E2) 1 mg versus placebo was performed in 24 mildly hypertensive postmenopausal women taking enalapril maleate 10 mg twice daily. Potassium levels were obtained every other day for a total of 2 weeks in all subjects. Mean serum potassium levels in the DRSP/E2 treatment group relative to baseline were 0.22 mEq/L higher than those in the placebo group. Serum potassium concentrations also were measured at multiple timepoints over 24 hours at baseline and on Day 14. On Day 14, the ratios for serum potassium C_{max} and AUC in the DRSP/E2 group to those in the placebo group were 0.955 (90% CI: 0.914, 0.999) and 1.010 (90% CI: 0.944, 1.080), respectively. No patient in either treatment group developed hyperkalemia (serum potassium concentrations >5.5 mEq/L).

Drug-Herb Interactions: Herbal products containing St. John's Wort (hypericum perforatum) may induce hepatic enzymes (cytochrome P450) and p-glycoprotein transporter and may reduce the effectiveness of contraceptive steroids. This may also result in breakthrough bleeding.

Drug-Laboratory Test Interactions: Results of laboratory tests should be interpreted with the knowledge that the patient is taking an oral contraceptive. The following laboratory tests are modified:

Liver Function Tests: Aspartate serum transaminase (AST): variously reported elevations. Alkaline phosphatase and gamma glutamine transaminase (GGT): slightly elevated.

Coagulation Tests: Minimal elevation of test values reported for such parameters as prothrombin and factors VII, VIII, IX, and X.

Thyroid Function Tests: Protein binding of thyroxine is increased as indicated by increased total serum thyroxine concentrations and decreased T3 resin uptake.

Lipoproteins: Small changes of unproven clinical significance may occur in lipoprotein cholesterol fractions.

Gonadotropins: LH and FSH levels are suppressed by the use of oral contraceptives. Wait two weeks after discontinuing the use of oral contraceptives before measurements are made.

Glucose Tolerance: Oral glucose tolerance remained unchanged or was slightly decreased.

Tissue Specimens: Pathologists should be advised of oral contraceptive therapy when specimens obtained from surgical procedures and Pap smears are submitted for examination.

Metabolic Interactions: Metabolism of drospirenone (DRSP) and potential effects of DRSP on hepatic cytochrome P450 (CYP) enzymes have been investigated in in vitro and in vivo studies (see Action and Clinical Pharmacology, Pharmacokinetics, Metabolism). In in vitro studies DRSP did not affect turnover of model substrates of CYP1A2 and CYP2D6, but had an inhibitory influence on the turnover of model substrates of CYP1A1, CYP2C9, CYP2C19 and CYP3A4 with CYP2C19 being the most sensitive enzyme. The potential effect of DRSP on CYP2C19 activity was investigated in a clinical pharmacokinetic study using omeprazole as a marker substrate. In the study with 24 postmenopausal women (including 12 women with homozygous [wild type] CYP2C19 genotype and 12 women with heterozygous CYP2C19 genotype), the daily oral administration of 3 mg DRSP for 14 days did not affect the oral clearance of omeprazole (40 mg, single oral dose). Based on the available results of in vivo and in vitro studies, it can be concluded that, at clinical dose level, DRSP shows little propensity to interact to a significant extent with cytochrome P450 enzymes.

Noncontraceptive Benefits of Oral Contraceptives: Several health advantages other than contraception have been reported.

1. Combination oral contraceptives reduce the incidence of cancer of the endometrium and ovaries.
2. Oral contraceptives reduce the likelihood of developing benign breast disease and, as a result, decrease the incidence of breast biopsies.
3. Oral contraceptives reduce the likelihood of development of functional ovarian cysts.

4. Pill users have less menstrual blood loss and have more regular cycles, thereby reducing the chance of developing iron-deficiency anemia.
5. The use of oral contraceptives may decrease the severity of dysmenorrhea and premenstrual syndrome and may improve acne vulgaris, hirsutism, and other androgen-mediated disorders.
6. Oral contraceptives decrease the incidence of acute pelvic inflammatory disease and, thereby, reduce as well the incidence of ectopic pregnancy.
7. Oral contraceptives have potential beneficial effects on endometriosis.

DOSAGE AND ADMINISTRATION: Tablets must be taken in the order directed on the package every day at about the same time. The patient may begin using YASMIN (drospirenone and ethinyl estradiol) on Day 1 of her menstrual cycle (ie, the first day of menstrual flow), on Day 5, or on the first Sunday after her period begins. If the patient's period begins on Sunday, she should start that same day. If YASMIN tablets are taken later than Day 1 when first starting medication, an additional (barrier) method of birth control is recommended for the first seven days of use.

YASMIN 21 (21 Day Regimen): One hormone-containing yellow tablet is to be taken daily for 21 consecutive days. Tablets are then discontinued for 7 consecutive days. Withdrawal bleeding usually occurs within 2 to 3 days following discontinuation.

The patient begins each subsequent course of YASMIN 21 tablets on the same day of the week that she began her first course. She begins taking her next course on the 8th day after discontinuation, regardless of whether or not withdrawal bleeding is still in progress.

YASMIN 28 (28 Day Regimen): One hormone-containing yellow tablet is to be taken daily for 21 consecutive days, followed by one hormone-free white tablet daily for 7 consecutive days. Withdrawal bleeding usually occurs within 2 to 3 days following the last hormone-containing yellow tablet (i.e., while the patient is taking the hormone-free white tablets).

The patient begins each subsequent course of YASMIN 28 tablets on the same day of the week that she began her first course. She begins taking her next course immediately after completion of the last course, regardless of whether or not withdrawal bleeding is still in progress. There is no need for the patient to count days between cycles because there are no "off-tablet days".

Management of Missed Tablets: The patient should be instructed to use Table 4 if she misses one or more of her birth control pills. She should be told to match the number of pills missed with the appropriate starting time for her dosing regimen.

Table 4: YASMIN

Management of Missed Tablets

Sunday Start	Other Than Sunday Start
Miss One Pill at Any Time	**Miss One Pill at Any Time**
Take it as soon as you remember, and take the next pill at the usual time. This means that you might take two pills in one day.	Take it as soon as you remember, and take the next pill at the usual time. This means that you might take two pills in one day.
Miss Two Pills in a Row	**Miss Two Pills in a Row**
First Two Weeks 1. Take two pills the day you remember and two pills the next day. 2. Then take one pill a day until you finish the pack. 3. Use a back-up (barrier) method of birth control if you have sex in the seven days after you miss the pills. **Third Week** 1. Keep taking one pill a day until Sunday. 2. On Sunday, safely discard the rest of the pack and start a new pack that day. 3. Use a back-up (barrier) method of birth control if you have sex in the seven days after you miss the pills. 4. You may not have a period this month. **If you miss two periods in a row, call your doctor or clinic.**	**First Two Weeks** 1. Take two pills the day you remember and two pills the next day. 2. Then take one pill a day until you finish the pack. 3. Use a back-up (barrier) method of birth control if you have sex in the seven days after you miss the pills. **Third Week** 1. Safely dispose of the rest of the pill pack and start a new pack that same day. 2. Use a back-up (barrier) method of birth control if you have sex in the seven days after you miss the pills. 3. You may not have a period this month. **If you miss two periods in a row, call your doctor or clinic.**
Miss Three or More Pills in a Row	**Miss Three or More Pills in a Row**
Anytime in the cycle 1. Keep taking one pill a day until Sunday. 2. On Sunday, safely discard the rest of the pack and start a new pack that day. 3. Use a back-up (barrier) method of birth control if you have sex in the seven days after you miss the pills. 4. You may not have a period this month. **If you miss two periods in a row, call your doctor or clinic.**	**Anytime in the cycle** 1. Safely dispose of the rest of the pill pack and start a new pack that same day. 2. Use a back-up (barrier) method of birth control if you have sex in the seven days after you miss the pills. 3. You may not have a period this month. **If you miss two periods in a row, call your doctor or clinic.**

Patients Taking YASMIN 28: If the patient forgets any of the seven hormone-free white pills in Week 4, she should be advised to safely dispose of the pills she missed, and then to keep taking one pill each day until the pack is empty. A back-up method of birth control is not required.

Special Notes on Administration: Switching from another combined hormonal contraceptive (combined oral contraceptive (COC), vaginal ring, or transdermal patch): The patient should start YASMIN on the day she would normally start her next pack of combined oral contraceptive. In case a vaginal ring or transdermal patch has been used, the woman should start using YASMIN preferably on the day of removal, but at the latest when the next application would have been due.

Switching from a progestogen-only method (mini-pill, injection) or from a Progestogen-releasing Intrauterine System (IUS): The patient may switch from the mini-pill to YASMIN on any day of her cycle. Patients using a progestogen injection should start YASMIN on the day the next injection is due. Patients using an IUS should start YASMIN on the day the IUS is removed. In all cases, the patient should be advised to use an additional (barrier) method for the first 7 days of YASMIN use.

Following First Trimester Abortion: The patient may start using YASMIN immediately. When doing so, she need not take additional contraceptive measures.

Following Delivery or Second Trimester Abortion: Patients should be advised to start YASMIN on Day 21 to 28 after delivery or second trimester abortion, after consulting with their physician. When starting later, the patient should be advised to use an additional (barrier) method for the first seven days of YASMIN use. However, if intercourse has already occurred, pregnancy should be excluded before the actual start of use or the woman should be advised to wait for her next menstrual period prior to starting YASMIN. When the tablets are administered in the postpartum period, the increased risk of thromboembolic disease associated with the postpartum period must be considered.

Withdrawal/Breakthrough Bleeding: Withdrawal bleeding usually occurs within 3 days following the last hormone-containing yellow tablet. If spotting or breakthrough bleeding occurs while taking YASMIN, the patient should be instructed to continue taking YASMIN as instructed and by the regimen described above. She should be instructed that this type of bleeding is usually transient and without significance; however, if the bleeding is persistent or prolonged, the patient should be advised to consult her physician.

Although the occurrence of pregnancy is unlikely if YASMIN is taken according to directions, if withdrawal bleeding does not occur, the possibility of pregnancy must be considered. If the patient has not adhered to the prescribed dosing schedule (missed one or more hormone-containing tablets or started taking them on a day later than she should have), the probability of pregnancy should be considered at the time of the first missed period and appropriate diagnostic measures taken before the medication is resumed. If the patient has adhered to the prescribed regimen and misses two consecutive periods, pregnancy should be ruled out before continuing the contraceptive regimen.

Advice in Case of Vomiting: If vomiting occurs within 3 to 4 hours after a tablet is taken, absorption may not be complete. In such an event, the advice concerning management of missed pills is applicable.

OVERDOSAGE:
There have been no reports of overdose with YASMIN (drospirenone and ethinyl estradiol). Overdosage may cause nausea and vomiting, and withdrawal bleeding may occur in females. There are no antidotes and further treatment should be symptomatic, based on the knowledge of the pharmacological action of the constituents. Drospirenone is a spironolactone analogue which has antimineralocorticoid properties. Serum concentration of potassium and sodium and evidence of metabolic acidosis should be monitored in cases of overdose. Liver function tests should be conducted, particularly transaminase levels, 2 to 3 weeks after consumption.

For management of a suspected drug overdose, contact your regional Poison Control Centre. See the *CPS* Directory section for a list of Poison Control Centres.

ACTION AND CLINICAL PHARMACOLOGY: Mechanism of Action: YASMIN is a monophasic, combination oral contraceptive that contains the active ingredients drospirenone and ethinyl estradiol. Combination oral contraceptives act by suppression of gonadotropins. Although the primary mechanism of this action is inhibition of ovulation, other alterations include changes in the cervical mucus (which increases the difficulty of sperm entry into the uterus) and the endometrium (which reduces the likelihood of implantation).

Drospirenone is a spironolactone analogue with antimineralocorticoid activity. Preclinical studies in animals and in vitro have shown that drospirenone has no androgenic, estrogenic, glucocorticoid and antiglucocorticoid activity. Preclinical studies in animals have also shown that drospirenone has antiandrogenic activity.

Estrogen-containing combinations such as YASMIN increase the blood level of sex-hormone-binding-globulin (SHBG), which is capable of binding and thus inactivating androgens such as testosterone. Moreover, the anti-androgenic activity of drospirenone partially counteracts the effects of endogenous androgens, blocking the binding of dihydrotestosterone (DHT) at the receptor level, which makes it a suitable option in the treatment of acne. Drospirenone may also help to reduce edema of the wall of the sebaceous follicle during the second half of the menstrual cycle, which is partly responsible for the flare-up of inflammatory lesions at this cycle phase.

Pharmacodynamics: Drospirenone inhibits ovulation and follicular development at an oral threshold dose of 2 mg. Drospirenone 3 mg, in combination with ethinyl estradiol 0.030 mg, was found to be optimal for inhibition of ovulation and cycle control.

Drospirenone exhibited aldosterone antagonist activity at doses as low as 2 mg/day in healthy volunteers. Plasma renin activity and plasma aldosterone concentrations were increased, as was the excretion of aldosterone metabolites. The excretion of Na^+ was transiently increased by drospirenone (2 or 3 mg) alone or in combination with ethinyl estradiol (0.030 mg). Serum Na^+ and K^+ concentrations remained unchanged. The potency of drospirenone was 6.6 times higher on average than that of spironolactone, using the Na^+/K^+ urinary ratio as the primary indicator of potency of the aldosterone antagonistic effect.

Drospirenone (2, 3 or 4 mg) in combination with ethinyl estradiol (0.030 mg) displayed a favourable effect on the lipid profile with an increase in HDL and a slight decrease in LDL. Total cholesterol remained unchanged. In addition, oral glucose tolerance remained unchanged or was slightly decreased.

Drospirenone had no effect on the biosynthesis of sex hormone binding globulin (SHBG), and when administered in conjunction with ethinyl estradiol (0.030 mg), resulted in SHBG and corticosteroid binding globulin increases consistent with the dosage of ethinyl estradiol.

In vitro, drospirenone bound with low affinity to SHBG and did not bind at all to corticosteroid binding globulin (CBG).

Pharmacokinetics:

Table 5: YASMIN 21/YASMIN 28

Mean Pharmacokinetic Parameters of YASMIN (Drospirenone 3 mg and Ethinyl Estradiol 0.030 mg)

		Drospirenone Mean (%CV) Values			
Cycle/Day	**No. of Subjects**	**C_{max} (ng/mL)**	**t_{max} (h)**	**AUC $_{(0-24h)}$ (ng·h/mL)**	**$t_{½}$ (h)**
1/1	12	36.9 (13)	1.7 (47)	288 (25)	NA
1/21	12	87.5 (59)	1.7 (20)	827 (23)	30.9 (44)
6/21	12	84.2 (19)	1.8 (19)	930 (19)	32.5 (38)
9/21	12	81.3 (19)	1.6 (38)	957 (23)	31.4 (39)
13/21	12	78.7 (18)	1.6 (26)	968 (24)	31.1 (36)
		Ethinyl Estradiol Mean (%CV) Values			
Cycle/Day	**No. of Subjects**	**C_{max} (pg/mL)**	**t_{max} (h)**	**AUC $_{(0-24h)}$ (pg·h/mL)**	**$t_{½}$ (h)**
1/1	11	53.5 (43)	1.9 (45)	280.3 (87)	NA
1/21	11	92.1 (35)	1.5 (40)	461.3 (94)	NA
6/21	11	99.1 (45)	1.5 (47)	346.4 (74)	NA
9/21	11	87.0 (43)	1.5 (42)	485.3 (92)	NA
13/21	10	90.5 (45)	1.6 (38)	469.5 (83)	NA

Legend: NA=Not available.

Absorption: The absolute bioavailability of drospirenone (DRSP) from a single entity tablet is about 76%. The absolute bioavailability of ethinyl estradiol (EE) is approximately 40% as a result of presystemic conjugation and first-pass metabolism. The absolute bioavailability of YASMIN which is a combination tablet of drospirenone and ethinyl estradiol has not been evaluated. Serum concentrations of DRSP and EE reached peak levels within 1-3 hours after administration of YASMIN. After single-dose administration of YASMIN, the relative bioavailability, compared to a suspension, was 107% and 117% for DRSP and EE, respectively.

The pharmacokinetics of DRSP are dose proportional following single doses ranging from 1-10 mg. Following daily dosing of YASMIN, steady state DRSP concentrations were observed after 10 days. There was about 2- to 3-fold accumulation in serum C_{max} and AUC $_{(0-24h)}$ values of DRSP following multiple-dose administration of YASMIN (see Table 5).

For EE, steady-state conditions are reported during the second half of a treatment cycle. Following daily administration of YASMIN serum C_{max} and AUC$_{(0-24h)}$ values of EE accumulate by a factor of about 1.5 to 2.0.

Effect of Food: The rate of absorption of DRSP and EE following single administration of two YASMIN tablets was slower under fed conditions with the serum C_{max} being reduced about 40% for both components. The extent of absorption of DRSP, however, remained unchanged. In contrast the extent of absorption of EE was reduced by about 20% under fed conditions.

Distribution: DRSP and EE serum levels decline in two phases. The apparent volume of distribution of DRSP is approximately 4 L/kg and that of EE is reported to be approximately 4 5 L/kg.

DRSP does not bind to sex hormone-binding globulin (SHBG) or corticosteroid-binding globulin (CBG) but binds about 97% to other serum proteins. Multiple dosing over 3 cycles resulted in no change in the free fraction (as measured at trough levels). EE is reported to be highly, but nonspecifically, bound to serum albumin (approximately 98.5%) and induces an increase in the serum concentrations of both SHBG and CBG. EE-induced effects on SHBG and CBG were not affected by variation of the DRSP dosage in the range of 2 to 3 mg.

Metabolism: The two main metabolites of DRSP found in human plasma were identified to be the acid form of DRSP generated by opening of the lactone ring and the 4,5-dihydrodrospirenone-3-sulfate. These metabolites were shown not to be pharmacologically active. In in vitro studies with human liver microsomes, DRSP was metabolized only to a minor extent mainly by cytochrome P450 3A4 (CYP3A4).

EE has been reported to be subject to presystemic conjugation in both small bowel mucosa and the liver. Metabolism occurs primarily by aromatic hydroxylation but a wide variety of hydroxylated and methylated metabolites are formed. These are present as free metabolites and as conjugates with glucuronide and sulfate. CYP3A4 in the liver is responsible for the 2-hydroxylation which is the major oxidative reaction. The 2-hydroxy metabolite is further transformed by methylation and glucuronidation prior to urinary and fecal excretion.

Excretion: DRSP serum levels are characterized by a terminal disposition phase half-life of approximately 30 hours after both single- and multiple-dose regimens. Excretion of DRSP was nearly complete after ten days and amounts excreted were slightly higher in feces compared to urine. DRSP was extensively metabolized and only trace amounts of unchanged DRSP were excreted in urine and feces. At least 20 different metabolites were observed in urine and feces. About 38% to 47% of the metabolites in urine were glucuronide and sulfate conjugates. In feces, about 17% to 20% of the metabolites were excreted as glucuronides and sulfates.

For EE, the terminal disposition phase half-life has been reported to be approximately 24 hours. EE is not excreted unchanged. EE is excreted in the urine and feces as glucuronide and sulfate conjugates and undergoes enterohepatic circulation.

Special Populations and Conditions: Pediatrics: The safety and efficacy of YASMIN has not been established in women under the age of 16 years. Use of this product before menarche is not indicated.

Geriatrics: YASMIN is not indicated for use in postmenopausal women.

Race: The effect of race on the disposition of YASMIN has not been evaluated.

Hepatic Insufficiency: YASMIN is contraindicated in patients with hepatic dysfunction (also see Warnings and Precautions). The mean terminal half-life of DRSP for women with moderate hepatic impairment was 1.8 times greater than for women with normal hepatic function.

Renal Insufficiency: YASMIN is contraindicated in patients with renal insufficiency (also see Warnings and Precautions).

The effect of renal insufficiency on the pharmacokinetics of DRSP (3 mg daily for 14 days) and the effect of DRSP on serum potassium levels were investigated in female subjects (n=28, age 30-65) with normal renal function and mild and moderate renal impairment. All subjects were on a low potassium diet. During the study 7 subjects continued the use of potassium-sparing drugs for the treatment of the underlying illness. On the 14th day (steady-state) of DRSP treatment, the serum DRSP levels in the group with mild renal impairment (creatinine clearance CLcr, 50-80 mL/min) were comparable to those in the group with normal renal function (CLcr, >80 mL/min). The serum DRSP levels were on average 37% higher in the group with moderate renal impairment (CLcr, 30-50 mL/min) compared to those in the group with normal renal function. DRSP treatment was well tolerated by all groups. DRSP treatment did not show any clinically significant effect on serum potassium concentration. Although hyperkalemia was not observed in the study, in five of the seven subjects who continued use of potassium-sparing drugs during the study, mean serum potassium levels increased by up to 0.33 mEq/L. Therefore, potential exists for hyperkalemia to occur in subjects with renal impairment whose serum potassium is in the upper reference range and who are concomitantly using potassium sparing drugs.

STORAGE AND STABILITY: Store in original packaging between 15 and 30°C.

Medicines should not be disposed of via wastewater or household waste. Ask your pharmacist how to dispose of medicines no longer required. These measures will help to protect the environment.

SPECIAL HANDLING INSTRUCTIONS: There are no special handling instructions.

INFORMATION FOR THE PATIENT: Published in e-CPS, available by subscription at www.e-cps.ca.

DOSAGE FORMS, COMPOSITION AND PACKAGING: YASMIN 21: Each hormone-containing yellow, round, film-coated tablet contains: 3.0 mg drospirenone and 0.030 mg ethinyl estradiol. Nonmedicinal ingredients: cornstarch, hydroxypropylmethyl cellulose, lactose monohydrate, magnesium stearate, modified starch, polyethylene glycol, povidone, talc, titanium dioxide and yellow ferric oxide. Blister packs containing 21 hormone-containing yellow film-coated tablets.

YASMIN 28: Each hormone-containing yellow, round, film-coated tablet contains: 3.0 mg drospirenone and 0.030 mg ethinyl estradiol. The white tablets are hormone-free. Nonmedicinal ingredients for both hormone-containing and hormone-free tablets: cornstarch, hydroxypropyl methylcellulose, lactose monohydrate, magnesium stearate, povidone, talc and titanium dioxide. Hormone-containing tablets also contain the following nonmedicinal ingredients: modified starch, polyethylene glycol and yellow ferric oxide. Blister packs containing 21 hormone-containing yellow and 7 hormone-free white, film-coated tablets.

(Shown in Product Identification Section)

Yaz® Ⓟ

drospirenone—ethinyl estradiol

Oral Contraceptive—Acne Therapy

Bayer

Date of Revision: June 3, 2010

SUMMARY PRODUCT INFORMATION:

Route of Administration	Dosage Form/ Strength	Clinically Relevant Nonmedicinal Ingredients
Oral	Tablet/3.0 mg drospirenone and 0.020 mg ethinyl estradiol	Lactose monohydrate For a complete listing see Dosage Forms, Composition and Packaging.

INDICATIONS AND CLINICAL USE: YAZ (drospirenone and ethinyl estradiol) is indicated for:

- Conception control
- Treatment of moderate acne vulgaris in women ≥14 years of age who have no known contraindications to oral contraceptive therapy, desire contraception, and have achieved menarche

CONTRAINDICATIONS: YAZ should not be used in women with:

- a history of or actual thrombophlebitis or thromboembolic disorders
- a history of or actual cerebrovascular disorders
- a history of or actual myocardial infarction or coronary artery disease
- valvular heart disease with complications
- a history of or actual prodromi of a thrombosis (e.g., transient ischemic attack, angina pectoris)
- presence of severe or multiple risk factor(s) for arterial or venous thrombosis:
  - severe hypertension (persistent values of ≥160/100 mmHg)
  - hereditary or acquired predisposition for venous or arterial thrombosis, such as Factor V Leiden mutation and activated protein C (APC-) resistance, antithrombin-III-deficiency, protein C deficiency, protein S deficiency, hyperhomocysteinemia and antiphospholipid-antibodies (anticardiolipin antibodies, lupus anticoagulant)
  - severe dyslipoproteinemia
  - heavy smoking (>15 cigarettes per day) and over age 35
  - diabetes mellitus with vascular involvement
  - major surgery associated with an increased risk of postoperative thromboembolism
  - prolonged immobilization
- active liver disease or history of, or actual benign or malignant liver tumors
- known or suspected carcinoma of the breast
- carcinoma of the endometrium or other known or suspected estrogen-dependent neoplasia
- undiagnosed abnormal vaginal bleeding
- steroid-dependent jaundice, cholestatic jaundice, history of jaundice in pregnancy
- any ocular lesion arising from ophthalmic vascular disease, such as partial or complete loss of vision or defect in visual fields
- known or suspected pregnancy
- current or history of migraine with focal aura
- history of or actual pancreatitis if associated with severe hypertriglyceridemia
- renal insufficiency
- hepatic dysfunction
- adrenal insufficiency
- hypersensitivity to this drug or to any ingredient in the formulation or component of the container. For a complete listing, see Dosage Forms, Composition and Packaging.

WARNINGS AND PRECAUTIONS:

> **Serious Warnings and Precautions**
> Cigarette smoking increases the risk of serious adverse effects on the heart and blood vessels. This risk increases with age and becomes significant in oral contraceptive users older than 35 years of age. Women should be counselled not to smoke (see Warnings and Precautions, Cardiovascular).
> Hormonal contraceptives **do not protect** against sexually transmitted infections (STIs) including HIV/AIDS. While using hormonal contraceptives, it is advisable to use latex or polyurethane condoms **in combination with** hormonal contraceptives to protect against STIs.

General: Discontinue Medication at the Earliest Manifestation of:

A. **Thromboembolic and Cardiovascular Disorders** such as thrombophlebitis, pulmonary embolism, cerebrovascular disorders, myocardial ischemia, mesenteric thrombosis, and retinal thrombosis.
B. **Conditions that Predispose to Venous Stasis and to Vascular Thrombosis** (e.g., immobilization after accidents or confinement to bed during long-term illness). Other nonhormonal methods of contraception should be used until regular activities are resumed. For use of oral contraceptives when surgery is contemplated, see Warnings and Precautions, Peri-operative Considerations.
C. **Visual Defects—Partial or Complete**
D. **Papilledema, or Ophthalmic Vascular Lesions**
E. **Severe Headache of Unknown Etiology or Worsening of Pre-existing Migraine Headache**
F. **Increase in Epileptic Seizures**

The following information is provided from studies of combination oral contraceptives (COCs).

The use of combination hormonal contraceptives is associated with increased risks of several serious conditions including myocardial infarction, thromboembolism, stroke, hepatic neoplasia, and gallbladder disease, although the risk of serious morbidity and mortality is small in healthy women without underlying risk factors. The risk of morbidity and mortality increases significantly if associated with the presence of other risk factors such as hypertension, hyperlipidemias, obesity, and diabetes. Other medical conditions which have been associated with adverse circulatory events include systemic lupus erythematosus, hemolytic uremic syndrome, chronic inflammatory bowel disease, (Crohn's disease or ulcerative colitis), sickle cell disease, valvular heart disease, and atrial fibrillation.

The following conditions have been reported to occur or deteriorate with both pregnancy and COC use, although a direct association with COCs has not been firmly established: porphyria, systemic lupus erythematosus, hemolytic uremic syndrome, Sydenham's chorea, herpes gestationis, and otosclerosis-related hearing loss.

The information contained in this section is principally from studies carried out in women who used combination oral contraceptives with higher formulations of estrogens and progestins than those in common use today. The effect of long-term use of combination hormonal contraceptives with lower doses of both estrogen and progestin administered orally remains to be determined.

YAZ contains 3 mg of the progestin drospirenone (DRSP) that has antimineralocorticoid activity, including the potential for hyperkalemia in high-risk patients, comparable to a 25 mg dose of spironolactone. YAZ should not be used in patients with conditions that predispose to hyperkalemia (e.g., renal insufficiency, hepatic dysfunction, and adrenal insufficiency). Women receiving daily, long-term treatment for chronic conditions or diseases with medications that may increase serum potassium should have their serum potassium level checked during the first treatment cycle. Drugs that may increase serum potassium include ACE inhibitors, angiotensin-II receptor antagonists, potassium-sparing diuretics, heparin, aldosterone antagonists, and NSAIDs.

Carcinogenesis and Mutagenesis: Breast Cancer: Increasing age and a strong family history are the most significant risk factors for the development of breast cancer. Other established risk factors include obesity, nulliparity, and late age for first full-term pregnancy. The identified groups of women that may be at increased risk of developing breast cancer before menopause are long-term users of oral contraceptives (more than 8 years) and starters at early age. In a few women, the use of oral contraceptives may accelerate the growth of an existing but undiagnosed breast cancer. Since any potential increased risk related to oral contraceptive use is small, there is no reason to change prescribing habits at present.

Women receiving oral contraceptives should be instructed in self-examination of their breasts. Their physicians should be notified whenever any masses are detected. A yearly clinical breast examination is also recommended, because, if breast cancer should develop, drugs that contain estrogen may cause a rapid progression.

Cervical Cancer: The most important risk factor for cervical cancer is persistent human papillomavirus infection. Some epidemiological studies have indicated that long-term use of COCs may further contribute to this increased risk, but there continues to be controversy about the extent to which this finding is attributable to confounding effects, e.g., cervical screening and sexual behaviour including use of barrier contraceptives.

Hepatocellular Carcinoma: Hepatocellular carcinoma may be associated with oral contraceptives. The risk appears to increase with duration of hormonal contraceptive use. However, the attributable risk (the excess incidence) of liver cancers in oral contraceptive users is extremely small. A liver tumor should be considered in the differential diagnosis when severe upper abdominal pain, liver enlargement or signs of intra-abdominal hemorrhage occur in women taking COCs.

Cardiovascular: Predisposing Factors for Coronary Artery Disease: Cigarette smoking increases the risk of serious cardiovascular side effects and mortality. Birth control pills increase this risk, especially with increasing age. Convincing data are available to support an upper age limit of 35 years for oral contraceptive use by women who smoke.

Other women who are independently at high risk for cardiovascular disease include those with diabetes, hypertension, abnormal lipid profile, or a family history of these. Whether oral contraceptives accentuate this risk is unclear.

In low-risk, nonsmoking women of any age, the benefits of oral contraceptive use outweigh the possible cardiovascular risks associated with low-dose formulations. Consequently, oral contraceptives may be prescribed for these women up to the age of menopause.

Hypertension: Patients with essential hypertension whose blood pressure is well-controlled may be given hormonal contraceptives, but only under close supervision. If a significant elevation of blood pressure in previously normotensive or hypertensive subjects occurs at any time during the administration of the drug, cessation of medication is necessary.

Endocrine and Metabolism: Diabetes: Current low-dose oral contraceptives exert minimal impact on glucose metabolism. Diabetic patients, or those with a family history of diabetes, should be observed closely to detect any worsening of carbohydrate metabolism. Patients predisposed to diabetes who can be kept under close supervision may be given oral contraceptives. Young diabetic patients whose disease is of recent origin, well-controlled, and not associated with hypertension or other signs of vascular disease such as ocular fundal changes, should be monitored more frequently while using oral contraceptives.

Lipid and Other Metabolic Effects: A small proportion of women will have adverse lipid changes while on oral contraceptives. Alternative contraception should be used in women with uncontrolled dyslipidemia (see also Contraindications). Elevations of plasma triglycerides may lead to pancreatitis and other complications.

Gastrointestinal: Published epidemiological studies indicate a possible association of COC use and the development of Crohn's disease and ulcerative colitis, although this has not been firmly established.

Genitourinary: Vaginal Bleeding: Persistent irregular vaginal bleeding requires assessment to exclude underlying pathology.

Fibroids: Patients with fibroids (leiomyomata) should be carefully observed. Sudden enlargement, pain, or tenderness requires discontinuation of the use of oral contraceptives.

Hematologic: Epidemiological studies have suggested an association between the use of COCs and an increased risk of arterial and venous thrombotic and thromboembolic diseases such as myocardial infarction, deep venous thrombosis, pulmonary embolism, and of cerebrovascular accidents. These events occur rarely.

The use of any combined oral contraceptive carries an increased risk of VTE compared with no use. The excess risk of VTE is highest during the first year a woman ever uses a combined oral contraceptive or restarts (following a 4-week or greater pill-free interval) the same or a different COC. Data from a large, prospective 3-armed cohort study suggest that this increased risk is mainly present during the first 3 months. VTE is fatal in 1% to 2% of cases.

A large, prospective 3-armed cohort study has shown that the frequency of VTE diagnosis ranges from about 8 to 10 per 10 000 woman-years in users of oral contraceptives with low estrogen content (<50 µg ethinyl estradiol). The most recent data suggest that the frequency of VTE diagnosis is approximately 4.4 per 10 000 woman-years in nonpregnant, non-COC users and ranges from 20 to 30 per 10 000 pregnant women or postpartum.

Overall the risk for venous thromboembolism (VTE) in users of oral contraceptives with low estrogen content (<50 µg ethinyl estradiol) is two- to three-fold higher than for nonusers of COCs who are not pregnant and remains lower than the risk associated with pregnancy and delivery.

Venous thromboembolism (VTE), manifesting as deep venous thrombosis and/or pulmonary embolism, may occur during the use of all COCs.

Extremely rarely, thrombosis has been reported to occur in other blood vessels (eg, hepatic, mesenteric, renal, cerebral, or retinal veins and arteries) in COC users. There is no consensus as to whether the occurrence of these events is associated with the use of COCs.

Symptoms of deep venous thrombosis (DVT) can include: unilateral swelling of the leg or along a vein in the leg; pain or tenderness in the leg, which may be felt only when standing or walking; increased warmth in the affected leg; red or discolored skin on the leg.

Symptoms of pulmonary embolism (PE) can include: sudden onset of unexplained shortness of breath or rapid breathing; sudden coughing which may bring up blood; sharp chest pain which may increase with deep breathing; sense of anxiety; severe light headedness or dizziness; rapid or irregular heartbeat. Some of these symptoms (eg, "shortness of breath", "coughing") are nonspecific and might be misinterpreted as more common or less severe events (eg, respiratory tract infections).

The risk for arterial thromboembolism (ATE) in users of oral contraceptives with low estrogen content (<50 µg ethinyl estradiol) ranges from about 1 to 3 cases per 10 000 woman-years. An arterial thromboembolic event (ATE) can include cerebrovascular accident, vascular occlusion, or myocardial infarction (MI). Symptoms of a cerebrovascular accident can include: sudden numbness or weakness of the face, arm, or leg, especially on one side of the body; sudden confusion, trouble speaking or understanding; sudden trouble seeing in one or both eyes; sudden trouble walking, dizziness, loss of balance or coordination; sudden, severe or prolonged headache with no known cause; loss of consciousness or fainting with or without seizure. Other signs of vascular occlusion can include: sudden pain, swelling, and slight blue discoloration of an extremity; acute abdomen.

Symptoms of MI can include: pain, discomfort, pressure, heaviness, sensation of squeezing or fullness in the chest, arm, or below the breastbone; discomfort radiating to the back, jaw, throat, arm, stomach; fullness, indigestion or choking feeling; sweating, nausea, vomiting, or dizziness; extreme weakness, anxiety, or shortness of breath; rapid or irregular heartbeats.

Arterial thromboembolic events may be fatal.

Other Risk Factors for Venous or Arterial Thromboembolism or of a Cerebrovascular Accident: Other generalized risk factors for venous or arterial thromboembolism include but are not limited to age, severe obesity (body mass index >30 kg/m^2), a personal history, a positive family history (the occurrence of VTE/ATE in a direct relative at a relatively early age may indicate genetic predisposition and systemic lupus erythematosus.

If a hereditary or acquired predisposition for venous or arterial thromboembolism is suspected, the woman should be referred to a specialist for advice before deciding on any COC use. The risk of VTE/ATE may be temporarily increased with prolonged immobilization, major surgery, or trauma. In these situations, it is advisable to discontinue COC use (in the case of elective surgery at least four weeks in advance) and not to resume COC use until two weeks after complete remobilization. Also, patients with varicose veins and leg cast should be closely supervised. Other risk factors may include smoking (with heavier smoking and increasing age, the risk further increases, especially in women over 35 years of age), dyslipoproteinemia, hypertension, migraine, valvular heart disease, and atrial fibrillation.

Biochemical factors that may be indicative of hereditary or acquired predisposition for venous or arterial thrombosis include Activated Protein C (APC) resistance, hyperhomocysteinemia, antithrombin-III deficiency, protein C deficiency, protein S deficiency, antiphospholipid antibodies (anticardiolipin antibodies, lupus anticoagulant).

When considering risk/benefit, the physician should take into account that adequate treatment of a condition may reduce the associated risk of thrombosis and that the risk associated with pregnancy is higher than that associated with low-dose COCs (<0.05 mg ethinyl estradiol).

Hepatic/Biliary/Pancreatic: In some cases of elevated liver enzymes reported during clinical trials with YAZ, a contributory role of YAZ could not be ruled out. YAZ is contraindicated in patients with active liver disease (see Contraindications and Drug Interactions, Drug-Laboratory Test Interactions).

Acute or chronic disturbances of liver function may necessitate the discontinuation of COC use until markers of liver function return to normal.

Jaundice: Patients who have had jaundice should be given oral contraceptives with great care and under close observation. Oral contraceptive-related cholestasis has been described in women with a history of pregnancy-related cholestasis. Women with a history of cholestasis may have the condition recur with subsequent hormonal contraceptive use.

The development of severe generalized pruritus or icterus requires that the medication be withdrawn until the problem is resolved.

If a patient develops jaundice that proves to be cholestatic in type, the use of oral contraceptives should not be resumed. In patients taking hormonal contraceptives, changes in the composition of the bile may occur and an increased incidence of gallstones has been reported.

Gallbladder Disease: Patients taking oral contraceptives have a greater risk of developing gallbladder disease requiring surgery within the first year of use. The risk may double after 4 or 5 years.

Hepatic Nodules: Hepatic nodules (adenoma and focal nodular hyperplasia) have been reported, particularly in long-term users of oral contraceptives. Although these lesions are extremely rare, they have caused fatal intra-abdominal hemorrhage and should be considered in women presenting with an abdominal mass, acute abdominal pain, or evidence of intra-abdominal bleeding.

Immune: Angioedema: Exogenous estrogens may induce or exacerbate symptoms of angioedema, in particular, in women with hereditary angioedema.

Neurologic: Migraine and Headache: The onset or exacerbation of migraine or the development of headache of a new pattern that is recurrent, persistent or severe, requires discontinuation of hormonal contraceptives and evaluation of the cause. Women with migraine headaches who take oral contraceptives may be at increased risk of stroke (see Contraindications).

Ophthalmologic: Patients who are pregnant or are taking oral contraceptives may experience corneal edema that may cause visual disturbances and changes in tolerance to contact lenses, especially of the rigid type. Soft contact lenses usually do not cause disturbances. If visual changes or alterations in tolerance to contact lenses occur, temporary or permanent cessation of wear may be advised.

Peri-operative Considerations: There is an increased risk of thromboembolic complications in oral contraceptive users after major surgery. If feasible, oral contraceptives should be discontinued and an alternative method substituted at least 1 month prior to **major** elective surgery. Oral contraceptive use should not be resumed until the first menstrual period after hospital discharge following surgery.

Psychiatric: Patients with a history of emotional disturbances, especially the depressive type, may be more prone to have a recurrence of depression while taking oral contraceptives. In cases of a serious recurrence, a trial of an alternate method of contraception should be made, which may help to clarify the possible relationship. Women with premenstrual syndrome (PMS) may have a varied response to oral contraceptives, ranging from symptomatic improvement to worsening of the condition.

Renal: Fluid Retention: Hormonal contraceptives may cause some degree of fluid retention. They should be prescribed with caution and only with careful monitoring in patients with conditions which might be aggravated by fluid retention.

Sexual Function/Reproduction: Return to Fertility: After discontinuing oral contraceptive therapy, the patient should delay pregnancy until at least 1 normal spontaneous menstrual cycle has occurred in order to date the pregnancy. An alternate contraceptive method should be used during this time.

Amenorrhea: In some women, withdrawal bleeding may not occur during the tablet-free interval. If the COC has been taken according to directions, it is unlikely that the woman is pregnant. However, if the COC has not been taken according to directions prior to the first missed withdrawal bleed, or if two withdrawal bleeds are missed, pregnancy must be ruled out before COC use is continued.

Women having a history of oligomenorrhea, secondary amenorrhea, or irregular cycles may remain anovulatory or become amenorrheic following discontinuation of estrogen-progestin combination therapy.

Amenorrhea, especially if associated with breast secretion, that continues for 6 months or more after withdrawal, warrants a careful assessment of hypothalamic-pituitary function.

Reduced Efficacy: The efficacy of COCs may be reduced in the event of missed tablets, gastrointestinal disturbances or concomitant medication (see Drug Interactions).

Skin: Chloasma may occasionally occur with use of COCs, especially in women with a history of chloasma gravidarum. Women with a tendency to chloasma should avoid exposure to the sun or ultraviolet radiation while taking COCs.

Special Populations: Pregnant Women: Oral contraceptives should not be taken by pregnant women. If pregnancy occurs during treatment with YAZ, further intake must be stopped. However, if conception accidentally occurs while taking the pill, there is no conclusive evidence that the estrogen and progestin contained in the oral contraceptive will damage the developing child. One infant was born with esophageal atresia during treatment with YASMIN, an OC of similar composition but with different dose and regimen. The causal association is unknown.

Nursing Women: In breast-feeding women, the use of oral contraceptives results in the hormonal components being excreted in breast milk and may reduce its quantity and quality. If the use of oral contraceptives is initiated after the establishment of lactation, there does not appear to be any effect on the quantity and quality of the milk. There is no evidence that low-dose oral contraceptives are harmful to the nursing infant.

If possible, the nursing mother should be advised not to use oral contraceptives but to use other forms of contraception until she has completely weaned her child.

After oral administration of YASMIN, an OC of similar composition but with different dose and regimen, about 0.02% of the drospirenone dose was excreted into the breast milk of postpartum women within 24 hours. This results in a maximal daily dose of about 3 µg drospirenone in an infant.

Pediatrics: The safety and efficacy of YAZ has not been established in women under the age of 14 years. Use of this product before menarche is not indicated.

Geriatrics: YAZ is not indicated for use in postmenopausal women.

Monitoring and Laboratory Tests: Physical Examination and Follow-up: Before oral contraceptives are used, a thorough history and physical examination should be performed, including a blood pressure determination and the family case history carefully noted. In addition, disturbances of the clotting system must be ruled out if any members of the family have suffered from thromboembolic diseases (e.g., deep vein thrombosis, stroke, myocardial infarction) at a young age. Breasts, liver, extremities, and pelvic organs should be examined and a Papanicolaou (PAP) smear should be taken if the patient has been sexually active.

The first follow-up visit should be done 3 months after oral contraceptives are prescribed. Thereafter, examinations should be performed at least once a year, or more frequently if indicated. At each annual visit, examination should include those procedures that were done at the initial visit as outlined above or per recommendations of the Canadian Task Force on the Periodic Health Examination.

ADVERSE REACTIONS: Adverse Drug Reaction Overview: An increased risk of the following serious adverse reactions has been associated with the use of oral contraceptives: benign hepatic tumors; cerebral hemorrhage; cerebral thrombosis; congenital anomalies; gallbladder disease; hypertension; mesenteric thrombosis; myocardial infarction; neuro-ocular lesions (e.g., retinal thrombosis); pulmonary embolism; thrombophlebitis.

The following adverse reactions also have been reported in patients receiving oral contraceptives: nausea and vomiting, usually the most common adverse reaction, occurs in approximately 10% or fewer of patients during the first cycle. The following other reactions, as a general rule, are seen less frequently or only occasionally: abdominal pain; amenorrhea during and after treatment; auditory disturbances; breakthrough bleeding; breast changes (tenderness, enlargement and secretion); cataracts; changes in appetite; change in corneal curvature (steepening); changes in libido; change in menstrual flow; change in weight (increase or decrease); chloasma or melasma which may persist; cholestatic jaundice; chorea; cystitis-like syndrome; mental depression; diarrhea; dizziness; dysmenorrhea; edema; endocervical hyperplasia; erythema multiforme; erythema nodosum; gastrointestinal symptoms (such as abdominal cramps and bloating); headache; hemolytic uremic syndrome; hemorrhagic eruption; hirsutism; hypersensitivity; impaired renal function; increase in size of uterine leiomyomata; intolerance to contact lenses; loss of scalp hair; migraine; nervousness; optic neuritis; pancreatitis; porphyria; possible diminution in lactation when given immediately postpartum; premenstrual-like syndrome; rash (allergic); Raynaud's phenomenon; reduced tolerance to carbohydrates; retinal thrombosis; rhinitis; spotting; temporary infertility after discontinuation of treatment; urticaria; vaginal candidiasis; vaginal discharge; vaginitis.

Clinical Trial Adverse Drug Reactions: Because clinical trials are conducted under very specific conditions the adverse reaction rates observed in the clinical trials may not reflect the rates observed in practice and should not be compared to the rates in the clinical trials of another drug. Adverse drug reaction information from clinical trials is useful for identifying drug-related adverse events and for approximating rates.

The clinical development programs were conducted independently for each of the 2 indications and utilized indication-specific inclusion criteria, study designs, and settings. Thus, the safety results of the studies are presented separately and are not pooled.

The following adverse drug reactions were reported at a frequency ≥1% in pivotal clinical trials using YAZ as an oral contraceptive:

Table 1: YAZ

Adverse Drug Reactions With Frequency of ≥1% in Pivotal OC Clinical Trials With YAZ (N=2438)

HARTS Body System	HARTS Preferred Term	n	%
Digestive System/General	Nausea	48	2.0
Nervous System/General	Headache	118	4.8
Nervous System/Central Nervous System/Brain	Emotional lability	28	1.1
Skin and Appendages/Dermatose/Acneform	Acne	24	1.0
Skin and Appendages/Breast Disorders	Breast pain	106	4.3
Urogenital System/Female Genital Disorders/ Menstrual Disorders	Amenorrhea	61	2.5
	Intermenstrual bleeding	110	4.5

Legend: HARTS=Hoechst Adverse Reaction Terminology System; N=total number; n=number of subjects; OC=oral contraception.

The following adverse drug reactions were reported at a frequency ≥1% in pivotal clinical trials using YAZ in the treatment of moderate acne vulgaris:

Table 2: YAZ

Adverse Drug Reactions With Frequency of ≥1% in Pivotal Moderate Acne Vulgaris Clinical Trials With YAZ (N=536)

HARTS Body System	HARTS Preferred Term	n	%
Digestive System/General	Nausea	22	4.1
	Vomiting	7	1.3
Nervous System/General	Headache	24	4.5
Nervous System/Central Nervous System/Brain	Emotional lability	12	2.2
	Depression	7	1.3
Skin and Appendages/Breast Disorders	Breast pain	8	1.5
Urogenital System/Female Genital Disorders/ Menstrual Disorders	Dysmenorrhea	8	1.5
	Metrorrhagia	53	9.9
	Menorrhagia	14	2.6
	Menstrual disorder	8	1.5

Legend: HARTS=Hoechst Adverse Reaction Terminology System; N=total number; n=number of subjects.

Less Common Clinical Trial Adverse Drug Reactions: The following adverse drug reactions were seen at a frequency of <1% and ≥0.1% in pivotal clinical trials using YAZ as an oral contraceptive:

Body as a Whole: abdominal pain, asthenia, back pain, pain in extremity, pelvic pain.

Cardiovascular System: hypertension, migraine, varicose vein.

Digestive System: diarrhea, dyspepsia, flatulence, gastritis, vomiting.

Metabolic and Nutritional Disorders: weight gain, edema, peripheral edema.

Musculoskeletal System: muscle cramps.

Nervous System: dizziness, paresthesia, sweating increased, depression, libido decreased, nervousness, somnolence.

Skin and Appendages: breast enlargement, acne, pruritus, fibrocystic breast, rash.

Urogenital System: hypomenorrhea, leukorrhea, vaginal dryness, vaginal moniliasis, dysmenorrhea, metrorrhagia, vaginal hemorrhage, menstrual disorder, PAP smear suspicious, vaginitis, menorrhagia.

The following adverse drug reactions were seen at a frequency of <1% and ≥0.1% in pivotal clinical trials using YAZ in the treatment of moderate acne vulgaris:

Body as a Whole: abdominal pain, asthenia, malaise.

Cardiovascular System: hypertension, migraine.

Urogenital System: amenorrhea, leukorrhea, PAP smear suspicious, uterine enlargement, vaginal moniliasis.

The following adverse drug reactions were seen at a frequency of <0.1% and ≥0.01% in pivotal clinical trials using YAZ as an oral contraceptive:

Body as a Whole: abdomen enlarged, accidental injury, allergic reaction, cyst, face edema, hernia, infection, moniliasis.

Cardiovascular System: phlebitis, syncope, tachycardia, vascular disorder.

Digestive System: biliary pain, cholecystitis, constipation, gastrointestinal disorder, gastrointestinal fullness, increased appetite, liver function test abnormal, oral moniliasis.

Endocrine System: endocrine disorder.

Metabolic and Nutritional Disorders: generalized edema, ALT increased, weight loss.

Nervous System: hot flashes, insomnia, vertigo.

Respiratory System: epistaxis.

Skin and Appendages: alopecia, breast neoplasm, chloasma, dermatitis acneiform, dry skin, eczema, erythema nodosum, hypertrichosis, skin disorder, skin striae.

Special Senses: conjunctivitis, dry eye, eye disorder.

Urogenital System: anorgasmia, cervix neoplasm, dyspareunia, endometrial disorder, ovarian cyst, vulvovaginitis, withdrawal bleeding.

Post-Market Adverse Drug Reactions: The following unexpected adverse events have also been reported very rarely in users of YAZ, but a causal relationship has not been established: hot/cold sensations, muscle spasms, and muscle twitching.

DRUG INTERACTIONS: Overview: The concurrent administration of oral contraceptives with other drugs may lead to breakthrough bleeding and/or may result in an altered response to either agent (see Table 3 and Table 4). Reduced effectiveness of the oral contraceptive, should it occur, is more likely with the low-dose formulations. It is important to ascertain all drugs that a patient is taking, both prescription and nonprescription, before oral contraceptives are prescribed.

Drug-Drug Interactions:

Table 3: YAZ

Drugs Which May Decrease the Efficacy of Oral Contraceptives

Class of Compound	Drug	Proposed Mechanism	Suggested Management
Antacids		Decreased intestinal absorption of progestins.	Dose 2 hours apart.
Antibiotics	Ampicillin Cotrimoxazole Penicillin	Enterohepatic circulation disturbance, intestinal hurry.	For short course, use additional method or use another drug. For long course, use another method.
	Rifabutin Rifampin	Increased metabolism of progestins. Suspected acceleration of estrogen metabolism.	Use another method.
	Chloramphenicol Metronidazole Neomycin Nitrofurantoin Sulfonamides Tetracyclines	Induction of hepatic microsomal enzymes. Also disturbance of enterohepatic circulation.	For short course, use additional method or use another drug. For long course, use another method.
	Troleandomycin	May retard metabolism of oral contraceptives, increasing the risk of cholestatic jaundice.	
Anticonvulsants	Carbamazepine Ethosuximide Felbamate Lamotrigine Oxcarbazepine Phenobarbital Phenytoin Primidone Topiramate	Induction of hepatic microsomal enzymes. Rapid metabolism of estrogen and increased binding of progestin and ethinyl estradiol to SHBG.	Use higher dose oral contraceptives (50 µg ethinyl estradiol), another drug or another method.
Antifungals	Griseofulvin	Stimulation of hepatic metabolism of contraceptive steroids may occur.	Use another method.
Cholesterol Lowering Agents	Clofibrate	Reduces elevated serum triglycerides and cholesterol; this reduces oral contraceptive efficacy.	Use another method.
HIV Protease Inhibitors	Ritonavir	Induction of hepatic microsomal enzymes.	Use another drug or another method.
Non-nucleoside Reverse Transcriptase Inhibitors	Nevirapine	Induction of hepatic microsomal enzymes.	Use another drug or another method.
Sedatives and Hypnotics	Barbiturates Benzodiazepines Chloral hydrate Glutethimide Meprobamate	Induction of hepatic microsomal enzymes.	For short course, use additional method or another drug. For long course, use another method or higher dose oral contraceptives.
Other Drugs	Antihistamines Analgesics Antimigraine preparations Phenylbutazone preparations Vitamin E	Reduced oral contraceptive efficacy has been reported. Remains to be confirmed.	

Oral contraceptives may interfere with the metabolism of other drugs. Accordingly, plasma and tissue concentrations may either increase (e.g., cyclosporine) or decrease (e.g., lamotrigine).

Table 4: YAZ

Modification of Other Drug Action by Oral Contraceptives

Class of Compound	Drug	Modification of Drug Action	Suggested Management
Alcohol		Possible increased levels of ethanol or acetaldehyde.	Use with caution.
Alpha-II Adrenoreceptor Agents	Clonidine	Sedation effect increased.	Use with caution.
Anticoagulants	All	Oral contraceptives increase clotting factors, decrease efficacy. However, oral contraceptives may potentiate action in some patients.	Use another method.
Anticonvulsants	All	Estrogens may increase risk of seizures.	Use another method.
	Lamotrigine	Decreased lamotrigine levels, may lead to breakthrough seizures.	Use another method.
Antidiabetic Drugs	Oral hypoglycemics and insulin	Oral contraceptives may impair glucose tolerance and increase blood glucose.	Use low-dose estrogen and progestin oral contraceptive or another method. Monitor blood glucose.
Antihypertensive Agents	Guanethidine and methyldopa	Estrogen component causes sodium retention, progestin has no effect.	Use low-dose estrogen oral contraceptive or use another method.
	Beta blockers	Increased drug effect (decreased metabolism).	Adjust dose of drug if necessary. Monitor cardiovascular status.
Antipyretics	Acetaminophen	Increased metabolism and renal clearance.	Dose of drug may have to be increased.
	Antipyrine	Impaired metabolism.	Decrease dose of drug.
	ASA	Effects of ASA may be decreased by the short-term use of oral contraceptives.	Patients on chronic ASA therapy may require an increase in ASA dosage.
Aminocaproic Acid		Theoretically, a hypercoagulable state may occur because oral contraceptives augment clotting factors.	Avoid concomitant use.
Betamimetic Agents	Isoproterenol	Estrogen causes decreased response to these drugs.	Adjust dose of drug as necessary. Discontinuing oral contraceptives can result in excessive drug activity.
Caffeine		The actions of caffeine may be enhanced as oral contraceptives may impair the hepatic metabolism of caffeine.	Use with caution.
Cholesterol Lowering Agents	Clofibrate	Its action may be antagonized by oral contraceptives. Oral contraceptives may also increase metabolism of clofibrate.	May need to increase dose of clofibrate.
Corticosteroids	Prednisone	Markedly increased serum levels.	Possible need for decrease in dose.
Cyclosporine		May lead to an increase in cyclosporine levels and hepatotoxicity.	Monitor hepatic function. The cyclosporine dose may have to be decreased.
Folic Acid		Oral contraceptives have been reported to impair folate metabolism.	May need to increase dietary intake, or supplement.
Meperidine		Possible increased analgesia and CNS depression due to decreased metabolism of meperidine.	Use combination with caution.
Phenothiazine Tranquilizers	All phenothiazines, reserpine and similar drugs	Estrogen potentiates the hyperprolactinemia effect of these drugs.	Use other drugs or lower dose oral contraceptives. If galactorrhea or hyperprolactinemia occurs, use other method.
Sedatives and Hypnotics	Chlordiazepoxide Lorazepam Oxazepam Diazepam	Increased effect (increased metabolism).	Use with caution.
Theophylline	All	Decreased oxidation, leading to possible toxicity.	Use with caution. Monitor theophylline levels.

(cont'd)

Table 4: YAZ *(cont'd)*
Modification of Other Drug Action by Oral Contraceptives

Class of Compound	Drug	Modification of Drug Action	Suggested Management
Tricyclic Antidepressants	Clomipramine (possibly others)	Increased side effects: e.g., depression.	Use with caution.
Vitamin B_{12}		Oral contraceptives have been reported to reduce serum levels of Vitamin B_{12}.	May need to increase dietary intake, or supplement.

Several of the anti-HIV protease inhibitors (e.g., ritonavir) and nonnucleoside reverse transcriptase inhibitors (e.g., nevirapine) have been studied with coadministration of oral combination hormonal contraceptives; significant changes (increase and decrease) in the mean AUC of the estrogen and progestin and the potential to affect hepatic metabolism have been noted in some cases. The efficacy and safety of oral contraceptive products may be affected. Healthcare providers should refer to the label of the individual anti-HIV protease inhibitor for further drug-drug interaction information.

No formal drug-drug interaction studies have been conducted with ethinyl estradiol/drospirenone.

Interactions With Drugs That Have the Potential to Increase Serum Potassium: There is a potential for an increase in serum potassium in women taking YAZ with other drugs (see Warnings and Precautions). Of note, occasional or chronic use of NSAID medication was not restricted in any of the YAZ clinical trials.

A drug-drug interaction study of DRSP 3 mg/estradiol 1 mg versus placebo was performed in 24 mildly hypertensive postmenopausal women taking enalapril maleate 10 mg twice daily. Potassium levels were obtained every other day for a total of 2 weeks in all subjects. Mean serum potassium levels in the DRSP/estradiol treatment group relative to baseline were 0.22 mEq/L higher than those in the placebo group. Serum potassium concentrations also were measured at multiple timepoints over 24 hours at baseline and on day 14. On day 14, the ratios for serum potassium C_{max} and AUC in the DRSP/estradiol group to those in the placebo group were 0.955 (90% CI: 0.914, 0.999) and 1.010 (90% CI: 0.944, 1.080), respectively. No patient in either treatment group developed hyperkalemia (serum potassium concentrations >5.5 mEq/L).

Drug-Food Interactions: Interactions with food have not been established.

Drug-Herb Interactions: Herbal products containing St. John's Wort (Hypericum perforatum) may induce hepatic enzymes (cytochrome P450) and p-glycoprotein transporter and may reduce the effectiveness of contraceptive steroids. This may also result in breakthrough bleeding.

Drug-Laboratory Test Interactions: Results of laboratory tests should be interpreted with the knowledge that the patient is taking an oral contraceptive. The following laboratory tests are modified:

A. **Liver Function Tests:** Aspartate serum transaminase (AST)—variously reported elevations Alkaline phosphatase and gamma glutamine transaminase (GGT)—slightly elevated.
B. **Coagulation Tests:** Minimal elevation of test values reported for such parameters as prothrombin and factors VII, VIII, IX, and X.
C. **Thyroid Function Tests:** Protein binding of thyroxine is increased as indicated by increased total serum thyroxine concentrations and decreased T_3 resin uptake.
D. **Lipoproteins:** Small changes of unproven clinical significance may occur in lipoprotein cholesterol fractions.
E. **Gonadotropins:** LH and FSH levels are suppressed by the use of oral contraceptives. Wait 2 weeks after discontinuing the use of oral contraceptives before measurements are made.
F. **Glucose Tolerance:** Oral glucose tolerance remained unchanged or was slightly decreased.

Tissue Specimens: Pathologists should be advised of oral contraceptive therapy when specimens obtained from surgical procedures and PAP smears are submitted for examination.

Drug-Lifestyle Interactions: No studies on the effects of YAZ on the ability to drive or use machines have been performed.

Metabolic Interactions: Metabolism of drospirenone (DRSP) and potential effects of DRSP on hepatic cytochrome P450 (CYP) enzymes have been investigated in in vitro and in vivo studies (see Action and Clinical Pharmacology, Pharmacokinetics, Metabolism). In in vitro studies, DRSP did not affect turnover of model substrates of CYP1A2 and CYP2D6, but had an inhibitory influence on the turnover of model substrates of CYP1A1, CYP2C9, CYP2C19, and CYP3A4, with CYP2C19 being the most sensitive enzyme. The potential effect of DRSP on CYP2C19 activity was investigated in a clinical pharmacokinetic study using omeprazole as a marker substrate. In the study with 24 postmenopausal women (including 12 women with homozygous [wild type] CYP2C19 genotype and 12 women with heterozygous CYP2C19 genotype), the daily oral administration of 3 mg DRSP for 14 days did not affect the oral clearance of omeprazole (40 mg, single oral dose). Based on the available results of in vivo and in vitro studies, it can be concluded that at clinical dose levels DRSP shows little propensity to interact to a significant extent with cytochrome P450 enzymes.

Noncontraceptive Benefits of Oral Contraceptives: Several health advantages other than contraception have been reported:

1. Combination oral contraceptives reduce the incidence of cancer of the endometrium and ovaries.
2. Oral contraceptives reduce the likelihood of developing benign breast disease and, as a result, decrease the incidence of breast biopsies.
3. Oral contraceptives reduce the likelihood of development of functional ovarian cysts.
4. Pill users have less menstrual blood loss and have more regular cycles, thereby reducing the chance of developing iron-deficiency anemia.
5. The use of oral contraceptives may decrease the severity of dysmenorrhea and premenstrual syndrome, and may improve acne vulgaris, hirsutism, and other androgen-mediated disorders.
6. Oral contraceptives decrease the incidence of acute pelvic inflammatory disease and, thereby, reduce as well the incidence of ectopic pregnancy.
7. Oral contraceptives have potential beneficial effects on endometriosis.

DOSAGE AND ADMINISTRATION:

Tablets must be taken in the order directed on the package every day at about the same time. The patient may begin using YAZ (drospirenone and ethinyl estradiol) on day 1 of her menstrual cycle (i.e., the first day of menstrual flow) or on the first Sunday after her period begins. If the patient's period begins on Sunday, she should start that same day. If YAZ tablets are taken later than day 1 when first starting medication, an additional (barrier) method of birth control is recommended for the first 7 days of use.

One hormone-containing light pink tablet is to be taken daily for 24 consecutive days, followed by 1 hormone-free white tablet daily for 4 consecutive days. Withdrawal bleeding usually occurs within 2 to 3 days following administration of the last hormone-containing light pink tablet (ie, while the patient is taking the hormone-free white tablets).

The patient begins each subsequent course of YAZ tablets on the same day of the week that she began her first course. She begins taking her next course immediately after completion of the last course, regardless of whether or not withdrawal bleeding is still in progress.

Management of Missed Tablets: The patient should be instructed to use Table 5 if she misses 1 or more of her birth control pills. She should be told to match the number of pills missed with the appropriate starting time for her dosing regimen.

If the patient forgets any of the 4 hormone-free white pills in week 4, she should be advised to safely dispose of the pills she missed, and then to keep taking 1 pill each day until the pack is empty. A back-up method of birth control is not required.

Special Notes on Administration: Switching from Another Combined Hormonal Contraceptive (combined oral contraceptive (COC), vaginal ring, or transdermal patch): The patient should start YAZ on the day she would normally start her next pack of combined oral contraceptive. In case a vaginal ring or transdermal patch has been used, the woman should start using YAZ preferably on the day of removal, but at the latest when the next application would have been due.

Switching from a Progestin-only Method (mini-pill, injection) or from a Progestin-releasing Intrauterine System (IUS): The patient may switch from the mini-pill to YAZ on any day of her cycle. Patients using a progestin injection should start YAZ on the day the next injection is due. Patients using an IUS should start YAZ on the day the IUS is removed. In all cases, the patient should be advised to use an additional (barrier) method for the first 7 days of YAZ use.

Following First Trimester Abortion: The patient may start using YAZ immediately. When doing so, she need not take additional contraceptive measures.

Following Delivery or Second Trimester Abortion: Patients should be advised to start YAZ on day 21 to 28 after delivery or second trimester abortion, after consulting with their physician. When starting later, the patient should be advised to use an additional (barrier) method for the first 7 days of YAZ use. However, if intercourse has already occurred, pregnancy should be excluded before the actual start of use, or the woman should be advised to wait for her next menstrual period prior to starting YAZ. When the tablets are administered in the postpartum period, the increased risk of thromboembolic disease associated with the postpartum period must be considered.

Withdrawal/Breakthrough Bleeding: Withdrawal bleeding usually occurs within 3 days following the last hormone-containing light pink tablet. If spotting or breakthrough bleeding occurs while taking YAZ, the patient should be instructed to continue taking YAZ as prescribed and by the regimen described above. She should be instructed that this type of bleeding is usually transient and without significance; however, if the bleeding is persistent or prolonged, the patient should be advised to consult her physician.

Although the occurrence of pregnancy is unlikely if YAZ is taken according to directions, if withdrawal bleeding does not occur, the possibility of pregnancy must be considered. If the patient has not adhered to the prescribed dosing schedule (missed 1 or more hormone-containing tablets or started taking them on a day later than she should have), the probability of pregnancy should be considered at the time of the first missed period and appropriate diagnostic measures taken before the medication is resumed. If the patient has adhered to the prescribed regimen and misses 2 consecutive periods, pregnancy should be ruled out before continuing the contraceptive regimen.

Advice in Case of Vomiting: If vomiting occurs within 3 to 4 hours after a tablet is taken, absorption may not be complete. In such an event, the advice concerning management of missed pills is applicable.

Table 5: YAZ
Management of Missed Pills

Sunday Start	Other than Sunday Start
Miss One Pill at Any Time	**Miss One Pill at Any Time**
Take it as soon as you remember, and take the next pill at the usual time. This means that you might take two pills in one day.	Take it as soon as you remember, and take the next pill at the usual time. This means that you might take two pills in one day.
Miss Two Pills in a Row	**Miss Two Pills in a Row**
First Two Weeks 1. Take two pills the day you remember and two pills the next day. 2. Then take one pill a day until you finish the pack. 3. Use a back-up (barrier) method of birth control if you have sex in the seven days after you miss the pills. **Third and Fourth Weeks** 1. Keep taking one pill a day until Sunday. 2. On Sunday, safely discard the rest of the pack and start a new pack that day. 3. Use a back-up (barrier) method of birth control if you have sex in the seven days after you miss the pills. 4. You may not have a period this month. **If you miss two periods in a row, call your doctor or clinic.**	**First Two Weeks** 1. Take two pills the day you remember and two pills the next day. 2. Then take one pill a day until you finish the pack. 3. Use a back-up (barrier) method of birth control if you have sex in the seven days after you miss the pills. **Third and Fourth Weeks** 1. Safely dispose of the rest of the pill pack and start a new pack that same day. 2. Use a back-up (barrier) method of birth control if you have sex in the seven days after you miss the pills. 3. You may not have a period this month. **If you miss two periods in a row, call your doctor or clinic.**
Miss Three or More Pills in a Row	**Miss Three or More Pills in a Row**
Anytime in the Cycle 1. Keep taking one pill a day until Sunday. 2. On Sunday, safely discard the rest of the pack and start a new pack that day. 3. Use a back-up (barrier) method of birth control if you have sex in the seven days after you miss the pills. 4. You may not have a period this month. **If you miss two periods in a row, call your doctor or clinic.**	**Anytime in the Cycle** 1. Safely dispose of the rest of the pill pack and start a new pack that same day. 2. Use a back-up (barrier) method of birth control if you have sex in the seven days after you miss the pills. 3. You may not have a period this month. **If you miss two periods in a row, call your doctor or clinic.**

OVERDOSAGE:

There have been no reports of overdose with YAZ (drospirenone and ethinyl estradiol). Overdosage may cause nausea and vomiting, and withdrawal bleeding may occur in females. There are no antidotes and further treatment should be symptomatic based on the knowledge of the pharmacological action of the constituents. Drospirenone is a spironolactone analogue which has antimineralocorticoid properties. Serum concentration of potassium and sodium and evidence of metabolic acidosis should be monitored in cases of overdose. Liver function tests should be conducted, particularly transaminase levels, 2 to 3 weeks after consumption.

For management of a suspected drug overdose, contact your regional Poison Control Centre. See the *CPS Directory* section for a list of Poison Control Centres.

ACTION AND CLINICAL PHARMACOLOGY: Mechanism of Action: YAZ is a monophasic, combination oral contraceptive that contains the progestin drospirenone (3.0 mg) and a low dose of the estrogen ethinyl estradiol (0.020 mg). Combination oral contraceptives act by suppression of gonadotropins. Although the primary mechanism of this action is inhibition of ovulation, other alterations include changes in the cervical mucus (which increases the difficulty of sperm entry into the uterus) and the endometrium (which reduces the likelihood of implantation).

Drospirenone is a spironolactone analogue with antimineralocorticoid activity. Preclinical studies in animals and in vitro have shown that drospirenone has no androgenic, estrogenic, glucocorticoid, and antiglucocorticoid activity. Preclinical studies in animals have also shown that drospirenone has antiandrogenic activity.

Estrogen-containing combinations such as YAZ increase the blood level of sex hormone binding globulin (SHBG), which is capable of binding and thus inactivating androgens such as testosterone. Moreover, the antiandrogenic activity of drospirenone partially counteracts the effects of endogenous androgens, blocking the binding of dihydrotestosterone (DHT) at the receptor level, which makes it a suitable option in the treatment of acne. Drospirenone may also help to reduce edema of the wall of the sebaceous follicle during the second half of the menstrual cycle, which is partly responsible for the flare-up of inflammatory lesions at this cycle phase.

Pharmacodynamics: Drospirenone inhibits ovulation and follicular development at an oral threshold dose of 2 mg. Drospirenone 3 mg in combination with ethinyl estradiol was found to be optimal for inhibition of ovulation and cycle control. Administration of 3 extra days of hormone (YAZ 24 day active versus a 21-day active of the same combined oral contraceptive) results in additional suppression of the ovary and of follicular development. This was observed in a study where hormone-containing pills of each regimen were intentionally missed on the first 3 days of the cycle and subsequent follicular development was monitored.

Drospirenone exhibited aldosterone antagonist activity at doses as low as 2 mg/day in healthy volunteers. Plasma renin activity and plasma aldosterone concentrations were increased, as was the excretion of aldosterone metabolites. The excretion of Na^+ was transiently increased by drospirenone (2 or 3 mg) alone or in combination with ethinyl estradiol. Serum Na^+ and K^+ concentrations remained unchanged. The potency of drospirenone was 6.6 times higher on average than that of spironolactone, using the Na^+/K^+ urinary ratio as the primary indicator of potency of the aldosterone antagonistic effect.

Drospirenone (2, 3, or 4 mg) in combination with ethinyl estradiol (0.020 mg) displayed a favourable effect on the lipid profile with an increase in HDL and a slight decrease in LDL. Total cholesterol remained unchanged. In addition, oral glucose tolerance was slightly increased, but remained within the reference range.

Drospirenone had no effect on the biosynthesis of SHBG, and when administered in conjunction with ethinyl estradiol (0.020 mg), resulted in SHBG and corticosteroid binding globulin increases consistent with the dosage of ethinyl estradiol.

In vitro, drospirenone bound with low affinity to SHBG and did not bind at all to corticosteroid binding globulin (CBG).

Pharmacokinetics:

Table 6: YAZ

Summary of Pharmacokinetic Parameters[a] (drospirenone 3 mg and ethinyl estradiol 0.020 mg) in Healthy Young Women

Cycle/Day	No. of Subjects	C_{max} (ng/mL)		t_{max} (h)		$AUC_{(0\text{-}24h)}$ (ng·h/mL)		$t_{½}$ (h)	
Drospirenone									
1/1	23	38.4	(25.20%)	1.5	(1–2)	268	(18.90%)	nd	
1/21	23	70.3	(14.50%)	1.5	(1–2)	763	(17.40%)	30.8	(21.90%)
Ethinyl Estradiol									
1/1	23	32.8	(44.90%)	1.5	(1–2.2)	108	(51.80%)	nd	
1/21	23	45.1	(34.70%)	1.5	(1–2)	220	(57.40%)	nd	

[a] The geometric mean is given for all parameters except t_{max}, with the geometric coefficient of variation in parentheses. For t_{max}, the median is given, with the range in parentheses.

Legend: AUC=area under the curve; C_{max}=maximum concentration; h=hour; mL=millilitre; nd=not determined; ng=nanogram; $t_{1/2}$=elimination half-life; t_{max}=time of maximum concentration.

Absorption: The absolute bioavailability of DRSP from a single entity tablet is about 76%. The absolute bioavailability of EE is approximately 40% as a result of presystemic conjugation and first-pass metabolism. The absolute bioavailability of YAZ which is a combination tablet of drospirenone and ethinyl estradiol stabilized by betadex as a clathrate (molecular inclusion complex) has not been evaluated. The bioavailability of EE is similar when dosed via a betadex clathrate formulation compared to when it is dosed as a free steroid. Serum concentrations of DRSP and EE reached peak levels within 1 to 2 hours after administration of YAZ. After single dose administration of YAZ, the relative bioavailability compared to a suspension was 107% and 97% for DRSP and EE, respectively.

The pharmacokinetics of DRSP are dose proportional following single doses ranging from 1-10 mg. Following daily dosing of YAZ, steady-state DRSP concentrations were observed after 8 days. There was about 2- to 3-fold accumulation in serum C_{max} and $AUC_{(0\text{-}24h)}$ values of DRSP following multiple-dose administration of YAZ.

For EE, steady-state conditions are reported during the second half of a treatment cycle. Following daily administration of YAZ, serum C_{max} and $AUC_{(0\text{-}24h)}$ values of EE accumulate by a factor of about 1.5 to 2.0 (see Table 6).

Effect of Food: The rate of absorption of DRSP and EE following single administration of 2 tablets, each containing 3 mg DRSP and 0.030 mg EE was slower under fed conditions, with the serum C_{max} being reduced about 40% for both components. The extent of absorption of DRSP, however, remained unchanged. In contrast the extent of absorption of EE was reduced by about 20% under fed conditions.

Distribution: DRSP and EE serum levels decline in 2 phases. The apparent volume of distribution of DRSP is approximately 4 L/kg, and that of EE is reported to be approximately 4 to 5 L/kg.

DRSP does not bind to SHBG or CBG, but binds about 97% to other serum proteins. Multiple dosing over 3 cycles resulted in no change in the free fraction (as measured at trough levels). EE is reported to be highly but nonspecifically bound to serum albumin (approximately 98.5%) and induces an increase in the serum concentrations of both SHBG and CBG. EE induced effects on SHBG and CBG were not affected by variation of the DRSP dosage in the range of 2 to 3 mg.

Metabolism: The 2 main metabolites of DRSP found in human plasma were identified to be the acid form of DRSP generated by opening of the lactone ring and the 4,5-dihydrodrospirenone-3-sulfate. These metabolites were shown not to be pharmacologically active. In in vitro studies with human liver microsomes, DRSP was metabolized only to a minor extent, mainly by cytochrome P450 3A4 (CYP3A4).

EE has been reported to be subject to presystemic conjugation in both small bowel mucosa and the liver. Metabolism occurs primarily by aromatic hydroxylation, but a wide variety of hydroxylated and methylated metabolites are formed. These are present as free metabolites and as conjugates with glucuronide and sulfate. CYP3A4 in the liver are responsible for the 2-hydroxylation which is the major oxidative reaction. The 2-hydroxy metabolite is further transformed by methylation and glucuronidation prior to urinary and fecal excretion.

Excretion: DRSP serum levels are characterized by a terminal disposition phase half-life of approximately 30 hours after both single- and multiple-dose regimens. Excretion of DRSP was nearly complete after 10 days and amounts excreted were slightly higher in feces compared to urine. DRSP was extensively metabolized and only trace amounts of unchanged DRSP were excreted in urine and feces. At least 20 different metabolites were observed in urine and feces. About 38% to 47% of the metabolites in urine were glucuronide and sulfate conjugates. In feces, about 17% to 20% of the metabolites were excreted as glucuronides and sulfates.

For EE, the terminal disposition phase half-life has been reported to be approximately 24 hours. EE is not excreted unchanged. EE is excreted in the urine and feces as glucuronide and sulfate conjugates and undergoes enterohepatic circulation.

Special Populations and Conditions: Pediatrics: The safety and efficacy of YAZ has not been established in women under the age of 14 years. Use of this product before menarche is not indicated.

Geriatrics: YAZ is not indicated for use in postmenopausal women.

Race: No clinically significant difference was observed between the pharmacokinetics of DRSP or EE in Japanese versus Caucasian women (aged 20-35 years) when YAZ was administered daily for 21 days. The effect of race on the disposition of YAZ has not been evaluated.

Hepatic Insufficiency: YAZ is contraindicated in patients with hepatic dysfunction (see also Contraindications and Warnings and Precautions). The mean exposure to DRSP in women with moderate hepatic impairment is approximately 3 times higher than the exposure in women with normal hepatic function. The mean terminal half-life of DRSP for women with moderate hepatic impairment was 1.8 times greater than for women with normal hepatic function. YAZ has not been studied in women with severe hepatic impairment.

Renal Insufficiency: YAZ is contraindicated in patients with renal insufficiency (see also Contraindications and Warnings and Precautions).

The effect of renal insufficiency on the pharmacokinetics of DRSP (3 mg daily for 14 days) and the effect of DRSP on serum potassium levels were investigated in female subjects (n=28, age 30-65) with normal renal function and mild and moderate renal impairment. All subjects were on a low potassium diet. During the study, 7 subjects continued the use of potassium-sparing drugs for the treatment of the underlying illness. On the 14th day (steady-state) of DRSP treatment, the serum DRSP levels in the group with mild renal impairment (creatinine clearance CL_{cr}, 50-80 mL/min) were comparable to those in the group with normal renal function (CL_{cr}, >80 mL/min). The serum DRSP levels were on average 37% higher in the group with moderate renal impairment (CL_{cr}, 30-50 mL/min) compared to those in the group with normal renal function. DRSP treatment was well tolerated by all groups. DRSP treatment did not show any clinically significant effect on serum potassium concentration. Although hyperkalemia was not observed in the study, in 5 of the 7 subjects who continued use of potassium-sparing drugs during the study, mean serum potassium levels increased by up to 0.33 mEq/L. Therefore, potential exists for hyperkalemia to occur in subjects with renal impairment whose serum potassium is in the upper reference range and who are concomitantly using potassium sparing drugs.

STORAGE AND STABILITY: Store in original packaging between 15 and 30°C.

Medicines should not be disposed of via wastewater or household waste. Ask your pharmacist how to dispose of medicines no longer required. These measures will help to protect the environment.

SPECIAL HANDLING INSTRUCTIONS: There are no special handling instructions.

INFORMATION FOR THE PATIENT: Published in e-CPS, available by subscription at www.e-cps.ca.

DOSAGE FORMS, COMPOSITION AND PACKAGING: Each hormone-containing, light pink, film-coated tablet contains: drospirenone 3.0 mg and ethinyl estradiol 0.020 mg stabilized by betadex as a clathrate (molecular inclusion complex). The white tablets are hormone-free. Nonmedicinal ingredients for hormone-containing tablets: β-cyclodextrin, cornstarch, hydroxypropyl methylcellulose, lactose monohydrate, magnesium stearate, red ferric oxide, talc and titanium dioxide. Nonmedicinal ingredients for hormone-free tablets: cornstarch, hydroxypropyl methylcellulose, lactose monohydrate, magnesium stearate, povidone, talc and titanium dioxide. Blister packs contains 24 hormone-containing, light pink and 4 hormone-free white, film-coated, round tablets.

(Shown in Product Identification Section)

Yohimbine-Odan™ Ⓟ

yohimbine HCl

Sympatholytic

Odan

SUPPLIED: 2 mg: Each round, powder blue, uncoated, scored, embossed tablet, engraved "O/2.0" contains: yohimbine HCl 2 mg. Nonmedicinal ingredients: cellulose, FD&C Blue #1, magnesium stearate and sodium starch glycolate. Gluten-, lactose- and tartrazine-free. White plastic bottles of 100 and 500.

5.4 mg: Each oval, pink, uncoated, scored, embossed tablet, engraved "O/5.4" contains: yohimbine HCl 5.4 mg. Nonmedicinal ingredients: cellulose, FD&C Red #3, magnesium stearate and sodium starch glycolate. Gluten-, lactose- and tartrazine-free. White plastic bottles of 100 and 500.

6 mg: Each round, pink, uncoated, scored tablet, engraved "Yohimbine O-6" contains: yohimbine HCl 6 mg. Nonmedicinal ingredients: cellulose, FD&C Red #3, lactose and magnesium stearate. Gluten- and tartrazine-free. White plastic bottles of 100.

Yondelis™ Ⓟ

trabectedin

Antineoplastic Agent

Janssen-Ortho

Date of Preparation: May 13, 2010

SUMMARY PRODUCT INFORMATION:

Route of Administration	Dosage Form/ Strength	Clinically Relevant Nonmedicinal Ingredients
Intravenous Through Central Line	Sterile lyophilized powder for injection/ 1 mg	None For a complete listing see Dosage Forms, Composition and Packaging.

INDICATIONS AND CLINICAL USE: YONDELIS (trabectedin) in combination with CAELYX (pegylated liposomal doxorubicin hydrochloride [PLD]) is indicated for the treatment of patients with platinum-sensitive ovarian cancer for whom one first-line platinum-based chemotherapy regimen, including adjuvant therapy, has failed, and who are not expected to benefit, are ineligible or not willing to receive retreatment with platinum-based chemotherapy.

Approval of YONDELIS in combination with CAELYX is based on progression-free survival (PFS) benefit in patients with relapsed ovarian cancer. A prolongation of overall survival or quality of life benefit has not been demonstrated.

Geriatrics (>65 years of age): No relevant differences in the safety profile or effectiveness were seen in this patient population (see Dosage and Administration, Geriatrics (>65 years of age)). Dose adjustments based uniquely on age criteria are not routinely recommended.

Pediatrics (<18 years of age): The safety and efficacy of YONDELIS in pediatric patients have not been established. Therefore, this medicinal product should not be used in children and adolescents.

CONTRAINDICATIONS:

- Patients who are hypersensitive to YONDELIS (trabectedin) or to any ingredient in the formulation or component of the container. For a complete listing, see Dosage Forms, Composition and Packaging.
- YONDELIS should not be administered to nursing mothers (see Warnings and Precautions, Special Populations).
- YONDELIS should not be administered to patients with an active serious or uncontrolled infection.

WARNINGS AND PRECAUTIONS:

Serious Warnings and Precautions

YONDELIS (trabectedin) should be prescribed by a qualified healthcare professional who is experienced in the use of antineoplastic therapy.

YONDELIS must not be used in patients with elevated bilirubin levels (see Special Populations, Hepatic Impairment).

The following are clinically significant adverse events:

- Hepatotoxicity (see Hepatic/Biliary/Pancreatic).
- Rhabdomyolysis (see Rhabdomyolysis and Severe CPK Elevations (>5×ULN)).
- Febrile Neutropenia and Sepsis (see Hematologic).
- Pulmonary embolism (see Pulmonary Embolism).
- Injection site reactions (see Injection Site Reactions).

Please refer to the Product Monograph for CAELYX for information on its Warnings and Precautions.

General: Caution should be taken if medicinal products associated with hepatotoxicity are administered concomitantly with YONDELIS, since the risk of hepatotoxicity may be increased. The concomitant use of YONDELIS with alcohol must be avoided.

Carcinogenesis and Mutagenesis: Long-term carcinogenicity studies have not been performed. YONDELIS is genotoxic both in vitro and in vivo.

Cardiovascular: Special attention must be given to the risk of myocardial damage from cumulative doses of doxorubicin HCl. Please refer to the Product Monograph for CAELYX for additional information on cardiovascular events.

Clinically significant symptomatic cardiac adverse events, defined as cardiac-related adverse events of Grade 2 or higher, were observed in both treatment arms (3% in the YONDELIS + CAELYX arm and 2% in the CAELYX monotherapy arm). Congestive heart failure events (including left ventricular dysfunction, cardiac failure, cardiac failure congestive and ventricular dysfunction) in the YONDELIS + CAELYX arm were 2% (n=6) and <1% (n=1) in the CAELYX monotherapy arm.

A multigated acquisition (MUGA) scan or 2-D echocardiogram should be performed prior to treatment with YONDELIS in combination with CAELYX, and patients with a left ventricular ejection fraction below the normal limit for the institution should not be treated.

In the pivotal phase 3 trial, 1 case of QTc prolongation was reported in the YONDELIS + CAELYX group (n=333). A QT/QTc prolongation study has been completed but results are not yet available.

Pulmonary Embolism: There were 17 (5%) and 8 (2%) cases of pulmonary embolism reported in the YONDELIS + CAELYX arm and in the CAELYX monotherapy arm, respectively.

Gastrointestinal: Grade 3 or 4 vomiting and nausea were reported commonly. All patients must be premedicated with corticosteroids, such as dexamethasone, to protect the liver and as antiemetic medication. Additional anti-emetics may be administered as needed (see Dosage and Administration, Recommended Dose and Dosage Adjustment).

Hematologic: Grade 3 or 4 neutropenia has been very commonly reported and associated with YONDELIS combination therapy with CAELYX. Neutropenia was associated with complications such as febrile neutropenia, sepsis and infections, some of which were fatal. Neutrophil nadirs occurred at a median of 15 days and recovered within a week. Twenty-seven subjects (8%) and 7 subjects (2%) had febrile neutropenia in the YONDELIS + CAELYX combination arm and the CAELYX monotherapy arm, respectively. Three (1.2%) subjects in the combination arm had deaths associated with neutropenia (neutropenic sepsis, sepsis and febrile neutropenia) and one subject in the CAELYX monotherapy arm died due to sepsis. Colony-stimulating growth factors have been used to manage neutropenia. One hundred and forty (42%) of subjects in the combination arm and 57 subjects (17%) in the CAELYX monotherapy arm were treated with colony-stimulation growth factors.

Grades 3 or 4 thrombocytopenia associated with YONDELIS therapy have been very commonly reported. In the pivotal study, Grade 3 or 4 abnormalities in platelet counts were observed for 77 subjects (23%) in the YONDELIS + CAELYX combination arm and 14 subjects (4%) in the CAELYX monotherapy arm. Bleeding-related adverse events were reported in a similar percent of subjects in the YONDELIS + CAELYX (9%) and CAELYX (8%) arms.

A full blood cell count including differential and platelet count must be performed at baseline, weekly for the first two cycles and then once between cycles (see Dosage and Administration, Recommended Dose and Dosage Adjustment). YONDELIS should not be administered to patients with baseline neutrophil counts of less than 1500 cells/mm³ and platelets count of less than 100 000 cells/mm³. If severe neutropenia (ANC<500 cells/mm³) lasting more than 5 days or associated with fever or infection occur, dose reduction is recommended (see Dosage and Administration, Dose Adjustments During Treatment).

Hepatic/Biliary/Pancreatic: Reversible acute increases in alanine aminotransferase (ALT) and aspartate aminotransferase (AST) have been reported in patients treated with YONDELIS in combination with CAELYX. Grade 3/4 transaminase elevations occurred in ≤51% of patients, grade 4 occurred in <5%. The median time to the occurrence of ALT or AST increase to grade 3/4 was 8 days. Elevated levels decreased to below grade 3/4 in about 8 days. Transaminase elevations were non-cumulative and decreased in magnitude and incidence with each subsequent cycle. YONDELIS must not be used in patients with elevated bilirubin at the time of initiation of cycle. Patients with increases in AST, ALT and alkaline phosphatase between cycles may necessitate a dose reduction (see Dosage and Administration, Dose Adjustments During Treatment).

Monitoring of alkaline phosphatase, bilirubin, and aminotransferases (AST and ALT) should occur prior to each cycle of therapy, weekly during the first two cycles of therapy, and at least once between treatments in subsequent cycles (see Monitoring and Laboratory Tests).

Injection Site Reactions: Administration through a central venous line is required (see Dosage and Administration, Dosing Considerations). Patients may develop a potentially severe injection site reaction when YONDELIS is administered through a peripheral venous line.

There have been few reported cases of YONDELIS extravasation, with subsequent tissue necrosis requiring debridement. There is no specific antidote for extravasation of YONDELIS. Extravasation should be managed by local standard practice.

The percentage of catheter related ADRs were 14% vs. 3% in the YONDELIS in combination with CAELYX arm vs. CAELYX arm alone, respectively.

Rhabdomyolysis and Severe CPK Elevations (>5×ULN): YONDELIS must not be used in patients with CPK >2.5 ULN (see Dosage and Administration, Recommended Dose and Dosage Adjustment). Rhabdomyolysis has been uncommonly reported, usually in association with myelotoxicity, severe liver function test abnormalities or renal failure. Severe CPK elevations were observed in 2% of patients treated with YONDELIS in combination with CAELYX. Therefore, CPK should be closely monitored routinely during therapy and especially whenever a patient may be experiencing any of these toxicities or muscle weakness or muscle pain. CPK should be monitored weekly during the first two cycles of therapy and at least once between treatment and subsequent cycles. If rhabdomyolysis occurs, supportive measures such as parenteral hydration, urine alkalinisation and dialysis should be promptly established, as indicated. Treatment with YONDELIS should be discontinued until the patient fully recovers.

Caution should be taken if medicinal products associated with rhabdomyolysis (e.g., statins) are administered concomitantly with YONDELIS, since the risk of rhabdomyolysis may be increased.

Renal: Creatinine clearance must be monitored prior to and during treatment. YONDELIS must not be used in patients treated in combination with CAELYX with creatinine clearance <60 mL/min (see Dosage and Administration, Recommended Dose and Dosage Adjustment).

Special Populations: Pregnant Women: No sufficient clinical data on exposed pregnancies are available. However, based on its known mechanism of action, YONDELIS may cause serious birth defects when administered during pregnancy. YONDELIS should not be used during pregnancy unless clearly necessary. If it is used during pregnancy, the patient must be informed of the potential risk to the fetus and be monitored carefully. If YONDELIS is used at the end of pregnancy, potential adverse reactions should be monitored carefully in the newborns.

Reproduction: Women of childbearing potential must use effective contraception during treatment and 3 months thereafter, and immediately inform the treating physician if a pregnancy occurs.

YONDELIS can have genotoxic effects. If pregnancy occurs during treatment genetic counselling should be considered. Genetic counselling is also recommended for patients wishing to have children after therapy.

Nursing Women: It is not known whether YONDELIS is excreted in human milk. The excretion of YONDELIS in milk has not been studied in animals. Breast-feeding is contraindicated during treatment and 3 months thereafter (see Contraindications).

Geriatrics (>65 years of age): Of the 1132 patients from single agent clinical trials from an integrated safety analysis in several tumour types, 19% were over 65 years. No relevant differences in the safety profile or effectiveness were seen in this patient population. Of the 672 patients with ovarian cancer who received YONDELIS in combination with CAELYX, 24% were 65 years of age or older and 6% were over 75 years. No difference in safety was observed in this patient population. In this study, a multivariate analysis of progression-free survival, age over 65 years did not affect the outcome. Results from population pharmacokinetic analyses indicate that the plasma clearance and distribution volume of YONDELIS are not influenced by age. Therefore, dose adjustments based uniquely on age criteria are not routinely recommended.

Pediatrics (<18 years of age): The safety and efficacy of YONDELIS in pediatric patients have not yet been established. Therefore, YONDELIS should not be used in children and adolescents.

Renal Impairment: Studies including patients with renal insufficiency (creatinine clearance <60 mL/min) have not been conducted in patients with ovarian cancer treated with YONDELIS in combination with CAELYX and therefore YONDELIS must not be used in this patient population (see Dosage and Administration). The pharmacokinetics of YONDELIS are not expected to be impacted by mild or moderate renal impairment (see Action and Clinical Pharmacology, Renal Insufficiency).

Hepatic Impairment: Patients with elevated bilirubin at the time of initiation of cycle must not be treated with YONDELIS.

Patients must meet specific criteria on hepatic function parameters to start treatment with YONDELIS:

- Bilirubin ≤ upper limit of normal (ULN)
- Alkaline phosphatase of non-osseous origin ≤2.5×ULN (consider hepatic isoenzymes 5 nucleotidase or GGT, to distinguish if the elevation could be osseous in origin)
- Albumin ≥25 g/L
- Alanine aminotransferase (ALT) and aspartate aminotransferase (AST) ≤2.5×ULN

The use of YONDELIS in patients with impaired hepatic function has not been adequately studied. Since systemic exposure to YONDELIS may be increased due to hepatic impairment and therefore the risk of hepatotoxicity might be increased, the use of YONDELIS in patients with clinically relevant liver diseases, such as active chronic hepatitis, is not recommended (see Dosage and Administration, Recommended Dose and Dosage Adjustment).

Monitoring and Laboratory Tests: Prior to each treatment cycle, patients must fulfill the following baseline criteria:

- Absolute neutrophil count (ANC) ≥1500/mm³
- Platelets count ≥100 000/mm³
- Hemoglobin ≥9 g/dL
- Bilirubin ≤ ULN
- Alkaline phosphatase of non-osseous origin ≤2.5×ULN
- Aminotransferases (AST and ALT) ≤2.5×ULN
- Albumin ≥25 g/L
- Serum creatinine ≤1.5 mg/dL (≤132.6 μmol/L) or creatinine clearance ≥60 mL/min
- CPK ≤2.5×ULN

Monitoring of hematological (a full blood count including differential and platelet count) and biochemical parameters (alkaline phosphatase, bilirubin, CPK, and aminotransferases [AST and ALT]) should occur at baseline and weekly during the first two cycles of therapy, and at least once between treatments in subsequent cycles. If any of the following events occur at any time between cycles, the YONDELIS and CAELYX dose must be reduced (see Dosage and Administration):

- ANC <500/mm³ lasting for more than 5 days or associated with fever or infection
- Platelets count <25 000/mm³
- Increase of bilirubin >ULN
- Alkaline phosphatase of non-osseous origin >2.5×ULN
- Increase of aminotransferases (AST or ALT) >5×ULN, which has not recovered by day 21; any other grade 3 or 4 adverse reactions (such as nausea, vomiting, fatigue)

ADVERSE REACTIONS: Adverse Drug Reaction Overview: Adverse drug reactions (ADRs) are adverse events that are considered to be reasonably associated with the use of YONDELIS (trabectedin) based on a comprehensive assessment of available adverse event information.

YONDELIS in Combination with CAELYX in Advanced Ovarian Cancer: The most common ADRs, reported in ≥20% of patients treated with YONDELIS in combination with CAELYX were neutropenia, leukopenia, anemia, thrombocytopenia, nausea, vomiting, diarrhea, hand-foot syndrome, fatigue, alanine aminotransferase increased, aspartate aminotransferase increased, blood alkaline phosphatase increased, constipation, abdominal pain and stomatitis.

In the pivotal study, ADRs leading to dose adjustment and cycle delays occurred in 43% and 65% of patients in the YONDELIS + CAELYX combination arm, and in 35% and 37% of patients in the CAELYX monotherapy arm, respectively. ADRs that led to treatment termination occurred in 17% of subjects in the YONDELIS + CAELYX combination arm and 9% of subjects in the CAELYX monotherapy arm. The most common adverse drug reaction, reported ≥5% leading to drug discontinuation, was neutropenia.

Clinical Trial Adverse Drug Reactions: The following safety profile of YONDELIS in combination with CAELYX is based on the evaluation of a phase 3 clinical trial OVA 301 of 663 patients with advanced relapsed ovarian cancer who received either CAELYX (30 mg/m²) followed by YONDELIS (1.1 mg/m²) every 3 weeks or CAELYX alone (50 mg/m²) every 4 weeks. The combination of YONDELIS with CAELYX was given to 333 patients in this trial. In the combination arm, the median number of cycles given was 6.0 cycles (range: 1 to 21) for a median of 19 weeks. In the CAELYX only arm, the median number of cycles given was 5.0 cycles (range: 1 to 22) for a median of 20 weeks. Most ADRs were managed with dose reductions or delays.

Adverse reactions reported among patients treated with YONDELIS in combination with CAELYX during clinical studies that occurred at a rate ≥1% are shown in Table 1.

Table 1: YONDELIS

Adverse Drug Reactions in ≥1% of Patients with Ovarian Cancer Treated with YONDELIS in Combination with CAELYX

Adverse Drug Reaction System Organ Class Preferred Term	YONDELIS + CAELYX (n=333) %			CAELYX (n=330) %		
	Any (%)	Grade 3	Grade 4	Any (%)	Grade 3	Grade 4
Infections and Infestations						
Neutropenic infection	1	1	0	0	0	0
Neutropenic sepsis	1	<1	<1	0	0	0
Blood and Lymphatic System Disorders						
Neutropenia	77	29	34	38	14	8
Leukopenia	48	25	8	26	7	3
Anemia	48	10	3	25	5	1
Thrombocytopenia	36	10	8	8	2	1
Febrile neutropenia	8	6	2	2	2	<1
Pancytopenia	2	2	1	0	0	0
Bone marrow failure	2	<1	1	<1	<1	0
Granulocytopenia	2	1	<1	0	0	0
Metabolism and Nutrition Disorders						
Dehydration	5	2	1	5	2	0
Hypokalemia	11	4	<1	8	1	0
Anorexia	32	2	0	26	3	<1
Psychiatric Disorders						
Insomnia	10	0	0	5	0	0
Nervous System Disorders						
Headache	16	1	0	8	<1	0
Peripheral sensory neuropathy	5	0	0	3	0	0
Dysgeusia	5	<1	0	3	0	0
Syncope	2	2	0	<1	0	0
Cardiac Disorders						
Palpitations	4	<1	0	0	0	0
Left ventricular dysfunction[a]	1	<1	0	0	0	0
Respiratory, Thoracic and Mediastinal Disorders						
Dyspnea	15	3	<1	10	2	<1
Cough	12	0	0	12	0	0
Pulmonary embolism	5	1	2	2	1	1
Pulmonary edema	1	0	0	0	0	0
Gastrointestinal Disorders						
Nausea	74	10	0	42	4	0
Vomiting	56	12	<1	30	4	0
Constipation	32	2	0	28	2	0
Diarrhea	26	2	0	19	2	0
Abdominal Pain	20	1	0	33	5	<1
Stomatitis	20	1	0	33	5	<1
Dyspepsia	13	<1	0	11	1	0
Hepatobiliary Disorders						
Hyperbilirubinemia	16	1	0	7	1	0
Hepatotoxicity	2	1	0	<1	0	0
Skin and Subcutaneous Tissue Disorders						

(cont'd)

Table 1: YONDELIS *(cont'd)*

Adverse Drug Reactions in ≥1% of Patients with Ovarian Cancer Treated with YONDELIS in Combination with CAELYX

Adverse Drug Reaction System Organ Class Preferred Term	YONDELIS + CAELYX (n=333) %			CAELYX (n=330) %		
	Any (%)	Grade 3	Grade 4	Any (%)	Grade 3	Grade 4
Hand-foot syndrome[b]	24	4	0	54	18	1
Skin hyperpigmentation	6	0	0	3	0	0
Alopecia	12	0	0	14	<1	0
Rash	11	0	0	17	1	0
Musculoskeletal, Connective Tissue, and Bone Disorders						
Musculoskeletal pain	4	<1	0	3	<1	0
Myalgia	5	<1	0	3	0	0
Renal and Urinary Disorders						
Renal failure acute	2	1	<1	1	1	0
General Disorders and Administration Site Conditions						
Pyrexia	20	1	0	13	1	0
Fatigue	46	8	<1	36	5	<1
Asthenia	17	2	0	12	2	0
Mucosal inflammation	12	2	0	19	6	0
Edema peripheral	9	1	0	8	0	<1
Edema	3	<1	0	1	0	0
Catheter site pain	3	0	0	0	0	0
Catheter site erythema	2	0	0	0	0	0
Catheter site inflammation	2	0	0	1	0	0

[a] All patients reporting left ventricular dysfunction, after discontinuation of study therapy improved.
[b] For patients who experience hand-foot syndrome, the CAELYX dose should be modified as described in the CAELYX Product Monograph.

Hepatotoxicity: Administration of YONDELIS + CAELYX commonly results in reversible liver transaminase elevations. Dexamethasone pre-medication appeared to decrease the frequency and severity of transaminase elevations. In Study OVA-301, 3 (0.9%) subjects fulfilled Hy's Law criteria for predicting severe liver toxicity, but none of these 3 subjects developed severe liver toxicity. This finding was similar to the experience with 19 YONDELIS single agent Phase 2 studies (14 cases (1.2%) met the definition of Hy's Law but none of these cases developed severe liver toxicity).
Pulmonary Embolism: There were 17 (5%) and 8 (2%) cases of pulmonary embolism reported in the YONDELIS + CAELYX arm and in the CAELYX monotherapy arm, respectively.
Febrile Neutropenia: Twenty-seven subjects (8%) had febrile neutropenia in the combination arm and 7 subjects (2%) in CAELYX monotherapy arm. Three (1.2%) subjects in the combination arm had deaths associated with neutropenia (neutropenic sepsis, sepsis and febrile neutropenia) and one subject in the CAELYX monotherapy arm died due to sepsis.
Congestive Heart Failure: Congestive heart failure events (including left ventricular dysfunction, cardiac failure, cardiac failure congestive and ventricular dysfunction) were 2% (n=6) in the YONDELIS + CAELYX arm and <1% (n=1) in the CAELYX monotherapy arm.
Less Common Clinical Trial Adverse Drug Reactions (<1%): Rhabdomyolysis: Rhabdomyolysis has been uncommonly reported and severe CPK elevations were observed in 2% of patients treated with YONDELIS in combination with CAELYX, usually in association with myelotoxicity, severe liver function test abnormalities or renal failure.
Additional Data from Clinical Trials: In a phase 2 single agent study with YONDELIS in 59 subjects with ovarian cancer, reported adverse events with the frequency greater than 10% included arthralgia (12%), phlebitis (15%) and weight increase (20%). In the pivotal study (Study OVA-301), the incidence of arthralgia, phlebitis, and weight increase was 6%, 2%, and 1%, respectively in the combination arm. In a second phase 2 single agent ovarian cancer study in 107 subjects, hypophosphatemia and parasthesia were reported in 34% and 11% of subjects, respectively. In the pivotal phase 3 study, the incidence of hypophosphatemia and paresthesia was 1% and 3%, respectively in the combination arm.
Abnormal Hematologic and Clinical Chemistry Findings: See Table 2.

Table 2: YONDELIS

Abnormal Hematologic and Clinical Chemistry Findings (Laboratory Values)

Lab Type Lab Test Name	YONDELIS/CAELYX (N=333) (%)			CAELYX (N=330) (%)		
	Any	Grade 3	Grade 4	Any	Grade 3	Grade 4
Hematology						
Hemoglobin	95	13	6	82	6	2
Neutrophils	92	30	42	74	20	10
Platelets	64	12	11	27	2	2
WBC	95	45	18	82	16	4
Chemistry						
Alkaline phosphatase	61	2	0	42	1	0
ALT	96	46	5	36	2	0
AST	89	12	2	43	1	<1

(cont'd)

Table 2: YONDELIS *(cont'd)*

Abnormal Hematologic and Clinical Chemistry Findings (Laboratory Values)

Lab Type Lab Test Name	YONDELIS/CAELYX (N=333) (%)			CAELYX (N=330) (%)		
	Any	Grade 3	Grade 4	Any	Grade 3	Grade 4
Bilirubin	25	<1	0	13	<1	0
Creatine kinase	22	1	1	14	0	0
Creatinine	28	<1	<1	25	1	0
Potassium (low)	42	8	1	28	3	1

DRUG INTERACTIONS: Drug-Drug Interactions: Effects of Other Substances on YONDELIS: A population analysis based on sparse-sampling data from a Phase 3 study demonstrated that the plasma clearance of trabectedin was decreased by approximately 31% in 86 patients who were co-administered CAELYX 30 mg/m² compared to 745 patients enrolled in 14 studies who received trabectedin alone. Data from a separate Phase I study, in which full pharmacokinetic profiles for trabectedin were obtained for 16 patients who received trabectedin 0.9 to 1.3 mg/m² in combination with CAELYX 30 mg/m², indicated a comparable (i.e., a mean difference of 16%) plasma clearance of trabectedin as for the same doses of trabectedin given as a single agent. Results of both analyses are provided to show the degree of change in the clearance values of trabectedin that may be observed upon co-administration of this drug with pegylated liposomal doxorubicin.

Since trabectedin is metabolized mainly by CYP3A4, the concentrations of trabectedin in plasma are likely to be increased in patients who are co-administered drugs that potently inhibit the activity of this isoenzyme (e.g. oral ketoconazole, fluconazole, ritonavir, clarithromycin or aprepitant). Co-administration of YONDELIS with potent inhibitors of CYP3A4 is not recommended.

Results from the population pharmacokinetic analyses (n=831 subjects) indicated that the plasma clearance of trabectedin was 19% higher in patients who received any concomitant dexamethasone administration relative to those who did not. The co-administration with potent inducers of CYP3A4 (e.g., rifampicin, phenobarbital, St. John's Wort) may also further increase the metabolic clearance of trabectedin.

Preclinical data have demonstrated that trabectedin is a substrate of P-glycoprotein (P-gp). Concomitant administration of inhibitors of P-gp, e.g. cyclosporine and verapamil, may alter trabectedin distribution or elimination. The clinical relevance of this interaction, e.g. for CNS toxicity, has not been established and caution should be exercised when concomitantly administering YONDELIS with inhibitors of P-gp.

Trabectedin is highly bound to human plasma protein. In vitro, plasma protein binding of trabectedin was not affected by 14 prototypical drugs (valproic acid, ceftazidime, cloxacillin, erythromycin, warfarin, diazepam, tamoxifen, digitoxin, ondansetron, paracetamol, diclofenac, acetylsalicylic acid, propranolol) that bind to albumin and α1-acid glycoprotein and a slight (28%) increase in the free concentration of trabectedin only occurred with the highest tested concentrations of phenytoin (400 μM).
Impact of YONDELIS on Co-Administered Drugs: In vitro, trabectedin does not induce or inhibit major cytochrome P450 enzymes.

A population analysis based on sparse-sampling data from a Phase 3 study demonstrated that the plasma pharmacokinetics of PLD 30 mg/m² are similar when co-administered with trabectedin 1.1 mg/m² (86 patients) and when given alone (80 patients).
Drug-Lifestyle Interactions: No studies on the effects of the ability to drive and to use machines have been performed. However, fatigue or asthenia has been reported in patients receiving YONDELIS. Patients who experience any of these events during therapy must not drive or operate machines.

The concomitant use of YONDELIS with alcohol must be avoided due to hepatotoxicity of the medicinal product.

DOSAGE AND ADMINISTRATION: Dosing Considerations: Treatment must be administered under the supervision of a physician experienced in the use of antineoplastic agents. Its use should be confined to personnel specialized in the administration of cytotoxic agents.

Administration through a central venous line is required.
Recommended Dose and Dosage Adjustment: YONDELIS (trabectedin) is used in combination with CAELYX (PLD) every three weeks. YONDELIS is administered at a dose of 1.1 mg/m² as a 3 hour intravenous infusion after CAELYX 30 mg/m², as a 90 minute intravenous infusion.

For CAELYX dosage administration instructions, see CAELYX Product Monograph.

All patients must be premedicated with corticosteroids such as dexamethasone 20 mg IV, 30 minutes before each YONDELIS infusion; not only as anti-emetic prophylaxis, but also because it appears to provide hepatoprotective effects. Additional anti-emetics may be administered as needed.

The following criteria are required to allow treatment with YONDELIS:

- Absolute neutrophil count (ANC) ≥1500/mm³
- Platelet count ≥100 000/mm³
- Hemoglobin ≥9 g/dL
- Bilirubin ≤ upper limit of normal (ULN)
- Alkaline phosphatase of non-osseous origin ≤2.5×ULN (consider hepatic isoenzymes 5 nucleotidase or GGT, to distinguish if the elevation could be osseous in origin)
- Albumin ≥25 g/L
- Alanine aminotransferase (ALT) and Aspartate aminotransferase (AST) ≤2.5×ULN
- Serum creatinine ≤1.5 mg/dL (≤132.6 μmol/L) or creatinine clearance ≥60 mL/min
- Creatine phosphokinase (CPK) ≤2.5 ULN

The same criteria as above (except if CPK >2.5×ULN) must be met prior to initiation of next cycles. Otherwise treatment must be delayed for up to 3 weeks until the criteria are met. If these toxicities persist beyond 3 weeks, treatment discontinuation should be considered.

The same dose should be given for all cycles provided that no grade 3-4 toxicities are seen and the patient fulfils the re-treatment criteria.
Dose Adjustments During Treatment: Prior to re-treatment, patients must fulfill the baseline criteria defined above. If any of the following events occur at any time between cycles, the YONDELIS and CAELYX dose must be reduced one level, according to Table 3, for subsequent cycles:

- ANC <500/mm³ lasting for more than 5 days or associated with fever or infection
- Platelets count <25 000/mm³
- Increase of bilirubin > ULN
- Alkaline phosphatase of non-osseous origin >2.5×ULN
- Increase of aminotransferases (AST or ALT) >5×ULN, which has not recovered by day 21; any other grade 3 or 4 adverse reactions (such as nausea, vomiting, fatigue)

Once a dose has been reduced because of toxicity, dose escalation in the subsequent cycles is not recommended. If any of these toxicities reappear in subsequent cycles in a patient exhibiting clinical benefit, the YONDELIS and CAELYX dose may be further reduced as per Table 3 when YONDELIS is used in combination therapy with CAELYX. In the event that further dose reductions are necessary, treatment discontinuation should be considered.

For additional CAELYX dosage adjustments, see the CAELYX Product Monograph.
Duration of Treatment: In clinical trials, there were no pre-defined limits to the number of cycles administered. Treatment continued whilst clinical benefit was noted. YONDELIS has been administered for 6 or more cycles in 52% of patients treated with combination dose and schedule. Combination regimen has been used for up to 21 cycles. No cumulative toxicities have been observed in patients treated with multiple cycles.
Patients with Impaired Hepatic Function: Patients with elevated bilirubin at the time of initiation of cycle must not be treated with YONDELIS.

Patients with hepatic impairment may be at increased risk for toxicity since systemic exposure may be increased. Recommendations for a starting dose in these patients cannot be made because the use of YONDELIS in patients with impaired hepatic function has not been adequately studied. Use of YONDELIS is not recommended in this patient population. Patients must meet specific criteria on hepatic function parameters to start treatment with YONDELIS (see Warnings and Precautions, Special Populations).

Table 3: YONDELIS

Dose Modification Table for YONDELIS in Combination with CAELYX for Ovarian Cancer and CAELYX

	YONDELIS	CAELYX
Starting dose	1.1 mg/m²	30 mg/m²
First reduction	0.9 mg/m²	25 mg/m²
Second reduction	0.75 mg/m²	20 mg/m²

Patients with Impaired Renal Function: Studies including patients with renal insufficiency (creatinine clearance <60 mL/min in combination therapy for ovarian cancer) have not been conducted and therefore YONDELIS must not be used in this patient population (see Warnings and Precautions, Special Populations).

Pediatrics (<18 years of age) : The safety and efficacy of YONDELIS in pediatric patients have not yet been established. Therefore, YONDELIS should not be used in children and adolescents (see Warnings and Precautions, Special Populations).

Geriatrics (>65 years of age): Dose adjustments based uniquely on age criteria are not routinely recommended (see Warnings and Precautions, Special Populations).

Administration: YONDELIS reconstitution and dilution of the reconstituted solution must be conducted under aseptic conditions in a manner consistent with recommended safe procedures for handling cytotoxic compounds. Each vial containing 1 mg of YONDELIS is reconstituted with 20 mL of sterile water for injections. The solution obtained has a concentration of 0.05 mg/mL and is for single use only.

Reconstitution: A syringe is used to inject 20 mL of sterile water for injections into the 1 mg vial. Shake the vial until complete dissolution. The reconstituted solution results in a clear, colourless to brownish yellow solution, essentially free of visible particles.

This reconstituted solution contains 0.05 mg/mL of YONDELIS. It requires further dilution and is for single-use only.

Strength	Vial Size	Volume of Diluent to be Added to Vial	Nominal Concentration per mL
1.0 mg	25 mL	20 mL sterile water for injection	0.05 mg/mL

Instructions for dilution: The reconstituted solution should be diluted with sodium chloride 9 mg/mL (0.9%) solution for infusion or glucose 50 mg/mL (5%) solution for infusion. The required volume should be calculated as follows:

$$\text{Volume (mL)} = \frac{\text{BSA (m}^2\text{) x individual dose (mg/m}^2\text{)}}{0.05\ \text{mg/mL}}$$

BSA = Body Surface Area

The appropriate amount of solution should be withdrawn from the vial and added to an infusion bag containing 500 mL of normal saline 0.9% solution for infusion or dextrose 5% solution for infusion if administration is to be made through a central venous line.

After administration of the CAELYX infusion, the intravenous line should be flushed well with 5% dextrose in water (D_5W) before administration of YONDELIS. CAELYX must not be mixed with saline.

YONDELIS must not be mixed or diluted with medicinal products except those mentioned above.

Parenteral drug products should be inspected visually for particulate matter and discoloration prior to administration, whenever solution and container permit. After reconstitution and dilution, chemical and physical stability has been demonstrated for 30 hours up to 25°C. The reconstituted solution should be diluted and used immediately. The total elapsed time between initial reconstitution and end of treatment should not be longer than 30 hours.

OVERDOSAGE:

There is limited data on the effects of YONDELIS overdose. The major anticipated toxicities are gastrointestinal, bone marrow suppression and hepatic toxicity. There is no specific antidote for YONDELIS currently available. In the event of an overdose, patients should be closely monitored and symptomatic supportive care measures instituted as required.

> For management of a suspected drug overdose, contact your regional Poison Control Centre. See the *CPS* Directory section for a list of Poison Control Centres.

ACTION AND CLINICAL PHARMACOLOGY: Mechanism of Action: Trabectedin binds to the minor groove of DNA, bending the helix to the major groove. This binding to DNA triggers a cascade of events affecting several transcription factors, DNA binding proteins, and DNA repair pathways, resulting in perturbation of the cell cycle.

Pharmacodynamics: Trabectedin has been shown to exert antiproliferative in vitro and in vivo activity against a range of human tumour cell lines and experimental tumours, including malignancies such as sarcoma, breast, non-small cell lung, ovarian and melanoma.

In vitro and in vivo xenograft models have shown additive or synergistic effects when trabectedin was combined with doxorubicin in several cell lines but the combination study with ovarian cells has not been carried out.

Pharmacokinetics: Systemic exposure after intravenous administration as a constant rate intravenous infusion is dose proportional at doses up to and including 1.8 mg/m². The pharmacokinetic profile of trabectedin is consistent with a multiple compartment disposition model, including a terminal half-life in plasma of 175 hours. The concentrations of trabectedin in plasma do not accumulate when administered every 3 weeks.

Distribution: Trabectedin has a large volume of distribution (greater than 5000 L), consistent with extensive distribution into peripheral tissues.

Trabectedin is highly bound to plasma proteins. The mean free (unbound) fraction in plasma is 2.23% and 2.72% at a total plasma concentration of 10 ng/mL and 100 ng/mL, respectively.

Metabolism: Trabectedin is extensively metabolized. Cytochrome P450 3A4 is the major cytochrome P450 isozyme responsible for the oxidative metabolism of trabectedin at clinically relevant concentrations. The contribution of other P450 enzymes to the metabolism of trabectedin cannot be ruled-out. No appreciable glucuronidation of trabectedin has been observed.

Excretion: The mean (SD) recovery of total radioactivity was 58% (17%), and 5.8% (1.73%) in the feces (24 days) and urine (10 days), respectively, after a dose of radio-labelled trabectedin was administered to 8 cancer patients. Negligible quantities (<1% of the dose) of unchanged drug are excreted in the feces and in urine. The clearance of trabectedin in whole blood is approximately 35 L/h. This value is approximately one-half the rate of human hepatic blood flow. Thus the trabectedin extraction ratio can be considered moderate. The inter-patient variability of the population estimate for plasma clearance of trabectedin was 49% and intra-patient variability was 28%.

Special Populations and Conditions: A population pharmacokinetic analysis indicated that the plasma clearance of trabectedin is not influenced by total body weight (range: 36 to 148 kg), body surface area (range: 0.9 to 2.8 m²), age (range: 19 to 83 years), or gender.

Race: The effects of race and ethnicity on trabectedin pharmacokinetics have not been studied.

Hepatic Insufficiency: The clearance of trabectedin may be decreased in patients with hepatic impairment resulting in higher concentrations of trabectedin in plasma. The effect of hepatic impairment on the pharmacokinetics of trabectedin has not been sufficiently studied and the use of YONDELIS is not recommended in this patient population. Patients with elevated bilirubin levels must not be treated with YONDELIS.

Renal Insufficiency: There is no relevant influence of renal function measured by creatinine clearance on trabectedin pharmacokinetics within the range of values (≥30.3 mL/min) present in the patients included in the clinical studies. No data are available in patients with a creatinine clearance of less than 30.3 mL/min. The low recovery (<9% in all studied patients) of total radioactivity in the urine after a single dose of ^{14}C-labelled trabectedin suggests that renal impairment would have little influence on the elimination of trabectedin or its metabolites.

STORAGE AND STABILITY: Store unopened vials in a refrigerator (2-8°C).

After reconstitution, chemical and physical stability has been demonstrated for 30 hours up to 25°C.

From a microbiological point of view, the reconstituted solution should be diluted and used immediately. If not diluted and used immediately, in-use storage times and conditions prior to use of the reconstituted product are the responsibility of the user and would normally not be longer than 24 hours at 2 to 8°C, unless reconstitution has taken place in controlled and validated aseptic conditions.

After dilution, chemical and physical stability has been demonstrated for 30 hours up to 25°C. The total hold time between initial reconstitution and end of treatment should not be longer than 30 hours.

SPECIAL HANDLING INSTRUCTIONS: YONDELIS (trabectedin) is a cytotoxic anticancer medicinal product and, as with other potentially toxic compounds, caution should be exercised during handling. Procedures for proper handling and disposal of cytotoxic medicinal products must be followed. YONDELIS should be handled and disposed of in a manner consistent with other anticancer drugs. Accidental contact with the skin, eyes or mucous membranes must be treated immediately with copious amounts of water.

Any unused product or waste material should be disposed of in accordance with local requirements for cytotoxic medicinal products.

No incompatibilities have been observed between YONDELIS and polyvinylchloride (PVC) and polyethylene (PE) bags and tubing, and titanium implantable vascular access systems.

INFORMATION FOR THE PATIENT: Published in e-CPS, available by subscription at www.e-cps.ca.

DOSAGE FORMS, COMPOSITION AND PACKAGING: Each vial of sterile lyophilized white to off white powder contains: trabectedin 1 mg. Nonmedicinal ingredients: phosphoric acid, potassium dihydrogen phosphate, potassium hydroxide and sucrose. Individually cartoned vials of 25 mL.

Z

Zaditor® ℞
ketotifen fumarate
Anti-allergy Agent

Novartis Pharmaceuticals

Date of Revision: March 30, 2009

SUMMARY PRODUCT INFORMATION:

Route of Administration	Dosage Form/ Strength	Clinically Relevant Nonmedicinal Ingredients
Topical (instillation)	Ophthalmic Solution 0.025% as ketotifen	Preservative benzalkonium chloride 0.01% For a complete listing see Dosage Forms, Composition and Packaging.

INDICATIONS AND CLINICAL USE: ZADITOR (ketotifen fumarate ophthalmic solution) is indicated for:
- treatment of allergic conjunctivitis.

CONTRAINDICATIONS:
- Patients who are hypersensitive to this drug or to any ingredient in the formulation or component of the container. For a complete listing, see Dosage Forms, Composition and Packaging.

WARNINGS AND PRECAUTIONS: General: For topical use only. Not for injection or oral use.

As with all ophthalmic preparations containing benzalkonium chloride, patients are advised not to instill ZADITOR (ketotifen fumarate ophthalmic solution) while wearing soft (hydrophilic) contact lenses. Wearers of soft contact lenses should be instructed to remove lenses prior to instillation of drops and to wait at least ten minutes after instilling ZADITOR before they insert their contact lenses.

To prevent contaminating the dropper tip and solution, care should be taken not to touch the eyelids or surrounding areas with the dropper tip of the bottle. Keep the bottle tightly closed when not in use.

Special Populations: Pregnant Women: There are no clinical trials on the use of ZADITOR (ketotifen fumarate ophthalmic solution) in pregnant or nursing women, therefore, ZADITOR should not be used during pregnancy, except if the benefit justifies the potential risk to the foetus.

Pediatrics (>3 years of age): ZADITOR is indicated for use in pediatric patients over the age of 3 years.

ADVERSE REACTIONS: Adverse Drug Reaction Overview: In controlled clinical studies with ZADITOR (ketotifen fumarate ophthalmic solution), conjunctival injection was the most common ocular adverse reaction related to therapy, with a reported incidence of 7.0%. Headache was the most common non-ocular adverse reaction related to therapy, with a reported incidence of 1.5%. The occurrence of these side effects were generally mild and did not result in discontinuation or interruption of trial medication.

The following ocular adverse reactions related to therapy were reported at an incidence of less than 3%.

Itching, dry eyes, burning or stinging, eyelid disorder and discharge.

DRUG INTERACTIONS: Overview: If ZADITOR (ketotifen fumarate ophthalmic solution) is used concomitantly with other eye medications, patients should be advised to wait at least 5 minutes between the medications.

DOSAGE AND ADMINISTRATION: Recommended Dose and Dosage Adjustment: The recommended dose is one drop in the affected eye(s) every 8 to 12 hours.

OVERDOSAGE:
Oral ingestion of the contents of a 5 mL bottle would be equivalent to 1.25 mg of ketotifen fumarate. Clinical results have shown no serious signs or symptoms after the ingestion of up to 20 mg of ketotifen fumarate.

> For management of a suspected drug overdose, CPhA recommends that you contact your **regional Poison Control Centre**. See the *CPS* Directory section for a list of Poison Control Centres.

ACTION AND CLINICAL PHARMACOLOGY: Mechanism of Action: Ketotifen is a fast acting non-competitive histamine antagonist (H1-receptor). In addition, ketotifen inhibits the release of mediators from mast cells involved in hypersensitivity reactions. Decreased chemotaxis and activation of eosinophils has also been demonstrated. Additionally, ketotifen attenuates the effects of PAF and inhibits cAMP phosphodiesterase.

In human conjunctival allergen challenge studies, ZADITOR (ketotifen fumarate ophthalmic solution) was significantly more effective than placebo in preventing ocular itching and redness associated with allergic conjunctivitis. The effect was seen within minutes after administration and lasted up to 12 hours.

Pharmacodynamics: In human conjunctival allergen challenge studies, ZADITOR was significantly more effective than placebo in preventing ocular itching and redness associated with allergic conjunctivitis. The effect was seen within minutes after administration and lasted up to 12 hours.

In a placebo-controlled clinical study designed to evaluate safety, ZADITOR, administered four times a day for 6 weeks, was shown to be safe and well-tolerated in subjects aged 3 years and older.

STORAGE AND STABILITY: Store between 4 and 25°C.

INFORMATION FOR THE PATIENT: Published in e-CPS, available by subscription at www.e-cps.ca.

DOSAGE FORMS, COMPOSITION AND PACKAGING: Each mL of clear ophthalmic solution contains: ketotifen fumarate 0.345 mg equivalent to ketotifen 0.25 mg. Nonmedicinal ingredients: benzalkonium chloride, glycerol, hydrochloric acid/sodium hydroxide and purified water. Multi dose white plastic bottles of 5 mL with controlled dropper tips.

Zanaflex® ℞
tizanidine HCl
Antispastic

Paladin

Date of Preparation: January 25, 1999
Date of Revision: July 7, 2009

SUMMARY PRODUCT INFORMATION:

Route of Administration	Dosage Form/ Strength	Clinically Relevant Nonmedicinal Ingredients
Oral	Tablet 4 mg	Anhydrous lactose For a complete listing see Dosage Forms, Composition and Packaging.

INDICATIONS AND CLINICAL USE: Adults: Zanaflex (tizanidine HCl) is a short-acting drug for the management of spasticity.
Geriatrics: Evidence from clinical studies and experience suggests that use in the geriatric population may be associated with differences in safety or effectiveness and a brief discussion can be found in the appropriate sections (Warnings and Precautions and Action and Clinical Pharmacology).
Pediatrics (<18 years of age): No data are available.

CONTRAINDICATIONS: Patients who are hypersensitive to this drug or to any ingredient in the formulation or component of the container. For a complete listing, see Dosage Forms, Composition and Packaging.

Coadministration of tizanidine with moderate and potent CYP1A2 inhibitors such as fluvoxamine or ciprofloxacin is contraindicated (see Warnings and Precautions).

Zanaflex is contraindicated in patients for whom spasticity is needed to maintain function, such as maintenance of upright posture and balance in locomotion.

WARNINGS AND PRECAUTIONS: General: Hypotension: Tizanidine HCl is an α_2-adrenergic agonist (like clonidine) and can produce hypotension. In a single dose study where blood pressure was monitored closely after dosing, two thirds of patients treated with 8 mg of Zanaflex had a 20% reduction in either the diastolic or systolic BP. The reduction was seen within 1 hour after dosing, peaked 2 to 3 hours after dosing and was associated, at times, with bradycardia, orthostatic hypotension, lightheadedness/dizziness and rarely syncope. The hypotensive effect is dose related and has been measured following single doses of ≥2 mg.

The chance of significant hypotension may possibly be minimized by titration of the dose and by focusing attention on signs and symptoms of hypotension prior to dose advancement. In addition, patients moving from a supine to a fixed upright position may be at increased risk for hypotensive and orthostatic effects.

Caution is advised when Zanaflex is to be used in patients who have a history of orthostatic hypotension or labile blood pressure or who are receiving concurrent antihypertensive therapy. Zanaflex should not be used with other α_2-adrenergic agonists.

Risk of Liver Injury: Zanaflex use occasionally causes drug induced liver injury, most often hepatocellular in type. In controlled clinical studies, approximately 5% of patients treated with Zanaflex had elevations of liver function tests (ALT, AST) to greater than 3 times the upper limit of normal (or 2 times if baseline levels were elevated). The patients usually remain asymptomatic despite increased aminotransferases. In occasional symptomatic cases, nausea, vomiting, anorexia and jaundice have been reported. The onset of the elevated liver enzymes typically occurred within the first 6 months of treatment with Zanaflex and most resolved rapidly upon drug withdrawal with no reported residual problems. In postmarketing experience, three deaths associated with liver failure have been reported in patients treated with tizanidine, including one case of fatal fulminant hepatitis.

Monitoring of aminotransferase levels is recommended during the first 6 months of treatment (e.g., baseline, 1, 3 and 6 months) and periodically thereafter, based on clinical status. Because of the potential toxic hepatic effect of tizanidine, the drug should be used only with extreme caution in patients with impaired hepatic function.

Sedation: In the multiple dose, controlled clinical studies, 48% of patients receiving any dose of Zanaflex reported sedation as an adverse event. In 10% of these cases, the sedation was rated as severe compared to <1% in the placebo treated patients. Sedation may interfere with every day activity.

The effect appears to be dose related. In a single dose study, 92% of the patients receiving 16 mg, when asked, reported that they were drowsy during the 6-hour study. This compares to 76% of the patients on 8 mg and 35% of the patients on placebo. Patients began noting this effect 30 minutes following dosing. The effect peaked 1.5 hours following dosing. Of the patients who received a single dose of 16 mg, 51% continued to report drowsiness 6 hours following dosing compared to 13% in the patients receiving placebo or 8 mg of Zanaflex.

In the multiple dose studies, the prevalence of patients with sedation peaked following the first week of titration and then remained stable for the duration of the maintenance phase of the study.

Hallucinations: Zanaflex use has been associated with hallucinations. Formed, visual hallucinations or delusions have been reported in 5 of 170 patients (3%) in two North American controlled clinical studies. Most of the patients were aware that the events were unreal. One patient developed psychoses in association with the hallucinations. One patient continued to have problems for at least 2 weeks following discontinuation of Zanaflex. Dosage reduction or discontinuation should be considered for patients who experience hallucinations while receiving Zanaflex. Particular caution should be observed if Zanaflex is administered to patients with a prior history of psychotic illness.

Limited Database for Chronic Use of Single Doses Above 8 mg and Multiple Doses Above 24 mg per Day: Clinical experience with long-term use of Zanaflex at single doses of 8 to 16 mg or total daily doses of 24 to 36 mg is limited. Approximately 75 patients have been exposed to individual doses of 12 mg or more for at least one year and approximately 80 patients have been exposed to total daily doses of 30 to 36 mg/day for at least one year. There is essentially no long-term experience with single, daytime doses of 16 mg. Because long-term clinical study experience at high doses is limited, only those adverse events with a relatively high incidence are likely to have been identified.

Discontinuation of Treatment with Zanaflex: If therapy needs to be discontinued, especially in patients who have been receiving high doses for long periods, the dose should be decreased slowly to minimize the risk of withdrawal and rebound hypertension, tachycardia, and hypertonia.

The following additional precautions are listed alphabetically.

Carcinogenesis and Mutagenesis: Only animal carcinogenesis data and mutagenesis data from in vitro and in vivo assays are available.

Cardiovascular: Prolongation of the QT interval and bradycardia were noted in chronic toxicity studies in dogs at doses equal to the maximum human dose on a mg/m² basis. ECG evaluation was not performed in the controlled clinical studies. There have been post-market reports of QT prolongation and a small number of reports of torsades de pointes, none of them fatal, during Zanaflex treatment.

Caution should be exercised when Zanaflex is prescribed with drugs known to prolong the QT interval.

Tizanidine HCl can produce hypotension associated, at times, with bradycardia and orthostatic hypotension, dizziness and rarely syncope (see Warnings and Precautions, General).

Dependence/Tolerance: Monkeys were shown to self-administer tizanidine in a dose-dependent manner, and abrupt cessation of tizanidine produced transient signs of withdrawal at doses >35 times the maximum recommended human dose on a mg/m² basis. These transient withdrawal signs (increased locomotion, body twitching, and aversive behavior toward the observer) were not reversed by naloxone administration. Tizanidine is closely related to clonidine, which is often abused in combination with narcotics and is known to cause symptoms of rebound upon abrupt withdrawal. There have been cases of rebound symptoms reported on sudden withdrawal of tizanidine. Some of the case reports suggest that these patients were also misusing opioids. Withdrawal symptoms included but were not limited to: hypertension, tachycardia, hypertonia, convulsions, tremor, and anxiety. As with clonidine, withdrawal is expected to be more likely in cases where high doses are used, especially for prolonged periods. There have been also reports of tizanidine abuse and dependence, most of them with concomitant use of opioids, benzodiazepines, other hypnotics or multiple analgesics. The potential for tizanidine abuse should be monitored, especially in patients simultaneously using opioids or benzodiazepines.

Drug Interaction with CYP1A2 Inhibitors: Concomitant use of tizanidine and moderate or potent CYP450 1A2 inhibitors is contraindicated (see Contraindications). Concomitant use of tizanidine with fluvoxamine, a potent CYP450 1A2 inhibitor in man, resulted in a 33-fold increase in the tizanidine AUC by fluvoxamine; concomitant use of tizanidine with ciprofloxacin, another CYP1A2 inhibitor, resulted in a 10-fold increase in tizanidine AUC; in both studies, clinically significant hypotension resulted along with somnolence, dizziness and decreased psychomotor performance (see Drug Interactions). Coadministration of tizanidine with other inhibitors of CYP1A2 such as antiarrhythmics (amiodarone, mexiletine, propafenone), cimetidine, other fluoroquinolones (norfloxacin, moxifloxacin), and ticlopidine should be avoided or used with caution.

Hepatic/Biliary/Pancreatic: Zanaflex use occasionally causes drug induced liver injury, most often hepatocellular in type (see Warnings and Precautions, General).

Information to Be Provided to the Patient: Patients should be advised of the limited clinical experience with Zanaflex both in regard to duration of use and the higher doses required to reduce muscle tone (see Warnings and Precautions, General).

Because of the possibility of Zanaflex lowering blood pressure, patients should be warned about the risk of clinically significant orthostatic hypotension (see Warnings and Precautions, General).

Because of the possibility of sedation, patients should be warned about performing activities requiring alertness, such as driving a vehicle or operating machinery (see Warnings and Precautions, General). Patients should also be instructed that the sedation may be additive when Zanaflex is taken in conjunction with drugs (baclofen, benzodiazepines) or substances (e.g., alcohol) that act as CNS depressants.

Neurologic: Zanaflex use has been associated with sedation (see Warnings and Precautions, General).

Zanaflex use has been associated with hallucinations (see Warnings and Precautions, General).

Ophthalmologic: Dose-related retinal degeneration and corneal opacities have been found in animal studies at doses equivalent to approximately the maximum recommended dose on a mg/m² basis. There have been no reports of corneal opacities or retinal degeneration in the clinical studies.

Renal: Zanaflex should be used with caution in patients with renal insufficiency (Clcr <25 mL/min), as clearance is reduced by more than 50%. In these patients, during titration, the individual doses should be reduced. If higher doses are required, individual doses rather than dosing frequency should be increased. These patients should be monitored closely for onset or increase in severity of the common adverse events (dry mouth, somnolence, asthenia and dizziness) as indicators of potential overdose.

Special Populations: Use in Women Taking Oral Contraceptives: Zanaflex should be used with caution in women taking oral contraceptives; as clearance of tizanidine is reduced by approximately 50% in such patients. In these patients, during titration, the individual doses should be reduced.

Pregnant Women: The effect of Zanaflex on labor and delivery in humans is unknown.

Reproduction studies performed in rats at a dose of 3 mg/kg, equal to the maximum recommended human dose on a mg/m² basis and in rabbits at 30 mg/kg, 16 times the maximum recommended human dose on a mg/m² basis did not show evidence of teratogenicity. Tizanidine at doses equal to and up to 8 times the maximum recommended human dose on a mg/m² basis increased gestation duration in rats. Prenatal and postnatal pup loss was increased and developmental retardation occurred. Postimplantation loss was increased in rabbits at doses of 1 mg/kg or greater, equal to or greater than 0.5 times the maximum recommended human dose on a mg/m² basis. Zanaflex has not been studied in pregnant women. Zanaflex should be given to pregnant women only if the potential benefit clearly outweighs the potential risk to mother and child.

Nursing Women: It is not known whether Zanaflex is excreted in human milk, although as a lipid soluble drug, it might be expected to pass into breast milk.

Pediatrics (<18 years of age): There are no adequate and well-controlled studies to document the safety and efficacy of Zanaflex in children under 18 years in age.

Geriatrics: Zanaflex should be used with caution in elderly patients because clearance is decreased four-fold.

ADVERSE REACTIONS: Adverse Drug Reaction Overview: In multiple dose, placebo-controlled clinical studies, 264 patients were treated with Zanaflex (tizanidine HCl) and 261 with placebo. Adverse events, including severe adverse events, were more frequently reported with Zanaflex than with placebo.

Common Adverse Events Leading to Discontinuation: Forty-five of 264 (17%) patients receiving Zanaflex and 13 of 261 (5%) patients receiving placebo in three multiple dose, placebo-controlled clinical studies discontinued treatment for adverse events. When patients withdrew from the study, they frequently had more than one reason for discontinuing. The adverse events most frequently leading to withdrawal of Zanaflex treated patients in the controlled clinical studies were asthenia (weakness, fatigue and/or tiredness) (3%), somnolence (3%), dry mouth (3%), increased spasm or tone (2%) and dizziness (2%).

Most Frequent Adverse Clinical Events Seen in Association with the Use of Tizanidine: In multiple-dose, placebo-controlled clinical studies involving 264 patients with spasticity, the most frequent adverse events were dry mouth, somnolence/sedation, asthenia (weakness, fatigue and/or tiredness) and dizziness. Three quarters of the patients rated the events as mild to moderate and one quarter of the patients rated the events as being severe. These events appeared to be dose related.

Clinical Trial Adverse Drug Reactions: Because clinical trials are conducted under very specific conditions the adverse reaction rates observed in the clinical trials may not reflect the rates observed in practice and should not be compared to the rates in the clinical trials of another drug. Adverse drug reaction information from clinical trials is useful for identifying drug-related adverse events and for approximating rates.

The events cited reflect experience gained under closely monitored conditions of clinical studies in a highly selected patient population. In actual clinical practice or in other clinical studies, these frequency estimates may not apply, as the conditions of use, reporting behavior, and the kinds of patients treated may differ. Table 1 lists treatment emergent signs and symptoms that were reported in greater than 2% of patients in three multiple dose, placebo-controlled studies who received Zanaflex where the frequency in the Zanaflex group was at least as common as in the placebo group. These events are not necessarily related to Zanaflex treatment. For comparison purposes, the corresponding frequency of the event (per 100 patients) among placebo treated patients is also provided.

Table 1: Zanaflex

Multiple Dose, Placebo-Controlled Studies (Frequent (>2%) Adverse Events Reported for Which Zanaflex Incidence is Greater than Placebo)

	Zanaflex n=264 (%)	Placebo n=261 (%)
Dry Mouth	49	10
Somnolence	48	10
Asthenia[a]	41	16
Dizziness	16	4
Urinary Tract Infection	10	7
Infection	6	5
Constipation	4	1
Liver Function Tests Abnormal	3	<1
Vomiting	3	0
Speech Disorder	3	0
Amblyopia (blurred vision)	3	<1
Urinary Frequency	3	2
Flu Syndrome	3	2
ALT Increased	3	<1
Dyskinesia	3	0
Nervousness	3	<1
Pharyngitis	3	1
Rhinitis	3	2

[a] Weakness, fatigue and/or tiredness.

In the single dose, placebo-controlled study involving 142 patients with spasticity, the patients were specifically asked if they had experienced any of the four most common adverse events dry mouth, somnolence (drowsiness), asthenia (weakness, fatigue and/or tiredness), and dizziness. In addition, hypotension and bradycardia were observed. The occurrence of these adverse events is summarized in Table 2. Other events were, in general, reported at a rate of 2% or less.

Table 2: Zanaflex

Single Dose, Placebo-Controlled Study (Common Adverse Events Reported)

	Zanaflex 8 mg n=45 (%)	Zanaflex 16 mg n=49 (%)	Placebo n=48 (%)
Somnolence	78	92	31
Dry Mouth	76	88	35
Asthenia[a]	67	78	40
Dizziness	22	45	4
Hypotension	16	33	0
Bradycardia	2	10	0

[a] Weakness, fatigue and/or tiredness.

Other Adverse Events Observed During the Evaluation of Tizanidine: Zanaflex was administered to 1187 patients in additional clinical studies where adverse event information was available. The conditions and duration of exposure varied greatly, and included (in overlapping categories) double-blind and open-label studies, uncontrolled and controlled studies, inpatient and outpatient studies, and titration studies. Untoward events associated with this exposure were recorded by clinical investigators using terminology of their own choosing. Consequently, it is not possible to provide a meaningful estimate of the proportion of individuals experiencing adverse events without first grouping similar types of untoward events into a smaller number of standardized event categories.

In the tabulations that follow, reported adverse events were classified using a standard COSTART-based dictionary terminology. The frequencies presented, therefore, represent the proportion of the 1187 patients exposed to Zanaflex who experienced an event of the type cited on at least one occasion while receiving tizanidine. All reported events are included except those already listed in Table 1. If the COSTART term for an event was so general as to be uninformative, it was replaced with a more informative term. It is important to emphasize that, although the events reported occurred during treatment with Zanaflex, they were not necessarily caused by it.

Events are further categorized by body system and listed in order of decreasing frequency according to the following definitions: frequent adverse events are those occurring on one or more occasions in at least 1/100 patients (only those not already listed in the tabulated results from placebo-controlled studies appear in this listing); infrequent adverse events are those occurring in 1/100 to 1/1000 patients.

Body as a Whole: Frequent: fever; Infrequent: allergic reaction, moniliasis, malaise, abscess, neck pain, sepsis, cellulitis, death, overdose; Rare: carcinoma, congenital anomaly, suicide attempt.

Cardiovascular System: Infrequent: vasodilatation, postural hypotension, syncope, migraine, arrhythmia; Rare: angina pectoris, coronary artery disorder, heart failure, myocardial infarct, phlebitis, pulmonary embolus, ventricular extrasystoles, ventricular tachycardia.

Digestive System: Frequent: abdomen pain, diarrhea, dyspepsia; Infrequent: dysphagia, cholelithiasis, fecal impaction, flatulence, gastrointestinal hemorrhage, hepatitis, melena; Rare: gastroenteritis, hematemesis, hepatoma, intestinal obstruction, liver damage.

Hemic and Lymphatic System: Infrequent: ecchymosis, hypercholesteremia, anemia, hyperlipemia, leukopenia, leukocytosis, sepsis; Rare: petechia, purpura, thrombocythemia, thrombocytopenia.

Metabolic and Nutritional System: Infrequent: edema, hypothyroidism, weight loss; Rare: adrenal cortex insufficiency, hyperglycemia, hypokalemia, hyponatremia, hypoproteinemia, respiratory acidosis.

Musculoskeletal System: Frequent: myasthenia, back pain; Infrequent: pathological fracture, arthralgia, arthritis, bursitis.

Nervous System: Frequent: depression, anxiety, paresthesia; Infrequent: tremor, emotional lability, convulsion, paralysis, thinking abnormal, vertigo, abnormal dreams, agitation, depersonalization, euphoria, migraine, stupor, dysautonomia, neuralgia; Rare: dementia, hemiplegia, neuropathy.

Respiratory System: Infrequent: sinusitis, pneumonia, bronchitis; Rare: asthma.

Skin and Appendages: Frequent: rash, sweating, skin ulcer; Infrequent: pruritus, dry skin, acne, alopecia, urticaria; Rare: exfoliative dermatitis, herpes simplex, herpes zoster, skin carcinoma.

Special Senses: Infrequent: ear pain, tinnitus, deafness, glaucoma, conjunctivitis, eye pain, optic neuritis, otitis media, retinal hemorrhage, visual field defect; Rare: iritis, keratitis, optic atrophy.

Urogenital System: Infrequent: urinary urgency, cystitis, menorrhagia, pyelonephritis, urinary retention, kidney calculus, uterine fibroids enlarged, vaginal moniliasis, vaginitis; Rare: albuminuria, glycosuria, hematuria, metrorrhagia.

Post-Market Adverse Drug Reactions: Table 3 includes events determined to be medically significant and/or potentially life threatening and assessed as associated with the use of Zanaflex or the possible relationship to Zanaflex cannot be completely excluded.

Table 3: Zanaflex

Post-Market Spontaneous Adverse Event Reports

Adverse Event	Frequency			
	≥1%	<1% and ≥0.1%	<0.1% and ≥0.01%	<0.01%
Blood and Lymphatic System Disorders				
Agranulocytosis				X
Disseminated Intravascular Coagulation				X
Cardiac Disorders				
Tachycardia				X
Pulmonary Oedema				X
Cardiac Arrest				X
Torsades de Pointes				X
Cardiorespiratory Arrest				X
Ventricular Fibrillation				X
General Disorders and Administration Site Conditions				
Pyrexia				X

(cont'd)

Table 3: **Zanaflex** *(cont'd)*

Post-Market Spontaneous Adverse Event Reports

Adverse Event	Frequency ≥1%	<1% and ≥0.1%	<0.1% and ≥0.01%	<0.01%
Hepatobiliary Disorders				
Hepatic Function Abnormal				X
Hepatitis				X
Hepatic Disorder				X
Jaundice				X
Hepatic Failure				X
Hepatic Necrosis				X
Hepatitis Fulminant				X
Hepatic Fibrosis				X
Hepatic Cirrhosis				X
Immune System Disorders				
Anaphylactic Shock				X
Investigations				
Electrocardiogram QT Prolonged				X
Musculoskeletal and Connective Tissue Disorders				
Rhabdomyolysis				X
Nervous System Disorders				
Loss of Consciousness				X
Cerebrovascular Accident				X
Cerebral Infarction				X
Psychiatric Disorders				
Confusional State				X
Renal and Urinary Disorders				
Renal Failure Acute				X
Renal Failure				X
Respiratory, Thoracic and Mediastinal Disorders				
Dyspnea				X
Skin and Subcutaneous Tissue Disorders				
Erythema Multiforme				X
Vascular Disorders				
Shock				X
Circulatory Collapse				X

In post-marketing experience, nausea has also been reported at a frequency of <0.1% and ≥0.01%.

DRUG INTERACTIONS:

> **Serious Drug Interactions**
> - **Moderate or potent CYP1A2 inhibitors such as fluvoxamine and ciprofloxacin (see Contraindications).**

Overview: In vitro studies of cytochrome P450 isoenzymes using human liver microsomes indicate that neither tizanidine nor its major metabolites are likely to affect the metabolism of other drugs metabolized by cytochrome P450 isoenzymes. There are reports of drug interaction of tizanidine and CYP1A2 inhibitors, such as oral contraceptives, fluvoxamine, fluoroquinolones, and others.

Acetaminophen: Zanaflex delayed the T_{max} of acetaminophen by 16 minutes. Acetaminophen did not affect the pharmacokinetics of Zanaflex.

Alcohol: Alcohol increased the AUC of Zanaflex by approximately 20% while also increasing its C_{max} by approximately 15%. This was associated with an increase in side effects of Zanaflex. The CNS depressant effects of Zanaflex and alcohol are additive.

Oral Contraceptives: No specific pharmacokinetic study was conducted to investigate interaction between oral contraceptives and Zanaflex, but retrospective analysis of population pharmacokinetic data following single and multiple dose administration of 4 mg Zanaflex showed that women concurrently taking oral contraceptives had 50% lower clearance of Zanaflex than women not on oral contraceptives.

Antihypertensives: In placebo-controlled clinical trials, Zanaflex has been administered concomitantly with antihypertensive medications in 30 patients. The addition of Zanaflex to antihypertensive therapy was associated with a 20-30% increase in the incidence of clinically significant decreases in systolic or diastolic blood pressure compared with both placebo plus antihypertensive (N=36) and Zanaflex alone (N=226).

Concurrent use of antihypertensive and Zanaflex therapy also resulted in an increase in reports of orthostatic hypotension. Lower initial doses and cautious dose titration should be considered when Zanaflex is to be administered to patients receiving antihypertensive therapy or if antihypertensive therapy is to be initiated in a patient receiving Zanaflex.

Fluvoxamine and Other CYP1A2 Inhibitors: Zanaflex should not be used together with moderate and potent CYP1A2 inhibitors such as fluvoxamine and ciprofloxacin (see Contraindications). Concomitant use of tizanidine with fluvoxamine, a potent CYP450 1A2 inhibitor in man, resulted in a 33-fold increase in the tizanidine AUC by fluvoxamine in 10 healthy male subjects. Concomitant use of tizanidine with ciprofloxacin resulted in a 10-fold increase in tizanidine AUC in 10 healthy male subjects. In both studies, clinically significant hypotension resulted along with somnolence, dizziness and decreased psychomotor performance. Coadministration of tizanidine with other inhibitors of CYP1A2 such as antiarrhythmics (amiodarone, mexiletine, propafenone), cimetidine, other fluoroquinolones (norfloxacin, moxifloxacin), oral contraceptives, and ticlopidine should be avoided or used in caution (see also Warnings and Precautions, Drug Interaction with CYP1A2 Inhibitors).

Drugs Known to Prolong the QT Interval: Prolongation of the QT interval and bradycardia were noted in chronic toxicity studies in dogs at doses equal to the maximum human dose on a mg/m² basis. ECG evaluation was not performed in the controlled clinical studies. There have been post-market reports of QT prolongation and a small number of reports of torsades de pointes, none of them fatal, during Zanaflex treatment. **Zanaflex should be used with caution in patients taking drugs known to prolong the QT interval.**

Drug-Food Interactions: Administering tizanidine with food increases the C_{max}, the time to peak concentration, and the extent of absorption of tizanidine (see Action and Clinical Pharmacology). These pharmacokinetic differences may result in clinically significant differences when switching between fed or fasted states, such as changed incidence of adverse events or delayed/more rapid onset of activity, depending on the nature of the switch (see Dosage and Administration).

DOSAGE AND ADMINISTRATION: Dosing Considerations:

- Administration of tizanidine with food increases the C_{max}, the time to peak concentration, and the extent of absorption of tizanidine. These pharmacokinetic differences may result in clinically significant differences when switching between fed or fasted states, such as changed incidence of adverse events or delayed/more rapid onset of activity, depending on the nature of the switch. For this reason, the prescriber should recommend patients to always take tizanidine the same way with regard to fed and fasted state (see Action and Clinical Pharmacology).
- If therapy needs to be discontinued, especially in patients who have been receiving high doses for long periods, the dose should be decreased slowly to minimize the risk of withdrawal and rebound hypertension, tachycardia, and hypertonia.

Recommended Dose and Dosage Adjustment: A single oral dose of 8 mg of Zanaflex (tizanidine HCl) reduces muscle tone in patients with spasticity for a period of several hours. The effect peaks at approximately 1 to 2 hours and dissipates between 3 to 6 hours. Zanaflex dosing should be scheduled such that the peak effect coincides with activities for which relief of spasticity is most desirable. Effects are dose-related.

Although single doses of less than 8 mg have not been demonstrated to be effective in controlled clinical studies, the dose-related nature of Zanaflex's common adverse events, particularly blood pressure reduction, make it prudent to begin treatment with single oral doses of 2 mg. Increase the dose gradually (2 to 4 mg steps) to optimum effect (satisfactory reduction of muscle tone at a tolerated dose).

The dose can be repeated at 6 to 8 hour intervals, as needed, to a maximum of three doses in 24 hours. The total daily dose should not exceed 36 mg.

Experience with single doses exceeding 8 mg and daily doses exceeding 24 mg is limited. There is essentially no experience with repeated, single, daytime doses greater than 12 mg or total daily doses greater than 36 mg (see Warnings and Precautions).

OVERDOSAGE:
There have been cases of tizanidine overdose reported in post-marketing experience. Most of these were intentional overdoses, about a quarter have resulted in fatality, and in at least half of these cases, other CNS depressants were involved. The majority of cases involved depressed consciousness (somnolence, stupor, or coma), depressed cardiovascular function (bradycardia, hypotension), and depressed respiratory function (respiratory depression or failure).

Should overdosage occur, basic steps to ensure the adequacy of an airway and the monitoring of cardiovascular and respiratory systems should be undertaken. For the most recent information concerning the management of overdose, contact a poison control center.

> For management of a suspected drug overdose, CPhA recommends that you contact your **regional Poison Control Centre**. See the *CPS* Directory section for a list of Poison Control Centres.

ACTION AND CLINICAL PHARMACOLOGY: Mechanism of Action: Tizanidine is an agonist at α_2-adrenergic receptor sites and presumably reduces spasticity by increasing presynaptic inhibition of motor neurons. In animal models, tizanidine has no direct effect on skeletal muscle fibers or the neuromuscular junction, and no major effect on monosynaptic spinal reflexes. The effects of tizanidine are greatest on polysynaptic pathways. The overall effect of these actions is thought to reduce facilitation of spinal motor neurons.

The imidazoline chemical structure of tizanidine is related to that of the anti-hypertensive drug clonidine and other α_2-adrenergic agonists. Pharmacological studies in animals show similarities between the two compounds, but tizanidine was found to have one-tenth to one-fiftieth (1/50) of the potency of clonidine in lowering blood pressure.

Pharmacokinetics: Absorption: Following oral administration, tizanidine is essentially completely absorbed and has a half-life of approximately 2 hours. Following administration of tizanidine peak plasma concentrations occurred at approximately 1 hour after dosing. Food increases the mean C_{max} by approximately 30% and increases the median time to peak concentration by approximately 25 minutes, from 1 hour to 1 hour and 25 minutes. Food increases the extent of absorption of tizanidine by approximately 30%. Tizanidine has linear pharmacokinetics over a dose of 1 to 20 mg.

Metabolism: The absolute oral bioavailability of tizanidine is approximately 40%, due to extensive first-pass metabolism in the liver; approximately 95% of an administered dose is metabolized. Tizanidine metabolites are not known to be active; their half-lives range from 20 to 40 hours.

Distribution: Tizanidine is widely distributed throughout the body; mean steady state volume of distribution is 2.4 L/kg following intravenous administration in healthy adult volunteers. Tizanidine is approximately 30% bound to plasma proteins, independent of concentration over the therapeutic range.

Excretion: Following single and multiple oral dosing of ^{14}C-tizanidine, an average of 60% and 20% of total radioactivity was recovered in the urine and feces, respectively.

Special Populations and Conditions: Age Effects: No specific pharmacokinetic study was conducted to investigate age effects. Cross study comparison of pharmacokinetic data, following single dose administration of 6 mg Zanaflex showed that younger subjects cleared the drug four times faster than the elderly subjects. Zanaflex has not been evaluated in children (see Warnings and Precautions).

Gender: No specific pharmacokinetic study was conducted to investigate gender effects. Retrospective analysis of pharmacokinetic data, however, following single and multiple dose administration of 4 mg Zanaflex showed that gender had no effect on the pharmacokinetics of Zanaflex.

Race: Pharmacokinetic differences due to race have not been studied.

Hepatic Insufficiency: Pharmacokinetic differences due to hepatic impairment have not been studied (see Warnings and Precautions).

Renal Insufficiency: Zanaflex clearance is reduced by more than 50% in elderly patients with renal insufficiency (creatinine clearance <25 mL/min) compared to healthy elderly subjects; this would be expected to lead to a longer duration of clinical effect. Zanaflex should be used with caution in renally impaired patients (see Warnings and Precautions).

STORAGE AND STABILITY: The product should be stored at 15-30°C. Dispense in containers with child resistant closure.

INFORMATION FOR THE PATIENT: Published in e-CPS, available by subscription at www.e-cps.ca.

DOSAGE FORMS, COMPOSITION AND PACKAGING: Each white tablet, embossed with "A594" on one side and cross-scored on the other, contains: tizanidine HCl 4.576 mg equivalent to 4 mg tizanidine base. Nonmedicinal ingredients: anhydrous lactose, microcrystalline cellulose, silicon dioxide colloidal and stearic acid. Bottles of 150.

(Shown in Product Identification Section)

Zanosar™ P

streptozocin

Antineoplastic

Pfizer

Date of Revision: March 30, 2009

> **Caution: Streptozocin should be administered under the supervision of a physician experienced in the use of cancer chemotherapeutic agents (see Warnings and Precautions). Renal, hepatic and bone marrow/hematologic evaluations should be done at regular intervals. Renal toxicity is dose related and cumulative and may be fatal.**

PHARMACOLOGY: Streptozocin inhibits DNA synthesis in bacterial and mammalian cells. In bacterial cells, a specific interaction with cytosine moieties leads to degradation of DNA. The biochemical mechanism leading to mammalian cell death has not been definitively established; levels required to kill cells are considerably lower than those required to inhibit DNA synthesis or to inhibit several of the enzymes involved in DNA synthesis.

Streptozocin inhibits the progression of cells into mitosis but the agent does not appear to be specifically lethal to cells in a single phase of the cell cycle.

It is active in the L1210 leukemic mouse over a fairly wide range of parenteral dosage schedules. In many experimental animal species, streptozocin induces a diabetes that resembles human hyperglycemic non-ketotic diabetes mellitus. This phenomenon, which has been extensively studied, is consequent upon histopathologic alteration of pancreatic islet beta cells.

The metabolism of streptozocin has not been fully studied. When given i.v. to mice or dogs, it disappears from the blood very rapidly. In all species tested, it concentrates in the liver and kidney. Less than 10% of the drug (or metabolites containing an N-nitrosourea group) is excreted by the kidney. Metabolic products have not been identified.

INDICATIONS: For the treatment of metastatic islet cell carcinoma of the pancreas. Responses have been obtained with both functional and nonfunctional carcinomas. Because of its inherent renal toxicity, therapy with this drug should be limited to patients with symptomatic or progressive metastatic disease.

CONTRAINDICATIONS: In patients with known hypersensitivity to the drug.

Pre-existing renal disease is a strong contraindication to its use. Use of the drug in such a patient must be judged by the physician in terms of the potential benefit as opposed to the known risk.

WARNINGS: Streptozocin should be administered under the supervision of a physician experienced in the use of cancer chemotherapeutic agents.

Renal Function: Many patients treated with streptozocin have experienced renal toxicity as evidenced by azotemia, anuria, hypophosphatemia, glycosuria and renal tubular acidosis. Such toxicity is dose-related and cumulative and may be severe or fatal. Renal function must be monitored before and after each course of therapy. Serial urinalysis, blood urea nitrogen, plasma creatinine, serum electrolytes and creatinine clearance should be obtained prior to, at least weekly during, and 4 weeks after drug administration. Serial urinalysis is particularly important for the early detection of proteinuria and should be quantitated with a 24 hour collection when proteinuria is detected.

Mild proteinuria and hypophosphatemia are the first signs of renal toxicity and may herald further deterioration of renal function. Reduction of the dose or discontinuation of treatment is suggested in the presence of significant renal toxicity.

This drug should not be used in combination with or concomitantly with other potential nephrotoxins.

During therapy, a patient need not be hospitalized but should have access to a facility with laboratory and supportive resources sufficient to monitor drug tolerance and to protect and maintain a patient compromised by drug toxicity.

Other toxicities are nausea and vomiting, which may be severe and at times treatment-limiting. In addition, liver dysfunction, diarrhea, and bone marrow/hematological changes have been observed in some patients.

Effects at Site of Injection: Care should be taken to avoid extravasation of the drug, since under such conditions severe local tissue necrosis will occur.

Immunosuppressant Effects/Increased Susceptibility to Infections: Administration of live or live-attenuated vaccines in patients immunocompromised by chemotherapeutic agents including streptozocin may result in serious or fatal infections. Vaccination with a live vaccine should be avoided in patients receiving streptozocin. Killed or inactivated vaccines may be administered; however, the response to such vaccines may be diminished.

Mutagenesis, Carcinogenesis, Impairment of Fertility: Streptozocin is mutagenic in bacteria, plants and mammalian cells. When administered parenterally, it has been shown to induce renal tumors in rats and to induce liver tumors and other tumors in hamsters. Stomach and pancreatic tumors were observed in rats treated orally with streptozocin. Streptozocin has also been shown to be carcinogenic in mice.

Streptozocin adversely affected fertility when administered to male and female rats.

When exposed dermally, some rats developed benign tumors at the site of application of streptozocin. Consequently, streptozocin may pose a carcinogenic hazard following topical exposure if not properly handled. If streptozocin powder or solution contacts the skin or mucosae, immediately wash the affected area with soap and water (see Dosage, Handling Instructions).

PRECAUTIONS: Patient Follow-up: Patients must be monitored closely, particularly for evidence of renal, hepatic, and bone marrow/hematopoietic toxicity. Serial urinalysis, blood urea nitrogen, and plasma creatinine levels, and creatinine clearance should be done prior to and at least once weekly during and for 4 weeks after drug administration (see Warnings, Renal Function).

Similarly, complete blood counts and liver function studies should be done weekly. Reduction of the dose or discontinuation of therapy is suggested in response to the appearance of significant renal, hepatic, or bone marrow/hematopoietic abnormalities, but must be weighed against the possible benefit of continued therapy of clinically progressive disease.

Storage Limitations: After reconstitution, the solution may be stored in a refrigerator for 48 hours. However, this formulation contains no preservatives, and is not intended as a multiple-dose vial. (See Storage under Dosage).

Drug Interactions: When streptozocin is used in combination with antineoplastic drugs with similar cytotoxic effects, additive toxicity is likely to occur.

Streptozocin has been reported to prolong the elimination half-life of doxorubicin leading to increased severe bone marrow suppression. In case of concomitant administration of the two drugs, a reduction of doxorubicin dosage should be considered.

The administration of amphotericin B with antineoplastic drugs, including streptozocin, may increase the risk of nephrotoxicity, hypotension and bronchospasm. If it is necessary to give this combination of agents, a close monitoring of blood pressure as well as renal and pulmonary function is advisable.

The concurrent use of streptozocin and phenytoin has been reported in one case to result in reduced streptozocin cytotoxicity.

Concomitant use of steroids with streptozocin may result in severe hyperglycemia.

Pregnancy: Safe use during pregnancy has not been established. Streptozocin is mutagenic in bacteria and plants. By analogy with other nitrosoureas, it would be expected to exhibit teratogenic effects in animals.

When administered to pregnant monkeys, it appears promptly in the fetal circulation. It has been shown to induce renal tumors in rats, and liver and other tumors in hamsters. The physician must judge the possible benefit to the patient against these known toxic effects when considering the advisability of therapy in males or females who may contemplate the initiation of pregnancy or in pregnant females.

Reproduction studies revealed that streptozocin is teratogenic in the rat and has abortifacient effects in rabbits. There are no studies in pregnant women.

Streptozocin should be used during pregnancy only if the potential benefit justifies the potential risk to the fetus. Women of childbearing potential who are to undergo streptozocin therapy should be informed of the potential hazard to the fetus and should be advised to avoid becoming pregnant during treatment.

Lactation: It is not known whether streptozocin is excreted in human milk. Because many drugs are excreted in human milk and because of the potential for serious adverse reactions in nursing infants, nursing should be discontinued in patients receiving streptozocin.

Children: No data on treatment of children are available.

Effects on Patients Ability to Operate a Vehicle or Machinery: On the basis of reported adverse reactions (i.e. confusion, lethargy), streptozocin may potentially increase the risk of injury while driving or operating machinery.

ADVERSE EFFECTS: Renal and Urinary Disorders: (See Warnings.)

Renal toxicity is the most serious and dose-limiting adverse effect of streptozocin treatment, occurring in approximately 25 to 75% of treated patients. Streptozocin-induced nephrotoxicity is cumulative and **may be severe or fatal**. Increase of BUN, anuria, proteinuria, hypophosphatemia, hyperchloremia, and proximal renal tubular acidosis which may be associated with a Falconi-like syndrome evidenced by glycosuria, acetonuria and aminoaciduria are manifestations of glomerular and tubular function abnormalities. Hypokalemia and hypocalcemia have also occurred. Hypophosphatemia and mild proteinuria appear to be the earliest signs of nephrotoxicity, whereas increase of BUN and serum creatinine concentrations usually develop later following continued treatment with the drug.

Although mild renal adverse effects may be reversible following discontinuation of streptozocin, nephrotoxicity may be irreversible and fatalities associated with chronic renal failure may occur if therapy with the drug is continued after nephrotoxicity is observed.

Cases of nephrogenic diabetes insipidus following streptozocin therapy have been reported. One had spontaneous recovery and the second responded to indomethacin.

Gastrointestinal Disorders: Most patients have experienced severe nausea and vomiting, occasionally requiring discontinuation of drug therapy. Nausea and vomiting usually begin within 1 to 4 hours following administration of streptozocin and may persist for 24 hours or longer. Incidence and severity of nausea and vomiting may be reduced with 5-day continuous i.v. infusion. Conventional antiemetics (e.g., phenothiazines) are usually only minimally effective in preventing or reducing streptozocin-induced nausea and vomiting. Some patients experienced diarrhea. Increases in serum bilirubin concentration and hypoalbuminemia have also been reported.

Hepatobiliary Disorders: Severe and fatal hepatic effects have occurred rarely (see Investigations).

Metabolic and Nutrition Disorders: Mild to moderate abnormalities of glucose tolerance have been noted in some patients but these have generally been reversible. Insulin shock with severe hypoglycemia has occurred rarely during streptozocin therapy in patients with insulinomas, usually within 24 hours after administration of the drug.

Blood and Lymphatic System Disorders: Bone marrow/hematological toxicity has been rare, most often involving mild decreases in hematocrit values. However, **fatal hematological toxicity, resulting from leukopenia (leading to sepsis) and from thrombocytopenia has been observed**. Mild to moderate myelosuppression, which may be manifested as leukopenia/neutropenia, thrombocytopenia and anemia (decreased hematocrit and hemoglobin concentration) occurs in 10 to 20% of patients receiving the drug. Myelosuppression may be cumulative and may be more severe in patients previously treated with other antineoplastic agents or radiation therapy. Leukocyte and platelets nadirs generally occur 1 to 2 weeks following treatment with the drug. Asymptomatic eosinophilia, which disappeared following discontinuance of streptozocin, has also been reported.

Investigations: Transient increases in serum concentrations of AST, ALT, LDH and/or alkaline phosphatase have been reported. Increases in serum bilirubin concentration and hypoalbuminemia have also been reported.

General Disorders and Administration: Severe necrosis has been reported following extravasation of the drug. A burning sensation, extending from the site of injection up the arm, has been reported in some patients especially following i.v. push administration. Pyrexia has occurred rarely.

Nervous System Disorders/Psychiatric Disorders: Confusion, lethargy and depression, have been reported in a limited number of patients receiving continuous i.v. infusion for 5 days. Adverse CNS effects have not been associated with other regimens.

OVERDOSE:

Treatment: No specific antidote is known, thus every possible measure should be taken to avoid an overdose; this includes full awareness of the potential danger of an overdose, careful calculation of the dose to be administered and availability of adequate diagnostic and treatment facilities.

For management of a suspected drug overdose, CPhA recommends that you contact your **regional Poison Control Centre**. See the *CPS* Directory section for a list of Poison Control Centres.

DOSAGE: Streptozocin should be administered i.v. It is not active orally. Although it has been administered intra-arterially, this is not recommended pending further evaluation of the possibility that adverse renal effects may be evoked more readily by this route of administration.

Dosage Schedules: Two different dosage schedules have been employed successfully:

Daily Schedule: The recommended dose for daily i.v. administration is 500 mg/m² of body surface area for 5 consecutive days every 6 weeks until maximum benefit or until treatment-limiting toxicity is observed. Dose escalation on this schedule is not recommended.

Weekly Schedule: The recommended initial dose for weekly i.v. administration in 1000 mg/m² of body surface area at weekly intervals for the first 2 courses (weeks). In subsequent courses, drug doses may be escalated in patients who have not achieved a therapeutic response and who have not experienced significant toxicity with the previous course of treatment. However, **a single dose of 1500 mg/m² body surface area should not be exceeded** as a greater dose may cause azotemia.

When administered on this schedule, the median time to onset of response is about 17 days and the median time to maximum response is about 35 days. The median **total** dose to onset of response is about 2000 mg/m² body surface area and the median **total** dose to maximum response is about 4000 mg/m² body surface area.

When streptozocin is used in combination with other chemotherapeutic agents, reduction of dosage is often necessary.

The ideal duration of maintenance therapy has not yet been clearly established for either of the above schedules.

For patients with functional tumors, serial monitoring of fasting insulin levels allows a determination of biochemical response to therapy. For patients with either functional or non-functional tumors, response to therapy can be determined by measurable reductions of tumor size (reduction of organomegaly, masses, or lymph nodes).

Stability and Storage: Unopened vials should be stored at refrigeration temperatures (2 to 8°C) and protected from light (preferably stored in carton).

The total storage time for streptozocin after reconstitution should not exceed 48 hours at refrigeration temperatures (2 to 8°C) or 24 hours at room temperature (below 25°C). However, since this product contains no preservatives and is not intended as a multiple-dose vial and in order to avoid the risk of microbial contamination, it is recommended that the solution be used as soon as possible and within 12 hours from reconstitution.

Further dilution of the reconstituted solution with 500 mL of Sodium Chloride Injection USP does not alter the solution stability.

Incompatibilities: Streptozocin has been reported to be incompatible with allopurinol in sodium chloride 0.9% solution, resulting in drug precipitation. Aztreonam or piperacillin/tazobactam diluted in 5% dextrose cause solution colour changes and are to be considered incompatible.

Reconstituted Solutions: Reconstitute with 9.5 mL of Dextrose Injection USP, Sterile Water for Injection USP, or Sodium Chloride Injection USP. The resulting pale-gold solution will contain 100 mg of streptozocin and 22 mg of citric acid per mL. Where more dilute infusion solutions are desirable, further dilution in the above vehicles is recommended. When reconstituted as directed, the pH of the solution will be between 3.5 and 4.5.

Special Instructions: Handling: The following precautionary measures are recommended in proceeding with the preparation and handling of cytotoxic agents such as streptozocin.

1. Pregnant staff should be excluded from working with this drug.
2. Personnel should be trained in good technique for reconstitution and handling.
3. The procedure should be carried out in a vertical laminar flow hood (biological Safety Cabinet—Class II). The work surface should be protected by disposable, plastic-backed, absorbent paper.
4. Personnel should wear: PVC gloves, safety glasses, disposable gowns and masks.
5. All items used for reconstitution, administration or cleaning, including gloves, should be placed in high-risk waste-disposal bags for high-temperature incineration.

Streptozocin waste should be deactivated by reaction with hydrobromic acid in glacial acetic acid or by oxidation with a solution of potassium permanganate in sulfuric acid.

SUPPLIED: Each off-white to pale yellow colored freeze-dried cake contains: streptozocin 1 g and citric acid anhydrous 220 mg. When necessary, pH was adjusted with hydrochloric acid and/or sodium hydroxide. Vials of 1 g. Store unopened vials at refrigeration temperatures (2 to 8°C) and protected from light (preferably stored in carton).

Zantac® Ⓟ

ranitidine HCl

Histamine H2-Receptor Antagonist

GlaxoSmithKline

Date of Revision: August 12, 2010

PHARMACOLOGY: Ranitidine is an antagonist of histamine at gastric H_2-receptor sites. Thus, ranitidine inhibits both basal gastric secretion and gastric acid secretion induced by histamine, pentagastrin and other secretagogues. On a weight basis, ranitidine is between 4 and 9 times more potent than cimetidine. Inhibition of gastric acid secretion has been observed following i.v., intraduodenal and oral administration of ranitidine. This response is dose-related, a maximum response being achieved at an oral dose of 300 mg/day.

Pepsin secretion is also inhibited but secretion of gastric mucus is not affected. Ranitidine does not alter the secretion of bicarbonate or enzymes from the pancreas in response to secretin and pancreozymin.

Ranitidine is rapidly absorbed after oral administration of 150 mg ranitidine, peak plasma concentrations (300 to 550 ng/mL) occurred after 1 to 3 hours. Two distinct peaks or a plateau in the absorption phase result from reabsorption of drug excreted into the intestine. These plasma concentrations are not significantly influenced by the presence of food in the stomach at the time of the oral administration nor by regular doses of antacids.

Bioavailability of oral ranitidine is approximately 50% to 60%. Serum protein binding of ranitidine in man is in the range of 10 to 19%. The elimination half-life is approximately 2 to 3 hours. The principal route of excretion is the urine (40% recovery of free and metabolized drug in 24 hours).

There is a significant linear correlation between the dose administered and the inhibitory effect upon gastric acid secretion for oral doses up to 300 mg. A plasma ranitidine concentration of 50 ng/mL has an inhibitory effect upon stimulated gastric acid secretion of approximately 50%. Estimates of the IC_{50} range from 36 to 94 ng/mL. Following the administration of 150 mg ranitidine orally, plasma concentrations in excess of this lasted for more than 8 hours, and after 12 hours, the plasma concentrations were sufficiently high to have a significant inhibitory effect upon gastric acid secretion. In patients with duodenal ulcer, 150 mg oral ranitidine every 12 hours significantly reduced mean 24-hour hydrogen ion activity by 69% and nocturnal gastric acid output by 90%. Furthermore, 300 mg ranitidine given at night is as effective in reducing 24-hour intragastric acidity as 150 mg ranitidine given orally twice daily.

Following administration of 50 mg ranitidine injection i.m., plasma concentrations in excess of 100 ng/mL were achieved within 5 minutes and remained above this level for 4 to 6 hours.

I.V. infusion (rate: 0.125 mg/kg/hour) produced a rise of intragastric pH between 5.6 and 7 after 2 hours and maintained this level over the 24-hour period, when administered to seriously ill patients. The volume of gastric secretion was reduced by more than 55%. Doubling the infusion rate to 0.25 mg/kg/hour produced no further increase in gastric acid inhibition.

A single 50 mg i.v. bolus dose of ranitidine injection produced significant acid inhibition 8 to 9 hours after administration. When 13 seriously ill patients with 2 or more risk factors (shock, sepsis, respiratory failure, jaundice, renal insufficiency or peritonitis) were treated with a 50 mg i.v. bolus dose of ranitidine injection followed by a continuous infusion of 0.2 mg/kg/hour, the number of "at risk" days (gastric pH less than 3.5 at 3 consecutive 4-hour aliquots) was approximately half that of placebo-treated patients.

Tablets: In respect of both 24-hour acidity and nocturnal acid output, oral ranitidine 150 mg twice daily was superior to cimetidine 200 mg 3 times daily and 400 mg at night ($p<0.001$ and <0.05, respectively).

Treatment of volunteers with oral ranitidine 150 mg twice daily for 7 days did not cause bacterial overgrowth in the stomach.

Volunteers treated with an oral dose of ranitidine have reported no significant gastrointestinal or CNS side effects; moreover, pulse rate, blood pressure, ECG and EEG were not significantly affected in man following ranitidine administration.

In healthy human volunteers and patients, ranitidine, when administered orally, did not influence plasma levels of the following hormones: cortisol, testosterone, estrogens, growth hormone, follicle stimulating hormone, luteinizing hormone, thyroid stimulating hormone, aldosterone or gastrin; although, like cimetidine, ranitidine reduced vasopressin output. Treatment for up to 6 weeks with ranitidine 150 mg twice daily by mouth did not affect the human hypothalamic-pituitary-testicular-ovarian or -adrenal axes.

Injection: I.M. ranitidine is fully bioavailable in comparison to i.v. ranitidine. The median elimination half-life of ranitidine injection 50 mg, administered i.v. or i.m., was found to be 2.3 hours (range 120 to 160 minutes). In comparison, the elimination half-life following oral administration is approximately 2 to 3 hours. However, the half-life of ranitidine in patients with renal dysfunction is prolonged. In a study of 27 patients with renal dysfunction (plasma creatinine concentration greater than 300 μmol/L), therapeutic plasma levels of ranitidine were shown to be achieved without risk of drug accumulation, if half the normal dose of the drug was administered.

Ranitidine injection is well tolerated following i.v. administration at dose levels of up to 100 mg q.i.d. It is evident that these levels are in excess of those recommended for normal clinical use.

At 50 mg i.v., ranitidine injection had no effect on prolactin levels. Only at the 300 mg i.v. dose level was there an increase in prolactin secretion, which was equivalent to that produced by 200 mg of cimetidine administered i.v.

Patients Over 50 Years of Age: In patients over 50 years of age, half-life is prolonged (3 to 4 hours) and clearance is reduced, consistent with the age-related decline of renal function. However, systemic exposure and accumulation are 50% higher. This difference exceeds the effect of declining renal function, and indicates increased bioavailability in older patients.

INDICATIONS: ZANTAC (ranitidine hydrochloride) Tablets, Injection, and Oral Solution are indicated for the treatment of duodenal ulcer, benign gastric ulcer, reflux esophagitis, post-operative peptic ulcer, Zollinger-Ellison Syndrome, and other conditions where reduction of gastric secretion and acid output is desirable. These include the following:

- the treatment of nonsteroidal anti-inflammatory drug (NSAID)-induced lesions, both ulcers and erosions, and their gastrointestinal (GI) symptoms and the prevention of their recurrence;
- the prophylaxis of GI hemorrhage from stress ulceration in seriously ill patients;
- the prophylaxis of recurrent hemorrhage from bleeding ulcers;
- the prevention of Acid Aspiration Syndrome (Mendelson's Syndrome) from general anesthesia in patients considered to be at risk for this, including obstetrical patients in labor, and obese patients.

In addition, ZANTAC is indicated for the prophylaxis and maintenance treatment of duodenal or benign gastric ulcer in patients with a history of recurrent ulceration.

CONTRAINDICATIONS: ZANTAC (ranitidine hydrochloride) is contraindicated for patients known to have hypersensitivity to ranitidine or to any ingredient in the formulation. For a complete listing, see Supplied.

WARNINGS: Gastric Ulcer: Treatment with a histamine H_2-antagonist may mask symptoms associated with carcinoma of the stomach and, therefore, may delay diagnosis of that condition. Accordingly, where gastric ulcer is suspected, the possibility of malignancy should be excluded before therapy with ZANTAC (ranitidine hydrochloride) is instituted.

Concomitant NSAID Use: Regular supervision of patients who are taking NSAIDs concomitantly with ZANTAC is recommended, especially in the elderly and those with a history of peptic ulcer. Baseline endoscopic and histological evaluation is necessary to rule out gastric carcinoma.

Patients with a History of Acute Porphyria: Rare clinical reports suggest that ranitidine may precipitate acute porphyric attacks. Therefore, ranitidine should be avoided in patients with a history of acute porphyria.

Pregnancy: The safety of ZANTAC in the treatment of conditions where a controlled reduction of gastric secretion is required during pregnancy has not been established. Reproduction studies performed in rats and rabbits have revealed no evidence of ZANTAC induced impaired fertility or harm to the fetus. Ranitidine crosses the placenta. Nevertheless, if the administration of ZANTAC is considered to be necessary, its use requires that the potential benefits be weighed against possible hazards to the patient and to the fetus.

Lactation: ZANTAC is secreted in breast milk in lactating mothers, but the clinical significance of this has not been fully evaluated. Like other drugs, ZANTAC should only be used during nursing if considered essential.

Children: Experience with ZANTAC in children is limited. It has, however, been used successfully in children aged 8 to 18 years in oral doses up to 150 mg twice daily.

PRECAUTIONS: General: Injection: Bradycardia in association with rapid administration of ZANTAC (ranitidine hydrochloride) Injection has been reported rarely, usually in patients with factors predisposing to cardiac rhythm disturbances. Recommended rates of administration should not be exceeded (see Adverse Effects and Dosage).

The use of higher than recommended doses of IV H_2-antagonists has been associated with rises in liver enzymes when treatment has been extended beyond five days.

Impaired Renal Function: ZANTAC is excreted via the kidneys and, in the presence of renal impairment, plasma levels of ZANTAC are increased and elimination prolonged. Accordingly, it is recommended in such patients, to decrease the dosage of ZANTAC by one-half. Accumulation of ZANTAC with resulting elevated plasma concentrations will occur in patients with renal impairment (creatinine clearance less than 50 mL/min); a recommended daily dose of oral ranitidine in such patients should be 150 mg.

Drug Interactions: Ranitidine has the potential to affect the absorption, metabolism or renal excretion of other drugs. The altered pharmacokinetics may necessitate dosage adjustment of the affected drug or discontinuation of treatment.

Interactions occur by several mechanisms including:

1) Inhibition of Cytochrome P450-linked Mixed Function Oxygenase System: Ranitidine at usual therapeutic doses does not potentiate the actions of drugs which are inactivated by this enzyme system such as diazepam, lidocaine, phenytoin, propranolol and theophylline.

There have been reports of altered prothrombin time with coumarin anticoagulants (e.g. warfarin). Due to the narrow therapeutic index, close monitoring of increased or decreased prothrombin time is recommended during concurrent treatment with ranitidine.

2) Competition for Renal Tubular Secretion: Since ranitidine is partially eliminated by the cationic system, it may affect the clearance of other drugs eliminated by this route. High doses of ranitidine (e.g., such as those used in the treatment of Zollinger-Ellison syndrome) may reduce the excretion of procainamide and N-acetylprocainamide resulting in increased plasma levels of these drugs.

3) Alteration of Gastric pH: The bioavailability of certain drugs may be affected. This can result in either an increase in absorption (e.g. triazolam, midazolam) or a decrease in absorption (e.g. ketoconazole, atazanavir, delaviridine, gefitnib).

Sporadic cases of drug interactions have been reported in elderly patients involving both hypoglycemic drugs and theophylline. The significance of these reports cannot be determined at present, as controlled clinical trials with theophylline and ZANTAC have not shown interaction.

If high doses (2 g) of sucralfate are coadministered with ZANTAC, the absorption of ZANTAC may be reduced. This effect is not seen if sucralfate is taken at least 2 hours after ZANTAC administration.

Special Populations: In patients such as the elderly, persons with chronic lung disease, diabetes or the immunocompromised, there may be an increased risk of developing community acquired pneumonia. A large epidemiological study showed an increased risk of developing community acquired pneumonia in current users of H_2-receptor antagonists versus those who had stopped treatment, with an observed adjusted relative risk increase of 1.63 (95% CI, 1.07-2.48).

Geriatrics: Since malignancy is more common in the elderly, particular consideration must be given to this before therapy with ZANTAC is instituted. Elderly patients receiving NSAIDs concomitantly with ZANTAC should be closely supervised.

As with all medication in the elderly, when prescribing ZANTAC, consideration should be given to the patient's concurrent drug therapy. Sporadic cases of drug interaction have been reported in elderly patients involving both hypoglycemic drugs and theophylline. The significance of these reports cannot be determined at present, as controlled clinical trials with theophylline and ZANTAC have not shown interaction. Elderly patients may be at increased risk for confusional states and depression.

ADVERSE EFFECTS: Tablets, Injection and Oral Solution: The following adverse reactions have been reported as events in clinical trials or in the routine management of patients treated with ZANTAC (ranitidine hydrochloride). A cause and effect relationship to ZANTAC is not always established.

Central Nervous System: headache, sometimes severe; malaise; dizziness; somnolence; insomnia; vertigo; and reversible blurred vision suggestive of a change in accommodation. Isolated cases of reversible mental confusion, agitation, depression, and hallucinations have been reported, predominantly in severely ill elderly patients. In addition, reversible involuntary movement disorders have been reported rarely.

Cardiovascular: Isolated reports of tachycardia, bradycardia, premature ventricular beats, and AV block have been noted. Asystole has been reported in very few individuals with and without predisposing conditions following i.v. administration and has not been reported following oral administration of ZANTAC (see Precautions and Dosage).

Gastrointestinal: constipation, diarrhea, nausea/vomiting and abdominal discomfort/pain.

Hepatic: In normal volunteers, transient and reversible ALT and AST values were increased to at least twice the pretreatment levels in 6 of 12 subjects receiving ranitidine 100 mg q.i.d. i.v. for 7 days, and in 4 of 24 subjects receiving 50 mg q.i.d. i.v. for 5 days. Therefore, it may be prudent to monitor AST and ALT in patients receiving i.v. treatment for 5 days or longer and in those with pre-existing liver diseases. With oral administration, there have been occasional reports of hepatitis, hepatocellular or hepatocanalicular or mixed, with or without jaundice. In such circumstances, ranitidine should be discontinued immediately. These are usually reversible, but in exceedingly rare circumstances, death has occurred.

Renal: Very rare cases of acute interstitial nephritis have been reported.

Musculoskeletal: rare reports of arthralgia and myalgia.

Hematologic: Blood count changes (leukopenia, thrombocytopenia) have occurred in a few patients. These are usually reversible. Rare cases of agranulocytosis or pancytopenia, sometimes with marrow hypoplasia or aplasia, have been reported.

Endocrine: No clinically significant interference with endocrine or gonadal function has been reported. There have been a few reports of breast symptoms and breast conditions (such as gynaecomastia and galactorrhoea).

Dermatologic: rash, including cases suggestive of mild erythema multiforme. Rare cases of vasculitis and alopecia have been reported.

Other: Rare cases of hypersensitivity reactions (including chest pain, bronchospasm, fever, rash, eosinophilia, anaphylaxis, urticaria, angioneurotic edema, hypotension) and small increases in serum creatinine have occasionally occurred after a single dose. Acute pancreatitis and reversible impotence have been reported rarely.

OVERDOSE:

Symptoms: There is no experience to date with deliberate overdosage.

Treatment: The usual measures to remove unabsorbed drug from the gastrointestinal tract (including activated charcoal or syrup of ipecac), clinical monitoring and supportive therapy should be employed.

For management of a suspected drug overdose, contact your **regional Poison Control Centre**. See the *CPS* Directory section for a list of Poison Control Centres.

DOSAGE: Tablet, and Oral Solution Administration: Duodenal Ulcer and Benign Gastric Ulcer: 300 mg once daily at bedtime or 150 mg twice daily taken in the morning and before retiring. It is not necessary to time the dose in relation to meals. In most cases of duodenal ulcer and benign gastric ulcer, healing will occur in 4 weeks. In the small number of patients whose ulcers may not have fully healed, these are likely to respond to a further 4-week course of treatment. In the treatment of duodenal ulcers, 300 mg twice daily for 4 weeks may be of benefit when more rapid healing is desired.

Maintenance Therapy: Duodenal Ulcers, Benign Gastric Ulcers: Patients who have responded to short-term therapy, particularly those with a history of recurrent ulcer, may benefit from chronic maintenance therapy at a reduced oral tablet dosage of 150 mg once daily at bedtime.

In the management of duodenal ulcers, smoking is associated with a higher rate of ulcer relapse (up to 9.2 times higher in one trial), and such patients should be advised to stop smoking. In those patients who fail to comply with such advice, 300 mg nightly provides additional therapeutic benefit over the 150 mg once daily dosage regimen.

Reflux Esophagitis: Acute Treatment: 300 mg once daily at bedtime, or alternatively 150 mg twice daily, taken in the morning and before retiring, for up to 8 weeks. In patients with moderate to severe esophagitis, the dosage of ranitidine may be increased to 150 mg 4 times daily for up to 12 weeks.

Long-term Management: For the long-term management of reflux esophagitis, the recommended adult oral dose is 150 mg twice daily.

Postoperative Peptic Ulcer: 150 mg twice daily, taken in the morning and before retiring.

Pathological Hypersecretory Conditions (Zollinger-Ellison Syndrome): 150 mg 3 times daily may be administered initially. In some patients, it may be necessary to administer 150 mg doses more frequently. Doses should be adjusted to individual patient needs. Doses up to 6 g/day have been well tolerated.

Treatment of NSAID-induced Lesions (both ulcers and erosions) and their Gastrointestinal Symptoms and Prevention of their Recurrence: In ulcers following NSAID therapy or associated with continued NSAIDs, 150 mg twice daily for 8 to 12 weeks may be necessary. For the prevention of NSAID-associated ulcer recurrence, 150 mg twice daily may be given concomitantly with nonsteroidal anti-inflammatory drug therapy.

Prophylaxis of Acid Aspiration Syndrome (AAS): 150 mg the evening prior to anesthesia induction is recommended; however, 150 mg 2 hours before anesthesia induction is also effective. Alternatively, ZANTAC Injection may be used. For the prevention of AAS in pre-partum patients who elect for anesthesia, 150 mg every 6 hours may be employed, but if general anesthesia is warranted, a non-particulate oral antacid (e.g., sodium citrate) could supplement ZANTAC therapy. In an emergency situation, the use of alkalis, antacids, and meticulous anesthetic technique is still necessary, as ZANTAC does not affect the pH and volume of the existing gastric content.

Prophylaxis of Hemorrhage from Stress Ulceration in Seriously Ill Patients or Prophylaxis of Recurrent Hemorrhage in Patients Bleeding from Peptic Ulceration who Are Currently Managed by I.V. ZANTAC: An oral dose of 150 mg twice daily may be substituted for the injection once oral feeding commences.

If necessary, ZANTAC Oral Solution may be administered by orogastric or nasogastric tube as an alternative.

Note: A 150 mg dose of ranitidine is equivalent to 10 mL of ZANTAC Oral Solution, and 300 mg ranitidine is equivalent to 20 mL of ZANTAC Oral Solution.

Geriatrics: For all conditions listed above, the drug dosage for the elderly who are seriously ill should start at the lowest recommended dose and be adjusted as necessary with close supervision.

Patients over 50 years of age (see Pharmacology, Patients Over 50 Years of Age).

Parenteral Administration: In some hospitalized patients with pathological hypersecretory conditions or intractable duodenal ulcers, or in patients unable to take oral medication, ZANTAC may be administered parenterally according to the following recommendations:

I.M. Injection: 50 mg (2 mL) every 6 to 8 hours (no dilution is required).

I.V. Injection: 50 mg (2 mL) every 6 to 8 hours. Dilute ZANTAC Injection, 50 mg in compatible i.v. solution (see Parenteral Administration, Dilution of Parenteral Products) to a total volume of 20 mL and inject over a period of **not less than 5 minutes** (see Precautions). Parenteral administration may continue until oral feeding is commenced and if there is still a risk, oral ZANTAC may then commence.

Intermittent I.V. Infusion: 50 mg (2 mL) every 6 to 8 hours. Dilute ZANTAC Injection 50 mg in 100 mL of compatible i.v. solution (see Parenteral Administration, Dilution of Parenteral Products) and infuse over 15 to 20 minutes. In some patients, it may be necessary to increase dosage. When this is required, the increases should be made by more frequent administration of a 50 mg dose, but generally should not exceed 400 mg/day.

In the prophylaxis of upper gastrointestinal hemorrhage from stress ulceration in seriously ill patients, a primary dose of 50 mg as a slow (over a period of not less than 5 minutes) i.v. injection followed by a continuous i.v. infusion of 0.125 to 0.250 mg/kg/hour may be preferred (see Precautions). The higher infusion concentration (0.25 mg/kg/hour) should be reserved for patients who are unresponsive to a lower concentration (0.125 mg/kg/hour).

In the prophylaxis of hemorrhage from stress ulceration in seriously ill patients or prophylaxis of recurrent hemorrhage in patients bleeding from peptic ulceration, parenteral administration may continue until oral feeding is commenced and if there is still a risk, oral ZANTAC may then commence.

For patients considered at risk of developing Acid Aspiration Syndrome (Mendelson's Syndrome): 50 mg by i.m. or slow (over a period of not less than 5 minutes) i.v. injection 45 to 60 minutes before induction of general anesthesia. In an emergency situation, the use of alkalis, antacids, and meticulous anesthetic technique is still necessary, as ZANTAC does not affect the pH and volume of the existing gastric content.

Dilution of Parenteral Products: I.M. Injection: No dilution is required.

I.V. Injection: ZANTAC Injection for i.v. injection should be diluted to 20 mL (2.5 mg/mL) with one of the recommended diluents listed below.

Intermittent I.V. Infusion: ZANTAC Injection for intermittent i.v. infusion should be diluted to 100 mL (0.5 mg/mL) with one of the recommended diluents listed below. ZANTAC Injection is compatible in polyvinyl chloride infusion bags and in glass with the following intravenous fluids: 0.9% sodium chloride; 5% dextrose; 0.18% sodium chloride and 4% dextrose; 4.2% sodium bicarbonate; Hartmann's solution. Admixtures of ZANTAC Injection with 0.18% sodium chloride and 4% dextrose or 4.2% sodium bicarbonate or Hartmann's solution should be discarded after 24 hours. Although i.v. admixtures of ZANTAC Injection with 5% dextrose or 0.9% sodium chloride may often be physically and chemically stable for longer periods, due to microbiological considerations they are usually recommended for use within the maximum 72 hours when refrigerated (2 to 8°C) followed by 24 hours at room temperature.

Hospitals and institutions that have recognized admixture programs and use validated aseptic techniques for preparation of i.v. solutions may extend the storage time for ZANTAC Injection in admixture with 5% Dextrose Injection or 0.9% Sodium Chloride Injection in polyvinyl chloride infusion bags, in concentrations of up to 2 mg/mL, to 35 days when stored under refrigeration at 2 to 8°C.

Note: As with all parenteral drug products, intravenous admixtures should be inspected visually for clarity, particulate matter, precipitate, discolouration and leakage prior to administration, whenever solution and container permit. Solutions showing haziness, particulate matter, precipitate, or discolouration or leakage should not be used.

SUPPLIED: Injection: Each mL of solution for i.v. or i.m. injection contains: ranitidine HCl 28 mg (equivalent to ranitidine anhydrous free base 25 mg) in sterile water for injection. Nonmedicinal ingredients: disodium hydrogen orthophosphate, phenol (5 mg/mL) and potassium dihydrogen orthophosphate. Unit dose colorless glass vials of 2 mL, packages of 10. Multidose colorless glass vials of 40 mL, packages of 1. Store between 2 and 25°C. Protect from light. ZANTAC Injection should not be autoclaved.

Oral Solution: Each 10 mL of clear, peppermint-flavored solution contains: ranitidine HCl 168 mg (equivalent to ranitidine anhydrous free base 150 mg). Nonmedicinal ingredients: alcohol (7.5% w/v), butylparaben, dibasic sodium phosphate, flavor mint, hydroxypropyl methylcellulose, monobasic potassium phosphate, propylparaben, sodium chloride, sodium cyclamate and sorbitol. Bottles of 300 mL. Store at or below 25°C. Protect from light. Keep out of reach of children.

Tablets: 150 mg: Each white, round, biconvex, film-coated tablet engraved ZANTAC 150 on one face and GLAXO on the other contains: ranitidine HCl 168 mg (equivalent to ranitidine anhydrous free base 150 mg). Nonmedicinal ingredients: magnesium stearate and microcrystalline cellulose; film-coating suspension: hydroxypropyl methylcellulose, titanium dioxide and triacetin. Gluten- and tartrazine-free. Foil packs of 60. Bottles of 100 and 500. Store between 2 and 30°C. Protect from light.

300 mg: Each white, capsule-shaped, film-coated tablet engraved ZANTAC 300 on one face and GLAXO on the other contains: ranitidine HCl 336 mg (equivalent to ranitidine anhydrous free base 300 mg). Nonmedicinal ingredients: croscarmellose sodium, magnesium stearate and microcrystalline cellulose; film-coating suspension: hydroxypropyl methylcellulose, titanium dioxide and triacetin. Gluten- and tartrazine-free. Foil packs of 30. Bottles of 60. Store between 2 and 30°C. Protect from light.

(Shown in Product Identification Section)

Zantac®
ranitidine HCl
Histamine H2-Receptor Antagonist

McNeil Consumer Healthcare

Zantac® Maximum Strength Non-Prescription
ranitidine HCl
Histamine H2-Receptor Antagonist

McNeil Consumer Healthcare

Date of Preparation: July 19, 2001
Date of Revision: November 15, 2007

PHARMACOLOGY: Ranitidine is an antagonist of histamine at gastric H_2-receptor sites. Thus, ranitidine inhibits both basal gastric secretion and gastric acid secretion induced by histamine, pentagastrin and other secretagogues. Inhibition of gastric acid secretion has been observed following intravenous, intraduodenal and oral administration of ranitidine. This response is dose-related, a maximum response being achieved at an oral dose of 300 mg/day.

Pepsin secretion is also inhibited but secretion of gastric mucus is not affected. Ranitidine does not alter the secretion of bicarbonate or enzymes from the pancreas in response to secretin and pancreozymin.

Ranitidine is rapidly absorbed after oral administration, peak plasma concentrations being achieved within 2 to 3 hours. These plasma concentrations are not significantly influenced by the presence of food in the stomach at the time of the oral administration nor by regular doses of antacids.

Bioavailability of oral ranitidine is approximately 50%. Serum protein binding of ranitidine in man is in the range 10 to 19%. The elimination half-life is approximately 3 hours. The principal route of excretion is the urine (40% recovery of free and metabolized drug in 24 hours).

There is a significant linear correlation between the dose administered and the inhibitory effect upon gastric acid secretion for single oral doses up to 300 mg. In healthy subjects a single 75 mg dose of ranitidine significantly reduced meal-stimulated intragastric acidity ($[H^+]$ AUC) compared with placebo. The effect of ranitidine on intragastric acidity and pH is also dose-related.

The important pharmacologic activity of ranitidine is inhibition of gastric acid and fluid secretion in basal and stimulated states, which increases the pH and decreases the volume of secretions. A single 75 mg dose, compared to placebo, has an early onset of action; significantly elevating gastric pH within one hour, and lasting for up to 13 hours post dosing. After correcting for onset of action (within one hour), the duration of acid suppression for ranitidine 75 mg is up to 12 hours (i.e. all day or all night). In the same multicentre, randomized, cross-over study, the onset of acid suppression effect for ranitidine 75 mg was statistically superior to famotidine 10 mg at only one and two hours post-dosing. The duration and degree of acid suppression of ranitidine 75 mg (63.1%, n=75) were superior to cimetidine 200 mg (37.8%, n=52) over the 10 hour daytime evaluation period. See Table 1 and Table 2.

Table 1: Zantac

Summary of Weighted Mean Hydrogen Ion Activity (H^+AUC mmol/L·h)

Time Period	Placebo N=75 Subjects	Ranitidine 75 mg N=75 Subjects	Cimetidine 200 mg N=52 Subjects	Famotidine 10 mg N=22 Subjects
Total (20 h)	30.89	18.21[a,b]	25.08[a]	19.32[a]
Day (11:00h-22:30h)	32.76	18.19[a,b]	22.06[a]	13.23[a]
Night (22:30h-08:30h)	28.83	23.23[a,b]	28.09	25.41[a]

[a] $p<0.05$ compared with paired placebo group.
[b] $p<0.05$ compared with paired cimetidine group.

Table 2: Zantac

Changes in Intragastric Acidity and pH

	Median Percentage Decrease in Acidity			Median Intragastric pH	
	Total	Day[a]	Night[a]	Day[a]	Night[a]
Ranitidine 75 mg (N=75)	44.1%[b]	63.1%[b]	21.2%[b]	2.10[c]	1.80[c]
Famotidine 10 mg (N=22)	38.9%	58.9%	20.1%	2.06[c]	1.90
Cimetidine 200 mg (N=52)	23.0%	37.8%	1.8%	1.69[c]	1.77
Placebo (N=75)				1.48	1.70

[a] Day=12:30h to 22:30h; night=22:30h to 8:30h.
[b] $p<0.05$ compared with paired cimetidine group.
[c] $p<0.05$ compared with paired placebo group.

In a large, multicentre, dose-ranging, placebo-controlled trial in patients with episodic heartburn, a single 75 mg dose relieved symptoms within 30 minutes and provided relief for the duration of the 4 hour evaluation period.

Volunteers treated with an oral dose of ranitidine have reported no significant gastrointestinal or central nervous system side effects; moreover pulse rate, blood pressure, electrocardiogram and electroencephalogram are not significantly affected in man following ranitidine administration.

In healthy human volunteers and patients, ranitidine, when administered orally did not influence plasma levels of the following hormones: cortisol, testosterone, oestrogens, growth hormone, follicle-stimulating hormone, luteinizing hormone, thyroid-stimulating hormone, aldosterone or gastrin; although like cimetidine, ranitidine reduced vasopressin output. Treatment for up to 6 weeks with ranitidine 150 mg twice daily by mouth did not affect the human hypothalamic-pituitary-testicular-ovarian or -adrenal axes.

The safety and efficacy of 75 mg ranitidine for treatment of episodic heartburn were established in two large replicate Phase III studies involving 2985 patients. These two pivotal studies demonstrated that one ranitidine 75 mg tablet was statistically and clinically superior to placebo in providing relief of episodic heartburn beginning at 30 minutes.

In two subsequent heartburn treatment trials evaluating total pain relief, both the 75 mg and 150 mg strengths of ranitidine were demonstrated to be statistically significantly superior to placebo as shown in Table 3.

Table 3 presents pooled data for the primary efficacy variable of total pain relief for the first treated episode (TOTPAR) along with its associated p values.

Table 3: Zantac Maximum Strength Non-Prescription

Pooled Treatment Data Primary Variable (Intent-to-treat subjects)

Efficacy Variable	Ranitidine 150 mg (N=637)	Ranitidine 75 mg (N=637)	Placebo (N=635)	Ranitidine 75 mg vs Placebo (p value)	Ranitidine 150 mg vs Placebo (p value)	Ranitidine 150 mg vs Ranitidine 75 mg (p value)
TOTPAR for 1st drug treated episode (mean)	20.8	20.4	18.3	<0.001	0.004	0.673

The safety and efficacy of 150 mg ranitidine for the prevention or reduction of severity of meal-induced heartburn when taken immediately before consuming food and beverages anticipated to provoke heartburn was studied in two pivotal and one supporting large replicate Phase III well-controlled, multi-center, double-blind, randomized, placebo-controlled studies involving 2,484 patients. The results of the 2 pivotal and supporting studies are summarized in Table 4.

Table 4: Zantac Maximum Strength Non-Prescription

Pooled Prevention Data for Key Efficacy Variables (Intent-to-treat subjects) Pivotal Studies

Efficacy Variable	Ranitidine 150 mg (N=518)	Ranitidine 75 mg (N=524)	Placebo (N=521)
Treatment meal AUC (mm·hr)	87.0±3.96[a,b]	91.1±3.84[a,c]	107.5±4.17
Reduction in treatment meal AUC (%)	49.1±2.44[a]	44.0±2.29[a,d]	32.7±2.93
Treatment meal peak heartburn severity (mm)	40.2±1.29[a]	41.6±1.23[a,e]	47.0±1.28
Peak heartburn reduction (%)	42.6±1.78[a]	38.7±1.73[a,f]	31.2±1.79
Largest consecutive time points with no heartburn	5.3±0.24[a]	4.7±0.23	4.2±0.22

[a] $p<0.05$ versus placebo.
[b] $p<0.05$ versus ranitidine 75 mg.
[c] N=520.
[d] N=518.
[e] N=521.
[f] N=519.

Table 5: Zantac Maximum Strength Non-Prescription

Prevention Data for Key Efficacy Variables (Intent-to-treat subjects) Supporting Study

Efficacy Variable	Ranitidine 150 mg (N=306)	Ranitidine 75 mg (N=309)	Placebo (N=306)
Treatment meal AUC (mm·hr)	94.6±5.91	88.6±4.97	98.8±4.83
Reduction in treatment meal AUC (%)	45.4±3.08	43.4±3.20	39.2±3.05
Treatment meal peak heartburn severity (mm)	42.4±1.80	43.4±1.60	46.8±1.61
Peak heartburn reduction (%)	39.7±2.47	37.4±2.30	32.8±2.29

(cont'd)

Table 5: Zantac Maximum Strength Non-Prescription *(cont'd)*

Prevention Data for Key Efficacy Variables (Intent-to-treat subjects) Supporting Study

Efficacy Variable	Ranitidine 150 mg (N=306)	Ranitidine 75 mg (N=309)	Placebo (N=306)
Largest consecutive time points with no heartburn	5.5±0.32[a]	5.2±0.30	4.4±0.29

[a] p≤0.05 versus placebo.

In pooled data of the 2 studies reflected in Table 4, ranitidine 150 mg was effective in preventing meal-related heartburn. Ranitidine 75 mg was statistically significantly better than placebo for the primary endpoint in one of the 2 pivotal clinical trials and in the pooled analysis, but was less consistently effective than ranitidine 150 mg in the prevention pivotal trials.

INDICATIONS: Zantac Tablets are indicated for fast and effective relief, treatment, and prevention, day or night, of the burning and discomfort of acid indigestion (dyspepsia), heartburn, hyperacidity, sour stomach, and upset stomach associated with excess stomach acid. These symptoms may be brought on by consuming food and beverages.

CONTRAINDICATIONS: Zantac (ranitidine hydrochloride) is contraindicated for patients known to have hypersensitivity to any component of the preparation.

WARNINGS: Gastric Carcinoma: Treatment with a histamine H_2-antagonist may mask symptoms associated with carcinoma of the stomach and, therefore, may delay diagnosis of that condition. Accordingly, patients should be advised to consult a physician if they have difficulty swallowing or persistent abdominal discomfort or if symptoms get worse or persist for more than 2 weeks.
Use in Patients with a History of Acute Porphyria: Rare clinical reports suggest that ranitidine may precipitate acute porphyric attacks. Therefore, ranitidine should be avoided in patients with a history of acute porphyria.
Pregnancy: The safety of Zantac in the treatment of conditions where a controlled reduction of gastric secretion is required during pregnancy has not been established. Reproduction studies performed in rats and rabbits at higher doses have revealed no evidence of ranitidine induced impaired fertility or harm to the fetus. Nevertheless, if the administration of ranitidine is considered to be necessary, its use requires that the potential benefits be weighed against possible hazards to the patient and to the fetus.
Lactation: Ranitidine is secreted in breast milk in lactating mothers but the clinical significance of this has not been fully evaluated. Women who are breast feeding are advised to speak with their doctor before taking Zantac Tablets.

PRECAUTIONS: Use in Impaired Renal Function: Ranitidine is excreted via the kidneys and, in the presence of severe renal impairment, plasma levels of ranitidine are increased and elimination prolonged. Accordingly, Zantac should be used under physician supervision for these patients.
Drug Interactions: Although ranitidine has been reported to bind weakly to cytochrome P450 in vitro, recommended doses of the drug do not inhibit the action of the hepatic cytochrome P450-linked oxygenase enzymes. A review of selected publications of controlled clinical drug interaction studies, at the level of hepatic elimination has indicated ranitidine is unlikely to cause clinically significant potentiation of actions of drugs which are inactivated by the hepatic cytochrome P450 enzyme system; these drugs may include: diazepam, phenytoin, propranolol, theophylline, and warfarin. Sporadic cases (approximately 1 case per 4 million patient treatments) of drug interactions have been reported in elderly patients involving both hypoglycaemic drugs and theophylline. The significance of these reports can not be determined at present, as controlled clinical trials have not shown interactions. These reports are based on use for prescription indications and dosage. Patients consuming NSAIDs may have dyspepsia as a side effect of these medicines and should consult a physician or a pharmacist before taking Zantac.
Antacids: Concurrent administration of high-dose antacids (75 mEq) with ranitidine is not recommended. The absorption of ranitidine may be decreased. Patients should be cautioned not to take antacids within ½ to 1 hour of ranitidine ingestion.
Ketoconazole: Simultaneous administration of ketoconazole and ranitidine may result in reduction of the absorption of ketoconazole by some mechanism as yet unidentified (e.g., a pH dependent effect on absorption or a change of volume of distribution). Patients should be cautioned not to take ranitidine for at least 2 hours after ketoconazole. These reports are based on use of prescription indications and dosage.
Sucralfate: If high doses of sucralfate (two grams) are co-administered with Zantac, the absorption of Zantac may be reduced. This effect is not seen if sucralfate is taken at least two hours after Zantac administration. These reports are based on use of prescription indications and dosage.
Procainamide: Ranitidine is believed to compete for active renal tubular secretion and/or inhibit the absorption of procainamide. Data indicates adjustment of procainamide doses in the elderly, patients with renal insufficiency, and patients receiving high doses of ranitidine is warranted. These reports are based on use for prescription indications and dosage.
Interactions with the following drugs have been reported with prescription strength ranitidine: Alendronate, amoxicillin, clavulanic acid, cefditoren, cefpodoxime, ceftibuten, delavirdine, dicumarol, diltiazem, enoxacin, fluvastatin, fosphenytoin, gefitinib, glyburide, itraconazole metformin, midazolam, miglitol, nisoldipine, pancreatin, pancrelipase, pancuronium, pentoxifylline, sucralfate, tolazoline, triamterene, triazolam, tubocurarine.
In a ranitidine-triazolam drug-drug interaction study, triazolam plasma concentrations were higher during b.i.d. dosing of ranitidine than triazolam given alone. The mean area under the triazolam concentration-time curve (AUC) values in 18- to 60-year-old subjects were 10% and 28% higher following administration of 75-mg and 150-mg ranitidine tablets, respectively, than triazolam given alone. In subjects older than 60 years of age, the mean AUC values were approximately 30% higher following administration of 75-mg and 150-mg ranitidine tablets. It appears that there were no changes in pharmacokinetics of triazolam and (alpha)-hydroxytriazolam, a major metabolite, and in their elimination. Reduced gastric acidity due to ranitidine may have resulted in an increase in the availability of triazolam. The clinical significance of this triazolam and ranitidine pharmacokinetic interaction is unknown.
Ethanol: Consumption of moderate amounts of alcohol is unlikely to result in clinically important alterations in blood alcohol concentrations and/or alcohol metabolism. The co-administration of a single oral dose of ranitidine 75 mg and ethanol 0.15 g/Kg has no clinically relevant effect on ethanol pharmacokinetics as shown in a double-blind placebo-controlled, crossover study in 25 healthy subjects.
Geriatrics: Since malignancy is more common in the elderly, particular consideration must be given to this before therapy with Zantac is instituted. Elderly patients receiving NSAIDs concomitantly with Zantac should be closely supervised. As with all medication, in the elderly, consideration should be given to concurrent drug therapy.

ADVERSE EFFECTS: Zantac (ranitidine) has been shown to be generally very well tolerated. In various clinical trials involving either 75 mg or 150 mg of Zantac the adverse reaction rates were comparable with the most frequently reported adverse events being: headache, nausea, vomiting, and diarrhea: common [frequent] >1% and <10%. Overall adverse event incidence among ranitidine-treated subjects was comparable to that seen in placebo-treated subjects, (no statistical difference) independent of demographic characteristics.
The following adverse reactions have been reported as events in clinical trials, in post-marketing surveillance, or in the routine management of patients treated with prescription doses of ZANTAC (ranitidine hydrochloride). The majority of these events have been observed following oral administration of higher prescription doses of ranitidine, and a causal relationship to ZANTAC has not always been established.
Central Nervous System: headache, sometimes severe; malaise; dizziness; somnolence; insomnia; vertigo; dystonia; and reversible blurred vision suggestive of a change in accommodation. Isolated cases of reversible mental confusion, delusion, delirium, mania, agitation, depression, hallucinations have been reported, predominantly in severely ill elderly patients.
Cardiovascular: As with other H_2 receptor antagonists, there have been rare reports of arrhythmias such as tachycardia, premature ventricular beats, bradycardia, and atrioventricular block.
Gastrointestinal: constipation, diarrhea, nausea/vomiting and abdominal discomfort/pain. Rebound hypersecretion has been reported upon withdrawal of ranitidine therapy.
Hepatic: Transient and reversible changes in liver function tests can occur (increase in ALT and AST values). With oral administration, there have been occasional reports of hepatitis, hepatocellular or hepatocanalicular or mixed with or without jaundice and cholestatic jaundice. In such circumstances, ranitidine should be discontinued immediately. These are usually reversible, but in exceedingly rare circumstances, death has occurred.
Musculoskeletal: Rare reports of arthralgia and myalgia.
Hematologic: Blood count changes (anemia, leukopenia, thrombocytopenia) have occurred in a few patients. These are usually reversible. Rare cases of agranulocytosis, pancytopenia, or neutropenia, sometimes with marrow hypoplasia or aplasia have been reported.
Endocrine: No clinically significant interference with endocrine or gonadal function has been reported. There have been rare reports of breast symptoms in men taking ranitidine.
Dermatologic: rash, including cases suggestive of mild erythema multiforme. Alopecia, contact dermatitis, photosensitivity.
Other: Rare cases of hypersensitivity reactions (including angina, chest pain, bronchospasm, fever, rash, eosinophilia, anaphylaxis, urticaria, angioneurotic edema, hypotension) and small increases in serum creatinine have occasionally occurred after a single dose. Acute pancreatitis, meningitis, nephrotoxicity has been reported rarely. Rare cases of reversible involuntary motor disturbances and intraocular pressure changes have been reported.

OVERDOSE:
Symptoms: There is no experience to date with deliberate overdosage.
Treatment: The usual measures to remove unabsorbed drug from the gastrointestinal tract (including activated charcoal or syrup of ipecac), clinical monitoring and supportive therapy should be employed. Also, if need be, the drug can be removed from the plasma by haemodialysis. Up to 6 g per day has been administered without untoward effect.

For management of a suspected drug overdose, CPhA recommends that you contact your **regional Poison Control Centre**. See the *CPS* Directory section for a list of Poison Control Centres.

DOSAGE: Adults and Children 16 Years of Age and Older: One tablet should be taken when symptoms appear, day or night. If symptoms persist for more than 1 hour or return after 1 hour, a second tablet may be taken. The maximum dosage is 2 tablets (150 mg ranitidine for the 75 mg strength tablet or 300 mg for the 150 mg strength tablet) in a 24 hour period.
For prevention of symptoms brought on by consuming food or beverages, 1 tablet should be taken 30 to 60 minutes before eating a meal or consuming beverages expected to cause symptoms.
Patients are advised to consult their physician if symptoms get worse or continue after 14 days of treatment.
Children Under 16 Years: Children under 16 years of age should be supervised by a physician.

INFORMATION FOR THE PATIENT: Published in e-CPS, available by subscription at www.e-cps.ca.

SUPPLIED: Zantac: Each pink, five-sided, biconvex, film-coated tablet, with "Z" engraved on one side and "75" on the other, contains: ranitidine HCl 84 mg equivalent to ranitidine anhydrous free base 75 mg. Nonmedicinal ingredients: tablet: magnesium stearate and microcrystalline cellulose; film-coating: hypromellose, iron oxide, titanium dioxide and triacetin. Gluten-, sodium- and sucrose-free. Blister packs of 4, 10 and 30. Bottles of 60 and 124. Store between 15 and 30°C. Avoid excessive humidity.
Zantac Maximum Strength Non-Prescription: Each dark pink, five-sided, biconvex, film-coated tablet with "Z" engraved on one side and "150" on the other, contains: ranitidine HCl 168 mg (ranitidine 150 mg anhydrous free base). Nonmedicinal ingredients: tablet: magnesium stearate and microcrystalline cellulose; film-coating: hypromellose, iron oxide, titanium dioxide and triacetin. Also contains synthetic red iron oxide. Gluten-, sodium- and sucrose-free. Blister packs of 3, 8 and 24. Bottles of 50 and 95. Store between 15 and 30°C. Avoid excessive humidity.

Zap®

star anise oil (Illicium verum)

Head Lice Treatment

PendoPharm

SUPPLIED: Each pack contains: a spray-on lotion and a rigid fine-toothed comb specially designed to remove lice and their eggs (nits). Spray contains enough lotion for up to 8 applications. Medicinal ingredient: star anise oil (Illicium verum). Nonmedicinal ingredients: caprylic/capric triglyceride (fractionated coconut oil), isopropyl alcohol, Cananga odorata (Ylang-Ylang) flower oil. Plastic bottles of 60 mL. Spray contains enough lotion for up to 8 applications. Store at room temperature (15-30°C). Caution: flammable. For external use only.

The reader is invited to consult CPhA's monograph **Thiazide Diuretics**.

Zaroxolyn® Pr

metolazone

Diuretic—Antihypertensive

sanofi-aventis

Date of Revision: December 15, 2006

PHARMACOLOGY: Metolazone is a diuretic antihypertensive drug for the treatment of edema.
Metolazone is a quinazoline diuretic, with properties generally similar to the thiazide diuretics. The actions of metolazone result from interference with the renal tubular mechanism of electrolyte reabsorption. Metolazone acts primarily to inhibit sodium reabsorption at the cortical diluting site and to a lesser extent in the proximal convoluted tubule. Sodium and chloride ions are excreted in approximately equivalent amounts. The increased delivery of sodium to the distal-tubular exchange site results in increased potassium excretion.
Metolazone does not inhibit carbonic anhydrase. A proximal action has been shown in humans by increased excretion of phosphate and magnesium ions, and by a markedly increased fractional excretion of sodium in patients with severely compromised glomerular filtration.
The antihypertensive mechanism of action of metolazone is not fully understood but is presumed to be related to its saluretic and diuretic properties.
Pharmacokinetics: Metolazone is absorbed rapidly; however, rate and extent of absorption is dependent on the formulation. Table 1 shows that bioavailability of metolazone is different from Mykrox (another product containing metolazone).

Table 1: Zaroxolyn

Pharmacokinetic Variables of Metolazone[a]

Formulation	0-48h AUC ng·h/mL	0-∞ AUC ng·h/mL	C_{MAX} ng/mL	T_{MAX} h
Metolazone soln 2.5 mg	230.59 (61.96)	235.4 (61.50)	37.50 (9.91)	1.25 (0.44)
Mykrox 2.5 mg	199.40 (36.38)	209.4 (41.00)	18.75 (2.58)	3.17 (1.03)
Zaroxolyn 2.5 mg	99.74 (28.97)	127.0 (37.08)	3.63 (0.87)	7.67 (6.65)

[a] Values presented are means (±SD).

Clinical studies have shown that 90 to 95% of metolazone is bound to red blood cells and plasma protein. The prolonged duration of action of metolazone is attributed to its protein binding and allows for once a day dosing. Only a small amount of metolazone is metabolized. Most of the drug is excreted in the unconverted form in the urine.
When metolazone is given, diuresis and saluresis usually begin within one hour and persist for 24 hours depending on the dose. The effect may be prolonged beyond 24 hours particularly at the higher recommended dosages.

INDICATIONS: For the treatment of edema accompanying congestive heart failure and edema accompanying renal diseases including the nephrotic syndrome, and states of diminished renal function. Metolazone (2.5 mg) has also been used in the management of mild to moderate essential hypertension, alone or in combination with other antihypertensive drugs of a different class.

CONTRAINDICATIONS: In anuria, in hepatic coma or pre-coma, and in cases of known allergy and hypersensitivity to metolazone.

WARNINGS: Rarely, the rapid onset of severe hyponatremia and/or hypokalemia has been reported following initial doses of thiazide and non-thiazide diuretics. When symptoms consistent with severe electrolyte imbalance appear rapidly, the drug should be discontinued and supportive measures should be initiated immediately. The appropriateness of therapy with this class of drug should be carefully re-evaluated.

Hypokalemia may occur, with consequent weakness, cramps, and cardiac arrhythmias. Hypokalemia is a particular hazard in digitalized patients or those who have had or have a ventricular arrhythmia; dangerous or fatal arrhythmias may be precipitated. Serum potassium should be determined at regular intervals, and dose reduction, potassium supplementation or addition of a potassium-sparing diuretic instituted if indicated. Hypokalemia is dose-related (see Precautions).

Azotemia and hyperuricemia may be noted or precipitated during the administration of metolazone. Infrequently, gouty attacks have been reported in persons with a history of gout. If azotemia and oliguria worsen during treatment of patients with severe renal disease, metolazone should be discontinued.

Unusually large or prolonged losses of fluid and electrolytes may result when metolazone is administered concomitantly to patients receiving furosemide.

Particular care must be taken, especially during initial therapy, when metolazone is used with other antihypertensive drugs of a different class to avoid excessive reduction in blood pressure (see Precautions, Drug Interactions).

PRECAUTIONS: All patients receiving metolazone should have serum electrolytes measured at appropriate intervals and be observed for clinical signs of fluid and/or electrolyte imbalance; namely, hyponatremia, hypochloremic alkalosis, and hypokalemia. Serum and urine electrolyte determinations are particularly important when the patient is vomiting excessively, has severe diarrhea, or is receiving parenteral fluids.

The risk of hypokalemia is increased when larger doses are used; when diuresis is rapid; when severe liver disease is present; when corticosteroids are given concomitantly; when oral intake of potassium is inadequate or when excess potassium is being lost extrarenally, such as with vomiting or diarrhea.

Hyponatremia may occur at any time during long-term therapy and, on rare occasions, may be life-threatening (see Warnings).

Warning signs of electrolyte imbalance irrespective of cause are: dryness of mouth; thirst; weakness; lethargy; drowsiness; restlessness; muscle pains or cramps; muscular fatigue; hypotension; oliguria; tachycardia; and gastrointestinal disturbances such as nausea and vomiting.

Use of diuretics similar to metolazone have been associated, on rare occasions, with pathologic changes in the parathyroid glands. This possibility should be kept in mind with clinical use of metolazone. Hypercalcemia has been noted in a few patients.

Sulfonamide derivatives have been reported to exacerbate or activate systemic lupus erythematosus.

Orthostatic hypotension may occur; this may be potentiated by alcohol, barbiturates, narcotics, or concurrent therapy with other antihypertensive drugs.

Special caution should be used in treating patients with severe hepatic disease since metolazone may induce metabolic alkalosis in cases of potassium depletion which may precipitate episodes of hepatic encephalopathy (see Contraindications).

Caution should be observed when administering metolazone to patients with severely impaired renal function. As most of the drug is excreted by the renal route, cumulative effects may be seen (see Contraindications).

Metolazone may raise blood glucose concentrations, possibly causing hyperglycemia and glycosuria in patients with diabetes or latent diabetes.

Laboratory Tests: Periodic determination of serum electrolytes; blood urea nitrogen; uric acid; and glucose levels should be assessed at appropriate intervals during metolazone therapy (see Warnings).

Drug Interactions: Alcohol, barbiturates, or narcotics: See Precautions.

Antihypertensives: See Warnings and Precautions. When metolazone is used with other antihypertensive drugs, particular care must be taken, especially during initial therapy. Dosage of other antihypertensive agents, especially the ganglionic blockers and quanethidine, should be reduced. Hydralazine in therapeutic doses may interfere with the natruretic action of metolazone.

Corticosteroids or ACTH Therapy: May increase the risk of hypokalemia and increase salt and water retention.

Curariform Drugs: Diuretic-induced hypokalemia may enhance neuromuscular blocking effects of curariform drugs (such as tubocurarine). The most serious effect would be respiratory depression which could proceed to apnea. Accordingly, it is advisable to discontinue metolazone tablets 3 days before elective surgery.

Digitalis: See Warnings.

Drugs Used to Treat Gout: See Warnings. Dosage adjustment of the gout medication may be necessary to control hyperuricemia and gout.

Furosemide and Other Loop Diuretics: See Warnings. Unusually large or prolonged losses of fluids and electrolytes may result.

Insulin and Oral Antidiabetic Agents: Adjustment of dosage may be necessary. See Precautions.

Lithium: See Warnings.

Methenamine: Efficacy may be decreased due to urinary alkalizing effect of metolazone.

Salicylates and Other NSAIDs: May antagonize natruretic, diuretic and antihypertensive effects of metolazone. Patients should be monitored carefully.

Sympathomimetics: May decrease the antihypertensive effect of metolazone. Metolazone may decrease arterial responsiveness to norepinephrine, but this diminution is not sufficient to preclude effectiveness of the pressor agent for therapeutic use.

Pregnancy: Since metolazone crosses the placenta and appears in cord blood, its administration to women of childbearing age requires that the potential benefits of the drug be weighed against its possible hazards to the fetus. The potential effects on the fetus include fetal or neonatal jaundice, thrombocytopenia, and possibly other adverse reactions which have occurred in the adult. However, teratogenic studies in mice, rats and rabbits have not shown teratologic effects in these animals.

Lactation: Metolazone appears in breast milk. Thus, it is possible that the effects of metolazone may occur in the newborn under these circumstances. If the use of metolazone is deemed essential for a nursing mother, the patient should stop nursing.

Children: Safety and effectiveness in children have not been established; therefore, metolazone is not recommended for use in the pediatric age group.

ADVERSE EFFECTS: The following adverse reactions have been reported. Several are single or comparably rare occurrences. Adverse reactions are listed in decreasing order of severity within body systems.

Cardiovascular: chest pain/discomfort, orthostatic hypotension, excessive volume depletion, hemoconcentration, venous thrombosis, palpitations.

Central and Peripheral Nervous System: syncope, neuropathy, vertigo, paresthesias, psychotic depression, impotence, dizziness/lightheadedness, drowsiness, fatigue, weakness, restlessness (sometimes resulting in insomnia), headache.

Dermatologic/Hypersensitivity: necrotizing angitis (cutaneous vasculitis), purpura, dermatitis (photosensitivity), urticaria and skin rashes.

Gastrointestinal: hepatitis: intrahepatic cholestatic jaundice, pancreatitis, vomiting, nausea, epigastric distress, diarrhea, constipation, anorexia, abdominal bloating.

Hematologic: aplastic/hypoplastic anemia, agranulocytosis, leukopenia.

Metabolic: hypokalemia, hyponatremia, hyperuricemia, hypochloremia, hypochloremic alkalosis, hyperglycemia, glycosuria, increase in serum urea nitrogen (BUN) or creatinine, hypophosphatemia (see Warnings and Precautions).

Musculoskeletal: joint pain, acute gouty attacks, muscle cramps or spasm.

Other: transient blurred vision, chills.

In addition, adverse reactions reported with similar antihypertensive diuretics, but which have not been reported to date for metolazone, include: bitter taste, dry mouth, sialadenitis, xanthopsia, respiratory distress (including pneumonitis), thrombocytopenia and anaphylactic reactions. These reactions should be considered as possible occurrences with clinical usage of metolazone.

Whenever adverse reactions are moderate or severe, metolazone dosage should be reduced or therapy withdrawn.

OVERDOSE:

Symptoms: Orthostatic hypotension, dizziness, drowsiness, syncope, diuresis with accompanying electrolyte abnormalities, hemoconcentration and hemodynamic changes due to plasma volume depletion may occur. In some instances, depressed respiration may be observed. At high doses, lethargy of varying degree may appear and may progress to coma within a few hours. Also, gastrointestinal irritation and hypermotility may occur. Temporary elevation of BUN has been reported, especially in patients with impairment of renal function.

Treatment: There is no specific antidote available, but immediate evacuation of the stomach contents is advised. Care should be taken when evacuating the gastric contents to prevent aspiration, especially in the stuporous or comatose patient. Dialysis is not likely to be effective. Supportive measures should be initiated as required to maintain hydration, electrolyte balance, respiration and cardiovascular and renal functions.

Serum electrolyte change, and cardiovascular and renal functions, should be closely monitored.

For management of a suspected drug overdose, CPhA recommends that you contact your **regional Poison Control Centre**. See the *CPS* Directory section for a list of Poison Control Centres.

DOSAGE: Effective dosage of metolazone should be individualized according to indications and patient response. A single daily dose is recommended. Therapy with metolazone should be titrated to gain an initial therapeutic response and to determine the minimal dose possible to maintain the desired therapeutic response.

Usual Dosages: Edema: Edema of cardiac failure: 5 to 10 mg, once daily. Edema of renal disease: 5 to 20 mg, once daily.

Treatment of Edematous States: The time interval for the initial dosage to show effect may vary; diuresis and saluresis usually begin within 1 hour and persist for 12 to 24 hours, depending on dosage. When a desired therapeutic effect has been obtained, it may be advisable to reduce the dose, if possible. The daily dose depends on the severity of the patient's condition, sodium intake and responsiveness. A decision to change the daily dose should be based upon the results of thorough clinical and laboratory determinations. If antihypertensive drugs or diuretics are given concurrently with metolazone, more careful dosage adjustment may be necessary. For patients with congestive cardiac failure who tend to experience paroxysmal nocturnal dyspnea, it is usually advisable to employ a dosage near the upper end of the range to ensure prolongation of diuresis and saluresis for a full 24-hour period.

Hypertension: Mild to moderate essential hypertension: 2.5 to 5 mg, once daily.

Treatment of Hypertension: The time interval required for the initial dosage regimen of metolazone to show effect may vary from 3 to 4 days to 3 to 6 weeks in the treatment of elevated blood pressure. Doses should be adjusted at appropriate intervals to achieve maximum therapeutic effect.

SUPPLIED: Each pink, slightly biconvex tablet, debossed with its numeric strength on one side and "ZAROXOLYN" on the other contains: metolazone 2.5 mg. Nonmedicinal ingredients: cellulose, D&C Red #33 aluminum lake and magnesium stearate. Alcohol-, gluten-, lactose-, paraben-, sucrose- and tartrazine-free. HDPE bottles of 100. Store at room temperature and protect from light. Dispense from tight, light-resistant containers.

(Shown in Product Identification Section)

Zavesca® Ⓟ

miglustat

Glucosylceramide Synthase Inhibitor

Actelion

Date of Revision: March 3, 2010

SUMMARY PRODUCT INFORMATION:

Route of Administration	Dosage Form/ Strength	Nonmedicinal Ingredients
Oral	Capsule, 100 mg	See Dosage Forms, Composition and Packaging.

INDICATIONS AND CLINICAL USE: ZAVESCA (miglustat) is indicated for the treatment of adult patients with mild to moderate Type 1 Gaucher disease for whom enzyme replacement therapy is not a therapeutic option (e.g. due to constraints such as allergy, hypersensitivity, or poor venous access).

ZAVESCA is indicated to slow the progression of some of the neurological manifestations in patients with Niemann-Pick Type C disease.

Geriatrics: There is no experience with the use of ZAVESCA in patients over the age of 70.

Pediatrics: There is no experience with the use of ZAVESCA in patients with type 1 Gaucher disease under the age of 18. Patients below 4 years of age were not enrolled in the prospective study of ZAVESCA in Niemann-Pick type C disease.

CONTRAINDICATIONS: ZAVESCA is contraindicated in patients who are hypersensitive to miglustat or to any excipient in the formulation.

ZAVESCA is contraindicated in women who are or may become pregnant. If ZAVESCA is administered to women of reproductive potential, they should be informed of the potential hazard to the foetus. See Warnings and Precautions.

WARNINGS AND PRECAUTIONS: Therapy should be directed by physicians knowledgeable in the management of patients with Gaucher disease or Niemann-Pick Type C disease, as appropriate.

The consumer information should be reviewed with the patient.

General: Severe Gaucher Disease: The safety and efficacy of ZAVESCA have not been specifically evaluated in patients with severe Gaucher disease.

Switching from Enzyme Replacement Therapy to ZAVESCA in Gaucher Disease: Switching to ZAVESCA should be considered only for patients who have had their disease well stabilized on enzyme replacement therapy.

Niemann-Pick Type C Disease: The benefit of treatment with ZAVESCA for neurological manifestations in patients with Niemann-Pick Type C disease should be evaluated on a regular basis to assess the benefit of continuing therapy with ZAVESCA.

Gastrointestinal: Gastrointestinal events, mainly diarrhea, have been observed in more than 85% of patients, either at the outset of treatment or intermittently during treatment. The mechanism is probably inhibition of disaccharidases in the gastrointestinal tract. The majority of cases are mild and are expected to resolve spontaneously on therapy. In clinical practice, diarrhea has been observed to respond to diet modification (reduction of lactose and other carbohydrate intake), to taking ZAVESCA away from meals, and/or to anti-diarrheal medication such as loperamide. In some patients, temporary dose reduction may be necessary. Discontinuation may be necessary if symptoms persist or become severe. Patients with chronic diarrhea or other persistent gastrointestinal events that do not respond to these interventions should be investigated according to clinical practice. ZAVESCA has not been evaluated in patients with a history of significant gastrointestinal disease, including inflammatory bowel disease.

Hematologic: Mild reductions in platelet counts without association to bleeding were observed in some patients with Niemann-Pick Type C disease treated with ZAVESCA. In patients included in the clinical trial, 40%-50% of patients had platelet counts below the lower limit of normal at baseline. Monitoring of platelet counts is recommended in these patients.

Sexual Function/Reproduction: Patients should be informed of the potential hazard to the foetus.

Females: See Contraindications. ZAVESCA is contraindicated in women who are or may become pregnant. All females should have a pregnancy test before using ZAVESCA. Women of child bearing potential taking ZAVESCA should use a reliable method of contraception.

Males: Male patients should maintain reliable contraceptive methods while taking ZAVESCA and should be informed that it may affect the semen. Female partners of male patients treated with ZAVESCA should also consider reliable contraception.

Studies in rats have shown that miglustat adversely affects spermatogenesis, sperm parameters and reduces fertility. These effects were seen at doses that gave similar exposure as the proposed human therapeutic dose.

Until further information is available, it is advised that before seeking to conceive, male patients should cease ZAVESCA and maintain reliable contraceptive methods for three months thereafter.

Renal: ZAVESCA should be used with caution in patients with renal impairment.

Miglustat is known to be substantially excreted by the kidney, and the risk of adverse reactions to this drug may be greater in patients with impaired renal function. The clearance of miglustat is decreased by 40 to 60% in patients with mild to moderate renal impairment, and up to 70% in patients with severe renal impairment. As a result of this, dose reductions are recommended for those patients with mild to moderate renal impairment, the reduction being dependent upon the level of their creatinine clearance adjustment. For those patients with severe renal impairment, treatment with miglustat is not recommended. Since elderly patients are more likely to have decreased renal function, care should be taken in dose selection, and it may be useful to monitor renal function.

Neurologic: Cases of peripheral neuropathy and tremor have been reported in patients treated with ZAVESCA with or without concurrent conditions such as vitamin B_{12} deficiency and monoclonal gammopathy. Peripheral neuropathy seems to be more common in patients with type 1 Gaucher disease compared to the general population.

All patients should undergo baseline and repeat neurological evaluation. Patients who develop symptoms such as numbness and tingling should have a careful re-assessment of risk-benefit.

Hepatic/Biliary/Pancreatic: ZAVESCA has not been evaluated in patients with moderate to severe hepatic impairment.

Carcinogenesis and Mutagenesis: Miglustat was not mutagenic or clastogenic in a battery of in vitro and in vivo assays including the bacterial reverse mutation (Ames), chromosomal aberration (in human lymphocytes), gene mutation in mammalian cells (Chinese hamster ovary), and mouse micronucleus tests. ZAVESCA causes an increased incidence of interstitial cell adenomas in male rats. In both male and female mice, the administration of ZAVESCA resulted in an increased incidence of inflammatory, hyperplastic and neoplastic lesions in the large intestine.

Dependence/Tolerance: The dependence potential of ZAVESCA has not been evaluated in human studies.

Special Populations: Pregnant Women: There are no adequate and well-controlled studies of miglustat in pregnant women. ZAVESCA should not be used during pregnancy. See Contraindications.

Nursing Women: ZAVESCA should not be used in nursing mothers unless the potential benefit justifies the potential risk to the infant.

Pediatrics: There is no experience with the use of ZAVESCA in patients with Type 1 Gaucher disease under the age of 18. Patients below 4 years of age were not enrolled in the prospective study of ZAVESCA in Niemann-Pick Type C disease. See Dosage and Administration.

Reduced growth has been reported in some pediatric patients with Niemann-Pick Type C disease in the early phase of treatment with ZAVESCA where the initial reduced weight gain may be accompanied or followed by reduced height gain. Growth should be monitored in pediatric and juvenile patients during treatment with ZAVESCA; the benefit/risk balance should be reassessed on an individual basis for continuation of therapy.

Geriatrics: Clinical studies of ZAVESCA did not include sufficient numbers of patients aged 65 and over to determine whether they respond differently from younger patients. Other reported clinical experience has not identified differences in responses between the elderly and younger patients. In general, dose selection for an elderly patient should be cautious, usually starting at the low end of the dosing range, reflecting the greater frequency of decreased hepatic, renal, and cardiac function and of concomitant disease or other drug therapy.

Monitoring and Laboratory Tests: Patients with Type 1 Gaucher disease should have their disease status regularly monitored by assessment of spleen and liver volumes and hematologic analysis. Regular monitoring of vitamin B_{12} level is recommended because of the high prevalence of vitamin B_{12} deficiency in patients with Type 1 Gaucher disease. Monitoring of platelet counts and renal function is recommended in patients treated for Niemann-Pick Type C disease with ZAVESCA (see Warnings and Precautions, Hematologic and Renal).

ZAVESCA has not been evaluated in patients with a history of or in the presence of cataracts. Regular follow-up is recommended in these patients.

Occupational Hazards: No studies on the effects on the ability to drive or to use machinery have been performed. Dizziness has been reported as a very common adverse event and patients suffering from dizziness should not drive or operate machinery.

ADVERSE REACTIONS: Adverse Drug Reaction Overview: Type 1 Gaucher Disease: All 80 patients with Type 1 Gaucher disease in the combined data set from the clinical studies reported at least one adverse event during their treatment period. These events appeared at the outset of treatment or occurred intermittently during treatment. The most frequent (very common) adverse events were diarrhea (69 patients, 86%), weight decrease (51 patients, 64%), flatulence (36 patients, 45%), and abdominal pain (34 patients, 43%). Tremor was reported by 18 patients (23%). Headache, nausea, and dizziness were reported by 10-20% of patients. The majority of cases were mild or moderate in severity, and resolved spontaneously, after dose reduction, or upon treatment discontinuation. See Warnings and Precautions. All other treatment-related adverse events (constipation, paresthesia, generalized weakness, cramps, loss of appetite, visual disturbance, and thrombocytopenia) were reported by <10% of patients.

Fourteen (18%) of the 80 patients exposed to ZAVESCA for up to 42 months withdrew from the study due to an adverse event. The most frequent adverse events leading to withdrawal were associated with gastrointestinal (diarrhea, flatulence, abdominal pain) or neurological symptoms (tremor, headache, dizziness and paresthesia). With regard to all patients enrolled during the first 6 months of treatment, withdrawals due to adverse events were more common in the 100 mg TID ZAVESCA treatment group (9 patients, 11%) than in the 50 mg TID ZAVESCA (5 patients, 6%) or Combination (2 patients, 3%) treatment groups.

Twenty-three (29%) patients had an adverse event that resulted in a dose reduction. The most common of these adverse events were diarrhea, weight loss, and tremor. During the first 6 months of treatment, dose reductions due to adverse events were more common in the combination treatment group than in the 100 mg TID ZAVESCA and 50 mg TID ZAVESCA treatment groups. The percentage of patients who had dose reductions due to an adverse event was similar in the 100 mg TID and 50 mg TID ZAVESCA treatment groups (6% and 4%, respectively).

Niemann-Pick Type C Disease: Of the 40 Niemann-Pick Type C patients, 97.5% (39 patients) experienced at least one adverse event during their treatment period. The most frequently occurring adverse events were diarrhea in 82.5% (33 patients), weight decrease in 60.0% (24 patients), tremor in 57.5% (23 patients), and flatulence in 55% (22 patients).

Nine patients withdrew from the study because of an adverse event including two from the pediatric population.

Serious Adverse Drug Reactions: Three non-fatal serious adverse events reported by two patients were considered to be related to ZAVESCA (neuritis and neuropathy; neuropathy) and these events occurred after 65 weeks of treatment (one event occurred 2.5 months after ZAVESCA discontinuation).

In patients with Type 1 Gaucher disease, isolated additional serious adverse drug reactions were reported from ongoing studies and include the following: gastrointestinal polyposis, and cerebellar syndrome.

In patients with Niemann-Pick Type C disease, 11 patients reported a total of 23 serious adverse events. The most frequent serious adverse events were infections and infestations and gastrointestinal disorders. None of the serious adverse events leading to discontinuation was considered related to ZAVESCA treatment.

Clinical Trial Adverse Drug Reactions: Because clinical trials are conducted under very specific conditions the adverse reaction rates observed in the clinical trials may not reflect the rates observed in practice and should not be compared to the rates in the clinical trials of another drug. Adverse drug reaction information from clinical trials is useful for identifying drug-related adverse events and for approximating rates.

Type 1 Gaucher Disease: Information presented in this section represents ZAVESCA-treated patients from the primary (0-12 months) and extension (12-42 months) phases of study OGT 918-001, and ZAVESCA-treated patients from the primary (0-6 months) and extension (6-24 months) phases of studies OGT 918-003 and OGT 918-004. A total of 80 patients were treated with ZAVESCA and were included in the safety population. This included 28 patients from study OGT 918-001 (100 mg TID), 18 patients from study OGT 918-003 (50 mg TID), and 33 patients from study OGT 918-004 (100 mg TID). Patients exposed to ZAVESCA in study OGT 918-004 included those patients who were treated with ZAVESCA 100 mg TID (12 patients) or with combination therapy ZAVESCA 100 mg TID and Cerezyme (12 patients), as well as 10 patients who switched to ZAVESCA 100 mg TID during the extension phase (6-12 months) following treatment with Cerezyme alone during the primary phase of the study (0-6 months).

Adverse reactions by WHO body system and preferred term with an incidence of >1 patient treated with miglustat are presented in Table 1.

Table 1: ZAVESCA

Adverse Reactions by WHO Body System and Preferred Term Occurring in Type 1 Gaucher Disease Patients with an Incidence of >1 Patient Treated with Miglustat

Adverse Reaction	ZAVESCA n=80[a] n (%)
Gastrointestinal	
Diarrhea	69 (86)
Flatulence	36 (45)
Abdominal pain	34 (43)
Nausea	9 (11)
Constipation	7 (9)
Vomiting	3 (4)
Anorexia	2 (3)
Dyspepsia	2 (3)
Dry mouth	2 (3)
Metabolic and Nutritional Disorders	

(cont'd)

Table 1: ZAVESCA *(cont'd)*

Adverse Reactions by WHO Body System and Preferred Term Occurring in Type 1 Gaucher Disease Patients with an Incidence of >1 Patient Treated with Miglustat

Adverse Reaction	ZAVESCA n=80[a] n (%)
Weight decrease	51 (64)
Central and Peripheral Nervous Systems	
Tremor	18 (23)
Headache	12 (15)
Dizziness	8 (10)
Paresthesia	6 (8)
Neuropathy	3 (4)
Vertigo	2 (3)
Body as a Whole	
Generalized weakness	4 (5)
Influenza like symptoms	2 (3)
Fatigue	2 (3)
Abdominal distension	2 (3)
Musculoskeletal Disorders	
Muscle cramps	7 (9)
Cramps	4 (5)
Psychiatric Disorders	
Appetite absent	4 (5)
Vision Disorders	
Visual disturbance	4 (4)
Platelet, Bleeding, and Clotting Disorders	
Thrombocytopenia	4 (5)

[a] Patients include those from the primary (0-12 months) and extension (12-42 months) phases of Study OGT 918-001, and the primary (0-6 months) and extension (6-24 months) phases of Studies OGT 918-003 and OGT 918-004.

Niemann-Pick Type C Disease: The safety information of ZAVESCA in Niemann-Pick Type C disease presented in this section comes from a prospective open-label clinical trial. The clinical trial included 29 adult and juvenile patients in a 12-month controlled period, followed by extension therapy for an average total duration of 3.9 years and up to 5.6 years. In addition 12 pediatric patients were enrolled in an uncontrolled substudy for an overall average duration of 3.1 years and up to 4.4 years. Among the 40 patients exposed to ZAVESCA in the trial 14 patients were treated for more than 3 years. The usual dose of ZAVESCA in adult patients was 200 mg t.i.d., and was adjusted according to body surface area in pediatric patients.

Adverse events by WHO body system and preferred term with an incidence of >1 patient treated with miglustat are presented in Table 2 and Table 3.

Table 2: ZAVESCA

Adverse Events by WHO Body System and Preferred Term Occurring in Niemann-Pick Type C patients with an Incidence of >1 Patient Treated with Miglustat, Juvenile and Adult Patients

	Miglustat (N=20)[a] n (%)	No Treatment (N=9)[a] n (%)
Gastrointestinal System		
Diarrhea	17 (85)	4 (44)
Flatulence	14 (70)	0 (0)
Abdominal pain	9 (45)	0 (0)
Nausea	7 (35)	1 (11)
Vomiting	6 (30)	0 (0)
Abdominal distension	4 (20)	0 (0)
Abdominal discomfort	3 (15)	0 (0)
Central and Peripheral Nervous Systems		
Tremor	11 (55)	2 (22)
Headache	9 (45)	3 (33)
Gait spastic	5 (25)	1 (11)
Paresthesia	4 (20)	1 (11)
Dysphagia	4 (20)	4 (44)
Intention tremor	3 (15)	0 (0)

(cont'd)

Table 2: ZAVESCA *(cont'd)*

Adverse Events by WHO Body System and Preferred Term Occurring in Niemann-Pick Type C patients with an Incidence of >1 Patient Treated with Miglustat, Juvenile and Adult Patients

	Miglustat (N=20)[a] n (%)	No Treatment (N=9)[a] n (%)
Dystonia	3 (15)	2 (22)
Sensory loss	2 (10)	1 (11)
Gait abnormal	2 (10)	4 (44)
Dysarthria	2 (10)	1 (11)
Clonic convulsion	2 (10)	0 (0)
Ataxia	2 (10)	1 (11)
Investigations		
Weight decreased	13 (65)	0 (0)
Infections and Infestations		
Nasopharyngitis	7 (35)	3 (33)
Psychiatric Disorders		
Depression	4 (20)	0 (0)
Insomnia	6 (30)	0 (0)
Agitation	3 (15)	0 (0)
Sleep disorder	2 (10)	0 (0)
General Disorders and Administration Site Conditions		
Fatigue	7 (35)	1 (11)
Peripheral coldness	2 (10)	0 (0)
Fall	2 (10)	2 (22)
Influenza like illness	2 (10)	0 (0)
Injury, Poisoning and Procedural Complications		
Laceration	3 (15)	1 (11)
Contusion	3 (15)	0 (0)
Metabolism and Nutrition Disorders		
Appetite decreased	5 (25)	0 (0)
Musculoskeletal Disorders		
Pain in limb	2 (10)	2 (22)
Arthralgia	3 (15)	0 (0)
Muscle cramps	2 (10)	0 (0)

[a] Patients include those from the primary (0-12 months) phase of Study OGT 918-007 in juvenile and adult patients.

Table 3: ZAVESCA

Adverse Events by WHO Body System and Preferred Term Occurring in Niemann-Pick Type C Patients with an Incidence of >1 Patient Treated with Miglustat, Pediatric Patients

	Miglustat (N=12)[a] n (%)
Gastointestinal System	
Diarrhea	8 (67)
Vomiting	4 (33)
Flatulence	4 (33)
Abdominal pain	2 (17)
Central and Peripheral Nervous Systems	
Gait abnormal	4 (33)
Hyperreflexia	3 (25)
Dysphagia	3 (25)
Ataxia	3 (25)
Tremor aggravated	2 (17)
Tremor	2 (17)

(cont'd)

Table 3: ZAVESCA *(cont'd)*

Adverse Events by WHO Body System and Preferred Term Occurring in Niemann-Pick Type C Patients with an Incidence of >1 Patient Treated with Miglustat, Pediatric Patients

	Miglustat (N=12)[a] n (%)
Supranuclear palsy	2 (17)
Gait spastic	2 (17)
Dystonia	2 (17)
Headache	2 (17)
Saccadic eye movement	2 (17)
Investigations	
Weight decreased	3 (25)
Infections and Infestations	
Nasopharyngitis	4 (33)
Sinusitis	3 (25)
Respiratory tract infection	2 (17)
Gastroenteritis viral	2 (17)
Ear infection	2 (17)
General Disorders and Administration Site Conditions	
Fatigue	5 (42)
Lethargy	2 (17)
Fall	2 (17)
Dehydration	2 (17)
Respiratory, Thoracic and Mediastinal Disorders	
Cough	4 (33)
Epistaxis	2 (17)
Injury, Poisoning and Procedural Complications	
Laceration	2 (17)

[a] Patients include those from the primary (0-12 months) phase of Study OGT 918-007 in pediatric patients.

Gastrointestinal: Diarrhea: Diarrhea have been reported in approximately 85% of patients treated with ZAVESCA. See Warnings and Precautions.

Weight Loss: Weight loss has been observed in approximately 65% of patients. The greatest effect was at 12 months, with a mean weight loss of 6-7% of body weight.

Neurological: Approximately 30% of patients in clinical trials in Type 1 Gaucher and Niemann-Pick Type C diseases reported tremor on treatment. In Type 1 Gaucher disease, these tremors were described as an exaggerated physiological tremor of the hands. Tremor usually began within the first month, and in many cases resolved during treatment. Dose reduction may ameliorate the tremor, usually within days, but discontinuation of treatment may sometimes be required.

Cases of peripheral neuropathy have been reported in patients treated with ZAVESCA with or without concurrent conditions such as vitamin B12 deficiency and monoclonal gammopathy. Peripheral neuropathy seems to be more common in patients with type 1 Gaucher disease compared to the general population. All patients should undergo baseline and repeat neurological evaluation. Patients who develop symptoms such as numbness and tingling should have a careful re-assessment of risk-benefit.

In an observational study including 103 patients not exposed to ZAVESCA, a total of 11 adult Type 1 Gaucher disease patients (11%) had peripheral polyneuropathy at baseline, suggesting a higher prevalence than in the general population. These data are consistent with a 10% prevalence of peripheral neuropathy previously reported in a cohort of Gaucher patients either naïve or treated with enzyme replacement therapy. See Warnings and Precautions, Neurologic.

Less Common Clinical Trial Adverse Drug Reactions <1%: There were no adverse drug reactions reported with a prevalence of <1%.

Abnormal Hematologic and Clinical Chemistry Findings: In clinical trials in Type 1 Gaucher disease, there were few notable changes in mean hematology and coagulation values during treatment. Parameters that changed by more than 10% between Baseline and Months 6, 12, and 18 were limited to: eosinophils at Months 6 (+19.8%), 12 (+21.7%), and 18 (+23.1%); basophils at Months 6 (+36.2%) and 18 (−31.7%); and partial thromboplastin time at Month 6 (+36.2%). It would be expected that hemoglobin, hematocrit, red blood count and platelets would increase over time as this is the intended treatment effect of the drug. These expected increases are seen from Month 24 onwards for these parameters: RBC count at Month 30 (+10.5%); platelets at Months 24 (+25.7%), 30 (+29.1%), and 36 (+33.1%); and hematocrit at Months 24 (+10.8%), 30 (+13.0%) and 36 (+12.4%). The only other parameters that changed by more than 10% between Baseline and Months 24, 30, and 36 were: lymphocytes at Months 24 (+14.2%) and 30 (+21.1%); monocytes at Months 24 (+10.8%) and 30 (+15.7%); basophils at Months 24 (−27.6%), 30 (−51.9%), and 36 (−39.8%).

In patients with Niemann-Pick Type C disease, the median of platelet counts at treatment start was around 160×10^9/L and slightly decreased below 150×10^9/L during the first year of treatment. After that, the median platelet count remained stable above 130×10^9/L. Of note, 39% of the patients already had platelet counts below the lower limit of normal at screening. Reduced platelet count is a common finding in Niemann-Pick Type C disease.

Post-Market Adverse Drug Reactions: The reporting rate for the most commonly reported events was 18.5% for diarrhea, 12.3% for weight decrease, 8.6% for tremor, 4.4% for unspecified neurological symptoms, 3.3% for memory impairment, and 2.6% for convulsions.

DRUG INTERACTIONS: Overview: Miglustat does not inhibit the metabolism of various substrates of cytochrome P450 enzymes and miglustat is not metabolised by these enzymes. Consequently, significant interactions are unlikely with drugs that are substrates/inducers/inhibitors of cytochrome P450 enzymes. No significant drug interactions have been seen with miglustat that would affect the dosing recommendations for ZAVESCA.

Drug-Drug Interactions: Imiglucerase (Cerezyme): Drug interaction between ZAVESCA (miglustat 100 mg orally three times daily) and Cerezyme (imiglucerase; 7.5 or 15 U/kg/day) was assessed in Cerezyme stabilized Type 1 Gaucher patients after one month of coadministration. There was no significant effect of Cerezyme on the pharmacokinetics of miglustat, with the coadministration of Cerezyme and miglustat resulting in a 22% reduction in C_{max} and a 14% reduction in AUC of miglustat. Limited data indicate that ZAVESCA has no or little effects on the pharmacokinetics of Cerezyme.

Loperamide: A population pharmacokinetic analysis indicated that concomitant Loperamide administration during clinical trials did not alter the pharmacokinetics of miglustat.

There is no change in the dosing recommendations when ZAVESCA is coadministered with Cerezyme and/or Loperamide.

Drug-Food Interactions: Coadministration of ZAVESCA with food results in a decrease in the rate of absorption of miglustat but has no statistically significant effect on the extent of absorption of miglustat.
Drug-Herb Interactions: Interactions with herbal products have not been established.
Drug-Laboratory Test Interactions: Interactions with laboratory tests have not been established.

DOSAGE AND ADMINISTRATION: Dosing Considerations: Dose selection may need to be adjusted for patients with mild or moderate renal impairment. Use in patients with severe renal impairment is not recommended.
Recommended Dose and Dosage Adjustment: Dosage in Type 1 Gaucher Disease: Adults: The recommended dose for the treatment of patients with Type 1 Gaucher disease is one 100 mg capsule administered orally three times a day at regular intervals. Capsules should be swallowed whole with water.
Pediatrics (under 18 years of age): There is only limited experience with ZAVESCA in patients under the age of 18 years.
Dosage in Niemann-Pick Type C Disease: Adults and Juvenile (12-17 years old): The recommended dose for the treatment of adult and juvenile patients with Niemann-Pick Type C disease is 200 mg three times a day.
Pediatrics (under 12 years of age): Patients below 4 years of age were not enrolled in the prospective study of ZAVESCA in Niemann-Pick Type C disease. Dosing in patients under the age of 12 should be adjusted on the basis of body surface area (BSA, mg/m²) as illustrated in Table 4.

Table 4: ZAVESCA

Dosing Adjustment in Patients Under the Age of 12

Body Surface Area (m^2)	Recommended Dose
>1.25	200 mg three times a day
>0.88–1.25	200 mg twice a day
>0.73–0.88	100 mg three times a day
>0.47–0.73	100 mg twice a day
≤0.47	100 mg once a day

Temporary dose reduction may be necessary in some patients because of diarrhea.

The benefit to the patient of treatment with ZAVESCA should be evaluated on a regular basis.

ZAVESCA can be taken with or without food. The risk of diarrhea may be reduced if ZAVESCA is taken between meals. See Warnings and Precautions.
Elderly: There is only limited experience with ZAVESCA in patients over the age of 65 years and the use of this drug is not recommended in these patient groups.
Renal Impairment: Pharmacokinetic data indicate increased systemic exposure to miglustat in patients with renal impairment. In patients with mild renal impairment (adjusted creatinine clearance 0.83-1.2 mL/s or 50-70 mL/min/1.73 m²) ZAVESCA administration should commence at a dose of 100 mg twice per day in patients with Type 1 Gaucher disease and at a dose of 200 mg twice per day (adjusted for body surface area in patients below the age of 12) in patients with Niemann-Pick Type C disease. In patients with moderate renal impairment (adjusted creatinine clearance of 0.5-0.83 mL/s or 30-50 mL/min/1.73 m²), ZAVESCA administration should commence at a dose of 100 mg once per day in patients with Type 1 Gaucher disease and at a dose of 100 mg twice per day (adjusted for body surface area in patients below the age of 12) in patients with Niemann-Pick Type C disease. Use in patients with severe renal impairment (creatinine clearance of <0.5 mL/sec or 30 mL/min/1.73 m²) is not recommended. In patients with renal impairment continued monitoring and appropriate dosage adjustment is recommended.
Hepatic Impairment: ZAVESCA has not been evaluated in patients with moderate to severe hepatic impairment. No metabolites of miglustat have been detected in animals or in humans either in vivo or in vitro. Miglustat is known to be substantially excreted by the kidney. There is no evidence to suggest that the dose of ZAVESCA should be altered in patients with hepatic impairment.
Missed Dose: If a scheduled dose of ZAVESCA is missed, a double dose should not be taken to make up for the forgotten individual dose. The patient should take the next capsule at the usual scheduled time.

OVERDOSAGE:
In the clinical development program for ZAVESCA , no patient experienced an overdose of study drug. However, ZAVESCA has been administered at doses of up to 3000 mg/day (approximately 10 times the recommended dose administered to Gaucher patients) for up to six months in Human Immunodeficiency Virus (HIV)-positive patients. Adverse events observed in the HIV studies included granulocytopenia, dizziness, and paresthesia. Leukopenia and neutropenia have also been observed in a similar group of patients receiving 800 mg/day or above.

For management of a suspected drug overdose, contact your regional Poison Control Centre. See the *CPS* Directory section for a list of Poison Control Centres.

ACTION AND CLINICAL PHARMACOLOGY: Mechanism of Action/Pharmacodynamics: Miglustat functions as a competitive and reversible inhibitor of the enzyme glucosylceramide synthase, the initial enzyme in a series of reactions which results in the synthesis of most glycosphingolipids. The goal of treatment with ZAVESCA is to reduce the rate of glycosphingolipid biosynthesis so that the amount of glycosphingolipid substrate is reduced to a level which allows the residual activity of the deficient glucocerebrosidase enzyme to be more effective (substrate reduction therapy). Miglustat crosses the blood-brain barrier.
Pharmacokinetics: Pharmacokinetic Parameters in Patients with Type 1 Gaucher Disease: See Table 5.

Table 5: ZAVESCA

Summary of ZAVESCA's Pharmacokinetic Parameters in Patients with Type 1 Gaucher Disease and Niemann-Pick Type C disease

	C_{max}	$t_{1/2}$	$AUC_{0\text{-}6h}$	Clearance	Volume of Distribution
Adult patients with Type 1 Gaucher disease Single dose (100 mg)	862 ng/mL	7.3 h	3746 ng·h/mL	11.8–13.8 L/h	83–105 L
Adult patients with Type 1 Gaucher disease Month 1 (100 mg, 3 times daily)	1922 ng/mL	6.4 h	8911 ng·h/mL	—	—
Juvenile/adults patients (over 12 years) with Nieman-Pick Type C disease Month 1 (200 mg, 3 times daily)	2698 ng/mL	3.0 h (t_{max})	16 412 ($AUC_{0\text{-}8h}$)	—	—
Pediatric patients (under 12 years) with Niemann-Pick Type C disease					
Month 1 (200 mg, 3 times daily)	2075 ng/mL	4.0 h (t_{max})	11 975 ($AUC_{0\text{-}8h}$)	—	—
Month 1 (200 mg, 2 times daily)	3289 ng/mL	3.54 h (t_{max})	18 792 ($AUC_{0\text{-}8h}$)	—	—
Month 1 (200 mg, once daily)	2223 ng/mL	4.0 h (t_{max})	15 866 ($AUC_{0\text{-}8h}$)	—	—

Absorption: In healthy subjects miglustat is rapidly absorbed following oral administration, with a t_{max} of approximately 2 to 2.5 hours. Coadministration of ZAVESCA with food results in a decrease in the rate of absorption of miglustat (C_{max} was decreased by 36% and t_{max} delayed 2 hours) but has no statistically significant effect on the extent of absorption of miglustat (AUC decreased by 14%). Miglustat exhibits linear, dose-proportional pharmacokinetics over a wide dose range (approximately 50-1120 mg single doses). Miglustat's pharmacokinetics remain stable after repeated dosing three times daily for up to 12 months. The pharmacokinetics of miglustat is similar in adult Type 1 Gaucher disease patients and Niemann-Pick Type C disease patients when compared to healthy subjects. Pharmacokinetic data were obtained in pediatric patients with Type 3 Gaucher disease aged 3-15 years, and patients with Niemann-Pick Type C disease aged 5-16 years. Dosing in children at 200 mg t.i.d. adjusted for body surface area resulted in C_{max} and AUCτ values which were approximately two-fold those attained after 100 mg t.i.d. in Type 1 Gaucher disease patients, consistent with the doselinear pharmacokinetics of miglustat. At steady state, the concentration of miglustat in cerebrospinal fluid of six Type 3 Gaucher disease patients was 31.4-67.2% of that in plasma. No significant relationships or trends were noted between miglustat pharmacokinetic parameters and demographic variables (age, gender, and body mass index).
Distribution: Mean apparent volume of distribution of miglustat is 83-105 L in Gaucher patients, indicating that miglustat distributes into extravascular tissues. Miglustat does not bind to plasma proteins.
Metabolism: No metabolites of miglustat were detected in vitro or in vivo. Miglustat is excreted unchanged in urine.
Excretion: The major route of excretion of miglustat is renal. Renal impairment has a significant effect on the pharmacokinetics of miglustat, resulting in increased systemic exposure to miglustat in such patients.
Special Populations and Conditions: Geriatrics: The pharmacokinetics of miglustat have not been evaluated in patients over the age of 65 years.
Gender: No significant relationship or trend was noted between miglustat pharmacokinetic parameters and gender.
Race: Ethnic differences in miglustat pharmacokinetics have not been evaluated in Gaucher patients. Based on a cross analysis study, the apparent oral clearance of miglustat in patients of Ashkenazi Jewish descent was not statistically different to that in others (1 Asian and 15 Caucasians).
Hepatic Insufficiency: ZAVESCA has not been evaluated in patients with moderate to severe hepatic impairment. See Dosage and Administration.
Renal Insufficiency: Limited data in patients with Fabry disease and impaired renal function indicate that oral clearance (CL/F) decreases with decreasing renal function. While the numbers of patients with mild to moderate renal impairment were small, the data suggest an approximate decrease in CL/F of 40% and 60%, respectively, in mild and moderate renal impairment, justifying the need to decrease the dose of ZAVESCA in such patients. See Dosage and Administration.

Data in severe renal impairment are limited to two patients with creatinine clearance in the range 0.3-0.48 mL/s (18-29 mL/min). These data suggest a decrease in CL/F up to 70% in patients with severe renal impairment. Treatment with miglustat in patients with severe renal impairment is therefore not recommended. See Warnings and Precautions and Dosage and Administration.

STORAGE AND STABILITY: ZAVESCA should be stored at room temperature between 15-30°C. Protect from moisture.

SPECIAL HANDLING INSTRUCTIONS: There are no special handling requirements for ZAVESCA.

INFORMATION FOR THE PATIENT: Published in e-CPS, available by subscription at www.e-cps.ca.

DOSAGE FORMS, COMPOSITION AND PACKAGING: Each white, opaque, hard capsule, with "OGT 918" printed in black on the cap and "100" printed in black on the body, contains: miglustat 100 mg. Nonmedicinal ingredients: magnesium stearate, povidone (K30) and sodium starch glycolate; capsule shell: black iron oxide (E172), gelatin, potassium hydroxide, propylene glycol, titanium dioxide (E171), shellac and water. Boxes of 5 blister cards of 18 capsules each (90 capsules/box).

(Shown in Product Identification Section)

ZeaSORB®
cellulose—chloroxylenol—aluminum dihydroxyallantoinate
Antibacterial—Antifungal

Stiefel, a GSK company

SUPPLIED: Each g of powder contains: 0.5% p-chloro-m-xylenol, aluminum dihydroxyallantoinate 0.2%. Nonmedicinal ingredients: fragrance, imidurea, microporous cellulose, starch acrylic copolymer and talcum. Sifter top plastic containers of 50 g.

ZeaSORB® AF
tolnaftate
Topical Antifungal

Stiefel, a GSK company

SUPPLIED: Each g of powder contains: tolnaftate USP 1%. Nonmedicinal ingredients: aluminum dihydroxyallantoinate, fragrance, imidurea, microporous cellulose, parachlorometaxylenol, starch acrylic copolymer and talcum. Sifter top plastic containers of 50 g.

Zeldox™ Ⓟ
ziprasidone HCl
Antipsychotic

Pfizer

Date of Revision: December 18, 2008

SUMMARY PRODUCT INFORMATION:

Route of Administration	Dosage Form/ Strength	All Nonmedicinal Ingredients
Oral	Capsules 20, 40, 60, and 80 mg	Lactose monohydrate, magnesium stearate, pregelatinized starch, and gelatin capsules

INDICATIONS AND CLINICAL USE: Schizophrenia: ZELDOX (ziprasidone hydrochloride) is indicated for the treatment of schizophrenia and related psychotic disorders. The prescriber should consider the finding of ziprasidone's greater capacity to prolong the QT/QTc interval compared to other antipsychotic drugs (see Contraindications and Warnings and Precautions).

The efficacy of ziprasidone was established in short-term (4- and 6-week) controlled trials of schizophrenic inpatients.

ZELDOX has been shown to be effective in maintaining clinical improvement during long-term therapy (1-year). The physician who elects to use ZELDOX for extended periods should periodically re-evaluate the long-term usefulness of the drug for the individual patient.

Bipolar Disorder: ZELDOX (ziprasidone hydrochloride) is indicated for the treatment of acute manic or mixed episodes associated with bipolar disorder. The prescriber should consider the finding of ziprasidone's greater capacity to prolong the QT/QTc interval compared to other antipsychotic drugs (see Contraindications and Warnings and Precautions).

The efficacy of ziprasidone in acute mania was established in 2 placebo-controlled, double-blind, 3-week studies which compared ziprasidone with placebo and 1 double-blind, 12-week (3-week placebo-controlled, active comparator acute phase and 9-week active comparator phase) study which compared ziprasidone to haloperidol and placebo, in patients meeting DSM-IV criteria for Bipolar I Disorder.

The effectiveness of ZELDOX for longer-term use and for prophylactic use in mania has not been systematically evaluated in controlled clinical trials. Therefore, physicians who elect to use ziprasidone for extended periods should periodically re-evaluate the long-term risks and benefits of the drug for the individual patient.

Geriatrics (>65 years of age): ZELDOX is not indicated in elderly patients with dementia (see Warnings and Precautions, Serious Warnings and Precautions Box and Action and Clinical Pharmacology, Special Populations and Conditions). Caution should be used when treating geriatric patients with ZELDOX. See Action and Clinical Pharmacology, Special Populations and Conditions and Dosage and Administration.

Pediatrics (<18 years of age): The safety and efficacy of ZELDOX in children under the age of 18 years have not been established.

CONTRAINDICATIONS:

- **QT Prolongation:** Because of ziprasidone's dose-related prolongation of the QT interval and the known association of fatal arrhythmias with QT prolongation by some other drugs, ziprasidone is contraindicated in patients with:
  - known history of QT prolongation (including congenital long QT syndrome);
  - recent acute myocardial infarction; or
  - uncompensated heart failure (see Warnings and Precautions).

  Pharmacokinetic/pharmacodynamic studies between ziprasidone and other drugs that prolong the QT interval have not been performed. An additive effect of ziprasidone and other drugs that prolong the QT interval cannot be excluded. Therefore, ziprasidone should not be given with dofetilide, sotalol, quinidine, other Class Ia and III anti-arrhythmias, mesoridazine, thioridazine, chlorpromazine, droperidol, pimozide, sparfloxacin, gatifloxacin, moxifloxacin, halofantrine, mefloquine, pentamidine, arsenic trioxide, levomethadyl acetate, dolasetron mesylate, probucol or tacrolimus. Ziprasidone is also contraindicated with drugs that have demonstrated QT prolongation as one of their pharmacodynamic effects and have this effect described in their respective Product Monograph as a contraindication or a warning (see Warnings and Precautions).
- Patients who are hypersensitive to ziprasidone or to any ingredient in the formulation or component of the container. For a complete listing see Dosage Forms, Composition and Packaging.

WARNINGS AND PRECAUTIONS:

> **Serious Warnings and Precautions**
>
> **Increased Mortality in Elderly Patients with Dementia: Elderly patients with dementia treated with atypical antipsychotic drugs are at an increased risk of death compared to placebo. Analyses of 13 placebo-controlled trials with various antipsychotics (modal duration of 10 weeks) in these patients showed a mean 1.6-fold increase in the death rate in the drug-treated patients. Although the causes of death were varied, most of the deaths appeared to be either cardiovascular (e.g., heart failure, sudden death) or infectious (e.g., pneumonia) in nature (see Warnings and Precautions, Special Populations, Use in Geriatric Patients with Dementia).**

QT Prolongation: (See also Contraindications.)

ZELDOX (ziprasidone hydrochloride) is associated with moderate QT/QTC interval prolongation, as described in the subsections below.

Recommendations Regarding Risk Factors for QT Prolongation: Many drugs that cause QT/QTc prolongation are suspected to increase the risk of a rare, potentially fatal polymorphic ventricular tachyarrhythmia known as torsades de pointes. Generally, the risk of torsades de pointes increases with magnitude of the QT/QTc prolongation produced by the drug.

Torsades may be asymptomatic or experienced by the patient as dizziness, palpitations, syncope or seizures. If sustained, torsades de pointes can progress to ventricular fibrillation and sudden cardiac death.

As per Health Canada's QT/QTc Guidelines, in the general population, certain circumstances may increase the risk of the occurrence of torsades de pointes in association with the use of drugs that prolong the QT/QTc interval, including (1) bradycardia; (2) electrolyte disturbances (e.g., hypokalemia, hypomagnesemia, or hypocalcemia); (3) concomitant use of other drugs that prolong the QT/QTc interval; (4) presence of congenital prolongation of the QT interval; (5) family history of sudden cardiac death at <50 years; (6) personal history of cardiac disease or arrhythmias; (7) acute neurological events, e.g., stroke; (8) being female or 65 years of age or older; (9) nutritional deficits e.g., eating disorders; (10) diabetes mellitus. Therefore:

- Ziprasidone should not be used in combination with other drugs that are known to prolong the QT/QTc interval (see Contraindications). Additionally, clinicians should be alert to the identification of other drugs that have been consistently observed to prolong the QT/QTc interval. Such drugs should not be prescribed with ziprasidone.
- Ziprasidone should also not be used in patients with congenital long QT syndrome, or in patients with a history of cardiac arrhythmias, with recent acute myocardial infarction, or with uncompensated heart failure (see Contraindications).
- If patients with stable cardiac disease are treated, an ECG review should be considered before treatment is started.
- Persistently prolonged QT/QTc intervals may also increase the risk of further prolongation and arrhythmia, but it is not clear that routine screening ECG measures are effective in detecting such patients. Rather, if cardiac symptoms, such as palpitations, vertigo, syncope or seizures occur then the possibility of a malignant cardiac arrhythmia should be considered and a cardiac evaluation including an ECG should be performed. If the QTc interval for a patient is >500 msec, then it is recommended that the treatment be stopped.
- It is recommended that patients being considered for ziprasidone treatment who are at risk for significant electrolyte disturbances (e.g., diuretic therapy, protracted diarrhea or vomiting, water intoxication, eating disorder, and alcoholism), have baseline serum potassium and magnesium measurements performed and levels corrected if necessary. Hypokalemia (and/or hypomagnesemia) may increase the risk of QT prolongation and arrhythmia. It is essential to periodically monitor serum electrolytes in patients for whom diuretic therapy is introduced during ziprasidone treatment.
- Patients receiving treatment with drugs that prolong the QT/QTc interval should be counselled appropriately, regarding risk factors, symptoms suggestive of arrhythmia and risk management strategies.

Description of Data:

1. **Studies Specifically Designed to Assess QT Prolongation: a) Comparative study (128-054): Six anti-psychotics:** A study directly comparing the QT/QTc prolonging effect of ziprasidone with several other drugs effective in the treatment of schizophrenia was conducted in patient volunteers (n=28-35 per drug). In the first phase of the trial, ECGs were obtained at the time of maximum plasma concentration when the drug was administered alone. In the second phase of the trial, ECGs were obtained at the time of maximum plasma concentration while the drug was co-administered with an inhibitor of the CYP450 metabolism of the drug.

   In the first phase of the study, the mean change in QTc from baseline was calculated for each drug, using a sample-based correction that makes adjustments for the effect of heart rate on the QT interval. The mean increase in QTc from baseline for ziprasidone (baseline correction) at 160 mg/day was 15.9 msec, which was approximately 9 to 14 msec greater than for four of the comparator drugs (haloperidol at 15 mg/day [7.1 msec], quetiapine at 750 mg/day [5.7 msec], risperidone at 16 mg/day [3.6 msec], and olanzapine at 20 mg/day [1.7 msec], but was approximately 14 msec less than the prolongation observed for thioridazine at 300 mg/day [30.1 msec].

   In the second phase of the study, the effect of ziprasidone on QTc length (16.6 msec) was not augmented by the presence of a metabolic inhibitor (ketoconazole 200 mg BID). The mean increase for the other comparator drugs was haloperidol [13.3 msec], quetiapine [8.0 msec], olanzapine [3.0 msec], and risperidone [2.6 msec], compared to thioridazine [29.6 msec].

   b) QT Effects at 2x maximum recommended ziprasidone dose: A study examining the effect of 3 doses of orally administered ziprasidone (including twice the recommended clinical dose, n=29) and haloperidol (the highest dose level was comparably high, n=30) on the QTc interval was conducted in clinically stable patients with schizophrenia and schizoaffective disorder. The study comprised 4 consecutive periods, including drug tapering (phase 1), wash out (phase 2), drug therapy (phase 3) followed by the study drug wash out and initiation of outpatient drug therapy (phase 4). Serial baseline electrocardiograms (ECGs) were collected under controlled conditions on the last day (day 0) of period 2 at times matched to those collected during study drug administration (phase 3) at the time of estimated peak drug exposure. At each steady-state dose level, three ECGs and a pharmacokinetic sample were collected at the predicted time of peak exposure to administered drug (T_{max}). One of the three ECG's was collected at T_{max} and the other two were collected one hour on either side of T_{max}.

   The mean increase in QTc from baseline for ziprasidone at 40 mg/day was 4.5 msec, and at 160 mg/day was 19.5 msec (comparable to the study described above). A further increase in dose to 320 mg/day (twice the maximum recommended clinical dose) led to an increase in QTc of 22.5 msec, which was only 3 msec more than after 160 mg/day in this study, suggesting a plateau. In comparison, there was no mean QTc increase apparent at the lowest haloperidol dose (2.5 mg/day). At the 2 higher doses of haloperidol, (15 and 30 mg/day), mean QTc increases ranged from 6.6 to 7.2 msec. No subject in either treatment group experienced a QTc interval ≥450 msec or an increase from baseline of ≥75 msec.
2. **Data from Non-QT specific ziprasidone studies:** In placebo-controlled trials, ziprasidone increased the QTc interval compared to placebo by approximately 10 msec at the highest recommended daily dose of 160 mg, which was the basis for subsequent QT-specific studies. The clinical trial data for ziprasidone did not reveal an excess risk of mortality for ziprasidone compared to other antipsychotic drugs or placebo.

   Electrocardiogram readings revealing QTc intervals exceeding the potentially clinically relevant threshold of 500 msec in clinical trials with ziprasidone occurred in: 2/3266 (0.06%) patients receiving ZELDOX (ziprasidone hydrochloride) and 1/538 (0.19%) patients receiving placebo. One patient had a history of prolonged QTc and a screening measurement of 489 msec; QTc was 503 msec during ziprasidone treatment. The other patient, who was receiving ziprasidone for more that 6.5 years without interruption, had a QTc of 503 msec at week 189, and 435 msec 19 weeks later, while maintained on the same oral dose of ziprasidone. There were confounding factors that contributed to the occurrence of these cases.
3. **Post-Marketing Data (see also Adverse Reactions, Post-Market Adverse Drug Reactions): Torsades de Pointes:** There have been rare post-marketing reports of torsades de pointes (in the presence of multiple confounding factors) (see Adverse Reactions, Post-Market Adverse Drug Reactions). Torsades de pointes have not been observed in association with the use of ziprasidone at recommended doses in clinical trials, but experience is too limited to rule out increased risk.

   Analysis of Post-Marketing Data: In view of the clinical trial data demonstrating a moderate QT prolongation effect of ZELDOX, a review of 5-year, post-marketing spontaneous data from the FDA AERS database was conducted using a set of heart-related search terms.

   Small elevations in spontaneous reporting rates were observed for ziprasidone compared with two other atypical antipsychotics, for both fatal cases, and "all" cases (i.e., fatal plus non-fatal).

   Accumulated case reports should not be used as a basis for determining the incidence of a reaction or estimating risk for a particular product, as neither the total number of reactions occurring, nor the number of patients exposed to the health product is known. Because of the multiple factors that influence reporting, quantitative comparisons of health product safety cannot be made from the data. Comparison of reporting rates cannot be employed to confirm or refute a hypothesis, due to well-known, inherent limitations with spontaneous reporting of adverse events.

General: Body Temperature Regulation: Disruption of the body's ability to reduce core body temperature has been attributed to antipsychotic agents. Appropriate care is advised when prescribing ziprasidone for patients who will be experiencing conditions which may contribute to an elevation in core body temperature, e.g., exercising strenuously, exposure to extreme heat, receiving concomitant medication with anticholinergic activity, or being subject to dehydration.

Cardiovascular: See also Contraindications and Warnings and Precautions, regarding QT prolongation.

Orthostatic Hypotension: Ziprasidone may induce orthostatic hypotension associated with dizziness, tachycardia and, in some patients, syncope, especially during the initial dose-titration period, probably reflecting its α_1-adrenergic antagonist properties. Syncope was reported in 0.6% (22/3834) of the patients treated with ziprasidone.

Ziprasidone should be used with particular caution in patients with known cardiovascular disease (history of myocardial infarction or ischemic heart disease, heart failure or conduction abnormalities), cerebrovascular disease or conditions which would predispose patients to hypotension (dehydration, hypovolemia and treatment with antihypertensive medications). Patients with a history of clinically significant cardiac disorders were excluded from the trials.

Dependence/Tolerance: ZELDOX has not been systematically studied, in animals or humans, for its potential for abuse, tolerance or physical dependence. While clinical trials did not reveal any tendency for drugseeking behaviour, these observations were not systematic and it is not possible to predict on the basis of this limited experience the extent to which ZELDOX will be misused, diverted and/or abused once marketed. Consequently, patients should be evaluated carefully for a history of drug abuse, and such patients should be observed closely for signs of ZELDOX misuse or abuse (e.g., development of tolerance, increases in dose, drug-seeking behaviour).

Endocrine and Metabolism: Hyperglycemia: As with some other antipsychotics, hyperglycemia, exacerbation of pre-existing diabetes, and diabetic coma have been reported very rarely during the use of ZELDOX. However, no causal relationship with ZELDOX has been established (see Adverse Reactions, Post-Market Adverse Drug Reactions).

Assessment of the relationship between atypical antipsychotic use and glucose abnormalities is complicated by the possibility of an increased background risk of diabetes mellitus in patients with schizophrenia and the increasing incidence of diabetes mellitus in the general population. Given these confounders, and that there is no data in drug-naïve patients, the relationship between atypical antipsychotic use and hyperglycemia-related adverse events is not completely understood. However, epidemiological studies, which did not include ZELDOX, suggest an increased risk of treatment-emergent hyperglycemia-related adverse events in patients treated with the atypical antipsychotics. Because ZELDOX was not marketed at the time these studies were performed, it is not known if ZELDOX is associated with this increased risk. Precise risk estimates for hyperglycemia-related adverse events in patients treated with atypical antipsychotics are not available.

Any patient treated with atypical antipsychotics should be monitored for symptoms of hyperglycemia, including polydipsia, polyuria, polyphagia, and weakness. Patients who develop symptoms of hyperglycemia during treatment with atypical antipsychotics should undergo fasting blood glucose testing. In some cases, hyperglycemia has resolved when the atypical antipsychotic was discontinued; however, some patients required continuation of anti-diabetic treatment despite discontinuation of the suspect drug. Patients with risk factors for diabetes mellitus (e.g., obesity, family history of diabetes) who are starting treatment with atypical antipsychotics should undergo fasting blood glucose testing at the beginning of treatment and periodically during treatment. Patients with an established diagnosis of diabetes mellitus who are started on atypical antipsychotics should be monitored regularly for worsening of glucose control.

Hyperprolactinemia: As with other drugs that antagonize dopamine D_2 receptors, and/or serotonin 5-HT_2 receptors, ZELDOX may elevate prolactin levels in humans. Elevations associated with ZELDOX treatment are generally mild and may decline during administration.

Increased prolactin levels were also observed in animal studies with this compound, and were associated with an increase in mammary gland neoplasia in mice; a similar effect was not observed in rats.

Tissue culture experiments indicate that approximately one-third of human breast cancers are prolactin-dependent in vitro, ZELDOX should only be administered to patients with previously detected breast cancer if the benefits outweigh the potential risks.

Although disturbances such as galactorrhea, amenorrhea, gynecomastia, and impotence have been reported with prolactin-elevating compounds, the clinical significance of elevated serum prolactin levels is unknown for most patients. Caution should be exercised when considering ziprasidone treatment in patients with pituitary tumors. Neither clinical studies nor epidemiological studies conducted to date have shown an association between chronic administration of this class of drugs and tumorigenesis in humans. The available evidence is considered too limited to be conclusive at this time.

Genitourinary: Priapism: Very rare cases of priapism have been reported with ZELDOX. This adverse reaction, as with other psychotropic drugs, did not appear to be dose-dependent and did not correlate with duration of treatment. The likely mechanism of action of priapism is a relative decrease in sympathetic tone. Severe priapism may require surgical intervention.

Hepatic/Biliary/Pancreatic: See Warnings and Precautions, Special Populations, Hepatic Impairment.

Neurologic: Neuroleptic Malignant Syndrome (NMS): A potentially fatal symptom complex sometimes referred to as NMS has been reported in association with the administration of antipsychotic drugs, including ZELDOX.

Clinical manifestations of NMS are hyperpyrexia, muscle rigidity, altered mental status, and evidence of autonomic instability (irregular pulse or blood pressure, tachycardia, diaphoresis, and cardiac dysrhythmia). Additional signs may include elevated creatinine phosphokinase, myoglobinuria (rhabdomyolysis), and acute renal failure.

In arriving at a diagnosis, it is important to identify cases where the clinical presentation includes both serious medical illness (e.g., pneumonia, systemic infection, etc.), and untreated or inadequately treated extrapyramidal signs and symptoms (EPS). Other important considerations in the differential diagnosis include central anticholinergic toxicity, heat stroke, drug fever, and primary central nervous system pathology.

The management of NMS should include: 1) immediate discontinuation of antipsychotic drugs including ZELDOX and other drugs not essential to concurrent therapy; 2) intensive symptomatic treatment and medical monitoring; and 3) treatment of any concomitant serious medical problems for which specific treatments are available. There is no general agreement about specific pharmacological treatment regimens for uncomplicated NMS.

If a patient requires antipsychotic drug treatment after recovery from NMS, the potential reintroduction of drug therapy should be carefully considered. The patient should be carefully monitored, since recurrences of NMS have been reported.

Tardive Dyskinesia (TD): A syndrome consisting of potentially irreversible, involuntary and disabling dyskinetic movements may develop in patients treated with antipsychotic drugs. Although the prevalence of the tardive dyskinesia syndrome appears to be highest among the elderly, especially elderly women, it is impossible to rely upon prevalence estimates to predict, at the inception of antipsychotic treatment, which patients are likely to develop the tardive dyskinesia syndrome. Whether antipsychotic drug products differ in their potential to cause tardive dyskinesia is unknown.

The risk of developing tardive dyskinesia, and the likelihood that it will become irreversible are believed to increase as the duration of treatment and the total cumulative dose of antipsychotic drugs administered to the patient increase. However, the syndrome can develop, although much less commonly, after relatively brief treatment periods at low doses.

There is no known treatment for established cases of tardive dyskinesia, although the syndrome may remit, partially or completely, if antipsychotic treatment is withdrawn. Antipsychotic treatment itself however may suppress (or partially suppress) the signs and symptoms of the tardive dyskinesia syndrome and thereby may possibly mask the underlying process. The effect that symptomatic suppression has upon the long-term course of the tardive dyskinesia syndrome is unknown.

Given these considerations, ZELDOX should be prescribed in a manner that is most likely to minimize the occurrence of tardive dyskinesia. Chronic antipsychotic treatment should generally be reserved for patients who 1) suffer from a chronic illness that is known to respond to antipsychotic drugs, and 2) for whom alternative, equally effective but potentially less harmful treatments are not available or appropriate. In patients who do require chronic treatment, the smallest dose and the shortest duration of treatment producing a satisfactory clinical response should be sought. The need for continued treatment should be reassessed periodically.

If signs and symptoms of tardive dyskinesia appear in a patient on ZELDOX, drug discontinuation should be considered. However, some patients may require treatment with ZELDOX despite the presence of the tardive dyskinesia syndrome.

Potential Effect on Cognitive and Motor Performance: Somnolence was a commonly reported adverse event in patients treated with ZELDOX. In the 4- and 6-week placebo-controlled trials, somnolence was reported in 14% of patients compared to 7% of placebo patients. Since ziprasidone has the potential to impair judgment, thinking, or motor skills, patients should be cautioned about performing activities requiring mental alertness, such as operating a motor vehicle (including automobiles) or operating hazardous machinery, until they are reasonably certain that ziprasidone therapy does not affect them adversely.

Seizures: During clinical trials, seizures occurred in 0.4% of patients treated with ziprasidone. There were confounding factors that may have contributed to the occurrence of seizures in many of these cases. Nevertheless, as with other antipsychotic drugs, ziprasidone should be used cautiously in patients with a history of seizures or with conditions that potentially lower the seizure threshold, e.g., Alzheimer's dementia. Conditions that lower the seizure threshold may be more prevalent in a population of 65 years or older.

Psychiatric: Suicide: The possibility of a suicide attempt is inherent in psychotic illness, and thus close supervision and appropriate clinical management of high-risk patients should accompany drug therapy.

Prescriptions for ZELDOX should be written for the smallest quantity of capsules consistent with good patient management, in order to reduce the risk of overdose.

Renal: Dose adjustments are not required for patients with renal impairment (see Action and Clinical Pharmacology, Special Populations and Conditions, Renal Insufficiency).

Serotonergic Syndrome: In isolated cases, there have been reports of serotonin syndrome temporally associated with the therapeutic use of ziprasidone in combination with other serotonergic medicinal products such as SSRIs. The features of serotonin syndrome can include confusion, agitation, fever, sweating, ataxia, hyperreflexia, myoclonus and diarrhea.

Skin: Rash: In pre-marketing trials with ziprasidone, about 5% of patients developed rash (173/3834) and/or urticaria (12/3834), with discontinuation in about one-sixth of these cases. The occurrence of rash was related to dose of ziprasidone, although the finding might also be explained by the longer exposure time in the higher dose patients. Several patients with rash had signs and symptoms of associated systemic illness, e.g., elevated white blood cells (WBC). Most patients improved promptly with adjunctive treatment with antihistamines or steroids and/or upon discontinuation of ziprasidone, and all patients experiencing these events were reported to recover completely. Upon appearance of rash for which an alternative etiology cannot be identified, ziprasidone should be discontinued.

Special Populations: Pregnant Women: There are no adequate and well-controlled studies in pregnant women. Patients should be advised to notify their physician if they become pregnant or intend to become pregnant. ZELDOX should be used during pregnancy only if the potential benefit justifies the potential risk to the fetus.

In animal studies, ziprasidone demonstrated developmental toxicity, including possible teratogenic effects at doses similar to human therapeutic doses. When ziprasidone was administered to pregnant rabbits during the period of organogenesis, an increased incidence of fetal structural abnormalities (ventricular septal defects and other cardiovascular malformations and kidney alterations) was observed at a dose of 30 mg/kg/day (3 times the maximum recommended human dose (MRHD) of 200 mg/day on a mg/m² basis). There was no evidence to suggest that these developmental effects were secondary to maternal toxicity. The developmental no-effect dose was 10 mg/kg/day (equivalent to the MRHD on an mg/m² basis).

In rats, embryofetal toxicity (decreased fetal weights, delayed skeletal ossification) was observed following administration of 10 to 160 mg/kg/day (0.5 to 8 times the MRHD on a mg/m² basis) during organogenesis or throughout gestation, but there was no evidence of teratogenicity. Doses of 40 and 160 mg/kg/day (2 and 8 times the MRHD on a mg/m² basis) were associated with maternal toxicity. The developmental no-effect dose was 5 mg/kg/day (0.2 times the MRHD on a mg/m² basis).

There was an increase in the number of pups born dead and a decrease in postnatal survival through the first 4 days of lactation among the offspring of female rats treated during gestation and lactation with doses of 10 mg/kg/day (0.5 times the MRHD on a mg/m² basis) or greater. Offspring developmental delays and neurobehavioral functional impairment were observed at doses of 5 mg/kg/day (0.2 times the MRHD on a mg/m² basis) or greater. A no-effect level was not established for these effects.

Labor and Delivery: The effect of ZELDOX on labor and delivery in humans is unknown.

Nursing Women: It is not known whether, and if so in what amount, ziprasidone or its metabolites are excreted in human milk. It is recommended that women taking ZELDOX should not breast-feed.

Pediatrics (<18 years of age): The safety and efficacy of ZELDOX in children under the age of 18 years have not been established.

Geriatrics (>65 years of age): The number of patients 65 years or older with schizophrenia or related disorders, exposed to ZELDOX during clinical trials was limited (n=109). In general, there was no indication of any different tolerability of ziprasidone or for reduced clearance of ziprasidone in the elderly compared to younger adults. Nevertheless, geriatric patients generally have decreased cardiac, hepatic and renal function, and more frequent use of concomitant medication. The presence of multiple factors that might increase the pharmacodynamic response to ziprasidone, or cause poorer tolerance or orthostasis, should lead to consideration of a lower starting dose, slower titration, and careful monitoring during the initial dosing period for elderly patients.

Use in Geriatric Patients with Dementia: Overall Mortality: Elderly patients with dementia treated with atypical antipsychotic drugs have an increased mortality compared to placebo in a meta-analysis of 13 controlled trials of various atypical antipsychotic drugs. ZELDOX is not indicated in elderly patients with dementia.

Dysphagia: Esophageal dysmotility and aspiration have been associated with antipsychotic drug use. Aspiration pneumonia is a common cause of morbidity and mortality in elderly patients, in particular those with advanced Alzheimer's dementia. Ziprasidone and other antipsychotic drugs should be used cautiously in patients at risk for aspiration pneumonia.

Use in Patients with Concomitant Illness: Ziprasidone has not been evaluated or used to any appreciable extent in patients with a recent history of myocardial infarction or unstable heart disease. Patients with these diagnoses were excluded from pre-marketing clinical studies. Because of the risks of QT/QTc prolongation and orthostatic hypotension with ziprasidone, caution should be observed in cardiac patients (see Contraindications, as well as QT Prolongation and Cardiovascular, Orthostatic Hypotension).

Hepatic Impairment: In patients with hepatic insufficiency, lower doses should be considered (see Dosage and Administration, Hepatic Impairment and Action and Clinical Pharmacology, Special Populations and Conditions, Hepatic Insufficiency).

Renal Impairment: Dose adjustments are not required for patients with renal impairment (see Action and Clinical pharmacology, Special Populations and Conditions, Renal Insufficiency).

Monitoring and Laboratory Tests: Patients being considered for ziprasidone treatment that are at risk of significant electrolyte disturbances should have baseline serum potassium and magnesium measurements. Low serum potassium and magnesium should be repleted before proceeding with treatment. Patients who are started on diuretics during ziprasidone therapy need periodic monitoring of serum potassium and magnesium. Ziprasidone should be discontinued in patients who are found to have persistent QTc measurements >500 msec (see Warnings and Precautions).

ADVERSE REACTIONS: Adverse Drug Reaction Overview: The stated frequencies of adverse events represent the proportion of individuals who experienced, at least once, a treatment-emergent adverse event of the type listed. An event was considered treatment-emergent if it occurred for the first time or worsened while receiving therapy following baseline evaluation.

Clinical Trial Adverse Drug Reactions: Because clinical trials are conducted under very specific conditions, the adverse reaction rates observed in the clinical trials may not reflect the rates observed in practice and should not be compared to the rates in the clinical trials of another drug. Adverse drug reaction information from clinical trials is useful for identifying drug-related adverse events and for approximating rates.

Adverse Events Observed in Short-Term, Placebo-Controlled Trials: The following findings are based on a pool of two 6-week, and two 4-week placebo-controlled trials for schizophrenia and a pool of three 3-week flexible dose trials for bipolar mania in which ziprasidone was administered in doses ranging from 10 to 200 mg/day.

Schizophrenia: Adverse Events Associated with Discontinuation of Treatment in Short-Term, Placebo-Controlled Trials: A total of 4.1% (29/702) of patients treated with ZELDOX (ziprasidone hydrochloride) in shortterm, placebo-controlled studies discontinued treatment due to an adverse event, compared with 2.2% (6/273) on placebo and 8.2% (7/85) on the active control drug. The most common event associated with dropout was rash, including 7 dropouts for rash among ziprasidone patients (1%) compared to no placebo patients (see Warnings and Precautions, Skin, Rash).

Adverse Events Occurring at an Incidence of 1% or more in Short-Term, Placebo-Controlled Trials (up to 6 weeks): Table 1 enumerates the incidence, rounded to the nearest percent, of treatment-emergent adverse events that occurred during acute therapy (up to 6 weeks) in predominantly schizophrenic patients, including only those events that occurred in 1% or more of patients treated with ziprasidone and for which the incidence in patients treated with ziprasidone was greater than the incidence in placebo-treated patients.

Table 1: ZELDOX

Treatment-Emergent Adverse Event Incidence in Short-Term Placebo-Controlled Trials—Schizophrenia

	Percentage of Patients Reporting	
Body System	**ZELDOX (n=702)**	**Placebo (n=273)**
Body as a Whole		
Asthenia	5	3
Accidental injury	4	2
Chest pain	3	2
Cardiovascular		
Tachycardia	2	1
Postural hypotension	1	0
Digestive		
Nausea	10	7
Constipation	9	8
Dyspepsia	8	7
Diarrhea	5	4
Dry mouth	4	2
Anorexia	2	1
Musculoskeletal		
Myalgia	1	0
Nervous		
Extrapyramidal symptoms[a]	14	8
Somnolence	14	7
Akathisia	8	7
Dizziness[b]	8	6
Respiratory		
Respiratory tract infection	8	3
Rhinitis	4	2
Cough increased	3	1
Skin and Appendages		
Rash	4	3
Fungal dermatitis	2	1
Special Senses		
Abnormal vision	3	2

[a] Extrapyramidal Symptoms includes the following adverse event terms: extrapyramidal syndrome, hypertonia, dystonia, dyskinesia, hypokinesia, tremor, paralysis and twitching. None of these adverse events occurred individually at an incidence greater than 5% in schizophrenia trials.

[b] Dizziness includes the adverse event terms dizziness and lightheadedness.

Explorations for interactions on the basis of gender did not reveal any clinically meaningful differences in the adverse event occurrence on the basis of this demographic factor.

Commonly Observed Adverse Events in Short-Term, Placebo-Controlled Trials: In the schizophrenia studies, the most commonly observed adverse events associated with the use of ziprasidone (incidence of 5% or greater) and observed at a rate on ziprasidone at least twice that of placebo were somnolence (14%), extrapyramidal symptoms (14%), and respiratory tract infection (8%).

Dose Dependency of Adverse Events in Short-Term, Placebo-Controlled Trials: An analysis for dose response in the schizophrenia 4-study pool revealed an apparent relation of adverse event to dose for the following events: asthenia, postural hypotension, anorexia, dry mouth, increased salivation, arthralgia, anxiety, dizziness, dystonia, hypertonia, somnolence, tremor, rhinitis, rash, and abnormal vision.

Extrapyramidal Symptoms (EPS)—Schizophrenia: The incidence of reported EPS for ziprasidone-treated patients in the short-term, placebocontrolled trials was 14% vs. 8% for placebo. Medications to treat EPS and movement disorders were allowed, but if clinically meaningful movement disorder side effects were observed by the clinician or volunteered by the subject, or if a clinically meaningful movement disorder, present at screening, increased in severity or required the administration of anticholinergics or propanolol, these symptoms and their severity were recorded as adverse event. Objectively collected data from those trials on the Simpson Angus Rating Scale (for EPS) and the Barnes Akathisia Scale (for akathisia) did not generally show a difference between ziprasidone and placebo.

Vital Sign Changes: ZELDOX is associated with orthostatic hypotension (see Warnings and Precautions, Cardiovascular, Orthostatic Hypotension).

ECG Changes: Ziprasidone is associated with an increase in the QTc interval (see Warnings and Precautions, QT Prolongation). In schizophrenia trials, ziprasidone was associated with a mean increase in heart rate of 1.4 beats per minute compared to a 0.2 beats per minute decrease among placebo patients.

Weight Gain: The proportions of patients meeting a weight gain criterion of ≥7% of body weight were compared in a pool of four 4- and 6- week placebo-controlled schizophrenia clinical trials, revealing a statistically significantly greater incidence of weight gain for ziprasidone (10%) compared to placebo (4%). A median weight gain of 0.5 kg was observed in ziprasidone patients compared to no median weight change in placebo patients. In this set of clinical trials, weight gain was reported as an adverse event in 0.4% of ziprasidone and 0.4% of placebo patients.

During long-term therapy with ziprasidone, a categorization of patients at baseline on the basis of body mass index (BMI) revealed the greatest mean weight gain and highest incidence of clinically significant weight gain (>7% of body weight) in patients with low BMI (<23) compared to normal (23-27) or overweight patients (>27). There was a mean weight gain of 1.4 kg for those patients with a "low" baseline BMI, no mean change for patients with a "normal" BMI, and a 1.3 kg mean weight loss for patients who entered the program with a "high" BMI.

Less Common Clinical Trial Adverse Drug Reactions (<1%)—Schizophrenia: Other Adverse Events Observed During the Pre-Marketing Evaluation of Oral ZELDOX: All reported treatment-emergent events are included except those already listed in Table 1 or in other sections. It is important to emphasize that, although the events reported occurred during treatment with ZELDOX capsules, they were not necessarily caused by the therapy.

The adverse events are categorized by body system and listed in order of decreasing frequency according to the following definitions: frequent adverse events are those occurring in at least 1/100 patients (only those not already listed in the tabulated results from placebo-controlled trials appear in this listing); infrequent adverse events are those occurring in 1/100 to 1/1000 patients; rare events are those occurring in fewer than 1/1000 patients.

Body as a Whole: Frequent: abdominal pain, flu syndrome, fever, accidental fall, face edema, chills, photosensitivity reaction, flank pain, hypothermia, motor vehicle accident. Rare: feeling hot.

Cardiovascular System: Frequent: hypertension; Infrequent: bradycardia, angina pectoris, atrial fibrillation. Rare: first degree AV block, bundle branch block, phlebitis, pulmonary embolus, cardiomegaly, cerebral infarct, cerebrovascular accident, deep thrombophlebitis, myocarditis, thrombophlebitis.

Digestive System: Frequent: vomiting; Infrequent: rectal hemorrhage, dysphagia, tongue edema. Rare: gum hemorrhage, jaundice, fecal impaction, gamma glutamyl transpeptidase increased, hematemesis, cholestatic jaundice, hepatitis, hepatomegaly, leukoplakia of mouth, fatty liver deposit, melena.

Endocrine: Rare: hypothyroidism, hyperthyroidism, thyroiditis.

Hemic and Lymphatic System: Infrequent: anemia, ecchymosis, leukocytosis, leukopenia, eosinophilia, lymphadenopathy. Rare: thrombocytopenia, hypochromic anemia, lymphocytosis, monocytosis, basophilia, lymphedema, polycythemia, thrombocythemia.

Metabolic and Nutritional Disorders: Infrequent: thirst, transaminase increased, peripheral edema, hyperglycemia, creatine phosphokinase increased, alkaline phosphatase increased, hypercholesteremia, dehydration, lactic dehydrogenase increased, albuminuria, hypokalemia. Rare: BUN increased, creatinine increased, hyperlipemia, hypocholesteremia, hyperkalemia, hypochloremia, hypoglycemia, hyponatremia, hypoproteinemia, glucose tolerance decreased, gout, hyperchloremia, hyperuricemia, hypocalcemia, hypoglycemic reaction, hypomagnesemia, ketosis, respiratory alkalosis.

Musculoskeletal System: Infrequent: tenosynovitis. Rare: myopathy.

Nervous System: Frequent: agitation, tremor, dyskinesia, hostility, paresthesia, confusion, vertigo, hypokinesia, hyperkinesia, abnormal gait, oculogyric crisis, hypesthesia, ataxia, amnesia, cogwheel rigidity, delirium, hypotonia, akinesia, dysarthria, withdrawal syndrome, buccoglossal syndrome, choreoathetosis, diplopia, incoordination, neuropathy. Rare: myoclonus, nystagmus, torticollis, circumoral paresthesia, opisthotonos, reflexes increased, trismus.

Respiratory System: Frequent: dyspnea; Infrequent: pneumonia, epistaxis. Rare: hemoptysis, laryngismus.

Skin and Appendages: Infrequent: maculopapular rash, urticaria, alopecia, eczema, exfoliative dermatitis, contact dermatitis, vesiculobullous rash.

Special Senses: Infrequent: conjunctivitis, dry eyes, tinnitus, blepharitis, cataract, photophobia. Rare: eye hemorrhage, visual field defect, keratitis, keratoconjunctivitis.

Urogenital System: Infrequent: impotence, abnormal ejaculation, amenorrhea, hematuria, menorrhagia, female lactation, polyuria, urinary retention, metrorrhagia, male sexual dysfunction, anorgasmia, glycosuria. Rare: gynecomastia, vaginal hemorrhage, nocturia, oliguria, female sexual dysfunction, uterine hemorrhage.

Bipolar Mania: Adverse Events Associated with Discontinuation of Treatment in Short-Term, Placebo-Controlled Trials: For ziprasidone-treated subjects in short-term, placebo controlled studies 5.5% (25/457) discontinued treatment due to AEs, compared with 3.1% (7/224) on placebo. The most common events associated with dropout (>0.5%) in the ziprasidone-treated patients were events affecting the nervous system (17/457; 3.7%), the digestive system (5/457; 1.1%), and body as a whole (4/457; 0.9%).

Adverse Events Occurring at an Incidence of 2% or more in Short-Term, Placebo-Controlled Bipolar Trials: Table 2 enumerates the incidence of treatment-emergent adverse events that occurred during therapy in bipolar patients, including only those events that occurred in 2% or more of patients treated with ziprasidone and for which the incidence in patients treated with ziprasidone was greater than the incidence in placebo-treated patients.

Table 2: ZELDOX

Treatment-Emergent, Adverse Event Incidence in Short-Term (up to 3 weeks), Placebo-Controlled Trials—Bipolar Mania

Body System and COSTART Preferred Term	Ziprasidone (n=457)	Placebo (n=224)
Body as a Whole		
Headache	67 (14.7%)	31 (13.8%)
Asthenia	21 (4.6%)	3 (1.3%)
Pain	15 (3.3%)	5 (2.2%)
Accidental injury	14 (3.1%)	3 (1.3%)
Cardiovascular		
Hypertension	10 (2.2%)	3 (1.3%)
Digestive		
Nausea	32 (7.0%)	13 (5.8%)
Dyspepsia	30 (6.6%)	11 (4.9%)
Constipation	25 (5.5%)	11 (4.9%)
Diarrhea	17 (3.7%)	7 (3.1%)
Vomiting	17 (3.7%)	5 (2.2%)
Tooth disorder	17 (3.7%)	5 (2.2%)

(cont'd)

Table 2: ZELDOX *(cont'd)*

Treatment-Emergent, Adverse Event Incidence in Short-Term (up to 3 weeks), Placebo-Controlled Trials—Bipolar Mania

Body System and COSTART Preferred Term	Ziprasidone (n=457)	Placebo (n=224)
Dry mouth	16 (3.5%)	6 (2.7%)
Increased salivation	12 (2.6%)	1 (0.4%)
Nervous		
Somnolence	104 (22.8%)	19 (8.5%)
Extrapyramidal syndrome	62 (13.6%)	11 (4.9%)
Akathisia	59 (12.9%)	10 (4.5%)
Dizziness	49 (10.7%)	9 (4.0%)
Dystonia	32 (7.0%)	3 (1.3%)
Tremor	23 (5.0%)	6 (2.7%)
Hypertonia	22 (4.8%)	3 (1.3%)
Agitation	19 (4.2%)	9 (4.0%)
Anxiety	17 (3.7%)	6 (2.7%)
Dyskinesia	11 (2.4%)	1 (0.4%)
Respiratory		
Pharyngitis	10 (2.2%)	1 (0.4%)
Skin and Appendages		
Pruritus	15 (3.3%)	5 (2.2%)
Special Senses		
Abnormal vision	18 (3.9%)	4 (1.8%)

Commonly Observed Adverse Events in Short-Term, Placebo-Controlled Trials: In bipolar mania clinical trials, the most common adverse reactions associated with the use of ziprasidone (incidence of 5% or greater) and observed at a rate on ziprasidone at least twice that of placebo were somnolence, akathisia, dizziness, dystonia, and extrapyramidal syndrome.

ECG Changes: Ziprasidone is associated with an increase in the QTc interval (see Warnings and Precautions, QT Prolongation).

Extrapyramidal Symptoms (EPS)—Bipolar Mania: The incidence of reported extrapyramidal syndrome and other EPS-related adverse events in the short-term, placebo-controlled trials was greater for ziprasidone-treated patients. Medications to treat EPS and movement disorders were allowed; but if clinically meaningful movement disorder side effects were observed by the clinician or volunteered by the subject, or if a clinically meaningful movement disorder present at screening increased in severity or required the administration of anticholinergics or propanolol, these symptoms and their severity were recorded as adverse events. EPS-related adverse events in all studies were usually mild, dose-related and reversible upon dose reduction and/or administration of antiparkinsonian medication. Objectively collected data from those trials on the Simpson Angus Rating Scale (for EPS) and the Barnes Akathisia Scale (for akathisia) did not generally show a difference between ziprasidone and placebo.

Less Common Clinical Trial Adverse Drug Reactions (<1%)—Bipolar Disorder: All reported treatment-emergent events are included except those already listed in Table 2 or in other sections. It is important to emphasize that, although the events reported occurred during treatment with ZELDOX capsules, they were not necessarily caused by the therapy.

The adverse events are categorized by body system and listed in order of decreasing frequency according to the following definitions: frequent adverse events are those occurring in at least 1/100 patients (only those not already listed in the tabulated results from placebo-controlled trials appear in this listing); infrequent adverse events are those occurring in 1/100 to 1/1000 patients; rare events are those occurring in fewer than 1/1000 patients.

Body as a Whole: Frequent: abdominal pain, back pain, neck pain; Infrequent: chest pain, infection, abscess, face edema, fever, flu syndrome, hot flushes, allergic reaction, cellulitis, chest pain substernal, chills infection bacterial, lab test abnormal, suicidal ideation.

Cardiovascular System: Infrequent: hypotension, tachycardia, palpitation, bundle branch block, migraine, bradycardia, hemorrhage, pallor, postural hypotension, QT interval prolonged, syncope.

Digestive System: Frequent: gastritis, flatulence, tongue edema, dysphagia, anorexia; Infrequent: increased appetite, gastroenteritis, duodenitis, fecal impaction, gingivitis, gum hemorrhage, mouth ulceration, periodontitis, stomach ulcer.

Hemic and Lymphatic System: Infrequent: bruise, leukopenia.

Metabolic and Nutritional Disorders: Infrequent: edema, peripheral edema, thirst, hypocalcemia, respiratory alkalosis, ALT increased, weight gain, weight loss.

Musculoskeletal System: Frequent: myalgia; Infrequent: arthralgia, joint disorder, leg cramps, myasthenia, bone pain, arthrosis, bone fracture accidental, myopathy, painful swelling.

Nervous System: Frequent: Insomnia, paralysis, depression, speech disorder, abnormal dreams, abnormal gait, hypesthesia, oculogyric crisis; Infrequent: manic reaction, muscular hypertonia, thinking abnormal, hypokinesia, withdrawal syndrome, bipolar affective disorder—manic, grand mal convulsion, nervousness, twitching, vertigo, amnesia, apathy, ataxia, bipolar affective disorder—depressive, confusion, delusions, depersonalization, hallucinations, hyperkinesia, manic depressive reaction, paresthesia, personality disorder, sleep disorder, torticollis, trismus.

Respiratory System: Frequent: respiratory tract infection, dyspnea, rhinitis, cough increased, respiratory disorder; Infrequent: asthma, sinusitis, bronchitis, hiccup, hypoxia.

Skin and Appendages: Frequent: rash, fungal dermatitis. Infrequent: sweating, acne, maculopapular rash, dry skin, urticaria, alopecia, dermatitis, exfoliative dermatitis, herpes simplex, skin disorder.

Special Senses: Frequent: ear pain; Infrequent:photophobia, conjunctivitis, tinnitus, ear disorder, otitis media, dry eyes, otitis externa.

Urogenital System: Frequent: vaginitis, dysmenorrhea; Infrequent: urinary frequency, polyuria, urinary tract infection, dysparеunia, female lactation, mastitis female, uterine spasm, dysuria, penile erection, urinary incontinence, anorgasmia, breast pain.

Post-Market Adverse Drug Reactions: Adverse event reports not listed above that have been received from spontaneous post-marketing reports for ZELDOX since market introduction are shown below (no causal relationship with ziprasidone has been established).

Cardiac Disorders: tachycardia, torsades de pointes (in the presence of multiple confounding factors—see Warnings and Precautions).

Gastrointestinal Disorders: dysphagia, swollen tongue.

Immune System Disorders: allergic reaction.

Metabolic and Nutritional Disorders: diabetic coma, lipids abnormal.

Nervous System Disorders: facial droop, neuroleptic malignant syndrome, serotonin syndrome (alone or in combination with serotonergic medicinal products), tardive dyskinesia.

Psychiatric Disorders: insomnia, mania/hypomania.

Renal and Urinary Disorders: enuresis, urinary incontinence.

Reproductive System and Breast Disorders: galactorrhea, priapism.

Skin and subcutaneous Tissue Disorders: angioedema, rash, Stevens-Johnson Syndrome.
Vascular Disorders: postural hypotension, syncope.

DRUG INTERACTIONS: Overview: Drug-drug interactions can be pharmacodynamic (combined pharmacologic effects) or pharmacokinetic (alteration of plasma levels). The risks of using ziprasidone in combination with other drugs have been evaluated as described below. Based upon the pharmacodynamic and pharmacokinetic profile of ziprasidone, possible interactions could be anticipated:

Pharmacodynamic Interactions:

1. Ziprasidone should not be used with any drug that prolongs the QT interval (see Contraindications and Warnings and Precautions).
2. Given the primary CNS effects of ziprasidone, caution should be used when it is taken in combination with other centrally acting drugs.
3. Because of its potential for inducing hypotension, ziprasidone may enhance the effects of certain antihypertensive agents.
4. Ziprasidone may antagonize the effects of levodopa and dopamine agonists.

Pharmacokinetic Interactions: Drug-Drug Interactions: Effect of Other Drugs on ZELDOX (ziprasidone hydrochloride): Ketoconazole: Ketoconazole, a potent inhibitor of CYP3A4, at a dose of 400 mg per day for 5 days, increased the AUC and C_{max} of ziprasidone (80 mg BID) by approximately 35-40%. The serum concentration of S-methyl-dihydroziprasidone, at the expected T_{max} of ziprasidone, was increased by 55% during ketoconazole treatment. No additional QTc prolongation was observed. Other potent inhibitors of CYP 3A4 would be expected to have similar effects.

Coadministration of potent CYP3A4 inhibitors has the potential of increasing ziprasidone serum concentrations. The clinical importance of this potential has not been clearly defined.

Carbamazepine: Carbamazepine is an inducer of CYP3A4; administration of 200 mg BID for 25 days resulted in a decrease of approximately 36% in the AUC of ziprasidone (20 mg BID). This effect may be greater when higher doses of carbamazepine are administered.

Valproate, Lamotrigine: Ziprasidone has not been studied for drug interaction with valproate or lamotrigine.

Cimetidine: Cimetidine at a dose of 800 mg QD for 2 days did not affect pharmacokinetics of ziprasidone (single 40 mg dose).

Antacids: The coadministration of 30 mL of Maalox with ziprasidone (single 40 mg dose) did not affect the pharmacokinetics of ziprasidone.

Benztropine, Propranolol, or Lorazepam: Population pharmacokinetic analysis of schizophrenic patients enrolled in controlled clinical trials has not revealed evidence of clinically significant pharmacokinetic interaction with benztropine, propranolol, or lorazepam.

Effect of ZELDOX on Other Drugs: Summary re: Potential for Effect on Cytochrome P450: In vitro studies revealed little potential for ziprasidone to interfere with the metabolism of drugs cleared primarily by CYP1A2, CYP2C9, CYP2C19, CYP2D6 and CYP3A4. Consistent with these in vitro results, studies in normal healthy volunteers showed that ziprasidone did not alter the metabolism of dextromethorphan, a CYP2D6 model substrate, nor of ethinyl estradiol, a CYP3A4 substrate. Thus, ziprasidone is unlikely to cause clinically important drug interactions mediated by these enzymes (see Action and Clinical Pharmacology, Pharmacokinetics).

Protein Binding: The in vitro plasma protein binding of ziprasidone was not altered by warfarin or propranolol, two highly protein-bound drugs, nor did ziprasidone alter the binding of these drugs in human plasma. Thus, the potential for drug interactions with ziprasidone due to displacement appears to be minimal.

Dextromethorphan: Consistent with in vitro results, a study in normal healthy volunteers showed that ziprasidone did not alter the metabolism of dextromethorphan, a CYP2D6 model substrate, to its major metabolite, dextrorphan. There was no statistically significant change in the urinary dextromethorphan/dextrorphan ratio.

Oral Contraceptives: Ziprasidone, at a dose of 20 mg BID, did not affect the pharmacokinetics of concomitantly administered oral contraceptives, ethinylestradiol (0.03 mg), a CYP3A4 substrate, or levonorgestrel (0.15 mg) progesterone components.

Lithium: Ziprasidone, at a dose of 40 mg BID, administered concomitantly with lithium at a dose of 450 mg BID for 7 days did not affect the steady-state level or renal clearance of lithium.

As ziprasidone and lithium are associated with cardiac conduction changes, the combination may pose a risk for pharmacodynamic interaction, including arrhythmias.

CNS Drugs/Alcohol: Given the primary CNS effects of ziprasidone, caution should be used when it is taken in combination with other centrally acting drugs, including alcohol.

Drug-Food Interactions: The absorption of ziprasidone is increased up to two-fold in the presence of food.

Drug-Herb Interactions: Interactions with herbal products have not been established.

Drug-Laboratory Test Interactions: Interactions with laboratory tests have not been established.

Drug-Lifestyle Interactions: Smoking: Based on in vitro studies utilizing human liver enzymes, ziprasidone is a substrate for CYP1A2, however, the contribution of this pathway is minor. Consistent with these in vitro results, population pharmacokinetic evaluation has not revealed any significant pharmacokinetic differences between smokers and nonsmokers.

DOSAGE AND ADMINISTRATION: Dosing Considerations: The absorption of ziprasidone is increased up to two-fold in the presence of food. ZELDOX (ziprasidone hydrochloride) should be administered with food. See also: Warnings and Precautions, QT Prolongation, Recommendations Regarding Risk Factors for QT Prolongation.

Recommended Dose and Dosage Adjustment: Schizophrenia: Initial Treatment: ZELDOX may be administered at an initial daily dose of 40 mg BID with food. However, individual patients may benefit from an initial dose of 20 mg BID. Daily dosage may subsequently be adjusted on the basis of clinical status up to 80 mg BID. Dosage adjustments, if indicated, should generally occur at intervals of not less than 2 days, since steady-state is achieved within 1 to 3 days.

Efficacy in schizophrenia was studied in a dose range of 20 to 100 mg BID in short-term, placebo-controlled clinical trials. There were trends toward dose response within the range of 20 to 80 mg BID, but results were not consistent. An increase to a dose greater than 80 mg BID is not generally recommended. The safety of doses above 100 mg BID has not been systematically evaluated in clinical trials.

Maintenance Treatment: It is recommended that responding patients with schizophrenia be continued on ZELDOX at the lowest dose needed to maintain remission. The efficacy of ZELDOX 20, 40, or 80 mg BID in maintenance treatment has been established over a 12-month treatment period.

Patients should be periodically reassessed to determine the need for maintenance treatment. While there is no body of evidence available to answer the question of how long the patient should be treated with ZELDOX, the effectiveness of maintenance treatment is well established for many other antipsychotic drugs.

Bipolar Disorder : Bipolar Mania: Initial Treatment: Oral ziprasidone should be administered at an initial daily dose of 40 mg BID with food. The dose should then be increased to 60 mg or 80 mg BID on the second day of treatment and subsequently adjusted on the basis of toleration and efficacy within the range 40-80 mg BID. In the flexible-dose clinical trials, the mean daily dose administered was approximately 120 mg.

Maintenance Treatment: There is no body of evidence available from controlled trials to guide a clinician in the longer-term management of a patient who improves during treatment of mania with ziprasidone. While it is generally agreed that pharmacological treatment beyond an acute response in mania is desirable, both for maintenance of the initial response and for prevention of new manic episodes, there are no systematically obtained data to support the use of ziprasidone in such longer-term treatment (i.e., beyond 3 weeks).

Dosage in Special Populations: Dosage adjustments are generally not required on the basis of age, gender, race, or renal impairment.

Hepatic Impairment: Lower doses should be considered for hepatic insufficiency, considering that <1% of ziprasidone is cleared renally, and there is a lack of experience with ziprasidone in patients with severe hepatic impairment.

Missed Dose: The missed dose should be taken at the next scheduled dose. Doses should not be doubled.

OVERDOSAGE:

Symptoms: In premarketing trials, accidental or intentional overdosage of ziprasidone was documented in 10 patients. All of these patients survived without sequelae. In the patient taking the largest confirmed amount, 3240 mg, the only symptoms reported were minimal sedation, slurring of speech, and transitory hypertension (200/95).

In post-marketing use, the most common adverse events reported in association with ziprasidone overdose generally included extrapyramidal symptoms, somnolence, tremor, and anxiety. Hypertension, hypotension, diarrhea, tachycardia, and prolongation of the QTc and QRS intervals have also been reported.

Treatment: There is no specific antidote to ziprasidone, and it is not dialyzable. The possibility of multiple drug involvement should be considered.

In case of acute overdosage, establish and maintain an airway and ensure adequate oxygenation and ventilation. Intravenous access should be established and gastric lavage (after intubation, if patient is unconscious) and administration of activated charcoal together with a laxative should be considered. The possibility of obtundation, seizure, or dystonic reaction of the head and neck following overdose may create a risk of aspiration with induced emesis.

Cardiovascular monitoring should commence immediately and should include continuous electrocardiographic monitoring to detect possible arrhythmias. If antiarrhythmic therapy is administered, disopyramide, procainamide, and quinidine carry a theoretical hazard of additive QT-prolonging effects that might be additive to those of ziprasidone.

Hypotension and circulatory collapse should be treated with appropriate measures such as intravenous fluids. If sympathomimetic agents are used for vascular support, epinephrine and dopamine should not be used, since beta stimulation combined with α_1-antagonism associated with ziprasidone may worsen hypotension. Similarly, it is reasonable to expect that the alpha-adrenergic-blocking properties of bretylium might be additive to those of ziprasidone, resulting in problematic hypotension.

In cases of severe extrapyramidal symptoms, anticholinergic medication should be administered.

Close medical supervision and monitoring should continue until the patient recovers.

> For management of a suspected drug overdose, CPhA recommends that you contact your **regional Poison Control Centre**. See the *CPS* Directory section for a list of Poison Control Centres.

ACTION AND CLINICAL PHARMACOLOGY: ZELDOX (ziprasidone hydrochloride) is an atypical antipsychotic agent for oral administration.

Mechanism of Action: The mechanism of action of ziprasidone, as with other drugs having efficacy in schizophrenia, is unknown. However, it has been proposed that the efficacy of this drug in schizophrenia is mediated through a combination of dopamine type 2 (D_2) and serotonin type 2 ($5HT_2$) antagonism.

Antagonism at receptors other than dopamine and $5HT_2$ with similar receptor affinities may explain some of the other therapeutic and side effects of ziprasidone. Antagonism of histamine H_1 receptors may explain the somnolence observed with ziprasidone. Antagonism of α_1-adrenergic receptors may explain the orthostatic hypotension observed with ziprasidone.

Pharmacodynamics: Ziprasidone exhibited high in vitro binding affinity for the dopamine D_2 and D_3, the serotonin 5-HT_{2A}, 5-HT_{2C}, 5-HT_{1A}, 5-HT_{1D}, and α_1-adrenergic receptors (K_i=4.8, 7.2, 0.4, 1.3, 3.4, 2, and 10 nM, respectively), and moderate affinity for the histamine H_1 receptor (K_i=47 nM). Ziprasidone functioned as an antagonist at the D_2, 5-HT_{2A}, and 5-HT_{1D} receptors, and as an agonist at the 5-HT_{1A} receptor.

Ziprasidone inhibited synaptic reuptake of serotonin and norepinephrine. No appreciable affinity was exhibited for other receptor/binding sites tested, including the cholinergic muscarinic receptor (IC_{50} >1 μM).

Pharmacokinetics: Overview: The multiple-dose pharmacokinetics of ziprasidone are dose-proportional within the proposed clinical dose range, and ziprasidone accumulation is predictable with multiple dosing. Steady-state is attained within 1-3 days when dosing as recommended. The mean terminal phase half-life after multiple dosing in normal volunteers and schizophrenic patients is between 6 and 10 hours, with a range of individual values from 3 to 18 hours.

Ziprasidone's activity is primarily due to the parent drug. Ziprasidone is extensively metabolized after oral administration with only a small amount excreted in the urine (<1%) or feces (<4%) as unchanged drug. Ziprasidone is unlikely to interfere with the metabolism of drugs metabolized by cytochrome P450 enzymes.

Absorption: Following oral administration of multiple doses of ziprasidone with food, peak serum concentrations typically occur 6 to 8 hours post-dose. The absolute bioavailability of a 20 mg dose under fed conditions is approximately 60%. The absorption of ziprasidone is increased up to two-fold in the presence of food.

Distribution: Ziprasidone has a mean apparent volume of distribution of 1.5 L/kg. Twice daily dosing generally leads to attainment of steady state within 1-3 days.

Ziprasidone is greater than 99% bound to plasma proteins, binding primarily to albumin and α_1- acid glycoprotein. The in vitro plasma protein binding of ziprasidone was not altered by warfarin or propranolol, two highly protein-bound drugs, nor did ziprasidone alter the binding of these drugs in human plasma. Thus, the potential for drug interactions with ziprasidone due to displacement is minimal.

Metabolism: Ziprasidone is extensively metabolized after oral administration with only a small amount excreted in the urine (<1%) or feces (<4%) as unchanged drug. Unchanged ziprasidone represents about 44% of total drug-related material in serum.

Ziprasidone is primarily cleared via three metabolic routes to yield four major circulating metabolites, benzisothiazolepiperazine (BITP) sulphoxide; BITP-sulphone; ziprasidone sulphoxide; and S-methyldihydroziprasidone.

In vitro studies using human liver subcellular fractions indicate that S-methyldihydroziprasidone is generated in two steps. The data indicate that the reduction reaction is mediated by aldehyde oxidase and the subsequent methylation is mediated by thiol methyltransferase. In vitro studies using human liver microsomes and recombinant enzymes indicate that CYP3A4 is the major CYP contributing to the oxidative metabolism of ziprasidone. CYP1A2 may contribute to a much lesser extent.

Based on in vivo abundance of excretory metabolites, less than one-third of ziprasidone metabolic clearance is mediated by cytochrome P450 catalyzed oxidation and approximately two-thirds via reduction by aldehyde oxidase. There are no known clinically relevant inhibitors or inducers of aldehyde oxidase.

Excretion: The mean terminal phase half-life after multiple dosing in normal volunteers and schizophrenic patients is between 6 and 10 hours, with a range of individual values from 3 to 18 hours. Approximately 20% of ziprasidone dose is excreted in the urine, with approximately 66% being eliminated in the feces. S-methyldihydroziprasidone is mainly eliminated by biliary excretion and CYP3A4 metabolism. The sulphoxide is eliminated through renal excretion and by secondary metabolism catalyzed by CYP3A4.

Special Populations and Conditions: Pediatrics: Safety and efficacy of ZELDOX in children have not been established.

Age and Gender: In a multiple-dose (8 days of treatment) study involving n=32 subjects, there was no difference in the pharmacokinetics of ziprasidone between men and women or between elderly (>65 years) and young (18 to 45 years) subjects. Additionally, population pharmacokinetic evaluation of patients in controlled trials has revealed no evidence of clinically significant age or gender-related differences in the pharmacokinetics of ziprasidone. Dosage modifications for age or gender are, therefore, not recommended.

Race: No specific pharmacokinetic study was conducted to investigate the effects of race. Population pharmacokinetic evaluation has revealed no evidence of clinically significant race-related differences in the pharmacokinetics of ziprasidone. Dosage modifications for race are, therefore, not recommended.

Hepatic Insufficiency: As ziprasidone is cleared substantially by the liver, the presence of hepatic impairment would be expected to increase the AUC of ziprasidone; a multiple-dose study at the lowest therapeutic dose of 20 mg BID for 5 days in subjects with clinically significant (Childs-Pugh Class A and B) cirrhosis (n=13) revealed an increase in AUC_{0-12} of 19% and 34% respectively, compared to a matched control group (n=13). A half-life of 7.1 hours was observed in subjects with cirrhosis compared to 4.8 hours in the control group. The effect of liver impairment on the serum concentrations of the metabolites is unknown.

Renal Insufficiency: Because ziprasidone is highly metabolized with less than 1% of the drug excreted unchanged, renal impairment alone is unlikely to have a major impact on the pharmacokinetics of ziprasidone. The pharmacokinetic characteristics of ziprasidone following 8 days of treatment with 20 mg BID were similar among subjects with varying degrees of renal impairment (n=27), and subjects with normal renal function (n=9), indicating that dosage adjustment based upon the degree of renal impairment is not required. Ziprasidone is not removed by hemodialysis.

STORAGE AND STABILITY: Store at controlled room temperature between 15-30°C.

INFORMATION FOR THE PATIENT: Published in e-CPS, available by subscription at www.e-cps.ca.

DOSAGE FORMS, COMPOSITION AND PACKAGING: 20 mg: Each size #4 blue/white hard gelatin capsule, imprinted in black with "Pfizer" and "396" or "ZDX 20", contains: ziprasidone hydrochloride, monohydrate equivalent to 20 mg of ziprasidone. Nonmedicinal ingredients: lactose monohydrate, magnesium stearate and pregelatinized starch. HDPE bottles of 100. Blisters of 10 and 30.

40 mg: Each size #4 blue/blue hard gelatin capsule, imprinted in black with "Pfizer" and "397" or "ZDX 40", contains: ziprasidone hydrochloride, monohydrate equivalent to 40 mg of ziprasidone. Nonmedicinal ingredients: lactose monohydrate, magnesium stearate and pregelatinized starch. HDPE bottles of 100. Blisters of 10 and 30.

60 mg: Each size #3 white/white hard gelatin capsule, imprinted in black with "Pfizer" and "398" or "ZDX 60", contains: ziprasidone hydrochloride, monohydrate equivalent to 60 mg of ziprasidone. Nonmedicinal ingredients: lactose monohydrate, magnesium stearate and pregelatinized starch. HDPE bottles of 100. Blisters of 10 and 30.

80 mg: Each size #2 blue/white hard gelatin capsule, imprinted in black with "Pfizer" and "399" or "ZDX 80", contains: ziprasidone hydrochloride, monohydrate equivalent to 80 mg of ziprasidone. Nonmedicinal ingredients: lactose monohydrate, magnesium stearate and pregelatinized starch. HDPE bottles of 100. Blisters of 10 and 30.

(Shown in Product Identification Section)

Zemuron® Ⓟ

rocuronium bromide

Nondepolarizing Skeletal Neuromuscular Blocking Agent

Schering-Plough

Date of Revision: July 15, 2010

SUMMARY PRODUCT INFORMATION:

Route of Administration	Dosage Form/ Strength	All Nonmedicinal Ingredients
Intravenous	Solution for Injection/10 mg/mL	Sodium acetate trihydrate, sodium chloride, water for injection, nitrogen. May contain sodium hydroxide and/or glacial acetic acid to adjust the pH to approximately 4.0.

INDICATIONS AND CLINICAL USE: ZEMURON (rocuronium bromide) is indicated as an adjunct to general anesthesia to facilitate routine endotracheal intubation or rapid sequence (initiated at 60-90 seconds post-administration) intubation to provide skeletal muscle relaxation during surgery or mechanical ventilation.

Rocuronium bromide is a non-depolarizing neuromuscular blocking agent with a rapid to intermediate onset and an intermediate duration of action depending on dose.

Geriatrics (>65 years of age): Lower maintenance doses and infusion rates are recommended as the duration of neuromuscular blockade tends to be longer in the elderly. For details, see Dosage and Administration, Geriatrics.

Pediatrics (≤18 years of age): ZEMURON is indicated for routine adjunct use in all pediatric patients, including term neonates and infants. Caution is advised in selecting the dosage for intubation and maintenance in neonates and infants because of limited controlled safety and efficacy data. ZEMURON is not recommended for rapid sequence intubation in pediatric patients. For details, see Dosage and Administration, Pediatrics.

CONTRAINDICATIONS: Patients who are hypersensitive to this drug or to any ingredient in the formulation or component of the container. For a complete listing, see Dosage Forms, Composition and Packaging.

WARNINGS AND PRECAUTIONS:

Serious Warnings and Precautions

ZEMURON (rocuronium bromide) should be administered in carefully adjusted dosage by or under the supervision of experienced clinicians who are familiar with its actions and the possible complications of its use. The drug should not be administered unless personnel and facilities for resuscitation and life support (tracheal intubation, artificial ventilation, oxygen therapy), and an antagonist of ZEMURON are immediately available. It is recommended that an adequate neuromuscular monitoring device be used to measure neuromuscular function during the administration of ZEMURON in order to monitor drug effect, determine the need for additional doses, and confirm recovery from neuromuscular blockade.

ZEMURON has no known effect on consciousness, pain threshold, thinking, or memory. To avoid distress to the patient, neuromuscular blockade should not be induced before unconsciousness.

General: Neuromuscular Blockade: Since ZEMURON causes paralysis of the respiratory muscles, ventilatory support is mandatory for patients treated with this drug until adequate spontaneous respiration is restored. As with all neuromuscular blocking agents, it is important to anticipate intubation difficulties, particularly when used as part of a Rapid Sequence Intubation technique.

Residual Neuromuscular Blockade: As with other neuromuscular blocking agents, residual neuromuscular blockade has been reported for ZEMURON. In order to prevent complications resulting from residual neuromuscular blockade, it is recommended to extubate only after the patient has recovered sufficiently from neuromuscular blockade. Other factors which could cause residual neuromuscular blockade after extubation in the post-operative phase (such as drug interactions or patient condition) should also be considered. The use of a reversal agent should be considered, especially in those cases where residual neuromuscular blockade is more likely to occur.

Hypothermia: Hypothermia reduces the requirement for the neuromuscular blocking agent.

Carcinogenesis and Mutagenesis: No human data are available.

Cardiovascular: Electrocardiogram (ECG) Monitoring: The overall analysis of ECG data from two clinical pharmacology studies in pediatric patients indicates that the combined use of rocuronium with general anesthetic agents may prolong the QTc interval. Some of the prolongation may reach clinical significance. Routine ECG monitoring is recommended, especially in pediatric patients. The routine precautions for treating arrhythmia should be taken into consideration.

Delayed Onset of Action: Conditions associated with prolonged circulation time such as cardiovascular disease, old age and oedematous state resulting in an increased volume of distribution, may contribute to a slower onset of action. The duration of action may also be prolonged due to a reduced plasma clearance.

Pulmonary Vascular Resistance: ZEMURON may be associated with increased pulmonary vascular resistance, so caution is appropriate in patients with pulmonary hypertension or valvular heart disease.

Endocrine and Metabolism: Obesity: Like other neuromuscular blocking agents, ZEMURON may exhibit a prolonged duration and a prolonged spontaneous recovery in obese patients, when the administered doses are calculated on actual body weight. See Dosage and Administration and Action and Clinical Pharmacology.

Hepatic/Biliary/Pancreatic: Because rocuronium is excreted in urine and bile, it should be used with caution in patients with hepatic impairment. In these patient groups prolongation of action has been observed with doses of 0.6 mg/kg rocuronium bromide. See Dosage and Administration and Action and Clinical Pharmacology.

Intensive Care Unit (ICU): Whenever the use of ZEMURON, or any neuromuscular blocking agent, is contemplated in the ICU, it is recommended that a peripheral nerve stimulator be used continuously to monitor neuromuscular transmission during administration and recovery. In addition, patients should receive adequate analgesia and sedation. Furthermore, additional doses of ZEMURON or any other neuromuscular blocking agent should not be given before there is a definite response to the first twitch. If no response is elicited, infusion administration should be discontinued until a response returns.

Long-Term Use in the ICU: To reduce the possibility of prolonged neuromuscular blockade and other complications that might occur following long-term use in the ICU, ZEMURON or any other neuromuscular relaxant should be administered in carefully adjusted doses by or under the supervision of experienced clinicians who are familiar with its actions and with appropriate peripheral nerve stimulator muscle monitoring techniques.

In rare cases, long-term use of neuromuscular blocking drugs to facilitate mechanical ventilation in ICU settings has been associated with prolonged paralysis and/or skeletal muscle weakness that is first noted during attempts to wean patients from the ventilator. In these patients, the actions of the neuromuscular blocking agent may be enhanced by other drugs (e.g., broad spectrum antibiotics, narcotics and/or steroids) or by conditions such as acid-base or electrolyte imbalance, hypoxic episodes of varying duration, or extreme debilitation. Additionally, patients immobilized for extended periods frequently develop symptoms consistent with disuse muscle atrophy. Recovery may vary from regaining movement and strength in all muscles to initial recovery of movement of the facial muscles and small muscles of the extremities then to the remaining muscles. In rare cases, recovery may involve an extended period of time or even require rehabilitation. Therefore, when there is a need for long-term mechanical ventilation, the benefits-to-risk ratio of neuromuscular blockade must be considered. The syndrome of critical illness polyneuropathy associated with sepsis and multiorgan failure may be associated with prolonged skeletal muscle paralysis, but can also occur without the use of muscle relaxants. Thus, the role of muscle relaxants in the etiology of prolonged paralysis in the ICU is not known with certainty.

Myopathy: After long term administration of other non-depolarizing neuromuscular blocking agents in the ICU alone or in combination with corticosteroid therapy, myopathy has been reported. Therefore, for patients receiving both neuromuscular blocking agents and corticosteroids, the period of use of the neuromuscular blocking agent should be limited as much as possible.

Neurologic: Neuromuscular Disease: In patients with myasthenia gravis or myasthenic (Eaton-Lambert) syndrome, small doses of non-depolarizing neuromuscular blocking agents may have profound effects. In such patients, a peripheral nerve stimulator and use of a small test dose may be of value in monitoring the response to administration of muscle relaxants. For patients having conditions in which prolonged neuromuscular blockade is a possibility (e.g., neuromuscular disease, carcinomatosis, severe cachexia, or debilitation), a peripheral nerve stimulator and use of a small test dose may be of particular value in assessing and monitoring dosage requirements.

Peri-Operative Considerations: Potentiation of Neuromuscular Blockade: Hypokalaemia (e.g. after severe vomiting, diarrhea and diuretic therapy), hypermagnesemia, hypocalcemia (after massive transfusions), hypoproteinemia, dehydration, acidosis, hypercapnia, cachexia, and debilitation.

Severe electrolyte disturbances, altered blood pH or dehydration should therefore be corrected when possible.

Rapid Sequence Induction of Anesthesia: Endotracheal intubation during rapid sequence induction has not been adequately studied at time points of less than 60 seconds post-administration of rocuronium bromide.

The experience with rocuronium bromide in rapid sequence induction in pediatric patients is limited. Rocuronium bromide is therefore not recommended for facilitating tracheal intubation conditions during rapid sequence induction in pediatric patients.

Clinical experience indicates that rocuronium bromide is often unsuitable for facilitating endotracheal intubation during rapid sequence induction in Cesarean section patients. Therefore it is not recommended for rapid sequence induction in obstetric patients. See Special Populations.

Renal: Because rocuronium is excreted in urine and bile, it should be used with caution in patients with severe renal impairment (creatinine clearance <30 mL/min). In these patient groups prolongation of action has been observed with doses of 0.6 mg/kg rocuronium bromide.

Sensitivity/Resistance: Anaphylaxis: Anaphylactic reactions can occur following the administration of neuromuscular blocking agents. These reactions have, in some cases (including cases with ZEMURON) been life threatening. Precautions, like the immediate availability of appropriate emergency treatment, for treating such reactions should always be taken. Particularly in the case of previous anaphylactic reactions to neuromuscular blocking agents, special precautions should be taken since allergic cross-reactivity to neuromuscular blocking agents has been reported.

Burns: Patients with burns are known to develop resistance to non-depolarizing neuromuscular blocking agents. It is recommended that the dose is titrated to response.

Special Populations: Pregnant Women: For rocuronium bromide, no clinical data on exposed pregnancies are available. Animal studies do not indicate direct or indirect harmful effects with respect to pregnancy, embryonal/foetal development, parturition or postnatal development. ZEMURON should be used during pregnancy only if the potential benefit justifies the potential risk to the fetus.

Use in Obstetrics (Cesarean section): Intubating conditions were poor or inadequate in 5 of 13 women receiving 3-4 mg/kg thiopental when intubation was attempted 60 seconds after administering 0.6 mg/kg (600 μg/kg) rocuronium bromide. Therefore, ZEMURON is not recommended for rapid sequence intubation in Cesarean section patients. The possibility of respiratory depression in the neonate should always be considered following a Cesarean section during which a neuromuscular blocking agent has been administered.

Nursing Women: It is unknown whether ZEMURON is excreted in human breast milk. Animal studies have shown insignificant levels of rocuronium bromide in breast milk. ZEMURON should be given to lactating women only when the attending physician decides that the benefits outweigh the risks.

Pediatrics: Caution is advised in selecting intubation and maintenance dosage in neonates and infants because of limited controlled safety and efficacy data. ZEMURON is not recommended for facilitating intubation during rapid sequence induction in pediatric patients. ZEMURON is not recommended for facilitating mechanical ventilation in the intensive care unit in pediatric patients because of insufficient safety and efficacy data. See Dosage and Administration, Pediatrics.

The overall analysis of ECG data in two clinical pharmacological studies in pediatric patients indicates that the combined use of ZEMURON with general anesthetic agents can prolong the QTc interval. The data also suggest that ZEMURON may increase heart rate. However, it was not possible to conclusively identify an effect of ZEMURON independent of that of anesthesia and other factors. Additionally, when examining plasma levels of ZEMURON in correlation to QTc interval prolongation, no relationship was observed. See Warnings and Precautions, Cardiovascular, Electrocardiogram (ECG) Monitoring and Adverse Reactions, Clinical Trial Adverse Drug Reactions.

Geriatrics: Lower maintenance doses and infusion rates are recommended for the elderly. ZEMURON is not recommended for the facilitation of mechanical ventilation in the intensive care in geriatric patients due to a lack of data on safety and efficacy. See Dosage and Administration, Geriatrics.

ADVERSE REACTIONS: Adverse Drug Reaction Overview: Although very rare, severe anaphylactic reactions to neuromuscular blocking agents, including ZEMURON, have been reported. Anaphylactic/anaphylactoid reactions are: bronchospasm, cardiovascular changes (e.g. hypotension, tachycardia, circulatory collapse—shock), and cutaneous changes (e.g. angioedema, urticaria). These reactions have, in some cases, been fatal. Due to the possible severity of these reactions, one should always assume they may occur and take the necessary precautions.

Since neuromuscular blocking agents are known to be capable of inducing histamine release both locally at the site of injection and systemically, the possible occurrence of itching and erythematous reactions at the site of injection and/or generalized histaminoid (anaphylactoid) reactions (see also under anaphylactic reactions above) should always be taken into consideration when administering these drugs.

In clinical studies only a slight increase in mean plasma histamine levels has been observed following rapid bolus administration of 0.3-0.9 mg/kg rocuronium bromide.

Prolonged Neuromuscular Blockade: The most frequent adverse reaction to nondepolarizing blocking agents as a class consists of an extension of the drug's pharmacological action beyond the time period needed. This may vary from skeletal muscle weakness to profound and prolonged skeletal muscle paralysis resulting in respiratory insufficiency or apnea.

Myopathy: Myopathy has been reported after the use of various neuromuscular blocking agents in the ICU in combination with corticosteroids (see Warning and Precautions, Long-Term Use in the ICU).

Local Injection Site Reactions: During rapid sequence induction of anesthesia, pain on injection has been reported, especially when the patient has not yet completely lost consciousness and particularly when propofol is used as the induction agent. In clinical studies, pain on injection has been noted in 16% of the patients who underwent rapid sequence induction of anesthesia with propofol and in less than 0.5% of the patients who underwent rapid sequence induction of anesthesia with fentanyl and thiopental.

Clinical Trial Adverse Drug Reactions: Because clinical trials are conducted under very specific conditions the adverse reaction rates observed in the clinical trials may not reflect the rates observed in practice and should not be compared to the rates in the clinical trials of another drug. Adverse drug reaction information from clinical trials is useful for identifying drug-related adverse events and for approximating rates.

The patients exposed in North American clinical studies (n=1137) provide the basis for calculation of adverse event rates. The following adverse reactions were reported in patients administered rocuronium bromide and the incidences of these adverse reactions were less than 1%:

Cardiovascular: arrhythmia, abnormal electrocardiogram, tachycardia.

Digestive: nausea, vomiting.

Respiratory: asthma (bronchospasm, wheezing, or rhonchi), hiccup.

Skin and Appendages: rash, injection site oedema, pruritus.

A meta-analysis of 11 clinical studies in pediatric patients (n=704) with rocuronium bromide (up to 1 mg/kg) showed that tachycardia was identified as adverse drug reaction with a frequency of 1.4%.

Approximately 5% pediatric patients reported QTcB longer than 500 msec in two rocuronium clinical pharmacological studies under general anesthesia and during surgery. Prolonged QTc intervals were observed both before and after rocuronium injection. However, a relationship between the plasma rocuronium concentrations and specific QTc intervals was not identified after rocuronium intubation doses of 0.45, 0.6, or 1.0 mg/kg.

Post-Market Adverse Drug Reactions: The information included in this section is based on post-marketing data and clinical trials (see Table 1).

The most commonly occurring adverse drug reactions include injection site pain/reaction, changes in vital signs and prolonged neuromuscular blockade. The most frequently reported serious adverse drug reactions during post-marketing surveillance is 'anaphylactic and anaphylactoid reactions' and associated symptoms.

DRUG INTERACTIONS: Drug-Drug Interactions: No formal clinical interaction studies have been conducted in adults or in pediatrics with rocuronium bromide and other drugs commonly used for anesthesia. Based on post-market clinical studies and experience, the following drugs have been shown to influence the magnitude and/or duration of action of non-depolarizing neuromuscular blocking agents:

Antibiotics: Antibiotics from several classes may enhance or prolong the neuromuscular blockade produced by rocuronium regardless of their route of parenteral administration (e.g. intravenous, intraperitoneal). Antibiotics such as aminoglycoside, lincosamide and polypeptide antibiotics, acylamino-penicillin antibiotics have been shown to increase the effect of rocuronium. Residual neuromuscular blockade has been reported after post-operative administration of: aminoglycoside, lincosamide, polypeptide and acylamino-penicillin antibiotics.

Anticonvulsants: Prior chronic administration of phenytoin or carbamazepine has been shown to decrease the effect of rocuronium. Increased effect of rocuronium has been shown with acute administration of phenytoin.

Table 1: ZEMURON

Post-Market Adverse Drug Reactions

	Preferred Term[a]	
MedDRA SOC	**Uncommon (≥1/1000 and <1/100)/ Rare[b] (≥1/10 000 and <1/1000)**	**Very Rare (<1/10 000)**
Immune System Disorders		Hypersensitivity
		Anaphylactic reaction
		Anaphylactoid reaction
		Anaphylactic shock
		Anaphylactoid shock
Nervous System Disorders		Flaccid paralysis
Cardiac Disorders	Tachycardia	
Vascular Disorders	Hypotension	Circulatory collapse and shock
		Flushing
Respiratory, Thoracic and Mediastinal Disorders		Bronchospasm
Skin and Subcutaneous Tissue Disorders		Angioneurotic oedema
		Urticaria
		Rash
		Erythematous rash
Musculoskeletal and Connective Tissue Disorders		Muscular weakness[c]
		Steroid myopathy[c]
General Disorders and Administration Site Conditions	Drug ineffective	Face oedema
	Drug effect/therapeutic response decreased	
	Drug effect/therapeutic response increased	
	Injection site pain	
	Injection site reaction	
Injury, Poisoning and Procedural Complications	Prolonged neuromuscular blockade	Airway complication of anaesthesia
	Delayed recovery from anesthesia	

[a] Frequencies are estimates derived from post-marketing surveillance reports and data from the general literature.
[b] Post-marketing surveillance data cannot give precise incidence figures. For that reason, the reporting frequency was divided over two rather than five categories.
[c] After long-term use in the ICU.
MedDRA version 8.1.

Corticosteroids: Long-term concomitant use of corticosteroids and ZEMURON in the ICU may result in prolonged duration of neuromuscular blockade or myopathy.
Inhalation Anesthetics: Halogenated volatile anesthetics potentiate the neuromuscular blockade of ZEMURON during induction and maintenance. Reversal of the blockade with anticholinesterase inhibitors could also be inhibited.
Local Anesthetics: Local anesthetics used during combined regional and general anesthesia have been shown to increase the duration of the neuromuscular blockade and decrease requirements of neuromuscular blocking agents.
Other Drugs: Increased effect of rocuronium has been shown with: acute administration of β-blocking agents, calcium channel blocking agents, diuretics, intravenous lidocaine, magnesium salts, lithium salts, procainamide, or quinidine and its isomer quinine. Residual neuromuscular blockade has been reported after post-operative administration of: quinidine, quinine and magnesium salts.
Other Non-Depolarizing Neuromuscular Blocking Agents: Administration of other non-depolarizing neuromuscular blocking agents in combination with ZEMURON may produce attenuation or potentiation of the neuromuscular blockade, depending on the order of administration and the neuromuscular blocking agent used.
Protease Inhibitors: Protease inhibitors (gabexate, ulinastatin) have been shown to decrease the effect of ZEMURON.
Succinylcholine: If rocuronium bromide is given following administration of succinylcholine, it should not be given until recovery from succinylcholine has been observed. The median duration of action of rocuronium bromide 0.6 mg/kg administered after a 1 mg/kg dose of succinylcholine when T1 returned to 75% of control was 36 minutes (range 14-57, n=12) vs. 28 minutes (17-51, n=12) without succinylcholine.

Succinylcholine given after the administration of ZEMURON may produce potentiation or attenuation of the neuromuscular blocking effect of ZEMURON.

It is not recommended to use a small dose of rocuronium bromide before an intubation dose of succinylcholine to reduce muscle fasciculation produced by succinylcholine.

DOSAGE AND ADMINISTRATION: Dosing Considerations: ZEMURON should be administered only by intravenous route. This drug should be administered by or under the supervision of experienced clinicians familiar with the use of neuromuscular blocking agents.

To avoid distress to the patient, ZEMURON should not be administered before unconsciousness has been induced. It should not be mixed in the same syringe or administered simultaneously through the same needle with alkaline solutions (e.g., barbiturate solutions).

As with other neuromuscular blocking agents, doses of ZEMURON should be individualized in each patient. The method of anesthesia and the expected duration of surgery, the method of sedation and the expected duration of mechanical ventilation, the possible interaction with other drugs that are administered concomitantly, and the condition of the patient should be taken into account when determining the dose. A peripheral nerve stimulator should be used to measure neuromuscular function during administration of ZEMURON in order to monitor drug effect, to determine the need for additional doses, and to confirm recovery from neuromuscular blockade.

Inhalational anesthetics do potentiate the neuromuscular blocking effects of ZEMURON. This potentiation however, becomes clinically relevant in the course of anesthesia, when the volatile agents have reached the tissue concentrations required for this interaction. Consequently, the choice of an intubating dose of rocuronium bromide should not, therefore, be reduced below 0.45 mg/kg if routine tracheal intubation is to be performed or below 0.60 mg/kg if rapid intubation is to be performed. Yet adjustments with ZEMURON should be made by administering smaller maintenance doses at less frequent intervals or by using lower infusion rates of ZEMURON during long lasting procedures (longer than 1 hour) under inhalational anesthesia (see Drug Interactions, Drug-Drug Interactions). Otherwise increases in the clinical duration (25-35%) and recovery time (20-70%) of neuromuscular blockade may be apparent in the presence of a halogenated inhalation agent.

Continuous infusion or intermittent bolus dosing to support long term mechanical ventilation has not been studied sufficiently to support dosage recommendations.

Recommended Dose and Dosage Adjustment: Adults: The following dosage recommendations may serve as a general guideline for tracheal intubation and muscle relaxation for short to long lasting surgical procedures.
Endotracheal Intubation: Routine Endotracheal Intubation: The recommended initial dose regardless of anesthetic regimen is 0.6 mg/kg rocuronium bromide. Neuromuscular blockade sufficient for intubation (80% blockade or greater) is attained in a median (range) time of 1 (0.4-6) minute(s) and most patients have intubation completed within 2 minutes. Maximum blockade is achieved in most patients in less than 3 minutes. This dose may be expected to provide 31 (15-85) minutes of surgical relaxation under opioid/N_2O/O_2 anesthesia. Under halothane, isoflurane, and enflurane anesthesia, some extension of the period of clinical relaxation should be expected (see Drug Interactions).
Endotracheal Intubation during Rapid Sequence Induction: In appropriately pre-medicated and adequately anesthetized patients, 0.60-1.2 mg/kg (600-1200 µg/kg) rocuronium bromide will provide good or excellent intubating conditions in most patients in 60-90 seconds.
Use of Lower or Higher Doses: A lower dose of rocuronium bromide (0.45 mg/kg) may be used. Neuromuscular blockade sufficient for intubation (80% blockade or greater) is attained in a median (range) time of 1.3 (0.8-6.2) minute(s) and most patients have intubation completed within 1.6 (1.0-7.0) minutes. Maximum blockade is achieved in most patients in 3.0 (1.3-8.2) minutes. This dose may be expected to provide 22 (12-31) minutes of clinical relaxation under opioid/N_2O/O_2 anesthesia. Patients receiving this low dose of 0.45 mg/kg who achieve less than 90% blockade (about 16% of these patients) may have a more rapid time to 25% recovery, 12 to 15 minutes.

A large bolus dose of 0.9 or 1.2 mg/kg may be administered under opioid/N_2O/O_2 anesthesia when necessary. These doses will provide >80% blockade in most patients in 1.1 and 0.7 minutes, respectively, with maximum blockade occurring in most patients in 1.4 and 1.0 minute, respectively. Doses of 0.9 and 1.2 mg/kg may be expected to provide 58 (27-111) and 67 (38-160) minutes of clinical relaxation under opioid/N_2O/O_2 anesthesia, respectively.

A high bolus dose of 1.6 or 2.0 mg/kg may be used when necessary. These doses resulted in good to excellent intubation conditions and excellent intubation conditions within 60 seconds after rocuronium bromide administration, respectively. Doses of 1.6 or 2.0 mg/kg may be expected to provide 76 (55-97) and 110 (80-160) minutes of clinical relaxation under alfentanyl/thiopental anesthesia.
Maintenance Dosing: Maintenance doses of 0.1, 0.15, and 0.2 mg/kg (100, 150, and 200 µg/kg) of rocuronium bromide administered at 25% recovery of control T1, provide a median 12, 17, and 24 minutes of clinically effective neuromuscular blockade during opioid/N_2O/O_2 anesthesia. Smaller or less frequent bolus maintenance doses (0.075-0.1 mg/kg rocuronium bromide) should be considered during anesthesia with a halogenated inhalation agents. Subsequent dosing should be guided based on the clinical duration following initial dose or prior maintenance dose and only when twitch height has recovered to 25% of control twitch height or when 2 to 3 responses to train-of-four stimulation are present. Cumulative effect with repetitive maintenance dosing has been observed but it is of minor clinical significance.
Continuous Infusion: After evidence of early spontaneous recovery (<10% of control T1) from initial doses of rocuronium bromide, a continuous infusion can be initiated to maintain a 90% suppression of twitch response or to maintain 1 to 2 responses to train-of-four stimulation. In adults under intravenous anesthesia, the infusion rate required to maintain neuromuscular blockade at this level ranges from 0.3-0.6 mg/kg/h and under inhalational anesthesia the infusion rate ranges from 0.3-0.4 mg/kg/h. Continuous monitoring of neuromuscular blockade is recommended since infusion rate requirements vary from patient to patient and with the anesthetic method used.

Initiation of the infusion after substantial return of neuromuscular function (more than 10% of control T1), may necessitate additional bolus doses to maintain adequate blockade for surgery.

Spontaneous recovery and reversal of neuromuscular blockade following discontinuation of rocuronium bromide infusion may be expected to proceed at rates similar to those following comparable total doses administered by repetitive bolus injections.

Infusion solutions of ZEMURON can be prepared by mixing ZEMURON with an appropriate infusion solution (see Dosage and Administration, Administration). Unused portions of infusion solutions should be discarded.
Pediatrics: Caution is advised in selecting intubation and maintenance dosages in neonates (0-1 month) and infants (1-3 months) because of limited controlled safety and efficacy data. ZEMURON is not recommended for rapid sequence intubation in pediatric patients because of insufficient safety and efficacy data.
Routine Endotracheal Intubation: The recommended initial intubation dose of ZEMURON is 0.6 mg/kg, however, a lower dose of 0.45 mg/kg may be used depending on the underlying pathology of the patient, use of other drugs, the surgical procedure planned, anesthetic technique and the age of the patient.
Halothane Anesthesia: Initial doses of 0.6 mg/kg (600 µg/kg) in children (3 months-12 years) under halothane anesthesia produce 100% neuromuscular blockade and excellent to good intubating conditions within approximately 60 to 90 seconds. This dose will provide approximately 25-30 minutes of clinical relaxation in children aged 1 to 12 years receiving halothane anesthesia. For infants aged 3-12 months, the duration of action of a 0.6 mg/kg dose is longer than in older pediatric patients, averaging 42 minutes under conditions of halothane anesthesia.
Sevoflurane (induction) and Isoflurane/Nitrous Oxide (maintenance): For sevoflurane induction ZEMURON doses of 0.45 mg/kg and 0.6 mg/kg in general produce excellent to good intubating conditions within 75 seconds in all pediatric ages. The time to maximum block for an intubating dose was approximately 60 seconds on average across all pediatric groups, longest in neonates (0-28 days) (70-80 seconds), and shortest in infants (1-3 months) (40-50 seconds). The duration of clinical relaxation following an intubating dose is shortest in children (2 years-11 years) and approximately 2-fold longer in neonates and infants.

For sevoflurane (induction), the time to maximum block for an intubating dose was shortest in infants (28 days up to 3 months) and longest in neonates (birth to less than 28 days). The duration of clinical relaxation following an intubating dose is shortest in children (greater than 2 years up to 11 years) and longest in infants.
Maintenance Doses: The recommended maintenance dose for pediatric patients of all age groups are similar to those in adults.
Halothane Anesthesia: When halothane is used for general anesthesia in pediatric patients aged 4-13 years, maintenance doses of 0.075-0.125 mg/kg (75-125 µg/kg), administered upon return of T_1 to 25% of control provide surgical relaxation for a median of 7-10 minutes.
Sevoflurane (induction) and Isoflurane/Nitrous Oxide (maintenance): When sevoflurane is used for induction and isoflurane/nitrous oxide for maintenance of general anesthesia, maintenance dosing of ZEMURON can be administered as bolus doses of 0.15 mg/kg at reappearance of T_3 in all pediatric age groups. Maintenance dosing can also be administered at the reappearance of T_2 at a rate of 7-10 µg/kg/min with the lowest dose requirement for neonates and the highest dose requirement for children.
Continuous Infusion: For continuous infusion in infants (3-23 months), children (2-11 years) and adolescents (12-18 years) the same infusion rates as for adults are recommended. Although for children (2-11 years) higher infusion rates might be necessary.

A continuous infusion of rocuronium bromide initiated at a rate of 0.012 mg/kg/min (12 µg/kg/min) upon return of T1 to 10% of control has been demonstrated to maintain neuromuscular blockade at 89-99% in children receiving halothane anesthesia.
Geriatrics: The recommended intubation dose is 0.6 mg/kg rocuronium bromide for the elderly. A dose of 0.6 mg/kg should be considered for Rapid Sequence Induction of anesthesia in the elderly in whom a prolonged duration of action is expected. The recommended maintenance dose for these patients is 0.075-0.1 mg/kg rocuronium bromide, and the recommended infusion rate is 0.3-0.4 mg/kg/h, regardless of the anesthetic technique used.

Geriatric patients exhibited a slightly prolonged median duration of surgical relaxation after an equivalent dose to younger adults. Following doses of 0.6, 0.9, and 1.2 mg/kg, the median (range) duration was 46 (22-73), 62 (49-75), and 94 (64-138) minutes under opioid/N_2O/O_2 anesthesia, respectively. No differences in duration of neuromuscular blockade following maintenance doses of rocuronium bromide were observed between elderly and younger subjects. Other reported clinical experience has not identified differences in response between elderly and younger patients, but greater sensitivity of some older individuals cannot be ruled out. See Action and Clinical Pharmacology.
Patients with Hepatic or Renal Impairment: The recommended intubation dose for patients with hepatic or renal impairment during routine anesthesia is 0.6 mg/kg rocuronium bromide. A dose of 0.6 mg/kg should be considered for Rapid Sequence Induction of anesthesia in these patients in whom a prolonged duration of action is expected. The recommended maintenance dose for these patients is 0.075-0.1 mg/kg rocuronium bromide, and the recommended infusion rate is 0.3-0.4 mg/kg/h regardless of the anesthetic technique used (see also Continuous Infusion).

When compared with patients with normal hepatic or renal function, no differences in onset time were observed in patients with hepatic or renal impairment at a dose of 0.6 mg/kg rocuronium bromide. The mean duration of surgical relaxation may have a greater variation in patients with renal impairment. It is about 1.5 times longer in patients with hepatic impairment.

Obese Patients: When used in obese patients (defined as patients with a body weight of 30% or more above ideal body weight) doses should be reduced taking into account ideal body weight.

Administration: ZEMURON is administered intravenously either as a bolus injection or as a continuous infusion.

Do not use ZEMURON if solution contains particles or is not clear.

Compatibility: Compatibility studies with the following infusion fluids have been performed. In nominal concentrations of 0.5 mg/mL and 2.0 mg/mL ZEMURON is compatible in solution with: 0.9% Sodium Chloride Injection, USP; 5% Dextrose Injection, USP; 5% Dextrose and 0.9% Sodium Chloride Injection, USP; Sterile Water for Injection, USP; Lactated Ringer's Solution.

Administration should be begun immediately after mixing, and should be completed within 24 hours. Unused solutions should be discarded.

Incompatibility: ZEMURON (rocuronium bromide), which has an acidic pH (pH: 3.8-4.2), should not be mixed with alkaline solutions (e.g. barbiturate solutions) in the same syringe or administered simultaneously during intravenous infusion through the same needle. If ZEMURON is administered via the same infusion line that is also used for other drugs, it is important that this infusion line is adequately flushed (e.g. with 0.9 % NaCl) between administration of ZEMURON and drugs for which incompatibility with ZEMURON has been demonstrated or for which compatibility with ZEMURON has not been established.

Incompatibility has been documented for ZEMURON when added to solutions containing the following drugs: amphotericin, amoxicillin, azathioprine, cefazolin, cloxacillin, dexamethasone, diazepam, enoximone, erythromycin, famotidine, furosemide, hydrocortisone sodium succinate, insulin, methohexital, methylprednisolone, prednisolone sodium succinate, thiopental, trimethoprim and vancomycin. ZEMURON is also incompatible with Intralipid.

Antagonism of Neuromuscular Blockade: Antagonists (such as neostigmine, edrophonium and pyridostigmine) should not be administered prior to the demonstration of some spontaneous recovery from neuromuscular blockage (reappearance of T_2 or first signs of functional recovery). The use of an adequate neuromuscular monitoring device to document recovery and antagonism of neuromuscular blockade is recommended. The time required for anticholinesterase mediated recovery is longer for reversals attempted at deeper levels of blockade.

Patients should be evaluated for adequate functional evidence of antagonism, e.g., 5 second head lift, adequate phonation, ventilation and upper airway maintenance. Ventilation must be supported until no longer required.

Antagonism by acetylcholinesterase inhibiting agents may be delayed in the presence of debilitation, carcinomatosis, and concomitant use of certain broad spectrum antibiotics, or anesthetic agents and other drugs which enhance neuromuscular blockade or depress respiratory function (see Drug Interactions). Under such circumstances the management is the same as that of prolonged neuromuscular blockade (see Overdosage).

OVERDOSAGE:

The possibility of iatrogenic overdosage can be minimized by carefully monitoring the muscle twitch response to peripheral nerve stimulation. In the event of overdosage and prolonged neuromuscular blockade, the patient should continue to receive ventilatory support and sedation. Adequate monitoring of vital organ function is recommended for the period of paralysis and during an extended period post recovery. Upon start of spontaneous recovery an acetylcholinesterase inhibitor (e.g. neostigmine, edrophonium, pyridostigmine) should be administered in adequate doses. When administration of an acetylcholinesterase inhibiting agent fails to reverse the neuromuscular effects of ZEMURON, ventilation must be continued until adequate spontaneous breathing is restored. Repeated dosage of an acetylcholinesterase inhibitor can be dangerous.

> For management of a suspected drug overdose, contact your regional Poison Control Centre. See the *CPS* Directory section for a list of Poison Control Centres.

ACTION AND CLINICAL PHARMACOLOGY: Mechanism of Action: ZEMURON (rocuronium bromide) is a nondepolarizing neuromuscular blocking agent with a rapid to intermediate onset and intermediate duration depending on dose. It acts by competing for cholinergic receptors at the motor end-plate. This action is antagonized by acetylcholinesterase inhibitors, such as neostigmine and edrophonium.

Pharmacodynamics: Pharmacodynamic Effects: The ED_{95} (dose required to produce 95% suppression of the first [T1] mechanomyographic (MMG) response of the thumb to indirect supramaximal train-of-four stimulation of the ulnar nerve) is approximately 0.3 mg/kg (300 μg/kg) in adults receiving opioid/N_2O/O_2 anesthesia. The ED_{95} in infants is lower than in adults and children (0.25, 0.35 and 0.40 mg/kg, respectively). With high doses of 2 mg/kg, clinical duration is 110 minutes. At equipotent doses, rocuronium has approximately the same clinically effective duration of action as vecuronium. However, the onset of action is approximately 40% shorter for rocuronium than for vecuronium at doses of 2 to 3 times the ED_{95}.

The median pharmacodynamic parameter values for rocuronium bromide over a range of doses are presented in Table 2 and Table 3.

Table 2: ZEMURON

Pharmacodynamic Parameter Values for the Initial Dose of Rocuronium Bromide Administered During Opioid/N_2O/O_2 Anesthesia (Adults) and Halothane Anesthesia (Children). Median [Range]

Rocuronium Bromide Dose Administered Over 5 sec.	Time to ≥80% Block (min)	Time to Maximum Block (min)	Clinical Duration (min)	Peak Effect (% of Control T_1)
Adults 18 to 64 yrs				
0.45 mg/kg (n=50)	1.3 [0.8–6.2]	3.0 [1.3–8.2]	22 [12–31]	2.5 [0–25]
0.6 mg/kg (n=142)	1.0 [0.4–6.0]	1.8 [0.6–13.0]	31 [15–85]	0 [0–9.7]
0.9 mg/kg (n=20)	1.1 [0.3–3.8]	1.4 [0.8–6.2]	58 [27–111]	0 [0–7]
1.2 mg/kg (n=18)	0.7 [0.4–1.7]	1.0 [0.6–4.7]	67 [38–160]	0 [0–4]
Geriatrics 65 to 78 yrs				
0.6 mg/kg (n=31)	2.3 [1.0–8.3]	3.7 [1.3–11.3]	46 [22–73]	0 [0–7]
0.9 mg/kg (n=5)	2.0 [1.0–3.0]	2.5 [1.2–5.0]	62 [49–75]	0 [0–0]
1.2 mg/kg (n=7)	1.0 [0.8–3.5]	1.3 [1.2–4.7]	94 [64–138]	0 [0–0]
Pediatric				
3 mo–1 yr				
0.6 mg/kg (n=17)	—	0.8 [0.3–3]	41 [24–68]	0 [0–0]
0.8 mg/kg (n=9)	—	0.7 [0.5–0.8]	40 [27–70]	0 [0–3]
1–12 yrs				
0.6 mg/kg (n=27)	0.8 [0.4–2]	1.0 [0.5–3.3]	26 [17–39]	0 [0–0]
0.8 mg/kg (n=18)	—	0.5 [0.3–1.0]	30 [17–56]	0 [0–0]

Clinical duration=time until return to 25% of control T_1.

Patients receiving doses of 0.45 mg/kg who achieved less than 90% block (16% of these patients) had about 12 to 15 minutes to 25% recovery.

Legend: n= the number of patients who had Time to Maximum block recorded.

Table 3: ZEMURON

Intubating Conditions in Patients with Intubation Initiated at 60 to 70 Seconds. Percent, Median [Range]

Rocuronium Bromide Dose (mg/kg) Administered Over 5 sec	Percent of Patients with Excellent[b] or Good[c] Intubating Conditions	Time to Completion of Intubation (min)
Adults[a] 18–64 yrs		
0.45 (n=43)	86%	1.6 [1.0–7.0]
0.6 (n=51)	96%	1.6 [1.0–3.2]
Pediatric 3 mo–1 yr		
0.6 (n=18)	100%	1.0 [1.0–1.5]
Pediatric 1–4 yrs		
0.6 (n=12)	100%	1.0 [0.5–2.3]

[a] Excludes patients undergoing Cesarean section.

[b] Excellent Intubating Conditions=jaw relaxed, vocal cords apart & immobile, no diaphragmatic movement.

[c] Good Intubating Conditions=jaw relaxed, vocal cords apart & immobile, some diaphragmatic movement.

Intubation Conditions: A dose of 0.60 mg/kg (2×ED_{95}) rocuronium bromide administered following the induction of thiopental/narcotic anesthesia in adults or halothane anesthesia in children generally produces good or excellent conditions for tracheal intubation initiated at 60-70 seconds post-administration (see Table 3). After administration of 0.45 mg/kg rocuronium bromide, following intravenous anesthesia (thiopental and fentanyl) in adults, acceptable intubation conditions are present after 90 seconds.

Rapid Sequence Induction of Anesthesia: During rapid sequence induction of anesthesia, following a dose of 1.0 mg/kg rocuronium bromide, adequate intubation conditions are achieved within 60 seconds in 93% of the patients with propofol anesthesia and 96% of the patients with fentanyl/thiopental anesthesia. Of these, 70% are rated excellent. The surgical relaxation with this dose approaches 1 hour, at which time the neuromuscular blockade may be reversed when functional recovery is evident. Following a dose of 0.6 mg/kg rocuronium bromide, adequate intubation conditions are achieved within 60 seconds in 81% and 75% of the patients during a rapid sequence induction technique with propofol or fentanyl/thiopental, respectively.

Maintenance Doses: In adult patients under opioid/N_2O/O_2 anesthesia, the median clinical duration (time from injection of the maintenance dose at a T1 of 25% of control to a return to 25% of the control T1) of maintenance doses of 0.1, 0.15 and 0.2 mg/kg (100, 150 and 200 μg/kg) of rocuronium bromide is 12 minutes (range 2-31 minutes), 17 minutes (range 6-50 minutes), and 24 minutes (range 7-69 minutes), respectively. Repeated maintenance doses results in insignificant increases in the median time of clinical duration (2-4 minutes) between the first and fifth consecutive dose. The median rate of spontaneous recovery of T1 from 25 to 75% (n=182), following the final maintenance dose of rocuronium bromide, is 13 minutes (4-84 minutes).

Inhalation Anesthetics: The duration of the neuromuscular blocking action of rocuronium bromide may be enhanced by approximately 30% in the presence of potent inhalation anesthetics. The median clinical duration of a dose of 0.6 mg/kg was 30, 38, and 42 minutes under opioid/N_2O/O_2, enflurane and isoflurane maintenance anesthesia, respectively. During 1-2 hr of infusion, the infusion rate of rocuronium bromide required to maintain about 95% blockade was decreased by as much as 40% under enflurane and isoflurane anesthesia (see Drug Interactions, Inhalation Anesthetics).

Obstetrics: Rocuronium bromide 0.6 mg/kg (600 μg/kg) was administered with thiopental, 3-4 mg/kg (n=13) or 4-6 mg/kg (n=42), for rapid sequence induction of anesthesia for Cesarean section. The umbilical venous plasma concentrations were 18% of maternal concentrations at delivery. No neonate had APGAR scores of <7 at 5 minutes post-delivery. Intubating conditions were poor or inadequate in 5 of 13 women receiving 3-4 mg/kg thiopental when intubation was attempted 60 seconds after drug injection. Therefore, ZEMURON is not recommended for rapid sequence induction in Cesarean section patients.

Pediatrics: Halothane Anesthesia: Children (1-13 years of age) under halothane anesthesia are less sensitive to rocuronium bromide (ED_{50} approximately 0.18 mg/kg [180 μg/kg], ED_{95} 0.35-0.4 mg/kg [350-400 μg/kg]) than adults on a mg/kg (μg/kg) basis. The onset time and duration of blockade are shorter in children (1-13 years) than in adults (see Table 2). The clinical duration of action of 0.6 and 0.8 mg/kg doses of rocuronium bromide are approximately 30-60% longer in infants aged 3 months to 1 year than in children aged 1-13 years (see Table 2). During halothane anesthesia, at doses of 0.6 mg/kg (600 μg/kg) of rocuronium bromide, the median onset time is 60 seconds (30-200 sec.) and the clinical duration is 26 min. (17-39 min.). Maintenance doses of 0.1 or 0.125 mg/kg (100 or 125 μg/kg) rocuronium bromide in children under halothane anesthesia provided a median clinical duration of 7 and 10 minutes, respectively. The median rate of spontaneous recovery of T1 from 25-75% was 9.5 minutes (4-29 minutes).

Table 4 presents the time to onset and clinical duration for the initial dose of ZEMURON (rocuronium bromide) injection under opioid/nitrous oxide/oxygen anesthesia in adults and geriatric patients, and under halothane anesthesia in pediatric patients.

Table 4: ZEMURON

Median (Range) Time to Onset and Clinical Duration Following Initial (Intubating) Dose During Opioid/Nitrous Oxide/Oxygen Anesthesia (Adults) and Halothane Anesthesia (Pediatric Patients)

ZEMURON Dose (mg/kg) Administered Over 5 sec	Time to ≥80% Block (min)	Time to Maximum Block (min)	Clinical Duration (min)
Adults 18 to 64 yrs			
0.45 (n=50)	1.3 (0.8–6.2)	3.0 (1.3–8.2)	22 (12–31)
0.6 (n=142)	1.0 (0.4–6.0)	1.8 (0.6–13.0)	31 (15–85)
0.9 (n=20)	1.1 (0.3–3.8)	1.4 (0.8–6.2)	58 (27–111)
1.2 (n=18)	0.7 (0.4–1.7)	1.0 (0.6–4.7)	67 (38–160)
Geriatric ≥65 yrs			
0.6 (n=31)	2.3 (1.0–8.3)	3.7 (1.3–11.3)	46 (22–73)
0.9 (n=5)	2.0 (1.0–3.0)	2.5 (1.2–5.0)	62 (49–75)
1.2 (n=7)	1.0 (0.8–3.5)	1.3 (1.2–4.7)	94 (64–138)
Infants 3 mo to 1 yr			
0.6 (n=17)	—	0.8 (0.3–3.0)	41 (24–68)
0.8 (n=9)	—	0.7 (0.5–0.8)	40 (27–70)
Pediatric 1 to 12 yrs			
0.6 (n=27)	0.8 (0.4–2.0)	1.0 (0.5–3.3)	26 (17–39)

(cont'd)

Table 4: ZEMURON *(cont'd)*

Median (Range) Time to Onset and Clinical Duration Following Initial (Intubating) Dose During Opioid/Nitrous Oxide/Oxygen Anesthesia (Adults) and Halothane Anesthesia (Pediatric Patients)

ZEMURON Dose (mg/kg) Administered Over 5 sec	Time to ≥80% Block (min)	Time to Maximum Block (min)	Clinical Duration (min)
0.8 (n=18)	—	0.5 (0.3–1.0)	30 (17–56)

Legend: n=the number of patients who had time to maximum block recorded.
Clinical duration=time until return to 25% of control T_1. Patients receiving doses of 0.45 mg/kg who achieved less than 90% block (16% of these patients) had about 12 to 15 minutes to 25% recovery.

Sevoflurane (induction) and Isoflurane/Nitrous Oxide (maintenance): Comparison between pediatric age groups showed that the mean onset time in term newborn infants and adolescents (1.0 min.) is slightly longer than in infants, toddlers and children (0.4, 0.6 and 0.8 min., respectively).

Comparing between pediatric age groups demonstrated that mean time to reappearance of T_3 was prolonged in term neonates and infants (56.7 and 60.7 min., respectively) when compared to toddlers, children and adolescents (45.4, 37.6 and 42.9 min., respectively).

Table 5 presents the time to onset and clinical duration for the initial dose of ZEMURON (rocuronium bromide) Injection under sevoflurane (induction) and isoflurane/nitrous oxide (maintenance) anesthesia in pediatric patients.

Table 5: ZEMURON

Median (Range) Time to Onset and Clinical Duration Following Initial (Intubating) Dose During Sevoflurane (induction) and Isoflurane/Nitrous Oxide (maintenance) Anesthesia (Pediatric Patients)

ZEMURON Dose (mg/kg) Administered Over 5 sec	Time to Maximum Block (min)	Time to Reappearance T_3 (min)
Neonates birth to <28 days		
0.45 (n=5)	1.1 (0.6–2.2)	40.3 (32.5–62.6)
0.6 (n=10)	1.0 (0.2–2.1)	49.7 (16.6–119.0)
1 (n=6)	0.6 (0.3–1.8)	114.4 (92.6–136.3)
Infants 28 days to ≤3 mo		
0.45 (n=9)	0.5 (0.4–1.3)	49.1 (13.5–79.9)
0.6 (n=11)	0.4 (0.2–0.8)	59.8 (32.3–87.8)
1 (n=5)	0.3 (0.2–0.7)	103.3 (90.8–155.4)
Toddlers >3 mo to ≤2 yrs		
0.45 (n=17)	0.8 (0.3–1.9)	39.2 (16.9–59.4)
0.6 (n=29)	0.6 (0.2–1.6)	44.2 (18.9–68.8)
1 (n=15)	0.5 (0.2–1.5)	72.0 (36.2–128.2)
Children >2 yrs to ≤11 yrs		
0.45 (n=14)	0.9 (0.4–1.9)	21.5 (17.5–38.0)
0.6 (n=37)	0.8 (0.3–1.7)	36.7 (20.1–65.9)
1 (n=16)	0.7 (0.4–1.2)	53.1 (31.2–89.9)
Adolescents >11 to ≤17 yrs		
0.45 (n=18)	1.0 (0.5–1.7)	37.5 (18.3–65.7)
0.6 (n=31)	0.9 (0.2–2.1)	41.4 (16.3–91.2)
1 (n=14)	0.7 (0.5–1.2)	67.1 (25.6–93.8)

Legend: n=the number of patients with the highest number of observations for time to maximum block or reappearance T_3.

Geriatrics: The duration of action of maintenance doses of 0.15 mg/kg rocuronium bromide might be somewhat longer under enflurane and isoflurane anesthesia in geriatric patients (approximately 20 minutes) than in adults under intravenous anesthesia (approximately 13 minutes). No accumulation of effect (progressive increase in duration of action) with repetitive maintenance dosing at the recommended level has been observed.
Hepatic Insufficiency: The influence of hepatic impairment on the pharmacodynamics of a 0.60 mg/kg dose of rocuronium bromide was investigated in a study in which 9 patients with alcoholic cirrhosis were compared to 10 patients with normal hepatic function. Relative to the normal group, the patients with hepatic impairment exhibited an increased clinical duration of action (60 versus 42 min). The recovery index (time for recovery from 25-75% T_1 suppression) was also prolonged in the cirrhotic patients (53 versus 20 min).
Renal Insufficiency: Three single centre clinical trials have been performed to compare the pharmacodynamic characteristics of a 0.6 mg/kg dose of rocuronium bromide in patients having normal renal function (n=31) to those for patients (n=30) having renal impairment undergoing kidney transplantation or AV shunt/peritoneal catheter implantation surgery for haemodialysis while receiving steady-state isoflurane anesthesia. The pharmacodynamic characteristics of ZEMURON were not altered in a consistent manner in the patients with renal impairment although clinical duration and recovery times were more variable than in patients with normal renal function.
Hemodynamics: Rocuronium has a weak vagus blocking effect and little effect on sympathetic ganglionic transmission. In most clinical trials, the monitoring of haemodynamic parameters during the period immediately following the administration of ZEMURON was confounded by laryngoscopy and intubation; events associated with elevations of heart rate and mean arterial blood pressure may result from multiple factors, including rocuronium bromide administration. In one study in which a six minute period was permitted to elapse between the administration of rocuronium bromide at 0.6, 0.9, and 1.2 mg/kg doses and subsequent intubation, no dose-dependent changes in heart rate or mean arterial pressure were observed. Infrequently clinical signs of histamine release (0.8%) have been reported in clinical trials.
Intensive Care Unit: Following continuous infusion in the Intensive Care Unit, the time to recovery of the train-of-four ratio to 0.7 depends on the level of blockade at the end of the infusion. After a continuous infusion for 20 hours or more the median time between return of T_2 to train-of-four stimulation and recovery of the train-of-four ratio to 0.7 approximates 1.5 (1-5) hours in patients without multiple organ failure and 4 (1-25) hours in patients with multiple organ failure.
Cardiovascular Surgery: In patients scheduled for cardiovascular surgery the most common cardiovascular changes during the onset of maximum blockade following 0.6-0.9 mg/kg ZEMURON are a slight increase in heart rate up to 9% and an increase in mean arterial blood pressure up to 16% from the control values.
Antagonism of Neuromuscular Blockade: Once spontaneous recovery has started (reappearance of T_2 or first signs of clinical recovery), the neuromuscular blockade produced by ZEMURON is readily reversed with various anticholinesterase agents, e.g., neostigmine, edrophonium or pyridostigmine.

Pharmacokinetics: The pharmacokinetic characteristics of intravenously administered ZEMURON are best described by a three compartment open model. The comparative population estimates for adult and geriatric surgical patients, pediatric patients and patients with renal impairment undergoing cadaver renal transplantation, and patients with hepatic cirrhosis are presented in Table 6, Table 7 and Table 8.

Table 6: ZEMURON

Summary of ZEMURON's Pharmacokinetic Parameters in Adult and Geriatric Patients Receiving a Single 0.6 mg/kg Dose During Opioid/N_2O/O_2 Anesthesia

	C_{max}	$t_{1/2}$ (h)	AUC	Clearance (L/kg/h)	Volume of Distribution (L/kg)
Adults					
(27–58 yr, n=22)	NA	1.4±0.4	NA	0.25±0.08	0.25±0.04
Geriatrics					
(65–78 yr, n=20)	NA	1.5±0.4	NA	0.21±0.06	0.22±0.03

Data are presented as mean±SD.

Pediatrics: The terminal half-life and other pharmacokinetic parameters of rocuronium in these pediatric patients are presented in Table 7.

Table 7: ZEMURON

Summary of ZEMURON's Pharmacokinetic Parameters in Pediatric Patients Receiving a Single 0.8 mg/kg Dose During Halothane Anesthesia

	C_{max}	$t_{1/2}$ (h)	AUC	Clearance (L/kg/h)	Volume of Distribution (L/kg)
Pediatrics					
(3–<12 mo, n=6)	NA	1.3±0.5	NA	0.35±0.08	0.30±0.04
(1–<3 yr, n=5)	NA	1.1±0.7	NA	0.32±0.07	0.26±0.06
(3–<8 yr, n=7)	NA	0.8±0.3	NA	0.44±0.16	0.21±0.03

Data are presented as mean±SD.

Pharmacokinetics of rocuronium bromide in pediatric patients (n=146) with ages ranging from 0 to 17 years were evaluated using a population analysis of the pooled pharmacokinetic datasets from two clinical trials under sevoflurane (induction) and isoflurane/nitrous oxide (maintenance) anesthesia. All pharmacokinetic parameters were found to be linearly proportional to body weight illustrated by a similar clearance ($L.hr^{-1}.kg^{-1}$). The volume of distribution ($L.kg^{-1}$) and elimination half-life (h) decrease with age (years). The pharmacokinetic parameters of typical pediatrics within each age group are summarized in Table 8.

Table 8: ZEMURON

Pharmacokinetic Parameters of Rocuronium in Pediatric Patients During Sevoflurane (induction) and Isoflurane/Nitrous Oxide (maintenance) Anesthesia

PK Parameter	Term newborn infants (0–27 days)	Infants (28 days–2 months)	Toddlers (3–23 months)	Children (2–11 years)	Adolescents (11–17 years)
Clearance ($L.hr^{-1}kg^{-1}$)	0.293	0.293	0.293	0.293	0.293
Volume of Distribution at Steady State ($L.kg^{-1}$)	0.424	0.295	0.232	0.177	0.174
Elimination Half-Life (hr)	1.1	0.9	0.8	0.7	0.7

Renal and Hepatic Impairment: See Table 9.

Table 9: ZEMURON

Summary of ZEMURON's Pharmacokinetic Parameters in Renal Transplant Patients and Hepatic Dysfunction Patients Receiving a Single 0.6 mg/kg Dose During Isoflurane Anesthesia

	C_{max}	$t_{1/2}$ (h)	AUC	Clearance (L/kg/h)	Volume of Distribution (L/kg)
Normal Renal and Hepatic Function					
(23–65 yr, n=10)	NA	2.4±0.8[a]	NA	0.16±0.05[a]	0.26±0.03
Renal Transplant Patients					
(21–45 yr, n=10)	NA	2.4±1.1	NA	0.13±0.04	0.34±0.11
Hepatic Dysfunction Patients					
(31–67 yr, n=9)	NA	4.3±2.6	NA	0.13±0.06	0.53±0.14

[a] Differences in the calculated $T_{1/2}\beta$ and C_L between this study and the study in adults vs. geriatrics (≥65 yr) are related to the different sample populations and anesthetic techniques.
Data are presented as mean±SD.

Distribution: The placental transfer of ZEMURON was investigated in two studies involving a total of 17 neonates born to women receiving 0.6 mg/kg rocuronium bromide during Cesarean section. The mean umbilical venous to maternal venous plasma ratio ranged from 16-22% in these studies.
Metabolism: Following administration of a single 1.0 mg/kg bolus dose to 10 adult patients, metabolites in the plasma or urine were either absent or below the limit of detection (5 ng/mL).
Excretion: Studies in cats and dogs indicate that rocuronium is eliminated primarily by the liver. In cats cumulative excretion 6 hours after a $6 \times ED_{90}$ dose was 9% in the urine and 54% in the bile. Consistent with the limited role of the kidney in the elimination of rocuronium, renal pedicle ligation did not substantially alter its time course in cats although clearance was significantly reduced. In contrast, hepatic exclusion in the cat significantly increased the duration of action of rocuronium, suggestive of a substantial role for the liver in the elimination of this compound.

Clinical data showed that following administration of a single 1.0 mg/kg bolus dose to 10 adult patients, total urinary excretion was 33% over a 24 hr period. Of this, 65% was recovered during the first 2 hours and 94% over the first 6 hours.

If ZEMURON is administered as a continuous infusion to facilitate mechanical ventilation for 20 hours or more, the mean elimination half-life and the mean (apparent) volume of distribution at steady state are increased. A large between-patient variability is found in controlled clinical studies, related to nature and extent of (multiple) organ failure and individual patient characteristics. In patients with multiple organ failure, a mean (±SD) elimination half-life of 21.5 (±3.3) hours, a (apparent) volume of distribution at steady state of 1.5 (±0.8) $L.kg^{-1}$ and a plasma clearance of 2.1 (±0.8) $mL.kg^{-1}.min^{-1}$ were found.

STORAGE AND STABILITY: ZEMURON should be stored under refrigeration (2-8°C) until ready to use. To facilitate use in the operating room, the unopened vials may be stored up to 90 days at room temperature (15-30°C). Use punctured vials of ZEMURON within 30 days.

After dilution with infusion fluids (see Dosage and Administration, Administration), chemical and physical in-use stability has been demonstrated for 72 hours at 30°C. From a microbiological point of view, the diluted product should be used immediately. If not used immediately, in-use storage times and conditions prior to use are the responsibility of the user/administrator and would normally not be longer than 24 hours at 2 to 8°C, unless dilution has taken place in controlled and validated aseptic conditions.

SPECIAL HANDLING INSTRUCTIONS: Any unused product or waste material should be disposed of in accordance with local requirements.

INFORMATION FOR THE PATIENT: Published in e-CPS, available by subscription at www.e-cps.ca.

DOSAGE FORMS, COMPOSITION AND PACKAGING: Each mL of a colorless to slightly yellow/brown, sterile non-pyrogenic solution for injection or infusion contains: rocuronium bromide 10 mg, sodium acetate, trihydrate 2 mg, sodium chloride approx. 3.3 mg, water for injection q.s. to 1 mL and nitrogen (present). May contain sodium hydroxide and/or glacial acetic acid to adjust the pH to approximately 4.0. Preservative-free. Multidose vials of 5 mL, boxes of 10. The rubber stopper of the vial does not contain latex.

Zerit™ Ⓟ

stavudine

Antiretroviral Agent

Bristol-Myers Squibb

Date of Preparation: March 14, 1996
Date of Revision: August 5, 2010

SUMMARY PRODUCT INFORMATION:

Route of Administration	Dosage Form/ Strength	Clinically Relevant Nonmedicinal Ingredients
Oral	Capsules 15, 20, 30 and 40 mg	Lactose For a complete listing, see Dosage Forms, Composition and Packaging.

INDICATIONS AND CLINICAL USE: ZERIT (stavudine), in combination with other antiretroviral agents, is indicated for the treatment of HIV-1 infection.

CONTRAINDICATIONS: ZERIT (stavudine) is contraindicated in patients with clinically significant hypersensitivity to stavudine or to any of the components contained in the formulation. For a complete listing, see Dosage Forms, Composition and Packaging.

WARNINGS AND PRECAUTIONS:

Serious Warnings and Precautions

Lactic Acidosis/Severe Hepatomegaly with Steatosis/Hepatic Failure: Lactic acidosis and severe hepatomegaly with steatosis, including fatal cases, have been reported with the use of nucleoside analogues alone or in combination, including stavudine and other antiretroviral agents. Although relative rates of lactic acidosis have not been assessed in prospective well-controlled trials, longitudinal cohort and retrospective studies suggest that this infrequent event may be more often associated with antiretroviral combinations containing stavudine. Female gender, obesity, and prolonged nucleoside exposure may be risk factors. Fatal lactic acidosis has been reported in pregnant women who received the combination of stavudine and didanosine with other antiretroviral agents. The combination of stavudine and didanosine should be used with caution during pregnancy and is recommended only if the potential benefit clearly outweighs the potential risk (see Warnings and Precautions, Pregnant Women).

Particular caution should be exercised when administering ZERIT to any patient with known risk factors for liver disease; however, cases of lactic acidosis have also been reported in patients with no known risk factors. Generalized fatigue, digestive symptoms (nausea, vomiting, abdominal pain, and sudden unexplained weight loss); respiratory symptoms (tachypnea and dyspnea); or neurologic symptoms (including motor weakness, see Neurologic) might be indicative of the development of symptomatic hyperlactatemia or lactic acidosis syndrome. Symptoms associated with hyperlactatemia may continue or worsen following discontinuation of antiretroviral therapy.

Treatment with ZERIT should be suspended in any patient who develops clinical or laboratory findings suggestive of lactic acidosis or pronounced hepatotoxicity (which may include hepatomegaly and steatosis even in the absence of marked transaminase elevations).

An increased risk of hepatotoxicity may occur in patients treated with ZERIT in combination with didanosine and hydroxyurea compared to when ZERIT is used alone. Deaths attributed to hepatotoxicity have occurred in patients receiving this combination. Patients treated with this combination should be closely monitored for signs of liver toxicity.

Neurologic: Motor weakness (which was fatal in some cases) has been reported rarely in patients receiving combination antiretroviral therapy including ZERIT. Most of these cases occurred in the setting of symptomatic hyperlactatemia or lactic acidosis syndrome. The evolution of motor weakness may mimic the clinical presentation of Guillain-Barré syndrome (including respiratory failure). If motor weakness develops in a patient receiving ZERIT, the drug should be discontinued. Symptoms may continue or worsen following discontinuation of therapy.

Peripheral neuropathy, manifested by numbness, tingling, or pain in the hands or feet, has been reported in patients receiving ZERIT therapy. Peripheral neuropathy, which is dose related, has occurred more frequently in patients with advanced HIV disease, a history of neuropathy, or concurrent neurotoxic drug therapy, including didanosine (see Adverse Reactions).

Peripheral neuropathy, which was severe in some cases, has been reported in HIV-infected patients receiving hydroxyurea in combination with antiretroviral agents, including didanosine with or without stavudine.

Pancreatic: Fatal and nonfatal pancreatitis have occurred during therapy when ZERIT was part of a combination regimen that included didanosine or didanosine and hydroxyurea, in both treatment-naive and treatment-experienced patients, regardless of degree of immunosuppression. This combination of ZERIT and didanosine and any other agents that are toxic to the pancreas should be suspended in patients with suspected pancreatitis. Reinstitution of ZERIT after a confirmed diagnosis of pancreatitis should be undertaken with particular caution and close patient monitoring. The new regimen should contain neither didanosine nor hydroxyurea.

General: Patients receiving ZERIT (stavudine) or any other antiretroviral therapy may continue to develop opportunistic infections and other complications of HIV infection and, therefore, should remain under close clinical observation by physicians experienced in the treatment of patients with HIV disease and associated complications.

Renal: In HIV-infected patients with renal impairment, renal clearance and apparent oral clearance of stavudine was decreased. The terminal elimination half-life ($t_{1/2}$) was prolonged up to 8 hours. C_{max} and T_{max} were not significantly affected by reduced renal function. Based on these preliminary observations, it is recommended that stavudine dosage be modified in patients with reduced creatinine clearance (≤50 mL/min) (see Dosage and Administration).

Immune: Immune Reconstitution Syndrome: During the initial phase of treatment, patients responding to antiretroviral therapy may develop an inflammatory response to indolent or residual opportunistic infections (such as MAC, CMV, PCP, and TB), which may necessitate further evaluation and treatment.

Hepatic: Hepatitis or liver failure, which was fatal in some cases, have been reported with ZERIT. Hepatotoxicity and hepatic failure resulting in death were reported during postmarketing surveillance in HIV-infected patients treated with antiretroviral agents in combination with hydroxyurea. Fatal hepatic events were reported most often in patients treated with the combination of hydroxyurea, didanosine, and stavudine. This combination should be avoided.

The safety and efficacy of ZERIT have not been established in patients with significant underlying liver disorders. During combination antiretroviral therapy, patients with preexisting liver dysfunction, including chronic active hepatitis, have an increased frequency of liver function abnormalities, including severe and potentially fatal hepatic adverse events, and should be monitored according to standard practice. If there is evidence of worsening liver disease in such patients, interruption or discontinuation of treatment must be considered.

Fat Redistribution: Redistribution/accumulation of body fat including central obesity, dorsocervical fat enlargement (buffalo hump), peripheral wasting, facial wasting, breast enlargement, and "cushingoid appearance" have been observed in patients receiving antiretroviral therapy. In randomized controlled trials of treatment-naive patients, clinical lipoatrophy or lipodystrophy developed in a higher proportion of patients treated with stavudine compared to other nucleosides (tenofovir or abacavir). Dual energy x-ray absorptiometry (DEXA) scans demonstrated overall limb fat loss in stavudine treated patients compared to limb fat gain or no change in patients treated with other nucleosides (abacavir, tenofovir or zidovudine). The incidence and severity of lipoatrophy or lipodystrophy are cumulative over time with stavudine-containing regimens. In clinical trials, switching from stavudine to other nucleosides (tenofovir or abacavir) resulted in increases in limb fat with modest to no improvements in clinical lipoatrophy. Given the potential risks of using ZERIT including lipoatrophy or lipodystrophy, a benefit-risk assessment for each patient should be made and an alternative antiretroviral carefully considered. Patients receiving ZERIT should be monitored for symptoms of lipoatrophy or lipodystrophy including a clinical examination to evaluate for physical signs of fat redistribution. Patients should be routinely questioned about body changes related to lipoatrophy or lipodystrophy.

Carcinogenesis, Mutagenesis, Impairment of Fertility: In 2-year carcinogenicity studies in mice and rats, stavudine was noncarcinogenic at doses which produced exposures (AUC) 39 and 168 times, respectively, human exposure at the recommended clinical dose. Benign and malignant liver tumors in mice and rats and malignant urinary bladder tumors in male rats occurred at levels of exposure 250 (mice) and 732 (rats) times human exposure at the recommended clinical dose.

Stavudine was not mutagenic in the Ames, *E. coli* reverse mutation, or the CHO/HGPRT mammalian cell forward gene mutation assays, with and without metabolic activation. Stavudine produced positive results in the in vitro human lymphocyte clastogenesis and mouse fibroblast assays, and in the in vivo mouse micronucleus test. In the in vitro assays, stavudine elevated the frequency of chromosome aberrations in human lymphocytes (concentrations of 25 to 250 µg/mL, without metabolic activation) and increased the frequency of transformed foci in mouse fibroblast cells (concentrations of 25 to 2500 µg/mL, with and without metabolic activation). In the in vivo micronucleus assay, stavudine was clastogenic in bone marrow cells following oral stavudine administration to mice at dosages of 600 to 2000 mg/kg/day for 3 days.

No evidence of impaired fertility was seen in rats with exposures (based on C_{max}) up to 216 times that observed following a clinical dosage of 1 mg/kg/day.

Special Populations: Pregnant Women: There are no adequate and well-controlled studies of stavudine in pregnant women. Stavudine should be used during pregnancy only if the potential benefit justifies the potential risk.

Fatal lactic acidosis has been reported in pregnant women who received the combination of stavudine and didanosine with other antiretroviral agents. It is not known if pregnancy augments the risk of lactic acidosis/hepatic steatosis syndrome reported in nonpregnant individuals receiving nucleoside analogues (see Warnings and Precautions, Serious Warnings and Precautions Box, Lactic Acidosis/Severe Hepatomegaly with Steatosis/Hepatic Failure). **The combination of stavudine and didanosine should be used with caution during pregnancy and is recommended only if the potential benefit clearly outweighs the potential risk.** Health care providers caring for HIV-infected pregnant women receiving stavudine should be alert for early diagnosis of lactic acidosis/hepatic steatosis syndrome.

Reproduction studies have been performed in rats and rabbits with exposures (based on C_{max}) up to 399 and 183 times, respectively, of that seen at a clinical dosage of 1 mg/kg/day and have revealed no evidence of teratogenicity or impaired fertility. A slight post-implantation loss was noted at 216 times the human exposure with no effect noted at approximately 135 times the human exposure. The incidence in fetuses of a common skeletal variation, unossified or incomplete ossification of sternebra, was increased in rats at 399 times human exposure while no effect was observed at 216 times human exposure. An increase in early rat neonatal mortality (birth to 4 days of age) occurred at 399 times the human exposure, while survival of neonates was unaffected at approximately 135 times the human exposure. A study in rats showed that stavudine is transferred to the fetus through the placenta. The concentration in fetal tissue was approximately one-half the concentration in maternal plasma. Stavudine has been shown to cross the human placenta in an ex vivo term model. Animal reproduction studies are not always predictive of human response.

Nursing Women: Studies in which lactating rats were administered a single dose (5 or 100 mg/kg) of stavudine demonstrated that stavudine is readily excreted into breast milk.

Although it is not known whether ZERIT is excreted in human milk, there exists the potential for adverse effects from stavudine in nursing infants. Because of both the potential for HIV transmission and the potential for serious adverse reactions in nursing infants, **mothers should be instructed not to breast-feed if they are receiving ZERIT.**

Pediatrics: The safety and effectiveness of ZERIT have been established in pediatric patients supported by evidence from adequate and well-controlled studies of stavudine in adults with additional data concerning safety and pharmacokinetics in pediatric patients.

Patients should be monitored for clinically significant elevations of hepatic transaminases. If these elevations develop on treatment, ZERIT therapy should be interrupted. If the hepatic transaminase values return to pretherapy levels, resumption of treatment may be considered using a dosage schedule of 1 mg/kg/day, not to exceed the recommended adult dose of 20 mg twice daily.

One open-label, phase I trial enrolled 38 subjects aged 5 weeks to 15 years; 9 had received no prior antiretroviral therapy and 29 had received zidovudine for a median duration of 104 weeks. Patients in this trial received ZERIT in initial doses ranging from 0.125 to 4.0 mg/kg/day with an average dose of 1.7 mg/kg/day for a median duration of 84 weeks (range 8-140 weeks). A second open-label trial, initiated to provide stavudine for children who had failed or were intolerant of alternative antiretroviral therapy, enrolled 51 subjects aged 8 months to 18 years who had received prolonged zidovudine and didanosine. These patients were treated with ZERIT at a dose of 2 mg/kg/day, for a median duration of 33 weeks (range 2 days - 82 weeks).

A multi-centre, randomized, double-blind trial (Study ACTG 240) evaluated ZERIT [d4t] (2 mg/kg/day) versus zidovudine [ZDV] (200 mg QID) in the treatment of HIV-infected pediatric patients who had received ≤6 weeks of prior antiretroviral therapy. Two hundred and sixteen subjects, with a median baseline CD4 cell count of 1000 cells/mm³, were enrolled. CD4 cell counts were better maintained on ZERIT treatment as compared with ZDV ($p<0.05$). Patients on ZDV experienced more neutropenia (19%) versus patients on ZERIT (7%) ($p<0.01$). No differences were observed in any other laboratory parameters, signs or symptoms.

Geriatrics: Clinical studies of ZERIT did not include sufficient numbers of patients aged 65 years and over to determine whether they respond differently than younger patients. Greater sensitivity of some older individuals to the effects of ZERIT cannot be ruled out.

In a monotherapy Expanded Access Program for patients with advanced HIV infection, peripheral neuropathy or peripheral neuropathic symptoms were observed in 15 of 40 (38%) elderly patients receiving 40 mg b.i.d. and 8 of 51 (16%) elderly patients receiving 20 mg b.i.d. Of the approximately 12 000 patients enrolled in the Expanded Access Program, peripheral neuropathy or peripheral neuropathic symptoms developed in 30% of patients receiving 40 mg b.i.d. and 25% of patients receiving 20 mg b.i.d. Elderly patients should be closely monitored for signs and symptoms of peripheral neuropathy.

Stavudine is known to be substantially excreted by the kidney, and the risk of toxic reactions to this drug may be greater in patients with impaired renal function. Because elderly patients are more likely to have decreased renal function, it may be useful to monitor renal function. Dose adjustment is recommended for patients with renal impairment (see Dosage and Administration, Recommended Dose and Dosage Adjustment).

Lactose Intolerance: ZERIT capsules contain lactose (120 and 240 mg depending on capsule strength). This amount is probably insufficient to induce specific symptoms of intolerance.

Monitoring and Laboratory Tests: Complete blood counts and clinical laboratory tests should be performed prior to initiating ZERIT therapy and at appropriate intervals thereafter.

Moderate elevations of mean corpuscular volume may be observed in patients taking ZERIT and may provide an indication of treatment compliance.

ADVERSE REACTIONS: Adult Patients: Adverse Drug Reaction Overview: A total of 202 patients in two clinical studies were treated with combination therapy that included stavudine in the regimen. The most clinically relevant serious adverse events, regardless of relationship to study treatment in these two clinical studies, included lactic acidosis, pancreatitis, hepatic dysfunction and peripheral neuropathy.

The most common adverse events in the stavudine-containing regimens of the combination therapy clinical studies, regardless of grade or relationship to study treatment, included asthenia, diarrhea, dry skin, headache, increased cough, nausea, pharyngitis, rash and vomiting. In total, 31 out of the 202 patients in the stavudine-containing regimens from these two clinical studies, discontinued study medication due to adverse events.

Clinical Trial Adverse Drug Reactions: Because clinical trials are conducted under very specific conditions the adverse drug reaction rates observed in the clinical trials may not reflect the rates observed in practice and should not be compared to the rates in the clinical trials of another drug. Adverse drug reaction information from clinical trials is useful for identifying drug-related adverse events and for approximating rates.

Many of the serious clinical adverse events reported from patients receiving stavudine in clinical trials were consistent with the course of HIV infection. Concurrent therapy with other medications was permitted in these trials. Therefore, it is difficult to distinguish which events were related to stavudine, the disease itself, or other therapies.

When ZERIT is used in combination with other agents with similar toxicities, the incidence of adverse events may be higher than when ZERIT is used alone. Pancreatitis, peripheral neuropathy, and liver function abnormalities occur more frequently in patients treated with the combination of ZERIT and didanosine.

Fatal pancreatitis and hepatotoxicity may occur more frequently in patients treated with ZERIT in combination with didanosine and hydroxyurea (see Warnings and Precautions).

Lactic Acidosis: Fatal lactic acidosis has occurred in patients treated with ZERIT in combination with other antiretroviral agents. Patients with suspected lactic acidosis should immediately suspend therapy with ZERIT. Permanent discontinuation of ZERIT should be considered for patients with confirmed lactic acidosis.

Peripheral Neuropathy: ZERIT therapy has rarely been associated with motor weakness, occurring predominantly in the setting of lactic acidosis. If motor weakness develops, ZERIT should be discontinued.

ZERIT (stavudine) therapy has also been associated with peripheral sensory neuropathy, which can be severe, is dose related, and occurs more frequently in patients being treated with neurotoxic drug therapy, including didanosine, in patients with advanced HIV infection, or in patients who have previously experienced peripheral neuropathy.

Patients should be monitored for the development of neuropathy, which is usually manifested by numbness, tingling, or pain in the feet or hands. Stavudine-related peripheral neuropathy may resolve if therapy is withdrawn promptly. In some cases, symptoms may worsen temporarily following discontinuation of therapy. If symptoms resolve completely, patients may tolerate resumption of treatment at one-half the dose (see Dosage and Administration). If neuropathy recurs after resumption of ZERIT, permanent discontinuation of ZERIT should be considered.

Pancreatitis: Pancreatitis resulting in death was observed in patients treated with ZERIT plus didanosine, with or without hydroxyurea, in controlled clinical studies and in postmarketing reports.

Pancreatitis was generally attributed to advanced disease or to prior or concurrent treatment with medications known to be associated with pancreatitis. The occurrences were not dose-related, and were occasionally fatal. Patients with a history of pancreatitis appear to be at increased risk for recurrence (see Warnings and Precautions).

Table 1: ZERIT

Clinical Adverse Events[a] in START 1[b] Studies with a Frequency of >5% in at Least One Treatment Group (Combination Therapy)

Adverse Events	Percent of Patients START 1 ZERIT + lamivudine + indinavir n=100[c]	zidovudine + lamivudine + indinavir n=102
Digestive System		
Nausea	43	63
Diarrhea	34	16
Vomiting	18	33
Pain Abdomen	21	14
Dyspepsia	5	8
Anorexia	12	9
Disorder Gastrointestinal	3	9
Body as a Whole		
Asthenia	25	26
Headache	25	26
Pain Back	23	20
Infection	17	16
Fever	14	11
Pain	15	9
Flu Syndrome	8	6
Accidental Injury	6	6
Infection Fungal	7	5
Chills	7	1
Respiratory System		
Pharyngitis	28	24
Cough Increased	21	16
Rhinitis	18	6
Sinusitis	13	7
Bronchitis	6	7
Skin/Appendages		
Rash	18	13
Dry Skin	11	12
Acne	5	6
Nervous System		
Peripheral Neurologic Symptoms/Neuropathy	8	7

(cont'd)

Table 1: ZERIT *(cont'd)*

Clinical Adverse Events[a] in START 1[b] Studies with a Frequency of >5% in at Least One Treatment Group (Combination Therapy)

Adverse Events	Percent of Patients START 1 ZERIT + lamivudine + indinavir n=100[c]	zidovudine + lamivudine + indinavir n=102
Depression	8	12
Insomnia	6	9
Dizziness	5	7
Metabolic/Nutritional System		
Bilirubinemia	9	4
Weight Decreased	4	8
Urogenital System		
Dysuria	9	6
Hematuria	10	4
Calculus Kidney	7	5
Special Senses		
Taste Perversion	6	10
Conjunctivitis	6	4
Musculoskeletal System		
Arthralgia	7	5
Myalgia	7	2

[a] Any severity, regardless of relationship to study regimen.
[b] START 1 compared triple combination regimens in 202 treatment-naive patients. Patients received either ZERIT (40 mg b.i.d.) plus lamivudine plus indinavir or zidovudine plus lamivudine plus indinavir.
[c] Duration of stavudine therapy=48 weeks.

Table 2: ZERIT

Clinical Adverse Events[a] in START 2[b] Studies with a Frequency of >5% in at Least One Treatment Group (Combination Therapy)

Adverse Events	Percent of Patients START 2 ZERIT + didanosine + indinavir n=102[c]	zidovudine + lamivudine + indinavir n=103
Digestive System		
Nausea	53	67
Diarrhea	45	39
Vomiting	30	35
Pain Abdomen	20	24
Flatulence	14	14
Dyspepsia	10	11
Anorexia	7	12
Dry Mouth	8	6
Eructation	4	8
Constipation	4	7
Ulcer Mouth	6	4
Body as a Whole		
Asthenia	32	38
Headache	46	37
Pain Back	11	13
Infection	23	18
Fever	20	8
Pain	17	24
Flu Syndrome	10	8

(cont'd)

Table 2: ZERIT *(cont'd)*

Clinical Adverse Events[a] in START 2[b] Studies with a Frequency of >5% in at Least One Treatment Group (Combination Therapy)

	Percent of Patients	
	START 2	
Adverse Events	**ZERIT + didanosine + indinavir n=102[c]**	**zidovudine + lamivudine + indinavir n=103**
Accidental Injury	6	8
Infection Fungal	6	5
Chills	7	5
Lesion	3	6
Respiratory System		
Pharyngitis	37	28
Cough Increased	27	20
Rhinitis	22	16
Sinusitis	17	7
Bronchitis	3	6
Disorder Lung	6	0
Skin/Appendages		
Rash	30	18
Dry Skin	33	23
Acne	6	2
Pruritus	13	11
Sweating	9	6
Nervous System		
Peripheral Neurologic Symptoms/Neuropathy	21	10
Depression	12	12
Insomnia	7	4
Dizziness	11	9
Metabolic/Nutritional System		
Bilirubinemia	7	3
Urogenital System		
Dysuria	2	6
Hematuria	7	8
Infection Urinary Tract	4	7
Special Senses		
Taste Perversion	12	21
Musculoskeletal System		
Arthralgia	9	12
Myalgia	10	6

[a] Any severity, regardless of relationship to study regimen.
[b] START 2 compared two triple-combination regimens in 205 treatment-naive patients. Patients received either ZERIT (40 mg b.i.d.) plus didanosine plus indinavir or zidovudine plus lamivudine plus indinavir.
[c] Duration of stavudine therapy=48 weeks.

Laboratory Abnormalities: Selected laboratory abnormalities reported in two controlled combination studies are provided in Table 3 and Table 4.

Table 3: ZERIT

Selected Laboratory Abnormalities in START 1 and START Studies (Grades 3-4)

	Percent of Patients			
	START 1		START 2	
Parameter	**ZERIT + lamivudine + indinavir n=100**	**zidovudine + lamivudine + indinavir n=102**	**ZERIT + didanosine + indinavir n=102**	**zidovudine + lamivudine + indinavir n=103**
Bilirubin (>2.6×ULN)	7	6	16	8
AST (>5×ULN)	5	2	7	7
ALT (>5×ULN)	6	2	8	5
GGT (>5×ULN)	2	2	5	2
Lipase (>2×ULN)	6	3	5	5
Amylase (>2×ULN)	4	<1	8	2

(cont'd)

Legend: ULN=upper limit of normal.

Table 4: ZERIT

Selected Laboratory Abnormalities in START 1 and START 2 Studies (All Grades)

	Percent of Patients			
	START 1		START 2	
Parameter	**ZERIT + lamivudine + indinavir n=100**	**zidovudine + lamivudine + indinavir n=102**	**ZERIT + didanosine + indinavir n=102**	**zidovudine + lamivudine + indinavir n=103**
Total Bilirubin	65	60	68	55
AST	42	20	53	20
ALT	40	20	50	18
GGT	15	8	28	12
Lipase	27	12	26	19
Amylase	21	19	31	17

Post-Market Adverse Drug Reactions: The following events have been identified during post-approval use of ZERIT. Because they are reported voluntarily from a population of unknown size, estimates of frequency cannot be made. These events have been chosen for inclusion due to their seriousness, frequency of reporting, causal connection to ZERIT, or a combination of these factors.
Body as a Whole: abdominal pain, allergic reactions, chills/fever, redistribution/accumulation of body fat, lipoatrophy/lipodystrophy (see Warnings and Precautions, Fat Redistribution).
Digestive Disorders: anorexia.
Exocrine Gland Disorders: pancreatitis [including fatal cases (see Warnings and Precautions)].
Hematologic Disorders: anemia, neutropenia, leukopenia, macrocytosis, and thrombocytopenia.
Liver: lactic acidosis and hepatic steatosis [including fatal cases (see Warnings and Precautions)], hepatitis and liver failure [including fatal cases (see Warnings and Precautions)].
Metabolic Disorders: diabetes mellitus, hyperglycemia.
Musculoskeletal: myalgia.
Nervous System: insomnia, severe motor weakness (most often reported in the setting of symptomatic hyperlactatemia or lactic acidosis, including fatal cases, see Warnings and Precautions).
Pediatric Patients: Adverse reactions and serious laboratory abnormalities in pediatric patients were similar in type and frequency to those seen in adult patients.

DRUG INTERACTIONS: Drug-Drug Interactions: Zidovudine may competitively inhibit the intracellular phosphorylation of stavudine (see Action and Clinical Pharmacology). Therefore, use of zidovudine in combination with ZERIT is not recommended. In vitro data indicate that the phosphorylation of stavudine is also inhibited at relevant concentrations by doxorubicin and ribavirin; therefore coadministration of stavudine with either doxorubicin or ribavirin should be undertaken with caution.

No pharmacokinetic interactions were observed between ZERIT and didanosine, lamivudine (3TC), or nelfinavir when co-administered in clinical trials.

Stavudine does not inhibit the major cytochrome P450 isoforms CYP1A2, CYP2C9, CYP2C19, CYP2D6, and CYP3A4; therefore, it is unlikely that clinically significant drug interactions will occur with drugs metabolized through these pathways.

Drug-Food Interactions: ZERIT (stavudine) may be taken without regard to meals. Absorption of stavudine was assessed in a study of 16 asymptomatic HIV-infected patients. Each patient received a 70 mg oral dose of ZERIT in the fasting state, 1 hour before a standardized meal, and immediately after a standardized meal. The results indicate that systemic exposure to stavudine is not reduced when ZERIT is taken with food. Although the rate of absorption decreased, the extent of absorption was not significantly (p=0.27) affected by the presence of food when ZERIT was taken immediately after a meal. Mean (±SD) C_{max} of stavudine was reduced from 1.44 (±0.49) µg/mL in the fasting state to 0.75 (±0.16) µg/mL after a meal, and the median time to achieve C_{max} was prolonged from 0.6 to 1.5 hours. However, mean (±SD) $AUC_{0-\infty}$ values were 2.50 (±0.71) µg·hr/mL and 2.31 (±0.55) µg·hr/mL in the fasting state and after a meal, respectively, indicating that systemic exposure was similar with or without the presence of food.

Drug-Herb Interactions: Interactions with herbs have not been established.

DOSAGE AND ADMINISTRATION:

Recommended Dose and Dosage Adjustment: Adults: The interval between oral doses should be 12 hours. ZERIT (stavudine) may be taken with or without food. The recommended doses are based on body weight, as outlined in Table 5.

Table 5: ZERIT

Adult Dosing

Patient Weight	ZERIT Dosage
<60 kg	30 mg b.i.d.
≥60 kg	40 mg b.i.d.

Dosage Adjustment: Renal Impairment: Adults: The following dose adjustments are recommended in adult patients with renal impairment: see Table 6.

Table 6: ZERIT

Recommended ZERIT Dosing Modifications for Subjects with Renal Impairment

Creatinine Clearance (mL/min)	Recommended ZERIT Dose by Patient Weight	
	≥60 kg	<60 kg
>50[a]	40 mg every 12 hours[a]	30 mg every 12 hours[a]
26–50	20 mg every 12 hours	15 mg every 12 hours
<25[b]	20 mg every 24 hours	15 mg every 24 hours

[a] Normal dose, no adjustment necessary.
[b] For patients undergoing hemodialysis, the daily dose of ZERIT should be administered after the completion of a scheduled hemodialysis session. On nondialysis days, ZERIT should be administered at the same time of day as it is on dialysis days.

Hepatic Impairment: Adults: Dosing adjustment is not necessary in subjects with stable hepatic impairment. In the event of rapidly elevating aminotransferase levels, treatment with ZERIT should be suspended.
Peripheral Neuropathy: Clinical symptoms of peripheral neuropathy which is usually characterized by numbness, tingling or pain in the feet or hands should prompt interruption of ZERIT treatment and evaluation of the patient. These symptoms may be difficult to detect in children (see Warnings and Precautions). If symptoms develop, ZERIT should be interrupted. Symptoms may resolve if therapy is withdrawn promptly. Some patients may experience a temporary worsening of symptoms following discontinuation of therapy. If symptoms resolve completely, resumption of treatment may be considered. If a reduced dose is warranted, use one-half the recommended dose.

OVERDOSAGE:
There is no known antidote for ZERIT (stavudine) overdosage. Experience with adults treated with 12 to 24 times the recommended daily dosage revealed no acute toxicity. Patients may benefit from administration of activated charcoal. Stavudine can be removed by hemodialysis, the mean±SD hemodialysis clearance of stavudine is 120±18 mL/min. It is not known whether stavudine is eliminated by peritoneal dialysis.

For management of a suspected drug overdose, contact your regional Poison Control Centre. See the *CPS* Directory section for a list of Poison Control Centres.

ACTION AND CLINICAL PHARMACOLOGY: Mechanism of Action: ZERIT (stavudine), also known as d4T, is a synthetic thymidine nucleoside analogue active against the Human Immunodeficiency Virus (HIV).

In vitro studies demonstrate that stavudine is converted to the triphosphate by cellular kinases. The 5′-triphosphate is the active form of the drug. In cell culture studies with two different cell lines, stavudine triphosphate had an intracellular half-life of 3.5 hours. Stavudine triphosphate has been shown to be a potent competitive inhibitor of HIV reverse transcriptase (ki=0.0083 to 0.032 μM). In addition, both stavudine triphosphate and the natural substrate, thymidine triphosphate, are used by HIV reverse transcriptase in vitro for incorporation into the nascent DNA chain. Stavudine lacks the 3′-hydroxyl group necessary for DNA elongation and once incorporated into DNA, functions as a DNA chain terminator in vitro. Both the inhibition of binding of thymidine triphosphate to reverse transcriptase and DNA chain termination may be partially responsible for inhibition of HIV replication in vitro. In addition to the inhibitory effect on HIV reverse transcriptase, stavudine triphosphate exhibits some inhibitory effect on DNA polymerase beta and gamma, and markedly reduces the syntheses of mitochondrial DNA.

Clinically, ZERIT has been studied in various combinations with other classes of anti-retroviral drugs, including didanosine, lamivudine (3TC), ritonavir, nelfinavir, saquinavir, indinavir, and hydroxyurea. However, zidovudine in combination with ZERIT is not recommended (see Warnings and Precautions, Drug Interactions). Both drugs are phosphorylated by the same cellular enzyme (thymidine kinase), which may preferentially phosphorylate zidovudine, thereby decreasing the phosphorylation of stavudine to its active triphosphate form.

Based on in vitro testing, the activation of stavudine has also been shown to be inhibited by other drugs. Among the several drugs tested, the only ones that may interfere with stavudine phosphorylation at relevant concentrations are doxorubicin and ribavirin, but not other drugs used in the therapy of HIV infection which are similarly phosphorylated. The clinical significance of this is unknown.

Clinical trials supporting the use of ZERIT in appropriate antiretroviral regimens for the treatment of HIV-infected patients, demonstrated, overall, greatest inhibition of HIV RNA levels and greatest increase in CD4 cell counts with triple-combination regimens.
Drug Resistance: HIV isolates with reduced susceptibility to stavudine have been selected in vitro and were also obtained from patients treated with stavudine. Phenotypic analysis of HIV-1 isolates from 61 patients receiving prolonged (6-29 months) stavudine monotherapy showed that post-therapy isolates from four patients exhibited EC_{50} values more than 4-fold (range 7- to 16-fold) higher than the average pretreatment susceptibility of baseline isolates. Of these, HIV-1 isolates from one patient contained the zidovudine-resistance-associated mutation T215Y and K219E, and isolates from another patient contained the multiple-nucleoside- resistance-associated mutation Q151M. Mutations in the RT gene of HIV-1 isolates from the other two patients were not detected. The genetic basis for stavudine susceptibility changes has not been identified.
Cross-resistance: Cross-resistance among HIV-1 reverse transcriptase inhibitors has been observed. Five of 11 stavudine post-treatment isolates developed moderate resistance to zidovudine (9- to 176-fold) and 3 of those 11 isolates developed moderate resistance to didanosine (7- to 29-fold). Several studies have demonstrated that prolonged stavudine treatment can select and/or maintain thymidine analogue mutations (TAMs) associated with zidovudine resistance. The decrease of susceptibility in cell culture is subtle requiring two or more TAMs (generally M41L and T215Y) before stavudine susceptibility is decreased (>1.5 fold). These TAMs are seen at a similar frequency with stavudine and zidovudine in virological treatment. The clinical relevance of these findings suggests that stavudine should be avoided in the presence of thymidine analogue mutations, especially M41L and T215Y.
Pharmacokinetics in Adults: The pharmacokinetics of stavudine have been evaluated in HIV-infected adult and pediatric patients (refer to Table 7). Peak plasma concentrations (C_{max}) and area under the plasma concentration-time curve (AUC) increased in proportion to dose after both single and multiple doses ranging from 0.03 to 4 mg/kg. There was no significant accumulation of stavudine with repeated administration every 6, 8, or 12 hours.

Table 7: ZERIT

Mean±SD Pharmacokinetic Parameters of Stavudine in Adult and Pediatric HIV-infected Patients

Parameter	Adult Patients	n	Pediatric Patients	n
Oral bioavailability (F)	86.4±18.2%	25	76.9±31.7%	20
Volume of distribution[a](VD)	58±21 L	44	18.5±9.2 L/m²	21
Apparent oral volume of distribution[b](VD/F)	66±22 L	71	not determined	—
Ratio of CSF: plasma concentrations (as %)[c]	not determined	—	59±35%	8
Total body clearance[a](CL)	8.2±2.3 mL/min/kg	44	247±94 mL/min/m²	21
Apparent oral clearance[b](CL/F)	8.0±2.6 mL/min/kg	113	333±87 mL/min/m²	20
Elimination half-life ($T_{1/2}$), i.v. dose[a]	1.15±0.35 h	44	1.11±0.28 h	21
Elimination half-life ($T_{1/2}$), oral dose[b]	1.44±0.30 h	115	0.96±0.26 h	20

(cont'd)

Table 7: ZERIT *(cont'd)*

Mean±SD Pharmacokinetic Parameters of Stavudine in Adult and Pediatric HIV-infected Patients

Parameter	Adult Patients	n	Pediatric Patients	n
Urinary recovery of stavudine (% of dose)	39±23%	88	34±16%	19

[a] Following 1 hour i.v. infusion.
[b] Following single oral dose.
[c] Following multiple oral doses.

Absorption: Following oral administration, stavudine is rapidly absorbed, with peak plasma concentrations occurring within 1 hour after dosing. The systemic exposure to stavudine is the same following administration as capsules or solution.
Distribution: Binding of stavudine to serum proteins was negligible over the concentration range of 0.01 to 11.4 μg/mL. Stavudine distributes equally between red blood cells and plasma.
Metabolism: The metabolic fate of stavudine has not been elucidated in humans.
Excretion: Renal elimination accounted for about 40% of the overall clearance regardless of the route of administration. The mean renal clearance was about twice the average endogenous creatinine clearance, indicating active tubular secretion in addition to glomerular filtration.

STORAGE AND STABILITY: ZERIT capsules should be stored at room temperature (15° to 30°C) and protected from excessive moisture. Keep bottles tightly closed.

INFORMATION FOR THE PATIENT: Published in e-CPS, available by subscription at www.e-cps.ca.

DOSAGE FORMS, COMPOSITION AND PACKAGING: 15 mg: Each light yellow and dark red capsule, imprinted with "BMS 1964" and "15", contains: stavudine 15 mg. Nonmedicinal ingredients: lactose, magnesium stearate, microcrystalline cellulose and sodium starch glycolate; capsule shell: gelatin, printing ink, silicon dioxide, sodium lauryl sulfate, titanium dioxide and yellow and red iron oxides. Bottles of 60.
20 mg: Each light brown capsule, imprinted with "BMS 1965" and "20", contains: stavudine 20 mg. Nonmedicinal ingredients: lactose, magnesium stearate, microcrystalline cellulose and sodium starch glycolate; capsule shell: gelatin, black iron oxide (20 mg only), printing ink, silicon dioxide, sodium lauryl sulfate, titanium dioxide and yellow and red iron oxides. Bottles of 60.
30 mg: Each light orange and dark orange capsule, imprinted with "BMS 1966" and "30", contains: stavudine 30 mg. Nonmedicinal ingredients: lactose, magnesium stearate, microcrystalline cellulose and sodium starch glycolate; capsule shell: gelatin, printing ink, silicon dioxide, sodium lauryl sulfate, titanium dioxide and yellow and red iron oxides. Bottles of 60.
40 mg: Each dark orange capsule, imprinted with "BMS 1967" and "40" contains: stavudine 40 mg. Nonmedicinal ingredients: lactose, magnesium stearate, microcrystalline cellulose and sodium starch glycolate; capsule shell: gelatin, printing ink, silicon dioxide, sodium lauryl sulfate, titanium dioxide and yellow and red iron oxides. Bottles of 60.

(Shown in Product Identification Section)

The reader is invited to consult CPhA's monograph **ACE Inhibitors.**

Zestoretic®

lisinopril—hydrochlorothiazide

Angiotensin Converting Enzyme Inhibitor—Diuretic

AstraZeneca

Date of Revision: October 21, 2009

PHARMACOLOGY: ZESTORETIC (lisinopril and hydrochlorothiazide) combines the action of an angiotensin converting enzyme inhibitor, lisinopril, and a diuretic, hydrochlorothiazide.
Lisinopril: Angiotensin converting enzyme (ACE) is a peptidyl dipeptidase which catalyzes the conversion of angiotensin I to the pressor substance, angiotensin II. Inhibition of ACE results in decreased plasma angiotensin II, which leads to increased plasma renin activity (due to removal of negative feedback of renin release) and decreased aldosterone secretion. Although the latter decrease is small, it results in a small increase in serum potassium. In patients treated with lisinopril plus a thiazide diuretic, there was essentially no change in serum potassium (see Precautions). ACE is identical to kininase II. Thus, lisinopril may also block the degradation of bradykinin, a potent vasodilator peptide. However, the role that this plays in the therapeutic effects of lisinopril is unknown.

While the mechanism through which lisinopril lowers blood pressure is believed to be primarily the suppression of the renin-angiotensin-aldosterone system, lisinopril also lowers blood pressure in patients with low-renin hypertension. However, black hypertensive patients (usually a low-renin hypertensive population) have a smaller average response to lisinopril monotherapy than non-black patients.

When lisinopril is given together with thiazide-type diuretics, its blood pressure lowering effect is approximately additive.
Hydrochlorothiazide: Hydrochlorothiazide is a diuretic and antihypertensive which interferes with the renal tubular mechanism of electrolyte reabsorption. It increases excretion of sodium and chloride in approximately equivalent amounts. Natriuresis may be accompanied by some loss of potassium and bicarbonate. While this compound is predominantly a saluretic agent, in vitro studies have shown that it has a carbonic anhydrase inhibitory action which seems to be relatively specific for the renal tubular mechanism. It does not appear to be concentrated in erythrocytes or the brain in sufficient amounts to influence the activity of carbonic anhydrase in those tissues.

Hydrochlorothiazide is useful in the treatment of hypertension. It may be used alone or as an adjunct to other antihypertensive drugs. Hydrochlorothiazide does not affect normal blood pressure. The mechanism of its antihypertensive action is not known. Lowering of the sodium content of arteriolar smooth muscle cells and diminished response to norepinephrine have been postulated.
Pharmacokinetics: Lisinopril: Following oral administration of lisinopril, peak serum concentrations occur within about 7 hours. Declining serum concentrations exhibit a prolonged terminal phase which does not contribute to drug accumulation. This terminal phase probably represents saturable binding to ACE and is not proportional to dose. Lisinopril does not bind to plasma proteins other than ACE.

Lisinopril does not undergo metabolism and is excreted unchanged entirely in the urine. Based on urinary recovery, the extent of absorption of lisinopril is approximately 25%, with large inter-subject variability (6-60%) at all doses tested (5-80 mg).

Lisinopril absorption is not influenced by the presence of food in the gastrointestinal tract.

Upon multiple dosing, lisinopril exhibits an effective half-life of accumulation of 12 hours.

In a study in elderly healthy subjects (65 years and above), a single dose of lisinopril 20 mg produced higher serum concentrations and higher values for the area under the plasma curve than those seen in young healthy adults given a similar dose. In another study, single daily doses of lisinopril 5 mg were given for 7 consecutive days to young and elderly healthy volunteers. Maximum serum concentrations of lisinopril on Day 7 were higher in the elderly volunteers than in the young.

Impaired renal function decreases elimination of lisinopril. This decrease becomes clinically important when the glomerular filtration rate is below 30 mL/min (see Precautions, Renal Impairment and Dosage).

Lisinopril can be removed by dialysis.

Studies in rats indicate that lisinopril crosses the blood-brain barrier poorly.
Hydrochlorothiazide: Hydrochlorothiazide is not metabolized but is eliminated rapidly by the kidney. The plasma half-life is 5.6-14.8 hours when the plasma levels can be followed for at least 24 hours. At least 61% of the oral dose is eliminated unchanged within 24 hours. Hydrochlorothiazide crosses the placental but not the blood-brain barrier and is excreted in breast milk.

Onset of the diuretic action following oral administration occurs in 2 hours and the peak action in about 4 hours. Diuretic activity lasts about 6 to 12 hours.
Lisinopril-Hydrochlorothiazide: Concomitant administration of lisinopril and hydrochlorothiazide has little, or no effect on the bioavailability of either drug. The combination tablet is bioequivalent to concomitant administration of the separate entities.

Pharmacodynamics: Lisinopril: Administration of lisinopril to patients with hypertension results in a reduction of both supine and standing blood pressure. Abrupt withdrawal of lisinopril has not been associated with a rapid increase in blood pressure. In most patients studied, after oral administration of an individual dose of lisinopril, the onset of antihypertensive activity is seen at one hour with peak reduction of blood pressure achieved by 6 hours. Although an antihypertensive effect was observed 24 hours after dosing with recommended single daily doses, the effect was more consistent and the mean effect was considerably larger in some studies with doses of 20 mg or more than with lower doses. However, at all doses studied, the mean antihypertensive effect was substantially smaller 24 hours after dosing than it was 6 hours after dosing. On occasion, achievement of optimal blood pressure reduction may require 2 to 4 weeks of therapy.

In hemodynamic studies in patients with essential hypertension, blood pressure reduction was accompanied by a reduction in peripheral arterial resistance with little or no change in cardiac output and in heart rate. In a study in nine hypertensive patients, following administration of lisinopril, there was an increase in mean renal blood flow that was not significant. Data from several small studies are inconsistent with respect to the effect of lisinopril on glomerular filtration rate in hypertensive patients with normal renal function, but suggest that changes, if any, are not large.

INDICATIONS: ZESTORETIC (lisinopril and hydrochlorothiazide) is indicated for the treatment of essential hypertension in patients for whom combination therapy is appropriate.

In using ZESTORETIC, consideration should be given to the risk of angioedema (see Warnings, Angioedema).

Lisinopril should normally be used in those patients in whom treatment with diuretic or betablocker was found ineffective or has been associated with unacceptable adverse effects.

ZESTORETIC is not indicated for initial therapy. Patients in whom lisinopril and diuretic are initiated simultaneously can develop symptomatic hypotension (see Precautions, Drug Interactions).

Patients should be titrated on the individual drugs. If the fixed combination represents the dosage determined by this titration, the use of ZESTORETIC may be more convenient in the management of patients. If during maintenance therapy dosage adjustment is necessary, it is advisable to use individual drugs.

CONTRAINDICATIONS: ZESTORETIC (lisinopril and hydrochlorothiazide) is contraindicated in patients who:

- are hypersensitive to any component of this product;
- have a known allergy to angiotensin converting enzyme inhibitors;
- have a history of angioneurotic edema relating to previous treatment with an angiotensin converting enzyme inhibitor;
- have hereditary or idiopathic angioneurotic edema, and because of the hydrochlorothiazide component, in patients who have anuria;
- hypersensitivity to other sulfonamide-derived drugs.

WARNINGS:

Serious Warnings and Precautions
When used in pregnancy, ACE inhibitors can cause injury or even death of the developing fetus. When pregnancy is detected, ZESTORETIC should be discontinued as soon as possible (see Warnings, Pregnancy, and Information to Be Provided to the Patient).

Angioedema: Angioedema has been uncommonly reported in patients treated with ZESTORETIC (lisinopril and hydrochlorothiazide) and may occur at any time during therapy. Angioedema associated with laryngeal or tongue edema and/or shock may be fatal. If angioedema occurs, ZESTORETIC should be promptly discontinued and the patient should be treated, and observed until the swelling subsides. Where swelling is confined only to the tongue, without respiratory distress, patients may require prolonged observation since treatment with antihistamines and corticosteroids may not be sufficient.

However, where there is involvement of the tongue, glottis or larynx, likely to cause airway obstruction, and especially in cases where there has been a history of airway surgery, emergency therapy should be administered promptly when indicated. This includes giving subcutaneous adrenaline/epinephrine (0.5 mL 1:1000) and/or maintaining a patent airway. The patient should be under close medical supervision until the complete and sustained symptom resolution has occurred.

The incidence of angioedema during ACE inhibitor therapy has been reported to be higher in black than in non-black patients.

Patients with a history of angioedema unrelated to ACE inhibitor therapy may be at increased risk of angioedema while receiving an ACE inhibitor (see Contraindications).

Hypotension: Symptomatic hypotension has occurred after administration of lisinopril, usually after the first or second dose or when the dose was increased. It is more likely to occur in patients who are volume depleted by diuretic therapy, dietary salt restriction, dialysis, diarrhea, or vomiting. Therefore, ZESTORETIC should not be used to start therapy or when a dose change is needed. Severe hypotension is also a risk in renin-dependant renovascular hypertension; ZESTORETIC is not indicated for this condition (see Indications). In patients with ischemic heart or cerebrovascular disease, an excessive fall in blood pressure could result in a myocardial infarction or cerebrovascular accident (see Adverse Effects). Because blood pressure could potentially fall, patients at risk for hypotension should start lisinopril therapy under very close medical supervision, usually in a hospital. Such patients should be followed closely for the first two weeks of treatment and whenever the dose of lisinopril and/or hydrochlorothiazide is increased. In patients with severe congestive heart failure, with or without associated renal insufficiency, excessive hypotension has been observed and may be associated with oliguria and/or progressive azotemia, and rarely with acute renal failure and/or death.

If hypotension occurs, the patient should be placed in supine position and, if necessary, receive an intravenous infusion of normal saline. A transient hypotensive response may not be a contraindication to further doses. These can usually be given to hypertensive patients without difficulty once the blood pressure has increased after volume expansion. Reinstitution of therapy at reduced dosages, or re-institution with either component alone, should be considered.

Neutropenia/Agranulocytosis: Agranulocytosis and bone marrow depression have been caused by angiotensin converting enzyme inhibitors. Several cases of agranulocytosis and neutropenia have been reported in which a causal relationship to lisinopril cannot be excluded. Current experience with the drug shows the incidence to be rare. Periodic monitoring of white blood cell counts should be considered, especially in patients with collagen vascular disease and renal disease.

Azotemia: Azotemia may be precipitated or increased by hydrochlorothiazide. Cumulative effects of the drug may develop in patients with impaired renal function. If increasing azotemia and oliguria occur during treatment of severe progressive renal disease, the diuretic should be discontinued.

Patients with Impaired Liver Function: Hepatitis (with very rare progression to hepatic failure), jaundice (hepatocellular and/or cholestatic), marked elevations of liver enzymes and/or serum bilirubin have occurred during therapy with lisinopril in patients with or without pre-existing liver abnormalities. In most cases the changes were reversed on discontinuation of the drug, and appropriate medical follow up.

Should the patient receiving ZESTORETIC experience any unexplained symptoms (see Precautions, Information to Be Provided to the Patient), particularly during the first weeks or months of treatment, it is recommended that a full set of liver function tests and any other necessary investigation be carried out. Discontinuation of ZESTORETIC should be considered when appropriate.

There are no adequate studies in patients with cirrhosis and/or liver dysfunction. ZESTORETIC should be used with particular caution in patients with pre-existing liver abnormalities. In such patients baseline liver function tests should be obtained before administration of the drug and close monitoring of response and metabolic effects should apply.

Thiazides should be used with caution in patients with impaired hepatic function or progressive liver disease, since minor alterations of fluid and electrolyte balance may precipitate hepatic coma.

Hypersensitivity Reactions: Sensitivity reactions to hydrochlorothiazide may occur in patients with or without a history of allergy or bronchial asthma.

The possibility of exacerbation or activation of systemic lupus erythematosus has been reported in patients treated with hydrochlorothiazide.

Pregnancy: ACE inhibitors can cause fetal and neonatal morbidity and mortality when administered to pregnant women. When pregnancy is detected, ZESTORETIC should be discontinued as soon as possible.

The use of ACE inhibitors during the second and third trimesters of pregnancy has been associated with fetal and neonatal injury including hypotension, neonatal skull hypoplasia, anuria, reversible or irreversible renal failure, and death. Oligohydramnios has also been reported, presumably resulting from decreased fetal renal function, associated with fetal limb contractures, craniofacial deformation, and hypoplastic lung development.

Prematurity, and patent ductus arteriosus and other structural cardiac malformations, as well as neurologic malformations, have also been reported following exposure in the first trimester of pregnancy.

Infants with a history of in utero exposure to ACE inhibitors should be closely observed for hypotension, oliguria, and hyperkalemia. If oliguria occurs, attention should be directed towards support of blood pressure and renal perfusion. Exchange transfusion or dialysis may be required as a means of reversing hypotension and/or substituting for impaired renal function; however, limited experience with those procedures has not been associated with significant clinical benefit.

Lisinopril, has been removed from the neonatal circulation by peritoneal dialysis.

Animal Data: Lisinopril was not teratogenic in mice treated on days 6-15 of gestation with up to 1000 mg/kg/day (625 times the maximum recommended human dose). There was an increase in fetal resorptions at doses down to 100 mg/kg; at doses of 1000 mg/kg, this was prevented by saline supplementation. There was no fetotoxicity or teratogenicity in rats treated with up to 300 mg/kg/day (188 times the maximum recommended dose) of lisinopril at days 6-17 of gestation. In rats receiving lisinopril from day 15 of gestation through day 21 postpartum, there was an increased incidence in pup deaths on days 2-7 postpartum and a lower average body weight of pups on day 21 postpartum. The increase in pup deaths and decrease in pup weight did not occur with maternal saline supplementation.

Lisinopril, at doses up to 1 mg/kg/day, was not teratogenic when given throughout the organogenic period in saline supplemented rabbits. Saline supplementation (physiologic saline in place of tap water) was used to eliminate maternotoxic effects and enable evaluation of the teratogenic potential at the highest possible dosage level. The rabbit has been shown to be extremely sensitive to angiotensin converting enzyme inhibitors (captopril and enalapril) with maternal and fetotoxic effects apparent at or below the recommended therapeutic dosage levels in man.

Fetotoxicity was demonstrated in rabbits by an increase incidence of fetal resorptions at an oral dose of lisinopril of 1 mg/kg/day and by an increased incidence of incomplete ossification at the lowest dose tested (0.1 mg/kg/day). A single intravenous dose of 15 mg/kg of lisinopril administered to pregnant rabbits on gestation days 16, 21 or 26 resulted in 88% to 100% fetal death.

By whole body autoradiography, radioactivity was found in the placenta following administration of labelled lisinopril to pregnant rats, but none was found in the fetuses.

Lactation: The presence of concentrations of ACE inhibitor has been reported in human milk. Use of ACE inhibitors is not recommended during breast-feeding.

Race: Angiotensin converting inhibitors cause a higher rate of angioedema in black patients than in non black patients.

The antihypertensive effect of angiotensin converting enzyme inhibitors is generally lower in black patients (usually a low-renin hypertensive population) than in non-black patients.

PRECAUTIONS: Renal Impairment: As a consequence of inhibiting the renin-angiotensin-aldosterone system, changes in renal function have been seen in susceptible individuals. In patients whose renal function may depend on the activity of the renin-angiotensin-aldosterone system, such as patients with bilateral renal artery stenosis, unilateral renal artery stenosis to a solitary kidney, or severe congestive heart failure, treatment with agents that inhibit this system has been associated with oliguria, progressive azotemia, and rarely, acute renal failure and/or death. In susceptible patients, concomitant diuretic use may further increase risk.

Use of ZESTORETIC (lisinopril and hydrochlorothiazide) should include appropriate assessment of renal function.

Thiazides may not be appropriate diuretics for use in patients with renal impairment and are ineffective at creatinine clearance values of 30 mL/min or below i.e., moderate or severe renal insufficiency (see Dosage, Dosage Adjustment in Renal Impairment).

Anaphylactoid Reactions During Membrane Exposure: Anaphylactoid reactions have been reported in patients dialysed with high-flux membranes (e.g.: polyacrylonitrile [PAN] and during low density lipoproteins (LDL) apheresis with dextran sulphate) and treated concomitantly with an ACE inhibitor.

Dialysis should be stopped immediately if symptoms such as nausea, abdominal cramps, burning, angioedema, shortness of breath and severe hypotension occur. Symptoms are not relieved by antihistamines. In these patients consideration should be given to using a different type of dialysis membrane or a different class of antihypertensive agent.

Anaphylactoid Reactions During Desensitization: There have been isolated reports of patients experiencing sustained life threatening anaphylactoid reactions while receiving ACE inhibitors during desensitizing treatment with hymenoptera (bees, wasps) venom. In the same patients, these reactions have been avoided when ACE inhibitors were temporarily withheld for at least 24 hours, but they have reappeared upon inadvertent rechallenge.

Hyperkalemia: In clinical trials hyperkalemia (serum potassium >5.7 mEq/L) occurred in approximately 1.4% of hypertensive patients. In most cases these were isolated values which resolved despite continued therapy. Hyperkalemia was not a cause of discontinuation of therapy. Risk factors for the development of hyperkalemia may include renal insufficiency, diabetes mellitus, and the concomitant use of potassium-sparing diuretics, potassium supplements and/or potassium-containing salt substitutes (see Precautions, Drug Interactions).

Valvular Stenosis, Hypertrophic Cardiomyopathy: There is concern on theoretical grounds that patients with aortic stenosis might be at particular risk of decreased coronary perfusion when treated with vasodilators because they do not develop as much after load reduction.

ZESTORETIC should be given with caution to patients with aortic or hypertrophic cardiomyopathy.

Metabolism: Thiazide therapy may impair glucose tolerance. Dosage adjustment of hypoglycemic agents may be required (see Precautions, Drug Interactions).

Hyperuricemia may occur, or acute gout may be precipitated, in certain patients receiving thiazide therapy.

Thiazides may decrease serum PBI levels without signs of thyroid disturbance.

Thiazides have been shown to increase excretion of magnesium; this may result in hypomagnesemia.

Thiazides may decrease urinary calcium excretion. Thiazides may cause intermittent and slight elevation of serum calcium in the absence of known disorders of calcium metabolism. Marked hypercalcemia may be evidence of hidden hyperparathyroidism. Thiazides should be discontinued before carrying out tests for parathyroid function. Increases in cholesterol, triglyceride and glucose levels may be associated with thiazide diuretic therapy.

Surgery/Anesthesia: In patients undergoing major surgery or during anesthesia with agents that produce hypotension, lisinopril blocks angiotensin II formation, secondary to compensatory renin release. If hypotension occurs and is considered to be due to this mechanism, it can be corrected by volume expansion (see Precautions, Drug Interactions).

Cough: A dry, persistent cough, which usually disappears only after withdrawal or lowering of the dose of ZESTORETIC, has been reported.

Such possibility should be considered as part of the differential diagnosis of the cough.

Geriatrics: In general, blood pressure response and adverse experiences were similar in younger and older patients given similar doses of lisinopril. Pharmacokinetic studies, however, indicate that maximum blood levels and area under the plasma concentration time curve (AUC) are doubled in older patients so that dosage adjustments should be made with particular caution.

Children: ZESTORETIC has not been studied in children and, therefore, use in this age group is not recommended.

Occupational Hazards: Ability to drive and use machines: Dizziness or tiredness may occur during treatment with ZESTORETIC.

Drug Interactions: Hypotension: Patients on Diuretic Therapy: Patients on diuretics and especially those in whom diuretic therapy was recently instituted, may occasionally experience an excessive reduction of blood pressure after initiation of therapy with lisinopril. The possibility of hypotensive effects with lisinopril can be minimized by either discontinuing the diuretic or increasing the salt intake prior to initiation of treatment with lisinopril (see Warnings, and Dosage).

Hypotension: Patients on Antihypertensive Therapy: When lisinopril is given to patients already treated with other antihypertensive agents, further falls in blood pressure may occur.

Potassium Supplements, potassium-sparing agents or potassium-containing salt substitutes: Since lisinopril decreases aldosterone production, elevation of serum potassium may occur. Potassium sparing diuretics such as spironolactone, triamterene or amiloride, or potassium supplements should be given only for documented hypokalemia and with caution and with frequent monitoring of serum potassium since they may lead to a significant increase in serum potassium. Salt substitutes which contain potassium should also be used with caution.

Agents Causing Renin Release: The antihypertensive effect of ZESTORETIC is augmented by antihypertensive agents that cause renin release (e.g. diuretics).

Agents Affecting Sympathetic Activity: Agents affecting sympathetic activity (e.g., ganglionic blocking agents or adrenergic neuron blocking agents) may be used with caution. Beta-adrenergic blocking drugs add some further antihypertensive effect to lisinopril.

Lithium: Lithium generally should not be given with diuretics or ACE inhibitors. Diuretic agents and ACE inhibitors reduce the renal clearance of lithium and add a high risk of lithium toxicity.

Gold: Nitritoid reactions (symptoms of vasodilatation including flushing, nausea, dizziness and hypotension, which can be very severe) following injectable gold (for example, sodium aurothiomalate) have been reported more frequently in patients receiving ACE inhibitor therapy.

d-tubocurarine: Thiazide drugs may increase the responsiveness to tubocurarine.

Insulin and Oral Hypoglycemic Agents: Insulin and oral hypoglycemic agents requirements in diabetic patients may be increased, decreased or unchanged. Previously latent diabetes mellitus may become manifest during thiazide administration (see Precautions, Metabolism).

Alcohol, Barbiturates, Or Narcotics: Potentiation of orthostatic hypotension may occur.

Corticosteroids, ACTH: Intensified electrolyte depletion, particularly hypokalemia may occur.

Pressor Amines (e.g. norepinephrine): Possible decreased response to pressor amines but not sufficient to preclude their use.

Non Steroidal Anti-inflammatory Drugs: In some patients, the administration of a non-steroidal anti-inflammatory agent can reduce the diuretic, natriuretic, and antihypertensive effects of loop, potassium-sparing and thiazide diuretics. Therefore, when ZESTORETIC and non-steroidal antiinflammatory agents are used concomitantly, the patient should be observed closely to determine if the desired effect of the diuretic is obtained.

In some patients with compromised renal function, lisinopril co-administration with nonsteroidal anti-inflammatory drugs (NSAIDS) may produce further renal function deterioration.

Indomethacin may diminish the antihypertensive efficacy of concomitantly administered lisinopril and hydrochlorothiazide.

Information to Be Provided to the Patient:

Serious Warning and Precautions

ZESTORETIC should not be used during pregnancy. Patients should be advised to stop the medication and contact their physician as soon as possible if they discover that they are pregnant while taking ZESTORETIC.

Angioedema: Angioedema, including laryngeal, may occur during treatment with ZESTORETIC. Patients should be so advised and told to report immediately any signs or symptoms suggesting angioedema (swelling of face, extremities, eyes, lips, tongue, difficulty in breathing) and to take no more drug until they have consulted with the prescribing physician.

Hypotension: Patients should be cautioned to report lightheadedness especially during the first few days of therapy. If actual syncope occurs, the patients should be told to discontinue the drug until they have consulted with the prescribing physician.

All patients should be cautioned that excessive perspiration and dehydration may lead to an excessive fall in blood pressure because of reduction in fluid volume. Other causes of volume depletion such as vomiting or diarrhoea may also lead to a fall in blood pressure; patients should be advised to consult with their physician.

Neutropenia: Patients should be told to report promptly any indication of infection (e.g., sore throat, fever) which may be a sign of neutropenia.

Impaired Liver Function: Patients should be advised to return to the physician if he/she experiences any symptoms possibly related to liver dysfunction. This would include "viral-like symptoms" in the first weeks to months of therapy (such as fever, malaise, muscle pain, rash or adenopathy which are possible indicators of hypersensitivity reactions), or if abdominal pain, nausea or vomiting, loss of appetite, jaundice, itching or any other unexplained symptoms occur during therapy.

You are pregnant, breast-feeding or thinking of becoming pregnant? Taking ZESTORETIC during pregnancy can cause injury and even death to your baby. This medicine should not be used during pregnancy. If you become pregnant while taking ZESTORETIC, stop the medication and report to your doctor as soon as possible. It is possible that ZESTORETIC passes into breast milk. You should not breast-feed while taking ZESTORETIC.

Note: As with many other drugs, certain advice to patients being treated with ZESTORETIC is warranted. This information is intended to aid in the safe and effective use of this medication. It is not a disclosure of all possible adverse or intended events.

ADVERSE EFFECTS: In clinical trials involving 930 patients, including 100 patients treated for 50 weeks or more, the most severe clinical adverse reactions were syncope (0.8%), and hypotension (1.9%). The most frequent clinical adverse reactions were: dizziness (7.5%), headache (5.2%), cough (3.9%), fatigue (3.7%) and orthostatic effects (3.2%).

Discontinuation of treatment due to adverse reactions occurred in 4.4% of patients, mainly because of dizziness, cough, fatigue or muscle cramps.

Adverse reactions that have occurred in clinical trials or in marketing experience are those which have been previously reported with lisinopril and hydrochlorothiazide when used separately for the treatment of hypertension.

Adverse reactions occurring in hypertensive patients treated with lisinopril and hydrochlorothiazide in controlled trials are shown in Table 1.

Adverse Reactions in Controlled Clinical Trials:

Table 1: ZESTORETIC

Incidence of Adverse Reactions Occurring in Patients Treated with ZESTORETIC in Controlled Clinical Trials

	Lisinopril 2633 Patients (%)	Lisinopril Plus Hydrochlorothiazide 930 Patients (%)
Cardiovascular		
Hypotension	0.8	1.9
Orthostatic Effects	0.9	3.2
Chest Pain	1.1	1.0
Syncope	0.2	0.8
Angina	0.3	0.1
Edema	0.6	0.1
Palpitation	0.8	0.9
Rhythm Disturbances	0.5	0.1
Chest Discomfort	—	0.6
Gastrointestinal		
Diarrhea	1.8	2.5
Nausea	1.9	2.2
Vomiting	1.1	1.4
Dyspepsia	0.5	1.3
Anorexia	0.4	0.2
Constipation	0.2	0.3
Flatulence	0.3	0.2
Abdominal Pain	1.4	0.9
Dry mouth	0.5	0.2
Nervous System		
Dizziness	4.4	7.5
Headache	5.6	5.2
Paresthesia	0.5	1.5
Depression	0.7	0.5
Somnolence	0.8	0.4
Insomnia	0.3	0.2
Vertigo	0.2	0.9
Respiratory		
Cough	3.0	3.9
Dyspnea	0.4	0.4
Upper Respiratory Infection	2.1	2.2
Dermatologic		
Rash	1.0	1.2
Pruritus	0.5	0.4
Flushing	0.3	0.8
Angioedema	0.1	—[a]
Musculoskeletal		
Muscle Cramps	0.5	2.0
Back Pain	0.5	0.8
Shoulder Pain	0.2	0.5
Other		
Fatigue	—	3.7
Asthenia	2.7	1.8
Decreased Libido	0.2	1.0
Fever	0.3	0.5
Impotence	0.7	1.2
Gout	0.2	0.2

[a] See ZESTORETIC (Marketing Experience Only).

Abnormal Laboratory Findings: Hypokalemia, Hyperkalemia: (See Precautions, Hyperkalemia, and Drug Interactions).

Creatinine, Blood Urea Nitrogen: Minor increases in blood urea nitrogen (3.8%) and serum creatinine (4.2%) were observed in patients with essential hypertension treated with ZESTORETIC. More marked increases have also been reported and were more likely to occur in patients with bilateral renal artery stenosis (see Precautions, Renal Impairment).

Increases in blood urea nitrogen and serum creatinine, usually reversible upon discontinuation of therapy, were observed in 1.1 and 1.6% of patients respectively with essential hypertension treated with lisinopril alone.

Serum Uric Acid, Glucose, Magnesium, Cholesterol, Triglycerides and Calcium: (See Precautions, Metabolism).

Hemoglobin and Hematocrit: Small decreases in hemoglobin and hematocrit (mean decreases of approximately 0.5 g percent and 1.5 vol percent, respectively) occurred frequently in hypertensive patients treated with ZESTORETIC but were rarely of clinical importance unless another cause of anemia coexisted. In clinical trials, 0.4% of patients discontinued therapy due to anemia. Rarely, hemolytic anemia has been reported.

Agranulocytosis and bone marrow depression, manifested as anemia, cytopenia or leukopenia, have been caused by angiotensin converting enzyme inhibitors, including lisinopril. Several cases of agranulocytosis and neutropenia have been reported in which a causal relationship to lisinopril cannot be excluded (see Warnings, Neutropenia/Agranulocytosis).

Post-Marketing Experience: The following undesirable effects have been observed and reported during treatment with ZESTORETIC with the following frequencies: Very common (≥10%), common (≥1%, <10%), uncommon (≥0.1%, <1%), rare (≥0.01%, <0.1%), very rare (<0.01%) including isolated reports.

Blood and Lymphatic System Disorders: Rare: anaemia. Very rare: agranulocytosis, bone marrow depression, thrombocytopenia, leucopenia, hemolytic anaemia (see Warnings, Neutropenia/Agranulocytosis).

Endocrine Disorders: Rare: inappropriate antidiuretic hormone secretion.

Metabolism and Nutrition Disorders: Uncommon: gout. Rare: hyperkalemia (see Precautions, Hyperkalemia), hypokalemia, hyperuricemia, hyperglycemia (see Precautions, Metabolism).

Nervous System and Psychiatric Disorders: Common: dizziness, headache, paraesthesia. Uncommon: depressive symptoms. Rare: olfactory disturbance.

Cardiac and Vascular Disorders: Common: orthostatic effects (including hypotension), syncope. Uncommon: palpitations.

Respiratory, Thoracic and Mediastinal Disorders: Common: cough (see Precautions, Cough).

Gastrointestinal Disorders: Common: diarrhoea, nausea, vomiting. Uncommon: dry mouth. Rare: pancreatitis. Very rare: intestinal angioedema.

Hepato-biliary Disorders: Very rare: hepatitis—either hepatocellular or cholestatic, jaundice, hepatic failure. Very rarely, it has been reported that in some patients the undesirable development of hepatitis has progressed to hepatic failure. Patients receiving ZESTORETIC who develop jaundice or marked elevation of hepatic enzymes should discontinue ZESTORETIC and receive appropriate medical follow up (see Warnings, Patients with Impaired Liver Function).

Skin and Subcutaneous Tissue Disorders: Common: rash. Uncommon: hypersensitivity/angioneurotic oedema: angioneurotic oedema of the face, extremities, lips, tongue, glottis and/or larynx (see Warnings, Angioedema). Very rare: cutaneous pseudolymphoma.

A symptom complex has been reported which may include one or more of the following: fever, vasculitis, myalgia, arthralgia/arthritis, a positive antinuclear antibodies (ANA), elevated red blood cell sedimentation rate (ESR), eosinophilia and leucocytosis, rash, photosensitivity or other dermatological manifestation may occur.

Musculoskeletal, Connective Tissue And Bone Disorders: Common: muscle cramps. Rare: muscle weakness.

Reproductive System and Breast Disorders: Common: impotence.

General Disorders and Administration Site Conditions: Common: fatigue, asthenia. Uncommon: chest discomfort.

Investigations: Common: increases in blood urea, increases in serum creatinine (see Precautions, Renal Impairment), increases in liver enzymes (see Warnings, Patients with Impaired Liver Function), decreases in haemoglobin. Uncommon: decreases in haematocrit. Rare: increases in serum bilirubin (see Warnings, Patients with Impaired Liver Function).

Lisinopril: Myocardial infarction or cerebrovascular accident possibly secondary to excessive hypotension in high risk patients, tachycardia, abdominal pain and indigestion, mood alterations, mental confusion and vertigo have occurred; as with other angiotensin converting enzyme inhibitors, taste disturbance and sleep disturbance have been reported; bronchospasm, rhinitis, sinusitis, alopecia, urticaria, diapheresis, pruritus, psoriasis and severe skin disorders (including pemphigus, toxic epidermal necrolysis, Steven-Johnson Syndrome and erythema multiforme), have been reported; hyponatraemia, uraemia, oliguria/anuria, renal dysfunction, acute renal failure, pancreatitis; rarely, haemolytic anaemia has been reported.

Hydrochlorothiazide: anorexia, gastric irritation, constipation, jaundice (intrahepatic cholestatic jaundice), pancreatitis, sialoadenitis, vertigo, xanthopsia, leucopenia, agranulocytosis, thrombocytopenia, aplastic anemia, haemolytic anaemia, purpura, photosensitivity, urticaria, necrotizing angiitis (vasculitis) (cutaneaous vasculitis), fever, respiratory distress including pneumonitis and pulmonary oedema, anaphylactic reactions, hyperglycaemia, glycosuria, hyperuricemia, electrolyte imbalance including hyponatremia, muscle spasm, restlessness, transient blurred vision, renal failure, renal dysfunction and interstitial nephritis.

OVERDOSE:

Symptoms: No specific information is available on the treatment of overdosage with ZESTORETIC (lisinopril and hydrochlorothiazide). Treatment is symptomatic and supportive. Therapy with ZESTORETIC should be discontinued and the patient observed closely. Suggested measures include induction of emesis and/or gastric lavage, if ingestion is recent, and correction of dehydration, electrolyte imbalance and hypotension by established procedures.

Lisinopril: Overdose symptoms include severe hypotension, electrolyte disturbances and renal failure. Overdosed patients should be kept under very close observation. Therapeutic measures depend on the nature and severity of symptoms. Measures to prevent absorption and methods to speed elimination should be employed. If severe hypotension occurs, place the patient in the shock position and infuse intravenous normal saline immediately. Vasopressors including angiotensin II may be considered if fluid replacement is inadequate or contraindicated. Circulating lisinopril may be removed by hemodialysis. Avoid high-flux polyacrylonitrile dialysis membranes (see Precautions, Anaphylactoid Reactions During Membrane Exposure). Serum electrolytes and creatinine should be monitored frequently.

Hydrochlorothiazide: The most common signs and symptoms observed are those caused by electrolyte depletion (hypokalemia, hypochloremia, hyponatremia) and dehydration resulting from excessive diuresis. If digitalis has also been administered, hypokalemia may accentuate cardiac arrhythmias.

Treatment: See Symptoms.

> For management of a suspected drug overdose, contact your **regional Poison Control Centre**. See the *CPS* Directory section for a list of Poison Control Centres.

DOSAGE: Essential hypertension: Dosage must be individualized. The fixed combination is not for initial therapy. The dose of ZESTORETIC (lisinopril and hydrochlorothiazide) should be determined by the titration of the individual components. ZESTORETIC should be taken at the same time each day.

Once the patient has been successfully titrated with the individual components as described below, either one ZESTORETIC 10/12.5 mg or one or two 20/12.5 mg or 20/25 mg tablets once daily may be substituted if the titrated doses are the same as those in the fixed combination. (See Indications and Warnings.)

Patients usually do not require doses in excess of 50 mg of hydrochlorothiazide daily, particularly when combined with antihypertensive agents.

For lisinopril monotherapy the recommended initial dose in patients not on diuretics is 10 mg of lisinopril once a day. Dosage should be adjusted according to blood pressure response. The usual dosage range of lisinopril is 10 to 40 mg administered in a single daily dose. The antihypertensive effect may diminish toward the end of the dosing interval regardless of the administered dose, but most commonly with a dose of 10 mg daily. This can be evaluated by measuring blood pressure just prior to dosing to determine whether satisfactory control is being maintained for 24 hours. If it is not, an increase in dose should be considered. The maximum dose used in long-term controlled clinical trials was 80 mg/day.

If blood pressure is not controlled with lisinopril alone, a low dose of a diuretic may be added. Hydrochlorothiazide 12.5 mg has been shown to provide an additive effect. After the addition of a diuretic, it may be possible to reduce the dose of lisinopril.

Diuretic Treated Patients: In patients who are currently being treated with a diuretic, symptomatic hypotension occasionally may occur following the initial dose of lisinopril. The diuretic should if possible, be discontinued for two to three days before beginning therapy with lisinopril to reduce the likelihood of hypotension (see Warnings, Hypotension). The dosage of lisinopril should be adjusted according to blood pressure response.

If the patient's blood pressure is not controlled with lisinopril alone, diuretic therapy may be resumed as described above.

If the diuretic cannot be discontinued, an initial dose of 5 mg of lisinopril alone should be administered and the patient remain under medical supervision for at least two hours, and until blood pressure has stabilized for at least an additional hour (see Warnings, Hypotension, and Precautions, Drug Interactions).

Dosage Adjustment in Renal Impairment: In patients with creatinine clearance greater than 30 mL/min the usual dose titration of the individual components is required.

Anaphylactoid reactions have been reported in patients dialysed with high-flux membranes (e.g.: polyacrylonitrile [PAN] and during low density lipoproteins (LDL) apheresis with dextran sulphate and treated concomitantly with an ACE inhibitor. (See Precautions, Anaphylactoid Reactions during membrane exposure.)

For patients with creatinine clearance between 10 and 30 mL/min the starting dose of lisinopril is 2.5-5.0 mg/day. The dosage may then be titrated upward until blood pressure is controlled or to a maximum of 40 mg daily.

When concomitant diuretic therapy is required in patients with severe renal impairment (creatinine clearance <10 mL/min), a loop diuretic, rather than a thiazide diuretic is preferred for use with lisinopril. Therefore, for patients with severe renal dysfunction the lisinoprilhydrochlorothiazide combination tablet is not recommended.

SUPPLIED: 10/12.5: Each peach, round, biconvex tablet, with "Zt" over "10" intagliated on one side and blank on the other side, contains: lisinopril 10 mg and hydrochlorothiazide 12.5 mg. Nonmedicinal ingredients: calcium hydrogen phosphate dihydrate, corn starch, magnesium stearate, mannitol, pregelatinized starch, red iron oxide and yellow iron oxide. Bottles of 100. Calendar packs of 30. Store at controlled room temperature 15 to 30°C. Keep container tightly closed. Protect from light.

20/12.5: Each white, round, biconvex tablet, with "Zestoretic" intagliated on one side and blank on the other side, contains: lisinopril 20 mg and hydrochlorothiazide 12.5 mg. Nonmedicinal ingredients: calcium hydrogen phosphate dihydrate, corn starch, magnesium stearate, mannitol, pregelatinized starch. Bottles of 100. Calendar packs of 30. Store at controlled room temperature 15 to 30°C. Keep container tightly closed. Protect from light.

20/25: Each peach, round, biconvex tablet, with "Zestoretic" intagliated on one side and blank on the other side, contains: lisinopril 20 mg and hydrochlorothiazide 25 mg. Nonmedicinal ingredients: calcium hydrogen phosphate dihydrate, corn starch, magnesium stearate, mannitol, pregelatinized starch, red iron oxide and yellow iron oxide. Bottles of 100. Calendar packs of 30. Store at controlled room temperature 15 to 30°C. Keep container tightly closed. Protect from light.

(Shown in Product Identification Section)

> The reader is invited to consult CPhA's monograph **ACE Inhibitors**.

Zestril®

lisinopril

Angiotensin Converting Enzyme Inhibitor

AstraZeneca

Date of Revision: November 17, 2009

PHARMACOLOGY: ZESTRIL (lisinopril) is an ACE inhibitor which is used in the treatment of hypertension, congestive heart failure and following myocardial infarction in hemodynamically stable patients.

Angiotensin converting enzyme (ACE) is a peptidyl dipeptidase which catalyzes the conversion of angiotensin I to the pressor substance, angiotensin II. Inhibition of ACE results in decreased plasma angiotensin II, which leads to increased plasma renin activity (due to removal of negative feedback of renin release) and decreased aldosterone secretion. Although the latter decrease is small, it results in a small increase in serum K^+. In patients treated with ZESTRIL and a thiazide diuretic there was essentially no change in serum potassium (see Precautions).

ACE is identical to kininase II. Thus, ZESTRIL may also block the degradation of bradykinin, a potent vasodilator peptide. However, the role that this plays in the therapeutic effects of ZESTRIL is unknown.

While the mechanism through which ZESTRIL lowers blood pressure is believed to be primarily the suppression of the renin-angiotensin-aldosterone system, ZESTRIL also lowers blood pressure in patients with low-renin hypertension.

Administration of ZESTRIL to patients with hypertension results in a reduction of both supine and standing blood pressure. Abrupt withdrawal of ZESTRIL has not been associated with a rapid increase in blood pressure. In most patients studied, after oral administration of an individual dose of lisinopril, the onset of antihypertensive activity is seen at one hour with peak reduction of blood pressure achieved by 6 hours. Although an antihypertensive effect was observed 24 hours after dosing with recommended single daily doses, the effect was more consistent and the mean effect was considerably larger in some studies with doses of 20 mg or more than with lower doses. However, at all doses studied, the mean antihypertensive effect was substantially smaller 24 hours after dosing than it was 6 hours after dosing. On occasion, achievement of optimal blood pressure reduction may require 2 to 4 weeks of therapy.

In hemodynamic studies in patients with essential hypertension, blood pressure reduction was accompanied by a reduction in peripheral arterial resistance with little or no change in cardiac output and in heart rate. In a study in nine hypertensive patients, following administration of ZESTRIL, there was an increase in mean renal blood flow that was not significant. Data from several small studies are inconsistent with respect to the effect of ZESTRIL on glomerular filtration rate in hypertensive patients with normal renal function, but suggest that changes, if any, are not large.

When ZESTRIL is given together with thiazide-type diuretics, its blood pressure lowering effect is approximately additive.

Administration of ZESTRIL to patients with congestive heart failure reduces afterload and preload of the heart, resulting in an increase in cardiac output, without reflex tachycardia. Exercise tolerance is improved.

In the Assessment of Treatment with Lisinopril and Survival Study (ATLAS) higher doses of ZESTRIL up to 35 mg once daily reduced the risk of the combined outcome of mortality and hospitalization in patients with chronic congestive heart failure. The ATLAS study was an international, multicenter, double-blind, parallel group clinical trial which evaluated the effects of low doses, 2.5 mg-5.0 mg, versus high doses, 32.5 mg-35.0 mg ZESTRIL on mortality and morbidity in patients with chronic congestive heart failure. A total of 1596 patients were randomized into the low dose and 1568 into the high dose groups. Patients entered into the ATLAS study were NYHA Class II, III, or IV, were treated with diuretics for at least 60 days prior to entry into the study, and had a left ventricular ejection fraction (LVEF) ≤30%. Class II patients were eligible only if they were hospitalized or received emergency room treatment in the previous six months. Prior treatment with ACE inhibitors and digoxin was permitted, and patients were permitted routine therapies, other than ACE inhibitors, for the duration of the study. The median follow-up period was 46 months. The protocol excluded patients with recent cardiac surgery, unstable coronary artery disease, unstable ventricular arrhythmias, unstable CHF, or a non-CHF disorder that may have limited survival during the course of the trial. Overall, 77% of patients were NYHA class III; 89% had previous ACE inhibitor treatment. For the principal secondary endpoint, all-cause mortality and all-cause hospitalization, high dose ZESTRIL was associated with an 11.6% (p=0.002) risk reduction over low dose (2.5 and 5 mg). High dose ZESTRIL was also associated with an 8.4% risk reduction in all-cause mortality and cardiovascular hospitalizations (p=0.036). The total number of hospitalizations per patient for heart failure was reduced by 23.2% (p=0.002).

Pharmacokinetics: After oral administration of ZESTRIL (lisinopril), peak serum concentrations of lisinopril occur within approximately 7 hours, although patients with recent myocardial infarction have demonstrated an increase in time to peak serum concentration to about 8 to 10 hours. Declining serum concentrations exhibit a prolonged terminal phase which does not contribute to drug accumulation. This terminal phase probably represents saturable binding to ACE and is not proportional to dose. Lisinopril does not bind serum proteins other than ACE.

Lisinopril does not undergo metabolism and is excreted unchanged entirely in the urine. Based on urinary recovery, the extent of absorption of lisinopril is approximately 25%, with large inter-subject variability (6-60%) at all doses tested (5-80 mg).

Lisinopril absorption is not influenced by the presence of food in the gastrointestinal tract.

Following multiple doses of lisinopril, the effective half-life of accumulation is 12 hours.

In a study in elderly healthy subjects (65 years and above), a single dose of lisinopril 20 mg produced higher serum concentrations and higher values for the area under the plasma curve than those seen in young healthy adults given a similar dose. In another study, single daily doses of lisinopril 5 mg were given for 7 consecutive days to young and elderly healthy volunteers and to elderly patients with congestive heart failure. Maximum serum concentrations of lisinopril on Day 7 were higher in the elderly volunteers than in the young, and still higher in the elderly patients with congestive heart failure. Renal clearance of lisinopril was decreased in the elderly, particularly in the presence of congestive heart failure.

Impaired renal function decreases elimination of lisinopril. This decrease becomes clinically important when the glomerular filtration rate is below 30 mL/min (see Precautions, Impaired Renal Function, and Dosage).

Lisinopril can be removed by dialysis.

Studies in rats indicate that lisinopril crosses the blood-brain barrier poorly.

INDICATIONS: Hypertension: ZESTRIL (lisinopril) is indicated in the treatment of essential hypertension and in renovascular hypertension. It may be used alone or concomitantly with thiazide diuretics. A great majority of patients (>80%) with severe hypertension required combination therapy. ZESTRIL has been used concomitantly with beta-blockers and calcium antagonists, but the data on such use are limited.

ZESTRIL should normally be used in those patients in whom treatment with diuretic or beta blocker was found ineffective or has been associated with unacceptable adverse effects. ZESTRIL can also be tried as an initial agent in those patients in whom use of diuretics and/or beta blockers is contraindicated or in patients with medical conditions in which these drugs frequently cause serious adverse effects.

Heart Failure: ZESTRIL is indicated in the management of symptomatic congestive heart failure as adjunctive treatment with diuretics, and where appropriate, digitalis. Treatment with ZESTRIL should be initiated under close medical supervision, usually in a hospital.

High doses of ZESTRIL reduce the risk of the combined outcomes of mortality and hospitalization (see Pharmacology and Dosage).

Treatment Following Acute Myocardial Infarction: ZESTRIL is indicated in the treatment of hemodynamically stable patients as early as within 24 hours following acute myocardial infarction, to improve survival. Patients should receive, as appropriate, the standard recommended treatments such as thrombolytics, ASA and betablocker(s).

Therapy with ZESTRIL should be reassessed after 6 weeks. If there is no evidence of symptomatic or asymptomatic left ventricular dysfunction, treatment with ZESTRIL can be stopped.

ZESTRIL should not be used if systolic blood pressure is less than 100 mmHg, if clinically relevant renal failure is present, or if there is a history of bilateral stenosis of the renal arteries (see Precautions, Hypotension Following Acute Myocardial Infarction, Renal Impairment).

General: In using ZESTRIL, attention should be given to the risk of angioedema (see Warnings, Angioedema).

CONTRAINDICATIONS: ZESTRIL (lisinopril) is contraindicated in patients who:

- are hypersensitive to any component of this product;
- have a known allergy to angiotensin converting enzyme inhibitors;
- have a history of angioneurotic edema relating to previous treatment with an angiotensin-converting enzyme inhibitor;
- have hereditary or idiopathic angioneurotic edema.

WARNINGS:

> **Serious Warnings and Precautions**
> **When used in pregnancy, ACE inhibitors can cause injury or even death of the developing fetus. When pregnancy is detected, ZESTRIL should be discontinued as soon as possible (see Warnings, Pregnancy, and Information to Be Provided to the Patient).**

Angioedema: Angioedema has been uncommonly reported in patients treated with ZESTRIL (lisinopril) and may occur at any time during therapy. Angioedema associated with laryngeal or tongue oedema and/or shock may be fatal. If angioedema occurs, ZESTRIL should be promptly discontinued and the patient should be treated, and observed until the swelling subsides. Where swelling is confined only to the tongue, without respiratory distress, patients may require prolonged observation since treatment with antihistamines and corticosteroids may not be sufficient. However, where there is involvement of the tongue, glottis or larynx, likely to cause airway obstruction, and especially in cases where there has been a history of airway surgery, emergency therapy should be administered promptly when indicated. This includes giving subcutaneous adrenaline (0.5 mL 1:1000), and/or maintaining a patent airway. The patient should be under close medical supervision until complete and sustained symptom resolution has occurred.

The incidence of angioedema during ACE inhibitor therapy has been reported to be higher in black than in non-black patients.

Patients with a history of angioedema unrelated to ACE inhibitor therapy may be at increased risk of angioedema while receiving an ACE inhibitor (see Contraindications).

Hypotension: Symptomatic hypotension has occurred after administration of ZESTRIL, usually after the first or second dose or when the dose was increased. It is more likely to occur in patients who are volume depleted by diuretic therapy, dietary salt restriction, dialysis, diarrhea, vomiting, or possibly in patients with renin-dependant renovascular hypertension (see Dosage).

In patients with severe congestive heart failure, with or without associated renal insufficiency, excessive hypotension has been observed and may be associated with oliguria and/or progressive azotemia, and rarely with acute renal failure and/or death. Because blood pressure could potentially fall, patients at risk for hypotension should start therapy under very close medical supervision, usually in a hospital. Such patients should be followed closely for the first two weeks of treatment and whenever the dose of lisinopril and/or diuretic is increased. Similar considerations apply to patients with ischemic heart or cerebrovascular disease in whom an excessive fall in blood pressure could result in a myocardial infarction or cerebrovascular accident (see Adverse Effects).

If hypotension occurs, the patient should be placed in supine position and, if necessary, receive an intravenous infusion of normal saline. A transient hypotensive response may not be a contraindication to further doses. These can usually be given to hypertensive patients without difficulty once the blood pressure has increased after volume expansion. However, lower ZESTRIL doses and/or reduced concomitant diuretic therapy should be considered.

If hypotension occurs during treatment following acute myocardial infarction, consideration should be given to ZESTRIL discontinuation (see Adverse Effects and Dosage, Treatment Following Acute Myocardial Infarction).

In some patients with congestive heart failure who have normal or low blood pressure, additional lowering of systemic blood pressure may occur with ZESTRIL. If hypotension occurs, a reduction of dose or discontinuation of therapy should be considered.

Neutropenia/Agranulocytosis: Agranulocytosis and bone marrow depression have been caused by angiotensin converting enzyme inhibitors. Several cases of agranulocytosis and neutropenia have been reported in which a causal relationship to lisinopril cannot be excluded. Current experience with the drug shows the incidence to be rare. Periodic monitoring of white blood cell counts should be considered, especially in patients with collagen vascular disease and renal disease.

Pregnancy: ACE inhibitors can cause fetal and neonatal morbidity and mortality when administered to pregnant women. When pregnancy is detected, ZESTRIL should be discontinued as soon as possible.

The use of ACE inhibitors during the second and third trimesters of pregnancy has been associated with fetal and neonatal injury including hypotension, neonatal skull hypoplasia, anuria, reversible or irreversible renal failure, and death. Oligohydramnios has also been reported, presumably resulting from decreased fetal renal function, associated with fetal limb contractures, craniofacial deformation, and hypoplastic lung development.

Prematurity, and patent ductus arteriosus and other structural cardiac malformations, as well as neurologic malformations, have also been reported following exposure in the first trimester of pregnancy.

Infants with a history of in utero exposure to ACE inhibitors should be closely observed for hypotension, oliguria, and hyperkalemia. If oliguria occurs, attention should be directed towards support of blood pressure and renal perfusion. Exchange transfusion or dialysis may be required as a means of reversing hypotension and/or substituting for impaired renal function; however, limited experience with those procedures has not been associated with significant clinical benefit.

Lisinopril has been removed from the neonatal circulation by peritoneal dialysis.

Animal Data: Lisinopril was not teratogenic in mice treated on days 6-15 of gestation with up to 1000 mg/kg/day (625 times the maximum recommended human dose). There was an increase in fetal resorptions at doses down to 100 mg/kg; at doses of 1000 mg/kg, this was prevented by saline supplementation. There was no fetotoxicity or teratogenicity in rats treated with up to 300 mg/kg/day (188 times the maximum recommended dose) of lisinopril at days 6-17 of gestation. In rats receiving lisinopril from day 15 of gestation through day 21 postpartum, there was an increased incidence in pup deaths on days 2-7 postpartum and a lower average body weight of pups on day 21 postpartum. The increase in pup deaths and decrease in pup weight did not occur with maternal saline supplementation.

Lisinopril, at doses up to 1 mg/kg/day, was not teratogenic when given throughout the organogenic period in saline supplemented rabbits. Saline supplementation (physiologic saline in place of tap water) was used to eliminate maternotoxic effects and enable evaluation of the teratogenic potential at the highest possible dosage level. The rabbit has been shown to be extremely sensitive to angiotensin converting enzyme inhibitors (captopril and enalapril) with maternal and fetotoxic effects apparent at or below the recommended therapeutic dosage levels in man.

Fetotoxicity was demonstrated in rabbits by an increased incidence of fetal resorptions at an oral dose of lisinopril of 1 mg/kg/day and by an increased incidence of incomplete ossification at the lowest dose tested (0.1 mg/kg/day). A single intravenous dose of 15 mg/kg of lisinopril administered to pregnant rabbits on gestation days 16, 21 or 26 resulted in 88% to 100% fetal death.

By whole body autoradiography, radioactivity was found in the placenta following administration of labeled lisinopril to pregnant rats, but none was found in the fetuses.

Lactation: The presence of concentrations of ACE inhibitor has been reported in human milk. Use of ACE inhibitors is not recommended during breast-feeding.

Race: Angiotensin converting inhibitors cause a higher rate of angioedema in black patients than in non black patients.

The antihypertensive effect of angiotensin converting enzyme inhibitors is generally lower in black patients (usually a low-renin hypertensive population) than in non-black patients.

PRECAUTIONS: Renal Impairment: As a consequence of inhibiting the renin-angiotensin-aldosterone system, changes in renal function have been seen in susceptible individuals. In patients whose renal function may depend on the activity of the renin-angiotensin-aldosterone system, such as patients with bilateral renal artery stenosis, unilateral renal artery stenosis to a solitary kidney, or severe congestive heart failure, treatment with agents that inhibit this system has been associated with oliguria, progressive azotemia, and rarely, acute renal failure and/or death. In susceptible patients, concomitant diuretic use may further increase risk.

In acute myocardial infarction, treatment with lisinopril should not be initiated in patients with evidence of renal dysfunction, defined as serum creatinine concentration exceeding 177 µmol/L and/or proteinuria exceeding 500 mg/24 h. If renal dysfunction develops during treatment with ZESTRIL (serum creatinine concentration exceeding 265 µmol/L or a doubling from the pre-treatment value), then the physician should consider withdrawal of ZESTRIL.

Use of ZESTRIL (lisinopril) should include appropriate assessment of renal function.

Hypotension Following Acute Myocardial Infarction: Lisinopril treatment following acute myocardial infarction must not be initiated in patients at risk of further serious hemodynamic deterioration after vasodilator treatment.

These include patients with systolic blood pressure of 100 mmHg or lower or those in cardiogenic shock.

During the first 3 days following the infarction, dosage reduction should occur if systolic blood pressure is between 100 and 120 mmHg (see Dosage, Treatment Following Acute Myocardial Infarction).

Patients with myocardial infarction in the GISSI-3 study treated with ZESTRIL, had a higher (9.0% vs 3.7%) incidence of persistent hypotension (systolic blood pressure less than 90 mmHg for more than 1 hour) than placebo.

Diabetic Patients: In diabetic patients treated with oral antidiabetic agents or insulin, glycemic control should be closely monitored during the first month of treatment with ZESTRIL. (See Precautions, Drug Interactions.)

Anaphylactoid Reactions During Membrane Exposure: Anaphylactoid reactions have been reported in patients dialysed with high-flux membranes [e.g.: polyacrylonitrile (PAN) and during low-density lipoproteins (LDL) apheresis with dextran sulphate] and treated concomitantly with an ACE inhibitor. Dialysis should be stopped immediately if symptoms such as nausea, abdominal cramps, burning, angioedema, shortness of breath and severe hypotension occur. Symptoms are not relieved by antihistamines. In these patients consideration should be given to using a different type of dialysis membrane or a different class of antihypertensive agent.

Anaphylactoid Reactions During Desensitization: There have been isolated reports of patients experiencing sustained life threatening anaphylactoid reactions while receiving ACE inhibitors during desensitizing treatment with hymenoptera (bees, wasps) venom. In the same patients, these reactions have been avoided when ACE inhibitors were temporarily withheld for at least 24 hours, but they have reappeared upon inadvertent rechallenge.

Hyperkalemia: In clinical trials with daily doses of 2.5 to 20 mg, hyperkalemia (serum potassium >5.7 mEq/L) occurred in approximately 2.2% of hypertensive patients and 4.0% of patients with congestive heart failure. In most cases these were isolated values which resolved despite continued therapy. Hyperkalemia was a cause of discontinuation of therapy in approximately 0.1% of hypertensive patients.

As shown in the ATLAS trial (see Pharmacology), high dose (up to 35 mg) versus low dose (up to 5 mg) treatment may predispose CHF patients to hyperkalemia (6.4% versus 3.5%). This event was manageable and rarely led to treatment withdrawal. Therapy discontinuation rates due to hyperkalemia for high versus low dose were 0.4% versus 0.1%, respectively. Risk factors for the development of hyperkalemia may include renal insufficiency, diabetes mellitus, and the concomitant use of potassium-sparing diuretics, potassium supplements and/or potassium-containing salt substitutes (see Precautions, Drug Interactions).

Valvular Stenosis, Hypertrophic Cardiomyopathy: There is concern on theoretical grounds that patients with aortic stenosis or hypertrophic cardiomyopathy might be at particular risk of decreased coronary perfusion when treated with vasodilators.

ZESTRIL should be given with caution to these patients.

Surgery/Anesthesia: In patients undergoing major surgery or during anesthesia with agents that produce hypotension, lisinopril blocks angiotensin II formation, secondary to compensatory renin release. If hypotension occurs and is considered to be due to this mechanism, it can be corrected by volume expansion.

Patients with Impaired Liver Function: Hepatitis, either hepatocellular or cholestatic, jaundice, marked elevations of liver enzymes and/or serum bilirubin have occurred during therapy with ZESTRIL in patients with or without pre-existing liver abnormalities (see Adverse Effects). Very rarely, it has been reported that in some patients the undesirable development of hepatitis has progressed to hepatic failure. Patients receiving Zestril who develop jaundice or marketed elevation of hepatic enzymes should discontinue Zestril and receive appropriate medical follow-up (see Precautions, Patients with Impaired Liver Function). Should the patient receiving ZESTRIL experience any unexplained symptoms (see Information to Be Provided to the Patient), particularly during the first weeks or months of treatment, it is recommended that a full set of liver function tests and any other necessary investigation be carried out. Discontinuation of ZESTRIL should be considered when appropriate.

There are no adequate studies in patients with cirrhosis and/or liver dysfunction. ZESTRIL should be used with particular caution in patients with pre-existing liver abnormalities. In such patients baseline liver function tests should be obtained before administration of the drug and close monitoring of response and metabolic effects should apply.

Cough: A dry, persistent cough, which usually disappears only after withdrawal or lowering of the dose of ZESTRIL, has been reported.

Such a possibility should be considered as part of the differential diagnosis of the cough.

Children: Safety and effectiveness in children have not been established.

Occupation Hazards: Ability to drive and use machines: dizziness or tiredness may occur during treatment with ZESTRIL.

Drug Interactions: Hypotension: Patients on Diuretic Therapy: Patients on diuretics and especially those in whom diuretic therapy was recently instituted, may occasionally experience an excessive reduction of blood pressure after initiation of therapy with lisinopril. The possibility of symptomatic hypotension with lisinopril can be minimized by discontinuing the diuretic prior to initiation of treatment with lisinopril and/or lowering the initial dose of lisinopril (see Warnings, Hypotension and Dosage).

Hypotension: Patients on Antihypertensive Therapy: When lisinopril is given to patients already treated with other antihypertensive agents, further falls in blood pressure may also occur.

Potassium Supplements, potassium-sparing agents or potassium-containing salt substitutes: Since lisinopril decreases aldosterone production, elevation of serum potassium may occur. Potassium sparing diuretics such as spironolactone, triamterene or amiloride, or potassium supplements should be given only for documented hypokalemia and with caution and with frequent monitoring of serum potassium since they may lead to a significant increase in serum potassium. Potassium-containing salt substitutes should also be used with caution.

Agents Causing Renin Release: The antihypertensive effect of ZESTRIL is augmented by antihypertensive agents that cause renin release (e.g. diuretics).

Agents Affecting Sympathetic Activity: Agents affecting sympathetic activity (e.g., ganglionic blocking agents or adrenergic neuron blocking agents) may be used with caution. Beta-adrenergic blocking drugs add some further antihypertensive effect to lisinopril.

NSAIDS: In some patients with compromised renal function, lisinopril co-administration with nonsteroidal anti-inflammatory drugs (NSAIDs) may produce further renal function deterioration.

Indomethacin may diminish the antihypertensive efficacy of concomitantly administered ZESTRIL.

Lithium Salts: As with other drugs which eliminate sodium, lithium elimination may be reduced. Therefore, the serum lithium levels should be monitored carefully if lithium salts are to be administered.

Gold: Nitritoid reactions (symptoms of vasodilatation including flushing, nausea, dizziness and hypotension, which can be very severe) following injectable gold (for example, sodium aurothiomalate) have been reported more frequently in patients receiving ACE inhibitor therapy.

Antidiabetics: Epidemiological studies have suggested that concomitant administration of ACE inhibitors and antidiabetic medicines (insulins, oral hypoglycaemic agents) may cause an increased blood glucose lowering effect with risk of hypoglycemia. This phenomenon appeared to be more likely to occur during the first weeks of combined treatment and in patients with renal impairment.

Information to Be Provided to the Patient:

Serious Warning and Precautions
ZESTRIL should not be used during pregnancy. Patients should be advised to stop the medication and contact their physician as soon as possible if they discover that they are pregnant while taking ZESTRIL.

Angioedema: Angioedema, including laryngeal edema and, may occur especially following the first dose of lisinopril. Patients should be so advised and told to report immediately any signs or symptoms suggesting angioedema (swelling of face, extremities, eyes, lips, tongue, difficulty in breathing) and to take no more drug until they have consulted with the prescribing physician.

Hypotension: Patients should be cautioned to report light headedness especially during the first few days of therapy. If actual syncope occurs, the patients should be told to discontinue the drug until they have consulted with the prescribing physician.

All patients should be cautioned that excessive perspiration and dehydration may lead to an excessive fall in blood pressure because of reduction in fluid volume. Other causes of volume depletion such as vomiting or diarrhea may also lead to a fall in blood pressure; patients should be advised to consult with their physician.

Neutropenia: Patients should be told to report promptly any indication of infection (e.g., sore throat, fever) which may be a sign of neutropenia.

Impaired Liver Function: Patients should be advised to return to the physician if he/she experiences any symptoms possibly related to liver dysfunction. This would include "viral-like symptoms" in the first weeks to months of therapy (such as fever, malaise, muscle pain, rash or adenopathy which are possible indicators of hypersensitivity reactions), or if abdominal pain, nausea or vomiting, loss of appetite, jaundice, itching or any other unexplained symptoms occur during therapy.

Hyperkalemia: Patients should be told not to use salt substitutes containing potassium without consulting their physician.

You are pregnant, breast-feeding or thinking of becoming pregnant? Taking ZESTRIL during pregnancy can cause injury and even death to your baby. This medicine should not be used during pregnancy. If you become pregnant while taking ZESTRIL, stop the medication and report to your doctor as soon as possible. It is possible that ZESTRIL passes into breast milk. You should not breast-feed while taking ZESTRIL.

Note: As with many other drugs, certain advice to patients being treated with ZESTRIL is warranted. This information is intended to aid in the safe and effective use of this medication. It is not a disclosure of all possible adverse or intended effects.

ADVERSE EFFECTS: In controlled clinical trials involving 3269 patients, 2633 patients with hypertension and 636 patients with congestive heart failure, excluding the ATLAS CHF study patients (see Pharmacology), the most frequent clinical adverse reactions were: dizziness (4.4%), headache (5.6%), asthenia/fatigue (2.7%), diarrhea (1.8%) and cough (3.0%), all of which were more frequent than in placebo-treated patients. Discontinuation of therapy was required in 5.9% of patients.

For adverse reactions which occurred in hypertensive patients and patients with congestive heart failure treated with ZESTRIL (lisinopril) in controlled clinical trials, comparative incidence data are listed in Table 1.

Adverse Events in Controlled Clinical Trials:

Table 1: ZESTRIL

Incidence of Adverse Reactions Occurring in Patients Treated with ZESTRIL in Controlled Clinical Trials

	Hypertension n=2633 (%)	Congestive Heart Failure n=636 (%)
Cardiovascular		
Hypotension	0.8	5.2
Orthostatic Effects	0.9	1.3
Chest Pain	1.1	7.4
Angina	0.3	3.8
Edema	0.6	2.5
Palpitation	0.8	1.9
Rhythm Disturbances	0.5	0.6

(cont'd)

Table 1: ZESTRIL *(cont'd)*

Incidence of Adverse Reactions Occurring in Patients Treated with ZESTRIL in Controlled Clinical Trials

	Hypertension n=2633 (%)	Congestive Heart Failure n=636 (%)
Gastrointestinal		
Diarrhea	1.8	6.1
Nausea	1.9	4.9
Vomiting	1.1	2.4
Dyspepsia	0.5	1.9
Anorexia	0.4	1.4
Constipation	0.2	0.8
Flatulence	0.3	0.5
Nervous System		
Dizziness	4.4	14.2
Headache	5.6	4.6
Paresthesia	0.5	2.8
Depression	0.7	1.1
Somnolence	0.8	0.6
Insomnia	0.3	2.4
Vertigo	0.2	0.2
Respiratory		
Cough	3.0	6.4
Dyspnea	0.4	7.4
Orthopnea	0.1	0.9
Dermatologic		
Rash	1.0	5.0
Pruritus	0.5	1.4
Musculoskeletal		
Muscle Cramps	0.5	2.2
Back Pain	0.5	1.7
Leg Pain	0.1	1.3
Shoulder Pain	0.2	0.8
Other		
Asthenia/Fatigue	2.7	7.1
Blurred Vision	0.3	1.1
Fever	0.3	1.1
Flushing	0.3	0.3
Gout	0.2	1.7
Decreased Libido	0.2	0.2
Malaise	0.3	1.1

Angioedema: Angioedema has been reported in patients receiving ZESTRIL (0.1%). In very rare cases, intestinal angioedema has been reported (see Warnings, Angioedema).

Hypotension: In hypertensive patients, hypotension occurred in 0.8% and syncope occurred in 0.2% of patients. Hypotension or syncope was a cause for discontinuation of therapy in 0.3% of hypertensive patients (see Warnings, Hypotension).

In patients with congestive heart failure, hypotension occurred in 5.2% and syncope occurred in 1.7% of patients. Hypotension and dizziness were causes for discontinuation of therapy in 1.7% of these patients.

As shown in the ATLAS trial (see Pharmacology), high dose (up to 35 mg) versus low dose (up to 5 mg) treatment may predispose patients to hypotension-related symptoms such as: dizziness (18.9% versus 12.1%), syncope (7.0% versus 5.1%), and hypotension (10.8% versus 6.7%). These events were manageable and rarely led to treatment withdrawal. Therapy discontinuation rates for high versus low dose were: dizziness 0.3 and 0%, hypotension 0.8% and 0.6%, and for syncope 0.3% and 0.3%, respectively.

Treatment Following Acute Myocardial Infarction: In a controlled, open trial, involving 19,394 acute myocardial infarction patients (GISSI-3; see Indications, Treatment Following Acute Myocardial Infarction), comparing lisinopril alone, transdermal glycerol trinitrate, lisinopril and transdermal glycerol trinitrate, or control (no treatment), the most frequent in-hospital adverse events were as follows: see Table 2.

Laboratory Test Findings: Serum Electrolytes: Hyperkalemia (see Precautions, Hyperkalemia).

Creatinine, Blood Urea Nitrogen: Increases in blood urea nitrogen and serum creatinine, usually reversible upon discontinuation of therapy, were observed in 1.1 and 1.6% of patients respectively with essential hypertension treated with ZESTRIL alone. Increases were more common in patients receiving concomitant diuretics and in patients with renal artery stenosis (see Precautions, Renal Impairment). In patients with congestive heart failure on 2.5 to 20 mg lisinopril and concomitant diuretic therapy, reversible increases in blood urea nitrogen (14.5%) and serum creatinine (11.2%) were observed in approximately 12.0% of patients. Frequently, these abnormalities resolved when the dosage of the diuretic was decreased.

As shown in the ATLAS trial (see Pharmacology), high dose (up to 35 mg) versus low dose (up to 5 mg) treatment may predispose patients to increased serum creatinine (9.9% versus 7.0%). This event was manageable and rarely led to treatment withdrawal. Therapy discontinuation rates due to increased serum creatinine for high versus low dose were 0.3% versus 0.4%, respectively.

Table 2: ZESTRIL

Adverse Events—Treatment Following Acute Myocardial Infarction

Event	Control n=4729	Lisinopril n=4713	Lisinopril + GTN n=4722	GTN Alone n=4731
Persistent Hypertension	3.6	8.8	9.3	3.9
Shock	2.5	2.8	2.2	1.9
Renal Dysfunction	1.1	2.4	2.4	1.1
Stroke	0.6	0.6	0.9	0.8
Re-infarction	2.2	2.2	2.2	1.9
Hemorrhagic Events	1.2	1.3	1.1	0.9
Post-infarction Angina	13.2	13.9	12.3	11.8
Ventricular Fibrillation	3.1	2.5	2.4	2.2
Sustained Ventricular Tachycardia	2.5	2.1	1.8	2.3
Atrial Flutter or Fibrillation	6.4	6.3	5.3	5.7
Complete Atrioventricular Block	2.4	2.9	2.5	2.1
Asystole	1.2	1.2	1.3	1.2
Intraventricular Septal Rupture	0.3	0.4	0.2	0.2
Papillary Muscle Rupture	0.3	0.4	0.5	0.4
Late CHF (>4 days)	4.5	4.5	4.2	4.2

Hematology: Decreases in hemoglobin and hematocrit (mean decreases of approximately 0.9 g % and 0.6 vol %, respectively) occurred frequently in patients treated with ZESTRIL but were rarely of clinical importance in patients without some other cause of anemia. Rarely, hemolytic anemia has been reported.

Agranulocytosis and bone marrow depression, manifested as anemia, cytopenia or leukopenia, have been caused by angiotensin converting enzyme inhibitors, including lisinopril. Several cases of agranulocytosis and neutropenia have been reported in which a causal relationship to lisinopril cannot be excluded (see Warnings, Neutropenia/Agranulocytosis).

Hepatic: Elevations of liver enzymes and/or serum bilirubin have occurred (see Precautions, Patients with Impaired Liver Function).

Discontinuations: Overall, 1.0% of patients discontinued therapy due to laboratory adverse experiences, principally elevations in blood urea nitrogen (0.8%), serum creatinine (0.1%) and serum potassium (0.1%).

Post-Marketing Experience: The following undesirable effects have been observed and reported during treatment with ZESTRIL with the following frequencies: Very common (≥10%), common (≥1%, <10%), uncommon (≥0.1%, <1%), rare (≥0.01%, <0.1%), very rare (<0.01%) including isolated reports.

Blood and Lymphatic System Disorders: Very rare: bone marrow depression, anemia thrombocytopenia, leucopenia, agranulocytosis, hemolytic anemia (see Warnings, Neutropenia/Agranulocytosis).

Endocrine Disorders: Rare: inappropriate antidiuretic hormone secretion.

Metabolism and Nutrition Disorders: Uncommon: hyperkalemia (see Precautions, Hyperkalemia). Rare: hyponatremia. Very rare: hypoglycemia (see Precautions, Diabetic Patients).

Nervous System and Psychiatric Disorders: Common: dizziness, headache. Uncommon: mood alterations (including depressive symptoms), paraesthesia, vertigo, taste disturbance, sleep disturbances. Rare: mental confusions, olfactory disturbance.

Cardiac and Vascular Disorders: Common: orthostatic effects (including hypotension) (see Warnings, Hypotension), syncope (frequency refers to congestive heart failure patient population, frequency in hypertensive patient population is "uncommon"). Uncommon: myocardial infarction or cerebrovascular accident (both possibly secondary to excessive hypotension in high risk patients, see Precautions, Hypotension Following Acute Myocardial Infarction), palpitations, tachycardia.

Respiratory Thoracic and Mediastinal Disorders: Common: cough. Uncommon: rhinitis. Very rare: bronchospasm, sinusitis.

Gastrointestinal Disorders: Common: diarrhea, vomiting. Uncommon: nausea, abdominal pain and indigestion. Rare: dry mouth. Very rare: pancreatitis, intestinal angioedema (see Warnings, Angioedema and Adverse Effects, Angioedema).

Hepato-biliary Disorders: Very rare: hepatitis—either hepatocellular or cholestatic, jaundice, hepatic failure. Very rarely it has been reported that in some patients the undesirable development of hepatitis has progressed to hepatic failure. Patients receiving Zestril who develop jaundice or marketed elevation of hepatic enzymes should discontinue Zestril and receive appropriate medical follow-up (see Precautions, Patients with Impaired Liver Function).

Skin and Subcutaneous Tissue Disorders: Uncommon: rash, pruritus, hypersensitivity/angioneurotic edema: angioneurotic edema of the face, extremities, lips, tongue, glottis, and/or larynx (see Warnings, Angioedema). Rare: urticaria, alopecia, psoriasis. Very rare: diaphoresis, pemphigus, toxic epidermal necrolysis, Steven-Johnson Syndrome, erythema multiforme, cutaneous pseudolymphoma.

A symptom complex has been reported which may include one or more of the following: fever, vasculitis, myalgia, arthralgia/arthritis, a positive antinuclear antibodies (ANA), elevated red blood cell sedimentation rate (ESR), oesinophilia and leukocytosis. Rash, photosensitivity or other dermatological manifestations may occur.

Renal and Urinary Disorders: Common: renal dysfunction. Rare: uremia, acute renal failure. Very rare: oliguria/anuria (see Precautions, Renal Impairment).

Reproductive System and Breast Disorders: Uncommon: impotence.

General Disorders and Administration Site Conditions: Uncommon: fatigue, asthenia.

Investigations: Uncommon: increases in blood urea, increases in serum creatinine (see Precautions, Renal Impairment), increases in liver enzymes (see Precautions, Patients with Impaired Liver Function). Rare: decreases in hemoglobin, decreases in hematocrit, increases in serum bilirubin (see Precautions, Patients with Impaired Liver Function).

OVERDOSE:

Symptoms: Overdose symptoms include severe hypotension, electrolyte disturbances, and renal failure.

Treatment: Overdosed patients should be kept under very close observation. Therapeutic measures depend on the nature and severity of symptoms. Measures to prevent absorption and methods to speed elimination should be employed. If severe hypotension occurs, place the patient in the shock position and infuse intravenous normal saline immediately. Vasopressors including angiotensin II may be considered if fluid replacement is inadequate or contraindicated. Circulating lisinopril may be removed by hemodialysis. Avoid high-flux polyacrylonitrile dialysis membranes (see Precautions, Anaphylactoid Reactions during membrane exposure). Serum electrolytes and creatinine should be monitored frequently.

For management of a suspected drug overdose, contact your **regional Poison Control Centre**. See the *CPS* Directory section for a list of Poison Control Centres.

DOSAGE: Since absorption of ZESTRIL tablets (lisinopril) is not affected by food, the tablets may be administered before, during or after meals. ZESTRIL should be administered in a single daily dose. ZESTRIL should be taken at the same time each day.

Dosage must be individualized and should be adjusted according to blood pressure response.

Essential Hypertension: In patients with essential hypertension, not on diuretic therapy, the usual recommended starting dose is 10 mg once a day. The usual dosage range is 10 to 40 mg per day, administered in a single daily dose. The antihypertensive effect may diminish toward the end of the dosing interval regardless of the administered dose, but most commonly with a dose of 10 mg daily. This can be evaluated by measuring blood pressure just prior to dosing to determine whether satisfactory control is being maintained for 24 hours. If it is not, an increase in dose should be considered. The maximum dose used in long-term controlled clinical trials was 80 mg/day. If blood pressure is not controlled with ZESTRIL alone, a low dose of diuretic may be added. Hydrochlorothiazide 12.5 mg has been shown to provide an additive effect. After the addition of diuretic, it may be possible to reduce the dose of ZESTRIL.

Diuretic Treated Patients: In hypertensive patients who are currently being treated with a diuretic, symptomatic hypotension may occur occasionally following the initial dose of ZESTRIL. The diuretic should be discontinued, if possible, for two to three days before beginning therapy with ZESTRIL to reduce the likelihood of hypotension (see Warnings). The dosage of ZESTRIL should be adjusted according to blood pressure response. If the patient's blood pressure is not controlled with ZESTRIL alone, diuretic therapy may be resumed as described above.

If the diuretic cannot be discontinued, an initial dose of 5 mg should be used under medical supervision for at least two hours and until blood pressure has stabilized for at least an additional hour (see Warnings, Hypotension and Precautions, Drug Interactions).

A lower starting dose is required in the presence of renal impairment, in patients in whom diuretic therapy cannot be discontinued, patients who are volume and/or salt-depleted for any reason, and in patients with renovascular hypertension.

Dosage Adjustment in Renal Impairment: Dosage in patients with renal impairment should be based on creatinine clearance as outlined in Table 3.

Table 3: ZESTRIL

Dosage Adjustment in Renal Impairment

Creatinine Clearance		Starting Dose mg/day
mL/s	**(mL/min)**	
0.5–1.17	31–70	5–10
0.17–0.5	10–30	2.5–5
<0.17 (including patients on dialysis)	<10 (including patients on dialysis)	2.5[a]

[a] Dosage and/or frequency of administration should be adjusted depending on the blood pressure response.

The dosage may be titrated upward until blood pressure is controlled or to a maximum of 40 mg daily.

Anaphylactoid reactions have been reported in patients dialysed with high-flux membranes (e.g.:polyacrylonitrile [PAN]and during low-density lipoproteins (LDL) apheresis with dextran suphate) and treated concomitantly with an ACE inhibitor (see Precautions, Anaphylactoid Reactions during membrane exposure).

Geriatrics: In general, blood pressure response and adverse experiences were similar in younger and older patients given similar doses of ZESTRIL. Pharmacokinetic studies, however, indicate that maximum blood levels and area under the plasma concentration time curve (AUC) are doubled in older patients so that dosage adjustments should be made with particular caution.

Renovascular Hypertension: Some patients with renovascular hypertension, especially those with bilateral renal artery stenosis or stenosis of the artery to a solitary kidney, may develop an exaggerated response to the first dose of ZESTRIL. In these patients, treatment should be started at low doses (2.5 or 5 mg), under close medical supervision. Thereafter, the dosage may be adjusted according to the blood pressure response. Doses should be carefully titrated.

Congestive Heart Failure: ZESTRIL is to be used in conjunction with diuretics, and where appropriate digitalis. Therapy must be initiated under close medical supervision, usually in a hospital. Blood pressure and renal function should be monitored, both before and during treatment with ZESTRIL, because severe hypotension and, more rarely, consequent renal failure have been reported (see Warnings, Hypotension and Precautions, Renal Impairment).

Initiation of therapy requires consideration of recent diuretic therapy and the possibility of severe salt/volume depletion. If possible, the dose of diuretic should be reduced before beginning treatment.

The recommended initial dose is 2.5 mg per day. The ZESTRIL dose should be increased: by increments of no greater than 10 mg; at intervals of no less than 2 weeks, up to a maximum of 35 mg once daily. Dose adjustment should be based on the individual patient's tolerance and clinical response.

Treatment Following Acute Myocardial Infarction: Treatment with ZESTRIL may be started as early as within 24 hours following the onset of symptoms in hemodynamically stable patients. Patients should receive, as appropriate, the standard recommended treatments such as thrombolytics, ASA and beta-blocker(s) (see Indications, Treatment Following Acute Myocardial Infarction).

The first dose of ZESTRIL is 5 mg given orally, followed by 5 mg after 24 hours, 10 mg after 48 hours and then 10 mg once daily thereafter.

Patients with a low systolic blood pressure (between 100 and 120 mmHg) when treatment is started or during the first 3 days after the infarct should be given a lower dose—2.5 mg orally. Treatment with ZESTRIL must not be initiated in patients who are at risk of serious hemodynamic deterioration (see Precautions, Hypotension Following Acute Myocardial Infarction). After three days, if hypotension occurs (systolic blood pressure less than or equal to 100 mmHg), a daily maintenance dose of 5 mg may be given with temporary reductions to 2.5 mg if needed. If prolonged hypotension occurs (systolic blood pressure less than 90 mmHg for more than 1 hour), ZESTRIL should be withdrawn.

Renal function should be assessed before and during therapy with ZESTRIL (see Precautions, Renal Impairment).

Dosing should normally continue for six weeks. At that time, patients with signs or symptoms of heart failure should continue with ZESTRIL (see Dosage, Congestive Heart Failure).

ZESTRIL is compatible with intravenous or transdermal glyceryl trinitrate.

SUPPLIED: 5 mg: Each pink, round, biconvex uncoated tablet, embossed with the number "5" within a heart-shaped symbol on one side and scored on the reverse side, contains: lisinopril 5 mg. Nonmedicinal ingredients: calcium hydrogen phosphate dihydrate, cornstarch, magnesium stearate, mannitol, pregelatinized cornstarch and red iron oxide. Bottles of 100 and calendar packs of 30. Store between 15 and 30°C.

10 mg: Each pink, round, biconvex, uncoated tablet, embossed with the number "10" within a heart-shaped symbol on one side and blank on the reverse side, contains: lisinopril 10 mg. Nonmedicinal ingredients: calcium hydrogen phosphate dihydrate, cornstarch, magnesium stearate, mannitol, pregelatinized cornstarch and red iron oxide. Bottles of 100 and calendar packs of 30. Store between 15 and 30°C.

20 mg: Each pink, round, biconvex, uncoated tablet, embossed with the number "20" within a heart-shaped symbol on one side and blank on the reverse side, contains: lisinopril 20 mg. Nonmedicinal ingredients: calcium hydrogen phosphate dihydrate, cornstarch, magnesium stearate, mannitol, pregelatinized cornstarch and red iron oxide. Bottles of 100 and calendar packs of 30. Store between 15 and 30°C.

(Shown in Product Identification Section)

Zevalin®

ibritumomab tiuxetan

Therapeutic Radiopharmaceutical

Bayer

Date of Revision: December 23, 2009

SUMMARY PRODUCT INFORMATION:

Route of Administration	Dosage Form/ Strength	Clinically Relevant Nonmedicinal Ingredients
Intravenous	Kit for the preparation of ^{90}Y-ibritumomab tiuxetan/3.2 mg ibritumomab tiuxetan in 2 mL 0.9% sodium chloride solution (1.6 mg/mL)	Human serum albumin For a complete listing see Dosage Forms, Composition and Packaging.

DESCRIPTION: The ZEVALIN (ibritumomab tiuxetan) kit provides the non-radioactive components for the radiolabeling of ibritumomab tiuxetan with yttrium-90 (^{90}Y). Each ZEVALIN kit contains the following components: one ZEVALIN vial containing 3.2 mg of ibritumomab tiuxetan (murine IgG_1 monoclonal antibody produced in a Chinese Hamster Ovary (CHO) cell line by recombinant DNA technology and conjugated to the chelating agent MX-DTPA) in 2 mL of 0.9% sodium chloride solution; one 50 mM sodium acetate vial; one formulation buffer vial; one empty reaction vial and four identification labels.

Physical Characteristics: Yttrium-90 decays by emission of beta particles, with a physical half life of 64.1 hours (2.67 days). The product of radioactive decay is non-radioactive zirconium-90. The range of beta particles in soft tissue ($_{\chi 90}$) is 5 mm. Radiation emission data for ^{90}Y are summarized in Table 1.

Table 1: ZEVALIN

Principal ^{90}Y Radiation Emission Data

Radiation	Mean % per Disintegration	Mean Energy (keV)
Beta minus	100	750–935

External Radiation: The exposure rate for 37 MBq (1 mCi) of ^{90}Y is 8.3×10^{-3} Ci/kg/h (32 R/h) at the mouth of an open ^{90}Y vial. Adequate shielding should be used with this beta emitter, in accordance with institutional good radiation safety practices.

To allow correction for physical decay of ^{90}Y, the fractions that remain at selected intervals before and after the time of calibration are shown in Table 2.

Table 2: ZEVALIN

Physical Decay Chart: ^{90}Y Half-life 2.67 Days (64.1 hours)

Calibration Time (h)	Fraction Remaining	Calibration Time (h)	Fraction Remaining
−36	1.48	0	1.00
−24	1.30	1	0.99
−12	1.14	2	0.98
−8	1.09	3	0.97
−7	1.08	4	0.96
−6	1.07	5	0.95
−5	1.06	6	0.94
−4	1.04	7	0.93
−3	1.03	8	0.92
−2	1.02	12	0.88
−1	1.01	24	0.77
0	1.00	36	0.68

INDICATIONS AND CLINICAL USE: ZEVALIN (ibritumomab tiuxetan), as part of the ZEVALIN therapeutic regimen, is indicated for the treatment of patients with relapsed or refractory low-grade or follicular, CD20 positive, B-cell non-Hodgkin's lymphoma, including patients with rituximab-refractory follicular non-Hodgkin's lymphoma.

CONTRAINDICATIONS: ZEVALIN (ibritumomab tiuxetan) is contraindicated in patients with known type I hypersensitivity or anaphylactic reactions to murine proteins or to any component of the ZEVALIN therapeutic regimen, including yttrium chloride and rituximab. ZEVALIN is also contraindicated in pregnant or nursing women (see Warnings and Precautions, Special Populations).

WARNINGS AND PRECAUTIONS:

Serious Warnings and Precautions

^{90}Y-ZEVALIN (ibritumomab tiuxetan) is a radiopharmaceutical and should be used only by physicians and other professionals qualified by training and experienced in the safe use and handling of radionuclides (see Dosage and Administration, Instructions for Preparation and Use).

Fatal Infusion Reactions with Rituximab: Deaths have occurred within 24 hours of rituximab infusion, an essential component of the ZEVALIN therapeutic regimen. Approximately 80% of fatal infusion reactions occurred in association with the first rituximab infusion. These fatalities were associated with an infusion reaction symptom complex that included hypoxia, pulmonary infiltrates, acute respiratory distress syndrome, myocardial infarction, ventricular fibrillation or cardiogenic shock. Patients who develop severe infusion reactions should have rituximab and ^{90}Y-ZEVALIN infusions discontinued and receive medical treatment (see Warnings and Precautions, Sensitivity/Resistance and Adverse Reactions).

Prolonged and Severe Cytopenias: ^{90}Y-ZEVALIN administration can result in severe and prolonged cytopenias, especially when administered after prior radiation or multiple chemotherapies. The risk of hematological toxicity may be increased when ZEVALIN is administered shortly (<4 months) after prior therapy with fludarabine-containing regimens (see Drug Interactions). The ZEVALIN therapeutic regimen should not be administered to patients with ≥25% lymphoma marrow involvement and/or impaired bone marrow reserve (see Warnings and Precautions, Hematologic and Adverse Reactions).

Severe Mucocutaneous Reactions: Severe mucocutaneous reactions, some with fatal outcome, have been reported in association with the ZEVALIN therapeutic regimen, which includes rituximab and ^{90}Y-ZEVALIN. Patients who develop a severe mucocutaneous reaction should have rituximab and ^{90}Y-ZEVALIN infusions discontinued and receive medical treatment (see Warnings and Precautions, Skin and Adverse Reactions).

Dosing: The prescribed, measured and administered dose of ^{90}Y-ZEVALIN should not exceed the absolute maximum allowable dose of 32.0 mCi (1200 MBq) (see Dosage and Administration).

General: ^{90}Y-ZEVALIN should be administered under the supervision of a health professional who is experienced in the use of radiopharmaceuticals (for radiopharmaceutical precautions see Dosage and Administration, Instructions for Preparation and Use). Appropriate management of therapy and complications is only possible when adequate diagnostic and treatment facilities are readily available.

ZEVALIN may be received, used and administered only by authorized persons in designated clinical settings. Its receipt, storage, use, transfer and disposal are subject to the regulations and/or appropriate licences of local competent official organizations.

As in the use of any other radioactive material, care should be taken to minimize radiation exposure to patients consistent with proper patient management, and to minimize radiation exposure to occupational workers.

Because the ZEVALIN therapeutic regimen includes the use of rituximab (see Dosage and Administration), please also consult the prescribing information for RITUXAN (rituximab) and follow instructions carefully.

The ZEVALIN therapeutic regimen is intended as a single course treatment. The safety and toxicity profile from multiple courses of the ZEVALIN therapeutic regimen or of other forms of therapeutic irradiation preceding, following or in combination with the ZEVALIN therapeutic regimen have not been established.

^{90}Y-ZEVALIN solution must not be administered to patients who are likely to develop life-threatening hematological toxicity signs.

Carcinogenesis and Mutagenesis: Out of 349 patients treated with the ZEVALIN therapeutic regimen, three cases of acute myelogenous leukemia and two cases of myelodysplastic syndrome have been reported following the ZEVALIN therapeutic regimen (see Adverse Reactions).

No long-term animal studies have been performed to establish the carcinogenic or mutagenic potential of the ZEVALIN therapeutic regimen. However, radiation is a potential carcinogen or mutagen.

Contamination: The contents of the ZEVALIN kit are not radioactive. However, during and after radiolabeling of ZEVALIN with ^{90}Y, care should be taken to minimize radiation exposure to patients and to medical personnel, consistent with institutional good radiation safety practices and patient management procedures.

General Disorders and Administration Site Conditions: Close monitoring for evidence of extravasation during the injection of ZEVALIN is required in order to avoid radiation-associated tissue damage. If any signs or symptoms of extravasation have occurred, the infusion should be immediately terminated and restarted in another vein. If possible extravasation is suspected, the physician should be informed.

Hematologic: The most common severe adverse events reported with the ZEVALIN therapeutic regimen were thrombocytopenia (61% of patients with platelet counts <50 000 cells/mm^3) and neutropenia (57% of patients with absolute neutrophil count [ANC] <1000 cells/mm^3) in patients with ≥150 000 platelets/mm^3 prior to treatment. Both incidences of severe thrombocytopenia and neutropenia increased to 78% and 74% for patients with mild thrombocytopenia at baseline (platelet count of 100 000 to 149 000 cells/mm^3). For all patients, the median time to nadir was seven to nine weeks and the median duration of cytopenias was 22-35 days. In <5% of cases, patients experienced severe cytopenia that extended beyond the prospectively defined protocol treatment period of 12 weeks following administration of the ZEVALIN therapeutic regimen. Some of these patients eventually recovered from cytopenia, while others experienced progressive disease, received further anti-cancer therapy or died of their lymphoma without having recovered from cytopenia. The cytopenias may have influenced subsequent treatment decisions (see Adverse Reactions).

Hemorrhage, including fatal cerebral hemorrhage, and severe infections, some with fatal outcome, have occurred in a minority of patients in clinical studies and in post-marketing experience. Careful monitoring for and management of cytopenias and their complications (eg, febrile neutropenia, hemorrhage) for up to three months after use of the ZEVALIN therapeutic regimen are necessary. Caution should be exercised in treating patients with drugs that interfere with platelet function or coagulation (eg, ASA, NSAIDs and COX-2 inhibitors) following the ZEVALIN therapeutic regimen, and patients receiving such agents should be closely monitored.

The ZEVALIN therapeutic regimen should not be administered to patients with ≥25% lymphoma marrow involvement and/or impaired bone marrow reserve, eg, due to prior myeloablative therapies; platelet count <100 000 cells/mm^3; neutrophil count <1500 cells/mm^3; hypocellular bone marrow (≤15% cellularity or marked reduction in bone marrow precursors) or to patients with a history of failed stem cell collection as safety and efficacy have not been established.

The risk of hematological toxicity may be increased after prior therapy with fludarabine-containing regimens (for details see Drug Interactions, Drug-Drug Interactions).

Special caution is required with respect to bone marrow depletion. In most patients administration of ZEVALIN (after pretreatment with rituximab) results in severe and prolonged cytopenia which is generally reversible (see Adverse Reactions, Abnormal Hematologic and Clinical Chemistry Findings). Complete blood cell and platelet counts must be monitored weekly following ZEVALIN treatment until levels recover or as clinically indicated.

Immune: The safety and efficacy of immunization with any vaccine, particularly live viral vaccines, following the ZEVALIN therapeutic regimen have not been studied. Due to the potential risk of developing viral infections, it is not recommended to administer live viral vaccines to patients who have recently received ZEVALIN (see Drug Interactions, Drug-Drug Interactions). A potentially limited ability of patients to generate a primary or anamnestic humoral response to any vaccine following ZEVALIN treatment has to be taken into consideration.

Patients must not receive growth factor treatment such as G-CSF for 3 weeks prior to ZEVALIN administration as well as for 2 weeks following completion of the treatment in order to assess the adequate bone marrow reserve correctly and because of the potential sensitivity of rapidly dividing myeloid cells to radiation (see Drug Interactions, Drug-Drug Interactions).

Neurologic: This product contains albumin, a derivative of human blood. Based on effective donor screening and product manufacturing processes, it carries an extremely remote risk for transmission of viral diseases. A theoretical risk for transmission of Creutzfeldt-Jakob disease (CJD) is also considered extremely remote. No cases of transmission of viral diseases or CJD have ever been identified for albumin.

ZEVALIN could affect the ability to drive and to use machines, as dizziness has been reported as a common side effect.

Sensitivity/Resistance: Infusion reactions may occur during or following ZEVALIN administration after pretreatment with rituximab. Signs and symptoms of infusion reactions may include dizziness, cough, nausea, vomiting, rash, pruritus, tachycardia, asthenia, pyrexia, and rigors (see Adverse Reactions). In case of a potential severe infusion reaction, treatment must be stopped immediately.

Hypersensitivity reactions following ZEVALIN administration are commonly observed. Severe hypersensitivity reactions including anaphylaxis occur in less than 1% of patients (see Adverse Reactions, Immunogenicity). In case of hypersensitivity reactions, ZEVALIN infusion must be stopped immediately. Medications for the treatment of hypersensitivity reactions, eg, epinephrine, antihistamines and corticosteroids, should be available for immediate use in the event of an allergic reaction during administration of the ZEVALIN therapeutic regimen. Patients who have received murine-derived proteins before ZEVALIN treatment should be screened for human anti-mouse antibodies.

Patients with evidence of HAMA have not been studied and may be at increased risk of allergic or serious hypersensitivity reactions during ZEVALIN therapeutic regimen administration.

After the use of ZEVALIN, patients should generally be tested for HAMA before any further treatment with mouse-derived proteins.

Sexual Function/Reproduction: The ZEVALIN therapeutic regimen results in a significant radiation dose to the testes. The radiation dose to the ovaries has not been established. There have been no studies to evaluate whether the ZEVALIN therapeutic regimen causes hypogonadism, premature menopause, azoospermia and/or mutagenic alterations to germ cells. There is a potential risk that ionizing radiation by ^{90}Y-ZEVALIN could cause toxic effects on the male and female gonads. Therefore it is recommended that women of childbearing potential, as well as males, use effective contraceptive methods during and up to 12 months following the ZEVALIN therapeutic regimen. Patients planning to have children should be informed accordingly.

Skin: Severe mucocutaneous skin reactions of erythema multiforme (including Stevens-Johnson syndrome) have been reported postmarketing with the administration of ZEVALIN after pretreatment with rituximab. The onset of the reactions varied from days to months. Although the incidence is rare, the fatality associated with the administration of the ZEVALIN therapeutic regimen that included renal failure progressing to death (observed in one report of postmarketing experience) is clinically relevant. In patients experiencing a severe mucocutaneous reaction, treatment must be discontinued.

Special Populations: Pregnant Women: ^{90}Y-ZEVALIN can cause fetal harm when administered to a pregnant woman. There are no adequate and well-controlled studies in pregnant women. Since IgGs are known to cross the placenta and because of the significant risk associated with the use of radiation, ZEVALIN is contraindicated during pregnancy (see Contraindications). Pregnancy must be excluded before the start of treatment in women.

Nursing Women: It is not known whether ZEVALIN is excreted in human milk. Since maternal IgGs are excreted in human milk and because of the unknown potential for absorption and immunosuppression in the infant, women must not breastfeed during treatment and for 12 months following treatment. Formula feeding should be substituted for breastfeeding.

Pediatrics (<18 years of age): The safety and effectiveness of the ZEVALIN therapeutic regimen in children have not been established.

Geriatrics (>65 years of age): Of 349 patients treated with the ZEVALIN therapeutic regimen in clinical studies, 38% (132 patients) were 65 years of age or over, while 12% (41 patients) were 75 years of age or over. No overall differences in safety or effectiveness were observed between these subjects and younger subjects, but greater sensitivity of some older individuals cannot be ruled out.

Patients with CNS Lymphoma: Patients with follicular NHL may present with CNS involvement. These patients were excluded from clinical trials because they require different treatment modalities. Since ZEVALIN may not cross the blood brain barrier, the efficacy has not been established in these patients. The use of ZEVALIN is therefore not recommended in NHL patients with CNS involvement.

Patients with Renal Impairment: The safety and effectiveness in patients with renal impairment have not been established.

Patients with Hepatic Impairment: The safety and effectiveness in patients with hepatic impairment have not been established.

Monitoring and Laboratory Tests: Complete blood counts (CBCs) and platelet counts should be obtained weekly following the ZEVALIN therapeutic regimen and should continue until levels recover. CBCs and platelet counts should be monitored more frequently in patients who develop severe cytopenia, or as clinically indicated.

ADVERSE REACTIONS: Adverse Drug Reaction Overview: Safety data, except where indicated, are based upon 349 patients treated in five clinical studies with the ZEVALIN (ibritumomab tiuxetan) therapeutic regimen (see Dosage and Administration). Because the ZEVALIN therapeutic regimen includes the use of rituximab, please also consult the prescribing information for RITUXAN (rituximab) for adverse reactions observed with rituximab alone.

The most serious adverse reactions caused by the ZEVALIN therapeutic regimen include infections (predominantly bacterial in origin), allergic reactions (bronchospasm and angioedema), hemorrhage while thrombocytopenic (resulting in death), and severe and prolonged cytopenias. Severe mucocutaneous reactions were also reported in postmarketing surveillance. In addition, patients who have received the ZEVALIN therapeutic regimen have developed myeloid malignancies and dysplasias. Fatal infusion reactions have occurred following the infusion of rituximab. Please refer to the Warnings and Precautions for detailed descriptions of these reactions.

The most common toxicities reported were neutropenia, thrombocytopenia, leukocytopenia, anemia, infections, fever, asthenia, chills, gastrointestinal symptoms (nausea, vomiting, abdominal pain and diarrhea), increased cough, dyspnea, dizziness, arthralgia, anorexia, anxiety and ecchymosis. Hematologic toxicity was often severe and prolonged, whereas most non-hematologic toxicity was mild in severity.

Clinical Trial Adverse Drug Reactions: Table 3 and Table 4 list adverse events that occurred in ≥5% of patients and in ≥1% and <5% of patients, respectively. A more detailed description of the incidence and duration of hematologic toxicities, according to baseline platelet count (as an indicator of bone marrow reserve), is provided in Table 5, Severe Hematologic Toxicity.

Because clinical trials are conducted under very specific conditions, the adverse reaction rates observed in the clinical trials may not reflect the rates observed in practice and should not be compared to the rates in the clinical trials of another drug. Adverse drug reaction information from clinical trials is useful for identifying drug-related adverse events and for approximating rates.

Table 3: ZEVALIN

Incidence of Adverse Events in ≥5% of Patients Receiving the ZEVALIN Therapeutic Regimen[a] (N=349)

	All Grades %	Grade 3/4 %
Any Adverse Event	**99**	**89**
Body as a Whole	**80**	**12**
Asthenia	43	3
Infection	29	5
Chills	24	<1
Fever	17	1
Abdominal Pain	16	3
Pain	13	1
Headache	12	1
Throat Irritation	10	0
Back Pain	8	1
Flushing	6	0
Cardiovascular System	**17**	**3**
Hypotension	6	1
Digestive System	**48**	**3**
Nausea	31	1
Vomiting	12	0
Diarrhea	9	<1
Anorexia	8	0
Abdominal Enlargement	5	0
Constipation	5	0
Hemic and Lymphatic System	**98**	**86**
Thrombocytopenia	95	63
Neutropenia	77	60
Anemia	61	17
Ecchymosis	7	<1
Metabolic and Nutritional Disorders	**23**	**3**
Peripheral Edema	8	1
Angioedema	5	<1
Musculoskeletal System	**18**	**1**
Arthralgia	7	1
Myalgia	7	<1
Nervous System	**27**	**2**
Dizziness	10	<1
Insomnia	5	0

(cont'd)

Table 3: ZEVALIN *(cont'd)*

Incidence of Adverse Events in ≥5% of Patients Receiving the ZEVALIN Therapeutic Regimen[a] (N=349)

	All Grades %	Grade 3/4 %
Respiratory System	**36**	**3**
Dyspnea	14	2
Increased Cough	10	0
Rhinitis	6	0
Bronchospasm	5	0
Skin and Appendages	**28**	**1**
Pruritus	9	<1
Rash	8	<1
Special Senses	**7**	**<1**
Urogenital System	**6**	**<1**

[a] Adverse events were followed for a period of 12 weeks following the first rituximab infusion of the ZEVALIN therapeutic regimen.
Note: All adverse events are included, regardless of causality.

The following adverse events were reported in ≥1% and <5% of patients.

Table 4: ZEVALIN

Incidence of Adverse Events in ≥1% and <5% of Patients Receiving the ZEVALIN Therapeutic Regimen[a] (N=349)

	%
Body as a Whole	
Chest Pain	4.3
Enlarged Abdomen	2.9
Pain Neck	2.6
Malaise	2.3
Allergic Reaction	2.0
Cellulitis	1.7
Flu Syndrome	1.7
Tumour Pain	1.7
Sepsis	1.4
Moniliasis	1.1
Axilla Pain	1.1
Injection Site Pain	1.1
Cardiovascular System	
Tachycardia	2.9
Hypertension	2.3
Palpitation	1.1
Digestive System	
Dyspepsia	3.7
Dry Mouth	2.0
Melena	2.0
Gastrointestinal Disorder	1.7
Stomatitis	1.7
Rectal Hemorrhage	1.4
Oral Moniliasis	1.4
Dysphagia	1.1
Gastrointestinal Hemorrhage	1.1
Gum Hemorrhage	1.1
Hemic and Lymphatic System	
Petechia	3.4
Febrile Neutropenia	2.6
Pancytopenia	2.0
Lymphadenopathy	1.1

(cont'd)

Table 4: ZEVALIN *(cont'd)*

Incidence of Adverse Events in ≥1% and <5% of Patients Receiving the ZEVALIN Therapeutic Regimen[a] (N=349)

	%
Metabolic and Nutritional Disorders	
Increased Lactic Dehydrogenase	3.7
Hyperglycemia	2.9
Dehydration	2.3
Increased AST	2.3
Increased BUN	2.0
Increased Alkaline Phosphatase	2.0
Hypocalcemia	1.7
Increased ALT	1.7
Increased Creatinine	1.4
Edema	1.4
Decreased Weight	1.4
Hypokalemia	1.1
Hypoproteinemia	1.1
Musculoskeletal System	
Bone Pain	2.6
Leg Cramps	2.0
Myasthenia	1.4
Nervous System	
Anxiety	3.7
Hypesthesia	2.6
Paresthesia	2.6
Depression	2.3
Somnolence	2.0
Agitation	1.1
Vasodilation	1.1
Respiratory System	
Sinusitis	4.9
Epistaxis	2.9
Bronchitis	1.7
Pneumonia	1.7
Voice Alteration	1.7
Pleural Effusion	1.4
Pharyngitis	1.1
Skin and Appendages	
Urticaria	4.0
Sweats	3.7
Night Sweats	3.2
Skin Disorder	2.3
Herpes Simplex	1.7
Herpes Zoster	1.1
Special Senses	
Conjunctivitis	2.9
Alopecia	1.1
Abnormal Vision	1.1
Urogenital System	
Dysuria	1.1

(cont'd)

Table 4: ZEVALIN (cont'd)

Incidence of Adverse Events in ≥1% and <5% of Patients Receiving the ZEVALIN Therapeutic Regimen[a] (N=349)

	%
Urinary Incontinence	1.1

[a] Adverse events were followed for a period of 12 weeks following the first rituximab infusion of the ZEVALIN therapeutic regimen.
Note: All adverse events are included, regardless of causality.

Severe or life-threatening adverse events occurring in 1% to 5% of patients consisted of pancytopenia (2%), allergic reaction (1%), gastrointestinal hemorrhage (1%), melena (1%), tumour pain (1%) and apnea (1%). The following severe or life-threatening events occurred in <1% of patients: angioedema, tachycardia, urticaria, arthritis, lung edema, pulmonary embolus, encephalopathy, hematemesis, subdural hematoma and vaginal hemorrhage. Fatal outcome has been observed with the following events either in clinical trials or in postmarketing experience: anemia, pancytopenia, hemorrhage while thrombocytopenic, infection, pneumonia, sepsis, myelodysplastic syndrome/acute myelogenous leukemia, severe mucocutaneous skin reactions, and intracranial hemorrhage while thrombocytopenic.

Abnormal Hematologic and Clinical Chemistry Findings: Hematologic toxicity was the most frequently observed adverse event in clinical trials and is dose-limiting. Thrombocytopenia, leukocytopenia, neutropenia and anemia have been reported very commonly as adverse drug reactions. Also, febrile neutropenia, pancytopenia and lymphocytopenia have been reported as common adverse drug reactions. Table 5 presents the incidence and duration of severe hematologic toxicity for patients with a normal baseline platelet count (≥150 000 cells/mm³) treated with the ZEVALIN therapeutic regimen and patients with mild thrombocytopenia (platelet count 100 000 to 149 000 cells/mm³) at baseline who were treated with a modified ZEVALIN therapeutic regimen that included a lower specific activity ^{90}Y-ZEVALIN dose at 0.3 mCi/kg (11 MBq/kg).

Table 5: ZEVALIN

Severe Hematologic Toxicity Observed in Clinical Trials with ZEVALIN

	ZEVALIN Therapeutic Regimen Using 0.4 mCi/kg ^{90}Y Dose (15 MBq/kg)	Modified ZEVALIN Therapeutic Regimen Using 0.3 mCi/kg ^{90}Y Dose (11 MBq/kg)
ANC		
Median nadir (cells/mm³)	800	600
Per patient incidence: ANC <1000 cells/mm³	57%	74%
Per patient incidence: ANC <500 cells/mm³	30%	35%
Median duration (days)[a]: ANC <1000 cells/mm³	22	29
Platelets		
Median nadir (cells/mm³)	41 000	24 000
Per patient incidence: platelets <50 000 cells/mm³	61%	78%
Per patient incidence: platelets <10 000 cells/mm³	10%	14%
Median duration (days)[b]: platelets <50 000 cells/mm³	24	35

[a] Median duration of neutropenia for patients with ANC <1000 cells/mm³ (date from last laboratory value showing ANC ≥1000 cells/mm³ to date of first laboratory value following nadir showing ANC ≥1000 cells/mm³, censored at initiation of next treatment or death).
[b] Median duration of thrombocytopenia for patients with platelets <50 000 cells/mm³ (date from last laboratory value showing platelet count ≥50 000 cells/mm³ to date of first laboratory value following nadir showing platelet count ≥50 000 cells/mm³, censored at initiation of next treatment or death).

Median time to ANC nadir was 62 days, to platelet nadir, 53 days, and to hemoglobin nadir, 68 days. In clinical trials with the indication of relapsed and refractory NHL, grade 3 or 4 thrombocytopenia was reported with median times to recovery of 13 and 21 days and grade 3 or 4 neutropenia with median times to recovery of 8 and 14 days. Information on growth factor use and platelet transfusions is based on 211 patients for whom data were collected. Filgrastim was given to 13% of patients and erythropoietin to 8%. Platelet transfusions were given to 22% of patients and red blood cell transfusions to 20%.

Infections and Infestations: During the first three months after initiating the ZEVALIN therapeutic regimen, 29% of patients developed infections. Three percent of patients developed serious infections comprising urinary tract infection, febrile neutropenia, sepsis, pneumonia, cellulitis, colitis, diarrhea, osteomyelitis and upper respiratory tract infection. Life-threatening infections were reported in 2% of patients, including sepsis, empyema, pneumonia, febrile neutropenia, fever, and biliary stent-associated cholangitis. During follow-up from three months to four years after the start of treatment with ZEVALIN, 6% of patients developed infections. Two percent of patients had serious infections comprising urinary tract infection, bacterial or viral pneumonia, febrile neutropenia, perihilar infiltrate, pericarditis and intravenous drug-associated viral hepatitis. One percent of patients had life-threatening infections that included bacterial pneumonia, respiratory disease and sepsis. Some of these infectious events have been associated with a fatal outcome. Infections may be bacterial, fungal or viral, including reactivation of latent viruses.

Secondary Malignancies: A total of 2% of patients developed secondary malignancies following the ZEVALIN therapeutic regimen. One patient developed a grade 1 meningioma, three developed acute myelogenous leukemia, and two developed a myelodysplastic syndrome. The onset of a second cancer was 8-34 months following the ZEVALIN therapeutic regimen and 4-14 years following the patients' diagnosis of NHL.

Immunogenicity: Hypersensitivity reactions following ZEVALIN administration are commonly observed. Severe (grade 3/4) hypersensitivity reactions including anaphylaxis occur in less than 1% of patients (see Warnings and Precautions, Immune).

Of 211 patients who received the ZEVALIN therapeutic regimen in clinical trials and who were followed for 90 days, there were eight (3.8%) patients with evidence of human anti-mouse antibodies (HAMA) (n=5) or human anti-chimeric antibodies (HACA) (n=4) at any time during the course of the study. Two patients had low titers of HAMA prior to initiation of the ZEVALIN therapeutic regimen; one remained positive without an increase in titer while the other had a negative titer post-treatment. Three patients had evidence of HACA responses prior to initiation of the ZEVALIN therapeutic regimen; one had a marked increase in HACA titer while the other two had negative titers post-treatment. Of the three patients who had negative HAMA or HACA titers prior to the ZEVALIN therapeutic regimen, two developed HAMA in absence of HACA titers, and one had both HAMA and HACA positive titers post-treatment. Evidence of immunogenicity may be masked in patients who are lymphopenic. There has not been adequate evaluation of HAMA and HACA at delayed timepoints, concurrent with the recovery from lymphopenia at 6-12 months, to establish whether masking of the immunogenicity at early timepoints occurs. The data reflect the percentage of patients whose test results were considered positive for antibodies to ibritumomab or rituximab using kinetic enzyme immunoassays to ibritumomab and rituximab. The observed incidence of antibody positivity in an assay is highly dependent on the sensitivity and specificity of the assay and may be influenced by several factors including sample handling and concomitant medications. Comparisons of the incidence of HAMA/HACA with the ZEVALIN therapeutic regimen to the incidence of antibodies with other products may be misleading.

Post-Market Adverse Drug Reactions: Skin and Subcutaneous Tissue Disorders: Severe mucocutaneous skin reactions of erythema multiforme (including Stevens-Johnson syndrome) have been reported (3 reports/3757 commercially treated patients=0.08%) with the administration of ZEVALIN after pretreatment with rituximab. Although the incidence is rare, the fatality associated with the administration of ZEVALIN after pretreatment with rituximab that included renal failure progressing to death (observed in one report of postmarketing experience) is clinically relevant.

General Disorders and Administration Site Conditions: Reports of extravasation with subsequent infusion site reaction, such as infusion site dermatitis, infusion site desquamation, and infusion site ulcer, have been received.

ZEVALIN-associated radiation might cause damage to lymphoma-surrounding tissue and complications due to lymphoma swelling.

DRUG INTERACTIONS: Drug-Drug Interactions: No formal drug interaction studies have been performed with ZEVALIN. Due to the frequent occurrence of severe and prolonged thrombocytopenia, the potential benefits of medications that interfere with platelet function and/or anticoagulation should be weighed against the potential increased risks of bleeding and hemorrhage. Patients receiving medications that interfere with platelet function or coagulation (eg, ASA, NSAIDs and COX-2 inhibitors) should have more frequent laboratory monitoring for thrombocytopenia. In addition, the transfusion practices for such patients may need to be modified given the increased risk of bleeding.

In a clinical trial it has been shown that the use of fludarabine-containing regimens within 4 months before ZEVALIN treatment may increase the risk of hematological toxicity (see also Warnings and Precautions, Hematologic).

Growth factor treatment such as G-CSF must not be given to patients for 3 weeks prior to ZEVALIN administration as well as for 2 weeks following completion of the treatment (see Warnings and Precautions, Immune).

The safety and efficacy of immunization with any vaccine, particularly live viral vaccines, following therapy with ZEVALIN have not been studied (see Warnings and Precautions, Immune).

Drug-Food Interactions: Interactions with food have not been established.

Drug-Herb Interactions: Interactions with herbal products have not been established.

Drug-Laboratory Test Interactions: Interactions with laboratory tests have not been established.

DOSAGE AND ADMINISTRATION: Dosing Considerations: The prescribed, measured and administered dose of ^{90}Y-ZEVALIN must not exceed the absolute maximum allowable dose of 32.0 mCi (1200 MBq), regardless of the patient's body weight. Do not give ^{90}Y-ZEVALIN to patients with a platelet count <100 000/mm³ (see Warnings and Precautions).

Recommended Dose and Dosage Adjustment: The ZEVALIN (ibritumomab tiuxetan) therapeutic regimen is administered in two steps: step 1 is a single intravenous infusion of 250 mg/m² of rituximab (not included in the ZEVALIN kit). Step 2 follows step 1 by seven to nine days and consists of a second infusion of 250 mg/m² of rituximab shortly (within 4 hours) prior to 0.4 mCi/kg of ^{90}Y-ZEVALIN administered as a ten-minute IV push.

ZEVALIN Therapeutic Regimen Dose Modification in Patients with Mild Thrombocytopenia: The ^{90}Y-ZEVALIN dose should be reduced to 0.3 mCi/kg (11 MBq/kg) for patients with a baseline platelet count between 100 000 and 149 000 cells/mm³.

Note that the dose of rituximab is lower when used as part of the ZEVALIN therapeutic regimen, as compared to the dose of rituximab when used as a single agent. Do not administer rituximab as an intravenous push or bolus.

Hypersensitivity reactions may occur. Premedication, consisting of acetaminophen and diphenhydramine, should be considered before each infusion of rituximab (see Warnings and Precautions).

ZEVALIN is supplied as a kit that contains all of the non-radioactive ingredients necessary to produce a single-unit dose of ZEVALIN for labeling with ^{90}Y for therapy.

^{90}Y chloride sterile solution will be shipped directly from the manufacturer upon placement of an order for the ZEVALIN kit. Rituximab must be ordered separately and is available through hospital pharmacies.

^{90}Y-ZEVALIN is a radiopharmaceutical and should be used only by physicians and other professionals qualified by training and experienced in the safe use and handling of radionuclides. **Changing the ratio of any of the reactants in the radiolabeling process may adversely affect therapeutic results and is not recommended. ^{90}Y-ZEVALIN should not be used in the absence of the rituximab pre-dose.**

Data on the retreatment of patients with ^{90}Y-ZEVALIN are not available.

Administration: The patient dose should be measured by a suitable radioactivity calibration system prior to administration.

The ^{90}Y-ZEVALIN solution must be prepared according to the section Dosage and Administration, Instructions for Preparation and Use.

Before administration to the patient, the percent radioincorporation of the prepared ^{90}Y-ZEVALIN must be checked according to the procedure outlined in Dosage and Administration, Directions for Quality Control.

If the average radiochemical purity is less than 95%, the preparation must not be administered.

The prepared infusion solution must be given as a slow intravenous administration over 10 minutes. The infusion must not be administered as an intravenous bolus.

No incompatibilities have been observed between ZEVALIN and infusion sets.

Step 1: First rituximab infusion: Rituximab at a dose of 250 mg/m² should be administered intravenously at an initial rate of 50 mg/h. Rituximab should not be mixed or diluted with other drugs. If hypersensitivity or infusion-related events do not occur, escalate the infusion rate in 50 mg/h increments every 30 minutes, to a maximum of 400 mg/h. If hypersensitivity or an infusion-related event develops, the infusion should be temporarily slowed or interrupted (see Warnings and Precautions). The infusion can continue at one-half the previous rate upon improvement of patient symptoms. Refer to the prescribing information of rituximab for detailed guidance on its use.

Step 2: Step 2 of the ZEVALIN therapeutic regimen is initiated seven to nine days following step 1 administration.

Second rituximab infusion: Rituximab at a dose of 250 mg/m² is administered intravenously at an initial rate of 100 mg/h (50 mg/h if infusion-related events were documented during the first rituximab administration) and increased by 100 mg/h increments at 30-minute intervals, to a maximum of 400 mg/h, as tolerated.

^{90}Y-ZEVALIN injection: Within four hours following completion of the rituximab dose, ^{90}Y-ZEVALIN at a dose of 0.4 mCi/kg (15 MBq/kg) actual body weight for patients with a platelet count ≥150 000 cells/mm³, and 0.3 mCi/kg (11 MBq/kg) actual body weight for patients with a platelet count of 100 000 to 149 000 cells/mm³ is injected intravenously over a period of ten minutes. ^{90}Y-ZEVALIN may be infused directly by stopping the flow from an infusion bag and administering it directly into the line. A 0.2 or 0.22-micrometer low-protein-binding membrane filter should be in line between the syringe and the infusion port prior to injection of ^{90}Y-ZEVALIN. After injection, the line should be flushed with at least 10 mL of 0.9% sodium chloride solution. Precautions should be taken to avoid extravasation. A free-flowing intravenous line should be established prior to ^{90}Y-ZEVALIN injection. Close monitoring for evidence of extravasation during the injection of ^{90}Y-ZEVALIN is required. If any signs or symptoms of extravasation occur, the infusion should be immediately terminated and restarted in another vein.

Instructions for Preparation and Use: The ZEVALIN carton is to be used by a qualified specialist to prepare a single dose of ^{90}Y-ZEVALIN for therapy. **Changing the ratio of any of the reactants in the radiolabeling process may adversely affect therapeutic results and is not recommended. ZEVALIN must not be mixed with other drugs.**

Read all directions thoroughly and assemble all materials before starting the radiolabeling procedure.

The patient dose should be measured by a suitable radioactivity calibration system immediately prior to administration. The dose calibrator must be operated in accordance with the manufacturer's specifications and quality control for the measurement of ^{90}Y.

Proper aseptic technique and precautions for handling radioactive materials should be employed. Waterproof gloves should be utilized during the preparation and determination of radiochemical purity of ^{90}Y-ZEVALIN. Appropriate shielding should be used during radiolabeling and use of a syringe shield is recommended during administration to the patient. The administration of radiopharmaceuticals creates risks for other persons from external radiation or contamination from spills of urine, vomiting, etc. Radiation protection precaution in accordance with local regulations must therefore be taken. Any unused product or waste material should be disposed of in accordance with local requirements. Contaminated materials must be disposed of as radioactive waste by the authorized route.

The radiolabeling of ZEVALIN shall be done according to the following directions.

Required materials not supplied in the carton:

A. ^{90}Y chloride sterile solution (^{90}Y chloride)
B. Three sterile 1-mL syringes
C. One sterile 3-mL syringe
D. Two sterile 10-mL syringes with 18-20 G needles
E. Instant thin-layer chromatographic silica gel strips (ITLC-SG)
F. 0.9% sodium chloride aqueous solution for the chromatography solvent
G. Suitable radioactivity counting apparatus
H. Developing chamber for chromatography
I. Membrane filter, 0.22-micrometer, low-protein-binding
J. Vial and syringe shield

Method:

1. Sterile, pyrogen-free ^{90}Y chloride must be used for the preparation of ^{90}Y-ZEVALIN. The use of high purity ^{90}Y chloride is required.
2. Before radiolabeling, allow the contents of the refrigerated carton to reach room temperature. Note: The ZEVALIN vial contains a protein solution that may develop translucent particulates. These particulates will be removed by filtration prior to administration.
3. Clean the rubber stoppers of all of the vials in the kit and the ^{90}Y chloride vial with a suitable alcohol swab and allow to air-dry.
4. Place the empty reaction vial in a suitable dispensing shield (pre-warmed to room temperature). To avoid the build-up of excessive pressure during the procedure, use a 10-mL syringe to withdraw 10 mL of air from the reaction vial.
5. Prior to initiating the radiolabeling reaction, determine the amount of each component needed according to the directions below:
   a. Calculate the volume of ^{90}Y chloride that is equivalent to 40 mCi based on the activity concentration of the ^{90}Y chloride stock. Use the certificate of analysis provided by the manufacturer of the ^{90}Y chloride for this calculation.
   b. The volume of 50 mM sodium acetate solution needed is equal to the volume of ^{90}Y chloride solution determined in step 5.a. above, multiplied by a factor of 1.2. (The 50 mM sodium acetate is used to adjust the pH for the radiolabeling reaction.)
   c. Calculate the volume of formulation buffer needed to bring the reaction vial contents to a final volume of 10 mL. This is the volume of formulation buffer needed to protect the labeled product from radiolysis and to terminate the labeling reaction. For example: The volume of ibritumomab tiuxetan required is 1.3 mL. If the volume of ^{90}Y chloride equivalent to 40 mCi is calculated to be 0.5 mL, then 0.6 mL of sodium acetate (0.5 mL multiplied by a factor of 1.2) is required. Therefore, the amount of formulation buffer needed is 7.6 mL (i.e., 10 mL—1.3 mL—0.5 mL—0.6 mL).
6. With a sterile 1-mL syringe, transfer the calculated volume of 50 mM sodium acetate to the empty reaction vial. Coat the entire inner surface of the reaction vial by gentle inversion or rolling.
7. Transfer 40 mCi of ^{90}Y chloride to the reaction vial with a sterile 1-mL syringe. Mix the two solutions and coat the entire inner surface of the reaction vial by gentle inversion or rolling.
8. With a sterile 3-mL syringe, transfer 1.3 mL of ZEVALIN (ibritumomab tiuxetan) to the reaction vial. Coat the entire surface of the reaction vial by gentle inversion or rolling. **Do not shake or agitate the vial contents, since this will cause foaming and denaturation of the protein.**
9. Allow the labeling reaction to proceed at room temperature for five minutes. Allowing the labeling reaction to proceed for a longer or shorter time may result in inadequate labeling.
10. **Immediately** after the five-minute incubation period, using a sterile 10-mL syringe with a large bore needle (18 G-20 G), transfer the calculated volume of formulation buffer from step 5.c. to the reaction vial, terminating incubation. Gently add the formulation buffer down the side of the reaction vial. If necessary to normalize air pressure, withdraw an equal volume of air. Coat the entire inner surface of the reaction vial by gentle inversion or rolling. Do not shake or agitate the vial contents. Avoid foaming.
11. Using the supplied labels, record the patient identification information, the date and time of preparation, the total activity and volume, and the date and time of expiration, and affix these labels to the reaction vial and shielded reaction vial container.
12. Calculate the volume required for a ^{90}Y-ZEVALIN dose of 0.4 mCi/kg (15 MBq/kg) of actual body weight for patients with a normal platelet count, and 0.3 mCi/kg (11 MBq/kg) of actual body weight for patients with a platelet count of 100 000-149 000 cells/mm^3. **The prescribed, measured and administered dose of ^{90}Y-ZEVALIN must not exceed the absolute maximum allowable dose of 32.0 mCi (1200 MBq), regardless of the patient's body weight.** Withdraw the required volume from the reaction vial contents into a sterile 10-mL syringe with a large bore needle (18 G-20 G). Assay the syringe and contents in a dose calibrator. The dose calibrator must be operated in accordance with the manufacturer's specifications and quality control for the measurement of ^{90}Y. The syringe should contain the dose of ^{90}Y-ZEVALIN to be administered to the patient and should be within 10% of the actual prescribed dose of ^{90}Y-ZEVALIN, not to exceed a maximum dose of 32.0 mCi. Do not exceed ±10% of the prescribed dose. Using the supplied labels, record the patient identification information, the date and time of preparation, the total activity and volume added, and the date and time of expiration, and affix these labels to the syringe and shielded unit dose container.
13. Determine radiochemical purity. See Directions for Quality Control that follow these Instructions for Preparation and Use.
14. ^{90}Y-ZEVALIN should be stored under refrigeration between 2 and 8°C until use and administered within eight hours of radiolabeling.
15. See Dosage and Administration, Administration, Step 2.
16. Discard vials, needles and syringes in accordance with regulations governing radioactive and biohazardous waste.

^{90}Y-ZEVALIN is suitable for administration on an outpatient basis. Beyond the use of vial and syringe shields for preparation and injection, no special shielding is necessary.

Directions for Quality Control: Procedure for Determining Radiochemical Purity (RCP):

1. At room temperature, place a small drop of ^{90}Y-ZEVALIN at the origin of an ITLC-SG strip.
2. Place the ITLC-SG strip into a chromatography chamber with the origin at the bottom and the solvent front at the top. Allow the solvent (0.9% NaCl) to migrate at least 5 cm from the bottom of the strip. Remove the strip from the chamber and cut the strip in half. Count each half of the ITLC-SG strip for one minute (CPM) with a suitable counting apparatus.
3. Calculate the percentage of RCP as follows:

$$\% \text{ RCP} = \frac{\text{CPM bottom half}}{\text{CPM bottom half + CPM top half}} \times 100$$

4. If the radiochemical purity is <95%, the ITLC procedure should be repeated. If repeat testing confirms that radiochemical purity is <95%, the preparation should not be administered.

Radiation Dosimetry: Based upon dosimetry studies with ^{111}In-ZEVALIN, the estimated radiation dosimetry for individual organs following administration of ^{90}Y-ZEVALIN at activities of 15 MBq/kg and 11 MBq/kg was calculated according to Medical Internal Radiation Dosimetry (MIRD) (see Table 6). The estimated radiation-absorbed doses to normal organs were substantially below recognized upper safety limits. Individual patient dosimetry results were not predictive for ^{90}Y-ZEVALIN toxicity and, accordingly, general performance of dosimetry is not recommended.

Table 6: ZEVALIN

Estimated Radiation Absorbed Doses From ^{90}Y-ZEVALIN

	^{90}Y-ZEVALIN mGy/MBq	
Organ	**Median**	**Range**
Spleen[a]	9.4	1.8–20.0
Liver[a]	4.8	2.9 –8.1
Lower large intestinal wall[a]	4.7	3.1–8.2
Upper large intestinal wall[a]	3.6	2.0–6.7
Heart wall[a]	2.9	1.5–3.2
Lungs[a]	2.0	1.2–3.4
Testes[a]	1.5	1.0–4.3
Small intestine[a]	1.4	0.8–2.1
Red marrow[b]	1.3	0.6–1.8
Urinary bladder wall[c]	0.9	0.7–1.3
Bone surfaces[b]	0.9	0.5–1.2
Ovaries[c]	0.4	0.3–0.5
Uterus[c]	0.4	0.3–0.5
Adrenals[c]	0.3	0.2–0.5
Brain[c]	0.3	0.2–0.5
Breasts[c]	0.3	0.2–0.5
Gallbladder wall[c]	0.3	0.2–0.5
Muscle[c]	0.3	0.2–0.5
Pancreas[c]	0.3	0.2–0.5
Skin[c]	0.3	0.2–0.5
Stomach[c]	0.3	0.2–0.5
Thymus[c]	0.3	0.2–0.5
Thyroid[c]	0.3	0.2–0.5
Kidneys[a]	0.1	0.0–0.3
Total body[c]	0.5	0.4–0.7

[a] Organ region of interest.
[b] Sacrum region of interest.
[c] Whole body region of interest.

The effective dose equivalent for ^{90}Y in a 70 kg adult resulting from an intravenously injected activity of 1 GBq of unbound ^{90}Y is 700 mSv (worst case).

OVERDOSAGE:
Doses as high as 0.52 mCi/kg (19.2 MBq/kg) of ^{90}Y-ZEVALIN (ibritumomab tiuxetan) were administered in ZEVALIN therapeutic regimen clinical trials and severe hematological toxicities were observed. No fatalities or second organ injury resulting from overdosage administrations were documented. However, single doses up to 50 mCi (1850 MBq) of ^{90}Y-ZEVALIN and multiple doses of 20 mCi (740 MBq) followed by 40 mCi (1480 MBq) of ^{90}Y-ZEVALIN were studied in a limited number of subjects. In these trials, some patients required autologous stem cell support to manage hematological toxicity. Patients recovered from these toxicity signs, and overdoses were not associated with serious or fatal outcome.

There is no known specific antidote for ^{90}Y-ZEVALIN overdosage. Treatment consists of discontinuation of ZEVALIN and supportive therapy, which may include growth factors. If available, autologous stem cell support should be administered to manage hematological toxicity.

For management of a suspected drug overdose, CPhA recommends that you contact your **regional Poison Control Centre**. See the *CPS* Directory section for a list of Poison Control Centres.

ACTION AND CLINICAL PHARMACOLOGY: ZEVALIN (ibritumomab tiuxetan) is composed of a murine IgG_1 monoclonal antibody (ibritumomab) covalently bound to the chelating agent tiuxetan. Unlabeled ZEVALIN is chelated with ^{90}Y chloride sterile solution before intravenous administration to prepare ^{90}Y-ZEVALIN, the active therapeutic agent.

Mechanism of Action: Ibritumomab reacts specifically with the CD20 antigen, which is present in approximately 93% of patients with B-cell NHL. The CD20 antigen is found on the surface of both normal and malignant B lymphocytes, but not on hematopoietic stem cells, pro-B-cells, normal plasma cells or other normal tissue.

The complementarity-determining regions of ibritumomab bind to the CD20 antigen on the target B lymphocytes, and the long β-energy pathlength of ^{90}Y (χ_{90}=5mm) allows neighbouring tumour cells in the range (100-200 cell diameters) of the β emissions to be killed without direct binding of the antibody. The binding of an anti-CD20 antibody combined with an effective cell-killing mechanism provides a highly selective method for the elimination of malignant B-cells and still allows the progenitor B-cells to regenerate the immune system normally.

Pharmacodynamics: In clinical studies, administration of the ZEVALIN therapeutic regimen resulted in sustained depletion of circulating B-cells. At four weeks, the median number of circulating B-cells was zero (range: 0 to 1084 cells/mm^3). B-cell recovery began at approximately 12 weeks following treatment, and the median level of B-cells was within the normal range (32 to 341 cells/mm^3) by nine months after treatment. Median serum levels of IgG and IgA remained within the normal range throughout the period of B-cell depletion. Median IgM serum levels dropped below normal (median 49 mg/dL, range 13 to 3990 mg/dL) after treatment and recovered to normal values by six months post-therapy.

Pharmacokinetics: The small quantities of ^{90}Y-ZEVALIN (approximately 2.1 mg) in a typical administration are not optimally targeted to tumours unless measures are taken to block or deplete CD20 binding sites, including those on circulating lymphocytes, and in normal or involved tissues with large numbers of B-cells and high blood flow (such as the spleen and liver). Rituximab administered prior to ZEVALIN treatment is used to optimize biodistribution. In patients in which an injection of ^{111}In-ZEVALIN (used for imaging purposes) was preceded by a single infusion of rituximab at either 100 mg/m^2 or 250 mg/m^2, known disease sites were imaged in both groups without accumulation of ^{111}In-ZEVALIN in normal organs. No substantial qualitative or quantitative differences in imaging were observed between the two rituximab doses, however the higher dose of 250 mg/m^2 was chosen since it would likely lead to an enhanced therapeutic effect.

In pharmacokinetic studies of patients receiving the ZEVALIN therapeutic regimen, the mean effective half-life for ^{90}Y activity in blood was 30 hours and the mean area under the fraction of injected activity (FIA) vs. time curve in blood was 39 hours. Over seven days, a median of 7.2% of the injected activity was excreted in urine.

Under conditions corresponding to the recommended treatment regimen, the kinetics of ZEVALIN fit a linear and noncompartmental model. The physical half-life of ^{90}Y is 64.1 hours (2.7 days), with rapid decay to stable and nontoxic zirconium-90. The minor amounts of unbound circulating radioactivity are eliminated in urine with a median effective half-life in blood of 27.1 hours and a median area under the curve (AUC) of 27.5 hours. Approximately 5.7% (range 3.2% to 8.9%) of the injected dose is eliminated in urine over a period of seven days, with 80% of this elimination complete within four days. This corresponds to a total urinary elimination of 2 mCi or less of the total radioisotope over a period of a few days.

Results of dosimetry measurements performed in 179 patients indicate that radiation doses delivered to normal organs and marrow by ^{90}Y-ZEVALIN at the recommended maximum dose of 0.4 mCi are significantly below exposure levels that would justify clinical concern (2000 cGy to normal organs; 300 cGy to marrow).

The correlation between myelotoxicity and red marrow dose was examined by the use of scatter plots and correlation analyses, comparing the blood cell nadir (neutrophils or platelets) and the recovery time versus the radiation dose to marrow. These data demonstrate a poor correlation between radiation dose to marrow and hematologic toxicity.

STORAGE AND STABILITY: After radiolabeling, an immediate use is recommended. Chemical and physical in-use stability has been demonstrated for 8 hours at 2 to 8°C and protected from light.

Store the ZEVALIN kit under refrigeration between 2 and 8°C in its original packaging to protect from light. Do not freeze. Administer within 8 hours of radiolabeling.

SPECIAL HANDLING INSTRUCTIONS: As in the use of any other radioactive material, care should be taken to minimize radiation exposure to patients consistent with proper patient management, and to minimize radiation exposure to occupational workers.

INFORMATION FOR THE PATIENT: Published in e-CPS, available by subscription at www.e-cps.ca.

DOSAGE FORMS, COMPOSITION AND PACKAGING: The ZEVALIN (ibritumomab tiuxetan) kit provides the non-radioactive components for the radiolabeling of ibritumomab tiuxetan with ^{90}Y.

^{90}Y chloride sterile solution will be shipped directly from the manufacturer upon placement of an order for the ZEVALIN kit. Rituximab must be ordered separately, and is available through hospital pharmacies.

Each ZEVALIN kit contains: one ZEVALIN vial containing 3.2 mg of ibritumomab tiuxetan in 2 mL of normal saline solution, as a clear, colourless solution that may contain translucent particles; one 50 mM sodium acetate vial containing 13.6 mg of sodium acetate trihydrate in 2 mL of Water for Injection as a clear, colourless solution; one formulation buffer vial containing 750 mg of human serum albumin, 76 mg of sodium chloride, 21 mg of sodium phosphate dibasic dodecahydrate, 4 mg of pentetic acid, 2 mg of potassium phosphate monobasic and 2 mg of potassium chloride in 10 mL of Water for Injection adjusted to pH 7.1 with either sodium hydroxide or hydrochloric acid as a yellow to amber coloured solution; one empty reaction vial and four identification labels. The contents of all vials are sterile, pyrogen free and contain no preservatives. The final formulation after radiolabeling contains 2.08 mg ^{90}Y-ibritumomab tiuxetan in a total volume of 10 mL.

Ziagen® ℞
abacavir sulfate
Antiretroviral Agent

ViiV Healthcare ULC

Date of Revision: April 23, 2010

SUMMARY PRODUCT INFORMATION:

Route of Administration	Dosage Form/ Strength	Clinically Relevant Nonmedicinal Ingredients
Oral	Tablet/300 mg abacavir	None For a complete listing see Dosage Forms, Composition and Packaging.
	Oral Solution/20 mg/mL abacavir	Propylene glycol For a complete listing see Dosage Forms, Composition and Packaging.

INDICATIONS AND CLINICAL USE: ZIAGEN (abacavir sulfate) is indicated in:

- antiretroviral combination therapy for the treatment of Human Immunodeficiency Virus (HIV) infection.

This indication is based on analyses of surrogate markers in controlled studies of up to 48 weeks in duration. The demonstration of the benefit of ZIAGEN is mainly based on results of studies in treatment naïve patients on combination therapy conducted with lamivudine and zidovudine. In patients with high viral load (>100 000 copies/mL) choice of therapy needs special consideration.

In one controlled study (CNA30021), more patients taking ZIAGEN 600 mg once daily had severe hypersensitivity reactions than patients taking ZIAGEN 300 mg twice daily (see Warnings and Precautions, Adverse Reactions and Dosage and Administration).

ZIAGEN is one of multiple products containing abacavir. Before starting ZIAGEN, review medical history for prior exposure to any abacavir-containing product in order to avoid reintroduction in a patient with a history of hypersensitivity to abacavir.

CONTRAINDICATIONS: ZIAGEN (abacavir sulfate) tablets and oral solution are contraindicated in patients:

- with previously demonstrated hypersensitivity to abacavir, or any of the other components of the product (see Warnings and Precautions and Dosage Forms, Composition and Packaging).
- with moderate or severe hepatic impairment since the pharmacokinetics have not been studied in this patient group.

WARNINGS AND PRECAUTIONS:

Serious Warnings and Precautions

- **Fatal Hypersensitivity Reactions:** Fatal hypersensitivity reactions have been associated with therapy with ZIAGEN (abacavir sulfate). Therapy ZIAGEN should be discontinued in patients developing signs or symptoms of hypersensitivity in 2 or more of the following groups: 1) fever, 2) rash, 3) gastrointestinal (including nausea, vomiting, diarrhea or abdominal pain, 4) constitutional (including generalized malaise, fatigue or achiness, 5) respiratory (including pharyngitis, dyspnea, cough and abnormal chest x-ray findings, predominantly infiltrates, which can be localized). (see Warnings and Precautions, Hypersensitivity Reactions to Abacavir). To minimize the risk of a life threatening hypersensitivity reaction, ZIAGEN should be permanently discontinued if hypersensitivity cannot be ruled out, even when other diagnoses are possible (acute onset of respiratory diseases, gastroenteritis or reactions to other medications).

  The symptoms of a hypersensitivity reaction can occur at any time during treatment with abacavir, but usually occur within the first six weeks of therapy. **ZIAGEN or any other medicinal product containing abacavir (e.g. KIVEXA, TRIZIVIR), must never be restarted following a hypersensitivity reaction, as more severe symptoms will recur within hours and may include life-threatening hypotension and death.** Severe or fatal hypersensitivity reactions can occur within hours after ZIAGEN re-introduction in patients who have no identified history or undiagnosed symptoms of hypersensitivity during their initial period of use of ZIAGEN.

  Patients who carry the HLA-B*5701 allele are at a significant increased risk for experiencing a hypersensitivity reaction to abacavir. Prior to initiating therapy with abacavir, it is recommended that screening for HLA-B*5701 status be undertaken. Screening is also recommended prior to re-initiation of abacavir in patients of unknown HLA-B*5701 status who have previously tolerated abacavir. Use of abacavir in patients known to carry the HLA-B*5701 allele is not recommended.

  Cases of abacavir hypersensitivity have occurred in patients who are HLA-B*5701 negative. The clinical diagnosis of suspected hypersensitivity to abacavir remains the basis for clinical decision making in all patients. Therefore, it is important to permanently discontinue abacavir and not rechallenge with abacavir if hypersensitivity cannot be ruled out, regardless of the presence or absence of the HLA-B*5701 allele due to the potential for a severe or even fatal reaction (see Warnings and Precautions, Hypersensitivity Reaction, Risk Factors: HLA-B*5701 Allele).
- **Lactic Acidosis and Severe Hepatomegaly with Steatosis:** Lactic acidosis and severe hepatomegaly with steatosis, including fatal cases, have been reported with the use of nucleoside analogues alone or in combination, including ZIAGEN and other antiretrovirals. A majority of these cases have been in women. Obesity and prolonged nucleoside exposure may be risk factors. However, cases have also been reported in patients with no known risk factors. Treatment with ZIAGEN should be suspended in any patient who develops clinical or laboratory findings suggestive of lactic acidosis or pronounced hepatotoxicity (which may include hepatomegaly and steatosis even in the absence of marked transaminase elevations) (see Warnings and Precautions, Hepatic/Biliary/Pancreatic).

General: ZIAGEN (abacavir sulfate) should always be used in combination with other antiretroviral agents. When antiretroviral regimens are changed due to loss of virologic response, ZIAGEN should not be added as a single agent.

Hypersensitivity Reactions: Serious and sometimes fatal hypersensitivity reactions have been associated with therapy with ZIAGEN (see Boxed Serious Warnings and Precautions). Patients who carry the HLA-B*5701 allele are at a significantly increased risk for experiencing a hypersensitivity reaction to abacavir.

Discontinue ZIAGEN as soon as a hypersensitivity reaction is suspected. To minimize the risk of a life-threatening hypersensitivity reaction, permanently discontinue ZIAGEN if hypersensitivity cannot be ruled out, even when other diagnoses are possible (e.g. acute onset respiratory diseases such as pneumonia, bronchitis, pharyngitis, or influenza; gastroenteritis; or reactions to other medications). If symptoms consistent with hypersensitivity are not identified, reintroduction can be undertaken with continued monitoring for symptoms of a hypersensitivity reaction. Make patients aware that a hypersensitivity reaction can occur with reintroduction of ZIAGEN or any other abacavir containing product and that reintroduction of ZIAGEN or any other abacavir containing product needs to be undertaken only if medical care can be readily accessed by the patient or others.

Following a hypersensitivity reaction to abacavir, **never** restart ZIAGEN or any other abacavir containing product because more severe symptoms can occur within hours and may include life-threatening hypotension and death.

Regardless of a patient's HLA-B*5701 status, if therapy with ZIAGEN or any other medicinal product containing abacavir has been discontinued and restarting therapy is under consideration, the reason for discontinuation should be evaluated to ensure that the patient did not have symptoms of a hypersensitivity reaction. If a hypersensitivity reaction cannot be ruled out, ZIAGEN or any other medicinal product containing abacavir (e.g. KIVEXA, TRIZIVIR) should not be restarted.

Overall, in clinical trials conducted before the introduction of screening for the HLA-B*5701 allele, hypersensitivity to abacavir was reported in approximately 8% of 2670 patients (n=206) in 9 clinical trials (range: 2% to 9%) with enrolment from November 1999 to February 2002. Data on time to onset and symptoms of suspected hypersensitivity in the nine studies were collected on a detailed data collection module. This reaction is characterized by the appearance of symptoms indicating multi-organ/body-system involvement. Symptoms can occur at any time during therapy; however they usually appear within the first 6 weeks (median time to onset 11 days) of initiation of treatment with ZIAGEN (see Adverse Reactions). See Figure 1.

Figure 1: ZIAGEN

Hypersensitivity Related Symptoms Reported with ≥10% Frequency in Clinical Trials (n=206 Patients)

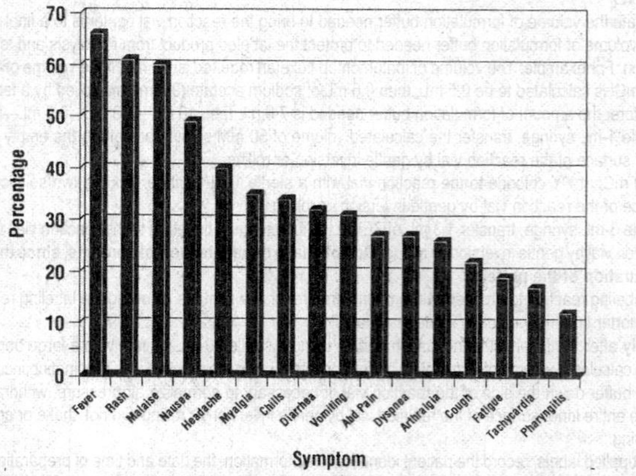

In controlled study (CNA 30021), more patients taking ZIAGEN 600 mg once daily had severe hypersensitivity reactions than patients taking ZIAGEN 300 mg twice daily (see Dosage and Administration). In this study, 4 patients (11%) receiving ZIAGEN 600 mg once daily experienced hypotension with a hypersensitivity reaction compared with 0 patients receiving ZIAGEN 300 mg twice daily.

A warning card with information for the patient about this hypersensitivity reaction is included in the ZIAGEN pack (see Information for the Patient, Warning Card).

Risk Factors: HLA-B*5701 Allele: Studies have shown that carriage of the HLA-B*5701 allele is associated with a significantly increased risk of a hypersensitivity reaction to abacavir. CNA106030 (PREDICT-1), a randomized, double blind study, evaluated the clinical utility of prospective HLA-B*5701 screening on the incidence of abacavir hypersensitivity reaction in abacavir-naïve HIV-1 infected adults (n=1650). In this study, use of pre-therapy screening for the HLA-B*5701 allele and exclusion of subjects with this allele reduced the incidence of clinically suspected abacavir hypersensitivity reactions from 7.8% (66/847) to 3.4% (27/803) (p<0.0001). Based on this study, it is estimated that 61% of patients with the HLA-B*5701 allele will develop a clinically suspected hypersensitivity reaction during the course of abacavir treatment compared with 4% of patients who do not have the HLA-B*5701 allele.

Screening for carriage of the HLA-B*5701 allele is recommended prior to initiating treatment with abacavir. Screening is also recommended prior to re-initiating abacavir in patients of unknown HLA-B*5701 status who have previously tolerated abacavir. For HLA-B*5701-positive patients, initiating or re-initiating treatment with an abacavir containing regimen is not recommended and should be considered only with close medical supervision and under exceptional circumstances where potential benefit outweighs the risk.

Skin patch testing is used as a research tool and should not be used to aid in the clinical diagnosis of abacavir hypersensitivity.

In any patient treated with abacavir, the clinical diagnosis of a hypersensitivity reaction must remain the basis of clinical decision making. Even in the absence of the HLA- B*5701 allele, it is important to permanently discontinue abacavir and not rechallenge with abacavir if a hypersensitivity reaction cannot be ruled out on clinical grounds, due to the potential for a severe or even fatal reaction.

Carcinogenesis and Mutagenesis: Abacavir induced chromosomal aberrations both in the presence and absence of metabolic activation in an in vitro cytogenetic study in human lymphocytes. Abacavir was mutagenic in the absence of metabolic activation, although it was not mutagenic in the presence of metabolic activation in an L5178Y mouse lymphoma assay. At systemic exposures approximately nine times higher than that in humans at the therapeutic dose, abacavir was clastogenic in males and not clastogenic in females in an in vivo mouse bone marrow micronucleus assay.

Abacavir was not mutagenic in bacterial mutagenicity assays in the presence and absence of metabolic activation.

Carcinogenicity studies with orally administered abacavir in mice and rats showed an increase in the incidence of malignant and non-malignant tumours. Malignant tumours occurred in the preputial gland of males and the clitoral gland of females of both species, and in the liver, urinary bladder, lymph nodes and subcutis of female rats. The majority of these tumours occurred at the highest abacavir dose in mice and rats, which corresponds to 24-32 times the expected systemic exposure in humans.

Cardiovascular: The results of a prospective, observational, epidemiological study designed to investigate the rate of myocardial infarction in patients on combination antiretroviral therapy (N=33 347) suggest that current or recent use (within the past 6 months) of abacavir may be associated with a potential increased risk of myocardial infarction. This elevated risk does not appear to increase further over time, and no excess risk was present in patients who had stopped taking abacavir more than 6 months previously. The relative risk of myocardial infarction was estimated to be 1.9 (95% CI 1.47-2.45). The absolute myocardial infarction rate was 6.1/1000 patient years of exposure for those recently exposed to abacavir compared to an absolute myocardial infarction rate of 2.6/1000 patient years of exposure for those not recently exposed. In addition, the absolute myocardial infarction rate ranged from 3.4 to 3.7/1000 patient years of exposure for patients recently exposed to other NRTIs (i.e. zidovudine, stavudine and lamivudine).

In a pooled analysis of GSK sponsored clinical trials (N=9639), no increased risk of myocardial infarction was observed with abacavir use. At this time, though the available data do not allow a definitive conclusion regarding the association between the use of abacavir and an increased risk of myocardial infarction, it is recommended that physicians discuss the potential benefits and risks of abacavir with their patients.

As a precaution, the underlying risk of coronary heart disease should be considered when prescribing antiretroviral therapies, including abacavir, and action taken to minimize all modifiable risk factors (e.g. hypertension, hyperlipidemia, diabetes mellitus and smoking).

Endocrine and Metabolism: Fat Redistribution: Redistribution/accumulation of body fat including central obesity, dorsocervical fat enlargement ("buffalo hump"), peripheral wasting, facial wasting, breast enlargement, and "cushingoid appearance" have been observed in patients receiving antiretroviral therapy. The mechanism and long-term consequences of these events are currently unknown. A causal relationship has not been established.

Hepatic/Biliary/Pancreatic: Lactic Acidosis/Severe Hepatomegaly with Steatosis: Lactic acidosis and severe hepatomegaly with steatosis, including fatal cases, have been reported with the use of nucleoside analogues either alone or in combination, including abacavir and other antiretrovirals. A majority of these cases have been in women.

Clinical features which may be indicative of the development of lactic acidosis include generalised weakness, anorexia and sudden unexplained weight loss, gastrointestinal symptoms and respiratory symptoms (dyspnea and tachypnea).

Obesity and prolonged nucleoside exposure may be risk factors. Particular caution should be exercised when administering ZIAGEN to any patient with known risk factors for liver disease; however, cases have also been reported in patients with no known risk factors. Treatment with ZIAGEN should be suspended in any patient who develops clinical or laboratory findings suggestive of lactic acidosis or pronounced hepatotoxicity (which may include hepatomegaly and steatosis even in the absence of marked transaminase elevations).

Impaired Hepatic Function: Abacavir is contraindicated in patients with moderate to severe hepatic impairment and dose reduction is required in patients with mild hepatic impairment.

Abacavir is metabolized primarily by the liver. The pharmacokinetics of abacavir have been studied in patients with mild hepatic impairment (Child-Pugh score 5-6) who had confirmed cirrhosis. The results showed that there was a mean increase of 1.89 fold in the abacavir AUC, and 1.58 fold in the half-life of abacavir. The AUCs of the metabolites were not modified by the liver disease. However, the rates of formation and elimination of these were decreased. The pharmacokinetics have not been studied in patients with moderate or severe hepatic impairment, therefore ZIAGEN is contraindicated in these patient groups. Once daily ZIAGEN 600 mg dosing has not been studied in the patients with impaired hepatic function and is not recommended for use in this population (see Dosage and Administration, Impaired Hepatic Function).

Immune: Therapy Experienced Patients: In clinical trials, patients with prolonged prior nucleoside reverse transcriptase inhibitor (NRTI) exposure or who had HIV-1 isolates that contained multiple mutations conferring resistance to NRTIs had limited response to abacavir. The potential for cross resistance between abacavir and other NRTIs should be considered when choosing new therapeutic regimens in therapy experienced patients.

In heavily pre-treated NRTI patients, the reduction in viral load with ZIAGEN was very low. The degree of viral load reduction as part of a new combination regimen will depend on the nature and duration of prior therapy which may have selected for HIV-1 variants with cross resistance to abacavir.

Immune Reconstitution Syndrome: During the initial phase of treatment, patients responding to antiretroviral therapy may develop an inflammatory response to indolent or residual opportunistic infections (such as MAC, CMV, PCP and TB), which may necessitate further evaluation and treatment.

Renal: Preliminary data from a single dose pharmacokinetic study of ZIAGEN in 6 end-stage renal disease patients has demonstrated that abacavir concentrations were similar to those with normal renal function. The two major metabolites (5'-glucuronide and 5'-carboxylate metabolites) are likely to accumulate but are considered inactive. No dosing modification of ZIAGEN is recommended in patients with renal dysfunction. However, ZIAGEN should be avoided in patients with end-stage renal disease. Once daily ZIAGEN 600 mg dosing has not been studied in the patients with impaired renal function and is not recommended for use in this population.

Respiratory: Severe respiratory symptoms, some indicative of adult respiratory distress syndrome (ARDS), occur in a small proportion of hypersensitivity reaction cases. ARDS or respiratory failure appears more likely to occur in a rechallenge situation.

Special Populations: Pregnant Women: There are no adequate and well controlled studies in pregnant women. ZIAGEN should be used during pregnancy only if the potential benefits outweigh the risk.

There have been reports of mild, transient elevations in serum lactate levels, which may be due to mitochondrial dysfunction, in neonates and infants exposed in utero or peri-partum to nucleoside reverse transcriptase inhibitors (NRTIs). The clinical relevance of transient elevations in serum lactate is unknown. There have also been very rare reports on developmental delay, seizures and other neurological disease. However, a causal relationship between these events and NRTI exposure in utero or peri-partum has not been established. These findings do not affect current recommendations to use antiretroviral therapy in pregnant women to prevent vertical transmission of HIV.

Studies in pregnant rats showed that abacavir is transferred to the fetus through the placenta. Developmental toxicity (depressed fetal body weight and reduced crown-rump length) and increased incidences of fetal anasarca and skeletal malformations were observed when rats were treated with abacavir at doses of 1000 mg/kg during organogenesis. This dose produced 35 times the human exposure, based on AUC.

In a fertility study, evidence of toxicity to the developing embryo and fetuses (increased resorptions, decreased fetal body weights) occurred only at 500 mg/kg per day. The offspring of female rats treated with abacavir at 500 mg/kg (beginning at embryo implantation and ending at weaning) showed increased incidence of stillbirth and lower body weights throughout life. In the rabbit, there was no evidence of drug-related developmental toxicity and no increases in fetal malformations at doses up to 700 mg/kg (8.5 times the human exposure at the recommended dose, based on AUC).

Antiretroviral Pregnancy Registry: To monitor maternal-fetal outcomes of pregnant women exposed to ZIAGEN, an Antiretroviral Pregnancy Registry has been established. Physicians are encouraged to register patients by calling ViiV Healthcare ULC's Drug Safety Department (1-877-393-8448).

Nursing Women: It is recommended that HIV infected women do not breastfeed their infants under any circumstances in order to avoid transmission of HIV. It is therefore recommended that mothers do not breastfeed their babies while receiving treatment with ZIAGEN.

Abacavir and its metabolites are secreted into the milk of lactating rats. It is expected that these will also be secreted into human milk, although this has not been confirmed. There is no data available on the safety of ZIAGEN when administered to babies less than three months old.

Pediatrics: Abacavir is rapidly and well absorbed from the oral solution when administered to children. The overall pharmacokinetic parameters in children are comparable to adults, with greater variability in plasma concentrations. The recommended dose for children from 3 months to 12 years old is 8 mg/kg twice daily. This will provide slightly higher mean plasma concentrations in children, ensuring that the majority will achieve a therapeutic concentration equivalent to 300 mg twice daily in adults. There are insufficient safety data to recommend the use of ZIAGEN in infants less than three months old.

Geriatrics: Clinical studies of ZIAGEN did not include sufficient numbers of patients aged 65 and over to determine whether they respond differently from younger patients. Other reported clinical experience has not identified differences in responses between the elderly and younger patients. In general, dose selection for an elderly patient should be cautious, reflecting the greater frequency of decreased hepatic, renal, or cardiac function, and of concomitant disease or other drug therapy. Once-daily ZIAGEN 600 mg dosing has not been studied in the elderly and is not recommended for use in this population.

Use of Once Daily ZIAGEN in Patients with Comorbid Conditions and in the Elderly: A ZIAGEN 600 mg OD regimen should not be used in patients over 65 years of age, or in patients with comorbid conditions such as hepatic or renal failure, as this dosing regimen has not been studied in this population.

ADVERSE REACTIONS: Adverse Drug Reaction Overview: Hypersensitivity Reactions: Fatal hypersensitivity reactions have been associated with therapy with ZIAGEN (abacavir sulfate).

Therapy with ZIAGEN or any other medicinal product containing abacavir **must not** be restarted following a hypersensitivity reaction because more severe symptoms will recur within hours and may include life-threatening hypotension and death. Patients developing signs or symptoms of hypersensitivity should discontinue treatment as soon as a hypersensitivity reaction is first suspected, and must seek medical evaluation immediately. To avoid a delay in diagnosis and minimize the risk of a life-threatening hypersensitivity reaction, ZIAGEN should be permanently discontinued if hypersensitivity cannot be ruled out, even when other diagnoses are possible (respiratory diseases, flu-like illness, gastroenteritis or reactions to other medications). ZIAGEN or any other medicinal product containing abacavir should not be restarted even if a recurrence of symptoms occurs following rechallenge with alternative medication(s).

Severe or fatal hypersensitivity reactions can occur within hours after ZIAGEN reintroduction in patients who have no identified history or unrecognized symptoms of hypersensitivity during their initial period of use of ZIAGEN (see Warnings and Precautions).

Regardless of a patient's HLA-B*5701 status, if therapy with ZIAGEN or any other medicinal product containing abacavir has been discontinued and restarting therapy is under consideration, the reason for discontinuation should be evaluated to ensure that the patient did not have symptoms of a hypersensitivity reaction. If a hypersensitivity reaction cannot be ruled out, ZIAGEN or any other medicinal product containing abacavir (e.g. KIVEXA, TRIZIVIR) should not be restarted.

Clinical Trial Adverse Drug Reactions: Because clinical trials are conducted under very specific conditions the adverse reaction rates observed in the clinical trials may not reflect the rates observed in practice and should not be compared to the rates in the clinical trials of another drug. Adverse drug reaction information from clinical trials is useful for identifying drug-related adverse events and for approximating rates.

Overall, in clinical trials conducted before the introduction of screening for the HLA-B*5701 allele, hypersensitivity to abacavir was reported in approximately 8% of patients in 9 clinical trials (range: 2% to 9%). This reaction is characterized by the appearance of symptoms indicating multi-organ/body-system involvement. Symptoms can occur at any time during therapy however they usually appear within the first six weeks (median time to onset 11 days) of initiation of treatment with abacavir.

In controlled study (CNA30021), more patients taking ZIAGEN 600 mg once daily had severe hypersensitivity reactions than patients taking ZIAGEN 300 mg twice daily (see Warnings and Precautions and Dosage and Administration).

Almost all patients developing hypersensitivity reactions will have fever and/or rash (usually maculopapular or urticarial) as part of the syndrome, however reactions have occurred without rash or fever.

The signs and symptoms of this hypersensitivity reaction are listed below. Those reported **in at least 10% of patients** with a hypersensitivity reaction are in bold text.

Gastrointestinal Tract: abdominal pain, diarrhea, mouth ulceration, **nausea, vomiting**.
Hematological: lymphopenia.
Liver/Pancreas: elevated liver function tests, hepatic failure.
Miscellaneous: anaphylaxis, conjunctivitis, edema, **fatigue**, **fever**, hypotension, lymphadenopathy, **malaise**.
Musculoskeletal: arthralgia, elevated creatine phosphokinase, **myalgia**, rarely myolysis.
Neurological/Psychiatric: headache, paraesthesia.
Respiratory Tract: adult respiratory distress syndrome, **cough, dyspnea**, respiratory failure, sore throat.
Skin: rash (usually maculopapular or urticarial).
Urology: elevated creatinine, renal failure.

Some patients who experienced a hypersensitivity reaction were initially thought to have acute onset or worsening respiratory disease. The diagnosis of a hypersensitivity reaction should be carefully considered for patients presenting with symptoms of acute onset respiratory diseases, even if alternative respiratory diagnoses (pneumonia, bronchitis, pharyngitis) or flu-like illness, gastroenteritis or reactions to other medications are possible.

Symptoms worsen with continued therapy, and usually resolve upon discontinuation of ZIAGEN.

Restarting ZIAGEN or any other medicinal product containing abacavir following a hypersensitivity reaction results in a prompt return of symptoms within hours. This recurrence of the hypersensitivity reaction may be more severe than on initial presentation, and may include life-threatening hypotension and death. Regardless of their HLA-B*5701 status, patients who develop this hypersensitivity reaction must discontinue ZIAGEN and must never be rechallenged with ZIAGEN or any other medicinal product containing abacavir (e.g. KIVEXA, TRIZIVIR).

For many of the other adverse events reported, it is unclear whether they are related to ZIAGEN, to the wide range of medicinal products used in the management of HIV disease or as a result of the disease process.

Many of the events listed (nausea, vomiting, diarrhea, fever, fatigue, rash) occur commonly as part of abacavir hypersensitivity. Therefore, patients with any of these symptoms should be carefully evaluated for the presence of this hypersensitivity reaction.

The majority of the events listed below have not been treatment limiting. Care however, must be taken to eliminate the possibility of a hypersensitivity reaction if any of these symptoms occur.

The following convention has been used for classification: very common (>1/10), common (>1/100, <1/10), uncommon (>1/1000, <1/100), rare (>1/10 000, <1/1000) very rare (<1/10 000).

Gastrointestinal: Common: diarrhea, nausea, vomiting. Rare: pancreatitis has been reported, but a causal relationship to ZIAGEN treatment is uncertain.

Metabolism and Nutrition Disorders: Common: anorexia, hyperlactatemia. Rare: lactic acidosis (see Warnings and Precautions).

Nervous System Disorders: Common: headache.

Others: Common: fatigue, fever, lethargy.

Skin and Subcutaneous Tissue Disorders: Common: rash (without systemic symptoms). Very rare: erythema multiforme, Stevens-Johnson syndrome and toxic epidermal necrolysis.

Cases of lactic acidosis, sometimes fatal, usually associated with severe hepatomegaly and hepatic steatosis, have been reported with the use of nucleoside analogues.

In controlled clinical studies laboratory abnormalities related to ZIAGEN treatment were uncommon, with no differences in incidence observed between ZIAGEN-treated patients and the control arms.

ZIAGEN Once Daily vs. ZIAGEN Twice Daily (Study CNA30021): Treatment emergent clinical adverse reactions (rated by the investigator as at least moderate) with a ≥5% frequency during therapy with ZIAGEN 600 mg once daily and efavirenz 600 mg once daily from Study 30021 were similar. For hypersensitivity reactions, patients receiving ZIAGEN once daily showed a rate of 9% in comparison to a rate of 7% for patients receiving ZIAGEN twice daily. However, patients receiving ZIAGEN 600 mg once daily, experienced a significantly higher incidence of severe drug hypersensitivity reactions and severe diarrhea compared to patients who received ZIAGEN 300 mg twice daily. Five percent (5%) of patients receiving ZIAGEN 600 mg once daily had severe drug hypersensitivity reactions compared to 2% of patients receiving ZIAGEN 300 mg twice daily. Two percent (2%) of patients receiving ZIAGEN 600 mg once daily had severe diarrhea while none of the patients receiving ZIAGEN 300 mg twice daily had this event.

Post-Market Adverse Drug Reactions: In addition to adverse events reported from clinical trials, the following events have been identified during use of abacavir in clinical practice. Because they are reported voluntarily from a population of unknown size, estimates of frequency cannot be made. These events have been chosen for inclusion due to either their seriousness, frequency of reporting, potential causal connection to abacavir, or a combination of these factors.

Body as a Whole: redistribution/accumulation of body fat (see Warnings and Precautions, Endocrine and Metabolism).

Hepatic: lactic acidosis and hepatic steatosis (see Warnings and Precautions, Hepatic/Biliary/Pancreatic).

Skin: Suspected Stevens-Johnson syndrome (SJS) and toxic epidermal necrolysis (TEN) have been reported in patients receiving abacavir primarily in combination with medications known to be associated with SJS and TEN, respectively. Because of the overlap of the clinical signs and symptoms between hypersensitivity to abacavir, SJS and TEN, and the possibility of multiple drug sensitivities in some patients, abacavir should be discontinued and not restarted in such cases. There have been reports of erythema multiforme with abacavir use.

Other Warnings: A patient with a diagnosis of AIDS dementia and a history of seizure disorder experienced a seizure 3 days after stopping ZIAGEN therapy. In the absence of an autopsy, a definitive diagnosis could not be adequately made, and a possible relationship to abacavir therefore could not be ruled out.

DRUG INTERACTIONS: Overview: Based on the results of in vitro experiments and the known major metabolic pathways of abacavir sulfate, the potential for drug interactions involving abacavir sulfate is low. Abacavir sulfate shows low potential to inhibit metabolism mediated by the cytochrome P450 3A4 enzyme. It has also been shown in vitro not to interact with drugs that are metabolized by CYP3A4, CYP2C9 or CYP2D6 enzymes. Induction of hepatic metabolism has not been observed in clinical studies. Therefore, there is little potential for drug interactions with antiretroviral protease inhibitors and other drugs metabolized by major P450 enzymes. Clinical studies have shown that there are no clinically significant interactions between abacavir sulfate, zidovudine, and lamivudine.

Drug-Drug Interactions: The drugs listed in Table 1 are based on either drug interaction case reports or studies, or potential interactions due to the expected magnitude and seriousness of the interaction (i.e. those identified as contraindicated).

Table 1: ZIAGEN

Established or Potential Drug-Drug Interactions

Proper Name	Effect	Clinical Comment
Ethanol	In men, the metabolism of abacavir sulfate is altered.	In men, the metabolism of abacavir sulfate is altered by concomitant ethanol resulting in an increase in AUC of abacavir of about 41%. The clinical significance of this is unknown. In men, abacavir sulfate has no effect on the metabolism of ethanol. This interaction has not been studied in women.
Methadone	Changes in abacavir pharmacokinetics.	In a pharmacokinetic study, coadministration of 600 mg abacavir twice daily and methadone showed a 35% reduction in abacavir C_{max} and a 1 hour delay, but AUC was unchanged. The changes in abacavir pharmacokinetics are not considered clinically relevant. In this study abacavir increased methadone systemic clearance by 22%. This change is not considered clinically relevant for the majority of patients, however occasionally methadone retitration may be required.
Retinoids	Interaction with elimination is possible.	Retinoid compounds such as isotretinoin, are eliminated via alcohol dehydrogenase. Interaction with abacavir is possible but has not been studied.

DOSAGE AND ADMINISTRATION: ZIAGEN (abacavir sulfate) is available as an oral solution for use in children and for those patients for whom tablets are inappropriate.

Dosing Considerations: An Information for the Patient Leaflet and Warning Card that provide information about recognition of hypersensitivity reactions should be dispensed with each new prescription and refill.

ZIAGEN can be taken with or without food.

Recommended Dose and Dosage Adjustment: Adults: The recommended oral dose of ZIAGEN for adults is 600 mg daily administered as either 300 mg twice daily or 600 mg once daily, in combination with other antiretroviral agents. The use of 600 mg once daily may be associated with a higher incidence of severe hypersensitivity reactions.

The use of once daily ZIAGEN 600 mg has not been studied in patients less than 18 years of age.

The use of once daily ZIAGEN 600 mg has not been studied in elderly patients or patients with comorbid conditions.

Adolescents Over 12 Years of Age: The recommended dose of ZIAGEN is 300 mg (one tablet or 15 mL of oral solution) twice daily in combination with other antiretroviral agents.

Adolescents and Pediatric Patients (over three months of age to age 12): The recommended oral dose of ZIAGEN for adolescent and pediatric patients 3 months up to 12 years of age is 8 mg/kg twice daily (up to a maximum of 300 mg twice daily) in combination with other antiretroviral agents.

Children Less Than Three Months of Age: There are insufficient data to recommend the use of ZIAGEN in infants less than three months old (see Warnings and Precautions, Pediatrics).

Change in Regimen: Patients changing to the once daily regimen should take 300 mg twice a day and switch to 600 mg once a day the following morning. Where an evening once daily regimen is preferred, 300 mg of ZIAGEN should be taken on the first morning only, followed by 600 mg in the evening. When changing back to a twice daily regimen, patients should complete the day's treatment and start 300 mg twice a day the following morning.

Patients, guardians and caregivers of pediatric patients must be made aware of the potential signs and symptoms of a hypersensitivity reaction to abacavir and that abacavir must be stopped and never restarted following a possible hypersensitivity reaction (see Warnings and Precautions and Adverse Reactions).

Renal Impairment: No dosage adjustment of ZIAGEN is necessary in patients with renal dysfunction. However, ZIAGEN should be avoided in patients with end-stage renal disease. The use of ZIAGEN 600 mg once daily has not been studied in patients with renal impairment and is not recommended for use in this population (see Warnings and Precautions, Renal).

Hepatic Impairment: Abacavir is primarily metabolized by the liver. The recommended dose of ZIAGEN in patients with mild hepatic impairment (Child-Pugh score 5-6) who have confirmed cirrhosis is 200 mg twice a day. To enable dose reduction ZIAGEN oral solution should be used for the treatment of these patients. ZIAGEN is contraindicated in patients with moderate or severe hepatic impairment, as the pharmacokinetics have not been studied in these patient groups. (See Contraindications and Warnings and Precautions, Impaired Hepatic Function.)

Missed Dose: If the patient forgets to take their medicine, they should take it as soon as they remember. Then continue as before. Patients should not take a double dose to make up for forgotten individual doses. If a patient stops therapy with ZIAGEN because of side effects or illness, they must check with their doctor before restarting therapy to make sure that symptoms of a hypersensitivity reaction have not been missed.

OVERDOSAGE:

There is no known antidote for ZIAGEN (abacavir sulfate).

If overdosage occurs, the patient should be monitored, and standard supportive treatment applied as required. Although no data is available, administration of activated charcoal may be used to aid in the removal of unabsorbed drug. It is not known whether abacavir sulfate can be removed by peritoneal dialysis or hemodialysis.

Limited data are available on the consequences of ingestion of acute overdoses in humans. Single doses up to 1200 mg and daily doses up to 1800 mg of abacavir sulfate have been administered to patients in clinical studies. No unexpected adverse reactions were reported. The effects of higher doses are not known. No specific signs or symptoms have been identified following such overdose.

For management of a suspected drug overdose, contact your regional Poison Control Centre. See the *CPS* Directory section for a list of Poison Control Centres.

ACTION AND CLINICAL PHARMACOLOGY: Mechanism of Action: Abacavir is a nucleoside analogue reverse transcriptase inhibitor. Abacavir is metabolized intracellularly to the active moiety, carbovir 5'-triphosphate (TP), a potent, selective inhibitor of HIV-1 and HIV-2, including HIV-1 isolates with reduced susceptibility to zidovudine, lamivudine, zalcitabine, didanosine and nevirapine. In vitro studies have demonstrated that its mechanism of action in relation to HIV is inhibition of the HIV reverse transcriptase enzyme, an event which results in chain termination and interruption of the viral replication cycle. Abacavir shows synergy in vitro in combination with nevirapine or zidovudine. It has been shown to be additive in combination with didanosine, zalcitabine, lamivudine and stavudine.

Pharmacokinetics: Absorption: Abacavir sulfate is rapidly and well absorbed following oral administration. The absolute bioavailability of oral abacavir sulfate in adults is about 83%. Following oral administration, the mean time (t_{max}) to maximal serum concentrations of abacavir is about 1.5 hours for the tablet formulation and about 1.0 hour for the solution formulation. There are no differences observed between the AUC for the tablet or solution. At 300 mg twice daily, the steady state C_{max} of abacavir sulfate tablets is approximately 3 µg/mL, and the AUC over a dosing interval of 12 hours is approximately 6 µg·h/mL. The C_{max} value for the oral solution is slightly higher than the tablet.

Food delayed absorption and decreased C_{max} but did not affect overall plasma concentrations (AUC). Therefore ZIAGEN can be taken with or without food.

In a study of 20 HIV-infected patients receiving abacavir 300 mg twice daily, with only one 300 mg dose taken prior to the 24 h sampling period, the geometric mean terminal carbovir-TP intracellular half-life at steady-state was 20.6 h, compared to the geometric mean abacavir plasma half-life in this study of 2.6 h. The steady state pharmacokinetic properties of abacavir 600 mg once daily was compared to abacavir 300 mg twice daily in a crossover study in 27 HIV-infected patients. Intracellular carbovir triphosphate exposures in peripheral blood mononuclear cells were higher for abacavir 600 mg once daily with respect to $AUC_{24,ss}$ (32 %, higher), $C_{max24,ss}$ (99% higher) and trough values (18% higher), compared to the 300 mg twice daily regimen. These data support the use of abacavir 600 mg once daily for the treatment of HIV-infected patients. Additionally, the efficacy and safety of this combination given once daily has been demonstrated in a pivotal clinical study.

STORAGE AND STABILITY: Tablets: ZIAGEN tablets should be stored between 15 and 30°C.
Oral Solution: ZIAGEN oral solution should be stored between 15 and 25°C.

SPECIAL HANDLING INSTRUCTIONS: Not applicable.

INFORMATION FOR THE PATIENT: Published in e-CPS, available by subscription at www.e-cps.ca.

DOSAGE FORMS, COMPOSITION AND PACKAGING: Oral Solution: Each mL of clear to opalescent, yellowish, strawberry-banana flavored liquid, contains: abacavir sulfate equivalent to abacavir 20 mg. Nonmedicinal ingredients: artificial strawberry and banana flavors, citric acid (anhydrous), hydrochloric acid, methylparaben, propylene glycol, propylparaben, saccharin sodium, sodium citrate (dihydrate), sodium hydroxide and sorbitol solution. Bottles of 240 mL.

Tablets: Each yellow, biconvex, capsule-shaped, film-coated tablet, scored and embossed with "GX 623" on both sides, contains: abacavir sulfate equivalent to abacavir 300 mg. Nonmedicinal ingredients: colloidal silicon dioxide, hydroxypropyl methylcellulose, magnesium stearate, microcrystalline cellulose, polysorbate 80, sodium starch glycolate, titanium dioxide, triacetin and yellow iron oxide. Bottles of 60.

(Shown in Product Identification Section)

Zinecard® Ⓟ

dexrazoxane

Cardioprotective Agent

Pfizer

Date of Revision: April 8, 2009

Caution: ZINECARD (dexrazoxane) is a potent drug and should be used only by physicians experienced with cancer chemotherapy drugs (see Warnings and Precautions). Blood counts and hepatic function tests should be performed regularly due to the possibility of additive myelosuppressive effects. ZINECARD should not be administered in a dose that exceeds 500 mg/m².

PHARMACOLOGY: ZINECARD (dexrazoxane) is a cyclic derivative of EDTA which, unlike EDTA, readily penetrates cell membranes. ZINECARD was shown to be able to protect the myocardium from anthracycline-induced cardiotoxicity. The mechanism by which ZINECARD exerts its cardioprotective activity is not fully understood. Results of laboratory studies suggest that dexrazoxane is converted intracellularly to an open-ringed chelating agent which interferes with iron-mediated free radical generation thought to be responsible, in part, for anthracycline-induced cardiotoxicity.

The efficacy of ZINECARD in preventing/reducing the incidence and severity of doxorubicin-induced cardiomyopathy was demonstrated in a series of prospective studies. In these studies, patients were treated with a doxorubicin-containing regimen and either ZINECARD or placebo starting with the first course of chemotherapy. Cardiac function was assessed by measurement of the left ventricular ejection fraction (LVEF) utilizing resting multigated nuclear medicine (MUGA) scans and by clinical evaluations. Patients receiving ZINECARD had significantly smaller mean decreases from baseline in LVEF and lower incidences of congestive heart failure than the control group. The difference in decline from baseline in LVEF was evident beginning with a cumulative doxorubicin dose of 150 mg/m² and reached statistical significance in patients who received ≥400 mg/m² of doxorubicin. The studies also assessed the effect of the addition of ZINECARD on the antitumor efficacy of the chemotherapy regimens.

In one of the studies (the largest of the breast cancer studies) patients with advanced breast cancer receiving fluorouracil, Adriamycin and cyclophosphamide (FAC) with ZINECARD had a lower response rate and a shorter time to progression than patients on the control arm although the survival of the patients who did or did not receive ZINECARD with FAC was similar. It appears that ZINECARD may potentiate doxorubicin toxicity in some patients, thus causing increased early dropout rate or decreased dose-intensity. More non-responders dropped out by course 3 in the ZINECARD arm. The non-responders correlated to dose delays due to additive myelotoxicity.

Two of the randomized breast cancer studies evaluating the efficacy and safety of FAC with either ZINECARD or placebo were amended to allow patients on the placebo arm who had attained a cumulative dose of doxorubicin of 300 mg/m² (6 courses of FAC) to receive FAC with open-label ZINECARD for each subsequent course.

Most of these patients had already experienced a partial or complete response or have stable disease. Analyses of these amended studies indicate that significant though not complete cardioprotection can be obtained with the administration of ZINECARD only after an accumulated dose of 300 mg/m² of doxorubicin. In addition, the time to tumor progression and survival of these 2 groups of patients were also compared. Results demonstrate significantly longer overall survival for the group of patients who received ZINECARD starting with the seventh course of FAC treatment.

INDICATIONS: ZINECARD (dexrazoxane) is indicated for reducing (preventing) the incidence and severity of cardiotoxicity associated with doxorubicin administration for the treatment of breast cancer in patients who have already experienced a partial response or at least maintain stable disease.

ZINECARD should be used only with chemotherapy regimens containing doxorubicin.

ZINECARD should be used only after tolerance to a full dose doxorubicin has been established (see Precautions).

CONTRAINDICATIONS: ZINECARD (dexrazoxane) should not be used as a chemotherapeutic agent.

WARNINGS: ZINECARD may add to the myelosuppression caused by chemotherapeutic agents. ZINECARD may interfere with the antitumor activity of chemotherapeutic agents. There is some evidence that the use of dexrazoxane concurrently with the initiation of fluorouracil, doxorubicin and cyclophosphamide (FAC) therapy interferes with the antitumor efficacy of the regimen, and this use is not recommended.

ZINECARD should only be used in those patients who have received a cumulative doxorubicin dose of 300 mg/m² and are continuing with doxorubicin therapy.

Although clinical studies have shown that patients receiving FAC with ZINECARD may receive a higher cumulative dose of doxorubicin before experiencing cardiac toxicity than patients receiving FAC without ZINECARD, the use of ZINECARD in patients who have already received a cumulative dose of doxorubicin of 300 mg/m² without ZINECARD, does not eliminate the potential for anthracycline induced cardiac toxicity. Therefore, cardiac function should be carefully monitored.

Pregnancy: ZINECARD should be used during pregnancy only if the potential benefit justifies the potential risk to the fetus. There is no conclusive information about dexrazoxane adversely affecting human fertility, or causing teratogenesis; however, in rats and rabbits, it is teratogenic and embryotoxic. Therefore, women of childbearing potential should be advised to practice effective contraception.

Lactation: Mothers should be advised not to breast-feed while undergoing therapy with ZINECARD (see Precautions).

Children: Safety and effectiveness in children have not been established.

PRECAUTIONS: General: In controlled studies, a slightly higher incidence of infection associated with granulocytopenia occurred in patients receiving ZINECARD. As ZINECARD will always be used with cytotoxic drugs, patients should be monitored closely. While the myelosuppressive effects of ZINECARD at the recommended dose are considered to be mild, additive effects upon the myelosuppressive activity of chemotherapeutic agents may occur.

ZINECARD should be administered only after the tolerance of the patient to the full dose of doxorubicin-containing chemotherapeutic regimen has been determined. ZINECARD should be given only when there is no need for dose reduction or dose delay, of the chemotherapeutic regimen due to myelosuppression or other toxicities, in 2 consecutive courses.

Currently, the only clinical experience with late administration is in patients who were crossed-over from placebo and received ZINECARD after 6 courses of chemotherapy. ZINECARD was found to retain its cardioprotective effect in these patients. However, an incidence of up to 20% of cardiovascular events was seen prior to the initiation of ZINECARD administration. Therefore, the administration of ZINECARD should not be delayed beyond the 7th course of therapy.

Laboratory Tests: As ZINECARD may add to the myelosuppressive effects of cytotoxic drugs, frequent complete blood counts, including one prior to each treatment, are recommended (see Adverse Effects).

Drug Interactions: Based on a kinetic study, ZINECARD does not appear to influence the pharmacokinetics of doxorubicin.

Lactation: It is not known whether this drug is excreted in human milk. Because many drugs are excreted in human milk and because of the potential for serious adverse reactions in nursing infants from dexrazoxane, it is recommended that nursing be **discontinued during treatment.**

Geriatrics: Clinical studies of ZINECARD did not include sufficient numbers of subjects 65 and over to determine whether they respond differently from younger subjects. Other reported clinical experience has not identified differences in responses between the elderly and younger patients. In general, elderly patients should be treated with caution due to the greater frequency of decreased hepatic, renal, or cardiac function, and concomitant disease or other drug therapy.

Patients with Moderate or Severe Renal Insufficiency: Greater exposure to dexrazoxane may occur in patients with compromised renal function. The ZINECARD dose should be reduced by 50% in patients with creatinine clearance values <40 mL/min (see Dosage).

Hepatic Insufficiency: The pharmacokinetics of ZINECARD have not been evaluated in patients with hepatic impairment. The ZINECARD dose is dependent upon the dose of doxorubicin. Since a doxorubicin dose reduction is recommended in the presence of hyperbilirubinemia, the ZINECARD dosage is proportionately reduced in patients with hepatic impairment (see Dosage).

ADVERSE EFFECTS: ZINECARD (dexrazoxane) at a dose of 500 mg/m² has been administered in combination with fluorouracil, doxorubicin, and cyclophosphamide (FAC) or cyclophosphamide, doxorubicin and vincristine (CAV) in randomized placebo controlled double-blind studies to patients with either metastatic breast cancer (FAC) or extensive disease small cell lung cancer (CAV). The dose of doxorubicin was 50 mg/m² in each of the trials. Courses were repeated every 3 weeks provided recovery from toxicity had occurred. Table 1 lists the incidence of clinical adverse experiences for patients receiving either ZINECARD or placebo in the breast cancer studies.

Table 1: ZINECARD
Incidence of Clinical Adverse Experiences

Adverse Experience	Percentage of Breast Cancer Patients with Adverse Experience	
	FAC+ZINECARD N=244	FAC+Placebo N=280
Alopecia	94%	96%
Nausea	82	89
Vomiting	63	77
Fatigue/Malaise	62	64
Anorexia	50	52
Stomatitis	36	45
Fever	35	33
Infection and/or Sepsis	31	28

(cont'd)

Table 1: ZINECARD *(cont'd)*

Incidence of Clinical Adverse Experiences

	Percentage of Breast Cancer Patients with Adverse Experience	
Adverse Experience	**FAC+ZINECARD N=244**	**FAC+Placebo N=280**
Diarrhea	22	24
Neurotoxicity	16	13
Pain on Injection	11	4
Streaking/Erythema	7	5
Dysphagia	6	10
Phlebitis	5	5
Esophagitis	5	9
Urticaria	4	2
Hemorrhage	2	2
Extravasation	2	1
Recall Skin Reaction	1	2
CHF	1	5

The only adverse experience that was observed in 5% more patients on FAC+ZINECARD than on FAC+placebo was pain on injection. However, the early drop-out rate for patients receiving ZINECARD was higher than for patients receiving placebo.

Myelosuppression: Eighty-eight percent (88%) of breast cancer patients receiving FAC+500 mg/m² ZINECARD and 85% of patients receiving FAC+placebo experienced Grade 3 or 4 granulocytopenia. Ten percent (10%) of patients receiving FAC+ZINECARD and 9% of patients receiving FAC+placebo experienced Grade 3 or 4 thrombocytopenia at some time while on study.

The median decline in hemoglobin levels from baseline was 2.6 g/dL for patients receiving FAC+ZINECARD or FAC+placebo.

Hepatic and Renal: Very few patients receiving FAC+ZINECARD or FAC+placebo experienced marked abnormalities in hepatic or renal function tests; the frequency and severity of abnormalities in bilirubin, alkaline phosphatase, LDH, BUN, and creatinine levels were similar.

OVERDOSE:

Symptoms: There have been no instances of drug overdose in the clinical studies sponsored by either Pharmacia Corporation or the National Cancer Institute, U.S.A. The maximum dose administered during the cardioprotection trials was 1000 mg/m² every 3 weeks.

Treatment: Disposition studies with ZINECARD (dexrazoxane) have not been conducted in cancer patients undergoing dialysis. However, retention of a significant dose fraction (>0.4) of the unchanged drug in the plasma pool, minimal tissue partitioning or binding, and availability of greater than 90% of the systemic drug levels in the unbound form suggest that its toxicity and efficacy would be altered by its removal using conventional peritoneal or hemodialysis.

There is no known antidote. Instances of suspected overdose should be managed with good supportive care until resolution of myelosuppression and related conditions is complete. Management of overdose should include treatment of infections, fluid regulation, and maintenance of nutritional requirements.

For management of a suspected drug overdose, CPhA recommends that you contact your **regional Poison Control Centre**. See the *CPS* Directory section for a list of Poison Control Centres.

DOSAGE: ZINECARD (dexrazoxane) should be reconstituted with M/6 Sodium Lactate Injection, USP, to give a concentration of 10 mg ZINECARD for each mL of sodium lactate. The reconstituted solution should be given by slow i.v. push or rapid drip i.v. infusion from an empty i.v. bag to which the solution has been added. No further dilution is necessary. ZINECARD should be given as a single administration, at any point, within a time period of 30 minutes before to 15 minutes after the start of doxorubicin administration.

The recommended dosage ratio of ZINECARD: doxorubicin is 10:1 (e.g. 500 mg/m² ZINECARD: 50 mg/m² doxorubicin) (see Precautions). Since a doxorubicin dose reduction is recommended in the presence of hyperbilirubinemia, the ZINECARD dosage should be proportionately reduced in patients with hepatic impairment to maintain the 10:1 ratio of dexrazoxane:doxorubicin.

In patients with moderate to severe renal dysfunction (creatinine clearance values <40 mL/min), the recommended dosage ratio of ZINECARD:doxorubicin is 5:1 (eg. 250 mg/m² ZINECARD:50 mg/m² doxorubicin). Creatinine clearance can be determined from a 24-hour urinary creatinine collection or estimated using the Crockcroft-Gault equation (assuming stable renal function).

$$\text{ClCr} = \frac{[140-\text{age (years)}] \times \text{weight (kg)}}{72 \times \text{serum creatinine (mg/dL)}}$$

For females, multiply the result by 0.85.

ZINECARD should be administered only after the tolerance of the patient to the full dose of doxorubicin-containing chemotherapeutic regimen has been determined. ZINECARD should be given only when there is no need for dose reduction or dose delay, of the chemotherapeutic regimen due to myelosuppression or other toxicities, in 2 consecutive courses.

ZINECARD should be given only to patients who have already experienced partial response or at least maintained stable disease.

Reconstituted Solutions: See Table 2.

Recommended Diluent for Reconstitution: M/6 Sodium Lactate Injection, USP (supplied in the carton with ZINECARD).

Table 2: ZINECARD

Reconstitution Table

Vial Size	Diluent Added to Vial (mL)	Approximate Available Volume (mL)	Nominal Concentration
250 mg	25	25	10
500 mg	50	50	10

Storage: The reconstituted solution should be stored for a maximum of 6 hours under refrigeration, 2 to 8°C. Unused solutions should be discarded.

Incompatibility: Unless specific compatibility data are available, ZINECARD should not be mixed with other drugs.

Guidelines for Safe Preparation and Handling: Caution in the handling and preparation of the reconstituted solution must be exercised and the use of gloves is recommended. If ZINECARD (dexrazoxane) powder or solution contacts the skin or mucosae, immediately wash thoroughly with soap and water.

Procedures normally used for proper handling and disposal of anticancer drugs should be considered for use with ZINECARD. However, there is no general agreement that all of the procedures recommended in the guidelines are necessary or appropriate.

Preparation and Handling: 1. Preparation of the reconstituted solutions should be done in a vertical laminar flow hood (Biological Safety Cabinet—Class II).

2. Personnel handling dexrazoxane solutions should wear PVC gloves, safety glasses and protective clothing such as disposable gowns and masks. If dexrazoxane solutions contact the skin or mucosa, the area should be washed with soap and water immediately.

3. Personnel regularly involved in the preparation and handling of antineoplastics should have blood examinations on a regular basis.

Disposal: 1. Avoid contact with skin and inhalation of airborne particles by use of PVC gloves and disposable gowns and masks.

2. All needles, syringes, vials and other materials which have come in contact with dexrazoxane should be segregated in plastic bags, sealed, and marked as hazardous waste. Incinerate at 1000°C or higher. Sealed containers may explode if a tight seal exists.

3. If incineration is not available, dexrazoxane may be detoxified by adding sodium hypochlorite solution (household bleach) to the vial, in sufficient quantity to decolorize the dexrazoxane, care being taken to vent the vial to avoid a pressure build-up of the chlorine gas which is generated. Dispose of detoxified vials in a safe manner.

Needles, Syringes, Disposable and Nondisposable Equipment: Rinse equipment with an appropriate quantity of sodium hypochlorite solution. Discard the solution in the sewer system with running water and discard disposable equipment in a safe manner. Thoroughly wash nondisposable equipment in soap and water.

Spillage/Contamination: Wear gloves, mask, protective clothing. Treat spilled liquid with sodium hypochlorite solution. Carefully absorb solution with gauze pads or towels, wash area with water and absorb with gauze or towels again and place in polyethylene bag; seal, double bag and mark as hazardous waste. Disposal of waste by incineration or by other methods approved for hazardous materials. Personnel involved in clean-up should wash with soap and water.

SUPPLIED: 250 mg: Each single dose vial contains: dexrazoxane 250 mg. pH is adjusted with hydrochloric acid, NF. Also contains a 25 mL vial of M/6 sodium lactate injection USP. Each mL contains: anhydrous sodium lactate 18.6 mg in Water for Injection. pH is adjusted with sodium hydroxide NF and/or hydrochloric acid NF. Store at controlled room temperature, 15 to 30°C.

500 mg: Each single dose vial contains: dexrazoxane 500 mg. pH is adjusted with hydrochloric acid, NF. Also contains a 50 mL vial of M/6 sodium lactate injection USP. Each mL contains: anhydrous sodium lactate 18.6 mg in Water for Injection. pH is adjusted with sodium hydroxide NF and/or hydrochloric acid NF. Store at controlled room temperature, 15 to 30°C.

Zithromax™ Ⓟ

azithromycin dihydrate

Antibiotic

Pfizer

Date of Preparation: May 13, 1994
Date of Revision: August 15, 2007

PHARMACOLOGY: ZITHROMAX (azithromycin dihydrate), a macrolide antibiotic of the azalide subclass, exerts its antibacterial action by binding to the 50s ribosomal subunits of susceptible bacteria and suppressing protein synthesis.

Following oral administration, azithromycin is rapidly absorbed (T_{max}=2 to 3 hours) and distributed widely throughout the body. Rapid movement of azithromycin from blood into tissue results in significantly higher azithromycin concentrations in tissue than in plasma (up to 50 times the maximum observed concentration in plasma). The absolute bioavailability is approximately 37%. When azithromycin suspension was administered with food to 28 adult healthy male subjects, the rate of absorption (C_{max}) was increased by 56% while the extent of absorption (AUC) was unchanged.

Food does not affect the absorption of azithromycin in the tablet dosage form. Azithromycin tablets and powder for oral suspension can be taken with or without food.

Pharmacokinetics: Adults: Plasma concentrations of azithromycin decline in a polyphasic pattern, resulting in an average terminal half-life of 68 hours. The prolonged half-life is likely due to extensive uptake and subsequent release of drug from tissues. Over the dose range of 250 to 1000 mg orally, the serum concentrations are related to dose. The long tissue half-life and large volume of distribution result from intracytoplasmic uptake and storage in lysosomal phospholipid complexes.

In adults, the following pharmacokinetic data have been reported: See Table 1.

Table 1: ZITHROMAX

Pharmacokinetic Data in Adults

Dose/Dosage Form	Subjects	C_{max} (µg/mL)	T_{max} (h)	AUC (µ·h/mL)	$T_{1/2}$ (h)
500 mg/250 mg tablet	12; fasted	0.34	2.1	2.49[a]	—
500 mg/250 mg table	12; fed	0.41	2.3	2.40[a]	—
1200 mg/600 mg tablet	12; fasted	0.66	2.5	6.8[b]	40

[a] 0-48 h.
[b] 0-last.

Biliary excretion of azithromycin, predominantly as unchanged drug, is a main route of elimination. Over the course of a week, approximately 6% of the administered dose appears as unchanged drug in the urine.

I.V. Administration: In patients hospitalized with community-acquired pneumonia (CAP) receiving single daily 1-hour i.v. infusions for 2 to 5 days of 500 mg azithromycin at a concentration of 2 mg/mL, the median maximum concentration (C_{max}) achieved was 3.00 µg/mL (range: 1.70 to 6.00 µg/mL) while the 24-hour trough level was 0.18 µg/mL (range: 0.07 to 0.60 µg/mL) and the AUC_{24} was 8.50 µg·h/mL (range: 5.10 to 19.60 µg·h/mL). The median C_{max}, 24-hour trough and AUC_{24} values were 1.20 µg/mL (range: 0.89 to 1.36 µg/mL), 0.18 µg/mL (range: 0.15 to 0.21 µg/mL) and 7.98 µg·h/mL (range: 6.45 to 9.80 µg·h/mL), respectively, in normal volunteers receiving a 3-hour i.v. infusion of 500 mg azithromycin at a concentration of 1 mg/mL. Similar pharmacokinetic values were obtained in patients hospitalized with CAP that received the same 3-hour dosage regimen for 2 to 5 days. See Table 2.

The average Cl_t and Vd values were 10.18 mL/min/kg and 33.3 L/kg, respectively, in 18 normal volunteers receiving 1000 to 4000 mg doses given as 1 mg/mL over 2 hours.

Comparison of the plasma pharmacokinetic parameters following the 1st and 5th daily doses of 500 mg i.v. azithromycin shows only an 8% increase in C_{max} but a 61% increase in AUC_{24} reflecting the 3-fold rise in C_{24} trough levels.

In a multiple-dose study in 12 normal volunteers utilizing a 500 mg (1 mg/mL) 1-hour i.v. dosage regimen for 5 days, the amount of administered azithromycin dose excreted in the urine in 24 hours was about 11% after the first dose and 14% after the 5th dose. These values are greater than the reported 6% excreted unchanged in urine after oral azithromycin administration.

Special Populations: Pediatric Pharmacokinetics: Pharmacokinetics in children receiving a total dose of 30 mg/kg: Table 3 shows mean pharmacokinetic parameters on day 5 in children 1 to 5 years and 5 to 15 years of age when azithromycin oral suspension was dosed in the absence of food at a total dose of 30 mg/kg delivered as 10 mg/kg on day 1 and 5 mg/kg on days 2 to 5.

Table 2: ZITHROMAX

Plasma Concentrations (µg/mL) After the Last Daily I.V. Infusion of 500 mg Azithromycin (median [range])

	Time after starting infusion (h)								
Concentration + Duration	0.5	1	2	3	4	6	8	12	24
2 mg/mL,	2.42	2.65	0.63	0.34	0.32	0.19	0.22	0.16	0.18
1 h[a]	(1.71–5.12)	(1.94–6.03)	(0.21–1.07)	(0.18–0.87)	(0.16–0.69)	(0.12–0.58)	(0.10–0.61)	(0.09–0.46)	(0.07–0.60)
1 mg/mL,	0.87	1.03	1.16	1.17	0.32	0.29	0.27	0.22	0.18
3 h[b]	(0.76–1.16)	(0.83–1.19)	(0.87–1.36)	(0.86–1.35)	(0.26–0.47)	(0.23–0.35)	(0.23–0.34)	(0.17–0.26)	(0.15–0.21)

[a] 500 mg (2 mg/mL) for 2-5 days in CAP patients.
[b] 500 mg (1 mg/mL) for 5 days in healthy subjects.

Table 3: ZITHROMAX

Pharmacokinetic Parameters on Day 5 at Dosage 10 mg/kg (Day 1) and 5 mg/kg (Days 2 to 5)

Age 1–5			Age 5–15		
C_{max} (µg/mL)	T_{max} (h)	$AUC_{0\text{-}24}$ (µg·h/mL)	C_{max} (µg/mL)	T_{max} (h)	$AUC_{0\text{-}24}$ (µg·h/mL)
0.216	1.9	1.822	0.383	2.4	3.109

Pharmacokinetics in children given a total dose of 30 mg/kg delivered as a single dose have not been studied.

Pharmacokinetics in children receiving a 60 mg/kg total dose: Two clinical studies enrolled 35 and 33 children respectively aged 3 to 16 years with pharyngitis/tonsillitis to determine the pharmacokinetics and safety of azithromycin for oral suspension in children when given 60 mg/kg in divided doses delivered as 20 mg/kg/day over 3 days or 12 mg/kg/day over 5 days with a maximum daily dose of 500 mg.

Table 4 shows pharmacokinetic data in the subset of children who received a total dose of 60 mg/kg. In both studies azithromycin concentrations were determined over a 24 hour period following the last daily dose.

Table 4: ZITHROMAX

Pharmacokinetics in Children Receiving a 60 mg/kg Total Dose

	3-Day Regimen (20 mg/kg×3 days)	5-Day Regimen (12 mg/kg×5 days)
n	11[b]	17[b]
C_{max} (µg/mL)	1.05± 44[a]	0.534±0.361[a]
T_{max} (h)	3±2.0[a]	2.2±0.8[a]
$AUC_{0\text{-}24}$ (µg/h/mL)	7.92±2.87[a]	3.94±1.90[a]

[a] Arithmetic means.
[b] Maximum weight for 3 day regimen was ≤25 kg and for 5 day regimen was ≤41.7 kg.

Similarity of overall exposure ($AUC_{0\text{-}\infty}$) between the 3 and the 5 day regimen is unknown.

Geriatrics: When studied in healthy elderly subjects from age 65 to 85 years, the pharmacokinetic parameters of azithromycin in elderly men were similar to those in young adults; however, in elderly women, although higher peak concentrations (increased by 30 to 50%) were observed, no significant accumulation occurred.

Renal Insufficiency: Azithromycin pharmacokinetics were investigated in 42 adults (21 to 85 years of age) with varying degrees of renal impairment. Following the oral administration of a single 1000 mg dose of azithromycin, mean C_{max} and $AUC_{0\text{-}120}$ increased by 5.1% and 4.2%, respectively in subjects with mild to moderate renal impairment (GFR 10 to 80 mL/min) compared to subjects with normal renal function (GFR >80 mL/min). The mean C_{max} and $AUC_{0\text{-}120}$ increased 61% and 35%, respectively in subjects with severe renal impairment (GFR <10 mL/min) compared to subjects with normal renal function (GFR >80 mL/min) (see Dosage).

Hepatic Insufficiency: In patients with mild to moderate hepatic impairment, there is no evidence of a marked change in serum pharmacokinetics of oral ZITHROMAX compared to those with normal hepatic function. In these patients urinary recovery of azithromycin appears to increase. Hence no dose adjustment is recommended for patients with mild to moderate hepatic impairment. Nonetheless, since the liver is the principal route of elimination for azithromycin, the use of oral ZITHROMAX preparations should be undertaken with caution in patients with impaired hepatic function.

INDICATIONS: Oral Administration: ZITHROMAX (azithromycin dihydrate) is indicated for treatment of mild to moderate infections caused by susceptible strains of the designated microorganisms in the following diseases and specific conditions. As recommended dosages, durations of therapy, and applicable patient populations vary among these infections, see Dosage for specific dosing recommendations.

Because some strains are resistant to azithromycin, when applicable, appropriate culture and susceptibility tests should be initiated before treatment to determine the causative organism and its susceptibility to azithromycin. Therapy with ZITHROMAX may be initiated before results of these tests are known; once the results become available, antibiotic treatment should be adjusted accordingly.

Adults: Treatment: Pharyngitis and Tonsillitis: Pharyngitis and tonsillitis caused by *S. pyogenes* (group A β-hemolytic streptococci) occurring in individuals who cannot use first line therapy.

Note: Penicillin is the usual drug of choice in the treatment of *S. pyogenes* pharyngitis, including the prophylaxis of rheumatic fever. ZITHROMAX is often effective in the eradication of susceptible strains of streptococci from the oropharynx. However, data establishing the efficacy of ZITHROMAX in the subsequent prevention of rheumatic fever are not available at present.

Acute Bacterial Exacerbations of Chronic Obstructive Pulmonary Disease: Acute bacterial exacerbations of chronic obstructive pulmonary diseases caused by *H. influenzae, M. catarrhalis*, or *S. pneumoniae*.

Community-acquired Pneumonia: Community-acquired pneumonia caused by *S. pneumoniae, H. influenzae, M. pneumoniae* or *C. pneumoniae* in patients for whom oral therapy is appropriate.

Azithromycin should not be used in patients with pneumonia who are judged to be inappropriate for oral therapy because of moderate to severe illness or risk factors such as any of the following: patients with cystic fibrosis, patients with nosocomially acquired infections, patients with known or suspected bacteremia, patients requiring hospitalization, elderly or debilitated patients, or patients with significant underlying health problems that may compromise their ability to respond to their illness (including immunodeficiency or functional asplenia).

Uncomplicated Skin and Skin Structure Infections: Uncomplicated skin and skin structure infections caused by *S. aureus, S. pyogenes* or *S. agalactiae*.

Genitourinary Tract Infections: Urethritis and cervicitis due to *N. gonorrhoeae* or *C. trachomatis*. Genital ulcer disease in men due to *H. ducreyi* (chancroid). Due to the small number of women included in clinical trials, the efficacy of azithromycin in the treatment of chancroid in women has not been established. Patients should have a serologic test for syphilis and appropriate cultures for gonorrhea performed at the time of diagnosis. Appropriate antimicrobial therapy and follow-up tests for these diseases should be initiated if infection is confirmed.

Prevention of Disseminated *M. Avium* Complex (MAC) Disease: ZITHROMAX, taken at a dose of 1200 mg weekly, alone or in combination with rifabutin at its approved dose, is indicated for the prevention of disseminated *M. avium* complex (MAC) disease in persons with advanced HIV infections.

Children: (see Dosage and Precautions, Children).

Treatment: Acute Otitis Media: Acute otitis media caused by *H. influenzae* (β-lactamase positive and negative strains), *M. catarrhalis* or *S. pneumoniae*. (For specific dosage recommendation, see Dosage.)

Pharyngitis and Tonsillitis: Pharyngitis and tonsillitis caused by *S. pyogenes* (group A β-hemolytic streptococci) occurring in individuals who cannot use first line therapy. (For specific dosage recommendation, see Dosage.)

Note: Penicillin is the usual drug of choice in the treatment of *S. pyogenes* pharyngitis, including the prophylaxis of rheumatic fever. ZITHROMAX is often effective in the eradication of susceptible strains of streptococci from the oropharynx. However, data establishing the efficacy of ZITHROMAX in the subsequent prevention of rheumatic fever are not available at present.

Community-acquired Pneumonia: Community-acquired pneumonia caused by *H. influenzae,S. pneumoniae, M. pneumoniae* or *C. pneumoniae* in patients for whom oral therapy is appropriate. (For specific dosage recommendation, see Dosage.)

Azithromycin should not be used in patients with pneumonia who are judged to be inappropriate for outpatient oral therapy because of moderate to severe illness or risk factors such as any of the following: patients with cystic fibrosis, patients with nosocomially acquired infections, patients with known or suspected bacteremia, patients requiring hospitalization, or patients with significant underlying health problems that may compromise their ability to respond to their illness (including immunodeficiency or functional asplenia).

Safety and effectiveness for pneumonia due to *H. influenzae* and *S. pneumoniae* were not documented bacteriologically in the pediatric clinical trial due to difficulty in obtaining specimens. Use of azithromycin for these two microorganisms is supported, however, by evidence from adequate and well-controlled studies in adults.

Injection: ZITHROMAX for injection is indicated for the treatment of patients with infections caused by susceptible strains of the designated microorganisms in the conditions listed below.

ZITHROMAX for Injection should be followed by oral administration of ZITHROMAX as required (see Dosage).

Adults: Lower Respiratory Tract: Community-acquired pneumonia (CAP) due to *C. pneumoniae, H. influenzae, M. catarrhalis, L. pneumophila, M. pneumoniae* or *S. pneumoniae* in patients who require initial i.v. therapy.

Genitourinary Tract: Pelvic inflammatory disease (PID) due to *C. trachomatis, N. gonorrhoeae* or *M. hominis* in patients who require initial i.v. therapy. If anaerobic organisms are suspected of contributing to the infection, an antimicrobial agent with anaerobic activity should be administered in combination with ZITHROMAX.

Patients should have a serologic test for syphilis performed at the time of diagnosis. Appropriate antimicrobial therapy and follow-up tests for this disease should be initiated if infection is confirmed.

Because some strains are resistant to azithromycin, appropriate culture and susceptibility tests should be initiated before treatment to determine the causative organism and its susceptibility to azithromycin. Therapy with ZITHROMAX may be initiated before results of these tests are known; once the results become available, antibiotic treatment should be adjusted accordingly.

CONTRAINDICATIONS: ZITHROMAX (azithromycin dihydrate) is contraindicated in patients with hypersensitivity to azithromycin, erythromycin, any macrolide or ketolide antibacterial agents, or to any excipient listed in Supplied.

WARNINGS: Serious allergic reactions, including angioedema, anaphylaxis and dermatological reactions including Steven's Johnson syndrome and toxic epidermolysis have been reported rarely (with rare reports of fatalities), in patients on ZITHROMAX (azithromycin dihydrate) therapy (see Contraindications). Allergic reactions may occur during and soon after treatment with ZITHROMAX. Despite initially successful symptomatic treatment of the allergic symptoms, when symptomatic therapy was discontinued, the allergic symptoms recurred soon thereafter in some patients without further azithromycin exposure. These patients required prolonged periods of observation and symptomatic treatment. If an allergic reaction occurs, the drug should be discontinued and appropriate therapy should be instituted. Physicians should be aware that reappearance of the allergic symptoms may occur when symptomatic therapy is discontinued.

Pseudomembranous colitis has been reported with nearly all antibacterial agents including ZITHROMAX and may range in severity from mild to life-threatening. Therefore, it is important to consider this diagnosis in patients who present with diarrhea subsequent to the administration of antibacterial agents. Treatment with antibacterial agents alters the normal flora of the colon and may permit overgrowth of clostridia. Studies indicate that a toxin produced by *C. difficile* is a primary cause of "antibiotic-associated colitis". After the diagnosis of pseudomembranous colitis has been established, therapeutic measures should be initiated. Mild cases of pseudomembranous colitis usually respond to discontinuation of the drug alone. In moderate to severe cases, consideration should be given to management with fluids and electrolytes, protein supplementation, and treatment with an antibacterial drug clinically effective against *C. difficile*.

In the absence of data on the metabolism and pharmacokinetics in patients with lysosomal lipid storage diseases (e.g.,Tay-Sachs disease, Niemann-Pick disease) the use of azithromycin in these patients is not recommended.

Rare cases of acute hepatic necrosis requiring liver transplant or causing death have been reported in patients following treatment with oral azithromycin.

I.M. use of azithromycin is not recommended; extravasation of drug into the tissues may cause tissue injury.

Intravenous Administration: Azithromycin for injection should be reconstituted and diluted as directed and administered as an intravenous infusion over not less than 60 minutes. **Do not administer as an intravenous bolus or an intramuscular injection** (see Dosage, ZITHROMAX for Intravenous Injection).

PRECAUTIONS: General: Since liver is the major route of elimination for ZITHROMAX (azithromycin dihydrate), the use of oral ZITHROMAX preparations should be undertaken with caution in patients with impaired hepatic function.

Due to limited data in subjects with GFR <10 mL/min, caution should be exercised when prescribing oral azithromycin in these patients (see Pharmacology, Special Populations, Renal Insufficiency).

Due to the lack of data, ZITHROMAX for injection should be used with caution in patients with hepatic and/or renal impairment (including patients on dialysis).

ZITHROMAX for injection should be reconstituted and diluted as directed and administered as an i.v. infusion over at least 60 minutes (see Dosage).

Local injection site reactions have been reported with the i.v. administration of ZITHROMAX. The incidence and severity of these reactions were the same when 500 mg azithromycin was given over 1 hour (2 mg/mL as 250 mL infusion) (see Adverse Effects). All volunteers who received infusate concentrations above 2 mg/mL experienced local i.v. site reactions, therefore, higher concentrations should be avoided.

Prolonged cardiac repolarisation and QT interval, imparting a risk of developing cardiac arrythmia and torsades de pointes, have been seen in treatment with other macrolides. A similar effect has been reported with azithromycin and can not be completely ruled out. There is information that 'QT Related Adverse Events' may occur in some patients receiving azithromycin, although these adverse events have not been reported in clinical trials with azithromycin. There have been spontaneous reports from post-marketing experience of prolonged QT interval and torsades de pointes (see Adverse Effects, Postmarketing Experience). These include but are not limited to: one AIDS patient dosed at 750 mg to 1 g daily experienced prolonged QT interval and torsades de pointes; a patient with previous history of arrythmias who experienced torsades de pointes and subsequent myocardial infarction following a course of azithromycin therapy; and a pediatric case report of prolonged QT interval experienced at a therapeutic dose of azithromycin which reversed to normal upon discontinuation.

Pregnancy: There are no adequate and well-controlled studies in pregnant women. In animal studies at doses up to moderately maternally toxic dose concentrations (i.e., 200 mg/kg/day), no evidence of harm to the fetus due to azithromycin was found. ZITHROMAX should not be used during pregnancy unless the expected benefit to the mother outweighs any potential risk to the fetus.

Lactation: There are no data on secretion in breast milk. Azithromycin should not be used in the treatment of lactating women unless the expected benefit to the mother outweighs any potential risk to the infant. Because azithromycin may accumulate in breast milk over time with continued ZITHROMAX therapy, if the lactating mother is treated with ZITHROMAX, the breast milk should be expressed and discarded during treatment.

Children: (See Pharmacology, Indications and Dosage.)

Acute Otitis Media: Safety and efficacy in the treatment of children with otitis media under 6 months of age have not been established (see Dosage).

Community-acquired Pneumonia: Safety and efficacy in the treatment of children with community-acquired pneumonia under 6 months of age have not been established (see Dosage).

Pharyngitis and Tonsillitis: Safety and efficacy in the treatment of children with pharyngitis and tonsillitis under 2 years of age have not been established (see Dosage).

Studies evaluating the use of repeated courses of therapy have not been conducted. Safety data with the use of ZITHROMAX at doses higher than proposed and for durations longer than recommended are limited to a small number of immunocompromised children who underwent chronic treatment.

In animal studies, treatment with azithromycin is associated with accumulation in various tissues, including the extra-cranial neural ganglia (i.e., retina and sympathetic nervous system). Tissue accumulation is both dose and time dependent, and is associated microscopically with the development of phospholipidosis (intra-lysosomal drug phospholipid complexes). The only evidence in animals that azithromycin is associated with alterations of intracellular phospholipid metabolism has been the documentation of small increases in phospholipid content after prolonged treatment (6 months) or exaggerated doses. Phospholipidosis has been observed at total cumulative doses only 2 multiples of the clinical dose. One month after withdrawal of treatment the concentration of azithromycin and the presence of phospholipidosis in tissue, including the retina, is at or near predose levels.

No data exist in humans in regard to the extent of accumulation, duration of exposure, metabolism or excretory mechanisms of azithromycin in neural tissue such as the retina and the cochlea. Rare cases of hearing loss have been reported (see Adverse Effects).

No data are available on the metabolism and pharmacokinetics of azithromycin in children with lysosomal lipid storage diseases (see Warnings).

The safety and effectiveness of ZITHROMAX for Injection in children or adolescents under 16 years have not been established.

Prevention of Disseminated *M. Avium* Complex (MAC) Disease: Safety and efficacy of ZITHROMAX for the prevention of MAC in children have not been established. Limited safety data are available for 24 children 5 months to 14 years of age (mean 4.6 years) who received ZITHROMAX for treatment of opportunistic infections. The mean duration of therapy was 186.7 days (range 13 to 710 days) at doses of <5 to 20 mg/kg/day. Adverse events were similar to those observed in the adult population, most of which involved the GI tract. While none of these children prematurely discontinued treatment due to a side effect, one child discontinued due to a laboratory abnormality (eosinophilia). Based on available pediatric pharmacokinetic data, a dose of 20 mg/kg in children would provide drug exposure similar to the 1200 mg adult dose but with a higher C_{max}.

Geriatrics: The pharmacokinetics in elderly volunteers (age 65 to 85) were similar to those in younger volunteers (age 18 to 40) for the 5-day oral therapeutic regimen. Dosage adjustment does not appear to be necessary for elderly patients with normal renal and hepatic function receiving treatment with this dosage regimen. Pharmacokinetic studies with i.v. azithromycin have not been performed in the elderly. Based on clinical trials, there appear to be no significant differences in safety or tolerance of i.v. azithromycin between elderly (age 65) and younger subjects (ages 16 to 64).

Drug Interactions: Antacids: Aluminum and magnesium containing antacids (Maalox) reduce the peak serum levels but not the extent of azithromycin absorption. ZITHROMAX and these drugs should not be taken simultaneously.

Atorvastatin: In healthy volunteers, co-administration of atorvastatin (10 mg daily) and azithromycin (500 mg daily) did not alter plasma concentrations of atorvastatin (based on HMG CoA-reductase inhibition assay).

Carbamazepine: In pharmacokinetic interaction study in healthy volunteers, no significant effect was observed on the plasma levels of carbamazepine or its active metabolite in patients receiving concomitant ZITHROMAX.

Cetirizine: In healthy male volunteers, co-administration of a 5-day regimen of azithromycin with cetirizine 20 mg at steady-state resulted in no pharmacokinetic interaction and no significant changes in the QT interval.

Cimetidine: Administration of cimetidine (800 mg) 2 hours prior to ZITHROMAX had no effect on azithromycin absorption.

Coumarin-Type Oral Anticoagulants: In clinical trials, ZITHROMAX did not affect the prothrombin time response to a single dose of warfarin.

During the post-marketing period, there have been reports of potentiated anticoagulation subsequent to coadministration of azithromycin and coumarin-type oral anticoagulants.

Although a causal relationship has not been established, prudent medical practice dictates careful monitoring of prothrombin time in all patients treated with ZITHROMAX and warfarin concomitantly. Concurrent use of macrolides and warfarin in clinical practice has been associated with increased anticoagulant effects.

Cyclosporine: In a pharmacokinetic study with healthy volunteers that were administered a 500 mg/day oral dose of azithromycin for 3 days and were then administered a single 10 mg/kg oral dose of cyclosporine, the resulting cyclosporine C_{max} and AUC_{0-5} were found to be significantly elevated. Consequently, caution should be exercised before considering concurrent administration of these drugs. If coadministration of these drugs is necessary, cyclosporine levels should be monitored and the dose adjusted accordingly.

Didanosine: Daily doses of 1200 mg ZITHROMAX had no effect on the pharmacokinetics of didanosine.

Efavirenz: When administered at a dose of 400 mg for seven days produced a 22% increase in the C_{max} of azithromycin administered as a 600 mg single dose. AUC was not affected.

Administration of a single 600 mg dose of azithromycin had no effect on the pharmacokinetics of efavirenz given at 400 mg doses for seven days.

Fluconazole: A single dose of 1200 mg azithromycin did not alter the pharmacokinetics of a single 800 mg oral dose of fluconazole.

Total exposure and half-life of 1200 mg azithromycin were unchanged and C_{max} had a clinically insignificant decrease (18%) by coadministration with 800 mg fluconazole.

Indinavir: A single dose of 1200 mg azithromycin had no significant effect on the pharmacokinetics of indinavir (800 mg indinavir t.i.d. for 5 days).

Midazolam: In healthy volunteers (N=12), co-administration of azithromycin 500 mg/day for 3 days did not cause clinically significant changes in the pharmacokinetics and pharmacodynamics of a single 15 mg dose of midazolam.

Nelfinavir: Coadministration of a single dose of 1200 mg azithromycin with steady-state nelfinavir (750 mg t.i.d.) produced an approximately 16% decrease in mean AUC_{0-8} of nelfinavir and its M8 metabolite. C_{max} was not affected.

Coadministration of nelfinavir (750 mg t.i.d.) at steady-state with a single dose of 1200 mg azithromycin increased the mean $AUC_{0-\infty}$ of azithromycin by 113% and mean C_{max} by 136%.

Dose adjustment of azithromycin is not recommended. However, close monitoring for known side effects of azithromycin, when administered in conjunction with nelfinavir, is warranted.

Rifabutin: Co-administration of ZITHROMAX and rifabutin did not affect the serum concentrations of either drug.

Sildenafil: In normal healthy male volunteers, there was no evidence of a statistically significant effect of azithromycin (500 mg daily for 3 days) on the AUC, C_{max}, T_{max}, elimination rate constant, or subsequent half-life of sildenafil or its principal circulating metabolite.

Theophylline: Concurrent use of macrolides and theophylline has been associated with increases in the serum concentrations of theophylline. ZITHROMAX did not affect the pharmacokinetics of theophylline administered either as a single i.v. infusion or multiple oral doses at a recommended dose of 300 mg every 12 hours. There is one postmarketing report of supraventricular tachycardia associated with an elevated theophylline serum level that developed soon after initiation of treatment with ZITHROMAX. Until further data are available, prudent medical practice dictates careful monitoring of plasma theophylline levels in patients receiving ZITHROMAX and theophylline concomitantly.

Trimethoprim/Sulfamethoxazole: Following administration of trimethoprim/sulfamethoxazole DS (160 mg/800 mg) for 7 days to healthy subjects, coadministration of 1200 mg azithromycin on Day 7 had no significant effects on peak concentrations or total exposure or urinary excretion of either trimethoprim or sulfamethoxazole.

Serum concentrations of azithromycin following administration of a single 1200 mg dose after administration of trimethoprim/sulfamethoxazole DS for 7 days were similar to those produced following a 1200 mg dose of azithromycin in other studies.

Zidovudine: Single 1 g doses and multiple 1200 mg or 600 mg doses of ZITHROMAX did not affect the plasma pharmacokinetics or urinary excretion of zidovudine or its glucuronide metabolite. However, administration of ZITHROMAX increased the concentrations of phosphorylated zidovudine in peripheral blood mononuclear cells.

Concomitant Therapy: The following drug interactions have not been reported in clinical trials with ZITHROMAX and no specific drug interaction studies have been performed to evaluate potential drug-drug interactions. Nonetheless, they have been observed with macrolide products, and there have been rare spontaneously reported cases with ZITHROMAX and some of these drugs, in postmarketing experience. Until further data are developed regarding drug interactions, when ZITHROMAX and these drugs are used concomitantly, careful monitoring of patients is advised both during and for a short period following therapy:

Digoxin: elevation of digoxin levels.

Disopyramide: increase in pharmacological effects.

Ergotamine or dihydroergotamine: acute ergot toxicity characterized by severe peripheral vasospasm and dysesthesia.

Triazolam: decreases in the clearance of triazolam and increases in the pharmacologic effect of triazolam.

Drugs Metabolized by the Cytochrome P450 System: elevations of serum hexobarbital, cisapride, and phenytoin levels.

Antihistamines: prolongation of QT intervals, palpitations or cardiac arrhythmias with concomitant administration of astemizole or terfenadine.

No data are available on the concomitant clinical use of ZITHROMAX and gentamicin or other amphiphilic drugs which have been reported to alter intracellular lipid metabolism.

ADVERSE EFFECTS: General: The majority of side effects observed in controlled clinical trials involving patients (adults and children) treated with oral ZITHROMAX (azithromycin dihydrate) were of a mild and transient nature. Approximately 0.7% of both adult patients (n=3812) and children (n=2878) from the 5-day multiple dose clinical trials discontinued ZITHROMAX therapy because of drug related side effects. Among adults receiving ZITHROMAX i.v., 1.2% of CAP, and 2% of PID patients discontinued treatment. Discontinuation rates were slightly higher for PID patients receiving concomitant metronidazole therapy (4%).

In adults given 500 mg/day for 3 days, the discontinuation rate due to treatment-related side effects was 0.4%. In clinical trials in children given 30 mg/kg, orally either as a single dose (n= 487) or over 3 days, (n=1729) discontinuation from therapy due to treatment-related side effects was approximately 1%.

Most of the side effects leading to discontinuation in patients on oral or i.v. therapy were related to the GI tract, e.g., nausea, vomiting, diarrhea, along with abdominal pain, rashes and increases in aminotransferases and/or alkaline phosphatase levels in adult patients receiving i.v. ZITHROMAX. Potentially serious treatment-related side effects including angioedema and cholestatic jaundice occurred in less than 1% of patients.

Oral Regimen: Adults: Multiple-dose Regimen: In adult patients, the most common treatment-related side effects in patients receiving the 3 or 5 day oral multiple-dose regimens of ZITHROMAX were related to the GI system with diarrhea/loose stools (4-5%), abdominal pain (2-3%), vomiting (1%) and nausea (3-4%).

Treatment related side effects that occurred with a frequency of 1% or less include:

Cardiovascular: hypertension.

Gastrointestinal: dry mouth, esophagitis, gastroenteritis, rectal hemorrhage, cholestatic jaundice.

Genitourinary: menorrhagia, urinary frequency, vaginitis.

Special Senses: conjunctivitis.

Nervous System: dizziness.

Allergic: pruritus.

Single 1 g Dose Regimen: In adult patients (n=904), side effects that occurred on the single 1 g dosing regimen of ZITHROMAX with a frequency greater than 1% included diarrhea (6.1%), nausea (4.9%), abdominal pain (4.9%), vomiting (1.7%), vaginitis (1.3%), loose stools (1.2%), and dyspepsia (1.1%).

Single 2 g Dose Regimen: Overall, the most common side effects in patients receiving a single 2 g dose of ZITHROMAX were related to the GI system. Side effects that occurred in patients in this study with a frequency of a 1% or greater included nausea (18.2%), diarrhea/loose stools (13.8%), vomiting (6.7%), abdominal pain (6.7%), vaginitis (2.2%), dyspepsia (1.1%), and dizziness (1.3%). The majority of these complaints were mild in nature.

Prevention of *M. Avium* Complex (MAC) Disease: Chronic therapy with ZITHROMAX 1200 mg weekly regimen: The nature of side effects seen with the 1200 mg weekly dosing regimen for the prevention of *M. avium* complex infection in severely immunocompromised HIV-infected patients were similar to those seen with short-term dosing regimens. See Table 5.

Table 5: ZITHROMAX

Incidence[a] (%) of Treatment-related[b] Adverse Events[c] in HIV-Infected Patients Receiving Prophylaxis for Disseminated MAC

	Study 155		Study 174		
	Placebo (n=91)	Azithromycin 1200 mg Weekly (n=89)	Azithromycin 1200 mg Weekly (n=233)	Rifabutin 300 mg Daily (n=236)	Azithromycin and Rifabutin (n=224)
Mean Duration of Therapy (days)	303.8	402.9	315	296.1	344.4
Discontinuation of Therapy (%)	2.3	8.2	13.5	15.9	22.7
Autonomic Nervous System					
Mouth Dry	0	0	0	3.0	2.7
CNS					
Dizziness	0	1.1	3.9	1.7	0.4
Headache	0	0	3.0	5.5	4.5
Gastrointestinal					
Diarrhea	15.4	52.8	50.2	19.1	50.9
Loose Stools	6.6	19.1	12.9	3.0	9.4
Abdominal Pain	6.6	27	32.2	12.3	31.7
Dyspepsia	1.1	9	4.7	1.7	1.8
Flatulence	4.4	9	10.7	5.1	5.8
Nausea	11	32.6	27.0	16.5	28.1
Vomiting	1.1	6.7	9.0	3.8	5.8
General					
Fever	1.1	0	2.1	4.2	4.9
Fatigue	0	2.2	3.9	2.1	3.1
Malaise	0	1.1	0.4	0	2.2
Musculoskeletal					

(cont'd)

Table 5: ZITHROMAX *(cont'd)*

Incidence[a] (%) of Treatment-related[b] Adverse Events[c] in HIV-Infected Patients Receiving Prophylaxis for Disseminated MAC

	Study 155		Study 174		
	Placebo (n=91)	**Azithromycin 1200 mg Weekly (n=89)**	**Azithromycin 1200 mg Weekly (n=233)**	**Rifabutin 300 mg Daily (n=236)**	**Azithromycin and Rifabutin (n=224)**
Mean Duration of Therapy (days)	303.8	402.9	315	296.1	344.4
Discontinuation of Therapy (%)	2.3	8.2	13.5	15.9	22.7
Arthralgia	0	0	3.0	4.2	7.1
Psychiatric					
Anorexia	1.1	0	2.1	2.1	3.1
Skin and Appendages					
Pruritus	3.3	0	3.9	3.4	7.6
Rash	3.2	3.4	8.1	9.4	11.1
Skin Discoloration	0	0	0	2.1	2.2
Special Senses					
Tinnitus	4.4	3.4	0.9	1.3	0.9
Hearing Decreased	2.2	1.1	0.9	0.4	0
Taste Perversion	0	0	1.3	2.5	1.3

a Reflects the occurrence of 1 event during the entire treatment period.
b Includes those events considered possibly or probably related to study drug.
c >2% adverse event rates for any group.

Side effects related to the GI tract were seen more frequently in patients receiving azithromycin than in those receiving placebo or rifabutin. In one of the studies, 86% of diarrheal episodes were mild to moderate in nature with discontinuation of therapy for this reason occurring in only 9/233 (3.8%) of patients.

I.V./Oral Regimen: Adults: The most common side effects (greater than 1%) in adult patients who received sequential i.v./oral ZITHROMAX in studies of **community-acquired pneumonia** were related to the GI system: diarrhea/loose stools (4.3%), nausea (3.9%), abdominal pain (2.7%), and vomiting (1.4%). Approximately 12% of patients experienced a side effect related to the i.v. infusion; most common were pain at the site and/or during the infusion (6.5%) and local inflammation (3.1%).

In adult women who received sequential i.v./oral ZITHROMAX in studies of **pelvic inflammatory disease**, the most common side effects (greater than 1%) were related to the GI system. Diarrhea (8.5%) and nausea (6.6%) were most frequently reported, followed by vaginitis (2.8%), abdominal pain (1.9%), anorexia (1.9%), rash and pruritus (1.9%). When azithromycin was coadministered with metronidazole in these studies, a higher proportion of women experienced side effects of nausea (10.3%), abdominal pain (3.7%), vomiting (2.8%) and application site reaction, stomatitis, dizziness, or dyspnea (all at 1.9%).

Side effects that occurred with a frequency of 1% or less included:
Gastrointestinal: dyspepsia, flatulence, mucositis, oral moniliasis, and gastritis.
Nervous System: headache, somnolence.
Allergic: bronchospasm.
Special Senses: taste perversion.
Oral Regimen: Children: Single and Multiple-dose regimens: In children enrolled in controlled clinical trials in acute otitis media and S. pyogenes pharyngitis, the type of side effects were comparable to those seen in adults (see below).

Different side effect incidence rates for the dosage regimens recommended in children were observed:
Acute Otitis Media: For the recommended total dosage regimen of 30 mg/kg, the most frequent side effects (≥1%) attributed to treatment were diarrhea, abdominal pain, vomiting, nausea and rash. The incidence, based on dosing regimen, is described in Table 6.

Table 6: ZITHROMAX

Incidence of Treatment-related Adverse Events in Acute Otitis Media

Regimen	Subjects	Overall ADR Incidence	Diarrhea	Abdominal Pain	Vomiting	Nausea	Rash
1-Day	487	14%	4%	1%	5%	1%	1%
3-Day	1395	7%	3%	2%	1%	<1%	<1%
5-Day	1888	6%	2%	1%	1%	1%	<1%

Community-acquired Pneumonia: For the recommended total dosage regimen of 30 mg/kg, the most frequent side effects attributed to treatment were diarrhea/loose stools, abdominal pain, vomiting/nausea and rash. The incidence is described in Table 7.

Table 7: ZITHROMAX

Incidence of Treatment-related Adverse Events in Community-acquired Pneumonia

Dosage Regimen	Subjects	Overall ADR Incidence	Diarrhea/ Loose stools	Abdominal Pain	Vomitin	Nausea	Rash
5-Day	323	12%	5.8%	1.9%	1.9%	1.9%	1.6%

Pharyngitis/Tonsillitis: For the recommended total dosage regimen of 60 mg/kg, the most frequent side effects attributed to treatment were diarrhea, vomiting, abdominal pain, nausea and headache. The incidence is described in Table 8.
Side effects that occurred with a frequency of 1% or less in patients included the following:
Cardiovascular: palpitations, chest pain.
Gastrointestinal: dyspepsia, flatulence, melena, constipation, anorexia, enteritis, loose stools, oral moniliasis and gastritis.
Genitourinary: monilia, vaginitis and nephritis.
Hematologic and Lymphatic: anemia, leukopenia.
Nervous System: dizziness, vertigo, somnolence, agitation, nervousness, insomnia and hyperkinesia.
General: fatigue, face edema, fever, fungal infection, pain and malaise.
Respiratory: cough increased, pharyngitis, pleural effusion and rhinitis.
Skin and Appendages: eczema, fungal dermatitis, sweating and vesiculobullous rash.
Allergic: allergic reaction, photosensitivity, angioedema, erythema multiforme, pruritus and urticaria.
Liver/Biliary: liver function test abnormal, jaundice and cholestatic jaundice.

Table 8: ZITHROMAX

Incidence of Treatment-related Adverse Events in Pharyngitis/Tonsillitis

Regimen	Subjects	Overall ADR Incidence	Diarrhea	Abdominal Pain	Vomiting	Nausea	Rash	Headache
5-Day	447	17%	5%	3%	6%	2%	<1%	1%

Postmarketing Experience: The following adverse experiences have been reported in patients under conditions (e.g., open trials, marketing experience) where a causal relationship is uncertain or in patients treated with significantly higher than the recommended doses for prolonged periods:
Allergic: arthralgia, edema, anaphylaxis (with rare reports of fatalities), serum sickness, urticaria, vasculitis, angioedema, pruritus.
Cardiovascular: Cardiac arrhythmias (including ventricular tachycardia), palpitations, hypotension. There have been rare reports of QT prolongation and torsades de pointes in patients receiving therapeutic doses of azithromycin, including a pediatric case report of QT interval prolongation which reversed to normal upon discontinuation (see Precautions).
Gastrointestinal: anorexia, constipation, dehydration, vomiting/diarrhea rarely resulting in dehydration, pancreatitis, pseudomembranous colitis, rare reports of tongue discoloration.
General: asthenia, paresthesia, fatigue, muscle pain.
Genitourinary: interstitial nephritis, acute renal failure, nephrotic syndrome, vaginitis.
Hematopoietic: thrombocytopenia.
Liver/Biliary: abnormal liver function including drug-induced hepatitis and cholestatic jaundice have been reported. There have also been rare cases of hepatic necrosis and hepatic failure, which have rarely resulted in death.
Nervous System: aggressive reaction, anxiety, dizziness, hyperactivity, seizure, convulsions, nervousness, agitation and syncope.
Skin/Appendages: serious skin reactions including erythema multiforme, exfoliative dermatitis, Stevens-Johnson syndrome, toxic epidermal necrolysis.
Special Senses: hearing disturbances including hearing loss, deafness and/or tinnitus, vertigo, taste/smell perversion and/or loss, abnormal vision.
Laboratory Abnormalities: Oral Therapy: Treatment: Adults: Clinically significant abnormalities (irrespective of drug relationship) occurring during the clinical trials in patients were reported as follows:
With an incidence of greater than 1%: decreased hemoglobin, hematocrit, lymphocytes, monocytes, albumin and blood glucose, elevated serum creatine phosphokinase, potassium, ALT, GGT and AST, BUN, creatinine, blood glucose, platelet count, eosinophils and monocytes.
With an incidence of less than 1%: leukopenia, neutropenia, decreased platelet count, elevated serum alkaline phosphatase, bilirubin, LDH and phosphate.

The majority of subjects with elevated serum creatine also had abnormal values at baseline.

When follow-up was provided, changes in laboratory tests appeared to be reversible.

In multiple-dose clinical trials involving more than 4500 patients, 3 patients discontinued therapy because of treatment-related liver enzyme abnormalities, one for treatment-related elevated transaminases and triglycerides and one because of a renal function abnormality.
Prevention of *M. Avium* Complex (MAC) Disease: In these immunocompromised patients with advanced HIV infection, it was sometimes necessary to assess laboratory abnormalities developing on study with additional criteria if baseline values were outside the normal range. See Table 9.

Table 9: ZITHROMAX

Prophylaxis Against Disseminated MAC Abnormal Laboratory Values

		Study 155		Study 174		
Criteria[a]		**Placebo (n=88)**	**Azithromycin 1200 mg Weekly (n=89)**	**Azithromycin 1200 mg Weekly (n=208)**	**Rifabutin 300 mg Daily (n=205)**	**Azithromycin and Rifabutin (n=199)**
Hemoglobin	<0.8×LLN[b]	31%	30%	19%	26%	21%
Platelet Count	<0.75×LLN	19%	16%	11%	10%	16%
WBC Count	<0.75×LLN	48%	49%	60%	53%	60%
Neutrophils	<0.5×LLN	16%	28%	23%	20%	29%
	<500/mm³	6%	13%	5%	6%	8%
AST	>2.0×ULN[c]	28%	39%	33%	18%	30%
	>200 U/L	10%	8%	8%	3%	6%
ALT	>2.0×ULN	24%	34%	31%	15%	27%
	>250 U/L	2%	6%	8%	2%	6%

a Secondary criteria also applied if baseline abnormal, as follows: Hemoglobin, 10% decrease; Platelet, 20% decrease; WBC count, 25% decrease; Neutrophils, 50% decrease; AST, 50% increase; ALT, 50% increase.
b Lower limit of normal.
c Upper limit of normal.

In a phase I drug interaction study performed in normal volunteers, 1 of 6 subjects given the combination of azithromycin and rifabutin, 1 of 7 given rifabutin alone and 0 of 6 given azithromycin alone developed a clinically significant neutropenia (<500 cells/mm³).
Treatment: Children: 1-, 3- and 5-Day Regimens: Laboratory data collected from 64 subjects receiving azithromycin in comparative clinical trials employing the 1-day regimen (30 mg/kg as a single dose), 1198 and 169 subjects receiving azithromycin respectively employing the two 3-day regimens (30 mg/kg or 60 mg/kg in divided doses over 3 days) were similar for regimens of azithromycin and all comparators combined, with most clinically significant laboratory abnormalities occurring at incidences of 1 to 5%. Similar results were obtained in subjects receiving the two 5-day regimens. Overall, 1948 and 421 patients were exposed to 30 mg/kg or 60 mg/kg, respectively in divided doses over 5 days. The data collected in the subset of azithromycin patients assessed for laboratory abnormalities were similar to those in all comparators combined with most clinically significant laboratory abnormalities occurring at incidences of 1 to 5%. In a single centre clinical trial, a decrease in absolute neutrophils was observed in the range of 21 to 29% for azithromycin regimens of 30 mg/kg given either as a single dose or over 3 days, as well as the comparator. No patients had significant neutropenia defined as an absolute neutrophil count <500 cells/mm³.

In clinical trials involving approximately 4700 pediatric patients, no patients discontinued therapy because of treatment-related laboratory abnormalities.
I.V. Therapy: With an incidence of 4 to 6%, elevated ALT, AST, and creatinine.

With an incidence of 1 to 3%, elevated LDH and bilirubin.

With an incidence of less than 1%, leukopenia, neutropenia, decreased platelet count, and elevated serum alkaline phosphatase.

In multiple-dose clinical trials involving more than 750 patients treated with sequential i.v./oral ZITHROMAX less than 2% of patients discontinued therapy because of treatment-related liver enzyme abnormalities.

When follow-up was provided, changes in laboratory tests appeared to be reversible for both oral and i.v. dosing.

OVERDOSE:

Symptoms: Up to 15 g cumulative dose of ZITHROMAX (azithromycin dihydrate) over 10 days has been administered in clinical trials without apparent adverse effect.

Adverse events experienced in higher than recommended doses were similar to those seen at normal doses.

Treatment: In the event of overdosage, general symptomatic and supportive measures are indicated as required.

For management of a suspected drug overdose, CPhA recommends that you contact your **regional Poison Control Centre**. See the *CPS* Directory section for a list of Poison Control Centres.

DOSAGE: General: Hepatic Impairment: In patients with mild to moderate hepatic impairment, there is no evidence of a marked change in serum pharmacokinetics of oral ZITHROMAX compared to those with normal hepatic function. In these patients urinary recovery of azithromycin appears to increase. Hence no dose adjustment is recommended for patients with mild to moderate hepatic impairment. Nonetheless, since the liver is the principal route of elimination for azithromycin, the use of oral ZITHROMAX preparations should be undertaken with caution in patients with impaired hepatic function.

Renal Impairment: No dosage adjustment of oral ZITHROMAX preparations is recommended for subjects with mild to moderate (GFR 10 to 80 mL/min) renal impairment. The mean AUC_{0-120} was similar in subjects with GFR 10 to 80 mL/min compared to subjects with normal renal function, whereas it increased 35% in subjects with GFR <10 mL/min compared to subjects with normal renal function. Caution should be exercised when azithromycin is administered to subjects with severe renal impairment (see Pharmacology, Special Populations, Renal Insufficiency and Precautions).

Due to the lack of data, ZITHROMAX for Injection should be used with caution in patients with hepatic and/or renal impairment (including patients on dialysis).

Oral Therapy: Adults: Dosing in Relation to Food: Tablets: ZITHROMAX tablets can be taken with or without food.

Upper and Lower Respiratory Infections/Skin and Skin Structure Infections: The recommended dose of ZITHROMAX for individuals 16 years of age or older in the treatment of mild to moderate acute bacterial exacerbations of chronic obstructive pulmonary disease due to the indicated organisms is: either 500 mg per day for 3 days or 500 mg as a single dose on the first day followed by 250 mg once daily on days 2 through 5 for a total dose of 1.5 g. The recommended dose of ZITHROMAX for the treatment of community-acquired pneumonia of mild severity, uncomplicated skin and skin structure infections, and for pharyngitis/tonsillitis (as second-line therapy) due to the indicated organisms is 500 mg as a single dose on the first day followed by 250 mg once daily on days 2 through 5 for a total dose of 1.5 g.

Genitourinary Infections: The recommended dose of ZITHROMAX for the treatment of genital ulcer disease due to *H. ducreyi* (chancroid) and nongonococcal urethritis and cervicitis due to *C. trachomatis* is: a single 1 g (1000 mg) oral dose of ZITHROMAX. This dose can be administered as four 250 mg tablets.

The recommended dose of ZITHROMAX for the treatment of urethritis and cervicitis due to *N. gonorrhoeae* is: a single 2 g (2000 mg) dose of ZITHROMAX. This dose can be administered as eight 250 mg tablets.

For Prevention of Disseminated *M. Avium* Complex (MAC) Disease: The recommended dose of ZITHROMAX for the prevention of disseminated *M. avium* complex (MAC) disease is 1200 mg (two 600 mg tablets) taken once weekly. This dose of ZITHROMAX may be continued with the approved dosage regimen of rifabutin.

Children: Dosing in Relation to Food: Powder for Oral Suspension: ZITHROMAX powder for oral suspension can be taken with or without food (see Pharmacology).

Pediatric Dosing Guidelines: The recommended **total** dose for children is 30 mg/kg for otitis media and community-acquired pneumonia. For pharyngitis/tonsillitis, the recommended **total** dose is 60 mg/kg.

Table 10: ZITHROMAX

Pediatric Dosing Guidelines

Indication	1-Day	3-Day	5-Day
Acute Otitis Media	30 mg/kg	10 mg/kg/day	Day 1: 10 mg/kg Day 2–5: 5 mg/kg
Pharyngitis/Tonsillitis			12 mg/kg/day
Community-Acquired Pneumonia			Day 1: 10 mg/kg Day 2–5: 5 mg/kg

Acute Otitis Media: The recommended dose of ZITHROMAX oral suspension for the treatment of children with acute otitis media is 30 mg/kg given as a single dose (not to exceed 1500 mg) or 10 mg/kg once daily for 3 days (not to exceed 500 mg/day) or 10 mg/kg as a single dose on the first day (not to exceed 500 mg/day) followed by 5 mg/kg/day on days 2 through 5 (not to exceed 250 mg/day) (see Table 10, Table 11 and Table 12 respectively).

The safety of redosing azithromycin in children who vomit after receiving 30 mg/kg as a single dose has not been established. In clinical studies involving 487 patients with acute otitis media given a single 30 mg/kg dose of azithromycin, 8 patients who vomited within 30 minutes of dosing were redosed at the same total dose.

Community-Acquired Pneumonia: The recommended dose of ZITHROMAX for oral suspension for the treatment of children with community-acquired pneumonia is 10 mg/kg as a single dose on the first day (not to exceed 500 mg/day) followed by 5 mg/kg on days 2 through 5 (not to exceed 250 mg/day) (see Table 13).

Effectiveness of the 3-day or 1-day regimen in children with community-acquired pneumonia has not been established.

Pharyngitis and Tonsillitis: The recommended dose for children with pharyngitis and tonsillitis is 12 mg/kg once daily for 5 days (not to exceed 500 mg/day) (see Table 14).

Table 11: ZITHROMAX

Pediatric Dosage Guidelines Based on Body Weight

Otitis Media: (1-Day Regimen)[a] Dosing Calculated on 30 mg/kg as a Single Dose Age 6 Months and Above, see Precautions, Children			
Weight kg	**200 mg/5 mL Day 1**	**Total mL per Treatment Course**	**Total mg per Treatment Course**
5	3.75 mL (3/4 tsp)	3.75 mL	150 mg
10	7.5 mL (1½ tsp)	7.5 mL	300 mg
20	15 mL (3 tsp)	15 mL	600 mg
30	22.5 mL (4½ tsp)	22.5 mL	900 mg

(cont'd)

Table 11: ZITHROMAX *(cont'd)*

Pediatric Dosage Guidelines Based on Body Weight

Otitis Media: (1-Day Regimen)[a] Dosing Calculated on 30 mg/kg as a Single Dose Age 6 Months and Above, see Precautions, Children			
Weight kg	**200 mg/5 mL Day 1**	**Total mL per Treatment Course**	**Total mg per Treatment Course**
40	30 mL (6 tsp)	30 mL	1200 mg
50 and above	37.5 mL (7½ tsp)	37.5 mL	1500 mg

[a] Effectiveness of the 1-day regimen in children with community-acquired pneumonia has not been established.

Table 12: ZITHROMAX

Pediatric Dosage Guidelines Based on Body Weight

Otitis Media: (3-day Regimen)[a] Dosing Calculated on 10 mg/kg/day Age 6 Months and Above, see Precautions, Children				
Weight kg	**100 mg/5 mL Day 1-3**	**200 mg/5 mL Day 1-3**	**Total mL per Treatment Course**	**Total mg per Treatment Course**
5	2.5 mL (1/2 tsp)		7.5 mL	150 mg
10	5 mL (1 tsp)		15 mL	300 mg
20		5 mL (1 tsp)	15 mL	600 mg
30		7.5 mL (1½ tsp)	22.5 mL	900 mg
40		10 mL (2 tsp)	30 mL	1200 mg
50 and above		12.5 mL (2½ tsp)	37.5 mL	1500 mg

[a] Effectiveness of the 3-day regimen in children with community-acquired pneumonia has not been established.

Table 13: ZITHROMAX

Pediatric Dosage Guidelines Based on Body Weight

Acute Otitis Media or Community-acquired Pneumonia Age 6 Months and Above, see Precautions, Children 5-Day Regimen						
Dosing Calculated on 10 mg/kg on Day 1 Dose, Followed by 5 mg/kg on Days 2 to 5						
Weight kg	**100 mg/5 mL Suspension**		**200 mg/5 mL Suspension**		**Total mL per Treatment Course**	**Total mg per Treatment Course**
	Day 1	**Days 2-5**	**Day 1**	**Days 2-5**		
5	2.5 mL (½ tsp)	1.25 mL (¼ tsp)			7.5 mL	150 mg
10	5 mL (1tsp)	2.5 mL (½ tsp)			15 mL	300 mg
20			5 mL (1 tsp)	2.5 mL (½ tsp)	15 mL	600 mg
30			7.5 mL (1½ tsp)	3.75 mL (¾ tsp)	22.5 mL	900 mg
40			10 mL (2 tsp)	5 mL (1 tsp)	30 mL	1200 mg
50 and above			12.5mL (2½ tsp)	6.25 mL (1¼ tsp)	37.5 mL	1500 mg

Table 14: ZITHROMAX

Pediatric Dosage Guidelines Based on Body Weight

Pharyngitis and Tonsillitis: (5-Day Regimen) Age 2 years and Above see, Precautions, Children			
Dosing Calculated on 12 mg/kg Once daily Days 1 to 5			
Weight kg	**200 mg/5 mL Suspension Day 1-5**	**Total mL per Treatment Course**	**Total mg per Treatment Course**
8	2.5 mL (½ tsp)	12.5 mL	500 mg
17	5 mL (1 tsp)	25 mL	1000 mg
25	7.5 mL (1½ tsp)	37.5 mL	1500 mg

(cont'd)

Table 14: ZITHROMAX *(cont'd)*

Pediatric Dosage Guidelines Based on Body Weight

Pharyngitis and Tonsillitis: (5-Day Regimen) Age 2 years and Above see, Precautions, Children			
Dosing Calculated on 12 mg/kg Once daily Days 1 to 5			
Weight kg	**200 mg/5 mL Suspension Day 1-5**	**Total mL per Treatment Course**	**Total mg per Treatment Course**
33	10 mL (2 tsp)	50 mL	2000 mg
40	12.5 mL (2 ½ tsp)	62.5 mL	2500 mg

I.V. Injection: Adults: ZITHROMAX for injection must be reconstituted and diluted as directed, and administered as an i.v. infusion over at least 60 minutes. **Do not administer as an intravenous bolus or an intramuscular injection (see Warnings).** I.V. therapy should be followed by oral ZITHROMAX. The timing of the switch to oral therapy should be done at the discretion of the physician and in accordance with clinical response.

The infusate concentration and rate of infusion for ZITHROMAX should be either 1 mg/mL over 3 hours, or 2 mg/mL over 1 hour.

Community-acquired Pneumonia in Patients Who Require Initial I.V. Therapy: The recommended dose is 500 mg i.v. as a single daily infusion for at least 2 days followed by oral therapy at 500 mg daily to complete a 7- to 10-day course of therapy.

Pelvic Inflammatory Disease: The recommended dose is 500 mg i.v. as a single daily infusion for at least 1 day followed by oral therapy at 250 mg daily to complete a 7-day course of therapy. Note: If anaerobic organisms are suspected of contributing to the infection, an antimicrobial agent with anaerobic activity should be administered in combination with ZITHROMAX.

Reconstitution Directions: Powder for Oral Suspension: Tap bottle to loosen powder. Add the directed volume of water. Shake well before each use. Oversized bottle provides shake space. Keep tightly closed. Table 15 indicates the volume of water to be used for reconstitution:

Table 15: ZITHROMAX

Volume of Water to be Used for Reconstitution

Amount of Water to be Added	Nominal Volume After Reconstitution (Azithromycin content)	Azithromycin Concentration After Reconstitution
9 mL (300 mg bottle)	15 mL (300 mg bottle)	100 mg/5 mL
9 mL (600 mg bottle)	15 mL (600 mg bottle)	200 mg/5 mL
12 mL (900 mg bottle)	22.5 mL (900 mg bottle)	200 mg/5 mL

Use only the dosing device provided to measure the correct amount of suspension (see Supplied). The dosing device may need to be filled multiple times to provide the complete dose prescribed. Rinse the device with water after the complete daily dose has been administered.

Following constitution, and for use with the oral syringe, the supplied plastic stopper should be inserted into the neck of the bottle then sealed with the original closure.

ZITHROMAX for Injection: See Table 16.

Table 16: ZITHROMAX

Reconstitution of ZITHROMAX for Injection

Strength	Reconstitution Solution	Volume to be Added	Approximate Volume Available	Nominal Concentration
500 mg	Sterile Water for Injection	4.8 mL	5 mL	100 mg/mL

Prepare the initial solution of ZITHROMAX for injection by adding 4.8 mL of Sterile Water for Injection to the 500 mg vial. Shake the vial until all of the drug is dissolved. Since the vial is evacuated, it is recommended that a standard 5 mL (nonautomated) syringe be used to ensure that the exact volume of 4.8 mL is dispensed. Each mL of reconstituted solution contains azithromycin dihydrate equivalent to 100 mg azithromycin. Reconstituted solution is stable for 24 hours when stored below 30°C. **The reconstituted solution must be further diluted prior to administration.**

Dilution of Reconstituted Solution: To provide azithromycin over a concentration range of 1 to 2 mg/mL, transfer 5 mL of the 100 mg/mL azithromycin solution into the appropriate amount of the following diluents: See Table 17.

Table 17: ZITHROMAX

Dilution of Reconstituted Solution

Final Infusion Concentration (mg/mL)	Amount of Diluent (mL)
1 mg/mL	500 mL
2 mg/mL	250 mL
Appropriate Diluents	
0.9% Sodium Chloride Injection 5% Dextrose in Water for Injection 0.45% Sodium Chloride Injection Lactated Ringer's Injection 5% Dextrose in 0.45% Sodium Chloride Injection with 20 mEq Potassium Chloride 5% Dextrose in Lactated Ringer's Injection 5% Dextrose in 0.3% Sodium Chloride Injection 5% Dextrose in 0.45% Sodium Chloride Injection Normosol-M in 5% Dextrose	

Diluted solutions prepared in this manner are stable for 24 hours at or below room temperature (30°C), or for 72 hours if stored under refrigeration (5°C). As with all parenteral drug products, i.v. admixtures should be inspected visually for clarity, particulate matter, precipitate, discoloration and leakage prior to administration, whenever solution and container permit. Solutions showing haziness, particulate matter, precipitate, discoloration or leakage should be discarded.

Only limited data are available on the compatibility of ZITHROMAX for Injection with other i.v. substances, therefore additives or other medications should not be added to ZITHROMAX for Injection or infused simultaneously through the same i.v. line. If the same i.v. line is used for sequential infusion of several different drugs, the line should be flushed before and after infusion of ZITHROMAX for Injection with an infusion solution compatible with ZITHROMAX for Injection and with any other drug(s) administered via the common line. If ZITHROMAX for Injection is to be given concomitantly with another drug, each drug should be given separately in accordance with the recommended dosage and route of administration for each drug.

INFORMATION FOR THE PATIENT: Published in e-CPS, available by subscription at www.e-cps.ca.

SUPPLIED: Injection: Each single dose vial contains: azithromycin dihydrate in a lyophilized form equivalent to azithromycin 500 mg. Nonmedicinal ingredients: anhydrous citric acid and sodium hydroxide for pH adjustment. After reconstitution, each mL contains azithromycin dihydrate equivalent to 100 mg azithromycin (see Dosage, Reconstitution Directions). Cartons of 10 single dose vials. Dry powder: Store at controlled room temperature (15 to 30°C). Diluted solution: Stable for 24 hours at or below 30°C, or for 72 hours if stored under refrigeration (5°C). For single use only. Discard any unused portion after use.

Tablets: 250 mg: Each pink, film-coated, modified capsular-shaped ZITHROMAX tablet, engraved "Pfizer" on the upper face, "306" or scored on the lower face, contains: azithromycin dihydrate equivalent to 250 mg of azithromycin. Nonmedicinal ingredients: anhydrous calcium phosphate dibasic, D&C Red #30 aluminum lake, hypromellose, lactose, magnesium stearate, pregelatinized starch, sodium croscarmellose, sodium lauryl sulfate, titanium dioxide and triacetin. The tablets are packaged in white plastic (high density polyethylene) bottles of 30 and 100 or in a single treatment package (Z-PAK) of 6 blister-packaged tablets per box. Store at controlled room temperature between 15 and 30°C.

600 mg: Each white, film-coated, modified capsular-shaped tablet, engraved on front with "Pfizer", "308" or scored on the lower face, contains: azithromycin dihydrate equivalent to 600 mg azithromycin. Nonmedicinal ingredients: anhydrous calcium phosphate dibasic, hypromellose, lactose, magnesium stearate, pregelatinized starch, sodium croscarmellose, sodium lauryl sulfate, titanium dioxide and triacetin. White plastic (high density polyethylene) bottles of 30 and 100 tablets. Store at controlled room temperature between 15 and 30°C.

Powder for Oral Suspension: After reconstitution, each bottle of cherry-flavored suspension contains: azithromycin dihydrate equivalent to: 300 mg/15 mL (100 mg/5 mL) or 600 mg/15 mL (200 mg/5 mL); or 900 mg/22.5 mL (200 mg/5 mL). Nonmedicinal ingredients: artificial flavors, FD&C Red #40, sodium phosphate, tribasic, sucrose, hydroxypropyl cellulose and xanthan gum. The 300 mg bottle (100 mg/5 mL) is supplied with a plastic stopper and a calibrated syringe. The 600 mg bottle (200 mg/5 mL) and the 900 mg bottle (200 mg/5 mL) are supplied with a plastic stopper, and a calibrated syringe and dosing cup. Dry powder: Store at controlled room temperature (15 to 30°C). Reconstituted suspension: Store between 5 and 30°C. Discard unused portion after 10 days.

(Shown in Product Identification Section)

The reader is invited to consult CPhA's monograph **HMG-CoA Reductase Inhibitors**.

Zocor®

simvastatin

Lipid Metabolism Regulator

Merck Frosst

Date of Revision: July 16, 2010

SUMMARY PRODUCT INFORMATION:

Route of Administration	Dosage Form/Strength	All Nonmedicinal Ingredients
Oral	Tablet 5 mg, 10 mg, 20 mg, 40 mg, 80 mg	Ascorbic acid, butylated hydroxyanisole, citric acid monohydrate, hydroxypropyl cellulose, hydroxypropyl methylcellulose, lactose monohydrate, magnesium stearate, microcrystalline cellulose, pregelatinized starch, talc, titanium dioxide. Tablets ZOCOR 5 mg, 10 mg and 20 mg contain yellow ferric oxide. Tablets ZOCOR 10 mg, 20 mg, 40 mg and 80 mg also contain red ferric oxide.

INDICATIONS AND CLINICAL USE: In patients at high risk of coronary events, because of existing Coronary Heart Disease (CHD) or other occlusive arterial disease, or being over the age of 40 years with a diagnosis of diabetes, ZOCOR (simvastatin) is indicated to:

- reduce the risk of total mortality, by reducing CHD deaths;
- reduce the risk of myocardial infarction;
- reduce the risk of ischemic stroke.

This indication applies to patients at high risk of coronary events, regardless of lipid status.

In hypercholesterolemic patients with coronary heart disease, ZOCOR slows the progression of coronary atherosclerosis, including reducing the development of new lesions and new total occlusions.

Hyperlipidemia: ZOCOR is indicated as an adjunct to diet, at least equivalent to the American Heart Association (AHA) Step 1 diet, for the reduction of elevated total cholesterol (total-C) and Low-Density Lipoprotein-cholesterol (LDL-C), apolipoprotein B (apo B), and triglycerides (TG) levels in patients with primary hypercholesterolemia (Type IIa)*, or combined (mixed) hyperlipidemia (Type IIb)* when the response to diet and other nonpharmacological measures alone has been inadequate. ZOCOR (5-80 mg/day) reduces the levels of total cholesterol (19-36%), LDL-cholesterol (26-47%), apolipoprotein B (19-38%), and triglycerides (12-33%), in patients with mild to severe hyperlipidemia (Fredrickson Types IIa and IIb). ZOCOR also raises HDL-cholesterol (8-16%) and therefore lowers the LDL-C/HDL-C and total-C/HDL-C ratios.

Limited data is available in homozygous familial hypercholesterolemia (FH). In a controlled clinical study with 12 patients, ZOCOR (40 and 80 mg/day) reduced elevated total cholesterol (12% and 23%), LDL-cholesterol (14% and 25%), and apolipoprotein B (14% and 17%), respectively. One patient with absent LDL-cholesterol receptor function had an LDL-cholesterol reduction of 41% with the 80 mg/day dose.

After establishing that the elevation in plasma lipids represents a primary disorder not due to underlying conditions such as poorly-controlled diabetes mellitus, hypothyroidism, the nephrotic syndrome, liver disease, or dysproteinemias, it should ideally be determined that patients for whom treatment with ZOCOR is being considered have an elevated LDL-C level as the cause for an elevated total serum cholesterol. This may be particularly relevant for patients with total triglycerides over 4.52 mmol/L (400 mg/dL) or with markedly elevated HDL-C values, where non-LDL fractions may contribute significantly to total cholesterol levels without apparent increase in cardiovascular risk. In most patients LDL-C may be estimated according to the following equation:

LDL-C (mmol/L)	=	Total cholesterol−[(0.37×triglycerides)+HDL-C]†
LDL-C (mg/dL)	=	Total cholesterol−[(0.16×triglycerides)+HDL-C]

When total triglycerides are greater than 4.52 mmol/L (400 mg/dL) this equation is less accurate. In such patients, LDL-cholesterol may be obtained by ultra centrifugation.

Pediatric Patients with Heterozygous Familial Hypercholesterolemia: ZOCOR is indicated as an adjunct to diet to reduce total-C, LDL-C, TG, and Apo B levels in adolescent boys and girls who are at least one year post-menarche, 10-17 years of age, with heterozygous familial hypercholesterolemia (HeFH).

* A disorder of lipid metabolism characterized by elevated serum cholesterol levels in association with normal triglyceride levels (Type IIa) or with increased triglyceride levels (Type IIb). Fredrickson DS, Levy RI, Lees RS. Fat transport in lipoproteins - An integrated approach to mechanisms and disorders. N Engl J Med 1967;276:148-56.

† DeLong DM, et al. A comparison of methods. JAMA 1986;256:2372-77.

CONTRAINDICATIONS:

- Patients who are hypersensitive to this drug or to any ingredient in the formulation. For a complete listing, see Dosage Forms, Composition and Packaging.
- Active liver disease or unexplained persistent elevations of serum transaminases.
- Pregnant and nursing women. Cholesterol and other products of cholesterol biosynthesis are essential components for fetal development (including synthesis of steroids and cell membranes). ZOCOR should be administered to women of childbearing age only when such patients are highly unlikely to conceive and have been informed of the possible harm. If the patient becomes pregnant while taking ZOCOR, the drug should be discontinued immediately and the patient appraised of the potential harm to the fetus. Atherosclerosis being a chronic process, discontinuation of lipid metabolism regulating drugs during pregnancy should have little impact on the outcome of long-term therapy of primary hypercholesterolemia (see Warnings and Precautions, Pregnant Women and Nursing Women).

WARNINGS AND PRECAUTIONS: Warnings and precautions are listed in alphabetical order.

General: Before instituting therapy with ZOCOR, an attempt should be made to control hypercholesterolemia with appropriate diet and exercise, weight reduction in overweight and obese patients, and to treat other underlying medical problems (see Indications and Clinical Use). The patient should be advised to inform subsequent physicians of the prior use of ZOCOR or any other lipid-lowering agent.

In primary prevention intervention the effects of simvastatin-induced changes in lipoprotein levels, including reduction of serum cholesterol, on cardiovascular morbidity or mortality or total mortality have not been established.

Endocrine and Metabolism: Effect on CoQ_{10} Levels (Ubiquinone): Significant decreases in circulating CoQ_{10} levels in patients treated with ZOCOR and other statins have been observed. The clinical significance of a potential long-term statin-induced deficiency of CoQ_{10} has not been established.

Effect on Lipoprotein(a): In some patients, the beneficial effect of lowered total cholesterol and LDL-C levels may be partly blunted by a concomitant increase in the Lipoprotein(a) [Lp(a)] level. Further research is currently ongoing to elucidate the significance of Lp(a) plasma level variations. Therefore, until further experience is obtained, it is suggested, when feasible, that Lp(a) measurements be carried out in patients placed on therapy with ZOCOR.

Endocrine: HMG-CoA reductase inhibitors interfere with cholesterol synthesis and as such might theoretically blunt adrenal and/or gonadal steroid production. Clinical studies with simvastatin and other HMG-CoA reductase inhibitors have suggested that these agents do not reduce plasma cortisol concentration or impair adrenal reserve and do not reduce basal plasma testosterone concentration. However, the effects of HMG-CoA reductase inhibitors on male fertility have not been studied in adequate numbers of patients. The effects, if any, on the pituitary-gonadal axis in premenopausal women are unknown.

Patients treated with simvastatin who develop clinical evidence of endocrine dysfunction should be evaluated appropriately. Caution should be exercised if an HMG-CoA reductase inhibitor or other agent used to lower cholesterol levels is administered to patients receiving other drugs (e.g. ketoconazole, spironolactone, or cimetidine) that may decrease the levels of endogenous steroid hormones (see Drug Interactions, Overview).

Hepatic/Biliary/Pancreatic: In clinical studies, marked persistent increases (to more than 3 times the ULN) in serum transaminases have occurred in 1% of adult patients who received ZOCOR (see Adverse Reactions, Laboratory Tests). When the drug was interrupted or discontinued in these patients, the transaminase levels usually fell slowly to pretreatment levels. The increases were not associated with jaundice or other clinical signs or symptoms. There was no evidence of hypersensitivity. Some of these patients had abnormal liver function tests prior to therapy with simvastatin and/or consumed substantial quantities of alcohol.

In the Scandinavian Simvastatin Survival Study (4S), the number of patients with more than one transaminase elevation to >3 times the ULN, over the course of the study, was not significantly different between the simvastatin and placebo groups (14 [0.7%] vs 12 [0.6%]). The frequency of single elevations of ALT to 3 times the ULN was significantly higher in the simvastatin group in the first year of the study (20 vs 8, p=0.023), but not thereafter. Elevated transaminases resulted in the discontinuation of 8 patients from therapy in the simvastatin group (n=2221) and 5 in the placebo group (n=2223). Of the 1986 simvastatin treated patients in 4S with normal liver function tests (LFTs) at baseline, only 8 (0.4%) developed consecutive LFT elevations to >3 times the ULN and/or were discontinued due to transaminase elevations during the 5.4 years (median follow-up) of the study. All of the patients in this study received a starting dose of 20 mg of simvastatin; 37% were titrated to 40 mg.

In 2 controlled clinical studies in 1105 patients, the 6-month incidence of persistent hepatic transaminase elevations considered drug-related was 0.7% and 1.8% at the 40 and 80 mg dose, respectively.

In HPS (Heart Protection Study), in which 20,536 patients were randomized to receive ZOCOR 40 mg/day or placebo, the incidences of elevated transaminases (>3×ULN confirmed by repeat test) were 0.21% (n=21) for patients treated with ZOCOR and 0.09% (n=9) for patients treated with placebo.

It is recommended that liver function tests be performed at baseline and thereafter when clinically indicated. Patients titrated to the 80 mg dose should receive an additional test prior to titration, 3 months after titration to the 80 mg dose, and periodically thereafter (e.g., semi-annually) for the first year of treatment. Special attention should be paid to patients who develop elevated serum transaminase levels, and in these patients, measurements should be repeated promptly and then performed more frequently.

If the transaminase levels show evidence of progression, particularly if they rise to three times the ULN and are persistent, the drug should be discontinued.

ZOCOR, as well as other HMG-CoA reductase inhibitors, should be used with caution in patients who consume substantial quantities of alcohol and/or have a past history of liver disease. Active liver disease or unexplained persistent transaminase elevations are contraindications to the use of ZOCOR; if such a condition should develop during therapy, the drug should be discontinued.

Moderate (less than three times the ULN) elevations of serum transaminases have been reported following therapy with ZOCOR (see Adverse Reactions). These changes were not specific to ZOCOR and were also observed with comparative lipid-lowering agents. They generally appeared within the first 3 months after initiation of therapy with simvastatin, were often transient, were not accompanied by any symptom and did not require interruption of treatment.

Muscle Effects: Myopathy/Rhabdomyolysis: Effects on skeletal muscle such as myalgia, myopathy and, rarely, rhabdomyolysis have been reported in patients treated with ZOCOR.

Rare cases of rhabdomyolysis with acute renal failure secondary to myoglobinuria, have been reported with ZOCOR and with other HMG-CoA reductase inhibitors.

Myopathy, defined as muscle pain or muscle weakness in conjunction with increases in creatine phosphokinase (CK) values to greater than ten times the upper limit of normal (ULN), should be considered in any patient with diffuse myalgias, muscle tenderness or weakness, and/or a marked elevation of CK. Patients should be advised to report promptly any unexplained muscle pain, tenderness or weakness, particularly if associated with malaise or fever. Patients who develop any signs or symptoms suggestive of myopathy should have their CK levels measured. ZOCOR therapy should be immediately discontinued if markedly elevated CK levels are measured or myopathy is diagnosed or suspected. Myopathy sometimes takes the form of rhabdomyolysis with or without acute renal failure secondary to myoglobinuria, and rare fatalities have occurred. The risk of myopathy is increased by high levels of HMG-CoA reductase inhibitory activity in plasma.

In the Scandinavian Simvastatin Survival Study, there was one case of myopathy among 1399 patients taking simvastatin 20 mg and no cases among 822 patients taking 40 mg daily for a median duration of 5.4 years. In two 6-month controlled clinical studies, there was one case of myopathy among 436 patients taking 40 mg and 5 cases among 669 patients taking 80 mg. The risk of myopathy is increased by concomitant therapy with certain drugs, some of which were excluded by the designs of these studies.

Pre-disposing Factors for Myopathy/Rhabdomyolysis: ZOCOR, as with other HMG-CoA reductase inhibitors, should be prescribed with caution in patients with pre-disposing factors for myopathy/rhabdomyolysis. Such factors include: personal or family history of hereditary muscular disorders; previous history of muscle toxicity with another HMG-CoA reductase inhibitor; concomitant use of a fibrate or niacin (nicotinic acid); uncontrolled hypothyroidism; alcohol abuse; excessive physical exercise; age ≥65 years; female gender; renal impairment; hepatic impairment; diabetes with hepatic fatty change; surgery and trauma; frailty; situations where an increase in plasma levels of active ingredient may occur (see Drug Interactions).

ZOCOR therapy should be temporarily withheld or discontinued in any patient with an acute serious condition suggestive of myopathy or predisposing to the development of rhabdomyolysis (e.g. sepsis, hypotension, major surgery, trauma, severe metabolic endocrine and electrolyte disorders, or uncontrolled seizures).

Myopathy/Rhabdomyolysis Caused by Drug Interactions: Pharmacokinetic Interactions: The use of HMG-CoA reductase inhibitors has been associated with severe myopathy, including rhabdomyolysis, which may be more frequent when they are coadministered with drugs that inhibit certain metabolic pathways in the cytochrome P-450 system. Simvastatin is metabolized by the cytochrome P-450 isoform 3A4 and as such may interact with agents which inhibit this enzyme (see Warnings and Precautions, Myopathy/Rhabdomyolysis and Drug Interactions, Overview).

The risk of myopathy/rhabdomyolysis is increased by concomitant use of simvastatin with the following:

- **Potent inhibitors of CYP3A4: e.g., the antifungal azoles itraconazole, and ketoconazole, the antibiotics erythromycin, clarithromycin and telithromycin, the HIV protease inhibitors, or the antidepressant nefazodone, particularly with higher doses of simvastatin** (see Drug Interactions).

Other Drugs:

- **Gemfibrozil or other fibrates (except fenofibrate), particularly with higher doses of simvastatin** (see Drug Interactions). When simvastatin and fenofibrate are given concomitantly, there is no evidence that the risk of myopathy exceeds the sum of the individual risks of each agent.
- **Cyclosporine or danazol** particularly with higher doses of simvastatin (see Drug Interactions).
- **Amiodarone with higher doses of simvastatin** (see Drug Interactions). In a clinical trial, myopathy was reported in 6% of patients receiving simvastatin 80 mg and amiodarone.
- **Calcium channel blockers**
  - **Verapamil with higher doses of simvastatin** (see Drug Interactions).
  - **Diltiazem:** In a clinical trial, patients on diltiazem treated concomitantly with simvastatin 80 mg had an increased risk of myopathy. In clinical studies, the risk of myopathy in patients taking simvastatin 40 mg with diltiazem was similar to that in patients taking simvastatin 40 mg without diltiazem (see Drug Interactions).
  - **Amlodipine:** In a clinical trial, patients on amlodipine treated concomitantly with simvastatin 80 mg had a slightly increased risk of myopathy. The risk of myopathy in patients taking simvastatin 40 mg was not increased by concomitant amlodipine (see Drug Interactions).
- **Fusidic acid (oral or iv):** Patients on fusidic acid (oral or iv) treated concomitantly with simvastatin may have an increased risk of myopathy (see Drug Interactions).
- **Niacin (≥1 g/day):** Myopathy, including rhabdomyolysis, has occurred in patients who were receiving coadministration of ZOCOR and other HMG-CoA reductase inhibitors with niacin, particularly in subjects with pre-existing renal insufficiency (see Drug Interactions).

As with other HMG-CoA reductase inhibitors, the risk of myopathy/rhabdomyolysis is dose related. In a clinical trial database in which 41 413 patients were treated with ZOCOR 24 747 (approximately 60%) of whom were enrolled in studies with a median follow-up of at least 4 years, the incidence of myopathy was approximately 0.03%, 0.08% and 0.61% at 20, 40 and 80 mg/day, respectively. In these trials, patients were carefully monitored and some interacting medicinal products were excluded.

In a clinical trial in which patients with a history of myocardial infarction were treated with ZOCOR 80 mg/day (mean follow-up 6.7 years), the incidence of myopathy was approximately 1.0% compared with 0.02% for patients on 20 mg/day. Approximately half of these myopathy cases occurred during the first year of treatment. The incidence of myopathy during each subsequent year of treatment was approximately 0.1%.

Reducing the Risk of Myopathy/Rhabdomyolysis: 1. General measures: All patients starting therapy with simvastatin, or whose dose of simvastatin is being increased, should be advised of the risk of myopathy and told to report promptly any unexplained muscle pain, tenderness or weakness. Simvastatin therapy should be discontinued immediately if myopathy is diagnosed or suspected. The presence of these symptoms, and a CK level >10 times the upper limit of normal indicates myopathy. In most cases, when patients were promptly discontinued from treatment, muscle symptoms and CK increases resolved. Periodic CK determinations may be considered in patients starting therapy with simvastatin or whose dose is being increased. Periodic CK determinations are recommended for patients titrating to the 80 mg dose. There is no assurance that such monitoring will prevent myopathy.

Many of the patients who have developed rhabdomyolysis on therapy with simvastatin have had complicated medical histories, including renal insufficiency usually as a consequence of long-standing diabetes mellitus. Such patients merit closer monitoring. Therapy with simvastatin should be temporarily stopped a few days prior to elective major surgery and when any major medical or surgical condition supervenes.

2. Measures to reduce the risk of myopathy/rhabdomyolysis caused by drug interactions (see above): Use of simvastatin concomitantly with potent CYP3A4 inhibitors (e.g., itraconazole, ketoconazole, erythromycin, clarithromycin, telithromycin, HIV protease inhibitors, or nefazodone) should be avoided. If treatment with itraconazole, ketoconazole, erythromycin, clarithromycin or telithromycin is unavoidable, therapy with simvastatin should be suspended during the course of treatment. Concomitant use with other medicines labeled as having a potent inhibitory effect on CYP3A4 at therapeutic doses should be avoided unless the benefits of combined therapy outweigh the increased risk.

The dose of simvastatin should not exceed 10 mg daily in patients receiving concomitant medication with cyclosporine, danazol, gemfibrozil, or other fibrates (except fenofibrate). The combined use of simvastatin with gemfibrozil should be avoided unless the benefits are likely to outweigh the increased risk of this drug combination. The benefits of the use of simvastatin in patients receiving other fibrates (except fenofibrate), cyclosporine, or danazol should be carefully weighed against the risks of these drug combinations. Caution should be used when prescribing fenofibrate with simvastatin, as either agent can cause myopathy when given alone. Addition of fibrates to simvastatin typically provides little additional reduction in LDL-C, but further reductions of TG and further increases in HDL-C may be obtained. Combinations of fibrate with simvastatin have been used without myopathy in small, short-term clinical studies with careful monitoring.

The dose of simvastatin should not exceed 20 mg daily in patients receiving concomitant medication with amiodarone or verapamil. The combined use of simvastatin at doses higher than 20 mg daily with amiodarone or verapamil should be avoided unless the clinical benefit is likely to outweigh the increased risk of myopathy.

The dose of simvastatin should not exceed 40 mg daily in patients receiving concomitant medication with diltiazem, unless the clinical benefit is likely to outweigh the increased risk of myopathy.

Caution should be used when prescribing amlodipine with simvastatin 80 mg as there is a slight increase in the risk of myopathy with concomitant use.

The dose of simvastatin should not exceed 40 mg daily in Chinese patients receiving concomitant medication with niacin (≥1 g/day). Interim safety data of an ongoing, double blind, randomised cardiovascular outcome study has shown that the incidence of myopathy was higher in Chinese patients versus non-Chinese patients.

Patients on fusidic acid (oral or iv) and simvastatin should be closely monitored for symptoms and/or signs of myopathy. Temporary suspension of simvastatin treatment may be considered.

Ophthalmologic: Current long-term data from clinical studies do not indicate an adverse effect of simvastatin on the human lens.

Renal: ZOCOR does not undergo significant renal excretion, modification of dosage should not be necessary in patients with moderate renal insufficiency. In patients with severe renal insufficiency (creatinine clearance <30 mL/min), dosages above 10 mg/day should be carefully considered and, if deemed necessary, implemented cautiously. This recommendation is based on studies with lovastatin (see Warnings and Precautions, Myopathy/Rhabdomyolysis).

Higher dosages (40-80 mg/day) required for some patients with severe hypercholesterolemia are associated with increased plasma levels of simvastatin. **Caution should be exercised in such patients who are also significantly renally impaired or are concomitantly administered P-450 inhibitors (see Warnings and Precautions, Myopathy/Rhabdomyolysis and Drug Interactions).**

Skin: In few instances eosinophilia and skin eruptions appear to be associated with simvastatin treatment. If hypersensitivity is suspected, ZOCOR should be discontinued.

Special Populations: Pregnant Women: ZOCOR is contraindicated during pregnancy.

Safety in pregnant women has not been established. No controlled clinical trials with simvastatin have been conducted in pregnant women. Rare reports of congenital anomalies following intrauterine exposure to HMG-CoA reductase inhibitors have been received. However, in an analysis of approximately 200 prospectively followed pregnancies exposed during the first trimester to ZOCOR or another closely related HMG-CoA reductase inhibitor, the incidence of congenital anomalies was comparable to that seen in the general population. This number of pregnancies was statistically sufficient to exclude a 2.5-fold or greater increase in congenital anomalies over the background incidence.

Although there is no evidence that the incidence of congenital anomalies in offspring of patients taking ZOCOR or another closely related HMG-CoA reductase inhibitor differs from that observed in the general population, maternal treatment with ZOCOR may reduce the fetal levels of mevalonate which is a precursor of cholesterol biosynthesis. Atherosclerosis is a chronic process, and ordinarily discontinuation of lipid-lowering drugs during pregnancy should have little impact on the long-term risk associated with primary hypercholesterolemia. For these reasons, ZOCOR should not be used in women who are pregnant, trying to become pregnant or suspect they are pregnant. Treatment with ZOCOR should be suspended for the duration of pregnancy or until it has been determined that the woman is not pregnant (see Contraindications).

Nursing Women: It is not known whether simvastatin or its metabolites are excreted in human milk. Because many drugs are excreted in human milk and because of the potential for serious adverse reactions, women taking ZOCOR should not nurse (see Contraindications).

Pediatrics: Safety and effectiveness of simvastatin in patients 10-17 years of age with heterozygous familial hypercholesterolemia have been evaluated in a controlled clinical trial in adolescent boys and in girls who were at least one year post-menarche. Patients treated with simvastatin had an adverse experience profile generally similar to that of patients treated with placebo. **Doses greater than 40 mg have not been studied in this population.** In this limited controlled study, there was no detectable effect on growth or sexual maturation in the adolescent boys or girls, or any effect on menstrual cycle length in girls. (See Dosage and Administration; Adverse Reactions; Action and Clinical Pharmacology.) Adolescent females should be counseled on appropriate contraceptive methods while on simvastatin therapy (see Contraindications; Warnings and Precautions, Special Populations, Pregnant Women). Simvastatin has not been studied in patients younger than 10 years of age, nor in pre-menarchal girls.

Geriatrics (>65 years of age): For patients over the age of 65 years who received simvastatin in controlled clinical studies, efficacy, as assessed by reduction in total and LDL-cholesterol levels, appeared similar to that seen in the population as a whole, and there was no apparent increase in the overall frequency and severity of clinical or laboratory adverse findings. However, in a clinical trial of patients treated with simvastatin 80 mg/day, patients ≥65 years of age had an increased risk of myopathy compared to patients <65 years of age.

Higher dosages (40-80 mg/day) required for some patients with severe hypercholesterolemia are associated with increased plasma levels of simvastatin. **Caution should be exercised in such patients who are also elderly or are concomitantly administered P-450 inhibitors (see Warnings and Precautions, Myopathy/Rhabdomyolysis and Drug Interactions).**

Elderly patients may be more susceptible to myopathy (see Warnings and Precautions, Pre-disposing Factors for Myopathy/Rhabdomyolysis).

Monitoring and Laboratory Tests: In the differential diagnosis of chest pain in a patient on therapy with ZOCOR cardiac and noncardiac fractions of serum transaminase and creatine phosphokinase levels should be determined.

ADVERSE REACTIONS: Adverse Drug Reaction Overview: Based on experience in a total of over 2300 patients, of whom more than 1200 were treated for one year and over 230 for 2 years or more, ZOCOR is generally well tolerated and adverse reactions are usually mild and transient.

In pre-marketing controlled clinical studies, 1.0% of patients were withdrawn due to adverse experiences attributable to ZOCOR.

Adverse experiences occurring at an incidence of ≥0.5% of 2361 patients treated with ZOCOR in pre-marketing controlled clinical studies and reported to be possibly, probably or definitely drug related are shown in Table 1.

Table 1: ZOCOR

Adverse Experiences Occurring in Patients Treated with ZOCOR in Pre-marketing Controlled Clinical Studies

	ZOCOR (n=2361) (%)
Gastrointestinal	
Abdominal Pain	2.2
Acid Regurgitation	0.5
Constipation	2.5
Dyspepsia	0.6
Diarrhea	0.8
Flatulence	2.0
Nausea	1.1
Nervous System	
Headache	1.0
Skin	
Rash	0.7
Miscellaneous	
Asthenia	0.8

In the Scandinavian Simvastatin Survival Study (4S) involving 4444 patients treated with 20-40 mg/day of ZOCOR (n=2221) or placebo (n=2223), the safety and tolerability profiles were comparable between groups over the median 5.4 years of the study.

Ophthalmologic: See Warnings and Precautions, Ophthalmologic.

Laboratory Tests: Marked persistent increases of serum transaminases (ALT, AST) have been noted (see Warnings and Precautions).

About 5.0% of patients had elevations of creatine phosphokinase (CK) levels three or more times the normal value on one or more occasions. This was attributable to the noncardiac fraction of CK. Myopathy has been reported rarely (see Warnings and Precautions, Myopathy/Rhabdomyolysis and Drug Interactions, Drug-Laboratory Interactions).

Uncontrolled Clinical Studies or Post-market Adverse Drug Reactions: The following additional adverse reactions were reported either in uncontrolled clinical studies or in post-marketing experience with ZOCOR, regardless of causality assessment.

Gastrointestinal: vomiting.

Hematologic: anemia, leukopenia, purpura.

Hepatic/Pancreatic: hepatitis. Hepatic failure with fatal or liver transplant outcome have been reported. Jaundice, pancreatitis.

Laboratory Tests: Elevated alkaline phosphatase and γ-glutamyl transpeptidase have been reported.

Muscular: rhabdomyolysis, muscle cramps, myalgia.

Neurologic: dizziness, paresthesia, peripheral neuropathy. Peripheral neuropathy with muscle weakness or sensory disturbance has been reported. Memory impairment.

Psychiatric: depression, insomnia.

Sensitivity: An apparent hypersensitivity syndrome has been reported rarely which has included some of the following features:

Angioedema	Flushing
Arthralgia	Lupus-like Syndrome
Arthritis	Malaise
Dermatomyositis	Photosensitivity
Dyspnea	Polymyalgia Rheumatica
Eosinophilia	Thrombocytopenia
ESR Increased	Urticaria
Fever	Vasculitis

Skin: erythema multiforme including Stevens-Johnson Syndrome, rash, pruritus, alopecia.

Others: Although the following adverse reactions were not observed in clinical studies with ZOCOR, they have been reported following treatment with other HMG-CoA reductase inhibitors: anorexia, psychic disturbances including anxiety, hypospermia and gynecomastia.

Pediatric Patients (ages 10-17 years): In a study involving pediatric patients 10-17 years of age with heterozygous familial hypercholesterolemia (n=175), the safety and tolerability profile of the group treated with ZOCOR was generally similar to that of the group treated with placebo (see Warnings and Precautions, Pediatrics; Action and Clinical Pharmacology).

DRUG INTERACTIONS: Overview: CYP3A4 Interactions: Simvastatin itself is a substrate for CYP3A4. However, simvastatin has no CYP3A4 inhibitory activity; therefore, it is not expected to affect plasma levels of other drugs metabolized by CYP3A4. Potent inhibitors of CYP3A4 increase the risk of myopathy by increasing the plasma levels of HMG-CoA reductase inhibitory activity during simvastatin therapy. These include itraconazole, ketoconazole, erythromycin, clarithromycin, telithromycin, HIV protease inhibitors, and nefazodone (see Warnings and Precautions, Myopathy/Rhabdomyolysis Caused by Drug Interactions).

Drug-Drug Interactions: Interactions with Lipid-Lowering Drugs that Can Cause Myopathy when Given Alone: The risk of myopathy may also be increased by the following lipid-lowering drugs that are not potent inhibitors of CYP3A4, but which can cause myopathy when given alone (see below and Warnings and Precautions).

- **Gemfibrozil:** The risk of myopathy/rhabdomyolysis is increased by gemfibrozil (see Dosage and Administration).
- **Other Fibrates (except fenofibrate):** These drugs (except fenofibrate) increase the risk of myopathy when given concomitantly with simvastatin, probably because they can produce myopathy when given alone (see Warnings and Precautions, Myopathy/Rhabdomyolysis Caused by Drug Interactions). When simvastatin and fenofibrate are given concomitantly, there is no evidence that the risk of myopathy exceeds the sum of the individual risks of each agent.

Concomitant Therapy with Other Lipid Metabolism Regulators:

- **Bile Acid Sequestrants (Cholestyramine):** Preliminary evidence suggests that the cholesterol-lowering effects of ZOCOR and the bile acid sequestrant, cholestyramine, are additive.

  When ZOCOR is used concurrently with cholestyramine or any other resin, an interval of at least two hours should be maintained between the two drugs, since the absorption of ZOCOR may be impaired by the resin.

Other Drugs:

- **Erythromycin, Clarithromycin, and Telithromycin:** (See Warnings and Precautions, Measures to reduce the risk of myopathy/rhabdomyolysis caused by drug interactions.)
- **Coumarin Anticoagulants:** In two clinical studies, one in normal volunteers and the other in hypercholesterolemic patients, simvastatin 20-40 mg/day modestly potentiated the effect of coumarin anticoagulants: the prothrombin time, reported as International Normalized Ratios (INR), increased from a baseline of 1.7 to 1.8 and from 2.6 to 3.4 in the volunteer and patient studies, respectively. In patients taking coumarin anticoagulants, prothrombin time should be determined before starting simvastatin and frequently enough during early therapy to ensure that no significant alteration of prothrombin time occurs. Once a stable prothrombin time has been documented, prothrombin times can be monitored at the intervals usually recommended for patients on coumarin anticoagulants. If the dose of simvastatin is changed, the same procedure should be repeated. Simvastatin therapy has not been associated with bleeding or with changes in prothrombin time in patients not taking anticoagulants.
- **Cyclosporine or Danazol:** The risk of myopathy/rhabdomyolysis is increased by concomitant administration of cyclosporine or danazol particularly with higher doses of simvastatin (see Warnings and Precautions, Myopathy/Rhabdomyolysis Caused by Drug Interactions).
- **Digoxin:** Concomitant administration of ZOCOR and digoxin in normal volunteers resulted in a slight elevation (<0.3 ng/mL) in drug concentrations (as measured by a digoxin radioimmunoassay) in plasma compared to concomitant administration of placebo and digoxin.
- **Amiodarone:** The risk of myopathy/rhabdomyolysis is increased by concomitant administration of amiodarone with higher doses of simvastatin (see Warnings and Precautions, Myopathy/Rhabdomyolysis Caused by Drug Interactions). In an ongoing clinical trial, myopathy has been reported in 6% of patients receiving simvastatin 80 mg and amiodarone.
- **Calcium channel Blockers:**
  - **Verapamil: The risk of myopathy/rhabdomyolysis is increased by concomitant administration of verapamil with higher doses of simvastatin** (see Warnings and Precautions, Myopathy/Rhabdomyolysis Caused by Drug Interactions). In an analysis of clinical trials involving 33 796 patients treated with simvastatin 20 to 80 mg, the incidence of myopathy was higher in patients receiving verapamil and simvastatin (0.54%) than in patients taking simvastatin without a calcium channel blocker (0.10%).
  - **Diltiazem:** The risk of myopathy/rhabdomyolysis is increased by concomitant administration of diltiazem with simvastatin 80 mg. In clinical studies, the risk of myopathy in patients taking simvastatin 40 mg with diltiazem was similar to that in patients taking simvastatin 40 mg without diltiazem (see Warnings and Precautions, Myopathy/Rhabdomyolysis Caused by Drug Interactions).
  - **Amlodipine:** Patients on amlodipine treated concomitantly with simvastatin 80 mg have a slightly increased risk of myopathy (see Warnings and Precautions, Myopathy/Rhabdomyolysis Caused by Drug Interactions).
- **Niacin (nicotinic acid) (≥1 g/day):** Cases of myopathy/rhabdomyolysis have been observed with simvastatin coadministered with lipid modifying doses (≥1 g/day) of niacin (see Warnings and Precautions, Myopathy/Rhabdomyolysis Caused by Drug Interactions).
- **Fusidic Acid (oral or iv):** Patients on fusidic acid (oral or iv) treated concomitantly with simvastatin may have an increased risk of myopathy/rhabdomyolysis (see Warnings and Precautions, Myopathy/Rhabdomyolysis Caused by Drug Interactions).
- **Other Concomitant Therapy:** In clinical studies, ZOCOR was used concomitantly with angiotensin converting enzyme (ACE) inhibitors, beta-blockers, diuretics and nonsteroidal anti-inflammatory drugs (NSAIDs) without evidence, to date, of clinically significant adverse interactions.

Drug-Food Interactions: Grapefruit juice contains one or more components that inhibit CYP3A4 and can increase the plasma levels of drugs metabolized by CYP3A4. The effect of typical consumption (one 250-mL glass daily) is minimal (13% increase in active plasma HMG-CoA reductase inhibitory activity as measured by the area under the concentration-time curve) and of no clinical relevance. However, very large quantities (over 1 liter daily) significantly increase the plasma levels of HMG-CoA reductase inhibitory activity during simvastatin therapy and should be avoided (see Warnings and Precautions, Myopathy/Rhabdomyolysis Caused by Drug Interactions).

Drug-Laboratory Interactions: ZOCOR may elevate serum transaminase and creatine phosphokinase levels (from skeletal muscles) (see Adverse Reactions, Laboratory Tests).

DOSAGE AND ADMINISTRATION: Dosing Considerations: Patients should be placed on a standard cholesterol-lowering diet before receiving ZOCOR, and should continue on this diet during treatment with ZOCOR. If appropriate, a program of weight control and physical exercise should be implemented.

Prior to initiating therapy with ZOCOR, secondary causes for elevations in plasma lipid levels should be excluded. A lipid profile should also be performed.

- **Patients at high risk of coronary events, because of existing Coronary Heart Disease (CHD) or other occlusive arterial disease, or being over the age of 40 years with a diagnosis of diabetes:** The usual starting dose of ZOCOR is 40 mg/day given as a single dose in the evening. Drug therapy can be initiated simultaneously with diet and exercise.
- **Patients with hyperlipidemia (who are not in the risk categories above):** The usual starting dose is 10 mg/day given as a single dose in the evening. Patients who require a large reduction in LDL-C (more than 45%) may be started at 40 mg/day given as a single dose in the evening. Patients with mild to moderate hypercholesterolemia can be treated with a starting dose of 5 mg of ZOCOR. Adjustments of dosage, if required, should be made as specified above.
- **Cholesterol levels should be monitored periodically and consideration should be given to reducing the dosage of ZOCOR if cholesterol levels fall below the desired range.**
- **Concomitant therapy with other lipid metabolism regulators:** If ZOCOR is used with gemfibrozil, the dose of ZOCOR should not exceed 10 mg/day (see Drug Interactions, Concomitant Therapy with Other Lipid Metabolism Regulators.)
- In patients taking cyclosporine, danazol, therapy should begin at 5 mg/day and not exceed 10 mg/day.
- In patients taking amiodarone or verapamil concomitantly with ZOCOR, the dose of ZOCOR should not exceed 20 mg/day (see Warnings and Precautions, Measures to reduce the risk of myopathy/rhabdomyolysis caused by drug interactions and Drug Interactions).
- In patients taking diltiazem concomitantly with ZOCOR, the dose of ZOCOR should not exceed 40 mg/day (see Warnings and Precautions, Measures to reduce the risk of myopathy/rhabdomyolysis caused by drug interactions and Drug Interactions).
- The dosage of ZOCOR should be individualized according to baseline LDL-C, total-C/HDL-C ratio and/or TG levels to achieve the recommended desired lipid values at the lowest possible dose and the patient response. Lipid levels should be monitored periodically and, if necessary, the dose of ZOCOR adjusted based on desired lipid levels.

Recommended Dose and Dosage Adjustment: The recommended dose range for most patients is 10 to 40 mg/day. The maximum dose is 80 mg/day, which should be used only for those patients who have not achieved their LDL-C goal utilizing the 40 mg dose (see Warnings and Precautions, Myopathy/Rhabdomyolysis). Adjustments of dosage, if required, should be made at intervals of not less than 4 weeks, to a maximum of 80 mg/day given as a single dose in the evening.

Dosage in Pediatric Patients (10-17 years of age) with Heterozygous Familial Hypercholesterolemia: The recommended usual starting dose is 10 mg once a day in the evening. The recommended dosing range is 10-40 mg/day; the maximum recommended dose is 40 mg/day. Doses should be individualized according to the recommended goal of therapy (see Action and Clinical Pharmacology).

Dosage in Renal Insufficiency: Because ZOCOR does not undergo significant renal excretion, modification of dosage should not be necessary in patients with mild to moderate renal insufficiency. However, caution should be exercised when ZOCOR is administered to patients with severe renal insufficiency; such patients should be started at 5 mg/day and be closely monitored (see Warnings and Precautions, Muscle Effects and Renal).

Missed Dose: If a tablet is missed at its usual time, it should be taken as soon as possible. But, if it is too close to the time of the next dose: only the prescribed dose should be taken at the appointed time. **A double dose should not be taken.**

OVERDOSAGE: A few cases of overdosage have been reported; the maximum dose taken was 3.6 g. All patients recovered without sequelae. General measures should be adopted.

> For management of a suspected drug overdose, contact your regional Poison Control Centre. See the *CPS* Directory section for a list of Poison Control Centres.

ACTION AND CLINICAL PHARMACOLOGY: Mechanism of Action: ZOCOR is a lipid-lowering agent derived synthetically from a fermentation product of *A. terreus*.

After oral ingestion, ZOCOR, which is an inactive lactone, is hydrolyzed to the corresponding β-hydroxyacid form. This principal metabolite is a specific inhibitor of 3 hydroxy-3-methylglutaryl-coenzyme A (HMG-CoA) reductase. This enzyme catalyzes the conversion of HMG-CoA to mevalonate, which is an early and rate-limiting step in the biosynthesis of cholesterol.

Pharmacodynamics: ZOCOR reduces cholesterol production by the liver and induces some changes in cholesterol transport and disposition in the blood and tissues. The mechanism(s) of this effect is believed to involve both reduction of the synthesis of Low-Density Lipoprotein (LDL), and an increase in LDL catabolism as a result of induction of the hepatic LDL receptors.

Pharmacokinetics: ZOCOR has complex pharmacokinetic characteristics.

Metabolism: Simvastatin is metabolized by the microsomal hepatic enzyme system (cytochrome P-450 isoform 3A4). The major active metabolites present in human plasma are the β-hydroxyacid of simvastatin and four other active metabolites.

STORAGE AND STABILITY: ZOCOR should be stored at room temperature (15-30°C).

INFORMATION FOR THE PATIENT: Published in e-CPS, available by subscription at www.e-cps.ca.

DOSAGE FORMS, COMPOSITION AND PACKAGING: 5 mg: Each buff, oval-shaped biconvex, film-coated tablet, engraved MSD 726 on one side and ZOCOR 5 on the other, contains: simvastatin 5 mg. Nonmedicinal ingredients: ascorbic acid, butylated hydroxyanisole, citric acid monohydrate, hydroxypropyl cellulose, hydroxypropyl methylcellulose, lactose monohydrate, magnesium stearate, microcrystalline cellulose, pregelatinized starch, talc, titanium dioxide and yellow ferric oxide. Blister packages of 28.

10 mg: Each peach, oval-shaped biconvex, film-coated tablet, engraved MSD 735 on one side and plain on the other, contains: simvastatin 10 mg. Nonmedicinal ingredients: ascorbic acid, butylated hydroxyanisole, citric acid monohydrate, hydroxypropyl cellulose, hydroxypropyl methylcellulose, lactose monohydrate, magnesium stearate, microcrystalline cellulose, pregelatinized starch, red ferric oxide, talc, titanium dioxide and yellow ferric oxide. Blister packages of 28.

20 mg: Each tan, oval-shaped biconvex, film-coated tablet, engraved MSD 740 on one side and plain on the other, contains: simvastatin 20 mg. Nonmedicinal ingredients: ascorbic acid, butylated hydroxyanisole, citric acid monohydrate, hydroxypropyl cellulose, hydroxypropyl methylcellulose, lactose monohydrate, magnesium stearate, microcrystalline cellulose, pregelatinized starch, red ferric oxide, talc, titanium dioxide and yellow ferric oxide. Blister packages of 28. High density polyethylene bottles of 100.

40 mg: Each brick-red, oval-shaped biconvex, film-coated tablet, engraved MSD 749 on one side and plain on the other, contains: simvastatin 40 mg. Nonmedicinal ingredients: ascorbic acid, butylated hydroxyanisole, citric acid monohydrate, hydroxypropyl cellulose, hydroxypropyl methylcellulose, lactose monohydrate, magnesium stearate, microcrystalline cellulose, pregelatinized starch, red ferric oxide, talc and titanium dioxide. Blister packages of 28.

80 mg: Each brick-red, capsule-shaped, film-coated tablet, engraved 543 on one side and 80 on the other, contains: simvastatin 80 mg. Nonmedicinal ingredients: ascorbic acid, butylated hydroxyanisole, citric acid monohydrate, hydroxypropyl cellulose, hydroxypropyl methylcellulose, lactose monohydrate, magnesium stearate, microcrystalline cellulose, pregelatinized starch, red ferric oxide, talc and titanium dioxide. Blister packages of 28.

(Shown in Product Identification Section)

Zofran® Ⓟ

ondansetron HCl dihydrate

Antiemetic

GlaxoSmithKline

Zofran® ODT Ⓟ

ondansetron

Antiemetic

GlaxoSmithKline

Date of Revision: March 1, 2010

SUMMARY PRODUCT INFORMATION:

Route of Administration	Dosage Form/Strength	Nonmedicinal Ingredients
Oral	Tablets/4 mg and 8 mg ondansetron (as hydrochloride dihydrate)	Lactose, magnesium stearate, methyl hydroxypropyl cellulose, microcrystalline cellulose, Opadry yellow or Opaspray yellow (containing titanium dioxide and iron oxide yellow) and pregelatinised starch
	Oral solution/4 mg/5 mL ondansetron (as hydrochloride dihydrate)	Citric acid, sodium benzoate, sodium citrate dihydrate, sorbitol, strawberry flavour
	ODT Oral Disintegrating tablets/4 mg and 8 mg ondansetron	Aspartame, gelatin, mannitol, sodium methyl hydroxybenzoate, sodium propyl hydroxybenzoate, and strawberry flavour
Intravenous	Injection/2 mg/mL ondansetron (as hydrochloride dihydrate)	2 mL or 4 mL ampoule: citric acid monohydrate, sodium chloride, sodium citrate 20 mL vial: citric acid monohydrate, methylparaben, propylparaben, sodium chloride, sodium citrate

INDICATIONS AND CLINICAL USE: Adults: ZOFRAN (ondansetron hydrochloride; and ondansetron) is indicated for:

- the prevention of nausea and vomiting associated with emetogenic chemotherapy, including high dose cisplatin, and radiotherapy.
- the prevention and treatment of post-operative nausea and vomiting.

Pediatrics (<18 years of age): Post-Chemotherapy: Clinical experience of ZOFRAN in children is currently limited, however, ZOFRAN was effective and well tolerated when given to children 4-12 years of age (see Dosage and Administration). ZOFRAN is not indicated for the treatment of children 3 years of age or younger.

Post-Radiotherapy: Safety and efficacy of ZOFRAN in any age group in this population following radiotherapy has not been established and is therefore not indicated for use in this population.

Post-Operative Nausea and Vomiting: Safety and efficacy of ZOFRAN in any age group in this population for the prevention and treatment of post-operative nausea and vomiting has not been established and is not indicated for use in this group.

Geriatrics (>65 years of age): Post-Chemotherapy and Radiotherapy: Efficacy and tolerance of ZOFRAN were similar to that observed in younger adults (see Dosage and Administration).

Post-Operative Nausea and Vomiting: Clinical experience in the use of ZOFRAN in the prevention and treatment of post-operative nausea and vomiting is limited and is not indicated for use in this population.

CONTRAINDICATIONS:

- ZOFRAN (ondansetron hydrochloride; and ondansetron) is contraindicated in patients with a history of hypersensitivity to the drug or any components of its formulations. For a complete listing, see Dosage Forms, Composition and Packaging.

WARNINGS AND PRECAUTIONS: General: Cross-reactive hypersensitivity has been reported between different 5-HT_3 antagonists. Patients who have experienced hypersensitivity reactions to one 5-HT_3 antagonist have experienced more severe reactions upon being challenged with another drug of the same class. The use of a different 5-HT_3 receptor antagonist is not recommended as a replacement in cases in which a patient has experienced even a mild hypersensitivity type reaction to another 5-HT_3 antagonist.

Rarely and predomininantly with intravenous ondansetron, transient ECG changes including QT interval prolongation have been reported (see Post-Market Adverse Drug Reactions).

ZOFRAN ODT (ondansetron) contains aspartame and therefore should be taken with caution in patients with phenylketonuria.

ZOFRAN (ondansetron hydrochloride) is not effective in preventing motion-induced nausea and vomiting.

Hepatic/Biliary/Pancreatic: There is no experience in patients who are clinically jaundiced. The clearance of an 8 mg intravenous dose of ZOFRAN was significantly reduced and the serum half-life significantly prolonged in subjects with severe impairment of hepatic function. In patients with moderate or severe impairment of hepatic function, reductions in dosage are therefore recommended and a total daily dose of 8 mg should not be exceeded. This may be given as a single intravenous or oral dose. As ondansetron is known to increase large bowel transit time, patients with signs of subacute intestinal obstruction should be monitored following administration.

Ondansetron does not itself appear to induce or inhibit the cytochrome P450 drug-metabolizing enzyme system of the liver. Because ondansetron is metabolised by hepatic cytochrome P450 drug-metabolizing enzymes, inducers or inhibitors of these enzymes may change the clearance and, hence, the half-life of ondansetron. On the basis of available data no dosage adjustment is recommended for patients on these drugs.

Special Populations: Pregnant Women: The safety of ondansetron for use in human pregnancy has not been established. Ondansetron is not teratogenic in animals. However, as animal studies are not always predictive of human response, the use of ondansetron in pregnancy is not recommended.

Nursing Women: Ondansetron is excreted in the milk of lactating rats. It is not known if it is excreted in human milk, however, nursing is not recommended during treatment with ondansetron.

Pediatrics (<3 years of age): Insufficient information is available to provide dosage recommendations for children 3 years of age or younger.

ADVERSE REACTIONS: Clinical Trial Adverse Drug Reactions: Because clinical trials are conducted under very specific conditions the adverse reaction rates observed in the clinical trials may not reflect the rates observed in practice and should not be compared to the rates in the clinical trials of another drug. Adverse drug reaction information from clinical trials is useful for identifying drug-related adverse events and for approximating rates.

ZOFRAN (ondansetron hydrochloride; and ondansetron) has been administered to over 2500 patients worldwide in controlled clinical trials and has been well tolerated.

The most frequent adverse events reported in controlled clinical trials were headache (11%) and constipation (4%). Other adverse events include sensations of flushing or warmth (<1%).

Cardiovascular: There have been rare reports of tachycardia, angina (chest pain), bradycardia, hypotension, syncope and electrocardiographic alterations.

Central Nervous System: There have been rare reports of seizures. Movement disorders and dyskinesia have been reported in two large clinical trials of ondansetron at a rate of 0.1-0.3%.

Dermatological: Rash has occurred in approximately 1% of patients receiving ondansetron.

Hypersensitivity: Rare cases of immediate hypersensitivity reactions sometimes severe, including anaphylaxis, bronchospasm, urticaria and angioedema have been reported.

Local Reactions: Pain, redness and burning at the site of injection have been reported.

Metabolic: There were transient increases of AST and ALT of over twice the upper limit of normal in approximately 5% of patients. These increases did not appear to be related to dose or duration of therapy. There have been reports of liver failure and death in patients with cancer receiving concurrent medications including potentially hepatotoxic cytotoxic chemotherapy and antibiotics. The etiology of the liver failure is unclear. There have been rare reports of hypokalemia.

Other: There have been reports of abdominal pain, weakness and xerostomia.

Special Senses: Rare cases of transient visual disturbances (e.g. blurred vision) have been reported during or shortly after intravenous administration of ondansetron, particularly at rates equal to or greater than 30 mg in 15 minutes.

Post-Market Adverse Drug Reactions: Over 250 million patient treatment days of ZOFRAN have been supplied since the launch of the product worldwide. The following events have been spontaneously reported during post-approval use of ZOFRAN, although the link to ondansetron cannot always be clearly established.

The adverse event profiles in children and adolescents were comparable to that seen in adults.

General Disorders: Rare cases of hypersensitivity reactions, such as, laryngeal edema, stridor, laryngospasm and cardiopulmonary arrest have also been reported.

Cardiovascular Disorders: There have been rare reports (<0.01%) of myocardial infarction, myocardial ischemia, angina, chest pain with or without ST segment depression, arrhythmias (including ventricular or supraventricular tachycardia, premature ventricular contractions, and atrial fibrillation), electrocardiographic alterations (including second degree heart block), palpitations and syncope.

Rarely and predominantly with intravenous ondansetron, transient ECG changes including QT interval prolongation have been reported (see Warnings and Precautions).

Eye Disorder: There have been very rare cases of transient blindness following ondansetron treatment, generally within the recommended dosing range and predominantly during intravenous administration.

The majority of blindness cases reported resolved within 20 minutes. Although most patients had received chemotherapeutic agents, including cisplatin a few cases of transient blindness occurred following ondansetron administration for the treatment of post-operative nausea or vomiting and in the absence of cisplatin treatment. Some cases of transient blindness were reported as cortical in origin.

Hepatobiliary Disorders: Occasional asymptomatic increases in liver function tests have been reported.

Nervous System Disorders: Transient episodes of dizziness (<0.01%) have been reported during or upon completion of IV infusion of ondansetron.

Uncommon reports (<1%) suggestive of extrapyramidal reactions including oculogyric crisis/dystonic reactions (e.g. oro-facial dyskinesia, opisthotonos, tremor, etc.), movement disorders and dyskinesia have been reported without definitive evidence of persistent clinical sequelae.

Respiratory, Thoracic and Mediastinal Disorders: There have also been rare reports of hiccups.

Very rare reports have been received for bullous skin and mucosal reactions (including Stevens-Johnson syndrome and toxic epidermal necrolysis). These reports have occurred in patients taking other medications that can be associated with bullous skin and mucosal reactions.

DRUG INTERACTIONS: Drug-Drug Interactions: Specific studies have shown that there are no pharmacokinetic interactions when ondansetron is administered with alcohol, temazepam, frusemide, tramadol or propofol.

Ondansetron is metabolised by multiple hepatic cytochrome P450 enzymes: CYP3A4, CYP2D6 and CYP1A2. Despite the multiplicity of metabolic enzymes capable of metabolising ondansetron which can compensate for an increase or decrease in enzyme activity, it was found that patients treated with inducers of CYP3A4 (i.e. phenytoin, carbamazepine, and rifampicin) demonstrated an increase in oral clearance of ondansetron and a decrease in ondansetron blood concentrations. No effect in ondansetron clearance secondary to enzyme inhibition or reduced activity (e.g. CYP2D6 genetic deficiency) has been identified to date.

Data from small studies indicate that ondansetron may reduce the analgesic effect of tramadol.

DOSAGE AND ADMINISTRATION: Dosing Considerations: Chemotherapy Induced Nausea and Vomiting: ZOFRAN (ondansetron hydrochloride; and ondansetron) should be given as an initial dose prior to chemotherapy, followed by a dosage regimen tailored to the anticipated severity of emetic response caused by different cancer treatments. The route of administration and dose of ZOFRAN should be flexible in the range of 8-32 mg a day. The selection of dose regimen should be determined by the severity of the emetogenic challenge (see Recommended Dose and Dosage Adjustment).

Recommended Dose and Dosage Adjustment: Chemotherapy Induced Nausea and Vomiting: Use in Adults: Highly Emetogenic Chemotherapy (e.g. regimens containing cisplatin): ZOFRAN has been shown to be effective in the following dose schedules for the prevention of emesis during the first 24 hours following chemotherapy:
Initial Dose: ZOFRAN 8 mg infused intravenously over 15 minutes given 30 minutes prior to chemotherapy.
or
ZOFRAN 8 mg infused intravenously over 15 minutes, given 30 minutes prior to chemotherapy, followed by 1 mg/h by continuous infusion for up to 24 hours.
or
ZOFRAN 32 mg diluted in 50-100 mL of saline or other compatible infusion fluid and infused over not less than 15 minutes*, given 30 minutes prior to chemotherapy.
Post-chemotherapy: After the first 24 hours, ZOFRAN 8 mg orally every 8† hours for up to 5 days.

No significant differences in terms of emesis control or grade of nausea have been demonstrated between the 32 mg single dose, the 8 mg single dose, or the 8 mg dose followed by the 24 hour 1 mg/h continuous infusion.

However, in some studies conducted in patients receiving medium or high doses of cisplatin chemotherapy, the 32 mg single dose has demonstrated a statistically significant superiority over the 8 mg single dose with regard to control of emesis.

The efficacy of ZOFRAN in highly emetogenic chemotherapy may be enhanced by the addition of a single intravenous dose of dexamethasone sodium phosphate, 20 mg administered prior to chemotherapy.

Less Emetogenic Chemotherapy (e.g. regimens containing cyclophosphamide, doxorubicin, epirubicin, fluorouracil and carboplatin): Initial Dose: ZOFRAN 8 mg infused intravenously over 15 minutes, given 30 minutes prior to chemotherapy; or ZOFRAN 8 mg orally 1 to 2 hours prior to chemotherapy.
Post-chemotherapy: ZOFRAN 8 mg orally twice daily for up to 5 days.
Use in Children: Clinical experience of ZOFRAN in children is currently limited however, ZOFRAN was effective and well tolerated when given to children 4-12 years of age. ZOFRAN injection should be given intravenously at a dose of 3-5 mg/m² over 15 minutes immediately before chemotherapy. After therapy, ZOFRAN 4 mg should be given orally every 8 hours† for up to 5 days. For children 3 years of age and younger, there is insufficient information available to make dosage recommendations (see Indications and Clinical Use).
Use in Elderly: Efficacy and tolerance in patients aged over 65 years were similar to that seen in younger adults indicating no need to alter dosage schedules in this population.
Radiotherapy Induced Nausea and Vomiting: Use in Adults: Initial Dose: ZOFRAN 8 mg orally 1 to 2 hours before radiotherapy.
Post-radiotherapy: ZOFRAN 8 mg orally every 8 hours† for up to 5 days after a course of treatment.
Use in Children: There is no experience in clinical studies in this population.
Use in Elderly: Efficacy and tolerance in patients aged over 65 years were similar to that seen in younger adults indicating no need to alter dosage schedules in this population.
Post-Operative Nausea and Vomiting: Use in Adults: For prevention of post-operative nausea and vomiting ZOFRAN may be administered as a single dose of 16 mg given orally one hour prior to anaesthesia. Alternatively, a single dose of 4 mg may be given by slow intravenous injection at induction of anaesthesia.

For the treatment of established post-operative nausea and vomiting, a single dose of 4 mg given by slow intravenous injection is recommended.
Use in Children: There is no experience in the use of ZOFRAN in the prevention and treatment of post-operative nausea and vomiting in children (see Indications and Clinical Use).
Use in Elderly: There is limited experience in the use of ZOFRAN in the prevention and treatment of post-operative nausea and vomiting in the elderly (see Indications and Clinical Use).
Patients with Renal/Hepatic Impairment: Use in Patients with Impaired Renal Function: No alteration of daily dosage, frequency of dosing, or route of administration is required.
Use in Patients with Impaired Hepatic Function: The clearance of an 8 mg intravenous dose of ZOFRAN was significantly reduced and the serum half-life significantly prolonged in subjects with severe impairment of hepatic function. In patients with moderate or severe impairment of hepatic function, reductions in dosage are therefore recommended and a total daily dose of 8 mg should not be exceeded. This may be given as a single intravenous or oral dose.

No studies have been conducted to date in patients with jaundice.
Patients with Poor Sparteine/Debrisoquine Metabolism: The elimination half-life and plasma levels of a single 8 mg intravenous dose of ondansetron did not differ between subjects classified as poor and extensive metabolisers of sparteine and debrisoquine. No alteration of daily dosage or frequency of dosing is recommended for patients known to be poor metabolisers of sparteine and debrisoquine.
Administration: Administration of Intravenous Infusion Solutions: Compatibility with Intravenous Solutions: ZOFRAN Injection is compatible with the following solutions:
For Ampoules: 0.9% w/v Sodium Chloride Injection; 5% w/v Dextrose Injection; 10% w/v Mannitol Injection; Ringers Injection; 0.3% w/v Potassium Chloride and 0.9% w/v Sodium Chloride Injection; 0.3% w/v Potassium Chloride and 5% w/v Dextrose Injection.
For Vials: 5% w/v Dextrose Injection; 0.9% w/v Sodium Chloride Injection; 5% w/v Dextrose and 0.9% w/v Sodium Chloride Injection; 5% w/v Dextrose and 0.45% w/v Sodium Chloride Injection; 3% w/v Sodium Chloride Injection.
Compatibility with Other Drugs: ZOFRAN Injection should not be administered in the same syringe or infusion with any other medication with the exception of dexamethasone (see below). ZOFRAN may be administered by intravenous infusion at 1 mg/hour, e.g. from an infusion bag or syringe pump.

The following drugs may be administered via the Y-site of the administration set, for ondansetron concentrations of 16 to 160 μg/mL. If the concentrations of cytotoxic drugs required are higher than indicated below, they should be administered through a separate intravenous line.
For Ampoules and Vials: Cisplatin: concentrations up to 0.48 mg/mL administered over 1 to 8 hours.
Dexamethasone: admixtures containing 8 mg of ondansetron and 20 mg of dexamethasone phosphate, in 50 mL of 5% dextrose infusion fluid stored in 50 mL polyvinyl chloride infusion bags, have been shown to be physically and chemically stable for up to two days at room temperature or up to seven days at 2-8°C. In addition, these same admixtures have demonstrated compatibility with Continu-Flo administration sets.

In a clinical study (Cunningham et al, 1989) ondansetron (standard dosing regimen) was given to patients receiving cisplatin or non-cisplatin chemotherapy. Eight patients who continued to experience nausea and vomiting were given dexamethasone in addition to ondansetron. In every case there was an improvement in the control of emesis and all patients preferred the combination of ondansetron and dexamethasone.
For Ampoules: 5-Fluorouracil: concentrations up to 0.8 mg/mL, administered at rates of at least 20 mL/hour. Higher concentrations of 5-fluorouracil may cause precipitation of ondansetron. The 5-fluorouracil infusion may contain up to 0.045% w/v magnesium chloride.
Carboplatin: concentrations of 0.18 mg/mL-9.9 mg/mL, administered over 10-60 minutes.
Ceftazidime: bolus IV doses, over approximately 5 minutes, of 250-2000 mg reconstituted with Water for Injections BP.
Cyclophosphamide: bolus IV doses over approximately 5 minutes, of 100-1000 mg, reconstituted with Water for Injections BP 5 mL per 100 mg cyclophosphamide.
Doxorubicin and Epirubicin: bolus IV doses, over approximately 5 minutes, of 10-100 mg as a 2 mg/mL solution. Lyophilized powder presentations can be reconstituted with 0.9% Sodium Chloride Injection USP.
Etoposide: concentrations of 0.144 mg/mL-0.25 mg/mL, administered over 30-60 minutes.

OVERDOSAGE:
At present there is little information concerning overdosage with ondansetron. Individual doses of 84 mg and 145 mg and total daily doses as large as 252 mg have been administered with only mild side effects. There is no specific antidote for ondansetron, therefore, in cases of suspected overdosage, symptomatic and supportive therapy should be given as appropriate.

The use of Ipecac to treat overdosage with ondansetron is not recommended as patients are unlikely to respond due to the anti emetic action of ondansetron itself.

"Sudden blindness" (amaurosis) of 2 to 3 minutes duration plus severe constipation occurred in one patient that was administered 72 mg of ondansetron intravenously as a single dose. Hypotension (and faintness) occurred in another patient that took 48 mg of oral ondansetron. Following infusion of 32 mg over only a 4-minute period, a vasovagal episode with transient second degree heart block was observed. In all instances, the events resolved completely.

For management of a suspected drug overdose, contact your regional Poison Control Centre. See the *CPS* Directory section for a list of Poison Control Centres.

ACTION AND CLINICAL PHARMACOLOGY: Mechanism of Action: ZOFRAN (ondansetron hydrochloride; and ondansetron) is a selective antagonist of the serotonin receptor subtype, $5\text{-}HT_3$. Its precise mode of action in the control of chemotherapy induced nausea and vomiting is not known.

Cytotoxic chemotherapy and radiotherapy are associated with the release of serotonin (5-HT) from enterochromaffin cells of the small intestine, presumably initiating a vomiting reflex through stimulation of $5\text{-}HT_3$ receptors located on vagal afferents. Ondansetron may block the initiation of this reflex. Activation of vagal afferents may also cause a central release of serotonin from the chemoreceptor trigger zone of the area postrema, located on the floor of the fourth ventricle. Thus, the antiemetic effect of ondansetron is probably due to the selective antagonism of $5\text{-}HT_3$ receptors on neurons located in either the peripheral or central nervous systems, or both.

The mechanisms of ondansetron's antiemetic action in post-operative nausea and vomiting are not known.
Pharmacodynamics: In vitro metabolism studies have shown that ondansetron is a substrate for human hepatic cytochrome P450 enzymes, including CYP1A2, CYP2D6 and CYP3A4. In terms of overall ondansetron turnover, CYP3A4 played the predominant role. Because of the multiplicity of metabolic enzymes capable of metabolising ondansetron, it is likely that inhibition or loss of one enzyme (e.g. CYP2D6 enzyme deficiency) will be compensated by others and may result in little change in overall rates of ondansetron clearance.
Pharmacokinetics: Pharmacokinetic studies in human volunteers showed peak plasma levels of 20-30 ng/mL at around 1½ hours after an 8 mg oral dose of ondansetron. An 8 mg infusion of ondansetron resulted in peak plasma levels of 80-100 ng/mL. Repeat dosing of an 8 mg tablet every 8 hours for 6 days increased the peak plasma value to 40 ng/mL. A continuous intravenous infusion of 1 mg/hour after the initial 8 mg loading dose of ondansetron maintained plasma levels over 30 ng/mL during the following 24 hour period.

The absolute bioavailability of ondansetron in humans was approximately 60% and the plasma protein binding was approximately 73%.

Following oral or IV administration, ondansetron is extensively metabolised and excreted in the urine and faeces. In humans, less than 10% of the dose is excreted unchanged in the urine. The major urinary metabolites are glucuronide conjugates (45%), sulphate conjugates (20%) and hydroxylation products (10%).

The half-life of ondansetron after either an 8 mg oral dose or intravenous dose was approximately 3-4 hours and may be extended to 6-8 hours in the elderly.

In a pharmacokinetic study of 16 epileptic patients maintained chronically on carbamazepine or phenytoin, reduction in AUC, C_{max} and $T_{½}$ of ondansetron was observed. This resulted in a significant increase in clearance. However, on the basis of available data, no dosage adjustment is recommended (see Warnings and Precautions).
STORAGE AND STABILITY: ZOFRAN (ondansetron hydrochloride; and ondansetron) Tablets, Oral Solution, Injection and ODT orally disintegrating tablets should be stored below 30°C.

ZOFRAN Oral Solution should be stored upright and should not be refrigerated.

ZOFRAN Injection should not be frozen and should be protected from light. ZOFRAN Injection must not be autoclaved.
Stability and Storage of Diluted Solutions: Compatibility studies have been undertaken in polyvinyl chloride infusion bags, polyvinyl chloride administration sets and polypropylene syringes. Dilutions of ondansetron in sodium chloride 0.9% w/v or in dextrose 5% w/v have been demonstrated to be stable in polypropylene syringes. It is considered that ondansetron injection diluted with other compatible infusion fluids would be stable in polypropylene syringes.

Intravenous solutions should be prepared at the time of infusion. ZOFRAN Injection, in ampoules and vials, when diluted with the recommended intravenous solutions, should be used within 24 hours if stored at room temperature or used within 72 hours if stored in a refrigerator, due to possible microbial contamination during preparation.

Hospitals and institutions that have recognized admixture programs and use validated aseptic techniques for preparation of intravenous solutions, may extend the storage time for ZOFRAN Injection in admixture with 5% Dextrose Injection and dexamethasone phosphate Injection (concentration of 0.34 mg/mL) in Viaflex bags, at a concentration of 0.14 mg/mL, to 7 days when stored under refrigeration at 2 to 8°C‡.
INFORMATION FOR THE PATIENT: Published in e-CPS, available by subscription at www.e-cps.ca.
SPECIAL HANDLING INSTRUCTIONS: Ampoule Opening Instructions for ZOFRAN Injection (2 mL and 4 mL ampoules): Ampoules are equipped with One Point Cut opening system and must be opened using the following instructions:
- Hold the bottom part of the ampoule in one hand with the dot facing you.
- Place the other hand on the top of the ampoule positioning the thumb on the dot. Snap the top of the ampoule **away from you.**

DOSAGE FORMS, COMPOSITION AND PACKAGING: ZOFRAN: Injection: Each mL contains: ondansetron 2 mg/mL (as hydrochloride dihydrate) for i.v. use. Nonmedicinal ingredients: citric acid monohydrate, methyl- and propylparaben (vials only), sodium citrate and sodium chloride. Ampuls of 2 mL (4 mg) and 4 mL (8 mg). Boxes of 5. Vials of 20 mL (40 mg), packed in individual cartons.
Oral Solution: Each 5 mL contains: ondansetron 4 mg (as hydrochloride dihydrate). Nonmedicinal ingredients: citric acid, sodium citrate dihydrate, sodium benzoate, sorbitol solution and strawberry flavor. Sucrose-free. Sweetened with sorbitol. Bottles of 50 mL.
Tablets: 4 mg: Each oval-shaped, yellow film-coated tablet, engraved "4" on one face and "GLAXO" on the other, contains: ondansetron 4 mg (as hydrochloride dihydrate). Nonmedicinal ingredients: lactose, magnesium stearate, methyl hydroxypropyl cellulose, microcrystalline cellulose, Opadry yellow or Opaspray yellow (containing titanium dioxide and iron oxide yellow) and pregelatinized starch. Gluten- and tartrazine-free. Unit dosed blister packs of 10. Tamper-evident polypropylene containers of 100.
8 mg: Each oval-shaped, yellow, film-coated tablet, engraved "8" on one face and "GLAXO" on the other, contains: ondansetron 8 mg (as hydrochloride dihydrate). Nonmedicinal ingredients: lactose, magnesium stearate, methyl hydroxypropyl cellulose, microcrystalline cellulose, Opadry yellow or Opaspray yellow (containing titanium dioxide and iron oxide yellow) and pregelatinized starch. Gluten- and tartrazine-free. Unit dosed blister packs of 10. Tamper-evident polypropylene containers of 100.
ZOFRAN ODT: 4 mg: Each white, round, plano-convex orally disintegrating tablet, with no markings on either side, contains: ondansetron (base) 4 mg. Nonmedicinal ingredients: aspartame, gelatin, mannitol, sodium methyl hydroxybenzoate, sodium propyl hydroxybenzoate and strawberry flavor. Double-foil blister packs with a peelable, aluminum foil laminate lidding, in paperboard cartons with 2 x 5 orally disintegrating tablets per blister.
8 mg: Each white, round, plano-convex orally disintegrating tablet, with no markings on either side, contains: ondansetron (base) 8 mg. Nonmedicinal ingredients: aspartame, gelatin, mannitol, sodium methyl hydroxybenzoate, sodium propyl hydroxybenzoate and strawberry flavor. Double-foil blister packs with a peelable, aluminum foil laminate lidding, in paperboard cartons with 2 x 5 orally disintegrating tablets per blister.

(Shown in Product Identification Section)

* Infusion of 32 mg ZOFRAN for injection should take place over a period of not less than 15 minutes, because of increased risk of blurred vision.

† The efficacy of twice daily dosage regimens for the treatment of post-chemotherapy emesis has been established only in adult patients receiving less emetogenic chemotherapy. The appropriateness of twice versus three times daily dosage regimens for other patient groups should be based on an assessment of the needs and responsiveness of the individual patient.

‡ As with all parenteral drug products, intravenous admixtures should be inspected visually for clarity, particulate matter, precipitate, discolouration and leakage prior to administration, whenever solution and container permit. Solutions showing haziness, particulate matter, precipitate, or discolouration or leakage should not be used.

Zoladex® 3.6 mg Ⓟ

goserelin acetate

Luteinizing Hormone-Releasing Hormone (LHRH) Analog

AstraZeneca

Date of Preparation: February 2, 2000
Date of Revision: June 24, 2010

SUMMARY PRODUCT INFORMATION:

Route of Administration	Dosage Form/ Strength	Clinically Relevant Nonmedicinal Ingredients
Subcutaneous injection	Depot/3.6 mg goserelin	Lactide-glycolide copolymer For a complete listing see Dosage Forms, Composition and Packaging.

INDICATIONS AND CLINICAL USE: ZOLADEX (goserelin acetate) is indicated for a number of hormone-dependent conditions as shown in Prostate Cancer, Breast Cancer and Benign Conditions:

Prostate Cancer:
- ZOLADEX is indicated for the palliative treatment of patients with hormone-dependent advanced carcinoma of the prostate (Stage M1 according to the Tumour-Node-Metastasis [TNM] classification system or Stage D2 according to the American Urologic Association [AUA] classification).
- ZOLADEX is indicated for use in combination with a non-steroidal antiandrogen and radiation therapy for the management of locally advanced (T3, T4) or bulky Stage T2b, T2c carcinoma of the prostate. Treatment with ZOLADEX and a non-steroidal antiandrogen should start 8 weeks prior to initiating radiation therapy and continue until completion of the radiation therapy.
- ZOLADEX as adjuvant hormone therapy to external beam irradiation for patients with locally advanced prostate cancer (Stage T3-T4).

Breast Cancer:
- ZOLADEX is indicated as an alternative to standard adjuvant chemotherapy in pre- and perimenopausal women with early breast cancer who are unsuitable for, intolerant to, or decline chemotherapy, and whose tumour contains estrogen and/or progesterone receptors.
- ZOLADEX is indicated for the palliative treatment of advanced breast cancer in pre- and perimenopausal women whose tumour contains estrogen and/or progesterone receptors.

Benign Conditions:
- ZOLADEX is indicated for the hormonal management of endometriosis, including pain relief and reduction of endometriotic lesions. Experience with ZOLADEX for the management of endometriosis has been limited to women 18 years of age and older, treated for 6 months.
- ZOLADEX is indicated for use as an endometrial thinning agent prior to endometrial ablation.

Pediatrics: The safety and effectiveness of ZOLADEX in children has not been established.

CONTRAINDICATIONS:
- Patients who are hypersensitive to this drug or to any ingredient in the formulation or component of the container. For a complete listing, see Dosage Forms, Composition and Packaging.
- Women having undiagnosed abnormal vaginal bleeding.

Pregnancy: ZOLADEX should not be used during pregnancy. As with other LHRH agonists it is not known whether ZOLADEX causes fetal abnormalities in humans. Women of child bearing potential should be carefully examined before treatment to exclude pregnancy. Non-hormonal methods of contraception should be employed during therapy (see Warnings and Precautions).
Lactation: The use of ZOLADEX during breast feeding is not recommended.

WARNINGS AND PRECAUTIONS: General: Initially, ZOLADEX (goserelin acetate) transiently increases serum testosterone in males and serum estradiol concentrations in females and other gonadal hormones. Although not necessarily related, isolated cases of short-term worsening of signs and symptoms have been reported during the first four weeks of therapy. Worsening of the clinical condition may occasionally require discontinuation of therapy and/or surgical intervention.
Effect on Ability to Drive a Vehicle and Use Machinery: There is no evidence that ZOLADEX results in impairment of ability to drive or operate machinery.
Dependence/Tolerance: There have been no reports of drug dependence following the use of ZOLADEX.
Endocrine and Metabolism: Males: Induced Hypogonadism: Suppression of pituitary gonadotropins and gonadal hormone production will occur with continued administration of ZOLADEX. These changes have been observed to reverse on discontinuation of therapy. However, whether the clinical symptoms of induced hypogonadism will reverse in all patients has not yet been established.
Metabolic: Impaired glucose tolerance has been observed in males using LHRH agonists. This may manifest as diabetes or loss of glycaemic control in those with pre-existing diabetes mellitus. Consideration should therefore be given to monitoring blood glucose.
Genitourinary: Males: Patients with Genitourinary Tract Symptoms: During the first month of therapy with ZOLADEX, patients at risk of developing ureteric obstruction should be closely monitored.
Ureteric obstruction may develop in male patients with a history of obstructive uropathy. If spinal cord compression or renal impairment due to ureteric obstruction are present, or develop, specific standard treatment of these complications should be instituted.
Immune: Antibody formation has not been observed during administration of ZOLADEX. Local reactions, such as mild bruising have been related to the trauma of the injection itself and not to the copolymer material of the depot or to the prolonged presence of ZOLADEX at the site of depot injection.
Musculoskeletal: Patients with Vertebral Metastases: During the first month of therapy with ZOLADEX, patients with vertebral metastases who are thought to be at particular risk of spinal cord compression should be closely monitored.
Changes in Bone Density: The use of LHRH agonists may cause a reduction in bone mineral density. In men and women, some bone loss can be anticipated as part of the natural aging process. It may also be expected to occur during medically induced hypo-androgenic state caused by long term ZOLADEX treatment.
Data from studies of ZOLADEX suggest that some recovery of bone mineral may occur on cessation of therapy.
In patients with major risk factors for decreased bone mineral content such as chronic alcohol and/or tobacco use, presumed or strong family history of osteoporosis or chronic use of drugs that can reduce bone mass such as corticosteroids or anticonvulsants, ZOLADEX may pose an additional risk. In these patients the risks and benefits must be weighed carefully before therapy with ZOLADEX is initiated. In women being treated for endometriosis, the use of ZOLADEX for longer than the recommended six months or in the presence of other known risk factors for decreased bone mineral content may cause additional bone loss.
Worsening of bone pain and other signs and symptoms have been reported infrequently in males and to a lesser extent in females during the first month of therapy with ZOLADEX (goserelin acetate). In men, by around 21 days after the first depot injection, testosterone concentrations have typically decreased to within the castrate range and remain suppressed with treatment every 28 days. It is unclear whether there is any relationship between these clinical events and the initial rise in serum testosterone or estradiol levels observed during the first few days following administration of the first depot injection.
In those who reported an increase in bone pain, the pain ranged in intensity from mild to severe and required either symptomatic management, including non-narcotic analgesics or in some severe cases, narcotic analgesics.
Sexual Function/Reproduction: Fertility: Suppression of serum estradiol will induce amenorrhea in the majority of patients after the first four weeks of treatment especially if started during the menstrual phase of the cycle. During early treatment with ZOLADEX some women may experience vaginal bleeding of variable duration and intensity. Such bleeding may represent estrogen withdrawal bleeding and is expected to stop spontaneously. Amenorrhea is expected to be maintained until 4 weeks after the last dose of ZOLADEX.
Menses usually resumed within 8 weeks following completion of therapy. Rarely, some women may enter the natural menopause during treatment with LHRH analogues and do not resume menses on cessation of therapy.
Time to return of menses after cessation of therapy with ZOLADEX may be prolonged in some patients.
A non-hormonal method of contraception should be used during treatment. Patients should be advised that if they miss or postpone a dose of ZOLADEX, ovulation may occur with the potential for conception. If a patient becomes pregnant during treatment, she should discontinue treatment and consult her physician.
Duration of Endometriosis Treatment: The safety of treatment, as well as re-treatment, beyond 6 months with ZOLADEX has not been established.
Endometrial Thinning: The use of ZOLADEX may cause an increase in cervical resistance. Therefore, care should be taken when dilating the cervix.
Special Populations: Pregnant Women: ZOLADEX should not be used in pregnancy as there is a theoretical risk of abortion or fetal abnormality if LHRH agonists are used during pregnancy. Potentially fertile women should be examined carefully before treatment to exclude pregnancy. Non-hormonal methods of contraception should be employed during therapy until menses resume.
Nursing Women: The use of ZOLADEX during breast feeding is not recommended.
Pediatrics: The safety and effectiveness of ZOLADEX in children has not been established.
Geriatrics: The labelling reflects the safety and effectiveness of ZOLADEX in the population over 65 years of age.
Monitoring and Laboratory Tests: Monitoring of Patients: During therapy with ZOLADEX, patients should be routinely monitored by physical examinations and appropriate laboratory tests. In prostate cancer patients tumour markers such as prostatic acid phosphatase (PAP), prostatic specific antigen (PSA) or acid phosphatase could be monitored. Additionally, if deemed appropriate by the physician, serum testosterone or serum estradiol may be monitored; however, this is not routinely required.
In prostate cancer patients, an assessment of bone lesions may require the use of bone scans. Prostatic lesions may be monitored by ultrasonography and/or CT scan in addition to digital rectal examination. The status of obstructive uropathy in males may be assessed and/or diagnosed using intravenous pyelography, ultrasonography or CT scan.
Impaired glucose tolerance has been observed in males using LHRH agonists. This may manifest as diabetes or loss of glycaemic control in those with pre-existing diabetes mellitus. Consideration should therefore be given to monitoring blood glucose.

Effect on Laboratory Tests: Although serum testosterone or serum estradiol may be elevated during the first few days after administration of the first depot, they return to normal within one week, and are suppressed by the end of three weeks. They remain suppressed throughout therapy with ZOLADEX.
Prostate cancer tumour markers (PSA and PAP), are not routinely monitored in the first few days of therapy; however, if the cancer is responsive to ZOLADEX therapy, then these levels, if elevated prior to the commencement of treatment, are usually reduced by the end of the first month.
Renal function tests, blood urea nitrogen and creatinine may rarely be elevated during the first few days of therapy in prostate cancer patients before returning to normal.
Diagnostic Interference: Administration of ZOLADEX in therapeutic doses results in suppression of the pituitary-gonadal system. Normal function is usually restored approximately 8 weeks after the last dose of ZOLADEX. Diagnostic tests of pituitary-gonadal function conducted during the treatment and within 8 weeks after discontinuation of ZOLADEX therapy may therefore be misleading.

ADVERSE REACTIONS: Adverse Drug Reaction Overview: The adverse effects seen with ZOLADEX (goserelin acetate) are due primarily to its pharmacologic action of sex hormone suppression and may give rise to certain expected effects that vary by sex.
Adverse events that have been observed at an equal frequency in both males and females follow. Very common adverse events (≥10%) consist of: decreased libido, hot flush, and hyperhidrosis. These are pharmacological effects which seldom require withdrawal of therapy. Common adverse reactions (≥1% to <10%) are: paraesthesia, abnormal blood pressure, rash and decrease in bone density. Drug hypersensitivity was reported uncommonly (≥0.1% to <1). Anaphylactic reaction has been reported rarely (≥0.01% to <0.1). Cases of pituitary tumours and psychotic disorder have also been occasionally reported during post-marketed use. As with other agents in this class, cases of pituitary hemorrhage have occasionally been reported following initial administration of ZOLADEX during post-marketed use.
Abnormal blood pressure, manifest as hypotension or hypertension are commonly observed in patients administered ZOLADEX. The changes are usually transient, resolving either during continued therapy or after cessation of therapy with ZOLADEX. Such changes have rarely required medical intervention including withdrawal of ZOLADEX treatment.
In males, erectile dysfunction was reported very commonly (≥10%). Commonly reported adverse reactions (≥1% to <10%) consist of: impaired glucose tolerance, spinal cord compression, bone pain, gynecomastia, cardiac failure and injection site reaction. Uncommon adverse reactions (≥0.1% to <1) are: arthralgia, ureteric obstruction and breast tenderness.
Heart failure was commonly reported (5%) in patients receiving ZOLADEX for prostate cancer treatment in clinical studies. Myocardial infarction and cardiac failure were observed in a pharmaco-epidemiology study of LHRH agonists and/or anti-androgens used in the treatment of prostate cancer. The risks for these cardiovascular adverse events appear to be increased when LHRH agonists are used in combination with anti-androgens.
In females, very common adverse reactions (≥10%) consist of: vulvovaginal dryness, breast enlargement and injection site reaction. Common adverse reactions (≥1% to <10%) are: mood alteration including depression, headache, arthralgia and tumour flare/tumor pain. Hypercalcemia occurs at an uncommon frequency (≥0.1% to <1%). Rare (≥0.01% to <0.1) cases of ovarian cyst have been reported. Degeneration of uterine fibroid occurs at an unknown frequency.
Following the administration of ZOLADEX, skin rashes have been reported as generally mild, often regressing without discontinuation of therapy.
Initially, prostate cancer patients may experience a temporary increase in bone pain, which can be managed symptomatically.
The use of LHRH agonists may cause a reduction in bone mineral density (see Warnings and Precautions).
Clinical Trial Adverse Drug Reactions: Prostate Cancer Patients: Five hundred and eighteen (518) prostate patients who had not been previously treated and who entered into 14 open multicentre studies were monitored for adverse reactions to ZOLADEX. The mean duration of treatment in these patients was 23 weeks.
The following reports from these clinical trials are considered to be possibly related to treatment with ZOLADEX: hot flush (51%), decreased libido (53%), decreased erections (57%), breast tenderness (3%), gynecomastia (2%), local intolerance at injection site (pain, erythema) (4%), and skin rash including erythema and urticaria (1.9%).
Also in these clinical studies, an initial rise in mean serum testosterone levels occurred during the first few days of treatment with ZOLADEX. In a few instances, patients experienced a worsening of signs and symptoms, during the first month after initiation of therapy (see Warnings and Precautions). For these patients, this was usually an increase in bone pain (4.2%), however, isolated cases of ureteric obstruction (1.1%) and/or spinal cord compression (1.2%) have also been reported during the initial four weeks of ZOLADEX therapy. The relationship of these observations to ZOLADEX is unknown.
The potential for exacerbation of signs and symptoms during the first few weeks of treatment is a concern particularly in male patients with impending neurologic compromise and in patients with severe obstructive uropathy (see Warnings and Precautions).
The most frequently reported (greater than 5%) adverse experiences during treatment with a LHRH-agonist in combination with flutamide are listed in Table 1. For comparison, adverse experiences seen with a LHRH-agonist and placebo are also listed in Table 1.

Table 1: ZOLADEX

Adverse Events (greater than 5%) Reported During Treatment with a LHRH-agonist in Combination with Flutamide

	(n=294) Flutamide+LHRH-agonist % All	(n=285) Placebo+LHRH-agonist % All
Hot flush	61	57
Loss of libido	36	31
Impotence	33	29
Diarrhea	12	4
Nausea/Vomiting	11	10
Gynecomastia	9	11
Other	7	9
Other gastrointestinal	6	4

As shown in Table 1, for both treatment groups, the most frequently occurring adverse experiences (hot flush, loss of libido, impotence) were those known to be associated with low serum androgen levels and known to occur with LHRH-agonists alone.
The only notable difference between these treatment groups was the higher incidence of diarrhea in the flutamide+LHRH-agonist group (12%) as compared to the placebo+LHRH-agonist group (4%). The cases of diarrhea reported were severe in less than 1% of the patients. In addition, the following adverse reactions were reported during treatment with flutamide+LHRH-agonist. No causal relatedness of these reactions to drug treatment has been made, and some of the adverse experiences reported are those that commonly occur in elderly patients.
Cardiovascular System: hypertension in 1% of patients. Rarely, thrombophlebitis, pulmonary embolism, and myocardial infarction.
Central Nervous System: CNS (drowsiness/confusion/depression/anxiety/nervousness) reactions occurred in 1% of patients. Rarely insomnia, tiredness, headache, dizziness, weakness, malaise, blurred vision and decreased libido have been reported.
Endocrine System: gynecomastia in 9% of patients. Rarely breast tenderness sometimes accompanied by galactorrhoea.
Gastrointestinal System: Nausea/vomiting occurred in 11%; diarrhea 12%, anorexia 4%, and other GI disorders occurred in 6% of patients. Increased appetite, indigestion and constipation have also been reported.
Hematopoietic System: Anaemia occurred in 6% of patients, leukopenia 3%, and thrombocytopenia 1%.
Liver and Biliary System: Clinically evident hepatitis and jaundice occurred in <1% of patients.
Skin: Irritation at the injection site and rash occurred in 3% of patients. Photosensitivity reactions have been reported in five patients.

Other: Pruritus, ecchymosis, herpes zoster, thirst, lymphedema, lupus-like syndrome, hematuria, reduced sperm counts have been reported rarely in long-term treatment. Edema occurred in 4% of patients; neuromuscular, genitourinary symptoms occurred in 2% of patients. Pulmonary symptoms occurred in <1% of patients.

Advanced Breast Cancer Patients: The adverse event profile for women with advanced breast cancer treated with ZOLADEX is consistent with the profile described for women treated with ZOLADEX for endometriosis. In very rare instances, breast cancer patients with bony metastases have developed hypercalcemia on initiation of therapy. In a controlled clinical trial (SWOG-8692) comparing ZOLADEX with oophorectomy in premenopausal and perimenopausal women with advanced breast cancer, the following events were reported at a frequency of 5% or greater in either treatment group regardless of causality. See Table 2.

Table 2: ZOLADEX

Adverse Reactions—Advanced Breast Cancer Patients

	Advanced Breast Cancer Patients	
Adverse Reactions	**ZOLADEX n=57 %**	**Oophorectomy n=55 %**
Hot flush	70	47
Tumour flare	23	4
Nausea	11	7
Edema	5	0
Malaise/fatigue/lethargy	5	2
Vomiting	4	7

In the Phase II clinical trial program in 333 pre- and perimenopausal women with advanced breast cancer, hot flush and decreased libido were assessed by specific patient inquiry. Hot flush occurred in 75.9 % of the 203 women in whom they were not present at baseline and decreased libido occurred in 47.7% of the 194 women with libido present at baseline. These events reflect the pharmacological actions of ZOLADEX.

Injection site reaction was reported in less than 1% of patients.

Early Breast Cancer Patients: The most frequently recorded possible adverse drug reactions, regardless of causality, for pre- and perimenopausal women aged ≤50 years with early breast cancer who received ZOLADEX (N=803) in an open randomized trial (ZEBRA) were headache (5.5%), pain (3.4%) and bone pain (3.4%).

Patients in the study who received ZOLADEX experienced higher incidences of the effects caused by estradiol suppression, e.g. hot flush, vulvovaginal dryness/soreness, and loss of libido, than those experienced in the cyclophosphamide, methotrexate and 5-fluorouracil (CMF) comparator treatment group. Within 6 months of completing ZOLADEX therapy, these incidences had decreased to below those seen in the CMF patients.

Table 3 lists the frequencies ≥1% of adverse drug reactions considered 'extremely likely' or 'probably' related to trial therapy (ZEBRA Trial, median follow-up of 7.5 years).

Table 3: ZOLADEX

Frequencies ≥1% of Adverse Drug Reactions (By COSTART Term) Considered "Extremely Likely" or "Probably" Related to Trial Therapy

	Number (%) of Patients	
Body System and COSTART Term[a,b]	**ZOLADEX (N=803)**	**CMF (N=802)**
Whole Body		
Headache	24 (3.0)	7 (0.9)
Pain	9 (1.1)	2 (0.2)
Asthenia	5 (0.6)	8 (1.0)
Cardiovascular		
Hypertension	14 (1.7)	1 (0.1)
Digestive		
Vomiting	4 (0.5)	84 (10.5)
Nausea	3 (0.4)	62 (7.7)
Hemic and Lymphatic		
Leukopenia	0 (0.0)	70 (8.7)
Metabolic and Nutritional		
Weight gain	13 (1.6)	13 (1.6)
ALT increased	1 (0.1)	9 (1.1)
Musculoskeletal		
Bone pain	17 (2.1)	3 (0.4)
Osteoporosis	11 (1.4)	4 (0.5)
Skin and Appendages		
Rash	4 (0.5)	8 (1.0)
Special Senses		
Conjunctivitis	1 (0.1)	9 (1.1)
Urogenital		

(cont'd)

Table 3: ZOLADEX *(cont'd)*

Frequencies ≥1% of Adverse Drug Reactions (By COSTART Term) Considered "Extremely Likely" or "Probably" Related to Trial Therapy

	Number (%) of Patients	
Body System and COSTART Term[a,b]	**ZOLADEX (N=803)**	**CMF (N=802)**
Metrorrhagia	10 (1.2)	1 (0.1)

[a] A patient may have had more than one adverse event that was considered "extremely likely" or "probably" related to trial therapy.

[b] Thirteen (1.6%) patients who received ZOLADEX, and 0 (0.0%) patients, who received CMF, recorded possible adverse reactions considered "extremely likely" or "probably" related to trial therapy that could not be attributed to a COSTART term.

Legend: ALT: Alanine aminotransferase; COSTART: Coding Symbols for Thesaurus of Adverse Reaction Terms.

Benign Conditions: In controlled clinical trials, comparing ZOLADEX every 28 days with danazol daily for the treatment of endometriosis, the following events elicited by direct questioning were reported at a frequency of 5% or more: see Table 4.

Table 4: ZOLADEX

Adverse Reactions Reported in Endometriosis Trials

	Endometriosis Trials	
Adverse Reactions	**ZOLADEX Treated n=411 %**	**Danazol Treated n=207 %**
Hot Flush	96	67
Vaginitis (Vulvovaginal Dryness)	75	43
Headache	75	63
Emotional Lability (Mood Swings)	60	56
Libido Decreased	61	44
Hyperhidrosis	45	30
Depression	54	48
Acne	42	55
Breast Atrophy	33	42
Seborrhea	26	52
Peripheral Edema	21	34
Breast Enlargement	18	15
Pelvic Symptoms	18	23
Pain	17	16
Dyspareunia	14	5
Libido Increased	12	19
Infection	13	11
Asthenia	11	13
Nausea	8	14
Hirsutism	7	15
Insomnia	11	4
Breast Pain	7	4
Abdominal Pain	7	7
Back Pain	7	13
Flu Syndrome	5	5
Dizziness	6	4
Application Site Reaction	6	—
Voice Alterations	3	8
Pharyngitis	5	2
Hair Disorders	4	11
Myalgia	3	11
Nervousness	3	5
Weight Gain	3	23
Leg Cramps	2	6
Increased Appetite	2	5
Pruritus	2	6
Hypertonia	1	10

From the endometriosis trials and other supporting safety studies, other adverse reactions, not listed above, elicited at a frequency of 1% or more are shown below. The relationship of these possible adverse reactions to therapy with ZOLADEX is unknown.

Body as a Whole: allergic reaction, chest pain, fever, malaise.
Cardiovascular: hemorrhage, hypertension, migraine, palpitations, tachycardia.
Digestive: anorexia, constipation, diarrhea, dry mouth, dyspepsia, flatulence.
Hemic and Lymphatic: ecchymosis.
Metabolic and Nutritional: edema.
Musculoskeletal: arthralgia, joint disorder.
Nervous: anxiety, parasthesia, somnolence, thinking abnormal.
Respiratory: bronchitis, cough increased, epistaxis, pharyngitis, rhinitis, sinusitis.
Skin: alopecia, dry skin, rash, pruritus, skin discoloration.
Special Senses: amblyopia, dry eyes.
Urogenital: dysmenorrhea, urinary frequency, urinary tract infection, vaginal hemorrhage.

In women with fibroids, degeneration of uterine fibroid may occur.

As with other LHRH agonists, there have been reports of ovarian cyst formation.

Changes in Bone Mineral Density: After 6 months of ZOLADEX treatment, 97 female patients treated with ZOLADEX for endometriosis showed an average 4.6% decrease of vertebral trabecular bone mineral density (BMD) as compared to pretreatment values. BMD was measured by dual-photon absorptiometry or dual energy x-ray absorptiometry. Forty-four of these patients were assessed for BMD loss 6 months after the completion (post-therapy) of the 6-month therapy period. Data from these patients showed an average 2.6% BMD loss compared to pretreatment values. Nine of the 97 patients were assessed for BMD at 12 months post-therapy. Data from these patients showed an average decrease of 2.5% in BMD compared to pretreatment values. These data suggest a possibility of partial reversibility.

In the ZEBRA study, a subgroup of patients were investigated for possible changes to bone mineral during their breast cancer treatment which consisted of 6 cycles of CMF or 2 years of ZOLADEX. The percentage change from baseline in BMD was assessed at 1, 2 and 3 years for both the lumbar spine and the femoral neck. Figure 1 and Figure 2 show that patients in both treatment groups lose bone mineral and continue to do so between 1 and 2 years following the start of treatment. However, by 3 years, one year after the end of ZOLADEX treatment, patients in the ZOLADEX group show partial recovery of bone mineral. The percentage change from baseline at both the lumbar spine and femoral neck at 3 years was less in the ZOLADEX than in the CMF group.

Figure 1: ZOLADEX

Percentage Change From Baseline in BMD (means ± SEM)—Lumbar Spine. Numbers of Patients are Shown in Parentheses

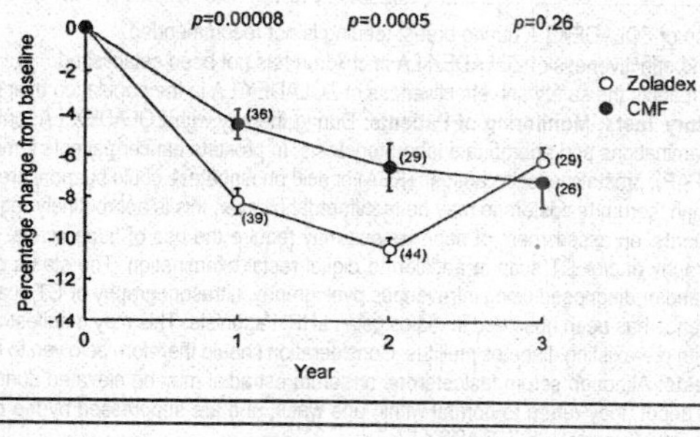

Figure 2: ZOLADEX

Percentage Change From Baseline in BMD (means ± SEM)—Neck of Femur. Numbers of Patients are Shown in Parentheses

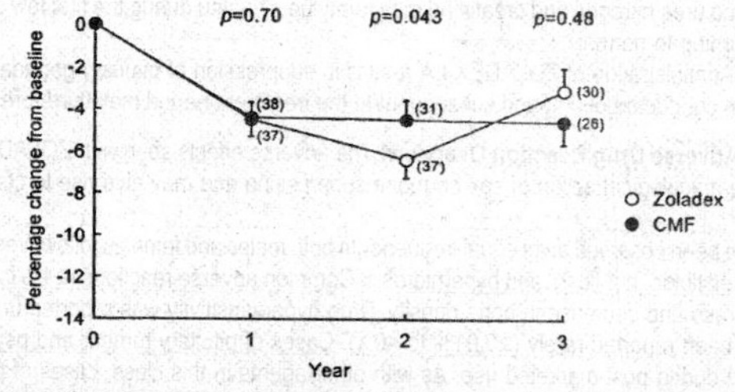

Less Common Clinical Trial Adverse Drug Reactions (<1%): When 942 male patients treated with ZOLADEX are considered, the adverse reactions listed below were reported to occur in less than 1% of patients with the exception of bone pain (2.9%), increased alkaline phosphatase (2.4%) and nausea/vomiting (1.4%).

Possible adverse reactions reported in the 942 male patients were as follows:

Cardiovascular: thrombophlebitis, pulmonary embolism, edema, tachycardia, atrial fibrillation, angina pectoris, congestive cardiac failure, hypertension, myocardial infarction, deep vein thrombosis, palpitations, cerebrovascular accident, central retinal vein thrombosis.
Dermatologic: pruritus, skin rashes including erythema, eczema and urticaria, worsening of ecchymoses and hair growth.
Gastrointestinal: dry mouth/thirst, polydipsia, nausea, vomiting, hematemesis, diarrhea, pain in abdomen, constipation, anorexia, flatulence, intolerance to alcohol, gingival atrophy.
Hematologic/Lymphatic: neutropenia, neutrophilia, lymphocytopenia, lymphocytosis, lowered protein/albumin and palpable lymph nodes.
Musculoskeletal: bone pain, signs and symptoms of spinal cord compression, (eg., paresthesia, paraparesis, paraplegia), muscular fatigue, myopathy, pain (other than bone), hyperesthesia, arthritis, suprapubic pain, polyarthralgia and neurological troubles with lower limbs.
Central Nervous System: vertigo, headaches, blackouts, flashes of light, decreased/blurred vision, glaucoma, drowsiness, lassitude, lethargy, malaise, disorientation, mental confusion, sensitivity to noise, taste disturbance.
Urogenital: renal impairment, renal tract obstruction, urinary retention, chronic renal failure, hydronephrosis, nocturia, testicular atrophy.
Laboratory Values: elevation of liver function test parameters, (eg., gamma GT, alanine aminotransferase, aspartate aminotransferase, and bilirubin), raised alkaline phosphatase, serum calcium and hyperkalemia.
Miscellaneous: fever, sore throat, influenza, herpes zoster, gangrene, decreased appetite.

Abnormal Hematologic and Clinical Chemistry Findings: Plasma Enzymes: Elevations of liver enzymes (AST, ALT) have been reported in less than 1% of all female patients. There was no other evidence of abnormal liver function. Causality between these changes and ZOLADEX have not been established.

Lipids: In a controlled trial, ZOLADEX therapy resulted in a minor, but statistically significant effect on serum lipids. In patients treated for endometriosis at 6 months following initiation of therapy, ZOLADEX treatment resulted in mean increases in LDL cholesterol of 0.55 mmol/L and HDL cholesterol of 0.07 mmol/L. Triglycerides increased by 0.09 mmol/L as well as total cholesterol by 0.65 mmol/L. At the end of 6 months of treatment, HDL cholesterol fractions (HDL2 and HDL3) were increased by 0.05 mmol/L and 0.02 mmol/L, respectively.

In the pivotal trials for endometrial thinning (n=258), the adverse reaction profile for ZOLADEX was similar to that seen in the endometriosis trials, however the frequency was generally lower.

DRUG INTERACTIONS: Drug-Drug Interactions: There are no known drug-drug interactions requiring dose adjustment.
Drug-Food Interactions: Interactions with particular foods have not been established.
Drug-Herb Interactions: Interactions with herbal products have not been established.
Drug-Laboratory Test Interactions: Interactions with laboratory tests have not been established.

DOSAGE AND ADMINISTRATION: Dosing Considerations: General: Although, isolated cases of vaginal spotting or bleeding during treatment have been reported, this is not associated with lack of pharmacodynamic effect in most instances. The majority of patients become amenorrheic within 8 weeks of starting treatment. In the small number of women who experience continued menstrual bleeding, estradiol blood levels should be measured. If menstrual bleeding persists and estradiol measurements correspond to postmenopausal values, appropriate diagnostic measures should be undertaken to rule out an intrauterine pathology.

Recommended Dose and Dosage Adjustment: Breast Cancer: ZOLADEX depot, containing goserelin acetate equivalent to 3.6 mg goserelin, should be administered subcutaneously every 28 days into the anterior abdominal wall following the procedure recommended on the package leaflet (see Instructions for Use).

Available data to date demonstrates that two years of adjuvant ZOLADEX therapy, 3.6 mg every 28 days, has been found to be at least equivalent to standard CMF regimens in terms of overall survival and equivalent to CMF in terms of disease-free survival in pre- and perimenopausal patients with early breast cancer and whose tumour is estrogen receptor-positive.

Prostate Cancer: When ZOLADEX is given in combination with a non-steroidal antiandrogen and radiotherapy for patients with Stage T2b-T4 prostatic carcinoma, treatment should be started 8 weeks prior to initiating radiotherapy and should continue until completion of the radiation therapy. A treatment regimen using a ZOLADEX 3.6 mg depot 8 weeks before radiotherapy, followed in 28 days by the ZOLADEX LA (10.8 mg) depot, can be administered by injection subcutaneously into the anterior abdominal wall.

Alternatively, four injections of the ZOLADEX 3.6 mg depot subcutaneously into the anterior abdominal wall can be administered at 28 day intervals, two depots preceding and two during radiotherapy until completion of the radiation therapy.

Endometriosis: One depot of ZOLADEX containing goserelin acetate equivalent to 3.6 mg goserelin, should be injected subcutaneously into the anterior abdominal wall every 28 days following the procedure recommended on the instruction card (see Instructions for Use on card attached to sterile pouch).

Endometrial Thinning: For use as an endometrial thinning agent prior to endometrial ablation, ZOLADEX should be administered by subcutaneous injection into the anterior abdominal wall as two 3.6 mg depots, four weeks apart, with surgery planned for between 0 and 2 weeks after the second depot injection.

Renal Impairment: In clinical studies, subjects with impaired renal function (creatinine clearance <20 mL/min) had a mean serum elimination half-life of 12.1 hours for ZOLADEX compared to 4.2 hours for male subjects with normal renal function (creatinine clearance >70 mL/min). This increase of approximately 8 hours in serum half-life is insufficient to warrant extending the 28-day dosing interval of the 3.6 mg depot, but will lead to modestly higher serum concentrations of the drug in such patients. No dose adjustment, therefore, is necessary for patients with renal failure.

Hepatic Impairment: Hepatic impairment does not compromise the clearance of ZOLADEX, therefore, a dosage adjustment is not needed for patients with hepatic impairment.

Geriatrics: No dosage adjustment is necessary in the elderly.

Pediatrics: The safety and effectiveness of ZOLADEX in children has not been established.

Administration: ZOLADEX 3.6 mg Step by Step Directions for Use (see package insert for illustrations): Caution: Do not depress plunger until Step 5. Read all instructions before use.

1. Put the patient in a comfortable position with the upper part of the body slightly raised. Swab abdominal injection site.
2. Remove the syringe from the opened foil pouch and hold the syringe at a slight angle to the light. Check that at least part of the ZOLADEX depot is visible.
3. Grasp the plastic safety tab and pull away from the syringe and discard. Remove needle cover. **Unlike liquid injections, there is no need to remove air bubbles as attempts to do so may displace the depot.**
4. Holding the syringe around the protective sleeve, pinch the patient's skin and insert the needle at a slight angle (30 to 45 degrees) to the skin. With the opening of the needle facing up, insert needle into the subcutaneous tissue of the anterior abdominal wall below the navel line, until the protective sleeve touches the patient's skin.

Do not penetrate into muscle or peritoneum. Incorrect grip and angle of administration is shown.

5. Moving your hand back to the finger grip, depress the plunger **fully**, until you can depress no more, to discharge the ZOLADEX depot and to activate the protective sleeve. You may hear a 'click' and will feel the protective sleeve automatically begin to slide to cover the needle. If the plunger is not depressed fully the protective sleeve will **not** activate.
6. Holding the syringe as shown, withdraw the needle and allow protective sleeve to continue to slide and cover needle. Dispose of the syringe in an approved sharps collector.

OVERDOSAGE:
The pharmacologic properties of ZOLADEX (goserelin acetate) and its mode of delivery make accidental or intentional overdosage unlikely. There is limited experience of overdosage in humans. In cases where ZOLADEX has unintentionally been readministered early or given at a higher dose than recommended, no clinically relevant adverse effects have been seen. Animal studies indicate that no increased pharmacologic effect would occur in man with higher doses or more frequent administration than those recommended. Subcutaneous doses of the drug as high as 1 mg/kg/day in rats and dogs produced no non-endocrine related sequelae; this dose is approximately 400 times that proposed for human use. If overdosage occurs, this should be managed symptomatically.

For management of a suspected drug overdose, contact your regional Poison Control Centre. See the *CPS Directory* section for a list of Poison Control Centres.

ACTION AND CLINICAL PHARMACOLOGY: Mechanism of Action: ZOLADEX (goserelin acetate) is a synthetic decapeptide analog of gonadotropin releasing hormone (GnRH or LHRH). When given acutely, goserelin acetate releases luteinizing hormone (LH) from the pituitary gland. However, following chronic administration, goserelin acetate is a potent inhibitor of gonadotropin production resulting in gonadal and consequently, accessory sex organ regression. This effect is the basis for the inhibition of growth of chemically-induced rat mammary tumours and transplantable rat prostate and pituitary tumours.

In animals and man, following an initial stimulation of pituitary LH secretion and a transient elevation in serum testosterone in males and serum estradiol in females, chronic administration results in inhibition of gonadotropin secretion.

In men, approximately 21 days after the initiation of therapy, a sustained suppression of pituitary LH results in the reduction of serum testosterone levels to a range normally seen in surgically castrated men, and of serum estradiol to levels comparable with those observed in post-menopausal women. This suppression of testosterone and estradiol is then maintained as long as therapy is continued.

When used in women this suppression of serum estradiol is associated with endometrial thinning, suppression of follicular development within the ovary and a response in hormone dependent breast cancer (tumours that are estrogen receptor (ER)—positive and/or progesterone receptor (Pg R)—positive), and endometriosis. Suppression of serum estradiol will induce amenorrhea in the majority of patients after the first four weeks of treatment especially if started during the menstrual phase of the cycle. During early treatment with ZOLADEX some women may experience vaginal bleeding of variable duration and intensity. Such bleeding may represent estrogen withdrawal bleeding and is expected to stop spontaneously. Amenorrhea is expected to be maintained until 4 weeks after the last dose of ZOLADEX.

ZOLADEX is a depot formulation of goserelin acetate dispersed in a cylindrical rod of biodegradable and biocompatible blend of high and low molecular weight range D-L Lactide-glycolide copolymer.

The bioavailability of goserelin acetate from ZOLADEX depot is almost complete. When injected subcutaneously, goserelin is released continuously over at least 28 days.

Administration of a depot every four weeks ensures that effective concentrations are maintained with no accumulation.

ZOLADEX is poorly protein bound and has a serum elimination half-life of about 4.2 hours in male subjects and 2.3 hours in female subjects with normal renal function. Although the half-life is increased in patients with impaired renal function, this has minimal effects, and hence, no change from a monthly dosing schedule is necessary. There is no significant change in the clearance of ZOLADEX in patients with hepatic impairment with normal renal function.

Pharmacodynamics: Daily doses of goserelin acetate of 25 to 500 µg in the aqueous formulation induce pituitary desensitization to endogenous and exogenous LHRH and after 7 to 21 days depress serum LH and testosterone. These findings indicate the locus of effect of goserelin acetate in man is at the pituitary gland. Initially, ZOLADEX like other LHRH agonists transiently increases serum testosterone concentrations.

In women, serum estradiol concentrations are suppressed by around 4 weeks after the first depot injection and remain suppressed until the end of the treatment period. In patients with estradiol already suppressed by an LHRH analogue, suppression is maintained on the change of therapy to ZOLADEX. Suppression of estradiol is associated with a response in endometriosis and will result in amenorrhoea in the majority of patients. Administration of goserelin acetate in a depot formulation every 28 days results in suppression of serum testosterone concentrations to that usually seen in the surgically castrate range and suppression of serum estradiol levels comparable to those seen postmenopausally.

Pharmacokinetics: Administration of ZOLADEX, in accordance with the dosage recommendations, ensures that exposure to goserelin is maintained with no clinically significant accumulation.

ZOLADEX is poorly protein bound and has a serum elimination half-life of about 4.2 hours in male subjects and 2.3 hours in female subjects with normal renal function. Although the half-life is increased in patients with impaired renal function absolute clearance is still relatively rapid. The existence of a non-renal, presumably hepatic, clearance and the absence of an increased incidence of possible adverse reactions in such patients implies that no adjustment in the proposed dosage regimen is necessary in patients with renal impairment. There is no significant change in the clearance of ZOLADEX in patients with hepatic impairment with normal renal function. The depot formulation of goserelin acetate releases drug continuously with peak serum concentrations occurring approximately two weeks after administration. Comparison of the pharmacokinetic profile of the 3.6 mg depot formulation with that of daily injections of goserelin acetate in the aqueous formulation at doses of 250 µg/day, indicated good bioavailability of the goserelin acetate depot formulation.

There is no evidence of drug accumulation when goserelin acetate depot is administered every 28 days.

Special Populations and Conditions: Pediatrics: The safety and effectiveness of ZOLADEX in children has not been established.

Geriatrics: No dosage adjustment is necessary in the elderly (see Dosage and Administration).

Hepatic Insufficiency: There is no significant change in pharmacokinetics in patients with hepatic failure. Hepatic impairment does not compromise the clearance of ZOLADEX, therefore a dosage adjustment is not needed for patients with hepatic impairment (see Dosage and Administration).

Renal Insufficiency: In patients with impaired renal function, the serum half-life is increased (serum half-life is 2-4 hours in patients with normal renal function). When ZOLADEX is given, as recommended, this change will not lead to any accumulation hence, no change in dosing is necessary (see Dosage and Administration).

STORAGE AND STABILITY: Protect from light and moisture. Store in the intact package between 2 and 25°C.

INFORMATION FOR THE PATIENT: Published in e-CPS, available by subscription at www.e-cps.ca.

DOSAGE FORMS, COMPOSITION AND PACKAGING: Each depot contains: goserelin acetate equivalent to goserelin 3.6 mg. The depot is supplied as a cylindrical rod of biodegradable and biocompatible D-L Lactide-glycolide copolymer and is presented in a sterile ready-to-use syringe with a 16 gauge needle for a single s.c. injection. This single-dose syringe is assembled with a protective sleeve (SafeSystem) in a sealed, sterile pouch that contains a desiccant. Instructions for administration, once every 28 days, are attached.

(Shown in Product Identification Section)

Zoladex® LA ℞

goserelin acetate

Luteinizing Hormone-Releasing Hormone (LHRH) Analog

AstraZeneca

Date of Preparation: February 2, 2000
Date of Revision: June 24, 2010

SUMMARY PRODUCT INFORMATION:

Route of Administration	Dosage Form/ Strength	Clinically Relevant Nonmedicinal Ingredients
Subcutaneous injection	Depot/10.8 mg goserelin	Lactide-glycolide copolymer For a complete listing see Dosage Forms, Composition and Packaging.

INDICATIONS AND CLINICAL USE: Prostate Cancer:

- ZOLADEX LA (goserelin acetate) is indicated for the palliative treatment of patients with hormone-dependent advanced carcinoma of the prostate (Stage M1 according to the Tumour-Node-Metastasis [TNM] classification system or Stage D2 according to the American Urologic Association [AUA] classification).
- ZOLADEX LA is indicated for use in combination with a non-steroidal antiandrogen and radiation therapy for the management of locally advanced (T3, T4) or bulky Stage T2b, T2c carcinoma of the prostate. Treatment with ZOLADEX LA and a non-steroidal antiandrogen should start 8 weeks prior to initiating radiation therapy and continue until completion of the radiation therapy.
- ZOLADEX LA as adjuvant hormone therapy to external beam irradiation for patients with locally advanced prostate cancer (Stage T3-T4).

Benign Conditions:

- ZOLADEX LA is indicated for the hormonal management of endometriosis, including pain relief and reduction of endometriotic lesions. Experience with ZOLADEX for the management of endometriosis has been limited to women 18 years of age and older, treated for 6 months.

Pediatrics: The safety and effectiveness of ZOLADEX LA in children has not been established.

CONTRAINDICATIONS:

- Patients who are hypersensitive to this drug or to any ingredient in the formulation or components of the container. For a complete listing, see Dosage Forms, Composition and Packaging.
- Women having undiagnosed abnormal vaginal bleeding.

Pregnancy: ZOLADEX LA should not be used during pregnancy. As with other LHRH agonists it is not known whether ZOLADEX LA causes fetal abnormalities in humans. Women of child bearing potential should be carefully examined before treatment to exclude pregnancy. Non-hormonal methods of contraception should be employed during therapy (see Warnings and Precautions).

Lactation: The use of ZOLADEX LA during breast feeding is not recommended.

WARNINGS AND PRECAUTIONS: General: Initially, ZOLADEX LA (goserelin acetate) transiently increases serum testosterone in males and serum estradiol concentrations in females. Although not necessarily related, isolated cases of short-term worsening of signs and symptoms have been reported during the first four weeks of therapy. Worsening of the clinical condition may occasionally require discontinuation of therapy and/or surgical intervention.

In women, ZOLADEX LA is only indicated for use in endometriosis. For female patients requiring treatment with goserelin for other conditions, refer to the prescribing information for ZOLADEX (3.6 mg depot).

Effect on Ability to Drive a Vehicle and Use Machinery: There is no evidence that ZOLADEX LA results in impairment of ability to drive or operate machinery.

Dependence/Tolerance: There have been no reports of drug dependence following the use of ZOLADEX LA.

Endocrine and Metabolism: Males: Induced Hypogonadism: Suppression of pituitary gonadotropins and gonadal hormone production will occur with continued administration of ZOLADEX. These changes have been observed to reverse on discontinuation of therapy. However, whether the clinical symptoms of induced hypogonadism will reverse in all patients has not yet been established.

Metabolic: Impaired glucose tolerance has been observed in males using LHRH agonists. This may manifest as diabetes or loss of glycaemic control in those with pre-existing diabetes mellitus. Consideration should therefore be given to monitoring blood glucose.

Genitourinary: Males: Patients with Genitourinary Tract Symptoms: During the first month of therapy with ZOLADEX LA, patients at risk of developing ureteric obstruction should be closely monitored.

Ureteric obstruction may develop in male patients with a history of obstructive uropathy. If spinal cord compression or renal impairment due to ureteric obstruction are present, or develop, specific standard treatment of these complications should be instituted.

Immune: Antibody formation has not been observed during administration of ZOLADEX LA. Local reactions, such as mild bruising have been related to the trauma of the injection itself and not to the copolymer material of the depot or to the prolonged presence of ZOLADEX at the site of depot injection.

Musculoskeletal: Patients with Vertebral Metastases: During the first month of therapy with ZOLADEX LA, patients with vertebral metastases who are thought to be of particular risk of spinal cord compression should be closely monitored.

Changes in Bone Density: The use of LHRH agonists may cause a reduction in bone mineral density. In men and women, some bone loss can be anticipated as part of the natural aging process. It may also be expected to occur during medically induced hypo-androgenic state caused by long term ZOLADEX LA treatment.

While specific data from the use of ZOLADEX LA are not currently available, data from studies of ZOLADEX suggest that some recovery of bone mineral may occur on cessation of therapy.

In patients with major risk factors for decreased bone mineral content such as chronic alcohol and/or tobacco use, presumed or strong family history of osteoporosis or chronic use of drugs that can reduce bone mass such as corticosteroids or anticonvulsants, ZOLADEX LA may pose an additional risk. In these patients the risks and benefits must be weighed carefully before ZOLADEX LA therapy is initiated. In women being treated for endometriosis, the use of ZOLADEX for longer than the recommended six months or in the presence of other known risk factors for decreased bone mineral content may cause additional bone loss.

Worsening of bone pain and other signs and symptoms have been reported infrequently in males and to a lesser extent in females during the first month of therapy with ZOLADEX LA. Initially, ZOLADEX LA like other LHRH agonists transiently increases serum testosterone concentrations. In men by around 21 days after the first depot injection, testosterone concentrations have typically decreased to within the castrate range and remain suppressed with treatment every 3 months. It is unclear whether there is any relationship between these clinical events and the initial rise in serum testosterone or estradiol levels observed during the first few days following administration of the first depot injection.

In those who reported an increase in bone pain, the pain ranged in intensity from mild to severe and required either symptomatic management, including non-narcotic analgesics or in some severe cases, narcotic analgesics.

Sexual Function/Reproduction: Fertility: Suppression of serum estradiol will induce amenorrhea in the majority of patients after the first four weeks of treatment especially if started during the menstrual phase of the cycle. During early treatment with ZOLADEX LA some women may experience vaginal bleeding of variable duration and intensity. Such bleeding may represent estrogen withdrawal bleeding and is expected to stop spontaneously. Amenorrhea is expected to be maintained until 12 weeks after the last dose of ZOLADEX LA. Rarely, some women may enter the natural menopause during treatment with LHRH analogues and do not resume menses on cessation of therapy.

Time to return of menses after cessation of therapy with ZOLADEX LA may be prolonged in some patients.

A non-hormonal method of contraception should be used during treatment. Patients should be advised that if they miss or postpone a dose of ZOLADEX LA, ovulation may occur with the potential for conception. If a patient becomes pregnant during treatment, she should discontinue treatment and consult her physician.

Duration of Endometriosis Treatment: The safety of treatment, as well as re-treatment, beyond 6 months with ZOLADEX LA has not been established.

The use of ZOLADEX LA may cause an increase in cervical resistance and care should be taken when dilating the cervix.

Special Populations: Pregnant Women: ZOLADEX LA should not be used in pregnancy as there is a theoretical risk of abortion or fetal abnormality if LHRH agonists are used during pregnancy. Potentially fertile women should be examined carefully before treatment to exclude pregnancy. Non-hormonal methods of contraception should be employed during therapy until menses resume.

Nursing Women: The use of ZOLADEX LA during breast feeding is not recommended.

Pediatrics: The safety and effectiveness of ZOLADEX LA in children has not been established.

Geriatrics: The labelling reflects the safety and effectiveness of ZOLADEX LA in the population over 65 years of age.

Monitoring and Laboratory Tests: Monitoring of Patients: During therapy with ZOLADEX LA, patients should be routinely monitored by physical examinations and appropriate laboratory tests. In prostate cancer patients tumour markers such as prostatic acid phosphatase (PAP), prostatic specific antigen (PSA) or acid phosphatase could be monitored. Additionally, if deemed appropriate by the physician, serum testosterone may be monitored; however, this is not routinely required.

In prostate cancer patients, an assessment of bone lesions may require the use of bone scans. Prostatic lesions may be monitored by ultrasonography and/or CT scan in addition to digital rectal examination. The status of obstructive uropathy in males may be assessed and/or diagnosed using intravenous pyelography, ultrasonography or CT scan.

Impaired glucose tolerance has been observed in males using LHRH agonists. This may manifest as diabetes or loss of glycaemic control in those with pre-existing diabetes mellitus. Consideration should therefore be given to monitoring blood glucose.

Effect on Laboratory Tests: Although serum testosterone or serum estradiol may be elevated during the first few days after administration of the first depot, they return to normal within one week, and are suppressed by the end of three weeks. They remain suppressed throughout therapy with ZOLADEX LA.

Prostate cancer tumour markers (PSA and PAP), are not routinely monitored in the first few days of therapy; however, if the cancer is responsive to ZOLADEX LA therapy, then these levels, if elevated prior to the commencement of treatment, are usually reduced by the end of the first month.

Renal function tests, blood urea nitrogen and creatinine may rarely be elevated during the first few days of therapy in prostate cancer patients before returning to normal.

Diagnostic Interference: Administration of ZOLADEX LA results in suppression of pituitary-gonadal system. Diagnostic tests of pituitary-gonadal function conducted during and subsequent to the treatment period may therefore be misleading.

ADVERSE REACTIONS: Adverse Drug Reaction Overview: The adverse effects seen with ZOLADEX LA (goserelin acetate) are due primarily to its pharmacological action of sex hormone suppression and may give rise to certain expected effects that vary by sex.

Adverse events that have been observed at an equal frequency in both males and females follow. Very common adverse events (≥10%) consist of: decreased libido, hot flush, and hyperhidrosis. Common adverse reactions (≥1% to <10%) are: paraesthesia, abnormal blood pressure, rash and decrease in bone density. Drug hypersensitivity was reported uncommonly (≥0.1% to <1). Anaphylactic reaction has been reported rarely (≥0.01% to <0.1). Cases of pituitary tumour and psychotic disorder have also been occasionally reported during post-marketed use. As with other agents in this class, cases of pituitary hemorrhage have occasionally been reported following initial administration of ZOLADEX during post-marketed use.

Abnormal blood pressure, manifest as hypotension or hypertension, are commonly observed in patients administered ZOLADEX LA. The changes are usually transient, resolving either during continued therapy or after cessation of therapy with ZOLADEX LA. Such changes have rarely required medical intervention including withdrawal of ZOLADEX LA treatment.

In males, erectile dysfunction was reported very commonly (≥10%). Commonly reported adverse reactions (≥1% to <10%) consist of: impaired glucose tolerance, spinal cord compression, bone pain, gynecomastia, cardiac failure and injection site reaction. Uncommon adverse reactions (≥0.1% to <1) are: arthralgia, ureteric obstruction and breast tenderness.

Heart failure was commonly reported (1.9%) in patients after the first 12 weeks following ZOLADEX LA administration for prostate cancer treatment in clinical studies. Myocardial infarction and heart failure were observed in a pharmaco-epidemiology study of LHRH agonists and/or anti-androgens used in the treatment of prostate cancer. The risks for these cardiovascular adverse events appear to be increased when LHRH agonists are used in combination with anti-androgens.

In females, very common adverse reactions (≥10%) consist of: vulvovaginal dryness, breast enlargement and injection site reaction. Common adverse reactions (≥1% to <10%) are: mood alteration including depression, headache, arthralgia and tumour flare/tumor pain. Rare (≥0.01% to <0.1) cases of ovarian cyst have been reported. Degeneration of uterine fibroid occurs at an unknown frequency.

Following the administration of ZOLADEX LA, skin rashes have been reported as generally mild, often regressing without discontinuation of therapy.

Initially, prostate cancer patients may experience a temporary increase in bone pain, which can be managed symptomatically.

The use of LHRH agonists may cause a reduction in bone mineral density (see Warnings and Precautions).

Clinical Trial Adverse Drug Reactions: Prostate Cancer Patients: Pharmacological effects include hot flush, hyperhidrosis and erectile dysfunction, seldom requiring withdrawal of therapy. Gynecomastia and breast tenderness have been noted infrequently. Initially, prostate cancer patients may experience a temporary increase in bone pain, which can be managed symptomatically. Isolated cases of spinal cord compression have been recorded.

The potential for exacerbation of signs and symptoms during the first few weeks of treatment is a concern particularly in male patients with impending neurologic compromise and in patients with severe obstructive uropathy (see Warnings and Precautions). Following the administration of ZOLADEX 3.6 mg depot, isolated cases of ureteric obstruction have been recorded.

Two controlled clinical trials were conducted with 157 patients, comparing treatment with ZOLADEX LA (10.8 mg) versus ZOLADEX 3.6 mg depots. During the comparative phase, patients were randomised to receive either a single 10.8 mg depot or three consecutive 3.6 mg depots (one every 4 weeks) over this initial 12 week period. The only adverse event reported in greater than 5% of these patients during this phase, was hot flush, with the ZOLADEX LA (10.8 mg) group having an incidence of 47% and the ZOLADEX 3.6 mg group having 48%.

From weeks 12-48 all patients were treated with one ZOLADEX LA depot every 12 weeks. During this noncomparative phase, the following adverse events, were reported in greater than 5% of patients; hot flush [vasodilation] (63.7%), general pain (14%), gynaecomastia (8.3%), pelvic pain (5.7%), bone pain (5.7%) and asthenia (5.1%).

The following adverse events reported in greater than 1%, but less than 5% of 157 patients treated with ZOLADEX LA depot every 12 weeks are tabulated below. Some of these would be expected in a proportion of the elderly population. See Table 1.

Table 1: ZOLADEX LA

Adverse Events in Controlled Studies with an Incidence of ≥1% but Less Than 5%

	Weeks 0 to 12		Week 12 Onwards	
	ZOLADEX 10.8 mg (n=78)		ZOLADEX 10.8 mg (n=157)[a]	
Body System/Adverse Events	**N**	**(%)**	**N**	**(%)**
Whole Body				
Abdominal pain	0	(0.0)	2	(1.3)
Aggravation reaction	0	(0.0)	5	(3.2)
Back pain	0	(0.0)	2	(1.3)
Flu syndrome	1	(1.3)	0	(0.0)
Headache	0	(0.0)	3	(1.9)
Infection	0	(0.0)	2	(1.3)
Sepsis	0	(0.0)	4	(2.5)
Cardiovascular				
Angina pectoris	1	(1.3)	1	(0.6)
Cerebral ischemia	0	(0.0)	2	(1.3)
Cerebrovascular accident	0	(0.0)	2	(1.3)
Heart failure	0	(0.0)	3	(1.9)
Pulmonary embolus	0	(0.0)	2	(1.3)
Varicose veins	1	(1.3)	0	(0.0)
Digestive				
Diarrhoea	1	(1.3)	4	(2.5)
Hematemesis	1	(1.3)	0	(0.0)
Endocrine System				
Diabetes mellitus	0	(0.0)	2	(1.3)
Hemic and Lymphatic				
Anemia	0	(0.0)	3	(1.9)
Metabolic and Nutritional				
Peripheral oedema	2	(2.6)	5	(3.2)
Nervous System				
Dizziness	0	(0.0)	5	(3.2)
Paresthesia	2	(2.6)	2	(1.3)
Urinary retention	0	(0.0)	2	(1.3)
Respiratory System				
Cough increased	0	(0.0)	4	(2.5)
Dyspnoea	0	(0.0)	6	(3.8)
Pneumonia	0	(0.0)	2	(1.3)
Skin and Appendages				
Herpes Simplex	1	(1.3)	1	(0.6)
Pruritus	0	(0.0)	2	(1.3)
Urogenital				
Bladder neoplasm	1	(1.3)	1	(0.6)
Breast pain	2	(2.6)	7	(4.5)
Hematuria	1	(1.3)	3	(1.9)
Impotence	2	(2.6)	2	(1.3)
Urinary frequency	0	(0.0)	2	(1.3)
Urinary incontinence	0	(0.0)	2	(1.3)
Urinary tract disorder	1	(1.3)	5	(3.2)
Urinary tract infection	3	(3.8)	7	(4.5)
Urination impaired	0	(0.0)	3	(1.9)

(cont'd)

Table 1: ZOLADEX LA *(cont'd)*

Adverse Events in Controlled Studies with an Incidence of ≥1% but Less Than 5%

[a] Adverse events occurring in the comparative phase of these studies (Weeks 0 to 12) are presented separately to data from the non-comparative phase (Week 12 onwards), as the differences in the two periods of observation made a direct comparison inappropriate.

In a controlled clinical trial conducted with 58 patients, ZOLADEX LA 10.8 mg was administered every 13 weeks (3 months). Adverse events were consistent with the results of earlier trials. The following adverse events were reported in 10% or more patients; hot flush [vasodilation] (67%), general pain (31%), pelvic pain (22%), back pain (16%), insomnia (16%), hyperhidrosis (14%), hypertension (12%), constipation (12%), urinary frequency (12%), and nocturia (10%).

The most frequently reported (greater than 5%) adverse experiences during treatment with a LHRH-agonist in combination with flutamide are listed in the table below. For comparison, adverse experiences seen with a LHRH-agonist and placebo are also listed in Table 2.

Table 2: ZOLADEX LA

Adverse Events (greater than 5%) Reported During Treatment with a LHRH-agonist in Combination with Flutamide

	Flutamide+LHRH-agonist (n=294) % All	Placebo+LHRH-agonist (n=285) % All
Hot flush	61	57
Loss of libido	36	31
Impotence	33	29
Diarrhea	12	4
Nausea/vomiting	11	10
Gynecomastia	9	11
Other	7	9
Other gastrointestinal	6	4

As shown in Table 2, for both treatment groups, the most frequently occurring adverse experiences (hot flush, loss of libido, impotence) were those known to be associated with low serum androgen levels and known to occur with LHRH-agonists alone.

The only notable difference between these treatment groups was the higher incidence of diarrhea in the flutamide+LHRH-agonist group (12%) as compared to the placebo+LHRH-agonist group (4%). The cases of diarrhea reported were severe in less than 1% of the patients. In addition, the following adverse reactions were reported during treatment with flutamide+LHRH-agonist. No causal relatedness of these reactions to drug treatment has been made, and some of the adverse experiences reported are those that commonly occur in elderly patients.

Cardiovascular System: hypertension in 1% of patients. Rarely thrombophlebitis, pulmonary embolism, and myocardial infarction.

Central Nervous System: CNS (drowsiness/confusion/depression/anxiety/nervousness) reactions occurred in 1% of patients. Rarely insomnia, tiredness, headache, dizziness, weakness, malaise, blurred vision and decreased libido have been reported.

Endocrine System: gynecomastia in 9% of patients. Rarely breast tenderness sometimes accompanied by galactorrhoea.

Gastrointestinal System: Nausea/vomiting occurred in 11%, diarrhea 12%, anorexia 4%, and other GI disorders occurred in 6% of patients. Increased appetite, indigestion and constipation have also been reported.

Hematopoietic System: Anaemia occurred in 6% of patients, leukopenia 3%, and thrombocytopenia 1%.

Liver and Biliary System: Clinically evident hepatitis and jaundice occurred in <1% of patients.

Skin: Irritation at the injection site and rash occurred in 3% of patients. Photosensitivity reactions have been reported in five patients.

Other: Pruritus, ecchymosis, herpes zoster, thirst, lymphedema, lupus-like syndrome, hematuria, reduced sperm counts have been reported rarely in long-term treatment. Edema occurred in 4% of patients; neuromuscular, genitourinary symptoms occurred in 2% of patients. Pulmonary symptoms occurred in <1% of patients.

Benign Conditions: Pharmacological effects of ZOLADEX LA treatment in women include hot flush and hyperhidrosis, and decreased libido, seldom requiring withdrawal from therapy. Headaches, mood alteration including depression, vulvovaginal dryness and breast enlargement have been noted infrequently. In women with fibroids, degeneration of uterine fibroids may occur.

As with other LHRH agonists, there have been reports of ovarian cyst formation.

Abnormal Hematologic and Clinical Chemistry Findings: Plasma Enzymes: Elevations of liver enzymes (AST, ALT) have been reported in less than 1% of all female patients. There was no other evidence of abnormal liver function. Causality between these changes and ZOLADEX LA have not been established.

Lipids: In a controlled trial, ZOLADEX therapy resulted in a minor, but statistically significant effect on serum lipids. In patients treated for endometriosis at 6 months following initiation of therapy, ZOLADEX treatment resulted in mean increases in LDL cholesterol of 0.55 mmol/L and HDL cholesterol of 0.07 mmol/L. Triglycerides increased by 0.09 mmol/L as well as total cholesterol by 0.65 mmol/L. At the end of 6 months of treatment, HDL cholesterol fractions (HDL2 and HDL3) were increased by 0.05 mmol/L and 0.02 mmol/L, respectively.

DRUG INTERACTIONS: Drug-Drug Interactions: There are no known drug-drug interactions requiring dose adjustment.
Drug-Food Interactions: Interactions with particular foods have not been established.
Drug-Herb Interactions: Interactions with herbal products have not been established.
Drug-Laboratory Test Interactions: Interactions with laboratory tests have not been established.

DOSAGE AND ADMINISTRATION: Dosing Considerations: General: Although, isolated cases of vaginal spotting or bleeding during treatment have been reported, this is not associated with lack of pharmacodynamic effect in most instances. The majority of patients become amenorrheic within 8 weeks of starting treatment. In the small number of women who experience continued menstrual bleeding, estradiol blood levels should be measured. If menstrual bleeding persists and estradiol measurements correspond to postmenopausal values, appropriate diagnostic measures should be undertaken to rule out an intrauterine pathology.

Recommended Dose and Dosage Adjustment: Prostate Cancer: One depot of ZOLADEX LA containing goserelin acetate equivalent to 10.8 mg goserelin, should be injected subcutaneously into the anterior abdominal wall every 3 months (**13 weeks**) following the procedure recommended on the instruction card (see Instructions for Use on card attached to sterile pouch). While the 3-month (**13 week**) schedule should be adhered to, a delay of a few days is permissible.

If in exceptional circumstances repeat dosing does not occur at 3 months, data indicate that castrate levels of testosterone are maintained for up to 16 weeks in the majority of patients.

When ZOLADEX LA is given in combination with a non-steroidal antiandrogen and radiotherapy for patients with Stage T2b-T4 prostatic carcinoma, treatment should be started 8 weeks prior to initiating radiotherapy and should continue until completion of the radiation therapy. A treatment regimen using a ZOLADEX 3.6 mg depot 8 weeks before radiotherapy, followed in 28 days by the ZOLADEX LA (10.8 mg) depot until completion of the radiation therapy, can be administered.

Endometriosis: One depot of ZOLADEX LA containing goserelin acetate equivalent to 10.8 mg goserelin, should be injected subcutaneously into the anterior abdominal wall every 12 weeks following the procedure recommended on the instruction card (see Instructions for Use on card attached to sterile pouch). While the 12-week schedule should be adhered to, a delay of a few days is permissible.

Renal Impairment: In clinical studies, subjects with impaired renal function (creatinine clearance <20 mL/min), had a mean serum elimination half-life of 12.1 hours for ZOLADEX compared to 4.2 hours for male subjects with normal renal function (creatinine clearance >70 mL/min). When ZOLADEX LA is given, as recommended, this change will not lead to any accumulation hence, no change in dosing is necessary for patients with renal failure.

Hepatic Impairment: Hepatic impairment does not compromise the clearance of ZOLADEX LA, therefore a dosage adjustment is not needed for patients with hepatic impairment.

Geriatrics: No dosage adjustment is necessary in the elderly.

Pediatrics: The safety and effectiveness of ZOLADEX LA in children has not been established. (See Warnings and Precautions.)

Administration: ZOLADEX LA 10.8 mg Step by Step Directions for Use (see package insert for illustrations): Caution: Do not depress plunger until Step 5. Read all instructions before use.

1. Put the patient in a comfortable position with the upper part of the body slightly raised. Swab abdominal injection site.
2. Remove the syringe from the opened foil pouch and hold the syringe at a slight angle to the light. Check that at least part of the ZOLADEX depot is visible.
3. Grasp the plastic safety tab and pull away from the syringe and discard. Remove needle cover. **Unlike liquid injections, there is no need to remove air bubbles as attempts to do so may displace the depot.**
4. Holding the syringe around the protective sleeve, pinch the patient's skin and insert the needle at a slight angle (30 to 45 degrees) to the skin. With the opening of the needle facing up, insert needle into the subcutaneous tissue of the anterior abdominal wall below the navel line, until the protective sleeve touches the patient's skin.

> Do not penetrate into muscle or peritoneum.

5. Moving your hand back to the finger grip, depress the plunger **fully**, until you can depress no more, to discharge the ZOLADEX depot and to activate the protective sleeve. You may hear a "click" and will feel the protective sleeve automatically begin to slide to cover the needle. If the plunger is not depressed fully the protective sleeve will **not** activate.
6. Holding the syringe as shown, withdraw the needle and allow protective sleeve to continue to slide and cover needle. Dispose of the syringe in an approved sharps collector.

OVERDOSAGE:

The pharmacologic properties of ZOLADEX LA (goserelin acetate) and its mode of delivery make accidental or intentional overdosage unlikely. There is limited experience of overdosage in humans. In cases where ZOLADEX LA has unintentionally been readministered early or given at a higher dose than recommended, no clinically relevant adverse effects have been seen. Animal studies indicate that no increased pharmacologic effect would occur in man with higher doses or more frequent administration than those recommended. Subcutaneous doses of the drug as high as 1 mg/kg/day in rats and dogs produced no non-endocrine related sequelae; this dose is approximately 400 times that proposed for human use. If overdosage occurs, this should be managed symptomatically.

> For management of a suspected drug overdose, contact your regional Poison Control Centre. See the *CPS* Directory section for a list of Poison Control Centres.

ACTION AND CLINICAL PHARMACOLOGY: Mechanism of Action: ZOLADEX LA (goserelin acetate) is a synthetic decapeptide analog of gonadotropin releasing hormone (GnRH or LHRH). When given acutely, goserelin acetate stimulates the release of pituitary luteinizing hormone (LH) from the pituitary gland. However, following chronic administration, goserelin acetate is a potent inhibitor of gonadotropin production resulting in gonadal and consequently, accessory sex organ regression. This effect is the basis for the inhibition of growth of chemically-induced rat mammary tumours and transplantable rat prostate and pituitary tumours.

In animals and man, following an initial stimulation of pituitary LH secretion and a transient elevation in serum testosterone in males and serum estradiol in females, chronic administration results in inhibition of gonadotropin secretion.

In men, approximately 21 days after the initiation of therapy, a sustained suppression of pituitary LH results in the reduction in serum testosterone levels to a range normally seen in surgically castrated men, and of serum estradiol to levels comparable with those observed in post-menopausal women. This suppression of testosterone and estradiol is then maintained on repeat administration of ZOLADEX LA as long as therapy is continued.

In women, serum estradiol concentrations are suppressed by around 4 weeks after the first depot injection and remain suppressed until the end of the treatment period. In patients with estradiol already suppressed by an LHRH analogue, suppression is maintained on the change of therapy to ZOLADEX LA. Suppression of estradiol is associated with a response in endometriosis and will result in amenorrhea in the majority of patients. During early treatment with ZOLADEX LA some women may experience vaginal bleeding of variable duration and intensity. Such bleeding may represents estrogen withdrawal bleeding and is expected to stop spontaneously. Amenorrhea is expected to be maintained until 12 weeks after the last dose of ZOLADEX LA.

ZOLADEX LA is a depot formulation of goserelin acetate dispersed in a cylindrical rod of biodegradable and biocompatible blend of high and low molecular weight range D-L Lactide-glycolide copolymer.

Administration of ZOLADEX LA, in accordance with the dosage recommendations, ensures that exposure to goserelin is maintained with no clinically significant accumulation.

ZOLADEX LA is poorly protein bound and has a serum elimination half-life of about 4.2 hours in male subjects and 2.3 hours in female subjects with normal renal function. Although the half-life is increased in patients with impaired renal function, this has minimal effects, and since, for the compound given, as recommended, in a 10.8 mg depot formulation, this change will not lead to any accumulation, no change in dosing is necessary in these patients. There is no significant change in the clearance of ZOLADEX LA in patients with hepatic impairment with normal renal function (see Pharmacokinetics).

Pharmacodynamics: Daily doses of goserelin acetate of 25 to 500 µg in the aqueous formulation induce pituitary desensitization to endogenous and exogenous LHRH and after 7 to 21 days depress serum LH and testosterone. These findings indicate the locus of effect of goserelin acetate in man is at the pituitary gland. Initially, ZOLADEX LA like other LHRH agonists transiently increases serum testosterone concentrations.

In men by around 21 days after the first ZOLADEX LA depot injection, testosterone concentrations have typically fallen to within the castrate range and remain suppressed with treatment every 3 months. In clinical trials using ZOLADEX LA for 48 weeks, suppression of serum testosterone to castrate levels has been maintained for the duration of therapy. Data exists which indicates that in the majority of patients (over 90%), serum testosterone levels remain suppressed to within the castrate range for up to 13 weeks (3 months).

In women, serum estradiol concentrations are suppressed by around 4 weeks after the first depot injection and remain suppressed until the end of the treatment period. In patients with estradiol already suppressed by an LHRH analogue, suppression is maintained on the change of therapy to ZOLADEX LA. Suppression of estradiol is associated with a response in endometriosis and will result in amenorrhoea in the majority of patients.

Pharmacokinetics: Administration of ZOLADEX LA, in accordance with the dosage recommendations, ensures that exposure to goserelin is maintained with no clinically significant accumulation.

ZOLADEX LA is poorly protein bound and has a serum elimination half-life of about 4.2 hours in male subjects and 2.3 hours in female subjects with normal renal function. Although the half-life is increased in patients with impaired renal function absolute clearance is still relatively rapid. The existence of a non-renal, presumably hepatic, clearance and the absence of an increased incidence of possible adverse reactions in such patients implies that no adjustment in the proposed dosage regimen is necessary in patients with renal impairment. There is no significant change in the clearance of ZOLADEX LA in patients with hepatic impairment with normal renal function. The ZOLADEX LA (10.8 mg) depot formulation of goserelin acetate releases drug continuously with peak serum concentrations occurring approximately two hours after administration.

Special Populations and Conditions: Pediatrics: The safety and effectiveness of ZOLADEX LA in children has not been established (see Warnings and Precautions).

Geriatrics: No dosage adjustment is necessary in the elderly (see Dosage and Administration).

Hepatic Insufficiency: There is no significant change in pharmacokinetics in patients with hepatic failure. Hepatic impairment does not compromise the clearance of ZOLADEX LA, therefore a dosage adjustment is not needed for patients with hepatic impairment (see Dosage and Administration).

Renal Insufficiency: In patients with impaired renal function, the serum half-life is increased (serum half-life is 2-4 hours in patients with normal renal function). When ZOLADEX LA is given, as recommended, this change will not lead to any accumulation hence, no change in dosing is necessary (see Dosage and Administration).

STORAGE AND STABILITY: Protect from light and moisture. Store in the intact package between 2 and 25°C.

INFORMATION FOR THE PATIENT: Published in e-CPS, available by subscription at www.e-cps.ca.

DOSAGE FORMS, COMPOSITION AND PACKAGING: Each depot contains: goserelin acetate equivalent to goserelin 10.8 mg. The depot is supplied as a cylindrical rod of biodegradable and biocompatible D-L Lactide-glycolide copolymer and is presented in a sterile ready-to-use syringe with a 14 gauge needle for a single s.c. injection. The single-dose syringe is assembled with a protective sleeve (SafeSystem) in a sealed, sterile pouch that contains a desiccant. Instructions for administration are attached.

(Shown in Product Identification Section)

Zolinza® Ⓟ

vorinostat

Histone Deacetylase Inhibitor—Antineoplastic Agent

Merck Frosst

Date of Revision: March 29, 2010

SUMMARY PRODUCT INFORMATION:

Route of Administration	Dosage Form/ Strength	Clinically Relevant Nonmedicinal Ingredients
Oral	Capsules 100 mg	Gelatin For a complete listing see Dosage Forms, Composition and Packaging.

INDICATIONS AND CLINICAL USE: ZOLINZA is indicated for the treatment of cutaneous manifestations in patients with advanced cutaneous T-cell lymphoma (CTCL) who have progressive, persistent or recurrent disease subsequent to prior systemic therapies.

The indication was approved based on response rate demonstrated in a single-arm phase II study.

Geriatrics (≥65 years of age): In clinical studies, the efficacy and safety of ZOLINZA in the elderly (≥65 years) were comparable to those seen in younger patients (<65 years).

Pediatrics: The safety and effectiveness of ZOLINZA in pediatric patients have not been studied.

CONTRAINDICATIONS:

- Patients who are hypersensitive to this drug or to any ingredient in the formulation. For a complete listing, see Dosage Forms, Composition and Packaging.
- Patients who have severe hepatic impairment (total bilirubin ≥3× ULN).

WARNINGS AND PRECAUTIONS:

> **Serious Warnings and Precautions**
> ZOLINZA should be administered under the supervision of a physician experienced with the use of chemotherapy and with treatment of cutaneous T-cell lymphoma.
> The following are clinically important adverse events:
> - Thromboembolism including fatal cases
> - Thrombocytopenia and anemia

Cardiovascular: Thromboembolism: Pulmonary embolism and deep vein thrombosis have been reported as drug-related adverse experiences in clinical trials with ZOLINZA. In the pivotal study in patients with CTCL treated with vorinostat 400 mg once daily (median duration of exposure ~4 months), the reported incidence of pulmonary embolism was 4.7% (4/86) and of deep vein thrombosis was 1.2% (1/86). In all completed and ongoing studies of vorinostat monotherapy in patients with CTCL, the proportion of patients with a venous thromboembolic event was 6.8% (10/147). In greater than 1000 patients with hematologic malignancies and solid tumors who have been treated with vorinostat as monotherapy, or in combination with other chemotherapy agents, in completed and ongoing clinical studies, the proportion of patients that experienced a venous thromboembolic event was approximately 5.0 %. In addition, there was an increase in the incidence of venous thromboembolic events in a randomized, double-blind study of patients with advanced non-small cell lung cancer who received vorinostat (400 mg once daily) in combination with chemotherapy (carboplatin and paclitaxel) as compared to patients who received chemotherapy alone. In this study, deep venous thrombosis and/or pulmonary embolism was reported in 6.5% (8/124) of patients in the vorinostat/chemotherapy treatment arm compared to 2.4% (3/124) of patients in the placebo/chemotherapy treatment arm.

Physicians should closely monitor patients for signs and symptoms of these events, particularly in patients with a prior history of thromboembolic events (see Adverse Reactions, Serious Drug-Related Adverse Events).

QT/QTc Prolongation: ZOLINZA is associated with QT/QTc interval prolongation (see Warnings and Precautions, Monitoring and Laboratory Tests and Action and Clinical Pharmacology, Cardiac Electrophysiology). Many drugs that cause QT/QTc prolongation are suspected to increase the risk of torsade de pointes.

Torsade de pointes is a polymorphic ventricular tachyarrhythmia. Generally, the risk of torsade de pointes increases with the magnitude of QT/QTc prolongation produced by the drug. Torsade de pointes may be asymptomatic or experienced by the patient as dizziness, palpitations, syncope, or seizures. If sustained, torsade de pointes can progress to ventricular fibrillation and sudden cardiac death.

Particular care should be exercised when administering ZOLINZA to patients who are suspected to be at an increased risk of experiencing torsade de pointes during treatment with a QT/QTc-prolonging drug. Risk factors for torsade de pointes in the general population include, but are not limited to, the following: female gender; age 65 years or older; baseline prolongation of the QT/QTc interval; presence of genetic variants affecting cardiac ion channels or regulatory proteins, especially congenital long QT syndromes; family history of sudden cardiac death at <50 years; cardiac disease (e.g., myocardial ischemia or infarction, congestive heart failure, left ventricular hypertrophy, cardiomyopathy, conduction system disease); history of arrhythmias (especially ventricular arrhythmias, atrial fibrillation, or recent conversion from atrial fibrillation); electrolyte disturbances (e.g., hypokalemia, hypomagnesemia, hypocalcemia); bradycardia (<50 beats per minute); acute neurological events (e.g., intracranial or subarachnoid haemorrhage, stroke, intracranial trauma); nutritional deficits (e.g., eating disorders, extreme diets); diabetes mellitus; and autonomic neuropathy.

Physicians who prescribe drugs that prolong the QT/QTc interval should counsel their patients concerning the nature and implications of the ECG changes, underlying diseases and disorders that are considered to represent risk factors, demonstrated and predicted drug-drug interactions, symptoms suggestive of arrhythmia, risk management strategies, and other information relevant to the use of the drug.

Heart Rate: ZOLINZA has been associated with increases in heart rate (see Action and Clinical Pharmacology, Cardiac Electrophysiology). Increases in heart rate may lead to worsening of cardiac conditions in patients with a history of ischemic heart disease or tachyarrhythmias. Caution should be observed in this patient population.

Drug Interactions: Other Histone Deacetylase (HDAC) Inhibitors: Severe thrombocytopenia and gastrointestinal bleeding have been reported with concomitant use of ZOLINZA and other HDAC inhibitors (e.g., valproic acid). Concurrent use of ZOLINZA with other HDAC inhibitors is not recommended (see Drug Interactions, Drug-Drug Interactions).

Coumarin-Derivative Anticoagulants: Physicians should carefully monitor PT and INR in patients concurrently administered ZOLINZA and coumarin-derivatives (see Drug Interactions, Drug-Drug Interactions).

Endocrine and Metabolism: Hyperglycemia: Hyperglycemia has been observed commonly in patients receiving ZOLINZA (see Adverse Reactions, Abnormal Hematologic and Clinical Chemistry Findings). Serum glucose should be monitored, especially in diabetic or potentially diabetic patients. Adjustment of diet and/or anti-hyperglycemic therapy may be necessary. Dose reduction or interruption may be considered in patients who develop severe hyperglycemia during ZOLINZA treatment.

Gastrointestinal: Gastrointestinal disturbances, including nausea, vomiting and diarrhea have been reported very commonly in patients treated with ZOLINZA (see Adverse Reactions) which may require the use of antiemetic and antidiarrheal medications. Women may experience more nausea, diarrhea and dysguesia than men.

Dehydration: Dehydration has been reported as a common serious drug-related adverse experience in clinical trials. Fluid and electrolyte replacement should be administered to prevent dehydration (see Adverse Reactions). Patients should be instructed to drink at least 2 L/day of fluids for adequate hydration. Pre-existing nausea, vomiting, and diarrhea should be adequately controlled before beginning therapy with ZOLINZA.

Hematologic: Treatment with ZOLINZA is associated with dose-related thrombocytopenia and anemia. If platelet counts and/or hemoglobin are severely reduced (platelets $<25\times10^3/mm^3$ and/or hemoglobin <6.5 g/dL) during treatment with ZOLINZA, the dose should be modified or therapy discontinued (see Warnings and Precautions, Monitoring and Laboratory Tests; Adverse Reactions and Dosage and Administration).

Special Populations: Hepatic Impairment: ZOLINZA was studied in a limited number of patients with hepatic impairment. Based on these results, ZOLINZA is not recommended in patients with moderate hepatic impairment (total bilirubin 1.5×-3× ULN). ZOLINZA is contraindicated in patients with severe hepatic impairment (total bilirubin >3× ULN). See Contraindications and Action and Clinical Pharmacology, Special Populations and Conditions, Hepatic Insufficiency.

Renal Impairment: ZOLINZA has not been studied in patients with renal impairment. Although negligible amount of vorinostat was excreted via the kidney, over 50% of the vorinostat dose was recovered as two major metabolites in the urine (see Action and Clinical Pharmacology). Patients with renal impairment should be treated with caution.

Pregnant Women: There are no adequate and well-controlled studies in pregnant women using ZOLINZA. In rats and rabbits administered vorinostat at dosages up to 50 and 150 mg/kg/day, respectively (below the human exposure based on AUC_{0-24}), treatment-related developmental effects including decreased mean live fetal weights, limited sites of incomplete ossifications and limited numbers of skeletal variations at the highest doses of vorinostat tested were observed. An increased incidence of gallbladder malformations was observed in rabbits. The no observed effect level was 15 and 20 mg/kg/day in rats and rabbits, respectively.

Women of childbearing potential should be advised to avoid pregnancy while on ZOLINZA. If ZOLINZA is used during pregnancy, or if the patient becomes pregnant while taking this drug, the patient should be apprised of the potential hazard to the fetus.

Nursing Women: It is not known whether this drug is excreted in human milk. Because many drugs are excreted in human milk and because of the potential for serious adverse reactions in nursing infants from ZOLINZA, women should be advised against breast-feeding while taking ZOLINZA.

Pediatrics: The safety and effectiveness of ZOLINZA in pediatric patients have not been studied.

Geriatrics (≥65 years of age): In clinical studies, the safety of ZOLINZA in the elderly (≥65 years) were comparable to those seen in younger patients (<65 years). No dosage adjustment is necessary in elderly patients.

Monitoring and Laboratory Tests: Careful monitoring of blood cell counts and chemistry tests, including electrolytes, glucose and serum creatinine, should be performed every 2 weeks during the first 2 months of therapy and monthly thereafter. Electrolyte monitoring should include potassium, magnesium and calcium. Baseline and periodic ECGs should be performed during treatment (see Warnings and Precautions, Cardiovascular, QT/QTc Prolongation).

ZOLINZA should be administered with particular caution in patients with congenital long QT syndrome, and patients taking anti-arrhythmic medicines or other medicinal products that lead to QT prolongation. Hypokalemia or hypomagnesemia should be corrected prior to administration of ZOLINZA, and consideration should be given to monitoring potassium and magnesium in symptomatic patients (e.g., patients with nausea, vomiting, diarrhea, fluid imbalance or cardiac symptoms).

ADVERSE REACTIONS: Adverse Drug Reaction Overview: The safety of ZOLINZA was evaluated in 107 CTCL patients in two single-arm clinical studies in which 86 patients received 400 mg once daily.

The most common drug-related adverse experiences in patients on 400 mg once daily could be classified into 4 symptom complexes: gastrointestinal symptoms (diarrhea, nausea, anorexia, weight decreased, vomiting, constipation, decreased appetite), constitutional symptoms (fatigue, chills), hematologic abnormalities (thrombocytopenia, anemia), and taste disorders (dysgeusia, dry mouth).

Table 1: ZOLINZA

Drug-related Clinical or Laboratory Adverse Experiences Occurring in CTCL Patients (Incidence ≥5%)

	ZOLINZA 400 mg Once Daily (N=86)			
	All Grades		Grade 3-5[a]	
Adverse Experiences	n	%	n	%
Fatigue	39	(45.3)	2	(2.3)
Diarrhea	40	(46.5)	0	(0.0)
Nausea	33	(38.4)	3	(3.5)
Dysgeusia	20	(23.3)	0	(0.0)
Thrombocytopenia	22	(25.6)	5	(5.8)
Anorexia	20	(23.3)	2	(2.3)
Weight Decreased	17	(19.8)	1	(1.2)
Dry Mouth	14	(16.3)	0	(0.0)
Vomiting	10	(11.6)	0	(0.0)
Blood Creatinine Increased	11	(12.8)	0	(0.0)
Alopecia	14	(16.3	0	(0.0)
Decreased Appetite	10	(11.6	1	(1.2)
Muscle Spasms	14	(16.3	2	(2.3)
Anemia	11	(12.8)	2	(2.3)
Constipation	9	(10.5)	0	(0.0)
Chills	9	(10.5)	1	(1.2)
Dizziness	6	(7.0)	1	(1.2)
Abdominal Pain	7	(8.1)	1	(1.2)
Proteinuria	7	(8.1)	0	(0.0)
Dyspnea	6	(7.0)	0	(0.0)
Headache	5	(5.8)	0	(0.0)

[a] None of these adverse experiences were Grade 5.

Clinical Trial Adverse Drug Reactions: Common Clinical Trial Adverse Drug Reactions (≥5%): Table 1 summarizes the specific drug-related adverse experiences by frequency and National Cancer Institute-Common Terminology Criteria for Adverse Events (NCI-CTCAE, version 3.0) Grade in the CTCL patients who received 400 mg once daily.

Serious Drug-Related Adverse Events: The most common serious drug-related adverse experiences in the 86 CTCL patients in two clinical studies receiving 400 mg once daily of ZOLINZA were pulmonary embolism, reported in 4.7% (4/86) of patients and anemia reported in 2.3% (2/86) of patients. There were single experiences of thrombocytopenia, death (of unknown cause), ischemic stroke, deep vein thrombosis, gastrointestinal hemorrhage, streptococcal bacteremia, dehydration, and syncope.

Three cases (4.1%, 3/74) of squamous cell carcinoma, not considered drug related by the investigator, were reported as serious clinical adverse experiences in the pivotal study.

Dose Modifications and Discontinuations: Of the CTCL patients who received the 400-mg once daily dose, 10.5% (9/86) of patients required a dose modification of ZOLINZA due to adverse experiences. These adverse experiences included increased serum creatinine, decreased appetite, hypokalemia, leukopenia, nausea, neutropenia, thrombocytopenia and vomiting. The median time to the first adverse experience resulting in dose reduction was 42 days (range 17 to 263 days).

Of the CTCL patients who received the 400-mg once daily dose, 10.5% (9/86) of patients discontinued ZOLINZA due to drug-related adverse experiences. These adverse experiences included anemia, angioneurotic edema, asthenia, chest pain, death, deep vein thrombosis, ischemic stroke, lethargy, pulmonary embolism and skin lesion.

Dehydration: Based on reports of dehydration as a serious drug-related adverse experience in clinical trials, patients were instructed to drink at least 2 L/day of fluids for adequate hydration. After these precautions were implemented, the incidence of dehydration decreased (see Warnings and Precautions, Gastrointestinal and Monitoring and Laboratory Tests).

Abnormal Hematologic and Clinical Chemistry Findings: Laboratory abnormalities were reported in the 86 patients who received the 400 mg dose and one patient who received a 350-mg dose.

Increased serum glucose was detected by laboratory safety tests in 69% (60/87) of CTCL patients, but was severe (Grade 3) in only 5 of these. Hyperglycemia was reported as a drug-related adverse experience in 4.7% (4/86) of CTCL patients who received the 400-mg once daily dose (see Warnings and Precautions, Endocrine and Metabolism).

Transient, non-severe increases in serum creatinine were detected in 47.1% (41/87) of CTCL patients.

Proteinuria was detected as a laboratory abnormality in 38 of 74 (51.4%) patients tested. The clinical significance of this finding is unknown.

Adverse Experiences in Non-CTCL Patients: In addition to the 107 CTCL patients, 312 patients with malignancies other than CTCL received ZOLINZA as monotherapy or in combination with other anti-cancer therapies. Drug-related adverse experiences reported in non-CTCL patients were generally similar to those reported in CTCL patients. However, the frequencies of individual adverse experiences were higher in the non-CTCL population. Drug-related serious adverse experiences reported in the non-CTCL population which were not observed in the CTCL population included single experiences of blurred vision, deafness, dysphagia, asthenia, abdominal pain, diverticulitis, hyponatremia, non-small cell lung cancer, tumor hemorrhage, Guillain-Barré syndrome, renal failure, urinary retention, cough, hemoptysis, hypertension and vasculitis.

DRUG INTERACTIONS: Overview: Clinical studies to evaluate drug-drug interactions of ZOLINZA have not been conducted. In animal models and in vitro human systems, the major pathways of metabolism of vorinostat involve glucuronidation and hydrolysis followed by β-oxidation. It is possible that vorinostat may interact with drugs metabolized via the same pathways.

Drug-Drug Interactions: See Table 2.

Table 2: ZOLINZA

Established or Potential Drug-Drug Interactions

Vorinostat with	Ref	Effect	Clinical comment
Coumarin-Derivative Anticoagulants	CT	Prolongation of prothrombin time (PT) and International Normalized Ratio (INR) were observed infrequently in patients receiving ZOLINZA concomitantly with coumarin-derivative anticoagulants.	Physicians should carefully monitor PT and INR in patients concurrently administered ZOLINZA and coumarin derivatives.
Other HDAC Inhibitors	CT	Severe (Grade 4) thrombocytopenia with associated gastrointestinal bleeding and anemia has been reported with the concomitant use of ZOLINZA and valproic acid.	ZOLINZA should not be administered concomitantly with other HDAC inhibitors (e.g., valproic acid) as class-specific adverse reactions may be additive.
Other QT/QTc Prolonging Drugs[a]	T	Concomitant use of ZOLINZA with another QTc prolonging drug may have an additive effect on QTc interval.	The concomitant use of ZOLINZA with another QT/QTc-prolonging drug should be avoided to the extent possible.
Drugs that disrupt electrolyte levels[b]	T	Electrolyte imbalance such as hypokalemia increases risk of QTc interval prolongation	The use of ZOLINZA with drugs disrupting electrolyte level is discouraged.

[a] For additional information see Other QT/QTc Prolonging Drugs.
[b] For additional information see Drugs that Disrupt Electrolyte Levels.
Legend: C=case study; CT=clinical trial; T=theoretical.

Other QT/QTc Prolonging Drugs: The concomitant use of ZOLINZA with another QT/QTc-prolonging drug should be avoided to the extent possible. Drugs that have been associated with QT/QTc interval prolongation and/or torsade de pointes include, but are not limited to, the examples in the following list. Chemical/pharmacological classes are listed if some, although not necessarily all, class members have been implicated in QT/QTc prolongation and/or torsade de pointes:

Class IA antiarrhythmics (e.g., quinidine, procainamide, disopyramide); Class III antiarrhythmics (e.g., amiodarone, sotalol, ibutilide); Class 1C antiarrhythmics (e.g., flecainide, propafenone); anthracyclines, including a history of prior treatment (e.g., doxorubicin, epirubicin); tyrosine kinase inhibitors (e.g., sunitinib, nilotinib, lapatinib); antipsychotics (e.g., chlorpromazine, pimozide, haloperidol, droperidol, ziprasidone); antidepressants (e.g., fluoxetine, venlafaxine, tricyclic/tetracyclic antidepressants e.g., amitriptyline, imipramine, maprotiline); opioids (e.g., methadone); macrolide antibiotics and analogues (e.g., erythromycin, clarithromycin, telithromycin); quinolone antibiotics (e.g., moxifloxacin, levofloxacin); pentamidine; antimalarials (e.g., quinine, chloroquine); azole antifungals (e.g., ketoconazole, fluconazole, voriconazole); domperidone; 5-HT_3 receptor antagonists (e.g., dolasetron, ondansetron); tacrolimus; beta-2 adrenoceptor agonists (e.g., salbutamol, formoterol).

Drugs that Disrupt Electrolyte Levels: Drugs that can disrupt electrolyte levels include, but is not limited to, the following: loop, thiazide, and related diuretics; laxatives and enemas; amphotericin B; high dose corticosteroids.

Drug-Food Interactions: Following a single dose 400 mg vorinostat administration, a high-fat meal was associated with a 38% increase in the systemic exposure of vorinostat and a modest decrease in the rate of absorption (2.5 hour delay in median T_{max}). The mean apparent $t_{½}$ and C_{max} were similar between the fasted and fed states (see Action and Clinical Pharmacology, Pharmacokinetics, Absorption).

Drug-Herb Interactions: Interactions with herbal products have not been established.

Drug-Laboratory Test Interactions: Interactions with laboratory tests have not been established.

Drug-Lifestyle Interactions: Dizziness and syncope have been reported in patients receiving ZOLINZA, which may affect a patient's ability to drive or operate machinery (see Adverse Reactions).

DOSAGE AND ADMINISTRATION: Dosing Considerations:

- Patients should be instructed to drink at least 2 L/day of fluid to prevent dehydration.
- ZOLINZA has not been studied in patients <18 years of age.

Recommended Dose and Dosage Adjustment: The recommended dose is 400 mg orally once daily with food.

ZOLINZA should be withheld in the presence of Grade 3-4 drug-related toxicity until the toxicity resolves to Grade 1 or less with the exception of Grade 3 anemia and thrombocytopenia. After recovering from drug-related toxicity, subsequent doses may be reduced to 300 mg orally once daily with food. The dose schedule may be further reduced to 300 mg once daily with food for 5 consecutive days each week, as necessary.

Treatment may be continued as long as there is no evidence of progressive disease or unacceptable toxicity.

Hepatic Impairment: ZOLINZA is contraindicated in patients with severe hepatic impairment (total bilirubin ≥3× ULN, see Contraindications) and is not recommended in patients with moderate hepatic impairment (total bilirubin 1.5×-3× ULN, see Warnings and Precautions, Special Populations, Hepatic Impairment).

Renal Impairment: ZOLINZA has not been studied in patients with renal impairment. Caution should be taken when ZOLINZA is administered in patients with renal impairment (see Warnings and Precautions, Special Populations, Renal Impairment, Action and Clinical Pharmacology, Special Populations and Conditions).

Geriatric Population: No dosage adjustment is necessary for the elderly (see Warnings and Precautions, Special Populations, Geriatrics (≥65 years of age)).

Missed Dose: If a dose is missed, it should be taken as soon as possible. If the patient does not remember until it is nearly time for the next dose, the patient should skip the missed dose and go back to the regular schedule. A double dose of ZOLINZA should not be taken.

OVERDOSAGE:

No specific information is available on the treatment of overdosage of ZOLINZA.

In clinical studies, the frequencies of more severe thrombocytopenia, anemia, fatigue and thromboembolic events were increased at doses higher than 400 mg once daily of ZOLINZA.

The pharmacological effects may be prolonged after serum levels of active vorinostat are no longer present. It is not known if vorinostat is dialyzable.

In the event of overdose, it is reasonable to employ the usual supportive measures, e.g., remove unabsorbed material from the gastrointestinal tract, employ clinical monitoring, and institute supportive therapy, if required.

For management of a suspected drug overdose, contact your regional Poison Control Centre. See the *CPS* Directory section for a list of Poison Control Centres.

ACTION AND CLINICAL PHARMACOLOGY: Mechanism of Action: ZOLINZA is a histone deacetylase (HDAC) inhibitor. HDACs catalyze the removal of acetyl groups from the lysine residues of proteins, including histones and transcription factors.

Vorinostat is a potent inhibitor of histone deacetylases HDAC1, HDAC2 and HDAC3 (Class I) and HDAC6 (Class II) (IC_{50}<86 nM). These enzymes catalyze the removal of acetyl groups from the lysine residues of proteins, including histones. The anti-neoplastic effect of vorinostat is attributed to the inhibition of HDAC activity and subsequent accumulation of acetylated proteins, including histones. Histone acetylation results in transcriptional activation of genes, including tumor suppressor genes, whose expression leads to induction of differentiation, apoptosis and/or inhibition of tumor growth.

Vorinostat induces apoptosis and inhibits cell growth in a wide variety of transformed cells in culture. In human colon carcinoma cells, inhibition of cell proliferation was observed at concentrations of vorinostat that cause the accumulation of acetylated histones. In vivo, vorinostat demonstrates anti-neoplastic activity in rodent tumour models including xenograft models of human prostate, breast and colon carcinoma. Overall, tumour regression was not observed. Rather, vorinostat mediated a decrease in tumour growth rate.

Cardiac Electrophysiology: The effect of ZOLINZA on cardiac electrophysiology was studied in a placebo controlled, two period crossover study in which patients with relapsed or refractory cancer (N=24, 12M/12F) were randomised to receive single doses of ZOLINZA 800 mg and placebo. The QT data were corrected for heart rate using the Fridericia formula (QTcF correction factor 0.33) and a study population-specific correction (QTcP correction factor 0.49). The maximum increase was 13.06 ms (90% CI 9.32, 16.81 ms) for QTcP at 4 hours post-dosing and 6.51 ms (90% CI 3.19, 9.82 ms) for QTcF at 24 hours post-dosing.

The magnitude of QTc prolongation observed in a clinical trial will depend on the study conditions, such as the subject population, the dose and duration of treatment, the equipment used, and the methods employed for reading the ECGs and analysing the QTc data. For this reason, QTc data from different clinical trials are not suitable for direct comparison in terms of magnitude of effect.

Heart rate increases were observed in the ZOLINZA 800 mg treatment arm from 2 to 12 hours post-dosing, with a mean maximum increase of 8.32 bpm (90% CI 5.02, 11.63 bpm) at 3 hours post-dosing (see Figure 2).

Figure 1: ZOLINZA

Placebo-Adjusted Means and 90% Confidence Intervals for Change-From-Baseline QTc Interval (msec) After Administration of Single-Dose 800-mg Vorinostat to Male and Female Patients with Advanced Cancer (N=24)

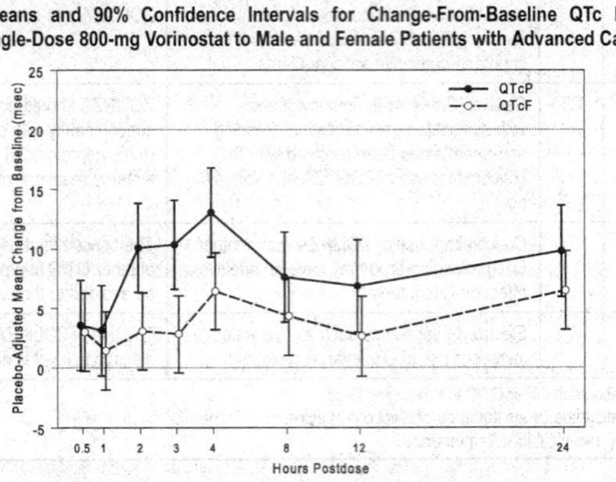

QTcP values are corrected for heart rate using a study population-specific correction ($QTc=QT/RR^{0.49}$).
QTcP vs RR slope : −0.005, 95% CI −0.022, 0.012.
QTcF values are corrected for heart rate using a Fridericia's correction ($QTc=QT/RR^{0.33}$).
QTcF vs RR slope: 0.074, 95% CI 0.057, 0.091.

Figure 2: ZOLINZA

Placebo-Adjusted Means and 90% Confidence Intervals for Change-From-Baseline Heart Rate (beats/min) After Administration of Single-Dose 800-mg Vorinostat to Male and Female Patients with Advanced Cancer (N=24)

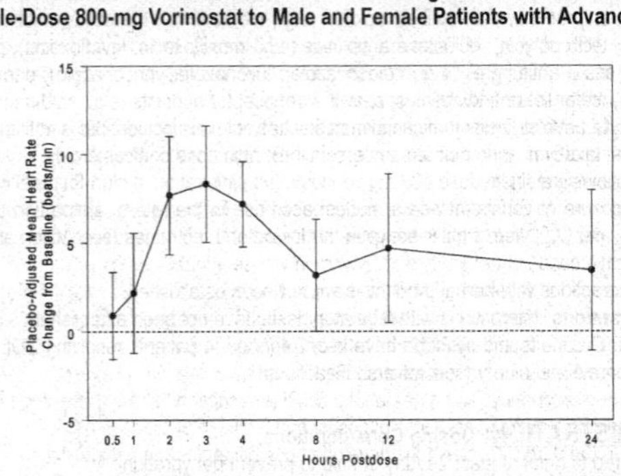

Pharmacokinetics: The pharmacokinetic parameters of vorinostat following a single and multiple doses of 400 mg in patients with cancer are shown in Table 3.

Absorption: The pharmacokinetics of vorinostat were evaluated in 23 patients with cancer. After oral administration of a single 400 mg dose of vorinostat with a high-fat meal, the mean area under the curve (AUC), peak serum concentration (C_{max}), and the median time to maximum concentration (T_{max}) were approximately 5.33 µM·hr, 1.02 µM and 4.00 hours, respectively.

In the fasted state, oral administration of a single 400 mg dose of vorinostat resulted in a mean AUC and C_{max} and median T_{max} of 3.87 µM·hr, 1.12 µM and 1.50 hours, respectively. Oral administration of vorinostat with a high-fat meal resulted in a 38% increase in mean AUC and a modest decrease in the rate of absorption (T_{max} delayed 2.5 hours) compared to the fasted state. Oral administration of multiple 400 mg doses of vorinostat with food resulted in a further 21% increase in mean AUC with C_{max} and T_{max} comparable to those following a single dose under fed state.

Distribution: Vorinostat is approximately 71% bound to human plasma proteins over the concentration range of 0.5 to 50 µg/mL.

Metabolism: The major pathways of vorinostat metabolism involve glucuronidation to form O-glucuronide vorinostat and hydrolysis followed by β-oxidation to form 4-anilino-4-oxobutanoic acid. Human serum levels were measured and, compared to vorinostat, the mean steady state serum exposures of O-glucuronide vorinostat and 4-anilino-4-oxobutanoic acid are approximately 4-fold and 13-fold higher, respectively. Both metabolites are pharmacologically inactive.

In vitro studies using human liver microsomes indicate negligible biotransformation by cytochromes P450 (CYP).

Table 3: ZOLINZA

Summary Statistics for Vorinostat Pharmacokinetic Parameters Following Single and Multiple Doses of Vorinostat 400 mg Daily in Male and Female Cancer Patients

Dose/Diet	C_{max} µM (Geometric mean [95% CI])	AUC µM·hr[a] (Geometric mean [95% CI])	T_{max} hr (Median [range])	$t_{½}$ hr (Harmonic mean [jackknife standard deviation])	f_e[b,c] (Arithmetic mean)
400 mg Single Dose Fasted (N=23)	1.12 [0.94, 1.33]	3.87 [3.31, 4.52]	1.5 [0.5, 10]	1.74 [0.78]	0.0021
400 mg Single Dose Fed (N=20)	1.02 [0.85, 1.23]	5.33 [4.53, 6.28]	4.0 [2.0, 10]	1.44 [0.65]	0.003
400 mg Multiple Dose Fed (N=14) 22 Days Once Daily	1.13 [0.91, 1.41]	6.46 [5.42, 7.69]	4.21 [0.5, 14]	1.34 [0.58]	0.0037

a AUC_{0-inf} is reported for single dose data; $AUC_{0-24 hr.}$ is reported for multiple doses. AUC_{0-inf} ~AUC_{0-24hr}.
b Arithmetic mean (single dose fasted N=22, single dose fed N=21, multiple dose fed N=12).
c Fraction excreted unchanged in urine.

Excretion: Vorinostat is eliminated predominantly through metabolism and vorinostat accounted for less than 1% of the dose recovered as unchanged drug in urine. The mean urinary recovery of two major pharmacologically inactive metabolites at steady state was 16±5.8% of vorinostat dose as the O-glucuronide of vorinostat, and 36±8.6% of vorinostat dose as 4-anilino-4-oxobutanoic acid. Total urinary recovery of these two metabolites averaged 52±13.3% of vorinostat dose. The mean terminal half-life ($t_{½}$) was ~2.0 hours for both vorinostat and the O-glucuronide metabolite, while that of the 4-anilino-4-oxobutanoic acid metabolite was 11 hours.

Drug Interactions with Additional Pharmacokinetic Data: No formal clinical studies have been conducted to evaluate drug interactions with vorinostat. In animal models and in vitro human systems, the major pathways of metabolism of vorinostat involve glucuronidation and hydrolysis followed by β-oxidation. It is possible that vorinostat may interact with drugs metabolized via the same pathways.

Vorinostat inhibits CYP drug metabolizing enzymes (CYP1A2, 2B6, 2C8, 2C9, 2C19, 2D6 and 3A4) in human liver microsomes only at high concentrations (IC_{50} >75 µM). Using primary human hepatocytes, CYP1A1, 1A2, 2B6, 2C9, 2C19 and 3A4 activities were evaluated. Decreased CYP2C9 and 3A4 activities were observed at concentrations higher (≥10 µM) than pharmacologically relevant. Overall, vorinostat is not expected to affect the pharmacokinetics of other agents. As vorinostat is not eliminated via the CYP pathways, it is anticipated that vorinostat will not be subject to drug-drug interactions when co-administered with drugs that are known CYP inhibitors or inducers.

In vitro studies indicate that vorinostat is not a substrate of human P-glycoprotein (P-gp). In addition, vorinostat has no inhibitory effect on human P-gp-mediated transport of vinblastine (a marker P-gp substrate) at concentrations of up to 100 µM. Thus, vorinostat is not likely to inhibit P-gp at the pharmacologically relevant serum concentration of 2 µM (C_{max}) in humans.

Special Populations and Conditions: Based upon an exploratory analysis of limited data, gender, race, and age do not appear to have meaningful effects on the pharmacokinetics of vorinostat.

Pediatrics: Vorinostat was not evaluated in patients <18 years of age.

Geriatrics: Of the total number of patients with CTCL in trials (N=107), 46 percent were 65 years of age and over, while 15 percent were 75 years of age and over. No overall differences in safety or effectiveness were observed between these subjects and younger subjects, and other reported clinical experience has not identified differences in responses between the elderly and younger patients, but greater sensitivity of some older individuals cannot be ruled out.

Hepatic Insufficiency: At doses of 100 and 200 mg QD of vorinostat, patients with severe (total bilirubin ≥3× ULN) and moderate (total bilirubin 1.5-3× ULN) hepatic dysfunction, respectively, had a higher incidence of adverse experiences and dose-limiting toxicities compared with patients with no hepatic dysfunction (see Contraindications and Warnings and Precautions).

Renal Insufficiency: Vorinostat was not evaluated in patients with renal impairment. Vorinostat is eliminated predominantly through metabolism with less than 1% of the dose recovered as unchanged drug in the urine. Total recovery of the two major pharmacologically inactive metabolites in the urine, however, averaged approximately 52% of the oral dose.

STORAGE AND STABILITY: Store at room temperature (15-30°C).

SPECIAL HANDLING INSTRUCTIONS: Direct contact of the powder in ZOLINZA capsules with the skin or mucous membranes should be avoided. If such contact occurs, wash thoroughly. ZOLINZA capsules should not be opened or crushed.

INFORMATION FOR THE PATIENT: Published in e-CPS, available by subscription at www.e-cps.ca.

DOSAGE FORMS, COMPOSITION AND PACKAGING: Each white, opaque, hard gelatin capsule with "568" over "100 mg" printed within radial bar in black ink on the capsule body, contains: vorinostat 100 mg. Nonmedicinal ingredients: magnesium stearate, microcrystalline cellulose and sodium croscarmellose; capsule shell: gelatin, titanium dioxide and may contain sodium lauryl sulfate. High density polyethylene bottles of 120.

(Shown in Product Identification Section)

The reader is invited to consult CPhA's monograph **Selective Serotonin Reuptake Inhibitors.**

Zoloft® 🅿

sertraline HCl

Antidepressant—Antipanic—Antiobsessional

Pfizer

Date of Preparation: January 28, 1992
Date of Revision: May 18, 2010

PHARMACOLOGY: The mechanism of action of sertraline is presumed to be linked to its ability to inhibit the neuronal reuptake of serotonin. It has only very weak effects on norepinephrine and dopamine neuronal reuptake. At clinical doses, sertraline blocks the uptake of serotonin into human platelets.

Like most clinically effective antidepressants, sertraline downregulates brain norepinephrine and serotonin receptors in animals. In receptor binding studies, sertraline has no significant affinity for adrenergic ($alpha_1$, $alpha_2$ & beta), cholinergic, GABA, dopaminergic, histaminergic, serotonergic (5-HT1A, 5-HT1B, 5-HT2) or benzodiazepine binding sites.

In placebo-controlled studies in normal volunteers, ZOLOFT (sertraline hydrochloride) did not cause sedation and did not interfere with psychomotor performance.

Pharmacokinetics: Following multiple oral once-daily doses of 200 mg, the mean peak plasma concentration (C_{max}) of sertraline is 0.19 µg/mL occurring between 6 to 8 hours post-dose. The area under the plasma concentration time curve is 2.8 mg·hr/L. For desmethylsertraline, C_{max} is 0.14 µg/mL, the half-life 65 hours and the area under the curve 2.3 mg·hr/L. Following single or multiple oral once-daily doses of 50 to 400 mg/day the average terminal elimination half-life is approximately 26 hours. Linear dose proportionality has been demonstrated over the clinical dose range of 50 to 200 mg/day.

Food appears to increase the bioavailability by about 40%: it is recommended that ZOLOFT be administered with meals.

Sertraline is extensively metabolized to N-desmethylsertraline, which shows negligible pharmacological activity. Both sertraline and N-desmethylsertraline undergo oxidative deamination and subsequent reduction, hydroxylation and glucuronide conjugation. Biliary excretion of metabolites is significant. Approximately 98% of sertraline is plasma protein bound. The interactions between sertraline and other highly protein bound drugs have not been fully evaluated (see Precautions).

The pharmacokinetics of sertraline itself appear to be similar in young and elderly subjects. Plasma levels of N-desmethylsertraline show a 3-fold elevation in the elderly following multiple dosing, however, the clinical significance of this observation is not known.

Analyses for gender effects on outcome did not suggest any differential responsiveness on the basis of sex.

Liver and Renal Disease: The pharmacokinetics of sertraline in patients with significant hepatic or renal dysfunction have been determined (see Precautions and Dosage).

Clinical Trials: Panic Disorder: Four placebo-controlled clinical trials have been performed to investigate the efficacy of ZOLOFT in panic disorder: two flexible dose studies and two fixed dose studies. At the last week of treatment (week 10 or 12), both flexible dose studies and one of the fixed dose studies showed statistically significant differences from placebo in favour of ZOLOFT in terms of mean change from baseline in the total number of full panic attacks (last observation carried forward analysis). As the flexible dose studies were of identical protocol, data for these investigations can be pooled. The mean number of full panic attacks at baseline was 6.2/week (N=167) in the ZOLOFT group and 5.4/week in the placebo group (N=175). At week 10 (last observation carried forward analysis), the mean changes from baseline were −4.9/week and −2.5/week for the ZOLOFT and placebo groups, respectively. The proportion of patients having no panic attacks at the final evaluation was 57% in the placebo group and 69% in the ZOLOFT group. The mean daily dose administered at the last week of treatment was approximately 120 mg (range: 25-200 mg) in the flexible dose studies. No clear dose-dependency has been demonstrated over the 50 to 200 mg/day dose range investigated in the fixed dose studies.

Obsessive-Compulsive Disorder: Five placebo-controlled clinical trials, in adults, of 8 to 16 weeks in duration have been performed to investigate the efficacy of ZOLOFT in obsessive-compulsive disorder: four flexible dose studies (50-200 mg/day) and one fixed dose study (50, 100, & 200 mg/day). Results for three of the four flexible dose studies and the 50 and 200 mg dose groups of the fixed dose study were supportive of differences from placebo in favour of ZOLOFT in terms of mean change from baseline to endpoint on the Yale-Brown Obsessive-Compulsive Scale and/or the National Institute of Mental Health Obsessive-Compulsive Scale (last observation carried forward analysis). No clear dose-dependency was demonstrated over the 50 to 200 mg/day dose range investigated in the fixed dose studies. In the flexible dose studies, the mean daily dose administered at the last week of treatment ranged from 124-180 mg.

One placebo-controlled clinical trial of 12 weeks duration, was performed in children and adolescents aged 6-17 years, to investigate the efficacy of ZOLOFT in obsessive-compulsive disorder. The study used flexible dosing, starting with 25 mg/day in children 6-12 years old (ZOLOFT n=53, placebo n=54) and with 50 mg/day in adolescents 13-17 years old (ZOLOFT n=39, placebo n=41). In both age groups, ZOLOFT was titrated up to a maximum 200 mg/day, over 4 weeks, as tolerated. The mean dose for completers (74/92 ZOLOFT treated patients) was 178 mg/day. Results showed statistically significant differences from placebo in favour of ZOLOFT in terms of mean change from baseline to endpoint (last observation carried forward analysis) on the Children's Yale-Brown Obsessive Compulsive Scale (p=0.005), the National Institute of Mental Health Obsessive-Compulsive Scale (p=0.019) and the Clinical Global Impresssion Improvement Rating Scale (p=0.002).

The long term safety, including effects on growth and development, in patients under 18 years of age, has not been established.

INDICATIONS: Depression: ZOLOFT (sertraline hydrochloride) is indicated for the symptomatic relief of depressive illness. However, the antidepressant action of ZOLOFT in hospitalized depressed patients has not been adequately studied.

A placebo-controlled European study carried out over 44 weeks, in patients who were responders to ZOLOFT has indicated that ZOLOFT may be useful in continuation treatment, suppressing reemergence of depressive symptoms.

However, because of methodological limitations, these findings on continuation treatment have to be considered tentative at this time.

Panic Disorder: ZOLOFT is indicated for the symptomatic relief of panic disorder, with or without agoraphobia. The efficacy of ZOLOFT was established in 10-week and 12-week controlled trials of patients with panic disorder as defined according to DSM-III-R criteria.

The effectiveness of ZOLOFT in long-term use for the symptomatic relief of panic disorder (i.e., for more than 12 weeks) has not been systematically evaluated in placebo-controlled trials. Therefore, the physician who elects to use ZOLOFT for extended periods should periodically reevaluate the long-term usefulness of the drug for the individual patient.

Obsessive-Compulsive Disorder: ZOLOFT is indicated for the symptomatic relief of obsessive-compulsive disorder (OCD). The obsessions or compulsions must be experienced as intrusive, markedly distressing, time-consuming, or significantly interfering with the person's social or occupational functioning.

The effectiveness of ZOLOFT in long-term use for the symptomatic relief of OCD (i.e., for more than 12 weeks) has not been systematically evaluated in placebo-controlled trials. Therefore, the physician who elects to use ZOLOFT for extended periods should periodically reevaluate the long-term usefulness of the drug for the individual patient.

CONTRAINDICATIONS: ZOLOFT (sertraline hydrochloride) is contraindicated in patients with known hypersensitivity to the drug.

Monoamine Oxidase Inhibitors: Cases of serious, sometimes fatal, reactions have been reported in patients receiving ZOLOFT (sertraline hydrochloride) in combination with a monoamine oxidase inhibitor (MAOI), including the selective MAOI, selegiline and the reversible MAOI (reversible inhibitor of monoamine oxidase-RIMA), moclobemide and linezolid, an antibiotic which is a reversible non-selective MAOI. Some cases presented with features resembling the serotonin syndrome. Similar cases, have been reported with other antidepressants during combined treatment with an MAOI and in patients who have recently discontinued an antidepressant and have been started on an MAOI. Symptoms of a drug interaction between an SSRI and an MAOI include: hyperthermia, rigidity, myoclonus, autonomic instability with possible rapid fluctuations of vital signs, mental status changes that include confusion, irritability, and extreme agitation progressing to delirium and coma. Therefore, ZOLOFT should not be used in combination with an MAOI, or within 14 days of discontinuing treatment with an MAOI. Similarly, at least 14 days should elapse after discontinuing ZOLOFT treatment before starting an MAOI.

Pimozide: The concomitant use of ZOLOFT and pimozide is contraindicated as ZOLOFT has been shown to increase plasma pimozide levels. Elevation of pimozide blood concentration may result in QT interval prolongation and severe arrhythmias including torsades de pointes (see Precautions and Information for the Patient).

WARNINGS: Potential Association with Behavioral and Emotional Changes, Including Self-harm: Pediatrics: Placebo-Controlled Clinical Trial Data:

- **Recent analyses of placebo-controlled clinical trial safety databases from SSRI and other newer antidepressants suggest that use of these drugs in patients under the age of 18 may be associated with behavioral and emotional changes, including an increased risk of suicidal ideation and behavior over that of placebo.**
- **The small denominators in the clinical trial database, as well as the variability in placebo rates, preclude reliable conclusions on the relative safety profiles among these drugs.**

Adults and Pediatrics: Additional Data:

- **There are clinical trial and post-marketing reports with SSRIs and other newer antidepressants, in both pediatrics and adults, of severe agitation-type adverse events coupled with self-harm or harm to others. The agitation-type adverse events include: akathisia, agitation, disinhibition, emotional lability, hostility, aggression, depersonalization. In some cases, the events occurred within several weeks of starting treatment.**

Rigorous clinical monitoring for suicidal ideation or other indicators of potential for suicidal behavior is advised in patients of all ages. This include monitoring for agitation-type emotional and behavioral changes.

Discontinuation Symptoms: **Patients currently taking ZOLOFT should not be discontinued abruptly, due to risk of discontinuation symptoms. At the time that a medical decision is made to discontinue an SSRI or other newer antidepressant drug, a gradual reduction in the dose rather than an abrupt cessation is recommended.**

Monoamine Oxidase Inhibitors: See Contraindications.

PRECAUTIONS: Serotonin Syndrome/Neuroleptic Malignant Syndrome: On rare occasions serotonin syndrome or neuroleptic malignant syndrome-like events have occured in association with treatment of ZOLOFT, particularly when given in combination with other serotonergic and/or neuroleptic/antipsychotic drugs. As these syndromes may result in potentially life-threatening conditions, treatment with ZOLOFT should be discontinued if patients develop a combination of symptoms possibly including hyperthermia, rigidity, myoclonus, autonomic instability with possible rapid fluctuations of vital signs, mental status changes including confusion, irritability, extreme agitation progressing to delirium and coma and supportive symptomatic treatment should be initiated. Due to the risk of serotonergic syndrome or neuroleptic malignant syndrome ZOLOFT should not be used in combination with MAO inhibitors or serotonin-precursors (such as L-tryptophan, oxitriptan) and should be used with caution in patients receiving other serotonergic drugs (triptans, lithium, tramadol, St. John's Wort, most tricyclic antidepressants) or neuroleptics/antipsychotics (see Contraindications and Drug Interactions).

Activation of Mania/Hypomania: During clinical testing in depressed patients, hypomania or mania occurred in approximately 0.6% of ZOLOFT (sertraline hydrochloride) treated patients. Activation of mania/hypomania has also been reported in a small proportion of patients with Major Affective Disorder treated with other marketed antidepressants.

Seizure: ZOLOFT has not been evaluated in patients with seizure disorders. These patients were excluded from clinical studies during the product's premarket testing. No seizures were observed among approximately 3000 patients treated with ZOLOFT in the development program for depression. However, 4 patients out of approximately 1800 (220 <18 years of age) exposed during the development program for obsessive-compulsive disorder experienced seizures representing a crude incidence of 0.2%. Three of these patients were adolescents, two with a seizure disorder and one with a family history of seizure disorder, none of whom were receiving anticonvulsant medication. Accordingly, ZOLOFT should be introduced with care in patients with a seizure disorder.

Suicide: The possibility of a suicide attempt is inherent in depression and may persist until significant remission occurs. Therefore, high risk patients should be closely supervised throughout therapy and consideration should be given to the possible need for hospitalization. It should be noted that a causal role for SSRIs and other antidepressants in inducing self-harm or harm to others has not been established. In order to minimize the opportunity for overdosage, prescriptions for ZOLOFT should be written for the smallest quantity of drug consistent with good patient management (see Warnings, **Potential Association with Behavioral and Emotional Changes, Including Self-harm**).

Because of the well-established co-morbidity between both obsessive-compulsive disorder and depression and panic disorder and depression, the same precautions should be observed when treating patients with obsessive-compulsive disorder and panic disorder.

Discontinuation of Treatment with ZOLOFT: When discontinuing treatment, patients should be monitored for symptoms which may be associated with discontinuation (e.g. dizziness, abnormal dreams, sensory disturbances (including paresthesias and electric shock sensations), agitation, anxiety, fatigue, confusion, headache, tremor, nausea, vomiting and sweating or other symptoms which may be of clinical significance (see Adverse Effects). A gradual reduction in the dosage over several weeks, rather than abrupt cessation is recommended whenever possible. If intolerable symptoms occur following a decrease in the dose or upon discontinuation of treatment, dose titration should be managed on the basis of the patient's clinical response (see Adverse Effects and Dosage).

Abnormal Bleeding: SSRIs and SNRIs, including sertraline hydrochloride, may increase the risk of bleeding events. Concomitant use of aspirin, nonsteroidal anti-inflammatory drugs, warfarin, and other anticoagulants may add to this risk. Case reports and epidemiological studies (case-control and cohort design) have demonstrated an association between use of drugs that interfere with serotonin reuptake and the occurrence of gastrointestinal bleeding. Bleeding events related to SSRIs and SNRIs have ranged from ecchymoses, hematomas, epistaxis, and petechiae to life-threatening hemorrhages.

Patients should be cautioned about the risk of bleeding associated with the concomitant use of Sertraline hydrochloride and NSAIDs, aspirin, or other drugs that affect coagulation.

Hyponatremia: Hyponatremia may occur as a result of treatment with SSRIs or SNRIs including sertraline. In many cases, hyponatremia appears to be the result of a syndrome of inappropriate antidiuretic hormone secretion (SIADH). Cases of serum sodium levels lower than 110 mmol/L have been reported. Elderly patients may be at greater risk of developing hyponatremia with SSRIs and SNRIs. Also patients taking diuretics or who are otherwise volume-depleted may be at greater risk (see Geriatrics). Discontinuation of sertraline should be considered in patients with symptomatic hyponatremia and appropriate medical intervention should be instituted.

Signs and symptoms of hyponatremia include headache, difficulty concentrating, memory impairment, confusion, weakness and unsteadiness which may lead to falls. Signs and symptoms associated with more severe and/or acute cases have included hallucination, syncope, seizure, coma, respiratory arrest, and death.

Occupational Hazards: Any psychoactive drug may impair judgment, thinking, or motor skills, and patients should be advised to avoid driving a car or operating hazardous machinery until they are reasonably certain that the drug treatment does not affect them adversely.

Patients with Concomitant Illness: General: Clinical experience with ZOLOFT in patients with certain concomitant systemic illnesses is limited. Caution is advisable in using ZOLOFT in patients with diseases or conditions that could affect metabolism or hemodynamic responses.

Cardiovascular Conditions: ZOLOFT has not been evaluated or used to any appreciable extent in patients with a recent history of myocardial infarction or unstable heart disease. However, the electrocardiograms of 1006 patients who received ZOLOFT in double-blind trials were evaluated and the data indicate that ZOLOFT is not associated with the development of clinically significant ECG abnormalities.

In placebo-controlled trials, the frequency of clinically noticeable changes (±15-20 mmHg) in blood pressure was similar in patients treated with either ZOLOFT or placebo.

Hepatic Dysfunction: Sertraline is extensively metabolized by the liver. A single dose pharmacokinetic study in subjects with mild, stable cirrhosis demonstrated a prolonged elimination half-life and increased AUC in comparison to normal subjects. The use of sertraline in patients with hepatic disease must be approached with caution. If sertraline is administered to patients with hepatic impairment, a lower or less frequent dose should be considered (see Pharmacology and Dosage).

Renal Dysfunction: ZOLOFT is extensively metabolized and excretion of unchanged drug in the urine is a minor route of elimination. In patients with mild to moderate renal impairment (creatinine clearance 30-60 mL/min) or moderate to severe renal impairment (creatinine clearance 10-29 mL/min), multiple-dose pharmacokinetic parameters (AUC_{0-24} or C_{max}) were not significantly different compared with controls. Half-lives were similar and there were no differences in plasma protein binding in all groups studied. This study indicates that, as expected from the low renal excretion of sertraline, sertraline dosing does not have to be adjusted based on the degree of renal impairment.

Carcinogenesis: In carcinogenicity studies in CD-1 mice, sertraline at doses up to 40 mg/kg produces a dose related increase in the incidence of liver adenomas in male mice. Liver adenomas have a very variable rate of spontaneous occurrence in the CD-1 mouse. The clinical significance of these findings is unknown.

Pregnancy: The safety of ZOLOFT during pregnancy and lactation has not been established and therefore, it should not be used in women of childbearing potential or nursing mothers, unless, in the opinion of the physician, the potential benefits to the patient outweigh the possible hazards to the fetus.

Exposure during late pregnancy to SSRIs may have an increased risk for persistent pulmonary hypertension of the newborn (PPHN). PPHN occurs in 1-2 per 1000 live births in the general population and is associated with substantial neonatal morbidity and mortality. In a retrospective case-control study of 377 women whose infants were born with PPHN and 836 women whose infants were born healthy, the risk for developing PPHN was approximately six-fold higher for infants exposed to SSRIs after the 20th week of gestation compared to infants who had not been exposed to antidepressants during pregnancy. A study of 831 324 infants born in Sweden in 1997-2005 found a PPHN risk ratio of 2.4 (95% CI 1.2-4.3) associated with patient-reported maternal use of SSRIs "in early pregnancy" and a PPHN risk ratio of 3.6 (95% CI 1.2-8.3) associated with a combination of patient-reported maternal use of SSRIs "in early pregnancy" and an antenatal SSRI prescription "in later pregnancy."

Post-marketing reports indicate that some neonates exposed to ZOLOFT, SSRIs (Selective Serotonin Reuptake Inhibitors), or newer antidepressants late in the third trimester have developed complications requiring prolonged hospitalization, respiratory support, and tube feeding. Such complications can arise immediately upon delivery. Reported clinical findings have included respiratory distress, cyanosis, apnea, seizures, temperature instability, feeding difficulty, vomiting, hypoglycemia, hypotonia, hypertonia, hyperreflexia, tremor jitteriness, irritability and constant crying. These features are consistent with either a direct toxic effect of SSRIs and other newer antidepressants, or, possibly, a drug discontinuation syndrome. It should be noted that, in some cases, the clinical picture is consistent with serotonin syndrome (see Precautions, Monoamine Oxidase Inhibitors). When treating a pregnant woman with ZOLOFT during the third trimester, the physician should carefully consider the potential risks and benefits of treatment. (See Dosage.)

Lactation: See Pregnancy.

Labor and Delivery: The effect of ZOLOFT on labor and delivery in humans is unknown.

Children: The safety and effectiveness of ZOLOFT in children below the age of 18 have not been established.

Geriatrics: 462 elderly patients (≥65 years) with depressive illness have participated in multiple dose therapeutic studies with ZOLOFT. The pattern of adverse reactions in the elderly was comparable to that in younger patients.

Hyponatremia: Several cases of hyponatremia have been reported and appeared to be reversible when sertraline was discontinued. Some cases were possibly due to the syndrome of inappropriate antidiuretic hormone secretion. The majority of these occurrences have been in elderly individuals, some in patients taking diuretics or who were otherwise volume depleted.
Platelet Function: There have been rare reports of altered platelet function and/or abnormal results from laboratory studies in patients taking ZOLOFT. While there have been reports of abnormal bleeding or purpura in several patients taking ZOLOFT, it is unclear whether ZOLOFT had a causative role.
Drug Interactions: CNS Active Drugs: ZOLOFT (200 mg daily) did not potentiate the effects of carbamazepine, haloperidol or phenytoin on cognitive and psychomotor performance in healthy subjects, however the risk of using ZOLOFT in combination with other CNS active drugs has not been systematically evaluated. Consequently, caution is advised if the concomitant administration of ZOLOFT and such drugs is required.
Pimozide: In a controlled study of a single dose (2 mg) of pimozide, 200 mg sertraline (q.d.) co-administration to steady state was associated with a mean increase in pimozide AUC and C_{max} of about 40%. Although these increases were not identified in the trial as being associated with clinically important effects on QT intervals, the trial design was not optimal for the investigation of pharmacodynamic effects in the clinical setting. For ethical considerations, a trial with higher doses could not be done. Since the highest recommended pimozide dose (12 mg) has not been evaluated in combination with sertraline, the effect on QT interval and PK parameters at doses higher than 2 mg at this time are not known. While the mechanism of this interaction is unknown, due to the narrow therapeutic index of pimozide and due to the interaction noted at a low dose of pimozide, concomitant administration of ZOLOFT and pimozide is contraindicated (see Contraindications and Information for the Patient).
Serotonergic Drugs: There is limited controlled experience regarding the optimal timing of switching from other antidepressants and antipanic agents to sertraline. Care and prudent medical judgment should be exercised when switching, particularly from long-acting agents. The duration of washout period which should intervene before switching from one selective serotonin reuptake inhibitor (SSRI) or Tricyclic Antidepressants (TCAs) etc. to another has not been established.

Co-administration with tryptophan, TCAs and other antidepressants may lead to a higher incidence of serotonin-associated side effects.

Rare postmarketing reports describe patients with weakness, hyperreflexia, and incoordination following the combined use of a selective serotonin reuptake inhibitor (SSRI) and 5-HT_1 agonists (triptans). If concomitant treatment with ZOLOFT and a triptan (e.g., almotriptan, sumatriptan, rizatriptan, naratriptan, zolmitriptan), tricyclic antidepressants, or other drugs with serotonergic activity (including but not limited to fenfluramine and tryptophan) is clinically warranted and appropriate observation of the patient for acute and long-term adverse events is advised.
St. John's Wort: In common with other SSRIs, pharmacodynamic interactions between ZOLOFT and the herbal remedy St. John's Wort may occur and may result in an increase in undesirable effects.
Lithium: In placebo-controlled trials in normal volunteers, the co-administration of sertraline with lithium did not significantly alter lithium pharmacokinetics, but did result in an increase in tremor relative to placebo, indicating a possible pharmacodynamic interaction. When co-administering sertraline with medications, such as lithium, which may act via serotonergic mechanisms, patients should be appropriately monitored.
Phenytoin: It is recommended that plasma phenytoin concentrations be monitored following initiations of sertraline therapy, with appropriate adjustments to the phenytoin dose. The pharmacokinetic and pharmacodynamic effects have not been adequately characterized.
Monoamine Oxidase Inhibitors: See Contraindications.
Drugs Metabolized by P450 System: Drugs Metabolized by P450 3A4: In two separate in vivo interaction studies, sertraline was co-administered with cytochrome P450 3A4 substrates, terfenadine or carbamazepine, under steady-state conditions. The results of these studies demonstrated that sertraline co-administration did not increase plasma concentrations of terfenadine or carbamazepine. These data suggest that sertraline's extent of inhibition of P450 3A4 activity is not likely to be of clinical significance.
Drugs Metabolized by P450 2D6: Many antidepressants, e.g., the SSRIs, including sertraline and most tricyclic antidepressants, inhibit the biochemical activity of the drug metabolizing isozyme, cytochrome P450 2D6 (debrisoquin hydroxylase), and thus may increase the plasma concentration of co-administered drugs that are metabolized primarily by 2D6 and which have a narrow therapeutic index, e.g., the tricyclic antidepressants and the type Ic antiarrhythmics, propafenone and flecainide. There is variability among the antidepressants in the extent of clinically important P450 2D6 inhibition. In two drug interaction clinical trials using desipramine and the recommended starting SSRI doses in normal volunteers, the effect of ZOLOFT was compared to two other SSRIs. In the first study, mean desipramine steady state AUC (24) increased by 23% and 380% during coadministration with ZOLOFT and the comparative SSRI, respectively. In a second study using a different comparative SSRI, mean desipramine steady state AUC (24) increased by 37% and 421% during coadministration with ZOLOFT and the comparative SSRI, respectively. These trial results indicate that the effect of ZOLOFT was significantly less pronounced than that of the two comparative SSRIs. Nevertheless, concomitant use of a drug metabolized by P450 2D6 with ZOLOFT, may require lower doses than are usually prescribed for the other drug. Furthermore, whenever ZOLOFT is withdrawn from co-therapy, an increased dose of the co-administered drug may be required.
Electroconvulsive Therapy: There are no clinical studies with the combined use of electroconvulsive therapy (ECT) and ZOLOFT.
Alcohol: Although ZOLOFT did not potentiate the cognitive and psychomotor effects of alcohol in experiments with normal subjects, the concomitant use of ZOLOFT and alcohol in depressed, panic disorder or OCD patients has not been studied and is not recommended.
Hypoglycemic Drugs: There are no controlled clinical trials with ZOLOFT in diabetic patients treated with insulin or oral hypoglycemic drugs.

In a placebo-controlled trial in normal volunteers, the administration of ZOLOFT for 22 days (dose of ZOLOFT was 200 mg/day for the final 13 days), caused a statistically significant 16% decrease in the clearance of tolbutamide following an i.v. dose of 1000 mg. In a placebo-controlled study in normal volunteers, glibenclamide (5 mg) was given before and after administration of sertraline (200 mg/day final dose) to steady state or placebo. No significant changes were observed in the **total** plasma concentration of glibenclamide.

Hypoglycemia requiring dextrose infusion was observed in one patient treated with ZOLOFT, glibenclamide, haloperidol, bisacodyl, aspirin and flucloxacillin. The causal relationship to ZOLOFT treatment was not firmly established. Nevertheless, close monitoring of glycemia in patients treated with ZOLOFT and oral hypoglycemic drugs or insulin is recommended.
Digoxin: In a parallel placebo controlled trial in normal volunteers (10 subjects per group), the administration of ZOLOFT for 17 days (dose of ZOLOFT: 200 mg for the last 10 days) did not cause changes in the total plasma concentrations of digoxin except a decrease of T_{max} as compared to baseline.
Beta-Blockers: There is no experience with the use of ZOLOFT in hypertensive patients controlled by beta-blockers. In a placebo-controlled crossover study in normal volunteers, the effect of ZOLOFT on the β-adrenergic blocking activity of atenolol was assessed. The mean CD25's (the doses of isoproterenol required to increase heart rate by 25 bpm, the chronotropic dose 25 or CD25) and the average decreases in heart rate seen with atenolol during exercise test were not statistically different in the ZOLOFT versus the placebo group. These data suggest that ZOLOFT does not alter the β-blocking action of atenolol.
Cimetidine: In a placebo-controlled crossover study in normal volunteers, the potential of cimetidine to alter the disposition of a single 100 mg dose of ZOLOFT was assessed. The mean sertraline C_{max} and AUC were significantly higher in the cimetidine-treated group, as were the mean desmethylsertraline T_{max} and AUC. These data suggest that concomitant administration of cimetidine may inhibit the metabolism of sertraline and its metabolite, desmethylsertraline, and may result in a decrease in the clearance and first pass metabolism of sertraline, with a possible increase in drug-related side effects.
Diazepam: In a normal volunteer, double-blind, placebo-controlled study comparing the disposition of intravenously administered diazepam before and after administration of sertraline (200 mg/day final dose) to steady state or placebo, there was a statistically significant 13% decrease relative to baseline in diazepam clearance for the sertraline group over that of the placebo group. These changes are of unknown clinical significance.
Warfarin: In a placebo-controlled study in healthy men comparing prothrombin time AUC (0-120 hr) following single dosing with warfarin (0.75 mg/kg) before and after dosing to steady state with either sertraline (200 mg/day final dose) or placebo, there was a statistically significant mean increase in prothrombin time of 8% relative to baseline for sertraline compared to a 1% decrease for placebo. The normalization of prothrombin time for the sertraline group was delayed compared to the placebo group. The clinical significance of these changes are unknown. Accordingly, prothrombin time should be carefully monitored when sertraline therapy is initiated or stopped in patients receiving warfarin.

Because sertraline is highly bound to plasma protein, the administration of ZOLOFT to a patient taking another drug which is tightly bound to protein may cause a shift in plasma concentrations potentially resulting in an adverse effect. Conversely adverse effects may result from displacement of protein bound sertraline by other tightly bound drugs.
Microsomal Enzyme Induction: ZOLOFT was shown to induce hepatic enzymes as determined by the decrease of the antipyrine half-life. This degree of induction reflects a clinically insignificant change in hepatic metabolism.
Physical and Psychological Dependence: In a placebo-controlled, double-blind, randomized study of the comparative abuse liability of ZOLOFT, alprazolam, and d-amphetamine in humans, ZOLOFT did not produce the positive subjective effects indicative of abuse potential, such as euphoria or drug liking, that were observed with the other two drugs. Premarketing clinical experience with ZOLOFT did not reveal any drug-seeking behavior. In animal studies ZOLOFT does not demonstrate stimulant or barbiturate-like (depressant) abuse potential. As with any CNS active drug, however, physicians should carefully evaluate patients for history of drug abuse and follow such patients closely, observing them for signs of ZOLOFT misuse or abuse (e.g. development of tolerance, incrementation of dose, drug-seeking behavior).

ADVERSE EFFECTS: Depression: In clinical development programs, ZOLOFT (sertraline hydrochloride) has been evaluated in 1902 subjects with depression. The most commonly observed adverse events associated with the use of ZOLOFT were: gastrointestinal complaints, including nausea, diarrhea/loose stools and dyspepsia; male sexual dysfunction (primarily ejaculatory delay); insomnia and somnolence; tremor; increased sweating and dry mouth; and dizziness. In the fixed dose placebo controlled study, the overall incidence of side effects was dose related with a majority occurring in the patients treated with 200 mg dose.

The discontinuation rate due to adverse events was 15% in 2710 subjects who received ZOLOFT in premarketing multiple dose clinical trials. The more common events (reported by at least 1% of subjects) associated with discontinuation included agitation, insomnia, male sexual dysfunction (primarily ejaculatory delay), somnolence, dizziness, headache, tremor, anorexia, diarrhea/loose stools, nausea and fatigue.
Incidence in Controlled Clinical Trials: Table 1 enumerates adverse events that occurred at a frequency of 1% or more among ZOLOFT patients who participated in controlled trials comparing titrated ZOLOFT with placebo.

Table 1: ZOLOFT
Treatment-emergent Adverse Experience Incidence in Placebo-controlled Clinical Trials in Adults[a]

Adverse Experience	Percent of Patients Reporting	
	ZOLOFT (N=861)	**Placebo (N=853)**
Autonomic Nervous System Disorders		
Mouth Dry	16.3	9.3
Sweating Increased	8.4	2.9
Cardiovascular		
Palpitations	3.5	1.6
Chest Pain	1.0	1.6
Central and Peripheral Nervous System Disorders		
Headache	20.3	19.0
Dizziness	11.7	6.7
Tremor	10.7	2.7
Paresthesia	2.0	1.8
Hypoesthesia	1.7	0.6
Twitching	1.4	0.1
Hypertonia	1.3	0.4
Disorders of Skin and Appendages		
Rash	2.1	1.5
Gastrointestinal Disorders		
Nausea	26.1	11.8
Diarrhea/Loose Stools	17.7	9.3
Constipation	8.4	6.3
Dyspepsia	6.0	2.8
Vomiting	3.8	1.8
Flatulence	3.3	2.5
Anorexia	2.8	1.6
Abdominal Pain	2.4	2.2
Appetite Increased	1.3	0.9
General		
Fatigue	10.6	8.1
Hot Flushes	2.2	0.5
Fever	1.6	0.6
Back Pain	1.5	0.9
Metabolic and Nutritional Disorders		
Thirst	1.4	0.9
Musculoskeletal System Disorders		
Myalgia	1.7	1.5
Psychiatric Disorders		
Insomnia	16.4	8.8
Sexual Dysfunction-Male[b]	15.5	2.2

(cont'd)

Table 1: ZOLOFT *(cont'd)*

Treatment-emergent Adverse Experience Incidence in Placebo-controlled Clinical Trials in Adults[a]

	Percent of Patients Reporting	
Adverse Experience	**ZOLOFT (N=861)**	**Placebo (N=853)**
Somnolence	13.4	5.9
Agitation	5.6	4.0
Nervousness	3.4	1.9
Anxiety	2.6	1.3
Yawning	1.9	0.2
Sexual Dysfunction-Female[c]	1.7	0.2
Concentration Impaired	1.3	0.5
Reproduction		
Menstrual Disorder[c]	1	0.5
Respiratory System Disorders		
Rhinitis	2.0	1.5
Pharyngitis	1.2	0.9
Special Senses		
Vision Abnormal	4.2	2.1
Tinnitus	1.4	1.1
Taste Perversion	1.2	0.7
Urinary System Disorders		
Micturition Frequency	2.0	1.2
Micturition Disorder	1.4	0.5

[a] Events reported by at least 1% of patients treated with Zoloft are included.
[b] % based on male patients only: 271 ZOLOFT and 271 placebo patients. Male sexual dysfunction can be broken down into the categories of decreased libido, impotence and ejaculatory delay. In this data set, the percentages of males in the ZOLOFT group with these complaints are 4.8%, 4.8% and 8.9%, respectively. It should be noted that since some ZOLOFT patients reported more than one category of male sexual dysfunction, the incidence of each category of male sexual dysfunction combined is larger than the incidence for the general category of male sexual dysfunction, in which each patient is counted only once.
[c] % based on female patient only: 590 ZOLOFT and 582 placebo patients.

Panic Disorder: In placebo-controlled clinical trials, 430 patients with panic disorder were treated with ZOLOFT in doses of 25-200 mg/day. During treatment, most patients received doses of 50-200 mg/day. Adverse events observed at an incidence of at least 5% for ZOLOFT and at an incidence that was twice or more the incidence among placebo-treated patients included: diarrhea, ejaculation failure (primarily ejaculatory delay), anorexia, constipation, libido decreased, agitation, and tremor.

In the total safety data base for panic disorder, 14% of patients discontinued treatment due to an adverse event. The most common events leading to discontinuation were nausea (2.6%), insomnia (2.3%), somnolence (2.3%), and agitation (2.1%).

Obsessive-Compulsive Disorder: In placebo-controlled clinical trials for OCD, adverse events observed at an incidence of at least 5% for ZOLOFT and at an incidence that was twice or more the incidence among placebo-treated patients included: nausea, insomnia, diarrhea, decreased libido, anorexia, dyspepsia, ejaculation failure (primarily ejaculatory delay), tremor, and increased sweating.

In placebo-controlled clinical trials for OCD, 10% of patients treated with ZOLOFT discontinued treatment due to an adverse event. The most common events leading to discontinuation were nausea (2.8%), insomnia (2.6%), and diarrhea (2.1%).

Incidence in Controlled Clinical Trials: Table 2 enumerates adverse events that occurred at a frequency of 2% or more among patients on ZOLOFT who participated in controlled trials comparing ZOLOFT with placebo in the treatment of panic disorder and obsessive-compulsive disorder. Only those adverse events which occurred at higher rate during ZOLOFT treatment than during placebo treatment are included.

Table 2: ZOLOFT

Treatment-emergent Adverse Experience Incidence in Placebo-controlled Clinical Trials for Panic and Obsessive-compulsive Disorder in Adults[a]

	Percent of Patients Reporting			
	Panic Disorder		Obsessive-compulsive Disorder	
Adverse Experience	**ZOLOFT (N=430)**	**Placebo (N=275)**	**ZOLOFT (N=533)**	**Placebo (N=373)**
Autonomic Nervous System Disorders				
Mouth Dry	15	10	14	9
Sweating Increased	5	1	6	1
Cardiovascular				
Palpitations	—	—	3	2
Chest Pain	—	—	3	2
Central and Peripheral Nervous System				
Tremor	5	1	8	1
Paresthesia	4	3	3	1
Headache	—	—	30	24
Dizziness	—	—	17	9
Hypertonia	—	—	2	1
Disorders of Skin and Appendages				
Rash	4	3	2	1
Gastrointestinal Disorders				
Nausea	29	18	30	11
Diarrhea	20	9	24	10
Dyspepsia	10	8	10	4
Constipation	7	3	6	4
Anorexia	7	2	11	2
Vomiting	6	3	3	1
Flatulence	—	—	4	1
Appetite Increased	—	—	3	1
General				
Fatigue	11	6	14	10
Hot Flushes	3	1	2	1
Pain	—	—	3	1
Back Pain	—	—	2	1
Metabolic and Nutritional Disorders				
Weight Increase	—	—	3	0
Musculoskeletal System Disorders				
Arthralgia	2	1	—	—
Psychiatric Disorders				
Insomnia	25	18	28	12
Somnolence	15	9	15	8
Nervousness	9	5	7	6
Libido Decreased	7	1	11	2
Agitation	6	2	6	3
Anxiety	4	3	8	6
Concentration Impaired	3	0	—	—
Depersonalization	2	1	3	1
Paroniria	—	—	2	1
Respiratory System Disorders				
Pharyngitis	—	—	4	2
Special Senses				
Tinnitus	4	3	—	—
Vision Abnormal	—	—	4	2
Taste Perversion	—	—	3	1
Urogenital				
Ejaculation Failure[b]	19	1	17	2
Impotence[c]	2	1	5	1

(cont'd)

[a] Events reported by at least 2% of patients treated with ZOLOFT are included, except for the following events which had an incidence on placebo greater than or equal to ZOLOFT [Panic Disorder]: headache, dizziness, malaise, abdominal pain, respiratory disorder, pharyngitis, flatulence, vision abnormal, pain, upper respiratory tract infection, and paroniria. [OCD]: abdominal pain, respiratory disorder, depression, and amnesia.
[b] Primarily ejaculatory delay; % based on male patients only: Panic Disorder: 216 ZOLOFT and 134 placebo patients, OCD: 296 ZOLOFT and 219 placebo patients.
[c] % based on male patients only: Panic Disorder: 216 ZOLOFT and 134 placebo patients, OCD: 296 ZOLOFT and 219 placebo patients.

Suicidality-related Adverse Events from Clinical Trials in Major Depressive Disorder in the Pediatric Population: In the safety analysis from controlled clinical trials in children and adolescents with major depressive disorder aged 6 to 17 years, both the number and percentage of patients for whom suicide attempts were reported was the same for the sertraline arm (2/189, 1.1%) as for the placebo arm (2/184, 1.1%), while the corresponding event rates of suicide attempts were 1.1% (2 attempts in 2/189 patients) in sertraline-treated patients versus 1.6% in placebo-treated patients (3 attempts in 2/184 patients). For the additional category of "other events possibly related to self-harm", which includes suicidal ideation and self-injurious behaviors such as cutting, event rates were 2.1% (4 events in 189 patients) in sertraline-treated patients and 0% in placebo-treated patients.

Overall, the total reported event rates for both suicide attempts and other events possibly related to self-harm are as follows: 3.2% or 6/189 for sertraline versus 1.6% or 3/184 for placebo (see Warnings, **Potential Association with Behavioral and Emotional Changes, Including Self-harm**).

Other Events Observed During the Premarketing Evaluation of ZOLOFT (sertraline hydrochloride): During its premarketing assessment, multiple doses of ZOLOFT were administered to 2710 subjects. The conditions and duration of exposure to ZOLOFT varied greatly, and included (in overlapping categories) clinical pharmacology studies, open and double-blind studies, uncontrolled and controlled studies, inpatient and outpatient studies, fixed-dose and titration studies, and studies for indications other than depression. Untoward events associated with this exposure were recorded by clinical investigators using terminology of their own choosing. Consequently, it is not possible to provide a meaningful estimate of the proportion of individuals experiencing adverse events without first grouping similar types of untoward events into a smaller number of standardized event categories.

All events are included except those already listed in the previous table or in the Precautions section, and those reported in terms so general as to be uninformative.

It is important to emphasize that although the events reported occurred during treatment with ZOLOFT, they were not necessarily caused by it.

Autonomic Nervous System Disorders: Infrequent: flushing, mydriasis, increased saliva, cold clammy skin; Rare: pallor.

Cardiovascular: Infrequent: postural dizziness, hypertension, hypotension, postural hypotension, edema, dependent edema, periorbital edema, peripheral edema, peripheral ischemia, syncope, tachycardia; Rare: precordial chest pain, substernal chest pain, aggravated hypertension, myocardial infarction, varicose veins.

Central and Peripheral Nervous System Disorders: Frequent: confusion; Infrequent: ataxia, abnormal coordination, abnormal gait, hyperesthesia, hyperkinesia, hypokinesia, migraine, nystagmus, vertigo; Rare: local anesthesia, coma, convulsions, dyskinesia, dysphonia, hyporeflexia, hypotonia, ptosis.

Disorders of Skin and Appendages: Infrequent: acne, alopecia, pruritus, erythematous rash, maculopapular rash, dry skin; Rare: bullous eruption, dermatitis, erythema multiforme, abnormal hair texture, hypertrichosis, photosensitivity reaction, follicular rash, skin discoloration, abnormal skin odor, urticaria.

Endocrine Disorders: Rare: exophthalmos, gynecomastia.

Gastrointestinal Disorders: Infrequent: dysphagia, eructation; Rare: diverticulitis, fecal incontinence, gastritis, gastroenteritis, glossitis, gum hyperplasia, hemorrhoids, hiccup, gastrointestinal bleeding, melena, hemorrhagic peptic ulcer, proctitis, stomatitis, ulcerative stomatitis, tenesmus, tongue edema, tongue ulceration.

General: Frequent: allergic reaction, allergy, asthenia; Infrequent: malaise, generalized edema, rigors, weight decrease, weight increase; Rare: enlarged abdomen, halitosis, otitis media, aphthous stomatitis.

Hematopoietic and Lymphatic: Infrequent: lymphadenopathy, purpura; Rare: anemia, anterior chamber eye hemorrhage.

Metabolic and Nutritional Disorders: Rare: dehydration, hypercholesterolemia, hypoglycemia.

Musculoskeletal System Disorders: Infrequent: arthralgia, arthrosis, dystonia, muscle cramps, muscle weakness; Rare: hernia.

Psychiatric Disorders: Infrequent: abnormal dreams, aggressive reaction, amnesia, apathy, delusion, depersonalization, depression, aggravated depression, emotional lability, euphoria, hallucination, neurosis, paranoid reaction, suicide attempt (including suicidal ideation), teeth-grinding, abnormal thinking; Rare: hysteria, somnambulism, withdrawal reactions.

Reproductive: Infrequent: dysmenorrhea*, intermenstrual bleeding*. Rare: amenorrhea*, balanoposthitis†, breast enlargement*, female breast pain*, leukorrhea*, menorrhagia*, atrophic vaginitis*.

Respiratory System Disorders: Infrequent: bronchospasm, coughing, dyspnea, epistaxis; Rare: bradypnea, hyperventilation, sinusitis, stridor.

Special Senses: Infrequent: abnormal accommodation, conjunctivitis, diplopia, earache, eye pain, xerophthalmia; Rare: abnormal lacrimation, photophobia, visual field defect.

Urinary System Disorders: Infrequent: dysuria, face edema, nocturia, polyuria, urinary incontinence; Rare: enuresis, oliguria, renal pain, urinary retention.

Laboratory Tests: In man, asymptomatic elevations in serum hepatic transaminases (AST and ALT) to a value ≥3 times the upper limit of normal have been reported infrequently (approximately 0.6% and 1.1%, respectively) in association with ZOLOFT administration. The proportion of patients having these elevations was greater in the ZOLOFT group than in the placebo group. These hepatic enzyme elevations usually occurred within the first 1 to 9 weeks of drug treatment and promptly diminished upon drug discontinuation.

ZOLOFT therapy was associated with small mean increases in total cholesterol (approximately 3%) and triglycerides (approximately 5%).

Uricosuric Effect: ZOLOFT is associated with a small mean decrease in serum uric acid (approximately 7%) of no apparent clinical importance.

Other Events Observed During the Postmarketing Evaluation of ZOLOFT: Adverse events not listed above which have been reported in temporal association with ZOLOFT since market introduction include: muscle contractions involuntary, acute renal failure, anaphylactoid reaction, angioedema, blindness, optic neuritis, cataract, increased coagulation times, bradycardia, AV block, atrial arrhythmias, QT-interval prolongation, ventricular tachycardia (including torsades de pointes-type arrhythmias), hypothyroidism, syndrome of inappropriate ADH secretion, agranulocytosis, aplastic anemia, pancytopenia, hematuria, leukopenia, thrombocytopenia, lupus-like syndrome, serum sickness, hyperglycemia, priapism, galactorrhea, hyperprolactinemia, neuroleptic malignant syndrome-like events, extrapyramidal symptoms, oculogyric crisis, serotonin syndrome, psychosis, pulmonary hypertension, severe skin reactions, which potentially can be fatal, such as Stevens-Johnson Syndrome, epidermal necrolysis, vasculitis, photosensitivity and other severe cutaneous disorders, rare reports of pancreatitis, and liver events.

The causal relationship between ZOLOFT treatment and the emergence of these events has not been established. The clinical features of hepatic events (which in the majority of cases appeared to be reversible with discontinuation of ZOLOFT) occurring in one or more patients include: elevated enzymes, increased bilirubin, hepatomegaly, hepatitis, jaundice, abdominal pain, vomiting, liver failure and death. There have been spontaneous reports of symptoms such as dizziness, paresthesia, nausea, headache, anxiety, fatigue, and agitation following the discontinuation of ZOLOFT treatment.

Adverse Reactions Following Discontinuation of Treatment (or Dose Reduction): There have been reports of adverse reactions upon the discontinuation of ZOLOFT (particularly when abrupt), including but not limited to the following: dizziness, abnormal dreams, sensory disturbances (including paresthesias and electric shock sensations), agitation, anxiety, fatigue, confusion, headache, tremor, nausea, vomiting and sweating or other symptoms which may be of clinical significance (see Precautions and Dosage).

Patients should be monitored for these or any other symptoms. A gradual reduction in the dosage over several weeks, rather than abrupt cessation is recommended whenever possible. If intolerable symptoms occur following a decrease in the dosage or upon discontinuation of treatment, dose titration should be managed on the basis of the patient's clinical response. These events are generally self-limiting. Symptoms associated with discontinuation have been reported for other selective serotonin reuptake inhibitors (see Precautions and Dosage).

OVERDOSE:

On the evidence available, sertraline has a wide margin of safety in overdose. Of 1027 cases of overdose involving sertraline hydrochloride worldwide, alone or with other drugs, there were 72 deaths (circa 1999).

Reported overdoses of sertraline alone of up to 13.5 g have been documented. However, an overdose of 2.5 g of sertraline alone had a fatal outcome.

Symptoms: Symptoms of overdose include serotonin-mediated side effects such as somnolence, gastrointestinal disturbance (such as nausea, vomiting, diarrhea), tachycardia, tremor, agitation and dizziness, ECG changes, anxiety and dilated pupils. Less frequently reported was coma.

Other important adverse events reported with sertraline hydrochloride overdose (single or multiple drugs) include alopecia, decreased libido, ejaculation disorder, fatigue, insomnia, bradycardia, bundle branch block, coma, convulsions, delirium, hallucinations, hypertension, hypotension, manic reaction, pancreatitis, QT-interval prolongation, serotonin syndrome, stupor and syncope.

* % based on female subjects only: 1705.

† % based on male subjects only: 1005.

Treatment: Establish and maintain an airway, and ensure adequate oxygenation and ventilation, if necessary. Activated charcoal, which may be used with sorbitol, may be as or more effective than lavage, and should be considered in treating overdose. Induction of emesis is not recommended.

Treatment was primary supportive and included monitoring and use of activated charcoal, gastric lavage or cathartics and hydration.

Gastric lavage with a large-bore orogastric tube with appropriate airway protection, if needed, may be indicated if performed soon after ingestion, or in symptomatic patients.

Cardiac and vital signs monitoring are recommended along with general symptomatic and supportive measures. There are no specific antidotes for ZOLOFT.

Due to the large volume of distribution of ZOLOFT, forced diuresis, dialysis, hemoperfusion, and exchange transfusion are unlikely to be of benefit.

In managing overdosage, the possibility of multiple drug involvement must be considered. The physician should consider contacting a poison control center for additional information on the treatment of any overdose.

> For management of a suspected drug overdose, contact your regional Poison Control Centre. See the *CPS* Directory section for a list of Poison Control Centres.

DOSAGE: ZOLOFT (sertraline hydrochloride) is not indicated for use in children under 18 years of age (see Warnings, Potential Association with Behavioral and Emotional Changes, Including Self-harm).

General: ZOLOFT should be administered with food once daily preferably with the evening meal, or, if administration in the morning is desired, with breakfast.

Initial Treatment: Depression and Obsessive-Compulsive Disorder: As no clear dose-response relationship has been demonstrated over a range of 50-200 mg/day, a dose of 50 mg/day is recommended as the initial dose.

Panic Disorder: ZOLOFT treatment should be initiated with a dose of 25 mg once daily. After one week, the dose should be increased to 50 mg once daily depending on tolerability and clinical response. No clear dose-response relationship has been demonstrated over a range of 50-200 mg/day.

Titration: In depression, OCD and panic disorder, a gradual increase in dosage may be considered if no clinical improvement is observed. Based on pharmacokinetic parameters, steady-state sertraline plasma levels are achieved after approximately 1 week of once daily dosing; accordingly, dose changes, if necessary, should be made at intervals of at least one week. Doses should not exceed a maximum of 200 mg/day.

The full therapeutic response may be delayed until 4 weeks of treatment or longer. Increasing the dosage rapidly does not normally shorten this latent period and may increase the incidence of side effects.

Maintenance: During long-term therapy for any indication, the dosage should be maintained at the lowest effective dose and patients should be periodically reassessed to determine the need for continued treatment.

Hepatic Impairment: As with many other medications, ZOLOFT should be used with caution in patients with hepatic impairment (see Precautions).

Children: **(see Warnings, Potential Association with Behavioral and Emotional Changes, Including Self-harm).**

Treatment of Pregnant Women During the Third Trimester: Post-marketing reports indicate that some neonates exposed to ZOLOFT, SSRIs, or other newer antidepressants late in the third trimester have developed complications requiring prolonged hospitalization, respiratory support, and tube feeding (see Precautions). When treating a pregnant woman with ZOLOFT during the third trimester, the physician should carefully consider the potential risks and benefits of treatment. The physician may consider tapering ZOLOFT in the third trimester.

Switching Patients to or from a Monoamine Oxidase Inhibitor: At least 14 days should elapse between discontinuation of an MAOI and initiation of therapy with ZOLOFT. In addition, at least 14 days should be allowed after stopping ZOLOFT before starting an MAOI (see Contraindications).

Discontinuation of ZOLOFT Treatment: Symptoms associated with the discontinuation or dosage reduction of ZOLOFT have been reported. Patients should be monitored for these and other symptoms when discontinuing treatment or during dosage reduction (see Precautions and Adverse Effects).

A gradual reduction in the dose over several weeks rather than abrupt cessation is recommended whenever possible. If intolerable symptoms occur following a decrease in the dose or upon discontinuation of treatment, dose titration should be managed on the basis of the patient's clinical response (see Precautions and Adverse Effects).

INFORMATION FOR THE PATIENT: Published in e-CPS, available by subscription at www.e-cps.ca.

SUPPLIED: 25 mg: Each yellow capsule contains: sertraline HCl equivalent to 25 mg of sertraline. Nonmedicinal ingredients: cornstarch, lactose (anhydrous), magnesium stearate and sodium lauryl sulfate; capsule shell: D&C Yellow No. 10, FD&C Yellow No. 6, gelatin and titanium dioxide. Gluten- and tartrazine-free. Opaque high density polyethylene bottles of 100. Store at controlled room temperature between 15 and 30°C.

50 mg: Each white and yellow capsule contains: sertraline HCl equivalent to 50 mg of sertraline. Nonmedicinal ingredients: cornstarch, lactose (anhydrous), magnesium stearate and sodium lauryl sulfate; capsule shell: D&C Yellow No. 10, FD&C Yellow No. 6, gelatin and titanium dioxide. Gluten- and tartrazine-free. Opaque high density polyethylene bottles of 100 and 250. Store at controlled room temperature between 15 and 30°C.

100 mg: Each orange capsule contains: sertraline HCl equivalent to 100 mg of sertraline. Nonmedicinal ingredients: cornstarch, lactose (anhydrous), magnesium stearate and sodium lauryl sulfate; capsule shell: D&C Yellow No. 10, FD&C Red No. 40, gelatin and titanium dioxide. Gluten- and tartrazine-free. Opaque high density polyethylene bottles of 100. Store at controlled room temperature between 15 and 30°C.

(Shown in Product Identification Section)

Zometa® Concentrate Ⓟ

zoledronic acid

Bone Metabolism Regulator

Novartis Pharmaceuticals

Date of Preparation: August 16, 2000

Date of Revision: September 1, 2009

SUMMARY PRODUCT INFORMATION:

Route of Administration	Dosage Form/ Strength	Clinically Relevant Nonmedicinal Ingredients
Intravenous injection	Concentrate: 4 mg zoledronic acid/5 mL[a]	Concentrate: mannitol, sodium citrate and water For a complete listing see Dosage Forms, Composition and Packaging.

[a] This corresponds to 4.264 mg zoledronic acid monohydrate.

INDICATIONS AND CLINICAL USE: Tumor-Induced Hypercalcemia (TIH): ZOMETA (zoledronic acid for injection) is indicated for the treatment of Tumor-Induced Hypercalcemia following adequate saline rehydration. Prior to treatment with ZOMETA, renal excretion of excess calcium should be promoted by restoring and maintaining adequate fluid balance and urine output.

Bone Metastases of Solid Tumors and Osteolytic Lesions of Multiple Myeloma: ZOMETA is indicated for the treatment of patients with documented bone metastases from solid tumors (including prostate cancer, breast cancer, lung cancer, renal cell carcinoma and other solid tumors) and patients with osteolytic lesions of multiple myeloma in conjunction with standard care in order to prevent or delay potential complications from the bone lesions (see Warnings and Precautions, Deterioration in Renal Function).

CONTRAINDICATIONS: ZOMETA (zoledronic acid for injection) is contraindicated in pregnancy, breast-feeding women and patients with clinically significant hypersensitivity to zoledronic acid or other bisphosphonates, or any of the excipients in the formulation of ZOMETA (see Dosage Forms, Composition and Packaging).

WARNINGS AND PRECAUTIONS:

Serious Warnings and Precautions
- **Osteonecrosis of the jaw (ONJ)** (See Warnings And Precautions, General)
- **Renal dysfunction** (See Warnings And Precautions, Renal)
- The use of ZOMETA is **not recommended in patients with severe renal impairment** (See Warnings And Precautions, Special Populations)
- Single doses of ZOMETA should not exceed 4 mg and the duration of the infusion should be no less than 15 minutes. (See Warnings And Precautions, Renal and Dosage and Administration).

General: Drug Interactions : ZOMETA contains the same active ingredient that is found in ACLASTA (zoledronic acid). Patients being treated with ZOMETA should not be treated with ACLASTA concomitantly.

ZOMETA should not be given together with other bisphosphonates since the combined effects of these agents are unknown.

ZOMETA is eliminated by renal excretion. Caution is indicated when zoledronic acid is administered in conjunction with drugs that are potentially nephrotoxic (e.g. aminoglycosides, other antineoplastic agents, ASA, NSAIDs), or that can significantly impact renal function (e.g. diuretics, ACE inhibitors, leading to dehydration).

ZOMETA should be used with extreme caution in conjunction with other antineoplastic agents that are either known to produce renal dysfunction (it is advised that renal function be monitored); or where the dose depends upon renal function (for example platinum-containing agents).

In multiple myeloma patients, the risk of renal dysfunction may be increased when ZOMETA is used in combination with thalidomide.

ZOMETA should not be mixed with calcium-containing intravenous infusions.

Effects on Ability to Drive or Use Machines: In rare cases, somnolence and/or dizziness may occur, in which case the patient should not drive, operate potentially dangerous machinery or engage in other activities that may be hazardous.

Musculoskeletal Pain: In post-marketing experience, severe and occasionally incapacitating bone, joint, and/or muscle pain have been reported in patients taking bisphosphonates. However, such reports have been infrequent. This category of drugs includes ZOMETA (zoledronic acid). The time to onset of symptoms varied from one day to several months after starting treatment. Most patients had relief of symptoms after stopping treatment. A subset had recurrence of symptoms when re-challenged with the same drug or another bisphosphonate.

Osteonecrosis of the Jaw: Osteonecrosis of the jaw (ONJ), has been reported in cancer patients treated with bisphosphonates, including ZOMETA. Although no causal relationship has been established, there is an association between bisphosphonate use and the development of ONJ. Post-marketing experience suggests a greater frequency of reports of ONJ based on tumour type (advanced breast cancer, multiple myeloma) and dental status (dental extractions, periodontal disease and local trauma including poorly fitting dentures); these are associated with a greater risk of developing ONJ. Cancer patients also receive other treatments that may play a role in the development of ONJ, such as chemotherapy and glucocorticosteroids. Many patients had signs of local infection including osteomyelitis.

Presentation of ONJ may include altered local sensation (hyperaesthesia or numbness), maxillofacial pain, "toothaches", denture sore spots, loose teeth, exposed bone in the oral cavity, impaired healing, recurrent or persistent soft tissue infection in the oral cavity and marked oral odour. The onset can be from months to years after commencing bisphosphonate therapy. Cancer patients should maintain good oral hygiene; it is recommended that advanced cancer patients be encouraged to have an oral examination of both hard and soft tissues, with preventive dentistry prior to treatment with bisphosphonates, and that such assessments continue at regularly scheduled intervals after bisphosphonate therapy is initiated. While on bisphosphonate treatment, these patients should avoid invasive dental procedures if possible. Biopsies are not recommended unless metastasis to the jaw is suspected. For patients who develop ONJ while on bisphosphonate therapy, dental surgery may exacerbate the condition. For patients requiring dental procedures, there is no data available to suggest whether discontinuation of bisphosphonate treatment reduces the risk of ONJ. Clinical judgment of the treating physician should guide the management plan of each patient based on individual benefit/risk assessment.

Tumor-Induced Hypercalcemia: It is essential in the initial treatment of tumor-induced hypercalcemia that intravenous rehydration be instituted to restore urine output. Patients should be hydrated adequately throughout treatment but overhydration must be avoided.

In patients with cardiac disease, especially in the elderly, additional saline overload may precipitate cardiac failure (left ventricular failure or congestive heart failure). Fever (influenza-like symptoms) may also contribute to this deterioration.

Carcinogenesis and Mutagenesis: In carcinogenicity studies, zoledronic acid was administered orally (gavage) to rats and mice for at least 104 weeks without evidence of carcinogenic potential. Chronic parenteral administration was not feasible given the potential of the compound to cause severe local irritation. The pharmacological bone changes (nonproliferative hyperostosis) typically observed following long term bisphosphonate administration to young animals with growing skeletons gave clear evidence of systemic exposure to zoledronic acid in both species at all doses.

Six mutagenicity studies were conducted with zoledronic acid: three Ames Assays (using *E. coli* and/or *S. typhimurium*), a gene mutation assay using V79 hamster cells, a cytogenetics test with Chinese hamster cells and an in vivo micronucleus assay in rats. There was no evidence of mutagenic potential.

Cardiovascular: Overall incidence of atrial fibrillation in a 3-year trial for post-menopausal osteoporosis using ACLASTA (zoledronic acid) 5 mg dose yearly, was 2.5% (96 out of 3862) and 1.9% (75 out of 3852) in patients receiving ACLASTA (zoledronic acid) and placebo, respectively. The rate of atrial fibrillation serious adverse events was 1.3% (51 out of 3862) and 0.6% (22 out of 3852) in patients receiving ACLASTA (zoledronic acid) and placebo, respectively. The increased incidence observed in this trial has not been observed in other clinical trials with zoledronic acid, including those with ZOMETA (zoledronic acid) 4 mg administered every 3-4 weeks in oncology patients. The mechanism behind the increased incidence of atrial fibrillation is unknown.

Hepatic/Biliary/Pancreatic : Hepatic Impairment: As only limited clinical data are available for patients with hepatic insufficiency, dosage recommendations cannot be given for this group.

Ophthalmologic: Ocular disturbances (conjunctivitis, uveitis, episcleritis, scleritis and orbital inflammation) have been reported with ZOMETA therapy. Patients with ocular events other than uncomplicated conjunctivitis should be referred to an ophthalmologist for evaluation. Treatment may need to be discontinued.

Peri-Operative Considerations : Patients treated with ZOMETA should avoid invasive dental procedures if possible. Biopsies are not recommended unless metastasis to the jaw is suspected. For patients who develop ONJ while on bisphosphonate therapy, dental surgery may exacerbate the condition. For patients requiring dental procedures, there is no data available to suggest whether discontinuation of bisphosphonate treatment reduces the risk of ONJ. Clinical judgment of the treating physician should guide the management plan of each patient based on individual benefit/risk assessment. (See also Warnings and Precautions, General, Osteonecrosis of the Jaw.)

Renal: Monitoring of renal function is recommended in all patients prior to the administration of each dose of ZOMETA.

Deterioration in Renal Function: Due to the risk of clinically significant deterioration in renal function, which may progress to renal failure, single doses of ZOMETA should not exceed 4 mg and the duration of the infusion should be no less than 15 minutes (See also Dosage and Administration).

Bisphosphonates, including ZOMETA have been associated with reports of renal dysfunction. **Factors that may increase the potential for deterioration in renal function include dehydration, pre-existing renal impairment, multiple cycles of ZOMETA or other bisphosphonates or using an infusion time shorter than currently recommended (the 4 mg dose is given as a single-dose intravenous infusion over not less than 15 minutes in not less than 100 mL diluent). Concomitant use of potentially nephrotoxic drugs (i.e. ASA, NSAIDS, diuretics, ACE inhibitors etc.) may also increase the potential for renal impairment. Renal function should be monitored appropriately during therapy with ZOMETA.** Renal deterioration, progression to renal failure (some with fatal outcome) and dialysis have been reported very rarely in cancer patients (e.g., those with hypercalcemia of malignancy and/or pre-existing renal disease) after the initial dose or a single dose of ZOMETA. Increases in serum creatinine may occur in some patients with chronic administration of ZOMETA at recommended doses. Patients with evidence of deterioration in renal function should be appropriately evaluated with consideration given as to whether the potential benefit of continued treatment with ZOMETA outweighs the possible risk.

ZOMETA should be used with extreme caution in conjunction with other antineoplastic agents that are either known to produce renal dysfunction (it is advised that renal function be monitored); or where the dose depends upon renal function (for example platinum-containing agents).

Respiratory: Patients with Asthma: While not observed in clinical trials with ZOMETA, administration of other bisphosphonates has been associated with bronchoconstriction in aspirin-sensitive asthmatic patients. ZOMETA should be used with caution in patients with aspirin-sensitive asthma.

Special Populations: Renal Impairment: ZOMETA is excreted exclusively via the kidney and the risk of adverse reactions may be greater in patients with impaired renal function. **The use of ZOMETA is not recommended in patients with severe renal impairment.** This recommendation is made in view of the potential impact of bisphosphonates including ZOMETA on renal function, the lack of extensive clinical safety data in patients with severe renal impairment at baseline (serum creatinine >400 µmol/L or >4.5 mg/dL in patients with tumour-induced hypercalcemia; and serum creatinine >265 µmol/L or >3.0 mg/dL in patients with bone metastases of solid tumours and osteolytic lesions of multiple myeloma) and only limited pharmacokinetic data in patients with severe renal impairment at baseline (creatinine clearance <30 mL/min).

Close monitoring of renal function is necessary in patients who are receiving concomitant drugs with nephrotoxic potential. Patients should have their serum creatinine levels assessed prior to each dose of ZOMETA.

Upon initiation of treatment in patients with bone metastases of solid tumors and osteolytic lesions of multiple myeloma, with mild-to-moderate renal impairment, lower doses of ZOMETA are recommended. In patients who show evidence of renal deterioration during treatment, appropriate evaluation should be carried out and consideration should be given as to whether the potential benefit outweighs the possible risk. If ZOMETA treatment is to be continued in these patients, ZOMETA should only be resumed when serum creatinine returns to within 10% of baseline (see Dosage and Administration).

Pregnant Women: ZOMETA should not be administered during pregnancy (see Contraindications). There is no clinical evidence to support the use of ZOMETA in pregnant women, and animal studies suggest ZOMETA may cause fetal harm when administered to a pregnant woman.

In animal reproduction studies zoledronic acid was administered subcutaneously to rats and rabbits. Teratogenicity manifested by external, visceral and skeletal malformations was observed in the rat at doses ≥0.2 mg/kg. There was also evidence of maternal toxicity at ≥0.2 mg/kg as well as fetal toxicity at 0.4 mg/kg. No teratological or embryo/fetal effects were observed in the rabbit. However, maternal toxicity was marked at ≥0.1 mg/kg due to decreased serum calcium. Bisphosphonates readily cross the placental barrier and are taken up into the developing fetal skeleton; thus, the teratogenicity observed in the rat was attributed to the compound's potency in lowering serum calcium and binding to fetal bone.

Nursing Women: ZOMETA should not be administered to breast-feeding women (see Contraindications). There is no clinical experience with ZOMETA in lactating women and it is not known whether ZOMETA passes into breast milk. A study in lactating rats has shown that another bisphosphonate AREDIA (pamidronate) passes into the milk. Mothers treated with ZOMETA should therefore not breast feed their infants.

Pediatrics: The safety and efficacy of ZOMETA in children have not been established. Until further experience is gained, ZOMETA can only be recommended for use in adult patients.

Geriatrics (>65 years of age): Controlled clinical studies of ZOMETA in TIH do not provide a sufficient number of geriatric subjects to determine whether patients 65 years and older respond differently. The median age in the two controlled clinical trials in patients with tumor-induced hypercalcemia was 61 years old (range: 21-87 years old).

Controlled clinical studies of ZOMETA in the treatment of bone metastases of solid tumors and osteolytic lesions of multiple myeloma in patients over age 65 revealed similar efficacy and safety compared to younger patients. The proportion of patients experiencing SREs is lower in the ZOMETA treatment group when compared to placebo and similar to AREDIA (pamidronate) 90 mg. Older patients generally had adverse events similar to those of the overall population. However, because of the greater frequency of decreased hepatic, renal, or cardiac function, and of concomitant disease or other drug therapy in elderly patients, ZOMETA should be administered with caution in this patient population.

Race: Japanese female subjects had substantially higher systemic exposure, i.e., 47% higher $AUC_{0\text{-}24h}$ and 39% higher C_{max} than the North American population (see Action and Clinical Pharmacology, Special Populations and Conditions, Race).

Monitoring and Laboratory Tests: Serum calcium, electrolytes, phosphate, magnesium and creatinine, and CBC, differential, and hematocrit/hemoglobin must be closely monitored in patients treated with ZOMETA.

Patients with anemia, leukopenia or thrombocytopenia should have regular hematology assessments. Occasional cases of mild, transient hypocalcemia, usually asymptomatic, have been reported. Symptomatic hypocalcemia occurs rarely and can be reversed with calcium gluconate. Patients who have undergone thyroid surgery may be particularly susceptible to develop hypocalcemia due to relative hypoparathyroidism.

In tumour-induced hypercalcemia, either ionized calcium or total serum calcium corrected (adjusted) for albumin should be monitored during treatment with ZOMETA. Serum calcium levels in patients who have hypercalcemia of malignancy may not reflect the severity of hypercalcemia, since hypoalbuminemia is commonly present. Corrected serum calcium values should be calculated using established algorithms, such as: Albumin-corrected serum calcium (CSC, mmol/L)=tCa+0.02 (mid-range albumin−measured albumin).

ADVERSE REACTIONS: Adverse Drug Reaction Overview: Adverse reactions to ZOMETA (zoledronic acid for injection) are usually mild and transient and similar to those reported for other bisphosphonates. Intravenous administration has been most commonly associated with fever. Occasionally, patients experience a flu-like syndrome consisting of fever, chills, bone pain and/or arthralgias and myalgias. In most cases, no specific treatment is required and the symptoms subside after 24 to 48 hours.

Gastrointestinal reactions such as nausea and vomiting have been reported following intravenous infusion of ZOMETA. Local reactions at the infusion site, such as redness or swelling, were observed infrequently.

Rare cases of rash, pruritus, and chest pain have been reported following treatment with ZOMETA.

As with other bisphosphonates, isolated cases of hypomagnesemia have been reported. Isolated cases of uveitis, episcleritis, and conjunctivitis have also been reported.

While not observed in clinical trials with ZOMETA, administration of other bisphosphonates has been associated with bronchoconstriction in acetylsalicylic acid-sensitive asthmatic patients.

Clinical Trial Adverse Drug Reactions: Tumor-Induced Hypercalcemia Clinical Trials : Patients with tumor-induced hypercalcemia may have numerous confounding medical conditions that make causality of adverse events difficult to assess due to the prevalence and wide variety of symptoms related to the underlying disease, its progression, and the side effects of cytotoxic chemotherapy.

In patients treated with ZOMETA, serum calcium may fall to asymptomatic hypocalcemic levels. This frequently leads to a reduction in renal calcium excretion which is accompanied by a fall in serum phosphate levels that does not require treatment.

Grade 3 [Common Toxicity Criteria (CTC)] serum creatinine was seen in 2.3% and 3.0% of patients receiving ZOMETA 4 mg and AREDIA (pamidronate) 90 mg, respectively in the clinical trials in tumor-induced hypercalcemia. Grade 4 (CTC) serum creatinine was seen in 0% and 1.0% in patients receiving ZOMETA 4 mg and AREDIA (pamidronate) 90 mg, respectively.

Table 1 lists the adverse experiences considered to be treatment related in the tumor-induced hypercalcemia trials.

Table 1: ZOMETA Concentrate

Treatment-related Adverse Experiences Reported in Tumor-induced Hypercalcemia Clinical Trials

	ZOMETA 4 mg % (N=86)	Aredia 90 mg % (N=103)
Fever	7.0	9.7
Hypocalcemia	5.8	1.9
Hypophosphatemia	3.5	1.0
Nausea	1.2	1.0
Pruritus	1.2	0
Skeletal Pain	1.2	1.0
Hypomagnesemia	1.2	0
Taste Perversion	1.2	0
Thirst	1.2	0
Pancytopenia	1.2	0

(cont'd)

Table 1: ZOMETA Concentrate *(cont'd)*

Treatment-related Adverse Experiences Reported in Tumor-induced Hypercalcemia Clinical Trials

	ZOMETA 4 mg % (N=86)	Aredia 90 mg % (N=103)
Arthralgia	1.2	0
Bradycardia	1.2	0
Confusion	1.2	0
Fatigue	1.2	0
Hallucination	1.2	0
Vomiting	1.2	0
Chest Pain	1.2	0

Bone Metastases of Solid Tumors and Osteolytic Lesions of Multiple Myeloma Clinical Trials : The adverse event data pertaining to bone metastases of solid tumors and osteolytic lesions of multiple myeloma are based upon the core and extension phases of the three pivotal controlled trials in this indication. These trials included 2042 safety evaluable patients treated with either ZOMETA 4 mg, AREDIA 90 mg or placebo. Of these 2042 patients who entered the core phase of the trials: 969 completed the core phase, 619 entered the safety extension phase, and 347 completed the extension phase. The median duration of exposure to ZOMETA 4 mg (core plus extension phases) was 10.5 months for patients with prostate cancer, 12.8 months for patients with breast cancer and multiple myeloma, and 4.0 months for patients with lung cancer and other solid tumors. The mean duration of exposure to ZOMETA 4 mg (core plus extension phases) was 11.8 months for patients with prostate cancer, 13.9 months for patients with breast cancer and multiple myeloma, and 5.7 months for patients with lung cancer and other solid tumors.

In general, ZOMETA was well tolerated across all studies for various tumor types in patients with bone metastases and in patients with multiple myeloma. The proportion of patients experiencing Grade 3 and Grade 4 laboratory abnormalities and adverse events were similar in patients treated with ZOMETA and AREDIA (pamidronate).

Grade 3 [Common Toxicity Criteria (CTC)] serum creatinine was seen in 1.3%, 1.5% and 1.7% of patients receiving ZOMETA 4mg, AREDIA 90 mg and placebo, respectively. Grade 4 (CTC) serum creatinine was in 0.4%, 0.4% and 0% of patients receiving ZOMETA 4 mg, AREDIA 90 mg and placebo, respectively.

The most commonly reported (>15%) adverse experiences occurred with similar frequencies in the ZOMETA, AREDIA and placebo treatment groups, and most of these adverse experiences may have been related to the underlying disease state or cancer therapy. Table 2 lists the adverse experiences which occurred in ≥15% of patients regardless of study drug relationship by preferred term and treatment group, in the bone metastases trials.

Table 2: ZOMETA Concentrate

Commonly Reported Adverse Experiences in Three Bone Metastases Clinical Trials

	ZOMETA 4 mg n (%)	Aredia 90 mg n (%)	Placebo n (%)
Patients Studied			
Total no. of patients studied	1031 (100)	556 (100)	455 (100)
Total no. of patients with an AE	1015 (98.4)	548 (98.6)	445 (97.8)
Adverse Events (preferred term)			
Bone Pain	55.2%	56.8%	62.4%
Nausea	46.2%	47.8%	37.6%
Fatigue	38.6%	43.2%	28.6%
Anemia	33.4%	31.5%	28.1%
Vomiting	32.3%	32.9%	26.8%
Pyrexia	31.8%	30.9%	19.6%
Constipation	31.0%	29.1%	38.2%
Dyspnea NOS	27.4%	27.9%	23.5%
Weakness	24.4%	19.4%	25.1%
Diarrhea NOS	24.2%	29.1%	18.2%
Myalgia	23.2%	25.7%	16.3%
Anorexia	22.4%	14.6%	23.1%
Cough	21.7%	23.2%	14.3%
Arthralgia	21.0%	23.6%	16.0%
Edema Lower Limb	20.9%	22.7%	18.5%
Malignant Neoplasm Aggravated	19.9%	17.4%	19.6%
Headache NOS	18.5%	26.8%	11.0%
Dizziness (excl. vertigo)	17.5%	16.4%	12.7%
Insomnia NEC	16.1%	20.0%	16.0%
Weight Decreased	15.9%	9.0%	13.4%
Back Pain	15.1%	19.1%	8.8%

(cont'd)

Table 2: ZOMETA Concentrate *(cont'd)*

Commonly Reported Adverse Experiences in Three Bone Metastases Clinical Trials

	ZOMETA 4 mg n (%)	Aredia 90 mg n (%)	Placebo n (%)
Paresthesia NEC	14.5%	15.3%	7.7%
Depression NEC	14.2%	17.1%	10.8%
Pain in Limb	13.9%	15.1%	11.4%

Legend: NOS=not otherwise specified; NEC=not elsewhere classified.

The adverse events occurring during the studies were generally of a type and frequency expected in patients with cancer and bone metastases, many of whom were undergoing antineoplastic therapy. Except for pyrexia, the absolute difference in the proportions of patients in the ZOMETA 4 mg group compared with the placebo group for any of the common adverse events did not exceed 10%. Pyrexia, or fever, may occur as part of an acute phase reaction with bisphosphonate administration.

Among less commonly occurring adverse events (<15% of patients in any group), hypocalcemia was reported in 4.7%, 2.5%, and 0.7% of patients in the ZOMETA 4 mg, AREDIA, and placebo groups, respectively. Hypokalemia was reported in 9.7%, 9.0%, and 4.8% of patients in the ZOMETA 4 mg, AREDIA, and placebo groups, respectively.

Hypotension: Based on the clinical trial experience, the frequency of nonserious hypotensive events is uncommon (between 0.1% and 1.0%).

Renal Dysfunction: In the bone metastases trials renal deterioration was defined as an increase of 44.2 μmol/L (0.5 mg/dL) for patients with normal baseline creatinine (<123.76 μmol/L or <1.4 mg/dL) or an increase of 88.4 μmol/L (1.0 mg/dL) for patients with an abnormal baseline creatinine (≥123.76 μmol/L or ≥1.4 mg/dL). The following are data on the incidence of renal deterioration in patients receiving ZOMETA 4 mg over 15 minutes in these trials (see Table 3).

Table 3: ZOMETA Concentrate

Percentage of Patients with Renal Function Deterioration Who Were Randomized Following the 15-Minute Infusion Amendment

Patient Population/Baseline Creatinine				
	ZOMETA 4 mg		Aredia 90 mg	
Multiple Myeloma and Breast Cancer	**n/N**	**(%)**	**n/N**	**(%)**
Normal	27/246	(11.0%)	23/246	(9.3%)
Abnormal	2/26	(7.7%)	2/22	(9.1%)
Total	29/272	(10.7%)	25/268	(9.3%)
	ZOMETA 4 mg		Placebo	
Solid Tumors	**n/N**	**(%)**	**n/N**	**(%)**
Normal	17/154	(11%)	10/143	(7%)
Abnormal	1/11	(9.1%)	1/20	(5%)
Total	18/165	(10.9%)	11/163	(6.7%)
	ZOMETA 4 mg		Placebo	
Prostate Cancer	**n/N**	**(%)**	**n/N**	**(%)**
Normal	12/82	(14.6%)	8/68	(11.8%)
Abnormal	4/10	(40%)	2/10	(20%)
Total	16/92	(17.4%)	10/78	(12.8%)

The risk of deterioration in renal function appeared to be related to time on study, whether patients were receiving ZOMETA (4 mg over 15 minutes), placebo, or AREDIA.

The frequency distribution of chemotherapy-associated adverse events by chemotherapy, renal involvement and treatment group for patients in the primary safety population is provided in Table 4. This includes patients who were administered at least one chemotherapeutic agent during the study (i.e. patients treated with only hormonal agents are not included). Each chemotherapeutic agent is classified in one of the three categories: renally excreted, nephrotoxic, or no renal involvement (see Table 5 and Table 6). For a chemotherapy that is both renally excreted and nephrotoxic, the agent is classified as nephrotoxic.

Patients receiving renally excreted drugs that were not nephrotoxic had a similar incidence of nausea for the ZOMETA and placebo treatment groups when compared to the nephrotoxic agents. Nausea was higher for the AREDIA treatment group for the nephrotoxic agents when compared to the agents that were not nephrotoxic and renally excreted. Vomiting, stomatitis and anorexia were similar for all of the treatment groups whether or not the agent was renally excreted or nephrotoxic. Alopecia was higher in all groups treated with nephrotoxic drugs when compared to renally excreted drugs.

Table 4: ZOMETA Concentrate

Frequency Distribution of Chemotoxicities (>1%) by Renal Involvement and Treatment Group for Patients Who Were Treated with at Least One Chemotherapy Agent (Safety Evaluable Patients)

	ZOMETA 4 mg	Aredia 90 mg	Placebo
Renal Involvement[a]			
Renally excreted Number of Patients	221	163	76
Total with Chemotoxicity	161 (72.9%)	100 (61.3%)	54 (71.1%)
Nausea	113 (51.1%)	68 (41.7%)	37 (48.7%)
Vomiting NOS	75 (33.9%)	48 (29.4%)	23 (30.3%)
Anorexia	55 (24.9%)	23 (14.1%)	28 (36.8%)
Appetite Decreased NOS	39 (17.6%)	16 (9.8%)	7 (9.2%)
Stomatitis	25 (11.3%)	21 (12.9%)	6 (7.9%)

(cont'd)

Table 4: ZOMETA Concentrate *(cont'd)*

Frequency Distribution of Chemotoxicities (>1%) by Renal Involvement and Treatment Group for Patients Who Were Treated with at Least One Chemotherapy Agent (Safety Evaluable Patients)

	ZOMETA 4 mg	Aredia 90 mg	Placebo
Alopecia	24 (10.9%)	18 (11.0%)	9 (11.8%)
Malaise	6 (2.7%)	3 (1.8%)	5 (6.6%)
Cachexia	4 (1.8%)	1 (0.6%)	3 (3.9%)
Gingivitis	3 (1.4%)	3 (1.8%)	0 (0.0%)
Mouth Ulceration	3 (1.4%)	2 (1.2%)	0 (0.0%)
Gingival Disorder NOS	0 (0.0%)	0 (0.0%)	1 (1.3%)
Malnutrition NOS	0 (0.0%)	2 (1.2%)	0 (0.0%)
Pallor	0 (0.0%)	0 (0.0%)	1 (1.3%)
Nephrotoxic			
Number of patients	471	248	164
Total with chemotoxicity	345 (73.2%)	191 (77.0%)	116 (70.7%)
Nausea	249 (52.9%)	136 (54.8%)	73 (44.5%)
Vomiting NOS	194 (41.2%)	99 (39.9)%	58 (35.4%)
Anorexia	117 (24.8%)	46 (18.5%)	48 (29.3%)
Alopecia	93 (19.7%)	54 (21.8%)	24 (14.6%)
Appetite Decreased NOS	63 (13.4%)	23 (9.3%)	17 (10.4%)
Stomatitis	59 (12.5%)	36 (14.5%)	7 (4.3%)
Malaise	18 (3.8%)	10 (4.0%)	8 (4.9%)
Mouth Ulceration	13 (2.8%)	5 (2.0%)	1 (0.6%)
Malnutrition NOS	6 (1.3%)	2 (0.8%)	1 (0.6%)
Pallor	6 (1.3%)	2 (0.8%)	2 (1.2%)
Gingivitis	5 (1.1%)	2 (0.8%)	0 (0.0%)
Cachexia	3 (0.6%)	0 (0.0%)	4 (2.4%)
No Renal Involvement			
Number of patients	0	1	0
Total with chemotoxicity	0 (0%)	1 (100%)	0 (0%)
Nausea	0 (0%)	1 (100%)	0 (0%)

[a] Each chemotherapeutic agent is classified in one of the three categories: renally excreted, nephrotoxic, or no renal involvement (see Table 5 and Table 6).

Legend: NOS=not otherwise specified.

Table 5: ZOMETA Concentrate

Listing of Chemotherapy Agents by Renal Involvement[a]—Renal Toxic

Preferred term	Preferred term
Adriamycin + Cyclophosphamide	M-VAC
Adriamycin + Vincristine + MTX	Methotrexate
Aldesleukin	Methotrexate Sodium
BCG Vaccine	Mitomycin
Carboplatin	Oxaliplatin
Cisplatin	Paclitaxel
Cyclophosphamide	Raltitrexed
Cyclophosphamide + 5-FU + Methotrexate	Streptozocin
Cyclophosphamide + 5-FU + Prednisolone	Strontium-89
Cyclophosphamide + Doxorubicin + 5-FU	Taxol + Carboplatin
Cyclophosphamide + Epirubicin	Tegafur
Dacarbazine	Tegafur Uracil
Etanercept	Teniposide
Gallium Nitrate	Thalidomide
Gemcitabine	Thiotepa
Gemcitabine Hydrochloride	Topotecan Hydrochloride

(cont'd)

Table 5: ZOMETA Concentrate *(cont'd)*

Listing of Chemotherapy Agents by Renal Involvement[a]—Renal Toxic

Preferred term	Preferred term
Hydroxycarbamide	Trastuzumab
Ifosfamide	Carboplatin + Etoposide
Interferon	CMF + Dexamethasone
Interferon Alfa	CMF + Tamoxifen
Interferon Beta	FAC + Tamoxifen Citrate
Interferon Gamma	Topotecan
Interferon Nos	EVCMF (Epirubicine + Vincri. + Cycloph. + MTX + 5FU)
Interleukin-2	

[a] David S. Fischer, M.Tish Knobf, Henry J. Durivage. The Cancer Chemotherapy Handbook, 5th edition. 1997.

Table 6: ZOMETA Concentrate

Listing of Chemotherapy Agents by Renal Involvement[a]—Renally Excreted

Preferred term	Preferred term
5-FU + Calciumfolinat	Flurouracil
Adriamycin + 5-FU	Formestane
Betamethasone	Irinotecan
Bethamethasone Sodium Phosphate	Irinotecan Hydrochloride
Bleomycin	Lomustine
Bleomycin Sulfate	Melphalan
Busulfan	Melphalan + Prednisolone
Capecitabine	Mitoxantrone
Carmustine	Mitoxantrone Hydrochloride
Cytarabine	Tropisetron Hydrochloride
Daunorubicin	Vinblastine
Dexrazoxane Hydrochloride	Vinblastine Sulfate
Docetaxel	Vincristine
Doxorubicin	Vincristine Sulfate
Doxorubicin Hydrochloride	Vindesine
Epirubicin	Vinorelbine
Epirubicin Hydrochloride	Vinorelbine Bitartrate
Etoposide	Vinorelbine Ditartrate
Exemestane	Pirarubicin
Floxuridine	

[a] David S. Fischer, M.Tish Knobf, Henry J. Durivage. The Cancer Chemotherapy Handbook, 5th edition. 1997.

Bone Metastases From Breast Cancer: Placebo-controlled Trial in Japanese Patients: In a placebo-controlled clinical study in breast cancer patients with bone metastases, 227 patients were evaluated for safety (114 ZOMETA and 113 placebo). Table 7 illustrates AEs that occurred more frequently in the ZOMETA arm compared to placebo. The adverse events occurring during the study were generally of a type and frequency expected in patients with cancer and bone metastases, many of whom were undergoing concurrent antineoplastic therapy.

Table 7: ZOMETA Concentrate

Most Commonly Reported AEs (incidence >10 %) Occurring More Frequently in the ZOMETA Arm Compared to Placebo

	ZOMETA 4 mg (n=114) n (%)	Placebo (n=113) n (%)
Pyrexia	63 (55.3)	37 (32.7)
Malaise	51 (44.7)	36 (31.9)
Headache NOS	34 (29.8)	32 (28.3)
Hypoesthesia	28 (24.6)	22 (19.5)
Arthralgia	24 (21.1)	18 (15.9)
Dyspnea NOS	21 (18.4)	15 (13.3)
Epigastric pain	19 (16.7)	8 (7.1)
Leukopenia NOS	17(14.9)	16(14.2)
Myalgia	15 (13.2)	13 (11.5)

(cont'd)

Table 7: ZOMETA Concentrate *(cont'd)*

Most Commonly Reported AEs (incidence >10 %) Occurring More Frequently in the ZOMETA Arm Compared to Placebo

	ZOMETA 4 mg (n=114) n (%)	Placebo (n=113) n (%)
Pruritus NOS	13 (11.4)	12 (10.6)
Edema lower limb	13 (11.4)	4 (3.5)
Anemia NOS	12 (10.5)	7 (6.2)
Pain NOS	12 (10.5)	11 (9.7)

Shows no. of subjects experiencing at least 1 AE in category in question.

Post-Market Adverse Drug Reactions: Cases of ONJ are uncommon. However, a large retrospective study of the frequency and risk factors for ONJ in cancer patients receiving intravenous bisphosphonates (Hoff, A. et al., 2008) indicated a higher proportion of reported cases in certain cancers, such as advanced breast cancer (1.2%) and multiple myeloma (2.4%), compared to the overall study population (0.72%). The majority of reported cases of ONJ are associated with invasive dental procedures (such as tooth extraction or dental surgery and local trauma including poorly fitting dentures) or periodontal disease. Many patients had signs of local infection including osteomyelitis.

Cases of anaphylactic reactions/shock, atrial fibrillation, hypotension leading to syncope or circulatory collapse (primarily in patients with underlying risk factors), somnolence, uveitis, episcleritis, scleritis and orbital inflammation as well as hypersensitivity reactions including cases of severe allergic reactions, bronchoconstriction and urticaria have also been reported. There were isolated reports that had ocular events with a bisphosphonate and had a re-occurrence when rechallenged with ZOMETA.

Spontaneously reported adverse drug reactions are presented below. Because these events are reported voluntarily from a population of uncertain size, it is not always possible to reliably estimate their frequency or clearly establish a causal relationship to ZOMETA exposure.

DRUG INTERACTIONS: Specific drug-drug interaction studies have not been conducted with ZOMETA. Zoledronic acid is not systemically metabolized and does not affect human cytochrome P450 enzymes in vitro. Zoledronic acid is not highly bound to plasma proteins (approximately 55%) and therefore, interactions resulting from displacement of highly protein-bound drugs are unlikely.

DOSAGE AND ADMINISTRATION

Dosing Considerations: Monitoring of renal function is recommended in all patients prior to the administration of each dose of ZOMETA.

Renal Impairment: ZOMETA is excreted exclusively via the kidney and the risk of adverse reactions may be greater in patients with impaired renal function.

ZOMETA has not been tested in patients with severe renal impairment (serum creatinine >400 µmol/L or >4.5 mg/dL in patients with tumor-induced hypercalcemia; and serum creatinine >265 µmol/L or >3.0 mg/dL in patients with bone metastases of solid tumors and osteolytic lesions of multiple myeloma). Therefore, its use is not recommended in this patient population.

Hepatic Impairment: As only limited clinical data are available for patients with hepatic insufficiency, dosage recommendations cannot be given for this group.

Recommended Dose and Dosage Adjustment: Tumor-Induced Hypercalcemia: The recommended dose of ZOMETA (zoledronic acid for injection) in hypercalcemia (albumin-corrected serum calcium ≥3.0 mmol/L (12 mg/dL)) is 4 mg. The 4 mg dose is given as a single-dose intravenous infusion over no less than 15 minutes following standard rehydration procedures.

> Albumin-corrected serum calcium (CSC, mmol/L)=tCa+0.02 (mid-range albumin−measured albumin).

Prior to treatment with ZOMETA (zoledronic acid for injection) renal excretion of excess calcium should be promoted by restoring and maintaining adequate fluid balance and urine output.

Patients who show complete or partial response initially may be retreated with ZOMETA 4 mg if serum calcium does not return to normal or does not remain normal after initial treatment although retreatment with ZOMETA 4 mg in TIH patients has not been assessed for efficacy and safety in prospective studies. It is recommended that at least one week must elapse before retreatment to allow for a full response to the initial dose. In addition, retreatment should be given to **only** those patients who can tolerate the standard rehydration procedures (i.e., 3 to 5 litres of fluids per day and more than 400 meq of sodium chloride per day). In any patient requiring repeated administration, serum BUN and creatinine must be evaluated and possible deterioration in renal function must be assessed prior to each re-administration (see Warnings and Precautions).

Dosage Adjustment: Mild to Moderate Renal Impairment: Dose reduction in patients with tumor-induced hypercalcemia with mild to moderate renal impairment is not recommended.

Bone Metastases of Solid Tumors and Osteolytic Lesions of Multiple Myeloma: The recommended dose of ZOMETA in patients with documented metastatic bone lesions from solid tumors and patients with osteolytic lesions of multiple myeloma for patients with creatinine clearance >60 mL/min is 4 mg, given as a single dose intravenous infusion over no less than 15 minutes every 3 to 4 weeks. In patients requiring antineoplastic therapy, ZOMETA should be administered either prior to or after this treatment. Patients will be required to take an oral calcium supplement of 500 mg and a multivitamin containing at least 400 IU of Vitamin D daily. If a patient has a prior history of hypercalcemia or develops hypercalcemia during treatment with calcium and Vitamin D supplementation, the patient is advised to discontinue taking calcium and Vitamin D.

ZOMETA has been used with cyclophosphamide, doxorubicin, paclitaxel, anastrozole, melphalan and tamoxifen. It has been given less frequently with docetaxel, dexamethasone, prednisone, carboplatin, letrozole, vinorelbine, cisplatin and gemcitabine.

Dosage Adjustment: Mild to Moderate Renal Impairment: ZOMETA has been used in patients with bone metastases of solid tumors and osteolytic lesions of multiple myeloma with mild to moderate renal impairment in clinical trials; their risk of renal deterioration was increased compared to that of patients with normal renal function. Therefore, if ZOMETA is to be administered to patients with mild to moderate renal impairment (defined as baseline creatinine clearance 30 mL/min to 60 mL/min), doses should be reduced. The following dosing recommendations are based on data from pharmacokinetic studies however, the efficacy and safety of adjusted dosing has not been prospectively assessed in clinical trials.

Upon treatment initiation, the recommended ZOMETA doses for patients with reduced renal function (mild and moderate renal impairment) are listed in Table 8. These doses are calculated based on pharmacokinetic data in order to achieve the same AUC as that achieved in patients with creatinine clearance of 75 mL/min (see Action and Clinical Pharmacology, Special Populations and Conditions, Renal Insufficiency). Creatinine clearance (CrCl) is calculated using the Cockcroft-Gault formula.

$$\text{CrCl (mL/min)} = \frac{1.2\ [140-\text{age (years)}]\times[\text{total body weight (kg)}]}{\text{serum creatinine } (\mu\text{mol/L})}\ \{\text{multiply by 0.85 for females}\}$$

Table 8: ZOMETA Concentrate

Recommended Doses for Patients with Reduced Renal Function

Baseline Creatinine Clearance (mL/min)	ZOMETA Recommended Dose[a]
>60	4.0 mg
50–60	3.5 mg
40–49	3.3 mg
30–39	3.0 mg

[a] Doses calculated assuming target AUC of 0.66 (mg·h/L) (CrCl=75 mL/min).

During treatment, serum creatinine should be measured before each ZOMETA dose and treatment should be withheld for renal deterioration. In the clinical studies, renal deterioration was defined as follows:

- For patients with normal baseline creatinine (<123 µmol/L or <1.4 mg/dL), an increase of 44 µmol/L or 0.5 mg/dL
- For patients with abnormal baseline creatinine (>123 µmol/L or >1.4 mg/dL), an increase of 88 µmol/L or 1.0 mg/dL

In the clinical studies, ZOMETA treatment was resumed only when the creatinine returned to within 10% of the baseline value. ZOMETA should be re-initiated at the same dose as that prior to treatment interruption.

Renal function should be monitored appropriately during therapy with ZOMETA. Patients with evidence of renal function deterioration should be appropriately evaluated and consideration should be given as to whether the potential benefit outweighs the possible risk.

Administration: Reconstitution: Method of Preparation: ZOMETA Concentrate: Vials of ZOMETA concentrate contain overfill allowing for the withdrawal of 5 mL of concentrate (equivalent to 4 mg zoledronic acid for injection). The content of the vials is withdrawn using a sterile syringe. This concentrate should immediately be diluted in 100 mL of sterile 0.9% Sodium Chloride Injection, USP, or 5% Dextrose Injection, USP. Do not store undiluted concentrate in a syringe, to avoid inadvertent injection. Any unused portion of ZOMETA concentrate should be discarded.

Reduced Doses for Patients with Baseline CrCl ≤60 mL/min: Withdraw an appropriate volume of the 5 mL—ZOMETA concentrate as needed:

4.4 mL for 3.5 mg dose
4.1 mL for 3.3 mg dose
3.8 mL for 3.0 mg dose

The withdrawn concentrate must be diluted in 100 mL of sterile 0.9% Sodium Chloride Injection, USP, or 5% Dextrose Injection, USP. The dose must be given as a single intravenous injection over no less than 15 minutes.

Incompatibilities: ZOMETA must not be mixed with calcium-containing infusion solutions, such as Lactated Ringer's solution, and should be administered as a single intravenous solution in a line separate from all other drugs.

Studies with glass bottles, as well as several types of infusion bags and infusion lines made from polyvinylchloride, polyethylene and polypropylene (prefilled with 0.9 % sodium chloride solution or 5 % glucose solution), showed no incompatibility with ZOMETA.

Stability of Diluted ZOMETA Solutions: If not used immediately after dilution with infusion media, for microbiological integrity, the solution should be refrigerated at 2°C - 8°C. The refrigerated solution should then be equilibrated to room temperature prior to administration. The total time between dilution, storage in the refrigerator and end of administration must not exceed 24 hours.

Strict adherence to the intravenous route is recommended for the parenteral administration of ZOMETA.

Note: Parenteral drug products should be inspected visually for particulate matter and discoloration prior to administration, whenever solution and container permit.

Store ZOMETA concentrate at 15-30°C.

OVERDOSAGE:

Clinical experience of acute overdose with ZOMETA (zoledronic acid for injection) is limited. There have been two patients who received maladministration of 32 mg of ZOMETA given over 5 minutes. Neither patient experienced any clinical or laboratory toxicity. Clinically relevant hypocalcemia should be corrected by intravenous administration of calcium gluconate.

In an open label study of ZOMETA 4 mg in breast cancer patients, a female patient received a single 48 mg dose of zoledronic acid in error. Two days after the overdose the patient experienced a single episode of hyperthermia (38°C), which resolved after treatment. All other evaluations were normal, and the patient was discharged seven days after the overdose.

A patient with Non-Hodgkin's Lymphoma received ZOMETA 4 mg daily on four successive days for a total dose of 16 mg. The patient developed paresthesia and abnormal liver function tests with increased GGT (nearly 100U/L, exact value unknown). The outcome of this case is not known.

Patients who have received doses higher than those recommended should be carefully monitored, since renal function impairment (including renal failure) and serum electrolyte (including calcium, phosphorus and magnesium) abnormalities have been observed.

> For management of a suspected drug overdose, contact your regional Poison Control Centre. See the *CPS* Directory section for a list of Poison Control Centres.

ACTION AND CLINICAL PHARMACOLOGY: Mechanism of Action: The principal pharmacologic action of ZOMETA (zoledronic acid for injection) is inhibition of bone resorption. Although the antiresorptive mechanism is not completely understood, several factors are thought to contribute to this action. Zoledronic acid accumulates in bone, where it blocks the resorption of mineralized bone and cartilage. In vitro, zoledronic acid inhibits osteoclastic activity and induces apoptosis in osteoclasts, as well as reducing the formation and recruitment of osteoclasts into bone. In vitro, zoledronic acid has a very large ratio between the desired inhibition of bone resorption and the adverse effects on bone mineralization. Zoledronic acid inhibits the osteoclastic hyperactivity and accelerated bone resorption induced by various stimulatory factors released by tumors. In long-term animal studies, doses of zoledronic acid similar to those recommended for the treatment of hypercalcemia inhibit bone resorption without adversely affecting the formation, mineralization, or mechanical properties of bone.

In addition to inhibiting osteoclastic bone resorption, zoledronic acid exerts direct anti-tumor effects on cultured human myeloma and breast cancer cells, inhibiting their proliferation and inducing apoptosis. Zoledronic acid also inhibits the proliferation of human endothelial cells in vitro and is anti-angiogenic in animal tumor models. In vitro zoledronic acid reduces the invasion of human breast cancer cells into the extracellular matrix.

Preclinical data suggest that low micromolar concentrations of zoledronic acid are cytostatic and pro-apoptotic in vitro to a range of human cancer cell lines (breast, prostate, lung, bladder, myeloma). This anti-tumor efficacy may be enhanced when used in combination with other anti-cancer drugs. Preclinical data suggest that zoledronic acid is also anti-proliferative for human fetal osteoblasts and promotes their differentiation, a property that may be potentially relevant for the treatment of bone metastases in prostate cancer. Zoledronic acid has been shown to inhibit the proliferation of human endothelial cells in vitro and is anti-angiogenic in vivo. Zoledronic acid at picomolar concentrations has been shown to inhibit tumor cell invasion through extracellular matrix in preclinical cancer models.

Pharmacodynamics: Clinical studies in TIH demonstrated that the effect of ZOMETA is characterized by decreases in serum calcium and urinary calcium excretion. Normalization of serum calcium by day 4 was greater for the ZOMETA 4 mg and 8 mg doses (45% and 56%, respectively) compared with AREDIA (pamidronate) 90 mg (33%).

Tumor-Induced Hypercalcemia: Osteoclastic hyperactivity resulting in excessive bone resorption is the underlying pathophysiologic derangement in tumor-induced hypercalcemia (TIH, hypercalcemia of malignancy) and metastatic bone disease. Excessive release of calcium into the blood as bone is resorbed results in polyuria and gastrointestinal disturbances, with progressive dehydration and decreasing glomerular filtration rate. This results in increased renal resorption of calcium, setting up a cycle of worsening systemic hypercalcemia. Correction of excessive bone resorption and adequate fluid administration to correct volume deficits are, therefore, essential to the management of hypercalcemia.

Most cases of hypercalcemia associated with malignancy occur in patients who have breast cancer, squamous-cell tumors of the lung or head and neck, renal cell carcinoma, and certain hematologic malignancies, such as multiple myeloma and some types of lymphomas. A few less common malignancies, including vasoactive intestinal-peptide-producing tumors and cholangiocarcinoma, have a high incidence of hypercalcemia as a metabolic complication. Patients who have tumor-induced hypercalcemia can generally be divided into two groups according to the pathophysiologic mechanism involved.

In humoral hypercalcemia, osteoclasts are activated and bone resorption is stimulated by factors such as parathyroid-hormone-related protein, which are elaborated by the tumor and circulate systemically. Humoral hypercalcemia usually occurs in squamous-cell malignancies of the lung or head and neck or in genitourinary tumors such as renal cell carcinoma or ovarian cancer. Skeletal metastases may be absent or minimal in these patients.

Extensive invasion of bone by tumor cells can also result in hypercalcemia due to local tumor products that stimulate bone resorption by osteoclasts. Tumors commonly associated with locally mediated hypercalcemia include breast cancer and multiple myeloma.

Total serum calcium levels in patients who have tumor-induced hypercalcemia may not reflect the severity of hypercalcemia, since concomitant hypoalbuminemia is commonly present. Ideally, ionized calcium levels should be used to diagnose and follow hypercalcemic conditions; however, these are not commonly or rapidly available in many clinical situations. Therefore, adjustment of the total serum calcium value for differences in albumin levels is often used in place of measurement of ionized calcium; several nomograms are in use for this type of calculation (see Dosage and Administration).

Bone Metastases of Solid Tumors and Osteolytic Lesions of Multiple Myeloma: Osteolytic bone lesions and metastases commonly occur in patients with multiple myeloma, breast cancer, non-small cell lung cancer, renal cell carcinoma and a variety of other solid tumors. Bone lesions associated with bone metastases from prostate carcinoma classically are osteoblastic in contrast to those from other carcinomas, which are usually osteolytic or mixed osteolytic/osteoblastic. Adenocarcinoma of the prostate spreads most commonly to the well vascularized areas of the skeleton such as the vertebral column, ribs, skull, and the proximal ends of the long bones. Prostate carcinoma cells have long been believed to gain access to the vertebral column and ribs via the Batson venous plexus, which is a low pressure, high volume plexus of vertebral veins that join the intercostal veins.

These bone changes in patients with evidence of osteolytic and osteoblastic skeletal destruction may cause severe bone pain that requires either radiation therapy or narcotic analgesics (or both) for symptomatic relief. These changes also cause pathologic fractures of bone in both the axial and appendicular skeleton. Axial skeletal fractures of the vertebral bodies may lead to spinal cord compression or vertebral body collapse with significant neurologic complications. Patients may also experience episode(s) of hypercalcemia.

Pharmacokinetics: Single or multiple (q 28 days) 5-minute or 15-minute infusions of 2, 4, 8 or 16 mg ZOMETA were given to 64 cancer patients with bone metastases. The post infusion decline of zoledronic acid concentrations in plasma was consistent with a triphasic process showing a rapid decrease from peak concentrations at end-of-infusion to <1% of C_{max} after 24 hours post infusion with population half-lives of $t_{½α}$ 0.24 hours and $t_{½β}$ 1.87 hours for the early disposition phases of the drug, followed by a prolonged period of very low concentrations in plasma between days 2 and 28 post infusion, with a terminal elimination half-life $t_{½γ}$ of 146 hours. The area under the plasma concentration versus time curve ($AUC_{0\text{-}24h}$) of zoledronic acid was linearly related to dose. The accumulation of zoledronic acid following a 28-day dosing schedule over 3 cycles was low, with mean $AUC_{0\text{-}24h}$ ratios cycles 2 and 3 versus 1 of 1.13±0.30 and 1.16±0.36, respectively.

In vitro and ex vivo studies showed low affinity of zoledronic acid for the cellular components of human blood. Binding to human plasma proteins was approximately 56% and independent of the concentration of zoledronic acid.

Zoledronic acid does not inhibit human P-450 enzymes in vitro. Zoledronic acid does not experience biotransformation. In animal studies <3% of the administered intravenous dose was found in the feces, with the balance either recovered in the urine or taken up by bone, indicating that the drug is eliminated intact via the kidney. Following an intravenous dose of 20 nCi ^{14}C-zoledronic acid in a cancer patient with bone metastases, the radioactivity excreted in the urine consisted solely of intact drug.

In 64 cancer patients with bone metastases on average (±s.d.) 39±16% of the administered dose was recovered in the urine within 24 hours, with only trace amounts of drug found in urine post day 2. The cumulative percent of drug excreted in the urine over 0-24 hours was independent of dose. The balance of drug not recovered in urine over 0-24 hours, representing drug presumably bound to bone tissue is slowly released back into the systemic circulation, giving rise to the observed prolonged low plasma concentrations days 2 to 28 post dose. The 0-24 h renal clearance of zoledronic acid was on average (±s.d.) 3.7±2.0 L/h.

Zoledronic acid clearance was reasonably independent of dose and demographic variables, with effects of body weight, gender, and race on clearance being within the bounds of the inter-patient variability of clearance, which was 36%.

Increasing the infusion time from 5 minutes to 15 minutes caused a 30% decrease in the zoledronic acid concentration at the end of the infusion, but had no effect on the area under the plasma concentration versus time curve.

Special Populations and Conditions: There are no pharmacokinetic data in patients with hypercalcemia.

Pediatrics: There are no pharmacokinetic data in pediatric patients (see Warnings and Precautions).

Geriatrics: The pharmacokinetics of ZOMETA were not affected by age in cancer patients with bone metastases aged 38 years to 84 years.

Race: The pharmacokinetics of 2 mg, 4 mg and 8 mg zoledronic acid have been evaluated in a Phase I study of Japanese patients with cancer and bone metastasis.

Japanese female subjects had substantially higher systemic exposure, i.e., 47% higher $AUC_{0\text{-}24h}$ and 39% higher C_{max} than the North American population (see Table 9) following a single dose intravenous of ZOMETA (4 mg over 15 minutes). The exposure of Japanese males were comparable to that of the North American population based on the limited data (n=4 and 1 for AUC and C_{max}, respectively).

Table 9: ZOMETA Concentrate

Comparative PK between Japanese and North American Population (mean±SD)

	Japan		North America	
	Female (n=14)	**Male (n=4 or 1)**	**Female (n=16)**	**Male (n=29)**
$AUC_{0\text{-}24h}$, ng·h/mL	154±38	118±40	114±22	100±32
C_{max}, ng·h/mL	111±22	64	87±20	77±28

Hepatic Insufficiency: There are no pharmacokinetic data in patients with impaired liver function. ZOMETA is not cleared by the liver, therefore impaired liver function may not affect the pharmacokinetics of ZOMETA.

Renal Insufficiency: Limited pharmacokinetic data are available for ZOMETA in patients with severe renal impairment (creatinine clearance <30 mL/min). The pharmacokinetic studies were conducted in cancer patients (n=64) typical of the target clinical population, showing renal function mainly in the range of normal to moderately impaired [mean (±s.d.) creatinine clearance 84±29 mL/min, range 22-143 mL/min]. In these 64 patients the renal clearance of zoledronic acid was found to closely correlate with creatinine clearance, representing in the mean (±s.d.) 75±33% of the creatinine clearance. Creatinine clearance is calculated by the Cockcroft-Gault formula (see Dosage and Administration):

$$\text{CrCl (mL/min)} = \frac{1.2\,[140-\text{age (years)}]\times[\text{total body weight (kg)}]}{\text{serum creatinine } (\mu\text{mol/L})} \quad \{\text{multiply by 0.85 for females}\}$$

Patients with mild renal impairment (creatinine clearance 50-80 mL/min) showed increases in plasma AUC of 26% to 36%, whereas patients with moderate renal impairment (creatinine clearance 30-50 mL/min) showed increases in plasma AUC of 27-41%, compared to patients with normal renal function (creatinine clearance >80 mL/min). However, there were no further increases in the systemic exposure after multiple doses in patients with impaired renal function (see Warnings and Precautions).

The population-derived relationship of ZOMETA clearance with creatinine clearance offers an algorithm for dose reduction in renal impairment. ZOMETA systemic clearance (CL) in individual patients can be calculated from the population clearance of ZOMETA and that individual's creatinine clearance, as $CL\ (L/h)=6.5\times(CLcr/90)^{0.4}$. This formula can be used to predict ZOMETA AUC in patients, where $CL=Dose/AUC_{0\text{-}\infty}$. The average $AUC_{0\text{-}24}$ in patients with normal renal function was 0.42 mg·h/L and the calculated $AUC_{0\text{-}\infty}$ for a patient with creatinine clearance of 75 mL/min was 0.66 mg·h/L following a 4 mg dose of ZOMETA.

STORAGE AND STABILITY: Store ZOMETA concentrate at 15-30°C.

After dilution with infusion media, the solution should be refrigerated at 2-8°C. The refrigerated solution should then be equilibrated to room temperature prior to administration. The total time between dilution, storage in the refrigerator, and end of administration must not exceed 24 hours.

ZOMETA must be kept out of the reach and sight of children and pets.

INFORMATION FOR THE PATIENT: Published in e-CPS, available by subscription at www.e-cps.ca.

DOSAGE FORMS, COMPOSITION AND PACKAGING: Each vial of concentrate contains: zoledronic acid sterile liquid concentrate 4 mg, this corresponds to zoledronic acid monohydrate 4.264 mg. Nonmedicinal ingredients: mannitol 220 mg per vial, USP, as bulking agent and sodium citrate as buffering agent and water for injection. Vials of 5 mL, cartons of 1.

(Shown in Product Identification Section)

Zomig® Ⓟ
zolmitriptan
Migraine Therapy

AstraZeneca

Zomig® Nasal Spray Ⓟ
zolmitriptan
Migraine Therapy

AstraZeneca

Zomig Rapimelt® Ⓟ
zolmitriptan
Migraine Therapy

AstraZeneca

Date of Preparation: August 20, 1998
Date of Revision: January 15, 2010

SUMMARY PRODUCT INFORMATION:

Product	Route of Administration	Dosage Form/ Strength	Clinically Relevant Nonmedicinal Ingredients[a]
ZOMIG	Oral	Conventional tablet/2.5 mg	Anhydrous lactose
ZOMIG RAPIMELT	Oral	Orally dispersible tablet/2.5 mg	None
ZOMIG Nasal Spray	Intranasal	Nasal spray/2.5 mg, 5 mg	None

[a] For a complete listing see Dosage Forms, Composition and Packaging.

INDICATIONS AND CLINICAL USE: Adults: ZOMIG (zolmitriptan) is indicated for the acute treatment of migraine attacks with or without aura.

ZOMIG is not intended for the prophylactic therapy of migraine or for use in the management of hemiplegic, basilar, or ophthalmoplegic migraine (see Contraindications). Safety and efficacy have not been established for cluster headache, which is present in an older, predominantly male population.

Pediatrics (<12 years of age): The safety and efficacy of ZOMIG have not been studied in children under 12 years of age. Use of the drug in this age group is, therefore, not recommended (see Warnings and Precautions, Special Populations).

Adolescents (12-17 years of age): The safety and efficacy of ZOMIG have not been established in patients 12-17 years of age. The use of ZOMIG in adolescents is, therefore, not recommended (see Warnings and Precautions, Special Populations).

Geriatrics (>65 years of age): The safety and efficacy of ZOMIG in patients over 65 years has not been established and its use in this age group is not recommended (see Warnings and Precautions, Special Populations).

CONTRAINDICATIONS: ZOMIG (zolmitriptan) is contraindicated under the following conditions:

- **in patients with history, symptoms, or signs of ischemic cardiac, cerebrovascular or peripheral vascular syndromes, valvular heart disease or cardiac arrhythmias (especially tachycardias). In addition, patients with other significant underlying cardiovascular diseases (e.g., atherosclerotic disease, congenital heart disease) should not receive ZOMIG. Ischemic cardiac syndromes include, but are not restricted to, angina pectoris of any type (e.g., stable angina of effort and vasospastic forms of angina such as the Prinzmetal's variant), all forms of myocardial infarction, and silent myocardial ischemia. Cerebrovascular syndromes include, but are not limited to, strokes of any type as well as transient ischemic attacks (TIAs). Peripheral vascular disease includes, but is not limited to, ischemic bowel disease, or Raynaud's syndrome (see Warnings and Precautions, Cardiovascular);**
- **in patients with uncontrolled or severe hypertension as ZOMIG can give rise to increases in blood pressure (see Warnings and Precautions, Hematologic);**
- **within 24 hours of treatment with another 5-HT_1 agonist, or an ergotaminecontaining or ergot-type medication like dihydroergotamine or methysergide (see Drug Interactions);**
- **in patients with hemiplegic, basilar or ophthalmoplegic migraine;**
- **concurrent administration of MAO inhibitors or use of zolmitriptan within 2 weeks of discontinuation of MAO inhibitor therapy (see Drug Interactions);**
- **in patients with hypersensitivity to zolmitriptan or any component of the formulation** (for a complete listing see Dosage Forms, Composition and Packaging).

WARNINGS AND PRECAUTIONS: General: ZOMIG (zolmitriptan) should only be used where a clear diagnosis of migraine has been established.

Lactose: Lactose is a nonmedicinal ingredient in ZOMIG tablets. Therefore, patients with rare hereditary problems of galactose intolerance (the Lapp lactase deficiency or glucose-galactose malabsorption) should not take ZOMIG tablets.

Psychomotor Effect: Although ZOMIG did not interfere with psychomotor performance in healthy volunteers, some patients in clinical trials experienced sedation with ZOMIG. Patients should thus be advised to avoid driving a car or operating hazardous machinery until they are reasonably certain that ZOMIG does not affect them adversely.

Cardiovascular: **Risk of Myocardial Ischemia and/or Infarction and Other Adverse Cardiac Events: ZOMIG has been associated with transient chest and/or neck pain and tightness which may resemble angina pectoris. Following the use of other 5-HT_1 agonists, in rare cases these symptoms have been identified as being the likely result of coronary vasospasm or myocardial ischemia. Rare cases of serious coronary events or arrhythmia have occurred following use of ZOMIG. In very rare cases angina pectoris has been reported.**

ZOMIG should not be given to patients who have documented ischemic or vasospastic coronary artery disease (see Contraindications). It is strongly recommended that ZOMIG not be given to patients in whom unrecognised coronary artery disease (CAD) is predicted by the presence of risk factors (e.g., hypertension, hypercholesterolemia, smoking, obesity, diabetes, strong family history of CAD, female who is surgically or physiologically postmenopausal, or male who is over 40 years of age) unless a cardiovascular evaluation provides satisfactory clinical evidence that the patient is reasonably free of coronary artery and ischemic myocardial disease or other significant underlying cardiovascular disease. The sensitivity of cardiac diagnostic procedures to detect cardiovascular disease or predisposition to coronary artery vasospasm is unknown. If, during the cardiovascular evaluation, the patient's medical history or electrocardiographic investigations reveal findings indicative of or consistent with coronary artery vasospasm or myocardial ischemia, ZOMIG should not be administered (see Contraindications).

These evaluations, however, may not identify every patient who has cardiac disease, and in very rare cases, serious cardiac events, such as myocardial infarction or coronary ischemia have occurred in patients without evidence of underlying cardiovascular disease.

For patients with risk factors predictive of CAD who are considered to have a satisfactory cardiovascular evaluation, the first dose of ZOMIG should be administered in the setting of a physician's office or similar medically staffed and equipped facility. Because cardiac ischemia can occur in the absence of clinical symptoms, consideration should be given to obtaining electrocardiograms in patients with risk factors during the interval immediately following ZOMIG administration on the first occasion of use.

However, an absence of drug-induced cardiovascular effects on the occasion of the initial dose does not preclude the possibility of such effects occurring with subsequent administrations.

Intermittent long-term users of ZOMIG, who have or acquire risk factors predictive of CAD, as described above, should receive periodic interval cardiovascular evaluations over the course of treatment.

If symptoms consistent with angina occur after the use of ZOMIG, ECG evaluation should be carried out to look for ischemic changes.

The systematic approach described above is intended to reduce the likelihood that patients with unrecognized cardiovascular disease will be inadvertently exposed to ZOMIG.

As with other $5HT_{1B/1D}$ agonists, atypical sensations over the precordium have been reported after the administration of zolmitriptan. Where such symptoms are thought to indicate ischemic heart disease, no further doses of zolmitriptan should be given and appropriate evaluation carried out.

Discomfort in the chest, neck, throat and jaw (including pain, pressure, heaviness and tightness) has been reported after administration of ZOMIG. Because 5-HT_1 agonists may cause coronary vasospasm, patients who experience signs or symptoms suggestive of angina following ZOMIG should be evaluated for the presence of CAD or a predisposition to variant angina before receiving additional doses, and should be monitored electrocardiographically if dosing is resumed and similar symptoms recur. Similarly, patients who experience other symptoms or signs suggestive of decreased arterial flow, such as ischemic bowel syndrome or Raynaud's syndrome following ZOMIG administration should be evaluated for atherosclerosis or predisposition to vasospasm (see Contraindications and Warnings and Precautions).

Cardiac Events and Fatalities Associated with 5-HT$_1$ Agonists: As with other triptans, zolmitriptan may cause coronary artery vasospasm. Serious adverse cardiac events, including acute myocardial infarction, life-threatening disturbances of cardiac rhythm, and death have been reported within a few hours following the administration of other 5-HT$_1$ agonists. Considering the extent of use of 5-HT$_1$ agonists in patients with migraine, the incidence of these events is extremely low.

Patients with symptomatic Wolff-Parkinson-White syndrome or arrhythmias associated with other cardiac accessory conduction pathway disorders should not receive ZOMIG.

Premarketing Experience with ZOMIG: Among the more than 2500 patients with migraine who participated in premarketing controlled clinical trials of ZOMIG conventional tablets, no deaths or serious cardiac events were reported. In premarketing controlled clinical trials of ZOMIG Nasal Spray, more than 1300 patients participated and there were no deaths or serious cardiac events to report.

Postmarketing Experience with ZOMIG: Serious cardiovascular events have been reported in association with the use of ZOMIG. The uncontrolled nature of postmarketing surveillance, however, makes it impossible to determine definitively the proportion of reported cases that were actually caused by ZOMIG or to reliably assess causation in individual cases.

Cerebrovascular Events and Fatalities with 5-HT$_1$ Agonists: Migraineurs may be at risk of certain cerebrovascular events. Cerebral haemorrhage, subarachnoid haemorrhage, stroke, and other cerebrovascular events have been reported in patients treated with 5-HT$_1$ agonists, and some have resulted in fatalities. In a number of cases, it appears possible that the cerebrovascular events were primary, the agonist having been administered in the incorrect belief that the symptoms were a consequence of migraine, when they were not. Before treating migraine headaches with ZOMIG in patients not previously diagnosed as migraineurs, and in migraineurs who present with atypical symptoms, care should be taken to exclude other potentially serious neurological conditions. If a patient does not respond to the first dose, the opportunity should be taken to review the diagnosis before a second dose is given. It should be noted that patients with migraine may be at increased risk of certain cerebrovascular events (e.g., stroke, haemorrhage, TIA).

Special Cardiovascular Pharmacology Studies with Another 5-HT$_1$ Agonist: In subjects (n=10) with suspected coronary artery disease undergoing angiography, a 5-HT$_1$ agonist at a subcutaneous dose of 1.5 mg produced an 8% increase in aortic blood pressure, an 18% increase in pulmonary artery blood pressure, and an 8% increase in systemic vascular resistance. In addition, mild chest pain or tightness was reported by four subjects. Clinically significant increases in blood pressure were experienced by three of the subjects (two of whom also had chest pain/discomfort). Diagnostic angiogram results revealed that 9 subjects had normal coronary arteries and 1 had insignificant coronary artery disease.

In an additional study with this same drug, migraine patients (n=35) free of cardiovascular disease were subjected to assessments of myocardial perfusion by positron emission tomography while receiving a subcutaneous 1.5 mg dose in the absence of a migraine attack. Reduced coronary vasodilatory reserve (~10%), increased coronary resistance (~20%), and decreased hyperaemic myocardial blood flow (~10%) were noted. The relevance of these findings to the use of the recommended oral dose of this 5-HT$_1$ agonist is not known.

Similar studies have not been done with ZOMIG. However, owing to the common pharmacodynamic actions of 5-HT$_1$ agonists, the possibility of cardiovascular effects of the nature described above should be considered for any agent of this pharmacological class.

Other Vasospasm-Related Events: 5-HT$_1$ agonists may cause vasospastic reactions other than coronary artery vasospasm. Peripheral vascular ischemia has been reported with 5-HT$_1$ agonists (see Adverse Reactions). Very rare reports of splenic infarction and gastrointestinal ischemic events including ischemic colitis, gastrointestinal infarction or necrosis, which may present as bloody diarrhea or abdominal pain, have been received.

Increased Blood Pressure: Significant elevation in blood pressure, including hypertensive crisis, has been reported on rare occasions in patients receiving other 5-HT$_1$ agonists with and without a history of hypertension. Very rarely these increases in blood pressure have been associated with significant clinical events. Isolated reports of chest pain, pulmonary edema, coronary vasospasm, transient cerebral ischemia, angina and subarachnoid hemorrhage have been received (see Contraindications). In patients with controlled hypertension, ZOMIG should be administered with caution, as transient increases in blood pressure and peripheral vascular resistance have been observed in a small portion of patients.

In pharmacodynamic studies, an increase of 1 and 5 mm Hg in the systolic and diastolic blood pressure, respectively, was seen in volunteers with 5 mg ZOMIG. In the headache trials, vital signs were measured only in a small, single-centre inpatient study, and no effect on blood pressure was seen. In a study of patients with moderate to severe liver disease, 7 of 27 patients experienced 20 to 80 mm Hg elevations in systolic or diastolic blood pressure after a 10 mg ZOMIG dose. Significant elevations in systemic blood pressure, including hypertensive crisis, have been reported on rare occasions in patients with and without a history of hypertension who received 5-HT$_1$ agonists. ZOMIG is contraindicated in patients with uncontrolled or severe hypertension (see Contraindications).

Dependence: The abuse potential of ZOMIG has not been assessed in clinical trials.

Endocrine and Metabolism: Phenylketonuria: Patients with phenylketonuria should be informed that ZOMIG RAPIMELT orally dispersible tablets contain phenylalanine (a component of aspartame). Each orally dispersible tablet contains 2.81 mg of phenylalanine.

Hepatic: ZOMIG should be administered with caution to patients with moderate or severe hepatic impairment, using a dose lower than 2.5 mg (see Action and Clinical Pharmacology and Dosage and Administration).

Immune: Rare hypersensitivity (anaphylaxis/anaphylactoid) reactions may occur in patients receiving 5-HT$_1$ agonists such as ZOMIG. Such reactions can be life threatening or fatal. In general, hypersensitivity reactions to drugs are more likely to occur in individuals with a history of sensitivity to multiple allergens. Owing to the possibility of cross-reactive hypersensitivity reactions, ZOMIG should not be used in patients having a history of hypersensitivity to chemically-related 5-HT$_1$ receptor agonists (see Adverse Events in Precautions and Adverse Reactions).

Neurologic: Care should be taken to exclude other potentially serious neurologic conditions before treating headache in patients not previously diagnosed with migraine or who experience a headache that is atypical for them. There have been rare reports where patients received 5-HT$_1$ agonists for severe headache that were subsequently shown to have been secondary to an evolving neurologic lesion. For newly diagnosed patients or patients presenting with atypical symptoms, the diagnosis of migraine should be reconsidered if no response is seen after the first dose of ZOMIG.

Seizures: Caution should be observed if ZOMIG is to be used in patients with a history of epilepsy or structural brain lesions, which lower the convulsion threshold.

Selective Serotonin Reuptake Inhibitors/Serotonin Norepinephrine Reuptake Inhibitors and Serotonin Syndrome: Cases of life-threatening serotonin syndrome have been reported during combined use of selective serotonin reuptake inhibitors (SSRIs)/serotonin norepinephrine reuptake inhibitors (SNRIs) and triptans. If concomitant treatment with ZOMIG and SSRIs (e.g., fluoxetine, paroxetine, sertraline) or SNRIs (e.g., venlafaxine) is clinically warranted, careful observation of the patient is advised, particularly during treatment initiation and dose increases. Serotonin syndrome symptoms may include mental status changes (e.g., agitation, hallucinations, coma), autonomic instability (e.g., tachycardia, labile blood pressure, hyperthermia), neuromuscular aberrations (e.g., hyperreflexia, incoordination) and/or gastrointestinal symptoms (e.g., nausea, vomiting, diarrhea) (see Drug Interactions).

Ophthalmologic: Binding to Melanin-Containing Tissues: When pigmented rats were given a single oral dose of 10 mg/kg of radiolabelled zolmitriptan, the radioactivity in the eye after 7 days, the latest time point examined, was still 75% of the values measured after 4 hours. This suggests that zolmitriptan and/or its metabolites may bind to the melanin of the eye. Because there could be accumulation in melanin rich tissues over time, it raises the possibility that zolmitriptan could cause toxicity in these tissues after extended use. However, no effects on the retina related to treatment with zolmitriptan were noted in any of the toxicity studies. No systematic monitoring of ophthalmologic function was undertaken in clinical trials, and no specific recommendations for ophthalmologic monitoring are offered, however, prescribers should be aware of the possibility of long-term ophthalmologic effects.

Preclinical Toxicology: Carcinogenicity: Carcinogenicity studies by oral gavage were carried out in rats and mice at doses up to 400 mg/kg/day. In mice the total exposure at the highest dose level was approximately 800 times that seen after a single 10 mg dose in humans and there was no effect on tumour type or incidence. In male rats at this dose level, where total exposure was approximately 3000 times that seen after a single 10 mg dose in humans, there was an increase in the incidence of thyroid follicular hyperplasia and benign adenomata. This has been shown to be due to an increase in thyroxine clearance caused by zolmitriptan at this dose level with a resultant chronic stimulation of the thyroid. There was no effect on tumour profile at the dose level of 100 mg/kg/day that gave an exposure multiple of approximately 800.

Mutagenicity: Zolmitriptan was mutagenic in an Ames test, in 2 of 5 strains of *S. typhimurium* tested, in the presence of, but not in the absence of, metabolic activation. It was not mutagenic in an in vitro mammalian gene cell mutation (CHO/HGPRT) assay. The nasal spray formulation was not mutagenic in two further Ames tests. Zolmitriptan was clastogenic in an in vitro human lymphocyte assay both in the absence of and the presence of metabolic activation. Zolmitriptan was not clastogenic in an in vivo mouse micronucleus assay. In three rat bone marrow micronucleus assays with the nasal spray formulation, the results overall were negative. In a mouse bone marrow micronucleus assay with the nasal spray formulation, there were sporadic increases in micronucleus erythrocytes, but the results were equivocal. Zolmitriptan was not genotoxic in an unscheduled DNA synthesis study.

Special Populations: Pregnant Women: Reproductive studies in male and female rats, at dose levels limited by toxicity, revealed no effect on fertility or reproduction.

Reproduction studies in rats and rabbits dosed during the period of organogenesis have been performed at levels limited by maternal toxicity. In rats dosed orally by gavage at 1200 mg/kg/day, giving a total exposure 3000-5000 times that seen following a single 10 mg dose in humans, there was a slight increase in early resorptions but no effect on fetal malformations. At a dose of 400 mg/kg/day in rats, an exposure multiple of approximately 1100, there were no effects of any kind on the fetus. The maximum achieved dose in rabbits was 30 mg/kg/day that gave a total exposure 30-40 times that seen following a single 10 mg dose in humans and there were no fetal effects.

The safety of ZOMIG for use during human pregnancy has not been established. ZOMIG should be used during pregnancy only if the potential benefit justifies the potential risk to the fetus.

Nursing Women: It is not known whether zolmitriptan and/or its metabolites are excreted in human milk. Because many drugs are excreted in human milk, caution should be exercised when considering the administration of ZOMIG to nursing women. Lactating rats dosed with zolmitriptan had milk levels equivalent to maternal plasma levels at 1 hour and 4 times higher than plasma levels at 4 hours.

Pediatrics (<12 years of age): The safety and efficacy of ZOMIG have not been studied in children under 12 years of age. Use of the drug in this age group is, therefore, not recommended.

Adolescents (12-17 years of age): Systemic exposure to the parent compound does not differ significantly between adolescents and adults, however exposure to the active metabolite is greater in adolescents (see Action and Clinical Pharmacology). The safety and efficacy of ZOMIG have not been established in patients 12-17 years of age. The use of ZOMIG in adolescents is, therefore, not recommended.

In a single randomized placebo-controlled study of 696 adolescent migraineurs (aged 12-17 years), the efficacy of ZOMIG tablets (2.5, 5 and 10 mg) was not established (see Adverse Reactions, Adverse Drug Reactions in Special Population).

Geriatrics (>65 years of age): The safety and efficacy of ZOMIG have not been studied in individuals over 65 years of age. The risk of adverse reactions to this drug may be greater in elderly patients as they are more likely to have decreased hepatic function, be at higher risk for CAD, and experience blood pressure increases that may be more pronounced. Clinical studies did not include patients over 65 year of age. Its use in this age group is, therefore, not recommended.

Special Disease Conditions: ZOMIG should be administered with caution to patients with diseases that may alter the absorption, metabolism, or excretion of drugs, such as impaired hepatic function (see Warnings and Precautions, Hepatic).

Monitoring and Laboratory Tests: Zolmitriptan is not known to interfere with commonly employed clinical laboratory tests.

ADVERSE REACTIONS: Serious cardiac events, including some that have been fatal, have occurred following the use of 5-HT$_1$ agonists. These events are extremely rare and most have been reported in patients with risk factors predictive of CAD. Events reported have included coronary artery vasospasm, transient myocardial ischemia, angina pectoris, myocardial infarction, ventricular tachycardia, and ventricular fibrillation (see Contraindications and Warnings and Precautions, General).

Clinical Trial Adverse Drug Reactions: Because clinical trials are conducted under very specific conditions the adverse reaction rates observed in the clinical trials may not reflect the rates observed in practice and should not be compared to the rates in the clinical trials of another drug. Adverse drug reaction information from clinical trials is useful for identifying drug-related adverse events and for approximating rates.

Experience in Controlled Clinical Trials with ZOMIG (zolmitriptan): Typical 5-HT$_1$ Agonist Adverse Reactions: As with other 5-HT$_1$ agonists, ZOMIG has been associated with sensations of heaviness, pressure, tightness or pain which may be intense. These may occur in any part of the body including the chest, throat, neck, jaw and upper limb. In very rare cases, as with other 5-HT$_1$ agonists, angina pectoris and myocardial infarction have been reported.

Transient increases in systemic blood pressure, have been reported in patients, with and without a history of hypertension. Very rarely these increases in blood pressure have been associated with significant clinical events. Isolated reports of chest pain, pulmonary edema, coronary vasospasm, transient cerebral ischemia, angina and subarachnoid hemorrhage have been received (see Warnings and Precautions, Cardiovascular, Increased Blood Pressure).

There have been rare reports of hypersensitivity reactions including urticaria and angioedema (see Warnings and Precautions, Immune).

Experience with ZOMIG Conventional Tablet (zolmitriptan): Acute Safety: In placebo controlled migraine trials, 1673 patients received at least one dose of ZOMIG. Table 1 lists adverse events that occurred in five placebo controlled clinical trials in migraine patients. Events that occurred at an incidence of 1% or more in any one of the ZOMIG 1 mg, 2.5 mg or 5 mg dose groups and that occurred at a higher incidence than in the placebo group are included. The events cited reflect experience gained under closely monitored conditions in clinical trials, in a highly selected patient population. In actual clinical practice or in other clinical trials, these frequency estimates may not apply, as the conditions of use, reporting behaviour, and the kinds of patients treated may differ.

Several of the adverse events appear dose related, notably paresthesia, sensation of heaviness or tightness in chest, neck, jaw and throat, dizziness, somnolence, and possibly asthenia and nausea.

Table 1: ZOMIG

Treatment-Emergent Adverse Events in 5 Single-Attack Placebo-Controlled Migraine Trials, Reported by ≥1% Patients Treated with ZOMIG

	Placebo	ZOMIG 1 mg	ZOMIG 2.5 mg	ZOMIG 5 mg
Number of patients	401	163	498	1012
Symptoms of Potential Cardiac Origin				
Neck/Throat/Jaw Sensations[a]	3.0%	6.1%	7.0%	10.9%
Chest/Thorax Sensations[a]	1.2%	1.8%	3.4%	3.8%
Upper Limb Sensations[a]	0.5%	2.4%	4.2%	4.1%
Palpitations	0.7%	0.0%	0.2%	2.2%
Other Body Systems: Neurological				
Dizziness	4.0%	5.5%	8.4%	9.5%
Nervousness	0.2%	0.0%	1.4%	0.7%
Somnolence	3.0%	4.9%	6.0%	7.7%
Thinking Abnormal	0.5%	0.0%	1.2%	0.3%
Tremor	0.7%	0.6%	1.0%	0.7%
Vertigo	0.0%	0.0%	0.0%	1.5%
Hyperesthesia	0.0%	0.0%	0.6%	1.1%
Digestive				

(cont'd)

Table 1: ZOMIG *(cont'd)*

Treatment-Emergent Adverse Events in 5 Single-Attack Placebo-Controlled Migraine Trials, Reported by ≥1% Patients Treated with ZOMIG

	Placebo	ZOMIG 1 mg	ZOMIG 2.5 mg	ZOMIG 5 mg
Diarrhea	0.5%	0.6%	1.0%	0.6%
Dry Mouth	1.7%	4.9%	3.2%	3.2%
Dyspepsia	0.5%	3.1%	1.6%	1.0%
Dysphagia	0.0%	0.0%	0.0%	1.8%
Nausea	3.7%	3.7%	9.0%	6.2%
Vomit	2.5%	0.6%	1.4%	1.5%
Miscellaneous				
Asthenia	3.2%	4.9%	3.2%	8.8%
Limb Sensations (upper and lower)[a]	0.7%	0.6%	0.4%	1.6%
Limb Sensations (lower)[a]	0.7%	1.2%	0.4%	1.8%
Sensations-Location Unspecified[a]	5.2%	4.9%	5.8%	9.2%
Abdominal Pain	1.7%	1.2%	0.6%	1.3%
Reaction Aggravated	1.0%	1.2%	1.0%	0.7%
Head/Face Sensations[a]	1.7%	6.7%	8.6%	10.9%
Myalgia	0.2%	0.0%	0.2%	1.3%
Myasthenia	0.2%	0.0%	0.6%	1.9%
Dyspnea	0.2%	0.6%	0.2%	1.2%
Rhinitis	0.2%	1.2%	1.2%	0.9%
Sweating	1.2%	0.0%	1.6%	2.5%
Taste Perversion	0.5%	2.5%	0.6%	0.7%

[a] The term sensation encompasses adverse events described as pain, discomfort, pressure, heaviness, tightness, heat/burning sensations, tingling and paresthesia.

ZOMIG is generally well tolerated. Across all doses, most adverse events were mild to moderate in severity as well as transient and self-limiting. The incidence of adverse events in controlled clinical trials was not affected by gender, weight, or age of patients; use of prophylactic medications; or presence of aura. There were insufficient data to assess the impact of race on the incidence of adverse events.

Long-Term Safety: In a long-term open label study in which patients were allowed to treat multiple migraine attacks for up to one year, 8% (167 of 2058) of patients withdrew from the study due to an adverse experience. In this study, migraine headaches could be treated with either a single 5 mg dose of ZOMIG, or an initial 5 mg dose followed by a second 5 mg dose if necessary (5+5 mg). The most common adverse events (defined as occurring at an incidence of at least 5%) recorded for the 5 mg and 5+5 mg doses, respectively, comprised, in descending order of frequency: neck/throat sensations* (16%, 15%), head/face sensations* (15%, 14%), asthenia (14%, 14%), sensations* location unspecified (12%, 11%), limb sensations* (11%, 11%), nausea (12%, 8%), dizziness (11%, 9%), somnolence (10%, 10%), chest/thorax sensations* (7%, 7%), dry mouth (4%, 5%), and hyperesthesia (5%, 4%). Due to the lack of a placebo arm in this study, the role of ZOMIG in causation cannot be reliably determined. The long term safety of a 2.5 mg dose was not assessed in this study.

Other Events: The frequencies of less commonly reported adverse clinical events are presented below. Because the reports include events observed in open and uncontrolled studies, the role of ZOMIG in their causation cannot be reliably determined. Furthermore, variability associated with adverse event reporting, the terminology used to describe adverse events, etc., limit the value of the quantitative frequency estimates provided. Event frequencies are calculated as the number of patients who used ZOMIG (n=4027) and reported an event divided by the total number of patients exposed to ZOMIG. All reported events are included except those already listed in the previous table, those too general to be informative, and those not reasonably associated with the use of the drug. Events are further classified within body system categories and enumerated in order of decreasing frequency using the following definitions: infrequent adverse events are those occurring in 1/100 to 1/1000 patients and rare adverse events are those occurring in fewer than 1/1000 patients.

Atypical Sensation: Infrequent was hyperesthesia.

General: Infrequent were allergy reaction, chills, facial edema, fever, malaise and photosensitivity.

Cardiovascular: Infrequent were arrhythmias, hypertension and syncope. Rare were bradycardia, extrasystoles, postural hypotension, QT prolongation, and thrombophlebitis. Rare reports of tachycardia, palpitations and transient increases in systemic blood pressure in patients with or without a history of hypertension (see Warnings and Precautions, Cardiovascular, Increased Blood Pressure).

Digestive: Infrequent were increased appetite, tongue edema, esophagitis, gastroenteritis, liver function abnormality and thirst. Rare were anorexia, constipation, gastritis, hematemesis, pancreatitis, melena and ulcer.

Hemic: Infrequent was ecchymosis. Rare were cyanosis, thrombocytopenia, eosinophilia and leucopenia.

Metabolic: Infrequent was edema. Rare were hyperglycemia and alkaline phosphatase increased.

Musculoskeletal: Infrequent were back pain, leg cramps and tenosynovitis. Rare were arthritis, tetany and twitching.

Neurological: Infrequent were agitation, anxiety, depression, emotional lability and insomnia. Rare were akathesia, amnesia, apathy, ataxia, dystonia, euphoria, hallucinations, cerebral ischemia, hyperkinesia, hypotonia, hypertonia, irritability and headache.

Respiratory: Infrequent were bronchitis, bronchospasm, epistaxis, hiccup, laryngitis and yawn. Rare were apnea and voice alteration.

Skin: Infrequent were pruritus, and rash. Rare reports were urticaria and angioedema.

Special Senses: Infrequent were dry eye, eye pain, hyperacusis, ear pain, parosmia, and tinnitus. Rare were diplopia and lacrimation.

Urogenital: Infrequent were hematuria, cystitis, polyuria, urinary frequency and urinary urgency. Rare were miscarriage and dysmenorrhea.

Experience in Controlled Clinical Trials with ZOMIG RAPIMELT (zolmitriptan): Acute Safety: In an international, placebo-controlled, double-blind trial to evaluate the efficacy and tolerability of ZOMIG RAPIMELT 2.5 mg in the acute treatment of adult patients with migraine, 231 patients received at least one dose of ZOMIG RAPIMELT. Most of the adverse events were of mild or moderate intensity, and no patients withdrew from the trial because of adverse events. The types of adverse events reported were consistent with known effects of this class of compound (5-HT$_{1B/1D}$) and were similar to those reported with the ZOMIG conventional tablet. The most frequently reported adverse events (>2%) for ZOMIG RAPIMELT 2.5 mg versus placebo, respectively, were asthenia (3% vs. 1%), tightness (3% vs. <1%), somnolence (3% vs. 2%), dizziness (3% vs. 1%), paresthesia (3% vs. 2%), hyperesthesia (2% vs. 0%), pharyngitis (2% vs. 0%), and nausea (2% vs. 1%).

* See footnote for Table 1.

Experience in Controlled Clinical Trials with ZOMIG Nasal Spray (zolmitriptan): Acute Safety: Among 1383 patients treating 3398 attacks with zolmitriptan nasal spray in a blinded placebo-controlled trial, there was a low withdrawal rate related to adverse events: 5 mg (1.3%), 2.5 mg (0%), 1 mg (0.8%) and placebo (0.4%). None of the withdrawals were due to a serious event. One patient was withdrawn due to abnormal ECG changes from baseline that were incidentally found 23 days after the last dose of ZOMIG Nasal Spray. The most common adverse events in clinical trials for ZOMIG Nasal Spray were: unusual taste, paresthesia, hyperesthesia, and dizziness. Table 2 lists the adverse events that occurred in ≥1% of the 1383 patients in the 2.5 mg tablet, placebo, 1 mg, 2.5 mg and 5 mg nasal spray dose groups of the controlled clinical trial.

Table 2: ZOMIG

Adverse Events in a Single Placebo-controlled Study, with an Incidence of ≥1% of Patients in any ZOMIG Nasal Spray Treatment Group by Body System

Body System and Adverse event (COSTART defined)[a]	Percentage of Patients				
	Tablet[d] 2.5 mg (N=233)	Placebo[b] (N=228)	ZOMIG Nasal Spray 1.0 mg (N=238)	ZOMIG Nasal Spray 2.5 mg (N=224)	ZOMIG Nasal Spray 5.0 mg (N=236)
Symptoms of Potential Cardiac Origin					
Pain Throat	1.3%	0.4%	0.0%	2.7%	2.1%
Pressure Throat	0.9%	0.0%	0.4%	0.0%	1.3%
Tightness Throat	1.3%	0.9%	1.3%	0.4%	1.7%
Tightness Neck	1.3%	0.0%	0.0%	0.0%	0.8%
Tightness Chest	1.3%	0.0%	0.8%	0.4%	0.8%
Palpitation	1.3%	0.4%	1.7%	1.3%	0.0%
Body/Abdomen					
Pain Abdominal	0.4%	0.9%	1.7%	1.3%	0.8%
Body/General					
Asthenia	2.1%	0.4%	0.4%	0.9%	2.1%
Heaviness Other	1.7%	0.0%	0.0%	0.9%	0.0%
Pain Local Specific	0.0%	0.4%	1.7%	0.9%	2.5%
Reaction Aggravation[c]	0.0%	2.2%	0.4%	0.9%	2.1%
Digestive					
Dry Mouth	1.3%	0.0%	1.7%	2.2%	1.3%
Nausea	1.3%	0.9%	1.3%	0.9%	1.7%
Nervous System/CNS					
Dizziness	1.7%	3.5%	2.9%	0.4%	0.0%
Insomnia	0.0%	0.0%	1.3%	1.3%	0.9%
Somnolence	0.4%	1.3%	0.8%	0.4%	1.7%
Nervous System/General					
Hyperesthesia	0.9%	0.0%	0.8%	0.4%	2.1%
Hypesthesia	1.3%	0.4%	0.4%	0.9%	0.8%
Nervous System/PNS					
Paresthesia	4.3%	3.9%	4.2%	3.1%	5.9%
Sensation Warm	2.1%	2.2%	0.4%	0.9%	0.0%
Respiratory					
Disorder or Discomfort of Nasal Cavity	0.9%	1.3%	2.1%	0.9%	1.3%
Special Senses					
Unusual Taste	1.3%	3.1%	7.6%	13.4%	16.9%

[a] The patient may have had more than 1 adverse event.
[b] The placebo treatment group included patients treated with placebo nasal spray and oral placebo.
[c] Events reported under this term includes increased nausea and increased headache.
[d] The incidences reported in this table are from one single placebo-controlled study. The treatment-emergent adverse events in five single-attack placebo-controlled migraine trials, reported by ≥1% patients treated with ZOMIG 1 mg, 2.5 mg and 5 mg tablets are listed in Table 1.

Local Adverse Reactions: Among 922 patients using an active zolmitriptan nasal spray to treat 2311 attacks in the controlled clinical study, approximately 3% noted local irritation or soreness at the site of administration. Adverse events of any kind, perceived in the nasopharynx (which may include systemic effects of triptans) were severe in about 1% of patients and approximately 60% resolved in 1 hour.

The adverse experience profile seen with ZOMIG Nasal Spray is similar to that seen with ZOMIG conventional tablets and ZOMIG RAPIMELT tablets, except for localized adverse events related to nasal dosing.

Overall Results of Clinical Trials: In a pool of 51 placebo-controlled and open labelled studies the above adverse events were reported at the described frequencies, with the exception of the following adverse events which were reported at a greater frequency. In total 17 301 patients with migraine were treated with ZOMIG, ZOMIG RAPIMELT or ZOMIG Nasal Spray. Events are classified within body system categories and enumerated in order of decreasing frequency using the following definitions: Common (frequent) adverse events were those occurring in 1/10 to 1/100 patients and uncommon (infrequent) adverse events are those occurring in 1/100 to 1/1000 patients.

Cardiac Disorders: Uncommon was tachycardia.

Nervous System Disorders: Common was headache.

Respiratory: Common was epistaxis for ZOMIG Nasal Spray only.
Vascular Disorders: Uncommon was transient increases in systemic blood pressure.

Sensations of heaviness, tightness, pain or pressure in the throat, neck, limbs or chest were common and consistent with those observed in Table 1 and Table 2.

Adverse Drug Reactions in Special Population: Adolescents (12-17 years of age): Table 3 lists the adverse events observed in a single randomized placebo-controlled study of 696 adolescent migraineurs aged 12-17 years (see Warnings and Precautions, Special Populations).

Table 3: ZOMIG

Adverse Events in a Single Placebo-controlled Adolescent Study, Reported by ≥1% of Patients Treated with ZOMIG

Body System and Adverse Event (COSTART term)	Percentage of Patients			
		ZOMIG		
	Placebo (N=176)	2.5 mg (N=171)	5 mg (N=174)	10 mg (N=178)
Cardiovascular				
Vasodilatation	0.6	0	2.9	3.9
Palpitation	0	0	1.1	0
Whole Body				
Tightness	1.1	2.9	5.7	11.2
Asthenia	1.1	1.8	1.1	5.1
Pain	0	1.8	1.7	5.1
Neck Pain	0	0.6	1.7	3.4
Abdominal Pain	0.6	1.2	0	1.7
Headache	0	1.2	2.9	1.1
Malaise	0	0	2.3	0.6
Pressure	0	1.8	0.6	0.6
Stiffness	0	0	0.6	2.8
Heaviness	1.1	0.6	0	1.1
Digestive				
Nausea	1.1	5.8	2.9	7.9
Vomiting	1.1	0.6	1.7	4.5
Dry Mouth	0.6	1.8	1.1	1.1
Nervous System				
Dizziness	2.3	4.7	4.6	9
Paresthesia	0	1.8	4.6	6.2
Somnolence	1.7	1.2	1.7	2.8
Hypertonia	0	0.6	1.7	1.1
Internasal Paresthesia	0	2.3	0.6	0
Tremor	0	0	0	1.7
Hyperesthesia	0	0	0	1.1
Respiratory System				
Pharyngitis	0.6	2.9	2.3	1.7
Dyspnea	0.6	0	1.1	0.6
Musculoskeletal				
Myalgia	0	0	1.1	0.6
Skin and Appendages				
Sweating	0	0	0	1.7
Special Senses				
Eye Pain	0	0.6	1.1	0.6
Amblyopia	0	0	0	1.1

Post-Market Adverse Drug Reactions: In addition to the adverse experiences reported during clinical testing of ZOMIG, the following adverse experiences have been reported in patients receiving marketed ZOMIG from worldwide use since approval. There are insufficient data to support an estimate of their incidence or to establish causality.

Serious adverse events have occurred during post-marketing surveillance following the use of ZOMIG oral tablets. These events are extremely rare and most have been reported in patients with risk factors predictive of CAD. Events reported have included coronary artery vasospasm, transient myocardial ischemia, angina pectoris and myocardial infarction (see Contraindications and Warnings and Precautions).

As with other 5-$HT_{1B/1D}$ agonists, there have been very rare reports of anaphylaxis or anaphylactoid reactions and gastrointestinal ischemic events including ischemic colitis, gastrointestinal infarction, splenic infarction, or necrosis, which may present as bloody diarrhea or abdominal pain.

Post-marketing experience with other triptans include a limited number of reports that describe pediatric (under 12 years of age) and adolescent (12-17 years of age) patients who have experienced clinically serious adverse events that are similar in nature to those reported as rare occurrences in adults.

DRUG INTERACTIONS: Drug-Drug Interactions: Ergot-Containing Drugs: Ergot-containing drugs have been reported to cause prolonged vasospastic reactions. Because there is a theoretical basis for these effects being additive, the use of ergot-containing or ergot-type medications (like dihydroergotamine or methysergide and zolmitriptan) within 24 hours of each other is contraindicated (see Contraindications).

Other 5-HT_1 Agonists: The administration of ZOMIG with other 5-HT_1 agonists has not been evaluated in migraine patients. As an increased risk of coronary vasospasm is a theoretical possibility with co-administration of 5-HT_1 agonists, use of these drugs within 24 hours of each other is contraindicated (see Contraindications).

All drug interaction studies with drugs listed below were performed in healthy volunteers using a single 10 mg dose of ZOMIG and a single dose of the other drug, except where otherwise noted.

MAO Inhibitors: In a limited number of subjects, following one week administration of 150 mg b.i.d. moclobemide, a specific MAO-A inhibitor, there was an increase of approximately 26% in both AUC and C_{max} for zolmitriptan and a 3-fold increase in the AUC and C_{max} of the active N-desmethyl metabolite. Administration of selegiline, a selective MAO-B inhibitor, at a dose of 10 mg/day for one week, had no effect on the pharmacokinetic parameters of zolmitriptan and the active N-desmethyl metabolite. The specificity of selegiline diminishes with higher doses and varies between patients. Therefore, co-administration of zolmitriptan in patients taking MAO inhibitors is contraindicated (see Contraindications).

Cimetidine and Other 1A2 Inhibitors: Following administration of cimetidine, a general P450 inhibitor, the half life and AUC of zolmitriptan and its active metabolite were approximately doubled. Patients taking cimetidine should not exceed a dose of 5 mg ZOMIG in any 24 hour period. Based on the overall interaction profile, an interaction with specific inhibitors of CYP 1A2 cannot be excluded. Therefore, the same dose reduction is recommended with compounds of this type, such as fluvoxamine and the quinolones (e.g., ciprofloxacin). Following the administration of rifampicin, no clinically relevant differences in the pharmacokinetics of zolmitriptan or its active metabolite were observed.

Oral Contraceptives: Retrospective analysis of pharmacokinetic data across studies indicated that mean plasma concentrations of zolmitriptan were generally greater in females taking oral contraceptives compared to those not taking oral contraceptives. Mean C_{max} and AUC of zolmitriptan were found to be higher by 30% and 50%, respectively, and T_{max} was delayed by 30 minutes in females taking oral contraceptives. The effect of ZOMIG on the pharmacokinetics of oral contraceptives has not been studied.

Propranolol: Propranolol, at a dose of 160 mg/day for 1 week increased the C_{max} and AUC of zolmitriptan by 1.5-fold. C_{max} and AUC of the N-desmethyl metabolite were reduced by 30% and 15%, respectively. There were no interactive effects on blood pressure or pulse rate following administration of propranolol with zolmitriptan.

Selective Serotonin Reuptake Inhibitors/Serotonin Norepinephrine Reuptake Inhibitors: Cases of life-threatening serotonin syndrome have been reported during combined use of selective serotonin reuptake inhibitors (SSRIs) or serotonin norepinephrine reuptake inhibitors (SNRIs) and triptans (see Warnings and Precautions).

The pharmacokinetics and effects of ZOMIG on blood pressure were unaffected by 4-week pre-treatment with oral fluoxetine (20 mg/day). The effects of zolmitriptan on fluoxetine metabolism were not assessed.

Acetaminophen: After concurrent administration of single 10 mg doses of ZOMIG and 1 g acetaminophen, there was no significant effect on the pharmacokinetics of ZOMIG. ZOMIG reduced the AUC and C_{max} of acetaminophen by 11% and 31% respectively and delayed the T_{max} of acetaminophen by 1 hour.

Metoclopramide: Metoclopramide (single 10 mg dose) had no effect on the pharmacokinetics of ZOMIG or its metabolites.

Xylometazoline: An in vivo drug interaction study with ZOMIG Nasal Spray indicated that 1 spray (100 µL dose) of xylometazoline (0.1% w/v), a decongestant, administered 30 minutes prior to a 5 mg nasal dose of zolmitriptan did not alter the pharmacokinetics of zolmitriptan.

DOSAGE AND ADMINISTRATION:

Dosing Considerations: The following general statements apply to all dosage formulations of ZOMIG.

ZOMIG (zolmitriptan) is recommended only for the acute treatment of migraine attacks. ZOMIG should not be used prophylactically.

The recommended adult starting dose for ZOMIG is 2.5 mg (see individual dosage forms under Dosage and Administration, Recommended Dose and Dosage Adjustment).

If the headache returns, the dose may be repeated after 2 hours. A dose should not be repeated, regardless of dosage form, within 2 hours. A total cumulative dose of 10 mg should not be exceeded in any 24 hour period.

Controlled trials have not established the effectiveness of a second dose if the initial dose is ineffective.

The safety of treating more than 3 migraine headaches with ZOMIG in a one month period remains to be established.

Hepatic Impairment: Patients with moderate to severe hepatic impairment have decreased clearance of zolmitriptan and significant elevation in blood pressure was observed in some patients. Use of a low dose (<2.5 mg) with blood pressure monitoring is recommended (see Action and Clinical Pharmacology and Warnings and Precautions, Hepatic).

Hypertension: ZOMIG should not be used in patients with uncontrolled or severe hypertension. Patients with mild to moderate hypertension should be treated cautiously at the lowest effective dose.

Cimetidine and Other 1A2 Inhibitors: Patients taking cimetidine and other 1A2 inhibitors should not exceed a dose of 5 mg ZOMIG in any 24 hour period (see Drug Interactions).

Recommended Dose and Dosage Adjustment: ZOMIG Conventional Tablets: Adults: The minimal effective single adult dose of ZOMIG is 1 mg. The recommended single dose is 2.5 mg. The 1 mg dose can be approximated by manually breaking a 2.5 mg conventional tablet in half.

In controlled clinical trials, single doses of 1 mg, 2.5 mg or 5 mg ZOMIG conventional tablets were shown to be effective in the acute treatment of migraine headaches. In the only direct comparison of the 2.5 and 5 mg doses, there was little added benefit from the higher dose, while side effects increased with 5 mg ZOMIG tablets (see Adverse Events, Table 1).

ZOMIG RAPIMELT: Adults: The minimal effective single adult dose of ZOMIG is 1 mg. The recommended single dose is 2.5 mg. **The ZOMIG RAPIMELT 2.5 mg orally dispersible tablet cannot be broken in half to approximate a 1 mg dose.**

The ZOMIG RAPIMELT orally dispersible tablet rapidly dissolves when placed on the tongue and is swallowed with the patient's saliva. ZOMIG RAPIMELT can be taken when water is not available thus allowing early administration of treatment for a migraine attack. This formulation may also be beneficial for patients who suffer from nausea and are unable to drink during a migraine attack, or for patients who do not like swallowing conventional tablets.

ZOMIG Nasal Spray: Adults: As stated for ZOMIG conventional tablets and ZOMIG RAPIMELT, the recommended initial starting dose of ZOMIG is 2.5 mg. For patients for whom a 2.5 mg dose of zolmitriptan is not optimally effective, a 5 mg dose of ZOMIG Nasal Spray is recommended.

In a controlled clinical trial, single doses of 0.5, 1.0, 2.5 and 5.0 mg ZOMIG Nasal Spray were shown to be effective in the acute treatment of migraine headaches. The 5 mg nasal spray dose provided significantly improved pain relief over 2.5 mg oral tablet (seen at 15, 30, 45, 60, and 120 minutes). The 2.5 mg dose of ZOMIG Nasal Spray did not provide any benefit over the 2.5 mg oral tablet.

ZOMIG Nasal Spray is administered as a single dose into one nostril. The nasal spray provides an alternative non-oral formulation of zolmitriptan to that of ZOMIG conventional tablets and ZOMIG RAPIMELT.

Administration: ZOMIG Conventional Tablets: The tablet should be swallowed with water.

ZOMIG RAPIMELT: The tablet should be placed on the tongue, where it will dissolve with the saliva. Water is not needed for the dispersible tablet.

ZOMIG Nasal Spray: The nasal spray should be administered into one nostril only. The device is a single dose unit and must not be primed before use. Patients should be advised to read the consumer information leaflet regarding the use of the nasal spray device prior to administration.

OVERDOSAGE:

There is no experience with clinical overdose. Volunteers receiving single 50 mg oral doses of ZOMIG (zolmitriptan) commonly experienced sedation.

The elimination half-life of zolmitriptan is 2.5-3 hours (see Action and Clinical Pharmacology), and therefore monitoring of patients after overdose with ZOMIG should continue for at least 15 hours or while symptoms or signs persist.

There is no specific antidote to zolmitriptan. In cases of severe intoxication, intensive care procedures are recommended, including establishing and maintaining a patent airway, ensuring adequate oxygenation and ventilation, and monitoring and support of the cardiovascular system.

It is unknown what effect hemodialysis or peritoneal dialysis has on the serum concentrations of zolmitriptan.

For management of a suspected drug overdose, CPhA recommends that you contact your **regional Poison Control Centre**. See the *CPS* Directory section for a list of Poison Control Centres.

ACTION AND CLINICAL PHARMACOLOGY: Mechanism of Action and Pharmacodynamics: ZOMIG (zolmitriptan) is a selective 5-hydroxytryptamine$_1$ (5-HT$_{1B/1D}$) receptor agonist. It exhibits a high affinity at human recombinant 5-HT$_{1B}$ and 5-HT$_{1D}$ receptors and modest affinity for 5-HT$_{1A}$ receptors. Zolmitriptan has no significant affinity (as measured by radioligand binding assays) or pharmacological activity at 5-HT$_2$, 5-HT$_3$, 5-HT$_4$, alpha$_1$, alpha$_2$, or beta$_1$, -adrenergic; H$_1$, H$_2$, histaminic; muscarinic; dopamine$_1$, or dopamine$_2$, receptors. The N-desmethyl metabolite of zolmitriptan also has high affinity for 5-HT$_{1B/1D}$ and modest affinity for 5-HT$_{1A}$ receptors.

It has been proposed that symptoms associated with migraine headaches arise from the activation of the trigemino-vascular system, which results in local cranial vasodilation and neurogenic inflammation involving the antidromic release of sensory neuropeptides [Vasoactive Intestinal Peptide (VIP), Substance P and calcitonin gene related peptide (CGRP)]. The therapeutic activity of zolmitriptan for the treatment of migraine headache is thought to be attributable to its agonist effects at 5-HT$_{1B/1D}$ receptors on the intracranial blood vessels, including the arterio-venous anastamoses, and sensory nerves of the trigeminal system which result in cranial vessel constriction and inhibition of pro-inflammatory neuropeptide release.

Pharmacokinetics: ZOMIG Conventional Tablets and ZOMIG RAPIMELT: Absorption and Bioavailability: In man, zolmitriptan is rapidly and well absorbed (at least 64%) after oral administration with peak plasma concentrations occurring in 2 hours. The mean absolute bioavailability of the parent compound is approximately 40%. Food has no significant effect on the bioavailability of zolmitriptan.

During a moderate to severe migraine attack in male and female patients, mean AUC$_{0-4}$ and C$_{max}$ for zolmitriptan were decreased by 40% and 25%, respectively and mean T$_{max}$ was delayed by one-half hour compared to the same patients during a migraine free period.

Plasma Kinetics and Disposition: When given as a single dose to healthy volunteers, zolmitriptan displayed linear kinetics over the dose range of 2.5 to 50 mg.

Distribution: The mean apparent volume of distribution is 7.0 L/kg. Plasma protein binding of zolmitriptan over the concentration range of 10-1000 ng/L is 25%.

There is no evidence of accumulation on multiple dosing with zolmitriptan up to doses of 10 mg.

Metabolism and Excretion: Zolmitriptan is eliminated largely by hepatic biotransformation followed by urinary excretion of the metabolites. The enzymes responsible for the metabolism of zolmitriptan remain to be fully characterized. The mean elimination half-life of zolmitriptan is approximately 2.5 to 3 hours. Mean total plasma clearance of zolmitriptan is 31.5 mL/min/kg, of which one-sixth is renal clearance. The renal clearance is greater than the glomerular filtration rate suggesting renal tubular secretion.

In a study in which radiolabelled zolmitriptan was orally administered to healthy volunteers, 64% and 30% of the administered ^{14}C-zolmitriptan dose was excreted in the urine and feces, respectively. About 8% of the dose was recovered in the urine as unchanged zolmitriptan. The indole acetic acid and N-oxide metabolites, which are inactive, accounted for 31% and 7% of the dose, respectively, while the active N-desmethyl metabolite accounted for 4% of the dose.

Conversion of zolmitriptan to the active N-desmethyl metabolite occurs such that metabolite concentrations are approximately two thirds that of zolmitriptan. Because the 5-HT$_{1B/1D}$ potency of the N-desmethyl metabolite is 2 to 6 times that of the parent, the metabolite may contribute a substantial portion of the overall effect after zolmitriptan administration. The half-life of the active N-desmethyl metabolite is 3 hours and the T$_{max}$ is approximately 2 to 3 hours.

ZOMIG Nasal Spray: Absorption: Zolmitriptan nasal spray is rapidly absorbed via the nasopharynx as detected in a Photon Emission Tomography (PET) study using [^{11}C]-zolmitriptan. Zolmitriptan was detected in plasma by 5 minutes and peak plasma concentration generally was achieved by 3 hours. (Approximately 40% of C$_{max}$ is achieved between 10-15 minutes after dosing). The time at which maximum plasma concentrations were observed was similar after single (1 day) or multiple (4 day) nasal dosing. Plasma concentrations of zolmitriptan are sustained for 4 to 6 hours after dosing. Zolmitriptan displays linear kinetics after multiple doses of 2.5 mg, 5 mg, or 10 mg. Increases in zolmitriptan and the N-desmethyl metabolite plasma concentrations were observed with multiple dosing but these were predictable from the single dose data and the dosing interval used in this study. The mean absolute bioavailability of ZOMIG Nasal Spray is approximately 41% and is similar to the tablet. The mean relative bioavailability of the nasal spray formulation is 102%, compared to the oral tablet.

Zolmitriptan and its active metabolite display dose proportionality after single or multiple dosing. Dose proportional increases in zolmitriptan and N-desmethyl metabolite C$_{max}$ and AUC were observed for 2.5 and 5 mg nasal spray doses. The pharmacokinetics for elimination of zolmitriptan and its active N-desmethyl metabolite are similar for all nasal spray dosages. The N-desmethyl metabolite is detected in plasma by 15 minutes and peak plasma concentration is generally achieved by 3 hours after administration.

Food has no significant effect on the bioavailability of zolmitriptan.

Distribution: Plasma protein binding of zolmitriptan is 25% over the concentration range of 10-1000 ng/mL. The mean (±SD) apparent volume of distribution for zolmitriptan nasal spray formulation is 8.3±3.6 L/kg.

Metabolism and Excretion: The mean elimination half-life for zolmitriptan and its active N-desmethyl metabolite following nasal spray administration are approximately 3 hours, which is similar to the half-life values seen after oral tablet administration. The half-life values were similar for zolmitriptan and the N-desmethyl metabolite after single (1 day) and multiple (4 day) nasal dosing.

Mean total plasma clearance is 25.9 mL/min/kg, of which one-sixth is renal clearance. The renal clearance is greater than the glomerular filtration rate suggesting renal tubular secretion.

The plasma concentrations and pharmacokinetics of zolmitriptan and the three major metabolites for the nasal spray and conventional tablet formulations are similar.

Special Populations and Conditions: Adolescents (12-17 years of age): In a single dose pharmacokinetic study of 5 mg zolmitriptan, systemic exposure to the parent compound was not found to differ significantly between adolescents and adults. However, plasma levels of the active metabolite were significantly greater (40-50%) in adolescents than adults.

Geriatrics (>65 years of age): Zolmitriptan pharmacokinetics in healthy elderly nonmigraineur (non-migraine sufferers) volunteers (age 65-76) were similar to those in younger non-migraineur volunteers (age 18-39).

Gender: Mean plasma concentrations of zolmitriptan were up to 1.5-fold greater in females than in males.

Race: The effect of race on the pharmacokinetics of zolmitriptan has not been systematically evaluated. Retrospective analysis of pharmacokinetic data between Japanese and Caucasian subjects revealed no significant differences.

Hepatic Insufficiency: A study to evaluate the effect of liver disease on the pharmacokinetics of zolmitriptan showed that the AUC and C$_{max}$ were increased by 94% and 50% respectively in patients with moderate liver disease and by 226% and 47% in patients with severe liver disease compared with healthy volunteers. Exposure to the metabolites, including the active N-desmethyl metabolite, was decreased. For the N-desmethyl metabolite, AUC and C$_{max}$ were reduced by 33% and 44% in patients with moderate liver disease and by 82% and 90% in patients with severe liver disease.

The effect of hepatic disease on the pharmacokinetics of zolmitriptan nasal spray has not been evaluated. Because of the similarity in exposure zolmitriptan tablets and nasal spray should have similar dosage adjustments and should be administered with caution in subjects with liver disease generally using doses less than 2.5 mg (see Warnings and Precautions).

The plasma half-life ($t_{½}$) of zolmitriptan was 4.7 hours in healthy volunteers, 7.3 hours in patients with moderate liver disease and 12 hours in those with severe liver disease. The corresponding $t_{½}$ values for the N-desmethyl metabolite were 5.7 hours, 7.5 hours and 7.8 hours respectively.

Seven out of 27 patients with hepatic impairment (4 with moderate and 3 with severe liver disease) experienced 20 to 80 mm Hg elevations in systolic and/or diastolic blood pressure after a 10 mg dose. Zomitriptan should be administered with caution in subjects with moderate or severe liver disease (see Warnings and Precautions, Hepatic and Dosage and Administration).

Renal Insufficiency: Following oral dosing in patients with severe renal impairment (ClCr ≥5-≤25 mL/min), clearance of zolmitriptan was reduced by 25% compared to normal (ClCr ≥70 mL/min). There was no significant change observed in the clearance of zolmitriptan in patients with moderate renal impairment (ClCr ≥26-≤50 mL/min). The effects of renal impairment on the pharmacokinetics of zolmitriptan nasal spray have not been evaluated.

Hypertension: No differences in the pharmacokinetics of zolmitriptan were noted in mild to moderate hypertensive volunteers compared to normotensive controls. In this study involving a limited number of patients, small dose-dependent increases in systolic and diastolic blood pressure (approximately 3 mm Hg) did not differ between mild/moderate hypertensives and normotensive controls.

STORAGE AND STABILITY: ZOMIG conventional tablets, ZOMIG RAPIMELT and ZOMIG Nasal Spray should be stored at room temperature between 15 and 30°C.

INFORMATION FOR THE PATIENT: Published in e-CPS, available by subscription at www.e-cps.ca.

DOSAGE FORMS, COMPOSITION AND PACKAGING: ZOMIG: Each yellow, round biconvex film-coated tablet, intagliated "Z" on one side, contains: zolmitriptan 2.5 mg. Nonmedicinal ingredients: anhydrous lactose, hydroxypropyl methylcellulose, magnesium stearate, microcrystalline cellulose, polyethylene glycol, sodium starch glycolate, titanium dioxide and yellow iron oxide. Blister packs of 3 and 6.

ZOMIG Nasal Spray: The ZOMIG Nasal Spray device is packaged in a carton and is a blue coloured plastic device with a grey protection cap, labelled to indicate the nominal dose. Patients should be cautioned to not remove the grey protection cap until prior to dosing. The ZOMIG Nasal Spray device is placed in a nostril and actuated to deliver a single dose, after which the device must be discarded. Patients should be cautioned to avoid spraying the contents of the device in their eyes. Nonmedicinal ingredients: citric acid, disodium phosphate (dodecahydrate or dihydrate) and purified water. Boxes of 6 single use nasal spray units.

Each ZOMIG Nasal Spray single dose unit spray supplies either 2.5 mg or 5 mg of zolmitriptan. The ZOMIG Nasal Spray unit must be discarded after use.

ZOMIG RAPIMELT: Each orally dispersible, white, round uncoated tablet, intagliated "Z" on one side with a beveled edge, contains: zolmitriptan 2.5 mg. Nonmedicinal ingredients: aspartame, citric acid, colloidal silicon dioxide, crospovidone, magnesium stearate, mannitol, microcrystalline cellulose, orange flavor and sodium bicarbonate. Blister packs of 2 and 6.

(Shown in Product Identification Section)

Zostavax®

zoster vaccine live, attenuated [Oka/Merck]

Live, Attenuated Virus Varicella-Zoster Vaccine

Merck Frosst

Date of Revision: February 9, 2010

SUMMARY PRODUCT INFORMATION:

Route of Administration	Dosage Form/ Strength	Clinically Relevant Nonmedicinal Ingredients
Subcutaneous Injection	Lyophilized powder reconstituted for injection Immunogen: varicella-zoster virus ≥19 400 PFU (plaque-forming units)	Hydrolyzed porcine gelatin and neomycin For a complete listing see Dosage Forms, Composition and Packaging.

DESCRIPTION: ZOSTAVAX (zoster vaccine live, attenuated [Oka/Merck]) is a live, attenuated virus vaccine (a lyophilized preparation of the Oka/Merck strain of varicella-zoster virus*).

INDICATIONS AND CLINICAL USE: ZOSTAVAX is indicated for the prevention of herpes zoster (shingles).

ZOSTAVAX is indicated for immunization of individuals 60 years of age or older. In a clinical trial of subjects 60 years of age or older, the overall efficacy of ZOSTAVAX against herpes zoster was 51%.

CONTRAINDICATIONS: History of hypersensitivity to any component of the vaccine, including gelatin.

History of anaphylactic/anaphylactoid reaction to neomycin (each dose of reconstituted vaccine contains trace quantities of neomycin). Neomycin allergy generally manifests as a contact dermatitis. However, a history of contact dermatitis due to neomycin is not a contraindication to receiving live virus vaccines.

Primary and acquired immunodeficiency states due to conditions such as: acute and chronic leukemias; lymphoma; other conditions affecting the bone marrow or lymphatic system; immunosuppression due to HIV/AIDS; cellular immune deficiencies.

Immunosuppressive therapy (including high-dose corticosteroids); however, ZOSTAVAX is not contraindicated for use in individuals who are receiving topical/inhaled corticosteroids or low-dose systemic corticosteroids or in patients who are receiving corticosteroids as replacement therapy, e.g., for adrenal insufficiency.

Active untreated tuberculosis.

Pregnancy (see Warnings and Precautions, Pregnant Women).

WARNINGS AND PRECAUTIONS: General: The health care provider should question the patient about reactions to a previous dose of any varicella-zoster virus (VZV)-containing vaccines (see Contraindications).

As with any vaccine, adequate treatment provisions, including epinephrine injection (1:1000), should be available for immediate use should an anaphylactic/anaphylactoid reaction occur.

Deferral of vaccination should be considered in the presence of fever >38.5°C.

ZOSTAVAX does not protect all individuals against the development of Herpes Zoster or its sequelae (see Action and Clinical Pharmacology).

The duration of protection beyond 4 years after vaccination with ZOSTAVAX is unknown. The need for revaccination has not been defined.

ZOSTAVAX has not been studied in individuals who have previously experienced an episode of herpes zoster.

Transmission: In clinical trials with ZOSTAVAX, transmission of the vaccine virus has not been reported. However, post-marketing experience with varicella vaccines suggests that transmission of vaccine virus may occur rarely between vaccinees who develop a varicella-like rash and susceptible contacts. Transmission of vaccine virus from varicella vaccine recipients without a VZV-like rash has been reported but has not been confirmed and is therefore a theoretical risk for vaccination with ZOSTAVAX.

Special Populations: Pregnant Women: There are no studies in pregnant women. It is also not known whether ZOSTAVAX can cause foetal harm when administered to a pregnant woman or can affect reproduction capacity. However naturally-occurring varicella-zoster virus infection is known to sometimes cause foetal harm. Therefore, ZOSTAVAX should not be administered to pregnant women; furthermore, pregnancy should be avoided for three months following vaccination (see Contraindications).

Nursing Women: It is not known whether VZV is secreted in human milk. Therefore, because some viruses are secreted in human milk, caution should be exercised if ZOSTAVAX is administered to a nursing woman.

Pediatrics: ZOSTAVAX is not recommended for use in this age group.

Geriatrics: The mean age of subjects enrolled in the largest (N=38 546) clinical study of ZOSTAVAX was 69 years (range 59-99 years). Of the 19 270 subjects who received ZOSTAVAX, 10 378 were 60-69 years of age, 7629 were 70-79 years of age, and 1263 were 80 years of age or older. ZOSTAVAX was demonstrated to be generally safe and effective in this population.

HIV-AIDS Patients: The safety and efficacy of ZOSTAVAX have not been established in adults who are known to be infected with HIV with or without evidence of immunosuppression (see Contraindications).

Immunocompromised Subjects: Data are not available regarding the use of ZOSTAVAX in immunocompromised subjects (see Contraindications).

ADVERSE REACTIONS: Adverse Drug Reaction Overview: In clinical trials, ZOSTAVAX has been evaluated for safety in more than 20 000 adults 50 years of age or older. ZOSTAVAX was generally well tolerated.

Clinical Trial Adverse Drug Reactions: In the largest of these trials, the Shingles Prevention Study (SPS), 38 546 subjects received a single dose of either ZOSTAVAX (n=19 270) or placebo (n=19 276) and were monitored for safety throughout the study. During the study, vaccine-related serious adverse experiences were reported for 2 subjects vaccinated with ZOSTAVAX (asthma exacerbation and polymyalgia rheumatica) and 3 subjects who received placebo (Goodpasture's syndrome, anaphylactic reaction, and polymyalgia rheumatica).

In the Adverse Event Monitoring Substudy, a subgroup of individuals from the SPS (n=3345 received ZOSTAVAX and n=3271 received placebo) were provided vaccination report cards to record adverse events occurring from Days 0 to 42 postvaccination in addition to undergoing routine safety monitoring throughout the study.

Table 1: ZOSTAVAX

Number of Subjects with ≥1 Serious Adverse Events (0-42 Days Postvaccination) in the Shingles Prevention Study

Cohort	ZOSTAVAX n/N %	Placebo n/N %	Relative Risk (95% CI)
Overall Study Cohort			
All ages	255/18 671 1.4%	254/18 717 1.4%	1.01 (0.85, 1.20)
60–69 years old	113/10 100 1.1%	101/10 095 1.0%	1.12 (0.86, 1.46)

(cont'd)

* Produced on human diploid cells (MRC-5).

Table 1: ZOSTAVAX *(cont'd)*

Number of Subjects with ≥1 Serious Adverse Events (0-42 Days Postvaccination) in the Shingles Prevention Study

Cohort	ZOSTAVAX n/N %	Placebo n/N %	Relative Risk (95% CI)
≥70 years old	142/8571 1.7%	153/8622 1.8%	0.93 (0.74, 1.17)
AE Monitoring Substudy Cohort			
All ages	64/3326 1.9%	41/3249 1.3%	1.53 (1.04, 2.25)
60–69 years old	22/1726 1.3%	18/1709 1.1%	1.21 (0.66, 2.23)
≥70 years old	42/1600 2.6%	23/1540 1.5%	1.76 (1.07, 2.89)

Legend: N=number of subjects in cohort with safety follow-up; n=number of subjects reporting an SAE 0-42 Days postvaccination.

The incidence of death was similar in the groups receiving ZOSTAVAX or placebo during the Days 0-42 postvaccination period: 14 deaths occurred in the group of subjects who received ZOSTAVAX and 16 deaths occurred in the group of subjects who received placebo. The most common reported cause of death was cardiovascular disease (10 in the group of subjects who received ZOSTAVAX, 8 in the group of subjects who received placebo). The overall incidence of death occurring at any time during the study was similar between vaccination groups: 793 deaths (4.1%) occurred in subjects who received ZOSTAVAX and 795 deaths (4.1%) in subjects who received placebo.

Vaccine-related injection-site and systemic adverse experiences reported at an incidence ≥1% are shown in Table 2. Most of these adverse experiences were reported as mild in intensity. The overall incidence of vaccine-related injection-site adverse experiences was significantly greater for subjects vaccinated with ZOSTAVAX versus subjects who received placebo (48% for ZOSTAVAX and 17% for placebo).

Table 2: ZOSTAVAX

Vaccine-Related Injection-Site and Systemic Adverse Experiences Reported in ≥1% of Adults Who Received ZOSTAVAX or Placebo (0-42 Days Postvaccination) in the Adverse Event Monitoring Substudy of the Shingles Prevention Study

Adverse Experience	ZOSTAVAX (N=3345) %	Placebo (N=3271) %
Injection Site		
Erythema[a]	35.6	6.9
Pain/tenderness[a]	34.3	8.6
Swelling[a]	26.1	4.5
Hematoma	1.6	1.4
Pruritus	7.1	1.0
Warmth	1.7	0.3
Systemic		
Headache	1.4	0.9

[a] Designates a solicited adverse experience. Injection-site adverse experiences were solicited only from Days 0-4 postvaccination.

The remainder of subjects in the SPS received routine safety monitoring, but were not provided report cards. The types of events reported in these patients were generally similar to the subgroup of patients in the Adverse Event Monitoring Substudy.

Within the 42-day postvaccination reporting period in the SPS, the number of reported noninjection-site zoster-like rashes among all subjects was small (17 for ZOSTAVAX, 36 for placebo; p=0.009). Of these 53 zoster-like rashes, 41 had specimens that were available and adequate for PCR testing. Wild-type VZV was detected in 25 (5 for ZOSTAVAX, 20 for placebo) of these specimens. The Oka/Merck strain of VZV was not detected from any of these specimens.

The number (n=59) of reported varicella-like rashes was also small. Of these varicella-like rashes, 10 had specimens that were available and adequate for PCR testing. VZV was not detected in any of these specimens. The results of virus testing in subjects with varicella-like and zoster-like rashes should be interpreted with caution due to the number of samples that were available for testing.

The numbers of subjects with elevated temperature (≥38.3°C) within 7 days post-vaccination were similar in the ZOSTAVAX and the placebo vaccination groups [6 (0.2%) vs. 8 (0.3%), respectively].

In other clinical trials conducted prior to the completion of the SPS, the reported rates of noninjection-site zoster-like and varicella-like rashes within 42 days postvaccination were also low in both zoster vaccine recipients and placebo recipients. Of the 17 reported noninjection-site zoster-like and varicella-like rashes, 10 specimens were available and adequate for PCR testing. The Oka/Merck strain was identified by PCR analysis from the lesion specimens of only two subjects who reported varicella-like rashes (onset on Day 8 and 17).

To address concerns for individuals with an unknown history of vaccination with ZOSTAVAX, the safety and tolerability of a second dose of ZOSTAVAX was evaluated. In a placebo-controlled, double-blind study, 98 adults 60 years of age or older received a second dose of ZOSTAVAX 42 days following the initial dose; the vaccine was generally well tolerated. The frequency of vaccine-related adverse experiences after the second dose of ZOSTAVAX was generally similar to that seen with the first dose.

Post-Market Adverse Drug Reactions: The following additional adverse reactions have been identified during post-marketing use of ZOSTAVAX. Because these reactions are reported voluntarily from a population of uncertain size, it is generally not possible to reliably estimate their frequency or establish a causal relationship to the vaccine.

Skin and Subcutaneous Tissue Disorders: rash.

Musculoskeletal and Connective Tissue Disorders: arthralgia; myalgia.

General Disorders and Administration Site Conditions: injection-site rash; injection-site urticaria; pyrexia; injection-site lymphadenopathy.

Immune System Disorders: hypersensitivity reactions including anaphylactic reactions.

DRUG INTERACTIONS: Overview: ZOSTAVAX must not be mixed with any other medicinal product in the same syringe. Other medicinal products must be given as separate injections and at different body sites.

Concurrent administration of ZOSTAVAX and antiviral medications known to be effective against VZV has not been evaluated.

Use with Other Vaccines: ZOSTAVAX and PNEUMOVAX 23 (pneumococcal vaccine, polyvalent, MSD Std.) should not be given concomitantly because concomitant use resulted in reduced immunogenicity of ZOSTAVAX.

DOSAGE AND ADMINISTRATION: Recommended Dose and Dosage Adjustment: For subcutaneous administration.

Do not inject intravascularly.

Individuals should receive a single dose consisting of the entire content of the vial (approximately 0.65 mL).

ZOSTAVAX is not a treatment for zoster or PHN. If an individual develops herpes zoster despite vaccination, active current standard of care treatment for herpes zoster should be considered.

At present, the duration of protection after vaccination with ZOSTAVAX is unknown. In the Shingles Prevention Study (SPS), protection was demonstrated through 4 years of follow-up. The need for revaccination has not yet been defined.

Reconstitute immediately upon removal from the freezer.

To reconstitute the vaccine, use only the diluent supplied, since it is free of preservatives or other antiviral substances which might inactivate the vaccine virus.

To reconstitute the vaccine, first withdraw the entire contents of the diluent vial into a syringe. To avoid excessive foaming, slowly inject all of the diluent in the syringe into the vial of lyophilized vaccine and gently agitate to mix thoroughly. Withdraw the entire contents into a syringe, and using a new needle, inject the total volume of reconstituted vaccine subcutaneously, preferably into the upper arm—deltoid region.

IT IS RECOMMENDED THAT THE VACCINE BE ADMINISTERED IMMEDIATELY AFTER RECONSTITUTION, TO MINIMIZE LOSS OF POTENCY. DISCARD RECONSTITUTED VACCINE IF IT IS NOT USED WITHIN 30 MINUTES.

Do not freeze reconstituted vaccine.

Caution: A sterile syringe free of preservatives, antiseptics, and detergents should be used for each injection and/or reconstitution of ZOSTAVAX because these substances may inactivate the vaccine virus.

It is important to use a separate sterile needle and syringe for each patient to prevent transfer of infectious agents from one individual to another.

Needles should be disposed of properly.

Parenteral drug products should be inspected visually for particulate matter and discoloration prior to administration, whenever solution and container permit. ZOSTAVAX when reconstituted is a semi-hazy to translucent, off-white to pale yellow liquid.

OVERDOSAGE:

There are no data with regard to overdose.

For management of a suspected drug overdose, CPhA recommends that you contact your **regional Poison Control Centre**. See the *CPS* Directory section for a list of Poison Control Centres.

ACTION AND CLINICAL PHARMACOLOGY: Herpes Zoster: Herpes zoster (HZ), known also as shingles or simply "zoster", is a manifestation of reactivation of VZV, which, as a primary infection, produces chickenpox (varicella).

Zoster is usually characterized by a unilateral, painful, vesicular cutaneous eruption with a dermatomal distribution. Although the blistering rash is the most distinctive feature of zoster, the most frequently debilitating symptom is pain, which may occur during the prodrome, the acute eruptive phase, and the postherpetic phase of the infection. During the acute eruptive phase, local pain has been reported to occur in up to 90% of immunocompetent individuals.

Anyone who has been infected with VZV, including those without a clinical history of varicella, is at risk for developing zoster, which is considered to be due to waning immunity to VZV. Nearly all adults are at risk for zoster.

The incidence and severity of zoster, as well as the frequency and severity of its complications, increase markedly with age, with two-thirds of the cases occurring in individuals older than 50 years of age. In recent studies, the lifetime risk of zoster has been estimated to be as high as 30% in the general population.

Zoster-associated hospitalization rates vary across countries and are estimated to range from 5 to 10 per 100 000 population for an average length of stay of 10 to 13 days. The proportion of zoster patients hospitalized increases with age, up to more than 10% in individuals over 65 years of age. Seventy to 80% of hospitalizations for zoster occur among immunocompetent individuals.

Zoster may be associated with serious complications such as PHN, scarring, bacterial superinfection, motor neuron palsies, pneumonia, encephalitis, Ramsay Hunt syndrome, visual impairment, hearing loss, and death.

Postherpetic Neuralgia: Postherpetic neuralgia (PHN) constitutes the most common serious complication and cause of zoster-associated morbidity in the immunocompetent host. In the SPS, where a highly specific definition of PHN was used, PHN complicated 12.5% of zoster cases in the placebo group.

PHN has been described as tender, burning, throbbing, stabbing, shooting and/or sharp pain that can persist for months or even years and can also lead to emotional distress. Allodynia (pain from an innocuous stimulus) is present in at least 90% of patients with PHN and is typically described as the most distressing and debilitating type of pain. Several definitions of PHN are widely used in the medical community, including pain persisting longer than 90 days after the onset of the rash.

Evaluation of Clinical Efficacy Afforded by ZOSTAVAX: In the Shingles Prevention Study (SPS), a placebo-controlled, double-blind clinical trial of ZOSTAVAX frozen formulation, 38 546 subjects 60 years of age or older were randomized to receive a single dose of either ZOSTAVAX (n=19 270) or placebo (n=19 276) and were followed for the development of zoster for a median of 3.1 years (range 31 days to 4.9 years). The study excluded people who were immunocompromised, anyone with a previous history of HZ, and those with conditions that might interfere with study evaluations, including people with cognitive impairment, severe hearing loss, those who were non-ambulatory and those whose survival was not considered to be at least 5 years. Randomization was stratified by age, 60-69 and ≥70 years of age. All suspected zoster cases were adjudicated by a clinical evaluation committee. Final determination of zoster cases was made by PCR, local culture, or the decision of the clinical evaluation committee, in that order. In both vaccination groups (ZOSTAVAX and placebo), subjects who developed zoster were given famciclovir, and, as necessary, pain medications. Severity of pain was evaluated according to a "worst pain" score on a 0-to-10 scale, using the Zoster Brief Pain Inventory (ZBPI), a validated questionnaire. A score of 3 or higher was considered clinically significant because it correlates with significant interference with Activities of Daily Living (ADL).

ZOSTAVAX significantly reduced the risk of developing zoster compared with placebo. The protective efficacy of ZOSTAVAX against zoster was 51% (95% CI: [44 to 58%], p<0.001).

STORAGE AND STABILITY: During shipment, to ensure that there is no loss of potency, the vaccine must be maintained at a temperature of −15°C or colder.

ZOSTAVAX **SHOULD BE STORED FROZEN** at an average temperature of −15°C or colder until it is reconstituted for **injection** (see Dosage and Administration). Any freezer, including frost-free, that has a separate sealed freezer door and reliably maintains an average temperature of −15°C or colder is acceptable for storing ZOSTAVAX. The diluent should be stored separately at room temperature (20 to 25°C) or in the refrigerator (2 to 8°C). Do not store the diluent in a freezer.

Before reconstitution, protect from light.

DISCARD IF RECONSTITUTED VACCINE IS NOT USED WITHIN 30 MINUTES.

DO NOT FREEZE THE RECONSTITUTED VACCINE.

INFORMATION FOR THE PATIENT: Published in e-CPS, available by subscription at www.e-cps.ca.

DOSAGE FORMS, COMPOSITION AND PACKAGING: ZOSTAVAX (zoster vaccine live, attenuated [Oka/Merck]) is supplied as a sterile, lyophilized white to off-white compact crystalline plug in a single-dose vial.

The diluent (Sterile Diluent for Merck & Co., Inc. live, attenuated, virus vaccines) is a sterile, clear, colourless fluid supplied separately in a single-dose vial.

After reconstitution, ZOSTAVAX is a semi-hazy to translucent, off-white to pale yellow liquid.

When reconstituted as directed, each single dose (0.65 mL) contains: varicella zoster virus, Oka/Merck strain (live, attenuated) ≥19 400 PFU†. Nonmedicinal ingredients: hydrolyzed porcine gelatin, monosodium L-glutamate monohydrate, potassium chloride, potassium phosphate monobasic, sodium chloride, sodium phosphate dibasic and sucrose. Preservative-free. The diluent is sterile water for injection. Manufacturing Process Residuals: The product also contains residual components of MRC-5 cells, and trace quantities of neomycin and bovine calf serum. 3 mL single-dose Type I glass vials. Each vial contains one dose of lyophilized vaccine (approximately 0.65 mL when reconstituted as directed). The diluent (0.7 mL) is supplied separately in 3 mL single-dose Type I glass vials. The container closure systems of ZOSTAVAX and the diluent are free of latex. ZOSTAVAX is available in packages of 1 single-dose vial. The diluent is also available in packages of 1 single-dose vial.

Zovirax® Cream Ⓟ

acyclovir

Antiviral Agent

GlaxoSmithKline

Date of Preparation: July 12, 2001
Date of Revision: March 21, 2007

† When reconstituted and stored at room temperature for up to 30 minutes.

PHARMACOLOGY: Acyclovir, a synthetic acyclic purine nucleoside analog, is a substrate with a high degree of specificity for herpes simplex and varicella-zoster specified thymidine kinase. Acyclovir is a poor substrate for host cell-specified thymidine kinase. Herpes simplex and varicella-zoster specified thymidine kinase transform acyclovir to its monophosphate, which is then transformed by a number of cellular enzymes to acyclovir diphosphate and acyclovir triphosphate. Acyclovir triphosphate is both an inhibitor of, and a substrate for, herpesvirus-specified DNA polymerase. Although the cellular α-DNA polymerase in infected cells may also be inhibited by acyclovir triphosphate, this occurs only at concentrations of acyclovir triphosphate which are higher than those which inhibit the herpesvirus-specified DNA polymerase. Acyclovir is selectively converted to its active form in herpesvirus-infected cells and is thus preferentially taken up by these cells. Acyclovir has demonstrated a very much lower toxic potential in vitro for normal uninfected cells because: 1) less is taken up; 2) less is converted to the active form; 3) cellular α-DNA polymerase has a lower sensitivity to the action of the active form of the drug. A combination of the thymidine kinase specificity, inhibition of DNA polymerase and premature termination of DNA synthesis results in inhibition of herpesvirus replication. No effect on latent non-replicating virus has been demonstrated. Inhibition of the virus reduces the period of viral shedding, limits the degree of spread and level of pathology, and thereby facilitates healing. During suppression, there is no evidence that acyclovir prevents neural migration of the virus. It aborts episodes of recurrent herpes due to inhibition of viral replication following reactivation.

INDICATIONS: For the topical management of initial episodes of genital herpes simplex infections. The prophylactic use of this preparation has not been established.

In the treatment of genital herpes, appropriate examinations should be performed to rule out other sexually transmitted diseases. Therapy should begin as early as possible after the start of an infection.

Two multicentre, double-blind, placebo-controlled studies were performed with acyclovir cream in immunocompetent patients with initial genital herpes. The cream was applied for up to 10 days or until healing had occurred. Results showed that acyclovir cream significantly reduced the duration of viral shedding, the formation of new lesions, the time to crusting and healing of lesions, and the duration of pain.

Whereas cutaneous lesions associated with herpes simplex infections are often pathognomonic, Tzanck smears prepared from lesion exudate or scrapings may assist in the diagnosis. Positive cultures for herpes simplex virus offer the only absolute means for confirmation of the diagnosis.

CONTRAINDICATIONS: For patients who develop hypersensitivity or chemical intolerance to acyclovir, valacyclovir or any of the components of the formulation, such as propylene glycol.

WARNINGS: Acyclovir cream is intended for topical use only and should not be used in the eye.

PRECAUTIONS: General: Acyclovir cream is not recommended for application to mucous membranes such as the mouth or vagina.

The recommended dosage, frequency of application and duration of treatment of acyclovir cream should not be exceeded (see Dosage).

There exist no data, at this time, which demonstrate that the use of acyclovir cream will prevent transmission of infection to other persons.

Since most cutaneous herpes simplex virus infections result from reactivation of latent virus, it is unlikely that acyclovir cream will prevent recurrence of infections when applied in the absence of signs and symptoms. Acyclovir cream should not be applied in an attempt to prevent recurrences; application should commence only at the earliest prodromal sign of disease onset.

Although clinically significant viral resistance associated with the use of acyclovir cream has not been observed, this possibility exists.

Sexual Function/ Reproduction: There is no information on the effect of acyclovir oral formulations on human female fertility. In a study of 20 male patients with normal sperm count, oral acyclovir administered at doses of up to 1 g per day for up to six months has been shown to have no clinically significant effect on sperm count, motility or morphology.

Pregnancy: Teratology studies carried out to date in animals have been negative in general. However, in a non-standard test in rats, there were fetal abnormalities such as head and tail anomalies, and maternal toxicity; since such studies are not always predictive of human response, acyclovir should not be used during pregnancy unless the physician feels the potential benefit justifies the risk of possible harm to the fetus. The potential for high concentrations of acyclovir to cause chromosome breaks in vitro should be taken into consideration in making this decision.

A postmarketing acyclovir pregnancy registry has documented pregnancy outcomes in women exposed to any formulation of acyclovir. The registry findings have not shown an increase in the number of birth defects amongst acyclovir-exposed subjects compared with the general population, and any birth defects showed no uniqueness or consistent pattern to suggest a common cause.

Lactation: Acyclovir, when given systemically, is known to be excreted into human milk. No information is available on levels of acyclovir which may appear in breast milk after administration of acyclovir cream. Caution should be exercised when acyclovir is administered to a nursing mother.

Children: Safety of use of acyclovir cream in children has not been established.

Drug Interactions: Clinical experience has identified no interactions resulting from topical or systemic administration of other drugs concomitantly with acyclovir cream.

ADVERSE EFFECTS: Because ulcerated genital lesions are characteristically tender and sensitive to any contact or manipulation, patients may experience discomfort upon application of acyclovir cream. Table 1 shows the number of initial genital herpes patients who reported adverse reactions in the 2 controlled clinical trials.

Table 1: Zovirax Cream

Adverse Effects

Adverse Reaction	Zovirax (n=54)	Placebo (n=47)
Burning/stinging on application	3	7
Rash	0	3
Itching	1	0
Retention of urine	2	2
Meningism	0	2
Paronychia	0	1
Total No. (%) of patients	6 (11%)	15 (32%)

Observed During Clinical Practice: Based on worldwide clinical practice experience in patients treated with acyclovir cream, the adverse events most commonly reported include contact dermatitis, application site reaction, eczema, allergic reaction, pain, and rash.

Less common events include pruritus, skin discoloration, urticaria, vesiculobullous rash, and facial edema.

There have been very rare reports of immediate hypersensitivity reactions including angioedema with topical acyclovir.

OVERDOSE:

Overdosage by topical application of acyclovir cream is unlikely because of limited transcutaneous absorption.

For management of a suspected drug overdose, CPhA recommends that you contact your **regional Poison Control Centre**. See the *CPS* Directory section for a list of Poison Control Centres.

DOSAGE: Apply liberally to the affected area 4 to 6 times daily for up to 10 days. A sufficient quantity of cream should be applied to adequately cover all lesions. A finger cot or rubber glove should be used while applying acyclovir cream, in order to prevent autoinoculation of other body sites or transmission of infection to other persons. **Therapy should be initiated as early as possible following onset of signs and symptoms.**

SUPPLIED: Each g of cream contains: acyclovir 50 mg. Nonmedicinal ingredients: cetostearyl alcohol, paraffin, poloxamer, propylene glycol and sodium lauryl sulfate. Tubes of 5 g. Store between 15 and 25°C and keep dry.

Zovirax® Ointment Pr

acyclovir

Antiviral Agent

GlaxoSmithKline

Date of Preparation: March 21, 2007

PHARMACOLOGY: Acyclovir, an acyclic nucleoside analog, is a substrate specific for herpesvirus-specified thymidine kinase. It inhibits replication of these viruses. Normal cellular thymidine kinase does not effectively utilize acyclovir as a substrate. Herpes virus-specified thymidine kinase transforms acyclovir to its monophosphate, which is then transformed by cellular enzymes to acyclovir diphosphate and acyclovir triphosphate. Acyclovir triphosphate is both an inhibitor of, and a substrate for, herpesvirus-specified DNA polymerase. Although the cellular α-DNA polymerase in infected cells may also be inhibited by acyclovir triphosphate, this occurs only at concentrations of acyclovir triphosphate which are higher than those which inhibit the herpesvirus-specified DNA polymerase. Acyclovir is preferentially taken up and selectively converted to its active form by herpesvirus-infected cells. Thus, acyclovir has a very much lower toxic potential for normal uninfected cells because: 1) less is taken up; 2) less is converted to the active form; 3) cellular α-DNA polymerase has a lower affinity for the active form of the drug.

INDICATIONS: For the management of initial episodes of genital herpes simplex infections. It is also indicated in the management of non life-threatening cutaneous herpes simplex virus infections in immunocompromised patients. The prophylactic use of this preparation has not been established.

In genital herpes, appropriate examinations should be performed to rule out other sexually transmitted diseases.

These indications are based on the results of a number of double-blind, placebo-controlled studies which examined changes in virus excretion, healing of lesions and relief of pain. Because of the wide biological variations inherent in herpes simplex infections, the following summary is presented merely to illustrate the spectrum of responses observed to date. As in the treatment of any infectious disease, the best response may be expected when therapy is begun at the earliest possible moment.

In immunocompromised patients, 93% were virus negative after 5 days of topical acyclovir therapy, whereas only 35% of placebo recipients were virus negative at the same time. In patients with herpes labialis, there was a significantly greater decrease in the amount of virus excreted after one day of therapy in those receiving acyclovir within 8 hours of the onset of cold sores when compared to identically treated placebo recipients.

Because complete re-epithelialization of herpes-disrupted integument necessitates recruitment of several complex repair mechanisms, the physician should be aware that the disappearance of visible lesions is somewhat variable and will occur later than the cessation of virus shedding. All immunocompromised patients who received topical acyclovir had healed their lesions 23 days after the initiation of a 10-day course of therapy; 75% of placebo patients had healed lesions at that point. Some placebo patients continued to have visible lesions for more than 30 days.

Pain associated with herpes infections is highly variable in frequency and intensity. 100% of the acyclovir-treated immunocompromised patients were pain-free by day 23 versus 70% of placebo-treated patients.

Whereas cutaneous lesions associated with herpes simplex infections are often pathognomonic, Tzanck smears prepared from lesions exudate or scrapings may assist in the diagnosis. Positive cultures for herpes simplex virus offer the only absolute means for confirmation of the diagnosis.

CONTRAINDICATIONS: Hypersensitivity or chemical intolerance to any of the components of the formulation, such as polyethylene glycol.

WARNINGS: 5% is intended for topical use only and should not be used in the eye or on mucous membranes.

PRECAUTIONS: General: The recommended dosage, frequency of application and duration of treatment of acyclovir ointment 5% should not be exceeded (see Dosage).

There exist no data, at this time, which demonstrate that the use of acyclovir ointment 5% will prevent transmission of infection to other persons.

Since most cutaneous herpes simplex virus infections result from reactivation of latent virus, is is unlikely that acyclovir ointment 5% will prevent recurrence of infections when applied in the absence of signs and symptoms. Acyclovir ointment 5% should not be applied in an attempt to prevent recurrences; application should commence only at the earliest prodromal sign of disease onset.

Although clinically significant viral resistance associated with the use of acyclovir ointment 5% has not been observed, this possibility exists.

Sexual Function/ Reproduction: There is no information on the effect of acyclovir oral formulations on human female fertility. In a study of 20 male patients with normal sperm count, oral acyclovir administered at doses of up to 1 g per day for up to six months has been shown to have no significant effect on sperm count, motility or morphology.

Lactation: Acyclovir, when given systemically, is known to be excreted into human milk. Although evidence suggests that absorption of acyclovir through the skin is minimal, caution should be exercised when acyclovir is administered to a nursing mother.

Pregnancy: All animal studies carried out to date on reproduction and teratology have been negative. However, since animal reproduction studies are not always predictive of human response, acyclovir ointment 5% should be used during pregnancy only if the physician feels the benefit will outweight the possible harm to the fetus.

A postmarketing acyclovir pregnancy registry has documented pregnancy outcomes in women exposed to any formulations of acyclovir. The registry findings have not shown an increase in the number of birth defects amongst acyclovir-exposed subjects compared with the general population, and any birth defects showed no uniqueness or consistent pattern to suggest a common cause.

Children: Safety of use of acyclovir ointment 5% in children has not been established.

Drug Interactions: Clinical experience has identified no known interactions resulting from topical or systemic administration of other drugs concomitantly with acyclovir ointment 5%.

ADVERSE EFFECTS: Because ulcerated genital lesions are characteristically tender and sensitive to any contact or manipulation, patients may experience discomfort upon application of ointment. In the controlled clinical trials, mild pain (including transient burning and stinging) was reported by 103 (28.3%) of 364 patients treated with acyclovir ointment 5% and by 115 (31.1%) of 370 patients treated with placebo; treatment was discontinued in 2 of these patients. Other local reactions among acyclovir-treated patients included pruritus in 15 (4.1%), rash in 1 (0.3%) and vulvitis in 1 (0.3%). Among the placebo-treated patients, pruritus was reported by 17 (4.6%) and rash by 1 (0.3%).

In all studies, there was no significant difference between the drug and placebo group in the rate or type of reported adverse reactions.

There have been very rare reports of immediate hypersensitivity reactions including angioedema with topical acyclovir.

OVERDOSE:

Overdosage by topical application of acyclovir ointment 5% is unlikely because of limited transcutaneous absorption.

For management of a suspected drug overdose, CPhA recommends that you contact your **regional Poison Control Centre**. See the *CPS* Directory section for a list of Poison Control Centres.

DOSAGE: Apply acyclovir ointment 5% liberally to the affected area 4 to 6 times daily for up to 10 days. A sufficient quantity of ointment should be applied to adequately cover all lesions. A finger cot or rubber glove should be used while applying acyclovir in order to prevent: (1) autoinoculation of other body sites or (2) transmission of infection to other persons. Therapy should be initiated as early as possible following onset of signs and symptoms.

SUPPLIED: Each g contains: acyclovir 50 mg in a polyethylene glycol base. Tubes of 4, 15 and 30 g. Store between 15 to 25°C and keep dry.

Zovirax® Oral ℞

acyclovir

Antiviral Agent

GlaxoSmithKline

Date of Revision: September 10, 2008

SUMMARY PRODUCT INFORMATION:

Route of Administration	Dosage Form/ Strength	Clinically Relevant Nonmedicinal Ingredients
Oral	Oral suspension 200 mg/5 mL Tablets 200 mg, 400 mg and 800 mg	ZOVIRAX 200 mg Tablets contain lactose. For a complete listing see Dosage Forms, Composition and Packaging.

INDICATIONS AND CLINICAL USE: ZOVIRAX (acyclovir) is indicated for the following conditions:

- The treatment of initial episodes of herpes genitalis.
- The suppression of unusually frequent recurrences of herpes genitalis (6 or more episodes per year).
- The acute treatment of herpes zoster (shingles) and varicella (chickenpox).

The results of clinical studies suggest that some patients with recurrent genital herpes may derive clinical benefit from the administration of oral ZOVIRAX if taken at the first sign of an impending episode. Those most likely to benefit are patients who experience severe, prolonged recurrences; such intermittent therapy may be more appropriate than suppressive therapy when these recurrences are infrequent.

Early treatment of acute herpes zoster (shingles) in immunocompetent individuals with oral ZOVIRAX resulted in decreased viral shedding; decreased time to healing; less dissemination; and alleviation of acute pain.

Treatment of varicella (chickenpox) in immunocompetent patients with oral ZOVIRAX reduced the total number of lesions, accelerated the progression of lesions to the crusted and healed stages, and decreased the number of residual hypopigmented lesions. In addition, ZOVIRAX decreased fever and constitutional symptoms associated with chickenpox.

The prophylactic use of acyclovir in chickenpox has not been established.

Geriatrics (≥65 years of age): Use in the geriatric population may be associated with differences in safety due to age-related changes in renal function and a brief discussion can be found in the appropriate sections (see Warnings and Precautions).

Pediatrics (<2 years old): No data is available.

CONTRAINDICATIONS: ZOVIRAX (acyclovir) is contraindicated for patients who develop hypersensitivity or who are hypersensitive to acyclovir, valacyclovir or any other components of the formulations of ZOVIRAX. For a complete listing, see Dosage Forms, Composition and Packaging.

WARNINGS AND PRECAUTIONS: General: Care should be taken to maintain adequate hydration in patients receiving high oral doses of acyclovir.

Suppressive therapy of herpes genitalis with ZOVIRAX (acyclovir) should be considered only for severely affected patients. Periodic evaluation of the need for continued suppressive therapy is recommended. In some patients, there is a tendency for the first recurrent episode to be more severe following cessation of suppressive therapy.

In severely immunocompromised patients, the physician should be aware that prolonged or repeated courses of acyclovir may result in selection of resistant viruses associated with infections which may not respond. Thrombotic thrombocytopenic purpura/haemolytic uremic syndrome (TTP/HUS), which has resulted in death, has occurred in immunocompromised patients receiving ZOVIRAX therapy.

The recommended dosage and length of treatment should not be exceeded (see Dosage and Administration). The decision to prescribe a course of suppressive therapy should be weighed in the light of our present knowledge about the long-term effects of ZOVIRAX and must clearly relate to the condition of the patient.

Whereas cutaneous lesions associated with herpes simplex infections are often pathognomonic, Tzanck smears prepared from lesion exudate or scrapings may assist in the diagnosis. Positive cultures for herpes simplex virus offer the only absolute means for confirmation of the diagnosis. Appropriate examinations should be performed to rule out other sexually transmitted diseases. All patients should be advised to take particular care to avoid potential transmission of virus if active lesions are present while they are on therapy. Genital herpes can also be transmitted in the absence of symptoms through asymptomatic viral shedding.

The clinical status of the patient and the adverse event profile of ZOVIRAX should be borne in mind when considering the patient's ability to drive or operate machinery. There have been no studies to investigate the effect of ZOVIRAX on driving performance or the ability to operate machinery. Further, a detrimental effect on such activities cannot be predicted from the pharmacology of the active substance.

Although chickenpox in otherwise healthy children is usually a self-limited disease of mild to moderate severity, adolescents and adults tend to have more severe disease. Treatment was initiated within 24 hours of the typical chickenpox rash in the controlled studies, and there is no information regarding the effects of treatment begun later in the disease course. It is unknown whether the treatment of chickenpox in childhood has any effect on long-term immunity. However, there is no evidence to indicate that treatment of chickenpox with ZOVIRAX would have any effect on either decreasing or increasing the incidence or severity of subsequent recurrences of herpes zoster (shingles) later in life.

Carcinogenesis and Mutagenesis: ZOVIRAX has caused mutagenesis in some acute studies at high concentrations of the drug.

Renal: Renal insufficiency or acute renal failure has been observed in patients taking ZOVIRAX at the recommended dosage and/or with no previous renal conditions and may be associated with renal pain (see Adverse Reactions, Post-Market Adverse Drug Reactions).

Acyclovir is eliminated by renal clearance, therefore the dose must be reduced in patients with renal impairment (see Dosage and Administration, Patients with Acute or Chronic Renal Impairment). Elderly patients are likely to have reduced renal function and therefore the need for dose reduction must be considered in this group of patients. Both elderly patients and patients with renal impairment are at increased risk of developing neurological side effects and should be closely monitored for evidence of these effects. In the reported cases, these reactions were generally reversible on discontinuation of treatment (see Adverse Reactions).

Caution should be exercised when administering to patients receiving potentially nephrotoxic agents since this may increase the risk of renal dysfunction.

Sexual Function/Reproduction: In a study of 20 male patients with normal sperm count, oral acyclovir administered at doses of up to 1 g per day for up to six months has been shown to have no clinically significant effect on sperm count, motility or morphology. There is no information on the effect of acyclovir oral formulations on human female fertility.

Special Populations: Pregnant Women: Teratology studies carried out to date in animals have been negative in general. However, in a non-standard test in rats, there were fetal abnormalities such as head and tail anomalies, and maternal toxicity; since such studies are not always predictive of human response, ZOVIRAX should not be used during pregnancy unless the physician feels the potential benefit justifies the risk of possible harm to the fetus. The potential for high concentrations of acyclovir to cause chromosome breaks in vitro should be taken into consideration in making this decision.

A post-marketing acyclovir pregnancy registry has documented pregnancy outcomes in women exposed to any formulation of ZOVIRAX. The registry findings have not shown an increase in the number of birth defects amongst subjects exposed to ZOVIRAX compared with the general population, and any birth defects showed no uniqueness or consistent pattern to suggest a common cause.

Nursing Women: Acyclovir concentrations have been documented in breast milk in 2 women following oral administration of acyclovir and ranged from 0.6 to 4.1 times corresponding plasma levels. These concentrations would potentially expose the nursing infant to a dose of acyclovir up to 0.3 mg/kg per day. Caution should therefore be exercised when ZOVIRAX is administered to a nursing woman.

Pediatrics: Safety and effectiveness in children less than 2 years of age have not been adequately studied.

Geriatrics: The possibility of renal impairment in the elderly must be considered and the dosage should be adjusted accordingly (see Warnings and Precautions, Renal and Dosage and Administration, Patients with Acute or Chronic Renal Impairment). Adequate hydration of elderly patients taking high oral doses of acyclovir should be maintained.

ADVERSE REACTIONS: Adverse Drug Reaction Overview: The most frequent adverse reactions associated with the use of ZOVIRAX (acyclovir) are headache and nausea.

Neurological side effects have also been reported in rare instances. Elderly patients and patients with a history of renal impairment are at increased risk of developing these effects. In the reported cases, these reactions were generally reversible on discontinuation of treatment (see Warnings and Precautions and Adverse Reactions, Post-Market Adverse Drug Reactions).

Clinical Trial Adverse Drug Reactions: Because clinical trials are conducted under very specific conditions the adverse reaction rates observed in the clinical trials may not reflect the rates observed in practice and should not be compared to the rates in the clinical trials of another drug. Adverse drug reaction information from clinical trials is useful for identifying drug-related adverse events and for approximating rates.

Treatment of Herpes Simplex: Short-term administration (5-10 days): The most frequent adverse reactions reported during clinical trials of treatment of genital herpes with oral ZOVIRAX in 298 patients are listed in Table 1.

Table 1: ZOVIRAX Oral

Adverse Reactions Reported in Clinical Trials of Treatment of Genital Herpes with Acyclovir

Adverse Reactions	Total	%
Nausea and/or Vomiting	8	2.7

Suppression of Herpes Simplex: Long-term administration: The most frequent adverse events reported in a clinical trial for the prevention of recurrences with continuous administration of 400 mg (two 200 mg capsules) 2 times daily are listed in Table 2.

Table 2: ZOVIRAX Oral

Adverse Reactions Reported in a Clinical Trial for the Prevention of Recurrences of Genital Herpes with Acyclovir

Adverse Reactions	1st Year (n=586) (%)	2nd Year (n=390) (%)	3rd Year (n=329) (%)
Nausea	4.8		
Diarrhea	2.4		
Headache	1.9	1.5	0.9
Rash	1.7	1.3	
Paresthesia		0.8	1.2
Asthenia			1.2

Evidence so far from clinical trials suggests that the severity and frequency of adverse events is unlikely to necessitate discontinuation of therapy.

Herpes Zoster: The most frequent adverse reactions reported during three clinical trials of treatment of herpes zoster (shingles) with 800 mg of oral ZOVIRAX 5 times daily for 7 or 10 days or placebo are listed in Table 3.

Table 3: ZOVIRAX Oral

Adverse Reactions Reported in Clinical Trials of Treatment of Herpes Zoster

Adverse Reactions	ZOVIRAX (n=323) (%)	Placebo (n=323) (%)
Malaise	11.5	11.1
Nausea	8.0	11.5
Headache	5.9	11.1
Vomiting	2.5	2.5
Diarrhea	1.5	0.3

Chickenpox: The most frequent adverse events reported during three clinical trials of treatment of chickenpox with oral ZOVIRAX or placebo are listed in Table 4.

Table 4: ZOVIRAX Oral

Adverse Reactions Reported in Clinical Trials of Treatment of Chickenpox

Adverse Reactions	ZOVIRAX (n=495) (%)	Placebo (n=498) (%)
Diarrhea	3.2	2.2

Less Common Clinical Trial Adverse Drug Reactions (<1%): Other adverse reactions reported in less than 1% of patients receiving ZOVIRAX in any clinical trial included: abdominal pain, anorexia, constipation, dizziness, edema, fatigue, flatulence, inguinal adenopathy, insomnia, leg pain, medication taste, skin rash, sore throat, spasmodic hand movement and urticaria.

Abnormal Hematologic and Clinical Chemistry Findings: No clinically significant changes in laboratory values have been observed in clinical trials for the treatment of chickenpox and zoster, and for the treatment and suppression of genital herpes with ZOVIRAX.

Post-Market Adverse Drug Reactions: The following events have been reported voluntarily during post-market use of ZOVIRAX in clinical practice. These events have been chosen for inclusion due to either their seriousness, frequency of reporting, potential causal connection to ZOVIRAX or a combination of these factors. Post-market adverse events are reported spontaneously from a population of unknown size, thus estimates of frequency cannot be made.

General: fever, headache, pain and peripheral edema.

Nervous: dizziness, paresthesia, agitation, confusion, tremor, ataxia, dysarthria, hallucinations, psychotic symptoms, convulsions, somnolence, encephalopathy and coma have been reported. These events are generally reversible and usually reported in patients with renal impairment, or with other predisposing factors (see Warnings and Precautions). These symptoms may be marked, particularly in older adults.

Digestive: diarrhea, gastrointestinal distress, nausea.

Hematological and Lymphatic: anaemia, leukopenia, lymphadenopathy and thrombocytopenia.

Hypersensitivity and Skin: alopecia, erythema multiforme, Stevens-Johnson syndrome, toxic epidermal necrolysis, rashes including photosensitivity, pruritus, urticaria, dyspnoea, angioedema and anaphylaxis.

Hepatobiliary Tract and Pancreas: reports of reversible hyperbilirubinemia and elevated liver related enzymes. Hepatitis and jaundice.

Musculoskeletal: myalgia.

Special Senses: visual abnormalities.

Urogenital: elevated blood creatinine and blood urea nitrogen (BUN). Acute renal failure, renal pain and hematuria have been reported. Renal pain may be associated with renal failure (see Warnings and Precautions).

DRUG INTERACTIONS: Drug-Drug Interactions: No clinically significant interactions have been identified.

Acyclovir is eliminated primarily unchanged in the urine via active renal tubular secretion. Any drugs administered concurrently that compete with this mechanism may increase acyclovir plasma concentrations. Probenecid and cimetidine increase the area under the curve (AUC) of acyclovir by this mechanism, and reduce acyclovir renal clearance. Similarly increases in plasma AUCs of acyclovir and of the inactive metabolite of mycophenolate mofetil, an immunosuppressant agent used in transplant patients have been shown when the drugs are coadministered. However, no dosage adjustment is necessary because of the wide therapeutic index of acyclovir.

Drug-Food Interactions: There is no known interaction with food (see Action and Clinical Pharmacology, Pharmacokinetics).

Drug-Herb Interactions: Interactions with herbal products have not been established.

Drug-Laboratory Test Interactions: Interactions with laboratory tests have not been established.

DOSAGE AND ADMINISTRATION: Dosing Considerations:

- The dosage of ZOVIRAX (acyclovir) should be reduced in patients with impaired renal function.
- Therapy should be initiated as soon as possible after a diagnosis of chickenpox or herpes zoster, or at the first sign or symptoms of an outbreak of genital herpes.
- The recommended dose and duration of use is dependent on the indication.

Recommended Dose and Dosage Adjustment: Treatment of Initial Infection of Herpes Genitalis: 200 mg (one 200 mg tablet or one teaspoonful of suspension [5 mL]) every 4 hours, 5 times daily for a total of 1 g daily for 10 days. Therapy should be initiated as early as possible following onset of signs and symptoms.

Suppressive Therapy for Recurrent Herpes Genitalis: The initial recommended dose is 200 mg (one 200 mg tablet or one teaspoonful of suspension [5 mL]) three times daily. This can be increased if breakthrough occurs up to a dosage of one 200 mg tablet or one teaspoonful [5 mL] of suspension, five times daily. If necessary, a dose of 400 mg (one 400 mg tablet [two 200 mg tablets] or two teaspoonfuls of suspension [10 mL]) given twice daily may be considered. Periodic re-evaluation of the need for therapy is recommended.

Administration of ZOVIRAX for intermittent therapy is 200 mg (one 200 mg tablet or one teaspoonful [5 mL] of suspension) every 4 hours 5 times daily for 5 days. Therapy should be initiated at the earliest sign or symptom (prodrome) of recurrence.

Treatment of Herpes Zoster: 800 mg (one 800 mg tablet, or 800 mg of another oral dosage form), every 4 hours, 5 times daily for 7 to 10 days. Treatment should be initiated within 72 hours of the onset of lesions. In clinical trials, the greatest benefit occurred when treatment was begun within 48 hours of the onset of lesions.

Treatment of Chickenpox: 20 mg/kg (not to exceed 800 mg) orally, 4 times daily for 5 days. Therapy should be initiated within 24 hours of the appearance of rash.

Patients with Acute or Chronic Renal Impairment: Caution is advised when administering acyclovir to patients with impaired renal function. Adequate hydration should be maintained.

Comprehensive pharmacokinetic studies have been completed following intravenous acyclovir infusions in patients with renal impairment.

Based on these studies, dosage adjustments are recommended in Table 5 for genital herpes and herpes zoster indications.

Table 5: ZOVIRAX Oral
Dosage Modification for Renal Impairment

Normal Dosage Regimen	Creatinine Clearance (mL/min/1.73 m²)	Adjusted Dosage Regimen	
		Dose (mg)	**Dosing Interval (hours)**
200 mg every 4 hours	>10	200	every 4 hours, 5×daily
	0–10	200	every 12 hours
400 mg every 12 hours	>10	400	every 12 hours
	0–10	200	every 12 hours
800 mg every 4 hours	>25	800	every 4 hours, 5×daily
	10–25	800	every 8 hours
	0–10	800	every 12 hours

Hemodialysis: For patients who require hemodialysis, the mean plasma half-life of acyclovir during hemodialysis is approximately 5 hours. This results in a 60% decrease in plasma concentrations following a six-hour dialysis period. Therefore, the patient's dosing schedule should be adjusted so that an additional dose is administered after each dialysis.

Peritoneal Dialysis: No supplement dose appears to be necessary after adjustment of the dosing interval.

Missed Dose: If a dose of ZOVIRAX is missed, the patient should be advised to take it as soon as he/she remembers, and then continue with the next dose at the proper time interval.

OVERDOSAGE:

Activated charcoal may be administered to aid in the removal of unabsorbed drug. General supportive measures are recommended.

Acyclovir is only partly absorbed in the gastrointestinal tract. Patients have ingested up to 20 g acyclovir on a single occasion, with no unexpected adverse effects. In clinical studies, the highest plasma concentration observed in a single patient at these doses was 10.0 µg/mL. Accidental, repeated overdoses of oral acyclovir over several days have been associated with gastrointestinal effects (such as nausea and vomiting) and neurological effects (headache and confusion).

Intravenous doses administered to humans have been as high as 1200 mg/m² (28 mg/kg) 3 times daily for up to 2 weeks. Peak plasma concentrations have reached 80 µg/mL. Overdosage of intravenous acyclovir has resulted in elevations of serum creatinine, blood urea nitrogen and subsequent renal failure. Neurological effects including confusion, hallucinations, agitation, seizures and coma have been described in association with intravenous overdosage.

Patients should be observed closely for signs of toxicity. Hemodialysis significantly enhances the removal of acyclovir from the blood and may, therefore be considered a management option in the event of symptomatic overdose. Precipitation of acyclovir in renal tubules may occur if the solubility (2.5 mg/mL) in the intratubular fluid is exceeded. In the event of renal failure and anuria, the patient may benefit from hemodialysis until renal function is restored (see Dosage and Administration).

> For management of a suspected drug overdose, contact your **regional Poison Control Centre**. See the *CPS* Directory section for a list of Poison Control Centres.

ACTION AND CLINICAL PHARMACOLOGY: Mechanism of Action: ZOVIRAX (acyclovir), a synthetic acyclic purine nucleoside analog, is a substrate with a high degree of specificity for herpes simplex and varicella-zoster specified thymidine kinase. Acyclovir is a poor substrate for host cell-specified thymidine kinase. Herpes simplex and varicella-zoster specified thymidine kinase transform acyclovir to its monophosphate which is then transformed by a number of cellular enzymes to acyclovir diphosphate and acyclovir triphosphate. Acyclovir triphosphate is both an inhibitor of, and a substrate for, herpesvirus-specified DNA polymerase. Although the cellular α-DNA polymerase in infected cells may also be inhibited by acyclovir triphosphate, this occurs only at concentrations of acyclovir triphosphate which are higher than those which inhibit the herpesvirus-specified DNA polymerase. Acyclovir is selectively converted to its active form in herpesvirus-infected cells and is thus preferentially taken up by these cells. Acyclovir has demonstrated a very much lower toxic potential in vitro for normal uninfected cells because: 1) less is taken up; 2) less is converted to the active form; 3) cellular α-DNA polymerase has a lower sensitivity to the action of the active form of the drug. A combination of the thymidine kinase specificity, inhibition of DNA polymerase and premature termination of DNA synthesis results in inhibition of herpes virus replication. No effect on latent non-replicating virus has been demonstrated. Inhibition of the virus reduces the period of viral shedding, limits the degree of spread and level of pathology, and thereby facilitates healing. During suppression there is no evidence that acyclovir prevents neural migration of the virus. It aborts episodes of recurrent herpes due to inhibition of viral replication following reactivation.

Pharmacokinetics: The pharmacokinetics of acyclovir after oral administration have been evaluated in 6 clinical studies involving 110 adult patients.

Absorption: In one study of 35 immunocompromised patients with herpes simplex or varicella-zoster infection given ZOVIRAX Capsules in doses of 200 to 1000 mg every 4 hours, 6 times daily for 5 days, the bioavailability was estimated to be 15 to 20%. In this study, steady-state plasma levels were reached by the second day of dosing. Mean steady-state peak and trough concentrations following the last 200 mg dose were 0.49 µg/mL (0.47 to 0.54 µg/mL) and 0.31 µg/mL (0.18 to 0.41 µg/mL), respectively and following the last 800 mg dose were 2.8 µg/mL (2.3 to 3.1 µg/mL) and 1.8 µg/mL (1.3 to 2.5 µg/mL). In another study, 20 immunocompetent patients with recurrent genital herpes simplex infections given ZOVIRAX Capsules in dose of 800 mg every 6 hours, 4 times daily for 5 days, the mean steady-state peak and trough concentrations were 1.4 µg/mL (0.66 to 1.8 µg/mL) and 0.55 µg/mL (0.14 to 1.1 µg/mL).

In a multiple-dose crossover study where 23 volunteers received ZOVIRAX as one 200 mg capsule, one 400 mg tablet and one 800 mg tablet 6 times daily, absorption decreased with increasing dose and the estimated bioavailabilities of acyclovir were 20, 15 and 10%, respectively. The decrease in bioavailability is believed to be a function of the dose and not the dosage form. It was demonstrated that acyclovir is not dose proportional over the dosing range 200 mg to 800 mg. In this study, steady-state peak and trough concentrations of acyclovir were 0.83 and 0.46 µg/mL, 1.21 and 0.63 µg/mL, and 1.61 and 0.83 µg/mL for the 200, 400 and 800 mg dosage regimens, respectively.

In another study in 6 volunteers, the influence of food on the absorption of acyclovir was not apparent.

A single oral dose bioavailability study in 23 normal volunteers showed that ZOVIRAX Capsules 200 mg are bioequivalent to 200 mg acyclovir in aqueous solution. In a separate study in 20 volunteers, it was shown that ZOVIRAX Suspension is bioequivalent to ZOVIRAX Capsules. In a different single-dose bioavailability/bioequivalence study in 24 volunteers, one ZOVIRAX 800 mg Tablet was demonstrated to be bioequivalent to four ZOVIRAX 200 mg Capsules.

Distribution: Plasma protein binding is relatively low (9 to 33%) and drug interactions involving binding site displacement are not anticipated.

Excretion: Following oral administration, the mean plasma half-life of acyclovir in volunteers and patients with normal renal function ranged from 2.5 to 3.3 hours. The mean renal excretion of unchanged drug accounts for 14.4% (8.6 to 19.8%) of the orally administered dose. The only urinary metabolite (identified by high performance liquid chromatography) is 9-[(carboxymethoxy)methyl]guanine.

Special Populations and Conditions: Pediatrics: In general, the pharmacokinetics of acyclovir in children is similar to adults. Mean half-life after oral doses of 300 mg/m² and 600 mg/m², in children aged 7 months to 7 years, was 2.6 hours (range 1.59 to 3.74 hours).

Orally administered acyclovir in children less than 2 years of age has not yet been fully studied.

Geriatrics: In the elderly, total body clearance falls with increasing age, associated with decreases in creatinine clearance, although there is little change in the terminal plasma half-life. Dosage reduction may be required in geriatric patients with reduced renal function (see Dosage and Administration).

Renal Insufficiency: The half-life and total body clearance of acyclovir are dependent on renal function.

A dosage adjustment is recommended for patients with reduced renal function (see Dosage and Administration).

STORAGE AND STABILITY: ZOVIRAX Tablets should be stored at controlled room temperature (15 to 25°C) in a dry place and protected from light.

ZOVIRAX Suspension should be stored at controlled room temperature (15 to 25°C).

INFORMATION FOR THE PATIENT: Published in e-CPS, available by subscription at www.e-cps.ca.

DOSAGE FORMS, COMPOSITION AND PACKAGING: Suspension: Each 5 mL of off-white, banana-flavored suspension contains: acyclovir 200 mg. Nonmedicinal ingredients: banana flavor, cellulose, glycerin, methylparaben, propylparaben, sorbitol, vanillin and water. Bottles of 475 mL.

Tablets: ZOVIRAX 200: Each blue, shield-shaped, beveled-edge, compressed tablet, imprinted "ZOVIRAX" on one side and a triangle on the reverse contains: acyclovir 200 mg. Nonmedicinal ingredients: cellulose, indigotine, lactose, magnesium stearate, povidone and sodium starch glycolate. Bottles of 100.

ZOVIRAX 400 WELLSTAT PAC: Each pink, shield-shaped, bevel-edged, compressed tablet, imprinted with "ZOVIRAX 400" on one side and a triangle on the reverse, contains: acyclovir 400 mg. Nonmedicinal ingredients: cellulose, magnesium stearate, povidone, iron oxide and sodium starch glycolate. Cartons of 56 blister-packed tablets.

ZOVIRAX 800 ZOSTAB PAC: Each blue, biconvex, elongated, scored, compressed tablet, imprinted with "ZOVIRAX 800" on one side, contains: acyclovir 800 mg. Nonmedicinal ingredients: cellulose, indigotine, povidone, magnesium stearate and sodium starch glycolate. Cartons of 50 blister-packed tablets.

(Shown in Product Identification Section)

Z-PAK™ (Zithromax™) Ⓟ

azithromycin dihydrate

Antibiotic

Pfizer

SUPPLIED: Each pink, film-coated, modified capsular-shaped tablet, engraved "Pfizer" on the upper face, "306" or scored on the lower face, contains: azithromycin dihydrate equivalent to azithromycin 250 mg. Nonmedicinal ingredients: anhydrous calcium phosphate dibasic, D&C Red #30 aluminum lake, hydroxypropyl methylcellulose, lactose, magnesium stearate, pregelatinized starch, sodium croscarmellose, sodium lauryl sulfate, titanium dioxide and triacetin. Single treatment package Z-PAK of 6 blister-packaged tablets per box. Store at controlled room temperature between 15 and 30°C.

Z-Plus®

menthol—zinc pyrithione

Antiseborrheic—Antidandruff

Dormer

SUPPLIED: Each mL of medicated shampoo and scalp cleanser contains: zinc pyrithione 2% w/w and menthol 0.3% w/w. Nonmedicinal ingredients: ammonium laureth sulfate, butylparaben, citric acid, dimethicone copolyol, FD&C Blue No. 1, fragrance, glycol distearate, hydroxypropyl methylcellulose, isopropylparaben, isobutylparaben, lauramide DEA, panthenol, polyquaternium-7, purified water, TEA-lauryl sulfate and titanium dioxide. Plastic bottles of 125 mL.

Zyban® Ⓟ

bupropion HCl

Smoking Cessation Aid

Biovail Pharmaceuticals

Date of Preparation: November 14, 2008
Date of Revision: February 4, 2009

PHARMACOLOGY: The mechanism by which ZYBAN (bupropion hydrochloride) enhances the ability of patients to abstain from smoking is unknown. However, it is presumed that this action is mediated by noradrenergic and/or dopaminergic mechanisms. ZYBAN is a weak inhibitor of the neuronal uptake of norepinephrine, serotonin, and dopamine, and does not inhibit monoamine oxidase. ZYBAN is chemically unrelated to nicotine or other agents currently used in the treatment of nicotine addiction.

Bupropion, initially developed as an antidepressant of the aminoketone class, is chemically unrelated to tricyclic, tetracyclic, selective serotonin re-uptake inhibitors or other known antidepressant agents. Its structure closely resembles that of diethylpropion; it is related to phenylethylamines.

Pharmacokinetics: Following oral administration of ZYBAN Tablets to healthy volunteers, peak plasma concentrations of bupropion are achieved within 3 hours. Food increased C_{max} and AUC of bupropion by 11% and 17%, respectively, indicating that there is no clinically significant food effect. In vitro tests indicate that bupropion is 84% bound to human albumin at plasma concentrations up to 200 µg/mL.

The mean elimination half-life (±SD) of bupropion after chronic dosing is 21 (±9) hours, and steady-state plasma concentrations of bupropion are reached within 5 days.

Three active metabolites have been identified. Bupropion and its metabolites exhibit linear kinetics following chronic administration of 150 to 300 mg/day. Plasma concentrations of the metabolites exceed those of the parent drug and may be clinically important.

The Nicotine Transdermal System (NTS) used in clinical trials did not appear to have effects on the pharmacokinetics of ZYBAN. Smokers and non-smokers appear to have similar pharmacokinetics of bupropion or its major metabolites.

Clinical Trials: The efficacy of ZYBAN as an aid to smoking cessation was demonstrated in 2 placebo-controlled, double-blind trials in nondepressed chronic cigarette smokers (n=1508, ≥15 cigarettes/day). In a third study, the efficacy of chronic administration (up to 1 year) of ZYBAN in preventing relapse to smoking was studied in a placebo-controlled, double-blind trial of nondepressed chronic cigarette smokers (n=432, ≥15 cigarettes/day). In these studies, ZYBAN was used in conjunction with individual smoking cessation counseling.

The first study was a dose-response trial conducted at 3 clinical centres. Patients in this study were treated for 7 weeks with 1 of 3 doses of bupropion (100, 150 or 300 mg/day) or placebo; quitting was defined as total abstinence during the last 4 weeks of treatment (weeks 4 through 7). Abstinence was determined by patient daily diaries and verified by carbon monoxide levels in expired air.

Table 1 shows a dose-dependent increase in the percentage of patients able to achieve 4-week abstinence (weeks 4 through 7). Treatment with ZYBAN at both 150 and 300 mg/day was significantly more effective than placebo, in this study. Treatment with ZYBAN (7 weeks at 300 mg/day) was more effective than placebo in helping patients maintain continuous abstinence through week 26 (6 months) of the study.

Table 1: ZYBAN

Dose-response Trial: Quit Rates by Treatment Group (Intent to Treat Analysis)

	Treatment Groups			
Abstinence From Week 4 Through Specified Week	**Placebo (n=151) % (95% CI)**	**ZYBAN 100 mg/day (n=153) % (95% CI)**	**ZYBAN 150 mg/day (n=153) % (95% CI)**	**ZYBAN 300 mg/day (n=156) % (95% CI)**
Week 7 (4-week quit)	17% (11–23)	22% (15–28)	27%[a] (20–35)	36%[a] (28–43)
Week 12	14% (8–19)	20% (13–26)	20% (14–27)	25%[a] (18–32)
Week 26	11% (6–16)	16% (11–22)	18% (12–24)	19%[a] (13–25)

a Significantly different from placebo (P≤0.05).

Quit rates are the proportions of all persons initially enrolled who abstained from week 4 of the study through the specified week.

The second study was a comparative trial conducted at four clinical centers. Four treatments were evaluated: ZYBAN 300 mg/day, HABITROL (nicotine transdermal system) (NTS) 21 mg/day, combination of ZYBAN 300 mg/day plus NTS 21 mg/day, and placebo. Patients were treated with ZYBAN for 9 weeks. Treatment with ZYBAN was initiated at 150 mg/day while the patient was still smoking and was increased after 3 days to 300 mg/day given as 150 mg twice daily. NTS 21 mg/day was added to treatment with ZYBAN after approximately 1 week when the patient reached the target quit date. During weeks 8 and 9 of the study, NTS was tapered to 14 and 7 mg/day, respectively. Quitting, defined as total abstinence during weeks 4 through 7, was determined by patient daily diaries and verified by expired air carbon monoxide levels.

In this study (see Table 2), patients treated with either ZYBAN or NTS achieved greater 4 week abstinence rates than patients treated with placebo. In addition, patients treated with the combination of ZYBAN and NTS achieved higher 4 week abstinence rates than patients treated with either of the individual active treatments alone, although only the comparison with NTS achieved statistical significance. Both ZYBAN and the combination of ZYBAN and NTS were more effective than placebo and NTS in helping patients maintain abstinence through week 52 of the study. Although the treatment combination of ZYBAN and NTS displayed the highest rates of continuous abstinence throughout the study, the quit rates for the combination were not significantly higher (P>0.05) than for ZYBAN alone. Quit rates for ZYBAN were similar in patients with and without prior quit attempts using nicotine replacement therapy.

Table 2: ZYBAN

Comparative Trial: Quit Rates by Treatment Group

	Treatment Groups			
Abstinence From Week 4 Through Specified Week	**Placebo (n=160) % (95% CI)**	**Nicotine Transdermal System (NTS) 21 mg/day (n=244) % (95% CI)**	**ZYBAN 300 mg/day (n=244) % (95% CI)**	**ZYBAN 300 mg/day and NTS 21 mg/day (n=245) % (95% CI)**
Week 7 (4-week quit)	23% (17–30)	36%[a] (30–42)	49%[a,c] (43–56)	58%[a,c] (51–64)
Week 12	20% (14–26)	29%[b] (23–34)	41%[a,c] (34–47)	48%[a,c] (42–54)
Week 26	13% (7–18)	18% (14–23)	30%[a,c] (24–35)	33%[a,c] (27–39)
Week 52	8% (3–12)	12% (8–16)	23%[a,c] (18–28)	28%[a,c] (23–34)

a P<0.01 vs placebo.
b P<0.05 vs placebo.
c P<0.01 vs NTS.

The third study was a long-term relapse prevention trial conducted at five clinical centers. Patients in this study received open-label ZYBAN 300 mg/day for 7 weeks. Patients who quit smoking while receiving ZYBAN were then randomized to ZYBAN 300 mg/day or placebo for a total study duration of 1 year. Abstinence from smoking was determined by patient self-report and verified by expired air carbon monoxide levels. Relapse was defined as the first cigarette smoked.

Results of this 1-year trial demonstrated statistically significantly less relapse to smoking for those patients taking ZYBAN compared to those taking placebo. The time for 50% of the patients to relapse to smoking was significantly longer for ZYBAN compared to placebo (32 weeks versus 20 weeks). Continuous abstinence rates were greater for those patients randomized to ZYBAN as compared to placebo through 6 months (P<0.05; 55% versus 44%). At 1 year, point prevalence abstinence rates only (abstinence from smoking for the 7 consecutive days preceding the clinic visit) were significantly higher for patients treated with ZYBAN compared to placebo-treated patients (P<0.01; 55% versus 42%).

Treatment with ZYBAN reduced some of the withdrawal symptoms compared to placebo: irritability, frustration, or anger; anxiety; difficulty concentrating; restlessness; and depressed mood or negative affect. Depending on the study and the measure used, treatment with ZYBAN showed evidence of reduction in craving for cigarettes or urge to smoke compared to placebo.

INDICATIONS: ZYBAN (bupropion hydrochloride) is indicated as smoking cessation treatment in conjunction with behavioural modification; nicotine replacement therapy may be used in addition to ZYBAN.

CONTRAINDICATIONS: To reduce the risk of seizures, ZYBAN (bupropion hydrochloride) is contraindicated in patients:

- **receiving WELLBUTRIN XL, WELLBUTRIN SR or any other medications that contain bupropion hydrochloride because the incidence of seizure is dose dependent see Warnings)**
- with a current seizure disorder (see Warnings)
- with a current or prior diagnosis of bulimia or anorexia nervosa because of a higher incidence of seizures (see Warnings) noted in patients treated for bulimia with the immediate release formulation of bupropion
- undergoing abrupt withdrawal from alcohol or benzodiazepines or other sedatives

To reduce risks due to drug interaction, the concomitant use of ZYBAN is contraindicated in patients currently taking:

- Monoamine oxidase (MAO) inhibitors.
- the antipsychotic thioridazine, since bupropion may inhibit thioridazine metabolism, thus causing an increase in thioridazine levels and a potential increased risk of thioridazine-related serious ventricular arrhythmias and sudden death.

At least 14 days should elapse between discontinuation of one drug and the start of another.

ZYBAN is contraindicated in patients who have shown an allergic response to bupropion or any other component of the formulation.

WARNINGS: Potential Association with the Occurrence of Behavioural and Emotional Changes, Including Self-Harm: Adult and Pediatric Reports of Agitation-Type Events: Although ZYBAN is not indicated for treatment of depression, it contains the same active ingredient—bupropion—as WELLBUTRIN SR and WELLBUTRIN XL antidepressant medications. Therefore, clinicians should be aware of the following information.

There are clinical trial and postmarketing reports with SSRIs and other newer antidepressants, including bupropion, in both pediatrics and adults, of severe agitation-type adverse events coupled with self-harm or harm to others. The agitation-type events include: akathisia, agitation, disinhibition, emotional lability, hostility, aggression, depersonalization. In some cases, the events occurred within several weeks of starting treatment.

Rigorous clinical monitoring for suicidal ideation or other indicators of potential for suicidal behaviour is advised in patients of all ages. This includes monitoring for agitation-type emotional and behavioural changes.

Seizures: Patients should be made aware that ZYBAN (bupropion hydrochloride) Tablets contain the same active ingredient found in WELLBUTRIN SR Sustained Release Tablets and WELLBUTRIN XL Extended Release Tablets, used to treat depression, and that ZYBAN should not be administered to patients already receiving a product containing bupropion hydrochloride (see Contraindications).

The use of bupropion is associated with a dose-dependent risk of seizures. **Clinicians should not prescribe doses over 300 mg/day for smoking cessation.** The risk of seizure is also related to patient factors, clinical situation, and concurrent medications, which must be considered in selection of patients for therapy with ZYBAN Tablets.

Seizures were not reported by patients participating in smoking cessation trials (n=1946). The seizure rate associated with doses of sustained-release bupropion up to 300 mg/day is approximately 0.1%. This incidence was prospectively determined during an 8-week treatment exposure in approximately 3100 depressed patients. Data for the immediate-release formulation of bupropion revealed a seizure incidence of approximately 0.4% in depressed patients treated at doses in a range of 300 to 450 mg/day. In addition, the estimated seizure incidence increases almost tenfold between 450 and 600 mg/day.

Predisposing Risk Factors for Seizures: The risk of seizure occurring with bupropion use appears to be associated with the presence of predisposing risk factors. Therefore extreme caution should be used when treating patients with predisposing factors which increase the risk of seizures, including: history of head trauma or prior seizure; central nervous system (CNS) tumour; the presence of severe hepatic impairment; excessive use of alcohol; addiction to opiates, cocaine, or stimulants; use of concomitant medications that lower seizure threshold, including but not limited to: antipsychotics, antidepressants, lithium, amantadine, theophylline, systemic steroids, quinolone antibiotics, and antimalarials; use of over-the-counter stimulants or anorectics; diabetes treated with oral hypoglycemics or insulin.

The above group of risk factors, including medications, should not be considered exhaustive; for each patient, all potential predisposing factors must be carefully considered.

In Order to Minimize the Risk of Seizure: The total daily dose of ZYBAN must not exceed 300 mg (the maximum recommended dose), and no single dose of ZYBAN may exceed 150 mg, in order to avoid high peak concentrations of bupropion and/or its metabolites.

If a Seizure Occurs: Patients should be warned that if they experience a seizure while taking ZYBAN, they should contact their doctor or be taken to a hospital emergency ward immediately, and should stop taking ZYBAN. Treatment should not be restarted if a patient has experienced a seizure while taking ZYBAN, WELLBUTRIN SR, or WELLBUTRIN XL.

Hepatic Impairment: The results of two single dose pharmacokinetic studies indicate that the clearance of bupropion is reduced in all subjects with Child-Pugh Grades C hepatic impairment, and in some subjects with milder forms of liver impairment. Given the risks associated with both peak bupropion levels and drug accumulation, ZYBAN is not recommended for use in patients with severe hepatic impairment. However, should clinical judgement deem it necessary, it should be used only with extreme caution at a reduced dose, to a maximum dose of 150 mg every other day.

All patients with hepatic impairment should be closely monitored for possible adverse effects (e.g., insomnia, dry mouth, seizures) that could indicate high drug or metabolite levels (see Dosage and Precautions).

Potential for Hepatotoxicity: In rats receiving large doses of bupropion chronically, there was an increase in incidence of hepatic hyperplastic nodules and hepatocellular hypertrophy. In dogs receiving large doses of bupropion chronically, various histologic changes were seen in the liver, and laboratory tests suggesting mild hepatocellular injury were noted.

PRECAUTIONS: General: Allergic Reactions: Anaphylactoid/anaphylactic reactions characterized by symptoms such as pruritus, urticaria, angioedema, and dyspnea have been reported at a rate of one to three per thousand in clinical trials. In addition, there have been rare spontaneous postmarketing reports of erythema multiforme, Stevens Johnson syndrome, and anaphylactic shock associated with bupropion. A patient should stop taking ZYBAN and consult a doctor if experiencing allergic or anaphylactoid/anaphylactic reactions (e.g., skin rash, pruritus, hives, chest pain, edema, and shortness of breath) during treatment.

Arthralgia, myalgia and fever have also been reported in association with rash and other symptoms suggestive of delayed hypersensitivity. These symptoms may resemble serum sickness.

Bupropion should be discontinued immediately if any hypersensitivity reactions are experienced. Symptoms of hypersensitivity should be treated in accordance with established medical practice. Clinicians should be aware that symptoms may persist beyond the discontinuation of bupropion, and clinical management should be provided accordingly. In post-market experience, there have been reports of hypersensitivity reactions in patients who consumed alcohol while taking bupropion. As the contribution of alcohol to these reactions has been established, patients should avoid alcohol when they are taking bupropion (see Alcohol Interaction).

Conditions that Predispose Patients to Seizures: To reduce the risk of seizures, ZYBAN is contraindicated in patients with specific conditions (see Contraindications), while extreme caution is recommended with other conditions (see Warnings).

Insomnia: In the dose response smoking cessation trial, 29% of patients treated with 150 mg/day of ZYBAN (bupropion hydrochloride) and 35% of patients treated with 300 mg/day of ZYBAN experienced insomnia, compared to 21% of placebo treated patients. Symptoms were sufficiently severe to require discontinuation of treatment in 0.6% of patients treated with ZYBAN and none of the patients treated with placebo.

In the comparative trial, 40% of the patients treated with 300 mg/day of ZYBAN, 28% of the patients treated with 21 mg/day of nicotine transdermal system (NTS), and 45% of the patients treated with the combination of ZYBAN and NTS experienced insomnia compared to 18% of placebo treated patients. Symptoms were sufficiently severe to require discontinuation of treatment in 0.8% of patients treated with ZYBAN and none of the patients in the other three treatment groups.

Insomnia may be minimized by avoiding bedtime doses and, if necessary, reduction in dose.

Agitation-type emotional and behavioural changes: Agitation-type changes are reported for ZYBAN, and monitoring for these indicators of potential suicidal behaviour is advised in patients of all ages given a newer antidepressant drug, including bupropion (see Warnings, Potential Association with the Occurrence of Behavioural and Emotional Changes, Including Self-Harm).

When reported in patients undergoing a smoking cessation attempt, such changes may be a symptom of nicotine withdrawal, along with depressed mood and related symptoms such as difficulty concentrating and anxiety.

Psychosis, Confusion, and Other Neuropsychiatric Phenomena: In clinical trials with ZYBAN conducted in nondepressed smokers, the incidence of neuropsychiatric side effects was generally comparable to placebo. Depressed patients treated with bupropion in depression trials have been reported to show a variety of neuropsychiatric signs and symptoms including delusions, hallucinations, psychosis, concentration disturbance, paranoia, and confusion. In some cases, these symptoms abated upon dose reduction and/or withdrawal of treatment.

Activation of Psychosis and/or Mania: Antidepressants can precipitate manic episodes in bipolar disorder patients during the depressed phase of their illness and may activate latent psychosis in other susceptible individuals. The sustained release formulation of bupropion is expected to pose similar risks. There were no reports of activation of psychosis or mania in clinical trials with ZYBAN conducted in nondepressed smokers.

Changes in Body Weight: Weight gain is a well-known side effect of smoking cessation and may either impede initiation of a quit attempt or precipitate relapse.

Treatment: In clinical trials where treatment was for 7 to 12 weeks, a trend for lower body weight gain in subjects treated with bupropion as compared to those treated with placebo was noted. This trend was not maintained. One year after bupropion discontinuation, a trend to lower body weight gain in patients previously treated with placebo was detected.

Maintenance: In the study of up to 1 year's treatment duration, patients treated with ZYBAN demonstrated significantly less weight gain (p≤0.05) than those patients treated with placebo throughout the study (3.6 kg vs 5.9 kg, respectively, at Week 52).
Cardiovascular Effects: In clinical practice, hypertension, in some cases severe, requiring acute treatment, has been reported in patients receiving bupropion alone and in combination with nicotine replacement therapy. These events have been observed in both patients with and without evidence of preexisting hypertension.

Data from a comparative study of ZYBAN, nicotine transdermal system (NTS), the combination of sustained-release bupropion plus NTS, and placebo as an aid to smoking cessation suggest a higher incidence of treatment-emergent hypertension in patients treated with the combination of ZYBAN and NTS. In this study, 6.1% of patients treated with the combination of ZYBAN and NTS had treatment-emergent hypertension compared to 2.5%, 1.6% and 3.1% of patients treated with ZYBAN, NTS, and placebo, respectively. The majority of these patients had evidence of preexisting hypertension. Three patients (1.2%) treated with the combination of ZYBAN and NTS and one patient (0.4%) treated with NTS had study medication discontinued due to hypertension compared to none of the patients treated with ZYBAN or placebo. Monitoring of blood pressure is recommended in patients who receive the combination of bupropion and nicotine replacement.

There is no clinical experience establishing the safety of ZYBAN in patients with a recent history of myocardial infarction or unstable heart disease. Therefore, care should be exercised if it is used in these groups. Bupropion was well tolerated in depressed patients who had previously developed orthostatic hypotension while receiving tricyclic antidepressants, and was also generally well tolerated in a group of 36 depressed inpatients with stable heart failure. However, bupropion was associated with a rise in supine blood pressure in the study of patients with stable heart failure, resulting in discontinuation of treatment in two patients for exacerbation of baseline hypertension.
Renal Impairment: There is no clinical experience establishing the safety of ZYBAN in patients with renal impairment. Bupropion is extensively metabolized in the liver to active metabolites, which are largely further metabolized before being excreted by the kidneys. ZYBAN should be used with caution in patients with renal impairment and a reduced frequency of dosing should be considered as bupropion and its metabolites may accumulate in such patients to a greater extent than usual. The patient should be closely monitored for possible adverse effects (e.g., insomnia, dry mouth, seizures) that could indicate high drug or metabolite levels.
Hepatic Impairment: Based on the variability reported for individual pharmacokinetic (PK) values of patients with mild hepatic impairment in a single dose pharmacokinetic study, patients with mild or moderate hepatic impairment should be initiated at 100 mg/day of bupropion. Bupropion is not recommended for patients with severe hepatic impairment (see Warnings and Dosage).

All patients with hepatic impairment should be closely monitored for possible adverse effects (e.g., insomnia, dry mouth, seizures) that could indicate high drug and metabolite levels (see Warnings and Dosage).
Occupational Hazards: Any psychoactive drug may impair judgment, thinking or motor skills. Therefore, subjects should be cautioned about operating hazardous machinery, including automobiles, until they are reasonably certain that the drug treatment does not affect their performance adversely.
Drug Interactions: In vitro studies indicate that bupropion is primarily metabolized to hydroxybupropion by Cytochrome P450IIB6 (CYP2B6) isoenzyme. Therefore the potential exists for a drug interaction between ZYBAN and drugs that affect the CYP2B6 isoenzyme metabolism (e.g., orphenadrine and cyclophosphamide). The threohydrobupropion metabolite of bupropion does not appear to be produced by the cytochrome P450 isoenzymes. Few systematic data have been collected on the metabolism of ZYBAN following concomitant administration with other drugs, or alternatively, the effect of concomitant administration of ZYBAN on the metabolism of other drugs.

Animal data indicate that bupropion may be an inducer of drug-metabolizing enzymes in humans. However, following chronic administration of bupropion, 100 mg t.i.d. to 8 healthy male volunteers for 14 days, there was no evidence of induction of its own metabolism. Bupropion is extensively metabolized. The coadministration of other drugs may affect its clinical activity. Carbamazepine, phenobarbital and phenytoin may induce the metabolism of bupropion. The effects of concomitant administration of cimetidine on the pharmacokinetics of bupropion and its active metabolites were studied in 24 healthy young male volunteers. Following oral administration of two 150 mg ZYBAN tablets with and without a single dose of 800 mg of cimetidine, there were no clinically relevant differences in C_{max}, t_{max}, half-life, and clearance of bupropion or hydroxybupropion, but there was a small but statistically significant increase in the combined threohydro and erythropropion AUC (16%) and C_{max} (32%).
Drugs Metabolized by Cytochrome P450IID6 (CYP2D6): Many drugs, including most antidepressants (SSRIs, many tricyclics), beta-blockers, antiarrhythmics, and antipsychotics are metabolized by the CYP2D6 isoenzyme. Although bupropion is not metabolized by this isoenzyme, bupropion and hydroxybupropion are inhibitors of the CYP2D6 isoenzyme in vitro. In a study of 15 male subjects (ages 19 to 35 years) who were extensive metabolizers of the CYP2D6 isoenzyme, daily doses of bupropion given as 150 mg twice daily followed by a single dose of 50 mg desipramine increased the C_{max}, AUC, and $t_{1/2}$ of desipramine by an average of approximately 2-, 5- and 2-fold, respectively. The effect was present for at least 7 days after the last dose of bupropion. Concomitant use of bupropion with other drugs metabolized by CYP2D6 has not been formally studied.
Coadministration of Thioridazine Contraindicated: Administration of the antipsychotic thioridazine alone produces prolongation of the QTc interval, which is associated with serious ventricular arrhythmias such as torsades de pointes, and sudden death. As this effect appears to be dose-related, it is anticipated that risk increases with inhibition of thioridazine metabolism. An in-vivo study suggests that drugs which inhibit CYP2D6 will elevate plasma levels of thioridazine. Therefore concomitant use of thioridazine with ZYBAN is contraindicated (see Contraindications).
Coadministration of Other Drugs Metabolized by CYP2D6 Isoenzyme: Coadministration of bupropion with other drugs that are metabolized by CYP2D6 isoenzyme including certain antidepressants (e.g., nortriptyline, imipramine, desipramine, paroxetine, fluoxetine, sertraline), antipsychotics (e.g., haloperidol, risperidone,), beta-blockers (e.g., metoprolol), and Type 1C antiarrhythmics (e.g., propafenone, flecainide), should be approached with caution and should be initiated at the lower end of the dose range of the concomitant medication. If bupropion is added to the treatment regimen of a patient already receiving a drug metabolized by CYP2D6, the need to decrease the dose of the original medication should be considered, particularly for those concomitant medications with a narrow therapeutic index.
MAO Inhibitors: Studies in animals demonstrate that the acute toxicity of bupropion is enhanced by the MAO inhibitor phenelzine (see Contraindications).
Cimetidine: The effects of concomitant administration of cimetidine on the pharmacokinetics of bupropion and its active metabolites were examined in a crossover study in 24 healthy young male volunteers, following oral administration of two 150 mg bupropion sustained release tablets with and without 800 mg of cimetidine. A single dose of cimetidine had no effect on single dose pharmacokinetic parameter estimates for bupropion, or hydroxybupropion, but caused a small statistically significant increase in the combined threohydro and erythrobupropion AUC (16%) and C_{max} (32%).
Levodopa and Amantadine: Limited clinical data suggest a higher incidence of neuropsychiatric adverse experiences, such as confusion, agitation and delirium, in patients receiving bupropion concurrently with either levodopa or amantadine. Tremor, ataxia and dizziness were also reported. Administration of ZYBAN to patients receiving either levodopa or amantadine concurrently should be undertaken with caution, using small initial doses and gradual dose increases.
Clopidogrel and Ticlopidine: Both clopidogrel and ticlopidine have been shown to significantly inhibit CYP2B6-catalysed bupropion hydroxylation. The mean area under the plasma concentration-time curve (AUC) of hydroxybupropion was reduced by 52% by clopidogrel and by 84% by ticlopidine. The AUC of bupropion was increased by 60% with clopidogrel and by 85% with ticlopidine. Therefore, concomitant administration of bupropion and either clopidogrel or ticlopidine may result in increased plasma concentrations of bupropion and reduced concentrations of hydroxybupropion. This may affect the efficacy of bupropion and may also increase the risk of concentration-dependent adverse events of bupropion, such as seizures (see Warnings, Seizures). Patients receiving drugs used to reduce blood clots (such as either clopidogrel and/or ticlopidine) are likely to require dose adjustments of bupropion.
Use of ZYBAN with Drugs that Predispose Patients to Seizures: Concurrent administration of ZYBAN with agents (e.g., antipsychotics, antidepressants, theophylline, lithium, amantadine, systemic steroids, etc.) that lower seizure threshold should be undertaken only with extreme caution (see Warnings). Low initial dosing and gradual dose increases should be employed.
Use of ZYBAN with other Drugs with CNS activity: The risks of bupropion in combination with other CNS-active drugs have not been systematically evaluated. Consequently, caution is advised if the concomitant administration of ZYBAN and such drugs is required.
Nicotine Transdermal System: See Precautions, Cardiovascular Effects.
Smoking Cessation: Physiological changes resulting from smoking cessation itself, with or without treatment with ZYBAN, may alter the pharmacokinetics of some concomitant medications, which may require dosage adjustment.
Alcohol Interactions: In post-marketing experience, there have been reports of adverse neuropsychiatric events or, reduced alcohol tolerance, in patients who were drinking alcohol during treatment with bupropion. Rarely, reports of fatal outcomes with this combination have been received, however a causal relationship has not been established. The consumption of alcohol during treatment with bupropion should be avoided (also see Warnings, Predisposing Risk Factor for Seizures).
Pregnancy: Teratogenic Effects: Teratology studies have been performed at doses up to 450 mg/kg in rats (approximately 14 times the MRHD on a mg/m² basis) and at doses up to 150 mg/kg in rabbits (approximately 10 times the MRHD on a mg/m² basis). There is no evidence of impaired fertility or harm to the fetus due to bupropion. There are no adequate and well-controlled studies in pregnant women. Because animal reproduction studies are not always predictive of human response, this drug should be used during pregnancy only if clearly needed. Pregnant smokers should be encouraged to attempt cessation using educational and behavioral interventions before pharmacological approaches are used.
Third Trimester: Postmarketing reports indicate that some neonates exposed to ZYBAN, SSRIs (Selective Serotonin Reuptake Inhibitors), or other newer anti-depressants late in the third trimester have developed complications requiring prolonged hospitalization, respiratory support, and tube feeding. Such complications can arise immediately upon delivery. Reported clinical findings have included respiratory distress, cyanosis, apnea, seizures, temperature instability, feeding difficulty, vomiting, hypoglycemia, hypotonia, hyperreflexia, tremor, jitteriness, irritability, and constant crying. The frequency of symptoms may vary with each drug. These features are consistent with either a direct toxic effect of SSRIs and other newer anti-depressants, or, possibly, a drug discontinuation syndrome. When treating a pregnant woman with ZYBAN during the third trimester, the physician should carefully consider the potential risks and benefits of treatment (see Dosage).
Labor and Delivery: The effect of ZYBAN on labor and delivery in humans is unknown.
Lactation: Bupropion and its metabolites are secreted in human milk. Because of the potential for serious adverse reactions in nursing infants from ZYBAN, a decision should be made whether to discontinue nursing or to discontinue the drug, taking into account the importance of the drug to the mother.
Children: Clinical trials with ZYBAN did not include individuals under the age of 18. Therefore, the safety and efficacy in a pediatric smoking population have not been established.
Geriatrics: Of the approximately 6000 patients who participated in clinical trials with bupropion sustained-release tablets (depression and smoking cessation studies), 275 were 65 and over and 47 were 75 and over. In addition, several hundred patients 65 and over participated in clinical trials using the immediate-release formulation of bupropion (depression studies). No overall differences in safety or effectiveness were observed between these subjects and younger subjects, and other reported clinical experience has not identified differences in responses between the elderly and younger patients, but greater sensitivity of some older individuals cannot be ruled out.

A single-dose pharmacokinetic study demonstrated that the disposition of bupropion and its metabolites in elderly subjects was similar to that of younger subjects; however, another single and multiple dose pharmacokinetic study has suggested that the elderly are at increased risk for accumulation of bupropion and its metabolites.

Bupropion is extensively metabolized in the liver to active metabolites, of which some are eliminated by the kidneys, while others are further metabolized before being excreted in urine. The risk of toxic reaction to this drug may be greater in patients with impaired renal function. Because elderly patients are more likely to have decreased renal function, care should be taken in dose selection, and it may be useful to monitor renal function (see Precautions, Renal Impairment and Dosage).

ADVERSE EFFECTS: The information included under Adverse Effects is based primarily on data from the dose-response trial and the comparative trial that evaluated ZYBAN (bupropion hydrochloride) for smoking cessation. Information on additional adverse events associated with the sustained-release formulation of bupropion is included in a separate section (see Other Events Observed During the Clinical Development and Postmarketing Experience of Bupropion).
Adverse Events Associated with Discontinuation of Treatment: Adverse events caused discontinuation of treatment in 8% of the 706 patients treated with ZYBAN and 5% of the 313 patients treated with placebo. The more common events leading to discontinuation of treatment with ZYBAN included nervous system disturbances (3.4%), primarily tremors, and skin disorders (2.4%), primarily rashes.
Incidence of Commonly Observed Adverse Events: The most commonly observed adverse events consistently associated with the use of ZYBAN were dry mouth and insomnia. The most commonly observed adverse events were defined as those that consistently occurred at a rate of five percentage points greater than that for placebo across clinical studies.
Dose Dependency of Adverse Events: The incidence of dry mouth and insomnia may be related to the dose of ZYBAN. The occurrence of these adverse events may be minimized by reducing the dose of ZYBAN. In addition, insomnia may be minimized by avoiding bedtime doses.
Adverse Events Occurring at an Incidence of 1% or More Among Patients Treated with ZYBAN: Table 3 enumerates selected treatment emergent adverse events from the dose response trial that occurred at an incidence of 1% or more and were more common in patients treated with ZYBAN compared to those treated with placebo. Table 4 enumerates selected treatment emergent adverse events from the comparative trial that occurred at an incidence of 1% or more and were more common in patients treated with ZYBAN, NTS, or the combination of ZYBAN and NTS compared to those treated with placebo. Reported adverse events were classified using a COSTART based dictionary.

Table 3: ZYBAN

Treatment-emergent Adverse Event Incidence in the Dose-response Trial[a]

Body System/ Adverse Experience	ZYBAN 100–300 mg/day (n=461) %	PBO (n=150) %
Body (General)		
Neck Pain	2	<1
Allergic Reaction	1	0
Cardiovascular		
Hot Flashes	1	0
Hypertension	1	<1
Digestive		
Dry Mouth	11	5
Increased Appetite	2	<1
Anorexia	1	<1
Musculoskeletal		
Arthralgia	4	3
Myalgia	2	1
Nervous System		
Insomnia	31	21
Dizziness	8	7
Tremor	2	1
Somnolence	2	1
Thinking Abnormality	1	0
Respiratory		
Bronchitis	2	0

(cont'd)

Table 3: ZYBAN *(cont'd)*

Treatment-emergent Adverse Event Incidence in the Dose-response Trial[a]

Body System/ Adverse Experience	ZYBAN 100–300 mg/day (n=461) %	PBO (n=150) %
Skin		
Pruritus	3	<1
Rash	3	<1
Dry Skin	2	0
Urticaria	1	0
Special Senses		
Taste Perversion	2	<1

[a] Selected adverse events with an incidence of at least 1% of patients treated with ZYBAN and more frequent than in the placebo group.

Table 4: ZYBAN

Treatment-emergent Adverse Event Incidences (%) in the Comparative Trial[a]

Adverse Experience	ZYBAN 300 mg/day (n=243) %	Nicotine Transdermal System (NTS) 21 mg/day (n=243) %	ZYBAN and NTS (n=244) %	Placebo (n=159) %
Body				
Abdominal Pain	3	4	1	1
Accidental Injury	2	2	1	1
Chest Pain	<1	1	3	1
Neck Pain	2	1	<1	0
Facial Edema	<1	0	1	0
Cardiovascular				
Hypertension	1	<1	2	0
Palpitations	2	0	1	0
Digestive				
Nausea	9	7	11	4
Dry Mouth	10	4	9	4
Constipation	8	4	9	3
Diarrhea	4	4	3	1
Anorexia	3	1	5	1
Mouth Ulcer	2	1	1	1
Thirst	<1	<1	2	0
Musculoskeletal				
Myalgia	4	3	5	3
Arthralgia	5	3	3	2
Nervous System				
Insomnia	40	28	45	18
Dream Abnormality	5	18	13	3
Anxiety	8	6	9	6
Disturbed Concentration	9	3	9	4
Dizziness	10	2	8	6
Nervousness	4	<1	2	2
Tremor	1	<1	2	0
Dysphoria	<1	1	2	1
Respiratory				
Rhinitis	12	11	9	8
Increased Cough	3	5	<1	1
Pharyngitis	3	2	3	0

(cont'd)

Table 4: ZYBAN *(cont'd)*

Treatment-emergent Adverse Event Incidences (%) in the Comparative Trial[a]

Adverse Experience	ZYBAN 300 mg/day (n=243) %	Nicotine Transdermal System (NTS) 21 mg/day (n=243) %	ZYBAN and NTS (n=244) %	Placebo (n=159) %
Sinusitis	2	2	2	1
Dyspnea	1	0	2	1
Epistaxis	2	1	1	0
Skin				
Application Site Reaction	11	17	15	7
Rash	4	3	3	2
Pruritus	3	1	5	1
Urticaria	2	0	2	0
Special Senses				
Taste Perversion	3	1	3	2
Tinnitus	1	0	<1	0

[a] Selected adverse events with an incidence of at least 1% of patients treated with ZYBAN, NTS, or the combination of ZYBAN and NTS and more frequent than in the placebo group.

In the relapse prevention study of up to 1 year in duration, ZYBAN was well tolerated. Adverse events were quantitatively and qualitatively similar to those observed in the dose-response and comparative trials.

Other Events Observed During the Clinical Development and Postmarketing Experience of Bupropion: Postmarketing reports suggest that the reintroduction of ZYBAN in patients who experienced a seizure is associated with a risk of seizure reoccurrence in some cases. Thus, patients should not restart ZYBAN therapy if they have had a seizure on either bupropion formulation (ZYBAN, WELLBUTRIN XL, or WELLBUTRIN SR). (See Warnings.)

In addition to the events noted above, the following events have been reported in clinical trials and postmarketing experience with the sustained-release formulation of bupropion in depressed patients and in nondepressed smokers, as well as in clinical trials and postmarketing clinical experience with the immediate-release formulation of bupropion.

Adverse events for which frequencies are provided below occurred in clinical trials with bupropion sustained release. The frequencies represent the proportion of patients who experienced a treatment emergent adverse event on at least one occasion in placebo controlled studies for depression (n=987) or smoking cessation (n=1013), or patients who experienced an adverse event requiring discontinuation of treatment in an open label surveillance study with bupropion sustained release tablets (n=3100). All treatment emergent adverse events are included except those listed in Table 3 and Table 4, those events listed in other safety related sections of the monograph, those adverse events subsumed under COSTART terms that are either overly general or excessively specific so as to be uninformative, those events not reasonably associated with the use of the drug, and those events that were not serious and occurred in fewer than two patients.

Events are further categorized by body system and listed in order of decreasing frequency according to the following definitions of frequency: Frequent adverse events are defined as those occurring in at least 1/100 patients. Infrequent adverse events are those occurring in 1/100 to 1/1000 patients, while rare events are those occurring in less than 1/1000 patients.

Adverse events for which frequencies are not provided occurred in clinical trials or postmarketing experience with bupropion. Only those adverse events not previously listed for sustained release bupropion are included. The extent to which these events may be associated with ZYBAN is unknown.

Body (General): Frequent were asthenia, fever, and headache. Infrequent were back pain, chills, inguinal hernia, musculoskeletal chest pain, pain, and photosensitivity. Rare was malaise.

Cardiovascular: Infrequent were flushing, migraine, postural hypotension, stroke, tachycardia, and vasodilation. Rare was syncope. Also observed were cardiovascular disorder, complete AV block, extrasystoles, hypotension, hypertension (in some cases severe, see Precautions, Cardiovascular Effects), myocardial infarction, phlebitis, and pulmonary embolism.

Digestive: Frequent were dyspepsia, flatulence, and vomiting. Infrequent were abnormal liver function, bruxism, dysphagia, gastric reflux, gingivitis, glossitis, jaundice, and stomatitis. Rare was edema of tongue. Also observed were colitis, esophagitis, gastrointestinal hemorrhage, gum hemorrhage, hepatitis, increased salivation, intestinal perforation, liver damage, pancreatitis, stomach ulcer, and stool abnormality.

Endocrine: Also observed were hyperglycemia, hypoglycemia and syndrome of inappropriate antidiuretic hormone.

Hemic and Lymphatic: Infrequent was ecchymosis. Also observed were anemia, leukocytosis, leukopenia, lymphadenopathy, pancytopenia, and thrombocytopenia.

Metabolic and Nutritional: Infrequent were edema, increased weight, and peripheral edema. Also observed was glycosuria.

Musculoskeletal: Infrequent were leg cramps and twitching. Also observed were arthritis and muscle rigidity/fever/rhabdomyolysis, and muscle weakness.

Nervous System: Frequent were agitation, depression, and irritability. Infrequent were abnormal coordination, CNS stimulation, confusion, decreased libido, decreased memory, depersonalization, emotional lability, hostility, hyperkinesia, hypertonia, hypesthesia, paresthesia, suicidal ideation and vertigo. Rare were amnesia, ataxia, derealization, hypomania and seizure. Also observed were abnormal electroencephalogram (EEG), akinesia, aphasia, coma, delirium, delusions, dysarthria, dyskinesia, dystonia, euphoria, extrapyramidal syndrome, hallucinations, hypokinesia, increased libido, manic reaction, neuralgia, neuropathy, paranoid reaction, and unmasking tardive dyskinesia.

Respiratory: Rare was bronchospasm. Also observed was pneumonia.

Skin/Hypersensitivity: Frequent was sweating. Infrequent was acne and dry skin. Rare was maculopapular rash. Also observed were alopecia, angioedema, erythema multiforme, exfoliative dermatitis, hirsutism, and Steven-Johnson syndrome. Arthralgia, myalgia and fever have also been reported in association with rash and other symptoms suggestive of delayed hypersensitivity. These symptoms may resemble serum sickness.

Special Senses: Frequent was amblyopia. Infrequent were accommodation abnormality and dry eye. Also observed were deafness, diplopia and mydriasis.

Urogenital: Frequent was urinary frequency. Infrequent were impotence, polyuria, and urinary urgency. Also observed were abnormal ejaculation, cystitis, dyspareunia, dysuria, gynecomastia, menopause, painful erection, prostate disorder, salpingitis, urinary incontinence, urinary retention, urinary tract disorder, and vaginitis.

ZYBAN (bupropion hydrochloride) is likely to have a low abuse potential.

OVERDOSE:

Symptoms: In addition to those events reported under Adverse Effects, overdose has resulted in symptoms including drowsiness, loss of consciousness and ECG changes such as conduction disturbances (including QRS prolongation) or arrhythmias.

There has been very limited experience with overdosage of the sustained-release formulation of bupropion; three such cases were reported during clinical trials in depressed patients. One patient ingested 3000 mg of bupropion sustained-release tablets and vomited quickly after the overdose; the patient experienced blurred vision and lightheadedness. A second patient ingested a "handful" of bupropion sustained-release tablets and experienced confusion, lethargy, nausea, jitteriness, and seizure. A third patient ingested 3600 mg of bupropion sustained-release tablets and a bottle of wine; the patient experienced nausea, visual hallucinations, and "grogginess". None of the patients experienced further sequelae.

There has been extensive experience with overdosages of the immediate-release formulation of bupropion. Thirteen overdoses occurred during clinical trials in depressed patients. Twelve patients ingested 850 to 4200 mg and recovered without significant sequelae. Another patient who ingested 9000 mg of immediate-release bupropion and 300 mg of tranylcypromine experienced a grand mal seizure and recovered without further sequelae.

Since introduction, overdoses of up to 17 500 mg of the immediate-release formulation of bupropion have been reported. Seizure was reported in approximately one-third of all cases. Other serious reactions reported with overdoses of the immediate-release formulation of bupropion alone included hallucinations, loss of consciousness, and sinus tachycardia. Fever, muscle rigidity, rhabdomyolysis, hypotension, stupor, coma, and respiratory failure have been reported when the immediate-release formulation of bupropion was part of multiple drug overdoses.

Although most patients recovered without sequelae, deaths associated with overdoses of the immediate-release formulation of bupropion alone have been reported rarely in patients ingesting massive doses of the drug. Multiple uncontrolled seizures, bradycardia, cardiac failure, and cardiac arrest prior to death were reported in these patients.

Treatment: In the event of overdose, hospitalisation is advised. Ensure an adequate airway, oxygenation, and ventilation. Monitor cardiac rhythm (ECG) and vital signs. EEG monitoring is also recommended for the first 48 hours post-ingestion. General supportive and symptomatic measures are also recommended. Induction of emesis is not recommended. Gastric lavage with a large-bore orogastric tube with appropriate airway protection, if needed, may be indicated if performed soon after ingestion or in symptomatic patients.

Activated charcoal should be administered. There is no experience with the use of forced diuresis, dialysis, hemoperfusion, or exchange transfusion in the management of bupropion overdoses. No specific antidotes for bupropion are known.

Due to the dose-related risk of seizures with ZYBAN, hospitalization following suspected overdose should be considered. Based on studies in animals, it is recommended that seizures be treated with intravenous benzodiazepine administration and other supportive measures, as appropriate.

In managing overdosage, consider the possibility of multiple drug involvement. The physician should consider contacting a Poison Control Centre for additional information on the treatment of any overdose. Telephone numbers for certified Poison Control Centres are listed in the *Compendium of Pharmaceuticals and Specialties (CPS)*.

For management of a suspected drug overdose, CPhA recommends that you contact your **regional Poison Control Centre**. See the *CPS* Directory section for a list of Poison Control Centres.

DOSAGE: ZYBAN (bupropion hydrochloride) is not indicated for use in children under 18 years of age.
Usual Dosage for Adults: The recommended and maximum dose of ZYBAN (bupropion hydrochloride) is 300 mg/day, given as 150 mg twice daily. Dosing should begin at 150 mg once daily for the first 3 days, followed by a dose increase to the recommended usual dose of 300 mg/day as necessary. There should be an interval of at least 8 hours between successive doses. **In order to minimize the risk of seizures (see Warnings), single doses of ZYBAN must not exceed 150 mg and** doses above 300 mg/day must not be used (see Warnings).

Treatment with ZYBAN should be initiated **while the patient is still smoking**, since approximately 1 week of treatment is required to achieve steady state blood levels of bupropion. Patients should set a "target quit date" within the first 2 weeks of treatment with ZYBAN, generally in the second week. Treatment with ZYBAN should be continued for 7 to 12 weeks; duration of treatment should be based on the relative benefits and risks for individual patients. If a patient has not made significant progress towards abstinence by the seventh week of therapy with ZYBAN, it is unlikely that he or she will quit during that attempt, and treatment should probably be discontinued. Dose tapering of ZYBAN is not required when discontinuing treatment. It is important that patients continue to receive counseling and support throughout treatment with ZYBAN, and for a period of time thereafter.

Maintenance: Nicotine dependence is a chronic condition. Many patients attempting to quit smoking experience multiple relapses. Systematic evaluation of ZYBAN 300 mg/day for the prevention of relapse demonstrated that treatment for up to 1 year was well tolerated and efficacious in preventing relapse (see Pharmacology). Whether to continue treatment with ZYBAN for periods longer than 12 weeks must be determined for individual patients.

Patients should be advised to swallow ZYBAN tablets whole with fluids, and not to chew, divide, crush or otherwise tamper with the tablets in any way that might affect the release rate of bupropion.

Missed Dose: ZYBAN should be taken at the same time each day and no more than the recommended dose should be taken each day. If the normal administration time has been missed, the dose should be skipped and administration resumed at the normal administration time of the following day.

Treatment of Pregnant Women During the Third Trimester: Postmarketing reports indicate that some neonates exposed to ZYBAN , SSRIs, or other newer anti-depressants late in the third trimester have developed complications requiring prolonged hospitalization, respiratory support, and tube feeding (see Precautions). When treating pregnant women with ZYBAN during the third trimester, the physician should carefully consider the potential risks and benefits of treatment. The physician may consider tapering ZYBAN in the third trimester.

Geriatrics: See Precautions, Geriatrics.

Dosage Adjustment for Patients with Impaired Hepatic Function: Mild and Moderate Hepatic Impairment: Given the variable pharmacokinetics of bupropion in patients with either mild or moderate hepatic impairment (Child-Pugh Grade A or B), treatment should be initiated at 100 mg/day of bupropion. Maintenance dose may be adjusted according to clinical response and tolerance. Caution should be exercised as there is no clinical experience with ZYBAN in hepatically impaired patients (see also Warnings and Precautions).

Severe Impairment: Given the risks associated with both peak bupropion levels and drug accumulation, ZYBAN is not recommended for use in patients with severe hepatic impairment. However, should clinical judgement deem it necessary, the drug should be used only with extreme caution (see also Warnings). The dose should not exceed 150 mg every other day in these patients. Any theoretical dose reduction for this patient population based on the findings of the pharmacokinetic studies may result in toxic drug levels in these patients (see Warnings).

Dosage Adjustment for Patients with Impaired Renal Function: ZYBAN should be used with caution in patients with renal impairment due to the potential for drug accumulation, and a reduced frequency of dosing should be considered (see Precautions, Renal Impairment).

Individualization of Therapy: Patients are more likely to quit smoking and remain abstinent if they are seen frequently and receive support from their physicians or other health care professionals. It is important to ensure that patients read the instructions provided to them and have their questions answered. Physicians should review the patient's overall smoking cessation program that includes treatment with ZYBAN. Patients should be advised of the importance of participating in the behavioural interventions, counseling, and/or support services to be used in conjunction with ZYBAN.

The goal of therapy with ZYBAN is complete abstinence. If a patient has not made significant progress towards abstinence by the seventh week of therapy with ZYBAN, it is unlikely that he or she will quit during that attempt, and treatment should be discontinued.

Patients who fail to quit smoking during an attempt may benefit from interventions to improve their chances for success on subsequent attempts. Patients who are unsuccessful should be evaluated to determine why they failed. A new quit attempt should be encouraged when factors that contributed to failure can be eliminated or reduced, and conditions are more favorable.

Combination Treatment with Bupropion and a Nicotine Transdermal System (NTS): ZYBAN may be prescribed in combination with NTS for smoking cessation. The prescriber should review the complete prescribing information for both ZYBAN and NTS before using combination treatment. Treatment with ZYBAN is initiated at 150mg/day while the patient is still smoking and increased after 3 days to 300mg/day given at 150 mg twice daily. Nicotine transdermal system (NTS) may be added to treatment with ZYBAN after approximately 1 week when the patient has reached the target quit date. During weeks 8 and 9, NTS should be tapered (see Pharmacology, Clinical Trials). Monitoring for treatment-emergent hypertension in patients treated with the combination of ZYBAN and NTS is recommended.

INFORMATION FOR THE PATIENT: Published in e-CPS, available by subscription at www.e-cps.ca.

SUPPLIED: Each purple, round, biconvex, film-coated, sustained-release tablet, printed "ZYBAN 150", contains: bupropion HCl 150 mg. Nonmedicinal ingredients: carnauba wax, cysteine hydrochloride, edible black ink, FD&C Blue No. 2 Lake, FD&C Red No. 40 Lake, hydroxypropyl methylcellulose, magnesium stearate, microcrystalline cellulose, polyethylene glycol, polysorbate 80 and titanium dioxide. Blister pack of 60. Store at 15 to 25°C. Store in a dry place, protected from light.

(Shown in Product Identification Section)

Zyclara™ Pr
imiquimod
Immune Response Modifier

Graceway

Date of Preparation: December 31, 2009

SUMMARY PRODUCT INFORMATION:

Route of Administration	Dosage Form/ Strength	Clinically Relevant Nonmedicinal Ingredients
Topical	Cream/9.4 mg imiquimod per 250 mg single-dose packet (3.75 % w/w)	For a complete listing see Dosage Forms, Composition and Packaging.

INDICATIONS AND CLINICAL USE: ZYCLARA cream is indicated for the topical field (area) treatment of multiple clinically typical visible or palpable actinic keratoses (AK), whether presenting at the start of therapy or revealed during therapy, of the face or balding scalp in adults.

Geriatrics (>65 years of age): No overall differences in safety or effectiveness were observed in clinical studies between the geriatric population and younger subjects (see Warnings and Precautions, Geriatrics (>65 years of age)).

Pediatrics: Safety and efficacy in patients below the age of 18 years have not been established (see Warnings and Precautions, Pediatrics (<18 years of age)).

Immunosuppressed: The safety and efficacy of ZYCLARA cream in immunosuppressed patients have not been established (see Warnings and Precautions, Immune).

CONTRAINDICATIONS: ZYCLARA cream is contraindicated in individuals with a history of sensitivity reactions to imiquimod or to any of the components in the formulation. It should be discontinued if hypersensitivity to any of its ingredients is noted (see Warnings and Precautions, Sensitivity/Resistance).

WARNINGS AND PRECAUTIONS: General: The efficacy of ZYCLARA cream in the prevention of squamous cell carcinoma (SCC) associated with AK has not been established.

The safety and efficacy of ZYCLARA cream topically applied to an area larger than the face or balding scalp (approximately 200 cm^2) has not been established. Therefore, topical application of ZYCLARA cream to larger areas is not recommended.

Systemic Reactions: Flu-like signs and symptoms may accompany, or even precede, local skin reactions and may include fatigue, nausea, fever, myalgias, arthralgias, and chills. An interruption of dosing or dose adjustment and an assessment of the patient should be considered (see Adverse Reactions).

Carcinogenesis and Mutagenesis: In a hairless mouse photocarcinogenicity study with solar ultraviolet light irradiation, imiquimod cream enhanced UVR-induced skin tumour development, but not beyond that of the vehicle cream. Vehicle cream alone enhanced ultraviolet induced skin tumour development. It is recommended that patients minimize or avoid natural or artificial sunlight exposure during treatment with ZYCLARA.

Immune: The safety and efficacy of ZYCLARA cream in immunosuppressed patients have not been established.

ZYCLARA topical cream should be used with caution in patients with pre-existing autoimmune conditions (including thyroiditis, multiple sclerosis, spondyloarthropathy, psoriasis, ulcerative colitis) (see Adverse Reactions, Post-Market Adverse Drug Reactions).

Sensitivity/Resistance: Hypersensitivity reactions (urticaria) and erythema multiforme have been reported in patients receiving imiquimod cream, however causality has not been established. ZYCLARA cream should be discontinued immediately if these events occur.

Skin: Local skin reactions such as erythema, scabbing/crusting, flaking/scaling/dryness, and edema are common.

Intense local skin reactions including erythema, scabbing/crusting and erosion/ulceration can occur after a few applications of ZYCLARA cream and may require an interruption of dosing (see Adverse Reactions and Dosage and Administration).

ZYCLARA cream has the potential to exacerbate inflammatory conditions of the skin, including chronic graft versus host disease.

Should a severe local skin reaction occur, the cream should be removed by washing the treatment area with mild soap and water and drying the area thoroughly. Treatment with ZYCLARA cream can be resumed after consultation with the treating physician, and once the skin reaction has subsided.

Exposure to sunlight (including sunlamps) should be avoided or minimized during use of ZYCLARA cream because of concern for heightened sunburn susceptibility. Patients should be warned to use protective clothing (e.g. hat) when using ZYCLARA cream. Patients with sunburn should be advised not to use ZYCLARA cream until fully recovered. Patients who may have considerable sun exposure, e.g., due to their occupation, and those patients with inherent sensitivity to sunlight should exercise caution when using ZYCLARA cream. Phototoxicity has not been adequately assessed for ZYCLARA cream. The enhancement of ultraviolet carcinogenicity is not necessarily dependent on phototoxic mechanisms. Imiquimod cream shortened the time to skin tumour formation in an animal photoco-carcinogenicity study. Therefore, it is prudent for patients to minimize or avoid natural or artificial sunlight exposure.

Special Populations: Pregnant Women: Imiquimod was not teratogenic in rat or rabbit teratology studies. In rats at a high maternally toxic dose (28 times human dose on a mg/m^2 basis), reduced pup weights and delayed ossification were observed. However, there are no adequate and well-controlled studies in pregnant women. Because animal reproduction studies are not always predictive of human response, this drug should be used during pregnancy only if the potential benefit justifies the potential risk to the fetus.

Nursing Women: It is not known whether topically applied imiquimod is excreted in human milk. Because many drugs are excreted in human milk, caution should be exercised when ZYCLARA cream is administered to nursing women.

Pediatrics (<18 years of age): Safety and efficacy in patients below the age of 18 years have not been established.

Geriatrics (>65 years of age): Of the 160 subjects treated with ZYCLARA cream in the clinical studies, 78 subjects were 65 years or older. No overall differences in safety or effectiveness were observed between these subject and younger subjects. No other clinical experience has identified differences in responses between the elderly and younger subjects, but greater sensitivity of some older individuals cannot be ruled out.

ADVERSE REACTIONS: Adverse Drug Reaction Overview: Clinical Trial Adverse Drug Reactions: The data described below reflect exposure to ZYCLARA cream or placebo in 319 subjects enrolled in two double-blind, placebo-controlled studies. Subjects applied ZYCLARA cream or placebo daily to the skin of the affected area (either the entire face or balding scalp) for two 2-week treatment cycles separated by a 2-week no treatment period. See Table 1 and Table 2.

Table 1: ZYCLARA

Adverse Reactions Occurring in >1% of ZYCLARA-Treated Subjects and at a Greater Frequency than with Placebo in the Combined Studies

Preferred Term	ZYCLARA Cream, 3.75% (N=160)	Placebo (N=159)
Headache	10 (6.3%)	5 (3.1%)
Application site pruritus	7 (4.4%)	1 (0.6%)
Fatigue	7 (4.4%)	0 (0%)
Nausea	6 (3.8%)	2 (1.3%)
Application site irritation	5 (3.1%)	0 (0%)
Application site pain	5 (3.1%)	0 (0%)
Pyrexia	5 (3.1%)	0 (0%)

(cont'd)

Table 1: ZYCLARA *(cont'd)*

Adverse Reactions Occurring in >1% of ZYCLARA-Treated Subjects and at a Greater Frequency than with Placebo in the Combined Studies

Preferred Term	ZYCLARA Cream, 3.75% (N=160)	Placebo (N=159)
Anorexia	4 (2.5%)	0 (0%)
Dizziness	4 (2.5%)	0 (0%)
Herpes simplex	4 (2.5%)	1 (0.6%)
Pain	4 (2.5%)	0 (0%)
Chest pain	3 (1.9%)	0 (0%)
Diarrhea	3 (1.9%)	0 (0%)
Lymphadenopathy	3 (1.9%)	0 (0%)
Application Site Swelling	2 (1.3%)	0 (0%)
Arthralgia	2 (1.3%)	0 (0%)
Blood glucose increased	2 (1.3%)	0 (0%)
Dermatitis	2 (1.3%)	0 (0%)
Food poisoning	2 (1.3%)	0 (0%)
Insomnia	2 (1.3%)	0 (0%)
Seborrhoeic keratosis	2 (1.3%)	0 (0%)
Squamous cell carcinoma	2 (1.3%)	1 (0.6%)
Vomiting	2 (1.3%)	1 (0.6%)

Table 2: ZYCLARA

Application Site Reactions in ZYCLARA-Treated Subjects as Assessed by the Investigator

Included Term	ZYCLARA Cream, 3.75%[a] (N=160)	Placebo[a] (N=159)
Any application site reaction	17 (10.6%)	2 (1.3%)
Application site pruritus	7 (4.4%)	1 (0.6%)
Application site irritation	5 (3.1%)	0 (0%)
Application site pain	5 (3.1%)	0 (0%)
Application site swelling	2 (1.3%)	0 (0%)
Application site paraesthesia	1 (0.6%)	1 (0.6%)
Application site scar	1 (0.6%)	0 (0%)

[a] Up to 2 packets daily.

Local skin reactions were collected independently of the adverse event "application site reaction" in an effort to provide a better picture of the specific types of local reactions that might be seen. The most frequently reported local skin reactions were erythema, flaking/scaling/dryness, and scabbing/crusting. The prevalence and severity of local skin reactions that occurred during controlled studies are shown in Table 3.

Table 3: ZYCLARA

Local Skin Reactions in the Treatment Area in ZYCLARA-Treated Subjects as Assessed by the Investigator

	ZYCLARA Cream, 3.75% (N=160)		Placebo (N=159)	
	All Grades	**Severe**	**All Grades**	**Severe**
Erythema	154 (96.3%)	40 (25.2%)	124 (78.0%)	0 (0.0%)
Edema	120 (75.0%)	9 (5.7%)	31 (19.5%)	0 (0.0%)
Weeping/Exudate	81 (50.6%)	9 (5.7%)	6 (3.8%)	0 (0.0%)
Flaking/Scaling/Dryness	147 (91.9%)	13 (8.2%)	123 (77.4%)	2 (1.3%)
Scabbing/Crusting	149 (93.1%)	22 (13.8%)	72 (45.3%)	0 (0.0%)
Erosion/Ulceration	99 (61.9%)	17 (10.7%)	14 (8.8%)	0 (0.0%)

Other adverse events observed in subjects treated with ZYCLARA cream in treatment regimens other than two 2-week treatment cycles include: application site bleeding, cheilitis, chills, herpes zoster, influenza-like illness, lethargy, myalgia, pancytopenia and pruritus.

Post-Market Adverse Drug Reactions: Rare reports have been received of either the onset or exacerbation of autoimmune conditions (including thyroiditis, multiple sclerosis, spondyloarthropathy, psoriasis, ulcerative colitis) in association with imiquimod 5% cream therapy.

DRUG INTERACTIONS: Overview: Interactions between ZYCLARA cream with other drugs have not been established.

DOSAGE AND ADMINISTRATION: Recommended Dose and Dosage Adjustment: ZYCLARA cream (up to 2 packets, 250 mg imiquimod cream per packet) should be applied once daily before bedtime to the skin of the affected treatment field (area) for two treatment cycles of 2 weeks each separated by a 2-week no-treatment period or as directed by physician.

Missed Dose: Each treatment cycle should not be extended beyond 2 weeks due to missed doses or rest periods.

Administration: Before applying the cream, the patient should wash the treatment area with mild soap and water and allow the area to dry thoroughly. ZYCLARA cream should be applied as a thin film to the entire treatment area and rubbed in until the cream is no longer visible. Up to 2 packets of ZYCLARA cream may be applied to the treatment area (face or scalp, but not both) at each daily application. Partially-used packets should be discarded and not reused. **ZYCLARA cream should be left on the skin for approximately 8 hours, after which time the cream should be removed by washing the area and the hands with mild soap and water.** The prescriber should demonstrate the proper application technique to maximize the benefit of ZYCLARA cream therapy.

Use of the cream in or near the eyes, lips and nostrils should be avoided. The application site is not to be occluded.

Local skin reactions in the treatment area are common (see Adverse Reactions). A rest period of several days and interruption of dosing may be considered if required by the patient's discomfort or severity of the local skin reaction. **However, each treatment cycle should not be extended beyond 2 weeks due to missed doses or rest periods.** Response to treatment cannot be adequately assessed until resolution of local skin reactions. Lesions that do not respond to treatment should be carefully re-evaluated and management reconsidered.

A transient increase in AK lesion counts may be observed during treatment due to the likely effect of imiquimod on subclinical lesions. The patient should continue dosing as prescribed.

OVERDOSAGE:
Overdosage of ZYCLARA cream in humans is unlikely due to minimal percutaneous absorption. Animal studies reveal a rabbit dermal lethal imiquimod dose of greater than 5000 mg/kg. Persistent **topical** overdosing of ZYCLARA cream could result in an increased incidence of severe local skin reactions and may increase the risk for systemic reactions.

The most clinically serious adverse event reported following multiple **oral** imiquimod doses of ≥200 mg was hypotension which resolved following oral or intravenous fluid administration.

For management of a suspected drug overdose, CPhA recommends that you contact your **regional Poison Control Centre**. See the *CPS* Directory section for a list of Poison Control Centres.

ACTION AND CLINICAL PHARMACOLOGY: Mechanism of Action: In vitro studies have demonstrated that imiquimod induces the release of interferon alpha (IFN-α) and other cytokines from human monocytes/macrophages and keratinocytes. The panel of cytokines induced varied with the cell's tissue origin. Topical in vivo application of imiquimod cream on mouse skin resulted in increased concentrations of IFN and tumour necrosis factor (TNF) compared with skin of untreated mice.

Pharmacodynamics: The mechanism of action of imiquimod in treating actinic keratosis (AK) lesions is unknown. While the following have been observed, the clinical significance of these observations in AK is not known. In a study of 58 patients with AK treated with imiquimod 3 times per week, the response of biomarkers sensitive to imiquimod after 16 weeks of dosing increased compared to the response after the first dose. For interleukin-1 antagonist, the median concentration observed following multiple dosing was <2-fold higher than that after single dose administration, for interferon-α was ≤3-fold, and for 2′5′-oligoadenylate synthetase was approximately 3-fold.

Pharmacokinetics: Percutaneous absorption of imiquimod has been studied through intact healthy skin, the skin of genital warts, and lesions of sun damaged skin. Percutaneous absorption of [^{14}C]imiquimod was minimal in a study involving six healthy subjects treated with a single topical application (5 mg) of [^{14}C]imiquimod in cream formulation. No radioactivity [^{14}C] was detected in the serum (lower limit of quantitation is 1 ng/mL) and <0.9% of the radiolabelled dose was excreted in the urine and feces following topical application.

ZYCLARA cream exhibited low systemic exposure to imiquimod and its metabolites when it was applied daily for 3 weeks (18.75 mg, 2 packets once daily) to the entire face and/or balding scalp (approximately 200 cm^2) of patients with AK (N=17). A mean (median) peak serum drug concentration at the end of week 3 was approximately 0.323 ng/mL. Steady-state levels were achieved in 2 weeks and T_{max} ranged between 6 and 9 hours.

The apparent half-life following topical dosing of 3.75% imiquimod cream was calculated as 29 hours after daily administration of 2 packets (18.75 mg) for 3 weeks.

Special Populations and Conditions: Age: No formal pharmacokinetic study was conducted to examine age related differences in the pharmacokinetic profile of ZYCLARA cream.

Gender: During 3 weeks of treatment, the C_{max} and AUC_{0-24} on Day 21 appeared to be similar in female and male subjects and lower in male subjects who applied ZYCLARA cream, to the balding scalp rather than the face.

STORAGE AND STABILITY: Store between 15 and 25°C. Avoid freezing.

INFORMATION FOR THE PATIENT: Published in e-CPS, available by subscription at www.e-cps.ca.

DOSAGE FORMS, COMPOSITION AND PACKAGING: Each g of cream contains: imiquimod 37.5 mg in an off-white to faintly yellow oil-in-water vanishing cream base. Nonmedicinal ingredients: benzyl alcohol, cetyl alcohol, glycerin, isostearic acid, methylparaben, polysorbate 60, propylparaben, purified water, sorbitan monostearate, stearyl alcohol, white petrolatum and xanthan gum. Single-use packets of 250 mg, boxes of 28 packets.

(Shown in Product Identification Section)

Zymar™ Pr
gatifloxacin
Antibacterial

Allergan

Date of Preparation: August 24, 2004

PHARMACOLOGY: Mechanism of Action: ZYMAR (gatifloxacin) ophthalmic solution 0.3% is a sterile solution for topical ophthalmic use. Gatifloxacin is an 8-methoxy synthetic fluoroquinolone antibacterial agent with in vitro activity against gram-negative and gram-positive, aerobic and anaerobic and clinically important atypical microorganisms.

The antibacterial action of gatifloxacin results from inhibition of DNA gyrase and topoisomerase IV. DNA gyrase is an essential enzyme that is involved in the replication, transcription and repair of bacterial DNA. Topoisomerase IV is an enzyme known to play a key role in the partitioning of the chromosomal DNA during bacterial cell division.

Pharmacokinetics: Ocular Administration: Gatifloxacin ophthalmic solutions 0.3% and 0.5% were administered to 1 eye of 6 healthy male subjects each. At all time points, serum gatifloxacin levels were below the lower limit of quantification (5 ng/mL) in all subjects. Pharmacokinetic parameters for ophthalmic dosing could not therefore be calculated. There is no human pharmacokinetic data available with respect to tear concentration following ocular administration.

Systemic Administration: Gatifloxacin is well absorbed from the gastrointestinal tract after oral administration and can be given without regard to food. The absolute bioavailability of gatifloxacin is 96%. Peak plasma concentrations of gatifloxacin usually occur 1-2 hours after oral dosing.

INDICATIONS: ZYMAR (gatifloxacin) ophthalmic solution 0.3% is indicated for the treatment of patients 1 year of age and older with bacterial conjunctivitis caused by susceptible strains of the following bacteria:

Aerobic Gram-positive Bacteria: *S. aureus, S. epidermidis, S. pneumoniae.*

Aerobic Gram-negative Bacteria: *H. influenzae.*

CONTRAINDICATIONS: ZYMAR (gatifloxacin) ophthalmic solution 0.3% is contraindicated in individuals who have shown hypersensitivity to gatifloxacin, to other quinolones, or to any of the components in this medication.

WARNINGS: Not for injection into the eye. For topical ophthalmic use only.

ZYMAR (gatifloxacin) ophthalmic solution 0.3% should not be injected subconjunctivally, nor should it be introduced directly into the anterior chamber of the eye.

In patients receiving systemic quinolones, serious and occasionally fatal hypersensitivity (anaphylactic) reactions, some following the first dose, have been reported. Some reactions were accompanied by cardiovascular collapse, loss of consciousness, angioedema (including laryngeal, pharyngeal or facial edema), airway obstruction, dyspnea, urticaria, and itching. If an allergic reaction to gatifloxacin occurs, discontinue the drug. Serious acute hypersensitivity reactions may require immediate emergency treatment. Oxygen and airway management should be administered as clinically indicated.

As with all antibiotics, serious and sometimes fatal events, some due to hypersensitivity and some due to uncertain etiology, have been reported in patients receiving systemic quinolone therapy. These events may be severe and generally occur following administration of multiple doses. Clinical manifestations may include one or more of the following: fever, rash or severe dermatologic reactions (e.g., toxic epidermal necrolysis, Stevens-Johnson syndrome); vasculitis, arthralgia, myalgia, serum sickness;

allergic pneumonitis, interstitial nephritis; acute renal insufficiency or failure; hepatitis, jaundice, acute hepatic necrosis or failure; anemia, including hemolytic and aplastic; thrombocytopenia, including thrombotic thrombocytopenic purpura; leukopenia; agranulocytosis; pancytopenia; and/or other hematologic abnormalities.

PRECAUTIONS: General: As with other anti-infectives, prolonged use of ZYMAR (gatifloxacin) ophthalmic solution 0.3% may result in overgrowth of nonsusceptible organisms, including fungi. If superinfection occurs discontinue use and institute alternative therapy. Whenever clinical judgment dictates, the patient should be examined with the aid of magnification, such as slit lamp biomicroscopy and, where appropriate, fluorescein staining.

Hypersensitivity: As with all topical ophthalmic drugs, there is a potential for a systemic reaction. Urticaria has been reported in patients receiving ZYMAR (see Adverse Effects).

Systemic quinolones have been associated with hypersensitivity reactions, even following a single dose.

Contact Lenses: Patients should not wear contact lenses while they have signs and symptoms of bacterial conjunctivitis.

Arthropathy: As with other members of the quinolone class, gatifloxacin has caused arthropathy and/or chondrodysplasia in juvenile rats and dogs when given systemically.

Arthrotoxic and osteotoxic potential of ZYMAR was not assessed in animals.

Drug Interactions: Specific drug interaction studies have not been conducted with ZYMAR ophthalmic solution. Limited information is available on the concurrent use of ZYMAR with other ophthalmic products.

Probenecid: Systemic administration of gatifloxacin (single oral 200 mg dose) with probenecid (500 mg BID×1 day) resulted in a 42% increase in AUC and 44% longer half-life of gatifloxacin.

Digoxin: Overall, only modest increases in C_{max} and AUC of digoxin were noted (12% and 19%, respectively) in 8 of 11 healthy volunteers who received concomitant administration of gatifloxacin (400 mg oral tablet, once daily for 7 days) and digoxin (0.25 mg orally, once daily for 7 days). In 3 of 11 subjects, however, a significant increase in digoxin concentrations was observed. In these 3 subjects, digoxin C_{max} increased by 18%, 29%, and 58% while digoxin AUC increased by 66%, 104%, and 79%, and digoxin clearance decreased by 40%, 51%, and 45%.

Systemic studies have also shown that gatifloxacin is chelated by polyvalent ions, such as iron, magnesium, zinc and aluminum.

No significant pharmacokinetic interactions occur when cimetidine, midazolam, theophylline, warfarin, or glyburide is administered concomitantly with oral gatifloxacin.

Pregnancy: There are no adequate and well-controlled studies of ZYMAR in pregnant women. This drug should not be used in pregnant women unless, in the physician's opinion, the potential benefit to the mother justifies the potential risk to the fetus.

ZYMAR solution has not been studied in pregnant animals. Oral and intravenous studies in pregnant animals indicate that gatifloxacin crosses the placenta and that reproductive and fetal effects occur at doses of ≥150 mg/kg/day, which cause maternal toxicity.

Lactation: It is not known whether gatifloxacin is excreted in human milk, although gatifloxacin has been shown to be excreted in the breast milk of rats. Because gatifloxacin may be excreted in human milk, a decision should be made either to discontinue nursing or to discontinue the administration of ZYMAR, taking into account the importance of ZYMAR therapy to the mother and the possible risk to the infant.

Children: The safety and efficacy of ZYMAR in infants below the age of one year have not been established. ZYMAR ophthalmic solution has been used to treat conjunctivitis in 14 infants between 1-2 years of age and 47 children between 3-12 years of age.

Elderly: No overall differences in safety or effectiveness have been observed between elderly and younger patients.

Information to Be Provided to the Patient: Physicians should instruct their patients to:

- avoid contaminating the applicator tip with material from the eye (or surrounding structures), fingers or other sources.
- refrain from wearing contact lenses if they have signs and symptoms of bacterial conjunctivitis.
- discontinue use of drug immediately and to contact their physician at the first sign of a rash or allergic reaction.

ADVERSE EFFECTS: In clinical studies 364 patients were treated with ZYMAR (gatifloxacin) ophthalmic solution 0.3% for up to 5 days. Treatment-related adverse events were reported for 14.6% (53/364) of patients. The most frequently reported treatment-related adverse events occurring in 0.5% to 5% of patients treated with gatifloxacin are listed in Table 1.

Table 1: ZYMAR

Percent of Patients in Phase 3 Trials with Treatment-Related Adverse Events Reported by 0.5% to 5% of Patients in the Active Treatment Arm

Body System Preferred Term	Gatifloxacin N=364 %
Ocular	
Superficial Punctate Keratitis	4.4
Eye Irritation	1.9
Dry Eye	1.6
Eyelid Edema	1.4
Lacrimation Increased	1.4
Visual Acuity Reduced	1.1
Eye Pain	0.8
Conjunctivitis Papillary	0.8
Eye Discharge	0.5
Other (Non Ocular)	
Erythema	0.8
Dermatitis, contact	0.5
Taste Disturbance	1.4
Rhinorrhoea	0.5
Edema	0.5

Other treatment-related adverse events occurring in less than 0.5% of patients included, conjunctival disorder, conjunctivitis, chemosis, conjunctival cyst, conjunctival hemorrhage, corneal deposits, eye disorder, photophobia, subepithelial opacities, blurred vision, dermatitis, generalized urticaria, nausea, sore throat, sneezing, dizziness, and iritis.

ZYMAR was discontinued due to an adverse event, either related or unrelated to the drug, in 1.6% (6/364) of patients.

Post-marketing Experience: Adverse events reported include macular edema, eye redness, eyelid edema, keratoconjunctivitis, blepharitis allergic, endophthalmitis, corneal disorder, eye irritation, uveitis, corneal ulcer, allergic reactions including pruritis and angioneurotic edema and neurological events including headache, tinnitus, tremor and oral parasthesia. Rare cases of corneal melts and perforation have been reported in patients with multiple confounding factors including preexisting large corneal ulcer, corneal thinning, undiagnosed dacryocystitis, and use of multiple topical medications. Thus, it is difficult to determine the relationship of the events to ZYMAR.

In one case, an elderly female with chronic conjunctivitis due to methicillin-resistant *S. aureus* and a history of dacrocystitis, reported corneal perforation. This patient was using multiple concomitant antibiotics and had demonstrated evidence of a corneal defect associated with the infection prior to using ZYMAR and continued using ZYMAR during a successful post operative repair healing period.

OVERDOSE:

Symptoms: A topical overdosage of ZYMAR (gatifloxacin) ophthalmic solution 0.3% is considered to be a remote possibility. Discontinue medication when heavy or protracted use is suspected. A topical overdosage may be flushed from the eye(s) with warm tap water.

If a 10 kg child swallowed the contents of a 5 mL bottle of ZYMAR (15 mg of drug) it would be exposed to 1.5 mg/kg of gatifloxacin. This is equivalent to 25% of the recommended adult systemic therapeutic dose of gatifloxacin of 400 mg/day for a 70 kg adult (6.0 mg/kg).

Treatment: See Symptoms.

For management of a suspected drug overdose, CPhA recommends that you contact your **regional Poison Control Centre**. See the *CPS* Directory section for a list of Poison Control Centres.

DOSAGE: The recommended dosage regimen for ZYMAR (gatifloxacin) ophthalmic solution 0.3% in the treatment of patients 1 year of age and older with bacterial conjunctivitis is:

Days 1 and 2: Instill one drop every two hours in the affected eye(s) while awake, up to 8 times daily.

Days 3 to 7: Instill one drop four times daily while awake.

Doses should be evenly spaced throughout the day.

INFORMATION FOR THE PATIENT: Published in e-CPS, available by subscription at www.e-cps.ca.

SUPPLIED: Each mL of sterile, clear, pale yellow colored, isotonic, unbuffered ophthalmic solution contains: gatifloxacin 3 mg/mL (0.3%). Nonmedicinal ingredients: benzalkonium chloride 0.005% (as preservative), edetate disodium, purified water and sodium chloride. May contain hydrochloric acid and/or sodium hydroxide to adjust pH (target pH of 6). White low density polyethylene bottles of 1, 2.5 and 5 mL with a controlled dropper tip and a tan, high density polyethylene (HIPS) cap. Store at 15 to 25°C. Protect from freezing.

Zyprexa® Ⓟ
olanzapine
Antipsychotic

Lilly

Zyprexa® Zydis® Ⓟ
olanzapine
Antipsychotic

Lilly

Zyprexa® IntraMuscular Ⓟ
olanzapine tartrate
Antipsychotic

Lilly

Date of Revision: February 23, 2009

SUMMARY PRODUCT INFORMATION:

Product	Route of Administration	Dosage Form/ Strength	All Nonmedicinal Ingredients
ZYPREXA	Oral	Tablets/2.5 mg, 5 mg, 7.5 mg, 10 mg, 15 mg, 20 mg	Tablets: carnauba wax, crospovidone, hydroxypropyl cellulose, hydroxypropyl methylcellulose, lactose, magnesium stearate, and microcrystalline cellulose Colour coating and ink contain some or all of the following ingredients: FD&C Blue No. 2 Aluminum Lake, polyethylene glycol, polysorbate 80, Synthetic Red Iron Oxide, titanium dioxide, triacetin
ZYPREXA Zydis	Oral	Orally disintegrating tablets/5 mg, 10 mg, 15 mg, 20 mg	Aspartame, gelatin, mannitol, sodium methyl paraben and sodium propyl paraben
ZYPREXA IntraMuscular	Intramuscular injection	Parenteral/10 mg per vial	Lactose, tartaric acid (hydrochloric acid and/or sodium hydroxide may have been added during manufacturing to adjust pH)

See Dosage Forms, Composition and Packaging for more information.

INDICATIONS AND CLINICAL USE: Adults: Oral Olanzapine: Schizophrenia and Related Disorders: ZYPREXA (olanzapine) is indicated for the acute and maintenance treatment of schizophrenia and related psychotic disorders. In controlled clinical trials, ZYPREXA was found to improve both positive and negative symptoms.

ZYPREXA has been shown to be effective in maintaining clinical improvement during 1-year of continuation therapy in patients who had shown an initial treatment response.

Bipolar Disorder: ZYPREXA (olanzapine) is indicated for the acute treatment of manic or mixed episodes in bipolar I disorder. Olanzapine may be used as monotherapy or cotherapy with agents commonly used in the treatment of acute bipolar disorder (e.g., lithium or divalproex sodium).

The efficacy of ZYPREXA as monotherapy maintenance treatment in bipolar patients with manic or mixed episodes who responded to acute treatment with ZYPREXA was demonstrated in two 1-year "time to relapse" trials.

The physician who elects to use ZYPREXA for extended periods should periodically re-evaluate the long-term usefulness of the drug for the individual patient (see Dosage and Administration).

Intramuscular Olanzapine: ZYPREXA IntraMuscular is indicated for the rapid control of agitation in patients with schizophrenia and related psychotic disorders, and bipolar mania. The efficacy of ZYPREXA IntraMuscular for the control of agitation was established in 2 short-term (24 hours) placebo-controlled trials in agitated inpatients with schizophrenia and one short-term (24 hours) placebo-controlled trial in agitated patients with mania associated with bipolar disorder.

Geriatrics (≥65 years): ZYPREXA is not indicated in elderly patients with dementia. See Warnings and Precautions—Serious Warnings and Precautions Box and Special Populations. Caution should be used when treating geriatric patients with ZYPREXA. See Action and Clinical Pharmacology, Warnings and Precautions, Special Populations, and Dosage and Administration.

Pediatrics (<18 years of age): The safety and efficacy of ZYPREXA have not been established in pediatric populations and its use is not recommended.

CONTRAINDICATIONS: ZYPREXA (olanzapine) is contraindicated in those patients with a known hypersensitivity to the drug or the excipients of the product. For a complete listing, see Dosage Forms, Composition and Packaging.

WARNINGS AND PRECAUTIONS:

Serious Warnings and Precautions
Increased Mortality in Elderly Patients with Dementia: Elderly patients with dementia treated with atypical antipsychotic drugs are at an increased risk of death compared to placebo. Analyses of thirteen placebo controlled trials with various atypical antipsychotics (modal duration of 10 weeks) in these patients showed a mean 1.6 fold increase in death rate in the drug-treated patients. Although the causes of death were varied, most of the deaths appeared to be either cardiovascular (e.g., heart failure, sudden death) or infectious (e.g., pneumonia) in nature. (See Warnings and Precautions, Special Populations, Use in Geriatric Patients with Dementia.)

General: Neuroleptic Malignant Syndrome: Neuroleptic Malignant Syndrome (NMS) has been reported very rarely (≤0.0025%) in pre-marketed and post-market surveillance. However, NMS is a potentially fatal symptom complex that has been reported in association with antipsychotic drugs. Clinical manifestations of NMS are hyperpyrexia, muscle rigidity, altered mental status, and evidence of autonomic instability (irregular pulse or blood pressure, tachycardia, diaphoresis, and cardiac dysrhythmia). Additional signs may include elevated creatine phosphokinase, myoglobinuria (rhabdomyolysis), and acute renal failure.

The management of NMS should include immediate discontinuation of all antipsychotic drugs including ZYPREXA, intensive monitoring of symptoms and treatment of any associated medical problems. There is no general agreement about specific pharmacological treatment for NMS. If a patient requires antipsychotic drug treatment after recovery from NMS, the re-introduction of therapy should be very carefully considered, since recurrence of NMS has been reported.

Weight Gain: Olanzapine was associated with weight gain during clinical trials. Clinically significant weight gain was observed across all baseline body mass index (BMI) categories (see Adverse Reactions, Other Adverse Events Observed During Clinical Trials with Oral and Intramuscular Olanzapine Across All Indications, Weight Changes). Using pooled data from patients treated with olanzapine over the dosage range of 5 mg to 20 mg per day mean gain was 5.4 kg. The mean change in weight was comparable for patients with schizophrenia and bipolar mania. A retrospective analysis of 573 patients receiving olanzapine for up to 3 years found that dose was not a significant predictor of greater long-term changes in weight.

In long-term studies (at least 48 weeks), both the magnitude of weight gain and the proportion of olanzapine-treated patients who had clinically significant weight gain were greater than in short-term studies. The percentage of patients who gained ≥25% of their baseline body weight with long-term exposure was very common (≥10%).

Body Temperature Regulation: Disruption of the body's ability to reduce core body temperature has been attributed to antipsychotic agents. Appropriate care is advised when prescribing ZYPREXA for patients who will be experiencing conditions which may contribute to an elevation of core temperature, e.g. exercising strenuously, exposure to extreme heat, receiving concomitant medication with anticholinergic activity, or being subject to dehydration.

Potential Effect on Cognitive and Motor Performance: Because ZYPREXA may cause somnolence, patients should be cautioned about operating hazardous machinery, including motor vehicles, until they are reasonably certain that ZYPREXA therapy does not affect them adversely.

Cardiovascular: Hypotension and Syncope: As with other drugs that have high alpha-1 adrenergic receptor blocking activity, ZYPREXA may induce orthostatic hypotension, tachycardia, dizziness, and sometimes syncope, especially at the initiation of treatment. In a clinical trial database of 2500 patients treated with oral ZYPREXA, syncope was reported in 0.6% (15/2500). The risk of orthostatic hypotension and syncope may be minimized by initiating therapy with 5 mg QD (see Dosage and Administration). A more gradual titration to the target dose should be considered if hypotension occurs.

Hypotension and/or syncope associated with bradycardia has been observed infrequently with ZYPREXA IntraMuscular.

Patients receiving intramuscular olanzapine should be closely observed for hypotension including postural hypotension, bradyarrhythmia and/or hypoventilation, particularly for the first 2 to 4 hours following injection. Patients should remain recumbent if dizzy or drowsy after injection until examination indicates that they are not experiencing hypotension including postural hypotension, bradyarrhythmia and/or hypoventilation.

Caution is necessary in patients who receive intramuscular olanzapine with other drugs having effects that can induce hypotension, bradycardia, respiratory or central nervous system depression. Concomitant administration of intramuscular olanzapine and parenteral benzodiazepine and/or other drugs with CNS depressant activity has been associated with post-marketing reports of serious adverse events, including fatalities and is therefore not recommended. If use of intramuscular olanzapine in combination with parenteral benzodiazepines is considered necessary, careful evaluation of clinical status for excessive sedation and cardiorespiratory depression is recommended (see Drug Interactions).

ZYPREXA should be used with particular caution in patients with known cardiovascular disease (history of myocardial infarction or ischemia, heart failure, or conduction abnormalities), cerebrovascular disease, and conditions which would predispose patients to hypotension (dehydration, hypovolemia, and treatment with antihypertensive medications).

Endocrine and Metabolism: Hyperglycaemia: As with some other antipsychotics, exacerbation of pre-existing diabetes and hyperglycaemia have been reported rarely and diabetic ketoacidosis and diabetic coma including some fatal cases have been reported very rarely during the use of ZYPREXA, sometimes in patients with no reported history of hyperglycaemia (see Adverse Reactions, Post-Market Adverse Drug Reactions). In some cases, a prior increase in body weight has been reported which may be a predisposing factor.

In clinical trials (up to 52 weeks) olanzapine was associated with a greater mean change in glucose relative to placebo. Treatment-emergent clinically significant changes in fasting glucose were observed in patients with or without evidence of glucose dysregulation at baseline (see Adverse Reactions, Other Adverse Events Observed During Clinical Trials with Oral and Intramuscular Olanzapine Across All Indications, Glucose Changes).

Assessment of the relationship between atypical antipsychotic use and glucose abnormalities is complicated by the possibility of an increased background risk of diabetes mellitus in patients with schizophrenia and the increasing incidence of diabetes mellitus in the general population. Given these confounders, the relationship between atypical antipsychotic use and hyperglycemia-related adverse events is not completely understood. However, epidemiological studies suggest an increased risk of treatment-emergent hyperglycemia-related adverse events in patients treated with the atypical antipsychotics. Precise risk estimates for hyperglycemia-related adverse events in patients treated with atypical antipsychotics are not available.

Any patient treated with atypical antipsychotics should be monitored for symptoms of hyperglycemia including polydipsia, polyuria, polyphagia, and weakness. Patients who develop symptoms of hyperglycemia during treatment with atypical antipsychotics should undergo fasting blood glucose testing. In some cases, hyperglycemia has resolved when the atypical antipsychotic was discontinued; however, some patients required continuation of anti-diabetic treatment despite discontinuation of the suspect drug. Patients with risk factors for diabetes mellitus (e.g., obesity, family history of diabetes) who are starting treatment with atypical antipsychotics should undergo fasting blood glucose testing at the beginning of treatment and periodically during treatment. Patients with an established diagnosis of diabetes mellitus who are started on atypical antipsychotics should be monitored regularly for worsening of glucose control.

Hyperprolactinemia: As with other drugs that block dopamine D_2 and/or serotonin 5-HT_2 receptors, olanzapine may elevate prolactin levels. Elevations associated with ZYPREXA treatment are generally mild, and may decline during continued administration.

Since tissue culture experiments indicate that approximately one third of human breast cancers are prolactin-dependent in vitro, ZYPREXA should only be administered to patients with previously detected breast cancer if the benefits outweigh the potential risks. Caution should also be exercised when considering ZYPREXA treatment in patients with pituitary tumours. Possible manifestations associated with elevated prolactin levels are amenorrhea, galactorrhea, and menorrhagia.

As is common with compounds which stimulate prolactin release, the administration of olanzapine resulted in an increase in the incidence of mammary neoplasms in both rats and mice. The physiological differences between rats and humans with regard to prolactin make the clinical significance of these findings unclear. To date, neither clinical nor epidemiological studies have shown an association between chronic administration of these drugs and mammary tumorigenesis.

Lipids: Increases in lipids have been observed in olanzapine-treated patients in placebo-controlled clinical trials. Treatment-emergent clinically significant changes in fasting lipids were observed in patients with or without evidence of dyslipidemia at baseline (see Adverse Reactions, Other Adverse Events Observed During Clinical Trials with Oral and Intramuscular Olanzapine Across All Indications, Lipids). Appropriate clinical monitoring is recommended, including baseline and follow-up lipid evaluations.

Gastrointestinal: Antiemetic Effect: Consistent with its dopamine antagonist effects, olanzapine may have an antiemetic effect. Such an effect may mask signs of toxicity due to overdosage of other drugs, or may mask symptoms of disease such as brain tumour or intestinal obstruction.

Genitourinary: Priapism: Rare cases of priapism have been reported with ZYPREXA. This adverse reaction, as with other psychotropic drugs, did not appear to be dose-dependent and did not correlate with the duration of treatment. The most likely mechanism of action of priapism is a relative decrease in sympathetic tone.

Hematologic: Hematologic Indices: In oral olanzapine clinical trials, there were no data to suggest ZYPREXA adversely affected bone marrow function, even in patients with a history of clozapine-associated neutropenia or leukopenia. ZYPREXA was associated with a 5.7% incidence of mainly transient treatment-emergent elevations of eosinophil counts above the normal range. Elevations were not associated with any symptoms, identifiable allergic phenomena, or changes in other hematologic indices. Rare cases of leukopenia have been reported with ZYPREXA. In case of symptoms of infection, WBC count and differential count should be considered.

Hepatic/Biliary Pancreatic: Transaminase Elevations: During pre-marketing clinical trials therapy with oral ZYPREXA was associated with elevation of hepatic transaminases, primarily ALT. Within a clinical trial database of 2280 ZYPREXA-treated patients, with baseline ALT levels ≤60 IU/L, 5.9% (134/2280) had treatment-emergent ALT elevations to >120 IU/L, 1.9% (44/2280) had elevations to >200 IU/L, and 0.2% (5/2280) had elevations to >400 IU/L. No patients had values in excess of 700 IU/L. None of the ZYPREXA-treated patients who had elevated transaminase values manifested clinical symptomatology associated with liver impairment. The majority of transaminase elevations were seen during the first six weeks of treatment. Most elevations were transient (66%) while patients continued on ZYPREXA therapy, or falling (11%) at the last available measurement. Of the 134 ZYPREXA-treated patients whose enzyme levels increased to >120 IU/L, 20 discontinued treatment (6 for hepatic, 14 for other reasons) while their ALT values were still rising. In 38 ZYPREXA-treated patients with baseline ALT >90 IU/L, none experienced an elevation to >400 IU/L.

Rare post-marketing reports of hepatitis have been received. Very rare cases of cholestatic or mixed liver injury have also been reported in the post-marketing period. Hepatic failure, including fatalities, has also been reported very rarely in the post-marketing period. See Adverse Reactions, Post-Market Adverse Drug Reactions.

Precaution should be exercised when using ZYPREXA in patients with pre-existing hepatic disorders, in patients who are being treated with potentially hepatotoxic drugs, or if treatment-emergent signs or symptoms of hepatic impairment appear.

For patients who have known or suspected abnormal hepatic function prior to starting ZYPREXA, standard clinical assessment including measurement of transaminase levels is recommended. Periodic clinical reassessment with transaminase levels is recommended for such patients, as well as for patients who develop any signs and symptoms suggestive of a new onset liver disorder during ZYPREXA therapy.

Neurologic: Tardive Dyskinesia: Tardive dyskinesia (TD), a syndrome consisting of potentially irreversible involuntary dyskinetic movements, is associated with the use of antipsychotic drugs. Tardive dyskinesia occurs more frequently in elderly patients; however, patients of any age can be affected. It is unknown whether antipsychotic drugs may differ in their potential to cause TD. However, during long-term, double-blind, extension schizophrenia maintenance trials (894 olanzapine-treated patients; median olanzapine treatment, 237 days), ZYPREXA was associated with a statistically significantly lower incidence of treatment-emergent dyskinesia compared to haloperidol. During long-term, double-blind, monotherapy extension bipolar maintenance trials (567 olanzapine-treated patients, for up to 1 year), there were no cases of TD in the ZYPREXA arms, as determined by either reported adverse events or the Abnormal Involuntary Movement Scale (AIMS). TD has been reported very rarely (≤0.0025%) in post-market surveillance.

The risk of developing tardive dyskinesia and the chance of it becoming irreversible are believed to increase as the duration of treatment and the cumulative dose of antipsychotic drug increase. However, the syndrome can develop, although less commonly, after relatively brief periods of treatment at low doses. There is no known treatment for established cases of TD. The syndrome may remit, partially or completely, if antipsychotic drug treatment is withdrawn. Antipsychotic drug treatment itself, however, may suppress the signs and symptoms of tardive dyskinesia, thereby masking the underlying process.

Given these considerations, ZYPREXA should be prescribed in a manner that is most likely to minimize the risk of tardive dyskinesia. As with any antipsychotic drug, ZYPREXA should be reserved for patients who appear to be receiving substantial benefit from the drug. In such patients the lowest effective dose and the shortest duration of treatment should be sought. The need for continued treatment should be reassessed periodically.

If signs or symptoms of tardive dyskinesia appear in a patient on ZYPREXA, drug discontinuation should be considered. However, some patients may benefit from continued treatment with ZYPREXA despite the presence of the syndrome.

Seizures: Conventional neuroleptics are known to lower seizure threshold. In clinical trials, seizures have occurred in a small number (0.9%, 22/2500) of ZYPREXA-treated patients. There were confounding factors that may have contributed to the occurrence of seizures in many of these cases. ZYPREXA should be used cautiously in patients who have a history of seizures or have conditions associated with seizure or have a lowered seizure threshold.

Psychiatric: Suicide: The possibility of suicide or attempted suicide is inherent in psychosis, and thus close supervision and appropriate clinical management of high-risk patients should accompany drug therapy.

Renal: Uric Acid: In the pre-marketing clinical trial database, oral ZYPREXA was associated with mild elevations of uric acid in some patients. However, only 1 ZYPREXA-treated patient experienced treatment-emergent gout, and the baseline uric acid concentration for this patient was at least as large as all concentrations observed while the patient was receiving ZYPREXA.

Special Populations: Pregnant Women: There are no adequate and well-controlled studies in pregnant women. Patients should be advised to notify their physician if they become pregnant or intend to become pregnant during treatment with ZYPREXA. Because human experience in pregnant females is limited, this drug should be used in pregnancy only if the potential benefit justifies the potential risk to the fetus.

Labor and Delivery: Parturition in rats was not affected by olanzapine. The effect of ZYPREXA on labour and delivery in humans is not known.

Nursing Women: In a study in lactating, healthy women, olanzapine was excreted in breast milk. Mean infant exposure (mg/kg) at steady state was estimated to be 1.8% of the maternal olanzapine dose (mg/kg). Patients should be advised not to breast feed an infant if they are taking ZYPREXA.

Pediatrics (<18 years of age): The safety and efficacy of ZYPREXA in children under the age of 18 years have not been established.

Geriatrics (≥65 years of age): The number of patients 65 years of age or over with schizophrenia or related disorders exposed to oral ZYPREXA during clinical trials was limited (N=44). Caution should thus be exercised with the use of ZYPREXA in the elderly patient, recognizing the more frequent hepatic, renal, central nervous system, and cardiovascular dysfunctions, and more frequent use of concomitant medication in this population (see Dosage and Administration).

Use in Geriatric Patients with Dementia: Overall Mortality: Elderly patients with dementia treated with atypical antipsychotic drugs showed increased mortality compared to placebo in a meta-analysis of 13 controlled trials of various atypical antipsychotic drugs. In five placebo-controlled trials with oral ZYPREXA in this population, the incidence of mortality was 3.5 % for ZYPREXA-treated patients compared to 1.5 % for placebo-treated patients. ZYPREXA is not indicated in elderly patients with dementia.

Dysphagia: Esophageal dysmotility and aspiration have been associated with antipsychotic drug use. Aspiration pneumonia is a common cause of morbidity and mortality in patients with advanced Alzheimer's disease. Olanzapine and other antipsychotic drugs should be used cautiously in patients at risk for aspiration pneumonia.

Cerebrovascular Adverse Events (CVAEs), Including Stroke, in Elderly Patients with Dementia: Cerebrovascular adverse events (e.g., stroke, transient ischemic attack), including fatalities, were reported in trials of olanzapine in elderly patients with dementia-related psychosis. In placebo-controlled studies, there was a higher incidence of CVAEs in patients treated with ZYPREXA compared to patients treated with placebo (1.3% vs. 0.4%, respectively see Adverse Reactions). ZYPREXA is not approved for the treatment of elderly patients with dementia.

There is insufficient evidence to determine whether CVAEs in elderly patients with dementia are associated specifically with ZYPREXA or all antipsychotic agents. Clinical trial data appear to suggest that patients with a dementia diagnosis of vascular or mixed type had a higher likelihood of experiencing CVAEs than other types of dementia.

The risks and benefits of the use of ZYPREXA in elderly patients with dementia should be assessed taking into account the risk predictors for CVAEs in the individual patient. Patients/caregivers should be advised to immediately report signs and symptoms of potential CVAEs, such as sudden weakness or numbness in the face, arms, or legs, and speech or vision problems.

Use in Patients with Other Concomitant Illness: Clinical experience with olanzapine in patients with concomitant illness is limited. Caution is thus advised when using ZYPREXA in patients with diseases or conditions that could affect the metabolism or the pharmacodynamic activity of olanzapine (see Dosage and Administration).

Use in Patients with Cardiac Disorders: ZYPREXA has not been evaluated in patients with a recent history of myocardial infarction or unstable heart disease. Patients with these conditions were excluded from pre-marketing clinical trials. Due to the more rapid and higher peak plasma concentrations following intramuscular compared to oral administration, particular caution is advised with the use of ZYPREXA IntraMuscular. ZYPREXA IntraMuscular should not be administered to patients with unstable medical conditions, such as acute or unstable cardiovascular conditions such as myocardial infarction, unstable angina pectoris, severe hypotension and/or bradycardia, or sick sinus syndrome. If the patient's medical history with regard to unstable medical conditions cannot be determined, the risks and benefits of IM olanzapine should be considered in relation to other alternative treatments.

Use in Patients with Diabetes and Risk Factors for Development of Diabetes: As with some other antipsychotics, exacerbation of pre-existing diabetes and hyperglycaemia have been reported rarely and diabetic ketoacidosis, and diabetic coma including some fatal cases have been reported very rarely during the use of ZYPREXA, sometimes in patients with no reported history of hyperglycaemia (see Adverse Reactions, Post-Market Adverse Drug Reactions). In some cases, a prior increase in body weight has been reported which may be a pre-disposing factor. Appropriate clinical monitoring is advisable in diabetic patients and in patients with risk factors for the development of diabetes mellitus.

Use in Patients with Renal and Hepatic Impairment: Small single-dose clinical pharmacology studies did not reveal any major alterations in olanzapine pharmacokinetics in subjects with renal or hepatic impairment. Given the limited clinical experience with ZYPREXA in patients with these conditions, caution should be exercised (see Dosage and Administration).

Other Concomitant Illnesses: As ZYPREXA demonstrated anticholinergic activity in vitro, caution is advised when prescribing for patients with symptomatic prostatic enlargement, narrow-angle glaucoma or paralytic ileus and related conditions.

In clinical trials, a single case of pre-existing intracranial hypertension was exacerbated.

ADVERSE REACTIONS: The stated frequencies of adverse events represent the proportion of individuals who experienced at least once, a treatment-emergent adverse event of the type listed. An event was considered treatment-emergent if it occurred for the first time or worsened while receiving therapy following baseline evaluation. It is important to emphasize that although the events were reported during therapy, they were not necessarily caused by the therapy.

Clinical Trial Adverse Drug Reactions: The prescriber should be aware that the figures in the tables and tabulations cannot be used to predict the incidence of side effects in the course of usual medical practice where patient characteristics and other factors differ from those that prevailed in the clinical trials. Similarly, the cited frequencies cannot be compared with figures obtained from other clinical investigations involving different treatments, uses, and investigators. The figures cited, however, do provide the prescribing physician with some basis for estimating the relative contribution of drug and nondrug factors to the side effect incidence in the populations studied.

Incidence of Adverse Events Associated with Discontinuation: Oral Administration: Schizophrenia and Related Disorders: In short-term, placebo-controlled trials, there was no statistically significant difference in rates of discontinuation of ZYPREXA or placebo attributed to adverse events. Overall, 5% of ZYPREXA-treated patients discontinued treatment for adverse events compared with 6% of placebo-treated patients. Discontinuations due to ALT elevations, however, were considered to be drug related (2% for olanzapine versus 0% for placebo) (see Warnings and Precautions, Renal).

Bipolar Disorder: Bipolar Mania: In short-term, placebo-controlled clinical trials, there was no difference overall in the incidence of discontinuation due to adverse events (2% for olanzapine versus 2% for placebo).

Bipolar Maintenance: In the long-term (1-year), placebo-controlled clinical trial, of the 225 ZYPREXA-treated patients, 16% (n=35) discontinued due to an adverse event, compared with 9% (n=12) of 136 placebo-treated patients.

In the long-term (1-year), active-controlled clinical trial, of the 217 ZYPREXA-treated patients, 19% (n=41) discontinued due to an adverse event, compared with 26% (n=55) of 214 lithium-treated patients.

All Short-Term Trials—Schizophrenia and Bipolar Mania Trials: In short-term, active-controlled clinical trials, of the 1796 oral ZYPREXA-treated patients in comparative clinical trials with haloperidol, 98 (5%) discontinued treatment for adverse events compared with 66 of 810 (8%) haloperidol-treated patients.

All Short-Term Trials—Overall Integrated Safety Database: In a pre-marketing clinical trial database of 2500 ZYPREXA-treated patients, 14.9% (372/2500) discontinued due to an adverse event. About half (183/372) of these discontinuations were associated with the underlying psychopathology. Other adverse events most commonly (incidence of 0.5%-0.6%) reported as the reason for discontinuation among olanzapine-treated patients were: ALT increased, unintended pregnancy, creatinine phosphokinase increased, and convulsion.

Intramuscular Administration: In short-term, placebo-controlled trials, there was little difference overall in the incidence of discontinuation due to adverse events (0.4%) for intramuscular olanzapine for injection vs. placebo (0%).

In short-term, active-controlled clinical trials, there was little difference overall in the incidence of discontinuations due to adverse events for patients treated with intramuscular olanzapine (0.6%) vs. intramuscular haloperidol-treated groups (1.8%).

In the overall integrated safety database, of the 722 patients treated with intramuscular olanzapine, a total of 5 (0.7%) discontinued due to adverse events. The adverse events leading to discontinuation were anxiety, maculopapular rash, agitation, hostility and tachycardia.

Incidence of Commonly Observed Adverse Events: Oral Administration: Schizophrenia and Related Disorders: In the schizophrenia placebo-controlled trials, the most commonly observed adverse events associated with the use of olanzapine (incidence of ≥5% and at least twice placebo) were: dizziness (11% for olanzapine vs 4% for placebo), constipation (9% vs 3%), ALT increased (8% vs 3%), personality disorder (8% vs 4%), weight gain (6% vs 1%), akathisia (5% vs 1%), and postural hypotension (5% vs 2%).

Bipolar Disorder: Bipolar Mania: In the bipolar mania monotherapy placebo-controlled trials, the most commonly observed adverse events associated with the use of olanzapine (incidence of ≥5% and at least twice placebo) were: somnolence (35% vs 13%), dry mouth (22% vs 7%), dizziness (18% vs 6%), asthenia (15% vs 6%), constipation (11% vs 5%), dyspepsia (11% vs 5%), increased appetite (6% vs 3%), and tremor (6% vs 3%).

In bipolar mania combination placebo-controlled trials, the most commonly observed adverse events associated with the combination of olanzapine and lithium or valproate (incidence of ≥5% and at least twice placebo) were: dry mouth (32% for olanzapine combination vs 9% for placebo), weight gain (26% vs 7%), increased appetite (24% vs 8%), dizziness (14% vs 7%), back pain (8% vs 4%), constipation (8% vs 4%), speech disorder (7% vs 1%), increased salivation (6% vs 2%), amnesia (5% vs 2%), and paresthesia (5% vs 2%). In addition to the latter list of adverse events identified during bipolar mania combination clinical trials tremor (≥10%) has also been identified.

Bipolar Maintenance: In the one-year 'time to relapse' placebo-controlled clinical trial in bipolar disorder, the most commonly observed adverse events associated with olanzapine (incidence of ≥5% and at least twice placebo) were: weight increased (8% for olanzapine vs 1.5% for placebo), headache NOS (6.7% vs 2.9%), fatigue (6.2% vs 1.5%), depression (5.8% vs 2.9%).

Other Indication Trials: Abnormal gait and falls have been observed very commonly (≥10%) in clinical trials with elderly patients with dementia-related psychosis. Also, urinary incontinence and pneumonia were commonly reported (≥1% and <10%) in these patients.

In clinical trials in patients with drug-induced (dopamine agonist) psychosis associated with Parkinson's disease, worsening of Parkinsonian symptomatology and hallucinations were reported very commonly and more frequently than with placebo.

Intramuscular Administration: There was one adverse event (somnolence) observed at an incidence of 5-6% or greater among intramuscular olanzapine 10 mg for injection-treated patients and not observed at an equivalent incidence among placebo-treated patients (olanzapine incidence at least twice that for placebo) during the placebo-controlled pre-marketing studies. The incidence of somnolence during the 24 hour IM treatment period in clinical trials in agitated patients with schizophrenia or bipolar mania was 6% for intramuscular olanzapine for injection and 3% for placebo.

Adverse Events Occurring at an Incidence of 1% or More Among Oral Olanzapine-Treated Patients: Certain portions of the discussion below relating to objective or numeric safety parameters are derived from studies in patients with schizophrenia and have not been duplicated for bipolar disorder trials. However, this information is also generally applicable to bipolar disorder. Table 1 enumerates the incidence of treatment-emergent adverse events, rounded to the nearest percent, that occurred during acute therapy (up to 6 weeks) of schizophrenia in 1% or more of patients treated with oral ZYPREXA (doses ≥2.5 mg/day) where the incidence in patients treated with ZYPREXA was greater than the incidence in placebo-treated patients.

Table 1: ZYPREXA

Schizophrenia Trials: Treatment-emergent Adverse Events Incidence in Placebo-controlled Clinical Trials with Oral Olanzapine—Acute Phase[a]

Body System/Adverse Event	Percentage of Patients Reporting Event	
	ZYPREXA (N=248)	Placebo (N=118)
Body as a Whole		
Headache	17%	15%
Pain	10%	9%
Fever	5%	3%
Abdominal Pain	4%	2%
Back Pain	4%	3%
Chest Pain	4%	2%
Neck Rigidity	2%	1%
Intentional Injury	1%	0%
Cardiovascular System		
Postural Hypotension	5%	2%
Tachycardia	4%	1%
Hypotension	2%	1%
Digestive System		
Constipation	9%	3%
Dry Mouth	7%	4%
Gamma Glutamyl Transpeptidase Increased	2%	1%
Increased Appetite	2%	1%
Hemic and Lymphatic		
Leukopenia	1%	0%
Metabolic and Nutritional Disorders		
ALT Increased	8%	3%
Weight Gain[b]	6%	1%
Edema	2%	0%
Peripheral Edema	2%	0%
AST Increased	2%	0%
Creatine Phosphokinase Increased	1%	0%
Musculoskeletal System		
Arthralgia	3%	2%
Joint Disorder	2%	1%
Twitching	2%	1%
Nervous System		
Somnolence[b]	26%	15%
Agitation	23%	17%
Insomnia	20%	19%
Nervousness	16%	14%
Hostility	15%	14%
Dizziness[b]	11%	4%
Anxiety	9%	8%
Personality Disorder	8%	4%
Akathisia[b]	5%	1%
Hypertonia	4%	3%
Speech Disorder	4%	1%
Tremor	4%	3%
Amnesia	2%	0%
Drug Dependence	2%	0%
Euphoria	2%	0%
Neurosis	1%	0%
Respiratory System		
Rhinitis	10%	6%
Cough Increased	5%	3%
Pharyngitis	5%	3%
Skin and Appendages		

(cont'd)

Table 1: ZYPREXA *(cont'd)*

Schizophrenia Trials: Treatment-emergent Adverse Events Incidence in Placebo-controlled Clinical Trials with Oral Olanzapine—Acute Phase[a]

	Percentage of Patients Reporting Event	
Body System/Adverse Event	**ZYPREXA (N=248)**	**Placebo (N=118)**
Fungal Dermatitis	2%	0%
Vesiculobullous Rash	2%	1%
Special Senses		
Amblyopia	5%	4%
Blepharitis	2%	1%
Eye Disorder	2%	1%
Corneal Lesion	1%	0%
Urogenital System		
Menstrual Disorder[c]	2%	0%

a The following events had an incidence equal to or less than placebo: abnormal dreams, accidental injury, anorexia, apathy, asthenia, cog-wheel rigidity, confusion, conjunctivitis, depression, diarrhea, dysmenorrhea[c], dyspepsia, ecchymosis, emotional lability, hallucinations, hyperkinesia, hypertension, hypokinesia, libido increased, myalgia, nausea, paranoid reaction, paresthesia, pruritus, rash, schizophrenic reaction, sweating, thinking abnormal, tooth caries, vaginitis[c], vomiting.
b Statistically significantly more frequent in patients treated with oral ZYPREXA than in patients treated with placebo.
c Denominator used was for females only (N=41 ZYPREXA; N=23 Placebo).

Adverse Events Occurring at an Incidence of 1% or More Among Intramuscular Olanzapine for Injection-Treated Patients: Table 2 enumerates the incidence, rounded to the nearest percent, of treatment-emergent adverse events that occurred in 1% or more of patients treated with intramuscular olanzapine for injection and with incidence greater than placebo who participated in the short-term, placebo-controlled trials in agitated patients with schizophrenia or bipolar mania.

Table 2: ZYPREXA

Treatment-Emergent Adverse Events: Incidence in Short-term (24 hour), Placebo-controlled Clinical Trials with Intramuscular Olanzapine for Injection in Agitated Patients with Schizophrenia or Bipolar Mania[a]

	Percentage of Patients Reporting Event	
Body System/Adverse Event	**Olanzapine (N=415)**	**Placebo (N=150)**
Body as a Whole		
Asthenia	2	1
Cardiovascular System		
Hypotension	2	0
Postural Hypotension	1	0
Nervous System		
Dizziness	4	2
Somnolence	6	3
Tremor	1	0

a Events reported by at least 1% of patients treated with olanzapine for injection, except the following events which had an incidence equal to or less than placebo: agitation, anxiety, dry mouth, headache, hypertension, insomnia, nervousness.

Other Adverse Events from Schizophrenia Trials: Certain portions of the discussion below relating to objective or numeric safety parameters, namely, vital sign changes, weight gain, laboratory changes, and ECG changes are derived from studies in patients with schizophrenia and have not been duplicated for bipolar mania. However, this information is also generally applicable to bipolar mania.

Weight Changes: During acute therapy (up to 6 weeks) in controlled clinical trials comparing ZYPREXA with placebo in the treatment of schizophrenia, the percentages of patients with weight gain ≥7% of baseline body weight at any time were 29% for ZYPREXA and 3% for placebo, which was a statistically significant difference. The average weight gain during acute therapy in patients treated with ZYPREXA was 2.8 kg. Clinically significant weight gain was observed across all baseline body mass index (BMI) categories. In long-term extension schizophrenia trials, there was an average gain of 5.4 kg, and 56% of olanzapine-treated patients with weight gain >7% of baseline body weight. In long-term extension bipolar maintenance trials, there was a mean weight gain of 3.8 kg, and with 31% of olanzapine-treated patients with weight gain >7% of baseline body weight (see Warnings and Precautions, Endocrine and Metabolism).

Vital Sign Changes: In placebo-controlled clinical trials, orthostatic hypotension (greater than 30 mm decrease in systolic blood pressure) occurred with an incidence of 5% in oral olanzapine-treated patients compared to 2% in placebo-treated patients (vital sign measurements collected only after 3-7 days of ZYPREXA treatment). Oral olanzapine was associated with a mean baseline to endpoint increase in heart rate of 2.4 beats per minute compared to no change among placebo-treated patients (see Warnings and Precautions, Cardiovascular).

Intramuscular olanzapine for injection was associated with bradycardia, hypotension, and tachycardia in clinical trials (see Warnings and Precautions, Cardiovascular).

Laboratory Changes: Olanzapine is associated with asymptomatic increases in ALT, AST, and GGT (see Warnings and Precautions, Hepatic/Biliary Pancreatic). Olanzapine is also associated with generally mild increases in serum prolactin, which usually decreases with continued drug treatment. Olanzapine is also associated with asymptomatic elevations of eosinophils and uric acid (see Warnings and Precautions, Renal), and with decreases in serum bicarbonate.

ECG Changes: Between-group comparisons for pooled placebo-controlled trials revealed no statistically significant olanzapine/placebo differences in the proportions of patients experiencing potentially important changes in ECG parameters, including QT, QTc, and PR intervals.

Other Adverse Events Observed During Clinical Trials with Oral and Intramuscular Olanzapine Across All Indications: The following discussion relates primarily to weight gain, lipids, and glucose changes observed during clinical trials across all indications.

Weight Changes: Weight gain has been very commonly observed in olanzapine-treated patients during clinical trials. In 13 placebo-controlled olanzapine monotherapy studies, 22.2% of olanzapine-treated patients gained ≥7% of their baseline body weight versus 3% of placebo-treated patients, with a median exposure of 8 weeks; 4.2% of olanzapine-treated patients gained ≥15% of their baseline weight versus 0.3% of placebo-treated patients, with a median exposure of 12 weeks. Clinically significant weight gain was observed across all baseline body mass index (BMI) categories.

In long-term studies (at least 48 weeks), both the magnitude of weight gain and the proportion of olanzapine-treated patients who had clinically significant weight gain were greater than in short-term studies. The percentage of patients who gained ≥25% of their baseline body weight with long-term exposure was very common (≥10%).

Lipids: In placebo-controlled clinical trials of up to 12 weeks in duration, olanzapine-treated patients had a greater mean increase in fasting total cholesterol, LDL cholesterol, and triglycerides compared to placebo-treated patients.

Mean increases in fasting lipid values (total cholesterol, LDL cholesterol, and triglycerides) were greater in patients without evidence of lipid dysregulation at baseline. However, for mean changes in fasting triglycerides, the difference between olanzapine and placebo was greater in patients with evidence of lipid dysregulation at baseline. Elevations in fasting triglyceride levels ≥11.3 mmol/L were uncommonly observed with olanzapine use (8 week median duration of exposure). See Table 3.

Table 3: ZYPREXA

Changes in Fasting Lipids Values from Adult Placebo-controlled Olanzapine Monotherapy Studies with Treatment Duration up to 12 Weeks

Laboratory Analyte	Olanzapine[a]	Placebo
Triglycerides: fasting normal to high (<1.70 mmol/L to ≥2.26 mmol/L)	9.2% (N=457)	4.4% (N=251)
Triglycerides: fasting borderline to high (≥1.70 mmol/L and <2.26 mmol/L to ≥2.26 mmol/L)	39.3% (N=135)	20.0% (N=65)
Cholesterol-Total: fasting normal to high (<5.18 mmol/L to ≥6.22 mmol/L)	2.8% (N=392)	2.4% (N=207)
Cholesterol-Total: fasting borderline to high (≥5.18 mmol/L and <6.22 mmol/L to ≥6.22 mmol/L)	23.0% (N=222)	12.5% (N=112)
LDL cholesterol: fasting normal to high (<2.59 mmol/L to ≥4.14 mmol/L)	0% (N=154)	1.2% (N=82)
LDL cholesterol: fasting borderline to high (≥2.59 mmol/L and <4.14 mmol/L to ≥4.14 mmol/L)	10.6% (N=302)	8.1% (N=173)

a Median duration of exposure 8 weeks.

For fasting HDL cholesterol, no statistically significant differences were observed between olanzapine-treated patients and placebo-treated patients (see Warnings and Precautions, Endocrine and Metabolism).

The proportion of patients who had changes in total cholesterol, LDL cholesterol or triglycerides from normal or borderline to high, or changes in HDL cholesterol from normal or borderline to low, was greater in long-term studies (at least 48 weeks) as compared with short-term studies. Treatment-emergent clinically significant changes in fasting lipids were observed in patients with or without evidence of dyslipidemia at baseline.

Glucose Changes: In clinical trials (up to 52 weeks) olanzapine was associated with a greater mean change in glucose relative to placebo.

The difference in mean changes between olanzapine and placebo was greater in patients with evidence of glucose dysregulation at baseline (including those patients diagnosed with diabetes mellitus or who met criteria suggestive of hyperglycemia), and these patients had a greater increase in HbA1c compared to placebo.

In patients with baseline normal fasting glucose levels (<5.5 mmol/L), 2.2% (N=543) of those treated with olanzapine (median exposure duration of 8 weeks) were found to have high glucose levels (≥6.99 mmol/L) during olanzapine treatment versus 3.4% (N=293) of those treated with placebo. In patients with baseline borderline fasting glucose levels (≥5.5 mmol/L and <6.99 mmol/L), 17.4% (N=178) of those treated with olanzapine (median exposure duration of 5 weeks) were found to have high glucose levels (≥6.99 mmol/L) during olanzapine treatment versus 11.5% (N=96) of those treated with placebo.

The proportion of patients who had a change in glucose level from normal or borderline at baseline to high increased over time. Treatment-emergent clinically significant changes in fasting glucose were observed in patients with or without evidence of glucose dysregulation at baseline.

Glycosuria was commonly reported in olanzapine-treated patients during clinical trials.

Vital Sign Changes: Bradycardia was uncommonly observed in clinical trials.

Photosensitivity Reactions: Photosensitivity reactions were uncommonly observed in clinical trials.

Dose-dependent Adverse Events: Dose-relatedness of adverse events was assessed using data from a clinical trial with a fixed dosage range. Table 4 enumerates the treatment-emergent adverse events in which there was a statistically significantly increasing dose response in this clinical trial.

Table 4: ZYPREXA

Schizophrenia Trials: Dose-dependent Adverse Events in a Fixed Dosage Range, Placebo-controlled Clinical Trial[a] of Oral Olanzapine

	Percentage of Patients Reporting Event			
Body System/Adverse Event	**Placebo (N=68)**	**ZYPREXA 5±2.5 mg/day (N=65)**	**ZYPREXA 10±2.5 mg/day (N=64)**	**ZYPREXA 15±2.5 mg/day (N=69)**
Digestive System				
Constipation	0%	6.2%	9.4%	14.5%
Nervous System				
Abnormal Dreams	0%	0%	1.6%	4.3%
Dizziness	2.9%	7.7%	9.4%	17.4%
Somnolence	16.2%	20.0%	29.7%	39.1%
Respiratory System				
Pharyngitis	1.5%	3.1%	1.6%	10.1%

a Fungal dermatitis was also reported with a statistically significantly increasing dose response, but is not included as a drug cause was remote.

Table 5 enumerates the treatment-emergent adverse events from one 8-week, randomized, double-blind, fixed-dose trial comparing 10 (N=199), 20 (N=200) and 40 (N=200) mg/day of olanzapine in patients with schizophrenia or schizoaffective disorder. Statistically significant differences among the 3 dose groups were observed for the following safety outcomes: fatigue, dizziness, prolactin elevation, and weight gain (mean change).

Incidence of Treatment-Emergent Extrapyramidal Symptoms: Table 6 enumerates the percentage of patients with treatment-emergent extrapyramidal symptoms as assessed by categorical analyses of formal rating scales during acute therapy in a controlled clinical trial comparing oral olanzapine at 3 fixed dosage ranges with placebo in the treatment of schizophrenia.

Table 5: ZYPREXA

Schizophrenia Trial: Dose-dependent Adverse Events in a Fixed Dose, Placebo-controlled Clinical Trial[a] of Oral Olanzapine

Adverse Event	ZYPREXA 10 mg/day (N=195)	ZYPREXA 20 mg/day (N=191)	ZYPREXA 40 mg/day (N=197)
Fatigue[b,c] (% reporting event)	1.5%	2.1%	6.6%
Dizziness[c] (% reporting event)	2.6%	1.6%	6.6%
Prolactin Elevation[b,c,d] (% reporting event)	31.2%	42.7%	61.1%
Prolactin Elevation[b,c] (mean change from baseline to endpoint)	−10.5 ng/mL	−1.7 ng/mL	4.9 ng/mL
Weight Gain ≥7% at any time (% reporting event)	14.0%	18.4%	20.5%
Weight Gain[b] (mean change from baseline to endpoint)	1.9 kg	2.3 kg	3.0 kg

[a] Study HGLF: 8-week, Phase IV, parallel, randomized, double-blind, fixed-dose study in patients with schizophrenia and schizoaffective disorder evaluating the dose-response efficacy and safety of olanzapine 10, 20, and 40 mg/day. Patients were titrated up to their randomized dose over 2 weeks.
[b] Significant difference between 10 vs. 40 mg/day.
[c] Significant difference between 20 vs. 40 mg/day.
[d] >24.2 ng/mL (female) or >18.77 ng/mL (male) at any time during the trial.

Table 6: ZYPREXA

Schizophrenia Trials: Treatment-emergent Extrapyramidal Symptoms Assessed by Rating Scales Incidence in a Fixed Dosage Range, Placebo-controlled Clinical Trial—Acute Phase[a]

	Percentage of Patients			
	Placebo	ZYPREXA 5±2.5 mg/day	ZYPREXA 10±2.5 mg/day	ZYPREXA 15±2.5 mg/day
Parkinsonism[b]	15%	14%	12%	14%
Akathisia[c]	23%	16%	19%	27%

[a] No statistically significant differences.
[b] Percentage of patients with a Simpson-Angus Scale total score ≥3.
[c] Percentage of patients with a Barnes Akathisia Scale global score ≥2.

Table 7 enumerates the percentage of patients with treatment-emergent extrapyramidal symptoms as assessed by spontaneously reported adverse events during acute therapy in the same controlled clinical trial comparing oral olanzapine at 3 fixed dosage ranges with placebo in the treatment of schizophrenia. Similar results were found during the long-term (up to 1-year) double-blind monotherapy extension bipolar maintenance trial comparing ZYPREXA with placebo; there was a higher statistical incidence of akathisia for combined doses of ZYPREXA versus placebo.

Table 7: ZYPREXA

Schizophrenia Trials: Treatment-emergent Extrapyramidal Symptoms Assessed by Adverse Events Incidence in an Oral Fixed Dosage Range, Placebo-controlled Clinical Trial—Acute Phase[a]

	Percentage of Patients Reporting Event			
Extrapyramidal Symptoms	Placebo (N=68)	ZYPREXA 5±2.5 mg/day (N=65)	ZYPREXA 10±2.5 mg/day (N=64)	ZYPREXA 15±2.5 mg/day (N=69)
Dystonic Events[b]	1%	3%	2%	3%
Parkinsonism Events[c]	10%	8%	14%	20%
Akathisia Events[d]	1%	5%	11%[a]	10%[a]
Dyskinetic Events[e]	4%	0%	2%	1%
Residual Events[f]	1%	2%	5%	1%
Any Extrapyramidal Event	16%	15%	25%	32%[a]

[a] Statistically significantly different from placebo.
[b] Patients with the following COSTART terms were counted in this category: dystonia, generalized spasm, neck rigidity, oculogyric crisis, opisthotonos, torticollis.
[c] Patients with the following COSTART terms were counted in this category: akinesia, cogwheel rigidity, extrapyramidal syndrome, hypertonia, hypokinesia, masked facies, tremor.
[d] Patients with the following COSTART terms were counted in this category: akathisia, hyperkinesia.
[e] Patients with the following COSTART terms were counted in this category: buccoglossal syndrome, choreoathetosis, dyskinesia, tardive dyskinesia.
[f] Patients with the following COSTART terms were counted in this category: movement disorder, myoclonus, twitching.

Table 8 enumerates the percentage of patients with treatment-emergent extrapyramidal symptoms as assessed by categorical analyses of formal rating scales during controlled clinical trials comparing fixed doses of intramuscular olanzapine for injection with placebo in agitation. Patients in each dose group could receive up to three injections during the trials. Patient assessments were conducted during the 24 hours following the initial dose of intramuscular olanzapine for injection. There were no statistically significant differences from placebo.

Table 9 enumerates the percentage of patients with treatment-emergent extrapyramidal symptoms as assessed by spontaneously reported adverse events in the same controlled clinical trial comparing fixed doses of intramuscular olanzapine for injection with placebo in agitated patients with schizophrenia. There were no statistically significant differences from placebo.

Other Investigational Trials: Cerebrovascular Adverse Events (CVAEs) in Elderly Patients with Dementia: Data from 5 placebo-controlled trials in elderly patients with dementia-related psychosis (Alzheimer's, vascular, and mixed; ZYPREXA n=1178 and placebo n=478) suggest that there was a higher incidence of CVAE in patients treated with ZYPREXA compared to patients treated with placebo (1.3% vs. 0.4%, respectively). Although the incidence of CVAE was not significantly different when analyzed with Fisher's Exact Test (p=0.177), the difference was found to be significant when simultaneously controlling for age, gender, and type of dementia using Poisson Regression (p=0.0428). Four patients died in the ZYPREXA group versus 1 patient in the placebo group. In open-label safety trials studied for up to 59 weeks in dementia patients (N=231), 7 cases of CVAEs, including 2 fatalities, were reported (see Warnings and Precautions).

Table 8: ZYPREXA IntraMuscular

Treatment-emergent Extrapyramidal Symptoms Assessed by Rating Scales Incidence in a Fixed Dose, Placebo-controlled Clinical Trial of Intramuscular Olanzapine for Injection in Agitated Patients with Schizophrenia[a]

	Percentage of Patients				
	Placebo	Olanzapine IM 2.5 mg	Olanzapine IM 5 mg	Olanzapine IM 7.5 mg	Olanzapine IM 10 mg
Parkinsonism[b]	0	0	0	0	3
Akathisia[c]	0	0	5	0	0

[a] No statistically significant differences.
[b] Percentage of patients with a Simpson-Angus Scale total score ≥3.
[c] Percentage of patients with a Barnes Akathisia Scale global score ≥2.

Table 9: ZYPREXA IntraMuscular

Treatment-emergent Extrapyramidal Symptoms Assessed by Adverse Events Incidence in a Fixed Dose, Placebo-controlled Clinical Trial of Intramuscular Olanzapine for Injection in Agitated Patients with Schizophrenia[a]

	Percentage of Patients Reporting Event				
	Placebo (N=45)	Olanzapine IM 2.5 mg (N=48)	Olanzapine IM 5 mg (N=45)	Olanzapine IM 7.5 mg (N=46)	Olanzapine IM 10 mg (N=46)
Dystonic Events[b]	0	0	0	0	0
Parkinsonism Events[c]	0	4	2	0	0
Akathisia Events[d]	0	2	0	0	0
Dyskinetic Events[e]	0	0	0	0	0
Residual Events[f]	0	0	0	0	0
Any Extrapyramidal Event	0	4	2	0	0

[a] No statistically significant differences.
[b] Patients with the following COSTART terms were counted in this category: dystonia, generalized spasm, neck rigidity, oculogyric crisis, opisthotonos, torticollis.
[c] Patients with the following COSTART terms were counted in this category: akinesia, cogwheel rigidity, extrapyramidal syndrome, hypertonia, hypokinesia, masked facies, tremor.
[d] Patients with the following COSTART terms were counted in this category: akathisia, hyperkinesia.
[e] Patients with the following COSTART terms were counted in this category: buccoglossal syndrome, choreoathetosis, dyskinesia, tardive dyskinesia.
[f] Patients with the following COSTART terms were counted in this category: movement disorder, myoclonus, twitching.

Data from these trials suggest that patients with a dementia diagnosis of vascular or mixed type had a 5-fold higher likelihood of experiencing CVAEs than patients with a diagnosis of Alzheimer's. There is insufficient information to determine whether CVAEs in elderly patients with dementia are associated specifically with ZYPREXA or all antipsychotic agents.

ZYPREXA is not approved for use in elderly patients with dementia.

Overall Mortality: Elderly patients with dementia treated with atypical antipsychotic drugs showed increased mortality compared to placebo in a meta-analysis of 13 controlled trials of various atypical antipsychotic drugs. In five placebo-controlled trials with oral ZYPREXA in this population, the incidence of mortality was 3.5 % for ZYPREXA-treated patients compared to 1.5 % for placebo-treated patients. ZYPREXA is not indicated in elderly patients with dementia.

Laboratory Changes: In 5 double-blind, placebo controlled clinical trials of elderly patients with dementia-related psychosis (n=1184 total in the olanzapine arms and n=478 total in placebo arms), olanzapine-treated patients showed significantly greater incidence rates compared to placebo-treated patients of low albumin (10.4% vs 5.5%, respectively), low hemoglobin (4.2% vs 1.8%) and low hematocrit (4.6% vs 2.4%). Of patients who had low albumin values, 3.6% in the olanzapine-treated group vs 1.4% in the placebo-treated also experienced a treatment-emergent respiratory infection. A causal relationship between the two adverse events has not been determined.

Adverse Events in Adolescent Patients (ages 13-17 years): The types of adverse events observed in adolescent patients treated with olanzapine were similar to those seen in adult patients. Although no clinical trials designed to compare adolescents to adults were conducted, the data from the adolescent trials were compared to those of the adult trials.

Mean increase in weight in adolescents (4.6 kg over 3 weeks median duration of exposure) was greater than in adults (2.6 kg over 7 weeks median duration of exposure).

In long-term studies (at least 24 weeks), both the magnitude of weight gain and the proportion of adolescent olanzapine-treated patients who had clinically significant weight gain were greater than in short-term studies and were greater than in adult patients with comparable exposures. With long-term exposure, approximately half of adolescent patients gained ≥15% and almost a third gained ≥25% of their baseline body weight. Among adolescent patients, mean weight gain was greatest in patients who were overweight or obese at baseline.

Increases in fasting glucose were similar in adolescents and adults treated with olanzapine; however, the difference between olanzapine and placebo groups was greater in adolescents compared to adults.

In long-term studies (at least 24 weeks), changes in glucose from normal at baseline to high were uncommon (<1% and ≥0.1%).

Increases in fasting total cholesterol, LDL cholesterol, and triglycerides were generally greater in adolescents than in adults treated with olanzapine. However, in short term trials, the differences between olanzapine and placebo were similar for adolescents and adults.

The proportion of treatment-emergent clinically significant changes in normal-to-high or borderline-to-high fasting total cholesterol, LDL cholesterol and triglycerides was greater in adolescents compared to adults, and the differences between olanzapine and placebo in these categories of laboratory values were also generally greater in adolescents. In long-term studies, treatment-emergent clinically significant changes in total cholesterol, LDL cholesterol, and triglycerides were observed in adolescents with or without evidence of dyslipidemia at baseline.

Table 10 summarizes core adverse drug reaction terms for olanzapine compared to placebo and their frequencies identified only during clinical trials in adolescent patients (ages 13 to 17 years). ZYPREXA is not indicated in adolescent patients (ages 13-17 years).

Table 10: ZYPREXA

Core Adverse Drug Reactions and Frequencies from Clinical Trials in Adolescent Patients (ages 13-17 years)

Body System/Adverse Reaction Term	Olanzapine		Placebo	
	Frequency	N	Frequency	N
Body as a Whole				
Weight gain ≥7% of baseline body weight (kg)[g]	40.6%	197	9.8%	112

(cont'd)

Table 10: ZYPREXA *(cont'd)*

Core Adverse Drug Reactions and Frequencies from Clinical Trials in Adolescent Patients (ages 13-17 years)

Body System/Adverse Reaction Term	Olanzapine		Placebo	
	Frequency	N	Frequency	N
Weight gain ≥15% of baseline body weight (kg)[h]	7.1%	197	2.7%	112
Digestive System				
Dry Mouth	6.15%	179	0%	89
Increased Appetite	24%	179	6%	89
Nervous System				
Sedation[a]	44.1%	179	9%	89
Clinical Chemistry				
ALT >3× ULN all randomized patients with ALT baseline ≤3× ULN[b]	12.1%	174	2.3%	87
AST—Increased[c]	27.6%	163	3.8%	79
Total bilirubin—Decreased[d]	22.1%	154	6.7%	75
GGT—Increased[e]	10.1%	169	1.2%	83
Prolactin—Increased[f]	47.4%	116	6.8%	59
Cholesterol—total, fasting normal to high (<4.40 mmol/L to ≥5.18 mmol/L)[i]	6.9%	87	2.3%	43
Cholesterol—total, fasting borderline to high (≥4.40 mmol/L and <5.18 mmol/L to ≥5.18 mmol/L)[i]	38.9%	36	7.7%	13
LDL cholesterol: fasting normal to high (<2.85 mmol/L to ≥3.37 mmol/L)	5.1%	98	4.5%	44
LDL cholesterol: fasting borderline to high (≥2.85 mmol/L and <3.37 mmol/L to ≥3.37 mmol/L)	48.3%	29	0%	9
Triglycerides, fasting normal to high (<1.02 mmol/L to >1.47 mmol/L)[i]	26.9%	67	10.7%	28
Triglycerides, fasting borderline to high (≥1.02 mmol/L and ≤1.47 mmol/L to >1.47 mmol/L)[i]	59.5%	37	35.3%	17
Glucose, fasting normal to high (<5.55 mmol/L to ≥6.99 mmol/L)[i]	0%	124	1.9%	53
Glucose, fasting borderline to high (≥5.55 mmol/L and <6.99 mmol/L to ≥6.99 mmol/L)[i]	14.3%	14	0%	13

a Represented cluster of MedDRA terms including: hypersomnia, lethargy, sedation, somnolence.
b Covance reference ranges:
Female: 13-≤17.999: Low: 6. High: 34 (U/L).
Male: 13-≤17.999: Low: 6. High: 43 (U/L).
c Covance reference ranges:
Female: 13-≤17.999: Low: 10. High: 40 (U/L).
Male: 13-≤17.999. Low: 10. High: 40 (U/L).
d Covance reference ranges:
Female: 13-≤17.999: Low: 3. High: 21 (mmol/L).
Male: 13-≤17.999: Low: 3. High: 21 (mmol/L).
e Covance reference ranges:
Female: 13-≤17.999: Low: 0. High: 33 (U/L).
Male: 13-≤17.999: Low: 0. High: 51 (U/L).
f Covance reference ranges for prolactin as published by Wiedemann and Jonetz-Mentzel (1993):
Female: 12 to 14 years: 2.52-16.90 ng/mL; 14 to 19 years: 4.20-39.00 ng/mL.
Male: 12 to 14 years: 2.84-24.00 ng/mL; 14 to 19 years: 2.76-16.10 ng/mL.
g Median duration of exposure was 4 weeks.
h Median duration of exposure was 19 weeks.
i Median duration of exposure was 3 weeks.
j Median duration of exposure was 5 weeks.

Post-Market Adverse Drug Reactions: Table 11 summarizes core adverse drug reaction terms and their frequencies identified from global post-marketing surveillance in addition to what was reported in clinical trials (see Clinical Trial Adverse Drug Reactions). A causal relationship between ZYPREXA and the emergence of these events has not been established.

Table 11: ZYPREXA

Core Adverse Drug Reactions Seen with Olanzapine Formulations[a]

Body System/Adverse Reaction Term	Frequency				
	≥10%	<10% and ≥1%	<1% and ≥0.1%	<0.1% and ≥0.01%	<0.01%
Body as a Whole					
Allergic Reaction[b]					X
Discontinuation Reaction[c]					X
Cardiovascular					
Venous Thromboembolism, Including Pulmonary Embolism and Deep Vein Thrombosis					X
Digestive System					
Pancreatitis					X
Hematologic					
Thrombocytopenia[d]					X
Leukopenia, Including Neutropenia				X	
Hepatobiliary Disorders					
Hepatitis				X	
Jaundice					X
Hepatic Failure					X
Metabolic					
Diabetic Coma					X
Diabetic Ketoacidosis[e]					X
Hypercholesterolemia[g]					X
Hyperglycaemia				X	
Hypertriglyceridemia[f,g]					X
Exacerbation of Pre-existing Diabetes				X	
Musculoskeletal System					
Rhabdomyolysis					X
Nervous System					
Seizures				X	
Skin and Appendages					
Alopecia					X
Rash				X	
Urogenital System					
Priapism					X
Laboratory Analytes					
Clinical Chemistry					
Alkaline Phosphatase–Increased					X
Total Bilirubin–Increased					X

a Adverse event identified from spontaneous post-marketing surveillance.
b e.g., maculopapular rash, anaphylactoid reaction, angioedema, pruritus, or urticaria.
c i.e., diaphoresis, nausea or vomiting.
d Including a case of thrombocytopenic purpura.
e COSTART term is diabetic acidosis.
f COSTART term is hyperlipemia.
g Random cholesterol levels of ≥6.22 mmol/L and random triglyceride levels of ≥11.30 mmol/L have been very rarely reported.

DRUG INTERACTIONS: Drug-Drug Interactions: Alcohol: Given the primary CNS effects of ZYPREXA, caution should be used when it is taken in combination with other centrally acting drugs and alcohol.

Levodopa and Dopamine Agonists: As it exhibits in vitro dopamine antagonism, ZYPREXA may antagonize the effects of levodopa and dopamine agonists.

Antihypertensive Agents: Because of its potential for inducing hypotension, olanzapine may enhance the effects of certain antihypertensive agents. Caution should be exercised in patients who receive medicinal products that can induce hypotension, bradycardia, or respiratory depression.

Potential for Other Drugs to Affect ZYPREXA: Carbamazepine: Concomitant carbamazepine therapy may induce the metabolism of olanzapine.

Activated Charcoal: The concomitant administration of activated charcoal reduced the oral bioavailability of ZYPREXA by 50% to 60%.

Antacids: Single doses of antacid (aluminium, magnesium) or cimetidine did not affect the oral bioavailability of ZYPREXA.

Valproate: Studies in vitro using human liver microsomes showed that olanzapine has little potential to inhibit the glucuronidation of valproate, which is the major metabolic pathway. Furthermore, valproate was found to have little effect on the metabolism of olanzapine in vitro. Daily concomitant in vivo administration of 10 mg olanzapine for 2 weeks did not affect steady state plasma concentrations of valproate. Therefore, concomitant olanzapine administration does not require dosage adjustment of valproate.

Fluoxetine: Fluoxetine (60 mg single dose or 60 mg daily for 8 days) causes a mean 16% increase in the maximum concentration of olanzapine and a mean 16% decrease in olanzapine clearance. The magnitude of the impact of this factor is small in comparison to the overall variability between individuals, and therefore dose modification is not routinely recommended.

CYP1A2 Inducers: Agents that induce CYP1A2 such as omeprazole may increase clearance of olanzapine.

CYP1A2 Inhibitors: Fluvoxamine, a specific CYP1A2 inhibitor, has been shown to significantly inhibit the metabolism of olanzapine. The mean increase in olanzapine C_{max} following fluvoxamine was 54% in female nonsmokers and 77% in male smokers. The mean increase in olanzapine AUC was 52% and 108%, respectively. A lower starting dose of olanzapine should be considered in patients who are using fluvoxamine or any other CYP1A2 inhibitors, such as ciprofloxacin or ketoconazole. A decrease in the dose of olanzapine should be considered if treatment with an inhibitor of CYP1A2 is initiated.

(cont'd)

Potential for ZYPREXA to Affect Other Drugs: Imipramine/Desipramine: In clinical trials with single doses of oral ZYPREXA, no inhibition of the metabolism of imipramine/desipramine (P450-CYP2D6) was evident.
Warfarin: In clinical trials with single doses of oral ZYPREXA, no inhibition of the metabolism of warfarin (P450 CYP2C9) was evident.
Diazepam: In clinical trials with single doses of oral ZYPREXA, no inhibition of the metabolism of diazepam (P450 CYP3A4) was evident.
Lithium or Biperiden: Oral ZYPREXA showed no interaction when coadministered with lithium or biperiden.
Drugs Metabolized via P450-CYP1A2, -CYP2C9, -CYP2C19, -CYP2D6, and -CYP3A4: In in vitro studies with human microsomes, olanzapine showed little potential to inhibit cytochromes P450-CYP1A2, -CYP2C9, -CYP2C19, -CYP2D6, and -CYP3A4. Olanzapine is thus unlikely to cause clinically important drug-drug interactions mediated through the metabolic routes outlined above. However, the possibility that olanzapine may alter the metabolism of other drugs, or that other drugs may alter the metabolism of olanzapine, should be considered when prescribing ZYPREXA.
Lorazepam: Simultaneous injection of intramuscular olanzapine and parenteral benzodiazepine is not recommended (see Warnings and Precautions). In a clinical pharmacokinetic/pharmacodynamic study, administration of intramuscular lorazepam (2 mg) two hours following intramuscular olanzapine (5 mg) did not significantly affect the pharmacokinetics of olanzapine, unconjugated lorazepam, or total lorazepam. Administration of intramuscular lorazepam two hours after injection of intramuscular olanzapine however, added to the somnolence observed with either drug alone.
Phenylketonurics: ZYPREXA Zydis contains phenylalanine (0.34, 0.45, 0.67, or 0.90 mg per 5, 10, 15, or 20 mg oral lyophilisate, respectively).
Drug-Food Interactions: Absorption of olanzapine is not affected by food.
Drug-Herb Interactions: Interactions with herbal products have not been identified.
Drug-Laboratory Interactions: Interactions with laboratory tests have not been identified.
Drug-Lifestyle Interactions: Smoking: Concomitant smoking may induce the metabolism of olanzapine.

DOSAGE AND ADMINISTRATION: Oral Administration: Schizophrenia and Related Disorders: Adults: ZYPREXA (olanzapine) should be administered on a once-a-day schedule without regard to meals, generally beginning with 5 to 10 mg, with a target dose of 10 mg/day within several days. Further dosage adjustments, if indicated, should generally occur at intervals of not less than 1 week, since steady state for ZYPREXA would not be achieved for approximately 1 week in the typical patient. When dosage adjustments are necessary, dose increments/decrements of 5 mg per day are recommended. An increase to a dose greater than target dose of 10 mg/day (i.e., to a dose of 15 mg/day or greater) is normally recommended only after clinical assessment.

In clinical trials a dose range of 5-20 mg/day was studied. Doses above 20 mg/day have been evaluated from a safety perspective (see Table 5 in Adverse Events, Dose-Dependent Adverse Events); however, efficacy at doses above 20 mg/day has not been systematically evaluated.
Maintenance Therapy in Schizophrenia: It is recommended that responding patients with schizophrenia be continued on ZYPREXA at the lowest dose needed to maintain remission. Patients should be reassessed periodically to determine the need for maintenance treatment. While there is no body of evidence available to answer the question of how long the patient should be treated with ZYPREXA, the effectiveness of maintenance treatment is well established for many other antipsychotic drugs.
Bipolar Disorder: Bipolar Mania: Adults: The recommended starting dose for olanzapine is 15 mg administered once a day in monotherapy and 10 mg daily in combination therapy.

It may be given without regard to meals as its absorption is not affected by food. The dosage range of olanzapine is from 5 mg to 20 mg per day. Daily dosage should be adjusted in response to clinical assessment.
Maintenance Therapy in Bipolar Disorder: Patients who have been receiving and responding to ZYPREXA for the treatment of acute manic or mixed episodes of bipolar disorder should initially continue maintenance therapy at the same dose. Subsequent daily dosage should be adjusted on the basis of clinical status within a range of 5-20 mg per day.

Patients should be periodically reassessed to determine the need for maintenance treatment and the appropriate dose for such treatment.
General Considerations for Oral Dosing in Special Populations: The Elderly or Debilitated Patient: In clinical trials, 44 patients with schizophrenia or related disorders who were 65 years of age or over were treated with ZYPREXA (5-20 mg daily) (see Warnings and Precautions, Special Populations). Given the limited experience with ZYPREXA in the elderly, and the higher incidence of concomitant illness and concomitant medication in this population, ZYPREXA should be used with caution.

The recommended starting dose is 5 mg in patients who are elderly, debilitated, who have a predisposition to hypotensive reactions, who otherwise exhibit a combination of factors that may result in slower metabolism of ZYPREXA (e.g., nonsmoking female patients), or who may be pharmacodynamically more sensitive to ZYPREXA. When indicated, dose escalation should be performed with caution in these patients.
Patients with Hepatic and/or Renal Impairment: As clinical experience is lacking in these patients, the lower initial starting dose and slower titration to initial target dose should be considered. Further dose escalation, when indicated, should be conservative (see Warnings and Precautions, Special Populations).
Missed Dose: If a patient misses a dose by a few hours, advise patient to take as soon as he/she remembers. If most of the day has passed, advise patient to wait until the next scheduled dose. Advise patients to not take 2 doses of ZYPREXA at once.
Administration of ZYPREXA Zydis: ZYPREXA Zydis orally disintegrating tablet is intended for oral administration only. It begins disintegrating in the mouth within seconds, allowing its contents to be subsequently swallowed with or without liquid.

The orally disintegrating tablet breaks easily and should be handled carefully, with dry hands. Direct contact with hands should be avoided if possible. One blister cell must be separated from the strip prior to peeling the blister backing. The blister backing should be carefully peeled back and the orally disintegrating tablet pushed out and placed directly in the mouth. The orally disintegrating tablet may also be stirred into 125 mL (4 ounces) of water, milk, coffee, orange juice or apple juice and the contents promptly consumed.
Intramuscular Administration: In clinical trials, individual doses of 5 mg, 7.5 mg and 10 mg of intramuscular olanzapine for injection have been shown to be effective in controlling agitation in patients with schizophrenia. Individual doses of more than 10 mg of intramuscular olanzapine have not been studied and are not recommended.
Usual Dose for Agitated Patients with Schizophrenia and Bipolar Mania: The usual initial dose for olanzapine injection is 10 mg, administered as a single intramuscular injection. A lower dose (5 mg or 7.5 mg) may be given, on the basis of individual clinical status.
Repeat and Maximum Dose: In clinical trials over a 24 hour period, a minority of patients required a second dose, and only a small percent of patients required a third dose of ZYPREXA IntraMuscular. Thus safety information on the use of repeated doses of ZYPREXA IntraMuscular is limited. Nevertheless, if warranted by the clinical situation, a second dose, 5-10 mg, may be administered 2 hours after the first injection. A third dose, if required, should be given no sooner than four hours after the second dose. The safety of total daily doses greater than 30 mg has not been evaluated in clinical trials.

The recommended maximum daily dose of olanzapine (oral and IM) is 20 mg, with no more than three injections in a 24 hour period.
General Considerations for Intramuscular Dosing in Special Populations: Elderly or Debilitated Patients: Lower doses (e.g. 2.5 mg) should be considered when clinical factors warrant.
Administration of ZYPREXA IntraMuscular: Zyprexa IntraMuscular is intended for intramuscular use only. Do not administer intravenously or subcutaneously. Inject slowly, deep into the muscle mass.

Concomitant administration of intramuscular olanzapine and parenteral benzodiazepine is not recommended (see Warnings and Precautions).

Parenteral drug products should be inspected visually for particulate matter and discolouration prior to administration, whenever solution and container permit.
Reconstitution: Directions for Preparation of ZYPREXA IntraMuscular with Sterile Water for Injection: Dissolve the contents of the vial using 2.1 mL of Sterile Water for Injection to provide a solution containing approximately 5 mg/mL of olanzapine. The resulting solution should appear clear and yellow. ZYPREXA IntraMuscular reconstituted with Sterile Water for Injection should be used immediately (within 1 hour) after reconstitution. **Discard any unused portion.**

Vial Size	Volume of Diluent to be Added to Vial	Approximate Available Volume	Nominal Concentration per mL
5 mL	2.1 mL of Sterile Water for Injection	2 mL	5 mg/mL

The following table provides injection volumes for delivering various doses of intramuscular olanzapine for injection reconstituted with Sterile Water for Injection.

Dose, mg olanzapine	Volume of Injection, mL
10	Withdraw total contents of vial
7.5	1.5
5	1
2.5	0.5

Physical Incompatibility Information: ZYPREXA IntraMuscular should be reconstituted only with Sterile Water for Injection. ZYPREXA IntraMuscular should not be combined in a syringe with diazepam injection because precipitation occurs when these products are mixed. Lorazepam injection should not be used to reconstitute ZYPREXA IntraMuscular as this combination results in a delayed reconstitution time. ZYPREXA IntraMuscular should not be combined in a syringe with haloperidol injection because the resulting low pH has been shown to degrade olanzapine over time.
Ongoing Therapy: If ongoing olanzapine therapy is clinically indicated, treatment with intramuscular olanzapine for injection should be discontinued and oral olanzapine may be initiated in a range of 5-20 mg/day as soon as clinically appropriate (see Dosage and Administration, Oral Administration).

OVERDOSAGE:
Signs and Symptoms: Very common symptoms reported in olanzapine overdose (≥10% incidence) include tachycardia, agitation/aggressiveness, dysarthria, various extrapyramidal symptoms, and reduced level of consciousness ranging from sedation to coma.

Other medically significant sequelae of olanzapine overdose include delirium, convulsion, possible neuroleptic malignant syndrome, respiratory depression, aspiration, hypertension or hypotension, cardiac arrhythmias (<2% of overdose cases) and cardiopulmonary arrest. Fatal outcomes have been reported for acute overdoses as low as 450 mg of oral olanzapine but survival has also been reported following acute overdose of approximately 2000 mg of oral olanzapine.
Management of Overdose: There is no specific antidote for olanzapine. Induction of emesis is not recommended. Standard procedures for management of overdose may be indicated (i.e. gastric lavage, administration of activated charcoal). The concomitant administration of activated charcoal was shown to reduce the oral bioavailability of olanzapine by 50 to 60%.

Symptomatic treatment and monitoring of vital organ function should be instituted according to clinical presentation, including treatment of hypotension and circulatory collapse and support of respiratory function. Do not use epinephrine, dopamine, or other sympathomimetic agents with beta-agonist activity since beta stimulation may worsen hypotension.

For management of a suspected drug overdose, contact your **regional Poison Control Centre**. See the *CPS* Directory section for a list of Poison Control Centres.

ACTION AND CLINICAL PHARMACOLOGY: Pharmacodynamics: Pharmacodynamic Properties: ZYPREXA (olanzapine), a thienobenzodiazepine, is an antipsychotic agent that demonstrates a broad pharmacologic profile across a number of receptor systems. Olanzapine displays high receptor affinity binding in vitro at dopamine D_1, D_3, D_4 (Ki=11-31 nM), 5-$HT_{2A/C}$ (Ki=4 and 11 nM, respectively), 5-HT_3, 5-HT_6, muscarinic M_1-M_5 (Ki=1.9-2.5 nM), adrenergic α_1 (Ki=19 nM), and histamine H_1 (Ki=7 nM) receptor subtypes. In a behavioural paradigm predictive of antipsychotic activity, olanzapine reduced conditioned avoidance response in rats at doses lower than 4 times those required to produce catalepsy. In a single dose (10 mg) PET study in healthy subjects, olanzapine produced higher 5-HT_{2A} than dopamine D_2 receptor occupancy. The percent of D_2 occupancy was less than the threshold value predictive of extrapyramidal events.

In animals olanzapine has been observed to produce a significant reduction in the firing of A10 dopaminergic cells. The number of spontaneously active A9 neurons either remained constant or was increased. This may explain the low incidence of extrapyramidal side effects with olanzapine usually associated with the typical antipsychotics.

Olanzapine also increases extracellular levels of dopamine in a regionally specific manner in the prefrontal cortex, similar to mood stabilizers, lithium and valproate.
Pharmacokinetics: Oral Administration: Absorption: ZYPREXA is well absorbed after oral administration, reaching peak plasma concentrations within 5 to 8 hours. The absorption is not affected by food.
Distribution: Plasma concentrations of orally administered olanzapine were linear and dose proportional in trials studying doses from 1 to 15 mg. The maximum plasma concentrations (C_{max}) of olanzapine after single oral doses of 5, 10 and 15 mg averaged 7, 14, and 21 ng/mL, respectively (20 ng/mL=0.064 µM). In young healthy volunteers, after once-a-day repeated dosing, steady-state C_{max} was approximately twice that achieved after a single dose (e.g. 23 ng/mL versus 12 ng/mL for a 10-mg dose). In the elderly, the steady state plasma concentration was approximately 3-fold higher than that achieved after a single dose (e.g. 16 ng/mL versus 5 ng/mL for a 5-mg dose). In both, young and elderly, steady-state concentrations of olanzapine were obtained after seven days of once daily dosing.

Over time and dosage range, pharmacokinetic parameters within an individual are very consistent. However, plasma concentrations, half-life and clearance of olanzapine may vary between individuals on the basis of smoking status, gender, and age (see Special Populations and Conditions). Data from pooled, single dose pharmacokinetic studies showed the half-life of olanzapine to range from 21 to 54 hours (5th to 95th percentile), and the apparent plasma clearance to range from 12 to 47 L/hr (5th to 95th percentile).

The plasma protein binding of olanzapine was about 93% over the concentration range of about 7 to about 1000 ng/mL. Olanzapine is bound predominantly to albumin and α_1-acid glycoprotein.
Metabolism: Olanzapine is metabolized in the liver by conjugative and oxidative pathways. The major circulating metabolite is the 10-N-glucuronide, which is pharmacologically inactive and does not pass the blood brain barrier. Cytochrome P450 isoforms CYP1A2 and CYP2D6 contribute to the formation of the N-desmethyl and 2-hydroxymethyl metabolites. Both metabolites exhibited significantly less in vivo pharmacological activity than olanzapine in animal studies. The predominant pharmacologic activity is from the parent olanzapine.

In vitro microsomal studies show that olanzapine is a weak inhibitor of CYP1A2 (Ki=36 µM), CYP2D6 (Ki=89 µM), and CYP3A4 (Ki=490 µM). Based upon these Ki values, little inhibition of these cytochrome P-450 enzymes is expected in vivo at concentrations below 5 µM (roughly 1500 ng/mL) because the olanzapine concentration will be less than 10% of its Ki value. In clinical studies, observed steady-state plasma concentrations of olanzapine are rarely >150 ng/mL (approximately 0.5 µM). Olanzapine is thus not likely to cause clinically important pharmacokinetic drug-drug interactions mediated through the metabolic routes outlined above. (See Drug Interactions.)
Elimination: After oral administration to healthy subjects, the mean terminal elimination half-life was 33 hours (21 to 54 hours for 5th to 95th percentile) and the mean olanzapine plasma clearance was 26 L/hr (12 to 47 L/hr for the 5th to 95th percentile). Olanzapine pharmacokinetics varied on the basis of smoking status, gender, and age. Table 12 summarizes these effects.

Table 12: ZYPREXA

Olanzapine Key Pharmacokinetics

Patient Characteristics	Half-Life (hours)	Plasma Clearance (L/h)
Nonsmoking	38.6	18.6
Smoking	30.4	27.7
Female	36.7	18.9
Male	32.3	27.3
Elderly (65 and older)	51.8	17.5
Nonelderly	33.8	18.2

Although smoking status, gender, and, to a lesser extent, age may affect olanzapine clearance and half-life, the magnitude of the impact of these single factors is small in comparison to the overall variability between individuals.

Pharmacokinetic studies demonstrate that ZYPREXA tablets and ZYPREXA ZYDIS dosage forms of olanzapine are bioequivalent. ZYPREXA ZYDIS orally disintegrating tablets can be used as an alternative to ZYPREXA tablets.

Intramuscular Administration: ZYPREXA IntraMuscular results in rapid absorption with peak plasma concentrations occurring within 15 to 45 minutes. The peak concentration is on average 4 to 5 fold higher than that of an equivalent oral dose. Area under the curve achieved after an intramuscular dose is equivalent to that achieved after oral administration of the same dose. The half-life observed after intramuscular administration is similar to that observed after oral dosing. The pharmacokinetics are linear over the clinical dosing range. Metabolic profiles after intramuscular administration are quantitatively similar and qualitatively identical to metabolic profiles after oral administration.

Special Populations and Conditions: Geriatrics: In a study involving 24 healthy subjects, the mean elimination half-life of olanzapine was about 1.5 times greater in elderly (>65 years) than in non-elderly subjects (≤65 years). Caution should be used in dosing the elderly, especially if there are other factors that might additively influence drug metabolism and/or pharmacodynamic sensitivity (see Dosage and Administration).

Gender: Clearance of olanzapine is approximately 30% lower in women than in men. There were, however, no apparent differences between men and women in effectiveness or adverse effects. Dosage modifications based on gender should not be needed.

Race: In a study of Caucasians, Japanese, and Chinese subjects, there were no differences in olanzapine pharmacokinetics among the three populations. Cytochrome P450 isoform CYP2D6 status does not affect the metabolism of olanzapine.

Hepatic Insufficiency: No differences in the single-dose pharmacokinetics of oral olanzapine were noted in subjects with clinically significant cirrhosis (who were mostly smokers) when compared to healthy subjects (all non-smokers). Multiple-dose studies in patients with hepatic impairment, however, have not been performed.

Renal Insufficiency: There was no significant difference in mean elimination half-life or olanzapine plasma clearance between subjects with severely impaired renal function compared to individuals with normal renal function. Approximately 57% of radiolabelled olanzapine is excreted in urine, principally as metabolites.

STORAGE AND STABILITY: ZYPREXA Tablets: Store tablets at 15-30°C. Protect from light and moisture.

ZYPREXA Zydis: Sensitive to light, keep tablets in the original package in a dry place at 15-30°C.

ZYPREXA IntraMuscular: Store ZYPREXA IntraMuscular (unconstituted) between 15-30°C.

Reconstituted ZYPREXA IntraMuscular may be stored at controlled room temperature 20-25°C [See USP] for up to 1 hour if necessary.

As with all parenteral drug products, reconstituted solutions should be inspected visually for clarity, particulate matter, precipitation, discolouration and leakage prior to administration, whenever solution and container permit. Solutions showing haziness, particulate matter, precipitate, discolouration or leakage should not be used. **Discard any unused portion of reconstituted ZYPREXA IntraMuscular.**

INFORMATION FOR THE PATIENT: Published in e-CPS, available by subscription at www.e-cps.ca.

DOSAGE FORMS, COMPOSITION AND PACKAGING: ZYPREXA: 2.5 mg: Each white, round, film-coated tablet, imprinted in blue ink with "LILLY" and the tablet identification code 4112, contains: olanzapine 2.5 mg (8 µmol). Nonmedicinal ingredients: carnauba wax, crospovidone, FD&C Blue No. 2 Aluminum Lake, hydroxypropyl cellulose, hydroxypropyl methylcellulose, lactose, magnesium stearate, microcrystalline cellulose, polyethylene glycol, polysorbate 80 and titanium dioxide. Amber HDPE bottles of 7 and 100.

5 mg: Each white, round, film-coated tablet, imprinted in blue ink with "LILLY" and the tablet identification code 4115, contains: olanzapine 5 mg (16 µmol). Nonmedicinal ingredients: carnauba wax, crospovidone, FD&C Blue No. 2 Aluminum Lake, hydroxypropyl cellulose, hydroxypropyl methylcellulose, lactose, magnesium stearate, microcrystalline cellulose, polyethylene glycol, polysorbate 80 and titanium dioxide. Amber HDPE bottles of 7 and 100.

7.5 mg: Each white, round, film-coated tablet, imprinted in blue ink with "LILLY" and the tablet identification code 4116, contains: olanzapine 7.5 mg (24 µmol), Nonmedicinal ingredients: carnauba wax, crospovidone, FD&C Blue No. 2 Aluminum Lake, hydroxypropyl cellulose, hydroxypropyl methylcellulose, lactose, magnesium stearate, microcrystalline cellulose, polyethylene glycol, polysorbate 80 and titanium dioxide. Amber HDPE bottles of 100.

10 mg: Each white, round, film-coated tablet, imprinted in blue ink with "LILLY" and the tablet identification code 4117, contains: olanzapine 10 mg (32 µmol). Nonmedicinal ingredients: carnauba wax, crospovidone, FD&C Blue No. 2 Aluminum Lake, hydroxypropyl cellulose, hydroxypropyl methylcellulose, lactose, magnesium stearate, microcrystalline cellulose, polyethylene glycol, polysorbate 80 and titanium dioxide. Amber HDPE bottles of 7 and 100.

15 mg: Each elliptical, film-coated light blue tablet, debossed with "LILLY" and the tablet identification code 4415, contains: olanzapine 15 mg (48 µmol). Nonmedicinal ingredients: carnauba wax, crospovidone, FD&C Blue No. 2 Aluminum Lake, hydroxypropyl cellulose, hydroxypropyl methylcellulose, lactose, magnesium stearate, microcrystalline cellulose, titanium dioxide and triacetin. Amber HDPE bottles of 7 and 100.

20 mg: Each elliptical, film-coated pink tablet, debossed with "LILLY" and the tablet identification code 4420, contains: olanzapine 20 mg (64 µmol). Nonmedicinal ingredients: carnauba wax, crospovidone, hydroxypropyl cellulose, hydroxypropyl methylcellulose, lactose, magnesium stearate, microcrystalline cellulose, polyethylene glycol, Synthetic Red Iron Oxide and titanium dioxide. Amber HDPE bottles of 100.

ZYPREXA Zydis: 5 mg: Each yellow, round, oral disintegrating tablet contains: olanzapine 5 mg (16 µmol). Nonmedicinal ingredients: aspartame, gelatin, mannitol, sodium methyl paraben and sodium propyl paraben. Aluminum blister strips in cartons of 7 and 28 tablets per carton.

10 mg: Each yellow, round, oral disintegrating tablet contains: olanzapine 10 mg (32 µmol). Nonmedicinal ingredients: aspartame, gelatin, mannitol, sodium methyl paraben and sodium propyl paraben. Aluminum blister strips in cartons of 7 and 28 tablets per carton.

15 mg: Each yellow, round, oral disintegrating tablet contains: olanzapine 15 mg (48 µmol). Nonmedicinal ingredients: aspartame, gelatin, mannitol, sodium methyl paraben and sodium propyl paraben. Aluminum blister strips in cartons of 7 and 28 tablets per carton.

20 mg: Each yellow, round, oral disintegrating tablet contains: olanzapine 20 mg (64 µmol). Nonmedicinal ingredients: aspartame, gelatin, mannitol, sodium methyl paraben and sodium propyl paraben. Aluminum blister strips in cartons of 28 tablets per carton.

ZYPREXA IntraMuscular: Each vial contains: olanzapine, as the tartrate, equivalent to olanzapine 10 mg. Nonmedicinal ingredients: lactose monohydrate and tartaric acid. Hydrochloric acid and/or sodium hydroxide may have been added during manufacturing to adjust pH. Single use 5 mL vials in packages of 1 (VL7597).

For reconstitution information, please refer to Dosage and Administration. ZYPREXA IntraMuscular is intended for intramuscular use only.

(Shown in Product Identification Section)

Zytram XL® Ⓟ

tramadol HCl

Opioid Analgesic

Purdue Pharma

Date of Revision: March 5, 2009

SUMMARY PRODUCT INFORMATION:

Route of Administration	Dosage Form/ Strength	All Nonmedicinal Ingredients
Oral	Controlled release tablets/150 mg, 200 mg, 300 mg, 400 mg	Hydrogenated vegetable oil, hypromellose, lactose, magnesium stearate, polyethylene glycol, talc, titanium dioxide

INDICATIONS AND CLINICAL USE: Adults: Zytram XL (tramadol HCl controlled release tablets) is indicated for:

- the management of moderate to moderately severe pain in adults who require continuous treatment for several days or more.

Geriatrics (>65 years of age): Healthy elderly subjects aged 65 to 75 years have plasma tramadol concentrations and elimination half-lives comparable to those observed in healthy subjects less than 65 years of age. Zytram XL should be administered with greater caution in patients over 75 years, due to the greater potential for adverse events in this population (see Warnings and Precautions and Dosage and Administration).

Pediatrics (<18 years of age): The safety and efficacy of Zytram XL has not been studied in the pediatric population. Therefore, use of Zytram XL tablets is not recommended in patients under 18 years of age.

CONTRAINDICATIONS:

- Patients who are hypersensitive to tramadol, opioids, or to any ingredient in the formulation.
- in any situation where opioids are contraindicated, including acute intoxication with alcohol, hypnotics, centrally acting analgesics, opioids, or psychotropic drugs. Tramadol may worsen central nervous system and respiratory depression in these patients;
- concomitant MAO inhibitors (or within 14 days of such therapy);
- severe renal or hepatic impairment (creatinine clearance of less than 30 mL/min and/or Child-Pugh Class C).

WARNINGS AND PRECAUTIONS: General: Zytram XL (tramadol HCl controlled release tablets) must be swallowed whole and should not be broken, chewed, dissolved or crushed, since this can lead to the rapid release of tramadol and absorption of a potentially fatal dose of tramadol.

Seizure Risk: Seizures have been reported in patients receiving tramadol within the recommended dosage range. Spontaneous post-marketing reports indicate that seizure risk is increased with doses of tramadol above the recommended range. Concomitant use of tramadol increases the seizure risk in patients taking: selective serotonin re-uptake inhibitors (SSRI antidepressants or anorectics); tricyclic antidepressants (TCAs), and other tricyclic compounds (e.g., cyclobenzaprine, promethazine, etc.); or opioids.

Administration of tramadol may enhance the seizure risk in patients taking: MAO inhibitors (see Contraindications); neuroleptics; or other drugs that reduce the seizure threshold.

Risk of convulsions may also increase in patients with epilepsy, those with a history of seizures, or in patients with a recognized risk for seizure (such as head trauma, metabolic disorders, alcohol and drug withdrawal, CNS infections). In tramadol overdose, naloxone administration may increase the risk of seizure.

Anaphylactoid Reactions: Serious and rarely fatal anaphylactoid reactions have been reported in patients receiving therapy with tramadol. When these rare reactions do occur it is often following the first dose. Other reported reactions include pruritus, hives, bronchospasm and angioedema. Patients with a history of anaphylactic reactions to codeine and other opioids may be at increased risk and therefore should not receive tramadol (see Contraindications).

Drug Abuse, Addiction and Dependence: Tramadol has a potential to cause psychic and physical dependence of the morphine-type (µ-opioid). The drug has been associated with craving, drug-seeking behaviour and tolerance development. Cases of abuse and dependence on tramadol have been reported. Zytram XL tablets should not be used in opioid-dependent patients. Tramadol can re-initiate physical dependence in patients who have been previously dependent or chronically using other opioids. In patients with a tendency to abuse drugs or a history of drug dependence, and in patients who are chronically using opioids, treatment with Zytram XL is not recommended.

Proper assessment of the patient, proper prescribing practices, periodic re-evaluation of therapy, and proper dispensing and storage are appropriate measures that help to limit abuse of opioid drugs.

A Risk Management program to support the safe and effective use of Zytram XL has been established. The following are considered to be the essential components of the Risk Management program:

a. Commitment to not emphasize or highlight the scheduling status of Zytram XL (i.e., not listed under a schedule to the CDSA) in its advertising or promotional activities;
b. Inclusion of a PAAB-approved fair balance statement in all Zytram XL advertising and promotional materials;
c. Provision of progress reports to TPD, MHPD and HECSB from a drug abuse surveillance program for Zytram XL;
d. Assurance that health-care education activities on pain management with Zytram XL include balanced, evidence-based and current information. Commitment to take reasonable actions to inform health-care professionals that there is Health Canada-approved patient information on benefits and risks, and to ensure that this information can be readily accessed through electronic and/or hard copy sources;
e. Reassessment of the risk management program 2 years post product launch.

Zytram XL is intended for oral use only. Zytram XL could be abused by breaking, crushing, chewing, snorting, or injecting the dissolved product. These practices will result in the uncontrolled delivery of the opioid and pose a significant risk to the abuser that could result in overdose and death. This risk is increased with concurrent abuse of alcohol and other substances. With parenteral abuse, the tablet excipients can be expected to result in local tissue necrosis, infection, pulmonary granulomas, and increased risk of endocarditis and valvular heart injury.

Zytram XL should not be used in opioid-dependent patients since it cannot suppress morphine withdrawal symptoms, even though it is an opioid agonist.

Abuse and addiction are separate and distinct from physical dependence and tolerance. In addition, abuse of opioids can occur in the absence of true addiction and is characterized by misuse for non-medical purposes, often in combination with other psychoactive substances. Tolerance as well as both physical and psychological dependence may develop upon repeated administration of opioids, and are not by themselves evidence of an addictive disorder or abuse.

Concerns about abuse, addiction, and diversion should not prevent the proper management of pain. The development of addiction to opioid analgesics in properly managed patients with pain has been reported to be rare. However, data are not available to establish the true incidence of addiction in chronic pain patients.

Careful record-keeping of prescribing information, including quantity, frequency, and renewal requests is strongly advised.

Withdrawal Symptoms: Withdrawal symptoms may occur following abrupt discontinuation of therapy. These symptoms may include anxiety, sweating, insomnia, rigors, pain, nausea, tremors, diarrhea, upper respiratory symptoms, piloerection and rarely hallucinations. Other symptoms that have been seen less frequently with tramadol discontinuation include: panic attacks, severe anxiety and paresthesias.

Patients on prolonged therapy should be withdrawn gradually from the drug if it is no longer required for pain control. Clinical experience suggests that withdrawal symptoms may be relieved by reinstitution of tramadol therapy followed by a gradual, tapered dose reduction of the medication combined with symptomatic support.

Risk of Overdosage: Serious potential consequences of overdosage with Zytram XL are central nervous system depression, respiratory depression and death. In treating an overdose, primary attention should be given to maintaining adequate ventilation along with general supportive treatment (see Overdosage).

Do not prescribe Zytram XL for patients who are suicidal or addiction prone.

Zytram XL should not be taken in doses higher than those recommended by the physician. The judicious prescribing of tramadol is essential to the safe use of this drug. With patients who are depressed or suicidal, consideration should be given to the use of non-narcotic analgesics. Patients should be cautioned about the concomitant use of tramadol products and alcohol because of potentially serious CNS-additive effects of these agents. Because of its added depressant effects, tramadol should be prescribed with caution for those patients whose medical condition requires the concomitant administration of sedatives, tranquilizers, muscle relaxants, antidepressants, or other CNS-depressant drugs. Patients should be advised of the additive depressant effects of these combinations.

Increased Intracranial Pressure or Head Trauma: Zytram XL should be used with caution in patients with increased intracranial pressure or head injury, since the respiratory depressant effects of opioid receptor agonism include carbon dioxide retention and secondary elevation of cerebrospinal fluid pressure, and such effects may be markedly exaggerated in these patients. Also, pupillary changes (miosis) from tramadol may obscure the existence, extent or course of intracranial pathology. Clinicians should also maintain a high index of suspicion for adverse drug reaction when evaluating altered mental status in these patients if they are receiving tramadol (see Warnings and Precautions, Respiratory Depression).

Respiratory Depression: Administer Zytram XL cautiously in patients at risk for respiratory depression. In these patients alternative non-opioid analgesics should be considered. When large doses of tramadol are administered with anesthetic medications or alcohol, respiratory depression may result. Respiratory depression should be treated as an overdose. If naloxone is to be administered, use cautiously because it may precipitate seizures (see Warnings and Precautions, Seizure Risk and Overdosage).

Interaction with Central Nervous System (CNS) Depressants: Zytram XL should be used with caution and in reduced dosages when administered to patients receiving CNS depressants such as alcohol, opioids, anesthetic agents, phenothiazines, tranquilizers or sedative hypnotics. Tramadol increases the risk of CNS and respiratory depression in these patients.

Zytram XL may be expected to have additive effects when used in conjunction with alcohol, other opioids, or illicit drugs that cause central nervous system depression.

"In Vitro" Dissolution Studies of Interaction with Alcohol: Increasing concentrations of alcohol in the dissolution medium, resulted in a slight decrease in the rate of release of tramadol from Zytram XL tablets. The clinical significance of the slight decrease in dissolution rate is unknown.

Use in Ambulatory Patients: Zytram XL may impair the mental and or physical abilities required for the performance of potentially hazardous tasks such as driving a car or operating machinery. The patient using this drug should be cautioned accordingly.

Use with Serotonin Re-uptake Inhibitors (SSRIs): Use Zytram XL with caution in patients taking SSRIs. Concomitant use of Zytram XL with SSRIs increases the risk of adverse events, including seizure and serotonin syndrome.

Acute Abdominal Conditions: As may occur with other analgesics, the administration of Zytram XL may complicate the clinical assessment of patients with acute abdominal conditions.

Use in Drug and Alcohol Addiction: Zytram XL is an opioid with no approved use in the management of addictive disorders. Its approved usage in individuals with drug or alcohol dependence, either active or in remission, is for the management of moderate to moderately severe chronic pain requiring continuous treatment with an opioid analgesic.

Carcinogenesis and Mutagenesis: The drug had no mutagenic effect in either the micro-nucleus test, which was carried out with mice, rats and hamsters administered two single oral and parenteral doses, or in the dominant-lethal test, in which mice were administered single and repeated oral and parenteral doses.

In carcinogenicity studies using tramadol, survival analysis did not show any statistically significant positive linear trend or differences in mortality among the placebo and tramadol treatment groups.

Special Populations: Pregnant Women: The safety of tramadol in pregnancy has not been established. Therefore, Zytram XL should not be used in pregnant women, prior to or during labour, unless in the opinion of the physician, the expected benefit to the patient outweighs the possible risk to the fetus.

Tramadol has been shown to cross the placenta. The mean ratio of serum tramadol in the umbilical veins compared to maternal veins was 0.83 for 40 women given tramadol during labour. Chronic use during pregnancy may lead to physical dependence and post-partum withdrawal symptoms in the newborn. Neonatal seizures, neonatal withdrawal syndrome, fetal death and stillbirth have been reported with tramadol hydrochloride during postmarketing reports with tramadol hydrochloride immediate-release products.

The effect of tramadol, if any, on the later growth, development and functional maturation of the child is unknown.

Nursing Women: Tramadol and its metabolites are found in small amounts in human breast milk. Since its safety in infants and newborns has not been studied, tramadol should not be administered for obstetrical preoperative medication, post delivery analgesia or at any time during breast-feeding.

Pediatrics (<18 years of age): The safety and efficacy of Zytram XL has not been studied in the pediatric population. Therefore, use of Zytram XL tablets is not recommended in patients under 18 years of age.

Geriatrics (>65 years of age): In general, dose selection for an elderly patient should be cautious, reflecting the greater frequency of decreased hepatic, renal or cardiac function; of concomitant disease and multiple drug therapy. The elimination half-life of tramadol may be prolonged in patients over 75 years, thereby increasing the potential for adverse events.

Renal Impairment: Zytram XL is contraindicated in patients with severe renal impairment. The elimination half-life of tramadol and its active metabolite may be prolonged in patients with renal impairment.

Hepatic/Biliary/Pancreatic Impairment: Zytram XL is contraindicated in patients with severe hepatic impairment. The elimination half-life of tramadol and its active metabolite may be prolonged in patients with hepatic impairment.

Monitoring and Laboratory Tests: Not applicable.

ADVERSE REACTIONS: Adverse Drug Reaction Overview: The pre-marketing development program for Zytram XL (tramadol HCl controlled release tablets) included exposure to a total of 1213 participants in seven randomized, double-blind controlled clinical trials (n=1028) and one six-month open-label trial (n=185). A summary of adverse events occurring at an incidence of 1% or more is given in Table 1, which includes all events, whether considered by the clinical investigator to be related to the study drug or not.

The most common adverse effects with Zytram XL are constipation, dizziness, headache, nausea, somnolence and vomiting. These are common effects associated with other drugs with opioid-agonist activity. Slower titration—a 7 day as compared to a 2 day schedule, may be an effective strategy to reduce adverse effects.

Clinical Trial Adverse Drug Reactions: Because clinical trials are conducted under very specific conditions the adverse reaction rates observed in the clinical trials may not reflect the rates observed in practice and should not be compared to the rates in the clinical trials of another drug. Adverse drug reaction information from clinical trials is useful for identifying drug-related adverse events and for approximating rates.

The stated frequencies of adverse events represent the proportion of individuals who experienced, at least once, a treatment-emergent adverse event of the type listed. An event was considered treatment emergent if it occurred for the first time or worsened while receiving therapy following baseline evaluation.

Table 1: Zytram XL

Adverse Events Reports in Zytram XL Clinical Trials (≥1%)

	Number of Patients	% of Patients n=1213
Body as a Whole		
Headache	132	10.9
Asthenia	93	7.7
Sweating	69	5.7
Pain	26	2.1
Central Nervous System		
Dizziness	214	17.6
Somnolence	191	15.7
Depression	12	1.0
Insomnia	24	2.0
Tremor	13	1.1
Vasodilation	24	2.0
Digestive System		
Constipation	274	22.6
Nausea	357	29.4
Vomiting	135	11.1
Diarrhea	54	4.5
Abdominal Pain	30	2.5
Anorexia	42	3.5
Dry Mouth	61	5.0
Dyspepsia	49	4.0
Flatulence	15	1.2
Respiratory System		
Cough Increased	11	1.0
Pharyngitis	17	1.4
Skin and Appendages		
Pruritus	27	2.2

Less Common Clinical Trial Adverse Drug Reactions (<1%): Body as a Whole: abnormal gait, accidental injury, back pain, chest pain, chills and fever, flu syndrome, infection, malaise, photosensitivity, syncope.

Cardiovascular: angina pectoris, arrhythmia, atrial flutter, hypertension, migraine, palpitation, peripheral vascular disorder, phlebitis, tachycardia.

Digestive: abnormal stools, bloating, diverticulitis, eructation, gastric motility reduced, gastritis, gastroenteritis, gastrointestinal hemorrhage, hiccup, irritable bowel syndrome, laryngitis, melena, pancreatitis, rectal disorder, rectal hemorrhage, thirst, tongue disorder, weight decrease.

Endocrine: abnormal ejaculation, impotence, libido decreased.

Hemolytic & Lymphatic: hemolytic anemia, liver function test abnormal.

Metabolic & Nutritional: alkaline phosphatase increased, hypercholesteremia, hyperglycemia, hyperlipemia, peripheral edema, hepatic enzymes increased.

Musculoskeletal: arthritis, arthrosis, bursitis, cramps, fatigue, gout, joint disorder, knee effusion, muscle pain, muscle weakness, myalgia, myopathy, pathological fracture, tendon disorder.

Nervous: abnormal coordination, abnormal dreams, abnormal thinking, amnesia, anxiety, apathy, ataxia, carpal tunnel syndrome, confusion, depersonalization, emotional lability, euphoria, hallucinations, hyperesthesia, hypertonia, loss of smell, malaise, myoclonus, nervousness, paresthesia, vertigo.

Respiratory: asthma, bronchospasm, dyspnea, epistaxis, hemoptysis, hyperventilation, pneumonia, respiratory disorder, rhinitis, sinusitis.

Skin: acne, dermatitis, dry skin, eczema, flushing, gooseflesh, herpes simplex, herpes zoster, purpura, rash, sebaceous cyst.

Special Senses: amblyopia, blepharitis, cellulitis, conjunctivitis, dry eyes, eustachian tube dysfunction, eye pain, halitosis, lacrimation disorder, otitis media, sore mouth, taste perversion, tinnitus, tooth disorder, vision abnormal.

Urogenital: albuminuria, calcium crystalluria, cystitis, dysuria, enlarged prostate, gynecomastia, hematuria, nocturia, polyuria, renal pain, urinary retention, urinary tract infection, urine abnormality, vaginal hemorrhage.

Abnormal Hematologic and Clinical Chemistry Findings: In clinical trials where clinical abnormalities were recorded (n=245), the following laboratory abnormalities were reported: ALT (3%), AST (2%), alkaline phosphatase (4%), creatinine (2%), BUN (4%), potassium (2%), sodium (1%), bilirubin (0.4%), basophils (0.4%), eosinophils (0.4%), lymphocytes (3%), monocytes (3%), neutrophils (1%), LDH (4%), RBC (3%), platelets (2%), WBC (2%), glucose (0.4%), triglycerides (1%) and TSH (0.4%).

Other Adverse Experiences Previously Reported in Clinical Trials or Post-Marketing Reports with Tramadol Hydrochloride: Adverse events which have been reported with the use of tramadol products include: allergic reactions (including anaphylaxis, angioneurotic edema and urticaria), bradycardia, convulsions, drug dependence, drug withdrawal (including agitation, anxiety, gastrointestinal symptoms, hyperkinesia, insomnia, nervousness, tremors), hyperactivity, hypoactivity, hypotension and respiratory depression. Other adverse events which have been reported with the use of tramadol products and for which a causal association has not been determined include: difficulty concentrating, hepatitis liver failure, pulmonary edema, Stevens-Johnson syndrome and suicidal tendency.

Serotonin syndrome (whose symptoms may include mental status change, hyperreflexia, fever, shivering, tremor, agitation, diaphoresis, seizures and coma) has been reported with tramadol when used concomitantly with other serotonergic agents such as SSRIs and MAOIs.

Drug Abuse, Addiction and Dependence: Tramadol may induce psychic and physical dependence of the morphine-type (μ-opioid) (see Warnings and Precautions, Drug Abuse, Addiction and Dependence). Dependence and abuse, including drug-seeking behaviour and taking illicit actions to obtain the drug are not limited to those patients with a prior history of opioid dependence. The risk in patients with substance abuse has been observed to be higher. Tramadol is associated with craving and tolerance development.

A Risk Management program to support the safe and effective use of Zytram XL has been established. The following are considered to be the essential components of the Risk Management program:

a. Commitment to not emphasize or highlight the scheduling status of Zytram XL (i.e., not listed under a schedule to the CDSA) in its advertising or promotional activities;
b. Inclusion of a PAAB-approved fair balance statement in all Zytram XL advertising and promotional materials;
c. Provision of progress reports to TPD, MHPD and HECSB from a drug abuse surveillance program for Zytram XL;
d. Assurance that health-care education activities on pain management with Zytram XL include balanced, evidence-based and current information. Commitment to take reasonable actions to inform health-care professionals that there is Health Canada-approved patient information on benefits and risks, and to ensure that this information can be readily accessed through electronic and/or hard copy sources;
e. Reassessment of the risk management program 2 years post product launch.

Withdrawal Symptoms: Withdrawal symptoms may occur if tramadol is discontinued abruptly. These symptoms may include: anxiety, sweating, insomnia, rigors, pain, nausea, tremors, diarrhea, upper respiratory symptoms, piloerection, and rarely, hallucinations. Other symptoms that have been seen less frequently with Zytram XL discontinuation include: panic attacks, severe anxiety, and paresthesias. Clinical experience suggests that withdrawal symptoms may be relieved by reinstitution of opioid therapy followed by a gradual, tapered dose reduction of the medication combined with symptomatic support.

DRUG INTERACTIONS: Overview: In vitro studies indicated that tramadol is unlikely to inhibit the CYP3A4-mediated metabolism of other drugs when tramadol is administered concomitantly at therapeutic doses. Tramadol does not appear to induce its own metabolism in humans, since observed maximal plasma concentrations after multiple oral doses are higher than expected based on single dose data. Tramadol is a mild inducer of selected drug metabolism pathways measured in animals.

Drug-Drug Interactions: MAO Inhibitors: Tramadol is contraindicated in patients receiving MAO inhibitors or who have used them within the previous 14 days (see Contraindications and Warnings and Precautions).

Drugs that Lower Seizure Threshold: Tramadol can increase the potential for selective serotonin re-uptake inhibitors (SSRIs), tricyclic anti-depressants (TCAs), anti-psychotics and other seizure threshold lowering drugs to cause convulsions (see Warnings and Precautions).

CNS Depressants: Concurrent administration of tramadol with other centrally acting drugs, including alcohol, centrally acting analgesics, opioids and psychotropic drugs may potentiate CNS depressant effects.

Carbamazepine: Patients taking carbamazepine may have a significantly reduced analgesic effect of tramadol. Since carbamazepine increases tramadol metabolism and because of the seizure risk associated with tramadol, concomitant administration of Zytram XL (tramadol HCl controlled release tablets) and carbamazepine is not recommended.

Quinidine: Tramadol is metabolized to M1 by the CYP2D6 isoenzyme. Quinidine is a selective inhibitor of that isoenzyme, so that concomitant administration of quinidine and tramadol results in increased concentrations of tramadol and reduced concentrations of M1. The clinical consequences of these findings are unknown. In vitro drug interaction studies in human liver microsomes indicate that tramadol has no effect on quinidine metabolism.

Inhibitors of CYP2D6: Inhibitors of CYP2D6 (e.g., quinidine, fluoxetine, paroxetine, amitriptyline) may inhibit the metabolism of tramadol, resulting in increased serum concentrations of tramadol and decreased concentrations of its O-demethylated metabolite (M1). Coadministration of quinidine did not diminish the analgesic effect of tramadol in human experimental pain models.

Inhibitors or Inducers of CYP3A4: Administration of CYP3A4 inhibitors, such as ketoconazole and erythromycin, or inducers, such as rifampin and St. John's Wort may affect the metabolism of tramadol, leading to altered tramadol exposure.

Cimetidine: Concomitant administration of tramadol and cimetidine is associated with a small prolongation of the half-life of tramadol, but no alteration of the Zytram XL dosage regimen is recommended.

Digoxin: Digoxin toxicity has occurred rarely during co-administration of digoxin and tramadol.

Protease Inhibitors, e.g., ritonavir: Co-administered ritonavir may increase the serum concentration of tramadol, resulting in tramadol toxicity.

Warfarin and Other Coumarin Anticoagulants: Alteration of the effect of warfarin, including elevation of prothrombin times, has been reported rarely during coadministration of warfarin and tramadol. While such changes have been generally of limited clinical significance for the individual products, periodic evaluation of prothrombin time should be performed when Zytram XL tablets and warfarin-like compounds are administered concurrently.

Drug-Food Interactions: In the presence of food, the availability and controlled-release properties of Zytram XL tablets were maintained with no evidence of dose dumping.

Drug-Herb Interactions: Interactions with herbal products have not been established.

Drug-Laboratory Test Interactions: Interactions with laboratory tests have not been established.

DOSAGE AND ADMINISTRATION: **Dosing Considerations:** Zytram XL (tramadol HCl controlled release tablets) is not recommended for minor pain, or acute short-term pain that may be treated adequately through lesser means where benefit does not outweigh the possible opioid-related side effects.

Due to possible differences in pharmacokinetic properties, Zytram XL tablets are not interchangeable with other tramadol-containing products.

The maximum recommended daily dose of Zytram XL should not be exceeded.

Zytram XL is contraindicated in patients with severe hepatic or renal impairment.

Administration: Zytram XL tablets must be swallowed whole and should not be broken, chewed, dissolved or crushed, since this can lead to the rapid release of tramadol and absorption of a potentially fatal dose of tramadol.

Recommended Dose and Dosage Adjustment: General: Zytram XL is designed to allow for once daily dosing, i.e., dosing at 24-hourly intervals. Treatment with Zytram XL should generally be initiated at the lowest available dose (150 mg).

As with all analgesic drugs, the dose of tramadol should be adjusted according to the severity of the pain and the clinical response of the individual patient. It is recommended that doses be slowly titrated—dosage adjustments generally separated by 7 days, to higher doses to minimize side effects.

The correct dosage for any individual patient is that which controls the pain for a full 24 hours, with no or tolerable side effects.

Patients Not Receiving Opioids at the Time of Initiation of Tramadol Treatment: The usual initial dose of Zytram XL for patients who have not previously received opioid analgesics is 150 mg q24h.

Patients Currently Receiving Other Tramadol Formulations: Patients currently receiving other oral immediate-release tramadol preparations may be transferred to Zytram XL tablets at the same or lowest nearest total daily tramadol dosage.

Adults: The usual initial dose is one 150 mg tablet daily. If adequate pain relief is not achieved, the dosage should be gradually titrated upwards. The maximum recommended daily dose is 400 mg.

Elderly Patients (>65 years old): Since the elimination half-life of tramadol may be prolonged in elderly patients, a starting dose of 150 mg daily is recommended. Upward dosage titration should be done with careful monitoring. Zytram XL should be administered with greater caution in patients over 75 years, due to the greater potential for adverse events in this population.

Pediatrics (<18 years old): The safety and efficacy of Zytram XL has not been studied in the pediatric population. Therefore, use of Zytram XL tablets is not recommended in patients under 18 years of age.

Patients with Renal or Hepatic Insufficiency: The elimination half-life of tramadol and its active metabolite may be prolonged in these patient populations. A starting dose of 150 mg daily is recommended. Upward dosage titration should be done with careful monitoring. Tramadol is contraindicated in patients with severe renal impairment and/or severe hepatic impairment. (creatinine clearance less than 30 mL/min and/or Child-Pugh Class C, see Contraindications).

Management of Breakthrough Pain: If episodes of breakthrough pain are encountered with appropriate adjustments of Zytram XL dose, acetaminophen, ibuprofen or tramadol may be given. If immediate release tramadol is used for breakthrough pain, the total daily dose of tramadol should not exceed 400 mg. Selection of breakthrough medication should be based on individual patient conditions. For patients whose dose has been titrated to the recommended maintenance dose, without attainment of adequate analgesia, the total daily dose may be increased, unless precluded by side effects.

Missed Dose: If a patient forgets to take one or more doses, they should take their next dose at the normal time and in the normal amount.

Discontinuation: Withdrawal symptoms may occur following abrupt discontinuation of therapy. These symptoms may include anxiety, sweating, insomnia, rigors, pain, nausea, tremors, diarrhea, upper respiratory symptoms, piloerection and rarely hallucinations. Other symptoms that have been seen less frequently with Zytram XL discontinuation include: panic attacks, severe anxiety, and paresthesias. Patients on prolonged therapy should be withdrawn gradually from the drug if it is no longer required for pain control.

OVERDOSAGE:

Deaths due to overdose have been reported with abuse and misuse of tramadol, by ingesting, inhaling, or injecting the crushed tablets. Review of case reports has indicated that the risk of fatal overdose is further increased when tramadol is abused concurrently with alcohol or other CNS depressants, including other opioids.

Symptoms of Overdose: Acute overdosage with tramadol can be manifested by respiratory depression, somnolence progressing to stupor or coma, skeletal muscle flaccidity, cold and clammy skin, constricted pupils, bradycardia, hypotension, and death.

Treatment of Overdose: In the treatment of tramadol overdosage, primary attention should be given to the re-establishment of a patent airway and institution of assisted or controlled ventilation. Supportive measures (including oxygen and vasopressors) should be employed in the management of circulatory shock and pulmonary edema accompanying overdose as indicated. Cardiac arrest or arrhythmias may require cardiac massage or defibrillation.

While naloxone will reverse some, but not all, symptoms caused by overdosage with tramadol, the risk of seizures is also increased with naloxone administration. Seizures may be controlled with diazepam.

Tramadol is minimally eliminated from the serum by hemodialysis or hemofiltration. Therefore treatment of acute tramadol intoxication with hemodialysis or hemofiltration alone is not appropriate.

Emptying of the gastric contents is useful to remove any unabsorbed drug.

> For management of a suspected drug overdose, CPhA recommends that you contact your **regional Poison Control Centre**. See the *CPS* Directory section for a list of Poison Control Centres.

ACTION AND CLINICAL PHARMACOLOGY: Mechanism of Action: Tramadol is a centrally acting synthetic opioid analgesic. Although its mode of action is not completely understood, from animal tests, at least two complementary mechanisms appear applicable: binding of parent and M1 metabolite to μ-opioid receptors and weak inhibition of reuptake of norepinephrine and serotonin.

Opioid activity is due to both low affinity binding of the parent compound and higher affinity binding of the O-demethylated metabolite M1 to μ-opioid receptors. In animal models, M1 is up to 6 times more potent than tramadol in producing analgesia and 200 times more potent in μ-opioid binding. Tramadol-induced analgesia is only partially antagonized by the opiate antagonist naloxone in several animal tests. The relative contribution of both tramadol and M1 to human analgesia is dependent upon the plasma concentrations of each compound.

Tramadol has been shown to inhibit reuptake of norepinephrine and serotonin in vitro, as have some other opioid analgesics. These mechanisms may contribute independently to the overall analgesic profile of tramadol. The relationship between exposure of tramadol and M1 and efficacy has not been evaluated in the Zytram XL (tramadol HCl controlled release tablets) clinical studies.

Apart from analgesia, tramadol administration may produce a constellation of symptoms (including dizziness, somnolence, nausea, constipation, sweating and pruritus) similar to that of other opioids. In contrast to morphine, tramadol has not been shown to cause histamine release. At therapeutic doses, tramadol has no effect on heart rate, left-ventricular function or cardiac index. Orthostatic hypotension has been observed.

Pharmacodynamics: The administration of naloxone only partially antagonizes tramadol's antinociceptive and analgesic effects in animals and man, indicating a contribution from non-opioid analgesic mechanisms. In animals and man the effect of tramadol is attenuated by the α2 adrenoceptor antagonist, yohimbine, and in animals, the serotonin antagonist rianserin reduces the antinociceptive effect of tramadol. This indicates the potential for a contribution to the analgesic effect of tramadol through modulation of monaminergic inhibitory pain pathways in the dorsal horn of the spinal cord, in addition to an opioidergic effect.

Pharmacokinetics: Absorption: Following oral administration of a single dose, tramadol is almost completely absorbed and the absolute bioavailability is approximately 70%. The elimination half life of tramadol is around 6 hours, although this is extended to around 16 hours as a result of prolonged absorption from the Zytram XL tablets.

Following administration of one Zytram XL tablet 200 mg in the fasting state, the mean peak plasma concentration (C_{max}) was 34% (dose adjusted) that of a 100 mg dose of tramadol given as an oral solution. This was associated with a more prolonged t_{max} (median 6 hours; range 4-8 hours) compared with the oral solution (median 1.5 hours; range 0.75-4 hours). The extent of absorption of tramadol from the Zytram XL tablet 200 mg was equivalent to that of the immediate release tramadol solution 100 mg, after dose adjustment. In the presence of food, the bioavailability and controlled release properties of Zytram XL tablets are maintained, with no evidence of dose-dumping.

In a single dose study, the dose-adjusted bioavailability of the 200 mg, 300 mg and 400 mg tablets were equivalent, confirming a linear pharmacokinetic response (in relation to both tramadol and O-desmethyltramadol) over this range of strengths.

In a steady state study, the dose adjusted bioavailability of the 150 mg and 200 mg tablets administered once-daily were equivalent. The bioavailability of all strengths of Zytram XL is therefore, dose-proportional. A steady-state study also confirmed that the Zytram XL tablet 150 mg provided an equivalent peak concentration and extent of absorption of tramadol as an immediate release capsule 50 mg administered 8-hourly.

Distribution: Tramadol has a great affinity for tissues (V_d=203±40 L) and the plasma protein binding is approximately 20%.

Metabolism: Tramadol is extensively metabolized after oral administration. The major metabolic pathways appear to be N- and O-demethylation and glucuronidation or sulfation in the liver. Only one metabolite (mono-O-desmethyltramadol—denoted M1) is pharmacologically active. Production of M1 is dependent on the CYP2D6 isoenzyme of cytochrome P-450.

Excretion: Approximately 30% of the dose is excreted in the urine as unchanged drug, whereas 60% of the dose is excreted as metabolites. The remainder is excreted either as unidentified or as unextractable metabolites.

Special Populations and Conditions: Pediatrics: The safety and efficacy of Zytram XL has not been studied in the pediatric population. Therefore, use of Zytram XL tablets is not recommended in patients under 18 years of age.

Geriatrics (>65 years of age): Healthy elderly subjects aged 65 to 75 years have plasma tramadol concentrations and elimination half-lives comparable to those observed in healthy subjects less than 65 years of age. In subjects over 75 years maximum serum concentrations are slightly elevated (208 vs 162 ng/mL) and the elimination half-life is slightly prolonged (7 vs 6 hours) compared to subjects 65 to 75 years of age. Adjustment of the daily dose is recommended for patients older than 75 years (see Dosage and Administration).

Gender: The absolute bioavailability of tramadol was 73% in males and 79% in females. The plasma clearance was 6.4 mL/min/kg in males and 5.7 mL/min/kg in females following a 100 mg IV dose of tramadol. Following a single oral dose, and after adjusting for body weight, females had a 12% higher peak tramadol concentration and a 35% higher area under the concentration-time curve compared to males. This difference may not be of any clinical significance.

Race: No data available.

Hepatic Insufficiency: Metabolism of tramadol and M1 is reduced in patients with advanced cirrhosis of the liver, resulting in a larger area under the serum-concentration time curve for tramadol and longer tramadol and M1 elimination half-lives (13 hours for tramadol and 19 hours for M1). Zytram XL is contraindicated in patients with severe hepatic impairment (Child-Pugh Class C) (see Contraindications).

Renal Insufficiency: Impaired renal function results in a decreased rate and extent of excretion of tramadol and its active metabolite M1. Zytram XL is contraindicated in patients with creatinine clearances of less than 30 mL/min (see Contraindications). The total amount of tramadol and M1 removed during a dialysis period is less than 7% of the administered dose.

Genetic Polymorphism: Not applicable.

STORAGE AND STABILITY: Store at room temperature (15-30°C).

SPECIAL HANDLING INSTRUCTIONS: Protect from light, moisture and high humidity. Keep in a safe place out of the reach of children.

INFORMATION FOR THE PATIENT: Published in e-CPS, available by subscription at www.e-cps.ca.

DOSAGE FORMS, COMPOSITION AND PACKAGING: 150 mg: Each white, film-coated, oval-shaped, controlled release tablet, plain on one side and T150 on the other, contains: tramadol HCl 150 mg. Nonmedicinal ingredients: hydrogenated vegetable oil, magnesium stearate and talc; film coating: hypromellose, lactose, polyethylene glycol and titanium dioxide. Opaque plastic bottles of 50.

200 mg: Each white, film-coated, oval-shaped, controlled release tablet, plain on one side and T200 on the other, contains: tramadol HCl 200 mg. Nonmedicinal ingredients: hydrogenated vegetable oil, magnesium stearate and talc; film coating: hypromellose, lactose, polyethylene glycol and titanium dioxide. Opaque plastic bottles of 50.

300 mg: Each white, film-coated, oval-shaped, controlled release tablet, plain on one side and T300 on the other, contains: tramadol HCl 300 mg. Nonmedicinal ingredients: hydrogenated vegetable oil, magnesium stearate and talc; film coating: hypromellose, lactose, polyethylene glycol and titanium dioxide. Opaque plastic bottles of 50.

400 mg: Each white, film-coated, oval-shaped, controlled release tablet, plain on one side and T400 on the other, contains: tramadol HCl 400 mg. Nonmedicinal ingredients: hydrogenated vegetable oil, magnesium stearate and talc; film coating: hypromellose, lactose, polyethylene glycol and titanium dioxide. Opaque plastic bottles of 50.

(Shown in Product Identification Section)

Zyvoxam® Ⓟ
linezolid
Antibacterial

Pfizer

Zyvoxam® I.V. Ⓟ
linezolid
Antibacterial

Pfizer

Date of Revision: September 23, 2005

SUMMARY PRODUCT INFORMATION:

Route of Administration	Dosage Form/ Strength	Clinically Relevant Nonmedicinal Ingredients
Oral	Tablet 600 mg	None For a complete listing see Dosage Forms, Composition and Packaging section.
Intravenous Injection	Intravenous injection 2 mg/mL	None For a complete listing see Dosage Forms, Composition and Packaging section.

INDICATIONS AND CLINICAL USE: ZYVOXAM (linezolid) Tablets and Injection are indicated for:

Treatment of adult patients with the following infections, when caused by susceptible strains of the designated micro-organisms:

Note: In infections where gram-negative and/or anaerobic pathogens are suspected or are known to also be present, ZYVOXAM should be used in combination with appropriate antibiotic(s) in order to provide adequate antimicrobial coverage. Once culture results become available antimicrobial therapy should be adjusted accordingly.

Vancomycin-resistant *E. faecium* (VREF) Infections: ZYVOXAM is indicated for the treatment of the following infections when due to VREF: Intra-abdominal, skin and skin-structure, and urinary tract infections (including cases associated with concurrent bacteremia).

Note: This indication for VREF is based on non-comparative studies.

Nosocomial pneumonia caused by *S. aureus* (methicillin-susceptible and -resistant strains), or *S. pneumoniae* (penicillin-susceptible strains only).

Community-acquired pneumonia caused by *S. pneumoniae* (penicillin-susceptible strains only) including cases with concurrent bacteremia or *S. aureus* (methicillin-susceptible and -resistant strains).

Complicated skin and skin structure infections including non-limb threatening diabetic foot infections, without concomitant osteomyelitis, caused by *S. aureus* (methicillin-susceptible and -resistant strains), *S. pyogenes*, or *S. agalactiae*.

Note: ZYVOXAM has not been studied in the treatment of necrotizing fasciitis or decubitus ulcers.

Uncomplicated skin and skin structure infections caused by *S. aureus* (methicillin-susceptible strains only) or *S. pyogenes*.

Due to concerns about inappropriate use of antibiotics leading to an increase in resistant organisms, prescribers should carefully consider alternatives before initiating treatment with ZYVOXAM in the outpatient setting.

Prior to instituting treatment with ZYVOXAM, appropriate specimens should be obtained for isolation of the causative organism(s) and for determination of susceptibility to ZYVOXAM.

If clinically indicated, treatment with ZYVOXAM may be started empirically before results of susceptibility testing are available. However, in infections where gram-negative and/or anaerobic pathogens are suspected or are known to be present, ZYVOXAM should be used in combination with an appropriate antibiotic in order to provide adequate antimicrobial coverage. Once culture results become available antimicrobial therapy should be adjusted accordingly.

CONTRAINDICATIONS:

- ZYVOXAM (linezolid) Tablets and Injection are contraindicated for use in patients who have known hypersensitivity to linezolid or any of the other product components.

WARNINGS AND PRECAUTIONS: General: The use of antibiotics may promote the overgrowth of nonsusceptible organisms. Should superinfection occur during therapy, appropriate measures should be taken.

ZYVOXAM (linezolid) Tablets and Injection have not been studied in patients with uncontrolled hypertension, pheochromocytoma, carcinoid syndrome, or untreated hyperthyroidism.

Large quantities of foods or beverages with high tyramine content should be avoided while taking ZYVOXAM (see Drug Interactions, Drug-Food Interactions for foods or beverages with high tyramine content).

The safety and efficacy of ZYVOXAM given for longer than 28 days have not been evaluated in controlled clinical trials.

Lactic acidosis has been reported with the use of ZYVOXAM. Patients who develop recurrent nausea or vomiting, unexplained acidosis, or a low bicarbonate level while receiving ZYVOXAM should receive immediate medical attention.

Drug Interactions: See also Drug Interactions, Drug-Drug Interactions.

Monoamine Oxidase Inhibition: ZYVOXAM is a reversible, nonselective inhibitor of monoamine oxidase. Therefore, linezolid has the potential for interaction with adrenergic and serotonergic agents.

Adrenergic Agents: Some individuals receiving ZYVOXAM may experience a reversible enhancement of the pressor response to indirect-acting sympathomimetic agents, vasopressor or dopaminergic agents. Commonly used drugs such as phenylpropanolamine and pseudoephedrine have been specifically studied. Initial doses of adrenergic agents, such as dopamine or epinephrine, should be reduced and titrated to achieve the desired response.

Serotonergic Agents: Very rare spontaneous reports of serotonin syndrome with co-administration of linezolid and serotonergic agents have been reported. Since there is limited experience with concomitant administration of linezolid and serotonergic agents, physicians should be alert to the possibility of signs and symptoms of serotonin syndrome (e.g., hyperpyrexia, and cognitive dysfunction) in patients receiving such concomitant therapy (see Drug Interactions, Drug-Drug Interactions, Serotonergic Agents).

Gastrointestinal: Pseudomembranous colitis: Pseudomembranous colitis has been reported with nearly all antibacterial agents, including linezolid, and may range in severity from mild to life-threatening. Therefore, it is important to consider this diagnosis in patients who present with diarrhea subsequent to the administration of any antibacterial agent.

Treatment with antibacterial agents alters the normal flora of the colon and may permit overgrowth of clostridia. Studies indicate that a toxin produced by *C. difficile* is a primary cause of "antibiotic-associated colitis".

After the diagnosis of pseudomembranous colitis has been established, appropriate therapeutic measures should be initiated. Mild cases of pseudomembranous colitis usually respond to drug discontinuation alone. In moderate to severe cases, consideration should be given to management with fluids and electrolytes, protein supplementation, and treatment with an antibacterial agent clinically effective against *C. difficile*.

Hematologic: Myelosuppression: Myelosuppression (anemia including pure red blood cell aplasia, leucopenia, pancytopenia, and thrombocytopenia) has been reported in patients receiving linezolid. In cases where the outcome is known, when linezolid was discontinued, the affected hematologic parameters have risen toward pretreatment levels. Complete blood counts should be monitored at least weekly in patients who receive linezolid, particularly in those who receive linezolid for longer than two weeks, patients who are at increased risk for bleeding, those with pre-existing myelosuppression, those receiving concomitant drugs that produce bone marrow suppression, or decreased hemoglobin levels or platelet counts or function, or those with a chronic infection who have received previous or concomitant antibiotic therapy. Discontinuation of therapy with linezolid should be considered in patients who develop or have worsening myelosuppression.

Animal Pharmacology: Dose- and time-dependent myelosuppression, as evidenced by bone marrow hypocellularity, decreased hematopoiesis, and decreased levels of circulating erythrocytes, leukocytes, and platelets, has been seen in animal studies. The hematopoietic effects occurred at doses of 40 and 80 mg/kg/day in dogs and rats, respectively (at exposures approximately 0.6 times in the dog and equal in the rat to the expected human exposure based on AUC). Hematopoietic effects were reversible, although in some studies reversal was incomplete within the duration of the recovery period.

Neurologic: Peripheral neuropathy has been reported primarily in patients treated for longer than the maximum recommended duration of 28 days with ZYVOXAM. When outcome was known, recovery was reported in only some cases following ZYVOXAM withdrawal.

If symptoms of peripheral neuropathy such as numbness, tingling, prickling sensations or burning pain occur, the continued use of ZYVOXAM should be weighed against the potential risk.

Convulsions have been reported to occur rarely in patients when treated with ZYVOXAM. In most of these cases, a history of seizures or risk factors for seizures was reported.

Ophthalmologic: Optic neuropathy has been reported in patients treated with ZYVOXAM, primarily those treated for longer than the maximum recommended duration of 28 days. When outcome was known, recovery was reported in some cases following ZYVOXAM withdrawal. In cases of optic neuropathy that progressed to loss of vision, patients were treated for longer than the maximum recommended duration. Visual blurring has been reported in some patients treated with ZYVOXAM for less than 28 days.

Visual function should be monitored in all patients taking ZYVOXAM for longer than the maximum recommended duration and in all patients reporting new visual symptoms regardless of length of therapy with ZYVOXAM. If patients experience symptoms of visual impairment, such as changes in visual acuity, changes in color vision, blurred vision, or visual field defect, prompt ophthalmologic evaluation is recommended. If optic neuropathy occurs, the continued use of ZYVOXAM in these patients should be weighed against the potential risks.

Special Populations: Pregnant Women: There are no adequate and well-controlled studies in pregnant women. ZYVOXAM should be used during pregnancy only if the potential benefit justifies the potential risk to the fetus.

Nursing Women: ZYVOXAM and its metabolites are excreted in the milk of lactating rats. Concentrations in milk were similar to those in maternal plasma. It is not known whether linezolid is excreted in human milk. Because many drugs are excreted in human milk, caution should be exercised when ZYVOXAM is administered to a nursing woman.

Pediatrics: Although it may be possible to extrapolate adult efficacy to pediatric patients, the appropriate dose and safety of ZYVOXAM have not been established in this population. Drug clearance of ZYVOXAM is increased in pediatric patients compared to adults, resulting in a shorter half-life (see Action and Clinical Pharmacology, Special Populations and Conditions, Pediatrics). Pediatric dosing regimens that provide a pharmacokinetic profile similar to adults have not been determined.

Geriatrics: Of the 2046 patients treated with ZYVOXAM in phase III comparator-controlled clinical trials, 589 (29%) were 65 years or older and 253 (12%) were 75 years or older. No overall differences in safety or effectiveness were observed between these patients and younger patients.

Monitoring and Laboratory Tests: Complete blood counts should be monitored at least weekly in patients who receive linezolid, particularly in those who receive linezolid for longer than two weeks, patients who are at increased risk for bleeding, those with pre-existing myelosuppression, those receiving concomitant drugs that produce bone marrow suppression, or decreased hemoglobin levels or platelet counts or function, or those with a chronic infection who have received previous or concomitant antibiotic therapy (see Warnings and Precautions, Hematologic, Myelosuppression).

Visual function should be monitored in all patients taking ZYVOXAM for longer than the maximum recommended duration and in all patients reporting new visual symptoms regardless of length of therapy with ZYVOXAM. If patients experience symptoms of visual impairment, such as changes in visual acuity, changes in color vision, blurred vision, or visual field defect, prompt ophthalmologic evaluation is recommended (see Warnings and Precautions, Ophthalmologic).

Information to Be Provided to the Patient: Patients should be advised that:

- They should inform their physician if they have a history of hypertension.
- They should inform their physician if taking medications containing sympathomimetic agents such as pseudoephedrine HCl, often found in cold remedies and decongestants.
- They should inform their physician if taking serotonin re-uptake inhibitors or other antidepressants.
- They should inform their physician if they experience changes in vision during therapy with linezolid.
- They should inform their physician if they experience numbness, tingling, prickling sensations or burning pain during therapy with linezolid.
- They should inform their physician if they have a history of seizures or convulsions.

ADVERSE REACTIONS: Adverse Drug Reaction Overview: The safety of ZYVOXAM (linezolid) Tablets and Injection were evaluated in 2046 patients enrolled in seven phase III comparator-controlled clinical trials, who were treated for up to 28 days. In these studies, 85% of the adverse events reported with ZYVOXAM were described as mild to moderate in intensity. The most common adverse events in patients treated with ZYVOXAM were diarrhea (incidence across studies: 2.8% to 11.0%), headache (incidence across studies: 0.5% to 11.3%), and nausea (incidence across studies: 3.4% to 9.6%).

Other adverse events reported in phase II and phase III studies included oral moniliasis, vaginal moniliasis, hypertension, dyspepsia, localized abdominal pain, pruritus, and tongue discoloration.

Clinical Trial Adverse Drug Reactions: Because clinical trials are conducted under very specific conditions the adverse reaction rates observed in the clinical trials may not reflect the rates observed in practice and should not be compared to the rates in the clinical trials of another drug. Adverse drug reaction information from clinical trials is useful for identifying drug-related adverse events and for approximating rates.

Phase III Clinical Trials: Table 1 shows the incidence of drug-related adverse events reported in at least 1% of patients in these trials by dose of ZYVOXAM.

Table 1: ZYVOXAM

Incidence of Drug-related Adverse Events Occurring in >1% of Patients Treated with ZYVOXAM in Comparator-controlled Clinical Trials

	Uncomplicated Skin and Skin Structure Infections		All Other Indications	
Adverse Event	ZYVOXAM 400 mg orally q12h (N=548)	Comparator (N=537)	ZYVOXAM 600 mg q12h (N=1498)	All Other Comparators (N=1464)
% of Patients with at Least 1 Drug-related Adverse Event	25.4	19.6	20.4	14.3
% of Patients Discontinuing due to Drug-related Adverse Events[a]	3.5	2.4	2.1	1.7
Diarrhea	5.3	4.8	4	2.7
Nausea	3.5	3.5	3.3	1.8
Headache	2.7	2.2	1.9	1
Taste Alteration	1.8	2	0.9	0.2
Vaginal Moniliasis	1.6	1.3	1	0.4
Fungal Infection	1.5	0.2	0.1	<0.1
Abnormal Liver Function Tests	0.4	0	1.3	0.5
Vomiting	0.9	0.4	1.2	0.4
Tongue Discoloration	1.1	0	0.2	0
Dizziness	1.1	1.5	0.4	0.3
Oral Moniliasis	0.4	0	1.1	0.4

[a] The most commonly reported drug-related adverse events leading to discontinuation in patients treated with ZYVOXAM were nausea, headache, diarrhea, and vomiting.

In controlled clinical trials, abdominal pain/cramp/distension and abnormal hematology tests were also reported occurring at an incidence of at least 1%.

Less Common Clinical Trial Adverse Drug Reactions (<1%): Adverse drug reactions that were possibly or probably related to ZYVOXAM with an incidence less than 1.0% but greater than 0.1% in controlled clinical trials were: see Table 2.

Table 2: ZYVOXAM

Adverse Drug Reactions with an Incidence <1.0% but >0.1% in Controlled Clinical Trials

Body System	Adverse Reactions
Metabolic and Nutritional	Amylase increased, hyperglycemia, hyponatremia, lipase high, serum creatine phosphokinase increased, AST increased and ALT increased
Special Senses	Blurred vision, tinnitus
Musculoskeletal	None
Hemic and Lymphatic	Eosinophilia, neutropenia, thrombocytopenia
Respiratory	None
Cardiovascular	Hypertension, phlebitis
Digestive	Constipation, dry mouth, dyspepsia, gastritis, glossitis, increased thirst, stomatitis and tongue discoloration
Nervous	Dizziness, hypesthesia, insomnia, paresthesia
Body as a Whole	Abdominal pain, chills, diaphoresis, fatigue, fungal infection, injection/vascular catheter site pain, and injection/vascular catheter site phlebitis/thrombophlebitis
Urogenital	Polyuria and vaginitis/vaginal infection
Skin	Dermatitis, moniliasis skin, pruritus, rash, and urticaria

In controlled clinical trials the pattern of drug related adverse reactions by body system with an incidence less than 1.0% but greater than 0.1% were similar to comparators.

Serious adverse reactions in controlled clinical trials considered possibly or probably related to ZYVOXAM treatment with an incidence less than 0.1% were, hypertension, kidney failure, liver function test abnormality, pancreatitis, thrombocytopenia, transient ischemic attacks and vomiting.

Phase IV Clinical Trials: In a phase IV comparator-controlled study (Study 113) of adult diabetic patients with clinically documented complicated skin and skin structure infections ("diabetic foot infections"), most drug-related adverse events were rated as mild or moderate in intensity; 13.0% were rated as severe, and with the exception of diarrhea (0.8%), each severe drug-related event was reported in no more than one patient. See Table 3.

Table 3: ZYVOXAM

Frequencies of Study-emergent Drug-related Adverse Events Reported for ≥1% of Patients in Either Treatment Group [Study 113, linezolid in the treatment of adult diabetic patients with clinically documented complicated skin and skin structure infections ("diabetic foot infections")]

COSTART Body System Classification	Adverse Event (Medically Equivalent Term[a])	Treatment Group: Linezolid N=241 n (%)[b]	Treatment Group: Comparator N=120 n (%)[b]
Total Reported	Patients reporting at least 1 drug-related AE	64 (26.6)	12 (10.0)
Digestive	Diarrhea	18 (7.5)	4 (3.3)
	Nausea	14 (5.8)	0
	Vomiting	4 (1.7)	1 (0.8)
	Dyspepsia	3 (1.2)	1 (0.8)
	Appetite decreased	3 (1.2)	0
Hemic and Lymphatic	Anemia	11 (4.6)	0
	Thrombocytopenia	9 (3.7)	0

a The information represents the number (%) of patients who reported a given study-emergent adverse event. Any patient with multiple reports of the same event was counted only once for that event.
b All percentages are based on the number of ITT patients.

Less Common Clinical Trial Adverse Drug Reactions (<1%): In Study 113, adverse drug reactions that were possibly or probably related to ZYVOXAM with an incidence less than 1.0% but greater than 0.1% were: see Table 4.

Table 4: ZYVOXAM

Adverse Drug Reactions That Were Possibly or Probably Related to ZYVOXAM with an Incidence <1.0% but >0.1%

Body System	Adverse Reactions
Metabolic and Nutritional	Healing abnormal, hypoglycemia, hypokalemia, LDH increased
Special Senses	Taste perversion
Musculoskeletal	None
Hemic and Lymphatic	Ecchymosis/bruise, neutropenia
Respiratory	Dyspnea
Cardiovascular	Congestive heart failure, peripheral vascular disorder
Digestive	Anorexia, biliary pain, *C. Difficile* colitis, cholestatic jaundice, disorder gastrointestinal NOS, disorder rectal, flatulence, gastrointestinal bleeding, monilia oral
Nervous	Disorientation, dizziness, somnolence
Body as a Whole	Abdominal cramp, abdominal pain localized, asthenia, disorder mucous membrane, fatigue, headache, fungal infection NOS, infection NEC, laboratory test abnormality other
Urogenital	None
Skin	Dermatitis, dermatitis fungal, erythema, rash, ulcer skin

Legend:
NEC=not elsewhere classified.
NOS=not elsewhere specified.

In Study 113, serious drug-related events were reported for seven patients in the linezolid treatment group: congestive heart failure, peripheral vascular disease; biliary pain and cholestatic jaundice; *C. difficile* colitis; gastrointestinal bleeding; anemia; and hypokalemia.

Phase III Clinical Trials: Abnormal Hematologic and Clinical Chemistry Findings: ZYVOXAM has been associated with thrombocytopenia when used in doses up to and including 600 mg every 12 hours for up to 28 days. In phase III comparator-controlled trials, the percentage of patients who developed a substantially low platelet count (defined as less than 75% of lower limit of normal and/or baseline) was 2.4% (range among studies: 0.3 to 10.0%) with ZYVOXAM and 1.5% (range among studies: 0.4 to 7.0%) with a comparator.

Thrombocytopenia associated with the use of ZYVOXAM appears to be dependent on duration of therapy (generally greater than 2 weeks of treatment). The platelet counts for most patients returned to the normal range/baseline during the follow-up period. No related clinical adverse events were identified in phase III clinical trials in patients developing thrombocytopenia. Bleeding events were identified in thrombocytopenic patients in a compassionate use program for ZYVOXAM; the role of linezolid in these events cannot be determined (see Warnings and Precautions).

Changes seen in other laboratory parameters, without regard to drug relationship, revealed no substantial differences between ZYVOXAM and the comparators. These changes were generally not clinically significant, did not lead to discontinuation of therapy, and were reversible. The incidence of patients with at least one substantially abnormal hematologic or serum chemistry value is presented in Table 5 and Table 6.

Table 5: ZYVOXAM

Percent of Patients Who Experienced at Least One Substantially Abnormal[a] Hematology Laboratory Value in Comparator-controlled Clinical Trials with ZYVOXAM

Laboratory Assay	Uncomplicated Skin and Skin Structure Infections: ZYVOXAM 400 mg q12h	Uncomplicated Skin and Skin Structure Infections: Comparator	All Other Indications: ZYVOXAM 600 mg q12h	All Other Indications: All Other Comparators
Hemoglobin (g/L)	0.9	0	7.1	6.6
Platelet Count (×10⁹/L)	0.7	0.8	3	1.8
WBC (×10⁹/L)	0.2	0.6	2.2	1.3
Neutrophils (×10⁹/L)	0	0.2	1.1	1.2

(cont'd)

Table 5: ZYVOXAM *(cont'd)*

a <75% (<50% for neutrophils) of Lower Limit of Normal (LLN) for values normal at baseline; <75% (<50% for neutrophils) of LLN and of baseline for values abnormal at baseline.

Table 6: ZYVOXAM

Percent of Patients Who Experienced at Least One Substantially Abnormal[a] Serum Chemistry Laboratory Value in Comparator-controlled Clinical Trials with ZYVOXAM

Laboratory Assay	Uncomplicated Skin and Skin Structure Infections: ZYVOXAM 400 mg q12h	Uncomplicated Skin and Skin Structure Infections: Comparator	All Other Indications: ZYVOXAM 600 mg q12h	All Other Indications: All Other Comparators
AST (U/L)	1.7	1.3	5.0	6.8
ALT (U/L)	1.7	1.7	9.6	9.3
LDH (U/L)	0.2	0.2	1.8	1.5
Alkaline Phosphatase (U/L)	0.2	0.2	3.5	3.1
Lipase (U/L)	2.8	2.6	4.3	4.2
Amylase (U/L)	0.2	0.2	2.4	2.0
Total Bilirubin (μmol/L)	0.2	0	0.9	1.1
BUN (mmol/L)	0.2	0	2.1	1.5
Creatinine (μmol/L)	0.2	0	0.2	0.6

a >2×Upper Limit of Normal (ULN) for values normal at baseline; >2×ULN and >2×baseline for values abnormal at baseline.

Phase IV Clinical Trials: Table 7 shows the frequencies of selected abnormal hematologic test values in Study 113 at End of Treatment.

Table 7: ZYVOXAM

Frequencies of Abnormal Values for Selected Hematology Assays at EOT [Study 113, linezolid in the treatment of adult diabetic patients with clinically documented complicated skin and skin structure infections ("diabetic foot infections")]

Hematology Assay	Clinically Significant Abnormal[a]/All abnormal values for assay: Linezolid n/N (%)	Comparator n/N (%)
Hemoglobin	9/111 (8.1)	1/52 (1.9)
Hematocrit	6/112 (5.4)	1/49 (2.0)
WBC	2/26 (7.7)	1/12 (8.3)
Platelet Count	9/43 (20.9)	3/16 (18.8)

a Abnormal values assessed by the investigator as clinically significant.
Legend:
EOT=end of treatment.
WBC=white blood count.

Table 8 summarizes abnormal chemistry values in Study 113 assessed at End of Treatment.

Table 8: ZYVOXAM

Frequencies of Abnormal Values for Selected Chemistry Assays at EOT[a] [Study 113, linezolid in the treatment of adult diabetic patients with clinically documented complicated skin and skin structure infections ("diabetic foot infections")]

Chemistry Assay	Clinically Significant Abnormal[a]/All abnormal values for assay: Linezolid n/N (%)	Comparator n/N (%)
ALT	3/32 (9.4)	1/15 (6.7)
AST	1/24 (4.2)	1/19 (5.3)
Bicarbonate	1/22 (4.5)	0/15
Lactic Dehydrogenase	3/38 (7.9)	0/16
Amylase	3/17 (17.6)	0/18

a Assessed by the investigator as clinically significant.
Legend:
ALT=alanine aminotransferase.
AST=aspartate aminotransferase.
EOT=end of treatment.

Post-market Adverse Drug Reactions: Myelosuppression (anemia including pure red blood cell aplasia, leukopenia, pancytopenia, and thrombocytopenia) has been reported during postmarketing use of ZYVOXAM (see Warnings and Precautions).

Peripheral neuropathy, and optic neuropathy sometimes progressing to loss of vision, have been reported in patients treated with linezolid. These reports have primarily been in patients treated for longer than the maximum recommended duration of 28 days (see Warnings and Precautions).

Lactic acidosis (see Warnings and Precautions, General), convulsions (see Warnings and Precautions, Neurologic), angioedema and anaphylaxis have been reported.

Very rare reports of bullous skin disorders such as those described as Stevens Johnson syndrome have been received.

Very rare spontaneous reports of serotonin syndrome with co-administration of linezolid and serotonergic agents have been reported (see Warnings and Precautions, Drug Interactions).

These events have been chosen for inclusion due to either their seriousness, frequency of reporting, possible causal connection to ZYVOXAM, or a combination of these factors. Because they are reported voluntarily from a population of unknown size, estimates of frequency cannot be made and causal relationship cannot be precisely established.

DRUG INTERACTIONS: Overview: Drugs Metabolized by Cytochrome P450: Linezolid is not an inducer of cytochrome P450 (CYP) in rats. It is not detectably metabolized by human cytochrome P450 and it does not inhibit the activities of clinically significant human CYP isoforms (1A2, 2C9, 2C19, 2D6, 2E1, 3A4). Therefore, no CYP450-induced drug interactions are expected with linezolid. Concurrent administration of linezolid does not substantially alter the pharmacokinetic characteristics of (S)-warfarin, which is extensively metabolized by CYP2C9. Drugs such as warfarin and phenytoin, which are CYP2C9 substrates, may be given with linezolid without changes in dosage regimen.

Drug-Drug Interactions: Monoamine Oxidase Inhibition: Linezolid is a mild reversible inhibitor of MAO-A and MAO B. Studies in healthy volunteers have examined the effect of linezolid on the pharmacodynamic responses to tyramine, sympathomimetic amines, and dextromethorphan.

Adrenergic Agents: A significant pressor response has been observed in normal adult subjects receiving linezolid and tyramine doses of more than 100 mg. Therefore, patients receiving linezolid need to avoid consuming large amounts of foods or beverages with high tyramine content (see Warnings and Precautions, Drug Interactions).

A reversible enhancement of the pressor response of either pseudoephedrine HCl (PSE) or phenylpropanolamine HCl (PPA) is observed when linezolid is administered to healthy normotensive subjects (see Warnings and Precautions, Drug Interactions). A similar study has not been conducted in hypertensive patients. The interaction studies conducted in normotensive subjects evaluated the blood pressure and heart rate effects of placebo, PPA or PSE alone, linezolid alone, and the combination of steady-state linezolid (600 mg q12h for 3 days) with two doses of PPA (25 mg) or PSE (60 mg) given 4 hours apart. Heart rate was not affected by any of the treatments. Blood pressure was increased with both combination treatments. Maximum blood pressure levels were seen 2 to 3 hours after the second dose of PPA or PSE, and returned to baseline 2 to 3 hours after peak.

Serotonergic Agents: A study to assess the potential interaction of linezolid with a serotonin reuptake inhibitor (dextromethorphan) was conducted in healthy volunteers. No significant differences were found in the pharmacodynamic measures of temperature, digit symbol substitution, nurse rated sedation, blood pressure, or pulse when subjects were administered dextromethorphan with or without linezolid. The effects of other serotonin reuptake inhibitors have not been studied. Very rare spontaneous reports of serotonin syndrome with co-administration of linezolid and serotonergic agents have been reported (see Warnings and Precautions, Drug Interactions).

Antibiotics: Aztreonam: The pharmacokinetics of linezolid or aztreonam are not altered when administered together.

Gentamicin: The pharmacokinetics of linezolid or gentamicin are not altered when administered together.

Antacids: No studies have been conducted with antacids and chelating agents. Based on the chemical structure, concurrent administration with these agents is not expected to affect absorption of linezolid.

Drug-Food Interactions: Large quantities of foods or beverages with high tyramine content should be avoided while taking ZYVOXAM. Quantities of tyramine consumed should be less than 100 mg per meal. Foods high in tyramine content include those that may have undergone protein changes by aging, fermentation, pickling, or smoking to improve flavor, such as aged cheeses (0 to 15 mg tyramine per 28 g); fermented or air-dried meats (0.1 to 8 mg tyramine per 28 g); sauerkraut (8 mg tyramine per 224 g); soy sauce (5 mg tyramine per 1 teaspoon); tap beers (4 mg tyramine per 360 mL); red wines (0 to 6 mg tyramine per 240 mL). The tyramine content of any protein-rich food may be increased if stored for long periods or improperly refrigerated.

Drug-Herb Interactions: Interactions with herbal products have not been established.

Drug-Laboratory Interactions: There are no reported drug-laboratory test interactions.

DOSAGE AND ADMINISTRATION:

Recommended Dose and Dosage Adjustment: The recommended dosage for the treatment of infections is described in Table 9. Doses are administered every 12 hours (q12h).

Table 9: ZYVOXAM

Dosage Guidelines for ZYVOXAM

Infection[a]	Dosage and Route of Administration	Recommended Duration of Treatment (consecutive days)
Vancomycin-resistant *E. faecium* infections, including concurrent bacteremia	600 mg IV or oral q12h	14 to 28
Nosocomial pneumonia	600 mg IV or oral q12h	10 to 14
Complicated skin and skin structure infections		
a) Except diabetic foot infections	600 mg IV or oral q12h	10 to 14
b) Non-limb threatening diabetic foot infections, without concomitant osteomyelitis	600 mg IV or oral q12h	14 to 28
Community-acquired pneumonia, including concurrent bacteremia	600 mg IV or oral q12h	10 to 14
Uncomplicated skin and skin structure infections	400 mg oral q12h	10 to 14

[a] Due to the designated pathogens (see Indications and Clinical Use).

Patients with infection due to MRSA should be treated with ZYVOXAM 600 mg q12h.

In controlled clinical trials, the protocol-defined duration of treatment for all infections ranged from 7 to 28 days. Total treatment duration was determined by the treating physician based on site and severity of the infection, and on the patient's clinical response.

No dose adjustment is necessary when switching from intravenous to oral administration. Patients whose therapy is started with ZYVOXAM Injection may be switched to ZYVOXAM Tablets at the discretion of the physician, when clinically indicated.

ZYVOXAM may be taken with or without food.

Missed Dose: If a dose is missed, it should be taken as soon as possible. However, if it is almost time for the next dose, the missed dose should be skipped and the regular dosing schedule resumed. Doses should not be doubled.

Administration: Intravenous: ZYVOXAM Injection should be administered by intravenous infusion over a period of 30 to 120 minutes. **Do not use this intravenous infusion bag in series connections.** Additives should not be introduced into this solution. If ZYVOXAM Injection is to be given concomitantly with another drug, each drug should be given separately in accordance with the recommended dosage and route of administration for each product.

If the same intravenous line is used for sequential infusion of several drugs, the line should be flushed before and after infusion of ZYVOXAM Injection with an infusion solution compatible with ZYVOXAM Injection and with any other drug(s) administered via this common line (see Compatible I.V. Solutions under Dosage and Administration).

ZYVOXAM Injection: ZYVOXAM Injection is supplied as a ready-to-use sterile isotonic solution for intravenous infusion. As with all parenteral drug products, intravenous solutions should be inspected visually for clarity, particulate matter, precipitate and leakage prior to administration, whenever solution and container permit. Solutions showing haziness, particulate matter, precipitate or leakage should not be used.

ZYVOXAM Injection may exhibit a yellow color that can intensify over time without adversely affecting potency. Discard unused portions.

Compatible I.V. Solutions: 5% Dextrose Injection, USP; 0.9% Sodium Chloride Injection, USP; and Lactated Ringer's Injection, USP.

Compatibility: Physical incompatibilities resulted when ZYVOXAM Injection was combined with the following drugs during simulated Y-site administration: amphotericin B, chlorpromazine HCl, diazepam, pentamidine isethionate, erythromycin lactobionate, phenytoin sodium, and trimethoprim-sulfamethoxazole. Additionally, chemical incompatibility resulted when ZYVOXAM Injection was combined with ceftriaxone sodium.

OVERDOSAGE:

In the event of overdosage, supportive care is advised, with maintenance of glomerular filtration. Hemodialysis may facilitate more rapid elimination of linezolid. In a phase I clinical trial, approximately 30% of a dose of linezolid was removed during a 3-hour hemodialysis session beginning 3 hours after the dose of ZYVOXAM was administered. Data are not available for removal of linezolid with peritoneal dialysis or hemoperfusion. Clinical signs of acute toxicity in animals were decreased activity and ataxia in rats and vomiting and tremors in dogs treated with 3000 mg/kg/day and 2000 mg/kg/day, respectively.

For management of a suspected drug overdose, CPhA recommends that you contact your **regional Poison Control Centre**. See the *CPS* Directory section for a list of Poison Control Centres.

ACTION AND CLINICAL PHARMACOLOGY: Mechanism of Action: Linezolid is a synthetic antibacterial agent of a new class of antibiotics, the oxazolidinones, with in vitro activity against aerobic gram-positive bacteria, certain gram-negative bacteria, and anaerobic microorganisms. Linezolid inhibits bacterial protein synthesis through a unique mechanism of action. Linezolid binds to sites on the bacterial 23S ribosomal RNA of the 50S subunit and prevents the formation of a functional 70S initiation complex, which is an essential component of the bacterial translation process. The mechanism of action of linezolid (oxazolidinones) differs from that of other antibiotic classes (e.g., aminoglycosides, beta-lactams, folic acid antagonists, glycopeptides, lincosamides, quinolones, rifamycins, streptogramins, tetracyclines, chloramphenicol). Therefore, cross-resistance between linezolid and the mentioned classes of antibiotics is unlikely. Linezolid is active against selected gram positive bacteria that are susceptible or resistant to these antibiotics. In vitro tests have shown that resistance to linezolid develops slowly via multiple-step mutations in the 23S ribosomal RNA and occurs at a frequency of 1×10^{-9} to 1×10^{-11}.

Pharmacokinetics: The mean pharmacokinetic parameters of linezolid after single and multiple oral and intravenous doses are summarized in Table 10. Plasma concentrations of linezolid at steady-state following oral dosing of 600 mg every 12 hours (q12h) are shown in Figure 1.

Table 10: ZYVOXAM

Mean (standard deviation) Pharmacokinetic Parameters of Linezolid

Dose of Linezolid	C_{max} (µg/mL)	C_{min} (µg/mL)	T_{max} (h)	AUC[a] (µg·h/mL)	$t_{1/2}$ (h)	CL (mL/min)
400 mg Tablet						
Single Dose[b] bid Dose	8.1 (1.83) 11 (4.37)	— 3.08 (2.25)	1.52 (1.01) 1.12 (0.47)	55.1 (25) 73.4 (33.5)	5.2 (1.5) 4.69 (1.7)	146 (67) 110 (49)
600 mg Tablet						
Single Dose bid Dose	12.7 (3.96) 21.2 (5.78)	— 6.15 (2.94)	1.28 (0.66) 1.03 (0.62)	91.4 (39.3) 138 (42.1)	4.26 (1.65) 5.4 (2.06)	127 (48) 80 (29)
600 mg I.V. Injection[c]						
Single Dose bid Dose	12.9 (1.6) 15.1 (2.52)	— 3.68 (2.36)	0.5 (0.1) 0.51 (0.03)	80.2 (33.3) 89.7 (31)	4.4 (2.4) 4.8 (1.7)	138 (39) 123 (40)
600 mg Oral Suspension						
Single Dose	11 (2.76)	—	0.97 (0.88)	80.8 (35.1)	4.6 (1.71)	141 (45)

[a] AUC for single dose=$AUC_{0-\infty}$; for multiple-dose=$AUC_{0-\tau}$.
[b] Data dose-normalized from 375 mg.
[c] Data dose-normalized from 625 mg.

Legend:
C_{max}=maximum plasma concentration.
C_{min}= minimum plasma concentration.
T_{max}=time to C_{max}.
AUC=area under concentration-time curve.
$t_{1/2}$=elimination half-life.
CL=systemic clearance.

The average minimum plasma concentrations (C_{min}) at steady state for oral administration of 400 or 600 mg linezolid every 12 hours were 3.08 and 6.15 µg/mL, respectively, and the corresponding average maximum concentrations (C_{max}) were 11.0 and 21.2 µg /mL, respectively. These results indicate that for these dose regimens, the C_{min} values are near or above the highest MIC_{90} (4 µg/mL) for target microorganisms.

Figure 1: ZYVOXAM

Plasma Concentrations of Linezolid at Steady-state Following Oral Dosing of 600 mg Every 12 Hours (Mean±Standard Deviation, n=16)

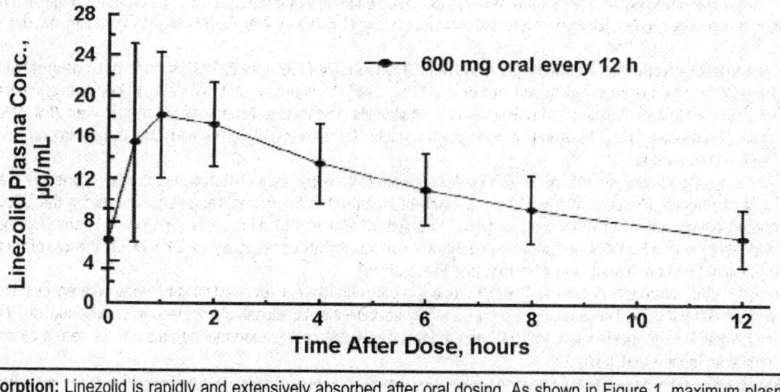

Absorption: Linezolid is rapidly and extensively absorbed after oral dosing. As shown in Figure 1, maximum plasma concentrations are reached approximately 1 to 2 hours after dosing, and the absolute bioavailability is approximately 100%. Therefore, linezolid may be given orally or intravenously without dose adjustment.

Linezolid may be administered without regard to the timing of meals. The time to reach the maximum concentration is delayed from 1.5 hours to 2.2 hours and C_{max} is decreased by about 17% when high fat food is given with linezolid. However, the total exposure measured as $AUC_{0-\infty}$ values is similar under both conditions.

Distribution: Animal and human pharmacokinetic studies have demonstrated that linezolid readily distributes to well-perfused tissues. The plasma protein binding of linezolid is approximately 31% and is concentration-independent. The volume of distribution of linezolid at steady-state averaged 40 to 50 L in healthy adult volunteers.

Linezolid concentrations have been determined in various fluids from a limited number of subjects in Phase I volunteer studies following multiple dosing of linezolid. The ratio of linezolid in saliva relative to plasma was 1.2 to 1 and for sweat relative to plasma was 0.55 to 1. The ratio for epithelial lining fluid was 4.5 to 1, and for alveolar cells of the lung was 0.15 to 1, when measured at steady-state C_{max}. In a small study of subjects with ventricular-peritoneal shunts and essentially non-inflamed meninges, the ratio of linezolid in cerebrospinal fluid to plasma at C_{max} was 0.7 to 1 after multiple dosing of linezolid.

Metabolism: Linezolid is primarily metabolized by oxidation of the morpholine ring, which results in two inactive ring-opened carboxylic acid metabolites: the aminoethoxyacetic acid metabolite (A), and the hydroxyethyl glycine metabolite (B). Formation of metabolite B is mediated by a non-enzymatic chemical oxidation mechanism in vitro. Linezolid is not an inducer of cytochrome

P450 (CYP) in rats, and it has been demonstrated from in vitro studies that linezolid is not detectably metabolized by human cytochrome P450 and it does not inhibit the activities of clinically significant human CYP isoforms (1A2, 2C9, 2C19, 2D6, 2E1, 3A4).

The lack of effect of linezolid to induce CYP2C9 was shown in a healthy volunteer study using warfarin as a metabolism probe.

Excretion: Nonrenal clearance accounts for approximately 65% of the total clearance of linezolid. Under steady-state conditions, approximately 30% of the dose appears in the urine as linezolid, 40% as metabolite B, and 10% as metabolite A. The renal clearance of linezolid is low (average 40 mL/min) and suggests net tubular reabsorption. Virtually no linezolid appears in the feces, while approximately 6% of the dose appears in the feces as metabolite B, and 3% as metabolite A.

A small degree of nonlinearity in clearance was observed with increasing doses of linezolid, which appears to be due to lower renal and nonrenal clearance of linezolid at higher concentrations. However, the difference in clearance was small and was not reflected in the apparent elimination half-life.

Special Populations and Conditions: Pediatrics: Currently, there are limited data on the pharmacokinetics of linezolid during multiple dosing in pediatric patients of all ages. No data have been collected in infants younger than 3 months of age.

Pharmacokinetic information indicates that pediatric patients dosed with 10 mg/kg IV have a similar C_{max} but a higher average clearance when corrected by body weight, and shorter apparent elimination half-life than adults receiving 625 mg of linezolid. Pediatric dosing regimens that provide a pharmacokinetic profile similar to adults have not been determined. Studies using doses higher than 10 mg/kg or dosing more frequently than every 12 hours have not been conducted in pediatric patients.

Geriatrics: The pharmacokinetics of linezolid are not significantly altered in elderly patients

Gender: Females have a slightly lower volume of distribution of linezolid than males. Plasma concentrations are higher in females than in males, which is partly due to body weight differences. After a 600 mg dose, mean oral clearance is approximately 38% lower in females than in males. However, there are no significant gender differences in mean apparent elimination-rate constant or half-life. Thus, drug exposure in females is not expected to substantially increase beyond levels known to be well tolerated. Therefore, dose adjustment by gender is not necessary.

Race: The total clearance of linezolid is not influenced by race. Therefore, dose adjustment is not necessary for different races.

Hepatic Insufficiency: The pharmacokinetics of linezolid are not altered in patients (n=7) with mild-to-moderate hepatic insufficiency (Child-Pugh class A or B). On the basis of the available information, no dose adjustment is recommended for patients with mild-to-moderate hepatic insufficiency. The pharmacokinetics of linezolid in patients with severe hepatic insufficiency have not been evaluated.

Renal Insufficiency: The pharmacokinetics of the parent drug linezolid are not altered in patients with any degree of renal insufficiency. However, the two primary metabolites of linezolid may accumulate in patients with renal insufficiency, with the amount of accumulation increasing with the severity of renal dysfunction (see Table 11). The clinical significance of accumulation of these two metabolites has not been determined in patients with severe renal insufficiency. Because similar plasma concentrations of linezolid are achieved regardless of renal function, no dose adjustment is recommended for patients with renal insufficiency. However, given the absence of information on the clinical significance of accumulation of the primary metabolites, use of linezolid in patients with renal insufficiency should be weighed against the potential risks of accumulation of these metabolites. Both linezolid and the two metabolites are eliminated by dialysis. No information is available on the effect of peritoneal dialysis on the pharmacokinetics of linezolid. Approximately 30% of a dose was eliminated in a 3-hour dialysis session beginning 3 hours after the dose of linezolid was administered; therefore, linezolid should be given after hemodialysis.

STORAGE AND STABILITY: Store ZYVOXAM Tablets at controlled room temperature between 15-30°C. Protect from light. Keep bottles tightly closed to protect from moisture.

Store ZYVOXAM Injection infusion bags in controlled room temperature between 15-30°C. Protect from light. Protect from freezing. Keep the infusion bags in the overwrap until ready to use. ZYVOXAM Injection may exhibit a yellow color that can intensify over time without adversely affecting potency.

Table 11: ZYVOXAM

Mean (Standard Deviation) AUCs and Elimination Half-lives of Linezolid and Metabolites A and B in Patients with Varying Degrees of Renal Insufficiency After a Single 600-mg Oral Dose of Linezolid

Parameter	Healthy Subjects CL_{cr}>80 mL/min	Moderate Renal Impairment 30<CL_{cr}<80 mL/min	Severe Renal Impairment 10<CL_{cr}<30 mL/min	Hemodialysis Dependent	
				Off Dialysis[a]	On Dialysis
Linezolid					
$AUC_{0-\infty}$, µg·h/mL	110 (22)	128 (53)	127 (66)	141 (45)	83 (23)
$t_{1/2}$ (h)	6.4 (2.2)	6.1 (1.7)	7.1 (3.7)	8.4 (2.7)	7 (1.8)
Metabolite A					
AUC_{0-48}, µg·h/mL	7.6 (1.9)	11.7 (4.3)	56.5 (30.6)	185 (124)	68.8 (23.9)
$t_{1/2}$ (h)	6.3 (2.1)	6.6 (2.3)	9 (4.6)	NA	NA
Metabolite B					
AUC_{0-48}, µg·h/mL	30.5 (6.2)	51.1 (38.5)	203 (92)	467 (102)	239 (44)
$t_{1/2}$ (h)	6.6 (2.7)	9.9 (7.4)	11 (3.9)	NA	NA

[a] Between hemodialysis sessions.

Legend:
NA=not applicable.

INFORMATION FOR THE PATIENT: Published in e-CPS, available by subscription at www.e-cps.ca.

DOSAGE FORMS, COMPOSITION AND PACKAGING: Injection: Each mL of sterile, isotonic solution for i.v. infusion, contains: linezolid 2 mg. Nonmedicinal ingredients: citric acid, dextrose, hydrochloric acid, sodium citrate, sodium hydroxide and water for injection. Latex- and PVC-free (bags and ports). Single use, ready-to-use flexible plastic infusion bags of 300 mL (600 mg), in a foil laminate overwrap.

Tablets: Each white, oval, film-coated, compressed tablet, printed with "ZYVOXAM 600mg" in red, contains: linezolid 600 mg. Nonmedicinal ingredients: ammonium hydroxide, carnauba wax, cornstarch, ethanol, ethyl acetate, hydroxypropylcellulose, hypromellose, iron oxide black, iron oxide red, magnesium stearate, microcrystalline cellulose, polyethylene glycol, propylene glycol, shellac, sodium starch glycolate, titanium dioxide and 2-ethoxyethanol. Bottles of 20.

(Shown in Product Identification Section)

Pr Pradax™
dabigatran etexilate

Dabigatran Etexilate 110mg and 150mg Capsules

Prescribing Summary

This is a condensed version of the Product Monograph. For complete information please refer to the Product Monograph available at www.boehringer-ingelheim.ca or by contacting Boehringer Ingelheim (Canada) Ltd., 5180 South Service Road, Burlington, Ontario, L7L 5H4.

Patient Selection Criteria

THERAPEUTIC CLASSIFICATION: Anticoagulant

INDICATIONS AND CLINICAL USE

- Prevention of stroke and systemic embolism in patients with atrial fibrillation, in whom anticoagulation is appropriate.

Geriatrics (>65 years of age): Clinical studies have been conducted in patients with a mean age >65 years. Safety and efficacy data are available (see CLINICAL TRIALS).

Pharmacokinetic studies in older subjects demonstrate an increase in exposure to dabigatran in most of those patients, usually in association with age-related decline of renal function (see WARNINGS AND PRECAUTIONS, Renal, and DOSAGE AND ADMINISTRATION, Renal Impairment).

Pediatrics (<18 years of age): The safety and efficacy of PRADAX have not been established in children less than 18 years of age. Therefore, PRADAX is not recommended in this patient population.

CONTRAINDICATIONS

- Severe renal impairment (CrCl <30mL/min)
- Hemorrhagic manifestations, bleeding diathesis, or patients with spontaneous or pharmacological impairment of hemostasis
- Lesions at risk of clinically significant bleeding, e.g., extensive cerebral infarction (hemorrhagic or ischemic) within the last 6 months, or active peptic ulcer disease with recent bleeding
- Concomitant treatment with strong P-glycoprotein (P-gp) inhibitors, i.e., oral ketoconazole (see DRUG INTERACTIONS)
- Known hypersensitivity to dabigatran or dabigatran etexilate or to any ingredient in the formulation or component of the container. For a complete listing, see the DOSAGE FORMS, COMPOSITION AND PACKAGING section of the Product Monograph.

Safety Information

WARNINGS AND PRECAUTIONS

The following Warnings and Precautions are listed in alphabetical order.

Bleeding

As with all anticoagulants, PRADAX should be used with caution in circumstances associated with an increased risk of bleeding. Bleeding can occur at any site during therapy with PRADAX. An unexplained fall in hemoglobin and/or hematocrit or blood pressure should lead to a search for a bleeding site. Patients at high risk of bleeding should not be prescribed PRADAX (see CONTRAINDICATIONS).

Close clinical surveillance (looking for signs of bleeding or anemia) is recommended throughout the treatment period, especially if risk factors are combined.

Table 1: Factors which increase hemorrhagic risk, as identified in clinical studies

Factors increasing dabigatran plasma levels	Moderate renal impairment (30-50 mL/min CrCl)
	P-glycoprotein-inhibitor comedication
Pharmacodynamic interactions	Acetylsalicylic acid
	NSAID
	Clopidogrel
Diseases/procedures with special hemorrhagic risks	Congenital or acquired coagulation disorders
	Thrombocytopenia or functional platelet defects
	Active ulcerative gastrointestinal disease
	Recent gastro-intestinal bleeding
	Recent biopsy or major trauma
	Recent intracranial hemorrhage
	Brain, spinal or ophthalmic surgery
	Bacterial endocarditis
Others	Age ≥75 years

The measurement of dabigatran-related anticoagulation may be helpful to avoid excessive high exposure to dabigatran in the presence of additional risk factors.

In patients who are bleeding, an aPTT test may be useful to assist in determining an excess of anticoagulant activity, despite its limited sensitivity. An aPTT >80 sec at trough, i.e., when the next dose is due, is associated with a higher risk of bleeding (see Monitoring and Laboratory Tests).

Should severe bleeding occur, treatment with PRADAX must be discontinued and the source of bleeding investigated promptly.

Agents that may enhance the risk of hemorrhage should not be administered concomitantly with PRADAX, or, if necessary, should only be administered with caution (see ACTION AND CLINICAL PHARMACOLOGY, Pharmacokinetic Interactions in the Product Monograph).

Treatments that should NOT be administered concomitantly with PRADAX due to increase in bleeding risk include: unfractionated heparin and heparin derivatives, low molecular weight heparins (LMWH), fondaparinux, bivalirudin, thrombolytic agents, GPIIb/IIIa receptor antagonists, ticlopidine, sulfinpyrazone, and vitamin K antagonists such as warfarin.

The concomitant use of PRADAX with the following treatments has not been studied and may increase the risk of bleeding: rivaroxaban, prasugrel, and the strong P-gp inhibitors itraconazole, tacrolimus, cyclosporine, ritonavir, tipranavir, nelfinavir and saquinavir.

Unfractionated heparin may be administered at doses necessary to maintain a patent central venous or arterial catheter.

In patients with atrial fibrillation treated for the prevention of stroke and systemic embolism, the co-administration of oral anti-platelet (including aspirin and clopidogrel) and NSAID therapies increases the risk of bleeding by about two-fold (see ACTION AND CLINICAL PHARMACOLOGY, Special Populations, *Pharmacokinetic Interactions*). If necessary, co-administration of low-dose ASA, i.e., ≤100 mg daily with PRADAX may be considered for other indications than stroke prevention in atrial fibrillation. Note that in the RELY trial, there is no evidence that the addition of ASA or clopidogrel to dabigatran, or its comparator warfarin, improved outcomes in respect to stroke (see CLINICAL TRIALS, Stroke Prevention in Atrial Fibrillation).

Treatment initiation with verapamil should be avoided in patients following orthopedic surgery who are already treated with PRADAX. Simultaneous initiation of treatment with PRADAX and verapamil should also be avoided at any time (see DRUG INTERACTIONS, *P-glycoprotein inhibitors*).

Interaction with P-gp inducers

The concomitant use of PRADAX with the strong P-gp inducer, rifampicin, reduces dabigatran plasma concentrations. Other P-gp inducers such as St. John's Wort or carbamazepine are also expected to reduce dabigatran plasma concentrations, and should be co-administered with caution (see DRUG INTERACTIONS and Special Populations).

Surgery/Procedural Interventions

Patients on PRADAX who undergo surgery or invasive procedures are at increased risk for bleeding. In these circumstances, temporary discontinuation of PRADAX may be required.

Pre-operative Phase

In advance of invasive or surgical procedures PRADAX should be stopped temporarily due to an increased risk of bleeding. If possible, PRADAX should be discontinued at least 24 hours before invasive or surgical procedures. In patients at higher risk of bleeding (see DOSAGE AND ADMINISTRATION) or in major surgery where complete hemostasis may be required, consider stopping PRADAX 2-4 days before surgery. Clearance of dabigatran in patients with renal insufficiency may take longer (see DOSAGE AND ADMINISTRATION, Renal). This should be considered in advance of any procedures.

PRADAX is contraindicated in patients with

severe renal dysfunction (CrCl <30 mL/min). Should acute renal failure occur before surgery is required, PRADAX should generally be stopped at least 5 days before major surgery.

If acute intervention is required, PRADAX should be temporarily discontinued, due to increased risk of bleeding. Surgery or procedural interventions should be delayed if possible until at least 12 hours after the last dose of PRADAX, with risk of bleeding weighed against the urgency of the needed intervention.

Peri-Operative Spinal/Epidural Anesthesia, Lumbar Puncture

Procedures such as spinal anesthesia may require complete hemostatic function.

In patients treated with PRADAX for VTE prevention following major orthopedic surgery and who undergo spinal or epidural anesthesia, or in whom lumbar puncture is performed in follow-up to surgery, the formation of spinal or epidural hematomas that may result in long-term or permanent paralysis cannot be excluded.

In the case of these peri-spinal procedures, administration of the first dose of PRADAX should occur after hemostasis has been obtained and no sooner than 2 hours following puncture or removal of catheters related to these procedures.

The risk of these rare events may be higher with post-operative use of indwelling epidural catheters or the concomitant use of other products affecting hemostasis. Accordingly, the use of PRADAX is not recommended in patients undergoing anesthesia with post-operative indwelling epidural catheters.

Post-Procedural Period

Resume treatment with PRADAX as soon as complete hemostasis is achieved.

Renal

PRADAX is contraindicated in cases of severe renal impairment (CrCl <30 mL/min). Patients who develop acute renal failure while on PRADAX should discontinue such treatment.

- *Patients with atrial fibrillation treated for prevention of stroke and systemic embolism:* Since no dose adjustment is necessary for most atrial fibrillation patients with moderate renal impairment (CrCl 30-50 mL/min), a standard daily dose of 300 mg, taken orally as one 150 mg capsule twice daily is recommended (see DOSAGE AND ADMINISTRATION, Renal Impairment).

Special Populations

Pregnant Women: Since there are no studies of PRADAX in pregnant women, the potential risk in these patients is unknown. Animal reproductive studies did not show any adverse effects on fertility or postnatal development of the neonate. Women of child-bearing potential should avoid pregnancy during treatment with PRADAX and when pregnant, women should not be treated with PRADAX unless the expected benefit is greater than the risk.

Nursing Women: Breast-feeding during treatment with PRADAX is not recommended. There are no clinical data available on the excretion of dabigatran into breast milk.

Geriatrics (>65 years of age): Pharmacokinetic studies in older subjects demonstrate an increase in drug exposure; especially in those patients with age-related decline of renal function (see WARNINGS AND PRECAUTIONS, Renal, and DOSAGE AND ADMINISTRATION, Renal Impairment).

- *Patients with atrial fibrillation treated for prevention of stroke and systemic embolism:* Patients aged 80 years and above should be treated with a daily dose of 220 mg taken orally as one 110 mg capsule twice daily. This alternate dosing may also be considered for other geriatric patients (see DOSAGE AND ADMINISTRATION, Elderly). Use with caution.

Pediatrics (<18 years of age): The safety and efficacy of PRADAX have not been established in children less than 18 years of age. Therefore, PRADAX is not recommended in this patient population.

Patients of low body weight (<50 kg): Since limited data are available in these patients, PRADAX should be used with caution.

Monitoring and Laboratory Tests

At recommended doses of PRADAX, dabigatran prolongs coagulation time as measured by the activated partial thromboplastin time (aPTT), thrombin time (TT) and ecarin clotting time (ECT). In patients who are bleeding due to excess activity of dabigatran, these coagulation tests would be expected to be elevated and may be helpful in assessing anticoagulant activity of dabigatran, if necessary (see ACTION AND CLINICAL PHARMACOLOGY, Pharmacodynamics). The aPTT is generally less sensitive to anticoagulant activity than either TT or ECT (see DRUG INTERACTIONS, Drug-Laboratory Interactions).

However, the aPTT test is widely available and provides an approximate indication of the anticoagulation intensity achieved with dabigatran. In patients who are bleeding, the aPTT test may be useful to assist in determining an excess of anticoagulant activity, despite its limited sensitivity. An aPTT greater than 80 sec at trough (when the next dose is due) is associated with a higher risk of bleeding. In circumstances where there is no excess of anticoagulant activity, the utility of aPTT is limited in monitoring anticoagulant status of patients taking PRADAX.

ADVERSE REACTIONS

The safety of PRADAX has been evaluated overall in 22,126 patients.

A total of 10,084 patients were exposed to at least one dose of dabigatran as study medication in four active-controlled clinical trials conducted to evaluate the safety and effectiveness of dabigatran etexilate in the prevention of venous thromboembolic events (VTE) following major elective orthopedic surgery. Of these, 5,419 were treated with 150 mg or 220 mg daily of PRADAX, while 389 received doses of less than 150 mg daily, and 1,168 received doses in excess of 220 mg daily.

In the RELY trial investigating the prevention of stroke and systemic embolism in patients with atrial fibrillation, a total of 12,042 patients were exposed to PRADAX. Of these, 6,059 were treated with 150 mg twice daily of dabigatran etexilate, while 5,983 received doses of 110 mg twice daily.

About 21% of patients with atrial fibrillation treated with dabigatran and about 16% of patients treated with warfarin for the prevention of stroke and systemic embolism (long-term treatment for up to 3 years) experienced adverse events considered related to treatment.

Bleeding

Bleeding is the most relevant side effect of PRADAX. Bleeding of any type or severity occurred in approximately 14% of patients treated short-term for elective hip or knee replacement surgery and in long-term treatment in 16.5% of patients with atrial fibrillation treated for the prevention of stroke and systemic embolism.

Although rare in frequency in clinical trials, major or severe bleeding may occur and, regardless of location, may lead to disabling, life-threatening or even fatal outcomes.

A summary description of major and total bleeding is provided in Table 2.

Table 2 shows the number of patients experiencing major and total bleeding event rates during the treatment period in the RELY study, conducted in patients with atrial fibrillation. In Table 2, the category of major bleeds includes both life-threatening and non-life threatening bleeds. Within life-threatening, intracranial bleeds is a subcategory of life-threatening bleeds. Intracranial bleeds include intracerebral (hemorrhagic stroke), subarachnoid and subdural bleeds. For this reason, these events may be counted in multiple categories.

Table 2: Frequency and annualized event rate (%) of bleeding events from the RELY trial

	Dabigatran etexilate 110 mg bid N (%)	Dabigatran etexilate 150 mg bid N (%)	Warfarin** N (%)
Patients randomized	6,015	6,076	6,022
Patient-years	11,899	12,033	11,794
Major bleeding event (MBE)*	342 (2.9)	399 (3.3)	421 (3.6)
Hazard ratio vs. warfarin (95% CI)	0.80 (0.70, 0.93)	0.93 (0.81, 1.07)	
p-value	0.0026	0.3146	
Life threatening MBE	147 (1.2)	179 (1.5)	218 (1.9)
Hazard ratio vs. warfarin (95% CI)	0.67 (0.54, 0.82)	0.80 (0.66, 0.98)	
p-value	0.0001	0.0305	
Intra-cranial hemorrhage (ICH)+	27 (0.2)	38 (0.3)	90 (0.8)
Hazard ratio vs. warfarin (95% CI)	0.30 (0.19, 0.45)	0.41 (0.28, 0.60)	
p-value	< 0.0001	< 0.0001	
Any bleeding event[a]	1,754 (14.7)	1,993 (16.6)	2,166 (18.4)
Hazard ratio vs. warfarin (95% CI)	0.78 (0.73, 0.83)	0.91 (0.85, 0.96)	
p-value	< 0.0001	0.0016	

*Adjudicated bleeds
**Dose-adjusted warfarin to an INR of 2.0 – 3.0
+ICH consists of adjudicated hemorrhagic stroke and subdural and/or subarachnoid hemorrhage.
[a]Investigator-reported bleeding events

Major bleeding fulfilled one or more of the following criteria:

- Bleeding associated with a reduction in hemoglobin of at least 20 grams per litre or leading to a transfusion of at least 2 units of blood or packed cells;
- Symptomatic bleeding in a critical area or organ: intraocular, intracranial, intraspinal or intramuscular with compartment syndrome, retroperitoneal bleeding, intra-articular bleeding or pericardial bleeding.

Major bleeds were classified as life-threatening if they fulfilled one or more of the following criteria:

- Fatal bleed; symptomatic intracranial bleed; reduction in hemoglobin of at least 50 grams per litre; transfusion of at least 4 units of blood or packed cells; a bleed associated with hypotension requiring the use of intravenous inotropic agents; a bleed that necessitated surgical intervention.

Clinical Trial Adverse Drug Reactions:

Because clinical trials are conducted under very specific conditions, the adverse reaction rates observed in the clinical trials may not reflect the rates observed in practice and should not be compared to the rates in the clinical trials of another drug. Adverse drug reaction information from clinical trials is useful for identifying drug-related adverse events and for approximating rates.

Table 3: Common Adverse Reactions observed in ≥1% of dabigatran-treated patients with atrial fibrillation in the active-controlled trial, RELY

	Dabigatran etexilate 110 mg N (%)	Dabigatran etexilate 150 mg N (%)	Warfarin N (%)
	5,983 (100)	6,059 (100)	5,998 (100)
Bleeding and anemia*	**599 (10.0)**	**747 (12.3)**	**825 (13.8)**
Anemia	73 (1.2)	97 (1.6)	74 (1.2)
Epistaxis	66 (1.1)	67 (1.1)	107 (1.8)
Gastrointestinal hemorrhage	196 (3.3)	277 (4.6)	155 (2.6)
Urogenital hemorrhage	66 (1.1)	84 (1.4)	96 (1.6)
Gastrointestinal disorders*	**735 (12.3)**	**772 (12.7)**	**220 (3.7)**
Abdominal pain	135 (2.3)	134 (2.2)	15 (0.3)
Diarrhea	75 (1.3)	71 (1.2)	11 (0.2)
Dyspepsia	250 (4.2)	234 (3.9)	13 (0.2)
Nausea	58 (1.0)	73 (1.2)	12 (0.2)

*Aggregate incidence presented for all adverse reactions within the body system, including those reactions occurring <1% and not listed in the Table above. Gastrointestinal adverse reactions occurred more often with dabigatran etexilate than warfarin. These were related to dyspepsia (including upper abdominal pain, abdominal pain, abdominal discomfort, epigastric discomfort), or gastritis-like symptoms (including GERD, esophagitis, erosive gastritis, gastric hemorrhage, hemorrhagic gastritis, hemorrhagic erosive gastritis, gastrointestinal ulcer).

Gastrointestinal (GI) hemorrhage occurred at a higher frequency with PRADAX compared to warfarin (see Table 3). GI adjudicated major bleeds were reported at 1.1%, 1.6%, and 1.1% (annualized rates) in the DE 110 mg, DE 150 mg and warfarin groups, respectively. GI life-threatening bleeds occurred with a frequency of 0.6%, 0.8% and 0.5% in the DE 110 mg, DE 150 mg and warfarin groups, respectively. Any GI bleeds occurred with a frequency of 5.4%, 6.1% and 4.0% in the DE 110 mg, DE 150 mg and warfarin groups, respectively. The underlying mechanism of the increased rate of GI bleeding has not been established (see CLINICAL TRIALS, Prevention of stroke and systemic embolism in patients with atrial fibrillation).

Allergic reactions or drug hypersensitivity including urticaria, bronchospasm, rash and pruritus have been reported in patients who received dabigatran etexilate. Rare cases of anaphylactic reactions have also been reported.

Less Common Clinical Trial Adverse Drug Reactions (<1%)

Observed with exposure to dabigatran 110 mg bid and 150 mg bid during the RELY trial, an active-controlled clinical trial for the prevention of stroke and systemic embolism in patients with atrial fibrillation:

Blood and lymphatic system disorders: thrombocytopenia
Vascular disorders: hematoma, hemorrhage
Gastrointestinal disorders: gastrointestinal ulcer, gastroesophagitis, gastro-esophageal reflux disease, vomiting, dysphagia
Hepatobiliary disorders: hepatic function abnormal/liver function test abnormal, hepatic enzyme increased
Skin and subcutaneous tissue disorders: skin hemorrhage, urticaria, rash, pruritus
Musculoskeletal and connective tissue and bone disorders: hemarthrosis
Renal and urinary disorders: hematuria
General disorders and administration site conditions: injection site hemorrhage, catheter site hemorrhage
Injury, poisoning and procedural complications: incision site hematoma, traumatic hematoma, incision site hemorrhage
Immune system disorder: drug hypersensitivity
Respiratory disorders: hemoptysis, bronchospasm
Nervous system disorders: intracranial hemorrhage

For abnormal liver function tests reported in the RE-LY trial, please see Table 5.

To report an adverse event, contact your Regional Adverse Reaction Monitoring Office at 1-866-234-2345, or contact: Boehringer Ingelheim (Canada) Ltd., 5180 South Service Rd., Burlington, ON L7L 5H4.

DRUG INTERACTIONS

Based on *in vitro* evaluation, neither dabigatran etexilate nor its active moiety, dabigatran, have been shown to be metabolized by the human cytochrome P450 system, nor did they exhibit effects on human CYP P450 isozymes.

Concomitant use of PRADAX with treatments that interfere with hemostasis or coagulation increases bleeding risk (see WARNINGS AND PRECAUTIONS, Bleeding). Co-administration of PRADAX with other anticoagulants has not been adequately studied and is not recommended.

In the RELY trial, conducted in patients with atrial fibrillation, a two-fold increase in major bleeding was seen in both dabigatran study treatment arms, as well as that of the comparator, warfarin, when ASA was administered concomitantly (see ACTION AND CLINICAL PHARMACOLOGY, Special Populations, *Pharmacokinetic Interactions* in the Product Monograph; CLINICAL TRIALS, Stroke Prevention in Atrial Fibrillation; and DOSAGE AND ADMINISTRATION).

Drug-Drug Interactions

Transporter interactions: Dabigatran etexilate, but not dabigatran, is a substrate with moderate affinity for the efflux P-glycoprotein (P-gp) transporter. Therefore, potent P-glycoprotein inducers or inhibitors may be expected to impact exposure to dabigatran.

P-glycoprotein inhibitors: P-gp inhibitors like verapamil, quinidine and amiodarone may be expected to increase systemic exposure to dabigatran, see Table 4 below. The strong P-glycoprotein inhibitor ketoconazole, when administered orally, is contraindicated (see CONTRAINDICATIONS). If not otherwise specifically described, close clinical surveillance (looking for signs of bleeding or anemia), along with a sense of caution is required when dabigatran is co-administered with strong P-glycoprotein inhibitors.

P-glycoprotein inducers: The concomitant use of PRADAX with the strong P-gp inducer rifampicin, reduces dabigatran plasma concentration. Other P-gp inducers such as carbamazepine and St John's Wort are also expected to reduce the systemic exposure of dabigatran. Less potent inducers such as tenofovir can potentially reduce systemic exposure. Caution is advised when co-administering these drug products.

P-glycoprotein substrates: Dabigatran etexilate is not expected to have a clinically meaningful interaction with P-glycoprotein substrates that do not also act as inhibitors or inducers of P-gp.

Table 4: Summary of Drug-Drug Interactions

Proper name	Ref*	Effect	Clinical comment
Amiodarone	CT	Dabigatran exposure in healthy subjects was increased by 60% in the presence of amiodarone (see ACTION AND CLINICAL PHARMACOLOGY, Special Populations, *Pharmacokinetic Interactions*).	Adjust dosing for patients treated for prevention of VTE after hip- or knee-replacement surgery to 150 mg daily PRADAX with amiodarone. Caution should be exercised.
			No dose adjustment is generally recommended for AF patients. Use with caution. Occasional testing of aPTT may be considered to rule out excessive anticoagulant effect.
Antacids (aluminium compounds, sodium bicarbonate, calcium and/or magnesium compounds, or combinations of these)	CT	In population PK analyses, a reduction in dabigatran exposure by 35% was seen over the first 24 hours following surgery. Thereafter, (>24 hours after surgery), a reduction of about 11% was observed.	Diminished clinical effect may occur, as may be expected for any drug resulting in an increase in gastric pH during PRADAX administration. PRADAX should be administered at least 2 hours before taking an antacid. Co-administration with PRADAX should be avoided within 24 hours after orthopedic surgery.
Atorvastatin	CT	When dabigatran etexilate was co-administered with atorvastatin, exposure of atorvastatin, and atorvastatin metabolites were not significantly changed. Dabigatran concentrations were decreased about 20%.	No dose adjustment is recommended.
Clarithromycin	CT	Dabigatran exposure in healthy subjects was increased by about 15% in the presence of clarithromycin (see ACTION AND CLINICAL PHARMACOLOGY, Special Populations, *Pharmacokinetic Interactions*).	No dose adjustment is recommended. Caution should be exercised.
Diclofenac	CT	When dabigatran etexilate was co-administered with diclofenac, pharmacokinetics of both drugs appeared unchanged.	No dose adjustment is recommended. Use with caution (see WARNINGS AND PRECAUTIONS, Bleeding, Table 2.)
Digoxin	CT	When dabigatran etexilate was co-administered with digoxin, no PK-interaction was observed.	No dose adjustment is recommended.
Ketoconazole	CT	Dabigatran exposure was increased 150% after single and multiple doses of ketoconazole (see ACTION AND CLINICAL PHARMACOLOGY, Special Populations, *Pharmacokinetic Interactions*).	**Co-administration with PRADAX is contraindicated.** (see CONTRAINDICATIONS).
Pantoprazole	CT	When dabigatran etexilate was co-administered with pantoprazole, a decrease in dabigatran AUC of about 30 % was observed. In the Phase III study, RELY, PPI co-medication did not result in lower trough levels and on average only slightly reduced post-dose concentrations (-11%) (see ACTION AND CLINICAL PHARMACOLOGY, Special Populations, *Pharmacokinetic Interactions*).	No dose adjustment is recommended. Diminished clinical effect may occur, as may be expected for any drug resulting in an increase in gastric pH during PRADAX administration.
Rifampicin	CT	After 7 days of treatment with 600 mg rifampicin qd total dabigatran AUC0-∞ and Cmax were reduced by 67% and 66% compared to the reference treatment, respectively (see ACTION AND CLINICAL PHARMACOLOGY, Special Populations, *Pharmacokinetic Interactions*).	Concomitant use of PRADAX with rifampicin should, in general, be avoided. Concomitant use would be expected to result in substantially diminished anticoagulant effect of PRADAX.
Verapamil	CT	When dabigatran etexilate, given at 150 mg once daily, was co-administered with moderate doses of oral verapamil, the Cmax and AUC of dabigatran were increased, but the magnitude of this change varied depending on the timing of administration and the formulation of verapamil used (see ACTION AND CLINICAL PHARMACOLOGY, Special Populations, *Pharmacokinetic Interactions*)	Dosing should be reduced to 150 mg PRADAX daily in patients treated for prevention of VTE after hip- or knee-replacement surgery who concomitantly receive dabigatran etexilate and verapamil. To minimize potential for interaction, PRADAX should be given at least two hours before verapamil. Caution should be exercised.
			Although no dose adjustment is recommended for AF patients, to minimize potential for interaction, PRADAX should be given at least two hours before verapamil. Caution should be exercised.
Quinidine	CT	Dabigatran exposure in healthy subjects was increased by 53 % in the presence of quinidine.	Adjust dosing for patients treated for prevention of VTE after hip- or knee-replacement surgery to 150 mg daily PRADAX. Caution should be exercised.
			Although no dose adjustment is recommended for AF patients, to minimize potential for interaction, PRADAX should be given at least two hours before quinidine, if possible. Caution should be exercised.

*C = Case Study; CT = Clinical Trial; T = Theoretical

Drug-Food Interactions

Food does not affect the bioavailability of PRADAX but delays the time-to-peak plasma concentrations by 2 hours.

Drug-Herb Interactions

Drug-herb interactions have not been investigated. Potent P-gp inducers such as St. John's Wort (Hypericum perforatum) may be expected to affect systemic exposure of dabigatran. Co-administration of these products is not recommended.

Drug-Laboratory Interactions

No single test (aPTT, TT, ECT) is adequate to reliably assess the anticoagulant activity of dabigatran following PRADAX administration. At therapeutic levels of dabigatran, thrombin time (TT) is the best measure of the pharmacodynamic effect of dabigatran because of its linear and sensitive relationship with dabigatran exposure (WARNINGS AND PRECAUTIONS, Monitoring and Laboratory Tests; ACTION AND CLINICAL PHARMACOLOGY, Pharmacodynamics, in the Product Monograph).

The aPTT test is widely available and provides an approximate indication of the anticoagulation intensity achieved with dabigatran. In patients who are bleeding, the aPTT test may be useful to assist in determining an excess of anticoagulant activity, despite its limited sensitivity. An aPTT greater than 80 sec at trough (when the next dose is due) is associated with a higher risk of bleeding.

Note that a PT (INR) test is not useful to assess the anticoagulant activity of PRADAX.

Drug-Lifestyle Interactions

No direct interaction between dabigatran etexilate and alcohol was demonstrated in animal models or has been hypothesized.

The effect of PRADAX on the ability to drive and use machines has not been investigated. However, no such interaction is to be expected.

Administration

DOSAGE AND ADMINISTRATION

PRADAX should be taken orally, with the entire capsule to be swallowed whole. The capsule should not be chewed, broken, or opened.

PRADAX should be taken regularly, as prescribed, to ensure optimal effectiveness. All temporary discontinuations should be avoided, unless medically indicated.

Recommended Dose and Dosage Adjustment

- *Prevention of stroke and systemic embolism in patients with atrial fibrillation:* The recommended dose of PRADAX is 300 mg daily, taken orally as one 150 mg capsule twice a day.

Elderly:

- *Prevention of stroke and systemic embolism in patients with atrial fibrillation:* Patients aged 80 years and above should be treated with a dose of 220 mg of PRADAX daily, taken orally as one 110 mg capsule twice a day (see WARNINGS AND PRECAUTIONS, Geriatrics, and CLINICAL TRIALS, Prevention of Stroke and Systemic Embolism in Patients with Atrial Fibrillation, Tables 24 and 25, in the Product Monograph).
- The usual recommended dose for most geriatric patients under the age of 80 years is 300 mg daily, taken orally as one 150 mg capsule twice a day (see CLINICAL TRIALS, Prevention of Stroke and Systemic Embolism in Patients with Atrial Fibrillation, Tables 24 and 25, in the Product Monograph). However, in geriatric patients, especially those over the age of 75 with at least one other risk factor for bleeding (see WARNINGS AND PRECAUTIONS, Bleeding, Table 2), the administration of a dose of 220 mg of PRADAX daily, taken orally as one 110 mg capsule twice a day, may be considered. It should be noted, however, that the effectiveness of stroke prevention may be expected to be lessened with this dosage regimen, compared to that of the usual one of 300 mg of PRADAX daily. As with any anticoagulant, caution is required when prescribing PRADAX to the elderly (see CONTRAINDICATIONS, and WARNINGS AND PRECAUTIONS, Bleeding).

Patients at risk of bleeding: *Prevention of stroke and systemic embolism in patients with atrial fibrillation:* Patients with an increased risk of bleeding (see WARNINGS AND PRECAUTIONS, Bleeding, Table 1), should be closely monitored clinically (looking for signs of bleeding or anemia). In such patients, a dose of 220 mg, given as 110 mg twice daily may be considered. A coagulation test, such as aPTT (see WARNINGS AND PRECAUTIONS, Monitoring and Laboratory Tests), may help to identify patients with an increased bleeding risk caused by excessive dabigatran exposure.

As for any anticoagulant, PRADAX is NOT indicated in patients at excessive risk of bleeding (see CONTRAINDICATIONS).

Renal impairment: Following oral dosing with dabigatran etexilate, there is a direct correlation of systemic exposure to dabigatran with degree of renal impairment (see WARNINGS AND PRECAUTIONS, Renal). The kidneys account for 85% of dabigatran clearance.

There are no data to support use in patients with severe renal impairment (CrCl <30 mL/min). Given the substantial increase in dabigatran exposure observed in this patient population, treatment with PRADAX is not recommended (see CONTRA-INDICATIONS, and ACTION AND CLINICAL PHARMACOLOGY, Renal Insufficiency).

- *Patients with atrial fibrillation treated for prevention of stroke and systemic embolism having moderate renal impairment (CrCl 30-50 mL/min):* No dose adjustment is recommended (see CLINICAL TRIALS, Prevention of Stroke and Systemic Embolism in Patients with Atrial Fibrillation, *Renal Impairment*). Patients with moderate renal impairment (CrCl 30-50 mL/min) should be treated with a daily dose of PRADAX at 300 mg taken orally as one 150 mg capsule twice daily, with caution. Regular assessment of renal status is required in these patients (see CONTRAINDICATIONS, WARNINGS AND PRECAUTIONS, Renal). A coagulation test, such as aPTT (see WARNINGS AND PRECAUTIONS, Monitoring and Laboratory Tests), may help to identify patients with an increased bleeding risk caused by excessive dabigatran exposure.

Creatinine clearance can be estimated using the Cockroft-Gault formula as follows:

Creatinine clearance (mL/min) =

$$\text{Males: } \frac{(140\text{-age (years)}) \times \text{weight (kg)}}{72 \times \text{serum creatinine (mg/100mL)}}$$

$$\text{Females: } \frac{0.85 \times (140\text{-age (years)}) \times \text{weight (kg)}}{72 \times \text{serum creatinine (mg/100mL)}}$$

P-glycoprotein inhibitors: P-gp inhibitors like verapamil, quinidine, and amiodarone may be expected to increase systemic exposure to dabigatran. Combination use with oral ketoconazole is contraindicated (see CONTRAINDICATIONS).

- *Patients with atrial fibrillation treated for prevention of stroke and systemic embolism:* No dose adjustment is recommended in patients concomitantly receiving amiodarone, quinidine or verapamil (see DRUG INTERACTIONS, Table 4, Summary of Drug-Drug Interactions; and ACTION AND CLINICAL PHARMACOLOGY, Special Populations, *Pharmacokinetic interactions* in the Product Monograph). Patients should be treated with a daily dose of 300 mg PRADAX taken orally as one 150 mg capsule twice daily. To minimize potential for interaction, PRADAX should be given at least two hours before verapamil (see ACTION AND CLINICAL PHARMACOLOGY, Special Populations, *Pharmacokinetic interactions* in the Product Monograph). Caution should be exercised. Close clinical surveillance is recommended.

Drugs that increase gastric pH, such as antacids, protein pump inhibitors (PPI): Diminished clinical effect for antacids may occur (see DRUG INTERACTIONS, Table 4, Summary of Drug-Drug Interactions). Although no dosage adjustment is generally necessary, administer PRADAX at least two hours before antacids, if possible, to minimize interaction potential. No dose adjustment is required for pantoprazole or other PPIs.

Concomitant antithrombotic use:
Concomitant use of ASA or clopidogrel with PRADAX in patients with atrial fibrillation approximately doubled the risk of major bleed, irrespective of dose of PRADAX used. A similar increase was noted with such concomitant use with the study comparator, warfarin. These observations contrasted with little apparent additional improvement in stroke and systemic embolic events with combined antithrombotic use and PRADAX (or warfarin). Concomitant use of PRADAX with an antithrombotic is not recommended for prevention of cardiogenic thromboembolic stroke in patients with atrial fibrillation. Concomitant use of ASA or other antiplatelet agents based on medical need to prevent myocardial infarction should be undertaken with caution. Close clinical surveillance is recommended.

Acute myocardial infarction (AMI):
Consideration should be given to discontinuing PRADAX in the setting of acute myocardial infarction should the treatment of myocardial infarction involve invasive procedures, such as percutaneous coronary revascularization, or coronary artery bypass surgery. Similar consideration should be given if thrombolytic therapy is to be initiated, because bleeding risk may increase. Patients with AMI should be treated according to current clinical guidelines for that disorder. In this setting, PRADAX may be resumed for the prevention of stroke and systemic embolism upon completion of these revascularization procedures.

Children: Since PRADAX has not been investigated in patients <18 years of age, treatment is not recommended.

Patient Body Weight: Population PK modelling shows that patients with a body weight of about 120 kg have about 20% lower drug exposure. Patients with a body weight of about 48 kg have about 25% higher drug exposure compared to patients with average weight. No dose adjustment deemed necessary.

Switching from PRADAX treatment to parenteral anticoagulant:

- In patients with atrial fibrillation treated for prevention of stroke and systemic embolism: wait **12 hours** after the last dose of PRADAX before switching to a parenteral anticoagulant.

Switching from parenteral anticoagulants treatment to PRADAX: If deemed medically appropriate, treatment with PRADAX should be initiated 0-2 hours prior to the time that the next dose of the alternate therapy would be due, or at the time of discontinuation in case of continuous treatment (e.g., intravenous unfractionated heparin, [UFH]).

Switching from Vitamin K antagonists to PRADAX: If deemed medically appropriate, PRADAX should only be started after Vitamin K antagonists have been discontinued, and the patient's INR is found to be below 2.0.

Cardioversion: Patients can be maintained on PRADAX while being cardioverted.

Missed Dose: *Prevention of stroke and systemic embolism in patients with atrial fibrillation:* If the prescribed dose of PRADAX is not taken at the scheduled time, the dose should be taken as soon as possible on the same day. A forgotten PRADAX dose may still be taken up to 6 hours prior to the next scheduled dose. From 6 hours prior to the next scheduled dose on, the missed dose should be omitted. Patients should not take a double dose to make up for missed individual doses. For optimal effect and safety, it is important to take PRADAX regularly twice a day, at approximately 12-hour intervals.

Administration
PRADAX may be taken with food, or on an empty stomach with water.

The capsule should be swallowed intact. It should not be opened, broken, or chewed (see ACTION AND CLINICAL PHARMACOLOGY in the full Product Monograph, Pharmacokinetics).

SUPPLEMENTAL PRODUCT INFORMATION

Adverse Reactions:

Liver Function Tests: In the long-term RELY study, observed abnormalities of liver function tests (LFT) are presented below in Table 5.

Table 5: Liver Function Tests in the RELY trial

	Dabigatran etexilate 110 mg twice daily N (%)	Dabigatran etexilate 150 mg twice daily N (%)	Warfarin N (%)
Total treated	5,983 (100.0)	6,059 (100.0)	5,999 (100.0)
ALT or AST >3xULN	118 (2.0)	106 (1.7)	125 (2.1)
ALT or AST >5xULN	36 (0.7)	45 (0.7)	50 (0.8)
ALT or AST >3xULN + Bilirubin >2xULN	11 (0.2)	14 (0.2)	21 (0.4)

OVERDOSAGE

There is no antidote to dabigatran etexilate or dabigatran. Doses of PRADAX beyond those recommended expose the patient to increased risk of bleeding. Excessive anticoagulation may require discontinuation of PRADAX. In the event of hemorrhagic complications, treatment must be discontinued and the source of bleeding investigated. Since dabigatran is excreted predominantly by the renal route, adequate diuresis must be maintained. Appropriate standard treatment, e.g., surgical hemostasis as indicated and blood volume replacement, should be undertaken. In addition, consideration may be given to the use of fresh whole blood or the transfusion of fresh frozen plasma.

As protein binding is low, dabigatran can be dialysed, although there is limited clinical experience in using dialysis in this setting. Activated prothrombin complex concentrates (e.g., FEIBA) or recombinant Factor VIIa or concentrates of coagulation factors II, IX or X, may be considered. There is some experimental evidence to support the role of these agents in reversing the anticoagulant effect of dabigatran but their usefulness in clinical settings has not yet been clearly demonstrated. Consideration should also be given to administration of platelet concentrates in cases where thrombocytopenia is present or long-acting antiplatelet drugs have been used. All symptomatic treatment should be given according to the physician's judgement.

For management of a suspected drug overdose, contact your regional Poison Control Centre.

Product Monograph is available upon request or at www.boehringer-ingelheim.ca

Boehringer Ingelheim (Canada) Ltd.
5180 South Service Road
Burlington, ON L7L 5H4

November 8, 2010

TARGIN®

Controlled release oxycodone/naloxone HCl tablets
10/5 mg, 20/10 mg, 40/20 mg

Prescribing Summary

Patient Selection Criteria

THERAPEUTIC CLASSIFICATION: Opioid Analgesic/Opiod Antagonist

INDICATIONS AND CLINICAL USE: Adults: Targin® (oxycodone hydrochloride/naloxone hydrochloride) is a controlled release tablet having a dual therapeutic effect. The oxycodone component in **Targin**® is indicated for the relief of moderate to severe pain in adults who require continuous around-the-clock opioid analgesia for several days or more. The naloxone component in **Targin**® is indicated for the relief of opioid-induced constipation (OIC). **Geriatrics (> 65 years of age):** In general, dose selection for an elderly patient should be cautious, usually starting at the low end of the dosing range, reflecting the greater frequency of decreased hepatic, renal, or cardiac function, concomitant disease and other drug therapy. The dosage should be adjusted to the intensity of the pain and the sensitivity of the individual patient. **Pediatrics (< 18 years of age):** The safety and efficacy of **Targin**® has not been studied in the pediatric population. Therefore, use of **Targin**® is not recommended in patients under 18 years of age.

CONTRAINDICATIONS:

Targin® (oxycodone hydrochloride/naloxone hydrochloride controlled release tablets) is contraindicated in:

- Patients who are hypersensitive to the active substances (oxycodone or naloxone) or other opioid analgesics or to any ingredient in the formulation. For a complete listing, see the **DOSAGE FORMS, COMPOSITION AND PACKAGING** section of the Product Monograph.
- In patients with known or suspected mechanical gastrointestinal obstruction (e.g., bowel obstruction, strictures) or any diseases/conditions that affect bowel transit (e.g., ileus of any type).
- Administration by the rectal route is contraindicated (see **WARNINGS AND PRECAUTIONS**).
- Patients with suspected surgical abdomen (e.g., acute appendicitis or pancreatitis).
- Patients with mild, intermittent or short duration pain that can be managed with other pain medications.
- The management of acute pain, including use in outpatient or day surgeries.
- The management of perioperative pain.
- Patients with acute asthma or other obstructive airway, and status asthmaticus.
- Patients with acute respiratory depression, elevated carbon dioxide levels in the blood, and cor pulmonale.
- Patients with acute alcoholism, delirium tremens, and convulsive disorders.
- Patients with severe CNS depression, increased cerebrospinal or intracranial pressure, and head injury.
- Patients taking monoamine oxidase (MAO) inhibitors (or within 14 days of such therapy).
- Women who are breast-feeding, pregnant, or during labour and delivery.
- Opioid-dependent patients and for narcotic withdrawal treatment.
- Patients with moderate to severe hepatic impairment (Child-Pugh Class B & C).

Safety Information

WARNINGS AND PRECAUTIONS:

General

Targin® (oxycodone hydrochloride/naloxone hydrochloride controlled release tablets) should be swallowed whole. Taking broken, chewed, dissolved or crushed Targin® tablets could lead to the rapid release and absorption of a potentially fatal dose of oxycodone.

Targin® should not be administered rectally due to the possible increased systemic availability of naloxone by this route and the potential for the occurrence of severe withdrawal effects (see CONTRAINDICATIONS). Targin® 40/20 mg tablets are for use in opioid tolerant patients only (see also DOSAGE AND ADMINISTRATION).

A single dose greater than 40 mg of oxycodone, or total daily doses greater than 80 mg of oxycodone, may cause fatal respiratory depression when administered to patients who are not tolerant to the respiratory depressant effects of opioids (see WARNINGS AND PRECAUTIONS and DRUG INTERACTIONS).

Patients for whom Targin® is prescribed should not give Targin® to anyone else as such inappropriate use may have severe medical consequences, including death.

Targin® should not be used to treat patients with constipation not related to opioid use.

Patients should be cautioned not to consume alcohol while taking **Targin**®, as it may increase the chance of experiencing dangerous side effects. There is no clinical experience in patients with cancer associated with peritoneal carcinomatosis or with sub-occlusive syndrome in advanced stages of digestive and pelvic cancers. Therefore, the use of **Targin**® in this population is not indicated. **Gastrointestinal** Diarrhea is a possible effect of naloxone. If severe or persistent diarrhea lasts for more than 3 days during treatment, patients should be advised to contact their physician. **Abuse of Opioid Formulations** If abused parenterally, intranasally or rectally by individuals dependent on opioid agonists, **Targin**® is expected to produce marked withdrawal symptoms – because of the systemic opioid receptor antagonist characteristics of naloxone by these routes – or to intensify withdrawal symptoms already present. **Targin**® consists of a dual polymer matrix intended for oral use only. Abuse can lead to overdose and death. This risk is increased when the tablets are crushed, dissolved, broken or chewed, and with concurrent consumption of alcohol or other CNS depressants. With parenteral abuse, the tablet excipients, especially talc, can be expected to result in local tissue necrosis, infection, pulmonary granulomas, and increased risk of endocarditis and valvular heart injury. **Dependence/Tolerance** As with other opioids, tolerance and physical dependence may develop upon repeated administration of **Targin**® and there is a potential for development of psychological dependence. **Targin**® tablets should therefore be prescribed and handled with the degree of caution appropriate to the use of a drug with abuse potential. Abuse and addiction are separate and distinct from physical dependence and tolerance. In addition, abuse of opioids can occur in the absence of true addiction and is characterized by misuse for non-medical purposes, often in combination with other psychoactive substances. Tolerance, as well as physical dependence, may develop upon repeated administration of opioids, and are not by themselves evidence of an addictive disorder or abuse. Concerns about abuse, addiction, and diversion should not prevent the proper management of pain. The development of addiction to opioid analgesics in properly managed patients with pain has been reported to be rare. However, data are not available to establish the true incidence of addiction in chronic pain patients. Opioids, such as oxycodone, should be used with particular care in patients with a history of alcohol and drug abuse. Drug abuse is usually not a problem in patients with pain in which opioids are appropriately indicated. Withdrawal symptoms may occur following abrupt discontinuation of therapy or upon administration of an opioid antagonist. Patients on prolonged therapy should be withdrawn gradually from the drug if it is no longer required for pain control. **Use in Drug and Alcohol Addiction Targin**® is an agonist/antagonist combination product with no approved use in the management of addictive disorders. **Neurologic Interaction with Other Central Nervous System Depressants:** Oxycodone should be used with caution and in a reduced dosage during concomitant administration of other opioid analgesics, general anaesthetics, phenothiazines and other tranquilizers, sedative-hypnotics, tricyclic antidepressants and other CNS depressants, including alcohol. Respiratory depression, hypotension and profound sedation or coma may result. Severe pain antagonizes the subjective and respiratory depressant actions of opioid analgesics. Should pain suddenly subside, these effects may rapidly become manifest. Patients who are scheduled for chordotomy or other interruption of pain transmission pathways should not receive **Targin**® within 24 hours of the procedure. **Head Injury:** The respiratory depressant effects of oxycodone, and the capacity to elevate cerebrospinal fluid pressure, may be greatly increased in the presence of an already elevated intracranial pressure produced by trauma. Also, oxycodone may produce confusion, miosis, vomiting and other side effects which obscure the clinical course of patients with head injury. In such patients, oxycodone must be used with extreme caution and only if it is judged essential. **Withdrawal Effects:** Withdrawal symptoms may occur following abrupt discontinuation of therapy. These symptoms may include body aches, diarrhea, gooseflesh, loss of appetite, nausea, nervousness or restlessness, runny nose, sneezing, tremors or shivering, stomach cramps, tachycardia, trouble with sleeping, unusual increase in sweating, palpitations, unexplained fever, weakness and yawning. Patients on prolonged therapy should be withdrawn gradually from the drug if it is no longer required for pain control. In patients who are appropriately treated with opioid analgesics and who undergo gradual withdrawal from the drug, these symptoms are usually mild. **Cardiovascular Targin**® should be used with caution in patients with pre-existing cardiovascular disease. Oxycodone administration may result in severe hypotension in patients whose ability to maintain adequate blood pressure is compromised by reduced blood volume or concurrent administration of drugs, such as phenothiazines or certain anaesthetics. Oxycodone may produce orthostatic hypotension in ambulatory patients. Oxycodone, like all opioid analgesics of the morphine-type, should be administered with caution to patients in circulatory shock, since vasodilation produced by the drug may further reduce cardiac output and blood pressure. **Respiratory Depression** Oxycodone should be used with extreme caution in patients with substantially decreased respiratory reserve, pre-existing respiratory depression, hypoxia or hypercapnia. Such patients are often less sensitive to the stimulatory effects of carbon dioxide (CO_2) on the respiratory centre and the respiratory depressant effects of oxycodone may reduce respiratory drive to the point of apnea. **Pre- and Post-Operative Use Targin® is contraindicated for perioperative use, within 24 hours before or after surgery. Targin® is not indicated for pain in the postoperative period if the pain is mild or not expected to persist for an extended period of time.** In the case of planned chordotomy or other pain-relieving operations, patients should not be treated with **Targin**® within 24 hours before or after the operation. Thereafter, if **Targin**® is to be continued after the patient recovers from the post-operative period, a new dose should be used in accordance with the changed need for pain relief. **Psychomotor Impairment Targin**® may impair the mental and/or physical abilities needed for certain potentially hazardous activities such as driving a car or operating machinery. Patients using **Targin**® should not drive or operate dangerous machinery unless they are tolerant to the effects of the drug. Patients should also be cautioned about the combined effects of **Targin**® with other CNS depressants, including other opioids, phenothiazines, sedative/hypnotics and alcohol. **Special Populations Special Risk Groups:** Oxycodone should be administered with caution and in a reduced dosage to debilitated patients, and in patients with Addison's disease, cholelithiasis, hypothyroidism, toxic psychosis, pancreatitis, prostatic hypertrophy or urethral stricture. **Nursing Women:** Oxycodone passes into the breast milk. It is not known whether naloxone is excreted in human milk. Since the safety of **Targin**® in infants and newborns has not been studied, **Targin**® is contraindicated in nursing mothers. **Pregnancy, Labour and Delivery:** Oxycodone and naloxone pass into the placenta. **Targin**® is contraindicated during pregnancy, labour and delivery due to impaired uterine contractility and the risk of neonatal respiratory depression. There are no adequate data from the use of **Targin**® in pregnant women or during childbirth. Animal studies have not been performed with oxycodone and naloxone in combination. While animal reproduction studies have revealed no evidence of harm to the fetus due to oxycodone, safe use in pregnancy has not been established. Long-term administration of oxycodone during pregnancy may lead to withdrawal symptoms in the newborn. **Geriatrics (> 65 years of age):** In general, dose selection for an elderly patient should be cautious, usually starting at the low end of the dosing range, reflecting the greater frequency of decreased hepatic, renal, or cardiac function, and of concomitant disease or other drug therapy. The dosage should be adjusted to the lowest **Targin**® dose which will achieve the overall treatment goal of satisfactory pain relief with acceptable side effects. **Pediatrics (< 18 years of age): Targin**® has not been studied in children and is not recommended for patients less than 18 years of age. The safety and efficacy of **Targin**® in children have not been established. **Hepatic Impairment:** A clinical trial has shown that plasma concentrations of both oxycodone and naloxone are elevated in patients with hepatic impairment. Naloxone concentrations were affected to a higher degree than oxycodone. The clinical relevance of this is under investigation. Caution must be exercised when administering **Targin**® to patients with mild hepatic impairment. **Targin® is contraindicated in patients with moderate and severe hepatic impairment** (see **CONTRAINDICATIONS**). **Renal Impairment:** A clinical trial has shown that plasma concentrations of both oxycodone and naloxone are elevated in patients with renal impairment. Naloxone concentrations were affected to a higher degree than oxycodone. The plasma concentrations obtained in patients with mild, moderate and severe renal impairment are comparable to those in mildly hepatic impaired patients. The clinical relevance of this is under investigation, but caution should be exercised when administering **Targin**® to patients with renal impairment. **"In Vitro" Dissolution Studies of Interaction with Alcohol** In-vitro data show that in presence of ethanol, at concentrations up to 40%, the controlled-release characteristics of the **Targin**® formulation were maintained and no breakdown of the controlled release mechanism was observed.

ADVERSE REACTIONS: Clinical Trial Adverse Drug Reactions The pre-marketing pivotal clinical program of **Targin**® (oxycodone hydrochloride/naloxone hydrochloride controlled release tablets) included exposure to 520 patients. A summary of adverse events occurring at an incidence of 1% or more is given below which includes all events, whether considered by the clinical investigator to be related to the study drug or not (see **CLINICAL TRIALS** for methodological details of the trials). Nausea was a very common adverse effect in patients taking **Targin**®. Nausea is a common effect associated with other drugs with opioid-agonist activity and tends to reduce with time. Adverse effects, including constipation, diarrhea, fatigue, headache and hyperhidrosis, often observed with other drugs with opioid-agonist activity, were also seen with **Targin**® treatment.

Adverse Event Reports in Targin® Pivotal Clinical Trials (≥1%)

(% of patients on **Targin**® (n = 520) / % of patients on Oxycodone CR (n = 446) / % of patients on Placebo * (n = 235): **Ear and labyrinth disorders:** vertigo 1.7/1.8/5.1. **Gastrointestinal disorders:** abdominal pain: 3.3/2.7/3.8; abdominal pain upper: 1.9/2.7/2.1; constipation: 6.5/10.5/8.9; diarrhea: 6.2/5.4/6.0; dry mouth: 2.5, 1.6, 2.1; dyspepsia: 1.4/3.4/3.0; flatulence: 1.2, 0.5, 0.9; nausea: 12.3/14.8/14.9; vomiting: 5.4/5.6/6.0. **General disorders and administrative site conditions:** asthenia: 1.4/0.0/0.9; chills: 1.2/0.7/0.9; drug withdrawal syndrome: 0.2/1.4/0.4; fatigue: 5.4/5.8/4.3; malaise: 0.2/0.7/1.7; edema peripheral: 1.7/1.8/0.0; pain: 2.3/1.6/2.1; pyrexia: 0.4/0.0/1.3. **Infections and infestations:** bronchitis: 1.5/1.1/0.0; cystitis: 0.2/1.4/1.3; gastroenteritis: 1.9/2.2/0.0; influenza: 1.2/1.6/0.4; nasopharyngitis: 2.9/4.7/4.3; sinusitis: 1.2/0.0/0.0; upper respiratory tract infection: 0.0/1.6/0.0; urinary tract infection: 3.5/2.2/1.3; viral infection: 1.5/1.4/1.3. **Injury, poisoning and procedural complications:** Contusion: 0.0/0.2/1.7. **Investigations:** blood cholesterol increased: 0.0/0.0/1.7; blood glucose increased: 1.9/0.2/0.4; blood triglycerides increased: 0.6/2.0/1.7; blood uric acid increased: 0.2/0.2/2.6; gamma-glutamyltransferase increased: 0.6/1.1/0.4; lymphocyte count decrease: 0.0/0.2/1.3. **Metabolism and nutrition disorders: anorexia:** 0.8/1.1/0.9; decreased appetite: 0.6/0.2/1.3; hyperglycemia: 1.2/1.4/0.0; hyperlipidemia: 1.2/0.2/0.0; hypertriglyceridemia: 1.4/0.2/1.3; hyperuricemia: 1.2/1.1/0.0. **Musculoskeletal and connective tissue disorders:** arthralgia: 1.5/2.2/2.1; back pain: 3.3/2.5/0.0; neck pain: 0.0/1.4/0.0; osteoarthritis: 1.2/1.6/0.0; pain in extremity: 1.5/1.1/0.0. **Nervous system disorders:** dizziness: 4.2/8.1/4.3; headache: 6.2/6.3/9.8; migraine: 1.4/0.2/0.4; sciatica: 1.5/0.0/0.0; somnolence: 1.2/1.1/0.0; tremor: 1.0/1.1/0.4. **Psychiatric disorders:** depression: 1.9/2.5/0.0; insomnia: 2.1/2.5/3.4; nervousness: 0.6/0.0/1.3; restlessness: 0.8/0.2/2.6; sleep disorder: 0.6/0.2/1.7. **Skin and subcutaneous tissue disorders:** hyperhidrosis: 6.5/4.3/6.4; pruritus: 2.9/4.0/3.0; rash: 1.2/0.5/0.0. **Vascular disorders:** hot flush: 1.0/2.0/0.9; hypertension: 0.6/1.4/1.7.

*** Placebo patients received immediate-release oxycodone or combination preparations with codeine 30mg as rescue medication in pivotal clinical trials.**

Less Common Clinical Trial Adverse Drug Reactions (< 1%): Other less common (< 1%) adverse drug reactions reported and considered in any way related to **Targin**® in randomized pivotal clinical trials are summarized in the Product Monograph **(see Adverse Reactions section in the Product Monograph)**.

To report a suspected adverse reaction, please contact:

Purdue Pharma
575 Granite Court
Pickering, ON
Canada L1W 3W8
Tel: 905-420-6400
1-800-387-5349

DRUG INTERACTIONS Overview Interaction with Central Nervous System (CNS) Depressants **Targin**® (oxycodone hydrochloride/naloxone hydrochloride controlled release tablets) should be dosed with caution and started in a reduced dosage (1/3 to 1/2 of the usual dosage) in patients who are currently taking other central nervous system depressants (e.g., alcohol, other opioids, sedatives, hypnotics, anti-depressants, sleeping aids, phenothiazines, neuroleptics, anti-histamines and anti-emetics), pyrazolidone and beta-blockers, as they may enhance the CNS-depressant effect (e.g., respiratory depression) of **Targin**®. Drug-Drug Interactions No interaction studies have been performed with **Targin**®. Administration with Mixed Activity Agonist/Antagonist Opioids Mixed activity agonist/antagonist opioid analgesics (i.e., pentazocine, nalbuphine, butorphanol, and buprenorphine) should be administered with caution to a patient who has received or is receiving a course of therapy with a pure μ-opioid agonist analgesic, such as the oxycodone in **Targin**®. In this situation, mixed activity agonist/antagonist analgesics may reduce the analgesic effect of oxycodone and/or may precipitate withdrawal symptoms in these patients. Drugs Metabolized by Cytochrome P450 Isozymes In vitro metabolism studies indicate that no clinically relevant interactions are to be expected between oxycodone and naloxone. At therapeutic concentrations, **Targin**® is not expected to cause clinically relevant interactions with other concomitantly administered drugs metabolized over the CYP isomers CYP1A2, CYP2A6, CYP2C9, CYP2C19, CYP2D6 and CYP2E1. Oxycodone is metabolized, in part, by CYP3A4 therefore caution is advised when **Targin**® is administered with CYP3A4 inhibitors/inducers. In addition, the likelihood of clinically relevant interactions between acetaminophen or acetylsalicylic acid and the combination of oxycodone and naloxone in therapeutic concentrations is minimal. MAO Inhibitors MAO inhibitors intensify the effects of opioid drugs which can cause anxiety, confusion and decrease respiration. **Targin**® is contraindicated in patients receiving MAO inhibitors or who have used them within the previous 14 days (see **CONTRAINDICATIONS**). Warfarin and Other Coumarin Anticoagulants Clinically relevant changes in International Normalized Ratio (INR or Quick-value) in both directions have been observed in individuals when oxycodone and coumarin anticoagulants are co-administered.

Administration

DOSAGE AND ADMINISTRATION: **Dosing Considerations:** **Targin® (oxycodone hydrochloride/naloxone hydrochloride controlled release tablets) should be swallowed whole. Taking broken, chewed, dissolved or crushed Targin® tablets could lead to the rapid release and absorption of a potentially fatal dose of oxycodone. Patients who are currently taking oral oxycodone can be switched to Targin® based on an equivalent oxycodone dose. For conversion from other opioids/opioid preparations, patients should be initiated on the lowest available Targin® strength, provided with adequate rescue medication, with dose titration to achieve satisfactory pain relief with acceptable side effects. Targin® doses must be individualized and should be assessed at regular intervals. Targin® 40/20 mg tablets are for use in opioid tolerant patients only. A single dose greater than 40 mg of oxycodone, or total daily doses greater than 80 mg of oxycodone, may cause fatal respiratory depression when administered to patients who are not tolerant to the respiratory depressant effects of opioids at equivalent doses (see WARNINGS AND PRECAUTIONS and DRUG INTERACTIONS). Targin® is contraindicated for rectal administration (see CONTRAINDICATIONS). Targin® is contraindicated in the perioperative period, within 24 hours before or after surgery. Targin® is not indicated for pain in the postoperative period if the pain is mild or not expected to persist for an extended period of time.** In the case of planned chordotomy or other pain-relieving operations, patients should not be treated with **Targin**® within 24 hours before or after the operation. Thereafter, if **Targin**® is to be continued after the patient recovers from the post-operative period, a new dose should be used in accordance with the changed need for pain relief. In steady-state studies, the analgesic efficacy of **Targin**® is equivalent to the OxyContin® controlled release oxycodone formulation. In clinical studies with **Targin**®, only patients who had previously been dosed on oxycodone were switched to **Targin**®. To date, there is no clinical experience evaluating switching from other analgesics to **Targin**®. **Targin**® doses must be individualized based upon the status of each patient and should be assessed at regular intervals after application. Proper optimization of doses scaled to the individual's pain should aim at the regular administration of the lowest dose of **Targin**® which provides pain relief. The dosage of the drug must be individualized according to the response and tolerance of the patient. **Targin**® should be taken at the determined dosage twice daily (every 12 hours) according to a fixed time schedule. **Single doses should not exceed 40 mg oxycodone and 20 mg naloxone. The maximum daily dose of Targin® is 80 mg oxycodone hydrochloride and 40 mg naloxone hydrochloride.** For patients requiring higher doses of **Targin**®, administration of supplemental controlled-release oxycodone at the same time intervals should be considered. In the case of supplemental oxycodone dosing, the beneficial effect of naloxone on bowel function may be impaired. In general, the lowest effective opioid analgesic dose should be selected. After discontinuation of therapy with **Targin**®, with a subsequent switch to another opioid, symptoms associated with reduced bowel motility can be expected. The controlled release tablets may be taken with or without food with sufficient liquid (with 4 to 6 oz. of water). The empty matrix tablet remnants may be visible in the stool. **Adults (over 18 years)** Patients Not Receiving Opioids at the Time of Initiation of **Targin**® Treatment (Opioid-Naïve) The usual initial adult dose for patients who have not previously received opioid analgesics is **Targin**® 10/5 mg every 12 hours. Patients Currently Receiving Opioids **Patients who are currently taking oxycodone can be switched to Targin® based on an equivalent oxycodone dose. Discontinue all other around-the-clock oxycodone analgesic medications when Targin® therapy is initiated.** In clinical studies with **Targin**®, only patients who had previously been dosed on oxycodone were switched to **Targin**®. Patients receiving other oral oxycodone formulations may be transferred to **Targin**® tablets at the same total daily dosage, equally divided into two 12-hourly **Targin**® tablet doses and reassessed with dose adjustments made accordingly. To date, there is no clinical experience to refer to for switching other opioid analgesics to **Targin**®. Patients already receiving oxycodone, and tolerant to the respiratory depressant effects, may be started on higher dose than the usual initial adult dose of 10/5 mg every 12 hours depending on their previous oxycodone dose. Not to exceed the maximum daily dose of **Targin**®, 80 mg oxycodone hydrochloride and 40 mg naloxone hydrochloride. **For conversion from other opioids/opioid preparations, discontinue all other round-the-clock opioid analgesic preparations. Patients should be initiated on the lowest available Targin® strength, provided with adequate rescue**

medication, with dose titration to achieve satisfactory pain relief with acceptable side effects. Targin® doses must be individualized and should be assessed at regular intervals. Targin® should be gradually titrated until adequate pain relief and acceptable side effects have been achieved. **The maximum daily dose of Targin® is 80 mg oxycodone hydrochloride and 40 mg naloxone hydrochloride.** Dose Titration Proper optimization of doses scaled to the relief of the individual's pain should aim at regular administration of the lowest dose of **Targin®** which will achieve the overall treatment goal of satisfactory pain relief with acceptable side effects. Dose adjustments may be made every 1-2 days until a stable dose is reached. Subsequent increases in **Targin®** dosage must be individualized according to the pain relief and tolerance of the patient with adequate rescue medication, as required (see Management of Breakthrough Pain section of the Product Monograph). **If breakthrough pain repeatedly occurs at the end of the dosing interval it is generally an indication for a dosage increase rather than more frequent administration. The maximum daily dose of Targin® is 80 mg oxycodone hydrochloride and 40 mg naloxone hydrochloride.** Management of Breakthrough Pain Some patients taking **Targin®** according to a fixed time schedule may require immediate-release analgesics as "rescue" medication for breakthrough pain. Immediate-release oxycodone or combination preparations with codeine 30 mg may be given. Alternatively, non-opioid analgesics may be used. **Targin®** is a controlled release formulation and therefore is not intended for use as rescue medication. For the treatment of breakthrough pain with an immediate-release opioid, a single dose of "rescue medication" should approximate one sixth of the equivalent daily dose of oxycodone hydrochloride. The need for more than two rescue medication doses per day (24 hours) is usually an indication that the dose of **Targin®** requires upward adjustment. This adjustment may be made every 1-2 days until a stable dose is reached. The aim is to establish a patient-specific 12 hour dose that will maintain adequate analgesia and minimize side effects for as long as pain therapy is necessary. Reducing the dosing frequency from every 12 hours is not recommended. **Managing Expected Opioid Adverse Experiences** Many patients receiving opioids, especially those who are opioid-naïve, will experience side effects. Clinical trials have shown that these effects are generally most bothersome during initial treatment and can be minimized by starting **Targin®** at 10/5 mg every 12 hours and gradually increasing the dose as needed. Other opioid related side effects such as sedation and nausea are usually self-limited and often do not persist beyond the first few days. If nausea persists and is unacceptable to the patient, treatment with anti-emetics or other modalities may relieve these symptoms and should be considered. **Missed Dose** If the patient forgets to take one or more doses, they should take their next dose at the next scheduled time and in the normal amount. **Discontinuation** Careful and regular monitoring are required to establish required maintenance of treatment. When the patient no longer requires therapy with **Targin®**, doses should be tapered gradually to prevent signs and symptoms of withdrawal in the physically dependent patient. Withdrawal symptoms may occur following abrupt discontinuation of therapy. These symptoms may include body aches, diarrhea, gooseflesh, loss of appetite, nausea, nervousness or restlessness, runny nose, sneezing, tremors or shivering, stomach cramps, tachycardia, trouble with sleeping, unusual increase in sweating, palpitations, unexplained fever, weakness and yawning. Patients on prolonged therapy should be withdrawn gradually from the drug if it is no longer required for pain control. In patients who are appropriately treated with opioid analgesics and who undergo gradual withdrawal from the drug, these symptoms are usually mild. If treatment discontinuation is required, the dose of opioid may be decreased as follows: one-half of the previous daily dose given every 12 hours or immediate release oxycodone every 6 hours for the first two days, followed by a 25% reduction every two days.

OVERDOSAGE (see Supplemental Product Information)

For management of suspected drug overdose, contact your Regional Poison Control Centre.

Study References

1. Pereira J, Bruera E *et al.* Alberta Hospice Palliative Care Resource Manual. A project of the Alberta Cancer Board with financial support provided by Alberta Cancer Foundation. Division of Palliative Care Medicine, University of Alberta, 2001:1-87.
2. Targin® Product Monograph, Purdue Pharma, March 2010.
3. Lowenstein O *et al.* Combined prolonged-release oxycodone and naloxone improves bowel function in patients receiving opioids for moderate-to-severe non-malignant chronic pain: a randomized controlled trial. *Expert Opin Pharmacother* 2009;10(4):531-543.

Supplemental Product Information

Information for Physicians to Convey to Patients

A patient information sheet should be provided when **Targin®** tablets are dispensed to the patient.

Patients receiving **Targin®** should be given the following instructions by the physician:

1. Patients should be informed that accidental ingestion or use by individuals (including children) other than the patient for whom it was originally prescribed, may lead to severe, even fatal, consequences.
2. Patients should be advised that **Targin®** contains oxycodone, an opioid pain medicine.
3. Patients should be advised that **Targin®** should only be taken as directed. The dose of **Targin®** should not be adjusted without consulting with a physician.
4. **Targin®** should be swallowed whole (not broken, chewed, dissolved or crushed) due to the risk of fatal oxycodone overdose.
5. Patients should be warned not to administer **Targin®** by the rectal route, as severe withdrawal effects may occur.
6. Diarrhea is a possible effect of naloxone. Patients should be advised to contact their physician if the diarrhea is severe or persistent.
7. Patients should be advised to report episodes of breakthrough pain and adverse experiences occurring during therapy. Individualization of dosage is essential to make optimal use of this medication.
8. Patients should not combine **Targin®** with alcohol or other central nervous system depressants (sleep aids, tranquilizers) because dangerous additive effects may occur resulting in serious injury or death.
9. Patients should be advised to consult their physician or pharmacist if other medications are being used or will be used with **Targin®**.
10. Patients should be advised that if they have been receiving treatment with **Targin®** and cessation of therapy is indicated, it may be appropriate to taper the **Targin®** dose, rather than abruptly discontinue it, due to the risk of precipitating withdrawal symptoms.
11. Patients should be advised of the most common adverse reactions that may occur while taking **Targin®**: nausea, constipation, diarrhea, hyperhidrosis, fatigue, vomiting, headache and dizziness.
12. Patients should be advised that **Targin®** may cause drowsiness, dizziness, or lightheadedness and may impair mental and/or physical ability required for the performance of potentially hazardous tasks (e.g., driving, operating machinery). Patients started on **Targin®** or patients whose dose has been adjusted should be advised not to drive a car or operate machinery unless they are tolerant to the effects of **Targin®**.
13. Patients should be advised that **Targin®** is a potential drug of abuse. They should protect it from theft or misuse.
14. Patients should be advised that **Targin®** should never be given to anyone other than the individual for whom it was prescribed.
15. Patients should be advised that **Targin®** 40/20 mg is for use only in individuals tolerant to the effect of equivalent doses of oxycodone.
16. Women of childbearing potential who become or are planning to become pregnant should be advised to consult a physician prior to initiating or continuing therapy with **Targin®**. Women who are breast-feeding or pregnant should not use **Targin®**.
17. Patients should be advised that they may pass empty matrix tablet remnants in the stool, and that this should not be a concern since the analgesic medication, oxycodone, has already been released.

ADVERSE REACTIONS

Post-Market Adverse Drug Reactions

In a two year non-interventional open-label, prospective, observational study (Study 9002) performed in Europe, 7,836 pain patients with severe pain for at least 4 months received **Targin®** and were monitored over a period of 4 weeks. Approximately 25% of the patients (n=1,963) were opioid naïve with the remaining 5,849 patients previously pre-treated with opioids. The most frequently reported adverse drug reactions in the total population were nausea (3.1%), constipation (3.1%), dizziness (2.4%), abdominal distension (1.9%), diarrhea (1.9%), abdominal pain (1.4%), vomiting (1.1%) and irregular bowel movements (1.1%). All these adverse drug reactions are consistent with the expected adverse event profile of the opioid analgesic class of drugs. **(see Adverse Reactions section in the Product Monograph).**

OVERDOSAGE

Symptoms

Depending on the history of the patient, an overdose of **Targin®** (oxycodone hydrochloride/naloxone hydrochloride controlled release tablets) may be manifested by symptoms that are either triggered by oxycodone (opioid receptor agonist) or by naloxone (opioid receptor antagonist).

Symptoms of oxycodone overdose include miosis, respiratory depression, somnolence progressing to stupor, skeletal muscle flaccidity, bradycardia as well as hypotension. Coma, non-cardiogenic pulmonary oedema and circulatory failure may occur in more severe cases and may lead to a fatal outcome.

Symptoms of a naloxone overdose alone are unlikely due to the low systemic availability of naloxone by the oral route. Withdrawal symptoms due to an overdose of naloxone should be treated symptomatically in a closely-supervised environment.

Treatment

Primary attention should be given to the establishment of adequate respiratory exchange through the provision of a patent airway and controlled or assisted ventilation. Clinical symptoms suggestive of an oxycodone overdose may be treated by the administration of opioid antagonists (e.g., naloxone 0.4-2 mg intravenously). Administration should be repeated at 2-3 minute intervals, as clinically necessary. It is also possible to apply an infusion of 2 mg naloxone in 500 mL of 0.9% sodium chloride or 5% dextrose (0.004 mg/mL naloxone). The infusion should run at a rate aligned to the previously administered bolus doses and to the patient's response.

Consideration may be given to gastric lavage.

Supportive measures (artificial ventilation, oxygen, vasopressors and infusions) should be employed, as necessary, to manage the circulatory shock accompanying an overdose. Cardiac arrest or arrhythmias may require cardiac massage or defibrillation. Artificial ventilation should be applied if necessary. Fluid and electrolyte metabolism should be maintained.

SPECIAL HANDLING INSTRUCTIONS: Store at Room Temperature (15-30°C). Keep in a cool dry place. Protect from light, heat and humidity. Keep **Targin®** out of sight and reach of children.

DOSAGE FORMS AND PACKAGING: Targin® 10/5 mg are white, oblong tablets with a film coating, marked OXN on one side and 10 on the other. **Targin®** 20/10 mg are pink, oblong tablets with a film coating, marked OXN on one side and 20 on the other. **Targin®** 40/20 mg are yellow, oblong tablets with a film coating, marked OXN on one side and 40 on the other. All strengths will be available in blisters (10s, 14s, 20s, 28s, 30s, 50s, 56s, 60s, 98s and 100s) and opaque plastic bottles of 50, 60, 100 and 250's (see **DOSAGE FORMS, COMPOSITION AND PACKAGING** in the Product Monograph).

Targin® is a registered Trademark of Purdue Pharma

Purdue Pharma Inc
General Partner of / commandité de
Purdue Pharma
Pickering, Ontario L1W 3W8
Member R&D
PURDUE
03/10

Toctino* (alitretinoin)

Prescribing Summary

Patient Selection Criteria

THERAPEUTIC CLASSIFICATION: Immunomodulator/Anti-inflammatory agent

INDICATIONS AND CLINICAL USE: TOCTINO* (alitretinoin) is indicated for the treatment of severe chronic hand eczema refractory to high potency topical corticosteroids in adults. TOCTINO* should only be prescribed by physicians knowledgeable in the use of retinoids systemically, who understand the risk of teratogenicity in females of childbearing potential (see CONTRAINDICATIONS and WARNINGS AND PRECAUTIONS: Serious Warnings and Precautions and Special Populations, Women of Childbearing Potential).

CONTRAINDICATIONS:

TOCTINO* (alitretinoin) is contraindicated in pregnancy.

- Females must not become pregnant while taking TOCTINO* and for at least one month after its discontinuation. TOCTINO* can cause severe birth defects in infants born to women who become pregnant during treatment with TOCTINO* in any amount, even for a short period of time. Potentially any exposed fetus can be affected. There are no accurate means of determining whether an exposed fetus has been affected (see WARNINGS AND PRECAUTIONS: Special populations, Women of childbearing potential). If pregnancy does occur during treatment with TOCTINO* or within one month after its discontinuation, TOCTINO* treatment must be immediately stopped and the physician and patient should discuss the desirability of continuing the pregnancy.
- TOCTINO* should only be prescribed by physicians knowledgeable in the use of retinoids systemically (see INDICATIONS AND CLINICAL USE).

TOCTINO* is contraindicated in breastfeeding women as well as in patients with: hepatic insufficiency; severe renal insufficiency; uncontrolled hypercholesterolemia; uncontrolled hypertriglyceridemia; uncontrolled hypothyroidism; hypervitaminosis A; hypersensitivity either to alitretinoin, to other retinoids or to any of the excipients, in particular in case of allergies to peanut or soya; with rare hereditary problems of fructose intolerance; receiving concomitant treatment with tetracyclines (see WARNINGS AND PRECAUTIONS).

SPECIAL POPULATIONS: Geriatrics (> 65 years of age): Clinical trial experience has not identified differences in responses between elderly and other patients. However clinical studies of TOCTINO* did not include sufficient numbers of subjects aged 65 years and over to determine with certainty whether they respond differently from younger subjects. Pediatrics: TOCTINO* is not recommended for use in patients under 18 years of age.

Safety Information

WARNINGS AND PRECAUTIONS

Serious Warnings and Precautions

Pregnancy Prevention: TOCTINO* (alitretinoin) is a known teratogen contraindicated in pregnancy (see boxed CONTRAINDICATIONS). Physicians should only prescribe TOCTINO* to females of childbearing potential if **ALL** the conditions described below under **"Conditions of use"** are met. In addition, when prescribing this drug to female patients of childbearing potential, physicians must use the TOCTINO* Pregnancy Prevention Program, which includes comprehensive information about the potential risks of this drug, a checklist for criteria which must be met prior to prescribing this drug to female patients of childbearing potential, detailed information on birth control options, a patient informed consent for review and signature, and monthly pregnancy reminders for physicians to use at each patient visit during the treatment period.

Neurologic: Treatment with systemic retinoids, including alitretinoin, has been associated with the occurrence of benign intracranial hypertension, some of which involved concomitant use of tetracyclines (see CONTRAINDICATIONS and WARNINGS AND PRECAUTIONS). Signs and symptoms of benign intracranial hypertension include headache, nausea and vomiting, visual disturbances and papilloedema. Patients who develop signs of benign intracranial hypertension should discontinue alitretinoin immediately (class effect).

Pregnancy Prevention and Conditions of Use: TOCTINO* is contraindicated in females of childbearing potential unless **ALL** of the following conditions apply:

1. The patient has severe chronic hand eczema that is refractory to high potency topical corticosteroids.
2. The patient is reliable in understanding and carrying out instructions.
3. The patient is able and willing to comply with the mandatory effective contraceptive measures.
4. The patient has received, and acknowledged understanding of, a careful oral and printed explanation of the hazards of fetal exposure to TOCTINO* and the risk of possible contraception failure.
5. The patient has been informed and understands the need to rapidly consult her physician if there is a risk of pregnancy.
6. The patient understands the need for rigorous follow-up on a monthly basis.
7. The patient uses effective contraception without any interruption for one month before beginning TOCTINO* therapy, during TOCTINO* therapy and for one month following discontinuation of TOCTINO* therapy. It is recommended that two reliable forms of contraception be used simultaneously.
8. The patient has had two negative pregnancy tests with a sensitivity of at least 25 mIU/mL before starting TOCTINO* therapy with the first pregnancy test conducted at initial assessment when the patient is qualified for TOCTINO* therapy by the physician. The patient has had a second serum or urine pregnancy test with a sensitivity of at least 25 mIU/mL with a negative result, performed in a licensed laboratory, within 11 days prior to initiating therapy. The patient has had two or three days of the next normal menstrual period before TOCTINO* therapy is initiated.
9. In the event of relapse treatment, the patient must also use the same uninterrupted and effective contraceptive measures one month prior to, during and for one month after TOCTINO*. (Re items 2 to 9, see WARNINGS AND PRECAUTIONS: Special Populations, Women of Childbearing Potential.) Even female patients who normally do not employ contraception due to a history of infertility, or claim absence of sexual activity must be advised to employ contraception while taking TOCTINO*, following the above guidelines. Even female patients who have amenorrhea must follow all the advice on effective contraception.

There is an extremely high risk that major human fetal abnormalities will occur if pregnancy occurs during treatment with TOCTINO* or up to one month following its discontinuation. Potentially any exposed fetus can be affected. Female patients of childbearing potential must not be given TOCTINO* until pregnancy is excluded. See SUPPLEMENTAL PRODUCT INFORMATION.

Pregnancy Tests: Female patients of childbearing potential must not be given TOCTINO* until pregnancy is excluded. It is mandatory that all female patients of childbearing potential treated with TOCTINO* have regular monthly pregnancy tests during treatment and one month after the discontinuation of treatment. The dates and results of pregnancy tests should be documented. See SUPPLEMENTAL PRODUCT INFORMATION.

Contraception: Effective contraception must be used for at least one month before starting TOCTINO* treatment, during treatment and for at least one month following the discontinuation of TOCTINO* treatment. See SUPPLEMENTAL PRODUCT INFORMATION.

Pregnancy: Pregnancy occurring during treatment with TOCTINO* and for one month after its discontinuation, carries the risk of fetal malformation and the increased risk of spontaneous abortion. (See CONTRAINDICATIONS as well as TOXICOLOGY: Reproduction and Teratology Studies in the Product Monograph.)

Breastfeeding Women: Alitretinoin is highly lipophilic, therefore the passage of alitretinoin into human milk is very likely. Due to the potential risk for the exposed child, the use of alitretinoin is contraindicated in breastfeeding mothers. (see CONTRAINDICATIONS).

Male Patients: Based on non-clinical findings, the male fertility may be compromised by treatment with TOCTINO*. Male patients should be reminded that they must not share their medication with anyone, particularly not females. See SUPPLEMENTAL PRODUCT INFORMATION.

General: TOCTINO* should not be prescribed if the patient's eczema (dermatitis) can be adequately controlled by standard measures, including skin protection, avoidance of allergens and irritants, and treatment with potent topical corticosteroids. Patients should be instructed never to give this medicinal product to another person and to return any unused capsules to their pharmacist at the end of treatment.

Blood Donations: Patients should not donate blood during therapy and for 1 month following discontinuation of TOCTINO* because of the potential risk to the foetus of a pregnant transfusion recipient.

Cardiovascular/Lipid Metabolism: Alitretinoin should be discontinued if hypertriglyceridemia cannot be controlled at an acceptable level or if symptoms of pancreatitis occur. Triglyceride levels in excess of 800 mg/dL (9 mmol/L) are sometimes associated with acute pancreatitis, which may be fatal. Patients at high risk for cardiac events should start on the lowest possible dose of altitretinoin and be carefully monitored due to increases in lipid levels. See SUPPLEMENTAL PRODUCT INFORMATION.

Gastrointestinal: Isotretinoin, which belongs to the same chemical class as alitretinoin, has been associated with inflammatory bowel disease (IBD), including regional ileitis, in patients without a history of intestinal disorders. If severe diarrhea is observed diagnosis of IBD should be considered. Patients experiencing abdominal pain, rectal bleeding or severe diarrhea should discontinue TOCTINO* immediately.

Psychiatric: Particular care needs to be taken in patients with a history of depression and patients on alitretinoin treatment should therefore be observed for signs of depression and referred for appropriate treatment if necessary. See SUPPLEMENTAL PRODUCT INFORMATION.

ADVERSE REACTIONS:

Adverse Drug Reaction Overview

The most frequent adverse drug reactions observed under alitretinoin therapy are headache (30 mg: 21%; 10 mg: 11%), and flushing (30 mg: 5.9%, 10 mg: 1.6%). The most common reason for discontinuation was headache (0.5% placebo, 1.4% 10 mg, 4.1% 30 mg), which typically occurred within the first 10 days of therapy, and was transient.

Adverse drug reactions with a frequency of ≥ 1% during clinical trials included: Skin and Subcutaneous Tissue Disorders – eczema, erythema, dry skin, dermatitis, pruritus, rash, alopecia; Nervous System Disorders – headache, dizziness; Infections and Infestations – nasopharyngitis, influenza, upper respiratory tract infection, pharyngitis, herpes simplex, rhinitis, folliculitis; Gastrointestinal Disorders – dry lip, dry mouth, nausea, cheilitis, diarrhoea, abdominal pain (upper), vomiting, dyspepsia; Musculoskeletal and Connective Tissue Disorders – back pain, arthralgia, myalgia, pain in extremity; General Disorders – fatigue; Eye Disorders – conjunctivitis, dry eye, abnormal eye sensation; Investigations – blood creatine phosphokinase increase, blood triglycerides increase, weight increase; Vascular Disorders – flushing, hypertension, hot flush; Psychiatric Disorders – depression, insomnia, sleep disorder; Respiratory, Thoracic and Mediastinal Disorders – pharyngolaryngeal pain; Metabolism and Nutrition Disorders – hypercholesterolaemia. For adverse events with a frequency of < 1%, see SUPPLEMENTAL PRODUCT INFORMATION.

To report an adverse event, you may notify Actelion Pharmaceuticals Canada Inc. at 1-866-531-4885 or Health Canada by phone: 1-866-234-2345 or fax 1-866-678-6789.

DRUG INTERACTIONS: See SUPPLEMENTAL PRODUCT INFORMATION.

Administration

Recommended Dose and Dosage Adjustment

The recommended dose range for TOCTINO* is 10 mg–30 mg once daily with a meal. The recommended start dose is 30 mg once daily. Dose reduction to 10 mg once daily may be considered in patients with unacceptable side effects. Patients at high risk for cardiac events should start on the lowest possible dose of alitretinoin and be carefully monitored due to increases in lipid levels (see WARNINGS AND PRECAUTIONS). In studies investigating 10 mg and 30 mg daily doses, both doses resulted in clearing of the disease. The 30 mg dose provided a more rapid response and a higher response rate. The 10 mg daily dose was associated with fewer adverse events (see ADVERSE REACTIONS and PART II, CLINICAL TRIALS of the Product Monograph). A treatment course of TOCTINO* may be given for 12 to 24 weeks depending on response. Discontinuation of therapy should be considered for patients who still have severe disease after the initial 12 weeks of treatment. In the event of relapse, patients may benefit from further treatment courses of TOCTINO*.

Children TOCTINO* is not recommended for use in patients under 18 years of age.

Missed Dose The missed dose should be taken as soon as it is remembered, and then the regular dosing schedule should be continued. Two doses of TOCTINO* should not be taken on the same day.

Administration The capsules should be taken once daily and must be taken with a meal.

SUPPLEMENTAL PRODUCT INFORMATION

WARNINGS AND PRECAUTIONS

SPECIAL POPULATIONS:

1. Women of childbearing potential – There is an extremely high risk that major human fetal abnormalities will occur if pregnancy occurs during treatment with TOCTINO* or up to one month following its discontinuation. Potentially any exposed fetus can be affected.

Pregnancy Tests: Female patients of childbearing potential must not be given TOCTINO* until pregnancy is excluded. The patient must have two negative pregnancy tests before starting TOCTINO* therapy with the first pregnancy test conducted at initial assessment when the patient is qualified for TOCTINO* therapy by the physician. A second pregnancy test must be performed within 11 days prior to starting TOCTINO* treatment. TOCTINO* treatment should start on the second or third day of the next normal menstrual period following this negative pregnancy test. It is mandatory that all female patients of childbearing potential treated with TOCTINO* have regular monthly pregnancy tests during treatment and one month after the discontinuation of treatment. The dates and results of pregnancy tests should be documented. These pregnancy tests will:

- Serve primarily to reinforce to the patient the necessity of avoiding pregnancy.
- In the event of accidental pregnancy, provide the physician and patient an immediate opportunity to discuss the serious risk to the fetus from this exposure to TOCTINO* and the desirability of continuing the pregnancy in view of the potential teratogenic effect of TOCTINO* (see CONTRAINDICATIONS and TOXICOLOGY: Reproduction and Teratology Studies of the Product Monograph).

Contraception: Effective contraception must be used for at least one month before starting TOCTINO* treatment, during treatment and for at least one month following the discontinuation of TOCTINO* treatment. It is recommended that two reliable forms of contraception be used simultaneously. At least 1 of these forms of contraception must be a primary form, unless the patient has undergone a hysterectomy. Effective forms of contraception include: tubal ligation, partner's vasectomy, intrauterine devices, birth control pills, and topical/injectable/insertable hormonal birth control products. Barrier forms of contraception include diaphragms, latex condoms, and cervical caps; each must be used with a spermicide. Any birth control method can fail. Therefore, it is critically important that women of childbearing potential use 2 effective forms of contraception simultaneously. Microdosed progesterone preparations (minipills) are not a suitable method of contraception during TOCTINO* therapy (see DRUG INTERACTIONS; Drug-Drug Interactions).

Patients should be prospectively cautioned not to self-medicate with the herbal supplement St. John's Wort because a possible interaction has been suggested with hormonal contraceptives based on reports of breakthrough bleeding on oral contraceptives shortly after starting St. John's Wort. Pregnancies have been reported by users of combined hormonal contraceptives who also used some form of St. John's Wort.

Pregnancy: Pregnancy occurring during treatment with TOCTINO* and for one month after its discontinuation, carries the risk of fetal malformation and the increased risk of spontaneous abortion (see CONTRAINDICATIONS and TOXICOLOGY: Reproduction and Teratology Studies of the Product Monograph). TOCTINO*, treatment must be stopped and the patient should be fully counselled regarding the serious risk to the fetus should they become pregnant while undergoing treatment. If pregnancy does occur during this time the physician and patient should discuss the desirability of continuing the pregnancy.

2. Male Patients – Small amounts of alitretinoin have been detected in the semen of healthy volunteers receiving 40 mg of alitretinoin and there is no indication of drug accumulation in semen. Assuming complete vaginal absorption of these amounts would have a negligible effect on the endogenous plasma levels of the female partner and therefore does not appear to pose a risk to the fetus if the partner is pregnant. Based on non-clinical findings, the male fertility may be compromised by treatment with TOCTINO*. Male patients should be reminded that they must not share their medication with anyone, particularly not females.

General: Carcinogenesis and Mutagenesis Alitretinoin was tested in 2-year carcinogenicity studies in rats and mice. Dose-related retinoid-specific toxicity was seen at higher doses, but no carcinogenic potential was noted.

Cardiovascular / Lipid Metabolism Alitretinoin has been associated with an increase in plasma cholesterol and triglyceride levels. Patients with increased tendency to develop hypertriglyceridemia include those with diabetes mellitus, obesity, increased alcohol intake and familial history. The cardiovascular consequences of hypertriglyceridemia are not well understood, but may increase the patient's risk status. Therefore, serum cholesterol and triglycerides (fasting values) should be monitored. Alitretinoin should be discontinued if hypertriglyceridemia cannot be controlled at an acceptable level or if symptoms of pancreatitis occur. Triglyceride levels in excess of 800 mg/dL (9 mmol/L) are sometimes associated with acute pancreatitis, which may be fatal. Patients at high risk for cardiac events should start on the lowest possible dose of altitretinoin and be carefully monitored due to increases in lipid levels.

Endocrine and Metabolism Changes in thyroid function tests have been observed in patients receiving alitretinoin, most often noted as a reversible reduction in thyroid stimulating hormone (TSH) levels and T4 [free thyroxine].

Hepatic/Biliary/Pancreatic Treatment with other systemic retinoids has been associated with transient and reversible increases in liver transaminases. In the event of persistent clinically relevant elevation of transaminase levels, reduction of the dose or discontinuation of treatment should be considered.

Musculo-skeletal and connective tissue disorders Treatment with other systemic retinoids has been associated with bone changes including premature epiphyseal closure, hyperostosis, and calcification of tendons and ligaments. Myalgia, arthralgia and increased serum creatinine phosphokinase values have been observed in patients treated with alitretinoin.

Neurologic Treatment with systemic retinoids, including alitretinoin, has been associated with the occurrence of benign intracranial hypertension, some of which involved concomitant use of tetracyclines (see CONTRAINDICATIONS and DRUG INTERACTIONS). Signs and symptoms of benign intracranial hypertension include headache, nausea and vomiting, visual disturbances and papilloedema. Patients who develop signs of benign intracranial hypertension should discontinue alitretinoin immediately.

Ophthamologic Treatment with alitretinoin has been associated with dry eyes. The symptoms usually resolve after discontinuation of therapy. Dry eyes can be helped by the application of a lubricating eye ointment or by the application of tear replacement therapy. Intolerance to contact lenses may occur which may necessitate the patient to wear glasses during treatment. Decreased night vision has been reported in patients treated with alitretinoin and other retinoids. These effects usually resolve after discontinuation of therapy. Patients should be advised of this potential problem and warned to be cautious when driving or operating machines.

Psychiatric Depression, aggravated depression, anxiety, aggressive tendencies, mood alterations, psychotic symptoms, and very rarely, suicidal ideation, suicide attempts and suicide have been reported in patients treated with systemic retinoids. Particular care needs to be taken in patients with a history of depression and patients on alitretinoin treatment should therefore be observed for signs of depression and referred for appropriate treatment if necessary. However, discontinuation of alitretinoin may be insufficient to alleviate symptoms and therefore further psychiatric or psychological evaluation may be necessary.

Skin The effects of UV light are enhanced by retinoid therapy, therefore patients should avoid excessive exposure to sunlight and the unsupervised use of sun lamps. Where necessary a sun-protection product with a high protection factor of at least SPF 15 should be used. Patients who experience dryness of the skin and lips should be advised to use a skin moisturizing ointment or cream and a lip balm.

Monitoring and Laboratory Tests Pregnancy tests: The patient should have two negative pregnancy tests (β-hCG in urine or serum) with a sensitivity of at least 25 mIU/mL before starting TOCTINO* therapy with the first pregnancy test conducted at initial assessment when the patient is qualified for TOCTINO* therapy by the physician. The patient then should have a second pregnancy test with a sensitivity of at least 25 mIU/mL with a negative result, performed in a licensed laboratory, within 11 days prior to initiating therapy. The patient must wait until the second or third day of their next normal menstrual period before starting TOCTINO*.

Pregnancy testing must be repeated monthly for pregnancy detection during TOCTINO* treatment and at one month after discontinuation of treatment. The dates and results of the pregnancy tests should be documented. The following tests are required before starting TOCTINO*, at first month, then as clinically indicated:

- Serum blood lipid determinations (under fasting conditions) should be performed before TOCTINO* is given and then at intervals (one month after the start of therapy) until the lipid response to TOCTINO* is established (which usually occurs within four weeks), and also at the end of treatment. (See WARNINGS AND PRECAUTIONS; General; Cardiovascular/Lipid Metabolism)
- Blood glucose level: patients with known or suspected diabetes should have periodic blood sugar determinations.

ADVERSE REACTIONS

Clinical Trial Adverse Drug Reactions – Headache was the most common AE and clearly showed a dose effect. Erythema and dry lips were also more frequent with alitretinoin 30 mg than with alitretinoin 10 mg. Additional AEs occurring with highest incidence in the 30 mg alitretinoin arm included dry skin, conjunctivitis, hypercholesterolemia, and flushing. Other commonly occurring AEs without strong apparent dose effect included nasopharyngitis, and eczema. All other treatment-emergent AEs were of similar frequency in the two alitretinoin groups and with the placebo group. Psychiatric effects, in particular depression, and mood changes and suicidal ideation, have been associated with retinoids. In alitretinoin clinical studies, patients have been monitored for depression using the CES-D (Center for Epidemiological Studies-Depression) score. Treatment with alitretinoin was not associated with changes in the CES-D score. The following adverse events were not observed in clinical trials with alitretinoin, but have been observed with other retinoids: Inflammatory bowel disease, diabetes mellitus, color blindness (color vision deficiencies), contact lens intolerance and decreased night vision. Changes in bone mineralization and extra-osseous calcifications have been associated with systemic retinoid treatment. In clinical studies with alitretinoin, degenerative changes of the spine and ligamentous calcifications were frequent findings in patients with chronic hand eczema before treatment (baseline), with minor progression in a small number of patients during treatment. These observations were consistent with age dependent degenerative changes.Assessments of bone density (DXA) did not indicate a dose dependent effect on bone mineralization. The most common laboratory changes consisted of increased levels of triglycerides (30 mg: 35.4%; 10 mg: 17.0%), increased cholesterol (30 mg: 27.8%; 10 mg 16.7%), decreased levels of thyroid stimulating hormone (TSH, 30 mg: 8.4%, 10 mg: 6.0%) and decreased levels of free T4 (30 mg: 10.5%; 10 mg: 2.9%).

Less Common Clinical Trial Adverse Drug Reactions (<1%) – Nervous system disorders: Benign intracranial hypertension; Eye disorders: Blurred vision, cataract; Vascular disorders: Vasculitis; Respiratory, thoracic and mediastinal disorders: Epistaxis; Skin and subcutaneous tissues disorders: Pruritus, rash, skin exfoliation, asteatotic eczema; Musculoskeletal and connective tissue disorders: exostosis, (hyperostosis), ankylosing spondylosis.The most frequent and relevant changes in individual laboratory values included elevated levels of fasting cholesterol and triglycerides with corresponding changes in high density lipoproteins (HDL) and low density lipoproteins (LDL), and lowered levels of thyroxin and TSH, predominantly in the 30 mg dose group. Other frequently reported changes were reductions in hemoglobin, hematocrit, and red blood cell (RBC) counts, which were more frequent in the 30 mg dose group. Elevated levels of creatinine phosphokinase were frequent in both alitretinoin groups.

DRUG INTERACTIONS

Overview Alitretinoin is metabolized by cytochrome P450 3A4 (CYP3A4). No drug interactions were observed when alitretinoin was co-administered with the oral contraceptive ethinyl estradiol and norgestimate. Co-administration with strong CYP3A4 or PgP inhibitors, such as ketoconazole, increases levels of alitretinoin, and dose reduction of alitretinoin may be considered in patients experiencing adverse events. Substrates of CYP3A4, such as cyclosporin or simvastatin, do not affect the pharmacokinetics of alitretinoin. Alitretinoin did not affect the pharmacokinetics of cyclosporin or ketoconazole. A slight reduction of simvastatin plasma levels was observed when co-administered with alitretinoin. Patients should not take vitamin A or other retinoids as concurrent medication due to the risk of developing hypervitaminosis A. Cases of benign intracranial hypertension (pseudotumor cerebri) have been reported with concomitant use of retinoids and tetracyclines. Therefore, concomitant treatment with tetracyclines must be avoided (see Serious Warnings and Precautions).

Drug-Drug Interactions

Table 3: Established or Potential Drug-Drug Interactions

	Ref	Effect	Clinical Comment
Simvastatin	CT	Decrease =16% in simvastatin levels	Dose adjustment of simvastatin during routine monitoring of CL and TG, if appropriate
Ketoconazole	CT	Increase ≈ 40% alitretinoin levels	Dose reduction of alitretinoin guided by the appearance of typical retinoids side effects such as headache and flushing

Legend: CT = Clinical Trial

Microdosed progesterone preparations (minipills) are not a suitable method of contraception during TOCTINO* therapy. An increased risk of liver toxicity may be seen if retinoids are taken concomitantly with methotrexate.

Drug-Food Interactions Clinical pharmacology studies with various formulations of alitretinoin demonstrated that when alitretinoin is taken with food, the systemic exposure is significantly enhanced. All subsequent clinical studies were done in a fed state. Therefore, alitretinoin must be taken with a meal.

SYMPTOMS AND TREATMENT OF OVERDOSE

For management of suspected overdose, contact your regional poison control centre.

Alitretinoin is a derivative of vitamin A. Alitretinoin has been administered in oncological clinical studies at dosages of more than the 10-fold of the therapeutic dosage given for chronic hand eczema. The toxicity observed was consistent with vitamin A toxicity, and included severe headache, diarrhea, facial flushing, hypertriglyceridaemia. These effects were reversible. Please contact the Poison Control Centre in case of overdose. The following precautions should be taken with all female patients of childbearing potential who have taken an overdose of TOCTINO*: 1. At the time of the overdose, a pregnancy test must be performed. 2. One complete menstrual cycle or one month after the overdose, a second pregnancy test must be performed. 3. Effective contraception must be used for at least one complete menstrual cycle after the overdose. Patients who present with a positive pregnancy test at the time of the overdose, or one complete menstrual cycle / one month after the overdose, should be fully counselled on the serious risk to the fetus from this exposure to TOCTINO* and the physician and the patient should discuss the desirability of continuing the pregnancy. (See CONTRAINDICATIONS, WARNINGS AND PRECAUTIONS, Special Populations, Women of Childbearing Potential, and TOXICOLOGY: Reproduction and Teratology Studies). Canadian Regional Poison Information Centres have been advised on the management of TOCTINO* overdoses and on the teratogenic potential of exposure to TOCTINO*.

STORAGE AND STABILITY TOCTINO* should be stored between 15 and 30 °C.

SPECIAL HANDLING INSTRUCTIONS Store in the original package. Keep the blister in the outer carton to protect from light.

DOSAGE FORMS, COMPOSITION AND PACKAGING 10 mg soft capsule: Each capsule contains 10 mg alitretinoin. The nonmedical ingredients are: Soybean oil, Partially hydrogenated soybean oil, Medium chain triglycerides, Yellow wax, DL-alpha-tocopherol. The capsule shell contains: Gelatin, Glycerol, Sorbitol, Water, Iron oxide.

30 mg soft capsule: Each capsule contains 30 mg alitretinoin. The nonmedical ingredients are: Soybean oil, Partially hydrogenated soybean oil, Medium chain triglycerides, Yellow wax, DL-alpha-tocopherol. The capsule shell contains: Gelatin, Glycerol, Sorbitol, Water, Iron oxide.

AVAILABILITY Capsules are available in blister packs of 10 capsules. Each box contains 3 blister packs.

REFERENCES: 1. TOCTINO* Product Monograph. Actelion Pharmaceuticals Canada Inc., October 2010. **2.** Ruzicka T, Lynde C, Jemec G *et al.* Efficacy and safety of oral alitretinoin in patients with severe chronic hand eczema refractory to topical corticosteroids: results of a randomised, double-blind, placebo-controlled, multicentre trial. *Br J Dermatol* April 2008;158(4):808-817.

Full Product Monograph available at Actelion Pharmaceuticals Canada Inc.
2550 Daniel-Johnson Blvd., Suite 701, Laval, Quebec H7T 2L1
Tel: 1-866-531-4885. www.toctino.ca
October 2010

TRA-10-31E_w/ref

ACTELION   Member R&D PAAB   Toctino* (alitretinoin)

BuTrans®

Buprenorphine transdermal delivery system

5 mcg/hr | 10 mcg/hr | 20 mcg/hr

Study References

1. BuTrans® Product Monograph, Purdue Pharma, February 2010.
2. Purdue Pharma, March 24, 2010.

Supplemental Product Information

Information for Physicians to Convey to Patients

A patient information sheet is included in the package of BuTrans® patches dispensed to the patient.

Patients receiving BuTrans® patches should be given the following instructions by the physician:

1. Patients should be informed that accidental ingestion or use by individuals (including children) other than the patient for whom it was originally prescribed, may lead to severe, even fatal, consequences.
2. Patients should be advised that BuTrans® patches contain buprenorphine, an opioid pain medicine.
3. Patients should be advised that each BuTrans® patch may be worn continuously for 7 days, and that each patch should be applied to a different skin site after removal of the previous transdermal patch.
4. Patients should be advised that the application sites should be rotated whenever a patch is replaced. After the patch is removed, a 3-week interval is required before the same site can be re-used as a strategy to prevent skin irritation and/or reduce the potential for increased drug absorption.
5. Patients should be advised that BuTrans® patches should be applied to intact, non-irritated and non-irradiated skin on a flat surface such as the upper chest, upper back, side of chest, or upper outer arm. Additionally, patients should be advised of the following:
   - If BuTrans® is part of an overall strategy to suitably manage pain in patients with cognitive impairment, the potential of each patient to remove the patch(es) and place them in the mouth or on others should be considered when recommending rotation sites;
   - Hair at the application site should be clipped (not shaved) prior to patch application;
   - If the site of BuTrans® application must be cleansed prior to application of the patch, do so with clear water;
   - Allow the skin to dry completely prior to patch application;
   - Do not use soaps, oils, lotions, alcohol, or any other agents that may irritate the skin or alter its characteristics.
6. Patients should be advised that BuTrans® should be applied immediately upon removal from the sealed package and after removal of the protective liner.

   Additionally, patients should be advised of the following:
   - The BuTrans® patch should not be used if the seal is broken, or if it is altered, cut, or damaged in any way prior to application. The transdermal patch should be pressed firmly in place with the palm of the hand for 30 seconds, making sure the contact is complete, especially around the edges;
   - The patch should **not** be folded.
7. Patients should be advised that while wearing the patch, they should avoid exposing the BuTrans® application site to direct external heat sources, such as:
   - heating pads;
   - electric blankets;
   - heat lamps;
   - saunas;
   - hot tubs;
   - heated water beds.
8. Patients should be advised that there is a potential for temperature-dependent increase in buprenorphine release from the patch that could result in an overdose of buprenorphine. If patients develop a high fever while wearing the patch they should contact their physician.
9. Patients should be advised that if they experience problems with adhesion of the BuTrans® patch, they may tape the edges of the patch with first aid tape.
10. Patients should be advised that if the patch falls off before 7 days a new patch may be applied to a different skin site.
11. When BuTrans® is no longer needed (used or unused), patients should be advised to fold the patch (so that the adhesive side adheres to itself) and immediately flush it down the toilet, or consult with a pharmacist about other disposal options.
12. Patients should be instructed that, if the drug adhesive layer accidentally contacts the skin other than the intended application site, the area should be washed clean with clear water and not soap, alcohol, or other chemicals, because these products may increase the ability of buprenorphine to go through the skin.
13. Patients should be advised that the dose of BuTrans® should NEVER be adjusted without the prescribing health care professional's instruction.
14. Patients should be advised that BuTrans® may impair mental and/or physical ability required for the performance of potentially hazardous tasks (e.g., driving, operating machinery).
15. Patients should be advised to refrain from any potentially dangerous activity when initially starting on BuTrans® or when their dose is being adjusted, until it is established that they have not been adversely affected.
16. Patients should be advised that BuTrans® should not be combined with alcohol or other centrally acting agents, such as: sleep medications, tranquilizers, sedatives and hypnotics because dangerous additive effects may occur, resulting in serious injury or death.
17. Patients should be advised to consult their physician or pharmacist if other medications are being, or will be, used with BuTrans®.
18. Patients should be advised of the potential for severe constipation.
19. Patients should be advised that if they have been receiving treatment with BuTrans® and cessation of therapy is indicated, it may be appropriate to taper the BuTrans® dose, rather than abruptly discontinue it, due to the risk of precipitating withdrawal symptoms. Withdrawal symptoms are generally milder than seen with full agonists, and begin after two days and may last up to two weeks.
20. Patients should be advised that BuTrans® contains buprenorphine, a drug with a potential for abuse.
21. Patients, family members and caregivers should be advised to protect BuTrans® from theft or misuse in the work or home environment.
22. Patients should be advised that BuTrans® should never be given to anyone other than the individual for whom it was prescribed because of the risk of death or other serious medical problems to that person, for whom it was not intended.
23. Patients should be instructed to keep BuTrans® in a secure place out of sight and reach of children due to the risk of **fatal respiratory depression.**
24. Women of childbearing potential who become or are planning to become pregnant should be advised to consult a physician prior to initiating or continuing therapy with BuTrans®.
25. Patients should be informed that, if the patch dislodges and accidentally sticks to the skin of another person, they should immediately take the patch off, wash the exposed area with water (and not soap, alcohol, or other chemicals, because these products may increase the ability of buprenorphine to go through the skin) and seek immediate medical attention for the accidentally exposed individual.

CELECOXIB

CELEBREX®

STUDY REFERENCES

1. IMS data, October 2009-September 2010. NSAID Market, monthly data, prescriptions.
2. Zhao SZ *et al.* Evaluation of the functional status aspects of health-related quality of life of patients with osteoarthritis treated with celecoxib. *Pharmacother* 1999;19:1269-78. Prospective, multicentre, randomized, double-blind, parallel-group, 12-week trial. Baseline measurements for CELEBREX®, naproxen and placebo, respectively were: total composite: 50.5, 52.9, 51.6; pain: 10.5, 11.0, 10.8; stiffness: 4.7, 5.0, 4.9; physical function: 35.4, 36.6, 36.0.
3. CELEBREX Product Monograph. Pfizer Canada Inc., April 2010. 12-week, double-blind, parallel-group study in 523 patients with OA or rheumatoid arthritis (RA) in whom baseline endoscopies revealed no ulcers. Patients were randomized to CELEBREX 200 mg BID or naproxen 500 mg BID.
4. Gimbel JS *et al.* Efficacy and tolerability of celecoxib versus hydrocodone/acetaminophen in the treatment of pain after ambulatory orthopaedic surgery in adults. *Clin Ther* 2001;23:228-41. Pooled data from two multicentre, randomized, placebo-controlled, double-blind, parallel-group trials of patients who had undergone uncomplicated orthopaedic surgery requiring open manipulation of bone periosteal elevation. In the initial 8-hour, single-dose study period, dosing was initiated within 24 hours after the end of anaesthesia. Pain assessments were conducted over the following 8-hour period. Pain intensity was reported by patients on a visual analog scale ranging from 0 to 3 (3 = worst pain). Pain intensity difference (PID) was derived by subtracting pain intensity scores at a specified timepoint from the baseline score.

CELECOXIB

CELEBREX®

FOSAVANCE®

alendronate sodium/cholecalciferol (Vitamin D_3)

References

1. British Columbia Ministry of Health Services. Expanded PharmaCare Coverage for Alendronate. January 18, 2010. Available at: http://www.health.gov.bc.ca/pharmacare/pdf/alend-prescriber.pdf, accessed June 21, 2010. **2.** Alberta Health and Wellness Drug Benefit List. Available at: https://www.ab.bluecross.ca/dbl/pdfs/ahwdbl_full_list.pdf. **3.** Saskatchewan Drug Formulary website. Available at: http://formulary.drugplan.health.gov.sk.ca/. **4.** Ontario Drug Benefit Formulary/Comparative Drug Index No. 41. UPDATE J. Effective June 23, 2009. Available at: http://www.health.gov.on.ca/english/providers/program/drugs/formulary/41_update_j_20090612.pdf, accessed on June 23, 2010. **5.** Liste des médicaments du Québec. Available at: https://www.prod.ramq.gouv.qc.ca/DPI/PO/Commun/PDF/Liste_Med/Liste_Med/liste_med_cor1_2010_06-01_en.pdf. **6.** New Brunswick Prescription Drug Program Formulary, March 10, 2010. Available at: http://www.gnb.ca/0212/pdf/NBPDP_Formulary/NBPDPFormularyMarch2010english.pdf. **7.** Nova Scotia Formulary. Available at: http://www.gov.ns.ca/health/Pharmacare/info_pro/pharmacists_bulletins/pharma_bulletins/Pharmacists%20Bulletin%2009-10.pdf. **8.** Newfoundland and Labrador Prescription Drug Program Coverage Status Table. March, 2010. **9.** Data on file, Merck Frosst Canada Ltd.: Product Monograph — FOSAVANCE®, 2009.

Humalog®

insulin lispro injection (rDNA origin)

Humalog® mix 25®

25% insulin lispro injection (rDNA origin)
75% insulin lispro protamine suspension

Humalog® mix 50®

50% insulin lispro injection (rDNA origin)
50% insulin lispro protamine suspension

Suspension for Injection, Lilly Standard

STUDY REFERENCES

1. Humalog®/Humalog® Mix25®/Humalog Mix50® Product Monograph, Eli Lilly Canada Inc. June 11, 2009.

LYRICA®

PREGABALIN

STUDY REFERENCES

References:

1. LYRICA Product Monograph, Pfizer Canada Inc., June 21, 2010.
2. Moulin DE *et al.* Pharmacological management of chronic neuropathic pain – consensus statement and guidelines from the Canadian Pain Society. *Pain Res Manage 2007*;12:13-21.
3. Arnold LM *et al.* A 14-week, randomized, double-blinded, placebo-controlled monotherapy trial of pregabalin in patients with fibromyalgia. *J Pain* 2008;9:792-805.

   14-week, randomized, double-blind, multiple-dose, placebo-controlled, multicentre study. 745 patients who had moderate-to-severe pain, i.e. mean baseline score (mean of the last 7 daily diary pain scores prior to study medication) of ≥4, and a diagnosis of fibromyalgia based on the ACR criteria. This study used an enriched population as placebo responders (≥30% reduction in mean pain scores) during the one-week run-in phase were discontinued and did not enter the double-blind phase. 1.6% of patients screened (n=19/1,195) were reported to be placebo responders. Patients were randomized to LYRICA 300 mg/day (n=183), 450 mg/day (n=190), 600 mg/day (n=188), or placebo (n=184). Patients were allowed to take acetaminophen up to 4 g/day as needed for pain relief. The number of completers was: LYRICA 300 mg/day (n=123), 450 mg/day (n=125), 600 mg/day (n=113), or placebo (n=125). The primary endpoint was the reduction in endpoint mean pain scores. Pain scores rated on 11-point numerical scale from 0 (no pain) to 10 (worst possible pain) during the past 24 hours. Mean baseline pain scores were 6.7 for LYRICA 300 mg/day, 6.7 for 450 mg/day, 6.8 for 600 mg/day, and 6.6 for placebo.
4. Crofford LJ *et al.* Fibromyalgia relapse evaluation and efficacy for durability of meaningful relief (FREEDOM): a 6-month, double-blind, placebo-controlled trial with pregabalin. *Pain* 2008;136:419-31.

   26-week, long-term relapse observation study. Patients who met the ACR criteria for fibromyalgia and who had a score of ≥40 on the pain Visual Analog Scale (VAS) were eligible to enter a 6-week, open-label, dose-optimization phase. During this phase, patients were titrated up to a total daily dose of 300 mg, 450 mg, or 600 mg. 566 LYRICA responders were randomized in the double-blind phase to either their optimized LYRICA dose (n=279) or to placebo (n=287). 38% of LYRICA responders completed 26 weeks of treatment vs 19% on placebo. The primary endpoint was time to loss of therapeutic response. Loss of therapeutic response was defined as having either a <30% reduction in pain VAS score, or worsening of symptoms necessitating alternate treatment. Responders were defined as having a ≥50% reduction in pain on the VAS and self-rating on the Patient Global Impression of Change scale of "much improved" or "very much improved".
5. Freynhagen R *et al.* Efficacy of pregabalin in neuropathic pain evaluated in a 12-week, randomised, double-blind, multicentre, placebo-controlled trial of flexible- and fixed-dose regimens. *Pain* 2005;115:254-63.

   In a 12-week, multicentre, randomized, double-blind, placebo-controlled study, 338 patients with either DPN (n=249) or PHN (n=89) were randomized to receive BID flexible-dose pregabalin (150-600 mg/day), fixed-dose pregabalin (600 mg/day) or placebo. In the flexible-dose arm, dose could be adjusted up or down over the first four weeks based on patients' individual response and tolerability. The primary efficacy measurement was mean pain score at endpoint, derived from ratings recorded by patients in a daily diary on an 11-point numerical pain rating scale (0=no pain, 10=worst possible pain). A significant difference in pain scores versus placebo was seen in the flexible dose range 150-600 mg/day ($p \leq 0.05$, weeks 2-3 and $p \leq 0.01$, weeks 4-12), and the fixed dose of 600 mg/day ($p \leq 0.05$, week 1 and $p \leq 0.01$, weeks 2-12).
6. Mease PJ *et al.* A randomized, double-blind, placebo-controlled, phase III trial of pregabalin in the treatment of patients with fibromyalgia. *J Rheumatol* 2008;35:502-14.

   Multicentre, double-blind, 13-week, randomized trial. 748 patients who met the ACR criteria for fibromyalgia and who had an average mean pain score of ≥4 on an 11-point numeric rating scale (NRS) during the baseline assessment were randomized to LYRICA 300 mg/day (n=185), 450 mg/day (n=183), 600 mg/day (n=190), or placebo (n=190). Patients were allowed to take acetaminophen up to 4 g/day as needed for pain relief. The number of completers was: LYRICA 300 mg/day (n=123), 450 mg/day (n=121), 600 mg/day (n=111), or placebo (n=130). The primary endpoint was the reduction in endpoint mean pain scores (mean of the last 7 daily pain scores while on study medication). Pain-related sleep difficulties were assessed using the Medical Outcomes Study-Sleep Scale (MOS-SS), a scale that runs from 0-100. Mean baseline MOS-SS score for overall sleep problem index was 65.0.

Pr MULTAQ™

dronedarone 400 mg

Study References

References: 1. MULTAQ™ Product Monograph, sanofi-aventis Canada Inc., July 31, 2009. **2.** Hohnloser S.H., et al. Effect of Dronedarone on Cardiovascular Events in Atrial Fibrillation. N Engl J Med 2009;360:668-678.

* In the double-blind, placebo-controlled ATHENA study, patients with paroxysmal or persistent AF or AFL were randomized to receive 400 mg dronedarone (*n*=2,301) or placebo (*n*=2,327) BID on top of usual therapy for up to 30 months maximum. Patients were to have at least one risk factor (including age, hypertension, diabetes, prior cerebrovascular accident, left atrium diameter ≥50 mm, or LVEF <0.40) together with AF/AFL and sinus rhythm both documented within the last 6 months. Patients could be in AF/AFL or in sinus rhythm after spontaneous conversion or following any procedures. As well, each patient needed 12-lead ECGs demonstrating AF/AFL and sinus rhythm within previous 6 months. Minimum treatment and follow-up was 12 months. Usual therapy may have included rate-control agents (e.g., beta-blockers, calcium antagonists, digoxin), antithrombotic agents (e.g., vitamin K antagonists, aspirin, other antiplatelet therapy), and/or other cardiovascular agents such as ACEIs/ARBs and statins.

† The safety profile of dronedarone 400 mg twice daily in patients with AF or AFL is based on 5 placebo-controlled studies: ATHENA, EURIDIS, ADONIS, ERATO, and DAFNE. In these studies, a total of 6,285 patients were randomized and treated. Of these, 3,282 patients were treated with dronedarone 400 mg twice daily and 2,875 received placebo. The mean exposure across studies was 12 months. In ATHENA, the maximum follow-up was 30 months.

Pr MULTAQ™

dronedarone 400 mg

Member R&D PAAB

sanofi aventis

Because health matters

Pr Protopic®

(tacrolimus 0.03%, 0.1% ointment)

Study References

1. PROTOPIC® Product Monograph, Astellas Pharma Canada, Inc. September 24, 2010.

A phase 3, 12-month, multicentre, randomized, vehicle-controlled study evaluating the efficacy of twice-weekly maintenance application of PROTOPIC 0.1% ointment in adult patients (≥ 16 years) with moderate to severe eczema. Patients with active disease entered an open-label period (OLP) during which they treated affected lesions with PROTOPIC ointment twice daily until improvement had reached a predefined score (Investigator's Global Assessment [IGA] ≤ 2, i.e. clear, almost clear or mild disease) for a maximum of 6 weeks. If patients did not respond to treatment, they were discontinued from the study. Thereafter, patients entered a double-blind disease control period (DCP) for up to 12 months. Patients were randomized to receive PROTOPIC 0.1% ointment or vehicle, once a day twice weekly on Mondays and Thursdays. If a disease exacerbation occurred, patients were treated with open-label PROTOPIC ointment twice daily for a maximum of 6 weeks until the IGA score returned to ≤ 2. Patients who did not achieve an IGA score of ≤ 2 were withdrawn from the study. Disease exacerbations (DE) were defined as an exacerbation requiring a "substantial therapeutic intervention," defined as a DE with an IGA of 3-5 (i.e. moderate, severe and very severe disease) on the first day of the flare, and requiring more than 7 days treatment.

Member R&D PAAB

astellas

Markham, Ontario L3R 9R9

SUTENT capsules
sunitinib malate

12.5 mg, 25 mg, 37.5§ mg, 50 mg sunitinib
Tyrosine Kinase Inhibitor
Anti-Tumour Agent
§ Not commercially available in Canada

Study References

1. Jewett M, Knox J, Kollmansberger C *et al.* The 2008 Kidney Cancer Forum, January 31–February 2, 2008. Consensus guideline: management of kidney cancer. Canadian Kidney Cancer Forum consensus statement. *Can Urol Assoc J* 2008;2(3):175–182. 2. Motzer RJ, Michaelson MD, Rosenberg J *et al.* Sunitinib efficacy against advanced renal cell carcinoma. *J Urol* 2007;178:1883–1887. 3. SUTENT® Product Monograph. Pfizer Canada Inc., April 2010. 4. Motzer RJ, Hutson TE, Tomczak P. Overall survival and updated results for sunitinib compared with interferon alfa in patients with metastatic renal cell carcinoma. *J Clin Oncol* 2009;27(22):3584–3590.

SUTENT® C.P. Pharmaceuticals International C.V., Owner/
Pfizer Canada Inc., Licensee

PAAB Member R&D

TARGIN®

Controlled release oxycodone/naloxone HCl tablets
10/5 mg, 20/10 mg, 40/20 mg

Study References

1. Pereira J, Bruera E *et al.* Alberta Hospice Palliative Care Resource Manual. A project of the Alberta Cancer Board with financial support provided by Alberta Cancer Foundation. Division of Palliative Care Medicine, University of Alberta, 2001:1-87.
2. Targin® Product Monograph, Purdue Pharma, March 2010.
3. Lowenstein O *et al.* Combined prolonged-release oxycodone and naloxone improves bowel function in patients receiving opioids for moderate-to-severe non-malignant chronic pain: a randomized controlled trial. *Expert Opin Pharmacother* 2009;10(4):531-543.

Purdue Pharma Inc
General Partner of / commandité de
Purdue Pharma
Pickering, Ontario L1W 3W8

Member R&D

03/10

PURDUE

Toctino* (alitretinoin)

REFERENCES: 1. TOCTINO* Product Monograph. Actelion Pharmaceuticals Canada Inc., October 2010. **2.** Ruzicka T, Lynde C, Jemec G *et al.* Efficacy and safety of oral alitretinoin in patients with severe chronic hand eczema refractory to topical corticosteroids: results of a randomised, double-blind, placebo-controlled, multicentre trial. *Br J Dermatol* April 2008;158(4):808-817.

Full Product Monograph available at Actelion Pharmaceuticals Canada Inc.
2550 Daniel-Johnson Blvd., Suite 701, Laval, Quebec H7T 2L1
Tel: 1-866-531-4885. www.toctino.ca
October 2010

* Trademark of Basilea Pharmaceutica AG, Basel, Switzerland; used under licence. TRA-10-31E_w/ref

ACTELION Member R&D PAAB Toctino* (alitretinoin)

ZOSTAVAX®
[zoster vaccine live, attenuated (Oka/Merck)]

10,06-a_136641
11-11-ZST-10-CDN-84130554c-SM

PRODUCT MONOGRAPH AVAILABLE AT
www.merck.ca
OR UPON REQUEST AT 1-800-567-2594

MERCK
Merck Frosst Canada Ltd., Kirkland, Quebec

Member R&D PAAB

Appendices and Glossaries

Appendices

Glossaries

Appendix 1: Narcotic and Controlled Drugs, Benzodiazepines and Other Targeted Substances

Table 1 summarizes the requirements for prescribing, dispensing and record-keeping for narcotics, controlled drugs, benzodiazepines and other targeted substances. This document is not intended to be a comprehensive review of the topic. The reader is therefore encouraged to seek additional and confirmatory information (e.g., Controlled Drugs and Substances Act, Narcotic Control Regulations, Food and Drug Regulations parts G and J, Benzodiazepines and Other Targeted Substances Regulations).
Reviewed 2010 by the Office of Controlled Substances, Health Canada.

Table 1: Narcotic and Controlled Drugs, Benzodiazepines and Other Targeted Substances: Summary of Requirements

Classification and Description	Legal Requirements
Narcotic Drugs[a] • 1 narcotic (e.g., cocaine, codeine, hydromorphone, ketamine, morphine) • 1 narcotic + 1 active non-narcotic ingredient (e.g., Novahistex DH, Tylenol No. 4) • All narcotics for parenteral use (e.g., fentanyl, pethidine) • All products containing hydrocodone, oxycodone, methadone or pentazocine • Dextropropoxyphene (e.g., Darvon-N, 642) • Nabilone (i.e., Cesamet)	• Written prescription required. • Verbal prescriptions not permitted. • Refills not permitted. • Written prescriptions may be prescribed to be dispensed in divided portions (part-fills) as indicated by the practitioner. • For part-fills, copies of prescriptions should be made in reference to the original prescription. Indicate on the original prescription: the new prescription number, the date of the part-fill, the quantity dispensed and the pharmacist's initials. • Transfers not permitted. • Record and retain all documents pertaining to all transactions for a period of at least 2 years, in a manner that permits an audit. • Sales reports required except for dextropropoxyphene, propoxyphene. • Report any loss or theft of narcotic drugs within 10 days after the discovery date to the Office of Controlled Substances at the address indicated on the forms.
Narcotic Preparations[a] • Verbal prescription narcotics: 1 narcotic + 2 or more active non-narcotic ingredients in a recognized therapeutic dose (e.g., Fiorinal-C¼, Fiorinal-C½, Robitussin AC, 282, 292, Tylenol No. 2, Tylenol No. 3) • Exempted codeine compounds: contain codeine up to 8 mg/solid dosage form or 20 mg/30 mL liquid + 2 or more active non-narcotic ingredients (e.g., Atasol-8)	• Written or verbal prescriptions permitted. • Refills not permitted. • Written or verbal prescriptions may be prescribed to be dispensed in divided portions (part-fills). • For part-fills, copies of prescriptions should be made in reference to the original prescription. Indicate on the original prescription: the new prescription number, the date of the part-fill, the quantity dispensed and the pharmacist's initials. • Transfers not permitted. • Exempted codeine compounds when dispensed pursuant to a prescription follow the same regulations as for verbal prescription narcotics. • Record and retain all documents pertaining to all transactions for a period of at least 2 years, in a manner that permits an audit. • Sales reports not required. • Report any loss or theft of narcotic drugs within 10 days after the discovery date to the Office of Controlled Substances at the address indicated on the forms.
Controlled Drugs[a] • Part I Amphetamines (e.g., Dexedrine, Adderall XR) Methylphenidate (e.g., Biphentin, Concerta, Ritalin) Pentobarbital Preparations: 1 controlled drug + 1 or more active noncontrolled ingredient(s) in a recognized therapeutic dose (e.g., Bellergal Spacetabs)	• Written or verbal prescriptions permitted. • Refills not permitted for verbal prescriptions. • Refills permitted for written prescriptions if the prescriber has indicated in writing the number of refills and dates for, or intervals between, refills. • Written or verbal prescriptions may be prescribed to be dispensed in divided portions (part-fills). • For refills and part-fills, copies of prescriptions should be made in reference to the original prescription. Indicate on the original prescription: the new prescription number, the date of the repeat or part-fill, the quantity dispensed and the pharmacist's initials. • Transfers not permitted. • Record and retain all documents pertaining to all transactions for a period of at least 2 years, in a manner that permits an audit. • Sales reports required except for controlled drug preparations. • Report any loss or theft of controlled drugs within 10 days after the discovery date to the Office of Controlled Substances at the address indicated on the forms.
• Part II Barbiturates (e.g., phenobarbital) Butorphanol Nalbuphine (e.g., Nubain Injection) Preparations: 1 controlled drug + 1 or more active noncontrolled ingredient(s) in a recognized therapeutic dose (e.g., Fiorinal) *(cont'd)*	• Written or verbal prescriptions permitted. • Refills permitted for written or verbal prescriptions if the prescriber has authorized in writing or verbally (at the time of issuance) the number of refills and dates for, or intervals between, refills. • Written or verbal prescriptions may be prescribed to be dispensed in divided portions (part-fills). • For refills and part-fills, copies of prescriptions should be made in reference to the original prescription. Indicate on the original prescription: the new prescription number, the date of the repeat or part-fill, the quantity dispensed and the pharmacist's initials. • Transfers not permitted. • Record and retain all documents pertaining to all transactions for a period of at least 2 years, in a manner that permits an audit. • Sales reports not required. • Report any loss or theft of controlled drugs within 10 days after the discovery date to the Office of Controlled Substances at the address indicated on the forms.

Appendix 1 *(cont'd)*

Table 1: Narcotic and Controlled Drugs, Benzodiazepines and Other Targeted Substances: Summary of Requirements *(cont'd)*

Classification and Description	Legal Requirements
Controlled Drugs[a] *(cont'd)* • Part III Anabolic steroids including: Testosterone (e.g., Androderm) Testosterone cypionate (e.g., Depo-Testosterone) Testosterone undecanoate (e.g., Andriol)	• Written or verbal prescriptions permitted. • Refills permitted for written or verbal prescriptions if the prescriber has authorized in writing or verbally (at the time of issuance) the number of refills and dates for, or intervals between, refills. • Written or verbal prescriptions may be prescribed to be dispensed in divided portions (part-fills). • For refills and part-fills, copies of prescriptions should be made in reference to the original prescription. Indicate on the original prescription: the new prescription number, the date of the repeat or part-fill, the quantity dispensed and the pharmacist's initials. • Transfers not permitted. • Record and retain all documents pertaining to all transactions for a period of at least 2 years, in a manner that permits an audit. • Sales reports not required. • Report the loss or theft of controlled drugs within 10 days after the discovery date to the Office of Controlled Substances at the address indicated on the forms.
Benzodiazepines and Other Targeted Substances[a] Alprazolam Bromazepam Chlordiazepoxide Clobazam Diazepam Ethchlorvynol Lorazepam Oxazepam Temazepam Triazolam Meprobamate	• Written and verbal prescriptions permitted. • Refills for written or verbal prescriptions permitted if indicated by prescriber and less than 1 year has elapsed since the day the prescription was issued by the practitioner. • Part-fills permitted as per prescriber's instructions. • For refills or part-fills of prescriptions, record the following information: date of the repeat or part-fill, prescription number, quantity dispensed and the pharmacist's initials. • Transfer of prescriptions permitted except for a prescription that has been already transferred. • Record and retain all documents pertaining to all transactions for a period of at least 2 years, in a manner that permits an audit. • Sales reports not required. • Report any loss or theft of benzodiazepines and other targeted substances within 10 days after the discovery date to the Office of Controlled Substances at the address indicated on the forms.

[a] The products noted are examples only.

Appendix 2: Special Access Programme

The following is an overview of Health Canada's Special Access Programme (SAP). This document is not intended to be a comprehensive review of the Programme.

Reviewed 2010 by the Special Access Programme, Health Canada (Alka Kurichh).

Mandate

The SAP considers requests from practitioners for access to non-marketed drugs for treatment, diagnosis or prevention of serious or life-threatening conditions when conventional therapies have been considered and ruled out, have failed, are unsuitable, and/or unavailable. The regulatory authority supporting the Programme is discretionary and a decision to authorize or deny a request is made on a case-by-case basis by taking into consideration the nature of the medical emergency, the availability of marketed alternatives and the information provided in support of the request regarding the use, safety and efficacy of the drug. This authority, however, does not extend to covering the cost of drugs and does not take into consideration the cost of marketed alternatives. If access is granted, the practitioner agrees to report on the use of the drug including any adverse events encountered with such use, and must account for all quantities received.

Important Considerations for Prescribing Practitioners

Authorization from SAP does not constitute an opinion or statement that a drug is safe, effective or of high pharmaceutical quality. The SAP does not conduct a comprehensive evaluation to ensure the validity of drug information or attestations of the manufacturer respecting safety, efficacy and quality. These are important factors for practitioners to consider when recommending the use of a drug and in making an appropriate risk/benefit decision in the best interests of the patient. The SAP strongly encourages practitioners treating individuals with drugs obtained through the Programme to seek informed consent before treatment.

Practitioners are encouraged to contact individual manufacturers to confirm the availability of a drug as well as to obtain the most up-to-date product information such as prescribing information and other data supporting the use of the drug. In all cases, the manufacturer has the final word on whether the drug will be supplied. The manufacturer also has the right to impose certain restrictions or conditions on the release of the drug to ensure that it is used in accordance with the latest information available. For instance, they may restrict the amount of product released, request further patient information, etc. All inquiries concerning the shipping, cost and/or payment of the drug should be directed to individual manufacturers.

Practitioners are required to provide both clinical justification for the use of the drug and the sources of scientific information supporting that justification. This requirement stems from Section C.08.010 of the *Food and Drug Regulations*, which requires the practitioner to provide data in their possession with respect to the use, safety and efficacy of the drug. This ensures that requests for access are evidence-based and appropriately supported.

In seeking and receiving access to a drug through the SAP, the practitioner agrees to provide both the SAP and the manufacturer with a report on the use of the drug, including information on adverse reactions and, on request, account for all quantities of drug received.

Requesting a Drug Product through the Special Access Programme

SAP Request Forms and associated instructions are available on the Health Canada website (see contact information below). There are two request forms and one reporting form: Form A is for a patient specific request, Form B is for a future use request and Form C is for reporting/patient follow-up. Each of the *SAP Request Forms* consists of two pages containing five sections. Practitioners are required to complete all five sections of the form for both new and repeat requests. The submission of an incomplete and or illegible copy will delay the review or lead to rejection of the application.

Submitting a Special Access Request Form

Fax completed forms to the SAP without an accompanying cover sheet. Reserve telephone calls for urgent requests requiring immediate attention. A completed form does not guarantee that a request will be authorized and additional information may be required during the review process. Every effort is made to process requests within 24 hours of receipt. However, given the mandate of the Programme and the volume of requests received, the SAP adopts a triage system to ensure that requests for drugs for life-threatening conditions take precedence over other less urgent matters. If a drug is new to the Programme, the total processing time may be extended, although every effort is made to contact the practitioner within 24 hours to discuss the process for handling new drugs.

After review, if an authorization is granted, the manufacturer is notified by telephone or fax. A Letter of Authorization is sent to the manufacturer and copied to the practitioner. Practitioners will be notified in the event that authorization is denied or if further information is required.

For further information on the Programme, refer to the SAP Guidance document and the Frequently Asked Questions (FAQs) found on the SAP website.

Special Access Programme Hours of Operation

SAP business hours are 8:30 am to 4:30 pm E.S.T., Monday to Friday. An on-call service is available after business hours for emergency situations by calling (613) 941-2108 and pressing 0. Calls to this number should be restricted to requests requiring immediate or overnight authorization.

SAP contact information:

Tel.: (613) 941-2108
Fax: (613) 941-3194
Email: SAPdrugs@hc-sc.gc.ca
Website: http://www.hc-sc.gc.ca/dhp-mps/acces/drugs-drogues/index_e.html

Appendix 3A: Adverse Events Following Immunization: Surveillance and Reporting

The following is a description of the Canadian Adverse Events Following Immunization Surveillance System (CAEFISS). This information is not intended to present a comprehensive review.

Reviewed 2010 by Vaccine Safety Section of the Public Health Agency of Canada (PHAC).

Surveillance of adverse events following immunization is carried out through a network linked to local, provincial and territorial public health authorities. The network is separate from the Canada Vigilance Program.

The following form (located in Appendix 3B) is the national Report of Adverse Events Following Immunization (AEFI) form which has been revised by the Vaccine Safety Section of PHAC in collaboration with the Federal/Provincial/Territorial Vaccine Vigilance Working Group. The revised form is accessible through the PHAC website in Portable Document Format (PDF): http://www.phac-aspc.gc.ca/im/pdf/hc4229e.pdf

The health care providers are requested to consult their local public health unit for specific reporting procedures in their jurisdiction. Jurisdictional contact information and AEFI User Guide (on how to complete an AEFI form), are accessible through the PHAC website: http://www.phac-aspc.gc.ca/im/ci-rp-eng.php

Background

Monitoring vaccine safety is of great importance: Public confidence in immunization programs depends on the safety and efficacy of vaccines. Vaccine safety surveillance is the responsibility not only of those who manufacture, regulate and administer vaccines, but also of all health care providers who provide advice to, and care for, individuals receiving vaccines. Health care providers provide a most valuable source of data and ensure the continued surveillance of vaccine safety by submitting case reports to public health authorities who evaluate and forward them to the PHAC for aggregation and analysis. With the case reports as the core, Canada has developed a strong program of safety monitoring, which includes interaction and/or participation with the following groups:

- The Advisory Committee on Causality Assessment (ACCA): meets regularly to review selected cases and to assess emerging vaccine safety issues.
- National Advisory Committee on Immunization (NACI): makes recommendations for the use of vaccines currently approved for use in humans in Canada; updates, reviews and publishes the *Canadian Immunization Guide*. The current Canadian Immunization Guide, 7th edition- 2006 is accessible through the PHAC website in Portable Document Format (PDF): http://www.phac-aspc.gc.ca/publicat/cig-gci/errarta-eng.php
- World Health Organization's International Drug Monitoring Program: collects drug safety data from more than 80 participating countries, thereby enhancing our ability to detect concerns.

Reporting adverse events following immunization is a vital component of the informed consent process: By reporting events of concern, health care professionals ensure continuous feedback on the impact of immunizations. Vaccine schedules have become increasingly complex and the messages from opponents of immunization are often well publicized. Therefore, counselling parents or patients about the safety of vaccines is becoming more difficult. The *Canadian Immunization Guide* incorporates a chapter on talking with patients about immunization. Refer to the *Suggested Readings* at the end of this section for further information on vaccines. Information on vaccine safety can also be found at http://www.phac-aspc.gc.ca/im/index-eng.php. The local public health unit should also be consulted for guidance.

Considerations When Reporting Adverse Events following Immunization

Health care providers should be vigilant, and are asked to report events that are felt to be related to immunization and that meet one or more of the following criteria:

- **Serious events:** those that are life threatening or result in death, require hospitalization or prolongation of an existing hospitalization, result in residual disability or cause congenital malformation.
- **Unexpected or unusual events:** those that are not listed/described in the local/regional product labelling (e.g. Package Insert or Summary of Product Characteristics.
- **Events that may influence subsequent immunizations:** those that may impact subsequent immunizations with the same vaccine or vaccines with similar components. The *Canadian Immunization Guide* outlines the absolute contraindications, and any precautions, to immunization with vaccines. These recommendations are evidence-based and sometimes differ from what is listed in the product monographs. If there is hesitation from either the parent/patient or the health care provider regarding the provision of subsequent doses, public health authorities can assist with a recommendation.

Suggested Readings

Canadian Coalition for Immunization Awareness & Promotion (CCIAP). *Vaccination information on the Internet: Can you trust what you read?* Available from: http://www.immunizationeducation. ca/documents/eng/InternetTips_Eng_1.pdf. Accessed November 25, 2008.

Gold R. *Your child's best shot: a parent's guide to vaccination.* 3rd ed. Ottawa (ON): Canadian Paediatric Society; 2006.

Grabenstein JD. *Immunofacts: vaccines and immunologic drugs.* St. Louis (MO): Facts and Comparisons; 2000.

National Advisory Committee on Immunization. *Canadian immunization guide.* 7th ed. Ottawa (ON): Public Health Agency of Canada; 2006. Available from: http://www.phac-aspc.gc.ca/publicat/cig-gci/index.html. Accessed November 25, 2008.

Plotkin SA, Orenstein WA, editors. *Vaccines.* 4th ed. Philadelphia (PA): WB Saunders; 2004.

References

1. Bentsi-Enchill A, Hardy M, Koch J et al. Adverse events temporally associated with vaccines-1992 report. *Can Commun Dis Rep* 1995;21(13):117-28.
2. Duclos P, Pless R, Koch J et al. Adverse events temporally associated with immunizing agents. *Can Fam Physician* 1993;39:1907-13.
3. Laboratory Centre for Disease Control. Proceedings of a workshop on post-marketing surveillance of vaccine-associated adverse events. *Can Dis Wkly Rep* 1991;17s4:1-9.
4. Scheifele DW, Halperin SA, Gold R et al. Assuring vaccine safety: a celebration of 10 years of progress with the IMPACT project. *Red Child Health* 2002;7:645-8.
5. Collet JP, MacDonald N, Cashman N et al. Monitoring signals for vaccine safety: the assessment of individual adverse event reports by an expert advisory committee. Advisory Committee on Causality Assessment. *Bull World Health Organ* 2000;78(2):178-85.

Appendix 3B

Public Health Agency of Canada / Agence de santé publique du Canada

REPORT OF ADVERSE EVENTS FOLLOWING IMMUNIZATION (AEFI)

INSTRUCTIONS: ***For more complete instructions and definitions, refer to the user guide at:***
http://www.phac-aspc.gc.ca/im/aefi-form-eng.php

Report events which have a temporal association with a vaccine and which cannot be clearly attributed to other causes. A causal relationship does not need to be proven, and submitting a report does not imply causality.

Of particular interest are those AEFIs which meet one or more of the following criteria:
a. Are of serious nature
b. Require urgent medical attention
c. Are unusual or unexpected events

Refer to the user guide, Background Information and for additional clarification.

NOTE:

- **The numbers below correspond to the numbered sections of the form.**
- **All dates should be captured in the following format: YYYY/MM/DD.**
- **When reporting an AEFI, check one of the boxes on the top right hand corner of the first page of the AEFI form to indicate whether it is an INITIAL or FOLLOW UP report. For all follow up reports, please specify the Unique Episode number.**

1a. The **"Unique episode number"** is assigned by the Province/Territory. Leave it blank unless authorized to assign it.
1b. The **"Region number"** is a number that corresponds to a given health unit. Leave it blank if it doesn't apply to your locale.
2. The "IMPACT LIN" is assigned by IMPACT nurse monitors (LIN: Local Inventory Number).
3. The information provided in this section is confidential and should not be sent to the Public Health Agency of Canada.
4a. Indicate the Province/Territory where the vaccine was administered, abbreviations may be used.
4c. Provide all information as requested in the table. For the "Dose #", provide the number in series (1, 2, 3, 4, or 5) if known. For the Influenza vaccine, unless a patient receives two doses in one season, the "Dose #" should be recorded as "1".
7a. Indicate the highest impact of the AEFI on the patient's daily activities as assessed by the patient or the parent/caregiver.
7c. Provide details of any investigations or treatments in section 10. If the patient was already in hospital when immunized and the immunization resulted in a longer hospital stay, indicate "Resulted in prolongation of existing hospitalization" and provide the number of days by which the patient's hospital stay was prolonged. For all hospitalizations, indicate the date of admission and discharge.
8. MOH/MHO: Medical Officer of Health, MD: Medical Doctor, RN: Registered Nurse.
9. Choose, from section 9 (AEFI details), the description that best fits the AEFI being reported. Make sure to record the time of onset and duration of signs/symptoms using the most appropriate time unit:
- If the interval is <1 hour, indicate in minutes;
- If it is ≥ 1 hour but <1 day; indicate in hours;
- If it is ≥1 day; indicate in days.

Report the time in one time unit only. Provide additional details of any investigation, therapy, and other information as appropriate in section 10.
11. This section is to be completed by the MOH/MHO, MD, RN or their designate who are assigned to provide public health recommendations according to the P/T best practices.
12. Information in this section is not collected by all P/Ts.

Return completed form to your local public health unit address at:

Alberta (AB)
British Columbia (BC)
Manitoba (MB)
New Brunswick (NB)
Newfoundland and Labrador (NL)
Northwest Territories (NT)
Nova Scotia (NS)
Nunavut (NU)
Ontario (ON)
Prince Edward Island (PE)
Quebec (QC)
Saskatchewan (SK)
Yukon (YT)
Public Health Agency of Canada (PHAC)

Canada

This reporting form has been formatted to conform to *CPS* page size. Source: *Report of adverse events following immunization*, Public Health Agency of Canada, 2010. © Reproduced with the permission of the Minister of Public Works and Government Services Canada, 2010.

Appendix 3B *(cont'd)*

Public Health Agency of Canada | Agence de santé publique du Canada

○ Initial report
○ Follow up report (Unique episode #)

REPORT OF ADVERSE EVENTS FOLLOWING IMMUNIZATION (AEFI)

1a. Unique episode #: **1b. Region #:** **2. IMPACT LIN:**

3. Patient Identification

First name: Last name: Health number:

Address of usual residence:
Province/Territory: Postal code: Phone: ( ) - (ext #:)

Information Source: First name: Last name: Relation to patient:

Contact info, if different:

4. Information at Time of Immunization and AEFI Onset

4a. At time of immunization
Province/Territory of immunization: ______
Date vaccine administered: YYYY / MM / DD (hr: am/pm)
Date of birth: YYYY / MM / DD **Age:** ______
Sex: ○ Male ○ Female ○ Other

4b. Medical history (up to the time of AEFI onset)
(Check all that apply and provide details in section 10)
❑ Concomitant medication(s)
❑ Known medical conditions/allergies
❑ Acute illness/injury

4c. Immunizing agent	Trade name	Manufacturer	Lot number	Dose #	Dosage/unit	Route	Site
					/		
					/		
					/		
					/		
					/		

5. Immunization Errors

Did this AEFI follow an incorrect immunization? ○ No ○ Unknown ○ **Yes**
(If **Yes**, *choose all that apply and provide details in section 10)*
❑ Given outside the recommended age limits ❑ Product expired
❑ Wrong vaccine given ❑ Incorrect route
❑ Dose exceeded that recommended for age ❑ Other, *specify:* ______

6. Previous AEFI

Did an AEFI follow a previous dose of any of the above immunizing agents (Table 4c)?
(Choose one of the following)
○ No ○ **Yes** *(Provide details in section 10)*
○ Unknown ○ Not applicable (no prior doses)

7. Impact of AEFI, Outcome, and Level of Care Obtained

7a. Highest impact of AEFI: *(Choose one of the following)*
○ Did not interfere with daily activities
○ Interfered with but did not prevent daily activities
○ Prevented daily activities

7b. Outcome at time of report:
○ Death ♦ Date: YYYY / MM / DD ○ Permanent disability/incapacity ♦
○ Not yet recovered ♦ ○ Fully recovered ○ Unknown
(Provide details in section 10 for items with ♦)

7c. Highest level of care obtained: *(Choose one of the following)*
○ Unknown ○ None ○ Telephone advice from a health professional ○ Non-urgent visit ○ Emergency visit
○ Required hospitalization (____ days) **OR** ○ Resulted in prolongation of existing hospitalization (by ____ days)
Date of hospital admission YYYY / MM / DD Date of hospital discharge YYYY / MM / DD

7d. Treatment received: ○ No ○ Unknown ○ Yes *(Provide details of all treatments including self treatment, in section 10)*

8. Reporter Information

Setting : ○ **Physician office** ○ **Public health** ○ **Hospital** ○ **Other, *specify:*** ______
Name: Phone: ( ) - (ext #:) Fax: ( ) -
Address:
City: Prov/Terr: Postal code: Date reported: YYYY / MM / DD
Signature: ______ ○ MD ○ RN ○ IMPACT ○ Other, *specify:* ______

Note: Discuss with patient or his/her parent/caregiver reason for reporting and confidentiality of information

Canada

Appendix 3B *(cont'd)*

Unique episode #: **Region #:** **IMPACT LIN:**

9. AEFI Details: Complete all sections as appropriate; for each, check all signs/symptoms that apply. Item(s) with asterisk (*) should be diagnosed by a physician. If not, provide sufficient information to support the selected item(s). Use Section 10 for additional information including, clinical details and test results.

❑ 9a. Local reaction at or near injection site
Interval: → __Min __Hrs __Days from immunization to onset of 1st symptom or sign
Duration: → __Min __Hrs __Days from onset of 1st symptom/sign to resolution of all symptoms/signs

❑ Infected abscess ❑ Sterile abscess ❑ Cellulitis ❑ Nodule ❑ Reaction crosses joint ❑ Lymphadenitis ❑ Other, *specify:* __________

For any injection site reaction indicated above, check all that apply below and provide details in section 10:
❑ Swelling ❑ Pain ❑ Tenderness ❑ Erythema ❑ Warmth ❑ Induration ❑ Rash ❑ Largest diameter of injection site reaction: ____ cm
Site(s) of reaction ______ (e.g. LA, RA) ❑ Palpable fluctuance ❑ Fluid collection shown by imaging technique (e.g. MRI, CT, ultrasound)
❑ Spontaneous/surgical drainage ❑ Microbial results ❑ Lymphangitic streaking ❑ Regional lymphadenopathy

❑ 9b. Allergic and Allergic-like events
Interval: → __Min __Hrs __Days from immunization to onset of 1st symptom or sign
Duration: → __Min __Hrs __Days from onset of 1st symptom/sign to resolution of all symptoms/signs

Chose one of the following: ○ **Anaphylaxis** ○ **Oculo-Respiratory Syndrome (ORS)** ○ **Other allergic events**
For a chosen event, check all that apply below and provide details in section 10:

Skin /mucosal	❑ Urticaria ❑ Erythema ❑ Pruritis ❑ Prickle sensation ❑ Rash *(For these events, specify site of reaction)* ANGIOEDEMA: ❑ Tongue ❑ Throat ❑ Uvula ❑ Larynx ❑ Lip ❑ Eyelids ❑ Face ❑ Limbs ❑ Other, *specify:* EYE(S): ❑ Red bilateral ❑ Red unilateral ❑ Itchy
Cardio-vascular	❑ Measured hypotension ❑ ↓central pulse volume ❑ Capillary refill time >3 sec ❑ Tachycardia ❑ ↓ or loss of consciousness (*Duration*) __________
Respiratory	❑ Sneezing ❑ Rhinorrhea ❑ Hoarse voice ❑ Sensation of throat closure ❑ Stridor ❑ Dry cough ❑ Tachypnea ❑ Wheezing ❑ Indrawing/retractions ❑ Grunting ❑ Cyanosis ❑ Sore throat ❑ Difficulty swallowing ❑ Difficulty breathing ❑ Chest tightness
Gastrointestinal	❑ Diarrhea ❑ Abdominal pain ❑ Nausea ❑ Vomiting

❑ 9c. Neurologic events
Interval: → __Min __Hrs __Days from immunization to onset of 1st symptom or sign
Duration: → __Min __Hrs __Days from onset of 1st symptom/sign to resolution of all symptoms/signs

❑ * **Meningitis** ❑ * **Encephalopathy/Encephalitis** ❑ * **Guillain-Barre Syndrome (GBS)** ❑ * **Bell's Palsy** ❑ * **Other Paralysis**
❑ **Seizure** ❑ * **Other neurologic diagnosis,** ***specify:*** ________________

For any neurologic event indicated above, check all that apply below and provide details in section 10:
❑ Depressed/altered level of consciousness, lethargy or personality change lasting ≥24hrs ❑ Focal or multifocal neurologic sign(s)
❑ Fever (≥38.0°C) ❑ CSF abnormality ❑ EEG abnormality ❑ EMG abnormality
❑ Neuroimaging abnormality ❑ Brain/spinal cord histopathologic abnormality
Seizure details: ❑ Witnessed by healthcare professional ○ Yes ○ No ○ Unknown
❑ Sudden loss of consciousness ○ Yes ○ No ○ Unknown
○ Focal **OR** ○ Generalized (*Specify:* ○ Tonic ○ Clonic ○ Tonic-Clonic ○ Atonic)
❑ Previous history of seizures (*Specify:* ❑ Febrile ❑ Afebrile ❑ Unknown type)

❑ 9d. Other defined events of interest
Interval: → __Min __Hrs __Days from immunization to onset of 1st symptom or sign
Duration: → __Min __Hrs __Days from onset of 1st symptom/sign to resolution of all symptoms/signs

For all selected defined events of interest below, provide details in section 10:

❑ **Hypotonic-Hyporesponsive Episode (age <2 years)** ❑ Limpness ❑ Pallor/cyanosis ❑ ↓responsiveness/unresponsiveness	❑***Thrombocytopenia** ❑ Platelet count $<150x10^9/L$ ❑ Petechial rash ❑ Other clinical evidence of bleeding
❑ **Persistent crying** (*Continuous and unaltered crying for ≥3 hours*)	❑ **Anaesthesia/Paraesthesia** (❑ Numbness ❑ Tingling ❑ Burning ❑ Formication ❑ Other, *specify:* ________________) ○ Generalized ○ Localized (*Site*) __________
❑ * **Intussusception**	
❑ **Arthritis** ❑ Joint redness ❑ Joint warm to touch ❑ Joint swelling ❑ Inflammatory changes in synovial fluid	❑ **Fever ≥38.0°C** (*Note: report* ***ONLY*** *if fever occurs in conjunction with a reportable event. For fever in a neurological event, use section 9c)*
❑ **Parotitis** (*Parotid gland swelling with pain and/or tenderness*)	
❑ **Rash** (*Non-allergic*) ○ Generalized ○ Localized (*Site*)________	❑ **Other severe or unusual event(s) not listed above**

This reporting form has been formatted to conform to *CPS* page size. Source: *Report of adverse events following immunization*, Public Health Agency of Canada, 2010. © Reproduced with the permission of the Minister of Public Works and Government Services Canada, 2010.

Appendix 3B *(cont'd)*

Unique episode #: **Region #:** **IMPACT LIN:**

10. Supplementary information *(Please indicate the section # when providing details. Please provide details of any investigation or treatment for the recorded AEFI).*

----

11. Recommendations for future immunization(s) according to the Provincial/Territorial best practices.
(Provide comments, use section 10 if extra space needed)

❑ No change to immunization schedule ❑ Expert referral, *specify:* ________ ❑ Determine protective antibody level	❑ Controlled setting for next immunization ❑ No further immunizations with: ______ *(specify)* ______ ❑ Active follow up for AEFI recurrence after next vaccine	❑ Other, *specify:* ______

Name: Professional status: ○ MOH/MHO ○ MD ○ RN ○ Other, *specify:* ______

Comments:

Phone: ( ) - (ext #:) Date: YYYY / MM / DD Signature: ______

12) Follow up information for a subsequent dose of same vaccine(s) *(Provide details in section 10)*

❑ Vaccine administered without AEFI ❑ Vaccine administered with recurrence of AEFI ❑ Vaccine administered, other AEFI observed
❑ Vaccine administered without information on AEFI ❑ Vaccine not administered

Appendix 4

Health Canada · Santé Canada

Canada Vigilance Adverse Reaction Reporting Form

Report of suspected adverse reactions to marketed health products in Canada

See instructions and information on adverse reaction reporting and confidentiality on Page 2.

Complete all mandatory items, marked by a *, and provide as much information as possible for the remaining items. PROTECTED WHEN COMPLETED – B**

A. Patient Information

1. Identifier

2. Age	3. Sex*	4. Height	5. Weight
☐ Years ______ ☐ Months	☐ Male ☐ Female	______ cm ______ feet	______ kg ______ lbs

B. Adverse Reaction

1. Outcome attributed to adverse reaction (Select all that apply)

- ☐ Death: (yyyy-mm-dd)
- ☐ Life-threatening
- ☐ Hospitalization
- ☐ Hospitalization – prolonged
- ☐ Disability
- ☐ Congenital malformation
- ☐ Required intervention to prevent damage/impairment
- ☐ Other:

2. Reaction date (yyyy-mm-dd)

3. Report date (yyyy-mm-dd)

4. Describe reaction or problem*

5. Relevant tests/laboratory data (including dates (yyyy-mm-dd))

6. Relevant history and pre-existing medical conditions (e.g. allergies, pregnancy, smoking/alcohol use, hepatic/renal dysfunction)

C. Suspected Health Product(s)

1. Name*, strength and manufacturer (if known)

#1

#2

2. Dose, frequency and route used

#1 | #2

3. Therapy dates (or duration)

#1 From (yyyy-mm-dd) - To (yyyy-mm-dd) | #2 From (yyyy-mm-dd) - To (yyyy-mm-dd)

4. Indication for use

#1 | #2

5. Reaction abated after use stopped or dose reduced

#1 ☐ Yes ☐ No ☐ Does not apply | #2 ☐ Yes ☐ No ☐ Does not apply

6. Lot #

#1

#2

7. Expiration

#1 (yyyy-mm-dd)

#2 (yyyy-mm-dd)

8. Reaction reappeared after reintroduction

#1 ☐ Yes ☐ No ☐ Does not apply | #2 ☐ Yes ☐ No ☐ Does not apply

9. Concomitant health products, excluding treatment of reaction (name, dose, frequency, route used and therapy dates (yyyy-mm-dd))

10. Treatment of reaction, including dates (yyyy-mm-dd)

D. Reporter Information

1. Name*, occupation, address, telephone number*

2. Health professional? ☐ Yes ☐ No

3. Reported to manufacturer? ☐ Yes ☐ No

** As per the Treasury Board of Canada Secretariat Government Security Policy.

A program of **MedEffect**™ **Canada**

HC Pub.: 100251 (September 2010)

Page 1 of 2

Canada

Appendix 4 *(cont'd)*

Instructions to Complete the Canada Vigilance Adverse Reaction Reporting Form

- Use this form only to report adverse reactions to Canadian marketed health products, including prescription and non-prescription medications; natural health products; biologically derived products such as vaccines and fractionated blood products; cells, tissues and organs; radiopharmaceuticals; and disinfectants and sanitizers with disinfectant claims.
- All sections of the form should be filled in as completely as possible. Use a separate form for each patient. Up to two suspected health products for a particular adverse reaction may be reported on one form. Attach an additional form if there are more than two suspected health products for the adverse reaction being reported. Additional pages may be attached if more space is required.
- For the "Identifier" box, provide some type of identifier that will allow you, the reporter, to readily locate the case if you are contacted for more information; do not use the patient's name. See the Confidentiality disclaimer at the bottom of this page.
- Any follow-up information for an adverse reaction that has already been reported can be submitted using a new form, indicating that it consists of follow-up information, including, if known, the date of the original report and the Adverse Reaction Number provided in the acknowledgement letter.
- **Reports can be faxed** to 1-866-678-6789 (toll-free) **or mailed** to: Canada Vigilance Program, Marketed Health Products Directorate, Health Canada, Postal Locator 0701E, Ottawa, Ontario K1A 0K9. Postage paid labels are available at www.healthcanada.gc.ca/medeffect or by calling 1-866-234-2345 (toll-free). Do not send reports by e-mail.

Information on Adverse Reaction Reporting

What is an adverse reaction?

An adverse reaction is a harmful and unintended response to a health product. This includes any undesirable patient effect suspected to be associated with health product use. Unintended effect, health product abuse, overdose, interaction (including drug-drug and drug-food interactions) and unusual lack of therapeutic efficacy are all considered to be reportable adverse reactions.

A serious adverse reaction is one that requires in-patient hospitalization or prolongation of existing hospitalization, causes congenital malformation, results in persistent or significant disability or incapacity, is life-threatening or results in death. Adverse reactions that require significant medical intervention to prevent one of these listed outcomes are also considered to be serious.

Which adverse reactions should be reported?

All suspected adverse reactions should be reported, especially those that are:

- *unexpected*, regardless of their severity, i.e., not consistent with product information or labelling; or
- *serious*, whether expected or not; or
- reactions to *recently marketed health products* (on the market for less than five years), regardless of their nature or severity.

Alternative ways to report

You can also report side effects to health products to the Canada Vigilance Program:

- By calling 1-866-234-2345 (toll-free)
- Online: www.healthcanada.gc.ca/medeffect

The Canada Vigilance Adverse Reaction Reporting Form is also available online at www.healthcanada.gc.ca/medeffect or at the back of the *Compendium of Pharmaceuticals and Specialties* (CPS).

Other Information

- Submission of a report does not constitute an admission that medical personnel or the product caused or contributed to the adverse reaction.
- Adverse reaction reports are, for the most part, only suspected associations. A temporal or possible association is sufficient for a report to be made. Reporting of an adverse reaction does not imply a definitive causal link.
- Health professionals and consumers may also report adverse reactions to the market authorization holder (MAH). Indicate on your adverse reaction report sent to Health Canada if a case was also reported to the product's MAH.

For additional information, contact a Canada Vigilance Regional Office by telephone at 1-866-234-2345 (toll-free) or:

Canada Vigilance Regional Office – British Columbia and Yukon
400-4595 Canada Way, Burnaby, BC V5G 1J9
CanadaVigilance_BC@hc-sc.gc.ca

Canada Vigilance Regional Office – Alberta and Northwest Territories
Suite 730, 9700 Jasper Ave, Edmonton, AB T5J 4C3
CanadaVigilance_AB@hc-sc.gc.ca

Canada Vigilance Regional Office – Saskatchewan
101 - 22nd Street East, Saskatoon, SK S7K 0E1
CanadaVigilance_SK@hc-sc.gc.ca

Canada Vigilance Regional Office – Manitoba
510 Lagimodière Blvd, Winnipeg, MB R2J 3Y1
CanadaVigilance_MB@hc-sc.gc.ca

Canada Vigilance Regional Office – Ontario and Nunavut
2301 Midland Ave, Toronto, ON M1P 4R7
CanadaVigilance_ON@hc-sc.gc.ca

Canada Vigilance Regional Office – Québec
1001 Saint-Laurent Street West, Longueuil, QC J4K 1C7
CanadaVigilance_QC@hc-sc.gc.ca

For New Brunswick, Nova Scotia, Prince Edward Island, Newfoundland and Labrador:

Canada Vigilance Regional Office – Atlantic
Suite 1625, 1505 Barrington St., Halifax, NS B3J 3Y6
CanadaVigilance_ATL@hc-sc.gc.ca

Confidentiality

Personal information collected, used or disclosed under the Canada Vigilance Program is confidential and protected. For the purposes of the Canada Vigilance Program, information related to the identity of a patient and/or reporter of the adverse reaction will be protected as personal information under the Privacy Act, and under the Access to Information Act, in the case of an access to information request. Provision of the information requested on this form is voluntary. Information from adverse reaction reports is maintained in a computerized database and used for the monitoring of marketed health products, which may contribute to the detection of potential product-related safety issues, as well as to the benefit-risk assessments of these products. For details about personal information collected under this program, visit the Government of Canada web site on Institution-Specific Personal Information Banks under Health Canada, Health Products and Food Branch, Branch Incident Reporting System, PIB # ppu 088 at: http://infosource.gc.ca/inst/shc/fed07-eng.asp (Health Products and Food Branch, Branch Incident Reporting System).

Page 2 of 2

Glossary of Medical Abbreviations

ACE	angiotensin converting enzyme
ACTH	adrenocorticotropic hormone
ADH	antidiuretic hormone
AHA	American Heart Association
AIDS	acquired immunodeficiency syndrome
ALT	alanine transferase (SGPT)
ANC	absolute neutrophil count
APTT	activated partial thromboplastin time
ASA	acetylsalicylic acid
AST	aspartate transferase (SGOT)
AUC	area under the concentration curve
AV	atrioventricular
b.i.d.	twice daily
BID	twice daily
BMI	body mass index
BMR	basal metabolic rate
BP	British Pharmacopoeia; blood pressure
BSA	body surface area
BSP	bromsulphalein
BUN	blood urea nitrogen
°C	degrees Celsius
^{14}C	radioactive carbon isotope of atomic weight 14
Ⓒ	controlled drug
CHF	congestive heart failure
CK	creatine kinase
cm	centimetre
CNS	central nervous system
COMT	catechol-o-methyltransferase
COPD	chronic obstructive pulmonary disease
CP	centipoise
CPK	creatine phosphokinase
CPR	cardiopulmonary resuscitation
CSD	Canadian Standard Drug
CSF	cerebrospinal fluid
CT	computed tomography
CVA	cerebrovascular accident
D&C	designation applied to dyes permitted for use in drugs and cosmetics
DIC	disseminated intravascular coagulation
dL	decilitre
DNA	deoxyribonucleic acid
DSA	digital subtraction angiography
ECG	electrocardiogram
ECT	electroconvulsive therapy
EEG	electroencephalogram
EENT	ear, eye, nose and throat
ERCP	endoscopic retrograde cholangiopancreatography
ESR	erythrocyte sedimentation rate
ET	endotracheal
FD&C	designation applied to dyes permitted for use in foods, drugs and cosmetics
FSH	follicle-stimulating hormone
g	gram
GFR	glomerular filtration rate
GGT	gamma-glutamyl transpeptidase, γ-glutamyltransferase
GI	gastrointestinal
G-6-PD	glucose-6-phosphate dehydrogenase
GVHD	graft-versus-host disease
h	hour/s
Hb	hemoglobin
hCG	human chorionic gonadotropin
HDPE	high density polyethylene
HIV	human immunodeficiency virus
HMG-CoA	hydroxy-methyl-glutaryl coenzyme A
hs	bedtime
HS	bedtime
^{131}I	radioactive iodine isotope of atomic weight 131
I.M. or i.m.	intramuscular
IM	intramuscular
INR	international normalized ratio
IOP	intraocular pressure
IU	international unit
IUD	intrauterine contraceptive device
I.V. or i.v.	intravenous
IV	intravenous
J	joule
kg	kilogram
L	litre
lb	pound
LE	lupus erythematosus
LGL	Lown-Ganong-Levine
LH	luteinizing hormone
μ	micron
μg	microgram
μL	microlitre
μm	micrometer
μmol	micromole
M	molar
MAO	monoamine oxidase
MAOI	monoamine oxidase inhibitor
mEq	milliequivalent
mg	milligram
MI	myocardial infarction
min	minim; minute
mIU	milli international unit
MJ	megajoule
mL	millilitre
mmHg	millimetre(s) of mercury
mmol	millimole
mOsm	milliosmole
MRI	magnetic resonance imaging
ms	millisecond
MS	multiple sclerosis
Ⓝ	narcotic
NF	National Formulary
ng	nanogram
nkat	nanokatal
NMS	neuroleptic malignant syndrome
NPN	nonprotein nitrogen
NSAID	nonsteroidal anti-inflammatory drug
NST	nonstress test
OHSS	ovarian hyperstimulation syndrome
oz	ounce
PABA	para-aminobenzoic acid
PBI	protein bound iodine
PBP	penicillin binding protein
pg	picogram (10^{-12})
PG	prostaglandin
pH	the logarithm, on the base 10, of the reciprocal of the hydrogenion concentration
pmol	picomole (10^{-12})
po	orally
PO	orally
ppm	parts per million
℞	prescription required
PR	rectally
PRA	plasma renin activity
prn	when needed
PRN	when needed
PSVT	paroxysmal supraventricular tachycardia
PT	prothrombin time
PTCA	percutaneous transluminal coronary angioplasty
q.i.d.	4 times daily
QID	4 times daily
®	registered trademark
RAI	radioactive iodine
r-hFSH	recombinant human follicle-stimulating hormone
RIA	radioimmunoassay
RNI	recommended nutrient intake
s	second
SA	sinoatrial
S.C. or s.c.	subcutaneous
SC	subcutaneous
SD	standard deviation
SGOT	serum glutamic oxaloacetic transaminase (AST)
SGPT	serum glutamic pyruvic transaminase (ALT)
SLE	systemic lupus erythematosus
SMA	sequential multiple analysis
SSPE	subacute sclerosing panencephalitis
SSRI	selective serotonin reuptake inhibitor
TS	target controlled substances
t.i.d.	3 times daily
TID	3 times daily
TM	trademark
TSH	thyroid-stimulating hormone
TT	thrombin time
ULN	upper limit of normal
USP	United States Pharmacopoeia
v/v	volume in volume
WBC	white blood cell
WHO	World Health Organization
WPW	Wolff-Parkinson-White
w/v	weight in volume
w/w	weight in weight

Glossary of Latin Prescription Terms

aa, ana	of each
a.c.	before meals (or food)
ad lib.	at pleasure
aeq., aequal.	equal
alb.	white
amp.	ampoule
aq. ad	water up to
aur. dext.	in (or to) the right ear
aur. laev. (or sinist.)	in (or to) the left ear
b.i.d. (or b.d.)	twice daily
c., c, cum	with
caps.	capsule
chart.	powder (wrapped)
collyr.	eye water
d.	day
d.t.d.	let such doses be sent
dos.	dose
et	and
ex (or in) aq.	in water
Ext.	extract
F., f., ft.	make, let it (them) be made
F.s.a.	make according to the art
fl.	fluid
flav.	yellow
fort.	strong
gtt.	drop(s)
h.s.	at bedtime
h.s.s.	to be taken at bedtime
ibid	in the same place
i.c.	between meals
idem	the same
lev.	light
liq.	solution, liquid
lin.	liniment
lot.	lotion
m.d., mod. dict.	as directed
m.d.a.	to be applied as directed
m.d.s.	to be taken as directed
M.D.S.	mix, dispense, label
m.d.u.	to be used as directed
M., ft. mist. (caps.) (ung.)	mix, let a mixture (capsule) (ointment) be made
mitis	mild
Mitte talis	send of such
moll.	soft
neb.	nebula, spray
ne rep., non rep.	do not repeat
no.	(in number)
nocte	(at) night
N.P., nom. prop.	by its proper name
O.	pint
ocul.	eye
oculent.	eye ointment
o.d.	in the right eye
o.h., om.h.	every hour
o.h. 2(ii), 3(iii), etc.	every two, three hours
o.l., o.s.	in the left eye
o.m., om.m., om. man.	every morning
o.n., om.n., om. noct.	every night
opt.	best
o.u.	in each eye
parv.	small
past.	paste or pastille
p.c.	after meals (food)
P.E.	powdered extract
per os	orally, by mouth
pil.	pill
pond.	heavy
P.P.A.	shake the bottle first
ppt.	precipitate(d)
pro	for
p.r.n.	when (as) required
pulv.	powder(ed)
q.d.	every day
q.2d.	every 2 days
q.i.d.	four times daily
qq.h. or q.h.	every hour
qq.2h. or q.2h.	every 2 hours
qq.q.h. or q.q.h. or q.4h.	every 4 hours
q.s.	a sufficient quantity
rep.	repeat
s.a.	according to art
s.n., suo nom.	by its own name
s.o.s.	if necessary
Sp., Spt.	spirit
s., sig., signa	label
ss., ss	one-half
stat.	at once
supp.	suppository
syr.	syrup
tab.	tablet
tal.	such
t.d.s.	to be taken three times daily
t.i.d. or t.d.	three times daily
t.i.d.a.c.	three times daily before meals
Tinct., Tr.	tincture
tuss.	cough
ung.	ointment
ut dict., u.d.	as directed

Glossary of Microorganism Abbreviations

The following microorganism abbreviations may appear in *CPS*.

Abbreviation	Full Name
Bacteria	
A. calcoaceticus	*Acinetobacter calcoaceticus*
A. bovis	*Actinomyces bovis*
A. israelii	*Actinomyces israelii*
A. aerogenes—see *E. aerogenes*	
A. faecalis	*Alcaligenes faecalis*
B. anthracis	*Bacillus anthracis*
B. polymyxa	*Bacillus polymyxa*
B. subtilis	*Bacillus subtilis*
B. bivius—see *P. bivia*	
B. distasonis	*Bacteroides distasonis*
B. forsythus	*Bacteroides forsythus*
B. fragilis	*Bacteroides fragilis*
B. funduliformis—see *F. necrophorum*	
B. melaninogenicus	*Bacteroides melaninogenicus*
B. ovatus	*Bacteroides ovatus*
B. thetaiotaomicron	*Bacteroides thetaiotaomicron*
B. uniformis	*Bacteroides uniformis*
B. ureolyticus	*Bacteroides ureolyticus*
B. vulgatus	*Bacteroides vulgatus*
B. bacilliformis	*Bartonella bacilliformis*
B. pertussis	*Bordetella pertussis*
B. burgdorferi	*Borrelia burgdorferi*
B. recurrentis	*Borrelia recurrentis*
B. catarrhalis—see *M. catarrhalis*	
B. melitensis	*Brucella melitensis*
B. cepacia	*Burkholderia cepacia*
C. granulomatis	*Calymmatobacterium granulomatis*
C. fetus	*Campylobacter fetus*
C. jejuni	*Campylobacter jejuni*
C. parvum	*Cryptosporidium parvum*
C. pneumoniae	*Chlamydophila pneumoniae*
C. psittaci	*Chlamydia psittaci*
C. trachomatis	*Chlamydia trachomatis*
C. diversus	*Citrobacter diversus*
C. freundii	*Citrobacter freundii*
C. botulinum	*Clostridium botulinum*
C. difficile	*Clostridium difficile*
C. perfringens	*Clostridium perfringens*
C. tetani	*Clostridium tetani*
C. acnes—see *P. acnes*	
C. diphtheriae	*Corynebacterium diphtheriae*
D. pneumoniae—see *S. pneumoniae*	
E. aerogenes	*Enterobacter aerogenes*
E. cloacae	*Enterobacter cloacae*
E. faecalis	*Enterococcus faecalis*
E. faecium	*Enterococcus faecium*
E. coli	*Escherichia coli*
E. lentum	*Eubacterium lentum*
F. nucleatum	*Fusobacterium nucleatum*
F. tularensis	*Francisella tularensis*
F. necrophorum	*Fusobacterium necrophorum*
G. vaginalis	*Gardnerella vaginalis*
H. aegyptius	*Haemophilus aegyptius*
H. ducreyi	*Haemophilus ducreyi*
H. influenzae	*Haemophilus influenzae*
H. parainfluenzae	*Haemophilus parainfluenzae*
H. pylori	*Helicobacter pylori*
K. oxytoca	*Klebsiella oxytoca*
K. pneumoniae	*Klebsiella pneumoniae*
L. acidophilus	*Lactobacillus acidophilus*
L. vaginalis	*Lactobacillus vaginalis*
L. pneumophila	*Legionella pneumophila*
L. canicola	*Leptospira canicola*
L. interrogans	*Leptospira interrogans*
L. monocytogenes	*Listeria monocytogenes*
M. furfur	*Malassezia furfur*
M. catarrhalis	*Moraxella catarrhalis*
M. lacunata	*Moraxella lacunata*
M. morganii	*Morganella morganii*
M. avium-intracellulare	*Mycobacterium avium-intracellulare*
M. bovis	*Mycobacterium bovis*
M. chelonae	*Mycobacterium chelonae*
M. genavense	*Mycobacterium genavense*
M. intracellulare	*Mycobacterium intracellulare*
M. kansasii	*Mycobacterium kansasii*
M. leprae	*Mycobacterium leprae*
M. marinum	*Mycobacterium marinum*
M. tuberculosis	*Mycobacterium tuberculosis*
M. xenopi	*Mycobacterium xenopi*
M. pneumoniae	*Mycoplasma pneumoniae*
N. catarrhalis—see *M. catarrhalis*	
N. gonorrhoeae	*Neisseria gonorrhoeae*
N. gonorrhoeae subsp	*Neisseria gonorrhoeae subspecies*
N. kochii	*Neisseria kochii*
N. meningitidis	*Neisseria meningitidis*
N. asteroides	*Nocardia asteroides*
N. brasiliensis	*Nocardia brasiliensis*
P. multocida	*Pasteurella multocida*
P. jiroveci	*Pneumocystis jiroveci*
P. asaccharolytica	*Porphyromonas asaccharolytica*
P. pestis—see *Y. pestis*	
P. gingivalis	*Porphyromonas gingivalis*
Pneumococcus—see *S. pneumoniae*	
P. bivia	*Prevotella bivia*
P. disiens	*Prevotella disiens*
P. intermedia	*Prevotella intermedia*
P. acnes	*Propionibacterium acnes*
P. mirabilis	*Proteus mirabilis*
P. vulgaris	*Proteus vulgaris*
P. rettgeri	*Providencia rettgeri*
P. stuartii	*Providencia stuartii*
P. aeruginosa	*Pseudomonas aeruginosa*
S. choleraesuis	*Salmonella choleraesuis*
S. enteritidis	*Salmonella enteritidis*
S. paratyphi	*Salmonella paratyphi*
S. typhi	*Salmonella typhi*
S. typhimurium	*Salmonella typhimurium*
S. marcescens	*Serratia marcescens*
S. boydii	*Shigella boydii*
S. dysenteriae	*Shigella dysenteriae*
S. flexneri	*Shigella flexneri*
S. sonnei	*Shigella sonnei*
S. minor	*Spirillum minor*
S. aureus	*Staphylococcus aureus*
S. epidermidis	*Staphylococcus epidermidis*
S. saprophyticus	*Staphylococcus saprophyticus*
S. maltophilia	*Stenotrophomonas maltophilia*
S. moniliformis	*Streptobacillus moniliformis*
S. agalactiae	*Streptococcus agalactiae*
S. anginosus	*Streptococcus anginosus*
S. bovis	*Streptococcus bovis*
S. faecalis—see *E. faecalis*	
S. milleri	*Streptococcus milleri*
S. mitior	*Streptococcus mitior*
S. mutans	*Streptococcus mutans*
S. pneumoniae	*Streptococcus pneumoniae*
S. pyogenes	*Streptococcus pyogenes*
S. sanguis	*Streptococcus sanguis*
S. viridans	*Streptococcus viridans*
S. erythreus	*Streptomyces erythreus*
S. somaliensis	*Streptomyces somaliensis*
S. tsukubaensis	*Streptomyces tsukubaensis*
T. pallidum	*Treponema pallidum*
T. pertenue	*Treponema pertenue*
T. whippelii	*Tropheryma whippelii*
U. urealyticum	*Ureaplasma urealyticum*
V. cholerae	*Vibrio cholerae*
X. maltophilia	*Xanthomonas maltophilia*
Y. enterocolitica	*Yersinia enterocolitica*
Y. pestis	*Yersinia pestis*
Y. pseudotuberculosis	*Yersinia pseudotuberculosis*
Fungi	
A. fumigatus	*Aspergillus fumigatus*
A. nidulans	*Aspergillus nidulans*
A. niger	*Aspergillus niger*
A. terreus	*Aspergillus terreus*
B. dermatitidis	*Blastomyces dermatitidis*
C. albicans	*Candida albicans*
C. glabrata	*Candida glabrata*

Glossary of Microorganism Abbreviations *(cont'd)*

Abbreviation	Full Name
Fungi *(cont'd)*	
C. immitis	*Coccidioides immitis*
C. krusei	*Candida krusei*
C. neoformans	*Cryptococcus neoformans*
E. floccosum	*Epidermophyton floccosum*
H. capsulatum	*Histoplasma capsulatum*
M. furfur	*Malassezia furfur*
M. audouini	*Microsporum audouini*
M. canis	*Microsporum canis*
M. gypseum	*Microsporum gypseum*
P. brasiliensis	*Paracoccidioides brasiliensis*
S. cerevisiae	*Saccharomyces cerevisiae*
T. crateriform	*Trichophyton crateriform*
T. gallinae	*Trichophyton gallinae*
T. interdigitale	*Trichophyton interdigitale*
T. megninii	*Trichophyton megninii*
T. mentagrophytes	*Trichophyton mentagrophytes*
T. rubrum	*Trichophyton rubrum*
T. schoenleinii	*Trichophyton schoenleinii*
T. sulfureum	*Trichophyton sulfureum*
T. tonsurans	*Trichophyton tonsurans*
T. verrucosum	*Trichophyton verrucosum*
T. violaceum	*Trichophyton violaceum*
Protozoa/Parasites	
C. cayetanesis	*Cyclospora cayetanesis*
C. sinensis	*Clonorchis sinensis*
C. parvum	*Crytosporidium parvum*
E. histolytica	*Entamoeba histolytica*
E. vermicularis	*Enterobius vermicularis*
G. lamblia	*Giardia lamblia*
I. belli	*Isospora belli*
O. viverrini	*Opisthorchis viverrini*
P. capitis	*Pediculus capitis*
P. carinii—see P. jiroveci	
P. falciparum	*Plasmodium falciparum*
P. jiroveci	*Pneumocystis jiroveci*
P. malariae	*Plasmodium malariae*
P. ovale	*Plasmodium ovale*
P. vivax	*Plasmodium vivax*
S. haematobium	*Schistosoma haematobium*
S. japonicum	*Schistosoma japonicum*
S. mansoni	*Schistosoma mansoni*
S. mekongi	*Schistosoma mekongi*
S. stercoralis	*Strongyloides stercoralis*
T. gondii	*Toxoplasma gondii*
T. solium	*Taenia solium*
T. vaginalis	*Trichomonas vaginalis*

Abbreviation	Full Name
Viruses	
CMV	Cytomegalovirus
EBV	Epstein-Barr virus
HCV	Hepatitis C virus
HAV	Hepatitis type A virus
HBV	Hepatitis type B virus
HSV	Herpes simplex virus
HIV	Human immunodeficiency virus
HTLV-1	Human T cell lymphotrophic retrovirus
HPV	Human papillomavirus
RSV	Respiratory syncytial virus
VZV	Varicella-zoster virus

Risk Factors for Drug Use During Pregnancy

Product monographs may refer to risk factors (A, B, C, D, X) for drug use during pregnancy. They are an indication of the level of risk that the drug poses to the fetus and are the definitions used by the Food and Drug Administration in the United States (Federal Register 1980;44:37434–67). The definitions are:

Category A:
Controlled studies in women fail to demonstrate a risk to the fetus in the first trimester (and there is no evidence of a risk in later trimesters), and the possibility of fetal harm appears remote.

Category B:
Either animal-reproduction studies have not demonstrated a fetal risk but there are no controlled studies in pregnant women or animal-reproduction studies have shown an adverse effect (other than a decrease in fertility) that was not confirmed in controlled studies in women in the first trimester (and there is no evidence of a risk in later trimesters).

Category C:
Either studies in animals have revealed adverse effects on the fetus (teratogenic or embryocidal or other) and there are no controlled studies in women or studies in women and animals are not available. Drugs should be given only if the potential benefit justifies the potential risk to the fetus.

Category D:
There is positive evidence of human fetal risk, but the benefits from use in pregnant women may be acceptable despite the risk (e.g., if the drug is needed in a life-threatening situation or for a serious disease for which safer drugs cannot be used or are ineffective).

Category X:
Studies in animals or human beings have demonstrated fetal abnormalities or there is evidence of fetal risk based on human experience or both, and the risk of the use of the drug in pregnant women clearly outweighs any possible benefit. The drug is contraindicated in women who are or may become pregnant.